THIRTY-EIGHTH EDITION

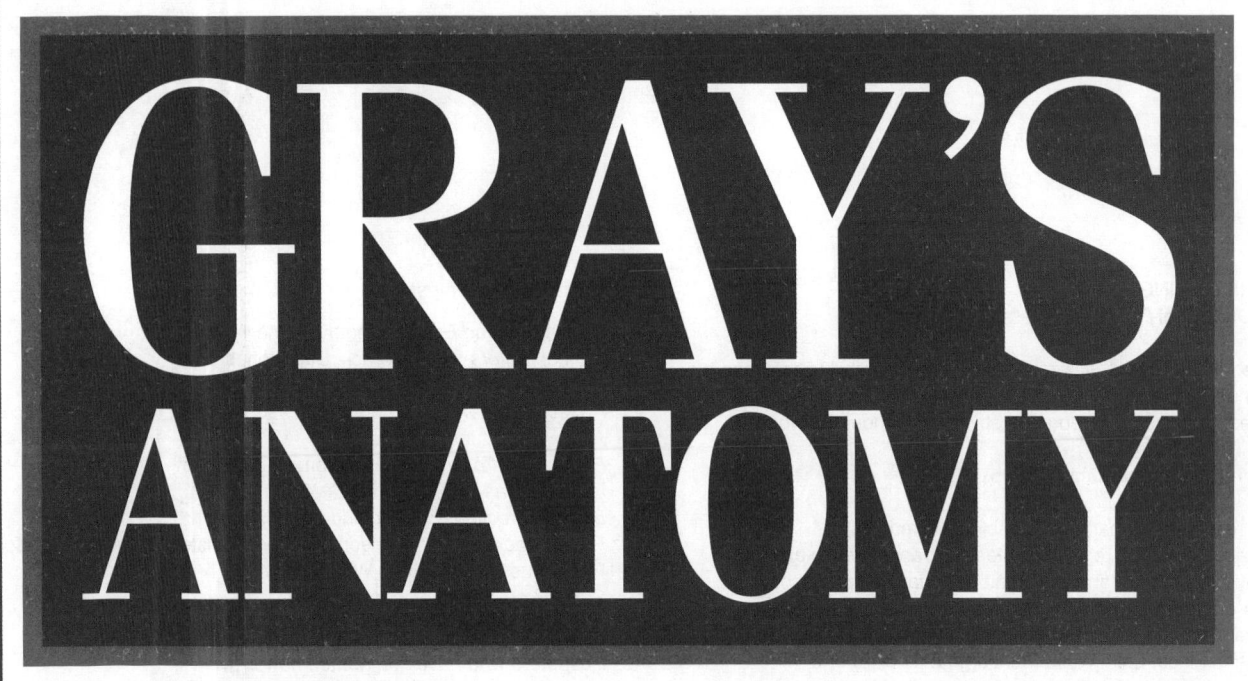

GRAY'S ANATOMY

THE ANATOMICAL BASIS OF MEDICINE AND SURGERY

CHAIRMAN OF THE EDITORIAL BOARD

The late **Peter L. Williams** DSc (Lond) MA MB BChir (Cantab) FRCS (Eng)

Emeritus Professor, University of London
Formerly Professor of Anatomy, Guy's Hospital Medical School, London

EDITORIAL BOARD

**Lawrence H. Bannister
Martin M. Berry
Patricia Collins
Mary Dyson
Julian E. Dussek
Mark W. J. Ferguson**

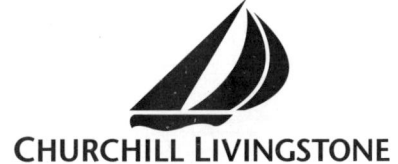

CHURCHILL LIVINGSTONE

NEW YORK EDINBURGH LONDON TOKYO MADRID AND MELBOURNE 1995

CHURCHILL LIVINGSTONE
Medical Division of Pearson Professional Limited

Distributed in the United States of America by Churchill Livingstone Inc., 650 Avenue of the Americas, New York, N.Y. 10011 and by associated companies, branches and representatives throughout the world.

ISBN 0–443–04560–7

British Library Cataloguing in Publication Data
A catalogue record for this book is available from the British Library.

Library of Congress Cataloging in Publication Data
A catalog record for this book is available from the Library of Congress.

For Churchill Livingstone

Commissioning Editor: Timothy Horne
Project Editors: Julia Merrick, Dilys Jones
Copy Editors: Therese Duriez, Kathleen Orr
Project Assistants: Graham Birnie, Isobel Black, Kim Craven, Nicola Haig, Alison Nicoll, Janice Urquhart
Project Controllers: Kay Hunston, Nancy Arnott
Design Management: Ian Dick
Design Direction: Erik Bigland
Proofreaders: Susan Ranson, Andrew Johnston, Elizabeth Lightfoot, Ian Ross, Russell Roy, Keith Whettam
Sales Promotion: Duncan Jones

Illustrators who have contributed new artwork

Andrew Bezear
Robert Britton
Peter Cox
Marks Creative
Patrick Elliott
Jenny Halstead
Dr A. A. van Horssen
Peter Jack
Peter Lamb
Gillian Lee
Lesley J. Skeates
Denise Smith
Philip Wilson

Photographers

Sarah-Jane Smith
Kevin Fitzpatrick

Printed in Great Britain

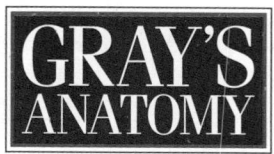

CONTENTS

CONTENTS

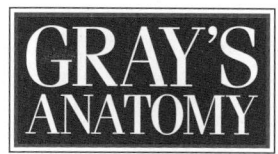

PREFACE

TO THE THIRTY-EIGHTH EDITION

With the publication of this the 38th edition of *Gray's Anatomy*, 137 years have elapsed since the first edition appeared. Although the human body remains the same, our understanding of it has changed immensely during this time, and continues to do so at an accelerating pace. The discipline of Anatomy has also changed out of all recognition because it is no longer just 'Descriptive and Applied'—as stated on the title pages until the last three editions—but is concerned with the whole of human morphology, its underlying principles and its relation to the larger world of scientific endeavour. This has been a major theme in the last three editions since 1971 under the highly innovative editorship of Professor Peter Williams and Professor Roger Warwick, who transformed the book in its scope and content and also its visual impact. In this work they were assisted by excellent illustrators, especially Richard Moore whose arresting imagery brought life and intellectual insight into a previously conventional, rather staid, low-key set of illustrations. This was complemented by Kevin Fitzpatrick's high quality colour photography, and later by artwork from Jenny Halstead and Kevin Marks who have continued in the tradition begun in the 35th edition. The vision of a transformed *Gray's Anatomy* was also shared by a number of contributors to the book, including Dr Mary Dyson and Dr Lawrence Bannister who became Assistant Editors in the 36th edition and then joint editors with Williams and Warwick in the 37th edition.

After the publication of the 37th edition in 1989, a momentous change in the editorship of *Gray's Anatomy* took place. The great proliferation of research information related to human morphology, and the increasingly heavy demands of academic life made it highly desirable to expand the editorship and the number of contributors to the book. Accordingly, the compilation of the 38th edition of *Gray's Anatomy* was begun in 1990 with the formation of an Editorial Board consisting of eight members under the Chairmanship of Professor Peter Williams. The traditional Sections of the book were increased in number and rearranged in a more appropriate manner; at the same time, new Section Editors were appointed to oversee their revision and to recruit specialist contributors.

Sadly, after a short illness, Professor Roger Warwick, who had been an enthusiastic and energetic co-editor for three earlier editions, and served only briefly on the new Editorial Board, died in September 1991. Another grievous loss was the death in October 1994 of Professor Peter Williams, who had devoted much of his professional life to *Gray's Anatomy*, and whose untiring advice and imagination had so much impact on the 38th as well as on previous editions. We were also saddened by the death in July 1994 of Professor John Pegington. His broad knowledge of clinical anatomy was a great asset; his specialist expertise in the skeletal system made him a natural choice to head his Section. We are grateful to Dr Roger Soames for editing the Skeletal System effectively in the limited time available.

The changes to the general organization of the 38th edition include the following. Completely new Sections have been added on Surface Anatomy and Neonatal Anatomy. Osteology and Arthrology are now fused into a single Section, the Skeletal System. The cellular aspects of the Introduction have been separated as Cells and Tissues, and the description of the skin, previously part of the Introduction, is combined with the breasts (in earlier editions considered with the female reproductive system) to form the Integumental System. Cellular aspects of blood and haemopoiesis, and of lymphoid tissue,

previously part of Angiology, have been combined in a separate Section, the Haemolymphoid System. Splanchnology has been split up into its component parts: the Respiratory, Alimentary, Urinary, Reproductive and Endocrine Systems. The names of the other Sections have been changed by adopting a more familiar and generally accepted terminology. Myology becomes Muscle; Angiology becomes Cardiovascular System; Neurology becomes Nervous System. The Introduction is now restricted to comments on the nature and historical development of Anatomy, on human evolution and on anatomical nomenclature. The Embryology and Development Section retains its title.

Section Editors have recruited additional contributors where appropriate, and have also introduced essays from invited academics and clinicians with specific expertise.

These essays have been distributed through the text to provide overviews of new or rapidly expanding areas of scientific research or important new clinical developments, and to relate the anatomical descriptions to wider areas of human biology. A list of contributors is given at the beginning of each Section. The entire text has been either rewritten or extensively revised, and there are many new illustrations; many of the original figures have also been updated. The Section Editors and contributors have worked hard to ensure that the text reflects modern advances, and that it is accessible to a wide variety of readers with varying backgrounds and interests.

All the changes instituted in this edition have been made in an attempt to assimilate the huge advances made in anatomical science since the last edition was published in 1989. We have summarized the explosion in knowledge resulting from the application of the techniques of molecular biology in all areas of our science, new findings from the application of modern non-invasive imaging methods, computer-assisted confocal microscopy, immunohistology and immuno-electron microscopy, computer-aided quantitative methods, and many other developments. Throughout we have been sensitive to Henry Gray's wishes that the book should address primarily the subject of human anatomy, and that it should serve the clinical world. However, over-specialization of the book has been resisted by retaining a wider backcloth of biological concerns beyond the old, historical boundaries of anatomy. Thus in the Introduction and in a number of other Sections, a brief account is given of the phylogenetic background of the human form and its systems, providing a context in which to describe their present condition. Many of the genes we carry have been conserved throughout the evolution of the animal kingdom, so that we see common patterns of development in such diverse forms as the fruit fly *Drosophila* and the human embryo which largely determine the mature human form. These approaches, we feel, are justified, and indeed are essential if we are ever to gain any real understanding of the human body's nature in all its complexity, and begin to answer the questions 'Who are we, and from whence did we come?'

L.H.B.
M.M.B.
P.C.
M.D.
J.E.D.
M.W.J.F.

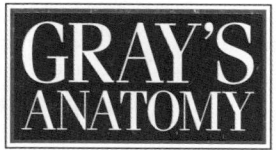

CONTRIBUTORS

Paul Aichroth MS FRCS
Consultant Orthopaedic Surgeon, Chelsea and Westminster
Hospital and Wellington Knee Surgery Unit, Wellington Hospital,
London

R. McN. Alexander DSc FRS
Professor of Zoology, University of Leeds, Leeds

Robert H. Anderson BSc MD FRCPath
Joseph Levy Professor of Paediatric Cardiac Morphology, National
Heart and Lung Institute; Honorary Consultant, Royal Brompton
Hospital, London

John Aplin MA PhD
Senior Lecturer in Biochemistry, Department of Obstetrics and
Gynaecology, University of Manchester, Manchester

Paul J. R. Barton BSc PhD
British Heart Foundation Senior Research Fellow; Senior Lecturer,
Department of Cardiothoracic Surgery, National Heart and Lung
Institute, London

Frank Billett PhD BSc
Visiting Research Fellow (Formerly Senior Lecturer), Department
of Biology, University of Southampton, Southampton

Alan Boyde PhD
Professor, Department of Anatomy and Developmental Biology,
University College London, London

A. S. Breathnach MSc MD
Emeritus Professor of Anatomy, University of London; Honorary
Senior Research Fellow, Division of Physiology and Institutional
Dermatology, United Medical and Dental Schools, St Thomas's
Campus, London

Nigel A. Brown BSc PhD
Head of Teratology, MRC Experimental Embryology and
Teratology Unit, and Senior Lecturer, Department of Child Health,
St George's Hospital Medical School, University of London,
London

J. C. Buckland-Wright BSc PhD
Reader in Radiological Anatomy, Division of Anatomy and Cell
Biology, United Medical and Dental Schools, Guy's Campus,
London

John Burn MD FRCP
Professor of Clinical Genetics, University of Newcastle upon Tyne,
Newcastle upon Tyne

Geoffrey Burnstock PhD DSc FAA MRCP (Hon) FRS
Professor and Head of Department of Anatomy and Developmental
Biology and Convenor, Centre for Neuroscience, University College
London, London

S. R. Butler MA PhD
Scientific Director, Burden Neurological Institute, Bristol

Arthur Butt BSc (Hons) MPhil PhD
Senior Lecturer in Physiology, Department of Physiology, United
Medical and Dental Schools, St Thomas's Campus, London

Malcolm B. Carpenter AB MD
Professor and Chairman Emeritus, Department of Anatomy, F.
Edward Hebert School of Medicine, Uniform Services University
of Health Science, Bethesda, Maryland

John Carroll BSc PhD
Scientist, MRC Experimental Embryology and Teratology Unit, St
George's Hospital Medical School, London

Alan Colchester BA BM BCh FRCP PhD
Senior Lecturer in Neurology, United Medical and Dental Schools,
Guy's Hospital, London

E. S. Crelin BA PhD
Professor of Anatomy, Department of Medicine, Yale University
School of Medicine, Newhaven, USA

H. Alan Crockard MB BCh BAO FRCS FRCS (Ed)
Consultant Neurosurgeon, National Hospital for Neurology and
Neurosurgery; Tutor, Surgical Workshop for Anatomical
Prosection, Royal College of Surgeons, London

Robin Huw Crompton BSc AM PhD
Lecturer in Anatomy, University of Liverpool, Liverpool
Editor-in-Chief *Folia Primatologica*

Michael J. Cullen MA DPhil (Oxon)
Principal Research Associate, School of Neurosciences, University
of Newcastle upon Tyne, Newcastle upon Tyne

Michael G. Daker BSc PhD
Senior Lecturer in Cytogenetics, Division of Medical and Molecular
Genetics, Guy's Hospital, London

Peter Dangerfield MD MBChB (St And)
University Lecturer and Honorary Clinical Lecturer, Departments
of Human Anatomy and Cell Biology and Orthopaedic and
Accident Surgery, University of Liverpool, Liverpool

Duncan R. Davidson PhD
Non-Clinical Scientist, Medical Research Council Human Genetics
Unit, Western General Hospital, Edinburgh

Michael H. Day MB BS DSc PhD
Senior Visiting Research Fellow, The Natural History Museum,
London

David Denison PhD FRCP
Emeritus Professor of Clinical Physiology, Royal Brompton
Hospital and The National Heart and Lung Institute, London

R. G. Edwards FRCOG FRS
Churchill College, Cambridge

Yvonne H. Edwards BSc (Hons) PhD
MRC Senior Staff, MRC Human Biochemical Genetics Unit,
University College London, London

D. A. Eisner MA DPhil
Professor of Veterinary Biology, Department of Veterinary
Preclinical Sciences, University of Liverpool, Liverpool

Susan E. Evans BSc PhD
Senior Lecturer, Department of Anatomy and Developmental Biology, University College London, London

Barry J. Everitt MA BSc PhD
Reader in Neuroscience, Department of Experimental Psychology, University of Cambridge, Cambridge

Heidi Felix PhD
Head of Research Laboratories, Ear, Nose and Throat Department, University Hospital, Zurich, Switzerland

Ian S. Fentiman MD FRCS
Consultant Surgeon, Guy's Hospital, London

Mark W. J. Ferguson BSc (Hons) BDS (Hons) PhD FFD RCSI
Professor and Dean, School of Biological Sciences, University of Manchester, Manchester

Anne Ferguson-Smith PhD
Wellcome/CRC Institute of Cancer and Developmental Biology, University of Cambridge, Cambridge

David Gaffan MA PhD
Medical Research Council External Scientific Staff, Department of Experimental Psychology, University of Oxford, Oxford

M. J. Gleeson MD FRCS
Professor and Consultant ENT Surgeon, Guy's Hospital, London

M. H. Glickstein BA PhD
Professor of Neuroscience, Department of Anatomy and Developmental Biology, University College London, London

Nicholas Goddard MB BS FRCS DipChirMain (Paris)
Consultant Orthopaedic Surgeon and Honorary Senior Lecturer, Royal Free Hospital and School of Medicine, London

Norman A. Gregson BSc PhD
Senior Lecturer, Division of Anatomy and Cell Biology, United Medical and Dental Schools, London

Michael M. Gunther MSc PhD
Department of Human Anatomy and Cell Biology, University of Liverpool, Liverpool

Sarah Guthrie MA PhD
Lecturer in Neuroanatomy, Division of Anatomy and Cell Biology, United Medical and Dental Schools, Guy's Hospital, London

Carole M. Hackney BSc (Hons) PhD
Reader, Department of Communication and Neuroscience, University of Keele, Keele

Wolfgang Hamann MD PhD (Hamburg)
Senior Lecturer and Honorary Consultant in Pain Relief, United Medical and Dental Schools of Guy's and St Thomas's Hospitals, London, and Director of Pain Relief Services, Lewisham Hospital, London

Paul J. Harrison MA BM BCh DM MRCPsych
Wellcome Senior Research Fellow in Clinical Science and Honorary Consultant Psychiatrist, University Departments of Psychiatry and Neuropathology, Oxford

R. Haskell FRCP, FDSRCS
Consultant Oral and Maxillofacial Surgeon, Guy's and St Thomas's Trust and Greenwich Healthcare Trust, London

Michael H. Hastings BSc PhD
University Lecturer in Anatomy, University of Cambridge, Cambridge

Basil Helal MCh (Orth) FRCS FRCSE
Emeritus Consultant, Royal National Orthopaedic Hospital, London; Honorary Consultant, The Royal London Hospital, London and Enfield Hospital Group, Enfield

Timothy R. Helliwell MD MRCPath
Senior Lecturer in Pathology, University of Liverpool; Consultant Histopathologist, Royal Liverpool University Hospital, Liverpool

Joe Herbert BSc MB ChB PhD
Reader in Neuroendocrinology, Department of Anatomy, University of Cambridge, Cambridge

Peter W. H. Holland MA PhD
Professor of Zoology, School of Animal and Microbial Sciences, University of Reading, Reading

Robin S. Howard MRCP PhD
Consultant Neurologist, National Hospital for Neurology and Neurosurgery and St Thomas's Hospital, London

Andrew Jackson MB BS FRCS
Consultant Orthopaedic Surgeon, St George's Hospital; Honorary Consultant, Royal National Orthopaedic Hospital, London

Martin H. Johnson MA PhD
Professor of Reproductive Sciences and Fellow of Christ's College, University of Cambridge, Cambridge

N. S. Jones BDS FRCS
Consultant Otorhinolaryngologist, University of Nottingham, Nottingham

Sheila J. Jones PhD
Professor of Anatomy, Department of Anatomy and Developmental Biology, University College London, London

Jack Joseph MD DSc FRCOG FCSLT (Hon)
Professor Emeritus, Guy's Hospital Medical School, University of London, London

Marion D. Kendall DSc PhD BSc
Professor of Histology, The Thymus Laboratory, The Babraham Institute, Cambridge and Department of Pharmacology, United Medical and Dental Schools, St Thomas's Campus London

Christopher Kennard PhD MB BS FRCP
Professor of Clinical Neurology, Charing Cross and Westminster Medical School, University of London; Honorary Consultant Neurologist, Charing Cross Hospital, London

Susan J. Kimber MA PhD
Senior Lecturer, School of Biological Sciences, University of Manchester, Manchester

Conrad A. King BSc MSc PhD
Senior Lecturer in Zoology, Department of Biology, University College London, London

William Niall Alexander Kirkpatrick BDS MBBS
Senior House Officer, Department of Plastic Surgery, Stoke Mandeville Hospital, Aylesbury

Leslie Klenerman ChM FRCS (Eng Ed)
Emeritus Professor of Orthopaedic and Accident Surgery, University of Liverpool, Liverpool

Anthony Lander MB BS DCH FRCS
Wellcome Research Fellow, Department of Child Health and MRC Experimental Embryology and Teratology Unit, St George's Hospital Medical School, London

N. M. Le Douarin
Professeur au Collège de France; Directeur de l'Institut d'Embryologie cellulaire et moléculaire du CNRS et du Collège de France, Nogent-sur-Marne, France

Roger N. Lemon BSc PhD MA (Cantab)
Professor and Head of Department, Sobell Department of Neurophysiology, Institute of Neurology, London

Olle Lindvall MD PhD
Professor of Neurology, University of Lund, Lund, Sweden

Douglas A. Luke BSc BDS PhD FDSRCS
Senior Lecturer in Anatomy, United Medical and Dental Schools, Guy's Campus, London

C. J. M. McCullough MA FRCS
Consultant Orthopaedic Surgeon, Northwick Park Hospital, Harrow

D. A. McGrouther MD FRCS
Professor of Plastic and Reconstructive Surgery, University College London Medical School, London

Stephen McMahon BSc PhD
Senior Lecturer, Department of Physiology, United Medical and Dental Schools, St Thomas's Hospital Medical School, London

Paul McMaster MA (Cantab) MB ChM (L'pool) FRCS (Eng & Edin)
Consultant General and Transplant Surgeon, Queen Elizabeth Hospital, Birmingham

Adrian Marston MA DM MCh FRCS MD
Emeritus Consultant Surgeon, The Middlesex Hospital and University College London Hospital Trust, University of London, London

Ivor Mason PhD BA
Senior Lecturer and Co-Director, Medical Research Council Brain Development Programme, Division of Anatomy and Cell Biology, United Medical and Dental Schools, Guy's Hospital, London

T. D. Matthews BSc MB BS DO FRCS FRCOphth
Research Fellow and Honorary Registrar, Charing Cross and Westminster Medical School, London

Pamela Milner BSc (Hons) PhD
Senior Research Fellow, Department of Anatomy and Developmental Biology, University College, London

Darius F. Mirza FRCS
Surgeon, Liver and Hepatobiliary Unit, Queen Elizabeth Hospital, Edgbaston, Birmingham

Barry Mitchell BSc PhD
Lecturer in Human Morphology, Faculty of Medicine, University of Southampton, Southampton

Isabella E. Moore DM MRCPath
Consultant Paediatric Pathologist, Department of Histopathology, Southampton University Hospitals NHS Trust, Southampton

Antoon F. M. Moorman PhD
Associate Professor in Anatomy and Embryology, Department of Anatomy and Embryology, Academic Medical Centre, University of Amsterdam, The Netherlands

John F. Morris BSc MB ChB MD MA
University Lecturer in Human Anatomy, University of Oxford; Wellcome–Franks Fellow and Tutor in Medical Studies, St Hugh's College, Oxford

Gonzalo Moscoso MB BS MD PhD
Senior Lecturer (Hon) in Early Human Development and Director, Early Human Development Research Unit, King's College Hospital School of Medicine and Dentistry, London

Richard L. Moss PhD
Professor and Chair of Physiology, Director, University of Wisconsin Cardiovascular Research Center, Department of Physiology, University of Wisconsin Medical School, Madison, USA

W. F. G. Muirhead-Allwood BSc (Hons) MB BS FRCS
Consultant Orthopaedic Surgeon, Royal National Orthopaedic Hospital Trust, Stanmore, The Whittington Hospital and King Edward VII's Hospital for Officers, London

Lars Neumann
Consultant Orthopaedic Surgeon, The Nottingham Shoulder and Elbow Unit, Nottingham City Hospital, Nottingham

M. D. O'Brien MD FRCP
Physician for Nervous Diseases, Department of Neurology, Guy's Hospital, London

Stephen C. O'Neill BSc (Hons) PhD
Lecturer, Veterinary Preclinical Sciences, University of Liverpool, Liverpool

W. J. Owen BSc MS FRCS
Consultant Surgeon, Guy's Hospital, London

Roger Parker MS FRCS
Clinical Anatomist, Department of Anatomy and Cell Biology, United Medical and Dental Schools, Guy's Hospital, London; Consultant Otolaryngologist, Royal Berkshire Hospital, Reading

Terence Partridge BSc PhD
Head of Muscle Cell Biology Unit, MRC Clinical Sciences Centre, Royal Postgraduate Medical School, Hammersmith Hospital, London

R. C. A. Pearson MA DPhil BM BCh (Oxon)
Professor of Neuroscience, Department of Biomedical Science, University of Sheffield, Sheffield

G. D. Perkin BA FRCP
Consultant Neurologist, Charing Cross Hospital, London and Hillingdon Hospital, Uxbridge

Marta E. Perry MUDr, LRCP, MRCS, PhD
Senior Lecturer, Division of Anatomy and Cell Biology, United Medical and Dental Schools, Guy's Campus, London

Terry M. Preston BSc
Senior Lecturer and Tutor, Biology Department, University College London, London

Sheila Rankin FRCR
Consultant Radiologist, Guy's Hospital, London

Geoffrey Raisman DM DPhil (Oxon)
Head, Laboratory of Neurobiology, National Institute for Medical Research, London

L. Rees MB BS
Lecturer, Division of Anatomy and Cell Biology, United Medical and Dental Schools, Guy's Campus, London

Charles H. Rodeck BSc MB BS DSc FRCOG
Professor and Head, Department of Obstetrics and Gynaecology, University College London Medical School, London

P. S. Rudland MA PhD MRCPath FIBiol
Professor of Biochemistry, University of Liverpool, Liverpool

Gordon L. Ruskell MS PhD DSc FBCO
Professor of Ocular Anatomy, City University, London

Brenda R. Russell PhD
Professor of Physiology, University of Illinois at Chicago, Chicago, USA

N. J. Saunders MD FRCS MRCOG
Consultant Obstetrician and Gynaecologist, Princess Anne Hospital, Southampton

John E. Scott BSc MSc PhD DSc
Professor, Chemical Morphology, Manchester University, Manchester

Robert A. Sells MB FRCS FRCS (Ed) MA
Director, Regional Transplant Unit; Consultant General Surgeon, Royal Liverpool University Hospital, Liverpool

Paul T. Sharpe BA PhD
Dickinson Professor of Craniofacial Biology, Department of Craniofacial Development, United Medical and Dental Schools, Guy's Hospital, London

Richard M. Sharpe BSc MSc PhD
MRC Special Appointment, MRC Reproductive Biology Unit, Centre for Reproductive Biology, Edinburgh

M. M. Sharr MRCP FRCS
Consultant Neurosurgeon, Guy's Hospital, London

P. S. Shepherd FRCP
Senior Lecturer and Honorary Consultant, Department of Immunology, United Medical and Dental Schools, Guy's Hospital, London

J. Victor Small PhD
Professor and Department Head, Institute of Molecular Biology of the Austrian Academy of Sciences, Salzburg, Austria

Kenneth J. Smith PhD
Reader in Neurology and Anatomy, Department of Neurology and Division of Anatomy, United Medical and Dental Schools, Guy's Campus, London

Moya Meredith Smith PhD DSc FLS
Reader in Comparative Odontology, United Medical and Dental Schools, Guy's Hospital, London

William A. Souter MB ChB (Hons) FRCS (Ed)
Consultant Orthopaedic Surgeon, Surgical Arthritis Unit, Princess Margaret Rose Orthopaedic Hospital, Edinburgh; Honorary Senior Lecturer, Department of Orthopaedics, University of Edinburgh, Edinburgh

John Maynard Stevens MB BS DRACR FRCR
Consultant Neuroradiologist, The National Hospital for Neurology and Neurosurgery and St Mary's Hospital, London

E. M. Tansey BSc PhD PhD
Historian of Modern Medical Science, Wellcome Institute for the History of Medicine, London

Cheryll Tickle MA PhD
Professor of Developmental Biology, Department of Anatomy and Developmental Biology, University College and Middlesex School of Medicine, London

John Trinick BSc PhD
Senior Research Fellow, Department of Veterinary Clinical Sciences, Bristol University, Bristol

Jan Voogd MD
Professor of Anatomy, Erasmus University, Rotterdam, The Netherlands

W. Angus Wallace FRCS (Ed) FRCS (Ed) (Orth)
Professor of Orthopaedic and Accident Surgery, The Nottingham Shoulder and Elbow Unit, Nottingham City Hospital, Nottingham

K. E. Webster BSc PhD MB BS
Professor of Anatomy and Human Biology and Head, Department of Anatomy and Human Biology, King's College London, London

Roy O. Weller BSc MD PhD FRCPath
Professor of Neuropathology, University of Southampton, Southampton; Consultant Neuropathologist to the Wessex Region

Colin Wendell-Smith AO MB BS PhD (Lond) LLD (Hon) (Tas) DObstRCOG FACE FRACOG
Emeritus Professor of Anatomy, University of Tasmania, Tasmania; Honorary Anatomist, Royal Hobart Hospital, Hobart, Tasmania, Australia

Michael Whitaker MA PhD
Professor of Cell Physiology, University College London, London

Bernard Wood BSc MB BS PhD
Derby Professor of Anatomy and Head, Department of Human Anatomy and Cell Biology, The University of Liverpool, Liverpool

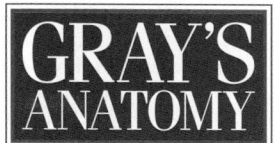

HISTORICAL ACCOUNT

BIOGRAPHY OF HENRY GRAY FRS FRCS (1827–61) by Peter L. Williams

William Gray, Henry's father, apparently an only child, was born in 1787, and for unascertained reasons entered the Royal Household where he was reared and subsequently became Deputy Treasurer to the Prince of Wales.

William Gray married Ann Walker in 1817 and throughout the reign of George IV they were accommodated at Windsor Castle. During this period they had four children, three sons and a daughter. Henry Gray, the original author of this book, was the second son; he had an older brother, a younger brother and a sister. The family remained at Windsor until 1830, when, with the accession of William IV, they took up residence at No. 8 Wilton Street, Belgrave Square, London, to be near to Buckingham Palace.

Robert Gray, Henry's younger brother, also studied medicine and became a naval surgeon; he died whilst at sea in his 22nd year. It is thought that their younger sister never married. Henry's older brother, Thomas William, studied law, becoming Attorney to the Queen's Bench in 1841, then in 1846 Solicitor to the High Court of Chancery. It was his third son, Charles, who developed smallpox in 1861, and it was whilst treating this nephew that Henry Gray contracted confluent smallpox which was to prove fatal.

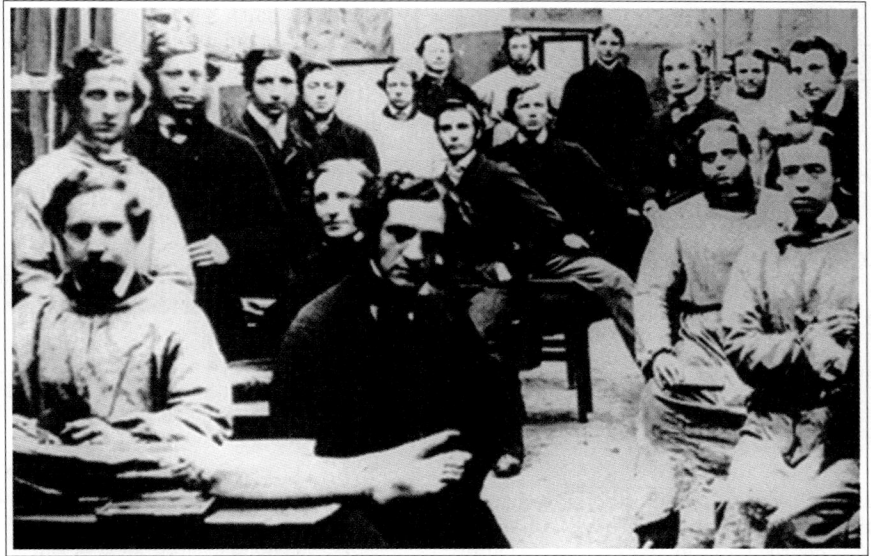

Henry Gray (centre) in the dissecting room of St George's Hospital in 1860.

Henry Gray was born in Windsor in 1827, but in 1830 No. 8 Wilton Street, Belgravia, became his home and he lived here for the rest of his relatively short life. Matriculating at 18 years of age, he entered St George's Hospital on 6 May 1845 as a 'perpetual student' (where his signature is preserved in the pupils' book). The hospital at that time held its Medical School partly in rooms rented in Kinnerton Street. Here the teaching of anatomy, chemistry, physiology, etc., was carried on, the lectures on medicine, surgery, and the clinical part of the curriculum were given at the hospital. Lecturers on anatomy in former days were in the habit of describing the premises (No. 75 Kinnerton Street, later the Animals' Hospital and Institute) as a diagrammatic representation, on a large scale, of the auditory canal and internal ear, with the main door, which was at the end of a short passage, compared to the tympanic membrane. Gray began to work at anatomy with much determination, probably

under Henry Charles Johnson, whose name is identified with St George's Hospital Medical School Prize in Anatomy. He pursued his study so diligently that in 1848, at the age of about 21, he was awarded the Triennial Prize of the Royal College of Surgeons for an essay on 'The Origin, Connection and Distribution of the Nerves of the Human Eye and its Appendages, illustrated by Comparative Dissections of the Eye in other Vertebrate Animals'. His earlier work showed exemplary blending of anatomy, physiology, embryology and neurology, applied to the special senses and ductless glands.

All who remembered Henry Gray as a student agree in describing him as a most painstaking and methodical worker, and one who learned his anatomy by the slow but invaluable method of making dissections for himself. He was awarded the MRCS on 11 February 1848.

In June 1850, Gray was appointed House Surgeon, and held the post for the usual year, 6 months under Robert Keate and Caesar Hawkins then 6 months under Edward Cutler and Thomas Tatum. On 3 June 1852 he was elected FRS, a rare distinction to be conferred on a man of 25. Having now come to be regarded as a very rising man, he returned to the dissecting-room, first as Demonstrator, then as Curator of the Museum, and Lecturer on Anatomy. He now devoted himself to the great work with which his name is identified. The first edition of the *Anatomy: Descriptive and Surgical*, was published by Parker & Son in 1858. In the preface, dated 1 August 1858, he 'gratefully acknowledges the great services he has derived in the execution of his work from the assistance of his friend, Doctor H. Vandyke Carter, late Demonstrator of Anatomy to St George's Hospital. All the drawings from which the engravings were made were executed by him. In the majority of cases they have been copied from or corrected by recent dissections made jointly by the author and Dr Carter.' Gray also thanks Timothy Holmes 'for his able assistance in correcting the proof-sheets.' Holmes, a polished scholar, probably improved the style in which the book was written, for Gray's own literary manner appears to have been very crude.

The book on its first appearance was praised by the *Lancet*, but

Certificate of election to a Fellowship of the Royal Society showing ten distinguished signatories.

accused by the *Medical Times* (1859, i, p. 241), in a scarifying article, of being largely a plagiarism from Quain and Sharpey's *Anatomy*, the textbook of the period. This charge Clinton Dent has sufficiently refuted:

'Undeniably many passages in Gray's work could be cited in which the phraseology and description closely resemble that of Quain and Sharpey's 'Anatomy'; but it is somewhat absurd in ordinary anatomical descriptions to accuse one writer of paraphrasing passages to be found in the work of another: forgetfulness of the source from which we are borrowing is an extremely common form of originality.'

In 1861 Caesar Hawkins and Edward Cutler, Surgeons, were succeeded by their Assistant Surgeons of St George's Hospital, and Gray became a candidate for the post of Assistant Surgeon, the other candidates being Timothy Holmes and Athol Johnson. Gray's election was regarded as certain, when he contracted smallpox while looking after his sick nephew, and died of its confluent variety on Thursday morning, 13 June 1861, after a very short illness. Burial, later in June, was at Highgate Cemetery. Other positions held by him at the time of his death were the Surgeoncies to the St George's and the St James's Dispensaries. Gray, at the time of his premature death at the age of 34, was engaged to be married.

His career had shown the highest promise and he was deeply mourned by his friends. Sir Benjamin Brodie, then growing blind, took up his pen almost for the last time to say to Charles Hawkins— 'I am most grieved about poor Gray. His death, just as he was on the point of realizing the reward of his labours, is a sad event indeed.... Gray is a great loss to the Hospital and the School. Who is there to take his place?' In the *Philosophical Transactions* was the paragraph, 'Mr Gray was, moreover, an accomplished and lucid teacher of anatomy, and much esteemed in private life, so that his early death was widely lamented by his professional brethren.'

It is idle to speculate whether Henry Gray would have reached the same distinction as a surgeon as he had in his earlier researches in physiology and avian embryology, and as an outstanding anatomist. However, he had already done sound work in pathology, and, indeed, at the time of his death he had made good progress with a work on 'Tumours', the manuscript of which, sadly, has been lost.

Over the decades, some misconceptions have become prevalent. The richly deserved, and increasingly widespread success of his textbook, *Anatomy: Descriptive and Surgical*, has been taken by many to assume that its contents reflected the intellectual scope of the man. It must be remembered that it was written for the needs of students and practitioners, especially in relation to practical surgery, many of whom were having to submit to the strictly prescribed sets of examinations then current. On the contrary, whilst he excelled in descriptive, often cadaveric, anatomy, many passages show his cognizance of the importance of (and differences in) living anatomy. Further, he had a profound interest in, and researched on, many other facets of the natural sciences, in addition to surgery, medicine, and pathology (see Table 1).

Without question, Henry Gray would have greatly enjoyed to participate in this great adventure, the 38th edition, in which so many of the finest minds and hands have been eager to co-operate in expanding, refining, and updating the work, on the existing foundation, to launch it towards the next millennium.

Table 1	Bibliography of Henry Gray
1848	The origin connexions and distribution of the nerves to the human eye and its appendages, illustrated by comparative dissections of the eye in other vertebrate animals. Original manuscript of this essay held by the Library of the Royal College of Surgeons
1850	On the development of the retina and optic nerve, and of the membranous labyrinth and auditory nerve. Philosophical Transactions of the Royal Society 140: 189–200
1852	On the development of the ductless glands in the chick. Philosophical Transactions of the Royal Society 142: 295–309
1853	On the structure and use of the spleen. Parker J W: London (A copy of this monograph is held by the Library of the Royal Society, London)
1853	An account of a dissection of an ovarian cyst which contained brain. Medico-Chirurgical Proceedings 36: 433–437
1856	On myeloid and myelo-cystic tumours of bone; their structure, pathology, and mode of diagnosis. Medico-Chirurgical Proceedings 39: 121–149
1858	Anatomy: Descriptive and Surgical. Parker J W: London
1860	Anatomy: Descriptive and Surgical. 2nd edition

A BRIEF HISTORY OF *GRAY'S ANATOMY* by E. M. Tansey

The first edition of Gray's *Anatomy: Descriptive and Surgical* appeared in 1858, towards the end of a particularly dynamic decade for medical science. During the 1850s Louis Pasteur demonstrated that fermentation depended on microorganisms; Hermann von Helmholtz measured the speed of nerve conduction; Thomas Addison described the adrenal insufficiency disease that now bears his name, and Gregor Mendel began experiments in his monastery garden that would ultimately reveal the laws of heredity. Intellectual seeds were being sown in the wider world also: Karl Marx published *The Communist Manifesto* in 1857 and Charles Darwin's *Origin of Species* appeared 2 years later. The latter's first suggestion of the theory of evolution through natural selection had been communicated, with a similar paper from Alfred Russell Wallace, to the Linnean Society of London in the summer of 1858. That was the same year in which Rudolph Virchow, developing Schwann and Schleiden's cell theory into a concept of disease creation, produced a new systematic approach to pathology, *Cellularpathologie*. Also that year the Medical Act was passed in Britain, which created the General Medical Council (GMC), the regulatory and licensing authority of the medical profession; and a young surgeon from St George's Hospital in London, Henry Gray, produced *Anatomy: Descriptive and Surgical*.

Three important themes in the recent history of medicine are thus exemplified by these events of 1858. Firstly, we see the increasing growth and vigour of scientific medicine, and the relevance of scientific research and theory, be it evolutionary Darwinism or cellular pathology, to medical practice. Secondly, the Medical Act emphasizes the growing professionalization of medical practice, and the concomitant moves towards regulated access and accredited training procedures, including the study of anatomy. Thirdly, Henry Gray acknowledges both the demands of the growing profession and the surge in scientific knowledge by producing a reliable educational text that satisfied the former and incorporated the latter.

Gray's book has now been in print for nearly 150 years, a remarkable record for any text, let alone one in the fast moving world of medical science. Throughout its long history the volume has been regularly revised and frequently reprinted; it has survived periods of stagnation to acquire a substantial reputation within worldwide academic circles; and it is one of the few medical texts known widely by name to the general public.

How then did a volume with the declared intention 'to furnish the Student and Practitioner with an accurate view of the anatomy of the Human Body ... especially ... practical surgery' achieve this position? For the purposes of analysis it is possible to determine four consecutive developmental stages: inception, consolidation, stasis and renaissance.

Inception

The first edition of *Anatomy: Descriptive and Surgical* focused on the macroscopical and topographical anatomy then deemed necessary for a practising surgeon, and won ready acclaim. The *Lancet* suggested that there was no work in any language of equal rank with Gray's *Anatomy*. The book was readily taken up in America, the first edition being produced there in 1859, and in 1860 a second British edition appeared, shortly before its young author died.

When Gray produced his first anatomy book it was less than 30 years after the passing of the Anatomy Act (1832), which had regulated the legal procurement of bodies for dissection by medical students. The removal of criminal associations from the subject thus encouraged the production of dissection guides and anatomy texts. Jones Quain had anticipated this with his *Elements of Descriptive and Practical Anatomy* in 1828, and G. V. Ellis' *Demonstrations of Anatomy* first appeared in 1840; both went through numerous editions, as did Cunningham's later *Manual* (1879) and *Textbook* (1902). However, what particularly distinguished Gray's book from its contemporaries was his emphasis on anatomical study as the practical basis of surgery, and the lavish use of woodcuts. As the *British Medical Journal*'s laudatory review emphasized: 'the power of the eye is, beyond all calculation, so much quicker in conveying intelligence than mere abstract reasoning', and it observed that the book would become **the** manual of anatomy. Longman acquired the rights to the work and after Gray's death organized a third edition under the supervision of Timothy Holmes, like Henry Gray a practising surgeon and anatomy teacher at St George's Hospital. Holmes and later editors continued the visual tradition by adding illustrations at a modest rate as the book passed through succeeding editions.

Until the end of the century the book continued to grow along the lines established by Gray. The editors remained practising surgeons, Holmes until 1880 (9th edition) and T. Pickering Pick, who succeeded him, both men regularly revising and updating the text and illustrations. The 5th edition (1869) was the first in which substantial alterations were introduced, as Holmes collected together the sections on General Anatomy (i.e. Microscopic Anatomy or Histology), which had been scattered throughout the text, to form an intro-

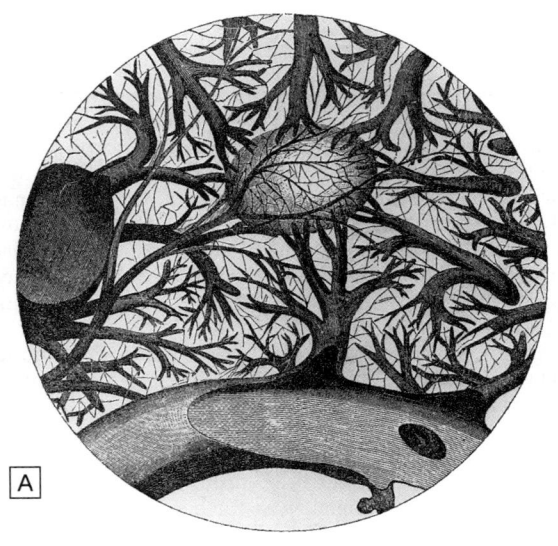

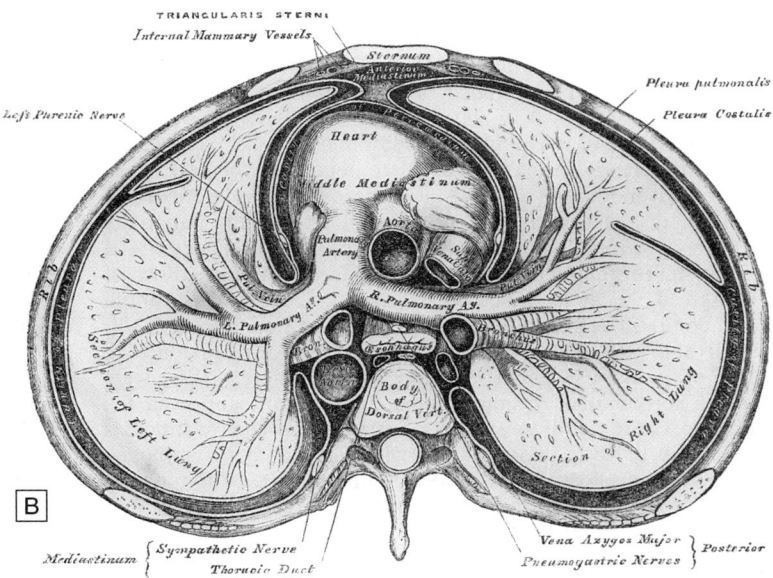

Illustrations from the first edition of *Anatomy: Descriptive and Surgical.* A. One of the splenic corpuscles showing its relations with the blood-vessels B. A transverse section of the thorax.

ductory section to the work as a whole. The chapter was, however, not fully integrated, being paginated separately from the main body of the work, until 1887 (11th edition), when Pickering Pick entirely rewrote the introductory section to encompass not only General Anatomy but also Development, changes he deemed necessary 'to keep pace with the ever-increasing activity of research in these branches of the science of Anatomy'.

Consolidation

Pick continued to update the work as a whole, although explicitly following Gray's original intention of producing a text for students of surgery. However, during the final decades of the nineteenth century medicine was becoming increasingly professionalized, a consequence of the 1851 Medical Registration Act and the Medical Act of 1858. The concomitant demands of medical education resulted in the creation of new academic departments and full-time, albeit few, teaching positions. Medical research and teaching could now provide careers for a limited number of men, and whole-time professional anatomists, rather than transient surgeons, appropriated much of the research and routine teaching of anatomy.

At the turn of the century a professional anatomist first became associated with *Gray's Anatomy*. From 1901 (15th edition) Robert Howden of Durham University served as joint editor with Pick, becoming sole editor from 1909 (17th edition) until 1926 (23rd edition). His influence was immediately apparent in a careful revision of the entire work, especially the section on Development, retitled 'Embryology', which he enriched with over 60 new illustrations; its content, however, remained strictly descriptive. He removed 'surgical' from the title and renamed it *Anatomy: Descriptive and Applied* (17th edition) to reflect the wider clinical relevance of anatomical knowledge, and employed specialist assistants to deal with the medical and surgical anatomy; a further step in this direction was the introduction of a chapter on Surface Anatomy in 1913 (18th edition). During Howden's editorship the number of figures almost doubled and colour was increasingly incorporated, a roll of innovation that excludes the routine replacement and maintenance of artwork from edition to edition. His successor was T. B. Johnston of Guy's Hospital, who began his 30-year association with the book in 1930 (24th edition), and who in 1938 (27th edition) first incorporated X-ray material in the volume formally entitled *Gray's Anatomy: Descriptive and Applied*.

Perhaps ironically, the acceptance of an eponymous title for the book occurred in the midst of battles to eradicate eponymous terminology from the text. Terminology disputes had raged for years, and one cynic has commented that anatomists would rather use each other's toothbrushes than employ their terminology. The twentieth century disputes have identifiable roots in the Nomenclature Committee of the Anatomische Gesellschaft, appointed in 1887 but still unable to reach agreement in 1895, when an unsatisfactory compromise, the Basle Nomina Anatomica (BNA), was produced. During the First World War Howden introduced the 'Basle' terminology in *Gray's*, although to temper objections from British anatomists he frequently included older, eponymous terms in parentheses.

After the First World War the Anatomical Society (of Great Britain and Ireland) formally decided to retain the older English terminology by modifying the BNA terms accordingly. The American Association of Anatomists preferred to adopt the internationally agreed 'Basle' terminology, and called on the British to cooperate in producing uniform nomenclature. With this appeal the editor of *Gray's* agreed, believing that English-speaking anatomists should share a common terminology. By the 26th edition (1935) T. B. Johnston had offered a compromise by incorporating the British Revision of the Basle Nomina Anatomica (BR), although these were sometimes accompanied by the original BNA terms, and even the appropriate Latin terms. A system of curved and square brackets was necessary to accommodate the variety of synonyms employed and an extensive Glossary was added. Although the editor 'hoped that the new terms will prove acceptable to instructed opinion and helpful to the uninitiated', the effect was stultifying.

Stasis

War-time paper shortages caused the Glossary to be excluded and the material on Surface Anatomy to be dispersed, and thus diluted,

within the general text. However, the 30th edition that emerged after the Second World War in 1949 showed a desire to return to the pre-war form and format. The strong adherence to the past became more apparent during the 1950s and 1960s as a succession of editors strove to keep an increasingly outmoded vehicle fresh. The difficulty of pruning 'dead wood' was acknowledged by the editors of the 31st edition (1954), and with the temptation of adding more and more detail, innovative changes between editions were slight. To accommodate these factual increases a disastrous editorial decision was made to print lengthy passages in small unattractive print. The volume became aesthetically unpleasing and intellectually tedious.

By this time a similar fate had befallen the American edition, which had been largely independent since its first editions and under different editorial hands, although the connections between the two remained extremely close until 1908. This was when the 17th edition appeared in America, a revision produced without reference to the English edition, although retaining the British numbering sequence. Subsequent editions were numbered in their own sequence and do not therefore correspond with the British editions. Two further editions were published before the First World War, although in 1913 the publishers took the unusual step of producing the 'local' American 19th edition edited by Edward Spitzka, and reproducing a 'New American from the 18th English' edited by Howden, which was not a commercial success. The experiment was not repeated and the American editors continued with their own revisions. By the 24th American edition (1942) *The Anatomy of the Human Body by Henry Gray* had a board of six associate editors with system responsibilities, and was a different production from its parent. To some extent these mechanisms delayed the earlier signs of age and weariness that troubled the original production, although by the 1960s the American edition too needed major refurbishment.

The necessity of completely modernizing the work had been recognized by D. V. Davies after completing the 34th, described by the *Lancet* as 'noble', edition. His unexpected death meant that such work was left to others. Peter Williams, Professor of Anatomy at Guy's Hospital, had been associated with *Gray's* since 1954: appointed by T. B. Johnson, he had assisted D. V. Davies on three editions (32nd to 34th edition). He was now joined by his colleague Roger Warwick to orchestrate and conduct the new production.

Renaissance

The 35th edition in 1973 marked the rebirth of the book, a remarkable production barely recognizable in appearance as *Gray's*, although in its comprehensive and authoritative content, it was the clear successor of the well-established tradition. Now simply entitled *Gray's Anatomy*, the book had increased in size by over one-third, a larger, double-column page format was used, and 600 more illustrations were added to an entirely rearranged text. The scholarly revision was further emphasized by the inclusion of a Bibliography of over 3000 references. Particularly striking were the specially designed illustrations, described by two early reviewers as 'garish' or 'pop-art', which were included alongside more conventional anatomical sections—an innovation in which the editors were clearly following Henry Gray's tradition of effective illustration. The text was markedly different from its predecessors. 'Anatomy' was interpreted in the broadest sense to include not only conventional morphological approaches, but also functional and experimental aspects. It succeeded in providing a coherent account of the structure of the human body from the ultrastructural to the macroscopic level, integrated with knowledge of development, growth and function. Detailed explorations of cytology, histology, embryology and neurology joined systematic topography in situating anatomy as a central discipline in the natural sciences.

The new *Gray's* was received with acclaim by its reviewers and its purchasers. The 35th edition sold over 200 000 copies world-wide, one-third in India, one-third in the United States and one-third in the rest of the world. The American sales indicate a particular triumph. The 35th was the first British edition, since the unfortunate experiment of 1913, to be successfully promoted alongside the American version. That achievement was further enhanced by the award of ELBS (Educational Low Priced Book Scheme) status for the 37th edition (1989), which enabled a subsidized volume to reach over 130 countries.

The editorial structure has also expanded. Five editorial assistants

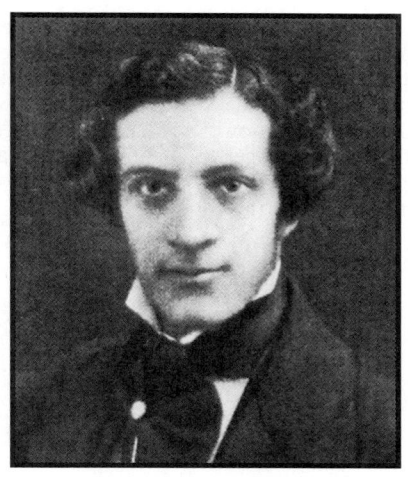

HENRY GRAY b. 1827 d. 1861

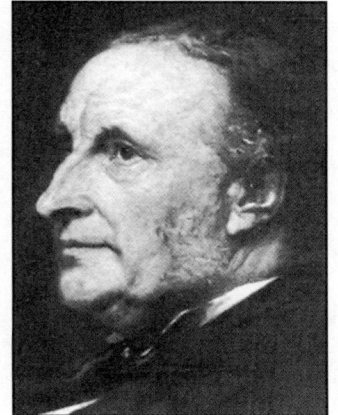

Timothy Holmes 1863–1880

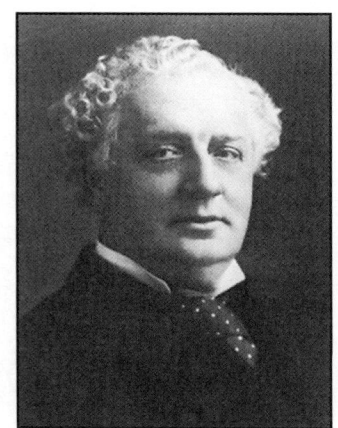

T. Pickering Pick 1883–1905

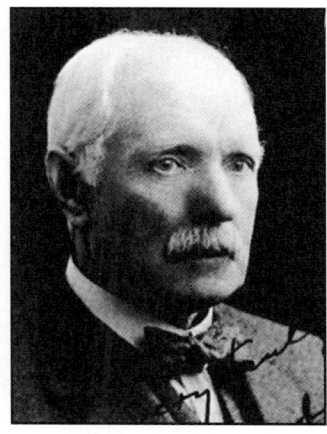

R. Howden 1901–1926

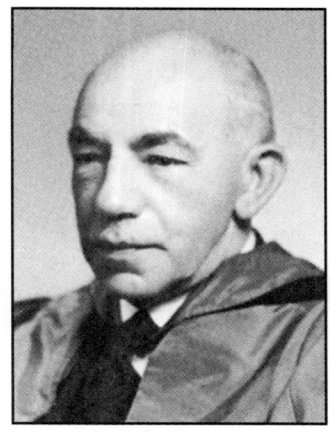

T. B. Johnston 1930–1958

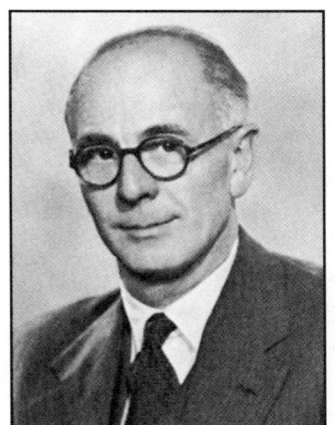

J. Whillis 1942–1954

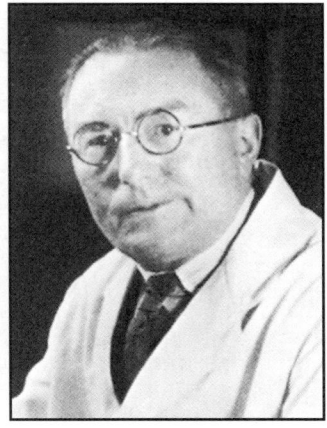

F. Davies 1958–1962

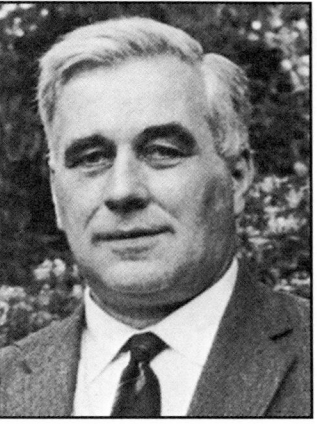

D. V. Davies 1958–1967

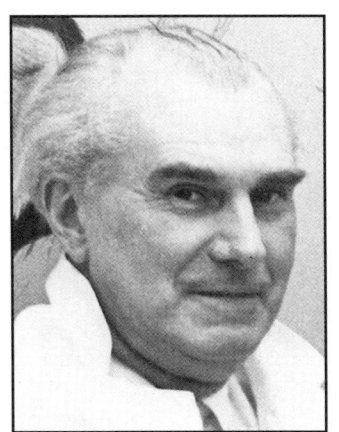

R. Warwick 1973–1989

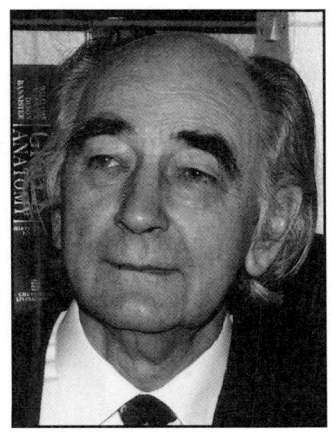

P. L. Williams 1973–1994

worked on the 35th edition, including Dr Lawrence Bannister, the first non-medical person to be appointed to contribute illustrated text to the publication. For the 36th edition he and Dr Mary Dyson, a fellow Reader in Anatomy at Guy's Hospital also trained in the zoological sciences, became associate editors and for the 37th edition they achieved co-editorial status with Peter Williams and Roger Warwick.

The preparation of this, 38th, edition has entailed yet further expansion and reorganization. There has been a substantial restructuring, with over a hundred contributors reporting via Section Editors to an editorial board chaired by Peter Williams, who, until his death, had been involved with the work for 40 years. *Gray's Anatomy* has been sold worldwide and has been translated into Spanish, Italian and Portuguese. The response of current readers to this edition is awaited with optimism.

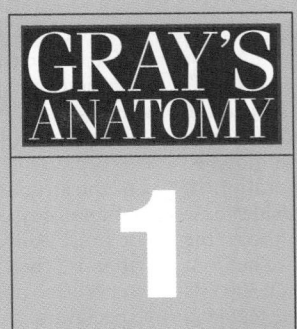

INTRODUCTION TO HUMAN ANATOMY

Section Editor: Lawrence H. Bannister

Contributor: Bernard A. Wood (Complete revision of Primate and human evolution)

WHAT IS ANATOMY?

The study of human anatomy, literally dissection, or the separation of the body into its parts, has signified many things to different cultures across the ages, and has been prompted by diverse motives: the need to cope with injury, disease and death, the generation of images for aesthetic, magical or religious purposes, and beside these practical preoccupations, a strong element of curiosity about the mysterious nature of human life and its mechanisms. The first recorded school of anatomy was in Alexandria (from about 300 BC to the second century AD) where the renowned anatomical teachers Herophilus and Erasistratus dissected the human body and described many of its structures. Before this time, dissection had been practised at various times in classical Greece, and also as part of the mummification process in Egypt during the previous two millennia, although little is known of how the dissectors interpreted what they found. The most influential anatomist in the ancient world was Galen (about 130–200 AD), a physician and prolific writer who studied anatomy at Alexandria and later worked in Rome. However, his anatomy was largely based on the dissection of animals rather than humans. Seriously flawed by many errors and misinterpretations, Galen's work became the received, unassailable text for anatomy, and seems to have exerted a deadening influence on the subject over the next 1300 years. Many terms used in modern anatomy have roots in Galen's work. Thereafter, anatomical literature of any consequence dates from the time of the Renaissance. Setting apart the extraordinary but until recently ignored studies by Leonardo da Vinci at the beginning of the sixteenth century, the foundation stone of modern anatomy is the work of Andreas Vesalius: *De Fabrica Corporis Humani*, published in 1543 when the author was aged 28 and teaching in Padua. This book had considerable impact because it was based on first-hand experience of human dissection rather than reliance on ancient texts, and, it must also be allowed, because of the imaginative and most striking quality of its excellent illustrations. After this epoch-making publication, anatomical science began to flourish, initially in the north Italian universities, then throughout Europe.

However, because of the social and religious attitudes surrounding the provision of bodies for dissection until recent times, the study of anatomy had many untoward resonances during the centuries that followed, some of them macabre, or anti-intellectual, others more benign. In England during the eighteenth century and later, the ultimate judicial threat to the wrong-doer was to be anatomized after execution. Throughout Europe, anatomists obtained their subjects for dissection largely from executions of criminals, from the poor houses, or, more often in Britain, from illicit graveyard exhumations. As medical science progressed during the nineteenth century and became more successful at treating the sick, the need for legally obtained cadavers was recognized and became carefully controlled by law. The sinister connotations of anatomy gradually faded as the benefits of a thorough medical training and the enlargement of medical knowledge became appreciated at large. So, for example, in Britain the bequeathal of one's body to medical schools after death eventually became an expression of personal philanthropy, often in gratitude for successful medical treatment in an earlier period of life. The anatomist became fully acceptable both socially, and, as the subject expanded beyond the confines of human topography, also academically. By the beginning of the twentieth century anatomy departments had generally achieved a high standing in the world of science, and prestigious university chairs in the subject attracted some of the best intellects into anatomical teaching and research.

The horizons of anatomy were also steadily expanding as specialized areas of study developed. From topographical anatomy new research fields arose: physical anthropology, palaeontology, comparative anatomy, biomechanics, kinesiology and radiological and other macroscopic imaging studies. At the microscopic level, histologists continued to explore a novel world of minute structures within the human body, and, as new instruments and methods of preparation were developed, anatomy forged ever-increasing links with biochemistry, physiology, genetics and physics. The complex changes of prenatal development were also discovered in embryological studies, and it became clear that much of adult anatomy can only be understood by knowing its prenatal history. In the study of the nervous system, neuroanatomy took its place as one of a battery of approaches needed for neurobiological exploration, complemented by neurophysiology, neuropharmacology, experimental psychology and, more recently, molecular biology and dynamic whole brain imaging.

Because of this immense ramification of interests and the blending of the structural approach with other disciplines, the proper territory of anatomy is at present hard to define. Clearly, for clinical purposes it must concern itself primarily with human topographic anatomy, that is, the clear and sufficiently detailed analysis of the body to serve the needs of surgeons, physicians and the various medical specialties. This was of course the central purpose of Henry Gray when he published the first edition of his *Anatomy*, and remains the chief focus of the 38th edition. But it is not sufficient merely to name the parts: anatomists have sometimes been criticized for a slavish attention to minutiae, and for the endless itemization and rotelearning of cadaveric structures with limited clinical importance. At its worst, anatomy could be a dingy subject, inhibitory to the intellect and hardly deserving the title of anatomical science.

Such views, sometimes expressed by senior personages who in their youth encountered oppressive anatomical regimes, have constrained many teaching departments into shunning the title of 'Anatomy' in favour of more progressive-sounding names. While these manoeuvres may be necessary to deflect prejudice and attract funding, it can be argued that too much apology is counterproductive. We should not make excuses, but celebrate, as we hope this book does, a discipline which is at the heart of modern life science, and, indeed, contributes richly to our general culture in so many ways. Anatomy is a timehonoured title encompassing a great range of endeavours, embracing all areas of knowledge relevant to the structural organization of the human body, and, like other branches of science, it is constantly changing as new research data transform our image of the body's dynamic organization. At the present time, anatomy is concerning itself more and more with the dynamic processes, the structure of the living rather than the dead: cadaveric dissection is of course essential to understand the architecture of the body, but it is important to add to this a knowledge of the structure of the living body. Computer-controlled imaging techniques are increasingly widening our appreciation of three-dimensional, living structure and may in the future be expected to play a major role in anatomical data acquisition, storage and communication as well as clinical diagnosis. The techniques of experimental embryology combined with microscopy, molecular biology and molecular genetics are also helping us to see how the adult body achieves its final form, why variations in structure appear and how the body regulates its microscopic arrangement in normal and regenerating tissues and organs.

Anatomy is part of the continuum of human knowledge. As in all areas of experience, it is possible to see human anatomy from what is essentially a reductionist viewpoint, to limit oneself to smaller and smaller areas of analysis and, of course, without such an approach all science drifts into meaningless generalization. The opposite, or one should say complementary, way of thinking, is holistic, integrative, looking for the connections between disparate areas of knowledge and larger patterns of organization or global significance. A balance between these two conceptual frameworks is clearly needed if science – 'things known' – is to be true to its name. So anatomy is not merely the separation of parts, the accurate description of bones, ligaments, muscles, vessels, nerves and so forth, but an attempt to grasp the totality of body structure, engaging many disciplines, constantly searching for underlying principles and viewing the living frame as an extraordinarily complex, labile entity with a temporal dimension, connected by evolutionary history to all other living organisms, expressing various morphologies as it develops, matures, reproduces, ages and dies, engaging in a plethora of integrated functions.

Furthermore, from a philosophical viewpoint, anatomy is not merely the structural biology of an animal species which happens to be human. Because we are self-aware, and the human body is the medium through which our experience of the world and our responses to it are transacted, the study of the human has a unique place in establishing the image we have of ourselves; ultimately the prosaic descriptions of the bones, muscles, blood vessels and neural pathways are the context of our experience of life.

In accordance with these views, in this Introduction we explore the setting of human anatomy with respect to the physical and biological worlds, before proceeding to the detailed descriptions of the body and its components.

ORIGIN OF LIFE ON EARTH

Our knowledge of human origins remains largely conjectural. It relies on fragmentary evidence from many different disciplines and is liable to major reassessment as new clues arrive, which they will no doubt continue to do and with increasing frequency. Relevant data arise from two major sources: the study of the fossilized remains of extinct forms, and comparative investigations of the anatomy, biochemistry and genetics of living species.

Of these, the first is the only reasonably direct means of establishing human ancestry; but because the fossil record is incomplete and it is difficult to interpret skeletal remains in their widely varying states of preservation, this approach has limitations. The more indirect comparative methods have also provided many useful clues about man's relationships, and the younger disciplines of molecular biology, particularly those dealing with molecular genetics, hold out great promise of unravelling the mechanisms by which the form and function of the human body are and were shaped. Of course the processes which gave rise to mankind have operated over immense periods of time, with widely varying influences of environment, both geological and biological. To understand the significance of these events we must also think of the physical forces which created the possibility of human emergence, of the preceding aeons and cosmic background from which life arose at first. Although these considerations may seem out of place in a textbook of anatomy, they are very relevant to our appreciation of the living substrate of the body, of its principles of construction and operation at all of its levels of organization including the cellular, tissue, developmental, systemic and integrated whole body grades, which are the themes of this book.

Present astronomical evidence points to emergence of the material universe from a single event 10–20 thousand million years ago, when the components of matter and perhaps with them the dimensions of space and time first appeared (1.1). In mathematical models of this event, it is envisaged that it occurred with unimaginable explosive force, generating temperatures of many millions of degrees and at first permitting the free existence of the fundamental, subatomic particles of matter. Within microseconds, as they began to cool, these assembled themselves into larger aggregates and finally atoms and then molecules of hydrogen. This matter expanded rapidly outwards and continues to do so even at the present time. From this singularity, the 'big bang', hydrogen molecules were first scattered fairly evenly in space but with some locational variations in density. Then under gravitational influences, they drifted together in denser clusters which eventually became massive and compact enough to convert the gravitational energy into temperatures sufficiently high to start thermonuclear fusion reactions and mass-energy conversion, so creating stars. (Currently, some theoreticians are even exchanging views of innovative, but speculative, mathematical models which may assist the approach to the problems of the prevailing conditions preceding, and at the inception of, the 'big bang'.)

Clusters of stars were drawn together into galaxies, and as they aged they sequentially, but asynchronously, passed through various changes in physical state, depending on their original dispersion and mass. At the enormous temperatures they generated, hydrogen atoms fused into progressively heavier atoms, forming the varieties of elements we know today. Some particularly massive stars became unstable and eventually exploded as supernovae, strewing the products of their fusion reactions into interstellar space where they cooled enough to form complex chemical compounds. It may have been that such material was captured by the gravitational fields of other stars, coalescing into larger masses which circled around them as planetary systems. Our Earth appears to have been formed in the solar system at about five thousand million years ago as a hot mass of rocks rich in elements such as carbon, silicon, oxygen, sulphur, chlorine and phosphorus, also many metals, especially sodium, calcium, potassium and iron. This world appears to have been at first highly volcanic but, as it began to cool, water vapour could

condense, forming the early seas, rivers and lakes, and generating the processes of erosion and sedimentary deposition which dominate the geology of our planet today. This early period was now cool enough to allow hitherto impossible chemical reactions in aqueous solution and the early water masses may have teemed with a wide variety of molecules in a dilute solution of inorganic ions. In particular, many carbon-based compounds were stable at these temperatures, yet could react with each other rapidly enough to create a rich carbon chemistry. It is likely that life arose in such an environment.

All matter, living or non-living, consists of the same basic subatomic units, and, varying quantitatively, many common atomic species. The most obvious distinction between the living and non-living is the dynamic level of molecular organization of this matter, that exhibited by the living being greater. Furthermore, development, growth and maintenance of living organisms involves a temporary increase in order, the ability to effect this increasing with the organism's level of complexity. Living organisms are usually ascribed a common series of attributes, for example the ability to sense and respond to environmental changes, to move, to grow and to reproduce. These vital attributes are considered further on page 20. To describe is not to define, however, and what distinguishes the living from the non-living eludes precise definition.

How living matter originated is still speculative. It is generally assumed, but rarely challenged among scientists, that life evolved exclusively on Earth from non-living matter. The commonest hypothesis is that when our planet had cooled sufficiently for the water vapour in its atmosphere to condense and begin to erode its rocks, the elements which dissolved in it combined to form simple inorganic molecules which, in response to solar energy, reacted chemically to produce the amino acid units of the enzymes essential to the life process. These interacted further, some evolving into 'living' self-replicating units, resembling viruses, in which the information necessary to ensure the accurate duplication of enzymes and other proteins was encoded in nucleic acids. Enclosure of some such units within proteolipid membranes might have produced the first unicellular organisms, perhaps like bacteria, each able to exert a measure of control over its internal environment, leading to increases in local order, longevity and reproductive capacity.

The results of experiments by Miller and Urey in 1953 suggested that amino acids could have been formed in the terrestrial atmosphere presumed to have existed some 4500 million years ago; this strengthens the hypothesis that life could have originated from non-living systems on Earth, but the next and literally vital evolutionary step, the chance interaction of these amino acids to form the proteinaceous enzymes necessary for self replication, has not been demonstrated. Lack of such a demonstration does not, of course, invalidate the hypothesis but equally the demonstration that amino acids could have formed in the then prevalent conditions does not prove that they actually did. An alternative hypothesis suggests that life may have originated extraterrestrially, and arrived as simple organisms in meteorites.

EVOLUTION OF LIFE ON EARTH

However life arose, many remain persuaded that it appears to have done so only once, since the highly complex macromolecules of differing living organisms and their metabolic interactions share too many common features to have arisen independently. (More strictly, whatever view of life's origin is envisaged, the 'only once' of the preceding paragraph should, perhaps, imply one common mechanism, whatever its possible multiplicity of sites and times.) The simplest living cells are the bacteria, blue-green algae and similar forms (collectively termed Prokaryotes), which have most of the essentials of other cells, except that they do not carry their genetic material in a nuclear compartment and, apart from the outer cell membrane, they lack membranous organelles. More complex cells (Eukaryotes) are likely to have arisen from these (however, see above) but differ from them in having nuclei containing larger quantities of genetic material in multiple chromosomes sequestered away from metabolic damage. Such cells needed a special (mitotic) apparatus to handle their more elaborate chromosomes at cell division and they also perfected ways of exchanging genes in meiosis

3

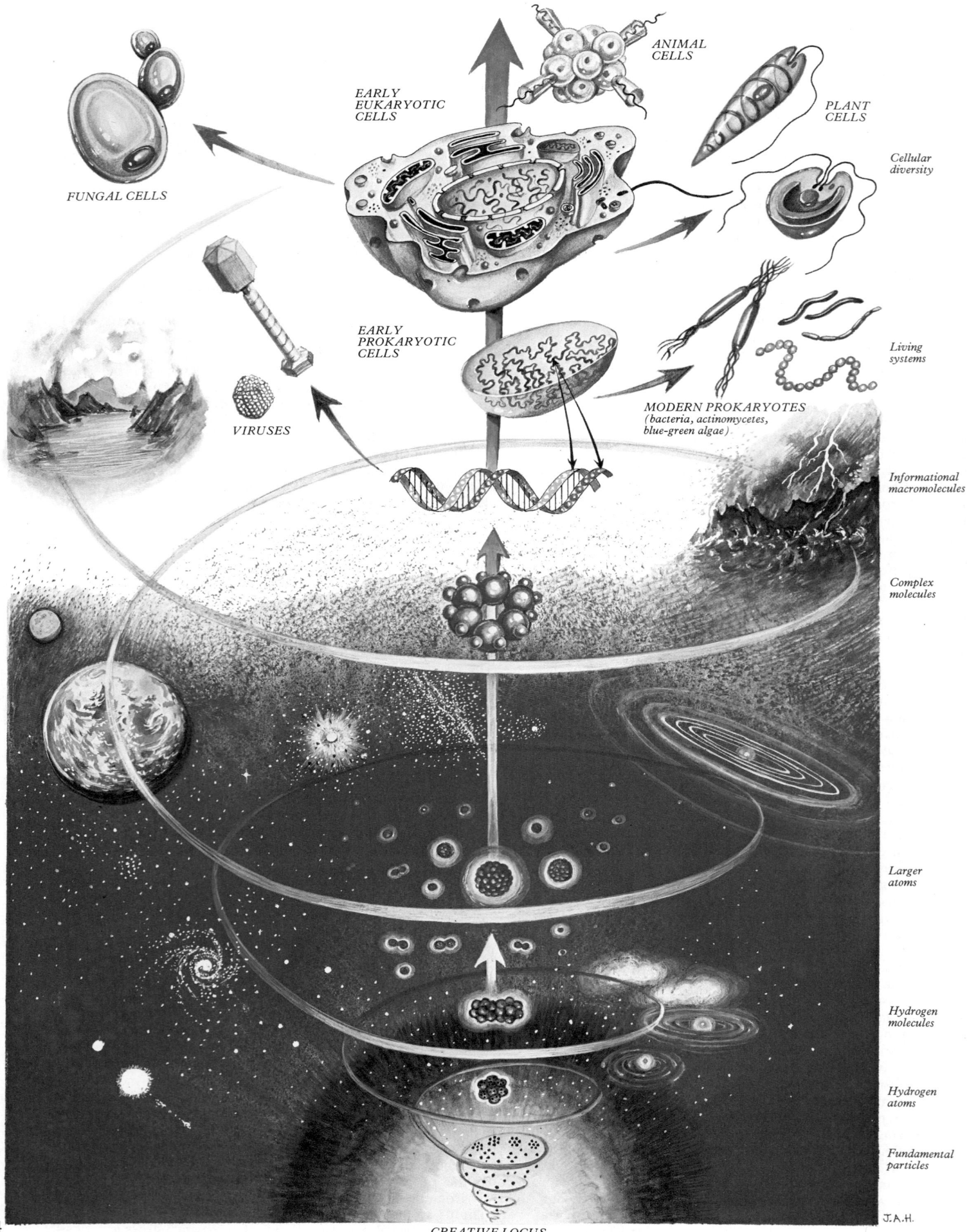

ANIMAL CELLS

EARLY EUKARYOTIC CELLS

PLANT CELLS

Cellular diversity

FUNGAL CELLS

EARLY PROKARYOTIC CELLS

Living systems

VIRUSES

MODERN PROKARYOTES (bacteria, actinomycetes, blue-green algae)

Informational macromolecules

Complex molecules

Larger atoms

Hydrogen molecules

Hydrogen atoms

Fundamental particles

J.A.H.

CREATIVE LOCUS

1.1 The origins of biological organization as envisaged from present cosmological, biochemical and palaeontological data.

which increased their variability and therefore the potential to exploit a variable environment. These cells also had complex membranous organelles within their cytoplasm so that different areas of the cell could be allocated to specialized functions. These developments appear to have been crucial because they allowed the formation of progressively more elaborate genetic material, structure and metabolism and consequently more complex form and function. It is likely that there were many different types of cell during this early experimental period, only some of them ancestral to the forms of life we know today, for example protozoa, unicellular algae, fungi, multicellular plants and animals (1.1, 2; see Vidal 1984). Some of these may have arisen as combinations of cells giving greater metabolic potential; thus both mitochondria and the chloroplasts of green plants have their own genetic apparatus distinct from the rest of the cell and may have arisen as independent organisms (see Margulis 1981). It is also likely that many of the earliest eukaryotes were able to use sunlight for their energy needs and had photosynthetic pigments. Certainly once the early nutrients in the environment had been depleted this would have been the only source of energy for the biological world, herbivorous and carnivorous animals depending for their supply of chemical energy on green plants. From this point onwards there must have been a great proliferation of different forms and the development of multicellular organisms in which different cells could carry out specialist tasks (see Romer 1968; Attenborough 1979).

ANIMAL KINGDOM: SELECTED PHYLA

The fossil record of these events begins with any clarity only when many of the major groups of invertebrates had already appeared, by about 500 million years ago, and the line of descent (1.2) can only be surmised. It is thought that the first truly multicellular animals (*Metazoa*) possessed two layers of cells (i.e. they were diploblastic), but that later a third layer was added giving an outer, ectodermal layer, a middle mesoderm and an inner endodermal lining to the gut (enteron). The outer layer provided an interface with the environment, the inner was concerned mainly with nutrition while the middle layer provided mechanical support, muscular systems and a route for nervous and circulatory systems. In the simplest *triploblasts*, such as flatworms (Platyhelminths), the mesoderm is usually a solid mass but in more complex forms it splits into an outer (somatic) and an inner (splanchnic or visceral) layer, the latter surrounding the gut which is thus free to move within the cavity (coelom) so formed within the mesoderm. In these animals (coelomates), an efficient vascular system is essential to convey nutrients absorbed in the gut across the coelom to the outer parts of the body and we find that they all possess propulsile heart-like structures as well as branching vascular channels. The freeing of the outer mesoderm from the gut also made further locomotor advances possible and many such animals are organized on a segmental pattern of repeated muscle blocks and attendant nerves and blood vessels which facilitate many different types of movement and specialized local body functions. This segmental pattern is fundamental to many groups of animals including ourselves and it is significant that at least some of the genetic mechanisms for generating segmentation and local specialization of segments (homiotic genes) appear to be much the same in both insects (e.g. *Drosophila*) and mammals.

From these segmented coelomates, which include annelid worms, arthropods, molluscs and echinoderms (i.e. starfish and their allies), are thought to have arisen the *chordate phylum*, possibly from an echinoderm-like stock. The simplest chordate-like animals we know today are aquatic filter-feeders such as sea-squirts (Urochordates) and the fish-like Cephalochordates (the lancelets *Branchiostoma* or *Amphioxus*). These filter their food from water through a series of slits flanked by supporting bars in their pharyngeal walls, which appear to be the forerunners of the embryonic pharyngeal clefts and arches of all vertebrates. Many of these primitive creatures also have hollow dorsal central nervous systems, derived perhaps by the invagination of superficial nerve nets such as those we see in starfish. They have bilateral symmetry and, at some stage in their lives, segmental muscle blocks grouped around a longitudinal stiff but flexible rod (notochord) permitting sinusoidal swimming movements. At least some of them also develop an additional embryonic group

of cells, the neural crest (see p. 234), which is of great significance in the development of many typical chordate features.

The origin of the true vertebrates from such groups appears to have been relatively late, the first well-preserved fossil forms, armour-plated fishes called Ostracoderms, occurring in Silurian rocks about 410 million years old, although fragments of fish-like scales also occur in much older strata. Ostracoderms lacked a true jaw mechanism (the agnathan condition) and were apparently rather poor swimmers, judging from the rudimentary state of their fins and the presence of only two semicircular canals in their inner ears. However, they had all of the typical vertebrate features including a brain and surrounding skull, a ventral heart and effective high-pressure blood system. Their pharyngeal arches supported gills and the clefts between them allowed the flow of water in a respiratory current. The heart pumped blood through a series of vessels lying in the pharyngeal arches, the basic number being six pairs. Although these were used for perfusion of the gills in respiratory gas exchange, they created a pattern which persists even in human embryonic development, where it is modified to form the great vessels leaving the heart (see p. 275). The modern cyclostomes (e.g. lampreys) are the descendants of these fishes.

The next advance was the modification of the most anterior pharyngeal arch to support the mouth, its ventral part becoming the mandibular arch (see p. 277); this allowed the development of more efficient and varied feeding (the gnathostome grade of organization) and teeth could be anchored to the jaw to increase its effectiveness. (For the upper jaw and teeth see p. 280 et seq., and p. 283.) Often the next (hyoidean) arch was used to support the first, as well as to contribute to the tongue apparatus. At the same time, swimming ability improved greatly with the formation of complex fins, a third semicircular canal and, no doubt, advances in brain organization to control movement more efficiently. These steps proved very successful and most later vertebrates arose from this stock. These early fishes included many different types, most of which became extinct although some, like the cartilaginous sharks and rays (Chondrichthyes), persisted and thrived. Another group of fishes, with bony skeletons (Osteichthyes) divided into a line leading to the majority of modern ray-finned fish and another, the Sarcopterygians, in which the fins were highly muscular and had an axial skeleton, a situation we see in modern lungfish and the Coelacanth *Latimeria*, anticipating the limbs of early terrestrial vertebrates. Some of these fishes may have been able to breathe air as well as to use their gills for respiration. Their upper jaws were fused with their brain case (neurocranium) to increase the skull's mechanical stability, and various plate-like bones derived from scales in the dermis reinforced the neurocranium, the skeleton of the jaws and other pharyngeal arches. These 'scale bones' correspond to the membrane bones of the human skull, while the more primitive neurocranial and viscerocranial elements are represented by its endochondral bones.

From such fishes emerged the earliest land-living vertebrates, during the Upper Devonian era about 270 million years ago. These were amphibians with many fish-like features but instead of pectoral and pelvic fins they had muscular limbs, each with five digits and a characteristic pattern of axial bones (the pentadactyl limb) as in all terrestrial vertebrates, or tetrapods. They were, therefore, able to move around on the swampy ground of the coal forests, where their remains became fossilized. Lacking gills except during larval life, they respired through diverticula of the oesophagus, i.e. simple lungs, a common method of accessory breathing even in fishes which live in tropical anoxic waters. Judging from the condition of modern amphibians such as salamanders, frogs and toads, these animals had hearts with partially divided ventricles, allowing them partial separation of blood for systemic and pulmonary circulations and, therefore, a more efficient respiratory transport permitting increased active movement. With the loss of gills, the arterial arcades of the pharyngeal arches were reduced in complexity and number and now were simple, but large, arteries leading to the head, body and lungs. Amphibians were, however, still depended on an aqueous environment since they laid their eggs in water and probably dehydrated easily through a relatively permeable skin.

Early reptiles probably emerged soon after the amphibia. Two major advances freed the new group from slavish dependence on water: the skin became keratinized and water resistant; reproduction could take place entirely on land as the young developed in an egg

5

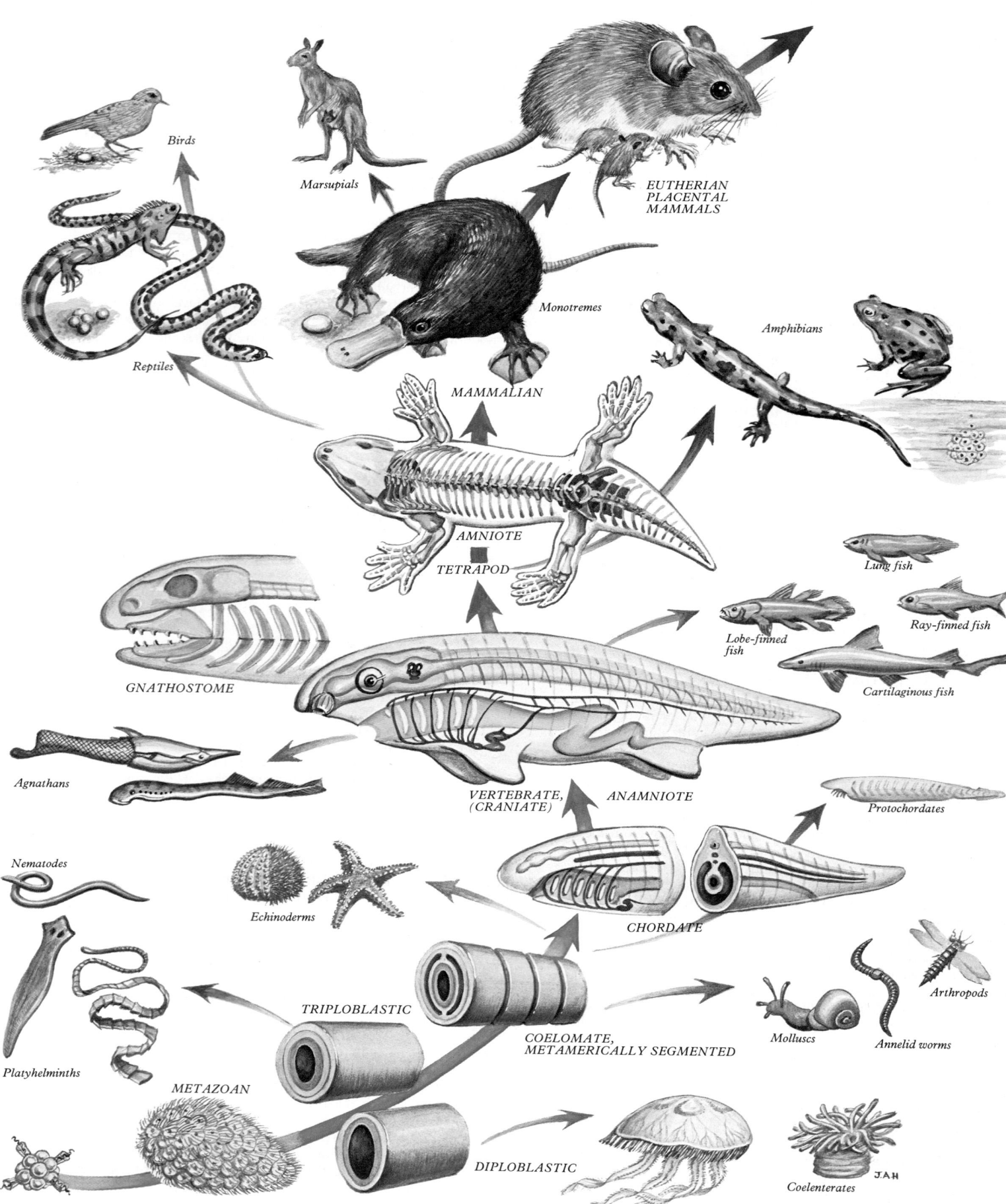

Birds

Marsupials

EUTHERIAN
PLACENTAL
MAMMALS

Monotremes

Amphibians

Reptiles

MAMMALIAN

AMNIOTE

TETRAPOD

Lung fish

Ray-finned fish

Lobe-finned
fish

Cartilaginous fish

GNATHOSTOME

Agnathans

VERTEBRATE,
(CRANIATE)

ANAMNIOTE

Protochordates

Nematodes

Echinoderms

CHORDATE

TRIPLOBLASTIC

COELOMATE,
METAMERICALLY SEGMENTED

Arthropods

Molluscs

Annelid worms

Platyhelminths

METAZOAN

DIPLOBLASTIC

Coelenterates

J.A.H

1.2 The relationships and different levels of organization of the major groups of animals leading to the mammalian class, based on currently available evidence.

enclosed in a shell which prevented water loss but allowed gaseous exchange. Within the shell the embryo floated in a fluid-filled space; the amniotic cavity and the membranes immediately surrounding it (amnion and chorion) acted as a gill. Except for the eggshell, these modifications were retained in all descendants of the reptiles including mammals.

Reptiles were now free to exploit the dry places of the earth as well as the humid ones and they became the dominant vertebrate group for many millions of years. Various internal changes took place including: complete separation of systemic and pulmonary circulations; the formation of a vena cava making the return of blood more efficient; development of a high-pressure kidney with more effective filtration; various modifications of the brain which increased its ability to analyse sensory data, organize motor activity and to establish more complex behaviour patterns in general.

Although many of the most successful reptilian groups such as the dinosaurs eventually became extinct, some persisted as the turtles, lizards, snakes and crocodiles of the present or became highly modified for flight, the birds. Another group of great significance comprised relatively unspecialized animals emerging quite early in reptilian history. These had a unique skull construction with a fossa in the middle of its lateral surface allowing the expansion of masticatory muscles, the Synapsid condition. Along this fossil line, several remarkable changes occurred. These included the expansion of the brain and its braincase, an alteration in the jaw mechanism so that several of the bones which hitherto had formed part of its articular mechanism became reduced in size, adapted for picking up auditory signals and progressively incorporated into the middle ear. Complex teeth of different types and with more than one cusp were also inserted into the jaws, a sign of more effective mastication, and a new, more robust joint formed between the mandibular condyle and the temporal bone. Locomotion was also modified by a rotation of the limbs bringing their intermediate and distal joints under the trunk, thus introducing an ability to lift the body off the ground, a change suggesting a cursorial habit commensurate with a high metabolic rate and, therefore, warm-bloodedness. (The manner of limb rotation and attendant modifications contrasts sharply in the fore- (upper), and hind- (lower) limbs: see pp. 613.) Hair probably covered their bodies in an insulating layer.

Such creatures coexisted with the ruling reptiles from the Permian era from about 200 million years ago and, when the latter became extinct, they replaced them as the dominant land vertebrates. By this time the full mammalian condition had been achieved, with a greatly expanded brain, fully functional temporomandibular joint, teeth specialized for different functions (incisors, molars, etc.) and showing the primitive pattern of mammalian cusps (see p. 1703). To judge from the nearest descendants of some of these early mammals, the Prototheria (Monotremes) of Australasia such as the Platypus, *Ornithorhynchus*, these creatures were certainly homeothermic, were covered in hair, suckled their young, although they still laid eggs, and had many other non-reptilian features such as a division of the trunk into a thorax and an abdomen, with a diaphragm allowing thoracic breathing. Their pharyngeal arterial arches were more streamlined, the third being developed only on the left to form the aorta. Such animals were obviously well equipped to deal with the wide variety of climatic conditions and of food sources available in a drastically changing environment. Their more advanced brains could no doubt enable them to exploit their environment more fully, and provide better maternal care. This development favoured the survival of offspring and permitted prolonged development after birth. Many different groups of such animals rapidly spread over the land masses; one of them, which dispensed with laying eggs by retaining the fetus in utero for the early part of its development, became dominant. These were the Metatheria (Marsupials), including the pouched forms such as the kangaroos and non-pouched species like the opossums. They had relatively larger and less 'reptilian' brains and a more effective feeding apparatus including highly specialized teeth. Again, from the many different types of marsupials a third mammalian group the Eutheria (Placentals) arose and, in turn, supplanted them. In these new mammals, the developing young were retained for much longer inside their mothers, attached, as were marsupial embryos, by a placenta which provided nutrition, respiratory exchange, removal of excretions, and other metabolic needs. The placenta of the Eutherians was much more elaborate and

effective than that of the marsupials, allowing birth at a very advanced stage of development and, in particular, permitting the brain to achieve considerable complexity before its use for survival in the outside world. These mammals rapidly replaced most of the other groups. This basic eutherian design which first emerged during the Cretaceous period about 120 million years ago, or possibly earlier, was extremely successful at adapting itself to many different evolutionary niches, radiating into the various mammalian forms we know today.

The closest living relatives of these early Eutheria are Insectivores such as the Shrews, small highly active animals with primitive tooth patterns and relatively unspecialized body form. It is thought that from species similar to these arose a group of animals which were ancestral to the Primates.

PRIMATE AND HUMAN EVOLUTION

Some two hundred and thirty species of living mammals are included within the order Primates. They are nearly all confined to tropical or subtropical forest habitats and span a wide range of body sizes, from the 100 g average body weight of the mouse lemur to the over 150 kg mean body weight of the gorilla. The features that unite them as primates are concentrated within the nervous and locomotor systems. They include:

- a relatively large brain for the size of the body;
- an emphasis on the visual system which is manifest by the relative size of the visual cortex, histological complexity of the primate retina, development of stereoscopic vision and greater bony protection for the eyeball;
- grasping hands and feet equipped with palms and soles which are padded and covered by ridges of skin and to which are attached spatulate nails and not claws.

CLASSIFICATION OF PRIMATES

Living primates sharing these attributes are usually arranged in one of two contrasting schemes (Table 1.1). One is based on the overall level of morphological specialization, or *grade*, and divides primates into Prosimians ('before apes and monkeys') and Simians ('apes and monkeys'); simian means 'snub-nosed'. The primate features of the simians are more clearly expressed, whereas the prosimians retain a suite of primitive features including an unfused mandibular (mental) symphysis, a persistent communication between the orbit and the temporal fossa, unfused frontal bones and the retention of a single claw, called a 'grooming claw', on the second manual digit. Prosimians comprise the lemurs, lorises and tarsiers, whereas monkeys from the New and Old Worlds, together with apes and modern humans, make up the living simians. The other classification of primates, according to *clades*, emphasizes on evolutionary history rather than an overall level of morphological complexity. The crucial difference between the two schemes is their treatment of the tarsiers. The cladistic scheme places special emphasis on the similarities between the retinae, orbits and placentae of the tarsiers and the simians and unites them in the suborder Haplorhini. The living lemurs and lorises then form a second infraorder, the Strepsirhini, which includes all living primates with a moist snout called a rhinarium.

EVOLUTION OF PRIMATES (1.3, 1.4)

Primate origins

Primates were among the first groups of eutherian mammals to differentiate, yet we have only scant evidence about their evolutionary history. How little we know can be judged from recent calculations which estimate that the 250 known species of fossil primates probably represent less than 5% of the primate species that have ever existed.

The first evidence for primate-like creatures comes from late Cretaceous and early Palaeocene rocks in North America, but recent discoveries in North Africa suggest that they were also present on that land mass during the Palaeocene. The earliest fossil evidence dates from 65 Myr and consists of teeth which resemble those of the living mouse lemur and dwarf bushbaby, and which suggest a

7

Table 1.1 Two classificatory schemes for the major groups of living primates. The two suborder schemes include 'clade-based' categories as well as the conventional 'grade-based' arrangement.

ORDER	SUBORDERS		INFRAORDERS	
	Grade	Clade		
	PROSIMII (prosimians)	STREPSIRHINI (strepsirhines)	LEMURIFORMES	LEMURS
			LORISIFORMES	LORISES
PRIMATES		HAPLORHINI (haplorhines)	TARSIIFORMES	TARSIERS
	ANTHROPOIDEA (simians/ anthropoids)		PLATYRRHINI	NEW WORLD MONKEYS (cebids, callitrichids, atelids)
			CATARRHINI	OLD WORLD MONKEYS (cercopithecids)
				APES/ HUMANS (hominoids)

creature with a body size little larger than a modern mouse. By 60 Myr ago these creatures, which belong to the infraorder Plesiadapiformes and which are usually referred to as plesiadapids, were diverse enough in North America to merit being assigned to at least four families. Although these animals were primitive in many respects, some scientists judged that the features they share with the later adapid primates from the Eocene are sufficient evidence to include the plesiadapids within the primate order. However other evidence, particularly from the skull, shows that the ear region of the plesiadapids was importantly different from that of living primates. In the latter the floor of the middle-ear cavity is formed from the petrosal bone, whereas in the plesiadapids it is formed from the entotympanic. Thus the plesiadapids are not included with 'primates of modern aspect' or 'euprimates', but are usually placed in a separate category of 'archaic' primates.

Recent commentators have suggested that the 'archaic' primates, the 'euprimates' both fossil and living, together with the tree shrews (Scandentia), bats (Chiroptera) and the flying lemurs (Dermoptera) should be grouped together as the Archonta. Relationships within that broad grouping have recently been further refined with only the flying lemurs, the 'euprimates' (both living and fossil) and the tree shrews included within the order Primates. It is interesting to note that this revives a much earlier proposal of Le Gros Clark that the tree shrews, or Scandentia, belonged within the order Primates. Whatever else one can conclude, it is evident that the early evolutionary history and relationships of the primates and their close relatives are far from resolved.

Eocene primates

The early Eocene fossil record is where the first sound evidence for 'euprimates' is encountered in the form of the lemur-like adapids and the tarsier-like omomyids. The shape of their teeth suggests that early 'euprimates' were adapted to eat varying proportions of fruit, leaves and insects. At one time or another both the omomyids and the adapids have been canvassed as ancestors of the later simians, but there is now an increasing realization that the omomyids and adapids may have been an evolutionary radiation quite distinct from the one which gave rise to the living primates. This is not as extraordinary as it sounds, for the disposition of the major land masses of the Eocene bore little resemblance to their present configuration. In early Eocene times Africa was separated from Europe and Asia by the Tethys sea and Eurasia, while North America formed Laurasia, an intermittently continuous subtropical landmass. South America was close enough to Africa at this time for land

mammals, including primates, to have crossed between them. The end of the Eocene was a period of substantial change in mammalian evolution. Many groups became extinct to the extent that palaeontologists call this time the 'great cut-off', or 'Grande Coupure'. The fossil record in the succeeding geological period is correspondingly sparse, hence its name, the Oligocene, meaning 'few fossils'.

The earliest loris-like creatures are known from the African Eocene but the origin of the modern lemurs is obscure. As for the third major component of the modern prosimians, the tarsiers, it can be concluded that unless northern hemisphere Eocene omomyid species like *Shoshonius* prove to be related to modern tarsiers, then the origins of the latter are probably to be found in the late Eocene or early Oligocene form *Afrotarsius*. Modern tarsiers are confined to Asian humid dipterocarp forest, the tarsiers and their forests having both apparently disappeared from Africa at the same time.

Evidence of early simian-grade primates comes from deposits in the Fayum depression of Egypt, the earliest of which may extend back into the Eocene as well as sampling the Oligocene (see below). Fossil remains of *Aegyptopithecus*, and other genera, provide sound evidence of cat-sized simians. Suspicions that the simians may have originated even earlier in the Eocene were initially fuelled by the discovery of remains belonging to *Amphipithecus* and *Pondaungia* from Burma. The more recent discovery of an incomplete set of cheek teeth from an Eocene site in Algeria, attributed to *Algeripithecus*, suggests that either the simians can be traced back to before 50 Myr, or that like the radiations of the adapids and omomyids, there was an Eocene radiation of creatures that resembled simians, but which were not themselves directly related to modern simians.

Recent discoveries of primates from a 45 Myr-old Eocene site in south-eastern China has added significant new information about primate evolution. Teeth virtually identical to those of the living tarsier confirm the antiquity of *Tarsius* and suggest that omomyids dispersed between North America and Asia in the middle Miocene. Evidence of a mandible attributed to a new family, *Eosimias*, suggests that Asia may have been an important centre for simian or anthropoid evolution. *Eosimias* with its unfused mandibular symphysis is amongst the most primitive simians known.

Origins of the monkeys and apes

Eleven genera of simians are now known from the African Oligocene and nearly all of them are best-documented from the extraordinarily rich Fayum region. This suggests that simians had undergone con-

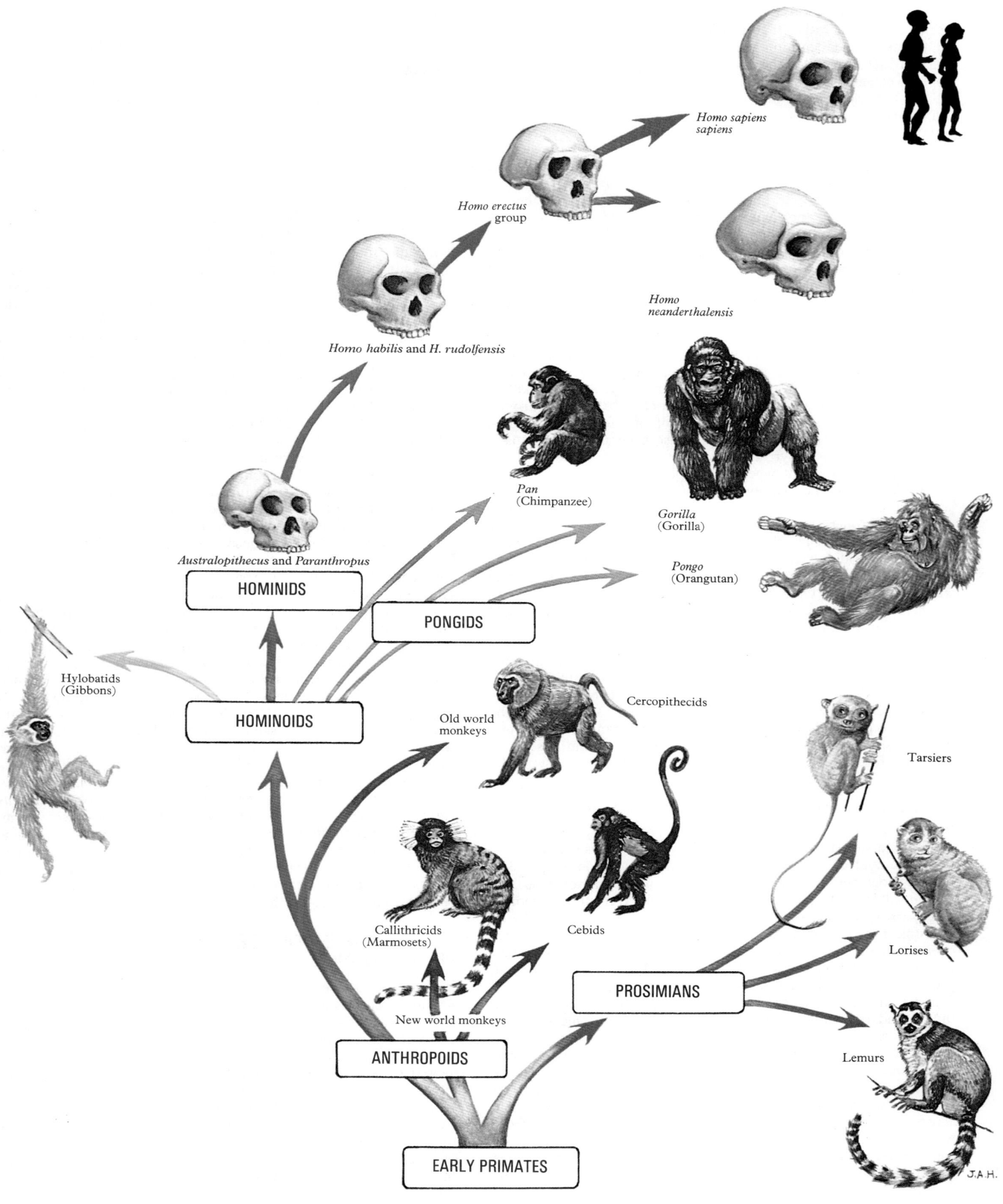

Homo sapiens sapiens

Homo erectus group

Homo neanderthalensis

Homo habilis and *H. rudolfensis*

Pan (Chimpanzee)

Gorilla (Gorilla)

Pongo (Orangutan)

Australopithecus and *Paranthropus*

HOMINIDS

PONGIDS

Hylobatids (Gibbons)

HOMINOIDS

Old world monkeys

Cercopithecids

Tarsiers

Callithricids (Marmosets)

Cebids

New world monkeys

PROSIMIANS

Lorises

ANTHROPOIDS

Lemurs

EARLY PRIMATES

J.A.H.

1.3 A simplified scheme outlining evolutionary relationships between *Homo sapiens* and other living euprimates. For simplicity and because of present uncertainties about classification, details of species of fossil primates have not been included (see text).

9

siderable diversification by this time. What features mark these fossil forms as simians rather than prosimians? The major differences are in the skull and dentition and include a reduced snout with the maxilla tucked beneath the anterior part of the brain case, a bony septum behind the orbit, a tall ascending mandibular ramus, fusion of the two elements of the frontal bone, and of the mandibular symphysis, closely-approximated and vertically-implanted incisors, square molar crowns and molarized premolars. Some genera like *Propliopithecus* resemble Old World monkeys, and others, such as *Aegyptopithecus*, have teeth which more closely resemble those of modern apes. *Aegyptopithecus* was apparently a frugivorous quadruped with a skeletal morphology which was adapted for climbing and leaping within the Oligocene rain forests. In many ways the early Old World simians more closely resembled living New World primates than contemporary Old World forms.

The New World Monkeys, or Platyrrhines, are a diverse group which has its own substantial evolutionary history. Apart from their geographical separation from the rest of the anthropoids they can be distinguished from the Old World simians, or Catarrhini, by their laterally-facing nostrils, hence the name of their infraorder, the 'flat-nosed' ones. In addition catarrhines have two fewer premolar teeth in each jaw than do the platyrrhines and they possess a tubular ectotympanic leading from the middle ear cavity. Also, unlike the platyrrhines, in the catarrhines there is a contact between the frontal and sphenoid bones in the wall of the temporal fossa. Catarrhines, with the exception of the gibbons, are also generally more sexually dimorphic than the platyrrhines.

Opinions differ about whether the platyrrhines evolved from a North American omomyid ancestor, or if they are derived from an early African ancestor at a time when the distance between Africa and South America was much less than it is today. The three Oligocene and the relatively few Miocene fossils from South America are each specialized enough to be related to one or other of the living platyrrhine subfamilies, implying that the major platyrrhine lineages may be up to 25 Myr old.

There are only two middle Miocene Old World monkey genera, but by 8 or 9 million years ago (late Miocene) the differentiation into the two main groups of living Old World monkeys, the Cercopithecinae (modern guenons, macaques, mangabeys and baboons) and the Colobinae (leaf-eating monkeys) was well-established. The fossil record suggests that the colobines most likely represent the primitive condition for the Old World monkey superfamily, the Cercopithecoidea. From this ancestral stock as many as 10 lineages evolved and exploited a wide range of habitats from deserts to montane forests. These fossil forms were generally substantially larger than their modern counterparts.

Evolutionary relationships within modern and fossil apes

The second superfamily within the Old World simians (catarrhines), the Hominoidea, is the group which includes modern apes and humans together with their fossil precursors. Hominoids became distinct at least 25 Myr ago. They began as a group of arboreal frugivores with body sizes much like those modern monkeys living in tropical forest habitats. Modern apes are characterized by specializations of the axial and postcranial skeletons. These include an elongated forelimb, features of the wrist and hand which facilitate pronation and supination, a mobile glenohumeral joint capable of extreme abduction, a craniocaudally-elongated scapula, a wide thorax and reduction in the length of the lumbar spine. There is good evidence to suggest that the modern apes are the impoverished representatives of a group that was much more numerous and taxonomically diverse during the middle and late Miocene. During this time, when forests were far more extensive in higher northern latitudes than they are today, fossil ape taxa were distributed widely across Europe and Asia. The discovery of a Miocene fossil ape from Namibia suggests that they also inhabited forests in the southern hemisphere. However, the late Miocene radiation of cercopithecoids which is described above, effectively replaced hominoids as the dominant primates in the Old World.

Modern and fossil apes and humans were traditionally divided by anthropologists into four families. One, the Oreopithecidae, is only known from the late Miocene fossil record. Whereas its teeth are Old World monkey-like, its postcranial skeleton is more ape-like. Its

taxonomic position is best left unresolved at present, but its strongest affinities are with the fossil and living great apes. The remaining three traditional hominoid families all have living representatives, namely (1) the gibbons and siamangs, sometimes known as the 'lesser apes', forming the Hylobatidae, (2) the gorillas, orang-utans and chimpanzees, making up the Pongidae, or pongids, and (3) modern humans, together with extinct species, within the genera *Homo*, *Australopithecus* and *Paranthropus*, together comprising the Hominidae, or hominids.

However, the application of molecular biological methods to the study of relationships within the superfamily, together with reassessments of the substantial Miocene fossil record of the apes, have prompted several reviews of this traditional scheme. One that uses the principles of phylogenetic analysis resolves the fossil and living apes into not four, but three families as follows.

The first and most primitive of the ape families, the Proconsulidae, is only known from fossil evidence. This exclusively African group apparently originated in the early Miocene and spans the period from 22 to about 17 Myr ago. Proconsul genera were apparently all arboreal quadrupeds with some adaptations for suspensory behaviour. The features they share with the other apes include the absence of a tail, an opposable thumb, specializations of the shoulder, low-crowned premolars and an increase in relative brain size compared with the Old World monkeys.

The second family corresponds to the Hylobatidae of the traditional scheme. There are no strong candidates for fossil representatives of the modern gibbons and siamangs, but *Lacopithecus* from the Miocene of China comes closest to being a gibbon ancestor.

The third family is the Hominidae, but in the new scheme this family incorporates at least three subfamilies. One, the Dryopithecinae is comprised of extinct taxa only. These include the Middle Miocene tribes of thick-enamelled apes, the Afropithecini and the Kenyapithecini, and the thin-enamelled Dryopithecini which are apparently little advanced beyond the proconsulids. The second subfamily, the Ponginae, incorporates the orang-utan and its subfossil representatives in the tribe Pongini, and its sister group comprises the fossil taxa belonging to the tribe Sivapithecini. The latter comprises remains discovered from the Middle and Late Miocene of Turkey and Pakistan and attributed to *Sivapithecus*. Two genera, *Rudapithecus* from Hungary and *Lufengpithecus* from China, may also be relatively unspecialized members of the sivapithecin group. To judge from its jaws and teeth, *Gigantopithecus* from Pakistan and China also belongs in the same subfamily. The third subfamily, the Homininae, comprises (1) the living gorilla subspecies, which are united in the tribe Gorillini; (2) making up the second tribe, the Hominini, are the two living chimpanzee species *Pan troglodytes* and *Pan paniscus*, and the genera *Ardipithecus*, *Australopithecus*, *Paranthropus* and *Homo*. Thus according to this new scheme, living forms that were traditionally referred to as pongids become 'pongins' (for the orang-utan) and 'gorillins' (for the gorilla). Fossil and living forms more closely related to modern humans than to any ape species, and which were (and usually still are) referred to as hominids become 'hominins' as do the two living chimpanzee species.

MOLECULAR EVIDENCE FOR HOMINOID RELATIONSHIPS

As indicated above, this very fundamental revision of hominoid taxonomy reflects molecular and other morphological evidence which suggests that the orang-utan is significantly different from the group which comprises gorillas, chimpanzees and modern humans. Molecular data can also be used to help estimate the time which has elapsed since each lineage became independent. Put another way, because molecular changes are generally neutral and occur at a steady rate, the degree of molecular difference can be used as a clock. The clock is not independent of palaeontological evidence, for the latter has to be used at some stage to calibrate the clock by establishing the age of one of the branching events. Conventionally this has been done using the separation of the Old World and New World simians and this suggests that Pongini (i.e. the lineage, or clade, to which the modern orang-utan belongs) separated from the African ape and modern human lineage around 12–14 Myr ago.

Evidence at the molecular level, be it at the level of proteins or down to the level of the base sequences of nuclear and mitochondrial

DNA, is providing stronger and stronger indications that the two modern chimpanzee species and modern humans are more closely related to each other than either is to modern gorillas. It is this evidence which underpins the revised taxonomy which places the latter taxon in the tribe Gorillini and the former taxa in the tribe Hominini. Traditional morphological evidence does not controvert the groupings suggested by the molecular evidence, but it must be said that it does not offer strong support either. The molecular clock suggests that the separation of the gorilla lineage was closely followed by the split between the lineages leading to chimpanzees and modern humans; estimated timings for the latter divergence vary from between 8 and 5 Myr ago. If the molecular data and dates are a reliable indication of evolutionary timing, then we should expect to find hominids no earlier than 8 or 9 Myr ago. (The old name 'hominids' will be used for simplicity to describe extinct forms which are more closely related to modern humans than to any other living taxon.)

Our knowledge of the evolutionary history of the subfamily Homininae would be greatly improved if we had any reliable fossil evidence for the lineages leading to modern gorillas and chimpanzees but, as yet, apart from an upper jaw dated to around 9 Myr ago, and which may represent the type of creature from which the modern gorilla evolved, no such evidence has been recovered.

HOMINID EVOLUTION (1.4)

With the exception of several isolated teeth from Ngorora and Lukeino in the Baringo region of Kenya (which, however, provide insufficient evidence for them to be reliably classified), the fossil mandibles from Lothagam and Tabarin, dating from around 5 Myr, offer the first evidence of creatures that may postdate the separation of the lineage leading to modern humans from that leading to the two modern chimpanzee species.

The first hominids–australopithecines (Table 1.2A)

The Lothagam and Tabarin mandibles, together with the more than 4 Myr-old remains from Aramis in Ethiopia, belong to the oldest australopithecine, initially called *Australopithecus ramidus*. Its thin enamel and small, simple deciduous molars are distinct from later, new australopithecines and probably justify the designation of a separate genus called *Ardipithecus*, for this material. The earliest australopithecine for which there is good evidence is *Australopithecus afarensis*. While aspects of the skull, teeth and postcranial skeleton of *A. afarensis* are ape-like, what sets it apart from the apes are its smaller canines, relatively enlarged molar teeth and a reorganized pelvic girdle and vertebral column which allowed an upright posture and a bipedal gait to be maintained with less muscular effort than is required by modern apes when they stand and walk bipedally. However, the brains of these early 'gracile' australopithecines were absolutely and relatively little larger than those of chimpanzees and the skeletons of their forelimbs and trunk are ape-like. The relatively primitive postcranial skeleton of *A. afarensis* suggests that the range of postures and locomotor modes it adopted probably embraced the

options exercised by modern chimpanzees, but with changes in the pelvic girdle indicating a greater emphasis on bipedal standing, walking and running. There is direct evidence of a bipedal gait in the form of footprints at Laetoli in Tanzania which date from between 3 and 4 Myr ago. This increased emphasis on bipedalism was probably prompted by modifications to the habitat consequent on climatic changes. The climate was becoming steadily more arid with the result that the woodland environment was breaking up, with groups of trees separated by sizeable patches of grassland. However, true savannah grassland did not appear until much closer to 2 Myr ago and these early australopithecines were likely to have lived near to dense tree cover.

Fossil evidence for *A. afarensis* is confined to East Africa. In southern Africa evidence of a hominid displaying a similar level of organization, but which belongs to a different species, was first discovered in 1924. This hominid, which was given the name *Australopithecus africanus*, has larger molar teeth and a shorter more strongly buttressed muzzle than its East African counterpart. These features have prompted some investigators to see it as ancestral to the temporally later 'robust' australopithecines, whereas other workers have stressed the ways in which *A. africanus* resembles, and could be ancestral to, the genus *Homo* (see below).

Three forms of 'robust' australopithecines are presently recognized. They all demonstrate, to a greater or lesser extent, what has been called a 'hypermasticatory trend', that is substantial enlargement of the molar teeth, molarization of the premolars and reduction in the size of the canines and incisors. These modifications have the effect of extending the length of the functional molar tooth row anteriorly, taking it closer to the front of the jaws. One of these 'robust' australopithecine species, *Paranthropus aethiopicus*, has enlarged molar teeth but retains a substantial muzzle. The other two, *Paranthropus robustus* from southern Africa, and especially *Paranthropus boisei* from East Africa, have tall, flat and wide faces which suggest that the masticatory muscles had been reorganized to concentrate chewing on the row of enlarged molar and molarized premolar teeth. These muscles are capable of generating substantial power. This could either have generated major point forces or was dissipated over the large surface area of the molar crowns. The more derived form of the East African 'robust' australopithecine, *P. boisei*, and the southern African form, *P. robustus*, appear in the fossil record around 2–2.3 Myr ago and may well represent one response of hominids to an acceleration in the rate of increase of aridity and cooling that was affecting the African continent at this time. The brains of the 'robust' australopithecines were similar in relative size to those of the 'gracile' australopithecines and what little we know of their locomotor skeleton suggests that they were occasional rather than habitual bipeds. Some workers have claimed that *P. robustus* manufactured stone artefacts, but the anatomical and the archaeological evidence is inconclusive. Despite their epithet 'robust', which was introduced to refer to their teeth, jaws and face, the 'robust' australopithecines were not especially large-bodied though they display a wide range of body size and *P. boisei* has a level of sexual dimorphism similar to that of the modern gorilla. There is no fossil

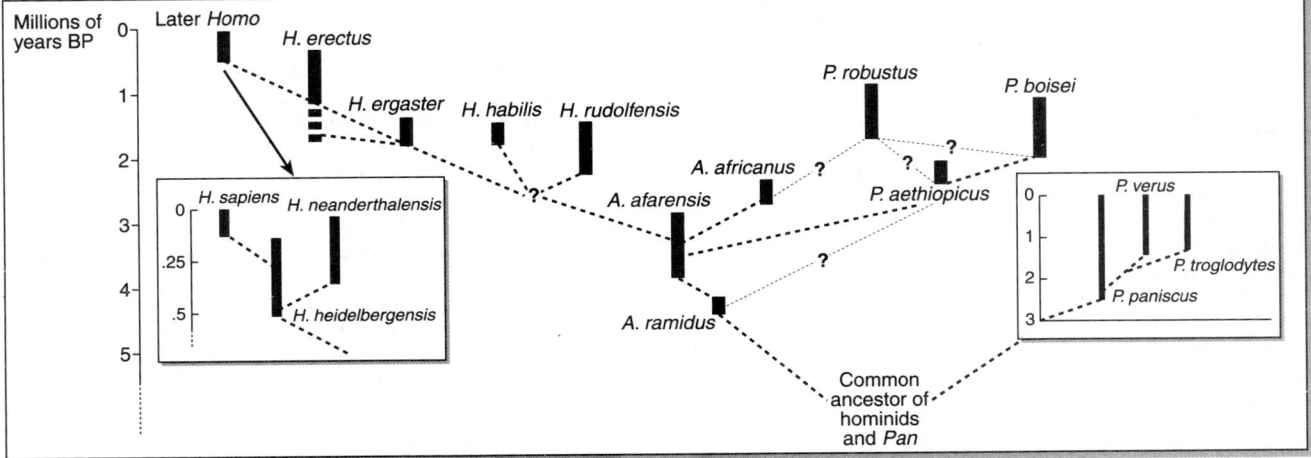

1.4   Phylogenetic scheme indicating probable relationships (dashed lines) and possible relationships (dotted lines) between hominid taxa. Note that the term 'H. sapiens' here includes more than one species (see text).

Table 1.2 Characteristics of Australopithecines and early human species

A. Australopithecines

	Australopithecus afarensis	Australopithecus africanus	Paranthropus aethiopecus boisei	Paranthropus robustus
Height (m)	1–1.5	1.1–1.4	1.2–1.4	1.1–1.3
Weight (kg)	30–50	30–50	35–50	30–40
Physique	Light build: some ape-like features (e.g. shape of thorax: long arms relative to legs: curved fingers and toes: marked to moderate sexual dimorphism)	Light build: probably relatively long arms: more 'human' features: probably less sexual dimorphism	Very heavy build: relatively long arms: marked sexual dimorphism	Heavy build: relatively long arms: moderate sexual dimorphism
Brain size (ml)	400–500	400–500	430–525	approx. 500
Skull form	Low, flat forehead: projecting face: prominent brow ridges	Higher forehead: shorter face: brow ridges less prominent	Prominent crests on top and back of skull: very long, flattish face: strong facial buttressing	Crest on top of skull: long, broad, flattish face: moderate facial buttressing
Jaws/teeth	Relatively large incisors and canines: gap between upper incisors and canines: moderate-sized molars	Small incisor-like canines: no gap between upper incisors and canines: larger molars	Very thick jaws: small incisors and canines: large, molar-like premolars: very large molars	Very thick jaws: small incisors and canines: large molar-like premolars: very large molars
Distribution	Eastern Africa	Southern Africa	Eastern Africa	Southern Africa
Known date (years ago)	>4–2.5 million	3.0–2.5 million	2.4–1.2 million	2–1 million

B. Homo

	Homo habilis	Homo rudolfensis	Homo erectus (including Homo ergaster)	'Archaic Homo sapiens'	Neanderthals	Early modern Homo sapiens
Height (m)	1–1.25	?	1.6–1.8	?	1.5–1.8	1.6–1.85
Weight (kg)	25–40	? 40–50	50–70	50–70	50–70	50–80
Physique	Relatively long arms: moderate sexual dimorphism	?	Robust but human skeleton: moderate sexual dimorphism	Robust but human skeleton: moderate sexual dimorphism	As 'archaic H. sapiens', but adapted for cold: moderate sexual dimorphism	Modern skeleton: ? adapted for warmth: moderate sexual dimorphism
Brain size (ml)	500–675	700–800	750–1250	1100–1400	1200–1750	1200–1600
Skull form	Higher forehead: relatively small face: obvious nasal margins	Flatter forehead: large wide midface	Flat, thick skull with large occipital and brow ridge	Higher skull: face less protruding	Reduced brow ridge: thinner skull: large nose: midface projection	Small or no brow ridge: shorter, high skull
Jaws/teeth	Smaller jaws: narrow molars	Robust jaw: large molars: molar-like premolars	More slender jaw: smaller teeth than H. habilis: reduced size of third molar	Similar to H. erectus but teeth may be even smaller	Similar to 'archaic H. sapiens': teeth smaller except for incisors: some chin development	Shorter jaws than Neanderthals: chin developed: teeth may be smaller
Distribution	Eastern (+southern?) Africa	Eastern Africa	Africa, Asia and Indonesia	Africa, Asia and Europe	Europe and western Asia	Africa and western Asia
Known date (years ago)	2–1.6 million	2.5–1.8 million	1.9–0.2 million	400 000–100 000	? 400 000–30 000	? 130 000→

evidence for either *P. robustus* or *P. boisei* later than about 1.3 Myr ago.

Early Homo (Table 1.2B)

Perhaps as early as 2.5 Myr, and certainly by 2 Myr ago, two new species of hominid appear in the fossil record of East Africa. One, *Homo rudolfensis*, best known from Koobi Fora in Kenya, has teeth which are much like those of the 'gracile' australopithecines with some evidence of molar-like premolars. However, its skull is much less ape-like than *Australopithecus* in that it has lost its muzzle and both the base and vault have broadened to accommodate a larger brain. No postcranial bones have been found associated with cranial material; thus there is no direct evidence about the posture and locomotion of *H. rudolfensis*. There is, however, direct evidence about the postcranial skeleton of the second early *Homo* species, *Homo habilis*, and this suggests that its posture and locomotion was little different to that of the australopithecines. What is different, however, is the skull which is advanced in both shape and brain

volume compared to those of the 'gracile' australopithecines. The molar and premolar teeth are small and narrow in *H. habilis*, but, to judge from the postcranial skeleton, the creatures themselves were small, so any dental reduction compared to *Australopithecus* may be more apparent than real. These two early species are placed within the genus *Homo* and not included in *Australopithecus* or *Paranthropus* for different reasons. The former taxon, *H. rudolfensis*, is assigned to *Homo* because of its substantially, around 50%, larger brain, while the latter taxon, *H. habilis*, is similarly assigned because of its reorganized cranium and a dentition which places less emphasis on the molars and premolars. To judge from postcranial evidence *H. habilis* was not a habitual biped, yet the position of the foramen magnum suggests that the base of the cranium had been modified to allow for truncal uprightness.

Homo erectus

Our own species, *Homo sapiens*, differs from the living apes in three major ways. Our brains are larger, our jaws and teeth are generally smaller and differently proportioned, whilst our postcranial skeleton is adapted for a habitual bipedal posture and gait. The first hominid species to demonstrate unambiguous signs of all three of these distinctive features is early African *Homo erectus*, which some workers call *Homo ergaster*. These remains date back to 1.9 Myr and are best known from sites in Kenya around Lake Turkana. The skull has a brain size little larger than that of *H. rudolfensis*, but the face, jaws and teeth are significantly smaller. The teeth are similar in size to those of *H. habilis*, but whereas the body size of the latter is estimated to be no larger than 40 kg, the body size of early African *H. erectus* or *H. ergaster* is closer to 60 kg. Thanks to the remarkable preservation of an associated skeleton found at West Turkana, KNM-WT 15000, the postcranial skeleton is well known. It shares many features of the pelvis and the femur with later *Homo* species. Its stature and proportions also resemble those of later *Homo* species and differ from the preceding australopithecines.

Although the earliest remains of *H. erectus* are found in East Africa, it is now more than a century ago that the first fossil evidence for *H. erectus* was found in Java (now Indonesia). Recent reports suggest that some of these remains may be as old as the African ones, and there is sound evidence that they are at least 1 Myr old. Subsequent discoveries in China at a cave that was then called Choukoutien, and which is now called Zhoukoudian, indicate that *H. erectus* survived in Asia as recently as 200 Kyr ago.

Emergence of modern humans

It is a paradox that the hominid species with which we should be the most familiar, namely *Homo sapiens*, is the least well defined. There is no type specimen of *H. sapiens* and because it is a polytypic taxon, a range of skull shapes and limb proportions have to be taken into account when considering whether fossil remains can be included within *H. sapiens*. When this is done the earliest evidence for what has come to be called 'anatomically modern' *H. sapiens* comes from Africa and the Near East at around 100 Kyr. It is at this time that we find evidence of skulls with vertical foreheads, tall and expanded parietal bones and a much reduced dentition. There is, however, a substantial collection of material which is more advanced than *H. erectus* yet which is not as derived as anatomically-modern *H. sapiens*. Such material is known from Africa (e.g. Ndutu and Kabwe), Europe (e.g. Mauer) and China (e.g. Dali and Jinnuishan). The best-known material in this 'archaic *Homo*' category are the remains which have been attributed to *Homo neanderthalensis*. This species has a characteristically-shaped cranial vault, its jaws, teeth and nose are set forward in the face and the skeleton is robust with large joint surfaces. At present the earliest evidence of Neanderthals comes from Spain at around 300–400 Kyr ago. The characteristic Neanderthal morphology is confined to Western Europe, the Near East and adjacent parts of Asia. Throughout most of the period from which Neanderthal remains have come the climate of these regions was cold and much of Europe was reduced to tundra. Neanderthals are generally interpreted as a species of the genus *Homo* which was adapted to these harsh, cold, conditions.

In other parts of the world comparable populations of archaic humans were not as morphologically distinct. Some workers emphasize regional continuity of morphology, pointing, for example, to features of the face which can be identified within Chinese populations of *H. erectus*, and then traced down through archaic humans to contemporary anatomically-modern human Chinese populations. These claims underpin the 'Regional Continuity' hypothesis which proposes that there was not a single origin for anatomically-modern humans but several regionally distinct centres of evolution. The proponents of this hypothesis do not claim that these regional centres were totally genetically isolated, but they do suggest that the effects of gene exchange between regions was relatively trivial compared to the 'vertical' transmission of genes through time. The alternative proposal, known as the 'Out of Africa' hypothesis, suggests that Africa was the single regional centre where the evolutionary change from an archaic human to an anatomically-modern human morphology took place. This hypothesis is based on both palaeontological and molecular anthropological evidence. The former consists of the early dates of the African evidence for anatomically-modern humans and the latter rests on interpretations of mitochondrial (mt) DNA sequences from individuals, sampling a wide range of modern human populations. Initial assessments of the mt DNA evidence saw it as providing strong evidence that mt DNA variation was greatest in Africans, the inference being that these were the longest established populations and thus the first region to evolve anatomically-modern human mt DNA. It has since been realized that the statistical methods used to draw these inferences were flawed. Recalculations have resulted in an interpretation which still places Africa as the regional centre of origin, but with a much wider range of time, perhaps as early as 300–400 Kyr, for the migration out of Africa.

New World and Australasia

Whereas the fossil record suggests that hominids have been part of the African faunal record for between 4 and 5 Myr and have been living in Asia for at least 1 Myr, the hominid fossil record has no great time depth in two other continents, America and Australasia. Opinions differ about how good the evidence is for hominid activity at sites in South America, but as yet the earliest sound evidence for hominids in the Americas is tool manufacture dated to at most a few tens of thousands of years ago. Modern human occupation of Australasia apparently has a greater antiquity than that, and dates of hominid sites in the coastal region of north-west Australia point to incursions of hominids from the Asian mainland as early as 60–70 Kyr. The incursions were facilitated by falls in sea level exposing extensive coastal shelves which, along with some island hopping, would have provided routes from Asia. Thus the entry of anatomically-modern human populations into mainland Australia substantially predates the appearance of anatomically-modern human populations in Western Europe.

There are morphological differences between geographically separated populations of modern humans, but they are relatively insignificant. Variation between groups of modern humans amounts to approximately 10% of the total genetic variation within and between modern human populations. Skull shape and limb proportions vary between regions, but most of this variation is climate-related, for example, the warmer the climate the relatively longer the limbs.

The inheritance of form and function from the different stages of evolution, culminating in the supreme development of mental self-awareness and abstract thought, is one of the greatest stories that science has to tell, although understood in only the barest outline. Here we study the functional anatomy of *H. sapiens*, a form which is not only complexly adapted to a multitude of present activities, but also bears within it legacies of its past; an awareness of this helps us to understand many of the otherwise inexplicable patterns expressed in the human frame, and perhaps to appreciate both its frailty and the most wonderfully effective complexity which it has attained.

For further reading on primate evolution, see Cartmill (1992) and Andrews (1992). For recent reviews of hominid evolution, see Stringer and Andrews (1988), Stringer (1990) and Wood (1992).

ANATOMICAL NOMENCLATURE

A subject such as anatomy, with its accent on description, necessarily requires a very large number of names for structure and processes. For effective communication such words should be as simple as possible and used with unfailing precision. Unfortunately both these aims have only been partially accomplished.

In the first place, as in other sciences, common words do not exist in any language for thousands of structures which require to be named, and the need for new names never ceases. For this reason the manufacture of new names has been based, like the Linnean classification, upon stems of Latin and Greek words. When Latin and often also Greek were a usual part of general education, the actual meanings of these stems were familiar. Even in these days, when classical education is the privilege of only a small minority, many of the words used are familiar because they have to some extent crept into ordinary language, sometimes with a little distortion: musculus, tendo, arteria, vena, cranium, etc. are so like their vernacular equivalents that use of the Latin form is easy.

Words derived from Latin and Greek have also the advantage of being suitable for international usage and efforts have been made to ensure uniform usage since 1895, when the Basle *Nomina Anatomica* was introduced. In 1950 at the Oxford (5th) International Congress of

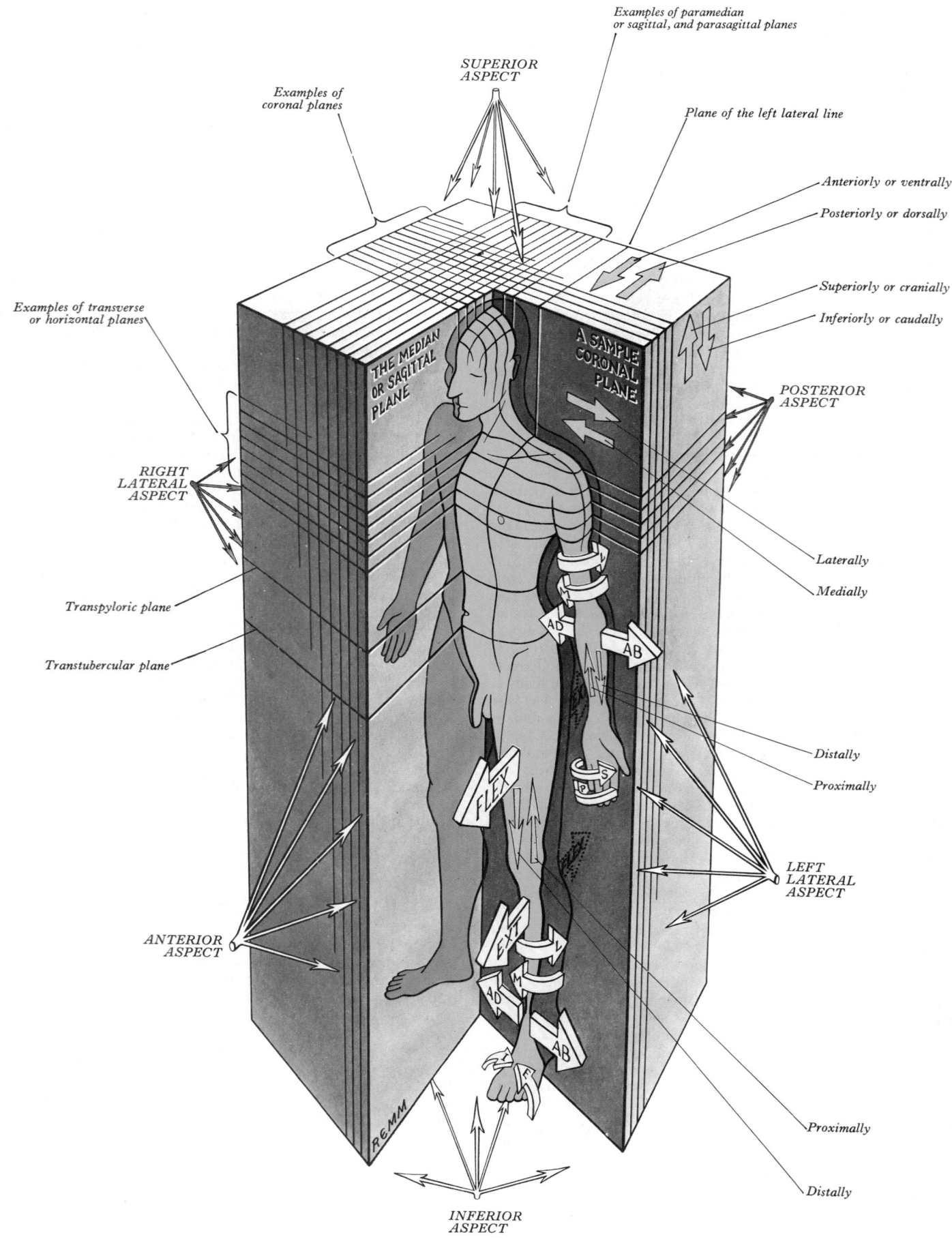

Examples of paramedian or sagittal, and parasagittal planes

SUPERIOR ASPECT

Examples of coronal planes

Plane of the left lateral line

Anteriorly or ventrally

Posteriorly or dorsally

Superiorly or cranially

Inferiorly or caudally

Examples of transverse or horizontal planes

THE MEDIAN OR SAGITTAL PLANE

A SAMPLE CORONAL PLANE

POSTERIOR ASPECT

RIGHT LATERAL ASPECT

Laterally

Medially

Transpyloric plane

Transtubercular plane

AD

AB

Distally

Proximally

FLEX

S

P

LEFT LATERAL ASPECT

ANTERIOR ASPECT

EXT

M

AD

AB

Proximally

I

E

Distally

INFERIOR ASPECT

1.5   The terminology widely used in descriptive anatomy. The abbreviations shown on the solid arrows: AD—adduction. AB—abduction, FLEX—flexion (of the thigh at the hip joint), EXT—extension (of the leg at the knee joint), M and L—medial and lateral rotation. P and S—pronation and supination. I and E—inversion and eversion.

Anatomists, a new body was instituted, the International Anatomical Nomenclature Committee, whose first Honorary Secretary was T B Johnston (one of our editorial predecessors; later Secretaries also included Roger Warwick, co-editor of the last three editions of *Gray's*.

It must be said at once that the officially and internationally agreed terms (see *Nomina Anatomica, Nomina Histologica, Nomina Embryologica*, 6th Edn 1992) are not always adhered to in textbooks or atlases. They are, of course, subject to revision at each quinquennial World Congress of Anatomists and doubtless many are still inept and many are far too complex. Who will stringently adhere to 'aponeurosis musculi bicipitis brachii' for what we in English call the 'bicipital aponeurosis'? Of course, each national language is permitted, and even encouraged, to vernacularize Latin terms, as long as the relation to the official Latin remains clear. No one expects a sudden reference to 'biceps femoris' when dealing with the arm, and hence 'biceps' for 'musculus biceps brachii' is safe to use, as long as no misunderstanding occurs.

This is the policy which we have adopted, not, unfortunately, with complete uniformity. We recognize the difficulty of pure Latinity for a large number of our readers and we prefer to anglicize Latin terms but to give the official form, at least once, in parentheses.

Coming also under the topic of nomenclature are the names of lines, planes and directions, used in describing structures. Conventionally the body is regarded as being in the so-called 'anatomical position' (**1.5**) whenever such descriptions are applied. This position might be called one of supplication—the body upright, facing forwards (anteriorly), with the palms also anterior. There may be only two real objections to this. In the natural standing position with pendant arms, the forearms are usually half pronated. It is hence sometimes more apposite to speak of radial and ulnar aspects of the forearm, rather than medial and lateral. However, some anatomists regret the rigid adherence to the full anatomical position both morphologically and, from some aspects, functionally. Close inspection reveals it as an energy consuming position, seldom actively adopted and involving some scapular rotation and adduction, full lateral rotation of the humerus, direct mediolateral disposition of the elbow joint's axis, full supination of forearm and hand and with the pollex laterally placed! From this stem the somewhat unexpected courses of the radial and ulnar nerves and the disposition of the carpal and digital flexors and extensors. It proves most instructive to compare these and other features with their arrangement in natural standing or in many habitual postures or complex 'precision' activities. (Prominent exceptions are placing objects in the mouth or, for examination, before the eyes.) Secondly, due to rotation of the leg at the hip in all but very primitive quadrupeds, the originally dorsal extensor aspect has become anterior or ventral with respect to the knee and ankle joints. Furthermore, the extensor and flexor aspects of the hip joint are the converse of those at the knee joint.

However, once a little comprehension of the broader facts of mammalian and hence human morphology is established, these difficulties are easily overcome. We have freely used the synonyms: anterior, ventral, flexor, palmar; also posterior, dorsal, extensor as apposite for the trunk and upper limb, but they are not always satisfactory synonyms; for example, the extensor aspect of the leg is **anterior** with respect to the knee and ankle joints and **superior** in the foot and digits; the plantar (flexor) aspect of the foot is, of course

inferior, and so on. (Further details and discussion of these problems may be found at appropriate locations throughout Sections 4 and 16.)

There is also a group of terms defining positions and directions along the axis of the body which is, of course, upright in humans. Structures which are nearer the head end, i.e. **cranial**, are officially **superior** and those nearer the tail end, i.e. **caudal**, are **inferior**. **Medial** and **lateral**, meaning nearer or further from the body's midline axis, are complemented by **median**, meaning in the vertical, anteroposterior (sagittal) midline plane. Other recognized planes are transverse (at right angles to the median axis, or the putative axes of limbs) and vertical (coronal), orthogonal to the sagittal plane.

The whole system can be equated with a cubical reference grid, anterior, posterior, superior, inferior, right and left aspects corresponding to the six faces of the cube, whose orthogonal sections are transverse, coronal and sagittal (**1.5**). Various degrees of obliquity must, of course, add slight complications, compound terms, for example posterolateral, being employed; but it is a well-tried system and most useful, as long as the somewhat artificial 'anatomical position' is kept clearly in mind.

A variety of other positional terms exist and are used occasionally in this text, for example, **distal** and **proximal** are useful in describing some structures in limbs, the datum point being the limb's attachment to the trunk. They are also sometimes used in connection with nerves, arteries, veins, lymphatics, bronchi and other branching structures. Other terms are often found appropriate, for example superficial, deep, radial and tangential.

We recognize that our readers may at first find some of these conventions unfamiliar and even irritating but familiarity with this positional system and reasonable adherence to it and its terms are as essential to clear, unambiguous communication (in clinical, academic and **all** such circumstances) as is the use of internationally recognized unequivocal terms for structures and processes.

The systematic basis of the present text

Gray's Anatomy was founded on the principle that to understand the body's construction it is necessary to analyse it in terms of its component systems as well as its regional topography. The book has remained true to this precept throughout its many editions. The systematic approach has considerable strengths: it provides a means of ready reference to each system, and can be clearly related to functional considerations as well as many clinical matters. Of course, this arrangement is to some extent an artificial separation of what in the body are intimately interdependent components, both during development and in the mature body. It is obvious that whilst there are indeed many clinical conditions where dysfunction of a particular system occurs, there are many others in which topographical nearness of different systems is the prime consideration, and that surgery, in particular, has a regional basis. Clearly what is needed is both a systematic account and a regional, topographical one. While it would require much more than a single volume to accomplish this goal, there are many areas in the present work where the regional anatomy of specific body areas is considered. This is most obvious in the new sections concerned with Surface Anatomy (Section 16) and Neonatal Anatomy and Growth (Section 4), but they also occur in relevant sections throughout the work, as an assiduous use of the index will demonstrate.

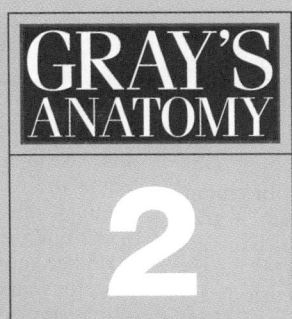

CELLS AND TISSUES

Section Editor: Lawrence H. Bannister

With contributions from Conrad King: Cytoskeleton; Terry Preston: Cell motility (essay); Ivor Mason: The nucleus and DNA; Michael Daker: Chromosomes and cell reproduction; John E. Scott: Connective tissue matrix

---

CELLS

INTRODUCTION

As already stated, it is the aim of Anatomy as a scientific discipline not only to describe the form of the body but to gain a true understanding of the biological principles and processes which underlie that form. The body is essentially a cellular structure: it begins its existence as a single cell, the fertilized ovum, it develops by multiplication and differentiation of cells, it matures as the cells and the substances they generate achieve their mature state; senescence is the decay and death the final cessation of cellular activities. It is, therefore, highly appropriate to consider the body's general construction in the context of its microscopic cellular anatomy.

The study of cells—cytology—and of their aggregations to form tissues and organs—histology—embraces many complementary approaches, including the study of cell and tissue structure, physiology, biochemistry, biophysics and biometrics, all of which disciplines have greatly contributed to and continue to enrich our comprehension of cellular life.

HISTORICAL BACKGROUND

In this section of *Gray's* we examine the nature of the cells—primarily their structure because this is the emphasis of anatomy, but also their molecular organization and physiological behaviour where these are relevant to their microanatomy. In the introduction to this section we first review briefly how the present state of knowledge was reached during the historical past, and next the structures of the chief components of cells in general are described, including their different membranous structures and filamentous systems, the genetic apparatus of the nucleus, and the manner in which cells reproduce and move. In the second part of the section the structure and biology of two types of multicellular assemblies (tissues), epithelia and general connective tissue are outlined. Other more specialized tissues are dealt with elsewhere in relation to the relevant systems: those of the skin in Section 5, cartilage and bone with the skeleton (Section 6), muscle tissues in Section 7, nervous tissue in Section 8, haemal and lymphoid tissue in 9, and endothelia in 10.

Our present view of the body's cellular organization has a history spanning at least three centuries (for accounts of this period see the works by Singer 1931, Singer & Underwood 1962, Taton 1966) and, like most scientific advances, it has closely followed developments in technology, in this case, chiefly the design and construction of optical equipment. Simple systems of multiple lenses were first made in the Netherlands during the early seventeenth century and these primitive microscopes gave access to a hitherto totally unknown world of minute objects. There followed the early period of graphic description of the microscopic features of many animals and plants, begun by the members of the Accademia dei Lincei (1609–1630) in Italy, whose number included, amongst others, Galileo, Cesi, Stelluti and Faber of Bambourg (the inventor of the term 'microscope').

During the second half of the seventeenth century, a number of scientists in different countries (the 'Classical Microscopists') carried out more comprehensive investigations of the world of microscopic biology, which were published as a series of beautifully illustrated monographs. In Bologna, Marcello Malpighi investigated a great range of microscopic objects and was the first to examine the microstructure of the skin, kidney and spleen and to establish that capillary networks intervened between arteries and veins. He also laid the earliest foundations of microscopic embryology. In London, Robert Hooke in his great treatise *Micrographia* (1665) delineated with meticulous care a great richness of microscopic life and first used the term 'cells', although these were actually the network of dead cell walls in cork wood. Anton van Leeuwenhoek in Delft, Nehemia Grew in London and Jan Swammerdam in the Netherlands and France also made great contributions to animal and plant microscopy during this period.

Thereafter, except for embryologists such as de Graaf, Stensen and Wolff, there were few major advances in microscopic investigation until the nineteenth century, when better microscopes began to be made, achromatic lenses appearing in about 1830 and, some-what later, immersion objectives. At this time there was a great increase in scientific activity in many disciplines and from this period come the first of the modern histologists such as Henle, Schwann, Deiters and Purkinje and later Remak, Ranvier, Leydig, Virchow, Metchinikov, Golgi and Hertwig, among many others. The work of Kölliker in Würzburg, in particular, was a major contribution to histology and this subject as a separate discipline dates from his publication of the first histology textbook in 1852.

However, these developments depended on new insights into the nature of biological organization. A major conceptual advance was the formulation of the cell theory, independently, by the botanist Schleiden in 1838 and the zoologist Schwann in 1839; by this time it was realized that the whole body is composed of aggregations of microscopic living units, cells, each with a nucleus and possessing a measure of independence as well as being subservient to the body as a whole. The physiology, mechanics and pathological reactions of the body reflect the properties and activities of the cells of which it is composed.

Some years before, the French anatomist Bichat (1771–1802) had coined the term 'tissues' (fabrics) to categorize the textures of the different parts of the body, distinguishing 21 different classes. Schwann reduced these to five (in modern times we have four; see however p. 67). In 1844 Owen used the term 'histology' for their study (from the Greek: *histos* = something woven). Different methods of preparation were now being used to demonstrate the microscopic structure of tissues; separation of tissues and cells by maceration and microdissection were largely supplanted by the more refined methods of wax sectioning and staining with dyes appropriated from the burgeoning dye-stuffs industry.

Developments in the theory and technology of lenses culminated in the design of a high resolution compound microscope by Abbé and its construction by Messrs. Zeiss at Jena in the 1870s, setting the field for a rapid expansion of cytology and histology as serious disciplines. Histology was now established as a major branch of Anatomy and, during the following few decades, most of what we know today as classic light microscope histology was established, including the elucidation of chromosome behaviour in mitosis, meiosis and fertilization and the exploration of the cellular structure of the nervous system. The first successes in the culture of cells in artificial media were also achieved during this period, initially in 1907 by Harrison in Baltimore and subsequently developed by Carrel in New York. In a later period, from about 1930–1950, other optical refinements were introduced to allow viewing of living cells, including dark field, phase, interference contrast and ultraviolet microscopy. However, by this time, histology had lost some of its initial impetus and had long since reached its theoretical limit of point-to-point resolution, i.e. twice the wavelength of visible light (about $0.2 \mu m$), limiting effective magnification to about a thousand times.

The renaissance of cell biology was heralded by the development in the 1950s of effective electron microscopy, increasing resolution a thousandfold and permitting useful magnifications of up to a million to be reached. An era of great activity followed, in which appropriate methods of tissue preparation were explored and applied to a wide variety of cells, tissues and organs. The result was the discovery of a great richness of structural detail which has revolutionized our understanding of cells and their functional roles. At the same time, cell fractionation methods for studying the biochemistry of organelles were being developed and used in combination with electron microscopy. The powerful techniques of X-ray diffraction were solving many problems of macromolecular structure, the most celebrated success being the double helical organization of deoxyribonucleic acid (DNA) demonstrated by Crick, Watson, Wilkins and Franklin in 1952, leading to the unravelling of the genetic code and its role in protein synthesis.

Various other methods have also proved of great value: for example, autoradiographic analysis, in which the positions of isotopically-labelled molecules assimilated and transported by cells can be detected in sectioned material by their effects on photographic emulsion; various immunological methods for detecting different types of complex molecules by means of specific antibody binding,

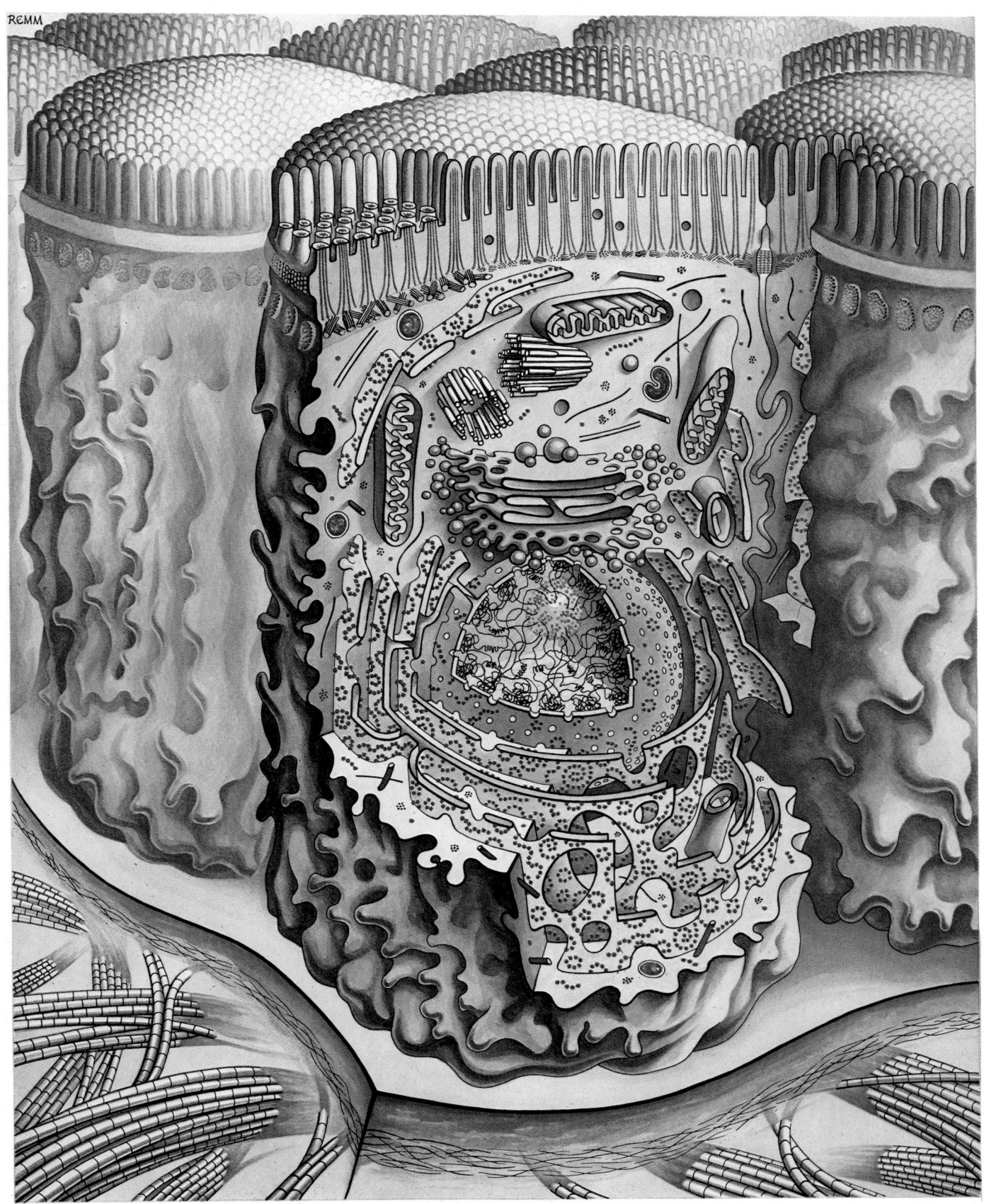

2.1 A three-dimensional reconstruction of some of the principal architectural features of an absorptive cell lying in the simple columnar epithelium of the small intestine. Part of the cell is cut away to expose the nuclear envelope (green); nuclear contents are the nucleolus (red) and chromosomes (black). Outside in the cytoplasm lie the endoplasmic reticulum (yellow) with ribosomes (red) in clusters; the Golgi apparatus (pink) is shown in a supranuclear position, various cytoplasmic vesicles including lysosomes (purple), microtubules (blue), microfilaments, and a centriole pair (grey) are also shown. The apical surface of the cell is covered with microvilli supported by microfilaments which are inserted into a filamentous terminal web. Junctional complexes are seen at the lateral borders of cells apically. A lamina basalis (purple) forms the boundary of the epithelium basally, and lies in close relation to the underlying reticulum and collagen.

greatly assisted by the production of monoclonal antibodies; other major contributions with special structural methods, including scanning electron microscopy to study the surfaces of cells, freeze-fracture or freeze-etching methods to expose the interiors of their membranes and related structures, microanalysis of the elemental composition of tissues and cells, computer-dependent analysis of light microscope images to visualize organelle behaviour in living cells, quantitative (stereological) analysis of cellular components and many other applications. Most recently, the growth of recombinant DNA technology to detect and determine the precise composition of particular genes and to follow their expression in the cell (see p. 52) has provided a particularly powerful set of tools not only for the analysis of cell function but also to synthesize cellular products for clinical and commercial use.

Inevitably, during the early decades of electron microscopy, a strong emphasis was placed on the description of microscopic structure, so that by the mid-1970s the forms and intracellular contents of most of the major cell types, tissues and organs of the body had been systematically investigated at the ultrastructural level. Since that time, a more experimental approach has prevailed and we are steadily gaining fresh insights into the principles governing the dynamic organization of cellular systems and their interactions. Many major problems remain to be solved and, judging from past experience, more have yet to be recognized. But at least many of the fundamental questions of biological existence are being addressed seriously and we can begin to expect a rich return from the investment of so much intellectual labour over the past century.

GENERAL ORGANIZATION OF CELLS

Before proceeding to describe detailed cellular structure, it is desirable to make a brief review of their general composition. The living matter of which cells are made, protoplasm, is composed mainly of water (70% or more by volume), with dissolved inorganic cations (ions of hydrogen, potassium, sodium, calcium, magnesium, iron, etc.) and anions (chloride, bicarbonate, hydroxyl, phosphate, sulphate, etc.), but is also permeated with assemblies of large organic molecules which compose the cellular structure and the system of enzymes and energy carriers providing the basis of living processes within cells. Of the large molecules, the most abundant are those of lipids, carbohydrates, proteins and nucleic acids. The first three of these provide structural materials and enzymes; nucleic acids are important in directing the activities of the cell and in passing on this ability to new cells and to subsequent generations. Numerous smaller organic molecules also abound in the protoplasm, engaged in the teeming biochemical traffic which comprises cell function.

The cell interior is relatively unstable in composition, and must be held ionically, osmotically and electrically within a narrow range for it to function effectively. However, each cell is also in a constant dynamic interchange with its external environment, including other cells, and continuous expenditure of energy is needed to maintain a steady internal state. If this is lost, the cell undergoes degeneration and eventually dies.

In the living state, most individual cells are greyish in appearance in transmitted light and each is bounded by a deformable, selectively

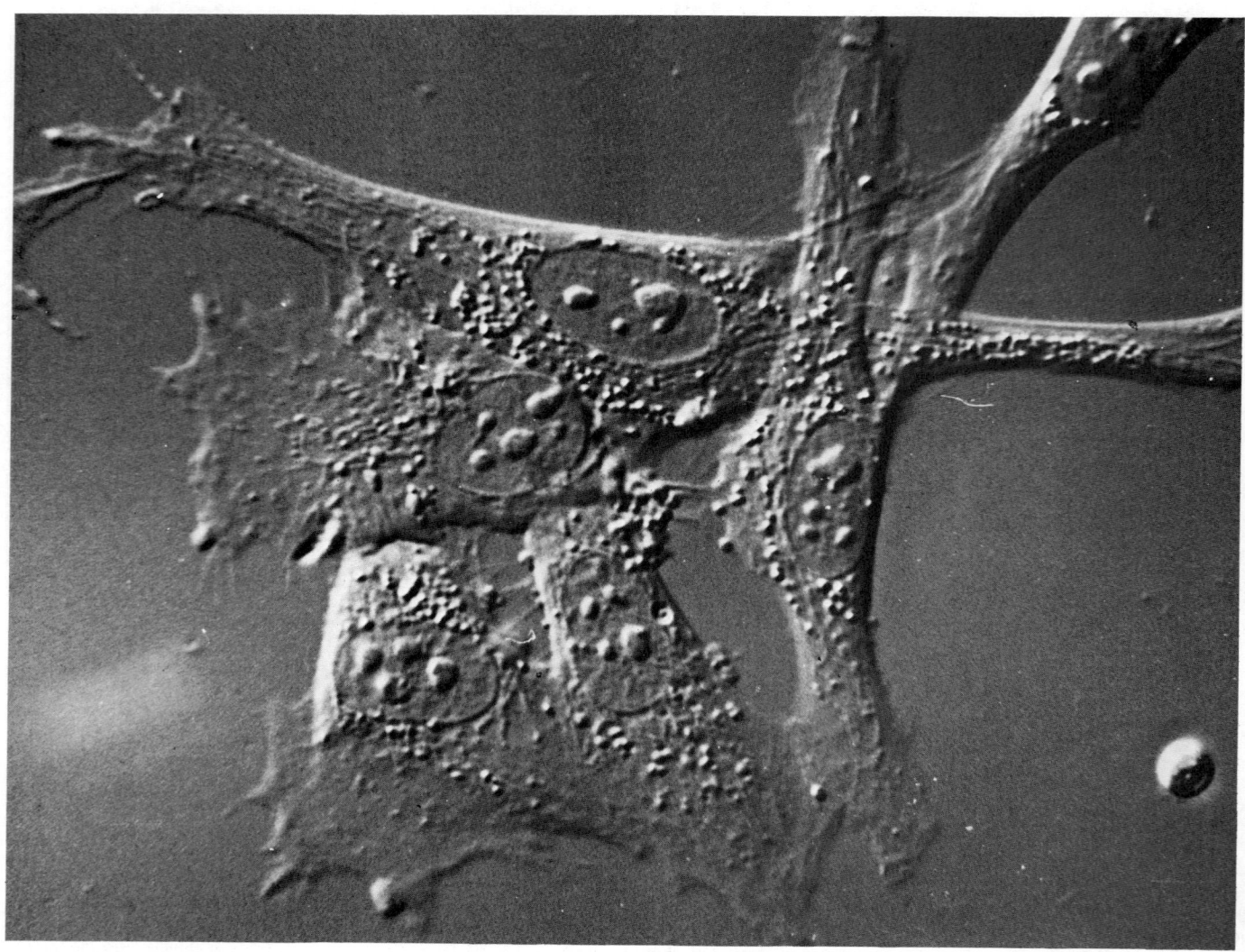

2.2 A high-power micrograph of living cells (fibroblasts in tissue culture), viewed by Normarski interference microscopy. Provided by the Paediatric Research Unit, Guy's Hospital Medical School, London. Magnification × 2000.

permeable membrane which separates it from the environment, and confers on cells many properties essential to the maintenance of life. Within, the physical properties of the cytoplasm vary from those of a stiff gel to a highly fluid state, depending on the presence of complex filamentous macromolecules and their interactive states. However, individual cells are composed of many distinctive assemblies of macromolecules which form centres of functional cooperation; these *organelles* will be described in some detail in this section, as an appreciation of their roles in cell activities is fundamental to an understanding of the organization of cells and their aggregates.

Cell size

Most mammalian cells lie within the size range 5–50 μm in diameter; for example, resting lymphocytes are amongst the smallest, at about 6 μm across, red blood cells are about 7.5 μm and columnar epithelial cells about 20 μm tall and 10 μm wide. Some cells are much larger than this: mature ova may be 80 μm across and megakaryocytes of the bone marrow over 200 μm in diameter. Large neurons and skeletal muscle cells have relatively enormous volumes because of their highly attenuated forms—some may be over a metre in length. Generally speaking, limitations of cell size are determined by problems with rates of diffusion, either of substances into and out of cells or within them. The major advantage of cellularity is that diffusion of materials over short distances of up to 50 μm is relatively rapid so that metabolic needs of active cells can be sustained easily and cellular aggregates react rapidly to the control systems of the body. As a cell increases in size, its mass increase outstrips its surface area unless its shape changes, since the mass varies by the cube of the diameter, whereas the area only increases by the square (see the discussion of this problem by Thompson 1942). Processes depending on the surface area (e.g. diffusion of gases, transport of nutrients, etc.), therefore, become increasingly difficult to maintain at adequate levels. The distance of the cell periphery from the nucleus also becomes greater, so that exertion of nuclear control on the cytoplasm becomes more problematical. In large cells these issues are to some extent overcome by increasing the relative surface area, either by folding or flattening, and nuclear control can be facilitated by creating more nuclei in each cell either by fusion of mononuclear cells (a *syncytium*), as in skeletal muscle, or more rarely by the multiplication of nuclei without corresponding cytoplasmic division (a *plasmodium*, in the human an unusual and irregular finding in some epithelial cells, e.g. hepatocytes, p. 1805). Intracellular diffusion can also be much accelerated by processes of active transport across membranes and directed by motile mechanisms within the fluid regions of the cell.

Motility. This is a characteristic of most cells, taking the form of movements of cytoplasm or specific organelles from one part of the cell to another (e.g. cytoplasmic streaming). It also includes the extension of parts of cells such as pseudopodia, ruffled borders filopodia and microvilli from the surface, locomotion of whole cells by complex streaming interactions with their environment (amoeboid locomotion, etc.) or the beating of flagella (p. 42), cell division, muscle contraction and ciliary beating which moves fluid over internal body surfaces. Cell movements are also involved in the uptake of materials from their environment (endocytosis,

phagocytosis) and the reciprocal passage of large molecular complexes out of cells (exocytosis, secretion).

Cell shape. The external appearances of cells vary widely (**2.1–4**) depending on their interactions with each other, their extracellular environment, and internal structures. Their surfaces are often highly folded when absorptive or transport functions are performed across its boundary, forming microvilli and other protrusions or infoldings, thus creating a large surface area for transport or diffusion.

Cells and tissues

Cells rarely operate independently of each other and tend to form aggregates by reciprocal adhesion, often assisted by the formation of special structural attachments. They may also communicate with each other either by releasing and detecting chemical messages diffusing through intercellular spaces or more rapidly by membrane contact, in many cases involving small, temporary transmembrane channels (p. 28). Cohesive or spatially aggregated groups of cells constitute *tissues* and more complex assemblies of tissues form functional systems such as the visceral *organs*, whose development and maintenance depend on as yet poorly understood cellular interactions.

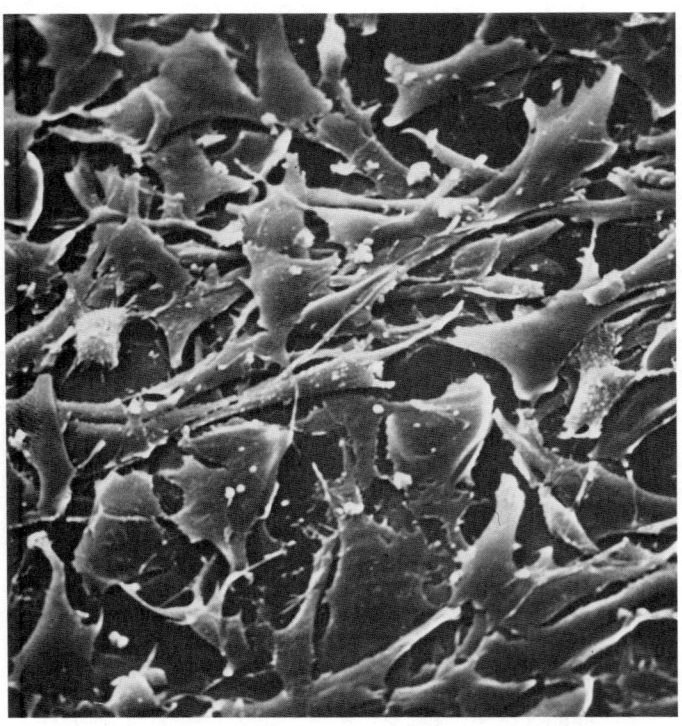

2.3   Flattened fibroblasts growing in tissue culture viewed with the scanning electron microscope. Material provided by L. Mallucci. Magnification × 500.

CELL STRUCTURE

Although great modifications of form and activities may take place in different cells during their development and maturation, a common pattern of organization can be seen in their structure and functions. In describing this pattern, as seen with the methods of electron microscopy coupled with many other techniques, we will consider first the outer parts of the cell, the *cytoplasm*, and then the central *nucleus*. Within the cytoplasm are present several distinct systems of organelles (**2.**1, 4, 5). These include a series of membrane-bound structures which form separate compartments within the cytoplasm, such as the endoplasmic reticula, Golgi complexes, lysosomes, peroxisomes, mitochondria and transport, secretory and storage vesicles. They also comprise various structures lying outside these membranous organelles in the portion of the cytoplasm known as the *cytosol*, including ribosomes, several types of filamentous protein assemblies (collectively, the *cytoskeleton*), some assisting to determine general cell shape or supporting special extensions of the cell surface (microvilli, cilia, flagella); others are involved in the assembly of new filamentous organelles (e.g. centrioles) or internal movements of the cytoplasm. Also in the cytosol lie many soluble proteins and metabolites of various kinds. The whole cell is bounded externally by a specialized membrane, the *plasma membrane*. Within the cytoplasm is the nucleus, a special membrane-lined compartment containing the genetic instructions of the cell, the chromosomes; other nuclear organelles lying in the nuclear sap, for example the nucleolus,

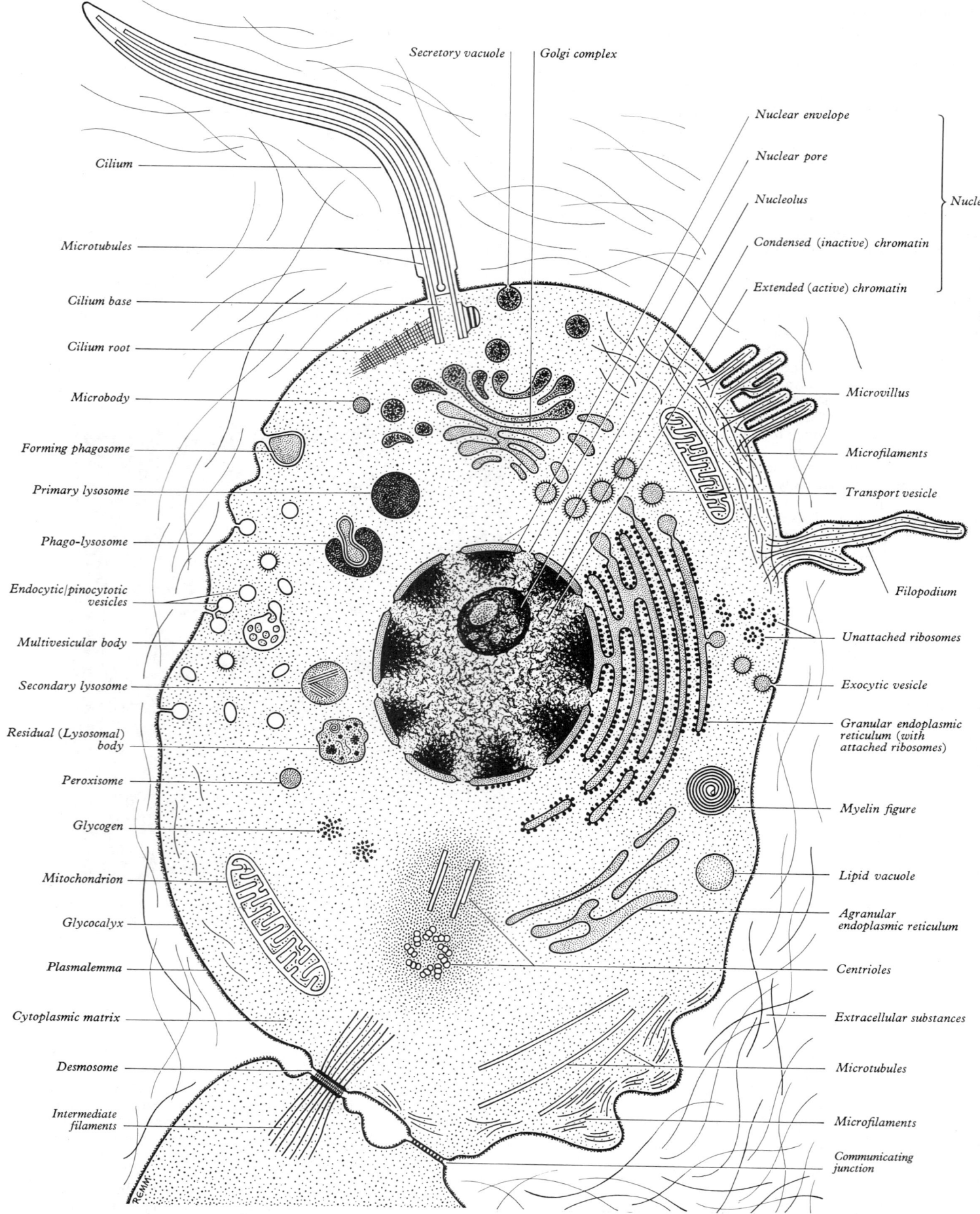

Secretory vacuole

Golgi complex

Cilium

Microtubules

Cilium base

Cilium root

Microbody

Forming phagosome

Primary lysosome

Phago-lysosome

Endocytic/pinocytotic vesicles

Multivesicular body

Secondary lysosome

Residual (Lysosomal) body

Peroxisome

Glycogen

Mitochondrion

Glycocalyx

Plasmalemma

Cytoplasmic matrix

Desmosome

Intermediate filaments

Nuclear envelope

Nuclear pore

Nucleolus

Condensed (inactive) chromatin

Extended (active) chromatin

Nucleus

Microvillus

Microfilaments

Transport vesicle

Filopodium

Unattached ribosomes

Exocytic vesicle

Granular endoplasmic reticulum (with attached ribosomes)

Myelin figure

Lipid vacuole

Agranular endoplasmic reticulum

Centrioles

Extracellular substances

Microtubules

Microfilaments

Communicating junction

2.4 A composite diagram showing the principal structures found within tissue cells. Only a proportion of the features illustrated will be present in any specific cell type.

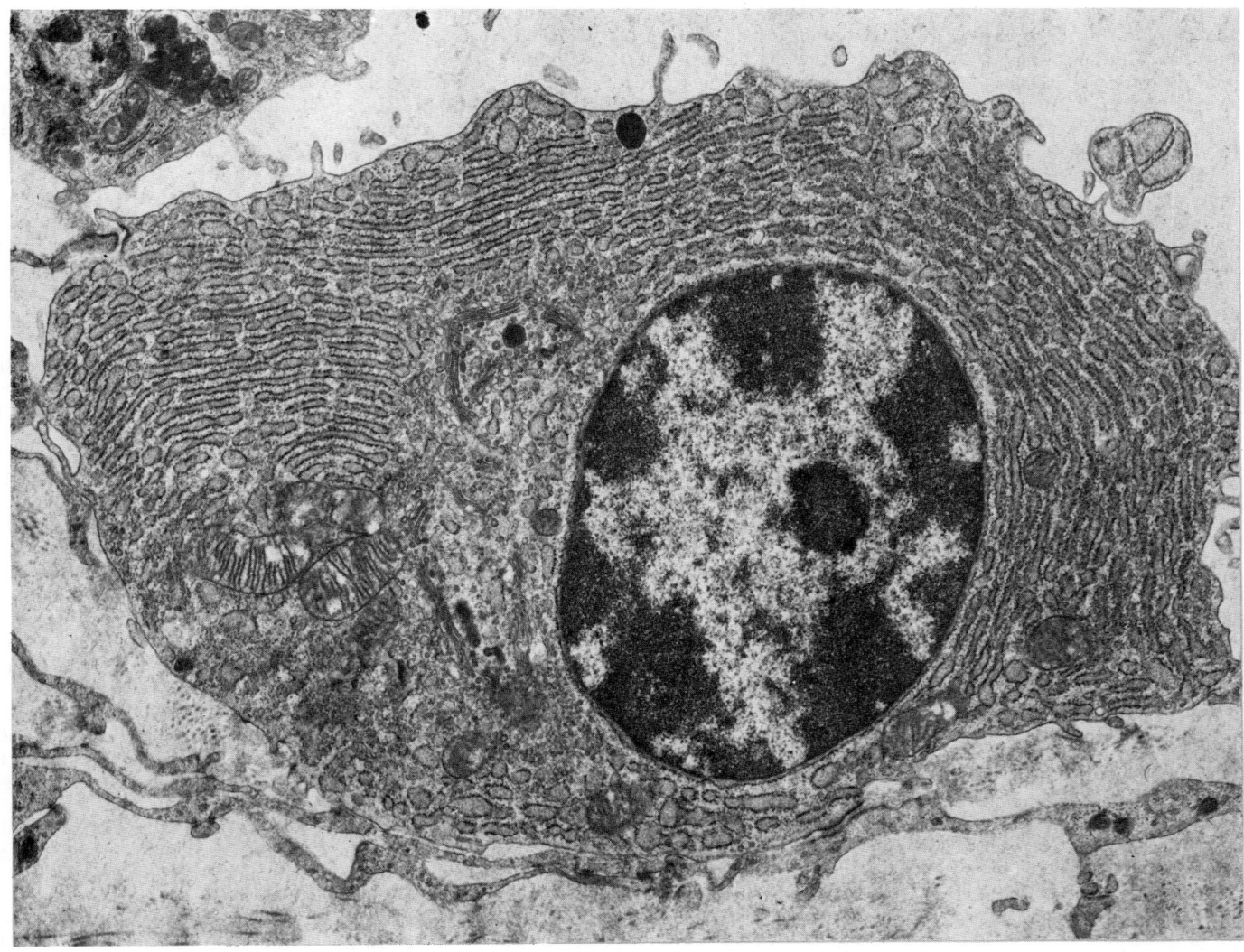

2.5 An electron micrograph of a protein-synthesizing cell (plasmacyte: mature B-lymphocyte) in section showing abundant rough endoplasmic reticulum, Golgi apparatus, mitochondria, lysosomes and a cell membrane with surface protrusions (filopodia). Magnification × 12 000.

are involved in the expression of these instructions. These different structures and an outline of their known activities will now be briefly described. For further details the reader is referred to other lengthier texts, such as those by Kristić (1984), Weiss (1983a), Fawcett (1994), Alberts et al (1994).

CYTOPLASM

MEMBRANE SYSTEMS OF THE CELL

With the advent of electron microscopy, it was confirmed that cells are bounded by a distinct membrane and internally are permeated by membrane-lined vacuoles and channels, forming a series of closed compartments within cells. Both external and internal membranes (*cytomembranes*) have many common features. All are composed of phospholipids and proteins, usually in an approximately 3:2 ratio, with a small amount of carbohydrate. The amount of lipid in an external membrane permits a layer two molecules thick to cover the cell surface. As long ago as 1925 Gorter and Grendel proposed that all cell membranes are bilayers of lipid, with the hydrophobic ends of each lipid molecule pointing towards the interior of the membrane and the hydrophilic ends pointing outwards. Later, Danielli and Davson (1935) suggested that the protein might line both sides of the lipid to form a protein/lipid sandwich, but more recently the *fluid mosaic* model was proposed and widely confirmed, in which the proteins are envisaged as embedded or floating in the lipid bilayer

(Singer & Nicolson 1972; see also Bretscher 1985). Some proteins, because of the extensive hydrophobic portions of their polypeptide chains, span the entire width of the membrane (*transmembrane proteins*) whilst others are only superficially attached. Carbohydrates in the form of oligosaccharides and polysaccharides are bound either to proteins (glycoproteins) or to lipids (glycolipids), projecting outwards from the surface of the membrane.

These features, deduced partly from biochemical and biophysical data, can be correlated with electron microscopic appearances. Membranes, suitably fixed and stained by heavy metals, show in section two densely stained layers separated by an electron-translucent zone (**2.**6), the total thickness being about 7.5 nm (the classic '*unit membrane*' of Robertson 1959), probably reflecting binding of stain by the 'heads' of the phospholipid molecules. Freeze-fractured and/or etched specimens in which the deeply frozen sample is cleaved to expose membrane interiors and of which a metal-shadowed carbon replica is then made and viewed by electron microscopy (**2.**6, 8), have also demonstrated a bilaminar structure in membranes. Cleavage planes usually pass along the midline of each membrane where the hydrophobic 'tails' of phospholipids meet. This method has also demonstrated intramembranous particles (IMPs) embedded in the lipid layers; these are in the 5–15 nm range and in most cases represent large transmembrane protein molecules or assemblies of such molecules. IMPs are distributed asymmetrically between the two half-membranes, usually adhering more to one face than the other. In plasma membranes (which form the cell surface), the **inner** or protoplasmic half-membrane carries most particles, exposed at its

23

externally-facing surface (the P face). The corresponding inwardly-directed (E) surface of the **external** half-membrane usually shows pits into which the particles fit (**2.6**, 8, 10). Not all the proteins of membranes are **visible** as particles, however; some are either too small or not compact enough to appear in this form and have, as yet, been demonstrated only biochemically. Where they have been identified, particles usually represent channels for the transmembrane passage of ions or molecules.

Biophysical measurements show the phospholipid bilayer to be highly fluid, allowing diffusion **along the plane** of the membrane at rates as high as 2 μm/second (Bretscher 1975). Thus proteins are able to move freely along such planes unless anchored from within the cell. Some internal membranes possess much more protein than the external cell membrane, for example the inner mitochondrial membrane which is rich in enzyme activity; the fluidity of such membranes is correspondingly much reduced.

The functions of cell membranes are many: they form boundaries selectively limiting diffusion and creating physiologically distinct compartments inside the cell, dividing those regions within the channel system (*vacuoplasm*) from those outside it (*cytosol* or *hyaloplasm*). Membranes actively control the passage of electrolytes and small organic molecules, generate bioelectric potentials and provide surfaces for the attachment of enzymes often associated with the movement of reaction products across membranes (*vectorial metabolism*). Membranes also serve as sites for the reception of external stimuli, including hormones and other chemical agents, and for the recognition and attachment of other cells. Conversely, they may alter the activities of other cells by transmitting to them chemical or physical messages of various kinds. Lastly, they can act as points of attachment of intracellular structures—the basis for locomotor activity and for cytoskeletal stability (p. 36).

Membranes within cells can, on occasion, fuse with each other and so form a potentially continuous system. However, there are barriers to the indiscriminate mixing of membrane components so that each maintains its unique chemical and functional features. Thus, although the membrane systems of a cell can be viewed as a single entity, they are highly distinctive and localized in their activities.

Cell membranes are synthesized by the granular endoplasmic reticulum (p. 30), usually in collaboration with the Golgi apparatus.

PLASMA MEMBRANE (PLASMALEMMA OR CELL MEMBRANE)

The plasma membrane differs from other membranes in that it forms the external boundary of the cell (**2.6**, 7) and, as such, possesses many distinctive structural features; for example, it bears a diffuse carbohydrate-rich coat, the *cell coat* or *glycocalyx*, externally. In certain sites it also forms *intercellular junctions* of various types with other cells or *adhesive plaques* and in some instances, hemi-desmosomes with extracellular structures (see p. 27). Within the cell, filaments of the cytoskeleton are also anchored to the plasma membrane proteins, immobilizing them or transmitting motile forces from within the cell to the cell surface and thus causing changes of cell shape or locomotion. The plasma membrane is **selectively permeable**, allowing the free passage of some gases and water but restricting the movements of larger ions such as those of sodium, potassium, calcium, chloride and bicarbonate to special proteinaceous channels, which can be opened or closed by the cell to regulate transmembrane traffic. The passage of many other substances such as glucose, amino acids and nucleic acid precursors is also limited to such routes. In most cases, each channel will only admit one species of ion or molecule; substances either move passively through these apertures along diffusion gradients, or by energy-consuming active transport. Movements of such materials into and out of the cell vary greatly, depending on their local concentrations, cell requirements, the availability of chemical energy, action of external hormones and neurotransmitters and many other factors. However, lipid-soluble substances may be able to pass through the lipidic portion of membranes directly so that, for example, steroid hormones can enter the cytoplasm without passing through protein channels. The uptake of larger molecules involves the invagination and rounding up of the plasma membrane to form small vacuoles termed *endocytic vesicles* (**2.4**), which are transported to other regions within the cell. The reverse process—extrusion of organic molecules—is achieved by *exocytic vesicles* which fuse with the plasma membrane and release their contents to the exterior.

The plasma membrane, like other cytomembranes, is in constant flux (see Pearse & Bretscher 1981), the whole surface being regularly changed by subtraction through endocytosis or the loss of components externally and by addition of new membrane from exocytic vesicles. Endocytosed membrane may either be degraded in the lysosomal system of the cell or components of it recycled back to the cell surface in vesicular form; there is thus a continual traffic between the cell interior and surface, allowing the cell to modify the properties of its plasma membrane in response to metabolic needs or to external stimuli, add new membrane during growth, repair surface damage, take in large molecular complexes from outside and engage in many other interactions with the cell environment.

The plasma membrane also has special roles in co-ordinating many cellular activities by signalling changes in the cell's environment to the cell interior and in maintaining the cell's shape and coherence. It therefore acts as a sensory surface, with a wide variety of special receptor molecules, some responding only to a narrow range of stimuli (e.g. the receptors for insulin, acetylcholine (ACh) and low density lipoprotein), others being activated by more general factors such as the contact with other cells or inorganic surfaces. Stimulation of the cell surface may result in changes in the bioelectric transmembrane potential causing fluxes of inorganic ions; this is most striking in the *excitable* plasma membranes of nerve and muscle cells in which the 'resting' voltage can change transiently from as much as 100 mV (negative inside) to 50 mV (positive inside) when suitably stimulated, a result of the opening and subsequent closure of channels selectively permeable to sodium and potassium (see p. 905).

Stimulation of surface receptors also often activates a 'second messenger' which may profoundly change the metabolism or motility of the whole cell. Adenylate cyclase, an enzyme associated with the plasma membrane of probably all nucleated cells, is prominent in this process; its activation results in changes in concentrations of cyclic adenosine monophosphate (cyclic AMP) within the cell, leading to alterations in DNA synthesis, gene expression, protein synthesis, actin and myosin interactions and many other intracellular events. Cyclic guanidine monophosphate (cyclic GMP) is controlled by similar enzyme systems and may have effects antagonistic to those of cyclic AMP. Some hormones and neurotransmitters act in this manner and it is probable that many types of intercellular communication use this or similar systems. Another mechanism of much current interest involves the phospholipid phosphoinositol and its derivatives in calcium-regulating processes within the cell, which lead to the activation of phosphokinases and phosphorylation of various cellular components, a step with far-reaching metabolic and structural consequences (see Berridge 1985).

Although these considerations apply to the plasma membranes of all cells, those of specialized cells are often highly developed in some particular respect. Thus, sensory membranes of retinal photoreceptors, derived from the plasma membrane, have numerous photoreceptive proteins embedded in their surfaces; the acetylcholine-receptive sole-plate membranes of skeletal muscle cells likewise are studded with protein particles able to bind the transmitter. Research in this field is indeed of great potential since it may reveal much about cellular functions in general and also give a deeper understanding of the actions of drugs on cells; the cell membrane is undoubtedly the primary target of a wide variety of chemotherapeutic agents, anaesthetics and other substances of medical importance.

The cell coat (glycocalyx)

As mentioned above, the cell coat forms an integral part of the plasma membrane, projecting as a diffuse filamentous layer 2–20 nm or more from the lipoprotein surface. It is composed of the carbohydrate portions of glycoproteins and glycolipids embedded in the plasma membrane (**2.6**, 7), consisting of much branched oligosaccharides and polysaccharides, the terminal residues of which are usually negatively charged sialic acids, such as n-acetyl neuraminic acid, but are also often rich in galactose residues. These and other carbohydrates can be readily demonstrated by electron microscopy, using dyes such as ruthenium red, or more specifically with plant-derived chemical probes termed *lectins* (e.g. concanavalin A, wheat germ agglutinin, phytohaemagglutinin) which bind to

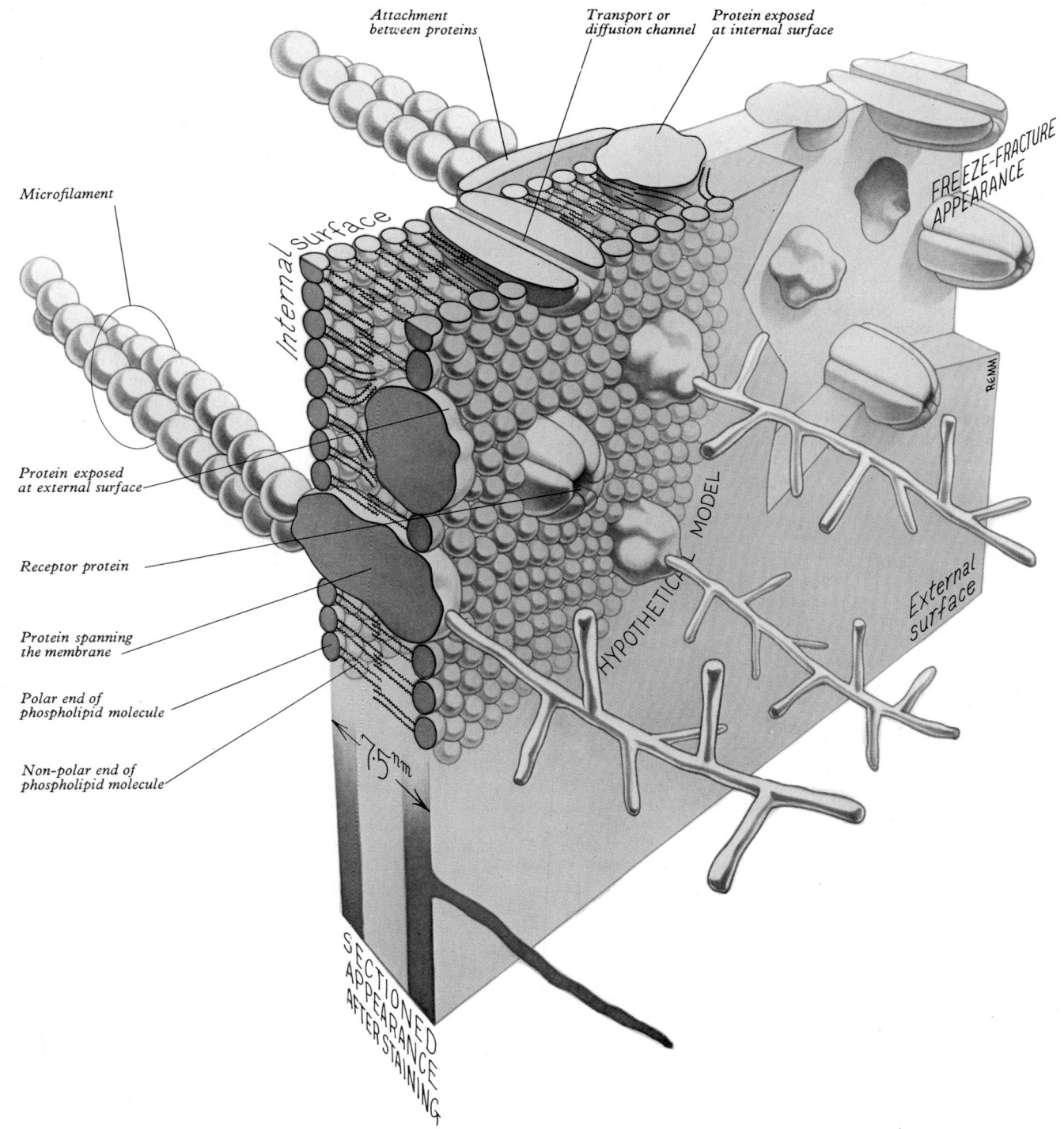

Attachment
between proteins

Transport or
diffusion channel

Protein exposed
at internal surface

FREEZE-FRACTURE
APPEARANCE

Microfilament

Internal surface

HYPOTHETICAL MODEL

External surface

Protein exposed
at external surface

Receptor protein

Protein spanning
the membrane

Polar end of
phospholipid molecule

Non-polar end of
phospholipid molecule

7.5 nm

SECTIONED
APPEARANCE
AFTER STAINING

2.6 The various 'appearances' of the plasma membrane as studied with different electron microscope techniques, including sectioning and freeze-fracturing together with current interpretations of the results of these and other biophysical methods. In this diagram, membrane proteins (green) are either confined to a single leaflet of the lipid bilayer, or they span both layers. Branched carbohydrate chains (grey) are shown attached to some transmembrane proteins on the external surface of the membrane, and a double helical actin filament (pink) is attached to the inside (left). The hydrophobic tails of the lipid molecules are shown as thin black lines and their hydrophilic heads as spheres: blue for the outer surface of the membrane and yellow for the inner surface. These various shapes are, of course, only schematic, as the various protein, lipid and carbohydrate molecules of which cell membranes are constituted have differing detailed shapes.

particular carbohydrate groups. By conjugating lectins with fluorescent molecules, or with electron microscopic tracers such as ferritin, horseradish peroxidase or colloidal gold, the surface carbohydrates can readily be visualized and even quantitated.

The precise composition of the glycocalyx varies with cell type; many tissue antigens are located in the coat, including the major histocompatibility antigen (MHC) systems and, in the case of erythrocytes, blood group antigens (p. 1410). Special adhesion molecules enabling cells to adhere selectively to other cells or extracellular material are also present and are of utmost importance in maintaining the integrity of cellular assemblies of all kinds (see p. 26). They are also vital to a wide range of developmental movements and interactions between cells, for example the formation of intercommunicating neural networks in the nervous system.

Because of the predominance of negatively-charged carbohydrates at cell surfaces, cells tend to repel each other if they approach too

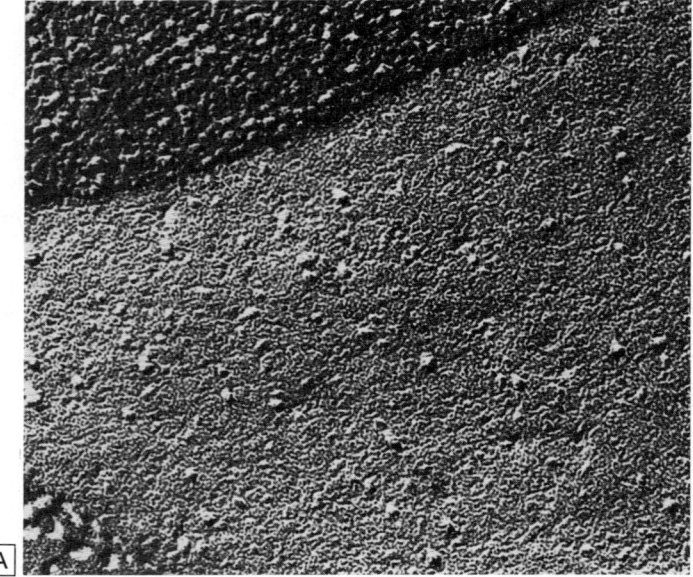

2.7 Electron micrograph of a section through the surface of a fibroblast stained with ruthenium red to show the thick glycocalyx. Magnification × 40 000.

closely. Thus, except at special junctions, there is a distance of at least 20 nm between the plasma membranes of adjacent cells. But some positively-charged molecules also exist at cell surfaces and can form intercellular links with negative charges across the intercellular gap.

Since the glycoproteins and glycolipids are usually free to move in the plane of the membrane, addition of lectins or antibodies can cause the aggregation of these carbohydrate-rich molecules which become cross-linked to form raft-like groups or 'patches'. If these are further aggregated by motile activities of the cell (an energy-dependent process), they may merge to form a 'cap' at one pole of the cell. In other cells (e.g. erythrocytes) the carbohydrate-rich molecules are prevented from wandering or forming patches by internal anchoring proteins (p. 38).

INTERCELLULAR AND EXTRACELLULAR CONTACTS

The plasma membrane is, of course, the surface which establishes contact with other cells and with the structural materials of its extracellular environment. Such contacts lead to a number of different interactions which have a profound effect on the biology of cells, affecting their shape, position, differentiation, metabolism, morphogenesis and ability to multiply, depending on the cell type and the organization of the surrounding extracellular materials. Contacts may be primarily adhesive, enabling cells to stick to each other and

to extracellular fibrils or other structures. They may also be involved in signalling between cells either directly by specialized contacts, or indirectly through extracellular macromolecules. In many instances, the same contacts subserve both adhesion and signalling. Contacts between cells can also be used in other ways, for example, to create diffusion barriers. Structurally there are two main classes of contact, both of them associated with cell adhesion molecules:

- those without any obvious ultrastructural features in the areas of contact
- those with ultrastructurally visible specializations.

'Unspecialized' adhesive contacts

Cells typically adhere to one another or to extracellular structures over extensive areas of their surface, although their lipid bilayers do not approach closer than about 20 nm, a distance determined by the net negative electrostatic potential of their surface carbohydrates, especially sialic acid which exerts a charge repulsion between adjacent plasma membranes. However, various transmembrane or membrane-anchored glycoproteins protrude externally from the plasma membrane and form adhesive contacts over such distances. These are termed cell adhesion molecules (CAMs) of which many types have been described, and more are continually being discovered. They include a number of categories, divisible broadly into those whose adhesive properties depend on the presence of calcium ions, and those which are calcium-independent (see also p. 111).

Calcium-dependent adhesion molecules. Three sub-types of these are known: the cadherins, selectins and integrins.

Cadherins. These are responsible for strong general intercellular adhesion; they are single-pass transmembrane proteins, with five domains on their external ends (four of them repeated) which are heavily glycosylated. At their cytoplasmic ends they are attached by intermediary proteins (*catenins*) to underlying cytoskeletal fibres (either actin or intermediate filaments). Different types of cell may possess different forms of cadherins, for example N-cadherins in nervous tissue, E-cadherins in epithelia, and P-cadherins in the placenta. These molecules bind to those of the same type in other cells (homophilic binding), so that cells of the same class adhere to each other preferentially, forming tissue groups or layers (as in epithelia), reforming these even after they have been disaggregated experimentally. For review, see Geiger and Ayalon (1992).

Selectins. These are another quite distinct form of adhesion molecule, found in leucocytes and other migratory cells. They are transmembrane glycoproteins which can bind, with a rather low affinity, to the carbohydrate groups on other cell surfaces to permit movement between the two, albeit rather restricted in speed, for

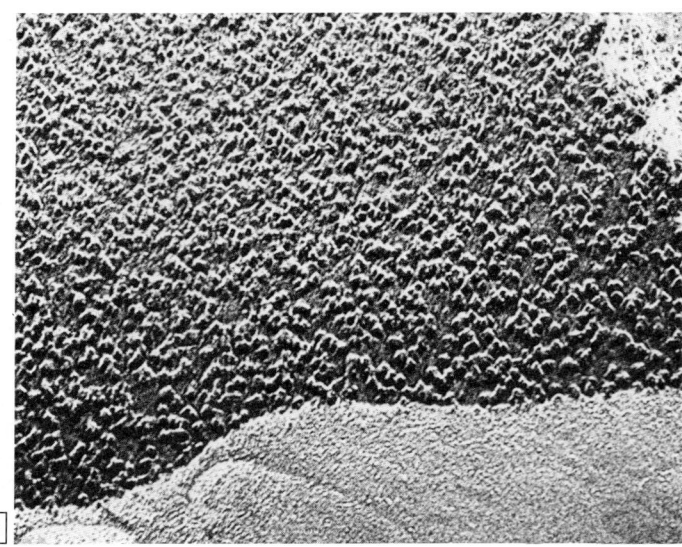

2.8 Electron micrographs of the plasma membrane of an erythrocyte prepared by freeze-fracturing. A shows the external (*E*) fracture face, bearing few particles and some pit-like depressions; in B the internal (*P*) fracture face is visible, showing numerous particles. Magnification × 80 000.

example the rolling adhesion of leucocytes on the walls of blood vessels (p. 1461). For review, see Haas & Plow (1994).

Integrins. These are glycoproteins which typically mediate adhesion between cells and extracellular tissue components, for example fibronectin, collagen, laminin. Each integrin molecule is formed of two subunits (α and β) each of which has several (or more) subtypes, whose combinations provide at least 20 specificities, each one directed to a particular extracellular molecule, or, at their other ends, anchored within the cell to a particular cytoskeletal component (see Rosen & Bertozzi 1994).

Calcium-independent adhesion molecules. Of these the best known are glycoproteins which have external domains similar to immunoglobulin molecules. They are mostly transmembrane proteins, but some of them are entirely external, either attached to the plasma membrane by glycosylphosphotidylinositol (GPI) anchor, or secreted as soluble components of the extracellular matrix. As with the cadherins, like binds to like, i.e. they are homophilic. Many different types have now been described in different tissues. Two well-researched groups are the *Neural Cell Adhesion Molecules* (*N-CAMs*), with nearly 20 known varieties currently, and the *Intercellular Adhesion Molecules* (*ICAMs*) expressed on leucocytes. These adhesion molecules are coexpressed with the calcium dependent classes; their distinctive roles are not entirely clear but it is thought that they may modulate intercellular adhesion; for example, the soluble form of N-CAM may bind to membrane-bound forms and so block intercellular adhesion. For a recent review, see Walsh & Doherty (1993).

Reduction of the normal adhesive properties of cells in malignant neoplasms favours their rapid local spread and the formation of secondary colonies (metastases) elsewhere.

For further reading on cell adhesion molecules and intercellular contacts, consult Alberts et al (1994), and see also p. 111.

Specialized junctional structures

Specialized junctional structures are localized regions of cell surfaces at cell–cell or cell–extracellular matrix where contacts occur, detectable with the electron microscope because of dense material attached to the internal and, often, external aspects of the plasma membrane. Three major classes exist: occluding, adhesive and communicating junctions.

The occluding junction (zonula occludens, tight junction). This type of junction creates diffusion barriers in continuous layers of cells, including epithelia, mesothelia and endothelia, preventing the passage of materials across the cellular layer through intercellular gaps. It forms a continuous belt (zonula) around the cell perimeter (near the luminal surface in the case of cuboidal or columnar cells; Pinto da Silva & Kachar 1982). At a zonula occludens the membranes of the adjacent cells come into contact, obliterating the gap between them. Freeze-etching shows that the contacts between the membranes lie along branching and anastomosing ridges formed by the incorporation of chains of protein particles within the membranes (**2.10, 11A**), distorting and stiffening them along the lines of contact.

This arrangement dictates that substances can only pass through the layer of cells provided with these junctions by diffusion or transport through their luminal membrane and cytoplasm, so that the cells can control the movements across the surfaces that they bound. Thus occluding junctions prevent the leakage of potentially toxic substances from the lumina of viscera into the surrounding tissues, retain colloids within the bloodstream and form important diffusion barriers in many other sites, for example the blood–brain barrier (p. 1221). This can be seen experimentally if colloidal tracers such as ferritin or horseradish peroxidase (HRP) are placed either in the lumen of an epithelium-lined cavity, or alternatively into the tissues beneath it. It is then found that the tracer cannot pass the line of occluding junctions in either direction.

A second, most important function of occluding junctions is to create regional differences in the plasma membranes of the cells which they enclose. It is known that in epithelia the composition of the apical plasma membranes of cells differs from that of their basolateral surfaces, allowing these regions to engage in special activities (e.g. directional transport of ions and uptake of macromolecules). Because the occluding junctions have high concentrations of fixed transmembrane proteins, they act as barriers to lipid and protein diffusion laterally within membranes. In this way,

specialized regions of membrane can be maintained in an appropriate position, for example the secretory surface of a gland cell or the ion-transporting surface of a kidney tubule cell (see Simons & Fuller 1985). For a recent review of tight junctions see Schneeberger & Lynch (1992).

Specialized adhesive contacts. These include intercellular and cell–extracellular matrix contacts where cells adhere strongly to each other or to adjacent matrix components. Intercellular contacts can be subdivided into *adhesive belts*, *adhesive strips*, and *adhesive spots* (*desmosomes*). In all of these there is a high concentration of CAMs which bind at their exposed ends to those of adjacent cells, and at their internal ends to cytoskeletal fibres via intermediary proteins. The latter create electron-dense undercoatings of the plasma membrane visible by electron microscopy, and which act to distribute tensional forces throughout the cell instead of just to the plasma membrane which is mechanically very weak. Cell–matrix junctions include *hemidesmosomes* and *focal spots*.

The adhesive belt (*zonula adherens*) (**5.9, 10.**) This is a continuous zone formed around the apical perimeters of epithelial, mesothelial and endothelial cells, parallel and just basal to the occluding belt (see above). High concentrations of cadherins occur here, their cytoplasmic ends anchored via the proteins vinculin and α-actinin to a layer of actin microfilaments which form a dense undercoat in this region. This helps to reinforce the rather weak intercellular attachment of the occluding belt and prevents its disruption when tissues are stretched. The gap between cell surfaces is about 20 nm, and no electron-dense material is usually observed in this space.

The adhesive strip (*fascia adherens*). This is a type of junction similar to the adhering belt but forming a limited anchoring strip or patch, anchoring together the surfaces of many types of cell: for example, smooth muscle cells, the intercalated discs of cardiac muscle cells (p. 768), between glial cells and neurons and many other situations. Again, these involve cadherins attached indirectly to actin filaments on the inner side of the membrane.

The desmosome (*macula adherens*). This is a limited plaque-like area of particularly strong intercellular contact where additional adhesion molecules occur (**2.9, 10**). It can be sited anywhere on the cell surface. The intercellular gap is about 25 nm, filled with electron-dense filamentous material running transversely across it and also marked by a series of densely staining bands running parallel to the cell surfaces. Within the cells on either side there is a dense undercoating of the plasma membrane, into which the ends of intermediate filaments are inserted (**2.9, 10**). These structures form strong anchorage points between cells, particularly where strong cohesion is needed, for example, in the stratum spinosum of the epidermis (p. 382) where they are extremely numerous and large. In some regions desmosomes are much smaller, for example between endothelial cells lining capillaries, and in fetal tissue.

The adhesion molecules of desmosomes include the integrins desmoglein I and II. In freeze-fracture preparations intramembranous particles and pits are present on both the P and E faces of the membranes, a characteristic feature of these structures (of unknown significance). For review see Garrod (1993), Koch & Franke (1994).

Hemidesmosomes. These are best known as anchoring junctions between the bases of epidermal cells and the extracellular structures of the underlying connective tissue (p. 382), although similar structures, less well defined, also occur in other situations. Ultrastructurally they resemble a single-sided desmosome, anchored on one side to the plasma membrane, and on the other to the basal lamina (**5.39**) and adjacent collagen fibrils. On the cytoplasmic side of the membrane there is a dense coat into which keratin filaments rather than actin filaments are inserted. Although they look very like desmosomes, they are chemically quite distinct, and also use integrins as their adhesion molecules rather than cadherins. As already noted, less highly structured attachments with a similar arrangement exist between many other cell types and their surrounding matrix, for example between smooth muscle cells and their matrix fibrils, between the ends of skeletal muscle cells and tendon fibres, etc. They range from large areas of apposition to small punctate attachments (focal adhesion plaques, see below).

Focal adhesion plaques. These are regions of local attachment between cells and the matrix, typically situated at or near the ends

27

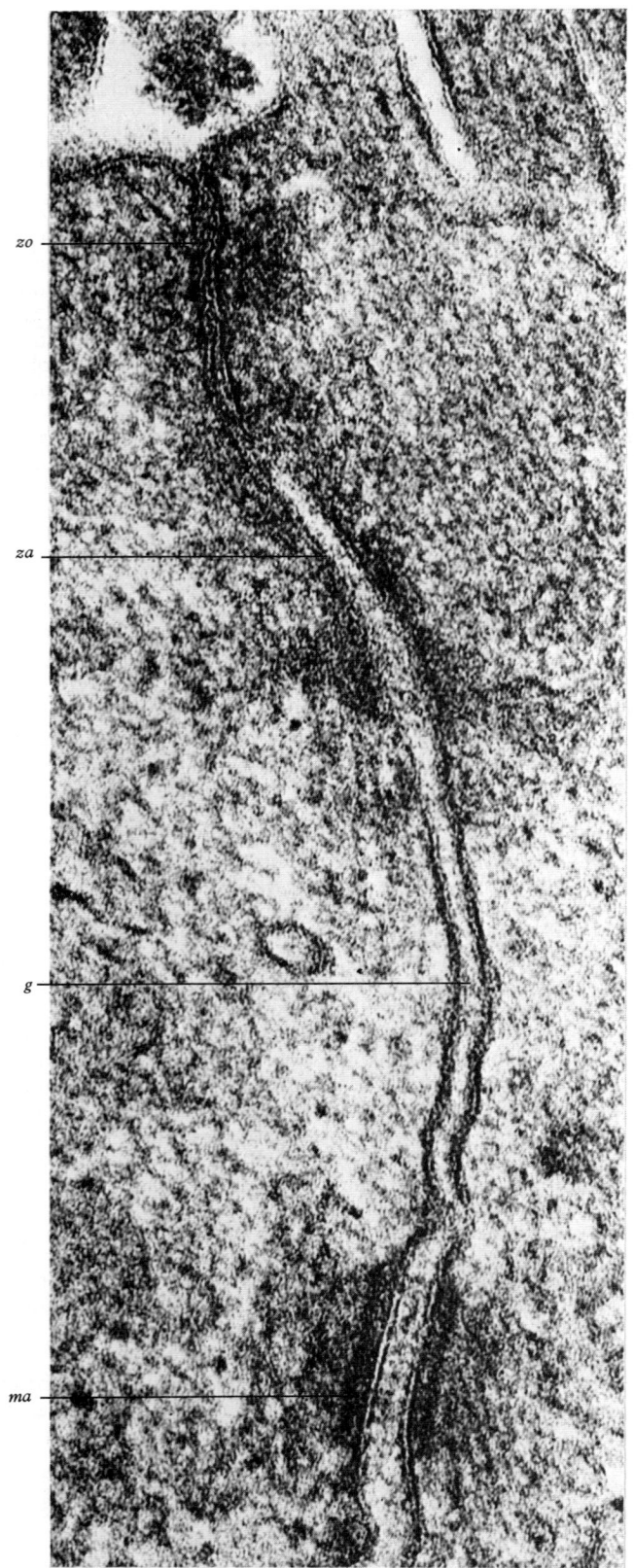

2.9 A high-power electron micrograph· of a junctional complex between two epithelial cells showing a zonula occludens (tight junction) (*zo*), a zonula adherens (*za*), a macula adherens (desmosome) (*ma*), and a normal intercellular gap (*g*). Magnification × 130 000.

continuity between these and the cytoskeleton of the cell so attached. Such adhesions are usually only short-lived, their formation and breakage being part of the locomotor activities of migratory cells. Although at first glance they appear to be simple attachments, research shows several protein systems to be involved in their formation and breakage, including various signalling complexes (e.g. tyrosine kinases and phosphorylases) which inform the cell of the extracellular contact and initiate cytoskeleton assembly.

Communicating junctions (gap junctions) (2.10, 12). When sectioned transversely, these superficially resemble occluding junctions but the two apposed lipid bilayers are separated by an apparent gap of 3 nm. Bridging this gap, the membranes have numerous protein channels whose external ends meet in the middle to create a series of minute pathways from one cell to the next. These channels may exist in only small numbers, when they may be difficult to detect structurally, although they lower the transcellular electrical resistance and can be discerned by measuring this with microelectrodes. Larger assemblies may number many thousands of channels, often packed in hexagonal arrays. Such junctions form limited attachment plaques (Goodenough & Revel 1970) rather than continuous zones, thereby allowing free passage of substances along the cleft between cells (unlike occluding junctions). They occur in numerous tissues including the liver, epidermis, connective tissues, cardiac muscle and smooth muscle (*nexuses*); they are also common in embryonic tissues. In the central nervous system they are found in the ependyma and between neuroglial cells, and they form electrical synapses between some types of neurons (see p. 932).

While communicating junctions form diffusion channels between cells, the size of their apertures limits intercellular movements to rather small molecules and ions (up to a molecular weight of about 1000 kDa); this includes sodium, potassium and calcium ions, various second messenger components and a number of metabolites, but not messenger RNA. In some excitable tissues (e.g. cardiac and smooth muscle), one cell can activate another by electrotonic current flow through communicating junctions without the intervention of a chemical transmitter, and this is also true of electrical synapses (p. 932). Elsewhere their functions are not certain; experimentally they have been shown to be permeable to various dyes and to form pathways with low resistance to the flow of ionic current. Communicating junctions probably permit metabolic cooperation between adjacent cells or groups of cells. Thus, in embryonic life, such junctions may aid the establishment of pattern and the co-ordinated differentiation of the whole blastula, within and between germ layers, or of more localized tissues (Fraser 1985). This may involve the movement of regulatory substances involved in gene blocking or gene repression and de-repression diffusing freely or creating morphogenetic gradients (see p. 113). Communicating junctions may also assist in the control of cell division since in damaged tissues they disappear while tissues undergo repair by mitosis, to reappear when regeneration ceases (Bennett 1973, Fusijawa et al 1976).

Freeze-fracturing and etching methods (Staehelin 1974) and computer-aided high resolution electron microscopy (Unwin & Ennis 1984) show hexagonal arrays of membrane particles on both sides of communicating junctions, each particle (or 'connection') composed of six protein subunits (nexins) surrounding a central channel (cf. 2.6, 10) which, when apposed to a similar unit in an adjacent cell, forms a small communicating passage between the two. Such particles may also exist in smaller numbers, or singly, elsewhere on the cell, so that intercellular communication may not be restricted to special junctional areas. Changes in pH and calcium ion concentrations, etc. can cause narrowing or closure of such channels, so intercellular communication can change with the metabolic alterations in the participating cells (Unwin & Zampighi 1980). The precise chemistry of the nexins varies in different tissues. For further reading, see Stauffer & Unwin (1992), Beyer (1993), Alberts et al (1994).

Junctional complexes. These are combinations of junctions found around the apical ends of epithelial cells (Farquhar & Palade 1963; 2.9, 10) where an occluding belt is flanked basally by an adhering belt and a line of desmosomes running around the circumference of the cell. This arrangement provides a diffusion barrier apically, reinforced mechanically by the other two components.

Other types of junction. Chemical synapses and neuromuscular junctions are specialized areas of intercellular adhesion where there

of actin filament bundles (stress filaments) which are anchored through intermediary proteins (desmoplakins, etc.) to the cytoplasmic domains of integrins. In turn these are attached at their external ends to collagen or other filamentous structures, so that there· is

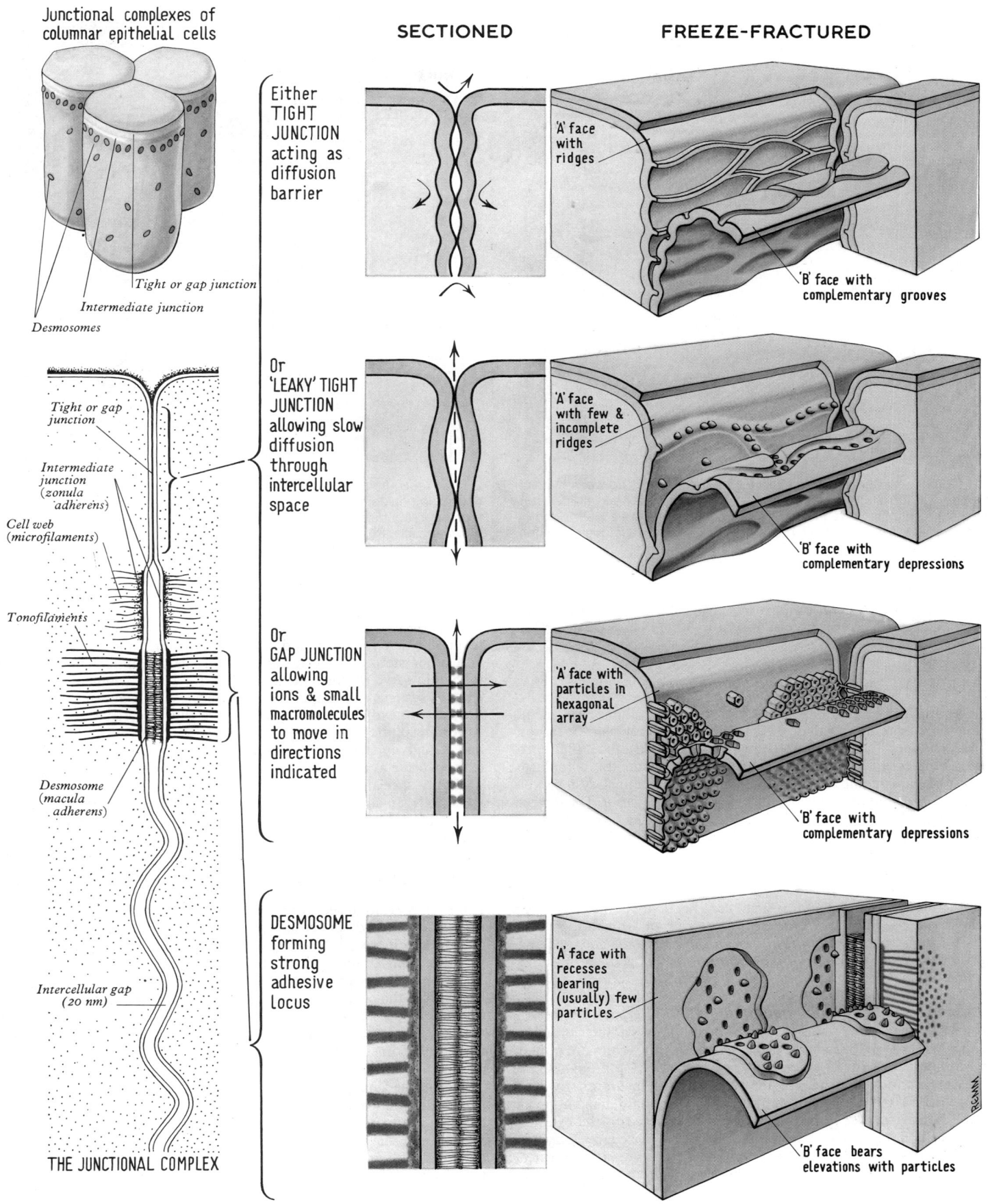

Junctional complexes of columnar epithelial cells

Tight or gap junction

Intermediate junction

Desmosomes

Tight or gap junction

Intermediate junction (zonula adherens)

Cell web (microfilaments)

Tonofilaments

Desmosome (macula adherens)

Intercellular gap (20 nm)

THE JUNCTIONAL COMPLEX

SECTIONED

FREEZE-FRACTURED

Either TIGHT JUNCTION acting as diffusion barrier

'A' face with ridges

'B' face with complementary grooves

Or 'LEAKY' TIGHT JUNCTION allowing slow diffusion through intercellular space

'A' face with few & incomplete ridges

'B' face with complementary depressions

Or GAP JUNCTION allowing ions & small macromolecules to move in directions indicated

'A' face with particles in hexagonal array

'B' face with complementary depressions

DESMOSOME forming strong adhesive locus

'A' face with recesses bearing (usually) few particles

'B' face bears elevations with particles

2.10 Schemata of various junctions commonly occurring between cells, showing current interpretations of the electron microscopic appearances seen after sectioning and with freeze-fracturing techniques. For clarity, the freeze-fracturing data are presented as though it were possible to separate and fold back the two leaflets of the plasma membrane to expose the intramembranous protein particles inserted on their two faces. The A face = the P fracture face and the B = the E fracture face in current terminology.

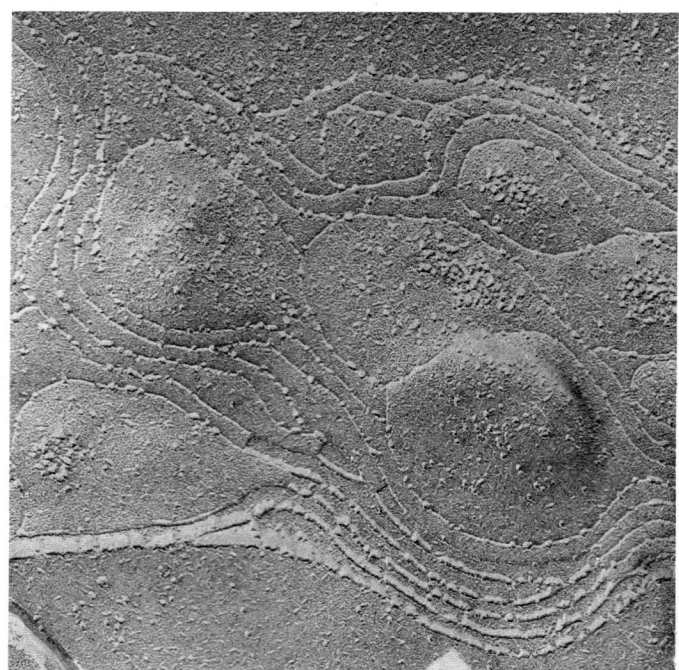

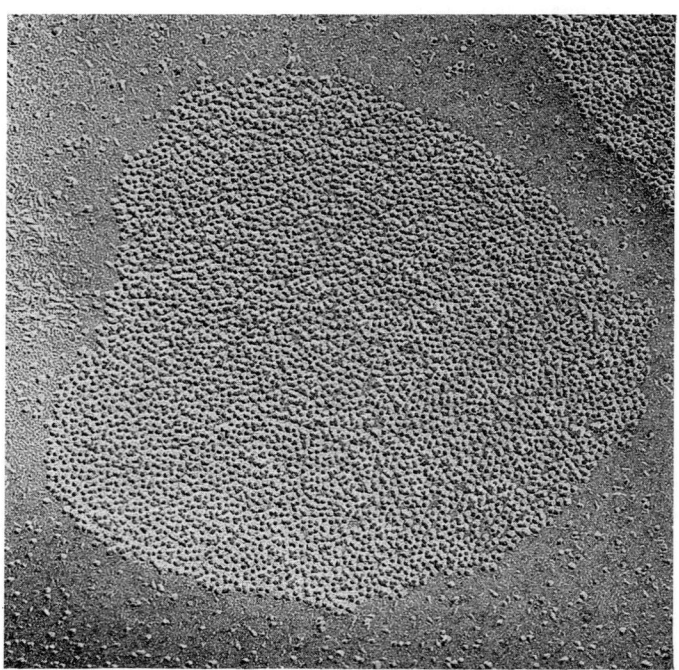

2.11 Freeze-fractured zonula occludens (tight junction) between two epidermal cells of fetal skin showing the anastomotic network of lines representing contacts between membranes. Compare with **2.10**. Provided by Andrew Kent, Department of Anatomy, UMDS, Guy's Campus, London. Magnification × 25 000.

2.12 Freeze-fractured communicating (gap) junctions between two developing epidermal cells. The tightly packed intramembranous particles represent channels for electrotonic coupling and diffusion of small molecules between cells. Provided by Andrew Kent, Department of Anatomy, UMDS, Guy's Campus, London. Magnification × 25 000.

is also secretion of neurotransmitters from one of the participants, and specialized receptor molecules on the other. They are described in Section 8 (pp. 935–937).

ENDOPLASMIC RETICULUM

The endoplasmic reticulum is the system of interconnecting membrane-lined channels (Palade 1975) within the cytoplasm (**2.13**A–C). These channels take various forms, including cisternae (flattened sacs), tubules and vesicles. The membranes divide the cytoplasm into two major compartments: that inside the channel system, the *vacuoloplasm*; and that outside, the *hyaloplasm* or *cytosol*. The former constitutes the space in which secretory products are stored or transported to the Golgi complex and cell exterior; the latter is made up of the colloidal proteins such as enzymes, carbohydrates and small protein molecules, together with ribosomes, and ribonucleic acid.

Structurally, the channel system can be divided into *granular (rough) endoplasmic reticulum*, to the exterior of which ribosomes are attached, and *agranular (smooth) endoplasmic reticulum*, lacking ribosomes. When cells are disrupted and centrifuged, both endoplasmic reticula break up into vesicles respectively termed *granular* and *agranular microsomes*.

Granular endoplasmic reticulum (GER). This can synthesize proteins, because of its attached ribosomes. Most of such proteins are passed **through** the membranes to which the ribosomes are bound and accumulate within the cisternae of this system although some intramembranous proteins are inserted into the membrane, where they remain. After passage from the GER, they remain in membrane-bound bodies such as lysosomes or else are secreted to the exterior of the cell. Some carbohydrates are also synthesized by enzymes within the cavities of the GER and may be attached to newly-formed protein (glycosylation). Vesicles are budded off from the GER (at a special ribosome-free region, the *transitional element*, for transport to the Golgi complex as part of the protein-targeting mechanism of the cell (see below).

In embryonic cells, endoplasmic reticulum is scant and ribosome clusters lie mostly unattached in the hyaloplasm. During differentiation, membranes usually increase greatly and ribosomes may become attached to form GER.

Agranular endoplasmic reticulum. This is associated with carbohydrate metabolism and many other metabolic processes, including detoxification and synthesis of lipids and of cholesterol and other steroids. The membranes of the agranular endoplasmic reticulum serve as convenient surfaces for the attachment of many enzyme systems (e.g. important detoxification mechanisms involving the enzyme cytochrome P_{450}) which are thus accessible to the substrates in solution within the cell. They also cooperate with the GER and Golgi apparatus to elaborate new membranes, the protein, carbohydrate and lipid components being added in different regions.

Highly specialized types of endoplasmic reticulum are present in some cells. In striated muscle cells the agranular endoplasmic reticulum (*sarcoplasmic reticulum*) stores calcium ions, which are liberated to initiate contraction on appropriate stimulation.

RIBOSOMES

Ribosomes (ribonucleoprotein particles) are granules about 15 nm across, composed of equal parts, by weight, of protein and (ribosomal) RNA (rRNA); they are responsible for the synthesis of proteins from amino acids (Palade 1955; Siekevitz & Palade 1960). Each ribosome is made of two subunits (Lake 1981), one slightly larger than the other, sedimenting in the centrifuge at different rates (in nucleated cells mainly at 60S and 40S, where S = the Svedberg unit of sedimentation rate, a function of density, shape, etc.; the whole ribosome sediments at 80S). The subunits can be further dissociated into about 73 different proteins (40 in the large subunit and 33 in the small), with structural and enzymatic functions. Three small rRNA strands (28, 5.8 and 5S), highly convoluted, lie in the large subunit, and one in the small subunit (18S). Most of these rRNA molecules are derived from the nucleolus (p. 55). The large and small subunits are separate from each other when not engaged in protein synthesis.

Ribosomes may be solitary, relatively inactive *monosomes*, or form groups (*polyribosomes* or *polysomes*) attached to messenger RNA (mRNA) which they translate during protein synthesis. Polysomes can be attached to membranes, constituting the GER (see above) or may lie free in the hyaloplasm where they synthesize proteins for use outside the channel system, including enzymes of the cytosol, structural proteins of the cell (e.g. actin, tubulin) and haemoglobin

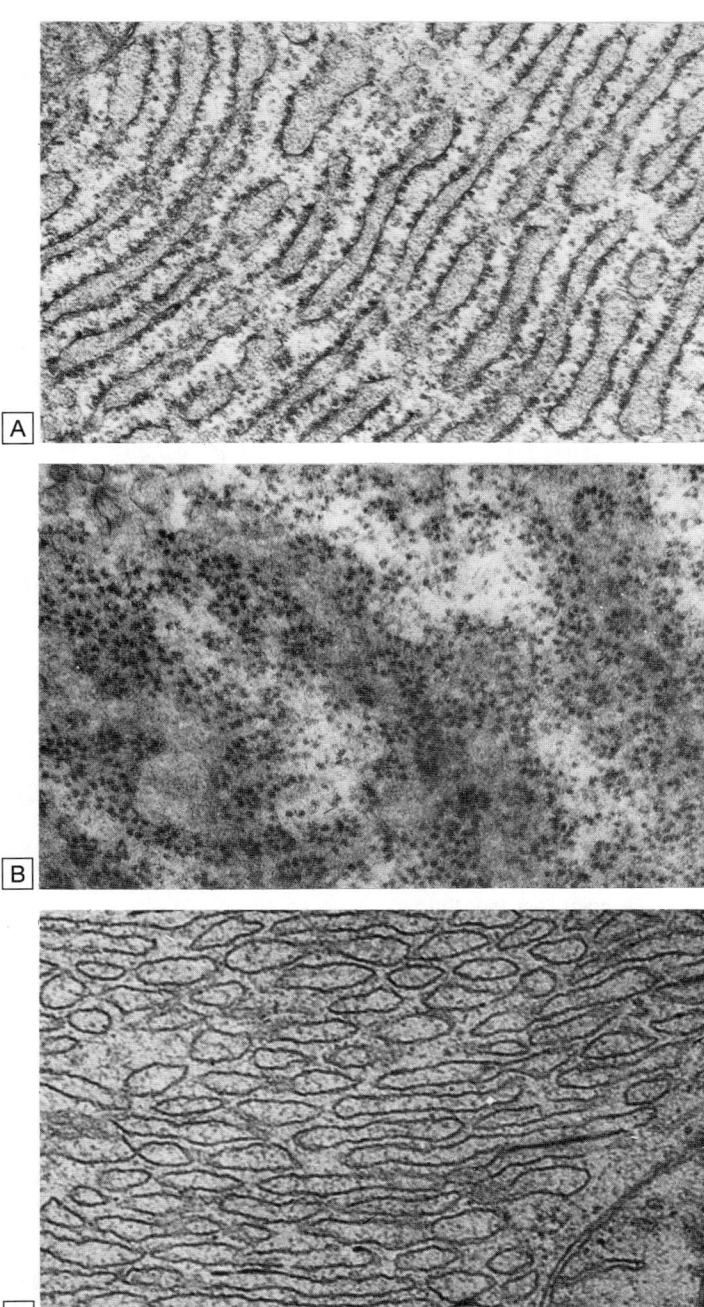

appropriate, attachment to the endoplasmic reticulum via an intermediate docking protein, directing the protein through its membrane into the cisternal cavity.

Subunit proteins of the ribosomes themselves are synthesized in the cytoplasm by other ribosomes. They then enter the nucleus where they bind to rRNA from the nucleolus to form the two major subunits; these then pass separately back into the cytoplasm and only associate to form a complete ribosome when they attach themselves to an mRNA molecule (Nomura 1984). When protein synthesis is over, the two subunits dissociate but may serve more than once. For further reading, see Merrick (1992), Alberts et al (1994).

Mitochondrial ribosomes differ from those of the general cytoplasm, being somewhat smaller (55S). They will be discussed later (see below). The ribosomes of fungi and prokaryote organisms such as bacteria are also smaller than those of the nucleated cells of animals (and plants), which may perhaps reflect the less complex regulatory mechanisms of these relatively primitive species.

GOLGI COMPLEX (GOLGI APPARATUS OR DICTYOSOME) (2.14, 15)

Beginning with the Italian Camillo Golgi, optical microscopists of the nineteenth and early twentieth centuries recognized a distinct cytoplasmic region near the nucleus, particularly prominent in secretory cells when stained with silver or other metallic salts. For many years it was considered a staining artefact, but with the advent of electron microscopy it was authenticated as a cellular organelle of considerable metabolic importance. Numerous biochemical and structural studies have since shown that the Golgi complex is part of the pathway by which proteins synthesized in the granular endoplasmic reticulum (GER) are modified chemically and targeted to the cell surface for secretion or for storage in membranous vesicles. The molecular details of these processes are still a topic of great research activity.

Ultrastructurally, the Golgi complex is a membranous organelle consisting of a stack of up to four flattened membranous cisternae, together with clusters of vesicles surrounding its surfaces (see Rambourg & Clermont 1990). Seen in vertical section, it is often cup-shaped, usually with the convex side nearest the nucleus. Small transport vesicles are received from the transitional elements of the GER at one face of the Golgi stack, the *cis-face* (or forming surface) where they deliver their contents to the first cisterna in the series by membrane fusion. The budding and transport of vesicles from the GER involves the addition of special *coat proteins* (COP) to the external aspects of the membranes (see Kreis and Pepperkok 1994). From the edges of this cisterna, the protein is transported to the next cisterna by vesicular budding and then fusion, and this process is repeated until the final cisterna at the *trans-face* (condensing surface) is reached. From this, larger vesicles are formed for delivery to other parts of the cell. According to the chemical events within them, the Golgi cisternae are divisible into three groups, forming the cis-, intermediate- and trans-compartments (see p. 32).

2.13 Ultrastructural details of the endoplasmic reticulum: A. rough endoplasmic reticulum; B. polysome groups attached to obliquely sectioned cisternae showing 'rosette' configuration; C. smooth endoplasmic reticulum. B provided by D R Turner, Guy's Hospital Medical School. Magnification × 30 000.

in erythroblasts. Some of the cytosolic products, however, include proteins which can be inserted directly into (or through) membranes of selected organelles, such as mitochondria and peroxisomes (see below).

In a mature polysome all the attachment sites of the mRNA are occupied as ribosomes move along it, synthesizing protein according to its instructions, so the number of ribosomes in a polysome indicates the length of the messenger RNA molecule and hence the size of the protein being made.

The two major subunits have separate roles in protein synthesis. The smaller is the site of attachment and translation of mRNA; the larger is responsible for the release of the new protein and, where

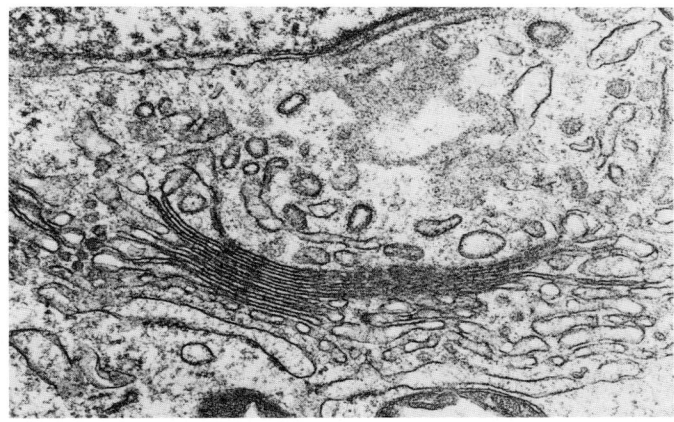

2.14 Electron micrograph of a Golgi apparatus in a spermatocyte showing the central multilamellar cisternae and clusters of peripheral vesicles. Magnification × 15 000.

In addition to these cisternae there are also other membranous structures which form an integral part of the Golgi complex, termed the *cis-Golgi* and *trans-Golgi networks*. The *cis*-Golgi network is a region of complex membranous channels interposed between the GER and the Golgi cis-face, receiving and transmitting vesicles in both directions. Many studies have shown that it acts to select appropriate proteins from the GER for delivery by vesicle to the Golgi stack, inappropriate proteins being similarly shuttled back to the GER. Thus, there is also a reverse process by which materials in the Golgi stack can be transported through this system back to the endoplasmic reticulum. The drug Brifeldin A causes the disintegration of the cis-Golgi network and blocks the transport of proteins to the Golgi complex (see Pelham 1991).

The trans-Golgi network (TNG), placed at the other side of the Golgi stack, is also a region of interconnected membrane channels engaged in protein sorting. Here, modified proteins processed in the Golgi cisternae are packaged selectively into vesicles and dispatched to different parts of the cell. The packaging depends on the detection by the TNG of particular amino acid sequences or other features of the proteins, leading to their enclosure in membranes of appropriate composition which will further modify their contents, for example, by extracting water to concentrate them, or pumping in protons to acidify their contents, depending on the type of protein. The membranes also contain specific signal proteins which may allocate them to microtubule-based transport pathways and to dock with appropriate targets elsewhere in the cell (see p. 39), including the plasma membrane in the case of secretory vesicles. Vesicle formation and budding at the TGN also involves the addition of *clathrin* and related proteins on their external surface to form coated vesicles (Robinson 1994).

Within the Golgi stack itself proteins undergo a series of sequential chemical modifications, already begun in the GER. These include changes in glycosyl groups, for example, removal of mannose, addition of N-acetyl glucosamine and sialic acid, sulphation of attached glycosaminoglycans (GAGs), and protein phosphorylation. Lipids formed in the endoplasmic reticulum are also routed for vesicle incorporation. A much studied route for modification and targeting is that of lysosomal enzymes. For retention within the cell it has been shown that a particular sequence of amino acids has to be present, and without these, proteins are immediately passed into the secretory channel and thence to the exterior. This step involves the addition of mannose-6-phosphate to the lysosomal protein by the cis-compartment of the Golgi complex. This is recognized by mannose-6-phosphate receptors associated with the TGN which sorts the enzymes into appriopriate vesicles which are then shuttled to the late endosome/lysosomes. Thus, lysosomal enzymes are selected for packaging in specific lysosomal-type membranes (see below).

There are various cytochemical markers for the Golgi complex including various specific proteins involved in its different components (Rothman 1981).

The role of the Golgi complex in the synthesis of primary lysosomes is a major part of its activities in some cells rich in these organelles, and a special region of the cell may be dedicated to their production e.g. the Golgi–endoplasmic reticulum–lysosome complex (GERL) of neurons (see Novikoff & Shin 1964).

In glandular cells with an apical secretory zone, the Golgi complex is positioned between the secretory surface and the nucleus; in fibroblasts, where secretory activity is more general, there are two or more groups of Golgi stacks and in liver cells up to 50. It is often closely associated with the centrosome, a region of the cell containing a centriole pair and related microtubules, a significant association considering the microtubule-mediated transport system and the anchoring of the Golgi complex itself to microtubules.

DEGRADATIVE VACUOLE SYSTEM: ENDOCYTIC VESICLES, ENDOSOMES AND LYSOSOMES

An important aspect of cell biology is the uptake of materials from the extracellular environment into membranous compartments within the cytoplasm and their delivery to membrane-lined channels and vacuoles where they are sorted. This system is linked to a second series of membranous compartments containing acid hydrolases which can process or degrade materials taken into the cell (*heterophagy*), and at the same time eliminate or inactivate unwanted

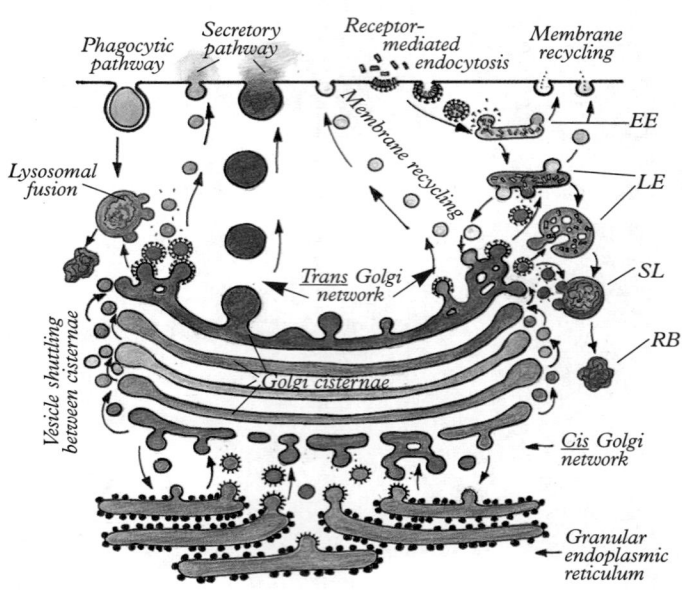

2.15 Diagram illustrating the major structural and functional features of the Golgi complex and its associated organelles. For further details, see the text. EE=early endosome; LE=late endosome; SL=secondary lysosome; RB=residual body.

structures originating within the cell, including organelles that are worn out, damaged or no longer relevant (*autophagy*; see Alberts et al 1994). Together these two systems create a complex dynamic network of small vesicles, tubules, flat cisternae and rounded vacuoles, with a constant traffic between its various elements. There is also a continual exchange of vesicles between this array and the Golgi complex which provides it with hydrolytic enzymes and receives back depleted vesicles for recharging.

The structures involved in the initial uptake from the exterior are small *endocytic vesicles* which take in (endocytose) macromolecules, fluids and small particles, or larger *phagosomes*, typical of specialist cells such as macrophages which take in large particles, for example bacteria and cell debris (*phagocytosis*).

Endocytic vesicles and early endosomes (2.15)

Many macromolecules required for cell metabolism are taken up from the extracellular fluid by the invagination of small areas of the plasma membrane and their separation into the cytoplasm of vesicles about 60 nm in diameter which contain extracellular fluid or macromolecules attached to the membrane surface (Rodman et al 1990). The uptake of fluid is termed *pinocytosis* (= cell drinking), and that of bound macromolecules is *receptor-mediated endocytosis*. Of course, fluid is taken into the cell whenever endocytosis occurs; but whether it can occur independently of receptor-mediated endocytosis is not clear. Endocytic vesicles are constantly being formed at the plasma membrane of most active cell types. In receptor-mediated endocytosis, receptor proteins spanning the plasma membrane bind molecules to be taken into the cell, by their externally exposed ends and this triggers a series of events on the inner side of the plasma membrane causing the membrane to bulge inwards locally as a small *coated pit* which deepens and finally pinches off into the cytoplasm as a *coated vesicle*. During this process the inner ends of the receptor molecules bind a series of proteins from the cytoplasm which cross-link them into a curved basket-like array, bending the membrane inwards and eventually separating it as a vesicle from the surface. The cytoplasmic proteins bringing this about are, first, small globular *adaptins* that bind to the internal ends of the receptor proteins, and second, the protein *clathrin* which cross-links adjacent adaptins to form a basket-like structure bending the membrane inwards into a sphere (see Robinson 1994). Individual clathrin molecules have a characteristic shape, consisting of three arms (a triskelion), and these can assemble themselves in a characteristic network composed of the adaptin/receptor complex, visible ultrastructurally in sections as a dense localized undercoating of the plasma membrane (hence the terms coated pit and coated vesicle); in freeze-etched preparations the basket-like appearance is most striking (Vigers et al 1986; Heuser 1989). The formation of coated vesicles is not dependent on an energy source. Once it is interiorized the coated vesicle rapidly sheds its coat of adaptin and clathrin, and fuses with a tubular cisterna termed an *early endosome*, where the receptor molecules release their bound ligands. From the early endosome, membrane and receptors can be recycled to the cell surface as *exocytic vesicles*, replenishing the plasma membrane ready for the next round of endocytic vesicle formation (Pryer et al 1992).

Phagosomes

Phagosomes are larger vesicles formed around large particles such as bacteria. They are also produced by the invagination of the plasma membrane, but the nature of this process is different from receptor-mediated endocytosis in that it needs chemical energy from the breakdown of adenosine 5'-triphosphate (ATP), and does not appear to involve clathrin. The particle to be phagocytosed adheres to the plasma membrane by receptor molecules of some kind, sometimes relatively non-specifically, but often involving an intermediate step, for example, bacteria may first be coated by antibodies or complement, and these are bound in turn by antibody or complement receptors at the surface of the phagocyte (see also p. 1415). The bacterium is then engulfed within the cell by invagination to produce a membrane-lined phagosomal vacuole. This process appears to depend on actin-myosin based motility (for further details see p. 43). Later, lysosomal enzymes are added to the phagosome to degrade its contents.

Late endosomes

After a brief sojourn in the early endosomes, materials can be passed on to *late endosomes*, a more deeply placed set of tubules, vesicles or cisternae. These also receive lysosomal enzymes via vesicles (small lysosomes) shuttling in from the Golgi complex (Machamer 1993). The pH of late endosomes is quite low (about 5.0) and this activates the lysosomal acid hydrolases to attack the endosomal contents; the products of hydrolysis are then passed through the membrane wall into the cytosol, or may be retained in the endosomes. Because there is a constant exchange between the late endosomes and the trans-Golgi (TNG) network (see above) particles introduced into the cell through this system may find their way to the Golgi apparatus. As more enzymes arrive, a late endosome may grow considerably in size by vesicle fusion, and the enzyme concentration may increase greatly; such large dense structures are classical *lysosomes*, as described first by de Duve (see de Duve & Wattiaux 1966; Bainton 1981). However, these large organelles do not appear in all cells, perhaps because in these the late endosomes deal very rapidly with endocytosed material. Late endosomes have a variety of forms, one being the *multivesicular body* (**2.**16) generated by the fusion of vesicles and/or tubules, the excess membrane being budded off internally in small cytoplasmic blebs (Holtzmann 1976).

Lysosomes

Lysosomes are dense spheroidal membrane-bounded bodies 80–800 nm in diameter (**2.**16), often with complex inclusions representing material undergoing hydrolysis (then sometimes termed *secondary lysosomes*). They contain acid hydrolases able to degrade a wide variety of substances. So far, more than 40 lysosomal enzymes have been described, including many varieties of proteases, lipases, carbohydrases, esterases and nucleases. The enzymes are strongly glycosylated, and are maintained at a low pH by proton pumps in the lysosomal membranes. They can be detected histochemically by

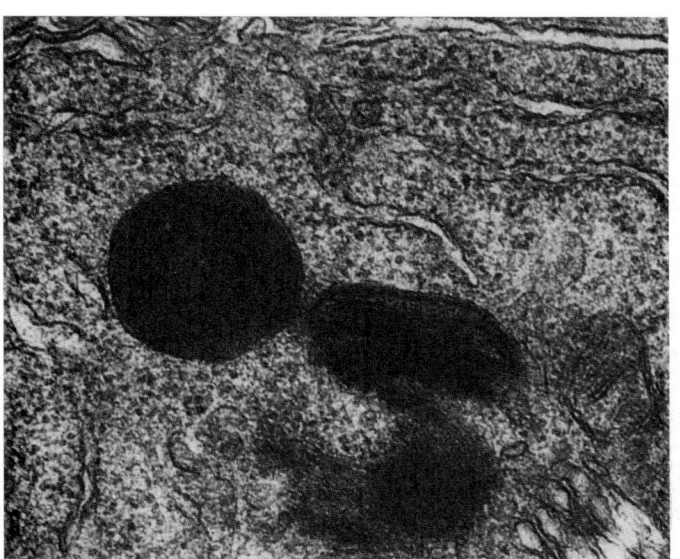

A

B

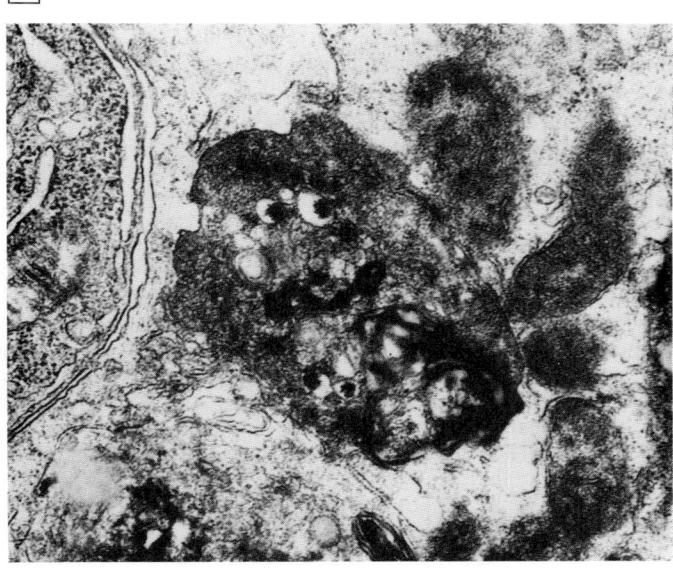

C

2.16 Electron micrographs of lysosomes in various stages: A. a group of lysosomes in an olfactory receptor cell showing small primary lysosomes (left), and larger secondary lysosomes containing lamellar débris; B. a multivesicular body with which endocytic vesicles are in the process of fusing; C. a residual body, the end stage of lysosomal hydrolysis of engulfed cellular organelles. All magnifications × 30 000.

various tests for such hydrolases; the enzyme *acid phosphatase* (β-glycerylphosphatase) has been widely used as a marker of lysosomes for light and electron microscopy, though it is not invariably present.

Lysosomes are numerous in cells active in phagocytosis of large particles such as bacteria, for example macrophages and neutrophil leucocytes, in which lysosomes are responsible for destroying phagocytosed bacteria. In these the phagosome containing the bacterium may fuse with several lysosomes (the term *phagolysosome* is given to a phagosome in the process of lysosomal fusion). Lysosomes are also well represented in cells with a high turnover of organelles, for example, exocrine gland cells and neurons, a process which is not entirely understood; worn out organelles such as old mitochondria and endoplasmic reticulum are marked in some way for demolition, a process seen in sections as a partial engulfment in a membranous cisterna (Dunn 1990). The organelle is then interiorized within a lysosome and rapidly degraded.

Material which has been attacked by hydrolases within late endosomes and lysosomes may be completely degraded to soluble end-products (e.g. proteins to amino acids) which can pass into the cell's metabolic pathway, but more usually some undigestible debris remains and the vesicle is then called a *residual body*. This may be passed in vesicles to the cell surface where it is ejected by exocytosis or it may persist inside the cell as an inert residual body. If the cell has a short lifespan these are dispersed when the cell dies, but in long-lived cells considerable numbers of residual bodies can accumulate within the cell ('*storage excretion*'), often fusing to form larger dense vacuoles with complex lamellar inclusions. As their contents are often darkly pigmented, this may change the colour of the tissue, as seen, for example, in neurons where the end-product of lysosomal digestion *lipofuscin* (neuromelanin or senility pigment: see p. 922) gives ageing brains a brownish-yellow coloration, and in the pigmentation of the olfactory epithelium due to the accumulation of residual bodies in the supporting cells of this tissue (p. 1322).

Lysosomal enzymes may also be secreted to the cell surface, either as part of a process to alter the extracellular matrix (as in osteoclast demolition of bone) or perhaps inadvertently through mistargeting by Golgi-derived lysosomal vesicles. Abnormal release of enzymes can cause tissue damage, as in certain types of arthritis. Normally, however, small amounts of lysosomes are retrieved by receptor-mediated endocytosis and returned to the endosomal system. Enzymes released by one cell can also, therefore, be taken up by other cells and incorporated into their own lysosomes.

Lysosomal membranes, normally impermeable to their enclosed enzymes, may allow the enzymes to leak. Exposure to ionizing radiations, or some carcinogens, silica, asbestos particles, anoxia, heat and many drugs causes such effects, with consequent cellular damage or death. Indeed, it was initially thought lysosomes played a major role in the self destruction of cells (hence the term 'suicide bags' for these organelles), and undoubtedly this does occur postmortem as their enzymes leak into the cytosol.

Some drugs, for example cortisone, can stabilize lysosomal membranes and may, therefore, inhibit many lysosomal activities including the secretion of enzymes, and their fusion with phagocytic vesicles.

Lysosomal storage diseases. If any of the lysosomal enzymes are defective because of gene mutations in their encoding, the materials which they normally degrade will accumulate within late endosomes and lysosomes. Many instances of such lysosomal storage diseases have been recorded; among them are syndromes in which profound morphogenetic changes occur; for example Tay-Sachs disease in which a faulty gangliosidase leads to the accumulation of glycolipid in neurons, causing death within childhood. In Hurler's syndrome, failure to metabolize certain glycosaminoglycans (GAGs) causes the accumulation of large amounts of matrix within connective tissue, distorting the growth of many parts of the body. For further reading, see Dice 1990, Alberts et al 1994.

PEROXISOMES

Peroxisomes (microbodies) are membrane-bound vacuoles (**2.4**), about 0.5–0.15 μm across, often with dense cores or crystalline interiors composed chiefly of high concentrations of the enzyme urate oxidase (de Duve 1973, 1983; Tolbert & Essner 1981). Large (0.5 μm) peroxisomes are particularly numerous in hepatocytes and

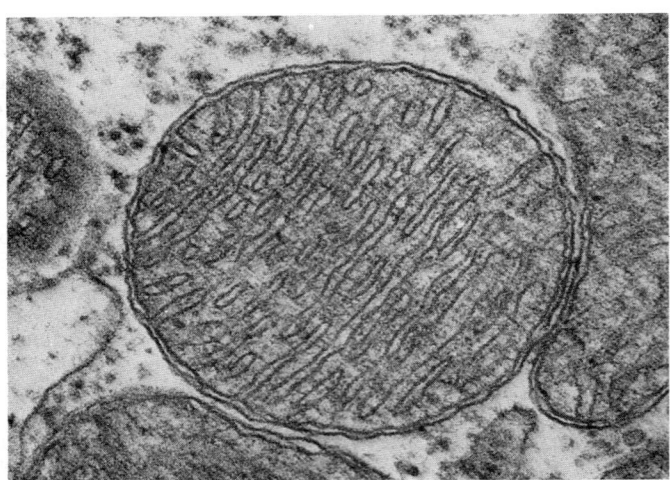

2.17 Electron micrograph showing details of mitochondrial structure: the outer membrane, the inner membrane folded to form cristae and their related intra-mitochondrial spaces are visible. Magnification × 30 000.

kidney tubule cells, but peroxisomes of some size are typical of all nucleated cell types. This organelle is important in the oxidative detoxification of various substances taken into or produced within cells, including ethanol and formaldehyde. Oxidation is carried out by a number of enzymes including D-amino acid oxidase and urate oxidase which generate hydrogen peroxide as a source of molecular oxygen. Excess amounts of hydrogen peroxide are broken down by another enzyme, *catalase*. Peroxisomes also oxidize fatty acid chains (β-oxidation).

The formation of peroxisomes is rather unusual in that their membranes appear to be derived only by the multiplication of previously existing peroxisomes, and their internal proteins are passed from the cytosol directly through channels in their membranes rather than by packaging from the granular endoplasmic reticulum (GER) and Golgi body. These features are also found in mitochondria (see below) although these possess some of their own genes, unlike peroxisomes which are coded for entirely in the nucleus. It has been suggested that, like mitochondria, peroxisomes originated as symbiotic prokaryote organisms which in the early history of eukaryotic cells were taken into the cytoplasm to provide oxygen-related metabolism, and transferred their genomes entirely to the nuclear chromosomes but retained a measure of self-replication in the formation of their membranes. A genetic abnormality in the translocation of proteins into peroxisomes leading to peroxisomal enzyme deficiencies is seen in the Zellweger syndrome, caused by a gene mutation in an integral membrane protein (peroxisome assembly factor-1) which is usually fatal shortly after birth in the homozygous condition (Shimozawa et al 1992; for further reading see Lazarow 1993).

MITOCHONDRIA

The mitochondrion is a membrane-bound organelle of great metabolic significance, the principal source of chemical energy in most cells (see e.g. Ernster & Schatz 1981; Tzagoloff 1982). Mitochondria are the site of the citric acid (Krebs') cycle and the electron transport pathway by which complex organic molecules are finally oxidized to carbon dioxide and water, a process which provides the energy to drive the production of adenosine 5'-triphosphate (ATP) from adenosine 5'-diphosphate (ADP) and inorganic phosphate (oxidative phosphorylation). The numbers of these organelles in a particular cell reflect its general energy requirements. In hepatocytes there may be as many as 2000, whereas in resting lymphocytes there may be only a few. Mature erythrocytes lack mitochondria altogether. Such cells rely mainly on glycolysis for their energy supplies. However, some very active cells, for example fast twitch skeletal muscle fibres (p. 754), have few mitochondria, and also use glycolysis for their energy requirements, allowing them to work rapidly but for only a limited duration. Mitochondria were first observed with the light microscope as long thin threads (mitochondrion = thread-like body), or alternatively as spherical or ellipsoidal bodies in the cytoplasm of most cells, particularly those with a high metabolic rate such as secretory cells in exocrine glands. In living cells viewed by bright field, phase contrast or interference microscopy, they appear highly labile, constantly changing shape and position, although usually attached to internal structures of the cell and sometimes moving linearly along definite pathways; they can divide and have also been seen to fuse (see Bereiter-Hahn 1990).

With the electron microscope (**2**.17) they are usually seen as elliptical bodies from 0.5–2.0 μm long. In some instances they may be larger than this, for example, in cardiac muscle cells. Each mitochondrion is lined by an outer and an inner membrane, separated by a variable gap termed the *intermembrane space*. Within the lumen, surrounded by the inner membrane, is the *mitochondrial matrix*. The outer membrane is smooth and sometimes attached to other organelles (e.g. microtubules), while the inner membrane is deeply folded to form incomplete transverse or longitudinal septa or tubular invaginations, *cristae mitochondriales*, which thus create a relatively large surface area of membrane. Cristae are more numerous and complex in cells with a high metabolic rate than in relatively inactive ones; in heart muscle, for instance, they are numerous and show complex pleats. In mitochondria of the lipocytes of brown fat (p. 77), cristae are particularly conspicuous but their chemical activities are diverted to the direct production of heat rather than ATP (see Nicholls & Rial 1984). Cristae of cells in the adrenal cortex are typically tubular. The significance of these different arrangements is not clear, although they may reflect tissue-specific differences in mitochondrial chemistry (see below). The permeability of the two membranes differs considerably; the outer membrane is freely permeable to many substances because of the presence of large non-specific channels formed by characteristic proteins (*porins*), whereas the inner membrane is permeable to only a narrow range of molecules. The presence of cardiolipin, an unusual phospholipid, in the inner membrane may contribute to this relative impermeability.

The mitochondrial matrix, of variable density and granularity, is an aqueous environment containing a multitude of enzymes in quite high concentrations, and filaments of mitochondrial DNA with the apparatus for transcription and translation of a set of genes unique to this organelle (mitochondrial messenger and transfer RNAs, mitochondrial ribosomes with ribosomal RNAs). The DNA forms a closed ring, about 5 μm across when extracted and spread out, and several identical copies are present in each mitochondrion. This DNA has a ratio between its nitrogen bases different from that of nuclear chromosomal DNA, and the RNA sequences also differ in the precise genetic code used in protein synthesis (Grivell 1983). The ribosomes are smaller and quite distinct from those of the rest of the cell and resemble those of bacteria.

Mitochondria are able to multiply by simple transverse division during interphase (Attardi & Schatz 1988), so that mitochondria are essentially self-replicating, and, like chloroplasts in plants, an instance of *cytoplasmic inheritance*. A rather limited number of proteins of the inner matrix and inner membrane are encoded by the small number of genes along the mitochondrial DNA (Anderson et al 1981). The great majority of mitochondrial proteins are encoded by nuclear genes and made in the cytosol then inserted through special channels in the mitochondrial membranes to reach their various destinations. Their membrane lipids are synthesized in the endoplasmic reticulum.

Since mitochondria are only formed from previously existing ones, it follows that all mitochondria in the body are in effect descended from those in the cytoplasm of the fertilized ovum. Further, it has recently been shown that these are entirely of maternal origin—the mitochondrion of the sperm is not incorporated into the ovum at fertilization (see Giles et al 1980), so that mitochondria (and any of their genetic variants) are passed only through the female line, a situation of much genetic interest.

The ribosomes and nucleic acids are, interestingly, similar to those of bacteria, prompting the suggestion that the far distant (1200 million years or more) ancestors of mitochondria were symbiotic oxygen-using bacteria which came into partnership with eukaryotic cells previously incapable of metabolizing the oxygen being produced by primitive plants; according to this view, the mitochondria lost their ability to lead an independent existence (see Margulis 1981)

and transferred most but not all of their genes to the nucleus of the host cell (for further reading, see Gray 1989).

Mitochondria are the principal site of a number of enzyme systems, particularly those of oxidative phosphorylation associated with the tricarboxylic acid (Krebs') cycle and cytochrome electron transport sequences of respiration. They are the chief sites where chemical energy is derived from breakdown of organic compounds in respiration to form high-energy organic phosphate compounds (particularly ATP and guanosine triphosphate, GTP) by an unusual chemical mechanism, the chemi-osmotic process (Mitchell 1961), entailing the pumping of hydrogen ions out of the mitochondria to drive the synthesis of ATP as the ions diffuse back into the matrix (Hatefi 1985). These energy-rich compounds pass to other parts of the cell where they fuel a wide variety of energy-consuming reactions. The various enzymes of the Krebs' cycle occur in the mitochondrial matrix, while those of the cytochrome system and oxidative phosphorylation are localized chiefly in the inner mitochondrial membrane. Some of these ATP-ases form large enzyme assemblies (ATP-synthase) in the inner membrane which are responsible for the final act of ATP synthesis; when mitochondria are hypotonically disrupted and negatively stained, these complexes become visible as minute lollipop-like structures consisting of spheres about 9 nm across, supported by stalks (elementary, submitochondrial or stalked particles). Further analysis including X-ray diffraction studies (Bianchet et al 1991) show that the heads of these particles consist of a cluster of 6 ATP-ase subunits and the stalks are H + carriers; only when they are assembled together can they synthesize ATP which requires the passage of H+ through the total assembly.

In addition to these structures, various inclusions have been described in the mitochondrial matrix of different tissues, including crystalline bodies and dense granules, the significance of which is uncertain.

It is interesting that these organelles are distributed within the cell according to regional energy requirements, for example, near the bases of cilia in ciliated epithelia, at the base of the cells of proximal convoluted renal tubules, where considerable active transport occurs, and around the proximal end of the flagellum in spermatozoa (p. 127). Mitochondria are concerned with many chemical reactions besides oxidative phosphorylation, some of them tissue-specific; for instance, various urea-forming enzymes are found in liver cell mitochondria, and a number of genetic diseases of mitochondria are known which exclusively affect particular tissues including skeletal muscle (mitochondrial myopathies) and nervous tissue (mitochondrial neuropathies). For further information on this topic see the reviews by Morgan-Hughes (1986) and Wallace (1992).

OTHER VESICLES AND VACUOLES

In addition to the membranous compartments of the Golgi-endosome/lysosome system there are various other membranous bodies present within cells. Some of these constitute part of the mechanism for internally translocating macromolecules; and are hence termed *transport vesicles*. Typically these are small (about 60 nm in diameter) similar to endocytic and exocytic vesicles (see above), which can properly be regarded as specialized transport vesicles. Also included in this class are *transcytotic vesicles* which begin as endocytic vesicles but instead of carrying their cargoes to an intracellular destination, they pass to another surface of the cell and discharge their contents into the extracellular space. Such vesicles are frequent in cells where macromolecules are transported across a cellular boundary, for example in endothelial cells lining blood vessels and lymphatics (p. 1461). An extreme example is found in the anterior chamber of the eye where considerable quantities of ocular fluid are taken up by modified endothelial cells in the canal of Schlemm in relatively huge transcytotic vacuoles and transported to the venous system (p. 1327).

Exocytosis, as already mentioned, is involved in the cycling of membranes and receptor molecules from endosomes and the Golgi apparatus to the surface of the cell. However, in secretory cells exocytic vesicles and larger secretory vacuoles form a major pathway from the Golgi complex to the exterior. Such structures may be secreted immediately or stored until the signal to secrete arrives, when they may be discharged in large quantities (e.g. the histamine-containing vacuoles of histaminocytes: mast cells, p. 79). In the synapses of many nerve cells exocytic vesicles contain neurotransmitters which are again stored in the presynaptic ending until an action potential arrives to trigger a very rapid but highly controlled release of their contents into the synaptic cleft (p. 932). The molecular rules governing these processes appear to be quite complex, and are quite poorly understood, but involve a number of separate processes: the transport of the vesicle to the surface, its recognition of the correct part of the plasma membrane and attachment to its inner surface ('docking'), then the fusion of the lipid bilayers of vesicles and plasma membrane and the release of the secreted material. In the systems which have been analysed in any detail it appears that these events are facilitated by various transmembrane proteins within the vesicle walls which act as signals for appropriate transport, docking and membrane fusion. For further reading, consult Alberts et al (1994).

Lipid vacuoles. These are spheroidal bodies of various sizes found within many cells, but especially prominent in the lipocytes of adipose tissue. They do not belong to the Golgi-related vacuolar system of the cell, and they are not membrane bound since they are really lipid droplets floating in the cytosol. In lipocytes they can attain truly impressive sizes—80 μm or more in diameter. Lipid vacuoles are often surrounded by cytoskeletal filaments which presumably help to stabilize them within cells and stop them from fusing with the membranes of other organelles including the plasma membrane. In lipocytes they function as stores of chemical energy, and as thermal and mechanical insulators, but in many other cells they may represent intermediates or end-products of other chemical pathways, for example in steroid synthesizing cells where they may be prominent features of the cytoplasm.

Cytosolic organelles

Surrounding the membranous compartments which constitute the various organelles described in the first part of this section is the aqueous cytosol. Within this compartment of the cell are various other, non-membranous organelles of great importance to its biology. They include a system of filamentous proteins known as the *cytoskeleton*, and may also variably contain a number of other inclusions, especially *storage granules* of various kinds. The structure of these will now be outlined.

CYTOSKELETON

The term cytoskeleton is used to denote a system of filamentous

intracellular proteins of different shapes and sizes which form a complex often interconnected network throughout the cytoplasm, sometimes invading the nucleus of the cell. Like the skeleton of the body, it performs many related tasks: it provides mechanical support to cell structures, maintaining cell shape and stiffness, enabling cells to adopt highly asymmetric or irregular profiles (e.g. in neurons) and, therefore, playing an important part in establishing their structural polarity; they can provide stiffness and support for projections from the cell's surface such as microvilli and cilia and anchor these into the cytoplasm. The cytoskeleton can also provide a system of coordinates which specify where and how many metabolic activities occur in the cell. It can do this by anchoring specific organelles in particular places: the Golgi apparatus near the nucleus and endoplasmic reticulum, for example, mitochondria near the sites of energy consumption, and ribosomes where specific proteins are needed. Besides these important functions, the cytoskeleton is supremely associated with motility, either within the cell, as seen, in the shuttling of vesicles and macromolecules from one cytoplasmic site to another, in the moving of chromosomes during mitosis, in embryonic morphogenesis, and, most remarkably of all, in the contraction of muscle cells which is caused by a highly specialized cytoskeleton.

The components of the cytoskeleton include several types of proteinaceous assemblies. The way in which movements are created by these structures and their importance both in the daily lives of cells and in more complex processes of development will be considered later (p. 43); here we will give a brief account of their form and composition. For general reviews of the cytoskeleton, see e.g. Amos & Amos (1991), Bray (1992), Kreis & Vale (1992), Alberts et al (1994), Fawcett (1994).

The roll-call of cytoskeletal structures is lengthening rapidly as molecular biology combined with electron microscopy, immunocytochemistry and in vitro observations of living cells continues to define new forms. The most extensive filamentous structures found in non-muscle cells are of three major types: microfilaments composed of actin, microtubules made of tubulin, and intermediate filaments composed of intermediate filament proteins. Other important components are shorter (generally) protein filaments which can bind to the foregoing types to link them together or generate movements. These include *actin-binding proteins*, among which are numbered myosin, a protein which in some cells can assemble into conspicuous thick filaments, and *microtubule-associated proteins*. There are also numerous other more minor filamentous proteins which play roles in many cell types, but are generally less well understood.

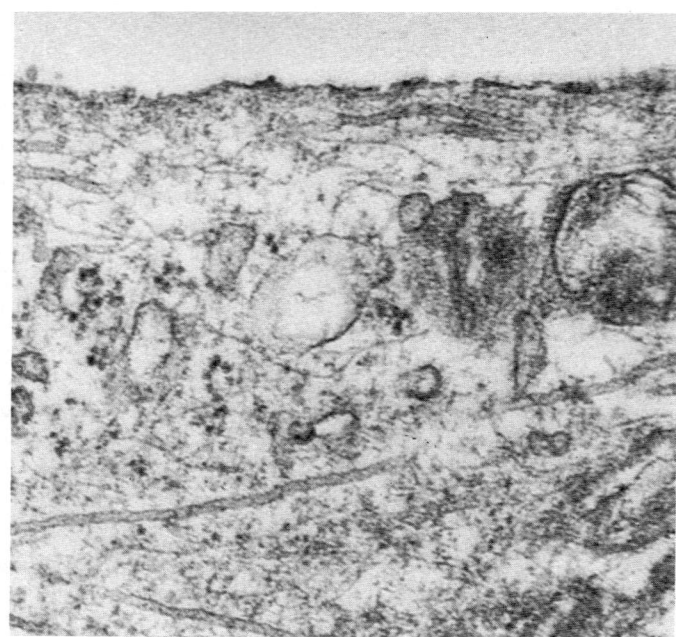

2.18 Electron micrograph of microtubules and microfilaments in a tangential section through a fibroblast. Magnification × 50 000.

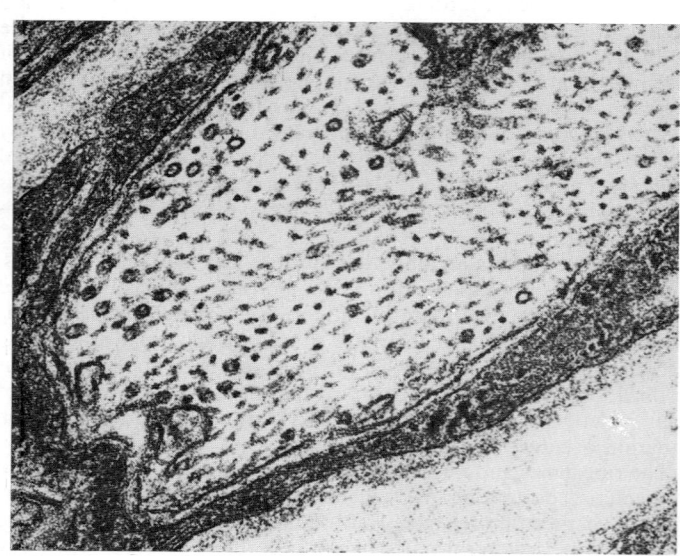

2.19 Microtubules and neurofilaments in a transverse/oblique section of part of a small nerve fibre. The microtubules have a circular cross-section whereas the smaller neurofilaments appear solid. Magnification × 50 000.

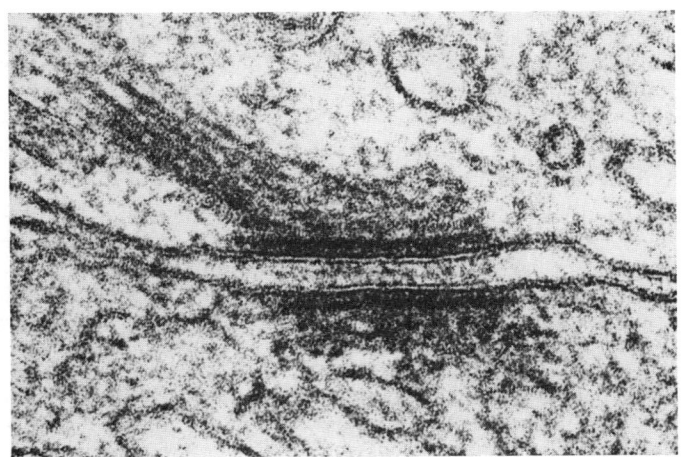

2.20 Intermediate filaments associated with a desmosome (macula adherens) between two epithelial cells. Magnification × 100 000.

ACTIN FILAMENTS (MICROFILAMENTS)

Actin filaments are well-defined filaments with a width of 6–8 nm (2.22), and a solid cross-section. Within most cell types actin constitutes the most abundant protein present and in some motile cells its concentration may exceed 200 μM (10 mg protein per ml). The filaments are formed by the ATP-dependent polymerization of actin monomer into a characteristic linear form in which the subunits are arranged in a single tight zig-zag helix to produce the superficial appearance of a double spiral with a distance of 13 subunits between turns (see Holmes et al 1990). The polymerized form is termed *F-actin* (fibrillar actin) and the unpolymerized form is *G-actin* (globular actin), with a molecular weight of 43 kDa. Each monomer has an asymmetric structure, so that when they are assembled the filament has a defined polarity, with a *plus* end favouring monomer addition, and *minus* end favouring monomer loss. If myosin derivatives are added to filamentous actin in a suitable medium they bind to it in a characteristic manner ('decoration'), attaching at a definite angle to give the appearance of a series of arrowheads pointing towards the *minus* end of the filament, and the barbs towards the *plus* end.

There is a dynamic equilibrium between G-actin and F-actin, and it is generally estimated that in most cells about 50% of the actin is in the polymerized state. The fungal toxin cytochalasin inhibits actin-dependent motility by binding to the plus end of F-actin, thereby disrupting this dynamic equilibrium.

Actin-binding proteins: molecules which modify actin organization

A wide variety of actin-binding proteins exist and these can modulate the form taken by actin within the cell. Such interactions are fundamental to the structure of cytoplasm and to cell shape since they regulate cytoplasmic viscosity (and therefore, can produce different microenvironments), connect filaments together in large groups, cause bundles to extend or contract, attach them to the

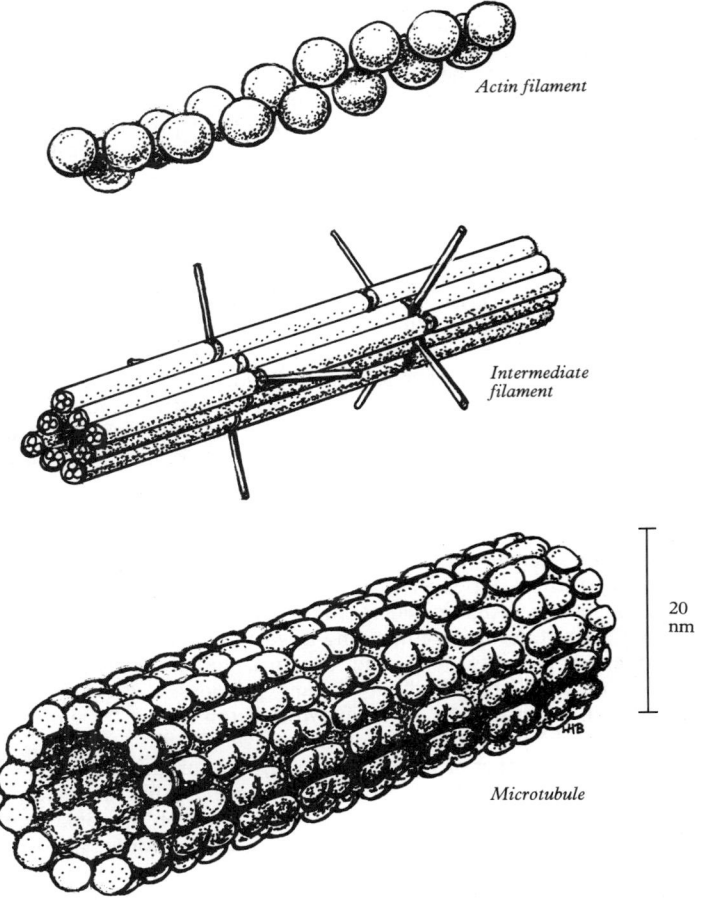

Actin filament

Intermediate filament

20 nm

Microtubule

2.22 The substructure of some major cytoskeletal components, including (top) an actin microfilament formed by polymerization of globular actin monomers; (middle) an intermediate filament composed in this example (e.g. vimentin) of eight sub-filaments, each containing two or three paired acidic and basic polypeptide chains, some extending laterally as side-arms; and (below) a microtubule composed of assemblies of tubulin dimers arranged in a tight helix.

2.21 Intermediate filaments, in this case composed of glial fibrillary acidic protein (GFAP), demonstrated in cultured retinal astrocytes with anti-GFAP antibodies coupled to rhodamine. Provided by Caroline Wigley, UMDS, Guy's Campus, London. Magnification × 5000.

plasma membrane and mediate actin-based motility. On the basis of these activities, they can be divided into bundling proteins, gel-forming proteins and severing proteins.

Bundling proteins tie actin filaments together in longitudinal arrays to form cables or core structures. These may be closely spaced, as in microvilli, microspikes and filopodia to tie parallel filaments tightly together, forming stiff bundles of filaments which are all orientated in the same direction. Included in this group are fimbrin, and villin (also classified as a severing protein). Other actin-bundling proteins form rather looser bundles of filaments which run anti-parallel to each other (with respect to their plus and minus ends). The proteins cross-linking these include α-actinin (also found in the Z-bands of striated muscles) and myosin II (see also below) which can form cross-links with ATP-dependent motor activity, causing adjacent actin filaments to slide on each other and thus either change the shape of cells or, if the actin bundles are anchored into the cell membrane at both ends, maintain a degree of active rigidity.

Gel-forming proteins interconnect adjacent actin filaments crossing each other at angles, to form filamentous meshworks (gels) composed of randomly orientated F-actin. Such networks are frequently found in the cortical regions of cells, for example fibroblasts, forming a semi-rigid zone from which most other organelles are excluded. The protein filamin is an example of such a molecule.

Severing proteins can bind to F-actin filaments and sever them, to produce profound changes within the actin cytoskeleton and in its coupling to the cell surface. Examples include gelsolin and severin.

OTHER ACTIN-BINDING PROTEINS

Actin cytoskeletons are attached to the plasma membrane either directly or indirectly through a variety of membrane-associated proteins which may also create links via transmembrane proteins to the extracellular matrix. Best known of these is the family of spectrin-like molecules which can bind to actin and also to each other and various membrane-associated proteins to create supportive, somewhat elastic networks beneath the plasma membrane. Spectrin is found in erythrocytes (p. 1405) but closely related molecules are present in many other cells: fodrin in nerve cells, and a sub-family of dystrophins in the sole plates of muscle cells (M-dystrophin: see p. 748) and nerve cells (P-dystrophin in cerebellar Purkinje cells, C-dystrophin in cortical neurons, eutrophin in many other cells). Other molecules directly or indirectly connecting these to integral plasma membrane proteins (e.g. integrins) and thence to focal adhesions are proteins such as ankyrin (which also bind actin directly), band 4.1, vinculin, talin, zyxin, paxillin and many others. The detailed chemistry and behaviour of these proteins is beyond the scope of the present account; for further information consult Bray (1992), Otto (1994). In addition to these various molecular species, myosin I and other 'unconventional' myosins (see below) have been shown to be important in connecting actin filaments to membranous structures including the plasma membrane, and transport vesicles within cells (see below), and finally, tropomyosin, an important regulatory protein of muscle fibres, is also present in non-muscle cells, where its function may be primarily to stabilize actin filaments against depolymerization (Pittenger et al 1994).

In conclusion to this consideration of actin it should be noted that the presence of networks containing large amounts of cellular actin, the interchangeability of F- and G-actins, and the existence of a wide variety of actin-binding proteins provides a very effective mechanism for modelling the actin cytoskeleton during the motility, growth and differentiation of a diverse range of cells.

There are a number of subtypes of actin, some primarily associated with cell plasma membranes; others lie deeper within the cytosol. Muscle cells contain particularly robust forms of microfilament. Actin binds to the protein myosin when an energy source (ATP) is available and when appropriately organized. This leads to various types of shearing movement which can produce cell motility of different kinds, including muscular contraction (p. 741). Actin microfilaments can be detected electron microscopically by incubating cells, made permeable to proteins, with heavy meromyosin which binds to actin and decorates the filaments with arrowhead formations. Actin can also be readily detected by labelling with anti-actin antibodies conjugated to a fluorescent dye for light microscopy; or to an electron-dense marker (e.g. colloidal gold) for electron

microscopy. It also binds the fungal derivative phalloidin which can be fluorescently labelled, too. The cytochalasins (fungal products) cause depolymerization of some actin microfilaments (see Spudich & Lin 1972), and, therefore, provide a valuable experimental tool in research into their functions.

MICROTUBULES

Microtubules are polymeric fibres with hollow cylinders about 24 nm in diameter (**2.18, 19, 22**), of varying length (some up to 70 μm in spermatozoan flagella). They are present in most cell types but are particularly abundant in neurons, leucocytes, blood platelets and in the mitotic spindles of dividing cells. They also form part of the structure of cilia, flagella and centrioles (see below). Helical microtubules occur in Schwann cells (p. 951) and oligodendrocytes. Massed parallel bundles of interconnected microtubules are found in the pillar cells supporting the sensory cells of the cochlea. Microtubules rarely show acute bends, indicating a degree of stiffness.

Microtubules are polymers of tubulin. There are two major forms of this protein α- and β-tubulins which before assembly occur together as dimers (see e.g. Soifer 1986) with a combined molecular weight of 100 kDa (50 kDa each). Each protein subunit is about 5 nm across and microtubules in transverse section are made up of a ring of such globular subunits, usually 13 in number, also arranged along the long axis in straight rows of alternating tubulins α and β, forming the wall of a cylinder (these rows can, therefore, be viewed as *protofilaments*). Each longitudinal row is slightly out of alignment with its neighbour, so that a spiral pattern of alternating α and β subunits appears when the microtubule is viewed from the side (Amos & Klug 1974). There is a dynamic equilibrium between the dimers and assembled microtubules; as with actin, asymmetries in the dimers create a directionality to the microtubule; tubulin is added preferentially to one end (plus), in contrast with the minus end which is relatively slow growing. It is, therefore, possible to add tubulin at one end while removing it at the other (a phenomenon called 'treadmilling', see also p. 61), in which case the microtubule will gradually shift its position longitudinally.

Various drugs (e.g. colcemid, vinblastine, griseofulvin, nicodazole) can cause microtubule depolymerization by binding the soluble tubulin dimers and so shifting the equilibrium towards the unpolymerized state. Microtubule demolition causes a wide variety of effects, including the inhibition of cell division because microtubules are present in the mitotic spindle (p. 61). Conversely, the drug taxol *stabilizes* microtubules to the extent that processes depending on their turnover no longer operate (e.g. some aspects of axoplasmic flow in neurons, so causing peripheral neuropathy).

Different microtubules have varying degrees of stability, for example those of cilia are generally unaffected by many anti-microtubule drugs, due to chemical modifications to their assembled structure. There are also differences between tissues, for example neurons have a special subclass. Tubulins associated with microtubule organizing centres (see below) include another type γ-tubulin. Polymerization requires phosphorylation of tubulins by GTP, and also a nucleation site such as the end of a pre-existing microtubule or a microtubule-organizing centre such as those surrounding (and including) centrioles, around which spindle microtubules polymerize during cell division (Pickett-Heaps 1975) and from which cilia can grow (see p. 43). In other instances such centres have no obvious structural basis, thus centrioles are not always essential to microtubule formation.

Microtubule-associated proteins (MAPs)

Within the cytoplasm or attached to the walls of the microtubules are various small proteins which can bind to assembled tubulins which may be either structural or associated with motility. *Structural MAPs* form cross-bridges between adjacent microtubules or between microtubules and other structures such as intermediate filaments, mitochondria and the plasma membrane, with lengths ranging from 50–185 nm. Such molecules include the well known MAPs found in neurons such as MAPs 1A and 1B present in neuronal dendrites and axons, MAPs 2A and 2B chiefly in dendrites, and *tau*, found only in axons. MAP 4 is the major MAP in many other cell types. Structural MAPs are implicated in various aspects of microtubule biology, including their formation, maintenance and demolition.

These molecules are, therefore, of considerable significance in cell morphogenesis, mitotic division, maintenance and modulation of cell shape and a plethora of cell activities dependent on microtubules (see the review of MAPs by Hirokawa 1994). *Motility-associated MAPs* are found in a number of situations where movement occurs over the surfaces of microtubules, for example the transport of cytoplasmic vesicles, bending of cilia and flagella and some movements of mitotic spindles. They include a large family of motor proteins, the best known of which are the dyneins and kinesins. Another protein, dynamin, has recently been demonstrated, (although now also shown to be involved in endocytosis) and to this should be added kinetochore proteins responsible for chromosomal movements in mitotic and meiotic anaphase (see p. 61). All of these molecules have binding sites for microtubules and the ability to actively slide along their surfaces. At the same time, kinesins and dyneins can also attach to membranous structures such as transport vesicles and thus convey them along microtubules for considerable distances, a vital mechanism for the selective targeting of materials made in one part of the cell to distant destinations. Such movements occur in both directions along microtubules: kinesin-dependent motion appears to be towards the *plus* ends of microtubules, for example from the cell body towards the axon terminals in neurons, and away from the centrosome in epithelial and other cells with a radial distribution of microtubules. Conversely, dynein-related movements appear to be in the opposite direction, i.e. to the *minus* ends of microtubules. Dyneins also form the arms of peripheral microtubules in cilia and flagella where they can form 'walking' cross-bridges to adjacent microtubule pairs and so generate shearing forces which cause the axonemal array of microtubules to bend and thus generate ciliary and flagellar beating movements. Besides the kinesins and dyneins, recent research has found a number of related motor proteins which can also interact with microtubules, for instance kinesin-related proteins which cross-link mitotic spindle microtubules to push the two centriolar poles apart during mitotic prophase, and it is probable that such molecules are of considerable importance in many other motile activities of cells.

INTERMEDIATE FILAMENTS

Intermediate filaments include a family of protein filaments about 10 nm thick, found in different cell types and often present in large numbers where structural strength is needed (**2.19–22**) or forming a scaffolding for the attachment of other structures. It has been shown by immunochemistry and other means that several families of intermediate filament occur, all with a broadly similar chemical structure. Chemically they can be divided into three major categories designated A, B and C, each subdivisible according to their detailed molecular structure, so that a total of 6 classes are currently recognized (see Table 2.1). The different types are characteristic of particular tissues or states of maturity so that they have come to be important indicators of cell origins or levels of differentiation, and of considerable value for histopathology. Of the different classes, *keratin* proteins are found in epithelia, keratin (or *cytokeratin*) filaments always being composed of combinations of Types I (acidic) and II (basic or neutral) keratins in equal parts. Bundles of keratin filaments in the epidermis were previously called tonofibrils or tonofilaments, reflecting their cable-like mechanical properties. About 15 types of acidic keratin proteins are known and the same number of basic or neutral types. Studies with specific monoclonal antibodies have distinguished many varieties of such filaments, even within keratinocytes; it is possible to discern a changing pattern of keratin chemistry as cells proceed from their basal positions in the epidermis to their fully mature flattened state in the stratum corneum where they are virtually solid plates of keratin filaments. Genetic abnormalities of keratins are known to affect the mechanical stability of epithelia: for example, the disease epidermolysis bullosa simplex which causes lysis of epidermal basal cells and, therefore, blistering when subject to mechanical stresses, is caused by defects in genes encoding keratins 5 and 14, whereas when keratins 1 and 10 are affected, cells in the stratum spinosum lyse to give intraepidermal blistering (epidermolyic hyperkeratosis). (For further information, see the reviews by Coulombe 1993.) *Vimentins* occur in mesenchyme-derived cells of connective tissue, *desmins* in muscle cells, *glial fibrillar acidic protein (GFAP)* in central nervous system glial cells and

Table 2.1		Classes of intermediate filament proteins		
Group	Type	Name	kDa	Tissues/cells
A	I	Keratins I (acidic)	40–70	Epithelia
	II	Keratins II (basic/neutral)	40–70	Epithelia
B	III	Vimentin	54	Mesenchyme derived
		Desmin	53	Muscle
		Glial fibrillary acidic protein (GFAP)	50	CNS glia, Olfactory glia
		Peripherin		Rods and cones Peripheral axons
	IV	Neurofilament NF-L NF-M NF-H Nestin Internexin	68 95 115	Neurons
C	V	Nuclear lamins I–III	65–75	All nuclei

olfactory glia, and *peripherin* in peripheral axons. *Neurofilaments* are a major cytoskeletal element of neurons, particularly in axons where they are the dominant protein. Neurofilaments are heteropolymers of low, medium and high molecular weight neurofilament proteins (NF-L, -M and -H respectively); NF-L is always present in combination with either NF-M or NF-H.

Abnormal neurofilament structures have been found in a number of neuropathological conditions. It is likely that genetic defects in these structures are important in a range of neurodegenerative diseases which show abnormal neurofilament assemblies. Although definitive evidence for this is not yet available, experiments on transgenic mice have shown that overexpression of the NF-L protein produces a neurological condition resembling the human motor neuron disease, amyotrophic lateral sclerosis (for reviews see Liem 1993; Lee & Cleveland 1994).

Other intermediate filament proteins include *nestin*, a molecule resembling neurofilament protein but forming intermediate filaments in neurectodermal stem cells. *Nuclear lamins* form intermediate filaments which line the inner surface of the nuclear envelope of all nucleated cells (see p. 47), providing a mechanical framework for the nucleus and acting as attachment sites for chromosomes. They are unusual in that they form a square lattice of regularly spaced crossing filaments rather than bundles, reflecting their unusual molecular composition.

The exact manner in which intermediate filament proteins polymerize to form linear filaments is much more complex than that of tubulin or actin, and has not been fully characterized. The individual intermediate filament proteins are chains with a middle a-helical region flanked on either side by non-helical domains. These proteins are coiled together as dimers which are themselves further coiled to create short rods about 45 nm long. These are assembled end to end or are diagonally staggered in echelon into subfibrils, and, usually, eight of these are rolled up into a hollow cylinder which constitutes the 10 nm intermediate filament itself. A cross-section of a single intermediate filament with this arrangement would, therefore, pass through 16 individual protein subunits, although in some filaments the number appears to vary from this. The non-coiled regions of the subunits are thought to project outwards as side arms which can link intermediate filaments into bundles or attach them to the other structures. The existence of various combinations of subunit proteins within one filament provides great chemical and functional diversity to these structures. The tightly linked structure makes the filaments very stable chemically, and indeed they are difficult to solubilize for chemical analysis, requiring 2M urea to bring them into solution. However, in the living cell they have also been shown to be quite dynamic, especially in immature cells, perhaps as a result of phosphorylation which tends to destabilize their structure.

For further information about intermediate filaments, see Stewart (1993), Alberts et al (1994), Heins and Aebi (1994).

MYOSINS

Although myosin can be considered as simply just another actin-binding protein, its importance in cell motility, especially muscle contraction, merits an extra comment. The myosin family is composed of several classes, the complexities of which are becoming apparent as more members are being discovered from the analysis of cDNA libraries. The chief characteristic of myosin molecules is the presence of a globular head consisting of a heavy and a light chain. The heavy chain bears an a-helical tail of varying length. The head has an ATP-ase activity and can bind to and move along actin filaments, so that myosins are *motor proteins*. The best-known class is myosin II, which occurs in muscle and in many non-muscle cells. Its molecules have two heads and two tails entwined to form a long rod; the rods can bind to each other to form the long *thick filaments*, as seen in striated and smooth muscle fibres, and in myoepithelial cells (p. 71) and myofibroblasts (p. 76). Myosin II molecules can also assemble into smaller groups, especially dimers which can cross-link individual actin microfilaments in stress fibres and other F-actin arrays. The ATP-dependent sliding of myosin on actin produces muscle contraction and also extension of microfilament bundles, as seen in the flattening of fibroblasts in culture or the contraction of the ring of actin and myosin around the cleavage furrow of dividing cells. There are a number of known subtypes of myosin II which assemble in different ways and have different dynamic properties. In skeletal muscle the myosin molecules form filaments about 120 nm thick, reversing their direction of assembly at the midpoint to produce a symmetrical arrangement of subunits (p. 739). In smooth muscle the molecules form thicker flattened ribbons and are orientated in different directions on either face of the ribbon (p. 774). These arrangements have important consequences for the detailed nature of the contractile force generated by the different types of muscle cell.

Other myosins of considerable importance to cell activities include a collection of various molecules known as *unconventional myosins*. An example of these is the *myosin I* subfamily, single-headed molecules with a tail of varying length. These are especially associated with membranes to which their tails can attach, and are implicated in the movements of membranes on actin filaments, for example, of vesicles which track along F-actin in a similar manner to kinesin and dynein-related movements along microtubules (p. 39). Other proposed functions of myosin I are the movements of membranes in phagocytosis, microspike formation in growth cones and other membrane-cytoskeleton related motility, as well as actin–actin sliding and attachment of actin to membranes (e.g. those of microvilli). Other myosins have recently been isolated, although the significance of this great diversity is not understood. For reviews of myosins, see Titus (1993).

VERY THIN FILAMENTS

A very heterogeneous group of filamentous structures with widths of 2–4 nm also occur in various cells. The two most widely studied forms, *titin* and *nebulin*, are found in striated muscles. These are relatively huge molecules with subunit weights of around a million, and native molecules are about 1 μm in length. Surprisingly, they constitute about 13% of the total protein of skeletal muscle. Their elastic properties are important for the proper functioning of muscle, and possibly for cells in general. For further details see Keller 1995; also page 747.

MICROVILLI

Microvilli are finger-like cell surface extensions (**2**.1, 23, 24) usually about 0.1 μm in diameter and up to about 2 μm long. When arranged in a regular parallel series, they constitute a *striated border*, as seen at the absorptive surfaces of the epithelial cells (enterocytes, see p. 1771) of the small intestine; when less regular, as in the gallbladder epithelium and proximal kidney tubules, the term *brush border* is applied.

Covered by plasma membrane, they are supported internally by closely packed bundles of actin microfilaments linked by cross-bridges of the actin-bundling proteins *villin* and *fimbrin* (see Mooseker 1985). Connecting the microfilaments to the plasma membrane are other bridges composed of *myosin I* and calmodulin. There is no evidence that the microvilli are motile, although it is possible that the myosin link to the plasma membrane generates movement in the latter to replace lost or degraded membrane components. The microfilament bundles of microvilli are implanted within the cell's apical cytoplasm amongst a transverse meshwork of transversely running microfilaments linked by spectrin, the *terminal web*, which

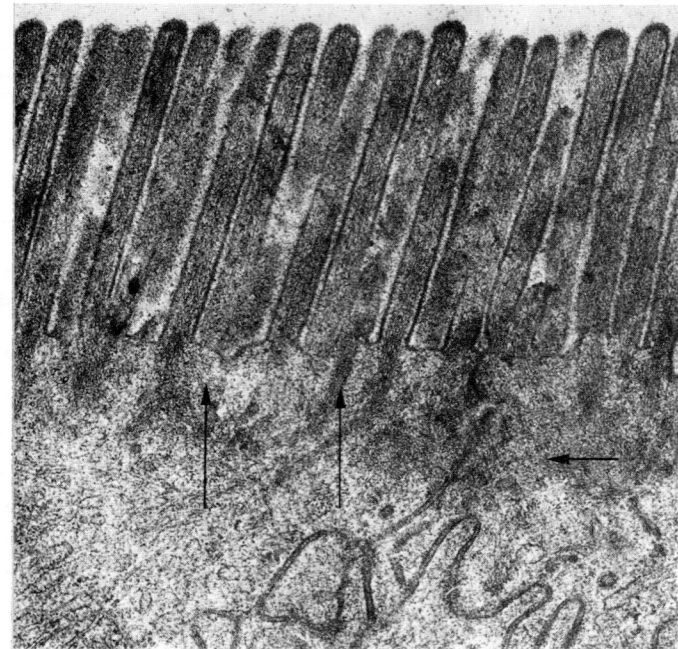

A

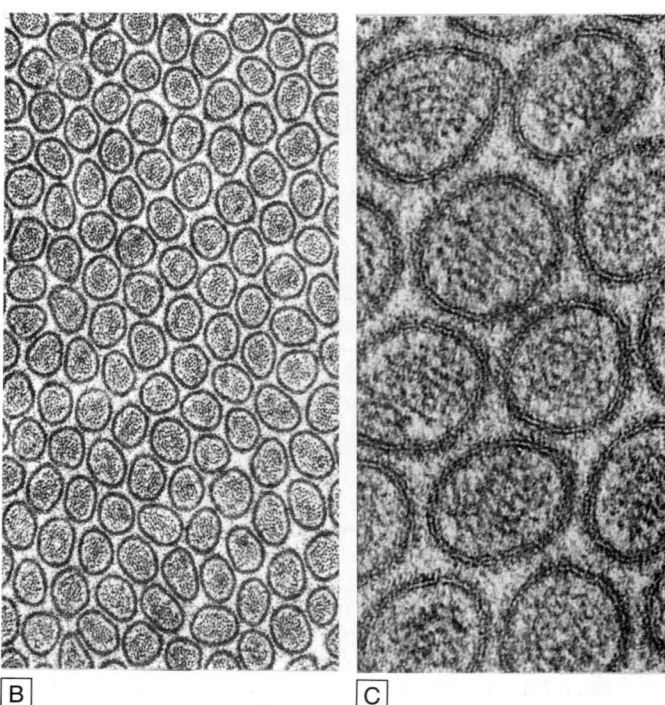

B   C

2.23 Electron micrographs of microvilli from a striated border of an absorptive columnar epithelial cell of the small intestine (compare with 2.67): A. vertical section showing microvilli with supporting microfilaments (long arrows) and terminal web (short arrow); B. horizontal section through cell surface cutting each microvillus transversely. Insert (c) shows the details of a few microvilli from B; note the bilayer structure of the plasma membrane and the fuzzy external cell coat. Magnifications: A and B × 20 000; c × 110 000.

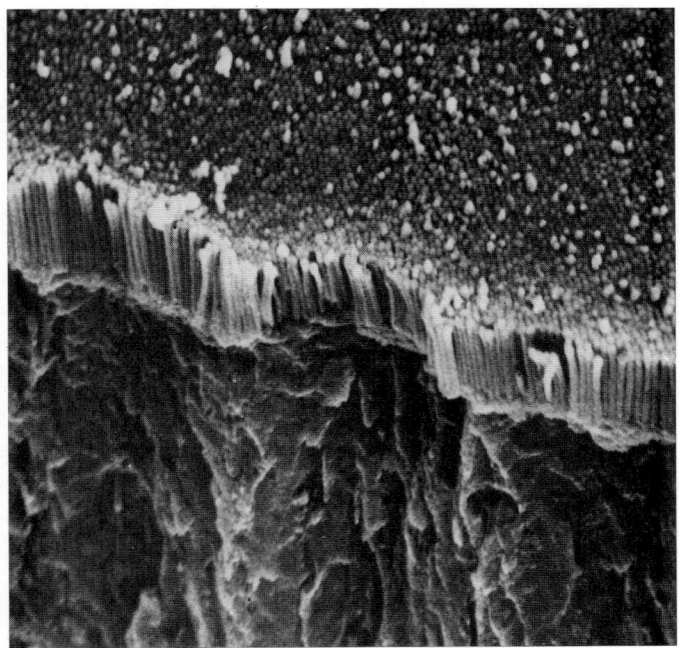

2.24 Scanning electron micrograph of a striated border from the small intestine showing numerous microvilli. The epithelium has been cut vertically to allow the microvilli to be viewed from the side as well as from above. Magnification × 6000.

a single cell, as in bronchial epithelium, or only one or two as with some mesothelial cells. Each male gamete possesses a single flagellum about 70 μm long.

By electron microscopy (2.25–27) each cilium or flagellum is seen to consist of a *shaft*, constituting most of its length, with a diameter of about 0.25 μm, a tapering *tip* and, at its base within the surface cytoplasm of the cell, a *kinetosome* (basal body, basal granule or blepharoplast) about 1 μm long (Gibbons & Grimstone 1960). The whole structure is bounded, except at its base, by plasma membrane. In freeze-fracture preparations chain-like groups of characteristic membrane particles, the *ciliary necklace*, surround the proximal end of the cilium (Gilula & Satir 1972). These particles may assist the control of ciliary beating. The core of the cilium is a cylinder of nine double microtubules (the axoneme), surrounding a central pair of single microtubules. At the base of the cilium (the kinetosome) each microtubule doublet, the two parts of which are designated the A and B subfibres, are twisted through 40° (2.25D, 26) and another microtubule, the C subfibre, is added. The central pair sometimes end above the cell surface in a dense sphere or axosome, beneath which lies a transverse partition or basal plate. Associated with the kinetosome are often one or more cross-banded filamentous rootlets and a plate-like basal foot, which probably help to anchor the cilium into the cytoplasm. At the apical end, the various microtubular elements do not all continue to the tip; the A subfibres are the first to end, then the B subfibres and, finally, the central pair terminate.

Within the shaft lie several filamentous structures associated with the microtubules, such as radial spokes which extend inwards from the outer microtubules towards the central pair. The outer doublet microtubules bear two rows of tangential dynein arms attached to the A subfibre of one doublet, pointing towards the B subfibre of

is also anchored around its edges to the zonula adherens. The protein myosin also occurs in the terminal web and is thought to bind to the actin to stiffen this part of the cell. In vitro this meshwork can be stimulated to contract, and this is thought to play a role in adjusting the extracellular space and the permeability of the tight junctions around the cell apex. At the apex of the microvillus, the free ends of microfilaments are inserted into a dense mass which includes the protein α-actinin (Mooseker & Tilney 1975).

Microvilli greatly multiply the area of surface (up to 40 times, in striated borders) and are found at sites of active absorption. In the small intestine, microvilli have a very thick glycocalyx (see p. 1771) which binds digestive enzymes, but the membranes themselves also carry disaccharidases synthesized in the cells which bear them, as well as various proteins which are channels for nutrient absorption. Irregular microvilli, filopodia, are also found on the surfaces of many types of cell, particularly free macrophages and fibroblasts. Again, these may be associated with transport processes, particularly phagocytosis, and with cell motility.

Large, regular microvilli are called *stereocilia* (a name unfortunately retained from pre-electron microscopy days when the distinction between these and true cilia was not understood). These are found on cochlear and vestibular receptor cells where they act as sensory transducers, and also occur in the absorptive epithelium of the epididymis. Transient microvillus-like structures found on developing or motile cells include elongate *microspikes* on axonal growth cones and on ruffled membranes at the leading edges of migratory cells (see 2.30).

CILIA AND FLAGELLA

Cilia and flagella are, typically, motile hair-like projections of the cell surface (cilium = eyelash, flagellum = whip), that create currents in the surrounding fluid or movements of the cell to which they are attached. Cilia occur on many internal surfaces of the body, particularly the epithelia of most of the respiratory tract, parts of the male and female reproductive tracts, the ependyma lining the central canal of the spinal cord and ventricles of the brain and the mesothelia of the peritoneal and plural cavities. They also occur at olfactory receptor and vestibular hair cell endings and, modified, as portions of the rods and cones of the retina; cilia are, in addition, present on many dividing tissue cells. Many cilia may be present on

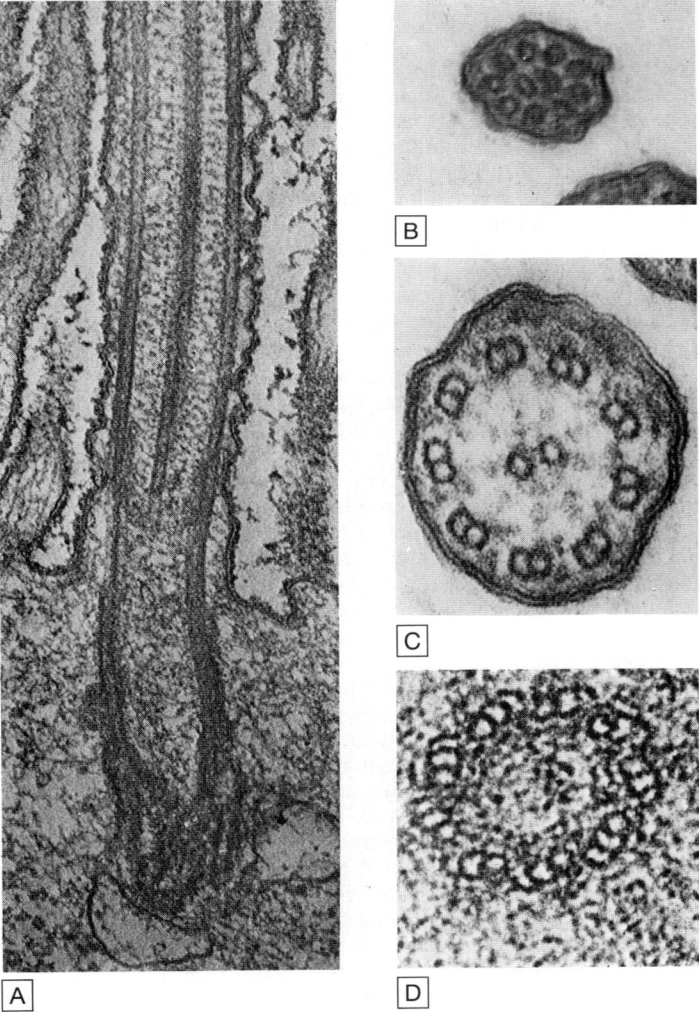

2.25 Electron micrographs of cilia cut (A) longitudinally, and (B, C, D) through the tip, shaft and base respectively. Magnifications: A × 50 000; B–D × 110 000.

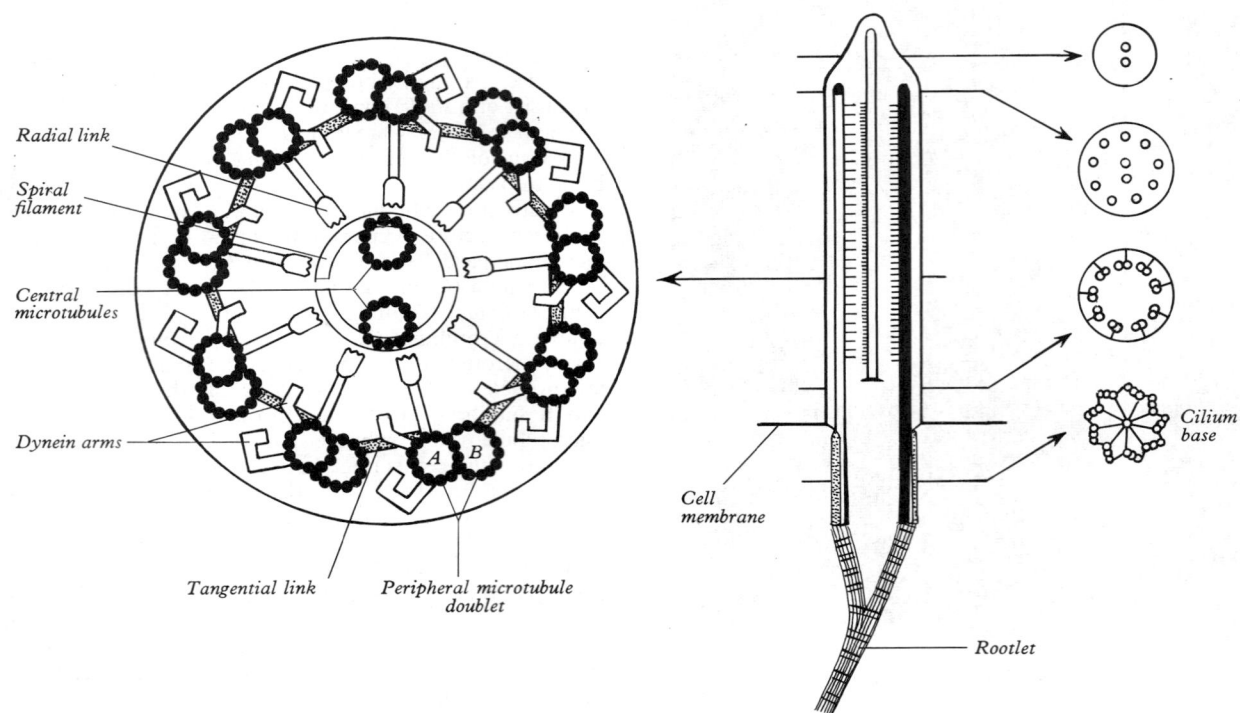

Radial link

Spiral filament

Central microtubules

Dynein arms

Tangential link

Peripheral microtubule doublet

Cell membrane

Cilium base

Rootlet

2.26 The internal structure of a cilium in longitudinal section (centre), the disposition of microtubules at various levels (right), and the detailed cross-sectional appearance of the shaft of the cilium (left). In the latter, hook-like dynein arms extend from the peripheral doublets and radial links with expanded heads project towards the central pair of microtubules. A filamentous spiral encircles the central pair. Adjacent peripheral doublet microtubules are also connected by tangential links. Redrawn from Sleigh (1977).

the adjacent doublet. Adjacent doublets are also linked by thin filaments. Other filaments partially encircle the central pair of microtubules, which are also united by ladder-like spokes. Because of the '9 + 2' pattern of tubules, there is a plane of symmetry which passes perpendicular to a line joining the central pair and corresponds to the direction of bending.

Movements of cilia and flagella (see Sleigh 1974, 1977), are similar in broad outline (**2.28**). Flagella move by rapid undulation passing from the attached to the free end. In human spermatozoa there is a helical component in this motion, although the precise form is hydrodynamically complex (see e.g. Brokaw 1975).

In cilia, the beating is planar, but asymmetrical. In the effective stroke, the cilium remains stiff except at the base where it bends to produce an oar-like stroke. Then follows the recovery stroke during which the bend passes from base to tip, returning the cilium to its initial position for the next cycle. The activity of groups of cilia is usually coupled so that the bending of one is rapidly followed by the bending of the next and so on, resulting in long travelling or metachronal waves (see also p. 1671). These pass over the tissue surface in the same direction as the effective stroke. Mechanical coupling of adjacent cilia is caused by their viscous interaction, the bending of one initiating beating of the next.

When a cilium bends, the microtubules do not change in length but slide on one another (Warner & Satir 1974). The 'arms' of peripheral doublets are made of a protein 'dynein' and slant towards the cilium base from their attached ends. Dynein has an ATP-ase activity, stimulated by magnesium ions, and causes mutual sliding of adjacent doublets by initially attaching sideways to the next pair then swinging upwards towards the tip of the cilium. The radial spokes and various other substructures appear to modify the form of the ciliary bending (Warner & Mitchell 1980). A group of genetic diseases is known in which the cilia beat either ineffectively or not at all (e.g. Cartagena's immotile cilium syndrome) and these cilia show various ultrastructural defects in their internal structure—lack of dynein arms, missing spokes, and so forth. Such patients suffer various respiratory problems due to the accumulation of particles in the lungs, and males are typically sterile due to loss of sperm motility. It is also intriguing that if cilia are immotile, about 50% of patients have an alimentary tract which is arranged as a mirror image of the usual pattern, i.e. it rotates in the opposite direction during early development, perhaps because cilia on its coelomic surface are involved in the initial choice of direction.

The cilia of olfactory receptors (p. 1321) show the typical '9 + 2' arrangement of subfibres, although dynein arms are apparently absent (Lidow & Menco 1984). Cilia of retinal rods and cones, however, lack the central pair of microtubules. Dividing cells of many tissues (e.g. the adrenal cortex) also show a small number of cilia which protrude from the cell surfaces into the intercellular spaces. Their function is unknown but they may represent some unavoidable, functionless by-product of cell division processes.

Cilia and flagella are formed by the polymerization of tubulin on centrioles, which are synthesized deep in the cell and then move to

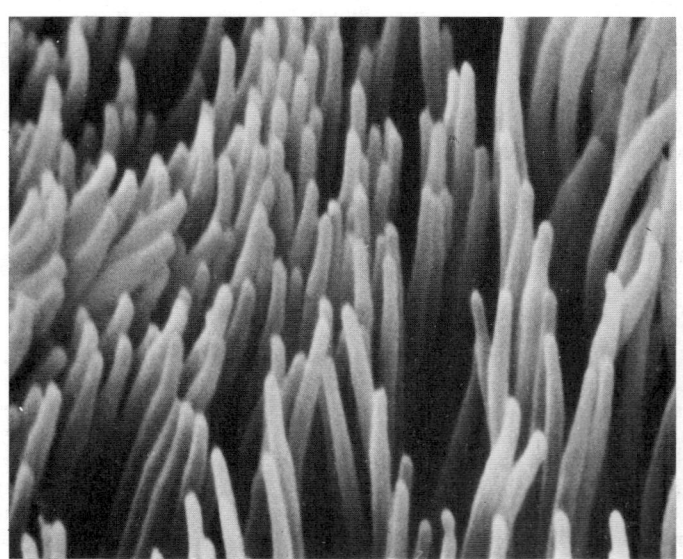

2.27 Scanning electron micrograph of the ciliated surface in the trachea. Magnification × 10 000.

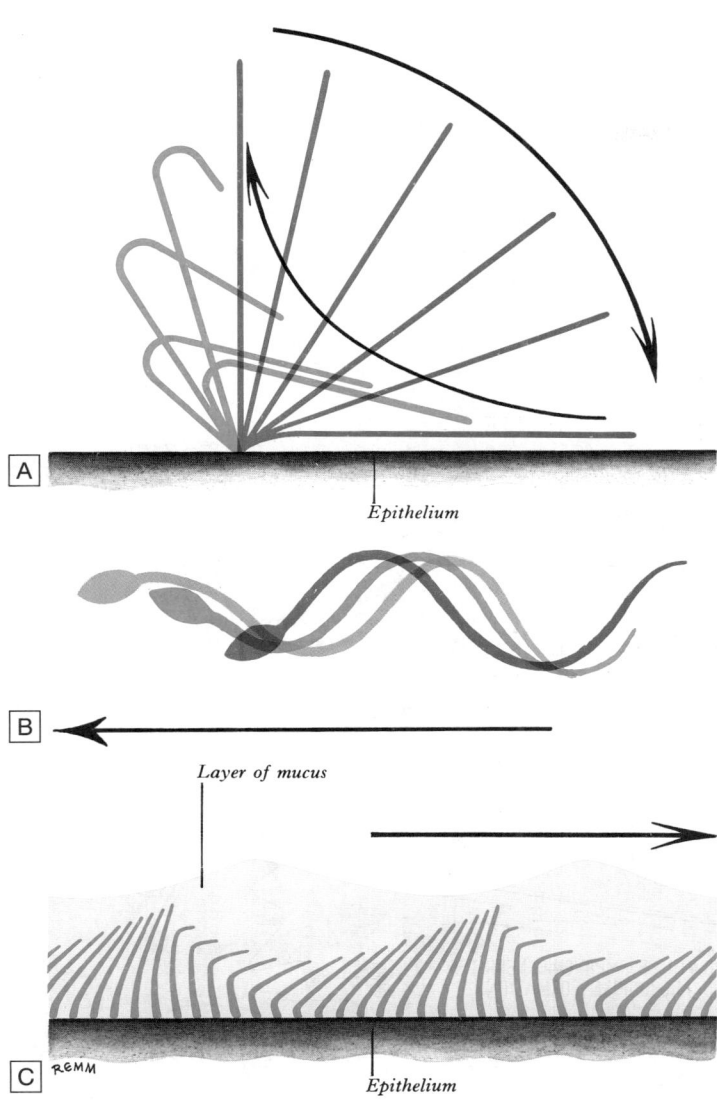

CENTRIOLES AND MICROTUBULE-ORGANIZING CENTRES

Centrioles are microtubular cylinders about 1 μm long by 0.25 μm in diameter (Johnson & Rosenbaum 1992), identical in structure with kinetosomes (see above) but not attached to cilia (2.1, 29). At least two centrioles occur in all cells capable of division (except during meiosis in the oöcyte, see p. 122), usually lying close and at right angles to each other, together often termed a *diplosome*, within a somewhat dense region of cytoplasm, the *centrosome*. Various filamentous or granular structures (centriolar satellites or pericentriolar bodies) surround them. This centriolar complex is a centre for microtubule assembly, for example in the generation of the spindle and aster microtubules during cell division, the sprouting of cilia and the provision of axonal and dendritic microtubules in developing neurons. It is also the source of cytoplasmic microtubules in various other cells, and its proximity to the Golgi complex provides that structure with a means of targeting its vesicular products to different parts of the cell (p. 32). Prior to cell division a new centriole forms near each old one and the resulting pairs are passed on to the two new cells (Rattner & Phillips 1973).

As noted above, microtubules are formed by tubulin assembly on a template, usually the *plus* end of a pre-existing microtubule. Although the microtubules of cilia are assembled directly on the ends of centrioles, spindle and other cytoplasmic microtubules grow from the surrounding centriolar satellites rather than centrioles themselves. The nature of this organizing capacity is not certain; in flowering plants spindle microtubules are formed without centrioles, so they may not be essential to this process. Centres at which microtubules are formed are termed *microtubule organizing centres*; it has recently been shown that these often contain a special form of tubulin (γ-tubulin) which may have special properties in facilitating tubulin assembly. For further details, see the reviews by Brinkley (1984), Oakley (1992) and Joshi (1994).

2.28 Diagram of ciliary (A) and flagellar (B) action. In A the effective stroke is shown in red and the recovery stroke in blue. In B successive movements of the sperm tail are indicated in red, blue and green; C represents a number of cilia in the respiratory tract showing the metachronal wave and the direction of mucus movement.

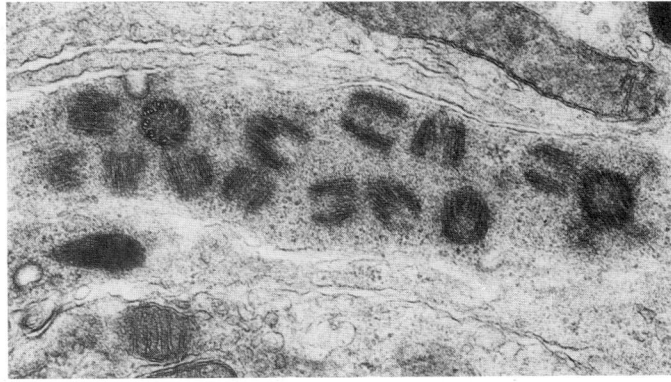

2.29 Transmission electron micrograph of a group of centrioles in a developing nerve cell dendrite. Provided by A Cuschieri, University of Malta. Magnification × 25 000.

lie immediately beneath the cell membrane before the cilia begin to sprout (Sorokin 1968; Staprans & Dirksen 1974). Once initiated, they grow by the addition of tubulin and other materials to the distal end.

Cell motility

Cell motility (see 2.30) plays a crucial role in the life of everyone from the act of conception until death. Embryogenesis is based upon the finely orchestrated movements of individual cells, which, responding to the particular instructions of their genes, divide, migrate and in concert with others may construct the neural tube or lay down the rudiments of the future endo-skeleton. After birth the activities of motile tissues, cardiac, skeletal and smooth muscle are the sole manifestations of an underlying ferment of cytoplasmic motor activities. Beyond the resolution of the human eye continue the activities of cell division, exocytosis, wound healing, blood clotting, circulation of lymphocytes and the patrolling of effector defence cells—macrophages and polymorpho-nuclear leucocytes. New developments in computer assisted microscopy now enable us to witness directly the gliding of single microtubules or even actin filaments and as a consequence make possible the best possible assay system for potential cell motors—that of motion itself (see Preston et al 1990).

Blood cells are carried through the vascular system as passengers at high velocity (from the arm to the foot in less than 1 minute). While the erythrocytes remain in this circuit, white cells need to activate their own motor apparatus to escape from the vascular space. Lymphocytes, in order to complete their assigned peregrinations

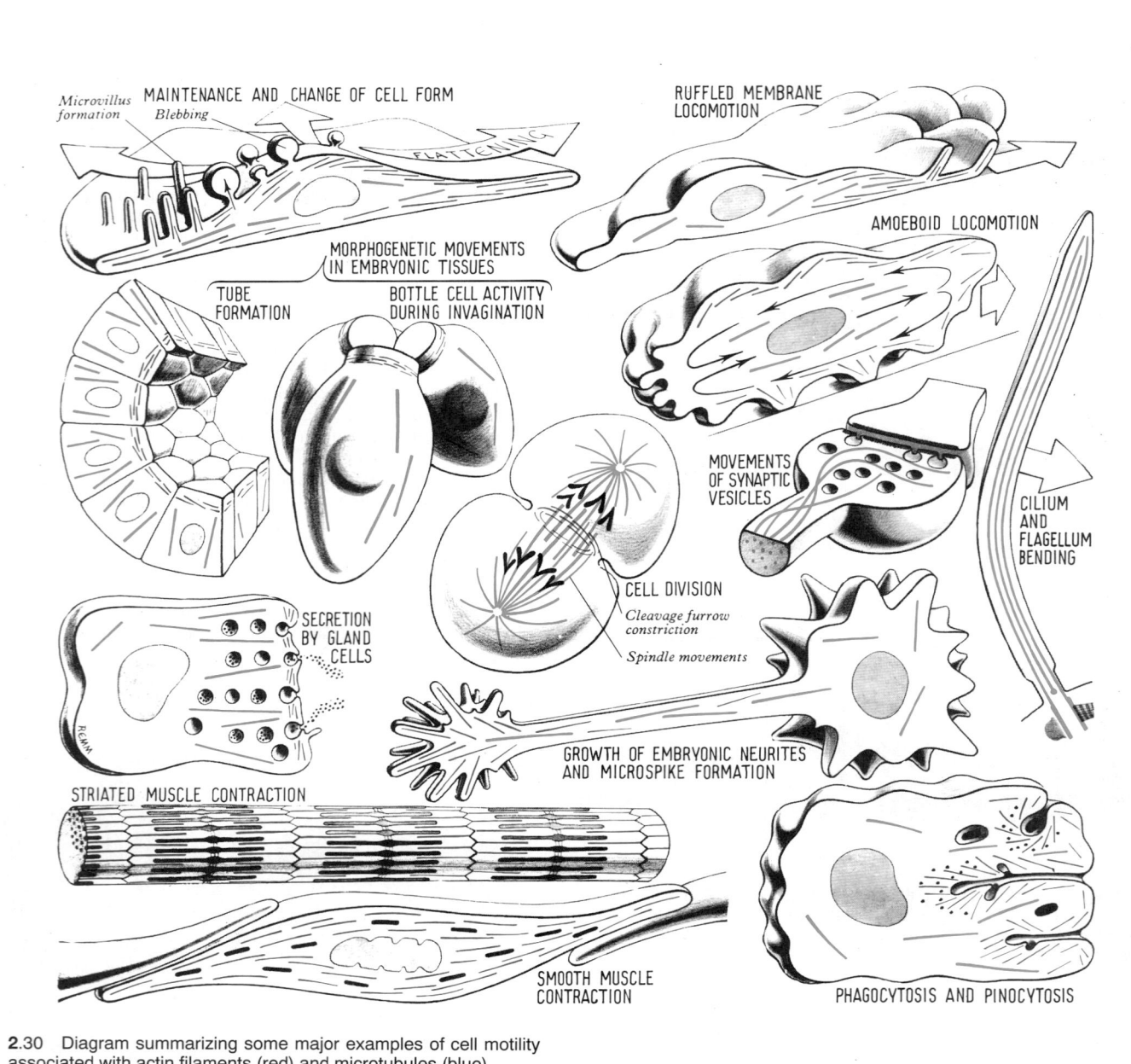

2.30 Diagram summarizing some major examples of cell motility associated with actin filaments (red) and microtubules (blue).

through the lymph vessels, need constantly to escape from and return to the vascular space. While the global transport speed is very high (hundreds of cell lengths per second) cells moving under their own power do so at extremely low velocity—in the range of $0.1 \mu m–10 \mu m.min^{-1}$.

The world as we perceive it, where inertial forces dominate, is experienced quite differently by cells. Being such small objects (diameter approximately $20 \mu m$) their activities are dominated by viscous forces—for them aqueous fluids are as syrup might be to us. Although this point may seem rather arcane it turns out that the motility of all cells has evolved to be reconciled to this restraint. What are the biochemical engines that enable cells to

overcome these viscous forces? There are two principal categories—those associated with F-actin (in concert with myosins) and those associated with microtubules (in concert with kinesins, dyneins)—unified by the following common features:

- The engine consists of two partners, a linear polymer with chemically distinct ends which acts as a cofactor and guide rail for a nucleotide triphosphatase (NTPase) whose substrate is usually ATP (Alberts & Miake-Lye 1992).
- Hydrolysis of each molecule of $NTP \to NDP + P_i$ is coupled to the production of mechanical force which moves the enzyme *unidirectionally* (this is dictated by the intrinsic polarity of F-actin or

microtubules) along its polymer partner a small, finite distance (ca. 20 nm).
- The force produced by each such cross-bridge cycle is infinitesimally small (ca. $1pN = 1 \times 10^{-12}$ N).
- The turnover rate of these NTP-ases is extremely slow (ca. 40 NTP molecules per second) compared with that of a cytosolic enzyme. It is a tribute to biological design that these unpromising performance characteristics, adequate for intracellular transport, have been amplified during evolution into that remarkable tension machine—skeletal muscle. Here the myosin II:F-actin ratio is very high. In non-muscle cells actin may reach concentrations of $200 \mu M$ whereas those of the myosins are of the

order of 2 μm; this speaks for different functions of myosins here.

The effects of the action of such 'ratchet' motors in cells depends upon the local cytoarchitecture and the relative abundance of the particular NTP-ase motor protein. Some antibiotics exert their effects by usurping a cell's intrinsic control over the integrity of its actin filaments or its microtubules. For example, the *Vinca* alkaloid vincristine can disrupt microtubules and block cell division, a property exploited in cancer chemotherapy. If the NTP-ase is coupled to a membrane-delimited vesicle (e.g. endocytotic or exocytotic vesicles, mitochondria) or a protein assemblage (as in axoplasmic transport) then this cargo can be shuttled through the cytoplasm towards its destined location. As far as microtubule highways are concerned there exist motors to carry cargo towards either the *minus* end or the *plus* end. Originally a clear-cut story it now is apparent that among the kinesin family there are members which can travel in either direction along microtubules.

When the NTP-ase is anchored to filaments then tension may be generated within the cell by F-actin-based stress fibres and transferred to the extracellular matrix, as in wound healing. During cell division the cytoskeleton disassembles causing cells to round up. The cleavage furrow, newly assembled from cortically anchored overlapping arrays of actin filaments with opposite polarities, is then constricted by the action of myosin II which in turn is thought to be regulated by complex cell cycle events. The motor may play a part in cell protrusive processes (filopodia, ruffles, lamellipodia) by interacting with the re-arranging F-actin cortical networks. In non-muscle cells the functions of cytoplasmic myosin II appear to be limited to cell cleavage, development of cortical tension and re-distribution of ligands bound to the cell surface in a process known as capping. Myosin II is not the motor for crawling cell locomotion, as gene deletion experiments with the slime mould *Dictyostelium* have demonstrated (Manstein et al 1989). The spotlight has now turned on the varied family of mini-myosins, e.g. myosin I (Hammer 1991), as putative force proteins to drive the F-actin cytoskeleton. However, other non-actin based locomotory systems may exist: the amoeboid sperm of nematode worms completes its crawling odyssey along the female tract without the benefit of an actin-based cytoskeleton, the components of which are specifically lost during gamete differentiation, suggesting that other mechanisms of cellular propulsion may be present in the animal kingdom, including perhaps mammals.

Swimming cells, such as sperm, perform work directly on the surrounding fluid by propagating waves along their axonemes; the resultant forces drive the sperm forwards in the bulk liquid phase. Epithelial cilia, in order to sweep mucus across their luminal surface, employ a simpler beat pattern. Each cycle is biphasic and consists of a rigid power stroke followed by a deeply arched recovery stroke. Since this latter is performed close to the epithelial surface within the stationary fluid boundary layer it avoids producing an equal and antagonistic thrust to that of the effector stroke. For both flagella and cilia, beating results from the conversion by locally imposed shear within the axoneme of the fundamental sliding force. This is generated by transient cross-bridge interactions between dynein arms irreversibly bound to the A tubule of the nine outer doublet microtubules and the wall of the B tubule belonging to the adjacent doublet (see also p. 42).

For crawling or amoeboid cells the situation is more complex than axoneme powered motility since locomotion is achieved only at the expense of a constant turnover or re-modelling of the cytoskeleton. Such a flux does indeed occur. The combination of sophisticated interference microscopy and computation has identified vectorial flow of material in the cytoplasm of living fibroblasts at speeds of up to $2 \, \mu m.s^{-1}$ (Brown & Dunn 1989). Motive force generation here is predicated on the actin-based cytoskeleton with its ability to switch rapidly and locally among its repertoire of macromolecular assemblies (e.g. cortical meshworks, filament bundles) and to interact cooperatively with myosin ATP-ases. Less transparent, however, is the fact that in order to progress, such cells need constantly to make and break attachments to their immediate substratum. Without traction the activities of their obvious motile components— pseudopodia, lamella or microspikes erupting anteriorly—would be rendered useless. Visible only by special optical methods are the differentiated points of substratum contact, termed focal adhesions, which mediate traction. This technique (reflection interference microscopy) has revealed points of considerable similarity in the formation and turnover of these substratum anchorage points on glass coverslips by cells as evolutionary distant as amoebae and mammalian fibroblasts.

In metazoan cells focal contacts consist of numerous proteins which integrate F-actin bundles (stress fibres) with cell surface adhesion receptors known as integrins (p. 27). This ensures the integration of the cytoskeleton with the extracellular environment ensuring a physical link between force production, cell protrusion and traction. Wound healing depends in part upon the tension generated by the stress fibres of concerted groups of fibroblasts pulling upon the collagen fibres of the extracellular matrix rather in the manner of the adductor muscles responsible for closing the shells of clams.

So far the biochemical regulatory mechanism(s) responsible for the integration of protrusion and traction remain(s) unknown yet some exciting glimpses are emerging. For some time it was known that there is an evident connection between serum growth factors, small guanine-nucleotide binding proteins (G-proteins) related to the products of the oncogene *Ras*, and actin cytoskeletons. Recent experiments have demonstrated that the molecular link between these extracellular signals and the actin cyto-architecture resides in a cascade of GTP-ases belonging to the *Ras* superfamily (Ridley & Hall 1992; Ridley et al 1992). Activation of one (Rac) at once induces ruffles **and** activates another GTP-binding protein (Rho) which stimulates stress fibre formation.

It has become clear that the diverse nature of the extracellular matrix provides not only a physical substratum for traction but also chemical cues which, in addition to possible soluble chemical messages, convert random walk behaviour into useful, directed locomotion. This is particularly important during embryogenesis. In adults most cells are sedentary, interacting with their neighbours and the extracellular matrix via specific cell surface receptors (Pullman & Bodmer 1992). However release from these restraints as a consequence of viral or chemical transformation may enable a cell to recommence the motile activities of its embryonic forebears (Hynes & Lander 1992) and to undertake cell division outside of normal control processes. Such antisocial behaviour, continuing unchecked, may result ultimately in metastasis and death through cancer. Lymphocytes, however, are professional wanderers constantly scanning the body for foreign invaders. Leaving the blood they move through lymphatic organs and tissues as adherent cells, enter the lymphatics as non-adhesive cells and, finally, return to the blood via the thoracic and right lymphatic duct. This complex migratory process attended by adhesive changes involves three distinct families of adhesion receptors at the cell surface: the immunoglobulin superfamily, the integrins and the selectins (which are important for the interaction of leucocytes with the vascular endothelium Springer 1990). The often fatal congenital leucocyte adhesion deficiency condition is due to a mutation affecting leucocyte integrins. Such compromised cells are unable to emigrate from the blood and thus fail to reach and destroy pathogens in tissues.

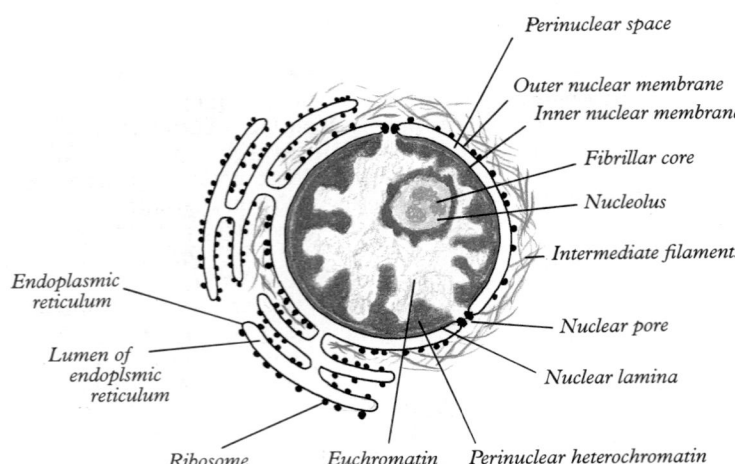

Perinuclear space

Outer nuclear membrane
Inner nuclear membrane

Fibrillar core

Nucleolus

Intermediate filaments

Nuclear pore

Nuclear lamina

Endoplasmic reticulum

Lumen of endoplsmic reticulum

Ribosome   Euchromatin   Perinuclear heterochromatin

2.31 Diagram showing the chief features of a typical nucleus and its relation to the granular endoplasmic reticulum. The nucleus is surrounded by two membranes which constitute the nuclear envelope, perforated by nuclear pores. The outer membrane is continuous with the endoplasmic reticulum, and associated externally with a loose network of cytoplasmic intermediate filaments. The inner nuclear membrane is coated internally by a more dense intermediate filament network of nuclear lamins which, in turn, is associated with dense perinuclear heterochromatin which is transcriptionally inactive. The core of the nucleus is filled with decondensed euchromatin which is active in transcription. Embedded in the euchromatin is the nucleolus which forms a nuclear subcompartment in which transcription of ribosomal RNA occurs.

NUCLEUS

The nucleus is the largest organelle within most eukaryotic cells and is one of the attributes that distinguishes eukaryotic from prokaryotic (e.g. bacterial) cells. It generally has a spherical or ellipsoid shape and, having a diameter of 3–10 μm, it can be observed through the light microscope in living cells in culture. A number of histological stains can be used to identify nuclei in tissue sections; many of these detect molecules that are largely confined to the nucleus such as deoxyribonucleic acid (DNA) and the basic histone proteins.

NUCLEAR ENVELOPE

The nucleus (**2.31**) is surrounded by two layers of membrane, each of which is a lipid bilayer, and which together form the nuclear envelope (**2.32, 33**). The outer membrane layer and the lumen between the two layers are continuous with the rough endoplasmic reticulum. Indeed, like the rough endoplasmic reticulum, the outer membrane of the nuclear envelope has many ribosomes engaged in protein synthesis attached to it. Proteins synthesized on these ribosomes pass

into the space between the two membrane layers which is called the perinuclear space. Intermediate filaments are associated with both the inner (nuclear) and outer (cytoplasmic) surfaces of the nuclear envelope. Within the nucleus these proteins form a dense 'shell' beneath the envelope called the *nuclear lamina* consisting of specialized nuclear forms of intermediate filament called *nuclear lamins*. These cross each other at right-angles to create a meshwork covering the nuclear envelope interior. Between these and the inner nuclear membrane there is another thin filamentous protein layer. The inner nuclear membrane skeleton determines the shape of the nucleus and reinforces its envelope mechanically, and the ends of chromosomes are anchored to the layer of lamins, as seen clearly during meiotic prophase (p. 50). Condensed chromatin (heterochromatin) also tends to aggregate against the nuclear envelope during interphase, presumably reflecting this terminal attachment. At the end of mitotic and meiotic prophase the lamin filaments disassemble, causing the vesiculation of the nuclear membranes, and, at the end of anaphase, the lamins reattach to the chromosomes and create a new nuclear compartment round which the nuclear membranes reform. A network of filamentous proteins, the *nuclear matrix*, is also present throughout the nucleus. The nuclear matrix is associated with newly-replicated DNA and, indeed, is enriched in enzymes of the replication machinery; it is also associated with genes being actively transcribed and may be involved in transcriptional regulation.

Nuclear pores allow transport across the nuclear envelope

The essential role of regulating the transport of molecules between the nucleus and the cytoplasm is performed by specialized nuclear pore structures which perforate the nuclear envelope. These structures act as highly selective, directional molecular filters allowing the entrance to the nucleus by proteins such as histones and gene regulatory proteins, which are synthesized in the cytoplasm but which function in the nucleus. They also permit the exit of molecules synthesized in the nucleus (e.g. ribosomal subunits, transfer RNAs and messenger RNAs) to the cytoplasm.

Under the electron microscope, nuclear pores appear as disc-like structures with an outer diameter of about 100 nm and an inner pore with a diameter of 9 nm (**2.33, 34**). The nuclear envelope of an active cell is crossed by up to 4000 of these structures. The nuclear pore complex has an octagonal symmetry and is constructed by the assembly of approximately 100 protein subunits (*nucleoporins*). The structure of the nuclear pore complex has been determined by computer-aided reconstruction of information from electron-micrographs although some details remain to be settled. The inner and outer nuclear membranes appear to fuse around the pore complex, but transfer of lipids and proteins between the two is prevented, possibly by the luminal subunits of the pore. The complex appears to consist of 3 major components:

- an *outer ring* of eight protein subunits attached to the membrane, with an equal number of spokes converging centrally on an *inner ring* or central plug

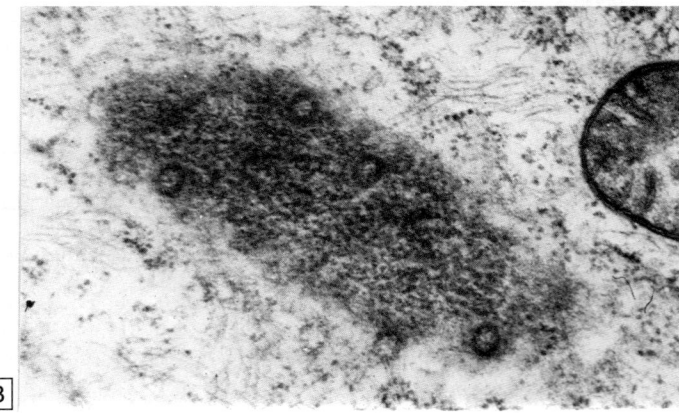

2.32A, B Electron micrograph of the nuclear envelope: A. in transverse section to show inner and outer membranes, and nuclear pores; B. in tangential section to show pore complexes (dense rings). Micrograph (B)

provided by M Dyson of Guy's Hospital Medical School. Magnification × 25 000.

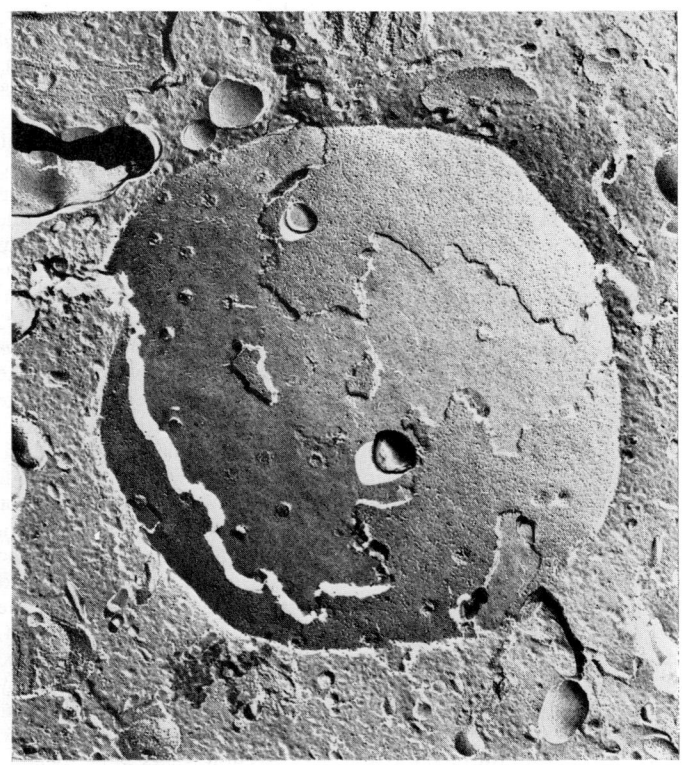

2.33 Freeze-fractured cell in which the fracture plane has passed through the nuclear envelope exposing portions of its two membranes and several nuclear pores. Magnification × 20 000.

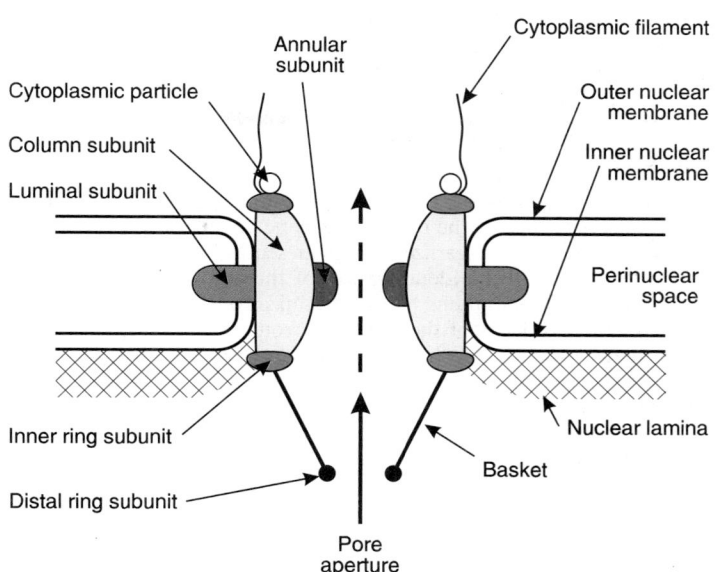

2.34 Diagram showing the structural organization of a nuclear pore. For details, see text.

- eight short filaments which extend from the outer ring outwards into the cytoplasm
- another set of eight filaments reaching inwards towards the interior of the nucleus, converging onto another, *distal ring* thus forming a truncated cone (**2.34**).

For further details, see Forbes 1992, Fabre and Hurt 1994. Note also, similarly arranged structures: *annulate lamellae* present in some cells (p. 122).

The pore is freely permeable to small molecules, ions and proteins up to about 17 kDa. Proteins of up to 60 kDa seem to be able to equilibrate slowly between the nucleus and cytoplasm across the pore but larger proteins are normally excluded. However, certain proteins are selectively transported into the nucleus and some of these, such as the DNA polymerases, are very large indeed. Proteins that are selectively transported into the nucleus possess a nuclear localization signal within their amino acid sequences. These signals are recognized by cytoplasmic proteins which facilitate the 'docking' of translocated proteins with the cytoplasmic surface of the pore. The amino acid sequences of nuclear localization signals vary considerably between different proteins, suggesting that there may be a large number of cytoplasmic proteins able to recognize them and bring them to the pore. Generally, nuclear localization signals are small, about 4 to 8 amino acids long, and contain a high proportion of the basic amino acids, arginine and lysine, and frequently proline residues also. Cytoplasmic proteins passively direct those proteins carrying a nuclear localization signal to the pore but translocation into the nucleus is energy dependent; that is, it requires the hydrolysis of ATP. In the absence of ATP or at low temperatures which do not allow its hydrolysis, prospective nuclear proteins accumulate at the pores but do not enter the nucleus. The ability of some proteins to enter the nucleus is further regulated by modifications or associations in the cytoplasm of the cell. For example, some gene regulatory proteins cannot enter the nucleus until they have been phosphorylated in the cytoplasm and this generally occurs in response to signals from outside the cell. Alternatively, steroid hormone receptors, which are gene regulatory proteins, associate with the cytoskeleton until they bind hormone molecules, whereupon they dissociate from the cytoskeleton and can be transported into the nucleus.

Transport also occurs from the nucleus to the cytoplasm. In particular, RNAs synthesized in the nucleus are transported through nuclear pores into the cytoplasm. There is a directionality to this process since labelled RNA injected into the nucleus will enter the cytoplasm, but if injected into the cytoplasm it does not enter the nucleus. However, the nature of the regulation of this directional transport is not understood.

Nuclear lamina

The nuclear lamina is a dense network of intermediate filament proteins which lines the inner nuclear membrane and provides a connecting link between the membrane and the nuclear heterochromatin. The nuclear lamina is typically about 30 nm thick and is constructed mainly from the association of 10 nm diameter filaments of a specialized class of intermediate filament proteins called nuclear lamins. Three lamin proteins have been identified, lamins A, B and C, but all arise from a single lamin gene through alternative splicing. Lamin B interacts directly with a receptor protein of 58 kDa embedded in the inner nuclear membrane. Lamins A and C do not associate with this receptor but instead bind to each other and to lamin B to form the dense meshwork of the nuclear lamina. The lamins also interact with proteins of the heterochromatin matrix, although the nature of these associations is not well understood. For further details, see Georgatos et al, 1994.

Regulation of the nuclear envelope and nuclear lamina during cell division

During early prophase of mitosis the nuclear envelope and its associated structures break down to allow the condensing chromosomes to assemble on the mitotic spindle and ultimately to separate. At the end of mitosis (telophase) nuclear envelopes must reform around the two daughter sets of chromosomes. In prophase the nuclear lamina breaks down and the nuclear envelope becomes dissociated into small vesicles which remain associated with the endoplasmic reticulum during the rest of mitosis. The breakdown of the nuclear lamina is triggered by the phosphorylation of the lamin proteins on serine residues which causes them to dissociate from one another. Lamins A and C become dispersed throughout the cytoplasm during cell division but lamin B remains bound to its receptor on the vesicular remnants of the nuclear envelope. A key regulatory enzyme of the cell cycle called M-phase promoting factor (MPF) which triggers the entry into prophase of mitosis also phosphorylates the lamins. The proteins of the nuclear pore complexes also seem to be disrupted during prophase.

The decondensation of chromosomes during telophase seems to act as a trigger for the reassembly of the nuclear envelope. The nuclear envelope vesicles fuse with one another and pore complexes are reformed. At the same time, serine phosphatase enzymes dephosphorylate the lamins allowing the nuclear lamina to reform.

HISTORICAL BACKGROUND OF MOLECULAR GENETICS

The nucleus contains the inheritable material (genetic code) which directs the activities of the cell. The genetic code is carried by DNA molecules which are organized in linear sequences in chromosomes inside the nucleus. The identification of the genetic material of the cell and the understanding of its organization and activity is the result of the synthesis of data derived from two separate branches of biological science: biochemistry and genetics. The recognition of DNA as the genetic material has a history which spans almost one hundred years, dating from the characterization of nucleic acids, of which DNA was probably the major component, from extracts of the nuclei of dead white blood cells by Friedrich Miescher in 1860s (Miescher 1871). However, half a century would pass before further biochemical analysis of the structure of DNA was performed, a large step in its determination as the genetic substance. In the intervening period, geneticists and cell biologists made the major contributions. These were underpinned by the momentous findings of Gregor Mendel. By studying genetic crosses between inbred strains of the garden pea, he discovered that certain characteristics, for example seed coat colour, were dominant if present in either of the parent plants; that is, they would appear in all of the offspring. Those characteristics that were masked by a dominant trait were called recessive. Mendel found that in a cross between inbred strains of pea in which one parent exhibited dominant and the other recessive characteristics for a particular feature, all of the first generation of offspring would show the dominant character. However, if the first generation offspring were then mated amongst themselves one quarter of their progeny had the recessive character. Mendel concluded that this would only be possible if each parent had two copies of the heritable unit (subsequently celled genes by Wilhelm Johannsen in 1909) for the trait and that each offspring inherited one unit from each parent. This could happen only if there was a segregation during gametogenesis such that each gamete only carried one unit. These conclusions are now known as Mendel's first law. In addition, Mendel showed that different traits such as seed colour and seed shape could be inherited independently of one another (independent assortment) and this became known as Mendel's second law. Although these remarkable experiments and the conclusions drawn from them were reported in 1865, it was not until 1900 that they were rediscovered and their significance realized.

During the late 1800s chromosomes were described by cytologists using the light microscope to study cells undergoing division. At the end of the division process it was found that the number of chromosomes present was identical in cells from the same species. Moreover, for a given species, individual chromosomes could be distinguished by their morphology (overall size, size of their arms, appearance after staining with histological dyes) and that each cell had two chromosomes of each morphological type. Prior to cell division each chromosome is copied (replicated) and the two copies called chromatids remain joined together at a single point called the centromere. Schneider and, subsequently, Flemming observed that during division (mitosis) the two sister chromatids divide longitudinally and are pulled apart. Later, Van Beneden reported that both daughter cells inherit one of each chromatid pair. In 1903, Walter Sutton made the crucial discovery that, in contrast to mitosis, during gametogenesis (meiosis) each gamete only inherits one chromosome of each morphological type. Thus the total chromosome number of the gamete (haploid chromosome number) is half that of a somatic cell (diploid chromosome number). Sutton proposed that the halving of chromosome numbers during meiosis could account for the distribution of traits described by Mendel in his first law. A simple prediction following from the idea that chromosomes might contain the Mendelian units of heredity (genes), is that genes located on the same chromosome should segregate together, i.e. should be inherited together in the progeny of a particular mating. This was first confirmed by the geneticist Thomas Hunt Morgan in 1909 by crossing strains of the fruit fly, *Drosophila melanogaster*. He found that in this animal the genes tend to segregate as four groups called

linkage groups. This correlated precisely with the presence of four visible chromosome pairs in the fruit fly; the correspondence of linkage group number and the number of chromosome pairs was subsequently confirmed by other workers for a variety of organisms including the Mendel's analytical subject *Pisum*, the pea plant.

What was the nature of the heritable information carried by the genes? The initial finding of relevance to this problem was reported by Archibald Garrod in 1909 who first linked the genetic information with protein function. Garrod determined that the human heritable disease alkaptonuria was the result of a rare recessive mutation which was inherited according to Mendelian rules. He proposed that the condition was due to an abnormality in an enzyme involved in the breakdown of the phenolic ring structure of the amino acids phenylalanine and tyrosine. It is now known that this hypothesis is correct; alkaptonuria is due to a mutation in the gene encoding the metabolic enzyme homogenistic acid oxidase. Further support came from studies in the fruit fly, the favoured tool of geneticists, in which genes which determine eye colour have been particularly well studied. Grafting experiments performed by Beadle and Ephrussi (1937) put eye tissue from the larvae of flies with light coloured 'vermilion' or 'cinnabar' eyes into normal (wild-type) larvae which develop with a darker red eye colour. They found that the grafted eyes adopted the darker colour characteristic of the host eye tissue and concluded that a metabolic product(s) of the host tissue had facilitated the development of normal pigmentation in the graft. By contrast, grafts between the two mutant strains did not adopt the wild-type coloration. They again proposed a connection between gene activity and metabolism; it has subsequently been found that the cinnabar and vermilion mutations are due to defects in enzymes which produce the red pigmentation of the fruit fly eye. A few years later, Beadle, together with Edward Tatum (1941), concluded from their studies of mutants of the mould *Neurospora crassa*, only able to grow with amino acid or vitamin supplements, that 'each gene controls the reproduction, specificity and function of a particular enzyme' (Tatum 1959). We now know that genes do indeed encode the amino acid sequence (primary structure) of proteins and, although not all proteins have enzymatic activities, genes thereby control the functions of their protein products.

The first demonstration that DNA is the genetic material of most organisms was achieved by Avery, MacLeod and McCarty in 1944 when they showed that purified DNA from a 'smooth' capsuled Streptococcus could transform a 'rough' strain to the smooth phenotype. The enzyme DNase, which degrades DNA, inhibited this process. Subsequently, Hershey and Chase found that only the DNA component of a bacterial virus entered its bacterium host, yet could direct the synthesis of new virus proteins and the assembly of viral particles. These two studies established that the DNA component of chromosomes was the genetic material. The structure of DNA was finally elucidated by Watson and Crick (1952) who deduced that it had a double-helical structure established by a precise base pairing of guanine with cytosine and thymine with adenine. This self-complementary structure immediately suggested a mechanism by which DNA could be replicated and how the information in DNA could be transcribed into ribonucleic acid (RNA). In the early 1960s the mechanism by which the genetic material is decoded was determined. Messenger RNA (mRNA) was discovered to be the intermediate between the genomic DNA and protein synthesis, and the genetic code by which units of three nucleotides (codons) specify a particular amino acid through a transfer RNA (tRNA) intermediate was unlocked. These discoveries underpinned the present era of molecular biology, and facilitated the analysis of the organization and regulation of the genetic material which is described below. For general reviews, see Lewis (1990), Lodish and Darnell (1990).

STRUCTURE OF DNA

Nearly all of the genetic material of eukaryotic cells is sequestered in the nucleus, the exceptions being certain other organelles such as mitochondria and the chloroplasts of plants which contain some DNA themselves (p. 34). The structure of the DNA molecule as discovered by Watson and Crick comprises two polynucleotide strands that are oriented in opposite directions, that is they are antiparallel (2.35). Each strand is a polymer of the four nucleotides: the purines—adenine and guanine—and the pyrimidines—cytosine and

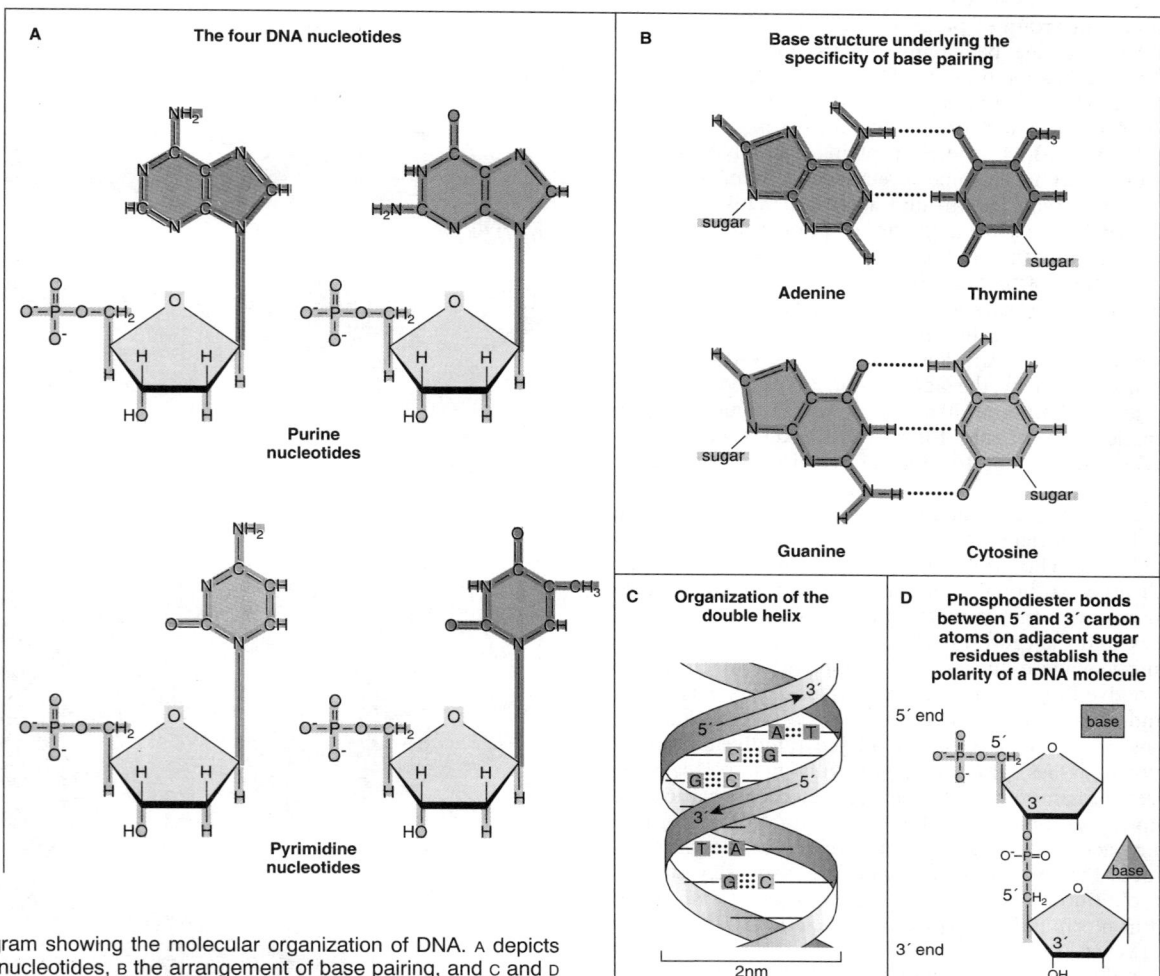

2.35A–D Diagram showing the molecular organization of DNA. A depicts the four deoxynucleotides, B the arrangement of base pairing, and C and D the construction of the DNA double helix.

thymine (**2.35A**, B). The nucleotides are held together by phosphodiester bonds which link the 5' carbon atom of the deoxyribose sugar to the 3' carbon of the next and this gives each DNA strand its polarity (**2.35D**). The two strands are held together by specific base-pairing interactions (guanine binds to cytosine and adenine to thymine) which involve both hydrogen bonds and Van der Waal's forces (**2.35B**). Therefore, every genome has an equal number of guanine and cytosine residues and an equal number of thymine and adenine residues and each strand is complementary in nucleotide sequence to its partner. The two chains together form a helical structure 2 nm in diameter with 3.4 nm between turns.

The structure of the DNA molecule immediately suggested a mechanism by which the genetic material could be replicated and passed between generations. Since each strand is complementary to the other, if the two strands are separated, each can serve as a template to make a new DNA strand which is identical to its original partner. This is indeed the process which occurs during DNA replication, with local separation of the two strands allowing DNA polymerases to synthesize DNA strands complementary to the two templates. This results in each of the parent strands being partnered by a newly-synthesized and complementary daughter molecule; this form of replication is called *semi-conservative replication*.

STRUCTURE OF EUKARYOTIC CHROMOSOMES

Organization of chromosomal DNA

The nuclear DNA of eukaryotic cells is organized into linear units called chromosomes. The DNA in a normal human diploid cell contains 6×10^9 nucleotide pairs which are organized in the form of 46 chromosomes (44 autosomes and 2 sex chromosomes). The largest human chromosome (number 1) contains approximately 2.5×10^8

nucleotide pairs and the smallest (the Y chromosome) about 5×10^7 nucleotide pairs. Each chromosomal DNA molecule contains a number of specialized nucleotide sequences which are associated with its replication and maintenance. Arranged along the length of the DNA molecule are a number of specific initiation sites for DNA synthesis during chromosomal replication called *replication origins*. There are many of these along each DNA molecule; during DNA replication they are not all used simultaneously but rather initiate synthesis in an ordered and sequential fashion. This suggests that there may be some differences amongst them.

Each DNA molecule contains a single *centromere region* through which the condensed chromosomal DNA associates with the mitotic spindle during mitosis (p. 58). During mitosis a discoidal structure called the *kinetochore*, composed of a complex array of proteins, associates with the centromeric region of DNA to attach it to the microtubular spindle. A third specialized type of nucleotide sequence defines the end of each chromosomal DNA molecule; these regions are enriched in guanosine and cytosine nucleotides and are called *telomeres*. They are not synthesized by the same DNA polymerase as the rest of the chromosome but by a specialized enzyme called telomerase which also folds the telomere into a specialized structure. The function of the telomere is to provide a template for priming the replication of the 'lagging' strand during DNA synthesis (see later) without which the terminal sequences of the chromosome would be progressively lost.

Chromatin

DNA is organized in chromosomes by a heterogeneous set of proteins to form a DNA-protein complex which is called *chromatin*. The protein constituents of chromatin are the *histones* and the *non-histone proteins*. The latter group of proteins is extremely heterogeneous and includes DNA and RNA polymerases, gene regulatory proteins and high-mobility group proteins (HMG proteins). However, the histones are the most abundant group of proteins in chromatin and they are primarily responsible for the 'packaging' of chromosomal DNA (see below). There are five histone proteins: H1, H2A, H2B, H3 and H4, and the last four of these combine to form a compact granule, the *nucleosome core*. A nucleosome core is a histone octomer comprising two each of the H2A, H2B, H3 and H4 proteins. The DNA molecule winds twice around each nucleosome core in such a manner that 146 nucleotide pairs are organized around it (**2.36**). This packaging organizes the DNA into a chromatin fibre 11 nm in diameter and gives this form of chromatin the appearance of 'beads-on-a-string' in electron micrographs, with each 'bead' separated by a length of DNA about 50 nucleotide pairs long. When chromatin is arranged with the string of beads fully extended it is termed euchromatin and in this condition it is actively transcribed to form RNA. Chromatin can also be highly folded by the aggregation of nucleosomes into spiral clusters (solenoids) about 30 nm thick rather than the 11 nm of the euchromatic form, or may form even thicker super-clusters. This is achieved by the binding together of H1 histones of adjacent nucleosomes.

The heterochromatin is characteristically located mainly around the periphery of the nucleus, except over the nuclear pores, and around the nucleolus. The two forms of chromatin can generally convert to each other, although some may be permanently hetero-chromatic, for example the inactive one of the two X chromo-somes in females, and the central part of each chromosome where it binds to the mitotic spindle during cell division (the centromere). In cells which are active in transcription the nucleus is typically rich in euchromatin and usually relatively large (an open face nucleus, e.g. in most neurons, many stem cells, and in the rapidly multiplying cells of embryonic tissues). In transcriptionally inactive cells the chromatin is predominantly in the condensed, heterochromatic state, and may comprise as much as 90% of the total. Examples of these are mature neutrophil leucocytes where the condensation of chromatin induces the formation of a multilobed densely staining nucleus, and in old fibrocytes. Extremely heterochromatic nuclei are also often seen in moribund cells (pyknotic nuclei). In most mature active cells, however, there is a more even mixture of the two, indicating that only a relatively small proportion of the DNA is being transcribed. A striking instance of this is seen in the mature B lymphocyte (plasmacyte) where much of the chromatin is in the condensed condition, arranged in regular masses around the per-imeter of the nucleus (**2.5**); although this cell is actively transcribing, most of its protein is of a single immunoglobulin type, so that much of its genome is in an inactive state.

The positioning of the nucleosomes on actively transcribed DNA is influenced by other DNA-binding proteins and also by the nucleotide sequence of the DNA itself. DNA sequences that are rich in adenosine and thymine bases are more easily folded around nucleosomes because they are more easily compressed. Nucleosomes are also frequently absent from the regulatory regions of genes (see below) as these regions have gene regulatory proteins associated with them which exclude the nucleosomes.

During mitosis the chromatin must be further condensed to form the familiar short chromosomes of the metaphase stage of division (p. 58). This shortening is achieved through four levels of close-packing of the chromatin. The euchromatin is organized by histone H1 into the coiled 'solenoid' of 30 nm diameter associated with heterochromatin and this structure is formed into loops of 300 nm diameter by another set of fibrillar *scaffold proteins*. In this state the chromatin is not transcriptionally active. The 300 nm loops are then themselves arranged in a helical structure 700 nm in diameter which is further condensed to produce the familiar mitotic chromosome structure of about 1.4 μm diameter. Overall this progressive folding of the chromosomal DNA by interactions with specific proteins can reduce approximately 5 cm of chromosomal DNA to a length of about 5 μm.

STRUCTURE AND REGULATION OF EUKARYOTIC GENES

The genetic information of the cell is expressed through an inter-mediate molecule, RNA, which in turn is translated into protein. RNA is copied from one strand of the DNA molecule by an RNA

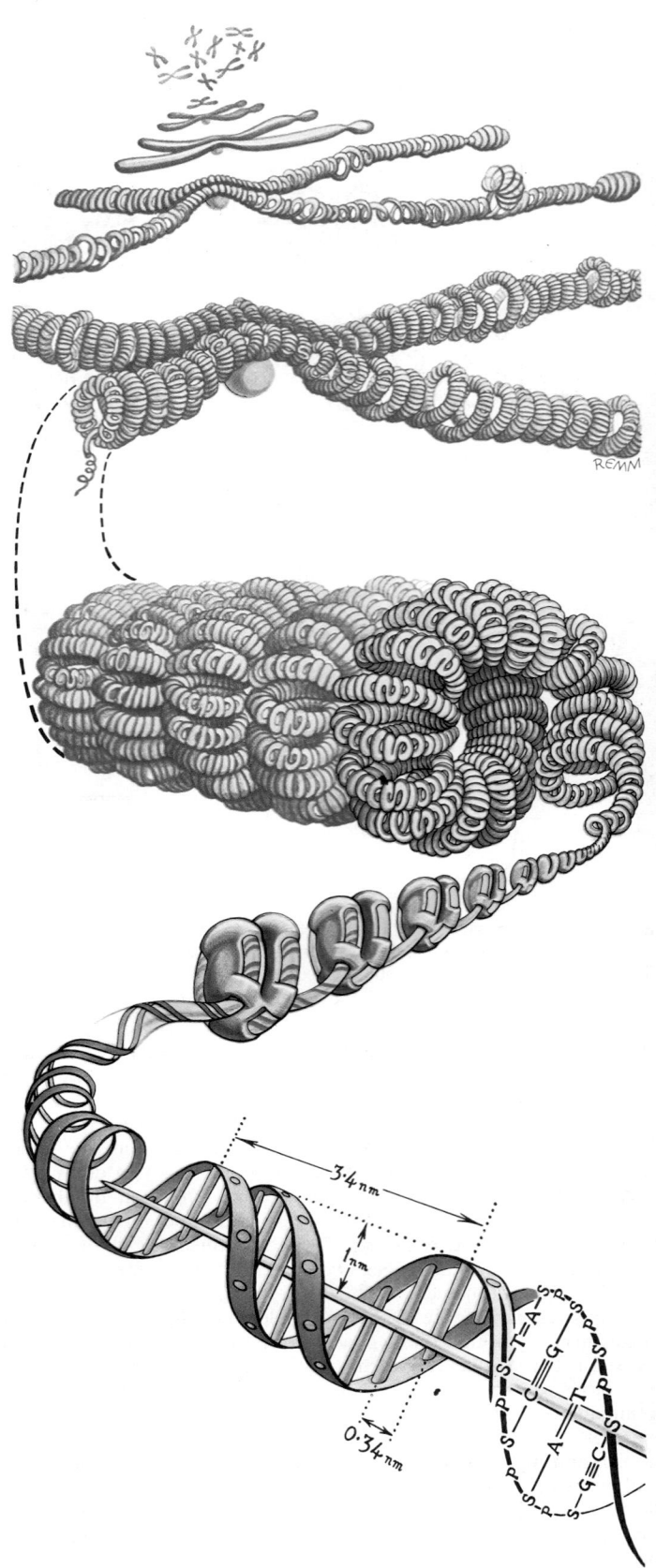

2.36 A possible model for the organization of DNA and protein in chro-mosomes during early metaphase in mitosis. Each chromosome consists of two chromatids united at the primary constriction where the centromere is also sited. In the exposed region of the DNA molecule, the chemical groups of the 'backbone' of each helix—S (sugar) P (phosphate)—and the bases—A (adenine), T (thymine), C (cytosine) and G (guanine)—are represented. Several nucleosomes are also depicted (see text). The 'coiled-coil' configuration of chromosomal DNA is represented only schematically and does not indicate the 'loop and backbone' arrangement which is thought to typify the metaphase chromosomes.

polymerase and thus is complementary to that strand. Like DNA, RNA is a linear polynucleotide sequence but differs from DNA in that the sugar residue of each nucleotide is ribose instead of deoxyribose, and the base uracil replaces thymine. Those RNA molecules that encode proteins are called *messenger RNAs* or *mRNAs*. Other RNAs include ribosomal RNAs (rRNAs) and transfer RNAs (tRNAs) that are involved in translation of proteins and small nuclear RNAs (snRNAs) which are involved in RNA splicing. The synthesis of a particular RNA is regulated by gene-regulatory proteins which interact with RNA polymerases. Such factors bind to specific sequences (regulatory sequences) at either end of or within the region of DNA encoding the transcribed RNA. A useful operational definition of what constitutes a gene is that a gene is a unit of transcription which includes the region of DNA from which the RNA is transcribed, with all of the regulatory sequences flanking it.

The protein-coding sequences of a particular gene are not continuous but are interrupted by non-coding regions called *introns*. These are present in the newly synthesized mRNA transcript but are removed in the nucleus by a process called *RNA splicing* to form the mature mRNA. This is further modified by 'capping' and frequently by 'polyadenylation' and sometimes its nucleotide composition is altered selectively (*editing*). A mature RNA transcript comprises a continuous region coding for protein, generally flanked by 'upstream' (5') and 'downstream' (3') non-coding sequences; the whole length represents the regions remaining after splicing-out of the introns and these are encoded by regions of the DNA called *exons*.

The mRNA is exported to the cytoplasm where it is *translated* by ribosomes into a linear sequence of amino acids, thereby forming a polypeptide chain. Each mRNA can be translated more than one thousand times, resulting in a considerable amplification during this step. The RNA carries a faithful transcript of the coding sequences of the gene. Amino acids are encoded by groups of three nucleotides, called *codons*. Each codon is also recognised by a specific tRNA, binding to it and carrying a particular amino acid from the cytosol, for example, the sequence AUG on the mRNA specifies the incorporation of methionine, and UAU specifies tyrosine; this is the *triplet code*. The complementary base triplet of the tRNA is termed an *anticodon*. Some codons do not specify the incorporation of an amino acid; these are called *stop codons* (UAA, UAG, UGA) because they result in the termination of protein synthesis and thus specify the position of the end of the protein. Proteins are frequently subject to further (*post-translational*) modification such as the addition of side chains, for example phosphate or sugar residues or cleavage by proteases.

2.37 illustrates the process of gene expression for a typical eukaryotic protein, and the levels at which it can be regulated. There is now considerable evidence that the expression of the product of a particular gene can be regulated during all of the steps between the initiation of transcription and the modification of its protein product. These events are described in detail below.

Structure and transcriptional regulation of protein-encoding eukaryotic genes

The structure of a hypothetical eukaryotic (i.e. non-bacterial) gene which encodes a protein is depicted in **2.**38 together with regulatory proteins involved in its transcription. Eukaryotic genes are transcribed by three RNA polymerases and each is associated with genes having a particular type of organization. RNA polymerase I only transcribes rRNA, polymerase II transcribes mRNAs and polymerase III transcribes tRNAs and some repetitive sequences in the genome. These RNA polymerases are all high molecular weight multiprotein complexes. Transcription of mRNA sequences begins when RNA polymerase II binds to a specific DNA sequence called the *promoter*. This causes the DNA helix to open up in the region of the promoter, allowing the polymerase access to the DNA strand which is complementary to the future mRNA sequence, and, therefore, serves as a template for it. The binding of the polymerase to the promoter sequence involves several associated proteins. The first of these, *transcription factor* (*TF*) *IID*, actually recognizes the promoter; this then associates with several other proteins including RNA polymerase II to form a complex. One of the accessory proteins phosphorylates the polymerase and this is thought to allow transcription to begin. In many genes the promoter region contains the nucleotide sequence TATA while in others it may be rich in guanosine and cytosine residues. Transcription is initiated about 30

nucleotides downstream of the promoter sequence, and continues until the polymerase complex dissociates from the DNA template at the transcription termination site to complete the primary mRNA transcript. The promoter determines the basal rate of transcription of a gene. RNA polymerase II synthesizes mRNA at a rate of about 30 nucleotides per second and RNA polymerase II molecules involved in the process of transcription can be observed by electron microscopy as dense granules. For many genes it seems that only one polymerase complex is present on a gene at a particular time; however, sometimes several complexes are seen on a gene, indicating that different genes are transcribed at different rates.

The rate of transcription is regulated by two mechanisms. The first is the accessibility of the gene to the proteins of the transcriptional machinery, that is, its organization in the chromatin, and the second is the availability of the gene regulatory proteins that control its expression. DNA regions undergoing active transcription are organized into the extended 11 nm diameter nucleosomal configuration that is characteristic of euchromatin and referred to as *active chromatin*. It is believed that the more condensed forms of chromatin do not allow polymerases and regulatory proteins access to the genes. The process by which DNA is converted from a condensed form to the less dense active form is not well understood. There is evidence that active chromatin may extend from the condensed chromatin as a loop, suggesting that specific DNA-protein interactions may identify and regulate the formation of such decondensed regions. These DNA regions may regulate the expression of a group of genes that are clustered adjacent to one another on the chromosome and become extended on the same loop. One such DNA element, the *locus control region*, appears to regulate the accessibility of the globin gene cluster for transcription in erythrocyte progenitor cells.

Gene regulatory proteins also influence gene expression. These proteins are frequently present in only a few copies per nucleus and in order to be able to find their target genes, their location in the nuclear matrix is likely to be precisely determined. A large number of these factors have now been identified; well-known examples include FOS, MYC, JUN, homeobox-containing proteins and 'zinc finger' proteins. Each gene regulatory protein binds to a specific DNA sequence that is generally between 6 and 10 nucleotides in length and such elements are called *enhancers*. Enhancers can perform two regulatory functions. The first is to confer cell type-specificity to the expression of a gene and the second is to regulate the rate of transcription. Enhancers can function to regulate the expression of a gene even when quite distantly removed from its promoter and they can be located before a transcription unit (upstream), after the transcription termination signal (downstream) or even within introns. The activity of some enhancer elements is absolutely required for transcription of a gene and their differential regulation can be mediated by the presence or absence of their associated gene regulatory proteins in different cell types. Different genes have multiple different associated enhancer elements but genes expressed in the same cell type (e.g. acetylcholine receptor and muscle myosin in muscle cells) often have the same enhancer elements associated with them. Enhancer elements also influence the rate of gene transcription, that is the number of RNA polymerase II molecules actively transcribing the gene at any one time. Most enhancers increase the rate of transcription of a gene, but some, called *repressors*, can downregulate expression or abolish it altogether. It is not clear precisely how the interaction of regulatory proteins with enhancer elements influences gene expression. It may be that the binding of the regulatory protein to its enhancer alters the local configuration of the chromatin, increasing the accessibility of the promoter elements to the polymerase II complex. Alternatively, perhaps the chromatin is folded to allow a direct interaction between the gene regulatory protein and the polymerase complex. Regulatory proteins appear to be able to associate with enhancer elements that are associated with nucleosomes and subsequently displace the nucleosome. By contrast, the factors associated with the formation of the polymerase II complex on the promoter cannot assemble on a promoter that is associated with a nucleosome, so it seems likely that one mechanism by which gene regulatory proteins and enhancer elements function is to displace nucleosomes from promoter sequences to allow the polymerase complex access (see Croston & Kadonga 1993).

In summary, the control region of a typical eukaryotic gene comprises:

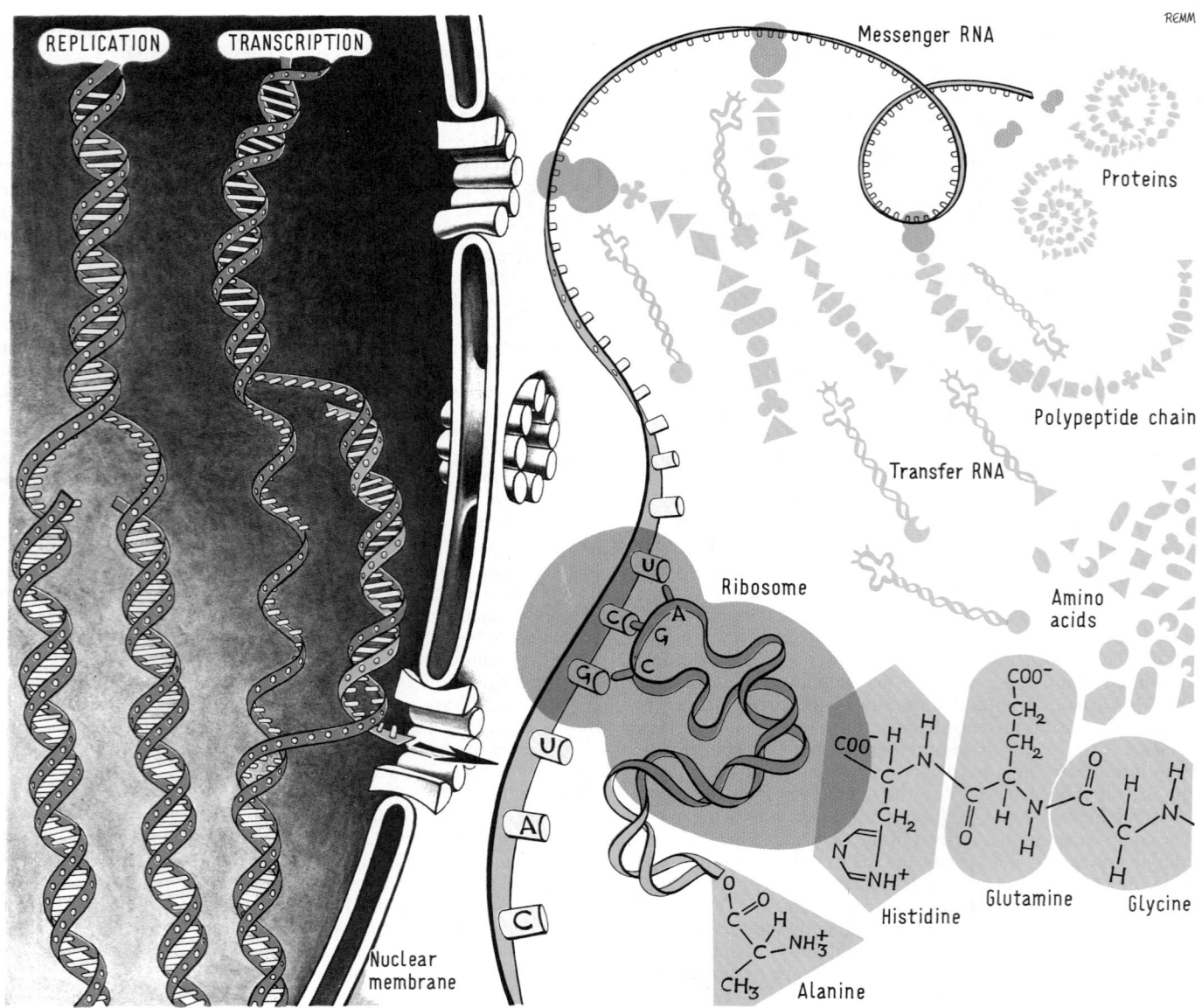

2.37A Schema showing the relation between DNA replication and DNA transcription (mRNA formation) leading to protein synthesis (right). For clarity, this simple schema omits RNA splicing, capping and polyadenylation and various other processes occurring during these events, as outlined in **2.37B**. Abbreviations of RNA bases: C—cytosine, G—guanine, U—uridine.

- a promoter to specify the transcription start site and confer the basal rate of transcription
- a number of enhancer elements which regulate transcription.

The accessibility of the gene regulatory sequences is determined by the configuration of the chromatin.

Regulation and processing of mRNA

The primary mRNA transcript generated from DNA by transcription is subsequently modified at both of its ends. The first modification is at the 5' end of the transcript, the end from which the RNA is synthesized, and this involves the addition of methylguanine 'cap'. This takes place soon after RNA synthesis has started, after only 20–30 nucleotides have been added to the extending nascent transcript. By contrast to the normal 5'–3' nucleotide bonding in RNA molecules the methylguanine cap is joined to the transcript by a 5'–5' linkage. The cap seems to play a role in the subsequent translation of the mRNA and also protects the transcript from degradation.

Most mRNAs have a poly(A) tail added to their 3' end. This tail is not added at the site at which transcription halts but at a specific cleavage site in the transcript, specified by the sequence AAUAAA, and occurs about 20 nucleotides downstream of it. Cleavage is followed by the addition of about 200 adenylic acid residues to the new 3' end of the transcript. The poly(A) tail appears to function to stabilize the mRNA, preventing its degradation, to facilitate its export through nuclear pores to the cytoplasm and to facilitate efficient translation. The poly(A) tail may influence RNA stability through its progressive shortening. The poly(A) tails of most cytoplasmic mRNAs gradually shorten with time until they reach about 30 residues when the mRNAs themselves disappear. This suggests that the loss of the tail suddenly exposes the RNA to RNase enzymes which degrade the transcript. It is noteworthy that short-lived transcripts exhibit accelerated rates of poly(A) loss.

Following transcription, introns are removed from the primary transcript by RNA splicing. This occurs in the nucleus, prior to export of the transcript to the cytoplasm. Introns themselves can vary in size between about 100 and 15 000 nucleotides. However, all introns have conserved sequences at either end which direct the splicing process (**2.39**). These comprise a 5' splice or donor site and a 3' splice or acceptor site. The mechanism by which introns are precisely excised is known; it involves the assembly of a multimolecular complex called the *spliceosome* on the intron sequences and the hydrolysis of ATP to provide energy. The spliceosome comprises several small nuclear ribonucleoprotein complexes (snRNPs). The first two of these, the U1 snRNP and U2 snRNP,

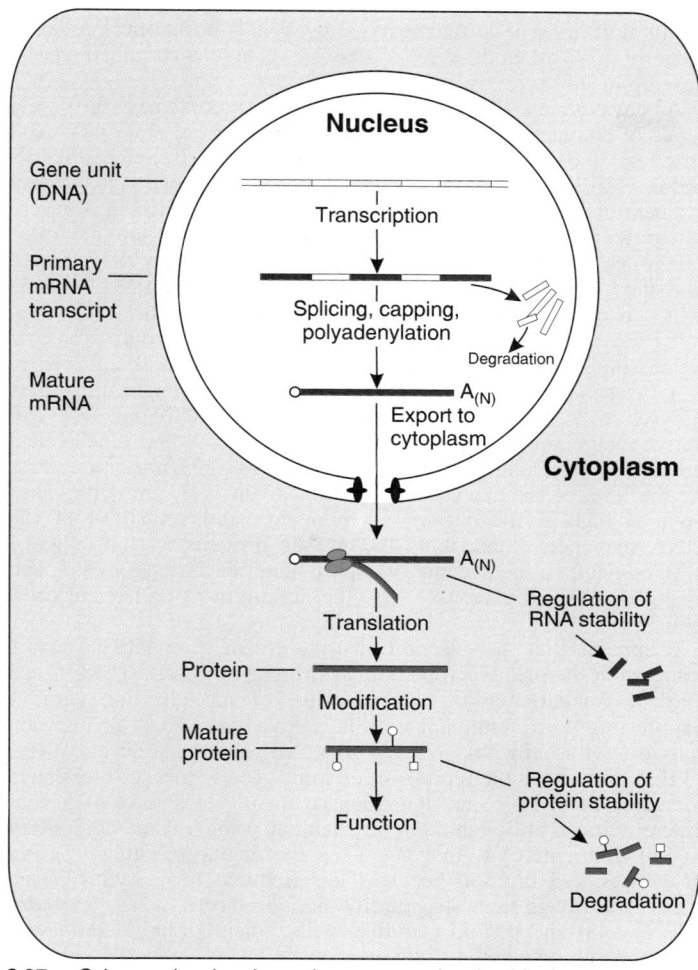

2.37B Schema showing the main processes involved in the production of protein from its encoding gene in the eukaryotic cell. Note that potentially regulation can occur at every step in this process.

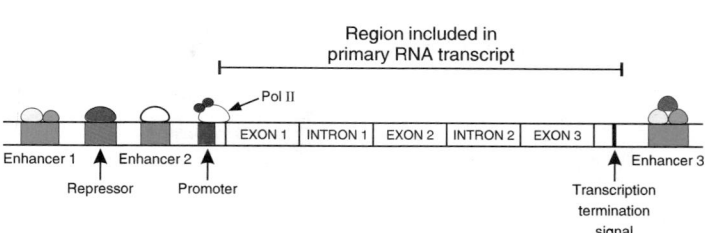

2.38 The structure of a typical eukaryotic gene transcribed by RNA polymerase II. The region included in the primary RNA transcript is indicated and includes three exons and two intron sequences. Transcription is initiated by a multiprotein complex including RNA polymerase II which binds to a specific sequence called the promotor which is located just upstream of the initiation site for transcription. Transcription is terminated at sequences downstream of exon 3 by the polymerase detaching from the DNA. Flanking the gene are a number of regulatory regions (enhancer and repressor elements) which influence the rate of gene transcription and can also inhibit or promote transcription in a tissue-specific manner. These function by binding specific gene regulatory proteins which regulate the association of the RNA polymerase II complex with the promotor.

assemble on the 5' donor site and the 'lariat' branch point within the intron respectively (see **2.39**). The binding of further RNPs brings the donor site and the branch site together and the 'A' residue at the branch site attacks and cleaves the donor splice site. The result of this is that the 5' end of the intron becomes covalently joined to the branch site A residue to form a lariat-like structure. The free 3' end of the upstream exon then attacks the splice acceptor site, cleaving it and ligating to the 5' end of the downstream exon. The spliceosome/intron complex is released and the intron is subsequently degraded. The removal of all of the introns from a precursor RNA seems to be required before the transcript can translocate to the cytoplasm through a nuclear pore.

RNA splicing can also alter the sequence of the protein encoded by a transcript, by specifically removing exons together with the introns flanking them. This process, called *alternative splicing*, frequently generates different protein isoforms in different cell types all of which are encoded by the same gene. Alternative splicing occurs in a highly regulated manner with repressor proteins preventing splicing at certain sites and activator proteins directing the splicing machinery to other splice sites.

As mentioned above, cytoplasmic mRNAs are subject to degradation by coexisting ribonucleases and the poly(A) tails seem to play a role in regulating this process. It has been observed that the transcripts of certain genes only exist in the cytoplasm for a few minutes whereas others are stable for more than a day. It has recently been shown that the sequence UAAAU is repeated several times in the 3' non-coding sequences of many short-lived mRNAs. This sequence may regulate the rapid loss of the poly(A) tails of such mRNAs. By contrast, the transferrin receptor transcript exhibits a different mode of regulation. It has binding sites in its 3' non-coding region for an iron-sensitive protein. Under conditions of low cytoplasmic iron concentration the protein is bound to the transferrin

mRNA and the transcript is stabilized. However, when iron levels are increased the protein dissociates from the mRNA and the latter is rapidly degraded. For a review of splicing, see Newman (1994).

Regulation of protein synthesis and stability

The translation of mRNA to form proteins occurs in the cytoplasm and is performed by ribosomes which are found either in the cytoplasm associated with the cytoskeleton or associated with the membranes of the endoplasmic reticulum and nucleus. Each ribosome comprises a small (40S) subunit and a large (60S) subunit. The 40S subunit contains an 18S rRNA molecule and about 30 proteins whereas the 60S subunit contains 28S, 5.8S and 5S rRNAs and about 50 proteins (see p. 30). The first translated codon of most proteins is AUG, which encodes a methionine amino acid, although CUG is sometimes used, a methionine still being the first residue incorporated. The 40S ribosome subunit first associates with the 5' cap of the mRNA and then scans along the mRNA for the first AUG (methionine) codon at which it may initiate protein synthesis. The choice of whether or not to initiate synthesis at this methionine depends on the nucleotide sequences around it. If the sequence is unfavourable the subunit scans further downstream to identify a suitable initiation site. The initiation of protein synthesis is regulated by a protein called *elongation initiation factor (eIF-2)*. In its active form this protein is in a complex with GTP and facilitates the binding of the first tRNA, methionyl initiator tRNA, to the 40S subunit. When this eIF-2/GTP/tRNA/40S complex binds to an appropriate AUG the GTP is hydrolyzed to GDP and the eIF-2 molecule dissociates from the complex allowing the 60S ribosomal complex to associate with its 40S partner and protein synthesis to occur.

Translation can also be regulated by *repressor proteins* that bind to mRNA sequences, located between the cap site and the AUG initiation codon. Such regulation occurs in the ferritin transcript in which an iron-responsive protein binds upstream of the AUG and prevents translation in conditions of low cytoplasmic iron concentration, but dissociates when iron levels increase, allowing translation to occur.

The newly-synthesized protein is frequently not produced in an active form but requires further modifications before becoming functional. This frequently involves precise folding, a process that often requires accessory proteins called *chaperonins*. Alternatively, it might require a secondary modification to the nascent polypeptide such as glycosylation or phosphorylation or even the cleavage of the

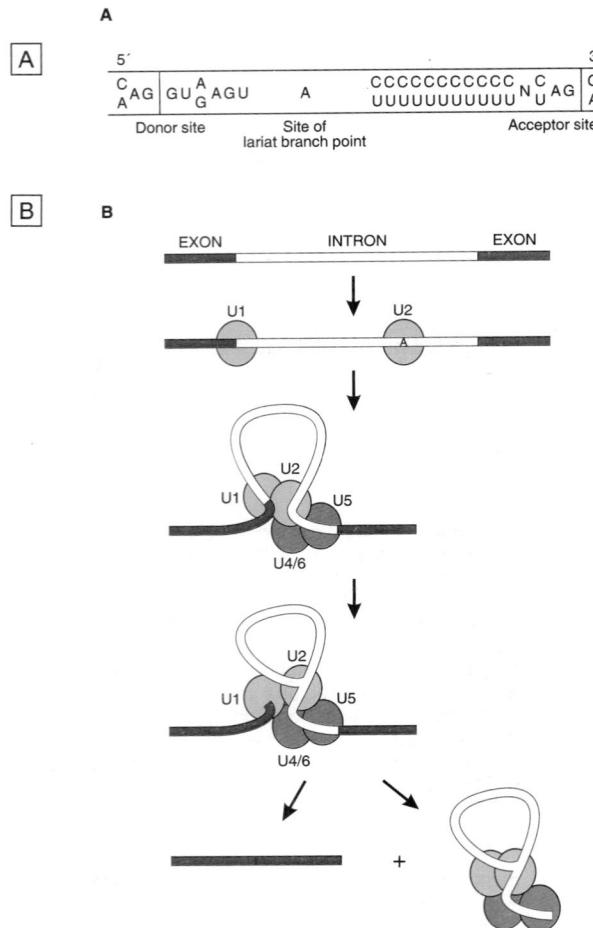

A

Donor site Site of lariat branch point Acceptor site

B

EXON INTRON EXON

2.39 RNA splicing. A shows the consensus sequences which regulate RNA splicing. B depicts the major steps in the splicing process. See text for details.

precursor by a specific protease to generate an active fragment. The latter process is used to generate the active molecule insulin from its inactive precursor pro-insulin.

The regulation of cytoplasmic protein stability is achieved by covalently attaching a small protein called *ubiquitin* to those proteins that are to be destroyed. There are several pathways by which ubiquitination can be achieved in the cytoplasm and each employs a different enzyme to conjugate ubiquitin to its target. However, all of these link ubiquitin molecules to lysine residues on the target protein. Thereafter, several further ubiquitin moieties are added to the first and this polyubiquitin complex is recognized by a large protein-degradation complex called the *proteasome*. Proteasomes occur throughout the cytoplasm and seem to be cylindrical structures with proteases in their central lumen into which the ubiquinated protein is fed. The protein is degraded to short peptides within the proteasome. Proteins identified for degradation include misfolded or damaged proteins but also short-lived proteins. The amino-terminal amino acid of mature proteins seems to have a major influence on their half-life. For example, proteins with an amino-terminal arginine are rapidly degraded whereas those with methionine, serine, threonine or valine are not. This phenomenon is known as the N-end rule. The modification of the amino-terminal residue by acetylation, sometimes called blocking, also seems to prolong the lifetime of the protein.

CELLULAR DIFFERENTIATION

Differential gene regulation as described above underlies cellular differentiation, the process by which specialized cell types are generated. Each differentiated cell type has its own characteristic repertoire of proteins which are associated with that cell's specialized function and whose expression is the result of differential gene regulation. The process of differentiation and the gene regulatory

events that underlie it are regulated by signals in the local environment of the cell and these processes are best exemplified in the developing embryo.

As development of an organism proceeds, its cells pass through a series of changes in gene expression, reflected in alterations of cell structure and behaviour (see also pp. 115–118). Initially, all cells possess rather similar properties but, as embryogenesis gathers momentum, they begin to diversify, first separating into broad categories (e.g. the principal germ layers, etc.) and then into narrower categories (tissues and subtypes of tissues) until finally they mature into the '*end cells*' of their particular lineage (Gurdon 1973). Some cells which are capable of giving rise to others throughout life (*stem cells*) never proceed to the ultimate point of this progression and retain some embryonic characteristics (p. 108) but in all cases there is a *sequential pattern of gene expression* which changes and limits the cell to a particular specialized range of activities. We can detect such changes as alterations in cell structure and biochemical properties, particularly in the types of proteins which are synthesized. At the level of the gene, differentiation of this kind must be based on a change in the pattern of repression and activation of the DNA sequences transcribing the specific proteins of that stage of development; in the lifetime of a particular cell lineage, many such changes will take place (see, e.g. the development of haemal cells, p. 1413).

It appears that the selection of a pattern of gene activity occurs some while before its expression in protein synthesis. Thus, a cell may be **committed** to a particular line of specialization without manifesting its commitment until later; once 'switched' in this way, cells are not usually able to revert to an earlier stage of development, so that an irreversible repression of some gene sequences must have occurred. Stem cells may remain permanently at a level of partial differentiation, although some of their offspring will be committed to full differentiation. In general, as the degree of differentiation progresses, cell division becomes less frequent (e.g. erythroblasts, p. 1413), although some structurally specialized cells such as Schwann cells (p. 948) and certain glandular cells, when suitably stimulated, may undergo repeated mitotic divisions.

What constitutes the appropriate stimulus for a cell line to differentiate at successive stages in development is one of the most fascinating of biological problems and one which also lies at the heart of many pathological transformations including carcinogenesis. In the embryo, differentiation depends upon a wide variety of circumstances (see p. 108), although in most cases chemical interactions between cells or between different regions of the same cell are thought to be of primary significance. The initiation of a particular pathway of cellular development may, however, also depend upon complex, competitive interactions between cells or upon the position which a cell occupies within a cell group (see discussion on 'positional information' on pp. 107, 108). In addition, differentiation may also depend upon some temporal sequence such as the number of previous cell divisions (pp. 107, 110). Even in mature tissues in which cell turnover occurs, similar mechanisms appear to ensure the final differentiation to a functional end cell. In some cases this is linked to the presence of a physiological stimulus as, for example, in the case of the 'B' lymphocytes which respond to exposure to an appropriate antigen by differentiating into plasma cells which secrete a neutralizing antibody. In other cases, particularly where a cell is part of a highly organized system, more subtle mechanisms must be present.

THE CELL CYCLE (2.40)

By definition, the cell cycle is that period of time between the birth of a cell, as a result of the division of its parent cell, and its own division to produce two daughter cells. The most immediately obvious events of the cell cycle observable by light microscopy are those of mitotic division—the condensation of chromosomes, their alignment and separation on the mitotic spindle, and the separation of the cell progeny. This process is described in detail later in this section (p. 58); it is designated the M phase of the cell cycle (see **2.43**), lasting for about 1–2 hours. However, the entire cell cycle takes considerably longer, between 20 and 24 hours in most adult tissues, and is divided into four distinct phases: G_1, S, G_2 and M. The combination of G_1, S and G_2 phases is known as interphase. At

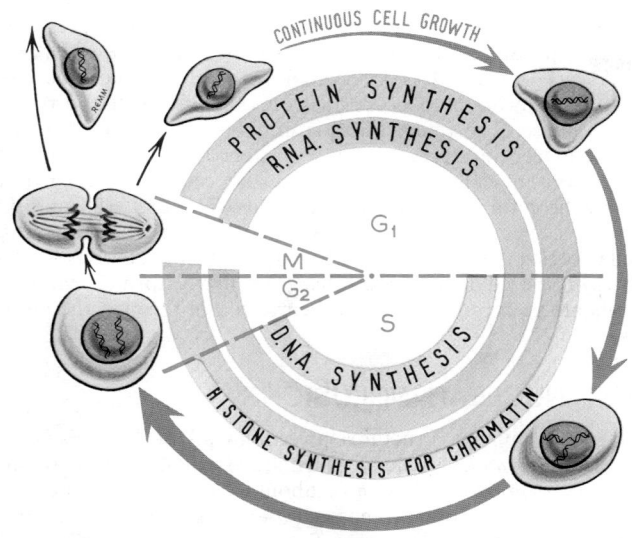

2.40   Diagram showing the major events of the cell cycle.

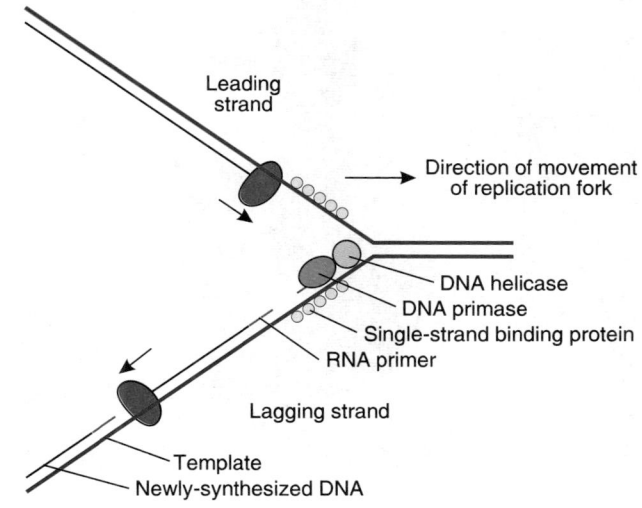

2.41   Schematic diagram depicting DNA synthesis at a replication fork. See text for details.

the end of the M phase, two separate daughter cells exist and each is now at the beginning of the G_1 *phase*; this is a period in which most of the metabolites required to complete another cell cycle are generated. It is also the period during which the cell makes the decision of whether to divide or not. Cells which no longer divide are described as *quiescent* and have entered a phase called G_0. During G_1, cells respond to growth factors directing the cell to complete another cycle and, once made, this decision is irreversible. Growth factors can also stimulate quiescent cells to leave G_0 and re-enter the cell cycle, whereas 'tumour supressor genes' block the cycle in G_1. Thus, G_1 is a crucial period during which the division of a cell is regulated and is also the interval during which oncogenes may function pathologically to cause uncontrolled cell division. DNA replication (described in detail below) occurs during *S phase*, at the end of which the DNA content of the cell has doubled. During G_2 *phase* the cell is preparing for division and this period ends with the breakdown of the nuclear envelope (see above) and the onset of chromosome condensation. The times taken for the S_1, G_2 and M phases are similar for most cell types, occupying about 6, 4 and 2 hours respectively, whereas the duration of G_1 shows considerable variation: it can be as short as 2 hours in rapidly-dividing cells, for example in embryonic tissues, or longer than 12 hours in some adult tissues.

The regulation of the transitions between the cell cycle phases is now becoming understood at the molecular level from studies of mammalian cells, frog oöcytes and, especially, yeast cells. At the transition between G_1 and S phase and between G_2 and M phase, members of a family of proteins called *cyclins* attain their maximum abundance in the cell. The G_1 cyclin progressively accumulates during G_1 and the M phase cyclin accumulates during late S phase and throughout G_2. High levels of cyclin proteins activate a family of protein kinase enzymes called p34 kinases which are present at constant levels during the cell cycle, although their state of activation varies. The activation of different p34 kinases regulates the transitions between G_1 and S and between G_2 and M. It is becoming clear that the activities of these enzymes and their cyclin activators are themselves subject to complex regulation; target proteins for phosphorylation by the p34 kinases are now being identified (see Murray & Hunt 1993).

DNA REPLICATION

The process of DNA replication is best understood in prokaryotic cells; however, there is increasing evidence that the process is fundamentally similar in mammalian cells. As discussed above, rep-

lication is initiated at specific regions of the chromosomal DNA called *replication origins* and this occurs during S phase of the cell cycle. Several initiator proteins bind to the replication origin and introduce a DNA helicase molecule to the origin. The helicase unwinds and separates the two strands of the parent DNA molecule to allow each to serve as a template for replication. The helicase also loads a DNA primase on to one strand, the leading strand, and this enzyme synthesizes a short RNA primer from which DNA synthesis is initiated on that strand. The region where DNA synthesis is ongoing appears as a Y-shape in electron micrographs and has been called the replication fork. In this region DNA synthesis is facilitated by base-pairing and is semi-conservative (see above). DNA replication is performed by a DNA polymerase which synthesizes DNA only in a 5' to 3' direction. Since the two template DNA strands have an opposite polarity, DNA is synthesized in a continuous manner on one strand, the leading strand, and in a series of discontinuous filling-in steps on the other, the lagging strand (**2**.41). DNA synthesis on the lagging strand is facilitated by the periodic synthesis of RNA primers by the primase enzyme associated with the helicase at the replication fork. These are produced every 200 nucleotides or so; each filling-in step removes the previous RNA primer and the newly-synthesized fragment is ligated to the end of the previous one. At the replication fork the DNA helicase hydrolyses ATP during the process by which it opens up the DNA duplex. As the strands separate, single-strand binding proteins associate with them to stabilize them in an open configuration for DNA synthesis. These proteins are removed by the passage of the polymerase across their associated DNA region (for more detail see Diffley 1994).

The process of DNA synthesis requires high fidelity and this is achieved by a number of mechanisms. Firstly, the polymerase cannot incorporate a new nucleotide on to a growing strand if the preceding nucleotide is incorrectly paired with its partner on the template strand. Such mismatched nucleotides are removed by a 'proof-reading' exonuclease activity which is associated with the polymerase itself. In addition, both bacterial and mammalian cells contain mismatch repair enzymes which detect replication errors by virtue of the distortions of the DNA helix that they produce. These enzymes can distinguish the new DNA strand from its template partner and specifically remove and replace the mismatched nucleotide from the newly-synthesized strand.

THE NUCLEOLUS (**2**.42)

The most prominent feature of an interphase nucleus is the presence of one or more spheroidal inclusions called nucleoli. For reviews,

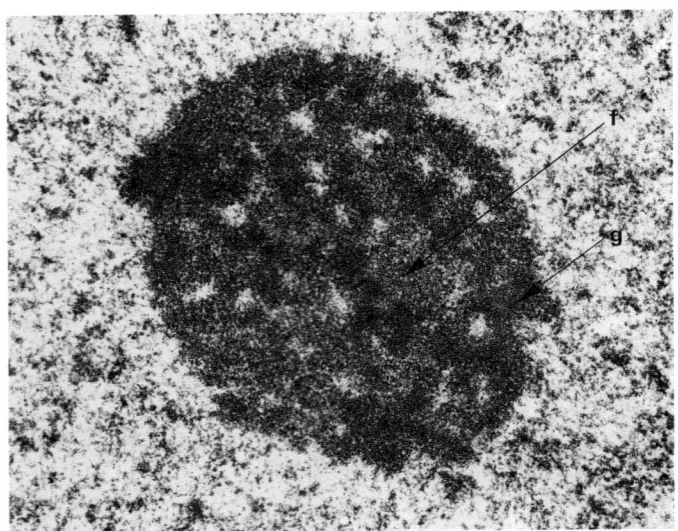

2.42 Electron micrograph of a nucleolus from a highly active cell, showing the pars filamentosa (f) enclosed in the darker pars granulosa (g). Magnification × 25 000.

see Scheer and Weisenberger (1994), Mélèse and Xue (1994). These are the site of most of the rRNA synthesis and ribosome subunit assembly. The number of nucleoli per nucleus varies between different species. Under the electron microscope the nucleolus comprises a pale fibrillar region containing non-transcribed DNA, dense fibrillar cores which are the sites of rRNA transcription, granular regions in which ribosome subunits are assembled and a diffuse nucleolar matrix. In man, there are 5 pairs of chromosomes which bear rRNA genes and these genes are organized in clusters of tandemly repeated units on each chromosome. Each rRNA unit is transcribed indi-

vidually by RNA polymerase I and the primary transcript does not contain any introns but encodes the 28S, 5.8S and 18S rRNA molecules. These rRNAs are separated by subsequent processing of the transcript. Since 5 different chromosomes carry the rRNA gene clusters each nucleolus is associated with 10 chromosomes in a diploid cell. During mitosis the nucleolus breaks down and reforms after telophase. The reformation is initiated by the onset of transcription in certain regions of the clusters on each chromosome. These regions are called nucleolar organizing centres and their fusion precedes the reformation of the nucleolus. The 28S, 18S and 5.8S rRNA molecules are assembled into their ribosomal subunits in the granular region of the nucleolus together with the 5S rRNA which is not synthesized in the nucleolus. The newly formed ribosomal subunits are then translocated to the cytoplasm through the nuclear pores.

OTHER NUCLEAR INCLUSIONS

Other less prominent structures present in all nuclei (Wischnitzer 1973) include *granules*, some of which are associated with chromatin margins (*perichromatin granules*), about 40 nm across, and others lying between the chromatin masses (*interchromatin granules*), about 20 nm across; the significance of these is unknown. *Perichromatin fibres* also occur at the margins of the chromatin. In addition, many other nuclear inclusions have been described as constant features of some cells or occurring occasionally, including fibrillar material, membranous structures and larger granules. In the prophase of the first meiotic division, long fibrillar *synaptonemal complexes* connect adjacent chromosomes (p. 61). Other structures which have been reported in different types of cell include membranous vesicles and lamellae, bundles of filaments, crystals and further varieties of granule. Some of these may represent symbiotic C viruses, common non-pathogenic inhabitants of mammalian nuclei. The nature of the other inclusions is obscure. The nucleoplasm also contains numerous enzymes, nucleotide precursors and proteins, only identifiable by cytochemical or biochemical means; these are, of course, involved in nuclear metabolism.

REPRODUCTION OF CELLS

During prenatal development most cells undergo repeated division as the body grows in size and complexity. As cells mature they differentiate in structure and function and may finally lose the ability to divide, as do neurons, or may persist permanently as stem cells capable of dividing throughout life, as in the haemopoietic tissue of bone marrow.

Rates of cell division vary considerably in different tissues (see e.g. Potten et al 1979; Lewin 1980; Lloyd et al 1982); in many epithelia subject to mechanical stress, the replacement of damaged cells by division of stem cells may be rapid, as seen for crypts between intestinal villi; it may also vary according to demand, as in healing of wounded skin, where cell proliferation rises to a peak and then returns to the normal replacement level. The rate of cell division is, therefore, tightly coupled to the demand for growth and replacement; where this coupling is faulty, tissues either fail to grow or replace their cells, or else they overgrow, giving rise to neoplasms.

The mechanism of normal control of cell division is complex and poorly understood. During early embryonic life, control appears to be local, involving the diffusion of metabolites from one cell group to another, so stimulating or inhibiting division of cells. At later stages, endocrine control is also involved. Several hormones affect cell division rates either generally (e.g. somatotrophic hormone) or locally (e.g. progesterone). Some hormones may act on division by affecting general metabolic rates (thyroid hormones) or protein synthesis (some corticosteroids and somatotrophic hormone). At least some of these effects may be mediated by the intracellular release of cyclic adenosine monophosphate (cyclic AMP) which inhibits synthesis of new DNA during the S phase.

In adult tissues, local control of cell division is an important factor in wound healing. A class of compounds termed *chalones*, which

inhibit cell division, has been isolated from normal tissue cells. A possible model for their action is that normal cells produce chalones which inhibit division of the cells in their locality; when some cells are damaged or destroyed, the concentration of chalones drops allowing cell division to occur until the normal levels are restored, when division is again inhibited.

TYPES OF CELL DIVISION

Two distinct events occur in cell division: division of the nucleus (*karyokinesis*) and of the cytoplasm (*cytokinesis*); they are usually, but not always, coupled. For reviews of these processes, consult Lewin (1980), Inoue (1981), Zimmerman and Forer (1981), Alberts et al (1994).

Nuclear division can occur in three ways. In the first, termed *amitotic* or *direct division*, nuclear material is distributed at random to the resultant cells. (This process, once thought to be common, is in fact restricted to pathological conditions.) In the other two modes of nuclear division, complex chromosomal manoeuvres take place (*indirect division*), comprising *mitosis* and *meiosis*.

Mitosis (**2**.43) occurs in most somatic cells and results in the distribution of identical copies of the parent cell's genome to the resulting cells. In *meiosis*, occurring in the divisions immediately before final production of gametes, the number of chromosomes is halved to the haploid number, so that at fertilization the diploid number is restored; some exchange of genetic material also occurs between homologous chromosomes, a *reassortment* of genes. This leads to further genetic variability in a population, the essence of evolution.

Mitosis and meiosis are alike in many respects, differing chiefly in

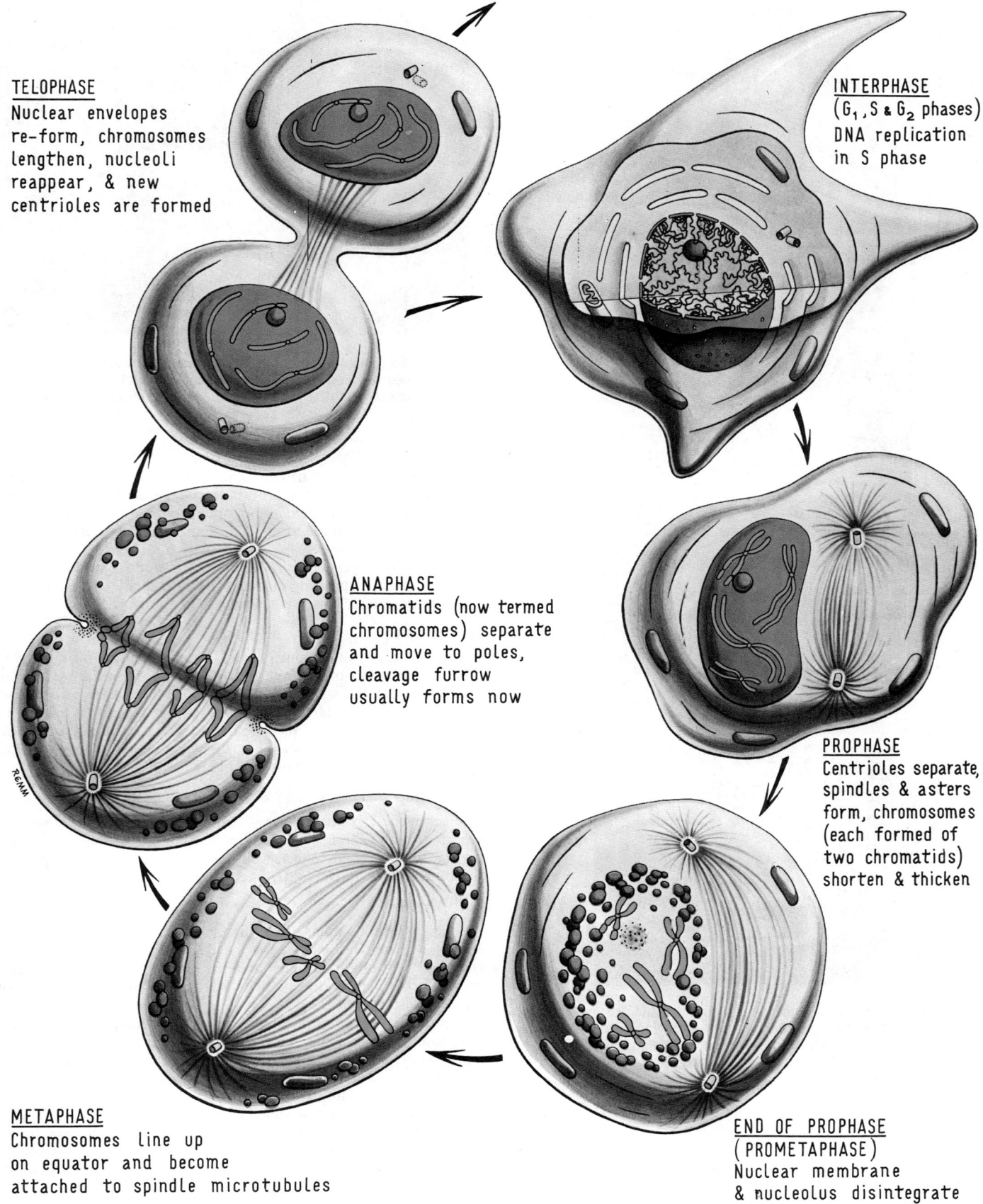

TELOPHASE
Nuclear envelopes
re-form, chromosomes
lengthen, nucleoli
reappear, & new
centrioles are formed

INTERPHASE
(G_1, S & G_2 phases)
DNA replication
in S phase

ANAPHASE
Chromatids (now termed
chromosomes) separate
and move to poles,
cleavage furrow
usually forms now

PROPHASE
Centrioles separate,
spindles & asters
form, chromosomes
(each formed of
two chromatids)
shorten & thicken

METAPHASE
Chromosomes line up
on equator and become
attached to spindle microtubules

END OF PROPHASE
(PROMETAPHASE)
Nuclear membrane
& nucleolus disintegrate

2.43   The main stages of the mitotic cycle of a somatic cell.

chromosomal behaviour during the early stages of cell division. In
meiosis two divisions occur in quick succession; the first of them is
unlike mitosis (*meiosis I, heterotypical* division) but the second more
like mitosis (*meiosis II, homotypical* division).

MITOSIS

As already stated, new DNA is synthesized during the S phase of
interphase, so that in diploid cells the **amount** of DNA has doubled by

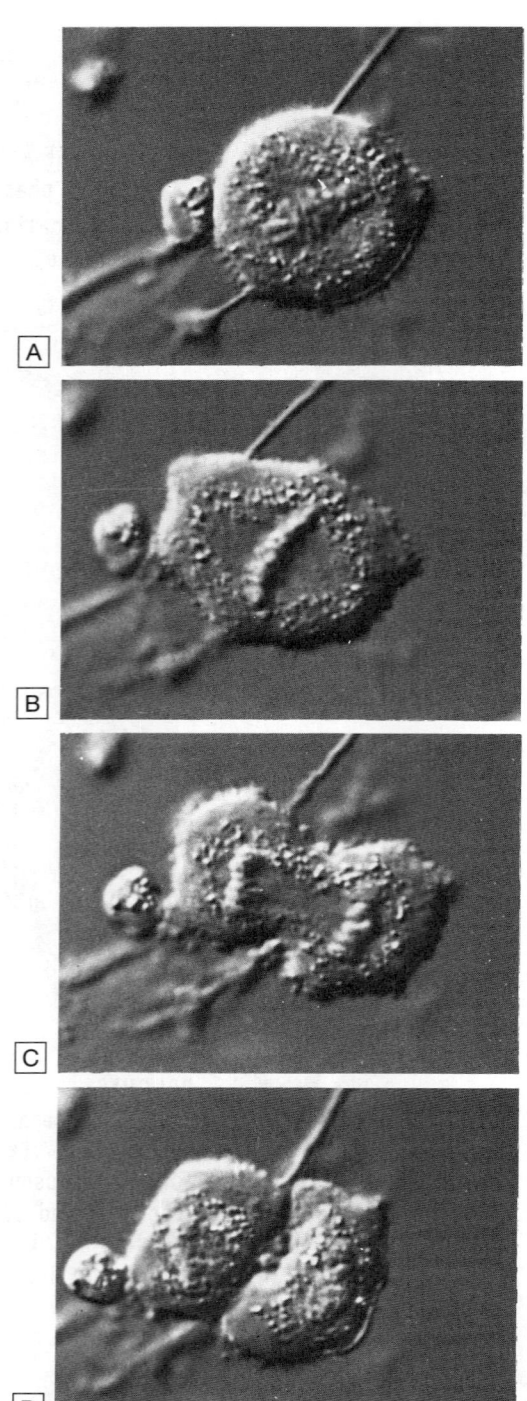

2.44   A series of micrographs taken at different stages of mitosis of a human fibroblast in tissue culture; compare with 2.43. Nomarski interference microscopy. A. Early metaphase; B. metaphase; C. anaphase; D. telophase. Provided by the Paediatric Research Unit, Guy's Hospital Medical School. Magnification × 1500.

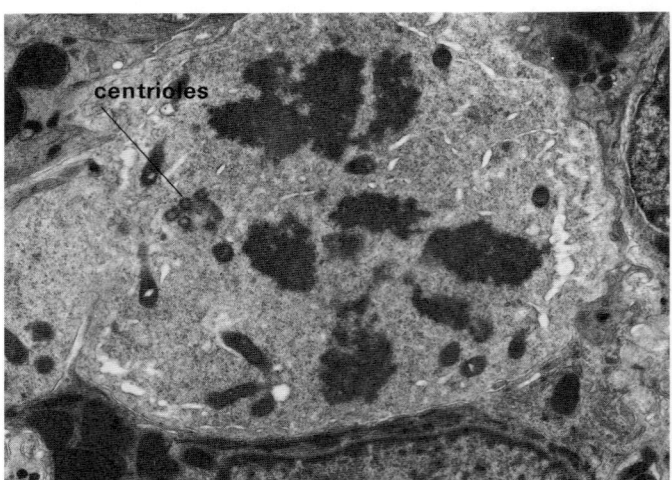

2.45   Electron micrograph of an epithelial cell in mitotic metaphase. The chromosomes are seen as blocks of dense material, and are sectioned approximately along the plane of the equator. Magnification × 10 000.

Outside the nucleus, centrioles begin to separate, moving to opposite poles of the cell; parallel microtubules are synthesized between them to create the *central spindle* and others radiate to form the *astral rays*, collectively termed asters. The spindle and two asters together constitute the *achromatic figure* or *diaster* (amphiaster).

As prophase proceeds, the nucleoli disappear and finally the nuclear envelope suddenly disintegrates into small vesicles to release the chromosomes. This event marks the end of prophase.

Metaphase

As the nuclear envelope disappears, the spindle microtubules invade the central region of the cell and the chromosomes move towards the equator of the spindle (*prometaphase*). Once they have arrived at this imaginary plane (the *metaphase* or *equatorial plate*), the chromosomes attach by their centromeres to spindle microtubules and are so arranged in a star-like ring when viewed from either pole of the cell or sectional across this plane (2.45).

Anaphase

The centromere in metaphase is a double structure; its halves now separate, both carrying an attached chromatid, so that the original chromosome has, in effect, split lengthwise into two new chromosomes. These move apart, one towards each pole.

Telophase

At the end of anaphase the chromosomes are grouped at each end of the cell, both aggregations being diploid in number. The chromosomes now re-extend and the nuclear envelope reappears, beginning as membranous vesicles at the ends of the chromosomes. Nucleoli also reappear.

Meanwhile, cytoplasmic division, which usually begins in early anaphase, is progressing. This process is accompanied at late metaphase by cytoplasmic movements involving the equal distribution of mitochondria and other organelles around the cell periphery. In anaphase an infolding of the cell equator begins and deepens as the *cleavage furrow* (Schroeder 1973). Small vacuoles form in the cytoplasm along the plane of cleavage and eventually the furrow divides the cell into two. Where the constriction meets the remains of the spindle, a dense region of cytoplasm, the *midbody*, is visible but eventually the new cells separate, each with its derived nucleus. The spindle remnant now disintegrates. While the cleavage furrow is active, a peripheral band of actin and myosin appears in the constricting zone and the contraction of this is probably responsible for furrow formation. During telophase the filaments of the cleavage furrow contract down on the remaining spindle microtubules to form the dense *midbody* which finally disappears.

Failure of *disjunction* and '*lagging*' of chromatids may sometimes occur, so that paired chromatids pass to the same pole. Of the two

the onset of mitosis to the tetraploid value, although the chromosome **number** is still diploid. During mitosis, this amount is halved between the two resulting cells, so that DNA quantity and chromosome number are now diploid in both. The nuclear changes which achieve this distribution can be divided into four phases: prophase, metaphase, anaphase and telophase (2.43, 44).

Prophase

The strands of chromatin, highly extended during interphase, begin to shorten, thicken and resolve themselves into recognizable chromosomes, each made up of two chromatids joined at the centromere.

STAGES OF MEIOSIS

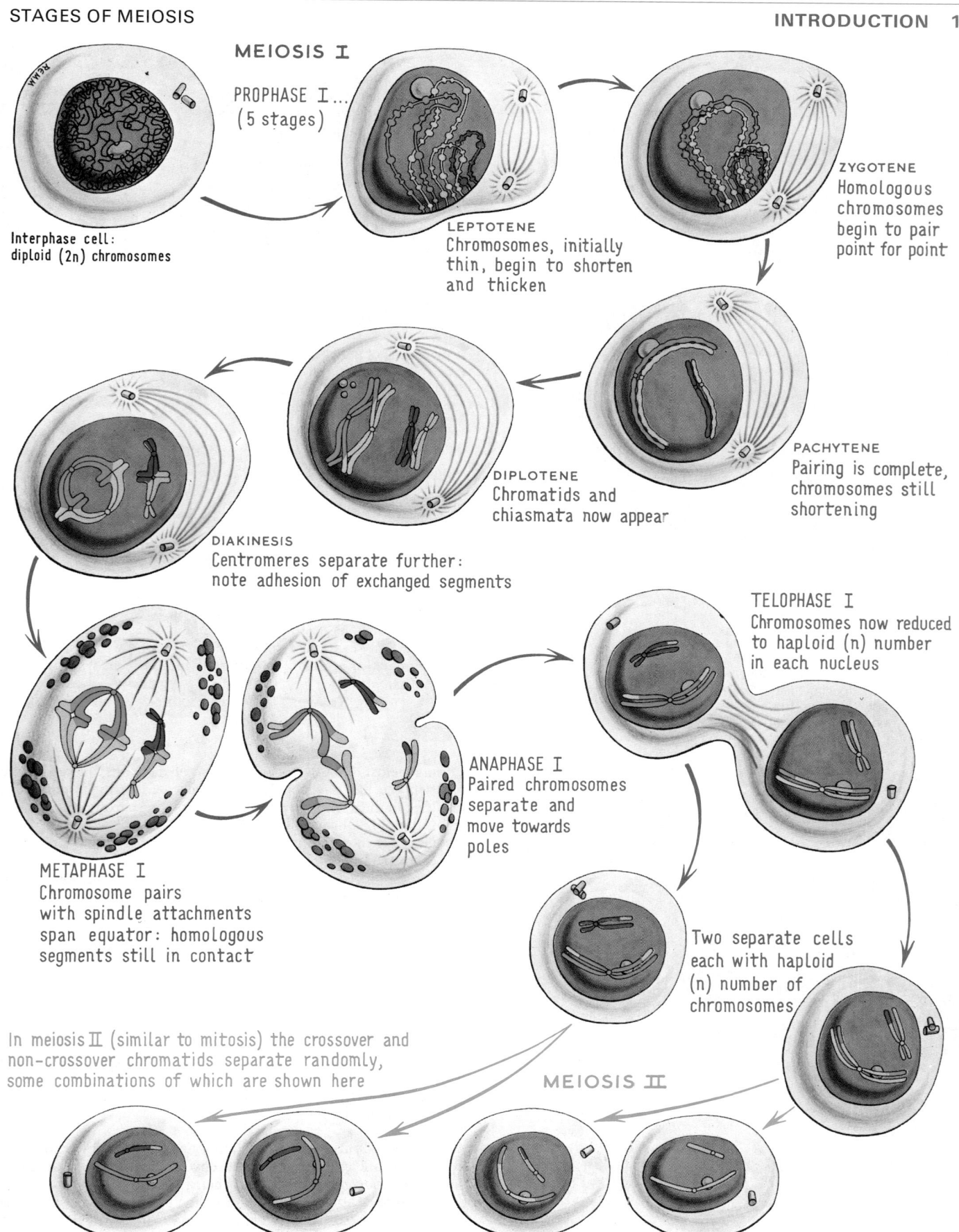

MEIOSIS I

PROPHASE I...
(5 stages)

Interphase cell:
diploid (2n) chromosomes

LEPTOTENE
Chromosomes, initially
thin, begin to shorten
and thicken

ZYGOTENE
Homologous
chromosomes
begin to pair
point for point

PACHYTENE
Pairing is complete,
chromosomes still
shortening

DIPLOTENE
Chromatids and
chiasmata now appear

DIAKINESIS
Centromeres separate further:
note adhesion of exchanged segments

METAPHASE I
Chromosome pairs
with spindle attachments
span equator: homologous
segments still in contact

ANAPHASE I
Paired chromosomes
separate and
move towards
poles

TELOPHASE I
Chromosomes now reduced
to haploid (n) number
in each nucleus

Two separate cells
each with haploid
(n) number of
chromosomes

In meiosis II (similar to mitosis) the crossover and
non-crossover chromatids separate randomly,
some combinations of which are shown here

MEIOSIS II

2.46   Chief stages in the meiotic cycle (male). For clarity only four chromosomes out of the total 46 are shown. Please note that the detailed
movements of chromosomes during different stages of Meiosis II are not
shown in this figure.

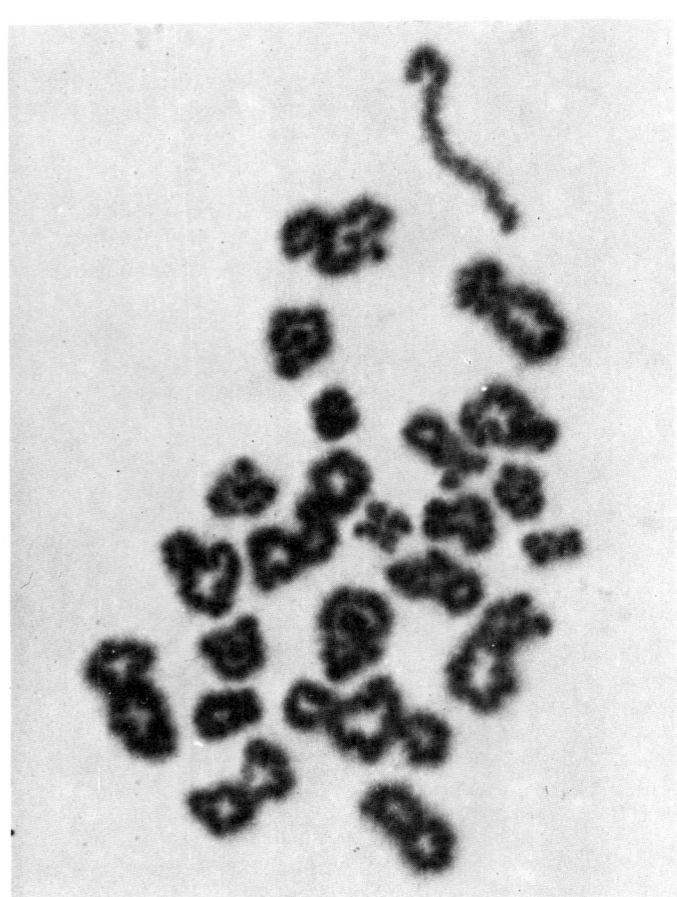

2.47 Photomicrograph of chromosomes from a human spermatocyte in late prophase (diakinesis) of the first meiotic division showing bivalents beginning to separate. Note the paired sex chromosomes (top) which are joined end to end. Provided by the Paediatric Research Unit, Guy's Hospital Medical School.

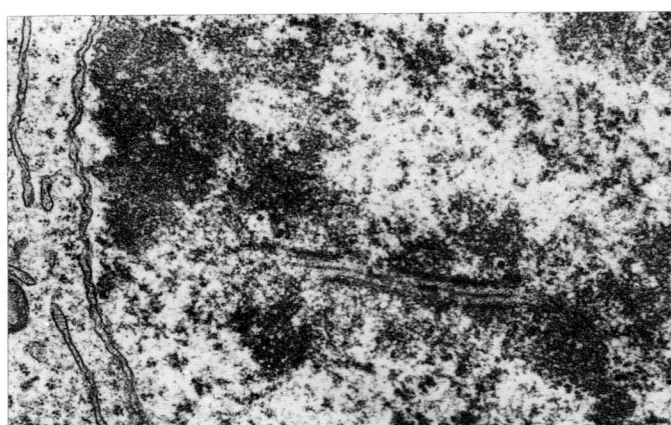

2.49 Detail of a synaptonemal complex in a cell similar to that shown in **2.39**. Note the masses of heterochromatin and the fibrillar core of the synaptonemal complex. **Magnification × 20 000.**

new cells, one will have more and the other fewer chromosomes than the diploid number (see p. 63). Exposure to ionizing radiation promotes such events and may, by chromosomal damage, inhibit mitosis altogether. A typical symptom of *radiation sickness* is the failure of epithelia to replace lost cells, with consequent ulceration ·of the skin and mucous membranes.

Mitosis can also be disrupted by several chemical agents, particularly colchicine and its derivatives colcemide, podophyllin and podophyllotoxin, and by viniblastine. These compounds inhibit or reverse spindle microtubule formation, so that mitosis is arrested in metaphase. This is useful in cytogenetic studies, since chromosomes are most easily examined in the metaphase condition, and also forms the rationale for attacking multiplying tumour cells with many types of cytotoxic drugs.

MEIOSIS

During meiosis (**2.46–49**) there are two cell divisions; in the interphase prior to the first division DNA is replicated in the usual manner, resulting in the tetraploid amount of DNA, the chromosomal number being diploid. During *meiosis I* the DNA is reduced to the diploid **amount** in each resultant cell, although the chromosome **number** is halved to the haploid value; in *meiosis II*, the DNA in each new cell formed is reduced to the haploid amount, the chromosome number remaining haploid. Details of this process differ for male and female lineages. For clarity, the process in the male will be dealt with first, as this demonstrates all the essential steps of meiosis. Differences in the female are described in Section 3.

MEIOSIS I

Prophase I

Prophase I is a long and complex phase which differs considerably from mitotic prophase and is customarily divided into five substages: the leptotene, zygotene, pachytene and diplotene stages and diakinesis (for details see Comings & Okada 1972; Whitehouse 1973; Moens 1974).

Leptotene stage. Chromosomes appear as individual threads attached at one end to the nuclear envelope and show characteristic beads (*chromomeres*) throughout their length.

Zygotene stage. Chromosomes have come together side by side in homologous pairs (a process which may already have occurred as early as telophase of the previous mitotic division). The homologous chromosomes pair point for point progressively, beginning at the attachment point to the nuclear envelope (Moens 1974), so that corresponding regions lie in contact. This process is *synapsis, conjugation* or *pairing*. Each pair is now a *bivalent*. In the case of the unequal X and Y sex chromosomes, which during zygotene and pachytene are sequestered in a secluded zone of the nucleus, the *sex*

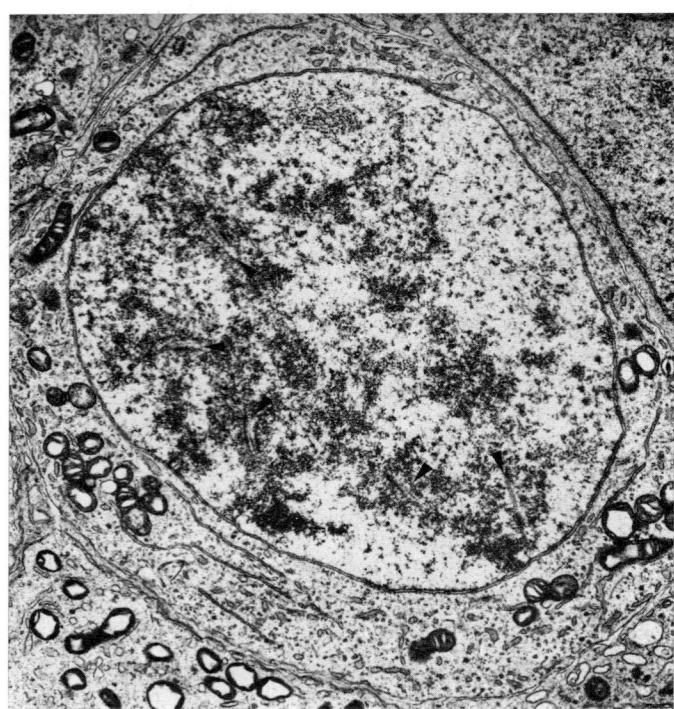

2.48 Electron micrograph of a primary spermatocyte (mouse) showing the nucleus in early prophase of the first meiotic division. Five synaptonemal complexes are visible (arrowheads). **Magnification × 10 000.**

vesicle (Solari & Tres 1967). Only limited *pairing segments* are homologous and these pair end to end (**2.47**); the remaining parts are *differential segments*. By electron microscopy, homologous chromosomes appear held together by a highly structured fibrillar band, the *synaptonemal complex* (**2.49**), which occupies the space (about 100 nm wide) between them (von Wettstein et al 1984, see also p. 56).

Pachytene stage. Spiralized shortening and thickening of each chromosome progresses and its two chromatids, joined at the centromere, become visible. Each bivalent pair, therefore, consists of four chromatids, forming a *tetrad*. Two chromatids, one from each bivalent chromosome, partially coil round each other, and during this stage it is probable that exchange of DNA (*crossing over* or *decussation*) occurs by breaking and rejoining, perhaps facilitated by the synaptonemal complex. Within the latter structure, regions of DNA exchange are marked by the presence of dense proteinaceous masses about 90 nm in diameter (*recombination nodules*) in which the processes of cutting and rejoining the adjacent DNA strands may occur.

Diplotene stage. Homologous pairs, now much shortened, separate except where crossing over has occurred (*chiasmata*). Sometimes chiasmata appear to move towards the ends of the chromatids (*terminalization*); at least one chiasma forms between each homologous pair and up to five have been observed (even up to 10 in some species). In human ovaries, primary oöcytes become diplotene by the fifth month in utero and each remains in this stage until the period prior to its ovulation (some for decades, and even up to 50 years).

Diakinesis. Remaining chiasmata finally resolve and the chromosomes, still as bivalents, become even shorter and thicker; they disperse, as bivalents, to lie against the nuclear envelope.

During prophase the nucleoli have disappeared and the spindle and asters have formed as in mitosis. At the end of prophase the nuclear envelope disappears and bivalent chromosomes move towards the equatorial plate (*prometaphase*).

Decussation. Exchange of genes between homologous chromosomes involves extraordinary precision whereby the DNA, at exactly corresponding positions on both, is severed and rejoined to the DNA of its corresponding partner. How this is achieved is not certain, although it has been proposed that the DNA double chains of the two exchanging chromatid segments are exchanged one at a time, perhaps with some remodelling of redundant DNA chains by partial dissolution and resynthesis in the correct position (Holliday 1964; Whitehouse & Hastings 1965). Such exchanges may occur during late zygotene and early pachytene (Whitehouse 1973), when there is some DNA synthesis; it is likely that the synaptonemal complex is an important mediator of genetic exchange.

Once segments of chromatid are exchanged and the chromosomes begin to separate, regions where crossing over has taken place become visible as chiasmata; these, therefore, represent a *past event* and chiasma formation is **not** synonymous with genetic recombination. After diakinesis the paired chromatids of a given chromosome adhere to each other more strongly than those of homologous chromosomes, even when exchange has occurred, producing the curious configurations which chromosomes adopt in metaphase of meiosis I (**2.49**).

Metaphase I

Metaphase I resembles mitotic metaphase except that the bodies attaching to the spindle microtubules are bivalents, not single chromosomes. These become arranged so that the homologous pairs lie parallel to the equatorial plate with one member on either side.

Anaphase and telophase I

Anaphase and telophase I also occur as in mitosis, except that in anaphase the centromeres do not split; thus, instead of the paired chromatids separating to move towards the poles, whole homologous chromosomes made up of two joined chromatids depart to opposite poles. Since positioning of bivalent pairs is random, assortment of maternal and paternal chromosomes in each telophase nucleus is also random.

During meiosis I, cytoplasmic division occurs as in mitosis to produce two new cells.

MEIOSIS II

Meiosis II commences after only a short interval during which no DNA synthesis occurs. This second division is more like mitosis, with separation of chromatids during anaphase; but in contrast to mitosis, the separating chromatids are genetically dissimilar. Cytoplasmic division also occurs and thus **four** cells result from meiosis I and II.

If cytoplasmic division fails during meiosis I, gametes with the diploid number of chromosomes result and thus give, at fertilization, a triploid zygote.

Other abnormalities, some of them viable, are produced by *non-disjunction* of chromosomes (p. 58), or by the *lagging* of individual chromosomes, during anaphase. These will be discussed later (p. 63). There is much evidence that, as maternal age increases, so does the frequency of such abnormalities.

Mechanism of chromosome movement during mitosis and meiosis

In both mitosis and meiosis the chromosomes undergo a predictable set of movements which bring them at first to the equator of the cell at metaphase, then translate them polewards in opposite directions during anaphase, to achieve equal distribution in the two cells formed at the end of cell division. Clearly, these events depend on the presence of spindle microtubules, since if these are made to depolymerize with antimicrotubule drugs such as colchicine, the chromosomes shorten but remain stationary, and separation is blocked. The molecular processes bringing about chromosome movements have been difficult to determine in spite of many intricate and inventive experiments to elucidate them. In the last few years some crucial observations have been made using micromanipulation and dissection of intact or isolated mitotic apparatuses. These studies show that there are at least three separate processes occurring during cell division. First there is the assembly of the mitotic spindle, with the separation of the centrioles. This entails the polymerization of tubulin on the microtubule-organizing centres (MTOCs) around the centrioles so that the fast growing (plus) ends of the microtubules are directed away from the centrioles, and the two sets are thus pointing towards each other. It is envisaged that the antiparallel microtubules push on each other, perhaps using dynein cross-bridges until the centrioles reach opposite poles of the cell. At this stage (late prophase/early metaphase) the spindle is composed of relatively stable microtubules stretching along much of the spindle's length, and also transient microtubules which grow rapidly from the poles towards the equator, then as rapidly shorten again by depolymerization. In the second stage, the nuclear envelope breaks down at the beginning of metaphase, freeing the chromosomes which can now be contacted by the transient microtubules; the attachment seems to be a random affair, but once a growing microtubule has touched the kinetochore in the centromeric region of a chromosome, it binds to it and stabilizes (for the time being). Up to 20 microtubules may attach themselves to a single kinetochore, some as yet unknown mechanism ensuring that (during mitosis) the two kinetochores of each chromosome (one for each chromatid) are attached to microtubules from opposite poles. During this stage the chromosomes move along the spindle until they reach the equator, when they stop. Lastly, during mitotic anaphase the two chromatids separate and it appears that the kinetochores now migrate along the surface of the microtubules to which they are attached towards their minus ends, i.e. polewards. This motion is energy-dependent, and resembles the kinesin- and dynein-based translation of vesicles along microtubules during interphase (p. 39). As the kinetochore and attached chromosome moves away from the equator the related microtubule bundle depolymerizes behind it so that it progressively shortens. Eventually, when the chromosomes have reached their final position, the spindle disintegrates entirely. Many details remain to be determined, including the events of the first meiotic division where four kinetochores (representing two chromosomes of two chromatids each) are presented to microtubules at the equator. For further reading, see Bloom (1993), Alberts et al (1994), Ault and Rieder (1994).

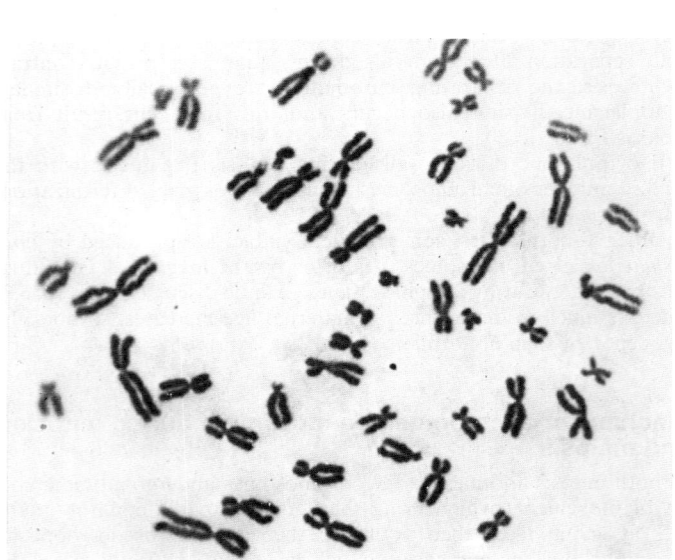

2.50 A spread preparation of metaphase chromosomes of a human fibroblast. Provided by the Paediatric Research Unit, Guy's Hospital Medical School.

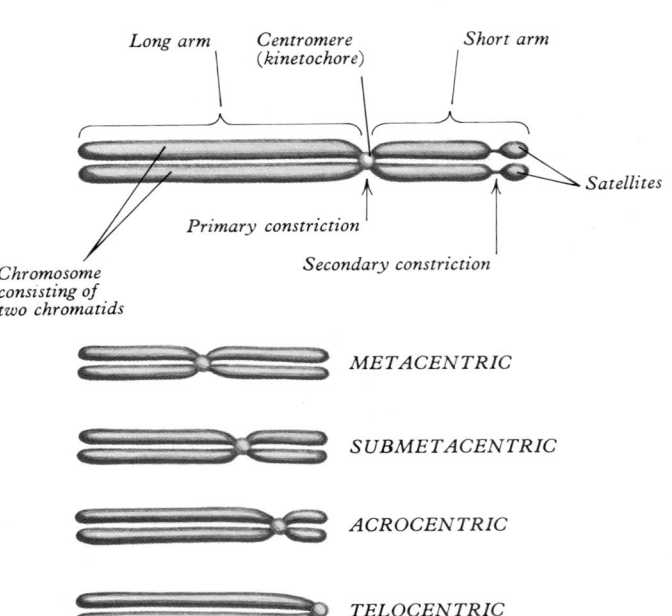

2.51 The major structural features of chromosomes seen in mitotic metaphase; the terminology of the different chromosomal regions is given together with the various major categories of chromosome, classified according to differences in the position of the primary constriction.

CLASSIFICATION OF HUMAN CHROMOSOMES

Since a number of genetic abnormalities can be directly related to the chromosomal pattern, the characterization or *karyotyping* of chromosomes is of considerable diagnostic importance. Their identifying features are most easily seen during metaphase, although recently prophase chromosomes have also been used for more detailed analysis (see below).

As a source of chromosomes, lymphocytes can be separated from blood samples or cells taken from other sources. For diagnosis of

2.52 Karyotype of G-banded chromosome from a normal male, produced using a computer image capture and analysis system. The insert (bottom right) shows the two x chromosomes from a female karyotype. (Karyotype prepared by Lisa Durvill Holmes, S.W. Regional Cytogenetics Centre, Bristol.)

fetal chromosome patterns, samples of amniotic fluid, containing fetal cells, can be aspirated from the uterus (amniocentesis) or for some purposes, a small piece of a chorionic villus (p. 338) removed from the placenta. Whatever their origin, the cells are cultured in vitro and stimulated to divide by treatment with phytohaemagglutinin or other chemicals. Mitosis is later interrupted at metaphase with spindle inhibitors and chromosomes dispersed by swelling the cells in hypotonic solutions followed by air drying, or squashing, to rupture the cells and flatten the chromosomes. These can then be stained to allow the identification of individual chromosomes by size, shape and distribution of stain (**2.50–52**). When large numbers of cells have to be examined for clinical purposes, automatic scanning light microscopy with computer control and analysis can greatly facilitate the identification of chromosomes and any abnormalities (**2.52**). Methods include: *general techniques* to show the obvious landmarks, for example length of arms, position of primary and secondary constrictions; and *banding techniques* to demonstrate differential staining patterns, characteristic for each chromosome type. Since the introduction of the first banding methods (Caspersson et al 1968), several methods have been developed, such as fluorescence staining with quinacrine mustard and related compounds (Q bands **2.56**), Giemsa staining after treatment with alkali (G bands), 'reverse-Giemsa' staining in which the light and dark areas are reversed (R bands) and the staining of constitutive heterochromatin with silver salts (C-banding **2.53**); T-banding methods stain the ends (telomeres) of chromosomes and other techniques can be used to demonstrate nucleolar organizing centres. In *high resolution banding*, chromosomes arrested in prophase are used (**2.54**), even greater detail being discernible in these more elongated forms (Yunis et al 1978).

By such methods, chromosomes can be classified by length, positions of primary and secondary constrictions, presence of satellites, number and positions of the transverse bands and the distribution of constitutive heterochromatin (see **2.52**). A system of numbering autosomal pairs of chromosomes in order of decreasing size, from 1 to 22, has been adopted according to the conventions agreed in London (1960) and Chicago (1964). Before the introduction of banding, some chromosomes were difficult to distinguish and thus were grouped together in seven categories (A–G) according to size and detailed shape and updated more recently (ISCN 1985). However, the later methods allow unambiguous identification and a classification agreed first in Paris (1972) is now generally accepted.

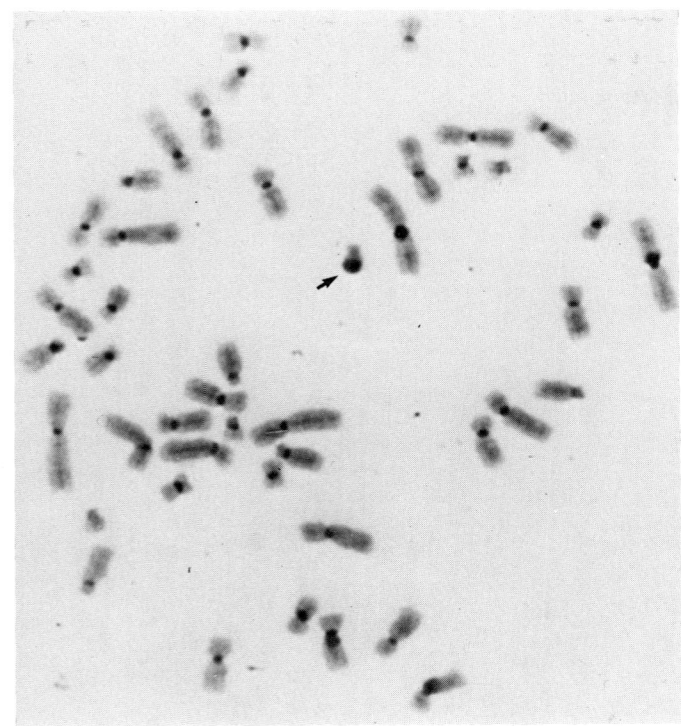

2.53 Human (male) metaphase spread stained with the C-banding method to show constitutive heterochromatin (dark spots) mainly centromeric in position. The arrow indicates the Y chromosome in which heterochromatin is situated terminally in the long arm. Provided by the Paediatric Research Unit, Guy's Hospital Medical School. Magnification × 1300.

Major categories of human chromosomes

A summary of the major classes of chromosomes is given below:

Group	
1–3 (A)	Large metacentric chromosomes
4–5 (B)	Large submetacentric chromosomes
6–12 + X (C)	Metacentrics of medium size
13–15 (D)	Medium-sized acrocentrics with satellites (and nucleolar organizing centres)
16–18 (E)	Shorter metacentrics (No. 16) or submetacentrics (Nos. 17 and 18)
19–20 (F)	Shortest metacentrics
21–22 + Y (G)	Short acrocentrics, 21 and 22 with satellites (and nucleolar organizing centres), Y without satellites

These advances also improved the recognition of abnormal chromosome patterns, but more recently the use of in situ hybridisation with DNA probes has transformed the identification of even very small abnormalities (see below).

SEX CHROMATIN

The interphase nuclei of female mammals differ from those of males in that a heterochromatic body is usually present on the inner face of the nuclear envelope in females (**2.57**). This structure, the *sex chromatin* or *Barr body* (Barr & Bertram 1949), may protrude from the surface of polymorphic nuclei (as a 'drumstick'). It is now regarded as one of the X chromosomes which is synthetically inert and thus heterochromatic, its euchromatic partner carrying out all necessary functions in RNA synthesis (Lyon 1962). The inert X chromosome also replicates later during interphase than its homologue.

CHROMOSOME ABNORMALITIES

Chromosome abnormalities can be numerical or structural in nature. Errors in chromosome number can arise in mitosis or meiosis through chromosome non-disjunction or lagging, to give cells that have an extra chromosome (i.e. the cells are *trisomic*), or have a missing chromosome (and are, therefore, *monosomic*). During mitosis, or in the second division of meiosis, these errors may result from the failure of sister chromatids to separate correctly at anaphase. Similarly, during the first division of meiosis, paired homologous chromosomes may fail to move separately to opposite poles during anaphase.

Autosomal trisomies (i.e. trisomies not involving the sex chromosomes) occur relatively frequently in live-born infants. Most frequently, these involve chromosomes 13, 18 and 21, giving rise to Patau, Edwards and Down syndromes respectively. Trisomy 21 is the most common, being associated with a birth frequency risk of 1 in 700 in the general population. This rises with increasing maternal age, and prenatal testing of fetuses of mothers over the age of 35 is normal practice. Autosomal monosomies are usually lethal and rarely occur.

Numerical abnormalities involving the sex chromosomes give rise to several well-recognized syndromes, including Turner syndrome (single X chromosome), Klinefelter syndrome (XXY, i.e. 47 chromosomes in total), also 47,XXX and 47,XYY. In general, abnormalities resulting from errors of sex chromosome number are less severe than those associated with autosomal trisomies. This is because all X chromosomes in excess of one are to a large extent rendered genetically inactive (Lyon hypothesis), while the Y chromosome is largely heterochromatic (non-transcribing) in nature and, therefore, additional Y chromosomes do not cause serious gene imbalance.

Any situation with extra or deficient chromosomes so that the number is not an exact multiple of the basic haploid number (n) may be referred to as *aneuploidy*. In contrast, extra whole chromosome sets over the normal diploid number (2n) are called *polyploids*. Some polyploids occur naturally in certain tissues such as the liver, and polyploids such as tetraploids (4n) and octaploids (8n) normally result from chromosome replication without subsequent cell division. Triploidy (3n) on the other hand, can only result from an abnormal conception (e.g. normal haploid egg fertilized by diploid sperm). Both triploid and tetraploid conceptions occur from time to time, but neither survive to give live-born infants. Chromosome disorders are found in about 20% of all conceptions, but the birth frequency is only about 6%. The majority of chromosomally abnormal fetuses are eliminated as early spontaneous abortions. In total, approximately 60% of all spontaneous abortions show a chromosome abnormality, half of which are in the form of a trisomy. Chromosome abnormalities may also be structural in nature. Deletions result in a

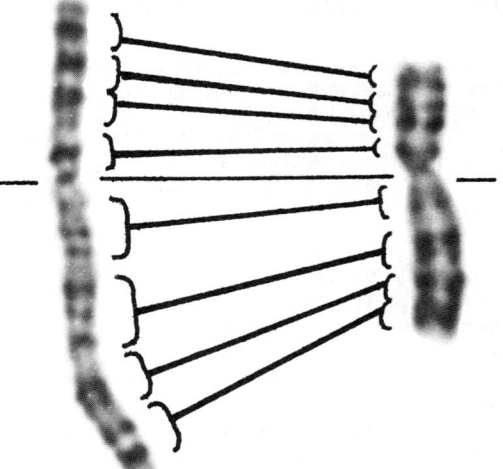

2.54 Two chromosomes (both chromosome number 2), showing Giemsa banding at different periods of mitosis. On the right the cell was arrested during metaphase when the chromosomes are shortest. On the left an earlier (late prophase—early metaphase) chromosome shows that the later bands are formed by the condensation of several sub-bands. Provided by the Paediatric Research Unit, Guy's Hospital Medical School. Magnification × 3700.

HUMAN KARYOTYPE CHROMOSOME NUMBER 2

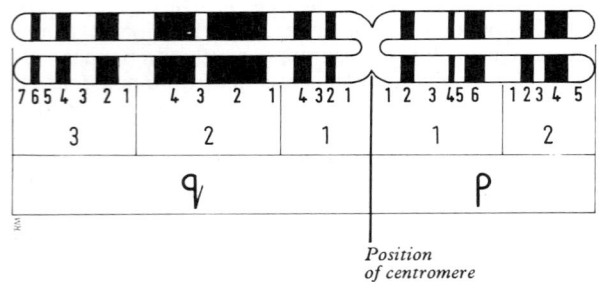

HUMAN KARYOTYPE
CHROMOSOME NUMBER 15

■ Positive staining Giemsa
and Quinacrine methods

□ Negative staining except
for reverse Giemsa method

▨ Variable staining

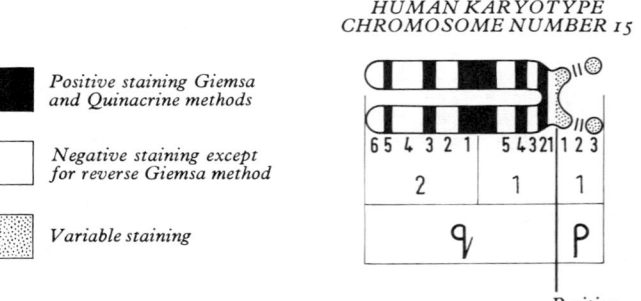

Position
of centromere

Position
of centromere

2.55 Nomenclature of the banding patterns in two human chromosome types, designated by the Paris Convention, for different staining techniques. (For details see text.)

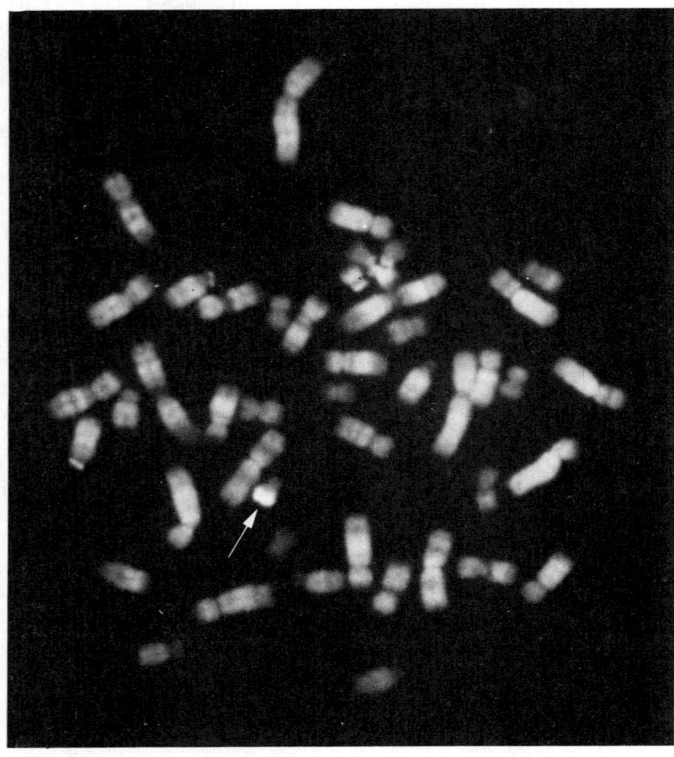

2.56 A chromosome spread from a normal human male cell, treated with a fluorescent dye (see text) and photographed using fluorescence microscopy. In addition to the terminal fluorescence of the long arm of the Y chromosome (arrow), bands which fluoresce less strongly are also present on the other chromosomes, providing a basis for their identification. Supplied by the Paediatric Research Unit, Guy's Hospital Medical School. Magnification × 1500.

2.57 Fibroblasts from a human female, in tissue culture, showing dense heterochromatic Barr bodies (arrows) lying close against the nuclear envelope. Kindly provided by the Paediatric Research Unit, Guy's Hospital Medical School. Magnification × 2000.

loss of chromosome material and are usually associated with an abnormal phenotype (e.g. Wolf syndrome and Cri-du-Chat syndrome, which show partial deletions of the short arms of chromosomes 4 and 5 respectively).

Other structural abnormalities include *inversions* and *translocations*. In the former, segments within a chromosome become inverted, while translocations involve an exchange of segments between different chromosomes. Neither of these in themselves necessarily results in a loss of genetic material, and hence individuals with such abnormalities (carriers) are usually phenotypically normal. A problem only arises during gametogenesis, when gametes which are chromosomally unbalanced may be produced. An important type of chromosome exchange constitute the Robertsonian translocations. These always involve acrocentric chromosomes (i.e. 13, 14, 15, 21 or 22). The breakpoints in the two chromosomes involved occur very close to their respective centromeres and the two long arms join to

form a translocation chromosome, while the short arms are usually lost. This is of no consequence as the acrocentric short arms are largely heterochromatic in nature and, therefore, 'genetically inert'; the only functional genes present on them code for certain ribosomal RNAs, and since the same genes are typically present on all other acrocentric chromosomes, their loss can be tolerated without causing any problems. One of the more frequent types of Robertsonian translocations involves chromosomes 14 and 21; in such cases, the balanced carriers are at risk of producing a Down syndrome infant due to abnormal segregation of the chromosomes at meiosis, i.e. the 14/21 translocation chromosome segregating with the normal chromosome 21, resulting in a gamete with two chromosome 21 long arms. Fertilization with a normal gamete will result in a conceptus that is effectively trisomic for chromosome 21.

Mention has already been made of high resolution banding. With this technique the relatively few, rather dense bands seen on

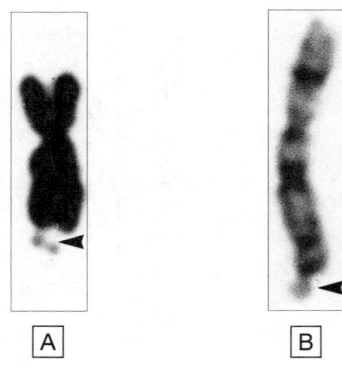

2.58 X chromosomes showing fragile site at Xq27.3 (arrows). A solid staining and B G-banded.

contracted chromosomes become resolved into sub-bands, enabling the chromosomes to be examined in greater detail (**2**.54). Much interest is currently directed at looking for relatively small deletions that can be associated with specific phenotypic abnormalities, and among the growing list of such disorders are Prader–Willi syndrome and Angelman syndrome, both of which may show the same small deletion in the long arm of chromosome 15 just below the centromere (see below).

The Fragile-X syndrome gives rise to one of the more common forms of inherited mental retardation. Cytogenetically, it is typified by the occurrence of a 'fragile site' near the distal end of the long arm of the X chromosome (Xq27.3) (**2**.58). Under certain conditions of culture the fragile site is normally expressed in a proportion of cells as chromatid or chromosome gaps, and until recently this phenomenon has been the basis of a cytogenetic diagnosis for this disorder. However, the results are sometimes inconclusive, par-

ticularly in females, and in this, and other areas of cytogenetics, increasing use is being made of molecular techniques to supplement, or even replace traditional methods. It is now known, for example, that the majority of individuals with Fragile-X syndrome have a mutation which involves a 'CGG' DNA sequence repeated a variable number of times. Over successive generations this triplet may become amplified until, at approximately 200 repeats, or more, it is no longer functional. In such individuals, the X chromosome fragility is expressed. The DNA analysis thus provides a highly accurate means for assessing the Fragile-X status of an individual and is becoming the accepted method of diagnosis for this disorder. In a similar way, increasing use is being made of molecular probes for the detection of small deletions; thus molecular defects of chromosome 15 have been observed for both Prader–Willi and Angelman syndromes where chromosome deletions have not been detectable at the light microscope level. Another microdeletion that has recently received considerable clinical attention involves the region q11.2 of chromosome 22. There appear to be a number of closely linked gene loci involved, so that there is a wide spectrum of phenotypes associated with deletions within this region. These include DiGeorge syndrome, velocardiofacial syndrome and conotruncal heart defects. **2**.59 demonstrates the use of chromosome 22-specific probes in the diagnosis of these conditions. Other probes that are chromosome-specific enable whole chromosomes to be 'painted' a specific colour using different fluorochromes and, in this way, small translocations can be highlighted very effectively (**2**.60, 61). Chromosome-specific probes can also be used to demonstrate the presence of individual chromosomes in interphase nuclei (**2**.62), a technique that clearly has potential for prenatal diagnostic screening for trisomies.

Imprinting and uniparental disomy

Prader–Willi syndrome (PWS) and Angelman syndrome (AS) show very distinct and contrasting features. At the same time, both have been observed to have apparently the same deletion of chromosome 15. In PWS it would seem that the deletion has invariably been inherited from the father but in AS, from the mother. These findings can be explained by the concept of 'imprinting'. This involves the differential 'switching off' of genes according to whether they have been transmitted by the mother or father. Although the observable

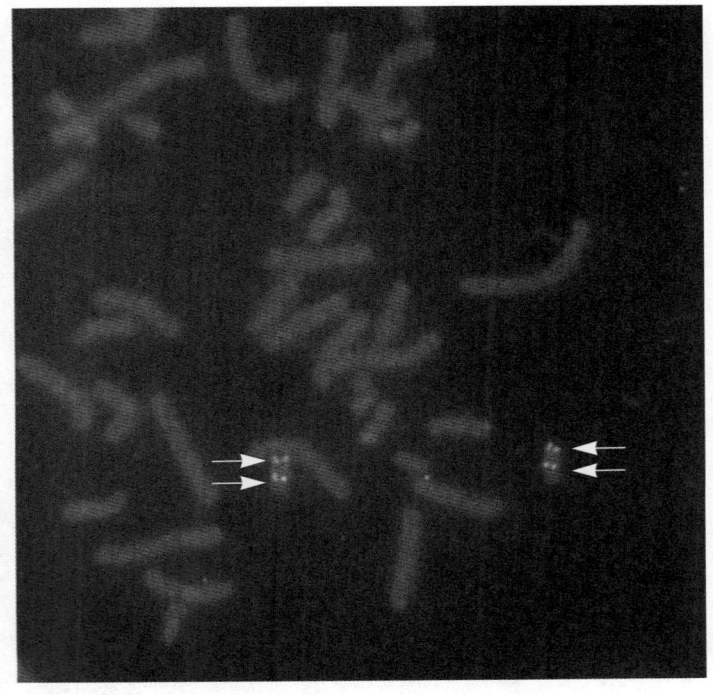
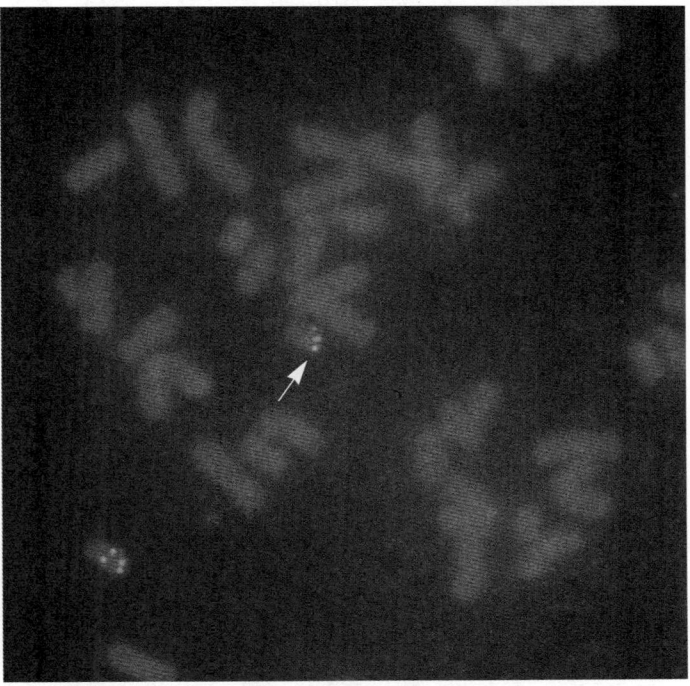

2.59A, B A. Metaphase spread showing chromosome 22-specific probes detected by FITC and counterstained with propidium iodide. The proximal signals (large arrow) are within the region q11.2. The more distal signals (small arrows) control probes confirming the identity of each homologue of chromosome 22. B. Metaphase spread from a patient with a deletion of the proximal signal in one homologue of chromosome 22.

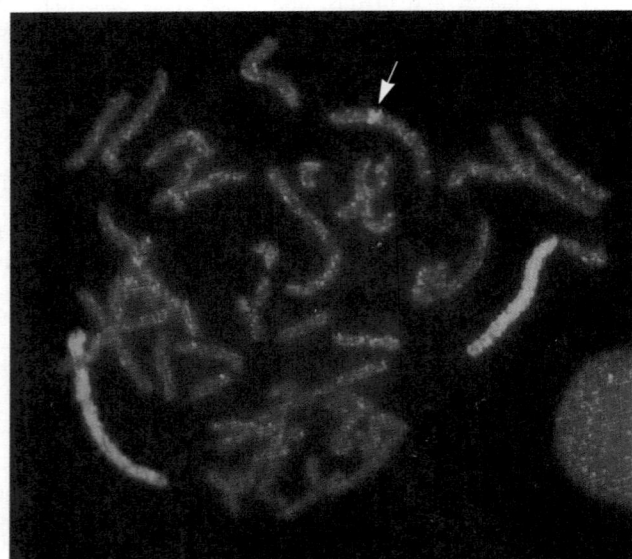

2.60 Metaphase spread using chromosome 2 paint (FITC labelled) to show an interstitial insertion of a small segment (arrowed) from the long arm of chromosome 2 into the long arm of chromosome 5. (This image was produced using a cooled CCD camera equipped with Smartcapture Software (Digital Scientific Limited, UK). The original slide was prepared by C. M. Mackie, Cytogenetics Laboratory, Guy's Hospital, London.)

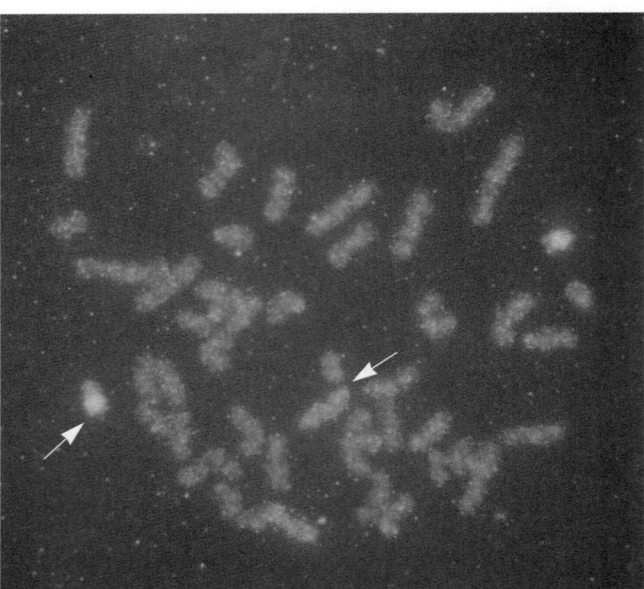

2.61 Metaphase spread using two-colour painting to show a small balanced translocation between chromosomes 11 and 22 (11 Texas Red; 22 FITC labelled). The distal region of the short arm of chromosome 11 (large arrow) can clearly be seen translocated onto the long arm of one of the homologues of chromosome 22. The very small segment of the chromosome 22 long arm involved in the reciprocal translocation is seen as a faint green signal on the end of the short arm of chromosome 11 (small arrow). (Photograph from a slide prepared by C. M. Mackie, Cytogenetics Laboratory, Guy's Hospital, London.)

chromosome deletion is small, it is most likely that the two syndromes are determined by different genes, and it is thought that PWS becomes manifest when the paternally derived chromosome 15 shows the deletion (and, therefore, lacks the gene(s) for normal development). Although the same gene or genes are present on the maternally derived chromosome 15, they are switched off—probably by DNA methylation. In the case of AS, the reverse situation exists, the paternally derived gene(s) being switched off, so that a deletion in the maternally derived chromosome 15 will result in the typical features of AS. The operation of this type of mechanism is further

substantiated by the fact that in a small percentage of PWS that lack visible cytological deletions, molecular studies have shown that the two homologues of chromosome 15 are both maternal in origin. Such an event is referred to as 'uniparental disomy', and could result from an early non-disjunctional event involving, say, the maternal 15 to give a trisomic situation. Subsequent loss of the paternal chromosome 15 then restores the disomic condition. As a consequence of imprinting, however, both these maternal chromosomes will have the gene(s) required for normal development switched off, and a PWS phenotype will result.

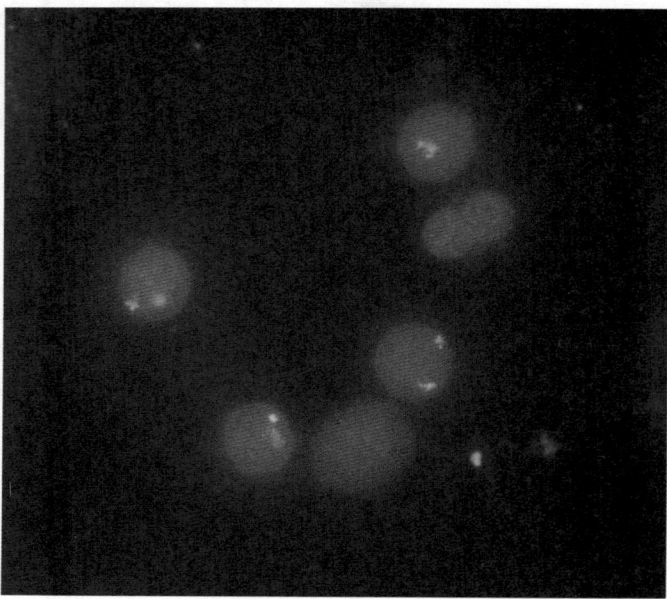

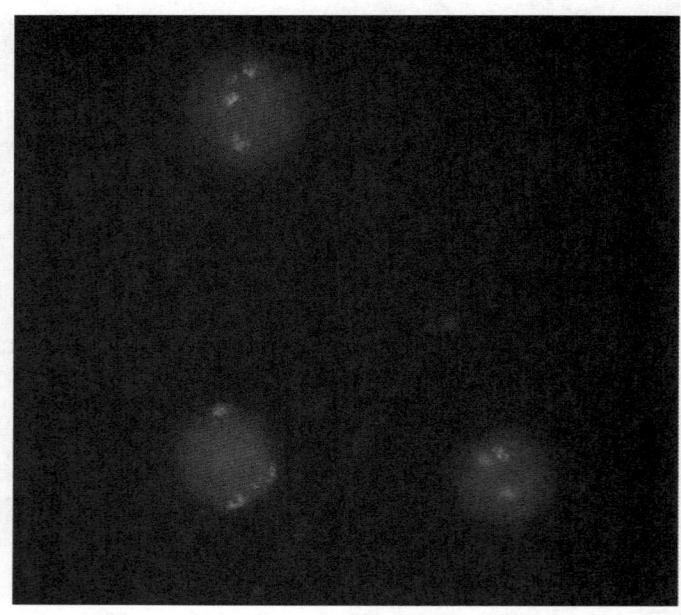

2.62 Identification of chromosome 18 in interphase nuclei using a centromeric probe detected with FITC and counterstained with propidium iodide.

A. *Normal*—two signals and B. *Trisomy 18*—three signals. (Photographs from slides prepared by C. M. Mackie, Cytogenetics Laboratory, Guy's Hospital.)

TISSUES

Introduction

Although some cells in the body are essentially migratory and therefore to some extent independent entities, most exist in aggregations which carry out similar or closely related functions, and which behave in a coordinated manner. Such groups are termed tissues. It would appear at first sight that there are innumerable tissues, each with its particular topographical territory, but extensive research has shown that they can be classified into a fairly small number of broad categories on the basis of their structure, behaviour and molecular properties. According to structure, most cell aggregates can be divided into four major types: *epithelia, connective tissues, muscle* and *nervous tissue*. Epithelia are essentially continuous layers of cells with little intercellular space which line surfaces (or are derived from such). In connective tissue the cells are embedded in intercellular substances which are typically abundant; muscle consists largely of specialised contractile cells, while nervous tissue consists of (1) cells specialised for conducting and transmitting electrochemically mediated information, and (2) of other cells which support those engaging in this activity. This simple scheme is of considerable value in predicting the behaviour of the constituent cells in both normal life and in pathological states, and in general, molecular studies have supported the concept. Thus, for example,

the intermediate filament proteins characteristic of all epithelia are (cyto)keratins, those of connective tissue are vimentins, desmins are typical of muscle; neurofilament and glial fibrillary acidic proteins characterise nervous tissue. However, as more and more molecular probes are used, the boundaries often begin to blur, and some cells have features of more than one tissue type, e.g. myofibroblasts, neuroepithelial receptors, ependymal cells of the central nervous system, etc. It is likely that eventually the simplified four tissues scheme will have to give way to a classification which reflects more closely the sequence of genomic events during the differentiation of individual cell lineages. Meanwhile the scheme, with all its anomalies, is most useful for descriptive purposes, and will be employed in the present account.

In this second part of the Cells and Tissues Section, two widespread tissues will be described: epithelia and 'general' or 'ordinary' connective tissue. Specialised skeletal connective tissue (cartilage, bone) are described with the skeleton (Section 6); muscle tissue with the muscles (Section 7); and nervous tissue with the nervous system (Section 8). Specialised defensive cells, also forming part of the general connective tissues, are considered with the haemolymphoid system (Section 9).

EPITHELIUM

The term *epithelium* is applied to the layer or layers of cells covering body surfaces. Strangely, this term originally referred to the cellular covering of the nipple (*thelos*) but has been extended to include the cellular covering of the body's exterior surface, and of all the body cavities opening on to it. Embryologically, epithelia are derived from the three germ layers. The ectoderm gives rise to the epidermis, glandular tissue of the breast, cornea and the junctional zones of the buccal cavity and anal canal. The endoderm forms the epithelial lining of the alimentary canal and its glands, most of the respiratory tract and the distal parts of the urogenital tract.

The epithelium-like cell layers lining internal cavities and the proximal parts of the urogenital tract stem from mesoderm and are variously known as *mesothelia*, lining the pericardial, pleural and peritoneal cavities, and *endothelia*, lining blood vessels and lymphatics. The term epithelium is retained for urinary and genital tract linings derived from mesoderm, however.

Epithelia function generally as selective barriers, aiding or preventing materials traversing the surfaces which they cover; some also protect underlying tissues against dehydration, chemical and mechanical damage; some elaborate and secrete materials into the spaces which they bound; others function as sensory surfaces. Indeed, many features of nervous tissue can be regarded as those of a modified epithelium.

Mesothelia and endothelia are classified as distinct from epithelia, as they are derived from mesenchymal cells rather than ectodermal or endodermal elements, and have some characteristic mesenchyme-derived features, for example, their cytoskeletal intermediate filaments are of the connective tissue type (vimentin) rather than the keratin filaments found in epithelia proper.

CHARACTERISTICS OF EPITHELIA

Epithelia (**2**.63) are predominantly cellular, that is, they possess little extracellular material. Intercellular junctions are usually numerous. Cell shape, typically polygonal, is partly determined by their cytoplasmic contents and partly by pressure from surrounding tissues, among other factors. The basal surface of an epithelium is in contact with a thin layer of filamentous protein and proteoglycan termed the *basal lamina*.

Epithelia can typically regenerate when injured, as seen most

dramatically in the liver, which can replace excised portions rapidly. Continuous replacement is also important where abrasion occurs and most epithelia covering external surfaces show a steady rate of cell division, which offsets loss of cells due to this cause. Perhaps because of this ability, tumours of epithelial origin (papillomata and carcinomata) are common.

Usually, blood vessels do not penetrate epithelia, diffusion from capillaries of neighbouring tissues providing nutrition. This limits the maximum thickness of living cell layers. Epithelia with their supporting connective tissue can often be removed surgically as one 'layer', collectively known as a *membrane*. Where the surface is moistened by mucous glands it is a *mucous membrane* or *mucosa*. (A similar layer of connective tissue covered by mesothelium is a *serous membrane* or *serosa*.)

CLASSIFICATION OF EPITHELIA (2.63)

Epithelia can be grouped into *unilaminar* (*simple*) epithelia—single layers of cells resting on a basal lamina; and *multilaminar* epithelia—that is, more than one cell thick. The latter includes: *replacing* or *stratified squamous* epithelia, in which superficial cells are constantly replaced from the basal layers; *urothelium* (*transitional epithelium*) serving special functions in the genito-urinary tract; and other multilaminar epithelia which, like urothelium, are replaced only very slowly under normal conditions. *Seminiferous epithelium* is a specialized tissue found in the testis.

UNILAMINAR (SIMPLE) EPITHELIA

Unilaminar epithelia may be further subdivided, according to the shape of their cells, into squamous, cuboidal, columnar and pseudo-stratified types. Cell shape is largely related to cell volume; where little cytoplasm is present, denoting few organelles and therefore a low metabolic activity, cells are squamous or low cuboidal. Highly active cells, for example ciliated and secretory forms, contain abundant mitochondria and endoplasmic reticulum and are typically tall cuboidal or columnar (although there are exceptions to this rule, e.g. kidney proximal convoluted tubule cells are cuboidal and bear many microvilli).

67

E P I T H E L I A L   T I S S U E S

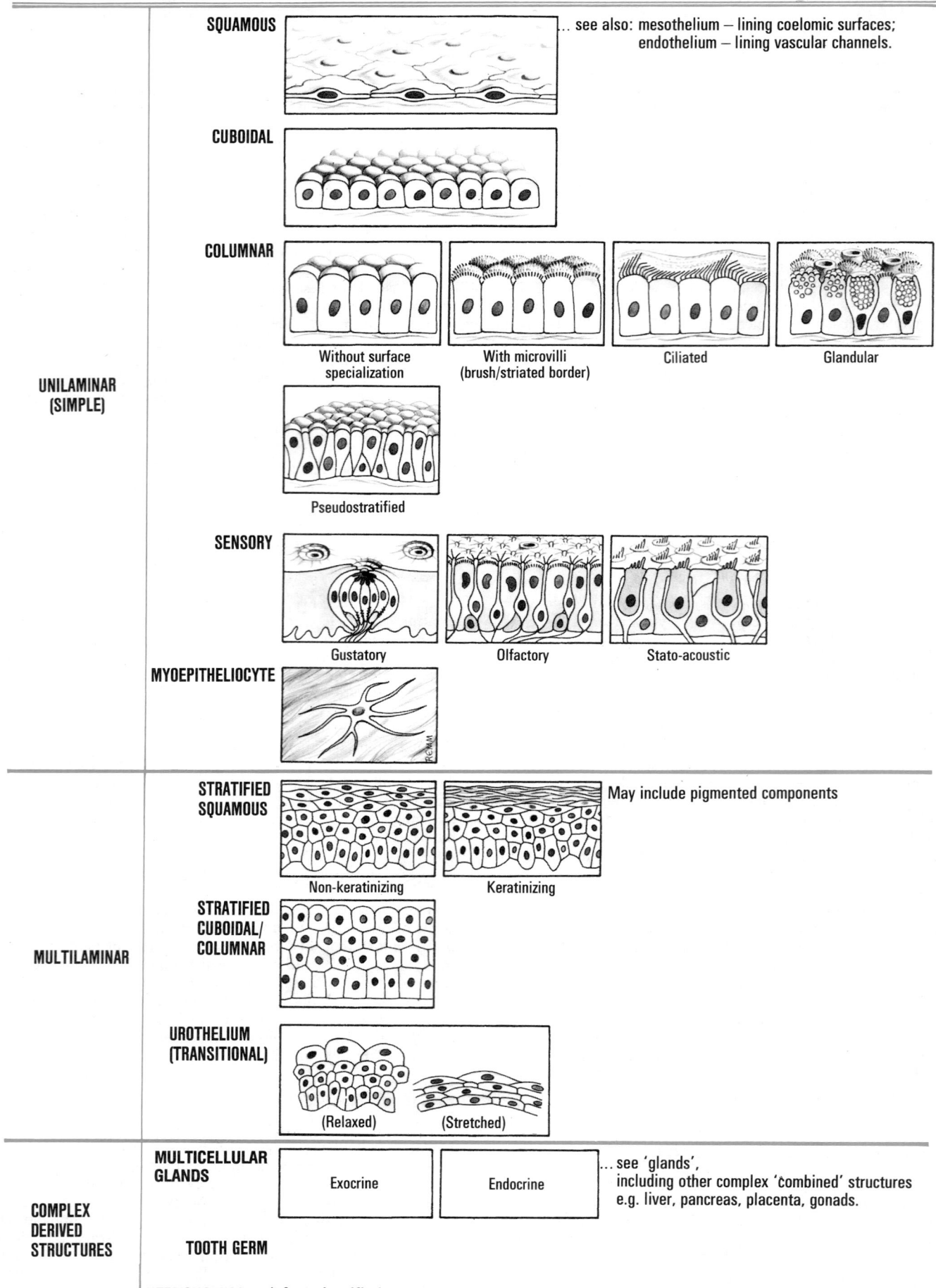

SQUAMOUS

... see also: mesothelium — lining coelomic surfaces;
endothelium — lining vascular channels.

CUBOIDAL

COLUMNAR

Without surface specialization | With microvilli (brush/striated border) | Ciliated | Glandular

UNILAMINAR (SIMPLE)

Pseudostratified

SENSORY

Gustatory | Olfactory | Stato-acoustic

MYOEPITHELIOCYTE

STRATIFIED SQUAMOUS

May include pigmented components

Non-keratinizing | Keratinizing

STRATIFIED CUBOIDAL/ COLUMNAR

MULTILAMINAR

UROTHELIUM (TRANSITIONAL)

(Relaxed) | (Stretched)

MULTICELLULAR GLANDS

Exocrine | Endocrine

... see 'glands',
including other complex 'combined' structures
e.g. liver, pancreas, placenta, gonads.

COMPLEX DERIVED STRUCTURES

TOOTH GERM

NERVOUS TISSUE (often classified as a separate tissue, but retains many characteristics of its epithelial origins).
SEMINIFEROUS EPITHELIUM

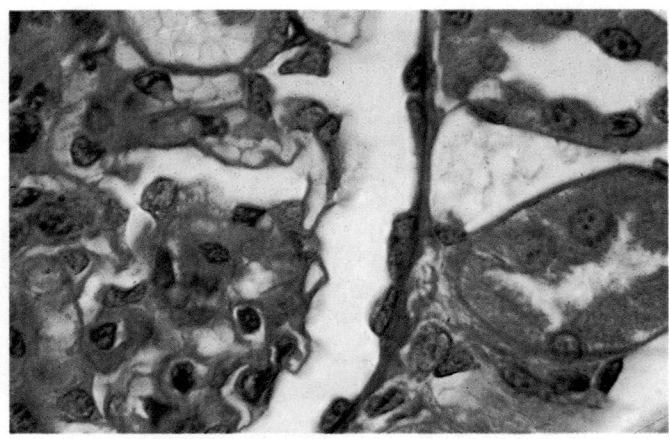

2.64 Part of a renal corpuscle showing vertically sectioned simple squamous epithelial cells in Bowman's capsule. Mallory's triple stain.

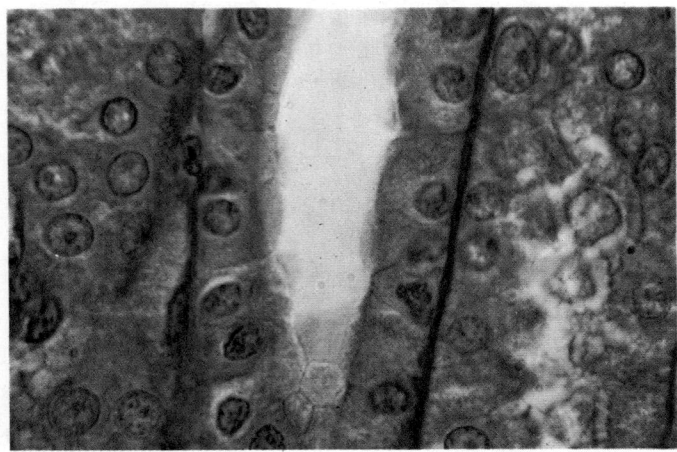

2.65 Simple cuboidal epithelium in renal collecting ducts. Masson's trichrome stain.

Unilaminar epithelia can also be subdivided into those which have special functions, i.e. those with cilia, microvilli (brush and striated borders), secretory vacuoles (in mucous and serous glandular cells) or sensory features. *Myoepitheliocytes*, which are contractile, occur as isolated cells associated with glandular structures, for example salivary glands and mammary glands.

SQUAMOUS (PAVEMENT) EPITHELIUM

Squamous epithelium is composed of flattened, interlocking, polygonal cells (*squames*). The cytoplasm may in places be only 0.1 μm thick and the nucleus usually bulges into the overlying space (**2.63**, 64). These cells line the alveoli of the lungs, renal corpuscles, the thin segments of the nephric tubules and various parts of the inner ear (see e.g. **8.495**).

Simple squamous epithelia may also be *tessellated*, the cells having sinuous interlocking borders rather than straight boundaries.

Because it is so thin, squamous epithelium allows rapid diffusion of gases and water but may also engage in active transport, as indicated by the numerous endocytic vesicles often seen in such cells. Occluding junctions between adjacent cells ensure that materials pass primarily *through* cells rather than between them.

CUBOIDAL AND COLUMNAR EPITHELIA

Cuboidal and columnar epithelia consist of regular rows of cylindrical cells (**2.65–67**). Cuboidal cells are square in vertical section, whereas columnar cells are taller than their diameter, and both are polygonal when sectioned horizontally. Commonly, microvilli are found on their free surfaces, providing a large absorptive area (p. 40), for example, the epithelium of the small intestine (columnar cells with a striated border), the gallbladder (columnar cells with a brush border) and proximal and distal convoluted tubules of the kidney (large cuboidal cells with brush borders). Ciliated columnar epithelium lines most of the respiratory tract (**2.68–70**) as far as the respiratory bronchioles (excepting the lower pharynx and vocal folds), some of the tympanic cavity and auditory tube, the uterine tube and patches in the cavity of the uterus and cervix, and efferent ductules of the testis.

Mucous glands also line the respiratory tract and cilia sweep a layer of viscous fluid and trapped dust particles, etc. from the lung towards the pharynx (the *mucociliary rejection current*), clearing the respiratory passages of inhaled particles. In the uterine tube, cilia may assist the passage of ova from the peritoneal cavity to the uterus.

Some columnar cells are glandular, their apices containing mucus or proteinaceous vacuoles, for example mucin-secreting and chief cells of the gastric epithelium. Often mucous cells lie among non-secretory ones, allowing expansion of the secretory apices to give a shape characteristic of these, the *goblet*, *chalice* or *calciform* cells (**2.67**), for example in the intestinal epithelium. For further details of glandular tissue, see page 73.

Mucus

Mucus is a viscous suspension of complex glycoproteins of various kinds, as well as many other secretory products of adjacent epithelial cells. All mucous glycoproteins (*mucins*) consist of filamentous *core proteins* to which are attached carbohydrate chains, usually branched, standing out from the core protein like bristles in a bottle brush; up to 600 such chains occur in human salivary mucus, so that the entire molecule is quite huge. Furthermore, such glycoproteins typically are linked by sulphydryl groups into tetramers, with molecular weights of 2 million or more. Carbohydrate residues include glucose, fucose, galactose and the negatively charged N-acetylglucosamine (sialic acid), particularly near the free ends of the chains. The terminals of some carbohydrate chains are identical with the blood group antigens of the ABO (ABH) group in about 80% of the population ('secretors', bearing the *secretor gene* S^e) and can be detected in salivary mucus with appropriate clinical tests. There is an interesting correlation between the absence of these antigens in mucus and proneness to gastric ulcers and it is possible that they

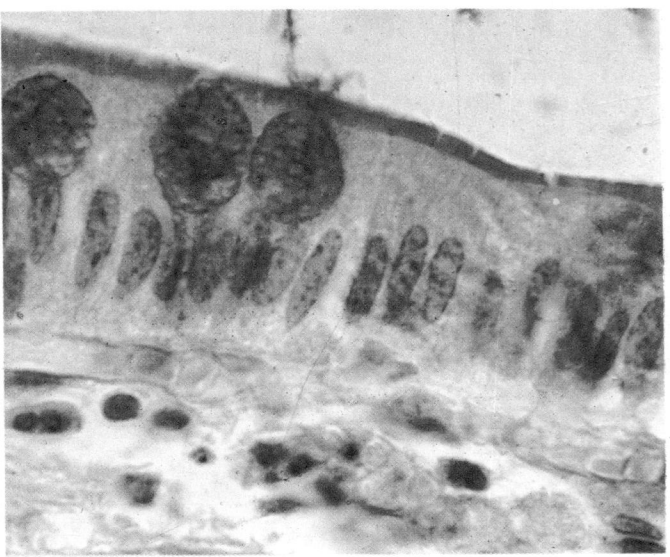

2.66 Simple columnar epithelium of the small intestine showing absorptive cells with a striated border and goblet cells. PAS-haematoxylin.

2.63 (*opposite*) Classification of the major types of epithelia and associated tissues described in the ensuing section.

69

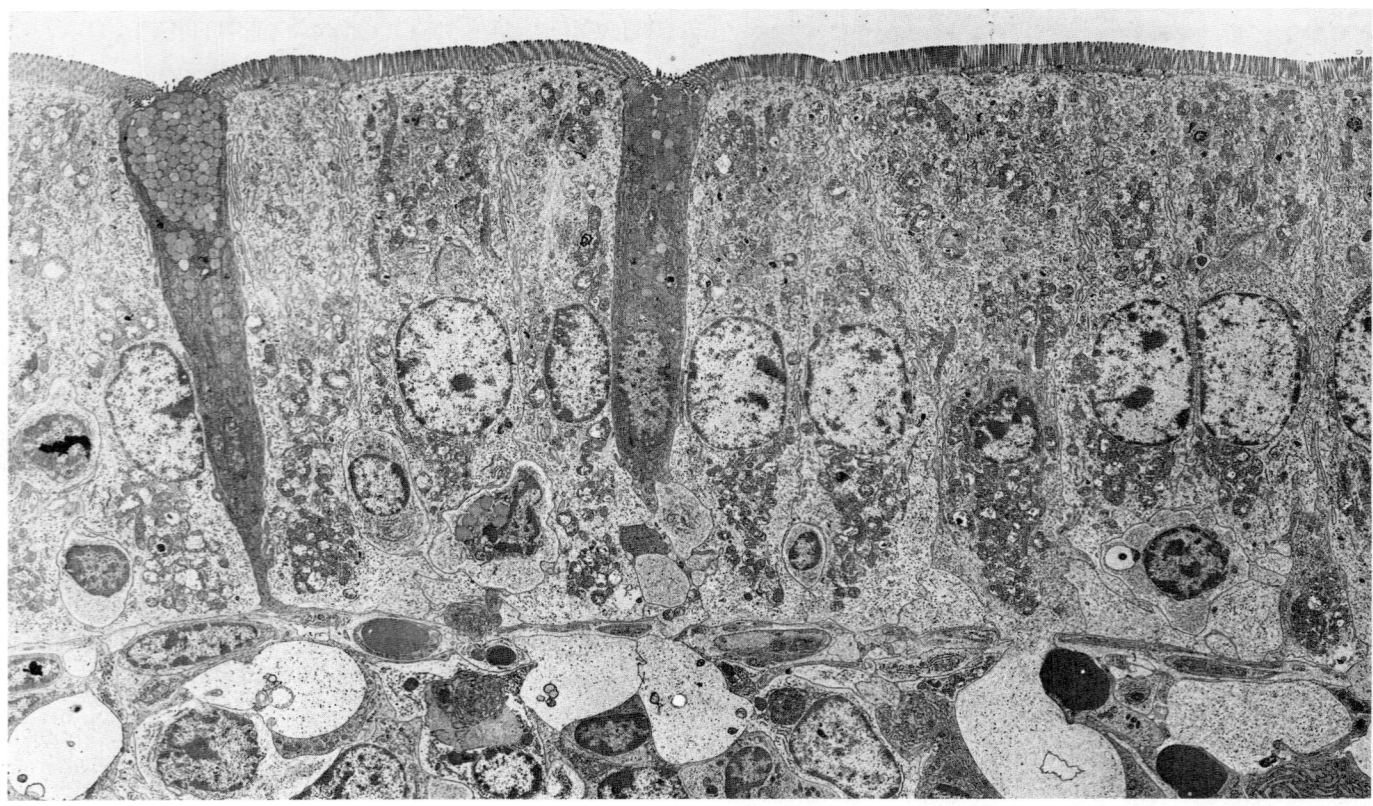

2.67 Low-power electron micrograph of a vertical section through simple columnar epithelium bearing microvilli; two goblet cells are also present. Note the presence of several small lymphocytes near the epithelial base.

Small intestine. Provided by Derrick Lovell, Guy's Hospital Medical School. Magnification × 8000.

confer protective properties on gastric and perhaps other types of mucus. The long polymeric carbohydrate chains bind water and so protect surfaces against drying; when in dilute suspension, their molecules can slide over one another with ease, providing good lubricating properties, and their negative charges also bind cations such as Na^+. In more concentrated states, they form viscous layers which protect the underlying tissues against damage.

Mucus is synthesized in a stepwise fashion (Peterson & Leblond 1964); protein synthesized in the granular endoplasmic reticulum is passed to the Golgi complex, where it is first conjugated with sulphated carbohydrates to form the glycoprotein, *mucinogen*, then exported in small dense vesicles which swell as they approach the cell surface and finally fuse with it to release the mucus.

PSEUDOSTRATIFIED EPITHELIUM

Pseudostratified epithelium is a simple columnar epithelium in which nuclei lie at different levels in a vertical section (**2**.63). Not all cells extend through the whole thickness of the epithelium, some constituting a basal cell layer, often mitotic and able to replace damaged mature cells. Migrating lymphocytes and mast cells within columnar epithelia may also give a pseudostratified appearance

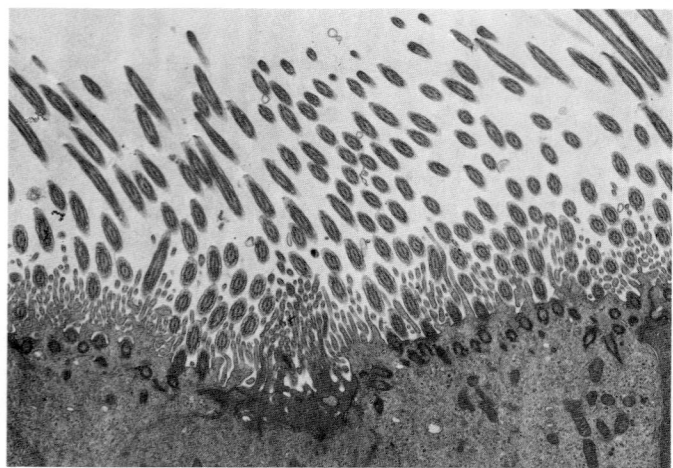

2.68   Detail of a group of cilia cut in various planes at the surface of a ciliated columnar epithelial cell from the upper respiratory tract. Note the presence of small microvilli interspersed between the cilia. Magnification × 7500.

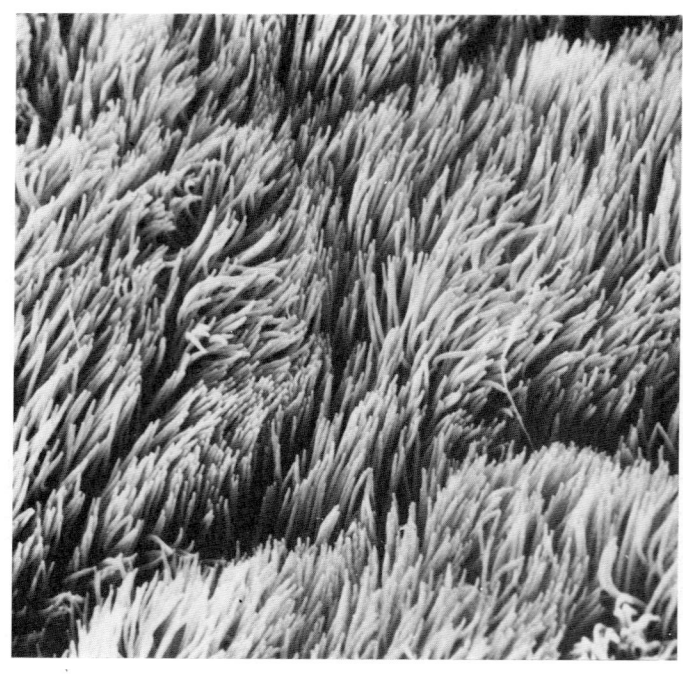

2.69   Low-power scanning electron micrograph of the ciliated surface of the trachea. Magnification × 3000.

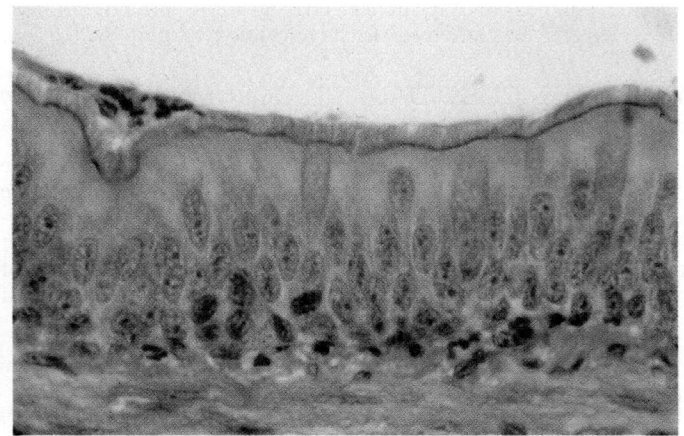

2.70 Simple ciliated pseudostratified epithelium at the surface of a bronchus showing a superficial layer of mucus entrapping some particles, and several goblet cells. PAS-haematoxylin. Magnification × 850.

because their nuclei are placed at different depths. Much of the ciliated lining of the respiratory tract is of the pseudostratified type (2.70), and so also are the sensory epithelium of the olfactory area (p. 1313) and parts of the male urethral lining (2.71).

SENSORY EPITHELIA

Sensory epithelia are restricted to special sense organs of the olfactory, gustatory and vestibulocochlear receptor systems. All of these contain sensory cells surrounded by supportive, non-receptive cells. Olfactory receptors are modified neurons, their axons passing directly to the brain, but the other types are specialized epithelial cells synapsing with terminals of afferent (and sometimes efferent) nerve fibres (see Nervous System, Section 8).

MYOEPITHELIOCYTES

Also sometimes termed *basket cells*, these are fusiform or stellate in shape, containing actin and myosin filaments; they contract when stimulated by nervous or neurohormonal signals (Abe et al 1981). They surround the secretory portions and ducts of some glands, for example mammary, lacrimal, salivary and sweat glands (Nagato et al 1980), lying within the basal laminae at the surface of these structures. Their contraction assists the initial flow of secretion into larger channels. Myoepitheliocytes are ultrastructurally similar to smooth muscle cells in the arrangement of their actin and myosin but they originate from ecto- or endoderm. They are considered further on page 780.

MULTILAMINAR EPITHELIA

Multilaminar epithelia are found at surfaces subjected to mechanical wear and tear or other potentially harmful conditions. They can be divided into those which continue to replace their surface cells from deeper layers (stratified squamous epithelia) and others where replacement is extremely slow except after injury.

STRATIFIED SQUAMOUS EPITHELIA

Stratified squamous epithelia are multilayered tissues in which there is a constant formation, maturation and loss of cells. Formed mitotically in the most basal layers, their cells move more superficially, changing from a cuboidal or columnar shape to a more flattened form, and eventually being shed from the surface. These epithelia occur in sites exposed to mechanical stresses and provide for a constant protection of the underlying tissues against mechanical, microbial and chemical damage. Typically, the cells are held together by numerous desmosomes to form strong continuous cellular sheets. The two major types of these epithelia are *keratinized* and *non-keratinized stratified squamous epithelia*.

Keratinized epithelium (2.72)

Keratinized epithelium is found at surfaces which are subject to drying as well as mechanical stresses or are exposed to high levels of abrasion. These include the entire epidermis, the mucocutaneous junctions of the lips, nostrils, distal anal canal, the outer surface of the tympanic membrane and parts of the oral lining—gingivae, hard palate and anterior dorsal tongue. Their cells, *keratinocytes*, are formed by the mitosis of basally-sited stem cells (the *stratum basale*) and gradually pass towards the surface in a column of moving cells. When newly formed, keratinocytes contain many ribosomes, mitochondria and other metabolically active organelles and have an extensive cytoskeleton of keratin filament bundles (tonofibrils), anchored into the plasma membrane at desmosomal contacts with neighbouring cells. The most basal layer of cells is also anchored to the basal lamina by hemidesmosomes (p. 27). As keratinocytes move away from the base, the cell surfaces become highly folded, tightly interlocking with those of adjacent cells to present a spiny appearance. These cells (*prickle cells*) together comprise the *stratum spinosum*. As they move more superficially they begin to flatten and synthesize other substances including a dense, basophilic protein, keratohyalin, which mingles with the keratin filaments and gives the cells of this layer (the *stratum granulosum*) a granular appearance. Simultaneously, the cells synthesize and secrete a glycolipid which coats the cell surface, forming a thick, adhesive, water-resistant lipidic cement between the flattened cells. At this stage the cells lose their nuclei, the keratin filaments become firmly embedded in the matrix protein and the cells are now dead, flattened plates (squames);

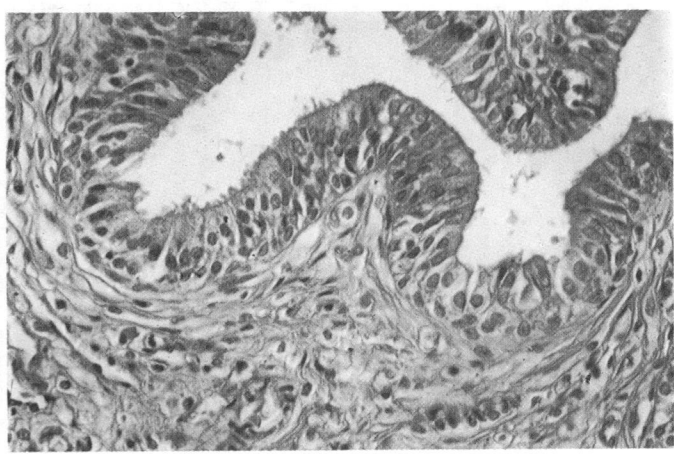

2.71 Pseudostratified epithelium from the male urethra. Haematoxylin and eosin. Magnification × 400.

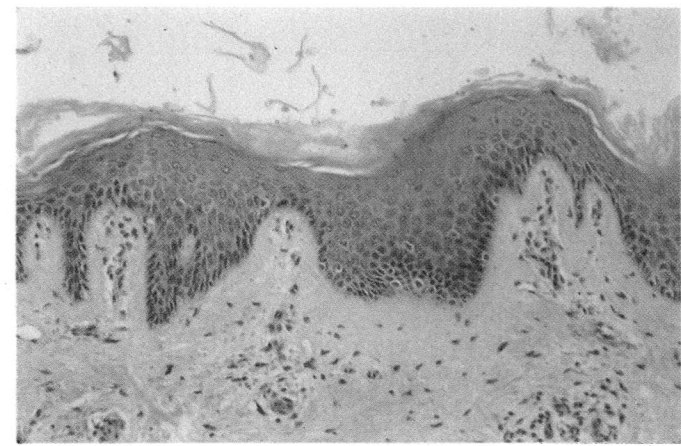

2.72 Section of keratinized stratified squamous epithelium forming the epidermis of the skin, in this example of the scalp. Note the presence of a superficial zone of anucleate keratinized cells. Connective tissue of the dermis underlies the epithelium. Haematoxylin and eosin. Magnification × 150.

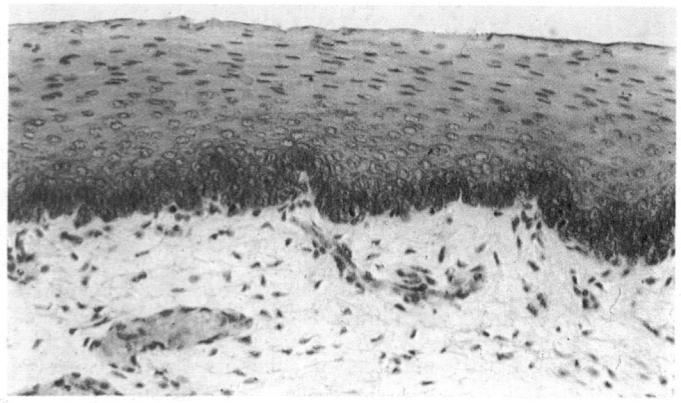

2.73 Non-keratinizing, stratified squamous epithelium from the human tongue. A vertical section stained with haematoxylin and eosin. Note the presence of nuclei in the surface cells. Magnification × 150.

initially these anucleate cells form a thin glassy stratum (*stratum lucidum*) which rapidly matures into the final condition of the external *stratum corneum*. The cells of this layer ('corneocytes') eventually flake off from the surface. For further information on these processes, see page 383.

This unusual combination of strongly coherent layers of living cells and more superficial strata made of plates of inert, mechanically robust protein complexes, interleaved with water-resistant lipid, makes this type of epithelium an excellent barrier against different types of injury and water loss.

Non-keratinizing epithelium

Non-keratinizing epithelium is present at surfaces subject to abrasion but protected from drying (**2.73**), including the buccal cavity (except for the areas noted above), oro- and laryngopharynx, oesophagus, part of the anal canal, vagina, distal uterine cervix, distal urethra, the conjunctiva and cornea, inner surfaces of eyelids and the vestibule of the nasal cavities. Characteristically, its cells go through the same transitions in general shape as seen in the keratinized type but do not fill completely with keratin or secrete glycolipid, and retain their nuclei until they desquamate at the surface. In sites where considerable abrasion occurs the epithelium is thicker and its more superficial cells may synthesize some keratin (*parakeratinized* epithelia in contrast to the fully, or *orthokeratinized*, state of keratinized epithelium), as, for example, in much of the buccal cavity (see p. 1687). Diets deficient in vitamin A may induce keratinization of such epithelia and excessive doses may lead to its transformation into mucus-secreting epithelium.

Cells gently removed by swabbing epithelial surfaces can be

collected, stained and examined for signs of pathological (e.g. cancerous) transformations (exfoliative cytology, e.g. p. 1875).

STRATIFIED CUBOIDAL AND COLUMNAR EPITHELIA

Two or more layers of cuboidal or columnar cells are typical of the walls of the larger ducts of some exocrine glands, such as the pancreas and salivary glands and the ducts of sweat glands, presumably affording more strength than a single layer. These are not continually replaced by basal mitoses and there is no progression of form from base to surface, although they can repair themselves if damaged.

UROTHELIUM (URINARY OR TRANSITIONAL EPITHELIUM)

Urothelium (**2.74–76**) lines much of the urinary tract, extending from the ends of the collecting ducts of the kidneys, through ureters and bladder to the proximal portion of the urethra. In males it covers the urethra as far as the ejaculatory ducts, then becomes intermittent, finally being replaced by pseudostratified epithelium in the membranous urethra (see also p. 1831). In females it also extends as far as the urogenital membrane. During development part of it is derived from mesoderm and part from ectoderm and endoderm. The epithelium appears to be 4–6 cells thick and lines organs which undergo considerable distension and contraction; it can, therefore, stretch greatly without losing its integrity. In stretching, the cells

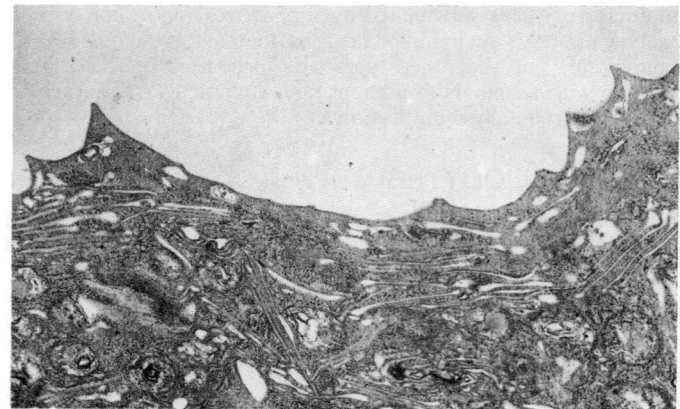

2.75 Transmission electron micrograph of the surface of the urothelium (transitional epithelium) lining the relaxed bladder. Note the angular profiles of the epithelial surface and the plate-like areas of membrane internalisation. Magnification × 15 000.

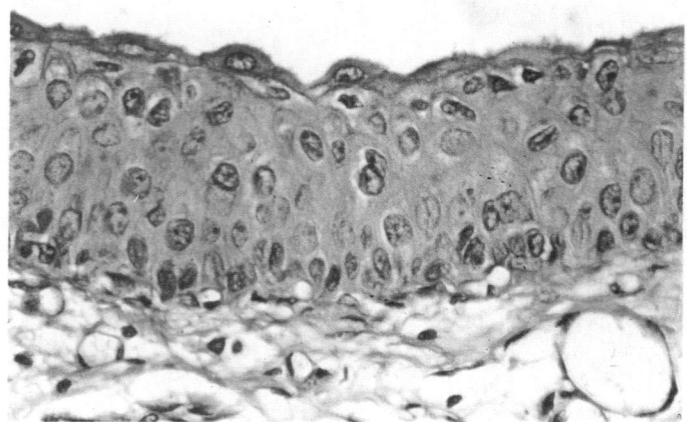

2.74 A vertical section through the surface of a ureter to show the urothelium lining its lumen, stained by Mallory's triple staining technique. Magnification × 600.

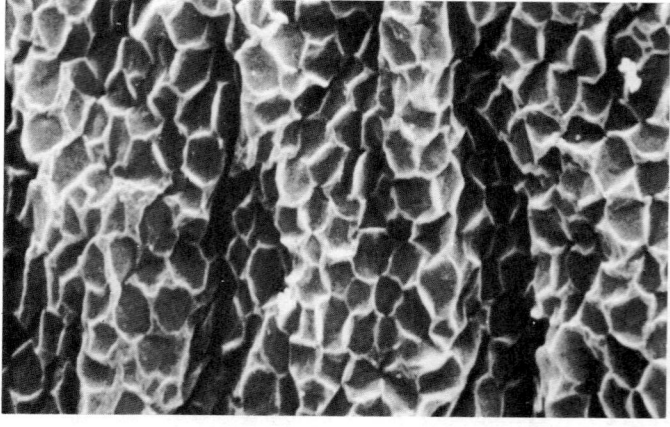

2.76 Scanning electron micrograph of the (relaxed) urothelial surface showing the plate-like arrangement of its plasma membrane. Magnification × 6000.

become flattened, without altering their positions relative to each other, since they are firmly connected by numerous desmosomes (see review by Hicks 1975). On close inspection, many cells are seen to be attached to the basal lamina of the epithelium by slender basal processes and it has been proposed that perhaps all cells, even the most superficial, are attached to the base; thus this tissue could be viewed as a type of specialized pseudostratified epithelium (see p. 1832), in which case it should be reclassified as a unilaminar epithelium (see Scheidegger 1980; Walton et al 1982). However, this view is not generally accepted.

The basally placed cells are cuboidal when relaxed, uninucleate (diploid) and basophilic with many ribosomes. More apically the cells progressively fuse to form larger, binucleate or uninucleate but polyploid cells. The surface cells are largest and may even be octoploid; their luminal surfaces are covered by a plasma membrane bearing plates of glycoprotein particles embedded in its lipid bilayer. These arrays stiffen the membrane so that, when the epithelium is in the relaxed state and the surface area of the cells is reduced, the glycoprotein-lipid plates are partially taken into the cytoplasm within vacuoles or diverticula, re-emerging on to the surface when its area increases once more through stretching (see Minsky & Chlapowski 1978).

These unusual membranes, together with the occluding junctions of the surface cells, form an effective barrier preventing urine from passing into the epithelium or beyond into the adjacent tissues. The urothelium, therefore, creates a protective lining to the urinary system which prevents its rather toxic contents from damaging surrounding structures.

Normally, cell turnover is very slow, cell division being restricted to the basal layer, and infrequent. When damaged, however, the epithelium regenerates quite rapidly (Annis 1962).

SEMINIFEROUS EPITHELIUM

Seminiferous epithelium is highly specialized and consists of a heterogenous population of cells forming the lineage of the spermatozoa, (spermatogonia, spermatocytes, spermatids), together with supporting cells (Sertoli cells). This epithelium is described further on page 1850.

GLANDS (2.77–79)

One of the features of many epithelia—their ability to alter the environment which they face by the directed transport of ions, water or macromolecules—is seen par excellence in glandular tissue. Here the metabolism and structural organization of the cells is specialized for the elaboration, transport and release of macromolecules, usually from the apical surface into neighbouring spaces or compartments. Such cells may exist as isolated individuals amongst other non-secretory cells, such as goblet cells in the absorptive lining of the small intestine, or may form highly coherent sheets of epithelium with a common secretory design, for example the mucous lining of the stomach and, in a highly folded configuration, the complex salivary glands. Glands may be broadly divided into:

- *exocrine glands* which secrete on to surfaces continuous with the body's exterior, including the alimentary tract, respiratory system, urinary and genital ducts, and their derivatives, and of course the integument itself;
- *endocrine glands* (ductless glands) which secrete hormones directly into the circulatory system which then conveys their secretions throughout the body to affect the activities of other cells.

Paracrine gland cells are similar to endocrine cells, but their

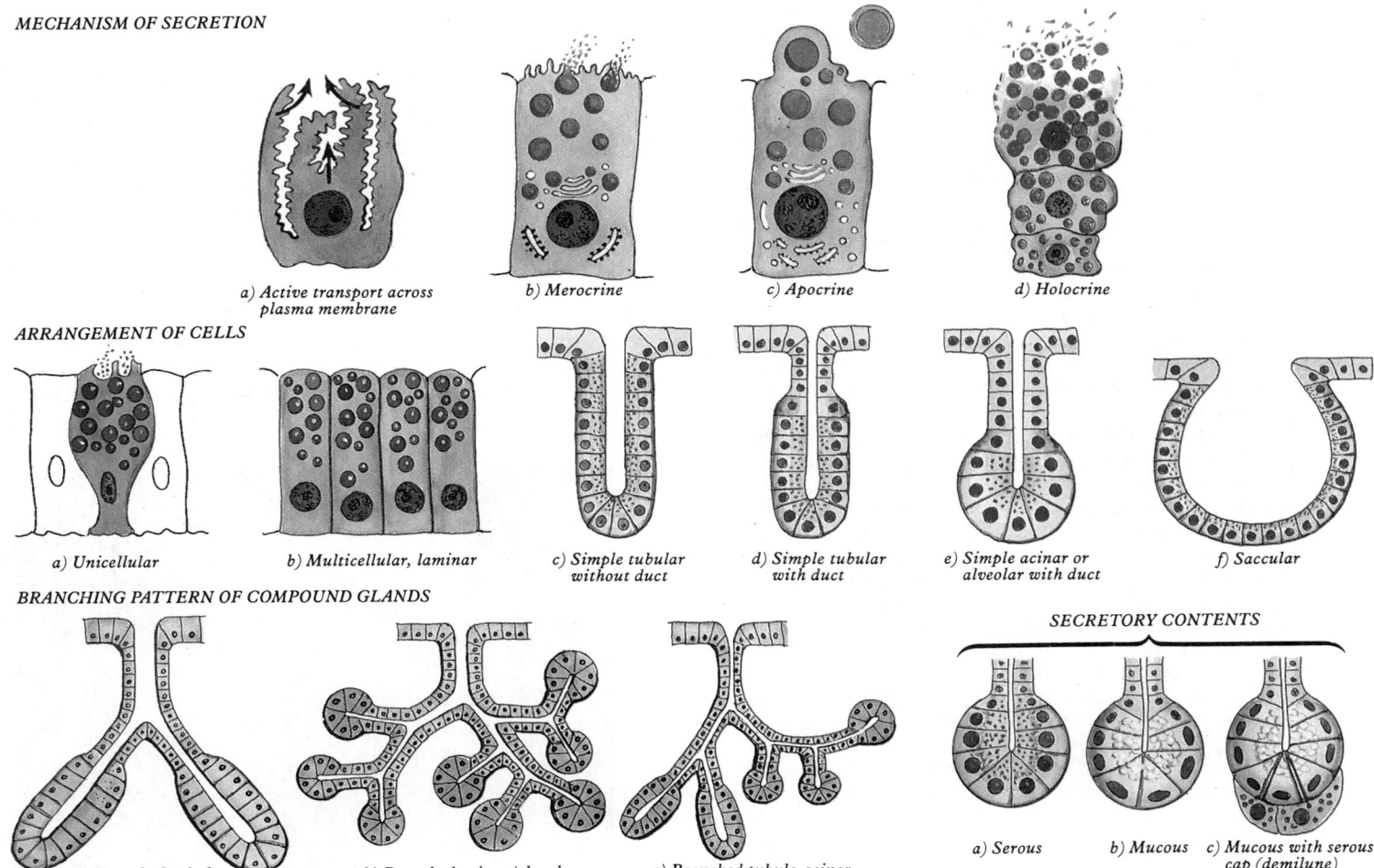

MECHANISM OF SECRETION

a) *Active transport across plasma membrane*   b) *Merocrine*   c) *Apocrine*   d) *Holocrine*

ARRANGEMENT OF CELLS

a) *Unicellular*   b) *Multicellular, laminar*   c) *Simple tubular without duct*   d) *Simple tubular with duct*   e) *Simple acinar or alveolar with duct*   f) *Saccular*

BRANCHING PATTERN OF COMPOUND GLANDS

a) *Branched tubular*   b) *Branched acinar/alveolar*   c) *Branched tubulo-acinar*

SECRETORY CONTENTS

a) *Serous*   b) *Mucous*   c) *Mucous with serous cap (demilune)*

2.77 Schema which shows the different types of glands classified by currently used methods.

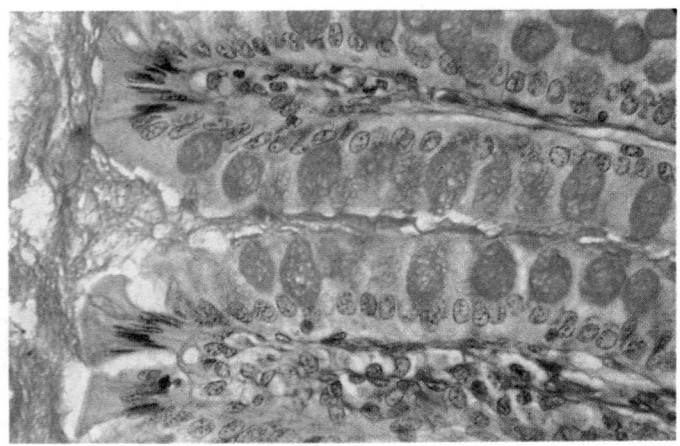

2.78 Section through part of a simple tubular gland (colon) stained with alcian blue to show mucous gland cells. Magnification × 500.

secretions diffuse locally to cellular targets in their immediate vicinity. In addition to strictly epithelial glands, some tissues derived from the nervous system are *neurosecretory*, including the adrenal medulla and neurohypophysis; these are considered further with other endocrine glands in Section 15.

Relation of gland cell structure to secretory products

Glandular cells of different types synthesize and release a wide variety of macromolecules and other materials, and their cellular organization reflects the chemical nature of their secretory products. At one end of the range, parietal cells lining the walls of gastric glands secrete hydrochloric acid, and various gland cells in the small intestine wall release bicarbonate, sodium and chloride ions and water. In a similar fashion, eccrine sweat glands in the skin secrete a very dilute solution of electrolytes derived from tissue fluid. These types of secretion involve small exocytic vesicles or proteinaceous channels in the plasma membrane rather than any elaborate secretory mechanism. More typically secretory are cells of the various glands lining the alimentary tract and its embryonic derivatives. These are mainly glycoprotein synthesizers such as mucous and zymogen cells. Their cytoplasm is characteristically rich in granular endoplasmic reticulum which synthesizes the protein component and begins its glycosylation, and is also well-endowed with Golgi complex components which complete glycosylation (and often sulphation) amongst other modifications of proteins destined for secretion. In some cells, for example mucin secretors (p. 69) the amounts of added carbohydrates are considerable, whereas in others, for example pancreatic acinar cells, the protein component predominates. Such cells are rich in cytoplasmic nucleic acids and therefore often appear very basophilic in stained light microscopic preparations although their secretory vacuoles may give different reactions. The secretory products are concentrated and packaged at the *trans-Golgi network* (TGN) into membranous vesicles which may be stored in the cytoplasm for later secretion, or more rarely, secreted immediately.

In endocrine cells secreting steroids, such as those of the adrenal cortex, gonads and placenta, the cytoplasmic organization is quite different: they are extremely rich in agranular (smooth) endoplasmic reticulum, and often, lipid droplets, which are related chemically to the pathways of steroid synthesis. Such cells are often quite eosinophilic by light microscopy, and may have conspicuous stainable lipid inclusions.

Types of secretory processes (2.77)

The mechanism of secretion also varies considerably. Where the secretions are initially packaged into vesicles, these are conveyed to the cell surface where they are discharged in a number of different ways. In *merocrine secretion*, by far the most common type, their membranes fuse with the plasma membrane to release their contents to the exterior. This apparently simple train of events involves a surprisingly complex set of molecular interactions; the directed movement of vesicles to a particular part of the cell—usually the

apex—appears to be at least partly due to microtubular transport, although where vesicles are large other mechanisms may also operate. Having arrived at the appropriate part of the cell surface, specialized transmembrane molecules in the secretory vacuole wall recognize marker proteins on the cytoplasmic side of the plasma membrane and bind to them (see also p. 32). This initiates interactions with other sets of proteins which cause the fusion of the two membranes and the consequent release of the vesicle contents. Membrane added to the cell surface by repeated vesicle fusion can be taken back into the cell by endocytosis and re-cycled for further secretory vesicles (see Pearse & Bretscher 1981). The stimulus for secretion varies with the type of cell, but often appears to involve a classic second messenger system such as the cyclic AMP pathway which causes internal calcium release in the cytoplasm, for example, in mucous cells.

In *holocrine glands*, such as the sebaceous glands in the skin, the cells first fill with secretory products (lipidic droplets in this instance) then disintegrate to liberate the accumulated mass of secretory vesicles. In *apocrine glands*, some of the apical cytoplasm is pinched off with the contained secretions. The best understood example of this is the secretion of milk lipid by mammary gland cells (p. 422), although only a minimal amount of cytoplasm is actually released in this case. Larger amounts of cytoplasm seem to be involved in secretion by specialized apocrine sweat glands in the axilla and genitoanal regions of the body. In some tissues there is a combination of different types of secretion. For instance, the parietal cells of the gastric glands also secrete a protein–intrinsic factor, presumably by the merocrine method; mammary gland cells secrete lipid by apocrine secretion but the milk protein casein in the merocrine mode. The mechanism by which steroid synthesizing cells release their products appears to be poorly understood, although it is possible that they pass directly through the plasma membrane because of their lipophilic properties.

Chemical classification of glands

Glands can be classified by their secretory products. Exocrine glands of some regions, for example the buccal cavity, are traditionally divided into:

- mucus-secreting or *mucous glands*, whose cells possess frothy cytoplasm with basal flattened nuclei and stain with metachromatic stains and periodic acid-Schiff (PAS) methods;
- *serous glands* where the cells have centrally placed nuclei, and eosinophilic granules in their cytoplasm, secreting mainly glycoproteins (including lysozyme, a bactericide, and digestive enzymes).

Some glands are entirely mucous (for instance the sublingual salivary glands), whilst others are mainly serous (the parotid salivary glands). The submandibular gland is mixed, some lobules being predominantly mucous and others serous. In some regions mucous

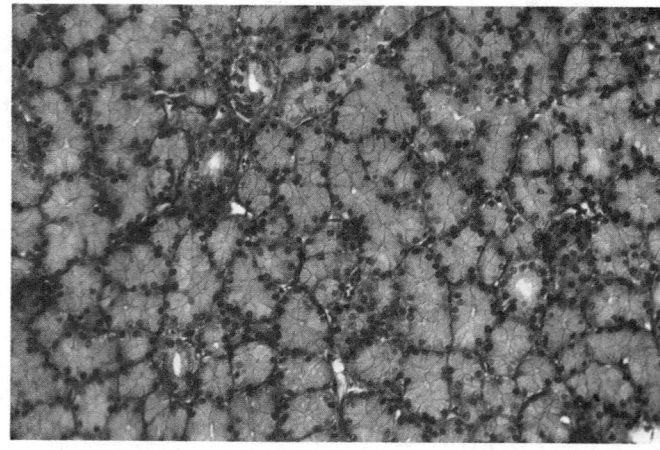

2.79 Section through a compound alveolar gland (nasopharynx), stained with periodic acid-Schiff to show mucus within secretory lobules. The connective tissue septa have been stained blue. Two small ducts are also visible. Magnification × 160.

acini are capped with crescents of serous cells (*serous demilunes*). While this simple approach to classification has some convenience for easy description, chemical analyses of glandular secretions shows that there is a great diversity of molecules made and secreted by these and other glands, and that complex mixtures often exist within the same cell. Regional variations also occur throughout the body, each part having its own particular set of secretions appropriate to local function, and meriting individual attention.

Morphology of glands (2.77)

Exocrine glands. These are either unicellular (e.g. goblet cells, p. 69) or multicellular. The latter may be in the form of simple sheets of secretory cells, for example at the surface of the stomach, or may be extended into diverticula of various shapes and extents. Such glands may be single units (*simple glands*) or branched, *compound glands*. Simple unbranched tubular glands exist in the walls of many of the hollow viscera, for example the small intestine and uterus, while some glands have expanded, flask-like ends (acini or alveoli). Such glands may consist entirely of secretory cells, or may have a blind-ending secretory portion leading through a non-secretory duct to the lumen of the viscus, in which case the ducts may modify the secretions as they pass along them. Glands with ducts may be branched (compound), sometimes forming elaborate ductal trees. Compound glands generally have acinar or alveolar secretory lobules, but the secretory units may alternatively be tubular or mixed tubulo-acinar. More than one type of secretory cell may occur within a particular secretory unit, or individual units may be specialized to just one type of secretion (e.g. mucous and serous acini of salivary glands). While the significance of these different types of geometry is not yet understood, they all constitute ways of creating a larger area for secretion than would be available at a simple secretory surface.

Endocrine glands. Secreting directly into the circulation, these tend to be grouped around rich beds of capillaries or sinusoids that are typically lined by endothelia possessing small apertures (fenestrated endothelia) which allow the rapid passage of macro-molecules through their walls. Endocrine cells may be arranged in *clumps* around vascular networks or *cords* between parallel vascular channels or as hollow balls or cells (*follicles*) surrounding their stored secretions. Isolated endocrine cells also exist scattered throughout the alimentary and respiratory tracts (the entero-endocrine system, p. 1787).

Control of secretion

The high metabolic rate of many glands is reflected in their rich vascular beds which can often be controlled by autonomic vasomotor nerves to modify glandular activity. Gland cells can also be controlled directly or indirectly by autonomic secretomotor fibres which may either form synapses on their bases (e.g. in the adrenal medulla) or release neuromediators in the vicinity of the glands to reach them by more distant diffusion, or alternatively to act indirectly by an intermediary, for example histamine released neurogenically from another cell, as in the gastric lining. Paracrine influences from enteroendocrine cells are also important in the alimentary and bronchial glands. In many endocrine glands, circulating hormones from the adenohypophysis stimulate synthesis and secretion by their target cells. Such signals, mostly detected by receptors at the cell surface and mediated by second messenger systems, may increase the synthetic activity of gland cells, and also cause them to discharge their secretions by exocytosis.

Secretions already released into ducts are expressed rapidly from certain glands by the contraction of associated myoepithelial cells enclosing the secretory units and smaller ducts. These may be under direct neural control, as in salivary glands, or, for example in the mammary gland, they respond to circulating hormones—oxytocin in this instance.

Secretory cycle. On close inspection, most glands show cells in varying stages of synthesis, secretion and depletion, and except in the case of holocrine secretory cells which die when they release their contents, there is typically a cycle of activity in which secretions are first synthesized, then stored until the signal is given to secrete. The cell may then rest briefly before recommencing synthesis of secretion. In certain instances, for example goblet cells, the cell has only a limited, programmed life span and may only secrete for a short period of time before its demise.

COMPLEX STRUCTURES DERIVED FROM EPITHELIUM

Complex structures include those organs which are largely derived from epithelia and retain their highly cellular nature; they often possess typical epithelial features such as secretory, absorptive and transport functions and include the liver, placenta, and the amelo-blasts lamina of the early tooth germ, responsible for secreting the tooth enamel (p. 1710). At the far end of this range, the highly cellular, neurectoderm-derived nervous system as a whole can be viewed as a highly elaborate epithelial structure.

CONNECTIVE TISSUES

INTRODUCTION

The connective tissues may be defined as that group of tissues predominantly composed of intercellular material (*matrix*), secreted mainly by its cells which are, therefore, usually widely spaced. Many of the special properties of connective tissues are determined by the composition of the matrix and their classification is also largely based on its characteristics. In some varieties, the cellular component eventually comes to dominate the tissue, although it begins with a high matrix : cell ratio, for example, adipose tissue. Connective tissues are derived from embryonic mesoderm or, in the head region, largely from neural crest (see p. 147).

Connective tissues play several essential roles in the body, both **structural**, since many of the extracellular elements possess special mechanical properties, and **defensive**, a role which has a cellular basis. They also often possess important trophic and morphogenetic roles in organizing and influencing the growth and differentiation of surrounding tissues. Structural connective tissues are conveniently divided into 'ordinary' (or 'general') types, distributed widely, and special *skeletal* types, namely cartilage and bone which are described elsewhere (pp. 443–451). A third variety, the *haemolymphoid tissues*, consists of the cells of the blood and lymphoid tissue and their precursors; these are often considered to be akin to other types of connective tissue because of their similar mesenchymal origins and also because the various defensive cells of the blood form part of a typical connective tissue cell population. However, for convenience, these tissues will be considered separately in another section (p. 1423).

Connective tissue is thus formed of *cells* and *extracellular matrix*. The matrix in turn is composed of *fibres* and a relatively amorphous *ground substance*. It is noteworthy that a number of cell types of connective tissue are derived from haemal tissue of the bone marrow or from lymphoid tissue, reaching the connective tissues via the circulating blood and migrating into them through their endothelial walls.

CELLS OF GENERAL CONNECTIVE TISSUE

Cells of general connective tissue can be conveniently separated into:

- the resident cell population (fibroblasts, adipocytes, persistent mesenchymal stem cells, etc.)

75

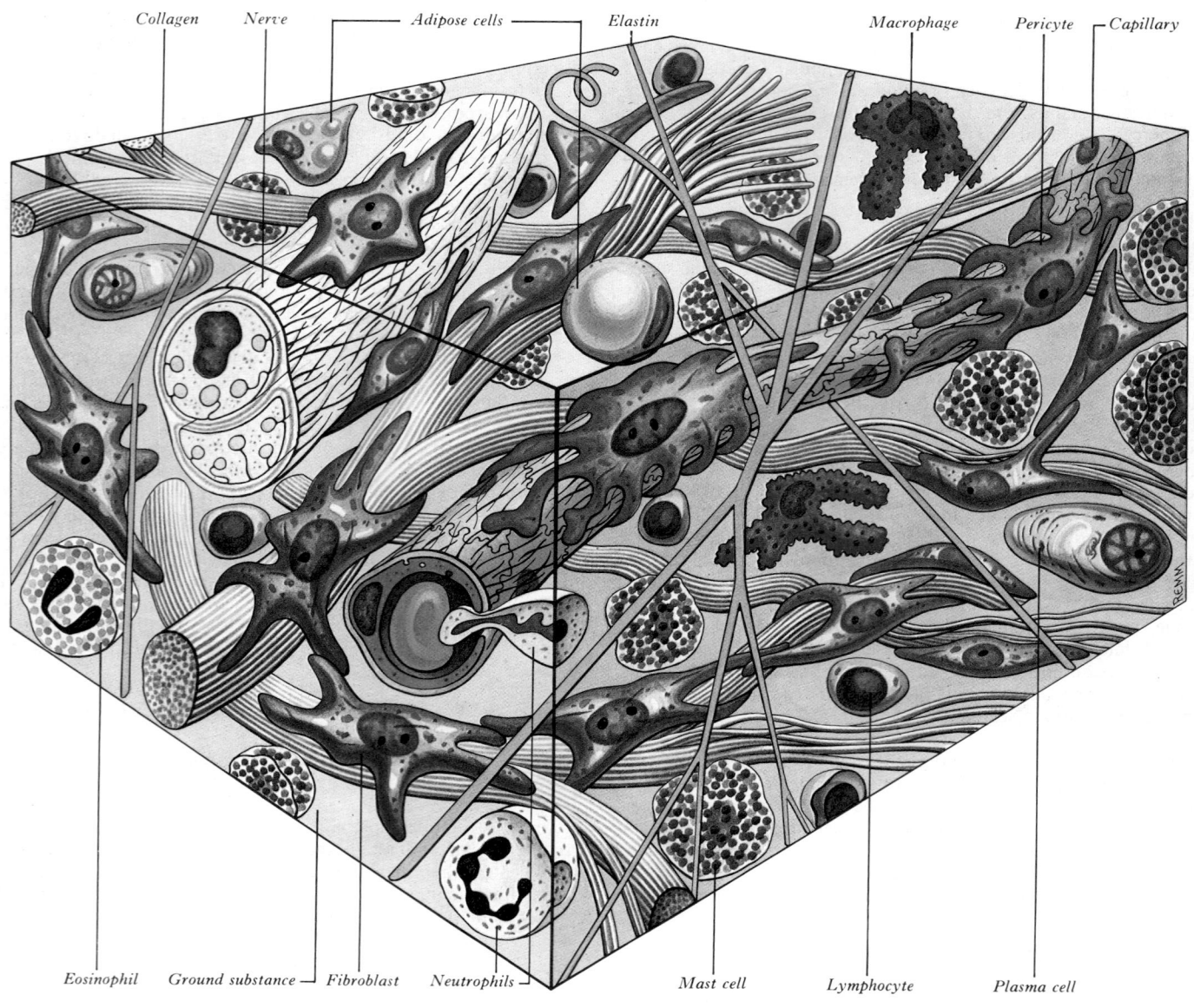

Collagen   Nerve   Adipose cells   Elastin   Macrophage   Pericyte   Capillary

Eosinophil   Ground substance   Fibroblast   Neutrophils   Mast cell   Lymphocyte   Plasma cell

2.80   Diagrammatic reconstruction of loose connective tissue showing the characteristic cell types, fibre and intercellular spaces.

● a fluctuating population of immigrant, wandering cells with various defensive functions (macrophages, lymphocytes, mast cells, neutrophils and eosinophils) which may change their activities, structures and numbers according to defensive demand.

A graphic summary of these cell types is presented in **2.80**. Embryologically, fibroblasts and adipocytes arise from relatively undifferentiated *mesenchymal stem cells*, some of which may remain in the tissues, providing a postnatal source of new cellular elements. As noted above, the other cells migrate into the tissue from bone marrow and lymphoid tissue.

FIBROBLASTS

Fibroblasts are usually the most numerous cells. They are flattened and irregular in outline, with branching processes; in profile they appear fusiform or spindle-shaped (**2.80, 81**). Fibroblasts synthesize most of the extracellular matrix of connective tissue and accordingly have all the features typical of cells actively engaged in synthesis and secretion of proteins. Their nuclei are relatively large, active or euchromatic (open-faced) and possess prominent nucleoli. In young and active cells the cytoplasm is abundant and basophilic because of the high concentration of rough endoplasmic reticulum (Hall 1968; Ross 1975; Hay 1981). In old and inactive fibroblasts (often termed *fibrocytes*) the cytoplasm is sparse, the endoplasmic reticulum scanty and the nucleus flattened and heterochromatic (close-faced).

In active fibroblasts, mitochondria are abundant and several sets of Golgi complexes are present.

Fibroblasts are usually adherent to the fibres (collagen and elastin) which they lay down. In some highly cellular structures, for example glands and lymphoid tissue, fibroblasts and delicate collagenous fibres (reticulin fibres) form fibrocellular networks often called *reticular tissue*. The fibroblasts may then be termed reticular cells, e.g. in the spleen (p. 1439).

Fibroblasts are particularly active during wound repair, multiplying and laying down a fibrous matrix which becomes invaded by numerous blood vessels (*granulation tissue*; see Ross 1968). Contraction of wounds (p. 413) is at least in part caused by the shortening of specialized contractile fibroblasts (*myofibroblasts*) which arise in such areas (Gabbiani et al 1973). Fibroblast activity is influenced by various factors such as steroid hormone levels, dietary content and prevalent mechanical stresses. In vitamin C deficiency there is an impairment of collagen formation.

ADIPOCYTES (LIPOCYTES, FAT CELLS)

Adipocytes occur singly or in groups in the meshes of many but not all connective tissues, being specially numerous in *adipose tissue* (**2.82, 83**; see also p. 88). When occurring singly the cells are oval or spherical in shape but when mutually compressed they are polygonal. They vary in diameter, averaging about 50 μm. Each cell consists of

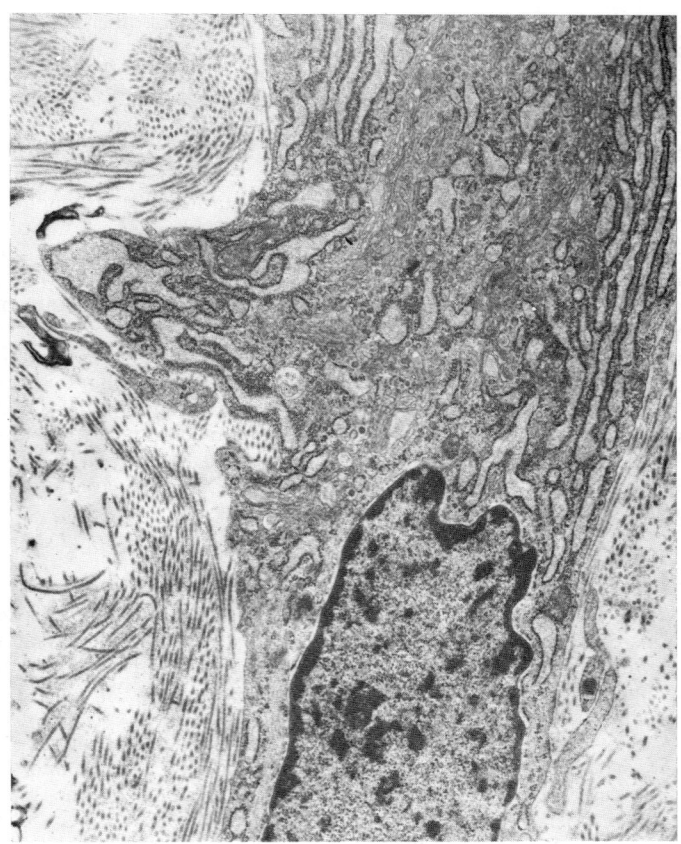

2.81 Transmission electron micrograph of part of a fibroblast. Note the abundant endoplasmic reticulum and extensive Golgi complex. Some extra-cellular collagen fibres are also visible. Magnification × 15 000.

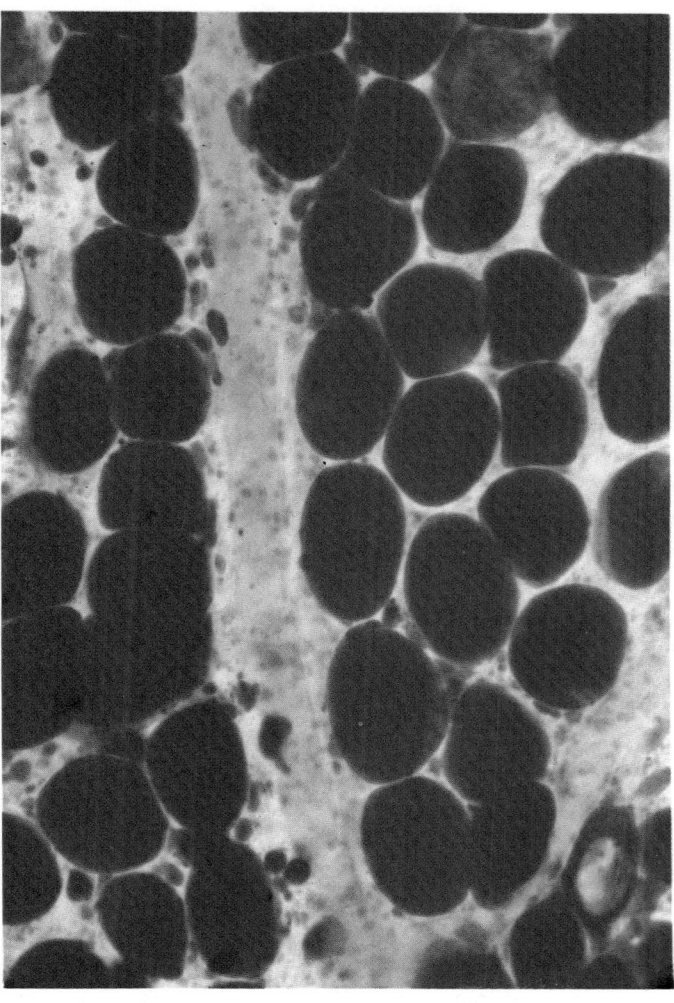

2.82 Adipocytes clustered around a blood vessel in a mesentery, stained as whole mount with Sudan red and mounted in an aqueous medium to avoid alcoholic extraction of lipid. Magnification × 175.

a peripheral rim of cytoplasm, in which the nucleus is embedded, surrounding a single large central globule of fat (see Slavin 1985). There is a slight accumulation of cytoplasm around the nucleus, which is oval in shape and appears compressed against the cell membrane by the lipid droplet, as does the Golgi complex. Ultra-structurally, lipid droplets are in direct contact with the surrounding cytoplasm without an enclosing membrane. Many cytoskeletal filaments are also seen around the lipid vacuole as well as some endoplasmic reticulum and mitochondria.

In sections not specially prepared to preserve fat this is usually dissolved out by the solvents used, particularly xylol; only the nucleus and the peripheral rim of cytoplasm surrounding a central empty space are left, so that the cell has a signet-ring appearance (**2.**83). The fat is fixed and stained by osmium tetroxide and specially coloured by alcoholic solutions of certain dyes, notably Sudan III, Sudan black and Scharlach R, which are more soluble in fat than in the solvent; lipid is conveniently demonstrated in frozen or cryostat sections (**2.**69). The fat consists of glycerol esters of oleic, palmitic and stearic acids.

Doubts exist as to whether fat cells are specifically and exclusively concerned with the storage, and perhaps the synthesis, of fat. Prior to the storage of fat within them they are stellate in shape and difficult to distinguish from fibroblasts and, when depleted of fat, they revert to this appearance. As fat accumulates the cells enlarge and become rounded, the fat first appearing as isolated small globules which later coalesce to form a single large droplet. Conversely, during depletion the single large globule diminishes in size and then breaks up into droplets while the cells become stellate in shape. Fat cells, however, seem to have a well-defined distribution within the body and there is evidence that they are indeed specific cells.

In most mammals which have been studied but especially in those which hibernate, certain deposits of fat are characterized by the presence of a large cell type in which the fat is present as several separate droplets and not as a single globule; their mitochondria also have unusually large and numerous cristae. These deposits of fat are often termed *brown* adipose tissue and are concerned with heat production, mediated by mitochondria. In many species they occur in the interscapular tissue, dorsally, in the subcutaneous tissue of the ventral thorax, axillae, renal capsule and posterior abdominal wall. In human neonates brown fat is present in the interscapular region and may be more widespread. Its importance in later years is

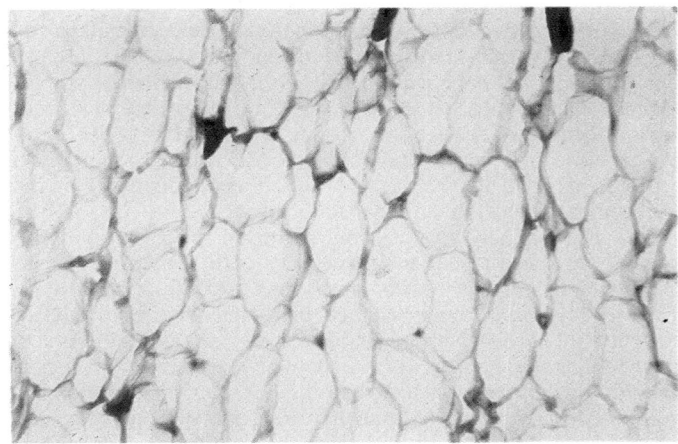

2.83 A group of subcutaneous adipocytes in section after processing for routine histology. Note that the lipid has been totally extracted leaving the cells with only a narrow rim of cytoplasm containing (where sectioned) a nucleus. Compare with **2.**82. Magnification × 125.

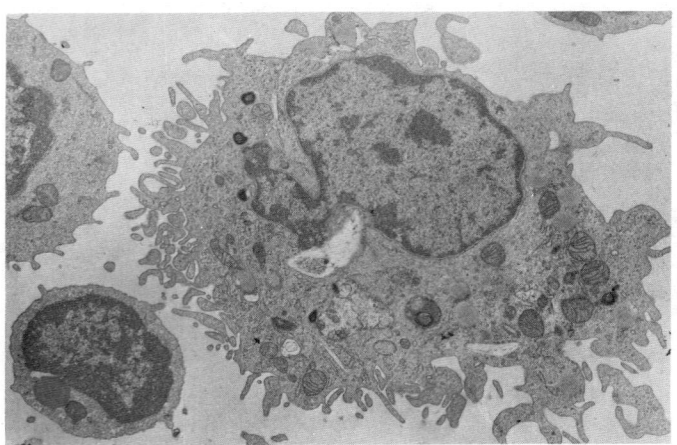

2.84 Electron micrograph of a macrophage (right) and a small lymphocyte (lower left). Magnification × 6000.

uncertain. (See Cannon & Nedergaard 1985 for a review of this subject.)

The mobilization of fat is under nervous or hormonal control and noradrenaline released at sympathetic nerve endings in adipose tissue is particularly important in this respect.

MACROPHAGES (HISTIOCYTES, CLASMATOCYTES)

Macrophages are also numerous in connective tissue where they may be either attached to matrix fibres (stationary, or fixed macrophages), when their shape is irregular with many filopodia (**2.84**); or they may be motile (nomadic macrophages) of a more rounded and regular form.

Macrophages are relatively large cells, about 15–20 μm in diameter, their nuclei usually indented and somewhat heterochromatic, with a prominent nucleolus. Their cytoplasm is mildly basophilic and typically has a 'frothy' appearance under the light microscope. These cells are important phagocytes, forming part of the *mononuclear phagocyte system* (p. 1414). They can engulf and digest particulate organic materials, such as bacteria and other foreign bodies, and are also able to dispose of dead or moribund cells prior to tissue regeneration. They are also the source of a number of important soluble secreted proteins which have a profound effect on many other cell types (see below). Macrophages are able to multiply mitotically to some extent in the connective tissues, but are derived from haemopoietic stem cells (p. 1414) in the bone marrow, circulating in the blood as monocytes before migrating through venule walls into their final extravascular sites.

Ultrastructurally, macrophages contain numerous lysosomes which digest ingested materials. Inert materials such as small particles of carbon or metals may also be taken up, a quality useful in demonstrating macrophages histologically, since their cytoplasm becomes filled with ingested particles if an experimental animal is previously injected with a suspension of India ink (**2.85**), trypan blue or lithium carmine (vital staining). Macrophages may also be separated magnetically from mixed cell samples by first treating them with iron carbamyl, which they endocytose.

These cells are also of great importance in many immunological aspects of defence and their interactions with numerous defensive cells in the regulation of the immune system are widespread. Antigens processed by macrophages can be presented with class MHC II molecules to lymphocytes to stimulate them, and so they can act as *antigen-presenting cells* (p. 1415). They may selectively phagocytose particles previously coated by antibodies (*opsonins*, see p. 1420) synthesized by lymphocytes and they are themselves sites for *homocytotropic antibody* attachment, which enables them to recognize and attack foreign substances (see also monocytes, p. 1405). They can also be stimulated into a high level of phagocytosis by soluble proteins, *cytokines* of various classes released by lymphocytes (p. 1420), and such *activated macrophages* may then synthesize and

release cytokines themselves to affect the behaviour of other defensive cells.

Many properties of connective tissue macrophages are similar to those of a number of specialized cell types in other sites, particularly: circulating monocytes, alveolar phagocytes in the lungs, littoral phagocytes in the lymph nodes, spleen and bone marrow, Kupffer cells of the liver sinusoids, microglial cells of the brain, Langerhans cells of the epidermis, dendritic and interdigitating cells of lymphoid tissue. Various cell-labelling experiments have shown that the precursors of these cells arise in the bone marrow as monocyte-like cells which then pass in the circulation to their final destinations, where, however, they may continue to divide. These cells constitute the mononuclear phagocyte system (p. 1414), the different categories apparently having distinctive functions, preferred sites of action and possessing different antigenic markers as well as many common ones.

All macrophages are capable of motility, when suitably stimulated. When grouped around a large foreign body, macrophages may also fuse together to form *syncytial giant cells* and *epithelioid cells*. These and other aspects of macrophage biology will be considered further in Section 9 (p. 1414).

LYMPHOCYTES

Whilst they are typically present in small numbers, these cells are numerous in general connective tissue only in pathological states, migrating from adjacent lymphoid tissue or from the circulation. The majority are small cells (6–8 μm) with rounded, highly heterochromatic or often deeply indented nuclei (p. 1405, and see **2.84**). When appropriately stimulated they enlarge, developing numerous ribosomes. Two major functional classes exist, termed 'B' and 'T' lymphocytes (see p. 1417). B-lymphocytes originate in the bone marrow, then pass to various lymphoid tissue sites where they proliferate. When antigenically stimulated, they undergo further mitotic divisions, then enlarge as they mature to form *plasmacytes* (plasma cells) which synthesize and secrete antibodies (immunoglobulins). Mature plasmacytes are rounded or ovoid, up to 15 μm across, and have extensive arrays of granular endoplasmic reticulum. Their nuclei are spherical and have a characteristic 'cartwheel' or 'clock-face' configuration of heterochromatin which is regularly distributed in peripheral clumps (**2.5**). The prominent Golgi complex is also seen with a light microscope as a pale region to one side of the nucleus, whilst the remaining cytoplasm is deeply basophilic due to the abundant endoplasmic reticulum. Mature plasmacytes are unable to divide.

T-lymphocytes stem from cell stocks initially formed by the bone marrow but later migrating to and multiplying within the thymus before passing into the peripheral lymphoid system where they continue to multiply. When antigenically stimulated, these cells enlarge and their cytoplasm becomes filled with 'free' polysome

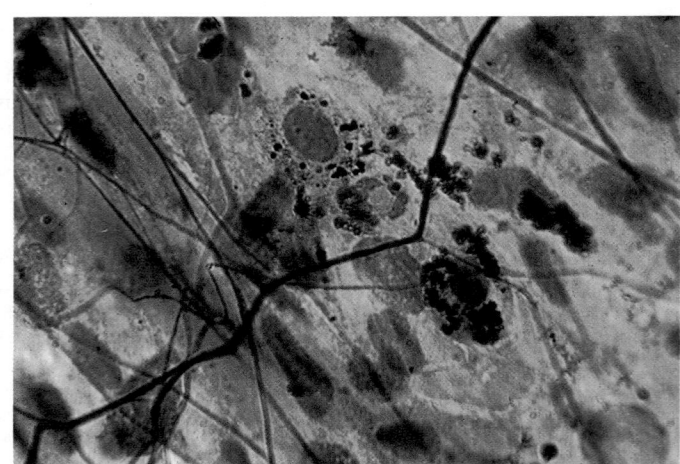

2.85 Loose connective tissue in the mesentery of a rabbit which had previously been injected intraperitoneally with India ink, showing fibroblasts and macrophages. The cytoplasm of the macrophages is full of phagocytosed particles, the collagen is stained pink and the elastin fibres black. Van Gieson's and Verhoeff's elastin stain. Magnification × 1000.

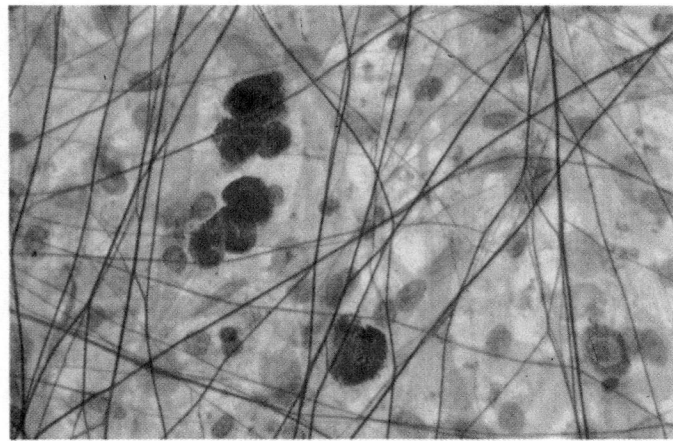

2.86 Mast cells (histaminocytes) in a whole mount spread of loose connective tissue (mesentery) stained with carmine-lithium carbonate to show mast cell granules. The network of elastin fibres has also been counterstained by the Verhoeff method. Magnification × 660.

clusters. The functions of T-lymphocytes are numerous and incompletely understood, but include the recognition and destruction of virus-infected cells, tumour cells, fungi, tissue and organ grafts, the modulation of B-lymphocytes and interactions with several other defensive cells. Different subsets of T-lymphocytes have distinctive roles in these activities.

Further details of the natural history of lymphocytes may be found on pages 1417–1423.

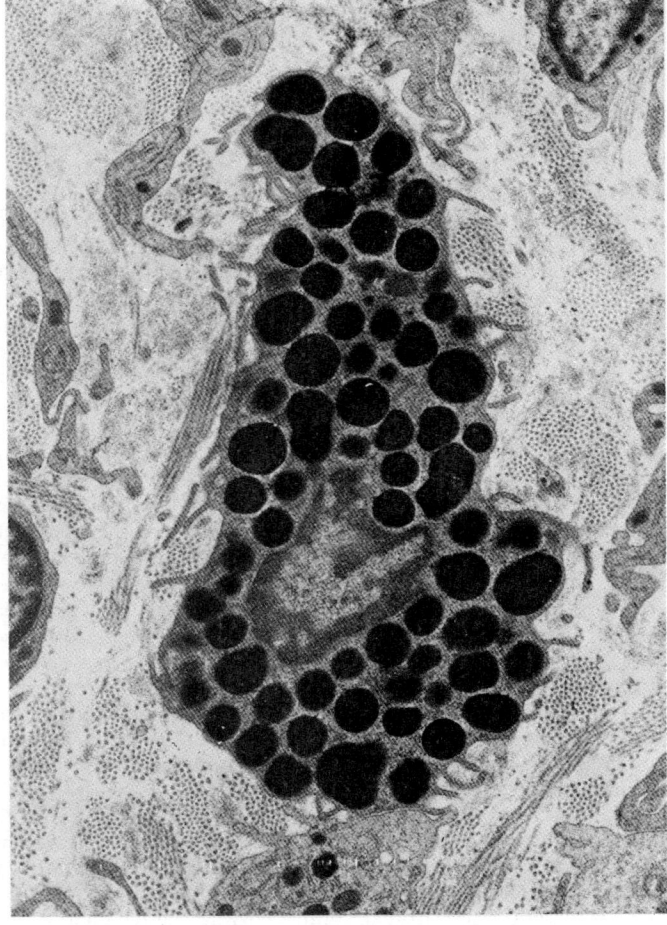

2.87 Electron micrograph of a mast cell showing the large densely staining membrane-bound cytoplasmic granules. Magnification × 6000.

MAST CELLS (MASTOCYTES, HISTAMINOCYTES)

Mast cells are important defensive cells which occur particularly in loose connective tissues and often in the fibrous capsules of certain organs such as the liver (see the review of this cell by Holgate 1983). They are characteristically numerous around blood vessels and nerves. Mast cells are round or oval, about 12 μm in diameter, with many filopodia extending from the cell surface (2.86, 87). The nucleus is centrally placed and relatively small, being surrounded by large numbers of prominent vesicles, a well-developed Golgi apparatus but scanty endoplasmic reticulum. The vesicles show a strongly positive reaction with the periodic acid-Schiff (PAS) stain for carbohydrates and with toluidine blue, methylene blue, azure A and alcian blue; they show strong *metachromatic* staining reactions (staining a colour different from the dye being used), also indicating an acid glycosaminoglycan content. Ultrastructurally the membrane-bounded vesicles (or 'granules') vary in size and shape (mean diameter about 0.5 μm) and have a rather heterogeneous content, differing with species. In man the vesicles usually contain dense osmiophilic material which may be finely granular, lamellar or in the form of membranous whorls; these variants may coexist in the same vesicle, which may also present in places a crystalline substructure. For these reasons they have sometimes been termed *compound granules* (2.88).

The available evidence points to the presence in mast cell granules of a wide variety of substances which can initiate and amplify a great range of defensive responses in the surrounding connective tissue, many of them associated with inflammation. The major granule components are the proteoglycan *heparin*, *histamine*, *tryptase*, *superoxide dismutase*, *aryl sulphatase*, *β-hexosaminidase* and various other enzymes; also present are *eosinophil chemotactic factors* (tetrapeptides) and *neutrophil chemotactic factors*. Mast cells may be disrupted to release some or all of their contents either by direct mechanical or chemical trauma, or following contact with particular antigens to which the body has previously been exposed (9.17). The latter may result from interaction between the antigen and *homocytotropic antibodies* of the IgE and IgG$_4$ classes associated with the mast cell plasma membrane and may give rise to local responses (e.g. urticaria), or generalized ones (anaphylactic shock) following the release of large amounts of histamine into the general circulation. They have thus been implicated in many of the phenomena occurring in inflammatory reactions, allergies and hypersensitivity states. The modes of action of their released mediators

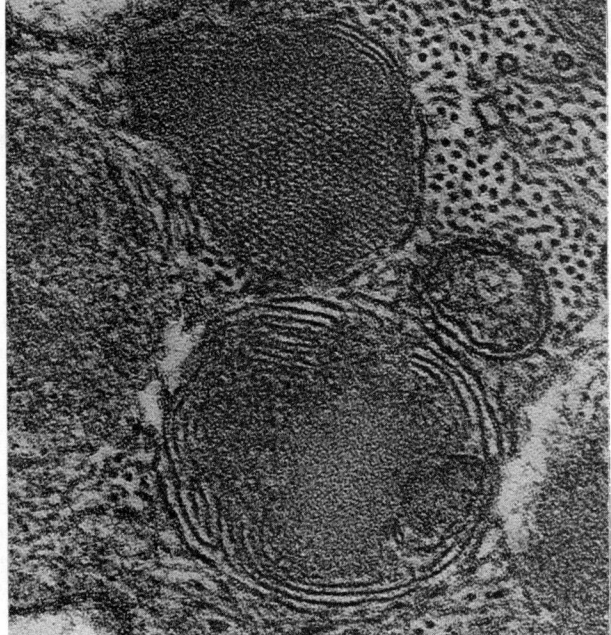

2.88 Higher magnification of part of a mast cell from human skin, showing the complex internal structure of its granules. Cross-sections of microtubules and intermediate filaments are also visible in this section. Magnification × 100 000.

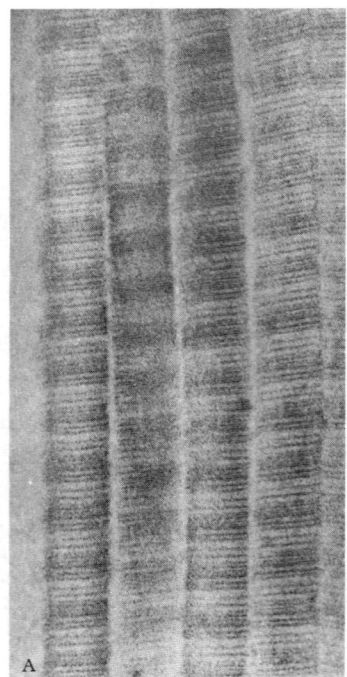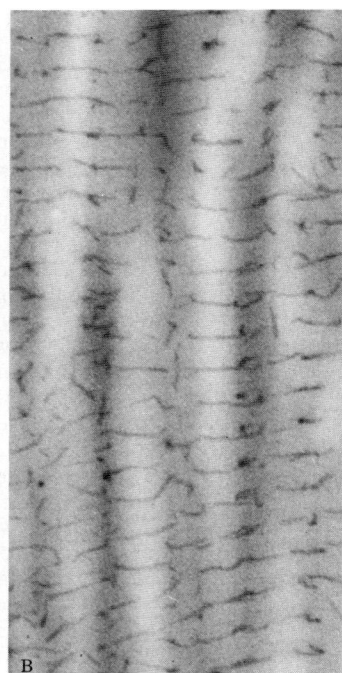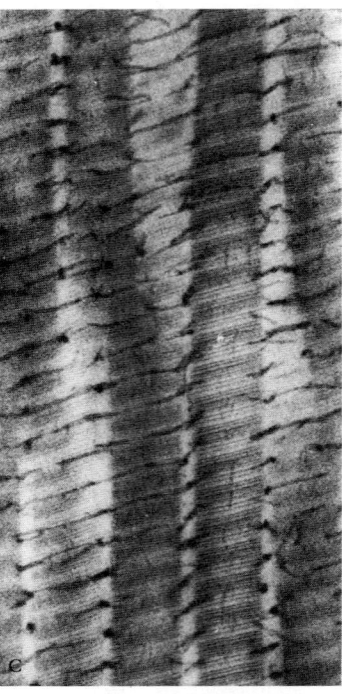

2.89A–C Transmission electron micrographs of skin collagen fibrils stained in different ways to demonstrate the banding pattern and the presence of associated proteoglycans. In A the fibres have been longitudinally sectioned and stained with uranyl acetate to show the characteristic major 64 nm repeat pattern with several sub-bands visible between. B has been stained with Cupromeronic blue demonstrating the filamentous proteoglycans encircling and interconnecting collagen fibrils. In C both stains have been used to show that the proteoglycan connections correspond to the 64 nm cross bands. Micrographs provided by J Scott and Marion Haigh, Department of Chemical Morphology, University of Manchester. Magnification: A × 100 000; B and C × 65 000.

are exceedingly complex and involve many chemical reactions which alter capillary permeability, can cause smooth muscle contraction, activate and attract various other defensive cells, activate platelets, inhibit clotting and lead to many other local or systemic reactions.

Mast cells closely resemble basophil leucocytes of the general circulation and it is widely considered that they arise from the bone marrow and pass to the tissues as basophils, migrating through the capillary and venule walls to their final destination. However, there are minor differences between the typical basophil and the mast cell in terms of their cytochemistry, which suggest either a different lineage for the two, or perhaps that the basophil matures into a mast cell when it reaches its extravascular environment. In connective tissues at least two subclasses of mast cells have been recognized, one resident in the mucosae of the alimentary and respiratory tracts, and others situated elsewhere. They differ in their detailed chemistry and their reactions to drugs (Friedmann 1986).

NEUTROPHIL AND EOSINOPHIL LEUCOCYTES

These are also immigrant cells from the circulation, frequently present (especially neutrophils) in small numbers, but increasing greatly in infected tissues, where they are important components of cellular defence. Neutrophils are highly phagocytic, especially towards bacteria, while the functions of eosinophils are less well understood. They are described further on pages 1402 and 1403.

PIGMENT CELLS (MELANOCYTES)

Pigment cells occur in the corium (dermis) of skin, especially in dark races, and in the iris and choroid of the eye. Although some of these cells may be able to synthesize melanin (or related pigments), in which case they are described as *melanocytes* (derived from neural crest origins), the majority contain pigment which they have engulfed after its release from melanocytes, being unable to synthesize it themselves. Such cells are called *chromatophores* (or *melanophores*, when melanin is the pigment involved); they are typically stellate in form and may represent modified fibroblasts. They are generally stellate cells with long processes and numerous dark brown or black granules, believed to be melanin, in their cytoplasm. Their function is generally to prevent light from reaching adjacent cells.

EXTRACELLULAR MATRIX (ECM)

The term extracellular matrix is applied to the sum total of extracellular substances within connective tissue (**2**.80). Essentially it consists of a system of insoluble protein fibrils and soluble complexes composed of carbohydrate polymers linked to protein molecules (i.e. they are proteoglycans) which bind water. Mechanically, the ECM has evolved to distribute the stresses of movement and gravity while at the same time maintaining the shape of the different components of the body. It also provides the physicochemical environment of the cells embedded in it, forming a framework to which they adhere and on which they can move, maintaining an appropriate porous, hydrated ionic mileu, through which metabolites and nutrients can diffuse freely. There are many complex interactions between the connective tissue cells and the ECM which operate in both directions: the cells continually synthesize, secrete, alter and degrade its components, but are themselves profoundly affected by their contacts which govern many aspects of cell metabolism, growth, reproduction and movement.

The insoluble fibrils are mainly of two types of structural proteins, namely: collagen and elastin, whilst the soluble polymers consist of long carbohydrate chains, linked to proteins. There is also an ever-growing number of small filamentous proteins which perform a variety of functions in connective tissue including cell/matrix adhesion and matrix/cell signalling; these include fibronectin, laminin, merosin and, in bone, osteonectin, as well as a number of other less well characterized proteins.

At the microscopic level, these different constituents are divisible into *fibrillar* and *interfibrillar* components (the latter corresponding to the *ground substance* of the older literature). The collagen fibres resist pulling forces, while the elastin provides a measure of resilience when it is present. The hydrated, soluble polymers of the interfibrillar material (proteoglycans and hyaluronan) generally form a stiff gel resisting compressive forces.

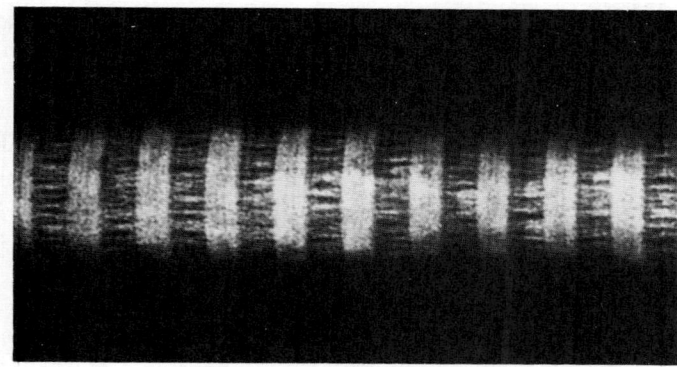

2.90 Portion of a Type I collagen fibril, negatively stained with phosphotungstate to show the substructure of longitudinal tropocollagen filaments and the banding pattern produced by this method. Dark areas represent hydrophilic sites including spaces between filaments. Notice that the banding appearance is different from the positively stained fibrils shown in **2**.89A. Magnification × 140 000.

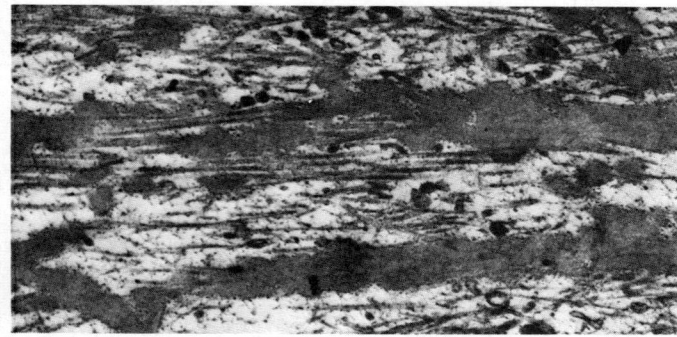

2.91 Developing elastin fibres and surrounding collagen fibres in a section stained with phosphotungstate. Notice the apparently amorphous appearance of the elastin. Provided by W. Jayaratnam. Magnification × 20 000.

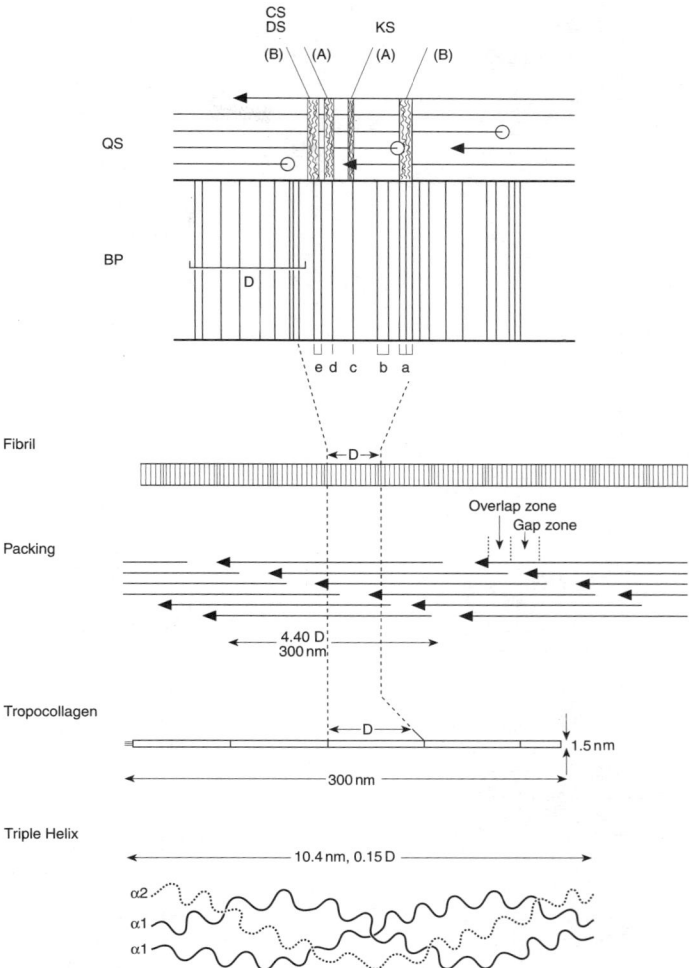

−Gly− Pro— Y — Gly− Pro−Hypro− Gly−X − Hypro − Gly−X − Hylys − Gly−X— Y −

2.92 The hierarchical organization of collagen, exemplified by Type I collagen. At the bottom is a typical sequence from an α chain of triplets of amino acids, each starting with glycine, and containing much hydroxyproline and proline. Next up, three α chains coil around each other to form a triple helix of the tropocollagen molecule, which can aggregate spontaneously in a quarter stagger array. The regular patterns of charged and non-polar amino acids appear as transverse bands after staining with heavy metals (see **2**.89B). At the top is the supramolecular aggregation of proteoglycans (PGs) with collagen fibres (see also **2**.98B). Small PDs (A and B) and PCS associate at d and e bands; the small PKSs (A and B) from corneal stroma are found at the a and c bands (see **2**.96A and text). Arrowheads denote the amino-terminal end of the polypeptide chains. The lower part of this figure is based on a scheme by M. E. Grant. Provided by J. E. Scott, Department of Chemical Morphology, University of Manchester.

The interfibrillar material contains most of the water, salts and diffusible substances in the tissue, and forms a minute meshwork providing intermolecular spaces with ready diffusional access of nutrients, gases, metabolites and signalling molecules to cells. Tissues which are specialized to resist tensile forces (e.g. that of tendons) are rich in fibrils, whereas those which elastically absorb compressive forces (e.g. cartilages) are rich in proteoglycans. In bone, mineral crystals take the place of most of the soluble polymers, endowing the tissue with incompressible rigidity.

COLLAGENS

Collagens (**2**.89–93) make up a very large proportion (about 30%) of all the proteins of the body, and consist of a wide range of related molecules which possess various roles in the organization and properties of connective (and some other) tissues. Their study is making rapid progress as the techniques of molecular biology are adding steadily to the number of recognized collagen classes. Collagens are classified using roman numerals to reflect the chronological order of their discovery. At least 14 types are now genetically characterized and others are being investigated.

The first collagen to be chemically and physically characterized was Type I, the most abundant of all the collagens and a constituent of the dermis, fasciae, bone, tendon, ligaments, blood vessels and the sclera of the eyeball. The characteristic collagen of cartilage and the vitreous body of the eye, with a slightly different chemical composition, is Type II, whilst Type III is present in several tissues including the dermis, and Type IV in basal laminae. The other types are widely distributed in various tissues (see Table 2.2). Five of the collagens (Types I, II, III, V and XI) form fibrils, while the rest are loosely described as non-fibrillar. Types IV, VIII and possibly X form sheets or meshworks rather than fibrils.

Chemically, all collagens have a number of features in common. Unlike most other proteins, they contain much hydroxyproline and all are composed of three polypeptides which to varying degrees are wound round each other to form triple helices. The formation of such helices depends on the reiteration of a glycine residue at every third amino acid position of each polypeptide chain, so that collagens also have a high glycine content. Very important post-translational modifications occur to the collagen chains within the endoplasmic reticulum and Golgi complexes of the cells synthesizing them, including the hydroxylation of proline to hydroxyproline, hydroxylation of lysine, and O-glycosylation of hydroxylysine by either galactose or glucosyl-galactose; after secretion the individual molecules are further cross-linked to form stable polymers. Functionally, collagens

Table 2.2   Collagen types and their distributions (based on van der Rest & Garrone, 1991)

Type	Former name	Good source	No. of α chain types	Mol mass: kDa	Molecular species
		Fibrillar collagens			
I	Collagen	Skin, bone, tendon	2	300	$[\alpha1(I)]_2\,\alpha2(I)$
		Dentine	1	300	$[\alpha1(I)]_3$
II	Cartilage collagen	Cartilage, vitreous body	1	300	$[\alpha1(II)]_3$
III		Skin, vessel walls	1	300	$[\alpha1(III)]_3$
V	A–B collagen	Hamster lung cultures	1	ca350	$[\alpha1(V)]_3$
		Fetal membranes	2	ca350	$[\alpha1(V)]_2\,\alpha2(V)$
		Placenta	3	ca350	$\alpha1(V)\,\alpha2(V)\,\alpha3(V)$
XI		Cartilage	3	ca300	$\alpha1(XI)\,\alpha2(XI)\,\alpha3(XI)$
		Non-fibrillar collagens			
FACIT collagens					
IX		Cartilage, vitreous body	3	ca250	$\alpha1(IX)\,\alpha2(IX)\,\alpha3(IX)$
XII		Embryonic tendon, periodontal ligament	1	ca700	$[\alpha1(XII)]_3$
XIV		Fetal skin, tendon	1	ca700	$[\alpha1(IV)]_3$
Meshwork-forming collagens					
IV		Basal laminae	2	ca400	$[\alpha1(IV)]_2\,\alpha2(IV)$
		Glomerular basal lamina	3	?	$\alpha3(IX)\,\alpha4(IX)\,\alpha5(IX)$
VIII		Descemet's membrane	2	?	$[\alpha1(VIII)]_2\,\alpha2(VIII)$
X		Epiphyseal plate	1	ca180	$[\alpha1(IV)]_3$
Other collagens					
VI	Intimal collagen	Skin, vessel walls, intervertebral discs	3	?	$\alpha1(VI)\,\alpha2(VI)\,\alpha3(VI)$
VII	LC collagen	Dermo-epidermal junction	1	?	$[\alpha1(VII)]_3$
XIII		Endothelial cell cultures	?	?	?

are structural proteins, unlike some other polymeric molecules with some similar chemical features, for example acetylcholinesterase (AChE) and the complement component C1q, which are non-structural.

Chemical nomenclature. Complete amino acid sequences of many of the collagen polypeptide chains are known. The polypeptides of collagen are called α chains and their individual amino acid composition is designated first with an arabic numeral to describe the subclass of chain and then with a roman numeral to denote the type of collagen they belong to. Thus the three polypeptides of Type I collagen comprise two $\alpha1(I)$ and one $\alpha2(I)$ chains, and the composition of the whole molecule is described as $[\alpha1(I)]_2\alpha2(I)$.

Type I collagen

Also known as 'collagen vulgaris', Type I collagen is very widely distributed. It forms inextensible fibrils in which collagen molecules are aligned side by side in a staggered fashion, with three-quarters of the length of each molecule in contact with neighbouring molecules, (**2.92**; the 'quarter-staggered array'). The 300 nm long molecules have a gap of about 40 nm between their ends; this arrangement is due to the amino acid sequences of adjacent molecules mutually interacting most stably with this degree of overlap.

The quarter-staggered array is strengthened by covalent cross-links between neighbouring molecules, formed at specific sites at the N and C terminal ends of each molecule. During synthesis, lysine residues are oxidized by lysyl oxidase, and the aldehydes thus produced undergo a series of reactions with the amino groups of lysine or hydroxylysine on nearby polypeptides to produce an array of aliphatic and heterocyclic (pyridinoline) cross-links that change in number and chemical composition with age.

The fibril has well-marked bands of charged and uncharged amino acids arranged across it that stain with heavy metals in a banding pattern, which is labelled in sequence a–e, repeated once every 65 nm (the D period). This pattern reflects the amino acid sequences of the collagen molecules in the quarter-staggered array. The asymmetrical a–e banding pattern can be parallel or anti-parallel on neighbouring collagen fibrils, in about equal numbers.

The banding pattern of longitudinally sectioned collagen I appears rather different from that of negatively stained fibrils (**2.89, 90**) because the negative stain occupies hydrated sites (e.g. the 'holes' between the ends of collagen molecules) whereas the dense lines in sectioned fibrils reflect the pattern of different amino acids, as described above.

Fibril diameters vary from tissue to tissue and with age. Developing

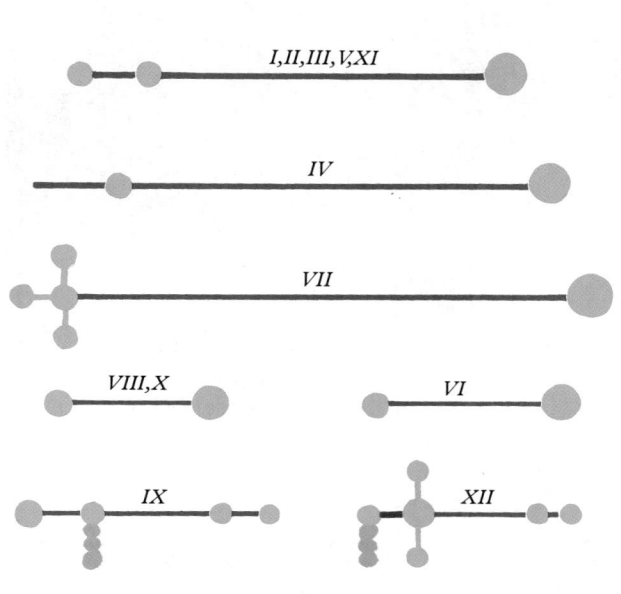

2.93 Molecular organization and relative dimensions of some major types of collagen. The triple helical chains are indicated in red, the globular domains in blue, and the acidic glycosaminoglycans in green.

tissues often have thinner fibrils than mature tissues. Corneal stroma fibrils are of uniform thin diameter, while tendon fibrils may be up to 20 times thicker and are quite variable. Tissues in which the fibrils are subject to high tensile loading tend to have thicker fibrils. Thick fibrils appear to be composites of uniform thin fibrils (protofibrils) which have a diameter of 8–12 nm. Among the factors which have been suggested to influence fibril diameters are the degree of glycosylation (which is greater in thin fibrils), the presence of minor collagens at the surface of the fibrils, the presence of extension peptides at the ends of the tropocollagen molecules and the type and concentration of ambient proteoglycan (Scott & Parry 1992). The polarity of neighbouring fibrils may influence the possibility of fusion of neighbouring fibrils, which probably cannot occur if they are anti-parallel.

The fibrils per se are relatively flexible but when mineralized (as in bone) or surrounded by high concentrations of proteoglycan (as in cartilage), the resulting fibre-reinforced composite materials are rigid. Collagen fibres often show regular patterns of light and dark along their length in polarized light, repeated about every 100 μm, probably reflecting the presence of crimps (or hinges) within the fibre, which provide a degree of reversible extensibility under tensile stress.

Fresh type I collagen fibres are white and glistening. They form bundles of various sizes, whose component fibres may leave one fascicle and interweave with others. They stain lightly with eosin, but can be strongly stained with aniline blue and with aldehyde fuchsin, as in van Gieson's method.

In many situations collagen fibrils are laid down in precise geometrical patterns, with successive layers alternating in direction, as in corneal stroma, where the high degree of order is essential for transparency. Other highly ordered tissues are the tendons, aponeuroses and ligaments.

Types II, III, V and XI collagens

Types II, III, V and XI collagens can aggregate to form fibrils, i.e. linear or one-dimensional structures. Their genes, and that of Type I collagen, are derived from a single ancestral gene. *Type II collagen* occurs in extremely thin (10 nm) short fibrils in the vitreous humour and in very thick fibrils in ageing human cartilage. The amino acid

sequence, banding pattern, cross-linking potential, polarity of fibrils, etc. are very similar to those of Type I collagen, as are also post-translational modifications (hydroxylation of proline and lysine and glycosylation). The fine fibrils in the vitreous are able to fuse into thicker aggregates in older tissue, possibly because of the breakdown of surrounding proteoglycan structure.

Type III collagen is very widely distributed, particularly in young and repairing tissue. It usually co-occurs with Type I collagen, and covalent links between Type I and Type III collagen have been demonstrated. In skin, many fibrils are probably composites of Types I and III collagens.

Types I, II and III collagens are made in the cell as procollagens, containing large globular portions at the N and C terminal ends of the triple helix (Table 2.2), which are removed by proteolysis before laying down in the tissue. In dermatosparaxis faulty processing leaves parts of the Type I globular domains uncleaved, resulting in malformed fibrils and hence in severe dysfunction of the tissue (skin).

Types IX and XI collagens

Types IX and XI collagens, the so-called *FACIT collagens* (fibril-associated collagens with interrupted triple helices), although not fibre forming per se, are associated with fibrillar collagens. Type IX collagen is found covalently linked to Type II collagen in cartilage, and may be covalently linked to Type II collagen in the vitreous. Type IX collagen is also a proteoglycan (see later), in that it has an attached chondroitin or dermatan sulphate chain, which in the case of the vitreous body in chickens is very long, but it may be much shorter in the human vitreous.

Type VII collagen

Type VII collagen is a linking or bridging collagen found in skin that forms a connection between the basal lamina and dermis. The absence of Type VII collagen is associated with the condition of epidermolysis bullosa.

Types IV and VIII collagens

In contrast to the fibrillar, i.e. linear or one-dimensionally aggregating collagens, these collagens can form meshworks (two or three dimensional aggregates) in the tissue. Their fundamental building units have flexible non-triple-helical portions which can reach out to their neighbours at a distance. Type IV collagen forms chicken-wire-like meshworks in the basal lamina that act as anchoring layers holding groups of cells together. Type VIII collagen forms meshworks in the Descemet's membrane of the cornea (p. 1325).

Reticulin fibres

Fine branching and anastomosing reticulin fibres form the supporting framework of many glands, the kidney and lymphoreticular tissue (lymph nodes, spleen etc. **9.32**)). They associate with basal laminae and are often found in the neighbourhood of collagen fibre bundles. Unlike collagen fibres reticulin takes up silver salts strongly but does not stain strongly with acid fuchsin. Reticulin shows a banding pattern similar to that of fibrillar collagens (**2.90**), and is chemically collagenous—possibly rich in Type III collagen.

Elastin

Elastin fibres are less widely distributed than collagen. They are yellowish in colour, branch and rejoin freely, and are usually thinner (10–20 nm) than collagen fibrils, although they can be thick, for example, in the ligamenta flava and ligamentum nuchae (**2.95**). Unlike collagen they show no banding pattern by electron microscopy. They stain with orcein, Weigert's resorcin fuchsin and with Verhoef's stain. They sometimes appear as sheets, as in the fenestrated elastic laminae of the aortic wall. Frequently co-occurring are thin filaments of *oxytalan* and *elaunin*, proteins with similar elastic properties but somewhat different staining reactions (Braverman & Fonferko 1982a,b).

Elastin-rich structures stretch easily with almost perfect recoil, the Young's modulus of elasticity being 6×10^6 (Bergel 1961), although they tend to calcify with age, and lose elasticity. Unstretched fibres show little or no birefringence, but become strongly birefringent on stretching (strain birefringence). This reflects increased order in the stretched elastin molecules, compared to the more random arrangement in unstretched fibres. Elastin is a protein of 70 kDa,

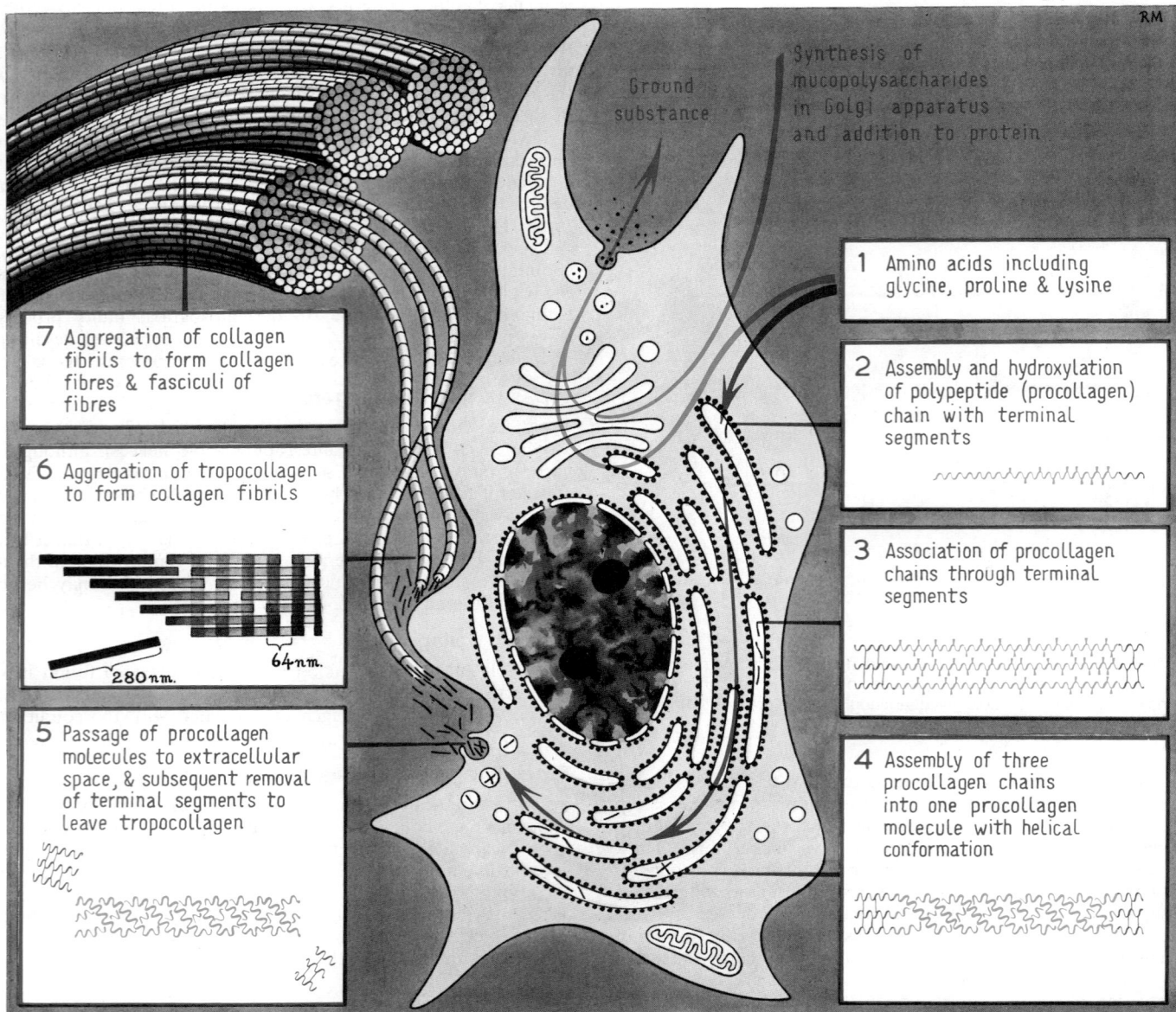

2.94 A schematic diagram showing the major steps in collagen synthesis by fibroblasts in connective tissue. For further details, see Olsen 1991.

rich in the hydrophobic amino acids valine and alanine (Sandberg et al 1981). The fibrils are highly cross-linked via two elastin-specific amino acids, desmosine and iso-desmosine, formed extracellularly from lysine residues, following oxidation by lysyl oxidase (similarly to cross-link formation in collagen, above). The rubber-like behaviour of elastin fibres springs from hydrophobic interactions between the amino acids valine, etc. which, in water, prefer to maintain a tightly packed arrangement, to which they revert after stretching forces have been removed.

Elastin is highly resistant to attack by acid and alkali, even at high temperatures. Elastases of pancreatic and bacterial origin can hydrolyze elastin (and other proteins).

GROUND (OR INTERFIBRILLAR) SUBSTANCE

The often-used term 'amorphous' ground substance is certainly a misnomer. There is considerable order in this compartment. Earlier views that fibrils were embedded in a jelly can be replaced with the concept that the collagen fibril controls the surrounding aqueous environment via specifically but non-covalently attached proteoglycan molecules, which then interact with each other via their glycan chains (Scott 1992).

Acid glycosaminoglycans (AGAGs)

The structural soluble polymers characteristic of the ECM are the acid glycosaminoglycans (AGAGs); these are unbranched chains of repeating disaccharide units, each unit carrying one or more negatively charged groups (carboxylate and/or sulphate esters). The anionic charge (fixed charge) is balanced by mobile cations (e.g. Na^+, K^+, etc.) from the interstitial fluid. Their polyanionic character endows the AGAGs with high osmotic activity (Donnan effects) and hence swelling pressure, which helps keep the fibrils apart and confers stiffness on the porous gel that they collectively create. It is also the property recognized by cationic dyes such as toluidine, Alcian and Cupromeronic blues, in the phenomenon termed basophilia.

The disaccharide units always contain a hexosamine residue (glucosamine, $GlcNH_2$ or galactosamine, $GalNH_2$), which in the interstial AGAGs is acetylated (thus, GlcNAc or GalNAc).

AGAGs are named according to the tissues in which they were first found: *hyal*uronan (vitreous body), *chondro*itins (cartilage), *derma*tan (skin), *kera*tan (cornea), *hepar*an (liver). This terminology is no longer relevant. 2.96A shows that most AGAGs are very widely distributed. Conversely, some corneas contain little or no keratan sulphate. The name of Karl Meyer is associated with the pioneering work in this field. For reviews, see Scott (1985, 1992).

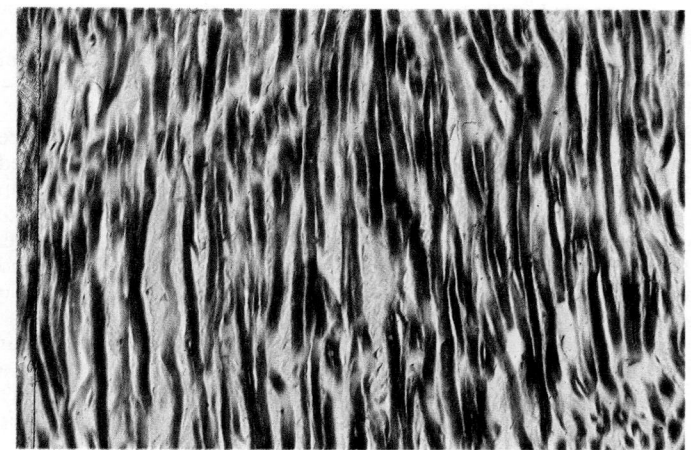

2.95 Longitudinal section through an elastic ligament of an ox showing elastin fibres (black) interspersed with collagen fibres. Verhoeff's and van Gieson's stains. Magnification × 200.

All AGAGs except hyaluronan (HA) are connected to specific amino-acid residues of protein cores, either via ether links to the hydroxyl groups of serine or threonine (O-linked) or to the amide group of asparagine (N-linked; **2.96A**). Sulphate groups are added to the polymer in patterns that vary from tissue to tissue, and with age. Most occur on the GlcNAc or GalNAc residues. Usually there is a higher density of sulphation at the non-reducing end (distal to the protein core) of the glycan chain.

All the interstitial AGAGs have the same pattern of glycosidic links, centred on the hexosamine residues, i.e. 1:3 Glc (or Gal) NAcβ1:4, which profoundly influences the potential shape or configuration (i.e. the secondary structures) the polymers can assume in solution. This confers similar potential to interact with each other on all members of the group of interstitial AGAGs. Keratan sulphate (KS) was for long thought to be quite different from the chondroitins, but in fact the polymer backbone (β1:4 Glcβ1:3 −> Gal) is identical in both (Scott 1992).

Though it is meaningful to speak of 'typical' structures for each GAG species, there are in principle large numbers of possible structures in a single chain, with a spectrum in each tissue and species. Dermatan sulphate (DS) is formed from CS4 by epimerization of GlcUA residues to L-iduronate, (L-IdoUA), to an extent which varies from tissue to tissue. Hyaluronan is the only AGAG with a constant chemical structure.

The second important group of AGAGs is based on the *heparan* polymer (α1:4, 1:4 linked glycan). The parameters which vary in the interstitial AGAGs (position and degree of sulphation, epimerization of GlcUA to L-IdoUA) also vary in these AGAGs. In addition, conversion of N-acetyl (acetamido) groups to sulphamato (-NSO$_3$, often incorrectly called N-sulphate) occurs to a variable extent.

Free AGAG chains are not normally found in ECM.

Hyaluronan (HA). This was formerly called hyaluronic acid (or hyaluronate, since only the salt exists at physiological pH) (for articles on HA see the book edited by Evered & Whelan 1989). The ending -an is standard for polysaccharides (glycans). HA is found in all ECM, and in most tissues, its molecules being relatively enormous. It is quantitatively important in embryonic and developing tissue.

In spite of a relatively simple structure consisting of an extremely long chain (as many as 25 000) of non-sulphated disaccharides, hyaluronan interacts specifically at low concentrations with many

Type of GAG chain	Abbreviation	Repeating disaccharide unit	Typical structure	Linkage to protein	Molecular mass (kDa)
Interstitial AGAGs					
		β1:4, 1:3 glycans			
Hyaluronan	HA	GlcUA–GlcNAc		No link to protein	1000
Chondroitin-4-sulphate	CS4	GlcUA–GalNAc		O-linked	10–50
Chondroitin-6-sulphate	CS6	GlcUA–GalNAc		O-linked	10–50
Keratan sulphate	KS	GlcNAc–Gal		N or O linked	3–25
Dermatan sulphate	DS	GlcUA or L–IdoUA } → GalNAc		O-linked	10–50
Membrane-associated AGAGs					
		α1:4, 1:4 glycans			
Heparan sulphate	HS	GlcUA or L–IdoUA } → { GlcNAc or 2-sulphamato-2-deoxy D-glucose		O-linked	7–40

Interstitial proteoglycans

Types of proteoglycan	Covalently linked AGAGs	Good sources	Molecular mass (kDa)	Shape	Location or function
Small	CS4, CS6 or DS or KS 1 or 2 chains	Cartilage, i.v. disc tendon, skin sclera cornea, i.v. disc cartilage	100		Collagen fibril associated
Large	CS and DS 5–10 chains	skin, sclera tendon	200		Interfibrillar, spacefilling
Very large	CS4, CS6 and KS 100 chains	cartilage, i.v. disc, blood vessels	1000–2000		Interfibrillar, spacefilling

2.96A Classification of acidic glycosaminoglycans (AGAGs) and proteoglycans of the extracellular matrix. The typical structure of the repeating disaccharide units (above) are, from top to bottom, hyaluronan, chondroitin 6-sulphate, and dermatan sulphate. The shapes of proteoglycans (below) are based on rotary shadowed preparations and are not to scale. Provided by J E Scott, Department of Chemical Morphology, University of Manchester.

types of cell that carry appropriate receptors, with important effects on their behaviour. It is the keystone in the aggregation of proteoglycans and link proteins that possess specific HA binding sites (e.g. laminin). The very large aggregates (>108 kDa) that are thus formed may be the essential compression-resisting units in cartilage. HA forms very viscous solutions which are probably the major lubricants in synovial joints. Because of its ability to bind water, in Wharton's jelly and vitreous humor (and in rooster comb) it participates in semi-rigid structures, co-operating with sparse but regular meshworks of thin collagen fibrils. These properties probably depend on its secondary structure and its ability to aggregate reversibly with itself, and with other molecules including interstitial AGAGs (Scott 1992).

Chondroitin-4- and -6-sulphates (CS4, CS6). These molecules, formerly chondroitin sulphates A and C, are found in all cartilages, often in very high total concentrations (>10% of the dry weight), and in most ECM. Most are mixed or hybrid AGAGs, pragmatically labelled according to the predominant component, i.e. -4- or -6-sulphate. The completely unsulphated form, chondroitin, occurs in small amounts if at all, but in, for example, cornea much of the CS4 is undersulphated, so that less than 20% of the GalNAc 4 positions carry a sulphate group. Conversely, an oversulphated CS, often called CS 'D', is found in fish cartilages, but not in significant amounts in human ECM.

CS chains are found attached to non-interstitial molecules, for example, the membrane glycoproteins CD44, syndecan and thrombomodulin.

The ability of CS6 chains to aggregate with each other may contribute to the semi-rigid gel structure in the vitreous body.

Keratan sulphates (KS). Although these are ECM components, they have very close relationships to the epithelial glyco-proteins, since they are polylactosamines. However, their polymer backbone (β1:3 Galβ1:4 Glc) is actually identical with that of the chondroitins (Scott 1992), and it appears that the cell can manufacture two almost identical polymers (KS and CS) by two different metabolic routes, possibly depending on the tissue oxygen tension. KS is present in increasing amounts with age in cartilages and intervertebral discs, and with thickness of the corneal stroma in mammals, to over 60% of the tissue AGAG (for articles on KS see the book edited by Greiling & Scott 1989).

Dermatan sulphate (DS). This is formed from CS4 by the epimerization of the D-GlcUA residues to L-IdoUA. The point at which CS becomes DS is a matter of definition, but over 10% conversion would qualify. There is, thus, a very close relationship between CS and DS, but the IdoUA ring is more flexible than GlcUA, which influences the overall shape of DS, and, therefore, interactions with other molecules. DS aggregates with itself in solution, and this phenomenon probably plays a part in the organization of most ECM (see below).

DS, unlike CS4, is not found in very high local concentrations in tissues.

Heparan sulphates. Although not structural in the sense that the interstitial AGAGs are (see below), heparan sulphates are important constituents of basement membranes, and also of membrane-associated proteoglycans, from which position they may interact directly with constituents of the ECM.

Proteoglycans (PG)

There is no accepted terminology for proteoglycans. The standard abbreviation is PG and the prefix indicating proteoglycan is P. Hence if the glycan (G) was DS, the relevant proteoglycan would be PDS, proteodermatan sulphate. The abbreviation DS PG is also in use for dermatan sulphate, but is not preferred on the grounds of brevity and consistency. A number of trivial names (e.g. decorin, aggrecan, perlecan, etc.) have been introduced to mark the acquisition of relevant cDNA sequences, but these contain little or no chemical information and are not logically consistent.

The existing classification of proteoglycans into three groups:- small, large and very large, is ad hoc, based on the size and shape of the protein core (Scott 1988) (see **2.96**A).

Small PGs (CS, DS, and KS). These have been found attached to a family of globular proteins of very similar size (~45 kDa), amino acid composition (i.e. leucine rich) and gene structure. The PGs appear on electron microscopy after rotary shadowing as tadpole-shaped, with the globular protein as the head and one or two glycan chains as the tail(s).

Large PGs. These molecules contain one or two globular protein domains connected via a polypeptide chain to which are attached 5–10 AGAG chains, mainly CS but also some DS.

Very large PGs. These are complex molecules with up to three globular regions linked by a polypeptide chain to which are attached about 100 CS and KS chains. An amino-terminal globular region contains the HA binding site. The protein contains a lectin-like sequence and sometimes an epidermal growth factor (EGF) sequence. The KS chains are mainly placed toward the amino-terminal end and the HA binding region. A number of oligosaccharides are also attached to the protein.

This PG is a large molecular complex, a space-filling molecule par excellence. It concentrates a very large amount of charge in a relatively small volume, which is further enhanced when it aggregates with HA and other similar PGs. The osmotic and electrostatic swelling forces are then maximized.

CS or DS chains are attached covalently to *Type IX* collagen, which, therefore, qualifies as an ECM proteoglycan.

SUPRAMOLECULAR ORGANIZATION IN ECM

Localization of ECM components

Progress in establishing supramolecular organization in ECM has depended on three kinds of reagents:

- specific antibodies to proteins such as the collagens, elastins, protein cores, and to AGAG chains that can be used immunohistochemically (macro-stains **2.89**B, C)
- electron dense reagents such as Cupromeronic blue that positively stain AGAGs in critical electrolyte concentration (CEC) techniques (mini-stains)
- enzymes such as keratanases 1 and 2, chondroitinases and dermatanases that specifically digest AGAGs, establishing or confirming identities of stained substrates.

Macro-stains are intrinsically more specific than mini-stains, although the CEC procedures give clear indications of degrees of sulphation, etc. which antibody based methods cannot do. The latter have intrinsically less resolving power at molecular levels, and cannot in general show the orientation, shape and size of the substrate, which, in principle, the mini-stains can. Mini-stains cannot specifically demonstrate proteins, but are well suited to morphometry of the AGAGs, while the converse is true of the macro-stains. Their properties are complementary (Scott 1985).

PROTEOGLYCAN: COLLAGEN INTERACTIONS

The small PGs have been shown by electron histochemistry (Cupromeronic blue in CEC methodology) to interact with Type I collagen-rich fibrils at specific binding sites. PDS binds at the d and e bands of the collagen, and PKS at the a and c bands. These bands are either in, or at the 'step' to the gap zone of the fibril (**2.89**, 92). Available evidence suggests that the PG protein interacts with collagen. Occupancy of a binding site is specific to a given PG. In the absence of this PG the site is not occupied (the one PG:one binding site hypothesis). Thus, the a and c bands are occupied only in the corneal stroma, since the stromal PKS is not present in significant amounts in other tissues. All soft (non-mineralized) tissues contain PDS which binds at the d and e bands (**2.92**). The relative rates of occupancy d/e and a/c vary with tissue and/or with species (Scott 1988).

The AGAG chains are oriented orthogonally to the collagen fibrils, sometimes completely encircling them (**2.89**B, C), and very frequently forming bridges between neighbouring fibrils. In the cornea as many as four fibrils are bridged by the same filament of AGAG. Evidence from morphometry and physical chemistry suggests that the AGAG chains are aggregated together in an antiparallel way, acting as a cross-linking structure between PG cores, which are attached to collagen fibrils (**2.96**B). Similar structures are seen in all soft connective tissue collagen fibril bundles. It is possible that the aggregated AGAGs act as yardsticks to space the fibrils according to the length of the AGAG chains. In the corneal stroma this length

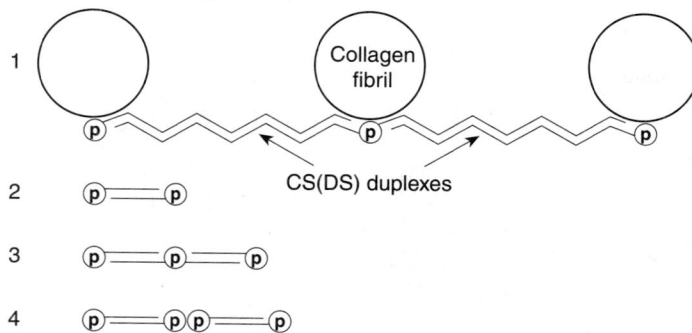

2.96B Schema of proteoglycan (PG)–collagen interactions in connective tissues, incorporating acidic glycosaminoglycan (AGAG) aggregates. In 1, collagen fibres depicted in cross section, are linked by duplexes (or higher aggregates) of antiparallel AGAG molecules, attached to PG protein cores (P), which are also associated with the collagen fibres at specific binding sites. The interfibrillar distance correlates with the length of the particular AGAG chain (being greater in the cornea and less in the skin) DS, KS and possibly CS6 can take part in such structures (Scott 1992; see also text). The molecular arrangements illustrated in 2–4 show various ways in which AGAGs containing 1 or 2 chains could form bridging structures. Provided by J E Scott, Department of Chemical Morphology, University of Manchester.

coincides with the observed fibril separation, which is very regular, as required for transparency and hence vision (Scott 1992).

PGs are seen inside thick collagen fibrils, regularly arrayed, but with their AGAG chains oriented along the fibril axis. It appears that these PGs are associated individually with one of the thin protofibrils that modularly comprise the fibril.

PG AGAGs in bone are not arrayed in the same orthogonal way as in, for example, tendon. They are absent from the gap zone. Since the gap zone is the site of first nucleation of mineralization, the AGAG may play some part in controlling calcification.

FILAMENTOUS PROTEINS WITH ADHESIVE PROPERTIES

Filamentous proteins with adhesive properties are structural proteins which include a range of molecules mediating adhesion between cells and the extracellular matrix (ECM), often in association with collagens, proteoglycans and other ECM components. All of them are glycosylated and are, therefore, glycoproteins. In general connective tissue, the best known are the protein families of the fibronectins (and osteonectin in bone), laminins and tenascins, but there is a rapidly growing list of other proteins or glycoproteins associated with extracellular adhesion, including the nidogens (entactins), perlecan, decoran, aggregan, etc. (see Alberts et al 1994). These molecules are complex structures with binding sites for various other ECM molecules and also for cell adhesion molecules (CAMs), especially the integrins (p. 27), enabling cells to selectively adhere to appropriate matrix structures (e.g. the basal lamina). They also constitute signalling molecules which are detected by cell surface receptors and initiate changes within the cytoplasm, for example to promote the formation of hemidesmomes or other areas of strong adhesion, reorganize the cytoskeleton, promote or inhibit locomotion and cell division, and to affect many other aspects of cell biology. At present there is much interest in the variability of these molecules as a potential means of signalling between the cells which lay them down and other cells which may contact them later, as a sort of patterned extracellular 'memory' which could specifically direct the morphogenesis and migrations of cells and tissues.

Fibronectin

Fibronectin is a large glycoprotein molecule consisting of a dimer held together by disulphide links, each subunit composed of a string of large repetitive domains joined by flexible regions, and bearing binding sites for collagen, heparin and cell surface receptors, especially integrins. It is, therefore, able to promote adhesion between all of these elements. In connective tissues the molecules are able to bind in an orderly fashion to cell surfaces to form short fibronectin

filaments. Other variants are passed into the circulation as plasma fibronectins. Many isoforms of fibronectin are known, generated by alternative splicing of mRNA from the very large, single gene encoding this molecular family. This variation provides a basis for selective adhesion of different cell types to the matrix both during development and in maturity. Those found in embryonic tissues are also expressed in wound repair, where they facilitate tissue proliferation and cell movements, but they revert to the adult form once this has been achieved.

Laminin

Laminin is a large (850 kDa) flexible cruciform molecule composed of three polypeptide chains (designated α, β, and γ, corresponding to the older names of A, B_1 and B_2) whose terminal two-thirds are wound round each other to form the stem of a cross, the free ends forming the upright and transverse members. The molecule bears binding sites for a number of other ECM molecules including heparan sulphate, Type IV collagen, entactin, and laminin receptor molecules situated in cell plasma membranes. There are many isoforms of the different chains, giving at least 18 types of laminin. Laminin molecules can assemble themselves into flat regular meshworks, forming part of the basal lamina (see below). For further details see Tryggvason (1993).

Tenascin

Tenascin is another large glycoprotein consisting of six subunits joined at one end to form a radiating structure like the spokes of a wheel. Although abundant in embryonic tissues, its adult distribution is restricted. It appears to be important in guiding cell migrations and axonal growth in early development, either promoting or inhibiting these depending on the cell and tenascin type (Erickson 1993). Like other adhesion molecules there is a family of tenascin molecules formed by alternative splicing of the tenascin gene, giving a large variety of forms by different combinations of subunits in the sixfold assembly of this molecule.

BASAL LAMINA AND BASEMENT MEMBRANE

Light microscopy showed many years ago that at the interface between connective and other tissues, for example between the dermis and epidermis, there is a narrow layer of cell-free matrix which typically stains strongly for carbohydrates with the PAS method, and for collagen (e.g. with van Gieson's stain). This was termed the *basement membrane*, and was envisaged as a homogeneous sheet of extracellular material to which adjacent tissues were attached. Electron microscopy modified this view, as it was found that the basement membrane is composed of two quite distinct components: a thin, finely fibrillar layer, the *basal lamina*, associated closely with the cell surface, and a more distant, variable *reticular lamina* of larger fibrils and ground substance (**2.97**). The basal lamina was also found to be present on its own or with a minimal reticular lamina in many other situations, for instance around Schwann cells, muscle cells, capillary endothelium and at the base of many epithelia.

The synthesis of the basal lamina components is not yet entirely settled. In situ studies of mRNA synthesis show that Type IV collagen is made by the cells in close contact with this structure, whereas nidogen is synthesized by connective tissue cells (Dziadek & Thomas 1993). For the basement membrane in skin, see page 382.

Basal lamina

Basal lamina is usually about 80 nm thick and consists of a fibrillar layer, the *lamina densa* (20–50 nm wide) separated from the plasma membrane of the adjacent cell by a narrow electron-lucent zone, the *lamina lucida* (see Inoue 1989). The lamina lucida shows granular or fibrillar features representing the presence of various proteoglycans, the extracellular domains of integrins and other small glycoproteins; in the basal lamina of the epidermis, this lamina (see p. 382) is crossed by hemidesmosomes anchored into the lamina densa. The lamina densa is a delicate network composed of laminin, Type IV collagen entactin (nidogen) and perlecan (a large heparan sulphate proteoglycan). These are thought to be assembled in the form of a flattened three-dimensional network where the laminin molecules form a hexagonal lattice rather like chicken wire, which the other molecules stabilize by cross-linking (see Yurchenco and O'Rear 1994).

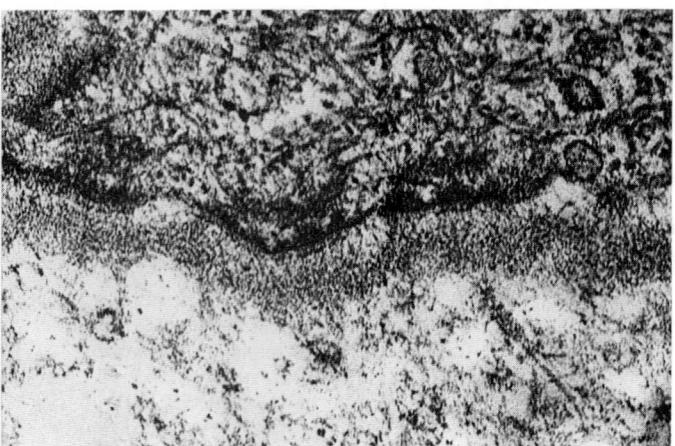

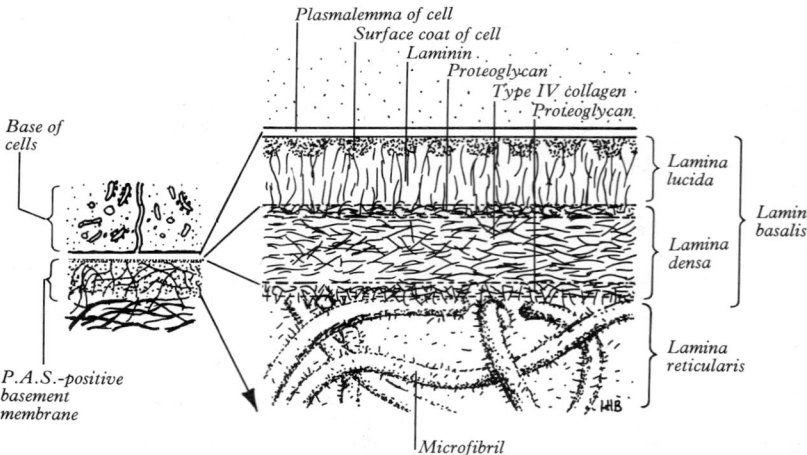

2.97A Section through the base of the epidermis (human) showing the basal lamina. Visible are the lamina lucida just below the dense plasmalemma of the overlying cell and the thick fuzzy lamina densa, below which is the paler area of the connective tissue matrix containing a few microfibrils in section. Also shown are several hemidesmosomes with filamentous connections crossing the lamina lucida. Magnification × 60 000.

2.97B Diagram showing the organization of the basement membrane components (compare **2.97A** and **5.39**).

Although all basal laminae have a similar form, their detailed organization and sizes vary with their tissue sites. At the epidermal–dermal junction, special glycoproteins are present in the lamina lucida, and hemidesmosomes also anchor the neighbouring keratinocytes to the lamina densa (see **5.39, 40**). The kidney glomerular basal lamina is unusual in having a lucent zone on both sides of the lamina densa (laminae rarae interna and externa) and in various other features associated with the specialized filtering functions of this structure (p. 1822). In some situations the basal lamina may be particularly thick and so, incidentally, easier to investigate, as in the glomerular membrane of the kidney, the lens capsule, the anterior limiting (Descemet's) membrane in the cornea and Reichert's membrane in the placenta of certain mammals (see Kefalides 1973; Heathcote & Grant 1981).

Reticular (or fibroreticular) lamina

The reticular lamina consists of dense matrix containing collagen filaments including (in skin) those of Type VII collagen (anchoring fibrils) which bind the lamina densa to the adjacent connective tissue. The high concentration of proteoglycans in this zone is responsible for the positive PAS reaction in light microscopic sections.

Functions of basal laminae

The basal laminae perform important roles in the biology of the tissues lying in contact with them. They form selectively permeable barriers between adjacent tissues in some cases (as in the glomerular filter of the kidney's retaining large molecules but allowing small ones to pass); they have mechanical functions, forming anchoring intermediaries between epithelial and connective tissues, assisting to stabilize and orientate the tissue layers; they also have profound instructive effects on the adjacent tissues, determining their polarity, rate of cell division, metabolism, movements and repair. In addition, they act as pathways for the migration and routing of growing cell processes, for example in regeneration in the peripheral nervous system after injury (p. 956) when basal lamina components guide the outgrowth of axons and the re-establishment of neuromuscular junctions. Changes in basal lamina thickness are also often associated with pathological conditions, as in the thickening of the glomerular membrane in glomerulonephritis and diabetes, although it may be difficult to allot causes and effects in such cases. For further reading on the structure and properties of the basal lamina see Inoue (1989), Farquhar (1991), Alberts et al (1994), Yurchenco and O'Rear (1994).

CLASSIFICATION OF CONNECTIVE TISSUES

The connective tissues differ considerably in appearance, consistency and composition in different regions according to the local functional requirements. These differences are related to the predominance or otherwise of one or other of the cell types, the concentration, arrangement and types of fibre and the character of the ground substance. On these bases, *general (ordinary) connective tissues* can be classified into *irregular* and *regular* types, distinguished by the absence or presence of a high degree of orientation in their fibrous elements.

IRREGULAR CONNECTIVE TISSUES

These can be further subdivided into *loose*, *dense* and *adipose*.

Loose (areolar) connective tissue

Loose connective tissue is the most generalized form (**2.80, 99**). It is extensively distributed and its chief use is to bind parts together, though allowing a considerable amount of movement to take place because of its elasticity. It occurs as the submucous coat in the digestive tract and as subserous tissue. It forms the subcutaneous tissue in regions where this is devoid of fat as in the eyelids, penis, the scrotum and labia. It is also found between muscles, vessels and nerves, forming their investing sheaths and connecting them with surrounding structures. It is present in the interior of organs, binding together the lobes and lobules of compound glands, various coats of the hollow viscera and muscle and nerve fibres.

Loose connective tissue consists of a meshwork of thin collagen and elastin fibres interlacing in all directions to give a measure of both elasticity and tensile strength. The large meshes contain the soft, pliable semifluid ground substance composed of proteoglycans, and the different connective tissue cells, scattered along the fibres or in the meshes. Occasional adipocytes, usually in small groups, are seen, particularly around blood vessels.

Dense irregular connective tissue

Dense irregular connective tissue is found in regions which experience considerable mechanical stress and where protection is given to ensheathed organs. The matrix contains a high proportion of collagen fibres which form thick bundles (**2.99**) interweaving in three dimensions and giving considerable strength. Active fibroblasts are few in number and most are flattened with heterochromatic nuclei. The vascular supply is limited, as might be expected.

Examples may be found in the reticular layer of the dermis, the connective tissue sheaths of muscle and nerves and the adventitia of large blood vessels. The capsules of various glands, the coverings of various organs such as the penis and testes, the sclera of the eye and periostea and perichondria are all composed of dense irregular connective tissue.

Adipose tissue

A few fat cells occur in loose connective tissue in most parts of the body. However, in adipose tissue (**2.82, 83**) they occur in great abundance and constitute the principal component. Adipose tissue occurs only in certain regions and this selective distribution suggests that the fat is deposited in genetically determined sites. It occurs in abundance in subcutaneous tissue, which is sometimes referred to as the *panniculus adiposus*, and around the kidneys, in the mesenteries and omenta, in the female breast, in the orbit behind the eyeball, in the marrow of bones deep to the plantar skin of the foot, and as localized pads in the synovial membrane of many joints. Its distribution in subcutaneous tissue shows characteristic age and sex differences.

Adipose tissue consists of adipocytes (p. 76) embedded in a vascular loose connective tissue, which is usually divided into lobules by stronger fibrous septa carrying the larger blood vessels, whence each lobule receives an independent blood supply. Within the lobules the fat cells are round or, when mutually compressed, polygonal. Loose connective tissue and septa both contain the other cellular components of fibrous tissue. Fat deposits serve as energy stores, sources of metabolic lipids, thermal insulation (subcutaneous fat), mechanical shock-absorbers (e.g. soles of the feet, palms of the hands, gluteal

fat, synovial membranes, etc.), and may also serve more complex, cosmetic or behavioural functions. In some regions the connective tissue framework of the fatty tissue often contains large amounts of elastic tissue and in emaciation these deposits, where mechanically important, tend to be spared until a late stage, for example, plantar and palmar superficial fasciae, and perirenal fat. In the newborn human, as in many adult lower mammals, there are areas of specialized

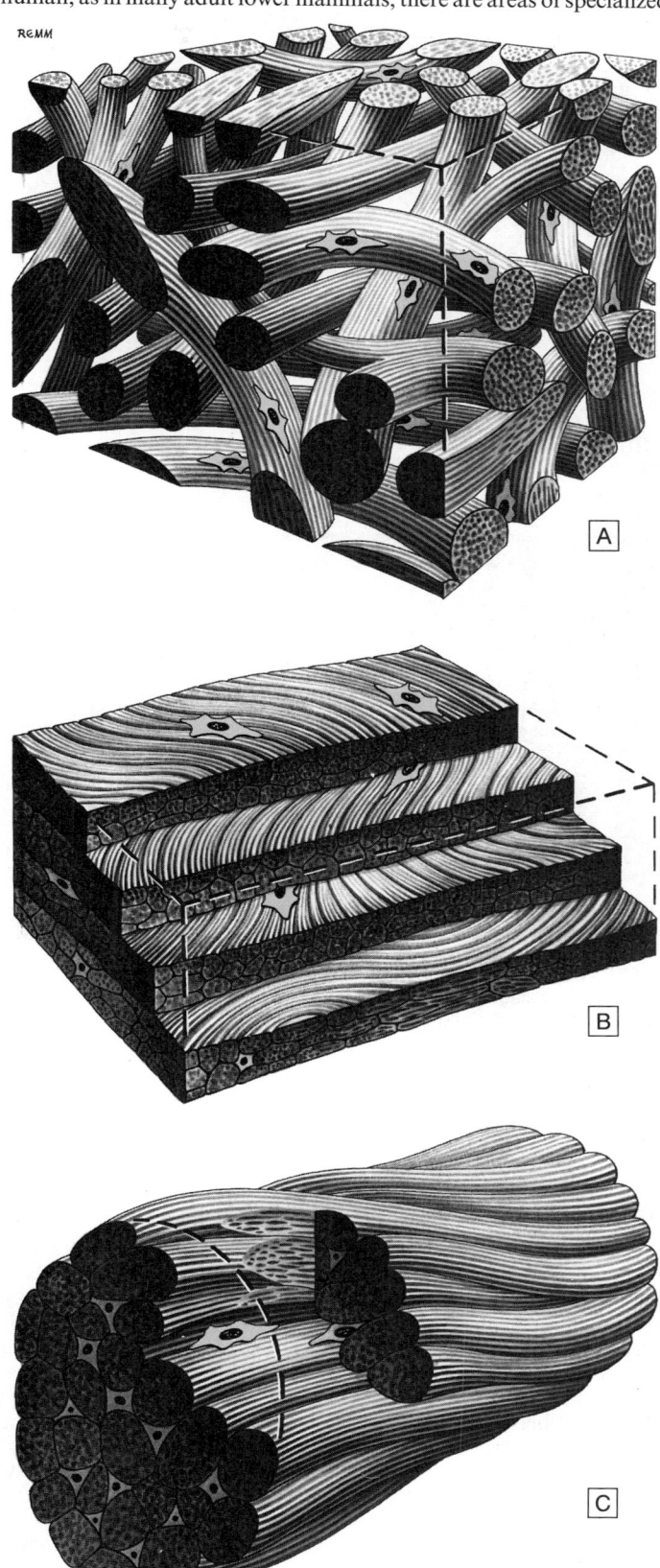

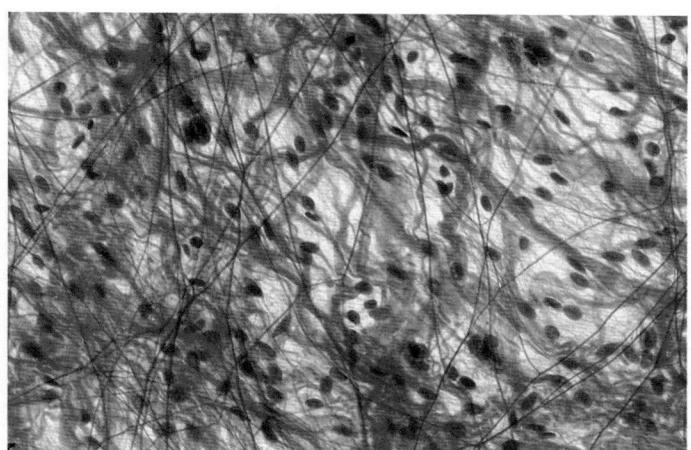

2.98 Loose connective tissue in the mesentery, viewed as a whole mount preparation stained to show the interwoven collagen fibres (red) and network of thin elastin fibres, with interspersed cells. Van Gieson/Verhoeff's stain. Magnification × 200.

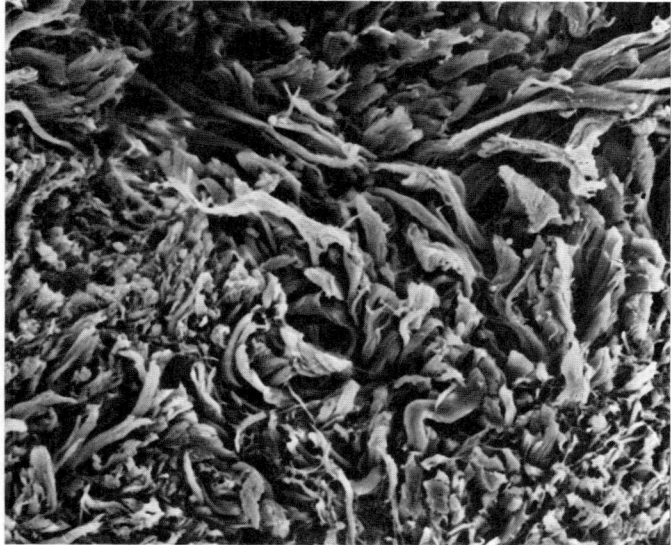

2.99 Scanning electron micrograph of dense irregular connective tissue (human dermis) showing the complex interwoven nature of its fibrous matrix. Magnification × 1000.

2.100 Three types of arrangement of collagen fibres in: (A) dense irregular connective tissue; (B) a ligament; (C) a tendon.

89

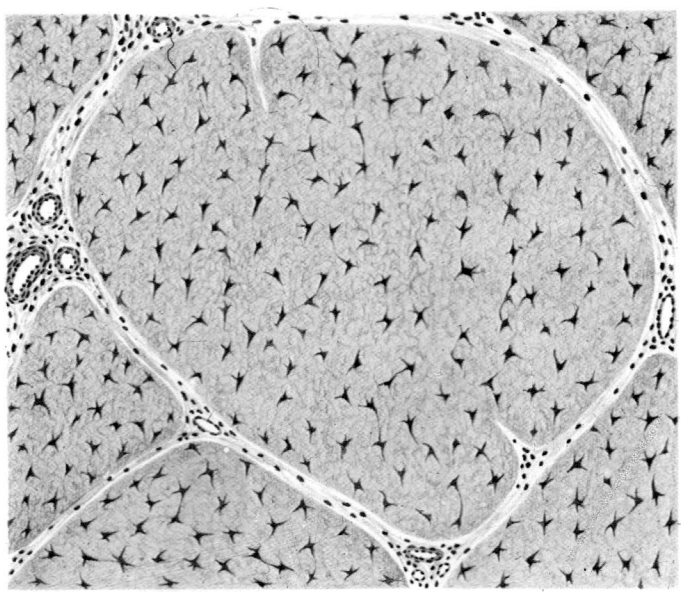

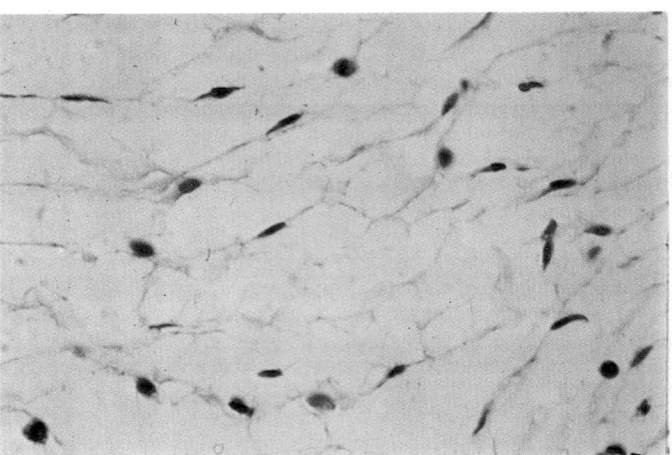

2.103   A section of fetal mesenchyme showing mucoid tissue sparsely populated with cells. Magnification × 500.

2.101   Transverse section of a tendon showing fibrocytes enclosed between bundles of collagen fibres.

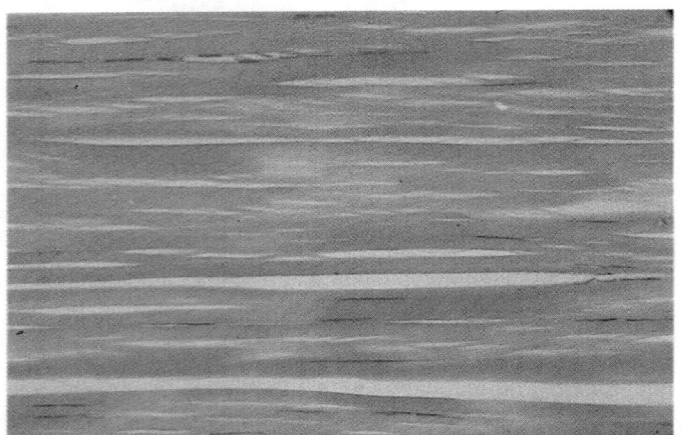

2.102   Longitudinal section through a tendon, showing the parallel organization of its collagen fibres. A few long, flattened fibrocyte nuclei are also visible. Haematoxylin and eosin. Magnification × 200.

brown fat, which is capable of generating heat by the breakdown of nutrients in unusual mitochondria (see also pp. 34, 77).

REGULAR CONNECTIVE TISSUES

Regular connective tissue includes those highly fibrous tissues with fibres regularly orientated, either to form sheets such as fasciae and aponeuroses, or thicker bundles as ligaments or tendons (**2**.100–102). The direction of the fibres within such structures is related to the stresses which they undergo but there is considerable interweaving of fibrous bundles, even within tendons, which increases their structural stability and resilience.

The fibroblasts which secrete the fibres may eventually become trapped within the fibrous structure, where they are compressed, and present highly angular outlines. Cross-sections of tendons show inactive fibroblasts with stellate profiles and small heterochromatic nuclei. Fibroblasts on the external surface may be active in continued fibre formation and they afford a pool of cells able to repair damage (see McMinn 1969).

Regular connective tissue is predominantly collagenous but in some ligaments elastic components also occur, as in the ligamenta flava of the vertebral laminae and in the vocal folds. Some elastin is also present between the collagen lamellae of many other ligaments and fasciae. In other sites, the collagen fibres may form precise geometrical patterns, as in the cornea (see p. 1326).

Mucoid tissue. This is a fetal or embryonic type of connective tissue (**2**.103), found chiefly as a stage in the development of connective tissue from mesenchyme. It exists in the 'jelly of Wharton', which forms the bulk of the umbilical cord, and consists of a copious matrix, largely made up of hydrated 'mucosubstances' and a fine meshwork of collagen fibres, in which nucleated cells with branching process (probably fibroblasts) are found (Boyd & Hamilton 1970). However, the stellate appearance of the cells in Wharton's jelly probably results from fixation and staining of excised cords which have suffered a haemodynamic collapse (Parry 1970). When this is avoided the cells are aligned and strap-like. Such findings may well apply to other situations in which mucoid tissue is found. Usually few fibres occur in typical mucoid tissue, though at birth the umbilical cord shows a considerable development of perivascular collagen fibres; after birth it is still to be seen in the pulp of a developing tooth. In the adult the vitreous body of the eye is a persistent form of mucoid tissue in which the fibres and cells are very few in number, and the nucleus pulposus of the intervertebral disc is similar.

Pigmented connective tissue. Such tissue, as occurs in the choroid and in the lamina fusca of the sclera of the eye, is composed of loose connective tissue, in which large numbers of pigment cells (melanocytes) are also present.

VESSELS AND NERVES OF CONNECTIVE TISSUE

Generally, few blood vessels supply the tissue itself, the numbers of cells and, therefore, the metabolic demand being relatively low, although many blood vessels may pass through en route for other tissues, as in loose connective tissue. In dense collagenous or elastic tissues the blood vessels usually run parallel to and between the longitudinal bundles, sending communicating branches across the bundles; in some of its forms, such as in the periosteum and dura mater, they are fairly numerous. *Lymphatic vessels* are very numerous in most forms of connective tissue, especially in the loose tissue beneath the skin and the mucous and serous surfaces. They also occur abundantly in the sheaths of tendons, as well as in the tendons themselves. *Nerve* endings of various kinds also terminate in connective tissues and provide sensory innervation detecting mechanical stresses, painful stimuli and thermal changes (see p. 965). In adipose tissue, sympathetic efferents are important in regulating the metabolism of adipose cells, especially the breakdown of lipid.

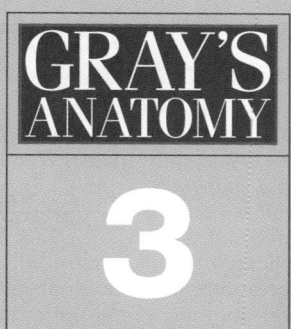

EMBRYOLOGY AND DEVELOPMENT

Section Editor: Patricia Collins

The basic developmental pattern of this chapter was laid down by the late Peter Williams; it has provided a sound foundation. The dramatic advances of molecular biology since the last edition have produced vast amounts of data on developing systems, synthesis of which has provided some insight into common embryonic processes occurring in all systems of the body. An account of the diverse development of each system has only been possible because of the specialist advice and help from many contributors, each experts in their fields. Significant portions of the text have been revised by Mark Ferguson, Sarah Guthrie, Frank Billett, Sue Kimber and John Aplin; and contributions have been gratefully received from Aidan Breathnach, Nigel Brown, Duncan Davidson, John Carroll, Nicole Le Douarin, Bob Edwards, Anne Ferguson-Smith, Tom Fleming, Peter Holland, Martin Johnson, Anthony Lander, Barry Mitchell, Isabella Moore, Antoon Moorman, Gonzalo Moscoso, Charles Roedeck, Paul Sharpe, Richard Sharpe, Cheryl Tickle and Michael Whitaker.

Illustrations have been provided by Kevin Marks, Peter Lamb, Peter Jack, Jenny Halstead, Mark Hay and Andrew Bezear and Denise Smith.

This chapter has evolved in its revision reflecting the changing and improving techniques now used for examining embryos. It has also grown by interstitial and accretionary growth, to encompass the increase in the depth and extent of our understanding of developmental processes.

Although the chapter has been written to provide the most up to date account of the subject as we go to press, I hope it is also accessible to a wide range of students who hopefully will become inspired by the subject and contribute to it in the future.

INTRODUCTION

The life cycle passes through phases, from gametes to zygote, embryo to fetus and finally juvenile to adult. Revolution of the cycle is ensured by the repetition of this sequence. In humans, gamete production occurs in the female during embryonic life and is completed prior to birth; in males gamete cell lines are stored during the embryonic and juvenile stage ready for further replication in adulthood. In terms of the propagation of individuals, the accurate copying of DNA during gametogenesis, the inclusion of variation in the code during meiosis and the successful production of a viable juvenile, which is able to pass on its DNA, are the major features of the cycle. The mechanisms which control phases of the cycle are contained within the genome and expression of genes and their products, in particular sequences, result in the morphological changes seen during embryo formation. Study of the interactions of molecules responsible for such morphological changes forms the basis of developmental biology. The embryology and development section is initially concerned with those basic features of development which are common to all multicellular (metazoan) animals, more especially chordate craniates, particularly as viewed in the light of their evolutionary history. The experimental work, genetic analysis and the concepts of the later 20th-century developmental biology are outlined. Following a description of the earliest assumption of embryonic morphology, the development of the human embryo is considered in detail in relation to the development of individual systems; in each case descriptions of embryonic morphology are supported by experimental evidence of the underlying molecular mechanisms. The consequences of error in developing systems are examined.

THE COMPARATIVE PRINCIPLE

There are two important, indeed fundamental, approaches to anatomical study which lead to a significantly deeper understanding of the structure of the human body not only at the gross and histological levels but also, increasingly, at the molecular level; these concern the **comparative** and **developmental** aspects, particularly through the study of craniate/vertebrate chordates and their subgroups the anamniotes and amniotes. The importance of both aspects is deeply rooted in the history of the discipline of anatomy.

The science of *comparative anatomy* was founded during the latter half of the 18th century and became established during the first half of the 19th century. A notable British contribution was made by the great physiologist and surgeon John Hunter (1728–93) whose vast collection of some 14 000 specimens, many of them fossils and skeletal structures, was subsequently sorted and catalogued by Richard Owen (1804–92) to form the basis of the Hunterian Museum of the Royal College of Surgeons. Owen was influenced greatly by the ideas of 'transcendental anatomy' and 'idealistic morphology' emanating especially from Germany (Goethe, 1739–1842) and France (Geoffroy Saint-Hilaire, 1772–1844) which fostered the notion that organisms were related through common anatomical design. Of particular interest is Owen's distinction between homologous (same basic design) and analogous (same function) structures; also noteworthy was his concept of a *vertebrate archetype*, which laid particular emphasis on the *segmental organization* of the skeleton. The theme of comparative anatomy, that there is a basic pattern to all vertebrate structure, was enhanced by the gradual realization that this pattern emerged during *embryonic development* in a relatively simple form. The concept of the *germ layers*, implying the invariant origin of tissues, initially formulated by Von Baer (1828), together with his emphasis that during development generalized structure precedes specific and specialized structure, cemented the link between the developmental and comparative aspects.

The publication of Darwin's *The Origin of Species by Natural Selection* (1859) provided the third, and critically important, element towards an enlightened approach to the study of human anatomy in general and to embryology in particular. Although the famous dictum of Haeckel (1874) that ontogeny (development) recapitulates phylogeny (evolution) encapsulates a view that is still regarded as controversial, nevertheless, it provides a useful guideline for the appreciation of the emergent pattern of the vertebrate embryo as it passes through phases shared by a common ancestor.

CONCEPTS AND TERMINOLOGY

Almost all of the terms which were employed to describe the development of chordates came into use during the second half of the 19th century. The acceptance of a generally understood, and internationally acceptable, terminology was essential to the emergence of embryology as a true **numerate, experimental science** in its own right. However, during the closing decades of the century important **concepts** became **embodied** in terms which implied support for the comparative principle based on the dominance of the germ layer theory and on the rarely questioned view that the embryological development of animals **recapitulated** important facets of their evolution.

An examination of the origin and meaning of the terms currently used to describe embryonic development reveals a list still dominated by 19th-century terminology. The familiar terms *morula*, *blastula* and *gastrula* derive from Haeckel's (1874) view that early stages of development correspond to a sequence whereby, during evolution, a simple multicellular mass of cells initially gave rise to a hollow sphere; subsequent invagination of part of the outer surface of the sphere produced a two-layered structure, designated by Haeckel as the *gastreae* stage of evolution, equivalent to the relatively simple gastrula stage of many marine organisms, for instance that of the sea urchin (p. 96). This initial invagination of embryonic cells was thus termed *gastrulation*. Although the progression envisaged by Haeckel was hypothetical, it is important to understand that it was driven by the evolutionary imperative and derived much of its plausibility from observations of embryos.

The notion that gastrulation is the most important phase of development is historically related to its association with the germ layer theory, particularly in relation to chordates. Basically this theory, originally formulated by Von Baer (1837) and later refined by the brothers Hertwig (1879–83), states that the structure of all **animals** above the level of coelenterates is derived from **three embryonic layers**, namely an outer *ectoderm*, an inner *endoderm* and an intervening *mesoderm*, each layer generating specific tissue components corresponding to the triploblastic design of the post-embryonic form. In vertebrates, for instance, it was envisaged that the ectoderm gave rise to the epidermis and the major part of the nervous system; the endoderm generated the epithelial lining of the gut and contributed to derived glandular structures as well as to the lining of the lungs; and the mesoderm formed the vascular system and much of the musculoskeletal structure.

Although the terms ectoderm, mesoderm and endoderm quickly became established and were, from the outset, commonly used to describe the germ layers, the terms *epiblast* or *ectoblast* (outer embryonic layer), *mesoblast* (middle embryonic layer) and *hypoblast* or *endoblast* (inner embryonic layer) were for many years recognized alternatives (Lankester 1877; Balfour 1888). Sedwick (1902) in fact suggested that the term mesoblast was **the** appropriate term for the middle layer of amniotes. Certainly in some ways the *'blast'* terminology is preferable; it retains the embryological connotation implicit in many other terms (e.g. *blastoderm, blastocyst, blastopore*) and clearly relates to the derived term *triploblastic*.

Currently the terms epiblast and hypoblast are used to describe the upper and lower cell layers of the *amniote* blastoderm respectively. Recently the term mesoblast has been reinstated both to describe the middle layer of amniote embryos and to designate mesenchymal cells produced from the primitive streak (Nakasuji 1992) (see also p. 124). In amniotes both *embryonic* and *extraembryonic* tissues (*membranes*) develop. The extraembryonic tissues are derived from both the epiblast and hypoblast, (see p. 98), whereas the embryonic tissues are derived from the epiblast alone. This critical division of cell lineages into embryonic and extraembryonic distinguishes the *amniota* from the *anamniota* where all the cells derived from the zygote are embryonic (see below).

Despite the subsequent modification of the germ layer theory and the rejection of the idea of the *invariant* fate of cells derived from particular layers, the fundamental insight that the theory provided towards an enlightened understanding of the relation between embryonic development, histology and gross anatomical structure cannot be underestimated. The 19th-century embryologists recognized a close association between the process of gastrulation and the formation of the middle embryonic layer. However, Balfour (1888) and others frequently made a distinction between the two processes, because in some embryos other methods of forming the middle layer were envisaged. Largely as a result of experimental studies (see below), the modern view of gastrulation is that of a *dynamic process* which shifts prospective cell populations at, or associated with, the surface of the early embryo to its interior, resulting in the *tripartite division* of material from which the basic structure of the embryo, and thus that of the adult, is derived. Although vertebrate eggs may differ greatly in size and thus undergo strikingly different cleavage patterns after fertilization, they achieve through gastrulation a remarkably similar result (see p. 100). It is in this context that gastrulation, as the essential **prerequisite** for the determination of triploblastic structure, may indeed be regarded as the single most important event in, and a vital concept of, embryonic development.

The use of the germ layers as a focus to describe early development has proved problematical in recent years due to the inflexibility of the terminology and its non-specific usage by the novice and the expert. The appeal of three layers from which all structures derive is enduring. However, it was known at the time the theory was gaining popularity that its focus on three layers was simplistic and misleading. The acceptance of other ways of deriving embryonic cells, apart from at gastrulation, for example by ingression of neural crest cells (see below), was slow. Changes in embryological terminology pertinent to the germ layers were not incorporated into many embryological texts, skewing the perceived value of some cell populations compared to others. The consequence has been that the words used to describe the middle layer of the embryo—mesoderm, mesoblast, and mesenchyme (see below)—are frequently used synonymously and without regard to changes in cell–cell contact and cell status; writers have ignored particularly the *transition from epithelium to free cells and vice versa*, such events being of significant importance during development. This vague use of terminology has inhibited the precise description of the origin and interaction of embryonic tissues.

It is apparent that the simple invagination of a sheet of epithelial cells by the deformation of a ball of cells will involve different cellular mechanisms from the separation of individual cells from an epithelium to a free state (as occurs at the primitive streak, see p. 142). Cells which were seen free in groups within an embryo, with copious extracellular matrix, were termed *mesenchyme* by Hertwig (1881) and were described by Lankester (1877) as *mesoblast*—'cells which wandered through the matrix between the inner and outer layers of the embryo'. Hay (1968) suggested the terms *primary mesenchyme* for those cells formed by ingression at the primitive streak, and *secondary mesenchyme* for those formed by ingression at other sites, for example the neural crest (see p. 147). She noted that the mesenchymal cells formed from the streak usually revert to an epithelial status when they reach their destination. Thus the populations of mesenchymal cells within a triploblastic embryo include, inter alia: mesenchymal cells which may differentiate along a connective tissue lineage, migrating epithelial cells which display a mesenchymal phenotype whilst migrating, and stem cells which may retain the ability to differentiate along different lines according to the local environmental influences. Recombinant experiments now allow mesenchyme populations to be exchanged to see if their site of origin is important in determining their final fate. Thus the specificity with which cells are termed assists understanding of their possible developmental fates.

A **clarification** of the terminology associated with the middle layer seems to be appropriate for the following reasons. Unlike the terms ectoderm and endoderm, which fittingly describe the outer and inner epithelial layers of the embryo, the term mesoderm, as currently used in *amniote development*, applies to an embryonic tissue which can be either epithelial or mesenchymal. The recognition of the importance of epithelial/mesenchymal interactions during development necessitates that the cellular arrangements within the embryo are described specifically. For this reason the term mesoblast is subsequently used in this section to denote a temporary, embryonic cell lineage, which will later generate **either** an epithelial **or** a free cell arrangement. The free cell arrangement will be termed *mesenchyme*; it will be designated according to its position or fate within the embryo. The *epithelial arrangement* will be specified with reference to its structure, prospective fate and location. In view of its dynamic nature mesenchyme should no longer be regarded as 'embryonic connective tissue'. The reader should note that the traditional term—mesoderm—will be retained in the brief account of prospective fate maps of blastulae and gastrulae in *anamniota*, and occasionally in other sections of this volume (for discussion see Collins & Billett 1995).

REPRODUCTION

Reproduction, the ability of an organism to reproduce a more or less exact replica of itself, is a fundamental feature of living material; it is a property which at the onset of the origin of life (see p. 3) would have established the boundary between systems with the attributes of life and their complex, non-living, biochemical precursors. The advent of cellularization, which conserved complexity, ensured its survival by replication but allowed the possibility of genetic variation (through mutational change) and laid the foundation for a primitive reproductive capacity capable of further evolution, initially by **asexual** means but ultimately by a **sexual** method.

Gametogenesis

Although asexual methods of reproduction are common among relatively simple animals, and are sometimes incorporated into the life cycle of more advanced forms (insects), sexual reproduction is found throughout the animal kingdom. A multicellular organism which reproduces sexually consists mainly of general body (*somatic*) cells which, although exhibiting extreme ranges of variation in size, shape and specific functional as well as morphological characteristics, all possess certain common features of their genetic apparatus. This contrasts with the highly distinctive differentiation process and genetic changes which occur within the *gonads* and result in the formation of mature *germ* cells or *gametes*. General somatic cells usually possess a full or *diploid number* of chromosomes, a half of which was originally derived from each parent. However, the *activity* and *expression* of the many different gene loci on the chromosomes varies in different cell types in adult tissues, and during development as differentiation occurs. The somatic cells which are capable of dividing do so by the process of mitosis (p. 57). Each chromosome, having first made a faithful replica of itself and thus of its genes, divides longitudinally and each resultant cell is again equipped with the diploid number of chromosomes which are replicas of those in the parent cell. During *gametogenesis*, however, a complex series of changes termed *meiosis* are set in train (p. 60). Essentially, during this, the original chromosome number is reduced to a half, the *haploid number*, in which a *recombination* of the genetic material has occurred. (Details are considered on p. 56.) The male gonad or *testis* produces many small motile gametes or *spermatozoa* in which the cytoplasmic machinery is much reduced; each consists of a nucleus bearing the genetic apparatus, the chromosomes, with a closely applied acrosome derived from a Golgi apparatus and succeeded by a long flagellum which is partly ensheathed by an energy-transforming mitochondrial sheath (p. 125). In contrast the female gonad or *ovary* produces fewer, larger, non-motile *ova* (eggs), their cytoplasm containing a variable quantity of food reserves (*yolk* or *deutoplasm*). The fusion of the gametes forms a *zygote* and restores the characteristic diploid chromosome number of the species. Most importantly, however, as the chromosomes are derived from parents which are genetically dissimilar, the sexual process fosters genetic variation, in contrast to the asexual method where it is limited to mutational change.

Influence of egg size and structure

The pattern of early development is greatly influenced by the size of the egg destined to become an embryo; this particularly affects the stages of cleavage and gastrulation (see below) (**3.1**). Depending almost exclusively on their yolk (nutritional reserve) content, eggs vary enormously in size, ranging from c.100 μm in diameter (e.g. for

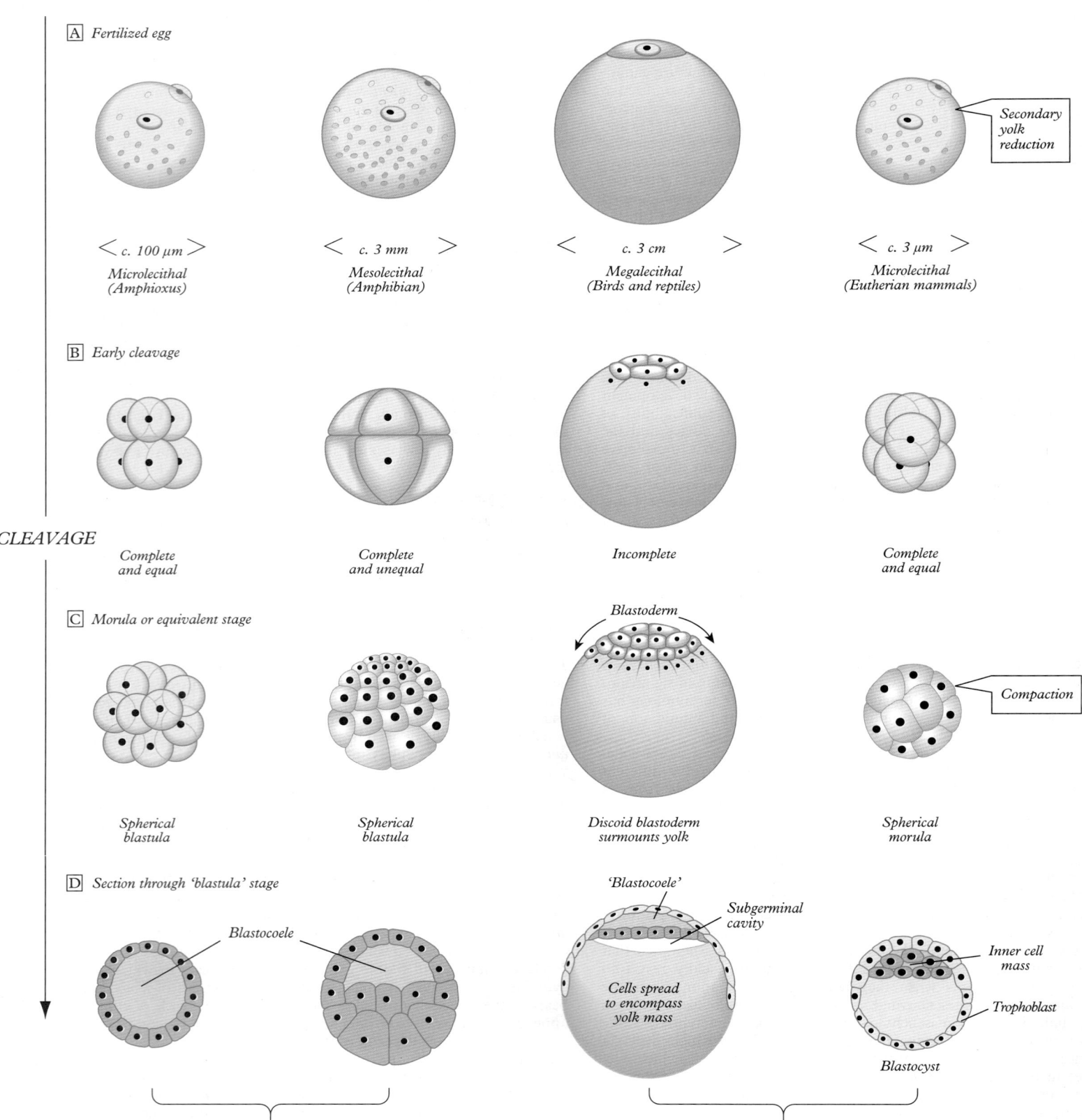

A Fertilized egg

< c. 100 μm >
Microlecithal
(Amphioxus)

< c. 3 mm >
Mesolecithal
(Amphibian)

< c. 3 cm >
Megalecithal
(Birds and reptiles)

< c. 3 μm >
Microlecithal
(Eutherian mammals)

Secondary yolk reduction

B Early cleavage

CLEAVAGE

Complete and equal

Complete and unequal

Incomplete

Complete and equal

C Morula or equivalent stage

Blastoderm

Compaction

Spherical blastula

Spherical blastula

Discoid blastoderm surmounts yolk

Spherical morula

D Section through 'blastula' stage

'Blastocoele'

Subgerminal cavity

Blastocoele

Cells spread to encompass yolk mass

Inner cell mass

Trophoblast

Blastocyst

In anamniotes (e.g. primitive chordates, ganoid fish and all amphibians) the whole blastula is transformed into an embryo.

In amniotes (reptiles, birds and mammals) the embryo is confined to an initially discoid part of the blastula or to an inner cell mass. The remainder forms supportive and protective *extraembryonic membranes*, i.e. amnion, chorion, yolk sac, allantois, and contributes to placental structures.

3.1 Early development of chordates I: egg size, yolk volume and distribution, cleavage pattern.

A–D. Variation in the pattern of cleavage in chordate embryos associated with differences in oöcyte size, yolk volume and distribution. The overall phylogenetic trend is from left to right and the developmental progression is from above downwards.

Note: (i) Blastocoelic development is not always associated with megalecithal eggs; the eggs of most modern boy fish (teleosts) are relatively small but exhibit a blastodermic type of development. (ii) The blastocoele of *Amphioxus* and amphibians is probably not homologous with the apparently similar spaces in birds and reptiles, and the blastocyst cavity of mammals.

sea urchins and mammals) to over 1 cm (most birds and many reptiles); if volumes are compared, related to the power of 3, the difference is obviously even more striking. This difference in size is concerned with such factors as the need to disperse the progeny as **quickly** as possible, through the agency of a larval form (e.g. teleosts and sea urchins), or the need to **sustain** embryonic development for as long as possible, in the virtually closed environment of a *cleidoic egg* (e.g. birds). In the first case large numbers of small eggs are produced by the female and fertilization is **external**, in the second only a few large eggs are produced, for which **internal** fertilization is a prerequisite. The situation among present-day reptiles, birds and mammals (collectively referred to as *amniotes*) is particularly relevant to that which now exists in man. Both birds and mammals evolved from reptilian precursors (see p. 5) who by their ability to lay eggs which could develop on land achieved complete independence of the general aqueous environment to which their amphibian ancestors were restricted. (Better eggs rather than stronger legs were essential for the conquest of land.) The problems posed by the closed environment of the egg, relating to the provision of a local aqueous milieu, respiration, efficient utilization of the stored yolk and the enforced storage of excretory products were solved by the evolution of *extraembryonic membranes* (see below). The reptilian precursors of the eutherian mammals at first retained their yolk-laden eggs and then utilized the existing membrane structures to make contact with the female parent, thus initiating the evolution of the varieties of *placentae* and complete dependence of embryonic development on the mother. Egg retention virtually eliminated the need for yolk with a consequent *secondary reduction* in the size of the egg to that now seen in mammals. This trend can be detected among a few present-day reptile groups, for example skinks. Thus although the eggs of mammals are **similar** in **size** to those of many marine invertebrates their evolutionary history has produced a **fundamental difference** in structure; this **must** be borne in mind when their development is considered.

Apart from size, embryonic development is determined, in a fundamental way, by the *intrinsic molecular structure* of the egg. In anamniotes, this structure is generated during oögenesis and subsequently modified by oöcyte maturation which transforms the diploid oöcyte into the haploid egg. This process confers a distinct *radial symmetry*, centred around the animal–vegetal axis, in many eggs. (A cephalocaudal axis in the case of insects.) The subsequent formation of a dorsoventral axis, usually by fertilization, establishes *bilateral symmetry*. The time of appearance, degree and reversibility of the appearance of this bilateral symmetry varies greatly between animal groups; in some cases the bilateral symmetry appears to be directly related to the point of sperm entry, but frequently it is not. The comparative and experimental evidence for the existence of this *inherent* symmetry, its relative fixity and lability, and especially the role of the egg cortex, was established many years ago. With the recent discovery of genes which determine polarity it remains an important focus of current research.

Egg structure provides the *heterogeneous cytoplasmic environment* which interacts with the *genetic programme* emanating from the zygote nucleus at the beginning of development. The subsequent progressive interaction and mutual modification of *cytoplasmic* and *nuclear components* was the basis of Morgan's (1934) explanation of the generation of diverse cell types during embryonic development.

The experimental analysis of the *causal mechanisms* of development (see p. 103) has revealed that *zygotes* exhibit some degree of segregation of cytoplasmic elements (determinants). However, the degree, precision and lability of this segregation varies greatly among animal groups. In some invertebrate eggs, for instance those of platyhelminthes, molluscs and annelids, a highly ordered structure is associated with a precise pattern of *spiral cleavage*, although in others, such as ascidians, it is not. With this type of egg structure the fate of the initial cleavage cells is fixed, and a cell separated at this stage results in the development of a partial embryo; cleavage of this kind is referred to as *determinate*, and proceeds to *mosaic development*. In contrast eggs possessing a more labile cytoplasmic structure are referred to as *indeterminate*; they undergo *regulative development*. Here each of the first few cells of the embryo has the capacity to form a complete although (obviously) smaller embryo (see p. 102). However, it is important to note that the implied distinction between the two types of egg structure is only one of

degree; even the most mosaic eggs retain some regulative capacity (conferred by polar lobe material) and similarly most regulative eggs possess some degree of mosaicism.

Fertilization

Fertilization, the fusion of egg and sperm, achieves many purposes: it restores the chromosomal complement of the species; it determines the chromosomal sex of the new individual possessing either XX or XY sex chromosomes; it fosters genetic variation (in contrast to the asexual method where the variation is limited to mutational change) because the chromosomes are derived from genetically dissimilar parents; and it also activates the developmental potential of the egg itself. The presence of an X or Y chromosome has far-reaching consequences on all body systems, especially in terms of embryonic growth rate and final size, on the later proportions of muscle and fat in the body and also on some brain and spinal cord nuclei. *Activation*, which can also be achieved artificially or parthenogenetically, initiates the first stage of the reproductive process, the formation of the embryo. The reproductive cycle is completed by the production of sexually mature individuals capable of forming gametes, ensuring the continuation of the species-specific replicative process.

For all vertebrates and most invertebrates the process of reproduction, leading to maturity, is a long and complicated one. It is not so with simpler organisms which may merely divide after reaching the requisite level of complexity; here the time between successive generations (the reproductive period) is short and favours a rapid increase in number (as in bacteria and protozoa). The reproduction of an organism can only be said to be complete when it is itself capable of, or participating in, the reproductive process. In metazoan animals three phases can be recognized. The first of these is *embryogenesis* (which is considered in the following section); it is followed by a period dominated by *growth* (see p. 365) and finally by the phase leading to *sexual maturity*.

EMBRYONIC DEVELOPMENT

Fertilized, activated eggs containing both male and female pronuclei are termed *zygotes*. All zygotes undergo, initially, similar developmental processes; these are *cleavage* and *gastrulation*. Those zygotes which develop in cleidoic eggs also produce *extraembryonic membranes* which enable the nutritive yolk to be supplied to the embryo, establish a respiratory exchange, allow waste products to be removed and permit an aqueous environment to develop around the embryo itself. Similar membranes develop in mammalian embryos but they are especially concerned with establishing a connection between the embryonic tissues and the maternal circulation, i.e. a *placenta*. Development to this end is termed *implantation*. Thus in mammals generally, and for man in particular, stages of embryonic development are also subdivided. A distinction is often made between development occurring before the zygote has established a firm connection with the mother; this is sometimes referred to as *preimplantation development* (a stage when manipulation of the zygote can occur; see p. 132), and subsequent development which is termed *postimplantation*. The earliest development of all embryos (postimplantation in mammals) is termed *primary embryogenesis*, a stage when cell populations are formed and massive cell migrations occur. Later, the development of organs and systems is referred to as *organogenesis*. When mammalian embryos reach a certain size, growth rather than morphogenesis occurs. The embryo is referred to as a *fetus*; this occurs at 56–57 postovulatory days in humans when the onset of bone marrow formation in the humerus can be seen (Streeter 1949); at this stage more than 90% of the named structures of the adult body have appeared. The term *conceptus* defines the embryo (or fetus) plus its associated extraembryonic (or fetal) membranes.

Cleavage

Cleavage is the process by which the first mitotic divisions of the zygote produce the founder cells of the embryo, and, in amniotes, also the cells which give rise to the extraembryonic membranes. The process, by dividing the large amount of egg cytoplasm between many smaller cells, restores the nuclear/cytoplasm ratio of the cells; little growth occurs during this time. The first cells formed by cleavage are called *blastomeres*. The pattern of cleavage differs between (and frequently within) the Classes: it depends upon the amount of yolk in the zygote and the factors within the cytoplasm which influence the timing of mitosis and the angle of the mitotic spindle. Divisions can occur through the *animal* and *vegetal poles* of the zygote—*meridionally*, or between the poles—*equatorially*; the divisions can also produce *equal* or *unequal*-sized daughter cells. In most species apart from mammals the rate of cell division and the position of the blastomeres is patterned by *maternal factors* in the cytoplasm; the genome of the zygote does not appear to function in these early stages. The differences in cleavage pattern will be briefly described (**3**.1).

In the **sea urchin** which has small (miolecithal) eggs and thus small zygotes, the first two cleavage planes pass meridionally and at right angles to each other; the third cleavage is equatorial. Subsequent cleavages, however, are different for those cells at the animal pole and those at the vegetal. Ultimately a hollow *blastula* (a ball of cells with a central cavity or *blastocoele*) will be formed. This cleavage pattern is described as *radial holoblastic* (complete) cleavage, the same as in *Amphioxus*.

The **amphibian** zygote is mesolecithal: it contains much more yolk concentrated in the vegetal pole, which prevents initial symmetric cleavages. In this class cleavage is unequal. Cleavage furrows extend from the animal to the vegetal pole but at differing rates, passing faster through the animal pole cytoplasm and more slowly through the vegetal pole yolk. The first two cleavage planes are meridional and the third is equatorial but forms above the yolk resulting in an unequal cytoplasmic distribution. Thus the embryo has four smaller cells at the animal pole and four larger cells at the vegetal. The cleavage pattern is still radial holoblastic.

In **reptiles** and **birds** the enormous amount of yolk in the megalecithal zygote allows cleavage to occur only in the *blastodisc* at the animal pole. Cleavage furrows appear on the blastodisc but do not penetrate the yolk. A single-layered *blastoderm* is initially produced; then equatorial cleavages divide the cells into a layer three to four cells thick. The yolky eggs of most fishes also develop in this way. As the zygote is not completely cleaved in these animals, cleavage is termed *meroblastic* and, in the case of reptiles, birds and most fish where only a blastodisc is present, cleavage is *discoid*.

Mammalian cleavage is very different from the other types of cleavage described. Mammalian zygotes are very small (average diameter 100 µm) being miolecithal due to the *secondary reduction* of yolk associated with viviparity. Despite this reduction in yolk, a polarity can be identified in the oöcyte prior to fertilization, by the eccentric position of the spindle and a lack of microvilli on the oölemma directly superjacent; this region is also the site of extrusion of the polar cells on completion of meiosis. It seems that sperm do not generally penetrate the oöcyte in this region; no symmetry appears to be conferred by sperm entry. After fertilization the male pronucleus moves through the (now) zygote cytoplasm towards the centre, as does the female pronucleus after its meiotic division is completed. Thus at the commencement of cleavage the two pronuclei are relatively central in the zygote. At present there is no firm evidence concerning the absence or presence of segregated developmental determinants in the human oöcyte cytoplasm.

Cleavage in mammals is slow in comparison to amphibians, each division being 12 to 24 hours apart (a frog zygote can divide into 37 000 cells in 43 hours). The first cleavage plane is meridional, as in other species. However, in the second cleavage only one cell divides meridionally; the other divides equatorially. Later the four blastomeres undergo rearrangement to bring the cleavage planes at right angles to each other. This type of cleavage is termed *rotational holoblastic* and appears to be peculiar to mammals (Gulyas 1975). The early cleaved cells do not divide synchronously, so there is often a 3-cell stage, or a 5-cell stage. Unlike most other animals, the zygote genome is activated during early cleavage in mammals so that these early cleavage planes are not controlled by maternal cytoplasmic determinants as in amphibian cleavage (see above). Following the third cleavage, i.e. at the 8-cell stage, the mammalian blastomeres, alone, undergo *compaction*, where the cells maximize their contact with each other, forming a compact ball of cells. The outer cells form tight junctions, whereas the inner cells form gap junctions. The outer cells also exhibit cellular polarity with distinct outer (polar) and inner (apolar) surfaces. The fourth cleavage division produces a 16-cell morula which has an outer layer of cells, termed *trophoblast*,

destined to form extraembryonic structures, especially the placenta, and an *inner cell mass* which will in part give rise to the embryo. The trophoblast cells secrete fluid into the morula producing a space and sequestering the inner cell mass to one side of the trophoblast. The structure so formed is the *blastocyst*; it is specific to mammalian development.

Gastrulation

Gastrulation is a process in which the cells of the blastula are rearranged into new positions to form a basic multilayered body plan of the embryo. During this process large cell populations move in concert to become apposed to other initially distant cell populations. Cell populations which will be found in certain positions **within** the embryo after gastrulation can be identified **on** the blastula surface before gastrulation begins; thus the embryonic layers, ectoderm, endoderm and mesoderm, can be mapped on the blastula surface of, for example, amphibians, and the prospective regions of certain tissues can be predicted in birds and mammals (**3**.3 indicates the time and stage at which gastrulation occurs in chick, rat, mouse and human embryos).

Invertebrate gastrulation. The simplest form of gastrulation entails the *invagination* of a roughly spherical, single-layered ball of cells (the *blastula*), to form a double-layered structure containing a new cavity, the *archenteron*. The initially circular rim through which invagination occurs is the *blastopore*. Sea urchin gastrulation is of this kind. In such embryos the archenteron expands forward to make contact with, and fuse with, a small depression, the *stomodeum*. In this way the 'mouth' of the pluteus larva of the sea urchin is formed. The original blastoporal opening of the archenteron remains as the 'anus' of the larval gut. In these embryos as soon as gastrulation starts mesenchyme cells form and break free from the invaginating inner wall of the *blastocoele*; these primary mesenchyme cells foster the deposition of calcite spicules which form the larval skeleton. A further population of mesenchyme cells is generated from the anterior region of the invaginating archenteron. Filopodial extensions of the mesenchyme cells assist the gastrulation process (these extensions traverse the mucopolysaccharide matrix enclosed in the blastocoele cavity and become attached to the inner wall of the blastula and by contraction drag the archenteron inwards (Gustafson & Kinnaider 1956; Gustafson & Wolpert 1961). It is important to note the association between the invagination of the archenteron and the internal proliferation of a mesenchyme cell lineage. (For details of sea urchin gastrulation see Gilbert 1991.)

Chordate gastrulation. The simplest form of this is seen in the development of *Amphioxus* (*Branchiostoma*); here, as in the sea urchin, a gastrula is formed by the invagination of a spherical blastula (**3**.2). However, unlike the sea urchin, the invagination process involves the movement of **defined** prospective areas of mesoderm and endoderm from the blastula surface to the interior as the archenteron is formed; also no free mesenchyme cells are proliferated into the blastocoelic space. At the end of gastrulation the roof and upper sides of the archenteron are formed by mesoderm, and the rest of the cavity is lined with endoderm. At the end of gastrulation, the mesodermal (chordamesodermal) roof of the archenteron, in contact with the overlying ectoderm, induces the formation of a *neural tube*. Then the margins of the endoderm (lateral to the chordamesoderm) pass medially where they meet and fuse in the mid-dorsal line, to form a rod-like *notochord* above and the roof of the true *enteron* (*embryonic gut*) below. Simultaneously a series of mesodermic evaginations form segmental *coelomic pouches*; these expand and fuse to form the *coelom* (**3**.2). Although these initial stages of the development of *Amphioxus* (a prototype chordate) serve as a good model for the early development of most vertebrates it must be remembered, however, that the formation of metamerically arranged coelomic pouches is an unusual feature. Moreover, no real head structure is formed in *Amphioxus* and it has an excretory system whose basic elements, solenocytes, resemble the flame cells of flat worms (Goodrich 1930). Above all a defining feature of vertebrate development, the *neural crest*, is missing (see below); this raises the possibility of the diphyletic origin of chordates (see Lovtrup 1974).

Amphibian gastrulation. The amphibian provides a better example of *vertebrate gastrulation*. The process involves invagination of predetermined regions of the blastula via a blastopore which is at first crescent-shaped with only a dorsal blastoporal lip; it then accrues

EARLY DEVELOPMENT OF CHORDATES II
GASTRULATION, NEURULATION, BASIC BODY PLAN

A AMPHIOXUS

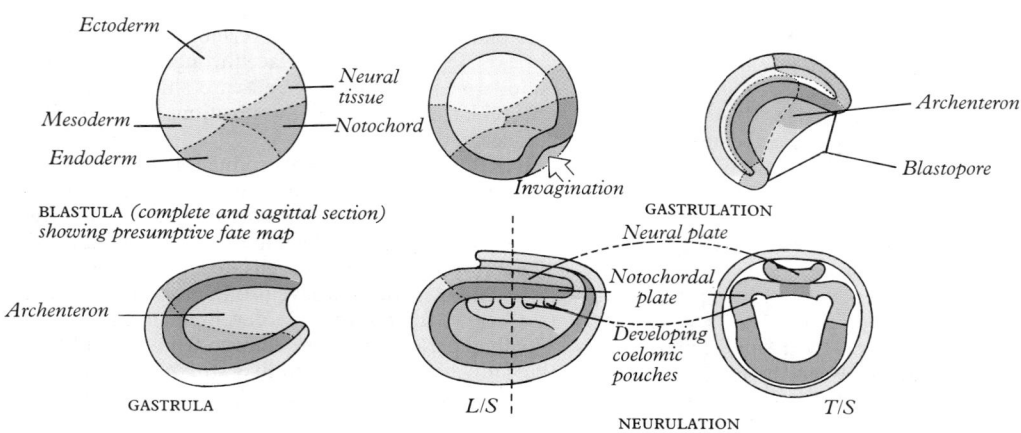

B AMPHIBIAN

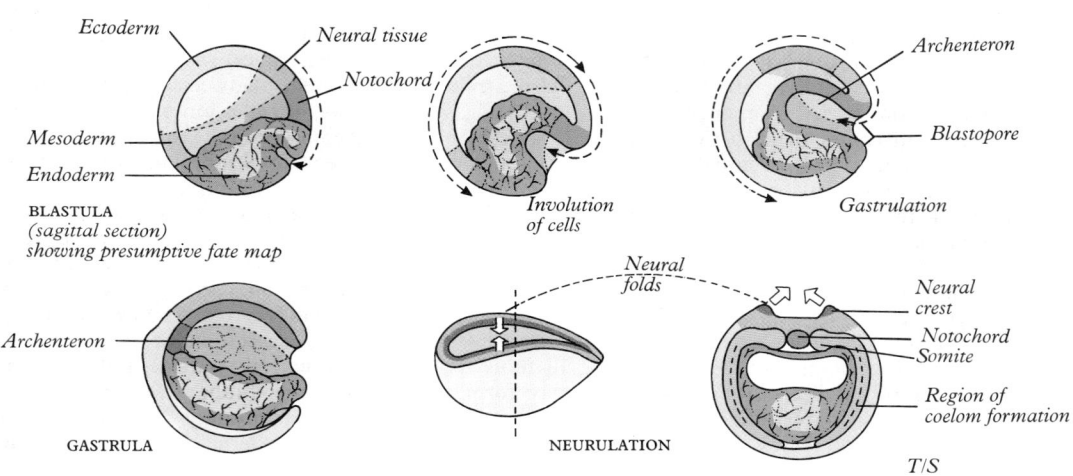

C BASIC BODY PLAN
(Head region)

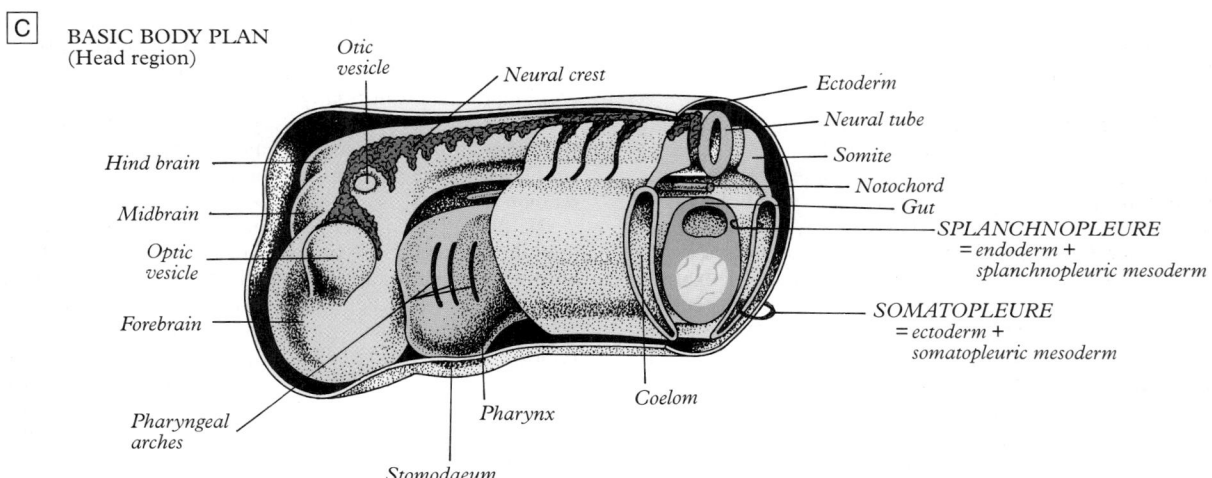

3.2 Early development of chordates II: gastrulation, neurulation, basic body plan.

A–B. Comparison of early development. Gastrulation, mesoderm formation

and neurulation in *Amphioxus* (A) and an amphibian (B).
c. Basic structure of a vertebrate embryo modified to show initial disposition of the neural crest mesenchyme. (After Waddington 1958.)

lateral borders becoming U-shaped; lastly a ventral border can be discerned and the blastopore presents, finally, a circular hole in the vegetative hemisphere. The amphibian blastula (generally) possesses two layers of cells over the animal hemisphere, including around the marginal zone near the equator, whereas the vegetal hemisphere is full of larger yolk-laden cells. Both layers of the animal hemisphere invaginate at the blastopore. The dynamic movements of chordamesodermal cells from the exterior to the interior via the dorsal lip of the blastopore, and of the mesoderm later via the lateral lips, are matched by a more passive inward movement of mesoderm and prospective endoderm via the ventral lip.

There are important differences in detail between the two major groups of amphibians which relate to the precise location of the prospective mesoderm and may reflect the diphyletic origin of the Class. In urodeles (newts and salamanders, e.g. *Amblystoma*) the prospective mesoderm is located on the surface of the blastula; in anurans (frogs and toads, e.g. *Xenopus*) it is located immediately beneath an outer layer of cells in an area corresponding to that seen in urodeles (Keller 1975; 1976). **3.2** presents the classic picture of gastrulation and its consequences in a typical urodele. The site of the dorsal lip of the blastopore is indicated by a small pigmented depression more or less at the boundary between the marginal zone and the yolk-laden vegetal cells; invagination to form the archenteron thus begins in the grey crescent area in a region of prospective endoderm. The invagination of the cranial endoderm is followed, progressively, by that of the chordamesoderm, and somitic and lateral plate mesoderm. This movement gradually involves the entire blastopore which is simply the morphological manifestation of the dynamic movement of cells from the surface to the interior. The invaginated chordamesoderm, which is located in the roof of the archenteron, becomes constricted lateromedially and extended craniocaudally through the intercalation of its component cells (Keller 1984). The remaining mesoderm comes to lie between the outer ectoderm and the inner endoderm which eventually lines most of the archenteron. The lateral components of the so-called 'mesodermal mantle' are arranged in the order expected from the disposition of their prospective precursors on the surface of the blastula.

The material first carried in at the dorsal lip forms the *prechordal plate* (Adlemann 1922, 1926; see also p. 147); it consists of mesoderm and foregut endoderm. The coelom, in amphibians, is formed by cavitation of the mesoderm; there are no coelomic pouches as seen in *Amphioxus*. Once the archenteron roof has been formed by the chordamesoderm its proximity to the overlying ectoderm initiates induction of the *neural plate* which rolls up and fuses into a neural tube. In amphibians neural populations are formed in the trunk and head from cells termed *neural crest*; these cells also give rise to mesenchymal populations in the head. Neural crest cells are found, prior to neurulation, between the neural plate and the surface ectoderm in all vertebrate embryos. (For a detailed account of amphibian gastrulation see Gilbert 1991.)

Reptilian and avian gastrulation. The presence of large amounts of yolk in the eggs of reptiles and birds not only confines cleavage to the blastoderm but either severely limits (reptiles) or completely prevents the formation of an archenteron. At the end of cleavage in these forms the blastoderm consists of two layers of cells, an upper *epiblast* and a lower *hypoblast* which is adjacent to the yolk. The predetermined cells which formed a spherical blastula in, for example, amphibians, is now represented in two dimensions on the epiblast of the flattened blastoderm. The outward sign of gastrulation is the formation of the *primitive streak* on the surface of the embryo; this represents a progressive, craniocaudal ingression of cells along the dorsal midline. Inasmuch as it represents a dynamic structure caused by the inward movement of *prospective mesoderm* and *endoderm* from the surface to the interior, the primitive streak of amniotes is analogous to the *blastopore* of amphibians. In reptiles, a tube-like structure is formed during gastrulation by the initial invagination of cells at the cranial end of a broad primitive streak. This structure, said to be lined entirely with mesoderm, is known as the *chordamesodermal canal*; it corresponds to the archenteron of amphibians. It is less obvious in most avian embryos, although a small pit at the cranial end of the primitive streak (Hensen's node), the site at which chordamesodermal cells invaginate to underlie the ectoderm, may be regarded as a remnant.

Mammalian gastrulation. The gastrulation movements seen in reptilian and avian embryos evolved as adaptations to eggs with large amounts of yolk. Interestingly these movements are retained in mammalian embryos even though there is a secondary reduction in the size of the eggs caused by the development of viviparity. The transformation of the mammalian embryonic cells, the *inner cell mass*, into a two-layered germinal disc composed of (as in avian embryos) epiblast and hypoblast corresponds to the end of cleavage (the blastula stage) of other vertebrate embryos. A primitive streak appears on the epiblast surface through which prospective embryonic endoderm and mesoblast cells are shifted (and/or generated) from the epiblast into their relative positions beneath the remaining surface ectoderm.

It is apparent that the production of a layered embryo by the invagination of a spherical blastula (amphibian) is superseded by a different mechanism in *blastodermic* gastrulation (reptiles and birds), some mechanisms of which are retained in mammalian gastrulation. The morphology of the cells formed by this latter ingression is different, as is the extensive production of extraembryonic structures (see below) for both in ovo development and in utero development. The final derivation of the embryo from a simple layer of epithelium, the induction of the primitive streak and the production of mesenchyme are all unlike the early types of gastrulation.

Extraembryonic membranes—the evolution of amniotes

Ancestral reptiles developed a mechanism of containing highly yolky eggs within a closed environment (the cleidoic egg). Embryos developing in such an environment produced not only the ectoderm and endoderm concerned with embryonic development but also extensions of these layers (membranes) which formed around the yolk to aid the transport of nutrients, between the embryo and the egg shell to allow gas transfer, as an extension of the gut to sequester waste products outside the embryo, and around the embryo to provide an aqueous environment for embryonic development. Thus the *extraembryonic membranes* were formed.

Four fundamental extraembryonic membranes develop. The *yolk sac* and the *allantois* are continuous with, and derived from, the embryonic endoderm and splanchnopleuric mesoderm. They become associated with extraembryonic blood vessels thus producing a *vascular splanchnopleure*. When yolk is present the vascularized yolk sac encloses and ensures the utilization of the stored material. The allantois serves to store excretory waste and, with the chorion, it may form a respiratory membrane. The *amnion* and *chorion* are developed from, and are in continuity with, the embryonic ectoderm and the somatopleuric mesoderm; they form an *avascular somatopleure*. The amnion and associated chorion provide an aqueous environment, physical protection, and, after secondary vascularization, a means of respiratory exchange with the exterior. The secondary vascularization of the chorion is by co-aptation and fusion of its internal aspect, depending on the Class and Species, on some combination of: a normally expanding yolk sac; a partially or wholly inverted yolk sac; or a (highly) variably expanded allantois. The production of the extraembryonic membranes is of such evolutionary significance that reptiles, birds and mammals are collectively termed *amniotes*.

Of the **egg-laying amniotes**, many present-day reptiles, all birds, and the prototheria (e.g. the duck-billed platypus) develop extraembryonic membranes as described above. As embryonic development proceeds (**3.3**), the amnion develops as folds from the ectodermal body wall which grow from the head, tail and lateral regions of the embryo; the folds fuse over the dorsal surface of the embryo to create a cavity into which amniotic fluid is secreted. The option of *viviparity* evolved through the retention of the egg by the mother; probably initially as a protection of the egg from predators. Subsequent loss of yolk and the consequent need to forge an efficient *physiological link* between embryo and mother led to the development of a *placenta* with components derived from the pre-existing extraembryonic structures and the maternal tissues. Metatherian mammals (marsupials) develop a yolk sac placenta in utero, based on a link between the yolk sac splanchnopleure and the maternal endometrium. However, the gestation length offered by this form of placentation is very short; consequently in these species, the young are born very immature, at a 'larval stage', with precociously developed lungs, mouth and upper limbs, allowing the newborn to

FORMATION OF EXTRA-EMBRYONIC MEMBRANES

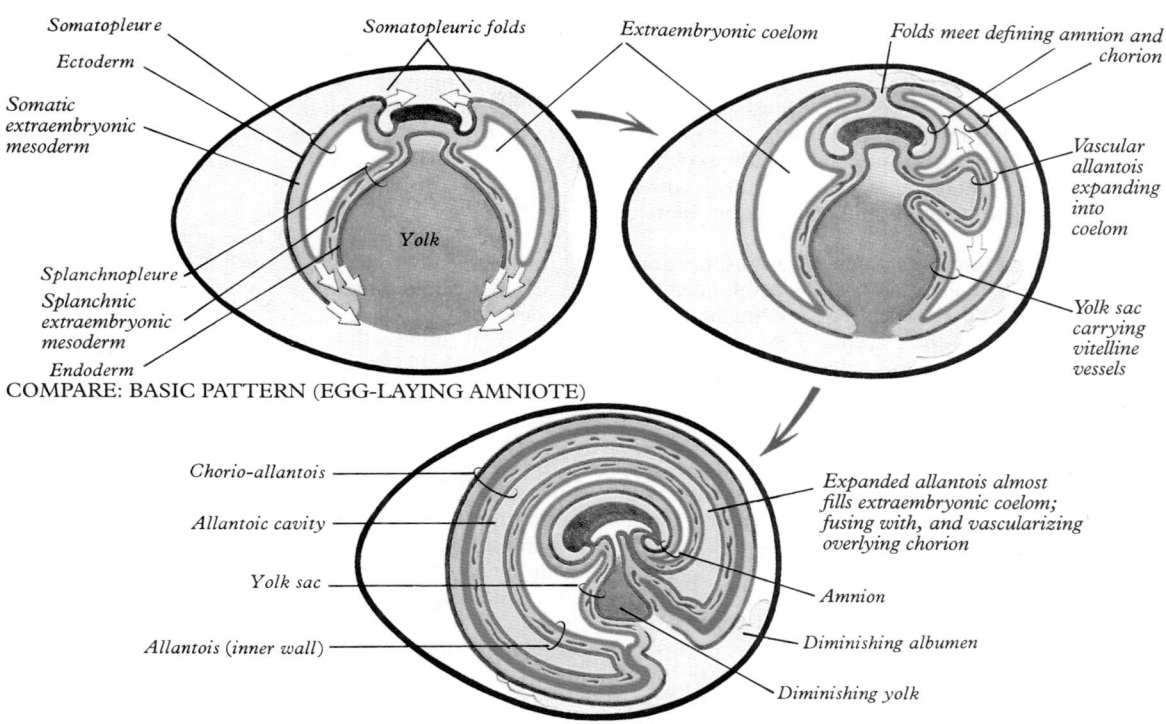

COMPARE: BASIC PATTERN (EGG-LAYING AMNIOTE)

WITH: EUTHERIAN MAMMALS—

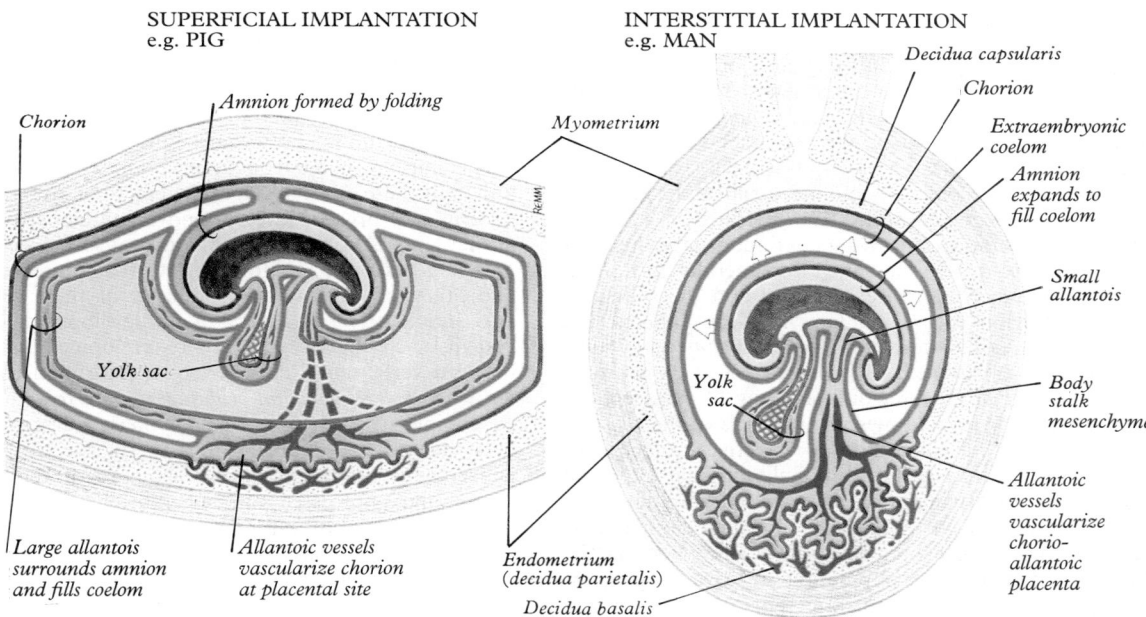

SUPERFICIAL IMPLANTATION
e.g. PIG

INTERSTITIAL IMPLANTATION
e.g. MAN

3.3 A generalized series of diagrams to allow comparison of the mode of formation of extraembryonic membranes in a megalecithal egg-laying amniote (e.g. chick) with that of a eutharian mammal exhibiting superficial implantation and a large allantois (e.g. pig), and a eutherian mammal showing interstitial implantation and a diminutive allantois (man). Note in each case the vascularization of the yolk sac, and the manner in which the expanded allantois (chick, pig) or its homologue in man, the body stalk mesoderm continuing from the small allantoic diverticulum, bear allantoic blood vessels which vascularize the overlying chorion. The latter is applied either to the shell or to the uterine decidua.

climb to the pouch and attach to the teat. The hind limbs are, however, still at an embryonic stage as are other systems of the body.

Eutherian mammals exploit the allantoic circulation which is no longer needed for respiratory purposes as it is in avian embryos. The allantoic (umbilical) vessels form a vascular link connecting the embryo to a specialized region of the chorion and the maternal circulation, i.e. the placenta. The variety of placental types need not concern us here (see p. 166); suffice it to say that superficial implantation as seen in the pig may be regarded as the primitive condition and interstitial implantation as seen in the mouse and man the most advanced (**3.**3). Note, however, that the extraembryonic membranes and the placentae of mouse and man are utterly different topographically.

During the time of implantation the outer layer of the blastocyst, the trophoblast, shows two different cell arrangements, a cellular *cytotrophoblast* and an external invasive *syncytiotrophoblast* composed of a multinucleate mass of cytoplasm which leads the implantation into the maternal endometrium. Later extraembryonic mesoblast from the inner cell mass forms a layer over the inner surface of the cytotrophoblast; it is this trilaminar layer which is termed the chorion.

In placental mammals the extraembryonic membranes develop **before** the embryonic tissues; they utilize new methods to ensure the survival of the embryo. The chorion in particular has different roles: it produces hormones which maintain the status of the maternal uterine endometrium; it (inter alia) produces cells which support the maternal vessels invaded by the implanting embryo; it suppresses the immune response of the mother to the implanted embryo (which bears paternal as well as maternal genes); and it affects other regions of the maternal body stimulating milk production later in development.

Because the readiness of the chorion to assume its various functions is paramount to the survival of the embryo, early development in mammals is especially related to development of the extraembryonic membranes and the establishment of the placenta. Thus the development of mammalian embryonic tissues lags behind the timescale of, for example, the chick (**3.**32). In the chick eggs are deposited and incubation commences about 24 hours after fertilization; developmental stages are related to incubation at 39.4°C. The notochord is formed after about 20 **hours'** incubation but the amnion is not formed until 60 hours' incubation. In human embryos the amnion is formed before any embryonic development has occurred, by about 10.5 **days**; the notochord forms later, at about 16 days.

Primary embryogenesis

Gastrulation, by moving cell populations from the surface of the blastula or blastoderm to the interior, and by specifically juxtaposing the chordamesoderm to the ectoderm, sets in train a series of developmental processes initially termed the *primary inductive interaction*. Such an interaction initiates a phase of morphogenesis which establishes a *basic axial structure*, common to all vertebrates. A number of events occur more or less simultaneously. The ectoderm on the dorsal surface of the embryo, in contact with the chordamesoderm, flattens to form the *neural plate* which becomes bounded by prominent folds. These *neural folds* rise up and join in the midline to form the *neural tube* medially and other neural populations, not involved in the fusion, the *neural crest* and *ectodermal placodes*, laterally. These neural populations are the precursors of the central and peripheral nervous systems. The mesoblast beneath the neural tube forms the *notochord* along the midline (axis) and paraxially segments into the paired *somites*, which are generated in a *craniocaudal progression*. The endoderm forms a continuous layer beneath the mesoblast which proliferates and migrates laterally forming a layer between the superjacent surface ectoderm and the subjacent gut endoderm. Starting in the region lateral to the somites, the mesoblast splits into two populations separated by the *intraembryonic coelom*, with those mesoblast cells adjacent to the coelom transforming into a *mesothelium*. The region consisting of surface ectoderm, underlying mesenchyme and mesothelium (the epithelial layer lining the intraembryonic coelem) is known collectively as the *somatopleure* (with both the mesenchymal population and coelomic epithelium (mesothelium) originating in the region being described as somatopleuric), whereas the region consisting of endoderm, underlying mesenchyme and mesothelium is known collectively as the *splanchnopleure* (the mesenchymal population and overlying mesothelium similarly is termed splanchnopleuric). Segmentally arranged *nephrogenic elements* develop at the junction between the somatopleuric and splanchnopleuric regions.

During these changes the embryo elongates and distinct trunk and head regions emerge. The rapid growth of the brain promotes head flexion and the lateral walls of the embryonic disc converge ventrally; thus a recognizable embryonic shape is formed. After head folding the gut can be delineated into fore, mid and hind portions; in amniotes the midgut is connected by a stalk to the yolk sac and the hindgut is connected by a stalk to the allantois. Later there are signs of division of the neural tube into fore-, mid- and hindbrain and about this time too, *neural crest cells* begin to proliferate and migrate internally, and away from their site of origin (at the fold between the surface ectoderm and neural ectoderm) to form neural populations in the trunk and major mesenchymal populations in the head which give rise to the *pharyngeal arches*.

At the end of this phase (**3.**4) vertebrate embryos are more alike than they are different. Despite original variations in egg size, pattern of cleavage and apparent differences in gastrulation, the end product is a remarkably similar body plan. This comparison remains valid at the beginning of *organogenesis* but from this time differences of structure soon arise as the development of the different genera diverge from the plan. These individual differences require specific study.

Embryonic convergence

Von Baer (1825) (see p. 92) recognized that all vertebrates pass through an embryonic stage which is remarkably similar among the group as a whole. This stage is attained after primary embryogenesis as described above and is distinguished by the presence of the pharyngeal arches; thus it has been termed the *pharyngula stage* (Ballard 1971, 1976). It features a basic body plan with three specified axes, a midline neural tube with an expanded cephalic region, a midline heart, a midline gut, a series of paired pharyngeal arches around the cephalic end of the gut and bilateral symmetry in the lateral structures. Similarity of appearance is matched by similarity in size so that at this stage the craniocaudal dimension of most vertebrate embryos averages around 7–8 mm. There is a striking difference, however, in the time it takes embryos to reach the pharyngula stage: for instance it takes 4–5 **days** in the case of birds (developing at about 39°C), but 4–5 **weeks** in the case of mammals. A comparable stage is reached in *Xenopus* (an amphibian), developing at a much **lower** temperature of about 23°C, after only 2–3 days.

Central to any discussion of the relation between phylogeny and ontogeny (see also p. 92) is the fact that convergence towards the pharyngula stage is achieved despite large differences in the developmental processes which precede, and the varying time it takes to reach, this body plan. The pharyngula stage can be considered to be a period of major developmental and evolutionary constraint. This concept can be explained in terms of the interactions of embryonic cells at the various stages of development. During early development there are relatively few interactions and few domains (local areas where interactions may occur); thus the embryo is free to develop and change with few constraints. Similarly, during organogenesis, although there are many local interactions progressing as the body systems and organs develop, and many embryonic domains, there are few interactions **between** the domains. However, at the pharyngula stage there are a number of critical cellular interactions occurring and, most importantly, the domains of these cellular interactions **must** interact. This imposes a major developmental constraint on the system, such that this stage of development is highly conserved between vertebrates. This period of maximum constraint has been termed the *developmental evolutionary hour glass* (**3.**4); it is imposed by complexity and it is the final phase during which the embryo must behave as a whole if it is to survive. During the early and later phases of development, each side of the pharyngula stage, evolutionary processes may generate change without detriment to the basic vertebrate structure; however, changes occurring at the pharyngula stage may prove lethal.

Ontogenetic change can give rise to phylogenetic change by a variety of mechanisms, such as a change of the embryonic source for forming the structure, in the embryonic processes specifying the structure (e.g. changes in pattern-generating mechanisms), in developmental sequence, and in the timing of developmental events. Even small changes in embryonic processes may result in major changes to adult morphology or function. This is the basis of saltatory evolutionary theory, whereby major morphological changes are thought to occur suddenly in the fossil record, as opposed to a more gradualistic change, which characterizes other morphological features. Development thus forms the basis for all evolutionary theory and studies. (For a detailed consideration of major associations between development and evolution see Hall 1992.)

'All that we call phylogeny is today, and ever has been, ontogeny itself. Ontogeny is, then, the primary, the secondary, the universal fact. It is ontogeny from which we depart and ontogeny to which we return. Phylogeny is but a name for the lineal sequences of ontogeny, viewed from the historical standpoint'.

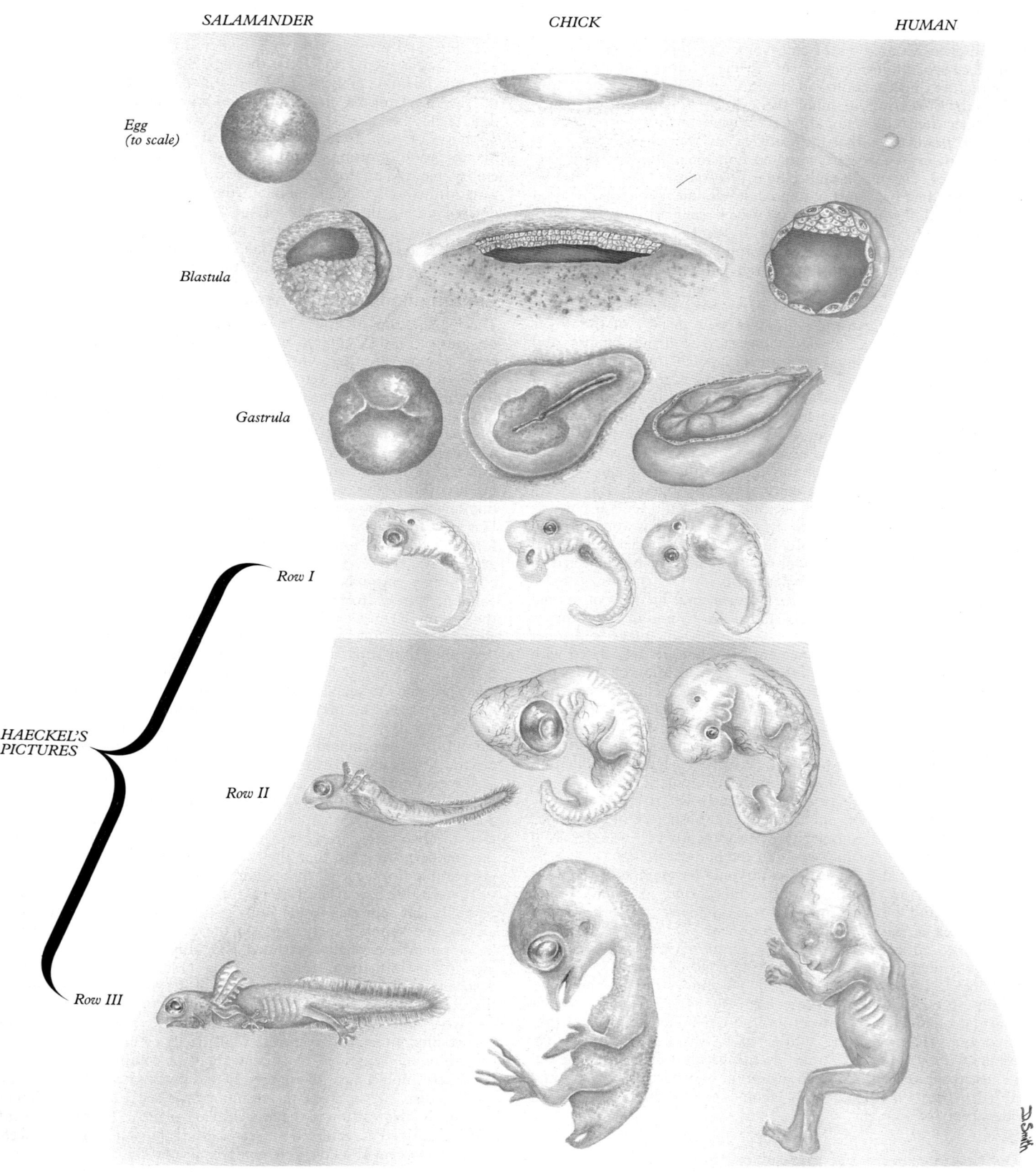

SALAMANDER

CHICK

HUMAN

*Egg
(to scale)*

Blastula

Gastrula

Row I

*HAECKEL'S
PICTURES*

Row II

Row III

3.4   The developmental evolutionary hourglass. This figure illustrates in 6 rows the disparate sizes of 3 types of vertebrate egg at the commencement of development, different organization of the earliest cell lineages in the blastula stage and differences in gastrulation (in the human the amnion has been removed to reveal the surface of the embryo). In row 4 the pharyngula stage is illustrated: here there is a remarkable similarity between the embryos at the time the body plan is formed; thereafter (rows 5 and 6) embryos becomes progressively different. The time at which embryos are similar is suggested to be a time of maximum developmental constraint (see text). (From Elinson 1987 with permission.)

Developmental biology—the analytical approach

A comprehensive analysis of embryonic development impinges on many facets of biological science, especially those concerned with cell structure and function and the molecular basis of gene action and control. Bearing in mind the cellular foundation of developmental systems this is not altogether surprising; what is sometimes forgotten, however, is that the study of the way in which embryos develop has, in recent years, initiated fundamental advances in our knowledge of gene action and cellular physiology.

The overriding problems of animal development concern the need to understand the mechanisms by which cellular diversity arises from the relatively simple structure of the egg, and how specific developmental pattern and precise morphological form is generated. These are of course problems shared with other developmental systems, notably plant development, regeneration and wound healing, and phenomena such as metaplasia, metastasis and senescence. In this context embryology is seen as part of the larger science of *developmental biology*. Concerned with the common and related problems associated with all the systems mentioned above, developmental biology has largely replaced the narrower discipline of embryology. The techniques currently available to the developmental biologist include electron microscopy, microsurgical manipulation, immunocytochemistry and probes for specific gene expression. A battery of such techniques is often employed to study a particular problem, although it is sometimes the case that the methods used seem to lose sight of the original aim of the investigation. It is always important to ask of any study not only what is its general purpose but what precise question within its chosen field it is attempting to answer. In some cases it is also necessary to consider the ethical dimension, for instance when embryos are either being subjected to microsurgery or gene transfer experiments.

A necessary prerequisite for the experimental analysis of animal development is an accurate and detailed description of the embryos under investigation. The emergence of embryology as a distinct science coincided with the refinement of techniques associated with light microscopy, thus facilitating the precise location of embryonic tissues and their progressive fate during development. Subsequently electron microscopy greatly enhanced this cellular level of description. What may be regarded as even more refined levels of description, virtually at the molecular level, are now available through the use of immunochemical techniques and gene probes. It is a combination of such techniques with those of micromanipulation experiments, devised many years ago, that has recently led to a significantly greater understanding of, inter alia, the establishment of embryonic axes (see p. 118), the complexity of head morphology (see p. 157) and basic patterning of the head and the body region.

The generally valid picture of embryonic development which we now have is mainly the result of a detailed study of relatively **few** animals. By and large, the material was originally chosen because it was, or became, easy to obtain and observe. Latterly attention has become focused, even more narrowly, on those embryos which have not only yielded a considerable body of knowledge in the recent past (e.g. chicks, *Xenopus*, *Drosophila*, the laboratory mouse), but have proved especially well suited to current trends of research in developmental biology. This concentration on a limited number of preferred types has been the subject of criticism in the past (e.g. Needham 1959) and also more recently (Raff 1992). The renewed interest in the relation between evolution and development (Gould 1977; Lovtrup 1984; Hall 1992) highlights the value of studying a wide variety of animals.

AN HISTORICAL PERSPECTIVE OF EXPERIMENTAL EMBRYOLOGY

The main areas of concern of developmental biologists today are inextricably linked with those topics which were of compelling interest to the embryologists of the past: How does the egg give rise to the embryo? What is the basis of cellular differentiation? What factors are involved in morphogenesis? What is the relation between development and evolution? More recent efforts to refine these

questions and provide satisfying answers to them are dealt with in a later section (p. 110). Here the significant earlier work which, by experimental analysis, achieved a fundamental understanding of the mechanisms involved in embryogenesis will be briefly described.

Many of the techniques described below, those of micromanipulation, grafting, translocation and deletion of fragments of embryonic tissue, together with necessary improvements in the general methods used to maintain the experimental material, were devised during the first half of the 20th century. The end of this period saw the beginning of a newer phase of experimentation involving nuclear transplantation and more refined methods of tracking the movement and disposition of embryonic cells.

Preformation and epigenesis

The explanation of how the apparently simple egg generates the obviously complex embryo was the source of a major controversy over several centuries. On one side were those who supported *preformation*; they believed that the egg contained a miniature adult form and that development was essentially a process of growth of a pre-existing structure. On the other side were the exponents of *epigenesis* who maintained that the embryo developed gradually from a relatively simple structure, analogous in some ways to the opening of a leaf or flower bud of a plant. Harvey (1578–1657), famous for his discovery of the circulation of the blood, was an early supporter of this epigenetic view, based on his observations of chick development. Harvey's dictum 'ex ovo omnia' now appears to be remarkably foresighted; more practical was his view that 'eggs cost little and are always and everywhere to be had'. Among preformationists controversy raged between the ovists, who believed that the egg contained the preformed embryo, and the spermists, who favoured the sperm. There was, in fact, dating from the time of Aristotle, a strong presumption to imagine semen as the active principle initiating development in a passive, featureless egg which merely provided the material for embryogenesis. In a male dominated society the spermists prevailed to such an extent that some of the early microscopists were convinced that they could actually detect homunculi in human sperm and drew some imaginative figures. Eventually with more careful, and less biased, observations the epigenetic view gained general acceptance. It can be maintained, however, that inasmuch as the genome contains essential molecular information for specific development and that many eggs contain predetermined cytoplasmic components, a preformationist input remains a valid concept. In fact, the two views are no longer regarded as incompatible; indeed the 'modern view' is that they are not only complementary but inseparable (for a recent discussion, see Hall 1992).

Towards the end of the 19th century a few embryologists adopted an analytical approach to the study of animal development. Importantly some simple experiments on the earliest (cleavage) stage of development eventually provided conclusive evidence against the idea of preformation. Initially, Roux (1888) demonstrated that destruction of one of the first two cells of the frog embryo produced the equivalent of half an embryo. Later work, however, which involved the complete separation of the first two cells gave one of two results: either two complete (half-sized) embryos were formed or one of the separated blastomeres gave a complete embryo and the other simply a mass of apparently undifferentiated cells (**3.5**). The striking disparity between the results of the separation experiment depends on the relation of the first cleavage plane to the grey crescent which is formed at fertilization (see p. 98). If the first cleavage **bisects** the grey crescent **two** complete embryos are produced; in a cleavage which confines the crescent to one blastomere only, and thus deprives the other of this feature, then only the former produces a complete embryo. The importance of this structural element is discussed below in relation to the discovery of the 'organizer'.

A complementary set of separation experiments, involving both 2- and 4-cell stages, was carried out by Hans Driesch (1891) using sea urchin eggs; the separated blastomeres produced half and quarter size larvae (**3.5**). Although Driesch claimed that even smaller larvae were obtainable from separated blastomeres of the 8-cell stage, subsequent work did not support this finding. Driesch's experimental results supported his theoretical view of development which contained an element of vitalism, now regarded as unacceptable. Driesch (1921) considered that every part of the egg cytoplasm was equipotential and that therefore the formation of an increasingly complex embryo was not possible unless this basic material was organized by a non-material agency; he called this organizing principle *entelechy*. This concept, derived from the Greek word meaning soul, was central to the philosophy of Aristotle (384–322 BC). It was in fact a key element in Aristotle's own view of animal development which he viewed as a succession of linked material events the organization of which was dependent on, and driven forward by, the non-material and all pervading *soul*.

Blastomeric potential

Both the amphibian and sea urchin investigations demonstrate that the initial blastomeres have the potential to form whole embryos; they thus possess a considerable capacity for regulation. They are not highly structured, confirming that in the original restricted sense there is no basis for preformation. Some eggs (ascidians, annelids and molluscs) are, or at fertilization become, highly structured. Separation of the early blastomeres of such 'mosaic eggs' give embryonic fragments which are compatible with a strictly determined cell lineage, but even in these cases it is possible to demonstrate some regulation of structure.

The first two cleavages of the sea urchin egg are meridional, are at right angles and, significantly, they do not cut across, but include, the animal–vegetal axis of the egg. The importance of this axis was highlighted by Hörstadius (1939) who demonstrated, for instance, that separation of the upper and lower halves of the 8-cell stage (cutting across the animal–vegetal axis) produced not half-sized complete larvae but two quite different but derived embryonic structures (**3**.5). Hörstadius suggested that a balanced interaction between animal and vegetal components of the egg was essential for the harmonious development of the larval structure and proved his hypothesis by an elegant series of combination experiments involving partial fragments derived from the animal and vegetal halves taken from the early cleavage stages of the embryo.

Numerous investigations have since focused attention on the importance of the *intrinsic axial structure* of the egg which becomes entrenched during cleavage. This has been demonstrated for many animals, and is related to the distribution of factors which appear to determine specific cell lineages (e.g. in *Xenopus* and ascidians); it also appears to underpin the linear-craniocaudal pattern of structure of the developing organism (e.g. in insects). Distinct, and experimentally demonstrable, polarity and the dependent early separation of cell lineages, is not, however, a feature of all types of eggs; notably the mammalian egg, which although similar in size and superficial appearance to that of the sea urchin, does not possess an equivalent polar structure. In this case cell lineage determination is delayed until the compacted 8-cell stage (see p. 134).

Nucleocytoplasmic interaction—nuclear transplantation

The central concept that progressive nucleocytoplasmic interaction provides a satisfactory explanation of embryonic development became generally accepted during the early part of the 20th century. The definitive form of this concept was formulated by Morgan (1934); it embodied the following elements. Initially, equipotential (genetically equivalent) nuclei are distributed during development in a *heterogeneous cytoplasm*; the cytoplasmic environment then modifies the *genetic activity of the nuclei*; the altered activity of the nuclei will in turn modify the surrounding cytoplasm; such reciprocal interactions result in the progressive differentiation of embryonic cells as development proceeds. The existence of a *heterogeneous egg cytoplasm* and its capacity to modify the activity of the early cleavage nuclei accords with the experiments described above. The nuclear transplantation experiments, described below, address the problem of nuclear equivalence and the permanency of any change imposed by the cytoplasmic environment.

By applying a hair loop constriction to a newly fertilized newt egg Spemann (1914) carried out what was in effect an in ovo nuclear transfer (**3**.5). The constriction confined the zygote nucleus to one half of the egg but did not prevent its division into 16–32 cells. At this stage one of the cleavage nuclei was allowed to enter the anucleate portion of the egg; cleavage followed in this portion and in some cases a second, twin, embryo was formed. Although, as would be expected, the relationship of the constriction to the grey crescent (see above) affected the outcome of the experiment it clearly demonstrated the *equivalence* of the early cleavage nuclei in amphibian embryos. This means that, provided they are not damaged by the experimental procedure, **any** of these nuclei can, in collaboration with the egg cytoplasm, programme the whole of development. Do nuclei retain this capacity beyond the early cleavage stage? Amphibian nuclear transplant experiments provided an unequivocal, and positive answer to this question.

Initially the technique for the isolation and physical transfer of animal cell nuclei was established using amoebae (Commandon & De Fonbrane 1939; Lorch & Daneilli 1950). Using a frog (*Rana pipiens*) a similar technique was used by Briggs and King (1952) to transfer nuclei from blastulae and gastrulae to enucleated eggs. Variable results were obtained, including a variety of abnormal embryos, but importantly, a few embryos went on to develop completely normally and to produce viable tadpoles (**3**.5). A significant extension of this work involved the serial transplantation of nuclei from the blastula to neurula stages obtained from an initial transplant (King & Briggs 1956). The derived clones showed persistent, and similar, patterns of normality, including some which produced a high percentage of normal embryos. Clearly a proportion of embryonic nuclei remained totipotent even in cells committed to differentiation. Using the South African clawed frog (*Xenopus laevis*) and a different technique involving ultraviolet radiation to enucleate the eggs, together with a genetically determined nuclear marker, to distinguish host from donor nuclei, Gurdon (1960) and his colleagues confirmed and considerably extended the original work, most notably to show that nuclei derived from the intestinal epithelium of feeding tadpoles could produce a few viable embryos following serial transplantation (Gurdon 1962). Even transplanted and serially transferred nuclei, derived from the keratinized cells of adult *Xenopus* epithelium have been used to produce living, but eventually moribund, tadpoles (Gurdon et al 1975). It could be imagined that these experiments on amphibian embryos might provide a route for the nuclear cloning of mammals, including man. Recent work (McGrath & Solter 1984) suggests that this is not even a remote possibility.

Significance of gastrulation

Although the dynamic nature of gastrulation and its association with the formation of mesoblast is implicit in much early descriptive work, the current view of gastrulation among chordates, i.e. one of coordinated cell movement leading to an inductive interaction between mesoblast and overlying ectoderm, and the consequent development of axial structure, derives from the experimental work carried out in the earlier part of this century. It was during this period that several important microsurgical procedures and cell marking techniques were developed.

The use of vital dyes (e.g. Bismarck brown, neutral red) applied to the surface of the amphibian blastula enabled Vogt (1929) to demonstrate that well-defined areas moved from the surface to the interior during gastrulation. In particular there was an active movement of prospective chordamesoderm over the dorsal and lateral lips of the blastopore during the formation of the archenteron and a more passive dragging in, ventrolaterally, of prospective endoderm (**3**.6). Graper (1929) demonstrated an apparently analogous shift of material from the epiblastic surface of the early chick embryo, using a combination of vital dyes and time lapse cinematography; this pioneering work was refined at a later date, particularly by Spratt (1946), using early chick blastoderms cultured in vitro. Such techniques initiated the detailed mapping of presumptive (prospective) areas (destined to give rise to particular tissues) on the surface of the chordate blastula or its blastoderm equivalent. Gastrulation was visualized as the process which ensured that these areas moved into the right place at the right time during this fundamental stage of embryogenesis.

The importance of gastrulation as the essential prerequisite for the generation of the characteristic axial structure of chordates was revealed by work which led to the discovery of *the organizer* associated with the dorsal lip of the blastopore of amphibian embryos. The fundamental contribution was made by Spemann (1918) who

Experimental analysis of development I

A   *Sea Urchin - Normal Development*

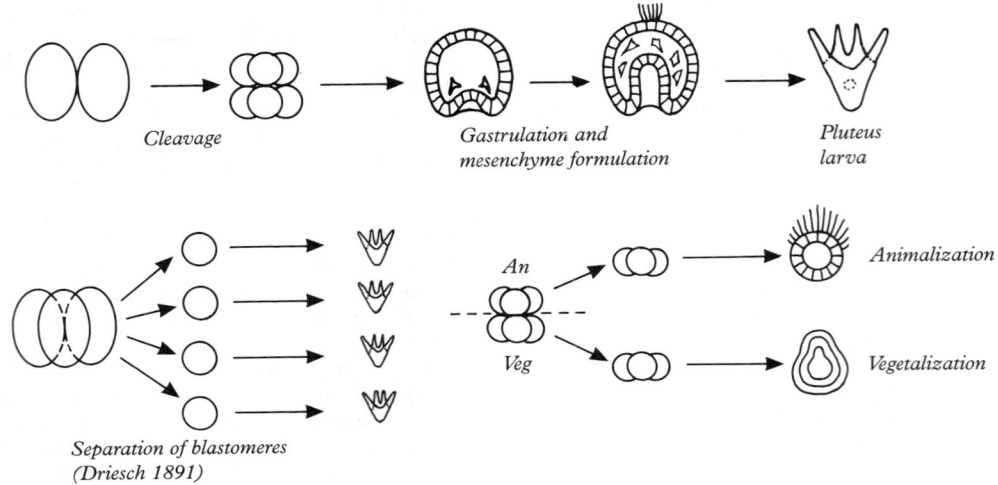

An   An
Veg   Veg

*Separation of blastomeres
(Driesch 1891)*

B   *Amphibia   Separation of blastomeres - significance of grey crescent (Spemann 1938)*

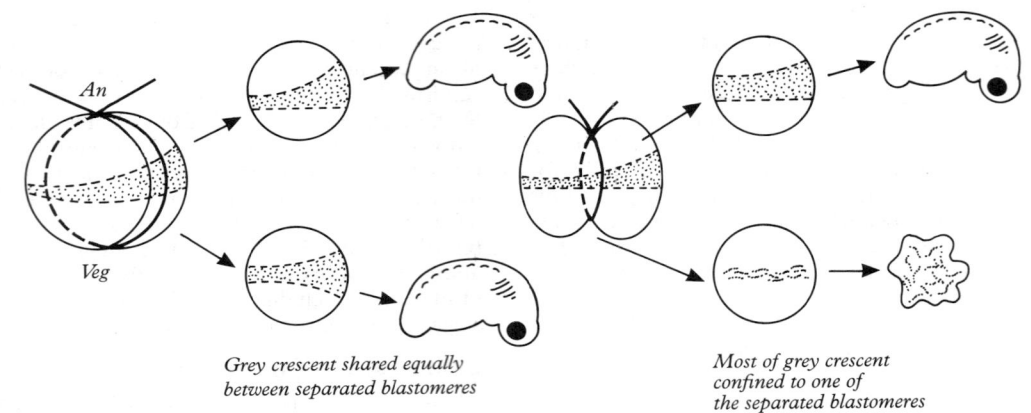

*Grey crescent shared equally
between separated blastomeres*

*Most of grey crescent
confined to one of
the separated blastomeres*

C   *Amphibia   Equvalence of nuclei to 16 cell stage (Spemann 1928)*

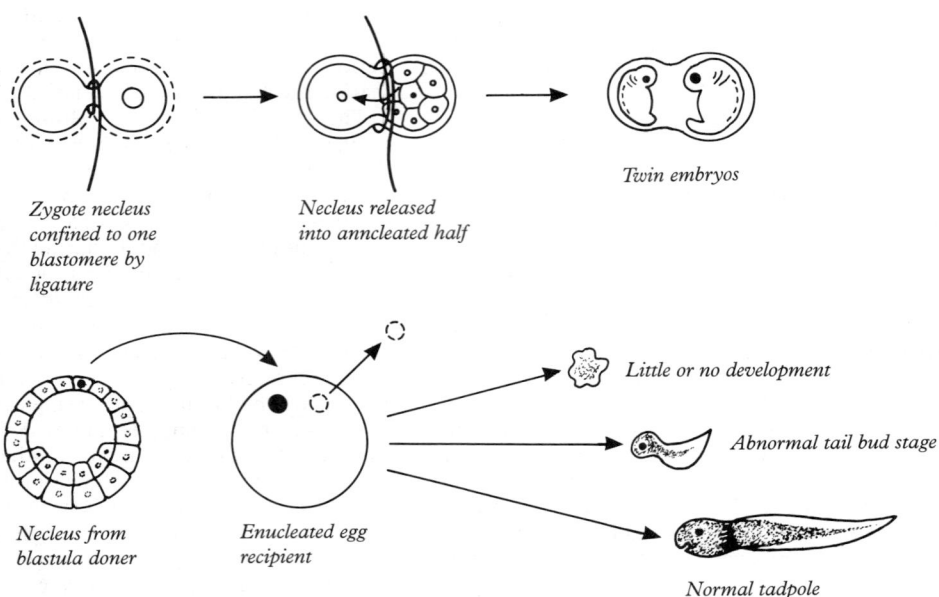

*Zygote necleus
confined to one
blastomere by
ligature*

*Necleus released
into anncleated half*

Twin embryos

*Necleus from
blastula doner*

*Enucleated egg
recipient*

Little or no development

Abnormal tail bud stage

Normal tadpole

3.5 Experimental analysis of development I: early work. Fundamental
observations and procedures. A, B. Importance of egg structure (Driesch,
1891; Horstadius, 1939; Spemann 1938). c. Equivalence of early cleavage
nuclei (Spemann, 1928). D. Nuclear transplantation (Briggs and King, 1952).

showed that when a small area taken from the blastoporal region of a newt embryo was grafted into another location (e.g. opposite the dorsal lip) it produced a *secondary embryonic axis*. As the amount of grafted material was small compared to the size of the induced structure it was clear that both the graft and the host tissue participated in its formation; in other words the graft organized the new structure. Elegant proof that this was the case was provided by using a *xenoplastic grafting* technique where the dorsal lip from **one species** of newt was grafted into the early gastrula of **another species** whose cells were distinguished by their pigment content (Spemann & Mangold 1924) (**3**.6). The discovery of the organizer opened up many (mostly productive) areas of research, including the discovery of an analogous region (Hensen's node) in the primitive streak stage of the chick embryo (Waddington 1932). A fruitless search for the chemical nature of the organizer eventually led to the discovery that even inorganic material could induce neural structures in gastrular ectoderm. Above all, however, it was the work of Spemann and others which established the concept of *primary embryonic induction*, namely, that it is the **contact** between the archenteron roof and overlying ectoderm, brought about by gastrulation, that **induces** the formation of the neural (medullary) plate and the corresponding axial organization of the mesoblast which lies beneath the prospective central nervous system (CNS). This is the major consequence of the complete invagination of the presumptive chordamesoderm which commences with the appearance of the dorsal lip of the blastopore in amphibian embryos or its equivalent in other chordates. **3**.6 illustrates some relatively simple experiments which demonstrate what is undeniably the most significant interaction of embryonic tissues during the development of vertebrate animals. (For a detailed account see Saxén & Toivonen 1962.)

Anamniote induction of mesoderm

Although the significance of the Spemann organizer in the formation of the chordate embryo cannot be underestimated it has been realized for a number of years that the associated primary induction, appropriately named at the time, is preceded by another fundamental inductive event which **predetermines** the basic mediolateral pattern of the prospective mesoderm. This concerns the interaction which takes place at the boundary between the vegetal yolk mass and the marginal zone (prospective endomesoderm) at the blastula stage of amphibian embryos. This concept of the early induction of mesoderm by the underlying vegetal cells, primary endoderm, was suggested by the work of Nieuwkoop (1973). The pattern of the induction is related to bilateral symmetry imposed on the amphibian egg (formation of the grey crescent) at fertilization; this leads to the distinction between a ventral influence (determining blood, mesothelium, etc.) and a dorsal influence (determining notochord and somites). A review by Nieuwkoop (1985) provides a valuable summary of the origin and importance of the inductive interactions during amphibian development. A similar mechanism to *mesodermal induction* may explain the influence of the *hypoblast* on the *epiblast* of amniote embryos (see p. 143). The demonstration of a key role for the vegetal domain of the egg (or a derived structure—the hypoblast) in chordate embryos relates to the well-known vegetal influence on early development, demonstrable for the eggs of several marine molluscs and annelids (Wilson 1904). There has been a resurgence of interest in mesoderm induction following the implication of growth factors.

Organogenesis and embryonic tissue interactions

In vertebrates the precursors of individual organs begin to make their appearance soon after the end of gastrulation and the subsequent formation of neural tube. The development of many of these systems is largely dependent on embryonic tissue interactions. In principle these so-called *secondary* and *tertiary inductions* resemble the primary induction inasmuch as they are dependent on the competence of the target tissue to respond to the inductive stimulus provided by a neighbouring one. The importance of these interactions is indicated in those sections which deal, in detail, with the development of specific organ systems in the human embryo; current views on the cytological and molecular basis of the mechanisms involved are also dealt with in a following section (see p. 110).

Of historical interest are the following significant discoveries: the influence of the developing optic cup on the formation of the lens in amphibian embryos (Spemann 1901; Lewis 1905); the role of the ancestral pronephric duct in the induction of mesonephric tubules (Waddington 1939) and the essential role of mesenchyme cells in limb formation.

Significance of the neural crest

Not all mesenchyme is derived from mesoderm invagination through the blastopore (amphibians) or mesoblast ingression through the primitive streak (amniotes). The most important alternative origin is the neural crest. The significance, migration and fate of the neural crest cells has been (His 1879; Katschenko 1888; Platt 1894), and is currently, of great interest (see p. 240). The importance of the neural crest cannot be underestimated; it appears to be a unique feature of vertebrates distinguishing them from their chordate ancestors (Gans & Northcutt 1983).

Pioneering experiments on amphibian embryos (Landacre 1911; Stone 1922, 1926; DuShane 1935) tracked the migration of the neural crest cells by excision and translocation of their sites of origin in the crest, established the distinction between *head* and *trunk crest cells*, and gradually defined the extent of the neural crest contribution to vertebrate development. Eventually detailed mapping of the head neural crest in urodele embryos enabled the origin of the branchial structures to be determined with great precision (Hörstadius & Sellman 1946). Examples of these early experiments, which contributed to a fundamental understanding of the significance of the neural crest, are illustrated in **3**.6. A detailed account of this work is given by Hörstadius (1950).

CURRENT CONCEPTS IN DEVELOPMENTAL BIOLOGY

Generation of cell diversity

Originating from a single but highly specialized cell, the zygote, the *generation of cell diversity* is an intrinsic feature of animal development. In mammals the adult organism contains in the region of 300 distinct cell phenotypes characteristically arranged to form specific organs and tissues. As in all animals above the level of sponges and coelenterates these cells may be classified according to function such as muscle, nerve, connective tissue and so on. In general, the lower the grade of organization the fewer cell types there are: coelenterates contain fewer than ten cell types, some of which perform a dual function, for example musculo-epithelial cells. Within a major animal group, such as the amniotes, a great variety of form and function is derived from similar embryonic cellular ingredients possessing broadly equivalent potential to develop into a fixed number of cell types. Any general theory of development must attempt to understand the factors causing the divergence of cell fate and the individual and collective role of cells as their phenotypes diverge; it further needs to acknowledge the constraints that evolution has apparently placed on the essential contribution of cells.

To this end it is important to appreciate the concept of a limited number of *basic cell types* from which all current diversity appears to be derived, both in development and in evolution (Willmer 1960; Lovtrup 1974). Observations on cultured cells derived from a variety of tissues led Willmer (1960) to the view that only three or four fundamental cell types existed. Based on their appearance and behaviour in culture, together with their potential to generate further diversity, he termed these cell types *amoebocytes*, *epitheliocytes*, *myxoblasts* and *myoblasts* (myxoblasts and myoblasts were thought to be variants of *mechanocytes*). Nerve cells were not included in the original classification. Such cell types are characteristic of the initial stages of development; for instance, mesenchyme cells (myxoblasts) and embryonic epithelia (epitheliocytes) feature prominently in the gastrulation process (see pp. 96 and 142). Lovtrup (1975, 1983, 1984) has refined and expanded the notion of basic cell type in an attempt to construct a logical and cell-based framework for epigenesis. His analysis emphasizes the importance of cytoskeletal elements (e.g. microtubules, microfilaments) and the role of extracellular material specifically associated with each of his proposed 'cell orders'. To avoid a perceived ambiguity in Willmer's classification, Lovtrup proposed an alternative nomenclature for the basic cell types. *Solocytes* (*s-cells*) are those cells which are capable of free movement and do not readily form stable aggregates; as they move they may

Experimental analysis of development II

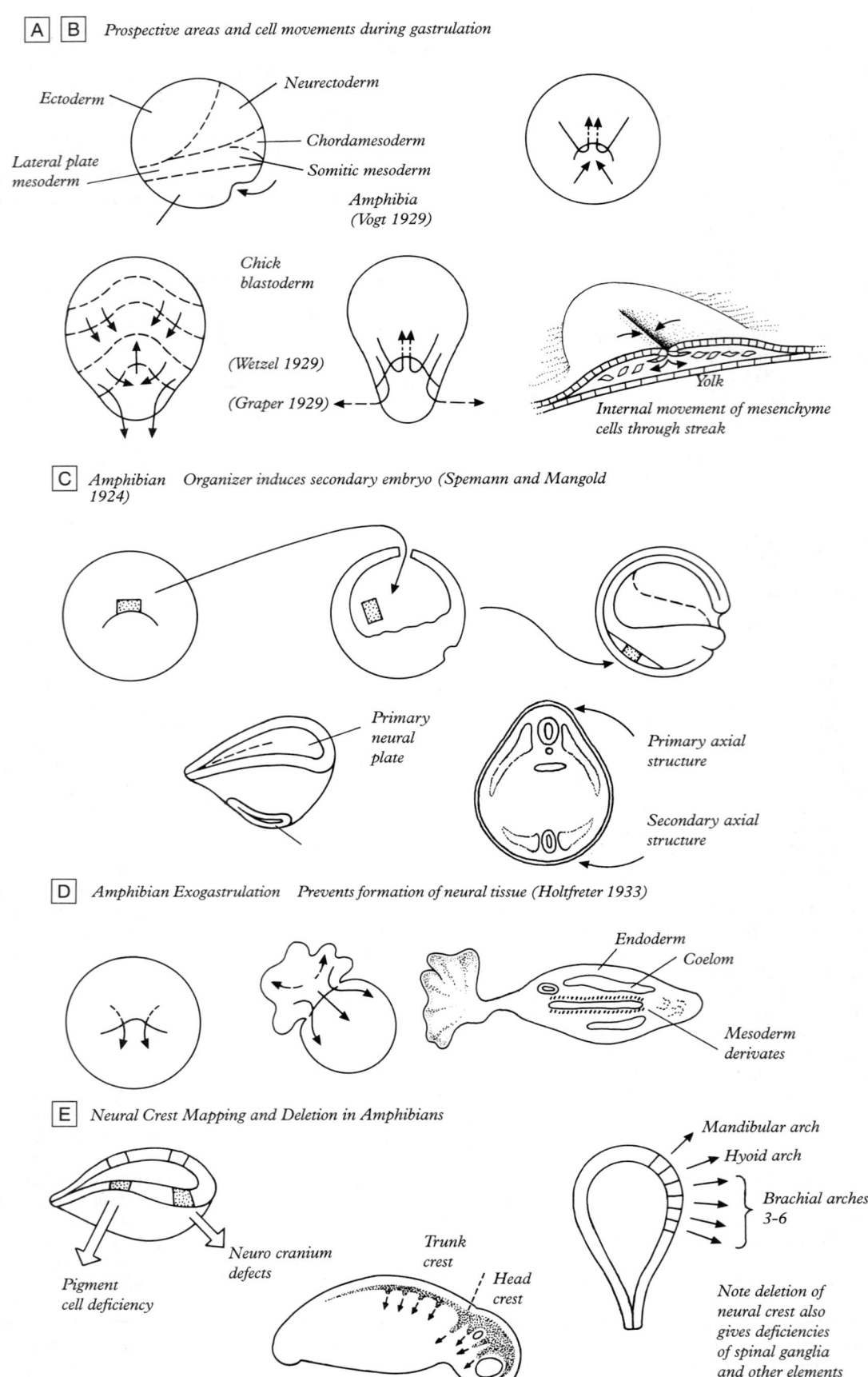

A B *Prospective areas and cell movements during gastrulation*

Ectoderm

Neurectoderm

Chordamesoderm

Somitic mesoderm

Lateral plate mesoderm

Amphibia (Vogt 1929)

Chick blastoderm

(Wetzel 1929)

(Graper 1929)

Yolk

Internal movement of mesenchyme cells through streak

C *Amphibian   Organizer induces secondary embryo (Spemann and Mangold 1924)*

Primary neural plate

Primary axial structure

Secondary axial structure

D *Amphibian Exogastrulation   Prevents formation of neural tissue (Holtfreter 1933)*

Endoderm

Coelom

Mesoderm derivates

E *Neural Crest Mapping and Deletion in Amphibians*

Neuro cranium defects

Pigment cell deficiency

Trunk crest

Head crest

Mandibular arch

Hyoid arch

Brachial arches 3-6

Note deletion of neural crest also gives deficiencies of spinal ganglia and other elements of nervous system

3.6 Experimental analysis of development II: early work. Fundamental observations and procedures. A, B. Mapping of presumptive areas; dynamic nature of gastrulation (Vogt, 1929; Graper, 1929). C, D. The organizer and primary induction (Spemann and Mangold, 1924; Holtfreter, 1933). E. Neural crest derivatives (Stone, 1922; 1926; Horstadius and Sellmann, 1946).

form either lobopodia (solo-lobocytes, sl-cells, i.e. amoebocytes) with short actin filaments or very long filopodia (solo-filocytes, sf-cells, i.e. myxoblasts) which contain cytoplasmic microtubules. *Colligocytes (c-cells)* are cells which, through their adhesiveness, form aggregates, typically epithelial; they also have two varieties, colligo-lobocytes and colligo-filocytes; the former contain microfilaments, the latter microtubules, corresponding to comparable s-cells. Solocytes produce extracellular matrix molecules, with heparan sulphate and hyaluronate being characteristic. (Løvtrup notes that hyaluronate is produced in the embryo particularly by mesenchymal cells; see also p. 153.) Solocytes form solid aggregates stabilized by short filopodia which form tight junctions with their neighbours. Colligocytes on the other hand produce a layer of reticular and fibrillar collagen within a matrix containing sulphated proteoglycans; they are adhesive and form junctional complexes. A limited number of transformations are possible between these conceptual cell types; namely solocytes can form aggregates (s-c transformation) and lobocytes can convert to filocytes. Ciliated or flagellated variants of each basic type are possible, giving a total of eight types altogether (**3.7**). Based on the analysis of the structure and function of this limited number of cell types, and paying due regard to the constraints imposed by evolution, Lovtrup provides a logical approach not only to the problem of cell diversity but to morphogenesis in general. (Despite the unusual terminology Lovtrup's views merit close attention, not least because they eliminate the need to relate the discussion of cell diversity to germ layer theory or to use terms which no longer seem appropriate to modern developmental biology. To quote Løvtrup (1983): '... it is difficult, or even impossible, to interpret and understand the processes of cell differentiation occurring in the embryo on the basis of terminology currently employed in cell biology'.)

Embryonic cells and tissues

The first cell divisions of an embryo are cleavage divisions, which repeatedly reduce the size of the cells (blastomeres), restoring the nucleus to cytoplasm ratio and resulting in cells of typical size. The arrangement of the cells within the morula produces differences between the cells because of their relative position, their exposure to the environment and their junctional connections to other cells. This results in the *differential* expression of cell morphology: for example the outer cells of the morula become polarized and exhibit apical microvilli; they acquire different junctional connections with their lateral neighbours compared to their connections with the cells in the centre of the morula; the outer cells act in concert as a cell population forming the earliest epithelium.

After gastrulation the arrangement of embryonic cells into tissues is apparent. Epithelial cells (Løvtrup's colligocytes), which form the upper and lower layers of the embryo, have apical–basal polarity, narrow intercellular clefts, juxtaluminal junctional complexes and a developed basal lamina composed of extracellular matrix proteins synthesized by the cells. The cells between the inner and outer epithelial layers are mesenchymal in arrangement. Mesenchymal cells (Løvtrup's solocytes) have no polarity; they have junctional complexes which are not juxtaluminal and they produce extracellular matrix molecules and fibres from the whole cell surface.

These two embryonic cell states are not necessarily immutable and *transition from epithelia to mesenchyme* and vice versa occurs during development. The causative factors of such changes in cell aggregation and contact are not clear and many different factors of a temporal or locally inductive nature may be involved. Transitional events during gastrulation and the early stages of development may be different from those occurring at the later stages of organogenesis. For example, it is likely that early mesenchymal populations are heterogeneous, containing migrating epithelial cells which **temporarily** express a mesenchymal appearance: the first cells to ingress at the primitive streak and migrate between the epiblast and hypoblast form epithelia at their destination (Bellairs 1987) in the epithelial somite (see p. 144) and the somatopleuric and splanchnopleuric coelomic epithelia (see p. 155). Similarly, splanchnopleuric mesenchyme forms endothelia generally throughout the embryo but may engage in this transition either early or late. However, the nephrogenic mesenchymal cells, produced from proliferation of the coelomic epithelium, form epithelial nephrons only during a specific time period.

Conversely, epithelial cells can reorganize their extracellular mat-

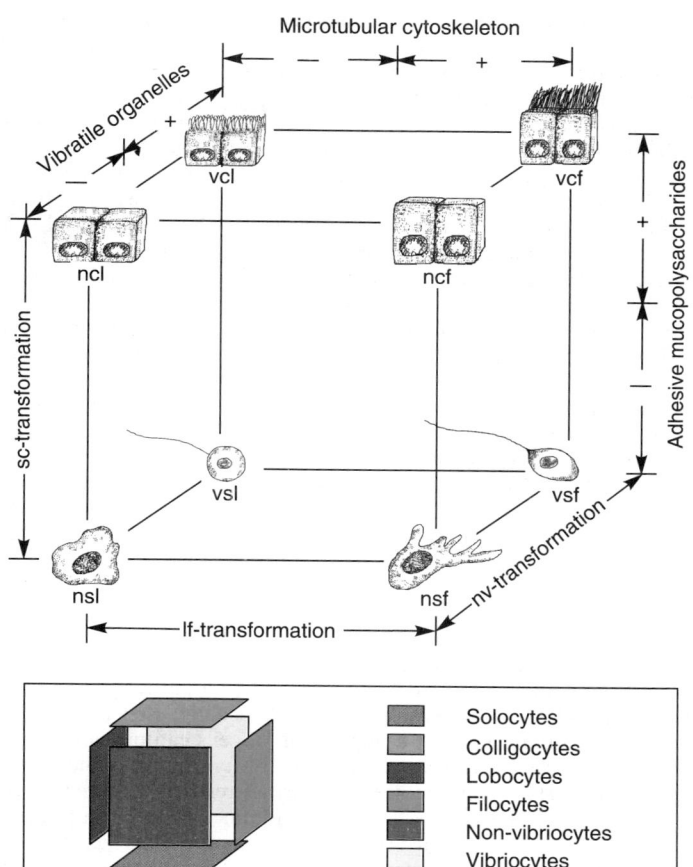

3.7 Lovtrup cell cube. Typical representatives of 8-cell orders are shown in the corners of the cube. The 4-cell orders located at the same face of the cube constitute a cell class. The lower face of the cube shows solocytes, the upper face the colligocytes, the left face the lobocytes, the right face the filocytes, the front face the non-vibriocytes and the back face the vivriocytes. Three transformations or differentiations required to form the several cell types are indicated. (After Løvtrup 1974 with permission.)

rices and transform into mesenchymal cells. This is seen in the most basic manner at the primitive streak and later in the formation and migration of the neural crest (Greenberg & Hay 1982; Hay 1989). Often cell proliferation of particular cell lines occurs at an epithelium, for example formation of intermediate mesenchyme from the proliferating coelomic epithelium and production of myogenic cells from the epithelial plate of the somite. However, a later specific example of transition from epithelium to mesenchyme occurs in the heart where endocardial epithelial cells become cardiac mesenchyme at the atrioventricular canal and the proximal outflow tract of the heart (see p. 300). This latter example is a locally induced transformation and different from the production of mesenchymal cells from a germinal epithelium.

DEVELOPMENTAL HIERARCHY

Much of the specification of the basic embryonic body plan is the result of a **hierarchy** of developmental decisions at different developmental times. The earliest embryonic cells may be described as *totipotent* meaning they have the capacity to become any cell of the adult body. (An alternative view is that the earliest cells are optimally differentiated for the stage of development they have reached, as they will be at any stage throughout development.) During development, cells respond to intrinsic or extrinsic cues by following a developmental pathway which will result in the *commitment* of those cells to a particular fate. In mammals, for instance, an early choice is made at about the 8-cell stage when some cells become committed to develop into extraembryonic tissues and others into embryonic tissues. Similar *binary choices* subsequently occur for both the extraembryonic cells and the embryonic cells. For the extraembryonic line, trophoblast cells become either cytotrophoblast or syncytiotrophoblast; the cytotrophoblast cells become either mural or polar trophoblast. For the embryonic line, inner cell mass cells become either hypoblast or epiblast; the hypoblast can become either visceral or parietal. (It is worth noting at this point that there is little to distinguish blastomeres before the 8-cell stage and few choices may be made before this time. At the time of compaction the outer cells of the morula express cell adhesion molecules, form junctions and exhibit apical microvilli. The connection of these cells results in a different environment for the cells in the centre of the morula. Thus different fates for the inner and outer populations of blastomeres can now be linked to cell signalling, interaction and response.)

3.37 shows the binary choices for particular early extraembryonic and embryonic cell fates. Within the embryo these choices focus from the general (e.g. ectoderm becomes neural plate, neural crest and surface ectoderm) to region specific (e.g. the latter cell populations become regions of the brain and spinal cord, regions of the autonomic nervous system or parts of the face and skull and epidermis respectively). Finally the tissues of the regions so formed develop very specifically into differentiated cell phenotypes, for example neurons, glia, osteocytes, fibrocytes, melanocytes, keratinocytes, etc.

Restriction and determination

As cells become committed to a particular fate they lose the ability to choose an alternative range of developmental pathways, i.e. they become *restricted*. The term restriction is usually used to refer to limitations in the ways that a population of cells can develop. Once restricted, cells are set on a particular pathway of development and after a number of binary choices (i.e. further restrictions) are said to be *determined*. Determined cells are programmed to follow a process of development which will lead to *differentiation*. The determined state is a heritable characteristic of cells; it is the final step in restriction. After a cell has become determined it will progress to a differentiated phenotype providing the environmental factors are suitable. For example, melanocytes normally express the black pigment melanin; for this they require the presence of tyrosine in the environmental medium. While the tyrosine is present the cells achieve their differentiated phenotype with black coloration. If, however, the cells are maintained in a tyrosine-free culture medium the cells can no longer synthesize melanin and they become pale; they no longer appear differentiated. If at a later time the tyrosine is replaced in the medium the cell line can once more synthesize melanin. This demonstrates that the *determined state* is *stable* and not dependent on the environment, whereas the *differentiated phenotype is labile*. This process is evident in the repair of a wound or fractured bone in an adult, as well as in an embryo.

The process of determination and differentiation within embryonic cell populations can be assessed by the ability of cell populations to produce specific proteins. All cells have a series of genes which code for proteins considered essential for cellular metabolism. Such genes and proteins have been termed *primary* (colloquially termed housekeeping genes and proteins) to illustrate their ubiquity. As cells become determined they synthesize proteins specific to their state of determination. These are termed *secondary* proteins, for example liver and kidney cells but not muscle produce arginase. At the most differentiated state cells produce *tertiary* proteins, those which no other cell line can synthesize, for example ovalbumin in oviduct cells or haemoglobin in erythrocytes (the genes and proteins in this case have been colloquially termed *luxury* to denote their speciality). Primary, secondary and tertiary proteins are an expression of stages of determination and differentiation, coded by a range of genes. Other gene products can be detected which, by their expression, *confer* a particular determination and differentiation pathway on undetermined, or even differentiated cells, i.e. establish a cell *lineage*. The genes coding for these products, which can *direct* the fate of cells faced with a binary choice, were termed 'switch genes' by Waddington (1940); they have since been identified. Their expression in cells allows two choices: the presence or absence of the gene product determines which lineage the cells generate. In vertebrates the *MyoD-1* (myoblast determination 1) gene found in myoblasts can change differentiated adipose cells, fibroblasts or hepatocytes transfected with the gene into a myocyte lineage.

Determination pathways

As populations of cells become progressively determined they can be described as *transient amplifying cells*, *progenitor cells*, *stem cells*, and *terminally differentiated cells*.

Transient amplifying cells. These are cells proliferating and producing equally determined cells; they undergo *proliferative cell mitoses*. At some stage transiently amplifying populations will, as a result of an inductive stimulus, enter a *quantal cell cycle* (Holtzer et al 1972). The cells, as a response to molecular signalling, undergo a *quantal mitosis* resulting in an increase in the restriction of **their** progeny, which continue to undergo proliferative mitoses at a progressive level of determination. The quantal mitosis corresponds to the time of binary choice (see above) when the commitment of the progeny is different from the parent.

Progenitor cells are already determined along a particular pathway; they may individually follow that differentiation pathway or may proliferate producing larger numbers of similarly determined progenitor cells which subsequently differentiate. Examples of progenitor cells are neuroblasts or myoblasts.

Stem cells are cells which individually, or as a population, can **both** produce determined progeny **and** reproduce themselves. It is generally thought that whereas proliferative cell division may be symmetric, giving derived cells with identical determination, stem cells undergo asymmetric divisions, whereby one daughter remains as a stem cell (i.e. retains the determination of the parent cell), while the other proceeds along a differentiation pathway (possibly leading to death). Stem cells are seen later in development and in adult life. It appears that differing combinations of growth factors can either maintain cells in a stem cell-like state, or cause them to differentiate.

Terminally differentiated cells. By their extreme specialization these cells can no longer divide, for example erythrocytes and neurons.

Programmed cell death or apoptosis. This is a particular variety of terminal differentiation where the final outcome is the death of individual cells or cell populations. Apoptosis is an effective mechanism for eliminating unwanted cells which die without rupture of the lyosomes and autolysis which would release their contents into the extracellular environment and cause inflammation. Programmed cell death is seen in the developing limb where cells die along the pre- and postaxial limits of the apical ectodermal ridge so limiting its extent (p. 290), and similarly between the digits allowing their separation (p. 290). Within the nervous system neuroblasts which project to abnormal targets and fail to receive the appropriate neurotrophic factors undergo programmed cell death.

Work on the nematode *Caenorhabditis elegans* has suggested that the cell death programme is normally **on** in all cells, and that cell death is prevented by an over-riding 'survival' programme (reviewed in Raff 1992). This survival programme often involves growth factors and highly conserved gene products, such as that encoded by *BCL-2* (Tomei & Cope 1991, 1994; Jacobson & Evan 1994). The idea that all cells are critically dependent on survival signals, such as those generated from growth factors or the extracellular matrix, is an attractive hypothesis. It provides a simple mechanism for eliminating cells which end up in abnormal locations during development. As different tissues might be expected to produce different sets of survival factors, a misplaced cell deprived of the specific signals it requires for survival would die. It is suggested that dependence on such survival signals may be a useful mechanism for controlling cell numbers in higher vertebrates, if cells are forced to compete with one another for limited amounts of such signalling molecules.

Measurements of determination

Examination and experimental perturbation of embryos of different stages allows the investigation of states of restriction and determination attained by particular cell populations. The addition of dyes or markers to cells within the living embryo, removal of local cell populations, growth of portions of embryonic tissue in culture, transplantation of portions of embryo to different places in the same embryo (homoplastic), or to different embryos (heteroplastic), recombination of embryonic tissues within and between Classes (xenoplastic) and the formation of chimeric embryos (especially quail–chick, see p. 221) all add information about the time at which, and the position in which, cell populations become determined.

The addition of dyes or markers to cells and cell populations allows their relative migrations to be followed. From the movements of labelled cells and the differentiation pathways they follow, a predictive *fate map* can be produced for a known stage in development (3.42). This method was used to examine gastrulation in the amphibian embryo (Vogt 1929; see p. 103) where vital dyes, added to populations of cells prior to gastrulation, permitted the visualization of their ingression at the blastopore. More recently the fate of much smaller populations of epiblast cells were demonstrated after ingression through the avian primitive node (Selleck & Stern 1991; see p. 143). The production of fate maps formed the basis of further experimentation in which regions of embryos (with a known fate) could be killed, removed, or transplanted to a different location, and the resultant differentiation of the cells could be compared to the normal developmental pathway elucidated by the fate map.

If cell populations of predicted fate are cultured in a neutral medium (i.e. one with no known inductive substances) they will differentiate. However, the final differentiation state may be different from that predicted from the fate map. The explantation and culture reveal an original state of commitment termed *specification*. The degree of specification of cell populations may differ from their determination because cell populations may be altered in the embryo by later inductive influences. However, these influences may need to be local and constant to increase restriction and determination in a cell population.

Clonal analysis is a special form of fate mapping in which a single cell is labelled. Subsequently at a later stage both the position and state of determination or differentiation of its progeny are identified (Slack 1991). Clonal analysis has been used to examine the fate of epiblast during gastrulation in the mouse (Lawson et al 1991; see p. 143) and to establish the degree of cell determination.

Developmental regulation

The concept of developmental regulation emerged from numerous experiments in which individual blastomeres were removed from embryos to see if they could independently produce a normal individual. If cytoplasmic segregation occurred as the zygote divided, then individual blastomeres would possess different cytoplasmic constituents and their fates would differ. This was the basis of *mosaic development*, where the early blastomeres have a strictly determined lineage based on their cytoplasmic constituents (see p. 141). Such embryos can never produce monozygotic twins because the cytoplasm of the zygote is regionally restricted even before the 2-cell stage.

However, the individual blastomeres of some embryos will each produce entire embryos if separated at an early stage, showing that instead of developing into a predicted embryonic part, each blastomere could regulate its development to produce a complete organism; this is termed *regulative development*. The phenomenon of regulation exhibits *global features* wherein a mass of cells reorganizes **as a whole**, suggesting avenues of cell–cell communication for sharing this meta-organizational information and plan.

The effects of regulation are well established but the mechanisms underlying such regulation are not yet understood. There is a strong presumption that the embryo, by some mechanism, has an indication of its own size and how big it should be for a particular developmental stage. Homeostatic mechanisms are deployed in order to seek and maintain this 'target size' in embryos where naturally occurring or experimental perturbations cause it to depart from the normal growth curve. Although extreme, this viewpoint is supported by observations on twinning and fusion experiments, catch-up growth and responses to inductive reprogramming (teratogenic insults; Snow 1989).

Twinning experiments. When first formed, twin embryos will be approximately half the normal size, as the process of twinning leads to the formation of two embryonic axes within a normal-sized blastocyst. Interestingly, the proportions of parts within these miniature embryonic primary axes are normal, and despite starting out at half the size, each fetus is of comparable size to a singleton fetus by the second trimester of pregnancy (Snow 1989). Twin fetuses thus go through a phase of accelerated growth during most of organogenesis although the mechanism by which this occurs is obscure. Monozygotic twins constitute a high risk group for susceptibility to malformation; although this may be due to their small initial size, it seems more likely that the risk is generated by the higher than normal growth rate that they experience at critical times in their early development (Snow 1989).

The phenomenon of twinning reveals important insights into aspects of normal development (Slack 1991). First, it excludes any model for regional specification based solely on the localization of determinants in the egg cytoplasm. Second, it shows that these cellular interactions are able to accommodate a change of *scale* in the pattern generating mechanism. Boundaries which would be formed $100\,\mu m$ apart in the normal embryo will be formed approximately $79\,\mu m$ apart in the twins (Slack 1991). Third, as alluded to above, twinning clearly demonstrates that the final size of an embryonic structure does not depend on the size of the original primordium, but rather on some, as yet unelucidated, mechanism which can stop growth, when a certain absolute size has been reached.

Fusion experiments. The converse of twinning is the fusion of two or more embryos to give one giant early embryo, or the increase in size of an embryo by the addition of cells injected into the blastocyst cavity (Snow 1989). In such cases normal development ensues, and has been reported for aggregates of 16 8-cell mouse embryos (Snow 1989). When born, these chimeric embryos are of normal size. The downward regulation in size of the embryo aggregates occurs shortly after implantation, between the appearance of the amniotic cavity and the primitive streak. The mechanism of size regulation seems to involve a lengthening of the cell cycle during this period (Snow 1989). Size regulation in these circumstances seems to be completed before the onset of organogenesis which is thus normal. The implications for normal development from these fusion experiments is similar to those outlined for twinning.

Catch-up growth. A region or regions of the embryo can be removed at varying stages of development without disturbing the pattern or the proportions of the fully formed embryo. This *defect regulation* involves a number of complex processes, including compensatory catch-up growth (Snow 1989). Although this may result in reconstitution of the deleted part, later disturbances in embryonic timing and cell division patterns may give rise to abnormalities, often at locations different from the site of the primary insult (MacKee & Ferguson 1984; Snow 1989).

Inductive reprogramming. In this example of developmental regulation, if a signalling centre, for example an apical ectodermal ridge of a developing limb, or the zone of polarizing activity in the limb bud, is grafted to an abnormal position, it can cause the surrounding tissue to follow a pathway of development which does not correspond to the fate map and is instead induced by the grafted signalling tissue (see p. 290). This mechanism is seen in experimental epithelial/mesenchymal recombinations (see below). A similar outcome can be achieved by the topical application of morphogens (see below), such as retinoic acid.

Regeneration. It is important not to confuse embryonic regulation with regeneration in adult or fetal tissues (Slack 1991). Regeneration involves the re-establishment of *regional differences* in the newly formed replacement parts, while regulation involves the re-establishment of a fate map on a partial domain of uncommitted tissue (Slack 1991). Regeneration occurs in many lower organisms, for example the formation of new heads and tails in transected flat worms, new apical and basal regions in transected hydra, or the replacement of a whole severed limb or tail, or appropriate part thereof, in adult amphibia. In general, regeneration follows one of two main types: *morphallaxis*, in which the whole re-forms by rearrangement and differentiation of the existing tissues without further growth, and *epimorphosis*, in which there is new growth of blastemal tissue, which subsequently matures into the full regenerate. Regeneration involves similar positional signalling cues to normal development, and may share some similar morphogens, for example retinoic acid and its receptors (Brockes 1994; see p. 116). An interesting form of embryonic response which is midway between embryonic regulation and regeneration is the phenomenon of scar-free dermal embryonic wound healing (Whitby & Ferguson 1991).

CELL AND TISSUE INTERACTIONS

It is clear from the existence of regulation and the differing differentiation pathways of cells in the early embryo, that interactions take place between the cells of the developing embryo. These cellular interactions provide the developmental integration and fine control necessary to achieve tissue specific morphogenesis. In the early embryo, such interactions may occur only if particular regions of the embryo are present, for example signalling centres or organizers (see p. 105). As the embryo matures, so interactions tend to occur between adjacent cell populations, for example epithelium and mesenchyme, and later between adjacent differentiating tissues, for example between nerves and muscle or muscle and skeletal elements. Tissue interactions result in changes or reorganization of one or both tissues; these changes would not occur in the absence of the tissue interactions. The process of tissue interaction is also called *induction*; one tissue is said to induce another. The ability of a tissue to respond to inductive signals is called *competence* (Waddington 1940). (Competence may be considered as a subset of *potency*. Potency is the total of all things a particular region of embryonic tissue can become if put into the appropriate environment. Competence includes all the outcomes achievable by that tissue **in response** to the environments present in the embryo at that particular stage.) Inductive interactions may be more or less complicated: only the induced tissue may change or both tissues may change and participate, as in morphogenesis, or, more commonly, several reciprocal inductive interactions may be required over a prolonged period of developmental time before a specific organ or tissue will form.

Types of interaction

Two types of cell and tissue interaction have been defined by Holtzer (1968): *permissive* and *instructive*.

In a *permissive interaction*, a signal from an apposing tissue is necessary for the successful self-differentiation of the responding tissue. This means a cell population (or the matrix molecules secreted by them) will maintain mitotic activity in an adjacent cell population. Since a variety of **different** cell populations may permit a **specific** cell population to undergo mitosis and cell differentiation, no specific instruction or signal, which may limit the developmental options of the responding tissue, is involved. Thus this signal does not influence the developmental pathway selected; there is no restriction. The responding tissue has the intrinsic capacity to develop and only needs appropriate environmental conditions to express this capacity. Permissive interactions often occur later in development, where a tissue whose fate has already been determined is maintained and stabilized by another.

An *instructive (directive) interaction* (induction) changes the cell type of the responding tissue (i.e. the cell population becomes restricted). Wessells (1977) proposed four general principles in most instructive interactions.

(1) In the presence of tissue A, responding tissue B develops in a certain way.

(2) In the absence of tissue A, responding tissue B does not develop in that way.

(3) In the absence of tissue A, but in the presence of tissue C, tissue B does not develop in that way.

(4) In the presence of tissue A, a tissue D, which would normally develop differently, is changed to develop like B.

An example of (4) above is the experimental association of chicken flank ectoderm with mouse mammary mesenchyme, resulting in the morphogenesis of mammary gland-like structures: chickens do not normally develop mammary glands (Sakakura 1983).

In an experimental context, instructive interactions have thus been more narrowly defined to describe the situation where the apposition of two dissimilar tissue types, which would not normally come in contact, results in one or other of those developing a unique morphology and gene expression, which would not normally be present (Sharpe & Ferguson 1988).

For any specific interaction, five basic questions can be asked:

- What is the tissue source for the inductive signal (i.e. where does the specificity reside)?
- What are the physicochemical properties of this signal?
- What is the mode of intercellular transmission?
- How do the responding cells process these signals?
- How do these signals result in the terminal differentiation of the cells and/or the morphogenesis of the tissue?

Many early experiments described the tissue source for the inductive signal, the responding tissue and the resultant morphogenetic effect. Recent advances have identified the nature of many of the

signals and analogous substances which have similar effects, the variety of cellular transmission of the signals and the receptors and the consequences of signalling to the target tissue.

As will also be evident, however, in the subsequent sections, at a mechanistic level it is unclear whether there are fundamental differences between instructive and permissive interactions: they are more likely easily identifiable experimental outcomes, depending upon the nature of the signalling molecule, its divergent effects on the two tissues and the state of competence of the responding tissue. Tissue interactions continue into adult life and are probably responsible for maintaining the functional heterogeneity of adult tissues and organs. For example, there is complex tissue heterogeneity with sharply compartmentalized boundaries in the oral cavity; the distinction between the attached gingiva of the gums, the alveolar mucosa of the floor of the mouth and the lips, the vermilion border and the skin, are sharp and distinct boundaries of specific epithelial and mesenchymal differentiation and are almost certainly maintained by continuing epithelial/mesenchymal interactions in adult life (for review see Sharpe & Ferguson 1988). Perturbation of these interactions throughout the body may underlie a wide variety of adult diseases, including susceptibility to cancer and proliferative disorders.

Epithelial/mesenchymal interactions

These are a specific subset of embryonic tissue interactions involving signalling between an epithelial tissue and a mesenchymal tissue. They are particularly common and important during embryonic development. They provide a mechanism for coordinating and fine tuning the development, for example mitotic rate, differentiative ability, etc, of the two tissues, which are key for successful morphogenesis. As with general tissue interactions, epithelial/mesenchymal interactions are often described as instructive or permissive.

Generally mesenchymal populations control the pattern of development, i.e. whether an arm or leg develops, or whether stomach or colon develops; however, epithelial cells often retain their original cytodifferentiation and may have an early profound effect on the underlying mesenchyme. Thus in a recombination of chick gut epithelium and mouse mesenchyme, or vice versa, whereas the patterning of the intestinal villi will be determined by the underlying mesenchyme, the epithelial cells will produce the enzymes associated with the relevant species, i.e. mouse epithelium will produce lactase and chick epithelium sucrase, regardless of the origin of the underlying mesenchyme (Haffen et al 1989). Further, within gut development there is the suggestion that the epithelium may first influence the mesenchyme thus conferring its morphogenetic properties; a similar effect may be seen in the early stages of formation of the base of the skull, where the neuroepithelium, by placing specific molecules in the basal lamina, can halt migration of subjacent mesenchymal cells and initiate their differentiation along a chondrogenic pathway (see p. 274). Thus there are temporally reciprocal interactions between the epithelium and mesenchyme, the epithelium signalling to the mesenchyme, which then in turn signals back to the epithelium, etc. Such sequential spatial and temporal reciprocal interactions have been termed *epigenetic cascades* (Hall 1992); they lead to the differentiation and morphogenesis of most tissues and organs (Sharpe & Ferguson 1988; Baird 1990; Hall 1992). An example of a reciprocal tissue interaction can be seen in mammalian tooth development summarized in **3.8**. Other examples of epithelial/mesenchymal interactions are used throughout the section to illustrate the mechanisms in each system. (For an excellent text on interactions consult Wessells 1977.)

Mechanisms of signalling

In theory, there are four principle mechanisms by which cellular interactions may be signalled: *direct cell–cell contact*, *cell adhesion molecules* and their receptors, *extracellular matrix molecules* and their receptors, and *growth factors* and their receptors. Many of these mechanisms interact and it is likely that combinations of them are involved in development. **3.9** illustrates diagrammatically some ways by which mesenchymal cells could signal to epithelial cells. An additional set of identical mechanisms could operate for epithelial to mesenchymal signalling. Clearly, these mechanisms would increase in complexity, for example by reciprocal interactions or by the divergent effects of a single molecule on epithelial and mesenchymal cells.

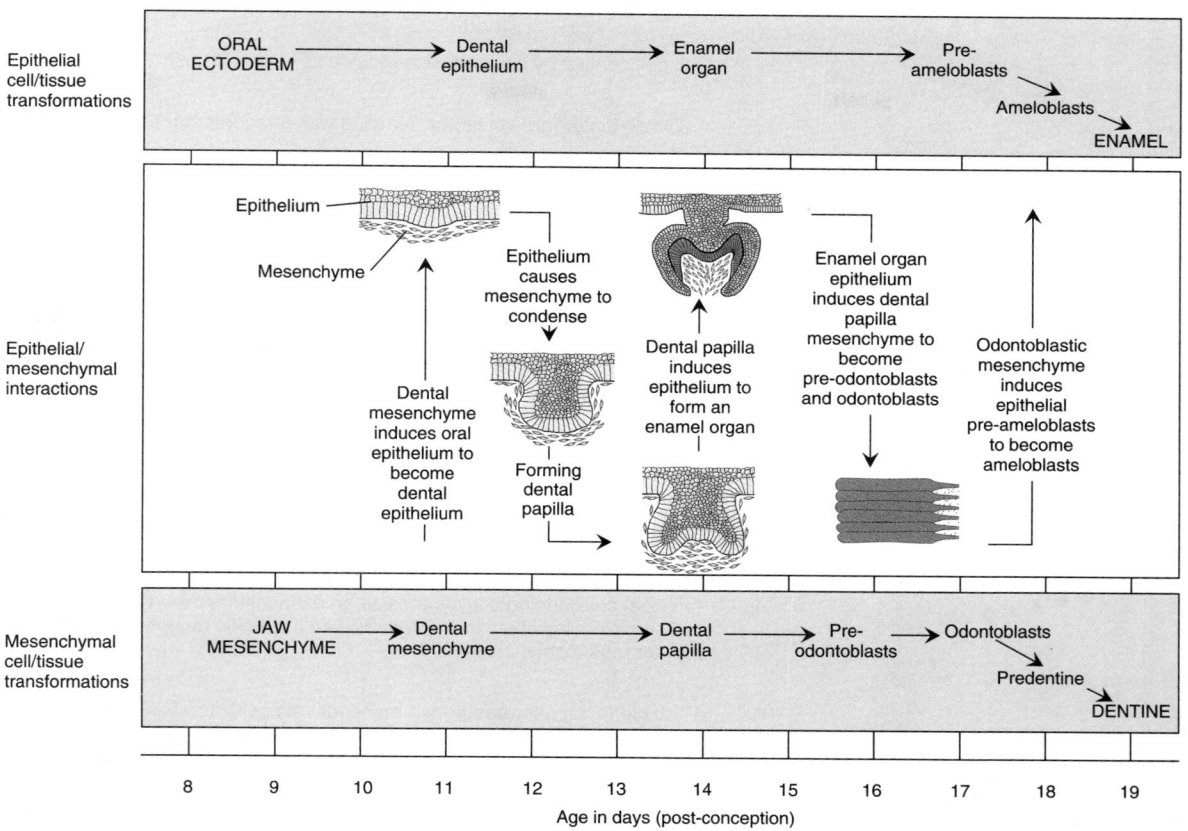

3.8 An example of reciprocal tissue interaction in mammalian tooth development. The sequence of epithelial/mesenchymal interactions involved in the development of teeth in the embryonic mouse. E8–19 represent age in days after conception. (After Lumsden 1987.)

Direct cell–cell contact. Gap junctions appear to be important for communication and transfer of information between cells. Antibodies to gap junctional proteins, experimentally injected into early amphibian embryos, appear to disrupt aspects of neural induction, and in mammalian embryos disruption of gap junctions at the 8-blastomere stage prevents compaction from occurring. It is suggested that gap junctional communication is involved in patterning (see below). The intercellular passage of dye between cells via gap junctions can be monitored, and the distribution of gap junctions both spatially and temporally can be studied in embryos by antibodies to *connexins*, constitutive proteins of gap junctions. Dye coupling of cells has been recorded as cells of the paraxial mesenchyme form epithelial somites, and between neuroepithelial cells within rhombomeres (Martinez et al 1992), and connexins have been noted between cardiac myocytes (Fromaget et al 1992) and in the media of the outflow tract of the heart (Minkoff et al 1993).

Endogenous electrical fields are also thought to have a role in cell–cell communication. Such fields have been demonstrated in a range of amphibian embryos and in vertebrate embryos during primitive streak ingression (Jaffe & Stern 1979; Winkel & Nuccitelli 1989); experiments in which endogenous currents were shunted out of embryos resulted in tail defects (Hotary & Robinson 1992). Neuroepithelial cells have been shown to be electrically coupled regardless of their position relative to interrhombomeric boundaries.

Cell adhesion molecules (CAMs or cadherins). These families of molecules which mediate adhesion between cells have been identified and their spatial and temporal distribution localized in the early embryo. They are thus candidates for signalling cellular interactions. Some of the most extensively studied CAMs include the *neural cell adhesion molecule* (*N-CAM*), first identified in nerve cells, *liver cell adhesion molecule* (*L-CAM*), first identified in the liver, *cell–cell adhesion molecule* (*C-CAM*) (Edelman 1986, 1988), and *substrate adhesion molecule* (*SAM*). Although Edelman (1988), in his morphoregulatory hypothesis of development, directly implicated the expression of CAMs and SAMs in embryonic induction, current evidence indicates that their expression may represent an early response of groups of cells to embryonic induction signals and that

such expression can modify the behaviour of groups of induced cells. To this extent cell adhesion molecules may be much more important in morphogenetic events.

Other molecules found in the extracellular matrix (see below), for example fibronectin and laminin inter alia, can modulate cell adhesion by their degree of glycosylation. Self-assembly or cross-linking by matrix molecules may affect cell adhesiveness by increasing the availability of binding sites or by obscuring them (Adams & Watt 1993).

Extracellular matrix molecules and their receptors. These are synthesized by both epithelial and mesenchymal cells. *Epithelial cells* produce a two-dimensional *basal lamina*. A variety of matrix molecules including *laminin*, *fibronectin*, *type IV collagen* and various *proteoglycans* are found in basal laminae. The particular molecules can vary during development according to spatial and temporal patterns resulting in changes in behaviour of the underlying mesenchymal cells (e.g. see development of skull, p. 271). *Mesenchymal cells* produce extracellular matrix molecules in three-dimensions. Those adjacent to an epithelial layer will contribute to it forming a *basement membrane* which secures the epithelial layer to the underlying tissue, whilst those cells deep within a mesenchymal population may synthesize *matrix molecules* (fibrillar or granular) to separate cells locally, open migration routes, or leave information within the matrix to act on cell populations passing at a later time (Nathan & Sporn 1991). Molecules of the extracellular matrix are complex; they include more than 19 individual types of *collagen* (some of which are capable of being individually spliced to give more than 100 variants (Mayne & Burgeson 1987), *proteoglycans* and *glycoproteins* (which come in a wide variety of forms, with and without binding proteins; Scott 1989, 1993; Knudson & Knudson 1993; Erickson 1993), and *elastic fibres* (Rosenbloom et al 1993). Of particular interest is *hyaluronic acid*, a glycosaminoglycan. Because of its vast capacity to bind water molecules it creates and structures the space between the mesenchymal cells, creating much of the overall shape of embryos. Experimental removal of hyaluronic acid prevents the formation of cell migration routes, removes the support for overlying epithelia, and disrupts the normal branching of glandular systems.

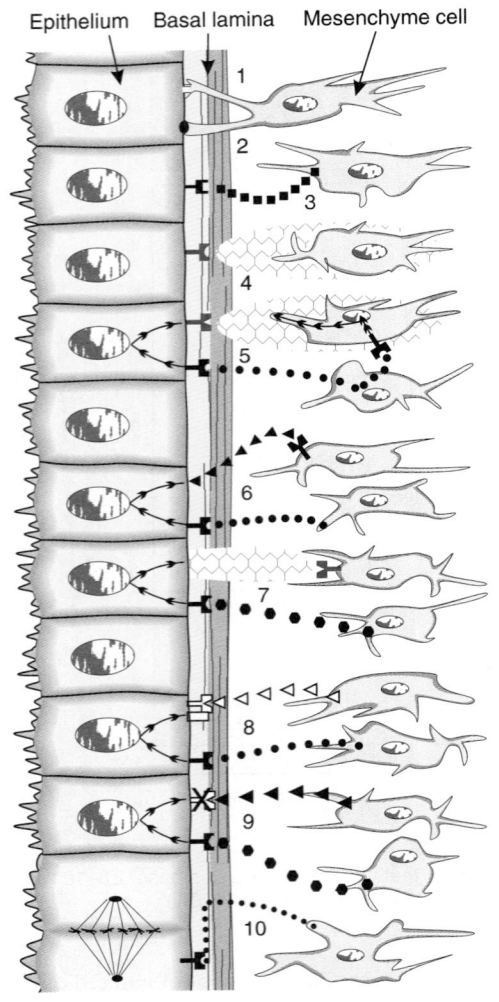

Epithelium Basal lamina Mesenchyme cell

1 Direct cell-cell contact by gap junctions.

2 Cell-cell contact by cell adhesion molecules.

3 A soluble factor (growth factor) reacting with a receptor for that factor on the epithelial cells.

4 Extracellular matrix molecule secreted by the mesenchyme cells interacting with a receptor on the epithelial cell.

5 A soluble factor (growth factor) secreted by a mesenchymal cell having a biphasic action interacting (i) with a receptor on an epithelial cell, causing it to express a specific extracellular matrix molecule receptor; (ii) with a receptor on a mesenchyme cell, causing it to secrete a specific extracellular matrix molecule which then interacts with the induced epithelial receptor.

6 A soluble factor (growth factor) secreted by a mesenchyme cell interacting with a receptor on an epithelial cell causing it to express a receptor, or secrete a factor, which interacts with another factor synthesized, or receptor expressed, by another mesenchyme cell.

7 A soluble factor secreted by a mesenchyme cell interacting with a receptor on an epithelial cell causing it to synthesize an extracellular matrix molecule (or a receptor for such a molecule) which then interacts with a specific receptor for that molecule on another mesenchyme cell.

8 A soluble factor secreted from a mesenchyme cell interacting with a receptor on an epithelial cell causing it to synthesize a molecule which stabilises or enhances the interaction between a mesenchymal derived factor and its epithelial receptor.

9 A soluble factor secreted by a mesenchyme cell interacting with a receptor on an epithelial cell causing the inhibition of synthesis/assembly of a factor or receptor.

10 A soluble factor secreted by a mesenchyme cell binding to the extracellular matrix of the basal lamina where it remains active and subsequently interacts with a receptor on an epithelial cell which appears at a later developmental time.

3.9 Illustrates the many ways by which mesenchyme cells could signal to epithelial cells. Precisely the same mechanisms can operate in reverse, i.e. epithelium to mesenchyme.

Fibronectin deposited extracellularly along a migration pathway will affect cells which touch it later, causing realignment of their intracellular actin filaments and thus their orientation; fibronectin induces cell migration. The receptors for extracellular matrix molecules like fibronectin and laminin were termed *integrins* (Horowitz 1986) because they integrate (via α and β subunits which span the cell membrane) extracellular proteins and intracellular cytoskeletal elements, allowing them to act together. The binding preference of integrins depends upon their combination of subunits and environmental conditions.

Mutations of the genes which code for extracellular matrix molecules give rise to a number of congenital disorders; for example mutations in type I collagen give rise to *osteogenesis imperfecta*; in type II collagen they produce disorders of cartilage; and in fibrillin they lead to Marfan's syndrome.

Although all molecules secreted into the spaces around the mesenchymal cells are technically extracellular matrix molecules, growth factors (see below) are distinguished from them. Growth factors (see below) and extracellular matrix molecules share numerous cooperative properties; indeed there are huge stores of growth factor proteins bound and sequestered to extracellular matrix molecules, particularly those of the basal laminae. Growth factors interact with extracellular matrix molecules in the following ways:

• Growth factors can bind to specific extracellular matrix molecules and remain active
• Specific extracellular matrix molecules bind and neutralize growth factors
• Extracellular matrix molecules have growth factor repeat sequences which may function as:

– building blocks
– sites of growth factor activity
– cell migration attachment sites
• There is cooperative secretion of extracellular matrix molecules and growth factors
• Growth factors stimulate extracellular matrix molecule biosynthesis
• Growth factors stimulate extracellular matrix receptor expression
• Extracellular matrix molecules down regulate synthesis of growth factors and/or their receptors.

It is believed that growth factor activation may be a key in signalling epithelial/mesenchymal interactions. (For an extensive review of extracellular matrix molecules see Adams & Watt 1993.)

Growth factors and their receptors. Large families of growth factors and their receptors have been identified at the molecular level and their spatial and temporal distributions have been mapped during embryogenesis. Examples of such families include the *epidermal growth factor family* (EGF), the *transforming growth factor beta family* (TGFβ) (which includes the bone morphogenetic proteins), the *fibroblast growth factor family* (FGF), the *insulin-like growth factor family* (IGFs), the *platelet derived growth factor family* (PDGF), etc. Growth factors can (despite their name) signal a wide variety of cellular effects, including stimulation or inhibition of growth, differentiation, migration, etc. (Sporn & Roberts 1990). Because each family of growth factors is so large, and because there are a similarly extensive number of receptors, the possible signalling combinations are considerable. Often, a single growth factor can bind with varying affinities to individual receptor family members. Some of these receptors are monogamous, recognizing only one

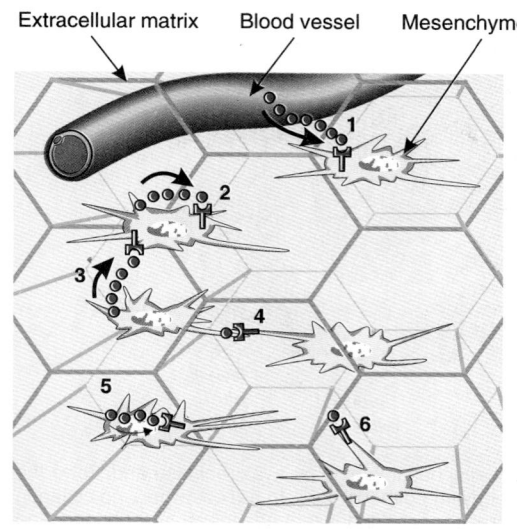

Extracellular matrix   Blood vessel   Mesenchyme cell

1   **Endocrine**   Delivery of growth factor by the bloodstream from a distant biosynthetic site to the target mesenchyme cell.

2   **Autocrine**   Synthesis of growth factor by the cell, its secretion, binding and activation of a surface receptor elsewhere on its own surface.

3   **Paracrine**   Synthesis of growth factor by the cell, its secretion and diffusion to an adjacent cell (or group of cells) where it binds to and activates a cell surface receptor.

4   **Juxtacrine**   Synthesis of growth factor by the cell. The growth factor remains on the cell surface and binds to and activates a receptor on an immediately adjacent cell.

5   **Intracrine**   Synthesis of growth factor within the cytoplasm of the cell. The growth factor moves to the nucleus and binds and activates its own nuclear receptors.

6   **Matricrine**   Synthesis and export of growth factor from the cell. The growth factor binds to the extracellular matrix where it remains active and subsequently binds to and activates a receptor for that growth factor on the same or a different cell.

3.10   Cells can also communicate by the reception, production and secretion of *growth factors*. A typical embryonic mesenchyme cell could receive and produce growth factors in this way.

isoform, whereas others are polygamous, recognizing all isoforms. The effects of any individual growth factor may therefore depend on which receptor isoform, or ratio of isoform receptors, are displayed on the cell surface. It is now clear that developmental information resides, not in any single molecule, but rather in the combination of molecules to which a cell is exposed. Thus, varying combinations of growth factors in varying concentrations can elicit quite different effects on similar cells (Jessell & Melton 1992).

Examples of the importance of growth factors in embryonic signalling are mentioned throughout the section in the context of the development of the individual systems where this is appropriate. Two examples are given here. Members of the FGF family and TGFβ family (principally *activins*) are involved in signalling mesoblast induction (Jessell & Melton 1992). For example, isolated amphibian blastocoele roofs (termed, animals caps) treated with activin form dorsomedial mesoderm structures whereas treatment with FGF results in ventral components; activin alone (in the absence of hypoblast) will induce primitive streak formation in the chick epiblast. Palatal differentiation into nasal pseudostratified ciliated columnar cells, oral stratified squamous cells or medial edge epithelial cell adhesion and migration by the underlying mesenchyme appears to be signalled by a variety of growth factors, for example *transforming growth factor alpha* (TGFa) (Dixon et al 1991), TGFβ1, 2 and 3 (Brunet et al 1994), IGFII (Ferguson et al 1992), FGF1 and 2 (Sharpe et al 1992).

Growth factors can be delivered to and act upon cells in a variety of fashions: *endocrine, autocrine, paracrine, intracrine, juxtacrine* and *matricrine* (**3**.10). Interestingly, many growth factors are secreted in a latent form, for example associated with a propeptide (latency associated peptide) in the case of TGFβ (Miyazono et al 1993; Taipale et al 1994) or attached to a binding protein, in the case of IGFs. Activity of the growth factor is dependent on dissociation from the binding protein or the latency associated protein, and therefore post-translational mechanisms of growth factor activation represent a critical control point for growth factor activity. Such activation mechanisms may involve *specific proteases* and/or *conformational changes* in the latency associated complex, by binding, for example, to a different receptor (in the case of TGFβ, binding of mannose-6-phosphate residues on the latency associated peptide, to the mannose-6-phosphate/IGFII receptor; Taipale et al 1994).

The specific activity of various growth factors may equally depend on stabilization of the growth factor at the receptor by an accessory molecule. A good example of this is the delivery and stabilization of the activity of FGF2 by heparin sulphate proteoglycan (Walker et al 1994). Such complexity in the signalling system means that for

most developing organs, there is at present only a rudimentary knowledge of the specifics of which combinations of signals give rise to which kinds of differentiation.

The diverse range of growth factors and their receptors, and their importance in developmental processes has been discussed by Ferguson (1994). He argues that the numerous growth factors and their receptors interact to give a smooth temporal integration of developmental events. Thus one growth factor may alter the synthesis of another growth factor, or its receptor (Sharpe et al 1992). If the signalling systems are both hierarchical and functionally redundant, with each developmental event having a window of operational viability that may be achieved by a principal mechanism with a number of parallel backup mechanisms, then, if there were a disturbance in any one system its effects would be minimized by a parallel backup system. Thus whilst one main mechanism for developmental processes might be sought, this may not necessarily be the way that evolution has optimized embryonic development. Survival of the embryo may be considered the driving force behind evolution, with generation of phenotypic variation also an important phylogenetic force. Ferguson suggests that both of these may be achieved by utilizing developmental mechanisms which are quite slack, with appropriate backups, or self-balancing programmes, which ensure smooth development of the embryo, its survival and the generation of variation.

Thus it seems that epithelial and mesenchymal cell populations can structure the space around them by secretion of particular matrix molecules or growth factors which can in turn organize the cells that contact them. The extracellular matrix is structured rather than random so that cell–matrix interactions and matrix–cell interactions control: the position of migration routes; whether cells migrate or not; whether cells begin differentiation or not. Matrix molecules thus propagate developmental instructions from cell to cell forming a far-reaching four- (spatial and temporal) dimensional communication mechanism.

MORPHOGENESIS AND PATTERN FORMATION

Morphogenesis may be described as the assumption of form by the whole, or part, of a developing embryo. As a term it is used to denote the movement of cell populations and the changing shape of an embryo particularly during early development. The most obvious examples of morphogenesis are the large migrations occurring during gastrulation; however, local examples include *branching morphogenesis*.

The development of branches from a tubular duct occur over a period of time. In this case an interaction between the proliferating

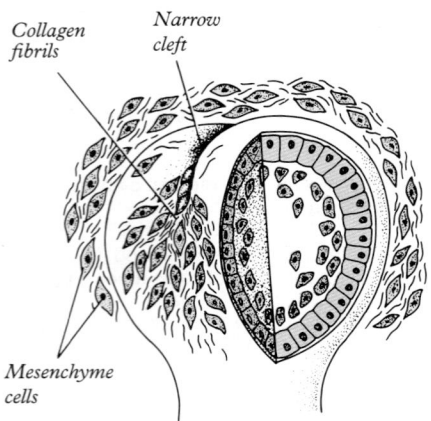

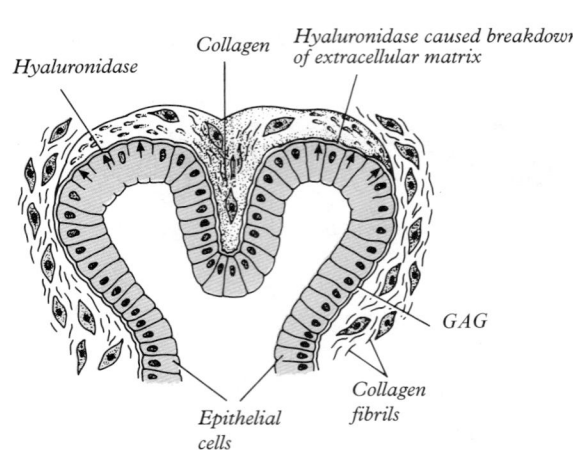

3.11   Branching of a tubular duct may occur as a result of an interaction between the proliferating epithelium of the duct and its surrounding mesenchyme and extracellular matrix. Mesenchymal cells initiate cleft formation by producing collagen III fibrils locally within the development clefts and hyaluronidase over other parts of the epithelium. Collagen III prevents local degradation of the epithelial basal lamina by hyaluronidase and slows the rate of mitosis of the overlying epithelial cells. In regions where no collagen III is produced, hyaluronidase breaks down the epithelial basal lamina and locally increases epithelial mitoses forming an expanded acinus. (From Gilbert 1991 with permission.)

epithelium of the duct and its surrounding mesenchyme and extracellular matrix results in a series of clefts which produce a characteristic branching pattern (**3**.11). Normally during tubular and acinar development hyaluronidase secreted by the underlying mesenchymal cells breaks down the basal lamina produced by the epithelial cells and this locally increases epithelial mitoses forming an expanding acinus. The mesenchyme then initiates cleft formation by producing collagen III fibrils within the putative clefts. (If the collagen is removed no clefts develop; if excess collagen is not removed, supernumerary clefts appear.) The collagen acts to protect the basal lamina from the effects of the hyaluronidase and thus the overlying epithelia have a locally reduced mitotic rate. The region of rapid mitoses at the tip of the acinus is thus split into two and two branches develop from this point. This mechanism of branching morphogenesis is seen throughout the systems, from lungs to kidney and including most glandular organs.

Pattern formation concerns the processes whereby the individual members of a mass of cells, initially apparently homogeneous, follow a number of **different** avenues of differentiation precisely related to each other in an orderly manner in space and time. The 'patterns' embraced by the term apply not only to regions of regular geometrical order, for example the crystalline lens, but also to asymmetrical structures such as the tetrapod limb. For such a process to occur individual cells must be informed of their position within the embryo and utilize that information for appropriate differentiation; thus *positional information* is a fundamental concept for explaining mechanisms of pattern formation (Wolpert 1989). The picturesque model adopted to present this hypothesis is the so-called 'French Flag Problem' (**3**.12). In this a line of communicating cells are considered to have three possibilities for differentiation: blue, white or red, and they form a correctly proportioned French Flag whatever the number of cells in the line and even if parts of the original line are removed. It is assumed that each cell is assigned a positional value by appropriate signals with respect to boundaries at the ends of the line (**3**.12). Such a hypothesis does not only explain proportionate differentiation, but also epimorphic and morphallaxic regeneration (see above). Thus positional information provides a unifying concept for understanding the development and regulation of a variety of patterns. The same signals and positional values may be used to specify different patterns; the differences arising from both developmental history and/or genetic constitution.

The essential features of a co-ordinate system to establish positional information are, *boundaries* with respect to which position is specified; a *scalar* which gives a measure of distance from the

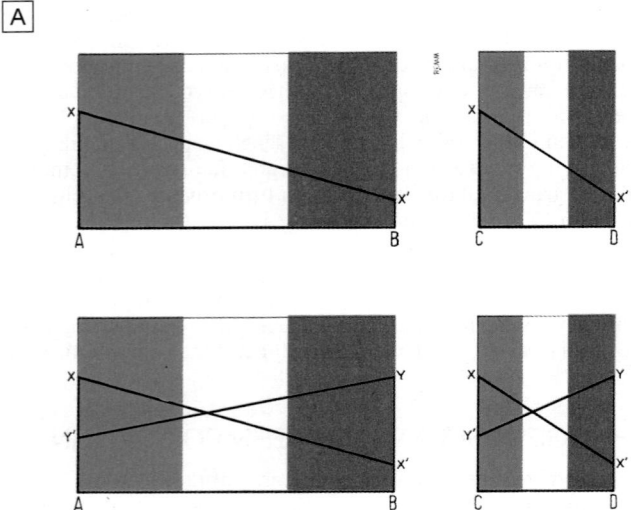

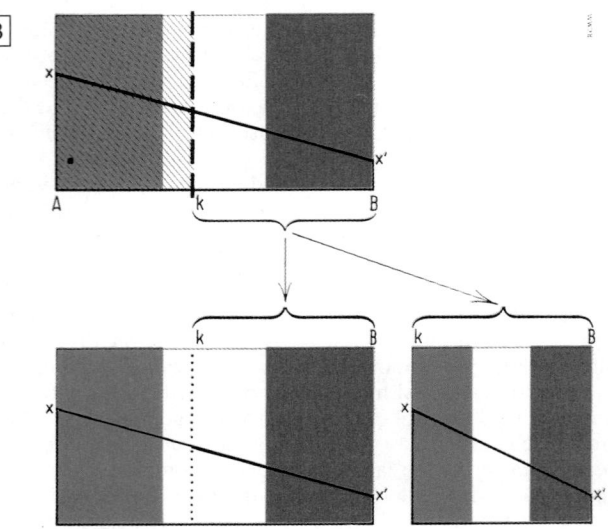

3.12A   Diagram illustrating one hypothesis concerning positional information in relation to pattern formation, by reference to the so-called 'French Flag' problem. A–B and C–D indicate long and short rows of cells respectively, X, X' and Y, Y' the concentrations of morphogenetically active substances. Above: X–X' shows the gradient of a single substance; below: X–X' and Y–Y' the gradients of two substances. In each case a similar triple differentiation occurs. See text for discussion. (Modified from and provided by L Wolpert 1971 a,b, 1978.)

3.12B   Diagram using the 'French Flag' analogy to illustrate application of the hypothesis of positional information advanced to explain regeneration, after ablation (cross-hatch) of part of an array of cells, either by morphallaxis (right) or by epimorphosis (left).

boundary; and *polarity* which specifies the direction in which position is measured from the boundary (Wolpert 1989). For a one-dimensional system, all the necessary features can be provided by a monotonic decrease in the concentration of a chemical (a morphogen), which could be set up with a localized source or by reaction diffusion. The concentration of chemical at any point then provides a scale or a measure of distance from the boundary and the slope of the concentration gradient effectively provides the polarity. Nearly all positional fields are small, none being longer than about 1 mm in maximum linear dimension, or about 50 cell diameters (most are much smaller). The time required to specify position appears to be in the order of hours (Wolpert 1989).

The term *morphogen* (first used by Turing 1952) was originally used in relation to pattern formation; the distribution of a morphogen reflected the resulting overt pattern. Its use has now been extended to include a concentration gradient that specifies position (as above), i.e. a *positional* signal (Wolpert 1989). This definition clearly distinguishes between a positional signal (morphogen) and an induction signal (see above) as the latter does not specify pattern. Differences between these types of signal (as discussed by Wolpert 1989) are as follows:

Positional signal	Inductive signal
Involves same or different tissues	Interaction between two different tissues
Specification of multiple cell states	Specification of one cell state
Graded response	All or none response
Larger range signal	Shorter range signal
Polarity	No polarity
Provided by or linked to boundary region	Relation to boundaries variable
Instructive	Instructive or permissive

The best example of a morphogen is the graded distribution of the protein encoded by the *bicoid* gene, which is the key regulator for patterning along the cephalocaudal axis of the Drosophila embryo (Nusslein-Volhard 1991; Lawrence 1992). The *goosecoid* gene (named because of its similarities to the Drosophila gooseberry and bicoid genes) serves the same function in vertebrate embryos (De Robertis et al 1992), and has been demonstrated in *Xenopus* and mouse (see p. 143). In vertebrates, *retinoids* (vitamin A derivatives) represent a major class of non-peptide growth factor signals that best fulfil the criteria for morphogens (Jessell & Melton 1992). In development of the limb (see p. 291) transplantation of the zone of polarizing activity from the postaxial border of the limb bud to the preaxial border results in mirror image skeletal duplication. This effect can be mimicked by applying retinoic acid to the preaxial mesenchyme (Tickle et al 1982), leading to the hypothesis that retinoic acid is the *endogenous polarizing signal* in the limb. It has been suggested that it acts by stimulating the local synthesis of TGFβ family members particularly BMP2 (Francis et al 1994).

THE MOLECULAR CONTROL OF EMBRYONIC MORPHOLOGY

Two related themes have emerged recently that have revolutionized our understanding of developmental processes: (1) that the control of embryonic morphology has been highly conserved in evolution between vertebrates and invertebrates; (2) that this control involves families of genes coding for proteins that act as transcriptional regulators.

Homeobox

The fruit fly Drosophila possesses eight *homeotic genes* which specify the structures developing on each body segment. There are two regions on Drosophila chromosome 3 that contain these genes: one region, the *Antennapedia complex* (*ANT-C*), contains five genes; the second, *Bithorax complex* (*BX-C*), contains three. The existence of these genes was determined by the study of *homeotic mutations* which result in conversion of one body part of the fly to another, for example legs developing on the head in place of antennae. The

mutations involved single genes which, when cloned, all had a highly conserved sequence of 183 base pairs (bp), coding for 61 amino acids at the C-terminus of the protein. This sequence was termed the *homeobox*. Investigation of its structure revealed that it formed a region in the protein that bound to DNA (reviewed by Scott 1989). One of the intriguing features of the homeotic genes is that the linear order of each gene, from the 3' end to the 5' end, is the same as its expression, along the cephalocaudal axis of the embryo, a feature referred to as *collinearity*. Further analysis of genes involved in the control of segmentation in the fly showed that many of them also contain homeobox sequences but with little else in common. Thus, many of the genes known from mutations to be essential for normal embryonic morphology had one small region in common (the homeobox) that codes for a DNA-binding function. This suggests that embryonic morphology in Drosophila is controlled overall by DNA-binding proteins that function as transcriptional regulators, controlling the expression of other genes. These other genes might consist of genes encoding structural proteins, growth factors, cell adhesion molecules, signalling molecules, cell surface proteins, extra-cellular matrix proteins, enzymes, etc. that act in concert to generate tissue morphogenesis.

Vertebrate *Hox* genes

The identification of genes containing homeoboxes in vertebrates raised the possibility that such genes might have similar functions in vertebrate embryos as in invertebrate embryos, assuming that evolutionary conservation of the homeobox implies an important role. Currently, 38 genes containing homeoboxes are known in mammals, and all show a high degree of similarity with the homeoboxes of the Drosophila homeotic genes. These genes are called *Hox* (murine) or *HOX* (human) and are found in four *clusters* known as A (mouse chromosome 6, human chromosome 7), B (mouse chromosome 11, human chromosome 17), C (mouse chromosome 15, human chromosome 12), and D (mouse chromosome 2, human chromosome 2). The *Hox* genes are numbered from 1 to 13, with 1 corresponding to a cephalic gene and 13 a more caudally placed gene. *Hox a-6*, *Hox b-6*, *Hox c-6* and *Hox d-6* are located at the same relative positions in their respective clusters and are referred to as a *paralogous group* (**3**.13) (Scott 1992).

It should be noted that an earlier nomenclature of *Hox* genes reflected their order of discovery rather than any logical system. The nomenclature described above was recommended by the Mouse and Human Gene Mapping Nomenclature Committees (Scott 1992). It provides a system that identifies all the *Hox* genes in their relative positions and allows some flexibility for the discovery of genes in other vertebrates. The Nomenclature Committee also noted that the term *Hox* should be used only for vertebrate genes related to the Drosophila *ANT-C* and *BX-C* gene clusters, by position in a complex, and by their sequence and expression along the cephalocaudal axis. Sequence similarity alone would not qualify for the use of the *Hox* name. Thus genes previously termed *Hox-7* and *Hox-8* are renamed *Ms x-1* and *Ms x-2* respectively.

All *Hox* genes have a number of features in common: they all have homeoboxes at their 3' ends that are related to Drosophila homeotic gene homeoboxes; they all have a single small intron of around 1 kb with the homeobox being in the second exon; they are all transcribed in the same direction; and they are all expressed in the embryonic nervous system, somites and limbs.

The outstanding feature of the *Hox* genes is their remarkable *conservation* with the fly homeotic genes. Based on amino acid sequence and cluster position, each paralogous group of *Hox* genes can be traced to a Drosophila homeotic gene. Thus, the *Hox* genes are *phylogenetically* related to the homeotic genes and have arisen via duplication of an original ancestral invertebrate cluster. Even more remarkable is that the collinearity of homeotic gene position and embryonic expression is also the same for *Hox* genes. Thus, the closer to the 3' end a gene is in a cluster, the more cephalic is its expression in the embryo (**3**.13). Paralogous genes, being related to the same ancestral gene, show similar cephalic expression domains, but interestingly have different dorsoventral domains in the developing CNS.

The level of evolutionary conservation between homeotic and *Hox* genes implies that they have similar functions and thus *Hox* genes might function to control morphology in mammalian embryogenesis.

115

Direct manipulation of *Hox* gene expression in murine embryos has shown this to be the case (see below).

Hox codes

Hox genes are expressed in developing ectodermal structures, such as the rhombomeres and neural crest, in a wide variety of mesenchymally derived organs such as the somites, heart, kidney, testis, etc. but not in any endodermally derived structures. The striking feature of *Hox* expression is that the genes have overlapping expression domains but with very distinct cephalic boundaries. Thus, at any point along the cephalocaudal axis of the embryo, cells of the CNS and paraxial mesenchyme (which later forms somites) have a characteristic complement of *Hox* gene expression. This complement of *Hox* genes (homeoproteins) is believed to form an *axial code* (*Hox code*) that specifies position along the cephalocaudal axis.

Hox codes have been identified in four different locations in the embryo:

- an *axial code*, specifying somites (Kessel & Gruss 1991)
- a *branchial code* specifying neuronal and neural crest development in the branchial region (Hunt & Krumlauf 1991; Hunt et al 1991a)
- an *organogenesis code* (a variation of the axial code) (Gaunt et al 1988)
- a *limb code* (Dollé et al 1989).

In all these regions, the overlapping domains of *Hox* gene expression have been interpreted as providing specific positional information (**3**.14). For example, in the hindbrain the cranial boundaries of expression of *Hox* genes correspond to the morphological boundaries, the rhombomeres (**3**.14A). The expression of *Hox* genes

in the rhombomeric neuroepithelium is believed to specify the rhombomeres and pattern the resulting motor neurons. This *Hox* gene expression is also carried over into the cranial neural crest cells according to their position of origin, imparting upon them positional information which will be used to determine their ultimate fates (**3**.14B; Hunt et al 1991b). (For further description of *Hox* gene expression in the rhombomeres see p. 228.)

The importance of the axial code in specification of somites is suggested by disruption of the *Hox c-8* gene which results in a transformation of the first lumbar vertebra into an extra thoracic vertebra (T14) complete with ribs (Le Mouellic et al 1992). In developing avian limb buds, ectopic expression of *Hox d-11* results in disruption of the digit pattern (Morgan et al 1992). This is most evident in the leg when *Hox d-11* is ectopically expressed in more preaxial regions resulting in a preaxial toe that looks like the adjacent index toe (Morgan et al 1992).

Retinoic acid and *Hox* codes

The teratogenic effects of retinoic acid (a derivative of vitamin A) have been extensively studied for over 25 years. Embryos (human and rodent) exposed to excess retinoic acid show abnormalities of many different organs, the most striking being craniofacial and limb defects (reviewed by Morris-Kay 1993). The most intriguing feature of craniofacial retinoic acid teratogenesis is that the abnormalities produced appear to originate from abnormal development of the hindbrain. This, together with the fact that *Hox* gene expression in cultures of embryonic carcinoma cells is sensitive to exogenous retinoic acid concentration, led to the conclusion that retinoic acid exerts its teratogenic effects on craniofacial development by par-

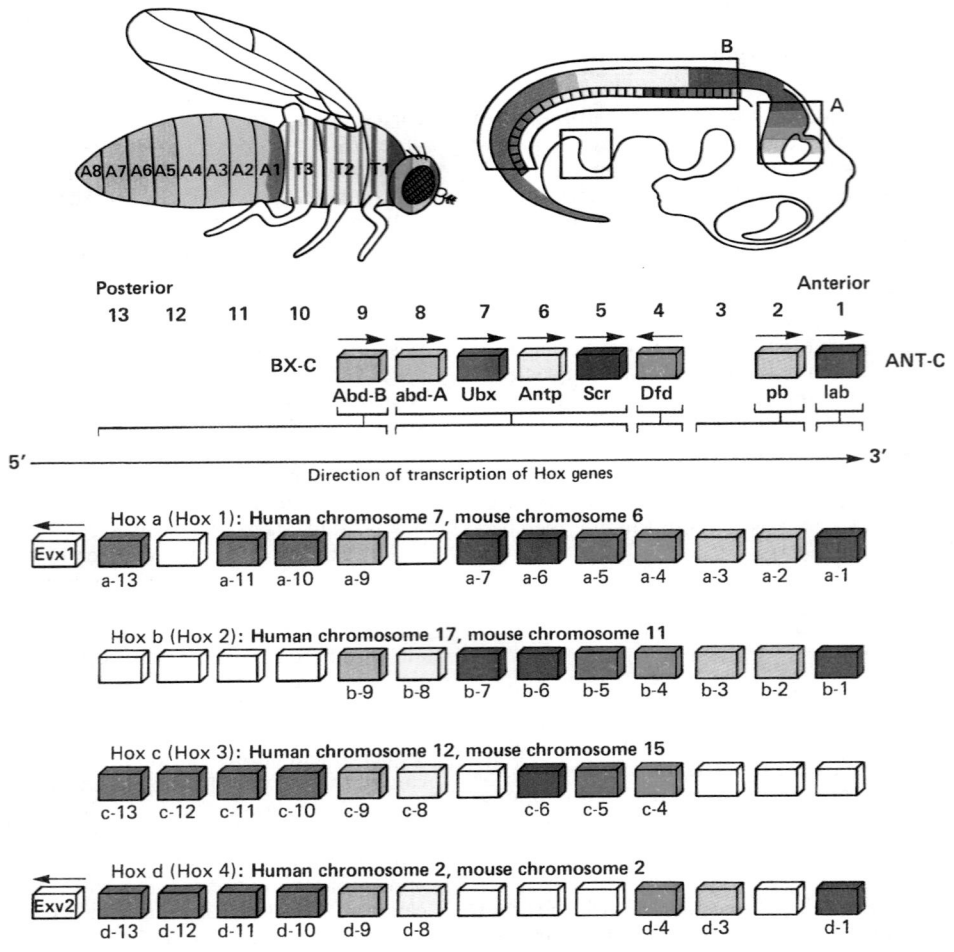

3.13   The mammalian *Hox* and *Drosophila* HOM-C gene complexes. This shows diagrammatically the relationships between the *Drosophila* homeotic (HOM-C) genes and the mammalian *Hox* genes. The genes are represented by boxes which are coloured to indicate evolutionary-related genes. The colours are also transposed onto the adult fly and midgestation stage mammalian embryo to represent their expression domains and show the evidence for colinearity.

The boxes A, B and C on the mammalian embryo are the regions enlarged in **3**.14. (Adapted from Coletta et al 1994.)

ticularly altering *Hox* gene expression (Simeone et al 1990). Retinoic acid induces a transformation of rhombomeres 2/3 into a 4/5 identity, with a corresponding transformation of the trigeminal motor cranial nerve into a facial motor cranial nerve (Marshall et al 1992). Neural crest cells derived from rhombomeres 2/3 also appear caudalized since they express *Hox* genes corresponding to 4/5.

Similar effects of excess retinoic acid on vertebral and limb development are also consistent with its affecting *Hox* gene expression and disrupting the *Hox* code. Caudal transformations of vertebrae along the complete body axis observed with retinoic acid administration are postulated to result from alteration of *Hox* gene expression (Kessel & Gruss 1991).

The limb *Hox* code with respect to the digit pattern consists of overlapping domains of the caudal *Hox d* genes (*Hox d-9–d-13*) (see p. 293 and **3.14B**). Implantation of retinoic acid soaked beads into the preaxial margin of the developing limb results in a mirror-image duplication of the digit pattern (see above) and duplication, in a mirror fashion, of the expression of *Hox d* genes consistent with their role in determining the digit pattern (Izpisua-Belmonte et al 1991).

Non-*Hox* homeobox genes

It is now clear that the *Hox* genes represent only one particular group of genes having homeoboxes and that there are many more homeobox genes that are **not** clustered and which are only related to *Hox* genes by virtue of having a homeobox. These homeobox genes are called by a variety of names, for example *Msx, Mox, Dlx, Otx*, Cdx, *Emx, Goosecoid*, etc.; they have widely varied expression patterns in embryos. The common feature of these genes is that on the whole their expression is unrelated to the cephalocaudal expression of

the *Hox* genes and they are often highly restricted to particular cells in developing organs. Whether any of these genes produce 'codes' for development of individual organs remains to be seen. Many of these genes, in common with *Hox* genes, are related to individual Drosophila homeobox genes but in vertebrates they are duplicated to varying extents. Thus, Drosophila has a single muscle specific homeobox (*msh*) gene, whereas mammals have three *msh*-related genes, *Ms x-1*, *Ms x-2* and *Ms x-3* (Hill et al 1989; Robert et al 1989; Holland 1991; MacKenzie et al 1991, 1992). Similarly, the Drosophila *distalless* gene has at least five related genes (*Dl x-1–5*) in mammals (Cohen et al 1989; Price et al 1991; Porteus et al 1991; Robinson et al 1991). It is probable that duplication of these genes occurred progressively during evolution of more complex body plans again demonstrating a link between morphology and homeobox genes.

Pax genes

Pax genes belong to a family of morphogenetic regulatory genes, initially identified by homology to the Drosophila segmentation gene '*paired*', which encodes DNA binding transcription factors (reviewed by Hastie 1991; Gruss & Walther 1992). A total of 9 genes have so far been identified containing this '*paired*'-box (a sequence seen in the '*paired*' gene), and four of this group also contain a homeobox (Walther et al 1991; Stapleton et al 1993). *PAX* genes have proved to be particularly interesting, largely because at least two of them, *PAX-3* and *PAX-6*, have been shown to be the genes that are mutated in two human genetic diseases, Waardenburg's syndrome (Baldwin et al 1992; Tassabehji et al 1992) and aniridia (Ton et al 1991; Jordan et al 1992) respectively. Waardenburg's syndrome is responsible for 2–3% of total congenital deafness and accompanying

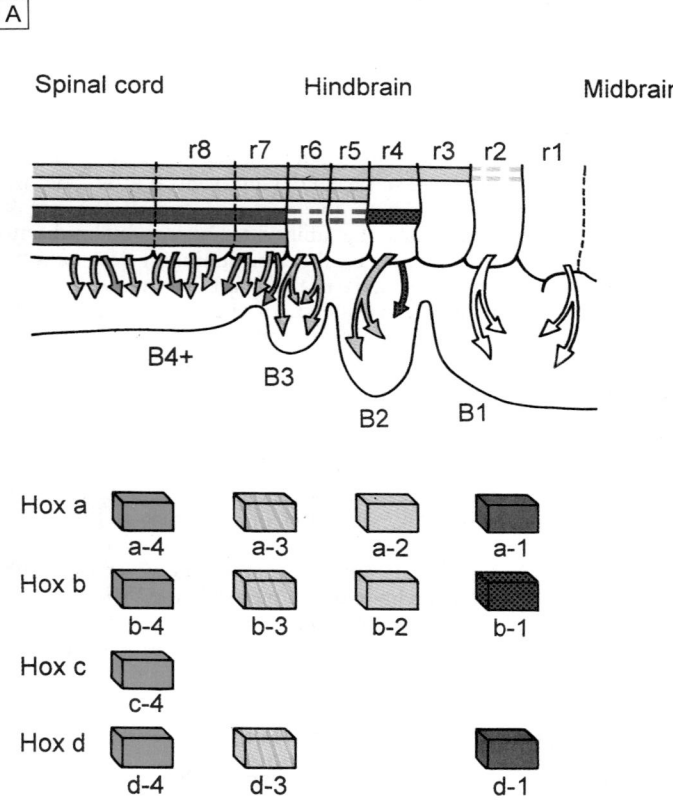

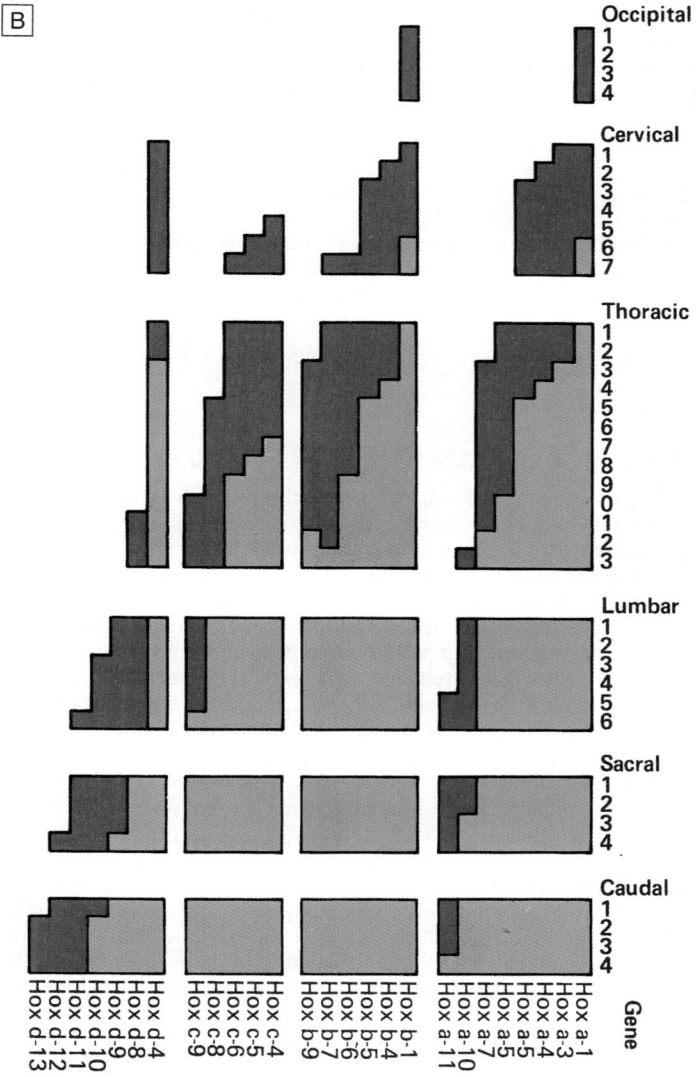

3.14A The branchial *Hox* code. Expression of the *Hox* genes in the developing hindbrain neuroectoderm is transferred to the migrating neural crest cells according to the position from which they originate. Thus the development of the structures derived from branchial arches 2–4 + may be specified by the combination of *Hox* genes expressed in the neural crest cells. Note that no *Hox* genes are expressed in neural crest cells that form the first pharyngeal arch.

3.14B The principle of this code is that different anterior-posterior domains of *Hox* gene expression in the somites (developing prevertebrae) specify a code which determined vertebral development. (Adapted from Kessel & Gruss 1991.)

features include dystopic canthorum and pigmentary disturbances such as frontal white blaze of hair (a disruption of neural crest cell development). The aniridia phenotype has a failure of iris development and abnormal retinal development. Both these conditions are autosomal dominant. Both syndromes have equivalent mutations in mice, namely *Splotch* (Waardenburg) and *Small eye* (aniridia) caused by mutations in the *Pax-3* (Epstein et al 1991) and *Pax-6* genes respectively. In common with the transgenic mutations in *Hox* genes, the *Pax* mutations only produce abnormalities in a *subset* of tissues where they are expressed. Thus, although both genes are expressed in the developing CNS, no major abnormalities are seen here in the mutants.

Transgenics, gene knock-outs and functional redundancy

A method for investigating the function of a particular gene during development is to knock out the gene using deletional mutations in embryonic stem cells, followed by the production of embryonic chimeras and subsequently transgenic animals carrying the null phenotype. A variation on such an approach is to construct a transgenic animal in which manipulation of the promoter region of the gene results in expression either in the wrong place and/or at the wrong time. As integration of exogenous genetic constructs within the genome is somewhat random, occasionally the construct inserts at a position where it disrupts an important host gene, thus creating an insertional mutant. In such mutants the inserted DNA acts as a marker so that subsequent cloning of the region surrounding it reveals the important host gene, for example in the case of x-linked cleft palate (Wilson et al 1993).

The function of a developmental gene can also be inferred from the distribution of its protein (as revealed by immunolocalization) or messenger RNA (as revealed by in situ hybridization) or by functional studies (such as addition or deletion of the gene product). In several instances, targeted disruption of a gene using transgenic knock-out approaches produces a phenotype similar to the one predicted from such expression studies (Satokata & Maas 1994). Other targeted inactivations result in early embryonic death, as clearly the gene product is required for early embryonic development: this can often be avoided by expressing the transgene from a tissue-specific promoter, which is active later in development (Werner et al 1993). However, one astonishing theme appears to be emerging, namely that the disruption of a supposedly important gene frequently produces a minimal or null phenotype, and apparently normal animals are born (Erickson 1993; Ferguson 1994).

GENERATION OF THE EMBRYONIC BODY PLAN

SPECIFICATION OF THE BODY AXES

Embryos may be considered to be constructed with three orthogonal spatial axes, plus a further temporal axis. In anamniotes the mechanisms by which the axes of the embryo are established are to some extent understood. Dorsoventral and cephalocaudal axes are specified by changes in the zygote cytoplasm at fertilization. In mammalian embryos axes cannot be specified at such early stages and it is only after the early extraembryonic structures have been formed and the inner cell mass can be seen that *embryonic axes* can be defined.

In amniotes, the *dorsoventral axis*, described as the first axis (Gurdon 1992), has been identified by the appearance of the epiblast. In reptilian and avian embryos the blastodisc layer of cells separates into two, the upper layer of which forms the epiblast. In mammals the future epiblast can be predicted when the hollow blastocyst has formed. The inner cell mass becomes (seemingly) randomly located on the inside of the trophectoderm and forms a population of epiblast cells subjacent to the trophoblast. This region implants first. It is not known whether the trophectoderm in contact with the inner cell mass initiates implantation so that the future dorsal surface of the embryo is closest to the disrupted maternal vessels at the implantation site, or whether the inner cell mass can travel around the inside of the trophoblast to gain a position subjacent to the implantation site once implantation has commenced; the latter has been suggested as likely (O'Rahilly & Muller 1987).

It is worth reflecting at this point that the whole **initially flat** embryonic disc may be conferred with axes; however, their subsequent orientation in the folded embryo, at the body plan stage, will be utterly different. Only a circumscribed central ellipse of the early embryonic disc will form dorsal structures in the folded embryo; the remainder of the disc, to its periphery, will form lateral and ventral structures. In mammalian embryos the peripheral edge of the disc will become constricted at the umbilicus. Thus, although the appearance of part of the epiblast is noted as the specification of the dorsal surface of the embryo, the inner layer, i.e. the hypoblast, is not by default a ventral embryonic structure.

It is not until the appearance of the primitive streak that a true primary axis is conferred on the embryo, the *cephalocaudal axis*. The underlying hypoblast cells, which do not contribute to the embryo proper, induce the streak formation **and** its orientation (see p. 142). If the hypoblast at the caudal region of the embryonic disc is rotated with respect to the overlying epiblast a new streak will form according to the new orientation of the hypoblast (Azar & Eyal-Giladi 1981).

At gastrulation ingression of epiblast through the primitive streak produces a population of mesoblast cells which, by the position through which they ingress, have axial and medial or lateral characteristics assigned to them. Cells ingressing through the primitive node will give rise to (axial) notochord cells and cells of the medial halves of the somites (as well as embryonic endoderm), whereas the lateral halves of the somites and the lateral plate mesenchyme come from epiblast populations either more caudally placed in the primitive streak or ingressing later. The axial and medial populations will remain as **dorsal** structures in the folded embryo, and the surface ectoderm above them will exhibit dorsal characteristics; the lateral plate mesenchyme will become **lateral** and **ventral** after embryonic folding, and the surface ectoderm above this population will gain ventral characteristics. Dorsoventral specification of the developing limbs appears to reside in the surface ectoderm, and may be so designated at this early stage. Thus the dorsoventral axis of the *folded embryo* is also specified by the passage of epiblast cells through the primitive streak.

Presumptive head structures and prospective dorsal mesoblast are located close to each other immediately adjacent to the primitive node, whereas cells destined to be caudal and ventral arise from the lateral epiblast and converge to the posterior end of the streak. However, the mesoblast has the ability to be regionalized into different dorsoventral cell types until the beginning of neurulation.

The third and last spatial axis is the *bilateral*, or *latero-lateral axis*. This is present as a consequence of the development of the former two axes. Initially the right and left halves of the embryonic body are bilaterally symmetric and in two places on each side of the body wall (somatopleure) lateral projections, the upper and lower limbs, develop.

With the last axis in play, the temporal, modification of the embryo relative to its original axes can be seen. The segmental arrangement of the cephalocaudal axis is very obvious in the early embryo and remains in many structures in adult life; so too dorsal embryonic structures remain dorsal and undergo relatively little change. The originally midline, ventral structures, however, especially those derived from splanchnopleuric mesenchyme, such as the cardiovascular system and the gut, are subject to extensive shifts, changing from a bilaterally symmetric arrangement to a whole body that is now chiral (see below).

SEGMENTATION IN THE EMBRYO

The identification of *Hox* genes which control the development of segments of *Drosophila* embryos in vertebrate embryos provides a framework to explain the segmental structures which develop during ontogeny, many of which are to be replaced by derived non-segmental arrangements later.

The grouping of vertebrates as a separate subphylum of chordata is based on the possession of a *segmented vertebral column*. (Repeating body segments of this nature are termed *metameric* implying a repetition of basically similar structures.) Evidence suggests that the developmental processes involved in forming vertebrae may be responsible for many of the other segmentally arranged tissues and systems including the peripheral nervous system (PNS), the cardiovascular system, and, to a limited extent, the patterning of skin appendages.

Vertebrae are formed from bilateral aggregations of mesenchymal cells derived from ingression of the epiblast at gastrulation (see pp. 100, 142). The cells migrate to lie lateral to the notochord where they are termed *paraxial mesenchyme*. As the embryo begins neurulation the paraxial mesenchyme segments to form discrete populations of cells termed *somites*. Cells ingressing through the lateral edges of the primitive node form the medial halves of the somite whereas cells ingressing through the cranial portion of the primitive streak form the lateral halves (see p. 143). The mesenchymal population of each somite undergoes a transformation to epithelium, with the cells forming gap junctions. Later the original medial portion of the epithelial somite reverts to mesenchyme to become the *sclerotome*, while the lateral part remains as the *epithelial plate of the somite* (also termed dermomyotome) which acts as a germinal epithelium for myogenic cells collectively termed the *myotome*. The cephalocaudal region of the embryo corresponding to individual somites is defined as the *fundamental metameric segment*, and thus the initial myotomes are segmental.

Sclerotomal cells migrate medially to surround the notochord. At this time differences are apparent between the cranial and caudal halves of the sclerotome. The cranial portion has binding sites for peanut lectin, cytotactin and tenascin. Individual vertebrae form from a fusion of the caudal half of one somite and the cranial half of the somite below (see also p. 266). The intersomitic cleft which thus develops (fissure of von Ebner) is a boundary zone. The reorganization of the sclerotomes along these lines results in the myotome of each somite spanning two adjacent vertebrae, i.e. each *segmental* somite contributes to cranial and caudal halves of two adjacent *intersegmental* vertebrae.

The myotomes generally produce two main muscular blocks, the *epaxial muscle group* which forms sequentially arranged erector spinae muscles, and the *hypaxial muscle group* which merges into a muscle mass to form the trunk muscles of the anterolateral body wall. The limbs and tongue muscles are formed by local myogenic populations arising from the ventrolateral edge of specific somites.

Motor neurons grow out from the CNS, and, with sensory axons from the neural crest cells of the dorsal root ganglia and autonomic axons, they *preferentially* migrate through the cranial portion of each sclerotome. Thus, in higher vertebrates, the subdivision of the sclerotome is responsible for generating the segmental arrangement of the PNS and ensures the exit of the spinal nerves between the vertebrae.

Each primitive dorsal aorta gives rise to paired, *ventral segmental arteries* which supply the gut, *lateral segmental arteries* to the mesonephros and bilateral *intersegmental arteries* to the body wall. These latter vessels persist almost unchanged in the thoracic and lumbar regions as the intercostal, subcostal and lumbar arteries. The venous drainage of the body is into intersegmental veins and the azygos system.

Characteristically a somite was described as giving rise to a segmental strip of dermis supplied by a sensory spinal nerve, thus giving rise to the term *dermatome* as used in medical practice. Another use of the term, to refer to a portion of a somite, is no longer used with an analogous meaning. The epithelial plate of the somite produces mainly myogenic cells which give rise to all of the voluntary muscle of the trunk and limbs. Some cells arise from the somites which contribute to the connective tissue of the dermis superjacent to the epaxial muscles and result in the patterning of the overlying epidermis. Patterning of the epidermis of the ventral part of the trunk and of the limbs is controlled by the somatopleuric mesenchyme (see p. 291).

The nephrogenic mesenchyme (see p. 199), which develops slightly later between the somites and the coelom, has been regarded as being segmentally influenced. The pronephros of lower vertebrates develops nephrostomes and nephrocoeles (characteristically joined to the somite lumen in some cases). However, more recent studies have shown that, apart from their segmental blood supply, the functional pronephroi and mesonephroi of reptilian embryos do not appear segmentally organized (Collins 1990) (mammalian embryos do not possess a functional pronephros).

Within the head, segmentation is also seen relative to the branchiomeric arches. Here the *Hox* genes have an overlapping expression of genes which coincide with the rhombomeric boundaries in the hindbrain. Specification of the neural tube, branchiomeric motor and sensory nerves, and neural crest mesenchyme appears to be controlled by the *Hox* genes, resulting in the typical arrangement of cartilage, nerve and blood vessels seen in each arch. Patterning of the arches is controlled by the neural crest mesenchyme.

Segmentation in the head and expression of the *Hox* genes is noted rostrally only as far as the rostral end of the paraxial mesenchyme and the notochord. Structures rostral to the notochord have been termed part of the prechordal or new skull; they are extensively derived from neural crest. The most rostral portions of the brain, however, have been shown to express a range of other genes (not associated with the *Hox* codes; see p. 255); generally they seem to have a nested arrangement similar to gene expression in the limb. Other studies have demonstrated a banding pattern of lineage within the cortex, with cells respecting a line between cortical and basal forebrain (see p. 255).

Thus the basic body plan of the embryo is drawn to segmental grid lines with boundaries between the segments maintained by different expression of genes and proteins, etc. which restrict cell migration in these regions. Organogenetic processes modify this initially segmental vertebrate body plan. The development of many systems illustrates either a retention of a segmental plan (e.g. spinal nerves, see p. 226) or its local replacement (e.g. the modifications of somatic intersegmental vessels by the development of longitudinal anastomoses, see p. 318). Abnormalities may result from improper specification of segments along the cephalocaudal axis as well as failure to produce the appropriately modified segmental plan.

LATERALIZATION IN THE EMBRYO

Externally the body appears symmetric about the midline but the viscera are *asymmetric* such that the body plan is not superimposable upon its mirror image. It is a puzzle that this asymmetry is *handed* (chiral) rather than random, that is, it is almost always asymmetric in the same direction. For example, the cardiac apex is directed towards the left and the liver lies to the right. When the structure or arrangement of one or more of the laterally asymmetric organs is abnormal it is thought that errors in the specification or interpretation of left–right information may have occurred in early embryogenesis. Defects of lateralization may be responsible for some congenital anomalies of the heart, bronchial branching, lung lobation, major vessels, portal venous anatomy, the spleen and gastrointestinal mesenteric attachments. The frequent association of these anomalies with one another strengthens the view that they are due to a common defect and that this defect is one of lateralization. However, there are other defects also commonly seen with these abnormalities whose association requires a different explanation since the pathology seems to be independent of positional information. For example, pathology is seen in the lungs, ears and sinuses in *primary ciliary dyskinesia* and in the kidneys, liver and pancreas in cases of *renal-hepatic-pancreatic-dysplasia* when associated with abnormal situs (Lurie et al 1991). Another non-lateralized association is agnathia (Pauli et al 1981), which may be due to an insult occurring at the stage when both sidedness is specified and the mandible first forms.

In primary ciliary dyskinesia, the clinical manifestations of recurrent chest infection, sinusitis and male infertility are well explained by the ciliary and flagella dyskinesia (Greenstone et al 1988), but the link with abnormal situs, which appears random, is not. Afzelius (1976) suggested that orientated embryonic cilia may establish visceral handedness and cells with single cilia have been noted in embryonic tissues including the murine primitive node and early notochord (Fujimoto & Yanagisawa 1983), but these embryonic cilia are likely to be immotile. Primary ciliary dyskinesia includes a heterogeneous collection of autosomal recessive ciliary dyskinesias in which most commonly there is a defect in *dynein*, a ciliary and intracellular motor protein. This has been suggested as a candidate component in the establishment of lateralization (Brown et al 1991) but sometimes in primary ciliary dyskinesia the dynein is normal yet there may still be situs inversus. Alternatively since the orientation of cilia in this condition shows greater variance than normal (Rautiainen et al 1990) it may be that a common mechanism is responsible for both the orientation of laterally asymmetric information and also for ciliary orientation.

119

Renal-hepatic-pancreatic dysplasia is sometimes associated with abnormal situs and it may be that two closely linked genes, one perhaps associated with tubule formation and another associated with the specification of situs, have both been disrupted. Whatever the mechanism, the association of these defects with abnormal situs provides clues to the developmental biology and cautions for the paediatrician and surgeon.

Abnormal situs

In amniotes, the organs develop from a bilaterally symmetric epiblast. The first overt morphological asymmetry is a greater convexity of the right border of the midline embryonic heart tube (Patten 1922). This precedes looping, also towards the right, which places the ventricles and vessels in the correct arrangement for later function and septation. That asymmetry is first apparent in the heart may be no more than a reflection that the heart is an early organ to develop from a previously covert asymmetry; however, abnormal lateralization of the cardiac segments has unquestionably serious consequences and abnormal situs may occur in more than one segment of the heart tube. For example, there can be mirror-image dextrocardia in which all segments are inverted, or transposition of the major vessels alone, or congenitally corrected transposition, or atrial isomerism. Clinically, the site of the atrial appendages provides the best guide to the associated cardiac and vascular anomalies (Anderson et al 1990), from which the prognosis is best predicted.

Dextral looping of the embryonic heart tube is highly conserved in vertebrates, but the mechanism of looping and its consistent handedness are not understood. Conservation of the direction of looping across the phyla suggests that similar genes and mechanisms may be involved.

A normal arrangement of the cardiac atria, ventricles, vessels and viscera is referred to as *situs solitus*. However, there is no agreed terminology for patterns which include abnormally lateralized organs. The terms *situs inversus, situs inversus partialis, situs indeterminus, heterotaxy* and *asplenia/polysplenia* or *splenic syndromes* have been used, often without definition. The abnormal arrangements are so varied and include almost all permutations of sidedness of the asymmetric organs that no single term provides a satisfactory description for any one case. An unpaired asymmetric organ such as the stomach may have one of three arrangements: *solitus* (the usual arrangement), *inversus* (mirror-image arrangement), or *ambiguous* (indeterminate). With paired organs that differ morphologically from their contralateral partner, such as atria, bronchi, lung lobes, arrangement may similarly be either usual or mirror image, but in addition, a situation of symmetry can occur. For example, there may be the same number of lung lobes on each side, or both atria may have the same sidedness, as assessed by the atrial appendages, either both left- or both right-sided in appearance. Such arrangements are called *isomerisms*.

When inversion or isomerism is found, the location of individual organs, vessels, cardiac segments and defects should be documented to provide a complete description in any one case, and uninformative terminology avoided.

Aetiology of lateralization

There are both genetic and environmental influences in the aetiology of abnormal lateralization. Autosomal recessive (Arnold et al 1983), an X-linked pattern (Mathias et al 1987), and possible autosomal dominant pedigrees (Nikawa et al 1983) have been described. In animals various teratogens can cause situs inversus, sometimes alone (Fujinaga 1992) but more often with other anomalies also (Fujinaga & Baden 1991). In both humans and some strains of mice, defects of lateralization are seen amongst the congenital anomalies of offspring of diabetic pregnancies. A mitochondral source of oxygen-free radicals during gastrulation has been suggested to play a role in this aetiology (Lander & Brown 1994).

In the mouse an autosomal recessive allele *inversus viscerum* (*iv*), causes situs inversus in just under half of the homozygotes, situs solitus with the same frequency and a few isomerisms and discordant inversions (Hummel & Chapman 1959). The spectrum of anomalies is very similar to the patterns of lateralized defects seen in man, including annular pancreas and preduodenal portal vein. The cardiac and splenic anomalies seen with the atrial isomerisms (Seo et al

1992) are also similar to human defects. The *iv* mutation lies near the immunoglobulin heavy-chain-constant-region complex (Igh-C) on chromosome 12 (syntectic to human chromosome 14q3) (Brueckner et al 1989; de Meeus et al 1992).

A second mutation *inv*, also recessive, has occurred in a transgenic mouse *OVE210* in which 100% situs inversus is reported in homozygous offspring (Yokoyama et al 1993). The flanking sequences map to chromosome 4. The defect is fatal in homozygotes before 7 days postnatal and dysplasia of the liver and renal tract contribute to death. It is not yet known if this model represents the renal-hepatic-pancreatic dysplasia seen in abnormal situs in humans. If it does, it is possible that two or more closely linked genes involved in situs and in tubule development have been disrupted by the transgene.

Cellular and molecular models of lateralization

The body plan is handed, i.e. it is chiral, but as yet it is not known where *handed* information comes from or the nature of the mechanism of its expression. One model (**3**.15) suggests handedness to be signalled by an orientated chiral molecule fixed with respect to the craniocaudal and dorsoventral axes. Brown and Wolpert (1990) illustrated this with a hypothetical chiral 'F' molecule that could align its vertical limb with polar microtubules arranged in the craniocaudal direction and normally to be fixed in a frontal plane so that its arms point to a specific side. They depicted the 'F' molecule in cells that have been polarized with respect to the midline. Each cell could then establish the side of the embryo on which it is situated. This then establishes handedness at the level of the tissues. To account for situations of random handedness, as is seen in primary ciliary dyskinesia and in the *iv/iv* mouse, Brown and Wolpert proposed a means of generating a left–right gradient across the embryo at random. A homogeneous distribution of a biochemical factor across the midline could become asymmetric by amplification of thermal noise through a reaction-diffusion mechanism (Kauffman et al 1978). In normal circumstances this amplification could be biased by the handed cellular asymmetry. Organs and tissues then interpret the gradient and express their sidedness accordingly. Absence of the 'F' molecule leads to randomization of the left–right gradient and a 50% incidence of situs inversus.

The Brown-Wolpert model was elaborated to explain the observation that abnormal situs is frequently seen in the right conjoined twin. They hypothesized that once a left–right difference is established a property becomes fixed on the right, such that after bisection left–right cannot be re-established in the right twin but the labile left side can respecify to give normal situs in the left twin.

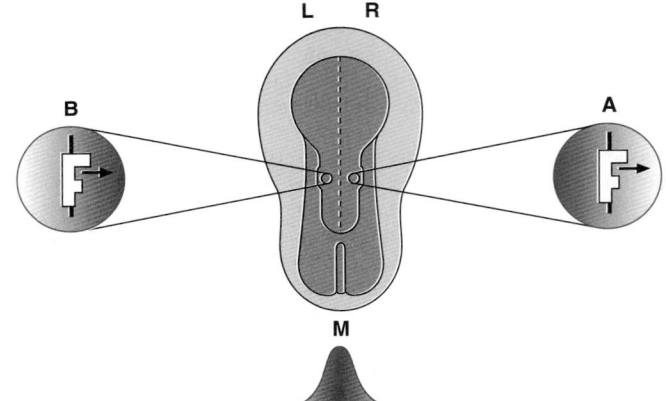

3.15 In this model cells are able to detect their own left from right with an orientated chiral molecule 'F' aligned with respect to the cephalocaudal and dorsoventral axes. The cell is also able to detect the direction of the midline by determining differences in concentration of a morphogen (M). If a cell's right-hand side is furthest from the midline the cell is on the right-hand side of the embryo (cell A), and in contrast if the cell's right-hand side is nearest the midline it is on the left-hand side of the embryo (cell B). A second mechanism is present that can amplify small random differences in some agent on one side of the midline. In this way a gradient from one side of the embryo to the other can be established at random. The cells A and B which now have different properties on the two sides are able to bias the gradient in a consistent direction. From this gradient tissues determine their situs. (Supplied by Lander & Brown.)

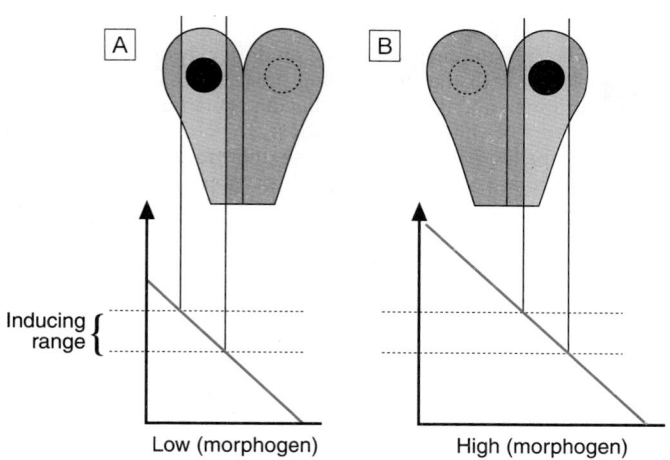

Low (morphogen)   High (morphogen)

3.16   A primary left-right gradient is established. A narrow range of sensitivity exists allowing (in A) a lateralized primordium to develop on the left-hand side. By only increasing the baseline of the gradient a lateralized primordium would develop on the opposite side (B). Inversion can therefore be generated without reversing the handedness of the primary asymmetry. (Supplied by Lander & Brown.)

A mutation leading to reversed orientation of the 'F' molecule may account for the 100% situs inversus seen in *inv/inv* mice. However, other mechanisms for producing 100% inversion without reversing the primary handed information have been proposed (Brown & Lander 1993; see **3**.16). Sequencing the genes for the normal alleles at *iv* and *inv* may illuminate steps in the establishment of situs but still may not tell us how it is specified.

Other examples of handedness

Other examples of handedness not linked with body plan handedness also occur in humans, for example handedness in cerebral dominance and hand preference. However, in these cases the incidence of left handedness in those with defects in situs is the same as in the general population. Animals are individually handed but this is random at the population level which may suggest that cerebral lateralization, important in the neurobiology of language, is quintessentially human (Corbalis 1989). Though not directly linked, similar mechanisms and homologous genes may be involved in the establishment of situs and cerebral lateralization.

That the organs are asymmetric may not be surprising but it is far from clear why or how they are asymmetric in the same direction, and why this should be so universal. It is clear that when lateralization is abnormal there are frequent cardiac, vascular, splenic and mesenteric anomalies of clinical importance. Correct lateralization seems to be of crucial importance to survival.

EARLY HUMAN DEVELOPMENT

FEMALE GAMETE

The life cycle of the mammalian oöcyte starts in early embryos, when the primordial germ cells first differentiate, and is culminated many years later when a mature cell is fertilized. The development of germ cells into fertile oöcytes can be divided into several distinct phases, including: establishing the germ cell population; oöcyte growth and meiotic maturation; and growth and development of the antral follicle (**3**.17).

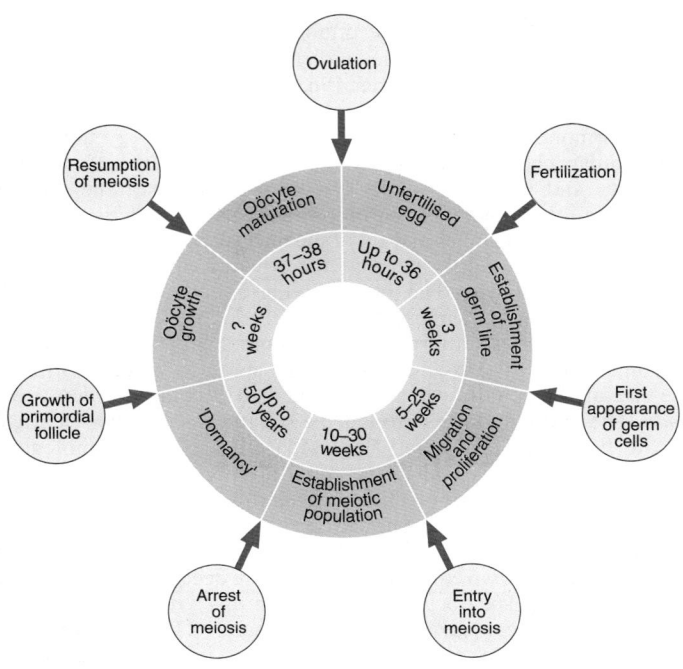

3.17   The life cycle of the human female germ cell. The approximate timings are for the human. The time taken for oöcyte growth in the human is not known but is thought to be several months. (Adapted with permission from McLaren 1988.)

Establishing the germ cell population

In mammals it is accepted that there is not a determined germ line as exists in drosophila and probably in frogs. The precise origin of the primordial germ cells in humans is not clear. In mice the germ cells are first recognized as a clump of about 40 alkaline positive cells in the extraembryonic mesoblast of 7.5 day old embryos (Ginsburg et al 1990). In humans of about 6 weeks postconception the germ cells migrate from their extragonadal site of origin to the gonadal ridges where they proliferate. By 8–10 weeks gestation about 600 000 oögonia populate the developing ovary (Baker 1963); from 12 weeks they begin their differentiation into primary oöcytes. The ovary is fully colonized in the fifth intrauterine month with maximal numbers reaching nearly 7 000 000 (Baker 1963). Primary oöcyte numbers then decrease so that by birth there are about 1 000 000 (4000 in mice) (Block 1953; Baker 1963; Baker 1972) (**3**.18). After birth a further degeneration occurs so that by puberty only 40 000 oöcytes remain (Pinkerton et al 1961) (**3**.18) and of these only 400 are ovulated during the reproductive lifespan of the female. This widespread degeneration is a feature of germ cell development in all mammals studied (Ingram 1962; Baker 1972) and appears to occur around pachytene, when crossing over takes place (see below). It has been suggested that meiotic pairing anomalies induce this atresia of fetal oöcytes (Speed 1988).

From an early time the oöcytes become enclosed by somatic cells of the fetal ovary, surrounded by a basement membrane. This forms a unit known as a *primordial follicle*. The development of the primordial follicles is the final stage in establishing the germ cell population in the ovary. As each follicle supports and nurtures the development of one oöcyte, the population of follicles established during development represent the sole irreplaceable source of oöcytes for the reproductive lifespan of the female.

Growth of the oöcyte

A primary oöcyte is distinguishable from other cells in the ovary by its large size, being about 35 μm in diameter in the human. An, as yet, unidentified signal triggers the initiation of growth of the primordial follicle. The first signs of growth are an enlargement of the oöcyte while the surrounding somatic cells, now termed *granulosa cells*, assume a cuboidal shape and begin to proliferate. The human oöcyte reaches a final diameter of 120–140 μm which represents an approximate 1000-fold increase in cell volume.

Number of germ
cells (x10^{-6})

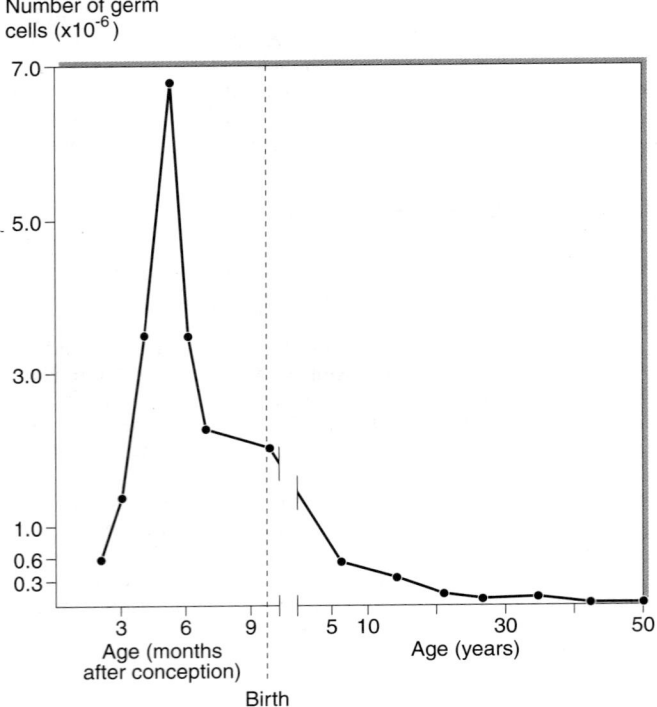

3.18 Changes in germ cell numbers in the human ovary with age. (From Baker 1972.)

Early after the initiation of oöcyte growth, patches of amorphous filamentous material appear between the oöcyte and the granulosa cells, eventually they completely surround the oöcyte forming the *zona pellucida*; its thickness increases with oöcyte growth. The zona pellucida is associated with all mammalian oöcytes, it forms a barrier, permeable to large macromolecules, between the oöcyte and the granulosa cells. Its main role appears to be at fertilization where it is responsible for the species-specific recognition of spermatozoa and also for triggering the acrosome reaction. The mouse oöcyte zona pellucida contains three glycoproteins ZP1, ZP2 and ZP3 all of which are produced by the oöcyte (Wassarman 1990 for review).

Although separated by the zona pellucida, the oöcyte and granulosa cells are dependent on the presence of each other for normal growth and differentiation. Communication between the two cell types is maintained by granulosa cell processes that pass through the zona pellucida and form gap-junctions with the plasma membrane of the oöcyte (Zamboni 1972; Anderson & Albertini 1976). Although not clearly established in the human, amino acids, other small metabolites, and regulatory molecules are known to pass between oöcytes and granulosa cells of other species (Moor et al, 1981; Heller, Cahill & Schultz 1981). This metabolic coupling allows the granulosa cells to contribute to the nutrition and regulation of the oöcyte. The oöcyte and granulosa cells are, however, interdependent and in the absence of an oöcyte the granulosa cells fail to develop further. This results in a 'streak ovary', seen in Turner's syndrome if the oöcytes degenerate, or in degenerating follicles if oöcytes are lost at later stages of folliculogenesis. Recent studies have demonstrated the importance of secreted factors from the oöcyte in regulating the proliferation and differentiation of the granulosa cells.

As the granulosa cells increase in number and form several layers, the oöcyte becomes increasingly isolated from the systemic and somatic influences of the ovary. During the growth of the follicle it becomes enveloped by a further layer of compressed, elongate cells thought to be derived from the ovarian stroma, the *theca folliculi* (**3.20**), which is separated from the granulosa cells by a basal lamina. At the time of antrum formation the theca differentiates into two layers, the *theca interna* and *theca externa*.

Cytological changes during oöcyte growth

The nucleus of the primary oöcyte is relatively large, vesicular, usually eccentric, with a prominent nucleolus (**3.**20, 21). The distinctive nature of the nucleus is reflected in the more common name *germinal vesicle*. The *oölemma* (plasma membrane) of small oöcytes is smooth and in close apposition with the surrounding pregranulosa cells. As oöcyte growth continues and the zona pellucida increases in thickness, a uniform cover of microvilli develops. In non-growing primary oöcytes, organelles are relatively sparse and are concentrated in the juxtanuclear region. As oöcyte growth progresses, the number and size of organelles increase and they disperse from the juxtanuclear zone through the cytoplasm. The Golgi apparatus is well developed and consists of parallel cisternae and numerous small vesicles; the latter also appear throughout the cytoplasm. Juxtanuclear anulate lamellae occur interspersed between spherical or slightly elongate mitochondria (Zamboni 1972). At first the endoplasmic reticulum is vesicular and displays few ribosomes which increase during oöcyte growth. Granular endoplasmic reticulum and free ribosomes, though not prominent, also increase. Lipid granules begin to appear; they are thought to correspond to the yolk platelets of earlier vertebrates but are smaller and less frequent in primates. Soon after oöcyte growth is initiated *cortical granules* begin to form from the Golgi apparatus; they are 500 nm electron dense granules, bound by a membrane (Gulyas 1980). As oöcyte growth nears completion the granules are distributed around the cortex in close proximity to the plasma membrane. The cortical granules are exocytosed at fertilization and are responsible for modifying the zona pellucida and plasma membrane to prevent further sperm penetration (Wassarman 1990).

Meiotic divisions of the oöcyte

From about 12 weeks gestation the oöcytes undergo a final series of DNA replication prior to entering the first meiotic division. Note that prophase of the first meiotic division is subdivided into five successive stages: leptotene, zygotene, pachytene, diplotene and diakinesis. During pachytene of first meiosis, the homologous chromosomes form bivalents and it is at this time that chiasmata form and recombination takes place (see p. 60). At entry into the final stage of the first meiotic prophase, *diplotene*, the pairing relaxes and the bivalents begin to separate, a process termed *desynapsis*. Oöcytes are arrested at diplotene, in the first meiotic prophase; they remain in this state, from about 20 weeks gestation, until stimulated to mature many years later. In rodents the chromatin becomes very diffuse, a state referred to as *dictyotene*. During dictyotene the bivalents separate further until they can no longer be traced, although some connections may remain. Thus the fully grown primary oöcyte contains the *diploid* number of double-stranded chromosomes and has been arrested at the diplotene (dictyotene in rodents) stage since before birth (Manotaya & Potter 1963; Ohno & Smith 1964).

The stimulation to resume meiosis is the midcycle surge of luteinizing hormone (LH; see p. 1866) which results in a number of intracellular changes first signified by the disappearance of the nucleolus and followed rapidly by the dissolution of the nuclear membrane. Homologous chromosomes have undergone condensation along the inner margin of the nuclear envelope and become arranged in homologous pairs at the equator of a spindle in the cortex of the oöcyte. The poles of the spindle in oöcytes lack centrioles and are composed of pericentriolar material (Szollozi 1972). As anaphase approaches, the homologous pairs of chromosomes move towards the poles of the spindle. A bulge forms at the site of the spindle which is destined to become the *first polar body*. The midbody forms around the spindle and initiates cleavage of the first polar body and final separation of the homologous chromosomes occurs. Unlike the equal division of the nucleus, the division of the cytoplasm is highly **unequal**, the polar body carrying with it its numerically equal chromosomal complement and an exiguous share of the cytoplasm. (The first polar body is occasionally seen to cleave into two equal fragments before degenerating sometime after ovulation.) The oöcyte resulting from this reduction division is known as the *secondary oöcyte*; it contains 23 double-stranded chromosomes (**3.**19). In the absence of an interphase the chromosomes are rearranged around the equator of a second spindle. At metaphase of the second meiotic division the secondary oöcyte arrests until fertilization or parthenogenetic activation stimulates the completion of meiosis which is marked by extrusion of the *second polar body*.

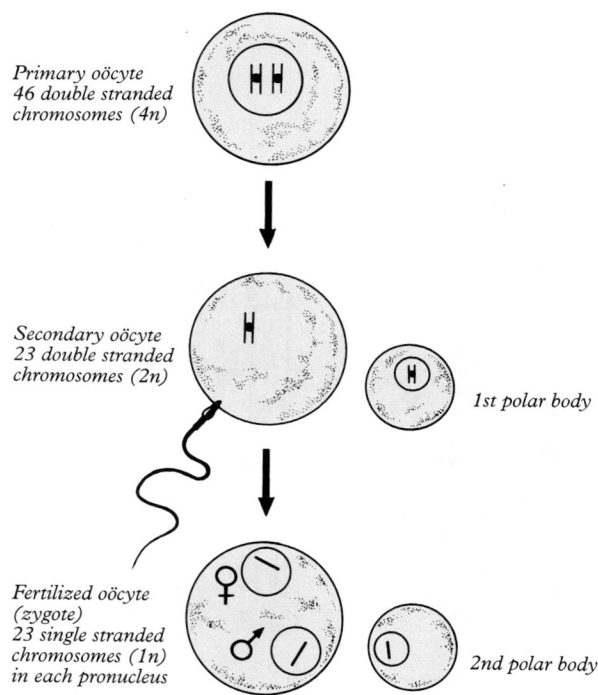

Primary oöcyte
46 double stranded
chromosomes (4n)

Secondary oöcyte
23 double stranded
chromosomes (2n)

1st polar body

Fertilized oöcyte
(zygote)
23 single stranded
chromosomes (1n)
in each pronucleus

2nd polar body

3.19   Diagram showing the reduction in the number of chromosomes during maturation of the human oöcyte. Fertilization occurs before the completion of meiosis. This is typical for most mammalian species while some invertebrates show slight differences. The first division is the reductive division. Note that during oögenesis meiosis yields only one gamete compared to 4 during spermatogenesis. For clarity, details of the events of crossing over are not included here but can be found on page 129.

The maturing primary oöcyte can produce some mRNA and rRNA. Its 'maternal' mRNA stores sustain it as it synthesizes various peptides during its final maturation from diakinesis through metaphase 1 to metaphase 2 in a period of about 37 hours. Meiotic maturation is regulated by a series of cell-cycle regulatory proteins similar to those in somatic cells. Resumption of meiosis and entry into metaphase I is associated with an increase in the activity of maturation promoting factor, a combination of $p34^{cdc2}$ and cyclin B. At exit from metaphase I and entry into the second meiotic division, there is a transient decrease in maturation promoting factor activity. Arrest of the oöcyte in metaphase II is associated with the stabilization of *maturation promoting factor* by *cytoctatic factor*, a component of which is the product of the *c-mos* proto-oncogene. Fertilization triggers the destruction of maturation promoting factor and cytoctatic factor allowing the oöcyte to re-enter the cell-cycle, resulting in completion of meiosis and entry into G_1 of the first mitotic division.

Since the sperm delivers its haploid set of chromosomes prior to the completion of meiosis, the mammalian oöcyte is **not** technically an *ovum* as it is never a haploid cell. This is different to other species, e.g. sea-urchins, where fertilization occurs after the oöcyte has extruded the second polar body and the ovum contains a single haploid pronucleus. Nevertheless, the term remains widely used for many stages of mammalian oögenesis and embryogenesis.

Development of the antral follicle and ovulation

Changes within the granulosa cell population, which form the primordial follicle, are concomitant with oöcyte growth. As the multi-laminar follicle grows, a fluid-filled antrum appears among its proliferating cells, gradually dividing them into an internal stratum, the *cumulus oöphorus*, and an external *stratum granulosum*. At one site the two populations maintain continuity (**3**.20) and are connected via an extensive network of gap-junctions (Gilula et al 1978; Larsen et al 1986). The fully grown primary oöcyte is situated in the cumulus. As the antrum expands with *liquor folliculi* (follicular fluid) the granulosa cells form an envelope around the antrum which gradually thins to about 5–6 cells (Zamboni et al 1972). The granulosa cells closest to the basement membrane are columnar in shape while those closest to the antrum are polygonal. In the granulosa cell layer there is an increasing abundance of mitochondria, granular endoplasmic reticulum and free ribosomes and their Golgi organelles become more prominent, indicating increasing steroidogenic activity. The primary oöcyte, which remains in the prolonged prophase of the first meiotic division, retains its microvilli and its complex interrelationship with the cumulus cells outside the zona pellucida (**3**.21). The cells immediately surrounding the oöcyte within the cumulus oöphorus are known as the *corona radiata*.

Ovulation is initiated by a surge of gonadotrophins which also stimulates the resumption of meiosis in the oöcyte. Just prior to ovulation, about 36 hours after the LH surge, the oöcyte extrudes the *second polar body* and arrests at metaphase of the second meiotic

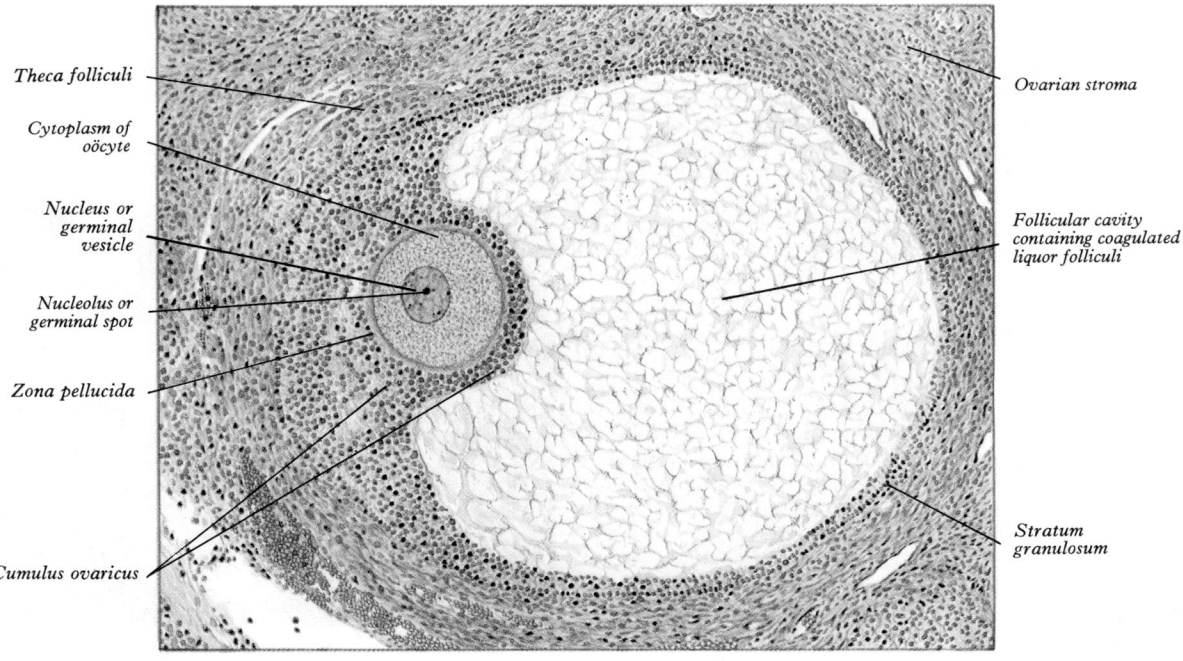

Theca folliculi

Cytoplasm of oöcyte

Nucleus or germinal vesicle

Nucleolus or germinal spot

Zona pellucida

Cumulus ovaricus

Ovarian stroma

Follicular cavity containing coagulated liquor folliculi

Stratum granulosum

3.20   Ovarian follicle from a woman aged 28 years. Haematoxylin and eosin. Magnification × c. 90.

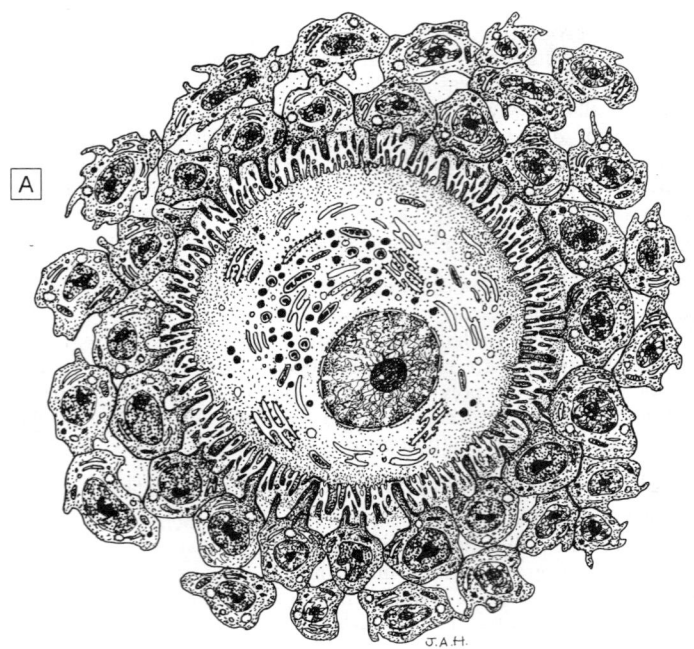

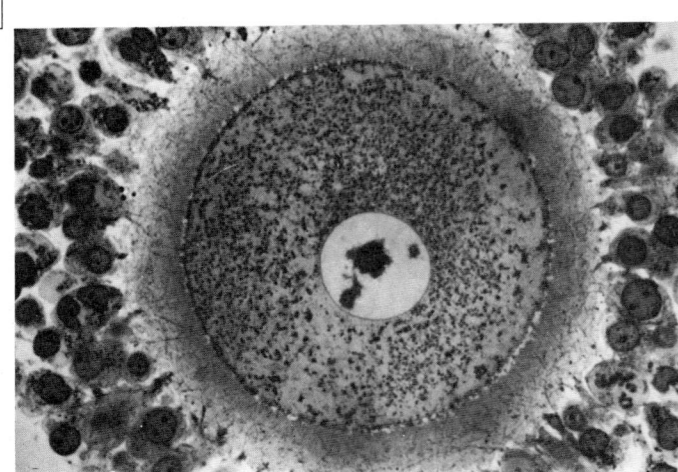

3.21A Drawing constructed from electron micrographs of a primary oöcyte surrounded by its zona pellucida, outside which are aggregated follicular cells of the corona radiata. Note extensive invasion of the zona by microvilli of the oöcyte interdigitating with cytoplasmic processes of the follicular cells. Where some of the latter approach the plasma membrane of the oöcyte, desmosomoid junctions are visible. Note the organelle-rich cytoplasm of the oöcyte. (Modified from Anderson & Beams 1960, with permission.)

3.21B Human oöcyte photographed in transverse section. Follicular cells surround it, the zona pellucida intervening. Epon-embedded, osmic-acid fixed, toluidine blue stained. Magnification × 550. (Baca & Zamboni 1967.)

division. At this stage the oöcyte is termed the *secondary oöcyte* (**3.22**) and is surrounded by a clear *perivitelline* space beneath the zona pellucida. Leading up to ovulation the processes of the cumulus cells are withdrawn from the zona. Coincident with the breakdown of the cumulus cell processes there is a decrease in gap-junctions throughout the follicle (Larsen et al 1986) and the cumulus oöphorus expands in a hyaluronic acid matrix.

Soon after the LH surge, the preovulatory follicle becomes hyperaemic and oedematous. A small area of the follicle and overlying ovarian cortex becomes thin and translucent. As ovulation ensues the surface of the ovary bulges and eventually tears, liberating the secondary oöcyte surrounded by the zona pellucida and corona radiata. The mechanism responsible for the thinning of the follicle wall is not precisely known but is thought to involve the activation of collagenolysis through increased plasmin production as well as serine proteases; acting together the tensile strength of the follicle wall is reduced and rupture occurs (Lipner 1988). The released secondary oöcyte and expanded corona radiata is rapidly collected from the peritoneal cavity by the fimbria of the oviduct and carried into the infundibulum by ciliary movements of its epithelium (Austin 1963). Unless fertilization occurs, the secondary oöcyte is discharged from the uterus in the debris of the next menstrual period: if it is fertilized, the zygote which results is retained and pregnancy begins. (For details of fertilization see p. 132.)

Oöcyte maturation in vivo and in vitro

Meiotic maturation refers to the development of the oöcyte from diplotene of meiosis I to metaphase II, where the oöcyte arrests, ready to undergo fertilization (see above). In addition to the nuclear events of maturation, the oöcyte becomes able to support the normal events of fertilization. This process is generally referred to as *cytoplasmic maturation* but very little is understood about the biochemical or molecular basis of these changes.

In vivo the preovulatory surge of gonadotrophins triggers meiotic maturation leading to germinal vesicle breakdown and progression to metaphase II (see above). Alternatively, mammalian oöcytes have the property that they can be stimulated to resume meiosis in vitro simply by removal of the oöcyte from the antral follicle (Pincus & Enzman 1935; Edwards 1965). This observation shows that the

follicle is responsible for maintaining the oöcyte in meiotic arrest, although the mechanism remains unclear. Due to the ability of cAMP to inhibit meiotic maturation in vitro (Cho et al 1974) much attention has been paid to its role as the endogenous regulator of meiotic maturation (see Schultz 1986). The signal transduction mechanisms by which the surge of gonadotrophins relieves the inhibition of meiosis is also unclear. Several mechanisms are possible. The LH surge may serve to deprive the oöcyte of inhibitory signals from the follicle, for example by causing the inhibition of gap-junctional communication. Alternatively it may generate a positive signal in the follicular cells that overrides follicular inhibition. Recent work favours the latter hypothesis since hormones can override cAMP maintained meiotic inhibition in vitro (Dekel & Beers 1978; Downs et al 1988) and because gap-junctions between the oöcyte and follicular cells remain until after meiotic maturation has resumed (Moor et al 1981; Eppig 1982).

The ability to undergo the normal events of fertilization is not a

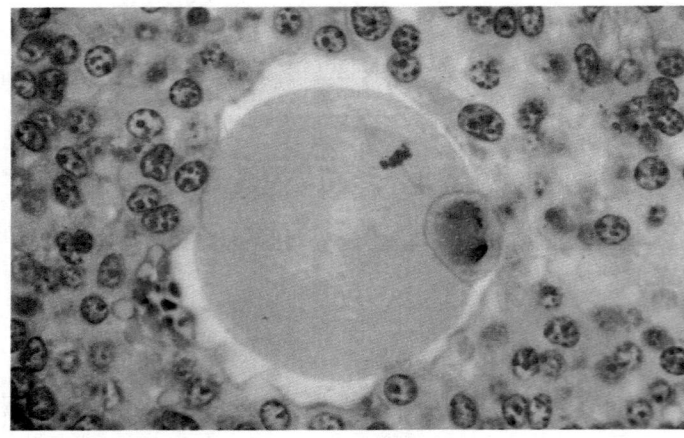

3.22 The mature secondary oöcyte surrounded by the expanded cumulus oöphorus. The chromosomes can be seen aligned on the metaphase spindle. Magnification × c. 500. (Photograph supplied by J Carroll.)

feature of all mammalian oöcytes. This property is acquired during meiotic maturation. Immature oöcytes with an intact germinal vesicle can be penetrated by sperm but fail to decondense the sperm head (Iwamatsu & Chang 1972). The ability to support full sperm head decondensation and pronuclear development is maximal once the oöcyte is arrested at metaphase II. Thus the final stages of oöcyte maturation are critical for the oöcyte to undergo fertilization and development. These changes apparently occur normally in vitro as some oöcytes matured in vitro have full development potential (Schroeder & Eppig 1984; Lu et al 1988; Cha et al 1991), although viability is generally lower than after maturation in vivo. The presence of follicle cells during meiotic maturation is necessary for normal cytoplasmic maturation (Stagmiller & Moor 1984) but the precise nature of oöcyte modifications and how they may be influenced by the somatic environment are unclear.

MALE GAMETE

Gametogenesis in the male exhibits both marked similarities and differences in comparison with the development of ova. During maturation there is the same reduction of chromosomes to the haploid number and genetic recombination, but in the testis there is a continuous formation of spermatocytes and spermatozoa during reproductive life, linked with the enormous number of gametes which are formed. In each ejaculate there are many times more spermatozoa than there are germ cells in both ovaries at their peak content before birth; whereas the latter is of the order of 10 to 12 million, a single ejaculation may contain 300 million spermatozoa, only one of which may fertilize an ovum. (The nomenclature of male gametes is not yet unified officially; spermatozoön, spermatoid, sperm and spermium are all used.)

Morphology of spermatozoa

A spermatozoön, or sperm (Rothschild 1957; Fawcett 1961a, 1975; Pikó 1969), is a smaller cell than an oöcyte, highly specialized to reach the latter and to carry to it its own haploid chromosome complement. Its expanded *caput* or *head* contains little cytoplasm and is connected by a short constricted *cervix* or *neck* to the *cauda* or *tail*. The latter is a flagellum of complex structure, usually divided into *middle*, *principal* and *end parts* or *pieces*. Volumetrically the tail much exceeds the head, which varies greatly in different species (Rothschild 1957; Phillips 1975), being ovoid or piriform in man, somewhat flattened at the tip in lateral profile, with a maximum length of about 4 μm and a maximum diameter of 3 μm. The tail, about 45–50 μm in length, displays a greater uniformity between species.

Head (3.23). This is an extreme example of chromatin concentration, consisting largely of a dense and visually uniform nucleus, with a distinct bilaminar nuclear membrane and a bilaminar *acrosomal cap* (head cap), the latter covering the terminal two-thirds of the nucleus and partly derived from the spermatid Golgi apparatus. The acrosomal cap is thin in a human spermatozoön but in other species it is often large and more complex in shape. The acrosome has been shown to contain several enzymes including acid phosphatase, hyaluronidase and a protease (*acrosomase*), which are probably involved in penetration of the oöcyte. The nucleus and acrosome are enveloped in a continuous plasma membrane without intervening cytoplasm (Fawcett & Burgos 1956; Anberg 1957). The chromatin is stabilized by disulphide bonds, as if to protect its genetic content during the spermatozoön's journey (Fawcett 1975). So densely packed is the chromatin that it appears homogeneous even under electron microscopy. It has a strong affinity for basic stains, consisting of about 40% (dry weight) deoxyribonucleic acid and a protein rich in arginine (Daoust & Clermont 1955). It is also resistant to physical stress, e.g. ultrasonication (Henle et al 1938), and to mechanical shear (Mann 1949). Defects in condensation of nuclear material may be visible under light microscopy as relatively clear areas or *nuclear vacuoles*. Attempts to discover structural details in the nucleus in a variety of species, by polarization microscopy, X-ray diffraction and freeze-fracturing techniques, have shown a lamellar structure which cannot yet be equated with chromosomal content. The human Y chromosome has been identified using fluorescence microscopy (**2.53**).

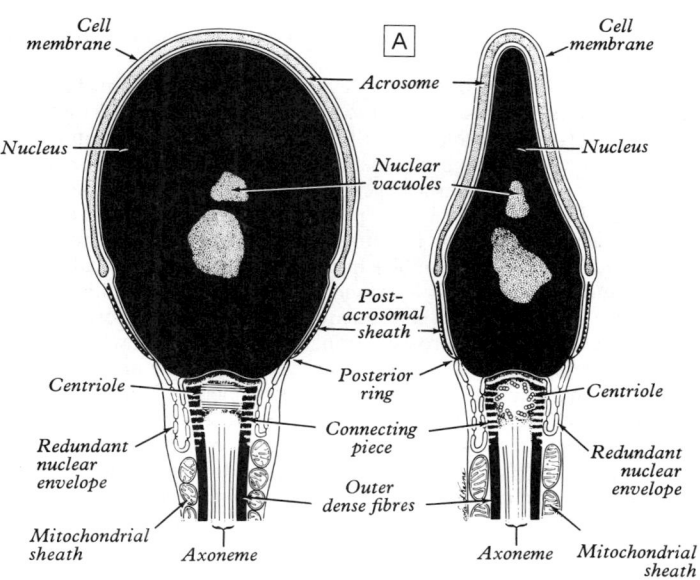

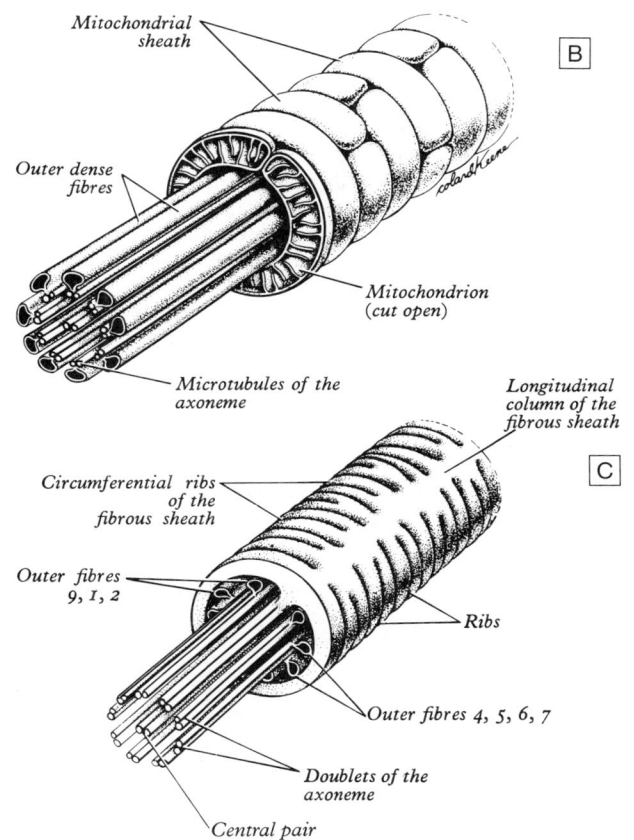

3.23 Diagrams of human spermatozoön showing: A. the head, viewed in its major (left) and minor (right) diameters; B. the middle part; C. the principal part or tail. (By courtesy of Fawcett & Hafez and C V Mosby.)

Between the head and the middle part of body of the spermatozoön is a slight constriction, the *neck*, about 0.3 μm long. In its centre (**3.23**), close to a shallow recess in the base of the nucleus, is a well-formed centriole, corresponding to the *proximal* centriole of the spermatid from which the spermatozoön differentiated (**3.25**). The axial filament complex (axoneme) is derived from the *distal* centriole, a funnel-shaped *connecting piece* or *basal body* from which the outer fibrils of the tail extend (see below). (The *nuclear recess*, or *implantation fossa*, is the region of attachment of the complex filamentary structure of the tail. It is continuous with the post-acrosomal part of the nuclear envelope concerned in fusion with the ovum and its nucleus.) A small amount of cytoplasm exists in the neck, covered by a plasma membrane continuous with that of the head and tail.

Middle part or piece. A long cylinder, about 1 μm in diameter and 7 μm long, it consists of an *axial bundle of microtubules (fibrils)* or *axoneme* (the axial 'filament' of light microscopy), surrounded by a *mitochondrial sheath* in which the mitochondria of the spermatid have become arranged in a helical manner (**3.23B**), the whole being enveloped by cytoplasm and a plasma membrane, as in the neck. The axoneme consists of a central pair of microtubules within a symmetrical set of nine doublet microtubules, as in a typical cilium (p. 41), and outside this is a second ring of nine coarser fibres, less symmetric in arrangement and unequal in size. These external fibres are also less regular in cross-sectional profile (see below), showing marked interspecific variations. They appear to be non-contractile despite showing a surface striation. Their function is obscure. The mitochondrial helix exhibits 10–14 turns (Reed & Reed 1948) but this sheath is subject to considerable variation in abnormal spermatozoa (Fujita et al 1970). The number of mitochondria seems excessive in some species, including *Homo sapiens*, when related to the energy requirements of the axonema. Their close relation to the external coarse fibres is suggestive but, as noted, these are apparently not contractile. At the caudal end of the middle part of the cell, immediately anterior to the tail, is an electron-dense body, the *annulus* (**3.25**). The mitochondria of the sheath are much compressed, but it is now certain that they retain their individuality (Fawcett & Ito 1965).

Principal part or tail. This is the motile part of the cell. Being about 40 μm long and 0.5 μm in diameter, it forms the greater part of the spermatozoön. The axial bundle of fibrils and the surrounding array of coarse fibres are continued uninterruptedly from the basal body through the mitochondrial sheath and through the whole length of the tail except for its terminal 5–7 μm, in which the axial bundle alone persists, the coarse fibres ceasing before them. It is only in this terminal *end part* or *piece* that the tail has the typical structure of a flagellum; the coarse fibres are peculiar to mammalian spermatozoa, which also display other specializations. External to the fibres and fibrils, coarse and fine, is a circumferentially orientated dense *fibrous sheath*, whose individual elements branch and reunite to form a tight reticulum. A small amount of cytoplasm and a plasma membrane complete the major elements in the structure of the tail. The finer details of the structure have been studied intensively in mammals such as the guinea-pig (Fawcett 1965) and, while there is little doubt that the human spermatozoön is highly similar (Pedersen 1969), the descriptions presented here are based perforce on appearances in the guinea-pig.

Spermatogenesis

This is the complex series of changes by which spermatogonia are transformed into spermatozoa, similar in some general features—particularly in reduction division and genetic recombination—to the evolution of ova from oögonia, but differing in the more profound morphological metamorphosis involved. Spermatogenesis may, for convenience, be divided into three phases. During the first, *spermatocytosis*, spermatogonia proliferate by mitotic division to replace themselves and to produce primary spermatocytes. In the second phase, *meiosis*, two successive maturation divisions, the first a true reduction division as in the case of the oöcyte, produce *secondary spermatocytes* and then *spermatids*, all with the haploid number of chromosomes. In the third phase, *spermiogenesis* or *spermateliosis*, the spermatids become spermatozoa; it is during this period that the greatest visible transformation of structure occurs (**3.24**).

Spermatogenesis is an orderly and complex sequence of events, with characteristic time constants and cell associations for each mammalian species. The details of these in the human testis will be discussed with that organ (p. 1851).

Spermatocytosis

During embryonic, fetal and perhaps also early postnatal life, *primordial germ cells* in the tubules of the testes divide mitotically to produce spermatogonia (Witschi 1948, 1951; Mintz 1960), from which, at and subsequent to puberty, the development of spermatocytes and spermatozoa commences. It is the cyclic divisions of these cells, the details of which have attracted much attention in recent years, that form the starting place for production of the huge numbers of spermatozoa discharged into the seminal plasma to form the seminal fluid. The series of changes involved do not occur in a synchronous manner in all seminiferous tubules at the same time, although they do in considerable parts of an individual tube, with variations in different mammalian species, including mankind. As the cycle of change from spermatogonia to spermatids proceeds at any particular locus in a tubule, a succession of varying cell associations can be observed and measured; the process is termed the *cycle of the seminiferous epithelium* (Clermont & Leblond 1955) (p. 1852).

In man, three types of spermatogonia can be distinguished and are termed: the *dark type A*, *light type A* and *type B* (Clermont 1963). Spermatogonia are large rounded cells, the three types showing little difference in size or in their cytoplasm, but the A series, light and dark, are distinguishable by their nucleoli which are eccentric and attached to the internal aspect of the nuclear membrane. The

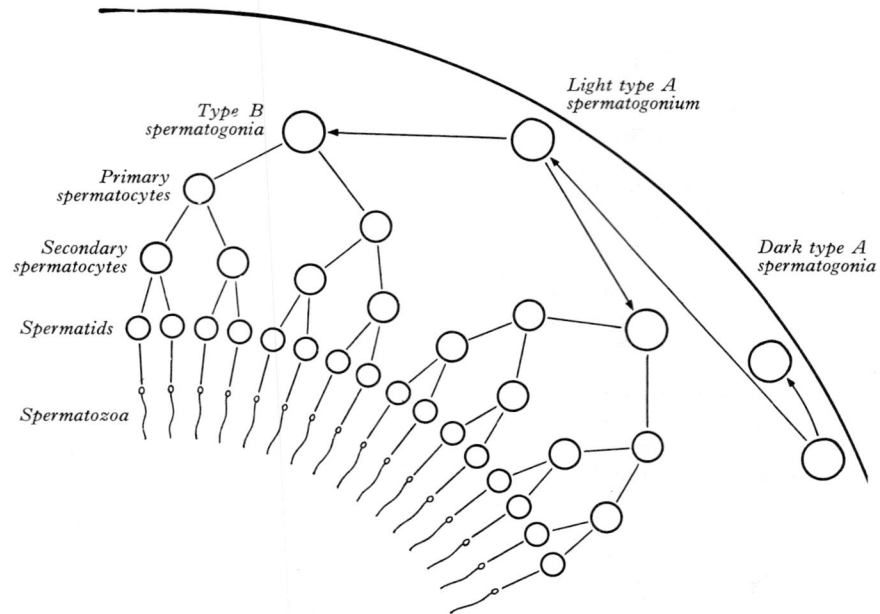

3.24 Diagram showing the stages in the maturation of the spermatozoön. The division of the primary spermatocyte is heterotypical; the remaining divisions are homotypical. Some have described a further division of sper-matids in the human testis, but this is unconfirmed—see text for further details and compare with illustration **8.194**.

type B spermatogonia have a more constantly spherical nucleus, in which the nucleolus is central in position. The dark type A is distinguished from the pale type A by its dark nucleoplasm and a large pale-staining nuclear vacuole. The dark type A is now considered, largely on morphological grounds, to be the progenitor or stem spermatogonium (Clermont 1963). Such cells, peripherally situated in the tubule and often in pairs, divide mitotically at the beginning of a seminiferous cycle, some to produce two further dark type A spermatogonia, thus replenishing the complement of stem cells, others into two light type A spermatogonia. Mitotic division of a light type A spermatogonium furnishes two type B spermatogonia. On theoretical grounds, it is probable that in man a larger series of spermatogonial divisions may occur, so that the ultimate spermatocyte progeny of a stem cell may in fact be more numerous than is here indicated (Clermont 1966). Each type B spermatogonium then divides again mitotically into two *resting primary spermatocytes* or preleptotene spermatocytes. The dark type A cells remain arranged along the basal lamina of the tubule, whereas the pale type A, type B spermatocytes and the spermatids derived from them lie closer to the lumen, into which the free end-product, spermatozoa, will be discharged. These events constitute spermatocytosis, which is now followed by meiosis.

Meiosis of spermatocytes

The primary spermatocytes soon enter the prophase of the *first maturation* (*reduction*) *division*, which is prolonged over several days through the successive stages of leptotene, zygotene, pachytene, diplotene and diakinesis (p. 61) (Clermont 1963, 1966). As the nuclear membrane now disappears in metaphase, the bivalent chromosomes are arranged on the equatorial plate, separating into two groups and moving to opposite poles in anaphase, followed in the usual manner by reformation of the nuclear membranes in telophase and division of the cell. These three phases occur much more rapidly than prophase and during the whole process there is a considerable increase of nuclear and cytoplasmic material, bringing the primary spermatocyte back to a size comparable with that of the stem spermatogonium. The two *secondary spermatocytes* thus formed contain, of course, the haploid number of chromosomes, this *first maturation division* being the one which is strictly speaking *meiotic*.

After a brief interphase each secondary spermatocyte now undergoes a *second maturation division*, which is by mitosis. The two resultant cells are spermatids and with their formation the phase of meiosis may be considered to end, being followed by their maturation into spermatozoa (spermiogenesis). Theoretically each primary spermatocyte may be expected to produce four spermatids but in mankind the yield is less than this, presumably because some spermatocytes degenerate during maturation.

Criticism of the traditional view that spermatids do not divide has been expressed (Roosen-Runge 1952) and tentative corroboration of this came from electron microscope and other studies (Fawcett et al 1959; Fawcett 1961b). These interpretations have subsequently been subjected to critical rescrutiny. Electron microscopy has also shown that the division of the cell body (cytokinesis) in spermatocytes may be delayed, so that fine cytoplasmic bridges remain, interconnecting such cells even beyond the stage of the next nuclear division (Fawcett et al 1959). These bridges, which may remain in the case of spermatids until a late phase in their transformation into spermatozoa, are short, devoid of spindle fibres or other remnants and are enclosed in annular thickenings of the plasma membrane. They probably permit interchange of organelles, may be involved in synchronization of development and may contribute to the mechanical stability of the spermatid-Sertoli cell complexes. Such cytoplasmic interconnection may also help to explain the formation of multinucleated masses when the seminiferous epithelium is injured, as in making teased preparations. Except where connected together by bridges the developing spermatids are very closely associated with Sertoli cells, whose processes are insinuated between them.

During the differentiation of some rodent spermatids a fusiform conglomeration of microtubules, the 'spindle-shaped body', appears between the annulus and fibrous sheath. The same structure has been observed in human spermatids; its functional significance is uncertain but an association with the development of the fibrous sheath has been suggested (Pedersen 1969; Wartenburg & Holstein 1975).

Spermiogenesis

During *spermiogenesis* (spermateliosis), spermatids go through a complex series of changes to become spermatozoa (**3.25**) and this

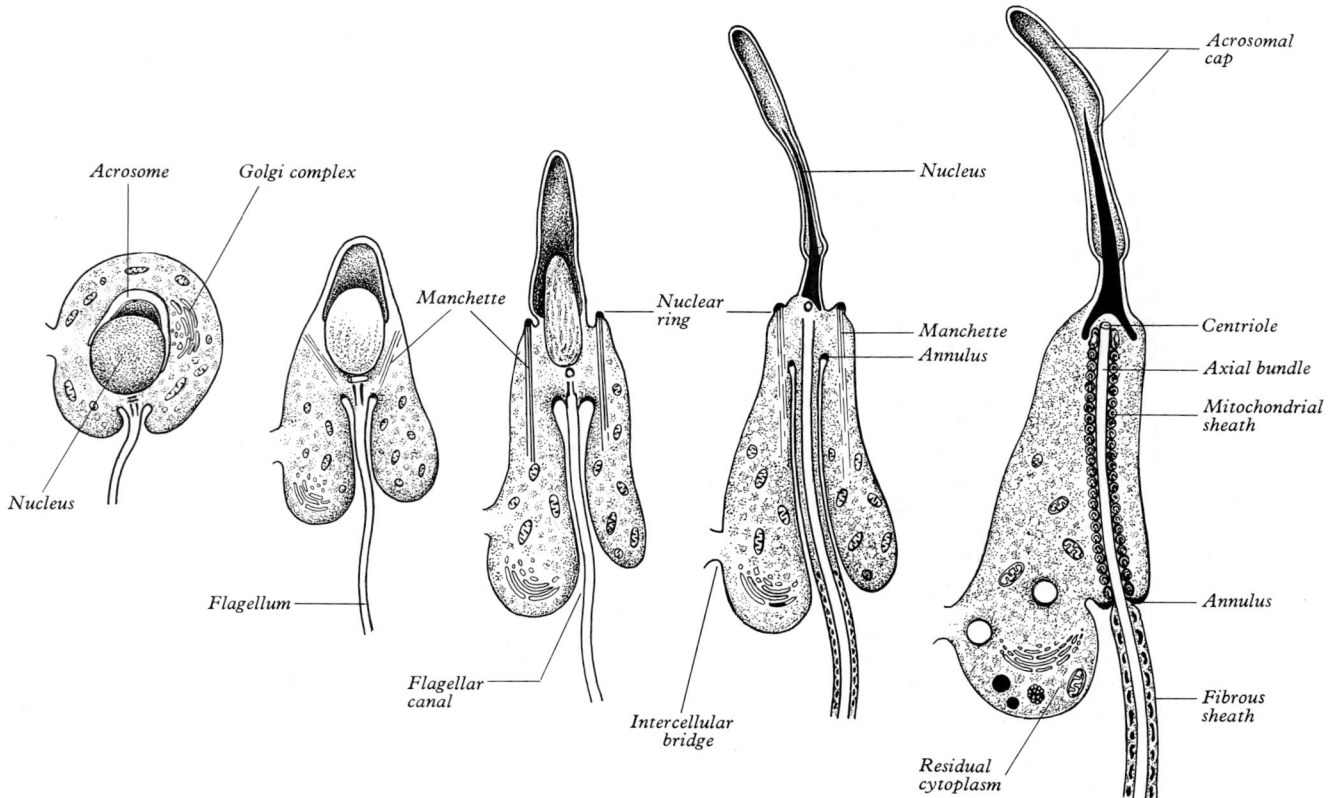

3.25 Differentiation of the spermatid (guinea pig), from left to right. Note nuclear condensation and elongation, appearance of the *manchette* and fibrous sheath, caudal movement of the annulus, and development of the mitochondrial sheath. (Modified after Fawcett in Bloom & Fawcett 1975.)

127

metamorphosis has been studied in particular by light microscopy, using preparations stained by the periodic-acid Schiff technique (PAS); (Clermont 1963). Electron microscopy has confirmed these observations (Fawcett & Burgos 1956). In the newly formed spermatid the Golgi apparatus (idiosome–Golgi complex) is large but otherwise typical, consisting of flattened membrane-enclosed vesicles, usually stacked in a parallel array, together with rounded minute vesicles which are possibly nipped off from the flattened variety, the whole complex being juxtanuclear. A few electron-dense homogeneous *paracrosomal granules*, which are intensely PAS-positive, develop in separate Golgi complex vesicles and the latter coalesce into a single large *acrosomal vesicle*, the separate granules fusing into a single spherical *acrosomal granule*. This vesicle, with its granule attached to its juxtanuclear wall, becomes adherent to the nuclear membrane over an area which will be anterior or 'leading' in the maturing spermatozoön. The granule flattens, but its central part bulges slightly into a shallow depression in the nucleus, which becomes progressively more ovoid (**3.25**). By successive absorption of further vesicles from the Golgi complex, the material in the acrosomal vesicle increases and the vesicle expands as a bilaminar cap over the anterior two-thirds of the nucleus. Coincident with these changes, the spermatid elongates and the Golgi complex and associated cytoplasm migrate to the posterior part of the cell, bringing the external wall of the acrosomal vesicle into contact with the plasma membrane at the anterior aspect of the cell. The acrosomal granule now spreads out between the layers of the vesicle until it is uniformly distributed and no longer a localized structure. When the centrioles begin to separate (see below), microtubules develop forming an inverted conical array, the *manchette*, perinuclear in position and expanding from the region of the acrosomal cap; its precise significance is not yet explained.

In the early spermatid the nucleus is of relatively low density, containing finely dispersed granules which aggregate into larger and denser masses as development proceeds. These finally agglomerate into a homogeneously dense mass, usually containing one or more regions of low electron-density and variable in size, position and shape—the *head vacuoles* (Fawcett & Burgos 1956). Correlated biochemical and ultrastructural studies indicate a considerable variation in the chromatin content of spermatozoa, this heterogeneity being more marked in mankind than other primates or rodents; it probably indicates a lower fertilizing power (Bedford et al 1973).

The two centrioles are near the posterior aspect of the nucleus from an early stage. One remains unmodified; the other becomes modified into the basal body of the spermatozoön (see p. 125). The annulus arises close to the latter (the distant centriole) but its origin from it is doubtful. The axial fibrils begin to develop from the basal body, extending 'caudally' into the cytoplasm of the cell as it becomes progressively more elongated. Only the proximal part of the bundle of fibrils remains surrounded by cytoplasm, to form the definitive middle part of the spermatozoön. In this, the mitochondria of the spermatid assemble to form the helical sheath. The detailed development of the fibrous sheath of the tail part is unknown. These changes complete what might be called the period of 'organogenesis' of the spermatid, whose further development into a spermatozoön is largely concerned with enlargement of the tail.

During the final maturation of spermatids into individual spermatozoa some of the cytoplasm is detached as a *residual body*. This contains some mitochondria, Golgi membranes and vesicles, RNA particles, lipid granules but of course no nucleus. Residual bodies are prominent when spermatozoa are being released into their tubule. They are engulfed by Sertoli cells, which accounts for the increase in lipid content of these cells at this period (Lacy 1960).

As already stated, there is a close relation between developing spermatids and Sertoli sustentacular cells. The spermatogonia are external or basal to the Sertoli cells in the tubule and the spermatocytes which develop from the former are embraced by Sertoli processes; the spermatids are even more deeply embedded in the supportive cells. (For further details see p. 1852.) These associations have been regarded as symbiotic, a single sustentacular cell being grouped with several spermatids. The Sertoli cells are phagocytic and absorb not only residual bodies but also degenerating germ cells. They have been attributed a metabolic role and may form, or at least transmit, hormones involved in the maturation of germ cells. Until released into the seminiferous tubule, spermatozoa are very

firmly held by the Sertoli cells. Their release is sometimes termed *spermiation* and is followed by rapid translation of the spermatozoa to the epididymis.

Maturation of spermatozoa

Maturation is a complex process which has received much attention. Spermatozoa show little independent motility while still in the male genital tract, though when removed from the epididymis they may display circular swimming movements or even directive movements if taken from the cauda epididymis near the beginning of the ductus deferens (Blandau & Rumery 1964). From the results of artificial insemination of rabbits with spermatozoa from the caput and cauda of the epididymis, it has been postulated that some form of maturation process takes place in this organ, during which the spermatozoön attains its specific pattern of motility (Gaddum 1968). Apart from these incomplete activities, spermatozoa are largely transported through the genital tract by ciliary action, by fluid currents set up by localized secretion and absorption and by muscular contractions. Associated with the maturation of spermatozoa in the genital tract in some mammals is the extrusion of a small mass of cytoplasm, the *kinoplasmic droplet* or *residual body*, which migrates backwards along the surface of the head and middle part of the spermatozoön before disappearing. It consists of membrane-enclosed cytoplasm containing fine tubules and vesicles (Bloom & Nicander 1961; Guraya 1963). Human spermatozoa have not been shown to undergo any demonstrable structural changes during passage through the epididymis, but there is evidence of an increase in sulphide cross-linking between proteins (Bedford & Calvin 1974). Moreover, restorative surgery after vasectomy indicates that at least part of the human epididymis is essential for motility (Bedford et al 1973).

Motility of spermatozoa. In cross-section the tail is oval and tapers caudally and its central area is typical of a flagellum or cilium. The surrounding coarse fibres are obovate or petal-shaped and unequal in size, one being consistently the largest. This is given the number 1 and the rest are numbered from this in a clockwise manner. These fibres are separated into two unequal groups by slender *longitudinal* columns in the fibrous sheath which interrupts its circumferential fibres and extend inwards to meet the coarse fibres numbered 3 and 8. This divides the interior of the tail into *major* and *minor compartments*, containing respectively coarse fibres 4, 5, 6 and 7, and 9, 1 and 2. The plane through the two columns also passes through the central pair of the axial bundle of fibrils and can be used as a reference datum for other structural details. For example, the transverse diameter of the head has been considered to lie at right angles to the plane of the columns, but it has now been shown in the guinea-pig that the angle between the two planes is 20–30° less than a right angle (Fawcett 1968). Such details may be instrumental in elucidating the motile activities of the tail. It is now generally accepted that the tail executes undulatory movements in one plane, but it has also been suggested that a helical component is superimposed upon this, there being perhaps two separable mechanisms, one involving flat waves travelling along the tail, the other associated with torsional activity (Gray 1958; Bishop 1962; Lindahl & Drevius 1964).

The latter variety of movement has been linked with the unequal size and distribution of the coarse fibrils; it has also been suggested that the central pair of fine fibrils act as axial stiffeners. The asymmetry of the spermatozoan head has also been invoked to explain supposed helical movement. However, it has to be admitted that the full details of the mechanisms of spermatozoal motility are unknown.

Some further details deserve mention. The dense outer fibres have been shown to exhibit an oblique or helical striation in replicas of dried whole mounts of rodent spermatozoa (Phillips & Olson 1975). The central axoneme (**3.23**), consisting of the usual ciliary pattern of nine double fibrils or 'doublets', has been intensively studied Fawcett 1975 for survey of literature). Each fibril is a microtubule, itself constructed of a regular number of protofibrils. Protein bridges connect adjoining doublets at regular intervals and radial links extend centrally to the central doublet of the axoneme.

As soon as they are ejaculated the spermatozoa display their full pattern of motility. The precise factors which trigger off these movements enabling human gametes to travel at a rate of 1.5–3 mm/min are not yet clear; but the other constituents of semen, derived from the epididymis and testis and from the seminal vesicle and prostate, are generally considered to exert an activating influence. The motility varies greatly in different species, disappearing in minutes in some fish but usually persisting in mammals for hours and even days when introduced into the female genital tract. Exact figures for its persistence in the human female are uncertain and are of doubtful value, since it is likely that, as in other mammals, human spermatozoa quickly lose their potency for fertilization, although still motile. They have been recovered in a motile state in human cervical mucus several days after insemination and will survive in this condition for as long as 7 days when implanted into such secretions in vitro. These survival periods may, however, be of little significance, in view of the speed with which spermatozoa reach the infundibulum of the uterine tube and the brevity of their fertilizing power. Spermatozoa have been shown to reach their tubal destination in a manner of minutes after ejaculation in some mammals and experiments on recently excised human uteri and tubes indicated a time of about 70 minutes (Brown 1944). The conclusion must be that factors other than their own motility are responsible for the transport of spermatozoa from the site of deposition in the vaginal fornix to the ovarian end of the uterine tube and there is considerable evidence that contraction of the uterine and tubal musculature is responsible (Bickers 1960).

It is not usually recognized that a spermatozoön must be adaptable to a wide range of environments in its long journey from the seminiferous tubule to the uterine tube, encountering major changes in the electrolyte and non-electrolyte constituents in the fluids with which it is successively surrounded. Nevertheless, a collectively vast amount of observation and experiment has been recorded in connection with the effects of the multitude of factors, both physical and chemical, in the natural media involved regarding the behaviour of these cells and particularly their motility and fertility (Nelson 1967; Mann 1967); e.g. the effects of respiratory gas tensions, reaction, various ions, antibodies, vitamins, hormones, inhibitory substances, temperature, different forms of radiation and other factors have been studied in remarkable detail, for which monographs and original papers must be consulted. The effects of low temperatures in preserving spermatozoa and perhaps prolonging their vitality have attracted much research in connection with artificial insemination, both in stock-breeding and in infertile human marriage. Mammalian semen, including that of human beings (Parkes 1952), can be stored at temperatures of about −70°C for weeks and even months, the motility and fertility of its suspended spermatozoa reappearing when the suspension is unfrozen. However, storage of human semen presents difficulties (Polge 1957).

Seminal plasma. The fluid component of *seminal fluid* or *semen*; it contains a remarkable array of substances, including muco-proteins, a dozen or more identified proteolytic enzymes, the bases spermine, glycerylphosphorylcholine and ergothioneine, a group of organic acids called prostaglandins (which have pharmaco-dynamic actions on the uterus and smooth muscle in general), acids such as citric, ascorbic, uric, lactic and pyruvic, and the sugars sorbitol, inositol and fructose. The fructose added to the fluid by the secretion of the seminal vesicle is an essential substrate in the anaerobic glycolysis by which spermatozoa survive the low oxygen tensions existing in semen itself and in the female genital tract. Prostaglandins are now believed to play a role, perhaps by modulation of neurotransmitter release, in the contraction/relaxation activity of the nonstriated muscle in the testicular capsule and interlobular septa adjacent to the seminiferous tubules (as suggested by von Euler 1936). Consult Ellis and Hargrove (1977) for literature.

Capacitation

After ejaculation into the female, the spermatozoa undergo the final step in their maturation, a process known as *capacitation*. It has been shown that spermatozoa are not able to fertilize ova until they have been within the genital tract of the female for a period of time, usually of hours but varying with the species (Austin 1951; Chang 1951; Austin & Walton 1960). The mechanism of capacitation, whereby the spermatozoön is activated to enter and fertilize the ovum, is still uncertain. A confusing array of findings with regard to the interactions of the two gametes immediately prior to this event have been described, unfortunately in widely different vertebrates and invertebrates. It is probable that hyaluronidase hastens the separation

of corona radiata cells from the ovum, and thus facilitates the spermatozoön's approach to the zona pellucida. The origin of hyaluronidase from the acrosomal cap is associated with subsequent loss of the cap (Leuchtenberger & Schrader 1950), at least in part (Austin & Bishop 1958). 'Capacitated' spermatozoa observed in the zona pellucida or perivitelline space have invariably lost most of their acrosomal material (Leuchtenberger & Schrader 1950; Pikó & Tyler 1964) and it is clear that capacitation is some process of activation which precedes penetration. Antigenic 'coating' substances on the surface of mammalian spermatozoa, including those of man (Weil 1965), have been recorded and it is possible that an immunological reaction may be involved. Interaction between a *fertilizin*, derived from the ovum or elsewhere in the female genital tract, and a spermatozoan *anti-fertilizin* has been associated with capacitation, but the interrelationship between the various events is still sub judice, as comprehensive reviews show (Metz & Monroy 1969; Chang & Hunter 1975). Capacitation may be regarded as the terminal event of maturation of the spermatozoön, prior to actual fertilization, for which it is preparation.

UNION OF THE GAMETES

Sexual reproduction is initiated by the fusion of distinct male and female gametes (sperm and egg respectively) produced by appropriately different parental forms. In some of the earliest organisms to propagate by sexual reproduction, such as primitive algae, the gametes are all alike, except presumably in their genetic content. The profound differences which have evolved in the gametes of the great majority of plants and animals—vertebrate and invertebrate—appear to depend on a conflict between adaptation for the carriage of nutrients for one gamete and improvement in motility for the other. The egg, by extruding genetic material at the meiotic divisions, accumulates cytoplasm and is considered immobile; during its development the sperm loses cytoplasm retaining only the nucleus, mitochondria, a propulsive tail and such organelles necessary for the production of enzymes for breaching the outer walls of the egg. This dimorphism of the gametes has in turn entailed the evolution of equally profound differences between the individuals producing the two kinds of gametes, males and females, in regard to the organs concerned in bringing together these dissimilar gametes and ensuring the development of their fused product, the *zygote*, until it is able to undertake a separate existence.

The central feature of reproduction in most plants and animals is the *fusion* of the gametes at fertilization. Fusion is the precursor of *syngamy*, when the two gamete pronuclei come together to reconstitute a diploid *zygote* nucleus. Syngamy is the second and final stage of the genetic assortment that accompanies (and is, no doubt, the reason for) sexual reproduction; the first stage is meiotic crossing over (recombination). Genetic sex is determined at syngamy by the presence or absence of the Y chromosome that determines the male sex in mammals and several other animal groups. The Y chromosome, if present, is necessarily contributed by the sperm which therefore determines the sex of the zygote. In most animals, phenotypic sex is female, unless active genes on the Y chromosome are present to trigger the active programme for male sex determination.

Although syngamy is essential for the maintenance of ploidy, other changes within the egg that are equally essential for normal development are triggered by fertilization. Mammalian gametes are fertilized when in the second meiotic metaphase: fertilization causes the cell division cycle to resume, completing meiosis and extruding the second set of redundant meiotic chromosomes as the second *polar body*. Thereafter, cell division (segmentation or cleavage) proceeds within the zona pellucida until the blastocyst stage (Howlett & Bolton 1985).

Parthenogenesis

A mature egg can contain all that is necessary to make a new being and can under some circumstances commence to develop. This is particularly evident in the cases of *natural* and *artificial parthenogenesis*. Natural parthenogenesis occurs quite widely, a good example being aphids, which produce parthenogenetic females to maximize generation overlap and thus population growth rate at

129

times of food abundance, reverting to sexual reproduction when food is scarce. Artificial parthenogenesis stimulates this potentiality of the egg to develop further without fertilization by a variety of mechanical, chemical and physico-chemical means, such as pricking of the egg or exposure to altered tonicity and chemicals. It has been successful in a wide variety of animals, though not in mammals where offspring rarely survive beyond the embryonic stage (underlining the point that the genetic contribution of the gamete nuclei to early development is small, but becomes important later). In the case of rabbits, viable parthenogenotes have been reported, but the observation has never been substantiated.

Parental imprinting

The presence of chromosomes from both parental origins is crucial for spatial organization and the controlled growth of cells, tissues and organs (Azim & Surani 1986). There is extensive evidence which suggests differential roles for paternal and maternal genomes during mammalian embryogenesis. Embryos in which the paternal pronucleus has been removed and replaced with a second maternal pronucleus develop to a relatively advanced stage, in the mouse, to form 25-somite embryos with very limited development of the

trophoblast and extraembryonic tissues. In contrast, embryos in which the maternal pronucleus has been replaced by a second paternal pronucleus develop very poorly, forming embryos of only 6–8 somites, but with extensive trophoblast. Thus it seems that the maternal genome is relatively more important for the development of the embryo, while the paternal genome is essential for the development of the extraembryonic tissues.

This *functional inequivalence* of homologous parental chromosomes is called *parental imprinting*. The process of parental imprinting causes the expression of particular genes to be dependent on their parental origin, with some genes being expressed only from the maternally inherited chromosome and others from the paternally inherited chromosome. These genes are called *imprinted genes*, they are believed to have inherited maternal or paternal specific *imprints* which affect their activity (**3.26**) (Surani et al 1986; Solter 1988). The mechanism of imprinting is thought to involve the acquisition of molecular signals attached to the DNA or chromatin which are known as *epigenetic modifications*. These modifications must have the following properties:

(1) They must be able to affect the transcription of the gene.

(2) They must be heritable in somatic cells over many cell divisions and not lost during chromosome replication.

(3) Most importantly, the imprints must be erased in the male and female germ lines during gametogenesis to allow new imprints to be set down which are specific to the parental origin of the newly formed gametes.

Methylation of some critical CpG dinucleotides in the DNA of

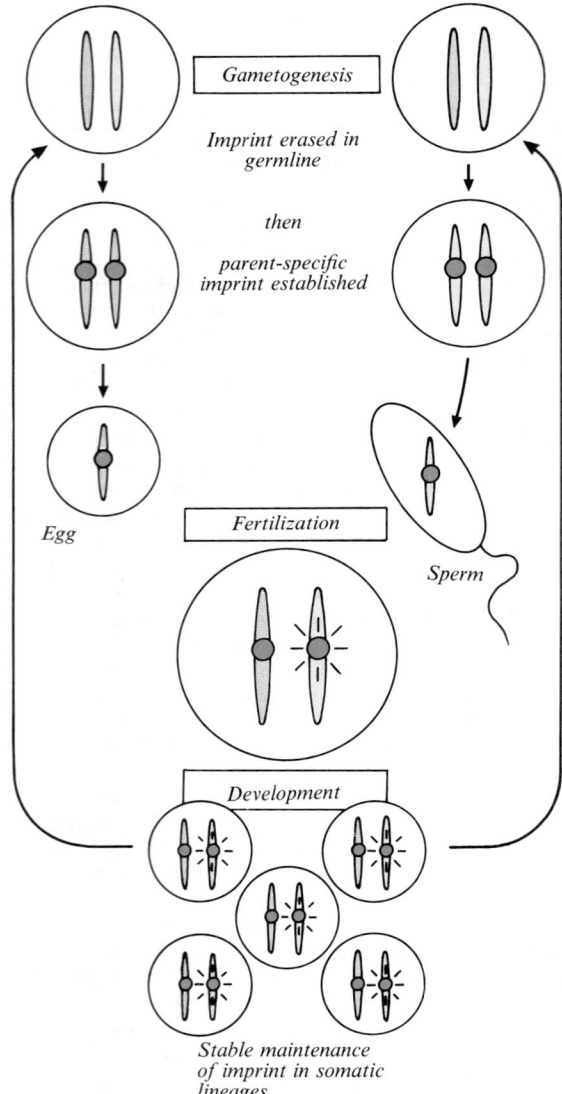

3.26 Heritability of parental imprints. Parental imprints are chromosome modifications which affect the activity of some genes. Imprints cause these genes to be expressed depending on their parental origins. Here, a maternally inherited chromosome (pink) carries an imprint circle (red circle) resulting in *repression* of a gene. The same gene on the paternally inherited chromosome (blue) is imprinted (green circle) allowing it to be *expressed*. After fertilization in the organism the imprint is stably inherited in the somatic lineages with the chromosomes remembering their parental origin. In the germline the imprint is erased and then re-established so that all the gametes will carry either the maternal or paternal specific imprint.

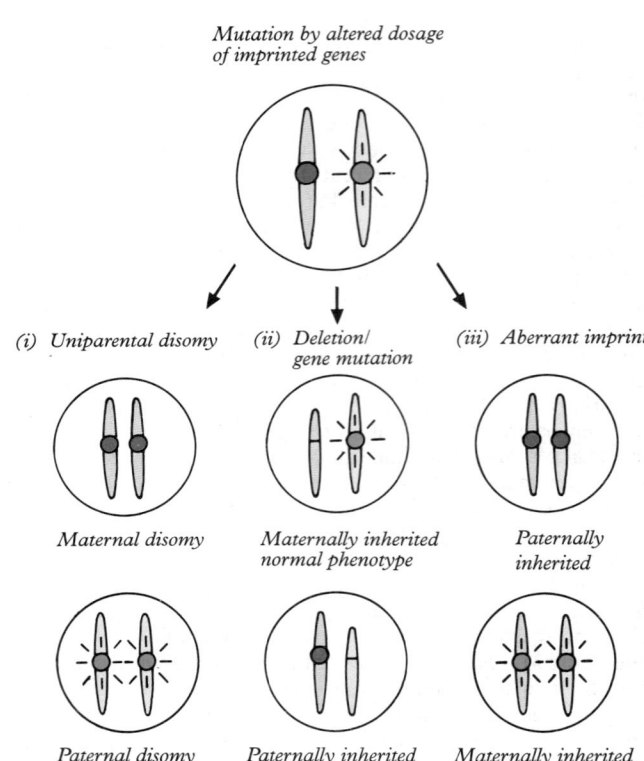

3.27 Mutation by altered dosage of imprinted genes. An imprint is inherited maternally (red circle) causing repression of a gene and expression of the paternally inherited copy.

(i) Uniparental disomy, an alteration in the dosage of the parental chromosomes, is maternal duplication/paternal deficiency (maternal disomy), or paternal duplication/maternal deficiency (paternal disomy). Thus both copies of the imprinted gene are repressed (the maternal disomy in this example) or expressed (the paternal disomy in this example);

(ii) Inheritance of a mutation such as a deletion will result in a mutant phenotype only if the mutation is in the active copy of the gene (paternal in this example). If the repressed allele is mutated a normal phenotype will result as the active copy is still intact;

(iii) Mutations may also cause the imprint modification itself to be perturbed such that an inappropriate modification occurs. Thus the chromosome no longer acts faithfully to its parental origin and the gene cannot exhibit appropriate imprinted activity.

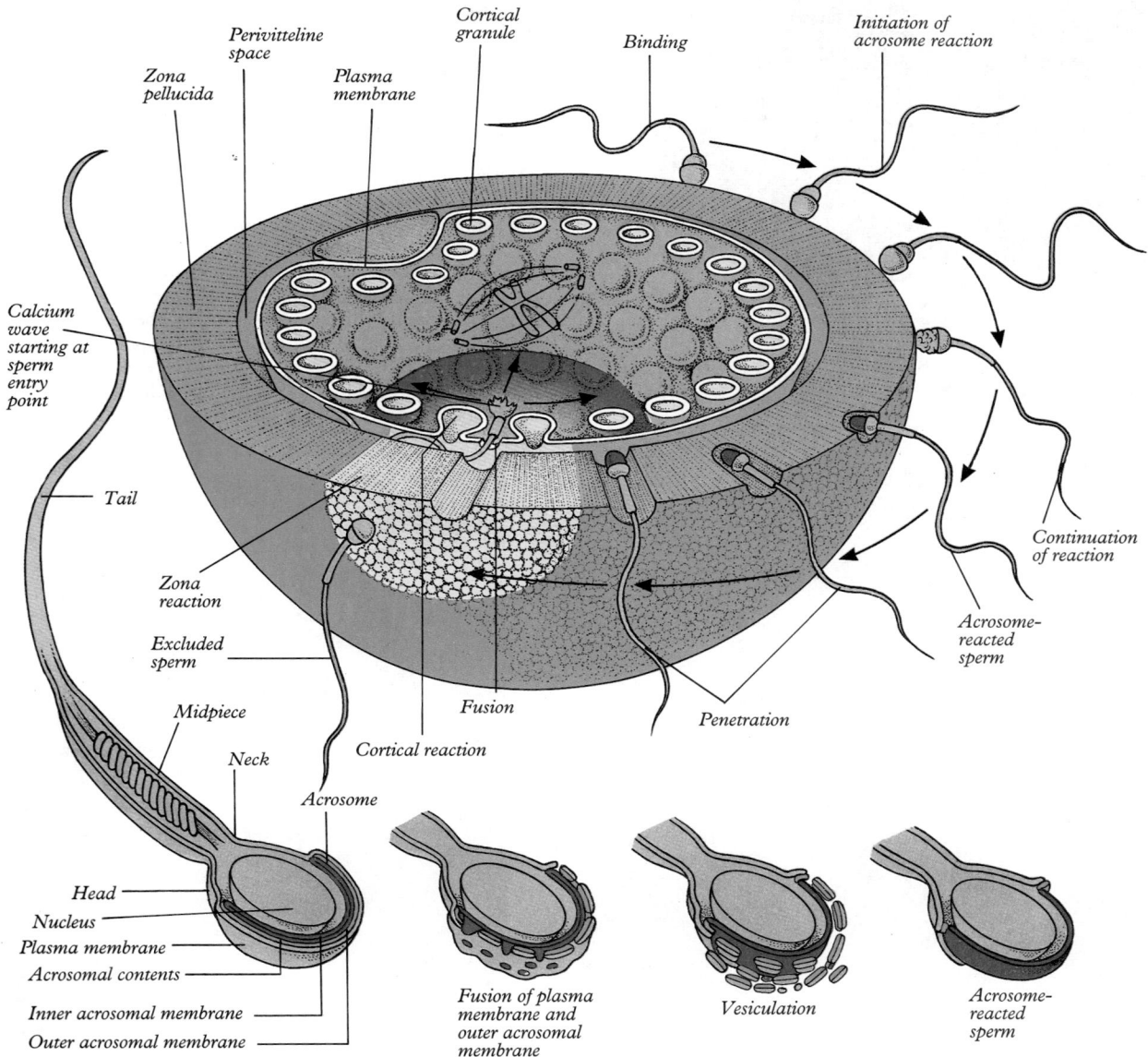

3.28 Fertilization pathway includes a succession of steps. After a sperm cell binds to the zona pellucida, what is called the acrosome reaction takes place (see detail at bottom). The outer membrane (blue) acrosome, an enzyme-rich organelle in the anterior of the sperm head, fuses at many points with the plasma membrane surrounding the sperm head. Then those fused membranes form vesicles, which are eventually sloughed off from the head, exposing the acrosomal enzymes (red). The enzymes digest a path through the zona pellucida, enabling the sperm to advance. Eventually the sperm meets and fuses with the egg's plasma membrane, fertilizing the egg. Completion of the pathway triggers the cortical and zona reactions. First enzyme-rich cortical granules in the egg's cytoplasm release their contents (yellow) into the zona pellucida, starting at the point of fusion and progressing right and left. Next, in the zona reaction, the enzymes modify the zona pellucida, transforming it into an impenetrable barrier to sperm as a guard against polyspermy (multiple fertilization). (Paul Wasserman in Scientific American Dec 1988, with permission of the publishers.)

imprinted genes is one type of epigenetic modification believed to be important in the imprinting process (Sasaki et al 1993).

The requirement for both parental genomes is limited to a subset of the chromosomes (Cattanach & Beechey 1993). This has become evident through the analysis of the individuals with uniparental duplications and corresponding deficiencies, *uniparental disomy*, of particular chromosomal regions. Uniparental disomy (3.27) can arise through meiotic and mitotic non-disjunction events and result in individuals completely disomic or exhibiting *mosaicism* of disomic and non-disomic cells. If imprinted genes reside on the affected chromosomes then the uniparental disomic cells will either express a double dose of the gene or have both copies repressed. For example, the gene encoding the embryonal mitogen insulin-like growth factor II is expressed from the paternally inherited chromosome and repressed when maternally inherited (DeChiara et al 1991). Thus individuals with maternal duplication/paternal deficiency, *maternal disomy*, of the chromosome carrying the insulin-like growth factor II gene do not express any of the growth factor. Mice with this deficiency are growth retarded (Ferguson-Smith et al 1991).

In humans, some conditions show parental origin effects in their patterns of inheritance and several imprinted disorders in man have been described. These disorders can be attributed to alterations in the dosage of imprinted genes either through chromosomal uniparental disomy, trisomy or mutations (e.g. deletions) involving the gene or the imprints. In these disorders, males and females are equally affected; however, manifestation of the disorder depends on the parental origin of the uniparental disomy or the sex of the parent from whom the mutation is inherited. Disorders exhibiting parental origin effects in their patterns of inheritance include the Beckwith-

131

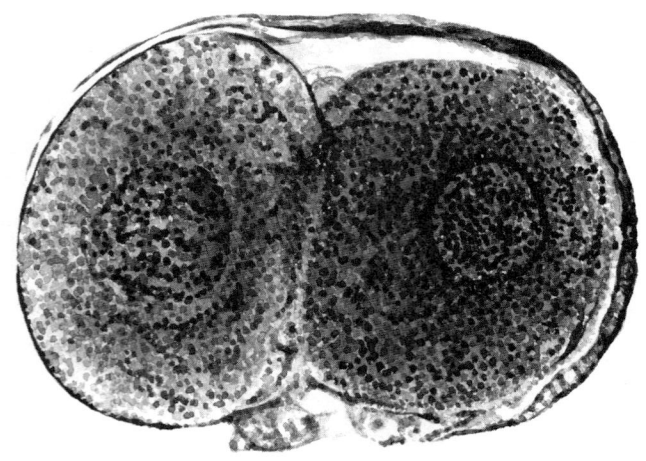

3.29 Early human cleavage: 2-blastomere stage recovered from the uterine tube. A polar cell is seen at each end of the cleavage plane. Magnification × c. 700. (Hertig et al 1954.)

Wiedermann syndrome (Wiedermann 1964; Eliot & Maher 1994), Prader-Willi syndrome (Holm et al 1993) and Angelman syndrome (Angelman 1965; Nichols et al 1992). Parental imprinting mutations are also implicated in the genesis of some tumour syndromes, notably Wilm's tumour and familial glomus tumours.

Fertilization

Fertilization normally occurs in the ampullary region of the uterine tube probably within 24 hours of ovulation. Very few spermatozoa reach the ampulla to achieve fertilization. They must undergo capacitation, still incompletely understood, which may involve modifications in membrane sterols or surface proteins. They traverse the cumulus oöphorus and corona radiata, then bind to specific glycoprotein receptors on the zona pellucida, ZP3 and ZP2. Interaction of ZP3 with the sperm head induces the *acrosome reaction*, in which fusion of membranes on the sperm head releases enzymes, such as acrosin, which help to digest the zona around the sperm head allowing the sperm to reach the perivitelline space. In the perivitelline space, the spermatozoön fuses with the oöcyte microvilli, possibly via two disintegrin peptides in the sperm head and integrin in the oölemma. Fusion of the sperm with the oölemma causes a

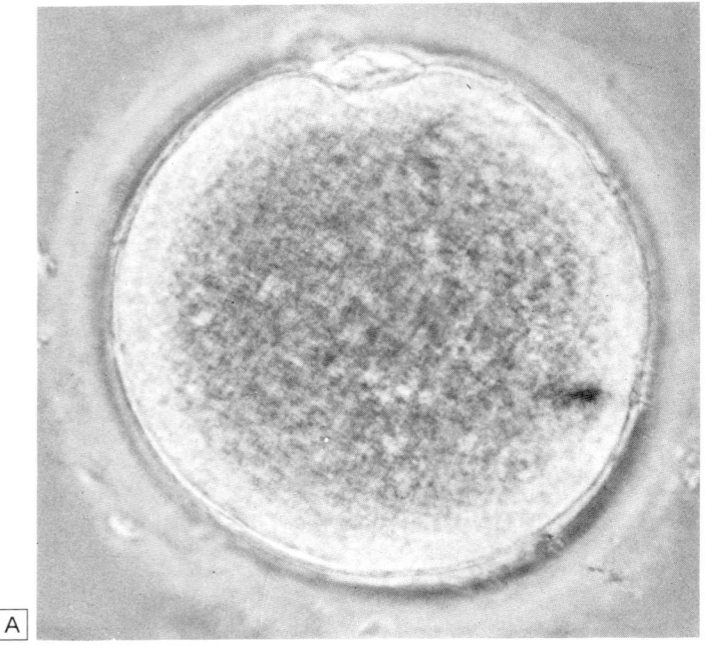

A

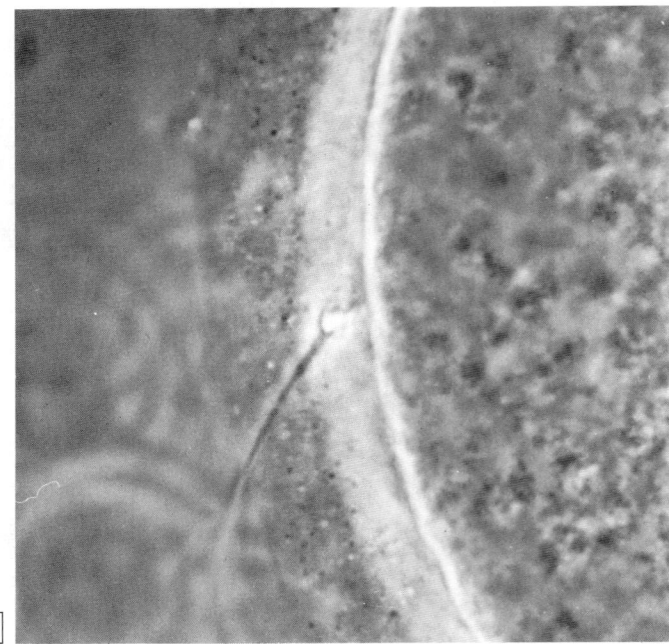

B

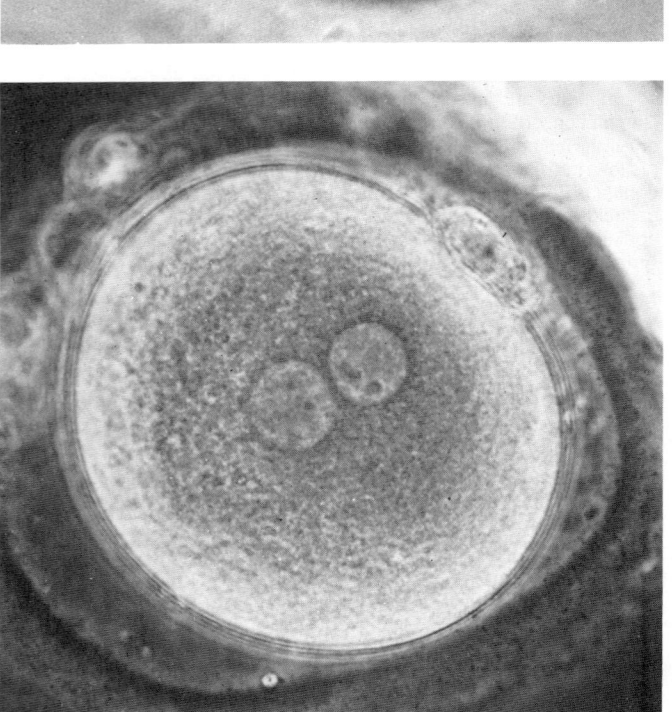

C

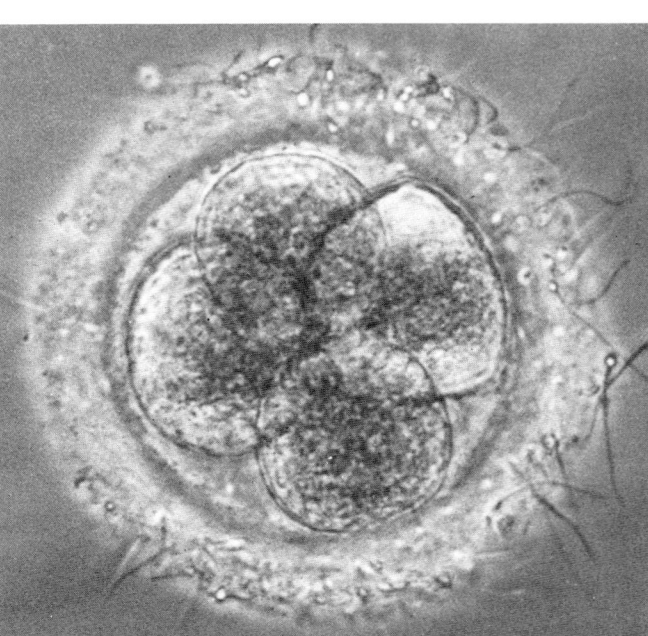

D

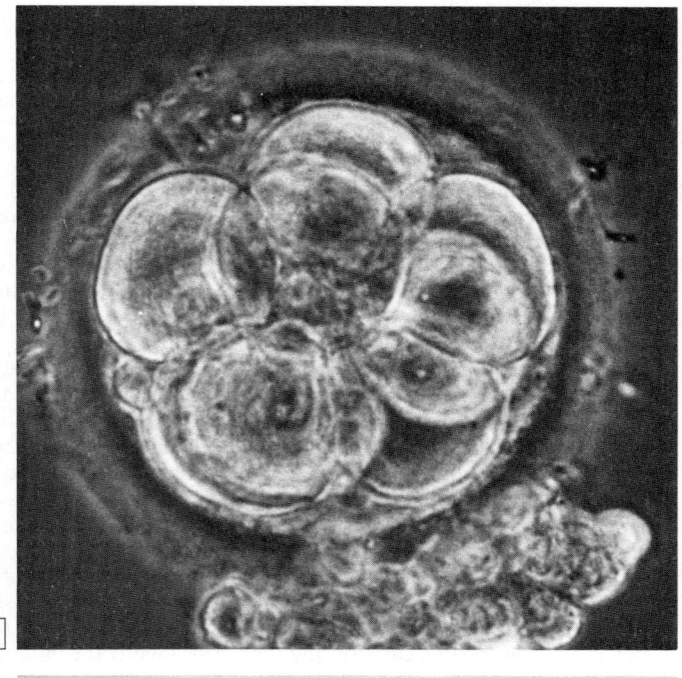

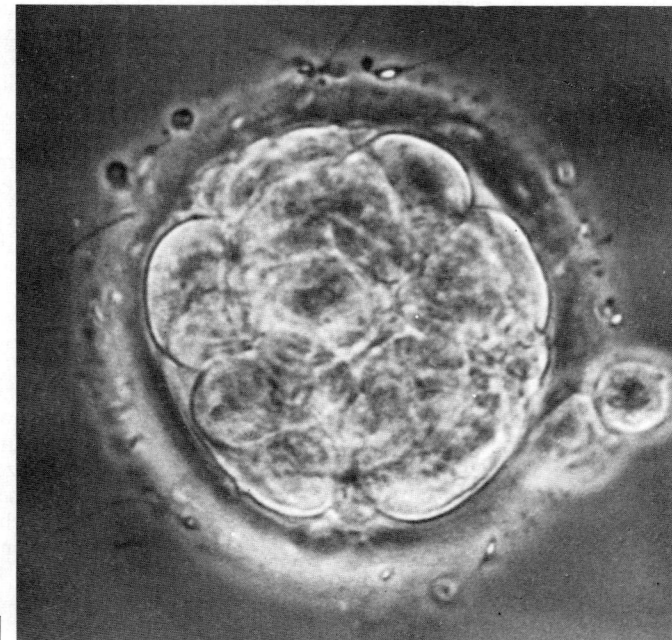

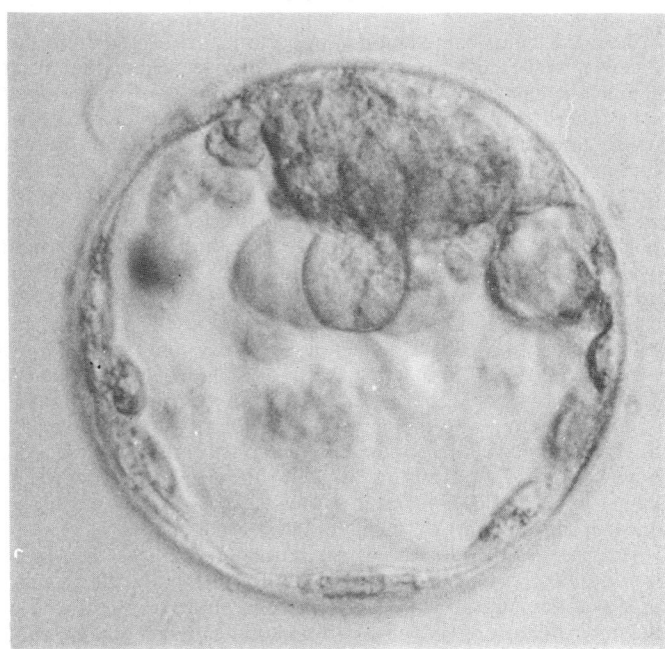

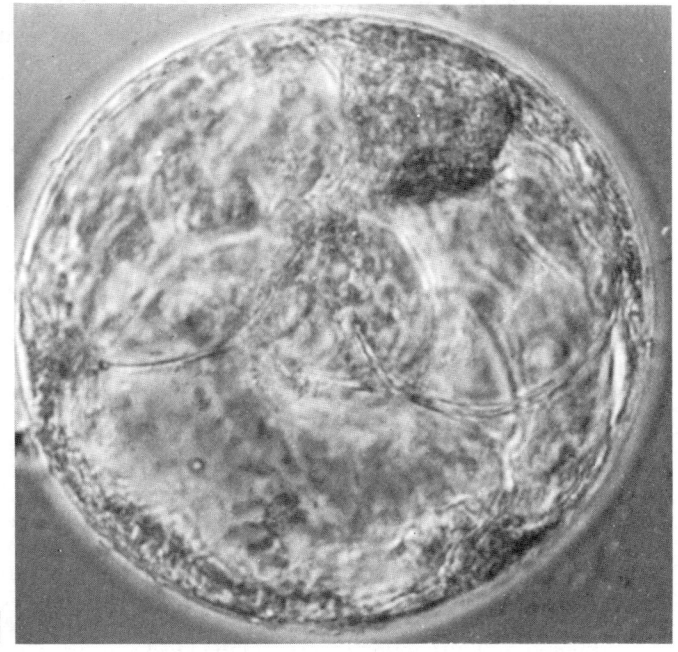

3.30A–H These are all photographs of living human specimens in tissue culture. These specimens were provided by R G Edwards of the Anatomy Department, Cambridge University; B, E, F and G are reproduced by courtesy of *Nature* and C by courtesy of the *Journal of Reproduction and Fertility*.

A. An unfertilized oöcyte surrounded by the zona pellucida; the first polar cell can be seen.

B. High magnification of the surface of an unfertilized living human oöcyte; the head of a spermatozoön is visible in the perivitelline space and its tail is beating outside the zona pellucida.

C. After penetration by the spermatozoön, the male and female pronuclei

can be seen near the centre of the 'ovum', whilst two polar cells lie beneath the zona pellucida.

D. Human cleavage—4-celled stage.

E. 8-celled stage.

F. 16-celled stage.

G. An early living human blastocyst. Note the blastocyst cavity, small flattened mural trophoblastic cells, and the projecting clump or large cells constituting the inner cell mass.

H. A blastocyst which has lost its zona pellucida and started to expand.

weak membrane depolarization and leads to a *calcium wave* which is triggered by the sperm at the site of fusion and crosses the egg within 5–20 seconds (see **3.28**). The calcium wave amplifies the local signal at the site of sperm–oöcyte interaction and distributes it throughout the oöcyte cytoplasm. The increase in calcium concentration is the signal that causes the oöcyte to resume cell division initiating the completion of meiosis II and setting off the developmental programme that leads to embryogenesis. All vertebrate, and some invertebrate, eggs initiate a calcium wave at fertilization.

The pulses of intracellular calcium that occur every few minutes for the first few hours of development also trigger the fusion of *cortical granules* with the oölemma. The cortical secretory granules release an enzyme that hydrolyses the ZP3 receptor on the zona pellucida and so prevents other sperm from binding and undergoing the acrosome reaction, thus establishing the *block to polyspermy*. The same cortical granule secretion may also modify the vitelline layer and oölemma, making them less susceptible to sperm–oöcyte fusion and providing a further level of polyspermy block.

The sperm head undergoes its protamine → histone transition as the second polar body is extruded. The two *pronuclei* grow, move together and condense in preparation for syngamy and cleavage after 24 hours (3.32). Nucleolar rRNA and perhaps some mRNA is synthesized in pronuclei, and a succeeding series of cleavage divisions produces eight even-sized blastomeres at 2.5 days, when embryonic mRNA is transcribed.

Several examples of cells, *oötids*, which contain male and female pronuclei have been described. Pronuclear fusion as such does not occur; the two pronuclear envelopes disappear and the two chromosome groups move together to assume positions on the first cleavage spindle. Thus there is no true zygote stage containing a membrane-bound nucleus.

Fertilization of human gametes in vitro (IVF) is very successful (3.28). Controlled ovarian stimulation, (e.g. with pituitary down-regulation with luteinizing hormone releasing hormone (LHRH); analogues followed by stimulation with menopausal gonadotrophins, enables many preovulatory oöcytes (often 10 or more) to be aspirated by laparoscopy or transvaginal ultrasound. Micromanipulation assists severe male infertility, especially by injecting a spermatozoön directly into the oöplasm to obtain 50% fertilizations. Genetic disease in embryos is being diagnosed by applying the polymerase chain reaction to polar bodies removed from oöcytes, or to one or more blastomeres excised from cleaving embryos or pieces of trophectoderm excised from blastocysts. Pronucleate and cleaving embryos are cryopreserved using propanediol or dimethylsulphoxide, and blastocysts using glycerol. Conception rates per cycle using ovarian stimulation, IVF and successive transfers of fresh and cryopreserved embryos far outstrip those obtained during non-assisted conception (Edwards & Brody 1993).

PREIMPLANTATION DEVELOPMENT

Cleavage

The first divisions of the fertilized oöcyte are termed cleavage. They distribute the cytoplasm approximately equally among daughter *blastomeres*, so although the cell number of the preimplantation embryo rises its total mass actually falls slightly (3.29, 30). The cell cycle is quite long, the first two cell cycles being around 24 hours each, thereafter reducing to 12 to 18 hours. Cell division is asynchronous and daughter cells may retain a cytoplasmic link through much of the immediately subsequent cell cycle via a midbody, due to the delayed completion of cytokinesis. No centrioles are present until the 16- to 32-cell stage, but amorphous pericentriolar material is present and serves to organize the mitotic spindles, which are characteristically more barrel than spindle shaped at these stages.

All cleavage divisions after fertilization are dependent upon continuing protein synthesis. In contrast, passage through the earliest cycles is independent of mRNA synthesis (to 2 cells in mouse, 4 cells in pig, 8 cells in human, 16 cells in cow and sheep), but thereafter the inhibition of transcription experimentally blocks further division and development, indicating that activation of the embryonic genome is required. There is also direct evidence for the synthesis of embryonically encoded proteins at this stage. At the same time as the embryo's genes first become both active and essential, the previously functional maternally derived mRNA is destroyed. However, protein made on these maternal templates does persist at least to the blastocyst stage. Interestingly, spontaneous developmental arrest of embryo culture in vitro seems to occur during the cell cycle of gene activation in all species studied including the human, but it is not caused by total failure of that activation process (Schultz 1993). The early cleavage stages, up to around the 8-cell stage, require pyruvate or lactate as metabolic substrates, but thereafter more glucose is metabolized and may be required (Leese 1991).

The earliest stage at which different types of cells can be identified within the cleaving embryo probably depends upon the species but tends to be around the 8- to 16-cell stage. It has been studied in most detail in the mouse embryo. Up to the early 8-cell stage of mouse embryogenesis, cells are essentially spherical, loosely touching each other, having no specialized intercellular junctions or significant extracellular matrix, and the cytoplasm of each being organized in a radially symmetric manner around a centrally located nucleus.

During the 8-cell stage, the process of *compaction* occurs in which cells:

- flatten on each other to maximize intercellular contact
- initiate formation of gap and focal tight junctions
- radically reorganize their cytoplasmic organization from radially symmetric to a highly asymmetric phenotype.

This latter process includes the migration of nuclei towards the centre of the embryo, redistribution of surface microvilli and an underlying mesh of microfilaments and microtubules to the exposed surface and the localization of endosomes beneath the apical cyto-skeletal mesh. As a result of the process of compaction, the embryo forms a primitive proto-epithelial cyst, with 8 polarized cells, their apices facing outward and their basolateral surfaces internally. The focal tight junctions, which align to become increasingly linear, are localized to the boundary between the apical and basolateral surfaces; gap junctions form between apposed basolateral surfaces and become functional (Fleming & Johnson 1988).

The process of compaction involves the cell surface and calcium dependent cell:cell adhesion glycoprotein E-cadherin (also called L-CAM or uvomorulin). Neutralization of its function disturbs all three elements of compaction. The whole process can function in the absence of both mRNA and protein synthesis. Post-translational controls are sufficient and seem to involve regulation through protein phosphorylation. Significantly, although E-cadherin is not synthesized and present on the surface of cleaving blastomeres, it first becomes phosphorylated early during the 8-cell stage at the initiation of compaction.

The process of compaction is important for the generation of cell diversity in the early embryo. As each polarized cell divides, it retains significant elements of its polar organization so that its daughter cells inherit cytocortical domains, the nature of which reflect their origin and organization in the parent 8-cell. Thus, if the axis of division is aligned approximately at right angles to the axis of cell polarity, the more superficially placed daughter cell inherits all the apical cytocortex and some of the basolateral cytocortex and is polar, whilst the more centrally placed cell inherits only basolateral cytocortex and is apolar. In contrast, if the axis of division is aligned approximately along the axis of the cell polarity, two polar daughter cells are formed. Thus, *2-cell populations* are formed in the 16-cell embryo that differ in phenotype (polar, apolar) and position (superficial, deep), and the number of cells in each population in any one embryo will be determined by the ratio of divisions along and at right angles to the axis of 8-cell polarity. The theoretical and observed limits of the polar to apolar ratio are 16:0 and 8:8. The outer, polar cells contribute largely to the trophectoderm whilst the inner, apolar cells contribute almost exclusively to the inner cell mass in most embryos (Johnson et al 1986).

In cleavage therefore, the generation of cell diversity, to either *trophectoderm* or *inner cell mass*, occurs in the 16-cell morula and precedes the formation of the blastocyst. During the 16-cell cycle, the outer polar cells continue to differentiate an epithelial phenotype, displaying further aspects of polarity and intercellular adhesion typical of epithelial cells, while the inner apolar cells remain symmetrically organized. During the next cell division (16- to 32-cell stage), a proportion of polar cells again divide differentiatively as in the previous cycle, each yielding one polar and one apolar progeny that enter respectively the trophectoderm and inner cell mass lineages. However, in this case, differentiative division is less common than at the 8- to 16-cell transition, yet has the important function of regulating an appropriate number of cells in the two tissues of the blastocyst. Thus, if differentiative divisions were relatively infrequent at the 8- to 16-cell transition, they will be more frequent at the 16- to 32-cell transition, and vice versa.

Following division to the 32-cell stage, the outer polar cells complete their differentiation into a functional epithelium, and display structurally complete zonular tight junctions and begin to form desmosomes. The nascent trophectoderm engages in vectorial fluid transport in the apical to basal direction to generate a cavity which expands in size during the 32- to 64-cell cycles converting the ball of cells to a sphere, the blastocyst. By the blastocyst stage, the diversification of the trophectoderm and inner cell mass lineages is complete and trophectoderm differentiative divisions no longer occur. In the late blastocyst, the trophectoderm is referred to as the *trophoblast*; it can be divided into *polar trophoblast* which lies in direct contact with the inner cell mass, and *mural trophoblast* which surrounds the blastocyst cavity (**3**.35).

Staging of embryos

Prenatal life can be divided into an embryonic period and a fetal period. The embryonic period covers the first 8 weeks of development (weeks following ovulation and fertilization resulting in pregnancy). The ages of early human embryos have been previously estimated by comparing their development with that of monkey embryos of known postovulatory ages. Because embryos develop at different rates and attain different final weights and sizes, a classification of human embryos into 23 stages occurring during the first 8 post-ovulatory weeks was developed, most successfully, by Streeter (Streeter 1942); a task continued today by O'Rahilly (O'Rahilly & Muller 1987). An embryo was initially staged by comparing its development to other embryos. The correlation of particular maternal menstrual histories and the known developmental ages of monkey embryos allowed the construction of growth tables so that the size of an embryo (specifically the greatest length) could be used to predict its presumed age in postovulatory days. Streeter believed such estimations could be ±1 day for any given stage. Within this staging system, which is more fully described for embryonic development on page 344, embryonic life commences with

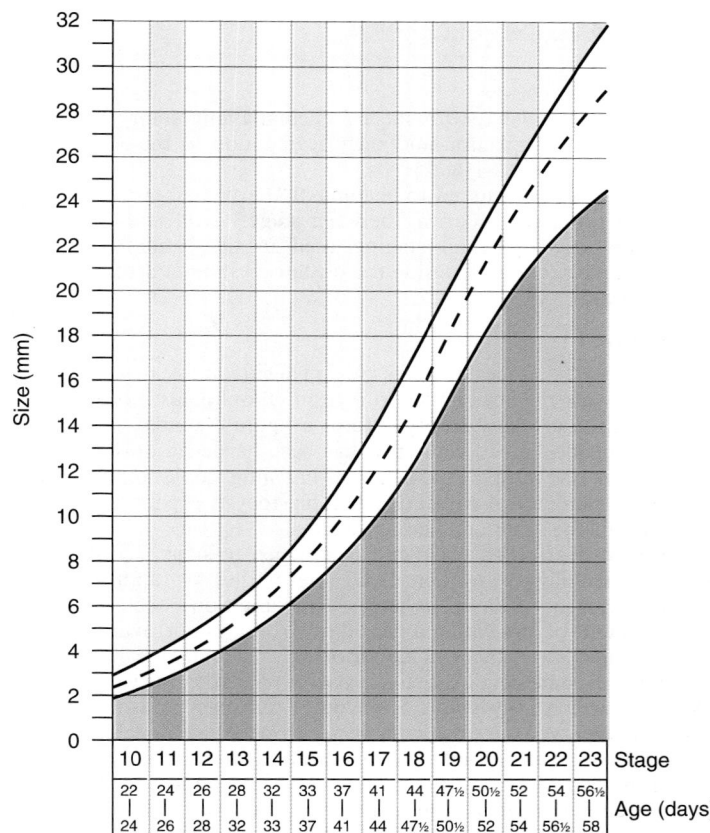

3.31   Chart of developmental stages 10–23. (Devised by Streeter 1942 and O'Rahilly & Muller 1987.)

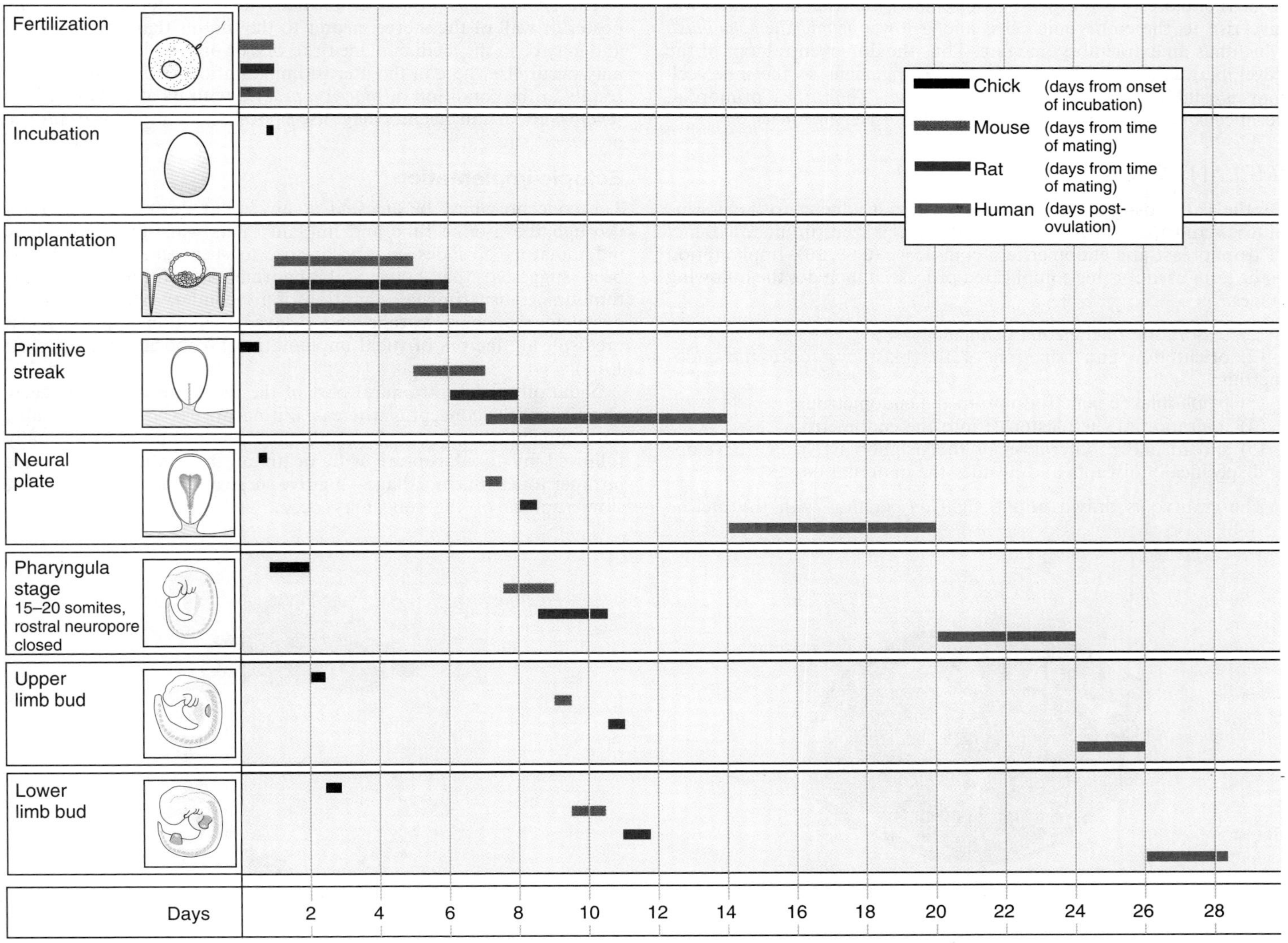

3.32   Within developmental biology evidence concerning the nature of developmental processes has come mainly from experiments on a number of vertebrate embryos. The most commonly used amniote embryos are chick, mouse and rat. This chart illustrates the comparative time scale of development of these animals and the human.

fertilization at stage 1, with stage 2 encompassing embryos from 2 cells, through compaction and early segregation to the appearance of the blastocoele (3.31, 3.32).

The reader is also urged to examine 3.37 which shows the developmental processes occurring between stages 1–10, and 4.1 which shows the developmental staging used in the Embryology and Development section alongside the obstetric estimation of gestation used clinically.

Blastocyst

The blastocyst 'hatches' from its zona pellucida at 6–7 days, possibly assisted by an enzyme similar to trypsin. Trophoblast oozes out of a small slit, and many embryos form a figure 8 shape, bisected by the zona pellucida, especially if it has been hardened during oöcyte maturation and cleavage. Such half-hatching could result in the formation of identical twins. Hatched blastocysts expand and differentiation of the inner cell mass proceeds.

The free unattached blastocyst is assigned to stage 3 of development (O'Rahilly & Muller 1987; see p. 140) at approximately 4 postovulatory days, whereas implantation (before villus development) occurs within a period of 7–12 days postovulation and over the next two stages of development. Two stage 3 blastocysts examined in some detail (Hertig et al 1954) include: one with 58 cells (3.33), of which only about 5 are inner cell mass and destined to form the embryo, the remainder being trophoblast, concerned with extraembryonic membranes and placentation; and another blastocyst consisting of 107 cells (3.34), of which 69 are mural trophoblast cells, 30 are polar trophoblast cells and 8 form the inner cell mass. Even at this early stage these 8 cells are already arranged into an upper layer (i.e. closest to the polar trophoblast), the *epiblast*, which will give rise to the embryonic cells, and a lower layer, the *hypoblast*, which has an extraembryonic fate. Thus the dorsoventral axis of the developing embryo and a bilaminar arrangement of the inner cell mass is established at or before implantation. (The earliest primordial germ cells may also be defined at this stage; Hertig 1968.)

IMPLANTATION

On the sixth postovulatory day the blastocyst adheres to the uterine mucosa and the events leading to the specialized, intimate contact of trophoblast and endometrium commence (3.35, 36). Implantation is the term used for this complicated process; it includes the following stages:

(1) dissolution of the zona pellucida
(2) orientation and adhesion of the blastocyst onto the endometrium
(3) trophoblastic penetration into the endometrium
(4) migration of the blastocyst into the endometrium
(5) spread and proliferation of the trophoblast, which envelops and specifically disrupts and invades the maternal tissues.

The embryo is drawn into a tight association with the uterine epithelium; uterine fluid is withdrawn by progesterone-sensitive pinopods, and short-range forces enable embryos to adhere to epithelia. The pentasaccharide lacto-N-fucopentose-1 on the epithelium and its receptor on the trophoblast could be specifically involved in adhesion. For details of placental development see page 166.

The trophoblast from stages 4 and 5 onwards has two distinct cell arrangements: *cytotrophoblast*, cuboidal cells which form the mural and polar trophoblast; and externally *syncytial trophoblast* (*syncytiotrophoblast*), a multinucleated mass of cytoplasm which forms initially in areas near the inner cell mass after apposition of the blastocyst to the uterine mucosa. It is the syncytial trophoblast which penetrates the uterine luminal epithelium. The uterine epithelial cell junctions are breached by flanges of syncytial trophoblast without apparent damage to the maternal cell membranes or disruption of the intercellular junctions; rather shared junctions are formed with many of the uterine epithelial cells (Enders et al 1983). As the blastocyst burrows more deeply into the endometrium syncytial trophoblast forms over the mural cytotrophoblast but never achieves the thickness of the syncytial trophoblast over the embryonic pole.

The youngest implanting human blastocyst recovered and described in detail (Hertig & Rock 1945, Carnegie embryo No. 8020 Stage 5a) shows an early stage in the process. The polar trophoblast displays an extensive syncytial development which projects into the endometrial stroma but syncytial lacunae have not yet developed. The blastocyst is not completely embedded and a portion of its wall at the abembryonic pole still projects into the uterine lumen. The age is believed to be 7 postovulatory days (Hertig & Rock 1945).

The *site of implantation* is normally in the endometrium of the posterior wall of the uterus, nearer to the fundus than to the cervix, and may be in the median plane or to one or other side. Implantation may occur elsewhere in the uterus; implantation near the internal os results in the condition of *placenta praevia* with its attendant risk of severe antipartum haemorrhage (see p. 1873), or in an *extrauterine* or *ectopic* site.

Ectopic implantation

The conceptus may be arrested at any point during its migration through the uterine tube and implant in its wall. Previous tubule inflammatory episodes may predispose to such tubal arrest. It has been suggested that congenital abnormalities of the tube, tubal tumours, transperitoneal migration of a secondary oöcyte from one ovary to the opposite tube and delayed ovulation are additional predisposing factors of tubal implantation (Woodruff & Pauerstein 1969).

Nidation of the intramural part of the tube often results in early abortion of the conceptus whereas, if it occurs elsewhere in the tube, development often proceeds for about 2 months and is then usually followed by tubal rupture with death of the embryo and severe intraperitoneal haemorrhage—a grave surgical emergency. However, slow rupture of the tube may occur, accompanied by a further

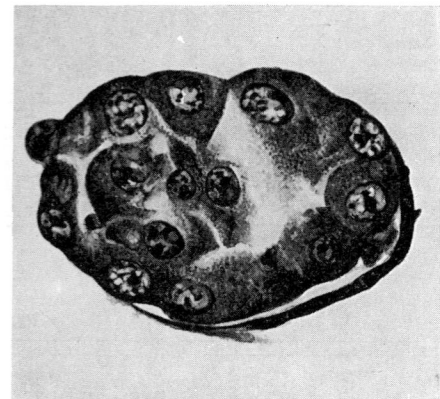

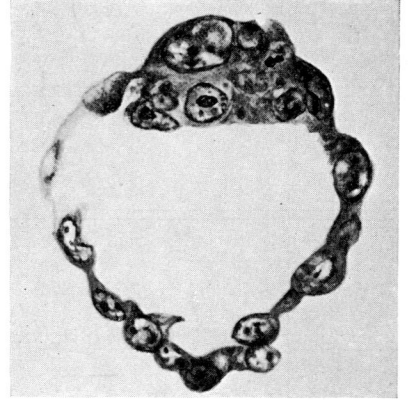

3.33 Section of a 58-cell human blastocyst recovered from the uterine cavity showing the zona pellucida, trophoblast and inner cell mass. Magnification × c. 510. (Hertig et al 1954.)

3.34 Section of a 107-cell human blastocyst recovered from the uterine cavity. The mural and polar trophoblastic cells and the inner cell mass can be distinguished. Magnification × c. 550. (Hertig et al 1954.)

implantation of the conceptus into any adjacent peritonealized surface (secondary abdominal pregnancy), which may lead to rupture of the surface with similar consequences.

Primary ovarian or *abdominal* pregnancies have also been described, in which it has been presumed that the fertilization occurred in the vicinity of the ovary; most cases, however, are probably of the secondary type following a slow tubal rupture or a slow extrusion of the conceptus through the abdominal ostium of the tube.

Apart from their important clinical implications, such conditions emphasize the interesting fact that the conceptus can implant successfully into tissues other than a normal progestational endometrium. Further, prolonged development can occur in such sites and is usually terminated by a mechanical or vascular accident and not by a fundamental nutritive or endocrine insufficiency or by an immune maternal response.

POSTIMPLANTATION DEVELOPMENT

The earliest developmental processes in mammalian embryos involve the production of the extraembryonic structures which will support and nourish the embryo during development. Production of these layers begins before implantation is complete. At present it is unclear where the extraembryonic cell lines arise. The trophoblast was considered to be a source but evidence now points to the inner cell mass as the site of origin. Figure **3**.37 shows the sequence of development of various tissues in the early embryo.

Amniotic cavity

Ultrastructural examination of rhesus monkey embryos at the equivalent of stage 5a show that the *epiblast* cells, which are closest to the implanting face of the trophoblast, have a definite polarity, being arranged in a radial manner with extensive junctions near the centre of the mass of cells, supported by supranuclear organelles (Enders et al 1986). A few epiblast cells are contiguous with cytotrophoblast cells; however, apart from this contact a basal lamina surrounds the now, initially, spherical cluster of epiblast cells isolating them from all other cells. Those epiblast cells adjacent to the hypoblast become taller and more columnar than those adjacent to the trophoblast; this causes the epiblast sphere to become flattened and the centre of the sphere to be shifted towards the polar trophoblast. Amniotic fluid accumulates at the eccentric centre of the now lenticular epiblast mass which is bordered by apical junctional complexes and microvilli. By day 10.5, in the rhesus monkey, there is a definitive *amniotic cavity* roofed by low cuboidal cells which possess irregular microvilli. The cells share short apical junctional complexes and associated desmosomes (Enders et al 1986) and rest on an underlying basal lamina. A demarcation between true amnion cells and those of the remaining definitive epiblast is clear. The columnar epiblast cells are arranged as a pseudostratified layer with microvilli, frequently a single cilium, clefted nuclei and large nucleoli; the cells have a distinct, continuous basal lamina. Cell division in the epiblast tends to occur near the apical surface, causing this region to become more crowded than the basal region. At the margins of the embryonic disc the amnion cells are contiguous with the epiblast; there is a gradation in cell size from columnar to low cuboidal within a two to three cell span (**3.38, 39**).

Yolk sac

The *hypoblast* just prior to implantation consists of a layer of squamous cells only slightly larger in extent than the epiblast. The cells exhibit polarity with apical microvilli facing the cavity of the blastocyst and apical junctional complexes, but they lack a basal lamina. During early implantation the hypoblast extends beyond the edges of the epiblast and can now be subdivided into those cells in contact with the epiblast basal lamina, the *visceral hypoblast*, and those cells in contact with the mural trophoblast, *parietal hypoblast*. The squamous parietal hypoblast cells may share adhesion junctions with the mural trophoblast and, rarely, gap junctions. The visceral hypoblast cells are cuboidal; they have a uniform apical surface towards the blastocyst cavity but irregular basal and lateral regions with flanges and projections underlying one another and extending into intercellular spaces. There is no basal lamina subjacent to the

visceral hypoblast and the distance between the hypoblast cells and the epiblast basal lamina is variable.

A series of modifications of the original blastocystic cavity develops beneath the hypoblast later than those developing above the epiblast. Whilst the amniotic cavity is enlarging within the sphere of epiblast cells, the parietal hypoblast cells are proliferating and spreading along the mural trophoblast until they extend most of the way around the circumference of the blastocyst converging towards the abembryonic pole; at the same time a space appears between the parietal hypoblast and the mural trophoblast limiting the circumference of the hypoblastic cavity. A variety of terms have been applied to the parietal hypoblast layer: extraembryonic hypoblast and later extraembryonic endoderm or the exocoelomic (Heuser's) membrane. The cavity which the layer initially surrounds is termed the *primary yolk sac*, although O'Rahilly and Muller (1987) commend the term *primary umbilical vesicle*. There is considerable confusion concerning the developmental state of the primary yolk sac before initiation of the later cavity, the secondary yolk sac, and in the way in which it forms (see Enders et al 1986). Enders et al conclude that the presence of a complete primary yolk sac cannot be determined from the material in the Carnegie collection or from their studies. The *secondary yolk sac* has been suggested to form in a variety of ways:

- from cavitation of visceral hypoblast (Hill 1932), a method similar to formation of the amnion
- rearrangement of proliferating visceral hypoblast (Heuser & Streeter 1941)
- folding of the parietal layer of the primary yolk sac into the secondary yolk sac (Luckett 1978).

Certainly numerous mitotic figures are seen in the visceral hypoblast preceding secondary yolk sac formation, and at the margin of the visceral portion hypoblast cells overlie one another and appear to indicate a reflection of the layer. Enders et al (1986) conclude that a central portion of the secondary yolk sac may derive from parietal hypoblast and the remainder from visceral but point out that the derivation of the cells may be of little significance as experimental work has shown that in the mouse differentiation of parietal and visceral hypoblast can be reversed (Hogan & Tilly 1981).

The visceral hypoblast cells may later have a focus of production in the posterior margin of the disc. The cells later induce the formation of the primitive streak thus establishing the axis of the embryonic disc (Azar & Eyal-Giladi 1979, 1981; Khaner & Eyal-Giladi 1989). With the later formation of the embryonic cell layers from the epiblast (see p. 142) the visceral hypoblast appears to be sequestered into the secondary yolk sac wall by the expansion of the newly formed embryonic endoderm beneath the epiblast (Tam & Beddington 1992).

It is necessary to point out at this juncture that the early embryonic bilaminar disc was thought to contain the outer layer—future skin—and inner layer—future gut lining—of the embryo, the ectoderm and endoderm. This was the basis of the germ layer theory. Experimental studies have now shown that all of the embryonic cell lines derive from the upper layer of the embryonic disc and that the lower layer has no embryonic fate. The terms epiblast and hypoblast are used to make this distinction between the earliest bilaminar disc layers and the later embryonic layers (see p. 92 for a full account of the embryonic nomenclature).

Descriptions of several human blastocysts at stages 5 and 6 (O'Rahilly & Muller 1987) are available (**3.36, 38, 39**). The trophoblast is now divisible into cytotrophoblast and syncytial trophoblast over the whole of the blastocyst; it is thickest over the embryonic pole but diminishes in thickness over the sides and is exceedingly thin over the abembryonic pole, the last part to be embedded. The syncytial trophoblast which invades and becomes incorporated into maternal vessels encloses numerous lacunae containing maternal blood (Enders et al 1983).

Extraembryonic tissues and coelom

By definition extraembryonic tissues encompass all tissues that do not contribute directly to the future body of the definitive embryo, and later, the fetus. At stage 5 embryos are implanted but not yet villous; they range from 7–12 days old. A feature of this stage is the first formation of extraembryonic mesoblast which will come to

137

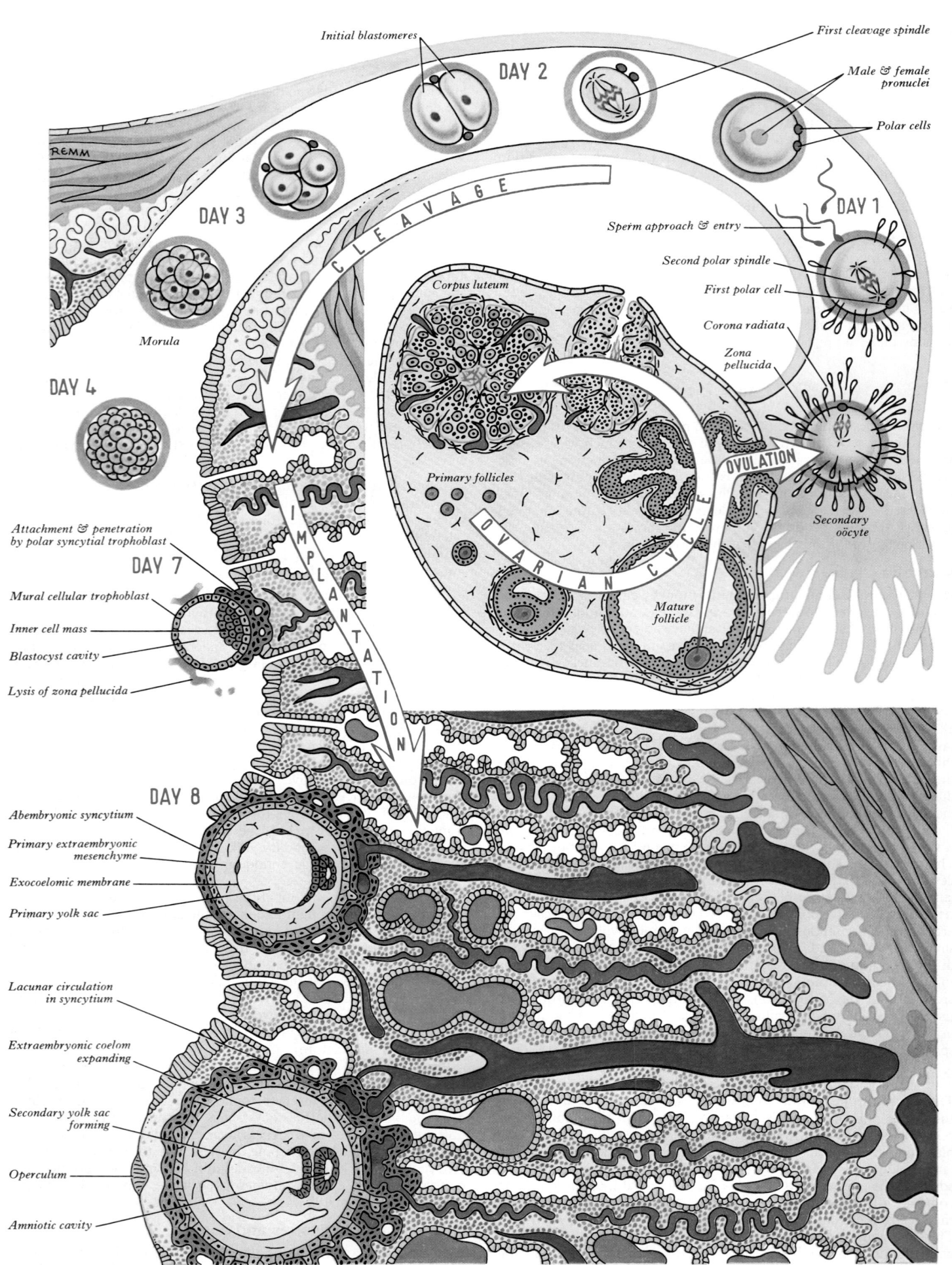

Initial blastomeres

DAY 2

First cleavage spindle

Male & female pronuclei

Polar cells

REMM

DAY 3

DAY 1

Sperm approach & entry

Second polar spindle

First polar cell

Corona radiata

Zona pellucida

Morula

CLEAVAGE

Corpus luteum

OVULATION

DAY 4

Primary follicles

OVARIAN CYCLE

Secondary oöcyte

Mature follicle

Attachment & penetration by polar syncytial trophoblast

IMPLANTATION

DAY 7

Mural cellular trophoblast

Inner cell mass

Blastocyst cavity

Lysis of zona pellucida

DAY 8

Abembryonic syncytium

Primary extraembryonic mesenchyme

Exocoelomic membrane

Primary yolk sac

Lacunar circulation in syncytium

Extraembryonic coelom expanding

Secondary yolk sac forming

Operculum

Amniotic cavity

3.35A   A composite schema of the major events in the varian cycle: ovulation, fertilization, tubal transport and cleavage, differentiation of blastocyst, implantation, early embryogenesis and incipient placentation. Consult text and references for further details and alternative views of formation of amnion, yolk sac and cytotrophoblast.

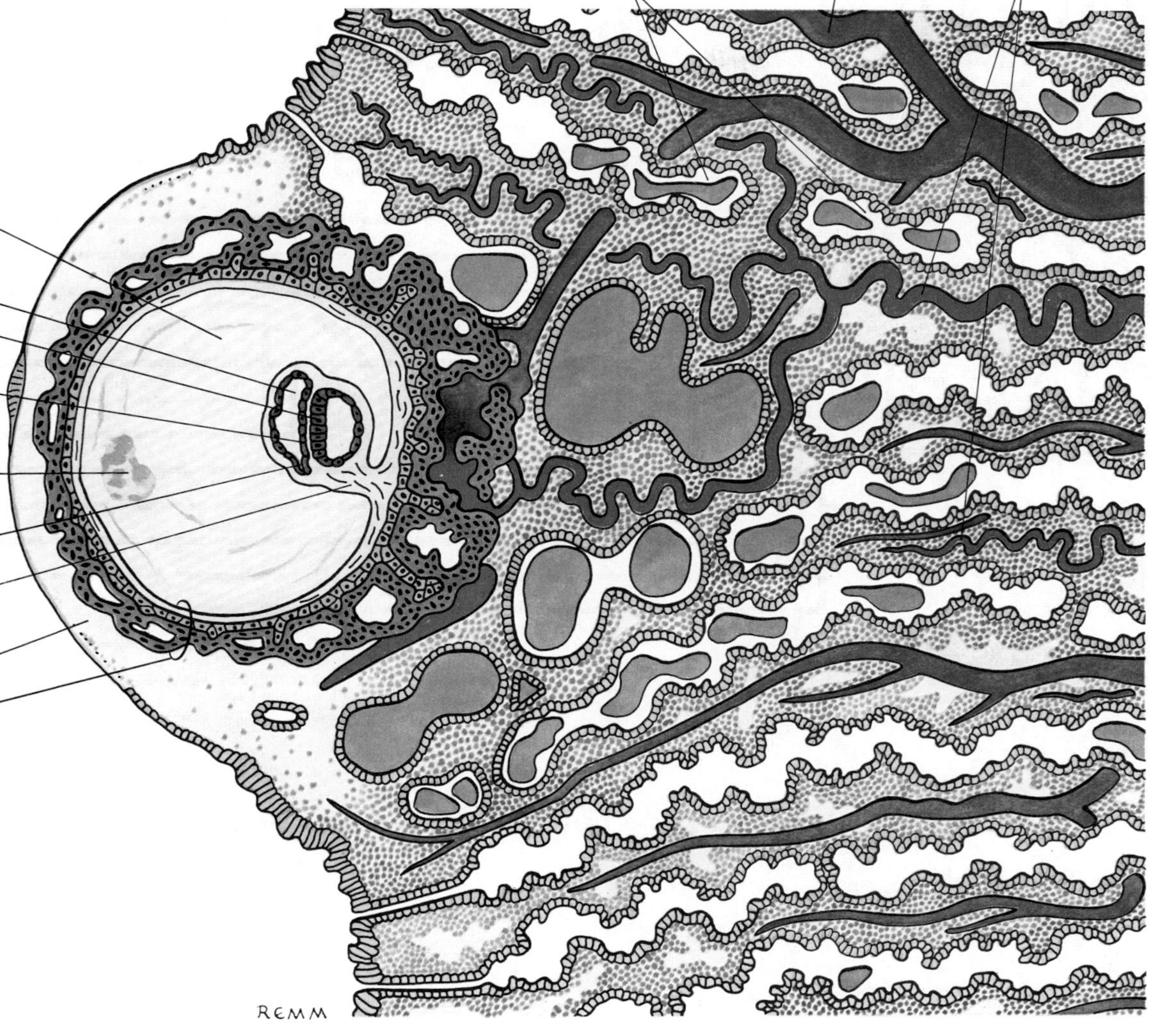

Dilated endometrial glands with secretory products

Endometrial vein

Spiral arteries

Expanded extraembryonic coelom (chorionic cavity)

Secondary yolk sac cavity

Embryonic ectoderm

Embryonic endoderm

Remnants of primary yolk sac

Allantoic diverticulum

Connecting stalk

Decidua capsularis

Chorion

REMM

3.35B Further expansion and differentiation of the blastocyst.

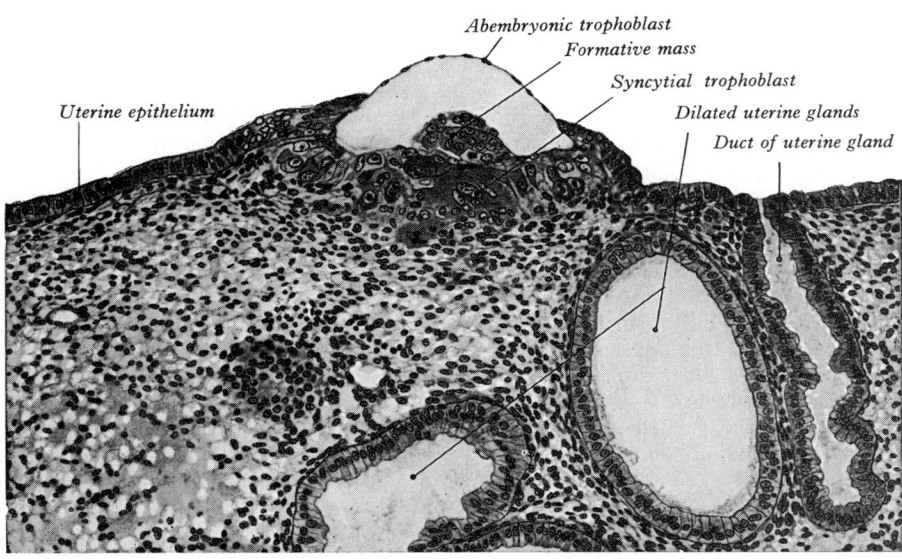

Abembryonic trophoblast

Formative mass

Syncytial trophoblast

Dilated uterine glands

Duct of uterine gland

Uterine epithelium

3.36 A human blastocyst (Carnegie 8020), fertilization age 7–7.5 days, in process of embedding in the uterine mucosa. In the actual specimen the abembryonic trophoblast had collapsed on the formative mass but, for clarity, it has been shown projecting into the uterine cavity. Magnification × c. 150. (Rock & Hertig 1942, 1944.)

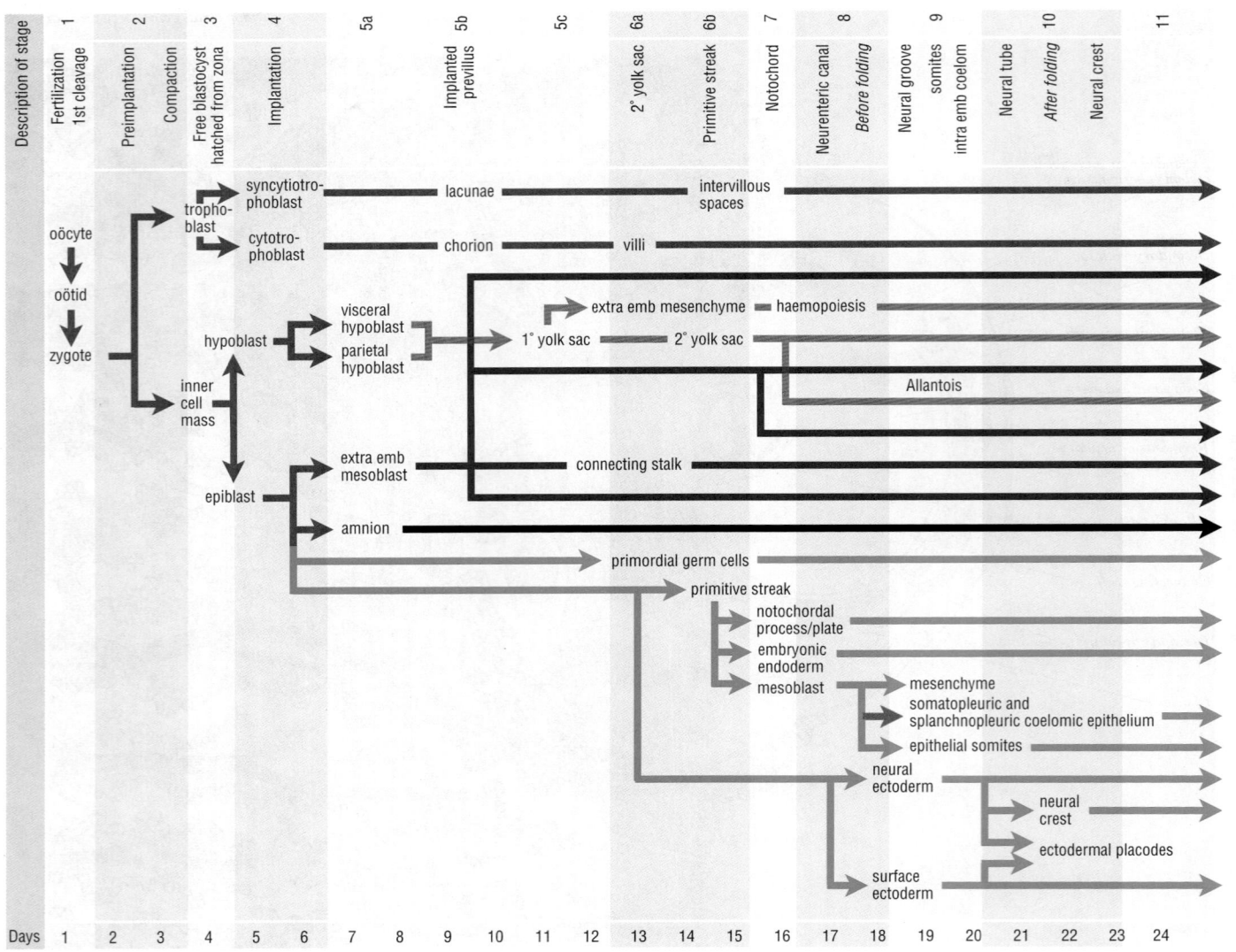

3.37 Chart to show the developmental processes occurring during the first 10 stages of development. In the early stages a series of binary choices determine the cell lineages. Generally the earliest stages are concerned with formation of the extraembryonic tissues, whereas the later stages see the formation of embryonic tissues.

cover the amnion, secondary yolk sac and the internal wall of the mural trophoblast and will form the connecting stalk of the embryo with its contained allanto-enteric diverticulum. The origin of this first mesoblastic extraembryonic layer is by no means clear. For many years it was thought to develop by delamination from the cytotrophoblast (Hertig & Rock 1949), although it was also suggested that it derived from the inner cell mass hypoblast (Heuser & Streeter 1941), or the caudal region of the epiblast (Luckett 1978). The fate of the first mesoblastic extraembryonic layer is at least two-fold and may in fact indicate more than one origin; it gives rise to both the layer known as extraembryonic *mesoblast*, arranged as a *mesothelium* with underlying *mesenchymal* cells; and also to *angioblastic tissue*, which forms the extraembryonic endothelia and blood cells. Recent investigators have disputed the idea of a trophoblastic origin of extraembryonic mesoblast after the observation that there is always a complete basal lamina underlying the trophoblast. The migration of cells out of an epithelium is usually associated with previous disruption of the basal lamina (Nichols 1985, 1986; Erickson 1986). The predominant layer of cells without a basal lamina in the blastocyst is the hypoblast. Enders and King (1988) have convincingly suggested that the earliest mesoblast derives from the parietal hypoblast which appears to form an extracellular structure corresponding to the *magma reticulare* between the mural trophoblast and the primary yolk sac in the stage 5 embryo. They have demonstrated the development of subhypoblastic cells into extraembryonic mesenchyme and into the earliest formed capillaries within developing

villi of the placental disc. They note that it is not clear whether the extraembryonic mesenchyme derives from later proliferation of the earliest subhypoblastic cells or from continuous seeding from the hypoblastic layer, as both cell groups are mitotically active.

Epiblast cells are known to produce extraembryonic mesoblast prior to the development of the primitive streak. This mesenchymatous tissue initially mushrooms beneath the cytotrophoblastic cells at the embryonic pole forming the cores of the developing villus stems, and villi, and the capillaries within them (for information on placentation see p. 157, and for intraembryonic blood vessels see below).

At approximately 13 postovulatory days the conceptus consists of an outer cytotrophoblast (mural trophoblast), clothed externally by labyrinthine syncytiotrophoblast, and the beginnings of an extraembryonic mesoblastic lining; these layers together constitute the *chorion*. The cavity of the blastocyst is now termed the *chorionic cavity* (**3.39**). The embryo proper, situated to one side of the chorion, consists of an epiblastic layer of pseudostratified columnar cells resting on a basal lamina, which is contiguous with a simple layer of amnion cells. The amnion cells are in contact with extraembryonic mesoblast which separates them from the cytotrophoblast. Beneath the epiblast is a layer of visceral hypoblast which is reflected at the edges of the epiblast to form a small cavity, the secondary yolk sac; this may also contain some of the original parietal hypoblast within its wall. The chorionic cavity is filled with diffuse extracellular matrix and extraembryonic mesenchyme cells which attach to the secondary

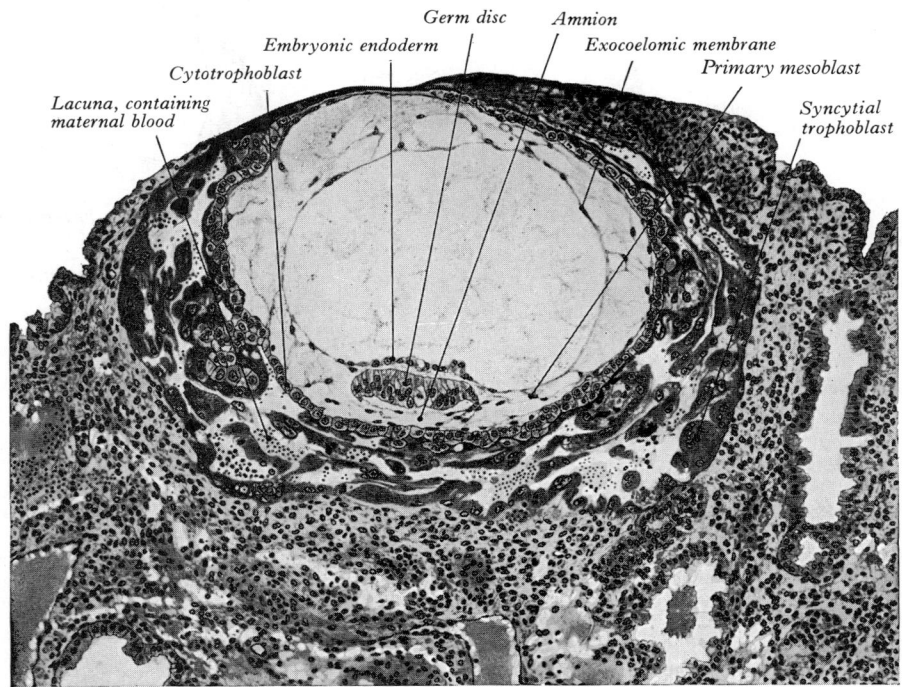

Lacuna, containing
maternal blood
Cytotrophoblast
Embryonic endoderm
Germ disc
Amnion
Exocoelomic membrane
Primary mesoblast
Syncytial
trophoblast

3.38 A human blastocyst (Carnegie 7700), fertilization age 12–12.5 days, embedded in the stratum compactum of the endometrium. Compare with **3.36**. Note lacunae in the syncytial trophoblast, many containing maternal blood; also that the primary yolk sac, surrounded by the exocoelomic mem-

brane, does not fill the blastocyst cavity. The cells of the germ disc are now columnar and form an ectodermal plate. (Drawn from a photomicrograph by A T Hertig.) Magnification × c. 105. (Hertig & Rock 1941.)

yolk sac wall to form a layer of extraembryonic mesenchyme covered with mesothelium. When the extraembryonic mesothelium has completely lined the mural trophoblast and covered both the amnion

Strands of
coagulum in
chorionic
cavity
Secondary
yolk sac
Large blood clot over the point of entry
Intervillous space
Ectodermal germ disc
Trophoblast
Cavity of amnion
Stratum
compactum

Villous stems (secondary grade of
differentiation—see text)
Uterine gland

3.39 An advanced human blastocyst, embedded in the stratum compactum; estimated age, 13.5 days. (Rock & Hertig 1942.)

and the secondary yolk sac the chorionic cavity can be termed the *extraembryonic coelom*.

Towards one end of the embryonic region the extraembryonic mesoblast surrounds a diverticulum of the visceral hypoblast, the allantois, which passes from the roof of the secondary yolk sac to the same plane as the amnion. Whereas initially extraembryonic mesoblast connects the amnion to the chorion over a wide area, with continued development and expansion of the extraembryonic coelom this attachment becomes increasingly circumvented to a *connecting stalk*, a permanent connection between the future *caudal end* of the embryonic disc and the chorion. The connecting stalk forms a pathway along which vascular anastomoses around the allantois establish communication with those of the chorion.

The conceptus at stage 5 consists of the walls of three cavities, amnion and yolk sac, connected at the embryonic bilaminar disc by the epithelial epiblast and visceral hypoblast, enclosed in a larger extraembryonic coelom (chorionic cavity). A fourth cavity, the *allantois*, will form as a hypoblastic diverticulum in stage 7. The 'bilaminar disc' commonly referred to in embryology texts does *not* yet possess the *definitive* embryonic ectoderm and endoderm layers which will give rise to embryonic structures. Only the epiblast will give rise to the embryo. All other layers produced so far are extraembryonic. The amnion and chorion (and surrounding mesoblast) are part of the *extraembryonic somatopleure* whereas the yolk sac, allantois and surrounding extraembryonic mesoblast constitute *extraembryonic splanchnopleure*. At the junctional zone surrounding the margins of the embryonic area, where the walls of the amnion and yolk sac converge, the somatopleuric and splanchnopleuric layers of extraembryonic mesoblast are continuous.

Formation of the embryonic tissues

At early stage 6 the epiblast is producing extraembryonic mesenchyme from its caudal margin. With the appearance of the *primitive streak* a process is begun whereby cells of the epiblast either pass deep to the epiblast layer to form the populations of cells within the embryo or they remain on the dorsal aspect of the embryo to become the embryonic ectoderm. The primitive streak marks the beginning of gastrulation, a period when gross alterations in morphology and complex rearrangements of cell populations occur. The epiblast will during this time give rise to a complex trilaminar structure with a

141

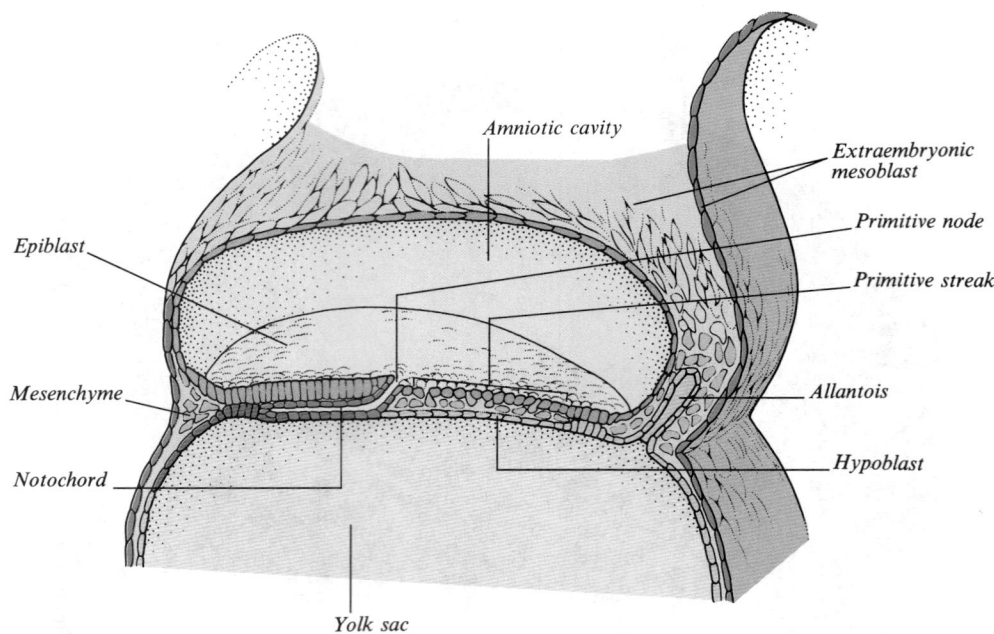

3.40 Diagram of a section through an early conceptus. Ingression of mesoblast is occurring at the primitive streak and the notochord is ingressing via Hensen's node.

defined craniocaudal axis. By the end of gastrulation, cell populations from different, often widely separated, regions of the embryonic disc will often become closely related and the embryonic shape will have been produced.

Primitive streak

Seen from the dorsal (epiblastic) aspect, at stage 6, the embryonic disc appears elongated. The primitive streak is first seen in the caudal region of the embryonic disc, orientated along its long axis, conferring the future craniocaudal axis of the embryo (**3.40, 41**). Although the future cranial and caudal regions of the embryo are well within the boundaries of the embryonic disc, it has become the practice to term the region of the disc closest to the streak caudal, and the region of the disc furthest from the streak cranial or rostral. With the development of the streak the terms medial and lateral can now be used. The primitive streak is a midline proliferative region of the epiblast where cells may break free from the epithelium and migrate **beneath the epiblast** (**3.41**). At the cranial end of the streak there is a curved ridge of cells termed the primitive node (see below) and, in the

midline of the node and streak, cells sink into a primitive groove prior to passing subjacent to the epiblast. *The relative dimensions of the primitive streak and the fates of the cells which pass through it change with the developmental stage.* Thus the streak extends half way along the disc in the stage 6 embryo, reaches its greatest relative length in stage 7 and its maximum length in stage 8. It is still present in stage 11 embryos but relatively few cells pass through it at this stage compared to the early stages.

The passage of epiblast cells through the primitive streak begins their transformation into all of the embryonic cell lines. In this way epiblast forms the embryonic endoderm, the notochord, the primordial germ cells and the mesoblast, as well as contributing extraembryonic mesoblast to the developing placenta. The epiblast cells which do not pass through the streak give rise to the neural and surface ectoderm of the embryo.

The primitive streak may be considered to be generally homologous with the blastopore of lower vertebrates (e.g. amphibia), with the nodal region corresponding to the dorsal lip. Experiments clearly show the lip of the blastopore to be a dynamic wave front

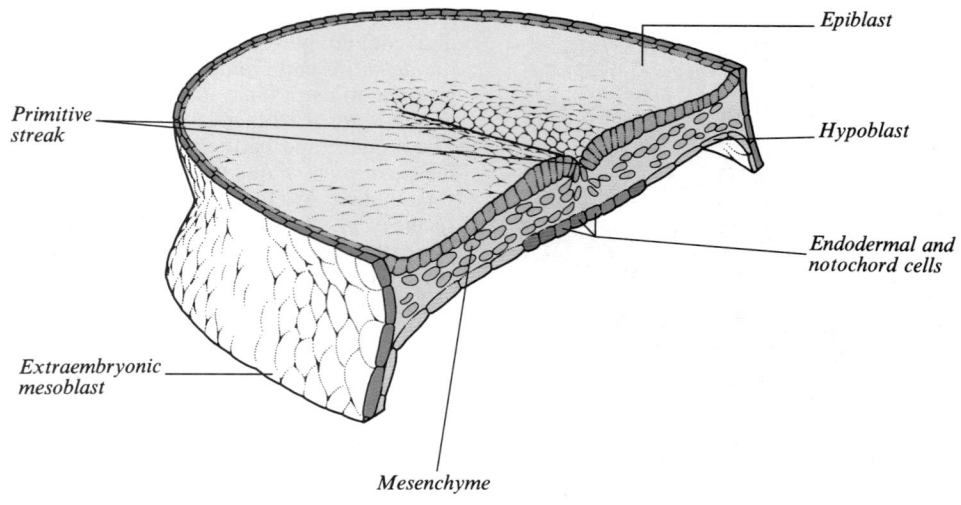

3.41 Diagram of a transverse section through the embryonic plate at the level of the primitive streak to show the early movement of mesoblast between the epiblast and underlying hypoblast.

on which cells are carried into the interior to form the roof of the archenteron, a situation analogous to ingression through the node of the prechordal plate and endoderm.

The primitive streak similarly may be considered analogous to the coapted, or fused, lateral lips of the blastopore. Finally, the cloacal membrane and its immediate environs are considered analogous to the ventral lip of the blastopore. This homology is strengthened by studies which suggest that both the primitive node and the primitive streak represent the 'organiser' of the amniote embryo (Tam & Beddington 1992). The dorsal lip of the blastopore was known many years ago to act as an organizer in amphibian embryos (Spemann & Mangold 1924). The experiments which have now demonstrated a homeobox gene, goosecoid, in *Xenopus* prior to dorsal lip formation, in the same position as Spemann's organizer, and have further demonstrated goosecoid expression in the cephalic end of the mouse primitive streak confirm this homology (De Robertis et al 1992).

At the primitive streak, epiblast cells undergo a period of intense proliferation, the rate of division being much faster than that of blastomeres during cleavage (Graham 1973). Streak formation is associated with:

- the local production of several cell layers
- extensive disruption of the basal lamina
- increase in adhesive plaques and gap junctions
- synthesis of vimentin and loss of cytokeratins by the emerging cells (Lawson et al 1991).

The process by which cells become part of the streak and then migrate away from it is termed *ingression*; it relies on a complete layer of visceral hypoblast beneath the epiblast basal lamina (Bellairs 1987) as well as loss of the epiblast basal lamina at the region of the streak. Azar and Eyal-Giladi (1979, 1981) have shown that the hypoblast induces the formation of the primitive streak. Further it has been demonstrated, in the chick, that the original caudal marginal zone, where the hypoblast cells are generated, prevents other regions of the hypoblast from forming hypoblastic cells and thereby other primitive streaks (Khaner & Eyal-Giladi 1989). Tam and Beddington (1992) provide other evidence to support this finding, noting that the hypoblast beneath the streak does not seem to be replaced by the embryonic endoderm, which sequesters the visceral hypoblast into the secondary yolk sac (see below), even at late streak stages.

Primitive node, or Hensen's node is the most rostral region of the primitive streak. It appears as a curved ridge of cells similar in shape to the top of an old-fashioned keyhole. Cells ingressing from the ridge pass into the primitive pit (the most rostral part of the primitive groove) and then migrate rostrally beneath the epiblast. The primitive node has been recorded in all stage 7 human embryos. At this time, early to midstreak stages, the primitive streak achieves its greatest relative length, about 50% of the total length of the embryonic disc. The primitive node produces axial cell populations,

the prechordal plate, notochord, embryonic endoderm and the medial halves of the somites.

Several workers have noted that in the chick, the node can induce the formation of an extra axis when grafted to a host embryo (Selleck & Stern 1992; Schoenwolf et al 1992), and further it can induce supernumerary digits when grafted into the anterior margin of developing limb buds, properties not seen in other regions of the epiblast. Removal of the node results in complete absence of the notochord and a loss of control of neurulation (O'Rahilly & Muller 1986).

Fate maps. Maps of the epiblast at the primitive streak stage have been derived for many vertebrates. They indicate the putative cell lines which derive from the epiblast layer and suggest that most, perhaps all, chordate embryos share a common strategy of early tissue allocation. The first fate maps of mammalian epiblast (Beddington 1981, 1982; Tam & Beddington 1987) illustrate the broad similarity in composition of the epiblast in a range of vertebrates. Studies of cell fate have shown that epiblast cells which will pass through the streak can be identified, randomly located within the epiblast layer, before their ingression (Stern & Canning 1990); that epiblast fate is determined at or before the time of ingression through the streak, suggesting that *passage through the streak* is the most important factor for future differentiation; and that the position of ingression, be it through the streak or node, directly affects the developmental fate of the cell (Lawson et al 1991). For a composite of the information on the position of ingression through the streak and node see **3**.42.

Time of ingression. The time at which epiblast cells pass through the streak will affect the future fate of the cells. There is an enormous rate of growth of the embryonic disc during the primitive streak stage. In the mouse the embryonic axis increases 3.5 fold in length between the prestreak and neural plate stages. At each stage of development the streak is slightly different, as is the embryo, therefore descriptions of streak stage embryos, and of cells ingressing through the streak must specify the stage of streak development. Often the primitive streak stage is subdivided into early, mid or late streak stages.

Position of ingression through the node or streak. This is also important in deciding the fate of particular cells. Passage through the streak is specified according to position, e.g. via the node, rostral, middle or caudal regions of the streak. Cells ingressing through the primitive node give rise to the axial cell lines, endoderm, notochord and the medial halves of the somites. The rostral portion of the primitive streak produces cells for the lateral halves of the somites, whereas the middle streak produces the lateral plate mesoblast. The next caudal portion of the streak gives rise to the primordial germ cells, which can be distinguished histologically and histochemically at midstreak stages, and the most caudal portion of the streak contributes cells to the extraembryonic mesoblast until the early

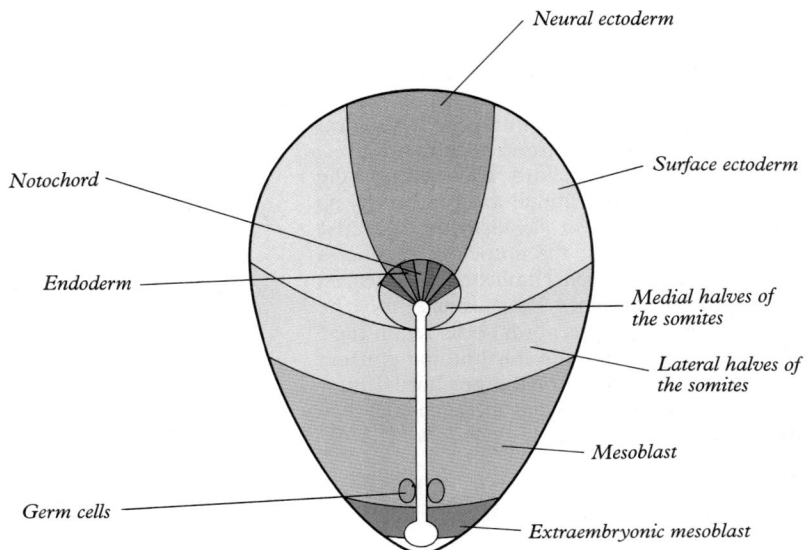

Neural ectoderm

Surface ectoderm

Notochord

Endoderm

Medial halves of the somites

Lateral halves of the somites

Mesoblast

Germ cells

Extraembryonic mesoblast

3.42 Diagram of the predictive fates of the epiblast cell population at the time the primitive streak is present.

somite stage. It is notable that most of the cells termed mesoblast, produced by ingression through the middle and rostral streak regions, differentiate into epithelia on reaching their initial destination (Bellairs 1987).

Embryonic endoderm

The earliest cells migrating through the primitive node and streak give rise to both the *embryonic endoderm* and the *notochord*. Definitive embryonic endoderm has been shown to be derived from epiblast cells located at the primitive node and rostral primitive streak by fate mapping and in situ labelling studies (Lawson et al 1991; Selleck & Stern 1991). It has been demonstrated, in the mouse, that by the midstreak stage the endodermal cells are beneath the epiblast mainly in the midline, interspersed with presumptive notochordal cells, forming the roof of the secondary yolk sac (Tam & Beddington 1992). The ingressing endoderm is suggested to displace the visceral hypoblast into the secondary yolk sac wall by a dramatic territorial expansion, probably brought about by a change in the morphology of these epithelial cells. The putative endoderm cells are cuboidal within the node and become squamous in the endoderm layer; this could result in a fourfold increase in the surface area covered by the cell population (Tam & Beddington 1992). However, a complete replacement of the visceral hypoblast has not yet been confirmed and there may be a mixed population of cells in the endodermal layer in the early stages. For the developmental fate of the embryonic endoderm see **3.43**.

Ingression of cells through the streak and node in the human is apparent at stage 6, and by stage 7 a population of endoderm and notochord cells is present beneath the epiblast (**3.41, 43**). From stages 6–11 the roof of the secondary yolk sac is formed by a midline population of cells, the notochordal plate, in direct lateral continuity with the endodermal cells. It is not until stage 11 that the definitive notochord is formed in the pharyngeal region and the endoderm cells can join across the midline.

Prechordal plate

The prechordal plate is defined as a localized thickening of the endoderm rostral to the notochordal process. As such it represents the first population of endoderm cells to ingress through the primitive node. There is some confusion over the limits and fate of the prechordal plate (sometimes prochordal plate). The term has been used to describe:

- an area of endoderm
- the buccopharyngeal membrane
- an accumulation of mesenchymal cells immediately rostral to the notochord believed to be derived from the endoderm (Adelmann 1922, 1926), a view which has been supported until quite recently (Noden 1988).

The majority of the endodermal and notochordal cells become epithelial after ingression, the endoderm forming the roof of the secondary yolk sac with a local, prechordal region up to 8 cells thick, while the notochordal cells form an epithelial rod between the epiblast and endoderm. (The epithelial prechordal plate forms the endodermal layer of the buccopharyngeal membrane, the pre-oral gut and probably all of the foregut.) A small group of cells, however, remain mesenchymal rostral to the notochord and beneath the epithelial endoderm; these form the most cranial axial mesenchyme population and they are termed *prechordal mesenchyme*. Wachtler and Jacob (1986) have demonstrated that the notochordal process is composed of determined myogenic cells immediately after its formation. The posterior portion becomes transformed into the chorda (notochord proper) whereas the prechordal cells retain their mesenchymal morphology and myogenic fate. Orthotopic grafting has demonstrated that cells leave the edges of the prechordal mesenchyme and migrate laterally into the periocular mesenchyme; they give rise to all the extrinsic ocular muscles (p. 154) (see also p. 274).

Notochordal process

The notochordal process in the stage 8 embryo can be described in three parts:

- a rostral part composed of a cell mass continuous with the prechordal mesenchyme

- a mid portion with cells arranged in a tube with a central notochordal canal
- a caudal portion which consists of a U-shaped arrangement of cells, the notochordal plate, contiguous with the embryonic endoderm.

In the latter arrangement the floor of the notochordal canal has broken down opening the notochordal canal to the secondary yolk sac. This groove and its connection to the primitive node is termed the neurenteric canal. The notochordal process has also been termed the head process, the chordamesoderm, or chorda. It has been suggested that the ingression of notochordal cells is matched by specification of overlying neural ectodermal cells and that both cell lines arise from a common progenitor cell. The notochordal plate is thus matched in length by the future neural floor plate (Jessell et al 1989; see also p. 146).

Notochordal plate

The notochordal plate roofs the secondary yolk sac and early gut until stage 11, at which time the pharyngeal region is the last to contain notochordal plate, the remainder of the plate having formed definitive notochord. The definitive notochord separates from the alimentary layer by a mechanism similar to formation of the neural tube (see p. 217). The most caudal part of the notochordal plate is in continuity with the primitive node, and here, as noted, there may be a transient connection between the amniotic cavity and the secondary yolk sac, the neurenteric canal. (The latter is so named because its upper opening is in the future caudal floor of the neural groove; its lower opening is into the archenteron. See also p. 98.)

Intraembryonic mesoblast (mesenchyme)

The morphology of cells passing through the primitive streak is well documented (Sanders 1986). Epiblast cells ingress through the cranial and middle parts of the streak individually, maintaining their apical epithelial contacts while elongating ventrally. The cells become flask-shaped with thin attenuated apical necks and broad basal regions. The basal and lateral surfaces form lamellipodia and filopodia and the apical contact is released. The cells are now free *mesoblast* cells, their fibroblastic, stellate morphology reflecting the release from the epithelial layer. Once through the streak the cells migrate away using as a substratum the basal lamina of the overlying epiblast and extracellular matrix. The cells contact one another by filopodia and lamellipodia, with which they also contact the basal lamina. Gap junctions have been observed between filopodia and cell bodies. With the appearance of the mesoblast, spaces form between the epiblast and visceral hypoblast which are filled with extracellular matrix rich in glycosaminoglycans. The migrating mesoblast has a leading edge of cells which open up the migration routes and the following cells seem to be pulled along behind in a coordinated mass movement.

Details of the embryological terminology can be found on page 93; however, it should be noted that the terms mesoblast and mesenchyme are being used in a specific manner and are not interchangeable. Previously, cells forming a population between the epiblast and hypoblast were termed mesoderm, or, more recently, mesenchyme. Hay (1968) commended the terms primary and secondary mesenchyme to distinguish between those cells arising from ingression through the streak and from neural crest ingression (see also p. 93). The primary mesenchymal cells will revert to epithelia at their destinations. However, whereas some primary mesenchymal cells may become epithelial within a short time frame, for example somites and lateral plate, other cells may differentiate into endothelium much later, or change to endothelium then back to mesenchyme once more. To cope with these conflicts in terminology the mixed population of epiblast cells which ingress through the primitive streak and come to lie between the epiblast and embryonic endoderm will be termed mesoblast until their fate as specific mesenchymal or epithelial populations is clear.

Primordial germ cells

Although early studies on human embryos have reported primordial germ cells and described their development from the early endoderm of the yolk sac and allantois it is now clear from animal experimentation that the primordial germ cells arise from epiblast ingres-

Endoderm epithelium

Primitive gut

Foregut — recesses, diverticula and glands of the pharynx.

General mucous glandular and duct-lining cells and the main follicular cells of the thyroid.

Epithelium of pharyngeal pouches (tonsil, middle ear cavity, thymus, parathyroids 3 & 4, C-cells of thyroid), adenoids, epithelial lining of the auditory tube, tympanic cavity, tympanic antrum, internal lamina of the tympanic membrane.

Respiratory tract — epithelial lining, secretory and duct-lining cells of the trachea, bronchi, bronchioles and alveolar sacs.

Epithelial lining, secretory and duct-lining cells of the oesophagus, stomach and duodenum.

Hepatocytes of liver, biliary tract, exocrine and endocrine cells of the pancreas.

Midgut — epithelial lining, glandular and duct-lining cells of the duodenum, jejunum, appendix, caecum, part of transverse colon.

Hindgut — epithelial lining, glandular and duct-lining cells of part of the transverse, descending and sigmoid colon, rectum, upper part of anal canal.

Allantois — urinary bladder, vagina, urethra, secretory cells of the prostate and urethral glands.

Coelomic wall epithelium

Walls of intraembryonic coelom

Primitive pericardium — myocardium, parietal pericardium.

Pericardio-peritoneal canals — visceral, parietal and mediastinal pleura, pleuroperitoneal membranes contributing to diaphragm.

Splanchnopleuric epithelium — visceral peritoneum of stomach, peritoneum of lesser and greater omenta, falciform ligament, lienorenal and gastrosplenic ligaments.

Somatopleuric epithelium — parietal peritoneum.

Primitive peritoneal cavity
Splanchnopleuric epithelium — visceral peritoneal covering of mid and hind gut, the mesentery, transverse and sigmoid mesocolon.

Pronephros, epithelial lining of mesonephric ducts, ductus deferens, epididymis, seminal vesicles, ejaculatory duct, ureters, vesical trigone.

Mullerian ducts, epithelial lining of uterine tubes, body and cervix of uterus, vagina, broad ligament of uterus.

Germinal epithelium of gonad (note the germ cells are not included on this chart because of their early sequestration into the extraembryonic tissues).

Germinal epithelium forming cortex of adrenal gland.

Somatopleuric epithelium - parietal peritoneum, tunica vaginalis of testis.

Mesenchyme

Paraxial mesenchyme
(somites and somitomeres)
Sclerotome — vertebrae and portions of the neurocranium, axial skeleton.
Myotome — all voluntary muscles of the head, trunk and limbs.
Dermatome — dermis of skin over dorsal regions.

Intermediate mesenchyme — connective tissue of gonads, mesonephric and metanephric nephrons, smooth muscle and connective tissues of the reproductive tracts.

Septum transversum — epicardium, fibrous pericardium, portion of diaphragm, oesophageal mesentery, sinusoids of liver, tissue within lesser omentum and falciform ligament.

Lateral plate mesenchyme
Splanchnopleuric layer — smooth muscle and connective tissues of respiratory tract and associated glands.

Smooth muscle and connective tissues of intestinal tract, associated glands and abdominal mesenteries.

Smooth muscle and connective tissue of blood vessels (also see below).

Somatopleuric layer — appendicular skeleton, connective tissue of limbs and trunk, including cartilage, ligaments and tendons.

Dermis of ventral body wall and limbs.

Mesenchyme of external genitalia.

Angiogenic mesenchyme
Endocardium of heart, endothelium of blood and lymphatic vessels, vessels of choroid plexus, sinusoids of liver and spleen, circulating blood cells, microglia, tissue macrophages.

Surface ectoderm epithelium

Ectodermal placodes
Adenohypophysis.

Cranial sensory ganglia of nerves V, VII, VIII, IX, X.

Olfactory receptor cells and olfactory epithelium.

Epithelial walls of the membranous labyrinth, the cochlear organ of Corti.

Lens of the eye.

Enamel organs of the teeth.

Cranial structures
Secretory and duct-lining cells of the lacrimal, nasal, labial, palatine, oral and salivary glands.

Epithelia of the cornea and conjunctiva.

Epithelial lining of the external acoustic meatus and external epithelium of the tympanic membrane.

Epithelial lining of the lacrimal canaliculi and nasolacrimal duct.

Epithelial lining of the paranasal sinuses, lips, cheeks, gums and palate.

Epidermal structures
Most of the cutaneous epidermal cells, the secretory, duct-lining and myoepithelial cells of the sweat, sebaceous and mammary glands.

Hairs and nails.

Proctodeal epithelium and epithelium of the terminal male urethra.

Neural plate epithelium

CNS — Brain and spinal cord
Neurohypophysis.

Prosencephalon (telencephalon and diencephalon) — cerebral hemispheres, basal nuclei.

Mesencephalon — cerebral peduncles, tectum, tegmentum.

Rhombencephalon (metencephalon and myelencephalon) — cerebellum, pons, medulla oblongata.

Spinal cord.

All cranial and spinal motor nerves.

All CNS neurons, including preganglionic efferent neurons, with somata within the CNS.

Astrocytes and oligodendrocytes

Ependyma lining the cerebral ventricles, aqueduct and central canal of brain and spinal cord, tanycytes covering the choroid plexuses, circumventricular cells.

Retina and optic nerve (II), epithelium of the iris, ciliary body and processes.

Neural crest

Neural derivatives
Sensory neurons of the cranial ganglia V, VII, VIII, IX, X.

Sensory neurons of the spinal dorsal root ganglia and their peripheral sensory receptors.

Satellite cells in all sensory ganglia.

Sympathetic ganglia and plexuses: neurons and satellite cells.

Parasympathetic ganglia and plexuses: neurons and satellite cells.

Enteric plexuses: neurons and glial cells.

Schwann cells of all the peripheral nerves.

Medulla of the adrenal gland. Chromaffin cells. Carotid body type I cells (and type II, satellite type cells).
Calcitonin-producing (C-cells).

Melanocytes.

Mesenchymal derivatives in the head
Frontal, parietal, squamous temporal, nasal, vomer, palatine bones, maxillae and mandible etc.

Meninges.

Choroid and sclera of eye.

Connective tissue of lacrimal, nasal, labial, palatine, oral and salivary glands.

Dentine of teeth.

Connective tissues of head, including cartilage, ligaments and tendons.

Connective tissues of thyroid gland and of the pharyngeal pouches, i.e. parathyroid glands, thymus.

Tunica media of the outflow tract of the heart and the great vessels.

3.43 Chart indicating the structures which will be derived from specific epithelial and mesenchymal populations in the early embryo.

sing at the caudal end of the primitive streak. Where these epiblast cells are located on the embryonic disc, i.e. from rostral regions which migrate to the streak or from local caudal regions, has not been elucidated. However, some studies have demonstrated *extremely early segregation* of the germ cells, when the epiblast layer consists of only 10–13 cells (Soriano & Jaenisch 1986). It is suggested that the primordial germ cells remain sequestered in the extraembryonic mesenchyme at the caudal end of the embryo until the embryonic endoderm has been produced and gastrulation completed (Ginsburg et al 1990), then with the folding of the embryo underway, the primordial germ cells begin their migration along the allantoic and hind gut endoderm. The formation of the tail fold brings the proximal portion of the allantois within the body reducing the final distance over which the cells migrate to the genital ridges.

Embryonic ectoderm

When the ingression of cells through the primitive streak is completed the cells remaining in the epiblast layer are termed embryonic ectoderm cells. This layer still contains a mixed population as both surface ectoderm cells and neural ectoderm cells are present. It is suggested that these cells were originally in the cranial half of the disc at the early streak stage, with the neural fated cells being closest to the streak and the surface ectoderm being most cranial (**3.42**). The process of neurulation resites most of the neuroepithelial cells (see below). For the developmental fates of the surface and neural ectoderm see **3.43**.

Trilaminar disc

The stage 8 embryo, of approximately 18–19 postovulatory days, has three layers present and can be termed the trilaminar disc. It is pear-shaped, broader cranially than caudally. The upper *epiblast* cells are tall, forming a pseudostratified columnar epithelial layer with a basal lamina, except at the primitive streak where the cells are ingressing to form the other layers. The more cranially placed epiblast will give rise to the surface ectoderm. The extent of the future neural plate can be assessed; it is correlated to the length and width of the notochordal plate directly beneath. The lower embryonic endoderm, a simple squamous layer with a developing basal lamina, is not always complete at this stage particularly in the midline caudal to the prechordal plate, which is still occupied by the notochordal process or plate.

The middle, mesoblast, layer is composed of free cells migrating cranially, laterally and caudally from the primitive streak. They produce extracellular matrix which separates the epiblast and endoderm of the embryonic area permitting their passage. The streams of mesoblast which pass in a cranial direction flank the notochordal plate, pass around the prechordal plate region and then converge medially to fuse in the midline beyond its cephalic border. This transmedian mass is the cardiogenic mesoblast in which the heart and pericardium are to develop. Around the extreme cephalic margin of the embryonic area, the cardiogenic mesoblast fuses with the junctional zone of extraembryonic mesoblast. This region will eventually form the septum transversum and primitive ventral mesentery of the foregut. Mesoblast passing laterally from the streak soon approaches and becomes confluent with the extraembryonic mesoblast around the margins of the disc, i.e. at the *junctional zone* where the splanchnic and somatic strata of extraembryonic mesoblast merge.

The mesoblast which streams caudally from the primitive streak skirts the margins of the cloacal membrane (see below) and then converges towards the caudal midline extremity of the embryonic disc to become continuous with the extraembryonic mesoblast of the connecting stalk. Thus the mesoblast extends between the epiblast and endoderm over all of the disc area except cranially at the prechordal plate (see p. 144), a portion of which will become the *buccopharyngeal membrane*, and caudally at the *cloacal membrane*. The cloacal membrane is a patch of thickened endoderm, similar to the prochordal plate, caudal to the primitive streak. At the present time it is not clear if the lower layer of the cloacal membrane consists of visceral hypoblast like the more cranial primitive streak, (the hypoblast is necessary for maintaining the streak), or if it is replaced by migrating embryonic endoderm, or if there is a region for ingression of endoderm at the caudal end of the streak similar to the node cranially.

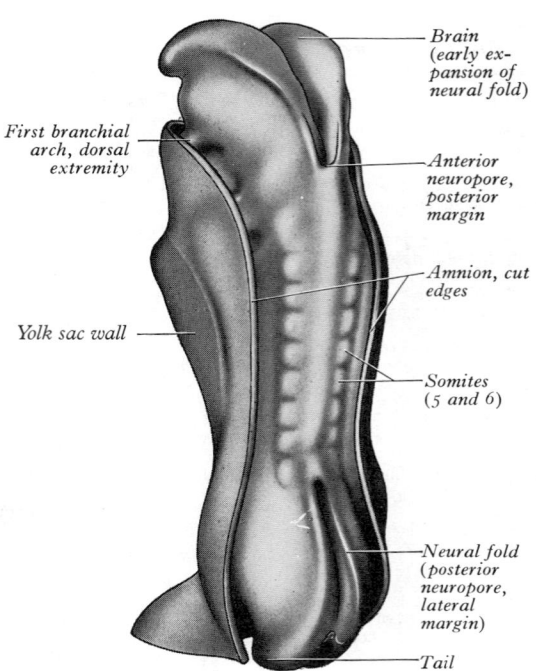

3.44 A human embryo, 2.1 mm long, with 9 somites: left lateral and dorsal aspects. Nearly all the yolk sac and the caudal amnion have been excised to show the tail region. (From a model by Eternod.)

Still further caudally the embryonic disc develops a midline diverticulum adjacent to the cloacal membrane, this diverticulum, the *allantois*, projects into the extraembryonic connecting stalk. There is little information concerning which cells form the allantois, i.e. whether it is composed of visceral hypoblast, parietal hypoblast or embryonic endoderm. The allantois later develops a rich anastomotic blood supply around it in the manner of the yolk sac.

Neurulation

Neurulation begins at stage 9 (**3.44**, **45**). The process, although continuous spatially and temporally, can be divided into four stages:

(1) local elongation of the ectoderm cells in a midline zone of the disc and their reorganization into a pseudostratified epithelium, the *neural plate*.
(2) reshaping of the neural plate.
(3) bending of the plate into a *neural groove*.
(4) closure of the neural groove into a *neural tube* from the midportion to its cranial and caudal ends with formation of a continuous surface ectoderm dorsal to the tube.

The regions of rostral and caudal fusion are termed rostral and caudal neuropores respectively.

The extent of the neural plate initially corresponds precisely in length to the underlying notochord and axial tissues; thus it extends from the cranial border of the primitive node to the buccopharyngeal membrane (**3.46**). Later it extends laterally beyond the notochord to cover the paraxial mesenchyme. Studies have suggested that the neural floor plate cells arise from a common progenitor cell which also provides the cell line for the notochord (Jessell et al 1989) (see also p. 226).

During the period of neurulation extensive changes are taking place in the embryonic mesoblast. Mesoblast cells migrate to their destinations, predetermined by their passage through the streak or node, and rapidly show differences in morphology and organization. Initially, two separate cell populations can be identified:

- a thickened medial portion which lies close to the notochord and elevating neural folds, the *paraxial mesenchyme*
- a flattened lateral portion which extends to the periphery of the embryonic area, the *lateral plate mesenchyme*; this mesenchyme is contiguous with the extraembryonic mesoderm which covers the amnion and yolk sac walls.

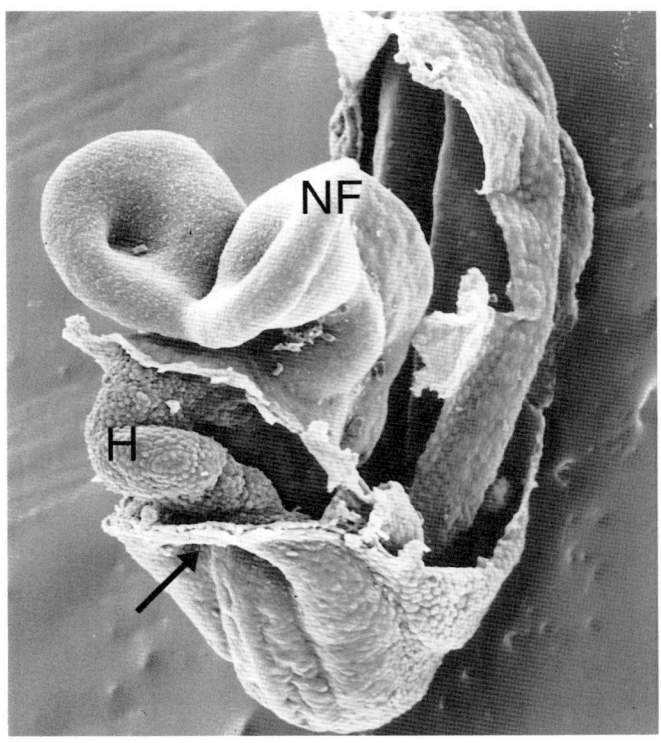

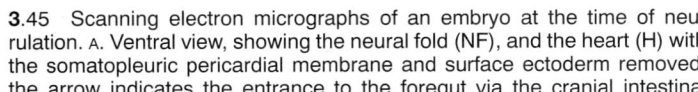

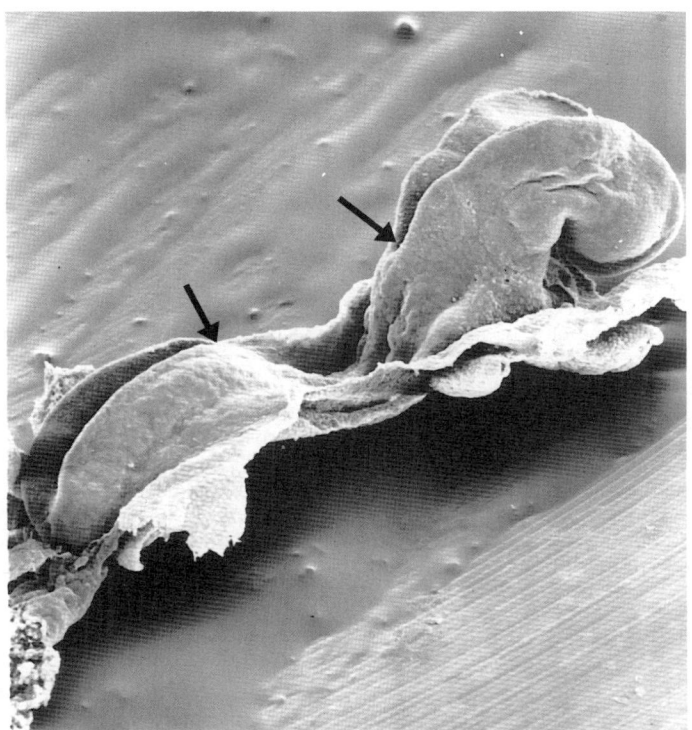

3.45 Scanning electron micrographs of an embryo at the time of neurulation. A. Ventral view, showing the neural fold (NF), and the heart (H) with the somatopleuric pericardial membrane and surface ectoderm removed; the arrow indicates the entrance to the foregut via the cranial intestinal portal. B. Dorsolateral view; the arrows indicate the extent of rostral (to the right) and caudal (to the left) neural tube formation. (Photographs by P Collins; printed by S Cox, Electron Microscopy Unit, Southampton General Hospital.)

The paraxial mesenchyme shows the earliest differentiation. When the neural folds fuse, initially at the level of the hindbrain and cervical cord, the paraxial mesenchyme forms segmental condensations each side of the neural tube, the epithelial somites. Between 4 and 12 pairs of somites are formed during stage 10, the most caudal somites being on a level with the caudal neuropore; they develop caudally from unsegmented mesenchyme at a rate which matches the caudal fusion of the neural tube (see somites below).

As the neural plate grows, its margins become raised as the *neural folds*. The neural folds become particularly prominent at the cranial end of the disc, the future forebrain. Here the folds are separated rostrally from each other by the terminal notch, which abuts the buccopharyngeal membrane. Three major divisions of the brain appear at this time, before the neural tube has formed. They are marked by two slight transverse constrictions on the surface ectoderm indicating a division into the prosencephalon or forebrain, the mesencephalon or midbrain and the rhombencephalon or hindbrain.

Neural tube formation. This is closely linked to changes in cell shape. The neural ectodermal cells become elongated and then wedge shaped. It has been suggested that the forces needed to shape the neural tube are intrinsic to the neurectoderm cells themselves; neurulation occurs as a result of the changes in shape of these cells generated by their cytoskeleton elements (Schoenwolf & Smith 1990). The entire neural plate is also elongating and has considerable cell proliferation at this time. The lateral mesenchymal cells and extracellular matrix provide support for the elevating folds and surface ectoderm and aid the alignment of the neural layers at fusion.

The neural groove deepens, its lateral then dorsal edges come into contact and fuse to convert the groove into a sagittal slit-like canal. The overlying surface ectodermal layers from each side likewise fuse over the neural tube. Neural tube fusion occurs first in the hindbrain or upper cervical region in the third week (stage 10, 22–23 post-ovulatory days). The fusion extends both rostrally and caudally until only a small opening is left at each end. These are the rostral and caudal neuropores; they close in the middle and latter ends of the fourth week respectively. The neural tube forms the central nervous system (CNS). After closure of the neural tube has commenced, ridges can be seen on the floor of the rhombencephalon: these are termed *rhombomeres* and they have significance for patterning of the brain and head region (for a more detailed account of neurulation see below).

Neural crest

Neural crest is the name given to a band of cells at the outermost edges of the neural plate, adjacent to the presumptive epidermis (3.46). Neural crest cells, from the head region, assume a mesenchymal morphology and begin migration prior to neural tube closure; in the trunk, the cells remove themselves from the epithelium as the neural tube closes. They lie on the dorsal part of the newly formed neural tube for some time before migration. Crest cells can migrate over considerable distances, they contribute a major population of mesenchyme to the head, and also to a wide range of different cell lines in the trunk. They are referred to either as neural crest cells or as ectomesenchyme, to note their derivation from the

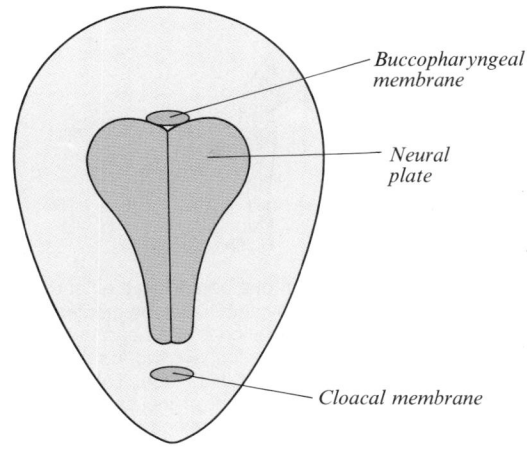

3.46 Diagram showing the extent and shape of the neural plate. The buccopharyngeal and cloacal membranes are indicated.

ectoderm. (Hay 1968 commended the term secondary mesenchyme.) They do not usually give rise to epithelial tissues. They give rise to much of the peripheral nervous system (PNS) (see below).

Ectodermal placodes. These make a significant contribution to the PNS and are intimately involved in the formation of the cranial sensory ganglia (see p. 224). After the neural crest cells have begun their migration and have passed beneath the placodal regions the surface ectoderm shows localized thickenings. In the lateral regions of the pharyngeal arches, at stage 10–11, cells remove themselves individually from the ectoderm and become associated with neural crest cells in the cranial sensory ganglia supplying these arches (see p. 224). Larger ectodermal placodes retain their epithelial nature and become closely associated with the neural tube. Two otic placodes are localized one on each side at the lateral region of the second pharyngeal arch; they give rise to the fluid filled labyrinth of the inner ear (see p. 262). One midline placode invaginates as the adenohypophysis (see p. 257) immediately rostral to the buccopharyngeal membrane. Prior to neurulation, the cells which will give rise to the adenohypophyseal placode lie in the midline, rostral neural fold (neural ridge) (**3.**100). There are a variety of non-neural placodes. The paired optic placodes give rise to the lens in each eye; similar specializations of the ectoderm in the head give rise to the outer coating of the teeth.

Folding of the embryo

In a diagrammatic representation of the disc viewed from the ectodermal aspect, all of the future external surface of the body is delimited. Each end of the gut tube is specified on the ectodermal surface at the buccopharyngeal and cloacal membranes, regions where the ectoderm and underlying endoderm are opposed without intervening mesoblast. In the midline between these membranes the neural tube will form from fusion of the lateral edges of the neural plate and the surface ectoderm will fuse in the midline to constitute the future skin of the back.

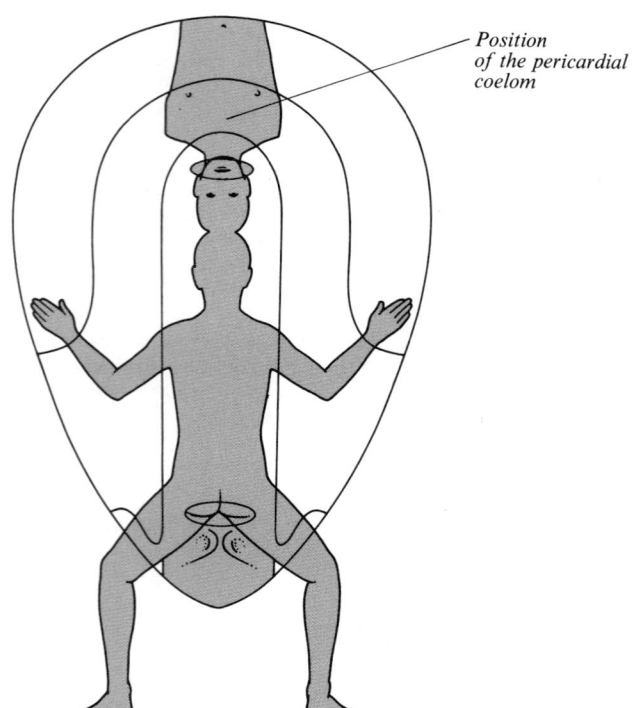

Position
of the pericardial
coelom

3.47 Diagrammatic representation of a person on the flat embryonic disc. The position of the central nervous system has been matched to the dimensions of the neural plate, and the position of the heart in the thorax to the position of the pericardial coelom. The limbs, although represented in this diagram, are not present on the disc at this stage. The usefulness of this diagram lies in its illustration of the extent of the anterior body wall both rostral to the buccopharyngeal membrane and caudal to the cloacal membrane. The future dorsal regions of the body are found medially on the disc, while the ventral regions of the body are situated laterally and peripherally on the disc. After head and tail folding and lateral folding the peripheral edge of the disc becomes constricted as the edge of the umbilicus.

The representation of a person on the trilaminar disc (**3.**47) shows to some extent the way in which the positions of the main body structures are already specified in the unfolded embryo. The portion of the disc between the buccopharyngeal membrane and the edge of the disc will become the anterior thoracic wall and the anterior abdominal wall cranial to the umbilicus. Further caudally, midway along the neural axis, the lateral portions of the disc will become the lateral and anterior abdominal walls of the trunk; that portion of the disc beyond the cloacal membrane will form the anterior abdominal wall caudal to the umbilicus. Thus the circumference of the disc, where the embryonic tissue meets the extraembryonic membranes, will become restricted to the connection between the anterior abdominal wall and the umbilical cord, i.e. the umbilicus.

Head folding begins at stage 9 when the fusing cranial neural plate rises above the surface ectoderm and the portion of the disc rostral to the buccopharyngeal membrane, containing the cardiogenic mesenchyme, moves to lie ventral to the developing brain. The prosencephalon and buccopharyngeal membrane are now the most rostral structures of the embryo. The previously flat region of endoderm, the prechordal plate, is now modified into a deep tube, the primitive foregut. Tail folding can be seen in stage 10 embryos when the whole embryo comes to rise above the level of the yolk sac. The similar movement of the part of the disc caudal to the cloacal membrane results in its repositioning ventral to the neural plate. Generally, as the embryo rises above the edges of the disc the lateral regions of the disc are drawn ventrally and medially, contributing to the lateral folding of the embryo. (For a full understanding of this process it is necessary to study the diagrams in **3.**48A–G)

Formation of the intraembryonic coelom

At and just before stage 9 (before formation of the head fold), vesicles appear between the mesenchymal cells cranial to the buccopharyngeal membrane and within the cranial lateral plate mesenchyme. At the periphery of the vesicles the mesenchymal cells develop junctional complexes and apical polarity, thus forming an epithelium. The vesicles become confluent forming a horseshoe-shaped tube, the *intraembryonic coelom*, which extends caudally to the level of the first somite and laterally into the lateral plate mesenchyme towards the extraembryonic mesenchyme; the intra- and extraembryonic coeloms do not communicate at this stage. The lateral plate mesenchyme thus develops somatopleuric coelomic epithelium subjacent to the ectoderm, and a splanchnopleuric coelomic epithelium next to the embryonic endoderm (**3.**49).

During development of the head fold the morphological movements which organize the foregut and buccopharyngeal membrane have a similarly profound effect on the shape of the intraembryonic coelom. The midline portion of the originally flat, horseshoe-shaped coelom moves ventrally leaving the caudal arms of the horseshoe in their original position. Thus the midline part of the coelom, which was originally just rostral to the buccopharyngeal membrane, comes to lie anterior (ventral) to the foregut (caudal to the buccopharyngeal membrane), and the two lateral extensions of the coelom pass close to the lateral walls of the foregut on each side: the caudal portions of the coelom (the two arms of the horseshoe), which in the unfolded disc communicated laterally with the extraembryonic coelom, turn 90° to lie lateral to the gut, communicating with the extraembryonic coelom ventrally.

Compartments of the coelom which will later in development give rise to the body cavities can already be seen; the midline ventral portion, caudal to the buccopharyngeal membrane, becomes the pericardial cavity, the canals lateral to the foregut (pericardioperitoneal canals) become the pleural cavities and the uppermost part of the peritoneal cavity, and the remaining portion of the coelom becomes the peritoneal cavity. By stage 11 the intraembryonic coelom within the lateral plate mesenchyme extends caudally to the level of the caudal wall of the yolk sac. The intra- and extraembryonic coeloms communicate widely each side of the midgut along the length of the embryo from the level of the 4th somite (**3.**50).

In the early embryo the intraembryonic coelom provides a route for the circulation of coelomic fluid which, with the beating of the heart tube, functions as a primitive circulation, taking nutritive fluid deep into the embryo, until superseded by the blood vascular system.

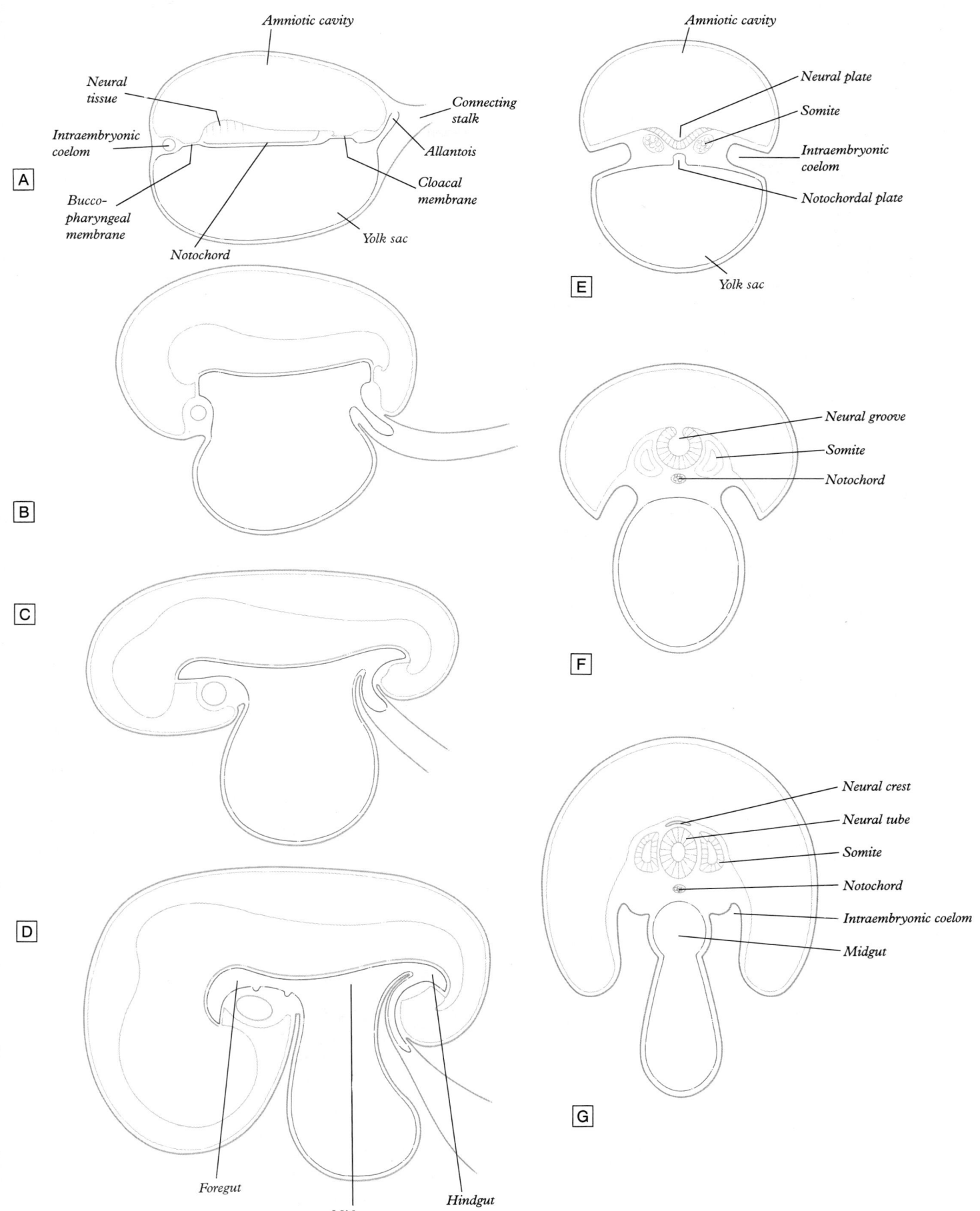

3.48 A series of diagrams to illustrate head and tail folding of the embryo, and lateral folding.

A–D. Midsagittal (longitudinal or axial) sections through the embryonic disc at successive stages; the relative positions of the buccopharyngeal and cloacal membranes have been maintained, thus the movement of the most rostral and caudal portions of the disc can be followed. As these portions of the disc move ventrally the, initially, widely open yolk sac becomes constricted and fore- and hindgut divisions can be seen; the midgut is that region which remains in wide connection to the yolk sac.

E–G. Transverse sections through the midpoint of the embryonic disc at successive stages to illustrate lateral folding. This occurs as neurulation proceeds.

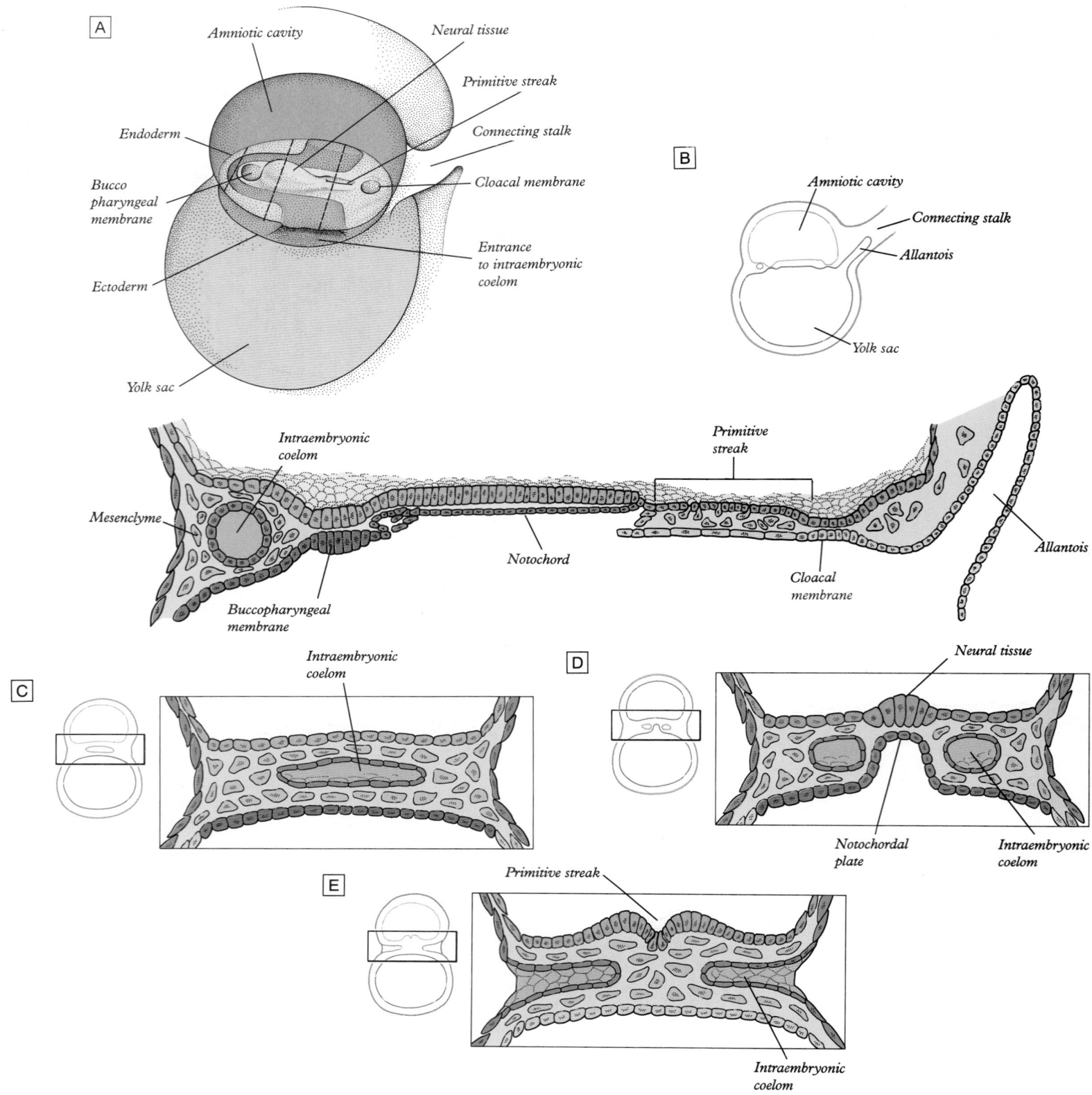

3.49 A. Diagram of an unfolding embryo showing the disposition of the intraembryonic coelom within the embryonic disc. The lines across the embryo show the level of transverse sections through the disc.

B. Longitudinal section through the disc. C, D, E. Transverse sections through the disc at the points indicated in (A).

In spite of the importance of the coelom in defining the body cavities, and of the coelomic epithelium in the production of the major mesenchymal populations of the trunk (3.51), only a few workers have considered the overall contribution of the coelom and its epithelium to the embryo (Streeter 1942; Langemeijer 1976). The coelom can be described as a single, tubular organ comparable to the neural tube in that it possesses a specialized wall that encloses a cavity. Certainly the proliferating coelomic epithelium has many

similarities to the neural ectoderm. It is pseudostratified columnar epithelium with an inner germinal layer from which cellular progeny migrate. Both epithelia after the germinal phase ultimately form the lining of a cavity, ependyma for the neural epithelium and mesothelium for the coelomic epithelium.

The coelomic epithelium like the neural epithelium produces cells destined for different fates from different sites and developmental times. It is noticeable that the coelomic cells (like the neural

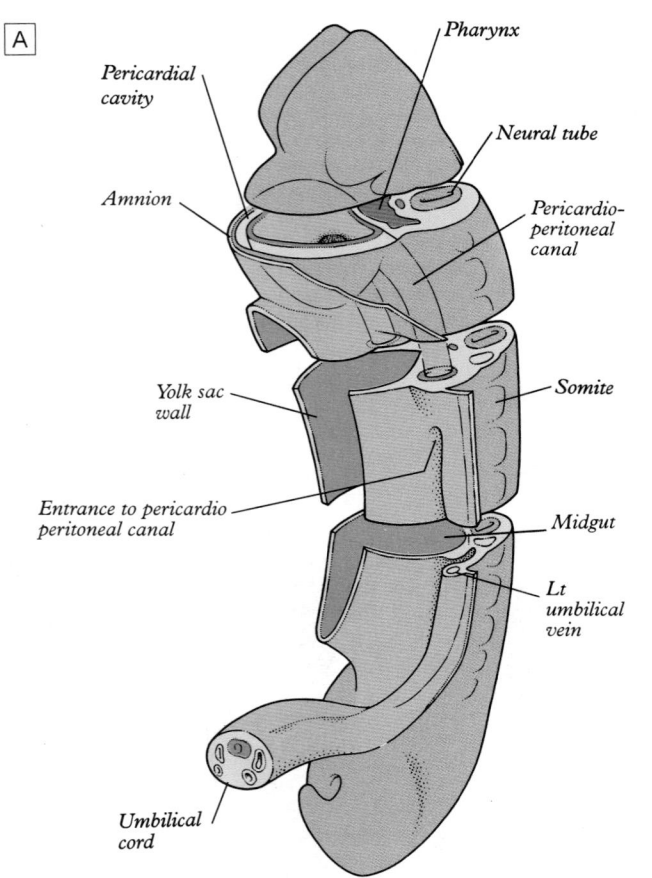

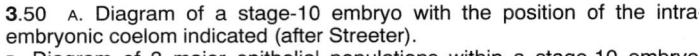

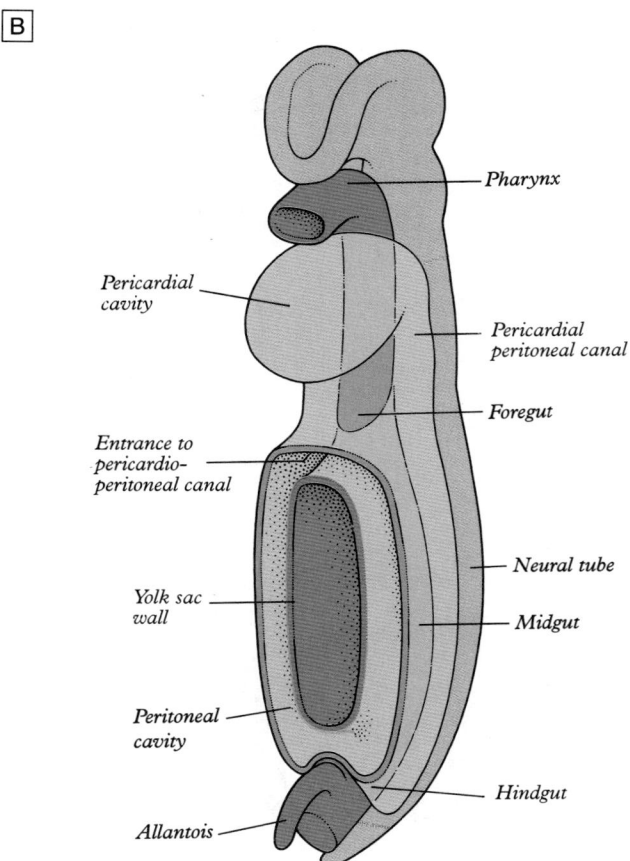

3.50   A. Diagram of a stage-10 embryo with the position of the intra-embryonic coelom indicated (after Streeter).
B. Diagram of 3 major epithelial populations within a stage-10 embryo,
viewed from a ventrolateral position. The neural tube lies dorsal to the gut; ventrally the intraembryonic coelom crosses the midline at the level of the foregut and hindgut, but is lateral to the midgut and a portion of the foregut.

epithelium) have apical epithelial specializations but tapering processes below which directly contact the underlying mesenchyme, there being no basal lamina. The possibility of the tapering processes forming directional signals for migrating progeny, similar to radial glia of the neural tube, has not been examined.

The proliferating coelomic epithelium produces two types of progeny: mesenchymal cells, either general or localized populations, and epithelial cells. The mesenchymal cells may become epithelial as their development fate; the epithelial derivatives, however, retain their epithelial differentiation.

General mesenchyme is produced from nearly all of the coelomic epithelium; it gives rise to the smooth muscle and connective tissue coats of tubes, e.g. of the gut, respiratory tract, reproductive and urinary tracts. Localized mesenchymal populations give rise to, among other structures: the septum transversum from the caudal pericardial region (forms part of the liver); a proliferation from the splanchnopleuric coelomic epithelium of the pleuroperitoneal canals dorsal to the stomach (forms part of the spleen); intermediate mesenchyme from the junction of the splanchnopleuric and somatopleuric coelomic epithelia (forms part of the early embryonic kidney).

Specific regions of the coelomic epithelium produce epithelial progeny which differentiate into structures as diverse as cardiac muscle, podocytes of the pronephric kidney (particularly in fish, avian and reptilian embryos), mesonephric epithelia, sustentacular cells which surround the primordial germ cells, and the epithelia lining the male and female reproductive tracts.

The coelomic channel and the primitive circulation which passes through it is of paramount importance up to stage 13. Whereas the superficial tissues of the embryo can receive nutrients via the amniotic sac and yolk sac fluids, the deeper tissues are, until the formation of the coelom, under conditions similar to tissue culture. From stage 10 however, exocoelomic fluid, propelled by the first contractions of the developing heart, is brought into contact with the deeply placed

mesenchyme. This early 'circulation' ensures an adequate supply of nutrients to the rapidly increasing amount of embryonic tissue, and meets most of the requirements of the deeper mesenchymal derivatives.

From stage 12 the endothelial system expands, filling rapidly with plasma which passes across the locally thinned coelomic epithelium into the large hepatocardiac channels which project into the pericardioperitoneal canals at the level of the 7th somite (O'Rahilly & Muller 1987).

With the formation of the coelomic epithelium and the intra-embryonic coelom the stage of gastrulation is over and organogenesis is underway. Just as the very early bilaminar disc could be viewed as an arrangement of three cavities (plus the allantois), now the same cavities can be examined after folding and the **embryonic** layers continuous with the walls of those cavities can be specified:

- the ectoderm and amnion line the amniotic cavity
- the embryonic endoderm and visceral endoderm line the yolk sac and allantois
- the intra- and extraembryonic coelomic epithelium lines the coelomic cavity, which consists of a large extraembryonic coelom continuous with a smaller intraembryonic coelom (**3.52**).

Each of these epithelia is supported by mesenchyme; all of the organs of the body will develop from interactions between one of these epithelial layers and its underlying mesenchyme. For an overview of the fate of the embryonic tissues see **3.43**.

Embryonic tissues

The cells of the embryo after gastrulation are arranged in two fundamental types of tissue, epithelial and mesenchymous and, despite regional modifications introduced as the various tissues develop, these types persist in large measure throughout life.

Epithelial tissues. These are tissues in which the cells are closely packed, with narrow intercellular clefts containing minimal extra-

151

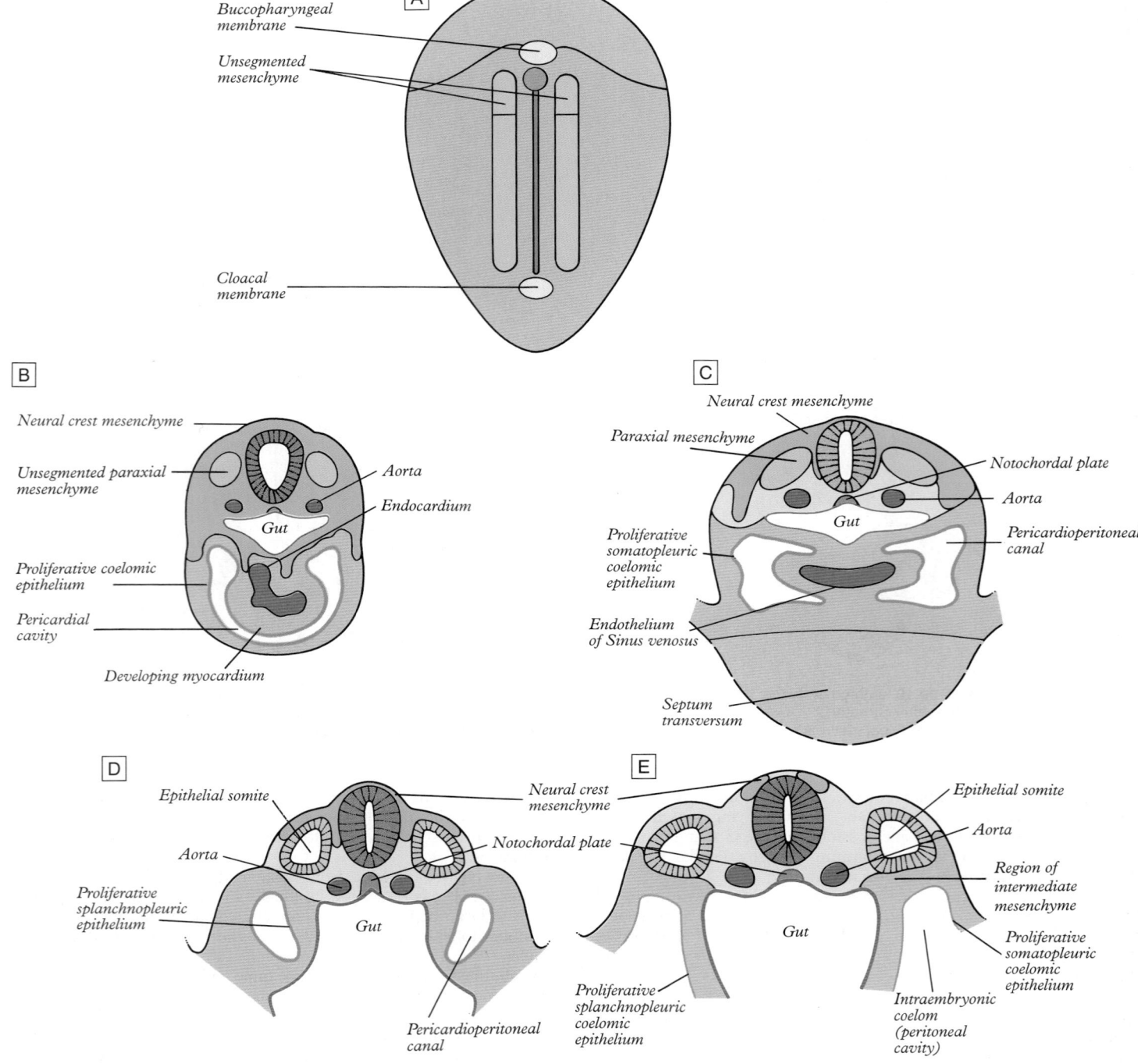

3.51   A. Diagrammatic representation of the mesoblast populations within the early embryonic disc.
B–E. A series of transverse sections, arranged cranial to caudal, from a stage-10 embryo. The populations of mesenchyme and the sites of mesenchymal proliferation are indicated.

cellular material, and a developed basal lamina containing specific proteins synthesized by the epithelium itself. The cells usually show juxtaluminal intercell surface specializations such as desmosomes, tight junctions, gap junctions, etc. (pp. 27–29), and specializations of the apical surface, which may exhibit microvilli or cilia. Characteristically epithelia clothe internal and external surfaces as simple or compound cellular sheets which separate phases of differing composition (e.g. the external environment and the subepithelial tissue fluids, intravascular and extravascular fluids, etc.). Traffic of materials in the intercellular clefts between cells is limited and passage occurs across the cells and their limiting membranes, which function as energy-dependent selective barriers, enhancing the passage of some materials and impeding the passage of others.

Historically the embryo was considered to be at the onset of organogenesis once three layers had been formed (see p. 92). However in the stage 11 embryo there are many more than three separate epithelial populations; they include surface ectoderm, the neural tube, notochord, embryonic endoderm, somites, somatopleuric and splanchnopleuric coelomic epithelia, epithelial ducts from intermediate mesenchyme and a range of endothelia. The majority of the derivatives of these layers retain their epithelial character throughout life; local invaginations produce glands and duct linings, which may retain their connection with their parent epithelia, although they may become detached as in the case of endocrine glands. Throughout development all epithelial tissues require underlying cells, sometimes in the form of other epithelial layers but more likely as free cells

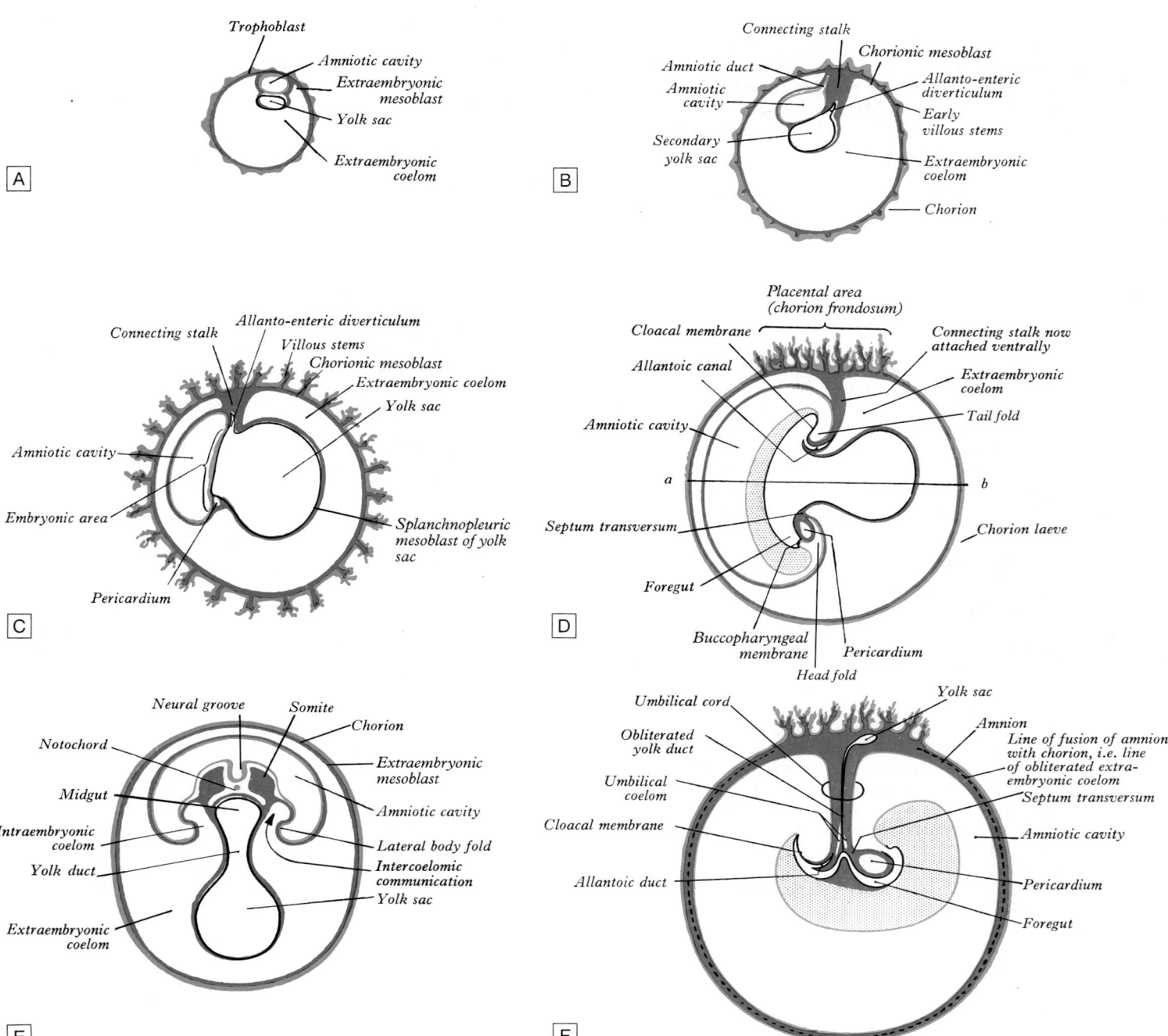

3.52 Diagrams showing: A. an early stage in development of the human blastocyst; B. the early formation of the allanto-enteric diverticulum and the definition of the connecting stalk; C. a later stage of the development. Observe that the heart occupies the most rostral part of the embryonic area and is separated from the prosencephalon by the buccopharyngeal membrane; D. formation of the head and tail folds, the expansion of the amnion and the delimitation of the umbilicus; E. a transverse section along the line *ab* in D. Observe that the intraembryonic coelom communicates freely with the extraembryonic coelom; F. a later stage in the development of the umbilical cord.

It should be noted that whilst these diagrams, from an earlier edition, are useful for showing the general changes in disposition of the embryo and extraembryonic membranes, the modern view of development of the villous stems has been revised. Consult text.

collectively termed mesenchyme to support them and engage in developmental processes.

Mesenchyme

This is a term first introduced over a century ago (Hertwig 1881) as an alternative to mesoblast. Mesenchyme cells have no polarity; they form junctional complexes which are not exclusively juxtaluminal and they produce extracellular matrix molecules and fibres from the whole cell surface. Mesenchymal populations form most of the tissue of the early embryo, occupying all the regions between the various epithelial layers described above.

Mesenchymal cells support epithelia throughout the developing body, both locally where they contribute to the basal lamina and smooth muscle of tubes, and generally where they differentiate into connective tissue (see p. 110). Specific mesenchymal populations control the patterning of local regions of epithelium.

The space beneath epithelia and between mesenchyme cells is filled with *extracellular matrix molecules* and *fibres*; these include localized molecules of the basal lamina (e.g. laminin, fibronectin, etc.) and much larger complex associations of collagen, glycosaminoglycans, proteoglycans and glycoproteins between the mesenchyme cells. The external shape changes of the embryo reflect different rates of

153

production of matrix molecules which support mesenchyme cells and their overlying epithelia; these molecules also provide migration routes for mesenchymal populations, and further, organize migrating cells by aligning intracellular proteins according to depositions of specific matrix molecules. Many of the signals for migration or differentiation are received from cells via matrix molecules, be they in the basal lamina, or in the matrix between cells. The presence or absence of certain matrix molecules may cause mesenchyme cells to migrate, or to stop migration and commence differentiation (see pp. 111, 112).

Subdivisions of the mesenchyme

The first mesoblast population of the trilaminar disc (termed primary mesenchyme by Hay (1968)) derives from epiblast cell ingression at the primitive node and streak. On reaching its final destination this mesoblast can be subdivided, by position, into populations of mesenchyme cells, i.e. *axial, paraxial* and *lateral plate* (**3.51A**). Local proliferation of these mesenchymal populations produces the enormous growth and expansion of the embryo. *Intermediate* mesenchyme develops slightly later between the paraxial mesenchyme and the lateral plate. A later, secondary, contribution of mesenchyme comes from neuroectoderm cells, i.e. the *neural crest*. Although the fate of much of the trunk neural crest is to form parts of the PNS, in the head crest cells contribute a significant population of ecto-mesenchyme which specifies the pattern of development in the viscerocranium.

Axial mesenchyme

The first epiblast cells to ingress through the primitive streak form the endoderm and notochord. These cells initially occupy a midline position with the earliest endodermal cells forming the prechordal plate, but later the notochordal cells remain medially and the endodermal cells flatten and spread laterally. A population of cells which remain mesenchymal just rostral to the notochordal plate are termed *prechordal mesenchyme* (**3.148**). These axial mesenchyme cells are tightly packed, unlike the more lateral paraxial cells, but are not contained in an extracellular sheath as is the notochord.

Adelmann (1927) described the development of the oculomotor muscles in the chick from mesenchyme formed from the prechordal plate. This was in conflict with later studies which suggested that extraocular muscles arose from small cavities in the mesenchyme each side of the diencephalon in mammals, the so-called preotic somites (Gilbert 1952, 1957)—a view supported by Meier (1986) and Noden (1983a) who suggested that the most cranial somitomeres (see below) develop into the extrinsic ocular muscles. However Adelmann's hypothesis has been confirmed by chimera experiments (Christ et al 1986; Wachtler & Jacob 1986), which showed that prechordal mesenchyme is displaced laterally at the time of head flexion and that the cells become integrated with those of the paraxial mesenchyme. Later this mesenchyme migrates to occupy the wall of the local head cysts where it provides the precursor cells for all of the extrinsic ocular muscles.

Notochord. Also called the chordamesoderm, this arises from epiblast cells of the medial part of the primitive node (Selleck & Stern 1991). It passes though several stages during development. The earliest notochordal cells are termed the notochordal process, or head process; they are intimately mixed with the endodermal cells. A canal has been identified in the notochordal process but seems not to be present in the notochordal plate, which remains from stage 8 to stage 11.

The development of the notochordal plate into notochord proceeds longitudinally from caudal to rostral, and the last areas to retain the plate are in the pharynx. The mechanism of notochordal formation is similar to, but a mirror image of, that of neurulation. The notochordal plate forms a deep groove; the vertical edges of the groove move medially and touch, then the endodermal epithelium from each side fuses ventral to the notochord. The definitive notochord is surrounded by a basal lamina which is in direct contact with the neural tube dorsally and the digestive epithelium ventrally.

The early notochordal process cells express myogenic markers transitorily as they migrate beneath the epiblast but later they become epithelial, forming junctions and an outer basal lamina. The cells swell, developing an internal pressure (turgor) which confers rigidity on the notochord.

The notochord has traditionally been thought of as the axial organizer of the embryonic disc. It is suggested, from amphibian and avian studies, that progenitor cells at the node provide cell lines for **both** the notochord and the overlying medial cells of the neural plate, termed the notoplate, or (neural) floor plate (Jessell et al 1989). Although once formed the two cell populations are functionally distinct, the notochord seems to be important for the maintenance and later development of the neural floor plate, and the extension of the neural floor plate depends on the presence of underlying notochordal cells (see p. 265). Later the notochord is not so influential in neural development but it has a specific role in vertebral development providing a focus for sclerotomal migration (see p. 510).

Notochordal cells in the rhesus monkey at stage 11–12 show well-developed Golgi apparatus, mitochondria, rough endoplasmic reticulum (RER) and coated vesicles (Wilson & Hendrickx 1990), with a well-developed basal lamina. However, in the pharyngeal region of 5-week embryos the notochordal and endodermal cells are closely opposed with cell processes passing from one layer to another at the site of the bursa pharyngea. Later the basal laminae are reformed as the notochord and endoderm layers separate and mesenchymal cells become interposed (Babic 1990). The notochordal cells maintain a neural crest free zone of about 85 µm around themselves (Pettway et al 1990) in early development.

Paraxial mesenchyme

Epiblast cells which migrate through the primitive node and rostral primitive streak during gastrulation form mesoblast cells which migrate to a position lateral to the notochord and beneath the developing neural plate. Cells ingressing through the primitive node form the medial part of this paraxial mesenchyme and cells ingressing through the rostral streak form the lateral part (**3.42**) (Selleck & Stern 1991). The paraxial mesenchyme extends cranially from the primitive streak to the prechordal plate immediately rostral to the notochord (**3.148**). Prior to somite formation it is also termed segmental plate in birds and unsegmented mesenchyme in mammals. Somitogenesis commences caudal to the otic vesicles each side of the rhombencephalon, thus somites are postotic. Paraxial mesenchyme rostral to the otic vesicle was not thought to segment; however, the appearance of somitomeres has been described.

Somitomeres. Experimental studies by Meier and colleagues reported in a series of papers (Meier 1979, etc.) have drawn attention to the appearance of the preotic unsegmented paraxial mesenchyme when examined with scanning electron microscope (SEM). The mesenchyme shows concentric rings of cell bodies and processes forming paired, bilaminar cylinders named *somitomeres* each side of the notochord and beneath the overlying neural plate. Somitomeres have been identified in a wide range of vertebrates; it is suggested that they are somite precursors prior to the compaction stage (see below).

The first pair of somitomeres to form lie either side of the prechordal plate with subsequent somitomeres separated across the midline by the notochord. In the chick the eighth somitomere, located just caudal to the otic vesicle, is the first to form a somite. All somitomeres caudal to this level develop into somites.

The first seven pairs of somitomeres which underlie the developing brain do not condense into somites; they remain in somitomeric pattern and later the mesenchyme cells disperse to form the basal portion of the skull and all of the striated muscle of the head (**3.148**). There is still dispute as to the origin of the so-called preotic somites which give rise to the musculature of the eye. Christ et al (1986) suggest they derive from mesenchyme arising from the prechordal plate.

Somitogenesis. As the neural folds elevate the somitomeres begin to condense forming discrete clusters of cells, the *somites*. This occurs initially at the eighth somitomere which is just caudal to the midpoint of the notochordal plate. The first somite so formed is the first occipital. Somites can be seen each side of the fusing neural tube in the human embryo from stage 9.

During somitogenesis the mesenchyme cells show changes in shape and in cell–cell adhesion becoming organized into epithelial somites. With development proceeding in a craniocaudal direction, the segmental plate is a transient and constantly changing structure, forming somites from its cranial end whilst mesenchyme, patterned into somitomeres, is being added to its caudal end by the regressing primitive streak (Packard & Meier 1983).

Experimental evidence has shown that somite induction occurs as the mesenchyme leaves the primitive streak, with cells being committed very early in development. Somites will form from cultured segmental plate with or without the presence of neural tube tissue or primitive node tissue (Packard & Jacobson 1976).

Somitogenesis (**3.131B**) entails five main stages (after Ede & El-Gadi 1986):

(1) The mesenchymal cells undergo *compaction*.

(2) The outer cells of the compacted somite block form a high columnar epithelium surrounding a central cavity. Some free mesenchyme cells may remain in the cavity.

(3) The ventral and ventromedial walls of the somite later revert to mesenchyme again, when they are termed the *sclerotome*.

(4) The mesenchyme cells of the sclerotome migrate ventrally and medially towards the notochord, meeting the sclerotomal cells from the other side of the body. These cells begin differentiation into chondroblasts forming the vertebral bodies (see p. 267).

(5) The remaining cells constitute the *epithelial plate of the somite*, also termed the *dermomyotome*. The dorsomedial lip of the epithelial plate folds back onto its lateral wall and the cells expand along the inside of the plate. The inner cells form myotubes and constitute the *myotome*. The dermomyotome and the definite myotome portion give rise to the hypaxial and epaxial muscles respectively.

Later cells migrating from the ventral edge of the epithelial plate of the occipital somites pass into the floor of the mouth to form the muscles of the tongue. Cells from the ventral edge of those somites opposite the developing limb buds migrate into the limbs to form the skeletal muscles of the limbs (Christ et al 1986).

Forty-four pairs of somites form caudal to the otic vesicle (postotic somites): 4 occipital, 8 cervical, 12 thoracic, 5 lumbar, 5 sacral and 8–10 coccygeal.

The somites give rise to the axial skeleton, i.e. the vertebral column and ribs from the sclerotome portion, and all the striated muscle in the body from the myotomes. Also they give rise to the muscles of the tongue, diaphragm and limbs from their ventrolateral edges (from those somites opposite the developing limbs), and the ventrolateral muscles of the trunk (from those somites between the limbs). The muscles of the head arise from the unsegmented somitomeres. Whereas the majority of the somites produce a similar range of derivatives, the most cranial and most caudal are different. The occipital somites and the cranial somitomeres are involved in formation of the base of the skull and most of the calvaria (see p. 271); the caudal somites regress early.

The somites, once formed, lie lateral to the neural tube. They cause bulges in the overlying ectoderm and can be readily identified in fresh and fixed embryos. Counting somites provides a method of staging embryos; the first somites are seen at Carnegie stage 9 but by stage 13 there are more than 30 somites and accurate enumeration is difficult. At the latter stages the limb buds provide an easier external feature for staging purposes.

Somites have a specific effect on the position of the developing spinal nerves, which preferentially grow through the cranial half of the sclerotome. Even if a portion of neural tube is turned through 180°, the nerves will deviate to grow through the cranial portion of the somite (Keynes & Stern 1986). Note that the spinal nerves are derived from two sources, the motor nerves from the neural tube, and the sensory nerves from the neural crest. The somites affect the developing nerves still further in that addition of an extra somite causes the production of an extra dorsal root ganglion from the neural crest, and removal of a somite prevents ganglion formation. (For more details see p. 226.)

Lateral plate

Lateral plate is the term for the early mesoblast population lateral to the paraxial mesenchyme; it is unsegmented. These mesoblastic cells, which arise from the middle of the primitive streak (primary mesenchyme), migrate cranially, laterally and caudally to their destinations where they revert to epithelium. They form a continuous layer which adheres to the ectoderm dorsally and the endoderm ventrally and faces a new intraembryonic cavity, the intraembryonic coelom, which, becoming confluent with the extraembryonic coelom,

provides a route for the circulation of coelomic fluid through the embryo. The epithelial coelomic wall thus formed becomes highly proliferative and rapidly produces a thick layer of mesenchymal cells deep to it. The mesenchymal population subjacent to the ectoderm is termed *somatopleuric mesenchyme*, and is produced by the somatopleuric coelomic epithelium. The mesenchymal population surrounding the endoderm is termed *splanchnopleuric mesenchyme*, and is produced by the splanchnopleuric coelomic epithelium.

It is important to note that these terms are only relevant caudal to the third visceral arch. Rostral to this there is a sparse mesenchymal population between the pharynx and the surface ectoderm (prior to migration of the head neural crest) with no landmarks to demarcate lateral from paraxial mesenchyme. This *unsplit lateral plate* forms the cricoid and arytenoid cartilages, the tracheal rings and the associated connective tissue (Noden 1988).

Somatopleuric mesenchyme (**3.51B–E**). This produces a mixed population of connective tissues and has a significant organizing effect opposite the limbs. Chick–quail chimera experiments have demonstrated that the pattern of limb development is controlled by the connective tissue cells, specifically by information contained in the somatopleuric mesenchyme (Kieny et al 1986). Regions of the limb are specified by interaction between the surface ectoderm (apical ectodermal ridge) and underlying somatopleuric mesenchyme; together these tissues form the progress zone of the limb (see p. 288). The somatopleuric mesenchyme in the limb bud further specifies the postaxial border of the developing limb. Muscles of the limbs derive from somitic precursor muscle cells (see above). The somatopleuric mesenchyme thus gives rise to the connective tissue elements of the appendicular skeleton, including the pectoral and pelvic girdles, the bones and cartilage of the limbs and their associated ligaments and tendons. Further, somatopleuric mesenchyme controls the pattern of development in the limbs, including the ectodermal specialities seen in proximal and distal parts of the limb, perhaps by mechanisms similar to the control of craniofacial development by cephalic neural crest (see below).

Splanchnopleuric mesenchyme (**3.51B–E**). Surrounding the developing gut and respiratory tubes, it contributes connective tissue cells to the lamina propria and submucosa; also smooth muscle cells to the muscularis mucosae and muscularis externa. It has a patterning role here also as in the limbs. Recombination experiments of endodermal epithelium combined with different mesenchymal populations have shown that the splanchnopleuric mesenchyme specifies the villus type in the gut, or the branching pattern in the respiratory tract.

Intermediate mesenchyme

This is a loose collection of mesenchyme cells found between the somites and the lateral plate (**3.51B–E**). Its development is closely related to the progress in differentiation of both the somites and the proliferating coelomic epithelium from which it derives. Intermediate mesenchyme is not present in the chick before somitogenesis and not prior to formation of the eighth somite. In embryos with eight to ten somites it is present lateral to the sixth, but does not extend cranially. The mesenchyme cells are arranged as layers, one continuous with the dorsal side of the paraxial mesenchyme and the somatopleure, the other with the ventral side of the paraxial mesenchyme and the splanchnopleure.

As development proceeds the intermediate mesenchyme forms a loosely packed cord of cells dorsolaterally which lengthens at the caudal end ultimately joining the cloaca. This is the precursor of the nephric duct. The cranial portion of this duct anlage, which gives rise to the pronephric duct in lower amniotes, degenerates whereas the middle part becomes epithelial and canalized forming the mesonephric duct.

In some amniotes the coelomic epithelium differentiates directly into specialized excretory cells, podocytes medially and a ciliated tract laterally which communicates with the nephric duct. In humans this pronephric stage is truncated and mesonephric tubules arise from proliferation and delamination of the coelomic epithelium along a strip each side of the median line. The mesonephric tubules once formed show early regional differentiation with one end forming podocytes and the other ciliated epithelium; they connect to the mesonephric duct.

The intermediate mesenchyme which forms the nephric system does not show the segmentation seen in the paraxial mesenchyme,

155

although it has for many years been described as a segmental structure.

As already noted, the intermediate mesenchyme develops from proliferating coelomic epithelium between the splanchnopleuric and the somatopleuric coelomic epithelia. In that region the coelomic epithelium and the underlying intermediate mesenchyme together contribute to the adrenal glands and the gonads.

Angioblastic mesenchyme

Mesoblastic cells give rise to the blood vascular and lymphatic systems of the embryo, forming the endothelial lining, the smooth muscle coat and the connective tissue adventitia (the latter may alternatively arise from splanchnopleuric mesenchyme). The vascular systems have to function precociously to fulfil the needs of the embryo as well as developing towards the vessel arrangements necessary for independent life after birth. The early endothelial channels form complex anastomotic links which may supply structures valuable to embryonic life or develop along redundant phylogenetic lines until converted to vessels appropriate for later stages of development.

The specific origin of endothelium is proving very difficult to establish in spite of the newer techniques of chimera production and immunocytochemical labelling. The rapidity with which embryos are vascularized is phenomenal and the constant modelling and remodelling of vessels compounds the difficulties of systematic study. Certainly during vascular reorganization the direction of blood flow in many vessels may reverse several times, causing obvious problems in deciding which vessels are veins and which arteries; in fact vessels may be both. It is only after the tunica media has developed that histological criteria can be used to identify the status of vessels.

Historically many theories were presented which supported the extraembryonic development of blood vessels. Blood islands appear in the yolk sac wall between the yolk sac endoderm and the extraembryonic mesoblast; these islands fuse to provide the early yolk sac circulation. Only after the formation of extraembryonic blood islands is vasculogenesis seen in the body of the embryo, giving rise to the hypothesis that all intraembryonic vessels are derived from extraembryonic, yolk sac endothelial populations that grow into the embryo. This hypothesis led to the conclusion that there are no angiogenic precursor cells within the embryo.

More recent immunological studies have demonstrated *angiogenic cells* within the early mesenchymal populations of the embryo; however they have not established the origin of these cells, i.e. whether or not they derive from yolk sac mesenchyme which has invaded the embryo. The earliest angioblastic cells are present in 1-somite chicks within the splanchnic mesenchyme around the margin of the entrance to the foregut. Later, labelled cells are present more caudally close to the endoderm of the mid- and hindgut. Later still, individual angioblasts are present in the head mesenchyme and somatopleuric mesenchyme. In a series of chimera experiments Noden (1991) has shown that ultimately all mesenchymal tissues, apart from notochord and prechordal plate, contain angioblastic cells. He notes that no ectodermal tissue, i.e. neuroepithelium and neural crest mesenchyme, contain endogenous endothelial cells. This means that crest derived mesenchyme of the face and jaw is dependent on adjacent mesenchyme for its angioblastic cells; whether this is paraxial or lateral plate mesenchyme is not clear.

Chimera experiments have further demonstrated the highly invasive nature of angioblastic cells. They are able to migrate in every direction throughout embryonic mesenchymal tissues; however, they do not enter the neural epithelium, forming instead a plexus of endothelial capillaries around the brain.

The ultimate position of endothelial vessels is believed to be patterned, like other tissues, by the mesenchymal populations of neural crest in the head, somatopleuric mesenchyme in the limbs and splanchnopleuric mesenchyme around the viscera.

Neural crest

The neural crest is the name given to a band of epithelial cells at the outermost edges of the neural plate, between the presumptive epidermis and the neural tube; these cells are committed to a neural crest lineage before the neural plate begins folding. As a further, separate origin of mesenchyme cells in the embryo, arising after the usual formation of mesoblast from the primitive streak, the neural

crest is unique. As an entity it has only a temporary existence. It develops at the time of closure of the neural tube and soon after the crest cells disperse (2.29c), in some cases migrating over considerable distances, to a variety of different developmental fates. The extent of their diversity encompasses

- the PNS apart from the somatic motor neurons, i.e. the neurons and glia of the sensory, autonomic and enteric nervous systems
- the medulla of the adrenal gland
- all the melanocytes found in the epidermis
- nearly all of the mesenchyme of the head including the viscerocranium (see below) and page 276
- the tunica media of the aortic arch arteries.

It is interesting to note that unlike mesoblast produced from the primitive streak, none of the cells that arise from the neural crest become arranged as epithelia.

Horstadius, in a classic work published in 1950, summarized the knowledge at that time, noting that descriptions of the neural crest were very rare in textbooks. Because the cells have such a range of diverse derivatives they have been in the past very difficult to follow developmentally. Horstadius noted that it was not possible to trace the migrations and ultimate fates of the neural crest cells with the experimental methods available then. In more recent years a technique of chimera production (Le Douarin & McLaren 1984) and antibody labelling has transformed this field of embryology and given significant insights into the most fundamental developmental processes and the fates of very specific regions of the neural crest.

Neural crest cells begin as ectodermal epithelial cells at the junction of the neural plate and presumptive epidermis. The crest cell population arising from the head is larger than that found at any trunk level and gives rise to a diverse array of connective tissues in addition to peripheral neuronal, glial and pigment cells. As both the development and fate of head and trunk neural crest cells are very different they will be considered separately.

Trunk neural crest. This is formed as the neural tube closes, initially in the cervical region, then proceeding caudally; thus various stages of crest development can be found in the more caudal regions of the embryo. As the neural tube begins to fuse dorsally in the midline the neural crest cells lose their epithelial characteristics and junctional connections and form a band of loosely arranged mesenchyme cells immediately dorsal to the neural tube and beneath the ectoderm. Initially the crest cells mostly have their long axis perpendicular to the long axis of the neural tube; later the cell population expands laterally and around the neural tube as a sheet.

Trunk neural crest cells migrate via three routes from their position dorsal to the neural tube (3.110):

- ventrally
- dorsolaterally
- in a rostrocaudal direction along the aorta.

After the epithelial somites dissociate to form the sclerotome and dermomyotome, the majority of the crest cells migrate ventrally passing either into the intersomitic space or through the rostral half of the dispersing sclerotome. These crest cells do not move medially towards the notochord but continue ventrally towards the adrenal medulla, or the region of the putative sympathetic trunk or the aorta. Other crest cells move a shorter distance between the neural tube and the posterior sclerotome; it is suggested that they get trapped in this position to form the dorsal root ganglia (Bronner-Fraser 1987).

In the second migration route, crest cells pass dorsolaterally between the ectoderm and the epithelial plate of the somite into the somatopleure where they eventually form the skin melanocytes.

Head neural crest. These cells, unlike in the trunk, migrate before the neural tube closes. Two populations of crest cells develop: those which retain a neuronal lineage and contribute to the somatic sensory and parasympathetic ganglia in the head and neck; and those which produce extensive mesenchymal populations. Each brain region has its own crest population which migrates around the sides of the neural tube in a dorsolateral migration to reach the ventral side of the head (3.148). Crest cells surround the prosencephalic and optic vesicles and occupy each of the pharyngeal arches. They provide mesenchyme cells which will produce the connective tissue in the viscerocranium and parts of the neurocranium. Thus all cartilage, bone, ligament, tendon, dermal components and glandular stroma in the head derives from the head neural crest.

Head

The head is one of the most complex regions of the vertebrate body and its development is correspondingly intricate. Head development is fundamentally similar in all vertebrate groups. It involves the migration of disparate cell populations, the transient contact between cells and cell populations and contact between cells and matrix environments. The development of the vertebrate head and the mechanisms by which such development occurs are closely connected to its evolution. Indeed study of the genetic regulation of head development is providing clues to the origin of the vertebrate line (for more details on evolution of the head see p. 287).

All vertebrates have a tripartite brain (with fore-, mid- and hindbrain) and morphological segmentation during hindbrain development. All vertebrates have essentially the same series of cranial nerves and ganglia, with the same connections to the CNS. Similarly the neurocranium of vertebrates is composed of paired sensory capsules surrounding their respective sense organs. Most significantly, all vertebrates have a significant portion of their skull and face rostral to the notochord. The developing tissue responsible for this 'prechordal' (Couly et al 1993) or 'new' head (Gans &

Northcutt 1983) is the (ectodermal) neural crest. Unlike its role in the trunk, where it contributes to the sensory and autonomic nervous system, in the head the neural crest produces a significant mesenchymal population which patterns the development of the pharyngeal arches, produces the vault of the skull, induces the migration of ectodermal placodes and contributes to the sensory ganglia and sense organs in the head.

The structures that are present in the head during development appear to be segmentally organized. This segmentation may be controlled by conserved homeotic genes which have been identified in a wide range of vertebrates. However, there are still many problems with interpretation of the developmental processes operating within the head. Axial tissues and those more laterally placed seem to be induced at different times and from different precursor populations; they do not mix. Yet, other cell populations can migrate through the boundaries between medial and lateral populations and may preferentially do so. Generally, the mechanisms of development in the head are different from those in the trunk. The extent of the difference is not as yet known. Figure **3**.148 shows diagrammatic representations of the structures present in the head of a stage 11 embryo arranged in register. It should be appreciated that the head undergoes a rostrocaudal development and that therefore the structures illustrated would not be present simultaneously.

NUTRITION OF THE EMBRYO

In early development the blastomeres derive their nourishment in part from stores laid down in the cytoplasm of the primary oöcyte. Such stores are possibly maintained at a high concentration but are not as extensive as those found in the yolk of most non-mammalian species. In addition it is assumed that the embryo derives nutrition from tubal and uterine secretions (Leese 1988, 1989). The cleaving embryo uses pyruvate rather than glucose as an energy substrate, but switches to the utilization of glucose at the blastocyst stage (Leese & Barton 1984; Hardy et al 1989). During the preimplantation phase new protein production occurs but there is also breakdown, resulting in a slight net decrease in protein content. Similarly, lipid metabolism shows considerable changes over the preimplantation period. As well as compounds that act as metabolic precursors, the uterine tube and uterus and their respective secretions contain cytokines. Receptors for some of these have been detected in the preimplantation embryos of experimental species (DiAugustine et al 1988; Heyner et al 1989; Pampfer et al 1991; McLachlan et al 1991; Harvey & Kaye 1991; Miyazawa 1992; Wiley et al 1992; Dardik et al 1992).

Subsequently, during the process of implantation, breakdown products stemming from lysed uterine tissues may also provide a source of nutrition. Then follows a period of about two weeks during which the embryonic disc is dependent on nutrients obtained from the fluid-filled cavities of the amnion, the coelom and the yolk sac. These fluids contain products arising as a result of absorption by trophoblast from lysed uterine tissues and extravasated maternal blood. However, at an early stage in development these sources of supply are much diminished. The lumen of the neural tube is isolated by closure of the neuropores, the extraembryonic coelom becomes, relatively, greatly reduced (**3**.52) and is later shut off from the intraembryonic coelom, and the obliteration of the yolk duct separates the yolk sac from the gut. Absorption of nutrients over the surface of the embryo becomes inadequate as the surface-to-volume ratio decreases. It therefore becomes imperative that some other source should be available at an early stage. This involves the maternal circulation coming into close, although indirect, apposition with the developing embryonic circulation.

The differentiating *angioblastic* mesenchyme, in which the embryonic vessels and erythrocytes develop, is probably first formed from the deepest layer of mesenchyme which clothes the endoderm of the yolk sac early in the third week (p. 140). Slightly later, angioblastic mesenchyme can also be recognized in the connecting stalk and mesenchyme of the chorion, and it then appears also within the embryonic area. Within the angioblastic mesenchyme spaces form

and the cells lining them differentiate into typical flattened endothelial cells. Neighbouring spaces join to form capillary plexuses. Meanwhile small localized groups of mesenchymal cells project into the spaces and become cut off to form *blood islands*, their cells differentiating into embryonic erythrocytes.

The vessels formed in the chorion soon establish an intimate relationship with the maternal circulation (**3**.55, p. 160). Vessels develop in the embryo as two longitudinal channels which, at their headward ends, invade the wall of the pericardium; the position and direction of the invasion changes with the progress of head fold formation. The two channels are the rudimentary right and left dorsal aortae and after folding their cranial ends curve ventrally in the lateral wall of the pharynx to reach the cranial end of the pericardium. Here they fuse, becoming continuous with the developing primitive tubular heart. Caudally the aortae traverse the connecting stalk as the rudimentary umbilical arteries and break up into capillaries in the chorion. The venules from the chorion converge on the stalk where they form the right and left umbilical veins, which run headwards in the somatopleure, close to the margin of the embryonic area, to reach the caudal end of the tubular heart.

The pericardial cavity never communicates directly with the extraembryonic coelom, and (before head folding) at its craniolateral limits the somatopleure and splanchnopleure are continuous (**3**.159A). With formation of the head fold the mesenchymal masses extending from the surface of the pericardium are altered in disposition or even reversed and the original cranial mass comes into intimate relation with the *ventral* wall of the foregut as far as the cranial rim of the cranial intestinal portal (**3**.52). After reversal, the caudal wall of the pericardium deepens dorsoventrally; the mesenchyme between it, the gut and proximal yolk stalk forms a sheet, which is the *septum transversum*. At this stage it is bounded on its headward surface by the pericardium and on its caudodorsal surface by the foregut. On its dorsolateral surface it is limited by the bilateral pericardioperitoneal canals, which connect the pericardium with the peritoneal cavity, and on its caudolateral surface by the single crescentic opening of the peritoneal cavity into the extraembryonic coelom. The umbilical and body wall veins, which run in the somatopleure, and the vitelline veins, which run in the splanchnopleure, meet in the junctional mesenchyme of the septum transversum and so gain the venous end of the heart. Through these various channels the early embryonic circulation is established (p. 312 et seq.). By the end of the third week the primitive cardiovascular system has been established and the heart has begun to beat so that the blood now circulates.

FETAL MEMBRANES AND PLACENTA

Allantois

The allanto-enteric diverticulum (**3.**52B, c) arises early in the third week as a solid, endodermal outgrowth from the dorsocaudal part of the yolk sac into the mesenchyme of the connecting stalk. (For discussion of the construction of the outgrowth, see p. 151.) It soon becomes canalized and, when the hindgut is developed, the proximal (enteric) part of the diverticulum is incorporated in its ventral wall and the distal (allantoic) part remains as the allantoic duct and is carried ventrally to open into the ventral aspect of the cloaca or terminal part of the hindgut (**3.**52). The diverticulum, lined with endoderm, is surrounded by mesenchyme of the connecting stalk, in which the umbilical vessels develop at a slightly later stage.

In reptiles, birds and many mammals the allantoic diverticulum develops into a stalked vesicle or diffuse cord which continues expanding into the extraembryonic coelom and forms a vascular organ to which the term *allantois* should perhaps be restricted. In birds it spreads over the dorsal surface of the embryo as a flattened sac between amnion and chorion (with which it fuses) and surrounds the yolk sac. It forms the chorio-allantoic circulation, allowing gas exchange across the shell membrane and absorption of nutrients from the yolk. With the formation of the amnion the embryo is, in most mammals, separated entirely from the chorion and is not united to the chorion again until the allantoic mesenchyme spreads to become applied to its inner surface. The human embryo, however, is never wholly separated from the chorion; its caudal end is joined to the latter by a thick band of mesenchyme, the *connecting stalk*, which accordingly is regarded as precociously formed *allantoic mesenchyme*.

Amnion

The amnion is a membranous sac that surrounds the embryo; it is developed in reptiles, birds and mammals (Amniota), but not in amphibia or fishes (Anamniota).

In the human embryo the amnion appears as a cavity within the inner cell mass adjacent to the overlying trophoblast. (For details see p. 137.) This cavity is roofed by a stratum of epithelial cells, and its floor is formed by the cells of the embryonic germ disc—continuity between the roof and floor being at the margin of the disc. The epithelial cells vary from tall columnar to flat and more squamous (Goto 1959). Fluid, the *liquor amnii*, occupies the amniotic cavity and increases steadily in volume as the sac gradually expands in the extraembryonic coelom (**3.**52); this continues until the coelom is obliterated, except for a small volume which is enclosed within the proximal part of the umbilical cord (the *umbilical coelom*).

Externally the amnion is covered with a thin layer of somatopleuric extraembryonic mesenchyme, which is continuous at the margins of the disc both with the splanchnopleuric extraembryonic mesenchyme covering the yolk sac and with the intraembryonic mesenchyme. Through the connecting stalk it is continuous also with the extraembryonic chorionic mesenchyme. It is commonly stated, based on morphological observations, that this extraembryonic mesenchyme is derived from the trophoblast. There is no experimental evidence for or against this in primates. In rodents, labelling studies have shown that it is derived from the embryonic ectoderm via the primitive streak (Gardner & Rossant 1979; Lawson & Pedersen 1992).

Connecting stalk and umbilical cord

The *connecting stalk* (**3.**52) is, as described above, a mass of precociously formed allantoic mesenchyme, which at first connects the caudal end of the embryonic area with the chorion. Proximally (its embryonic end) it surrounds the short allanto-enteric diverticulum but it is traversed throughout its length by the umbilical (allantoic) vessels. At first its dorsal surface is covered with the amnion and its ventral surface is bounded by the extraembryonic coelom. As a result of the folding of the embryo and distension of the amnion, the embryonic end of the connecting stalk comes to lie on the ventral surface of the embryo, and its mesenchyme approaches that covering the yolk sac and its stalk. With continued expansion of the amnion, the extraembryonic coelom is largely obliterated (**3.**52) and its only remaining part surrounds the elongating yolk stalk; this part still

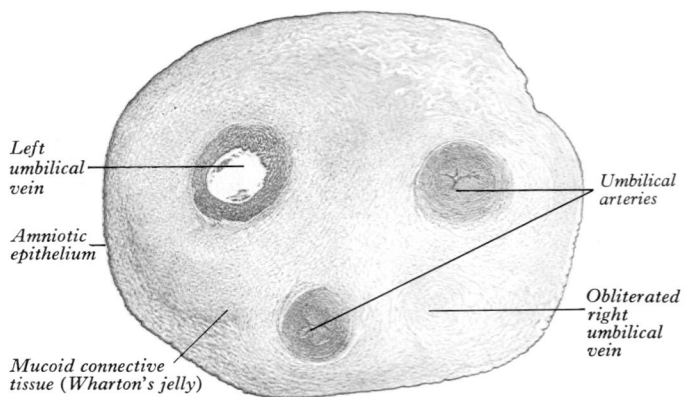

3.53 Transverse section through a human umbilical cord, stained with haematoxylin and eosin. Magnification × c. 8.

communicates freely through the umbilicus with the intraembryonic coelom. The mesenchyme-covered surfaces of the dome and folds of the expanding amnion now reach the chorion and converge on the connecting stalk and yolk stalk (and their vessels), and the umbilical cord is formed as they meet and the two mesenchymal compartments fuse (**3.**52) thus almost completely closing off the intraembryonic coelom. A limited exocoelomic recess persists in the embryonic end of the cord (*umbilical coelom*), retaining its communication with the intraembryonic coelom, and is involved in later enteric development (see below and p. 190).

The *umbilical cord* (**3.**53) thus consists of an outer covering of flattened amniotic epithelial cells, containing an interior mass of mesenchyme of diverse origins (see below). Embedded in the latter are two endodermal tubes—the yolk and allantoic ducts—their associated vitelline and allantoic (umbilical) blood vessels and, near its fetal end, the remains of the extraembryonic coelom mentioned above.

The *mesenchymal core* is derived from the somatopleuric extraembryonic mesenchymal covering the amniotic folds; the splanchnopleuric extraembryonic mesenchyme of the yolk stalk which carries the vitelline vessels and clothes the endodermal yolk duct; and similar allantoic mesenchyme of the connecting stalk which clothes the allantoic duct and carries initially two umbilical arteries and two umbilical veins. These various mesenchymal compartments fuse and are gradually transformed into the loose connective tissue (*Wharton's jelly*) which characterizes the more mature cord. The tissue consists of widely spaced elongated fibroblasts separated by an intercellular space filled with a copious matrix consisting of a delicate three-dimensional meshwork of fine collagen fibres surrounded by a dilute ground substance (Parry 1970). The latter contains a variety of hydrated glycosaminoglycans and is particularly rich in hyaluronic acid. In specimens which have been excised before fixation and staining, the fibroblasts present stellate profiles.

The part of the extraembryonic coelom (the *umbilical coelom*) included in the base of the umbilical cord acts as a sac which receives the normal *umbilical hernia* of the midgut, developing in the embryo between the sixth and tenth weeks (p. 190). After the disappearance of this hernia the extraembryonic coelomic sac is normally obliterated.

The yolk sac becomes located between the amnion and chorion as they fuse near the placental attachment of the cord (**3.**52, 54, 63). It continues to grow slowly and is sometimes found at term in this site, as a small vesicle usually less than 5 mm in diameter. The yolk stalk and its contained endodermal duct and accompanying vessels gradually elongate with growth in length of the umbilical cord. The duct and vessels slowly degenerate and they have usually disappeared by midpregnancy.

The endodermal allantoic duct, which is confined to the proximal end of the growing cord, also elongates and thins but may persist as an interrupted series of epithelial strands until term. At the umbilicus the proximal strand is often continuous with the median intraabdominal *urachus*, which in turn continues into the apex of the bladder (p. 201).

Usually, the embryonic right umbilical vein disappears in the early months of pregnancy (exceptionally only one artery may persist). The vessels of the umbilical cord are rarely straight but usually show a twisted conformation which may exist as either a right- or left-handed cylindrical helix. The number of turns involved may be relatively few or, at the other extreme, may even exceed 300. Their causation has been variously ascribed to unequal growth of the vessels, or to torsional forces imposed by fetal movements; their functional significance is obscure; perhaps their pulsations and contractions (see below) assist the venous return to the fetus in the umbilical vein. When fully developed the umbilical vessels, particularly the arteries, are provided with a strong muscular coat which contracts readily in response to mechanical stimuli. The outermost bundles pursue an interlacing spiral course so that, when they contract, they produce shortening of the vessel and thickening of the media, with folding of the interna and considerable narrowing of the lumen. This action may account for the periodic sharp constrictions of contour—the so-called *valves of Hoboken*—which often characterize these vessels.

When fully developed, the umbilical cord is on average some 50 cm long and 1–2 cm in diameter, but the length is subject to great variation (20–120 cm). Exceptionally short or long cords are associated with fetal problems and complications during labour as discussed by Benirschke and Kaufmann (1990). The cord usually attaches to the placenta but in a minority of cases velamentous insertion is observed (i.e. into the membranes) and may be associated with vulnerability to injury and attendant obstetric complications. This is discussed in detail by the same authors.

Implantation

As noted (p. 132), fertilization occurs in the lateral or ampullary part of the fallopian tube, and is followed around 26–40 hours later by the first cleavage. The dividing preimplantation embryo is conveyed along the tube to the uterine cavity by ciliary action of the tube aided by muscular tubal contractions; the journey occupies about 3 days. After entering the uterine lumen the morula develops an internal cavity and becomes a blastocyst, still surrounded by the zona pellucida. By this stage two distinctive groups of cells have emerged: one constitutes the *inner cell mass* which will form the embryo and contribute to the extraembryonic membranes; the second is the *trophectoderm*, flattened polyhedral cells surrounding the blastocyst cavity which have ultrastructural features typical of a transporting epithelium (Enders & Schlafke 1965; Lopata et al 1982). The cells covering the inner cell mass are known as *polar trophectoderm* and those surrounding the blastocyst cavity as *mural trophectoderm*. From these cells the trophoblast of the mature placenta is derived.

It has been suggested that the mesenchyme of the chorion is derived either from the trophoblast or the extraembryonic endoderm. Experimental evidence addressing this question is naturally lacking in the human but the mesoblastic layer of the murine chorion are derived from the embryonic ectoderm via the primitive streak (Rossant & Croy 1985; Rossant 1986). This is in agreement with the morphological observations of Luckett (1978) for the human.

Escape of the blastocyst from the zona is a prerequisite for its implantation in the uterine mucosa (see p. 136). This may involve the production of a trypsin-like enzyme and the presence of local weaknesses in the zona (Perona & Wasserman 1986; Lindenberg & Hyttel 1989). In the interval between ovulation and blastocyst arrival in the uterine cavity, preimplantation changes also occur in the uterine mucosa. These progestational changes are detailed later (p. 162).

The process of implantation involves an initial *attachment* of the polar trophectoderm to the endometrial luminal epithelium. Following this it *penetrates* the epithelium and underlying basal lamina and implants into the stroma, using a combination of motile and locally degradative activities.

A major problem in establishing the mechanism of the initial interaction is that in the earliest in situ implantation sites available for examination, implantation is already underway (Hertig et al 1956; Pijnenborg 1990). Early implantation in primates is initiated by a close approach of the trophoblastic plasma membrane to the tips of the microvilli and irregular surface protrusions of the uterine epithelial cells. The microvilli shorten and disappear and, for

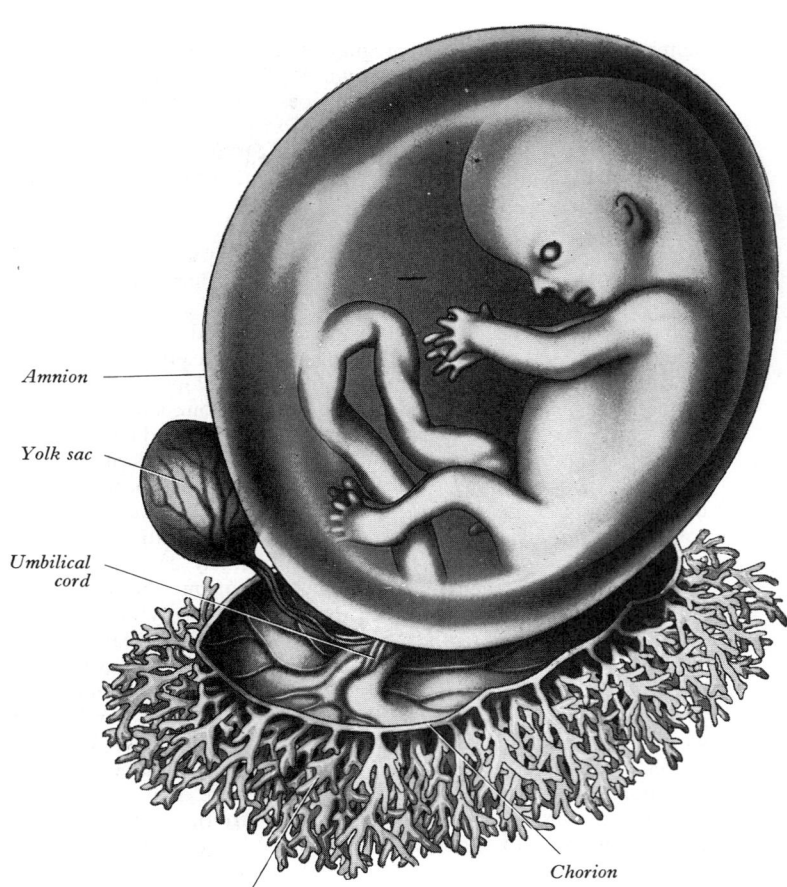

Amnion

Yolk sac

Umbilical cord

Chorion

Villous stems of chorion frondosum

3.54 A fetus of about 8 weeks, enclosed in the amnion, magnified about 2.5 diameters. A part of the chorion frondosum with its branching villous stems is shown in the lower part of the figure. The villous stems have been detached from the basal plate, which is not shown here.

a period, there is a close mutual apposition between the contours of the trophoblast and the uterine epithelial cell surface. From in vitro studies initial implantation in the human seems to involve attachment of trophectoderm to the endometrial epithelium followed by intrusion between the epithelial cells without their destruction (Lindenberg et al 1986, 1990). The syncytium sends finger-like projections between adjacent epithelial cells towards the underlying basal lamina, the two layers becoming closely interlocked by the formation of numerous tight junctions between them. Some authors have suggested that fusion between these two cell types may occur (Denker 1990).

The subepithelial basal lamina is penetrated by the trophoblast. There is evidence for production by preimplantation embryos of proteases that degrade basal lamina extracellular matrix molecules (Glass et al 1983) including type IV collagen (Behrendtsen et al 1992). In rodents it appears that the underlying stroma contributes to the local breakdown of the epithelial basal lamina and matrix (Blankenship & Given 1992). Implantation of the human blastocyst continues with erosion of maternal vascular endothelium and glandular epithelium and phagocytosis of secretory products until the blastocyst occupies an uneven *implantation cavity* in the stroma (*interstitial implantation*). It is not known precisely when syncytiotrophoblast first appears, but by the time contact is established with the stroma, the outermost cells are syncytial (Hertig et al 1956). In the early postimplantation phase, the maternal surface is resealed by a combination of re-epithelialization and formation of a plug that has been suggested to consist of fibrin.

Trophoblast and chorion

If fertilization and implantation are successfully accomplished, a hormone secreted by the syncytiotrophoblast, *human chorionic gonadotrophin* (hCG), prolongs the life of the corpus luteum, which continues to secrete progesterone and oestrogens during approximately the first 2 months of pregnancy. Thereafter these and other hormonal functions are the province of the definitive placenta (Devroey et al 1990). Menstruation does not occur and the endometrium, now known as the *decidua of pregnancy*, thickens further to form a suitable nidus for the conceptus. During the first few days after implantation, hCG appears in the urine where its presence is used as the basis for tests for early pregnancy.

The syncytiotrophoblast increases rapidly in thickness over the embryonic pole with a progressively thinner layer over the rest of the wall towards the abembryonic pole. As the blastocyst implants, the syncytiotrophoblast invades and digests the uterine tissues, including glands and the walls of maternal blood vessels (see **3.36**, 38 and Böving 1959, 1963). Microvillus-lined clefts and lacunar spaces develop in the syncytiotrophoblastic envelope (days 9–11 of pregnancy) and establish communications with one another. Early, many of them contain maternal blood (**3.36**, 38) derived from dilated uterine capillaries and veins, the walls of which have been partially destroyed. As the conceptus grows, the lacunar spaces enlarge, becoming confluent to form an initial *intervillous space*; their microvillous trophoblastic walls are converted at first into an irregular spongework or *labyrinth* (known inappropriately as primary villi; days 12–13). This is then invaded first with cytotrophoblast and then with mesenchyme (days 13–15) to form a radial array of *secondary placental villi*. Villous strands extend from the syncytial layer of the chorion across the intervillous space. On their embryonic aspect is a layer of cytotrophoblast, lined by vascularized fetal mesenchyme. The villous strands extend to the layer of peripheral trophoblast which is apposed directly to the excavated maternal tissues. Through spaces in the latter, extravasated maternal blood continues to enter the intervillous space. However, there is evidence that the maternal vascular circuit that connects the uterine arterial supply via the intervillous space to maternal veins is not fully functional until late in the first trimester (Hustin & Schaaps 1987).

As the intrasyncytial lacunae are developing, a *column* of proliferating cytotrophoblast extends from the *chorionic plate* and breaks through the syncytium to make direct contact with the maternal stroma (before day 15). Further cytotrophoblast proliferation then occurs laterally so that neighbouring outgrowths meet to form a spherical *cytotrophoblastic shell* around the conceptus (**3.35, 38, 55**). Capillaries form within the mesenchymal core (**3.55**) and establish connections with the radicles of the umbilical vessels in the general mesenchyme of the chorion. The heart now beats, establishing circulation between the yolk sac, the embryo and the chorio-allantoic placenta (days 18–22). Each villus now consists, from its base in the chorionic plate and throughout much of its extent, of a vascularized mesenchymal core, covered by a single (*Langhans*) layer of cytotrophoblast, which is again ensheathed by a layer of syncytium. These *tertiary* (or *mesenchymal*) villi proceed into a sequence of developmental changes continuing to term (see below). Near the maternal interface they contain no mesenchymal core but comprise a solid *cytotrophoblastic cell column*, continuous peripherally with the trophoblastic shell. At its periphery, the developing placenta thus consists of tertiary chorionic villi connected to the maternal stroma by cytotrophoblast columns—so-called *anchoring villi*.

Continuing growth of the cytotrophoblast columns occurs and single mononuclear cells detach from their distal tips and infiltrate the maternal decidua (Pijnenborg et al 1980, 1981, 1990). This process occurs in two phases: an initial infiltration of the basal decidua, with *interstitial extravillous trophoblast* tending to be more populous in the vicinity of maternal spiral arteries; and a second wave of migration by which the extravillous trophoblast reaches the inner one-third of the myometrium. At the same time, cytotrophoblast from the shell penetrates into and migrates along the inner walls of maternal spiral arteries (*endovascular extravillous trophoblast*), again penetrating by the 18th week as deep as the inner myometrial segments. The interstitially migrating cells appear to have the capacity to invade arteries from their periphery. The function (possibly the sole function) of this infiltrative behaviour by cytotrophoblast appears to be in the remodelling of the maternal arteries with loss of smooth muscle and associated elastic and collagenous matrix and its replacement with non-resistive fibrinoid, thus allowing for an expansion of the vessels and as much as a 20-fold increase in the flow of blood into the intervillous space. Common pregnancy pathologies including intrauterine growth retardation,

pre-eclampsia and spontaneous abortion are all associated with incomplete vascular remodelling probably arising from a failure of penetration by extravillous trophoblast (Khong 1991).

Expansion of the whole conceptus is accompanied by *radial growth* of the villi and, simultaneously, an integrated *tangential growth* with expansion of the trophoblastic shell and increased complexity and branching of the villous tree continuing to term. Eventually each stem forms a complex consisting of a single *trunk* (*truncus*) attached by its base to the chorion, from which arise distally, second and third order branches (intermediate and terminal villi; Castelluci et al 1990). *Terminal villi* are specialized for exchange between the fetal and maternal circulations (**3.56**). Each terminal villus commences as a syncytial outgrowth which, as it continues to grow, is invaded by cytotrophoblastic cells which then develop a core of fetal mesenchyme; this is finally vascularized by fetal capillaries (i.e. each villus passes through primary, secondary and tertiary grades of histological differentiation). Thus the germinal *cytotrophoblast*, by multiplicative growth, can continue to add additional cells which fuse with the overlying syncytium and allow the expansion of the haemochorial interface. The terminal villi continue to form and branch, within the confines of the definitive placenta (see below) throughout gestation, projecting in all directions into the intervillous space.

As these changes proceed, the intervillous space, at first spanned by the early villous stems and their branches, is increasingly permeated by growing free villi. It contains the circulating maternal blood, and is bounded:

- On its *fetal aspect* by a chorionic plate consisting of syncytial, cytotrophoblastic and mesenchymal layers of the chorion, the latter carrying radicles of the umbilical vessels and fusing laterally with the mesenchyme of the expanding amnion.
- On its maternal aspect by a *basal plate* consisting of *incomplete peripheral syncytium* with an outer *cytotrophoblastic shell* and *columns* extending deeper into the maternal decidual stroma. The trophoblast and adjacent decidua are enmeshed in layers of *fibrinoid* and basement membrane-like extracellular matrix to form a complex junctional zone (Enders 1968; Aplin 1991b; Damsky et al 1992). Where a discrete layer of fibrinoid is present between the trophoblastic shell and decidual stroma, this is known as *Nitabuch's layer*.
- Crossing it from chorionic to basal plates, the main trunks of the *villous stems* dividing into their intermediate and terminal villi; the trunk and its branches may be regarded as the essential structural, functional and growth unit of the developing placenta.

From the third week until about the second month of pregnancy the entire chorion is covered with villous stems which are thus continuous peripherally with the trophoblastic shell which is in close apposition with **both** the decidua capsularis and the decidua basalis. The villi adjacent to the basal decidua, however, are stouter, longer and show a greater profusion of terminal villi. As the conceptus continues to expand, the decidua capsularis is progressively compressed and thinned, the circulation through it is gradually reduced and, accordingly, the adjacent villi slowly atrophy and disappear. This process starts at the abembryonic pole and by the end of the third month the abembryonic hemisphere of the conceptus is largely denuded. Eventually the whole chorion apposed to the capsularis is smooth (the *chorion laeve*). In contrast, the villous stems of the disc-shaped region of chorion apposed to the decidua basalis increase greatly in size and complexity (the *chorion frondosum*), and together with the basalis constitute the *definitive placental site*.

Further consideration of the placenta must now be deferred until the preparation of the uterine tissues for the implantation and development of the blastocyst has been briefly described.

CYCLICAL CHANGES IN THE UTERUS

Throughout the period of reproductive life (i.e. from about the fifteenth to the forty-fifth year), except during pregnancy and lactation, a series of closely interrelated cyclical changes occur in the ovary, uterus and vagina. Each cycle extends over a period of about 28 days. In the ovarian cycle, which is described more fully elsewhere (pp. 122, 1865), one follicle usually reaches full maturity, ruptures and releases its secondary oöcyte during this period. The wall of the

NUTRITION THROUGHOUT GESTATION

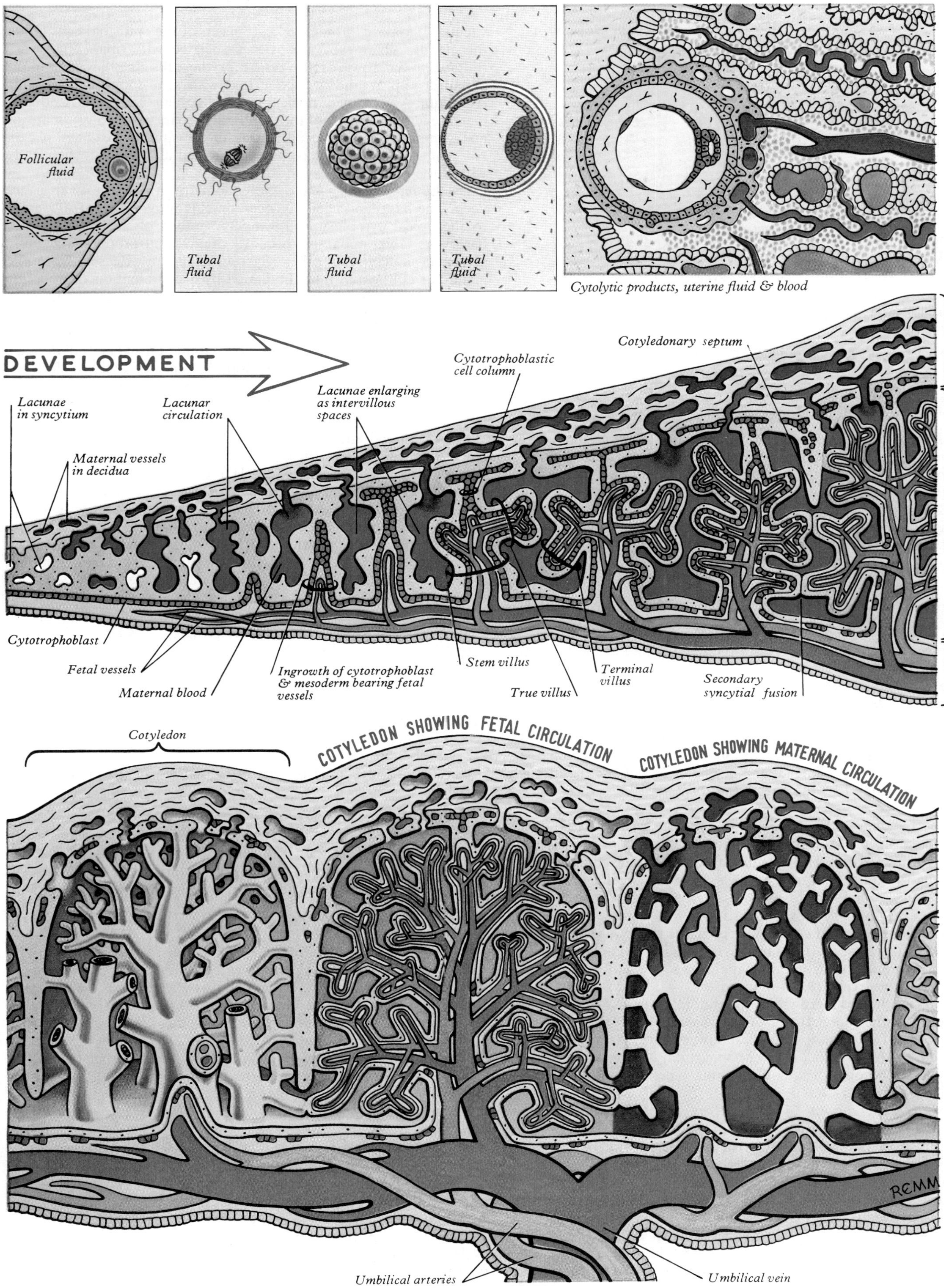

Follicular fluid

Tubal fluid

Tubal fluid

Tubal fluid

Cytolytic products, uterine fluid & blood

DEVELOPMENT

Basal plate

Cotyledonary septum

Cytotrophoblastic cell column

Lacunae in syncytium

Lacunar circulation

Lacunae enlarging as intervillous spaces

Maternal vessels in decidua

Villous labyrinth

Cytotrophoblast

Fetal vessels

Maternal blood

Ingrowth of cytotrophoblast & mesoderm bearing fetal vessels

Stem villus

True villus

Terminal villus

Secondary syncytial fusion

Chorionic plate

Cotyledon

COTYLEDON SHOWING FETAL CIRCULATION

COTYLEDON SHOWING MATERNAL CIRCULATION

Umbilical arteries

Umbilical vein

3.55 Nutrition of oöcyte, zygote, morula, free and implanted blastocyst, embryo and fetus throughout gestation. Embryonic and placental development proceed from left to right. Aspects of mature placental structure and circulation are shown below.

161

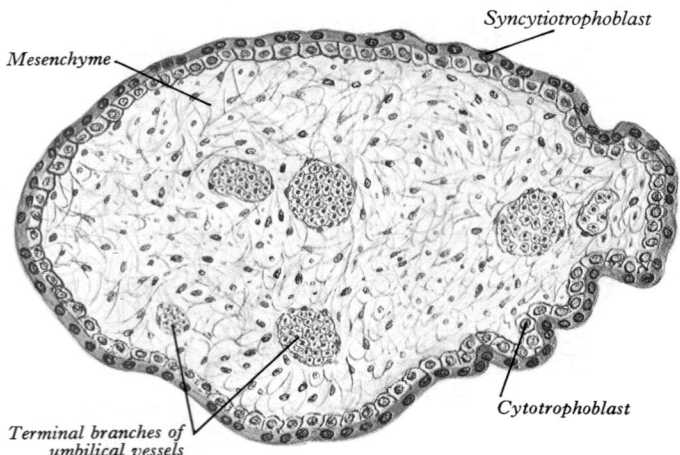

Mesenchyme

Syncytiotrophoblast

Terminal branches of umbilical vessels

Cytotrophoblast

3.56 Transverse section of a terminal villus stained with haematoxylin and eosin.

follice is then transformed into an important endocrine gland, the *corpus luteum* (p. 1865). About 10 days after ovulation the corpus luteum begins to regress, then ceases to function and is replaced by fibrous tissue.

The changes of the *uterine cycle* (*menstrual cycle*) chiefly involve the lining endometrium of the body and fundus of the uterus and may, for convenience, be divided into three phases:

- menstrual
- proliferative
- secretory (Noyes et al 1950; Wynn 1977; Cornillie et al 1985; Dockery et al 1988a, 1990; Aplin 1989; Buckley & Fox 1989).

The secretory phase coincides with the luteal phase of the ovarian cycle.

In the *menstrual* (*haemorrhagic*) *phase* the superficial part of the endometrium, next to the free surface, is shed piecemeal, leaving mainly the basal zone, adjacent to the uterine muscle (**3.57**). Approximately two-thirds to three-quarters of the thickness of the endometrium may be shed. Outwardly this phase is marked by a discharge of blood with necrotic epithelial and stromal debris from the uterus through the vagina. This discharge, the menstrual flow, lasts some 3–6 days.

In the early *proliferative phase*, and even before the menstrual flow ceases, the epithelium from the persisting basal parts of the uterine glands grows luminally over the denuded surface of the endometrium. Re-epithelialization is complete by days 5–6 after the start of menstruation. Initially the tissue is only 1–2 mm thick and lined by low cuboidal epithelium. The glands are straight and narrow with short columnar cells. The apical cell surface contains microvilli, and some ciliated cells are present. The stroma is dense and contains small numbers of lymphocytes amongst the larger population of mesenchymally-derived cells (**3.57**). During the 10–12 days of the proliferative phase there is a growth of the endometrium associated with the presence in the bloodstream of oestrogen. This is produced by the ovary (**3.58**) and acts through receptors present on both the stromal and epithelial cells of the endometrium. Mitoses are present and the glands become distinctly tortuous. Their lining epithelium becomes tall columnar (**3.57**).

Ovulation occurs about 14 days before the onset of the next menstrual flow. The changes occurring in the secretory phase depend upon the presence in the bloodstream of *progesterone* and *oestrogens*, secreted by the corpus luteum (**3.58**). Steroid receptors in the endometrium respond by activating a programme of new gene expression to produce, in the following 7 days, a highly regulated sequence of differentiative events presumably required to prepare the tissue for implantation (Dockery et al 1988a,b; Smith et al 1989; Aplin 1989, 1991a; Bell 1990). Part of the response is direct, but there is evidence that some of the effects may be mediated through growth factors (Nelson et al 1991; Tabibzadeh 1991). The first morphological effects of progesterone are evident 24–36 hours after ovulation. In the early secretory phase glycogen masses (known incorrectly as 'subnuclear

vacuoles') appear in the basal cytoplasm of the epithelial cells lining the glands, where they are often associated with lipid. Nuclei are thus displaced towards the centre of the cells (**3.59**). Giant mitochondria appear and are associated with semi-rough endoplasmic reticulum. A prominent nuclear channel system is present. A notable increase in polarization of the gland cells occurs with Golgi apparatus and secretory vesicles accumulating in the supranuclear cytoplasm. Nascent secretory products may be detected immunohistochemically within the gland cells.

By the *midsecretory phase* the endometrium may be up to 6 mm deep. The basal epithelial glycogen mass is progressively transferred to the apical cytoplasm, allowing the return of nuclei to the cell base. The Golgi apparatus becomes dilated and products including glycogen, mucin and other glycoproteins are released from the glandular epithelium into the lumen by a combination of apocrine and exocrine mechanisms, reaching a maximum approximately 6 days after ovulation (Smith et al 1989). These secretory changes are considerably less pronounced in the basal gland cells and the luminal epithelium than in the glandular cell population of the functionalis. In the late secretory phase glandular secretory activity declines. Production by gland cells of certain specific secretory products however is not observed until the mid- and late-secretory phases (Bell 1990).

Progestational effects on the stroma are also evident (Wienke et al 1968; Cornillie et al 1985; Aplin et al 1988; Dockery et al 1990). In the early secretory phase nuclear enlargement occurs and the packing density of the resident mesenchymal cells increases due in part to the increase in volume of gland lumens and onset of secretory activity in the epithelial compartment. In the midsecretory phase, a notable oedema appears with a corresponding decrease in the density of collagen fibrils. At the same time the endoplasmic reticulum and Golgi apparatus become more prominent, and there is evidence for new synthesis of collagen as well as its endocytosis and degradation.

In the late secretory phase decidual differentiation occurs in the superficial stromal cells surrounding blood vessels. This transformation includes rounding of the nucleus and an increase in the cytoplasmic volume with a concurrent increase and dilatation of the rough endoplasmic reticulum (RER) and Golgi systems and cytoplasmic accumulation of lipid droplets and glycogen. The cells begin to produce basal lamina components including laminin and type IV collagen. Features of the fully differentiated decidual cell are described in the next section.

Three strata can now be clearly recognized in the endometrium (**3.57**):

- *stratum compactum*, next to the free surface, in which the necks of the gland are but slightly expanded and the stromal cells show a distinct decidual reaction
- *stratum spongiosum*, where the uterine glands are tortuous, dilated and ultimately only separated from one another by a small amount of interglandular tissue
- a thin *stratum basale*, next to the uterine muscle, containing the tips of the uterine glands embedded in an unaltered stroma.

Towards the end of this period, as regression of the corpus luteum occurs, those parts of the stroma showing a decidual reaction and the glandular epithelium both undergo degenerative changes and the endometrium often diminishes in thickness. These degenerative changes precede the phase of bleeding.

During *menstruation*, blood escapes from the superficial vessels of the endometrium forming small haematomata beneath the surface epithelium which raise it. Blood and necrotic endometrium then begin to appear in the uterine lumen. The shedding of the endometrium starts at the surface and extends into the deeper layers. The amount of tissue lost is variable, but usually the stratum compactum and most of the spongiosum are desquamated.

The endometrium is regenerated from the stratum basale and that part of the spongy layer which remains, the surface epithelium being reformed with remarkable rapidity.

During the proliferative, early and midsecretory phases of the cycle, the bone-marrow derived cells present in endometrium are mainly macrophages and classic T cells, with very few B cells. In the late secretory phase, an unusual, large, granular lymphocyte population is recruited to the tissue (Starkey et al 1991) and is found mainly in the stromal compartment.

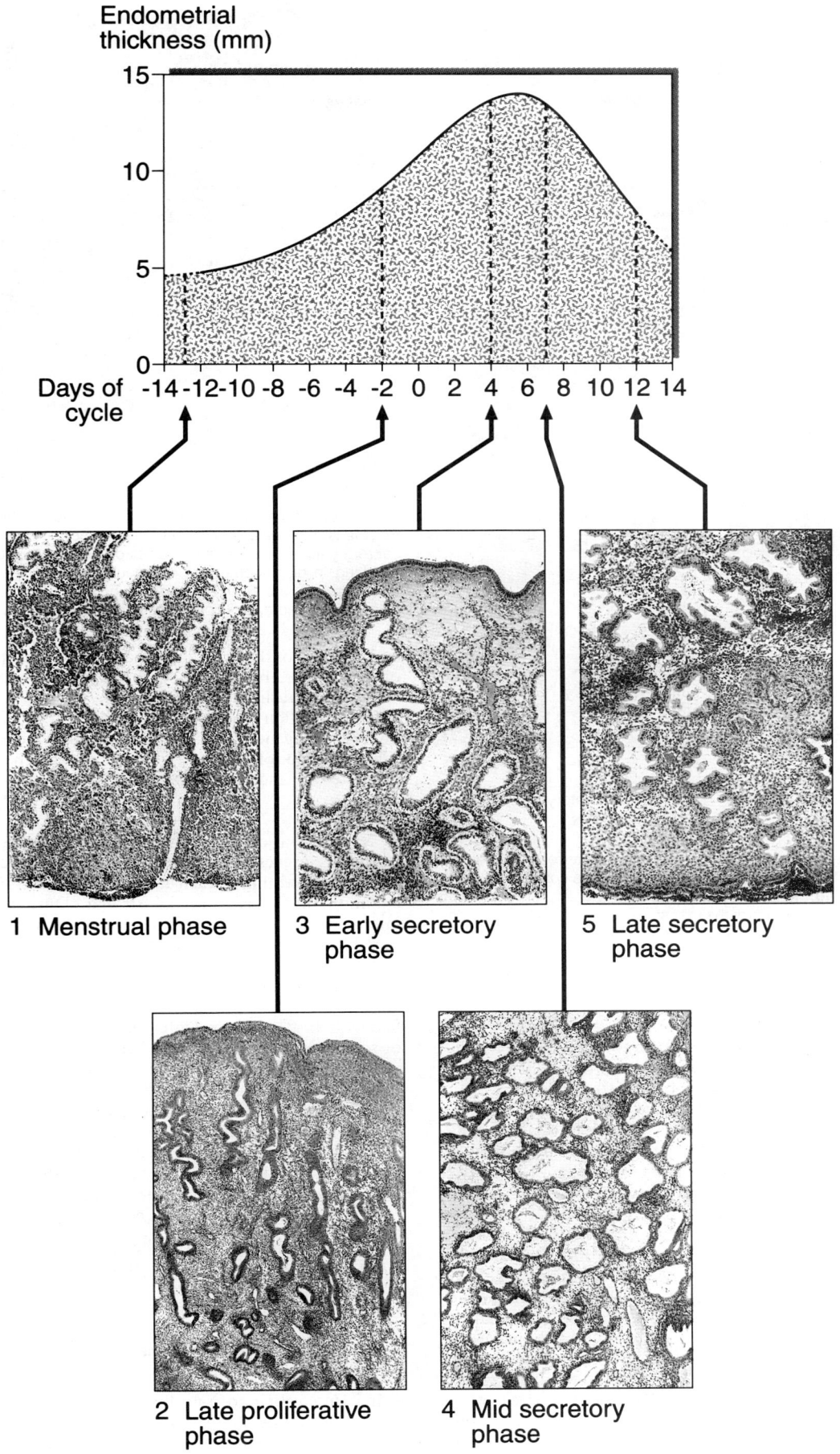

Endometrial thickness (mm)

Days of cycle

1 Menstrual phase

3 Early secretory phase

5 Late secretory phase

2 Late proliferative phase

4 Mid secretory phase

3.57 Stages in the menstrual cycle. The top panel shows the variation in thickness of endometrium during an idealized 28-day cycle in which ovulation occurs at day 0. Measurements were made by transvaginal ultrasound.

The five lower panels are histological sections of endometrium at the cycle times indicated. (From Buckley & Fox with permission of Chapman & Hall).

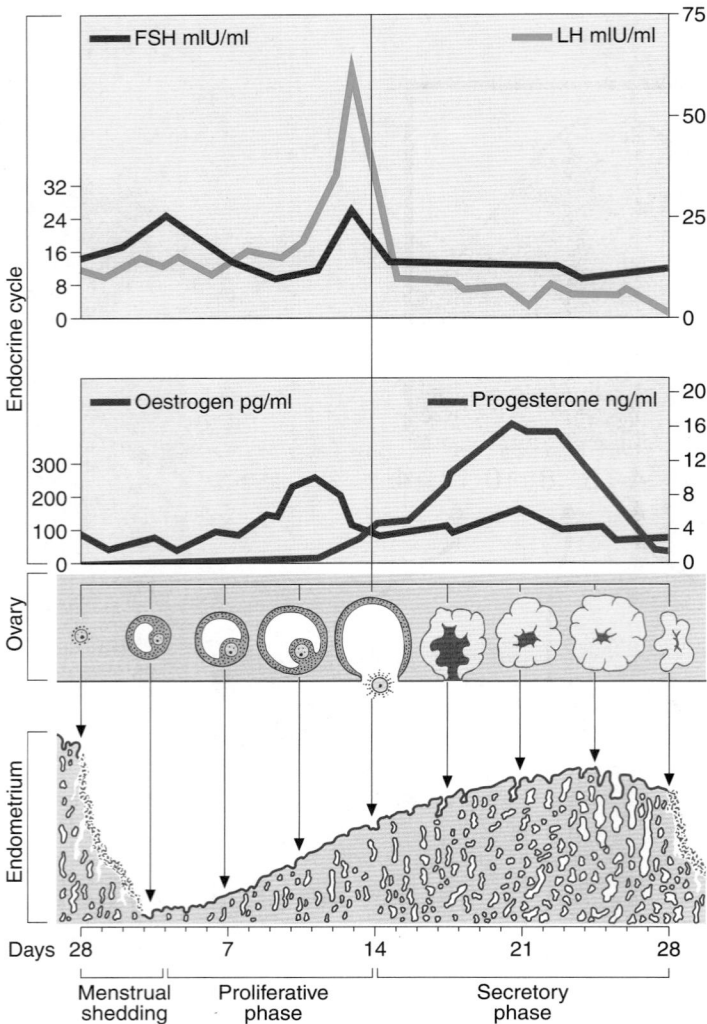

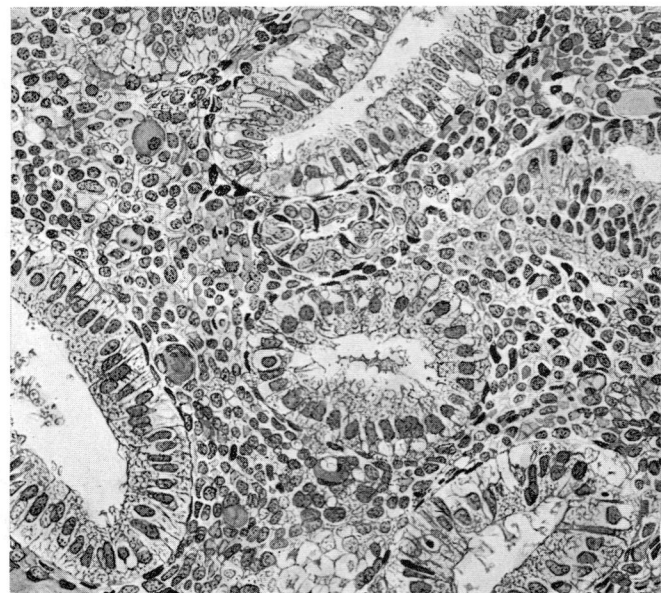

3.59 Section of human endometrium at about the seventeenth day of the menstrual cycle (early secretory phase) to show the accumulation of secretory material in the basal parts of the epithelial cells lining the glands, resulting in displacement of the nuclei towards the lumen of the gland. Magnification × c. 300. Stained with haematoxylin and eosin. (Lent by the Shattock Museum, St Thomas's Hospital Medical School.)

3.58 Composite diagram emphasizing some salient features of the female reproductive cycles. Note the (simplified) neuroendocrine control loops, the periodic changes during the non-pregnant state of the ovarian cycle with concomitant endometrial changes of the menstrual (uterine) cycle, variations in circulating plasma hormone levels, and the consequences of pregnancy. Neuroendocrine controls are further detailed elsewhere (pp. 1863, 1877). FSH = follicle stimulating hormone; LH = luteinizing hormone. (Modified from Wendell-Smith et al 1984.)

and anaemia of the superficial strata. During the periods of relaxation of the vessels, blood escapes from the devitalized capillaries and veins, thus causing the *menstrual haemorrhage.*

If fertilization of the ovum does not occur, the corpus luteum undergoes degeneration. The breakdown of the endometrium follows this cessation of function and is due to the reducing levels of progesterone and oestrogen (p. 1873).

Decidua

If fertilization occurs, chorionic gonadotrophin secreted by the conceptus rescues the corpus luteum and progesterone levels continue to rise, preventing menstruation and stimulating decidual differentiation of the endometrial stroma. During decidualization the interglandular tissue increases in quantity; it contains a substantial population of leucocytes (large granular lymphocytes, macrophages and T cells) distributed amongst large decidual cells. The latter are mesenchymally-derived stromal cells which have accumulated varying amounts of glycogen, lipid and vimentin-type intermediate filaments in their distended cytoplasm. They may contain one, two or sometimes three nuclei. The light microscopic appearance of these cells is rounded, but although they lack the long thin cytoplasmic projections typical of fibroblasts, the cell shape varies depending on the local packing density, which is widely variable. Frequently, rows of club-like cytoplasmic protrusions enclosing granules are found at the periphery. Outside the cell is a characteristic capsular basal lamina (Wynn 1974; Aplin 1989; Enders 1991).

Decidualization of the endometrial stroma occurs in humans regardless of the presence of a conceptus, as indicated by:

- the similar changes seen in the presence of an ectopic pregnancy
- the pseudodecidual changes observed in the late secretory phase of a non-conception cycle
- the decidualization observed after prolonged treatment with progesterone
- the ability of cultured stromal cells to decidualize in vitro in the presence of progesterone.

It is interesting to note that in rats, decidualization of stromal cells requires not only steroidal sensitization, but also an initiation signal from the embryo. Rats do not menstruate, but rather exhibit an oestrous cycle. The rather advanced differentiation achieved by the human stroma in the absence of a pregnancy may conceivably be related to the need for the seemingly wasteful sloughing of large parts of the tissue at menstruation.

The *vascular bed* of the endometrium undergoes significant changes during the menstrual cycle. The arteries to the endometrium arise from a *myometrial plexus* and consist of short *straight* vessels to the basal portion of the endometrium and more muscular *spiral* arteries to its superficial two-thirds. The capillary bed consists of an endothelium with a basal lamina that is discontinuous in the proliferative phase, becoming more distinct by midsecretory phase (Roberts et al 1992). Pericytes are present, some of which resemble smooth muscle cells, and these are sometimes enclosed within the basal lamina. The pericytes make contact with the endothelial cells by means of cytoplasmic extensions that project through the basal lamina. Enlargement of the pericytes is evident beginning in the early secretory phase and leading to a conspicuous cuff of cells in the mid- and late-secretory phases. The venous drainage, consisting of narrow perpendicular vessels which anastomose by cross branches, is common to both the superficial and basal layers of the endometrium. The arterial supply to the basal part of the endometrium remains unchanged during the menstrual cycle. The spiral arteries to the superficial strata, however, lengthen disproportionately, become increasingly coiled and their tips approach more closely the uterine epithelium during the secretory phase of the menstrual cycle. This leads to a slowing of the circulation in the superficial strata with some vasodilation. Immediately before the menstrual flow these vessels begin to constrict intermittently causing stasis of the blood

Decidual cells produce a range of secretory products (Bell 1986; Fazleabas et al 1991; Seppala et al 1992) including insulin-like growth factor, binding protein 1 and prolactin, which diffuse across the chorio-amnion and may be detected in amniotic fluid in the first trimester of pregnancy. They may also be internalized by trophoblast. These secretions probably play a role in the maintenance and growth of the conceptus in the early prehaemochorial phases of postimplantational development, when placentation is transiently *deciduochorial*. Decidualization also involves extensive remodelling of the stromal extracellular matrix. In addition to production of the capsular basal lamina, degradation and new synthesis of fibrillar collagen occur with a net decrease in the fibril density. Extracellular matrix, growth factors and protease inhibitors produced by the

decidua probably modulate the degradative activity of the trophoblast (Lala & Graham 1990; Librach et al 1991; Bischof et al 1992; Seppala et al 1992) and support placental morphogenesis and access of the placenta to the maternal blood supply. Thus formation of the haemochorial placenta requires a developmental progression specified in the trophoblast but dependent on the maternal environment for its correct expression. It also depends on the lack of immunological rejection of the semi-allogeneic conceptus, which is achieved by the absence of polymorphic histocompatibility antigens (HLA) on trophoblast but may also depend in some part on the specialized immune cell populations present in the decidua and their cytokine network (Starkey et al 1991).

Decidual differentiation is not evident in the stroma at the earliest

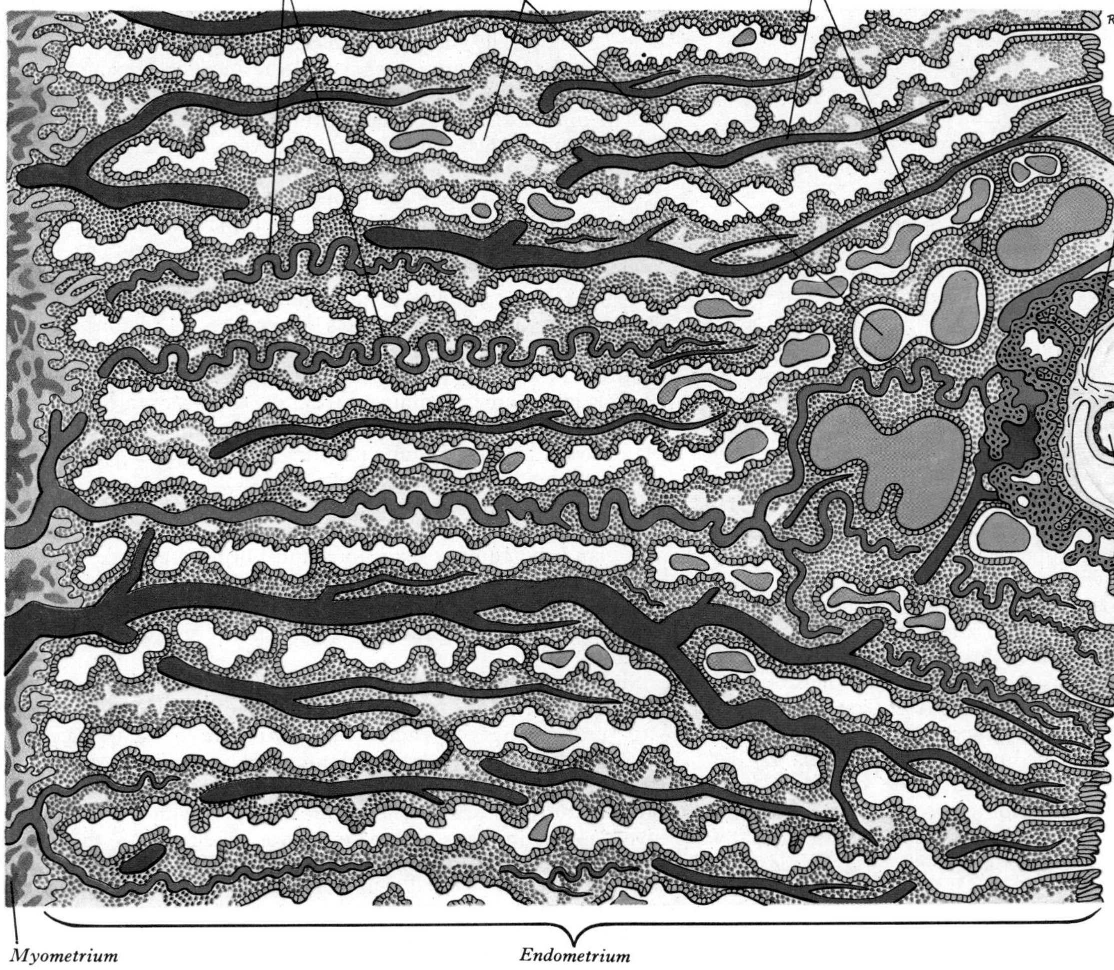

Spiral arteries   *Dilated uterine glands with secretory products*   *Endometrial veins*   REMM   *Connecting stalk*

Syncytiotrophoblast

Allantoic diverticulum

Trophoblastic lacuna

Cellular trophoblast

Decidua capsularis

Extra-embryonic mesoblast

Extraembryonic coelom

Yolk sac cavity

Amniotic cavity

UTERINE CAVITY

Myometrium   *Endometrium*

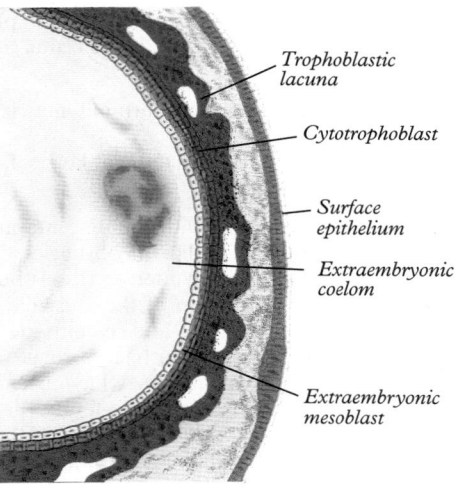

Trophoblastic lacuna

Cytotrophoblast

Surface epithelium

Extraembryonic coelom

Extraembryonic mesoblast

3.60 Diagram showing the general structure of the implanting blastocyst and its relationship to the tissues of the endometrium on the fifteenth day after fertilization. Note the arrangement and gradation in thickness of the syncytial trophoblast which has eroded the maternal tissues. Some of the deeper trophoblastic lacunae already contain maternal blood. Note also the active dilated uterine glands, the endometrial venous plexus, spiral arteries, and the stage of development of the cellular trophoblast, amnion, yolk sac, allantoic diverticulum, connecting stalk and the extraembryonic mesoblastic layers lining the extraembryonic coelom. For further details see text.

165

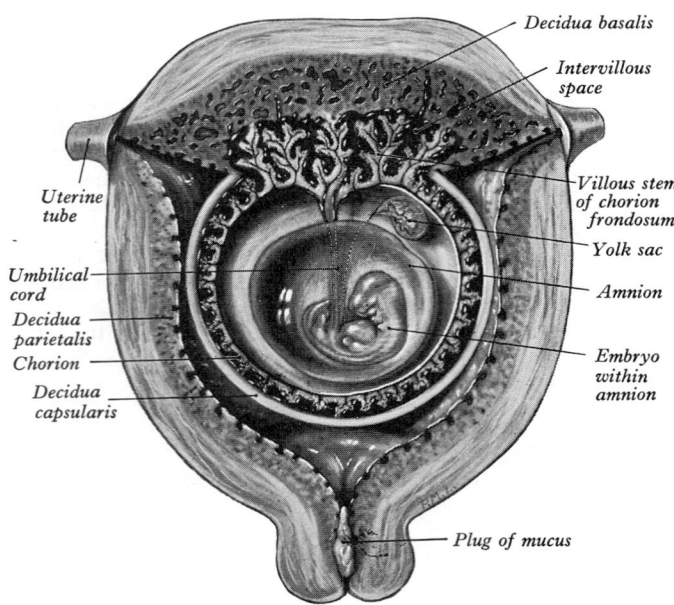

Decidua basalis

Intervillous space

Uterine tube

Villous stems of chorion frondosum

Yolk sac

Umbilical cord

Amnion

Decidua parietalis

Chorion

Embryo within amnion

Decidua capsularis

Plug of mucus

3.61 Plan of the gravid uterus in the second month. A placental site precisely in the uterine fundus as indicated in the plan is, however, rather unusual. (The dorsal, ventral or lateral wall of the corpus uteri is more usual.)

stages of implantation, and it may not be until a week later that fully differentiated cells are present (Enders 1991). Distinctive names are now applied to different regions of the decidua: the part covering the conceptus is the *decidua capsularis*, the part between the conceptus and the uterine muscular wall is the *decidua basalis*, and it is here that the placenta is subsequently developed; the part which lines the remainder of the body of the uterus is the *decidua parietalis* (**3**.61). However, there is no evidence that their respective resident maternal cell populations exhibit different properties in these various locations.

Coincidentally with the growth of the embryo and the expansion of the amnion (p. 142), the decidua capsularis is thinned and distended (**3**.60, 61) and the space between it and the decidua parietalis gradually obliterated. By the second month of pregnancy the three endometrial strata recognizable in the premenstrual phase, compactum, spongiosum and basale, are better differentiated and easily distinguished. In the spongiosum the glands are compressed and appear as oblique slit-like fissures lined by low cuboidal cells. By the beginning of the third month of pregnancy the capsularis and parietalis are in contact; by the fifth month the capsularis is greatly thinned, while during the succeeding months (**3**.62) it virtually disappears.

DEFINITION OF THE HUMAN PLACENTA

The human placenta is initially *labyrinthine* as the early villous stems are formed, but becomes secondarily *villous* with the development of generations of terminal villi. Maternal blood bathes the surfaces of the chorion which bound the intervillous space and it is thus defined as *haemochorial*, distinguishing it from the different grades of fusion between the maternal and fetal tissues which exist in many other mammals (*epitheliochorial*, *syndesmochorial*, *endotheliochorial* and others; Mossman 1987).

The chorion is vascularized by the allantoic blood vessels of the body stalk and the human placenta is termed *chorio-allantoic* (whereas in some mammals a *choriovitelline* placenta either exists alone or supplements the chorio-allantoic variety). Finally, the human placenta is said to be *deciduate* because maternal tissue is shed with the placenta and membranes at term as part of the afterbirth (see below).

An exhaustive account of the growth, dimensional changes, vasculature and haemodynamics, cell varieties, ultrastructure and histochemistry of the placenta, and the physiological aspects of placental transfer and its status as a metabolic store and endocrine gland, lies beyond the scope of the present volume. What follows is necessarily

an abbreviated account of selected topics and the interested reader should consult the profusion of original papers devoted to these subjects. The classic work of Boyd and Hamilton (1970) and the more recent volume of Benirschke and Kaufmann (1990) provide unrivalled sources of information and extensive bibliography. A survey of placental transfer mechanisms is to be found in Sibley and Boyd (1992).

The placenta at term

The expelled placenta (**3**.63) is a flattened discoidal mass with an approximately circular or oval outline, with an average volume of some 500 ml (range 200–950 ml), average weight about 500 g (range 200–800 g), average diameter 185 mm (range 150–200 mm), average thickness 23 mm (range 10–40 mm) and an average surface area of about 30 000 mm². Thickest at its centre (the original embryonic pole) it rapidly diminishes in thickness towards its periphery where it continues as the chorion laeve.

Macroscopically, its *fetal* or *inner surface*, covered by amnion, is smooth, shiny and transparent and the mottled appearance of the subjacent chorion, to which it is closely applied, can be seen through it. The umbilical cord is usually attached near the centre of the fetal surface, and branches of the umbilical vessels radiate out under the amnion from this point, the veins being deeper and larger than the arteries. Beneath the amnion and close to the attachment of the cord, the remains of the yolk sac can sometimes be identified as a minute vesicle, up to 5 mm in diameter, with a fine thread—a vestige of the yolk stalk—attached to it.

The *maternal surface* is finely granular and mapped into some 15–30 lobes by a series of fissures or grooves. The lobes are often somewhat loosely termed *cotyledons* (but see also below) and the grooves correspond to the bases of incomplete *placental septa* which become increasingly prominent from the third month onwards. They extend from the maternal aspect of the intervillous space (the basal plate) towards, but not quite reaching, the chorionic plate. The septa are complex structures comprising components of the cyto-trophoblastic shell and residual syncytium along with maternally derived material including decidual cells, occasional blood vessels and gland remnants, collagenous and fibrinoid extracellular matrix and, in the later months of pregnancy, foci of degeneration. The nature of the maternal surface of the expelled placenta is of course determined by the tissue plane of separation of the placenta at parturition.

Studies of the human placenta include morphometric analysis, surface architecture using scanning electron microscopy, ultra-structural studies of angioarchitecture and possible mechanisms whereby the maternal placental circulation is controlled. The ultra-structure of biopsies taken from placental uterine beds which were presumed to be normal has been reviewed (Wynn 1974). A detailed investigation into the connective tissue 'skeleton' of the placenta, with a helpful bibliography, has been provided by Ockleford and Wakely (1982).

Separation of the placenta

After delivery of the fetus the placenta becomes separated from the uterine wall and, together with the so-called 'membranes', is expelled as the *afterbirth*. Separation takes place along the plane of the stratum spongiosum and extends beyond the placental area, detaching:

- the villous placenta with associated fibrinoid matrix and small amounts of decidua basale
- the chorio-amnion together with a superficial layer of the decidua capsularis/parietalis.

The chorio-amnion is continuous with the placenta at its margin and constitutes the '*membranes*' familiar in obstetrics. The process of separation requires rupture of many uterine vessels but their torn ends are closed by the firm contraction of the muscular wall of the uterus after delivery of the placenta and membranes and thus, under normal circumstances, postpartum haemorrhage is limited in amount. When the placenta and membranes have been expelled, a thin layer of stratum spongiosum is left as a lining for the uterus, but it soon undergoes degeneration and is cast off in the early part of the puerperium. A new epithelial lining for the uterus is then regenerated from the remaining stratum basale.

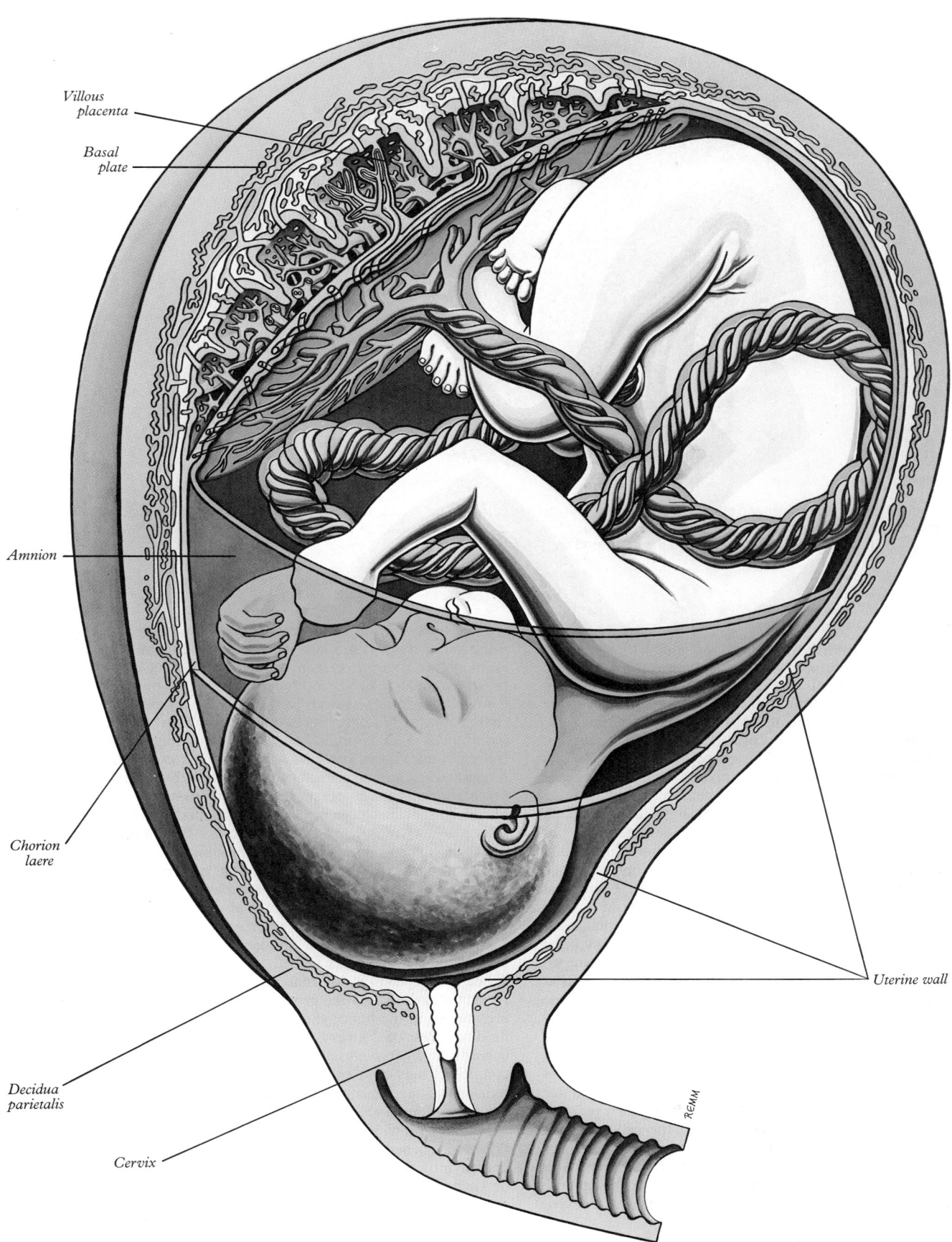

Villous placenta

Basal plate

Amnion

Chorion laere

Decidua parietalis

Cervix

Uterine wall

REMM

3.62 Diagram showing a full-term human fetus in utero, including a sectional view of the placenta, the amnion (mauve), chorion (green), uterine wall and cervix (yellow), the cervix with a plug of mucus in the cervical canal, the umbilical cord and its contained vessels, and the rugose vaginal wall. Note the characteristic flexed posture of the fetus and its limbs, and the overall position within the uterus which the fetus commonly occupies. (Other positions, although less frequent, are, however, also quite common.) Note also the single umbilical vein carrying oxygenated blood, the two umbilical arteries carrying deoxygenated blood, the arborization of these vessels in the chorionic plate (see through the overlying amnion) and their branches which pass into the villous stems. The latter span the intervillous space and there branch into intermediate and terminal villi; incomplete placental septa project from the basal plate towards the chorionic plate. See text for further details.

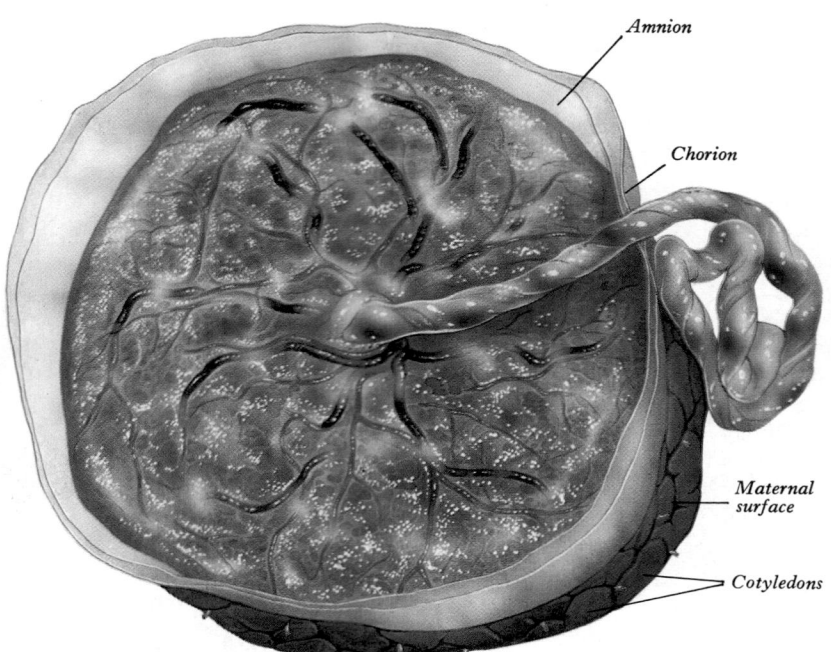

Amnion

Chorion

Maternal surface

Cotyledons

3.63   The fetal surface of a recently delivered placenta. The spiral umbilical vessels in the umbilical cord, and their radiating branches shine through the transparent amnion. The maternal surface is exposed in the lower and right corner of the figure. Note the fringes of amnion and chorion, the majority of which have been cut away near the placental margin. (Drawn from a coloured photograph provided by E F Gibberd.)

Chorio-amnion

Between the tenth and twelfth weeks of pregnancy the amniotic cavity expands and the chorion frondosum regresses to form the chorion laeve which is in turn apposed to the decidua capsularis. During the same period the amnion and chorion fuse to form the chorio-amnion, and this avascular membrane persists to term.

The inner surface of the amnion consists of a simple cuboidal epithelium with a microvillous apical surface beneath which is a cortical web of intermediate filaments and microfilaments. There are no tight junctional complexes between adjacent cells and cationic dyes penetrate between the cells as far as the basal lamina (King 1982). The intercellular clefts present scattered desmosomes, but elsewhere the clefts widen and contain interlacing microvilli. These features are consistent with selective permeability properties. The epithelium synthesizes and deposits extracellular matrix into the compact layer of acellular stroma located beneath the basal lamina, as well as the basal lamina itself (Lister 1968; Wynn & French 1968; Aplin et al 1985, 1986; Campbell et al 1990). The compact layer varies considerably in thickness between different specimens. Beneath the compact layer is a fibroblast layer and then a spongy layer that abuts the chorion laeve. It is likely that lateral movement of the amnion occurs relative to the chorion in response to mechanical stress, and that this is effectively lubricated by the spongy layer.

The chorion at term consists of an inner cellular layer containing fibroblasts and a reticular layer of fibroblasts and Hofbauer cells that resembles the mesenchyme of an intermediate villus. The outer layer consists of cytotrophoblast 3–10 cells deep resting on a pseudo-basal lamina that extends beneath and between the cells (Bourne 1963; Aplin & Campbell 1985). Obliterated villi are occasionally seen within the trophoblast layer and represent the remnants of villi present in the chorion frondosum of first trimester. Although the interface between the trophoblast and decidua parietalis is uneven, no trophoblast infiltration of the parietalis occurs.

The *liquor amnii* increases in quantity up to the sixth or seventh month and then diminishes slightly; at the end of pregnancy it is usually somewhat less than a litre. It provides a buoyant medium which supports the delicate tissues of the young embryo and allows free movement of the fetus during the later stages of pregnancy. It also diminishes the risk to the fetus of injury from without. It contains less than 2% of solids, including urea, inorganic salts, a small amount of protein and frequently a trace of sugar. The liquor is derived from multiple sources: secretions from amnion epithelium; filtration of fluid from maternal vessels via the parietal decidua and amniochorion; filtration from the fetal vessels via the chorionic plate or the umbilical cord; fetal urine. In early pregnancy, diffusion from intracorporeal vessels via fetal skin provides another source (Benirschke & Kaufmann 1990). In the early stages it resembles blood plasma in composition and is probably formed largely by transport across the amniotic membrane but as pregnancy advances it becomes progressively more dilute, partly by the addition of fetal urine. Glycoprotein secretions from amniotic epithelium include fibronectin. It has been shown experimentally that there is a considerable and rapid flux of water across the amniotic membrane. There is rapid exchange between the amniotic fluid and maternal and fetal circulations, probably via the placenta and fetal kidneys. By the end of the third month the expanding amnion has extensive contact with the chorion laeve and only these thin membranes separate the amniotic fluid from the decidua parietalis, the tissues and vessels of which provide another route for the exchange of water and dissolved substances (Plentl 1958; Bell 1986).

Secretory products of maternal decidua (see below), including prolactin and insulin-like growth factor binding protein (IGF-BP1), are present in the liquor (Seppala et al 1992). A volume of amniotic fluid in excess of 2 litres is generally considered to be abnormal and constitutes *hydramnios*. A deficiency is termed *oligamnios*. Both conditions may be associated with fetal abnormalities; for example, fetuses with agenesis of the kidneys or atresia of the lower urinary tract are often associated with oligamnios.

Fetal swallowing of amniotic fluid is a normal occurrence; the fluid is absorbed into the fetal circulation and passes the placental barrier into the maternal circulation. Cases of oesophageal atresia or anencephaly, in which swallowing is impossible or impaired, and open spina bifida are often associated with hydramnios. With these neural defects, impaired swallowing is accompanied by direct discharge of cerebrospinal fluid (CSF) into the amniotic liquor. In fetuses with spina bifida and some other neural tube defects the concentration of alphafetoprotein in the amniotic fluid is exceptionally high and is used to diagnose these abnormalities (Brock 1976). Fluid is also produced in the fetal lungs; however, most of this fluid remains in the lungs as a mechanical effect of the amniotic fluid pressure. Pulmonary hypoplasia at birth may be caused by severe congenital urinary obstruction (see p. 181).

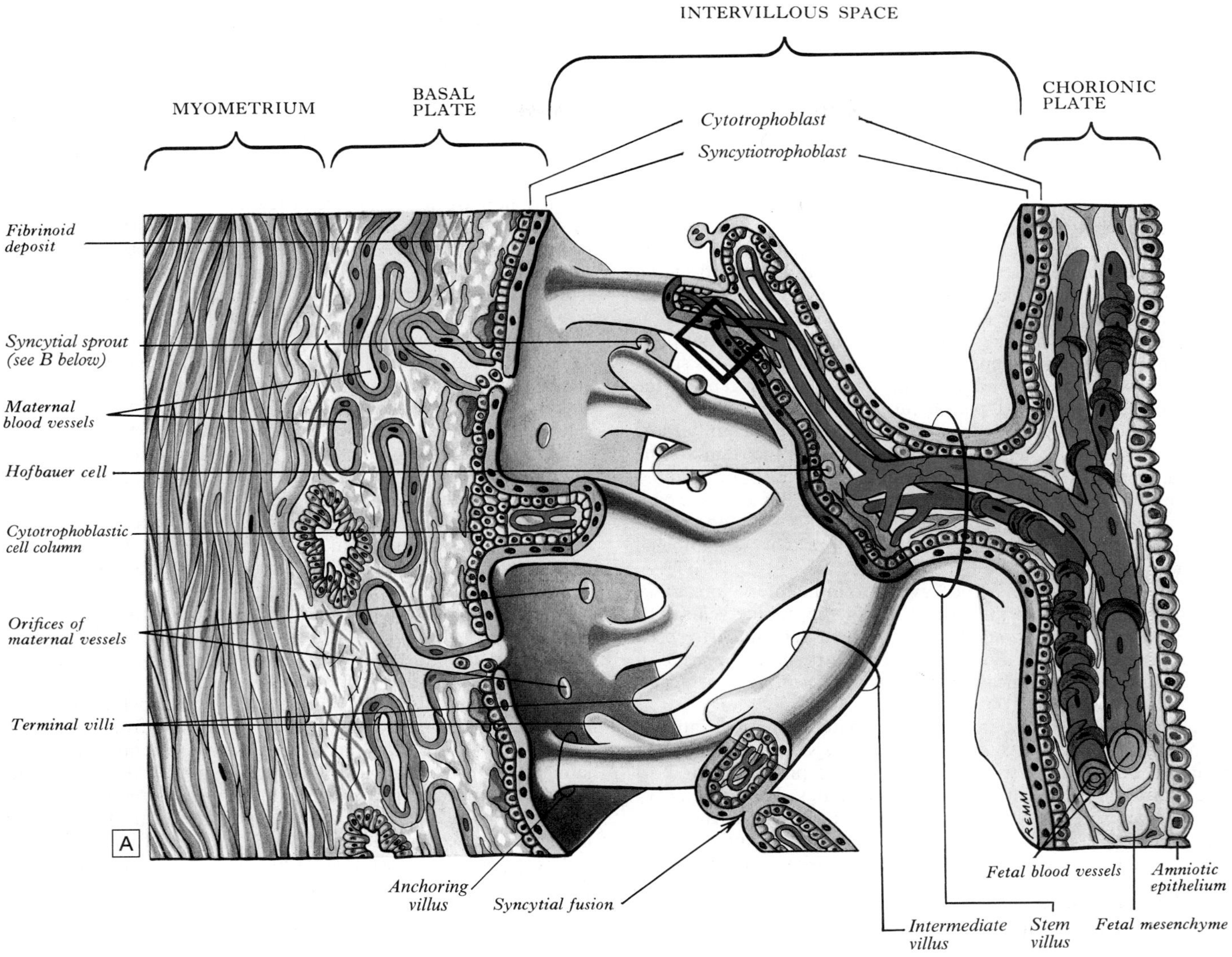

INTERVILLOUS SPACE

MYOMETRIUM   BASAL PLATE   *Cytotrophoblast*   CHORIONIC PLATE

Syncytiotrophoblast

Fibrinoid deposit

Syncytial sprout (see B below)

Maternal blood vessels

Hofbauer cell

Cytotrophoblastic cell column

Orifices of maternal vessels

Terminal villi

A

Anchoring villus   *Syncytial fusion*

Fetal blood vessels   *Amniotic epithelium*

Intermediate villus   *Stem villus*   *Fetal mesenchyme*

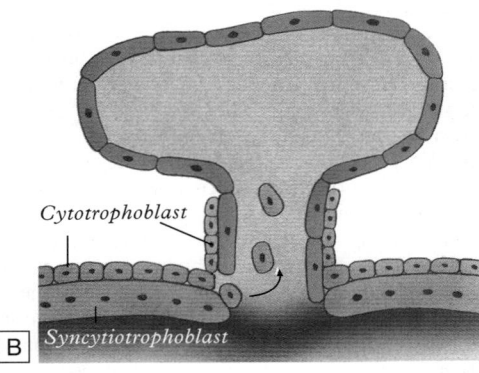

Cytotrophoblast

B   *Syncytiotrophoblast*

3.64B   A syncytial spout.

PLACENTAL TISSUES

These are arranged as a chorionic plate, a basal plate and, between the two, the villous stems, their branches and the intervillous space (**3.**55–64).

Chorionic plate. This is covered on its fetal aspect by the amniotic epithelium, on the stromal side of which is a connective tissue layer carrying the main branches of the umbilical vessels. Adjacent to this is a diminishing layer of cytotrophoblast and finally the inner syncytial wall of the intervillous space. The connective tissue layer derives from fusion between mesenchyme-covered surfaces of amnion and chorion and is more fibrous and less cellular than Wharton's jelly of the umbilical cord, except near the larger vessels. The latter radiate and branch from the cord attachment (with variations in the

3.64A   Schematic diagram to show the arrangement of the placental tissues. Note the chorionic and basal plates and the intervillous space spanned by a villous stem and its divisions. The sectioned surfaces show the disposition of the fetal and maternal blood vessels, the amniotic epithelium, the cellular and syncytial layers of trophoblast and the complex junctional zone between the fetal and maternal tissues in the basal plate containing deposits of fibrinoid material and isolated masses of peripheral syncytium. B Note also the presence of surface syncytial sprouts, a stromal trophoblastic bud and Hofbauer cells (large phagocytic cells) associated with a terminal villus, and syncytial fusion occurring between the tips of two terminal villi. See text for further details. The region enclosed in the larger rectangle is shown greatly enlarged in **3.**65.

branching pattern), until they reach the bases of the trunks of the villous stems, which the branches enter and then arborize within the intermediate and terminal villi. There is no anastomosis between vascular trees of adjacent stems but, in contrast, the two umbilical arteries are normally joined by some form of substantial transverse (Hyrtl's) anastomosis at, or just before they enter, the chorionic plate.

Basal plate. From the fetal to maternal aspect this consists of:

- the outer wall of the intervillous space comprising in different places syncytium, cytotrophoblast or fibrinoid matrix
- Rohr's stria of fibrinoid
- what remains of the cytotrophoblastic shell
- Nitabuch's stria of fibrinoid
- maternal decidua.

Nitabuch's stria and the basal decidua contain cytotrophoblast and multinucleate trophoblast giant cells originating from the mononuclear cytotrophoblast population that infiltrates the basal decidua during the first 18 weeks of pregnancy. These cells penetrate as far as the inner one-third of the myometrium, but can often be observed at or near the decidual–myometrial junction. They are not found in the parietal decidua nor the adjacent myometrium. Thus the placental-bed giant cell appears to be a differentiative end stage in the extravillous trophoblast lineage (Aplin 1991b).

The striae of fibrinoid are irregularly interconnected and variable in prominence. Strands pass from Nitabuch's stria into the adjacent decidua. The latter contains basal remnants of the endometrial glands, large and small decidual cells scattered in a connective tissue framework which also supports an extensive venous plexus.

Throughout the second half of pregnancy the basal plate is thinned and progressively modified, with a relative diminution of the decidual elements, and increasing deposition of fibrinoid and admixture of fetal and maternal derivatives.

Intervillous space. Through the various layers of the basal plate the maternal blood vessels approach and reach the intervillous space. The spiral arteries of the endometrium open through gaps in the cytotrophoblastic shell and peripheral syncytium. However, they probably do not open directly into the intervillous space until as late as the tenth week. At term, from the inner myometrium to the intervillous space, the walls of most spiral arteries consist of fibrinoid matrix within which cytotrophoblast is embedded. This allows expansion of the arterial diameter to give an increased flow of blood which is privileged in being independent of vasoconstrictors. Endothelial cells, where present, are often hypertrophic.

The veins which drain the blood away from the intervillous space pierce the basal plate and join tributaries of the uterine veins. The presence of a marginal venous sinus, which has hitherto been described as a constant feature, occupying the peripheral margin of the placenta and communicating freely with the intervillous space, has not been confirmed.

In the macaque monkey, radio-opaque material injected into the aorta passes in spurts or jets to the intervillous space and at sufficient pressure to drive it towards the chorion, thus preventing a short circuit of arterial blood into the venous openings. The openings of the coiled arteries show intermittent activity. Myometrial contractions alter the pressure in the intervillous space and promote placental venous drainage (Ramsey et al 1963; Martin 1965).

Placental lobes and lobules

The placental *lobes* are demarcated by the grooves on its maternal surface, and they correspond in large measure to the major branches of distribution of umbilical vessels, particularly well seen in specimens X-rayed after intravascular injection of radio-opaque media. However, the application of the term cotyledon to these major lobes does not correspond directly to its usage in comparative placentology, where cotyledon refers to scattered discontinuous patches of villous chorion interspersed with non-villous chorion (as found for example in cows).

The fetal cotyledon of the human placenta evidently corresponds to a major villous stem and its branches. Early in pregnancy, the chorion bears some 800–1000 of such stems but as pregnancy advances, with the formation of the chorion laeve and possibly some fusion between adjacent stems, the number is progressively reduced until only about 60 persist in the placental area in the last months of pregnancy.

Structure of a villus

Chorionic villi are the essential structures involved in exchanges between mother and fetus and, accordingly, the villous tissues separating fetal and maternal blood are of crucial functional importance. From the chorionic plate, progressive branching occurs into the villous tree, stem villi giving way to intermediate and terminal villi. For a complete description of the development and structure of the villous tree, readers are referred to Benirschke and Kaufmann (1990).

Each villus has a core of connective tissue containing collagen types I, III, V and VI as well as fibronectin. Cross-banded fibres (30–35 nm) of type I collagen are often found as bundles. Type III collagen is present as thinner (10–15 nm) beaded fibres forming a meshwork that often encases the larger fibres. Collagens V and VI are present as 6–10 nm fibres closely associated with collagens I and III. The basal lamina-associated molecules laminin and collagen type IV are present in the stroma in association with fetal vessels, as well as in the trophoblast basal lamina (Amenta et al 1986). Overlying

this matrix are ensheathing cyto- and syncytial trophoblast bathed by the maternal blood in the intervillous space (**3.55**, 64, 65, 66). Cohesion between the cells of the cytotrophoblast and also between this layer and the syncytium is provided by numerous desmosomes between their apposed plasma membranes.

In earlier stages, the cytotrophoblast forms an almost continuous layer on the basal lamina, but after the fourth month it gradually expends itself producing syncytium (Midgley et al 1963). As the cytotrophoblast decreases, the syncytium becomes directly adjacent to the basal lamina over an increasingly large area and becomes progressively thinner. A few cytotrophoblastic cells, usually disposed singly, persist until term. In the first and second trimester cytotrophoblastic sprouts are present, covered in syncytium, and represent a stage in the development of new villi. At the tips of anchoring villi cytotrophoblast columns extend from the villous basal lamina to the maternal decidual stroma as described previously.

The cells of the *villous cytotrophoblast* (*Langerhans cells*) are pale-staining with only a slight basophilia. Ultrastructurally, they show a rather electron-translucent cytoplasm, with relatively few organelles: clusters of ribosomes, narrow cisternae of rough endoplasmic reticulum, a number of large mitochondria, variable Golgi apparatus and intermediate filaments particularly in association with the desmosomes. Between the desmosomes, the membranes of adjacent cells are separated by about 20 nm. Sometimes the intercellular gap widens to accommodate microvillous projections from the cell surfaces; the gap occasionally contains patches of fibrinoid.

A smaller population of intermediate cytotrophoblast may also be found in the chorionic villi. This postmitotic population represents a state of partial differentition between the cytotrophoblast stem cell and the overlying syncytium (Jones & Fox 1991).

The syncytial cytoplasm is more strongly basophilic and possesses many ultrastructural features which distinguish it from the cytoplasm of the Langhans cells. Where the plasma membrane adjoins basal lamina it is often complexly infolded into the cytoplasm, whereas the surface bordering the intervillous space is set with numerous long microvilli, the cores of which show linear densities. These microvilli are responsible for the brush border of light microscopy.

The syncytial cytoplasm is exceedingly complex and more electron-dense than that of Langhans cells. It contains a wealth of free ribosomes, cisternae of granular endoplasmic reticulum, scattered representations of the Golgi complex, mitochondria, a cytoskeleton of microfilaments and a profusion of vesicles and vacuoles, some smooth and some coated, of a wide size range, numerous lysosomes, phagosomes and other electron-dense inclusions (Jones & Fox 1991). It is an intensely active tissue layer across which most transplacental transport must occur. It is also responsible for the secretion of a range of placental proteins into the maternal circulation. These include chorionic gonadotrophin, chorionic somatomammotrophin (formerly known as placental lactogen) and others.

Glycogen is held to be present in both layers of the trophoblast at all stages but it is not always possible to demonstrate it by histochemical means. Lipid droplets are also present in both layers and free in the core of the villus. In the trophoblast they are found principally within the cytoplasm but also occur extracellularly between cytotrophoblast and syncytium, or between the individual cells of the cytotrophoblast and also in the basal lamina. These droplets diminish in number with advancing age and may represent fat in transit from mother to fetus, or a pool of precursors for steroid synthesis. Membrane-bound granular bodies of moderate electron-density also occur in the cytoplasm, particularly in the syncytium. Some of these are probably secretion granules. The lysosomes and phagosomes are evidently concerned with the degradation of materials engulfed from the intervillous space.

On the free surface of the villus various types of specialization occur, though care must be taken to distinguish these from artifacts caused by tangential sectioning (Cantle et al 1987). In the immature placenta, syncytial sprouts are found representing the first stages of development of new terminal villi. These later become invaded by cytotrophoblast and villous mesenchyme. Occasionally, adjacent syncytial sprouts make contact and fuse to form slender syncytial bridges. Syncytial sprouts are also present in the term placenta, but here the enclosed nuclei are largely degenerative. Syncytial knots represent similar aggregates of degenerative nuclei, but here not associated with a projection from the villous surface. This may

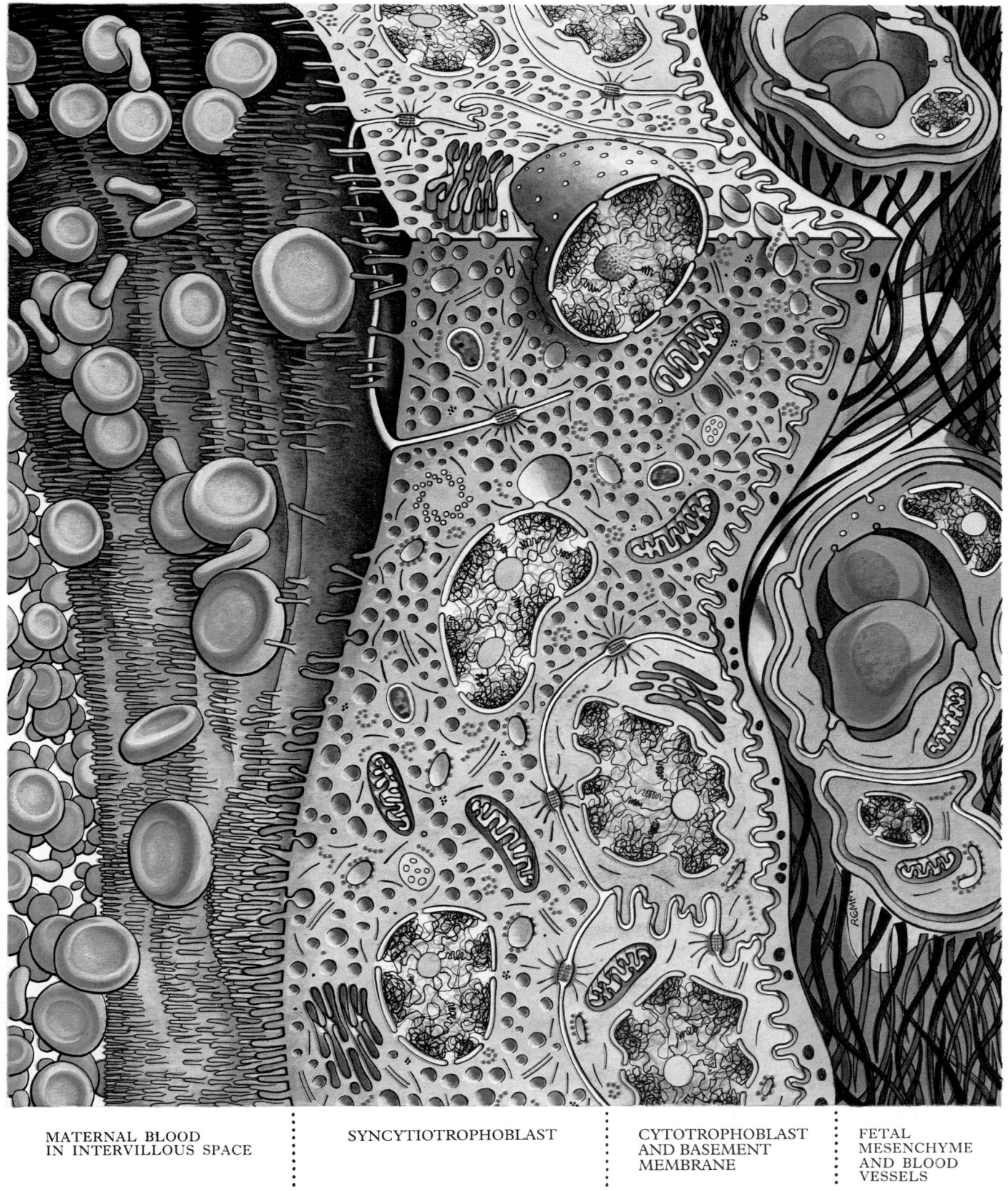

MATERNAL BLOOD
IN INTERVILLOUS SPACE

SYNCYTIOTROPHOBLAST

CYTOTROPHOBLAST
AND BASEMENT
MEMBRANE

FETAL
MESENCHYME
AND BLOOD
VESSELS

3.65   Schematic diagram showing the detailed ultrastructural features of the tissues (enclosed in a rectangle in **3**.64) which intervene between the maternal and fetal blood streams. Note the contrasting architecture of the syncytial and the cellular trophoblasts, and the substantial basement mem-brane and delicate fetal mesenchyme which separate the trophoblast from the fetal vessels. Contrast the nucleate fetal, and anucleate maternal ery-throcytes. For further description see text. (Based on data in Boyd & Hamilton 1970.)

represent a sequestration phenomenon involving removal of sen-escent nuclear material from adjacent metabolically active areas of syncytium. The sprouts may become detached, forming *maternal syncytial emboli* which pass to the lungs. It has been computed that there is a passage of some 100 000 of such sprouts daily into the maternal circulation. In the lungs they provoke little local reaction and apparently disappear by lysis but they may, on occasion, form foci for neoplastic growth.

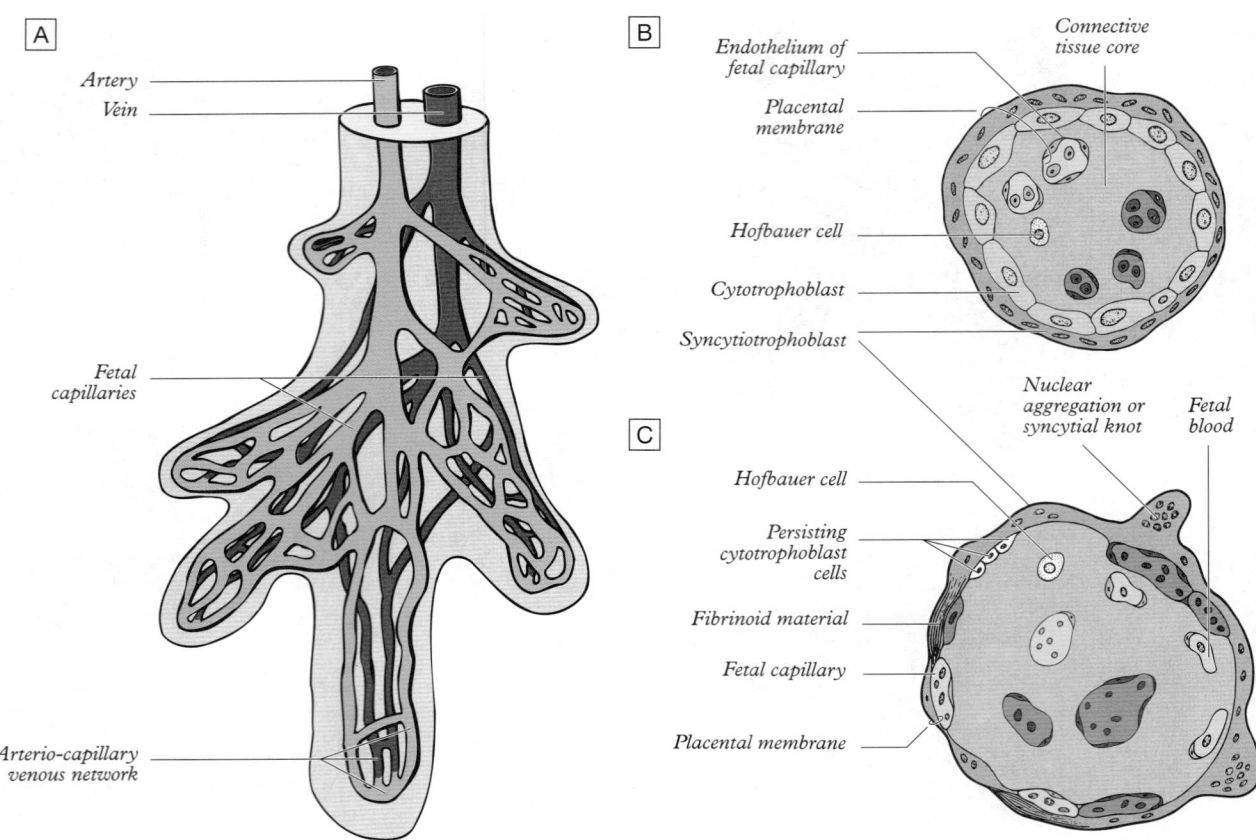

3.66A Drawing of a chorionic villus showing its arterio–capillary–venous system carrying fetal blood. The artery carries deoxygenated blood and waste products from the fetus, whereas the vein carries oxygenated blood and nutrients to the fetus. B, C. Drawings of sections through a chorionic villus at 10 weeks and at full term, respectively. The villi are bathed externally in maternal blood. The placental membrane, composed of fetal tissues, separates the maternal blood from the fetal blood. Note that this membrane becomes very thin towards the end of pregnancy. Hofbauer cells are probably phagocytic cells.

Fibrinoid deposits are frequently found on the villous surface in areas lacking syncytiotrophoblast; this appears to be a repair mechanism in which the fibrinoid forms a wound surface that is subsequently re-epithelialized by trophoblast (Nelson et al 1990). The extracellular matrix glycoprotein tenascin is localized in the stroma adjacent to these sites (Castelluci et al 1991).

The core of the villus contains small and large reticulum cells, fibroblasts, and large phagocytic *Hofbauer cells* which are more numerous in early pregnancy (Jones & Fox 1991). Early mesenchymal cells probably differentiate into small reticulum cells which in turn produce fibroblasts or large reticulum cells. The small reticulum cells appear to delimit a collagen-free stromal channel system through which Hofbauer cells migrate (Martinoli et al 1984). Mesenchymal collagen increases from a network of fine fibres in early mesenchymal villi to the densely fibrous stroma of stem villi of the second and third trimester. After about the 14th week, the stromal channels found in immature intermediate villi are infilled by collagen to give the fibrous stroma characteristic of the stem villus.

The fetal vessels include arterioles and capillaries. Their endothelial cells contain fine cytoplasmic filaments and they extend bulbous projections into the lumen. Pericytes may be found in close association with the capillary endothelium. From late first trimester the vessels are surrounded externally by a periendothelial basal lamina membrane. From the second trimester, and later in terminal villi, dilated thin-walled capillaries are found immediately adjacent to the villous trophoblast, the two basal laminae having apparently fused to produce a vasculo-syncytial interface.

Maturation and functions of the placenta

In the early stages of placental development the blood in the fetal vessels is separated from the maternal blood in the intervillous space by the fetal vascular endothelial cells, the connective tissue of the villus, the subepithelial basal lamina and its covering of cyto- and syncytial trophoblast. These constitute a *placental barrier* interposed between the bloodstreams, but it is a selectively permeable barrier and allows water, oxygen and other nutritive substances and hormones to pass from mother to fetus, and some of the products of excretion to pass from fetus to mother.

Throughout pregnancy, the placenta increases its surface area and thickness, with accompanying increases in the size, length and complexity of branching of the villous stems (Benirschke & Kaufmann 1990). At term, the placental diameter varies between 200–220 mm, the mean placental weight is 470 g, its mean thickness is 25 mm and the total villous surface area exceeds 10 m². The placental barrier becomes reduced in thickness during gestation. After the fourth month the villous syncytium comes into direct apposition to the subepithelial basal lamina over an increasing area (80% at term) and it also becomes thinner. The fetal capillaries approach the surface of the terminal villi and become dilated.

The mechanism of transfer of substances across the placental barrier is complex. The volume of maternal blood circulating through the intervillous space has been assessed at 500 ml per minute (Assali et al 1960). Simple diffusion suffices to explain gaseous exchange. Transfer of ions and other water soluble solutes is by paracellular diffusion, transcellular diffusion and transport, although the relative importance of each of these for most individual solutes is unknown, and the paracellular pathway is morphologically undefined. Glucose transfer involves facilitated diffusion and active transport mechanisms carry calcium and at least some amino acids. The fat-soluble and water-soluble vitamins are likely to pass the placental barrier with different degrees of facility, and indeed it is known that the water-soluble vitamins B and C pass readily. Water is interchanged between fetus and mother (in both directions) at about 3.5 litres per hour. The transfer of substances of high molecular weight such as complex sugars, some lipids, hormonal and non-hormonal proteins varies greatly in rate and degree, and is not so readily understood.

Energy-dependent selective transport mechanisms including receptor-mediated transcytosis are probably involved.

Lipids may be transported unchanged through and between the cells of the trophoblast to the core of the villus. The passage of maternal antibodies (immunoglobulins) across the placental barrier confers some degree of passive immunity on the fetus. In this instance it is widely accepted that transfer is by micropinocytosis. Investigation of transplacental mechanisms is complicated by the fact that the trophoblast itself is the site of synthesis and storage of certain substances, e.g. glycogen. For comprehensive reviews of placental transfer mechanisms consult Sibley and Boyd (1992) and Faber and Thornburg (1983).

The placenta is an important endocrine organ; some steroid hormones, various oestrogens, β endorphins, progesterone, hCG and human chorionic somatomammotropin (hCS)—also known as placental lactogen (hPL)—are synthesized and secreted by the syncytium. The trophoblast is rich in birefringent lipids and cytochemical methods show that it also contains enzyme systems which are associated with the synthesis of steroid hormones.

It has been suggested that leucocytes may migrate from the maternal blood through the placental barrier into the fetal capillaries. It has also been shown that some fetal and maternal red blood cells may cross the barrier (Dancis 1959). The former may have important consequences, for example in rhesus incompatibility (p. 1407).

The majority of drugs are small molecules that are sufficiently lipophilic to pass the barrier. Many are apparently tolerated by the fetus, but some may exert grave teratogenic effects on the developing embryo (e.g. thalidomide). A well-documented association exists between maternal alcohol ingestion and fetal abnormalities (Sadler 1990). Addiction of the fetus can occur to substances of maternal abuse such as cocaine and heroin.

Finally, a wide variety of bacteria, spirochaetes, protozoa and viruses (including human immunodeficiency virus, HIV) are known to pass the placental barrier from mother to fetus, although the mechanism of transfer is uncertain. The presence of maternal rubella in the early months of pregnancy is of especial importance in relation to the production of congenital anomalies (see p. 333).

Placental variations

As a rule the placenta is attached to the posterior wall of the uterus near the fundus, with its centre in or near the median plane. The site of attachment is determined by the point where the blastocyst becomes embedded but the factors on which this depends are not yet understood. The placenta may be attached at any point on the uterine wall, offering no complications to a normal labour unless it is so low down that it overlies the internal os uteri, in which case serious antepartum haemorrhage may occur, especially if it is nearly central in position. This occurs in about 0.5% of pregnancies and is known as *placenta praevia*. (*Extrauterine* sites of implantation are discussed on p. 136.)

The umbilical cord, although usually attached near the centre of the organ, may reach it at any point between its centre and margin, the latter known as a *battledore* placenta. Occasionally the cord fails to reach the placenta itself and ends in the membranes in its vicinity. With such a *velamentous insertion* of the cord, the larger branches of the umbilical vessels traverse the membranes before they reach and ramify on the placenta. A small *accessory* or *succenturiate* placental lobe is occasionally present, connected to the main organ by membranes and blood vessels; it may be retained in utero after delivery of the main placental mass and prolong postpartum haemorrhage. Occasionally other degrees of division occur (*bipartite* or *tripartite* placentae). Other variations include *placenta membranacea*, in which villous stems and their branches persist over the whole chorion, and *placenta circumvallata*, in which its margin is undercut by a deep groove. Pathological forms of adherence or penetration include *placenta accreta*, with exceptional adherence to the decidua basalis, *placenta increta*, in which the myometrium is invaded, and *placenta percreta*, when the invasion by placental tissue has passed completely through the uterine wall.

At birth, when ligature of the umbilical cord is delayed, the blood volume of the child is, on the average, appreciably greater than it is when the ligature is applied at the earliest possible moment (Yao et al 1969). It appears that in the former case much of the blood in the fetal placental vessels is transferred from the placenta to the fetus.

DEVELOPMENT OF INDIVIDUAL SYSTEMS

Embryonic development has so far been considered as a whole, but, as the definition of its structures proceeds, overall description becomes so complicated as to actually impede the clarity of appreciation of the events occurring. It is, hence, customary and convenient to limit attention to individual systems in their further development; but it must never be overlooked that the analysis of a whole organism into such divisions, however attractive on morphological and functional grounds, is largely a product of the sequential nature of human perception. Not only do the several systems into which we divide the organism develop simultaneously; they also interact and modify each other. This necessary interdependence is not only supported by the evidence of experimental embryology but is also emphatically demonstrated by the phenomena of growth anomalies, which cut across the artificial boundaries of systems in most instances. For these reasons it is most desirable that the development of any one individual system should be frequently related to others, especially those most closely associated with it (both spatiotemporally and causally).

So far the development of the embryo has been taken to an age of between 3 and 4 weeks, the stage of early somite formation, equivalent to Horizons X or XI on the scale established by the studies of Streeter and others (1942, 1945, 1948, 1949) and of stages 10–11 of O'Rahilly and Muller (1987). As it is notoriously difficult to age embryos with total accuracy, stages of development have been generally used in this section. A particular stage is not an alternative way of indicating the developmental age of an embryo: a stage conveys the developmental status of many of the systems in concert.

No one criterion could place a particular embryo within one stage or another: the stage is estimated from examination of a number of key structures throughout the body. Figure **3**.31 shows a graph of developmental stage and time.

The commencement of the development of the following systems begins at the body plan, pharyngula, stage (see p. 100). It is only partly constricted from the yolk sac, but the head and tail folds are well formed, with enclosure of the foregut and hindgut (proenteron and metenteron). The forebrain projection dominates the cranial end of the embryo; the buccopharyngeal membrane and cardiac prominence are caudal and ventral to this. The intraembryonic mesenchyme has begun to differentiate with the paraxial mesenchyme undergoing segmentation into somites. Neural groove closure is progressing to a neural tube and is separated from the dorsal aspect of the gut by the notochord. The earliest blood vessels have appeared and a primitive tubular heart occupies the pericardium. The chorionic circulation is soon to be established, after which the embryo rapidly becomes completely dependent for its requirements upon the maternal bloodstream. The intraembryonic part of the coelom consists of the transmedian pericardial cavity, leading dorsocaudally into right and left pericardioperitoneal canals (coelomic ducts). The canals occupy mesenchyme dorsal to the septum transversum, caudal to which they expand into the peritoneal cavity. This establishes, for a time, a free communication with the extraembryonic coelom (**3**.49, **50**). The development of all of the systems described in the remainder of this section begins at this stage.

RESPIRATORY AND GASTROINTESTINAL SYSTEMS

PRIMITIVE GUT

The primitive gut is divided, by head and tail folding, into three main compartments; the *foregut* extends from the buccopharyngeal membrane (a localized region where ectoderm and endoderm are in direct opposition see p. 146) to its opening, or continuation, into the central midgut region via the cranial intestinal portal (3.67). Foregut derivatives are: part of the buccal cavity, the pharynx (and numerous subregions), the respiratory system, the oesophagus, stomach, superior and proximal half of the descending part of the duodenum, the liver, gallbladder and biliary duct systems, the pancreas and ducts. The site of the original cranial intestinal portal is immediately caudal to the common hepatopancreatic ampulla and papilla. The *midgut* extends between the intestinal portals being, in the early embryo, in wide communication with the yolk sac. With constriction of the connection to the yolk sac the midgut becomes tubular and lengthens being destined to form the remaining duodenum, jejunum, ileum, caecum and appendix, ascending colon and much of the transverse colon. The *hindgut* extends from the region of the putative splenic flexure to (and a little beyond) the cloacal membrane (a caudal region where the ectoderm and endoderm are in direct opposition, see p. 146). Its gut derivatives are the descending colon, sigmoid colon, rectum and anal canal to the level of the anal valves. The caudoventral part of the hindgut is continuous with the allantois; it separates from the alimentary hindgut and contributes to the urinary bladder, urethra and associated glands.

At a cellular level the primitive embryonic gut is formed from three sources:

(1) The *splanchnopleuric coelomic epithelium*. Initially this is a proliferative epithelium which forms the splanchnopleuric mesenchymal populations; later it forms the outer, serosal or visceral epithelial layer.

(2) The *endodermal epithelium* forms the epithelium of the mucosa, the lining cells of adjoining ducts and the secretory cells of the associated glands.

(3) The intervening *splanchnopleuric mesenchyme* forms all of the structures and tissue between the epithelial layers, i.e. the outer connective tissue layers, the muscularis externa and submucosal connective tissue; the muscularis mucosae and lamina propria of the mucosa; and the local angiogenic tissue which gives rise to the blood and lymphatic vessels.

The splanchnopleuric mesenchyme provides by far the greatest cell mass to the primitive gut. Generally the splanchnopleuric mesenchyme patterns the development of the endodermal epithelium both spatially and temporally; it contributes to the external shape of the primitive gut structures and modifies the shape of the splanchnopleuric coelomic epithelium, and therefore of the coelom. (For the derivations of these tissues see p. 145.) The gut is innervated by migrating *neural crest* cells which form the *enteric plexuses*. Lymphoid tissue becomes incorporated into the embryonic gut, both by assimilation of individual cells within the epithelium of the mucosa, and also by colonization of the submucosa by germinal centres of lymphoid tissue.

PRIMITIVE FOREGUT

Buccal cavity

This derives from both ectodermal and endodermal regions. The rostral growth of the embryo and formation of the head fold causes the pericardial area and buccopharyngeal membrane to come to lie on the ventral surface of the embryo (p. 148). With further expansion of the forebrain dorsally, and bulging of the pericardium ventrally, together with enlargement of the facial prominences laterally, the buccopharyngeal membrane becomes depressed forming the base of a hollow, the *stomodeum* or *primitive buccal cavity* (3.68). At the end of the fourth week (stage 12) the membrane breaks down and a communication is established between the stomodeum and cranial end of the foregut (future oropharynx). No vestige of the membrane is evident in the adult, and this embryonic communication should

3.67 Diagram of the major epithelial populations within the early embryo. The early gut tube is close to the notochord and neural tube dorsally. The splanchnopleuric layer of the intraembryonic coelomic epithelium is in contact with the foregut ventrally and laterally, with the midgut laterally and with the hindgut ventrally and laterally.

Figure 3.67 labels: Pharynx, Pericardial cavity, Pericardio-peritoneal canals, Body wall, somatopleuric mesenchyme and coelomic epithelium, Epithelium of midgut, splanchnopleuric mesenchyme and coelomic epithelium, Allantois, Foregut, Midgut, Peritoneal cavity, Hindgut

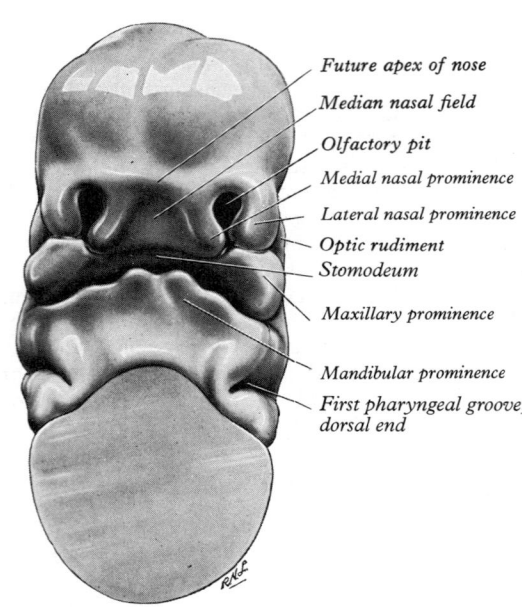

3.68 The head of a human embryo in the sixth week: ventral aspect. (From a model by K Peter.)

Figure 3.68 labels: Future apex of nose, Median nasal field, Olfactory pit, Medial nasal prominence, Lateral nasal prominence, Optic rudiment, Stomodeum, Maxillary prominence, Mandibular prominence, First pharyngeal groove, dorsal end

not be confused with the permanent oropharyngeal isthmus. The epithelium of the lips and gums, salivary glands and the enamel of the teeth are ectodermal in origin, from the stomodeal walls, but the epithelium of part of the tongue and adnexa, developed in the posterior floor of mouth and pharynx, is derived from endoderm. The development of the teeth and gums is described on page 1712.

The pharyngeal arches grow in a ventral direction and lie progressively between the stomodeum and pericardium; with the completion of the mandibular prominences and the development of the maxillary prominences (p. 277), the opening of the stomodeum assumes a pentagonal form, bounded cranially by the frontonasal prominence, caudally by the mandibular prominences and laterally by the maxillary prominences (3.68). With the inward growth and fusion of the palatine processes (3.146), the stomodeum is divided into a nasal and a buccal part. Along the free margins of the prominences bounding the mouth cavity appears a shallow groove, and the ectoderm in its floor thickens and invades the underlying mesenchyme; it divides into a medial *dental lamina* and a lateral *vestibular lamina*. The central cells of the latter degenerate and the furrow becomes deepened. It is now termed the *labiogingival groove* or *sulcus*; its inner wall contributes to the formation of the alveolar processes of the maxillae and the mandible and their gingivae, while its outer wall forms the lips and cheeks.

Structures in the wall of the oral cavity, i.e. *mucous glands, salivary glands, teeth* and *taste buds*, are formed by ectoderm/mesenchymal interactions. Similarly the buccal epithelium is so formed but results in a non-keratinized layer in contrast to the outer ectodermal layer which forms the keratinized layer of skin.

Teeth. These are formed by an ectoderm/mesenchyme interaction and are dealt with, more appropriately, under development of the viscerocranium (see p. 274).

Salivary glands. These arise from the epithelial lining of the mouth. The *parotid gland* can be recognized in human embryos 8+ mm long (stage 15) as an elongated furrow running dorsally from the angle of the mouth between the mandibular and maxillary prominences. The groove, which is converted into a tube, loses its connection with the epithelium of the mouth, except at its ventral end, and grows dorsally into the substance of the cheek. The tube persists as the *parotid duct* and its blind end proliferates in the local mesenchyme to form the gland. Subsequently the size of the oral fissure is reduced by partial fusion between the maxillary and mandibular prominences and the duct opens thereafter on the inside of the cheek at some distance from the angle of the mouth. The *submandibular gland* is identifiable in human embryos 13 mm long as an epithelial outgrowth from the floor of the *linguogingival groove* (see below) into the mesenchyme. It increases rapidly in size, giving off numerous branching processes which later acquire lumina. At first the connection of the submandibular outgrowth with the floor of the mouth lies at the side of the tongue, but the edges of the groove in which it opens come together, from behind forwards, and

form the tubular part of the *submandibular duct*. As a result, the orifice of the duct is shifted forwards till it is below the tip of the tongue, close to the median plane. The *sublingual gland* arises in embryos about 20 mm long as a number of small epithelial thickenings in the linguogingival groove and on the groove's lateral side, which later closes to form the submandibular duct. Each thickening canalizes separately; many of the multiple sublingual ducts open separately on the summit of the sublingual fold, others join the submandibular duct.

Tongue. This appears as a small median elevation, named the *median tongue bud (tuberculum impar)*, in the floor of the pharynx before the pharyngeal arches meet ventrally; it subsequently becomes incorporated in the anterior part of the tongue. A little later two oval *distal tongue buds (lingual swellings)* appear on the inner aspect of the mandibular prominences. They meet each other in front, and caudally they converge on the median tongue bud, with which they fuse (3.69). A sulcus forms along the ventral and lateral margins of this elevation and deepens, internal to the future alveolar process of the mandible, to form the *linguogingival groove*, while the elevation constitutes the anterior or buccal (presulcal) part of the tongue. Caudal to the median tongue bud, a second median elevation, the *hypobranchial eminence* (copula of His), forms in the floor of the pharynx, and the ventral ends of the fourth, the third and, later, the second pharyngeal arches converge into it. A transverse groove separates its caudal part to form the epiglottis, while ventrally it approaches the presulcal tongue rudiment, spreading in the form of a V, and forming the posterior or pharyngeal part of the tongue. In the process the third arch elements grow over and bury the elements of the second arch, excluding it from the tongue. As a result the mucous membrane of the pharyngeal part of the tongue receives its sensory supply from the glossopharyngeal, the nerve of the third arch. In the adult the union of the anterior and posterior parts of the tongue approximately corresponds to the angulated *sulcus terminalis*, its apex at the *foramen caecum*, a blind depression produced at the time of fusion of the constituent parts of the tongue, but also marking the site of ingrowth of the median rudiment of the thyroid gland.

At first the tongue consists of a mass of mesenchyme covered on its surface by ectoderm and endoderm. During the second month occipital myotomes migrate from the lateral aspects of the myelencephalon and invade the tongue to form its musculature. They pass ventrally round the pharynx to reach its floor accompanied by their nerve (the hypoglossal) (see p. 1256).

The composite character of the tongue is indicated by its innervation. Impulses from and to the anterior, buccal part are mediated by: (1) the lingual nerve, derived from the post-trematic nerve of the first arch (mandibular nerve) and (2) the chorda tympani, often held to be the pretrematic nerve to the first arch. The posterior, pharyngeal part of the tongue is innervated by the glossopharyngeal, the nerve of the third arch and its root, near the epiglottis, by the vagus.

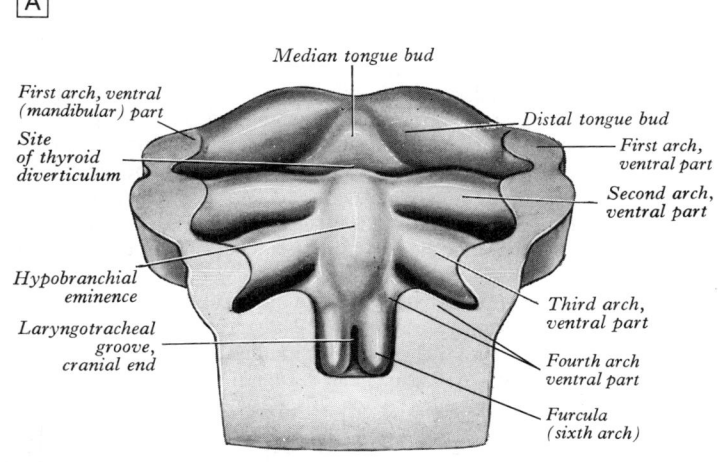

A

First arch, ventral (mandibular) part

Site of thyroid diverticulum

Median tongue bud

Distal tongue bud

First arch, ventral part

Second arch, ventral part

Hypobranchial eminence

Laryngotracheal groove, cranial end

Third arch, ventral part

Fourth arch ventral part

Furcula (sixth arch)

3.69A The floor of the pharynx of a human embryo at the beginning of the sixth week. (From a model by K Peter.)

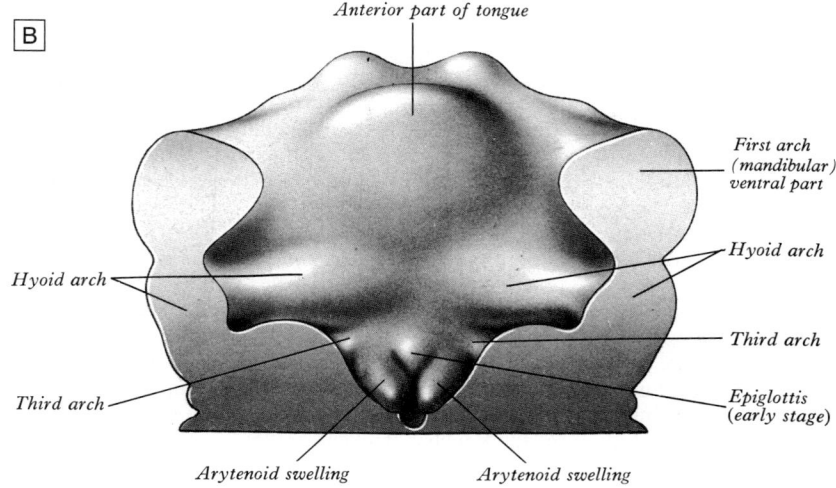

B

Anterior part of tongue

First arch (mandibular) ventral part

Hyoid arch

Third arch

Epiglottis (early stage)

Hyoid arch

Third arch

Arytenoid swelling

Arytenoid swelling

3.69B The floor of the pharynx of a human embryo, about 6 weeks old. (From a model by K Peter.)

The sulcus terminalis cannot be distinguished earlier than the 52-mm stage according to some observers. The vallate papillae appear at about the same time, increasing in number until the 170-mm stage. Serial reconstructions also suggest that the territory of the glossopharyngeal nerve extends considerably beyond these papillae.

Thyroid gland. This gland is first identifiable in embryos of about 20 somites, as a median thickening of endoderm in the floor of the pharynx between the first and second pharyngeal pouches and immediately dorsal to the aortic sac (Davis 1923). This area is later invaginated to form a median diverticulum which appears late in the fourth week in the furrow immediately caudal to the median tongue bud (**3.69**). It grows caudally as a tubular duct the tip of which bifurcates and subsequently the whole mass divides into a series of double cellular plates, from which the isthmus and the lateral lobes of the thyroid gland are developed. The *primary thyroid follicles* differentiate by reorganization and proliferation of the cells of these plates. *Secondary follicles* subsequently arise by budding and subdivision (Norris 1916). These primary and secondary endodermal cells are the progenitors of the follicular parenchyma proper. The claim that the fourth pharyngeal pouches contribute thyroid tissue to the lateral lobes of the gland was long disputed and perhaps seemed unlikely on the grounds of comparative embryology. (But see below—the *ultimobranchial body* and the derivation of *parafollicular* or *C cells*.)

The original diverticulum, its bifurcation and generations of follicles invade the hypobranchial neural crest mesenchyme. From the latter are derived the thin connective tissue capsule, thinner 'interlobular' septa and delicate perifollicular investments. These carry the main vascular, characteristic fenestrated capillaries, lymphatics and autonomic nerve supply.

The connection of the median diverticulum with the pharynx is termed the *thyroglossal duct*. The site of its initial continuation with the endodermal floor of the mouth is marked by the foramen caecum. From here it extends caudally in the median line ventral to the primordium of the hyoid bone, behind which it later forms a recurrent loop. The distal part of the duct commonly differentiates variably as the pyramidal lobe and levator muscle (or 'suspensory' fibrous band) of the thyroid. The remainder fragments and disappears, but the lingual part is often identifiable until late in fetal life and may branch and give rise to miniature salivary glands (Boyd 1964). Occasionally parts of the midline thyroglossal duct persist (occurring in lingual, suprahyoid, retrohyoid, or infrahyoid positions). They may form aberrant masses of thyroid tissue, cysts, fistulae or sinuses, usually in the midline (see p. 1892). A *lingual thyroid* situated at the junction of the buccal and pharyngeal parts of the tongue is not uncommon, but nodules of glandular tissue may also be found other than in the midline, e.g. laterally placed posterior to sternocleidomastoid, and, on occasion, below the level of the thyroid isthmus (see p. 1892).

Pharyngeal pouches

The development of the pharyngeal arches during stages 10 to 13 (see p. 187) causes morphological changes in the primitive rostral foregut resulting in a widened orifice at the putative mouth, rapidly narrowing caudally. The foregut rostrally is compressed dorsoventrally such that there is limited, or virtually no, true lateral wall. Between the individual arches, in the early stages, the ectoderm and endoderm are transiently closely apposed with little intervening mesenchyme. Externally such regions are termed *pharyngeal* (or *branchial*) *clefts*; internally they are referred to as *pharyngeal pouches*.

The close proximity of the ectoderm and endoderm is maintained between the first cleft and pouch which becomes the *tympanic membrane*, with minimal mesenchyme between the layers. The *first pouch* and, some maintain, part of the *second pouch*, i.e. its dorsal part, together expand as the *tubotympanic recess* which gives rise to the middle ear system (see below). The relationship between subsequent clefts and pouches diverges with mesenchyme intervening; the endoderm of the pouches thickens and evaginates into localized regions of neural crest and unsplit lateral plate mesenchyme.

The *second pouch* is much reduced in dimensions compared to the first and its ventral part is the focus of lymphoid development as the *palatine tonsil*. A generalized ring of lymphoid tissue develops in the primitive foregut at this region, resulting in the median pharyn-

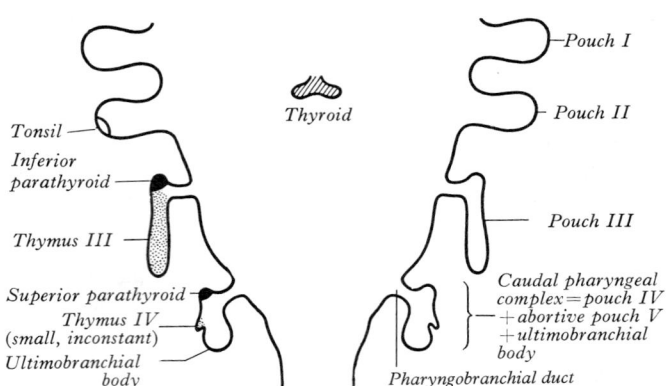

3.70   Scheme showing the development of the branchial epithelial bodies. The numbered sacs are the endodermal pharyngeal pouches.

geal *tonsil* (*adenoid*), the bilateral *tubal tonsils* and the *lingual tonsil* on the posterior part of the tongue.

The *third pouch* gives rise to the *thymus* ventrally and the *parathyroid III* dorsally, whereas the *fourth pouch* produces the *parathyroid IV* and an *ultimobranchial body*. The complex of the dorsal and ventral portions of the fourth pouch plus the lower ultimobranchial body is termed the *caudal pharyngeal complex* (**3**.70).

Tonsils. Derived from the ventral parts of the second pharyngeal pouches which lie between the tongue and the soft palate; the endoderm lining these pouches grows into the surrounding mesenchyme as a number of solid buds. These buds are excavated by degeneration and shedding of their central cells, and thus the tonsillar *fossulae* and *crypts* are formed. Lymphoid cells accumulate around the crypts and become grouped as lymphoid follicles. A slit-like *intratonsillar cleft* extends into the upper part of the tonsil and is possibly a remnant of the second pharyngeal pouch.

Thymus. Derived from the endoderm of the ventral part of the third pharyngeal pouch on each side (**3**.70), the thymus cannot be recognized prior to the differentiation of the inferior parathyroid glands (see below), which occurs when the embryo is 10–12 mm long (stage 16), but thereafter it is represented by two elongated diverticula which soon become solid cellular masses and grow caudally into the surrounding neural crest mesenchyme. Ventral to the aortic sac the two thymic rudiments meet and are subsequently united by connective tissue only; the rudiments themselves remain unfused. The connection with the third pouch is soon lost, but the stalk may persist for some time as a solid, cellular cord.

The development of thymic tissue from the ventral recess of the fourth pharyngeal pouch probably occurs in a proportion of embryos, although this has been denied by some authorities (Weller 1933; Norris 1938). Thymic tissue developing from this site is usually found near but outside the thyroid gland in close association with the superior parathyroid gland. An ectodermal contribution to the thymus, probably of placodal origin, occurs in some mammals but a similar contribution in man is conjectural (Garrett 1948).

Vascularized mesenchyme, including lymphoid stem cells, invades the cellular mass of the endodermal thymus and becomes partially lobulated. The cells of the cytoreticulum and the concentric corpuscles of the thymus are endodermal in origin. The epithelial character of these cells is more obvious in fetal life; some are even ciliated (Sebuwufu 1968). Lymphoid cells enter and colonize the thymus from the haemopoietic tissue stem cells during the third month.

At birth the thymus is large relative to total body weight. Its absolute weight increases in the first 2 years after birth, but its relative weight decreases. There is little change thereafter until about the seventh year, when rapid growth again occurs to reach a maximum at about 11 years. After this it begins to decline to an adult weight which is very variable but averages 12–15 g. In old age the gland shrinks still further, especially after wasting diseases. For this and other reasons it is rarely identifiable in the preserved cadaver of the aged (Keynes 1954; Lasi 1959; and p. 1429).

Parathyroid glands. These are also derivatives of the endoderm and adjacent mesenchyme. Prior to the appearance of the thymic rudiment from the third pharyngeal pouch, the epithelium on the dorsal aspect of the pouch and in the region of its duct-like connection with the cavity of the pharynx becomes differentiated as the primordium of the *inferior parathyroid gland*, recognizable by its cells, which stain more lightly than the other endodermal cells lining the pouch. Although the connection between the pouch and the pharynx is soon lost, the connection between the thymic and parathyroid rudiments persists for some time, and the latter passes caudally with the developing thymus. The *superior parathyroid glands* develop in a similar manner from the dorsal recess of the fourth pharyngeal pouches. They come into relation with, and appear anchored by, the lateral lobes of the thyroid gland and thus remain cranial to the parathyroid glands derived from the third pouch. The mesenchyme provides the connective tissue envelopment, vasculature including fenestrated capillaries and lymphatics; it is also a route for vasomotor nerves.

Ultimobranchial body. Already noted as an endodermal diverticular part of the *caudal pharyngeal complex* (**3**.70), it separates from the ectoderm of the fourth pharyngeal cleft and loses its connection with the pharynx by attenuation and rupture of the common pharyngobranchial duct. It becomes closely associated with the expanding lateral lobe of the thyroid gland, and the superior parathyroid (parathyroid IV) component of the complex lying dorsally and outside the thyroid gland. The remainder of the complex, which includes the ultimobranchial body and possibly some vestiges of the ventral recess of the fourth pharyngeal pouch and of the transitory fifth pharyngeal pouch, is enveloped by the thyroid gland. Although some controversy reigned, it is now strongly supported by evidence that the cells of the ultimobranchial body give·rise to the 'C' or parafollicular cells producing calcitonin in the thyroid gland of many if not all mammals (Halmi 1986). Calcitonin has been isolated from ultimobranchial tissue in vertebrates other than mammals (Copp et al 1967; Taylor 1968). The derivation of thyroid parafollicular cells has now been clearly demonstrated in embryonic sheep (Jordan et al 1973).

Pharynx

Study of the development of the head region has so far focused on local segmentation and the integration of nerves with neural crest derived connective tissue and paraxial mesenchyme, or somite, derived voluntary muscle. However, the mechanisms of formation of the pharynx, the role of the endoderm, and the specification of the junction between voluntary with involuntary muscle, are intimately related to the above and have still to be addressed, adding an increased level of complexity to the problem. The pharyngeal endoderm is in contact with mesenchyme and epithelia from many different sources e.g. neural crest, paraxial mesenchyme of the somitomeres, somites, lateral plate mesenchyme, which at this level is unsplit, cleft ectoderm, general endothelium and the outflow tract of the heart. The development of this region is likely then to be an interaction of all of these tissues in concert. The mechanism of formation of the pharynx is complex and intimately related to the development of the viscerocranium and laryngeal cartilages (p. 274). The inter-related roles of endoderm, neural crest, unsegmented paraxial mesenchyme, somites and splanchnopleuric mesenchyme in this region are not yet clear. It is likely that local development is controlled by *Hox* gene expression as seen in viscerocranial development (see **3**.148).

Whereas the distal foregut, midgut and hindgut are formed from three layers: a serous or adventitial layer, a layer of splanchnopleuric mesenchyme derived from the splanchnopleuric coelomic epithelium, and an inner endodermal epithelium, the proximal foregut has a mix of voluntary muscle around the upper pharynx blending, over the middle third of the oesophagus, into involuntary muscle of the lower oesophagus. The interface between the voluntary pharyngeal muscles and the gut involuntary muscles has not yet been clearly elucidated. A new mesenchymal population has been identified at the interface between the endoderm and the paraxial mesenchyme of the somitomeres and occipital somites (Noden 1991); it develops in a rostrocaudal and lateromedial sequence. Beginning as a sparse layer, it becomes denser prior to the formation of endothelial networks, ultimately forming a fenestrated mesenchymal monolayer between developing blood vessels and the endoderm. Later it expands between

the notochord and the roof of the foregut, and, it is suggested (Noden 1991), that it participates in the formation of pharyngeal and oesophageal smooth muscle and connective tissues. Further experimental studies are needed to confirm this; generally there is much in this region which requires extensive study.

As well as the pouch development described above, the endodermal aspect of the first (maxillomandibular) arch in its dorsal part contributes to the formation of the lateral wall of the nasopharynx in front of the orifice of the auditory tube. The ventral end of the first pouch becomes obliterated, but its dorsal end persists and deepens as the head enlarges. It remains close to the ectoderm of the dorsal end of the first cleft (see above) and, together with the adjoining lateral part of the pharynx and dorsal part of the second pharyngeal pouch, constitutes the *tubotympanic recess*, which forms the tympanic cavity and the auditory tube (p. 1370), and ultimately their extensions. The site of the second arch is partly indicated by the *palatoglossal arch*, but its dorsal end is separated from its ventral end by the forward growth of the third arch, which obliterates the intermediate part. Some believe that the site of the second pharyngeal pouch is represented by the *intratonsillar cleft*, around which the tonsil is developed. The third arch forms the *lateral glosso-epiglottic fold*, and its dorsal end takes part in the formation of the floor of the auditory tube. The ventral ends of the fourth arches fuse with the caudal part of the hypobranchial eminence and so contribute to the formation of the *epiglottis*. The adjoining portion becomes connected to the *arytenoid swelling* and may be identified in the *aryepiglottic fold*.

After the caudal part of the hypobranchial eminence has separated from the pharyngeal (posterior) part of the tongue (p. 175), it is in continuity with two linear ridges which appear in the ventral wall of the pharynx, the whole forming an inverted U, sometimes regarded as an independent formation, the *furcula* (of His). These vertical ridges have been identified as the sixth arches, placed very obliquely owing to the shortness of the pharyngeal floor compared with the greater extent of the roof. The ridges of the furcula are carried downwards on the ventral wall of the foregut and bound the median *laryngotracheal groove*, from which the lower part of the larynx, the trachea, bronchi and lungs are developed (see below). At the cranial end of the groove, paired arytenoid swellings arise which convert the slit-like upper aperture of the respiratory system into a T-shaped opening. The aryepiglottic folds (fourth arch derivatives) can be recognized at this stage.

RESPIRATORY SYSTEM

The development of the respiratory tree begins at stage 12 (approximately 26 days) when there is a sharp onset of epithelial proliferation within the foregut at regions of the endoderm tube destined to become the lungs, stomach, liver and dorsal pancreas (O'Rahilly & Muller 1986). The future *respiratory epithelium* bulges ventrally into the investing splanchnopleuric mesenchyme then grows caudally as a bulb-shaped tube (**3**.71). By stage 13 the caudal end of the tube has divided asymmetrically forming the future primary bronchi; with growth the right primary bronchus becomes orientated more caudally whereas the left extends more transversely. The *trachea* is clearly recognizable at stage 14. From this time the origin of the trachea remains close to its site of evagination from the future oesophagus, however, longitudinal growth of the trachea causes the region of the future carina to descend. Failure of separation of the trachea and oesophagus results in a *tracheo-oesophageal fistula* connecting one tube to the other. The condition also occurs if there is excessive ventral displacement of the dorsal wall of the foregut. This may result in an upper oesophageal segment which is separated from a thin distal tracheo-oesophageal fistule. The latter is usually in continuity with the lower oesophageal segment. Infants with this condition may appear to salivate excessively at birth, with or without respiratory distress (Beasley & Myers 1994).

Larynx. Formed from the cranial end of the respiratory diverticulum, the laryngotracheal groove, the larynx is bounded ventrally by the caudal part of the hypobranchial eminence (p. 175) and on each side by the ventral ends of the sixth arches. In the latter, two *arytenoid swellings* appear, one on each side of the groove (**3**.71A, B), and as they enlarge they approximate to each other and to the caudal part of the hypobranchial eminence (**3**.71A, B) from which the *epiglottis* is developed. The *opening* into the larynx, at first a vertical slit, is converted into a T-shaped cleft by the enlargement of the arytenoid swellings; the vertical limb of the T lies between the two swellings and its horizontal limb between them and the epiglottis. The arytenoid swellings differentiate into the *arytenoid* and *corniculate cartilages*, and the ridges joining them to the epiglottis become the definitive *aryepiglottic folds* in which the *cuneiform cartilages* are derived from the epiglottis. The *thyroid cartilage* is developed from

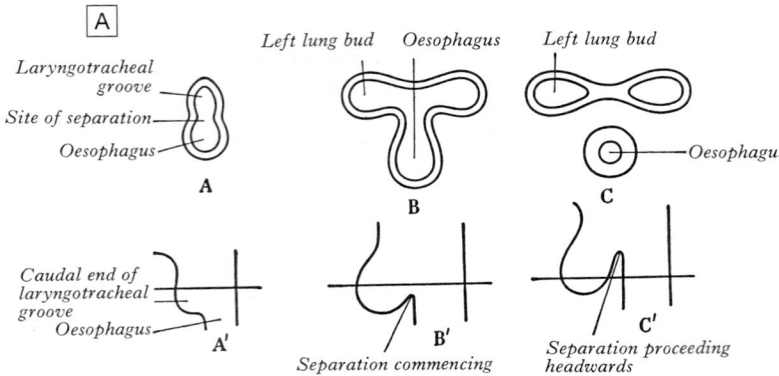

3.71A Diagrams to show the closure of the laryngotracheal groove and its separation from the oesophagus in the latter part of the fourth week. A, B and C represent transverse sections at the level shown in A¹, B¹ and C¹, which are outline drawings of the oesophageal region in three closely following stages. Left lateral aspect.

In A and A¹ the laryngotracheal groove communicates freely with the oesophagus.

In B¹ the lower end of the laryngotracheal groove has begun to close and to form right and left evaginations, which represent the earliest rudiments of the lung buds, seen in B.

In C¹ the separation of the laryngotracheal groove from the oesophagus has proceeded further in a headward direction, and in C the primitive lung buds are now freed from the oesophagus. (After Streeter 1948.)

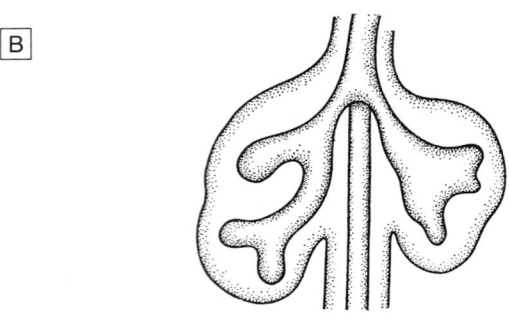

3.71B The lung buds from a human embryo, 11.8 mm long, showing commencing lobulation: ventral aspect. (After Streeter 1948.)

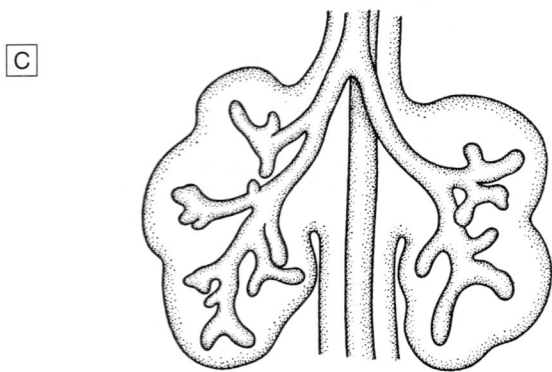

3.71C The lungs of a human embryo, in the early part of the sixth week. Right/left differences in lobation are evident. (After Streeter 1948.)

the ventral ends of the cartilages of the fourth, or fourth and fifth, pharyngeal arches; it appears as two lateral plates, each chondrified from two centres and united in the midventral line by a fibrous membrane in which an additional centre of chondrification develops. The *cricoid cartilage* arises from two cartilaginous centres, which soon unite ventrally, gradually extend and ultimately fuse on the dorsal surface of the tube as the cricoid lamina (see also p. 1638). For literature on the early development of the larynx, consult O'Rahilly and Tucker (1973).

Right and left lung buds. These grow dorsally, passing each side of the relatively smaller oesophagus and bulging into the laterally situated pericardio-peritoneal canals (3.67, 71). The parts of the latter accommodating the early lung buds may now be designated the *primary or primitive pleural coeloms*. The dramatic morphogenetic events whereby the primary pleural coelom and its contained developing lung, on each side, excavates and expands into the somatopleuric coelomic epithelium and mesenchyme, thus 'splitting' the primitive body wall into superficial and deep laminae, and forming the extensive *secondary or definitive pleural cavity* is considered further on page 180.

The investing mesenchyme surrounding the lung buds contains a mixed population of cells, some destined to pattern endodermal epithelium and others to produce the endothelial network which will surround the future airsacs; further mesenchymal cells will differentiate as the smooth muscle cells which surround both the respiratory tubes and the blood vessels. In stage 13 embryos, proliferation of the adjacent *splanchnopleuric coelomic epithelium* (of the primary pleural cavities) provides the *investing mesenchyme* which envelops the developing trachea and lung buds. The proliferative activity decreases in stage 14 and the mesenchyme becomes arranged in zones around the developing endoderm. At stage 15, angiogenetic mesenchyme is apparent around the primary bronchi; it forms an extensive capillary network around each lung bud, receiving blood from the developing sixth aortic arch artery and draining it into an anastomosis connected to the dorsal surface of the left atrium. After this stage the coelomic epithelium at the perimeter of the lung surface follows a differentiation pathway to form the *visceral pleura*.

At stage 15 differences in the histology of the oesophagus and the trachea can be seen. The oesophagus has a developing submucosa and muscular coats whereas the larger trachea has a connective tissue coat containing chondroblasts. The *lobar* or *secondary bronchi* can be seen at stage 16 and the *bronchopulmonary segments* are present at stage 17 when the lung enters the pseudoglandular phase of development. The trachea and oesophagus separate during stage 17.

Later stages of respiratory development see the repeated division of the bronchial tree to form the subsegmental bronchi. Stage 17 correlates to approximately 7 weeks when the embryo has achieved a crown rump length of about 12+ mm. The development of the lungs now moves into the fetal period (stage 23) and continues into the neonatal and postnatal periods. Various stages of lung development have been identified on the basis of the histological appearance of the lungs. They are:

- the pseudoglandular stage, from 7–17 weeks, when the lung resembles a tubulo-acinar gland
- the canalicular stage from 17–26 weeks
- the saccular stage from 24 weeks to birth
- the alveolar stage which begins before birth and continues into childhood perhaps up to 8 years of age although the time of completion of alveolar formation has not yet been established.

Pseudoglandular stage. This stage is described as extending approximately from weeks 7–17; it covers the development of the lower conducting airways and the appearance of the acinar structures. The growth and branching of the endoderm epithelium is controlled by the local investing splanchnopleuric mesenchyme as in most epithelial/mesenchymal interactions. The airways begin to differentiate during this stage, being lined proximally by high columnar epithelium and distally by cuboidal. Later the upper airways are lined with pseudostratified epithelium. Mucous glands develop by the 12th week and enlarge in the submucosa; secretory activity has been identified in the trachea at 14 weeks (Bucher & Reid 1961). The splanchnopleuric mesenchyme condenses around the epithelium and differentiates into smooth muscle and connective tissue cell types. Cartilage differentiation in the airways is poorly described; it is not clear if cartilage is synthesized in the pseudoglandular stage.

Canalicular stage (17–26 weeks). During this phase there are about three generations of branching after which the mesenchyme around the branching tips of the dividing respiratory tree decreases allowing the distal airspaces to widen. At 23 weeks longitudinal sections of the future distal regions show a sawtooth margin which may indicate the site of further acini. Peripheral growth is accompanied by an increase in the capillary network around the distal airspaces where, in many places, close contact is made with the respiratory cuboidal epithelium. At such contacts the respiratory epithelial cells decrease in height and begin to differentiate as type I pneumocytes. The cells which remain cuboidal are type II pneumocytes, which are believed to be the stem cells of the alveolar epithelium; they develop an increasing number of lamellar bodies which store surfactant from 6 months of gestation. With apposition of the capillary networks to the thin pneumocytes, and with reduction of the interstitial tissue of the lung gas exchange becomes possible.

Saccular stage (24 weeks to birth). At this stage thin walled terminal saccules are apparent, which will become alveolar ducts as development proceeds. There is a tremendous expansion of the prospective respiratory airspaces during this period which leads to a decrease in the interstitial tissue. The capillary networks become closely opposed as the airspaces get closer together. Invaginations termed secondary crests develop from the saccule walls. As a crest protrudes into a saccule, part of the capillary network becomes drawn in it. After the later expansion of the saccules on each side of the crest, a double capillary layer becomes annexed between the now alveolar walls. During the saccular stage elastin is deposited beneath the epithelium, an important step for future alveolar formation. The production of surfactant matures during this stage increasing the chances of the fetus to survive should it be born prematurely.

Alveolar stage. Exactly when the saccular structure of the lung can be termed alveolar is not yet clear, different workers having different definitions of what constitutes an alveolus. Thurlbeck (1992) notes that alveoli can be seen at 32 weeks and are present in all fetuses at 36 weeks which he recommends as the beginning of the alveolar stage, whereas Hislop et al (1986) suggested that the stage should commence at 28 weeks. As the distal airspaces expand during late gestation and continue after birth, there is a process of fusion of the capillary nets from one alveolus to the adjacent alveolus. Thus shortly after birth there is an extensive double capillary net. Fusion of these layers is apparent at 28 days postnatally and extensive at 1.5 years; it is probably complete by 5 years.

Interactions of early respiratory development

The control of the branching pattern of the respiratory tree resides with the *splanchnopleuric mesenchyme*. Recombination of tracheal mesenchyme with bronchial respiratory endoderm results in inhibition of bronchial branching, whereas recombination of bronchial mesenchyme with tracheal epithelium will induce bronchial outgrowths from the trachea (Wessels 1970; Hilfer et al 1985). Initially the tracheal mesenchyme is continuous with that surrounding the ventral wall of the oesophagus, but with lengthening and division of the tracheal bud and deviation of the lung buds dorsally, each bud becomes surrounded by its own specific mesenchyme thus permitting regional differences between the lungs, i.e. the number of lobes, or the degree of growth and maturity of a particular lung. Each lung develops by a process of dichotomous branching. For branching to occur a cleft must develop in the tip (or side) of the epithelial tube. The epithelium then evaginates each side of the cleft forming new branches which lengthen; the process is then repeated. Differences have been noted between the mesenchyme closely associated with the endoderm epithelium and that some distance away. At the tips of the developing epithelial buds the mesenchyme is flattened and densely packed; in contrast, along the side of the bud and in the clefts the mesenchyme forms an ordered row of cuboidal cells. Cells in both arrangements send processes towards the epithelial basal lamina which is thicker in the clefts, but so thinned as to be almost indistinguishable on the tips of the buds where the epithelium and mesenchymal cells form intimate contacts. Tenascin, an extracellular matrix molecule (also known as hexabrachion or cytotactin), is present in the budding and distal tip regions, but absent in the

clefts. Conversely fibronectin, an extracellular matrix molecule found commonly in basal laminae, is found in the clefts and along the sides of the developing bronchi, but not on the budding and distal tips (Abbott et al 1992); see also p. 114.

In extensive studies on lung development in mammals Ten Have-Opbroek (1991) has disputed that the pseudoglandular stage covers the development of the complete bronchial tree. He and his coworkers maintain that lung development can be divided into causally distinct bronchial and respiratory systems both of which proceed in the canalicular, saccular and alveolar stages. The epithelium of the developing bronchial system is columnar whereas in the respiratory system it is cuboidal. This latter epithelium is composed of precursors of the type II pneumocytes which exhibit early stages of multilamellar bodies. There is always a sharp demarcation between alveolar epithelium and bronchial epithelium throughout development, leading these workers to postulate that the bronchial and respiratory systems each originate from a different portion of the primordial respiratory diverticulum. The type II pneumocyte is the key cell in pulmonary acinus formation being the stem cell which produced type I pneumocytes and which ultimately matures into a surfactant producing cell. The cells at the distal end of the bronchial system are non-ciliated Clara cells which develop slowly prenatally.

Mesenchyme around the lung buds may be destined to become:

- the interstitial connective tissue of the lung
- endothelial networks (both blood vascular and lymphatic) and blood cells of the pulmonary and bronchial circulations
- smooth muscle cells which surround either the airways or the blood vessels.

Of the connective tissues line, lung fibroblasts retain an influence over the rate of cytodifferentiation and maturity of the lung epithelium. Lung fibroblasts from the pseudoglandular stage stimulate epithelial cell proliferation, whereas fibroblasts from the saccular stage promote differentiation (Caniggia et al 1991). From the saccular stage lung fibroblasts secrete an oligopeptide, fibroblast-pneumocyte factor (FPF), which stimulates neighbouring type II pneumocytes in the developing alveolar walls to produce the surfactant phospholipid, saturated phosphatidylcholine (SPC) contained in multilamellar bodies. In recent years premature babies and those who will be delivered preterm have been given cortisol, which binds to specific receptors in lung mesenchyme causing release of FPF, thus accelerating lung maturity.

There is an interesting sexual dimorphism in lung development. Androgens have been found to delay fetal lung maturation while stimulating fetal lung growth. Male type II cells are less mature than the female cells and this is thought to be due to delayed fibroblast maturation caused by androgens blocking the cortisol stimulation of FPFm RNA (Torday 1992).

The development of lung smooth muscle has been demonstrated by the use of antibodies against cytoskeletal and contractile proteins (Mitchell et al 1990). Initially the local lung mesenchyme is positive for vimentin filaments; however, this is later replaced by desmin in cells destined to become smooth muscle. The expression of both desmin and smooth muscle myosin indicates terminal differentiation of smooth muscle; however, α-smooth muscle actin-containing cells, which form a thick coat around the primitive airways, have been found to extend further than either the desmin or smooth muscle myosin-containing cells. It was noted that α-actin positive cells were found in regions of epithelial cleft formation, suggesting an association with branching morphogenesis.

Endothelial development is seen in the pseudoglandular stage when capillary networks form around the developing lung buds. These will become the capillary anastomoses around the future alveoli. The mesenchyme produces both the endothelium of the vessel tunica intima and the smooth muscle cells of the tunica media. Vimentin is noted in the smooth muscle cells around developing vessels in the pseudoglandular stage but this is replaced by desmin in the saccular stage.

Thoracic wall and pleural cavities

Whereas the preceding account describes the morphological and histological development of the respiratory tree, for the lungs to function they must be surrounded by a complete pleural cavity slightly larger than the capacity of the lungs. The development of the thoracic cage and the pleural cavities is therefore of vital importance for the functioning of the respiratory system.

At the same time as the splanchnopleuric mesenchyme is being produced from the proliferating coelomic epithelium so too is the somatopleuric. This latter mesenchyme is penetrated by the developing *ribs* which arise from the thoracic sclerotomes. In the midline the somatopleuric mesenchyme gives rise to the *sternum* and *costal cartilages* (see p. 538). The bony and cartilaginous cage provides insertions for the intercostal muscles which arise from the ventrolateral edge of the epithelial plate of the somites. The somatopleuric coelom epithelium after its proliferative phase gives rise to the parietal layer of pleura.

When the lung buds develop they project into the *pericardioperitoneal canals* subdividing them into *primary pleural coeloms* around the lung beds cranially, and paired *peritoneal coeloms* caudally which are continuous with the wider peritoneal coelom around the mid- and hindgut. The communications with the pericardial and peritoneal coeloms become the *pleuropericardial* and *pleuroperitoneal canals* respectively (3.72, 78). (When separation between these fluid-filled major coelomic regions is advancing towards completion, they are named the *pericardial, pleural* and *peritoneal cavities*; the serous walls of the latter are often called *sacs*. In early embryos the cavities retain substantial volumes of fluid and their walls are separate; they provide the route for a primitive type of circulation until superseded by the blood vascular system. In later fetal and postnatal life cavity walls are coapted, a mere microscopic film of serous fluid intervening.)

A curved elevation of tissue, the *pulmonary ridge*, develops on the lateral wall of the pleural coelom and partly encircles the pleuropericardial canal. The ridge is continuous with the dorsolateral edge of the septum transversum. The developing lung bud abuts on the ridge, which as a result divides into two diverging membranes meeting at the septum transversum. One is cranially placed and termed the *pleuropericardial membrane*; embedded within it the common cardinal vein and phrenic nerve reach the septum transversum by this route. The other membrane, caudally placed, is termed the *pleuroperitoneal membrane*. As the apical part of the lung forms it invades and **splits** the body wall and extends cranially on the **lateral aspect** of the common cardinal vein, carrying with it, or rather preceded by, an extension from the primary pleural coelom to form part of the *secondary* or *definitive pleural sac*. In this way the common cardinal vein and the phrenic nerve come to lie medially

in the mediastinum. The pleuropericardial canal, which lies medial to the vessel, is gradually narrowed to a slit, which is soon obliterated by the apposition and fusion of its margins (3.72). Its closure occurs early and is mainly effected by the growth and expansion of the surrounding viscera, heart and great vessels, lungs, trachea and oesophagus, and not by active growth of the pleuropericardial membrane across the opening to the root of the lung (3.72).

In addition to its extension in a cranial direction the lung and its associated visceral and parietal pleura also enlarge ventromedially and caudodorsally (see below). With the ventromedial extension, the lungs and pleurae therefore excavate and split the somatopleuric mesenchyme over the pericardium, separating the latter from the ventral and lateral thoracic walls (3.73). Thus the ventrolateral fibrous pericardium, parietal serous pericardium and mediastinal parietal pleura, although topographically deep, are *somatopleuric in origin*.

Separation of pleural and peritoneal cavities is effected by development of the diaphragm. The *septum transversum* is at first a condensation of mesenchyme, caudal to the pericardial cavity and extending from the ventral and lateral regions of the body wall to the foregut. Dorsal to it on each side is the relatively narrow *pleuroperitoneal canal*. The endodermal hepatic bud grows into the septum transversum, which then can be seen to consist of two parts. One, the *pars diaphragmatica*, is disposed in the transverse plane and lies over the convex cranial surface of the putative liver. The other, the *pars mesenterica*, lies initially in the median sagittal plane and is expanded by the developing liver. At this stage the liver is widely attached to the pars diaphragmatica and to the ventral abdominal wall. These attachments are the forerunners of the coronary and triangular ligaments and of the falciform ligament respectively. Medial to the pleuroperitoneal canals are the oesophagus and stomach with their dorsal mesentery, and, at the root of the latter, the dorsal aorta. Dorsolateral to the canals are the pleuroperitoneal membranes, which remain small; dorsally are the mesonephric ridges, suprarenals and gonads. Just as the enlargement of the pleural cavity cranially and ventrally is effected by a process of burrowing into the body wall, so its caudodorsal enlargement is effected in the same way. The expanding pleural cavities extend into the mesenchyme *dorsal* to the suprarenal glands, the gonads and (degenerating) mesonephric ridges. Thus somatopleuric mesenchyme is peeled off the dorsal body wall to form a substantial portion of the dorsolumbar part of the diaphragm. The pleuroperitoneal canal is closed by the fusion of its edges, which are carried together by growth of the

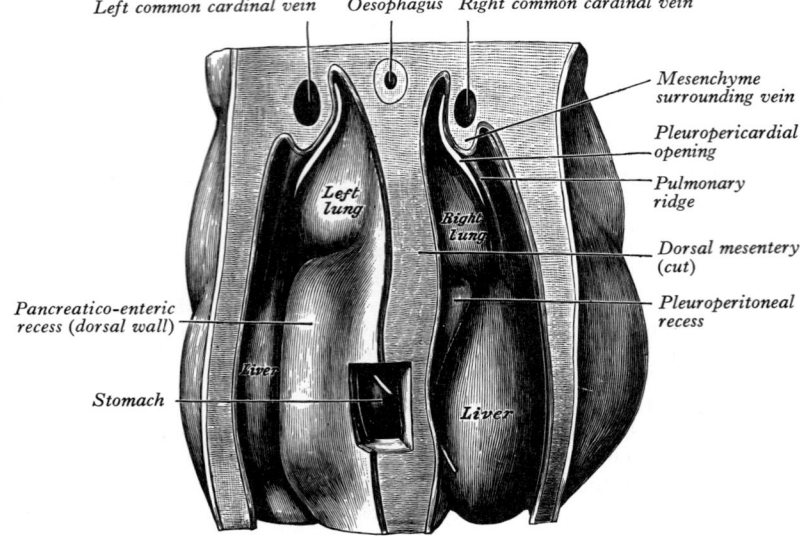

3.72 View, from the dorsal aspect, into the thoraco-abdominal part of the coelom of a human embryo, 6.8 mm long, in the fifth week. Note that the dorsal body wall, including the spinal cord, developing vertebral column, the dorsal aorta and the mesonephroi, has been removed. A window has been made in the dorsal wall of the pancreatico-enteric recess to expose the posterior surface of the stomach and a wire has been passed through the epiploic foramen. (After Piper.)

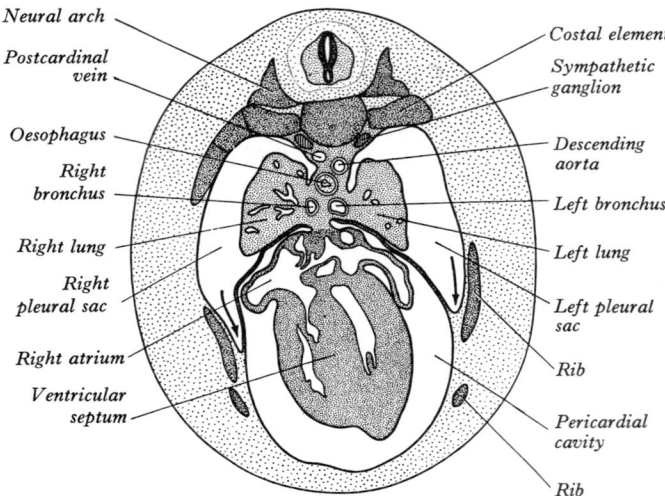

3.73 Transverse section of a 21 mm human embryo, showing how the pleural sacs extend ventrally on each side of the pericardium and split the body wall. The arrows indicate the directions of growth of the two secondary pleural sacs.

organs surrounding it and, in particular, that of the suprarenal, which carries the dorsal margin of the canal ventrally to meet the pars diaphragmatica of the septum transversum (Wells 1954). The right pleuroperitoneal canal closes earlier than the left. Hence it is on the left that an abnormal communication persisting between the pleural and peritoneal cavities is encountered more frequently.

While these changes occur, the septum transversum undergoes a progressive alteration in relative position. In a 2-mm human embryo, the dorsal border of the septum transversum lies opposite the second cervical segment but, as the embryo grows and the heart enlarges, it migrates caudally. At first the ventral border moves more rapidly than the dorsal, but after the embryo has attained a length of 5 mm it is the dorsal border which migrates more rapidly (3.112). When the dorsal border of the septum transversum lies opposite the fourth cervical segment, the phrenic nerve (C3, 4 and 5) and portions of the corresponding myotomes grow into it and accompany it in its later migrations. It is not until the end of the second month that the dorsal border of the septum transversum is opposite the last thoracic and first lumbar segments, the final position occupied by some of the dorsal attachments of the diaphragm and some derivatives of the pars mesenterica. However, the main derivatives of the pars diaphragmatica lie at considerably more cranial levels (see below and p. 270).

Formation of the diaphragm

The closure of the pleuroperitoneal openings completes a mainly mesenchymal partition which thereafter separates thoracic from abdominal viscera and forms the framework for the future diaphragm. This has a composite origin from many different mesenchyme sources. The sternal and costal parts are derived almost exclusively from the pars diaphragmatica of the septum transversum mesenchyme, with a small dorsolateral contribution from the pleuroperitoneal membranes and by excavation of the somatopleuric mesenchyme of the thoracic wall (costal part). Anterior to the oesophageal hiatus is a small contribution from the cranial oesophagophrenic continuation of the gastrohepatic part of the lesser omentum, both derived from the pars mesenterica of the septum transversum. Between the oesophageal and aortic hiatuses it is formed by the dorsal mesentery (strictly the dorsal meso-oesophagus but often, less precisely, included as part of the dorsal mesogastrium). The remainder of the lumbar part of the diaphragm is formed from mesenchyme around the abdominal aorta and more laterally from somatopleuric mesenchyme of the dorsal body wall behind the suprarenal, mesonephric ridge and gonad (Wells 1954). Some authorities consider that much greater areas of the adult diaphragm are derived from the pleuroperitoneal membranes and from the chest wall. Gaps between the lumbar and costal parts of the diaphragm are usually due to underdevelopment of the latter. Premitotic myoblasts, derived principally from the ventrolateral edges of the fourth cervical somites, invade the septum transversum (described on p. 270). They extend throughout the mesenchymal partition, giving rise to the muscular diaphragm (3.135) and its fibrous central tendon, or aponeurosis, with its trefoil shape, cruciform intersecting fibres and central nodal thickening. The caudal migration of the diaphragm during development has already been described (see above).

Maturation of the lungs

Whereas many fetal organs are able to grow to normal proportions even if they are in abnormal locations this is not the case for the lungs. Lung growth becomes impaired by restricted expansion and it is suggested that distension of the developing lung may provide a major stimulus to growth. Absence or impairment of fetal breathing movements is associated with pulmonary hypoplasia, as are defects affecting diaphragmatic activity. It is believed that normal fetal breathing movements increase the lung volume and stimulate growth of the distal airspaces. The mucous glands of the trachea and bronchi secrete a lung fluid during development. This fluid usually passes up the respiratory tract to mix with the amniotic fluid. Experimental ligation of the trachea results in accumulation of the fluid with the lung becoming much heavier than normal.

The relationship between lung fluid and amniotic fluid is far more complex than was previously thought. Pulmonary hypoplasia at birth is often associated with severe congenital urinary obstruction, as in Potter's syndrome. Thus there is a developmental link between

development of the lungs and the kidneys. In renal agenesis there is reduced bronchial branching as early as 12–14 weeks of gestation, before amniotic fluid is produced by the kidneys, suggesting a direct renal factor which supports lung development (Peters et al 1991). Later, the presence of amniotic fluid is necessary for normal fetal lung development. The fetal lung is a net fluid secretor; most of the fluid produced remains within the lungs as a mechanical effect of the amniotic fluid pressure; normally only a small amount of this fluid contributes to the amniotic fluid. Thus the normal functioning of the kidneys regulates the volume and pressure of the lung airway fluid and may in turn provide the pressure needed for expansion and enlargement of the bronchial and pulmonary systems. Interestingly, prolonged experimental lung drainage accelerates the maturity of the alveolar cells, possibly due to an inappropriate signal that birth is imminent (see also pp. 204, 335.

POSTPHARYNGEAL FOREGUT

Although the postdiaphragmatic gut is subdivided into three embryological portions, fore- mid- and hindgut, there are no corresponding fundamental morphological and cytological distinctions between the three parts. Thus the foregut produces a portion of the duodenum as does the midgut, and the midgut similarly produces large intestine as does the hindgut. The differences between portions of the gut develop as a result of interactions between the three embryonic tissue layers which give rise to the gut, namely:

- the endodermal inner epithelium
- the thick layer of splanchnopleuric mesenchyme
- the outer layer of proliferating splanchnopleuric coelomic epithelium.

The final layers of the gastrointestinal tract are derived as follows:

- The epithelial layer of the mucosa and connected ducts and glands are from the endodermal epithelium.
- The lamina propria and muscularis mucosa, the connective tissue of the submucosa, the muscularis externa and the external connective tissue are all from the splanchnopleuric mesenchyme.
- The outer peritoneal epithelium is from the splanchnopleuric coelomic epithelium.

Blood vessels and lymphatics develop from local populations of angiogenic mesenchyme throughout the gut, as do lymph nodes. Innervation of the gut is via the neural crest derived enteric and autonomic systems of nerves and plexuses. There is a craniocaudal developmental gradient along the gut with the stomach and small intestine developing in advance of the colon.

Oesophagus

The oesophagus can be distinguished from the stomach at stage 13 (embryo 5 mm). It elongates during successive stages and its absolute length increases more rapidly than the embryo as a whole. Cranially it is invested by splanchnopleuric mesenchyme posterior to the developing trachea, and more caudally between the developing lungs and pericardio-peritoneal canals posterior to the pericardium. Caudal to the pericardium, the terminal, pregastric segment of the oesophagus has a short thick *dorsal meso-oesophagus* (from splanchnopleuric mesenchyme), while ventrally it is enclosed in the cranial stratum of the septum transversum mesenchyme (i.e. a short *ventral meso-oesophagus*). Each of the above are continuous caudally with their respective primitive dorsal and ventral mesogastria (see p. 186). Thus the oesophagus has only limited areas related to a *primary* coelomic epithelium. However, note the subsequent development of the para-oesophageal right and left pneumato-enteric recesses (3.79), the relation of the ventral aspect of the middle third of the oesophagus to the oblique sinus of the pericardium, and the relation of its lateral walls in the lower thorax to the mediastinal pleura. All the foregoing are *secondary extensions* from the primary coelom.

The mucosa consists of two layers of cells by stage 15 (week 5), but the proliferation of the mucosa does not occlude the lumen at any time. The mucosa becomes ciliated at 10 weeks, and stratified squamous epithelium at the end of the 5th month; occasionally patches of ciliated epithelium may be present at birth. Circular muscle can be seen at stage 15 but longitudinal muscle has not been

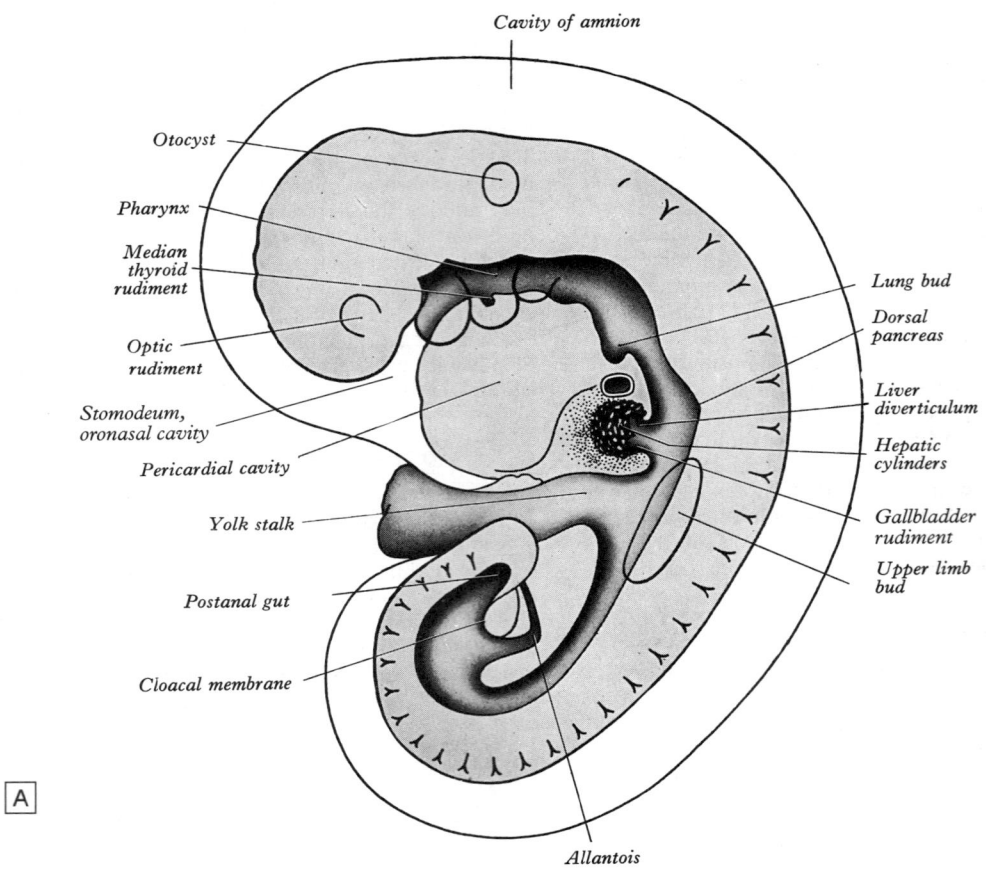

Cavity of amnion

Otocyst

Pharynx

Median
thyroid
rudiment

Optic
rudiment

Stomodeum,
oronasal cavity

Pericardial cavity

Yolk stalk

Postanal gut

Cloacal membrane

Lung bud

Dorsal
pancreas

Liver
diverticulum

Hepatic
cylinders

Gallbladder
rudiment

Upper limb
bud

A

Allantois

3.74A The digestive tube of a human embryo with 29 paired somites, a CR length of 3.4 mm and an estimated age of 27 days. Note pharyngeal development. Magnification × c. 25. (Streeter 1942.)

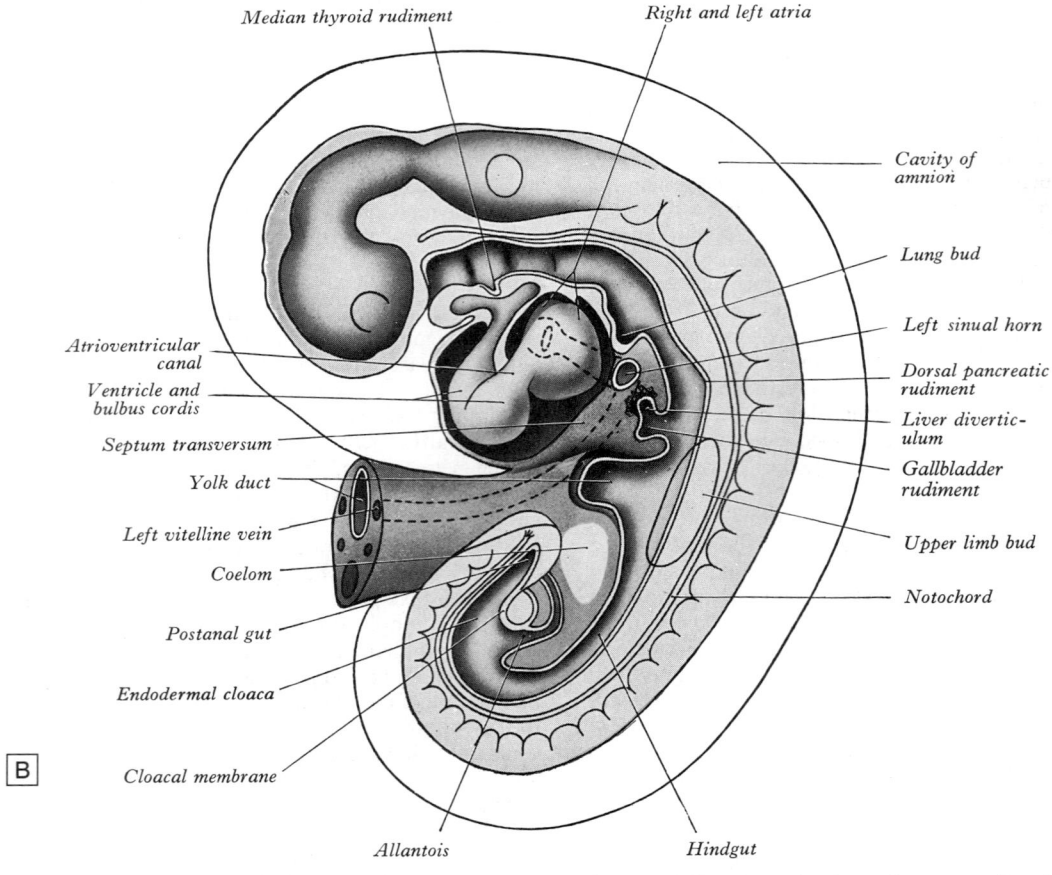

Median thyroid rudiment

Right and left atria

Cavity of
amnion

Lung bud

Left sinual horn

Dorsal pancreatic
rudiment

Liver divertic-
ulum

Gallbladder
rudiment

Upper limb bud

Notochord

Atrioventricular
canal

Ventricle and
bulbus cordis

Septum transversum

Yolk duct

Left vitelline vein

Coelom

Postanal gut

Endodermal cloaca

B

Cloacal membrane

Allantois

Hindgut

3.74B Composite diagram of a graphic reconstruction of a human embryo at the end of the fourth week. The alimentary canal and its outgrowths are shown in median section. The brain is shown in outline, but the spinal cord is omitted. The heart is shown in perspective, the left horn of the sinus venosus having been divided. The somites are indicated in outline. (After Streeter 1942.)

identified until stage 21. Neuroblasts can be demonstrated in the early stages; the myenteric plexuses have cholinesterase activity by 9.5 weeks and ganglion cells are differentiated by 13 weeks. It is suggested that the oesophagus is capable of peristalsis in the first trimester (Smith & Taylor 1972). Peristalsis along the oesophagus and at the lower oesophageal sphincter is immature at birth resulting in frequent regurgitation of food in the newborn period. The pressure at the lower oesophageal sphincter approaches that of the adult at 3–6 weeks of age.

Stomach

At the end of the fourth and beginning of the fifth week the stomach can be recognized as a fusiform dilation (**3**.74, 77) cranial to the wide opening of the midgut into the yolk sac. By the fifth week this opening has narrowed into a tubular vitelline intestinal duct (**3**.74, 75, 76), which soon loses its connection with the digestive tube (**3**.76). At this stage the stomach is median in position and separated cranially from the pericardium by the septum transversum (p. 151), which extends caudally on to the cranial side of the vitelline intestinal duct and ventrally to the somatopleure. Dorsally, the stomach is related to the aorta and, reflecting the presence of the pleuro-peritoneal canals on each side, is connected to the body wall by a short dorsal mesentery, the *dorsal mesogastrium* (**3**.79). The latter is directly continuous with the dorsal mesentery (mesenteron) of almost all of the remainder (except its caudal short segment) of the intestine. The liver develops as a hollow outgrowth from the ventral aspect of the foregut and grows cranially into the substance of the septum transversum (**3**.74, 76), this part of the septum (pars mesenterica) now being termed the ventral mesogastrium. The rest of the intestine has no ventral mesentery.

In human embryos of 10 mm, the characteristic gastric curvatures are already recognizable. (What follows in this paragraph is largely a summary of long-held traditional views of gastric and omental development. More recently close reappraisal of human embryonic serial sections has led to many major descriptive changes and alternative proposals, see p. 192.) Growth is more active along the dorsal border of the viscus; its convexity markedly increases and the rudimentary fundus appears. Because of more rapid growth of the dorsal border, the pyloric end of the stomach turns ventrally and the concave lesser curvature becomes apparent (**3**.76). The stomach is now **displaced** to the left of the median plane and apparently becomes physically **rotated**; thus its original right surface becomes dorsal and its left ventral. Accordingly the right vagus nerve is distributed mainly to the dorsal and the left mainly to the ventral surface of the organ. The dorsal mesogastrium increases in depth and becomes folded on itself; the ventral mesogastrium becomes more coronal than sagittal. The pancreatico-enteric recess (p. 186), hitherto usually described as a simple depression on the right side of the dorsal mesogastrium, becomes dorsal to the stomach and excavates downwards and to the left between the folded layers. It may now be termed the inferior recess of the *bursa omentalis*. Thus the stomach may be simplistically described as having two rotations. The first 90° clockwise, viewed from the cranial end, the second 90° clockwise about an anteroposterior axis. The displacement, morphological changes and apparent 'rotation' of the stomach have been attributed variously to its own and surrounding differential growth changes, extension of the pancreatico-enteric recess with changes in its mesenchymal walls, and pressure, particularly by the rapidly growing liver (Kanagasuntheram 1957). (As intimated, the account just given prevails in basic courses and textbooks and perhaps suffices for some purposes. For a more complete treatment see p. 192 et seq.)

Mucosal and submucosal development can be seen in the 8th to 9th weeks. No villi form in the stomach, unlike other regions of the gut, instead glandular pits can be seen in the body and fundus. These develop in the pylorus and cardia by weeks 10 and 11 when parietal cells can be demonstrated. *Acid secretion* has not been demonstrated in the fetal stomach before 32-week gestation, however *intrinsic factor* has been detected after 11 weeks. This increases from the 14th to 25th week until the pylorus, which contains a larger number of parietal cells than in the adult, also contains a relatively larger quantity of intrinsic factor. The significance of the early production of intrinsic factor and the late production of acid by the parietal cells is not known. Chief cells can be identified after weeks 12–13, although they cannot be demonstrated to contain pepsinogen until term. Also over the same period mucous neck cells can be seen which actively produce mucus from week 16. *Gastrin* producing cells have been demonstrated in the antrum between 19 and 20 weeks and gastrin levels have been measured in cord blood and in the plasma at term. Interestingly cord serum contains gastrin levels 2–3 times higher than those in maternal serum. (For an extensive account of gastric development see Grand et al 1976.)

The stomach muscularis externa develops its circular layer at 8–9 weeks when neural plexuses also develop in the body and fundus. The longitudinal muscle develops slightly later. The pyloric musculature is thicker than the rest of the stomach, although generally the thickness

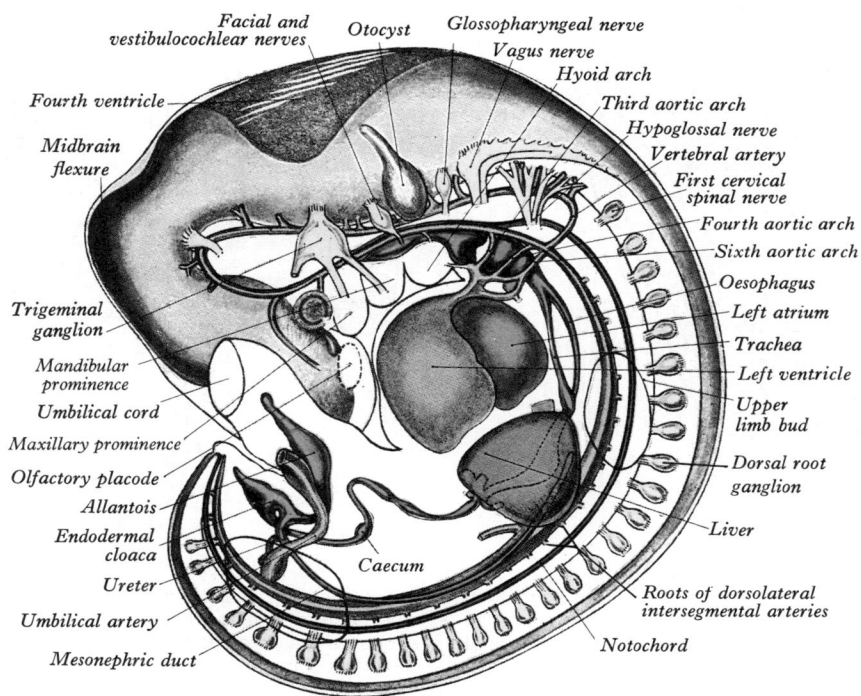

Facial and
vestibulocochlear nerves
Otocyst
Glossopharyngeal nerve
Vagus nerve
Hyoid arch
Fourth ventricle
Third aortic arch
Midbrain flexure
Hypoglossal nerve
Vertebral artery
First cervical spinal nerve
Fourth aortic arch
Sixth aortic arch
Trigeminal ganglion
Oesophagus
Left atrium
Mandibular prominence
Trachea
Left ventricle
Umbilical cord
Upper limb bud
Maxillary prominence
Olfactory placode
Dorsal root ganglion
Allantois
Endodermal cloaca
Ureter
Liver
Umbilical artery
Caecum
Roots of dorsolateral intersegmental arteries
Mesonephric duct
Notochord

3.75   A human embryo of 7 mm greatest length, in the fifth week: left lateral aspect. (After Thompson.)

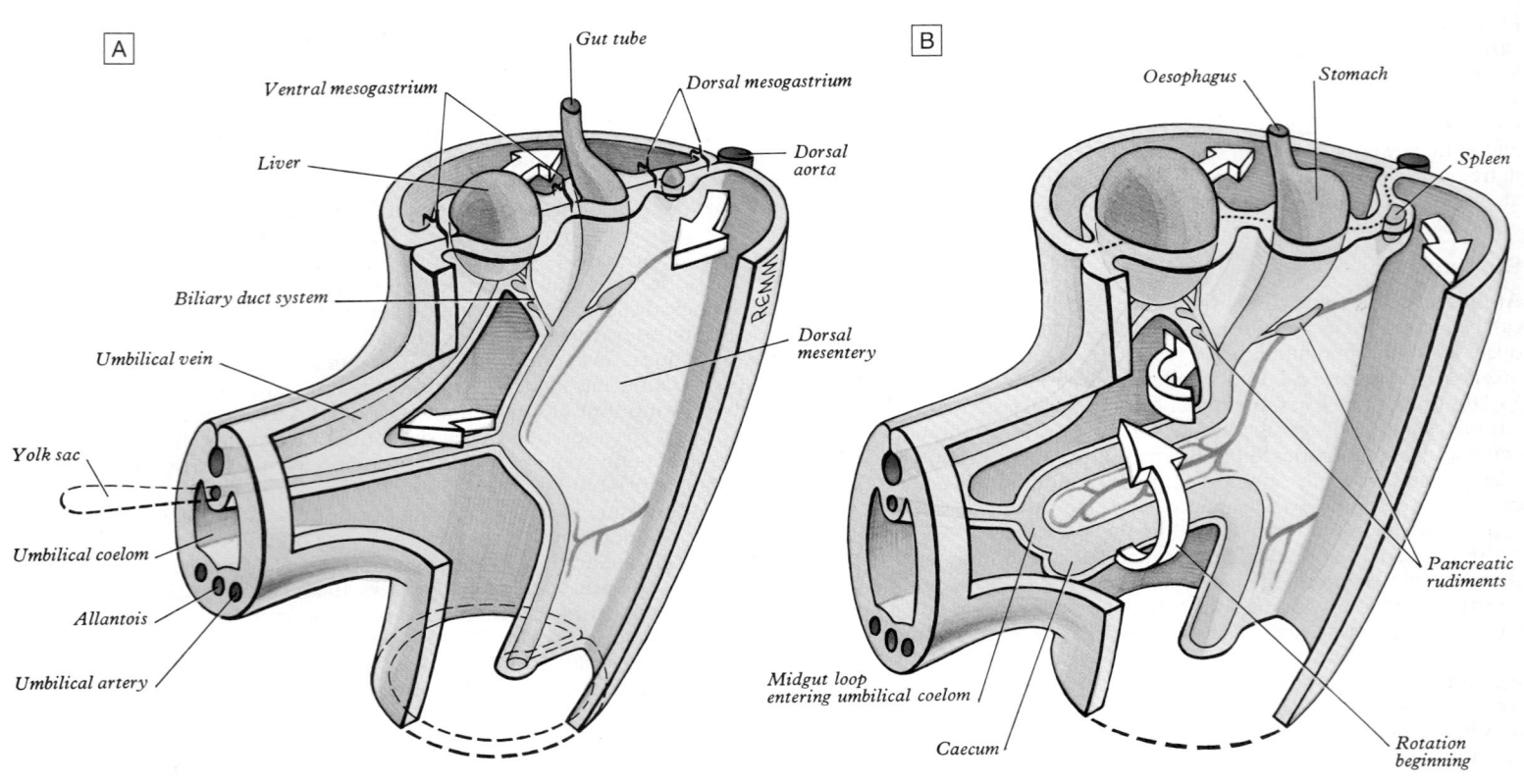

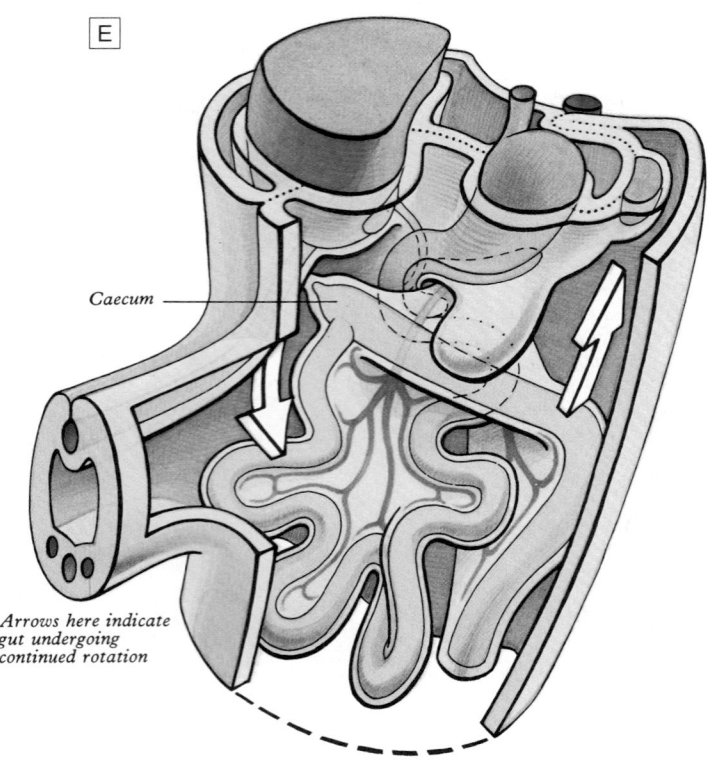

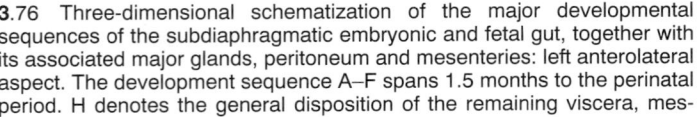

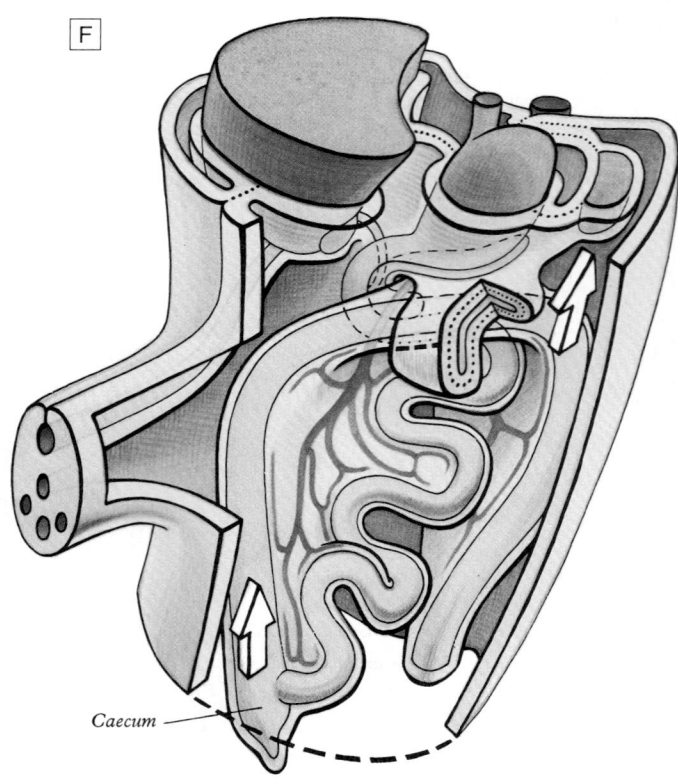

3.76   Three-dimensional schematization of the major developmental sequences of the subdiaphragmatic embryonic and fetal gut, together with its associated major glands, peritoneum and mesenteries: left anterolateral aspect. The development sequence A–F spans 1.5 months to the perinatal period. H denotes the general disposition of the remaining viscera, mes- enteric roots with their lines of attachment, and principal contained vessels, which approximate to the adult state for comparison. Some features of the sequence presented do not correspond to traditional descriptions. See text for further comment.

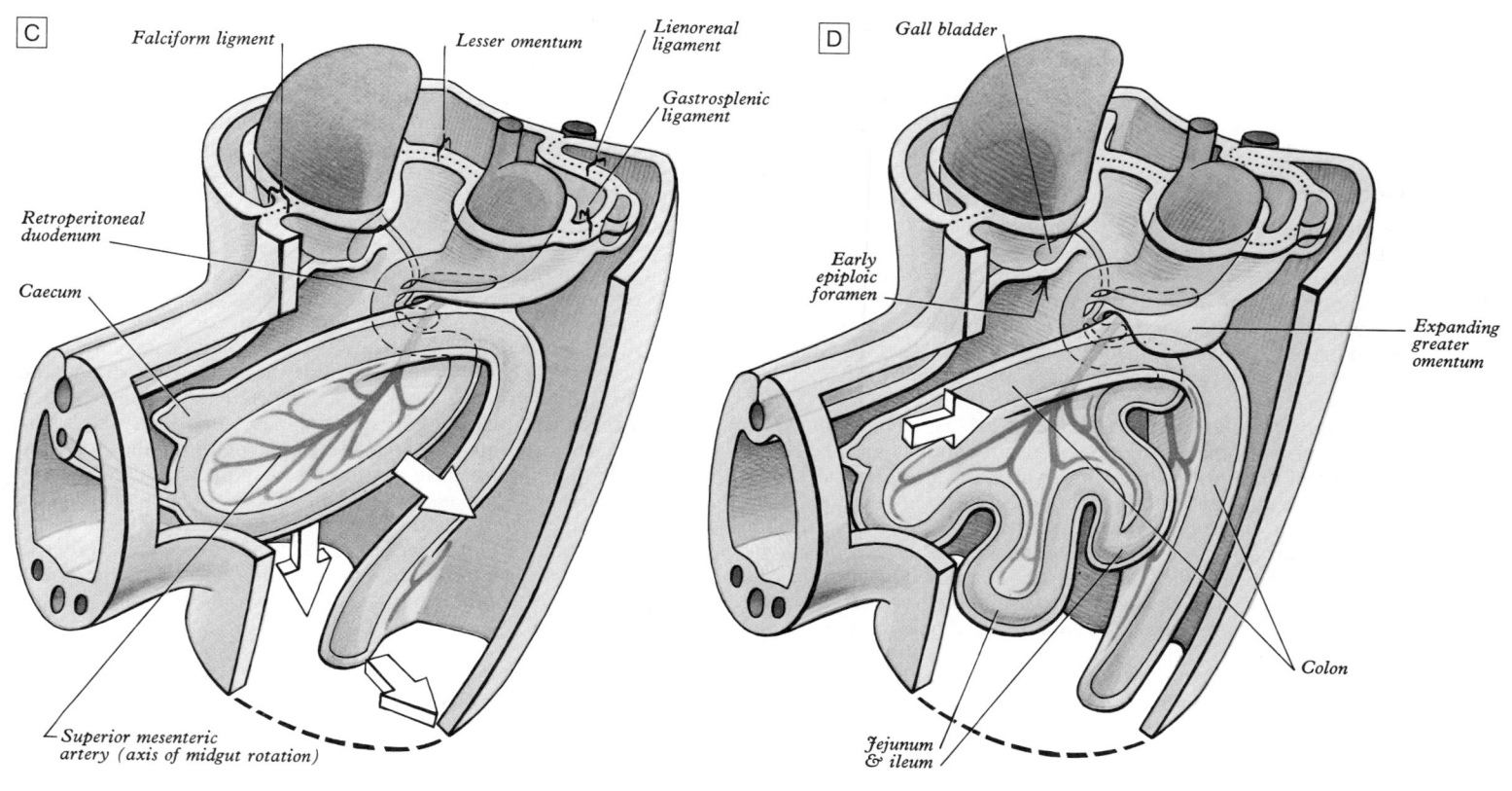

C

Falciform ligament

Lesser omentum

Lienorenal ligament

Gastrosplenic ligament

Retroperitoneal duodenum

Caecum

Superior mesenteric artery (axis of midgut rotation)

D

Gall bladder

Early epiploic foramen

Expanding greater omentum

Colon

Jejunum & ileum

G

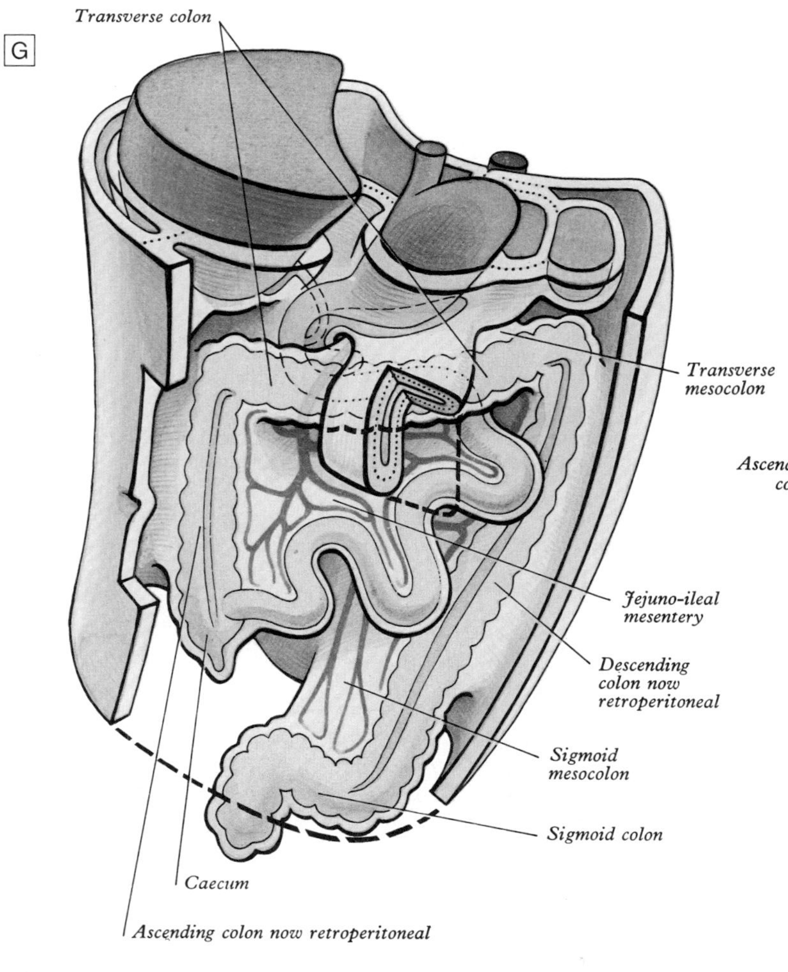

Transverse colon

Transverse mesocolon

Jejuno-ileal mesentery

Descending colon now retroperitoneal

Sigmoid mesocolon

Sigmoid colon

Caecum

Ascending colon now retroperitoneal

H

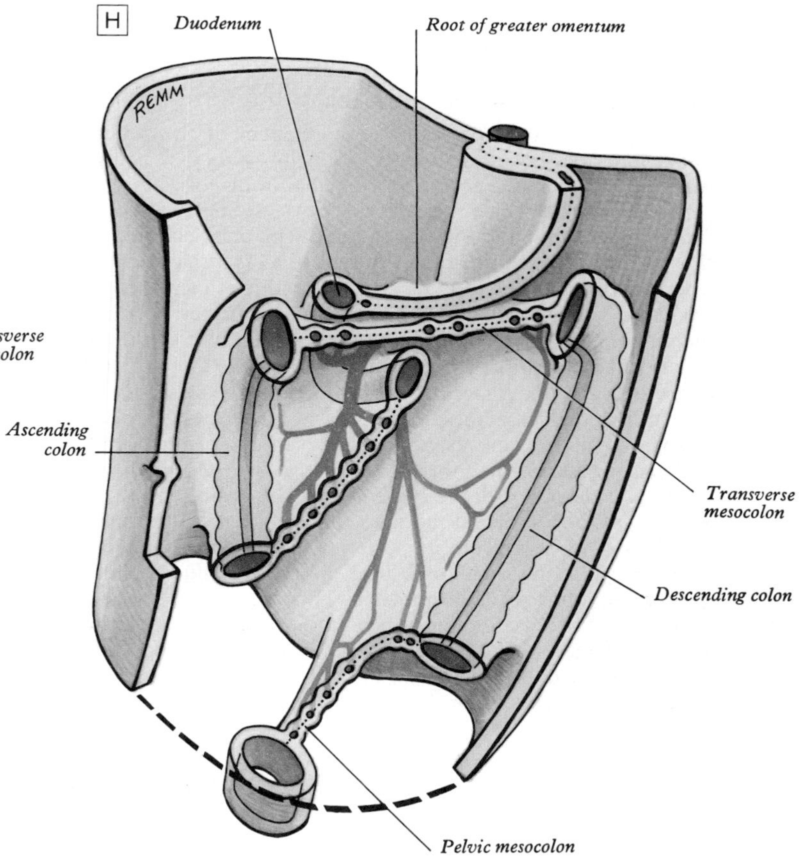

Duodenum

Root of greater omentum

REMM

Ascending colon

Transverse mesocolon

Descending colon

Pelvic mesocolon

of the total musculature of the stomach at term is reduced compared to the adult.

The serosa of the stomach derives from the splanchnopleuric coelomic epithelium (see above). No part of this serosa undergoes absorption; the original left side of the stomach serosa faces the greater sac, the right side the lesser sac (see below).

Duodenum

The duodenum is divided into four parts in the adult for descriptive purposes. From an embryological viewpoint the duodenum forms the caudal part of the foregut and the cranial part of the midgut. The importance of such a distinction lies with the presence of a ventral mesoduodenum (continuous cranially with the ventral mesogastrium), which is attached only to the foregut portion, and the derivation of the pancreas and liver, which from their origin are foregut structures.

Posteriorly the duodenum has a thick *dorsal mesoduodenum* which is continuous with the dorsal mesogastrium cranially and the dorsal mesentery of the midgut caudally. Anteriorly the extreme caudal edge of the ventral mesentery of the foregut extends onto the short initial segment of the duodenum. The liver arises as a diverticulum from the ventral surface of the duodenum at the foregut–midgut junction, i.e. initially where the midgut is continuous with the yolk sac wall (i.e. the cranial intestinal portal); the ventral pancreatic bud also arises from this diverticulum. The dorsal pancreatic bud evaginates posteriorly into the dorsal mesoduodenum slightly more cranially than the hepatic diverticulum. The 'rotations', differential growth, and cavitations related to the stomach and omenta cause corresponding movements in the duodenum which forms a duodenal loop directed to the right, with its original right side now adjacent to the posterior abdominal wall. This shift is compounded by the migration of the bile duct and ventral pancreatic duct around the duodenal wall; their origin shifts until it is found in the medial wall of the second part of the fully formed duodenum; the bile duct passes posteriorly to the duodenum and travels in the free edge of the ventral duodenum and ventral mesogastrium. Local adherence and then absorption of part of the duodenal serosa and the parietal peritoneum results in almost the whole of the duodenum becoming retroperitoneal apart from a short initial segment.

Dorsal and ventral mesenteries of the foregut

It is important to realize that the epithelium of the stomach and duodenum does not rotate relative to its investing mesenchyme. The rotation *includes* the coelomic epithelial walls of the pericardio-peritoneal canals, which are each side of the stomach and duodenum forming its serosa, and the elongating dorsal mesogastrium or much shorter dorsal mesoduodenum. A *ventral mesogastrium* can be seen when the distance between the stomach and liver increases. Whereas the *dorsal mesogastrium* takes origin from the posterior body wall in the midline, its connection to the greater curvature of the stomach, which lengthens as the stomach grows, becomes directed to the left as the stomach undergoes its first rotation. With the second rotation a portion of the dorsal mesogastrium now faces caudally. The ventral mesogastrium remains as a double layer of coelomic epithelium enclosing mesenchyme; this forms the *lesser omentum* (3.79; see below). Associated with the movement of the stomach is an extensive lengthening of the dorsal mesogastrium which becomes the *greater omentum*. This now, from its posterior origin, droops caudally over the small intestine then folds back anteriorly and ascends to the greater curvature of the stomach. Thus the greater omentum is composed of a fold containing, technically, four layers of peritoneum. The dorsal mesoduodenum is a much thicker structure; it fixes the position of the duodenum when the rest of the midgut and its dorsal mesentery elongate and pass into the umbilical cord. For a more detailed account of this process see page 197.

SPECIAL GLANDS OF THE POSTPHARYNGEAL FOREGUT

Pancreas

The pancreas develops from *two* evaginations of the foregut which fuse to form a single organ. A *dorsal pancreatic bud* can be seen in stage 13 embryos as a thickening of the endodermal tube which proliferates into the dorsal mesogastrium (3.77). A *ventral pancreatic bud* evaginates in close proximity to the liver primordium and cannot be clearly identified until stage 14 when it appears as an evagination of the bile duct itself. At stage 16 (5 weeks) differential growth of the wall of the duodenum results in movement of the ventral pancreatic bud and the bile duct to the right side and ultimately to a dorsal position. It is not clear whether there is a corresponding shift of mesenchyme during this rotation; however, the ventral pancreatic bud and the bile duct rotate from a position within the ventral mesogastrium (ventral mesoduodenum) to one in the dorsal mesogastrium (dorsal mesoduodenum) which is destined to become fixed onto the posterior abdominal wall. By stage 17 the ventral and dorsal pancreatic buds have fused, although the origin of the ventral bud from the bile duct is still clear. The developing pancreatic ducts usually fuse in such a way that most of the dorsal duct drains into the proximal part of the ventral duct (3.77). The proximal portion of the dorsal duct usually persists as an accessory duct. The fusion of the ducts takes place late in development or in the postnatal period: 85% of infants have patent accessory ducts as compared to 40% of adults. Fusion may not occur in 10% of individuals; here separate drainage into the duodenum is maintained (Githens 1989). Thus part of the head, the neck, body and tail of the pancreas derive from the dorsal pancreatic bud and the remainder of the head and

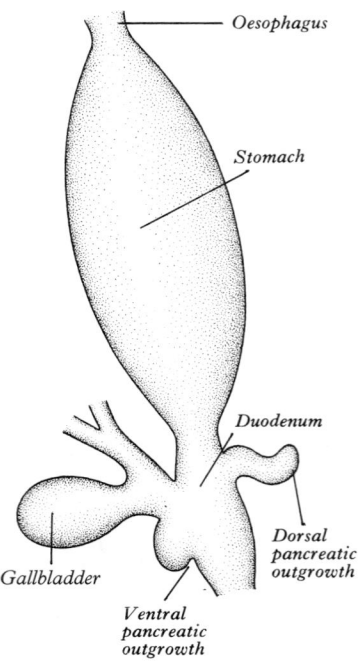

3.77A Diagram of an early stage in the development of the pancreas in a human embryo, 7.5 mm long; lateral view. (After Streeter.)

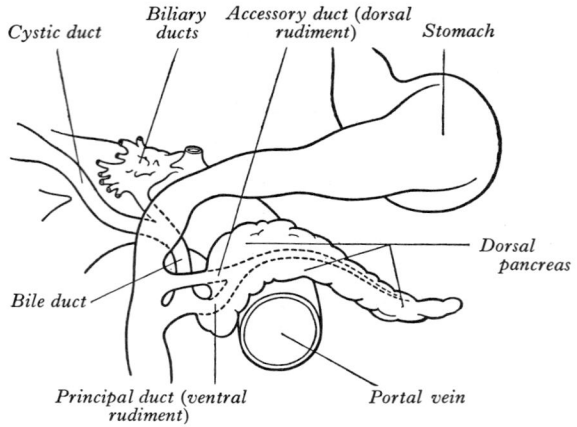

3.77B A later stage in the development of the pancreas in a human embryo, 14.5 mm long; ventral view. (After Streeter.)

uncinate process from the ventral bud. During the shift of the ventral bud the superior mesenteric vessels which are extending from the abdominal aorta become trapped between the head and uncinate process of the pancreas. Initially the body of the pancreas extends into the dorsal mesoduodenum and then cranially into the dorsal mesogastrium. As the stomach rotates, this portion of the dorsal mesogastrium is directed to the left forming the posterior wall of the lesser sac. The posterior layer of this portion of dorsal mesogastrium fuses with the parietal layer of the coelom wall (peritoneum) and the pancreas becomes mainly retroperitoneal. The region of fusion of the dorsal mesogastrium does not extend so far left as to include the tail of the pancreas which passes into the lienorenal ligament. The anterior border of the pancreas later provides the main line of attachment for the posterior leaves of the greater omentum.

The evaginations of pancreatic endoderm into the investing mesenchyme become tubular structures which branch progressively. The primitive duct epithelium provides the stem cell population for all the secretory cells of the pancreas. It gives rise to α cells which produce glucagon, β cells which produce insulin, and δ cells which produce somatostatin during weeks 8–10. Cells containing pancreatic polypeptide (PP) appear somewhat later. Initially these endocrine cells are located in the duct walls or in buds developing from them; later they accumulate in pancreatic islets. The dorsal bud gives rise to mostly α cells and the ventral bud to most of the PP cells. β cells develop from the duct epithelium throughout development and into the neonatal period. Later, in weeks 10–15, some of the primitive ducts differentiate into acinar cells. Zymogen granules or acinar cell markers can be detected at 12–16 weeks. The remaining primitive duct cells will differentiate into definitive ductal cells. In the fetus they develop microvilli and cilia but lack the lateral interdigitations seen in the adult. Branches of the main duct become interlobular ductules which terminate as blind ending acini or as tubular, acinar elements. The connective tissue between the ducts develops from the investing mesenchyme which, in the fetus, appears to be important in stimulating pancreatic proliferation and maintaining the relative proportions of acinar, α and β cells during development.

Liver

The liver is one of the most precocious embryonic organs; it functions as the main centre for haemopoiesis in the fetus. It develops from an endodermal evagination of the foregut and from the septum transversum mesenchyme, a region of unsplit lateral plate mesenchyme in the early embryo which receives mesenchyme cells from the proliferating coelomic epithelium in the protocardiac region. The development of the liver is intimately related to the development of the heart as the vitelline, followed by the umbilical, veins passing to the sinus venosus are disrupted by the septum transversum to form a hepatic plexus the forerunner of the hepatic sinusoids.

The developing liver can first be seen in the stage 11 embryo; the proliferation and bulging of the hepatic diverticulum stimulates the production of blood islands in the investing mesenchyme (**3.78**). By stage 12 the diverticulum has two parts: a caudal part, which will produce the cystic duct and gallbladder, and a cranial part which forms the liver biliary system (see also pancreatic anlage p. 186).

Around the cranial portion of the hepatic diverticulum the basal lamina disrupts progressively and individual epithelial cells migrate into the surrounding septum transversum mesenchyme (**3.79**). The previously smooth contour of the diverticulum merges into columnar extensions of endoderm, the so-called epithelial trabeculae, which stimulate the mesenchymal cells to form blood islands and endothelium. The advance of the endodermal epithelial cells promotes the conversion of more and more septum transversum mesenchyme into endothelium and blood cells with only a little remaining to form the scanty (human) liver capsule and interlobular connective tissue. This invasion by the hepatic epithelium is completed in stage 13 when it approaches the caudal surface of the pericardial cavity, with only a thin lamina of mesenchyme intervening which will give rise to part of the diaphragm.

During this early phase of development the liver is far more highly vascularized than the rest of the gut. The hepatic capillary plexus is connected bilaterally with the right and left vitelline veins and dorsolaterally they empty by multiple channels into enlarged hepatocardiac channels, which lead to the right and left horns of the sinus venosus; usually the channel on the right side is most developed. Both left and right channels bulge into the pericardio-peritoneal canals forming sites for the exchange of fluid from the coelom into the vascular channels (O'Rahilly & Muller 1986). The growth of the hepatic tissue in these regions is sometimes referred to as the left and right horns of the liver.

The liver remains proportionately large during its development forming a sizeable organ dorsal to the heart at stage 14, then more caudally placed by stage 16. By this stage hepatic ducts can be seen separating the hepatic epithelium from the extrahepatic biliary system, but even at stage 17 the ducts do not penetrate far into the liver. Later the lines of endodermal epithelial cells in continuity with the hepatic ducts differentiate into ductal cells following the developmental sequence of connective tissue differentiation around the portal vein and its branches.

The bile duct, which first has origin from the ventral wall of the foregut (now duodenum), migrates with the ventral pancreatic bud first to the right and then dorsomedially into the dorsal mesoduodenum.

As the liver enlarges, it projects more and more into the abdominal cavity. The medial coelomic epithelial walls around the liver constitute much of the ventral mesogastrium (but see below). The mesenchyme between these layers is in continuity with the septum transversum mesenchyme of the diaphragm superiorly. The coelomic epithelial layers of the ventral mesogastrium can almost approximate both anterior and posterior to the liver (a slender lamina of mesenchyme intervening), where they form the falciform ligament and the lesser omentum respectively; they form the visceral peritoneum where they are in contact with the liver. Cranially the liver remains in mesenchymal contact with the diaphragm and the epithelial leaves of the ventral mesogastrium are reflected onto the inferior surface of the diaphragm as the coronary and right and left triangular ligaments. (Strictly, the lesser omentum, in and near its free border, also includes the less extensive ventral mesoduodenum.) It is worth noting that as the ventral body wall develops, the falciform ligament, which attaches to the ventral body wall at the cranial intestinal portal, is drawn to the diminishing cranial rim of the umbilicus. Here it becomes increasingly oblique, curved and indeed 'falciform'. Whereas in the early embryo the connection between one pericardio-peritoneal canal and the other was directly across the ventral surface of the cranial midgut, immediately caudal to the developing primitive ventral mesogastrium, by stage 14 the passage from one side of the falciform ligament to the other necessitates passing below the greatly enlarged liver, or the curved lower edge of the falciform ligament, or lesser omentum. At 3 months the liver almost fills the abdominal cavity and its left lobe is nearly as large as its right. Later when the haematopoietic activity of the liver is assumed by the spleen and bone marrow the relative development of the liver changes and the left lobe actually undergoes some degeneration and becomes smaller than the right. The dominance of the right lobe is reflected in the large expanse of the coronary and right triangular ligaments, compared with the diminutive left triangular ligament (and their respective bare areas). Until birth the liver remains relatively larger than in the adult.

Experimental studies on the epithelial/mesenchymal interactions of liver development have demonstrated the specificity of the cell populations involved (Le Douarin 1975). They may be summarized as follows:

- Liver mesenchyme forms the endothelial cells of the liver and the endoderm forms the hepatocytes. If a mechanical barrier is inserted across the mesenchymal hepatic area just caudal to the endodermal outgrowth, liver tissue will develop normally cranial to the barrier where it is in contact with the endoderm; however, caudal to the barrier the mesenchyme will form endothelial cells and hepatic lobes, but there will be no hepatocytes present.
- Hepatic endoderm cells are incapable of differentiating into hepatocytes without hepatic mesenchyme. Cephalic and somitic mesenchyme is unable to promote differentiation of hepatic endoderm.
- Presumptive intestinal endoderm cells combined with hepatic mesenchyme do not produce hepatocytes.
- All derivatives of the lateral plate mesenchyme, both somatopleuric and splanchnopleuric mesenchyme, can promote the differentiation of hepatic endoderm, although not so strongly as hepatic mes-

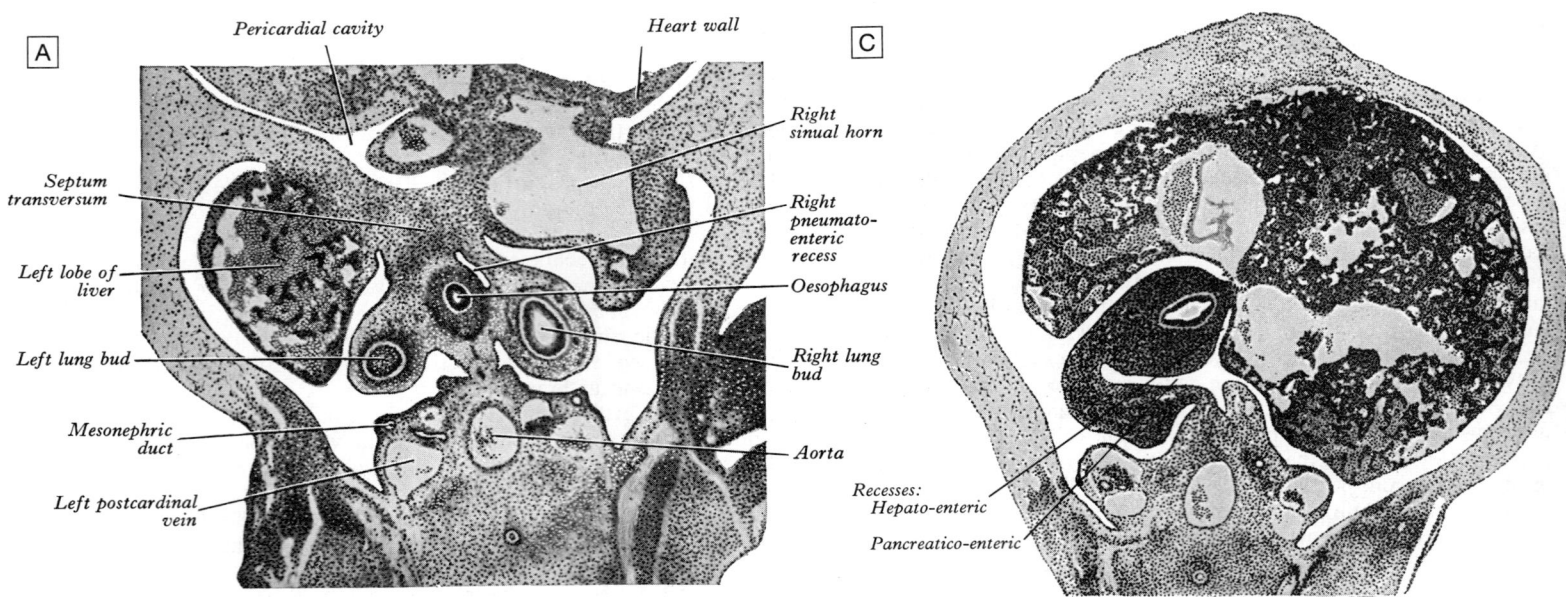

3.78A Transverse section of a human embryo, 8 mm long, showing the right pneumato-enteric recess.

3.78C Transverse section through the same embryo as **3**.187B, but 150 μm more caudally. Compare with the preceding figure and observe that the omental bursa (pancreatico-enteric recess) communicates with the general peritoneal cavity at this level.

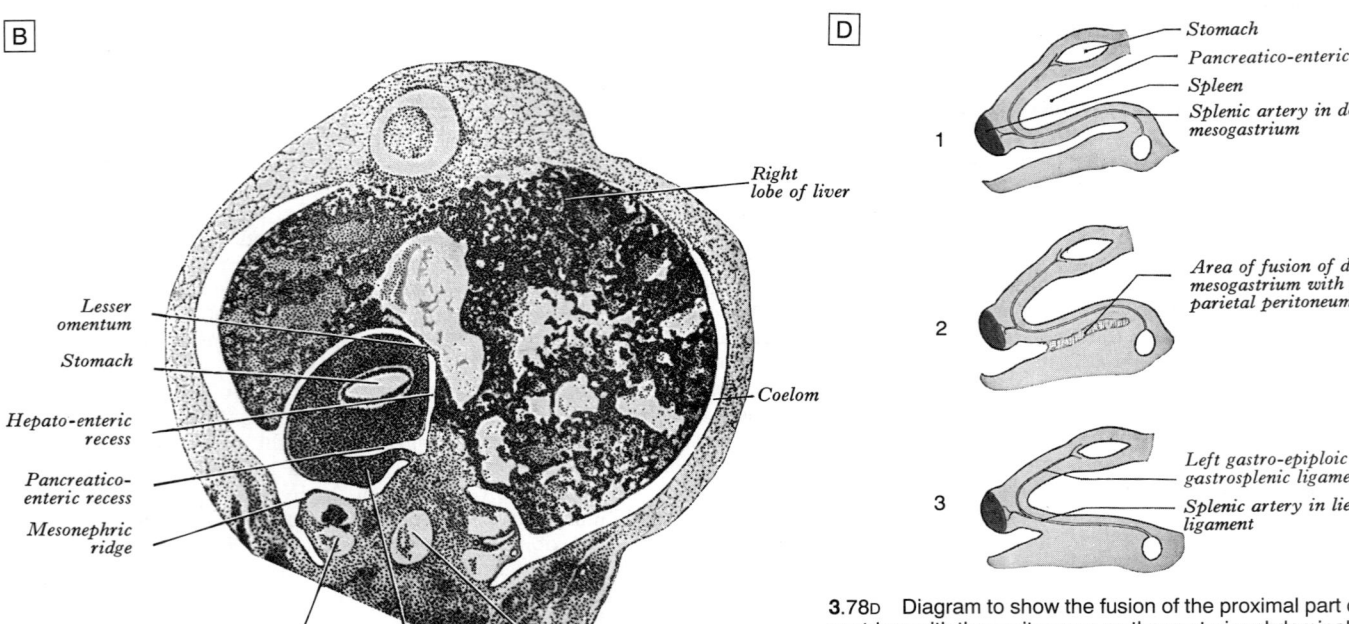

3.78B Transverse section through the same embryo as **3**.187A but 530 μm more caudally. Note that rotation of the stomach has taken place and that the sinusoidal spaces in the liver communicate freely with one another.

3.78D Diagram to show the fusion of the proximal part of the dorsal mesogastrium with the peritoneum on the posterior abdominal wall. Note also the conversion of the dorsal mesogastrium into the gastrosplenic and lienorenal ligaments. 1. represents a transverse section of an embryo in which the dorsal mesogastrium is still at the stage shown in A. 2. and 3. represent transverse sections of older embryos made at the same level (simplified, however, by retaining the shape and size of the stomach and spleen).

enchyme. Lateral plate mesenchyme will form blood sinusoids under these conditions.

It is inferred that matrix or cell surface properties are common throughout the lateral plate mesenchyme but are different from axial mesenchymal cells. Le Douarin (1975) suggests that the morphogenesis of the liver lobes are patterned by the septum transversum mesenchyme.

MIDGUT

The midgut forms the third and fourth parts of the duodenum, jejunum, ileum and two-thirds the way along the transverse colon; thus its development results in most of the small and a portion of the large intestine. In embryos of stages 10 and 11 it extends from the cranial to the caudal intestinal portals and communicates directly with the yolk sac over its entire length. Although it has a dorsal wall, at these stages the lateral walls have not yet formed. By stage 12 the connection with the yolk sac has narrowed such that the midgut has ventral walls cranially and caudally; this connection is reduced to a yolk stalk containing the vitello-intestinal duct during stage 13, at which time the yolk sac appears as a sphere in front of the embryo. Posterior to the midgut the splanchnopleuric coelomic epithelia converge forming the dorsal mesentery; ventrolaterally

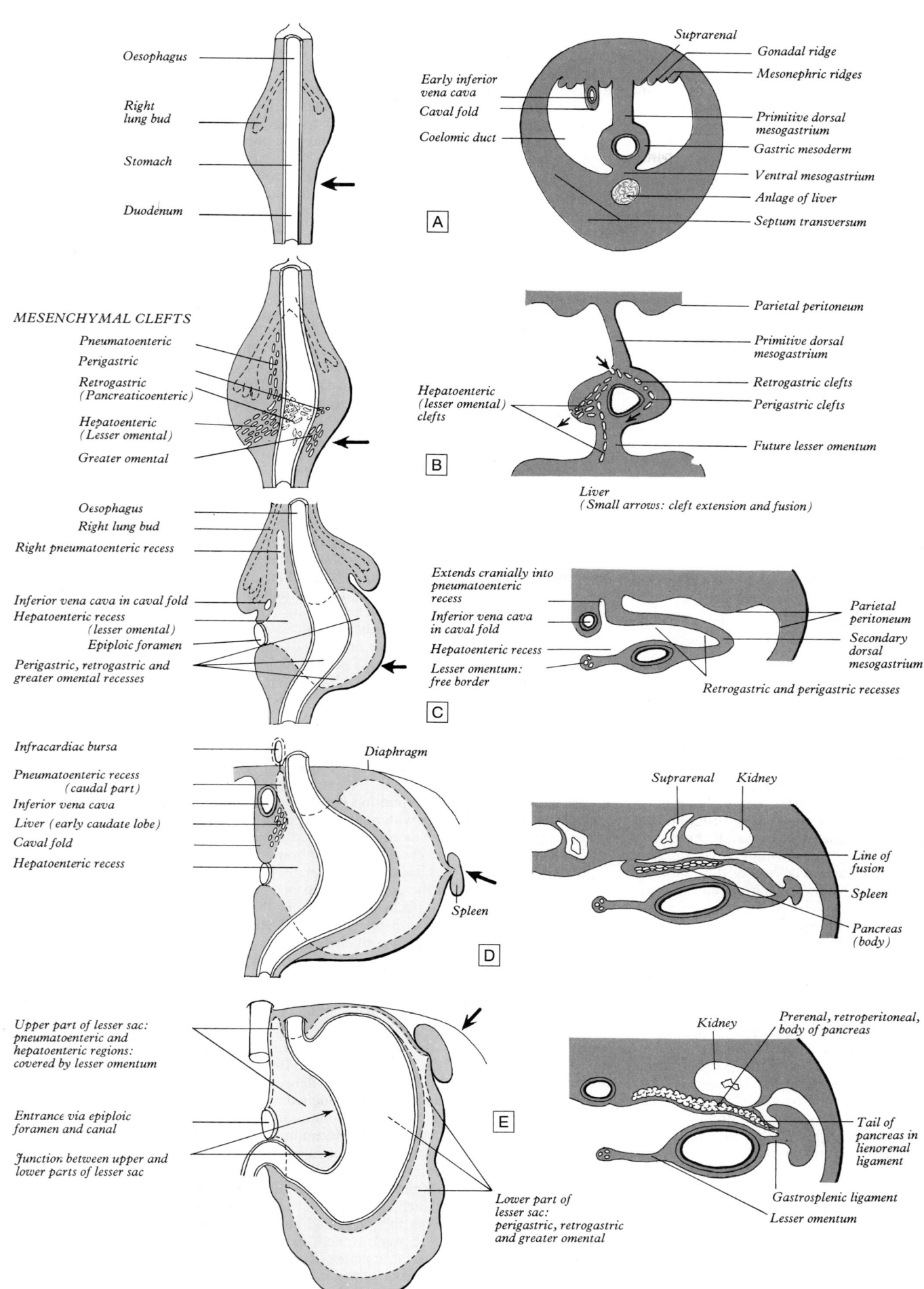

3.79 Development of the subdiaphragmatic foregut, its associated visceral and somatovisceral mesoderm and coelom, with particular reference to the terminal oesophagus, stomach, duodenum, spleen, the lesser sac of peritoneum and omenta: seen in semicoronal section (left column) and transverse section at the levels indicated (right column). This differs in some important respects from traditional accounts. The text furnishes further definitions, details and discussions.

the intraembryonic coelom is in wide communication with the extraembryonic coelom. At stage 14 the midgut has increased in length more than the axial length of the embryonic body and, with elongation of the dorsal mesentery, it bulges ventrally, deviating from the median plane.

Umbilical cord

The formation of the lateral body walls brings the zone of connection of ectoderm and amnion to the ventral part of the body. The embryo undergoes a rotation within the chorion so that it now has its ventral surface opposite the placenta. Amnion now covers the connecting stalk with its umbilical vessels and the elongating yolk stalk, thus limiting the previously wide connection of the intra- and extra-embryonic coeloms to a much narrower channel, an umbilica coelom, around the vitello-intestinal duct within the base of the forming umbilical cord.

The yolk stalk consists of:

- a central endodermal yolk duct
- a covering of splanchnopleuric extraembryonic mesenchyme (vitelline), which carries the vitelline arteries and veins
- a covering of splanchnopleuric coelomic epithelium.

The connecting stalk consists of:

- a central endodermal allanto-enteric duct (diverticulum)
- a covering of splanchnopleuric extraembryonic mesenchyme, conveying the umbilical (allantoic) vessels to and from the chorion
- a covering of splanchnopleuric coelomic epithelium.

Both the yolk stalk and the connecting stalk are enclosed by, from within and out:

- the somatopleuric coelomic epithelium
- the somatopleuric extraembryonic mesenchyme of the amnion
- the amniotic epithelial cells.

The mesenchymes of all three groups will fuse (see below), except in the embryonic base of the umbilical cord where it persists as the umbilical coelom. For more information on the umbilical cord see page 158.

Primary intestinal (or midgut) loop. This is present at stage 15 when a bulge, the *caecal bud*, can be discerned on the lower limb of the loop, caudal to the yolk stalk, which arises from the apex or summit of the loop (3.76). Later, the original proximal limb of the loop moves to the right and the distal limb to the left. Interestingly the longest portion of the dorsal mesentery is at the level of the yolk stalk; less relative lengthening occurs near the caudal end of the duodenum or the cranial half of the colon. The midgut extends into the umbilical coelom having already rotated through an angle of 90°, anticlockwise viewed from the ventral aspect. This relative position is roughly maintained so long as the protrusion persists, during which time the proximal limb which forms the small intestine elongates greatly, becoming coiled, and with its adjacent mesentery adopting a pleated appearance. The origin of the root of the mesentery is initially both median and vertical while at its intestinal attachment it is elongated (like a ruffle) and folded along a horizontal zone. The mesenteric sheet has spiralled with its contained vessels through 90°. The distal, colic, part of the loop elongates less rapidly and has no tendency to become coiled. By the time the fetus has attained a length of 40 mm (10 weeks), the peritoneal cavity has enlarged and the relative size of the liver and mesonephros is much less. The re-entry of the gut occurs rapidly and in a particular sequence during which it continues the process of *rotation*. The proximal loop returns first, with the jejunum mainly on the left and the ileum mainly on the right of the subhepatic abdominal cavity. Both coils of jejunum and ileum, however, as they re-enter the abdominal cavity slide inwards over the right aspect of the descending mesocolon, thus displacing the descending colon to the left and the transverse colon passes superiorly to the origin of the root of the mesentery. The caecum is the last to re-enter and at first lies on coils of ileum on the right. Later development of the colon leads to its elongation and to establishment of the hepatic and splenic flexures.

During the period when the midgut loop protrudes into the umbilical coelom the edges of the ventral body wall are becoming relatively closer, forming a more discrete root for the umbilical cord. Somatic mesenchyme, which will form the ventral body wall

musculature, migrates into the somatopleuric mesenchyme and passes ventrally toward the midline (see p. 270). When the midgut loop is abruptly returned to the abdominal cavity the more recognizable umbilical cord forms (see previously). The vitello-intestinal duct and vessels involute, the cranial end of the allantois becomes thinned and its lumen partially obliterated; it forms the urachus. The mesenchymal core of the umbilical cord is derived by coalescence from somatopleuric amniotic mesenchyme, splanchnopleuric vitello-intestinal (yolk sac) mesenchyme, and splanchnopleuric allantoic (connecting stalk) mesenchyme. These various layers become fused and are gradually transformed into the viscid, mucoid connective tissue (Wharton's jelly) which characterizes the more mature cord. The changes in the circulatory system result in a large cranially oriented left umbilical vein, the right umbilical vein regressing, and two spirally disposed umbilical arteries.

Mucosal development. The exact timing of the cellular morphogenesis of the gut is difficult to establish, especially as the gut undergoes a proximodistal gradient in maturation; developmental differences between parts of the small intestine or colon have not yet been correlated with age. The endodermal cells of the small intestine proliferate forming a layer some three to four cells thick with mitotic figures throughout. From 7 weeks (according to some accounts) blunt projections of the endoderm have begun to form in the duodenum and proximal jejunum; these are the developing villi which increase in length until in the duodenum the lumen becomes difficult to discern. The concept of occlusion of the lumen and recanalization which is described in many accounts of development does not match with the cytodifferentiation occurring in the gut epithelia. By 9 weeks the duodenum, jejunum and proximal ileum have villi and the remaining distal portion of ileum develops villi by 11 weeks. The villi are covered by a simple epithelium. Primitive crypts, epithelial downgrowths into the mesenchyme between the villi, appear between 10 and 12 weeks similarly along a craniocaudal progression. The morphological appearance of the small intestine is similar to the adult's by 16 weeks.

Whereas mitotic figures are initially seen throughout the endodermal layer of the small intestine prior to villus formation, by 10 to 12 weeks they are limited to the intervillous regions and the developing crypts. It is believed that the adult-like turnover of cells may exist when rounded-up cells can be observed at the villus tips, in position for exfoliation. The epithelial cells show an appropriate differentiation before 9 weeks when the absorptive enterocytes have microvilli at their apical borders. An apical tubular system appears at this time composed of deep invaginations of the apical plasma membrane and membrane-bound vesicles and tubules; there is also the appearance of many lysosomal elements (meconium corpuscles) in the apical cytoplasm. These latter features are more developed in the ileum than jejunum; they are most abundant at 16 weeks and diminish by 21 weeks. There are abundant deposits of glycogen in the fetal epithelial cells; it is suggested that prior to the appearance of hepatic glycogen the intestinal epithelium serves as a major glycogen store (Menard 1989). Goblet cells are present in small numbers by 8 weeks, Paneth cells differentiate at the base of the crypts in weeks 11 and 12 and enteroendocrine cells appear between weeks 9 and 11.

Meconium can be detected in the lumen of the intestine by the 16th week. It is derived from swallowed amniotic fluid which contains vernix and cellular debris, salivary, biliary, pancreatic and intestinal secretions and sloughed enterocytes. As the mixture passes along the gut, water and solutes are removed and cellular debris and proteins concentrated. Meconium contains enzymes from the pancreas and proximal intestine in higher concentrations in preterm than full-term babies (Koldovsky 1989).

Muscularis layer of the small intestine. This is derived from the splanchnopleuric mesenchyme as in other parts of the gut. At 26–30 weeks the gut shows contractions without regular periodicity; from 30–33 weeks repetitive groups of regular contractions were seen in preterm neonates (Ruckebusch 1989).

Serosa of the midgut. Possessing a dorsal mesentery alone, the movement of the root of this dorsal mesentery and the massive lengthening of its enteric border to match the longitudinal growth of the gut tube reflects the spiralizing of the midgut loop in the umbilical coelom. Specific regions of adherence of the serosa and parietal peritoneum result in the final disposition of parts of the small and large intestine in the peritoneal cavity. For an account of this see page 192.

PRIMITIVE HINDGUT

Just as the foregut has an extensive, ventral endodermal diverticulum which contributes to a system separate from the gut, so too the hindgut has a ventral diverticulum, the *allantois*, fated for a different system. However, unlike the respiratory diverticulum of the foregut the allantois is formed very early in development, prior even to formation of the embryonic endoderm and tail folding. With the reorganization of the caudal region of the embryo at stage 10, part of the allantois is drawn into the body cavity. The early embryonic hindgut thus consists of a dorsal tubular region extending from the caudal intestinal portal to the cloacal membrane, and a ventral blind-ending allantois extending from the cloacal region into the connecting stalk. The slightly dilated cavity, lined by endoderm, that cranially receives the enteric hindgut proper and the root of the allanto-enteric diverticulum is termed the *endodermal cloaca*. It is closed ventrally by the cloacal membrane (endoderm opposed to proctodeal ectoderm); it also has, transiently, a small recess of endoderm in the root of the tail, the *postanal gut*. As elsewhere, the hindgut, allantois and endodermal cloaca are encased in splanchnopleuric mesenchyme. Proliferation of the mesenchyme and endoderm in the angle of junction of hindgut and allantois produces a *urorectal septum*. Continued proliferation of the urorectal septum and elongation of the endodermal structures thrusts the endodermal epithelium towards the cloacal membrane with which it fuses centrally, separating the presumptive rectum and upper anal canal (dorsally) from the presumptive urinary bladder and urogenital sinus (ventrally) (**3.86**A–E). The cloacal membrane is thus divided into *anal* (dorsal) and *urogenital* (ventral) *membranes*. The nodal centre of division is the site of the future *perineal body*, the functional centre of the perineum.

DEVELOPMENT OF THE ENTERIC HINDGUT

The development of the large intestine, whether derived from mid- or hindgut seems to be similar. The proximal end of the colon can be first identified at stage 15 when an enlargement of a local portion of gut on the caudal limb of the midgut loop defines the developing *caecum*. An evagination of the distal portion of the caecum forms the *vermiform appendix* at stage 17. Apart from the embryonic studies of Streeter (1942 et seq) there is little information about the development of the large intestine in humans. A classic study by Johnson (1913) has not yet been superseded. The early endodermal lining of the colon appears stratified, with mitoses occurring throughout the layers. A series of longitudinal folds arise initially at the rectum and caecum and later in the regions of colon between these two points. The folds segment into villi with new villi forming between them while the developing mucosa invaginates into the underlying mesenchyme between the villi to form glands which increase in number by splitting longitudinally from the base upwards. The villous nature of the developing human colon has been confirmed (Bell & Williams 1982); the villi gradually diminish in size and are absent by the time of birth.

The similarity of development of the small and large intestines is further mirrored in the cytological differentiation. Fetal gut from 11 weeks shows dipeptidase activity in the colon as well as in the small intestine (Potter 1989). Throughout preterm development *meconium corpuscles* are seen in the colon as in the small intestine; they are believed to be the phagocytosed remains of neighbouring cells which have died as a result of programmed cell death.

There is little direct evidence of colonic function in the human fetus and neonate; however, the specific results of mammalian studies are being correlated to human studies where possible (Potter 1989). A number of distinct and important differences between the function of adult and fetal colon have been reported. The absorption of glucose and amino acids does not take place through the colonic mucosa in adult life; however, there is evidence of direct absorption of these nutrients during development. At birth the normal cycle of bile acids is not mature. In the adult, bile is secreted by the liver, stored in the gallbladder then secreted into the intestine where it is absorbed by the jejunum and ileum. In the fetus and neonate, the

transport of bile acids from the ileum by an active process does not occur, allowing bile salts to pass on into the colon. In the adult the presence of bile salts in the colon stimulates the secretion of water and electrolytes resulting in diarrhoeal syndrome; the fetal and neonatal colon however seems protected from this effect. The colon is not considered a site of significant nutrient absorption in the adult; however, neonates are unable to assimilate the full lactose load of a normal breast feed from the small intestine and a large proportion of it may be absorbed from the colon. Thus it is suggested that the colon fulfils a slightly different role in the preterm and neonatal period, conserving nutrient absorption and minimizing fluid loss until the neonate has adjusted to extrauterine life, oral feeding and the establishment of the symbiotic bacterial flora.

Muscularis layer of the colon. This is present and functioning by the 8th week, when peristaltic waves have been observed. The specific orientation of the longitudinal muscle layer into *taeniae coli* occurs in the 11th to 12th weeks when haustra appear. The enteric nerves are present in Meissner's and Auerbach's plexuses at 8 and 12 weeks respectively, with a craniocaudal migration of the nerves. A normal distribution of ganglion cells has been noted in preterm babies of 24 weeks, although there is a region devoid of ganglia just above the anal valves (Grand et al 1976). The puborectalis muscle appears in 20–30-mm embryos, following opening of the anal membrane.

Mesenchymal proliferation occurs around the rim of the ectodermal aspect of the anal membrane which thus comes to lie at the bottom of a depression, the *proctodeum*. With the absorption and disappearance of the anal membrane the anorectum communicates with the exterior. The lower part of the anal canal is formed from the proctodeal ectoderm and underlying mesenchyme, but its upper part is lined by endoderm. The line of union corresponds with the edges of the anal valves in the adult (p. 1780). In the fourth and fifth weeks a small part of the hindgut, the postanal gut, projects caudally beyond the anal membrane (towards the region of the tail); it usually disappears before the end of the fifth week. The dual origin of the anal canal is reflected by differences in arterial supply, venous and lymphatic drainage, innervation and epithelial specialization (summarized on p. 1782).

Lymphoid tissue in the developing gut

The neonatal gut becomes colonized by a range of bacterial flora, some of which exists in a symbiotic relationship with its host, some of which may be considered pathogenic. The gut therefore has a significant function in the defence of the body which can be seen in the development of the lymphoid tissues of the gut. Individual *lymphocytes* appear in the lamina propria of the gut from about week 12 of development and lymphoid aggregates, *Peyer's patches*, have been noted between 15 and 20 weeks; it is not clear whether these cells migrate in from distant sources or differentiate from the investing mesenchyme. The endodermal epithelium overlying the lymphoid aggregates is often distorted into a dome shape; the cells are a mixed population of enterocytes, endocrine cells, a reduced population of goblet cells and unique absorptive cells termed *M cells* (*membrane or microfold*). These latter cells are specialized to provide a mechanism for the transport of micro-organisms and intact macromolecules across the epithelium to the intraepithelial space and lamina propria where the underlying macrophages and lymphocytes are present. M cells have been observed in the fetus by 17 weeks (Moxey & Trier 1978); it is believed that they are formed by a specialized epithelial/mesenchymal interaction of the endoderm and underlying lymphoid type mesenchyme.

There are similarly specialized epithelial cells *between* the enterocytes. *Intraepithelial leucocytes* account for some 15% of the epithelial cells of the gut in the adult. They have been observed at 11 weeks' development, with a distribution of approximately three intraepithelial leucocytes per 100 gut epithelial cells (Orlic & Lev 1977). They are thought to be T and B lymphocytes. For an account of the very complex development of the immune cells of the gut consult Butzner and Befus (1989).

Innervation of the gut

The gut is innervated by the *enteric nervous system (ENS)* which unlike other components of the PNS, e.g. the automatic nervous system, can mediate reflex activity independently of control by the brain and spinal cord (see p. 235). The number of enteric neurons is very large, in the same order of magnitude as the number of neurons in the spinal cord (Furness & Costa 1980). The source of enteric neurons is from somite levels 1–7 and from 28 onwards. Crest cells invade the gut after migrating ventrally and via the dorsal mesentery. The glia cells associated with the gut have been identified as arising from similar levels; these cells are unlike Schwann cells and more closely resemble astrocytes. The precursors of enteric neurons colonize the bowel fairly rapidly in mammals (Gershon 1987); see also page 234.

DEVELOPMENT OF THE ALLANTOIC HINDGUT

After proliferation and migration of the *urorectal septum*, the cloacal region is divided into a dorsal portion, the putative rectum, and a ventral portion which can be subdivided into three regions:

- a cranial vesico-urethral canal, continuous above with the allantoic duct
- a middle, narrow channel, the pelvic portion
- a caudal, deep, phallic section, closed externally by the urogenital membrane (2.122).

The second and third parts together constitute the *urogenital sinus*. The paired mesonephric ducts, part of the urogenital system, fuse with the posterior wall of the urogenital sinus and become partially absorbed into its wall. They are incorporated over a triangular region with the developing ureters (which arise from the mesonephric ducts) at the two upper angles of the triangle, and the mesonephric ducts at the lower apex. The mesonephric ducts arise from coelomic epithelium derived from the intermediate mesenchyme; this mesonephric epithelium thus contributes to the trigone of the bladder and dorsal wall of the proximal (superior) half of the prostatic urethra, i.e. as far as the opening of the prostatic utricle and ejaculatory ducts (or its female homologue the whole female urethral dorsal wall). The remainder of the vesico-urethral part forms the body of the bladder and urethra; its apex is prolonged to the umbilicus as a narrow canal of variable length in the fibrous urachus.

Urethra

Although an endodermally derived structure, which is involved in a series of epithelial/mesenchymal interactions both with the local mesenchyme and with the ectoderm (in much the same way as the pharyngeal arches and facial primordia), the urethra is usually dealt with within the urogenital system. The same applies for the *prostate gland* and *vagina* (both outgrowths of the lower urogenital sinus or urethra), and the other smaller glandular structures developing around the body orifices. For details of these organs see pages 213–214.

It is worth noting at this stage that an interface between the endoderm and ectoderm occurs not only in the buccal region, but also at the proctodeum and the urethra. Specialized ectoderm/mesenchyme interactions produce folds and ridges that surround the ectoderm/endoderm junctions, which normally break down in utero. Generally epithelium which can be touched easily and has a somatic innervation is derived from ectoderm. In the buccal cavity and pharynx the ectoderm/endoderm zone is towards the posterior third of the tongue; touch here usually elicits the gag reflex, a protective response. In the anal canal the outer portion, distal to the anal valves, is ectodermally derived and somatically innervated; proximal to the valves the epithelium is endodermally derived and autonomically innervated. The urethra in the male is contained in the shaft of the penis with only a short invagination of ectoderm at the distal tip into the glans. In the female however the region of the early urethra remains open to form the vestibule into which the definitive urethra and vagina open. It is believed that these regions are invaded by ectoderm; they are innervated by somatic nerves.

Anomalies of the gut

Duodenal atresia is the most common small bowel obstruction. It occurs commonly because of the presence of a membrane across the lumen although 20% of cases are associated with annular pancreas. The diagnosis of this condition relies on the demonstration of the 'double-bubble sign' on ultrasound, due to the simultaneous distension of the stomach and the first portion of the duodenum.

Bowel atresia usually is not due to a problem with organogenesis but more likely due to a vascular insult during fetal life.

If the midgut loop fails to return to the abdominal cavity at the appropriate time a range of ventral defects can result ranging from minor to major. An *umbilical hernia* occurs when loops of gut protrude into a widened umbilical cord at term. The degree of protuberance may increase if the infant cries, raising the intra-abdominal pressure; however, these herniae resolve usually without treatment. *Omphalocoele* is a ventral wall defect with midline herniation of the intra-abdominal contents into the base of the umbilical cord. Herniated viscera are covered by the peritoneum internally and amnion externally. Omphalocoele range in size from a large umbilical hernia to a very large mass containing most of the visceral organs. *Gastroschisis* is a para-umbilical defect of the anterior abdominal wall associated with evisceration of the abdominal organs. The organs are not enclosed in membranes. Gastroschisis is thought to result from peri-umbilical ischaemia caused by vascular compromise of either the umbilical vein or arteries. Gastroschisis can be detected by prenatal ultrasonography (see p. 341).

Bladder and cloacal exstrophies are considered with development of the urogenital systems.

Imperforate anus is a term used to describe many different anorectal malformations. Minor anomalies are easily treated with an excellent prognosis; however, other defects are often associated with important anatomical deficiencies. The principal concern in all cases is the degree of bowel control, urinary control and in some cases sexual function which is compromised by the condition.

DEVELOPMENT OF THE BODY CAVITIES

PERITONEUM AND OMENTAL BURSA

Students addressing themselves de novo to topographical descriptions of the mature peritoneal cavity with its complex parietes, 'sessile' (or retroperitoneal) organs, peritonealized organs with their mesenteries (termed ligaments, folds or omenta in different locations), mesenteric contents and lines of reflexion and recesses, fossae, 'gutters', spaces and bursae, face a formidable task. Comprehension is often lacking, and much of what is merely rote retention quickly recedes. Preliminary study of a concise account of the development of an organ and its surroundings, or a survey of the whole region, is valuable; thus frequent cross reference should be made between any field of study of a mature organ, and its ontogeny.

The emergence of an embryonic disc and proliferation and spreading of intraembryonic mesoblast in the progressively pear-shaped, bilaterally symmetric, trilaminar embryo has been described (p. 142). The initial appearance of a median, rostrocaudally disposed protocardiac area, buccopharyngeal membrane, notochord, Hensen's node and primitive streak, is accompanied throughout the length of the notochord by laterally placed paraxial mesenchyme and lateral plate mesenchyme (the intermediate mesenchyme develops somewhat later). The embryonic plate is, at the disc margins, ringed by a band of extraembryonic mesoblast where somatopleure (amnion) and splanchnopleure are confluent; with growth, the band meets and fuses with the spreading lateral plate. The fusion of these three populations of mesoblast occurs at the *junctional zone*; the latter completely encircles the early embryonic plate periphery, but beyond the cranial tip of the notochord involves rostral streams of mesoblast from the primitive streak which skirt the buccopharyngeal membrane, meet in the protocardiac area and continue into a substantial part of the junctional zone. Caudally, mesoblast streams from the primitive streak, skirts the cloacal membrane and blends with the connecting stalk around its contained allantoic duct (p. 144). Median cavitation in the protocardiac area and its confluence with multiple clefts in each lateral plate forms a horseshoe-shaped *intraembryonic coelom* which is bounded dorsally by somatopleuric coelomic epithelium, ventrally by splanchnopleuric coelomic epithelium, medially by paraxial (later, intermediate) mesenchyme and, initially, rostrolaterally by the junctional zone (see below). Loss of the junctional zone in the caudal half of the embryonic margins establishes communication between intraembryonic and extraembryonic coeloms. Head, tail and lateral folding imposes craniocaudal reversal of the headward and tailward structures, assumption of embryonic form, circumscription of an umbilicus, enfoldment of a splanchnopleuric gut tube and definition of the primary body cavities and coelomic regions. The manner of their separation into definitive pericardial, pleural and peritoneal cavities has been described (see p. 180); particular emphasis is placed on the invasion and splitting of the somatopleure with expansion of the secondary pleural cavities, and submergence of the pericardium. The positional changes and multiple derivations of the diaphragm are discussed in musculoskeletal development (see p. 270). The intraembryonic encompassing of a splanchnopleuric gut tube, its allocation into foregut, midgut and hindgut regions and a summary of their derivatives have been considered (see above). Also the period of extrusion of the midgut loop into the umbilical exocoelom, concomitant differential growth and varying degrees of rotation of almost all parts of the subdiaphragmatic gut, return of the midgut loop, and profound serous membrane modifications are traced (pp. 190 et seq.).

Some repetition is unavoidable but, where apposite, brief summaries are appended to circumvent unacceptable degrees of crossreferencing; in other locations, further details and systematic names are given, when alternative morphogenetic events occur, but are infrequently mentioned in introductory accounts. Only those viscera developed in direct apposition to one of the primary coelomic regions, or a secondary extension of the latter, retain a partial or almost complete visceral serous cover. No coelomic cavitation occurs in the rostral and caudal ends of the embryo, i.e. the cranium, cervical vertebrae, buccal cavity, pharynx and their mural derivatives; similarly, the lower third of the rectum, anal canal, coextensive vagina and lower urinary tract. In all these cases, derived structures are embedded in unsplit *mixed somatovisceral mesenchyme*, often with accessions from the neural crest. (The possible classification of certain groups of **both** craniocervical **and** caudoperineal muscles and their nerves as 'special visceral' should be reviewed.) The cervicothoracic oesophagus is encased in prevertebral, retrotracheal and retrocardiac mesenchyme and develops no true dorsal or ventral mesentery. In the lower thorax the oesophagus inclines ventrally anterior to the descending thoracic aorta; the dorsocaudally sloping midline diaphragm between oesophageal and aortic orifices may be homologized with part of a *dorsal meso-oesophagus*; in the same manner, a ventral midline diaphragmatic strip may be considered a derivative of a *ventral meso-oesophagus*. At superior and intermediate thoracic levels parts of the lateral aspects of the oesophagus come into closer relation to the secondary, mediastinal, *parietal* pleura (p. 181).

The alimentary tube from the diaphragm to the commencement of the rectum possesses, throughout its length, initially, a sagittal dorsal mesentery; its line of continuity with the dorsal parietal peritoneum (i.e. its 'root' or 'line of reflexion') is, evidently, also midline. The abdominal foregut, from the diaphragm to the future hepatopancreatic duodenal papilla, also has a ventral mesentery. The latter extends from the ventrolateral margins of the abdominal oesophagus and, as yet 'unrotated', primitive stomach and proximal duodenum, cranially to the pars diaphragmatica of the septum transversum, anteriorly to the ventral abdominal wall to the level of the cranial rim of the umbilicus; caudally (between umbilicus and duodenum) it presents a crescentic free border. The midgut and hindgut have no ventral mesentery; thus the pleural and supraumbilical peritoneal cavities are initially (and transiently) bilaterally symmetrical above the umbilicus; below, the peritoneal cavity is freely continuous across the midline ventral to the gut.

A few general developmental points may be mentioned. Some organs, for example the lung, despite the extensive pulmonary growth and wide cavitation of a secondary pleural cavity, retain a relatively simple visceroparietal serous membrane disposition. The lung root, with its bronchial, neurovascular and lymphatic radicles is circumscribed by a comma-shaped line of reflexion, the dependent 'tail' or pulmonary ligament accommodating calibre variations in the contained tubes. Other organs with a single dorsal mesentery may undergo changes varying from slight to profound. Thus mesenteric changes are an integral accompaniment of alterations in their visceral contents including differential, sometimes asymmetric growth, regional or progressive degeneration, repositioning such as sequential extrusion, retrusion, rotation, spiralization and relative ascent or descent. The *parietovisceral line of reflexion* of the originally midline dorsal mesentery may become oblique (see the jejuno-ileal mesentery)

or transverse (see transverse mesocolon), angular (see sigmoid mesocolon) or complex and highly curved (see dorsal mesogastrium). In other locations, the events are more pronounced, the dorsal mesentery is lost entirely and the organ becomes 'sessile' or 'retroperitoneal', connective tissue only separating its external (usually posterior) surface from the abdominal parietes or the surface of another organ; the peritoneum is limited to some or all of its (usually) ventral and perhaps ventromedial and also ventrolateral surfaces. The resulting parietovisceral or intervisceral depressions or grooves are called pouches, fossae or gutters in different locations. The term *recess* has two distinct connotations, *embryological* (see below), and in *mature topography* where it denotes a peritonealized, blind-ended channel, extending from a major region of the peritoneal cavity, continuing in a retrovisceral or paravisceral position, and often partly enclosed by one or two vascularized (or avascular) peritoneal folds.

The movements of lines of reflexion, assumption of a retroperitoneal site and other changes, are often held to affect relatively large endodermal 'organs' encased in a **fine** layer of splanchnic mesenchyme which is continued to the parietes by an equally tenuous, but vascularized, mesentery. With growth and also shape and positional changes, part or the whole of the mesentery lies against the parietal peritoneum; their apposed surfaces fuse and are absorbed. Thus the line of reflexion is altered, or the organ becomes retroperitoneal; further, mesenteric neurovascular bundles lie ventral to structures derived primarily from the intermediate mesenchyme. Such mechanisms are significant throughout the subdiaphragmatic gut, but are predominant in the small and large intestine. However, such views fail to recognize the ability of all serous membranes to vary their thickness, lines of reflexion, disposition, 'space' enclosed and their channels of communication, by areal and thickness growth on one aspect combined with cavitation leading to expanding embryonic recess formation on the other. The ventral and dorsal foregut mesenteries are relatively large (composed of mesenchyme sandwiched between two layers of splanchnopleuric coelomic epithelium), compared with the slender endodermal tubes they encase. A complex series of recesses develop in the splanchnopleuric mesenchyme, become confluent, and with foregut rotation, differential growth of stomach, liver, pancreas and spleen, and completion of the diaphragm, the territories of the greater sac and lesser sac (omental bursa) are delimited, and the mesenteric complexes of these organs (omenta and 'ligaments') are defined (see below).

It is convenient to first consider the mesenteries of the small and large intestine after rotation and the principal growth patterns have been achieved and the developing pancreas is becoming retroperitoneal. Most of the duodenal loop encircles the head of the pancreas and is retroperitoneal, the peritoneum covering principally its ventral and convex aspects. Exceptions are a short initial segment of the superior (first) part; this is more completely peritonealized having the attachments of the right margins of the greater and lesser omenta; peritoneum is lacking when there is close apposition of the transverse colon to the descending (second) part, or where the latter is crossed by the root of the transverse mesocolon; also where *the* mesentery crosses the transverse (third) part, and descends across the ascending (fourth) part from its upper extremity at the duodenojejunal flexure. In addition to the main peritoneal relations of the duodenum just mentioned, one or more of up to six different *duodenal recesses* may develop. Their variations in shape and size, their intestinal, mesenteric and vascular relations and, when adequately recorded, their frequencies and disposition of their orifices are given on page 1744, and will not be repeated here.

The succeeding small intestine (jejunum and ileum) from the duodenojejunal flexure to the ileocaecal junction ('valve') undergoes, from a mesenteric standpoint, less modification of its embryonic form than other gut regions. Its early dorsal mesentery (no ventral component is present here, or caudally) is a continuous, single (but structurally bilaminar) sheet, with its parietal attachment—line of reflexion, or 'root'—in the midline. Usually, with development and the mechanisms mentioned above, the attachment of the root becomes an **oblique** narrow band from the left aspect of the second lumbar vertebra to the cranial aspect of the right sacro-iliac joint. Thus, from above downwards, it crosses the ascending and transverse parts of the duodenum, abdominal aorta, inferior vena cava, right psoas major and many structures related to these. For dimensions, contents and other details see pages 1765, 1772. Formal names—mesojejunum, meso-ileum—are seldom used; *the mesentery* is universal.

The caecum and vermiform appendix, as stated, arise as a diverticulum from the *antimesenteric* border of the caudal limb of the midgut loop and thus the caecum possesses no primitive mesocaecum. These regions of the gut undergo long periods of growth, often asymmetrical, and their final positions, dimensions and general topography show much variation (pp. 1774, 1775). The caecum is usually quite mobile with its lateral, medial, ventral, caudal and most of its dorsal surfaces clothed with visceral peritoneum. Peritoneum may be lacking dorsally near its continuation into the ascending colon. This arrangement is, however, usually complicated by the presence of two or three *caecal recesses*, bounded on one or more aspects by *local peritoneal folds* some of which carry vascular pedicles. For further details of the recesses (*superior* and *inferior ileocaecal* and *retrocaecal*) and folds (*lateral* and *medial parietocaecal*, *vascular caecal* and *ileocaecal*) see page 1744. The vermiform appendix is also almost wholly clothed with visceral peritoneum, derived from the diverging layers of its rather diminutive *mesoappendix*. The latter, of triangular profile, carrying the appendicular vessels, lymphatics and nerves, is further detailed on page 1743; it appears as a continuation of 'the' mesentery near its ileocaecal junction. Despite the opening remarks above, therefore, the mesoappendix should perhaps be regarded as a direct derivative of the primitive dorsal mesentery; on this view, a similar status for the vascular fold of the caecum should be considered. With approaching completion of differential growth, rotation and circumabdominal displacement of the colonic gut, until the fourth month, this part of the gut retains its primitive dorsal mesentery (mesocolon) throughout. Its original root is still vertical in the dorsal midline, from which it diverges widely, roughly as an incomplete, flattened pyramid, to reach its colonic border (at the future taenia mesocolica). During the fourth and fifth months substantial areas of the primitive mesocolon adhere to, then fuse with, the parietal peritoneum; thus some colonic segments become sessile while others have a shorter mesocolon with an (often profoundly) altered parietal line of attachment (root). In one series of 100 specimens studied (Treves 1885a, b) the most common arrangement occurred in about 50%; in these a transverse and a sigmoid mesocolon persisted and the sessile state affected the ascending colon, right (hepatic) flexure and the descending colon. In the remainder, either the ascending or descending, or both, colonic segments also retained a mesocolon (varying from a localized 'fold' to a complete mesocolon). When sessile, the ventral, medial and lateral aspects of the ascending or descending colon are clothed with peritoneum, the protrusion of the viscus producing medial and lateral peritoneal *paracolic gutters* on each side. The multiple topographical relationships of these parts of the colon and particularly the dorsal structures, with a mere fibro-areolar separation, are detailed on page 1745. This form of apposition to underlying structures proceeds from the ascending colon to include the right colic (hepatic) flexure, and thence continues antero-inferiorly to the left, thus involving the right-sided initial segment of the transverse colon. The right flexure is in contact with the caudal part of the ventrolateral surface of the right kidney, the colonic peritoneum passes cranially clothing this part of the kidney; sometimes reaching the rim of the right suprarenal. In either event, the peritoneum is next reflected ventrally as the lower layer of the coronary ligament to the dorsum of the right lobe of the liver: this renal peritoneum forms the floor of the *hepatorenal pouch* (of Morison). The pouch, in addition to its topographical relations with colon, kidney, suprarenal and liver, has clinically significant associations with the right lateral paracolic gutter, the epiploic foramen—its boundaries and their many contents—the vestibule of the mature omental bursa, the gallbladder and biliary ducts. (Numerous references are made to all the foregoing in Section 8). The right extremity of the transverse colon, as mentioned, is also sessile, fibro-areolar tissue separating it from the anterior aspect of the descending (second) part of the duodenum and the corresponding aspect of most of the head of the pancreas. The remainder of the transverse colon, up to and including the left (splenic) colic flexure, is almost completely peritonealized by the diverging layers of the *transverse mesocolon*. The root of the latter reaches the neck and whole extent of the anterior border of the body of the pancreas. The long axis of the definitive pancreas lies **obliquely**; also, the splenic

colonic flexure is considerably more rostral than the hepatic flexure; in accord, the root of the mesocolon curves obliquely upwards as it crosses the upper abdomen from right to left. As it expands, the postero-inferior wall of the greater omental part of the bursa omentalis (see below) gradually covers, becoming closely applied to, the transverse mesocolon and its contained colon, finally projecting beyond the latter. Craniocaudal adherence now occurs between the omental wall and the pericolonic and mesocolonic layers. In the mature condition, therefore, a cursory examination suggests that the transverse colon is connected to the posterior abdominal structures by a single mesenteric sheet; close inspection, however, shows this to be a compound structure, quadrilaminar in nature (p. 1743).

The left colic flexure receives much of its peritoneal covering from the left extremity of the transverse mesocolon; it is also often connected to the parietal peritoneum of the diaphragm over the tenth and eleventh ribs by a *phrenicocolic ligament*. The latter sometimes blends with a *presplenic fold* that radiates from the gastrosplenic ligament. The descending colon becomes sessile; it commences over the inferolateral border of the left kidney and first passes almost vertically in the depression between psoas major, quadratus lumborum and the aponeurotic origin of transversus abdominis, to the level of the iliac crest; here it inclines inferomedially crossing iliacus and psoas major to reach the brim of the true pelvis where it continues as the sigmoid colon. The numerous structures intervening between the posterior aspect of the descending colon and its fibromuscular 'bed' are detailed on page 1777. Contrary to often stated (but unsupported) assumptions, it has now been clearly demonstrated (Kanagasuntheram 1957) that the process of fusion and obliteration of both ascending and descending mesocolons commences laterally and progresses medially.

The sigmoid colon is ultimately most variable in its length and disposition, with numerous topographical relationships (p. 1777). It retains its dorsal mesocolon, but the initial midline dorsal attachment of its root is considerably modified in its definitive state. The latter is commonly described as an inverted V which is, however, asymmetric, and, other than the rectal termination of its right limb, lies wholly to the left of the midline. The apex of the V lies ventral to the bifurcation of the left common iliac artery; this separates it from the cranial part of the left sacro-iliac joint. The left limb of the V is shorter than the right and, bearing the inferior left colic (sigmoidal) vessels, is almost horizontal, inclining only slightly cranially as it is traced lateromedially from its origin to the apex. The right limb carries the superior rectal vessels; it is longer than the left and about 45° to the vertical, as it extends from the apex to its midline termination (at the cranial end of the rectum) on the ventral aspect of the third sacral vertebra. For details of the relationships and contents of the sigmoidal mesocolon, also the presence, form and age dependency of its associated *intersigmoid apical recess*, see pages 1743, 1744, 1778.

The rectum continues from the ventral aspect of the third sacral vertebra to its anorectal (perineal) flexure antero-inferior to the tip of the coccyx, the distance, of course, changing with age. All aspects are encased by mesenchyme; the early dorsally placed mass is named, by some authorities, the *dorsal mesorectum*. The latter does not form a true mesentery, however, but with progressive skeletal development it reduces to a woven fibroreolar sheet with patterned variations in thickness and fibre orientation. The sheet is closely applied to the ventral concavity of the sacrum and coccyx, with numerous fibromuscular and neurovascular elements enclosed (p. 1779). Thus, the rectum becomes sessile, visceral peritoneum being restricted to its lateral and ventral surfaces. With the disappearance of the postanal gut by the end of the fifth week, the ventrolateral peritoneum reaches the superior surface of the pelvic floor musculature, and this persists until late in the fourth month. In this period the ventral rectal peritoneum of the male is reflected to cover the posterior surface of the prostate and bladder trigone and associated structures; the female initially receives a reflexion covering almost the whole posterior aspect of the vagina, thence continuing over the uterus. Subsequently, the closely apposed walls of these deep peritoneal pouches fuse over much of their caudal extent, their mesothelia are lost, and the organs have an intervening, bilaminar (surgical separable), fibrous stratum. The latter is the masculine rectovesical fascia and posterior wall of the prostatic sheath; its female homologue is the posterior part of the fibrous envelope of the vagina, that intervenes between its middle two-fourths and the rectum. Thus the proximal third of the rectum has a peritoneal tunic ventrolaterally; the lateral extensions are triangular—deep proximally and tapering to an acute angle when the middle third of the rectum is reached. Thereafter, the middle third has peritoneum restricted to its ventral surface where it forms the posterior wall of the shallower rectovesical or rectovagino-uterine pouch. The remaining rectum and anal canal are subperitoneal.

The many additional peritoneal eminences, ridges, folds, grooves, fossae and pouches that on varying time scales characterize the true pelvis and lower abdomen simply reflect the growth patterns of the subjacent viscera, vessels, some nerves or features of the parietes. They are mentioned either in the following pages, or with the appropriate organ in other sections of this text.

Subdiaphragmatic foregut peritoneum

Subdiaphragmatic foregut peritoneum is complex in its definitive topography and, whilst having relatively simple symmetrical origins, becomes progressively more complicated during development. The latter involves rapidly changing three-dimensional arrays of serosal visceral surfaces, mesenchymal masses and mesenteric sheets. Difficulties are compounded by the (rather surprising) paucity of structural ontogenetic accounts, the obligatory absence of human experimental data, some slackening of surgical interest in topographical minutiae and the adoption of simplified basic instructional courses. Here a few paragraphs offer scant justice to the topic and space limitations permit only brief allusion to the (often 'investigator specific') variations in terminology commonly encountered. Classic investigations, reviews and bibliographies are found in Broman (1904, 1938); these may be contrasted with Kanagasuntheram (1957).

Some features have already been mentioned in other contexts, but will be summarized here to allow addition, deletion, criticism and suggested alternatives to the nomenclature and causal mechanisms invoked. (Throughout these and previous sections, reference should be made to 3.00A–H and 3.00A–E.)

The subdiaphragmatic foregut includes, sequentially, the presumptive short terminal oesophagus, stomach and proximal duodenum (as far as, and including, the hepatopancreatic anlage). These subregions of the foregut initially (3–4 mm CR length) constitute a continuous endodermal tube of roughly uniform calibre (but slightly flattened laterally in the gastric region), encased in a thick stratum of splanchnopleuric mesenchyme. The latter is linked from both its dorsal and ventral aspects with substantial blocks of splanchnopleuric mesenchyme that blend, respectively, with a wide dorsal midline strip of the body wall and diaphragm and the ventrolateral body wall and diaphragm, including the caudal base of the pericardium. Thus, at this early stage, the abdominal foregut with its associated mesenchymal masses comprises a thick sagittal septum, dividing the peritoneal coelom into right and left symmetric halves down to the level of the umbilicus. Until closure (p. 180), each half communicates with a pleural coelom via a small pleuroperitoneal canal. With the appearance of recognizable subregions of the foregut, and of the liver, pancreas and spleen, and the hepatopancreatic duct systems, each undergoes asymmetric differential growth (sometimes interpreted as physical 'rotation' of the whole organ—see below), expansion and relative displacement. Concurrently, the splanchnopleuric mesenchyme that encases each organ forms its muscularis and connective tissue framework. The outer splanchnopleuric coelomic epithelium, where present, forms its visceral peritoneal surfaces (serosa). The mesenchyme between organs (e.g. between stomach and liver, stomach and pancreas, stomach and spleen, spleen and left kidney) and that extending from a viscus to the parietes, increases in area and becomes relatively thinner, while its visceroparietal lines of attachment are altered, as are, necessarily, their topographical planes. These events follow the development of *multiple small clefts* within the thick mesenchyme; their coalescence and secondary opening into the primitive peritoneal cavity rapidly follows and then further expansion of the *developmental recess* so formed. (The sequence of events closely mimics the formation of the primary intraembryonic coelom in the protocardiac area and lateral plate mesenchyme (see p. 148). It is **not**, as commonly described, a simple depression followed by excavation into one of the thick mesenchymal strata from the primary peritoneal cavity. These morphogenetic changes result in a marked asymmetry of the upper abdominal

viscera, their mesenteries and associated subregions of the peritoneal cavity. The latter, although increasingly complex topographically, remains a single cavity with numerous intercommunicating regions, pouches and recesses. (The only small peritoneal sacs to separate completely from the main cavity are the *infracardiac bursa*—see below and p. 1751—and the *tunica vaginalis testis*.)

Human definitive peritoneum

The human definitive peritoneal cavity (there are extreme species specializations), is commonly described as comprising a *lesser sac* and a *greater sac* of peritoneum.

Lesser sac (or *definitive bursa omentalis*). This is compounded of a series of confluent recesses, mainly situated in the left, superior quadrant of the abdomen; however, it extends beyond the boundaries of the quadrant, crossing the median plane about 4 cm to the right and to a quite variable extent ventro-inferiorly. Briefly, it is intimately related to the retroperitoneal organs of the 'stomach bed', the transverse colon and its mesocolon, the postero-inferior surface of the stomach and mesenteries (omenta and ligaments) attached to its greater and lesser curvatures, the spleen and its ligaments, the caudate lobe and process of the liver and the diaphragm. (See below and p. 183 for details, also p. 197 for a discussion of the use of terms 'ligament' and 'omentum' in relation to peritoneal features.) A little above the centre of its right margin, the cavity of the lesser sac connects with that of the greater sac, i.e. the whole remainder of the peritoneal cavity, through a vertical slit, with apposed but easily separable walls, the epiploic foramen (p. 1738).

Greater sac. For practical convenience, this is often allocated into a number of subregions, or 'spaces': all, except two, are peritonealized, and all connect with neighbouring spaces, either by a wide direct or a more circuitous route. (In an overall peritoneal classification, as here, the cavity of the lesser sac and two extraperitoneal spaces are included.) The abdominal peritoneal cavity is (incompletely) divided by the transverse colon and its mesocolon into a *supracolic space* containing the foregut, its derivatives and mesenteries, and an *infracolic space* containing the midgut and hindgut with derivatives and mesenteries, already described. The supracolic space is subdivided into six: right and left *subphrenic*, *subhepatic* and *extraperitoneal* spaces. (The left subhepatic space is a rather inappropriate name for the omental bursa; the right extraperitoneal space is the 'bare area' of the liver; the left extraperitoneal space surrounds the left suprarenal and upper pole of left kidney.) The infracolic space is divided by the mesentery of the small intestine into **right** and **left** moieties, while external to the ascending and descending colon lie the *right* and *left lateral paracolic gutters*. All the latter are more or less directly continuous with the fossae and pouches of the lesser pelvis. (For further details of these various spaces see p. 1745 and throughout the account of the peritoneum in Gastrointestinal system.)

Abdominal foregut

Abdominal foregut and its associated splanchnopleuric mesenchyme has an ontogenetic history too complex to receive more than a brief summary here; also the origin, admixture and final fate of some masses remain uncertain in the absence of experimental data. However, the nomenclature employed is, in some cases, a misleading simplification merely handed on in successive accounts over many decades. Sometimes, unproven mechanisms are held to operate which, on close examination, could not result in the well-known definitive topography. Some additional terms and divergences from current morphogenetic accounts are included.

Early embryonic nomenclature is often confined to the mesenchymal masses lying dorsal and ventral to the foregut. However, the thick mesenchymes surrounding the wall of the gut itself are equally prominent morphogenetically. Although continuous with, they cannot be allocated quantitatively as parts of, the dorsal and ventral masses. It is useful, therefore, to refer to them simply as *oesophageal*, *gastric* and *duodenal splenchnopleuric mesenchymes*. Some of the latter areas are **compound** in the sense that by cavitation and cleavage they may provide part of their thickness as *secondary extensions* of surrounding primary mesenteries with new lines of visceral attachment and areal expansion. These processes also result in modification of parietal lines of reflexion and related peritoneal cavity.

Septum transversum

Septum transversum is the somewhat inappropriate name (but deeply ingrained in embryological literature) denoting all the mesenchyme that extends from the ventral aspect of the caudal foregut to the ventrolateral aspects of the supra-umbilical abdominal and lower thoracic walls; its rostral surfaces reach, and contribute to the caudal 'bases' of the pericardium and secondary pleural cavities; its caudal free surface arches from the duodenum to the cranial rim of the umbilicus. Dorsally it borders the pleuroperitoneal canals, is continuous with the foregut mesenchymes mentioned above, and contributes to the *caval fold* (see below). Some of these features have been encountered elsewhere (e.g. pp. 152, 180) and will only receive a brief summary here. After head fold formation, the most rostral part of the septum transversum has the common sinuatrial chamber of the heart embedded in it, each sinual horn of which receives the transeptal terminals of a vitelline, umbilical and common cardinal vein (for their fate see p. 180). As the pericardial cavity expands and the sinuatrial chamber 'rises' into it, septal mesenchyme follows (*pars pericardialis*) and condenses as the fibroserous diaphragmatic aspect of the pericardium. The intermediate stratum of septal mesenchyme (*pars diaphragmatica*) makes substantial contributions to the framework of the sternocostal parts of the diaphragm (**3.79**). Additional extensions occur into the mesenchymatous bed in which the subhepatic–hepatic–hepatocardiac parts of the inferior vena cava develop (p. 324) and in relation to the expanding liver. Thus the pars diaphragmatica alone truly merits the name septum transversum and even this is both incomplete (until closure of the pleuroperitoneal canals) and also, with expansion of the lungs, secondary pleural cavities, liver and stomach, soon becomes less 'transverse' as it develops a marked convexity towards the thorax. Strong fibrous continuity between the perinodal area of the central tendon of the diaphragm and the overlying fibrous pericardium persists. Midline strips of diaphragm ventral and dorsal to the oesophageal hiatus are held by some to be mesenteric in origin (see below): in the writers' view this merely adds confusion to an already complex terminology. Since this is their normal fate it seems preferable to term these the ventral and dorsal pars diaphragmatica of the oesophageal mesenchyme from the outset.

The remaining subdiapragmatic part of the septum 'transversum', as indicated, is designated the *pars mesenterica* and initially forms a sagitally placed ventral 'mesentery' for the foregut. Although a continuous sheet, thick subregions are recognized: a brief *ventral meso-oesophagus*, continuing into a more extensive *ventral mesogastrium*, the latter merging into a *ventral mesoduodenum* that has a caudal free border. Many (the majority of) accounts ignore these subregions and simply equate all derivatives of the ventral pars mesenterica as those of the ventral meso**gastrium**. Some confusion may occur, however, particularly with respect to the development and definitive courses of the main biliary ducts, hepatic artery, portal vein and attendant lymphatics and nerves, and to the hepatic and gastric serosae and mesenteries. As indicated, the mesenchymal modifications are correlated with the asymmetric growth patterns of the stomach, duodenum and liver (see pp. 183, 186 and below).

Abdominal foregut dorsal splanchnopleuric mesenchyme

Abdominal foregut dorsal splanchnopleuric mesenchyme commences rostrally as an oesophageal *dorsal pars diaphragmatica* which, as indicated, contributes a narrow midline strip extending between the oesophageal hiatus and the aortic orifice. The remainder, the *dorsal pars mesenterica*, again initially forms a midline sagittal dorsal septum of thick mesenchyme; its subregions (corresponding to the ventral ones) and parts of one continuous mesenchymal block are: a brief *dorsal meso-oesophagus*, a more extensive *dorsal mesogastrium* and a *dorsal mesoduodenum*. Their modifications are even more extensive than those of the ventral mesenteries and also have the additional complications of the developing pancreas and spleen. Further, many accounts ignore the subregions and collectively dub them **the** dorsal meso**gastrium**. This may lead to (perhaps minor) misplacement of the anlage of certain organs; however, the siting of the initiation of the lesser sac of peritoneum in the dorsal mesogastrium is both incorrect and confusing.

Caval fold

The caval fold is a linear eminence with divergent rostral and caudal ends that passes from the upper abdominal to the lower thoracic region and protrudes from the dorsal wall of the pleuroperitoneal canal. Cranially it becomes continuous, lateromedially, with the root of the pulmonary anlage and pleural coelom, the pars pericardialis of the septum transversum and the retrocardiac mediastinal mesenchyme. Caudally it forms an arch with *dorsal* and *ventral* horns; the dorsal merges with the primitive dorsal mesentery and the mesonephric ridge (and associated gonad and suprarenal); the ventral horn is confluent with the dorsal surface of the septal mesenchyme. Thus the fold is a zone where intestinal, mesenteric, intermediate, hepatic, pericardial, pulmonary and mediastinal mesenchymes meet and blend, and may justifiably be compared with the junctional zones of mesenchyme described elsewhere (p. 151). Contributions from septal mesenchyme are considered of particular importance by some authorities (Kanagasuntheram 1957). It provides a mesenchymal route for the upper abdominal, transdiaphragmatic and transpericardial parts of the inferior vena cava; it is also prominent in the development of parts of the liver, lesser sac of peritoneum and certain mesenteries. The left fold regresses whereas the right fold enlarges rapidly.

Lesser sac

The lesser sac (*definitive bursa omentalis*) has already been mentioned in terms of its general disposition and communication with the greater sac. Unfortunately considerable variation exists between the terminologies adopted by different authors, both during ontogeny and in adult topography. Development of the lesser sac is so intimately interlocked with additional ontogenetic features, particularly of the liver and stomach, their mesenteries, and secondary extensions of the greater sac, that these must receive brief mention.

Invasion of the ventral pars mesenterica by the hepatic and (transiently) the ventral pancreatic rudiment, followed by trifurcation of the primary hepatic anlage into right and left submasses and a caudal pars cystica, has been described (p. 187). Hepatic growth on the two sides is approximately equal in early fetal months, and the liver mass almost fills the ventral mesenchyme; but thick, short blocks of mesenchyme intervene between the liver and the foregut, diaphragm and supra-umbilical ventral body wall. Removal of the viscera at these symmetric stages reveals the cut edges of the mesothelium bordering the coelom and enclosing the wide areas of mesenchymal continuity. The latter has a large roughly circular central area with numerous tapering projections towards the abdomen: the obliquely cut mesenteries, caval folds, mesonephric and attendant ridges and the lateral rim of the pleuroperitoneal canals. The whole bears some resemblance to an inverted coronet, hence the name coronary ligament of the liver. (With growth and maturity the restricted use of the name is much less apposite.) Much of the mesenchymal mass surrounding the liver develops cavities that coalesce and open into the general coelomic cavity as extensions of the greater (and lesser) sacs of peritoneum. Thus almost all the ventrosuperior, visceral and some of the posterior aspects of the liver become peritonealized. The process involving the greater sac continues over the right lobe and ceases when the future superior and inferior layers of the coronary ligament and the right triangular ligament are defined. Those, plus a medial boundary provided by an extension of the lesser sac, enclose the 'bare area' of the liver where loose areolar tissue of septal origin persists. Due to asymmetric liver growth the same processes affecting the left lobe result in the smaller left triangular ligament. Where the superior layers of the coronary and left triangular ligaments meet they continue as a (bilaminar) ventral mesentery attached to the ventrosuperior aspects of the liver; its parietal attachment has a slight inclination to the right as it crosses the ventral diaphragm and then descends to the umbilicus. Its umbilicohepatic free caudal border, somewhat arched, carries the left umbilical vein (or, postnatally, the fibrous obliterated vein or *ligamentum teres*, with fine calibre para-umbilical veins); the whole structure constitutes the *falciform ligament*. Most of the latter may be considered the final ventral part of the ventral mesogastrium; its free border, however, has a ventral mesoduodenal origin.

As stated, the endodermal subdiaphragmatic foregut of the early embryo is a tube of almost uniform calibre, but with a slight fusiform gastric dilatation with a minimal degree of side-to-side flattening, encased in thick splanchnopleuric mesenchyme and splanchnopleuric coelomic epithelia (mesothelium). The mesenchyme is continuous with the primitive ventral and dorsal mesogastria and these indicate the sagittal positions of the *primitive* ventral and dorsal borders of the stomach. Many accounts state that the development of a ventrally directed concave *lesser curvature* and a more rapidly growing dorsocranially directed convex *greater curvature* and incipient *fundus* occur while the anlage is still sagittal. Thereafter, the whole miniature organ and attached mesogastria are supposed to physically rotate through almost 90° (see p. 190). On this view the original left surface becomes ventrosuperior and the primitive dorsal border is directed to the left as the greater curvature. The interpretation of various mesenteric and neurovascular sequelae were based on these assumptions. Inspection of closely-spaced series of embryos (Kanagasuntheram 1957, 1960) led to the suggestion that the morphogenetic changes in both stomach and duodenum and their attendant mesenteries were mainly, if not wholly, due to patterned differential growth rates and mesenchymal cleft formation and cleavage. Thus the stomach, initially a tube with slight lateral flattening, developed a linear zone of high proliferation along the length of the central part of its (original) left lateral wall. At first it became triangular in transverse section, with rounded angles and apex pointing to the left; further growth resulted in an elliptical profile. The ends of the sectional ellipse corresponded to the curvatures: the end directed to the right, and a little ventrally, to the lesser curvature and justifiably regarded as a modified primitive ventral border; the left end to the greater curvature, an entirely *new formation*. For a while the two primitive mesogastria are **both** attached near the emerging lesser curvature (the sites of the primitive dorsal and ventral borders). The profound changes involved in reaching the definitive state only supervene with the development of the lesser sac.

The *lesser sac* is the first indicated by the appearance of multiple clefts in the para-oesophageal mesenchyme on both left and right aspects of the oesophagus. Although they may become confluent, the left clefts are transitory and soon atrophy. The right clefts merge to form the *right pneumato-enteric recess* that extends from the oesophageal end of the lesser curvature as far as the caudal aspect of the right lung bud. At its gastric end it communicates with the general peritoneal cavity and lies **ventrolateral** to the gut; more rostrally it lies directly **lateral** to the oesophagus. It is **not**, as commonly stated, a simple progressive excavation of the right side of the **dorsal** mesogastrium. The right pneumato-enteric recess undergoes further extension, subdivision and modification mentioned below. From its caudal end a second process of cleft and cavity formation occurs producing the *hepato-enteric recess* that thins and expands the splanchnopleure between the liver and the stomach and proximal duodenum, and also reaches the diaphragm. The resulting, structurally bilaminar, mesenteric sheet is the *lesser omentum* and is derived from the small meso-oesophagus, the major part from the ventral mesogastrium, and the reduplicated strip including the free border from the ventral mesoduodenum. As differential growth of the duodenum occurs, the biliary duct is repositioned and most of the duodenum becomes sessile; the duodenal attachment of the free border and a continuous neighbouring strip of the lesser omentum becomes confined to the upper border of a short segment of its superior part. The free border, with contrasting growth and positioning of its attached viscera, gradually changes from the horizontal to the vertical. It carries the bile duct, portal vein and hepatic artery, and its hepatic end is reflected around the porta hepatis; an alternative name for this part of the lesser omentum is the *hepatoduodenal ligament*, and it forms the anterior wall of the epiploic foramen. The floor of the foramen is the initial segment of the superior part of the duodenum mentioned above, its posterior wall is the peritoneum covering the immediately subhepatic part of the inferior vena cava, and its roof the peritonealized caudate process of the liver. That major part of the lesser omentum from the lesser gastric curvature passes in an approximately coronal plant to reach the floor of the increasingly deep groove for the ductus venosus (postnatally the ligamentum venosum) on the hepatic dorsum. This part is sometimes called the *hepatogastric ligament*.

The pneumato-enteric recess continues to expand to the right into the substance of the caval fold, ceasing near the left margin of the hepatic part of the inferior vena cava; the latter remains extra-peritoneal, crossing the base of the now roughly triangular bare area of the liver (encompassed by coronary and right triangular ligaments) and this new expanded line of reflexion. With closure of the pleuro-peritoneal canals the rostral part of the right pneumato-enteric recess is sequestered by the diaphragm but often persists as a small serous sac in the right pulmonary ligament. The remaining caval fold mesenchyme to the left of the inferior vena cava, and forming the right wall of the upper part of the lesser sac, becomes completely invaded by embryonic hepatic tissue and is transformed into the caudate lobe of the liver. This smooth, vertically elongate mass projects into the cavity of the lesser sac, and both its posterior and much of its anterior surfaces are peritonealized because of the increasing depth of the groove for the ductus venosus and the attachment of the lesser omentum to its *floor*. The narrow isthmus of the *caudate process* connects its right inferior angle to the rest of the right lobe (and is the roof of the epiploic foramen). The parts of the lesser sac thus far described above and to the right of the lesser curvature of the stomach have received a plethora of names by different investigators; sometimes these stem from changing or contrasting views of ontogeny. A few prominent ones will be mentioned. Some regard the right rim only of the structures already listed as constituting the boundaries of the epiploic foramen. The narrow channel, a few centimetres long, passing to the left, and coextensive with the caudate process and peritonealized part of the initial duodenal segment, is called the *vestibule* of the lesser sac (but see below). The remaining, much more extensive part above the lesser curvature is termed, variously, the *upper (superior) part* (recess) of the lesser sac, the *hepatic part* of the lesser sac or finally the *hepato-enteric part of the pneumato-enteric recess*. Some authorities group all the foregoing under the general term *vestibule*; they are intimately related to the diaphragm and caudate lobe of the liver and coextensive with the lesser omentum. Varying use of the name vestibule partly reflects earlier, mistaken views of the ontogeny of the upper and lower parts of the lesser sac (about to be described). Much of the upper part was considered to be merely a part of the general peritoneal coelom 'captured' by differential growth and omental changes of plane, whereas fundamentally different mechanisms of excavation were considered to apply to the lower part, the '*true*' *omental bursa* of some authors. Current evidences suggest that the **same** array of developmental mechanisms, with only quantitative regional differences, apply to **all** coelomic regions. The general name omental bursa should be used with caution; both upper and lower parts have walls that are partly omental (lesser and greater omenta respectively); also neither part is functionally more nor less bursal than other coelomic regions—peritoneal, pleural or pericardial. Confusion stemming from the term 'recess' firmly established in embryology but, with different connotations, used sporadically in adult topography has been mentioned (p. 1744). Thus, the upper (superior) and lower (inferior) parts of the lesser sac seem preferable terms. Ultimately the junction between upper and lower parts is oblique, curving upwards as it passes from right to left; ventrally lies the gastric lesser curvature, dorsally the body of the pancreas. The left limit is a curved ridge of mesenchyme (future left *gastropancreatic fold*) carrying the left gastric artery and the right a curved ridge (future right *gastropancreatic fold*) carrying the common hepatic artery.

The *lower (inferior) part of the lesser sac* commences development at about 8–9 mm CR length—at this stage the early pneumato-enteric and hepato-enteric recesses are well established. Differential gastric growth is progressing (p. 183) giving an elliptical transverse sectional profile, with a right-sided lesser curvature, corresponding to the original ventral border of the gastric tube, to which the lesser omental gastric part of the ventral mesogastrium remains attached. As indicated, the greater curvature is a new formation, rapidly expanding, with its convex profile projecting mainly to the left, but also rostrally and caudally. It was emphasized that the original dorsal border of the gastric tube now traverses the dorsal aspect of the expanding rudiment, curving along a line near the *lesser* curvature; here, transiently, the *primitive* dorsal mesogastrium is attached. The latter blends with the thick layer of compound gastric mesenchyme clothing the posterior aspect and greater curvature of the miniature stomach; because of its thickness, the mesenchyme projects rostrally, caudally, and particularly to the left, beyond the 'new' greater curvature of the endodermal lining of the stomach. (It

197

may be noted that during these stages the geometries, and hence sectional profiles, of tissue strata and cavities are complex and change rapidly with varying levels of histological section and with time. Thus only a brief summary of some salient points can be attempted here. For details consult Kanagasuntheram 1957.) The processes already described in relation to the ventral mesenteries now supervene. Multiple clefts appear at various loci in the mesenchyme, with local mesenchyme to epithelial transition; each group of clefts rapidly coalesce to form (transiently) isolated closed spaces. The latter, by a continuation of the mechanism, soon join with each other and with the preformed upper part of the lesser sac, the newly formed epithelia joining the coelomic epithelium. The initial loci involve, firstly, the compound posterior gastric mesenchyme nearer the lesser curvature and along its zone of blending with the primitive dorsal mesogastrium; secondarily, in the dorsal mesoduodenum; thirdly, independently in the caudal rim where greater curvature mesenchyme and dorsal mesogastrium blend. As these cavities become confluent and their 'reniform' expansion follows, matches and then exceeds that of the gastric greater curvature, there are some major sequelae. The primitive dorsal mesogastrium increases in area not only by intrinsic growth, but as cavitation proceeds, by substantial additions from the dorsal lamella separated by cleavage of the posterior gastric mesenchyme: together these may conveniently be called the *secondary dorsal mesogastrium*. The *gastric attachment* of the latter changes as a set of somewhat spiral lines, longitudinally disposed, that move, with time, from near the lesser curvature towards, and finally reaching, the definitive greater curvature. The *parietal* mesogastrial and (cleaving) mesoduodenal *attachment* remains, for a time, in the dorsal midline, but subsequently undergoes profound changes. With the confluence of the cavities that collectively form the lower part of the lesser sac, its communication with the upper part, corresponding to the lesser gastric curvature and right and left gastropancreatic folds, becomes better defined. **Ventral** to the lower part of the cavity lies the postcleavage splanchnopleure covering the postero-inferior surface of the stomach and a short proximal segment of the duodenum. This ventral wall is continued beyond the greater curvature and duodenum as the splanchnopleuric strip of visceral attachment of the secondary dorsal mesogastrium and mesoduodenum. The radial width of the strip is relatively short rostrally (gastric fundus) and gradually increases along the descending left part of the greater curvature; it is longest throughout the remaining perimeter of the greater curvature as far as the duodenum, and this prominent part shows continued marginal (caudoventral and lateral) growth with extended internal cavitation (its walls constituting the expanding *greater omentum*). The **margins** of the cavity of the inferior part of the lesser sac are limited by the reflexed edges of the ventrally placed strata derived from the secondary dorsal mesogastrium just described. These converge, forming the splanchnopleuric dorsal wall, which is initially 'free' throughout except at its midline dorsal root. At roughly midgastric levels, encased in this dorsal wall, the pancreatic rudiment grows obliquely, its tail ultimately reaching the left limit of the lesser sac at the level of the junction between gastric fundus and body. (It may be mentioned that many earlier accounts held that the lower part of the lesser sac stemmed from a simple excavation of the dorsal mesogastrium—the pancreatico-enteric recess—with subsequent further extensions. This view has been discarded here.)

Centred on the dorsal mesogastrial region towards which growth of the pancreatic tail is directed, the anlage of the spleen appears in the coelomic epithelium and subjacent mesenchyme. As it expands into the upper left hypochondriac part of the *greater* sac, it retains its neurovascular pedicle and serous tunic, both of dorsal mesogastrial origin (pp. 1438, 1739).

The greater omentum and its contained extension of the lesser sac continue to grow both laterally, and particularly caudoventrally, covering and closely applied to the transverse mesocolon, transverse colon and inframesocolic and infracolic coils of small intestine. At this stage the quadrilaminar nature of the dependent part of the greater omentum is most easily appreciated. It will be recalled that 'simple' mesenteries, for example the mesentery of the jejuno-ileum, are bilaminar in that they possess two mesothelial surfaces (splanchnopleuric coelomic epithelium) enclosing a connective tissue core (from splanchnopleuric mesenchyme) which bears blood and lymphatic vessels, lymph nodes, nerves, adipose tissue and other cell

varieties. In the greater omentum, the gastric serosa covering its postero-inferior surface (single mesothelium) and the anterosuperior serosa (single mesothelium) converge, meeting at the greater curvature (and initial segment of the duodenum). The resulting bilaminar mesentery continues as the anterosuperior (or 'descending') stratum of the omentum which, on reaching the omental margins, is reflexed and 'returns' (or 'ascends') as its posterior bilaminar stratum to its parietal root. The two bilaminar strata are initially in fairly close contact caudally, but separated by a fine, fluid-containing, cleft-like extension of the lower part of the lesser sac. The posterior mesothelium of the posterior stratum makes equally close contact with the anterosuperior surface of the transverse colon (starting at its *taenia omentalis*) and with its transverse mesocolon.

At this stage, and subsequently, it is convenient to designate the lower part of the lesser sac as consisting of three *subregions*: retrogastric, perigastric and greater omental. The names are self-explanatory but their confines are all modified by various factors. Two phenomena are particularly prominent: gastric 'descent' relative to the liver, and fusion of peritoneal layers with altered lines of reflexion, adhesion of surfaces and loss of parts of cavities.

After the third month the hepatic growth diminishes, particularly the left lobe, and the whole organ recedes into the upper abdomen; meanwhile the stomach elongates and some descent occurs, despite its relatively fixed cranial and caudal ends. This causes the angular flexure of the stomach that persists postnatally: the concavity of the lesser curvature is now directed more precisely to the right, the lesser omentum is more exactly coronal and its free border vertical, ventral to the liver; the free border of the falciform ligament passes steeply rostrodorsally from umbilicus to liver. The mesenchymal dorsal wall of the lower part of the lesser sac, crossed obliquely by the growing pancreas, has hitherto remained free, with its original dorsal midline root. Substantial areas now fuse with adjacent peritonealized surfaces of retroperitoneal viscera, the parietes, or another mesenteric sheet or fold. In the latter case there occurs a variable loss of their apposed mesothelia and some continuity of their mesenchymal cores, but they remain surgically separable and no vascular anastomosis develops across the interzone. Above the pancreas the posterior secondary dorsomesogastrial wall of the sac becomes closely applied to the peritoneum covering the posterior abdominal wall and its sessile organs—the diaphragm, much of the left suprarenal gland, the ventromedial part of the upper pole of the left kidney, the initial part of the abdominal aorta, the coeliac trunk and its branches, and other vessels, nerves, and lymphatics. Their peritoneal surfaces fuse and, with some tissue loss, a **single** mesothelium covering these structures remains, intercalated as a new secondary dorsal wall for this part of the lesser sac. The pancreas, as indicated (p. 186), grows from the duodenal loop, penetrating the substance of the dorsal mesoduodenum and secondary dorsal mesogastrium, their mesenchymes and mesothelia initially clothing its whole surface, except where there exist peritoneal lines of reflexion. Its posterior peritoneum becomes closely applied to that covering all the posterior abdominal wall structures it crosses (prominently: the inferior vena cava, abdominal aorta, splenic vein, superior mesenteric vessels, inferior mesenteric vein, portal vein, left renal vessels, the caudal pole of the left suprarenal, a broad ventral band on the left kidney and various muscles, etc; see p. 1790). The intervening peritoneal mesothelia fuse and atrophy, the mesenchymal cores forming fascial sheaths and septa. The pancreas is now sessile and the peritoneum covering the upper left part of its head, neck and anterosuperior part of its body forms the central part of the dorsal wall of the lesser sac. The pancreatic tail remains peritonealized by a persisting part of the secondary dorsal mesogastrium as it curves from the ventral aspect of the left kidney towards the hilum of the spleen. (The infracolic parts of the pancreas are covered with greater sac peritoneum.) In the greater omental subregion of the lower part of the lesser sac two contrasting forms of mesenteric adhesion occur. The posterior 'returning' bilaminar stratum of the omentum undergoes partial fusion with the peritoneum of the transverse colon (at the taenia omentalis) and with its mesocolon. (They provide a great increase in the functional area of the stomach 'bed', p. 1755; also they remain surgically separable and no anastomosis occurs between omental and colic vessels.) In fetal life the greater omental cavity extends to the internal aspect of the lateral and caudal edges of the omentum. However, postnatally a slow but progressive fusion of the internal surfaces occurs with obliteration of the most dependent part of the cavity; this proceeds rostrally and, when mature, the cavity does not usually extend appreciably beyond the transverse colon. (The other fusions described above follow different patterns.) Transverse mesocolon–greater omentum fusion commences early while the umbilical hernia of the midgut has not returned; it is initiated between the right margin of the early greater omentum and near the root of the *presumptive* mesocolon, later spreading to the left. The pancreas becomes sessile mediolaterally (i.e. head, followed by neck and body from right to left). Paradoxically, in the suprapancreatic region, the direction of the process of fusion is reversed, progressing lateromedially from left to right. These events are wholly in accord with the numerous variations and anomalous visceral positioning and mesenteric arrangements that have been observed and recorded.

Correlated with the many facets of development of the lesser sac and its associated viscera, the original dorsal midline attachment to the parietes of the foregut dorsal mesentery is profoundly altered. However, despite the extensive areas of fusion, virtually the whole of the gastric greater curvature (other than a small suboesophageal area) and its topographical continuation, the inferior border of the first 2–3 cm of the duodenum, retain true mesenteric derivatives of the secondary dorsal mesogastrium and its continuation, the dorsal mesoduodenum. Thus, although regional names are given to assist identification and description, it must be emphasized that they are merely subregions of one continuous sheet; a short description of their 'root' or parietal line of reflexion is also given.

The upper (oesophagophrenic) part of the *lesser* omentum arches across the diaphragm and as this bilaminar mesentery approaches the oesophageal hiatus its laminae diverge, skirting the margins of the hiatus. They then descend for a limited distance and variable inclination, to enclose reciprocally-shaped areas on the dorsum of the gastric fundus and diaphragm. The area may be roughly triangular to quadrangular; it contains areolar tissue and constitutes the *bare area of the stomach* or, when large, the *left extraperitoneal space*. Its right lower angle is the base of the left gastropancreatic fold; its left lower angle reconstitutes the bilaminar mesentery. The root of the latter arches downwards and to the left across the diaphragm and suprarenal and gives the *gastrophrenic ligament* to the gastric fundus. Continuing to arch across the ventral surface of the upper part of the left kidney, its layers part to receive the pancreatic tail and initially extend to the hilum of the spleen as the *splenorenal* (*lienorenal*) *ligament*. The left half of this bilaminar 'ligament' provides an almost complete peritoneal tunic for the spleen (as indicated, projecting into the greater sac) then, reuniting with its fellow at the opposite rim of the splenic hilum, continues to the next part of the gastric greater curvature as the *gastrosplenic ligament*. The remaining major (perhaps two-thirds) of the gastric greater curvature and its short duodenal extension are the visceral attachment of the anterior, 'descending', bilaminar stratum of the greater omentum. Its returning, posterior, bilaminar stratum continues to its parietal root; the latter extends from the inferior limit assigned to the splenorenal ligament, continuing to curve caudally and to the right along the anterior border of the body of the pancreas, immediately cranial to the line of attachment of the transverse mesocolon. Crossing the neck of the pancreas, the same curve is followed for a few centimetres on to the gland's head; the omental root is then sharply recurved cranially and to the left, soon to reach the inferior border of the duodenum. Thus it reaches that part of the lesser sac provided by cleavage of the dorsal mesoduodenum from the greater sac, entering the epiploic foramen and traversing the epiploic canal between the caudate hepatic process and proximal duodenum, the lower right angle of the hepato-enteric recess, and crossing the right gastropancreatic fold, then descending behind the proximal duodenum to enter the right marginal strip enclosed by the greater omentum.

URINARY AND REPRODUCTIVE SYSTEMS

The urinary and reproductive organs are developed from *intermediate mesenchyme* (p. 155) and are intimately associated with one another especially in the earlier stages of their development. The urinary system develops ahead of the reproductive or genital system.

URINARY SYSTEM

The intermediate mesenchyme is found longitudinally placed in the trunk, subjacent to the somites (in the folded embryo), at the junction between the splanchnopleuric mesenchyme adjacent to the gut medially and the somatopleuric mesenchyme subjacent to the ectoderm laterally (**3.80**). Development of the intermediate mesenchyme progresses craniocaudally. In lower vertebrates the intermediate mesenchyme typically develops serial, segmental epithelial diverticuli termed *nephrotomes* each enclosing a cavity, the *nephrocoele*, and communicating with the coelom through a *peritoneal funnel*. The dorsal wall of each nephrotome evaginates as a *nephric tubule* communicating with the nephrocoele via a *nephrostome*. The dorsal tips of the earlier (cranial) developed nephric tubules bend caudally and fuse forming a longitudinal *primary excretory duct*, which grows caudally and curves ventrally to open into the cloaca. The more caudally placed and successively later developed tubules open secondarily into this duct or into tubular outgrowths from it. *Glomeruli*, specific arrangements of capillaries and overlying coelomic epithelium, arise from the ventral wall of the nephrocoele (*internal glomeruli*) or the roof of the coelom adjacent to the peritoneal funnels (*coelomic or external glomeruli*), or in both situations (**3.81**). An extensive area vascularized as a *glomus* rather than individual glomeruli can be seen in developing reptiles during organogenesis. In avian species external (pronephric, see below) glomeruli can be identified. Clusters of cells appropriately placed in mammalian embryos fail to differentiate into true glomeruli.

It has been customary to regard the renal excretory system as three organs, the *pronephros, mesonephros* and *metanephros*, suc-ceeding each other in time and space. The last to develop is retained as the permanent kidney. It is, however, difficult to provide reliable criteria that distinguish them as individual organs or to define their precise limits in the embryos of all animals. A functional pronephros with well-developed podocytes has been identified in chelonian embryos (Collins 1990) and in avian embryos (Jacob et al 1977); however, a pronephros cannot be distinguished as a separate organ in man. The earliest and most cranially situated nephric tubules are rudimentary, transient and regarded as marking the pronephric region, and the latter merges caudally without clear demarcation into the mesonephros. Human nephrotomes, with cavitation to form nephrocoeles which communicate with the coelom, are restricted to a few segments bordering the rostral limit of the intraembryonic coelom. Cranial to this (pronephric region) the intermediate mesenchyme develops irregular, transient, solid or vesicular balls of cells. Caudal to the level of the eighth to tenth somites the intermediate mesenchyme is termed the *nephrogenic cord*. This is connected at irregular intervals with the coelomic epithelium.

Primary excretory duct. This begins in stage 11 embryos of about 14 somites as a solid rod of cells in the dorsal part of the nephrogenic cord. Its cranial end is about the level of the ninth somite and its caudal tip merges with the undifferentiated mesenchyme of the cord. It differentiates before any nephric tubules; when the latter appear it is at first unconnected with them. In older embryos the duct has lengthened and its caudal end becomes detached from the nephrogenic cord to lie immediately beneath the ectoderm. From this level it grows caudally, independent of the nephrogenic mesenchyme, and then curves ventrally to reach the wall of the cloaca. It becomes canalized progressively from its caudal end to form a true duct which opens into the cloaca in embryos at stage 12. (Clearly, up to this stage, the name 'duct' is scarcely appropriate.)

Pronephros

The intermediate mesenchyme becomes visible in stage 10 embryos and the nephrogenic cord is distinguishable when 10 somites are

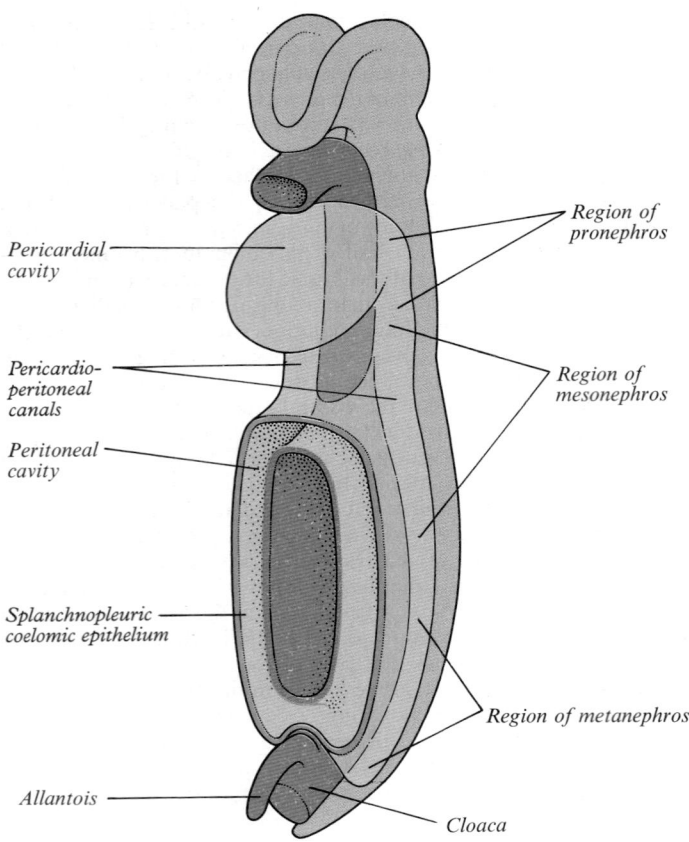

Pericardial cavity

Region of pronephros

Pericardio-peritoneal canals

Region of mesonephros

Peritoneal cavity

Splanchnopleuric coelomic epithelium

Region of metanephros

Allantois

Cloaca

3.80   Diagram of the major epithelial populations within the early embryo. The urogenital system arises from the proliferating coelomic epithelium at the dorsal wall of the intraembryonic coelom. The earliest nephric system, the pronephros, forms at the level of the pericardium and upper pericardio-peritoneal canals; the mesonephros, gonads and genital ducts form and project into the pericardio-peritoneal canals and the peritoneal cavity; the metanephros arises at the lowest levels of the peritoneal cavity.

present. The pronephros then is indicated as clusters of cells (rudimentary nephric tubules) in the nephrogenic mesenchyme (cord) (**3.**81). In regions cranial to the primary excretory duct these clusters develop no further. More caudally similar groups of cells appear and these become vesicular. The dorsal ends of the most caudal of these vesicles join the primary excretory duct, their central ends being connected with the coelomic epithelium by cellular strands probably representing rudimentary peritoneal funnels. Glomeruli are not developed in association with these cranially situated nephric tubules, which ultimately disappear. It is doubtful whether external glomeruli develop in human embryos. (For an overview and bibliographies concerning the early development of the human nephros consult Torrey 1954; O'Rahilly & Muecke 1972; O'Rahilly & Muller 1987.)

Mesonephros

From about stage 12 the primary excretory duct is termed the *mesonephric duct* (*Wolffian duct*); it lengthens and soon becomes connected to the cloaca. At this stage mesonephric tubules, developing from the intermediate mesenchyme between somite levels 8–20, begin to connect to the mesonephric duct; caudal to this there is a continuous ridge of nephrogenic mesenchyme to the level of somite 24. The mesonephric tubules are not metameric: there may be two or more mesonephric tubules opposite each somite.

Within the mesonephros, each tubule first appears as a condensation of mesenchyme cells which epithelialize and form a vesicle. One end of the vesicle grows towards and opens into the mesonephric duct, whilst the other dilates and invaginates; the outer stratum forms the *glomerular capsule*, while the inner cells differentiate into *mesonephric podocytes* which clothe the invaginating capillaries to form a glomerulus. The latter are supplied with blood through lateral

branches of the aorta (Streeter 1945). It is estimated that about 70–80 mesonephric tubules and a corresponding number of glomeruli develop. These tubules, however, are not present at the same time and it is rare to find more than 30–40 in an individual embryo, for the cranial tubules and glomeruli develop and atrophy before the development of those situated more caudally.

By the end of the sixth week each mesonephros is an elongated spindle-shaped organ which projects into the coelomic cavity, one on each side of the dorsal mesentery, from the level of the septum transversum to the third lumbar segment. This whole projection is the *mesonephric ridge* (Wolffian body); it develops subregions (see below), and the gonad is developed on its medial surface. There are striking similarities in structure between the mesonephros and the permanent kidney or metanephros, but the former's nephrons lack a segment corresponding to the descending limb of the loop of Henle (Leeson 1957; Davies & Routh 1957). The mesonephros is believed to produce urine by stage 17 (O'Rahilly & Muller 1987). A detailed comparison of the development and function of the mesonephros and metanephros in staged human embryos is lacking. In the chick no significant difference in the renal clearance of plasma sodium, potassium and magnesium ions were noted in 9-day embryos with functional mesonephric kidneys, and 15-day embryos with predominant metanephric kidneys; calcium clearance decreased over this time (Clarke et al 1993).

In stage 18 embryos (13–17 mm) the mesonephric ridge extends cranially to about the level of rib 9. In both sexes the cranial end of the mesonephros atrophies; in embryos of 20-mm length (stage 19) the organ is found only in the first three lumbar segments, although it may still possess as many as 26 tubules. The most cranial one or two tubules persist as the *rostral aberrant ductules*; the succeeding five or six tubules develop into the *efferent ductules of the testis* and the *lobules of the head of the epididymis* in the male, and the tubules of the *epoöphoron* in the female; the caudal tubules form the *caudal aberrant ductules* and the paradidymis in the male, and the *paroöphoron* in the female (see below).

Mesonephric duct. This runs caudally in the lateral part of the nephric ridge, at the caudal end of which it projects into the cavity of the coelom in the substance of a *mesonephric fold* (**3.**82–86). (Subsequently, with the neighbouring formation of the paramesonephric duct, they form the *tubal fold*—see below.) As the mesonephric ducts from each side approach the urogenital sinus the two folds fuse with each other, between the bladder ventrally and the rectum dorsally, forming across the cavity of the pelvis a transverse partition which is somewhat inaptly termed the *genital cord* (**3.**84). In the male the peritoneal fossa between the bladder and the genital cord becomes obliterated, but it persists in the female as the uterovesical pouch. The mesonephric duct itself becomes the canal of the *epididymis*, *ductus deferens* and *ejaculatory duct*. The *seminal vesicle* and the ampulla of the ductus deferens appear as a common swelling at the termination of the mesonephric duct during the end of the third and into the fourth month. This coincides with degeneration of the paramesonephric ducts, though no causal relation between the two has been established. Separation into two rudiments occurs at about 125-mm crown–heel length. The seminal vesicle elongates, its duct is delineated and hollow diverticula bud from its wall. About the sixth month (300-mm crown–heel length) the growth rate of both vesicle and ampulla is greatly increased; the cause is uncertain but may result from increased secretion of prolactin by the fetal or maternal hypophysis, or the effects of placental hormones. The tubules of the prostate show a similar increase of growth rate at the same time. In the female the mesonephric duct is vestigial, becoming the longitudinal duct of the epoöphoron.

Metanephros

Both the pronephros and the mesonephros are linear structures with stacks of tubules arranged along the craniocaudal axis of the embryo. This arrangement results in the production of hypotonic urine. The tubular arrangement in the metanephric kidney is fundamentally different: the tubules are arranged *concentrically* with the loops of Henle directed towards the renal pelvis. This arrangement allows different concentration gradients to develop within the kidney and results in the production of *hypertonic* urine. Thus metanephric nephrons do *not* join with the existing mesonephric duct but with an evagination of that duct which branches *dichotomously* resulting

PRIMITIVE VERTEBRATE EXCRETORY SYSTEM

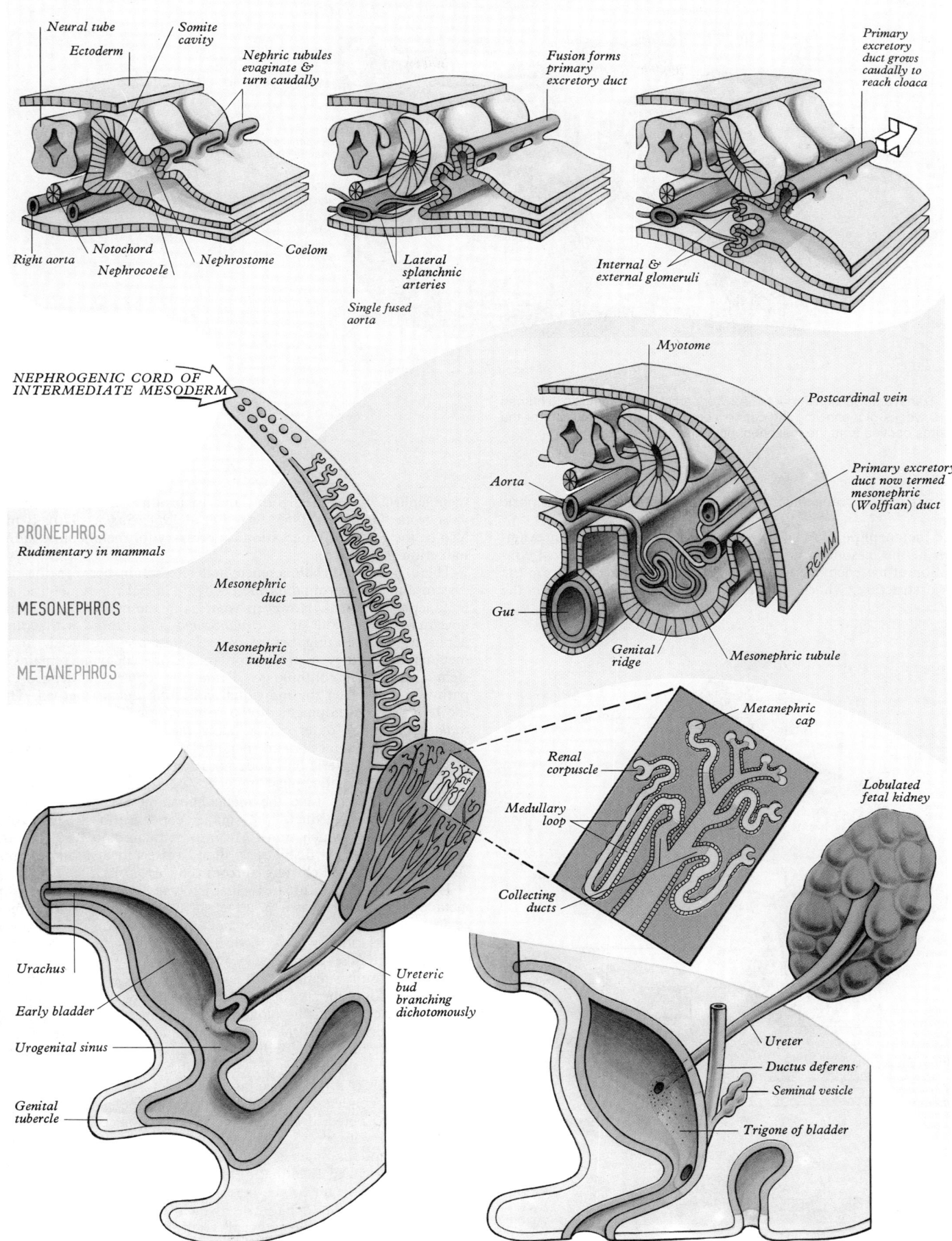

3.81 Principal features of the primitive vertebrate nephric system for comparison with the development of the human nephric system. It should be appreciated that a considerable period of embryonic and fetal life has been necessarily compressed into a single, static diagram. (Modified from Williams et al 1969.)

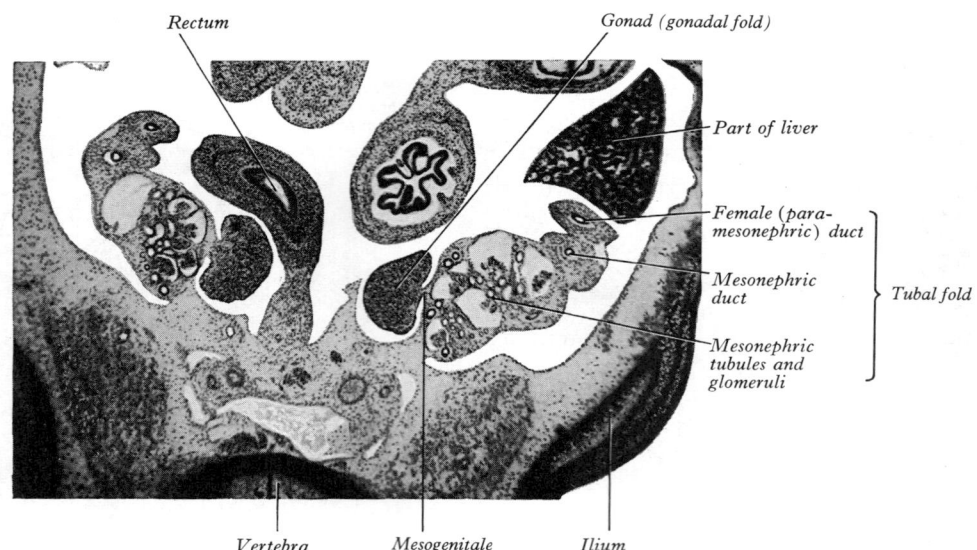

3.82   Transverse section through the lower part of the abdomen of a human fetus, 9 weeks old, showing the connections and relative positions of the structures derived from the mesonephric ridge.

in the particular arrangement of collecting ducts of the metanephric kidney.

The metanephric kidney develops from three sources: an evagination of the mesonephric duct, the *ureteric bud*, and a local condensation of mesenchyme termed the *metanephric blastema* form the nephric structure, while *angiogenic mesenchyme* migrates into the

Phallus

Ventral (vesico-urethral) part of cloaca

Mesonephric duct

Rectum

Caudal part of coelom

Ureter

Right common iliac vessels

Bifurcation of aorta and left common iliac artery

Sacrum

3.83   Transverse section of the tail end of a human embryo in the eighth week, CR length 22 mm. The projection from the dorsolateral aspect of the ventral portion of the cloaca marks the entry of the mesonephric duct. Stained with haematoxylin and eosin. Magnification × c. 20.

metanephric blastema slightly later to produce the glomeruli and vasa recta (Grobstein 1955; Saxen et al 1968; Saxen 1970). It may also be the case that innervation is necessary for metanephric kidney induction (see below).

There is an epithelial/mesenchymal interaction between the duct system and the surrounding mesenchyme in both mesonephric and metanephric systems. However, whereas in the mesonephric kidney development proceeds in a *craniocaudal progression*, with cranial nephrons degenerating before caudal ones are produced, in the metanephric kidney a proportion of the mesenchyme remains as stem cells which continue to divide and enter the nephrogenic pathway later when the individual collecting ducts lengthen. Thus the temporal development of the metanephric kidney is patterned *radially*, with the outer cortex being the last part to be formed. Generally the interactions in metanephric kidney development are as follows: the ureteric bud undergoes a series of *bifurcations* within the surrounding metanephric mesenchyme, forming smaller *ureteric ducts*. At the same time the metanephric mesenchyme condenses around the dividing ducts into smaller condensations. These form *S-shaped clusters* which transform into epithelia and fuse with the ureteric ducts at their distal ends. Blood vessels invade the proximal ends of the S-shaped clusters to form the *vascularized glomeruli*.

The ureteric bud bifurcates when it comes into contact with the metanephric blastema as a result of local extracellular matrix molecule synthesis by the mesenchyme. In metanephric culture, incubation of fetal kidneys in β-D-xyloside, an inhibitor of chrondroitin sulphate synthesis, dramatically inhibits ureteric bud branching. Both chondroitin sulphate proteoglycan synthesis and chondroitin sulphate glycosaminoglycan processing are necessary for the dichotomous branching of the ureteric bud (Fouser & Avner 1993). Subsequent divisions of the ureteric bud and the mesenchyme form the gross structure of the kidney with *major* and *minor calyces*, the distal branches of the ureteric ducts will form the *collecting ducts* of the kidney. As the collecting ducts elongate the metanephric mesenchyme condenses around them. An adhesion molecule, syndecan, can be detected between the mesenchymal cells in the condensate. The cells cease expression of N-CAM, fibronectin and collagen I and commence production of L-CAM (an adhesion molecule also called E cadherin) and the basal lamina constituents laminin and collagen IV. The mesenchymal clusters thus convert to small groups of epithelial cells which undergo complex morphogenetic changes. Each epithelial group elongates, forms a comma-shaped, then an S-shaped body which elongates further. It then fuses to a branch of the ureteric duct at its distal end while expanding as a dilated sac at the proximal end. The sac involutes with local cellular differentiation such that the outer cells become the *parietal*

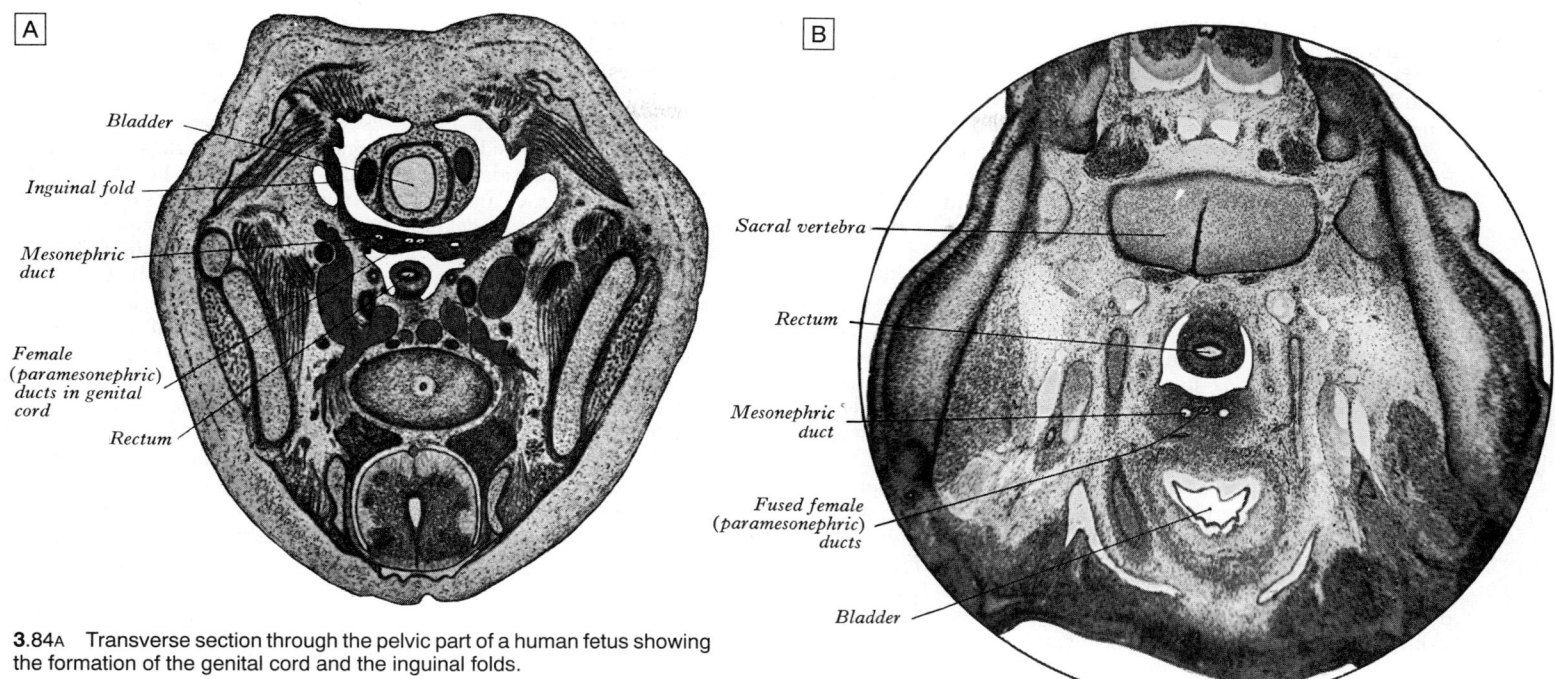

3.84A Transverse section through the pelvic part of a human fetus showing the formation of the genital cord and the inguinal folds.

3.84B Transverse section through the pelvis of a 9-week-old male human fetus, showing the approximation of the genital cord to the dorsal wall of the urogenital sinus.

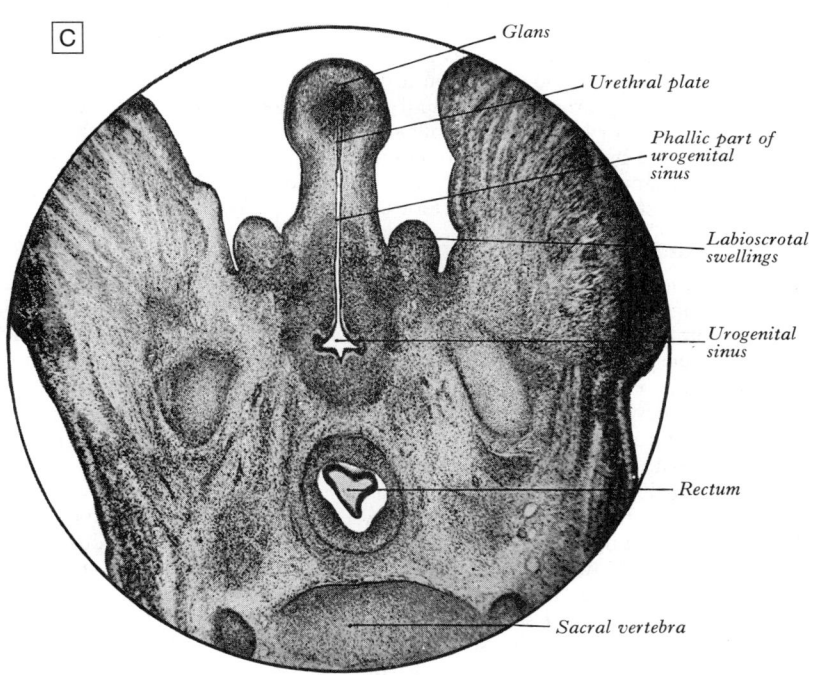

3.84C Transverse section through the lower part of the pelvis of a 9-week-old human fetus.

glomerular cells, while the inner ones become *visceral epithelial podocytes*. The podocytes develop in close proximity to invading capillaries which derive from *angiogenic mesenchyme* outside the nephrogenic mesenchyme (Ekblom et al 1982); this third source of mesenchyme produces the *endothelial* and *mesangial cells* within the glomerulus. Both the metanephric derived podocytes and the angiogenic mesenchyme produce fibronectin and other components of the glomerular basal lamina. The isoforms of type IV collagen within this layer follow a specific programme of maturation which occurs as the filtration of macromolecules from the plasma becomes restricted (Bard & Woolf 1992).

Platelet derived growth factor (PDGF) β-chain and the PDGF receptor β-subunit (PDGFR β) have been detected in developing human glomeruli between 54 and 105 days gestation. PDGF β-chain is localized in the differentiating epithelium of the glomerular vesicle during its comma and S-shaped stages, while PDGFR β is expressed in the undifferentiated metanephric blastema, vascular structures and interstitial cells. Both PDGF β-chain and PDGFR β are expressed by mesangial cells; this may promote further mesangial cell proliferation.

Metanephric mesenchyme will develop successfully in vitro making experimental perturbation of kidney development comparatively easy to evaluate. Early experimental studies demonstrated that other mesenchymal populations and also spinal cord were able to induce ureteric bud division and metanephric development. However, it has been demonstrated that nerves enter the developing kidney very early, via the ureter (Sariola et al 1989). If developing kidney rudiments are incubated with antisense oligonucleotides that neutralize nerve growth factor receptor (NGF-R) mRNA, nephrogenesis is completely blocked, leading to the conclusion that metanephric mesenchyme induction is a response to innervation (Sariola et al 1991). The powerful inductive effect of the spinal cord on metanephric mesenchyme may be demonstrating this same phenomenon.

All stages of nephron differentiation are present concurrently in the developing metanephric kidney. Antigens to the brush border of the renal tubule appear when the S-shaped body has formed. Tubules displaying this marker appear first in the inner cortical area.

At an early stage the metanephric kidney is **lobulated**, a condition which persists through fetal life but disappears during the first year after birth. Varying degrees of lobulation, however, on occasion, persist throughout life. The growth of left and right kidneys are well matched during development. Fetal kidney volume increases most during the second trimester in both sexes. However, in the third trimester male fetuses show greater values for renal volume than female fetuses (Sampaio 1992). The reason for this sex difference in renal development remains unknown; however, it has been shown

that kidneys from male rats are larger than those from females, attributed to both cellular hyperplasia and hypertrophy (Jean-Faucher et al 1987), and male fetuses are generally larger than females from 12 weeks postconception (Pedersen 1980).

Endocrine development of the kidney. In addition to its function as an excretory organ, the kidney is an endocrine organ producing hormones acting at sites within and without the kidney. The fetal kidney functions in utero producing *amniotic fluid*; however, *homeostasis* prior to birth is controlled by the *placenta*. Premature babies of less than 36 weeks have immature kidneys with incomplete differentiation of the cortical nephrons compromising their ability to maintain homeostasis. The problems of immaturity are further compounded by the effects of hypoxia and asphyxia which modify renal hormones; also the use of artificial ventilation has effects on renal haemodynamics and the renal hormones.

Hormones produced by the kidney are concerned with renal haemodynamics; they include the renin-angiotensin system, renal prostaglandins, the kallikrein-kinin system, and renal dopamine. *Renin* is found in both the smooth muscle cells of arterioles, inter-lobular arteries and branches of the renal artery, although it has also been described in the distal convoluted tubule cells; *kallikrein* has been demonstrated in rat fetal kidney (urinary kallikrein is lower in human newborns than in later life); *prostaglandins* have been demonstrated in the renal medulla and in large amounts in the renal tubule; *renal dopamine* has been identified in two sources, from the dopaminergic nerves and predominantly from the enzymatic conversion of levodopa (L-dopa) to dopamine in the early segments of the proximal convoluted tubule. Other hormones have been identified within the kidney; an antihypertensive lipid is produced in the interstitial cells of the renal medulla, and it also appears that histamine and serotonin can be synthesized by the kidney. Growth factors produced by human embryonic kidney cell include erythro-poietin, interleukin β and transforming growth factor-beta. The presence of erythropoietin and interleukin β in human embryonic kidney cells stimulates megakaryocyte maturation (Withy et al 1992). For a comprehensive account of this aspect of kidney development see Ballie (1992).

Ascent of the kidney. When it first appears, the metanephric renal rudiment is sacral but, as the ureteric outgrowth lengthens, it becomes positioned more and more cranially so that when the embryo has a length of some 13 mm its expanded pelvis lies on a level with the second lumbar vertebra. During this period the ascending kidney receives its blood supply *sequentially* from arteries in its immediate neighbourhood, e.g. the middle sacral and common iliac arteries; the definitive *renal artery* is not recognizable until the beginning of the third month. It arises from the most caudal of the three suprarenal arteries, all of which represent persistent meso-nephric or lateral splanchnic arteries (p. 318). Additional renal arter-ies are by no means uncommon. They may enter at the hilum or at the upper or lower pole of the gland, and they also represent persistent mesonephric arteries.

Anomalies of the urinary system

Anomalies of the urinary system are relatively common (3% of live births). *Renal agenesis* is the absence of one or both kidneys. In unilateral renal agenesis, the remaining kidney undergoes com-pensatory hypertrophy producing a nearly normal functional mass of renal tissue. Problems with kidney ascent can result in a *pelvic* kidney, or the kidneys may fuse together at their caudal poles resulting in a *horseshoe* kidney which cannot ascend out of the pelvic cavity because of the proximity to the inferior mesenteric artery which prevents further migration.

Several Hox genes and the Pax 2 gene have been identified in both developing and adult kidney associated with the collecting ducts and ureter. However, this area of research is still in its developmental stage. Genes associated with maldevelopment of the kidney have received further study to date, those associated with Wilm's tumour and renal cystic disease especially (see Bard & Woolf 1992; Fouser & Avner 1993). Many varieties of cystic renal disease occur, and a number of different classifications have been proposed (see Chis-holm & Williams 1982). For long it has been held that renal cysts in most, if not all, instances result from vesicular cell clumps retained after failure of fusion between the tips of branches from the ureteric diverticulum on the one hand, and metanephrogenic cap tissue on the other. Such a view is no longer considered tenable. It has been demonstrated, convincingly, that the cyst-like formations are wide dilatations of a part of otherwise continuous nephrons (Moffat 1982). *Adult polycystic renal disease*, the commonest form, is inherited as an autosomal dominant; in this condition the dilatations may affect any part of the nephron, from Bowman's capsule to collecting tubules. Less common is *infantile cystic renal disease*, inherited as a recessive trait where the proximal and distal tubules are dilated to some degree but the collecting ducts are grossly affected.

With the routine use of ultrasound as an aid to in utero diagnosis

of abnormalities, it has been shown that of the prevalence of 1–2 abnormal fetuses per 1000 ultrasound procedures, 20–30% are anomalies of the genitourinary tract. Such abnormalities can be detected as early as 12–15 weeks gestation. However, the decision to be made after such a diagnosis is by no means clear. Urinary obstruction is considered an abnormality yet transient modest obstruction is considered a normal component of the canalization of the urinary tract and has been reported in 10–20% of fetuses in the third trimester. A delay in canalization or in the rupture of the cloacal membrane can produce such a dilatation; similarly, the closure of the urachus at 32 weeks may be associated with high-resistance outflow for the system again resulting in transient obstruc-tion. The degree to which obstruction may cause renal parenchymal damage cannot be assessed in a developing kidney which may have primary nephrogenic dysgenesis (Grupe 1987).

The volume of *amniotic fluid* is used as an indicator of renal function. Too little amniotic fluid is termed *oligohydramnios*, too much, *hydramnios*. Although variation in the amount of amniotic fluid may suggest abnormalities of either the gut or kidneys, it is not always possible to correlate even severe oligohydramnios with renal dysfunction. There is an important relationship between the volume of amniotic fluid, lung development and maturity; oligohydramnios has been shown to be associated with pulmonary hypoplasia (see p. 181, Lung development).

Ureter

Further development of the ureter has attracted less attention than that of the kidney. The ureteric wall is highly permeable at an early stage (5 mm); its lumen becomes obliterated later (13–22 mm), to be subsequently recanalized. Both processes begin at intermediate levels of the ureter and proceed cranially and caudally. The recanalization is not associated with metanephric function, but possibly with the rapid elongation of the ureter in conformity with embryonic growth. Two fusiform enlargements appear at the lumbar and pelvic levels of the ureter; the lumbar enlargement during the fifth month, the pelvic not until the ninth month (the latter is inconstant). As a result the ureter shows a constriction at its upper end (*pelviureteric region*) and another as it crosses the pelvic brim. A third narrowing is always present at its lower end and is related to the growth of the bladder wall.

At first the caudal connection of the ureter is to the dorsomedial aspect of the mesonephric duct but, owing to differential growth, the connection becomes lateral to the duct. Thereafter the caudal end of the duct becomes incorporated in the developing bladder, and the orifice of the ureter opens separately into the bladder on the lateral side of the opening of the duct. Later the two orifices become separated still further and, although the ureter retains its point of entry into the bladder, the mesonephric duct opens into that part of the urogenital sinus which subsequently becomes the prostatic urethra.

REPRODUCTIVE SYSTEM

There are essentially four different cell lineages which contribute to the gonads:

- *proliferating coelomic epithelium* on the medial side of the meso-nephroi
- underlying *mesonephric mesenchyme*
- invading *angiogenic mesenchyme* already present in the meso-nephroi
- *primordial germ cells*, derived from the epiblast very early in development, which migrate later from their sequestration in the allantoic wall.

The *genital ducts* possess an external serosa derived from coelomic epithelium, a smooth muscle muscularis derived from underlying mesenchyme (similarity of the latter to splanchnopleuric mesenchyme has not yet been investigated), and an internal mucosa from either the *mesonephric duct* or from an invaginated tube of coelomic epithelium which forms the *paramesonephric* or *Mullerian duct*. The layers are invaded by angiogenic mesenchyme and by nerves.

Mesonephric and *paramesonephric* (*Mullerian*) ducts are produced

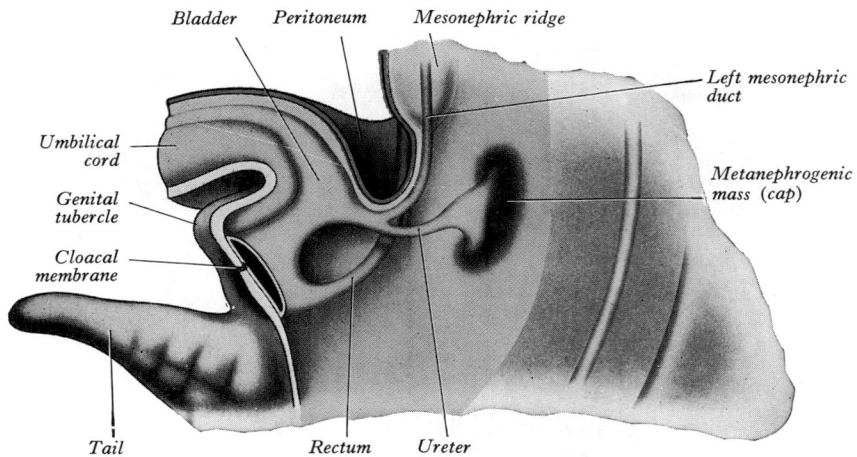

3.85 Schema, based on **3.86**D, to show the formation of the pelvis of the kidney and the metanephrogenic mass or cap.

in all embryos and at an early stage the gonadal development is termed *indifferent* or *ambisexual*. It was thought that development to one sexual phenotype or another occurred after migration of the primordial germ cells to the indifferent gonads. However, the development of male or female gonads, genital ducts and external genitalia is far more complicated, occurring as a result of a complex interplay between genetic expression, timing of development and the influence of sex hormones.

Early gonadal development (ambisexual or indifferent stage)

The formation of the gonads is first indicated by the appearance of an area of thickened coelomic epithelium on the medial side of the mesonephric ridge in the fifth week (**3.87, 88**). Elsewhere on the surface of the ridge the coelomic epithelium is one or two cells thick, but over this gonadal area it becomes many layered. The thickening rapidly extends in a longitudinal direction until it covers nearly the whole of the medial surface of the ridge. The thickened epithelium continues to proliferate, displacing the renal corpuscles of the mesonephros in a dorsolateral direction and itself forming a projection into the coelomic cavity, the *gonadal ridge*. Surface depressions form along the limits of the ridge which is thus connected to the mesonephros by an originally broad mesentery, the *mesogenitale*. In this way the mesonephric ridge becomes subdivided into a lateral part containing the mesonephric and paramesonephric ducts, which may be termed the *tubal fold*, and a medial part, termed the *gonadal fold*. The tubal fold also contains the nephric tubules and glomeruli at its base.

Up to the seventh week the ambisexual gonad possesses no sexually differentiating feature. From stage 15 the proliferating coelomic epithelium now forms a number of cellular *gonadal cords* (termed in some texts primary sex cords), separated by mesenchyme. These cords remain at the periphery of the primordium to form a cortex; more centrally a proliferation and labyrinthine cellular condensation of the mesenchyme of the mesonephros, including angiogenic mesenchyme, constitute a medulla.

Paramesonephric ducts

The paramesonephric (Mullerian) ducts initially develop in embryos of both sexes, but become dominant in the development of the **female** reproductive system; they are not detectable, however, until the embryo reaches a length of 10–12 mm (early sixth week). Development in the ambisexual period is followed by further details of the female duct maturation and finally brief notes of the limited male derivatives. Each commences as a linear invagination of the coelomic epithelium (the *paramesonephric groove*) on the lateral aspect of the mesonephric ridge near its cranial end, and its blind caudal end continues to grow caudally into the substance of the ridge as a solid rod of cells which acquires a lumen as it lengthens. Throughout the extent of the mesonephros it is *lateral* to the

mesonephric duct which acts as a guide for it. At the caudal end of the mesonephros (which it reaches in the eighth week), the paramesonephric duct turns medially (**3.89**) and crosses *ventral* to the mesonephric duct to enter the *genital cord* (**3.84**A, B), where it bends caudally in close apposition with its fellow of the opposite side. The two ducts reach the dorsal wall of the urogenital sinus during the third month, and their blind ends produce an elevation on it termed the *Mullerian sinus tubercle* (**3.89**). Each duct consists, at the end of the indifferent stage, of vertical cranial and caudal parts with an intermediate horizontal region.

In the female the cranial part forms the *uterine tube*, and its original coelomic invagination remains as the pelvic opening of the tube, the fimbriae becoming defined as the cranial end of the mesonephros degenerates. The caudal vertical parts of the two ducts fuse with each other (**3.87**B) to form the *uterovaginal primordium*. This gives rise to the lower part of the uterus and, as it enlarges, it takes in the horizontal parts to form the fundus and most of the body of the adult uterus. A constriction between the body of the uterus and the cervix can be found at 9 weeks. The stroma of the endometrium and the uterine musculature (myometrium) are developed from the surrounding mesenchyme of the genital cord.

At about 60 mm CR length an epithelial proliferation (the *sinu-vaginal bulb*) arises from the dorsal wall of the urogenital sinus in the region of the sinus tubercle, and its origin marks the site of the future hymen. Whether the epithelium involved in the proliferation is from the sinus (Bulmer 1957) or is epithelium of the mesonephric duct which has extended over the Mullerian tubercle (Vilas 1932; Meyer 1938; Forsberg 1963) is uncertain. The proliferation gradually extends cranially as a solid, anteroposteriorly flattened plate, inside the tubular mesodermal condensation of the uterovaginal primordium which will eventually become the fibromuscular *vaginal wall*. The caudal tip of the paramesonephric duct epithelium recedes until, at about the 140-mm stage, its junction with the sinus proliferation lies in the cervical canal.

Commencing from its caudal end, and gradually extending cranially through its whole extent, the solid plate formed by the sinus proliferation enlarges into a cylindrical structure; thereafter the central cells desquamate to establish the vaginal lumen. According to one view, the paramesonephric ducts do not directly contribute to the formation of the vagina (Frutiger 1969) but it has also been suggested that mesonephric and paramesonephric ducts are both concerned (Linkevich 1969). As the upper end of the vaginal plate enlarges it grows up to embrace the cervix, and then is excavated to produce the *vaginal fornices*. The urogenital sinus undergoes relative shortening craniocaudally to form the *vestibule*, which opens on the surface through the cleft between the genital folds. The lower end of the vaginal plate grows caudally so that in 105-mm embryos the vaginal rudiment approaches the vestibule. It was thought that tissue added to the vaginal plate was pushed cephalically from the caudal end of the vaginal plate; however, Witchi (1970) suggested that the

205

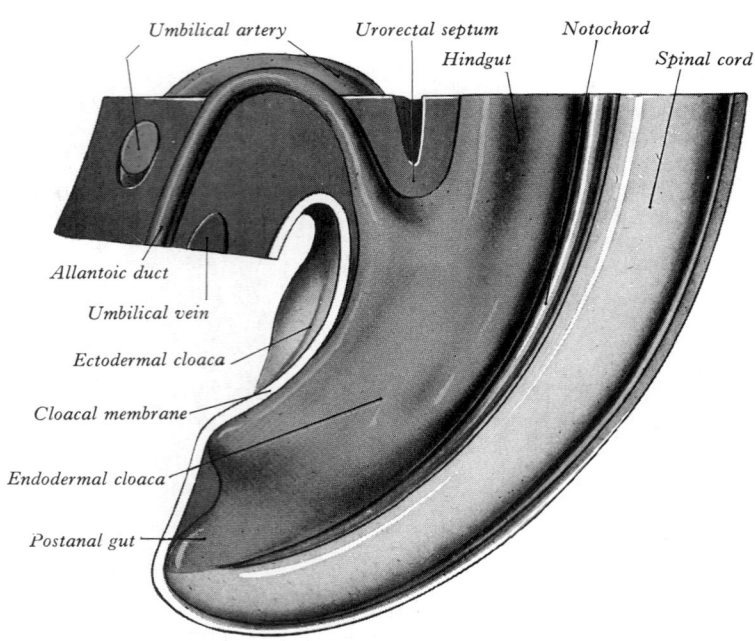

Umbilical artery   *Urorectal septum*   *Notochord*
Hindgut   *Spinal cord*

Allantoic duct

Umbilical vein

Ectodermal cloaca

Cloacal membrane

Endodermal cloaca

Postanal gut

3.86A   The tail end of a human embryo, about 4 weeks old. The model has been dissected to show the left lateral aspects of the spinal cord, notochord and endodermal cloaca. (After Keibel.)

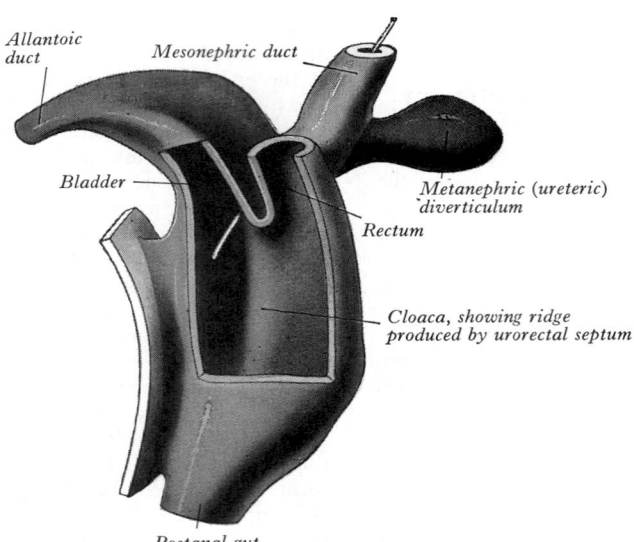

Allantoic duct   *Mesonephric duct*

Bladder

Metanephric (ureteric) diverticulum

Rectum

Cloaca, showing ridge produced by urorectal septum

Postanal gut

3.86B   The endodermal cloaca of a human embryo, near the end of the fifth week. A wire has been passed along the right mesonephric duct into the cloaca and a part of the left wall of the cloaca, including the left mesonephric duct, has been removed, together with the adjoining portions of the walls of the developing bladder and rectum. A piece of the ectoderm around the cloacal membrane has been left in situ and is uncoloured. (After Keibel.)

lower end of the vagina moves along the urethra to a separate opening in the vestibule. In fetuses of 162 mm the vaginal lumen is complete except at the cephalic end where the fornices are still solid; they are hollow by 170 mm. At approximately half way through gestation (180 mm) the genital canal is continuous with the exterior.

During the later months of fetal life the vaginal epithelium is enormously hypertrophied, apparently under the influence of maternal hormones, but after birth it assumes the inactive form of childhood (Fraenkel & Papanicolaou 1938).

The differing embryonic origins of the vaginal epithelium and uterine epithelium have been correlated with their dissimilar responses in adult life to stimulation with oestrogenic hormones (Zuckerman 1940).

In the male the paramesonephric duct mostly atrophies under the influence of *anti-Mullerian hormone* (AMH) (see p. 208) which is

released locally by the Sertoli cells of the testis (see below); thus persisting vestigial structures are most likely cranially and caudally at the limits of the local effects of AMH. A vestige of the cranial end of the duct persists as the *appendix testis* (p. 1848). The fused caudal ends of the two ducts are connected to the wall of the urogenital sinus by a solid *utricular cord* of cells. In this position it soon merges with a proliferation of sinus epithelium, the *sinu-utricular cord*, similar to, but less extensive than, the sinus proliferation in the female. This proliferating epithelium is claimed to be an intermingling of the endoderm of the urogenital sinus with the lining epithelia of the mesonephric and paramesonephric ducts, which have extended on to the surface of the sinus tubercle. As the sinu-utricular cord grows, so the utricular cord recedes from the tubercle. In the second half of fetal life the composite cord acquires a lumen and dilates to form the *prostatic utricle*, the lining of which consists

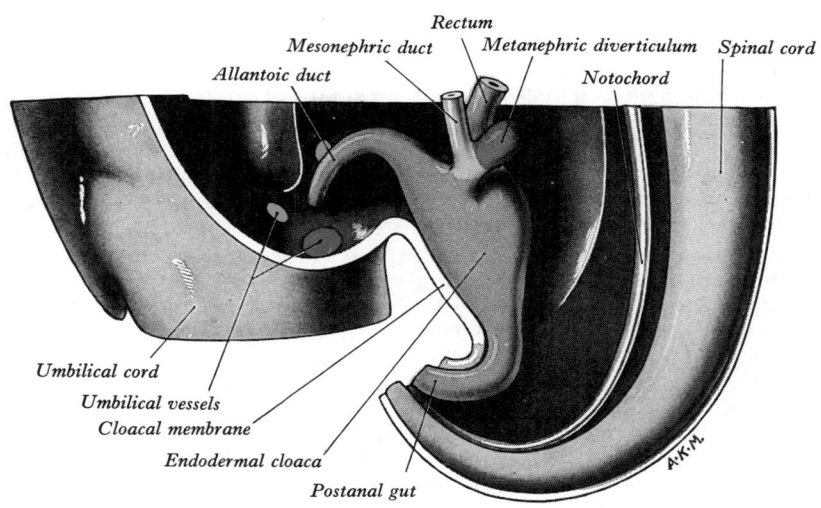

3.86c The caudal end of a human embryo, about 5 weeks old. (Drawn from a model by Keibel.)

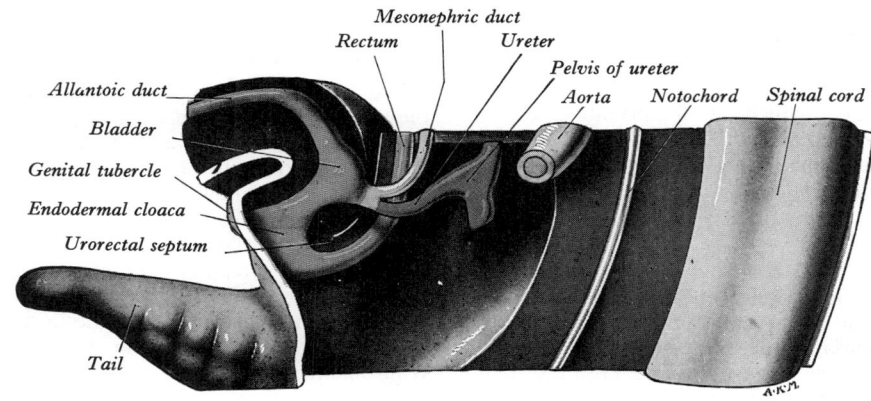

3.86d Part of the caudal end of a human embryo, about 6 weeks old. (Drawn from a model by Keibel, which has been partly dissected and is seen from the left side.)

of hyperplastic stratified squamous epithelium. The sinus tubercle becomes the *colliculus seminalis* (Vilas 1933; Glenister 1962).

Primordial germ cells

The primordial germ cells are formed very early from the epiblast, as demonstrated at the 2-somite stage in the chick (Clawson & Domm 1969). They are large cells, in comparison with most somatic cells, being from 12 to 20 μm in diameter, and characterized by vesicular nuclei with well-defined nuclear membranes and by a tendency to retain yolk inclusions long after these have disappeared from somatic cells. (For the ultrastructure of human primordial germ cells consult Fukuda 1976.) It is not yet established whether the primordial germ cells are derived from particular blastomeres during cleavage, if they constitute a clonal line from a single blastomere or are the product of a progressive concentration of the nucleus of the fertilized ovum by unequal partition of this at successive mitoses (Bounoure 1939). Primordial germ cells spend the early stages of development within the extraembryonic tissues near the end of the primitive streak and in the connecting stalk. In this situation they are away from the inductive influences affecting the majority of the somatic cells during early development.

Primordial germ cells can be identified in human embryos in stage 11 when the number of cells is probably not more than 20–30 (Hardisty 1967). When the tail fold has formed they appear within the endoderm and the splanchnopleuric mesenchyme and epithelium

of the hindgut as well as in the adjoining region of the wall of the yolk sac. By amoeboid movements and by growth displacement they migrate dorsocranially in the mesentery, passing around the dorsal angles of the coelom (medial coelomic bays) to reach the genital ridges from stage 15. It is believed that the genital ridges exert long-range effects on the migrating primordial germ cells which control their direction of migration and help support the primordial germ cell population.

In most vertebrates, mitosis in the germ cells is arrested after their early segregation to be renewed only when they reach the genital primordia. However, in mammals there is no such arrest and the cells proliferate both during and after migration to the mesonephric ridges; cells which do not complete this migration degenerate. After segregation the primordial germ cells are often termed *primary gonocytes*, which in turn divide for form secondary gonocytes. The distinction between the two generations is clear in most vertebrates, but the absence of mitotic arrest in mammals leads to a merging of the two stages.

While sexual differences in germ cell numbers occur in some vertebrate species, it is uncertain whether this represents an original difference at segregation or results from earlier and more rapid proliferation in one sex. No connection between numbers of primordial germ cells and fertility has been detected, but there is evidence that gross deficiency in number may affect individual fecundity (Hardisty 1967) (see also p. 211).

DEVELOPMENT OF THE GONADS

The factors which lead to formation of either testis or ovary are presented below and on page 210. The morphological events occurring in each type of gonadal development are presented first.

Testis

The majority of studies support the hypothesis that the seminiferous tubules are formed from lines of epithelial cells derived from the proliferating coelomic epithelium (but also see below). The epithelial cords (3.87) lengthen partly by additions from the coelomic epithelium and encroach on the medulla, where they unite with the network derived from the mesenchyme which ultimately becomes the *testicular rete*. The primordial germ cells are incorporated into the cords, which later become enlarged and canalized to form the seminiferous tubules (see Fukuda & Hedinger 1975). The cells derived from the surface of the early gonad form the *supporting cells* (of Sertoli). The *interstitial cells* of the testis are derived from mesenchyme and possibly also from coelomic epithelial cells which do not become incorporated into the tubules; they form, among other cells lines, the embryonic and fetal cells of Leydig which secrete testosterone. A later migration of mesenchyme beneath the coelomic epithelium forms the *tunica albuginea* of the testis. The cords of the rete testis, which canalize later, become connected to the glomerular capsules in the persisting part of the mesonephros. The rete cords ultimately become connected to the mesonephric duct by the five to twelve most cranial persisting mesonephric tubules and these become exceedingly convoluted and form the lobules of the head of the epididymis. The mesonephric duct, which was the primitive 'ureter' of the mesonephros, becomes the canal of the *epididymis* and the *ductus deferens* of the testis. The seminiferous tubules do not acquire lumina until the seventh month, but the tubules of the testicular rete do somewhat earlier.

Ovary

In its earliest stages, the ovary closely resembles the testis, although it is slower to differentiate its characteristically female features (3.87). Few, if any, of the gonadal cords invade the medulla, the majority remaining in the cortex, where they may be joined by a second proliferation from the epithelium overlying the gonad. In sections of the ovary in the third and subsequent months the cords appear as clusters of cells which may or may not contain primitive germ cells. These clusters are separated by fine septa of undifferentiated mesenchyme. An *ovarian rete* condenses in the medullary mesenchyme and some of its cords may form a junction with mesonephric glomeruli. The medulla subsequently regresses, and connective tissue and blood vessels from this region invade the cortex to form the stroma of the ovary. During this invasion the cortical cell clusters break into individual groups which surround the primordial germ cells, now *primary oöcytes*, which have entered the prophase of the first meiotic division. These cells were derived from a mitotic division of the primordial germ cells (*naked oögonia*). Their epithelial capsules consist of flattened *pregranulosa cells* derived from proliferations of coelomic epithelium (Gillman 1948). The ovary now has its *full complement* of primary oöcytes. The majority undergo atresia at various stages during their development, but the remainder resume development by completing the first meiotic division shortly before ovulation (see p. 123). The capsular cells at the same time enlarge and multiply to form the *stratum granulosum*, and as they do so they become surrounded by *thecal cells* which differentiate from the stroma.

Only the middle part of the gonadal ridge produces the ovary. Its cranial part is sterile and becomes the *suspensory ligament of the ovary* (infundibulopelvic fold of peritoneum). Its caudal region, also sterile, is incorporated in the *ovarian ligament*.

A study by Satoh (1991) disputes the origin of the cell lines responsible for production of the *gonadal supporting cells*, i.e. the Sertoli cells of the seminiferous tubules and the follicular cells of the ovary. After examination of serially sectioned human gonads from 5 weeks (stage 14) to 13 weeks gestational age, Satoh noted the initial proliferation of the *coelomic epithelium* which formed '*primary sex cords*'. He further identified epithelial cells subsequently emerging from the distal ends of the *mesonephric tubules* where the basal lamina is absent, terming these '*primordial sex cords*'; they branch

from the mesonephros towards the coelomic epithelium, although there is no continuity between these cells and the coelomic epithelium. He notes that the basal lamina of each primordial sex cord is contiguous with that of the mesonephros. He interprets the coelomic proliferation and production of the primary sex cords of coelomic cells as a preparation for the prominent protrusion of the gonad into the coelom which occurs rapidly, within half a day (from late week 5 to early week 6), after which the coelomic cells are arranged two or three cells deep with a basal lamina.

If the above description is upheld by other studies, the rete cords in the testis may be reinterpreted as outgrowths of the mesonephric tubules which are proliferating to produce the primordial sex cords. In ovarian development Satoh (1991) describes primordial sex cords, similar to those in the developing testis, originating from the mesonephros but notes they display an incomplete basal lamina. Later the primordial sex cords are displaced into the cortex. Satoh noted no secondary proliferation of the coelomic epithelium into the cortex of the ovary.

The extent of the mesonephric contribution to the gonads has been examined in the mouse and rabbit but as yet no clear conclusion as to the origin of the primary sex cords and Sertoli cells has been formed (Waternberg et al 1991; Buehr et al 1993). It is anticipated that immunohistochemical techniques will reveal the origin of the cells which ultimately surround the primordial germ cells. Further confirmation of this work is awaited with interest.

Sex determination in the embryo

It was believed that the gonads were indifferent or ambisexual until the arrival of the primordial germ cells in the gonadal ridge, when the sex of the embryo was 'turned on' by the presence of the male or female germ cells. It now seems that the germ cells may be essentially irrelevant to *testis determination*; embryos in which the genital ridges are devoid of germ cells may still have morphologically normal testis development (McLaren 1985). It is not clear if the germ cells are necessary for ovarian determination; however, they **are** required for the proper organization and differentiation of the ovary: their absence results in the development of 'streak gonads', where only lines of follicular cells can be seen, as in Turner's syndrome (see p. 122).

The processes of sex determination and differentiation are now seen to involve interacting pathways of gene activity which lead to the total patterning of the embryo to one or other sex. In one model of determination in humans, the female pathway is considered the default pathway; the Y chromosome of a male embryo diverts development into the testicular pathway and the resultant changes of the indifferent gonad to a testis produces a range of local and widely acting hormones which generate all the secondary sexual characteristics. (For a different model see Gilbert 1991.) The possession of a Y chromosome is usually associated with a male developmental pathway. The male determining region of the Y chromosome is located near its tip and termed the *testis-determining factor* (TDF). This is regarded by some workers as the 'master switch' which programmes the direction of sexual development. It is suggested that the TDF acts initially within the population of cells which will form the sex cords of the ambisexual gonad; these will differentiate into the support cells for the germ cells in both testis and ovary. TDF alters their subsequent development away from that of the female default pathway (i.e. into follicular cells) to that of Sertoli cells (Burgoyne et al 1988; Palmer & Burgoyne 1991). The Sertoli cells then influence the differentiation of the other cell types in the testicular pathway, e.g. Leydig cells appear some time later, and the connective tissue becomes organized into a male pattern. The germ cells are also affected by this environment when they arrive: they become enclosed within the Sertoli cells and thus enter mitotic arrest which is characteristic of spermatogenesis, instead of entering meiosis and meiotic arrest which is seen in oögenesis.

Subsequent differentiation into the male line is caused by the production of two factors: Sertoli cells make AMH (also called *Mullerian inhibiting substance* or MIS), which causes the regression of the Mullerian ducts (Josso & Picard 1986); Leydig cells produce testosterone which promotes the development of the mesonephric ducts (Grumbach & Ducharme 1960), sets into process the development of male external genitalia and sensitizes other tissues to testosterone (see below—descent of the testis). Thus the development

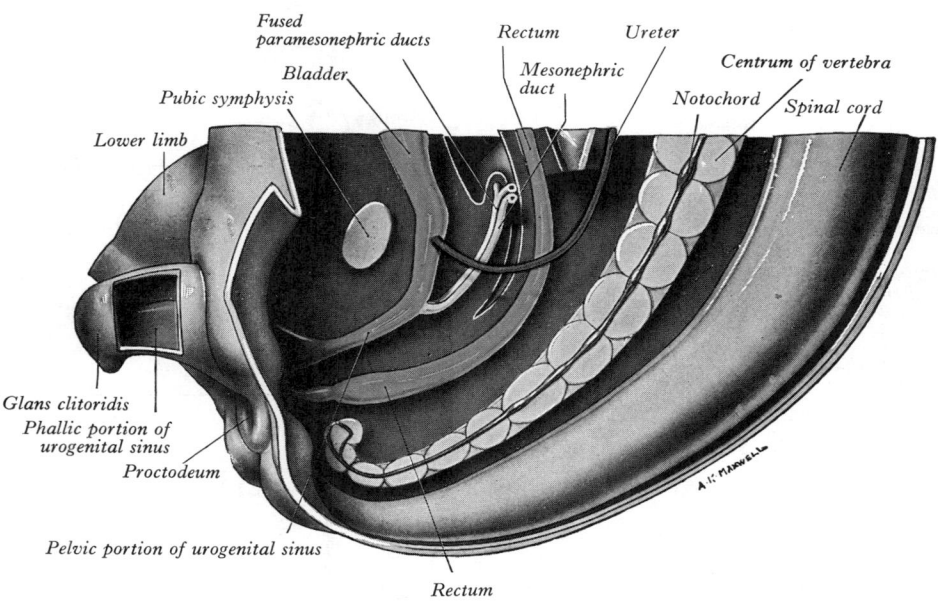

Fused paramesonephric ducts
Bladder
Pubic symphysis
Lower limb
Rectum
Mesonephric duct
Ureter
Centrum of vertebra
Notochord
Spinal cord
Glans clitoridis
Phallic portion of urogenital sinus
Proctodeum
Pelvic portion of urogenital sinus
Rectum

3.87A The tail end of a female human fetus, $8\frac{1}{2}$–9 weeks old. The model has been dissected from the left side to show the structures in and near the median plane. Note that the cloaca has now been separated into urogenital and intestinal segments. (After Keibel.)

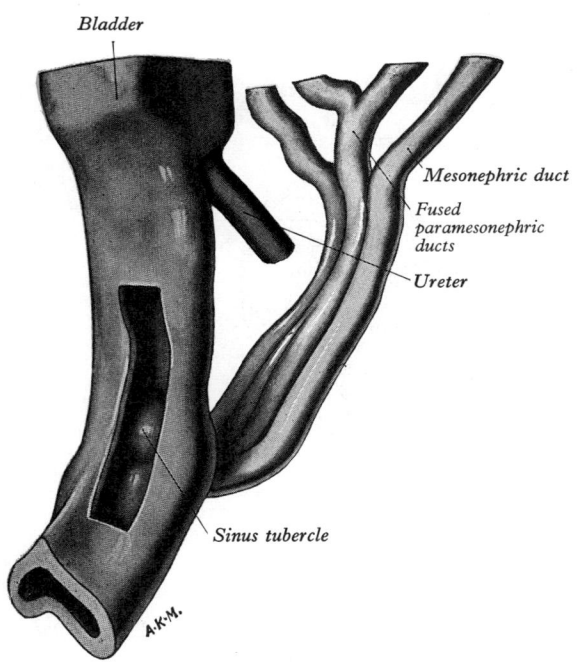

Bladder
Mesonephric duct
Fused paramesonephric ducts
Ureter
Sinus tubercle

3.87B Part of the vesico-urethral portion of the endodermal cloaca of a female human fetus, $8\frac{1}{2}$–9 weeks old. (Drawn from a model by Keibel.)

of male characteristics follows the expression of TDF, and female characteristics develop in its absence. Sex determination in mammals thus may be initiated by a signal which switches on TDF.

Further studies on the exact position of the TDF have been based on deletion mapping the Y chromosome in a class of XX males that arise from abnormal X:Y interchange at meiosis (Petit et al 1987). A conserved sequence that mapped to the Y chromosome of all mammals tested was found. The sequence formed part of a gene in the *Sex determining Region of the Y chromosome* and was thus termed SRY (see also p. 211). It is believed to be genetically and functionally equivalent to TDF. In the mouse, this gene (termed Sry) has been demonstrated, by cells in the genital ridge only, for a brief

period before testis differentiation. This gene has also been seen in mutant strains which lack germ cells, indicating that the gene is expressed in a somatic cell line within the genital ridge. The potential of the Sry gene was demonstrated by injecting it into fertilized mouse eggs which were reimplanted and allowed to develop. Examination of the gonads showed testes developing in chromosomal female animals indicating that Sry alone is able to initiate male development in a chromosomally female embryo (Koopman et al 1991). Interestingly it is also suggested that there must be other genes required for the development of the male phenotype that reside on chromosomes **other** than the Y (Lovell-Badge 1992).

Although the possession of a Y chromosome expressing SRY and TDF is, in many studies, seen as the fundamental cause of the switch to male phenotypic development, by initiating Sertoli cell differentiation, other studies have suggested that the possession of TDF **accelerates** the development of the gonads in XY embryos generally, so that testes are larger and more advanced than ovaries of the same age (Mittwoch 1988).

At the time of Sertoli cell differentiation in mice, the gonads of XY fetuses are on average 40% larger than their XX littermates, suggesting that the putative testes grow faster than putative ovaries before any morphological differentiation can be seen. Bovine male embryos generally develop to more advanced stages than do females during the first 8 days after insemination in vitro, well before gonadal differentiation (Xu et al 1992). Male human fetuses are generally bigger than females from 12 weeks gestation, and males are already slightly ahead of females at six weeks gestation just prior to testicular differentiation; it is suggested that this difference in the growth rate is encoded in the sex chromosomes (Pedersen 1980). Once gonadal development has commenced the difference in size between testes and ovaries becomes much greater than the difference between XY and XX fetuses as a whole. (Interestingly, the right gonad develops slightly ahead of the left, an observation which correlates with hermaphrodite development in which testes are more often on the right side and ovaries on the left.)

Mittwoch (1988) suggests that whereas in poikilotherms the sex of the embryo is determined by the temperature of incubation, homoiothermic animals have evolved a genetic mechanism to make sex determination independent of the environmental temperature. As mammals also have an in utero environment which receives female hormones from the mother, the accelerated development of the testis at the early embryological stages ensures arrest of meiosis of the germ cells and the production of local hormones which

INDIFFERENT STAGES

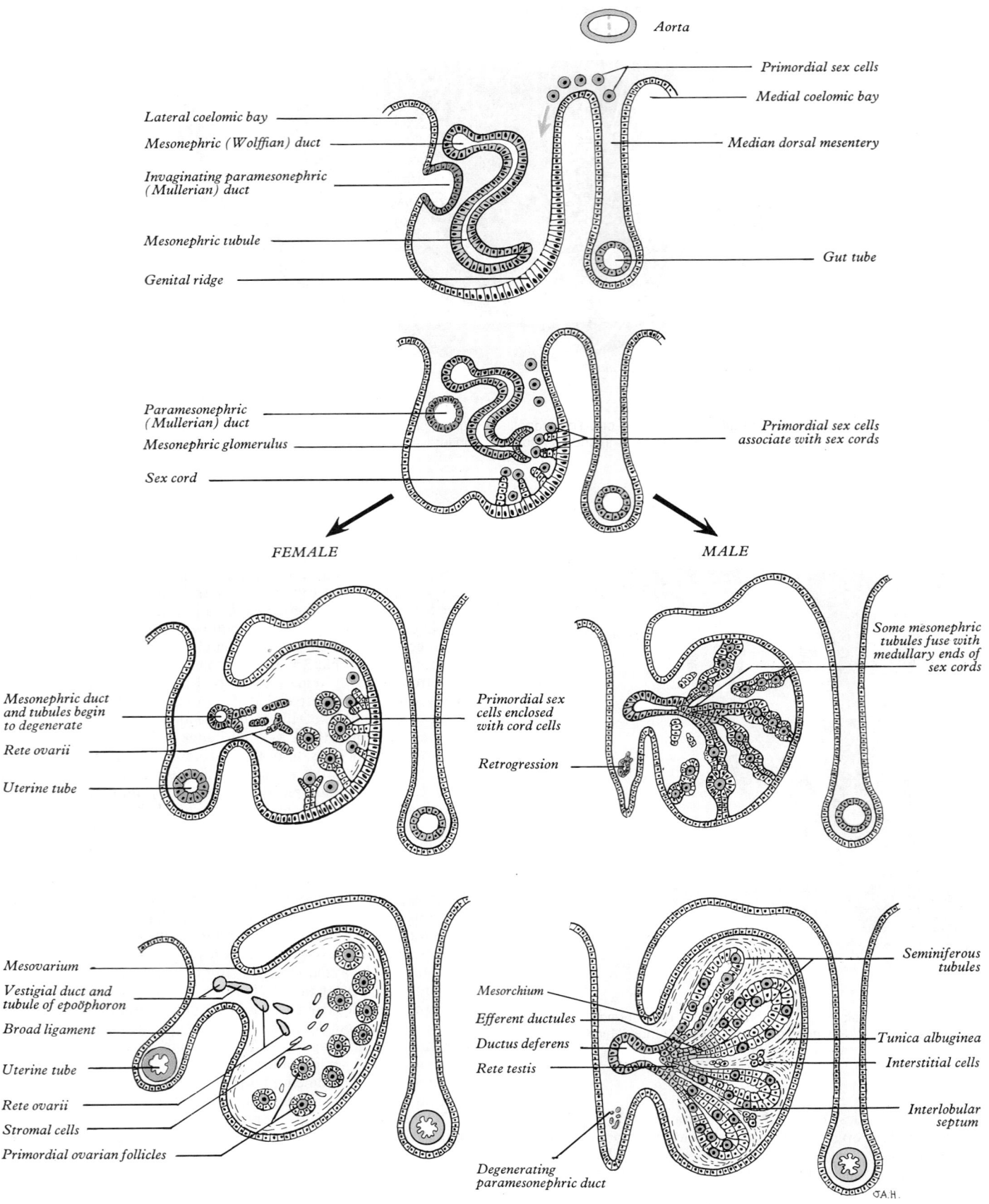

Aorta

Primordial sex cells

Medial coelomic bay

Lateral coelomic bay

Mesonephric (Wolffian) duct

Median dorsal mesentery

Invaginating paramesonephric (Mullerian) duct

Mesonephric tubule

Genital ridge

Gut tube

Paramesonephric (Mullerian) duct

Mesonephric glomerulus

Sex cord

Primordial sex cells associate with sex cords

FEMALE

MALE

Mesonephric duct and tubules begin to degenerate

Rete ovarii

Uterine tube

Primordial sex cells enclosed with cord cells

Some mesonephric tubules fuse with medullary ends of sex cords

Retrogression

Mesovarium

Vestigial duct and tubule of epoöphoron

Broad ligament

Uterine tube

Rete ovarii

Stromal cells

Primordial ovarian follicles

Seminiferous tubules

Mesorchium

Efferent ductules

Ductus deferens

Rete testis

Tunica albuginea

Interstitial cells

Interlobular septum

Degenerating paramesonephric duct

3.88   Schema of the development of the gonads and associated ducts as seen in transverse section. Note fate of primordial sex cells, mesonephric duct and tubules and paramesonephric duct in the two sexes.

masculinize the male embryo before the normal time for development of the reproductive tract and ovaries of the female.

The early expression of Sry has been demonstrated in the mouse embryo where two sex-determining regions, Sry and Zfy, are transcribed during preimplantation development, as early as the two-cell stage (Zwingman et al 1993).

The range of intersex conditions, of phenotypic sex which is not correlated to genotype, and the effect of multiple X chromosomes in males suggest that there may be many testis determining genes necessary for the male developmental pathway but only a single X chromosome for the female default pathway (Mittwoch 1992). Certainly once testicular differentiation and male hormone secretion have begun, other Y-chromosomal genes are required to maintain spermatogenesis and complete spermiogenesis. The impairment of oögenesis, by other chromosomal abnormalities, is much less severe than the impairment of spermatogenesis.

The source of the X chromosome may be an important factor in this paradigm; in mice a paternally derived X chromosome has been shown to have a retarding effect on development (Thornhill & Burgoyne 1993). More work in this area is awaited with interest.

Environmental effects on gonadal development

Disorders of development of the testis and reproductive tract in the male fetus are increasing in incidence. Testicular maldescent (cryptorchidism) and hypospadias appear to have doubled or trebled in incidence in the last 30–50 years, according to the best evidence (Giwercman & Skakkebaek 1992; Sharpe & Skakkebaek 1993), whilst testicular cancer has increased by an even greater margin to become now the commonest cancer of young men (Skakkebaek et al 1993). Although testicular cancer is primarily a disease of young men (95% of cases affect 15–45-year-old males) it is now established that this age-incidence reflects activation of pre-malignant carcinoma-in-situ (CIS) cells which are present at birth and which almost certainly arise during fetal life (Skakkebaek 1987; Skakkebaek et al 1993). Current opinion is that these CIS cells are primordial germ cells which have failed to develop normally. It is of interest that abnormalities of development of the testis and reproductive tract (e.g. gonadal dysgenesis, cryptorchidism, small testes) are important risk factors for the development of testicular cancer (Giwercman & Skakkebaek 1992; Brown et al 1992). However, the most dramatic change that appears to have occurred over the past 50 or so years is a fall in sperm counts in man of around 40–50% (Carlsen et al 1992). Although this dramatic decrease is obviously manifest only in adulthood, as with testicular cancer, the most likely explanation is impaired testicular development during fetal or childhood life (Sharpe 1993: Sharpe & Skakkebaek 1993).

The **Sertoli cells** are one of the first specialized somatic cells of the putative testis (see above); they briefly express Sex determining Region of the Y chromosome (SRY) before testis differentiation commences. Sertoli cells proliferate during these early stages and continue to do so for some or perhaps all of subsequent childhood life (Cortes et al 1987; Sharpe 1994); when replication ceases the Sertoli cells mature and cannot be reactivated. The importance of this period of Sertoli cell proliferation lies in the fact that each Sertoli cell can only support a fixed number of germ cells during their development into spermatozoa, i.e. the number of Sertoli cells produced at this time determines the maximal limit of sperm output (Sharpe 1994). Additionally, because it is the germ cells which comprise the bulk of the adult testis, then the number of Sertoli cells also predetermines the size to which the testes will grow; however, it should be kept in mind that factors which impair the process of spermatogenesis, resulting in the loss of germ cells, will also affect testicular size.

Studies in a range of laboratory and domestic animals have shown that differences in the number of Sertoli cells is the primary determinant of differences in testicular size and sperm output between species, between strains and between individuals (Sharpe 1994). The same is true for man: variation in Sertoli cell number is probably the most important factor in accounting for the enormous variation in sperm counts between individual men, whether fertile or infertile (MacLeod & Gold 1951; Carlsen et al 1992). Indeed, the available data for adult men indicates that Sertoli cell numbers vary across a 50-fold range (Johnson et al 1984). Although some of this variation may result from attrition of Sertoli cell numbers because of ageing (Johnson et al 1984), the major differences in Sertoli cell numbers will have been determined by events in fetal and/or childhood life (Sharpe 1994).

Sharpe (1994) has raised the question as to whether the reported 50% fall in sperm counts in men over the last half-century might be due to a secular decrease in the number of Sertoli cells. There are no data on comparative Sertoli cell numbers from 50 years ago. Alterations of Sertoli cell numbers, whether up or down, would not alter the quality of the spermatozoa produced and, histologically, such testes with lower Sertoli cell numbers could not be distinguished from those with higher numbers—only their overall size would be different (Sharpe 1994). Thus, the absence of any dramatic increase in the incidence of male infertility over the last half-century would not be inconsistent with a decease in Sertoli cell numbers over the same time period. However, other early events controlled by the Sertoli cells (testicular maldescent, masculinization, germ cell development) appear to be affecting an increasing proportion of human males. Comparable effects are also occurring in a range of wildlife (Colborn & Clements 1992), suggesting that environmental factors are most likely to blame. Sharpe (1994) suggests that *environmental oestrogens* may be the most likely causal agent, but warns that there is as yet no definitive proof that this is the case.

It is well established that administration of exogenous oestrogens to pregnant animals during the period when testicular differentiation and 'masculinization' are occurring in the male fetus will lead to abnormalities in these processes, resulting in increased risk of cryptorchidism and hypospadias at birth and smaller testes and reduced sperm counts in adult life (Arai et al 1983; Greco et al 1993; Sharpe & Skakkebaek 1993). The same is true for man, based on studies of the male offspring (Whitehead & Leiter 1981; Stillman 1982) of some of the 6 million women worldwide who were administered diethylstilboestrol (DES), in the period 1945–70, in the belief that it would prevent miscarriage. The basis for these oestrogen-induced abnormalities has not been fully worked out, but it is probably significant that testicular differentiation and masculinization are very early events occurring at a time when oestrogen levels in the maternal circulation are still relatively low (Tulchinsky et al 1972; Tulchinsky & Hobel 1973).

Sharpe and Skakkebaek (1993) suggest that there has been a generally increased human exposure to oestrogens over the past 50 years. This has been caused by changes in diet and body composition (more fat), leading to increased exposure of women to their own oestrogens (Adlercreutz 1990), and increased exposure to environmental oestrogens, the most important of which are a range of ubiquitous, pollutant chemicals which, when ingested, mimic the effects of oestrogens in the body by interacting with the receptors for oestradiol. Pesticides such as DDT (and its metabolite DDE) and other widely distributed compounds such as polychlorinated biphenyls (PCBs), though their use is now largely banned, continue to accumulate in living organisms because of their fat solubility. The bioaccumulation is a feature of many chlorinated hydrocarbons, several of which appear to be oestrogenic (Hileman 1993). More recently, degradation products of non-ionic surfactants (used widely in commercial detergents) have also been shown to be oestrogenic and these again are widely distributed, bioaccumulative and are present in some water sources and food chains (Clark et al 1992; Zoller 1993). It remains unknown whether the level of human exposure to such oestrogenic chemicals is sufficient to exert adverse effects on reproductive development of the early male fetus or developing child, but the increasing prevalence of such disorders in man and wildlife provides at least circumstantial support for this possibility (Sharpe & Skakkebaek 1993). More definitive evidence should become available in the next few years.

Sharpe (1994) urges that irrespective of whether increased human exposure to oestrogens is responsible for the increasing incidence of male reproductive abnormalities, it must be noted that reproductive ability of the adult human male is, to a considerable extent, predetermined by events in fetal life and/or childhood. He perceives a fairly urgent need for increased understanding of these early processes and their vulnerability to an altered hormonal milieu, in order that their importance in determining subsequent male fertility/infertility can be understood.

Descent of the gonads

Descent of the testis. This is **not** merely a simple migration. At first the testis lies on the dorsal abdominal wall, but, as it enlarges, its cranial end degenerates and the remaining organ therefore occupies a more caudal position. It is attached to the mesonephric fold by a peritoneal fold, the *mesorchium* (3.82) (the mesogenitale of the undifferentiated gonad), which contains the testicular vessels and nerves and a quantity of undifferentiated mesenchyme. In addition, it acquires a secondary attachment to the ventral abdominal wall, which has a considerable influence on its subsequent movements. At the point where the mesonephric fold bends medially to form the genital cord (p. 200), it becomes connected to the lower part of the ventral abdominal wall by an *inguinal fold* of peritoneum (3.84). The mesenchymal cells occupying the core of the inguinal fold condense as another cord, the *gubernaculum*, extending from the epidermal ectoderm which will later form the scrotum, through the inguinal fold and the mesorchium to the caudal pole of the testis. It traverses the site of the future inguinal canal, which is formed around it by the muscles of the abdominal wall as they differentiate. At the end of the second month the caudal part of the ventral abdominal wall is horizontal but, after the return of the intestine to the peritoneal cavity (p. 334), it grows in length and progressively becomes vertical. As a result, the umbilical artery pulls up a falciform peritoneal fold, as it runs ventrally from the dorsal to the ventral wall, and this forms the medial boundary of a peritoneal fossa into which the testis projects. This fossa is the *saccus vaginalis* or *lateral inguinal fossa* (p. 1737) and its lower end protrudes down the inguinal canal along the ventrosuperior aspect of the gubernaculum, as the *processus vaginalis*. The caudal pole of the testis is *retained* in apposition with the deep inguinal ring by the gubernaculum until the seventh month, when it abruptly and rapidly passes through the inguinal canal and gains the scrotum. As it descends it is necessarily accompanied by its peritoneal covering, and the adjoining peritoneum from the iliac fossa is drawn down into the processus vaginalis. The distal end of the processus vaginalis, into which the testis projects, forms the *tunica vaginalis testis* but the portion associated with the spermatic cord in the scrotum and in the inguinal canal normally becomes obliterated, usually leaving a fibrous remnant. Sometimes the remnant atrophies completely. Alternatively, its original cavity may persist in whole or in part and in any location. These variations may form the walls of hernial sacs or encysted fluid sites.

The mechanism of the descent of the testis has variously been ascribed, by different investigators, to shortening and active contraction of the gubernaculum, to increased intra-abdominal pressure, to a simple growth process and to the effect on the convex surface of the gland of the active contraction of the lower fibres of the internal oblique muscle, squeezing it through the canal. The gubernaculum precedes the testis both spatially and in rate of growth, forming a tapering column of soft tissue with the diminutive testis at its cranial pole. It continues to grow until the seventh month, by which time its caudal part has filled the future inguinal canal and has begun to expand the developing scrotum. In this it also precedes the processus vaginalis, but does not develop attachments to skin; nor is there any evidence that it produces the radiating extensions into the suprapubic, perineal and femoral sites, which are often used as explanations for the various forms of ectopia testis. By its soft consistency the gubernacular tissue (which in the early stage is formed mainly of hyaluronic acid) may offer a route of low resistance to the descending testis, and the cessation of its growth in the last two months of gestation, coupled with an accelerating rate of growth in the testis and epididymis, may also be a factor in testicular descent as far as the inguinal canal.

The mechanism of final, rapid descent into the scrotum is not yet clear. Endocrine effects seem certain, but this does not explain the actual agency. This account is based principally upon events as observed in porcine material by Backhouse and Butler (1960). A subsequent discussion of the problems of testicular descent and maldescent by Backhouse (1964) should be consulted. He had reviewed the literature since Hunter's original description (1762). Apparently the cremaster muscle develops in gubernacular mesenchyme and this may explain the development of the concept of the gubernaculum as a 'fibromuscular' ligament.

In the rat it has been shown that the gubernaculum is highly contractile during testicular descent. In the inguinoscrotal phase of descent the gubernaculum loses its hyaluronic acid, the cremasteric muscle develops and the processus vaginalis elongates. These processes are dependent on androgens, but attempts to isolate androgen receptors on the gubernaculum have, as yet, been unsuccessful. Division of the genitofemoral nerve, however, prevents both the inguinoscrotal testicular descent and differentiation and migration of the gubernaculum, suggesting that androgens acting on the nerve cell bodies of the genitofemoral nerve in the spinal cord could cause release of neurotransmitters from the nerve endings that might act as second messengers for androgens (Beasley & Hutson 1988). A peptide neurotransmitter, *calcitonin gene-related peptide* (CGRP), is present in the genitofemoral nerve and its cell bodies in the spinal cord. CGRP causes the gubernacula from newborn male mice to contract rhythmically; CGRP antagonists inhibit this contraction (Park & Hutson 1991). It is suggested that one of the effects of testosterone during gestation is to 'masculinize' the genitofemoral nerve by increasing the number of cells contributing to it. One cause of non-descent of the testes may be a result of insufficient testosterone during development resulting in a failure to produce enough nerve cells in the genitofemoral nerve; then, at the time of testicular migration, too little CGRP is produced to stimulate contractions in the gubernaculum and assist testicular descent.

Abnormalities of testicular descent. The testis may remain in the abdomen, or it may fail to reach the scrotum and may then lie in any of the following situations:

- in the perineum
- at the root of the penis
- at the superficial inguinal ring (p. 1855)
- in the upper part of the thigh.

These malpositions have been traditionally associated with certain additional extensions of gubernacular tissue. The largest extension normally passes to the scrotum while lesser extensions have been described as gaining attachment to the perineum, the root of the penis, the pubis, the inguinal ligament and the neighbourhood of the saphenous opening. The testis must follow the processus vaginalis and, should the latter for any reason follow any but the scrotal extension of the gubernaculum, malposition of the testis will result. It should be appreciated, however, that considerable doubt has now been expressed concerning these lesser expansions (previously the so-called 'tails of Lockwood'): possibly these reflect premature and abnormal fibrous partitioning of the gubernacular mesenchyme.

As noted, the processus vaginalis may remain completely patent, or its obliteration may be incomplete. When it retains a connection with the general peritoneal cavity it provides a preformed sac for a potential oblique inguinal hernia. It may be occluded at its upper end and may be shut off from the tunica vaginalis and yet remain patent in the intervening section. The patent portion may become distended with fluid, an *encysted hydrocoele* of the spermatic cord.

Descent of the ovary. This is less extensive than the testis. Like the testis, the ovary ultimately reaches a lower level than it occupies in the early months of fetal life but it does not leave the pelvis to enter the inguinal canal, except in certain anomalies. Connected to the medial aspect of the mesonephric fold by the *mesovarium* (homologous with the mesorchium), the ovary is also attached to the ventral abdominal wall through the medium of the inguinal fold. In this fold a mesenchymatous gubernaculum also develops but, as it traverses the mesonephric fold, it acquires an additional attachment to the lateral margin of the uterus near the entrance of the uterine tube. Its lower part, caudal to this uterine attachment, becomes the *round ligament of the uterus* and the part cranial to this the *ovarian ligament*, these structures together being homologous with the gubernaculum testis in the male. This new uterine attachment may be correlated with the restricted ovarian descent. At first the ovary is attached to the medial side of the mesonephric fold but, in accordance with the manner in which the two mesonephric folds form the genital cord (p. 200), its connection is finally to the posterior layer of the broad ligament of the uterus. The gubernaculum thus persists in the female, unlike the male, as **two** fibrous bands or ligaments on each side. The gubernaculum ovarii does not contract as a response to CGRP (see above).

The *saccus vaginalis* also appears in the female; its prolongation into the inguinal canal (sometimes termed the *canal of Nuck*) normally undergoes complete obliteration, but may remain patent and form the sac of a potential oblique inguinal hernia (p. 1788). *At birth* the ovary and the lateral end of the corresponding uterine tube lie above the pelvic brim, and they do not sink into the lesser pelvis until the latter enlarges sufficiently to contain both of them and the other pelvic viscera, including the bladder.

CLOACA AND EXTERNAL GENITALIA

Urinary bladder

The urinary bladder (**3.86**A–F) is derived partly from the so-called endodermal cloaca and partly from the caudal ends of the mesonephric ducts (**3.83, 86**A–F, **89**). The walls of the cloaca are composed of an endodermal lining encased in imtermediate mesenchyme. In contrast the mesonephric ducts are derived from an epithelium, from the intermediate mesenchyme continuous with the coelomic epithelium, encased in intermediate mesenchyme. After the separation of the rectum from the cloaca (p. 191), the ventral part of the cloaca becomes divided into three regions:

- a cranial *vesico-urethral canal*, continuous with the allantoic duct, into which the mesonephric ducts open
- a middle, narrow channel, the *pelvic* portion
- a caudal, deep, *phallic* section, closed externally by the urogenital membrane (**3.86**A–E).

The second and third parts together constitute the *urogenital sinus*. The ureter and the mesonephric duct come to open separately into the vesico-urethral part. The termination of the mesonephric duct then moves caudally to open into that part which will form the prostatic urethra. This occurs by the formation of a caudally directed loop of the duct behind the urogenital sinus, followed by absorption of the apposed walls. In this way the mesonephric duct contributes to the *trigone* of the bladder and dorsal wall of the proximal (superior) half of the *prostatic urethra*, i.e. as far as the opening of

the prostatic utricle and ejaculatory ducts (or its homologue the whole female urethral dorsal wall). The remainder of the vesico-urethral part forms the body of the bladder and urethra; its apex is prolonged to the umbilicus as a narrow canal, the *urachus*. In postnatal life the urachus is drawn downwards as the bladder descends but its upper end remains connected to one or both of the obliterated umbilical arteries. Its lumen persists throughout life and its lower end frequently communicates with the bladder near its apex (Begg 1930).

Cloacal malformations. These are much more variable in their anatomic form than other congenital malformations. Two varieties can be distinguished:

1. In *extroversion of the bladder* (*ectopia vesicae*) the lower part of the anterior abdominal wall is occupied by an irregularly oval area, covered with mucous membrane, on which the two ureters open (Wyburn 1937). Around its periphery this extroverted area, covered by urothelium, becomes continuous with the skin. This maldevelopment occurs after the separation of the ventral from the dorsal part of the cloaca. The urogenital membrane extends further cranially than it does in normal cases and the genital tubercle forms at its caudal limit. Rupture of the membrane thus throws the bladder open to the exterior.

2. In *extroversion of the cloaca* the condition is very similar, but is complicated by the presence of intestinal openings in the median plane. The urogenital sinus may remain with a high confluence of bladder, vagina *and* rectum. The cloacal membrane may be abnormally elongated and prematurely ruptured throughout its whole extent, prior to the formation of the urorectal septum, or, in some cases there may be only a small sinus opening externally at the skin. The anal musculature is often present but not associated with the anal canal. (For a comprehensive discussion of cloacal malformations and cloacal exstrophy see Ricketts et al 1991; Hendren 1992.)

Urethra

In the male the prostatic urethra proximal to the orifice of the prostatic utricle is derived from the vesico-urethral part of the cloaca and the incorporated caudal ends of the mesonephric ducts. The remainder of the prostatic part, the membranous part and probably the part within the bulb are all derived from the urogenital sinus. The succeeding section, as far as the glans, is formed by the fusion of the genital folds, while the section within the glans is formed from ectoderm (see below).

In the female the urethra is derived entirely from the vesico-urethral region of the cloaca (see above), including the dorsal region derived from the mesonephric ducts. It is homologous with the part of the prostatic urethra proximal to the orifices of the prostatic utricle and the ejaculatory ducts.

Urethral sphincter. This first forms as a mesenchymal condensation around the urethra in 12–15 mm (stage 18) embryos, after division of the cloaca. The mesenchyme proliferates becoming defined at the bladder neck in 31-mm embryos and along the anterior part of the urethra by 69 mm. The muscle fibres differentiate after 15 weeks gestation when both smooth and striated fibres can be seen. In females there is continuity between the smooth muscle of the urethral wall and of the bladder. In the male the muscle fibres are less abundant because of the local development of the prostate. Striated muscle fibres form around the smooth muscle initially in the anterior wall of the urethra and later they encircle the smooth muscle layer. The origin of the striated muscle is not known but could derive from the myogenic cells producing the puborectalis muscle. The smooth and striated components of the urethral sphincter are closely related but there is no mixing of fibres as seen in the anorectal sphincter (Bourdelat et al 1992).

Defects of the urethra. Defects due to arrests of development are not uncommon in the male. The urethra may open on the ventral (perineal) aspect of the penis at the base of the glans (see below), and the part of the urethra which is normally within the glans is absent. This constitutes the simplest form of *hypospadias*. In more severe cases the genital folds fail to fuse, and the urethra opens on the ventral aspect of a malformed penis just in front of the scrotum. A still greater degree of this malformation is accompanied by failure of the genital swellings to unite with each other. In these cases the scrotum is divided and, since the testes are also frequently unde-

INDIFFERENT STAGE

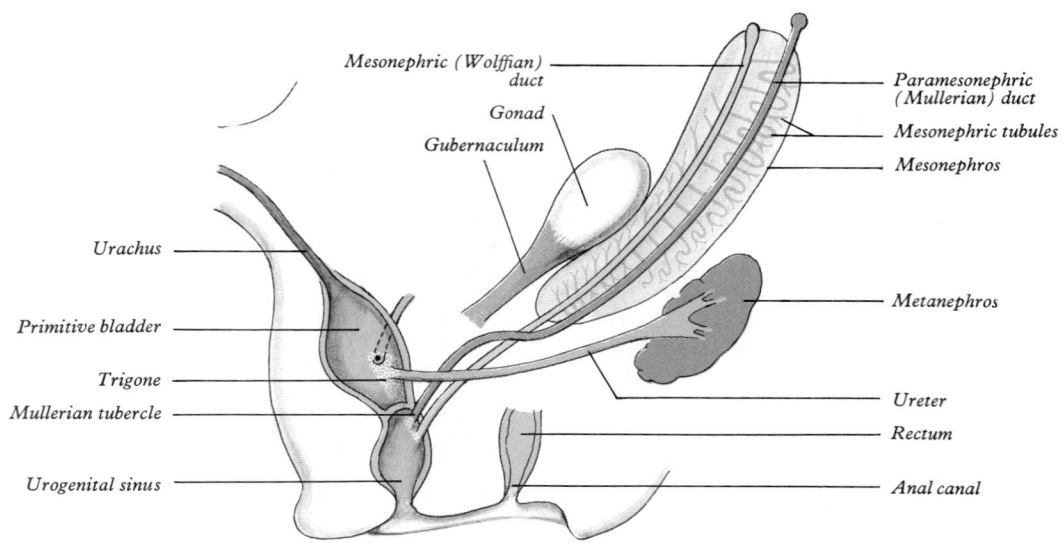

Mesonephric (Wolffian) duct
Gonad
Gubernaculum
Paramesonephric (Mullerian) duct
Mesonephric tubules
Mesonephros
Urachus
Primitive bladder
Trigone
Mullerian tubercle
Urogenital sinus
Metanephros
Ureter
Rectum
Anal canal

FEMALE   *MALE*

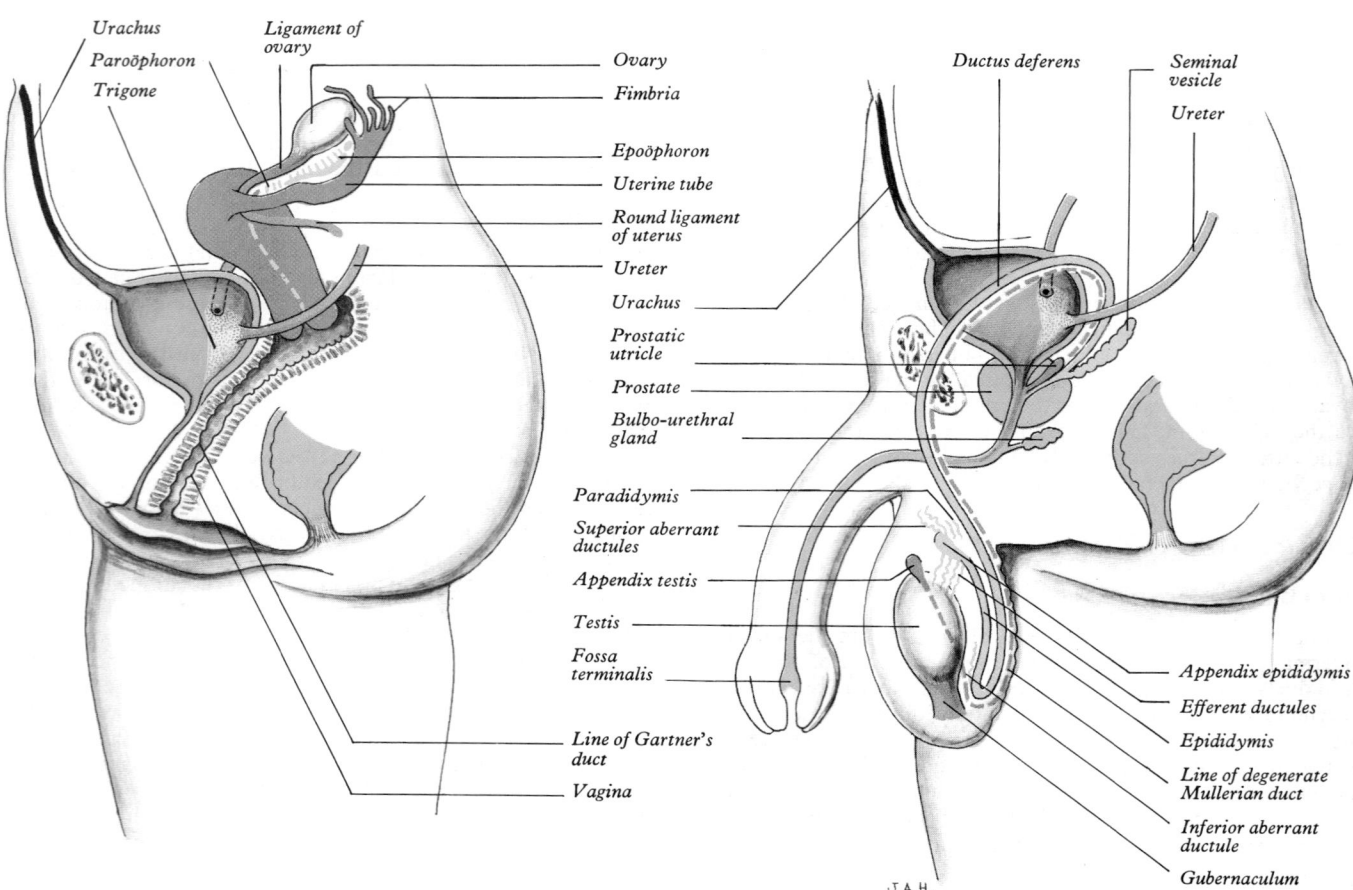

Urachus
Paroöphoron
Trigone
Ligament of ovary
Ovary
Fimbria
Epoöphoron
Uterine tube
Round ligament of uterus
Ureter
Urachus
Prostatic utricle
Prostate
Bulbo-urethral gland
Paradidymis
Superior aberrant ductules
Appendix testis
Testis
Fossa terminalis
Line of Gartner's duct
Vagina
Ductus deferens
Seminal vesicle
Ureter
Appendix epididymis
Efferent ductules
Epididymis
Line of degenerate Mullerian duct
Inferior aberrant ductule
Gubernaculum

J.A.H.

3.89   Disposition and fate of the mesonephric and paramesonephric ducts, mesonephric tubules, gonads and gubernaculum, primitive bladder and urogenital sinus, and ureters, as seen in the transformation from the indif-ferent stage to the definitive condition in the two sexes. (Modified from Williams et al 1969.)

scended, the resemblance to the labia majora is very striking. Male children suffering from this deformity are often mistaken for girls.

In *epispadias* the urethra opens on the dorsal aspect of the penis at its junction with the anterior abdominal wall. No satisfactory explanation has yet been suggested for this anomaly. For a genetic and epidemiological study of urinary tract malformations consult Bois et al (1975).

Prostate gland

The prostate arises during the third month from interactions between the urogenital sinus mesenchyme and the endoderm of the proximal part of the urethra. (In recombinant experiments in the rat, the sinus mesenchyme is capable of inducing glandular epithelium from adult bladder.) The earlier outgrowths, some 14–20 in number, arise from the endoderm around the whole circumference of the tube, but

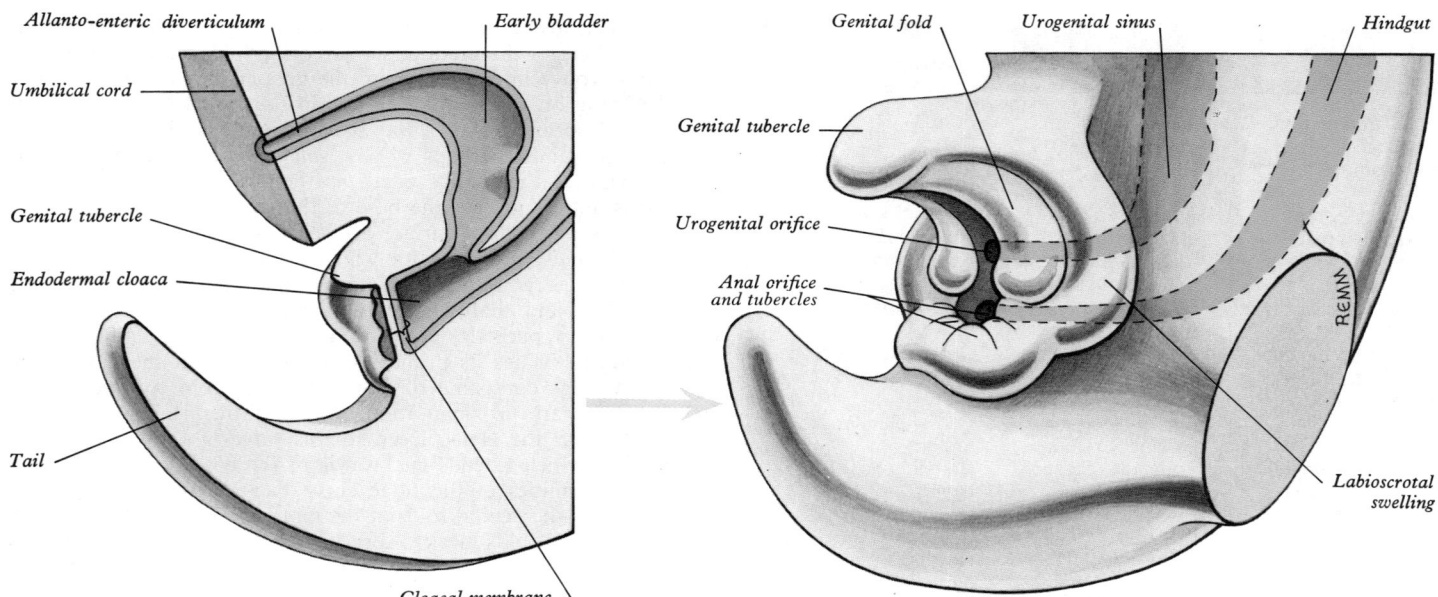

3.90 The development of the external genitalia from the indifferent stage to the definitive male and female conditions.

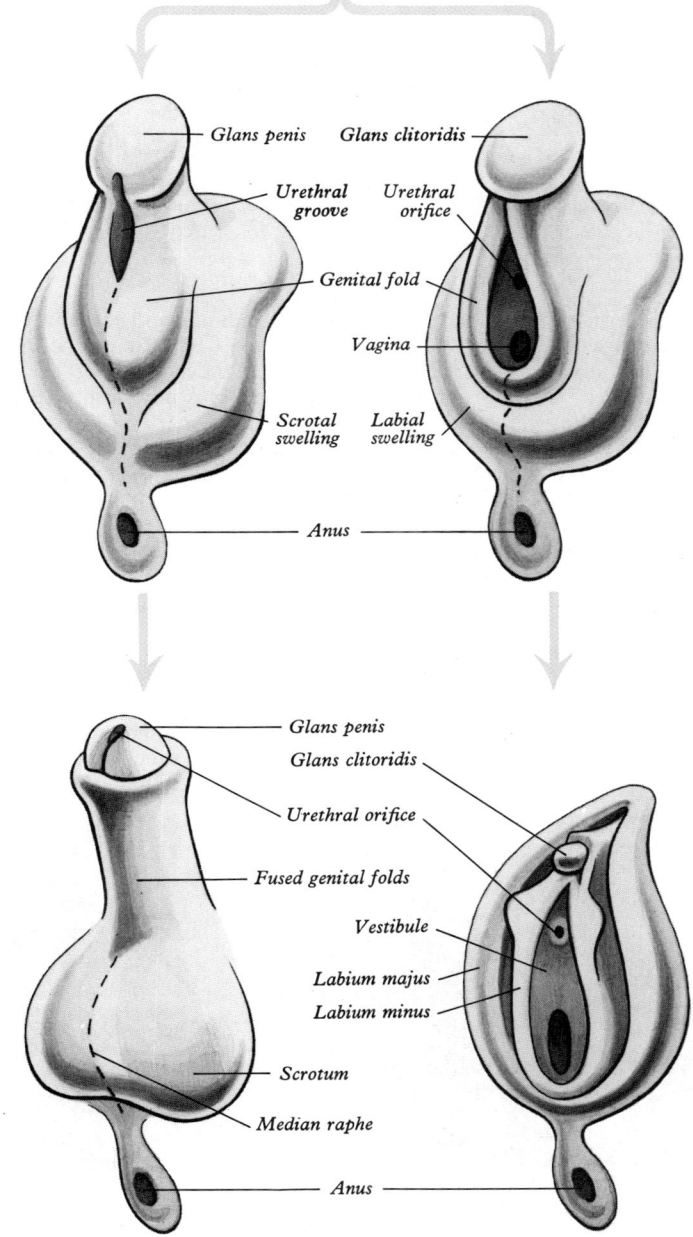

mainly on its lateral aspects and excluding the dorsal wall above the utricular plate. These outgrowths give rise to the *outer glandular zone* of the prostate (p. 1859). Later outgrowths from the dorsal wall above the mesonephric ducts arise from the epithelium of mixed urogenital, mesonephric and possibly paramesonephric origin covering the cranial end of the sinus tubercle. These produce the *internal zone* of glandular tissue. The outgrowths, which are at first solid, branch, become tubular and invade the surrounding mesenchyme, which is differentiating into non-striated muscle, associated blood and lymphatic vessels and connective tissues. The mesenchyme is invaded by autonomic nerves.

Similar outgrowths occur in the female but remain rudimentary. The urethral glands correspond to the mucosal glands around the upper part of the prostatic urethra and the para-urethral glands to the true prostatic glands of the external zone (Glenister 1962).

The *bulbo-urethral glands* in the male, and *greater vestibular glands* in the female, arise as diverticula from the epithelial lining of the urogenital sinus.

External genitalia

The external genital organs, like the gonads, pass through an indifferent state before distinguishing sexual characters appear (**3**.90). Patterning of the external genitalia may be achieved by mechanisms similar to those patterning the face and limb (see p. 294). Homologies of the parts of the urogenital septum are shown in Table **3**.1. From stage 13, *external genitalia primordia*, composed of underlying proliferating mesenchyme covered with ectoderm, arise around the cloacal membrane, between the primitive umbilical cord and the tail. During stage 15 the cloacal membrane is divided by the *urorectal septum* into a cranial *urogenital membrane* and a caudal *anal membrane*. Local ectodermal/mesenchymal interactions give rise to the anal sphincter which will develop without the presence of the urorectal septum or the anal canal. A surface elevation, the *genital tubercle*, appears at the cranial end of the urogenital membrane and two lateral ridges, the *genital or urethral folds*, form each side of the membrane. A distinct primordium which will become the *glans* of the penis or the *clitoris* can be recognized at the distal end of the genital tubercle. Elongation of the genital tubercle, urogenital membrane and the genital folds produces a *primitive phallus* (p. 180). As this structure grows it is described as having a cranial surface (analogous to the dorsum of the penis) and a caudal surface analogous to the perineal surface of both sexes. The urogenital sinus, contiguous with the internal aspect of the urogenital membrane, becomes attenuated within the elongating phallus forming the *primitive urethra*. The urogenital membrane breaks down at about stage 19 (20 mm, 6.5 weeks) allowing communication of ectoderm and

215

Table 3.1 Homologies of the parts of the urogenital system in male and female

Undifferentiated	Male	Female
Gonad	Testis	Ovary
Gubernacular cord	Gubernaculum testis	Ovarian and round ligaments
Mesonephros (Wolffian body)	Appendix of epididymis (?)	Appendices vesiculosae (?)
	Efferent ductules	Epoöphoron
	Lobules of epididymis	
	Paradidymis	Paroöphoron
	Aberrant ductules	
Mesonephric duct (Wolffian duct)	Duct of epididymis	Duct of epoöphoron
	Ductus deferens	
	Ejaculatory duct	
	Part of bladder and prostatic urethra	Part of bladder and urethra
Paramesonephric (or Mullerian) duct	Appendix of testis	Uterine tube
		Uterus
	Prostatic utricle	Vagina (?)
Allantoic duct	Urachus	Urachus
Cloaca: dorsal part	Rectum and upper part of anal canal	Rectum and upper part of anal canal
ventral	Most of bladder	Most of bladder and
part	Part of prostatic urethra	the urethra
urogenital	Prostatic urethra distal	
sinus	to utricle	
	Bulbo-urethral glands	Greater vestibular glands
	Rest of urethra to glans	Vestibule
Genital folds	Ventral penis	Labia minora
Genital tubercle	Glans penis	Clitoris
	Urethra in glans	

endoderm at the edges of the disrupted membrane and continuity of the urogenital sinus with the amniotic cavity. Urine can escape from the urinary tract from this time. The endodermal layer of the attenuated distal portion of the urogenital sinus now displayed on the caudal aspect of the phallus is termed the *urethral plate*. With proliferation of mesenchyme within the genital folds, the urethral plate sinks into the body of the phallus forming a *primary urethral groove*. The genital folds meet proximally in a transverse ridge immediately ventral to the anal membrane.

While these changes are in progress two *labioscrotal* (*genital*) *swellings* appear, one on each side of the base of the phallus; these extend caudally, separated from the genital folds by distinct grooves (**3.**90, 91).

Male genitalia. The growth of male external characteristics is stimulated by androgens regardless of the genetic sex. The male phallus enlarges to form the penis, its apex being the glans. The genital swellings meet each other ventral to the anus and unite to form the scrotum. The genital folds fuse with each other from behind

forwards enclosing the phallic part of the urogenital sinus behind to form the bulb of the urethra; similarly, the folds close the definitive urethral groove in front to form the greater part of the spongiose urethra. Fusion of the folds results in the formation of a median raphe and occurs in such a way that the lining of the postglandular urethra is mainly, perhaps wholly, *endodermal* in origin (Glenister 1954). Thus, as the phallus lengthens, the urogenital orifice is carried onwards until it reaches the base of the glans. From the tip of the phallus an ingrowth of surface *ectoderm* occurs within the glans to meet the penile urethra with which it fuses. Canalization of the ectoderm gives rise to a continuation of the urethra within the glans.

The glans and shaft of the penis are recognizable by the third month. The prepuce also begins to develop in the third month, when the urethra still has its primary external orifice at the base of the glans. A ridge consisting of a mesenchymal core covered by epithelium appears proximal to the neck of the penis and extends forwards over the glans. Deep to this ridge is a solid lamella of epithelium which extends backwards to the base of the glans. The ventral extremities of the ridge curve backwards to become continuous with the genital folds at the margins of the urethral orifice. As the urethral folds meet to form the terminal part of the urethra, the ventral horns of the ridge fuse to form the frenulum. Over the dorsum and sides of the glans, the epithelial lamella breaks down to form the preputial sac and thus free the prepuce from the surface of the glans. There-after the prepuce grows as a free fold of skin covering the terminal part of the glans. The preputial sac may not be complete until 6–12 months or more **after birth** and, even then, the presence of some connecting strands may still interfere with the retractability of the prepuce.

The mesenchymal core of the phallus is comparatively undifferentiated in the first 2 months, but during the third month the blastemata of the corpora cavernosa become defined. Nerves are present in the differentiating mesenchyme from the seventh week (Dail & Evan 1974).

Female genitalia. The female phallus, which exceeds the male in length in the early stages, becomes the clitoris. The genital swellings remain separate as the labia majora and the genital folds also remain separate, forming the labia minora. The perineal orifice of the urogenital sinus is retained as the cleft between the labia minora, above which the urethra and vagina open. The prepuce of the clitoris develops in the same way as its male homologue. By the fourth month the female external genitalia can no longer be masculinized by androgens.

Hormonal control of genital development

Development of the male phenotype requires fetal secretion of both testosterone and AMH, and development of the appropriate cytoplasmic testosterone-binding protein. Absence of the testosterone-binding protein results in XY individuals with testes and degenerated Mullerian ducts, but because they cannot respond to the circulating testosterone produced by their testes they develop female secondary sexual characteristics.

There is evidence that in certain tissues testosterone is converted into 5a-dihydrotestosterone, for example urogenital sinus and genital

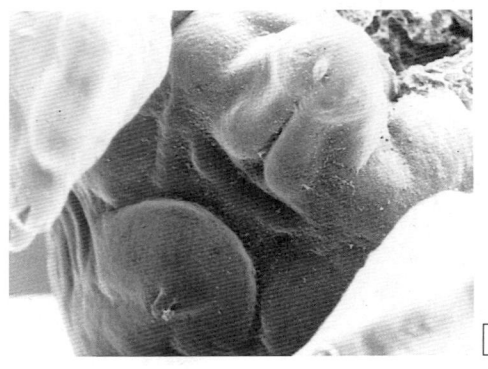 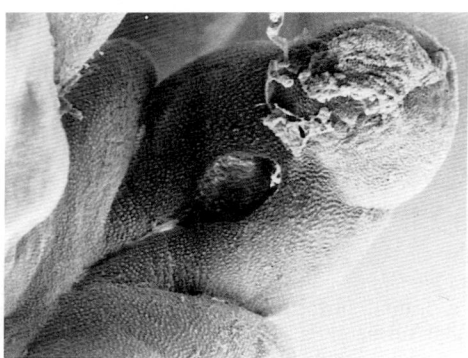 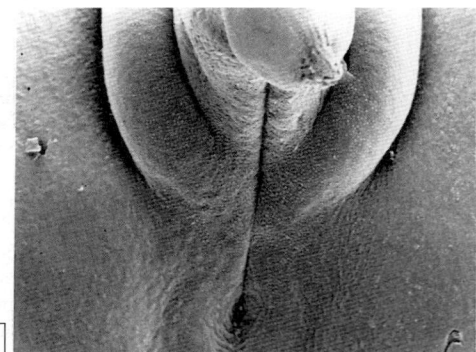

3.91 Scanning electron micrographs of early human external genitalia. A. Indifferent stage in a human embryo estimated as 42 postovulatory days. B. A human female embryo at 12 weeks development; note the genital folds are not fused. C. A human male embryo at 12 weeks; fusion of the genital folds has occurred. (Photographs by P Collins.)

swellings. In XY individuals with a genetic deficiency of the enzyme responsible for this conversion, functioning testes are present but also female external genitalia with an enlarged clitoris and a small vaginal pouch, suggesting that external genital development is under the control of 5α-dihydrotestosterone. Such individuals are usually raised as girls. However, at puberty the external genitalia become responsive to testosterone causing masculinization at this stage (Imperato-McGinley et al 1974).

It is apparent that the hormones produced by the fetal gonads act on targets other than internal and external genitalia; for example, the number of cell bodies contributing to the genitofemoral nerve is higher in males (see above), thus promoting descent of the testis. Sexual dimorphism has been noted in the brain of many species. The ability to detect testosterone receptors may elucidate many more sites of testosterone sensitivity than has been previously supposed.

NERVOUS SYSTEM AND SPECIAL SENSE ORGANS

The nervous system is divided into the *central nervous system* (CNS), which includes the brain and spinal cord, and the *peripheral nervous system* (PNS), which includes neuronal cell bodies outside the CNS and the nerves which take information to and from the brain and spinal cord. At a functional level those nerves which carry conscious sensations and innervate striated muscle (derived from axial and paraxial mesenchyme) are termed part of the *somatic nervous system*, whilst control of smooth muscle (derived from splanchnopleuric mesenchyme) resides with the *autonomic nervous system*, which is subdivided into *sympathetic* and *para-sympathetic* moieties.

The entire nervous system and the special sense organs originate from three sources each derived in turn from specific regions of the early epiblast generally termed neural ectoderm. The first source to be delineated is the *neural plate* which forms the CNS, the *somatic motor nerves* and the *preganglionic autonomic nerves*. The second source is from cells at the perimeter of the neural plate which remove themselves by epithelial/mesenchymal transition from the plate just prior to its fusion into a neural tube; these are the *neural crest cells* which form nearly all of the PNS, including the *somatic sensory nerves*, the *somatic* and *autonomic ganglia, postganglionic autonomic nerves* and *adrenal* and *chromaffin cells*; they also give rise to significant mesenchymal populations in the head. The third source is from *ectodermal placodes*; these are groups of cells which originate at the edge of the neural plate but remain in the surface ectoderm after neural tube formation undergoing epithelial/mesenchymal transition after the neural crest cells have commenced their migration. Ectodermal placodes contribute to the *somatic sensory ganglia* of the cranial nerves, to the *hypophysis*, the *inner ear* and, by a non-neuronal contribution, to the lens of the eye.

With the initiation of gastrulation, the first populations of epiblast cells to invaginate through the primitive streak form the prechordal plate, embryonic endoderm and notochord (see p. 144). These cells invaginate through the rostral end of the primitive streak (Hensen's node) and form a midline strip (chordamesoderm) subjacent to the overlying epiblast. Other epiblast cells passing through the lateral regions of Hensen's node, and the middle and caudal regions of the primitive streak, migrate laterally between the epiblast and the spreading embryonic endoderm and give rise to discrete populations of intraembryonic mesoblast. Those cells arising from Hensen's node and the rostral regions of the primitive streak remain close to the notochord as the paraxial mesenchyme, which later segments to form the somites; cells arising from the middle of the primitive streak migrate laterally, rostrally and caudally towards the edges of the embryonic disc and form the lateral plate mesenchyme (see p. 155). The epiblast cells remaining after gastrulation are designated surface ectoderm above the lateral plate mesenchyme and neurectoderm (neural plate) medially above the notochord and paraxial mesenchyme. Rostral to the notochord, prechordal mesenchyme forms a continuous mesenchymal network underlying the neurectoderm to which it is closely apposed.

The neural plate is a thickened epithelium, roughly oval but wider rostrally and narrowed caudally (**3.46**). The lateral edges of the plate become elevated as *neural folds* and approach one another to fuse in the dorsal midline as the *neural tube*. The early neural tube is coextensive with the notochord, stretching from the future cloacal membrane to the buccopharyngeal membrane. Studies on amphibian and avian embryos have suggested that Hensen's node gives rise not only to notochordal cells but also to the overlying midline region of

the neural plate which, after neurulation, will become the floor plate of the neural tube (Jessell et al 1989). The node does not, however, give rise to other regions of the neural plate. The notochord is important for the maintenance and later development of the floor plate of the neural tube (p. 226); axial extension of the floor plate in vitro requires the presence of underlying notochordal cells (Keller 1985). Extirpation of notochordal cells in amphibia prior to neural tube closure results in the absence of a floor plate, whereas removal of the notochord at a later stage does not affect floor plate development.

Despite the profound developmental modifications introduced by the secondary reduction of yolk in mammalian secondary oöcytes associated with viviparity (p. 95), it is widely assumed that similar *primary mechanisms* operate throughout the Chordata, including mankind. Certainly the requirement for cell interactions during early development, including neural induction, is conserved throughout many chordate groups. (For general reviews of neural induction consult Papalopulu & Kintner 1992; Ruiz i Altaba 1993.)

NEURAL TUBE

The physical process of *neurulation* occurs well after the onset of neural induction. The edges of the neural plate, which are continuous laterally with the surface ectoderm, roll up and fuse in the dorsal midline approximately at the cervical level (4th somite; **3.92**). Fusion then proceeds rostrally and caudally. Formation of the neural tube by elevation and fusion of the neural folds is termed *primary neurulation*. Secondary neurulation occurs in the lumbosacral region of the spinal cord in birds and mammals, and involves cavitation of a compact mass of cells. When the neural tube is closing, its walls consist of a single layer of columnar neural epithelial cells, the extremities of which abut on *internal* and *external limiting membranes*. The mechanism of rounding up of the neural plate into a neural tube has been studied particularly closely in amphibia (Burnside 1971). The columnar cells increase in length and develop numerous longitudinally disposed microtubules, whilst the borders of their luminal ends are firmly attached to adjacent cells by junctional complexes; the cytoplasmic aspect of the complexes being associated with a dense paraluminal web of microfilaments (see p. 28; also Watterson 1965). It is proposed that this disposition of organelles imparts a slight wedge conformation on at least some of the cells. In addition, nuclei assume basal positions that enhance cell wedging in two lateral and one medial 'hinge' regions, the latter being the floor plate (Schoenwolf & Smith, 1990). Together these factors result in neural groove and eventually neural tube formation. Soon, however, some of the peripheral cytoplasmic processes become detached from the (basal) external limiting membrane and rounded cells appear close to the inner membrane which, by their repeated mitotic division, form descendants which migrate outwards to take up an intermediate position in the wall of the tube. Histologically at this stage, therefore, the wall of the tube presents three zones or layers (**3.93, 94, 95**). The *internal ventricular zone* (variously termed the *germinal, primitive ependymal* or *matrix layer*) consists of the nucleated parts of the columnar cells and the round cells undergoing mitosis. The *mantle zone* (also termed *intermediate zone*) consists of the migrant cells from the divisions occurring in the deeper layer just described. The outer *marginal zone*, for a period, consists of the external cytoplasmic processes of some of the original columnar

217

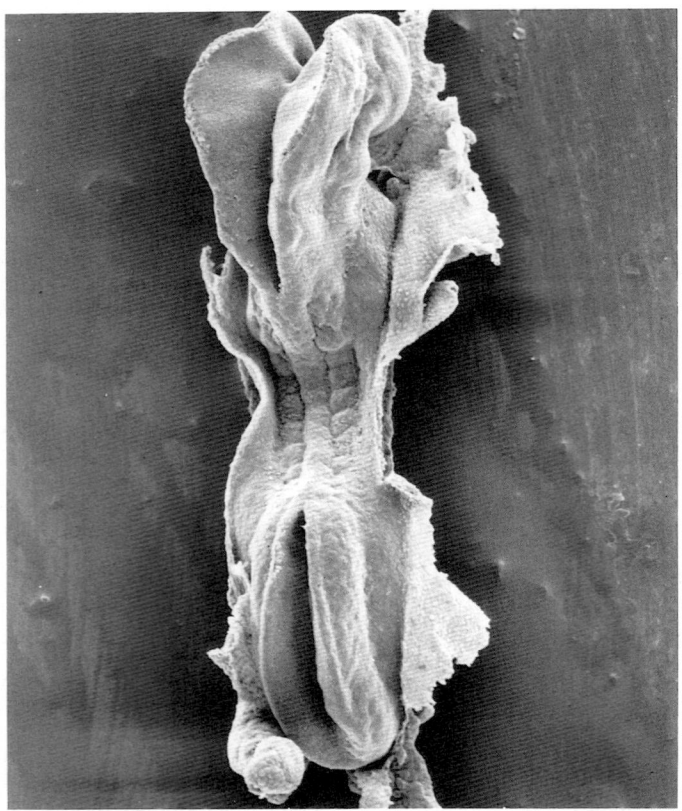

3.92 Scanning electron micrograph of a neurulating rat embryo comparable to a stage-10 human embryo (22–24 days). Somite formation occurs as neurulation proceeds caudally. (Photograph by P Collins; printed by S Cox, Electron Microscopy Unit, Southampton General Hospital.)

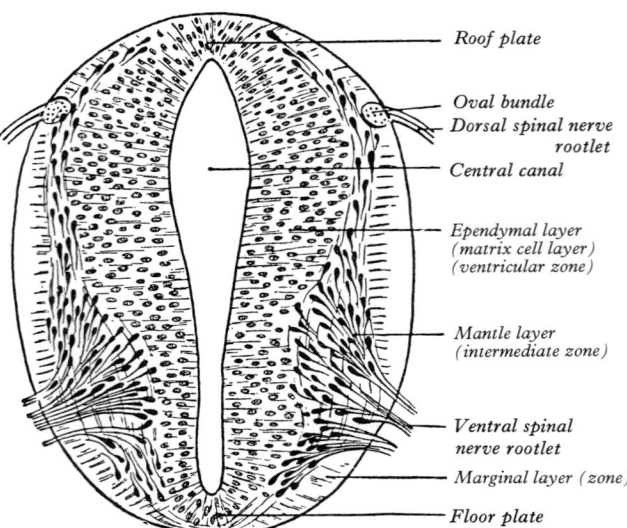

Roof plate
Oval bundle
Dorsal spinal nerve rootlet
Central canal
Ependymal layer (matrix cell layer) (ventricular zone)
Mantle layer (intermediate zone)
Ventral spinal nerve rootlet
Marginal layer (zone)
Floor plate

3.93 Transverse section through the developing spinal cord of a 4-week-old human embryo. Historically early terminology is retained; more recent terms are in parenthesis. (After His.)

cells, but it is soon invaded by tracts of axonal processes which grow from neuroblasts developing in the mantle zone, together with varieties of non-nervous cells (glial cells and later vascular endothelium and perivascular mesenchyme).

Prior to the closure of the neural tube the neural folds become expanded considerably in the head region as a first indication of a brain. Subsequent to the closure of the rostral neuropore (p. 146) these regional expansions form the three *primary cerebral vesicles* (**3**.96A–C). The term 'vesicle' may be rather a misnomer as it suggests an exaggerated view of these localized accelerations of growth in the wall of the brain (O'Rahilly & Gardner 1971). The bulging is not initially marked, and the vesicles are more likely gently fusiform tubes. The three regions are named (rostrocaudally) the *prosencephalon* or *forebrain*, the *mesencephalon* or *midbrain*, and the *rhombencephalon* or *hindbrain*, the latter being continuous caudally with the spinal cord. As a result of unequal growth of its different regions three flexures appear in the brain; two of these are concave ventrally and there are corresponding flexures of the head. The first of these flexures is associated with the formation of the head fold and forms ventral to the midbrain. Due to this *mesencephalic flexure* the forebrain bends in a ventral direction around the cephalic end of the notochord and foregut until its floor lies almost parallel with

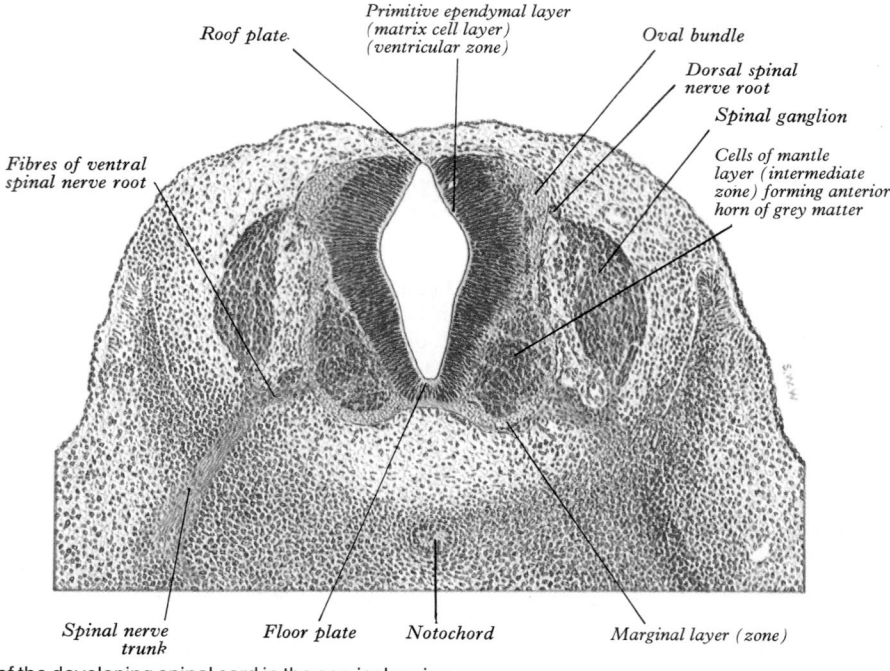

Primitive ependymal layer (matrix cell layer) (ventricular zone)
Roof plate
Oval bundle
Dorsal spinal nerve root
Spinal ganglion
Fibres of ventral spinal nerve root
Cells of mantle layer (intermediate zone) forming anterior horn of grey matter
Spinal nerve trunk
Floor plate
Notochord
Marginal layer (zone)

3.94 Transverse section of the developing spinal cord in the cervical region of a human embryo early in the sixth week, CR length 8 mm.

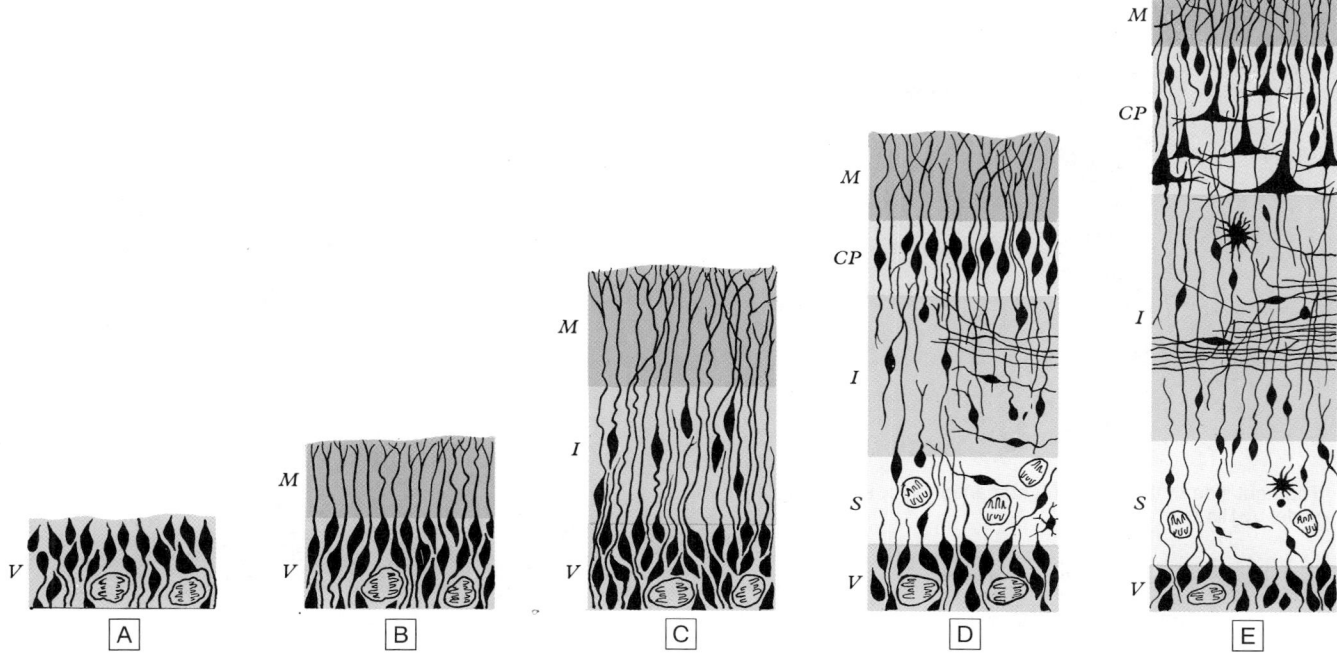

3.95 Schema of 5 sequential stages (A to E) in the development of part of the neural tube's wall in section to form cerebral cortex. Spinal cord development is limited to stages A to C. (Modified from Boulder Committee *initial* recommendations 1970.)

V = ventricular zone; M = marginal zone; I = intermediate zone (mantle zone); S = subventricular zone; CP = cortical plate. New research techniques led Rakic (1982) to advance many significant alterations and additions to these proposals: see p. 252 and **3**.123.

that of the hindbrain (**3**.96). The second bend appears at the junction of the hindbrain and spinal cord, the *cervical flexure* (**3**.96). This increases from the fifth to the end of the seventh week, by which time the hindbrain forms nearly a right angle with the spinal cord; after the seventh week, however, extension of the head takes place and the cervical flexure diminishes and eventually disappears. The third bend, the *pontine flexure*, is at the level of the future pons. It differs from the other two in that its convexity is directed ventrally and it does not substantially affect the outline of the head.

Concomitant with the development of the flexures, the regions of the brain enlarge allowing subdivisions of some of the original vesicles. The prosencephalon can be subdivided into two parts: the *telencephalon*, lateral evaginations of the early prosencephalon which will give rise to the cerebral hemispheres, and the *diencephalon*, the remaining midline portion of the prosencephalon. The mesencephalon remains undivided. The rhombencephalon is subdivided by the pontine flexure into the *metencephalon* rostrally which will give rise to the future pons and cerebellum and the *myelencephalon* caudally which will become the future medulla oblongata.

In addition to these gross divisions, the neural tube manifests a number of ridges and depressions which subdivide it further. Prominent among these are the serial bulges that appear very early in the rhombencephalon, before the main flexures of the neural tube develop. These bulges are termed *rhombomeres*, and apparently constitute the primary units of patterning in this region (see p. 125). Although bulges have also been observed in other brain regions, their developmental significance is only starting to be evaluated. For more recent accounts of the early development of the brain consult Bartelmez & Dekaban (1962), Jacobson (1970), Gaze (1970), Eccles (1973), Gottlieb (1973, 1974), Mark (1974), Rakic (1981, 1982), Smart (1982, 1983), Schoenwolf and Smith (1990).

During neurulation the neural tube becomes subdivided in the dorsoventral axis. In the ventral midline lies the *floor plate* (see **3**.93), a region containing non-neuronal cells that plays a role in patterning the dorsoventral axis, induces motor neurons, and, later, serves as a site for ventral commissures of nerve fibres. As the neural tube closes, cells arising from the edges of the neural folds form a distinct, transitory population in the dorsal midline outside the neural tube; this is the *neural crest*. This cell population lies between the neural tube and the surface ectoderm prior to migration to diverse locations throughout the embryo. Neural crest derivatives include the sensory

ganglia of the cranial and spinal nerves, the autonomic ganglia and nerves, the enteric nervous system, Schwann cells, pigment cells, odontoblasts, meninges and ectomesenchyme cells of the pharyngeal arches. The departure of the neural crest is followed by the formation of another specialized non-neuronal region dorsally, the *roof plate*, which, in some regions, forms dorsal commissures.

At first the neural tube caudal to the brain is oval in outline and its lumen is narrow and slit-like (**3**.93). As the lateral walls thicken, the lumen, now the central canal, widens in its dorsal part and is somewhat diamond-shaped on cross-section (**3**.93). The widening of the canal is associated with the development of a longitudinal *sulcus limitans* on each side. This divides the ventricular and mantle (intermediate) zones in each lateral wall into a *ventrolateral* or *basal lamina* and a *dorsolateral* or *alar lamina*. This separation indicates a fundamental functional difference. Within the spinal cord, the basal plate is concerned with motor function, containing the cell bodies of motor neurons of the anterior and lateral grey columns, while the alar plate receives sensory inflow from the dorsal root ganglia. Motor and sensory axons combine to form the segmentally arranged spinal nerves. In the head, the cranial nerves form a continuation to the series of spinal nerves, but are functionally and anatomically specialized. An important developmental contribution to the nervous system is also made by *neurogenic (ectodermal) placodes*, which are thickened regions of ectoderm in the head (see p. 257).

(The long held and widely used terms:

- roof plate
- floor plate
- alar lamina
- basal lamina

were changed to:

- dorsal lamina
- ventral lamina
- dorsolateral lamina
- ventrolateral lamina

in the *Nomina Embryologica* associated with the *Nomina Anatomica* (fourth edition) by the International Anatomical Nomenclature Committee (Tokyo 1975). The modified names are more apposite **throughout** the *early* neural tube (i.e. spinal cord and brainstem); however, these terms become much less appropriate in the rostral

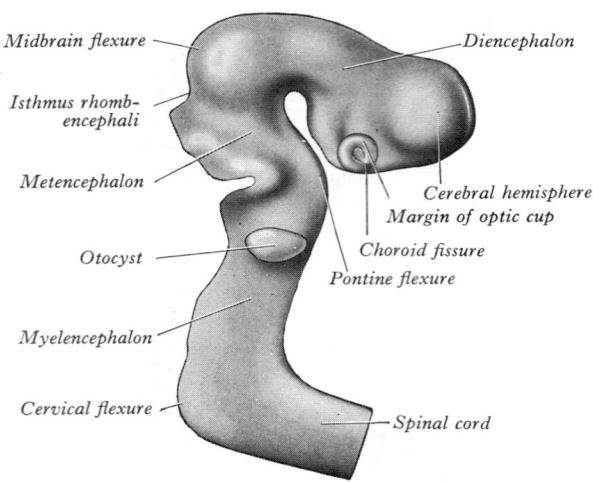

3.96A The right side of the brain of a human embryo, 9 mm long. (Drawn from a model by His.)

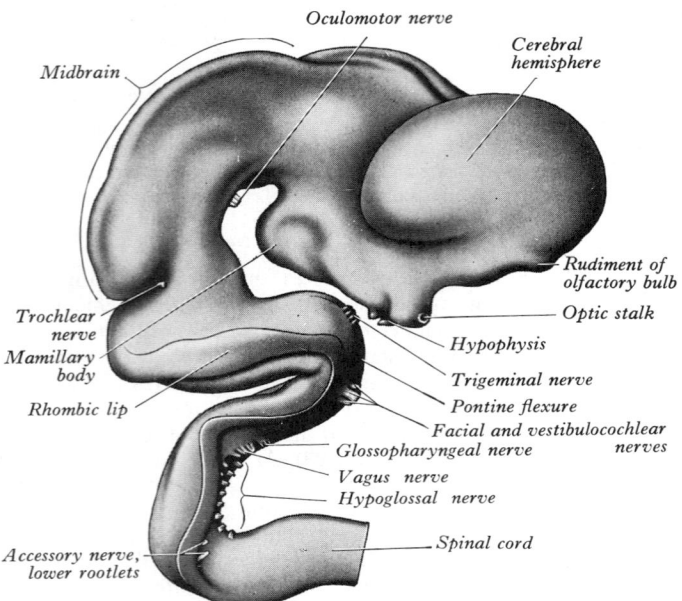

3.96c The right side of the brain of a human embryo, 13.6 mm long. The roof of the hindbrain has been removed. (From a model by His.)

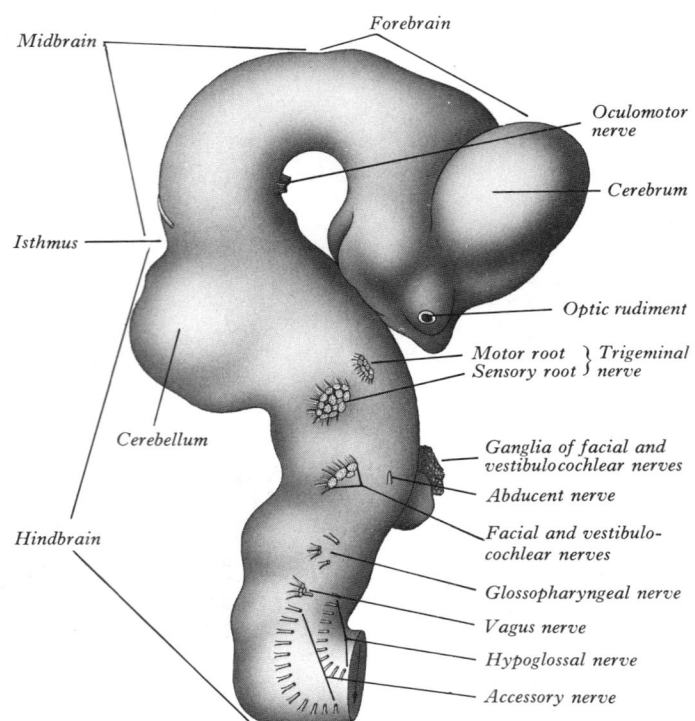

3.96B The brain of a human embryo about 10.2 mm long: right lateral surface. (From a model by His.)

half of the medulla oblongata and caudal half of the pons, with the profound positional changes accompanying the formation of the pontine flexure—**3.96A**. The older terminology is still retained by some research groups.)

Failure of neurulation produces the conditions of *craniorachischisis*, where the entire neural tube is unfused in the dorsal midline, *cranioschisis* or *anencephaly*, where the neural tube is fused dorsally to form the spinal cord but is not fused dorsally in the brain, and *spina bifida*, where local regions of the spinal cord, meninges and vertebrae may be malformed (p. 340, **3.197**). Anencephalic fetuses have severe disturbances in the shape, position and ossification of the basichondrocranium and in the course of the intracranial notochord.

NEURAL CREST

The neural crest is a **transient** structure found only in *vertebrate embryos*. It is derived from the lateral ridges of the neural plate (also called neural folds) and its appearance follows a craniocaudal gradient as the neural tube closes on the mediodorsal line. The neural crest in the chick was first described in 1868 by Wilhelm His

who called it *Zwischenstrand*, to emphasize its intermediate position between the neural tube and surface ectoderm. Wilhelm His also recognized that the neural crest was the origin of the spinal ganglia—hence the term *ganglion crest* that has also been used to designate this structure. The fact that the neural crest yields mesenchymal cells was first proposed at the turn of the century by Kastschenko (1888), Goronowitsch (1892) and later by Platt (1893) who showed that it contributes to the cartilage of pharyngeal arches and to the dentine of the teeth in lower vertebrates. Platt coined the term *mesectoderm* to designate the mesenchyme of ectodermal origin, a notion that challenged the current germ layer theory of von Baer (1828) (see p. 92).

Since these early times, the neural crest has attracted much attention from embryologists who, during the first half of this century, investigated the fate of this structure mainly in the amphibian embryo. The fact that neural crest cells migrate and settle in elected sites in the embryo, where they differentiate into a large variety of cell types, was deduced from ablation experiments, cell marking studies that involved the use of vital dyes, and experiments that relied on differences in cell size or pigmentation between related species of amphibians. However, none of these methods provided stable and specific markers so the migratory cells could only be distinguished for a short period of time. Nevertheless, the pluripotentiality of the neural crest was recognized and its role in contributing both to the PNS and to the facial skeleton was established.

A more precise cell marking technique was devised later by Weston (1963) and Chibon (1964) who labelled the DNA of migrating neural crest cells with tritiated thymidine (^{3}H-TdR). Owing to the rapid proliferation of embryonic cells the label is soon diluted so that it is not stable, and, furthermore, re-uptake of label released by dead cells compromised specificity. More recently methods based on the use of liposoluble carbocyanide dyes (diI, diO) have been used to label cell membranes in living cells. While easy to use and providing conspicuous labelling these methods also have the disadvantage of being neither precise nor stable.

Quail–chick chimeras

From the late sixties, up to recent years, most investigations on the neural crest have used the avian embryo. The introduction of the

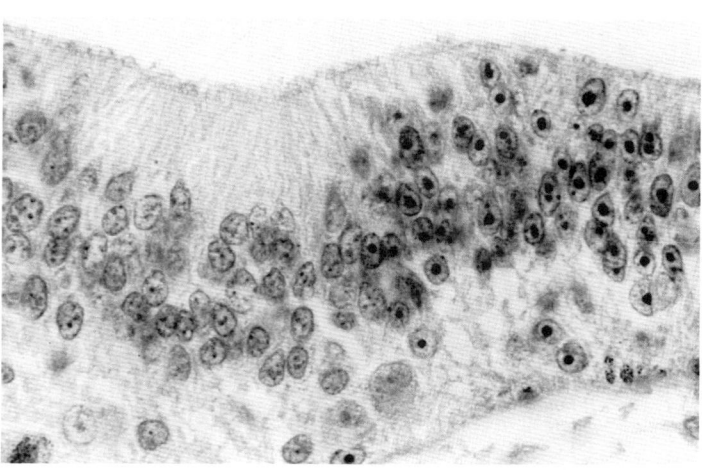

3.97 Neuroblasts of quail (right) and chick (left) stained by the Feulgen–Rossenbeck reaction. A large central mass of heterochromatin characterizes the quail nuclei. In chick cells, heterochromatin is distributed in small chromocentres. Magnification × 1276.

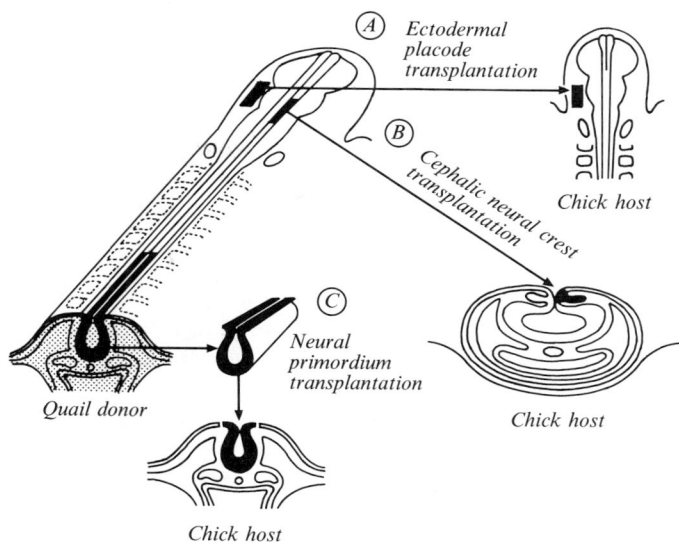

3.98 Diagram showing the experimental procedures that have been used to trace the cells of placodal (A) and neural crest (B, C) origin during PNS ontogeny in vivo.

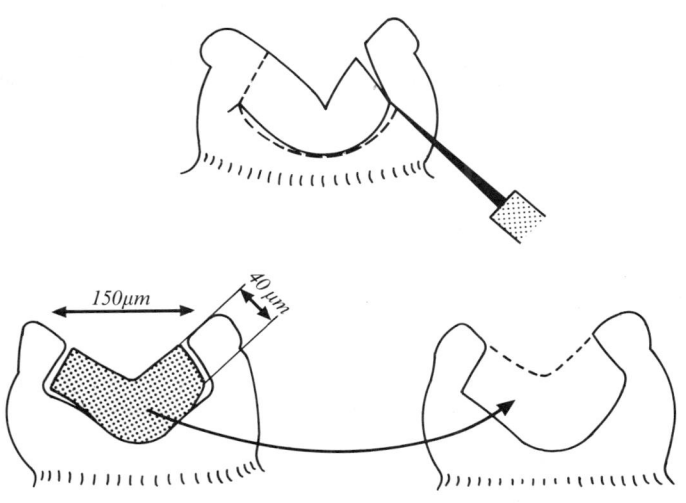

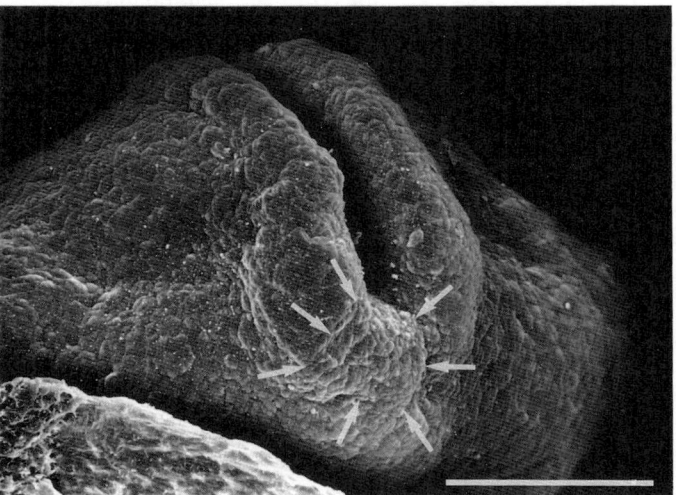

3.99 Isotopic graft of the quail rostral neural fold into a chick embryo at the early somitic stages. A. A fragment of the neural fold (about 150 × 40 μm) is removed in the chick and replaced by its counterpart from the quail. B. Three hours after the operation, the graft (the limits of which are underlined by the arrows) is well incorporated in the host's neural fold. Scale bar = 100 μm.

quail–chick marker system to neural crest embryology by Le Douarin (1969 et seq) has allowed the migration and fate of neural crest cells to be followed precisely up to the stage where they become fully differentiated. This technique is based on an observation by Le Douarin (1969), on the structure of the interphase nucleus in the Japanese quail. The cells of this species are characterized by the condensation of constitutive heterochromatin into a large mass, generally centronuclear, associated with the nucleolus. Although some variations in the distribution of heterochromatin and nucleolar RNA exist in the different cell types of the quail, this mass of heterochromatin is present in all embryonic and adult cell types of this species (Le Douarin 1973). Such a characteristic is rare in the animal kingdom (Le Douarin 1971); in most species the constitutive heterochromatin is evenly distributed in the nucleoplasm in small chromocentres as it is, for example, in the chick (**3.97**). Quail and chick cells can thus easily be distinguished by DNA staining or by electron microscopy where the large, DNA-rich nucleolus of the quail is easily recognizable. These species–species differences have been used to study the migration of embryonic cells and to analyse the contribution of cells of different embryonic origins to complex tissues or organs during ontogeny. Since the quail and the chick are closely related in taxonomy, the substitution of definite territories between embryos of these two species in ovo results in viable *chimeras* which develop normally and can hatch. Thus, when definite fragments of either the neural fold or the neural tube and associated neural crest of the quail are grafted *isotopically* or *isochronically* into the chick (or vice versa) the migration and fate of their constituent cells can be followed at any time after the operation (**3.98**). This approach has been systematically applied to the whole neuraxis to establish the fate map of the neural fold and to define the paths along which neural crest cells migrate. In addition to the nuclear marker, species specific antibodies and cDNA probes have been used to analyse the chimeras (Le Douarin 1993; Izpisua-Belmonte et al 1993).

Fate of the head neural fold

The neural fold establishes a **transition** between the neural ectoderm, i.e. the neural plate which becomes the brain and spinal cord, and the surface ectoderm which differentiates later into epidermis. Along most of the neuraxis, the cells forming the neural fold undergo an epithelial/mesenchymal transformation through which they acquire the migratory properties of neural crest cells. The *rostral prosencephalic neural fold*, however, does **not** generate neural crest. Quail–chick chimera recombination in embryos at the neurula stage (0–3 somites) (**3.99**), demonstrated that neural crest cells are produced along the neural axis rostrally as far as the diencephalon, at about the level from which the epiphysis arises. The rostral neural fold itself gives rise to the *hypophyseal placode*, i.e. the future Rathke's

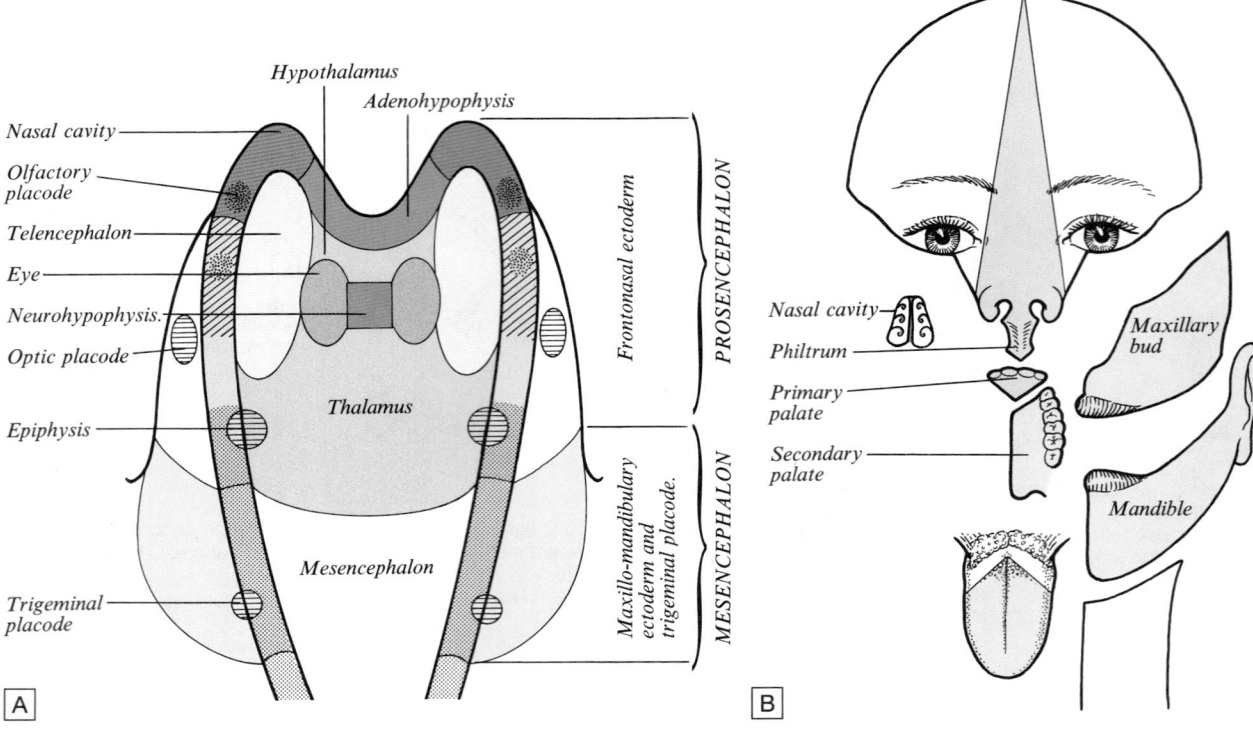

3.100 Fate map of the rostral region of the neural primordium as established by the quail–chick chimera system. A. The various territories yielding rostral head are indicated on the neural plate and neural fold of a 1–3 somite embryo. B. The results obtained in the avian embryo have been extrapolated to the human head. Thus, the neural fold area (green) yields the epithelium of the rostral roof of the mouth, the nasal cavities and part of the frontal area.

pouch, the *olfactory placodes* and associated *nasal epithelium*, including the roof of the nasopharynx and, more caudally, the skin of the upper lip (beak in chick) and the frontonasal area. Extrapolation to the human and the results obtained in quail–chick chimeras is represented in **3.100**.

Studies of the fate of the neural fold caudal to the mid-diencephalon revealed that the *frontal* and *parietal bones* are entirely of neural crest origin (Couly et al 1993) (see p. 274) as well as the *facial* and *hypobranchial skeleton* and part of the *optic* and *otic capsules* (Le Douarin 1982) (see p. 271).

By grafting cranial paraxial mesenchyme and the 6 rostral somites, Couly et al (1992, 1993) were able to delineate precisely the respective contributions to the skull of the somites, paraxial mesenchyme and of the neural crest. As represented on **3.101** for the chick, a region of the skull rostral to the extreme tip of the notochord can be distinguished; this region reaches the sella turcica and also a region caudal to this boundary. The former, the *achordal skull* is derived entirely from neural crest; the latter is derived from paraxial mesenchyme (cephalic or somitic) in its ventromedial part and is termed the *chordal skull* (see also p. 287).

Apart from the skull, the cephalic neural crest is the origin of several other derivatives (see derivative table p. 145). The overlapping developmental capacities of paraxial mesenchyme and neural crest is illustrated by the *meninges*. These are derived from the neural crest at the prosencephalic level (di- and telencephalon) and from paraxial mesenchyme for the rest of the CNS (see p. 256).

The *connective tissue component* of the glands derived from the buccal and pharyngeal epithelium, e.g. *salivary*, *thyroid*, *parathyroid* and *thymus* (see p. 176), and the *tunica media* and *externa* of the large blood vessels arising from the heart, are of neural crest origin (see p. 314), as are the *carotid body type I* and *type II cells* and the *calcitonin producing cells* (C-cells) that develop in the ultimobranchial bodies.

Although mesectoderm and mesenchyme share several developmental potentialities, that of yielding *vascular endothelial cells* is the strict reserve of the *mesenchyme* (see angioblastic mesenchyme pp. 156 and 299). That is why grafts of quail cephalic neural crest in chick embryos produce bones and connective tissues of donor type, but the vascular endothelium of all the vessels irrigating these tissues derives from the angioblastic mesenchyme of the host.

Neural crest and the PNS

Although the development of the spinal ganglia from neural crest has long been known, confusion existed regarding the origin of the PNS and the level of the neuraxis from which its various components emanate (Le Douarin & Teillet 1973; Le Douarin 1982). Using quail–chick chimeras, the fate maps of the PNS derivatives of the neural crest and of the placodal ectoderm, which contributes to the sensory ganglia of certain cranial nerves, were established (**3.102**).

A monoclonal antibody, NC1/HNK1, was found to label most avian neural crest cells at the time of their migration (Tucker et al 1984). It recognizes a glycosylated epitope carried by several surface molecules. Although it is not strictly specific for neural crest cells, even at migration time (the NC1/HNK1 epitope is lost by certain crest cells such as the mesectoderm, certain neurons and the melanocytes, but remains present on peripheral glia and neuronal subpopulations), the use of this antibody has been instrumental in showing that the *migration pattern* of neural crest cells in the trunk is **channelled by the somites**. It thus appears segmental although the crest cells exit uniformly along the whole neural tube. The crest cells are able to migrate, without impediment, between the somites and within the rostral sclerotomal half, but they cannot penetrate the caudal moiety of the sclerotomal mesenchyme (see p. 265). Thus the segmental distribution of the spinal and sympathetic ganglia is imposed on the neural crest cells by a prepattern that exists within the somitic paraxial mesenchyme (Rickman et al 1985; Kalchein & Teillet 1989).

Further experiments examined whether crest cells which were destined to form different parts of the PNS (**3.102**) were already restricted in their developmental potential. This could occur prior to migration, or be imposed subsequently by environmental cues to which they were exposed during migration or at their final destination. Quail neural crest cells were either transplanted before the onset of migration into *heterotopic* sites in the chick host, or developing quail peripheral ganglia were 'back transplanted' into the neural crest migration pathway of the chick.

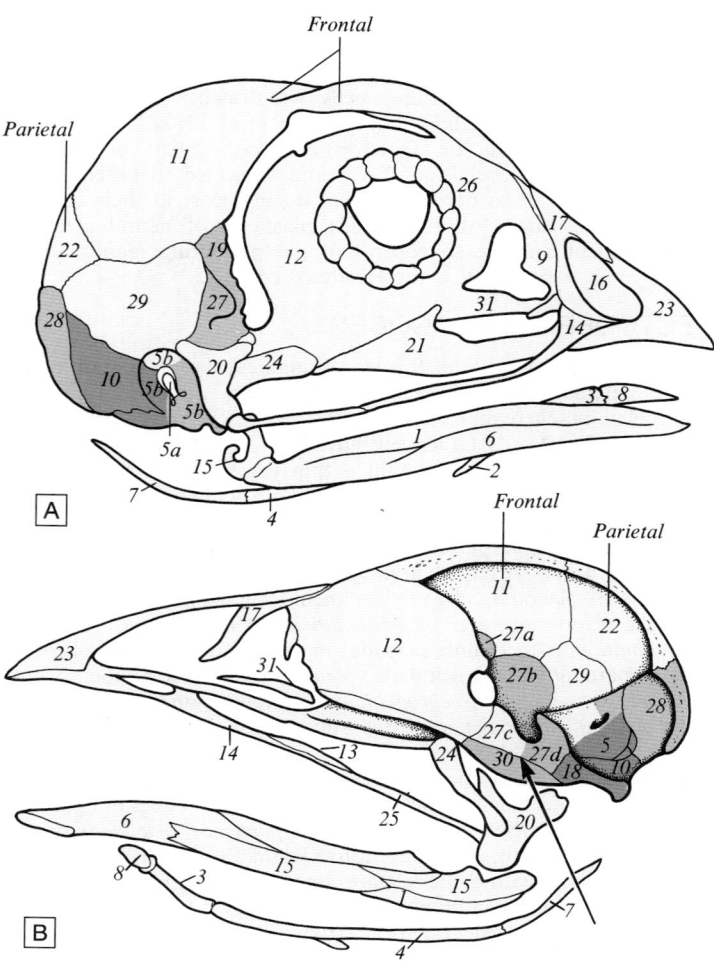

A Fate map   B Developmental potentials

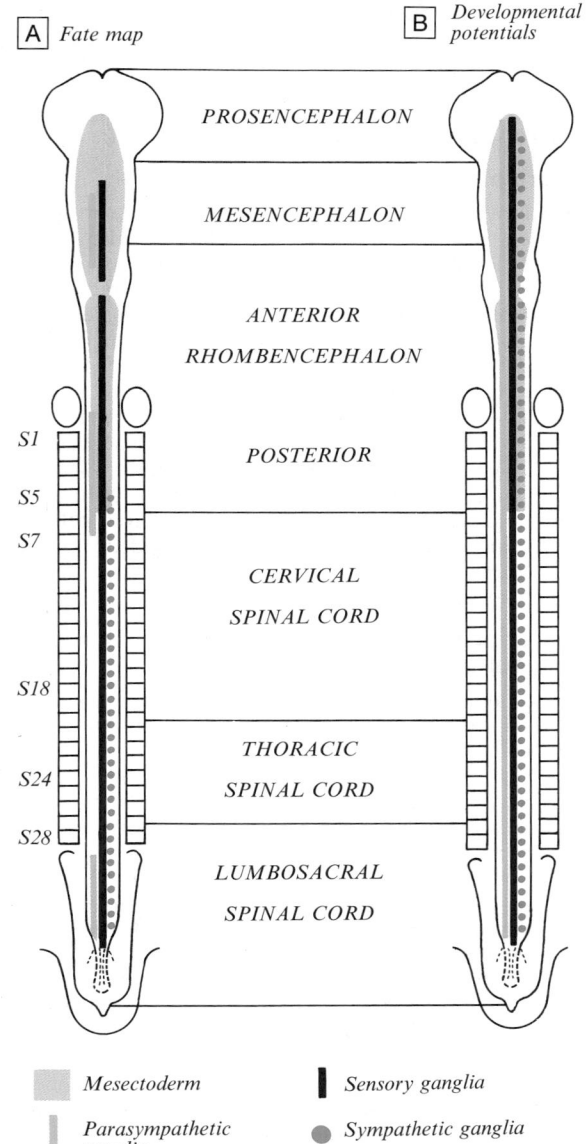

3.101 Schematic drawing of cephalic skeleton of bird. A. Right external view; B. right internal view. Yellow = skeleton of neural crest origin; red = skeleton of cephalic mesenchyme origin; purple = skeleton of somitic origin. (From Couly et al 1993.)

1 angular	18 occipital (basi)
2 basibranchial	19 postorbital
3 basihyal	20 quadrate
4 ceratobranchial	21 palatine
5 (a) columella and (b) otic capsule	22 parietal
6 dentary	23 premaxilla
7 epibranchial	24 pterygoid
8 entoglossum	25 quadratojugal
9 ethmoid	26 scleral ossicles
10 exoccipital	27 sphenoid: (a) orbitosphenoid; (b)
11 frontal	pleurosphenoid; (c) basipres-
12 interorbital septum	phenoid; (d) basipostsphenoid
13 jugal	28 supraoccipital
14 maxilla	29 squamosal
15 Meckel's cartilage	30 temporal
16 nasal capsule	31 vomer
17 nasal	

3.102A Fate map along the neural crest of the presumptive territories that yield the mesectoderm, the sensory, parasympathetic and sympathetic ganglia in normal development. B. Development potentials for the same cell types. If neural crest cells from any level of the neural axis are implanted into the appropriate sites of a host embryo, they can give rise to almost all the cell types forming the various kinds of PNS ganglia. This is not true, however, for the ectomesenchymal cells (also called mesectoderm) whose precursors are confined to the cephalic area of the crest down to the level of somite 5. S = somite.

Vagal neural crest. This normally gives rise to enteric ganglia but was transplanted into the neuraxis at the level (somites 18–24) from which the adrenal medulla, sympathetic and sensory ganglia are derived. The grafted quail cells followed the migration pathway appropriate to the *recipient* site. The cells reached the target organs (sympathetic ganglia and adrenal medulla) of the host where they differentiated into catecholamine producing cells and not into the enteric cholinergic neurons that would have been their normal fate. Similarly, when a neural primordium of the adrenomedullary level was transplanted into the vagal area, the grafted neural crest cells migrated to the gut where they differentiated into enteric ganglia; thus they did not express the adrenergic phenotype.

The back-transplantation approach showed that all types of peripheral ganglia contain, besides their characteristic neuronal and glial cell types, precursor cells that do not differentiate in these sites but can be led to do so if they are provided with appropriate environmental cues. Thus adrenergic cells can arise from sensory ganglia and from enteric plexuses in which this phenotype does not normally exist.

Neural crest derived glial cells provide another example. A surface glycoprotein of the immunoglobulin-like superfamily, the Schwann cell myelin protein (SMP), was found to be expressed exclusively by myelinating and non-myelinating Schwann cells in vivo (Dulac et al 1992). Neither the enteric glia nor the satellite cells of the peripheral ganglia carry this marker. The control of SMP gene expression by environmental cues and particularly its inhibition by the microenvironment of the gut of the dorsal root ganglion was demonstrated experimentally by changing the environment of the various types of glial cells. Thus enteric glia and sensory ganglia satellite cells synthesize SMP when they are withdrawn from their normal environment and cultured in vitro (Dulac & Le Douarin 1991; Cameron-Curry et al 1993).

It appears, therefore, that *precursors* of virtually all the cell types that compose the PNS are **present at every level** of the neuraxis (**3**.102). Therefore, the apparent regionalization of the fate map reflects the diversity of the embryonic rudiments to which the neural crest cells migrate rather than intrinsic restrictions that exist in the neural crest cell population before migration.

Factors promoting neural crest survival

Both survival and differentiation of sensory neuronal progenitors have been shown to depend on factors provided by the neural tube at the time the neural crest cells aggregate to form the dorsal root ganglia (E3–E4, i.e. days 3–4, in chick and quail embryos). Neurotrophins of the brain derived neurotrophic factor (BDNF) family along with the extracellular matrix protein, laminin, were shown to be responsible in this case (Kalcheim & Le Douarin 1986; Kalcheim et al 1987). Clearly other growth factors must play similar roles for the other types of neural crest derivatives. For example, basic fibroblastic growth factor (b-FGF) (Kalcheim 1989; Kalcheim & Neufeld 1990), insulin and insulin-like growth factor (IGF1) (Le Douarin & Smith 1988) were found to influence the differentiation of definite sets of neural crest derived cells at the early ontogenetic stages. Another example is provided by the *steel* factor and its receptor, c-kit, which play a decisive role in the differentiation of melanocytes (Williams et al 1992).

The pluripotentiality of neural crest cells analysed in clonal cultures

Culture conditions can be provided which allow neural crest cells to grow and express their developmental potentialities, even when seeded as single cells (Sieber-Blum & Cohen 1980; Baroffio et al 1988, 1991). This can be achieved in a culture medium which, ideally and in contrast to in vivo conditions, exerts minimal or no selective pressures on these cells but allows them to express their differentiating capacities without restriction.

Experiments involving either cephalic or truncal neural crest cells at the migratory stage showed that most of them are pluripotent, in that they yield clones that contain multiple phenotypes revealed by various markers. Thus different types of neurons can be identified by their morphology and their content of neurofilament proteins, neuropeptides or of enzymes for the synthesis of neurotransmitters. Glial cells react with antibodies that recognize glial surface molecules in vivo, such as HNK1, and Schwann cell myelin protein; melanocytes contain their own marker, melanin, and mesectodermal derivatives can be recognized when they differentiate into cartilage nodules or into desmin containing cells (Baroffio et al 1988; Ito & Sieber-Blum 1991). The abilities of individual neural crest cells to proliferate and differentiate, however, are highly variable. Some give rise to two and others to three or more phenotypes and the size of the clones varies greatly. A few cells give rise to clones in which only one cell type (e.g. neuronal or glial) can be detected and these are believed to arise from monopotent, fully committed precursors. The cells which give rise to clones in which all representatives of the neural crest are present, including mesectodermal derivatives such as cartilage, are found only in the cephalic area. Mesectodermal derivatives are commonly found associated with neural, glial and melanocytic cell types. This shows that, at the time of crest cell emigration, mesenchymal and neurectodermal lineages are not segregated in the neural crest as they are in the ectoderm and the mesoblast after gastrulation.

Thus it seems that the neural crest contains *totipotent stem cells* that are analogous to the hemopoietic stem cells which give rise to the multiple blood cell lineages (Anderson 1989). Such putative stem cells are only rarely seen during the migratory phase of the cephalic neural crest. It will be interesting to see if their frequency is higher at earlier stages of crest cell ontogeny.

Stem cells are characterized by their capacity for self renewal. Such self renewal has been demonstrated in rat neural crest (Stemple & Anderson 1992). In vivo labelling experiments in which chick premigratory single neural crest cells were either injected with a fluorescent dye (Bronner-Fraser & Fraser 1988, 1989), or infected with retroviruses (Frank & Sanes 1991) revealed that both clone size and cellular composition were variable. These results led to the notion that crest cell populations that reach their migratory destination are highly pluripotent. Only a small part of these potentialities will be realized in each neural crest derivative. Cells whose fate does not fit with the conditions encountered in a precision location will either die or remain quiescent. The latter alternative was demonstrated in experiments where neural crest cells, withdrawn from their normal environment such as the gut (Rothman et al 1987), various types of sensory ganglia (Le Douarin & Smith 1988) or the skin (Richardson & Sieber-Blum 1993) and subjected to different conditions, gave rise to derivatives that do not exist in their tissue of origin. Thus these studies suggest plasticity of neural crest cell development and assign control of the patterning mainly to the embryonic territories that the crest cells colonize.

ECTODERMAL PLACODES

The elevating neural folds formed during neurulation contain neural crest cells along most of the neural axis; these cells undergo epithelial/mesenchymal transition to acquire the migratory characteristics of crest cells. Other cells have been identified which originate in the neural folds but remain within the surface ectoderm after neurulation. These areas of neurepithelium within the surface ectoderm have been termed *ectodermal placodes*. Although the majority of the ectodermal placodes form nervous tissue, non-neurogenic placodes occur. After an appropriate inductive stimulus the local clusters of placodal cells remove themselves from the surrounding surface ectoderm either by *epithelial/mesenchymal transition* or by *invagination* of the whole placodal region to form a *vesicle* beneath the remaining surface ectoderm. *Neurogenic placodes* undergo both processes; paired *non-neurogenic placodes* invaginate to form the lens vesicles under the inductive influence of the optic vesicles (see p. 259).

The neural folds meet in the rostral midline adjacent to the buccopharyngeal membrane; this *rostral neural fold* does not generate neural crest but itself gives rise to the *hypophyseal placode* (Couly & Le Douarin 1985), i.e. the future Rathke's pouch (see p. 257), which remains within the surface ectoderm directly rostral to the buccopharyngeal membrane. The rostral neural fold also gives rise to the *olfactory placodes* (see p. 222), which remain as paired, laterally placed placodes, and to epithelium of the nasal cavity (**3**.100).

Further caudally, similar *neurogenic placodes* can be identified and divided into three categories, *ventrolateral* or *epibranchial*, *dorsolateral* and *intermediate* (**3**.103). The epibranchial placodes appear in the surface ectoderm immediately dorsal to the area of pharyngeal (branchial) cleft formation. The first epibranchial placode is located at the level of the first pharyngeal groove and contributes cells to the *distal* (*geniculate*) *ganglion* of the VIIth cranial nerve; the second and third epibranchial placodes contribute cells to the distal ganglia of cranial nerves IX (*petrosal*) and X (*nodose*) respectively. Generally these placodes thicken and cells begin to detach from the epithelium soon after the pharyngeal pouches have contacted the overlying ectoderm. Concurrently the neural crest cells reach and move beyond these lateral extensions of the pharynx. Cells budding off placodes show signs of early differentiation into neurons including the formation of neurites (D'Amico-Martel & Noden 1983). Epibranchial placodes may have their origins in the neurons innervating the taste buds in fishes.

Dorsolateral placodes may be related evolutionarily to the sensory receptors of the lateral line system of lower vertebrates. They are represented by the *otic placodes*, located lateral to the myelencephalon; they invaginate to form otic vesicles which become the *membranous labyrinth of the ear*. Neurons of the VIIIth nerve ganglia arise by budding off the ventromedial aspect of the otic cup after which they can be distinguished in the *acoustic* and *vestibular ganglia*.

Intermediate between the epibranchial and dorsolateral placodes are the *profundal* and *trigeminal placodes*. In man the profundal and trigeminal placodes are fused to form a single entity. Prospective neuroblasts migrate from foci dispersed throughout the surface ectoderm lateral and ventrolateral to the caudal mesencephalon and metencephalon to contribute to the distal portions of the trigeminal ganglia. (For a lucid account of placodal development see D'Amico-Martel & Noden 1983).

NEUROGLIA

Glial cells which support neurons in the CNS and PNS derive from three lineages, the *neuroectoderm* of the neural tube, the *neural crest*,

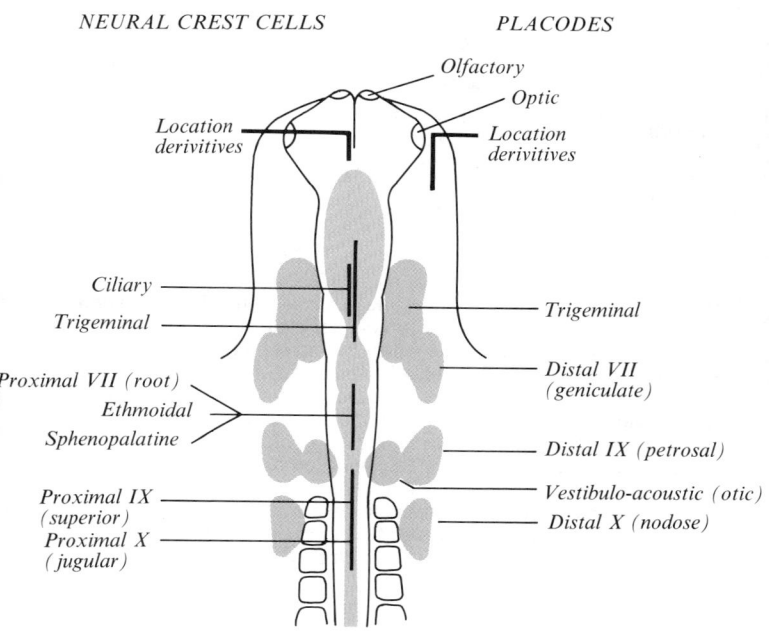

3.103 Diagram indicating the positions of neural crest and placodal cells in a 9.5-stage chick embryo. (From D'Amico Martell & Nodeh 1983.)

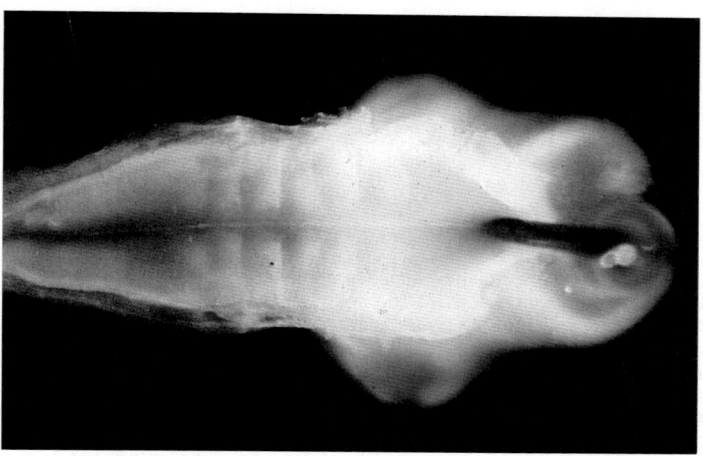

3.104 Photograph showing rhombomeric segmentation (Photograph supplied by Prof A Lumsden.)

and *angioblastic mesenchyme*. In the CNS, cells of the proliferating ventricular zone give rise to *astrocyte* and *oligodendrocyte* cell lines, the first a supporting and reactive cell in the CNS, the second responsible for myelination in the CNS. After the proliferative phase the cells remaining at the ventricular surface differentiate into *ependymal cells* which are specialized in many regions of the ventricular system as circumventricular organs (Collins and Woollam 1981). In the peripheral nervous system, neural crest cells produce *Schwann cells* which myelinate peripheral nerves, and also *astrocyte-like support cells* in the enteric nervous system (see p. 235). Angioblastic mesenchyme gives rise to a variety of blood cell types including the circulating monocytes which infiltrate the brain as *microglial cells* later in development.

The ventricular zone lining the early central canal of the spinal cord and the cavities of the brain give rise to at least two types of cell: glial fibrillary acidic protein (GFAP) positive and negative; many of their proliferative progeny migrate into the intermediate zone. The negative cells form neuroblasts which differentiate into neurons, and the positive cells glioblasts which differentiate first to form *primitive radial* varieties, and then generations of astroblasts and oligodendroblasts; the latter mature into astrocytes and oligodendrocytes (for their mature morphology and hypothesized functional roles, see p. 940). The earliest glioblasts' radial processes extend both outwards to form the outer limiting membrane deep to the pia mater and inwards, forming the inner limiting membrane around the central cavity. Their cell geometry may provide contact guidance paths for subsequent cell migrations, both neuroblastic and glioblastic. As the glioblasts differentiate into primitive neuroglia some lose their connections with both inner and outer limiting membranes. They may partially clothe the somata (between presumptive synaptic contacts) of neighbouring developing neuroblasts, or similarly enwrap intersynaptic surfaces of their neurites. (When many varieties of axon are involved, the encircling glial processes form internodal segments of myelin.) Further glial processes expand around intraneural capillaries as perivascular end-feet. Other glioblasts retain an attachment (or form new expansions) applied as pial end-feet to the innermost stratum of the meninges (pia mater)—this is the *pia intima* of some neurocytologists. Both strata may be termed *pia-glia*. In the developing rat brain, glioblasts which will develop into either oligodendrocytes or type-2 astrocytes are termed O-2A progenitors. They are known to express platelet derived growth factor (PDGF) receptors, unlike neurons, and can be stimulated to divide in culture by PDGF (Pringle et al 1992). Still other glioblasts remain lining the central canal and cavities of the brain as generalized or specialized ependymal cells, including tanycytes, but lose their

peripheral attachments. In some situations, as in the anterior median fissure of the spinal cord, the ependymal cells retain their attachments to both the inner and outer limiting membranes. Thus, in addition to functioning as perineuronal satellites, the glia provide cellular channels interconnecting extracerebral and intraventricular cerebrospinal fluid, the cerebral vascular bed, the intercellular crevices of the neuropil and the cytoplasm of all neural cell varieties. (For further comments see pp. 937–940.)

Microglia appear in the CNS after it has been penetrated by blood vessels and invade it in large numbers from certain restricted regions, whence they spread in what have picturesquely been called 'fountains of microglia', to extend deeply amongst the nervous elements.

MECHANISMS OF NEURAL DEVELOPMENT

Segmentation in the nervous system

Segmentation is conspicuous in man and other vertebrates in the serial arrangement of the vertebrae and axial muscles and in the periodicity of the spinal nerves. In the last century, the possibility that the neural tube might be divided into *segments* or *neuromeres* was entertained but some contended that bulges observed in the lateral walls of the neural tube were artifacts, or caused by mechanical deformation of the tube by adjacent structures. Recent years have seen a resurgence of interest in this subject, leading to a detailed evaluation of the significance of neuromeres. A series of eight prominent bulges which appear bilaterally in the rhombencephalic wall early in development have been termed *rhombomeres* (**3.**104). (While the term neuromere applies generally to putative 'segments' of the neural tube, the term rhombomere applies specifically to the rhombencephalon.) Rhombomeres have now been shown to constitute crucial *units of pattern formation*, based on the fact that many aspects of the patterning of neuronal populations and the elaboration of their axon tracts conform to a segmental plan. Domains of gene expression, for example those of the *Hox b* genes and the transcription factor *Krox 20*, abut rhombomere boundaries, and perhaps most importantly, single cell labelling experiments have revealed that cells within rhombomeres form segregated non-mixing populations. The neural crest also shows intrinsic segmentation in the hindbrain, being segregated into streams at its point of origin in the dorsal neural tube (Lumsden et al 1991). This may represent a mechanism whereby morphogenetic specification of the premigratory neural crest cells is conveyed to the pharyngeal arches. Although these segmental units lose their morphological prominence with subsequent development, they represent the fundamental ground plan of this part of the neuraxis, creating a series of semi-autonomous units within which local variations to patterning can then develop. The consequences of early segmentation for events later in development, such as the formation of definitive neuronal nuclei within the brainstem and of peripheral axonal projections remains to be explored.

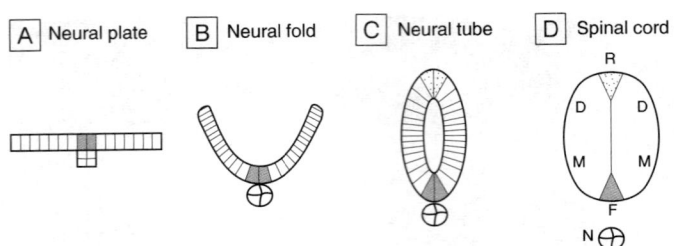

3.105A–D Diagrams to show successive stages in the development of the neural tube and spinal cord. A. The neural plate consists of epithelial cells. Cells at the midline of the neural plate are contacted directly by the notochord. More lateral regions of the neural plate overlie the paraxial mesenchyme (not shown). B. During neurulation, the neural plate bends at its midline elevating the lateral edges of the plate as the neural folds. Contact between the midline of the neural plate and the notochord is maintained at this stage. C. The neural tube is formed when the dorsal tips of the neural folds fuse. Cells in the region of fusion form a specialized group of dorsal midline cells, the *roof plate*. D. Cells at the ventral midline of the neural tube retain proximity to the notochord and differentiate into the *floor plate*. After neural tube closure neuroepithelial cells continue to proliferate and eventually differentiate into defined classes of neurons at different dorsoventral positions within the spinal cord. For example, sensory relay, commissural and other classes of dorsal neurons (D) differentiate near to the roof plate (R), and motor (M) neurons differentiate ventrally near to the floor plate (F), which by this time is no longer in contact with the notochord (N).

3.105E–H These figures summarize the results obtained from experiments in chick embryos in which a notochord or floor plate is grafted to the dorsal midline of the neural tube and in which the notochord is removed before neural tube closure. E. The normal condition, showing the ventral location of motor neurons (M) and the dorsal location of sensory relay neurons (D). F. Dorsal grafts of a notochord result in the induction of a floor plate at the dorsal midline and in the induction of ectopic dorsal motor neurons. G. Dorsal grafts of a floor plate also result in the induction of a new floor plate at the dorsal midline and in the induction of ectopic dorsal motor neurons. H. Removal of the notochord results in the elimination of the floor plate and the motor neurons and the expression of dorsal cells types (D) in the ventral region of the spinal cord. (After Jessell & Dodd 1992 with permission of W. B. Saunders.)

The appeal of segmentation as a fundamental principle in neural development rests on its theoretical attractiveness as a way of simplifying developmental problems, superimposing variations in regional identity on a basal, segmented pattern. In higher vertebrates, the diencephalic anlagen of various regions of the thalamus are found to exhibit distinctive patterns of histochemical staining, and to constitute domains of cell lineage restriction (Figdor & Stern 1993). The organization of the telencephalon is also reflected in domains of gene expression that abut sharp boundaries (reviewed in Puelles & Rubinstein 1993; Boncinelli 1993). However, substantial evidence that these regions employ segmentation in the same manner as the hindbrain has yet to accrue. It is also possible that while in the hindbrain rhombomeres are early units of patterning which are later obscured, those in the forebrain are later structures that constitute the definitive functional units. Recently, there have been many reports that the domains of expression of many presumed regulatory genes have sharp boundaries within the forebrain, some of which correspond with sulci identified in anatomical studies. Thus the subject of segmentation and its possible role in neural patterning in many brain regions is bound to continue to attract attention (see below).

The importance of *intrinsic segmentation* in the hindbrain is underlined by the absence of overt segmentation of the adjacent paraxial mesenchyme. While the somites are prominent segmented entities within the trunk, the mesenchyme of the head appears to be a single continuous block. Somitomeres have been identified lateral to the notochord by scanning electron microscope (Meier 1981; Meier & Packard 1984; see p. 154), but not all are convinced of their veracity. In the trunk, the sclerotomal mesenchyme (see p. 155) plays a role in segmenting the motor outflow and the emigration of the neural crest, and displays molecular heterogeneity. There is no evidence for this in the head; instead segmental properties are manifest in the neurectoderm. Moreover, ectomesenchyme cells seem to be specified with respect to their position prior to migration (Noden 1983a,b), and to be capable of patterning other structures, e.g. the muscles, in the arches into which they migrate. The emigration of neural crest cells from a particular axial level to the outlying arch is followed by axonal outgrowth of motor neurons from the same axial level, thus furnishing a mechanism whereby segmentation in the tube may be matched to that of the outlying structures.

In the spinal cord, however, there is no firm evidence for intrinsic segmentation. Instead, segmentation of the neural crest, motor axons, and thus eventually the spinal nerves, is dependent on the segmentation of the neighbouring somites. Experimental removal or intercalation of somites results in corresponding disturbances of pattern in these nervous structures (Keynes & Stern 1984, 1988). Both neural crest cell migration and motor axon outgrowth occur

through only the rostral and not the caudal sclerotome of each somite. The segmental emergence of crest cells that results ensures that dorsal root ganglia form only at intervals. The caudal sclerotome possesses inhibitory properties that deter neural crest cells and motor axons from entering (Davies et al 1990). This illustrates the general principle that the nervous system is closely interlocked, in terms of morphogenesis, with the 'periphery', i.e. surrounding non-nervous structures, and each is dependent upon the other for its effective structural and functional maturation.

Patterning of the brain and spinal cord

For more than a century experimental strategies have been devised to elucidate mechanisms that operate during the development of the nervous system. Whilst much has been established, answers to many fundamental questions still remain obscure. In recent years, the best efforts to understand the development of 'higher' vertebrates has perhaps come from work on the amphibian and chicken embryos, in which organisms embryological, biochemical and molecular techniques can be combined to greatest effect (see Detwiler 1936; Spemann 1938; Weiss 1950; Hughes 1968; Gottlieb 1974).

The generation of neural tissue involves an inductive signal from the underlying chordamesoderm (p. 295). Neural induction was discovered during experiments on the amphibian embryo by Spemann (1925). In the absence of this signal, ectoderm cells form epidermis; in its presence they form nervous tissue. Despite nearly 70 years having elapsed since the discovery of neural induction, the identity of the signal remains a mystery. Under experimental conditions a disappointingly wide variety of non-specific substances have been found to have a neural inductive influence in salamander and newt embryos, implying that the ectoderm is finely balanced between a neural and an epidermal fate (Spemann 1938; Hamburger 1988). Molecular biological approaches have, however, added impetus to these studies, and have identified some potential positive and negative regulators of neural induction. This work has concentrated on the frog embryo, *Xenopus laevis*, whose ectoderm is not so easily neuralized. The molecule *activin*, belonging to the transforming growth factor beta (TGFβ) family, is a known inducer of *mesoblastic tissue* (Smith 1987) and has been implicated in suppressing neural induction since in frog embryos, containing a truncated and nonfunctional activin receptor, neural tissue is overproduced (Hemmati-Brivanlou & Melton 1992). (For a discussion concerning the use of the term, mesoblast, see p. 93.) This finding might imply that neural differentiation is a default pathway, which activin normally acts to suppress. The suppressive effect of activin can only be blocked by *follistatin*, though this molecule is itself only a weak neural inducer (Hemmati-Brivanlou et al 1994). In addition another factor, *noggin*, has recently been isolated that can induce neural tissue from isolated ectoderm (Smith et al 1993). Hepatocyte growth factor/Scatter factor may also have the ability to induce neural tissue (Stern et al 1990). It is likely that in the future other candidate neural inducers will continue to be isolated; to elucidate the role of these various factors will require their inductive effect in culture to be placed in the context of their distribution and action in normal embryogenesis.

The first elements of the emerging neural pattern may be a **consequence** of neural induction. Neural induction is thus not solely a process that ensures neural differentiation, it is also involved in determining the regional pattern of the nervous system, before and during neural tube closure. Since neural inducing substance(s) have largely remained a mystery, attention has focused instead on the response of the induced neural tissue. Now, the abundance of region-specific molecular markers has renewed attempts to unravel the signals in regional induction.

Genes such as the *Hox* and *Pax* gene families, which encode transcription factor proteins and their homologues, cloned invertebrates, show intriguing expression patterns within the nervous system. Genes of the *Hox-b* cluster, for example, are expressed throughout the caudal neural tube, and up to discrete limits in the hindbrain that coincide with rhombomere boundaries. The ordering of these genes within a cluster on the chromosome (5'–3') is the same as the caudal to rostral limits of expression of consecutive genes. This characteristic pattern is surprisingly similar in fish, frogs, birds and mammals. Persuasive evidence is now accruing that *Hox* genes play a role in patterning not only of much of the neural tube but of much of the head region, consistent with their expression in neural crest cells, and within the pharyngeal arches (see p. 287). While these genes demarcate regions up to and including the hindbrain, those of the *Dlx*, *Otx* and *Emx* families are expressed in different rostrocaudal domains within the forebrain. Some *Pax* genes, on the other hand, are expressed in different dorso-ventral domains within the neural tube. *Pax-3* is expressed in the alar lamina, including the neural crest, while *Pax-6* is expressed in the intermediate plate. Both *Hox* and *Pax* genes have restricted expression patterns with respect to the rostrocaudal and the dorsoventral axes of the neural tube, consistent with roles in positional specification. (For reviews of the expression patterns of these genes see McGinnis & Krumlauf 1992; Krumlauf et al 1993; Puelles & Rubinstein 1993; Chalepakis et al 1993).

The expression of *Hox* genes and other molecular markers have been used to investigate the mechanisms of regional induction, particularly in the frog embryo. This work indicates that specification of the rostrocaudal axis probably occurs somewhat earlier than that of the dorsoventral axis. Earlier in the century, embryologists concentrated on the idea that regionalization of the mesoblast imposed a similar mosaic of positional values on the overlying neural plate. In amphibia, transplantation of various regions of mesoblast beneath the neural plate showed a regional induction. Caudal mesoblast induced spinal cord, whereas rostral mesoblast induced brain, as assessed by the morphology of the neuroepithelial vesicles (Mangold 1933). Supporting evidence for this hypothesis using contemporary methods has been scarce, however. One example is the finding that rostral mesoblast induces expression of the *engrailed* marker (expressed in the rostral neural tube) more frequently than does caudal mesoblast (Hemmati-Brivanlou & Harland 1990). Presently, the consensus view regarding the rostral axis is that the neural plate has considerable self-organizational properties. Signals from the mesoblast are undoubtedly required to elicit neural induction, but it is not necessary for regions of the mesoblast to underlie their corresponding neural counterpart in register to evince regionalization. Thus, for example pieces of tissue isolated prior to gastrulation in which the mesoblast and ectoderm lie in linear array exhibit a surprisingly accurate pattern of expression of *Hox* and other positional markers (Doniach et al 1992). Supporting evidence comes from experiments on amphibian exogastrulae, in which gastrulation fails and the mesoblast never underlies the neural plate. Exogastrulae exhibit the expression of a range of neural markers (Dixon & Kintner 1989; Ruiz i Altaba 1992). This implies that a signal travels in the *plane* of the neurectoderm, a possibility originally noted by Spemann (1938). In the same experimental system, patterns of expression of a *Dlx* gene in the forebrain were less faithfully rendered. The addition of prechordal mesoblast to the

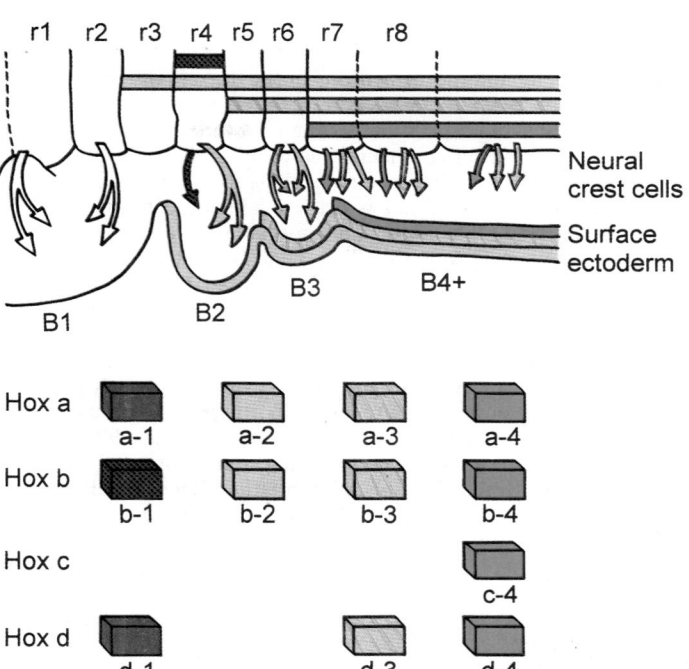

3.106A *Hox* gene expression domains in the branchiorhombomeric area in the mouse embryo at E 9.5. The arrows indicate neural crest cells migrating from the rhombencephalon and midbrain. At the former level they are shaded to indicate the *Hox* genes they express. The same combination of *Hox* gene is expressed in the rhombomeres and in the superficial ectoderm of the pharyngeal arches at the corresponding transverse levels. The 4 *Hox* clusters are represented below. (Modified from Hunt & Krumlauf 1992.)

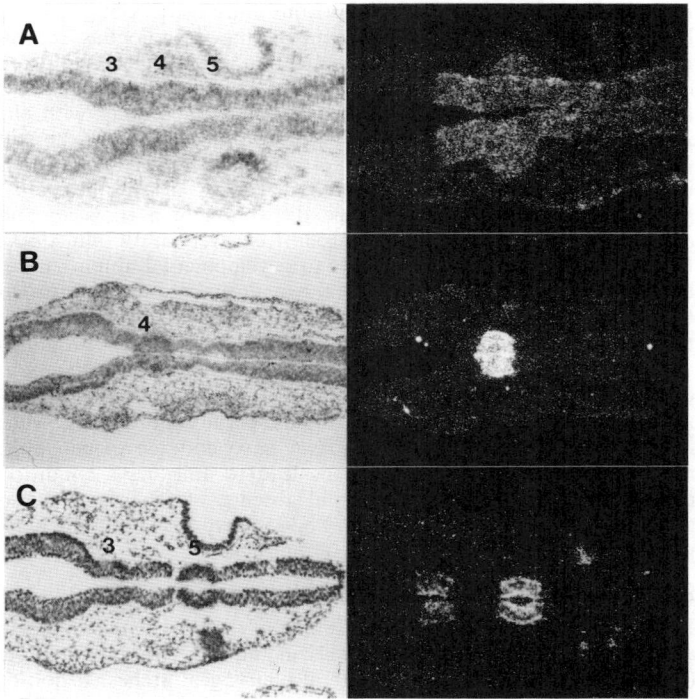

3.106B Expression patterns of regulatory genes in the mouse embryo hindbrain visualized by in situ hybridization. A = *Hox b-2* gene; B = *Hox b-1* gene; C = *Krox-20* gene. For each gene the left panel is a bright field photomicrograph; the right is taken under dark field illumination (white silver grains indicate expression). Cranial is to the left; numbers indicate rhombomeres. (Photographs supplied by D G Wilkinson.)

tissue pieces produced a better representation of the pattern, suggesting that patterning in more cranial regions requires additional signals to that travelling by the planar route (Papalopulu & Kintner 1993). Consistent with this is the observation that eyes (also forebrain structures) were never found in planar recombinations of ectoderm and mesoblast or in exogastrulae (Ruiz i Altaba 1992). Vertical apposition of the mesoblast is also required to promote differentiation of the floor plate and motor neurons in the dorsal part of the neural tube.

Whilst craniocaudal positional values are probably conferred on the neuroepithelium at the neural plate or early neural tube stage, dorsoventral positional values may become fixed later. The development of the dorsoventral axis is heavily influenced by the presence of the underlying notochord. The notochord induces the ventral midline of the neural tube, the floor plate (van Straaten et al 1988; Placzek et al 1990, see above). This specialized region consists of a strip of non-neural cells with distinctive adhesive and functional properties. Notably, it produces a chemoattractant that specifically directs the growth of commissural axons ventrally, to cross the floor plate and project contralaterally (Tessier-Lavigne et al 1988). Notochord and floor plate together participate in inducing the differentiation of the motor columns (Yamada et al 1991). Motor neuron differentiation occurs early, giving some grounds for the idea of a ventral to dorsal wave of differentiation. The notochord/floor plate complex may also be responsible for allotting the values of more dorsal cell types within the tube (3.105). For example, the dorsal domain of expression of *Pax-3* extends more ventrally in embryos experimentally deprived of notochord and floor plate, while grafting an extra notochord adjacent to the dorsal neural tube leads to a repression of *Pax-3* expression (Goulding et al 1993). Investigation of the conditions required for the generation of other neuronal groups has been hampered by the lack of cell-type-specific markers.

Evidence for the involvement in neural development of *Hox* and *Pax* genes has come from studies of animals mutant for members of these gene families. In the pharyngeal region of the head individual *Hox* genes are expressed within matching domains of the brain, the neural crest and the adjacent pharyngeal arches (see p. 238), giving rise to the idea that this might embody a code for patterning the region—*Hox code*. Transgenic 'knockout' mice have been generated by targeted disruption of *Hox* genes using homologous recombination in embryonic stem cells. Mice rendered deficient for *Hox a-3* showed defects in neural crest derived ganglia and derivatives of the third and fourth pharyngeal arches, corresponding with the pattern of normal gene expression (reviewed in Hunt & Krumlauf 1991). Knockouts of *Hox a-1* produced mice that showed disruptions in patterning of the hindbrain rhombomeres and also in the cranial ganglia, in a manner that reflected disruption of a transient and early phase of expression of the gene (reviewed in Wright 1993). Disruption of *Pax* genes also leads to developmental abnormalities in mice, and in the case of at least three genes these may be related to human diseases. For example, the gene *Pax-3* was found to have the same chromosomal localization as the mouse mutation *Splotch* and the affected locus in the human *Waardenburg's syndrome*, both of which are characterized by neural crest disturbances with pigmentation disturbances and occasional neural tube defects. Mice heterozygous for a mutation in *Pax-6* have underdeveloped eyes; mutations in the human *Pax-6* gene lead to aniridia, a condition characterized by complete or partial absence of the iris and also affecting the cornea, lens, retina and optic nerve (reviewed in Chalepakis et al 1993; see also p. 337).

Patterning of the branchiorhombomeric region

Intrinsic genetic control of the patterning of their derivatives appears also to exist in the neural crest cells in the branchiorhombomeric (the rhombencephalon plus the lateral pharyngeal arches) region of the body. The view that the neural crest itself possesses its own patterning capacities is supported by discoveries regarding the metameric organization of the hindbrain in vertebrates and its relation with the genetic control of its development by genes containing homeobox sequences with high degrees of homology with that of the Drosophila Antennapedia (Antp) homeogene (Hunt & Krumlauf 1992).

The expression of genes in the *Hox a, b, c* and *d* clusters (previously *Hox-1* to *4*) has been analysed in detail in the hindbrain and corresponding neural crest in the mouse (3.106). With few exceptions, the *Hox* genes expressed in the rhombomeres are **also** expressed in the neural crest at the same transverse levels. When neural crest cell migration is completed the same set of *Hox* genes is activated in the

surface ectoderm. Using the quail–chick marker system, Couly and Le Douarin (1990) distinguished, in the branchiorhombomeric region, a metameric disposition of ectodermal stripes or *ectomeres*. These include the rhombomeres, the neural folds which produce neural crest cells, and the surface ectoderm covering the pharyngeal arch colonized by the neural crest cells, arising from the same level. Taken together, these observations suggest that the positional information that controls pharyngeal arch patterning is first contained in the rhombencephalon and then transmitted to the pharyngeal area via neural crest cells. The fact that positional information is controlled by a combination of *Hox* gene expression was further demonstrated by targeted mutations in the mouse.

Disruption of *Hox a-3* gene mimics the Di George's syndrome, a congenital human disorder characterized by the absence (or near absence) of the thymus, parathyroids and thyroid, by the hypotrophy of the wall of the arteries derived from the aortic arches, and by subsequent conotruncal cardiac malformations. The *Hox a-3* nul mice also show reductions in the skeletal development of the jaws and hyoid cartilage and in the muscular and connective tissues of the pharynx and the tongue. The rhombencephalic neural crest provides the entire set of mesenchymal cells to the thymic, thyroid and parathyroid rudiments, and constitutes the whole musculoconnective wall of the arteries arising from the aortic arches (see p. 314). Moreover, it has been established (Auerbach 1960, 1961) that thymic histogenesis depends strictly upon induction of the epithelium by the mesenchyme. Similar interactions are critical as well for the other glandular structures of the buccopharyngeal area (Le Douarin 1968). It is therefore understandable that a developmental failure of the hindbrain neural crest accounts for all the Di George's syndrome anomalies and for most of those of the *Hox a-3/Hox a-3* mice.

In experimental mutation of the *Hox a-1* gene (Thomas & Capecchi 1990; McMahon & Bradley 1990; Lufkin et al 1991), the defects observed concerned the neural (and not the mesectodermal as for *Hox a-3*) derivatives of the neural crest and of the CNS at the level of rhombomeres 4–7. The morphogenesis of different neural crest derivatives corresponding either to the mesectodermal and/or the neural lineages therefore appear to be influenced by **different** sets of regulatory genes. Disruption of the *Hox a-2* gene has recently been shown to result in the homeotic transformation of skeletal elements derived from the second pharyngeal arch into more anterior structures corresponding to the 1st arch. This supports the contention that a combination of *Hox* genes (*Hox code*) is responsible for the patterning of neural crest hypobranchial derivatives and providing them with regional specification along the cranio-caudal axis of the body.

Histogenesis of the neural tube

The classic view of neural tube histogenesis was first propounded by Wilhelm His in 1890 and soon gained quite wide acceptance (e.g. Ramón y Cajal 1911). He proposed that subclasses of germinal cells were progenitors of particular classes of neurons and glial cells. Thus, almost from the first the wall of the tube was *stratified* and contained a variety of distinct cell types—*spongioblasts*, *neuroblasts* and *germinal cells*. Contemporaneously, the opposing view, that of *multipotential progenitors*, was also put forward (Vignal 1889; Koelliker 1887).

The round deeply placed germinal cells or *medulloblasts* (Glees 1963) were regarded by His as undifferentiated stem cells, which by repeated division gave further generations of both spongioblasts (glial progenitors) and neuroblasts. The primitive spongioblasts, originally elongate cells attached to both limiting membranes with their nuclei in the ventricular zone, were considered to differentiate into a number of *sustentacular cell* varieties. By losing contact with one or both limiting membranes, they would then differentiate into either astroblasts and astrocytes or oligodendroblasts and oligodendrocytes, or, retaining an internal attachment, into the definitive ependymal cells which line the central canal, and regionally specialized tanycytes (p. 939). The neural precursors, one of the cell types found in the mantle zone (intermediate zone), differentiated into the wide array of neurons. On this view, therefore, which constituted a *polyphyletic theory of neurogenesis*, the early neural epithelium was regarded as a *heterogeneous* grouping of cells with their various derivatives, developing **simultaneously**.

An opposing view, expounded by Schaper (1897a,b), interpreted the mitotic figures as synonymous with the neuroepithelial cells, simply seen in a different location and in different phases of the cell cycle. Not until the meticulous cytological studies of Sauer (1935a,b, 1936) did this theory gain wide acceptance. He maintained that the early neural epithelium, including the deeply placed ventricular mitotic zone, consists of a *homogeneous* population of pluripotent cells, the varying appearances merely reflecting different phases in a *proliferative cycle*, the sequence being termed by Sauer *interkinetic migration*. This proposal was essentially a *monophyletic theory of neurogenesis*. In subsequent years much experimental evidence based upon colchicine studies (e.g. Watterson et al 1956), spectro-photometric nuclear analysis (e.g. Sauer & Chittenden 1959) and upon autoradiographic studies following the distribution of cells at varying times after labelling with tritiated thymidine (e.g. Sidman et al 1959, Sidman 1970; Fujita 1963; Fujita & Fujita 1963) and ultrastructural studies (e.g. Hinds 1971) have supported the latter proposition. The scheme amplified by Fujita in a series of later publications is illustrated in **3**.107. The ependymal layer of earlier workers (termed by Fujita the *matrix layer*) is considered to be populated by a single basic type of *progenitor cell* and to exhibit three 'zones' (the M or mitotic, the I or intermediate, and the S or synthetic zones). As they pass through a complete intermitotic and mitotic cycle, the matrix cells show an 'elevator movement' progressively approaching and then receding from the internal limiting membrane. DNA replication occurs whilst the cells are extended and their nuclei occupy the S zone; they then enter a premitotic resting period whilst the cells shorten and their nuclei pass through the I zone. The cells now become rounded close to the internal limiting membrane (in the M zone) and undergo mitosis; thereafter they elongate again, their nuclei passing through the I zone during the postmitotic resting period, finally to enter the synthetic zone once again. The cells so formed may then either start another *proliferative cycle* or migrate outwards (i.e. radially) and differentiate into neurons as they approach and enter the adjacent stratum; possibly this differentiation is initiated as they pass through the I zone during the postmitotic resting period. The proliferative cycle continues with the production of clones of neurons, but this process eventually declines and is superseded by the production of *ependymal cell* and *macroglial cell* varieties.

Cumulative tritiated thymidine labelling studies have shown that an initial period of *symmetric division* is followed by a period of *asymmetric division*. At the last division, of course, two postmitotic daughters are produced. Later, the progeny of some of these divisions move away from the ventricle to form an intermediate (mantle) zone of neurons; others form a *subventricular zone* between the ventricular and intermediate layers, there continuing to multiply to provide further generations of neurons and glia. Both of these cell types subsequently migrate into the intermediate and marginal zones but in some regions of the nervous system (e.g. the cerebellar cortex, p. 261) some mitotic subventricular stem cells migrate across the entire neural wall to form a *subpial population*, thus establishing a new zone of cell division and differentiation. Many cells formed in this site remain subpial in position but others migrate back towards the ventricle through the developing nervous tissue, finishing their migrations in various definitive sites where they finally differentiate into neurons and macroglial cells.

It should be emphasized here that differences of opinion persist (and have increased in the last decade), concerning the precise details of these processes and the possible mechanisms involved. Further, considerable confusion has obtained between different neuro-embryologists in relation to the **terminology** to be adopted for the various 'layers' or 'zones' at different times and places in the developing neural tube. An international group of neurocytologists (the Boulder Committee 1970) proposed a less ambiguous nomenclature which is increasingly but not universally adopted. They termed the early pseudostratified neuroepithelium, in which the 'elevator movement' occurs, the *ventricular zone* (its further development is summarized below, on page 219, and in **3**.95). For an excellent review of the biological and terminological problems posed, and an extensive bibliography to the data indicated, consult Berry (1974), and for further comments on the natural history of neurons see page 921.

Figure **3**.95 summarizes the main stages of development of the neural tube and the nomenclature as **initially** proposed by the Boulder

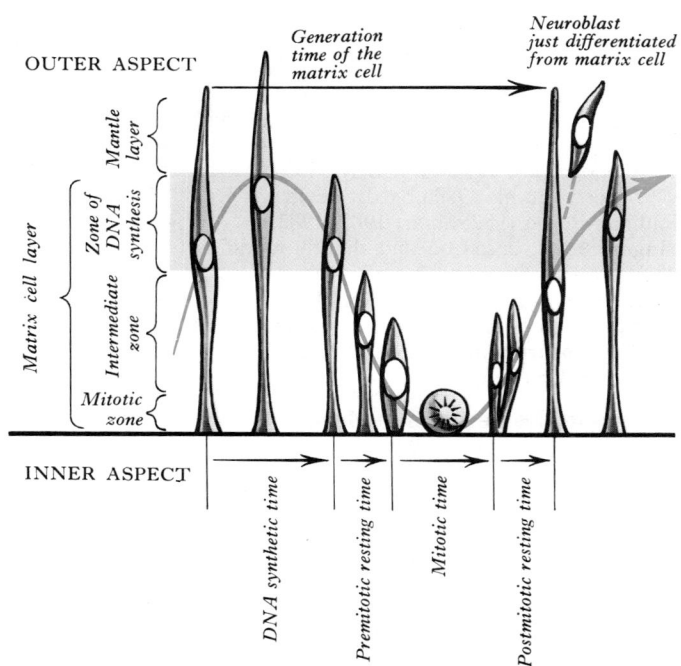

3.107 Diagram showing the cytogenetic cycle in the matrix cell layer and mantle layer in the wall of the developing neural tube. Note the various times and their associated time scales, through which the matrix cell nuclei pass during their postulated 'elevator movement' or 'interkinetic migration' which is described in greater detail in the text. (From S. Fujita, with permission of the author and the *Journal of Comparative Neurology*, 1963.)

Committee (1970), the complete series of stages A–E applying to the cerebral neocortex: only stages A–C are relevant in the context of the spinal cord. As detailed in the caption, it will be seen that the early pseudostratified *ventricular zone* (V) is followed by the sequential appearance of *marginal* (M), *intermediate* (I), *subventricular* (S) zones and, concurrently with the latter, the early *cortical plate* (CP) (see p. 252). It is unfortunate that this use of term **zone** for these major ontogenetic strata does **not** correspond to the M, I and S zones of Fujita detailed above (and in **3**.107), the latter applying to sub-divisions of the early neural tube only. More than a decade of research employing technical innovations induced Rakic (1982) to suggest a series of additional features and modifications of the original Boulder proposals. These are mentioned at various points in the text, and summarized in relation to the neocortex on page 252 and in **3**.123A–G.

Figure **3**.70 (based on the work of Berry & Rogers 1965; Berry 1974) may be noted here for comparison with **3**.123; it stems from labelling studies on the *pattern of migration* of neuroblasts in the developing neocortex in the rat and will be briefly mentioned later on page 253 et seq.

The following decade, and to the time of writing, has seen accelerating, enthusiastic application of newer, more refined techniques to these and related problems: in particular immuno-histochemistry and computer analysis of neurocellular geometry. This has resulted in reappraisal of some foregoing conclusions. The cytokinetics of the early pseudostratified neuroepithelium ('elevator' movement, or interkinetic migration) has been substantiated, as has the establishment of the principal zones proposed by the Boulder Committee. However, the latter has been modified (at least in the forebrain) by the recognition of an additional (though transient) stratum deep to the early cortical plate—the *subplate zone* (SP), see page 253—and many further features of cortical and subcortical maturation. Throughout most of the neuraxis, proliferative cell cycles are limited to the ventricular (V) and subventricular (S) zones, but their homogenous nature has been challenged. Immunocytochemical methods for demonstrating glial fibrillary acidic protein strongly suggest that **at least two** cell varieties are present in the early tubal neuroepithelium, perhaps in a precise mosaic pattern. (This may be classified as an *oligophyletic theory of neurogenesis*.) The early disposition of radial glial fibres is proposed by some to have a profound morphogenetic significance. The latter concerns not only their spatially ordered array, but the probability that they provide migration paths, by contact guidance, for at least the earlier generations of migratory neuroblasts, thus specifying their destinations. Neuronal geometry is further considered on pages 237, 243, 252. (See bibliographic reviews in Berry 1974, 1982; Schmitt & Worden 1979; Berry et al 1980a,b,c,d; Levitt & Rakic 1980; Rakic & Goldman-Rakic 1982; Smart 1982, 1983.)

Figure **3**.108, based on and slightly modified from Rakic (1981, 1982), is a simplified analysis of earlier and current theories of some cell varieties and lineages in neural tube histogenesis. In a recent presentation (Levitt et al 1981) some aspects of all earlier theories have been incorporated, others rejected. See caption and text above for further comment.

Lineage in the nervous system

Neurons come from two major embryonic sources: *central neurons* originate from the neural plate and tube whereas *ganglionic neurons* originate from the neural crest and placodes. The neural plate also provides ependymal and macroglial cells, while from the neural crest arise inter alia peripheral Schwann cells and chromaffin cells. Recently many difficulties in determining the origins and lineages of cells in the nervous system have been resolved by the use of autoradiography, microinjection or retroviral labelling of progenitor cells and cell culture.

During development, neurons are formed first, followed by glial cells. The timing of events differs in various parts of the CNS and between species. Most neurons are formed prenatally in mammals but some postnatal neurogenesis does occur, as in the case of the small granular cells of the cerebellum, olfactory bulb and hippocampus, and neurons of the cerebral cortex. Gliogenesis continues after birth in periventricular and other sites. Autoradiographic studies show that different classes of neurons develop at specific times. Large neurons such as *principal projection neurons* tend to

differentiate before small ones such as *local circuit neurons*. However, their subsequent migration appears independent of the times of their initial formation. Neurons can migrate extensively through populations of maturing, relatively static cells, to reach their destination; for example, cerebellar granule cells pass through a layer of Purkinje cells en route from the external pial layer to their final, central position. Later, the final form of their projections, cell volume and indeed their continuing survival depend on the establishment of patterns of functional connection (p. 255). For an account of glial cell development see page 225.

There are many questions regarding the factors determining the lineage of neural cells. For example, do individual progenitor cells give rise to both neurons and glia, and/or to different neuronal subtypes? Are there defined fields of progenitor cells that give rise to different regions of the CNS? Resolving these questions involves labelling a single progenitor cell, allowing development to proceed and then recording the positions and phenotypes of all labelled progeny, using specific antibodies or precise morphological criteria (e.g. at electron microscope level). Whilst in amphibia and avia direct cell injection of fluorescent lineage tracers is feasible, this is so far impossible in mammals, owing to the inaccessibility of the embryos in utero. Instead, lineage analyses have relied on the infection of progenitor cells in the ventricular zone of rodent embryos using replication defective retroviruses (Sanes et al 1986; Price et al 1987). The retroviral DNA incorporates into the genome of the infected cell providing an indelible marker that is transmitted to all progeny during cell division, but not to surrounding cells. Initial infective events are random, affording no control over the number or location of cells infected. Thus, defining single clones at later developmental times, when cell mixing may have taken place, is problematic. However, both the direct injection and retroviral techniques have yielded some information about lineage in various regions of the nervous system. In the optic tectum of avia, a single cell can give rise to **both** neurons and glia with diverse forms (Galileo et al 1990). A similar pattern was observed for the avian spinal cord, in which

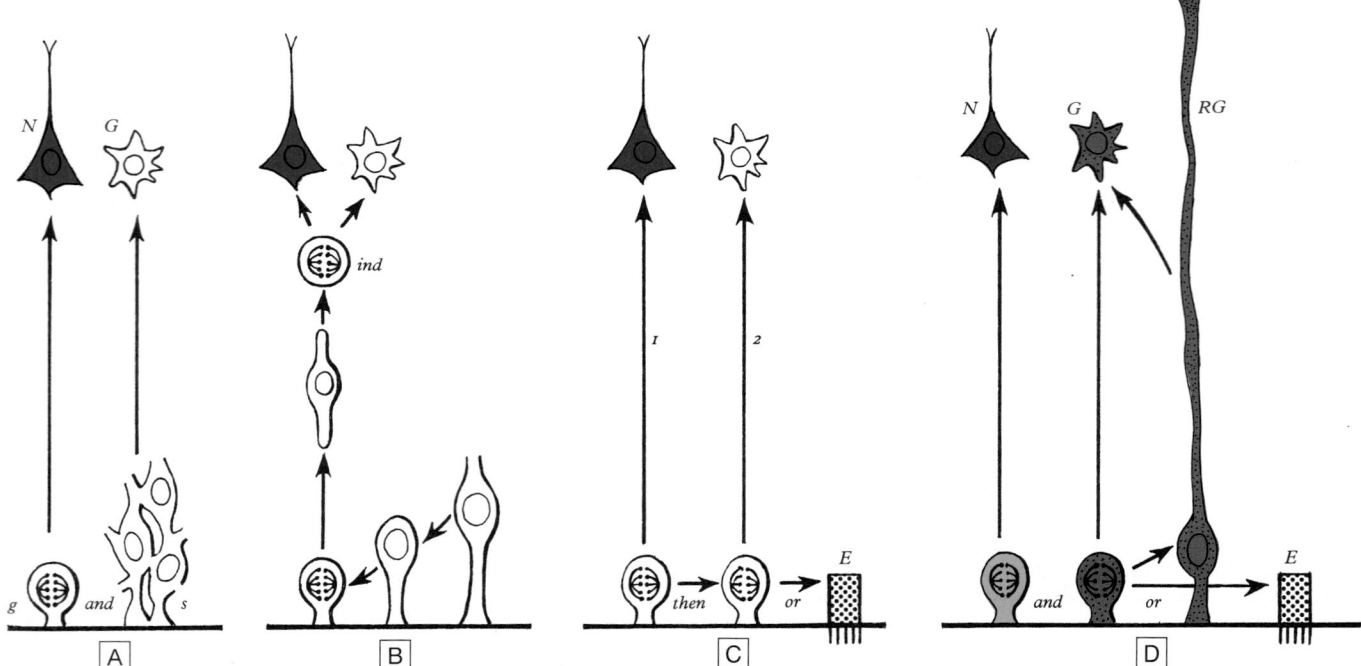

3.108 Simplified schemes of successively held theories of cell lineages during early neurogenesis.

A. His (1889) recognized two major cell varieties in the matrix layers (ventricular zone) lining the central canal and ventricles: spheroidal, proliferative, germinal cells (g), their progeny migrating to form neuroblasts (N) and neighbouring spongioblasts (s) whose progeny form varieties of glioblast (G).

B. Schaper (1897) held that ventricular zone mitoses gave outwardly migrating indifferent cells (ind), further division of which produced neuroblasts, glioblasts, or both.

c. Fujita (1963), using autoradiography, believed that a single proliferative type of matrix cell gave migratory generations *firstly* of neuroblasts, sec-

ondarily (later) of glioblasts; finally, the persistent remainder formed ependymal cells (E).

D. Currently, electron immunohistochemistry has demonstrated at least two distinct cell varieties, GFA (glial fibrillary acid protein) positive and negative, present in extremely early ventricular zones. The negative cells (blue) gave migratory neuroblasts (purple). The positive cells (magenta) gave: firstly, radial glioblasts (RG) that span the neural tube joining homologous internal and external points; later, directly or indirectly, generations of definitive glioblasts, and finally ependymal cells. The radial glial extensions probably provide contact guidance paths for echelons of neuroblast migration. (Modified after Rakic 1982.)

clones contained motor neurons and a range of other neurons such as interneurons and preganglionic autonomics, along with glia and ependymal cells (Leber et al 1990). Similarly, for the retina, experiments on rodents show that labelled cells produce a range of derivatives, consisting of any combination of rods, bipolar cells, amacrine cells and Muller glia (Turner & Cepko 1987). Furthermore, in the retina, cells were able to yield more than one cell type up to their terminal division. It should be noted that Muller glia resemble astrocytes, but are significantly different by morphological and molecular criteria; typical astrocytes are present in the retina but they have a different lineage, migrating from the optic nerve.

By contrast, information on lineage within the cortex has suggested some degree of lineage restriction. In one study, the majority of clones consisted of either neurons or glia (Walsh & Cepko 1992), while other authors found clones composed of either astrocytes, neurons or oligodendrocytes, or a mixture of the last two (Price & Thurlow 1988). An electron microscope study of the synaptic morphology and ultrastructure of retrovirally-marked cells has reported separate clones of pyramidal and non-pyramidal neurons, as well as of astrocytes and oligodendrocytes (Parnavelas et al 1992). These studies therefore tend to the conclusion that there are **separate** progenitors for different cell populations. There are two reasons why this conclusion might be called into question, however. First, this impression might be gained if the information gathered reflected events late in the lineage tree. Multipotent precursor cells might exist at early stages, but might not be detected, since the technical difficulties of introducing virus into the fetal ventricles precludes these experiments before E12 in the mouse of E14 in the rat. Secondly, recent studies suggest a much higher degree of cell dispersion tangentially within the cortex than has been suspected, making definitions of clonality problematic (see p. 255). Interestingly, a study in which progenitor cells were labelled in the chick hindbrain by direct cell injection yielded large clones of cells mostly with identical phenotypes and axonal projection patterns, implying early assignment of cell fate in this region.

Axonal growth and guidance

Initially neuroblasts are rotund or fusiform, their cytoplasm containing a prominent Golgi apparatus, many lysosomes, glycogen and numerous unattached ribosomes (Tennyson 1969). As maturation proceeds cells send out fine cytoplasmic processes; these contain neurofilaments, microtubules and other structures, often including centrioles at their bases where microtubules form (p. 31). Internally, endoplasmic reticulum cisternae appear and attached ribosomes and mitochondria proliferate but the glycogen content progressively diminishes. One process becomes the axon and other processes establish a dendritic tree. Axonal growth, studied in tissue culture, may be as much as 1 mm per day.

Ramón y Cajal (1890) was the first to recognize that the expanded end of an axon—the *growth cone*—is the principal sensory organ of the neuron. Subsequently, the growing tips of the neuroblasts have been studied in tissue culture (Harrison 1910; Speidel 1932, 1933; Pomerat et al 1967; Bray 1982; Letourneau 1985). Classically, the growth cone has been described as an expanded region that is constantly active, changing shape, extending and withdrawing small filopodia and lamellipodia that apparently 'explore' the local environment for a suitable surface along which extension may occur (Tennyson 1970; Bunge 1976; Pfenninger & Rees 1976; see 'Cell motility', p. 43). These processes are stabilized in one direction, determining the direction of future growth, and following consolidation of the growth cone, the exploratory behaviour recommences. This continuous cycle resembles the behaviour at the leading edge of migratory cells such as fibroblasts and neutrophils. The molecular basis of this behaviour is the scaffolding of microtubules and neurofilaments within the axon. Growing neuroblasts have a cortex rich in actin, associated with the plasma membrane, and a core of centrally-located microtubules and sometimes neurofilaments. The assembly of these components, along with the synthesis of new membrane, occurs in segments distal to the cell body and behind the growth cone, though some assembly of microtubules may take place near the cell body.

Indispensable to growth cone extension are products and organelles synthesized within the cell bodies that are passed outwards by proximodistal *axoplasmic flow* along the axons. Bulk axoplasmic

flow was first postulated following the experimental construction of nerves (Weiss & Hiscoe 1948), and since that time many intricate analyses of fast and slow components of *bidirectional flow systems* within axons have been made (Lubinska 1964, and see Neurosciences Research Programme 1968). The driving force of growth cone extension is uncertain. One possible mechanism is that tension applied to objects by the leading edge of the growth cone is mediated by actin, and that local accumulations of F-actin redirect the extension of microtubules. Under some culture conditions, growth cones can develop mechanical tension, pulling against other axons or the substratum to which they are attached. Possibly, tension in the growth cone acts as a messenger to mediate the assembly of cytoskeletal components. Adhesion to the substratum appears to be important for consolidation of the growth cone and elaboration of the cytoskeleton in that direction. However, growth is not simply proportional to adhesion, and axonal growth and guidance are likely to depend on a fine balance of cell surface and extracellular matrix molecules. For reviews on morphology, motility and directional growth of axons and their growth cones, consult James (1974), Rakic (1971a,b, 1981, 1982), Bentley and O'Connor (1994).

During development, the growing axons of neuroblasts navigate with precision over considerable distances, often pursuing complex courses to reach their targets. Eventually they make functional contact with their appropriate end organs (neuromuscular endings, secretomotor terminals, sensory corpuscles or synapses with other neurons). During the outgrowth of axonal processes from ventral motor neuroblasts to reach presumptive myoblasts in the limb buds, the earliest nerve fibres are known to cross appreciable distances over an apparently virgin landscape occupied by loose mesenchyme. A central problem for neurobiologists, therefore, has been understanding the mechanisms of axon guidance.

A vast research literature is now devoted to the issues of axonal pathfinding, e.g. '*The nerve growth cone*' edited by Letourneau et al (1990). Only the main ideas can be touched on here. Over the years two principal theories have emerged concerning the directional growth of nerve fibres—the *neurotropism* or *chemotropism hypothesis* of Ramón y Cajal (1919) and the principle of *contact-guidance* of Weiss (1941). The former, based initially upon observations on the innervation of epithelia, proposed that growing fibres were guided by some form of attraction, presumably chemical, which emanated from the target area to be innervated. The second view denied the existence of such attractive forces and, based upon many series of tissue culture experiments, held that pioneer axons were guided to their destination by preferential growth along pathways dictated exclusively by the structures with which the growth cone was in direct contact. After spending most of the century in the wilderness, however, the chemotropism idea of Ramón y Cajal has recently been borne out with relation to several aspects of neural development. The salient feature of chemotropism is that growth cones act as **sensors** to concentration gradients of molecules in the environment, and grow up the gradient towards the source, i.e. the target. This situation can be mimicked in vitro using an explant culture system in which tissue explants (neuroblasts of interest and target tissue) are placed at a distance in a three-dimensional collagen gel. In this system, stable gradients of substances diffusing from the target tissue may be established (Ebendahl 1977). Using this system, the developing epithelium of the face in the mouse, for example, has been shown to originate a chemoattractant that lures sensory afferents of the trigeminal system (Lumsden & Davies 1983, 1986) (**3.109**). In addition, the floor plate of the developing spinal cord has been found to exert a chemotropic effect on commissural axons that later cross it (Tessier-Lavigne et al 1988), while the developing pons produces a chemoattractant that elicits collateral budding from descending corticofugal fibres (Heffner et al 1990). Another possibility is that diffusible factors could also mediate chemorepulsion, deflecting growing axons from inappropriate areas, as has been shown to occur for olfactory axons, which avoid explants of septal tissue in culture (Pini 1993).

There is no doubt, however, that contact guidance mechanisms operate in parallel with neurotropism. Physical cues in the pathway may play a role, such as the pattern of spaces in the spinal cord of the newt, hypothesized to constitute a 'blueprint' for primary nervous pathways (Singer et al 1979). Adhesion to the structures the growth cone contacts also plays a role. Molecular dissection of the role of

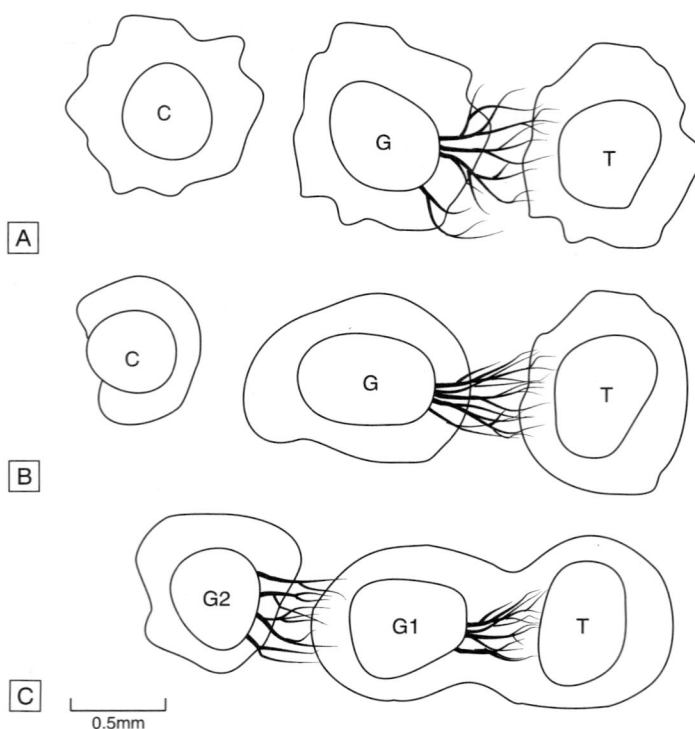

0.5mm

3.109A–C Cocultures of trigeminal ganglion (G) with control (C) and target (T) tissues after 48 hours. Neurite outgrowth is exclusively from the quadrant facing the target, and some neurites (especially in A) curve towards it. In (C) two ganglia G1 and G2 have been placed adjacent to the target; in both cases neurite outgrowth is exclusively from quadrants facing the target. (After Guthrie & Lumsden 1994 with permission.)

adhesion in growth cone navigation has led to the identification of several general classes of cell surface molecule. Among these are the *immunoglobulin superfamily*, which includes *neural cell adhesion molecule* (N-CAM) and *L1*, the *cadherins*, including *N-cadherin*, and the *integrin family*. The latter is a group of cell surface receptors that are molecular heterodimers which recognize and bind to components of the extracellular matrix, such as fibronectin, laminin and collagen. Thus, both cell–cell and cell–matrix interactions may be involved in axonal pathfinding. Evidence for the role of these molecules has been obtained from culture experiments in which substrata are coated with these molecules, from their immuno-localization in vivo, from perturbation experiments in which anti-bodies, enzymes or other agents are infused into embryos and axonal trajectories mapped, and studies of invertebrates mutant for various of these molecules. Retinal axons navigate to the optic tectum along pathways lined with the extracellular matrix molecule laminin (Cohen et al 1987), for example, while their fasciculation behaviour in the nerve, and defasciculation once they reach the tectum is governed to some extent by their levels and molecular expression of N-CAM (Schlosshauer et al 1984). Unravelling these processes is likely to prove complicated, however, for while molecules such as laminin may provide a permissive substratum for axon outgrowth, others such as tenascin exhibit growth-promoting or inhibitory properties (Spring et al 1989). In addition, the cell surface integrins comprise many different subtypes, which may recognize more than one extra-cellular matrix ligand.

The possible role played by *contact inhibition* in developmental processes has also been investigated in recent years. Culture experiments have shown that when chick peripheral sensory neurons and central neurons (retinal ganglion cells) are confronted, their motility is inhibited and they exhibit growth cone collapse (Kapfhammer et al 1986). This reduction or loss of growth cone structure may be analogous to contact paralysis of non-neuronal cells. Purification of fractions from embryonic brain has identified the protein *collapsin* as the active agent. The correct topographic arrangement of terminals in the optic tectum may also rely on such a mechanism. Axons from

temporal retina grow on membranes prepared from rostral tectum (their appropriate target) but fail to grow on those prepared from caudal tectum (their inappropriate target; Walter et al 1987). In addition, motor axons that grow from the spinal cord preferentially through the rostral portion of the sclerotome appear to avoid the caudal sclerotome due to contact inhibition. Glycoprotein fractions isolated from somites cause growth cone collapse that resembles that mediated by collapsin (Davies et al 1990).

Although many factors have been identified as having positive or negative effects on axonal growth and navigation, a crucial question is how direction might be specified. The attraction of chemotropism as a mechanism is that direction is provided by the gradient of chemotropic substance diffusing away from the target. However, there has also been considerable interest in the idea that gradients of adhesion might provide directional cues to growth cones—*hap-totaxis*. In culture, growth cones will grow preferentially along paths of greater adhesiveness (Letourneau 1975), but there is little firm evidence to suggest that such choices are made in vivo. In the moth wing epidermis, axon extension across distal or proximal regions that exhibit adhesive differences were proposed to reflect haptotactic phenomena (Nardi & Kafatos 1976). In reality very few axons may actually be pioneers, the majority growing on glial cells and pre-established axon fascicles, so that only the first few must respond to directional cues. At present, the consensus of opinion as to the mechanisms of axon guidance is that cues are multiple, with a different combination prevailing at different points in the pathway.

Once growth cones have arrived in their general target area, there is the additional problem of forming terminals and synapses. In recent years, much emphasis has been placed on the idea that patterns of connectivity depend on the death of inappropriate cells. Cell death during development coincides with the period of syn-aptogenesis, and present opinion favours the idea that it occurs due to failure of neurons to acquire a sufficient amount of a trophic factor (reviewed in Oppenheim et al 1992). Coincident firing of neighbouring neurons that have found the appropriate target region might be involved in eliciting release of factor(s), thus reinforcing correct connections. Such mechanisms may explain the numerical correspondence between neurons in a motor pool and the muscle fibres innervated (Tennyson 1969). If an axon fails to make the correct contacts, its parent soma atrophies and dies, probably as a result of toxic materials liberated within it. *Programmed cell death (apoptosis)* is a definable process with a morphology that is distinct from necrosis, and occurs in neurons (reviewed in Oppenheim 1991). Activation of a specific set of genes appears to be responsible for mediating cell death, while other genes can negate the apoptotic programme. Transfection of chick with the gene *Bcl-2* blocks cell death following withdrawal of trophic factors from some sensory neurons and sympathetic neurons (Garcia et al 1992; Allsopp et al 1993). On a subtler level, pruning of collaterals may give rise to mature neuronal architecture. The projections of pyramidal neurons from the motor and visual cortex, for example, start out with similar architecture, and the mature repertoire of targets is produced by pruning of collaterals leading to loss of projections to some targets (see p. 230).

The final growth of dendritic trees is also influenced by patterns of afferent connections and their activity; if deprived of afferents experimentally, dendrites fail to develop fully and, after a critical period, may become permanently affected even if functional inputs are restored, e.g. in the visual systems of young animals visually deprived (Blakemore 1974, 1991). Metabolic factors also affect the final branching patterns of dendrites, for example, thyroid deficiency in perinatal rats results in a small size and restricted branching of cortical neurons. This may be analogous to the mental retardation of cretinism (Eayrs 1955).

Once established, dendritic trees appear remarkably stable and partial deafferentation affects only dendritic spines or similar small details. If cells lose all afferent connections or are totally deprived of sensory input (see Guillery 1974), atrophy of much of the dendritic tree and even the whole neuron ensues, though different regions of the nervous system vary quantitatively in their response to such *anterograde transneuronal degeneration* (p. 920). Similar effects occur in *retrograde transneuronal degeneration*. As development proceeds plasticity is lost and soon after birth a neuron is a stable structure with a reduced rate of growth.

The role of trophic factors

The existence of maintenance factors in the nervous system was postulated in the case of the developing tetrapod limbs, from which such factors were thought to be conveyed to the CNS where they were capable of influencing the turnover of neuroblasts, i.e. the balance between the rate of proliferation and degeneration. Extirpation of the limb buds of chick embryos led to a massive reduction in numbers of motor and sensory neuroblasts implying that they were dependent on peripheral structures for their survival (Hamburger 1934). These ideas were given substance by the isolation and characterization of nerve growth factor (NGF) (Levi-Montalcini 1950, 1952, 1960, 1967; Cohen 1958; Cohen & Levi-Montalcini 1956; Levi-Montalcini & Chen 1971) from tissue and tumour extracts and snake venom. These authors demonstrated both in vivo and in vitro influences of NGF on the form and extent of nerve cell growth. Antibodies to NGF cause the death of neuronal subsets at times when they have reached their targets, and added NGF rescues neurons that would otherwise die. NGF is synthesized by various peripheral target organs of the nervous system (Levi-Montalcini & Angeletti 1968) from which it is taken into the nerve endings and transported back to the neuronal somata. It is necessary for the survival of many types of neuroblasts during early development and their axon and dendritic growth, and promotes the synthesis of neurotransmitters and enzymes. Since the discovery of NGF, several other trophic factors have been identified. Brain derived neurotrophic factor was purified, and subsequently neurotrophin-3 (NT-3) and NT- 4/5 were identified by molecular cloning. Neurotrophins exert their survival effects selectively on particular subsets of neurons, though some neurons can be supported by more than one neurotrophin (reviewed in Thoenen 1991). Extensive culture experiments have indicated that NGF is specific to *sensory ganglion cells* from the neural crest, *sympathetic postganglionic neurons* and *basal forebrain cholinergic neurons*. BDNF promotes the survival of *retinal ganglion cells, motor neurons, sensory proprioceptive* and *placode-derived neurons*, such as those of the nodose ganglion that are unresponsive to NGF. NT-3 has effects on motor neurons, and both placode and neural crest derived sensory neurons. Other growth factors found to influence the growth and survival of neural cells include the *fibroblast growth factors* (FGFs) and *ciliary neurotrophic factor* (CNTF), all of which are unrelated in sequence to the NGF family. Members of the FGF family support the survival of embryonic neuroblasts from many regions of the CNS. CNTF may control the proliferation and differentiation of sympathetic ganglion cells and astrocytes.

Each of the neurotrophins binds specifically to certain receptors on the cell surface. The receptor termed *p75* binds all the neurotrophins with similar affinity. By contrast, members of the family of receptor *tyrosine kinases* (Trks) bind with higher affinity and display binding preferences for particular neurotrophins. The presence of a Trk receptor seems to be required for p75 function. So far three Trk receptors have been identified. TrkA is the receptor for NGF, TrkB binds BDNF and NT-4/5, and TrkC binds NT-3. Possibilities of other interactions between factors and Trk receptors, such as an effect of NT-3 on TrkA and TrkB, have also been raised. Much progress in understanding the role of neurotrophins in vivo has recently been made by generating mice with null mutations of the Trk receptors and of the neurotrophins themselves. Homozygous TrkA mutant mice showed loss of small diameter temperature and pain afferents, and of sympathetic neurons (Smeyne et al 1994), corresponding to the neuronal subsets normally supported by NGF in culture. The exception were the cholinergic neurons in the basal forebrain, which were supported by NGF in culture, but whose numbers were unaffected in the null mutants. TrkB mutant mice showed loss of neurons in some sensory ganglia, particularly those receiving a placodal contribution, such as the vestibular ganglion. Motor neuron numbers were also reduced (Klein et al 1993). This implies an effect on the neuronal subsets normally dependent on BDNF. Interestingly, in BDNF mutant mice motor neuron numbers are approximately normal, implying that trophic effects on motor neurons may be mediated via binding of NT-4 to TrkB (Ernfors et al 1993). The results of the TrkC knockout showed a loss of neurons from dorsal root ganglia, particularly the large diameter afferents mediating proprioception (Klein et al 1994). This was consistent with observations of the survival-promoting effects of NT-3 on proprioceptive neurons in vitro, but it is not clear whether the other neuronal types supported by NT-3 in culture are also lost in the mutant.

Many uncertainties surround interpretations of these knockout experiments and their bearing on the role of these factors in vivo, for while TrkB and TrkC transcripts are widely distributed throughout the CNS, no gross defects centrally were seen in the TrkB and TrkC mutant mice. Although the neurotrophins were first envisaged as having their action via production by target organs, the situation has become considerably more complicated. Like NGF, BDNF and NT-3 are present in peripheral tissues, but unlike NGF, they are also expressed by motor and sensory neurons, raising the possibility of autocrine actions. In the future, new growth factors are likely to be identified and the full spectrum of their effects remains to be discovered. Nevertheless, the survival-promoting effects of BDNF and CNTF on motor neurons has led to the initiation of clinical trials with these molecules on patients with amyotrophic lateral sclerosis (neurotrophins reviewed in Loughlin & Fallon 1992; Lindsay et al 1994).

In addition to receiving trophic support from other tissues, nervous tissue also influences the metabolism of other tissues. This is true for many cell types, but neuronal effects are, however, perhaps more marked and far reaching. The most obvious example is the mutual dependence of motor neurons and muscles. If, during development, a nerve fails to connect with its muscle, both degenerate. But if the innervation of slow (red) or fast (white) skeletal muscles, each with peculiar functional properties, is exchanged, the muscles change structure and properties in accordance with innervation, indicating that nerve determines muscle type and not vice versa (Buller 1970, and see p. 904). However, in this case the type of muscle is apparently determined chiefly by the firing pattern of the efferent nerve fibre, rather than by any release of trophic chemical (Lømo & Westguard 1974). Trophic influences are clearest in lower vertebrates, in which a denervated limb rudiment fails to complete its development in the absence of nerve-mediated influences (Hamburger 1968). In higher vertebrates axons have trophic influence on the dendritic trees they innervate (p. 957), and on sensory structures. For example, the taste buds degenerate after denervation and regenerate only if the sensory nerves are present. Conversely, if auditory sensory cells are eliminated, the auditory neurons begin to degenerate and many eventually die, suggesting that in this case the trophic influence is the reverse of the usual situation. One recent example of such an interaction comes from mice mutant for the TrkC neurotrophin receptor, which show selective loss of 1a afferents to muscle spindles. In these mice the muscles are devoid of muscle spindles, presumably due to their deafferentation (Klein et al 1994). In addition to these presumably trophic effects, development is replete with examples of the nervous system influencing other tissues, such as the inductive influence of the optic vesicle on adjacent ectoderm resulting in the formation of a lens vesicle and the reciprocal influences of the developing lens and perioptic mesenchyme on the differentiation of the optic cup (p. 259).

PERIPHERAL NERVOUS SYSTEM

AUTONOMIC NERVOUS SYSTEM

The autonomic nervous system is, apart from the motor axons arising from the CNS, formed by the neural crest. This system includes the *sympathetic* and *parasympathetic neurons* in the peripheral *ganglia* with their accompanying glia, the *enteric nervous system* and glia, and the *adrenal medulla*.

In the trunk at neurulation, neural crest cells migrate from the neural epithelium to lie transitorily on the fused neural tube. Thereafter crest cells migrate laterally then ventrally to their respective destinations (3.110). Within the head the neural crest cells migrate prior to neural fusion producing a vast mesenchymal population as well as autonomic neurons.

The work of Le Douarin and co-workers has provided many data on the contribution of the neural crest in the development of the autonomic nervous system (Le Douarin 1982; Le Douarin 1990). Much of the work has been carried out on chick–quail chimeras (see p. 220) using histochemical markers to map the distribution of

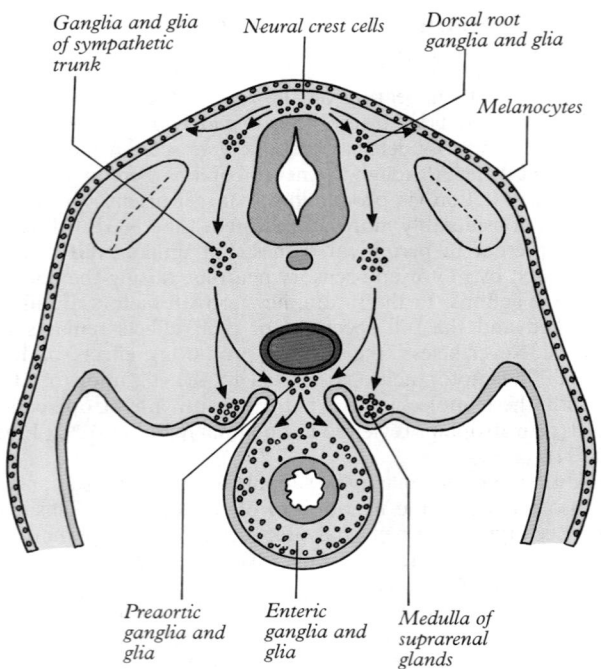

Ganglia and glia of sympathetic trunk

Neural crest cells

Dorsal root ganglia and glia

Melanocytes

Preaortic ganglia and glia

Enteric ganglia and glia

Medulla of suprarenal glands

3.110 Diagram showing the migration routes taken by neural crest cells in the trunk.

different categories of autonomic neurons. The results of this work have provided a map of four major regions of neural crest cell distribution to the autonomic nervous system, including *cranial*, *vagal*, *trunk* and *lumbosacral* crest. The cranial neural crest gives rise to the *cranial parasympathetic ganglia*, whereas the vagal neural crest gives rise to the *thoracic parasympathetic ganglia*. The trunk neural crest gives rise to the *sympathetic ganglia*, mainly the paravertebral ganglia, and *adrenomedullary cells*. This category is often referred to as being of the cells of the *sympathoadrenal lineage* (Patterson 1990; Carnahan & Patterson 1991; Scott-Duff et al 1991).

Neurons of the enteric nervous system are described as arising from the *vagal crest*, i.e. neural crest derived from *somite levels 1–7* (also see below), and *sacral crest*, caudal to the 28th somite. At all of these levels the crest cells are also differentiating into glial-like support cells alongside the neurons (**3.111**).

Parasympathetic ganglia

Cranial neural crest. In mammalian embryos, crest cells migrate from the region of the mesencephalon and rhombencephalon during the 4–10 somite stages (Nichols 1987; Chan & Tam 1988). By the 11 somite stage the wave of migration is greatest in the more caudal parts of the latter regions, with most in the rhombencephalon. In avian embryos, crest migration occurs at the level of the developing posterior mesencephalon and preotic myelencephalon during the 4 somite stage onwards (D'Amico-Martel & Noden 1983). The *ciliary ganglion* is formed by neural crest cells from the caudal third of the mesencephalon and the rostral metencephalon which migrate along or close to the ophthalmic branch of the trigeminal nerve. It may be reinforced by cells migrating from the nucleus of the oculomotor nerve along which a few scattered cells are always demonstrable in postnatal life. The *pterygopalatine ganglion* derives from preotic myelencephalic crest cells and may receive contributions from the ganglia of the trigeminal and facial nerves. The *otic* and *submandibular* ganglia also derive from myelencephalic neural crest and may have contributions from the glossopharyngeal and facial cranial nerves respectively (**2.29c**).

Vagal neural crest. Neural crest cells from the region located between the midotic placode and the caudal limit of somite 3 have been termed *cardiac neural crest*; they migrate through pharyngeal arches 3, 4, and 6 where they provide, inter alia, support for the embryonic aortic arch arteries, cells of the aorticopulmonary septum

and truncus, and cells which differentiate into the neural anlage of the *parasympathetic ganglia* of the heart. Sensory innervation of the heart is from the inferior ganglion of the vagus, which is derived from the nodose placodes (see p. 224). Neural crest cells migrating from the level of somites 1–7 (see above) are collectively termed vagal neural crest; they have been demonstrated to migrate to the gut along with sacral neural crest.

Sacral parasympathetic ganglia. These have attracted little recent attention; most studies have examined the development of the enteric nerves (see below).

Sympathetic ganglia

There is much variation in the timing of migration and differentiation of neural crest cells in the trunk region in different species, though the cells commencing migration first migrate furthest distally. In mammalian species, neural crest cells migrate ventrally during the 3–5 somite stage, to penetrate the underlying somites (Erikson et al 1989; Serbedzija et al 1990). Within a few hours the cells migrate further ventrally to the region of the future *paravertebral* and *prevertebral plexa*, notably forming the *sympathetic chain* of ganglia, as well as the major ganglia around the ventral visceral branches of the abdominal aorta (Serbedzija et al 1990). In avian embryos crest cells migrate preferentially through the rostral half of the somites to appear dorsolateral to the aorta. They spread paravertebrally as well as making contributions to the suprarenal medulla and paravertebral plexa (Le Douarin & Teillet 1974). The normal segmentation and size of the primary sympathetic ganglia in chicks have been found to depend on alternation of rostrocaudal characteristics of somites such that this positioning may regulate the direction of crest cells towards dorsal root ganglia and sympathetic ganglia (Goldstein & Kalcheim 1991). The local environment has been shown to be important in determining crest cell fate; after selective deletions of specific crest regions sympathetic ganglia still formed normally in the absence of dorsal root ganglia, thus implying that crest-derived precursors were uncommitted until receiving a stop signal (Scott 1984). Interestingly, in the quail embryo after crest cells have differentiated and formed dorsal root ganglia, there are dormant autonomic neuronal precursors in the dorsal root ganglia capable of differentiation into adrenergic cells. Furthermore, the differentiation of such cells is dependent on cell–cell interaction (Deville et al 1992).

Pre- and postganglionic cell differentiation and growth. It has been shown that there is cell specific recognition of postganglionic neurons and the growth cones of sympathetic preganglionic neurons they meet during their growth, and this may be important in guidance to their appropriate targets (Moorman & Hume 1990). The position of postganglionic neurons, and the exit point from the spinal cord of preganglionic neurons may influence the types of synaptic connections made, and the affinity for particular postganglionic neurons (Lichtmann et al 1979; Purves et al 1981). When a postganglionic neuroblast is in place it grows axons (and dendrites) and synaptogenesis follows (Rubin 1985a,b,c). In mammalian embryos the earliest axonal outgrowths from the superior cervical ganglion occur at about stage 15 (Rubin 1985a) and although the axon is the first cell process to appear, the position of the neurons does not apparently influence the appearance of the cell processes. There have been many studies of the innervation of peripheral targets (in rats) by sympathetic postganglionic nerves during postnatal life which have relied upon biochemical and immunohistological demonstration of neurotransmitter substances present (De Champlain et al 1970; Cochard et al 1979; Teitelman et al 1979). In this animal model, at an equivalent to human stage 17 (41 days), there will be many preganglionic axons in the superior cervical ganglion and they can influence electrical activity of postganglionic neurons (Rubin 1985c). By the time of birth, substantial numbers of functional synapses can be found in the superior cervical ganglion (Rubin 1985c), some 10% of the adult number (Smolen and Raisman 1980). Findings in the parasympathetic ganglia are somewhat similar. In the chick ciliary ganglion, for instance, postganglionic axons have been reported to grow in a similar manner towards their targets (Landmesser & Pillar 1974a), and there is a significant reduction in the numbers of ganglion cells during development, though synapses form on all cells present prior to death (Landmesser and Pillar 1974b), thus exhibiting a general phenomenon in ganglion maturation.

Phenotypic expression of differentiating autonomic neurons.

The elegant transplantation studies performed by Le Douarin's group have demonstrated that the local environment is the major factor which controls the appropriate differentiation of the presumptive autonomic ganglion neurons. The identity of the factors responsible for subsequent adrenergic, cholinergic or peptidergic phenotypic expression has yet to be elucidated, though fibronectin (Loring et al 1982; Sieber-Blum et al 1981) and basal lamina components molecules (Maxwell & Forbes 1987) have been suggested to initiate adrenergic phenotypic expression at the expense of melanocyte numbers. Cholinergic characteristics are acquired relatively early as shown by studies of premigratory neural crest cells (Le Blanc et al 1990) and the appropriate phenotypic expression may be promoted by cholinergic differentiation factor (Fukada 1985; Yamamori et al 1989) and ciliary neurotrophic factor (Lin et al 1989; Stöckli et al 1989). Schotzinger and Landis (1988) have demonstrated the development of a cholinergic phenotype by noradrenergic sympathetic neurons after innervation of a novel cholinergic target (sweat glands) in vivo. Neuropeptides are expressed by autonomic neurons in vitro and may be stimulated by various target tissue factors in sympathetic (Wong & Kessler 1987) and parasympathetic (Coulombe & Nishi 1991) neurons. Indeed, García-Arrasás et al (1986) point out that some neuropeptides are expressed more intensely during early stages of ganglion formation. At what stage coexistence of neuropeptides in synaptic vesicles of preganglionic nerves (e.g. Mitchell & Stauber 1993) and the chemical coding of pre- and postganglionic neurons occurs as in adult ganglion neurons (e.g. Mitchell et al 1993), is unknown.

A number of gene products are expressed on migrating neural crest cells, including the murine homeobox gene cluster *Hox-a* (Toth et al 1987; Galliot et al 1989), detected on dorsal root ganglion cells rather than sympathetic ganglia, *Hox-b* (Wilkinson et al 1989a; Holland & Hogan 1988) expressed in the nodose ganglia and in parts of the enteric nervous system, *Hox-c* (Breier et al 1988) in sympathetic ganglia, and (Robert et al 1989) on cephalic neural crest. Other gene products expressed by crest cells include the cellular oncogene c-ets 1 (Vandenbunder et al 1989) and the zinc finger gene *Krox-20* (Wilkinson et al 1989a) which is found on differentiating dorsal root and cranial ganglion cells. Two genes whose malexpression leads to abnormal development of neural crest-derived nervous system elements are *Hox a-4* which is associated with abnormal development of the enteric nervous system (Wolgemuth et al 1989), and *Hox a-1* which results in malformations of hindbrain development (Lufkin et al 1991; Chisaka et al 1992), and consequent derangements of cranial nerves.

Enteric nervous system

The enteric nervous system is different from the other components of the autonomic nervous system as, unlike the sympathetic and parasympathetic ganglia, the enteric nervous system can mediate reflex activity **independently** of control by the brain and spinal cord (Gershon 1987). The number of enteric neurons which develop is believed to be of the same magnitude as the number of neurons in the spinal cord (Furness & Costa 1980). The number of preganglionic fibres which supply the intestine, and therefore modulate the enteric neurons, are much fewer. This discrepancy led Langley (1921) to postulate that most of the enteric neurons receive no direct input from the CNS at all. (The position of neural crest contribution to the enteric nervous system is shown in **3**.111.)

It is worth noting at this point that enteric nerves have more in common with central nerves than peripheral nerves. Enteric nerves do **not** have the collagenous coats of extraenteric peripheral nerves, and, as in the CNS, there is no endoneurium within the enteric plexuses; rather the cells are supported by *glia* which closely resemble astrocytes and contain glial fibrillary acidic protein (GFAP). Although Schwann cells surrounding unmyelinated nerves also contain detectable amounts of GFAP, enteric glia contain more. Interestingly the enteric glia do not produce a surrounding basal lamina as do Schwann cells. Gershon (1987) reviews this field.

Chimeric experimentation has demonstrated that quail donor crest taken from axial levels, which do not normally supply the gut, and transplanted into the vagal regions of chick hosts produces an embryo with entirely quail enteric nerves. Thus the premigratory neural crest cells are not pre-patterned for specific axial levels; rather

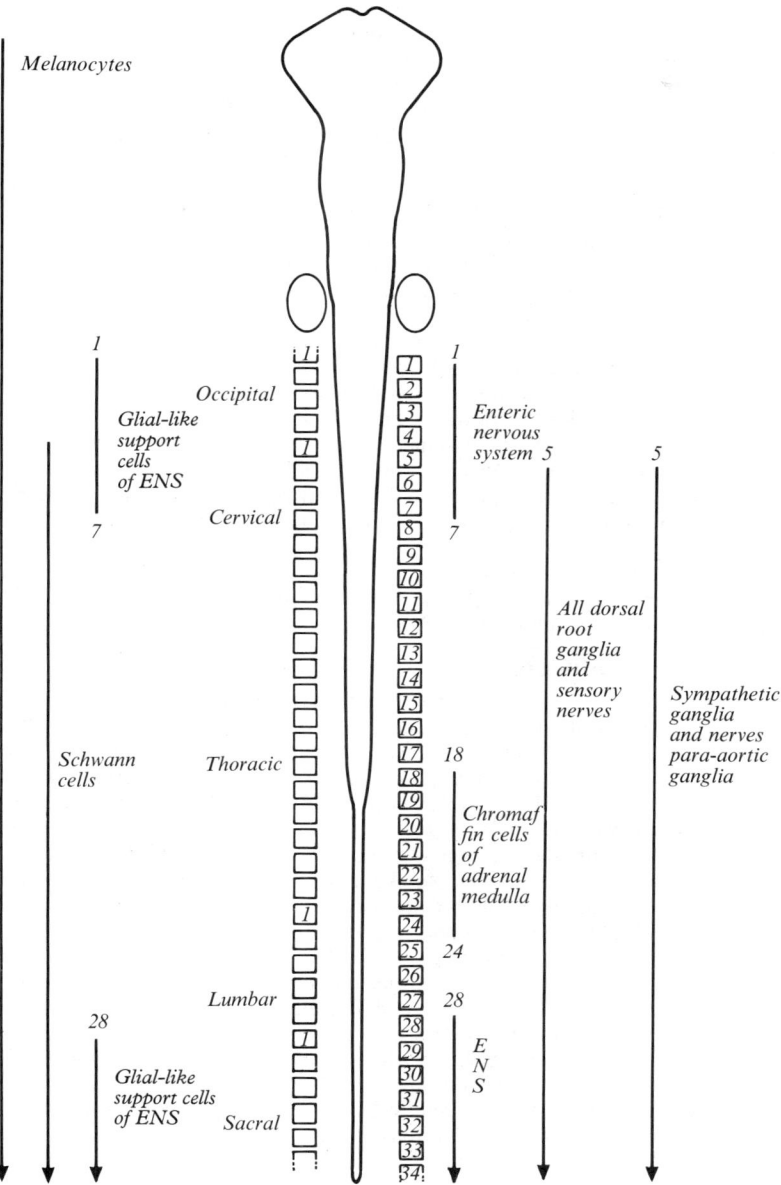

3.111   Diagram illustrating the derivatives of neural crest cells in the trunk. On the right of the diagram the somites are indicated and on the left the vertebral levels are indicated. The fate of crest cells arising at particular somite levels is shown.

they attain their axial value as they leave the neuraxis. Once within the gut wall there is a regionally specific pattern of enteric ganglia formation (Gabella 1981) suggested to be controlled by the local splanchnopleuric mesenchyme.

The most caudal derivatives of neural crest cells, from the lumbosacral region, form components of the pelvic plexus after migrating through the somites towards the level of the colon, rectum and cloaca. The cells come to lie initially within the developing mesentery and then transiently between the layers of the differentiating muscularis externa before finally, and later, forming a more substantial intramural plexus characteristic of the adult enteric nervous system. Of the neural crest cells that colonize the bowel, some of the foregut have been reported to acquire the ability to migrate outwards and colonize the developing pancreas, as the characteristic population of autonomic neurons (Kirchgessner et al 1992).

Hirschsprung's disease is suggested to result from a failure of neural crest cells to colonize the gut wall appropriately. The condition is characterized by a dilated segment of colon proximally and lack of peristalsis in the segment distal to the dilatation. Infants with Hirschsprung's disease show delay in the passage of meconium, constipation, vomiting and abdominal distension. Gershon (1987) has investigated a similar condition in the *ls/ls* mouse which develops congenital megacolon secondarily to aganglionosis of the terminal portion of the large bowel. The non-peristaltic portion of gut contains thick nerves in the adventitia, muscularis externa and submucosa but the number of cells in the submucosal plexus is reduced compared to normal mice. There are numerous aberrantly located ganglia outside the gut connected by axons to the nerves within the gut. Both the submucosal nerves and the aberrant ganglia have the characteristics of non-enteric neurons. Immunocytochemical studies of the enteric basal lamina have shown an increase in the amount of laminin, type IV collagen and heparan sulphate in the aganglionic gut. In normal mice laminin and type IV collagen are found beneath the mucosal and serosal epithelia and around the blood vessels. In the *ls/ls* mouse there is a broad zone of expression of these proteins around the entire outer gut mesenchyme, specifically of the aganglionic portion of bowel. Gershon (1987) suggests that the over-abundance of basal laminal components may prevent the neural crest cells from penetrating the gut wall; their new position outside the gut does not confer on them the environmental stimuli for enteric nerve differentiation so non-enteric development occurs in local ganglia adjacent to the gut.

In humans Hirschsprung's disease is often seen associated with other defects of neural crest development, e.g. Waardenburg type II syndrome which includes deafness and facial clefts with megacolon.

Chromaffin cells

Chromaffin cells are derived from the neural crest and found at numerous sites throughout the body. As well as the classic chromaffin cells of the *suprarenal medulla*, others in this group include the *bronchial neuroepithelial cells*, *dispersed epithelial endocrine cells* of the gut (formerly known as *argentaffin cells*), *carotid body cells*, and the *paraganglia*.

The sympathetic ganglia, suprarenal (adrenal) medulla and chromaffin cells are all derived from the cells of the *sympathoadrenal lineage* (Patterson 1990; Carnahan & Patterson 1991; Scott-Duff et al 1991). In the suprarenal medulla these cells differentiate into a number of types consisting of *small* and *intermediate-sized neuroblasts* or *sympathoblasts* and larger, initially rounded *phaeochromocytoblasts*. Molenaar et al (1990) have described the development of chromaffin cells in the suprarenal medulla in human fetuses aged 6–34 weeks. Using various markers two morphological cell types could be identified: large cells with pale nuclei from about 9 weeks, and clusters of small cells, appearing slightly later, at about 14 weeks. Their observations on the differential distribution of markers within these two cellular populations led them to conclude that the large cells were the progenitors of the chromaffin cells in the suprarenal medulla whilst the smaller cells were neuroblasts. The intermediate-sized neuroblasts differentiate into the typical *multipolar postganglionic sympathetic neurons* (which secrete noradrenaline at their terminals) of classic autonomic neuroanatomy. The smaller neuroblasts have been equated with the *small intensely fluorescent* (SIF) cells, types I and II. Both have been shown (at least in some species and sites) to be dopamine-storing and secreting cells. It is postulated that type I function as true interneurons, synapsing with the principal postganglionic neurons. Type II are thought to operate as local neuroendocrine cells, secreting dopamine into the ganglionic microcirculation. Both types of SIF cells probably modulate the principal preganglionic/postganglionic synaptic transmission. The large cells differentiate into masses of columnar or polyhedral *phaeochromocytes* (*classic chromaffin cells*) which secrete either adrenaline or noradrenaline. These cell masses are termed *paraganglia* and may be situated near, on the surface of, or embedded in the capsules of the ganglia of the sympathetic chain, or in some of the large autonomic plexuses. The largest members of the latter are the *para-aortic bodies* which lie along the sides of the abdominal aorta in relation to the inferior mesenteric artery. During childhood the para-aortic bodies and the paraganglia of the sympathetic chain partly degenerate and can no longer be isolated by gross dissection, but even in the adult chromaffin tissue can still be recognized microscopically in these various sites. It may be noted here that both the phaeochromocytes and the SIF cells, using a wider and more recent classification, are regarded as chromaffin; they belong to the amine precursor uptake and decarboxylation (APUD) series of cells and are paraneuronal in nature.

A pivotal role for glucocorticoids in the development of the chromaffin cell lineage has been emphasized by Hofmann et al (1989) and later by Michelsohn and Anderson (1992) who found that the development of the chromaffin phenotype involves two sequential, glucocorticoid-dependent events, and both appear to be mediated by the type II glucocorticoid receptor.

Enhancement of chromaffin cell process outgrowth, however, may be facilitated by various cell adhesion and extracellular matrix molecules (Poltorak et al 1990). Cell adhesion molecules play a major role in determination of tissue architecture during histogenesis of the suprarenal gland (Leon et al 1992). Two neural cell adhesion molecules N-CAM and L1 have been found to be expressed in the adult rat suprarenal gland. The expression of catecholamine synthesizing enzymes tyrosine hydroxylase and phenylethanolamine N-methyltransferase was correlated with the adhesion molecule expression. Groups of L1 and N-CAM positive cells were found to display different phenotypic expression of catecholamine synthesizing enzymes. Environmental factors also play an important role in the development of the physical and biochemical characteristics of chromaffin cells (Mizrachi et al 1990). Co-culture of human phaeochromocytoma cells with adrenal endothelial cells induced the tumour cells to acquire physical and biochemical characteristics of chromaffin cells, exhibiting similar organization as seen in vivo. The rapid transient increase in the change in the state of the proto-oncogene c-fos expression suggests that the mechanism(s) inducing the change in the state of the differentiation of tumour cells in co-culture with endothelial cells may be distinct from that described for the differentiation of chromaffin cells by glucocorticoids.

The differentiation of chromaffin cells appears not to be immutably fixed. Jousselin-Hosaja et al (1993) found that mouse suprarenal chromaffin cells can transform to neuron-like cholinergic phenotypes after being grafted into the hippocampus. Transdifferentiation of chromaffin cells to the neuron-like phenotype was also found to be induced after nerve growth factor application (de la Torre et al 1993).

The timing of the appearance of neurotransmitters and neuropeptides in chromaffin cells is not comprehensively established. In the avian sympathoadrenal system, however, 5HT-like immunoreactivity was found to be transiently expressed by chromaffin cells very early in development (E5–E8), disappearing almost entirely at more advanced embryonic stages (E10–E19) and in posthatched chicks where only a population of cells similar to mammalian SIF cells express immunoreactivity to 5HT (García-Arrasás & Martinez 1990). In relation to the development of catecholamine-synthesizing enzymes, in rat embryos, Anderson et al (1991) noted that sympathoadrenal precursors are first identifiable in primordial sympathetic ganglia at E11.5 when they express tyrosine hydroxylase. At this stage, the progenitors also coexpress neuronal markers, but also a series of chromaffin cell markers called *SA 1–5*. The observation of double labelled cells is consistent with the hypothesis that these cells represent a common progenitor to sympathetic neurons and suprarenal chromaffin cells. After E11.5, sympathetic ganglia no longer express chromaffin markers. Neuropeptides are also expressed by developing chromaffin cells. García-Arrasás et al (1992) have demonstrated the expression and development of neuropeptide Y (NPY)-like immunoreactivity in chromaffin cells of the chicken. They also found that NPY is coexpressed with somatostatin and serotonin. The expression of neuropeptides such as leucine enkephalin may be regulated by glucocorticoids and preganglionic nerves in suprarenal chromaffin cells (Henion & Landis 1992). These factors, therefore, participate in the generation of the mature neurochemical phenotypes present in the suprarenal medulla, both during development and in adults.

Suprarenal glands

Each suprarenal gland consists of a *cortex* derived from *coelomic epithelium* and a *medulla* into which *neural crest cells* migrate from somite levels 18–24 migrate (**3**.110, 111). The cortex is formed during the second month by a proliferation of the coelomic epithelium; cells pass into the underlying mesenchyme between the root of the dorsal mesogastrium and the mesonephros (Keene & Hewer 1927; Crowder 1957). The proliferating tissue extends from the level of the sixth to the twelfth thoracic segments. It is soon disorganized dorsomedially by invasion of neural crest cells which form the medulla and also by the development of venous sinusoids. The latter are joined by capillaries which arise from adjacent mesonephric arteries and penetrate the cortex in a radial manner. When proliferation of the coelomic epithelium ceases the cortex is enveloped ventrally, later dorsally, by a mesenchymal capsule derived from the mesonephros. The subcapsular nests of cortical cells are the rudiment of the *zona glomerulosa*. These nests proliferate cords of cells which pass deeply between the capillaries and sinusoids. The cells in these cords degenerate in an erratic fashion as they pass towards the medulla, becoming granular, eosinophilic and ultimately autolysed. These cords of degenerating cells constitute the *fetal cortex*, which undergoes a rapid degeneration during the first two weeks after birth with marked shrinkage of the gland. The *fascicular* and *reticular* zones of the adult cortex are proliferated from the glomerular zone after birth and are only fully differentiated by about the twelfth year.

SOMATIC NERVES

Spinal nerves

Each spinal nerve is connected to the spinal cord by a ventral root and a dorsal root. The fibres of the ventral roots grow out from cell bodies in the anterior and lateral parts of the mantle zone; these pass through the overlying marginal zone and external limiting membrane to enter the *myotomes* of the somites, or penetrate the latter, reaching the adjacent somatopleure, and in both sites ultimately form the α-, β- and γ-efferents. At appropriate levels these are accompanied by the outgrowing axons of preganglionic sympathetic neuroblasts (segments T1–L2), or preganglionic parasympathetic neuroblasts (S2–S4).

The fibres of the dorsal roots extend from the cells of the spinal ganglia. Before the neural groove is closed to form the neural tube, a ridge of neurectodermal cells, the *neural crest* (*ganglion ridge*), appears along the prominent margin of each neural fold. When the folds meet in the median plane the two neural crests fuse into a wedge-shaped mass along the line of closure of the tube. Neural crest cells are produced continuously along the length of the spinal cord, but gangliogenic cells migrate only into the rostral part of each somitic sclerotome where they condense and proliferate to form a bilateral series of oval-shaped *primordial spinal ganglia*. In addition to negative factors in the caudal sclerotome that deter neural crest

cells from entering (see p. 155), the rostral sclerotome has a mitogenic effect on the crest cells that settle within it (Goldstein et al 1990). From the ventral region of each ganglion a small part separates to form *sympatho-chromaffin cells* (p. 236), while the remainder becomes a *definitive* spinal ganglion. The spinal ganglia are arranged symmetrically at the sides of the neural tube and, except in the caudal region, are equal in number to the somites. The cells of the ganglia, like the cells of the mantle zone of the early neural tube, are glial and neuronal precursors. The glial precursors develop into the satellite cells, which become closely applied to the ganglionic nerve cell somata (perikarya), into Schwann cells, and possibly other cells. The neuroblasts, at first round or oval, soon become fusiform, with extremities gradually elongating into central and peripheral processes. The central processes grow into the neural tube, as the fibres of dorsal nerve roots, while the peripheral processes grow ventrolaterally to mingle with the fibres of the ventral root thus forming a *mixed spinal nerve*. As development proceeds the original bipolar form of the cells in the spinal ganglia changes; the two processes become approximated until they ultimately arise from a single stem in a T-shaped manner, to form a unipolar cell (sometimes, less appropriately, termed pseudo-unipolar). The bipolar form is, however, retained in the ganglion of the vestibulocochlear nerve.

The position of the early neural crest as a wedge-shaped mass along the line of tube closure noted above, and the identification of ganglionic cells in various positions in the wall of the early neural tube, and even within the central canal (Humphrey 1944, 1947), is strongly reminiscent of the developmental history of the *Rohon–Beard cells* in fish and amphibia (Rohon 1884; Beard 1896), which are thought to be important in the emergence of primitive locomotor patterns (Hughes 1968). In this regard, other investigators have claimed that in primitive chordates (Cyclostomes and Euselachians) the neural crest develops as an *evagination* of the dorsal region of the dorsolateral lamina of the late neural folds and early neural tube (Conel 1942). For a review of the origin, widespread migration and differentiation of neural crest cells see Weston (1970) Bellairs (1971) Leikola (1976) and page 220.

Cranial nerves

Cranial nerves may contain motor, sensory or both types of fibres. With the exception of the olfactory and optic nerves, the cranial nerves develop in a manner similar in some respects to components of the spinal nerves. The somata of motor neuroblasts originate

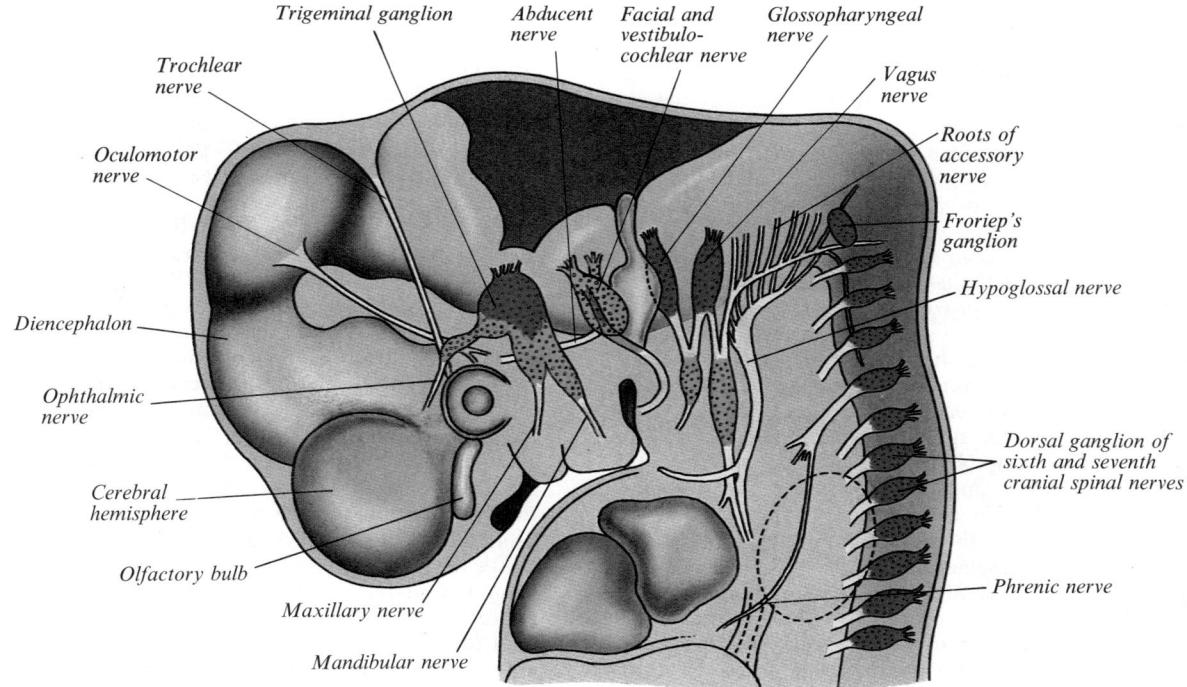

3.112 The brain and cranial nerves of a human embryo, 10.2 mm long. Note also the ganglia (stippled) associated with the trigeminal, facial vestibulocochlear, glossopharyngeal, vagus and spinal accessory nerves.

Froriep's ganglion, an occipital dorsal root ganglion, is inconstant and soon disappears. (After His.)

within the neuroepithelium, while those of sensory neuroblasts are derived from the neural crest and from ectodermal placodes.

The *motor fibres* of the cranial nerves to striated muscle are the axons of cells in the basal plate of the midbrain and hindbrain that grow outwards to their muscle fibres of distribution. The functional and morphological distinction between the neurons within these various nerves is based on the types of muscle innervated. In the trunk, the motor roots of the spinal nerves all emerge from the spinal cord close to the ventral midline to supply the muscles derived from the somites.

In the head the motor outflow is segregated into two pathways (**3.**112, 117). *General somatic efferent* neurons exit ventrally in a similar manner to those of the spinal cord, comprising the oculomotor, trochlear, abducens and hypoglossal nerves. Thus nerves III, IV, VI and XII parallel the organization of the somatic motor neurons in the spinal cord. The second motor component, *special branchial efferent*, comprises the accessory nerve and the motor parts of the trigeminal, facial, glossopharyngeal and vagus nerves, whose nerve exit points lie more dorsally than the somatic motor system.

The cranial nerves also contain a third class of efferent neurons, the *general visceral efferent* neurons (parasympathetic preganglionic) travelling in nerves III, VII, IX and X, which leave the hindbrain via the same exit points as the special branchial efferent fibres. All these three categories of motor neurons probably originate from the same region of the basal plate, adjacent to the floor plate. The definitive arrangement of nuclei then arises due to differential migration of neuronal somata. It is not known whether all these cell types share a common precursor within the rhombencephalon, though there is evidence that in the spinal cord somatic motor and preganglionic autonomic neurons are lineally related.

These motor neuron types have been thus designated according to the types of muscles or structures innervated. General somatic efferent nerves supply striated muscle now known to be derived from the *cranial (occipital) somites* and *prechordal mesenchyme*. Myogenic cells from the ventrolateral edge of the epithelial plate of occipital somites give rise to the intrinsic muscles of the tongue, while the prechordal mesenchyme gives rise to the extrinsic ocular muscles (see p. 274). Special branchial efferent nerves supply the *striated muscles developing within the pharyngeal (branchial) arches* (**3.**148). Chimeric experiments have shown that myogenic cells in the pharyngeal arches are derived solely from unsegmented paraxial mesenchyme, rostral to the somites, which migrates into the arch primordia (Noden 1983a; Couly et al 1992; see p. 275). Thus **all the voluntary muscles of the head originate from axial (prechordal) or paraxial mesenchyme** rendering the distinction between somatic efferent supply and branchial efferent supply somewhat artificial. However, the obviously special nature of the arch musculature, its patterning by the neural crest cells, its particularly rich innervation for both voluntary and reflex activity and the different origins from the basal plate of the branchial efferent nerves compared to the somatic efferent nerves, make the retention of a distinction between the two of value.

General visceral efferent neurons (parasympathetic preganglionic) innervate *glands of the head*, the *sphincter pupillae* and *ciliary muscles*, and the *thoracic and abdominal viscera*.

The *cranial sensory ganglia* are derived in part from the neural crest, and in part from cells of the ectodermal placodes (**3.**103, 112, 148; see p. 222). Generally, neurons distal to the brain derive from placodes while proximal ones derive from the neural crest (D'Amico-Martel & Noden 1980, **3.**148); supporting cells of all sensory ganglia arise from the neural crest (Noden 1978; D'Amico-Martel 1981). The most rostral sensory ganglion, the *trigeminal* (V) comprises both neural crest and placode-derived neurons that mediate *general somatic afferent* functions. In the case of more caudal cranial nerves (VII, IX and X) the same applies, but the two cell populations form **separate** ganglia in the case of each nerve. Analogous with the trigeminal, the proximal series of ganglia is neural crest derived (forming the proximal ganglion of VII, the *superior* ganglion of IX and the *jugular* ganglion of X) while the distal series derives from placodal cells (forming the *geniculate* ganglion of VII, the *petrosal* ganglion of IX and the *nodose* ganglion of X). These ganglia contain neurons that mediate *special*, *general visceral* and *somatic afferent* functions. The VIIth nerve has a *vestibular ganglion* containing both

crest and placodal cells and an acoustic ganglion from placodal neurons only; it conveys special somatic afferents.

Both neurons and supporting cells of the *cranial autonomic ganglia* in the head and the trunk originate from neural crest cells (Weston 1971; Le Douarin & Teillet 1974; see p. 223). Caudal to the ganglion of the vagal nerve the occipital region of the neural crest is concerned with the 'ganglia' of the accessory and hypoglossal nerves. Rudimentary ganglion cells may occur along the hypoglossal nerve in the human embryo; they undergo regression later. Ganglion cells are also found on the developing spinal root of the accessory nerve and these are believed to persist in the adult. The central processes of the cells of these various ganglia, where they persist, form some sensory roots of the cranial nerves and enter the alar lamina of the hindbrain; their peripheral processes join the efferent components of the nerve to be distributed to the various tissues innervated. Some incoming fibres from the facial, glossopharyngeal and vagal nerves collect to form an oval bundle, the *tractus solitarius*, on the lateral aspect of the myelencephalon. This bundle is the homologue of the oval bundle of the spinal cord, but in the hindbrain it becomes more deeply placed by the overgrowth, folding and subsequent fusion of tissue derived from the rhombic lip on the external aspect of the bundle.

CENTRAL NERVOUS SYSTEM

SPINAL CORD

In the future spinal cord the median *roof plate* (*dorsal lamina*) and *floor plate* (*ventral lamina*) of the neural tube do not participate in the cellular proliferation affecting the lateral walls and hence remain thin. Their cells contribute largely to the formation of the ependyma.

The neuroblasts of the *lateral* walls of the tube are large and at first round or oval (*apolar*). Soon they develop processes at opposite poles, becoming *bipolar neuroblasts*. One process is, however, withdrawn and the neuroblast becomes *unipolar*, although this is not invariably so in the case of the spinal cord. Further differentiation leads to the development of dendritic processes and they become typical multipolar neurons. In the developing cord they occur in small clusters representing clones of neurons. The development of a longitudinal *sulcus limitans* on each side of the central canal of the cord divides the ventricular and mantle zones in each lateral wall into a *basal* (*ventrolateral*) *lamina* or *plate* and an *alar* (*dorsolateral*) *lamina* or *plate* (**3.**113). This separation indicates a fundamental functional difference, for neural precursors in the basal lamina include the motor cells of the anterior (ventral) and lateral grey columns, while those of the alar lamina exclusively form 'interneurons' (those possessing both short and long axons), some of which receive the terminals of primary sensory neurons. Caudally the central canal of the cord exhibits a fusiform dilatation, the *terminal ventricle*.

Anterior (ventral) grey column

The cells of the ventricular zone are closely packed at this stage and arranged in radial columns (**3.**94). For experimental studies of radial migration patterns consult Berquist (1932, 1968), also bibliographies in Rakic (1981, 1982). Their disposition may be partly determined by contact guidance along the earliest *radial array* of glial fibres that traverse the **full thickness** of the early neuroepithelium. The cells of the intermediate (mantle) zone are more loosely scattered, and they increase in number at first in the region of the basal lamina. This enlargement outlines the *anterior (ventral) column* of the grey matter and causes a ventral projection on each side of the median plane, the floor plate remaining at the bottom of the shallow groove so produced. As growth proceeds these enlargements, further increased by the development of the *anterior funiculi* (regions of axons passing to and from the brain), encroach on the groove until it becomes converted into the slit-like anterior median fissure of the adult spinal cord (**3.**113). The axons of some of the neuroblasts in the anterior grey column traverse the marginal zone and emerge as bundles on the anterolateral aspect of the spinal cord as the *ventral spinal nerve rootlets*. These constitute, eventually, both the α-efferents which establish motor end plates on extrafusal striated muscle fibres and the γ-efferents which innervate the contractile polar regions of

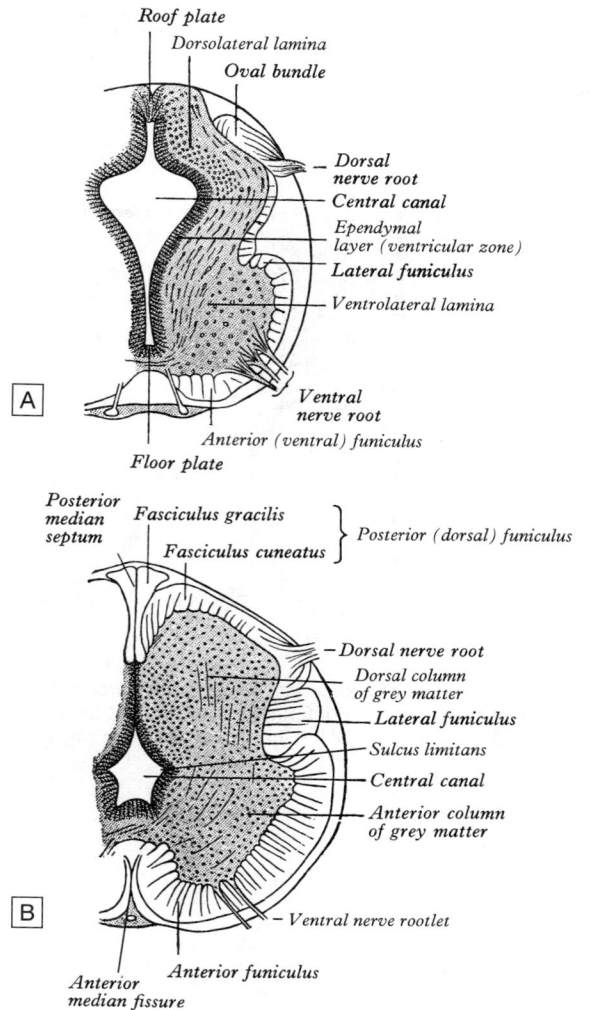

Roof plate
Dorsolateral lamina
Oval bundle

Dorsal nerve root
Central canal
Ependymal layer (ventricular zone)
Lateral funiculus
Ventrolateral lamina

A

Ventral nerve root
Anterior (ventral) funiculus
Floor plate

Posterior median septum
Fasciculus gracilis
Fasciculus cuneatus
} Posterior (dorsal) funiculus

Dorsal nerve root
Dorsal column of grey matter
Lateral funiculus
Sulcus limitans
Central canal
Anterior column of grey matter

B

Ventral nerve rootlet
Anterior funiculus
Anterior median fissure

3.113   Transverse sections through the developing spinal cord of human embryos: A. about 6 weeks old; B. about 3 months old. (After His.)

the intrafusal muscle fibres of the muscle spindles (p. 971). (The histogenesis of β-efferents is completely uncharted.)

Lateral grey column

In the thoracic and upper lumbar regions some intermediate (mantle) zone neuroblasts in the dorsal part of the basal plate outline a *lateral column*. Their axons join the emerging ventral nerve roots and pass as preganglionic fibres to the ganglia of the sympathetic trunk or related ganglia, the majority eventually myelinating to form *white rami communicantes*. The fibres constituting the rami establish synapses with the autonomic ganglionic neurons, and the axons of some of the latter proceed as postganglionic fibres to innervate smooth muscle cells, adipose tissue or glandular cells. Some of the preganglionic sympathetic efferent axons pass to the cells of the suprarenal medulla. The innervation of other 'chromaffin' tissues is less certain (but see the carotid body, p. 971). Similarly an autonomic lateral column is also laid down in the midsacral region and gives origin to the preganglionic para-sympathetic fibres of the pelvic splanchnic nerves.

The **changes** in cell number, position and density as seen in a longitudinal section of the chick spinal cord, based on investigations of Hamburger (1952), are illustrated in **3**.114. The anterior region of each basal plate forms at first a continuous column of cells throughout the length of the developing cord. In many forms this soon develops into two columns (on each side)—one medially placed, concerned with innervation of axial musculature, and a lateral one innervating the limbs. At limb levels the latter column enlarges enormously but regresses at other levels.

Thus the development of the cord involves an interplay between a number of fundamental processes which vary in prominence at different times and at different levels—cell *proliferation*, *migration*, followed either by progressive cell *growth* and *differentiation* or, in complete contrast, by cell *degeneration* and *death*. In the example quoted, cell proliferation persists as a prominent feature at the levels concerned with limb innervation, whilst at thoracic levels a *dorsomedial* migration of neuroblasts occurs to lay the foundation of the visceral efferent column. Further, save at limb levels, massive cell degenerations occur in the lateral 'motor' columns, whereas the medial columns, which innervate axial musculature, persist throughout the cord. The phenomenon of cell death and removal on a large scale, balanced against local proliferation and migration rates, has only been recognized relatively recently as a fundamental feature in many morphogenetic situations.

Thus, it has been shown, some ventrolateral laminal neuroblasts differentiate into the ventral horn neurons from which α-, β- and γ-efferent fibres arise, and these are accompanied at thoracic, upper lumbar and midsacral levels by preganglionic autonomic efferents from neuroblasts of the developing lateral horn. However, additionally, numerous interneurons develop in both these situations (including the well-studied Renshaw cells), but it is uncertain how many of these differentiate directly from ventrolateral lamina (basal plate) neuroblasts and how many migrate to their final positions from the dorsolateral lamina (alar plate).

In the human embryo, the definitive grouping of the ventral column cells, which characterizes the mature cord, occurs early, and by the fourteenth week (80 mm) all the major groups can be recognized (Romanes 1942, 1946, 1953, 1964).

As the anterior and lateral grey columns assume their final form the germinal cells in the ventral part of the ventricular zone gradually cease to proliferate and the layer becomes reduced in thickness until it ultimately forms the single-layered ependyma which lines the ventral part of the central canal of the spinal cord.

Posterior (dorsal) grey column

The posterior (dorsal) column is somewhat late in its development and, as a result, its ventricular zone is for a time much thicker in the dorsolateral lamina (alar plate) than it is in the ventrolateral lamina (basal plate) (**3**.94).

While the columns of grey matter are being defined, the dorsal region of the central canal becomes narrow and slit-like and its walls come into apposition and fuse with each other (**3**.113). In this way the central canal becomes relatively reduced in size and somewhat triangular in outline.

About the end of the fourth week advancing axonal sprouts invade the marginal zone. The first to develop are those destined to become short *intersegmental* fibres from the neuroblasts in the intermediate (mantle) zone, and also fibres of *dorsal roots* of spinal nerves which pass into the spinal cord from neuroblasts of the early spinal ganglia. The earlier dorsal root fibres that invade the dorsal marginal zone stem from **small** dorsal root ganglionic neuroblasts. By the sixth week the latter form a well-defined *oval bundle* near the peripheral part of the dorsolateral lamina (**3**.94, 113A); this bundle increases in size and, spreading towards the median plane, forms the *primitive posterior funiculus*; its constituent fibres are destined to be of fine calibre. Later, fibres derived from new populations of **large** dorsal root ganglionic neuroblasts join the dorsal root to become fibres of much larger calibre. As the posterior funiculi increase in thickness, their medial surfaces come into contact separated only by the *posterior medial septum*, which is ependymal in origin, neuroglial in nature. A more detailed analysis of the temporal sequence of modifications of the dorsal lamina (roof plate), posterior medial septum, and the lateral displacement of the *primitive posterior funiculus* with the later development of the fasciculus gracilis, based on a study of sectioned human embryos of 6–10 weeks and dissections of fetuses up to the end of the fourth month, has been provided by Hughes (1976). He proposed that the displaced primitive posterior funiculus may form the basis of the dorsolateral tract or fasciculus (of Lissauer), and also correlated the sequence, siting and calibre of the entrant dorsal root fibres with the changing size-distribution of the somata of the dorsal root ganglionic neuroblasts.

At about the third month long intersegmental fibres begin to appear and at about the fifth month corticospinal fibres. All nerve

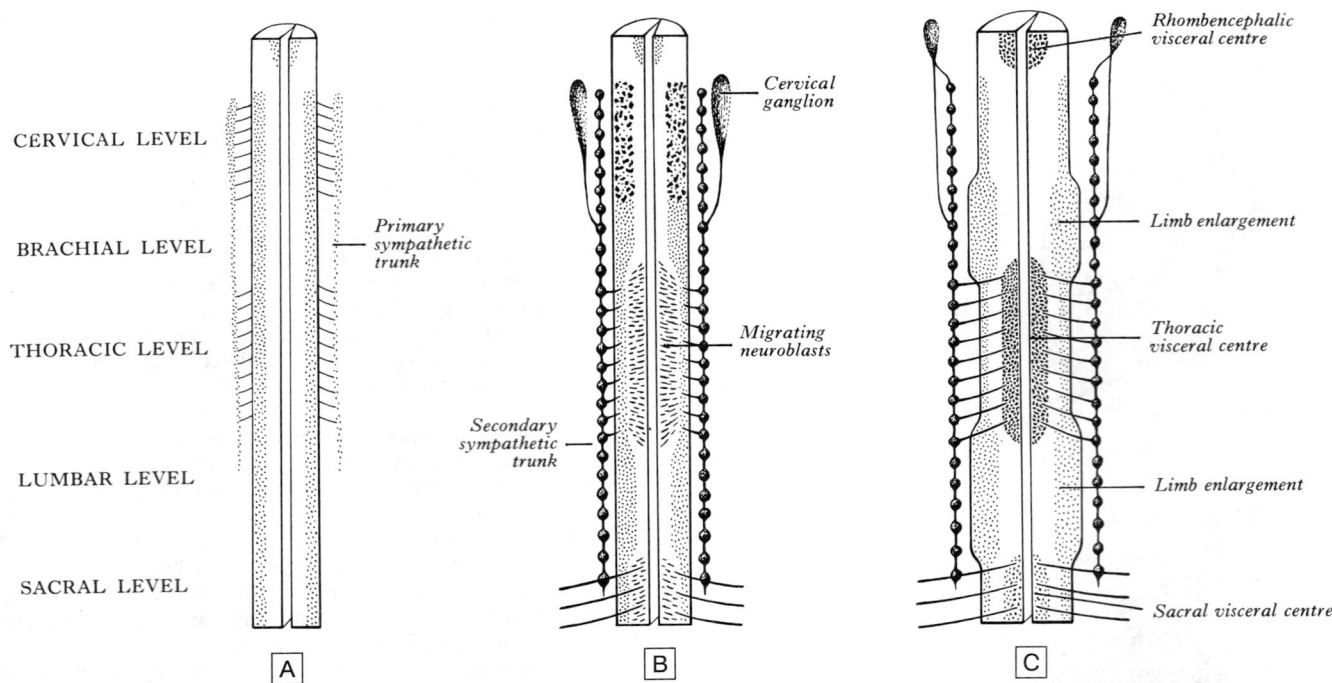

3.114 Diagrams illustrating the changing morphogenetic patterns in the developing neural tube of the chick seen in longitudinal section. Note the progression from A to C as the initial simple homogeneous columnar organization (A) is transformed into the definitive pattern (C). These changes follow variations in the turnover rate and differentiation rate of neuroblasts in different regions of the tube, combined with migration of neuroblasts in some regions and cell deaths in others. For further description see the text. (From V Hamburger, and by permission of the author and the New York Academy of Sciences.)

fibres are at first without myelin sheaths and different groups **commence** to develop sheaths at different times, e.g. the ventral and dorsal nerve roots about the fifth month, the corticospinal fibres after the ninth month. In peripheral nerves the myelin is formed by Schwann cells (derived from neural crest cells); in the CNS by oligodendrocytes (which develop from the ventricular zone of the neural tube). Myelination, of course, persists until overall growth of the CNS and PNS has ceased. Thus, in many sites, slow growth continues for long periods, even into the postpubertal years.

The cervical and lumbar enlargements first appear simultaneously with the development of their respective limb buds.

In early embryonic life the spinal cord occupies the **entire length** of the vertebral canal and the spinal nerves pass at right angles to the cord. After the embryo has attained a length of 30 mm the vertebral column begins to grow more rapidly than the spinal cord, the caudal end of which gradually becomes more cranial in the vertebral canal. Most of this relative rostral migration occurs during the first half of intrauterine life. By the twenty-fifth week the terminal ventricle of the spinal cord has altered in level from the second coccygeal vertebra to the third lumbar, a distance of nine segments, and there remain but two segments before the adult position is reached (Streeter 1919). As the change in level begins rostrally, the caudal end of the terminal ventricle, which has become adherent to the overlying ectoderm, remains in situ and the walls of the intermediate part of the ventricle and its covering pia mater become drawn out to form a delicate filament, the *filum terminale*. The separated portion of the terminal ventricle persists for a time but it usually disappears before birth. It does, however, occasionally give rise to congenital cysts in the neighbourhood of the coccyx. In the definitive state, the upper cervical spinal nerves retain their position roughly at right angles to the cord; proceeding caudally, however, the nerve roots lengthen and are progressively more oblique.

BRAIN

A summary list of the derivatives of the cerebral vesicles from caudal to rostral is given below:

Rhombencephalon (or hindbrain)	
1. Myelencephalon	Medulla oblongata
	Caudal part of the 4th ventricle
	Inferior cerebellar peduncles
2. Metencephalon	Pons
	Cerebellum
	Middle part of the 4th ventricle
	Middle cerebellar peduncles
3. Isthmus rhombencephali	Anterior medullary velum
	Superior cerebellar peduncles
	Rostral part of the 4th ventricle
Mesencephalon (or midbrain)	Cerebral peduncles
	Tegmentum
	Tectum
	Aqueduct
Prosencephalon (or forebrain)	
1. Diencephalon	Thalamus
	Metathalamus
	Subthalamus
	Epithalamus
	Caudal part of the hypothalamus
	Caudal part of the 3rd ventricle
2. Telencephalon	Rostral part of the hypothalamus
	Rostral part of the 3rd ventricle
	Central hemispheres
	Lateral ventricles
	Cortex (archaeocortex, palaeocortex, neocortex)
	Corpus striatum

Rhombencephalon

By the time the midbrain flexure appears, the hindbrain exceeds in length the combined extent of the other two brain vesicles. Rostrally it exhibits a constriction, the *isthmus rhombencephali* (**3**.96B), best viewed from the dorsal aspect. Ventrally the hindbrain is separated from the dorsal wall of the primitive pharynx only by the notochord, the two dorsal aortae and a small amount of mesenchyme; on each side it is closely related to the dorsal ends of the pharyngeal arches (3.141).

The pontine flexure appears to 'stretch' the thin, epithelial roof plate which becomes widened, the greatest increase in width corresponding to the region of maximum convexity, so that the outline of the roof plate becomes rhomboidal. By the same change the lateral walls become separated, particularly dorsally, and the cavity of the hindbrain, subsequently the fourth ventricle, becomes flattened and somewhat triangular on cross-section. The pontine flexure becomes increasingly acute until, at the end of the second month, the laminae of its cranial (metencephalic) and caudal (myelencephalic) slopes are opposed to each other (3.116c) and, at the same time, the lateral angles of the cavity extend to form the lateral recesses of the fourth ventricle.

About the end of the fourth week, when the pontine flexure is first discernible, a series of six transverse *rhombic grooves* appears in the ventrolateral lamina (basal plate) of the hindbrain. Between the grooves, the intervening masses of neural tissue are termed *rhombomeres* (see p. 219). These are closely associated with the pattern of the underlying motor nuclei of certain of the cranial nerves. The distribution of motor nuclei has been determined for avia and for rodents, but it is not known whether this pattern is conserved in humans. Rhombomere 1 contains the trochlear nucleus, rhombomeres 1, 2 and 3 contain the trigeminal nucleus, rhombomeres 4 and 5 the facial nucleus, rhombomeres 5 and 6 the abducens nuclei, rhombomeres 6 and 7 the glossopharyngeal nucleus, and rhombomeres 7 and 8 the vagus, accessory and hypoglossal nerves. Rhombomeric segmentation represents the ground plan of development in this region of the brainstem and is pivotal for the development of regional identity (see p. 229 and see also 3.148). With further morphogenesis, however, the obvious constrictions of the rhombomere boundaries disappear, and the medulla once again assumes a smooth contour. The differentiation of the lateral walls of the hindbrain into basal (ventrolateral) and alar (dorsolateral) plates has a similar significance to the corresponding differentiation in the lateral wall of the spinal cord (p. 238) and ventricular, mantle and marginal zones are formed in the same way.

Cells of the basal plate (ventrolateral lamina). These are often, in elementary accounts, simply termed 'motor' (but see below); they form **three** elongated, but interrupted, **columns** positioned ventrally and dorsally with an intermediate column between (3.115).

(1) The most *ventral column* is continuous with the anterior grey column of the spinal cord and will supply muscles considered 'myotomic' in origin. It is represented in the caudal part of the hindbrain by the hypoglossal nucleus, and it reappears at a higher level as the nuclei of the abducent, trochlear and oculomotor nerves, which are *somatic efferent nuclei*.

(2) The *intermediate column* is represented in the upper part of the spinal cord and caudal brainstem (medulla oblongata and pons) and is for the supply of branchial (pharyngeal) and postbranchial musculature. It is interrupted also, but the caudal brainstem part, which gives fibres to the ninth, tenth and eleventh cranial nerves, forms the elongated *nucleus ambiguus*. The latter continues into the cervical spinal cord as the origin of the spinal accessory nerve. At higher levels parts of this column give origin to the motor nuclei of the facial and trigeminal nerves. These three nuclei are termed *branchial (special visceral) efferent nuclei*.

(3) The most dorsal column of the basal plate (represented in the spinal cord by the lateral grey column) innervates viscera. It is interrupted also, its large caudal part forming some of the *dorsal nucleus* of the vagus and its cranial part the *salivatory nucleus*. These are termed *general visceral (general splanchnic) efferent nuclei* and their neurons give rise to preganglionic, parasympathetic nerve fibres.

It should be noted here that the neurons of the basal plate and their three columnar derivatives are only 'motor' in the sense that **some** of their number form either α, β or γ motor neurons, or preganglionic parasympathetic neurons. The remainder, which greatly outnumber the former, differentiate into functionally related interneurons and, in some loci, neuroendocrine cells.

Cell columns of the alar plate (dorsolateral lamina). These are also interrupted and give rise to *general visceral (general splanchnic) afferent, special visceral (special splanchnic) afferent, general somatic afferent* and *special somatic afferent* nuclei (their relative positions, in simplified transverse section, are shown in 3.115). The general visceral afferent column is represented by a part of the dorsal nucleus of the vagus (see also p. 1251), the special visceral afferent column by the nucleus of the tractus solitarius, the general somatic afferent column by the afferent nuclei of the trigeminal nerve (Brown 1974) and the special somatic afferent column by the nuclei of the vestibulocochlear nerve. (Again it should be noted here that the relatively simple functional independence of these afferent columns implied by the foregoing classification is, in the main, an aid to elementary learning. The emergent neurobiological mechanisms are in fact much more complex and less well understood). Although they tend to retain

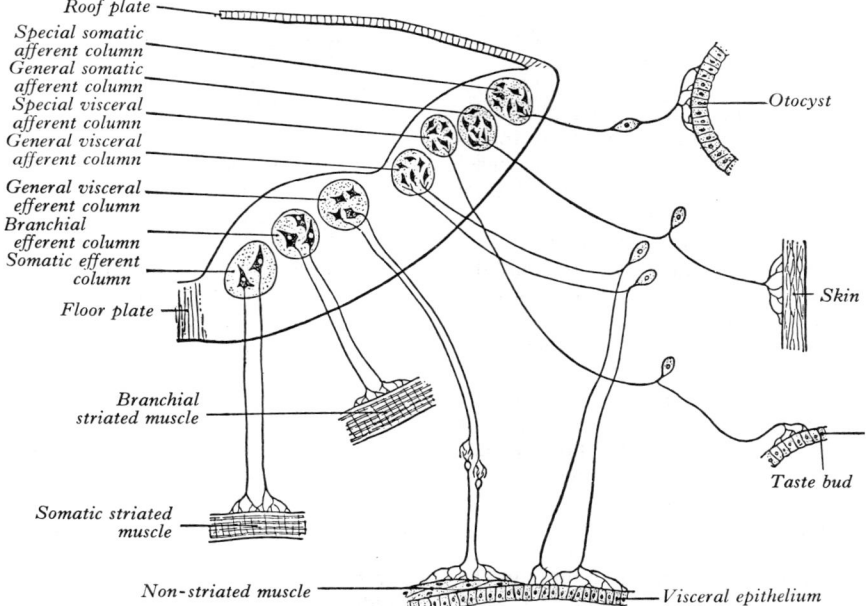

Roof plate
Special somatic afferent column
General somatic afferent column
Special visceral afferent column
General visceral afferent column
General visceral efferent column
Branchial efferent column
Somatic efferent column
Floor plate
Branchial striated muscle
Somatic striated muscle
Non-striated muscle
Otocyst
Skin
Taste bud
Visceral epithelium

3.115 Diagram of a transverse section through the developing hindbrain of a human embryo about 10.5 mm long, to show the relative positions of the columns of grey matter from which the nuclei associated with the different varieties of nerve components are derived. Note the postganglionic neurons associated with the general visceral efferent column, the bipolar neurons associated with the otocyst and the unipolar afferent neurons associated with the other alar lamina columns.

their primitive positions, some of these nuclei are later displaced by differential growth patterns and by the appearance and growth of neighbouring fibre tracts, and possibly by active migration. It has been suggested that a neuron tends to remain as near as possible to its predominant source of stimulation and that when the possibility of separation arises, owing to the development of neighbouring structures, it will migrate in the direction from which the greatest density of stimuli come. This phenomenon was termed neurobiotaxis (Kappers 1921, 1934). Cells can migrate in this way only by lengthening of their axons, which therefore trace the route taken by the cells on their transit. The curious courses of the fibres arising from the facial nucleus (p. 1243) and nucleus ambiguus have been held to illustrate this phenomenon. In the 10-mm embryo the facial nucleus lies in the floor of the fourth ventricle, occupying the position of the special visceral efferent column, and it is placed at a higher level than the abducent nucleus. As growth proceeds the facial nucleus migrates at first caudally and dorsally, relative to the sixth nerve nucleus, and then ventrally to reach its adult position. As it migrates, the axons to which its somata give rise elongate and their subsequent course is assumed to map out the pathway along which the facial nucleus has travelled. Similarly the nucleus ambiguus arises initially immediately deep to the ventricular floor, but in the adult it is more deeply placed and its efferent fibres first pass dorsally and medially before curving laterally to emerge at the surface of the medulla oblongata. Neurobiotaxis has been relatively well-documented for the case of branchial (special visceral) efferent and general visceral efferent neurons in the brainstem, whose somata are translocated dorsolaterally from the motor column towards their exit point and targets. Certainly the absence of placodal neurons which contribute to the trigeminal nerve results in the remaining crest derived neurons failing to undergo their normal migrations from medial to lateral positions in the floor of the metencephalon (Noden 1991).

Myelencephalon

The caudal slope of the embryonic hindbrain constitutes the myelencephalon, which develops into the medulla oblongata. The nuclei of the ninth, tenth, eleventh and twelfth cranial nerves develop in the situations already indicated and afferent fibres from the ganglia of the ninth and tenth nerves form an oval marginal bundle in the region overlying the alar (dorsolateral) lamina. The dorsal edge of this lamina throughout the rhombencephalon gives attachment to the thin expanded roof plate and is termed the *rhombic lip*. (The *inferior rhombic lip* is confined to the myelencephalon; the *superior rhombic lip* to the metencephalon.) As the walls of the rhombencephalon spread outwards, the rhombic lip protrudes as a lateral edge which becomes folded over the adjoining area. The rhombic lip may later become adherent to this area, and its cells migrate actively into the marginal zone of the basal plate. In this way the oval bundle which forms the *tractus solitarius* becomes buried. Alar plate cells which migrate from the rhombic lip are believed to give rise to the olivary and arcuate nuclei and the scattered grey matter of the nuclei pontis. While this migration is in progress the thin floor plate is invaded by fibres which cross the median plane (accompanied by neurons that cluster in and near this plane), and it becomes thickened to form the *median raphe*. Some of the migrating cells from the rhombic lip in this region do not reach the basal plate and form an oblique ridge across the dorsolateral aspect of the inferior cerebellar peduncle: the *corpus pontobulbare* (*nucleus of the circumolivary bundle*).

The lower (caudal half) part of the myelencephalon takes no part in the formation of the fourth ventricle and, in its development, it closely resembles the spinal cord. The nuclei, *gracilis* and *cuneatus*, and some reticular nuclei, are derived from the alar plate, and their efferent arcuate fibres and interspersed neurons play a large part in the formation of the median raphe.

At about the fourth month the descending *corticospinal fibres* invade the ventral part of the medulla oblongata to initiate the pyramids whilst dorsally, ascending fibres from the spinal cord, with olivocerebellar and parolivocerebellar fibres, external arcuate fibres, together with two-way reticulocerebellar and vestibulocerebellar interconnections, form the inferior cerebellar peduncle. (The reticular nuclei of the lower medulla probably have a dual origin from both basal and alar plates.)

Metencephalon

The rostral slope of the embryonic hindbrain is the metencephalon, from which both cerebellum and pons develop. Before formation of the pontine flexure the dorsolateral laminae of the metencephalon are parallel with one another. Subsequent to its formation the roof plate of the hindbrain becomes rhomboidal and the dorsal laminae of the metencephalon lie obliquely, being close at the cranial end of the fourth ventricle but widely separated at the level of its lateral angles. Accentuation of the flexure approximates the cranial angle of the ventricle to the caudal, and the alar plates of the metencephalon now lie almost horizontally.

Caudal to the developing cerebellum the roof of the fourth ventricle remains epithelial, covering an approximately triangular zone from the lateral angles of the rhomboid fossa to the median obex. Over this region nervous tissue fails to develop and vascular pia mater is closely applied to the subjacent ependyma. At each lateral angle and in the midline caudally the membranes break through forming the lateral and median apertures of the roof of the fourth ventricle. Subsequently, these are the principal routes by which cerebrospinal fluid, produced in the ventricles, escapes into the subarachnoid space. The vascular *pia mater* (*tela choroidea*), in an inverted V formation cranial to the apertures, invaginates the ependyma to form vascular fringes—the vertical and horizontal parts of the choroid plexuses of the fourth ventricle.

Cerebellum

The cerebellum consists of a cortex within which are buried a series of deep nuclei. This organization of the cerebellar cortex is similar to that of the cerebral cortex, except that the latter has six layers, while the former has only three. These are the *outer molecular layer*, the *Purkinje layer*, containing Purkinje cells which are the only output neurons of the cortex, and the *inner granular layer*.

Two rounded swellings develop which at first project partly into the ventricle (3.116B, C), forming the rudimentary cerebellar hemispheres. The most cranial part of the roof of the metencephalon originally separates the two swellings, but it becomes invaded by cells, which form the rudiments of the vermis. These cells were regarded as derivatives of both basal and alar plates (Baxter 1953). At a later stage, *extroversion of the cerebellum* occurs, with reduction of its *intraventricular* projection and an increasing dorsal *extraventricular prominence*. The cerebellum now consists of a bilobar (dumb-bell shaped) swelling stretched across the rostral part of the fourth ventricle (3.116), continuous rostrally with the anterior medullary velum, formed from the isthmus, and caudally with the epithelial roof of the myelencephalon. With growth a number of transverse grooves appear on the dorsal aspects of the cerebellar rudiment, as the precursors of the numerous fissures which characterize the surface of the mature cerebellum (3.117, also p. 243).

The *posterolateral fissure*, in its lateral parts, appears first, demarcating the then most caudal area from the rest of the cerebellar rudiment, enabling the *flocculi* to be identified. The lateral parts of this fissure extend medially, meet in the median plane and demarcate the nodule. The *flocculonodular lobes* can now be recognized and are the most caudal part of the cerebellum at this stage, but, owing to the growth of the adjoining areas, they progressively come to occupy the **anterior** part of the *inferior surface* in the adult. They are formed in proximity to the line of attachment of the epithelial roof, i.e. to the rhombic lip (p. 243 and 3.116, 117).

At the end of the third month a transverse sulcus appears on the rostral slope of the cerebellar rudiment and deepens to form the *fissura prima*, which cuts into the vermis and both hemispheres, separating the most cranial region to form the anterior lobe.

During the same period two short transverse grooves appear on the inferior vermis; the first is the *fissura secunda*, which demarcates the uvula, and the second the *prepyramidal fissure*, demarcating the pyramid (3.116B). The whole cerebellum now grows dorsally and the caudo-inferior aspects of the *hemispheres* expand much more than the inferior vermis, which therefore becomes buried at the bottom of a deep hollow—the *vallecula*. Meanwhile numerous additional fissures develop, which are approximately parallel to, and intervene between, the foregoing. They result in a relatively vast increase in surface area of the cerebellum but their precise positions and sys-

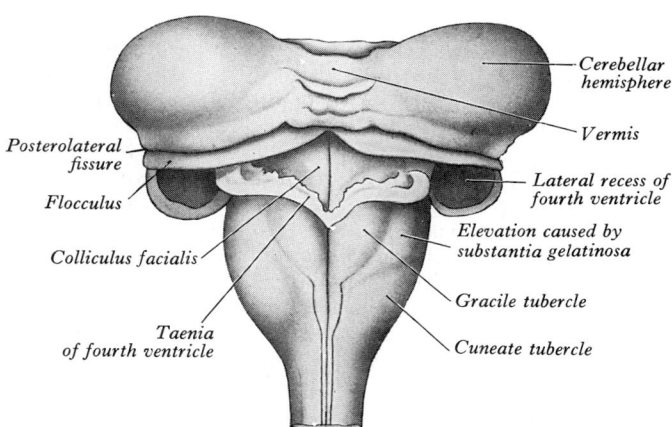

3.116A The cerebellum of a fetus in the fifth month. (After Kollmann.)

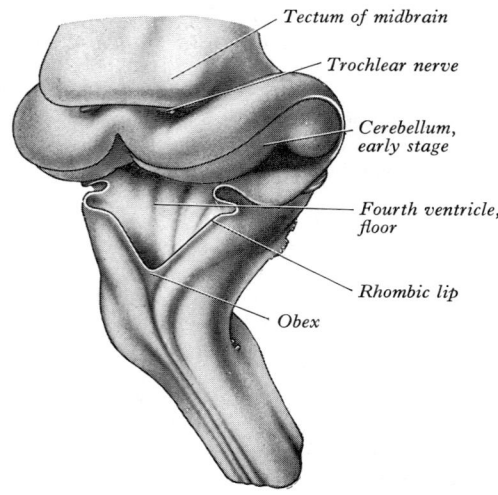

3.116B The dorsal aspect of the hindbrain of a human fetus about 3 months old: viewed from behind and partly from the right side. (From a model by His.)

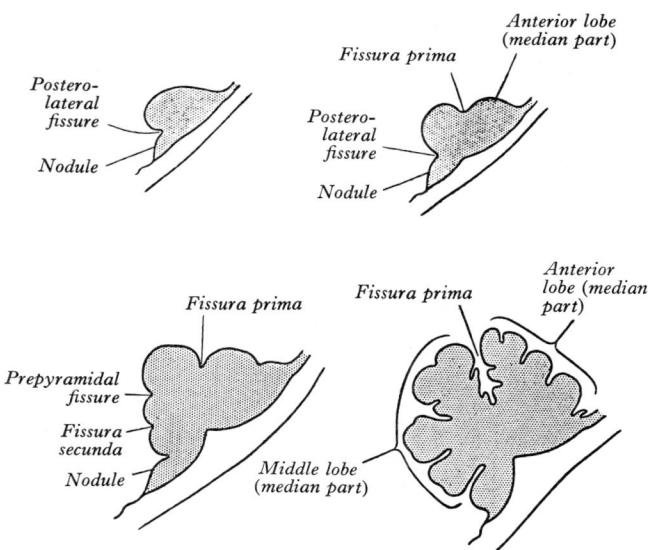

3.117 Median sagittal sections through the developing cerebellum, showing 4 different stages.

tematic names have limited functional or morphological significance. The most extensive of these develops into the *horizontal fissure*.

In many mammals a part of the hemisphere immediately rostral to the posterolateral fissure becomes defined as an entity; in some it forms a very prominent part of the cerebellum, termed the *paraflocculus*, but the relationship is purely topographical and, in contrast to the flocculus, the paraflocculus receives afferent connections mainly, but not entirely, from the cerebral cortex. It is uncertain whether any homologue of the paraflocculus exists in the human cerebellum or whether, as has been proposed, it is represented by some small patches of grey matter which are frequently present on the inferior surface of the middle cerebellar peduncle (Larsell 1947).

The emergence of arrays of principal fissures ('fissuration') and folia ('foliation') has been studied experimentally by a number of workers (Sievers et al 1981; Allen et al 1981). Proliferation of the external granular layer and its expansion relative to the white matter beneath appears to have a role in cortical folding. Other factors include outgrowth and differentiation of the fibres constituting the central white core, the Bergmann glia, the external granular ventricular zone, the pial/glial basal lamina and the pial fibroblasts. Selective experimental alteration of any of these elements alters or obliterates the folial pattern. (For these tissue components see below.)

Mammalian cerebellar histogenesis

Mammalian cerebellar histogenesis has been more completely described, both during normal ontogeny and after experimental intervention, than in any other part of the nervous system, due in large measure to its precisely ordered geometry and highly distinctive cell types. The connectivity, synaptology and electrophysiology of the latter have also been intensively studied, and some knowledge of these aspects is a prerequisite of any account of histogenesis (Section 8). Particularly valuable in histogenetic investigations have been nuclear labelling with tritiated thymidine, the analysis of genetic variants and the changes following surgical deafferentation, exposure to biochemically active agents, X-irradiation and virus diseases. Most studies have been confined to mice and rats, and whilst it seems probable that **qualitatively** similar cell migrations and contacts occur, **quantitative** findings and **ontogenetic timings** cannot, of course, be extrapolated to the human cerebellum. Only the briefest introduction can be entertained in this volume, and the interested reader should enter the literature by consulting such key references as Miale and Sidman (1961), Fujita (1963), Fujita et al (1966), Kornguth et al (1966, 1968), Mugnaini (1970), Eccles (1970), Hamori (1972), Altman (1972a,b,c), Eccles (1973), Swarz (1976), Swarz and del Cerro (1975, 1977), Berry (1982); Berry et al (1980a,b,c,d).

The early cerebellar rudiment consists of a pseudostratified epithelium showing interkinetic migration (p. 229) which soon develops the three basic zones—ventricular, mantle, and marginal—as elsewhere in the neural tube. The rudiment of the cerebellum originates from cells of the superior rhombic lip and adjacent dorsal part of the alar plate of the metencephalon and mesencephalon. Studies on avia have shown a hitherto unrecognized contribution to the cerebellum of the *mesencephalon*, due to the fact that at the isthmus, the dorsal part of the mesencephalon is displaced caudally and comes to overlie the myelencephalon (Hallonet et al 1990). The mesencephalon and metencephalon give rise to different cell populations within the cerebellum. The genetic control of cerebellar development is being investigated, and may depend upon the gene *Wnt-1*, whose expression domain forms an annulus, rostral to the isthmus; *Wnt-1* mutant mice have cerebellar defects (Thomas & Capecchi 1990).

The histogenesis of the cerebellum is complicated by the existence of **two** germinal zones, the first a ventricular zone lying beneath the developing cerebellar plate, the *internal germinal layer*, and the second coming to lie superficial to the mantle zone. The latter, termed the *external germinal layer*, is derived from cells migrating exclusively from the *metencephalic rhombic lip*. Initially, progenitor cells continue proliferating in the ventricular zone. Slightly later, spreading lateromedially from the rhombic lips to meet centrally in a subpial position (i.e. the most superficial part of the marginal zone), similarly uncommitted germinal cells proliferate forming the external germinal layer. Both layers continue *proliferative mitoses*, giving clonal progeny, until they are several cells thick. This *pro-*

liferative phase gradually diminishes with the onset of the *phase of neurogenesis*, and eventually overlaps and merges into a *phase of gliogenesis*. The generation of cell types in the cerebellum follows a precisely ordered time sequence. Specific neuronal varieties that characterize the deep cerebellar nuclei and cortex migrate to their definitive positions, develop axons and synaptic contacts, and mature (Altman & Bayer 1978; Berry et al 1980d). Similarly, as neurogenesis wanes, remaining germinal cells continue to give generations of committed glioblasts which although less well documented than the neuroblasts, also migrate to and mature in their definitive positions. The exception to this is the specialized, radially disposed *Bergmann glioblasts*, however, which are amongst the **first** cells to be committed in the early neuroepithelium and may provide contact guidance pathways for neuronal migration. The fate of each germinal layer will now briefly be reviewed.

Within the mantle layer, neurons differentiate in two strata, the superficial stratum giving rise to Purkinje cells of the cerebellar cortex and the deeper stratum giving rise to the neurons of the roof nuclei. Initially, *primitive Purkinje neuroblasts* and *primitive nuclear neuroblasts* emerge in approximately equal numbers, but whether this follows a series of symmetrical or asymmetrical mitoses is unknown. The nuclear neuroblasts remain embedded in the developing future white matter adjacent to the roof of the rostral part of the fourth ventricle. The main mass of nuclear neuroblasts then slowly subdivides into the primordial *fastigial, emboliform, globose* and *dentate deep cerebellar nuclei*, and the individual neuroblasts differentiate as either small intranuclear interneurons or the larger projection neurons. The axons of the latter invade the early cerebellar peduncles and pursue complex paths to their multiple destinations.

The Purkinje neuroblasts, in contrast, **migrate** superficially towards their definitive position in the expanding cortex, where they slowly mature into their highly characteristic form of somata and dendritic trees. As they migrate, the terminals of one process—the future axon—remain adjacent to, and ultimately in synaptic contact with, the nuclear neuroblasts, the remainder of the axon elongating as it 'trails' behind the advancing soma. The mature and developing Purkinje cell has been a favourite object for **quantitative** cytological and ultrastructural studies, both during normal ontogeny and after such experimental manipulations as suppression of granule cell (and therefore parallel fibre) development, or after prevention of climbing fibre growth (Hamori 1972 and p. 1036). The maturation of normal rat cerebellar cortical neurons has been described in normal development (Altman 1972b), and after experimental manipulation (Berry et al 1978, 1980a,b,c,d; Rakic 1981, 1982). When the formation of nuclear and Purkinje neurons has proceeded for some time, a number of the remaining cells of the ventricular zone give rise to generations of *Golgi neurons*, the small neurons of the roof nuclei and possibly some glia. These cells also migrate superficially to gradually occupy, and mature in, their definitive position and morphology.

The external germinal (also termed granular) layer, formed by migration of cells from the rhombic lip, is the origin of the *granule cells, basket cells, stellate cells* and probably some *glial cells*. These cells migrate centripetally to come to lie at varying depths within the developing cerebellum. Granule cells migrate through the molecular and Purkinje cell layers to form the *internal granular layer*. Basket and stellate cells, however, migrate only as far as the molecular layer. Basket cells migrate deeply to meet, and ultimately synapse with, the somata and axons of the ascending Purkinje neuroblasts, their axons passing transversely in the primordial cerebellar folia. Following more prolonged proliferation of the external granular layer vast numbers of granule cell neuroblasts are produced. Ramón y Cajal first described the migration of granule cells, based on Golgi preparations. He realized that the different morphologies of granule cells within different cortical layers represented a dynamic sequence. In the deeper part of the external granular layer the cells are bipolar, with two processes oriented parallel to the long axes of the folia, in a similar manner to the mature parallel fibres of the granule cells, each of which contacts many Purkinje cells. Cells at deeper levels possessed a third process oriented orthogonally, down which cells had apparently migrated into the molecular layer. The apparent mystery of this stereotyped vertical migration, despite obstructions, was solved by the discovery that external granule cells migrate inwards along the long radial processes of specialized glial cells—

the Bergmann glia (Mugnaini & Forstrønen 1967). The general significance of this mechanism in neural development was recognized by Rakic (1971a,b), who demonstrated the presence of radial glial cells in all parts of the primate brain. He considered that the migrating soma 'trailed' behind it an elongated axon which subsequently bifurcated to form the parallel fibre axons, whilst dividing axons passing in advance of the soma met the mossy afferents to form cerebellar glomeruli. The translocation of neuronal somata along glial processes has been studied extensively in culture, where neurons from the cerebellum or the cortex are equally able to migrate on glia derived from either region (reviewed in Hatten 1990). There appears to be a reciprocal dependence between neurons and glial cells, with the latter dependent on the neuron to arrest its division and promote its differentiation. A number of molecules may be involved in the migration, but antibodies against N-cadherin and integrin can disrupt the process. Mice mutant for the *weaver* (*wv*) gene develop with small cerebelli, due to loss of granule cells. Granule cells seem to be the primary site of action of *wv*, since *wv* mutant granule cells cannot migrate on wild-type glial cells (Hatten et al 1986); the gene encodes a membrane-associated ligand that induces neuronal differentiation (Gao et al 1992). The final generations of progenitor cells from the external germinal layer, relatively sparse and brief, occur whilst granule cell production is at its height; their progeny merely migrate locally and differentiate into outer stellate cells.

The origin of the cerebellar glial cells remains much more problematical and has been the subject of dispute for over a century. The view advanced by Obersteiner (1883) and Schaper (1897) was that the various macroglial cell varieties (Bergmann cells, astrocytes and oligodendrocytes) stemmed from final generations of germinal cells of both the internal and external germinal layers; this has received more recent experimental support (Fujita et al 1966; Fujita 1967; Meller et al 1969; Privat 1975). The second view proposed by Athias (1897) and Ramón y Cajal (1911) held that the macroglia were formed exclusively from the internal ventricular zone, and that the progeny of the external layer were solely the three varieties of neuroblast: this suggestion has been supported by the labelling studies of Swarz and del Cerro (1977). The consensus at the moment seems to be that both zones give rise to glia. But while the ventricular zone is responsible for the production of the early Bergmann glia, and of glial cells of the internal granular layer, glia of the molecular layer originate from the external granular layer. The microglial elements are exogenous, invading the cerebellar rudiment from the surrounding vasculature.

The remainder of the metencephalon becomes the pons, but little is known of the individual stages in the transformation. Ventricular, mantle and marginal zones are formed in the usual way, and the nuclei of the trigeminal, abducens and facial nerves develop in the mantle layer. It is possible that the grey matter of the formatio reticularis is derived from the basal plate and that of the nuclei pontis from the alar plate by the active migration of cells from the rhombic lip. However, about the fourth month the pons is invaded by corticopontine, corticobulbar and corticospinal fibres, becomes proportionately thicker, and takes on its adult appearance.

The region of the *isthmus rhombencephali* undergoes a series of changes notoriously difficult to interpret. As a result, however, the greater part of the region apparently becomes absorbed into the caudal end of the midbrain, only the roof plate, in which the anterior medullary velum is formed, and the dorsal parts of the alar plate, which become invaded by converging fibres of the superior cerebellar peduncles, remaining as recognizable derivatives in the adult. Note that originally the decussation of the trochlear nerves was **caudal** to the isthmus, but as the growth changes occur it is displaced in a rostral direction until it reaches its adult position.

Mesencephalon

The mesencephalon or midbrain, derived from the intermediate primary cerebral vesicle, persists for a time as a thin-walled tube enclosing a cavity of some size, separated from that of the prosencephalon by a slight constriction and from the rhombencephalon by the isthmus rhombencephali. Later, its cavity becomes relatively reduced in diameter, and in the adult brain it forms the *cerebral aqueduct*. The basal (ventrolateral) plate of the midbrain increases in thickness to form the *cerebral peduncles*, which are at first of small size, but enlarge rapidly after the fourth month, when their numerous fibre tracts begin to appear in the marginal zone (p. 1035 et seq). The neuroblasts of the basal plate give origin to the nuclei of the oculomotor nerve and some grey masses of the tegmentum, while the nucleus of the trochlear nerve remains in the region of the isthmus rhombencephali. The trigeminal mesencephalic nucleus originates from midbrain neural crest (Narayanan & Narayanan 1978). The cells of the dorsal part of the alar (dorsolateral) plates proliferate and invade the roof plate, which therefore thickens and is later divided into corpora bigemina by a median groove. Caudally this groove becomes a median ridge, which persists in the adult as the frenulum veli. The corpora bigemina are later subdivided into the *superior* and *inferior colliculi* by a transverse furrow. The *red nucleus*, *substantia nigra* and *reticular nuclei* of the midbrain *tegmentum* may first be defined at the end of the third month. Their origins are probably mixed from neuroblasts of both basal and alar plates.

The detailed histogenesis of the tectum and its main derivatives, the colliculi, will not be followed here, but in general the principles outlined for the cerebellar cortex (p. 243), the palaeopallium and neopallium (p. 253) also apply to this region. There exists a high degree of geometric order in the developing retinotectal projection (the equivalent of the retinogeniculate projection), and also a precise somatotopy in tectospinal projection. These facts, coupled with the ability of the fish and amphibian central nervous tracts to **regenerate** after severance, have led the retinotectal pathways to become classical sites for experimentation. Much interest has centred on two problems: how retinal axons reach the tectum, and how correct topographic connections are made. Many signals have been invoked to explain retinal ganglion axon guidance to the tectum. These may be pre-formed pathways, physical features, such as a pattern of holes and spaces at the optic nerve head (Silver & Sidman 1980), adhesive molecules in the pathway, such as neural cell adhesion molecules (Silver & Rutishauser 1984), and pre-existing axon tracts (Easter & Taylor 1989). However, the ability of ectopic axons to find the optic tectum when originating from supernumerary transplanted eyes has also suggested some globally-distributed positional information on the neuroepithelial surface, whose molecular identity has not been elucidated. The search for molecules in the specificity of termination sites on the tectum has been slightly more successful. Firstly, the results of perturbation experiments in amphibia led to the elaboration of a powerful theory of 'chemospecificity', in which positional cues on the surfaces of growing axons were envisaged to be shared with the appropriate target area on the tectum (Sperry 1963). The idea of a large number of unique markers was superseded by the idea that graded distributions of a few molecules might play the same role (Fraser 1980; Gierer 1981). In vitro, retinal temporal axons are found to prefer to grow on anterior tectal membranes and to avoid posterior membranes, corresponding with their termination site in vivo (Walter et al 1987). Other molecules have been identified that could mediate topographical matching via their distributions, for example the 'Trisler' molecule that is preferentially localized in dorsoposterior compared with ventro-anterior retina (Trisler et al 1981).

Prosencephalon

At an early stage, a transverse section through the forebrain shows the same parts as are displayed in similar sections of the spinal cord and medulla oblongata—thick lateral walls connected by thin floor and roof plates. Moreover, each lateral wall is divided into a dorsal area and a ventral area separated internally by the *hypothalamic sulcus*. This sulcus ends anteriorly at the medial end of the optic stalk (see below); in the fully developed brain, it persists as a slight groove extending from the interventricular foramen to the cerebral aqueduct. It is analogous to, if not the homologue of, the sulcus limitans. The thin roof plate remains epithelial, but invaginated by vascular mesenchyme, the tela choroidea of the choroid plexuses of the third ventricle. Later, the lateral margins of the tela undergo a similar invagination into the medial walls of the cerebral hemispheres (see below). The floor plate thickens, developing the nuclear masses of the hypothalamus and subthalamus.

At a very early period, before the closure of the rostral neuropore (p. 146), two lateral diverticula, the *optic vesicles*, appear, one on each side, about the level of the forebrain; for a time they communicate with its cavity by relatively wide openings. The distal parts of the optic vesicles expand, while the proximal parts become the tubular *optic stalks*. (Their further development is given on pp. 259–261.) The forebrain next grows, its tip curving ventrally, and two further diverticula rapidly expand from it, one on each side. These diverticula are rostrolateral to the optic stalks and subsequently form the *cerebral hemispheres*; their cavities are the rudiments of the lateral ventricles; they communicate with the median part of the forebrain cavity by relatively wide openings which ultimately become the interventricular foramina. The anterior limit of the median part of the forebrain consists of a thin sheet, the *lamina terminalis* (3.118A–c), which stretches from the interventricular foramina to the recess at the base of the optic stalks. The anterior part of the forebrain, including the rudiments of the cerebral hemispheres, is the *telencephalon* (*end-brain*), and the posterior part of the *diencephalon* (*between-brain*); both contribute to the formation of the third ventricle, although the latter predominates. The fate of the lamina terminalis is detailed below.

Diencephalon

The diencephalon is broadly divided by the hypothalamic sulcus into the *pars dorsalis diencephali* and *pars ventralis diencephali*; these, however, are composite, each contributing to diverse neural structures. The pars dorsalis develops into the (dorsal) thalamus and metathalamus along the immediate suprasulcal area of its lateral wall, whilst the highest dorsocaudal lateral wall and roof form the epithalamus. The *thalamus* (3.118A–c) is first visible as a thickening which involves the anterior part of the dorsal area (Cooper 1950). Caudal to the thalamus the lateral and medial geniculate bodies, or *metathalamus*, are recognizable at first as surface depressions on the internal aspect and as elevations on the external aspect of the lateral wall (Cooper 1945). With the enlargement of the thalami as smooth ovoid masses, they gradually narrow the wide interval between them into a vertically compressed cavity which forms the greater part of the third ventricle. After a time these medial surfaces may come into contact and become adherent over a variable area, the connection (single or multiple) constituting the *interthalamic adhesion*. The caudal growth of the thalamus excludes the geniculate bodies from the lateral wall of the third ventricle.

At first the lateral aspect of the developing thalamus is separated from the medial aspect of the cerebral hemisphere by a cleft, but with growth the cleft becomes obliterated (3.119) as the thalamus fuses with the part of the hemisphere in which the corpus striatum is developing. Later, with the development of the projection fibres (corticofugal and corticopetal) of the neocortex (p. 158), the thalamus becomes related to the internal capsule, which intervenes between it and the lateral part of the corpus striatum (lentiform nucleus). Ventral to the hypothalamic sulcus the lateral wall of the diencephalon, in addition to median derivatives of its floor plate, forms a large part of the hypothalamus and subthalamus.

The *epithalamus*, which includes the pineal gland, the posterior and habenular commissures and the trigonum habenulae, develops in association with the caudal part of the roof plate and the adjoining regions of the lateral walls of the diencephalon. At an early period (12–20 mm CR length) the epithalamus in the lateral wall projects into the third ventricle as a smooth ellipsoid mass, larger than the adjacent mass of the (dorsal) thalamus and separated from it by a well-defined *epithalamic sulcus*. In subsequent months growth of the thalamus rapidly overtakes that of the epithalamus; the intervening sulcus is obliterated. Thus, finally, structures of epithalamic origin are topographically relatively diminutive; in recent years, however, there has occurred a burgeoning of interest in, and understanding of, their functional roles (p. 1423). The *pineal gland* arises as a hollow outgrowth from the roof plate, immediately adjoining the mesencephalon. Its distal part becomes solid by cellular proliferation, but its proximal stalk remains hollow, containing the pineal recess of the third ventricle. In many reptiles the pineal outgrowth is double. The anterior outgrowth (*parapineal organ*) develops into the pineal or parietal eye (p. 1889) while the posterior outgrowth is glandular in character. It is the **posterior** outgrowth which is homologous with the pineal gland in man. The anterior outgrowth also develops in the human embryo but soon disappears entirely.

The *posterior commissure* is formed by fibres which invade the caudal wall of the pineal recess from both sides.

The *nucleus habenulae*, which is the most important constituent of

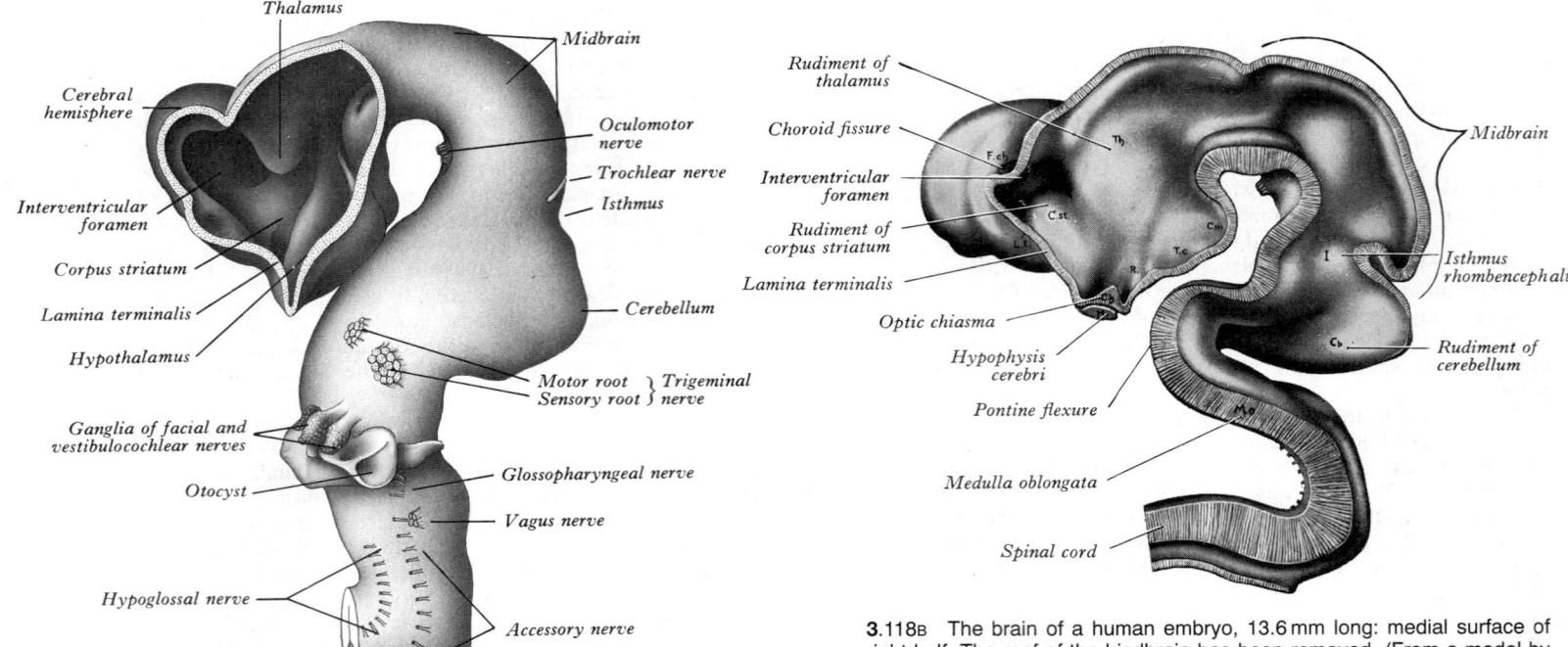

3.118A   The brain of a human embryo, about 10.2 mm long. (From a model by His.)

3.118B   The brain of a human embryo, 13.6 mm long: medial surface of right half. The roof of the hindbrain has been removed. (From a model by His.)

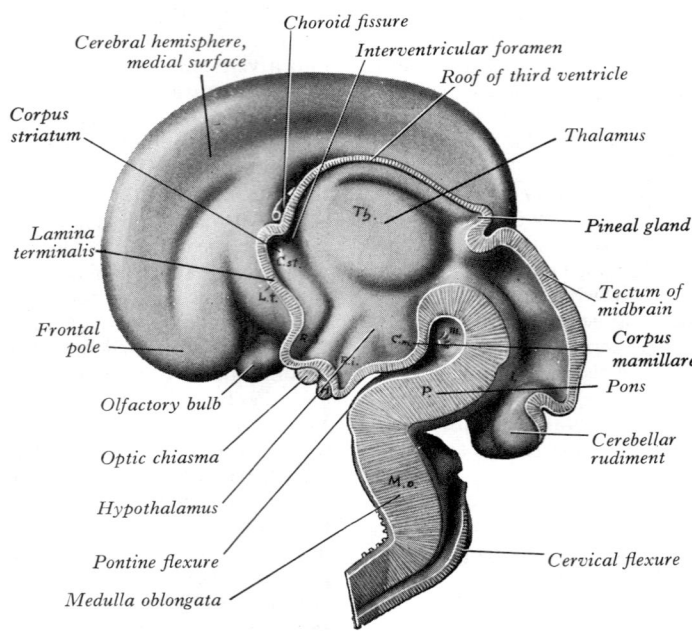

3.118C   Medial surface of the right half of the brain of a human fetus, about 3 months old.

the *trigonum habenulae,* is developed in the lateral wall of the diencephalon and is at first in close relationship with the geniculate bodies, from which it becomes separated by the dorsal growth of the thalamus. The *habenular commissure* develops in the cranial wall of the pineal recess.

The roof plate of the diencephalon, rostral to the pineal gland (and continuing over the median telencephalon) remains thin and epithelial in character and is subsequently invaginated by the choroid plexuses of the third ventricle. Before the development of the corpus callosum and the fornix it lies at the bottom of the longitudinal fissure; between and reaching the two cerebral hemispheres, it extends as far rostrally as the interventricular foramina and lamina terminalis. Here, and elsewhere, choroid plexuses develop by the close apposition of vascular pia mater and ependyma without intervening nervous tissue. With development, the vascular layer is infolded into the

ventricular cavity and develops a series of small villous projections, each covered by a cuboidal epithelium derived from the ependyma. The cuboidal cells carry numerous microvilli on their ventricular surfaces whilst basally their plasma membrane becomes complexly folded into the cell. The **early** choroid plexuses secrete a protein-rich cerebrospinal fluid into the ventricular system which may provide a nutritive medium for the primitive epithelial neural tissues. With increasing vascularity of the latter, however, the histochemical reactions of the cuboidal cells and the character of the fluid change to the adult type (Klosovskii 1963). It should also be noted that, in addition to choroid plexus formation, the remaining lining of the third ventricle does **not** simply form generalized ependymal cells. Many regions become highly specialized, developing concentrations of tanycytes or other modified cells, e.g. those of the *subfornical organ,* the *organum vasculosum (intercolumnar tubercle)* of the lamina

246

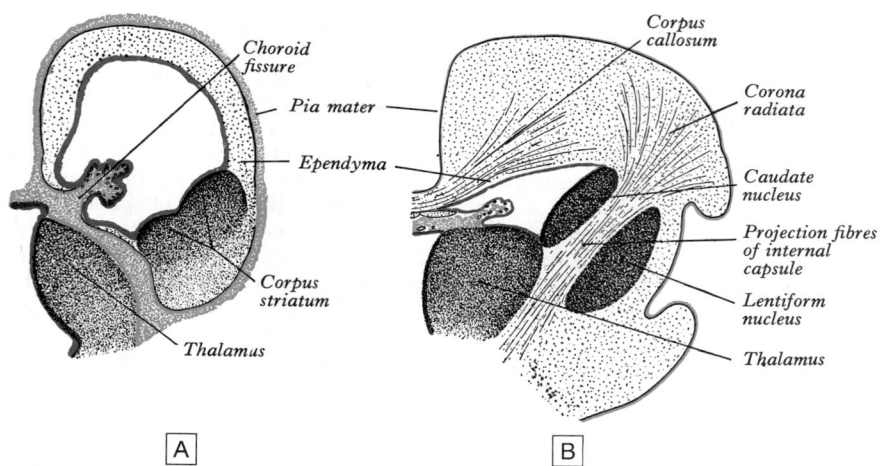

3.119 Diagrams illustrating transverse sections across the developing thalamus and cerebral hemisphere. Note that at the choroid fissure the vascular pia mater (blue) meets the ependyma (red) to form a choroid plexus. In (A) the lateral aspect of the thalamus is separated from the medial aspect of the hemisphere by an interval containing vascular mesenchyme.

In (B) this interval has disappeared; the expanded upper surface of the thalamus is covered by the ependyma of the lateral ventricle, and the approximation of the thalamus and the corpus striatum has provided a pathway for the projection fibres of the internal capsule. (Guthrie & Lumsden 1994 Neuroprotocols 4 Academic Press with permission.)

terminalis, the *subcommissural organ* and those lining the *pineal*, *suprapineal*, and *infundibular recesses* (Knigge et al 1975, Collins and Woollam 1981), collectively termed the *circumventricular organs*.

In addition to its subsulcal lateral walls, the floor of the pars ventralis diencephali takes part in the formation of the *hypothalamus*, including the mamillary bodies, the tuber cinereum and infundibulum of the hypophysis.

The *mamillary bodies* arise as a single thickening, which becomes divided by a median furrow during the third month. Anterior to them the *tuber cinereum* develops as a cellular proliferation which extends forwards as far as the infundibulum. In front of the tuber cinereum the floor of the diencephalon gives origin to a wide-mouthed diverticulum, which grows towards the stomodeal roof and comes into contact with the posterior aspect of a dorsally directed ingrowth from the stomodeum (Rathke's pouch, p. 257). These two diverticula together form the *hypophysis cerebri* (**3.128**). In the base of the neural outgrowth an extension of the third ventricle persists as the *infundibular recess*. The remaining caudolateral walls and floor of the ventral diencephalon are an extension of the midbrain tegmentum—the *subthalamus*. This forms the rostral limits of the red nucleus and substantia nigra, numerous reticular nuclei and a wealth of interweaving nerve fibre bundles, ascending, descending and oblique, with many origins and destinations.

The optic vesicles, which are described with the development of the eye (p. 259), are derived from the lateral wall of the prosencephalon before the telencephalon can be identified. They are usually regarded as derivatives of the diencephalon and the optic chiasma is often regarded as the boundary between diencephalon and telencephalon.

Telencephalon

The telencephalon (end-brain) consists of two lateral diverticula connected by a median region (the *telencephalon impar*). From the impar develops the anterior part of the cavity of the third ventricle, closed below and in front by the *lamina terminalis*. The lateral diverticula are outpouchings of the lateral walls of the telencephalon, which may correspond to the alar laminae, although this is uncertain; the cavities are the future lateral ventricles, and their walls the primordial nervous tissue of the *cerebral hemispheres*. The roof plate of the median part of the telencephalon remains thin and is, as noted, continuous behind with the roof plate of the diencephalon. In the floor plate and lateral walls of the prosencephalon, **ventral** to the primitive interventricular foramina, the **anterior** parts of the hypothalamus are developed; these include the optic chiasma, optic recess and related nuclei. The chiasma is formed by the meeting and partial decussation of the optic nerves in the ventral part of the lamina terminalis, and from it the optic tracts subsequently grow backwards to end in the diencephalon and midbrain.

Cerebral hemispheres

The cerebral hemispheres arise as diverticula of the lateral walls of the telencephalon, with which they remain in continuity around the margins of the initially relatively large interventricular foramina, except caudally, where they are continuous with the anterior part of the lateral wall of the diencephalon (**3.119**A, B); as growth proceeds the hemisphere enlarges forwards, upwards and backwards and acquires an oval outline, with medial and superolateral walls and a floor. As a result the medial surfaces approach, but are separated from each other by, a vascularized mesenchyme and pia mater that fills the *median longitudinal fissure*. At this stage the floor of the fissure is the epithelial roof plate of the telencephalon, which is directly continuous caudally with the epithelial roof plate of the diencephalon (**3.119**), as already stated above.

At the early oval stage of hemispheric development, regional names are given in accordance with their future principal derivatives. The rostromedial and ventral *floor* becomes linked with the forming olfactory apparatus and may be termed the primitive *olfactory lobe* (see below and p. 1317). The floor (ventral wall, or base) of the larger remainder of the hemisphere forms the anlage of the primitive corpus striatum and amygdaloid complex: hence this, including its associated rim of lateral and medial walls, is the *striate part of the hemisphere*. The rest of the hemisphere, the largest in surface area but initially possessing rather thin walls, medial, lateral, dorsal and caudal, is thus the *suprastriate part of the hemisphere*. The whole of the latter (except the interventricular foramen and its extension, the choroidal fissure) together with the superficial (subpial) zone of the striate part are the areas where histogenesis of named apparent variants of cerebral cortex (or pallium) occur. Further details, and comments on their plethora of terminologies and (often unsatisfactory) classifications, are furnished below.

The rostral end of the oval hemisphere becomes the definitive *frontal pole* but, as the hemisphere expands, its **original** posterior pole moves relatively in a caudoventral and lateral direction, curving thence towards the orbit in association with the growth of the caudate nucleus and numerous other structures to form the definitive *temporal pole*, and a **new** posterior part becomes evident which persists as the definitive *occipital* pole of the mature brain. The great expansion of the cerebral hemispheres is characteristic of mammals and especially of man, and in their subsequent growth they overlap, successively, the diencephalon and the mesencephalon and then meet the rostral surface of the cerebellum; the temporal lobes embrace the flanks of the brainstem.

The early diverticulum or anlage of the cerebral hemisphere contains initially a simple spheroidal *lateral ventricle* which is continuous with the third ventricle via the interventricular foramen, the rim of the latter being the site of the original evagination. With expansion and the assumption of an oval outline by the hemisphere, the ventricle becomes firstly roughly ellipsoid and then a curved cylinder, convex dorsally. The ends of the cylinder expand towards (but do not reach) the frontal and (temporary) occipital poles—differentiating and thickening neural tissues separate the ventricular cavities and pial surfaces at all points, except along the line of the choroidal fissure (see below). Pronounced changes in ventricular form accompany the emergence of a temporal pole; the original caudal end of the curved cylinder expands within its substance. This temporal extension passes ventrolaterally to encircle its side of the upper brainstem (cf. choroidal fissure below). Finally, from the root of the temporal extension another may develop in the substance of the definitive occipital pole, passing caudomedially; this is quite variable in size, often asymmetrical on the two sides; one or both may be absent. Although a continuous system of cavities, specific parts of the lateral ventricle are now given regional names: the *central part* (*body*) extends from the interventricular foramen to the level of the posterior edge (splenium) of the corpus callosum. From the body three *cornua* (*horns*) diverge—**anterior** towards the frontal pole, **posterior** towards the occipital pole and **inferior** towards the temporal pole.

It may be noted that at these early stages of hemispheric development the term pole is preferred, in most instances, to lobe; the latter are defined by specific surface topographical features which will appear over several months, and differential growth patterns persist for a considerable period.

About the fifth week a longitudinal groove appears in the anteromedial part of the floor of each ventricle. This groove deepens and forms a hollow diverticulum continuous with the hemisphere by a short stalk. The diverticulum becomes connected on its ventral or inferior surface to the *olfactory placode* (see p. 278), the cells of which give rise to the afferent axons of its sensory cells. These terminate in the walls of the diverticulum. As the head increases in size the diverticulum grows forwards and, subsequently losing its cavity, becomes converted into the solid *olfactory bulb*. The forward growth of the bulb is accompanied by elongation of its stalk, which forms the *olfactory tract*, and the part of the floor of the hemisphere to which the tract is attached constitutes the *piriform area* (see below). For comments on the accessory olfactory bulb see page 1317.

The pia mater which covers the epithelial roof of the third ventricle at this stage is itself covered with loosely arranged mesenchyme. In the meshes of this tissue numerous blood vessels develop and, as we have seen, on each side of the median plane these vessels subsequently invaginate the roof of the *third ventricle* to form its *choroid plexuses*. The lower part of the medial wall of the cerebral hemisphere, which immediately adjoins the epithelial roof of the interventricular foramen and the anterior extremity of the diencephalon, also remains epithelial, consisting of ependyma and pia mater, while elsewhere the walls of the hemispheres are thickening to form the *pallium*. The thin part of the medial wall of the hemisphere is invaginated by vascular tissue, continuous in front with the choroid plexus of the third ventricle and constituting the choroid plexus of the *lateral ventricle*. This invagination occurs along a line which arches upwards and backwards, parallel with and initially limited to the anterior and upper boundaries of the interventricular foramen; the curved indentation of the ventricular wall, where no nervous tissue develops between ependyma and pia mater, is termed the *choroid fissure* (**3.**118c, 119A, B). The subsequent assumption of the complex, but exquisite, definitive form of the choroidal fissure naturally depends on related growth patterns in neighbouring structures: some are particularly relevant. These are the relatively slow growth of the interventricular foramen, the secondary 'fusion' between the lateral diencephalon and medial hemisphere walls, the encompassing of the upper brainstem by the forward growth of the temporal lobe and its pole towards the apex of the orbit and the massive expansion of two great commissures of the cerebrum—the fornix and corpus callosum. (Many of these features are detailed further below and in the Neurology section.) Nevertheless, the choroidal fissure is now clearly a caudal extension of the (much reduced) interventricular foramen, which arches above the thalamus and in this region is only a few millimetres from the median plane. Near the caudal end of the thalamus it diverges ventrolaterally, its curve reaching and continuing in the medial wall of the temporal lobe over much of its length (i.e. to the tip of the inferior horn of the lateral ventricle). The upper

part of the arch is overhung by the corpus callosum and, throughout its convexity, is bordered by the fornix and its derivatives (see below). Thus, the extensive and helicoid disposition of the choroid plexus of the lateral ventricle is explained.

At first growth proceeds more actively in the floor and the adjoining part of the lateral wall of the developing hemisphere, and elevations formed by the rudimentary *corpus striatum* (**3.**118A) encroach on the cavity of the lateral ventricle (Cooper 1946). The head of the *caudate nucleus* appears as three successive parts, medial, lateral and intermediate, which produce elevations in the floor of the lateral ventricle. Caudally these merge to form the *tail* of the caudate nucleus and the *amygdaloid complex*. From the outset the latter are close to the temporal pole of the hemisphere and, when the occipital pole grows backwards and the general enlargement of the hemisphere carries the temporal pole downwards and forwards, the tail is continued from the *floor* of the central part (*body*) of the ventricle curving into the *roof* of its temporal extension, the future *inferior horn*, and the amygdaloid complex encapsulates its tip. Anteriorly the *head* of the caudate nucleus extends forwards to the floor of the interventricular foramen, where it is separated from the developing anterior end of the thalamus by a groove; later, the head expands in the floor of the anterior horn of the lateral ventricle. The *lentiform nucleus* develops from two laminae of cells, medial and lateral, which are continuous with both the medial and lateral parts of the caudate nucleus. The *internal capsule* appears first in the medial lamina and extends laterally through the outer lamina to the cortex. It divides the laminae into two, the internal parts joining the caudate nucleus and the external parts forming the lentiform nucleus. In the latter, which consists of two main parts, the remaining medial lamina cells give rise predominantly to the (medially placed) *globus pallidus* and the lateral to the (laterally placed) *putamen*. Subsequently the putamen expands concurrently with the intermediate part of the caudate nucleus (Hewitt 1958, 1961).

As the hemisphere enlarges, the caudal part of its medial surface overlaps and hides the lateral surface of the diencephalon (thalamic part), being separated from it by a narrow cleft occupied by vascular connective tissue. At this stage (about the end of the second month) a transverse section made caudal to the interventricular foramen passes from the third ventricular cavity successively through:

- the developing thalamus
- the narrow cleft just mentioned
- the thin medial wall of the hemisphere
- the cavity of the lateral ventricle, with the corpus striatum in its floor and lateral wall (**3.**119A).

As the thalamus increases in extent it acquires a superior in addition to medial and lateral surfaces, and the lateral part of its superior surface fuses with the thin medial wall of the hemisphere so that, finally, this part of the thalamus is covered with the ependyma of the lateral ventricle immediately ventral to the choroid fissure (**3.**119B). As a result the corpus striatum is approximated to the thalamus and separated from it only by a deep groove which becomes obliterated by increased growth along the line of contact. The lateral aspect of the thalamus is now in continuity with the medial aspect of the corpus striatum so that a secondary union between the diencephalon and the telencephalon is effected over a wide area, providing a route for the subsequent passage of projection fibres to and from the cortex.

Throughout the brainstem, as in the spinal cord, the *migration* and differentiation of neural progenitors to form nuclei is either minimal or limited, their progeny remaining immediately extra-ependymal or, partially displaced towards the pial exterior, being arrested deeply embedded in the myelinated fibre 'white matter' of the region. As noted, however, the 'roof-brain' of part of the fore-, mid- and hindbrains develops following an additional, fundamental pattern which results in a superficial layer of *grey matter*. The latter consists of neuronal somata, dendrites, the terminations of incoming (afferent) axons, the stems of (or the whole of) efferent axons, geometrically and functionally apposite glial cells and vasculature. Subsequent differentiation results in a highly organized subpial surface coat of grey matter termed the *cortex* (Latin: bark, e.g. of a tree) or *pallium* (Latin: pall, mantle or cloak). Pallium is used preferentially by neuroembryologists and some comparative zoologists; however, cortex is employed much more widely and will be used here. Neither term is used in the case of the mesencephalic tectum. In the cerebral hemisphere the superficial subpial regions of its wall, both striate and suprastriate (other than central areas of its medial wall, where secondary fusion with the diencephalon occurs and is encompassed by the lamina terminalis, interventricular foramen and curve of the choroid fissure), become invaded by migrating neuroblasts to form an elementary cerebral cortex. The cortical area which borders the lamina terminalis, the interventricular foramen, the convexity of the choroid fissure and continues into the diverging roots of the olfactory tract, has been simply termed the *limbic lobe* (or bordering lobe), together with its numerous subdivisions and connections (p. 1115 et seq), the *limbic system*. Its cortical derivatives possessing, some regard, a relatively elementary structure, have been termed the *allocortex* (other cortex).

The limbic lobe is the first part of the cortex to initiate differentiation (see below) and at first it forms a continuous, almost circular strip on the medial and inferior aspects of the hemisphere. Below and in front, where the stalk of the olfactory tract is attached, it constitutes a part of the *piriform area* (*palaeocortex* or *palaeopallium*). The portion outside the curve of the choroid fissure (3.120) constitutes the *hippocampal formation* (archaeocortex or *archaeopallium*). In this region the neural progenitors of the developing cortex proliferate and migrate (see below), and the wall of the hemisphere thickens and produces an elevation which projects into the medial side of the ventricle. This elevation is the *hippocampus* (Humphrey 1964, 1967). It appears first on the medial wall of the hemisphere in the area above and in front of the lamina terminalis (*paraterminal area*) and gradually extends backwards, curving into the region of the temporal pole where it adjoins the piriform area. The marginal zone in the neighbourhood of the hippocampus is invaded by neuroblasts forming the *dentate gyrus*. Both extend from the paraterminal area (see precommissural septum and prehippocampal rudiment) backwards above the choroid fissure and follow its curve downwards and forwards towards the temporal pole, where they continue into the piriform area. A shallow surface depression (which has been termed the *hippocampal sulcus*) grooves the medial surface of the hemisphere throughout the hippocampal formation.

The efferent fibres from the cells of the hippocampus collect along its medial edge and run forwards immediately above the choroid fissure. Anteriorly they turn ventrally and enter the lateral part of the lamina terminals to gain the hypothalamus, where they end in and around the mamillary body and neighbouring nuclei. These efferent hippocampal fibres form the *fimbria hippocampi* and the *fornix*. For the sources of afferent fibres to the hippocampus, hippocampal commissures and multiple subdivisions of the fornix.

The terms archaeocortex and palaeocortex as the two principal divisions of the *allocortex* focus on the acceptance by earlier neuroanatomists of the phylogenetically ancient nature of these regions. The remainder of the hemispheric surface, particularly in mammals, with a relatively vast expansion in primates, is, at least at some stage

in its history, a six-layered cortex, termed the *isocortex* (equal cortex) or *neocortex* (young cortex). Isocortex seems less appropriate, however, as all subregions showed fine structural differences. Furthermore, all three varieties of cortex are present simultaneously in an initial form in extant reptilia. Their relationship to piscine or amphibian ancestry remains controversial.

Development of the commissures

The development of the commissures effects a very profound alteration on the medial wall of the hemisphere. At the time of their appearance the two hemispheres are connected to each other by the median part of the telencephalon. The roof plate of this area remains epithelial, whilst its floor becomes invaded by the decussating fibres of the optic nerves and developing hypothalamic nuclei. These two routes are thus not available for the passage of commissural fibres passing from hemisphere to hemisphere across the median plane, and these fibres therefore pass through the anterior wall of the interventricular foramen, i.e. the lamina terminalis. The first com-

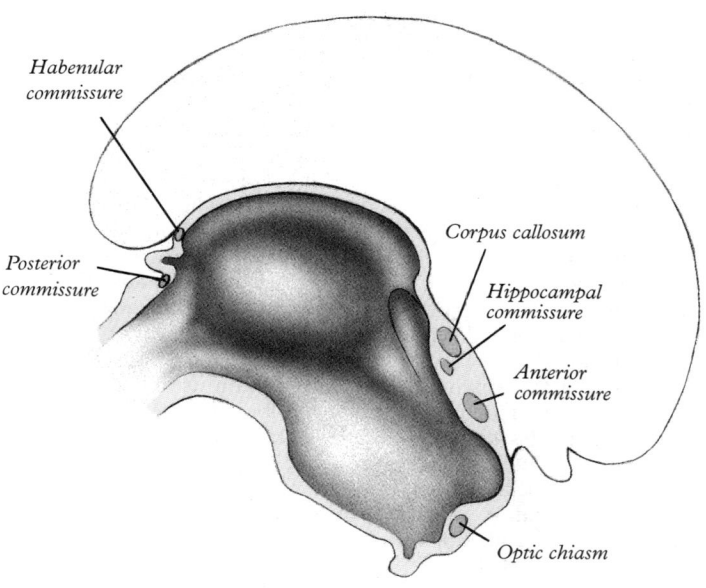

A   10 weeks

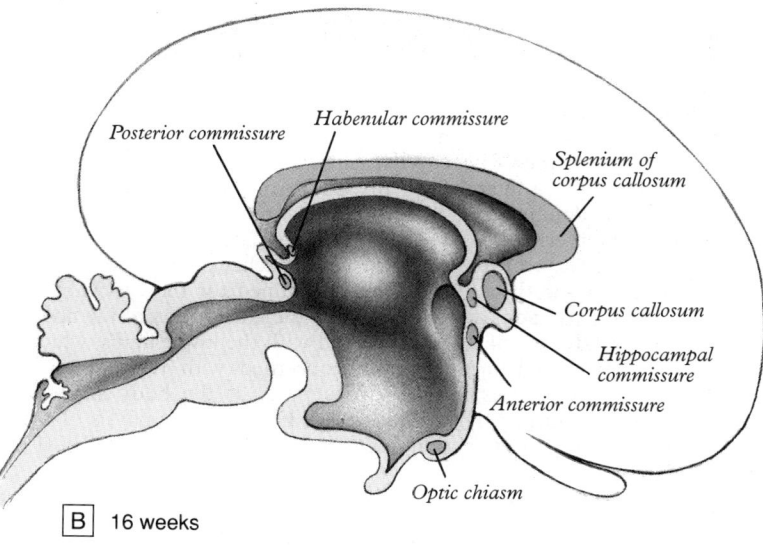

B   16 weeks

3.121 Formation of the commissures. The telencephalon gives rise to commissural tracts that integrate the activities of the left and right cerebral hemispheres. These include the anterior and hippocampal commissures and the corpus callosum. The small posterior and habenular commissures arise from the epithalamus. (From Larsen with permission.)

3.120 The brain of a human fetus, 4 months old: medial aspect of left half.

missures to develop are those associated with the palaeocortex and archaeocortex. Fibres of the olfactory tracts cross in the ventral or lower part of the lamina terminalis and, together with fibres from the piriform and prepiriform areas and the amygdaloid bodies, form the *anterior part* of the *anterior commissure*. In addition the two hippocampi become interconnected by transverse fibres which cross from fornix to fornix in the upper part of the lamina terminalis as the *commissure of the fornix*. Various other decussating fibre bundles (known as the *supraoptic commissures*, although they are not true commissures) develop in the lamina terminalis immediately dorsal to the optic chiasma, between it and the anterior commissure.

The commissures of the neocortex develop later and follow the pathways already established by the commissures of the limbic system. Fibres from the tentorial surface of the hemisphere join the anterior commissure and constitute its larger *posterior part*. All the other commissural fibres of the neocortex associate themselves closely with the commissure of the fornix and lie on its dorsal surface. These fibres increase enormously in number and the bundle rapidly outgrows its neighbours to form the corpus callosum (3.120, 121).

The *corpus callosum* originates as a thick mass connecting the two cerebral hemispheres around and above the anterior commissure. (This site has been called the precommissural area, but this use has been rejected here because of increasing use of the adjective precommissural to denote the position of parts of the limbic lobe— prehippocampal rudiment, septal areas and nuclei, strands of the fornix in relation to the anterior commissure of the mature brain.) The upper end of this neocortical commissural area extends backwards to form the trunk of the corpus callosum. The *rostrum* of the corpus callosum develops later and separates some of the rostral end of the limbic area from the remainder of the cerebral hemisphere. Further backward growth of the trunk of the corpus callosum then results in the entrapped part of the limbic area becoming stretched out to form the bilateral septum pellucidum (Hewitt 1962). As the corpus callosum grows backwards it extends above the choroid fissure, carrying the commissure of the fornix on its under surface. In this way a new floor is formed for the longitudinal fissure, and additional structures come to lie above the epithelial roof of the third ventricle. In its backward growth the corpus callosum invades the area hitherto occupied by the **upper** part of the archaeocortical hippocampal formation, and the corresponding parts of the dentate gyrus (3.120, 121) and hippocampus are reduced to vestiges—the *indusium griseum* and the *longitudinal striae*. However, the *postero-inferior* (temporal) archaeocortical regions of both dentate gyrus and hippocampus persist and **enlarge** because, with the forward growth of the temporal lobes, the brainstem presents a complete barrier to further extension of the corpus callosum in the median plane.

Neocortex

The growth of the *neocortex* and its enormous expansion are associated with the initial appearance of projection fibres (corticofugal and corticopetal) during the latter part of the third month. These fibres follow the pathway provided by the apposition of the lateral aspect of the thalamus with the medial aspect of the corpus striatum, and, as they do so, they (the *internal capsule*) divide the latter, almost completely, into a lateral part, the lentiform nucleus, and a medial part, the caudate nucleus; these two nuclei remain confluent only in their antero-inferior regions. The corticospinal tracts begin to develop in the ninth week of fetal life and have reached their caudal limits by the twenty-ninth week. The fibres destined for the cervical and upper thoracic regions and implicated in the innervation of the upper limb are in advance of those concerned with the lower limbs, which, in turn, are in advance of those concerned with the face. The appearance of reflexes in these three parts of the body shows a comparable sequence (Humphrey 1960). For further analysis of the development of the projection fibres and corpus striatum see Hewitt (1961, 1962).

The preceding emphasis on corticospinal projection fibres is a reflection of the limited information available to the earlier neuro-anatomists. It should be emphasized, however, that the majority of subcortical nuclear masses receive terminals from descending fibres of cortical origin. Furthermore, the foregoing are joined by thalamocortical, hypothalamocortical and other afferent ascending bundles, the whole complex constituting the internal capsule that divides the early corpus striatum. It should also be noted that the

internal capsular fibres pass **lateral** to the head and body of the caudate nucleus, the anterior cornu and central part of the lateral ventricle, the rostroventral extensions and body of the fornix, the dorsal thalamus and dorsal choroidal fissure; at similar levels they pass **medial** to the lentiform nucleus. With temporal lobe formation, the capsular fibres also lie medial to the inferior cornu of the lateral ventricle which has the amygdaloid complex capping its tip, the tail of the caudate nucleus in its roof, the hippocampus, dentate gyrus and fimbria of fornix in its floor, and temporal extension of the choroidal fissure in its medial wall.

At the end of the third month the superolateral surface of the cerebral hemisphere shows a slight depression anterosuperior to the temporal pole. This corresponds to the site of the corpus striatum in the floor and lateral wall of the ventricle, and its presence is due to the more rapid growth of the adjoining cortical regions. This *lateral cerebral fossa* gradually becomes overlapped and submerged, and is converted into the *lateral cerebral sulcus*; its floor becomes the *insula* (3.122A–G). The process, however, is not completed in its most anterior part until after birth. The presumptive neocortical areas that overlap the insula are termed the frontal, parietal and temporal *opercula*. The lentiform nucleus (lateral part of the corpus striatum) remains deep to and coextensive with the insula, the superficial zones of the latter transforming into varieties of cortex. Posteriorly the insula develops granular neocortex and an intermediate area forms agranular neocortex; finally the rostroventral area becomes similar to and continuous with the palaeocortex of the piriform area.

The growth changes in the temporal lobe which help to submerge the insula produce important changes in the olfactory and other neighbouring limbic areas. The olfactory tract, as it approaches the hemispheric floor, diverges into *lateral*, *medial* and (variable) *intermediate striae*. The medial stria is clothed with a thin archaeo-cortical *medial olfactory gyrus*: this curves up into further archaeo-cortical areas anterior to the lamina terminalis (paraterminal gyrus, prehippocampal rudiment, parolfactory gyrus, septal nuclei) and these continue into the indusium griseum. The lateral stria, clothed by the *lateral olfactory gyrus*, and, when present, the intermediate stria, terminate in the rostral parts of the *piriform area*. In brief, this includes the olfactory trigone and tubercle, anterior perforated substance and the uncus (hook) and entorhinal area of the anterior part of the future parahippocampal gyrus. Its lateral limit is indicated by the *rhinal sulcus*. (For details of the numerous subdivisions and putative interconnections of these areas, see p. 1115 et seq and 8.229– 250.)The forward growth of the temporal pole and the general expansion of the neopallium cause the lateral olfactory gyrus to bend laterally, the summit of the convexity lying at the antero-inferior corner of the developing insula (3.122A–G). During the fourth and fifth months much of the piriform area becomes submerged by the adjoining neopallium and in the adult only a part of it remains visible on the inferior aspect of the cerebrum.

Apart from the shallow hippocampal sulcus and the lateral cerebral fossa the surfaces of the hemisphere remain smooth and uninterrupted until early in the fourth month (3.122A–G). The parieto-occipital sulcus also appears about that time on the **medial** aspect of the hemisphere and its appearance seems associated with the increase in the splenial fibres of the corpus callosum. Over the same period the posterior part of the *calcarine sulcus* appears as a shallow groove extending forwards from a region near the occipital pole. It is a true infolding of the cortex in the long axis of the *striate area*, producing an elevation, the *calcar avis*, on the medial wall of the posterior horn of the ventricle.

During the fifth month the *sulcus cinguli* appears on the medial aspect of the hemisphere, but not until the sixth month do sulci appear on the inferior and superolateral aspects. The *central*, *precentral* and *postcentral sulci* appear, each in two parts, upper and lower, which usually coalesce shortly afterwards although they may remain discontinuous. The *superior* and *inferior frontal*, the *intra-parietal*, *occipital*, *superior* and *inferior temporal*, the *occipitotemporal*, *collateral* and *rhinal sulci* make their appearance during the same period, and by the end of the eighth month all the important sulci can be recognized (3.122A–G).

Histogenesis of the cortex

The histogenesis of the cortical (pallial) wall of the cerebral hemi-

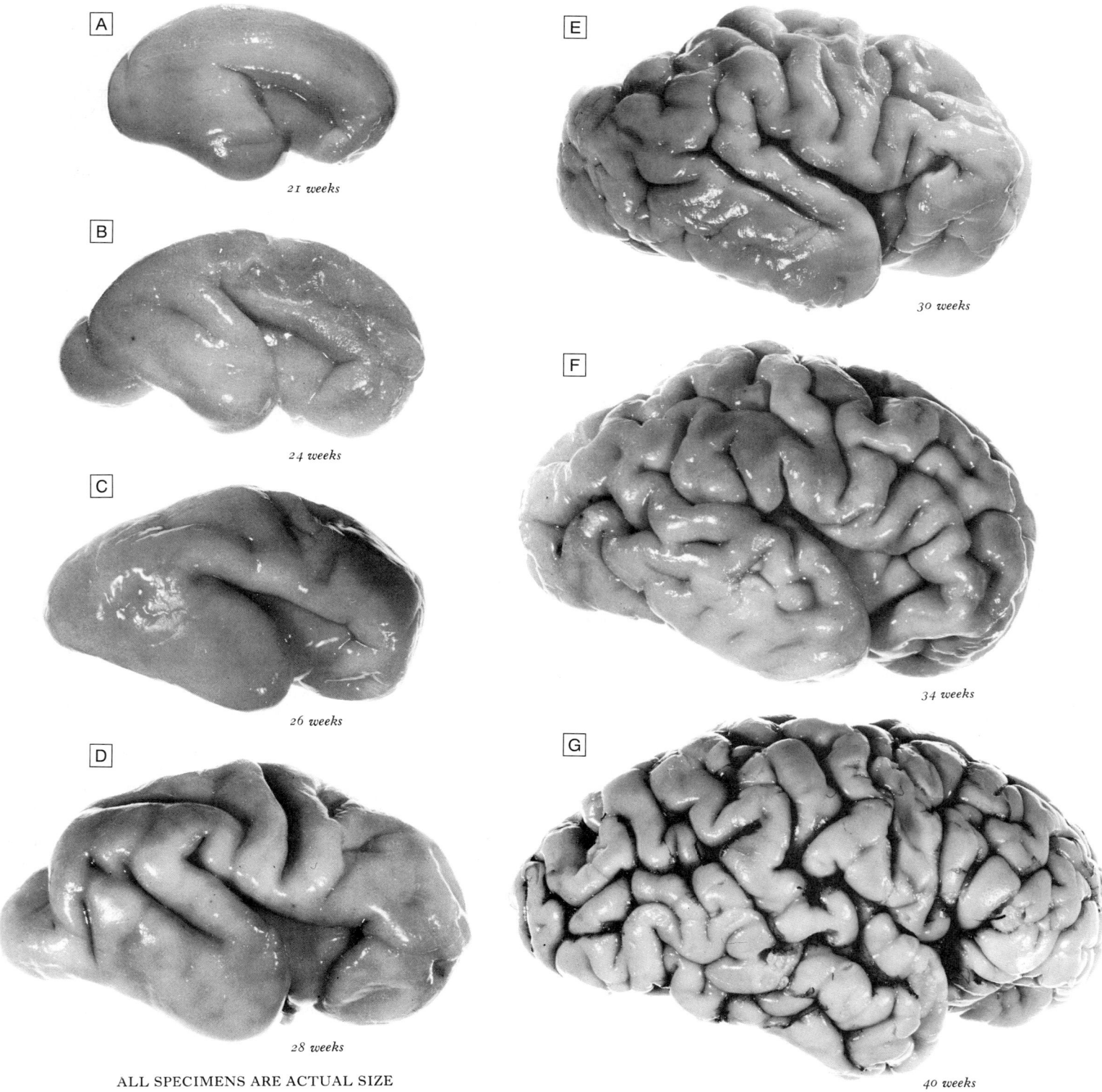

A 21 weeks

B 24 weeks

C 26 weeks

D 28 weeks

ALL SPECIMENS ARE ACTUAL SIZE

E 30 weeks

F 34 weeks

G 40 weeks

3.122 Series showing the superolateral surfaces of human fetal cerebral hemispheres at the ages indicated, demonstrating the changes in size, profile and the emerging pattern of cerebral sulci with increasing maturation. Note the changing prominence and relative positions of the frontal, occipital and particularly the temporal pole of the hemisphere. At the earliest stage (A) the lateral cerebral fossa is already obvious—its floor covers the developing corpus striatum in the depths of the hemisphere and progressively matures into the cortex of the insula. The fossa is bounded by overgrowing cortical regions, the frontal, temporal and parietal opercula, which gradually con-verge to bury the insula; their approximation forms the lateral cerebral sulcus. By the sixth month the central, pre- and postcentral, superior temporal, intraparietal and parieto-occipital sulci are all clearly visible. In the sub-sequent stages shown all the remaining principal and subsidiary sulci rapidly appear and by 40 weeks all the features which characterize the adult hemisphere in terms of surface topography are already present in miniature. (Photographs supplied by Dr Sabina Strick of the Maudsley Hospital, London.)

sphere has generated an impressive literature since the early 1930s. Nevertheless, because of the immense complexity, multiplicity of cell types and structural heterogeneity in different locations, descriptive and experimental analyses are less well understood and documented than those appertaining to the cerebellum, with its regular, geo-metrically ordered microstructure (p. 243). Only the briefest review of some basic principles, together with a few introductory key references, can be encompassed in this volume and the interested

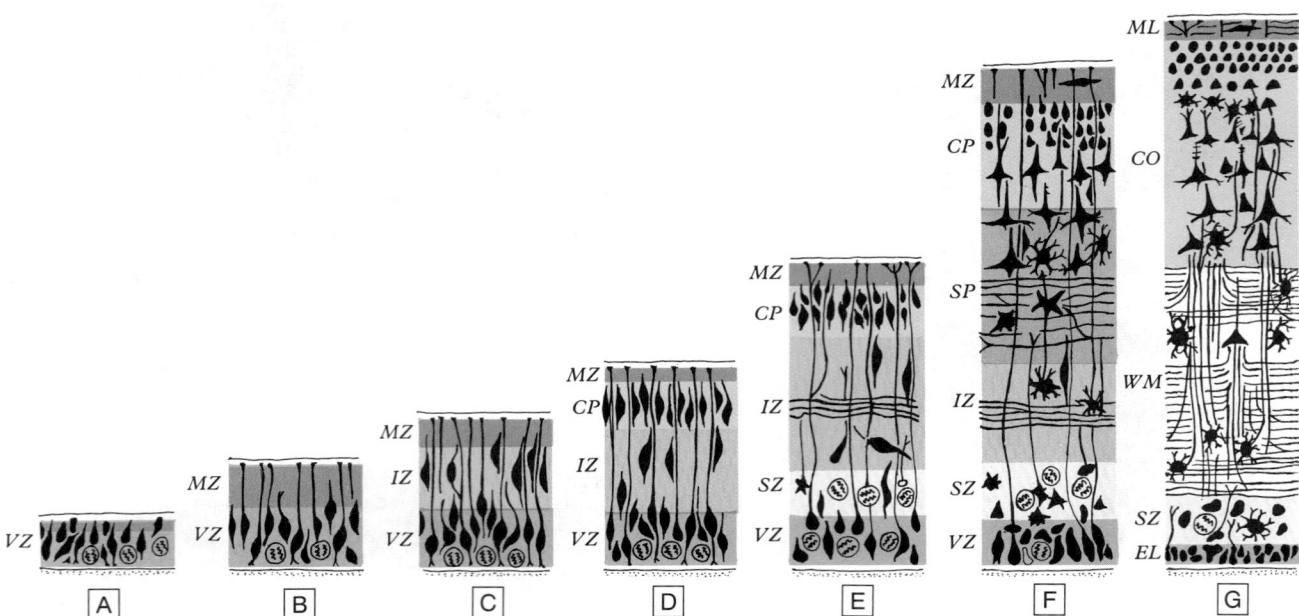

3.123 Formalized diagram of the laminar development of cerebral neo-cortex. The original proposals of the Boulder Committee (1970) have been revised, in the light of subsequent research, by Rakic (1982), with further additions and modifications in preparation for the present volume. See text for further comment. VZ = ventricular zone; MZ = marginal zone; IZ = intermediate zone (mantle zone); CP = cortical plate; SZ = subventricular zone; SP = subplate zone; CO = definitive neocortex; WM = white matter; EL = ependymal layer; ML = molecular layer.

reader will find it apposite to constantly cross-refer to the sections devoted to mature neuronal and cortical architecture (Section 6).

The wall of the earliest cerebral hemisphere, as elsewhere in the neural tube, consists of a pseudostratified epithelium, its cells exhibiting interkinetic migration as they proliferate to form clones of, it was assumed, as yet uncommitted germinal cells. The columnar cells elongate and (following the initial nomenclature proposed by the Boulder Committee, 1970 and **3**.123) their non-nucleated peripheral processes now constitute a *marginal zone*, whilst their nucleated, paraluminal and mitosing regions constitute the *ventricular zone*. Some of the mitotic progeny now leave the ventricular zone and migrate to occupy a *mantle (intermediate) zone*. This *proliferative phase* continues for a considerable period of fetal (and in some species postnatal) life but, as in the case of the cerebellar cortex, after a period groups of progenitor cells form, first, generations of definitive neurons and, later, glial cells which migrate to and mature in their final positions (see below for variant views). It must be appreciated, however, that these phases of proliferation, migration, differentiation and maturation are not precisely sequential for each cell variety but overlap each other in space and time.

The earliest migration of neuronal precursors from the ventricular and intermediate zones occurs radially until they approach, but do not reach, the pial surface, their somata becoming arranged as a transient *cortical plate*. Subsequently, proliferation wanes in the ventricular zone but for considerable periods persists in the immediately subjacent *subventricular zone*. From the pial surface inwards, therefore, there may now be defined the following zones: *marginal, cortical plate, subplate, mantle (intermediate), subventricular* and *ventricular*. Briefly, whilst the foregoing **terminology** is relatively recent it has for long been accepted that the marginal zone forms the outermost layer of the cerebral cortex, the neuroblasts of the cortical plate and subplate form the neurons of the remaining cortical laminae (the complexity, of course, varying in different locations and with further additions of neurons from the deeper zones), whilst the intermediate zone gradually transforms into the white matter of the hemisphere. Meanwhile other deep progenitor cells have been producing generations of glioblasts which also migrate into the more superficial layers. As proliferation wanes and finally ceases in the ventricular and subventricular zones their remaining cells differentiate into general or specialized ependymal cells, tanycytes or subependymal glial cells. Figure **3**.123A–F summarizes the modifications of the Boulder Committee's original proposals, suggested by Rakic (1982) in the light of more recent investigations.

As mentioned above, the phases of proliferation, neurogenesis and gliogenesis are by no means sequential as first envisaged but vary spatiotemporally with location and cell type. Further, the gliogenesis referred to was related to the (numerically largest) astrocyte and oligodendrocyte population of the mature tissue. However, as noted (p. 230), immunohistochemical studies of glial fibrillary acidic protein (GFAP) distribution showed a patterned array of GFAP-positive columnar cells in the earliest pseudostratified neuroepithelium of the neural tube including the walls of the rudimentary cerebral hemisphere. The positive cellular elements are interspersed with GFA-negative columnar cells, both undergoing interkinetic migration or proliferation. The GFAP-positive elements are presumptive glial cells which stretch radially across the full thickness of the wall of the telencephalon and provide contact guidance paths for the subsequent peripheral migration of neurons. Recent evidence suggests that these glial processes may be oriented in a manner that is far from strictly radial, and may instead branch extensively. The first groups of cells to migrate are destined for the deep cortical laminae, later groups passing through them to more superficial regions (see below). The subplate zone, a transient feature most prominent during midgestation, contains neurons surrounded by a dense neuropil: this subplate neuropil is the site of the most intense synaptogenesis in the cortex.

Thus, with growth, both radial and tangential, there occurs a great increase in cortical thickness and a vast increase in surface area.

Pioneering studies into cell migration in the developing mammalian *neocortex* were made by Tilney (1933), the technique available to him at this time being analysis of sections of Nissl stained tissue. Whilst it was clear that the subpial (marginal) zone formed the plexiform lamina (I), he considered that the remaining laminae stemmed from **three** quite distinct and **separate migrations** of neuroblasts up to the cortical plate. The first migration he thought differentiated into the external granular lamina (II) and the pyramidal lamina (III); the second migration forming the internal granular lamina IV; the third migration he held formed the ganglionic lamina V and the multiform lamina VI. On this view, therefore, the **outermost** layers were the **earliest** to be formed, with progressively deeper layers at successively later times.

The possibility of precisely the **reverse** sequence, progressing from *deep* to *superficial*, was first implied by the results of X-irradiation studies by Hicks et al (1959). Further irradiation studies (Berry & Eayrs 1966), and autoradiographic nuclear labelling studies (Berry & Rogers 1965; Berry 1974 and **3**.124) supported this contention. These

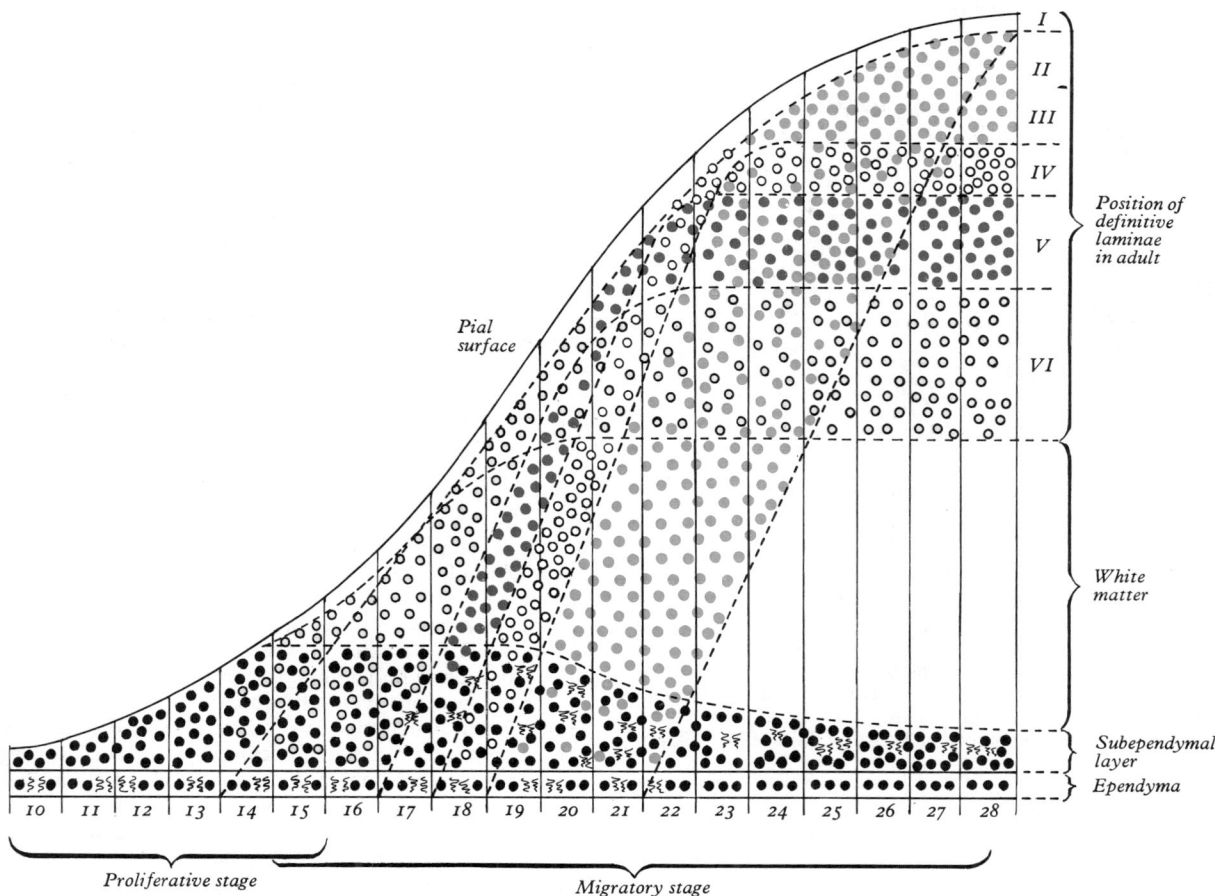

3.124 Schematic representation of the dynamics of neuroblast migrations during transformation of the early cranial neural tube to form the cerebral neocortex of the rat through days 10 to 28. Note the successive waves of migration.

Symbolic metaphase chromosomes = mitotic cells; full black discs = ventricular and subventricular zone neuroblasts; full yellow discs = infragranular neuroblasts destined for lamina VI; full magenta discs = infragranular neuroblasts destined for lamina V; open black circles = granular neuroblasts destined for lamina IV; full blue discs = supragranular neuroblasts destined for laminae III and II. (Redrawn and colour coded by permission from data provided by Professor M Berry (1974) of the Anatomy Department, Guy's Hospital Medical School, London.)

seminal investigations have, in the subsequent years, been amply confirmed in the rat (**3.125, 126**), mouse, opossum and golden hamster (Berry 1974, 1982; see also comments and bibliographies in: Smart 1982, 1983; Rakic & Goldman-Rakic 1982). Thus in these various mammals, apart from the pre-existing anlage of lamina I, the first laminae to be populated are VI and V, followed sequentially by laminae IV to II in 'inside–outside' fashion. Clearly, whilst the ontogenetic timings of migrations from these experimental sources are not directly appropriate to a volume on **human** anatomy, it is assumed from comparison of purely descriptive material that similar **patterns** of migration and elaboration occur in the human cortex. It should also be noted that, as yet only in the human cortex, a thin subpial lamina of densely staining cells, of unknown origin or destination, has been identified (Rabinowicz 1964, 1967; Brun 1965): they are not a prominent feature of cortical histogenesis but an analogy with the external germinal layer of the cerebellum has been suggested.

No attempt will be made here further to discuss neuroblast and glioblast differentiation, migration and maturation with the establishment of intercellular contacts. However, some general hypotheses may be mentioned, involving a comparison of ontogeny and phylogeny. Firstly, all parts of the neural tube, from the presumptive spinal cord to presumptive neocortex, pass through the stage of a pseudostratified epithelium and a proliferative phase, followed by differentiation of ventricular, mantle and marginal zones. Neuroblast migration, target cell contact and maturation (or, in some locations, *degeneration* and *cell death*), whilst **still confined** to the deeper reaches of the mantle zone, are the principal events in spinal cord development. Throughout the encephalon, however, the primary difference is the **continued migration** of neuroblasts and their

ultimate maturation far **beyond** the confines of the mantle zone, forming either nuclear masses, variously displaced from the ventricular and aqueductal channels, or, in the 'roof-brain' regions, reaching the subpial marginal zones forming, initially, a simple cortical plate of neuroblasts. The latter then differentiates into subzones, showing a tangential *laminar* organization, whilst in some

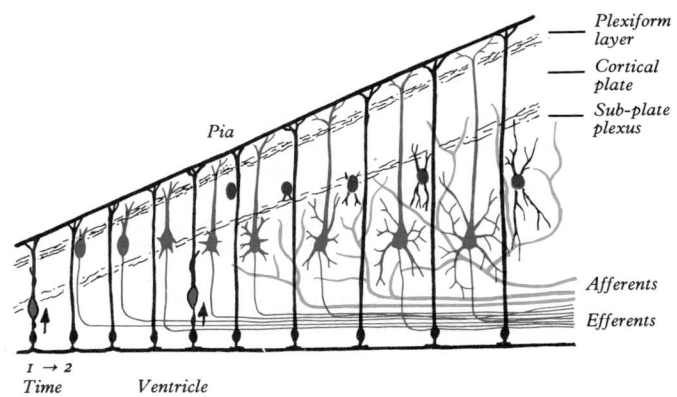

3.125 Diagram to show the manner of the initial stages of formation of apical and basal dendrites of pyramidal neurons, also of stellate neuron dendrites in the cortical plate. Note radial glial cells (black) extending from internal to external limiting membrane; these provide contact guidance paths for neuroblasts. 1. Migration of a presumptive pyramidal neuron (magenta). 2. Migration of a presumptive stellate neuron (purple). Time increments from left to right. (After Berry 1982.)

Superficial

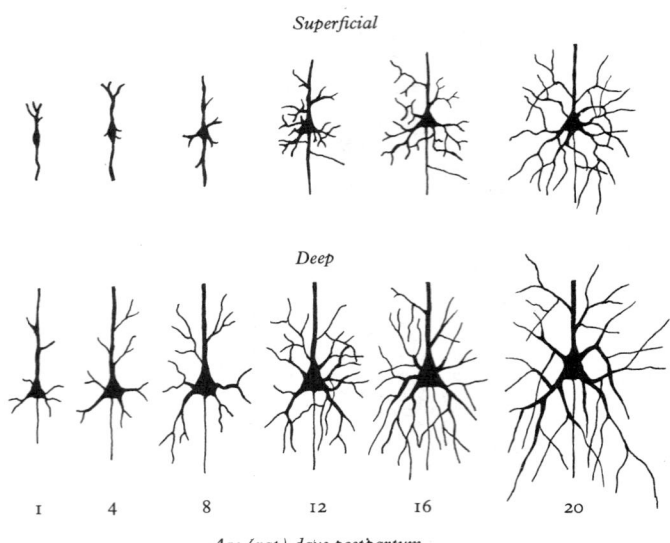

Deep

1   4   8   12   16   20

Age (rat) days postpartum

3.126   The temporal sequence of the initial appearance, growth and maturation, of basal and oblique dendrites by pyramidal neurons in the superficial and deep neocortical laminae of the rat. In the first postpartum week the deep neurons are well differentiated relative to the superficial neurons; the latter have only recently terminated their migration from the ventricular zone. Maturation of the superficial neurons relatively hastens in the second and third weeks, and by the twentieth postpartum day the degree of maturation of superficial and deep pyramidal neurons is the same. (After Berry 1982.)

locations there emerges a well-defined *columnar* (*modular*) radial organization. Such cortical dispositions are evident in the hemispheric forebrain, tectal midbrain and cerebellar hindbrain. In the pallial walls of the mammalian cerebral hemisphere, the phylogenetically **oldest** regions and the **first** to differentiate during ontogeny are those that **border** the interventricular foramen, and its extension the choroidal fissure, the lamina terminalis and piriform lobe. There exists an increasingly complex level of organization from three to six tangential laminae, passing from the dentate gyrus and cornu ammonis through the subiculum until the general neocortex is reached. (It may be noted that many investigators find the simple progression from three to six major laminae a gross oversimplification, and numerous subdivisions have been proposed, e.g. see cornu ammonis, p. 1124, and neocortex, p. 1141.) The **deepest** and phylogenetically oldest *tangential laminae* are the first to be populated by migrating progenitor cells, more superficial layers being added in sequence, their neuroblasts migrating **through** the older layers; the number of superadded laminae depends upon the location with respect to the choroidal fissure. These broad patterns have been demonstrated by nuclear labelling studies, not only in the neocortex but, with modifications, also in the dentate gyrus and hippocampus (see, e.g. Angevine 1975; Altman & Bayer 1975; Smart 1982).

Mechanisms of cortical development

Intense interest and research effort has been concentrated on elucidating the mechanisms of development of the mammalian cerebral cortex. In the 19th century two important ideas emerged. These were, firstly, that the cortex displayed *parcellation* into a number of functional areas, and secondly, that despite differences, these various areas were organized according to a common scheme. The science of phrenology claimed to allot functions to particular bumps on the surface of the brain, an idea that was proved broadly correct by surgical ablation experiments that showed loss of particular functions. Only later in the 19th century were attempts made to correlate histological with functional observations. Staining techniques made possible the visualization of differences in the sizes, shapes and distributions of cells in various cortical areas. Comparisons of the brains of various mammals also gave rise to the idea of functional and structural homology of cortical areas in different species. This may have led to the, perhaps, simplistic view that evolution simply adds new areas to an existing schema almost without modification, giving rise to the concepts of palaeocortex, archaeocortex and neo-

cortex. Nevertheless, it is clear that a common ground plan for the cerebral cortex exists among mammals, even if in humans extensive modifications have occurred. For example, the area given over to olfactory function is reduced, and association areas are massively expanded compared with the cortices of, say, rodents. In the present century, the mechanisms of development of the areal and the laminar organization of the cortex have been investigated, in addition to studies on the cellular mechanisms of neuronal migration within the cortex, and the developing pattern of connections. Only some of the central themes of the field of cortical development will be mentioned here.

The picture that is emerging of cortical development is one in which input plays a central role, and epigenetic interactions are crucial (see reviews: O'Leary 1989; McConnell 1992; Shatz 1992). Differences may exist in the timing and control of the emergence of the laminar and the areal organization. The neocortex, which constitutes 90% of the cortical area, goes through at least a period of its development when it contains 6 layers. Palaeocortex contains the olfactory areas, and the archaeocortex comprises the hippocampal formation. Within the 6-layered neocortex, each lamina has a distinct histology, function and connections. Layer 4 receives the major outputs from the thalamus, while layer 5 contains a high proportion of pyramidal neurons (large cells with prominent apical dendrites) with outputs to subcortical targets. Each of the layers are generated during a specific period of development in inside–outside fashion (p. 253). Rakic (1971) initially demonstrated the migration of neurons along radial glial processes, and the migratory behaviour of cortical neurons was subsequently investigated in vitro (Hatten 1990). Cortical neurons or cerebellar granule cells appear equally capable of migrating on hippocampal or cerebellar Bergmann glia, indicating conservation of migration mechanisms in different brain regions. Such neurons can migrate 10 times faster than in vivo, exhibiting close apposition and forming specialized junctions with the glial process and an active advancing process that extends and retracts. Antibodies to astrotactin may disrupt neuron–glia interactions (Edmondsen & Hatten 1987) and growth cones may secrete proteases that allow them to digest the extracellular matrix in their pathway (Krystosek & Seeds 1981).

Various lines of evidence point to the idea that the laminar fate of neurons is determined prior to migration. In the mutant *reeler* mouse, laminar formation is disrupted such that layers form in outside-in rather than inside-out array, yet axonal connections and neuronal properties appear normal (Caviness 1982). Laminar commitment was explored in heterochronic transplant experiments in the ferret. Since superficial cortical layers are generated later in development than deep ones, ventricular zone progenitor cells can be labelled and transplanted into host animals of a different age to investigate their laminar destination (McConnell & Kasnowski 1991). Cells from a brain in which layer 6 was being generated were labelled with 3H thymidine and transplanted into a brain in which layer 2/3 neurons were being generated. When the grafted cells had been allowed to complete their current round of division, they migrated to occupy laminae typical of their origin i.e. layer 6. When the cells were transplanted during S-phase of the cell cycle, however, so that they completed division in their new environment, the majority migrated into layer 2/3, appropriate to the host environment. Varying the time between labelling and injection showed that commitment to a particular cortical lamina occurs shortly after S-phase. This implies that cells acquire their laminar fate during certain phases of the cell cycle, depending on the environment, possibly since cells lie in the ventricular zone, adjacent to the forming white matter. Neurons of pre-existing laminae that have begun axonogenesis may provide a feedback on the forming cortical layers, providing a sort of developmental clock for histogenesis (reviewed in McConnell 1989, 1992).

In a plane perpendicular to its laminae, the cortex is divided up into a number of areas, displaying a hierarchy of organization. These include the primary areas, such as the motor cortex, the unimodal association areas concerned with the integration of information from one of the former, and multimodal association areas that integrate information from more than one modality. Besides these are the areas concerned with functions that are even less understood, such as the frontal lobes, concerned with goal-orientation responsibility and long-term planning. The primary areas are further divided up into somatotopic maps, while at the finest level, the cortex is known to consist of a series of 'columns', 50–500 μm wide. Within such a column, cells on a vertical traverse display common features of modality and electrophysiological responses to stimuli. Prominent examples of this organization are the ocular dominance columns of the visual cortex, with cells within a column all responding to visual stimuli received from one eye.

Controversy about the development of the prominent areal organization of the cortex may be seen as hinging on the dichotomy between the idea of a cortical 'protomap', and a gradually emerging pattern that may be largely dependent on afferent input. The former idea was originated by Rakic (1988). He proposed a mosaic of small groups of progenitor cells in the ventricular zone, each of which underwent radial migration to give rise to the segregated functional columns. This appealing idea could thus explain the whole hierarchy of cortical organization, and became predominant within the field, along with its implication that the migration of progenitor cells occurs without significant tangential movement.

Several lines of evidence now suggest that the radial unit idea of cortical development must be modified. This evidence comes from descriptive studies of the movement of progenitor cells in the developing cortex, and experimental approaches that involve transplantation of presumptive regions of cortex to other locations, after which their differentiation was examined. Experiments in which progenitor cells are marked using replication-incompetent retroviruses have been used extensively to investigate cell lineages and patterns of cell migration in the cerebral cortex. Retroviral particles in suspension are injected into the fetal ventricles, and infect progenitor cells close to the ventricular surface (Sanes et al 1986; Price et al 1987). Understanding patterns of cell migration in the cortex is essential for interpretation of these experiments, which has been controversial (see Guthrie 1992). Several progenitor cells are labelled in each brain, so that definition of their clonal progeny at a later time point must be based on the coherence and separation of clones from one another. In most studies, clones of cells are radially disposed, but there are often ambiguous outliers (Luskin et al 1988). Interpretation of such cells that may have migrated tangentially away from their point of origin is subjective. They may be considered as 'single cell clones', or as sibling cells that populate separate cortical radii (Walsh & Cepko 1988). In one study, the physical displacement of supposed clonal relatives implied that migration had occurred along the processes of cortical glia that may be obliquely-oriented (Austin & Cepko 1990).

An attempt to resolve the question of clonality was made by retroviral marking experiments in which progenitor cells were marked with unique genetic tags so that their progeny could be identified by molecular techniques, irrespective of migration paths (Walsh & Cepko 1992). Despite the necessity of sophisticated statistics to show the validity of this approach, this study yielded the interesting finding that cells of the same clone dispersed as much as 1.5 mm from each other (more than 10 times the diameter of a cortical column). Furthermore, clonal relatives could populate different functional areas such as motor, visual and somatosensory cortex, as well as several units (barrels) within the somatosensory cortex. Clones arising from retrovirally-marked precursors could also cross area boundaries in the hippocampus (Grove et al 1992). The presence of significant tangential dispersion in deep ventricular or subventricular zones has also been revealed by retroviral lineage experiments in which clonal dispersion was examined in the rat at various times after labelling (Walsh & Cepko 1993). The presence of an unsuspected degree of tangential movement was also described in cortical explant cultures, by directly injecting single cells with fluorescent dye and following them with time-lapse microscopy (Fishell et al 1993). While about 82% of cells moved in a radial or near radial direction, 13% of cells migrated rapidly in the tangential direction, often covering much larger distances than 500 μm, and making sharp right-angled turns from one pathway to the other. Interestingly, progenitor cells appeared to respect a line between the cortical and basal forebrain, raising the possibility of lineage restriction as a mechanism at least in the development of some forebrain regions. The weight of evidence now favours the idea of radial migration, with considerable tangential movement superimposed, at least of some cells. Nevertheless, some controversy exists, since in direct labelling experiments, cells could move tangentially 200 μm in 8 hours, whereas retroviral labelling

experiments showed tangential movement only occurring over the course of days. Analysis of transgenic mice in which a *lacZ* transgene is inserted into one of the X chromosomes may have helped to reconcile these views (Tan & Breen 1993). In hemizygous female embryos, the transgene is inactivated in half of the cells, leading to marking of 50% of cortical progenitors. In such animals, localization of the *lacZ* gene product showed the cortex to be patterned in alternating stripes of blue or white about 100–1000 μm wide. The banding pattern thus suggests population by groups of progenitor cells that have not dispersed widely in the tangential plane. However, in each of the stripes, about one-third of cells were the inappropriate colour, suggesting that a subpopulation had migrated tangentially.

Studies of cell migration are consistent with the idea that cortical areas might not be rigidly determined. Manipulations of the developing cortex by deafferentation or manipulation of inputs have been informative as to the state of commitment of cortical areas. In two independent sets of experiments, somatosensory or auditory cortex was induced to process visual information by misrouting retinal axons to somatosensory thalamus or auditory thalamus in the neonatal ferret (Sur et al 1988). In the first case, the lateral geniculate nucleus and the visual cortex were ablated and space was created in the medial geniculate by ablating the inferior colliculus. Amazingly, cells in the somatosensory or auditory cortex were visually driven, and receptive field and response properties resembled that seen in the visual cortex. This would seem to indicate that modality of a sensory thalamic nucleus or cortical area can be specified by inputs during development.

In the somatosensory cortex of the mouse, experiments on the cytoarchitectonic units termed 'barrels' have given much information on the specification of cortical areas. These units provide a one-to-one representation of sensory vibrissae on the muzzle, forming clusters of layer 4 neurons and thalamic afferents. Barrels can be detected by histochemical staining, but are only apparent during maturation, emerging out of what appears to be the uniform cortical plate. It is now well-established that the patterning of barrels is dependent on afferent input. Injury of individual vibrissae at birth leads to absence of the corresponding barrel (Van der Loos & Woolsey 1973). Furthermore, in strains of mice with abnormal sets of vibrissae, extra barrels are present in the cortex, but only if the anomalous vibrissa receives sufficient sensory axons (Walker & Van der Loos 1986). When pieces of visual cortex are transplanted into the position of somatosensory cortex, the characteristic barrel morphology develops (Schlaggar & O'Leary 1991). All this points to the importance of afferents in specifying cortical areas, tempered by the idea that some area-specific properties may be determined early on. Removal of an eye in primates leads to atrophy of area 17 of the visual cortex, due to lack of 50% of lateral geniculate neurons, the major input to this region. The drastic reduction in the size of area 17 is accompanied by a shift in the position of the area 17/18 boundary, and an area of cortex normally contained within area 17 takes on the appearance of area 18, pointing to some plasticity in the development of area-specific features. However, the laminar organization of area 17, the boundary between area 17 and 18, and the distribution of callosal projections from these areas are maintained (Dehay et al 1989).

Experiments on these questions, particularly in attempting to define the identity of transplanted regions, have suffered from a lack of area-specific markers. At present, the molecular markers available identify broader regions of the cortex, for example, the limbic system-associated membrane protein (LAMP) which is exclusive to limbic structures. Limbic regions transplanted elsewhere in the cortex maintain their expressions of this marker, perhaps arguing for early determination of this region (Barbe & Levitt 1991). Other markers are expressed differentially in the cortex relative to the adjacent forebrain areas (reviewed in Boncinelli 1994; Puelles & Rubinstein 1993). The genes *Emx-1* and *Emx-2* are expressed in neocortex but not the piriform cortex or basal ganglia, while *Dlx-1* and *Dlx-2* are expressed in the reciprocal pattern, in ventral forebrain regions including the basal ganglia (Bulfone et al 1993). *Emx-1* is expressed in the dorsal telencephalon, in a domain that is contained within that of *Emx-2*, which extends through the dorsal telencephalon and parts of the diencephalon. These expression domains are, in turn, contained within the expression domains of another gene, *Otx-1*, which is contained within that of *Otx-2* (Simeone et al 1992). Both these genes have expression domains that comprise dorsal, and most ventral domains of telencephalon, diencephalon and mesencephalon. Interestingly these 'nested' expression patterns appear during development in a sequence progressing from the most extensive domain to the least extensive, i.e. *Otx-2* is expressed first, followed by *Otx-1*, then *Emx-2*, then *Emx-1*. It is tempting to speculate, therefore, that these genes might be involved in the specification of cell fate in various brain regions.

The development of cortical projections has been investigated both in terms of laminar and area-specific connectivity. Recently, attention has focused on the idea that connections might be influenced by the existence of a transient population of subplate neurons. Studies by Marin-Padilla (1971) showed that the cortex develops within a preplate, consisting of corticopetal nerve fibres and the earliest generated neurons. This zone is then split by the arrival of cortical neurons into two zones, the subplate underneath the cortical plate, and the marginal zone at the pial surface. Subplate neurons extend axons via the internal capsule to the thalamus and superior colliculus at times before other cortical neurons have been born (McConnell et al 1989). Studies by Shatz and colleagues on the cat and the ferret have contended the subplate neurons to be a transient cell population that later dies. Thalamocortical afferents synapse with subplate neurons during their 'waiting period' prior to innervating their target in layer 4. Ablation of subplate neurons using kainic acid may cause thalamocortical afferents to fail to invade appropriate cortical areas (Ghosh & Shatz 1993). Axonal tracing studies in the rat, however, have contested the idea of a crucial role for subplate axons in thalamocortical connections. Labelling of axonal trajectories showed that subplate pathways to the internal capsule are established at about the same time as thalamocortical pathways to the thalamus, and that their trajectories in the cortex are separate (De Carlos & O'Leary 1992). More recently, the possibility that subplate axons may also play a role in the projection of cortical efferents from layer 5 and 6 has also been proposed. Examination of these axonal pathways following ablation of subplate neurons showed that in half the cases, cortical axons failed to invade their normal subcortical targets (McConnell et al 1994). In cultures of rat, visual cortical slices combined either with cortex or with thalamus subplate neurons were not detected; however, projections to the target tissue from the appropriate lamina were formed as in vivo (Bolz et al 1990). In cortex/thalamus cultures, corticofugal cells could be labelled even in the absence of corticopetal projections. The possibility that subplate axons showed regional specificity in their connections with particular thalamic nuclei was also tested in culture experiments by confronting visual cortex with a choice of appropriate (lateral geniculate nucleus) or inappropriate thalamic tissue (Molnar & Blakemore 1991), but no preference of projection was seen, making it unlikely that a selective chemotropism governs the trajectories of subplate axons.

A crucial question is the way in which region-specific projections are generated. Layer 5 neurons in various cortical areas extend axons to different repertoires of targets. For instance, layer 5 neurons of the visual cortex project to the tectum, pons and mesencephalic nuclei, while those in the motor cortex project to mesencephalic and pontine targets, the inferior olive and dorsal column nuclei and the spinal cord. An interesting feature of these cortical projections is that they arise by collateral formation (O'Leary & Terashima 1988) rather than by projection of the primary axon, or growth cone bifurcation. In the case of the corticopontine projection, collaterals are elicited by a diffusible, chemotrophic agent (Heffner et al 1990). Retrograde labelling of neurons at various times in development has shown that rather than being generated de novo, these patterns seem to arise by pruning of collaterals from a more widespread projection. So, visual cortical neurons possess a projection to the spinal cord early in development, which is later eliminated (O'Leary & Stanfield 1985). This later emergence of specific projections could arise either by intrinsic programming of the neurons to undergo this pruning, or position-dependent factors. Heterotopic transplantation experiments have now shown that the latter is the case (O'Leary & Stanfield 1989). When pieces of visual cortex were transplanted into motor areas, and the resulting layer 5 projections labelled at later times in development, projections to the spinal cord persisted, rather than being eliminated as in normal development. Neurons in pieces of motor cortex transplanted in the place of visual cortex lost their

collaterals in the same manner as the neurons of the host. Thus position plays an important role in the modelling of cortical projections, implying that the same classes of neurons exist in different tangential regions of the cortex. Presumably, the selective removal of inappropriate collaterals is governed by local factors at the site of axon termination rather than at the neuronal cell body. Nevertheless, some distinctions between neuronal classes may exist from an early stage, since cortical projection neurons are never found to possess callosal axons (Koester & O'Leary 1989). Interestingly, neurons destined to possess corticocortical axons may initially project to the opposite hemisphere, a projection that is later lost (Innocenti et al 1986). Elimination of axons to give rise to the mature distribution of callosal neurons may be affected by sensory inputs, since manipulation of thalamic inputs can lead to failure of this remodelling of callosal projections (Dehay et al 1989). Regressive events such as axon and synapse elimination and neuronal death thus play an important part in modelling the cortex. In rodents, for example, about 30% of cortical neurons die, with the number of cells in layer 4 being governed by thalamic input.

The critical role apparently played by thalamic input in organizing the regional differentiation of the cortex begs the question of how thalamic afferents are themselves organized. The possibility that each cortical area exerts a specific trophic or tropic influence on axons from the appropriate thalamic nucleus was examined in explant slice cultures in which the laminar origin of growing axons could be visualized. When portions of lateral geniculate nucleus were cultured with a 'choice' of occipital cortex and frontal cortex (appropriate and inappropriate targets respectively) no preference in the pattern of outgrowth was observed, although axons in both targets terminated correctly, in layer 4 (Molnar & Blakemore 1991). It seems unlikely, then, that a mosaic of region-specific, possibly diffusible factors directs the thalamocortical projection. Instead, it may be that thalamocortical and corticothalamic projections reach the internal capsule simultaneously to provide a mutual guidance mechanism. Factors in the local environment between thalamus and cortex that might lead to the specificity of projections have yet to be identified.

Perinatal brain

The state of differentiation at birth and at various postnatal stages, as seen in Golgi (metal impregnation) preparations, has been described in considerable detail elsewhere (Conel—a series of publications 1939–59). Gross nutritional deficiencies, selective neural ablation, endocrine imbalances, sensory deprivation, neurotropic viruses, vascular abnormalities and perinatal anoxia may all disturb the normal pattern of the cortex at birth. (See bibliographies in Rakic & Goldman-Rakic 1982.)

At birth the volume of the brain is approximately 25% of its volume in adult life. The greater part of the increase occurs during the first year, at the end of which the volume of the brain has increased to 75% of its adult volume. The growth can be accounted for partly by increase in the size of nerve cell somata, the profusion and dimensions of their dendritic trees, axons and their collaterals and by growth of the neuroglial cells and cerebral blood vessels, but it is the acquisition of myelin sheaths by the axons which is principally responsible for it. The great sensory pathways, visual, auditory and somatic, myelinate first, the motor fibres later. During the second and subsequent years, growth proceeds much more slowly; the brain attains adult size by the seventeenth or eighteenth year. This is largely due to continued myelination of various groups of nerve fibres.

MENINGES

The meningeal layers originate from paraxial mesenchyme in the trunk and caudal regions of the head, but from neural crest in regions rostral to the mesencephalon (the prechordal plate has also been suggested to make a contribution, see below). It may generally be the case that those skull bones which are formed from neural crest, e.g. the base of the skull rostral to the sella turcica, frontal, parietal and squamous temporal bones, overlie meninges which are also formed from crest cells. Certainly the work of Couly and Le Douarin (1991) supports the concept that the neural crest gives rise to the meninges over the prosencephalon.

The meninges may be divided in development into the *pachymeninx* (*dura mater*) and *leptomeninges* (*arachnoid layer*, subarachnoid space with arachnoid cells and fibres, and *pia mater*). All meningeal layers are derived from loose mesenchyme, which surrounds the developing neural tube, termed *meninx primitiva*, or *primary meninx*. (For a detailed account of the development of the meninges in the human consult O'Rahilly & Muller 1986.)

The first indication of *pia mater*, containing the plexus of blood vessels which forms on the neural surface, is seen in the stage 11 embryo (24 days) around the caudalmost part of the medulla; this extends to the mesencephalic level by stage 12. Mesenchymal cells projecting from the rostral end of the notochord, and those in the region of the prechordal plate, extend rostrally into the mesencephalic flexure and form the earliest cells of the *tentorium cerebelli*; O'Rahilly and Muller (1986b) note that at the beginning of its development the medial part of the tentorium is predominantly leptomeningeal. By stage 17 (41 days) *dura mater* can be seen in the basal areas where the future chondrocranium is also developing. The precursors of the venous sinuses lie within the pachymeninx at stage 19 (48 days), and by stage 20, cell populations in the region of the future *falx cerebri* are proliferating, although the dorsal regions of the brain are not yet covered with putative meninges.

By stage 23 (57 days) the dura is almost complete over the rhombencephalon and mesencephalon but is only present laterally around the prosencephalon. Subarachnoid spaces and most of the cisternae are present from this time after the *arachnoid mater* becomes separated from the primitive dura mater by the accumulation of cerebrospinal fluid, which now has a net movement out of the ventricular system. The medial part of the tentorium is becoming thinner. A dural component of the tentorium is seen from stage 19; the earlier developed medial portion disappears leaving a partial partition separating a subarachnoid area containing the telencephalon and diencephalon from one containing the cerebellum and rhombencephalon.

There is a very close relationship, during development, between the mesenchyme from which the cranial dura mater is formed and that which is chondrified and ossified, or ossified directly, to form the skull, and these layers are only clearly differentiated as the venous sinuses develop. (For an interesting study of pre- and postnatal growth of the tentorium cerebelli, with a mathematical analysis, see Klintworth 1967.) The relationship between the developing skull and the underlying dura mater continues during postnatal life while the bones of the calvaria are still growing.

The growth of the cranial vault is initiated from ossification centres within the desmocranial mesenchyme. A wave of osteodifferentiation moves radially outward from these centres stopping when adjacent bones meet, regions where sutures are induced to form. Once sutures are formed a second phase of development occurs in which growth of the cranial bones occurs at the sutural margins (Opperman et al 1993). Such growth forms most of the skull. It was proposed that the control of suture morphogenesis was sited in the dura mater and a variety of hypotheses have been generated to explain this process. One suggested that the dura mater contained fibre tracts which extended from fixed positions in the cranial base to sites of dural reflection underlying each of the cranial sutures. The tensional forces so generated would dictate the position of the sutures and locally inhibit precocious ossification. Other hypotheses support the concept of local factors in the calvaria which regulate suture morphogenesis. It has been shown clinically (and experimentally) that following removal of the entire calvaria the skull regenerates with sutures and bones developing in anatomically correct positions, suggesting that the dura can dictate suture position in regeneration of the neonatal calvaria. Markens (1975b) noted that transplantation of perinatal rat coronal suture blastema, in which the osteogenic fronts of the parietal and frontal bones had overlapped into adult host skulls, resulted in the formation of a suture which remained unossified up to 6 weeks in the host animal. Transplants of similar tissue from earlier stages did not give rise to sutures, suggesting that an osteo-inhibitory message, induced in the dura mater by the interaction between the suture blastema and the advancing osteogenic front, was responsible for maintaining the transplanted sutures. This finding has been confirmed by Opperman et al (1993) who found that in transplants of sutures in which the fetal dura mater was left intact a continuous fibrous suture remained between developing vault bones,

whereas in transplants in which the fetal dura mater was removed bony fusion occurred.

The presence of fetal dura is not required for the initial suture morphogenesis which appears to be controlled by mesenchymal cell proliferation and fibrous extracellular matrix synthesis induced by the overlapping of the advancing osteoinductive fronts of the calvarial bones. Opperman et al (1993) suggest that following overlap of the bone fronts a signal is transferred to the underlying dura inducing changes in localized regions beneath the sutures. Once a suture has formed, it serves as a primary site for cranial bone growth but requires constant interaction with the dura to avoid ossiferous obliteration.

ECTODERMAL PLACODES AND THE SPECIAL SENSE ORGANS

Many of the special sense organs and all of the sensory cranial nerves take origin from ectodermal placodes, regions of ectoderm containing neural progenitor cells which originate in the neural folds but remain in the surface ectoderm after neurulation (Couly & Le Douarin 1985; see p. 222). Generally the placodal cells undergo epithelial/mesenchymal transformation after an inductive stimulus, which may be given by the proximity of the neural tube or by subjacent migration of neural crest cells, and migrate deep to the surface ectoderm to join with crest cells. Ectodermal placodes are found rostrally as the *hypophyseal*, *olfactory* and *optic placodes*, giving rise to the *adenohypophysis*, *olfactory epithelium* and *lens of the eye* respectively. More caudally the placodal cells are arranged in three main groups: ventrolateral (epibranchial), dorsolateral and intermediate. Most groups give rise, with neural crest cells, to the cranial sensory ganglia; however, the dorsolateral placode—the *otic*—gives rise to the *membranous labyrinth of the ear*, to the *acoustic ganglion*, and, with neural crest cells, to the *vestibular ganglion*. Thus the ectodermal placodes provide a significant contribution to the special sense organs in the head.

PITUITARY GLAND (HYPOPHYSIS CEREBRI)

The hypophysis cerebri consists of the *adenohypophysis* and the *neurohypophysis* (consult p. 1883 for the varied usages of the older terms, anterior and posterior lobes, and of the more satisfactory terms adenohypophysis and neurohypophysis, and their subdivisions).

The adenohypophysis is derived, after neurulation, from placodal ectoderm of the stomodeal roof, and the neurohypophysis from the neurectoderm of the floor of the forebrain. However, chimera experimentation in chick embryos has revealed an early juxtaposition of the adenohypophyseal and neurohypophyseal populations prior to neurulation in the chick (Couly & Le Douarin 1985, 1987) and transplantation experiments have shown similar results in amphibian embryos (Kawamura & Kikuyama 1992). At this time the neural plate has raised lateral edges, the neural folds, containing putative neural crest cells and surface ectoderm, and a midline anterior neural ridge where the neural folds converge. The most rostral portion of the neural plate, which will form the hypothalamus, is in contact rostrally with the future adenohypophysis, in the anterior neural ridge, and caudally with the neurohypophysis, in the floor of the neural plate (see 3.100). After neurulation the cells of the anterior neural ridge remain in the ectoderm and form the hypophyseal placode which is in close apposition and adherent to the overlying forebrain. Neural crest mesenchyme later moves between the prosencephalon and surface ectoderm except at the region of the placode. Before rupture of the buccopharyngeal membrane, proliferation of the periplacodal mesenchyme results in the placode forming the roof and walls of a saccular depression. This hypophyseal recess (*pouch of Rathke; 3.127, 128*) is the rudiment of the adenohypophysis, lying immediately ventral to the dorsal border of the membrane, extending in front of the rostral tip of the notochord, and retaining contact with the ventral surface of the forebrain. It is constricted off by continued proliferation of the surrounding mesenchyme to form a closed vesicle, but remains for a time connected to the ectoderm of the stomodeum by a solid cord of cells, which can be traced down the posterior edge of the nasal septum. Masses of epithelial cells

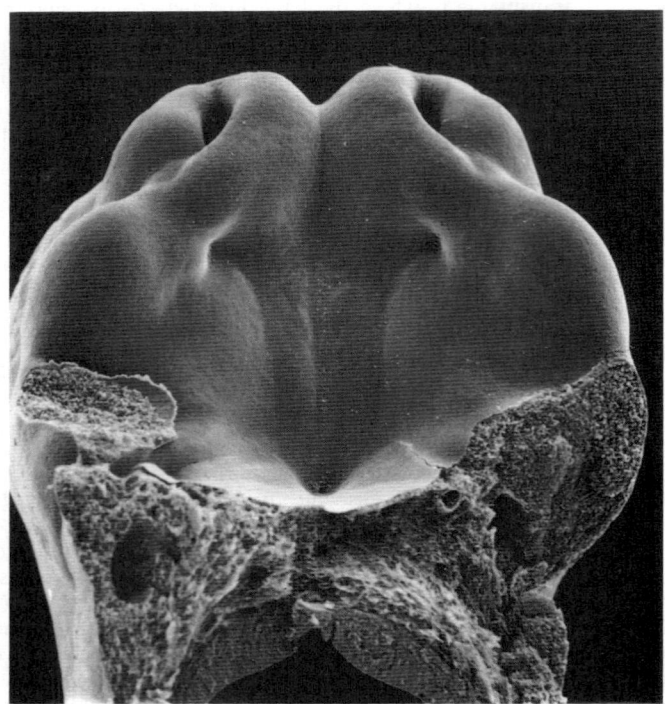

3.127   Scanning electron micrograph of the roof of the pharynx showing the invagination of placodal ectoderm to form the adenohypophysis (Rathke's pouch). (Photograph by P Collins; printed by S Cox, Electron Microscopy Unit, Southampton General Hospital.)

form mainly on each side and in the ventral wall of the vesicle, and the development of the adenohypophysis progresses by the ingrowth of a mesenchymal stroma. Differentiation of epithelial cells into stem cells and three differentiating types is said to be apparent during the early months of fetal development (Dubois 1967). It is also suggested that different types of cells arise in succession, and that they may be derived in differing proportions from different parts of the hypophyseal recess (Conklin 1968). A *cranio-pharyngeal canal*, which sometimes runs from the anterior part of the hypophyseal fossa of the sphenoid bone to the exterior of the skull, is often said to mark the original position of the hypophyseal recess (of Rathke). Traces of the stomodeal end of the recess are invariably present at the junction of the septum of the nose with the palate (see the *pharyngeal hypophysis*). Others have claimed, however, that the craniopharyngeal canal itself is a secondary formation caused by the growth of blood vessels, and is quite unconnected with the stalk of

the anterior lobe (Arey 1949). Just caudal to, but in contact with, the adenohypophyseal recess a hollow diverticulum elongates towards the stomodeum from the floor of the neural plate just caudal to the hypothalamus (**3.**128B); this region of neural outgrowth is the neurohypophysis. It forms an *infundibular sac*, the walls of which increase in thickness until the contained cavity is obliterated except at its upper end, where it persists as the *infundibular recess* of the third ventricle. Formed in this way the neurohypophysis becomes invested by the adenohypophysis which extends dorsally on each side of it. In addition, the adenohypophysis gives off two processes from its ventral wall which grow along the infundibulum and fuse to surround it, coming into relation with the tuber cinereum and constituting the *tuberal portion* of the hypophysis. The original cavity of Rathke's pouch remains first as a cleft, and later scattered vesicles, and can be identified readily in sagittal sections through the mature gland. The dorsal wall of Rathke's pouch, which remains thin, fuses with the adjoining part of the neurohypophysis as the *pars intermedia*.

A small endodermal diverticulum, named *Seessel's pouch*, projects towards the brain from the cranial end of the foregut, immediately caudal to the buccopharyngeal membrane. In some marsupials this pouch forms a part of the hypophysis, but in man it apparently disappears entirely.

NOSE

The early development of the olfactory placodes, external nose and nasal cavities have already been considered (p. 278).

The *olfactory nerve fibre bundles (fila olfactoria)* are developed from a proportion of the placodal cells which line the olfactory pits; these cells proliferate and give rise to *olfactory receptor cells*. Their central processes grow into the overlying olfactory bulb and thus form the axons of the olfactory nerves. It was claimed that the olfactory cells are from the first connected with the overlying brain by bridges of cytoplasm, within which the olfactory nerve fibres develop. More recent accounts, however, suggest that the earliest pioneer neurites are naked cytoplasmic processes which cross a mesenchyme-filled gap between the placode and the superjacent brain. Later these and subsequent generations of centrally directed neurites become enclothed in Schwann cell processes, presumably derived from the rostral neural crest (Pearson 1941; Van Campenhout 1956; Dejean et al 1958). Within the olfactory bulb the terminals of the olfactory axons divide repeatedly, and establish complex synaptic contacts with a number of neuroblast types in rudimentary *olfactory glomeruli* (p. 1116). The single dendrite extends towards the nasal cavity surface of the olfactory epithelium where, in most regions, slight expansion with surface specialization occurs (p. 1117).

The remaining placodal cells, with probable accessions from neighbouring rostral neural crest and mixed head mesenchyme, differentiate into columnar *supporting (sustentacular) cells*, rounded *basal cells* and, by invagination, the flattened *duct-lining* and polyhedral

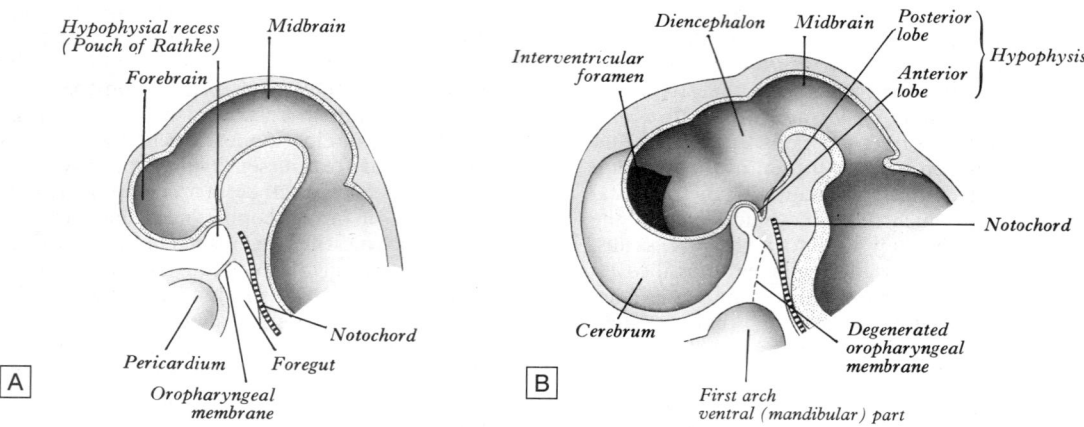

3.128   Schematic sagittal sections of heads of early embryos to show first stages in the development of the hypophysis.

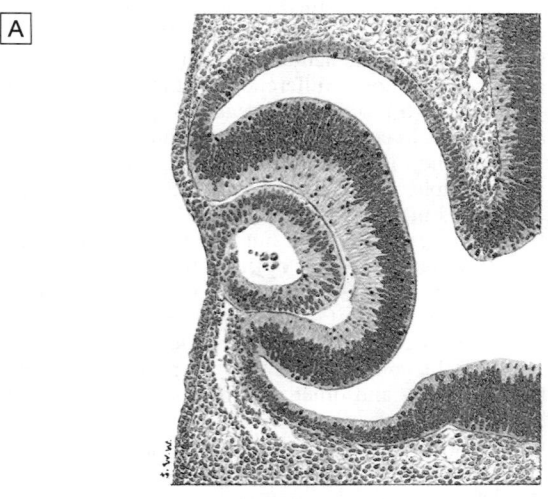

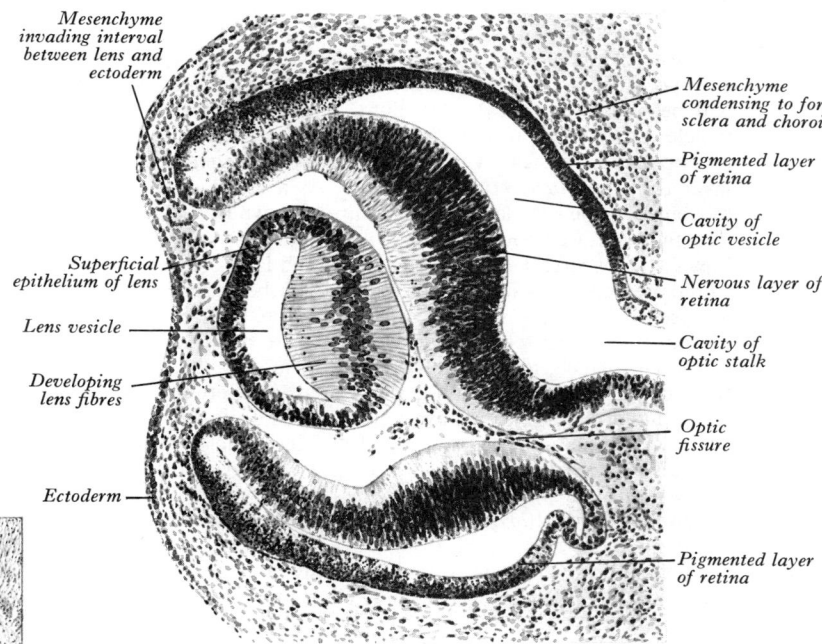

Mesenchyme invading interval between lens and ectoderm

Mesenchyme condensing to form sclera and choroid

Pigmented layer of retina

Cavity of optic vesicle

Superficial epithelium of lens

Nervous layer of retina

Lens vesicle

Cavity of optic stalk

Developing lens fibres

Optic fissure

Ectoderm

Pigmented layer of retina

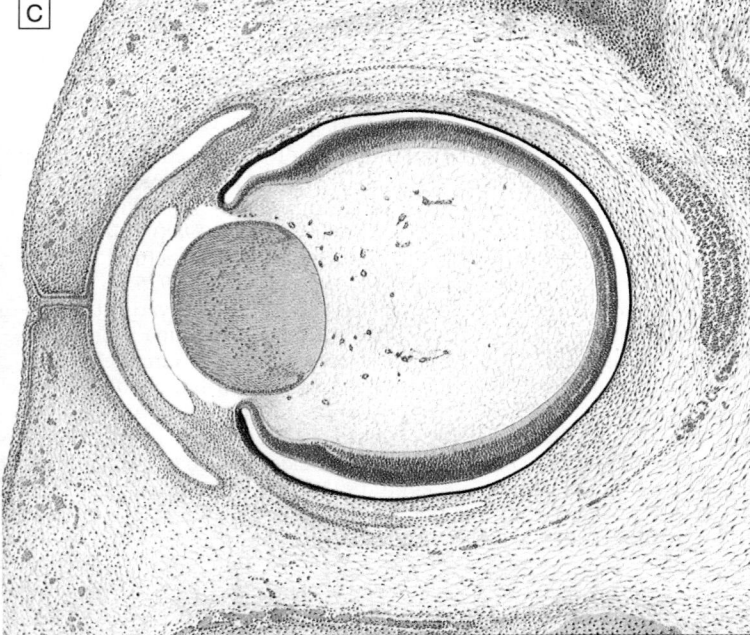

3.129A   Section through the developing eye of a human embryo, 8 mm CR length. The thick nervous and the thinner pigmented layers of the retina and the developing lens are shown. Stained with haematoxylin and eosin. Magnification × *c*. 114. (From material loaned by Professor R J Harrison.)

B. Section through the developing eye of a human embryo, 13.2 mm long. (Streeter 1948.)

C. Section through the eye of a human embryo of 40 mm CR length. Note the layers of the retina, developing lens, pupillary membrane, cornea, conjunctival sac, anterior and posterior aqueous chambers, the developing vitreous body, and condensing circumoptic mesenchyme and the fused eyelids. Stained with haematoxylin and eosin. Magnification × *c*. 62.

acinar cells of the glands of Bowman. Later, basal infiltration by lymphocytes occurs.

EYES

The formation of the eyes requires precisely co-ordinated development of tissues from three sources: the *neurectoderm of the forebrain* which forms the sensory retina and accessory pigmented structures, the *surface ectoderm* which forms the lens and cornea, and the intervening *neural crest mesenchyme* which contributes to the fibrous coats of the eye. Vascular tissue of the developing eye may form by local angiogenesis or vasculogenesis of angiogenetic mesenchyme (see p. 299). (General accounts of the development of the human eye are given by Mann 1964; O'Rahilly 1983; O'Rahilly & Muller 1987.)

Embryonic components of the eye

The first morphological sign of eye development is a thickening of the diencephalic neural folds at 22 days postovulation, when the embryo has 7–8 somites. This *optic primordium* extends on both sides of the neural plate, crossing the midline at the *primordium chiasmatis*. A slight transverse indentation, the *optic sulcus*, appears in the inner surface of the optic primordium on each side of the brain. During the period when the rostral neuropore closes, at about 24 days, the walls of the forebrain at the optic sulcus begin to evaginate, projecting laterally towards the surface ectoderm so that, by 25 days, the *optic vesicles* are formed. The lumen of each vesicle is continuous with that of the forebrain. Cells delaminate from the walls of the optic vesicle and, probably joined by head mesenchyme and cells derived from the mesencephalic neural crest, invest the vesicle in a sheath of mesenchyme. By 28 days, regional differentiation is apparent in each of the source tissues of the eye. The optic vesicle is visibly differentiated into its three primary parts: at the junction with the diencephalon a thick-walled region marks the future optic stalk; laterally, the tissue which will become the sensory retina forms a flat disc of thickened epithelium in close contact with the surface ectoderm; the thin-walled part of the vesicle which lies between these regions will later form the pigmented layer of the retina. The area of surface ectoderm that is closely apposed to the optic vesicle also thickens to form the *lens placode*. The mesenchymal sheath of the vesicle begins to show signs of angiogenesis. Evidence from the equivalent stage of mouse development shows that as the epithelial regions become morphologically distinct they are already differentiated at the molecular level. For example, the gene encoding the homeobox-containing transcription factor *Msx-2* is expressed in the future sensory retina and in the overlying surface ectoderm (Monaghan et al 1991) while *TRP-2/DT*, a gene encoding an early marker for melanoblasts, is expressed in the prospective pigmented retina (Steel et al 1992). Between 32 and 33 days postovulation, the lens placode and optic vesicle undergo co-ordinated morphogenesis.

259

The lens placode invaginates, forming a pit which pinches off from the surface ectoderm to form the *lens vesicle*. (Consult Zwaan & Hendriz 1973 for a detailed analysis of this process in the chick embryo.) The surface ectoderm reforms a continuous layer which will become the corneal epithelium. The lateral part of the optic vesicle also invaginates to form a cup, the inner layer of which (facing the lens vesicle) will become the *sensory retina*, and the outer layer the *pigmented retinal epithelium*. As a result of these folding movements, the two layers of the cup have what were their apical (lumenal) surfaces now facing one another across the much reduced lumen, the *intraretinal space*. The pigmented layer becomes attached to the mesenchymal sheath, but the junction between the pigmented and sensory layers is less firm and is the site of pathological detachment of the retina. The two layers are continuous at the lip of the cup which, at the end of the third month, grows round the front of the lens and forms the pigmented *iris*. Between the base of the cup and the brain, the narrow part of the optic vesicle forms the *optic stalk*. The anteroventral surface of the vesicle and distal part of the stalk are also infolded, forming a wide groove—the *choroid fissure*—through which mesenchyme extends with an associated artery, the *hyaloid artery*. As growth proceeds, the fissure closes, including the artery in the distal part of the stalk. Failure of the optic fissure to close is a rare anomaly and there is always a corresponding deficiency in the choroid and iris (*congenital coloboma*).

Early stages of eye development: mechanisms

Understanding of the mechanisms by which the tissues of the human eye become determined, then shaped and patterned, depends on experiments conducted on the embryos of other vertebrate species, notably the mouse, chick and various amphibia (reviewed by Saha et al 1992). These experiments provide general principles, but it should not be assumed that the conclusions can be applied directly to every detail of the human case. In particular, there appear to be significant differences between the different vertebrate classes as regards the developmental plasticity and capacity for regeneration of the tissues in the eye. The development of the eye involves a series of interactions between neighbouring tissues in the head. These interactions have been studied extensively in experimental tissue combinations, but much of the older literature is unreliable because of technical difficulties in separating the tissues cleanly, the lack of unambiguous host/graft markers to determine the origins of structures developed from the combined tissues and the lack of specific molecular indicators of tissue type by which to assay the resulting development. Studies in amphibia, using improved methods, have shown that the formation of the optic vesicle is a result of interactions between the mesenchyme of the head and the adjacent neurectoderm during gastrulation and neurulation. These interactions lead to the development of the potential to form optic vesicles throughout a broad anterior domain of neurectoderm. As a result of further interactions between mesenchyme and neurectoderm, this region becomes subdivided into bilateral domains at the future sites of the eyes. The parallel process of lens determination appears to depend on an inductive influence spreading through the surface ectoderm from the rostral neural plate. During a brief period of competence, this elicits a lens-forming area of the head (consult Grainger et al 1992 for a review). As the optic vesicle forms and contacts the potential lens ectoderm reciprocal interactions occur which are necessary for the complete development of both tissues.

Differentiation of the functional components of the eye

The developments described above bring the embryonic components of the eye into the spatial relationships necessary for the passage, focusing, and sensing of light. The next phase of development involves further patterning and cell-type differentiation in order to develop the specialized structures of the adult organ.

The *optic cup* becomes patterned, from the base to the rim, into regions with distinct functions (**3.**129A–C). The external stratum remains a rather thin layer of cells which, around 36 days, begin to acquire pigmented melanosomes and form the *pigmented epithelium of the retina*. In a parallel process which was already begun before invagination, the cells of the inner layer of the cup proliferate to form a thick epithelium. The inner layer forms neural tissue over the base and sides of the cup and non-neural tissue around the

lip. The non-neural epithelium is further differentiated into the components of the prospective iris at the rim and the ciliary body, a little further back adjacent to the neural area. The development of this pattern is reflected in regional differences in the expression of various genes which encode transcriptional regulators and are therefore likely to play key roles in controlling and coordinating development. Each of these genes is expressed prior to overt cell-type differentiation. For example, in the mouse embryo, the genes *Msx-2* and *Dlx-1* are expressed in the prospective neural retina and *Msx-1* in the ciliary epithelium. In mouse and human, *Pax-6* is expressed in the prospective ciliary and iris regions of the optic cup. Individuals heterozygous for mutations in *Pax-6* lack an iris, suggesting a causal role for this gene in the development of the iris. Each of these genes, in addition to being expressed in the eye, is also active at a variety of other specific sites in the embryo. This may, in part, account for the co-involvement of the eye and other organs in syndromes which result from single genetic lesions.

The developing neural retina. This comprises an outer *nuclear zone* and an inner *marginal zone*, devoid of nuclei. Around 36 days the cells of the nuclear zone invade the marginal zone, and by 44 days the nervous stratum of the retina consists of inner and outer *neuroblastic layers*. The inner neuroblastic layer gives rise to the ganglion cells, the amacrine cells and the somata of the 'fibrous' sustentacular cells (of Muller); the outer neuroblastic layer is the source of the horizontal and rod-and-cone bipolar neurons and probably the rod-and-cone cells, which first appear in the central part of the retina. By the eighth month all the named layers of the retina can be identified. However, the retinal photoreceptor cells continue to form after birth, generating an array of increasing resolution and sensitivity (Banks & Bennett 1988). (For bibliographies on retinal development, including ultrastructural studies, consult Spira & Hollenberg 1973; Fisher & Linberg 1975.)

Experiments on chick embryos indicate that the divergent differentiation of the pigmented and sensory layers of the retina depends on interactions mediated by diffusible molecules. For example, soluble factors from the retina elicit the polarized distribution of plasma membrane proteins and the formation of tight junctions in the pigmented epithelium (Rizzolo & Li 1993). Neural retinal differentiation appears to be mediated by fibroblast growth factors (Pittack et al 1991; Guillemot & Cepko 1992). Even after specific differentiation is under way in the pigmented epithelium, however, this tissue retains the potential to become neural retina and will do so if the embryonic retina is wounded.

The development of specific types of cell in the retina depends on cell interactions, rather than cell lineage. In the mouse, for example, a single retinal precursor cell can give rise to at least three different types of neuron or two types of neuron and a glial cell (Fields-Berry et al 1992) and, in frog embryos, the different types of cells in the retina can be generated without cell division (Harris & Hartenstein 1991). These interactions are mediated, at least in part, by diffusible factors which are likely to act over short range, coordinating the development of neighbouring cells (Wilkinson et al 1989; Watanabe & Raff 1992; Mudhar et al 1993). Fundamental aspects of the mechanisms by which cell signalling determines the pattern of neural cell differentiation are also becoming evident from studies which indicate the expression, in the mammalian retina, of genes that are known to be involved in spatial determination in invertebrates; examples are the mouse genes related to the Drosphila gene *Notch* (Reaume et al 1992) and *Achaete-Scute* (Guillemot & Joyner 1993).

Optic nerve develops from the optic stalk. The centre of the optic cup, where the optic fissure is deepest, will later form the *optic disc*. Here the neural retina is continuous with the corresponding invaginated cell layer of the optic stalk and, as a result, the developing nerve fibres of the ganglion cells pass directly into the wall of the stalk, converting it into the optic nerve. The fibres of the optic nerve begin to acquire their myelin sheaths shortly before birth, but the process is not completed until some time later. The *optic chiasma* is formed by the meeting and partial decussation of the fibres of the two optic nerves in the ventral part of the lamina terminalis at the junction of the telencephalon with the diencephalon in the floor of the third ventricle. Beyond the chiasma, the fibres are continued backwards as the optic tracts, principally to the lateral geniculate bodies and to the superior tectum.

The ciliary body is a compound structure; its epithelial components comprise the region of the inner layer of the retina between the iris and the neural retina together with the adjacent outer layer of pigmented epithelium. The cells in this region differentiate in close association with the surrounding mesenchyme to form highly vascularized folds that secrete fluid into the globe of the eye (reviewed in Bard 1990). The inner surface of the ciliary body also forms the site of attachment of the lens (see below), while the outer layer is associated with smooth muscle derived from mesenchymal cells in the choroid located between the anterior scleral condensation and the pigmented ciliary epithelium. This *ciliary muscle* functions to focus the lens.

The iris functions to regulate the aperture of the eye. It develops from the tip of the optic cup where the two layers remain thin and are associated with vascularized, muscular connective tissue. The muscles of the *sphincter* and *dilator pupillae* are unusual in being of neurectodermal origin, developed from the cells of the pupillary part of the optic cup. The mature colour of the iris develops after birth and depends on the relative contributions of the pigmented epithelium on the posterior surface of the iris and the chromatophore cells in the mesenchymal stroma of the iris. If only epithelial pigment is present, the eye appears blue; if there is an additional contribution from the chromatophores, the eye appears brown.

Lens. This is developed from the lens vesicle (**3.129A**). The vesicle is initially a ball of actively proliferating epithelium typically enclosing a clump of disintegrating cells. By 37 days, however, there is a clear difference between the thin anterior (i.e. outward facing) epithelium and the thickened posterior epithelium. Cells of the posterior wall lengthen greatly and fill the vesicle (**3.129B**, c) so that, by about 44 days the original cavity is reduced to a slit. The posterior cells become filled with a very high concentration of proteins (crystallins), which render them transparent. The cells themselves become densely packed within the lens as *primary lens fibres*. Cells at the equatorial region of the lens also elongate and add additional *secondary lens fibres* to the body of the lens in a process which continues into adult life. Characteristic ultrastructural changes during lens cell development have been described by Wulle and Lerche 1967. This process is sustained by continued proliferation of cells in the anterior epithelium. In the chick and mammal, the polarity and growth of the lens appear to depend on the differential distribution of soluble factors which promote either cell division or lens fibre differentiation and are present in the anterior chamber and vitreous humour respectively (Hyatt & Beebe 1993; Schultz et al 1993).

The developing lens is surrounded by a vascular mesenchymal condensation, the *vascular capsule*, the anterior part of which is named the *pupillary membrane*. The blood vessels supplying the posterior part of this capsule are derived from the *hyaloid artery*, those for the anterior part from the *anterior ciliary arteries*. By the sixth month all the vessels of the capsule are atrophied except the hyaloid artery, which becomes occluded during the eighth month of intrauterine life. The atrophy of both the hyaloid vasculature and the pupillary membrane appears to be an active process of programmed tissue remodelling dependent on macrophages (Lang & Bishop 1993). Prior to this, during the fourth month, the hyaloid artery gives off retinal branches and its proximal part persists in the adult as the *central artery of the retina*, together with its accompanying central vein (for details, consult Penfold et al 1990). The *hyaloid canal*, which carries the vessels through the vitreous, persists after the vessels have become occluded. In the newly born child it extends more or less horizontally from the optic disc to the posterior aspect of the lens but when the adult eye is examined with a slit-lamp it can be seen to follow a wavy, curvy course, sagging downwards as it passes forwards to the lens (Mann 1927). With the loss of its blood vessels the vascular capsule disappears and the lens becomes dependent for its nutrition on diffusion via the aqueous and vitreous humours. The lens remains enclosed, however, in the *lens capsule* which is a thickened basal lamina derived from the lens epithelium. Sometimes the pupillary membrane persists at birth, giving rise to *congenital atresia of the pupil.*

The vitreous body develops between the lens and the optic cup as a transparent, avascular gel of extracellular substance; the precise derivation of the vitreous is controversial. The lens rudiment and the optic vesicle are at first in contact, but after closure of the lens vesicle and formation of the optic cup they draw apart, remaining connected by a network of delicate cytoplasmic processes. This network, derived partly from cells of the lens and partly from those of the retina, is the *primitive vitreous body*. At first these cytoplasmic processes are connected to the whole of the neuroretinal area of the cup, but later they are limited to the ciliary region where, by a process of condensation, they form the basis of the suspensory ligaments of the *ciliary zonule*. The vascular mesenchyme which enters the cup through the choroidal fissure and around the equator of the lens associates locally with this reticular tissue and thus contributes to the formation of the vitreous body.

Aqueous chamber. This chamber of the eye develops in the space between the surface ectoderm and the lens which is invaded by mesenchymal cells of neural crest origin. The aqueous chamber initially appears as a cleft in this mesenchymal tissue. The mesenchyme superficial to the cleft forms the *substantia propria* of the cornea, which deep to the cleft forms the mesenchymal stroma of the iris and the pupillary membrane. Tangentially, this early cleft extends as far as the *iridocorneal angle* where communications are established with the sinus venosus sclerae. When the pupillary membrane disappears the cavity continues to form between the iris and the lens capsule as far as the zonular suspensory fibres. Thus the aqueous chamber is now divided by the iris into *anterior* and *posterior chambers*, communicating through the pupil. Their walls furnish the sites of production, and channels of circulation and reabsorption of the aqueous humour (p. 1349).

Cornea is induced in front of the anterior chamber by the lens and optic cup. The corneal epithelium is formed from the surface ectoderm and the epithelium of the anterior chamber from mesenchyme (O'Rahilly & Meyer 1959). Between the two is established a regular array of collagen fibres which serve to reduce scattering of light entering the eye (for a review of the process in the chick see Bard 1990).

Choroid and sclera. These differentiate as inner, vascular, and outer, fibrous, layers from the mesenchyme surrounding the optic cup. The blood vessels of the choroid develop from the fifteenth week and include the vasculature of the ciliary body. The choroid is continuous with the internal sheath of the optic nerve which is a part of the pia-arachnoid of the brain. Outside this, the sclera is continuous with the outer sheath of the optic nerve, and thus with the dura mater of the brain. The continuity of the subarachnoid space with the sheath of the optic nerve makes the optic disc and the venous return from the retina sensitive to pathological changes in the pressure of the cerebrospinal fluid.

Eyelids are formed as small cutaneous folds (**3.129c**). About the middle of the third month their edges come together and unite over the cornea, enclosing the *conjunctival sac*. They are usually said to remain united until about the end of the sixth month. When the eyelids open, the conjunctiva lines their inner surfaces and the white (scleral) region of the eye. For a detailed account consult Sevel (1988) and for an account of eyelid development in the mouse see Findlater et al (1993).

LACRIMAL APPARATUS

The epithelium of the alveoli and ducts of the *lacrimal gland* arise as a series of tubular buds from the ectoderm of the superior conjunctival fornix; these buds are arranged in two groups, one forming the gland proper and the other its palpebral process. The *lacrimal sac* and *nasolacrimal duct* are considered to be derived from the ectoderm in the nasomaxillary groove between the lateral nasal prominence and the maxillary prominence (p. 237). This thickens to form a solid cord of cells which sinks into the mesenchyme; during the third month the central cells of the cord break down and a lumen is acquired. In this way the nasolacrimal duct is established. The *lacrimal canaliculi* arise as buds from the upper part of the cord cells and, secondarily, establish openings (*punctua lacrimalia*) on the margins of the lids; the inferior canaliculus cuts off a small part of the lower eyelid to form the *lacrimal caruncle* and *plica semilunaris*. The epithelium of the cornea and conjunctiva is of ectodermal origin, as are also the eyelashes and the lining cells of the tarsal, ciliary and other glands which open on the margins of the eyelids. For general accounts of ocular developmental abnormalities consult Dejean et al (1958); Mann 1964; and Moore and Peroud (1993).

EARS

The rudiments of the *internal ears* appear shortly after those of the eyes as two patches of thickened, surface epithelium, *otic placodes*, lateral to the hindbrain (see p. 148). Each placode invaginates as an *otic pit* while at the same time giving cells to the *stato-acoustic (vestibulocochlear) ganglion* (**3.96A**). Studies have indicated that the vestibulocochlear ganglion is formed entirely by placodal cells and also that placodal cells populate the acoustic ganglion entirely and

the vestibular ganglion *with* a small contribution from neural crest cells (D'Amico-Martel & Noden 1983). The mouth of the pit then closes forming an initially piriform *otocyst* (*auditory* or *otic vesicle*) from which the epithelial lining of the *membranous labyrinth* is derived (**3.130A–F**). A vertical infolding of its wall progressively marks off a tubular diverticulum on the medial side, which differentiates into the *ductus* and *saccus endolymphaticus*, and they communicate via the ductus with the remainder of the vesicle—the *utriculosaccular chamber*—which is placed laterally. From the dorsal part of this

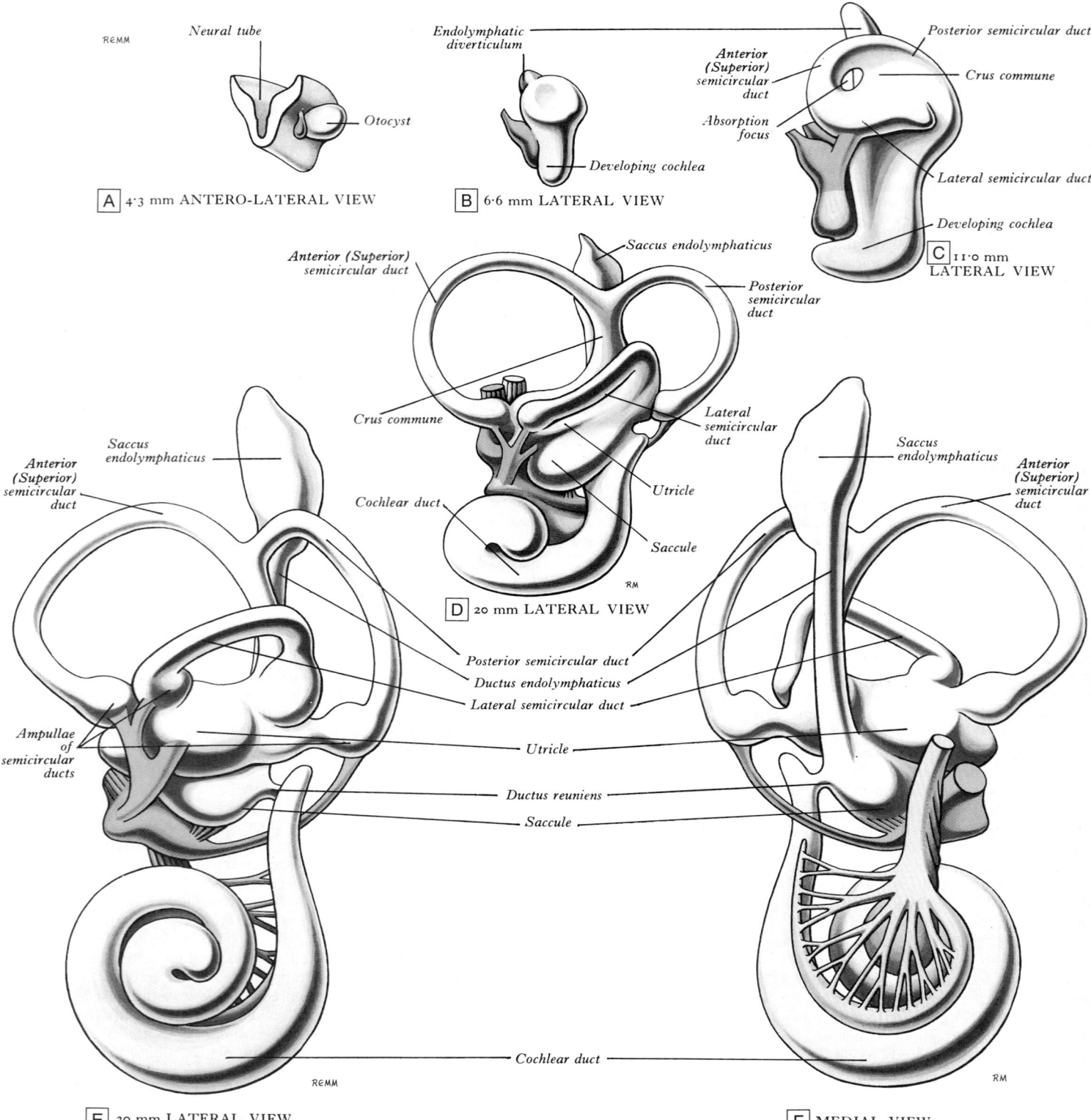

3.130 Diagrams showing the stages in the development of the membranous labyrinth from the otocyst, at the embryonic stages and viewed from the aspects indicated. Note also the relationship of the vestibular (orange) and cochlear (yellow) parts of the vestibulocochlear nerve. (From a series of models prepared by His.)

chamber three compressed diverticula appear as disc-like evaginations; the central parts of the walls of the discs coalesce and disappear while the peripheral portions of the discs persist as *semicircular ducts*; the anterior duct is completed first, and the lateral last. From the ventral part of the utriculosaccular chamber arises a medially directed evagination which progressively coils as the *cochlear duct*; its proximal extremity constricts as the *ductus reuniens*. The central part of the chamber now represents the membranous vestibule, divided into a smaller ventral *saccule* and a larger *utricle* mainly by horizontal infolding which extends from the lateral wall towards the opening of the ductus endolymphaticus, leaving only a narrow *utriculosaccular duct* between its divisions. This duct becomes acutely bent on itself, its apex being continuous with the ductus endolymphaticus. During this period the membranous labyrinth undergoes a rotation so that the long axis, originally vertical, becomes more or less horizontal (Bast & Anson 1949). Subsequently, otocyst derived cells, having contributed placodal cells to the vestibulocochlear ganglion, differentiate into the specialized paraneuronal hair cells of the utricle, saccule, ampullae of the semicircular ducts, and organ of Corti; they also differentiate into various specialized sustentacular cells and the unique epithelia of the stria vascularis and endolymphatic sac. The remainder form the general epithelial lining of the rest of the membranous labyrinth.

The mesenchyme surrounding the various parts of the epithelial labyrinth is converted into a *cartilaginous otic capsule*, and this is finally ossified to form most of the *bony labyrinth* of the internal ear. (Exceptions are the modiolus and osseous spiral lamina—see below.) For a time the cartilaginous capsule is incomplete and the cochlear, vestibular and facial ganglia are situated in the gap between its canalicular and cochlear parts. These ganglia are soon covered by an outgrowth of cartilage and at the same time the facial nerve is covered in by a growth of cartilage from the cochlear to the canalicular part of the capsule. In the embryonic connective tissue between the cartilaginous capsule and the epithelial wall of the labyrinth the perilymphatic spaces are developed. The rudiment of the *periotic cistern* or vestibular perilymphatic space can be seen in an embryo of from 30 to 40 mm in length in the reticulum between the saccule and the fenestra vestibuli. The scala tympani is next developed and begins opposite the fenestra cochleae; the scala vestibuli is the last to appear (Streeter 1917). The two scalae gradually extend along each side of the ductus cochlearis, and when they reach the tip of the ductus a communication, the *helicotrema*, is developed between them. The modiolus and the osseous spiral lamina of the cochlea are not preformed in cartilage but ossified directly from connective tissue.

Auditory tube and tympanic cavity. These are developed from a hollow, termed the *tubotympanic recess* (Frazer 1914), between the first and third pharyngeal arches, the floor of the recess consisting of the second arch and its limiting pouches. By the forward growth of the third arch the inner part of the recess is narrowed to form the tubal region, and the inner part of the second arch is excluded from this portion of the floor. The more lateral part of the recess subsequently develops into the *tympanic cavity* and the floor of this part forms the lateral wall of the tympanic cavity up to about the level of the chorda tympani nerve. From this it will be seen that the lateral wall of the tympanic cavity contains first and second arch elements, the first arch being limited to the part in front of the anterior process of the malleus. The second arch forms the outer wall behind this and turns on to the back wall to take in the tympanohyal region. Some observations, however, indicate that the tympanic cavity is derived wholly from the first pouch (Kanagasuntheram 1967). The tubotympanic recess is at first inferolateral to the cartilaginous otic capsule, but as the latter enlarges the relations become altered and the tympanic cavity becomes anterolateral. A cartilaginous process grows from the lateral part of the capsule to form the tegmen tympani and it curves caudally to form the lateral wall of the auditory tube. In this way, subsequent to ossification, the tympanic cavity and the proximal part of the auditory tube become included in the petrous region of the temporal bone. During the sixth or seventh month the mastoid antrum appears as a dorsal expansion of the tympanic cavity. Much of the cavity's

basic development thus occurs during *fetal* life (Bok 1966). A study of the posterior part of the tympanic cavity and in particular of the sinus tympani, a recess between the promontory and pyramid (p. 1373), emphasizes the late fetal development of this region (Bollobas & Hajdu 1975).

The opinion long held as to the development of the auditory ossicles was that the *malleus* derived from the dorsal end of the ventral mandibular (Meckel's) cartilage and the *incus* from the dorsal cartilage, probably corresponding to the quadrate bone of birds and reptiles. The *stapes* stems mainly from the dorsal end of the cartilage of the second (hyoid) arch, first as a ring (*annulus stapedis*) encircling the small stapedial artery (p. 314). The primordium of the stapedius muscle appears close to the artery and facial nerve at the end of the second month, and at almost the same time the tensor tympani begins to appear near the extremity of the tubotympanic recess (Candiollo & Levi 1969). Detailed analysis of early embryos concerning the *mesenchymal* origins of the blastemal ossicles, however, differs from the foregoing. Each ossicle has at least **two** distinct sources (see p. 277 and Hanson et al 1962).

At first the ossicles are embedded in the mesenchymal roof of the tympanic cavity and their extraneous origin is indicated in the adult by the covering which they receive from its mucous lining.

EXTERNAL EAR

The external acoustic meatus is developed from the dorsal end of the hyomandibular or first pharyngeal groove. Close to its dorsal extremity this groove extends inwards as a funnel-shaped *primary meatus* from which the cartilaginous part and a small area of the roof of the osseous meatus are developed. From this funnel-shaped tube a solid epidermal plug extends inwards along the floor of the tubotympanic recess; by the breaking down of the central cells of this plug the inner part of the meatus (*secondary meatus*) is produced, while its deepest ectodermal cells form the epidermal stratum of the *tympanic membrane*. The fibrous stratum of the membrane is formed from the mesenchyme between the meatal plate and the endodermal floor of the tubotympanic recess.

The development of the *auricle* is initiated by the appearance of six hillocks which form round the margins of the dorsal portion of the hyomandibular groove. Of the six, three are on the caudal edge of the mandibular arch and three on the cranial edge of the hyoid arch (**3.142**F). These hillocks appear at the 4 mm stage but they tend to become obscured as development proceeds and of those on the mandibular arch only the most ventral, which subsequently forms the *tragus*, can be identified throughout. The remainder of the auricle follows proliferation of the mesenchyme of the hyoid arch (Streeter 1922), which extends forwards round the dorsal end of the remains of the hyomandibular groove, forming a keel-like elevation—the forerunner of the *helix*. The contribution made by the mandibular arch to the auricle is greatest at the end of the second month; as growth continues, it is relatively reduced; eventually the area of skin supplied by the mandibular nerve extends little above the tragus. The lobule is the last part of the auricle to develop.

The rudiment of the eighth nerve appears in the fourth week as the *vestibulocochlear ganglion*, which lies between the otocyst and the wall of the hindbrain. At first it is fused with the ganglion of the facial nerve (*acousticofacial ganglion*) but later the two separate. The cells of the vestibulocochlear ganglion are mainly derived from the placodal ectoderm (see above); the ganglion divides into *vestibular* and *cochlear parts*, each associated with the corresponding division of the eighth nerve. The cells of these ganglia remain bipolar throughout life, each sending a proximal fibre into the brainstem, and a peripheral fibre to the internal ear. These neurons are also unusual in that many of their *somata* become enveloped in thin *myelin sheaths*.

The ganglionic fibres just described provide, of course, the afferent, sensory innervation of the labyrinthine hair cells. The latter soon become associated with the *outgrowing* axons from cells of the superior olivary complexes of the pons which provide an efferent innervation, the *olivocochlear bundle* (p. 1394). Development details are, however, lacking in mankind.

MUSCULOSKELETAL SYSTEM

The development of the musculoskeletal system is complex, requiring the coordinated integration of mesenchymal derivatives from different parts of the embryo and a variety of epithelial/mesenchymal interaction. Three distinct subpopulations of mesenchyme produce the majority of the system.

- *Paraxial mesenchyme* gives rise to the striated muscle throughout the head, trunk and limbs, virtually exclusively via the somites or preoccipital somitomeres (although axial mesenchyme from the prechordal plate produces the extrinsic eye muscles).
- *Somatopleuric mesenchyme* and a discrete portion of each somite, in the main, give rise to the skeletal elements, ligaments, tendons, fasciae, muscular and dermal connective tissue throughout the trunk and limbs. The former also patterns the development of the nerves, muscles and blood vessels in these locations.
- *Neural crest mesenchyme* produces the skeletal elements of the viscerocranium and much of the neurocranium, the ligaments, tendons, fasciae and muscular connective tissue throughout the head, including the meninges and dermal connective tissues. The neural crest also patterns the development of the nerves, muscles and blood vessels in these locations.

Germinal epithelia, which provide the populations of mesenchyme cells for these fates, are generated locally in the somites, each of which provides a discrete germinal epithelial plate for the production of myoblasts, and more extensively in the proliferating somatopleuric mesothelium. Neural crest cells proliferate as they migrate and also in situ. In all cases epithelial tissue close to the mesenchyme, often specifically ectoderm, contributes to the developmental processes by initiating some differentiation pathways and preventing others.

Because of the diversity of cell populations which contribute to the musculoskeletal system, its development will be considered in the following order:

(1) Development of the axial structures
—development of the musculoskeletal tissues of the trunk, i.e. the vertebral column and associated muscles. These structures are formed by the paraxial mesenchyme which surrounds the neural tube and notochord, and laterally by somatopleuric mesenchyme.
—development of the musculoskeletal tissues of the head, i.e. the skull and associated muscles. These structures are formed by several mesenchymal populations, i.e. a specialized portion of the axial musculoskeletal tissue, a mesenchymal population from the prechordal plate and a significant mesenchymal population from the ectodermal neural crest.

(2) Development of the appendicular structures
The musculoskeletal tissues of the limbs are formed from both somatopleuric mesenchyme and paraxial mesenchyme.

Our understanding of the general development of the connective and muscular tissues in the skeletal system has improved significantly with the advances in molecular biology and it is possible to see common developmental pathways which are followed by all myoblasts, chondroblasts or fibroblasts, etc. regardless of their site of origin. A brief account of some of these basic mechanisms may assist the interpretation of more specific events.

General development of connective tissue cells

The most fundamental facet of connective tissue differentiation is the production of mesenchymal condensations which, according to Atchley and Hall (1991), are the basic units from which morphology is constructed during development. Five developmental criteria identify a condensation:

- the number of stem cells
- the time of condensation initiation
- the mitotically active fraction
- the rate of cell division
- the rate of cell death.

These criteria may vary individually or in concert producing variability in developmental processes. A condensation is the first cellular product of epithelial/mesenchymal tissue interactions. (For

a general account of epithelial/mesenchymal interactions, see p. 110.) The formation of a mesenchymal condensation is associated with formation of gap junctions that allow intercellular communication followed by production of extracellular matrix molecules, if sufficient cells are associated within a condensation (Hall & Miyake 1992). The type and quantity of the matrix can induce and maintain production of further matrix molecules by competent cells. Particular matrix molecules are associated with specific developmental lineages and can be used to distinguish different cell fates, for example an osteogenic fate from a chondrogenic.

It is not yet clear how cells are committed to a connective tissue lineage; however, it has been shown that single mesenchyme cells will differentiate into chondroblasts if they are maintained in a rounded configuration. Connective tissue develops from mesenchyme of different origins, for example from somatopleuric mesenchyme, cephalic neural crest cells and parts of the somite (splanchnopleuric mesenchyme also in association with the viscera). The formation of cartilage has been extensively studied; however, less is known about the development of the widespread range of connective tissue or the origin of the osteoblastic lineage. Chondrogenesis is generally initiated from mesenchyme in response to an extracellular matrix mediated interaction, either via a basal lamina as in the sclerotomes (see below), or via an ectodermal mesenchymal interaction as in the limbs and facial processes (see below). Sclerotomal cells are already determined to a chondrogenic lineage, perhaps even before somite formation; interaction with the basal laminae of the notochord and neural tube enhances the differentiation process. The mesenchyme of the limb requires both the presence of an ectodermal sleeve early in development and then subsequent interaction with extracellular matrix products for both chondrogenic and fibrocyte differentiation. A high cell density in the core of the limb is required for chondrogenic differentiation whilst an antichondrogenic zone immediately beneath the ectoderm seems to prevent the differentiation of cartilage within the dermis and myogenic zone. Limb buds cultured in the coelomic cavity usually chondrify in their peripheral zones where the ectoderm is lacking or replaced by another kind of epithelium (Brand et al 1985). The ectoderm is believed to produce matrix molecules which encourage cell flattening and fibrogenic differentiation (Christ et al 1986). Expression of type II collagen in mesenchyme cells is often a sign of terminal differentiation along a chondrogenic lineage. The ultimate fate of such cells is production of type X collagen; when this occurs the cells hypertrophy and will ultimately die. Hypertrophied cells can start the mineralization process within the expanded cartilage lacunae. Regions of persistent cartilage, (e.g. trachea, pinna, etc.) do not permit the final differentiation fate of the cell line.

The factors promoting osteoblast development are not clear. Osteogenesis coincides with the vascularization of either a cartilage model, as in *endochondral ossification*, or of a mesenchymal condensation directly, as in *intramembranous ossification*. Ossification occurs at a much slower rate than chondrogenesis (for a fuller description of these processes see p. 471). Chondroclasts and osteoclasts have been identified in older developing limbs remodelling developing bone and cartilage; they may represent the same cell line in different locations (Jacob at al 1986). Adipocytes are also related to chondroblasts and osteoblasts and fibroblasts.

General development of skeletal muscle

A myogenic lineage, noted by the expression of myogenic determination factors, can be demonstrated transitorily in some cells shortly after their ingression through the primitive streak. The skeletal muscle found throughout the body is derived from the paraxial mesenchyme which segments to form the somites (see also development of the extrinsic ocular muscles).

Cells committed to a myogenic lineage will undergo a series of proliferative mitotic divisions prior to passage through a *terminal division* resulting in their restriction as *postmitotic myoblasts*. Postmitotic myoblasts can begin to transcribe the mRNAs for the major contractile proteins *actin* and *myosin* as well as a number of regulatory proteins of muscle contraction. Finally postmitotic myoblasts will assume a characteristic spindle shape and begin to fuse with one another, creating a tube-like *syncytium*, the *myotube*. (Interestingly myoblasts from different vertebrates will fuse to form hybrid myotubes.) Subsequent to fusion, *myofibrils* assemble in the periphery of the myotube. The early myofibrils develop the cross-striated organization first at the Z line, an *a*-actinin rich structure that anchors the actin filaments to form the I-Z-I complexes, and later in the A band region, occupied by the myosin filaments. Sarcomere formation proceeds from the periphery towards the centre of the myotubes. When this process is complete, the nuclei migrate from the centre to the periphery, and the syncytium is now called a *myofibre*. Myofibrils align laterally with one another, the sarcoplasmic reticulum and T-tubules become arranged in transverse orientation, and the myofibre continues to grow by splitting of myofibrils as well as by addition of new myofibrils.

During development at least three populations of myoblast are formed. Embryonic myoblasts give rise to primary myotubes and muscle fibres, and thus embryonic muscle. Subsequently smaller, secondary myotubes and muscle fibres arise from late myoblasts. Finally satellite cells which are also contained within the basal lamina differentiate. These latter cells may divide in postnatal life to provide new myoblasts to fuse with the muscle fibres ensuring growth of the muscle. For more information on subsets of muscle fibres consult Section 7.

The development of the central nervous system is crucial for normal formation of the *fetal* myoblast lineage. Formation of secondary fibres appears to be nerve dependent; the number of secondary fibres is reduced by denervation. It is suggested that secondary myotubes are initiated only at sites of innervation of primary myotubes.

AXIAL SKELETON AND MUSCLES

Somitogenesis

Cells destined to become paraxial mesenchyme ingress through the lateral aspect of the primitive node and rostral primitive streak (**3**.42); the mesenchyme cells thus formed retain contact with both the epiblast and hypoblast basal laminae as they migrate to their paraxial position and this persists for some time after reaching their destination.

After the onset of neurulation the paraxial mesenchyme caudal to the otic vesicle undergoes segmentation (**3**.131) in a craniocaudal progression forming discrete clusters of mesenchyme cells; this stage is termed *compaction*. In each tight cluster of paraxial mesenchyme the cells re-establish juxtaluminal junctions and organize themselves into an *epithelial somite*. The cells of the epithelial somite are polarized with respect to a central lumen which contains some mesenchymal core cells. The Golgi apparatus and mitotic figures are located in the apical region of the cells, as are actin and *a*-actinin; cilia develop on the free surface. The cells are joined by tight junctions and the basal surface rests on a basal lamina containing collagen, laminin, fibronectin and cytotactin (Keynes & Stern 1988). Processes from the somite cells pass through this basal lamina to contact the basal laminae of the neural tube and notochord (Hay 1968). A variety of cell adhesion molecules have been demonstrated in epithelial somites. It is worth noting that a single somite can be described as having six faces, like a cube; it is now apparent that each facet has a slightly different fate. Further, the position along the embryo may alter the developmental fate of parts of the somite.

The epithelial somite undergoes rapid development in the following manner: the cells of the ventromedial wall seem to be pulled towards the notochord, and despite extensive juxtaluminal junctions the cells break apart. The newly formed mesenchymal cells, collectively termed the *sclerotome*, migrate medially towards the notochord; they will give rise to the bones, joints and ligaments of the vertebral column (see below). The remaining cells of the somite are now termed the *epithelial plate of the somite* or the *dermomyotome*. This epithelium produces the cell lines which will give rise to (nearly) all the striated muscles of the body. Three separate myogenic lines can be seen. Firstly, cells produced along the *craniomedial edge of the epithelial plate* elongate from the cranial to the caudal edge on the underside of the basal lamina of the plate; they are collectively termed the *myotome*. (The latter term was previously used to describe *all* the

muscle forming cells of the somite; now it is usually restricted to cells deriving from the craniomedial edge.) They will give rise to the skeletal muscle dorsal to the vertebrae, the epaxial musculature (see below). Secondly, after initiation of the myotome, cells produced from the *ventrolateral edge of the epithelial plate*, opposite the limb bud, migrate into the developing limb to give rise to its skeletal muscle (see below). Lastly, the *remaining epithelial plate* (and underlying myotome cells) *grows into the flank region of the body*. The epithelial plate is still proliferating at the beginning of this stage. Later the epithelial plate cells revert to mesenchyme and processes from contiguous somites fuse to form a unified premuscular mass which gives rise to the ventrolateral muscles of the body wall (see below).

It was, for long, the case that once the myotome cells could be identified the remaining epithelial plate was termed the dermatome, its fate being described as forming the dermis of the skin. However, it is now clear that the epithelial plate continues to provide a significant source of myogenic precursor cells as it elongates into the body wall. Thus the detailed intimate relationship between the epithelial plate/dermatome, the generation of myogenic cells and the patterning of the epidermis of the skin is, as yet, by no means clear (see later). Studies describing a somitic contribution to the dermis, from the dermatome, localize it to the dermis over the epaxial muscles (Christ et al 1983), a much smaller distribution than the segmental portion of skin usually implied by this term.

The rate of somite formation has been estimated at approximately one pair every 3 hours (Menkes et al 1961; Chernoff & Lash 1981). The regularity of somite formation provides criteria for staging embryos; staging schemes have been developed both by Lash and Ostrovsky (1986) and by Ordahl (1993). Lash and Ostrosky describe five stages, from somitomere identification (see above) to the production of an epithelial somite distinct from the presegmental plate. Ordahl notes that morphogenetic events occur in successive somites at approximately the same rate. He designates the somite most recently formed from the segmental plate (stage 5 of Lash & Ostrovsky) as stage I, the next most recent as stage II, etc. After the embryo forms an additional somite, the ages of the previously formed somites increase by one roman numeral. In this conceptualization of somitogenesis compaction occurs at stage I; epithelialization at stages II to III; formation of mesenchymal sclerotome cells from stage V; myotome formation at stage VI; early migration of the ventrolateral lip of the epithelial plate and production of myotome cells can still be seen at stage X.

Differences have been identified in the fates of each of the six facets of a somite. Firstly the medial and lateral halves of the early epithelial somite have different origins and fates, later the cranial and caudal halves of the epithelial plate differ and finally the cranial and caudal halves of the sclerotome have different properties and fates. Experimental studies have shown that the precise developmental fates of these portions of the somite may be prescribed as the precursor cells ingress from the epiblast. Compaction and epithelialization may then shuffle these cells into their appropriate positions in the somite prior to migration.

Selleck and Stern (1991) have shown that the medial halves of somites are formed from cells migrating through the lateral portion of Hensen's node; the lateral halves derive from ingression through the primitive streak approximately 200 µm caudal to the node. The two somite halves do not seem to intermingle. The *medial half of the somite* produces both the *sclerotome* and the *myotome* (*epaxial musculature*); the *lateral half of the somite* provides the *hypaxial* and *limb musculature* (Ordahl & Le Douarin 1992; Ordahl 1993). (Interestingly the innervations of these muscle groups are provided by the posterior ramus of a spinal nerve for the epaxial muscles, and the ventral ramus for the hypaxial and limb muscles.) Of the other facets, the cranial portion of the epithelial plate is the site of origin of the myotome (see below). Differences in the craniocaudal fates of the portions of the somites have been studied in the development of the sclerotomes (see below).

Formation of the vertebrae from sclerotomes

The sclerotome forms from the ventromedial border of the epithelial somite. An *intrasegmental boundary* (fissure or cleft) appears within the *sclerotome* dividing it into loosely packed *cranial* and densely packed *caudal* halves; this boundary is initially filled with extracellular matrix and only few cells. The epithelial plate and later the myotome

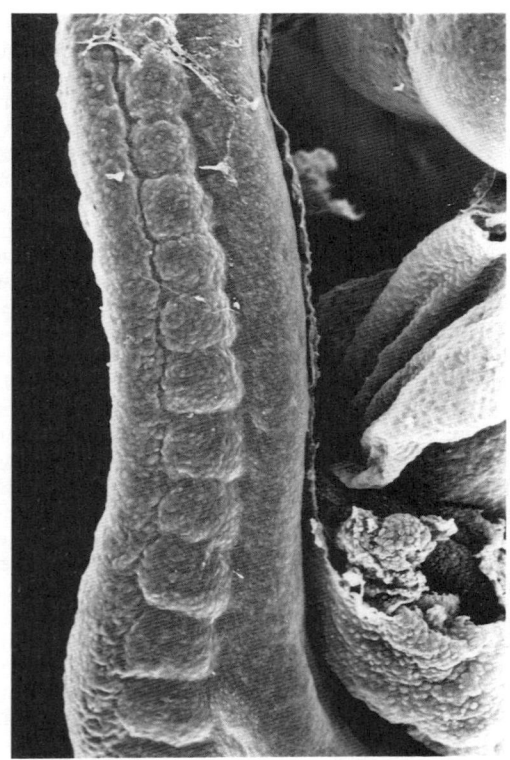

spans the two half-sclerotomes. The sclerotomal cells migrate towards the notochord which they surround, and with which they undergo a matrix-mediated interaction, differentiating chondrogenetically to form the cartilaginous precursor of the vertebral body. The peri-notochordal sheath transiently expresses type II collagen which is believed to initiate type II collagen expression, and thereafter a chondrogenic fate, in those mesenchyme cells which contact it (see also development of the chondrocranium, p. 274). Each *vertebra* is formed by the combination of much of the *caudal half of one bilateral pair of sclerotomes with much of the cranial half of the next caudal pair of sclerotomes.* Their fusion around the notochord produces the blastemal centrum of the vertebra (**3**.132; see also **3**.134). The mesenchyme adjoining the intrasegmental sclerotomic fissure now increases greatly in density forming a well-defined *perichordal disc.* This intervenes between the successive centra of two vertebrae and is the future annulus fibrosis of the intervertebral symphysis ('disc').

The boundary of the head and neck corresponds to the boundary between the 5th and 6th somites. The first true somite disappears early and somites 2–5 (occipital 1–4) fuse to form the basioccipital bone (see, however, preoccipital somitomeres). The vertebrae are formed from the 6th somite caudally, C1 being formed by the caudal

3.131A Scanning electron micrograph of a lateral view of an embryo showing the somites. The cranial somites are at the lower border and the more caudal somites are at the upper border. A change in size of the cranially more advanced somites is apparent. (Photograph by P Collins; printed by S Cox, Electron Microscopy Unit, Southampton General Hospital.)

Somitogenesis

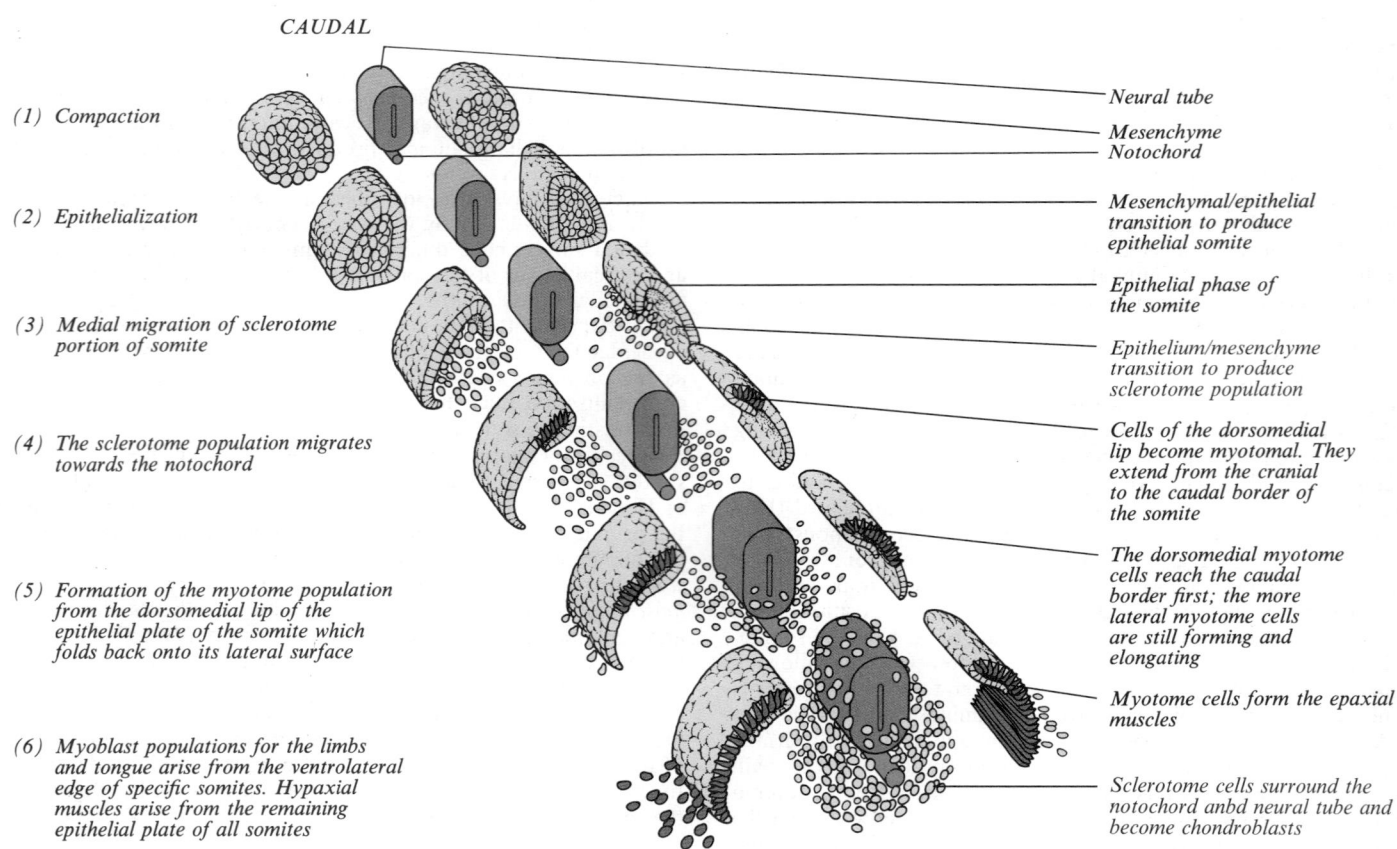

(1) *Compaction*

(2) *Epithelialization*

(3) *Medial migration of sclerotome portion of somite*

(4) *The sclerotome population migrates towards the notochord*

(5) *Formation of the myotome population from the dorsomedial lip of the epithelial plate of the somite which folds back onto its lateral surface*

(6) *Myoblast populations for the limbs and tongue arise from the ventrolateral edge of specific somites. Hypaxial muscles arise from the remaining epithelial plate of all somites*

CAUDAL

Neural tube

Mesenchyme
Notochord

Mesenchymal/epithelial transition to produce epithelial somite

Epithelial phase of the somite

Epithelium/mesenchyme transition to produce sclerotome population

Cells of the dorsomedial lip become myotomal. They extend from the cranial to the caudal border of the somite

The dorsomedial myotome cells reach the caudal border first; the more lateral myotome cells are still forming and elongating

Myotome cells form the epaxial muscles

Sclerotome cells surround the notochord anbd neural tube and become chondroblasts

CRANIAL

3.131B The stages of somitogenesis. Development proceeds in a cranio-caudal progression. The more cranially placed somites (at the lower right of the figure) are further developed than those caudally placed (at the upper left of the figure). The stages in somitogenesis are given on the left of the figure; more detailed information is given on the right.

half of occipital somite 4 and the cranial half of cervical somite 1 (**3**.132, 133). This shift of somite number and vertebral number accounts for the production of seven cervical vertebrae from eight cervical somites.

The basic pattern of a typical vertebra is initiated by this recombination of caudal and cranial sclerotome halves, followed by differential growth and sculpturing of the sclerotomal mesenchyme which encases the notochord and neural tube. This is the blastemal stage of vertebral development (**3**.134). As noted, the *centrum* encloses the notochord and lies ventral to the neural tube. From the dorsolateral angles of the centrum the neural arch curves to enclose the neural tube; from the zones of neurocentral confluence the arch comprises paired bilateral pedicles (ventrolaterally) and laminae (dorsolaterally) which coalesce in the midline dorsal to the neural tube. From the latter arises the anlage of the vertebral spine. On each side three further processes are delineated, projecting from the junction of pedicle and lamina cranially, caudally and laterally. The cranial and caudal projections are the blastemal *articular processes* (zygapophyses) and these become contiguous with reciprocal processes of adjacent vertebrae, their junctional zones the future zygapophyseal joints. The lateral projections are the true vertebral *transverse processes* (see below). Finally, growing anterolaterally from the ventral part of the pedicles, i.e. near the centrum, from the neighbouring perichordal disc, and, at most thoracic levels, with accessions from the next caudal adjacent pedicles, bilateral *costal processes* develop; these expand to meet the tips of the transverse processes. Note that the definitive vertebral *body* is compound, a median centrum and ventral expanded pedicle ends (bilateral) dorsolaterally.

In *cervical vertebrae* (**3**.134) the transverse process is dorsomedial to the foramen transversarium, while the costal process, corresponding to the head, neck and tubercle of a rib, limits the foramen ventrolaterally and dorsolaterally. The distal parts of these cervical costal processes do not normally develop; occasionally they do so in the case of the seventh cervical vertebra, even developing costo-

vertebral joints. Such *cervical ribs* may reach the sternum (p. 268). In the thoracic region the *thoracic costal processes* attain their maximum length as *the ribs* (see below). The extent of the transverse and costal processes of each vertebra can be compared in (**3**.134).

The *type* of vertebra is specified very early in development. If a group of thoracic somites is transplanted to the cervical region, ribs will still develop (Kieny et al 1972; Goldstein & Kalcheim 1992). Interestingly it is the sclerotome which is restricted; the myotome will produce muscle characteristic of the new location. At present the exact contribution of the caudal and rostral parts of the sclerotomes to the neural arches, pedicles and laminae and articular and transverse processes are not yet entirely clear (Bagnall et al 1988; Goldstein & Kalcheim 1992); similarly the exact origin of the intervertebral disc has not been established.

Condensation of the sclerotomal mesenchyme around the notochord can be seen in stage 15 human embryos as can right and left neural processes. Chondrification begins at stage 17, initiating the cartilaginous stage (**3**.134). Each centrum chondrifies from one cartilage anlage (Uhthoff 1990). Each half of a neural arch is chondrified from a centre starting in its base and extending ventrally into the pedicles, to meet, expand and blend with the centrum, and dorsally into the laminae. By stage 23 there are 33 or 34 cartilaginous vertebrae; however, the spinous processes have not yet developed giving a general appearance of total spina bifida occulta. Fusion of the spines does not occur until the fourth month. The transverse and articular processes are chondrified in continuity with the neural arches; intervening zones of mesenchyme which do not become cartilage mark the sites of their interarticular (zygapophyseal) joints and the complex of costovertebral joints, and synovial cavities appear later in these.

In general the thoracic spine develops ahead of the cervical and lumbar spine; however, towards the end of the second month ossification commences in the cartilaginous vertebrae in a craniocaudal progression. After 16 weeks it has progressed to L5 and ossification of each additional vertebra occurs over a period of 2–3

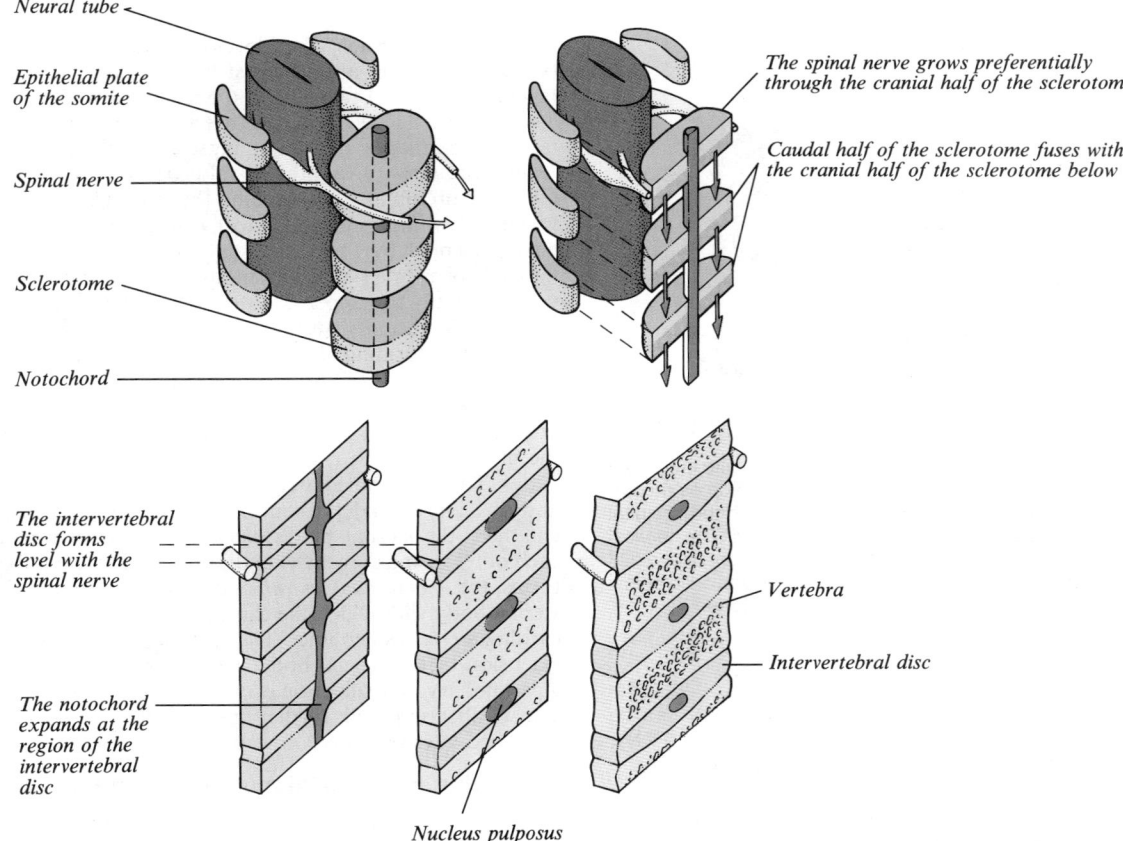

Neural tube

Epithelial plate of the somite

Spinal nerve

Sclerotome

Notochord

The spinal nerve grows preferentially through the cranial half of the sclerotome

Caudal half of the sclerotome fuses with the cranial half of the sclerotome below

The intervertebral disc forms level with the spinal nerve

The notochord expands at the region of the intervertebral disc

Vertebra

Intervertebral disc

Nucleus pulposus

3.132 Formation of vertebrae and intervertebral discs from the mesenchymal sclerotomes. Each vertebra is formed from the cranial half of one bilateral pair of chromosomes and the caudal half of the next pair of sclerotomes. The spinal nerves preferentially migrate through the cranial portion of the sclerotomes. (After Tuckmann-Daplessis & Hagel 1972).

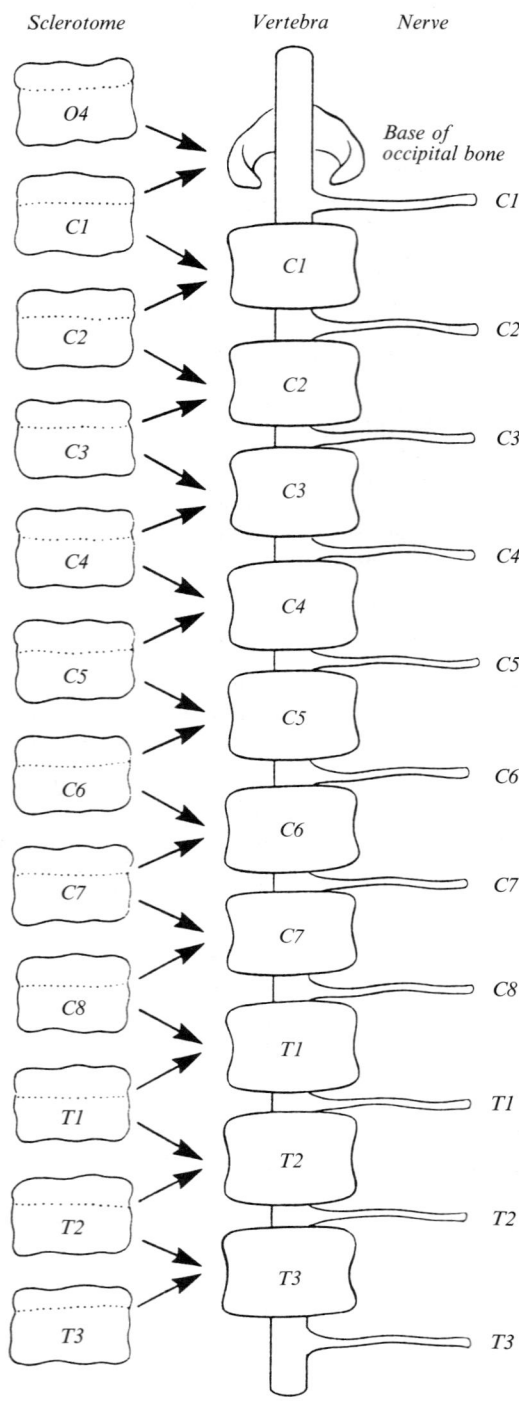

Sclerotome   *Vertebra*   *Nerve*

3.133 Contribution of the somites to the vertebrae. Each somite induces a ventral root to grow out from the spinal cord. When the sclerotomes recombine the cranial half of the first cervical sclerotome fuses with the occipital sclerotome above contributing to the occipital bone of the skull. The cervical nerves beginning with C1 exit above the corresponding vertebra. Nerve C8 exits below the last cervical vertebra (C7). After this level nerves arise below their vertebrae. (From Larsen, Embryology Churchill Livingstone.)

weeks with S2 being ossified by 22 weeks. In most cases S1 can be located at the level of the top of the iliac crest (Budorick 1991). Further details of ossification are described elsewhere (p. 471).

Intervertebral discs. Whereas the sclerotomal mesenchyme forming the body of the vertebrae replaces the notochordal tissue which it surrounds, between the developing vertebrae the notochord expands as localized aggregates of cells and matrix, thus forming the *nucleus pulposus* of the intervertebral disc (3.132, 134). This nucleus is surrounded by the intermediate part of each *perichordal disc*

which forms the annulus fibrosus and differentiates into an external laminated fibrous zone and an internal cuff around the nucleus pulposus. The inner zone contributes to the growth of the outer, and near the end of the second month of embryonic life it begins to merge with the notochordal tissue, being ultimately converted into fibrocartilage. After the sixth month of fetal life notochordal cells in the nucleus pulposus degenerate, being replaced by cells from the internal zone of the annulus fibrosus. This degeneration continues until the second decade of life, by which time all the notochordal cells have disappeared (p. 513). Thus, in the adult, notochordal vestiges are limited, at the most, to non-cellular matrix.

It is to be re-emphasized here that the original sclerotomes are coextensive with the individual *metameric body segments*, and that each sclerotomic fissure, perichordal disc, and finally the maturing intervertebral disc lies opposite the *centre* of each *fundamental body segment*. From this, it follows that the discs also correspond in level to (i.e. form the anterior boundary of) the intervertebral foramina, their contained mixed spinal nerves, ganglia, vessels and sheaths. Posteriorly, bounding the foramina are the capsules of the synovial interarticular (zygapophyseal) joints. Cranially and caudally lie the rims of the vertebral notches of adjacent vertebrae. Thus all the structures listed (and other associated ones) are often designated *segmental*, whereas because of their mode of development, vertebral bodies are designated *intersegmental*.

Ribs, costal cartilages and sternum

Ribs. These develop from the costal processes of the primitive vertebral arches, extending between the myotomic muscle plates. The development of ribs is usually limited to the thoracic vertebrae although ribs can arise occasionally from the seventh cervical vertebra. In the thoracic region (3.134) costal processes grow laterally to form a series of *precartilaginous ribs*. The transverse processes grow laterally behind the vertebral ends of the costal processes, at first connected by mesenchyme which later becomes differentiated into the ligaments and other tissues of the costotransverse joints. The capitular costovertebral joints are similarly formed from mesenchyme between the proximal end of the costal processes and the perichordal disc, and adjacent neural arch derived parts of usually two (sometimes one) vertebral bodies. Ribs 1–7 (vertebrosternal) curve round the body wall to reach the developing sternal plates. Ribs 8–10 (vertebrochondral) are progressively more oblique and shorter, only reaching the costal cartilage of the rib above and contributing to the costal margin. Ribs 11 and 12 are free (floating), with cone-shaped terminal cartilages providing muscle attachments (see p. 541). In *lumbar vertebrae* (3.134) the costal processes do not develop distally, but their proximal parts become the 'transverse processes' of these vertebrae, whose morphologically *true* transverse processes may be represented by their accessory processes (p. 526). Occasionally, movable ribs may develop in association with the first lumbar vertebra. Only the upper two or three *sacral costal processes* usually develop significantly (3.134). They fuse into the lateral mass of the sacrum, forming its ventral part. The *coccygeal vertebrae* are apparently devoid of costal processes.

Sternum. This is formed from bilateral condensations of *somatopleuric mesenchyme* (Gumpel-Pinot 1984) immediately ventral to the primordia of the clavicles and ribs; these are termed the sternal plates. They are immediately ventral to the rudiments of the clavicles and ribs, but are independent of them in their formation. As the ribs lengthen, the sternal plates *chondrify* and move medially towards each other fusing across the midline in a craniocaudal direction. This forms the *manubrium sterni* and four *sternebrae* which form the sternal body with which the clavicles and upper seven pairs of costal cartilages establish contact. The *xiphoid process* develops as a caudal extension of the sternal body. Hypertrophy of the cartilage cells as a preliminary to ossification occurs opposite future intercostal spaces. The ossification and further growth of the sternum and ribs is described later (see 6.123, and p 539).

Formation of the axial muscles from myotomes

Myogenic determination factors, MyoD, myogenin, Myf 5 and herculin/MRF 4 can first be detected in the medial half of the somite as early as stage II (Ordahl 1993), several hours prior to the onset of myotome formation. The *myotome* is formed in the following manner: cells of the epithelial plate are mainly orientated per-

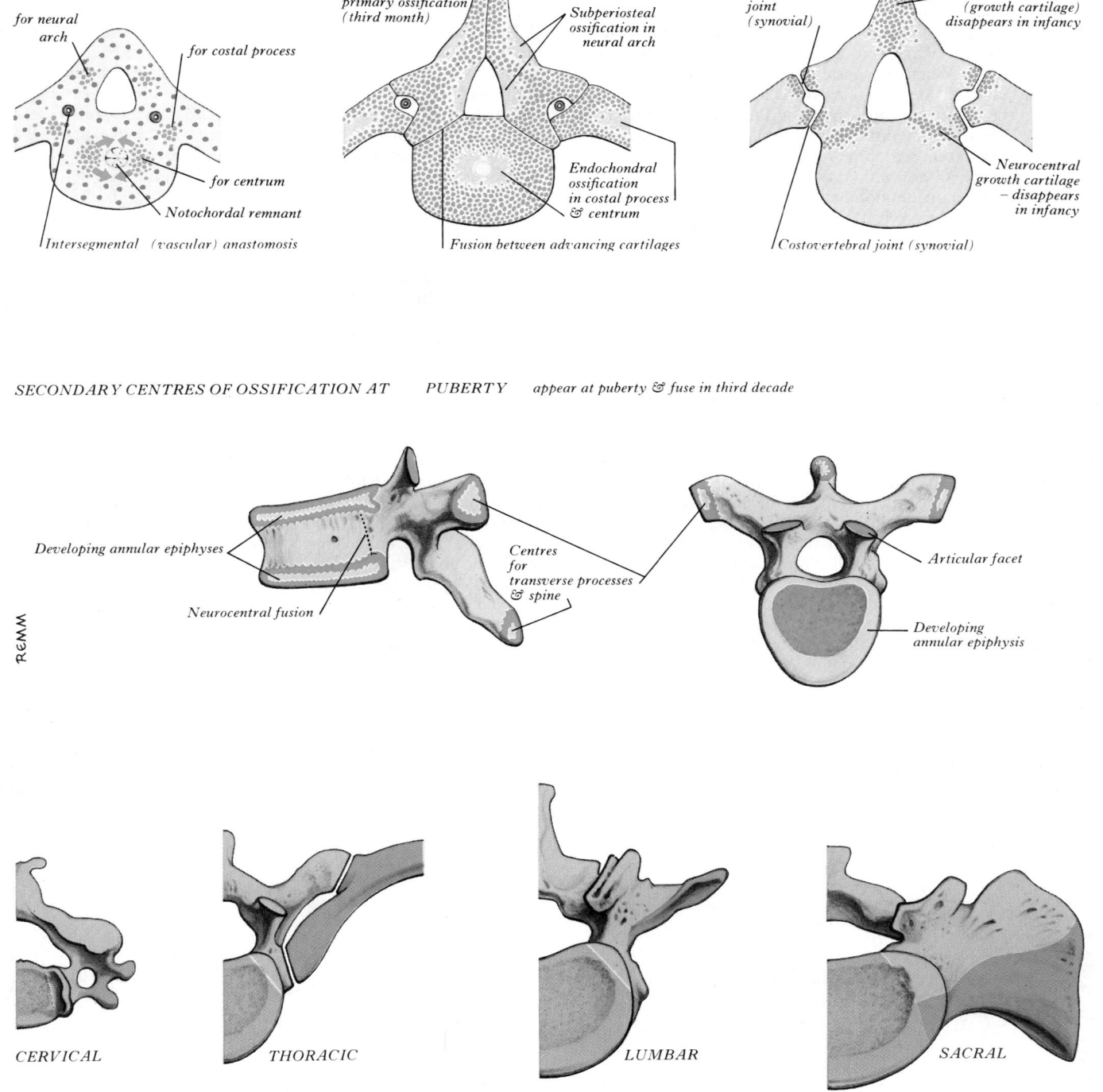

BLASTEMAL STAGE
with centres of chondrification

for neural arch

for costal process

for centrum

Notochordal remnant

Intersegmental (vascular) anastomosis

CARTILAGINOUS STAGE
with centres of primary ossification (third month)

Subperiosteal ossification in neural arch

Endochondral ossification in costal process & centrum

Fusion between advancing cartilages

OSSIFIC STAGE (perinatal)

Costotransverse joint (synovial)

Cartilaginous spine (growth cartilage) disappears in infancy

Neurocentral growth cartilage – disappears in infancy

Costovertebral joint (synovial)

SECONDARY CENTRES OF OSSIFICATION AT   *PUBERTY*   appear at puberty & fuse in third decade

Developing annular epiphyses

Neurocentral fusion

Centres for transverse processes & spine

Articular facet

Developing annular epiphysis

REMM

CERVICAL   *THORACIC*   *LUMBAR*   *SACRAL*

Parts of adult vertebrae derived from: CENTRA   *, NEURAL ARCHES*   *, COSTAL PROCESSES*   *of embryonic vertebrae*

3.134 Sequential diagrams of vertebral development through blastemal, cartilaginous and pre- and postnatal ossificatory stages. Bottom row indicates principal morphological parts of adult vertebrae.

pendicular to the back; however, the cells have different orientations according to their positions: they are transversely orientated along the dorsomedial edge and longitudinally orientated within the cranial edge of the epithelial plate (3.131). Myotome cells originate from the longitudinally orientated cells at the cranial edge of the epithelial plate. Individual cells are originally produced and anchored at the

269

craniomedial corner of the epithelial plate. Subsequently each sends a process to the caudal edge of the plate where it forms a second anchor point. Thus myotome formation continues caudally along the dorsomedial edge and laterally along the cranial edge. Each mononucleated, myotome cell thus becomes very elongated perpendicular to the cells of the epithelial plate. Development of subsequent cells produces a triangular shape of the myotome in its early formation. The growing myotome first reaches the caudal somite border on the medial side and later the ventrolateral edge (Kaehn et al 1988). When the vertebral bodies form, the future intervertebral fissure divides the sclerotome into rostral and caudal halves leaving the myotome fibres spanning the intervertebral joints and foramina. Thus the myotome derived muscles are always in a position to move adjacent vertebrae relative to each other.

Myotome cells are all *postmitotic embryonic myoblasts*; they fuse to form syncytia later in development (see above) to produce the *epaxial* musculature, the skeletal muscle dorsal to the vertebrae (erector spinae). The normal development of these myoblasts requires the presence of the neural tube (Christ 1970). It is also suggested that there is a possible interaction between precursor myotome cells and the medial neural crest cells which are commencing their migration at this time. The epaxial muscles are innervated by the dorsal ramus of each spinal nerve. The latter divides into its primary dorsal and ventral rami as it emerges from its intervertebral foramen (see above).

At much later stages *satellite cells* enter the myotome. Interestingly the development of endo-, peri- and epimysium in relation to the epaxial muscles has not been addressed; no population of connective tissue mesenchyme has yet been identified with this body region.

Ventrolateral trunk muscles. These are formed from the epithelial plate of the somite. After production of the myotome and the precursor myogenic cells of the limb, the remaining epithelial plate (and attached myotome) grows into the *flank somatopleuric mesenchyme*. At this stage the epithelial plate is still proliferating and producing myogenic precursor cells. The epithelial plate has a leading edge or process from which single cells or clusters of cells migrate in a ventral direction. It may be that these epithelial plate cells, which are in a more immature state of differentiation, act as *pioneer cells* for further cell movement (Jacob 1986). The previously segmented processes from adjacent epithelial plates form a *unified premuscular mass*. Both postmitotic myoblast cells and still dividing plate cells can be seen in the body wall; this may represent early and later forming myoblasts which will form heterokaryotic myotubes.

The *premuscular mass* subdivides into *abdominal muscle blastemata* for the *external* and *internal oblique* muscles, *transversus abdominis*

and *rectus abdominis*. At this time the number of somatopleural fibroblasts situated within the muscle-forming zone increases, and myotubes can be first seen. Lastly, there is a ventral shift of the already separated muscle blastemata within the growing abdominal wall to their definitive positions. During this process muscle differentiation continues and muscular connective tissue, tendons and aponeuroses develop.

The diaphragm. This is a partition between the thoracic and abdominal cavities; it derives from a variety of mesenchymal populations. Ventrally the *septum transversum mesenchyme* anchors the diaphragm to the anterior abdominal wall where it attaches to the xiphisternum and costal margin. The central portion of the diaphragm is formed from *splanchnopleuric mesenchyme* which surrounds the oesophagus and inferior vena cava and coats the pleuroperitoneal membranes. Laterally the diaphragm derives from the *somatopleuric mesenchyme* which is excavated by extension of the secondary pleural cavities into the costodiaphragmatic recesses. *Somitic myocytes* from the ventrolateral edge of the epithelial plate of somites C3, 4 and 5 migrate into the lateral regions of the diaphragm including the somatopleuric part. The central region becomes tendinous. The posterior attachment of the diaphragm descends to lower and lower positions until at the end of the second month it is opposite T12 or L1 (**3.135, 136**; see also p. 181).

Pelvic floor. This consists of the *ligamentous supports of the cervix*, and the *pelvic* and *urogenital diaphragms*, and constitutes another partition which traverses the body cavity. The dimensions of the pelvic cavity are much smaller than those at the caudal end of the thorax and the pelvic diaphragm is thus a smaller structure. Because of the irregular shape of the innominate bones the pelvic outlet has two planes which are filled by muscular groups arranged at different levels and directions. There is little information available about pelvic floor development in the human. The striated muscle derives from the somitic epithelial plates in a similar manner to the ventrolateral body wall. The *puborectalis* muscle appears in 20–30 mm embryos, following opening of the anal membrane, and striated muscle fibres can be seen at 15 weeks (Bourdelat 1992). Also at this time the smooth muscle of the urethral sphincter can be seen.

Upper and lower ends of the trunk. The upper and lower ends of the trunk are narrowed as a result of the development of axial structures cranially, and both axial and appendicular structures caudally. Cranially, the size of the ribs, the cervical pleura with its suprapleural membrane and the attached scalenus minimus muscle, together with the disposition of the other scaleni, create a narrow thoracic inlet which admits to the thorax only the contents of the root of the neck. Caudally, however, the pelvic outlet serves a dual

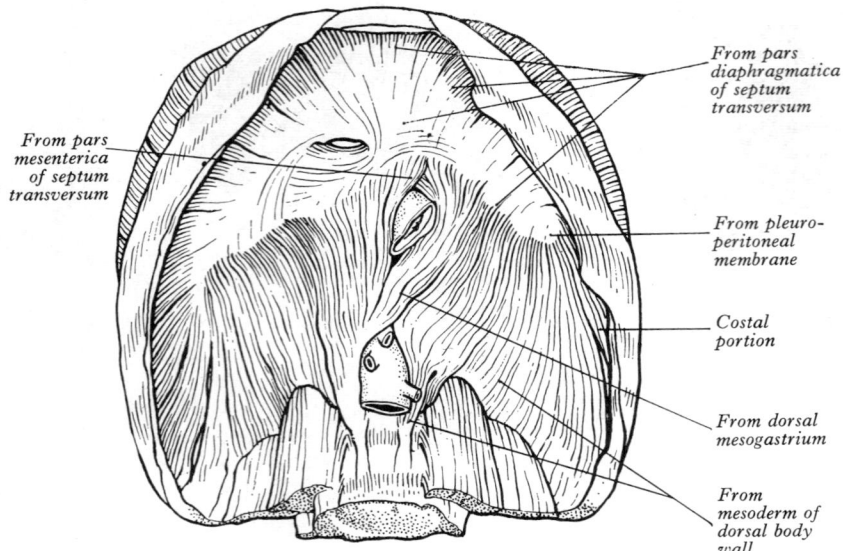

3.135 Inferior surface of the diaphragm showing the derivation of the different parts of its connective tissue framework. (After Wells 1954.)

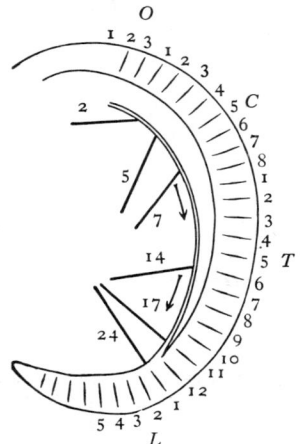

3.136 Schema showing stages in the descent of the dorsal attachment of the septum transversum. The numerals on the heavy lines indicate the length of the embryo in mm, and the position of the occipital, cervical, thoracic and lumbar segments is also shown. Note: straight lines ignore the true profile of the septum. (After Mall.)

function. It maintains the position of the pelvic organs and continence of the excretory organs by an arrangement of sphincter muscles. In addition, particularly with reference to the size of the human fetal head at term, the osteoligamentous boundary of the pelvic outlet, in the human, is relatively larger than that of all other quadrupeds; thus it requires a relatively extensive muscular and fibrous diaphragm.

HEAD

The head is composed of the skull surrounding the brain, and an outer covering of muscles, glands and skin. The skull has two distinct portions: that surrounding the brain and special sense organs—the *neurocranium*—and the lower face and jaws (also the palate, hyoid, epiglottis and larynx)—the *viscerocranium*. Each part derives from different mesenchymal populations and by different methods. The neurocranium develops from the *paraxial mesenchyme* in the head, i.e. the first five somites and the unsegmented somitomeres rostral to the first somite (Meier 1981), and from ectoderm via the *neural crest*. The basal portion of the skull is similar in structure and development to the vertebral column and is preformed in cartilage. The viscerocranium derives from ectoderm via invaginated head *neural crest* which streams into the developing arches forming all the connective tissue elements of the face. Bones of the viscerocranium form in the main from membranous ossification but there are cartilage models in each arch. The contribution of neural crest to the neurocranium in mammals is not yet clear, although it has been established in the chick that neural crest mesenchyme gives rise to the large bones lateral and dorsal to the brain by membranous ossification (Couly et al 1993). Lateral plate mesenchyme does not extend into the head (see p. 286).

NEUROCRANIUM

The bones of the skull (**3**.137) are developed in the mesenchyme which surrounds the cerebral vesicles but, before the osseous state is reached, the cranium passes through blastemal and cartilaginous stages like other parts of the skeleton. However, not all parts pass through a phase of chondrification; and hence the *chondrocranium* is incomplete, the remainder comprising the mesenchymatous, *blastemal desmocranium*. Most of the cranial vault and limited parts of its base are thus not preformed in cartilage. The mesenchymatous (membranous) and cartilaginous parts of the skull will, for convenience, be considered in sequence; they develop together and complement each other in forming the complete cranium, some of whose bones are composite structures derived from both sources. All elements, of course, pass first through a mesenchymatous phase (**3**.137).

The *blastemal skull* (desmocranium) begins to appear at the end of the first month as a condensation and thickening of the mesenchyme which surrounds the developing brain, forming localized masses which are the earliest distinguishable cranial elements. The first masses evident are in the occipital region, outlining the basilar (ventral) part of the occipital bone. These form an *occipital plate*, from which two extensions on each side grow laterally and spread to complete a foramen around each hypoglossal nerve. At the same time the mesenchymal condensation extends forwards, dorsal to the pharynx, to reach the primordium of the hypophysis, thus establishing the *clivus* of the cranial base and the *dorsum sellae* of the future sphenoid bone. Early in the second month it surrounds the developing stalk of the hypophysis and extends ventrally and rostrally between the two halves of the nasal cavity, where it forms the anlage of the ethmoid bone and of the nasal septum. The notochord traverses the ventral occipital plate obliquely, being at first near its dorsal surface and then lying ventrally, where it comes into close relationship to the epithelium of the dorsal wall of the pharynx, being for a time fused with it. It then re-enters the cranial base and runs rostrally to end just caudal to the hypophysis (**3**.137A).

During the fifth week bilateral *otocysts* (auditory vesicles) become enclosed within the *otic capsules*, which soon differentiate into dorsolateral *vestibular* and ventromedial *cochlear* parts, enveloping the primordia of the semicircular canals and the cochlea. Between these two regions the facial nerve lies in a deep groove. The otic capsules fuse with the lateral processes of the occipital plate, leaving a wide hiatus through which the internal jugular vein and the glossopharyngeal, vagus and accessory nerves pass. At this stage the mesenchyme around the developing hypophyseal stalk, which is forming the rudiment of the postsphenoid part of the sphenoid bone, spreads out laterally to form the future greater wings of this element. Smaller processes rostral to this indicate the sites of the lesser wings of the sphenoid, while other condensations reach the sides of the nasal cavity and also blend with the still mesenchymatous septum.

Basal regions of the skull

These are, in mammals, initially preformed in cartilage (**3**.137). This occurs primarily in three regions:

- caudally, in relation to the notochord
- intermediately, in relation to the hypophysis
- rostrally, between the orbits and the nasal cavities.

These may be named *parachordal*, *hypophyseal* and *interorbitonasal* regions. The *parachordal cartilage* is developed from paraxial mesenchyme related to the cranial end of the notochord and the first five (occipital) somites; caudally it exhibits traces of four primitive segments separated by the roots of the hypoglossal nerves. It is notable that the region of fusion between the rostral part of the occipital bones and the portion of the parachordal plate that is of somitomeric origin corresponds to the spheno-occipital synchondrosis, which is the site of growth for up to 20 years of age. The *otic capsule* is formed from three different sources (identified in the chick): the first somite, a portion of paraxial mesenchyme and neural crest mesenchyme (Couly et al 1993).

The *hypophyseal cartilage* ossifies to form the *postsphenoid part* of the *sphenoid bone*; it derives from both paraxial mesenchyme and neural crest in the chick (Couly 1993) (see also **3**.101). The paraxial mesenchyme contributes to the caudal part of the sella turcica, forming each side of the rostral end of the notochord, whereas the neural crest forms the more rostral portion of the sella turcica, and the region termed by Couly et al (1993) the *prechordal skeleton*. The interorbitonasal cartilage is perhaps to be equated with the trabeculae cranii of lower vertebrates and is usually known as the trabecular cartilage, which is a bilateral structure developing from two centres of chondrification. The *trabeculae cranii* and the *ethmoid* complex are of neural crest origin.

In the human embryo cranial chondrification begins in the second month; cartilaginous foci first appear in the occipital plate, one on each side of the notochord (parachordal cartilages); these later fuse at the end of the seventh week surrounding the notochord, whose oblique transit through the region has been mentioned (**3**.137A). The cartilaginous posterior part of the sphenoid is formed from two hypophyseal centres, flanking the stalk of the hypophysis and uniting at first behind, then in front, enclosing a *craniopharyngeal canal* containing the hypophyseal diverticulum. The canal is usually obliterated by the third month; its association with the derivation of the anterior lobe of the hypophysis from the pharyngeal diverticulum of Rathke has been denied.

The otic capsules, presphenoid, bases of the greater wings and lesser wings of the sphenoid, and finally the nasal capsules, in turn become chondrified. The whole nasal capsule is well developed by the end of the third month, consisting of a common median septal part (sometimes initially termed the *interorbitonasal septum*) and two lateral regions. The free caudal borders of the latter incurve to form the interior nasal conchae, which ossify during the fifth month and become separate elements. Posteriorly each lateral part of the nasal capsule becomes ossified as the ethmoidal labyrinth, bearing on its medial surface ridges the future middle and superior conchae. Part of the rest of the capsule remains cartilaginous as the septal and alar cartilages of the nose; part is replaced by the mesenchymatous vomer and nasal bones.

The ventral surface of the chondrocranium is associated with the cartilages of the pharyngeal arches, the development of which will be considered later (see p. 275 et seq). The bones of the cranial base which are thus preformed in cartilage (excepting the upper part of its squama), the petromastoid part of the temporal, the body, lesser wings and roots of the greater wings of the sphenoid, and the ethmoid. These constitute the cartilaginous part of the neurocranium. To summarize, therefore, the base of the skull—except for the orbital plates of the frontal and the lateral parts of the greater sphenoidal wings—is preformed in cartilage (**3**.137, see also **3**.101).

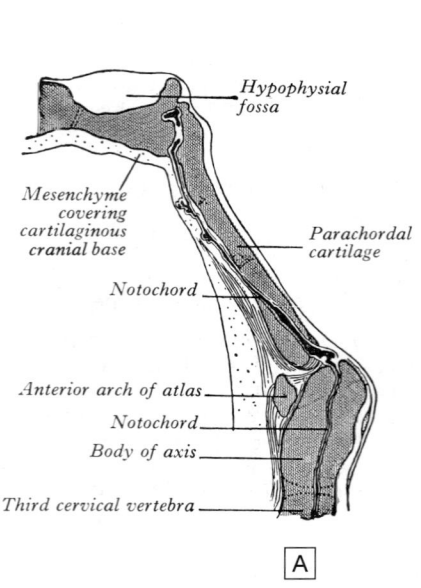

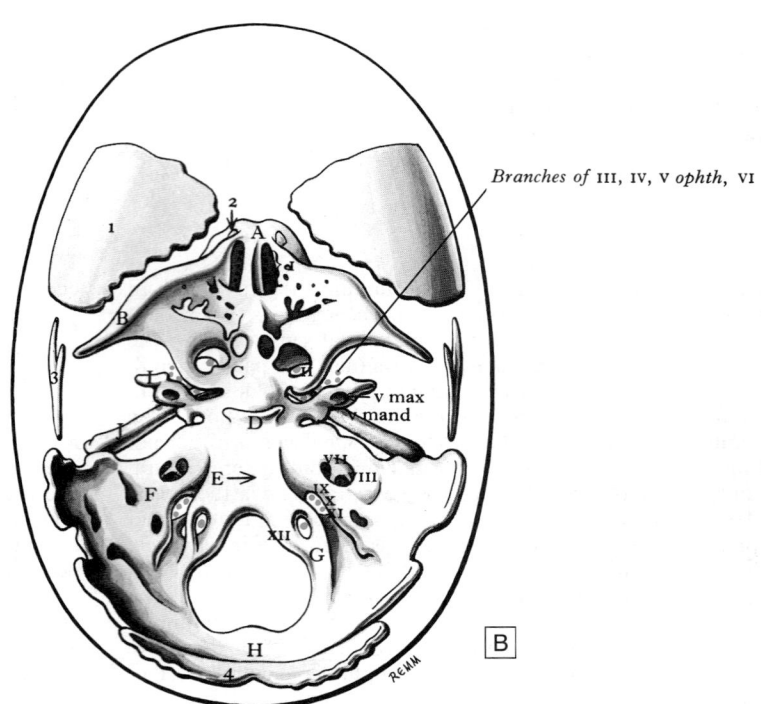

Key to chondral elements:

A   Nasal capsule
B   Orbitosphenoid
C   Presphenoid
D   Postsphenoid
E   Basi-occipital
F   Otic capsule
G   Exoccipital
H   Supra-occipital
I   Alisphenoid
J   Meckel's mandibular cartilage
K   Cartilage of malleus
L   Styloid cartilage
M   Hyoid cartilage
N   Thyroid cartilage
O   Cricoid cartilage
P   Arytenoid cartilage

Key to dermal (membrane) elements:

I   Frontal bone
2   Nasal bone
3   Squama of temporal bone
4   Squama of occipital bone
     (interparietal)
5   Parietal bone
6   Maxilla
7   Lacrimal bone
8   Zygomatic bone
9   Palatine bone
10   Vomer
11   Medial pterygoid plate
12   Tympanic ring
13   Mandible

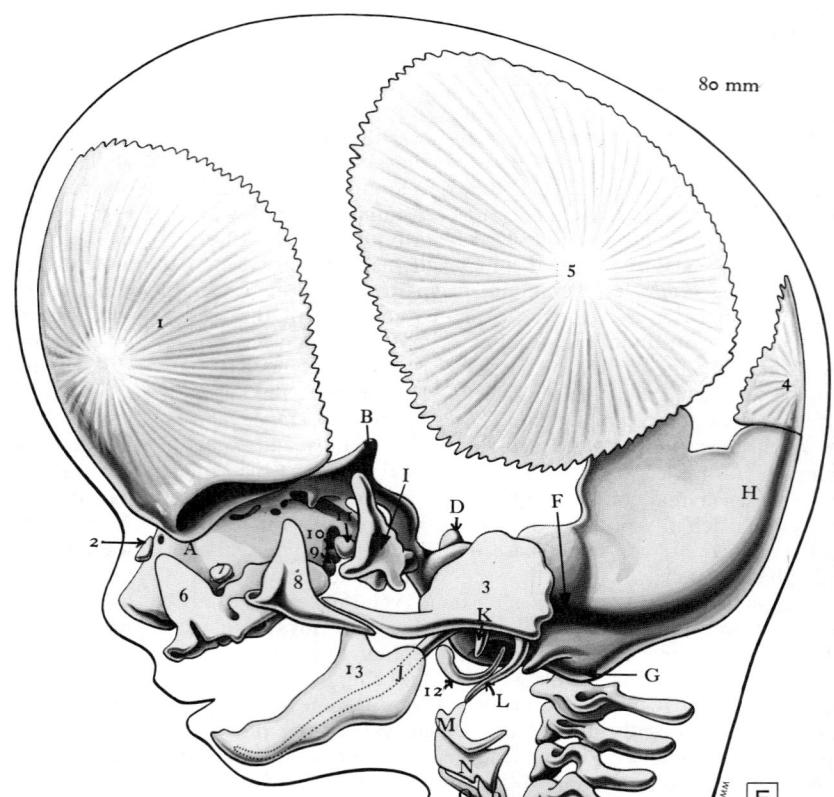

3.137   Representative stages in the development of the cranium. In all the diagrams the *chondrocranium* and cartilaginous stages of vertebrae are shown in blue, except where ossification is occurring and here the colour is green. The *desmocranium*, consisting of elements ossifying directly in mesenchyme, is shown in yellow. Cranial nerves are indicated by the appropriate roman numeral.

A. Sagittal section through the cranial end of the developing axial skeleton in an early human embryo of about 10 mm, showing the extent of the notochord. B. Key for diagram C. C. Superior aspect of cranium of human embryo at 40 mm. D. Lateral aspect of C. E. Key for diagram F. F. Lateral aspect of cranium of human embryo at 80 mm.

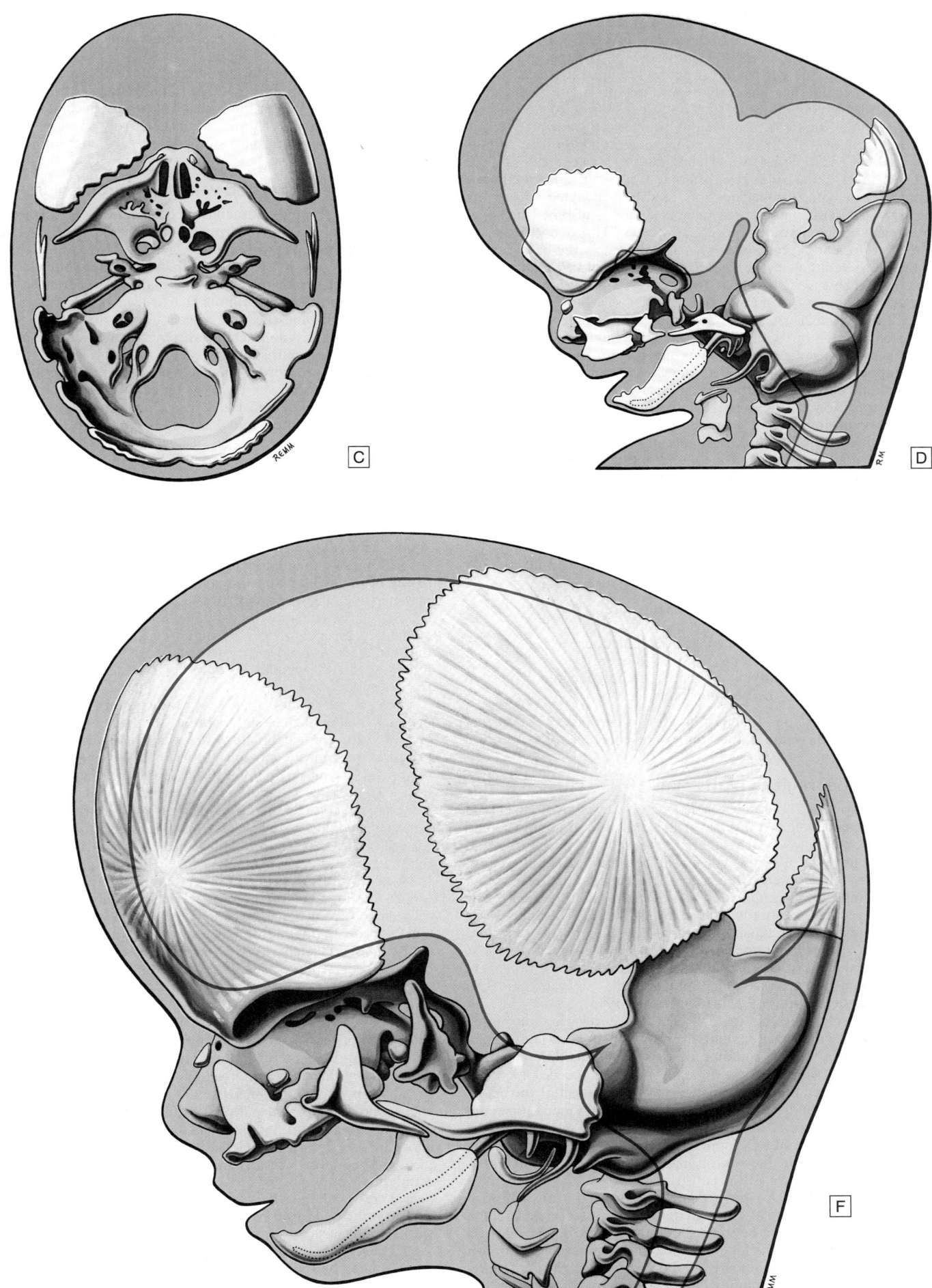

Specification of the pattern of the base of the skull may be caused by an epithelial/mesenchymal interaction involving the overlying neural tube. Thorogood (1988) proposed a 'flypaper model' of development for the cartilaginous neurocranium. The basal aspect of the neuroectoderm transiently expresses type II collagen around the olfactory regions, around the optic cups prior to and during invagination of the lens, around the otic vesicles, and on the ventrolateral surfaces of the diencephalon, mesencephalon and rhombencephalon (Thorogood 1988). The notochord also expresses type II collagen in its perichordal sheath. Some time later, after the neural expression of type II collagen has ceased, mesenchyme adjacent to the regions described above commences synthesis of type II collagen and begins differentiation into chondrocytes. Thorogood reasoned that the transient expression of type II collagen in the basal lamina of the neural epithelium causes localized arrest of cell migration of those mesenchyme cells which touch it, regardless of origin. (A similar mechanism is seen in the notochordal–sclerotome interaction; see p. 265.) At such sites cells accumulate and undergo a matrix-mediated interaction with the neural epithelium and differentiate along a chondrogenic lineage. Thus the pattern in which the cells are trapped, epigenetically determines the form of the chondrocranium. This has evolutionary implications, as slight alterations in the expression of the type II collagen by the neuroepithelium could have profound effects on the shape and form of the chondrocranium and on the whole skull, because the blastemal skull must connect to the plan initiated by the chondrocranium. This model could perhaps account for the diversity of skull shape seen in the vertebrates.

Ossification commences before the chondrocranium has fully developed, and as this change extends, bone overtakes cartilage until little of the chondrocranium remains. However, parts of it still exist at birth and small regions remain cartilaginous in the adult skull. At birth unossified chondrocranium still persists at:

- the alae, lateral nasal and septum of the nose
- the spheno-ethmoidal junction (p. 551)
- the spheno-occipital and sphenopetrous junctions (p. 551)
- the apex of the petrous bone (foramen lacerum)
- and also between ossifying elements of the sphenoid bone and between elements of the occipital bone.

Most of these regions function as growth cartilages. For further development of these areas and cranial bones in general see Section 6, Skeletal system.

Vault or upper regions of the skull

These first appear about the thirtieth day; they consist of curved plates of mesenchyme at the sides of the skull and gradually extend cranially to blend with each other; they also extend towards and reach the base of the skull, which will become part of the chondrocranium. The mesenchymatous (membranous) neurocranium, corresponding to the cranial vault, is not preformed in cartilage. Its elements, frequently described as dermal bones (p. 548), are the frontal bones, the parietals, the squamous parts of the temporal bones and the upper (interparietal) part of the occipital squama. It is now believed that the frontal, parietal and squamosal bones are formed from neural crest. Also the sutures of the calvarian and facial bones are made up of crest cells (Couly et al 1993).

There is a close association between the developing meninges, particularly the dura mater, and the calvarial bones. The dermal bones are formed by the initiation of a wave of osteodifferentiation moving radially from ossification centres within the desmocranial mesenchyme. When adjacent bones meet, proliferation of the osteogenic front ceases and sutures are induced to form. Once sutures are formed and the fibrous desmocranium is replaced by mineralized bone, a second phase of development occurs in which growth of the cranial bones occurs at the sutural margins (Opperman et al 1993). Such growth forms most of the calvaria.

Opperman et al (1993) have demonstrated that transplants of sutures in which the fetal dura mater is left intact results in a continuous fibrous suture between developing vault bones, whereas in transplants in which the fetal dura mater is removed bony fusion occurs. This interaction of underlying dura mater with the developing calvarial bones has been demonstrated experimentally, showing that the dura not only promotes the position and maintenance of sutures,

but also that dura can repattern both the reappearance and position of the bones and sutures of the cranial vault after removal of the calvaria in the neonate.

At the site of a developing suture the osteogenic fronts of two adjacent bones meet and overlap. Initially there is a highly cellular suture blastema between the bones which later becomes more dense and acellular. In the mature suture a narrow overlap of compact bone contains a dense, narrow band of cells continuous with the periosteum.

Musculature associated with the neurocranium

Most of the striated musculature of the head is formed during development of the viscerocranium when muscle masses, particularly from the second pharyngeal arch, migrate to cover parts of the neurocranium (see p. 284). However, two further sources of muscle provide myoblasts for the external ocular muscles and the tongue.

Extrinsic ocular muscles. All extrinsic ocular muscles derive from prechordal mesenchyme which lies at the rostral tip of the notochordal process and remains mesenchymal after the notochordal process becomes epithelial and gains a basal lamina (3.148). In early embryos prechordal mesenchyme migrates laterally towards the paraxial mesenchyme (p. 144). Its early myogenic properties in the head can be demonstrated by chimeric recombination, and further, if transplanted into limb buds it is able to develop into muscle tissue.

Early embryos develop bilateral cavities in the head, previously described as preotic somites. The walls of the premandibular head cavities are lined by flat or cylindrical cells which do not exhibit the characteristics of a germinal epithelium like the epithelial plate of the somite; also there is no basal lamina around the head cavities. As the oculomotor nerve grows down to the level of the head cavity a condensation of premuscle cells appears at the ventrolateral side of the head cavity. Later the head cavities are filled with ingrowing mesenchyme. The premuscular mass subdivides into the blastemata of the different muscles supplied by the oculomotor nerve (Wachtler & Jacob 1986). Similar events occur with respect to the intermediate head cavity (trochlear nerve and superior oblique muscle), and the caudal head cavity (abducent nerve and lateral rectus muscle).

There is no doubt that the head cavities are formed by a mesenchymal/epithelial shift similar to that seen in the somites. However, the epithelial plate of the somite is a germinal centre which produces postmitotic myoblasts destined for epaxial regions, and migratory premitotic myoblasts destined for the limbs and body wall. The head cavities may serve a similar purpose if a mesenchyme/epithelial shift is part of a maturation process for putative myoblasts; however, it may not need to provide a centre for cell replication: premitotic myoblasts differentiated directly from the prechordal mesenchyme may form the premuscular masses.

Muscles of the tongue. This development appears to be similar to the development of the muscles of the limb. Single, premitotic cells detach from the ventrolateral portion of the occipital somites and migrate to their ultimate positions (Wachtler & Jacob 1986) (3.131, 148). The connective tissue surrounding these muscles is derived from neural crest cells (Noden 1983).

VISCEROCRANIUM

The development of the viscerocranium is very complex. It involves the migration and interaction of epithelial populations derived from: the neural folds, surface ectoderm and endoderm; mesenchymal populations from the mesencephalic, metencephalic and myelencephalic neural crest, paraxial mesenchyme and angiogenic mesenchyme; and neural populations from the neural tube, neural crest and ectodermal placodes. Generally, the more rostral structures, i.e. face, palate, buccal cavity and nasal cavity, derive entirely from ectodermal populations (both epithelium and mesenchyme—via neural crest), whereas the caudal and related structures, i.e. pharynx and larynx, are derived from ectoderm, neural crest and interactions with endoderm.

The development of the face and neck is intimately related to the development of the brain and special sense organs; the reader is advised to refer to the development of the neural crest on pages 147 and 220, and of the head, page 157, and to 3.100, 101, 148.

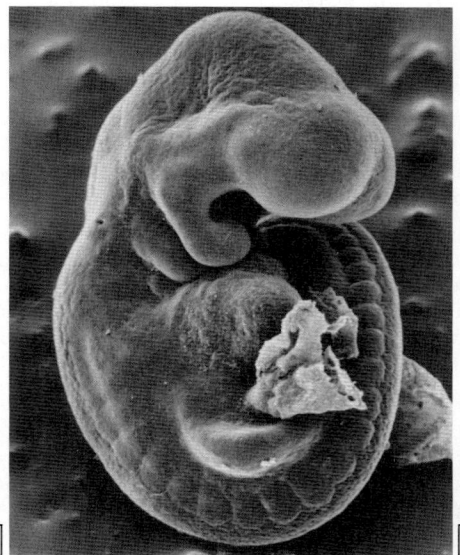 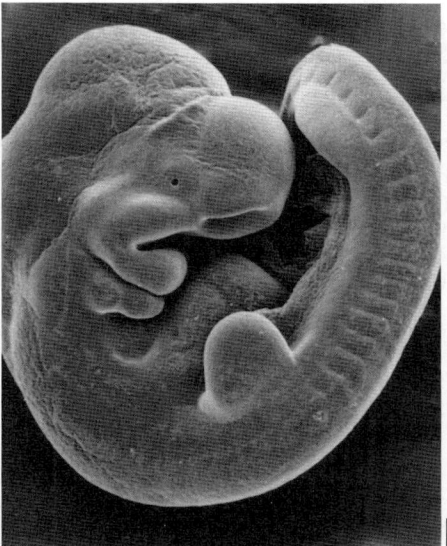 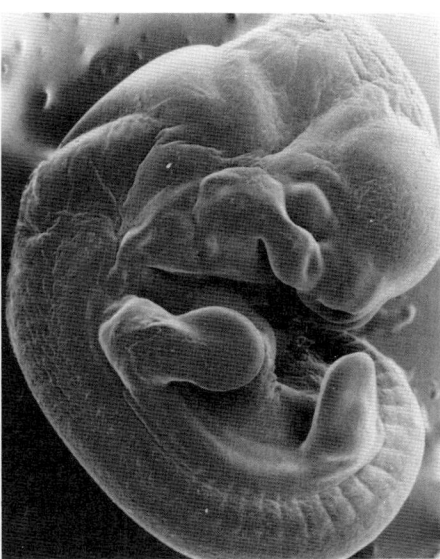

3.138   Series of scanning electron micrographs of rat embryos at days 11, 12 and 13: lateral view. A. Day 11, the pharyngula stage; the otic vesicle is still open but the lens vesicle has yet to invaginate; the first, second and third pharyngeal arches are present; an upper limb bud is present dorsal to the heart. B. Day 12, the lens vesicle has invaginated but is still open; the maxillary prominence has developed and is beneath the eye; the upper limb is becoming paddle-shaped and the lower limb is present. C. Day 13, the eyelids are beginning to develop; the maxillary prominence is merging with the lateral nasal prominence; both limb buds are well developed. The relative size and number of somites can be seen at each age. (Photographs by P Collins; printed by S Cox, Electron Microscopy Unit, Southampton General Hospital.)

All of the structures which give rise to the face and neck are segmentally organized during development; the hindbrain displays rhombomeres, the ectoderm—ectomeres and the paraxial mesenchyme—somitomeres. The overall segmentation of this region is related to the expression of axial genes in the head which have been conserved throughout evolution.

Vertebral pharyngeal apparatus

In all vertebrate embryos, after head fold formation the *stomodeum*, or primitive mouth, is bounded cranially by the projecting forebrain and caudally by the cardiac prominence (**3**.138). The mandibular region and the whole of the neck, which will subsequently intervene between mouth and developing thorax, are absent, but will be formed by the appearance and modification of six paired *branchial* (*gill*) *arches*, which develop in the lateral aspects of the head adjacent to the hindbrain (**3**.139, 140, 141). In the earliest vertebrates which were jawless (*Agnathia*), the branchial arches were a uniform series of bars behind the gill clefts; but long before the evolution of the terrestrial vertebrates, remarkable adaptations had occurred in them. Structures commonly regarded as the first pair of arches became the jaws, upper and lower, of the jaw-bearing vertebrates (*Gnathostomata*), including most fish; they are, therefore, usually named the *mandibular arches*. (The term 'mandibular arch' is widely used but not entirely appropriate because of the numerous maxillo-facial, nasal, otic and palatopharyngeal derivatives from its dorsal end.) It should, however, be noted that since this early identification, strong evidence has accumulated that, at least, a pair of *pre-mandibular arches* existed and have become adapted as the *trabeculae cranii* of subsequent vertebrate embryos. These are probably represented by the interorbitonasal cartilage of the human embryo (see p. 271) which forms a branchial element in the chondrocranium. The next (*postmandibular*) arch in the series is the *hyoid arch*; its skeletal derivatives form the varied hyoid elements present in all vertebrates with jaws. The most dorsal of the latter, the *hyomandibula*, is already present in cartilaginous fish as a strut between the skull and the primitive jaw joint, thereby reducing the cleft between the mandibular and hyoid arches to a small opening, the *spiracle*. The interesting further evolution of this region in land animals in connection with the auditory apparatus has been considered (p. 263). The hyoid arch also contributes to the formation of a gill cover, or *operculum*, in bony fish, and the remaining arches persist as the supports of the gill apparatus.

At first the arches produce rounded ridge-like prominences both of the overlying ectoderm and of the endodermal lining of the lateral walls and floor of the pharynx. In the furrows between these prominences the ectoderm and endoderm are in virtual contact. The thin membranes so formed break down permanently in gill-breathing vertebrates, transiently in reptile embryos, but persist in the tetrapods, in which open channels or 'true clefts' are not formed. However, the external *branchial grooves* which correspond to them are frequently, less appropriately, called *branchial clefts* and their internal counterparts are the *pharyngeal sacs* or *pouches*.

In gill-breathing vertebrates the exchange of respiratory gases is directly from solution in water to solution in blood. From the cranial end (arterial, but carrying deoxygenated blood) of the heart emerge two *ventral aortae* which traverse the ventral pharyngeal wall, sending branches curving dorsally into the branchial arches, where they feed capillary plexuses in the gills. These are drained by corresponding arteries, which join two *dorsal aortae* supplying the general circulation. As water is taken in through the mouth and passed back through the gill clefts, its dissolved oxygen diffuses through the pharyngeal endoderm and endothelium of the gills to reach the blood, carbon dioxide diffusing out of the latter into the water. This intimate relationship between the developing mouth, branchial apparatus and heart in water-breathing vertebrates is repeated in the embryos of their tetrapod descendants, but with many modifications necessary to changed respiratory function.

Although a description of the branchial apparatus is appropriate for water-breathing vertebrates, the application of this terminology to mammalian embryos is by no means universal. O'Rahilly and Muller (1992) consider the term *branchial* to be inappropriate for mammalian embryos. Similarly the term *visceral*, used synonymously to describe the arches, has been questioned by Noden (1991) who notes that 'visceral' suggests a primary relation between the arches and the internal pharyngeal tube that obscures the somatic function of most of the tissue within the arches. The region of the embryo containing the rostral foregut, surrounded by mesenchyme and ectoderm, constitutes the embryonic pharynx; the stage of development at which the arches are prominent has been termed the *pharyngula stage* (Ballard 1971, 1976; see p. 100). However, the appellation *pharyngeal* arches is also problematical as the first arch which forms most of the face is in the main composed of ectoderm alone, both on the outer and inner surfaces and within the arch (neural crest mesenchyme). Thus the first arch is technically not a pharyngeal structure, unlike the subsequent caudal arches which are composed of ectoderm externally, endoderm of the pharynx internally

275

and neural crest mesenchyme within the arches. This difference in origin of the first and subsequent arches is related to the evolution of the head and skull (see p. 287). For the purposes of the description of human embryology the term *pharyngeal* arches will be used; however, comparison with other species will involve the term branchial.

A typical pharyngeal arch

Generally each pharyngeal arch consists of an epithelial covering exteriorly and a mesenchymal core interiorly (3.139, 140, 141). The epithelium may be ectodermal entirely (as in the first arch), or ectoderm covering the external aspect of the arch and endoderm covering the internal aspect of the arch (as in the remaining arches). The mesenchyme within each arch derives from neural crest, paraxial and angiogenic mesenchymal populations. The motor and sensory

roots of a cranial nerve are associated with the epithelium and mesenchyme of each arch.

From these disparate cell populations each arch develops:

- region-specific *epithelial structures*
- a *skeletal element* from the neural crest mesenchyme
- associated *striated muscle* from the paraxial mesenchyme
- an *arch artery* from the angiogenic mesenchyme
- *motor* and *sensory* nerves specific to the arch.

The epithelia covering each arch is patterned by the underlying mesenchyme. Such patterning is specific for individual arches and results in such diverse specializations as: keratinized stratified squamous epithelium, hair, sweat, sebaceous and ceruminous glands; pseudostratified ciliated columnar epithelium, teeth, salivary, mucous

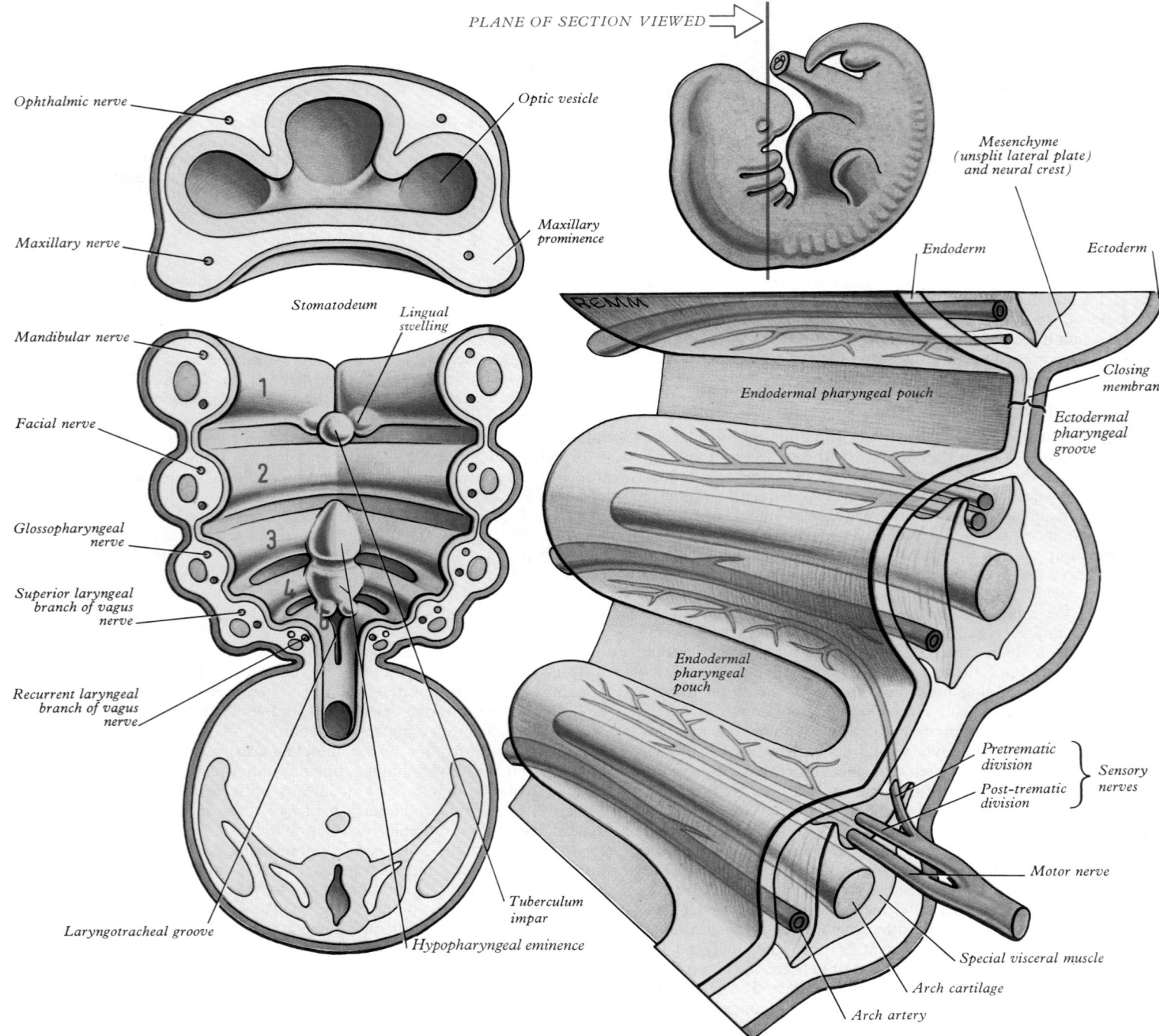

3.139 Schema of developing pharyngeal region showing (left) the pharyngeal floor and sectioned lateral walls, viewed from the dorsal aspect, and (right) details of generalized pharyngeal constituents, including arches,

endodermal pouches and ectodermal grooves. (Modified in part after Williams et al 1969.)

and lacrimal glands; the epithelia of glands such as the thyroid, parathyroids, thymus; and of the lymphoid tissues in the oro- and nasopharynx.

The skeletal element is formed from neural crest mesenchyme which condenses and subsequently chondrifies either wholly or in part of its length; if this change is complete the element extends dorsally until it comes into contact with the mesenchymatous cranial base lateral to the hindbrain. The arch cartilage, entirely or in part, may remain as cartilage, undergo endochondral ossification, be replaced completely by intramembranous ossification, or become ligamentous. Neural crest also gives rise to the *ligaments*, *tendons* and *connective tissue* in the arches and the *dermis* underlying the skin. Generally the neural crest controls the pattern of development of the arches and is itself programmed by the expression of *Hox* genes in the hindbrain (see p. 227).

The striated muscle of each arch, sometimes termed *branchial musculature* to denote its origin, derives from the unsegmented paraxial mesenchyme of the head, the somitomeres (see pp. 154, 285); the myoblasts may migrate great distances and lose connection with the skeletal elements in the arches which cease their original respiratory function. The identities of these muscle masses, where they assume new functions, can nevertheless be inferred by reference to their nerve supply.

An arch artery develops in each arch either by vasculogenesis, where angioblastic mesenchyme migrates into a region and initiates vessel development in situ, or by angiogenesis, where vessels develop by sprouting from the endothelium of pre-existing vessels (see p. 299). The paired arch arteries arise from the truncus arteriosus and pass laterally each side of the pharynx to join the dorsal aortae.

Nerves arise from the adjacent hindbrain (**3.96, 112**). They pass directly into the arches, which are ventral to it, by two methods. *Motor nerves* grow out from the basal plate of the midbrain and hindbrain to innervate the striated muscle in the arches. Generally these nerves are termed *special branchial efferent* noting their innervation of branchial musculature. *Sensory nerves* extend from cranial sensory ganglia which are derived in part from neural crest cells and in part from ectodermal placodes (see p. 237); they convey *general* and *special somatic afferent* axons. Within the arch a mixed nerve typically runs along the rostral border and is hence described as *post-trematic*, because it is behind or caudal to the cleft or trema rostral to the arch. A sensory branch from this principal post-trematic nerve passes to the immediately rostral arch where it runs close to the caudal border; it is thus *pretrematic* with respect to the cleft caudal to it (**3.139**). In the human embryo the pre- and post-trematic nerves cannot be identified with certainty.

DEVELOPMENT OF THE PHARYNGEAL ARCHES

The human circumoral *first pharyngeal arch* (**3.138, 139**) consists, on each side, of two main regions: a *ventral part* or *mandibular prominence* and a *dorsal part* or *maxillary prominence*. Each mandibular prominence, first seen at stage 10 (22 postovulatory days), grows ventromedially in the floor of the pharynx to meet its fellow in the midline, being situated between the primitive mouth and the cardiac (pericardial) prominence. The maxillary prominences are not seen until stage 13; their enlargement coincides with proliferation of neural crest mesenchyme between the ectoderm and prosencephalon forming the frontonasal prominence (see below). The enlargement of the first arch is particularly rostral to the site of the buccopharyngeal membrane; thus inner and outer aspects of this arch are covered with ectoderm. The *second* or *hyoid arches*, seen from stage 11, are caudal to the maxillomandibular; they similarly grow ventrally to meet and fuse in the midline. The *third arches* are seen at stage 12 (26 days) and the *fourth arches* by stage 13 (28 days); the latter especially are not prominent, being largely sunk in a depression produced by the caudal overlapping of the hyoid arch. The *fifth* and *sixth arches* cannot be recognized externally and can only be identified by the arrangement of the mesenchyme and by slight projections into the pharynx.

THE FIRST PHARYNGEAL ARCH

The first pharyngeal arch is sufficiently different, both in its structure and development, from the subsequent caudal arches for its separate

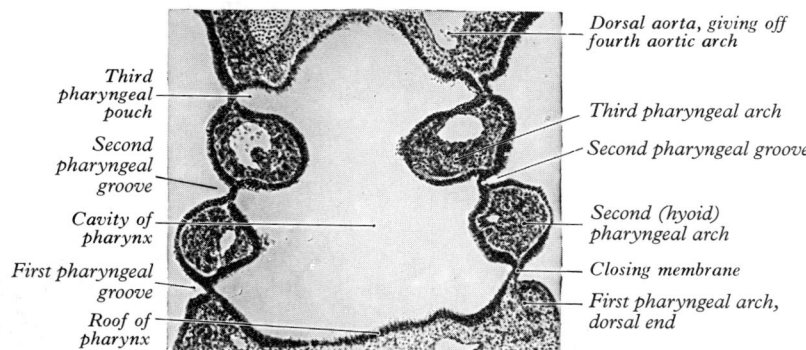

3.140 Oblique section through the pharynx of a human embryo of CR length 2 mm. Magnification × c. 50. (Norris 1938.)

examination. Unlike the other arches it possesses dorsal and ventral prominences, appearing C-shaped in lateral view (see **3.142**). The dorsal (maxillary) prominences interact with ectodermal epithelia and neural crest mesenchyme of the frontonasal prominence, and generally form more extensive skeletal structures than the other arches (see p. 284); particularly, these skeletal elements fuse with the chondrocranium. The first arch is completely clothed with ectoderm unlike the caudal arches which are dependent on the proximity of pharyngeal endoderm for their development. The ectoderm originates (in the 3-somite chick) from a territory lateral to the mesencephalic neural folds (see **3.145**). The mesencephalic folds themselves give rise to both the ectodermal placodal cells and neural crest cells which contribute to the trigeminal ganglion, and the mesenchymal population which streams into the mandibular and maxillary prominences.

The first arch contains on each side a dorsal and ventral cartilage. The former represents the *palatopterygoquadrate bar*, a prominent element in earlier vertebrates forming part of the upper jaw but much reduced in mammals. In human embryos its early appearance seems transient and its contribution to some permanent cranial structures, such as the maxilla, is uncertain (however, see below). The *ventral cartilage* (of Meckel, **3.143**) extends from the developing otic capsule into the mandibular prominence, meeting its fellow at its ventral end. The dorsal end of Meckel's cartilage becomes separated, and was often held to form the rudiments of both *malleus* and *incus*. However, there is strong palaeontological (Romer 1970) and comparative anatomical (Shute 1956) evidence that the incus is,

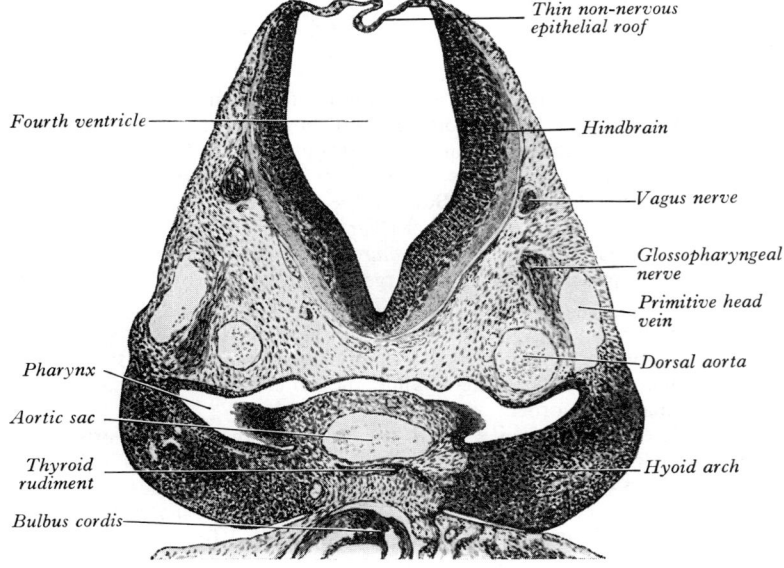

3.141 Oblique section through the head of a mole embryo, 4.5 mm long. The section passes through the hindbrain, the pharynx, the second (hyoid) and a part of the third pharyngeal arches.

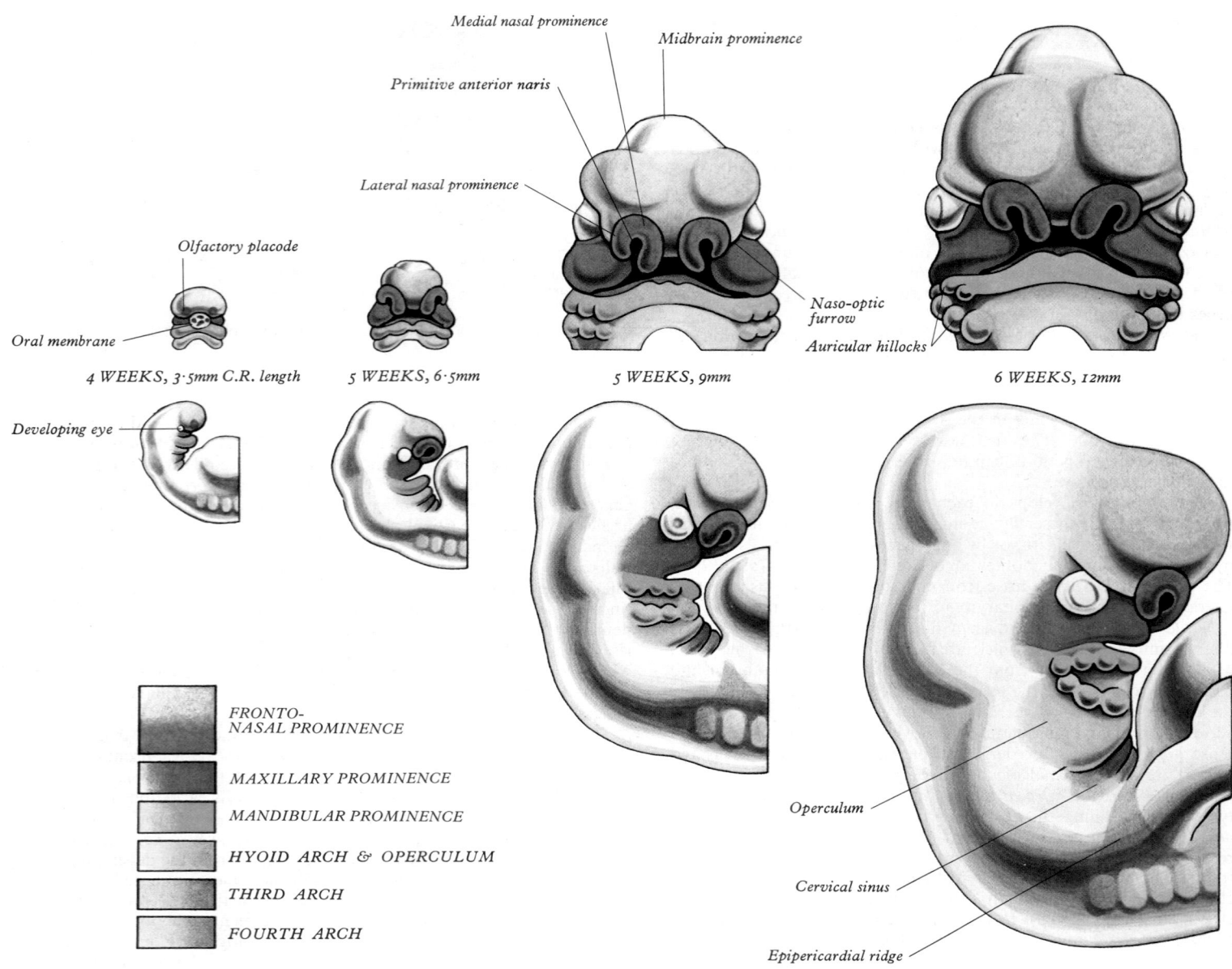

Medial nasal prominence

Midbrain prominence

Primitive anterior naris

Lateral nasal prominence

Olfactory placode

Naso-optic furrow

Oral membrane

Auricular hillocks

Developing eye

4 WEEKS, 3·5mm C.R. length

5 WEEKS, 6·5mm

5 WEEKS, 9mm

6 WEEKS, 12mm

FRONTO-NASAL PROMINENCE

MAXILLARY PROMINENCE

MANDIBULAR PROMINENCE

HYOID ARCH & OPERCULUM

THIRD ARCH

FOURTH ARCH

Operculum

Cervical sinus

Epipericardial ridge

3.142 Sequence of diagrams showing the superficial contributions of the facial prominences and pharyngeal elements to the development of the face, including the external nose, circumorbital structures, external acoustic meatus and pinna, and neck. All diagrams are drawn to scale. Note changes in general proportions and relative positions.

in part, to be regarded as a homologue of the *quadrate bone* of reptiles, and it is therefore probably more correctly regarded as a derivative of the palatopterygoquadrate cartilage. This cartilage may also contribute to the ala major of the sphenoid bone and the roots of its pterygoid plates. Beyond the rudiment of the malleus, the intermediate part of Meckel's cartilage disappears, but its sheath persists as the *anterior malleolar* and *sphenomandibular ligaments*. The ventral part, much the largest, is enveloped by the developing mesenchymatous mandible (p. 577); a small fraction of this, extending from the mental foramen almost to the site of the future symphysis, probably becomes ossified from invading mandibular tissue, into which it is incorporated, while the remainder of the cartilage is ultimately absorbed.

The cells which give rise to the muscle of the first arch arise from the paraxial mesenchyme localized to somitomeres 2 and 3 (Trainor et al 1994) (p. 285). The muscle mass of the mandibular part of the first arch forms the *tensor tympani*, *tensor veli palatini* and the *masticatory muscles*, including *mylohyoid* and the *anterior belly of digastric* (**3**.144). The tensor tympani retains its connection with the skeletal element of the arch through its attachments to the malleus, and the tensor veli palatini to the base of the medial pterygoid process, which may be derived from the dorsal cartilage of the first

arch, but the masticatory muscles transfer to the mandible, a dermal bone.

All these muscles are supplied by the mandibular nerve, the mixed 'post-trematic' nerve of the first arch.

Face

While the mandibular prominences are invading the floor of the pharynx, mesencephalic neural crest cells migrate rostrally and laterally between the prosencephalic neuroepithelium and the surface ectoderm to form the extensive *frontonasal prominence*. During the fifth week the sites of the *olfactory* or *nasal placodes* are established ventrolateral to the frontonasal prominence, dividing the latter, on each side, into *medial* and *lateral nasal prominences* or folds; the olfactory placodes originate from the neural folds (p. 222). The placodes are at first widely separated and coplanar with the surface ectoderm but, as the nasal prominences develop, they soon become depressed to form the *olfactory pits* (nasal sacs). The olfactory placodes are the anlage of the olfactory and vomeronasal epithelia, which derive from the rostral neural folds; these folds also give rise to the respiratory epithelia of the nasal cavity (see **3**.145). The lateral nasal prominences are the more evident (**3**.142, 146в), but the medial nasal prominences, still separated by the median remainder of the

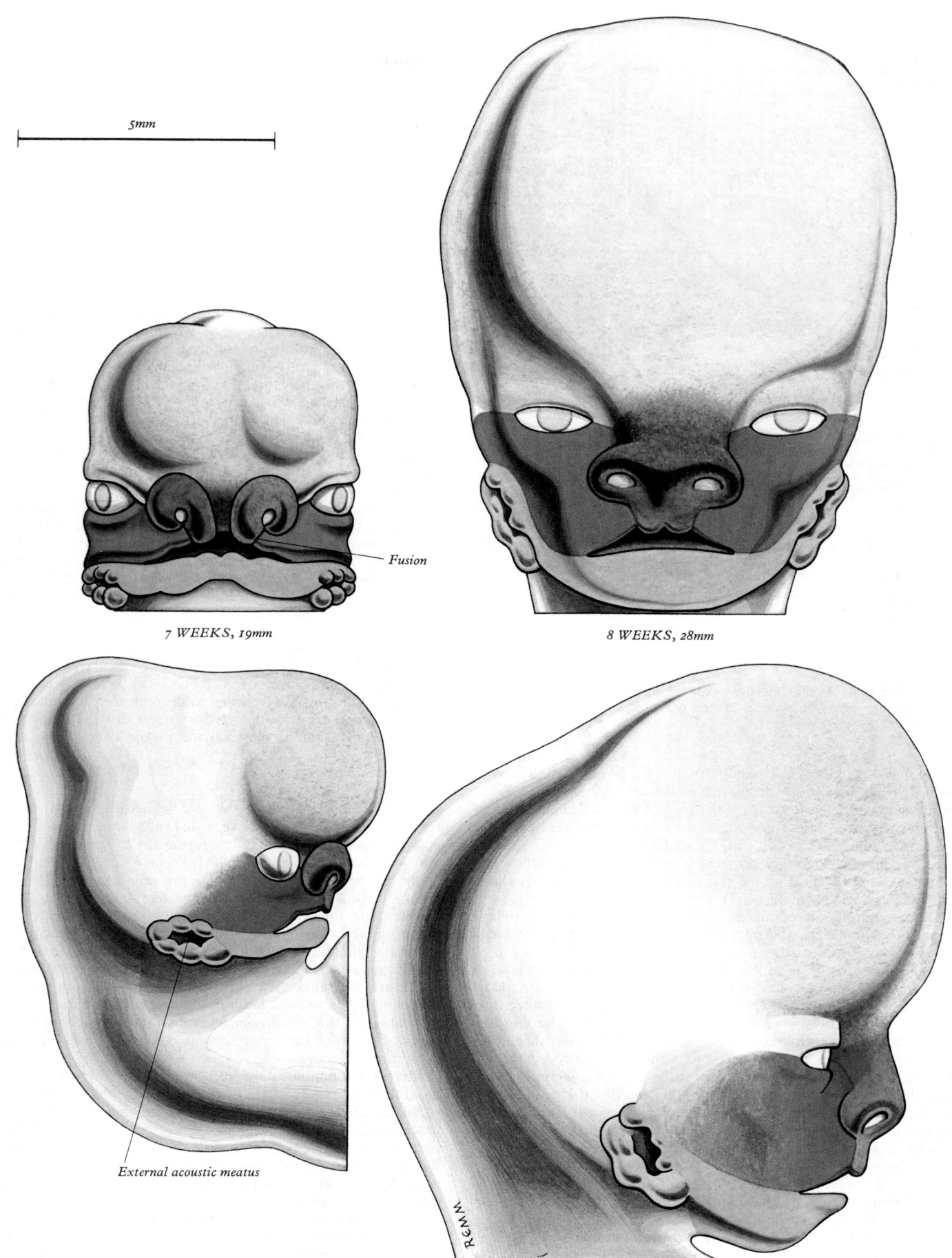

5mm

7 WEEKS, 19mm

8 WEEKS, 28mm

Fusion

External acoustic meatus

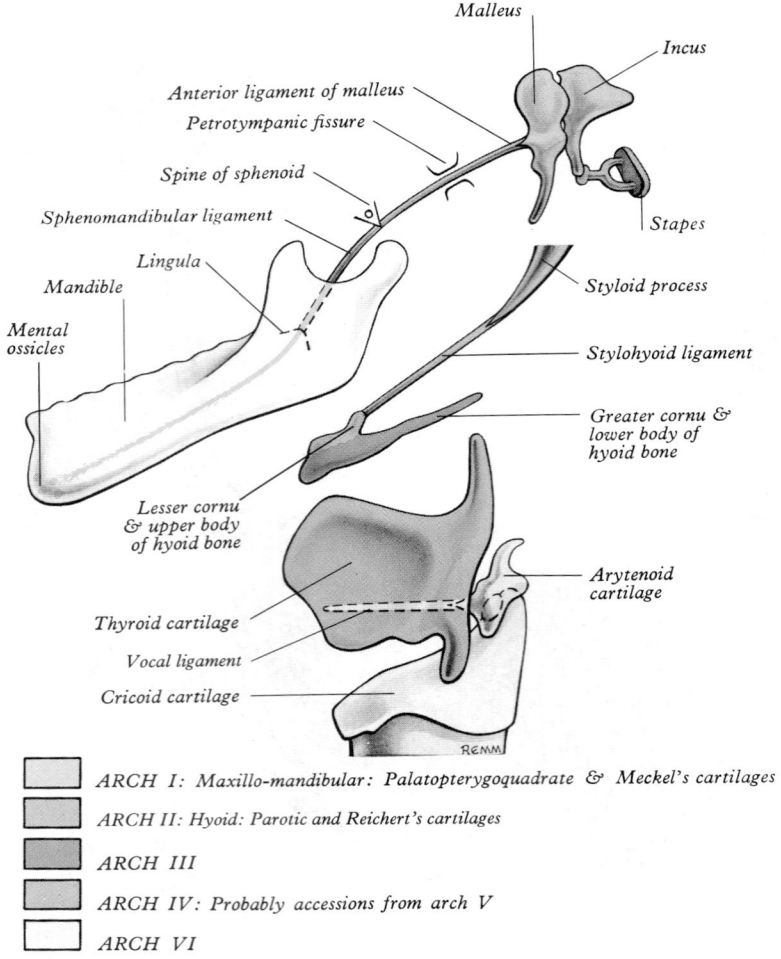

ARCH I: Maxillo-mandibular: Palatopterygoquadrate & Meckel's cartilages

ARCH II: Hyoid: Parotic and Reichert's cartilages

ARCH III

ARCH IV: Probably accessions from arch V

ARCH VI

3.143 Schema illustrating the skeletal derivatives (osseous and cartilaginous) of the pharyngeal arches (viscerocranium). (Modified from Williams et al 1969.)

frontonasal field, project caudally beyond the former. Extensions of mesenchyme from the medial prominence into the roof of the stomodeum proliferate to form the *premaxillary* fields. Each nasal sac has a ventral fold from which develops an epithelial *nasal fin* passing caudally to fuse with the stomodeal roof.

While these changes are progressing a somewhat triangular elevation swells ventrally from the cranial aspect of the dorsal region of each mandibular prominence. This is the *maxillary prominence*, and like the frontonasal prominence it consists of proliferating neural crest mesenchyme covered by ectoderm. Each maxillary prominence grows in a ventral direction and fuses with the lateral nasal prominence, the two being at first separated by a *nasomaxillary groove* (*naso-optic furrow*) (**3.142**; Streeter 1948). The opposed margins of the lateral nasal and maxillary prominences growing together thus establish continuity between the side of the future nose and the cheek (**3.142**). The ectoderm along the boundary between them does not entirely disappear; it gives rise to a solid cellular rod, which at first develops as a linear surface elevation, the *nasolacrimal ridge*, and then sinks into the mesenchyme (Politzer 1952). Its caudal end proliferates to connect with the caudal part of the lateral nasal wall, while its cranial extremity later connects with the developing conjunctival sac. The solid rod becomes canalized to form the *nasolacrimal duct* (**3.146B**).

(It should be noted that the epithelial folds and elevations due to loci of proliferation of underlying mesenchyme were long termed processes. The International Nomenclature Committee felt that this was not entirely appropriate and their revised term 'prominence' has been adopted here. Both terms are used in the literature.)

The relatively wide primitive mouth or *stomodeal fissure* is progressively reduced, and the epithelial and connective tissues of the cheek enlarged, by fusion between the adjacent surfaces of the

mandibular and maxillary prominences. This proceeds from the para-otic region to the angle of the definitive *oral fissure*.

Nasal cavity

The rounded apex of the triangular maxillary prominence extends beyond the lateral nasal prominence, crossing the caudal end of the olfactory pit to meet and fuse with the *premaxillary elevation* developing at the extremity of the frontonasal field. This closes off the lower or caudal edge of the olfactory pit, the upper part of the opening of which is thus defined as the primitive *external naris*. The growth of the surrounding mesenchyme leads to a deepening of the pit to become a primitive nasal cavity, or *nasal sac*, the epithelial wall of which, in the dorsocaudal part of its extent, the nasal fin, retains contiguity with the epithelium of the stomodeal roof. This contact area becomes progressively greater as growth continues, and the nasal fin is eroded, ultimately forming a thin layer, the *oronasal membrane* (**3.146A**), which also disappears later. Thereafter, the primitive nasal cavity communicates with the stomodeum through a primitive *internal naris* (*choana*), which is at this stage still well forward or ventrally situated in the stomodeal roof (Warbrick 1960). By these changes a new cranial boundary is set for the oral opening, consisting of the fused premaxillary and maxillary regions. This is the future upper lip, but it has not yet become separated from the deeper tissues which will form the maxillary alveolus. At the same time the nasal cavity acquires a floor through the fusion of the nasal prominences and the maxillary prominences. At this stage the two external nares are still widely separated by an area derived from the frontonasal field, but this separation becomes reduced by the fusion of the premaxillary mesenchyme from the two sides. According to some investigators the mesenchyme of the maxillary prominences invades the premaxillary regions, the mesenchyme of which is said to become buried, to form later the premaxilla or os incisivum (p. 574; Boyd 1933; Baxter 1953). The maxillary mesenchyme is thus considered by some to contribute substantially to the formation of the *philtrum* of the upper lip, thus accounting for its maxillary innervation. Others, however, maintain that the philtrum is derived wholly from premaxillary tissue (Keith 1948; King 1954; Warbrick 1960; Wood et al 1967) (see also **3.100**). The maxillary nerve primarily innervates the maxillary mesenchyme but apparently extends later into the territory of the frontonasal prominence. It should be added that some workers deny that sensory nerve distribution is a reliable guide to migration of mesenchyme in the case of the maxillary prominence.

Palate

Once the primitive nasal cavities are defined the ventral part of the roof of the oral cavity can be regarded as the *primitive palate* (*median palatine prominence*; **3.146A**). It is formed by the premaxillary regions and maxillary prominences, which become confluent and establish continuity with the thick median *nasal septal prominence* (*primitive nasal septum*). As the head grows in size, the region of mesenchyme between the forebrain and oral cavity increases greatly by proliferation and the nasal cavities deepen, extending towards the forebrain. Simultaneously they also extend dorsally from the primitive choanae as two narrow and deep grooves in the oral roof (**3.146**) which are separated by a partition. The grooves and the partition deepen together, and the latter becomes the *nasal septum*, continuous rostrally with the *primitive nasal septum* (**3.146B**). The broad dorsocaudal border of the nasal septum is at first in contact with the dorsum of the developing tongue (**3.146B**), the right and left nasal cavities still communicating freely with the mouth except where the nasal floor is already established ventrally by the primitive palate.

During Stage 17 (41 days) the internal aspects of the maxillary prominences produce *palatine processes* (*shelves*), which grow towards the midline but are for some time separated from each other by the tongue. At this stage the roof of the oral cavity projects ventrally beyond its floor and the tip of the developing tongue actually lies in contact with the cranial (superior) surface of the primitive palate. A coronal section dorsal to this shows the maxillary palatine processes contiguous with the sides of the tongue and bent into a vertical position on each side of it (**3.146B**). With further growth, the mandibular region and the tongue are carried forwards (ventrally), and the lingual tip passes round to the caudal surface of the primitive palate. At stage 23 (56–57 days) the palatine processes

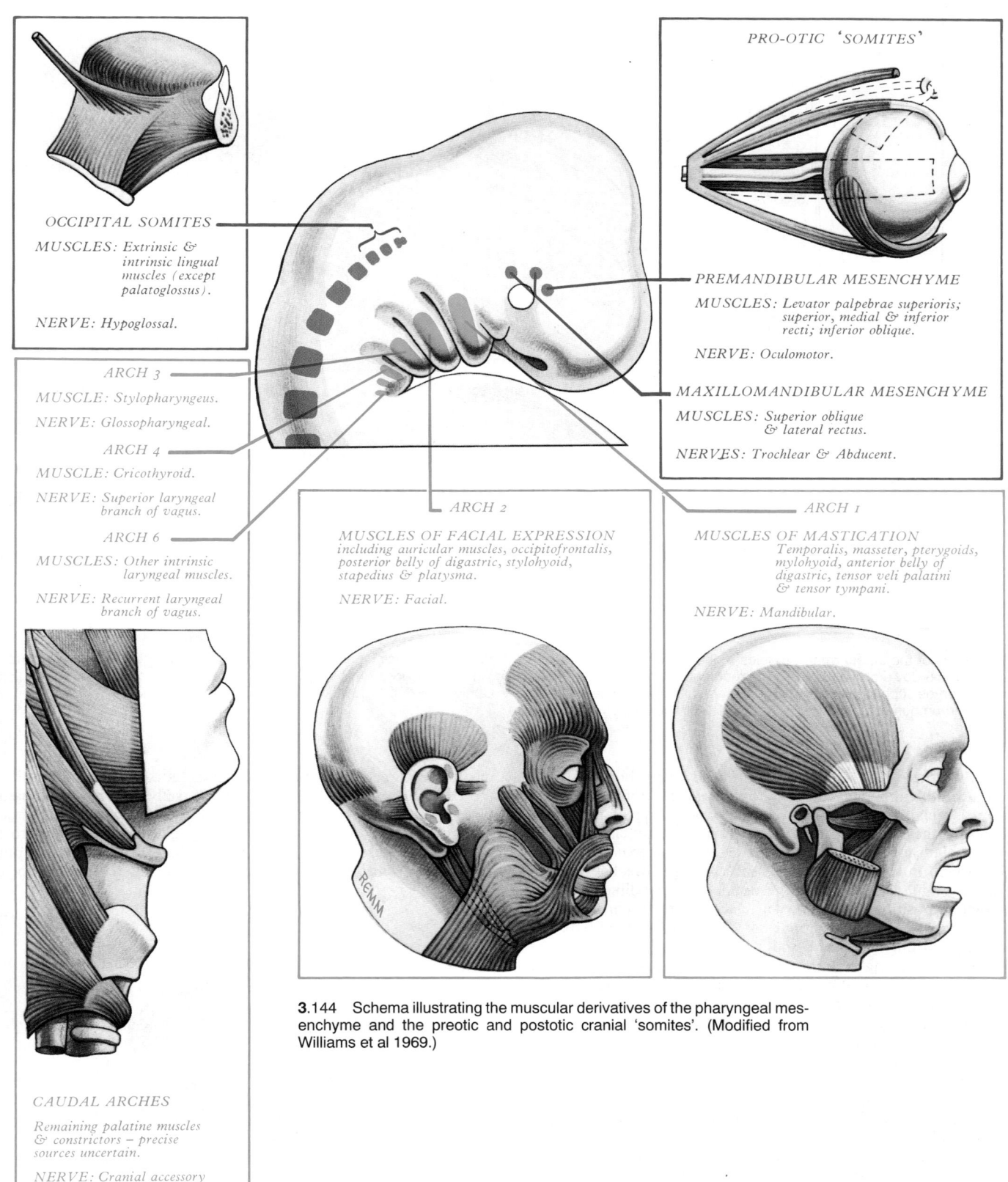

OCCIPITAL SOMITES

MUSCLES: Extrinsic &
  intrinsic lingual
  muscles (except
  palatoglossus).

NERVE: Hypoglossal.

PREMANDIBULAR MESENCHYME

MUSCLES: Levator palpebrae superioris;
  superior, medial & inferior
  recti; inferior oblique.

NERVE: Oculomotor.

ARCH 3

MUSCLE: Stylopharyngeus.

NERVE: Glossopharyngeal.

MAXILLOMANDIBULAR MESENCHYME

MUSCLES: Superior oblique
  & lateral rectus.

NERVES: Trochlear & Abducent.

ARCH 4

MUSCLE: Cricothyroid.

NERVE: Superior laryngeal
  branch of vagus.

ARCH 6

MUSCLES: Other intrinsic
  laryngeal muscles.

NERVE: Recurrent laryngeal
  branch of vagus.

ARCH 2

MUSCLES OF FACIAL EXPRESSION
including auricular muscles, occipitofrontalis,
posterior belly of digastric, stylohyoid,
stapedius & platysma.

NERVE: Facial.

ARCH 1

MUSCLES OF MASTICATION
  Temporalis, masseter, pterygoids,
  mylohyoid, anterior belly of
  digastric, tensor veli palatini
  & tensor tympani.

NERVE: Mandibular.

3.144   Schema illustrating the muscular derivatives of the pharyngeal mesenchyme and the preotic and postotic cranial 'somites'. (Modified from
Williams et al 1969.)

CAUDAL ARCHES

Remaining palatine muscles
& constrictors – precise
sources uncertain.

NERVE: Cranial accessory
  via branches of vagus.

rapidly elevate, assuming a horizontal position which allows them
to grow towards each other and thus to fuse (**3**.146c); this occurs
from before backwards.

  The change of position occurs very rapidly caused by the progressive region specific synthesis and accumulation of hyaluronic
acid within the palatal process mesenchyme. The hyaluronic acid
will bind up to 10 times its own weight of water, thus causing
swelling and expansion of the palatial shelves. This process is further
aided by the alignment of collagen fibrils and palatal mesenchymal
cells (the latter contract in response to acetylcholine and serotonin
which they secrete thus regulating the elevation of the shelves), and
by the epithelium which restrains the swelling. Once these forces are
in concert and exceed the resistance factors, the palatal shelves will
mechanically elevate. Such elevation occurs at a time of craniofacial

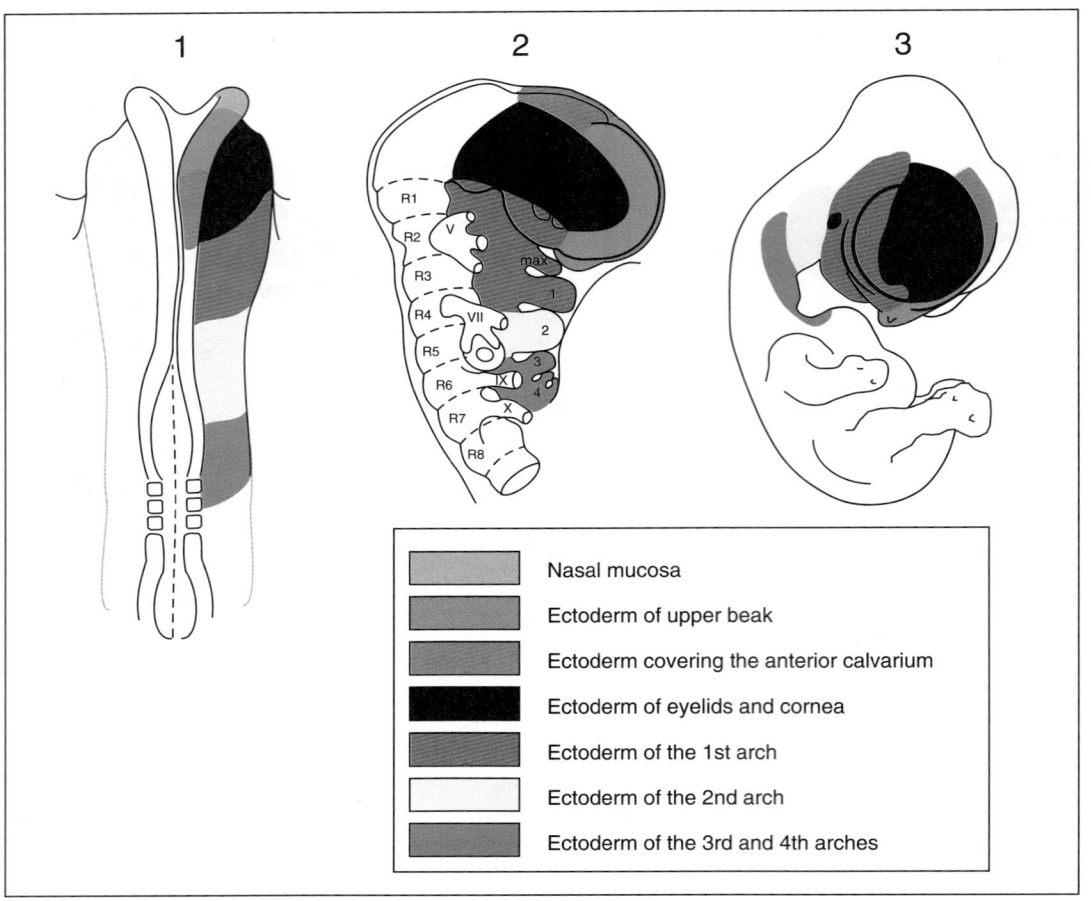

3.145   Growth of the ectodermal territories in the chick from the 3-somite stage (1) to the 8-day embryo (3). In (2) the rhombomeres are indicated and the cranial nerves supplying the pharyngeal arches; there is no neural crest outflow from rhombomeres 3 and 5. For further details see text. V = trigeminal nerve; VII = facial nerve; IX = glossopharyngeal nerve; X = vagus nerve; Max = maxillary prominence; the pharyngeal arches are indicated 1–4. (From Couly, Le Pouarin 1990 with permission.)

growth when there is constant growth in head height but almost no growth in head width. This latter factor is important: if palatal shelf elevation is delayed so that they elevate in a period of growth in facial width, the unfused processes are unable to touch physically and cleft palate may result. Other factors affecting palatal closure are the growth in length of the first arch cartilage (Meckel's) which allows the tongue to lower into the developing mandible. Further, the change in position of the maxilla relative to the anterior cranial base, which is maintained at about 84° during weeks 9 and 10, has the effect of lifting the head and upper jaw upwards from the mandible so permitting withdrawal of the tongue from between the palatal shelves and creating space for them to elevate. Mouth opening, tongue protrusion and hiccup movements have also been noted at this time; these movements and their associated pressure changes may assist palatal shelf elevation (Ferguson 1977, 1990, 1993). Generally in female embryos palatal shelf elevation occurs 7 days later than in males, making congenital cleft palate more likely in female embryos. After elevation the palatine processes grow medially along the inferior borders of the primitive choanae, uniting with them and with the margins of the median palatine prominence, except over a small area in the midline where a *nasopalatine canal* maintains connection between the nasal and oral cavities for some time and marks the future position of the incisive fossa. (The plates which form the early (primitive) palate are sometimes known as *median* palatine processes, the maxillary contributions being then named the *lateral* palatine processes.)

As the medial borders of the maxillary palatine processes fuse together, fusing also with the free border of the nasal septum, the nasal and oral cavities are progressively separated and the tongue is excluded from the former. The nasal cavities are thus extended dorsally and the choanae reach their final position, leaving the caudal edge of the nasal septum free in about its dorsal quarter as the

partition between them. Slightly later the dorsomedial extremities of the palatine processes, which extend dorsally beyond the choanae, fuse together rostrocaudally to form the future epithelia and connective tissues of the soft palate (3.146c). There is later an upgrowth of myogenic mesenchyme from the third and, probably, other pharyngeal arches into the palate and around the caudal margins of the

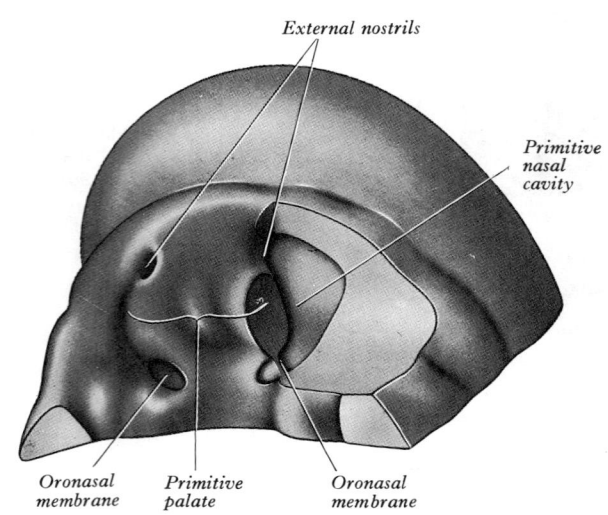

3.146A   Primitive palate of a human embryo in the seventh week. The figure shows the anterior part of the roof of the mouth; large parts of the left lateral nasal prominence and the left maxillary prominence have been removed to expose the left primitive nasal cavity. (From a model by K Peter.)

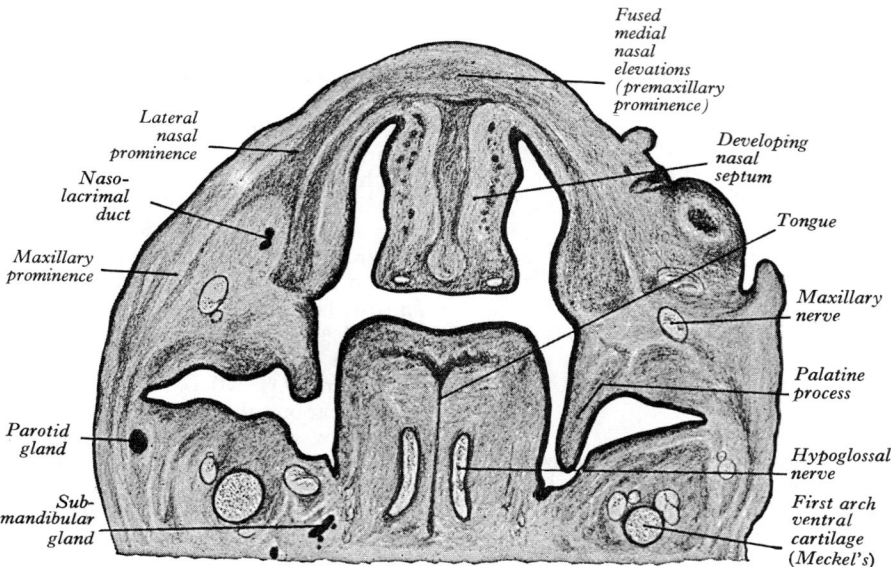

3.146B Oblique coronal section through the head of a human embryo 23 mm long. The nasal cavities communicate freely with the cavity of the mouth.

auditory tube, along a line corresponding in the final state to the palatopharyngeal arches (Baxter 1953).

On each side of the nasal septum, in a ventral or anterior position just above the primitive palate, placodal ectoderm is invaginated to form a pair of small diverticula, which extend dorsally and cranially into the septum. These are vestiges of the *vomeronasal organ* (**3.**146c), whose openings are close to the junction between the two premaxillae and the maxillae; they are always rudimentary in mankind, but are well-developed auxiliary olfactory organs in many vertebrates (pp. 1225, 1321). For bibliographies in the field of facial development consult Latham (1973).

Facial epithelium

The external ectoderm over the mandibular prominences becomes the skin of the face (**3.**147), and it also takes part in forming the tragus of the auricle (p. 1368). Its surface facial contribution is roughly triangular; the apex includes the tragus, the upper border extending to the lateral angle of the mouth and free border of lower lip; its lower border curves to follow the principal submandibular flexure line of the neck. The surface facial contribution of the maxillary prominence extends from the supratragic point to the lateral angles of eye and mouth, includes the lower eyelid and follows the paranasal line of the nasolacrimal duct, finally including a controversial amount of the upper lip.

The ectoderm on the arched, circumoral borders of both the mandibular and maxillary prominences, including the premaxilla medially, thickens along two curved parallel arches. The external thickening is the *labiogingival* or *vestibular lamina*, and the internal the *dental lamina*. The labiogingival lamina invades the subjacent mesenchyme and subsequently breaks down to form a sulcus (the vestibule) which separates the lower and upper lips from their adjacent gums. Within the mandibular prominence, the gum is separated from the tongue by the *linguogingival groove*. The dental lamina denote the sites of development of the enamel organs of the teeth.

Teeth. Teeth form from a series of epithelial/mesenchymal interactions along the dental lamina. In 27-mm embryos individual dental laminae expand into little ectodermal (dental) sacs surrounded by vascular mesenchyme. The ectoderm proliferates to form an *enamel organ* which surrounds a local portion of neural crest mesenchyme, the *dental papilla*; together this unit is a *tooth bud* or *germ*. The enamel organ initially forms a cap over the dental papilla then later it expands into a bell shape, the inner layer tightly adherent to the dental papilla and separated from the outer layer by accumulated glycosaminoglycans (GAGs). The inner cells of the enamel organ

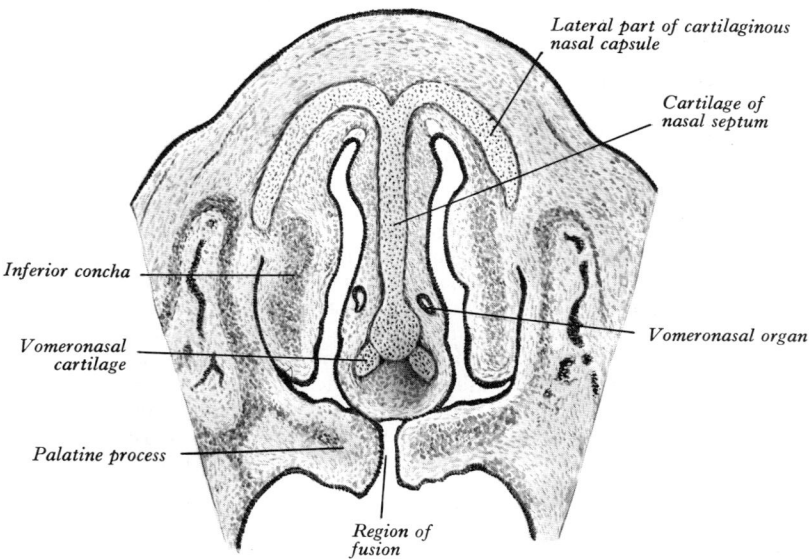

3.146c Coronal section through the nasal cavity of a human embryo 28 mm long. (After Kollmann.)

differentiate into *ameloblasts*, and the underlying mesenchymal cells into *odontoblasts*. Tooth development is further considered on page 111; the interactions associated with tooth development are considered below.

Both the deciduous and permanent teeth are formed as above. The permanent teeth develop in accessional positions from the lingual aspects of the existing tooth germ; however, the tooth germs for the 12 permanent molar teeth develop from posterior extensions of the dental laminae on each side of both jaws. Calcification begins in both deciduous and permanent teeth before birth; the deciduous teeth have well-developed crowns by full term, whereas the permanent teeth remain as tooth buds.

Just as the neural crest mesenchyme is responsible for the patterning of the pharyngeal arches, so it directs the pattern of tooth development. Thus, dental papilla mesenchyme is able to induce the formation of teeth in non-oral epithelium, and can specify the type of tooth produced, i.e. incisor or molar. Reciprocal interaction between the cells of the tooth germ in response to the extracellular

283

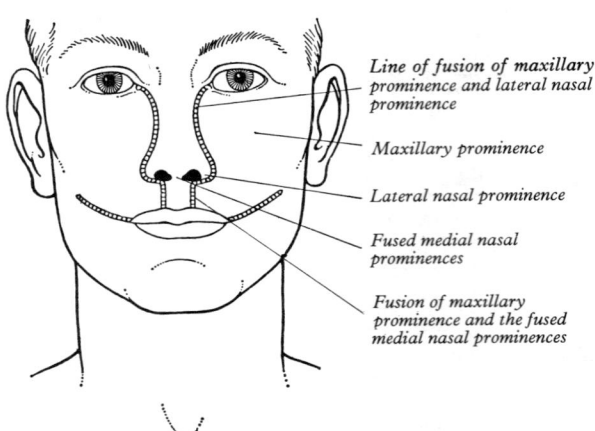

3.147 Diagram to show the parts of the adult face which are derived from the nasal elevations, and the maxillary and mandibular prominences.

Labels:
Line of fusion of maxillary prominence and lateral nasal prominence

Maxillary prominence

Lateral nasal prominence

Fused medial nasal prominences

Fusion of maxillary prominence and the fused medial nasal prominences

matrix they secrete occurs, i.e. secretion of predentin by odontoblasts stimulates the differentiation of the inner enamel organ into ameloblasts which secrete enamel.

When cranial neural crest is cultured alone it will differentiate into cartilage. If it is recombined with limb epithelium then cartilage and bone will form. However, when cranial neural crest is recombined with mandibular epithelium, salivary islands, hair and teeth form as well as cartilage and bone. Thus the mandibular epithelium is essential and specific for the development of teeth. At a local level, early (9–11.5 days) recombination of mouse mandibular epithelium and second arch mesenchyme results in teeth in 90% of cases, whereas the reverse recombination, second arch epithelium and mandibular arch mesenchyme, does not produce teeth. Later recombination experiments (11.5–12 days), where first arch mesenchyme is grafted with second arch epithelium, will produce teeth, leading to the conclusion that the crest mesenchyme becomes specified to produce teeth after day 12 (Kollar & Mina 1991). This specification can be changed experimentally. If presumptive incisor region of the mandibular epithelium is recombined with predetermined molar papillae from post-day 12 tooth germs, the shape of the teeth can be redefined by the epithelium and incisiform teeth develop.

The mesenchymal dental papilla can influence epithelia from different species; thus recombination of dental mesenchyme from 16–18-day mouse with oral epithelium from the mandibular epithelium of the chick resulted in tooth formation (Kollar & Fisher 1980). This is the more surprising as chicks do not normally develop teeth. Similarly recombination of chick arch mesenchyme and 10-day mandibular epithelium from the mouse resulted in tooth formation (Kollar & Mina 1991). In the latter case the epithelium initiated the dental papilla development.

Anomalies of facial development

Congenital malformations consequent upon arrest of development and failure of fusion of components in the formation of the face and palate are not uncommon. At the simplest, one maxillary prominence may fail completely to fuse with the corresponding premaxillary region (globular prominence), leading to a persistent fissure between the philtrum and lateral part of the upper lip on that side, *cleft lip* (less appropriately 'hare' lip). A similar but rare malformation follows failure of fusion between the maxillary prominence and the lateral nasal prominence, facial cleft, in which the nasolacrimal duct persists as an open furrow, a condition usually associated with cleft lip on the same side. The palatine processes may fail to fuse with each other and the nasal septum to variable degrees. In its severest form fusion is wholly lacking, leaving a wide fissure between the palatine processes through which the nasal septum is visible. On each side the premaxillary parts of the palate are separated from the maxillary palatine processes by clefts which are continuous ventrally with bilateral clefts in the upper lip. In such cases the philtrum is a separate entity, continuous cranially and dorsally with the nasal septum. The floor of the nasal cavity is deficient throughout its

extent and the choanae are not completed. Many varieties of milder degrees of cleft palate have been observed; the commonest type is unilateral, only one side of the nasal cavity being in communication with the mouth and the extent of the cleft being variable. In the mildest forms only the soft palate is cleft, or even merely the uvula. Such examples of arrested development may be associated with disturbances in embryonic nutrition during the second and the third months of gestation and the grosser varieties are usually coupled with malformations in other regions of the body (p. 333). In such cases the premaxillary region protrudes, with associated extension forwards of the nasal septum. For discussion see Latham (1973). Certain midline anomalies are rarely encountered, i.e. *median cleft lip* (true hare lip), *cleft nose* and *cleft lower jaw*. More common are minor degrees of *cleft chin* and *micrognathia*—underdevelopment of the lower jaw.

The further growth of the face during the fetal period has received little attention, although this period is by no means characterized entirely by incremental growth. It is during fetal life that human facial proportions develop (p. 371, Fig. 4.28). The facial and cranial parts display different patterns of growth, though each influences the other. For an interesting analysis of the data observed from 280 fetuses consult Lavelle (1974).

CAUDAL PHARYNGEAL ARCHES

Second pharyngeal arch

The ectoderm covering the outer aspect of the second pharyngeal arch originates from a strip of ectoderm lateral to the metencephalic neural fold (3.145), as does the otic placode (these placodal cells are located more laterally than the trigeminal placode in the 3-somite chick embryo). The cartilaginous element of the second arch (Reichert's cartilage) extends from the otic capsule to the midline on each side. Its dorsal end separates and becomes enclosed in the developing tympanic cavity as the *stapes*. Thereafter the cartilage gives rise to the *styloid process*, *stylohyoid ligament*, the *lesser cornu* and probably the *cranial rim* of the body of the *hyoid bone* (3.143).

The muscles of the second arch derive from somitomeres 4 and 5. For the most part the muscle mass migrates widely but retains its original nerve supply from the facial. The *stapedius*, *stylohyoid* and *posterior belly of digastric* remain attached to the hyoid skeleton, but the *facial musculature*, *platysma*, *auricular muscles* and *epicranius* all lose connection with it (3.144). Their migration is facilitated by the early obliteration of some of the first groove (cleft) and pouch (see below). (This cleft, the spiracle in fishes, is already much reduced in all but the earliest vertebrates.)

Third to sixth pharyngeal arches

The ectoderm adjacent to the myelencephalic neural fold, down to the level of somite 3, develops to cover the third and fourth pharyngeal arches, a much smaller distribution than that of the more rostral arches. The ectoderm in this region also gives rise to placodal cells which contribute to the petrosal and nodose ganglia. Chondrification does not occur in the dorsal parts of the skeletal elements of the third to sixth arches. The ventral cartilage of the third arch becomes the *greater cornu* of the *hyoid bone* and the *caudal part* of its *body*. (The whole of the body may be formed from the third arch cartilage.) Alternatively, the hyoid body may be derived from cartilage formed in the base of the hypobranchial eminence (p. 175) and thus from third arch tissue alone (Frazer 1926), acquiring its connection with the second arch cartilage secondarily.

The final adaptations of the cartilages of the skeletal elements in the fourth, fifth and sixth arches are a source of disagreement, but the following represents a fairly general view. The *thyroid cartilage* develops from the fourth and fifth arches, which may also give rise to the *arytenoid*, *corniculate* and *cuneiform cartilages*. The *cricoid cartilage* may be derived from the sixth arch cartilage, or it may be a modified tracheal ring. The *epiglottis* is developed in the substance of the hypobranchial eminence and probably not from 'true' branchial cartilage (3.144).

The paraxial mesenchyme from somitomeres 6 and 7 migrates to the third arch and somitomere 7 alone appears to invade the fourth arch (Trainor et al 1994). Somitomeric muscle was not identified in the sixth arch in the mouse. The muscle masses are adapted to form the musculature of the *pharynx, larynx* and *soft palate*. The *stylopharyngeus* can be attributed to the third and the *cricothyroid* to the fourth arch (**3.144**). The rest of the laryngeal muscles are derived from the sixth arch and used extensively for vocalization; thus they may not be represented to the same extent in non-human species. The precise origin of the remaining palatal muscles and the pharangeal constrictors is uncertain in man. A mixed origin, partly from paraxial mesenchyme and partly from adjacent myotomes, has been attributed to sternocleidomastoideus and trapezius (McKenzie 1955).

Nerves of the pharyngeal arches

The nerves of the pharyngeal arches immediately enter the dorsal ends of them (**3.139**). They are typically mixed, their motor component supplying the muscles of the arch and their sensory fibres innervating the skin and mucous membrane derived from the region. In fish the trunks of the nerves and their ganglia are close to the dorsal ends of the true clefts existing in these forms, each sending a post-trematic branch into its own arch and a pretrematic branch into the arch cranial to this. In mammals, some have claimed that both types of branch can be identified in the first arch, but only a single nerve can be identified with certainty in the second to sixth arches, with the exception of the fifth, the nerve of which is unknown and may have disappeared.

The trigeminal mandibular division is the post-trematic nerve of the first arch; the chorda tympani, or greater petrosal, has sometimes been regarded as its pretrematic nerve derived from the facial. The latter supplies the second arch, the glossopharyngeal the third, the superior laryngeal branch of the vagus the fourth and the latter's recurrent laryngeal branch the sixth. In lower vertebrates the fifth arch is also supplied by a vagal branch. Other branches that have, on occasion, been proposed as pretrematic are the tympanic branch of the glossopharyngeal and the auricular branch of the vagus. However, none of the foregoing fulfil sufficient criteria for them to be classified as pretrematic with confidence.

The difference in the courses of the recurrent laryngeal nerves can be explained by the development of the aortic arch arteries. In arches 1–5 the arch nerve enters rostral to its aortic arch artery. However, the nerve enters its sixth arch **caudal** to the aortic arch artery, retaining this position on the left side and hence being caudal to and looping round the ligamentum arteriosum in its final disposition. However, on the right, owing to the disappearance of the dorsal part of the sixth aortic arch artery and the whole of the fifth, the nerve loops round the caudal aspect of the **fourth** aortic arch artery, i.e. the subclavian artery.

Muscle of the pharyngeal arches

The muscles of the face and neck (**3.144**), sometimes described as branchiomeric because of their origin within the pharyngeal (branchial) arches, develop from a rostral continuation of the paraxial mesenchyme which, in the trunk, segments to form somites. Within the trunk somites give rise to medial skeletal elements: sclerotomes, which combine to form the vertebrae, lateral myotomic populations; myotomes, which form all of the striated muscle of the trunk and limbs; and limited dorsolateral connective tissue populations which contribute to the dermis over the dorsal surface dermatomes. Experimental quail–chick chimeras have permitted examination of the paraxial mesenchyme in the head to see if similar tripartite fates are available.

Although the paraxial mesenchyme in the head is unsegmented, a segmental pattern was described by Meier (1979) who noted seven *somitomeres* each side of the rostral notochord and beneath the overlying neural plate (see p. 154). Portions of paraxial mesenchyme, medial and lateral to the folding neural plate, were transplanted from quail embryos to chick and the fate of the cell populations followed (Couly et al 1992). At the 3-somite stage the cell density is much higher in the lateral paraxial mesenchyme than in the medial. Apart from the rostral regions of the medial paraxial mesenchyme, which in the avian embryo appeared to contribute to the ocular muscles (these in the main originate from prechordal mesenchyme; see p. 274), the medial mesenchyme gave rise to limited skeletal structures, for example part of the sphenoid and otic capsule, and connective tissues, including the mesencephalic and metencephalic meninges, but no muscles. In contrast, the lateral paraxial mes-

enchyme developed into the muscular lineages of the pharyngeal arches.

It is interesting that the fate of medial and lateral paraxial mesenchyme corresponds to the medial and lateral fates of the somites. The limited contribution to the dermis seen in the somites has no equivalence in the paraxial mesenchyme. In the head the dermis is formed by neural crest mesenchyme which also has the ability to develop calcified structures.

Prior to the formation of any skeletal elements in the arches, myoblasts migrate from the paraxial mesenchyme to the sites where overt muscle differentiation will occur and form premuscle condensations. The pattern of primary myotube alignment for any one muscle is specified by the surrounding neural crest mesenchyme and is not related to the source of the myoblasts. The rate and pattern of muscle maturation are closely associated with the development of the skeletal elements, such that muscles may attain attachments to one skeletal element but remain without additional attachments until the appropriate elements develop (McClearn & Noden 1988). Figure **3.148** shows the relationship between the somitomeres and the muscle masses migrating to each arch.

Pharyngeal grooves

Modification of the external contours of the arches occurs as the skeletal and muscular elements develop. The modification of the external *pharyngeal grooves* or (less appropriately) *clefts* produces the smooth contour of the neck. The concurrent development of the internal *pharyngeal pouches* also contributes to this process.

The first pharyngeal groove is obliterated ventrally, as in all but the most ancient vertebrates. In man its dorsal end deepens to form the epithelium of the external acoustic meatus and the external surface of the tympanic membrane. (For details see p. 262.)

At the dorsal ends of the first, second and fourth pharyngeal grooves thickened patches of ectoderm appear, the *epibranchial placodes*. These are closely related to the developing ganglia of the facial, glossopharyngeal and vagus nerves, to which they contribute (p. 224): these, and other placodal cells (*dorsolateral* and *suprabranchial*) also contribute to the trigeminal and vestibulocochlear ganglia (see **3.103**).

At the end of the fifth week the third and fourth arches are sunk in a retrohyoid depression, the *cervical sinus*. Cranially the sinus is bounded by the hyoid arch, dorsally by a ridge produced by ventral extensions from the occipital myotomes and by mesenchyme developing into sternocleidomastoid and trapezius. Caudally, the smaller *epipericardial ridge* separates the sinus from the pericardium and curves cranially near the midline and then with its fellow reaches the lingual swelling of the mandibular prominence and the hypobranchial eminence. Myoblasts from the occipital myotomes migrating to the tongue follow the epipericardial ridge together with the hypoglossal nerve. The long held view that the cervical sinus is obliterated by caudal growth of the hyoid arches to fuse with the cardiac elevation, excluding the succeeding arches from any part in the formation of the skin of the neck, has been criticized; an alternative view is that the sinus is reduced by gradual approximation of its walls from within outwards. It should be noted, however, that some contend that the surface course of the second groove persists as the curved submandibular *cervical flexure line*. Whatever the mechanism a smooth epidermal covering to the neck results with platysma (a second arch muscle), bounded both superficially and deep by superficial fascia, passing along the neck to the anterior thoracic wall.

Pharyngeal pouches

The first four pharyngeal pouches appear in sequence craniocaudally, and their endoderm approaches the ectoderm of the overlying pharyngeal grooves to form thin *closing membranes* (**3.139, 140**). The blind recesses of the second, third and fourth pouches are prolonged dorsally and ventrally as angular, wing-like diverticula. From the fourth a diverticulum grows caudoventrally and is at first demarcated from the pouch by a groove in which may occur a transient fifth aortic arch artery. From this diverticulum a fifth pouch may develop and establish a connection with the ectoderm. The remainder of this diverticulum is the *ultimobranchial body*. This, together with the fourth pouch and the transitory fifth, when present, constitute the *caudal pharyngeal complex*. Its communication with the cavity of the pharynx is the *common pharyngobranchial duct*. The ultimo-

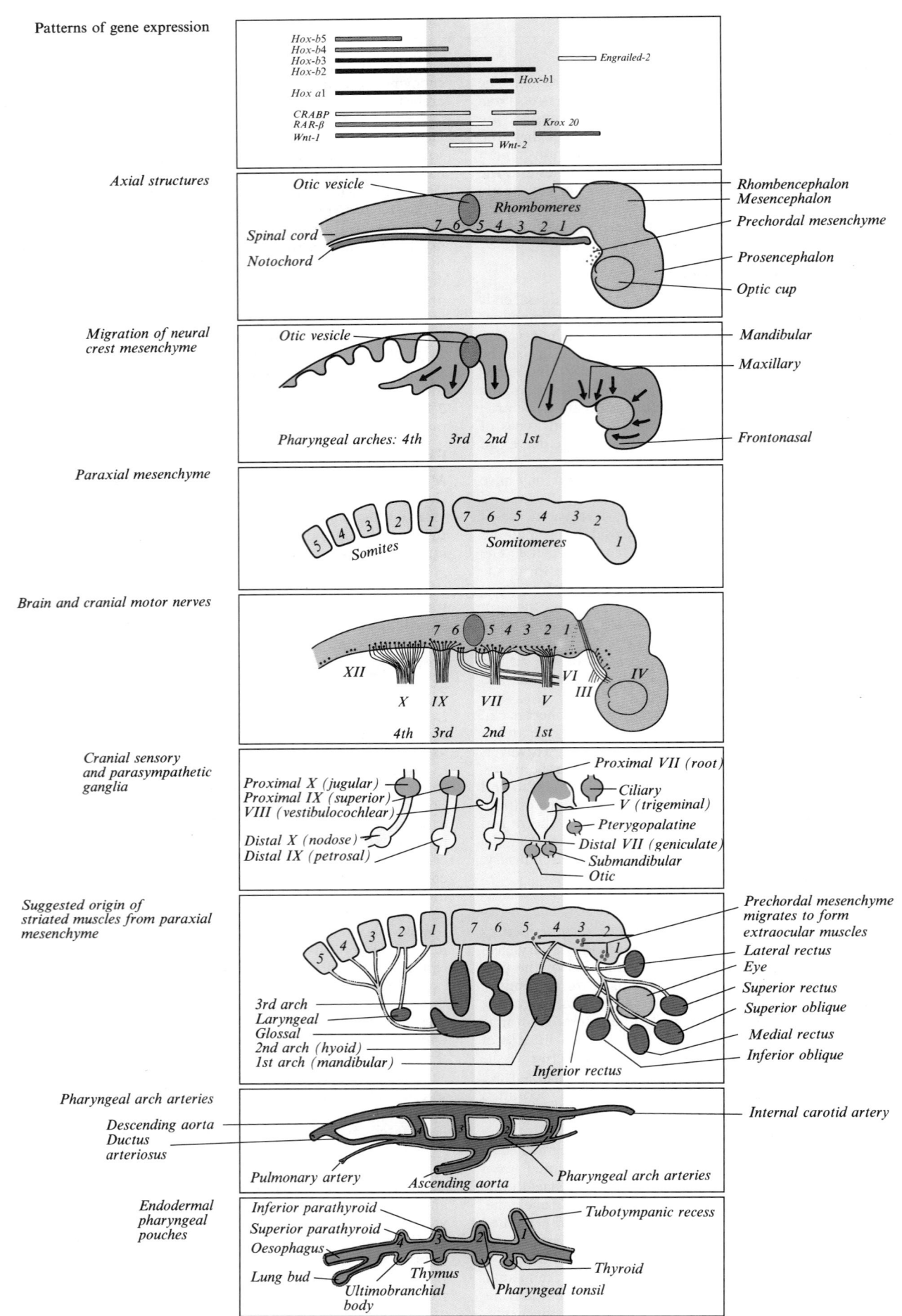

Patterns of gene expression

Hox-b5
Hox-b4
Hox-b3
Hox-b2
Hox a1
Hox-b1
Engrailed-2
CRABP
RAR-β
Krox 20
Wnt-1
Wnt-2

Axial structures

Otic vesicle
Rhombomeres
7 6 5 4 3 2 1
Spinal cord
Notochord
Rhombencephalon
Mesencephalon
Prechordal mesenchyme
Prosencephalon
Optic cup

Migration of neural crest mesenchyme

Otic vesicle
Mandibular
Maxillary
Pharyngeal arches: 4th 3rd 2nd 1st
Frontonasal

Paraxial mesenchyme

5 4 3 2 1 7 6 5 4 3 2 1
Somites
Somitomeres

Brain and cranial motor nerves

7 6 5 4 3 2 1
XII
X IX VII V
VI III IV
4th 3rd 2nd 1st

Cranial sensory and parasympathetic ganglia

Proximal X (jugular)
Proximal IX (superior)
VIII (vestibulocochlear)
Distal X (nodose)
Distal IX (petrosal)
Proximal VII (root)
Ciliary
V (trigeminal)
Pterygopalatine
Distal VII (geniculate)
Submandibular
Otic

Suggested origin of striated muscles from paraxial mesenchyme

5 4 3 2 1 7 6 5 4 3 2 1
3rd arch
Laryngeal
Glossal
2nd arch (hyoid)
1st arch (mandibular)
Inferior rectus
Prechordal mesenchyme migrates to form extraocular muscles
Lateral rectus
Eye
Superior rectus
Superior oblique
Medial rectus
Inferior oblique

Pharyngeal arch arteries

Descending aorta
Ductus arteriosus
Pulmonary artery
Ascending aorta
Pharyngeal arch arteries
Internal carotid artery

Endodermal pharyngeal pouches

Inferior parathyroid
Superior parathyroid
Oesophagus
Lung bud
Ultimobranchial body
Thymus
Pharyngeal tonsil
Tubotympanic recess
Thyroid

3.148 Schema illustrating the organization of the head and pharynx in an embryo at about stage 14. The individual tissue components have been separated but are aligned in register through the numbered zones. (After Noden.)

branchial body is almost a constant feature of vertebrate development (Watzka 1955). Its form in the human embryo, however, has been a matter of controversy. Apparently it is incorporated into the rest of the caudal pharyngeal complex and contributes to the development of the lateral thyroid rudiment (p. 177). Ultimobranchial bodies exist in the adults of many lower vertebrates and *calcitonin* has been isolated from such tissue (Copp et al 1967). There is thus a strong presumption that the parafollicular cells of the human thyroid gland, which are a source of calcitonin, are derived from ultimobranchial tissue.

The further development of the endodermal derivatives of the pharyngeal pouches is intimately associated with that of the mouth, pharynx and larynx, and is considered with them (p. 176).

Rhombomeres, *Hox* genes and arch development

It has been seen in the above accounts that the cranial neural crest proliferates to form a significant mesenchymal population in the head, face and pharyngeal arches which controls the pattern of development of the face and arches, specifying the position of muscles, nerves and blood vessels. Experimental studies have shown that if first arch (mandibular) crest is grafted into the hyoid (second) arch, mandibular structures form, suggesting that the differentiation pattern of the second arch paraxial mesenchyme and surface ectoderm was redefined by the new crest mesenchyme (Noden 1988). Other experiments on tooth development (see above) illustrate the same phenomenon. These experiments, however, do not suggest whether the crest cells gain their patterning ability before leaving the neural plate or afterwards during their migration to the arches.

The neural crest cells migrate from the neural folds of the diencephalon, mesencephalon, metencephalon and myelencephalon; crest cells do not arise from the prosencephalic neural folds. At the time of crest migration the hindbrain (rhombencephalon) is composed of a repeating pattern of bulges, the rhombomeres (see p. 241), segmental units seen in the brains of all developing vertebrates. Single-cell marking experiments show that rhombomeres operate as distinct compartments with lineage restriction. There are eight rhombomeres identified in the hindbrain. Labelling of crest cells along the neural folds prior to migration has revealed a relationship between the sites of emergence of the crest cells and the rhombomeric epithelium (Lumsden et al 1991). Neural crest cells originate from three discontinuous levels and migrate ventrally in three distinct streams (**3**.106A). Crest cells from rhombomeres 1 and 2 contribute to the trigeminal ganglion and produce first arch mesenchyme, crest cells from rhombomere 4 contribute to the facial and vestibulo-acoustic ganglion and produce second arch mesenchyme, while crest cells from rhombomere 6 contribute to the superior petrosal ganglion and produce third arch mesenchyme. Two axial levels, rhombomeres 3 and 5, do not contribute to the emergent neural crest. However, crest cells migrating from rhombomeres 3 and 5 have been isolated in vitro, suggesting that in vivo the even-numbered rhombomeres may exert a dominant negative effect upon the odd numbered, suppressing neural crest production (Graham et al 1993). Such suppression, by segregating the crest into three distinct streams, may ensure the specific filling of each of the pharyngeal arches and the correct development of each of the individual cranial ganglia. The specification of the neural crest thus occurs before it migrates from the neural folds.

The axial homeobox genes, *Hox-a* and *Hox-b* (see p. 228), are expressed in the rhombomeres and in neural crest cells from the point of origin, during migration and after migration has ceased. Each pharyngeal arch expresses a different combination of *Hox* genes in a segment restricted manner (Hunt et al 1991; **3**.106, 148). The exact relationship between *Hox* expression in the rhombomeres and later in the arches is not yet clear. For example, *Hox-b1* is delineated sharply in rhombomere 4 and later in arch 2; however, *Hox-b2* is expressed in all rhombomeres caudal from rhombomere 3, yet rhombomeres 3 and 5 do not produce migratory crest cells. Figure **3**.148 shows the extent of *Hox* expression in the rhombomeres, the neural crest and the surface ectoderm.

Disruptions of the *Hox* genes cause failure of normal crest cell proliferation and migration, producing anomalies similar to human congenital disorders, for example DiGeorge's syndrome (see p. 228).

Head development and evolution

The developmental mechanisms which operate within the trunk are different from those operating in the head: an observation which could be used to deduce that the head evolved by a different route from the other axial structures, using different cell populations which do not respond to, or differentiate earlier than, the inducers in the trunk region.

The vertebrate head is especially different from the 'cranial end' of its nearest relations, the cephalocaudates. They have, in common with vertebrates, segmented muscle blocks, a dorsal hollow nerve cord, gill slits and a notochord. However, they have no clear head, no obvious tripartite brain, no neural crest or ectodermal placodes, no paired sense organs or cranial ganglia. Amphioxus and other cephalocaudates may be considered to be distant relations of vertebrates; however, no link can be postulated that would demonstrate the gradual evolution of cephalization.

Until now, we have had few tools with which to examine the complexity and **comparative** nature of head development in extant species of vertebrates **and** cephalocaudates. The data now being generated by molecular biological studies on head development will have far-reaching effects and take much time to interpret.

A hypothesis of head evolution which is suggested by examination of the development of the head has been put forward by Gans and Northcutt (1983) and Northcutt and Gans (1983). They propose that the rostral part of the head, including the sense organs, prosencephalon, mesencephalon and surrounding skull, is derived from the neuroectoderm. Experimental studies have confirmed that the 'prechordal' skull, i.e. that part rostral to the notochord (Couly et al 1992), which surrounds the expanded rostral brain, is formed from neural crest, a population of neuroectoderm which invaginates between the neural tube and epidermal ectoderm, after neurulation. The neuroectoderm also gives rise to the sense organs via a series of ectodermal placodes, regions of neuroectoderm which do not separate from the epidermal ectoderm until the invaginated neural crest migrates beneath them. Between them, the cell populations produced by the neural crest and ectodermal placodes produce all of the sensory ganglia and sense organs within the head (the eyes, which are derived directly from the neural tube, are excluded from this group).

The neural crest also provides a new mesenchymal population which fulfils a role similar to that of the somatic and somatopleuric mesenchymes within the trunk. Specific interaction between the sclerotomal portion of the somite and the perinotochordal matrix promotes chondrogenesis around the notochord and neural tube resulting in the formation of the vertebrae. Condensations of somatopleuric mesenchyme within the limb have a chondrogenic fate when the cell density is high, and somatopleuric mesenchyme can be induced to follow this lineage in culture if the cells are arrested from migration and kept at high density. Neural crest cells, which never follow a chondrogenic pathway in the trunk, are able to differentiate into chondrocytes and other connective tissues in the head, and they are able to pattern the development of the facial primordia in the same manner as somatopleuric mesenchyme can pattern the limb. The mechanisms by which this occurs is not clear although the 'flypaper model', specifying the pattern of cranial chondrogenesis (Thorogood 1988), suggests that the neural crest responds to similar cues and in a similar manner as the sclerotomes (see p. 274).

It should be noted that the vertebrate head is formed not only by addition of neural crest in the rostral region but also by incorporation, in the caudal region, of an increasing number of vertebrae. The Agnatha have no vertebral contribution to the skull; the amphibians and selachians incorporate three occipital somites, whereas in the vertebrate skull all five occipital somites are included. This caudal enlargement contributes to the general increase in the volume of the skull around the expanding rhombencephalon at the same time as the crest-derived rostral portions of the skull surround the prosencephalon.

Mapping of the neural plate in the chick has shown that the prechordal skull is formed rostral to the adenohypophyseal placode from ectodermal and neural crest cells located in the neural folds. From rostral to caudal the neural folds produce the adenohypophysis (in the midline) and then on each side the olfactory ectodermal placode, the frontonasal ectoderm, the calvarial ectoderm and the cephalic neural crest (3.145). The ectoderm of the first pharyngeal arch is found lateral to the cephalic neural crest and it migrates rostrally and medially to contribute to the face (3.145). There is a neural crest-free gap over rhombomere 3 (see below) that separates presumptive frontonasal/maxillary/mandibular cells from the

second arch crest. Few or no crest cells are formed by neural folds at the level of the otic placode (rhombomere 5).

After neurulation, many structures present in the head of extant vertebrates are segmentally organized. For example, in the rhombencephalon there are ridges which divide the hindbrain into rhombomeres (3.148); subjacent paraxial mesenchyme is arranged as definitely segmented occipital somites and, more rostrally, possibly segmented somitomeres. More lateral and ventral locations contain the ectodermal placodes, the embryonic aortic arch arteries and the pharyngeal pouches. However, this segmentation is seen only caudal to the hypophysis, each side of the notochord. Thus the transient segmental nature of cephalic development is taking place in the 'ancestral' or 'old' head and brain. However, this paradigm is only partially supported by studies examining the expression of *Hox* genes in the developing brain.

Hox genes are expressed along the embryonic axis in invertebrate and vertebrate embryos. Recent cloning of *Hox* genes from cephalochordate embryos has shown an amphioxus *Hox* gene *Amphi-Hox-3* (Holland et al 1992) homologous to the mouse *Hox-2.7* gene. The rostral limit of expression of this gene in amphioxus is at the level of the 4/5 somite boundary at the neurula stage and at later stages within a spatially restricted domain

of the developing nerve cord. Homologous gene expression in vertebrate embryos corresponds to the rhombomere 4/5 boundary. Holland et al propose that the structures expressing these genes in the two body plans are homologous. They suggest that this evidence supports the hypothesis that the vertebrate head evolved by elaboration and expansion of a pre-existing cranial region rather than by production of a new rostral portion. The utilization of extensive neural crest populations in the head may have resulted because it was a source of mesenchyme which could be modified and adapted without simultaneous reorganization of the trunk; the developmental flexibility of the crest population could promote an evolutionary flexibility and produce the diversity seen in vertebrate species today.

Noden (1991) adds a note of caution to the general interpretation of the developmental processes within the head, especially with the eruption of molecular biological applications for studying embryonic development. He recognizes that our present understanding of the morphology of development, of the patterns of cell movement, commitment and interactions which lead to the spatial assembly of complex arrays, is as yet inadequate to provide a basis for interpreting molecular analysis. The resolution of these challenges in the understanding of head development is awaited with interest.

APPENDICULAR SKELETON AND MUSCLES

The appendicular skeleton and muscles arise from both paraxial mesenchyme (the epithelial somite) and lateral plate mesenchyme (somatopleuric).

Morphological changes in the limbs

The limbs develop via a continual series of complex epithelial/mesenchymal interactions initiated in the lateral body walls. The proliferating somatopleuric mesenchyme forms a ridge externally, ventrolateral to the somites, which extends caudally from the most caudal (sixth) pharyngeal arch, finally tapering towards the tail. Interaction of *specialized regions of the somatopleuric mesenchyme* with the overlying ectoderm gives rise to local, thickened regions of surface ectoderm and proliferation of the underlying mesenchyme; this specifies the position of the future limb buds. At the site of each putative limb the ectoderm forms a longitudinal ridge of high columnar epithelial cells, the *apical ectodermal ridge (AER)* (3.149, 150). The AER and the underlying, specialized somatopleuric mesenchyme are termed the *progress zone*; this remains at the distal tip of the limb until the digits are formed. The progress zone controls the orientation and progression of limb development and specifies the position of the skeletal elements. The somatopleuric mesenchyme controls the specific developmental fate of the overlying ectoderm and within the limb becomes the skeletal and connective tissue elements. Precursor muscle cells and neurons migrate into the limb somewhat later. Consistent with the craniocaudal progression of development, the upper limb develops in advance of the lower. The earliest signs of limb development are seen in stage 12 (26 days)

embryos. A ridge is visible along the lateral longitudinal axis of the body wall opposite somites 8–10, at the level of the entrance to the cranial intestinal portal; this is the upper limb bud. By stage 13 the lower limb bud is also visible.

The upper limb bud enlarges, protruding laterally from its elliptical base at the body wall as a flattened plate, with a curved border and an AER forming its distal tip; it also has initially equal and relatively flat *dorsal* and *ventral ectodermal surfaces*, and a somatopleuric mesenchymal core. For descriptive, experimental and conceptual purposes it has been necessary to define and name various 'axes', borders, surfaces and lines in relation to the bud (3.150). (However, some minor variation in *terminology* will be noted when human development is compared with basic tetrapod—amphibian, reptilian and also avian—development. Mechanisms, nevertheless, remain similar.) An imaginary line from the centre of the elliptical base of the bud, through the centre of its mesenchymal core, to the centre of the apical ectodermal ridge, defines the *proximodistal axis* of the bud (for long, in descriptive embryology, known simply as **the axis**). Named in relation to the latter, the limb border cranially placed is the *preaxial border* and that caudally placed is the *postaxial border*. (In tetrapods and birds, the latter are termed anterior and posterior borders, respectively; see below.) Any line passing through the limb bud from preaxial to postaxial border, (and orthogonal to the proximodistal axis) thus constitutes a *cranio-caudal axis*. The dorsal and ventral ectodermal surfaces thus clothe their respective aspects from preaxial to postaxial borders. Thus, any line passing from dorsal to ventral aspect (and orthogonal to both proximodistal and craniocaudal axes) constitutes a *dorsoventral axis*. (It should be noted here that the terms *dorsal* and *ventral axial lines* are to be used exclusively in relation to developing and definitive patterns of cutaneous innervation of the limbs and their associated levels of the trunk.

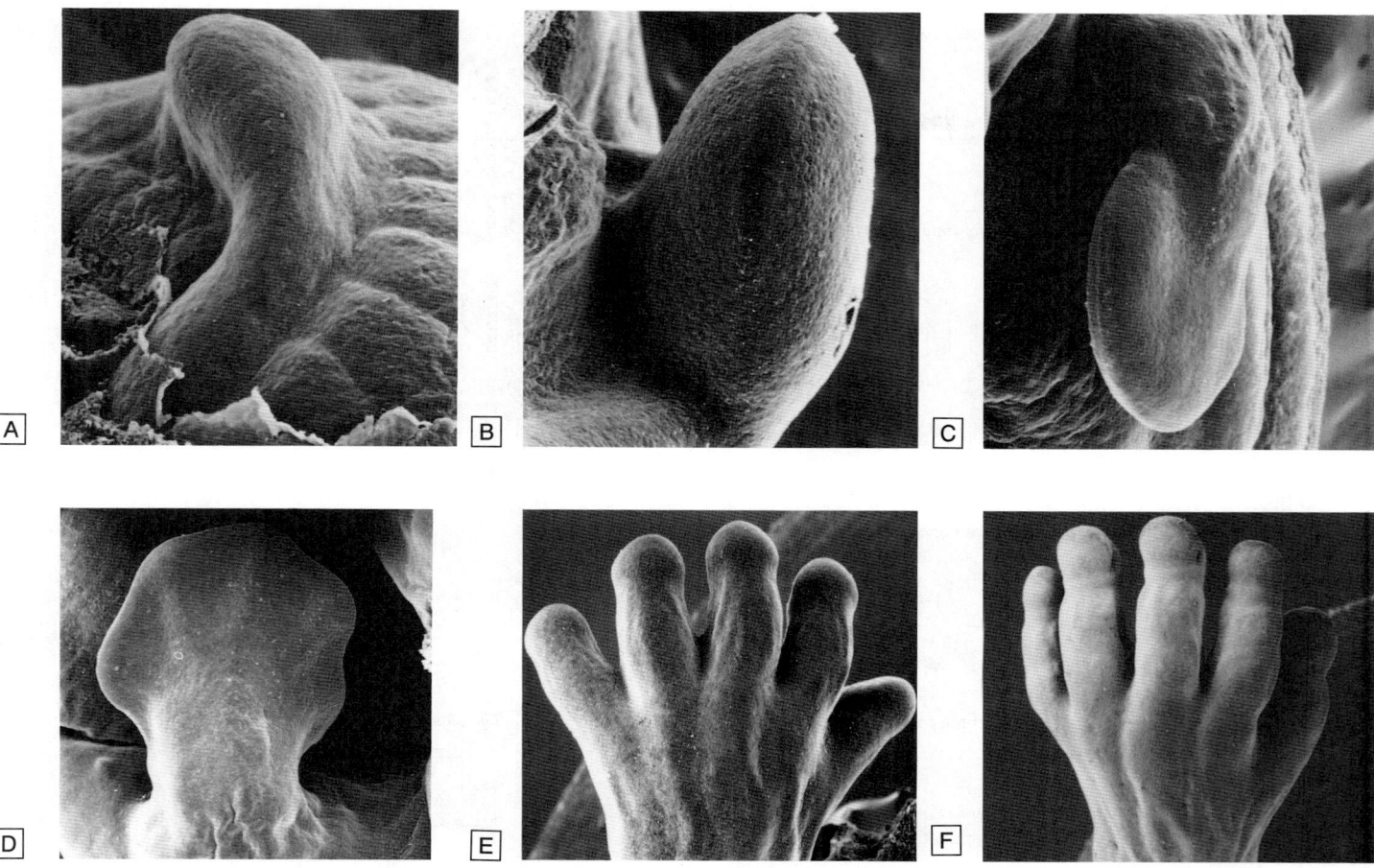

3.149 Series of scanning electron micrographs to show the development of the upper limb. A. The earliest limb bud viewed from the postaxial border. B. Limb bud viewed from postaxial border; the apical ectodermal ridge can be seen. C. Limb bud, ventrolateral view; the shoulder and elbow region are specified and a hand plate has formed. The apical ectodermal ridge is still obvious at the margin of the hand plate. D. Digital rays are present in the hand plate and the margin of the plate is becoming notched. E. The fingers are nearly separated and proliferations are commencing at the distal end of each digit to form the nail bed. F. The fingers each have tactile pads distally and nail development continues. (Photographs by P Collins; printed by S Cox, Electron Microscopy Unit, Southampton General Hospital.)

Early differential growth of parts of the limb bud result in two main changes to the originally symmetric axes of the limb:

(1) The dorsal aspect of the limb grows faster than the ventral; this causes the limb bud to curve around the body wall; the ventral surface of the limb which is closest to the body wall remains relatively flat but the dorsal surface bulges into the amniotic cavity; the originally laterally facing AER becomes increasingly directed ventrally.
(2) Slightly later the preaxial border grows faster than the postaxial, resulting in a further shift of the AER caudally rather than ventrally. These reorientations in the upper limb form the shoulder, arm and forearm; however, their effects cannot be seen until later (see below).

By stage 13 (28 days) the upper limb bud is curving ventrally while the lower limb bud is still directed laterally; in stage 14 embryos the preaxial border has started to lengthen in the upper limb but not yet in the lower. The upper limb at this stage is opposite the developing ventricles of the heart; the lower limb is closely associated with the wide umbilical cord. In stage 15 the upper limb can be subdivided into definite regions. The proximal portion of the limb still shows the dorsal bulge and ventral curve—this is the shoulder region and upper arm region; the next distal portion which was derived from the increase in the length of the preaxial border can now be identified as the forearm. The most distal portion is now expanded into a flattened hand plate.

At stage 16 the limbs appear much more substantial. The upper limb is sometimes close to the body wall and sometimes abducted; the lower limbs do not curve close to the body wall as the umbilical cord is very wide at this time. The hand plate has the first indications of digit rays and the lower limb has an early foot plate.

By stage 17 the upper limb has an elbow region and digit rays; in advanced members of this group the hand plate has a crenated rim indicating the beginning of tissue removal between the digits. The lower limb still has a flattened foot plate. Although a hip region can be seen there is no true knee as yet.

In stage 18 (44 days) embryos the foot plate has digit rays and there is further crenation of the hand plate between the digit rays. The lower limb appears to be flexed at the hip and abducted with the knee bent; this gives the appearance that the knee is facing laterally. There is very little skin of the thigh visible; the soles of the feet face the umbilical cord.

Changes during stages 19–23 are concerned with growth of the limbs and separation of the digits. The hands are now curving over the cardiac region. The distal phalangeal portions of the fingers enlarge at stage 21 forming the nail beds. This can be seen on the separated toes at stage 23. The feet can finally touch at stage 21 when the umbilical cord becomes proportionally smaller and the embryo larger.

Concepts of limb development

Limb development may be conceptualized as resulting from a series of ectodermal/mesenchymal interactions (3.150, 151). Such concepts are supported by experimental evidence from amphibian, avian and reptilian species which demonstrate a remarkable conservation of developmental processes. Chimeric experimentation has further revealed the specific fates of cell populations within the developing limb. The demonstration of conserved homeobox-containing genes in the developing limb (see below) may however require some

289

1. Axes of the limb

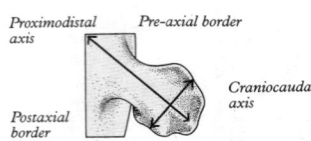

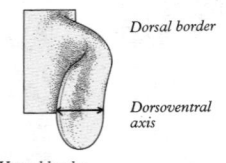

2. An apical ectodermal ridge (AER) is needed for limb outgrowth.

3. Only 'limb' mesenchyme can produce limb outgrowth.

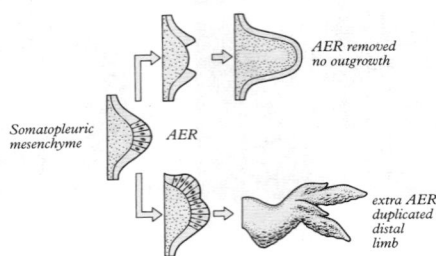

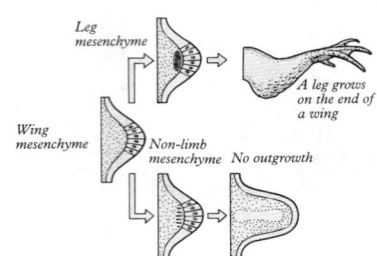

4. The AER and underlying mesenchyme = progress zone. This controls the time of limb development.

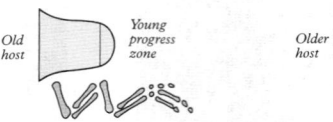

5. The zone of polarising activity (ZPA) specifies the postaxial border of the limb.

6. The ectodermal sleeve specifies the dorsal and ventral surfaces.

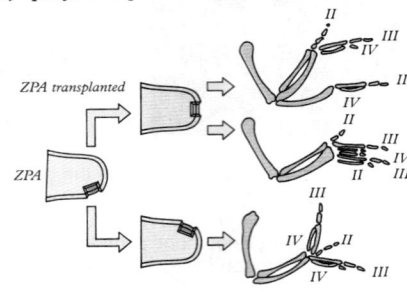

Transplantation of the ZPA into the AER or the pre-axial border produces distal limb reduplication. The digit closest to the ZPA is IV or V.

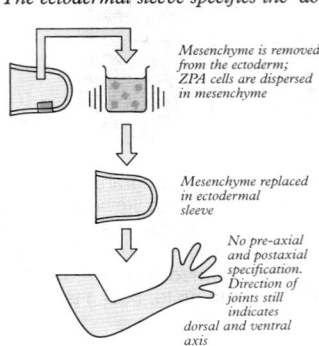

7. The length of the AER is controlled by necrotic zones.

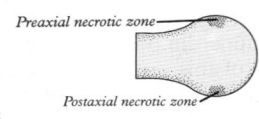

The number of digits is controlled by the length of the AER.

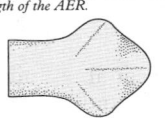

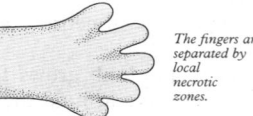

8. Hox expression in the limb.

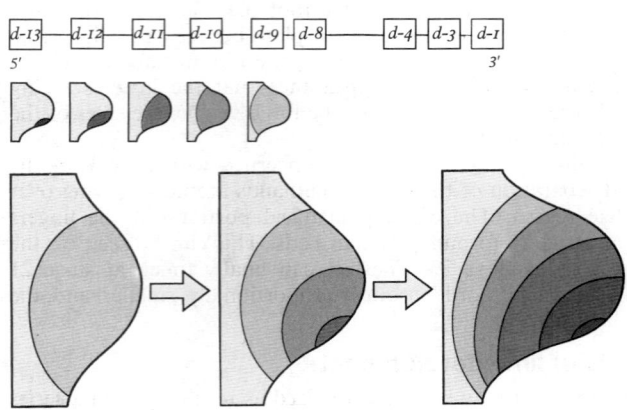

The Hox genes are expressed like nested dolls.

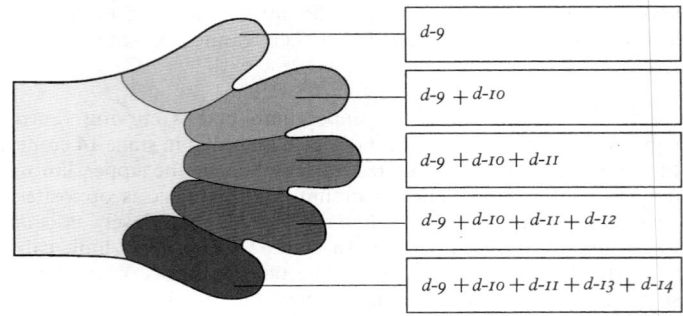

3.150 Schema illustrating the results of the major experimental studies on the developing limb. It should be noted that great strides have been made in identifying the factors responsible for the epithelial/mesenchymal interactions shown above. Fibroblast growth factor (FGF) can replace the apical ectodermal ridge and control limb outgrowth. FGF also maintains the ZPA. The gene *sonic hedgehog* (Shh), a homolog of the Drosophila segment polarity gene, has a polarizing activity in the limb and Shh colocalizes with ZPA activity. The interaction between the apical ectodermal ridge and the underlying mesenchyme can now be reinterpreted as an interaction between locally expressed Fgf4 (in the ridge) and Shh (in the mesenchyme). Retinoic acid also mimics the effect of ZPA activity and can induce expression of Fgf4. The lower schema, the *Hox* gene expression in the developing limb, may need reinterpretation in the light of these most recent advances. We look forward to this with interest.

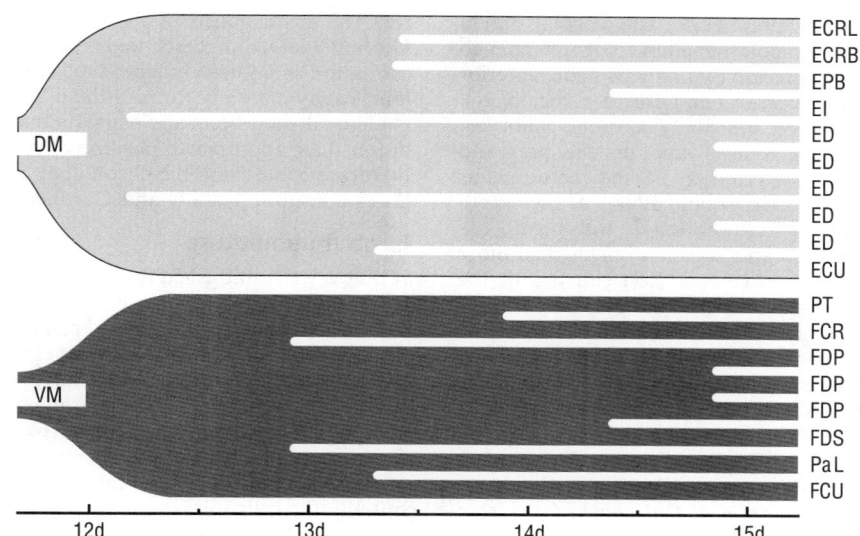

ECRL
ECRB
EPB
EI
ED
ED
ED
ED
ED
ECU

PT
FCR
FDP
FDP
FDP
FDS
PaL
FCU

DM

VM

12d   13d   14d   15d

3.151   Diagrammatic representation of the development of the dorsal and ventral muscle masses in the forearm. Changes in the extracellular environment induce local fusion of myoblasts and, from that point, division of the muscle mass. (After Kieny et al 1986.)

ECRL = extensor carpi radialis longus
ECRB = extensor carpi radialis brevis
EPB = extensor pollicis brevis
EIP = extensor indicis proprius
ED = extensor digitorum
ECU = extensor carpi ulnaris

PT = pronator teres
FCR = flexor carpi radialis
FDP = flexor digitorum profundus
FDS = flexor digitorum superficialis
Pa L = palmaris longus
FCU = flexor carpi ulnaris
d = days

reinterpretation of these concepts to reconcile the molecular model with the traditional model.

Progress zone (AER-mes). The outgrowth of a limb bud is controlled by the apical ectodermal ridge (AER) and the *underlying somatopleuric mesenchyme*. The epithelium seems to control the developmental stage of the limb and the somatopleuric mesenchyme controls the type of limb, interpreting the temporal information from the AER in a proximodistal developmental progression. These two tissue arrangements form the *progress zone*, a region which is believed to be the site where assignments are made to cell populations in the limb. As cells leave the progress zone, their *proximal/distal value* becomes fixed. Once the mesenchyme has been assigned it specifies the developmental pattern of the overlying ectoderm.

The work of Zwilling (1968), Saunders et al (1976), Hinchcliffe and Johnson (1980) has provided much evidence of limb morphogenesis. The knowledge may be summarized as follows:

- The AER and underlying mesenchyme provide the orientating influence for limb outgrowth. Removal of the AER results in cessation of limb development; insertion of a second AER results in two axes of development: there is duplication of distal structures from the graft onwards.
- Replacement of the underlying mesenchyme with any other mesenchyme results in no limb development: only 'limb' mesenchyme will promote limb bud formation; however, replacement of upper limb mesenchyme with lower limb mesenchyme does support limb growth but leads to the development of leg structures. In addition the leg mesenchyme will pass information back to the local ectoderm causing appropriate leg feather (in chick) development. It is reasoned that the mesenchyme beneath the AER provides an 'AER maintenance factor' which is essential to the function of the ridge.

The *temporal* nature of the information passing from the AER to the underlying mesenchyme was illustrated in a series of experiments by Summerbell (1974). A graft of a young limb bud to an older one with the progress zone removed results in duplication of limb elements. Conversely a graft of an old progress zone onto the stump of a younger limb produces a limb with intermediate sections missing (see **3**.150). The progress zone behaves independently as if no communication concerning positional values travels in a proximodistal direction. As cells leave the progress zone their proximodistal values are specified (**3**.150).

In grafting experiments only whole limb bones develop. Eight states of the progress zone can be described: i.e. humerus, ulnaradius, carpals I, carpals II, metacarpals, phalanges I, phalanges II,

phalanges III, each state taking approximately 8 hours. Summerbell and Lewis (1975) noted that the progress zone behaves like a clock whose ticks are cell-division cycles.

The precision with which skeletal growth occurs is often not appreciated. In calculating the growth in left limbs versus right limbs Summerbell et al (1973) concluded that the length of the left ulna of a limb did not vary by more than 5% of the length of the right.

Axes of the limb. The three developmental axes can be identified in the developing limb bud by stage 13 (**3**.150). These are, as noted above, the *proximodistal*, the *dorsoventral* and the *craniocaudal* axes. Each of the three principal axes seem to be specified by different mechanisms. The *proximodistal axis*, as mentioned previously, is controlled by the *progress zone* (i.e. the AER and subjacent somatopleuric mesenchyme). The *craniocaudal axis* is controlled by a small population of mesenchymal cells on the postaxial border of the limb bud, some distance from the AER; this mesenchyme is termed the *zone of polarizing activity* (ZPA). The ZPA specifies digit five; further away from the ZPA digits four, three, two and one develop.

If the ZPA is grafted beneath an AER, duplication of the limb occurs from that time onwards. If the ZPA is grafted onto the preaxial border of the limb a duplicated distal portion grows with the orientation reversed (**3**.150).

The *dorsoventral axis* of the limb appears to be controlled by the *ectoderm* of the limb. If the mesenchyme of a limb is removed and dissociated then repacked into the ectodermal sleeve, a limb will develop which has no anterior–posterior axis, i.e. the ZPA has been dispersed. However, the limb does have dorsal and ventral surfaces identified by the directions of the joints and position and type of hair.

Early skeletal elements of the limb. Formation of the cartilage elements of the limb has been suggested to be related to the shape of the limb and the conditions necessary for chondrogenesis. There is an *antichondrogenic zone* beneath the ectoderm of the limb which prevents chondrogenesis within the dermis and myogenic zones (p. 264). Foci of chondrogenesis occur in the **centre** of the limb bud where the cell density is highest, then the production of extracellular matrix by these cells encourages chondrogenic differentiation. In more distal portions of the limb, the limb bud widens forming first two centres of chondrogenesis, then later five centres. The AER is believed to control the width of the digital plate which in turn will reflect this width by the number of digits which develop. Zones on the cranial and caudal, or preaxial and postaxial borders of the limb which show preprogrammed cell death can be identified at the same time as the ZPA. These zones limit the length of the AER.

The experimentation concerning these zones was carried out in chick embryos. It is customary in anamniote embryology to refer to the craniocaudal axis as anteroposterior (with the human anterior and posterior surfaces being termed ventral and dorsal, respectively). This terminology has been retained for many amniote embryos, especially avian. Thus the special zones found on the pre- and postaxial borders of the limb are referred to, in the literature, as *anterior* and *posterior necrotic zones* (ANZ and PNZ). If the length of the AER becomes reduced then fewer digits will form—*oligodactyly*; if the AER is not reduced and becomes longer then more digits will form—*polydactyly*. This latter condition can permit the development of supernumerary digits on either the pre- or postaxial borders. There are other regions of cell death occurring between the digits which result in digital separation, but these occur later than the ANZ and PNZ. The cells between the digits are removed by macrophages. Note cells in the ANZ, PNZ and between the digits undergo apaptosis.

Most of the bones in the appendicular skeleton derive from somatopleuric mesenchyme. Within the upper limb, however, although the *clavicle* and *coracoid portion of the scapula* arise from somatopleuric mesenchyme, the *body and spine of the scapula* are believed to derive from the somites (Chevallier 1977). No recent studies yet dispute this finding.

Prechondroblasts are present in the upper limb at stage 13 and condensations of cartilage can be detected at stage 16 when the *humeral anlage* can be recognized. By stage 17, when the *radius* and *ulna* chondrify, the branched tips of the radial, median and ulnar nerves have migrated to the distal hand plate. The *carpal bones* chondrify at stage 18 when the hand plate shows notching of the digital rays. In the lower limb the *femur* and *tibia* have formed in cartilage and the sciatic nerve extends distally to the tibia by stage 18 (44 days).

The first evidence of bone formation is seen at the midpart of the diaphysis of long bones at 8 weeks. Vascular invasion of the cartilage matrix precedes the formation of a periosteal collar which extends proximally and distally until it reaches the future epiphyseal level where a *growth plate* will be established. By 10 weeks columns of chondrocytes can be seen at the epiphyseal level of most bones; however, only the lower end of the femur and upper end of the tibia develop ossification centres prior to birth (see p. 684). The pelvis forms from two hemipelves which each develop from one cartilaginous focus. Ossification of the pelvis commences with the ilium which undergoes endochondral ossification (similar to long bones) at 9.5 weeks.

Development of joints. Regions of developing cartilage are easily recognized in the developing limb as they have widely spaced cells surrounded by matrix. Between the developing skeletal elements the somatopleuric mesenchyme is more condensed forming plates of *interzonal mesenchyme* which mark the sites of future joints. Their development varies according to the type of joint formed.

In fibrous joints the interzone is converted into collagen, as the definitive connecting medium between the bones involved. In synchondroses it becomes (growth) cartilage of the modified hyaline type, whereas in symphyses the tissue is predominantly fibrocartilage, but retaining narrow para-osseous laminae of hyaline (growth) cartilage. The interzonal mesenchyme of developing synovial joints becomes trilaminar, due to the appearance of a more tenuous intermediate zone between two dense strata next to the cartilaginous ends of the skeletal elements of the region. As the skeletal elements chondrify and in part ossify, the dense strata of the interzonal mesenchyme also become cartilaginous and cavitation of the intermediate zone establishes the cavity or discontinuity of the joint. The loose mesenchyme around the cavity forms the synovial membrane and probably also gives rise to all other intra-articular structures, such as tendons, ligaments, discs and menisci. In joints containing discs or menisci and in compound articulations more than one cavity may appear initially, sometimes merging later into a complex single one. As development proceeds thickenings in the fibrous capsule can be recognized as the specializations peculiar to a particular joint. In some, however, such accessions to the fibrous capsule are derived from neighbouring tendons, muscles or cartilaginous elements.

Cavitation of the hip, shoulder and elbow joints has been reported at 7–8 weeks. The sacro-iliac joint can be recognized from 7 weeks, its development being slightly different from other synovial joints in

that the development of the ilium is ahead of that of the sacrum. Uhthoff (1990) suggests that the initial stages in the process of cavitation of joints is independent of movements but that a full, true joint cavity can only form in the presence of movements.

Generally the literature suggests that all musculoskeletal elements are in their appropriate positions by 10 weeks. For a review of the literature concerning the chronology of events in human embryonic limbs consult O'Rahilly and Gardner (1975) and Uhthoff (1990).

Limb musculature

It is now well established that all limb muscle precursor cells originate from the somites (Jacob et al 1986). These precursor cells are committed at an early stage and can be identified in the lateral halves of the somites (Selleck & Stern 1991; Ordahl 1993). After the mesenchymal sclerotome cells have migrated from the epithelial somite the remaining dorsolateral portion is termed the *epithelial plate* of the somite (3.131). Cells from the cranial edge of this plate form the axial musculature whereas cells from the *ventrolateral edge* of those somites opposite limb buds migrate into the limb anlagen. Initially the cells migrate as single mesenchyme-like cells, then later in groups; they are surrounded by a non-random, structured network of extracellular fibrils. The migrating cells branch at their leading ends into filopodia which are in contact with the extracellular fibrils or with other cells. It is thought that the orientation of the extracellular fibrils may direct the migration of the cells. The precursor muscle cells are, however, not competent to produce limb muscles prior to their migration into the limb, and it is thought that the somito–somatopleural migration is a time when precursor myogenic cells acquire their responsiveness to the somatopleuric connective tissue.

The proliferation of the limb bud is controlled at the distal tip where the somatopleuric mesenchyme and the overlying ectoderm form the AER (p. 291). The myogenic cells colonize the limb bud in a *proximodistal direction only*, and never reach the most distal portion of the limb where there seems to be a distal boundary for the muscle cells. The speed of migration of myogenic cells into the limb is considered to be constant, since the border of invasion seems to lag behind as soon as the rate of elongation of the limb bud becomes more pronounced. Myogenic cells are still indifferent regarding their region-specific determination when they first enter the limb. Myogenic cells from a limb will, if grafted into brachial or pelvic somites, assume the myogenic potentialities of the somites and give rise to normal wing or leg musculature. The muscle cells, unlike the somatopleuric mesenchyme, have no 'limbness'. Further, the muscle pattern developed in the limb reflects the pattern of the skeletal elements; duplication or lack of digits is accompanied by the duplication or lack of the corresponding muscles.

Two subpopulations of myogenic cells can be discerned in the limb bud. In the early buds there are mainly *replicating presumptive myoblasts*, considered to be *premitotic*, whereas in later stages there are also *postmitotic myoblasts*. It is interesting that the invading myoblasts are still replicating; this may be a prerequisite for the formation of the considerable amount of skeletal muscular tissue which will develop in the limbs.

The first myogenic cells to arrive in the limb form the principal *dorsal* and *ventral premuscular masses*; it is thought that all classes of tetrapods begin limb muscle development with these blocks which produce all the skeletal muscle in the limb. The blocks of premuscle undergo a spatiotemporal sequence of divisions and subdivisions as the limb lengthens which leads to the individualization of about 19 muscles (3.151) in the upper limb and 14 muscles in the lower limb. The splitting process in the mouse commences at day 12 and is completed by day 17 (Kieny et al 1986). Small changes in the extracellular environment of myoblasts are believed to induce local fusion of some cells and thus create a gap which divides the muscle mass into two. In the upper limb, the premuscle masses first divide into three masses, the next division gives rise to the muscles attached to the carpus, and the final division produces the long muscles of the digits. A similar pattern is seen in the lower limb (3.150). Thus the patterning of the musculature of the limb is controlled by the somatopleuric mesenchyme.

The axial development of the limb, particularly that controlled by the ZPA, also affects the formation of individual muscles from the premuscular mass, as, if the somatopleuric mesenchyme is dissociated and repacked in an ectodermal sleeve prior to myoblast migration, the muscle masses remain unsplit.

Each anatomical muscle appears as a composite structure; the muscle cells and myosatellite cells are of somitic origin; the connective tissue envelopes and the tendons are of somatopleuric origin. The precise way in which the muscles are anchored to the developing bones by the tendons is not clear.

Embryonic movements

Embryonic *movements* are vital for development of the musculo-skeletal system. As well as effects on the developing muscle they are necessary to align the trabeculae within the bones, the correct attachments of the tendons and the appropriate coiling of the constituent collagen fibres of the tendons. Simple movements of an extremity have been observed sporadically as early as the seventh week of gestation; combined movements of limb, trunk and head commence between 12 and 16 weeks of gestation. Fetal movements related to trunk and lower limb movements are perceived consistently by the mother from about 16 weeks gestation (quickening). Movements of the fetus are often slow, asymmetric twisting and stretching movements of the trunk and limbs, although there may be rapid, repetitive wide-amplitude limb movements. Movements of the embryo and fetus encourage normal skin growth and flexibility as well as the progressive maturation of the musculoskeletal system. It is noted that fetuses with dystrophies which prevent in utero movements develop webs of skin, *pterygia*, passing across the flexor aspects of joints which severely limit movements. A group of congenital disorders, collectively termed *multiple congenital contractures*, may result from genetic causes, limitations of embryonic and fetal joint mobility, or be secondary to muscular, connective tissue, skeletal or neurological abnormalities. These conditions may be recognized on prenatal ultrasound examination by the appearance of fixed, immobile limbs in bizarre positions, or by webbing in limb flexures. Specific syndromes, lethal multiple pterygium syndrome, and congenital muscular dystrophy have been described.

Hox genes in the developing limb

Study of the *Hox* gene clusters in limb development have provided

an evolutionary explanation of the tetrapod condition and of the pentate form (Tabin 1992). Early prognathostomes had only a *ventrolateral skin fold* extending along the length of the body axis from which paired fins evolved. Migration of somatopleuric mesenchyme into separate regions of the ventrolateral skin fold specified the position of the early paired appendages. The segments of the body prior to limb development express various *Hox* genes in overlapping preaxial to postaxial domains. The site of limb formation could have a number of overlapping *Hox* gene domains present in the somatopleuric mesenchyme of the lateral body wall; evolution of the limb from this mesenchyme would result in elongation of these domains which then overlap, not like stripes but rather as nested sets, like Russian dolls.

The pelvic girdle is suggested to have developed first with the pectoral girdle reactivating the same genetic programme later, both limbs using *Hox-a* and *Hox-d* genes. There is molecular evidence which suggests that the pectoral girdle may have evolved from a modified branchial arch (Zanger 1981). The base of the branchial arches expresses *Hox-C-6* which is also expressed in the extreme proximal, anterior region of the forelimb bud, but is not expressed in the hindlimb. This is of interest as chimera studies have shown that the scapula derives from somitic mesenchyme, while the clavicle, coracoid, sternum and pelvic girdles arise from somatopleuric mesenchyme (Gumpel-Pinot 1984).

Whereas both *Hox-a* and *Hox-d* are present in similar domains in the early limb bud, the *Hox-a* pattern shifts so that *Hox-a* genes show proximal/distal domains and *Hox-d* genes preaxial/postaxial domains. There are five genes in the *Hox-d* cluster which are expressed in the anterior/posterior axis. The nested arrangement of *Hox-d* genes means that the postaxial border of the limb has all *Hox-d* genes (*d*-13, *d*-12, *d*-11, *d*-10 and *d*-9) expressed; in the next anterior zone only four genes are expressed (*d*-12, *d*-11, *d*-10 and *d*-9), and so on until only *d*-9 is expressed. The five genes can specify five different types of digit. Polydactyly can be interpreted as duplication of an existing digit type but not the addition of a new type of digit. The genes do not however directly specify the digit structure, as the same *Hox* genes are expressed in both fore- and hindlimbs, and in homologous limbs of different species.

Similarities in the developmental mechanisms of facial primordia and limb buds

The proximodistal outgrowth which constitute both the facial primordia and the limb buds are controlled by similar epithelial/mesenchymal interactions and it seems that the local environmental factors which, for example, control the outgrowths of either face or limb will support the other tissue type. Recombination experiments have shown that limb apical ectodermal ridge ectoderm can be maintained by mesenchyme from the three types of facial primordia, i.e. frontonasal, maxillary and mandibular. Of the three types of facial primordia in the chick, frontonasal and maxillary most resemble the limb in that they both contain rods of cartilage and undergo polarized outgrowth. Recombination of frontonasal mesenchyme and younger limb apical ectodermal ridge promoted the development of a cartilage rod in the primordium, forming an outgrowth which resembled an upper beak to the extent that an egg tooth developed. Thus the ectodermal

signals from the limb were able to induce facial primordial development.

Reversed experiments, where limb mesenchyme was recombined with facial ectoderm also showed that supportive epithelial/mesenchymal interactions did occur. Interestingly both frontonasal epithelium and mandibular epithelium supported limb mesenchyme without any epithelial thickening, like an apical ectodermal ridge, which would normally be needed for proximodistal development of a limb. However, maxillary epithelium was not able to support limb outgrowth.

These experiments have demonstrated that the developmental signalling is similar but not identical in some facial primordia and the limb bud. One explanation for this could relate to the origin of the facial epithelium. The ectoderm covering the frontonasal process is derived from the neural fold of the prosencephalon (Couly & Le Douarin 1987), whereas the epithelium of the mandible and maxilla

originates from ectoderm lateral to the neural folds (Couly & Le Douarin 1990). The neural crest mesenchyme within the facial primordia also has different origins, arising from different neural levels (see p. 286).

The development of an egg tooth provides an epithelial marker for distal differentiation in the frontonasal primordium and suggests that a progress zone operates within the frontonasal mesenchyme, similar to that in the limb. Similar patterns of expression of *MSx1* and *MSx2* are seen in both limb buds and facial primordia. The expression of these genes has been shown to depend on proximodistal position within the limb and this may prove to be the same in the facial primordia.

It will be interesting to see if other ectodermal/mesenchymal primordia such as those which develop around the urogenital membrane and form the external genitalia have similar or different signalling mechanisms.

SKIN AND APPENDAGES

Skin is developed from the surface ectoderm and its underlying mesenchyme. *Surface ectoderm* gives rise to the keratinizing general surface epidermis and its appendages, the pilosebaceous units, sudoriferous glands and nail units. It should also be noted that interactions between ectoderm and mesenchyme also give rise to the internal epithelium of the buccal cavity and the teeth (see p. 283) and the nasal epithelia (see p. 280). The more differentiated descendants of ectodermal cells are known as *keratinocytes* because their most characteristic contents are fibrous proteins called *keratins*, and also to distinguish them from *non-keratinocytes*, immigrant cells of different developmental origin which constitute an important component of the epithelial sheet formed by the keratinocytes, and with which they have a relationship which has been loosely termed 'symbiotic' (see p. 395). The non-keratinocytes are: the *melanocytes* derived from the neural crest; the *Langerhans cells* of bone-marrow origin; and *lymphocytes*. The *Merkel cell* is also usually classed as a non-keratinocyte, although it is being increasingly regarded as a modified keratinocyte.

The *dermis*, composed of irregular connective tissue and some of the connective tissue sheaths of peripheral nerves, derives from somatopleuric mesenchyme, for the limbs and trunk, possibly somitic mesenchyme over the epaxial musculature, and from neural crest in the head. Angiogenic mesenchyme gives rise to the blood vessels of the dermis. Nerves and associated Schwann cells, of neural tube and neural crest origin, enter and traverse the dermis to reach their peripheral terminations during development.

EPIDERMIS AND APPENDAGES

General (interfollicular) epidermis

In the first 4–5 weeks, embryonic skin consists of a single layer of ectodermal cells overlying a mesenchyme containing cells of stellate dendritic appearance interconnected by slender processes, and sparsely distributed in a loosely arranged microfibrillar matrix (**3.152**). The interface between ectoderm (epidermis) and mesenchyme (dermis), known as the *Basement Membrane Zone* (BMZ), is an important site of mutual interactions upon which the maintenance of the two tissues depends both in prenatal and postnatal life (see below). Ectodermal cells, which characteristically contain glycogen deposits, contact each other at gap and tight junctions. The layer so formed soon develops into a bilaminar epithelium, the *epidermis*, when desmosomes also appear. The basal *germinative layer* gives rise to the definitive postnatal epidermis, and the superficial one to the *periderm*, a transient layer confined to fetal life. The periderm maintains itself and grows by the mitotic activity of its own cells, independent of those of the germinative layer, and expresses different keratin polypeptides. Originally flattened, the periderm cells increase in depth, with the central area containing the nucleus becoming elevated and projecting as a globular elevation towards the amniotic cavity (**3.153**). The plasma membrane develops numerous surface microvilli with an extraneous coat of glycosaminoglycans, and cytoplasmic vesicles become prominent deep to it. These developments reach a peak over the period 12–18 weeks, *at which time the periderm is a major source of the amniotic fluid* to which it may contribute glucose; it also has an absorptive function (Lane et al 1987). From about 20 weeks onwards, the globular protrusions become undermined and pinched off to float free in the amniotic fluid, and the now flattened periderm cells undergo a type of keratinization to form what is regarded as a temporary protective layer for the underlying developing epidermis proper, against an amniotic fluid of changing composition due to the accumulation of products of fetal renal excretion. Up to parturition, periderm squames continue to be cast off into the amniotic fluid, and they contribute to the *vernix caseosa*, a layer of cellular debris which covers the fetal skin at birth.

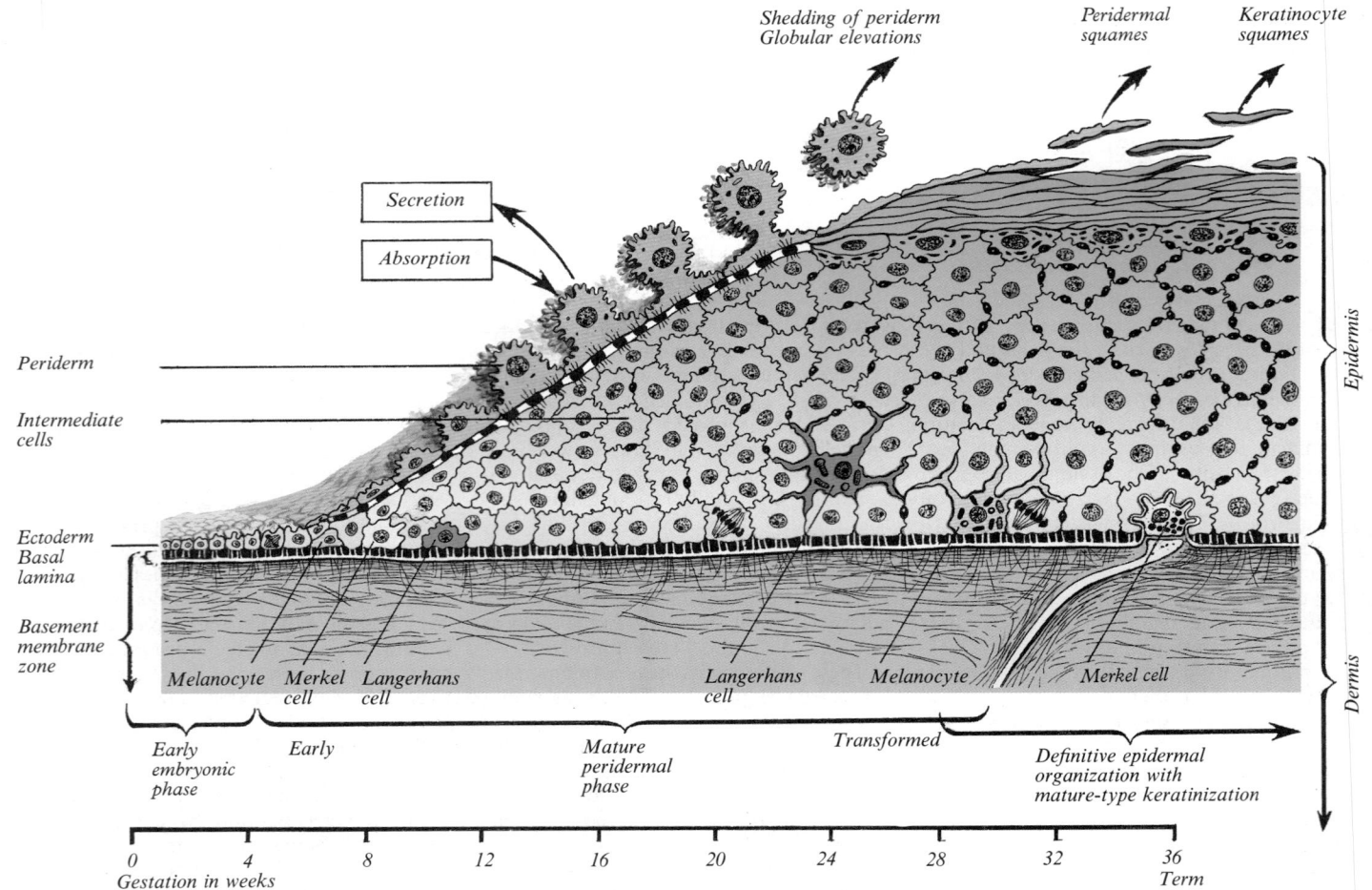

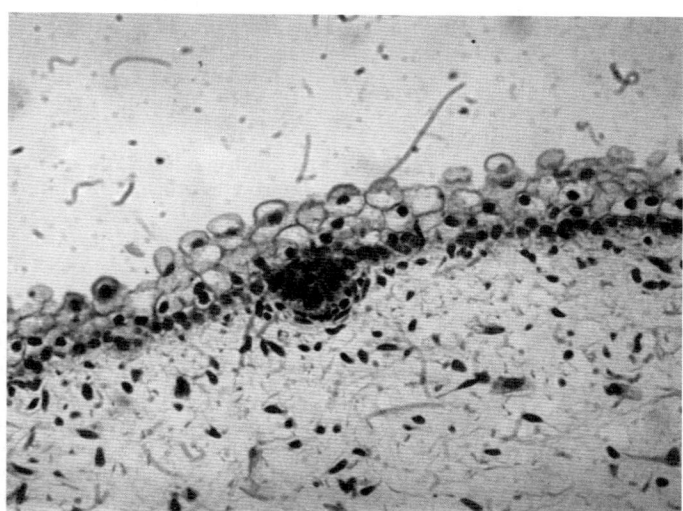

3.153 Bi-tri-laminar epidermis and underlying mesenchyme from skin of back of a 14-week-old fetus. Note globular elevations of superficial peri-dermal cells and, at one point, crowding of cells of the basal layer to form a hair germ, with underlying aggregation of mesenchymal cells to form a dermal papilla. Magnification × 329. (From Breathnach & Smith 1968 with permission.)

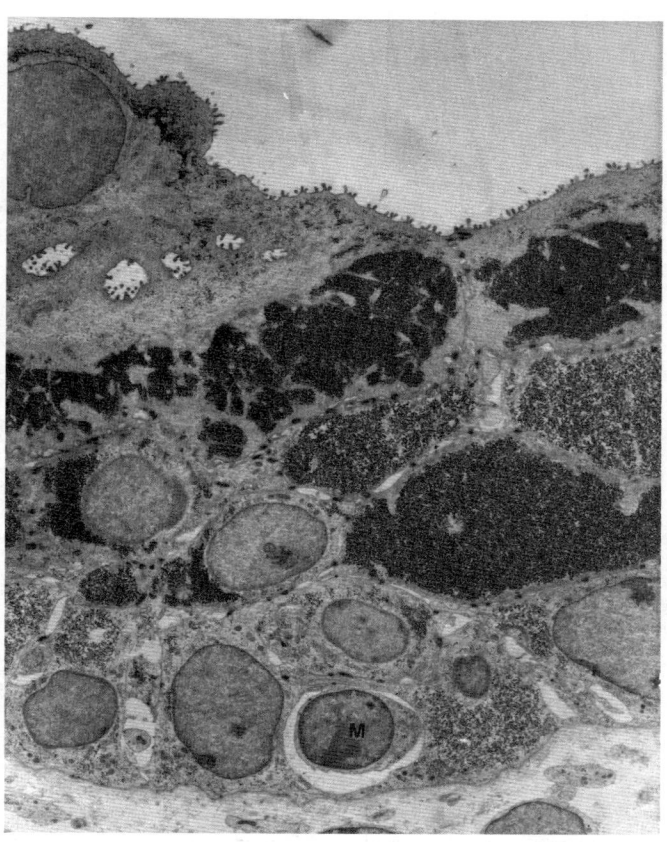

3.154 Epidermis from back skin of a 14-week fetus. There are several layers of intermediate cells between the germinative layer and the periderm, and a melanocyte (M) in the basal layer. There is now less glycogen in the basal layer cells; the globular protrusions of the periderm cells usually contain the nucleus and their surface microvilli are prominent. Magnification × 5000. (From Breathnach 1971 with permission.)

Proliferation in the germinative layer leads to a stratified appearance with successive layers of intermediate cells between it and the periderm. From an early stage, cells of all layers are packed with glycogen granules (**3**.154), presumably a source of energy during this early replicative stage of differentiation. Differentiation of these layers is not synchronous throughout all regions of the developing skin, being more advanced cranially than caudally, and on the body progressing from the midaxillary line ventrally. Reduction in glycogen content of the cells is associated with a shift towards biosynthetic activity connected with incipient *keratinization*, manifested by the presence of different enzymes and expression of keratins. Simple, low-weight keratins present from an early date are replaced by those of higher molecular weight associated with differentiation around 10–12 weeks, soon to be followed by profillagrin and fillagrin, and the appearance of keratohyalin granules among filamentous bundles of the uppermost intermediate layer cells at about 20 weeks (Moll et al 1982; Dale et al 1985). The first fully keratinized cells appear shortly afterward. By 24–26 weeks a definite stratum corneum exists in some areas, and by 30 weeks or so, apart from some lingering glycogen in intermediate cells, the interfollicular epidermis is essentially similar to that postnatally (see Breathnach 1971; Holbrook 1991, for further details).

Melanocytes. Of neural crest origin, these are present in the bilaminar epidermis of cephalic regions as early as 8 weeks (Sagebiel & Odland 1972). By 12–14 weeks they can reach a density of 2300 per mm^2 reducing to 800 per mm^2 just before birth (Holland et al 1989). Keratinocytes regulate the final ratio between themselves and melanocytes via growth factors, cell surface molecules and other signals (Scott & Haake 1991). Fetal melanocytes produce melanized melanosomes (see p. 389) and transfer them to keratinocytes, intrinsic activities clearly independent of ultra violet (u.v.) irradiation, and suggesting functions of melanin other than photoprotection.

Langerhans cells. These are of bone-marrow origin, are present in the epidermis by 5–6 weeks and are fully differentiated by 12–14 weeks (Breathnach & Wylie 1965). Their numbers increase at least partially by mitotic division in situ, but at 6 months are only 10–20% of those in the adult. It is not known if the Langerhans cell functions in immuno-surveillance in fetal skin.

Merkel cells. These appear in the glabrous epidermis of the palm and sole of the foot between 8 and 12 weeks (Moll et al 1986, 1989), and later in association with some hairs and with dermal axonal-Schwann-cell complexes. They are now thought to be modified keratinocytes rather than immigrants of neural crest origin (see p. 394).

Pilosebaceous unit

Pilosebaceous units develop at about 9 weeks, first in the regions of the eyebrows, lips, and chin, and at progressively later stages elsewhere, proceeding caudally. The first rudiment is a crowding of cells in the basal layer of the epidermis—the *pregerm*. Further proliferation and elongation of the cells leads to a *hair germ*, which protrudes downwards into the mesenchyme where it becomes associated with an aggregation of cells, the primitive *dermal papilla*. With continued downward growth, in a slanted anteroposterior direction, the hair germ becomes a *hair peg*, and when its bulbous lower end envelops the dermal papilla it is known as a *bulbous peg* (**3**.155). At this stage three swellings appear on the posterior wall. The uppermost is the rudiment of the *apocrine gland* (present only in some follicles), the middle forms the *sebaceous gland* and the lower one is the *bulb*, to which the *arrector pili muscle* (arising from underlying mesenchyme) later becomes attached. The cells of the lowermost region of the bulb, the *matrix*, divide actively and produce a pointed *hair cone*, which grows upwards to canalize a developing *hair tract*, along which the fully formed hair, derived by further differentiation of cells advancing from matrix, reaches the surface.

Four successive stages of hair follicle development have been noted by Muller et al (1991). Stage I is characterized by invagination of the epidermis into the dermis which occurs prior to week 11 of gestation; stage II corresponds to the hair germ (see above) and has been described during weeks 13–15 of gestation. The appearance of the putative sebaceous gland from about week 16 is characteristic of stage III, and stage IV is reached when the dermal sheath and the sebaceous glands are differentiated and the hair passes through the skin surface, at about week 18 of gestation.

Sebaceous glands develop independently of hair follicles in the nostrils, eyelids (as tarsal glands) and in the anal region. *Apocrine*

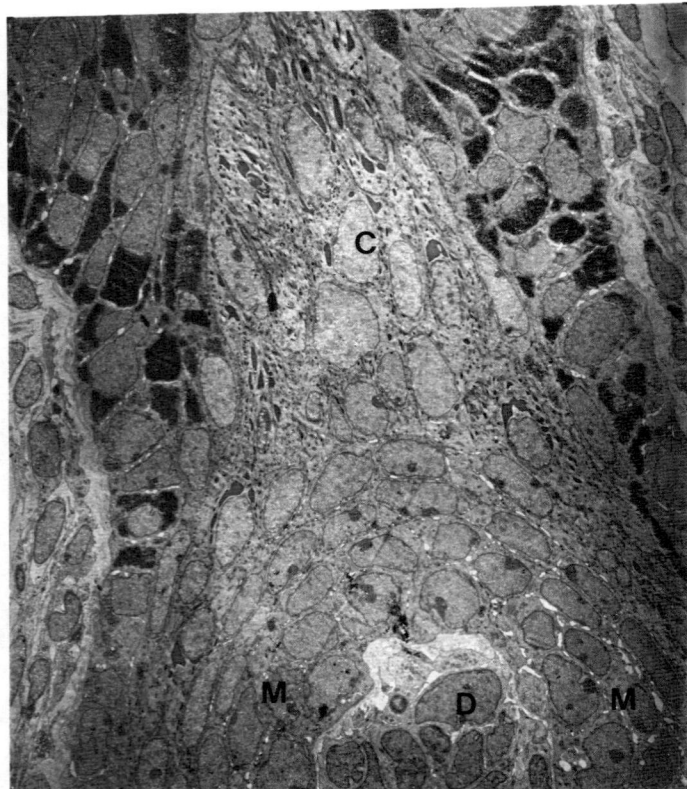

3.155 Longitudinal section of developing bulbous-peg stage hair follicle from scalp of a 15-week fetus. Cells of the dermal papilla (D) are now enveloped by matrix cell of the bulb (M), from which cells forming a conical hair cone (C) project apically, flanked by glycogen-containing cells of the outer root sheath. Magnification × 3600. (From Breathnach 1981 with permission.)

sweat glands are formed at the same time as eccrine glands (see below) and are at first distributed widely over the body; however, their number diminishes from 5 months' gestation resulting in the distribution seen in the adult (see p. 406). For further details of cellular events involved in ontogenetic differentiation of the hair and its sheaths, and of sebaceous and apocrine glands and the hair tract, see Sections 2 and 5. These processes are mirrored in the accelerated and compressed tempo of the differentiation of postnatal skin. Melanocytes are individually present at the hair-peg stage, and abundantly so and quite active in the bulbous peg. Langerhans cells have also been reported (Foster & Holbrook 1989).

Developing hair follicles are disposed in groups of three. Hairs produced prenatally are called *lanugo hairs*; they are short and downy, lack a medulla, and in certain parts of the body are arranged in a vortex-like manner into tracts. Late in pregnancy, lanugo hairs are replaced by *vellous hairs*, and these in turn by *intermediate hairs*, which are the predominant type until puberty. New follicles do not develop in postnatal skin.

Eccrine sweat glands

Eccrine sweat glands are one type of sudoriferous gland. Sweat gland rudiments appear in the second and third months as cell buds associated with the primary epidermal ridges of the finger and toe pads of terminal digits. They elongate into the dermis and by 16 weeks the lower end begins to form the *secretory coil*, within which, by 22 weeks, *secretory* and *myoepithelial* cells are evident. The solid cord of cells connecting the coil to the epidermis becomes the *intradermal duct*, and the lumina of both are formed by dissolution of desmosomal contacts between the cells (Holbrook 1991). The *intraepidermal duct* is foreshadowed by a coiled column of concentrically arranged inner and outer cells, within which, by fusion of lysosomal vacuoles, a lumen is formed which opens on the surface

at 22 weeks (Hashimoto et al 1965). As with hair follicles, no new eccrine glands develop postnatally. Sweating is said to be possible by 32 weeks, but clearly, has no functional significance in utero.

Mammary glands

Mammary glands are considered to be much modified sudoriferous glands and as such they are basically ingrowths from the ectoderm, which forms their ducts and alveoli, supported by vascularized connective tissue derived from the mesenchyme. In embryos of about the fifth or sixth week two ventral bands of thickened ectoderm, the *mammary ridges*, extend from axilla to the inguinal region, and in many mammals paired mammary glands develop at intervals along these ridges. In the human embryo the ridges are not prominent features, and only a single pair of glands develops in the pectoral region. The ridges disappear later in embryonic life, but before this the cranial third of each begins to show proliferation to form the two glandular rudiments. Supernumerary rudiments may form anywhere along the path of the mammary ridges and may develop into actual mammae or merely accessory or supernumerary nipples.

As each mammary primordium develops, its ectodermal ingrowth branches into 15–20 solid buds of ectoderm which will become the lactiferous ducts and their associated lobes of alveoli in the fully formed gland. These are surrounded by somatopleuric mesenchyme which forms the connective tissue, fat and vasculature and is invaded by the mammary nerves. By proliferation, elongation and further branching the alveoli are formed and the duct system defined. During the last two months of gestation the ducts become canalized and the epidermis at the point of original development of the gland forms a small *mammary pit*, into which the lactiferous tubules open. Perinatally the nipple is formed by mesenchymal proliferation. Should this fail the ducts open into shallow pits, a malformation known as inverted nipple. At birth the mammary glands are alike in their stage of development in both sexes, and in both some transient secretory activity may be observed, due presumably to circulating prolactin in the mother (Smith 1959). In males, thereafter, the mammary glands normally remain undeveloped; in females at puberty, in late pregnancy and during the period of lactation they undergo further, hormone dependent, developmental changes (pp. 418 et seq). For reviews of the prenatal histogenesis and ultrastructural appearances of mammary tissue consult Tobon and Salazar (1974): for postnatal reviews, pages 418 et seq.

Epidermal ridges

The epidermal ridges are foreshadowed as regularly spaced small downgrowths of epidermal cells which appear in finger and toe pads during the second and third months. They are known as *primary epidermal ridges*, separated by corresponding dermal ridges, and in the fifth month *secondary ridges* develop, the pattern becomes evident on the surface, and is finalized through further remodelling postnatally (Okajima 1975).

Nails

Fields of proliferative ectoderm appear on the tips of the terminal segments of the digits; they progressively reach a dorsal position, where at about 9 weeks a flattened *nail field* limited by *proximal*, *distal*, and *lateral nail grooves* is apparent. The nail field ultimately forms the *nail bed*, and the primordium of the nail is formed of a wedge of cells which grows diagonally, proximally and deeply into the mesenchyme from the proximal groove towards the underlying terminal phalanx. The deeper cells of this wedge form the primordium of the *matrix* which gives rise to the *nail plate*; this emerges from under a, now proximal, nail fold at about 14 weeks to grow distally over an already keratinized nail bed. The nail matrix is usually considered to have dorsal and ventral (intermediate) components, but there are conflicting opinions as to the extent to which each contributes to the nail, both in ontogeny and postnatally; it is generally agreed that the ventral matrix contributes the major part. It has been claimed that the nail bed additionally contributes up to 20% of the postnatal nail plate (Johnson et al 1991), but embryological studies to date are not clear on this matter. Most texts state that keratohyalin is not involved in the keratinization of nail, but certainly, up to at least 16 weeks, the dorsal matrix granulosa cells which are contributing keratinized cells to the nail plate and *eponychium* (*cuticle*) contain typical keratohyalin granules, and the cells of the ventral matrix next to the nail plate contain single and compound granules similar to those present in granulosa cells of oral epithelia (Breathnach 1971). Similar granules have recently been reported by Picardo et al (1992) in matrix cells of postnatal human toenail.

At 20 weeks, the nail plate entirely covers the nail field (nail bed), now limited distally by a *distal ridge*, which, when the plate projects beyond the tip, becomes the *hyponychium* beneath it. At birth, the histology of the main nail unit components is similar to that post-natally (Zaias 1990); the nail is long and overhanging, and easily falls off during cleansing.

Anomalous development of the epidermis and its derivatives is relatively common. Excessive or diminished growth, or even complete absence, may affect sebaceous or sudoriferous glands and hair, either locally or generally. Similarly, the epidermis may be excessively pigmented (*melanism*) or lack melanocytes (*albinism*). Excessive kera-tinization leads to *ichthyosis*. A *naevus* or 'mole' is a locus of excessive pigmentation. Ectodermal dysplasia is a rare condition characterized by fine blond and scanty hair, reduced or absent eyelash and eyebrows. The skin has deficient sweat and sebaceous glands. Teeth are usually peg- or cone-shaped; absence of major salivary glands may occur.

DERMIS

The mesenchymal cells underlying the surface ectoderm and early bi- and trilaminar epidermis contact each other by slender processes (**3.156**) to form an intercommunicating network. They secrete a matrix which is rich in ions, water, and macromolecules, proteoglycan/glycosaminoglycans, fibronectin, collagenous proteins of various types and elastin. Further development of these intrinsic components involves the differentiation of individual cell types, fibroblasts, endothelial cells, mast cells, etc., and the assembly of matrix components into organized fibrillar structures—collagen fibres and elastic fibres. During embryogenesis, the matrix is heterogeneous with regard to its biochemical and macromolecular components, both in terms of relative composition, and local and temporal distributions and gradients, so that it is essential to think of matrix differentiation as well as cytodifferentiation during development. Progressive alterations in matrix components underlie many mor-phological dispositions. The main glycosaminoglycans of embryonic

and fetal skin are glycuronic acid and dermatan sulfate. Collagens type I, III, V, and VI are distributed more or less uniformly regard-less of fetal age, with some local concentrations of III and V, the levels of which are higher than in postnatal skin. Collagens type IV and VII are predominantly found in the Basement Membrane Zone.

The progressive morphological differentiation of the dermis involves its separation from the subcutis at about the third month; changes in composition and size of collagen fibrils and their organ-ization into bundles amongst which cells become relatively fewer; downgrowth of epidermal appendages; the organization of nervous and vascular plexuses and the relatively late appearance of elastic networks. The papillary and reticular regions are said to be evident as early as 14 weeks, but the overall organization of the dermis continues postnatally (Holbrook 1991).

Blood vessels of the dermis. The dermal vasculature is generally thought to be developed in situ by transformation of angiogenetic mesenchymal cells. Closed endothelial-lined channels containing nucleated red cells are present by 6 weeks underneath the ectoderm (Breathnach 1971) and by the eighth week are arranged in a single plane parallel to the epidermis to form ultimately the subpapillary plexus (Johnson & Holbrook 1989). A second deeper horizontal plexus is evident by 50–70 days, and both extend by budding as development proceeds. From these plexuses the final patterns of arterioles, venules and capillaries (see p. 399) develop, and they are established shortly after birth. Pericytes are also developed from mesenchymal cells.

Lymphatic vessels. These are formed by mesenchymal cells which become organized to enclose pools of proteinaceous fluid leaking from developing capillaries (Ryan 1991).

EPITHELIAL/MESENCHYMAL INTERACTIONS IN DEVELOPING SKIN

Epidermal/mesenchymal (dermal) interactions involving mutual inductive mechanisms are important during development and post-natally (Sawyer & Fallon 1983). They occur at the interface between the two, the *basement membrane zone* (BMZ), the development of which may be considered in morphological, biochemical, and immunological terms.

The basement membrane zone, at the ectodermal stage, consists of the basal plasma membrane of the ectoderm cell, paralleled on the cytoplasmic side by a skein of microfilaments, and beneath it, a layer (0.1–0.2 μm) of microfibrillar-amorphous material deposited by the cell (**3.157**). At the bilaminar stage, a definite continuous

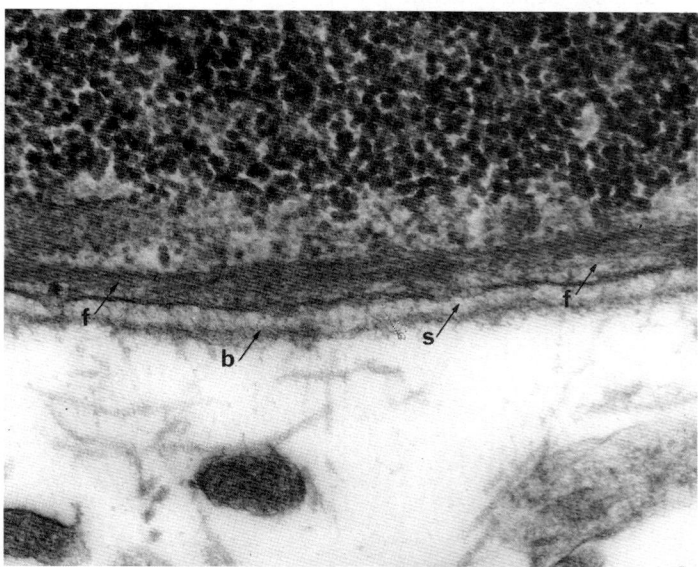

3.156 Mesenchymal cells from subepidermis of back skin of an 8-week fetus. Note numerous intercellular contacts by slender processes. Mag-nification × 10 800. (From Breathnach 1978 with permission.)

3.157 Interface between basal germinative cells of the bilaminar epidermis and mesenchyme of arm skin of a 6-week embryo. Note basal lamina (b), reticulo-filamentous material in lucid interval between the plasma membrane and basal lamina, and skein of filaments (s) paralleling the plasma mem-brane which lacks hemidesmosomes at this stage. The cytoplasm of the cell is packed with densely staining glycogen granules. Magnification × 105 000. (From Breathnach 1981 with permission.)

lamina densa is present, in the assembly of which fibronectin is involved, and it is separated from the basal plasma membrane by a lamina lucida traversed by loosely fibrillar material; similar filaments extend from the lamina densa into the mesenchymal matrix (**3**.157).

Hemidesmosomes begin to appear at 8 weeks as stratification starts, and anchoring fibrils at 9–10 weeks. By the end of the third month the basic morphology of the interfollicular BMZ is essentially similar to that postnatally (see p. 397). Immunocytochemical studies with monoclonal antibodies recognize the temporal onset of BMZ antigenic expression (Nazarro 1989). For example, GB3 antigens (associated with hemidesmosomes) and laminin are shown to be present in the lamina lucida at 6 weeks, and LDA-1 antigen and collagen type IV in the lamina densa at the same time. Antigen LH7:2, associated with anchoring fibrils, is present at 8 weeks. Bullous pemphigoid antigen (hemidesmosomes) and antigens AF-1, AF-2 (anchoring fibrils) and KF1 are expressed later, and the time of appearance of others is being regularly reported. These observations, combined with morphological ones, are of importance for prenatal diagnosis of genetically-determined diseases such as epidermolysis bullosa (Eady 1991).

The basal lamina provides a physical supporting substrate and attachment for the developing epidermis, and is thought to be selectively permeable to macromolecules and soluble factors regulating epidermal–dermal morphogenetic interactions. These have mainly been studied in other species, and in vitro (Sengel 1976; Woodley et al 1987), but it is likely that the general principles also apply in human development.

In the early stages of development the ectodermal/mesenchymal interactions contribute to the structuring of limb or facial primordia, e.g. the ectoderm promotes a chondrocyte free zone beneath it preventing chondrogenesis within the dermis and myogenic zones. Later, the dermis controls transformation of the ectoderm into

epidermis, and regulates its basal–apical polarization, differentiation, and stratification, by maintaining controlled proliferation of the basal layer cells. The epidermis, in turn, induces the dermis to start morphogenesis. Complicated interactions are involved in the morphogenesis of the epidermal appendages, e.g. hairs, scales, feathers, as revealed by intra-class and inter-class dermal–epidermal recombinations. These have shown that the presence or absence of appendages is due to a regional property of the underlying dermis, which also determines their type, distribution and pattern. The epidermis determines the class-specific morphology of appendages, their cephalocaudal polarization, and the species-specific amino acid composition of keratins. For example in the chick, when mesenchyme from the thigh is inserted beneath ectoderm that covers the proximal portion of an embryonic wing, the wing ectoderm forms leg feathers. In fact combination of mouse mesenchyme (which would normally cause the overlying ectoderm to form hair) with chick corneal epithelium (which would normally become curved and transparent) results in the first stages of feather formation. The ectoderm constructs the typical appendage of avian skin being unable to 'interpret' the mouse mesenchyme instructions to form the mammalian appendages—hair (Wessells 1977). Many 'informative' and 'permissive' messages and signals between epidermal cells and dermal cells and matrix are involved in these overall interactions. Matrix macromolecules including some of those of the basement membrane zone mentioned above, i.e. fibronectin, integrins (Buck & Horowitz 1987), cell adhesion molecules (cadherins), and soluble factors such as nerve growth factor, epidermal growth factor, retinoids and cyclic nucleotides have been suggested as mediators. There is evidence that calcium is involved as signal or messenger for some of the cell–substrate and cell–cell adhesive interactions involved (Fairley 1991). Similar interactions are also involved in wound healing and remodelling (see pp. 412, 416).

CARDIOVASCULAR SYSTEM

Endothelial development is morphologically first evident in the *extraembryonic tissues*. Here angioblastic tissue differentiates from extraembryonic mesenchyme in three regions:

- in the splanchnopleure of the yolk sac
- in the body stalk (containing the allantois)
- in the somatopleure of the chorion (Hertig 1935; Bloom & Bartelmez 1940).

It is suggested that the earliest endothelial cells differentiate from mesenchyme derived from the *parietal hypoblast* (Enders & King

1988; see p. 140). In the yolk sac and base of the body stalk, small, more or less spherical groups of cells are found early in the third week, termed *blood islands* (**3**.158). Stages of transformation of islands into blood-containing *vessels* are controversial in detail, but it is widely believed that peripheral cells of the islands flatten as the vascular endothelium, while the central cells transform into primitive red blood corpuscles (**3**.158B). Later these small blood-containing spaces merge forming a continuous network of fine vessels. In the chorionic end of the body stalk and extraembryonic mesoblast lining the chorion typical blood islands are not found, but some

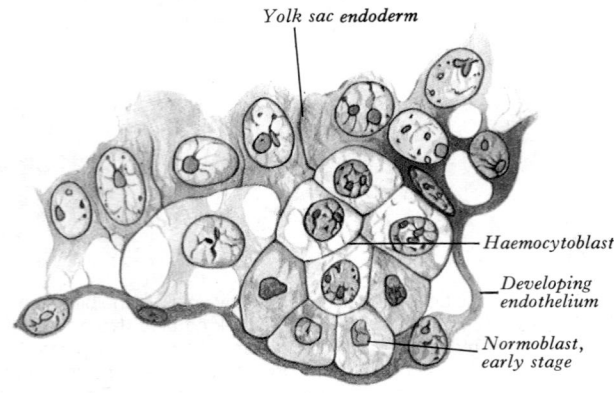

Yolk sac endoderm

Haemocytoblast

Developing endothelium

Normoblast, early stage

A

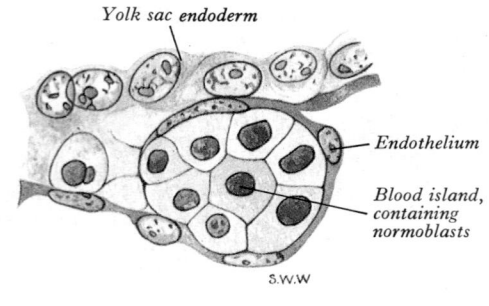

Yolk sac endoderm

Endothelium

Blood island, containing normoblasts

S.W.W

B

3.158 Part of a section through the wall of the yolk sac of an early human embryo to show: A. an early stage in the differentiation of angioblastic tissue;

B. a developing blood vessel including a blood island. (Hamilton et al 1962. Reproduced by permission of the authors and publishers.)

mesenchymal cells give rise to solid strands of *angioblasts*. Each strand contains two or three cells with rod-shaped nuclei arranged in a single row, which soon develops a space occupied by one or more nucleated haemoglobin-containing cells. These spaces coalesce to form blood vessels which are lined by endothelial derivatives of the mesenchyme; the precise source of their contained blood cells is uncertain. The earliest vessels, therefore, are formed at several separate centres; from the walls of these vessels buds grow out and become canalized, and thus converted into new vessels which join with those of neighbouring areas to form a close meshwork.

Intraembryonic blood vessels. These are first seen at the endoderm : mesenchyme interface within the lateral splanchnic mesenchyme at the caudolateral margins of the cranial intestinal portal. The origin of the intraembryonic angioblastic cells is not known, they may derive from migrating extraembryonic angioblastic cells, or a population of cells with angiogenic potential may be a product of one, or more, of the different types of intraembryonic mesenchyme. Chimeric experimentation has so far shown that all mesenchymal tissues, apart from notochord and prochordal plate, contain endogenous angioblastic cells, whereas no ectodermal tissues, i.e. neuroepithelium and neural crest mesenchyme, contain angiogenic cells (Noden 1991; see p. 156). Embryonic angioblasts are highly invasive, moving in every direction throughout embryonic mesenchymal tissue.

Prior to the establishment of the circulation, endothelial vessels are formed in two ways:

- by *vasculogenesis* (also termed *angioblastic vasculogenesis*), where new vessels develop in situ, e.g. endothelial heart tubes, dorsal aortae, umbilical and early vitelline vessels
- by *angiogenesis* (also termed *angiotrophic vasculogenesis*), where vessels develop by sprouting and branching from the endothelium of pre-existing vessels, e.g. as seen in most other vessel production.

Vasculogenesis has been subdivided into two successive phases (Poole & Coffin 1991); in type I, angioblasts arise in situ, as in the dorsal aorta; in type II, angioblasts migrate to the site of vessel development, as in the endocardium and postcardinal veins; angiogenesis continues from both these origins. (Early vascular patterns are described on pp. 222 and 230 et seq; see also **3**.180–189 and **3**.179A, B.) Once initiated, concurrent with the onset of somite formation, the development of blood vessels progresses at a phenomenal rate. During this time the direction of blood flow through a vessel may reverse; thus it cannot be designated artery or vein until the other tunics (media and externa) have started to develop. In the head and neck, 'cardiac neural crest' cells, i.e. crest cells originating between the midotic placode and the caudal limit of somite three, contribute to the supporting layers of the developing endothelium, particularly the tunica media. In the trunk, local mesenchyme (probably splanchnopleuric) serves that function. The subsequent development of the blood corpuscles is described on page 1407.

DEVELOPMENT OF THE HEART

EARLY CARDIAC DEVELOPMENT

In amniotes the heart is the earliest major organ to function. For obvious nutritive reasons it must not only accommodate a stream of blood but also begin to propel it. These early **functional** demands on the heart represent an important factor in the dynamics of its development. The early appearance of cardiac activity in the tubular hearts of chick and rat embryos was noted many years ago (e.g. Sabin 1920 et seq; Goss 1942). First manifested by arrhythmic and sporadic ventricular contractions, these are rapidly superseded by regular peristaltic activity propagated unidirectionally along the cardiac tube. In the account that follows, attention is necessarily concentrated upon the complex changes which transform a tube into a chambered septate human heart. It is also necessary to keep in mind that the early heart is only a few hundred micrometres (μm) in size and that at every stage the heart must be an effective circulatory pump.

The heart is formed from at least three sources:

- *angioblastic mesenchyme* lateral to the cranial intestinal portal
- *midline splanchnopleuric coelomic epithelium*; this is ventral to the foregut endoderm after the head-fold stage

- *neural crest cells* derived from the region between the otic vesicle and the caudal limit of somite three.

These sources will produce respectively:

- the endocardium and cardiac mesenchymal cells which produce the valvular tissue of the heart
- the myocardium, including the conducting tissue of the heart, and the specific matrix proteins associated with the developing heart, i.e. the cardiac jelly
- the aorticopulmonary septum and the media of the great vessels, and, possibly contributes to the conducting tissue of the heart.

Primitive cardiac myocytes can first be seen in the unfolded embryo, during the pre- and early somite period, as simple, cuboidal epithelial cells of the splanchnopleuric coelomic epithelium superjacent to the endoderm. Subsequently, elongated and flattened angioblastic mesenchymal cells differentiate from mesenchyme between the myocardial cells and the underlying endoderm. These groups of angioblastic cells are amongst the earliest intraembryonic vascular precursors to appear. They arise as single cells at the ventrolateral edges of the cranial intestinal portal and subsequently aggregate to form an epithelium, the *endocardium*, enclosing small cavities. The endocardial lined spaces coalesce in the vicinity of the developing foregut to establish bilateral, hollow tubular structures (**3**.159A, B). By stage 9, when the embryo has 3–4 somites, the head fold is apparent and the cardiac region of the embryo is undergoing reversal. The splanchnopleuric coelomic epithelium is now ventral to the foregut with the forming endocardial tubes dorsal.

It is worth noting here that the epicardium, as seen in the adult heart, is not present at this stage. Cardiac myocytes differentiate from the splanchnopleuric layer of coelomic epithelium which passes from right to left (in the folded embryo), ventral to and in contact with the primitive foregut; this layer is continuous on each side with the splanchnic walls of the pericardio-peritoneal canals. The somatopleuric coelomic epithelium at this point gives rise to the *parietal pericardium*. There is no visceral pericardial layer (unlike, e.g. the formation of visceral peritoneum; see p. 174). The *epicardium* is sometimes included in descriptions of the myocardium as epimyocardium; however, the epicardial layer proper develops later from septum transversum mesenchyme cells which spread over the myocardial tube.

The bilateral endocardial tubes become connected, merging to form one endocardial tube almost completely surrounded by putative myocardial cells; these, unlike the endocardium, form a continuous epithelium across the midline from the outset (**3**.1c, D). The endocardium is suspended by a primitive *dorsal mesocardium*. Using a monoclonal antibody specific for endothelial cell precursors (QH1), reactive cells have been demonstrated close to the basal surface of the endoderm just ventral to the foregut. It is suggested that this area may stabilize developing endothelium and promote fusion of the bilateral endothelial tubes. This portion of the endoderm remains in contact with the endocardium for some time via the dorsal mesocardium (Bolender & Markwald 1991).

The two endocardial tubes fuse across the midline progressively commencing at the arterial end (outflow tract) and extending to the venous end where the two putative atria are, initially, widely separated from each other. The single heart tube so formed is divided into, caudorostrally, the prospective left ventricle, prospective right ventricle and the outflow tract (see below). By stage 10 (22 days), the heart is thus composed of *inner* and *outer epithelial tubes*, the endocardium and myocardium respectively. These tubes become separated widely by a basal extracellular matrix secreted by the myocardial cells.

Extracellular matrix of the heart

The extracellular matrix of the heart, historically termed *cardiac jelly*, promotes occlusion of the tubular lumen during contraction, thus providing mechanical assistance for the generation of a blood flow; it also acts as a site for the deposition of inductive factors from the myocardial cells which may modify the differentiation of specific endocardial cells. It has been termed a gelatinoreticulum, a *myoepicardial reticulum* (**3**.159c, D) and more recently the *myocardial basement membrane* (Bolender & Markwald 1991); it is composed

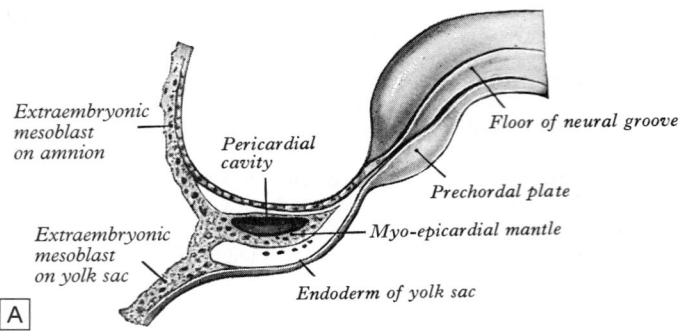

3.159A Median section through the cranial end of an early human embryo to show the position of the pericardium before the formation of the head fold. A few scattered angioblasts are seen between the cardiogenic plate and the yolk sac; they will ultimately form the endothelial heart tubes. (After C L Davis.)

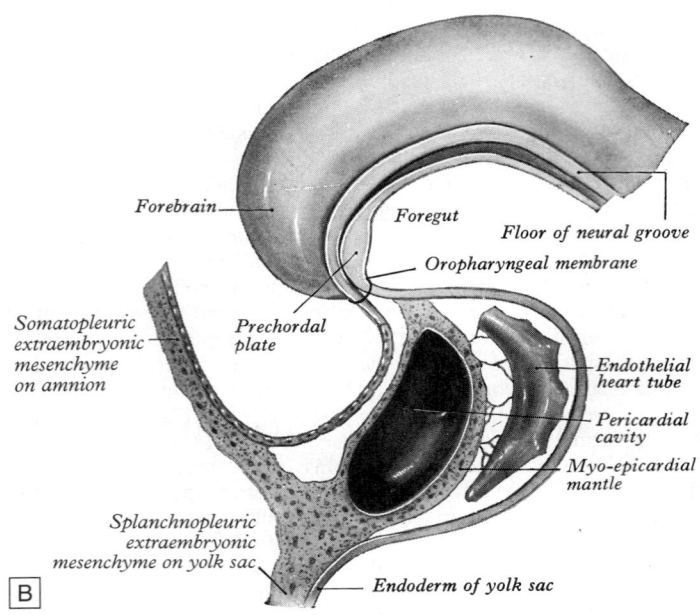

3.159B Median section through the cranial end of a young human embryo, showing the head fold in process of formation and its reversal effect on the position of the pericardium and endothelial heart; also intervening reticulum and myoepicardium.

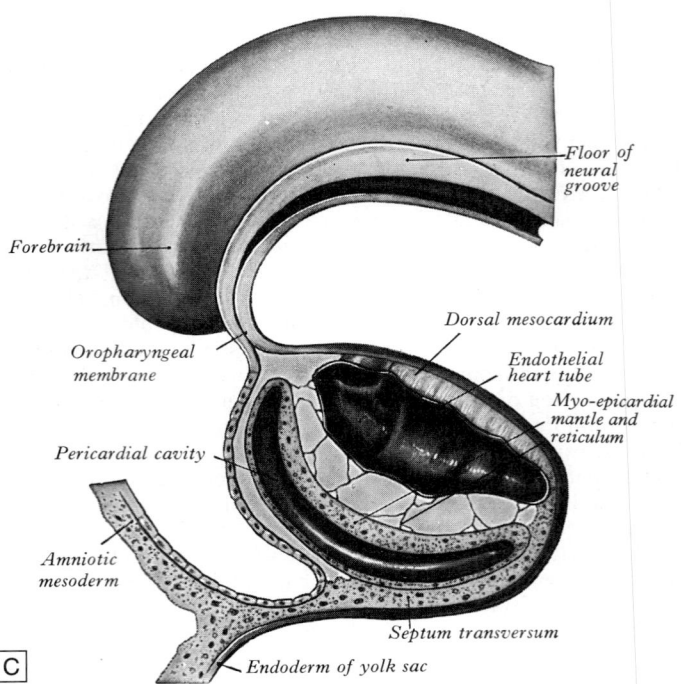

3.159C Median section through the cranial end of a young human embryo, after completion of the head fold and reversal of the pericardium.

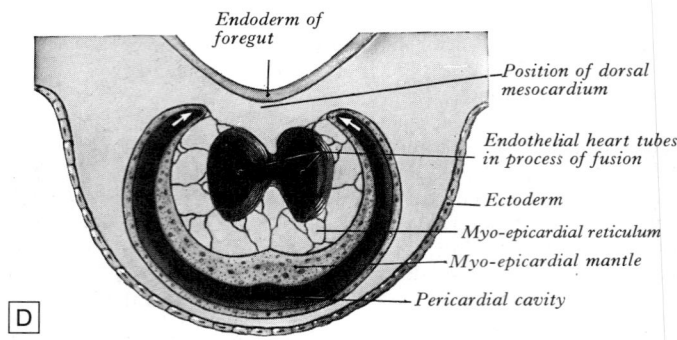

3.159D Horizontal section through the pericardium and developing heart of the embryo shown in C. The arrows indicate the directions in which the dorsolateral recesses of the pericardium deepen so as to define the transient dorsal mesocardium. (After C L Davis.)

of, inter alia, hyaluronic acid, hyaluronidase and fibronectin (see below). Endothelia generally show great diversity; subtle differences in morphology such as the presence or absence of fenestrations, or the extent of tight junctions, support the concept of *regional specificity of endothelia*. Within the heart the endocardium exhibits regional diversity with respect to its development potential. Inductive signals originating from the myocardial cells cause a *subset* of endocardial cells lining the atrioventricular canal and the proximal outflow tract to *transform into mesenchyme (cardiac mesenchyme)*, while the endocardial cells in other regions of the heart, for example in the ventricle, remain epithelial (Bolender & Markwald 1991). When activated by myocardial inductive factors the endocardial cells lose their cell–cell associations, showing decreased expression of N-CAM (a cell adhesion molecule, see p. 111) and increased expression of substrate adhesion molecules such as chondroitin sulfate and fibronectin, they undergo cytoskeletal rearrangements necessary for migration, and they express type I procollagen. Specific myocardial inductive factors have not yet been identified; proteins known to be present in the matrix include hyaluronic acid, hyaluronidase, fibronectin and putative cardiac adherons. The latter when fractionated and reapplied to an endothelial monolayer results in decreased expression of N-CAM, an event occurring prior to endocardial transformation to mesenchyme in situ.

The transformation of endocardium to mesenchyme may, perhaps, be the only example of a mesenchymal population derived from an endothelial lineage (Markwald et al 1990); the cells uniquely retain expression of the endothelial marker QH1. It is believed that the transformation is triggered by an intrinsic clock as a similar change occurs in vitro when atrioventricular endocardium is cultured with myocardium.

Formation of cardiac mesenchyme cells at the atrioventricular canal and the proximal outflow tract is followed by their migration into the myocardial basement membrane. Accumulation of mesenchyme and matrix in these regions produces protrusions, the *subendocardial cushions*, which bulge into the primary heart tube and support the valve function of the atrioventricular canal and outflow tract. The eventual fusion of opposing cushion tissue across the lumen of the atrioventricular canal forms a wedge of mesenchyme that serves to guide the union of the internal muscular septa. Interestingly the position of the subendocardial cushions corresponds to the future positions of the fibrous skeleton of the heart and the valves (**3.160**).

Simple heart tube

The simple heart tube elongates and develops an asymmetric twist. Aided by the position of the subendocardial cushions and the ventral

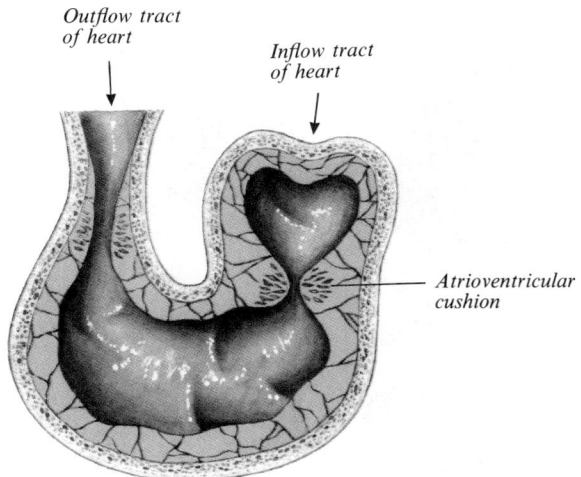

Outflow tract of heart

Inflow tract of heart

Atrioventricular cushion

3.160   Schematic section through the developing heart. Endocardial cells transform into cardiac mesenchyme in the atrioventricular canal and the proximal outflow tract.

fold of the heart a succession of cavities, joined by more constricted regions, begin to define the sinus venosus, atrium, ventricle and bulbus cordis (**3**.161–163, 164). Initially somewhat cylindrical, the cavities rapidly become more spherical (within 24 hours in the mouse). Coincidentally, cells of the myocardial mantle invade the subendocardial reticulum and form a complex network of inter-communicating *trabeculae*, external to but ultimately indenting and becoming clothed by endocardium. In many vertebrate groups the myocardium remains predominantly trabecular, but in birds and mammals compact layers of cardiac muscle develop external to the trabeculae. The latter also persist, however, but constitute a lesser volume of the propulsive tissue (see below).

These early events in cardiac development provide an approximate parallel between phylogeny and ontogeny. The evolution from a 'trabecular' heart to an organ with rounder chambers and a largely compacted myocardium is likely to be an expression of increased efficiency. An attempt to demonstrate this by mathematical analysis (Challice & Viragh 1973 et seq) provides some corroboration and also an explanation for the persistence of the internal trabeculation in the mammalian heart.

For discussions and bibliographies concerning experimental studies and the importance of haemodynamic influences on regional cardiac morphogenesis, consult Stalsberg and De Haan (1968), Bellairs (1971), Balinsky (1981), Orts-Llorca et al (1982), Bockman & Kirby (1990), Feinberg et al (1991).

GENERAL CARDIAC DEVELOPMENT

The *dorsal aortae* arise in situ as paired endothelial vessels. They extend caudally into the body stalk, establishing continuity with the umbilical arteries, which precede them in time of appearance. At their cranial ends the dorsal aortae curve ventrally round the sides of the foregut to reach the pericardium and become continuous with the cranial end of the endothelial heart tube, thus forming the first pair of aortic arches (**3**.161). In all vertebrates in which the heart and aortae are laid down **before** the formation of the head fold, the arteries communicate with the *caudal* end of the heart. When the head fold forms, as noted, the ends of the heart are **reversed** and the cranial ends of the dorsal aortae are curved forwards round the sides of the foregut as the first aortic arches.

A transverse groove appears on the surface of the heart tube about its middle, the junction of the *bulbus cordis* with the *ventricle*. The bulbus is cranial to the groove and continues as the first pair of aortic arches. The ventricle shows a second groove at its caudal end where it opens into a *common atrium*, which, initially, is embedded in the floor of the pericardium (the future *septum transversum*) and the chamber is disposed transversely. On each side the common atrium is joined caudally by a short venous trunk, formed by the union of the corresponding umbilical vein with veins issuing from the *vitelline* (yolk sac) *plexus*. These trunks represent the right and left *horns* of the *sinus venosus* (*sinual horns*) so that the common atrium may justifiably be termed a *common sinuatrial* (or *sinoatrial*) *chamber*. The umbilical and vitelline radicles of each sinual horn are soon joined laterally by a *common cardinal vein* (each the confluence of a *precardinal* and *postcardinal vein*; see p. 321).

At this point it should be noted that the regions of the early heart tube have over the years received many, often confusing names. Keith (1924) described, from caudorostrally, atrial, ventricular, bulbar and truncal components of the straight heart tube; Streeter (1942), described atrial, ventricular and bulbar portions only, but subdivided the bulbus into right ventricle, conus cordis and truncus arteriosus; Anderson et al (1978) described the ventriculobulbar portion as possessing two segments only, the primitive ventricle and the bulbus cordis, but they divided the ventricle into three parts, the inlet part—related to the atrioventricular valve, the trabecular portion, and the outlet part—which supports an arterial valve; Teal et al (1986) have recommended that the terms bulbus, conus and truncus be avoided completely, referring to the region between the trabeculated part of the right ventricle and the aortic sac as the outflow tract. Unfortunately the literature continues to retain all manifestations of the terminology including reference to the bulbus cordis/outflow tract as the conotruncus.

Early in the fourth week the heart tube undergoes a striking change. Hitherto the parietal pericardium has increased in length proportionally with the heart, but now the heart tube grows more rapidly and the bulboventricular tube bulges ventrally and caudally,

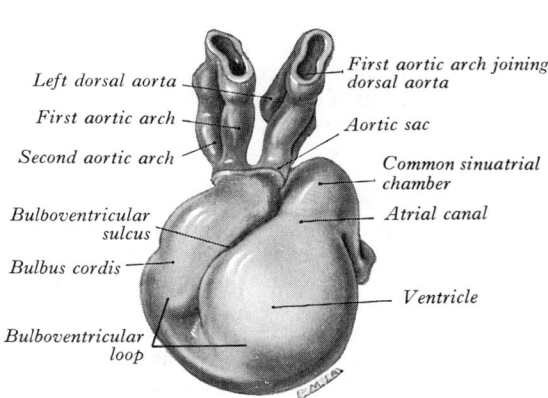

Left dorsal aorta

First aortic arch

Second aortic arch

Bulboventricular sulcus

Bulbus cordis

Bulboventricular loop

First aortic arch joining dorsal aorta

Aortic sac

Common sinuatrial chamber

Atrial canal

Ventricle

3.161   The heart of a 0.95 mm rabbit embryo, viewed from the ventral side. (Drawn from a model by G Born.)

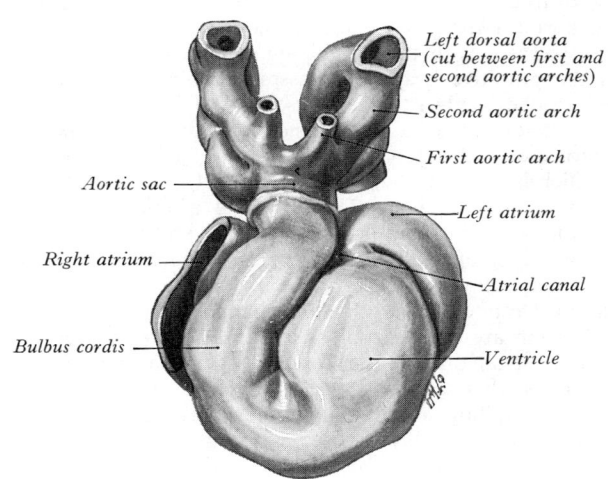

Left dorsal aorta (cut between first and second aortic arches)

Second aortic arch

First aortic arch

Aortic sac

Left atrium

Right atrium

Atrial canal

Bulbus cordis

Ventricle

3.162   The heart of a 1.7 mm rabbit embryo, viewed from the ventral side. (Drawn from a model by G Born.)

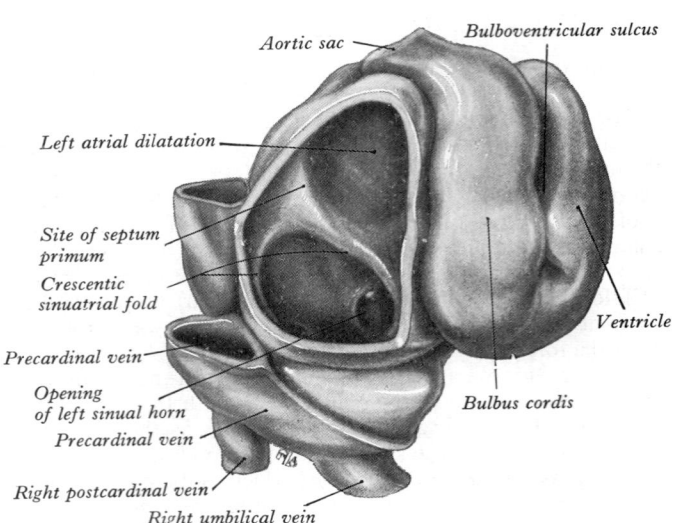

3.163 The heart shown in B, viewed from the right side and slightly from the ventral aspect. The right wall of the common sinuatrial chamber has been removed to show the interior. (Drawn from a model by G Born.)

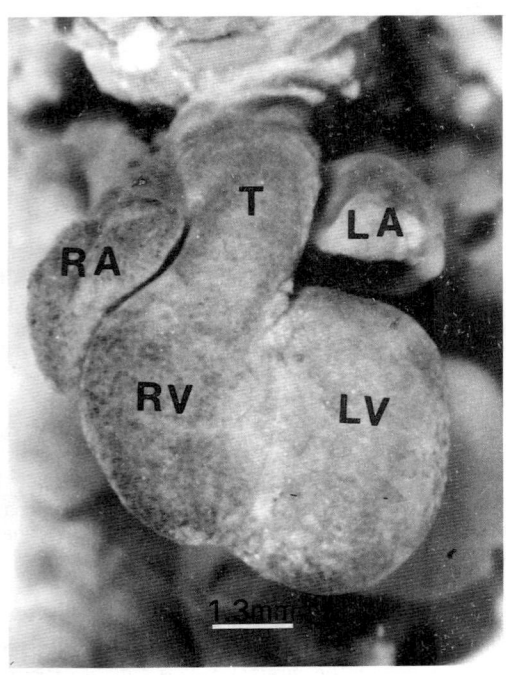

3.164 Human heart at 32 days (stage 15). Both atria are clearly visible. RA = right atrium; LA = left atrium; RV = right ventricle; LV = left ventricle; T = truncus arteriosus. Scale bar 1.3 mm.

forming a U-shaped loop; the bulbus cordis forming the right limb and the ventricle the left. The loop is conspicuous throughout the fourth and fifth weeks, and seen as a deep *bulboventricular sulcus* externally (**3**.161) and a corresponding *bulboventricular ridge* projects internally. Other factors often considered operative in determining the disposition of the loop are modifications in the tubular heart flow patterns, and coordinated ciliary action of the coelomic epithelium (Afzelius 1979).

Dorsolateral recesses of the splanchnopleuric pericardial layer adjacent to the myocardium deepen and approach one another (**3**.159D); their apposed walls fuse, completing a broad dorsal attachment between the edge of the myocardium and the parietal pericardium. This layer, the *dorsal mesocardium*, is transient, breaking down early in the fourth week and establishing a passage across the pericardial cavity from side to side dorsal to the heart. This persists as the *transverse sinus* of the pericardium. While these bulboventricular changes are occurring, the atrial part is also affected; the atrioventricular opening moves cranially and to the left, and both parts of the common atrial or sinuatrial chamber 'rise' or emerge from the mesenchyme of the septum transversum to grow cranially into the pericardial cavity dorsal to the ventricle. Owing to these changes the atrioventricular canal for a time connects the **left** part of the atrium to the ventricle and venous blood from the right side has to pass through both parts of the atrium.

At stage 10 (**3**.179A), about the middle of the fourth week, the bulbus cordis communicates with the dorsal aortae through the first pair of aortic arches, and both are connected with the capillary plexus associated with the developing cerebral vesicles. From this plexus the primitive head vein passes caudally, but ends blindly before it reaches the heart. The intersegmental arteries begin to grow out from the dorsal aorta on each side but have not yet established connections with their corresponding veins; and the postcardinal veins, which later drain the body wall caudal to the heart, are only in process of development. The umbilical arteries and veins are defined and, early in the fourth week, their terminals and radicles, respectively, link up with the capillaries which have developed in the chorionic villous stems, establishing the chorionic part of the circulation. Despite the fact that the channels for the remainder of the circulation are only partially established there is good ground for assuming, from observations made on living embryos by a variety of techniques, that the heart begins to contract about this time. Under the prevailing conditions, the effect can only be of an 'ebb and flow' nature, but this also serves to effect some movement in the nutritive fluid filling the pericardial cavity, coelomic ducts and exocoelom (p. 151), on which the embryo is still heavily dependent.

Towards the end of the fourth week the connection between the bulbus cordis and the first pair of aortic arches lengthens to form

the *truncus arteriosus*, and the cranial end of this vessel becomes connected to the dorsal aortae by a further five pairs of aortic arches. By this time the *venous drainage* of the body wall and neural tube has been established. On each side a *precardinal vein*, from the cranial end of the embryo, unites with a *postcardinal vein* from the caudal region to form the *common cardinal vein* (*duct of Cuvier*); the latter vessel opens close to the umbilical and vitelline veins into the dorsocaudal part of the common sinuatrial chamber (the three vessels on each side thus forming the right or left *sinual horn*).

As the chorionic circulation already exists the embryo can now exchange materials with the maternal blood in the intervillous space. This is not effected suddenly; initially the blood volume and its cellular content in the heart and vessels of the embryo is insufficient to enable it to take full advantage of this new source of nourishment, and until this is rectified, the embryo continues to draw upon the coelomic fluid.

The separation of a definitive *sinus venosus* from the *common atrium* completes the definition of the primitive chambers of the heart. A crescentic groove appears on the left wall of the sinuatrial chamber and rapidly deepens to the right. Hence the left horn of the sinus venosus loses its connection with the left part of the atrium and becomes linked to the right sinual horn by separation of the caudal part of the sinuatrial chamber; the latter now constitutes the *body of the sinus venosus*. At the same time the right sinual horn becomes more clearly demarcated from the right part of the atrium by a shallow groove, and its wide connection with the atrium (**3**.163) becomes relatively smaller (Foxon 1955). The right and left parts of the atrium grow cranially to occupy the dorsal part of the pericardial cavity, and later they bulge forwards, embracing the sides of the bulbus cordis (**3**.165).

The embryo has now reached a length of nearly 4 mm (**3**.179B). It possesses 28 somites and has almost completed the fourth week of development. From this stage onwards it is more convenient to deal with the individual chambers with only occasional reference to the development of the heart as a whole.

It must be noted that the above account of early cardiogenesis, though widely subscribed to, is not without its critics. In considering the many factors governing cardiac development—phylogenetic, ontogenetic, and physiological—the last is usually underestimated and the first is perhaps stated too dogmatically (Foxon 1955). Ontogenetic mechanisms must conform to the early demand for a functioning heart, and cardiogenesis is not necessarily a mere repetition of phylogenetic steps, which are themselves uncertain, however plausible they may seem (De Vries & Saunders 1962).

Sinus venosus

The right sinual horn increases rapidly in size at the expense of the left, due to the changes already outlined and to those occurring in the originally symmetric arrangement of the umbilical and vitelline veins by the development of the liver (3.186–8, p. 322). As a result the vitello-umbilical blood flow enters the right horn through a wide but short vessel, the *common hepatic vein*, which becomes the cranial end of the inferior vena cava. In addition, the right horn receives the right common cardinal vein (from the body wall of the right side) and the body of the sinus, which conveys the blood from the left horn and left common cardinal vein. Later, when *transverse connections* are established between the cardinal veins (3.189, 190), the blood from the body wall of the left side reaches the heart via the veins of the *right* side. The left common cardinal vein then becomes much reduced in size and forms the oblique vein of the left atrium and the fold of the left caval vein, while the left horn and the body of the sinus venosus persist as the *coronary sinus* (3.189B).

The right sinual horn opens into the right atrium through its dorsal and caudal walls. The orifice, elongated and often slit-like, is guarded by two muscular folds, the *right* and *left sinuatrial (venous) valves (valvules)* (3.165). These two valves meet cranially and become continuous with a fold which projects into the atrium from its roof, the *septum spurium*. Caudally the valves meet and fuse with the dorsal endocardial cushion of the atrial canal. The cranial part of the right sinuatrial valve loses its fold-like form, but its position is indicated in the adult heart by the crista terminalis of the right atrium; its caudal part forms the valve of the coronary sinus and most of the valve of the inferior vena cava. The medial (or left) end of the valve of the inferior vena cava is formed by a small fold continuous with the dorsal wall of the sinus venosus, the *sinus septum*. The latter intervenes between the orifice of the common hepatic vein and the opening of the body of the sinus. (In the mature heart see the *tendon of Tondaro* and *triangle of Koch*, p. 1477.)

The left venous valve blends with the right side of the atrial septum and usually no trace of it can be seen in the adult heart.

As the sinuatrial valves undergo these changes the right sinual horn becomes incorporated in the right atrium and expands to form its smooth dorsal wall, medial to the crista terminalis. This part of the adult atrium is termed the *sinus venarum*, the receiving chamber of the large venous orifices. The right half of the primitive atrium forms the internally ridged, more muscular, wall anterior to the crista terminalis and the right auricular appendage.

Right and left atria

As stated, the common atrium is derived from the cranial part of the sinuatrial chamber. It receives the opening of the sinus venosus dorsocaudally and to the right of the median plane, while it communicates ventrally with the ventricle through the atrioventricular canal, which has resumed its median position by the middle of the fifth week, thus permitting both right and left parts of the atrium to communicate with the common ventricular cavity. Dorsal and ventral swellings appear in the walls of the atrioventricular canal between the endothelial tube and the myoepicardial mantle. These, the *atrioventricular endocardial cushions*, consist of a core of myocardial basement membrane matrix and mesenchymal cells derived from the endocardium. They encroach on the canal and eventually fuse, leaving a relatively small orifice on each side. The fused tissue constitutes the *septum intermedium* (of His), which separates the two small right and left atrioventricular orifices and canals.

Internal separation into right and left atria is mainly effected by sequential growth of two septa (but with additional, less prominent structures). First the *septum primum* grows from the dorsocranial atrial wall as a crescentic fold (3.166A), separated from the left sinuatrial valve by the *interseptovalvular space*. The ventral horn of the crescent reaches the ventral atrioventricular cushion, the dorsal horn the dorsal cushion. Ventral and dorsal refer to the positions of the cushions after the atrium repositions to lie dorsal to the bulbus cordis. Strictly the cushions are ventrocranial and dorsocaudal in

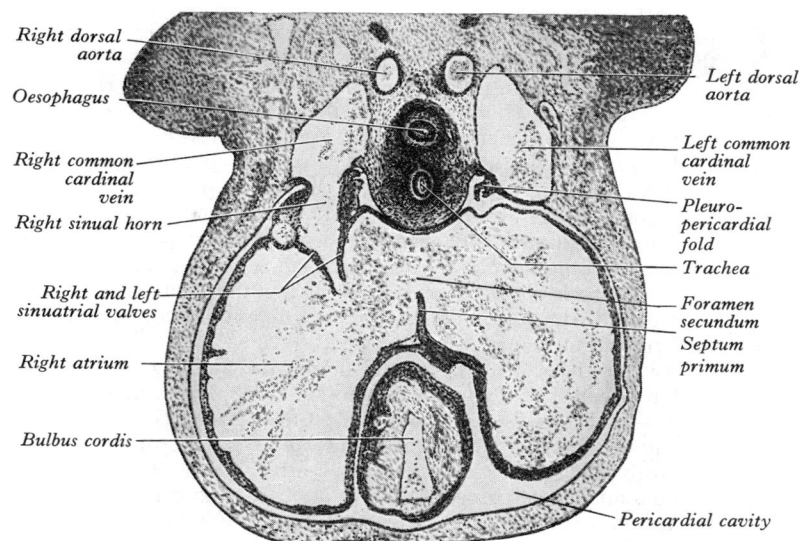

3.165 Transverse section of a human embryo, 8 mm long. Observe how the atria bulge forwards on each side of the bulbus cordis. The septum primum has broken down in its dorsal region and the two atria communicate through the ostium secundum or foramen ovale.

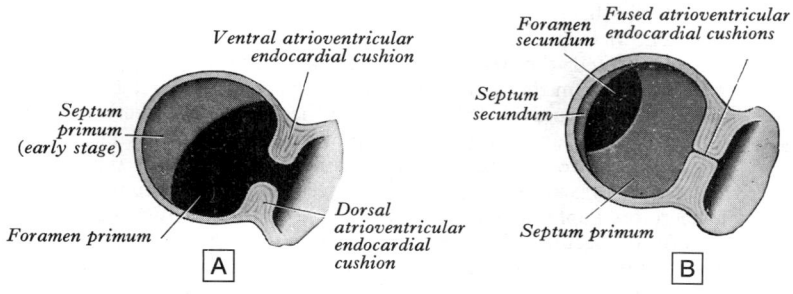

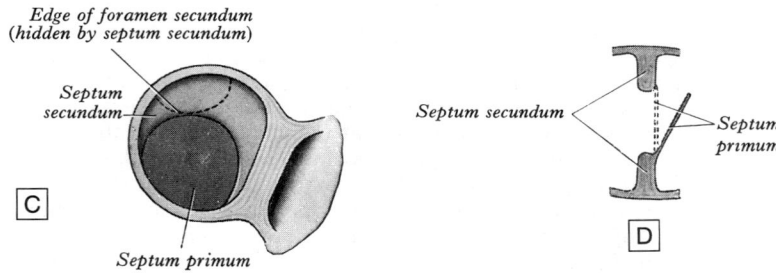

3.166 Diagrams representing three stages in the development of the atrial septum, viewed from the right side. The heart has been divided in its long axis to the right of its median plane and only the atria and the adjoining part of the ventricular cavity are depicted.

A. The septum primum has not yet obliterated the original communication between the two atria and the atrioventricular endocardial cushions have not yet fused.

B. The atrioventricular endocardial cushions have fused with each other and with the septum primum, which has broken down in its dorsal part. The foramen secundum, thus formed, subsequently moves to the position shown in C.

C. The septum secundum has formed and hides the foramen secundum, the margins of which are indicated by the curved, dotted line.

D. Section to show the valve-like character of the foramen secundum. When the pressure in the right atrium exceeds that in the left atrium, blood passes from the right to the left side of the heart, but when the two pressures are equal the septum primum assumes the position indicated by the dotted outline.

position, but ventral and dorsal are in general use and will be retained here. Ventral and caudal to the advancing edge of the septum the two atria communicate through the *foramen primum*

(3.166A). Free passage of blood from right to left atrium is essential throughout fetal life, as oxygenated blood from the placenta reaches the heart via the inferior vena cava (pp. 1500, 1503); therefore, as the foramen primum diminishes, the septum primum breaks down dorsally and a new right–left shunt, through the *foramen secundum*, is formed before the end of the fifth week. The foramen primum is finally occluded by fusion of the edge of the septum primum with the fused atrioventricular cushions, in the median plane. The foramen secundum enlarges, allowing sufficient free passage of blood from right to left atrium (**3**.166), and it persists throughout intrauterine life as **part** of the valvular *foramen ovale* in the progressively changing *interatrial septal complex* (see below). At first the foramen secundum is sited craniodorsally in the septum primum but it becomes modified until it is cranioventral.

Towards the end of the second month the muscular wall of the atrium becomes invaginated as another crescentic septum on the right side of the septum primum (**3**.166B, C). This, the *septum secundum*, involves more than the whole width of the inter-septovalvular space; thus the dorsal attachments of the septum primum and the left sinuatrial valve are carried into the interior of the atrium on its left and right surfaces respectively. The superior (ventrocranial) and inferior (dorsocaudal) horns of the septum secundum at first grow ventrally; the superior horn grows much more rapidly and fuses first with the septum intermedium; it is then continuous with the *sinus septum* (see above). Thus the free edge of the septum secundum (*crista dividens*) is at first directed caudoventrally and later caudally alone; it overlaps the foramen secundum (**3**.166C, D); thus the septum primum acts as a flap valve. Since the blood pressure is greater in the right atrium than in the left, the blood flows from right to left, but not conversely. The right–left flow occurs through the 'true', but somewhat misnamed *foramen ovale*, proceeding from the right atrium under the crescentic free border of the septum secundum, thence through the oblique cleft between the (parted) secondary and primary septal surfaces, to finally enter the left atrium through the foramen secundum. After birth the intra-atrial pressures are equalized and the free edge of the septum primum is therefore kept in contact with the left side of the septum secundum and fusion occurs. Not infrequently the fusion is incomplete, but the remaining cleft is usually small, valvular and has no functional significance. The initially free, crescentic margin of the septum secundum forms, after fusion, the *limbus fossae ovalis* and the septum primum the floor of the *fossa ovalis* of the adult heart. An alternative derivation of the septum secundum from a ridge developing to the right of the line of fusion between the confluent endocardial cushions and the septum primum has been advanced (Odgers 1934). The dorsal horn of the septum secundum is said to incorporate tissue derived from part of the left sinuatrial valve; its contribution, however, remains uncertain; sometimes, small vestigial remnants persist to maturity. Another view embodies the above suggestion, but regards the valve as of minor importance in this connection, describing, however, yet another ridge—the *septum accessorium*—contributing to the lower part of the dorsal border of the limbus (Christie 1963).

Early in the development of the septum primum a single, common *pulmonary vein*, suggested to develop from angiogenic cells positioned in the early dorsal mesocardium but in continuity with the endoderm, opens into the caudodorsal wall of the left atrium close to the septum. It is the union of a right and a left pulmonary vein, each formed by two small veins issuing in turn from each developing lung bud. Subsequently the common trunk and the two veins forming it expand and are incorporated in the left atrium to make up the greater part of its cavity. This expansion usually continues as far as the orifices of the four veins, which thus open separately into the left atrium; variations, however, are quite common. The left half of the primitive atrium is progressively restricted to the mature auricular appendage.

During the second month the two atria bulge ventrally one on each side of the bulbus cordis, which lies in a groove on their ventral surface (**3**.162, 165). These projecting parts of the atria form the auricular appendages of the adult heart.

Ventricles, bulbus cordis and truncus arteriosus

The process of separation of the ventricles is intimately related to that of the aortic and pulmonary orifices at the distal end of the bulbus (**3**.167–169) and also to the division of the truncus arteriosus into pulmonary and aortic channels. Their interdependence is such that the history of the truncus arteriosus is dealt with here, although strictly it takes no part in the formation of the heart itself. Bulbotruncal separation is conveniently considered before final interventricular septation and valve modelling. As intimated these complex events are the result of mutual interaction between factors controlling pattern formation, differential growth and the continuously changing blood-flow paths, volumes and pressures. This interplay moulds the grooves, ridges, outpouchings, valve complexes and varying myocardial thickness and architecture. Although described sequentially, many of these events occur simultaneously.

Blood enters the bulboventricular cavity through the right and left atrioventricular canals (ventricular *inflow tracts*) and is ejected through the proximal and distal bulbus (*outflow tracts*). Blood flow from the future left ventricle passes obliquely to the dorsal part of the bulbus, whereas right ventricular blood has a reverse inclination to the former and is expelled through the ventral part of the bulbus. These inclinations impose a mutually spiral flow on the two streams as they traverse the truncus.

Four endocardial cushions—ventral, dorsal, right and left—form in the distal part of the bulbus and the right and left cushions fuse to constitute a *distal bulbar septum*. This separates a ventral, *pulmonary orifice* from a dorsal, *aortic orifice*, and later the cushions divide and become modified to form the *semilunar valves* (see below).

The separation of the pulmonary trunk from the aorta is a more complicated process. Two ridge-like thickenings project into the interior of the truncus arteriosus between the entwined spiralized streams of blood. Proximally, the ridges project from the **lateral** walls of the vessel but, progressing distally, the right ridge passes obliquely on to the **ventral** and then the **left** wall, while the left ridge extends on to the **dorsal** wall and then the **right** wall (**3**.168). The ridges are therefore spiral and their fusion forms the *spiral aorticopulmonary septum*. Proximally this meets and fuses with the distal bulbar septum, and in accord with its spiral form the pulmonary trunk, which lies ventral to the aorta at its orifice, curves round to its left side as it ascends and finally lies dorsal to it (**3**.168). Distally the aorticopulmonary septum meets the dorsal wall of the aortic sac (see p. 312) cranial to the point where it is joined by the sixth pair of aortic arches, and thus the latter become branches of the pulmonary trunk while the remaining arches retain communication with the aorta (**3**.168).

The separation of the two ventricles from each other leaves the right ventricle in communication with the right atrium (inflow tract) and the pulmonary artery (outflow tract), and the left ventricle in communication with the left atrium (inflow tract) and the aorta (outflow tract). It involves a series of complex changes in which three distinct factors contribute to the formation of the *adult ventricular septum*:

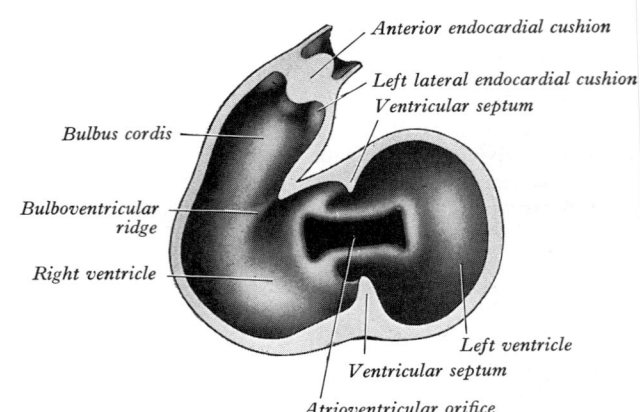

3.167 Diagram showing an early stage in the relations between the atrioventricular opening and ventricles, the cavity of the bulbus cordis and the bulboventricular ridge. The endocardial cushions at the distal end of the bulb are shown in a more differentiated state than they really exhibit at this stage. (After J E Frazer.)

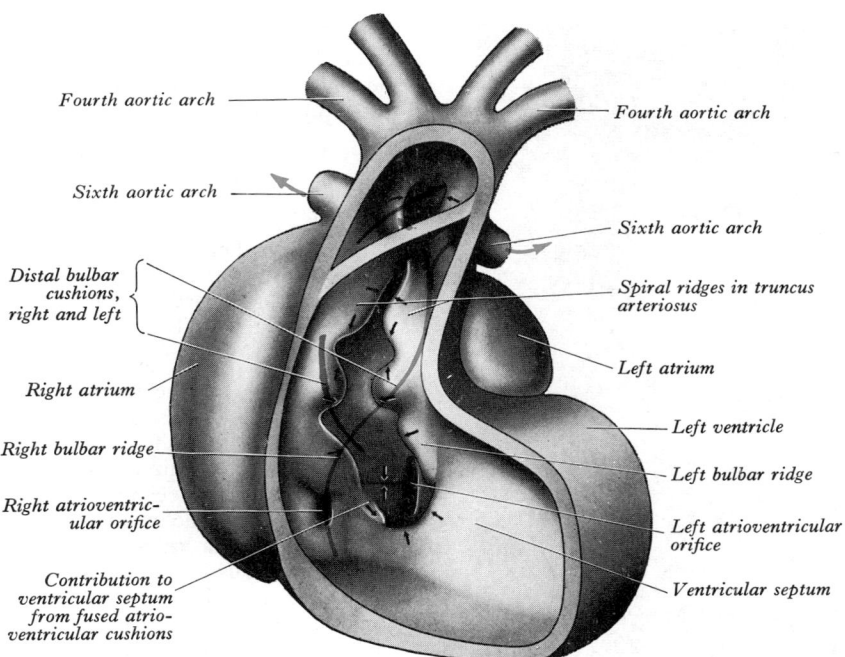

Fourth aortic arch

Sixth aortic arch

Distal bulbar
cushions,
right and left

Right atrium

Right bulbar ridge

Right atrioventric-
ular orifice

Contribution to
ventricular septum
from fused atrio-
ventricular cushions

Fourth aortic arch

Sixth aortic arch

Spiral ridges in truncus
arteriosus

Left atrium

Left ventricle

Left bulbar ridge

Left atrioventricular
orifice

Ventricular septum

3.168 Diagram to show the mode of formation of the septa which separate the aortic and pulmonary channels in the embryonic heart. The red arrow indicates the aortic channel and the blue arrow the pulmonary. The small black arrows indicate the direction of growth. (From a model by James Whillis.)

• the *fetal ventricular septum*
• the *proximal bulbar septum*
• the *atrioventricular endocardial cushions*.

Fetal ventricular septum

During the fifth week the right and left definitive ventricles appear as slight projections on the external surface of the primitive common ventricle. It is uncertain whether the right definitive ventricle is solely a derivative of the common ventricle, or of the caudal end of the primitive bulbus, or of both. In either event, the appearance of a caudal crescentic ridge in the inside of the heart indicates the separation between the two ventricles and, as the heart enlarges, this ridge deepens to form the early ventricular septum. The dorsal and ventral horns of the septum grow along the ventricular walls to meet and fuse with the corresponding endocardial cushions of the atrioventricular canal near their **right** extremities (**3.**167). The septum has a free sickle-shaped margin which, with the endocardial cushions, bounds a circular *interventricular foramen* (**3.**168) (sometimes delineated temporally as the interventricular foramen primum; **3.**170).

At first the bulboventricular junction is marked by a distinct notch on the outside of the heart (**3.**161) and inside is a corresponding *bulboventricular ridge*. The latter is between the atrioventricular orifice and the caudal part of the bulb (**3.**167) and its absorption is essential for the development of a four-chambered heart. Partly by absorption of the bulboventricular ridge and partly growth of the atrioventricular region, the **right** extremity of the atrioventricular canal comes to lie **caudal** to the orifice of the bulb (**3.**168). This alteration in relative positions of the structures concerned occurs while the ventricular septum is forming, paving the way for completion of ventricular partition (Wenink 1971, 1976).

Proximal bulbar septum

The proximal bulbar septum separates the bulbus cordis into pulmonary and aortic channels (*ventricular outflow tracts*), and is formed by the *right* and *left bulbar ridges*, which are in continuity with the corresponding distal bulbar endocardial cushions (which form the *distal bulbar septum*—see above). The ridges appear broad, shallow and less defined at their proximal and distal ends, but are somewhat taller and better defined in their midportion (**3.**170). The right bulbar ridge grows across the dorsal wall of the bulb and right extremity of the fused atrioventricular endocardial cushions to reach the dorsal horn of the free, crescentic edge of the ventricular septum and

obliterates the ventral or cranial part of the right atrioventricular orifice (**3.**168). The left bulbar ridge crosses the ventral wall of the bulb to reach the ventral or cranial horn of the ventricular septum. The bulbar ridges fuse thus separating the conus arteriosus of the right ventricle from the aortic vestibule; however, the caudal edge of the bulbar septum is still separated from the free crescentic edge of the ventricular septum by a diminishing interventricular channel (this has been termed the interventricular foramen secundum). The latter is closed by growth of tissue from the right extremity of the fused atrioventricular cushions (Odgers 1938) and this fuses, on its one aspect with the caudal border of the proximal bulbar septum and on its other with the margin of the ventricular septum. (A transitory interventricular foramen tertium has been described; it can be seen towards the end of the sixth week of gestation as an orifice 80 μm in its largest diameter. A dimple less than 40 μm in diameter is left for a brief period of time at the site of closure on the endocardial surface of the left ventricle.) The dorsal part of the bulb largely becomes absorbed, but its position is indicated by the dorsal wall of the aortic vestibule, which, however, is mainly formed by tissue extensions from the fused atrioventricular endocardial cushions.

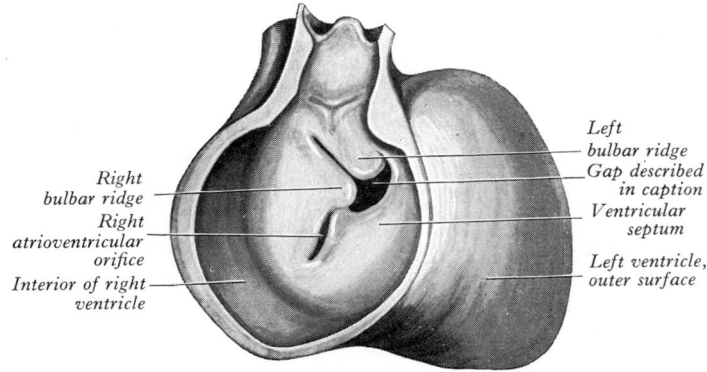

Right
bulbar ridge

Right
atrioventricular
orifice

Interior of right
ventricle

Left
bulbar ridge
Gap described
in caption
Ventricular
septum

Left ventricle,
outer surface

3.169 Diagram to show the part played by the fusion of the right and left bulbar ridges in the separation of the aortic and pulmonary channels. The darkly shaded area indicates the gap filled by the proliferation of cushion tissue (from the right extremity of the fused atrioventricular cushions) which establishes continuity between the proximal bulbar septum and the ventricular septum. Compare with **3.**168.

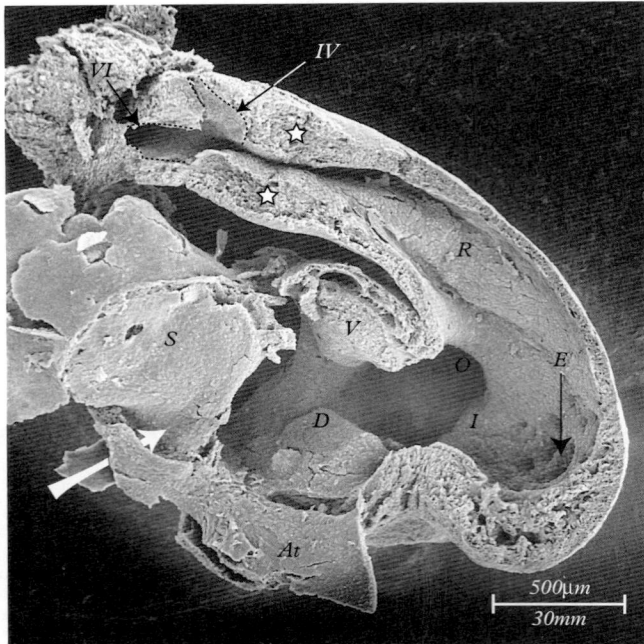

3.170   Human heart at 32 days (stage 15). The right lateral wall of the right atrium, right ventricle and the outflow tract have been removed. The septum primum (S) and the developing valve of the sinus venosus (open arrow) are at a distance from the unfused ventral (V) and dorsal (D) atrioventricular cushions. The interventricular foramen (primum) is open (circle). Its lower margin is made up by the developing interventricular septum (I). Note the left anterolateral ridge (R) and, at the distal margins of the truncus arteriosus, the valve swellings (*) of the putative aorta and pulmonary trunk. The swellings are in continuity with the IV and VI aortic arches. Magnification × 56.

Atrioventricular endocardial cushions

At their time of fusion the atrioventricular endocardial cushions are large relative to the size of the atrioventricular orifices. The atrial septal complex meets the approximate centre of the atrial surface of the cushions; the ventricular septum, however, meets them near their right margins. Thus a part of the fused cushions intervenes between the *right atrium* and the *left ventricle*, and it is this which forms the right wall of the aortic vestibule (*atrioventricular septum*, see **9**.34). The *membranous* part of the *interventricular septum*, continuous dorsally with the membranous *atrioventricular septum* in the completed heart (**3**.171), is also formed by proliferation of cushion tissue from the right extremity of the fused atrioventricular cushions. The persistence of an interventricular communication may follow anomalous development in this region. It may be noted that it is the craniodorsal part of the bulbar orifice, which lies above the ventricular septum, and normally becomes incorporated in the aortic

vestibule through which the left ventricle discharges into the truncal aortic channel. In some cases of persistent interventricular foramen the aortic orifice is described as 'overriding' the free upper border of the muscular interventricular septum (p. 1503).

Development of the fibrous skeleton of the heart

The *valve complexes of the heart*, four in number, arise in two main cardiac zones:

- the aortic and pulmonary valves at the distal bulbotruncal junction
- the mitral and tricuspid complexes extending from their inception between the atrioventricular junctions and loci on the interior of the ventricular walls.

Each commences as an internal endocardial projection of varying form enclosing cardiac mesenchyme (myocardial basement membrane matrix and mesenchymal cells). In some regions the mesenchymatous cells proliferate, transform into fibroblasts and produce a geometrically organized collagenous framework that varies with site and functional demands. Elsewhere the core is invaded by differentiating cardiac myoblasts.

Atrioventricular valves. These develop as shelf-like projections from the margins of the atrioventricular orifices, directed as almost complete conical sheets towards the ventricles, their advancing edges continuing, initially as trabecular ridges, deep into the ventricular cavity. With continued differential growth and excavation on their ventricular aspects, each sheet develops two (mitral) and three (tricuspid) marginal indentations, defining the principal *valve leaflets*, minor marginal indentations (clefts) subdividing some leaflets into scallops. Each leaflet develops functionally significant regional variations in surface texture; its core condenses as a collagenous lamina fibrosa. The latter blends at its atrioventricular base with the inappropriately named fibro-areolar valve 'annulus'—each a part of the complex, functionally crucial, fibrous 'skeleton' of the heart. The anterior leaflet of the tricuspid valve and both the anterolateral and posteromedial leaflets of the mitral valve appear at about the time when fusion of the atrioventricular cushions and bulbar ridges takes place. Delamination of the septal leaflet of the tricuspid valve, however, occurs after closure of the interventricular foramen during the seventh to eighth week of gestation (**3**.172).

Embryonic trabeculae. These start to emerge in the apical endocardial region of the primitive ventricles during stage 15 (32 days gestation). By stage 17 (42 days) well-developed embryonic trabeculae show a typical spatial orientation creating a number of ventricular sinuses and giving a sponge-like appearance to the internal relief of both ventricles (**3**.173). *Definitive trabeculae* are first observed about the 40th day of gestation, appearing initially in the walls of both ventricles at the level of the atrioventricular junction; they develop towards the apex of the heart (**3**.174). By 10 weeks gestation the trabeculae are fewer and confined to the apical region where they gradually disappear following a process of simplification, deletion and reabsorption. The remodelling process is accomplished without the intervention of macrophages or inflammatory cells in the immediate interstitium. Mesenchymal tissue surrounding the trabeculae passes between the margins of the valve leaflets, indentations, clefts and defined zones of the leaflet surface as the white,

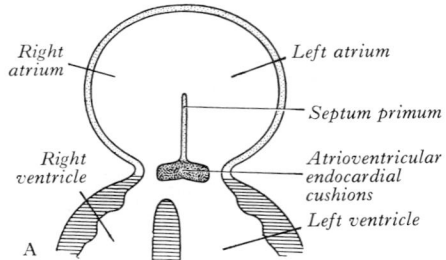

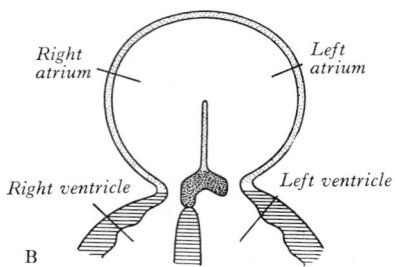

3.171   Diagram to show two stages in the formation of the adult ventricular septum. In (A) the right and left ventricles communicate with each other, but in (B) the interventricular communication has been closed by the fusion of the ventricular septum with the enlarged right extremity of the fused atrioventricular cushions. Note the position of the septum primum relative

to the fused atrioventricular cushions, and observe that in (B) cushion tissue intervenes between the two ventricles (membranous part of ventricular septum), and also between the *right* atrium and the *left* ventricle (atrioventricular septum).

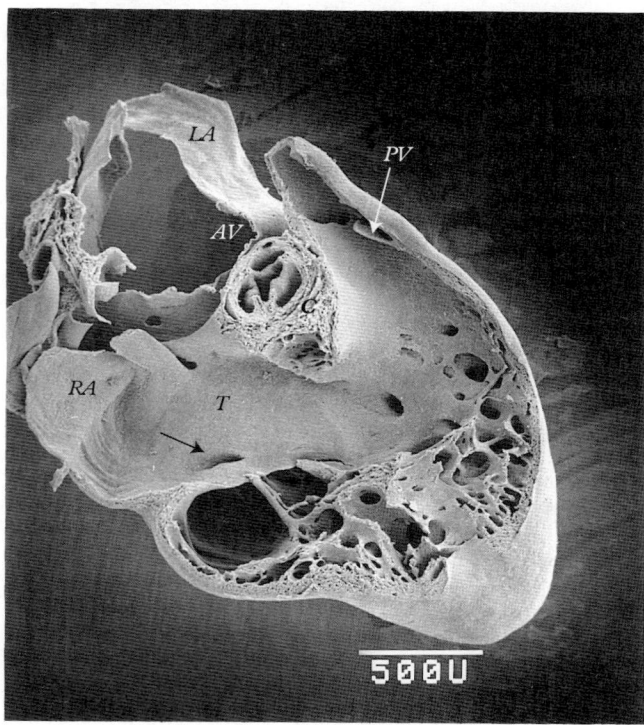

3.172   Septal aspect of the right ventricle of a human heart at 8 weeks gestation. Delamination of the septal leaflet of the tricuspid valve (T) is taking place. A cleft (arrow) has appeared marking the posterior margin of the septal leaflet. There are no clefts delineating the anterior margins in the region adjacent to the crista supraventricularis (C). Note the endocardial continuity instead. No tension apparatus is present. RA = right atrium; AV = aortic valve; LA = left atrium; PV = pulmonary valve. Magnification × 40.

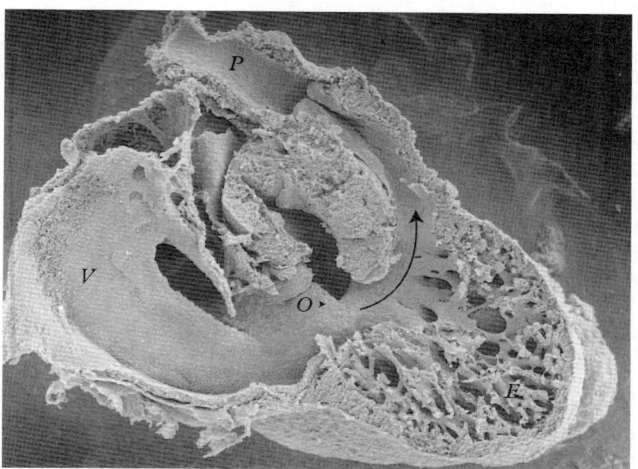

3.173   Human heart at 42 days gestation. The right lateral wall of the right atrium, right ventricle and the outflow tract have been removed. The valve of the sinus venosus (V) is prominent. There is no septal leaflet of the tricuspid valve guarding the inlet portion of the right ventricle. The parietal leaflet has been removed. The atrioventricular cushions are fused. Note the adjacent right lateral tubercles (open circle). A small interventricular foramen (secundum, see text) is indicated (open triangle). There is a well-developed right ventricular outflow tract (curved arrow). E = embryonic trabeculae; P = pulmonary trunk. Magnification × 50.

glistening, compacted, collagenous *chordae tendinae* and these converge towards the tip and sides of the single or grouped *papillary muscles* and blend with their connective tissue framework. The muscles are the ventricular ends of the original embryonic trabeculae and, whilst free throughout their length, their mural ends are confluent with mural ventricular musculature and receive a dense population of its nerves and specialized conducting tissues. (For details of the disposition, architecture and some functional implications of the cardiac valve complexes and fibrous skeleton see pp. 1481–1489.)

Aortic and pulmonary valves. These are formed from the four endocardial cushions which appear at the distal end of the bulbus cordis. The completion of the distal bulbar septum results in division of each lateral cushion into two; thus the number of thickenings is increased to six: three associated with the pulmonary orifice and three with the aortic. These are the rudiments of the aortic and pulmonary valves. Each cushion-derived intrusion grows and is excavated on its truncal aspect to form a semilunar valve cusp. Similar events affect the adjacent truncal or septal wall. Thus the pouches between the valves and the walls of the vessels gradually enlarge and form their related *sinuses*. The core of each cusp forms a collagenous lamina fibrosa, delicate and thin in each crescentic lunule, thick and compact in the central nodule, with marginal radiate and basal bands. The latter blend with the complex, scalloped, mural valve ring. Initially, one cusp of the pulmonary valve lies anteriorly and the other two posterolaterally, whereas one cusp of the aortic valve lies posteriorly and the other two anterolaterally. However, a rotation of the heart to the left before birth changes the orientation of the cusps of the pulmonary and aortic valves and this is reflected in the various schemes for the designation of these cusps in the mature heart (see pp. 1482–1488).

Development of cardiac muscle

Cardiac myocytes differentiate from the splanchnic coelomic cells of the pericardium. Myogenic activity begins at the beginning of stage 10, approximately 22 days gestation, when the embryo has about 4 somites. At this time the presumptive cardiac myocytes express myosin, actin, troponin and other contractile proteins. The cardiac myocytes do not fuse with their neighbours to form a syncytium as in skeletal muscle; rather they remain mononucleated, branched cells connected via intercellular junctions. For a detailed description of the development of cardiac muscle see page 770.

Concurrent with development of the contractile proteins of cardiac muscle, cardiac myocytes develop numerous *specific heart granules* which contain substances shown to induce natriuresis and diuresis, and a family of polypeptides generally known as *atrial natriuretic peptides*. Specific heart granules develop from the Golgi apparatus

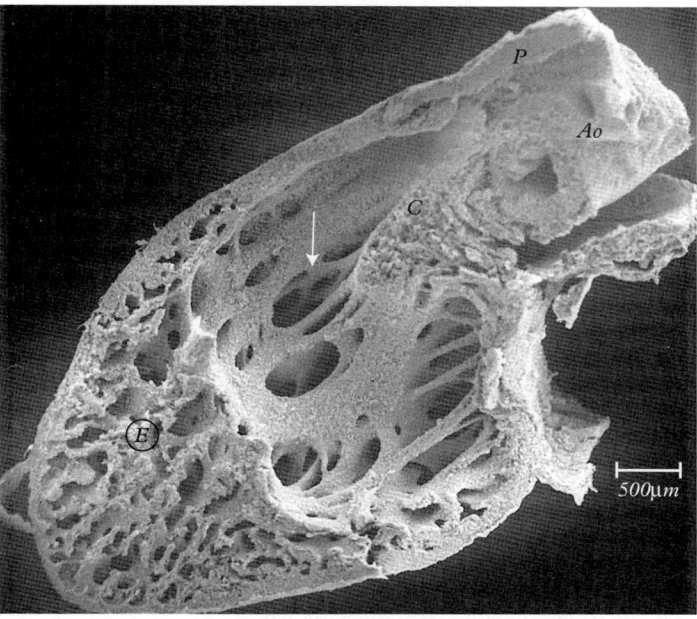

3.174   Parietal aspect of the right ventricle at 8 weeks gestation. The embryonic trabeculae (E) are confined to the lower half of the ventricular wall. An arrow shows the definitive trabeculae. Ao = aorta; P = pulmonary trunk; C = crista supraventricularis. Magnification × 45.

in both atria and ventricles during fetal life but become restricted to atrial muscle in the adult (Challice & Viragh 1973). Atrial natriuretic peptide is measurable when the heart is recognizably four-chambered. Within the atria almost all cells are capable of its synthesis (Navaratnam et al 1989).

Development of the conducting system of the heart

The development of the conducting system has been difficult to elucidate due to the inability of conventional histological staining methods to identify and delineate conducting tissues from other cardiac components during development. However, the recent descriptions of the patterns of expression of a number of markers for the conducting system such as HNK-1 (Nakagawa et al 1993) (which is identical to Leu-7; Ikeda et al 1990), GIN2 (Wessels et al 1992), neurofilament (Gorza & Vitadello 1989), connexin43 (van Kempen et al 1991) and *Msx-2* (*Hox-8*) (Chan-Thomas et al 1993) have brought more clarity to this field.

In the formed heart two types of myocardium have been distinguished. First, the *working myocardium* of atria and ventricles which is specialized in contraction. Second, the *conducting system* which is specialized in the coordinated propagation of the impulse over the myocardium (see p.1496 for its precise anatomy in the adult). The conducting system comprises: the *sinuatrial node*, where the impulse is generated, the *atrioventricular node*, responsible for the delayed transmission of the impulse from the atria to the ventricles, and the *atrioventricular bundle* and *left and right bundle branches*, by which the impulse is rapidly spread over the ventricles. This differentiation in the nomenclature between contracting and conducting cardiac myocytes has focused attention on morphological evidence for different cell lineages, yet the embryonic heart has a measurable electrical activity, as seen by electrocardiographic measurements (ECG), with no distinct conducting system. (For recent reviews see Lamers et al 1991; Moorman & Lamers 1994.)

Development of the nodes. The early heart tube is not segmented and, although a polarity can be observed along its craniocaudal axis, it is in essence a homogeneous tissue. Pacemaker activity is seen in the inflow tract from the earliest time (van Mierop 1967). Initially there is a poorly coupled pattern of excitation and contraction but this rapidly becomes a rhythmic activation pattern (Kamino 1991). Impulses so generated are *slowly propagated* leading to a peristaltoid form of contraction that is characteristic of the tubular heart (Patten & Kramer 1933). Indeed the slow propagation of the impulse is the predominant functional feature which distinguishes the myocardium of the early heart tube from that of the more advanced stages, leading to its description as *primary myocardium* (Moorman & Lamers 1994). It is suggested that the primary myocardium will give rise to both working myocardium and the conducting system (Patten 1956; Moorman & Lamers 1994), although some support the view that these myogenic lineages are separate and arise from different cell lines. Neural crest has been suggested to give rise to the conducting system, in some part due to the expression of HNK-1 and neurofilament in the conducting tissue (Gorza et al 1994). However, sinus node activity can be demonstrated prior to crest cell arrival in the heart and the expression of such markers may reflect the ambiguous neural and myocardial properties of the conducting system.

As development proceeds, segments of *fast-conducting* atrial and ventricular working myocardium differentiate within the slowly conducting primary myocardium (Arguello et al 1986; de Jong et al 1992). The resulting heart consists of five segments (3.175) displaying alternately slow and fast conduction; this is also reflected in the alternating levels of the major cardiac gap-junctional protein connexin43 in the consecutive segments (van Kempen et al 1991) and the appearance of an electrocardiographic output (van Mierop 1967). This architecture permits the pumping function of the embryonic heart in which no valves are present: the slowly conducting segments between the atrium and ventricle (atrioventricular canal), and ventricle and great arteries (outflow tract), contain the endocardial cushions which function as sphincteric valves. The segments persist until one-way valves have been sculpted from the endocardial cushions. The primary myocardium of the outflow tract regresses along with the formation of the semilunar valves and has virtually disappeared around the twelfth week of human development. The

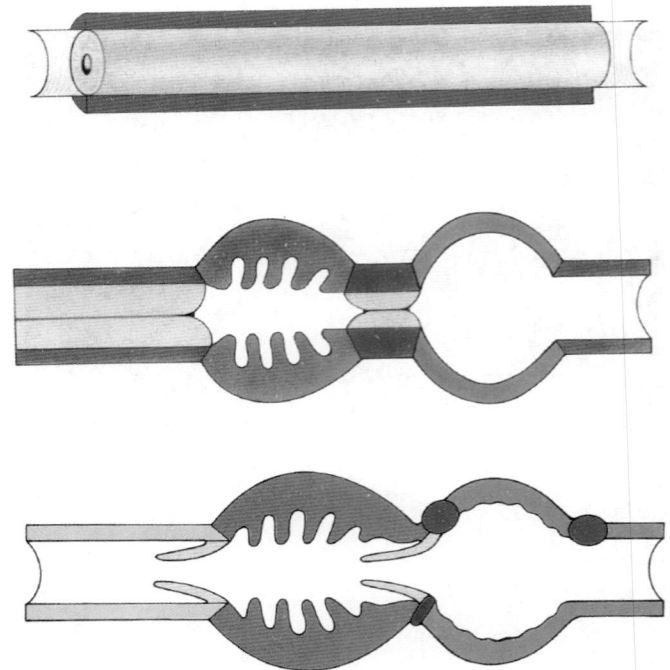

3.175 Schema of the development of cardiac segments in three 'prototypic' human stages showing the tubular heart at about 24 days (top) and 38 days (middle) of development, and the adult configuration (bottom). Blood flow is from right to left. Purple = primary myocardium; blue = atrial working myocardium; red = ventricular working myocardium; yellow = cushion/valvular tissue; green = no longer myocardium.

primary myocardium of the atrioventricular canal will become incorporated into the atria upon the formation of the atrioventricular valves from the ventricular inlets and the annulus fibrosus between 6 and 12 weeks of development; some persists as the, still slowly conducting, atrioventricular node.

Rings of *cardiac specialized tissue*, precursor tissue of the conducting system in the formed heart, have been thought to be present in the embryonic heart at the sinuatrial, atrioventricular, bulboventricular (interventricular) and bulbotruncal junctions (Wenink 1976; Anderson et al 1976), as in the '*four ring theory*'. However, it is crucial to realize that the primary myocardial, slowly conducting segments that remain after the formation of the atrial and ventricular segments should not be considered as newly formed rings. The presence of an *interventricular ring* has been immunohistochemically confirmed; it gives rise to the fast-conducting ventricular part of the conducting system encompassing the atrioventricular bundle and bundle branches (see below). Thus the conducting system of the formed heart encompasses two distinct functional components: the slowly conducting nodal component, consisting of persisting primary myocardium of the flanking segments, and the fast-conducting ventricular component, comprising the atrioventricular bundle and bundle branches.

The concept of cardiac specialized tissue may unintentionally suggest that it is a homogeneous tissue with a single function, being more specialized than other myocardium. However, it is contradictory to suggest that the nodal tissue which is reminiscent of primary myocardium is more specialized than the well-differentiated working myocardium.

Although since the discovery of the nodes attempts have been made to identify *internodal tracts* of specialized atrial cells (for review see Janse & Anderson 1974), as yet there is no convincing evidence to substantiate the presence of such tracts. Preferential conducting pathways in certain areas of the atrium can be accounted for by regional differences in the histological architecture and geometry of the atrial walls and septum (but see also page 1500).

Development of the ventricular conducting system. The development of the ventricular conducting system appears to have become essential, with the evolutionary emergence of two ventricles,

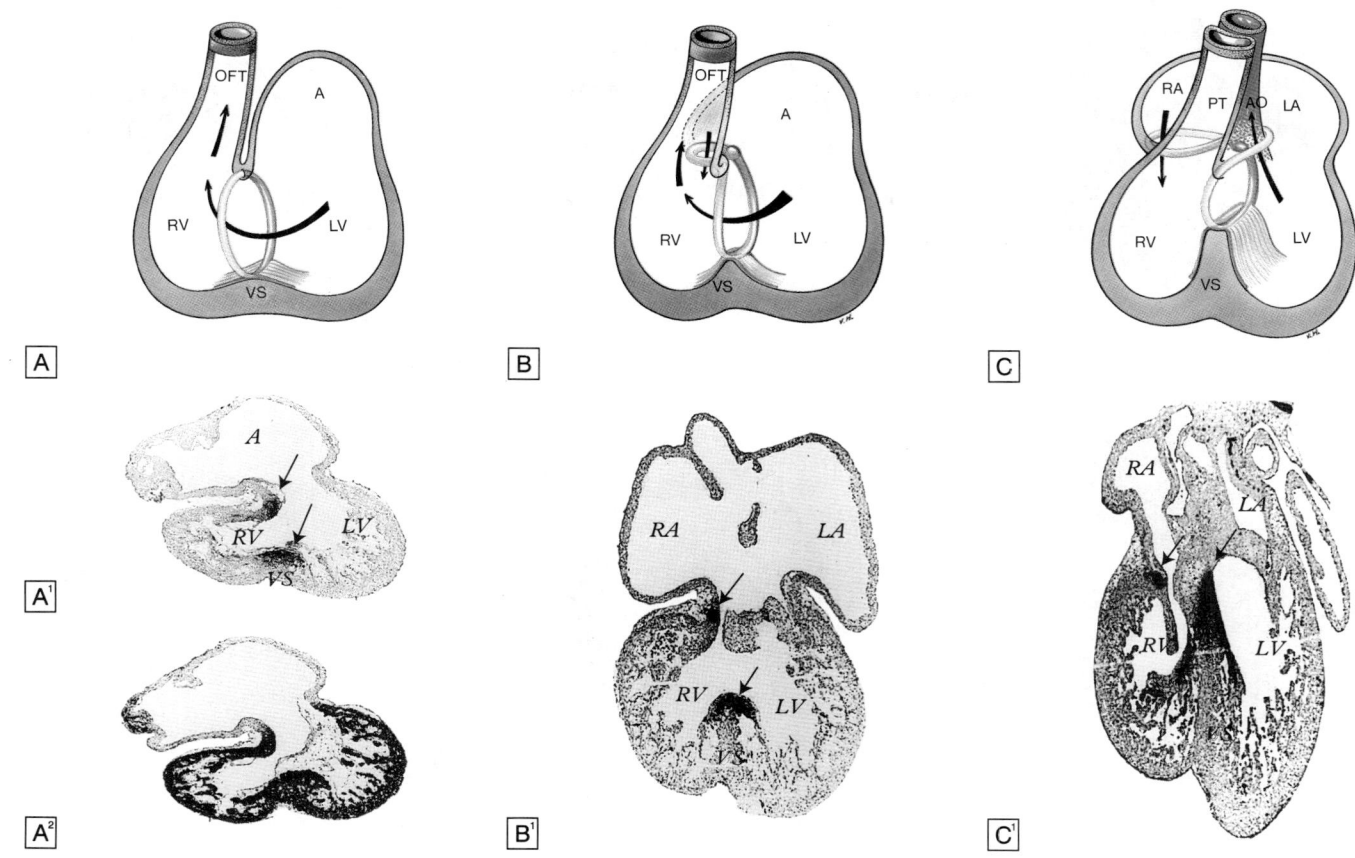

3.176   Development of the ventricular conducting system in the human heart. The upper sequence (A, B, C) shows schematic representations. The red part of the interventricular ring will give rise to the atrioventricular bundle and bundle branches, while the yellow part of the interventricular myocardium will not participate in the formation of the adult conducting system. The lower sequence (a–c) demonstrates immunohistochemical detection of GIN2, a marker for the developing conducting system.

A. At 5 weeks of development (a¹) expression of the neural marker is present in the interventricular myocardium, in the right atrioventricular junction and on top of the ventricular septum (arrowed); (a²) shows a serial section stained for the presence of ventricular myosin (beta myosin heavy chain) indicating that the neural marker is entirely expressed in the ventricular myocardium.

B. At 6 weeks of development the atrioventricular canal is expanding towards the right and the original interventricular myocardium becomes part of the right atrioventricular junction. In (b) expression of GIN2 is clearly present at the right atrioventricular junction and at the top of the ventricular septum (arrowed).

C. At 7 weeks of development the right atrium has become positioned entirely above the right ventricle and the outflow tract has expanded to the left; the left ventricle has gained access to the aorta. In (c) expression of GIN2 clearly identifies the right atrioventricular ring; the atrioventricular bundle and the bundle branches can be identified.

A = embryonic atrium; LV = embryonic left ventricle; RV = embryonic right ventricle; VS = developing ventricular septum; OFT = outflow tract; PT = pulmonary trunk; AO = aorta.

to guarantee simultaneous contraction of both ventricles. Hence the development of the ventricular conducting system is obligatorily associated with ventricular septation. In the early human embryo (stage 14, 5 weeks) (Wessels et al 1992; Ikeda et al 1992) and chick embryo (Chan-Thomas et al 1993) a myocardial ring can be identified encircling the foramen between the presumptive left and right ventricles on top and astride the developing ventricular septum (**3**.176). At this stage of development the atria are connected to the left ventricle only. The interventricular ring is a ventricular structure which, in the inner curvature of the ring, is also part of the myocardium of the atrioventricular canal. Between stages 16 and 19, as a result of the rightward expansion of the atrioventricular canal during subsequent stages, the right atrium gains access to the right ventricle, while, as a result of an apparent leftward expansion of the outflow tract, the left ventricle gains access to the subaortic outflow tract (**3**.177, 178). This entire process can be visualized by the expression of GIN2, one of the neuronal markers of cardiac myocytes. The atrioventricular bundle develops from the *dorsal portion of the interventricular ring* and is contiguous with the left and right bundle branches in the top of the ventricular septum. The anterior portion of this ring has been called the *septal branch*. This so-called 'third branch' of the atrioventricular bundle has been described as a 'dead-end tract' in some malformed hearts (Kurosawa & Becker

1985). It is not yet clear whether the GIN2-positive ring contributes to the formation of the atrioventricular node. As a consequence of the rightward expansion of the atrioventricular canal part of the GIN2-positive ring encircles the *right atrioventricular junction* and will end up in the lower rim of the atrium; this part of the ring is called the *right atrioventricular ring bundle* and has been demonstrated in fetal human hearts (Anderson & Taylor 1972; Anderson et al 1974). As a consequence of the apparent leftward expansion of the outflow tract, the GIN2-positive ring becomes positioned at the root and behind the subaortic outflow tract. This part is called the *retroaortic branch*. The septal branch, retroaortic branch and right atrioventricular ring bundle will disappear during normal development in mammals. Figure **3**.178 represents the entire system in the adult heart. As a rule basic processes are conserved in evolution. The presence of the entire system in adult chicken heart (Davies 1930) constitutes strong support for the unitary concept outlined.

The appreciation that the ventricular conducting system originates from a single interventricular ring provides a solid base to the understanding of the disposition of the conducting system in a number of congenital malformations (Anderson & Ho 1991). The concept accounts particularly well for the morphology and disposition of the atrioventricular node and bundle in hearts with straddling tricuspid valves, with double inlet left ventricles and

309

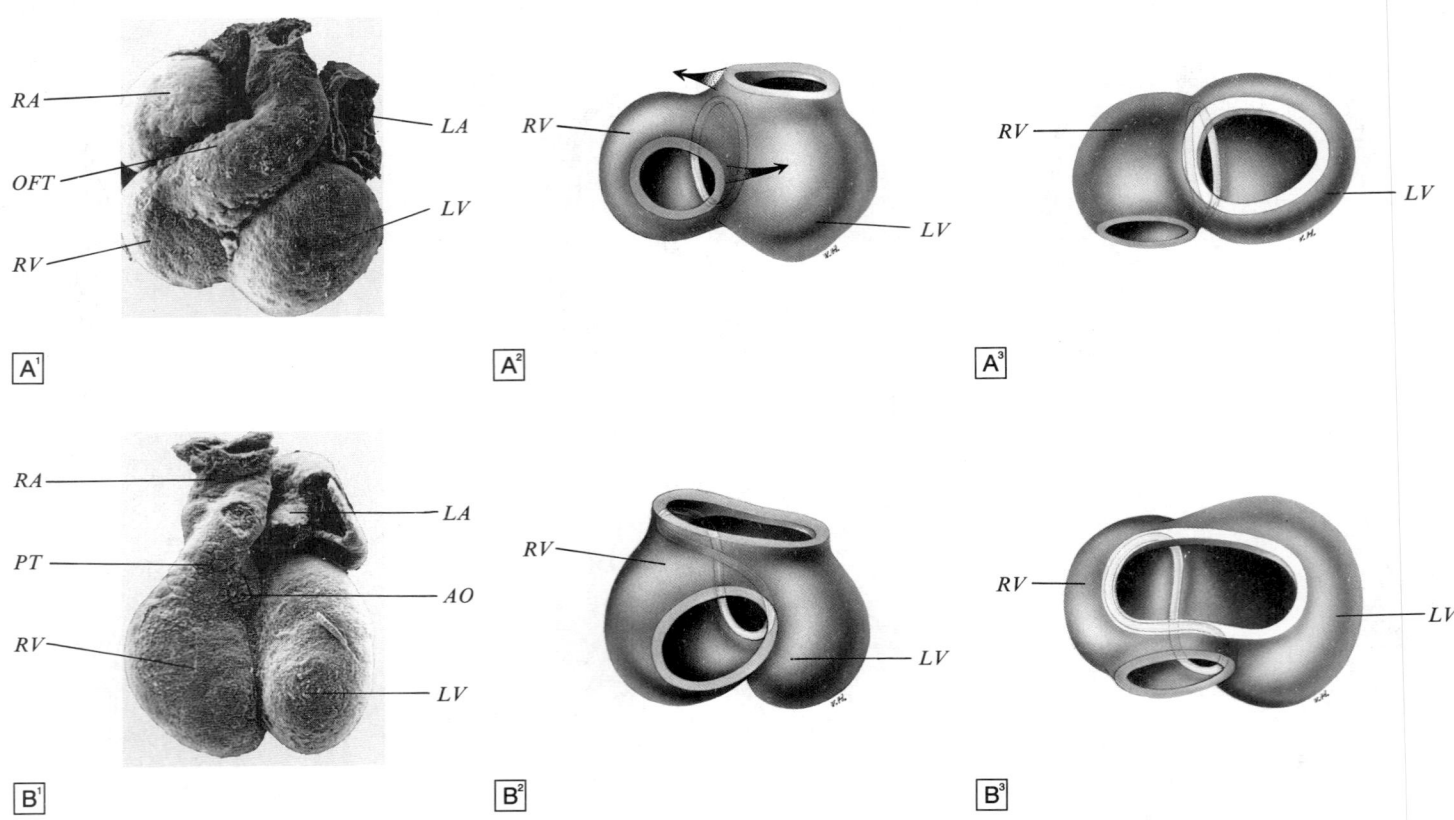

3.177A[1] Scanning electron micrograph of a heart at 5 weeks development; A[2]. schematic representation of the same heart, with atria and outflow tract removed. The arrows indicate the morphogenetic movements that will occur in the next stage, i.e. rightwards expansion of the atrioventricular canal and apparent leftwards expansion of the outflow tract. A[3]. The same scheme as in A[2], but turned 90° to permit an unobstructed view of the atrioventricular canal and of the developing ventricular septum. Note that the atrium (removed in this scheme) would be positioned entirely above the left ventricle.

  B[1]. Scanning electron micrograph of a heart at 7 weeks development;

B[2]. schematic representation of the same heart, with atria and outflow tract removed. The atrioventricular canal has expanded towards the right. B[3]. The same scheme as in B[2] but turned 90° to permit an unobstructed view in the atrioventricular canal and onto the developing ventricular septum. Note that the embryonic atrium has become positioned above the right and left ventricles.

  RA = right embryonic atrium; LA = left embryonic atrium; LV = left embryonic ventricle; RV = right embryonic ventricle; OFT = outflow tract; PT = pulmonary trunk; AO = aorta. (SEMs supplied by Prof. Dr Sc. Virágh, Budapest.)

with tricuspid atresia. The morphology of the latter heart defect is remarkably similar to the embryonic condition.

Fetal heart prior to birth

The development of the chambers of the heart has now been traced to a stage at which the main features of the adult heart are established. It is to be noted that the pattern has developed in such a way as to provide for the sudden establishment of the pulmonary circulation at birth (Dawes 1961, 1969), although it is adapted to the persistence of the placental circulation for the remainder of fetal life. The presence of the ductus venosus (p. 324) ensures that a substantial proportion of umbilical oxygenated blood gains the right atrium with a limited loss of oxygen to the liver. However, some umbilical blood and portal venous blood enters the hepatic sinusoids through venae advehentes; their drainage through venae revehentes (eventually the grouped hepatic veins) returns the blood to the hepatic segment of the inferior vena cava, some admixture occurring here. It was claimed that only minor further admixture of relatively oxygenated and deoxygenated blood occurs in the right atrium (Barclay et al 1939) and that nearly all the oxygenated blood passes through the foramen ovale into the left atrium, so gaining the left ventricle, aorta and systemic circulation. However, there is evidence for the opposing view that there is considerable mixing of the superior and inferior vena caval streams in the right atrium (Born et al 1954; Lind & Wergelius 1954). The inferior vena caval blood is directed by its valve towards the cleft ('foramen ovale') in the atrial septal complex. It has been estimated that about 75% passes through to the left atrium; the remainder mixes with the deoxygenated blood

from the superior vena cava; separation occurs at the crista dividens of the septum secundum. Because the transition from a placental to a pulmonary circulation occurs suddenly at birth, the right ventricle and the pulmonary trunk of the fetus are relatively large, although only a small amount of blood passes through the lung. Most of the blood expelled by the right ventricle to the pulmonary trunk passes through the ductus arteriosus to the descending aorta and therefore is under higher pressure than blood in the aorta. Thus the muscular wall of the right ventricle is thicker than the wall of the left, a condition which persists throughout fetal life but is progressively reversed postnatally. The origin of the carotid and subclavian arteries from the aorta above the junction with the ductus arteriosus may be correlated with the relatively rapid growth of the brain, demanding a copious blood supply, with the more advanced development of the upper limbs, relative to the lower, at birth, and the overall cephalocaudal gradient in the growth of the trunk.

EMBRYONIC CIRCULATION

In early development the arteries of the embryo are disproportionately large and their walls consist of little more than a single layer of endothelium. The cardiac orifices are also relatively large and the force of the cardiac contraction is weak. As a result, despite the rapid rate of contraction, the circulation is sluggish, but this is compensated for because the tissues are able to draw nourishment, not only from the capillaries but also from the large arteries. As the heart muscle thickens, compacts and strengthens, the

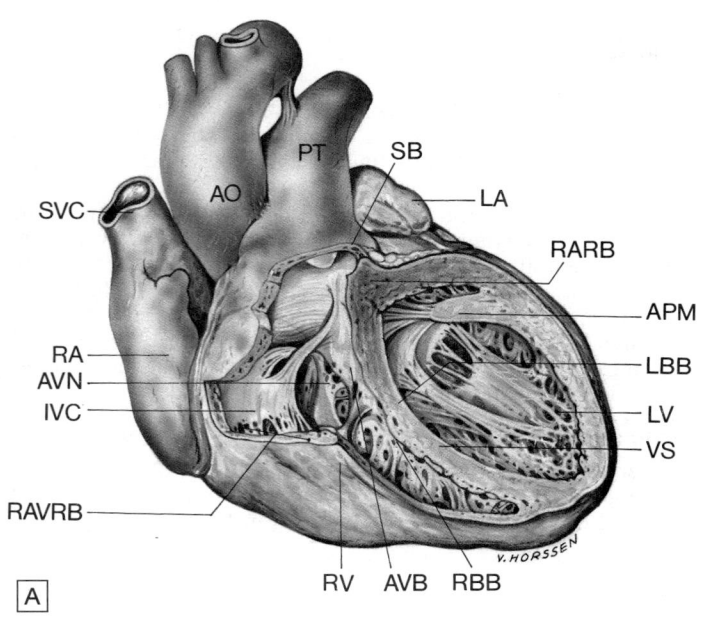

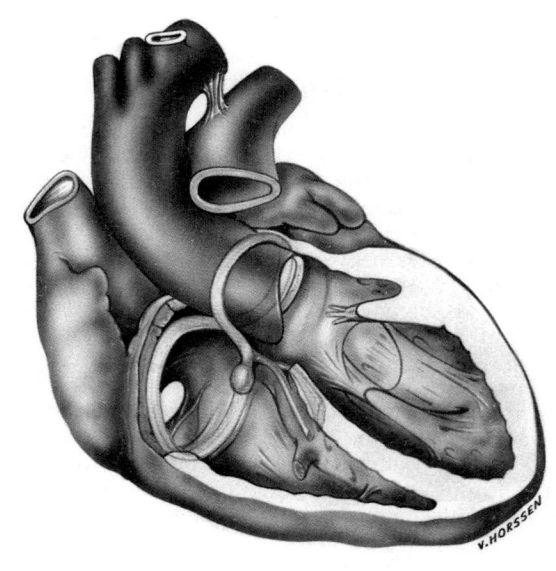

3.178   Position of the original interventricular myocardium in the formed heart. A. Heart with opened ventricles. B. Same heart with the pulmonary trunk removed and the position of the original ring indicated. The yellow parts have disappeared. SB = septal branch; LA = left atrium; RARB = retroaortic root branch; APM = anterior papillary muscle; LBB = left bundle branch; LV = left ventricle; VS = ventricular septum; RBB = right bundle branch; AVB = atrioventricular bundle; RV = right ventricle; RAVRB = right atrioventricular root bundle; IVC = atrioventricular vena cava; AVN = atrioventricular node; RA = right atrium; SVC = superior vena cava; AO = aorta; PT = pulmonary trunk.

cardiac orifices become both relatively and absolutely reduced in size, the valves increase their efficiency and the large arteries acquire their muscular walls and they too undergo a relative reduction in size. From this time onwards the embryo is dependent for its nourishment on the expanding capillary beds and henceforth the larger arteries' function becomes restricted to controllable distribution channels to keep its tissues constantly and appropriately supplied.

It will be noted that the heart commences to beat early, prior to the development of the conducting system, and that a circulation is established before a competent valvular mechanism.

It has been stated previously (see above) that the heart must meet the functional demands of the embryo as well as follow its appropriate developmental pathways, such as the physiology of the cardiovascular system and its regulation during development which is of particular importance. It is beyond the scope of this book to address this issue in detail; however, the following points are relevant to an appreciation of cardiovascular development.

In the early embryo growth is exponential, with the embryo doubling its weight about every 4 hours. This geometric growth needs a concomitant growth and increase in efficiency of the cardiovascular system to supply nutrients and oxygen, and to remove metabolic waste products, especially in regions of active growth and proliferation.

Cardiac output increases in proportion with the weight of the embryo. Cardiac rate increases with development; however, most of the increase in cardiac output results from a geometric increase in stroke volume. Noticeably, when dorsal aortic blood flow is matched to embryonic weight, blood flow remains constant over a more than 150-fold change in mass of the embryo. (For a discussion of early haemodynamics see Clarke 1991.)

Further development of the blood vessels

It is the case that the endodermal tissues, yolk sac (continuous with the splanchnopleure) and allantois, are primarily *vascular*, whereas the ectodermal tissues, chorion and amnion (somatopleure), are primarily *avascular*. The yolk sac and allantois secondarily vascularize the chorion in various ways, giving rise to the diverse varieties of placentae. Until recently it was not thought that any tissue interaction would be necessary for the process of intraembryonic

vasculogenesis. However, evidence now points to a permissive interaction between *endodermal* epithelia and mesenchymes that are *angioblastic*, i.e. capable of differentiating into endothelia in situ, for the initial production of the early blood vessels. Such angioblastic competence has been demonstrated among the ventral mesenchymes (splanchnopleuric) with which the endoderm interacts. Dorsal mesenchymal populations (which include somites and somatopleuric mesenchyme) are more likely to be vascularized by budding from established endothelia (an angiotrophic mechanism; Sherer 1991). Once the mechanism of angiogenesis has been determined by the presence of endoderm or not, the timing of endothelial differentiation is controlled by the angiogenic cells. The ultimate pattern of vessels formed is controlled by the surrounding, non-angiogenic, mesenchyme (Noden 1991) and blood vessels become morphologically specific for the organ in which they develop; they also become immunologically specific, expressing organ-specific proteins.

During embryonic *vasculogenesis* (angioblastic vasculogenesis) and *angiogenesis* (angiotrophic vasculogenesis, see p. 299), changes occur in the vascular extracellular matrix. All blood vessels seem to be initially surrounded by a fibronectin-rich matrix which is later incorporated into the basal lamina along with inter alia laminin, a particularly early constituent (Risau 1991). Several layers of fibronectin-expressing cells can be seen around the larger vessels (e.g. dorsal aortae).

Major restructuring changes take place during the early development of the circulation. Anastomoses appear and disappear, capillaries fuse and give rise to arteries or veins, and the direction of blood flow may reverse several times. It is suggested that the *mechanical stresses* that endothelial cells have to withstand cause the development of the larger vessels (Risau 1991). The *tunica media* of the vessels appears after a stable vascular pattern has formed. Thus medial differentiation of the dorsal aorta starts in that part where major vessels are connected. Generally, the endothelium does not synthesize a basal lamina in those regions where remodelling is active and similarly the mesenchyme around such endothelium does not express α-actin, laminin, etc. Appearance of these molecules is indicative of cessation of branching and differentiation of the media. It is unknown how pericytes and smooth muscle cell differentiation is induced.

The tunica media of the embryonic aortic arch arteries, with the exception of the ductus arteriosus, is formed by migrating *cardiac neural crest cells*. These cells produce the *elastic mediae* specific to these vessels (see p. 314).

DEVELOPMENT OF THE ARTERIES

Apart from the aortae none of the main vessels of the adult arise as single trunks in the embryo. Along the course of each vessel a capillary network is first laid down and by selection and enlargement of definite paths in this the larger arteries and veins are defined. The branches of main arteries are not always simple modifications of the vessels of a capillary network but arise as outgrowths from the enlarged stem.

As mentioned, subsequent to head fold formation each primitive aorta consists of ventral and dorsal parts which are continuous through the first embryonic aortic arch. The dorsal aortae run caudally, one on each side of the notochord, but in the fourth week they fuse from about the level of the fourth thoracic to that of the fourth lumbar segment to form a single definitive descending aorta. Although in many animals paired ventral aortae arise from the truncus arteriosus and course headwards on the ventral surface of the pharynx, in the human embryo the ventral aortae are fused and

form a dilated aortic sac (see **3**.179A and consult Congdon 1922). The first aortic arches run through the mandibular arches, and caudal to them five additional pairs are developed within the corresponding pharyngeal arches so that in all six pairs of aortic arches are formed (**3**.180A). The fifth arches are atypical and probably transient, at most, in mankind.

In fishes the aortic arches persist and give off branches to the gills, in which the blood is oxygenated. In mammals some of the arteries remain as permanent structures, while others disappear or are obliterated (**3**.180).

Caution should moderate unqualified use of the term *aortic arch(es)*. The *embryonic aortic arches* are paired bilateral series joining the ventral aortae (or their fused expanded homologue) with the dorsal aorta of its side after traversing the core of a pharyngeal arch. In contrast the *definitive aorta* consists of ascending aorta, aortic arch and descending (thoracic and abdominal) aorta—all parts of a single vessel in the mature state but derived from multiple embryonic sources. For one detailed analysis see **3**.180.

Aortic sac

This represents the fused, paired ventral aortae (**3**.179). As the embryo grows and the aorticopulmonary septum is formed, part of the caudal end of the sac is incorporated in the pulmonary trunk.

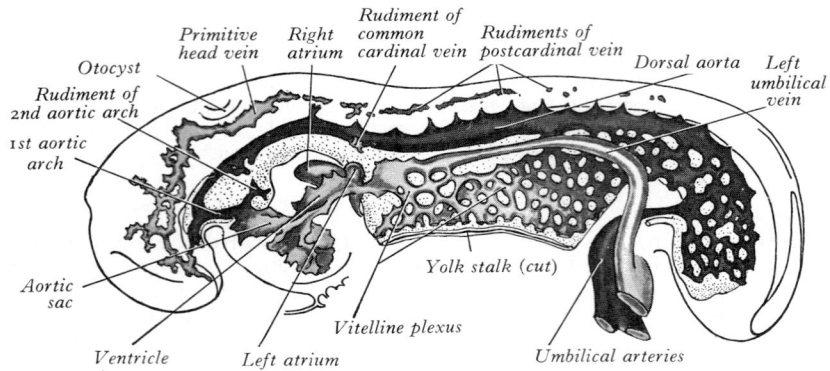

3.179A   The blood vascular system of a human embryo with 14 paired somites: estimated age, 23.5 days; CR length 2.4 mm. The arteries and veins are only in the process of development so that no true circulation is possible at this stage. Only the endothelial lining of the heart tube is shown. Magnification × *c*. 45. (Streeter 1942.)

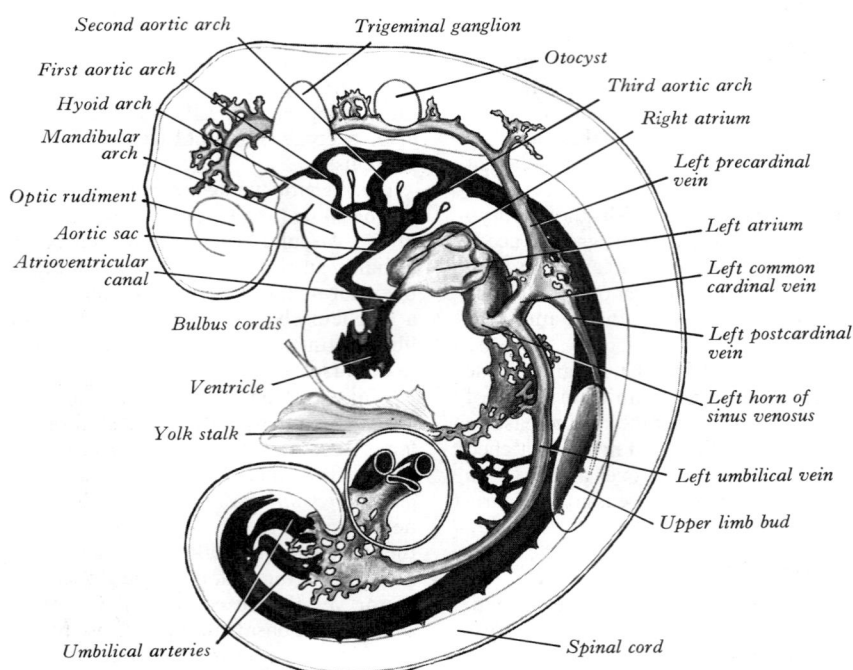

3.179B   Profile reconstruction of the blood vascular system of a human embryo having 28 somites: CR length 4 mm; estimated age 26 days. *Note*. Only the endothelial lining of the heart chambers is shown and, as the muscular wall has been omitted, the pericardial cavity appears much larger than the contained heart. Observe that the atrioventricular canal still connects the left atrium with the single ventricle. (Streeter 1942.)

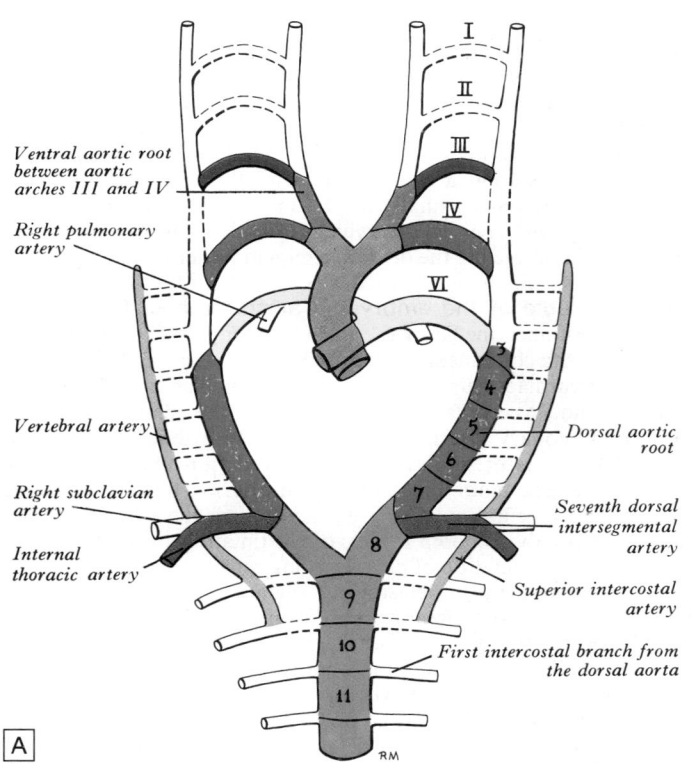

3.180A Schematic diagram showing the various components of the embryonic aortic arch complex in the human embryo. Structures which do not persist in normal development are indicated by interrupted lines. Roman numerals refer to the pharyngeal arches concerned; arabic numerals indicate the metameric body segments—somites.

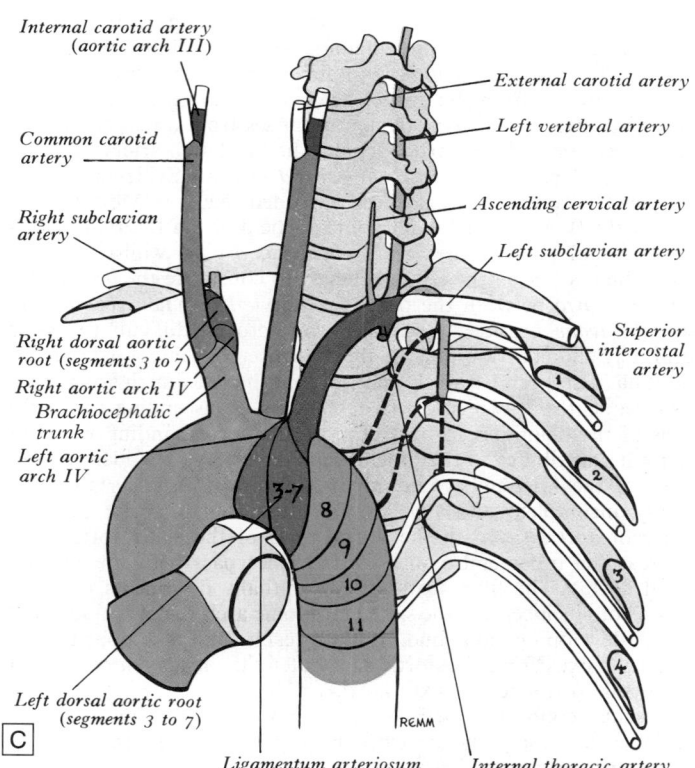

3.180C Diagram of the adult human aorta and its branches, left ventrolateral aspect, showing the position and relative sizes of the definitive contributions from the various embryonic components shown in A and B.

(Based on the work of A Barry, with permission of the author and *Anatomical Record*, **111**, 1951.)

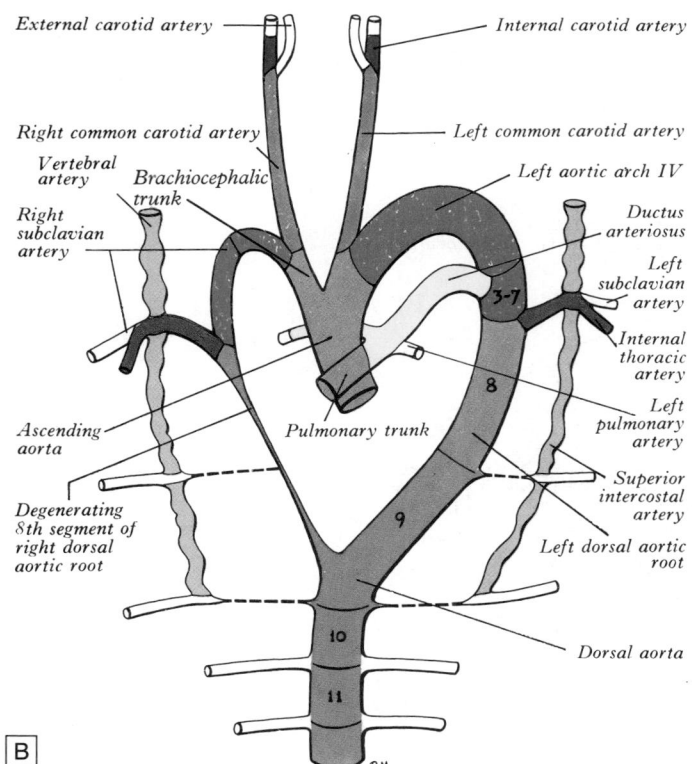

3.180B Diagrammatic ventral view of the aortic arch complex of a human embryo of 15 mm CR length. Note the asymmetry in the pattern that has developed by this stage. Compare with A and C.

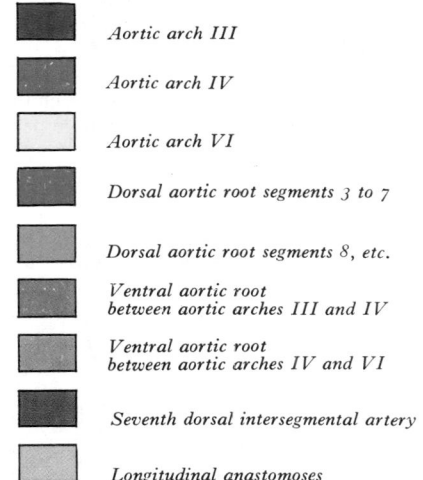

Aortic arch III

Aortic arch IV

Aortic arch VI

Dorsal aortic root segments 3 to 7

Dorsal aortic root segments 8, etc.

Ventral aortic root between aortic arches III and IV

Ventral aortic root between aortic arches IV and VI

Seventh dorsal intersegmental artery

Longitudinal anastomoses

The cranial end of the sac becomes drawn out into *right* and *left limbs* as the neck lengthens. The right limb becomes the brachiocephalic trunk and the left limb forms that part of the definitive arch of the aorta which lies between the origin of the brachiocephalic trunk and the left common carotid artery. The remainder of the sac contributes to the formation of the ascending arch of the aorta.

Embryonic aortic arches

The embryonic aortic arches (**3.**180), with the exception of the fifth, are developed in a craniocaudal sequence, but the more cranial are in process of disappearing before the caudal ones are completed. The first and second embryonic aortic arches are already dwindling by the time the third is established. The first disappears entirely. The

313

dorsal end of the second arch or *hyoid artery* remains as the stem of the *stapedial artery*, while the remainder of this arch also disappears (**3**.181). The *external carotid artery* first appears as a sprout which grows headward from the aortic sac close to the ventral end of the third arch artery. The *common carotid* arises from an elongation of the adjacent part of the aortic sac, and the third arch artery becomes the proximal part of the *internal carotid artery*. (Evidence against this view, however, has also been recorded: e.g. see Moffat 1959; Adams 1957). The fourth embryonic aortic arch on the right forms the proximal part of the *right subclavian artery*, whilst the corresponding vessel on the left is believed to constitute the *arch of the definitive aorta* between the origins of the *left common carotid* and *left subclavian arteries*. It has, however, proved difficult to assess accurately the contributions of the fourth embryonic aortic arches and it has also been variously claimed that the left fourth aortic arch is subsequently drawn into the descending or ascending (or both) limbs of the definitive aortic arch, and the corresponding vessel of the right contributes to the brachiocephalic artery. The identity and status of the fifth embryonic aortic arch artery is uncertain; it is usually incomplete and may connect the fourth aortic arch or subjacent aortic sac with the dorsal ends of the sixth aortic arch (whereas the other embryonic aortic arches pass between sac and dorsal aorta). The fifth aortic arch eventually disappears on both sides. From its inception the sixth embryonic arch vessel is associated with a developing lung bud. Initially each bud is supplied by a capillary plexus from the aortic sac. Later the plexus connects with the dorsal aorta and the sixth aortic arch is defined as a channel in the vascular connection between sac and dorsal aorta; however, this continues to supply the developing lung bud. When the aortico-pulmonary septum divides the *truncus arteriosus* into pulmonary trunk and ascending aorta the sixth aortic arches retain continuity with the former. On the right the ventral part of the sixth aortic arch persists as the stem of the right pulmonary artery, but its dorsal segment disappears, possibly due to a decreased blood flow resulting from partitioning of the aortic and pulmonary bloodstreams (Navaratnam 1963). On the left side the ventral part of the sixth aortic arch is absorbed into the pulmonary trunk, while its dorsal segment persists as the *ductus arteriosus*, which is functional during intrauterine life but becomes obliterated after birth, ultimately forming the fibrous *ligamentum arteriosum*. Postnatal *functional* closure nears completion within a few weeks but *structural* changes continue over many months (p. 107).

The transformation of the aortic arches described above is conditioned by environmental changes and results largely from changes in the pharynx and from the descent of the heart. The whole period of transformation can be divided, both temporally and spatially, into two phases, pharyngeal and postpharyngeal. In the *pharyngeal phase*, which lasts until about the 12 mm CR length stage (stage 17), the arrangement of the aortic arches resembles that in lower vertebrates. In this phase the course of the blood from the heart to the dorsal aorta follows a succession of different pathways—first arch, first and second arches, second and third arches, third and fourth aortic arches and finally third, fourth and sixth aortic arches. In the *postpharyngeal phase*, which extends onwards into, and beyond, intrauterine life the definitive human pattern and disposition of the vessels is finally established.

Tunica media of the embryonic aortic arches. In the early embryo, the tunica media of the third, fourth and sixth arches and the dorsal aorta contains smooth muscle cells that are not elastogenic and not of cardiac neural crest origin. The mediae of those vessels which do not receive a contribution from the neural crest, e.g. the intrapulmonary arteries or the subclavian arteries, continue to accumulate layers of smooth muscle derived from the surrounding mesenchyme. The embryonic aortic arch arteries, however, become surrounded by neural crest very early although there is initially no expression of either smooth muscle or elastin antigens by these cells. Later a larger population of crest cells migrates around these vessels and differentiates into an elastogenic phenotype. Neural crest cells differentiate in a downstream progression around the vessels, from the truncus arteriosus to the aortic arch arteries, until all of them are elastogenic. At the same time the original smooth muscle cells disappear along the great vessels to their first branch point (Rosenquist & Beall 1990). Ablation of the cardiac neural crest leads to changes in the embryonic aortic arch vessels: they may be absent, too large, too small, or aberrant in their connections and there is loss of bilateral symmetry. There is a significant decrease in the quantity of mesenchyme around these vessels resulting in direct apposition of endothelium and pharyngeal endodermal epithelium (Bockmann et al 1990). It should be noted that the *ductus arteriosus* (VIth aortic arch artery) and the *pulmonary arteries* have a *muscular tunica media* and not an elastic media as the other arch arteries. Thus just prior to, and after, birth the local action of prostaglandins can cause the ductus arteriosus to constrict and ultimately to close. *Coarctation of the aorta* is a condition in which the aorta is constricted, usually just above (preductal) or below (postductal) the entrance of the ductus arteriosus. An abnormal disposition of a smooth muscle media around the aorta at this point rather than an elastogenic media derived from the cardiac neural crest could result from an imperfect migration of crest cells into the aortic arch. The result would be an abnormal constriction of the aorta after birth.

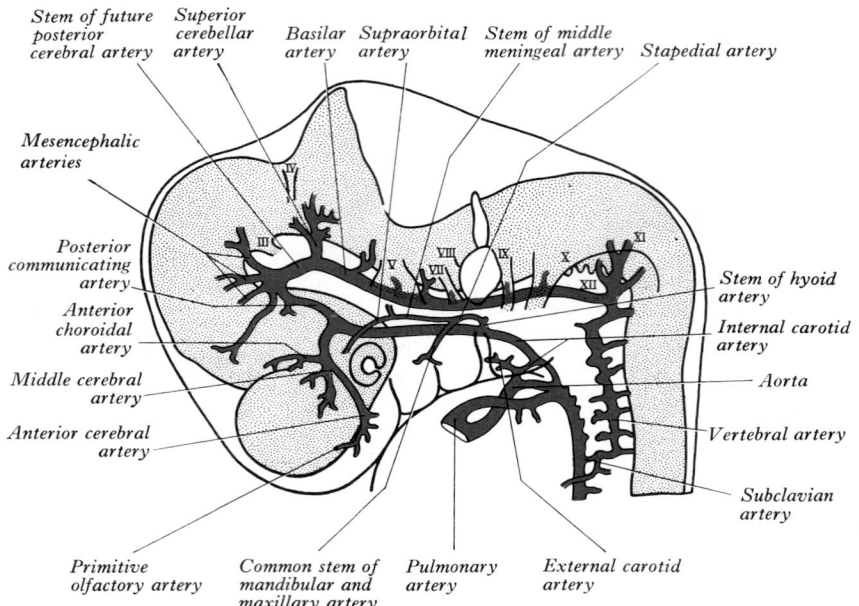

3.181 Diagram to show the origins of the main cranial arteries. (After Padget 1948.)

Cranial arteries

These develop in outline as follows (Padget 1948; **3**.181). The *internal carotid artery* is progressively formed from the third arch artery, the dorsal aorta cranial to this and a further forward continuation which differentiates, at the time of regression of the first and second aortic arches, from the capillary plexus extending to the walls of the forebrain and midbrain. At its anterior extremity this *primitive internal carotid* artery divides into *cranial* and *caudal* divisions, the former terminating as the *primitive olfactory artery*, supplying the developing regions implied, and the latter sweeping caudally to reach the ventral aspect of the midbrain, its terminal branches being the *primitive mesencephalic arteries*. Simultaneously bilateral longitudinal channels differentiate along the ventral surface of the hindbrain from a plexus fed by intersegmental and transitory presegmental branches of the dorsal aorta and its forward continuation. The most important of the presegmental branches is closely related to the fifth nerve— the *primitive trigeminal artery*. *Otic* and *hypoglossal* presegmental arteries also occur (Padget 1948); sometimes these persist. The longitudinal channels later connect, cranially, with the caudal divisions of the internal carotid arteries, each of which gives rise to an *anterior choroidal artery* supplying branches to diencephalon, including the telae choroideae, midbrain, and caudally with the vertebral arteries through the first cervical intersegmental arteries. Fusion of the longitudinal channels results in the formation of the *basilar artery*, whilst the caudal division of the internal carotid artery becomes the *posterior communicating artery* and the stem of the *posterior cerebral artery*. The remainder of the latter develops comparatively late, probably from the stem of the *posterior choroidal artery* which is annexed by the caudally expanding cerebral hemisphere, its distal portion becoming a *choroidal branch of the posterior cerebral artery*. Note that the posterior choroidal artery is supplying the tela choroidea at the future temporal end of the choroidal fissure, its rami advancing through the tela to become confluent with branches of the anterior choroidal artery (see above). In the rat, where the vascular pattern is essentially similar to that in man, this artery is derived from the posterior communicating artery, the common stem of origin of the posterior choroidal, mesencephalic and diencephalic arteries, together with a new channel formed in the plexus on the medial wall of the cerebral hemisphere initially supplied by the anterior choroidal artery (Moffat 1961a). The cranial division of the internal carotid artery gives rise to *anterior choroidal*, *middle cerebral* and *anterior cerebral arteries*, the stem of the primitive olfactory artery remaining as a small medial striate branch of the anterior cerebral artery. In the rat the primitive olfactory artery and its recurrent branch form the anterior cerebral artery, the territory of which is initially supplied by the primitive maxillary and the cranial ramus of the internal carotid arteries (Moffat 1961b). The *cerebellar arteries*, of which the superior is the first to differentiate, emerge from the capillary plexus on the wall of the rhombencephalon.

The source of the blood supply to the territory of the trigeminal nerve varies at different stages in development. When the first and second aortic arch arteries begin to regress, the supply to the corresponding arches is derived from a transient *ventral pharyngeal artery*, which grows from the aortic sac. It terminates by dividing into *mandibular* and *maxillary branches*. Later the *stapedial artery* develops from the dorsal stem of the second arch artery and passes through the condensed mesenchymal site of the future ring of the stapes to anastomose with the cranial end of the ventral pharyngeal artery thereby annexing its terminal distribution. The fully developed stapedial artery possesses three branches, *mandibular*, *maxillary* and *supraorbital*, which follow the divisions of the trigeminal nerve (**3**.181). The mandibular and maxillary branches diverge from a common stem. When the external carotid artery emerges from the base of the third arch it incorporates the stem of the ventral pharyngeal artery, and its maxillary branch communicates with the common trunk of origin of the maxillary and mandibular branches of the stapedial artery and annexes these vessels. The proximal part of the common trunk persists as the root of the *middle meningeal artery*. More distally the meningeal artery is derived from the proximal part of the supraorbital artery. The maxillary branch becomes the infraorbital artery and the mandibular branch forms the inferior alveolar artery.

When the definitive *ophthalmic artery* differentiates as a branch

from the terminal part of the internal carotid artery, it communicates with the supraorbital branch of the stapedial artery; distally this becomes the *lacrimal artery*. The latter retains an anastomotic connection with the middle meningeal artery. The dorsal stem of the original second arch artery remains as one or more *caroticotympanic branches* of the internal carotid artery.

At stage 20–23 (7–8 weeks), further expansion of the cerebral hemispheres produces the completion of the *circle of Willis*, with the development of the *anterior communicating arteries* by 8 weeks gestation. An annular network of meningeal arteries originates, mainly, from each middle cerebral artery and passes over each developing cerebral hemisphere; caudally similar meningeal branches arising from the *vertebral* and *basilar arteries* embrace the cerebellum and brainstem (Van den Bergh & Vander Eecken 1968). The further development of the telencephalon (see p. 247) somewhat obscures this early pattern over the cerebrum.

The meningeal arteries so formed have been classified into three groups, *paramedian*, *short circumferential* and *long circumferenital arteries*. They can be described both supratentorially and infratentorially; all give off fine side branches and end as *penetrating arteries*. Of the supratentorial vessels, the paramedian arteries have a short course prior to penetrating the cerebral neuropil (e.g. branches of the *anterior cerebral artery*); the short circumferential arteries have a slightly longer course before becoming penetrating arteries (e.g. the *striate artery*); the long circumferential arteries reach the dorsal surface of the hemispheres. Infratentorial meningeal arteries are very variable. The paramedian arteries, after arising from the basilar or vertebral arteries, penetrate the brainstem directly; the short circumferential arteries end at the lateral surface of the brain before penetration; the long circumferential arteries later form the range of cerebellar arteries. Note that these vessels arranged as a series of loops over the brain arise from the circle of Willis and brainstem vessels on the base of the brain.

At 16 weeks gestation, the *anterior*, *middle* and *posterior cerebral arteries* contributing to the formation of the circle of Willis are well established. The meningeal arteries arising from them display a simple pattern with little tortuosity and very few branches. With the increasing age of the fetus and acquisition of the gyral pattern on the surface of the brain, their tortuosity, diameter and number of branches increase. This branching pattern is completed by 28 weeks gestation and the number of branches does not increase further (Takashimá & Tanaka 1978). Numerous anastomoses (varying in size from 200–760 µm) occur between the meningeal arteries in the depths of the developing sulci, nearly always in the *cortical boundary zones* of the three main cerebral arteries supplying each hemisphere. The number, diameter and location of these anastomoses changes as fetal growth progresses due to a regression of the complex embryonic cerebral vascular system (see below). The boundary zones between the cerebral arteries may be the sites of inadequate perfusion in the premature infant.

Vascularization of the brain

The brain becomes vascularized by angiogenesis (angiotrophic vasculogenesis; see p. 298) rather than by direct invasion by angioblasts. Blood vessels form by sprouting from vessels in the pial plexus, which surrounds the neural tube from an early stage (Noden & Li 1991). In the quail vascularization begins in the hindbrain on day 4 of incubation. Using antibodies against endothelial cells, endothelial sprouts were seen to penetrate the neuroepithelium on each side of the midline at inter-rhombomeric junctions (see p. 225; Noden & Li 1991). These sprouts form branches which elongate at the junction between the ventricular and marginal zones; the branches project laterally within the inter-rhombomeric boundaries and longitudinally adjacent to the median floorplate. Subsequently, additional sprouts penetrate the inter-rhombomeric regions on the walls and floor of the hindbrain. Branches from the latter elongate towards and join the branches in the inter-rhombomeric junctions, forming primary vascular channels between rhombomeres and longitudinally on each side of the median floorplate (Noden 1991). Later additional sprouts invade the hindbrain within the rhombomeres, anastomosing in all directions.

The meningeal perforating branches pass into the brain parenchyma as *cortical*, *medullary* and *striate branches* (**3**.182). The cortical vessels supply the cortex via short branches which may form precapillary anastomoses, whereas the medullary branches supply the white matter. The latter converge towards the ventricle but rarely reach it; they often follow a tortuous course as they pass around nervous fascicles. The striate branches which penetrate into the brain through the anterior perforated substance (p. 1191), supply the basal nuclei and internal capsule via a sinuous course; they are larger than the medullary branches and the longest of them reach close to the ventricle. The periventricular region and basal nuclei are also supplied by branches from the *tela choroidea*; this develops from the early pial plexus but becomes medially and deeply placed as the telencephalon enlarges.

The cortical and medullary branches irrigate a series of cortico–subcortical cone-shaped areas, centred around a sulcus containing an artery. They supply a peripheral portion of the cerebrum and are grouped as *ventriculopetal arteries*. Striate branches, on the other hand, arborize close to the ventricle supplying a more central portion of the cerebrum; they, with branches from the tela choroidea, give rise to *ventriculofugal arteries*. The latter supply the ventricular zone (germinal matrix of the brain) and send branches towards the cortex. The ventriculopetal and ventriculofugal arteries run towards each other but they do not make any connections or anastomoses (3.182). The ventriculopetal vessels supply relatively more mature regions of the brain compared to the ventriculofugal, which are subject to constant remodelling and do not develop tunicae mediae until ventricular zone proliferation is completed. The *boundary zone* between these two systems (an outer centripetal and inner centrifugal) has practical implications related to the location of ischaemic lesions (periventricular leucomalacia, PVL) in the white matter of premature infant brains. The distribution of ischaemic lesions coincides with the demarcation zone between the centrifugal and centripetal vascular arterial systems (Wigglesworth & Pape 1978; also see below).

The same pattern of centripetal and centrifugal arteries develops around the fourth ventricle (Van den Bergh & Vander Eecken 1968). The ventriculofugal circulation is more extensive in the cerebellum than in the telencephalon. The arteries arise from the various cerebellar arteries and course, with the cerebellar peduncles, directly to the centre of the cerebellum by-passing the cortex. The ventriculopetal arteries derive from the meningeal vessels over the cerebellar surface and most terminate in the white substance.

At 24 weeks of gestation, there is a relatively well developed blood supply to the basal nuclei and internal capsule, through a prominent *Heubner's artery* (arteria recurrens anterior, see p. 1528), a branch of the anterior cerebral artery. The cortex and the white matter regions are rather poorly vascularized at this stage. Injection studies have demonstrated the distribution of arteries and veins on the lateral aspect of the cerebral hemispheres and shown that it is naturally affected by the formation of the Sylvian (lateral cerebral) fissure and development of cerebral sulci and gyri (Okudera et al 1988). Between 12 and 20 weeks gestation the middle cerebral artery and its branches are relatively straight with branching in an open-fan pattern. At the end of 20 weeks, the arteries become more curved as the opercula begin to appear and submerge the insular cortex. The area supplied by the middle cerebral artery becomes predominant when compared to the territories supplied by the anterior and posterior cerebral arteries. Early arterial anastomoses appear around 16 weeks gestation and increase in size with advancing age. The sites of anastomoses between the middle and anterior cerebral arteries move from the convexity of the brain towards the superior sagittal sinus. Anastomotic connections between the middle and posterior cerebral arteries shift towards the basal aspect of the brain.

By 32–34 weeks, marked involution of the ventricular zone (germinal matrix) takes place and the cortex acquires its complex gyral pattern and, associated with it, an increased vascular supply. The ventricular zone capillaries are gradually remodelled to blend with the capillaries of the caudate nucleus. Heubner's artery eventually supplies only a small area at the medial aspect of the head of the caudate nucleus. In the cortex, there is progressive elaboration of the cortical blood vessels (3.182), and towards the end of the third trimester, the balance of cerebral circulation shifts from a central, basal-nuclei oriented circulation to a circulation predominant in the cortex and the white matter (3.182). These changes in the pattern of cerebral circulation are of major significance in pathogenesis and distribution of hypoxic/ischaemic lesions in the developing human brain. In a *premature brain*, the majority of ischaemic lesions occur in the boundary zone between the centripetal and centrifugal arteries, in the periventricular white matter. In the *full-term infant* the cortical boundary zones and watershed areas between different arterial blood supplies are similar to those in adults.

Vessels of the ventricular zone (germinal matrix). It has been suggested that the germinal matrix (the region of the developing brain termed ventricular zone by the Bolder Committee, see p. 252, but often referred to clinically, somewhat imprecisely, as the germinal matrix) is particularly prone to ischaemic injury in the immature infant because of its unusual vascular architecture. A micro-angiographic study of the structure of the vessels in the peri-ventricular matrix (Takashima & Tanaka 1978) established that the germinal matrix is the end zone or border zone between the *cerebral arteries* and the *collection zone* of the *deep cerebral veins*. The subependymal veins (*septal, choroidal, thalamostriate* and *posterior terminal*, see p. 1204) flow **towards** the interventricular foramen with a sudden change of flow at the level of the foramen, where the veins recurve at an acute angle to form the paired *internal cerebral veins*. The capillary channels in the germinal matrix open at right angles, directly into the veins (Hambleton & Wigglesworth 1976). It has been postulated that these small vessels may be points of vascular rupture and the site of subependymal haemorrhage.

The capillary bed in the ventricular zone is supplied mainly by Heubner's artery and terminal branches of the lateral striate arteries from the middle cerebral artery (Wigglesworth 1980). As the highly cellular structure of the ventricular zone is a temporary feature, the vascular supply to this area displays some primitive features and has the capacity to remodel when, towards the end of gestation, the ventricular zone cells migrate and the remaining cells differentiate as ependyme (Wigglesworth & Pape 1980).

Some studies have shown that vessel density is relatively low in the ventricular zone and that this area may normally have a relatively low blood flow (Pasternak et al 1982). Immature vessels, without a complex basal lamina or glial sheet, have been described up to 26 weeks gestation in the zone (Larroche 1982), and it has been reported that the endothelium of these vessels is thinner than in the cortical vessels (Trommer et al 1987). In infants of less than 30 weeks gestation, the vessels in the ventricular zone contain no smooth muscle, collagen or elastic fibres (Haruda & Blanc 1981). Collagen and smooth muscle were seen in other regions after 30 weeks but were not detected in the remains of the zone (germinal matrix). The lack of these components could make the vessels in the ventricular zone vulnerable to changes in the intraluminal pressure and the lack of smooth muscle would debar them from participating in autoregulatory processes.

Hegedus and Molnar (1985) have shown that cerebral vessels in premature infants lack elastic fibres and have a disproportionately small amount of reticulin fibres. An electron microscopic study of the cortical and germinal plate blood vessels showed that in infants of between 25 and 32 weeks gestation the germinal matrix vessels consisted commonly of 1–2 endothelial cells with an occasional pericyte, and the capillary lumina were larger than those of the vessels in the cortex. In more mature infants the basal lamina was thicker and more irregular when compared to cortical vessels (Grunnet 1989).

Glial fibrillary acidic protein (GFAP) positive cells have been detected around blood vessels in the germinal matrix from 23 weeks gestation (Gould & Howard 1988). Glial cells may contribute to changes in the nature of endothelial intercellular junctions in brain capillaries (Tae-Cheng et al 1986).

Dorsal aortae

These persist on the cranial side of the third aortic arches as continuations of the internal carotid arteries (3.88A–C). The dorsal aorta between the third and fourth aortic arches, the *ductus caroticus*, diminishes and finally disappears; but from fourth arch to the origin of the seventh intersegmental artery the right dorsal aorta becomes part of the right subclavian artery (3.177). Caudal to the seventh intersegmental artery the right dorsal aorta disappears as far as the locus of fusion of thoracic aortae. After disappearance of the left ductus caroticus, the remainder persists to form the descending part of the arch of the aorta. Thence the fused right and left embryonic dorsal aortae persist as the definitive descending thoracic and abdominal aorta. A constriction, the *aortic isthmus*, is sometimes

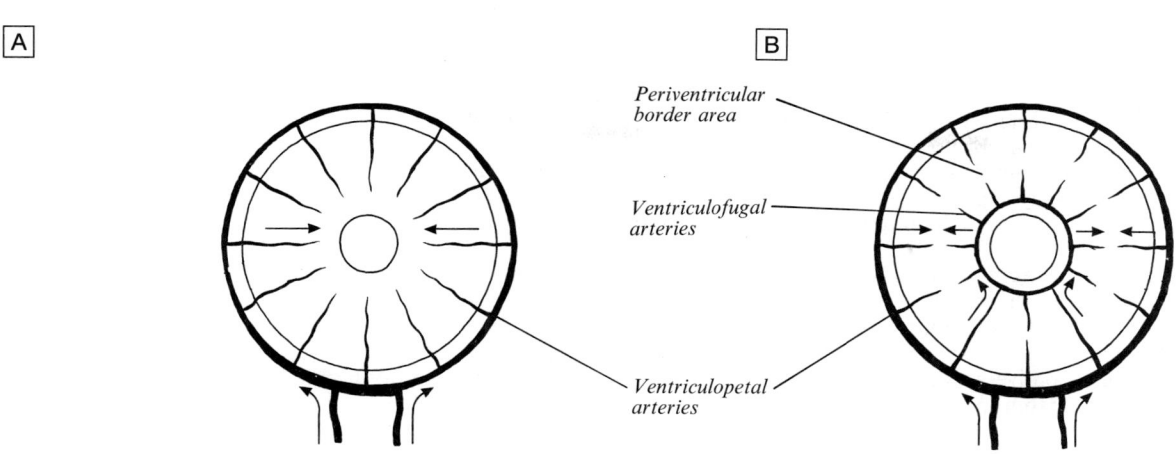

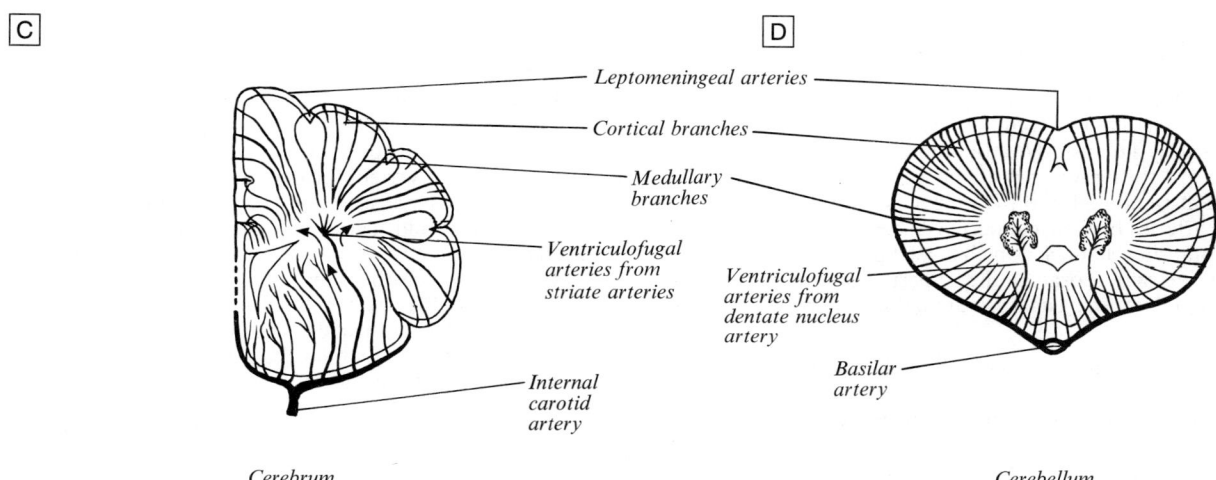

Cerebrum

Cerebellum

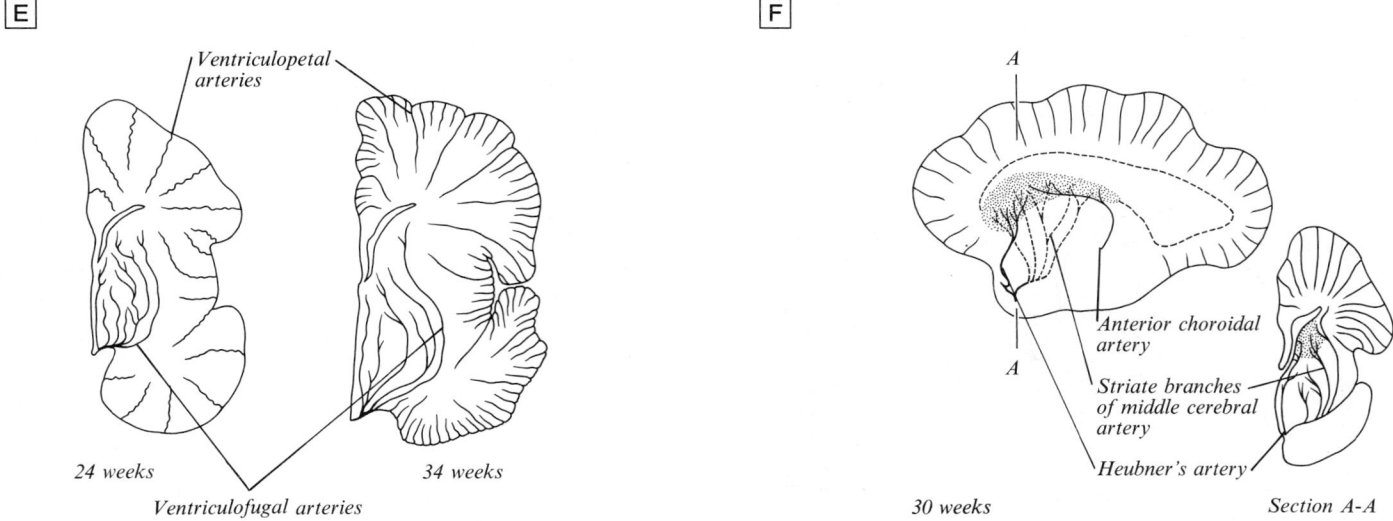

24 weeks

34 weeks

Ventriculofugal arteries

30 weeks

Section A-A

3.182 Schema of development of cerebral blood vessels. A. The brain is surrounded by a system of leptomeningeal arteries from afferent trunks at the base of the brain. Intracerebral arteries arise from this system and converge (ventriculopetally) towards the ventricle (the inner circle in this diagram). B. A few deep penetrating vessels supply the brain close to the ventricle and send ventriculofugal arteries towards the ventriculopetal vessels, without making anastomoses. Between these two systems there is a periventricular border area. C. The arrangement of ventriculopetal and ventriculofugal vessels around a cerebral hemisphere. D. The similar arrangement of vessels around the cerebellum. E. Changes in the arterial pattern of the human cerebrum between 24 and 34 weeks. F. Arterial supply to the basal ganglia at 30 weeks gestation. (For A–D see van den Berg & Eecken 1968; E and F from Hambleton & Wigglesworth 1976 with permission of the BMJ Publishing Group.)

317

present in the aorta between the final site of origin of the left subclavian artery and reception of the ductus arteriosus (see *coarctation* of the aorta, p. 1510).

In the adult, the right subclavian artery occasionally arises from the arch of the aorta distal to the origin of the left subclavian and then passes upwards and to the right behind the trachea and oesophagus. This condition is possibly explained by the persistence of the embryonic right dorsal aorta and the obliteration of the fourth aortic arch of the right side.

In birds the right fourth aortic arch is transformed into the definitive arch of the aorta; in reptiles the fourth arches of both sides persist and give rise to their characteristic double aortic arch. In both these classes, development of the heart and aortic arches is probably along phylogenetic lines so divergent from the mammalian pattern that comparisons may be inappropriate.

The heart originally lies ventral to the pharynx, immediately caudal to the stomodeum (**3.179**A); with the elongation of the neck and the development of the lungs it recedes within the thorax and, correspondingly, the vessels are drawn out and the original position of the fourth and sixth aortic arches is greatly modified. Thus, on the right the fourth aortic arch only recedes to the thoracic inlet, while on the left side it descends **into** the thorax. The recurrent laryngeal nerves (in contrast to the other arch nerves) originally pass to the larynx **caudal** to the sixth pair of aortic arches, and are therefore affected by the descent of these structures; thus in the adult the left nerve hooks round the ligamentum arteriosum **within** the thorax; on the right owing to the disappearance of the fifth and the dorsal part of the sixth aortic arch, the right recurrent laryngeal nerve hooks round the fourth aortic arch, i.e. the commencement of the right subclavian artery (i.e. just **above** the thoracic inlet).

At first the aortae are the only longitudinal vessels present, for their branches all run at right angles to the long axis of the embryo. later these transverse arteries become connected in certain situations by longitudinal anastomosing channels, which in part persist, forming such arteries as the internal thoracic, the superior and inferior epigastric, the gastro-epiploic, etc. Each primitive dorsal aorta gives off:

- ventral splanchnic arteries, paired segmental branches to the digestive tube
- lateral splanchnic arteries, paired segmental branches to the mesonephric ridge
- somatic arteries, intersegmental branches to the body wall.

Ventral splanchnic arteries. Originally paired vessels, these are distributed to the capillary plexus in the wall of the yolk sac. After fusion of the dorsal aortae they merge as unpaired trunks distributed to the increasingly defined and lengthening primitive digestive tube. Longitudinal anastomotic channels connect these branches along the dorsal and ventral aspects of the tube, forming dorsal and ventral splanchnic anastomoses (**3.183**; Ennabli & Niveiro 1967). These vessels obviate the need for so many 'subdiaphragmatic' ventral splanchnic arteries, and these are reduced to three: the coeliac trunk

and superior and inferior mesenteric arteries. As the viscera supplied descend into the abdomen their origins migrate caudally by differential growth; thus the origin of the coeliac artery is transferred from the level of the seventh cervical segment to the level of the twelfth thoracic, the superior mesenteric from the second thoracic to the first lumbar and the inferior mesenteric from the twelfth thoracic to the third lumbar. (Above the diaphragm, however, a variable number of ventral splanchnic arteries persist, usually four or five, supplying the thoracic oesophagus.) The dorsal splanchnic anastomosis persists in the gastro-epiploic, pancreaticoduodenal and the primary branches of the colic arteries, while the ventral splanchnic anastomosis forms the right and left gastric and the hepatic arteries. These arterial rearrangements have been investigated recently by angiography and explanatory haemodynamic hypotheses have been advanced (Barth et al 1976).

Lateral splanchnic arteries. These supply, on each side, the mesonephros, metanephros, the testis or ovary, and the suprarenal gland; all these structures develop, in whole or in part, from the intermediate mesenchyme of the mesonephric ridge (p. 200). One testicular or ovarian artery and three suprarenal arteries persist on each side. The phrenic artery branches from the most cranial suprarenal artery, and the renal artery arises from the most caudal. Additional renal arteries are frequently present and may be looked on as branches of persistent lateral splanchnic arteries.

Somatic arteries. *Intersegmental* in position, they persist, almost unchanged, in the thoracic and lumbar regions, as the posterior intercostal, subcostal and lumbar arteries. Each gives off a dorsal ramus which passes backwards in the intersegmental interval and divides into medial and lateral branches to supply the muscles and superficial tissues of the back (**3.183**). It also gives off a spinal branch, which enters the vertebral canal and divides into a series of branches to the tissues constituting the walls and joints of the osteoligamentous canal and neural branches to the spinal cord and spinal nerve roots (Somogyi et al 1973; Undi et al 1973). Having produced its dorsal branch the intersegmental artery runs ventrally in the body wall, gives off a lateral branch and terminates in muscular and cutaneous rami. Before their division, the stems of the somatic arteries, at thoracic and lumbar levels, provide small rami which enter the developing vertebral bodies.

Numerous longitudinal anastomoses link up the intersegmental arteries and their branches (**3.183**). On both sides a *postcostal anastomosis* connects their dorsal branches in the intervals between the necks of ribs and the vertebral transverse processes. This persists in the cervical region where it forms the greater part of the vertebral artery. A *post-transverse anastomosis* also connects the dorsal branches and forms the greater part of the deep cervical artery. A *precostal anastomosis* connects intersegmental arteries beyond the origins of their dorsal branches. The ascending cervical and the superior intercostal arteries are persistent parts of this vessel. Lastly, near the anterior median line intersegmental arteries are linked by a *ventral somatic anastomosis*. Most of these vessels persist bilaterally as the internal thoracic, the superior and inferior epigastric arteries.

Umbilical arteries at first are the direct caudal continuation of the primitive dorsal aortae and are present in the body stalk before any vitelline (yolk sac) or visceral branches emerge, indicating the dominance of the allantoic over the vitelline circulation in the human embryo. (On a comparative basis the umbilical vessels are chorio-allantoic and therefore 'somatovisceral'.) After the fusion of the dorsal aortae the umbilical arteries arise from their ventrolateral aspects and pass medial to the primary excretory duct (Wolffian) to the umbilicus. Later the proximal part of each umbilical artery is joined by a new vessel which leaves the aorta at its termination and passes lateral to the primary excretory duct. This, possibly the fifth lumbar intersegmental artery, constitutes the *dorsal root* of the umbilical artery (the original stem, the *ventral root*). The dorsal root gives off the axial artery of the lower limb, branches to the pelvic viscera and, more proximally, the external iliac artery. The ventral root disappears entirely, the umbilical artery now arising from that part of its dorsal root distal to the external iliac artery, i.e. the internal iliac artery.

Arteries of the limbs

The early limb bud receives blood via intersegmental arteries which contribute to a primitive capillary plexus. At the tip of the limb bud

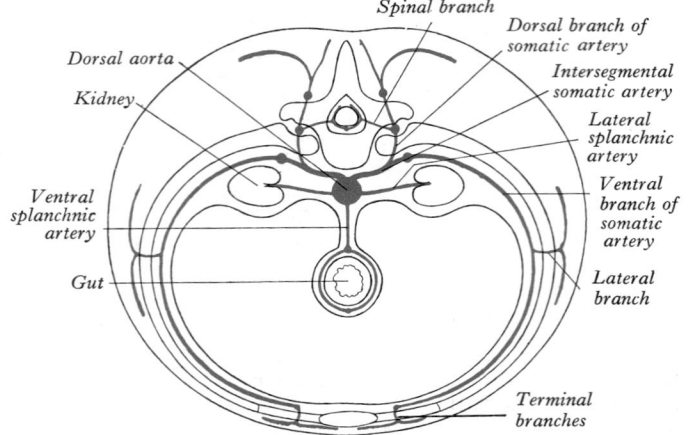

3.183 Diagram of the segmental and intersegmental arteries. Note the positions of the longitudinal anastomoses.

there is a *terminal plexus* that is constantly renewed in a distal direction as the limb grows. Later one main vessel supplies the limb and the terminal plexus; it is termed the *axial artery*. The terminal plexus is separated from the outer ectodermal sleeve of the limb by an *avascular zone* of mesenchyme. Experiments in which portions of ectoderm are implanted into a part of the limb that would otherwise be vascularized result in an avascular zone forming around the ectoderm. The avascular region contains an extracellular matrix consisting largely of hyaluronic acid. Removal of this hyaluronic acid by hyaluronidase results in vascularization of the tissue since partial degradation products of hyaluronic acid are angiogenic (Feinberg 1991). Thus ectodermal/mesenchymal interactions and extracellular matrix components are controlling the initial patterning of blood vessels within the limb. During these early stages of limb development the proximodistal regions of the limb are patterned by the *progress zone* beneath the *apical ectodermal ridge* (see p. 288), later after the main elements of the limb have developed the ectoderm and underlying mesenchyme interact to produce the epidermis and dermis (see p. 294). It may be that the early presence of the avascular zone ensures little interaction of these tissues until a later stage of development, thus preventing premature skin development.

The development of the vasculature in the limb precedes the morphological and molecular changes that occur within the limb mesenchyme. The differentiation of cartilage within the limb occurs only after local vascular regression begins, and only in areas with few or no capillaries. Regions of mesenchyme free of capillaries and at high cell density are the sites of chondrogenesis (see p. 291). Whether the presence, or lack, of blood vessels, by varying the supply of nutrients to the tissue can confer different local environmental stimuli for mesenchymal cells, thus resulting in heterogeneous differentiation of the tissue of the limb, or whether, on the other hand, the local environment is controlled by the diversity of the endothelial cells is not known. Similarly, it is not clear whether

inductive factors from the limb mesenchyme cause the changes in the blood vessel pattern.

In the *upper limb bud*, usually only one trunk, the subclavian, persists and it probably represents the lateral branch of the *seventh intersegmental artery*. Its main continuation (*axis artery*) to the upper limb (**3.**184), later the *axillary* and *brachial arteries*, passes into the forearm deep to the flexor muscle mass and terminates as a deep plexus in the developing hand. This vessel ultimately persists as the *anterior interosseous artery* and the *deep palmar arch*. A branch from the main trunk passes dorsally between the early radius and ulna as the *posterior interosseous artery*, while a second accompanies the median nerve into the hand, where it ends in a *superficial capillary plexus*. The *radial* and *ulnar arteries* are the latest arteries to appear in the forearm; at first the radial artery arises more proximally than the ulnar and crosses in front of the median nerve, supplying the biceps. Later, the radial artery establishes a new connection with the main trunk at or near the level of origin of the ulnar artery and the upper portion of its original stem usually disappears to a large extent (see also p. 1540). On reaching the hand the ulnar artery becomes linked up with the superficial palmar plexus, from which the *superficial palmar arch* is derived, while the median artery commonly loses its distal connections and is reduced to a small vessel. The radial artery passes to the dorsal surface of the hand but, after giving off dorsal digital branches, it traverses the first intermetacarpal space and joins the deep palmar arch.

Because of their multiple and plexiform sources, the temporal succession of emergence of principal arteries, anastomoses and peri-articular networks and functional dominance followed by regression of some paths, anomalies of the forelimb arterial tree are fairly common. In the main, such anomalous patterns present as: divergences in the mode and proximodistal level of branching; the presence of unusual compound arterial segments; aberrant vessels connecting other principal vessels, arcades or plexuses; and vessels occupying

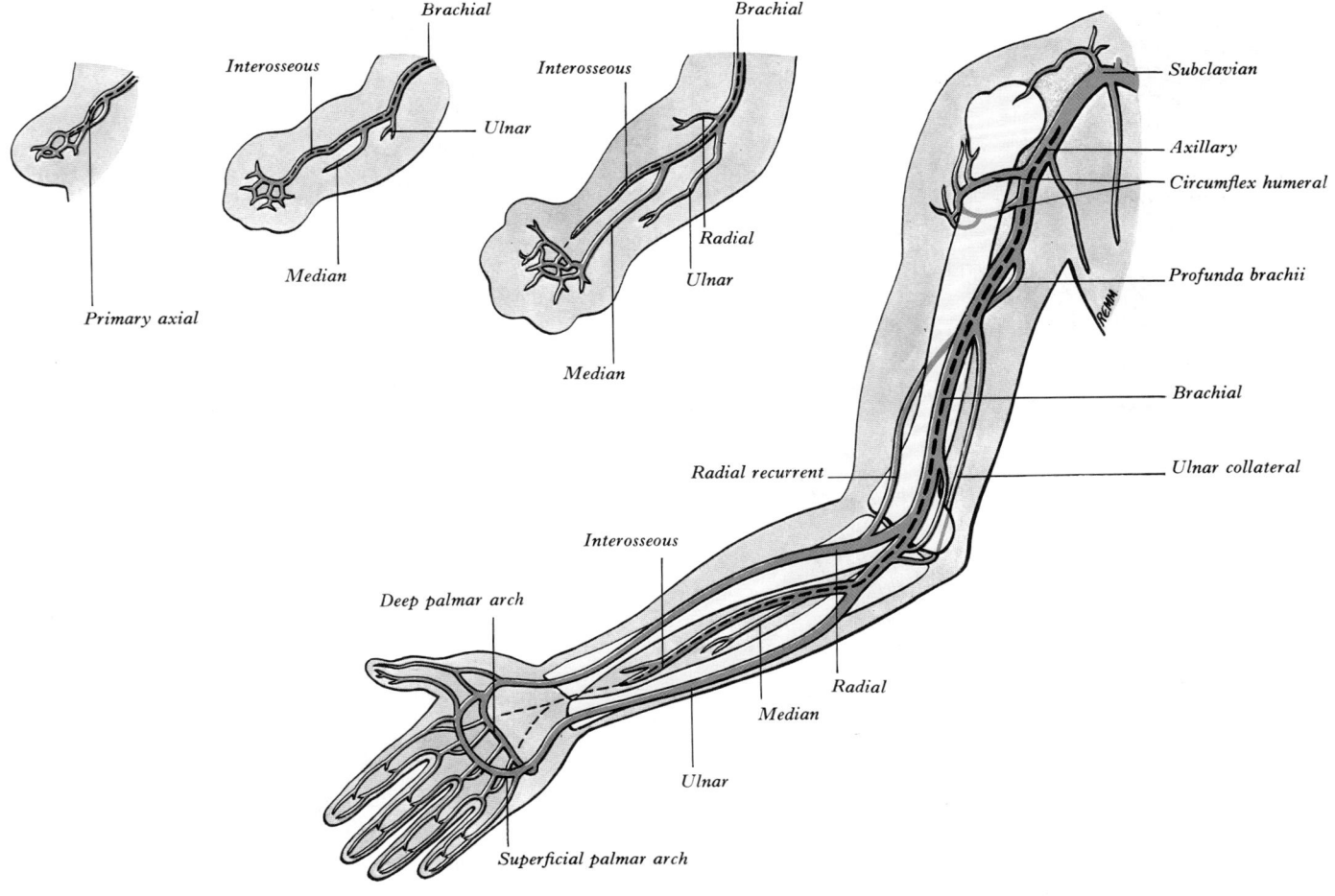

3.184   Stages in the development of the arteries of the arm. The original path of the axis artery is indicated by an interrupted line. (After Patten.)

exceptional tissue planes (e.g. superficial fascia instead of the usual subfascial route) or having unexpected neural, myological or osteo-ligamentous relationships. For example, see variations on pages 1539, 1541, 1543.

The *axial artery of the lower limb* (3.185) arises from the dorsal root of the umbilical artery, and courses along the **dorsal** surface of the thigh, knee and leg; below the knee it lies between tibia and popliteus and in the leg between the crural interosseous membrane and tibialis posterior. Ending distally in a *plantar network*, it gives off a perforating artery traversing the sinus tarsi to form a *dorsal network*. The *femoral artery* passes along the **ventral** surface of the thigh, opening a new channel to the lower limb. It arises from a capillary plexus, connected proximally with the femoral branches of the external iliac artery and distally with the axis artery. At the proximal margin of the popliteus the axis artery provides a *primitive posterior tibial* and a *primitive peroneal branch*, which run distally on the dorsal surface of that muscle and on tibialis posterior to gain the sole of the foot. At the distal border of popliteus the axis artery gives off a *perforating branch*, which passes ventrally between the tibia and the fibula and then courses to the dorsum of the foot,

forming the *anterior tibial artery* and *arteria dorsalis pedis*. The primitive peroneal artery communicates with the axis artery at the distal border of the popliteus and in its course in the leg (Senior 1919, 1920).

The femoral artery gradually increases in size and coincidentally most of the axis artery disappears; proximal to its communication with the femoral the root of the axis artery, however, persists as the *inferior gluteal artery* and the *arteria comitans nervi ischiadici*.

The proximal parts of the primitive posterior tibial and peroneal arteries fuse, but distally remain separate. Ultimately much of the primitive peroneal artery disappears, although a part of the axis artery is incorporated in the permanent peroneal artery. As in the forelimb (above) the same considerations apply to anomalies and variations.

DEVELOPMENT OF THE VEINS

Often, for convenience and apparent simplicity, the early embryonic veins are segregated into two groups, *visceral* and *somatic*. The visceral group comprises the derivatives of the vitelline and umbilical

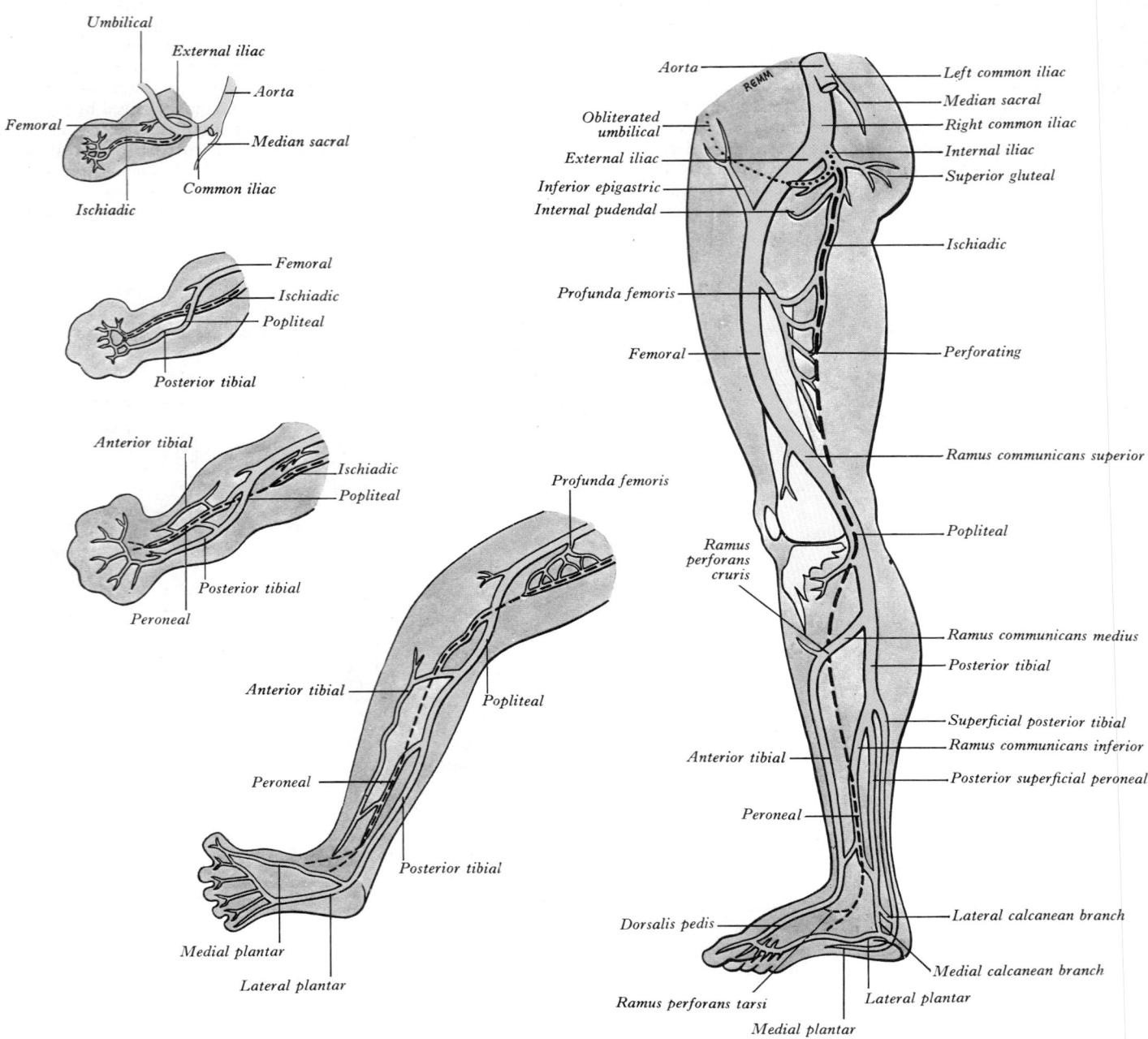

3.185 Stages in the development of the arteries of the leg. The original path of the axis artery is indicated by a dashed line. (After Senior.)

veins; the somatic group includes all remaining veins. Such a classification is a potentially misleading oversimplification, based on inadequate criteria. Many embryonic veins, with time, change the principal tissues they drain; others have some radicles from patently parietal tissues that become confluent with drainage channels that are clearly visceral, thus forming a compound vessel; finally some veins differentiate from contrasting mesenchymal layers at different points along their course (each having its distinct phylogenetic history).

Less confusion attaches to the recognition of three main groups of veins—the *vitelline, umbilical* and *cardinal* vein complexes; nevertheless, even here, some imprecision persists where, for instance, anastomoses or convergence of radicles from different groups occurs, where ontogenetically compound tissues are drained or when distinct developmental layers are traversed. The early embryonic veins develop initially with a symmetric bilateral array of channels; the **principal** events correlated with changes in this are the craniocaudal and mediolateral gradients in growth and differentiation of the nervous system, skeleton and musculature; diversion of cardiac venous return to the right with concomitant cardiac asymmetry; 'descent' of the heart and lungs; gut rotation and repositioning; and venous involvement by the developing liver, pancreas, spleen and mesonephric ridges. (Clearly, the temporospatial development sequences of **all** vascularized tissues are involved to varying, but less obvious, extents.) As noted, the primitive tubular symmetric heart receives its venous return through the right and left sinual horns (horns of the sinus venous). The horns are initially embedded in the mesenchyme of the septum transversum and each receives, most medially, the termination of the principal vitelline vein (but see below), more laterally, the umbilical vein and, most laterally, having encircled the pleuroperitoneal canal, the common cardinal vein. These cardiac inputs correspond, in large measure but not exclusively, with the groups of veins mentioned above.

Vitelline veins

The vitelline veins drain capillary plexuses developed in the splanchnopleuric mesenchyme of the secondary yolk sac. With head, tail and lateral fold formation, the upper recesses of the yolk sac are enclosed within the embryo as the splanchnopleuric gut tube extending from the stomodeal buccopharyngeal membrane to the proctodeal cloacal membrane. It may be emphasized that derivatives from **all** these levels possess a venous drainage, originally **vitelline in origin**, although many accounts are limited to the (mainly subdiaphragmatic–sacral) regions drained via the hepatic portal vein. The deep aspects of the maxillomandibular facial prominences, retrogingival oral cavity, the pharyngeal walls and their lymphoid and endocrine derivatives and the cervicothoracic oesphagus, all have drainage channels that connect with the *precardinal complex*, ultimately returning blood to the heart via the superior vena cava. Laryngeal and tracheobronchial veins also drain to the precardinal complex, whilst the capillary plexuses developed in the (splanchnopleuric) walls of the fine terminal respiratory passages and alveoli, converge on *pulmonary veins* of increasing calibre, finally making secondary connections with the left atrium of the heart and may be grouped with the vitelline systems. Even the heart, itself, first differentiates in splanchnopleure that, after head fold formation, forms the dorsal wall of the primitive pericardial cavity (floor of the rostral foregut) and may therefore be considered a highly specialized vitelline vascular derivative. Similarly at the caudal extremity of the splanchnopleuric gut tube (the future lower rectum and upper anal canal; p. 191) the vitelline venous drainage makes connections with the internal iliac radicles of the *postcardinal complex*.

The increasingly extensive remainder of the gut tube, from the gastric terminal segment of the future oesophagus to the upper rectum, is, as elsewhere, clothed with splanchnopleuric mesenchyme permeated by a capillary plexus; the latter drains into an anastomosing network of veins. The net is denser ventrally and in the central midgut region; for a while, it receives a leash of small veins from the definitive yolk sac that enter the embryo through the umbilicus, embedded in the yolk stalk. Later, in normal development, both stalk and vessels atrophy. Within the splanchnopleuric net, progressing rostrally, longitudinal channels anterolateral to the gut become increasingly well defined—the embryonic abdominal *vitelline veins*. Entering the septum transversum, the right and left vitelline

veins incline slightly, becoming parallel to the lateral aspects of the gut; they establish connections with capillary plexuses in the septal mesenchyme, then continue, finally curving to enter the medial part of the cardiac sinual horn of their corresponding side. The parts of the gut closely related to the presinual segments of the vitelline veins, just described, are the future subdiaphragmatic end of the oesophagus, primitive stomach, the superior (first) and descending (second) regions of the duodenum, and the remainder of the duodenal tube. The early septum transversum is a thick mass of mesenchyme filling the interval between the median foregut and ventral body wall, and extending from the primitive pericardium to the rostral lip of the umbilicus; in it somatopleuric and splanchnopleuric mesenchymes are confluent. When, later, the cardiac sinuatrium rises into the pericardium, the rostral part of the septum (*pars diaphragmatica*) is one of the multiple contributors to the framework of the definitive diaphragm; its caudal *pars mesenterica* provides ventral mesenteries, serous coats and mural tissues for the abdominal foregut, listed above. Where foregut continues into midgut (initially the rostral rim of the yolk stalk) the hepatic (and, transiently, ventral pancreatic) rudiments form as protrusions of the gut; the rapid and asymmetric invasion of the septum cranioventrally is correlated with profound modifications of the transeptal parts of the vitelline and umbilical veins, and the splanchnopleuric mesothelium, framework and mesenteries of the liver, stomach and duodenum (pp. 192–198). The stem of the earliest hepatic rudiment projects from the ventral wall of the future second (descending) part of the duodenum; whilst expansion of the body of the liver continues as indicated, with gut rotation and differential growth, the ultimate derivative of the stem, the common bile duct, curves posterior to the proximal duodenum to reach its termination through the left posteromedial aspect of the second part of the duodenum.

The principal ascending vitelline veins flanking the sides of the abdominal part of the foregut receive venules from its splanchnopleuric capillaries, and those of the septal mesenchyme. Within these venular nets, enlarged (but still plexiform) anastomoses connect the two vitelline veins. (For clarity these are represented diagrammatically as simple transverse channels, **3**.186.) A *subdiaphragmatic intervitelline anastomosis* develops in the rostral septal mesenchyme, lying a little caudal to the cardiac sinuatrial chamber, connecting the veins near their sinual terminations. (Sometimes termed *suprahepatic* because of the position of the hepatic primordium; with expansion of the latter the channel becomes partly *intrahepatic*.) The presumptive duodenum is crossed by three transverse *duodenal intervitelline anastomoses*; their relation to the gut tube alternates: the most cranial, the *subhepatic*, is ventral, the *intermediate* is dorsal and the *caudal* is ventral. It has become customary to describe the paraduodenal vitelline veins and their associated anastomoses as forming a figure 8. At this early stage when left and right embryonic veins are still symmetric, the cranial duodenal anastomosis becomes connected with the subdiaphragmatic anastomosis by a *median* longitudinal channel, the *primitive ductus venosus*, which is dorsal to the expanding hepatic primordium, but ventral to the gut. The further development of the vitelline veins and anastomoses is, as indicated, closely interlocked with rapid hepatic expansion and gut changes; also umbilical vein disposition and modification is closely involved, and their early emergence and arrangement must be outlined before an account of later asymmetries is undertaken. The latter differs in part from long held descriptions, following the detailed analyses of goat and human embryos by Dickson (1957).

Umbilical veins

The umbilical veins form by the convergence of venules draining the splanchnopleure of the extraembryonic allantois. Throughout *Amniota* the allantois arises as a diverticulum from the caudal yolk sac wall (later, the ventrorostral wall of the cloacal part of the hindgut, or future bladder). Its degree of vesicular, then sometimes saccular, expansion is extremely variable; on occasion it virtually fills the extraembryonic coelom; the human endodermal allantois is diminutive, projecting merely into the embryonic end of the connecting stalk. The latter is regarded by many as precociously formed allantoic mesenchyme, and the umbilical vessels as *allantoic* (with close affinities, because of their common phylogenetic history, with the vitelline vessels). In the human embryo the peripheral venules

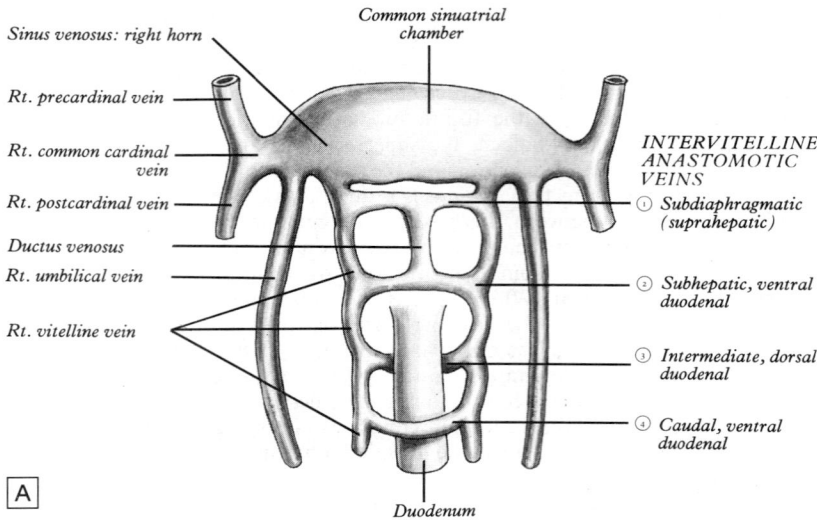

Sinus venosus: right horn

Common sinuatrial chamber

Rt. precardinal vein

Rt. common cardinal vein

Rt. postcardinal vein

Ductus venosus

Rt. umbilical vein

Rt. vitelline vein

INTERVITELLINE ANASTOMOTIC VEINS

① *Subdiaphragmatic (suprahepatic)*

② *Subhepatic, ventral duodenal*

③ *Intermediate, dorsal duodenal*

④ *Caudal, ventral duodenal*

A

Duodenum

B

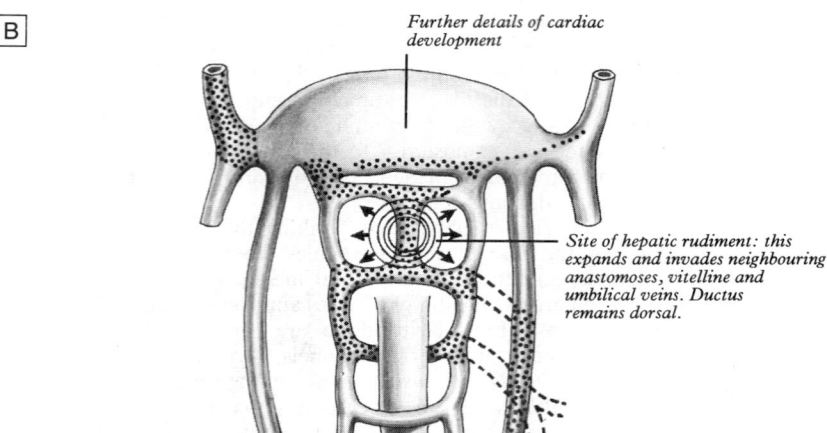

Further details of cardiac development

Site of hepatic rudiment: this expands and invades neighbouring anastomoses, vitelline and umbilical veins. Ductus remains dorsal.

Parts that persist, expand and modify into many main permanent channels (but see below)

New connexions forming further main permanent channels

Channels that either retrogress completely, form fibrous cords or vessels of fine calibre. Note: postnatally both the ductus venosus, and the left umbilical vein form substantial fibrous cords.

C

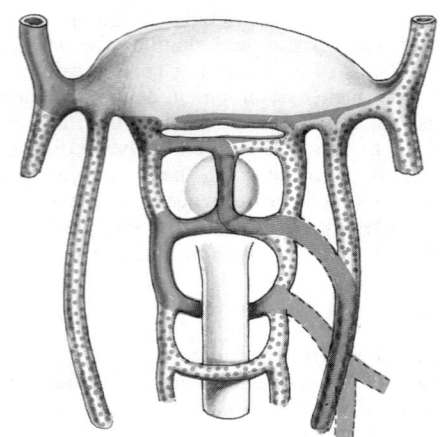

3.186 Development of the vitelline, umbilical and terminal cardinal vein complexes: the early symmetric condition. A. The topography and nomenclature of the veins forming the right and left sinual horns, the intervitelline anastomoses and the median ductus venosus. B. To assist understanding of later changes the symmetric pattern is used to indicate which segments persist or retrogress, the sites of formation of new channels and the intimately involved hepatic rudiment. C. A simplified representation of the subsequent main flow paths of oxygenated and deoxygenated blood.

drain the mesenchymal cores of the chorionic villous stems and terminal villi (extraembryonic *somatopleuric* structures); these are the radicles of a, usually single, *vena umbilicales impar* which traverses the compacting mixed mesenchyme of the umbilical cord to reach the caudal rim of the umbilicus. Here, the single cordal vein divides into primitive right and left umbilical veins; each curves rostrally in the somatopleuric lateral border of the umbilicus (i.e. where intraembryonic and extraembryonic or amniotic somatopleure are continuous), where it lies **lateral** to the communication between both the intraembryonic and extraembryonic coeloms. Rostrolateral to the umbilicus the two umbilical veins reach, enter and traverse the junctional mesenchyme of the septum transversum, connect with septal capillary plexuses, then continue, to enter their corresponding cardiac sinual horns (lateral to the terminations of the vitelline veins). This early symmetric disposition of the vitelline veins and anastomoses, umbilical and common cardinal veins and locus of the hepatic primordial complex is summarized in **3**.186.

Changes in the vitello-umbilical veins

Progressive changes in the vitello-umbilical veins are rapid, profound and closely linked with regional modifications of shape and position of the gut, expansion and invasion of venous channels by hepatic tissue, asymmetry of the heart and cardiac venous return. The principal events are summarized in **3**.186–188 and only brief textual allusions can be included here (see Dickson 1957 for details and bibliography).

From the pars hepatica of the ventral hepatopancreatic rudiment (p. 187) interconnected sheets and 'cords' of endodermal cells, the presumptive hepatocytes, penetrate the mesenchyme-filled spaces of the pre-existing septal capillary plexuses. Possibly, under the influence of the endodermal sheets, the plexuses become more profuse by the addition of angioblastic septal mesenchyme, which also forms masses of perivascular intrahepatic haemopoietic tissue. These processes extend along the plexiform connections of the vitelline, and later the umbilical veins until their intrahepatic (transeptal) zones themselves become largely plexiform—initially capillary in nature, but transforming into a mass of rather wider, irregular, sinusoidal vessels with a discontinuous endothelium containing many phagocytic cells (pp. 1802–1806). The lengths of vitelline veins involved in these processes are the intermediate parts of the segments extending from the subhepatic (cranioventral duodenal) to the suprahepatic (subdiaphragmatic) transverse intervitelline anastomoses and the corresponding lengths of the umbilical veins. Thus at this early stage the liver sinusoids are perfused by mixed blood reaching them through a series of branching vessels collectively called the *venae advehentes*, or *venae afferentes hepatis*; they are deoxygenated from the gut splanchnopleure via vitelline vein hepatic terminals and oxygenated from the placenta via hepatic terminals of the umbilical veins. Blood leaves the liver through four *venae revehentes* (*venae efferentes hepatis*): two on each side reach and open into their respective cardiac sinual horns. This full complement of four *hepatocardiac veins* is only transient, becoming reduced to one dominant, rapidly enlarging channel. As detailed below, the originally bilaterally symmetric cardinal vein complexes, both rostral and caudal, develop transverse or oblique anastomoses whereby the cardiac venous return is restricted to the definitive right atrium. (The pulmonary veins are the only major ones returning to the left atrium.) The increasingly deep inflexion of the left wall of the common sinuatrial chamber, separation of the left sinual horn and 'body' of the sinus venosus, movement to the right of the sinuatrial orifice, and right atrial inclusion of the right sinual horn have been noted (p. 293).

These cardiac and concomitant hepato-enteric changes are accompanied by events in supra-, intra- and subhepatic parts of the vitello-umbilical veins. Some vessels enlarge, persisting as definitive vessels to maturity and, in places, are joined later by other channels becoming defined in already established capillary plexuses. Other vessels retrogress, either disappearing completely or remaining as vestigial tags and occasionally vessels of fine calibre. Finally, some vessels of crucial importance in the circulatory patterns of embryonic and fetal life become obliterated **postnatally** and transformed to substantial fibrous cords. Both right and left umbilical hepatocardiac and the left vitelline hepatocardiac veins continue, for a time, to discharge blood into their sinual horns; however they begin to retrogress (**3**.186, 187). The right umbilical channel atrophies com-

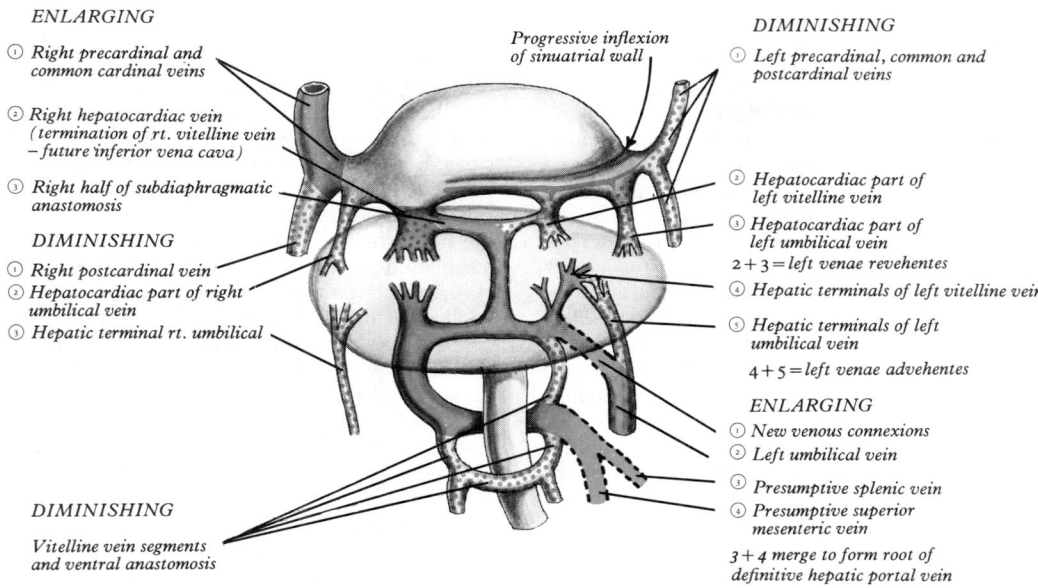

ENLARGING

① *Right precardinal and common cardinal veins*

② *Right hepatocardiac vein (termination of rt. vitelline vein – future inferior vena cava)*

③ *Right half of subdiaphragmatic anastomosis*

DIMINISHING

① *Right postcardinal vein*
② *Hepatocardiac part of right umbilical vein*
③ *Hepatic terminal rt. umbilical*

DIMINISHING

Vitelline vein segments and ventral anastomosis

Progressive inflexion of sinuatrial wall

DIMINISHING

① *Left precardinal, common and postcardinal veins*

② *Hepatocardiac part of left vitelline vein*
③ *Hepatocardiac part of left umbilical vein*
    2 + 3 = left venae revehentes
④ *Hepatic terminals of left vitelline vein*
⑤ *Hepatic terminals of left umbilical vein*
    4 + 5 = left venae advehentes

ENLARGING

① *New venous connexions*
② *Left umbilical vein*
③ *Presumptive splenic vein*
④ *Presumptive superior mesenteric vein*
    3 + 4 merge to form root of definitive hepatic portal vein

3.187   Development of the vitelline, umbilical and terminal cardinal vein complexes: a mid-stage of asymmetry has been reached between the early symmetric condition (**3**.186) and the definitive late prenatal state. Note the definition of the coronary sinus and the central role of the liver; compare homologous left- and right-sided vessels.

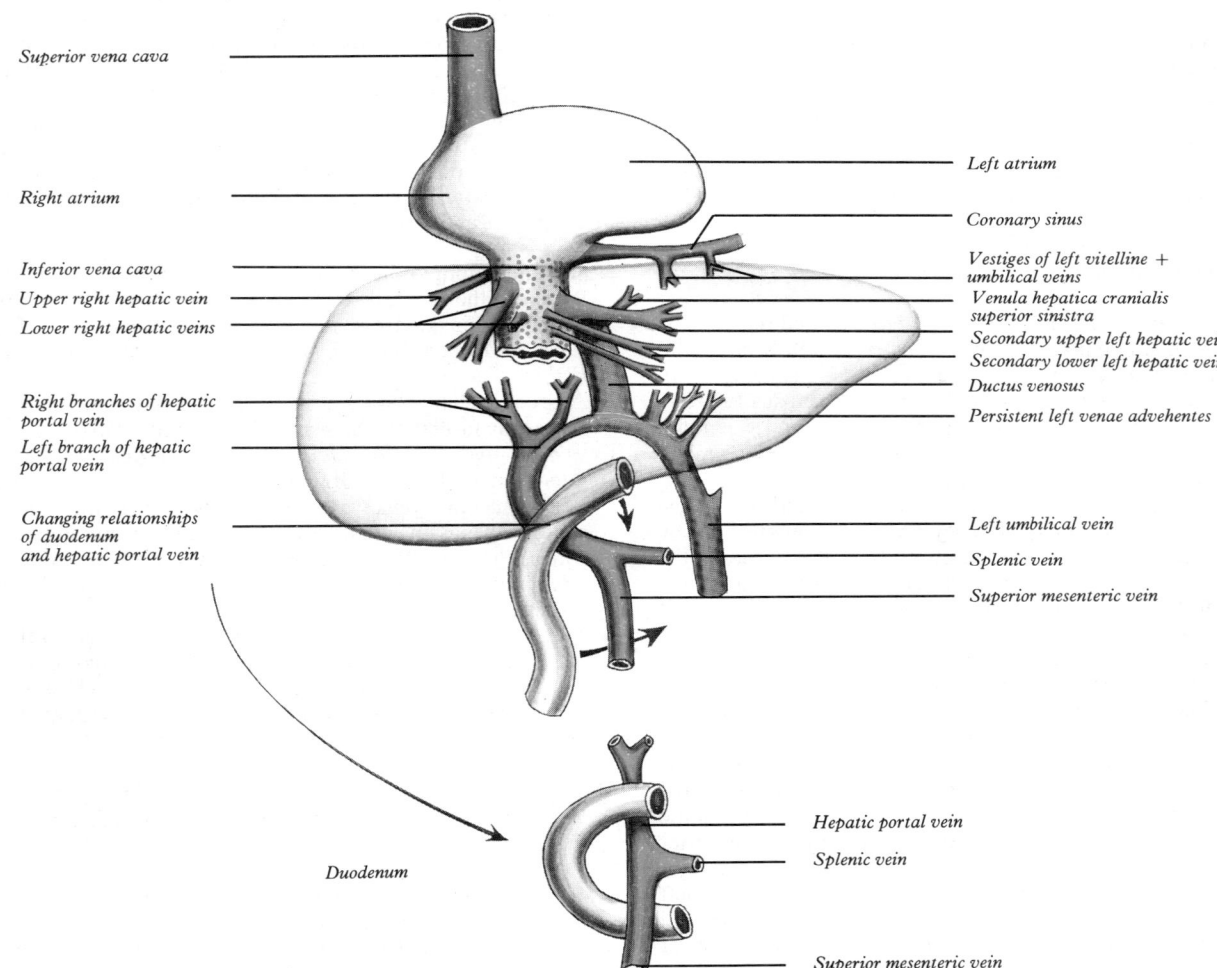

Superior vena cava

Right atrium

Inferior vena cava
Upper right hepatic vein
Lower right hepatic veins

Right branches of hepatic portal vein

Left branch of hepatic portal vein

Changing relationships of duodenum and hepatic portal vein

Duodenum

Left atrium

Coronary sinus

Vestiges of left vitelline + umbilical veins
Venula hepatica cranialis superior sinistra
Secondary upper left hepatic vein
Secondary lower left hepatic veins
Ductus venosus
Persistent left venae advehentes

Left umbilical vein
Splenic vein
Superior mesenteric vein

Hepatic portal vein
Splenic vein

Superior mesenteric vein

3.188   The condition of some main upper abdominal and intrathoracic right atrial terminal veins in the later prenatal months. Note the coronary sinus and attached vestiges, the terminations of the superior and inferior venae cavae; the grouped hepatic veins; the convergent formation and hepatic divarication of the hepatic portal vein, and the routes available for return of oxygenated left umbilical venous blood; also the changing disposition of the duodenal loop and its relationship to the definitive portal vein; the manner in which the left terminal branch of the latter establishes connections with the ductus venosus and the left umbilical vein. Return of placental blood to the fetal heart is along an (embryologically) complex path; **3**.186, 187 should assist clarification. See text for further details.

323

pletely; the left channels also disappear, but their cardiac terminals may, on occasion, be found as conical fibrous tags attached to the inferior wall of the coronary sinus. The right vitelline hepatocardiac vein continues enlarging and ultimately forms the terminal segment of the inferior vena cava. The latter receives the right venae revehentes and new channels draining the territories of the left venae revehentes; these collectively form the upper and lower groups of right and (secondary) left hepatic veins. The terminal caval segment also shows the orifice of the right half of the intervitelline subdiaphragmatic anastomosis (p. 321) and a large new connection with the right subcardinal vein (see below).

The hepatic terminals of the right and left duodenal parts of the vitelline veins are destined to form the corresponding branches of the *hepatic portal vein*, the left branch incorporating the cranial ventral intervitelline anastomosis. With rotation of the gut and formation of the duodenal loop. segments of the original vitelline veins and the caudal transverse anastomosis (indicated in **3**.186–188) atrophy, whilst new splanchnopleuric venous channels, the superior mesenteric and splenic veins, converge and join the left end of the dorsal intermediate anastomosis. The numerous other radicles of the portal vein and its principal branches, including the inferior mesenteric vein, are later formations.

For a period placental blood returns from the umbilicus via right and left umbilical veins, both discharging through venae advehentes into the hepatic sinusoids, where admixture with vitelline blood occurs. At approximately 7 mm CR length, the right umbilical vein retrogresses completely; the left umbilical vein retains some vessels discharging directly into the sinusoids, but new enlarging connections with the left half of the subhepatic intervitelline anastomosis emerge. The latter is the commencement of a *by-pass channel* for the majority of the placental blood, *which continues through the median ductus venosus* and finally the right half of the subdiaphragmatic anastomosis, to reach the termination of the inferior vena cava. Postnatally these channels are obliterated, with the resulting ligamentum teres extending from the umbilicus to the porta hepatis, whence, having established connections with the left branch of the portal vein, it continues as the ligamentum venosum to join an upper left hepatic vein, and terminates in the suprahepatic inferior vena cava.

Cardinal venous complexes

Cardinal venous complexes (**3**.189) are first represented by two large vessels on each side, the *precardinal* and *postcardinal veins*; the former drain the rostral part of the embryo, the latter its caudal region. The two veins on each side unite to form a short *common cardinal vein*, which passes ventrally, lateral to the pleuropericardial canal (p. 180), to open into the corresponding horn of the sinus venosus (**3**.179B). (The cardinal complexes are often, less appropriately, called parietal or somatic. In addition to drainage of the latter, they receive many radicles from splanchnopleuric structures.)

Owing to the rapid development of the head and brain the precardinal veins become enlarged. They are further augmented by the *subclavian* veins from the upper limb buds, and so become the chief tributaries of the common cardinal veins; these gradually assume an almost vertical position in association with the descent of the heart into the thorax. That part of the original precardinal vein rostral to the subclavian is now the *internal jugular vein*, and their confluence the *brachiocephalic vein* of each side. The right and left common cardinal veins are originally of the same diameter. By the development of a large oblique transverse connection, the *left brachiocephalic vein* carries blood across from the left to the right (**3**.179). The part of the original right precardinal vein between the junction of the two brachiocephalics and the azygos veins forms the upper part of the *superior vena cava*; the caudal part of the latter vessel (below the entrance of the azygos vein) is formed by the right common cardinal. Caudal to the transverse branching of the left brachiocephalic vein the left precardinal and left common cardinal veins largely atrophy, the former constituting the terminal part of the left superior intercostal vein, while the latter is represented by the ligament of the left vena cava and the oblique vein of the left atrium (**3**.189B). The remainder of the left superior intercostal vein is developed from the cranial end of the postcardinal vein and drains the second, third and, on occasion, the fourth intercostal veins. The oblique vein passes downwards across the back of the left atrium to open into the coronary sinus, which, as already indicated, represents

the persistent left horn of the sinus venosus. Right and left superior venae cavae are present in some animals, and occasionally persist in mankind.

The inferior vena cava (**3**.189) of the adult is a composite vessel, and the precise mode of development of its postrenal segment (caudal to the renal vein) is still somewhat uncertain. Its function is initially carried out by the right and left postcardinal veins, which receive the venous drainage of the lower limb buds and pelvis and run in the dorsal part of the mesonephric ridges, receiving tributaries from the body wall (*intersegmental veins*) and from the derivatives of the mesonephroi.

A second pair of longitudinal channels, the *subcardinal veins*, form in ventromedial parts of the mesonephric ridges and become connected to the postcardinal veins by a number of vessels traversing the medial part of the ridges. The subcardinal veins intercommunicate by a *pre-aortic anastomotic plexus*, which later constitutes the part of the *left renal vein* crossing anterior to the abdominal aorta.

The formation of an oblique transverse anastomosis between the iliac veins—which itself becomes the major part of the definitive *left common iliac vein*—diverts an increasing volume of blood into the right longitudinal veins, accounting for the ultimate disappearance of most of those on the left.

At its cranial end the subcardinal vein receives the *suprarenal vein* on each side, but on the right side it comes into intimate relationship with the liver. An extension of the vessel takes place in a cranial direction and meets and establishes continuity with a corresponding new formation which is growing caudally from the right vitelline hepatocardiac (common hepatic) vein. In this way on the right side a more direct route is established to the heart and the prerenal (cranial) segment of the inferior vena cava is defined.

The enlargement of the metanephros (p. 200) diverts the postcardinal vein from its course and the venous drainage of the mesonephric ridge is assumed by the subcardinal vein. At the same time new longitudinal channels appear and take over intersegmental venous drainage and the whole of the postcardinal vein disappears—except for its extreme cranial and caudal ends. There are at least three such channels on each side, in addition to the postcardinal and subcardinal already mentioned, but, so far as is known, only two of them persist as large vessels in the adult:

- A bilateral longitudinal channel forms dorsolateral to the aorta and **lateral** to the sympathetic trunk and takes over the intersegmental venous drainage from the posterior cardinal vein. This is the *supracardinal* or *thoracolumbar 'complex'*; alternatively *lateral sympathetic line vein*.
- A second channel forms on each side, also dorsolateral to the aorta but **medial** to the sympathetic trunk. This, the *azygos line vein* or *medial sympathetic line vein*, gradually takes over the intersegmental venous drainage from the thoracolumbar line. The intersegmental veins now obviously reach their longitudinal channel by passing medial to the autonomic trunk, the relationship which the lumbar and intercostal veins maintain thenceforth. Cranially the azygos lines join the persistent cranial ends of the posterior cardinal veins.
- Two *subcentral veins* are laid down directly dorsal to the aorta in the interval between the origins of the paired intersegmental arteries. These veins communicate freely with each other and with the azygos line veins, and these connections ultimately form the retro-aortic parts of the left lumbar veins and of the hemiazygos veins.
- Some authorities also recognize a *precostal* or *lumbocostal venous line*, anterior to the vertebrocostal element, and posterior to the supracardinal. A possible derivative is the ascending lumbar vein.

The thoracolumbar or supracardinal veins are, as indicated, lateral to the aorta and sympathetic trunks, which therefore intervene between them and the azygos lines. These veins communicate caudally with the iliac veins and cranially with the subcardinal veins in the neighbourhood of the pre-aortic intersubcardinal anastomosis. In addition, the supracardinal veins communicate freely with each other through the medium of the azygos lines and the subcentral veins. The most cranial of these connections, together with the supracardinal–subcardinal and the intersubcardinal anastomoses, complete a venous ring around the aorta below the origin of the

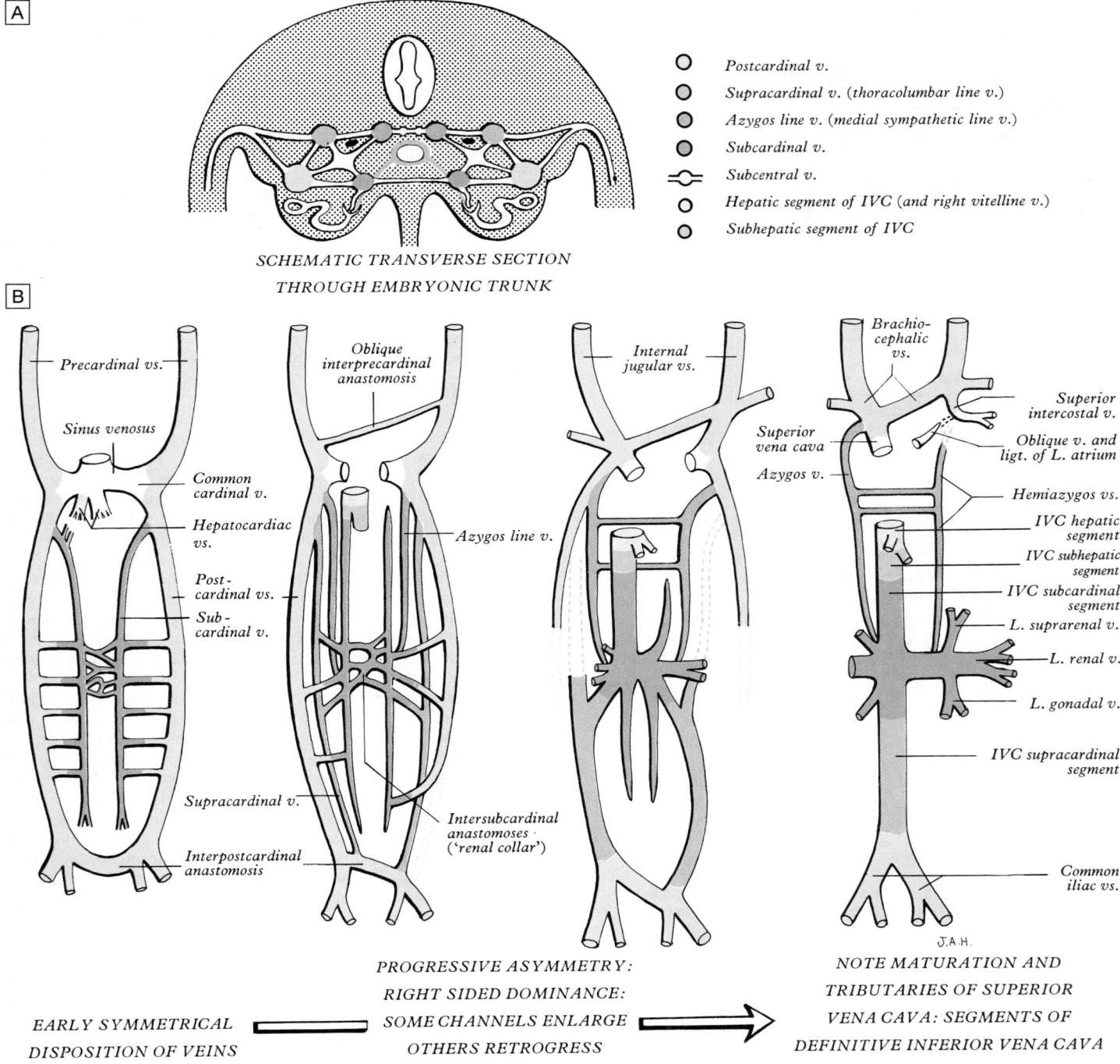

A. Schematic transverse section through embryonic trunk

Legend:
○ Postcardinal v.
○ Supracardinal v. (thoracolumbar line v.)
◐ Azygos line v. (medial sympathetic line v.)
◐ Subcardinal v.
⊷ Subcentral v.
○ Hepatic segment of IVC (and right vitelline v.)
○ Subhepatic segment of IVC

SCHEMATIC TRANSVERSE SECTION
THROUGH EMBRYONIC TRUNK

B.

EARLY SYMMETRICAL DISPOSITION OF VEINS

PROGRESSIVE ASYMMETRY: RIGHT SIDED DOMINANCE: SOME CHANNELS ENLARGE OTHERS RETROGRESS

NOTE MATURATION AND TRIBUTARIES OF SUPERIOR VENA CAVA: SEGMENTS OF DEFINITIVE INFERIOR VENA CAVA

3.189 Somatic venous development. A. Schematic section through the embryonic trunk. Principal longitudinal veins are colour-coded. Interconnections and intersegmental veins remain uncoloured. (Modified from Williams et al 1969.) B. Plan of development of principal somatic veins from the early symmetric state, through states of increasing asymmetry, to the definitive arrangement. (Modified from Williams et al 1969.)

superior mesenteric artery, termed the 'renal collar' (Huntington 1920).

The right supracardinal vein persists and forms the greater part of the postrenal segment of the inferior vena cava, the continuity of the vessel being maintained by the persistence of the anastomosis between the right supracardinal and the right subcardinal in the 'renal collar'. The left supracardinal disappears, but some of the 'renal collar' formed by the left supracardinal–subcardinal anastomosis persists in the left renal vein. It must be added that much confusion and disagreement exists with regard to the disposition, homologies and derivatives of the complicated array of longitudinal veins described above.

In summary, therefore, the inferior vena cava is formed from below upwards by:

- confluence of the common iliac veins
- a short segment of the right postcardinal vein
- postcardinal–supracardinal anastomosis
- part of the right supracardinal vein
- right supracardinal–subcardinal anastomosis
- right subcardinal vein
- a new anastomotic channel of double origin—the hepatic segment of the inferior vena cava
- the cardiac termination of the right vitelline hepatocardiac vein (common hepatic vein).

It should be noted that only the supracardinal part of the inferior vena cava receives the intersegmental venous drainage, and that the postrenal (caudal) segment of the inferior vena cava is on a plane

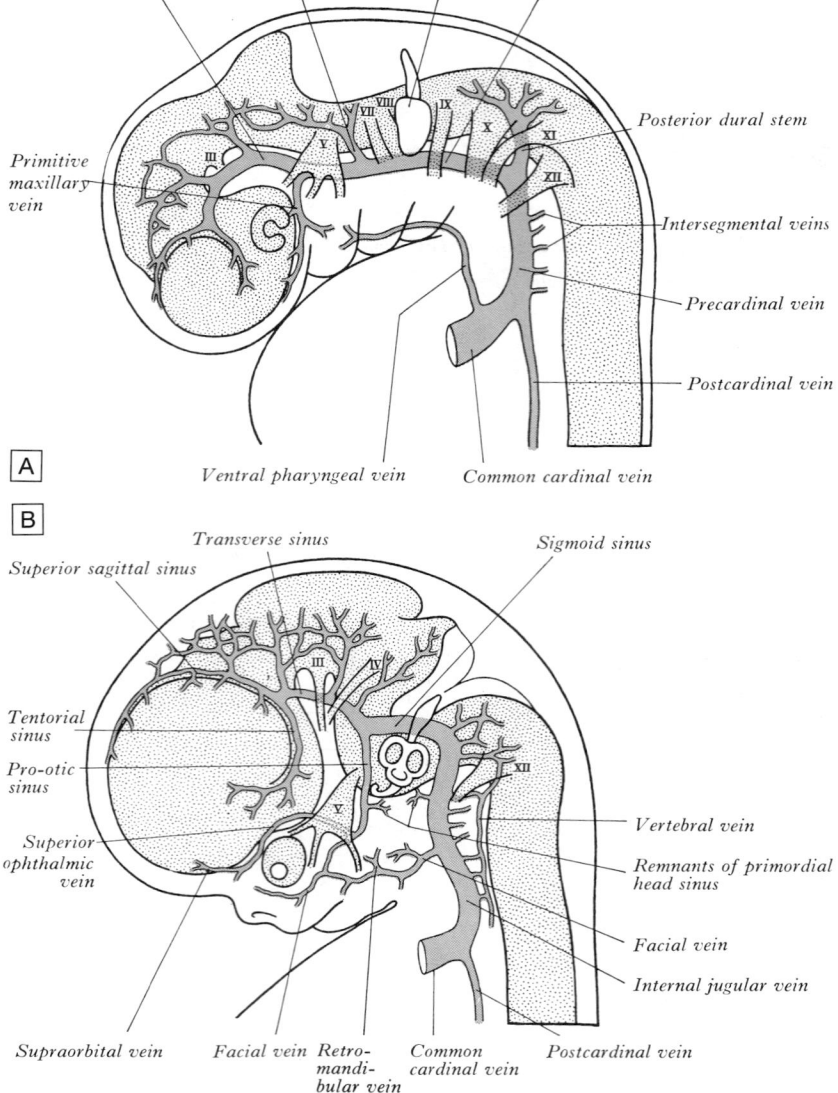

Anterior dural stem · Middle dural stem · Otocyst · Primary head sinus

Posterior dural stem

Primitive maxillary vein

Intersegmental veins

Precardinal vein

Postcardinal vein

[A]

Ventral pharyngeal vein · Common cardinal vein

[B]

Transverse sinus · Sigmoid sinus

Superior sagittal sinus

Tentorial sinus

Pro-otic sinus

Superior ophthalmic vein

Vertebral vein

Remnants of primordial head sinus

Facial vein

Internal jugular vein

Supraorbital vein · Facial vein · Retro-mandi-bular vein · Common cardinal vein · Postcardinal vein

3.190 Diagrams illustrating successive stages in the development of the veins of the head and neck at approximately 8 mm (A) and at approximately 24 mm CR length (B).

which lies dorsal to the plane of the prerenal (cranial) segment. Thus the right phrenic, suprarenal and renal arteries, which represent persistent mesonephric arteries, pass behind the inferior vena cava, while the testicular or ovarian, which has a similar development origin, passes anterior to it.

In some animals the right postcardinal vein constitutes a large part of the postrenal segment of the inferior vena cava. In these cases the right ureter, on leaving the kidney, passes medially dorsal to the vessel and then, curving round its medial side, crosses its ventral aspect. Rarely, a similar condition is found in the human subject, and indicates the persistence of the right postcardinal vein and failure of the right supracardinal to play its normal part in the development of the vessel.

The ultimate arrangement of some of the embryonic abdominal and thoracic longitudinal cardinal veins may be summarized:

● The terminal part of the left postcardinal vein forms the distal part of the left superior intercostal vein; on the right side its cranial end persists as the terminal part of the vena azygos.

● The caudal part of the subcardinal vein is in part incorporated in the testicular or ovarian vein (McClure & Butler 1925) and partly disappears. The cranial end of the right subcardinal vein is incorporated into the inferior vena cava and also forms the

right suprarenal vein. The left subcardinal vein, cranial to the intersubcardinal anastomosis, is incorporated into the left suprarenal vein. The renal and testicular or ovarian veins on both sides join the supracardinal–subcardinal anastomosis. On the left side this is connected directly to the part of the inferior vena cava which is of subcardinal status through an intersubcardinal anastomosis.

● The right supracardinal vein forms much of the postrenal (caudal) segment of the inferior vena cava. The left supracardinal vein disappears entirely.

● The right azygos line persists in its thoracic part to form all but the terminal part of the vena azygos. Its lumbar part can usually be identified as a small vessel which leaves the vena azygos on the body of the twelfth thoracic vertebra and descends on the vertebral column, deep to the right crus of the diaphragm, to join the posterior aspect of the inferior vena cava at the upper end of its postrenal segment. The left azygos line forms the hemiazygos veins.

● The subcentral veins give rise to the retro-aortic parts of the left lumbar veins and of the hemiazygos veins.

Veins of the head

The veins of the head have a complicated developmental history (**3**.190, and consult Markowski 1911; Streeter 1918; Padget 1957; Butler 1957, 1967; Browder & Kaplan 1976). The primary vessels consist of a close-meshed capillary plexus drained on each side by the precardinal vein, which is at first continuous cranially with a transitory *primordial hindbrain channel*, lying on the neural tube medial to the cranial nerve roots. This is soon replaced by the *primary head vein* which runs caudally from the medial side of the trigeminal ganglion, lateral to the facial and vestibulocochlear nerves and otocyst, then medial to the vagus nerve, to become continuous with the precardinal vein. A lateral anastomosis subsequently brings it lateral to the vagus nerve. The cranial part of the precardinal vein forms the internal jugular vein; its caudal moiety has already been described on page 324.

The primary capillary plexus of the head becomes separated into three fairly distinct strata by the differentiation of the skull and meninges. The superficial vessels, draining the integument and underlying soft parts, eventually discharge in large part into the *external jugular system*. They retain some connections with the deeper veins through so-called emissary veins. Deep to this is the *venous plexus of the dura mater*, from which the dural venous sinuses differentiate. This plexus converges on each side into *anterior*, *middle* and *posterior dural stems*. The anterior stem drains the prosencephalon and mesencephalon entering the primary head vein rostral to the trigeminal ganglion. The middle stem drains the metencephalon and empties into the primary head vein caudal to the trigeminal ganglion, while the posterior stem drains the myelencephalon into the commencement of the precardinal vein (**3**.98A, B). The deepest capillary stratum is the pial plexus from which the veins of the brain differentiate; it drains at the dorsolateral aspect of the neural tube into the adjacent dural venous plexus. In addition the primary head vein also receives, at its cranial end, the *primitive maxillary vein*, draining the maxillary prominence and region of the optic vesicle.

The vessels of the dural plexus undergo profound changes, largely accommodating the growth of the cartilaginous otic capsule of the membranous labyrinth and expansion of the cerebral hemispheres. With growth of the otic capsule the primary head vein is gradually reduced and a new channel joining anterior, middle and posterior dural stems appears dorsal to the cranial nerve ganglia and the capsule (Butler 1967). Where this new vessel joins the middle and posterior stems, together with the posterior dural stem itself, is formed the adult *sigmoid sinus* (**3**.190B).

Between the growing cerebral hemispheres and along the dorsal margins of the anterior and middle plexuses there forms a curtain of capillary veins, the *sagittal plexus*, in the position of the future falx cerebri. Rostrodorsally this plexus forms the *superior sagittal sinus* and is continuous behind with the anastomosis between the anterior and middle dural stems, which forms most of the *transverse sinus*. Ventrally the sagittal plexus differentiates into the *inferior sagittal* and *straight sinuses* and the *great cerebral vein*, and drains, more commonly, into the left transverse sinus. (For right/left variations in the terminations of sagittal and straight sinuses, and occurrence of a confluence, see p. 1583.)

The vessels along the ventrolateral edge of the developing cerebral hemisphere form the transitory *tentorial sinus*, which drains the convex surface of the cerebral hemisphere and basal ganglia, and the ventral aspect of the diencephalon, to the transverse sinus. With expansions of the cerebral hemispheres, and in particular the emergence of the temporal lobe, the tentorial sinus becomes elongated, attenuated and eventually disappears, and its territory is drained by enlarging anastomoses of pial vessels which become the *basal veins*, radicles of the great cerebral vein.

The anterior dural stem disappears and the caudal part of the primary head vein dwindles; it is represented in the adult by the *inferior petrosal sinus*. The cranial part of the primary head vein, medial to the trigeminal ganglion, persists and still receives the stem of the primitive maxillary vein. The latter has now lost most of its tributaries to the anterior facial vein, its stem becoming the main trunk of the *primitive supra-orbital vein*, which will form the *superior ophthalmic vein* of the adult. Thus, the main venous drainage of the orbit and its contents is now carried via the augmented middle dural stem, the *pro-otic sinus*, into the transverse sinus and at a later stage into the cavernous sinus. The *cavernous sinus* is formed from a secondary plexus, derived from the primary head vein and lying between the otic and basi-occipital cartilages. This forms the inferior petrosal sinus and drains through the primordial hindbrain channel into the internal jugular vein. The *superior petrosal sinus* arises later from a ventral metencephalic tributary of the pro-otic sinus; it communicates secondarily with the cavernous sinus (Butler 1957, 1967). The pro-otic sinus meanwhile has developed a new and more caudally situated stem draining into the sigmoid sinus; this new stem is the *petrosquamosal sinus* (p. 1584) and the pro-otic sinus becomes, with progressive ossification of the skull, diploic in position. The development of the venous drainage and portal system of the hypophysis cerebri is closely associated with that of the venous sinuses (Wislocki 1937; Niemineva 1950, see also p. 1883).

Cerebral veins. These can be identified from 16 weeks onwards; the *superior, middle, inferior, anterior* and *posterior cerebral veins* are developed and appear more tortuous than the meningeal arteries.

Veins draining the cortex, white matter and deeper structures are recognized in the midtrimester. *Subcortical veins* drain the deep white matter, deep cortical and subcortical superficial tissue; they terminate together, with *cortical veins* which drain the cortex, in the *meningeal veins*. The deep white matter and central nuclei are drained by longer veins, which meet and join subependymal veins from the ventricular zone. Anastomoses between various groups of cortical veins can be recognized by 16 weeks gestation. The *inferior anastomotic vein (of Labbe)*, an anastomosis between the middle cerebral and inferior cerebral veins, becomes recognizable at 20 weeks but the *superior anastomotic vein (of Trolard)*, connecting the superior and middle cerebral veins, appears not earlier than the end of 30 weeks.

Rapid cortical development is correlated with the regression of the middle cerebral vein and its tributaries and development of ascending and descending cortical veins and intraparenchymal (medullary) arteries and veins.

Cerebral venous drainage in a full-term baby is essentially composed of two principal venous arrays, the *superficial veins* and the *deep Galenic venous system* with anastomoses between these two systems persisting into adult life (Wigglesworth & Pape 1978).

Venous drainage of the face, scalp and neck. This becomes established after the development of the skull. The first identifiable vessel is the *ventral pharyngeal vein*, draining the massive mandibular and hyoid arches into the common cardinal vein. With the elongation of the neck its termination is transferred to the cranial part of the precardinal vein which later becomes the *internal jugular*. The ventral pharyngeal vein, receiving tributaries from the face and tongue, becomes the *linguofacial vein*. With development of the face the primitive maxillary vein extends its drainage into the territories of supply of the ophthalmic and mandibular division of the fifth nerve, including the pterygoid and temporal muscles, and over the lower jaw it anastomoses with the linguofacial vein. This anastomosis becomes the *facial vein*; it receives a strong *retromandibular vein* from the temporal region, and drains through the linguofacial vein into the internal jugular. The stem of the linguofacial vein is now the lower part of the facial vein, whilst the dwindling connection of the facial with the primitive maxillary becomes the *deep facial vein*. The *external jugular vein* is developed from a tributary of the cephalic

vein from the tissues of the neck and anastomoses secondarily with the anterior facial vein. At this stage the *cephalic vein* forms a venous ring around the clavicle from which it is connected with the caudal part of the precardinal. The deep segment of the venous ring forms the *subclavian vein* and receives the definitive external jugular vein. The superficial segment of the venous ring dwindles, but may persist in adult life (Padget 1957).

Veins of the limbs

At the tip of the early limb bud, blood in the terminal capillary plexus returns to the body via a *marginal vein* that develops along the pre- and postaxial borders of the limb. The marginal vein is separated from the overlying ectoderm by an avascular zone of mesenchyme (p. 319). As the limb enlarges the marginal vein can be subdivided into *pre-* and *postaxial veins* running along their respective borders. These latter vessels are the precursors of the superficial veins of the limb. Generally the preaxial (superficial) veins join to deep veins at the *proximal joint*, and the postaxial (superficial) veins join to deep veins at the *distal joint* of the limb. Deep veins develop in situ alongside the arteries.

In the upper limb the preaxial vein becomes the *cephalic vein*; it drains at the shoulder into the axillary vein. The postaxial vein becomes the *basilic vein*, which passes deep in the arm to continue as the axillary vein.

In the lower limb the preaxial vein becomes the *great saphenous vein* and drains at the saphenous opening into the femoral vein. The postaxial vein becomes the *short saphenous vein*; this passes deep to join the popliteal vein.

LYMPHATIC AND LYMPHOID SYSTEM

Two different views are current as to the initial stages in the development of the lymphatic system (Rusznyák et al 1960). According to the first view (Huntington 1908; McClure & Butler 1925) lymphatic spaces commence as clefts in the mesenchyme, and their lining cells take on the characteristics of endothelium (Kampmeier 1969). These spaces form capillary plexuses from which certain *lymph sacs*, to be noted later, are derived. The connections of the lymphatic and venous systems are regarded as entirely secondary. In contrast, however, according to Sabin (1912), the earliest lymph vessels arise as capillary offshoots from the endothelium of the veins, as capillary plexuses. These plexuses lose their connections with the venous system and become confluent to form lymph sacs. The balance of the evidence suggests that all but the earliest lymphatic channels originate independently of the venous system and only acquire connections with it at a later stage (Kampmeier 1969).

In the human embryo the lymph sacs from which the lymph vessels are derived are six in number: two paired (the *jugular* and the *posterior lymph sacs*) and two unpaired (the *retroperitoneal* and the *cisterna chyli*). In lower mammals an additional pair (the *subclavian*) is present, but in the human embryo these are merely extensions of the jugular sacs.

The position of the sacs is as follows (3.191):

- the *jugular*, the first to appear, at the junction of the subclavian vein with the precardinal, with later prolongations along the internal and external jugular veins
- the *posterior* encircling the left common iliac vein
- the *retroperitoneal*, in the root of the mesentery near the suprarenal glands
- the *cisterna chyli*, opposite the third and fourth lumbar vertebrae.

From the lymph sacs the lymph vessels bud out along lines corresponding more or less closely with the course of embryonic blood vessels, most commonly veins, but many arise de novo in the mesenchyme and establish connections with existing vessels. In the body wall and that of the intestine the deeper plexuses are the first to be developed; by continued growth of these, the vessels in the superficial layers are gradually formed.

The *thoracic duct* is, phylogenetically, a bilateral structure. In man it comprises the caudal part of the right vessel, a transverse anastomosis and the cranial part of the left vessel. According to the second view cited above, it is formed from anastomosing outgrowths from the jugular sacs and cisterna chyli. At its connection with the

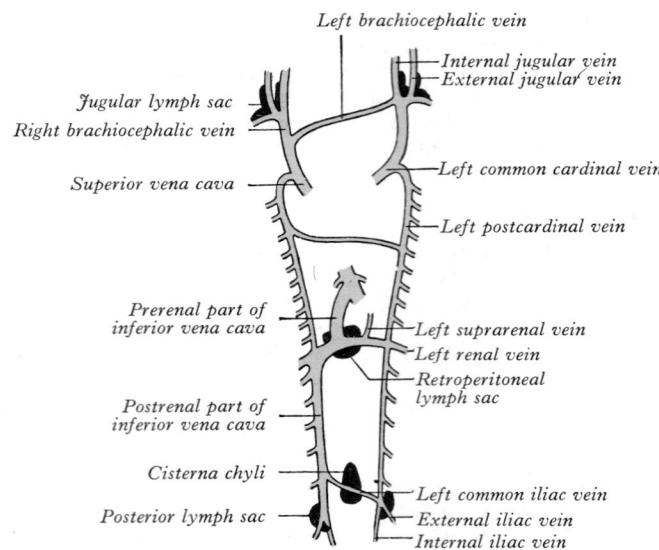

Left brachiocephalic vein

Internal jugular vein
External jugular vein

Jugular lymph sac
Right brachiocephalic vein

Superior vena cava

Left common cardinal vein

Left postcardinal vein

Prerenal part of inferior vena cava

Left suprarenal vein
Left renal vein
Retroperitoneal lymph sac

Postrenal part of inferior vena cava

Cisterna chyli

Posterior lymph sac

Left common iliac vein
External iliac vein
Internal iliac vein

3.191 Scheme showing the relative positions of the primary lymph sacs. (After F R Sabin.)

cisterna it is at first double, but the vessels soon join. Numerous valves are laid down in the duct during the fifth month, but many of them disappear prior to birth. Those which persist are formed in situations where the duct may be subjected to pressure, for example where it is crossed by the oesophagus and the aortic arch.

All the lymph sacs except the cisterna chyli (see p. 1609) are, at a later stage, divided by a number of slender connective tissue bridges. Subsequently they are invaded by lymphocytes and transformed into groups of lymph nodes, the lymph sinuses representing portions of the original cavity of the sac. The caudal part of the cisterna chyli is similarly converted, but its rostral part sometimes persists as a definitive cisterna; in many cases the cisterna chyli is plexiform (p. 1610). The siting of the major groups of lymph nodes follows a similar basic pattern amongst the mammals (Spira 1962).

Despite the wide array of labelling techniques for histology, there is a paucity of recent anatomical studies on the development of the

lymphatic system. Experimental studies have shown that loading of the vascular system with fluid increases the thoracic lymph duct flow in fetal sheep, suggesting that the rate of flow is an important safety factor against fetal oedema (Brace 1993).

Haemal lymph nodes are said to develop as mesenchymal condensations in close relation to blood vessels rather than lymphatics (Meyer 1917; Turner 1969a–d).

Spleen

The spleen (**3**.76, 78D, 79) appears about the sixth week as a localized thickening of the coelomic epithelium of the dorsal mesogastrium near its cranial end, and the proliferating cells invade the underlying angiogenetic mesenchyme, which becomes condensed and vascularized. The process occurs simultaneously in several adjoining areas which soon fuse to form a lobulated spleen of dual origin from coelomic epithelium and from mesenchyme of the dorsal mesogastrium. With enlargement, the spleen projects to the left so that its surfaces are covered by the peritoneum of the mesogastrium on its left aspect, thus forming a boundary of the general extrabursal (greater) sac. When fusion occurs between the dorsal wall of the bursa omentalis and the dorsal parietal peritoneum, fusion does not extend to the left as far as the spleen (**3**.78D, 79), which remains connected to the dorsal abdominal wall (left kidney and suprarenal) by a short lienorenal ligament, while its original connection with the stomach persists as the gastrosplenic ligament. The lienorenal ligament contains the tail of the pancreas. The earlier lobulated character of the spleen disappears, but is indicated by the presence of notches on its upper border in the adult.

The histogenesis of the spleen has attracted relatively little attention. For earlier accounts consult references (Sabin 1912; Thiel & Downey 1921; Lewis 1956; von Herrath 1958; Bloom & Fawcett 1975). The vascular reticulum is well developed at 8 to 9 weeks, with immature reticulocytes and numerous closely spaced thin-walled vascular loops. Differentiation of blood cells, macrophages, and of arteries, veins, capillaries and sinusoids has occurred by the eleventh to twelfth week. The capsule consists at first of cuboidal cells bearing cilia and microvilla (Weiss 1957).

The spleen is subject to various anomalies, including complete *agenesis*, multiple spleens or *polysplenia*, isolated small additional *spleniculi* and persistent lobulation. Attention has been directed to association of cardiac, pulmonary and other abnormalities with asplenia or polysplenia (Rose et al 1975).

For development of the thymus see page 176.

PRENATAL GROWTH IN FORM AND SIZE

The absolute size of neither embryo nor fetus affords a reliable indication of either its true age or stage of structural organization, even though graphs based on large numbers of observations have been constructed to provide averages. All such data suffer from the difficulty of equating dimensions and degree of differentiation with the actual time of conception, which can rarely, if ever, be established with complete exactness. The life of the individual really commences with fertilization, but the date of this cannot be exactly determined in mankind. It has long been customary to compute the age, whether in a normal birth or an abortion, from the first day of the last menstrual period of the mother but, since ovulation usually occurs near the fourteenth day of a period, this 'menstrual age' is about two weeks too much (see p. 92). Where a single coitus can be held to be responsible for conception, a 'coital age' can be established and the 'fertilization age' cannot be much less than this, because of the limited viability of both gametes; but it is usually held that the difference may be several days—a highly significant interval in the earlier stages of embryonic development. Even if the time of ovulation and coitus were known in instances of spontaneous abortion, not only would some uncertainty still persist with regard to the time of fertilization but there would also remain an indefinable period between the cessation of development and the actual recovery of the conceptus. With the legalization of abortion in some countries

the latter source of inaccuracy may be expected to become less important.

To overcome these difficulties early embryos have been graded or classified, on the basis of both internal and external features, into developmental stages or 'horizons' (**3**.192). Classic contributions in this field have been made by Lillie (1917), Streeter (1942, 1945, 1948, 1949), Hamilton (1944), Hertig et al (1956), Heuser & Corner (1957), and O'Rahilly and others between the years 1963 and 1987. Although it has become customary to describe these developmental levels as stages, the earlier descriptions are still accepted. However, Stages 1 to 9, covering the first three weeks of development, have been given a more reliable basis by O'Rahilly (1973), who has also gathered together the pertinent literature. Details on stages 1–23 are provided by O'Rahilly and Muller (1987), who describe developmental time in terms of postovulatory days. In each case the range is ± 1 day for stages 1–14; thereafter, the ages are greater than initially described by Streeter. Readers should consult the charts on pp. 45 and 50.

Stages 1 to 3. These occupy the first *4–5 days* after fertilization of the oöcyte in the ampulla of the uterine tube. The initial 24 hours (Stage 1) are occupied by fertilization, the dominant feature of which is the fusion of the male and female pronuclei. This is followed by the first mitotic division, which is the onset of segmentation, or cleavage, and is arbitrarily regarded as the transition from Stage 1 to Stage 2. Stage 2 is characterized by the continuation of cleavage, starting with two blastomeres and ending with about 12. During this stage the developing morula moves along the uterine tube, by mechanisms still not wholly understood, a journey occupying about four days. During the fourth day a segmentation cavity appears within the morula and this is taken as initiating Stage 3, which thus corresponds to the establishment of a free blastocyst.

Although comparatively few human embryos representing Stages 1 to 3 have been recovered (see p. 136 and consult O'Rahilly 1973), a considerable degree of agreement exists and, moreover, current observations of in vitro fertilization between human spermatozoa and ova (**3.**192A–H) support the earlier descriptions.

Stages 4 to 6. These are concerned with the endometrial attachment of the blastocyst, trophoblastic development, implantation, further development of the blastocyst and the appearance of the primitive streak (**3.**30, 35, 36, 38, 39). *Stage 4* corresponds to the *fifth and sixth postfertilization days*. The blastocyst, now in the uterine cavity, loses its zona pellucida and it begins the rapid but complex activities of orientation in respect of the endometrium, adhesion, penetration and the cellular proliferation of trophoblastic growth. This establishment of dependence on the maternal circulation for nutritional requirements is far more rapid in primates than in other mammals. *Stage 5* is reached when implantation has occurred, occupying the *seventh to twelfth days*; syncytiotrophoblastic and cytotrophoblastic strata have differentiated, the proamniotic cavity has appeared and a labyrinthine system of intercommunicating trophoblastic lacunae, through which the maternal blood ebbs and flows, has developed. A little later in Stage 5 the exocoelomic membrane has been identified. In Stage 6 chorionic villous stems become defined and begin to develop side branches almost at once, producing an increasingly complex intervillous space. A little later the primitive streak becomes apparent and differentiation of the embryonic area has commenced and may now be distinguished from the various extraembryonic tissues.

Because of the complexity of the events in Stages 5 and 6, both have been subdivided by some authorities. A much greater number of human embryos have been recovered which represent Stages 4 to 6.

Stages 7 to 9. Characterized by basic embryogenic changes, during *Stage 7* (*approximately sixteenth postovulatory day*) the primitive streak develops further and the notochordal ('head') process appears, together with the other mesenchymal strata. The chorion and amnion continue to develop, villous stems being generally distributed over the former but more pronounced at the embryonic pole. Haemopoetic foci appear in the wall of the definitive yolk sac, and the cloacal membrane and allanto-enteric diverticulum are defined. Associated with the latter primordial germ cells have been noted. In *Stage 8* (*seventeenth to nineteenth day*) the prechordal plate, primitive pit, neural groove and notochordal and neurenteric canals are all definable. By *Stage 9* (*nineteenth to twenty-first day*) the neural groove is deepening and the first somites begin to appear about midway along it. The cranial half of the groove, representing developing brain, begins to develop a cephalic flexure, optic primordia become visible and early head and tail folds have appeared, as Stage 10 is approached. The foregut is becoming defined, and early pharyngeal pouches may be identified. The embryo is now 1.5–2.0 mm in length.

Stages 10 to 12. Occupying *days 21–23, 23–25, 25–27* respectively, these stages feature continued formation of somites and, during this, the fourth week, head and tail folds are completed, the neural groove closes and primary cerebral vesicles appear. The cervical flexure can now be recognized, the optic vesicles form and the lental and otic placodes appear and become vesicular. The pharyngeal arches are appearing, lateral folds are more clearly defined and the cloacal membrane and hindgut are becoming distinct. Rudimentary limb buds appear and the heart tubes fuse into a common loop in which contractile activity commences. The primordia of the thyroid gland, lungs, liver, pancreas and mesonephric tubules are all identifiable. The embryo is about 4.0 mm in length.

Stages 13 to 15. Corresponding approximately to the *fifth week* of development (*28, 32* and *33 days*), at these stages the embryo grows from about 4 mm to 8 mm. It becomes markedly curved and its junction with the yolk sac relatively constricted. The cervical flexure is increased and the mesencephalic flexure is appearing. The

dorsolateral (alar) and ventrolateral (basal) laminae are differentiating, and the emerging corpus striatum, thalamus epithalamus and hypothalamus are loci of proliferating cells. The cranial and spinal nerves are developing, together with their ganglia, from the associated placodes and neural crest elements. The limb buds are elongating, displaying joint flexures; the rudimentary hands and feet are differentiating. The olfactory placodes, maxillary, mandibular and frontonasal prominences, tongue primordia and the hypophyseal pouch (of Rathke) are all appearing. The tubotympanic recesses are defined and the primordia of the thymus and parathyroid glands can be identified. In the developing heart the septum primum appears and its cornua define the foramen primum. The mesonephric ducts reach the cloaca and subsequently the metanephric (ureteric) buds appear and extend to the metanephrogenic masses of mesoderm in the sacral nephrogenic cord. The gonadal ridges, urorectal septum and genital tubercle are also developing.

Stages 16 to 20. Roughly equivalent to the sixth and seventh weeks, (*37, 41, 44, 47–48, 50–51 days*), by the end of these stages the embryo has a length of about 13–15 mm. Its curvature has further increased and its head and relatively long tail are in contact with the developing umbilical stump. The pontine flexure, cerebral hemispheres and cerebellum are developing. The upper limbs and the facial region are growing and differentiating rapidly; the palatal processes and primitive nasal prominences are apparent and the oronasal membrane ruptures. The liver produces a surface prominence between the cardiac region and the umbilical cord. Into the latter the midgut loop herniates and the appendix and caecum become distinguishable in it. The spleen develops, as do the paramesonephric (Mullerian) ducts. The foramen primum in the heart closes, with simultaneous opening of the foramen secundum and septation of the bulbus cordis. Cardiac muscle is differentiating. Haemopoiesis commences in the liver. Chondrification of many skeletal elements begins and ossification commences in mesenchymatous bones, the mandible and clavicles.

Stages 21 to 23. Completing the series (*52, 54, 56–67 days*), these stages represent the major part of the eighth week when the *formative* or *embryonic period* is regarded as coming to an end (**3.**192). During these stages there is a remarkable change in the external appearance of the embryo, for at the beginning of this period the individual still appears markedly 'embryonic', though clearly a primate, whereas at the end the form is most definitely human. The head is less flexed and the neck longer and clearly defined. The development of the face proceeds much further, with completion of the upper lip and nostrils, although the latter are plugged and the palate still incomplete. Enamel organs are developed from the dental laminae. The external ears and the eyelids are developing and the limbs elongate considerably, approaching much nearer their ultimate proportions and displaying well-formed hands and feet with separated digits. Early in this period the interventricular septum is completed. Skeletal and visceral muscle tissues begin to differentiate about this time, and generalized ossification occurs in enchondral bones. The onset of marrow formation in the humerus occurs at stage 23. This was adopted by Streeter (1949) as the conclusion of the embryonic and the beginning of the fetal period of prenatal life. Other systemic developments reached by this stage include vesicles in the metanephrogenic mass; the remainder of the nephrons and the collecting tubules of the kidneys are defined. The ovaries or testes are distinguishable and the paramesonephric (Mullerian) ducts are fusing to form the primordia of uterus and vagina. The external genitalia are further advanced and show sexual differentiation by the beginning of the eighth week. The cloacal membrane becomes perforate and the tail is retrogressing. By the end of the period the embryo possesses almost all the structural features, internal and external, characteristic of the human mammal and it now passes into the fetal period. The embryonic period, during which *patterned differentiation* occurs with consequent *organogenesis*, tends to overshadow the growth which accompanies these events. Very considerable increase in size has, however, occurred; from a single cell about 0.14 mm in diameter the embryo has become a most complex and functioning creature, consisting of millions of cells and with a length of about 30 mm or more, and it has increased in weight many thousands of times. During the *fetal period*, which occupies the third to tenth lunar months (**3.**193, 194), the accent is upon growth rather than differentiation but, of course, the latter continues throughout this period

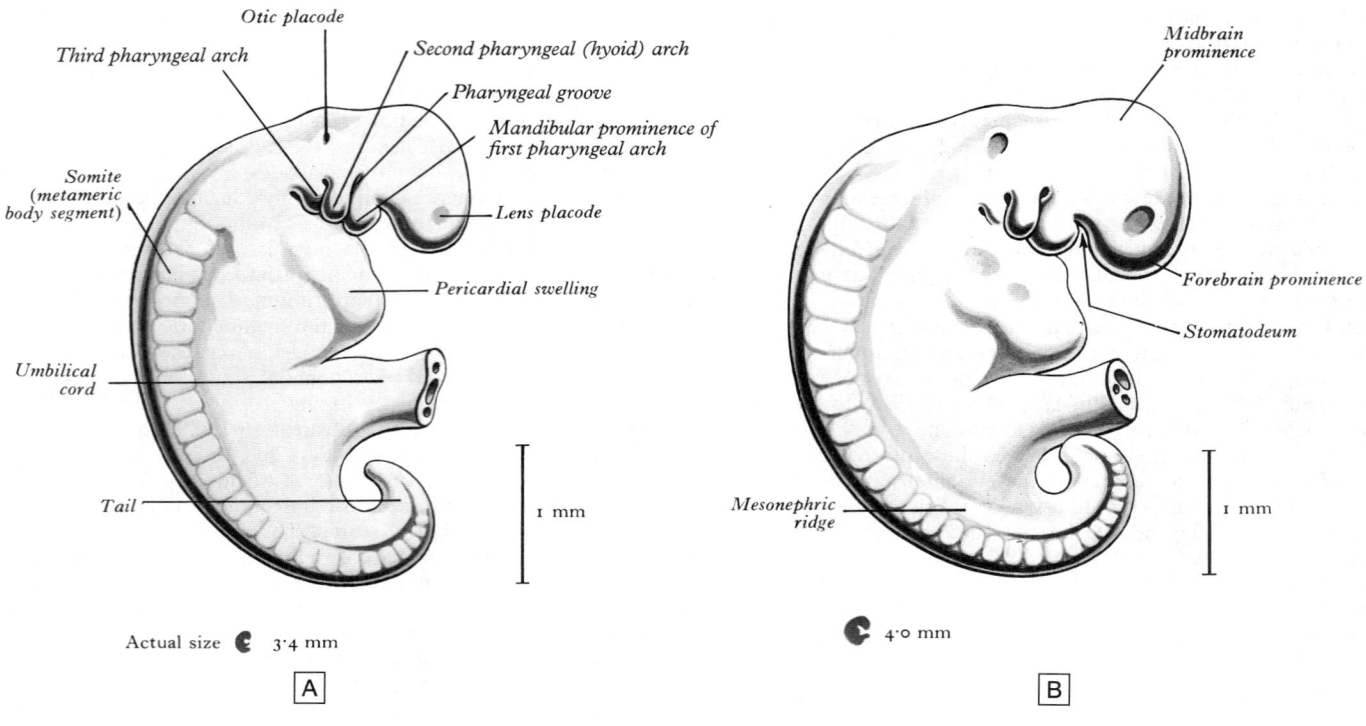

A

Third pharyngeal arch

Otic placode

Second pharyngeal (hyoid) arch

Pharyngeal groove

Mandibular prominence of first pharyngeal arch

Somite (metameric body segment)

Lens placode

Pericardial swelling

Umbilical cord

Tail

1 mm

Actual size 3·4 mm

B

Midbrain prominence

Forebrain prominence

Stomatodeum

Mesonephric ridge

1 mm

4·0 mm

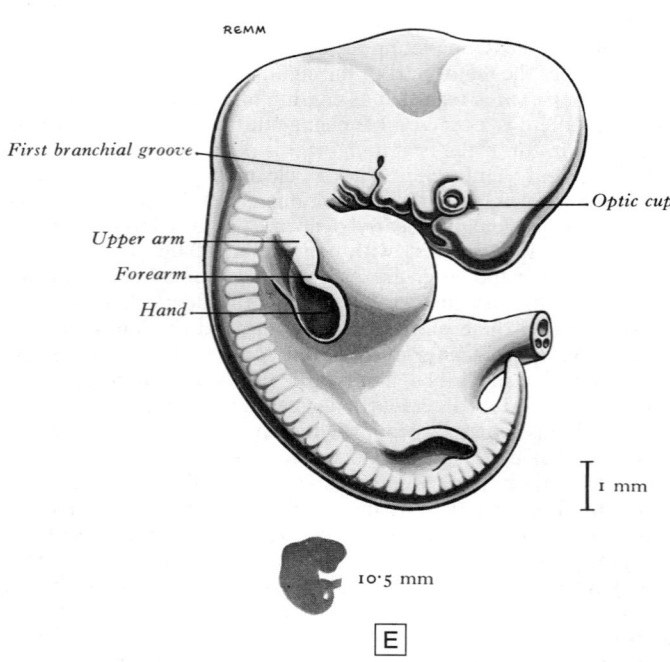
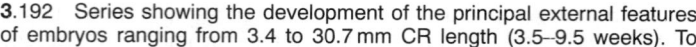

E

REMM

First branchial groove

Upper arm

Forearm

Hand

Optic cup

1 mm

10·5 mm

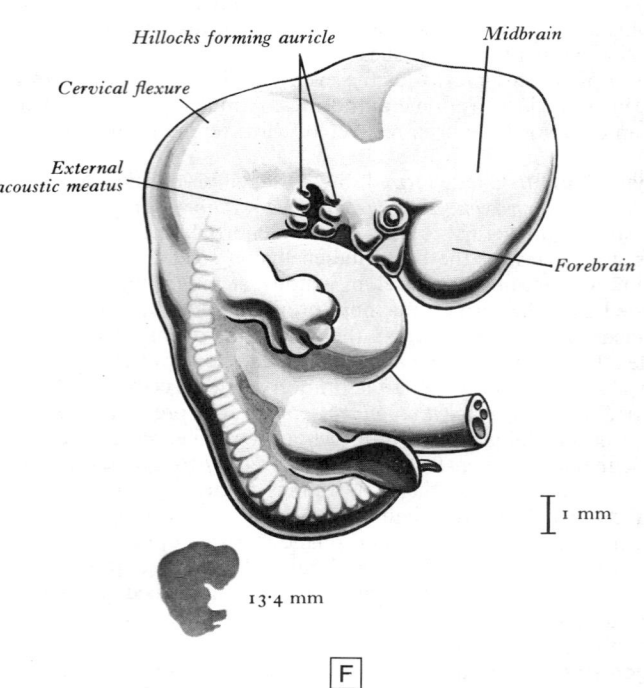

F

Hillocks forming auricle

Cervical flexure

External acoustic meatus

Midbrain

Forebrain

1 mm

13·4 mm

3.192   Series showing the development of the principal external features of embryos ranging from 3.4 to 30.7 mm CR length (3.5–9.5 weeks). To assist comparison a 1 mm scale is included in each case; the small silhouette is actual size.

and to a lesser degree after birth (and in some tissues, throughout life). During this period the overall rate of growth in length is greater but not markedly so; from the fourth to sixth weeks the rate is about 1 mm per day, with a maximum of about 2 mm during the fourth month. The increase in length in the fetal period is from 30/40 to about 500 mm, and the increase in weight from perhaps 2 or 3 g to more than 3000 g.

Third month. During this month head flexion decreases further and the neck becomes proportionately longer. The eyelids meet and fuse and will remain temporarily united until the sixth lunar month.

Nails appear on the digits and the upper limbs in general are comparatively accelerated in development. The umbilical protrusion of the gut is reduced—accompanying a proportionate augmentation of abdominal volume.

Fourth and fifth months. The covering of primary hair—the *lanugo* (see p. 405) appears during this month; the head and upper limbs are still disproportionately large and, although the trunk and lower limbs begin to catch up by increased rates of growth during the rest of uterine life, the same disproportion is present after birth and to a diminishing degree throughout childhood and on into the

330

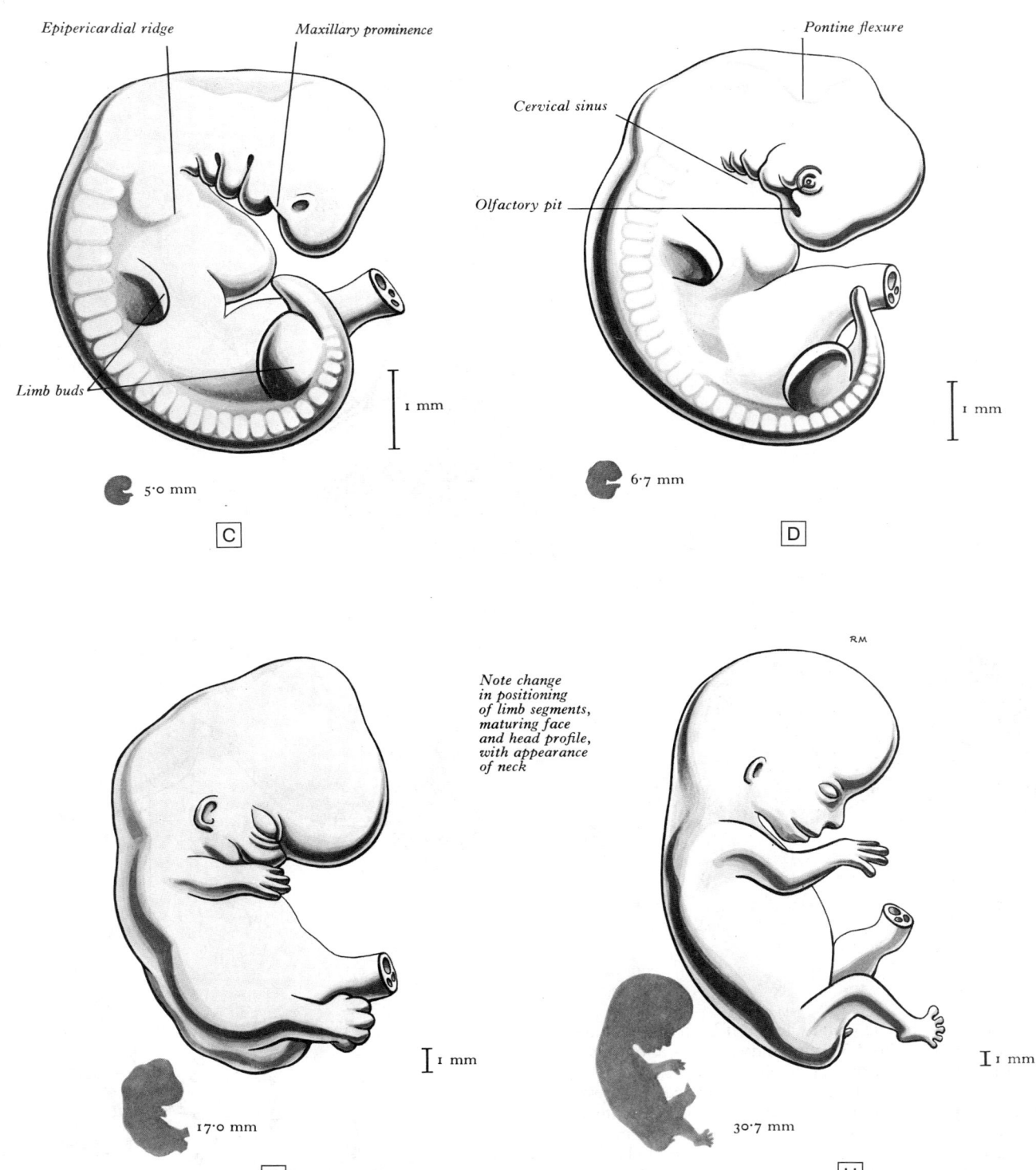

Epipericardial ridge

Maxillary prominence

Pontine flexure

Cervical sinus

Olfactory pit

Limb buds

1 mm

1 mm

5·0 mm

6·7 mm

C

D

Note change in positioning of limb segments, maturing face and head profile, with appearance of neck

RM

1 mm

1 mm

17·0 mm

30·7 mm

G

H

years of puberty. By the end of the fourth month the eyes have moved even further into an anteriorly directed position, but are still relatively wide apart. The external ear is approaching its characteristic form and is nearer its ultimate position, at the side of the head and no longer in the upper part of the neck. The total fetal length, including the lower limb, is now of the order of 230 mm. Its weight at the end of the *fifth month* is about 300 g, which will be increased more than tenfold during the second half of intrauterine life. Towards the end of this period sebaceous glands become active, and the sebum secreted blends with desquamated epidermal cells to form a cheesy covering to the skin, the *vernix caseosa*, usually considered to protect the former from maceration by the amniotic fluid. During this month the mother becomes conscious of fetal movement—so-called 'quickening'.

Sixth month. This month witnesses a further general change of bodily proportions and facial appearance towards those of the infant at birth. The lanugo darkens and the skin becomes markedly wrinkled, presumably through a disparity in the growth rates of cutaneous and subcutaneous tissues. The eyelids and eyebrows are now well developed. The vernix caseosa is more abundant. The length of the fetus is about 300 mm by the end of this month.

Seventh month. During this month the hair of the scalp is lengthening and the eyebrow hairs and the eyelashes are well-developed. The eyelids themselves separate and the pupillary membrane disappears. The body becomes more plump and rounded in contour and the skin loses its wrinkled appearance due to increased deposition of subcutaneous fat. Towards the end of this month the fetus is viable, without the technological assistance found in 'special

331

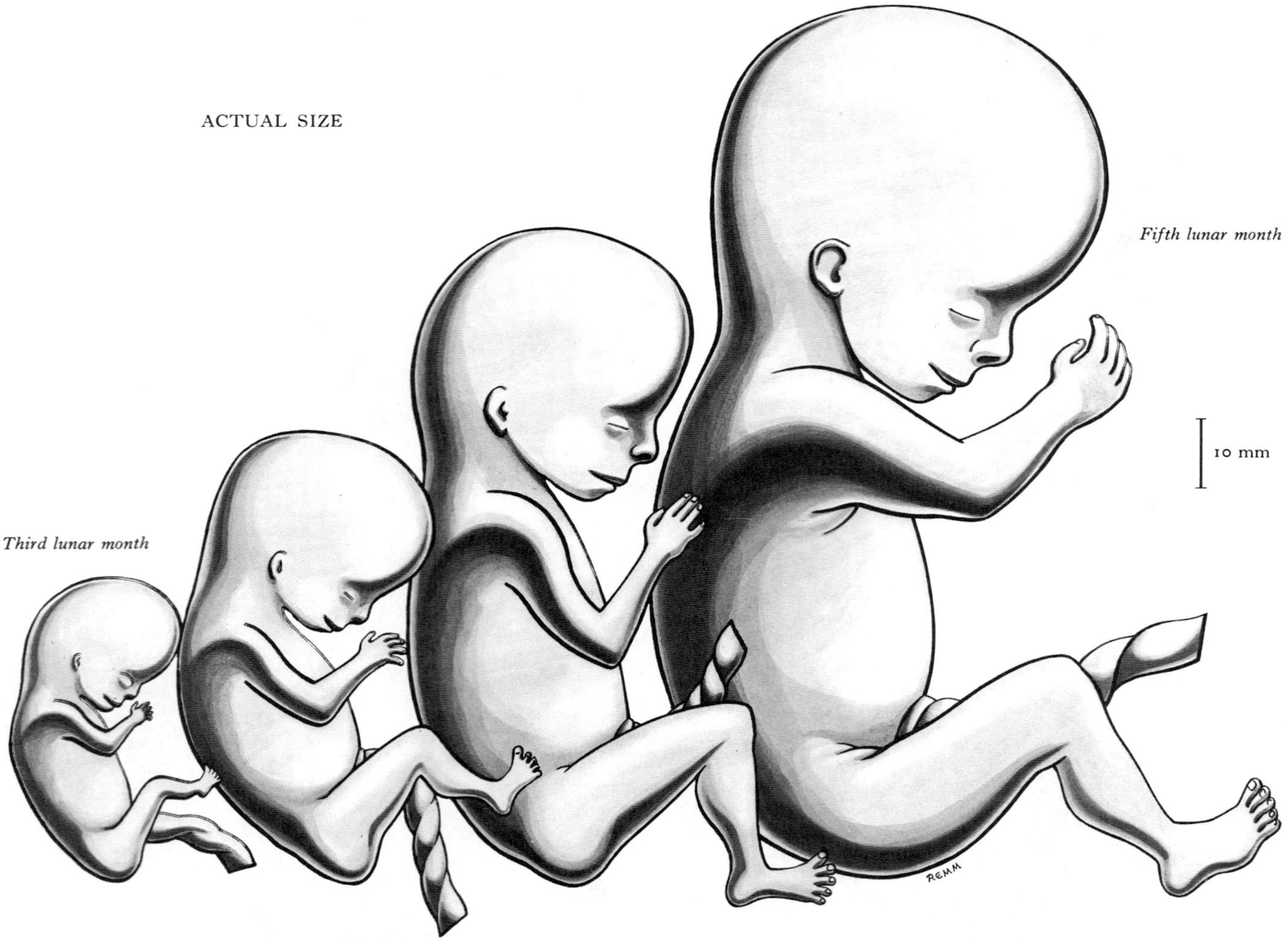

ACTUAL SIZE

Fifth lunar month

10 mm

Third lunar month

3.193   The progressive changes in fetal size and proportions during the third, fourth and fifth months.

baby units', and may be successfully raised if born prematurely. Its length has increased to about 350 mm and it weighs about 1.5 kg.

Remaining lunar months. Throughout the remaining lunar months of normal gestation the covering of vernix caseosa is prominent. There is a progressive loss of lanugo, except for the hairs on the eyelids, eyebrows and scalp. The bodily shape is becoming more infantile, but despite some acceleration in its growth the leg has not quite equalled the arm in length proportionately even at the time of birth. The thorax broadens relative to the head, and the infra-umbilical abdominal wall shows a relative areal increase, so that the umbilicus gradually becomes more centrally situated. Average lengths and weights for the eighth, ninth and tenth months are 40, 45 and 50 cm and 2, 2.5 and 3–3.5 kg.

Tenth lunar month. At the end of this month, just before birth, the lanugo has almost disappeared, the umbilicus is central and the testes, which begin to descend with the vaginal process of peritoneum during the seventh month and are approaching the scrotum in the ninth month, are usually scrotal in position. The ovaries are not yet in their final position at birth; although they have attained their final relationship to the uterine folds, they are still above the level of the pelvic brim.

The length of the period of gestation is regarded as nine calendar months in obstetric practice—approximately 270 days. It is usually about 266 days—10 lunar months less 14 days (see p. 344).

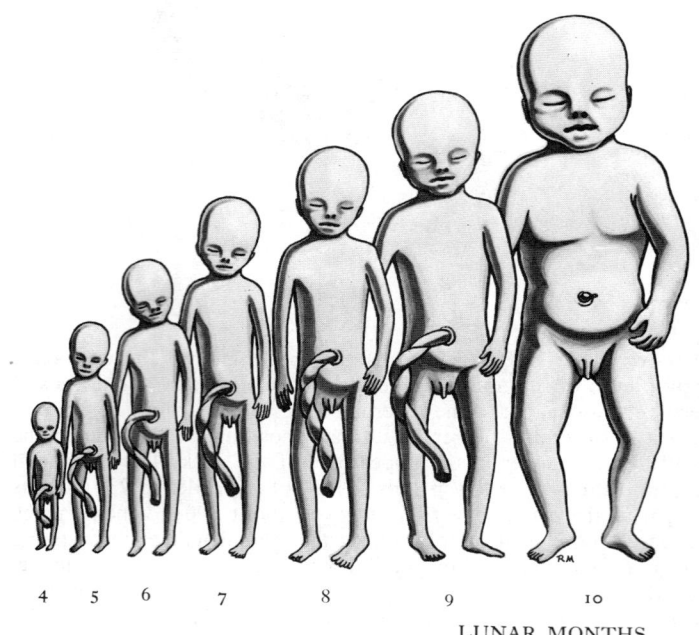

4   5   6   7   8   9   10

LUNAR MONTHS

3.194   Changes in *relative* size and bodily proportions at the fetal ages indicated.

CONGENITAL MALFORMATIONS AND PRENATAL DIAGNOSIS

INTRODUCTION

Infants have always been born with defects or anomalies. In early societies those surviving the neonatal period with developmental defects were often considered 'monsters'; they were viewed as throwbacks to undeveloped or underdeveloped types of humans, or thought to be a punishment to the mother or family. Records of human congenital malformations, in cave-paintings, sculptures and ultimately in writings, extend backwards into prehistory showing talipes, achondroplasia and conjoined twins, portrayed together with centaurs, sirens, mermaids and other fanciful creatures (Barrow 1971). The Hippocratic School identified hydrocephalus.

It was not until the seventeenth and eighteenth centuries that Harvey, Wolff, von Haller, the Hunters and their contemporaries, stimulated by the growing knowledge of embryology, initiated the *theory of embryonic arrest* to explain malformations. Saint-Hilaire experimented on developing chick embryos in the early nineteenth century, and with this approach the study of teratology (the origins and production of monsters) was consolidated as a science.

A commonly held belief that the experiences of the pregnant mother, usually visual, could influence her unborn offspring in an adverse manner is scarcely dead even today. However, that factors in the **maternal environment** may influence the embryo has proved true, but in a different sense, for Watson, as long ago as 1749, suggested that fetal disease, contracted by a transplacental route, might be a cause of congenital abnormality, citing variola as an example. This theory slowly dwindled, and was almost extinguished a century later by the authority of Virchow and His, whose views dominated teratological opinion through most of the second half of the nineteenth century. A contemporary, working in obscurity, was Mendel; as his work became known and genetics flowered into the twentieth century attention inevitably turned to the hereditary aspect of congenital defects (already foreshadowed by Paré and John Hunter, centuries earlier). In 1941 Gregg's observation that con-

genital cataract is associated with the infection of pregnant mothers by rubella revived interest in environmental factors.

Teratogenic causes

The expansion of experimental embryology has revealed a wide array of environmental agents capable of affecting normal development, including temperature variations, mechanical insult, variation in substances such as lithium and magnesium in culture media, exposure to irradiation, hypoxia, hypo- and hypervitaminosis, hormonal effects (especially with oestrogens and androgens), nutritional defects and exposure to various drugs and other chemicals. The identification of human teratogens may be said to have commenced with Gregg's demonstration of the effects of rubella virus. Other viral and bacterial maternal infections have since been implicated, especially cytomegalovirus and toxoplasmosis (see Table 3.2). But with the multiplication of drugs, for such purposes as abortion (aminopterin) and sedation (thalidomide), some of which have proved tragically teratogenic, teratological research has been much concentrated upon drugs.

A very large number of cytotoxic agents are now known, and many have been used as experimental teratogens, mostly on rodents. Some act as antimetabolites, amino-acid antagonists, antipurines or spindle toxins and most are highly selective in their effects, which are produced only by controlled dosage at specific periods during development. Wilson and Warkany (1965) formalized a methodology for screening drugs for teratogenicity in animals. Connors (1975) emphasized the complex array of variable parameters which help to determine whether an agent acts as a teratogen or not. These include embryonic age, the amount, route and mode of administration of the agent, placental and embryonic permeability, maternal or embryonic ability to inactivate the agent, the state of differentiation of target cells and their ability to recover. Sullivan (1975) reviewed the literature concerning teratogenic drugs taken by pregnant women, classifying them on their sites of action, whether directly on the

Table 3.2   Malformations caused by viral and bacterial maternal infections (Young 1992)

Teratogen	Critical period	Malformations
Rubella	Most affected if infection in first 6 weeks; very low risk >16 weeks	Congenital heart disease (especially patent ductus arteriosus), cataracts, microcephaly, mental handicap, sensorineural deafness, retinopathy, later insulin-dependent diabetes mellitus in 20%
Cytomegalovirus	Third or fourth month	Mental handicap or microcephaly occurs in 5–10% with congenital infection
Toxoplasmosis	12% risk at 6–17 weeks 60% risk at 17–28 weeks	Mental handicap, microcephaly, chorioretinitis
Alcohol	? First trimester	Mental handicap, microcephaly, congenital heart disease, renal anomaly, growth retardation, cleft palate, characteristic facies
Phenytoin (hydantoin)	First trimester; about 10% affected	Hypoplasia of distal phalanges, short nose, broad flat nasal bridge, ptosis, cleft lip and palate, mental handicap, later increased risk of malignancy, particularly neuroblastoma
Thalidomide	34–50 days from last menstrual period	Phocomelia, congenital heart disease, anal stenosis, atresia of external auditory meatus
Warfarin	Exposure at 6–9 weeks results in structural abnormalities in 30%; after 16 weeks mental handicap alone may be seen	Hypoplastic nose, upper airway difficulties, optic atrophy, stippled epiphyses, short distal phalanges, mental handicap
Chloroquine		Deafness, corneal opacities, chorioretinitis
Lithium		Congenital heart disease
Sodium valproate		Neural tube defect (1–2%), hypospadias, microstomia, small nose, long thin fingers

333

embryo (thalidomide, tetracycline antibiotics), on embryonic endocrine balance (oestrogens and androgens), on the placenta or on maternal tissues. These considerations are, of course, of intense clinical importance, but their contribution to explanations of teratogenic mechanisms is limited, except in so far as some drugs are known to be teratogenic at specific stages of development.

A chart of the known infectious and chemical teratogens is shown in Table 3.2.

Genetic causes

It has long been known that chromosomes and genes which regulate developmental processes may themselves be defective. The ways in which such defective chromosomes or genes may interact with other normal chromosomes, with the normal environmental conditions during development, or with abnormal environmental conditions, for example in infections or exposure to drugs, is not yet known. Study of such mechanisms forms the basis of genetic approaches to developmental perturbations and congenital malformations.

Genetic conditioning of congenital abnormalities whether structural, metabolic or behavioural has been the subject of very widespread research or observation. That alterations in the **number of chromosomes** can cause malformations was demonstrated in the 1950s, firstly when Tjio and Levan (1956) established the number of chromosomes in humans to be 46, and later in 1959 when Lejeune et al showed a tripling (trisomy) of chromosome 21.

From 1970 techniques became available for studying chromosomal banding and thus smaller aberrations of chromosomal structure. By 1989 in excess of 600 abnormalities of chromosomal structure had been described.

The first human anomaly to be identified as genetic was alkaptonuria (Garrod 1902), a rare condition in which patients have arthritis and urine which darkens on standing. It is now known to be a *single gene defect* causing deficiency of a single enzyme (homogentisic acid). Five enzyme defects had been identified by 1959 and that number had reached 200 by 1992. Genes can now be assigned to individual chromosomes. First those genes linked to the X chromosome were discovered. Later genes were mapped to the autosomes commencing with the thymidine kinase gene to chromosome 17 in 1967. So far 2316 genes have been mapped to their respective chromosomes and 40% of the Mendelian traits have been identified (Connor & Ferguson-Smith 1993).

The majority of congenital malformations seen in term neonates have not yet been linked either to specific chromosome aberrations or to single gene defects. This large group of malformations is believed to be caused by a number of pairs of genes producing additive effects which accrue until a threshold is passed; then morphological anomalies, which cannot be corrected by catch-up growth, result. Such malformations are termed *multifactorial disorders*. The number of genes involved is not known nor the mechanisms by which they interact with each other or the environment. More than 20 discontinuous multifactorial traits have been described; some cause congenital defects while others produce conditions seen commonly in adult life.

With the genetic and physical mapping reagents now becoming available considerable advances have been and are being made in the identification and localization of disease-genes. An impetus for this line of research was provided by The Human Genome Project (formally started in 1990), an international research effort to analyse the structure of human DNA and to determine the location of the estimated complement of about 100 000 human genes. So far about 2.3% of this total has been mapped. The Human Genome Project also includes the analysis of DNA from a set of non-human model species to provide comparative information about conserved gene action and how the human genome functions. For a review of the advances of the Human Genome Project see Guyer and Collins (1993).

Vulnerable periods of development

Information about the stage of gestation at which anomalies first appear has been obtained both by the correlation of malformations of particular organs and systems with the time at which those organs and systems develop, and by the direct experimental perturbation of development in animals to produce malformations similar to those seen in human infants. The time at which major organs develop can be indicated on a developmental scale (3.195). This allows examination of the state of development of each system at a given time.

Week	1	2	3	4	5	6	7	8	9	10	11	12
Crown-Rump Length: mm.			2	4	10	13	18	30				55
External appearance			Head & tail folding / pharyngeal arches			upper lip / palate		digits on hand / external ear	eyelids fuse			
Nervous system			neurulation / first neural crest cells	otic vesicle / optic cup		anterior lobe pituitary	posterior lobe pituitary / membranous labyrinth					
Respiratory				trachea / lung buds / primary bronchi			futher division of bronchi					
Gut			fore-mid hind-gut	thyroid liver / urorectal septum	pharyngeal pouches / dorsal & ventral pancreas / rotation of stomach		midgut loop rotating					midgut loop returns to abdomen
Kidney				mesonephroe / mesonephric duct / ureteric bud		metanephric nephrons / major calyces	minor calyces	kidneys ascend				
Genital			germ cells in allantoic wall / indifferent gonad		Mullerian ducts / testis differentiating / external genitalia indifferent			uterus & uterine tubes / vagina	testis at inguinal canal / prostate / external genitalia differeniating			
Cardiovascular		primative vascular system heart tube	septum primum / heart beats	septation of ventricles / spleen			septum secundum					
Musculoskeletal			somite period / 20 days...........................30 days / forelimb bud	forelimb digit rays / hind limb bud		cartilaginous part of skull	membranous part of skull				

3.195   Timetable of development. The development of individual systems can be seen progressing from left to right. To identify the systems and organs at risk at any time of development follow a vertical progression from top to bottom.

Although organogenesis is traditionally described for each system, all systems develop at the same time, within a very short period of the total gestation time. Thus, in **3**.195, it can be seen that little embryonic development occurs in the first two weeks (postovulatory) of gestation, when extraembryonic structures develop. Organogenesis occurs mainly between weeks 2 and 8, after which time tissue differentiation, growth and maturation continue to 38 weeks (see **3**.195).

Teratogenic insults may be embryotoxic or cause disruption of those systems undergoing major proliferative and morphological change. The time of the insult will be reflected in the systems affected. Genetic defects will affect earlier stages than teratogenic insults and may similarly result in abortion, but may also produce specific defects of tissue differentiation and genotypes with multiple anomalies which survive until term. Late malformations may be caused by mechanical effects.

Nomenclature

The identification of a developmental defect requires a description of the condition and an underlying knowledge of the development of the system or systems involved. In an attempt to standardize the descriptive terminology for birth defects, Spranger et al (1982) subdivided the all embracing title 'birth defect' into specific groups and recommended appropriate descriptive terms and their usage. The following terms were suggested:

- A *field defect* describes a collection of malformations affecting a developmental field, i.e. parts of an embryo which respond as a co-ordinated unit to a disturbance in development, or organs and tissues developing from a common origin, for example the neural crest. The latter may cause widespread (polytopic) effects.
- A *malformation* is defined as a primary structural defect of an organ or part of an organ resulting from an inherent abnormality in development, for example isolated, non-syndromal facial clefting or congenital heart disease.
- A *deformation* is a defect caused by an external mechanism affecting a normally formed organ or structure, for example talipes secondary to oligohydramnios.
- A *disruption* describes abnormal development as a result of external interference, which may be caused by: a *teratogen*—phenytoin causing distal limb hypoplasia; an *infection*—rubella causing cataracts; *trauma*—amniotic bands causing amputation.
- A *dysplasia* is defined as an abnormal organization of cells into a tissue, for example osteogenesis imperfecta. Many dysplasias are genetic and carry high recurrence risks for siblings and/or offspring, for example in skeletal defects like achondroplasia.
- A *sequence* describes multiple anomalies resulting from a single factor; for example, Potter sequence—here chronic leakage of amniotic fluid (or low urinary output)—leads to oligohydramnios which in turn leads to fetal compression causing talipes, dislocation of the hips, squashed facies and pulmonary hypoplasia.
- A *syndrome* is defined as a pattern of anomalies known to be causally related which do not constitute a sequence or a polytopic field defect. A syndrome can be caused by a chromosome abnormality, for example Down's syndrome; a single gene defect, for example Meckel syndrome; or an environmental agent, for example fetal alcohol syndrome.
- An *association* describes the non-random occurrence of multiple anomalies which fit none of the above definitions. Such associations are often described as an acronym; for example the VATER association includes Vertebral, Anal, Tracheo-Esophageal and Renal anomalies.

Congenital anomalies are also described as 'major' or 'minor'. A major defect is one which results in mortality or significant morbidity, whereas a minor defect would not affect normal life expectancy; an example of the latter would be a supernumerary nipple. However, it has been noted that the occurrence of an isolated minor malformation may indicate a more serious underlying problem, and that multiple minor malformations may be the only external features of an underlying syndrome (Young 1992).

Incidence

It may be stated with some veracity that defects of the genome account for the vast majority of spontaneous abortions in early pregnancy, defects seen at birth, defects in childhood and a range of adult disorders. The production of an appropriate genome is the first essential for an individual and later the satisfactory interaction of a particular genome with its environment can be described as 'health'. Thus examination of the statistics for congenital anomalies shows, in the main, the incidence of inappropriate genome production and the consequences of aberrant genome expression surviving to birth and childhood.

At least 15% of all recognized pregnancies result in spontaneous abortion before 12 weeks gestation, with 80% of spontaneously aborted embryos having major disturbances of development, often as a result of a non-viable cytogenetic abnormality (Young 1992). Chromosomal abnormalities occur in approximately 40% of unselected spontaneous abortions (Hsu 1986); of these autosomal trisomy accounts for 52%, monosomy X 19%, triploidy 16%, and tetraploidy 6%. Of the fetuses spontaneously aborted in the second trimester of pregnancy, up to 20 weeks gestation, 25% have morphological malformations.

The perinatal period extends from 28 weeks gestation to 7 days postnatally. Surveys indicate that approximately 25–30% of all perinatal deaths are caused by lethal congenital malformations. Neonatal deaths, up to 28 days postnatally, have a similar incidence (Young 1992).

Deaths from congenital malformations extend beyond the perinatal and neonatal periods into childhood making a significant contribution to childhood mortality. Population studies showed that in England and Wales in the period 1980–85, 27% of all deaths of infants under 1 year of age, 19% of all deaths of children aged 1–9 years and 7.5% of deaths of children aged 10–14 years were caused by congenital malformations.

From these figures it is apparent that at least 25–30% of human conceptions are malformed to some degree and that, generally, about 2–3% of all babies have at least one major malformation apparent at birth. The true incidence would also include malformations presenting later in life and would nearly double the value. Minor malformations of no medical or cosmetic significance are found in about 10% of the general population (Young 1992). For a summary of the incidence of malformations see Table 3.3.

It is beyond the scope of this text to give an in depth account of the thousands of defects now described. A selection of genome defects referred to in other parts of the embryology section will be outlined. The interested reader is recommended to study the list of some 385 diagnosable Mendelian disorders listed by Connor (1992).

Chromosomal defects

The defective separation of chromosomes at meiosis can result in tripling of individual chromosomes, *trisomy*. Apart from chromosome 1, each type of autosomal trisomy has been seen. Trisomy

Table 3.3 Overall incidence of malformations

	% Incidence
All babies	
Major malformations	
Apparent at birth	2–3
Apparent later	2
Minor malformations	10
Spontaneous miscarriages	
First trimester	85
Second trimester	25
Deaths in perinatal period	25
Deaths in first year of life	25
Deaths from 1 to 9 years	20
Deaths from 10 to 14 years	7.5

16 is especially frequent in conceptuses but rarely survives to late gestation. Fetuses with a triploid or tetraploid chromosome complement, in the main, abort before term. Sex chromosome trisomies rarely abort, whereas sex chromosome deletions (XO) often abort. Table 3.4 shows the main chromosomal anomalies.

Unbalanced deletions or duplications. Chromosomal defects are also seen in cases where a portion of one chromosome is translocated to another location. If the resulting conceptus receives the full complement of chromosomes the condition is said to be a *balanced translocation* and no defect will result. If on the other hand the conceptus receives either a gain or loss of chromosomal material the condition is said to be an *unbalanced translocation* and the conceptus will either abort or develop multiple dysmorphic features. A number of conditions resulting from an unbalanced chromosomal complement have been described; an example is the *Prader–Willi syndrome* caused by microdeletion at 15q11–13. Affected individuals have hypotonia and poor swallowing in the neonatal period; this improves with age and overeating and obesity develop. The external genitalia are hypoplastic.

Single gene defects

Single gene defects are inherited as autosomal dominant, autosomal recessive, X-linked dominant or X-linked recessive traits. A number of such gene defects are shown in Table 3.5 with the mode of inheritance and the chromosomal location of the gene where this is known.

X-linked gene defects. Vitamin D resistant rickets is an example of an X-linked dominant trait. Both males and females may be affected. In some other X-linked dominant conditions the affected males spontaneously abort.

X-linked recessive traits are more common; up to 368 have so far been identified and include:

- Duchenne muscular dystrophy (Xp21.2)
- Androgen insensitivity syndrome: testicular feminization, female phenotype, normal breast development, primary amenorrhoea, blind vaginal pouch, intra-abdominal testes
- Colour blindness: 3 Loci, blue (Ch7) and red and green (Xq28)
- Haemophilia: type A deficiency of factor VIII (Xq28); type B deficiency of factor IX (Xq27).

Multifactorial disorders

Multifactorial disorders account for the vast majority of anomalies detected in the fetal and neonatal period. In some cases some of the genes involved have been identified and correlated to specific developmental events.

DiGeorge's syndrome has a microdeletion at 22q11 in 15–20% of patients. The condition demonstrates a failure of neural crest migration particularly into pharyngeal arches 3 and 4. Clinical features include absence (or near absence) of the thymus, parathyroids and thyroid, hypoplasia of the wall of the arteries derived from the aortic arches, outflow track malformations, dysmorphic faces, fish-like mouth, down-slanting palpebral fissures. The condition can be induced experimentally in *Hox a–c* nul mice.

Hirschsprung's disease is inherited as a multifactorial trait. One in 5000–8000 neonates is affected, more females than males. It results from failure of the neural crest neurons to invade the gut wall leading to an aganglionic section (see p. 235).

Potter's sequence ensues from the absence of the kidneys and results in oligohydramnios, pulmonary hypoplasia, low set ears, squashed facies, talipes, amnion nodosum.

Wilm's tumour is nephroblastoma, diagnosed for 50% of cases within the first 3 years. It may be associated with microdeletions at 11p13. Patients also have aniridia, genitourinary malformations and mental and growth retardation. Wilm's tumour is often seen in

Table 3.4 The main chromosomal anomalies

Autosomal trisomy	Changes in sex chromosome number
Trisomy 13 (Patau's syndrome). Incidence is 1 in 5000 live births with a maternal age effect. Features include holoprosencephaly, sloping forehead, deafness, mental retardation, convulsions. Multiple eye anomalies (microphthalmia, colobomata), hyperteleorism, cleft lip, cleft palate, abnormal and low set ears. Clenched fists, rotation of thumbs, 'rocker bottom feet', cardiac defects. 50% of those affected die within the first month and only 10% survive beyond the first year. *Trisomy 18 (Edwards' syndrome).* Incidence is 1 in 3000 live births. 95% of affected fetuses abort spontaneously. Preponderance of females at birth. Features include narrow biparietal diameter, occipital prominence, mental retardation, short palpebral fissures, small mouth, low set ears, overlapping fingers, 'rocker bottom feet' or prominent heels, short sternum, cardiac defects. Birth weight is low and infants fail to thrive; 30% die within a month and only 10% survive beyond first year. *Trisomy 21 (Down's syndrome).* The overall incidence is 1 in 700 live births, with a much greater incidence at conception of which 60% abort spontaneously and about 20% are stillborn. The incidence increases with maternal age (1 in 300 for a 35-year-old mother, 1 in 22 for a 45-year-old mother). Generally the mother contributes the extra chromosome in 85% of cases and the father in 15% (Connor & Ferguson-Smith 1993). Features include mental retardation, short stature, stumpy limbs, brachycephalic skull. Typically the facies consists of open mouth, protruding fissured tongue, short nose, epicanthic folds and oblique palpebral fissures. The eyes have Brushfield spots. Hands and feet are broad with short fingers and toes. A single transverse palmar crease is often present (50%) and the little fingers are short and incurved (50%). A wide gap may be present between the first and second toes. Unless affected individuals suffer from serious cardiac malformations life expectancy is little reduced. Trisomy 21 accounts for about one-quarter of all moderate and severe mental handicap in children of school age. Affected people rarely reproduce; presenile dementia commonly occurs after 40 years of age.	*XXX.* Seen in 1 in 1000 females. Individuals appear clinically normal; 15–25% may have mild mental handicap. *XX Males.* 1 in 20 000 males may have a dislocation of the testis determining gene, Yp11.2 to Xp. Diagnosis may follow the prenatal prediction of a female infant, or patients may complain of infertility. This condition causes sterility, small testes and the endocrine feature of Klinefelter's syndrome. *XXY (Klinefelter's syndrome).* Birth incidence is 1 in 100 males; it results from non-disjunction with 47% of cases having a maternal origin for the extra X chromosome and 53% a paternal origin. This condition is the single commonest cause of hypogonadism and infertility in men. Testes do not produce the adult levels of testosterone which leads to poorly developed secondary sexual characteristics and gynaecomastia. *XYY.* Birth incidence is 1 in 1000 male births. The condition appears to be frequent in males in penal institutions for the mentally subnormal (20 in 1000). *XO (Turner's syndrome).* The incidence is 1 in 5000 female births with a much higher conception rate, 99% of which spontaneously abort. Monosomy X may arise from non-disjunction in either parent; in 80% of cases the maternal X is present. Features include hypogonadism; ovaries are absent or contain fibrous streaks but no Graafian follicles (streak ovary); short stature, no adolescent growth spurt, primary amenorrhoea. The neck may be webbed with a triangular fold of skin extending on each side from the mastoid outward towards the acromion. The chest is wide with an increased intermammary distance. The carrying angle may be increased. There is hypoplasia of the nails.

Table 3.5   Inheritance of single gene defects (Connor & Ferguson-Smith 1993)

Autosomal dominant genes	
Condition	Gene position
Achondroplasia. Short limbs especially proximally	
Apert syndrome. Craniosynostosis of calvarial sutures and bony syndactyly of digits	
Huntington's chorea. Late onset intellectual decline, seizures, myoclonus. CT scan shows caudate and putamen atrophy	Gene locus on 4p. Age dependent penetrance
Marfan's syndrome. Long limbs, lax joints, scoliosis. Lifespan 40–50 years	Mutations in fibrillin 1 gene on chromosome 15
Osteogenesis imperfecta. Brittle bones, 4 types described	Defect in collagen production due to genes on 7q & 17q
Treacher Collins' syndrome. Mandibulofacial dysostosis	Linkage to chromosome 5q demonstrated
Waardenburg's syndrome. White forelock, heterochromia iridis, deafness and telecanthus	Locus on 2q

Autosomal recessive genes	
Condition	Gene position
β-thalassaemia. Homozygotes have severe chronic anaemia due to ineffective erythropoiesis	Defect in β-globin gene cluster 11p identified, but at least 91 different point mutations produce the disorder
Cystic fibrosis. Pancreatic insufficiency; chronic lung disease secondary to recurrent infection	Mutations in cystic fibrosis transmembrane conductance regulator gene, 7q31
Friedreich's ataxia. Progressive ataxia, patients chairbound in second decade, death in third decade	Gene on 9q
Sickle cell anaemia. Blood film shows distorted erythrocytes. Some persistent fetal haemoglobin	Point mutation in amino-acid position 6 of β globin (E6V) which results in substitution of valine for glutamic acid
Congenital adrenal hyperplasia. Virilization of female, ambiguous genitalia. Neonatal vomiting, shock and death	Gene conversion or unequal crossing over of active cytochrome P450 genes, involved in steroid 21-hydroxylation, on Ch6
Mucopolysaccharidoses: Hurler's syndrome; Sanfilippo' syndrome; Morquio's disease; (Hunter's syndrome—X-linked recessive)	Deficiencies of specific enzymes
Phenylketonuria. Elevated blood and urine phenylalanine	Mutations in phenylalanine hydroxylase

patients with *Beckwith–Wiedemann syndrome* where a paternal deletion has been found at 11p15. Clinical features include macroglossia, anterior abdominal wall defects, high birth weight and hemihypertrophy.

Other congenital anomalies of the various body systems are considered to be of multifactorial origin; they are considered within the development of each system.

Mechanical effects

A number of congenital malformations are caused by mechanical effects, particularly the reduction of amniotic fluid and formation of amniotic bands. Oligohydramnios will cause pulmonary hypoplasia and positional defects such as talipes. Other types of deformation include congenital dislocation of the hip, congenital postural scoliosis, pterygia and mandibular asymmetry. The development of amniotic bands, strands of amnion produced by premature amniotic rupture, can cause limb amputations and, by adherence of such bands to other parts of the fetus, a variety of other defects including facial clefts.

TWINNING

Twinning occurs once in about every 80 births. Twins may be dizygotic (binovular or fraternal) or monozygotic (uniovular or identical), of which the former occurs more frequently.

Dizygotic twinning

Dizygotic twins result from multiple ovulations which can be induced by gonadotrophins or drugs such as clomiphene (commonly used in patients with infertility). There is increasing evidence that the trigger for spontaneous multiple ovulations is higher follicle-stimulating hormone (FSH) levels in twin-bearing mothers. Studies on the Nigerian Yoruba tribe, which has a high incidence of dizygotic twinning, has shown elevated levels of FSH and luteinizing hormone (LH) compared to Caucasians, whereas in Japanese women, with a very low twinning rate, the FSH and LH levels were significantly lower (Nylander 1973; Soma et al 1975). Studies of hormone levels during the first four days of menstruation in women who had at

least one set of twins, compared to those who had no twins, showed that FSH and oestradiol levels were both elevated in twin-bearing mothers (Martin et al 1984). Benirschke (1992) suggests that a gene may be responsible for higher FSH levels and thus be the cause of familial twinning. He notes that it is not yet clear whether the effect of increased FSH production seen in twin-bearing mothers is the result of a greater number of pituitary cells, more GNRH production or greater sensitivity of ovarian follicles.

Monozygotic twinning

Monozygotic twins arise from a single ovum fertilized by a single sperm. At some stage up to the establishment of the axis of the embryonic area and the development of the primitive streak the formative material separates into two parts, each of which gives rise to a complete embryo. The resultant twins have the same genotype, but the description 'identical twins' is best avoided as most monozygotic twins have differences in phenotypes.

Almost all studies on the incidence of monozygotic twinning have shown that it occurs with the same frequency over ages and populations (Benirschke 1992). No causative factor has been identified. Although experimentally the separation of blastomeres in early gestation can result in two or more individual embryos, only in the nine-banded armadillo do such divisions occur regularly. In this species division of the early conceptus results in monozygotic quadruplets. Division of the later stages of conception may occur; the process of hatching of the blastocyst from the zona pellucida may result in constriction of the emerging cells and separation into two discrete entities. Interestingly, identical twinning occurs more frequently after human in vitro fertilization (9 sets of identical twins amongst 600 IVF births; Edwards et al 1986). The most likely explanation for this is damage to the zona pellucida, resulting in abnormal hatching of the human embryo through the narrow artificial gaps and subsequent inner cell mass splitting (Alikani et al 1994). There is a gradual decrease in the average thickness of the zona pellucida with increasing maternal age, which may be causally related to the increase in frequency of monozygotic twinning with increased maternal age (Bulmer 1970; Alikani et al 1994).

It is thought that the ability of the early conceptus to regulate cell numbers and overall size is limited to the first 14 days of development. The precise time at which developmental regulation to produce twins ceases is unknown but is thought to correspond to this time span (Snow 1989). After twinning monozygotic embryos enter a period of intense catch-up growth. Despite starting out at half the size, each twin embryo or fetus is of comparable size to a singleton fetus in the second trimester of pregnancy, but declines in relative size in the last 10 weeks of pregnancy.

Late separation of twins from a single conceptus may result in conjoined twins; these may be equal as in some varieties of 'Siamese twins', or unequal as in acardia.

Placentae in twinning

The range of separation of the embryos is reflected in the separation of the extraembryonic membranes. The following types of placentation can occur (**3**.196):

- diamnionic, dichorionic separated
- diamnionic, dichorionic fused
- diamnionic, monochorionic
- monoamnionic, monochorionic.

The stage at which monozygotic twinning occurs will reflect the

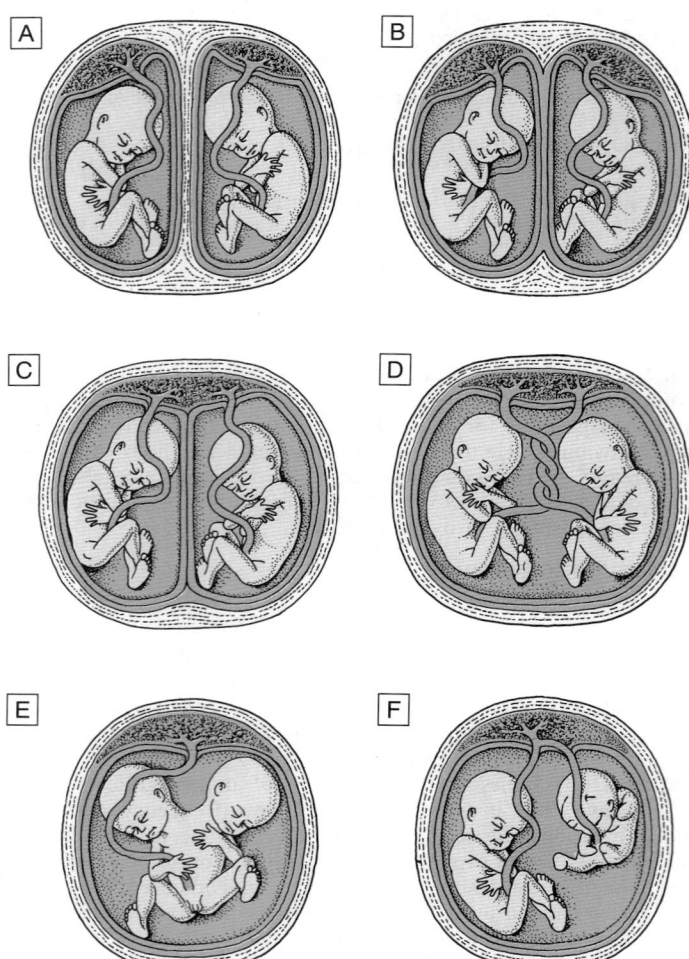

3.196 Schema of the relationships of the extraembryonic membranes in different types of twinning.

(A). Diamnionic, dichorionic separated, i.e. separation of the first two blastomeres results in separate implantation sites. (B). Diamnionic, dichorionic fused; here the chorionic membranes are fused but the fetuses occupy separate choria. (C). Diamnionic, monochorionic; reduplication of the inner cell mass can result in a single placenta and chorionic sacs but separate amniotic cavities. (D). Monoamnionic, monochorionic; duplication of the embryonic axis results in two embryos sharing a single placenta, chorion and amnion. (E). Incomplete separation of the embryonic axis results in conjoined twins ('Siamese twins'). (F). Unequal division of the embryonic axis or unequal division of the blood supply may result in an acardiac monster.

type of placentation seen. Monozygotic twinning may be diagnosed when monochorionic placentae are found, but only two-thirds of monozygotic twins have such placentae (with monoamnionic, monochorionic occurring in approximately 1–2% of twins). Of the dichorionic placentae, about 8% have been shown to be associated with monozygotic twins (Cameron 1968).

Monoamnionic, monochorionic placentae are associated with the highest perinatal mortality (>50%), caused both by entangling of the umbilical cords impeding the blood supply and by various vascular shunts between the placentae which may divert blood from one fetus to the other. Artery–artery anastomoses are the commonest followed by artery–vein anastomoses. If the shunting of blood across the placentae from one twin to the other is balanced by more than one vascular connection, development may proceed unimpaired. However, if this is not the case one twin may receive blood from the other leading to cardiac enlargement, increased urination and hydramnios in the recipient, and anaemia, oligohydramnios and atrophy in the donor.

Dizygotic twins have either completely separate chorionic sacs or sacs which have fused. Such placentae are separated by four membranes, two amnia and two choria; in addition such placentae have a ridge of firmer tissue at the base of the dividing membranes caused by the abutting of two expanding placental tissues against each other (Benirschke 1992). There may be size differences between diamnionic, dichorionic placentae because of intrauterine competition for space.

Sex ratio of twins

The sex of twins will be the same for monozygotic twins (which have the same genotype) and may be different for dizygotic twins. Interestingly there is an excess of like-sex pairs among dizygotic twins (James 1971). Monoamnionic, monochorionic, monozygotic twins are most likely to be female, as are acardiac twins. A prospective twin study in Belgium indicated that the proportion of males was reduced in monozygotic twins, irrespective of chorionic status, and there was a marked reduction of male monoamnionic, monochorionic twins compared to a random occurrence (Derom et al 1988). The male/female ratio for all monozygotic twins was 0.487, while for monoamnionic, monochorionic twins it was 0.231; dizygotic twins had a ratio of 0.518.

Multiple births

Multiple births greater than twinning, such as triplets or quadruplets, can arise from multiple ovulations, a single ovum, or both. It is most likely to be seen in women treated with drugs to stimulate ovulation.

For an excellent review of the types, frequency, inheritance and embryology of twinning, the diagnosis of their zygosity, the course and outcome of twin pregnancies, their possible evolutionary significance and some postnatal characteristics of twins, the interested reader should consult Bulmer (1970).

PRENATAL DIAGNOSIS AND TREATMENT

In the last 20 years a variety of techniques has been developed for the prenatal detection and diagnosis of many congenital disorders. They have entered into obstetric practice and are an important part of antenatal care. There are two broad types of testing for congenital disorders: screening and diagnostic.

Prenatal screening may be undertaken using biochemical, genetic or ultrasonic methods. Such methods will detect a subgroup of those tested who are at higher risk of having a disease or disorder than the original population screened. *Diagnostic tests* are usually more complex and their aim is to give a definitive answer, particularly if a suspicion of a problem has been raised by a screening test. They may be non-invasive, like a detailed high resolution ultrasound scan, but many are invasive providing samples of different fetal tissue for analysis.

Biochemical screening

Maternal blood samples may be taken at 16–18 weeks of pregnancy to screen for Down's syndrome and open neural tube defects. There are four main markers of Down's syndrome: advanced maternal age, raised maternal serum human chorionic gonadotrophin (hCG), low maternal serum unconjugated oestriol (uE_3), and low maternal serum alphafetoprotein (AFP). Of these the most discriminatory serum

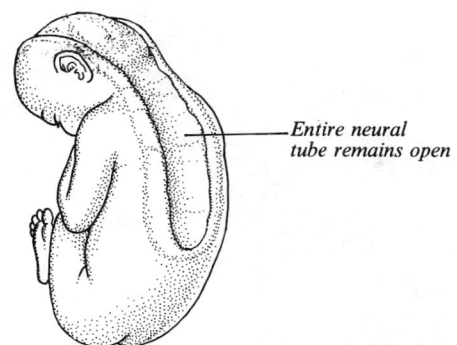

Entire neural tube remains open

Craniorachischisis

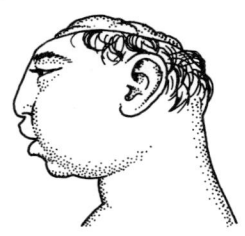

Anencephaly

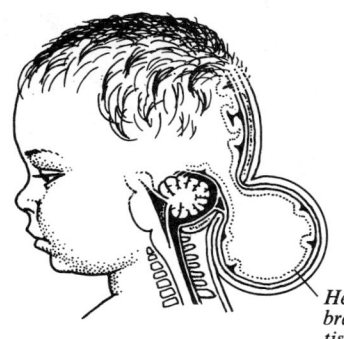

Herniated brain tissue

Meningoencephalocoele

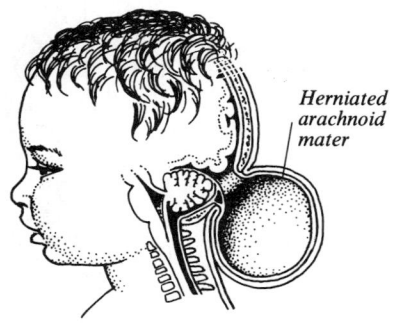

Herniated arachnoid mater

Cranial meningocoele

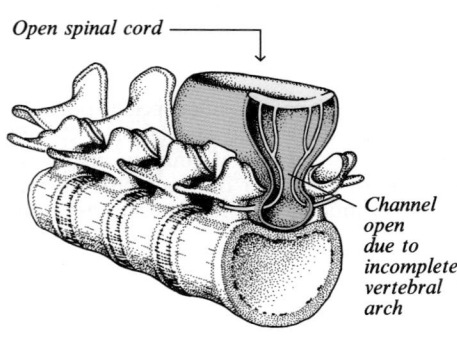

Open spinal cord

Channel open due to incomplete vertebral arch

Myelocoele

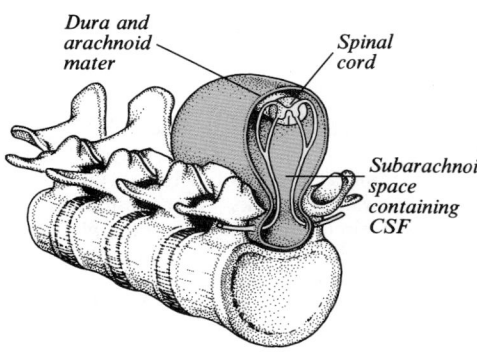

Dura and arachnoid mater

Spinal cord

Subarachnoid space containing CSF

Meningomyelocoele

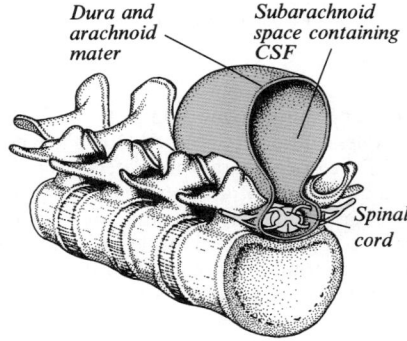

Dura and arachnoid mater

Subarachnoid space containing CSF

Spinal cord

Meningocoele

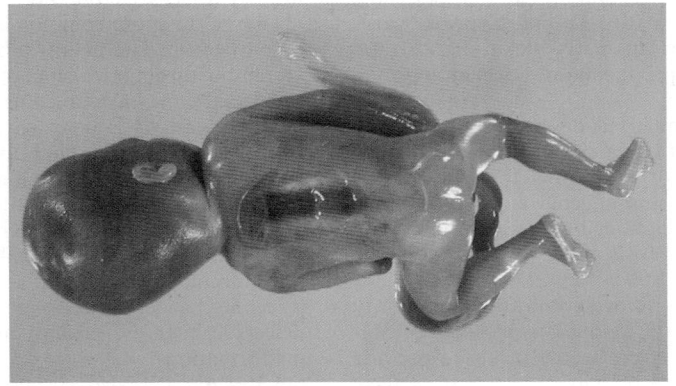

3.197 Some of the defects caused by failure of neural tube formation.
A. total failure of neurulation. B. failure of cranial neurulation. C. failure of spinal cord neurulation.

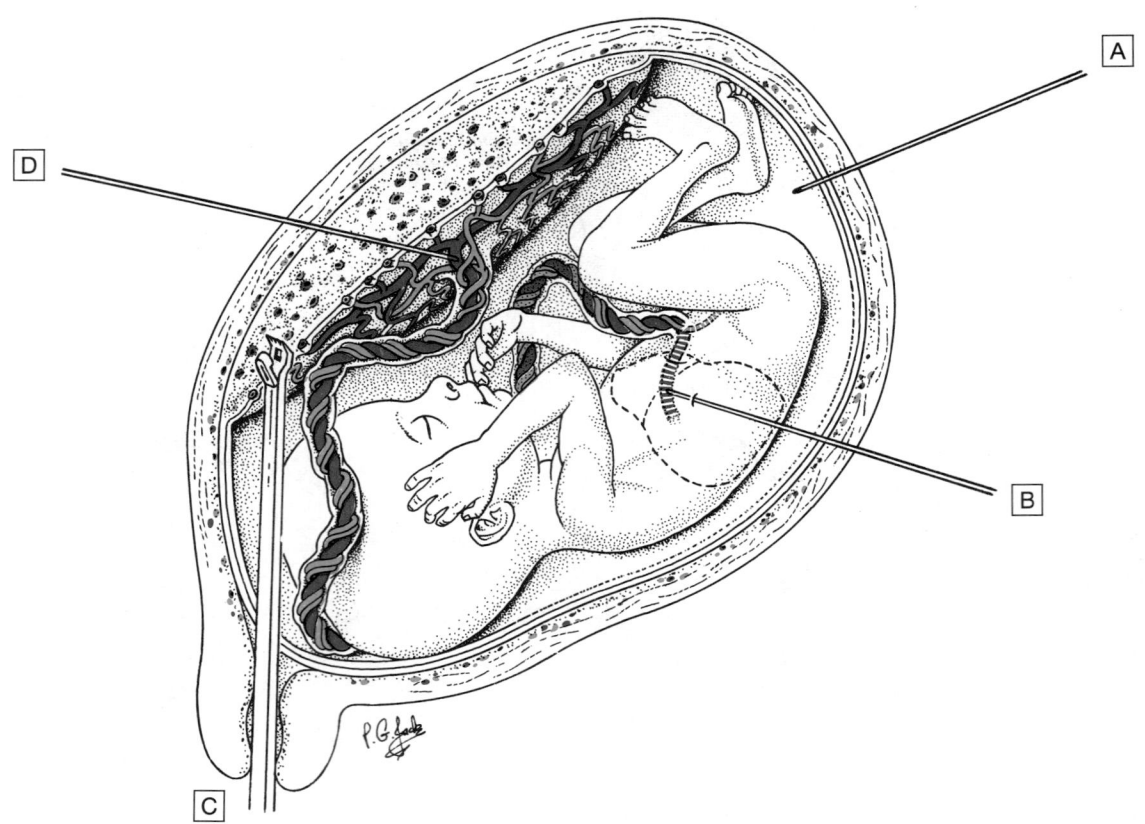

3.198   Diagram showing methods of fetal tissue sampling. (A) = needle in amniotic cavity to aspirate amniotic fluid (amniocentesis); (B) = needle into intrahepatic umbilical vein for fetal blood sampling. Note that the structures shown in this diagram are not to scale and that these procedures are not performed at the same gestational age; (C) = biopsy forceps passing through cervix into placenta (transcervical chorionic villus sampling); (D) = needle into umbilical vein at placental cord insertion to aspirate fetal blood sample.

marker for this condition is hCG. Examination of maternal blood samples will detect 60% of Down's syndrome.

Of the open neural tube defects, the most severe, craniorachischisis and anencephaly, are most easily detected by ultrasound. AFP leaks into the amniotic fluid and then into the maternal circulation in cases of open spina bifida. At 16–18 weeks levels of AFP in amniotic fluid are four times greater in open spina bifida than in unaffected pregnancies and there is a corresponding rise in AFP detected in the maternal serum. Such testing can detect 90% of cases, although the risk of false positives must be taken into account.

Genetic screening

As carriers of recessive disorders are not diseased, genetic screening affects future generations rather than the individuals tested. Diseases that are currently included in screening programmes are mainly inherited as autosomal recessive disorders. The genes responsible for such disorders are very common in the general population, especially in some subgroups; for example, up to 17% of Cypriots carry thalassaemia, and 23% of West Africans carry sickle cell disease. The chances of affected individuals producing an affected offspring is therefore higher in these groups.

Options open to carriers of an inherited disease are: to remain childless; to select a partner who is not a carrier of the same disease; to use artificial insemination by donor or another form of assisted reproduction; to ensure that only a non-affected embryo implants by preimplantation diagnosis on an eight-cell embryo; to terminate a pregnancy found by antenatal diagnosis to be affected (Chapple 1992).

To assist with such decisions early information about the newly formed conceptus is desirable. New techniques, especially of molecular cytogenetics, will be at the forefront in the future to provide such information. At present accurate diagnosis of genetic defects relies on the collection of fetal cells from amniocentesis, the culture of these cells and the analysis of metaphase chromosomes resulting in the production of a karyotype. This may take 16–20 days. The

use of DNA probes now permits the visualization of specific portions of chromatin in interphase. Detection of fetal sex, trisomy 18 and 13 can now be accomplished on examination of amniotic cells. It is suggested that the identification of a number of genetic defects will be possible via early chorionic examination in the future (Ferguson-Smith 1992).

Ultrasound screening

Ultrasonography is an imaging technique used for screening which can detect structural abnormalities and malformations. It can be performed and repeated without risk to mother or fetus and most women in the United Kingdom have such a scan at 18 to 20 weeks of pregnancy. Advanced ultrasonography requires high level skills and experience in the operator as well as knowledge of embryonic and fetal dysmorphology. A systematic anatomical survey of the head, face, brain, spinal cord, heart, chest, abdomen and its contents, urinary tract, skeleton and limbs is carried out.

One of the more common abnormalities that may be seen is spina bifida (**3**.197). The neural tube fails to close leaving a defect in the vertebrae, through which may protrude the meninges with or without the spinal cord (myelomeningocoele and meningocoele respectively). Often this lesion is detected by chance, or attention is drawn to it because associated cranial abnormalities may be seen, for example enlargement of the cerebral ventricles, or a lemon-shaped head due to concavity of the frontal bones. It may also present with an abnormal screening test, i.e. a raised maternal serum AFP. Spina bifida causes very severe handicap and most women with an affected fetus decide to terminate the pregnancy. The widespread use of screening has led to a 90% reduction in the incidence of neural tube defects at birth. Ultrasonography may detect up to 70% of all major malformations.

Ultrasound is also essential for the safe performance of all the invasive procedures. Such procedures are not without risk but in expert hands the fetal loss rate is increased by no more than 1–2%. The ultrasound scan reveals the intrauterine anatomy and enables the guidance of the instrument (needle or biopsy forceps) into the target, i.e. the amniotic cavity for amniocentesis, the placenta for chorionic villus sampling, the umbilical vein at the placental insertion of the umbilical cord or the intrahepatic tract of the umbilical vein for fetal blood sampling and the appropriate organ or structure for other tissues (**3**.198).

Prenatal treatment

A few of the abnormalities revealed by screening may be treated prenatally. Metabolic diseases and deficiencies have been treated, for example, by the administration of maternal corticosteroids for the prevention of respiratory distress in the premature infant, and by the administration of dexamethasone for congenital adrenal hyperplasia. Fetal cardiac arrhythmias can be treated by maternally administered agents.

One of the first fetal therapies, attributed to Liley (1963), was the intraperitoneal transfusion of blood for the treatment of severe erythrocyte alloimmunization. Access to the fetal circulation is now achieved by percutaneous umbilical blood sampling and intravascular transfusion using ultrasound guidance.

Fetal surgical techniques have developed recently, leading to a number of successful procedures which can promote normal growth during the latter part of pregnancy. Severe hydrothorax due to fluid in the pleural cavities causes pulmonary hypoplasia because pressure on the lungs and compression of the heart leads to heart failure and oedema (hydrops fetalis). These potentially fatal consequences can be prevented by placing a coiled catheter across the thoracic wall so that the hydrothorax can drain into the amniotic fluid and relieve the pressure in the chest. Urinary tract obstruction has been treated in utero, also hydrocephalus and, recently, congenital diaphragmatic herniae. At present many of these operations have limited success and are only appropriate for selected cases. For a review of fetal therapy, particularly the experiences of the Fetal Treatment Programme at the University of California, see Kuller and Golbus (1992).

Most malformations that are detected prenatally are definitively treated after birth. Often, however, awareness of the problem before birth leads to improved management and allows the parents to prepare themselves psychologically. In gastroschisis, for example, most of the gut has herniated through a small hole in the abdominal wall and floats freely in the amniotic fluid (**3**.199). Towards the end of the pregnancy the condition of the gut can deteriorate and the aim is to deliver the baby before this happens. Careful ultrasonographic monitoring is required to time this correctly so that the baby and its gut are in optimal condition for immediate postnatal surgery. In such circumstances the results are excellent.

With the rapidly increasing possibilities for prenatal diagnosis and treatment and the greater understanding provided by the basic sciences, the fetus is now regarded as a patient and is the focus of the new discipline of fetal medicine.

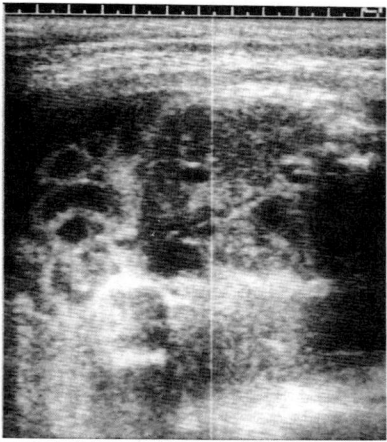

3.199 Ultrasound scan of cross section of fetal trunk with gastroschisis. Free loops of gut are seen floating in the amniotic fluid on the left.

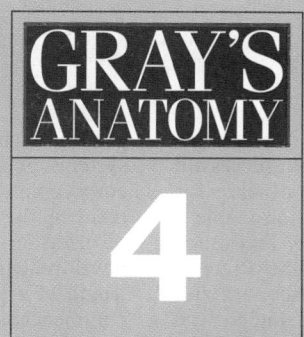

GRAY'S ANATOMY

4

NEONATAL ANATOMY AND GROWTH

Section Editor: Patricia Collins

Professor Edmund Crelin's publications provided much of the data for this chapter. The late Professor Peter Williams nurtured the inspiration, encouraged the development and supported the final birth of the chapter. Vitality has been added by two artists, Peter Jack and Peter Lamb; and Dr Mike Hall supplemented the whole with an essay on neonatal procedures. I am grateful to them all.

NEONATAL ANATOMY

Neonatology as a distinct discipline has a fairly recent origin. In Western societies technological advances have enabled successful management of full-term neonates to form the basis of care for preterm infants, many at ages which were considered non-viable a decade or two previously. Now, the study of neonatology very much overlaps the later stages of embryology and development. Preterm infants, although obviously past organogenetic processes, are still engaged in maturational processes with local interactions and pattern formation driving development at local and body system levels. The sudden release of such fetuses into a gaseous environment, of variable temperature, with full gravity and a range of micro-organisms, promotes the rapid maturation of some systems and the compensational growth, in terms of effect of gravity, or enteral feeding, or exposure to micro-organisms, of others. To understand this multitude of mechanisms operating within a newly delivered fetus, as much information concerning normal embryological and fetal development as possible is required. Today there are many texts on neonatal physiology but fewer which set out the basic differences between the anatomy of the full-term neonate and the adult. However, just as there are immense differences in the relations of some structures between the full-term neonate, child and adult, so there are also major differences between the 20 week gestation fetus and the 40 week fetus, just prior to birth. Thus the study of fetal anatomy at 20, 25, 30 and 35 weeks is vital for the investigative and life-saving procedures carried out on preterm infants today. This section has drawn together the available information on the anatomy of the full-term (40 week gestation, see below) neonate and added, where appropriate, notes on the preterm neonate. The reader is recommended to consult Crelin (1973) from which much of the basic anatomical information was acquired. Crelin notes particularly that the newborn infant is not a miniature adult; it is also important to note that very low-weight, early preterm, infants are similarly not the same as full-term infants.

Estimation of the developmental age of neonates

The development of embryos is described in terms of 'stages' (see p. 135), each stage being a time period during which a variety of systems or organs attain a particular stage of development. Such embryonic stages are based on a linear scale of development commencing at fertilization and ending at stage 23 (8 weeks after fertilization) when the embryo becomes a fetus. Using this scale, development averages 266 days, or 9.5 months. To estimate the **length of a pregnancy** to provide an estimated date of delivery, the commencement of gestation is traditionally determined **clinically** by counting from the date of the last menstrual period. Estimated in this manner it averages 280 days, or 10 lunar months (40 weeks). **4**.1 shows the two time scales used to depict embryonic development and the stage of pregnancy. Throughout the Embryology section, development is described from the time of fertilization, as depicted in the upper scale in **4**.1. However, when discussing fetal development and the gestational age of neonates, particularly those born before 40 weeks gestation (see below), the clinically estimated stage is invariably used in the literature. Thus in Neonatology and Growth descriptions of fetal stages and neonatal anatomy are related to the lower of the scales in **4**.1, the clinically derived weeks of pregnancy.

The period of pregnancy is often divided into thirds, termed *trimesters*. The first and second trimesters each cover a period of 12 weeks, and the third trimester covers the period from 24 weeks to delivery. Although the expected date of delivery is computed at 40 weeks of pregnancy, the *term* of the pregnancy, i.e. its completion resulting in delivery, is considered normal between 37 and 42 weeks. Neonates delivered before 37 weeks are called *preterm* (or *premature*) and after 42 weeks, *post term*. The period immediately prior to, and up to 7 days after, birth is termed the *perinatal period*; the commencement of the perinatal period is from the end of week 24 and infants born from this stage of pregnancy are classed as stillborn and contribute to the statistics of perinatal mortality if they die, whereas those fetuses which are delivered and die prior to this time are considered to be miscarriages of pregnancy. The technological advances in neonatal care can now assist the delivery and support of infants younger than 24 weeks. The *neonatal period* extends from birth to 28 days postnatally; it is divided into an early neonatal

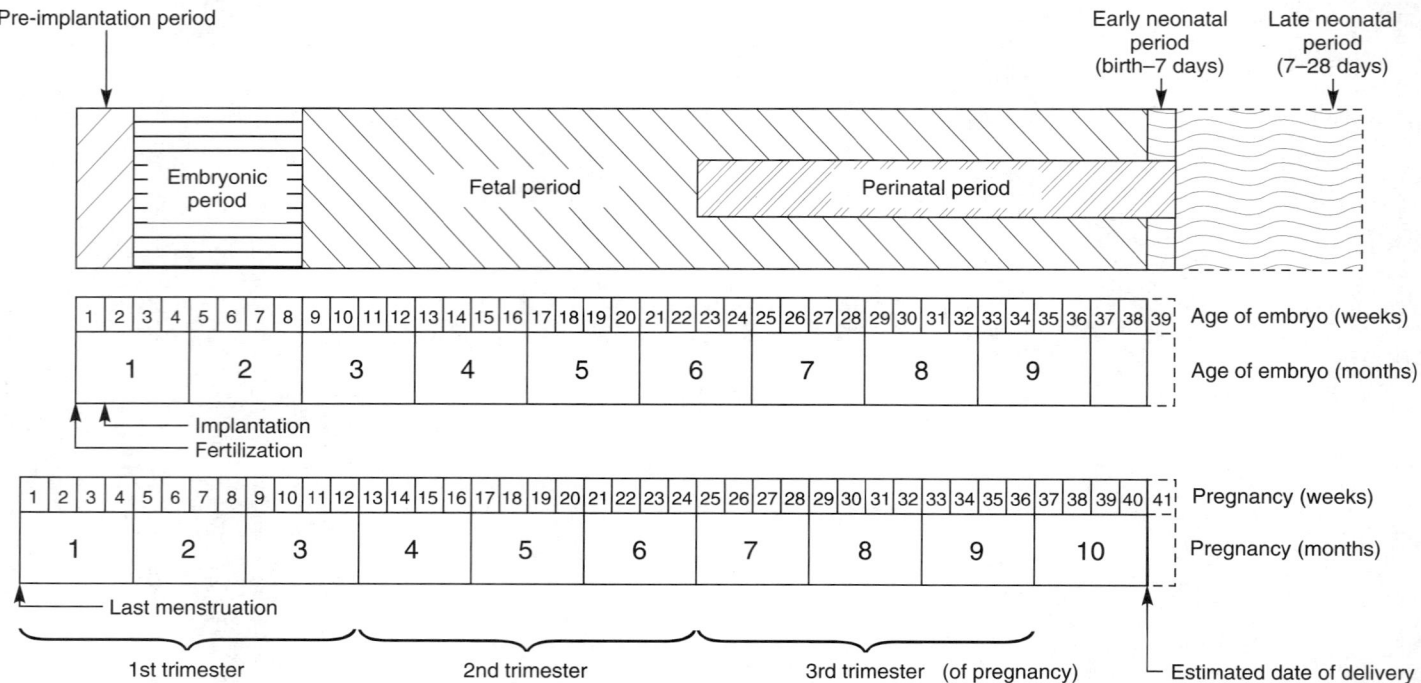

4.1   The two times scales used to depict human development. Embryonic development, in the upper scale, is counted from fertilization (or from ovulation, i.e. in postovulatory days; see O'Rahilly & Muller 1987). Times given for development in the Embryology and Development section are based on this scale. The clinical estimation of pregnancy is counted from the last menstrual period and is shown on the lower scale. Fetal ages given in the Neonatal Anatomy and Growth section will have been derived from the lower scale. Note that there is a two-week discrepancy between these scales. The perinatal period is very long as it includes all of the preterm deliveries.

STANDARD CHARTS OF PRENATAL GROWTH

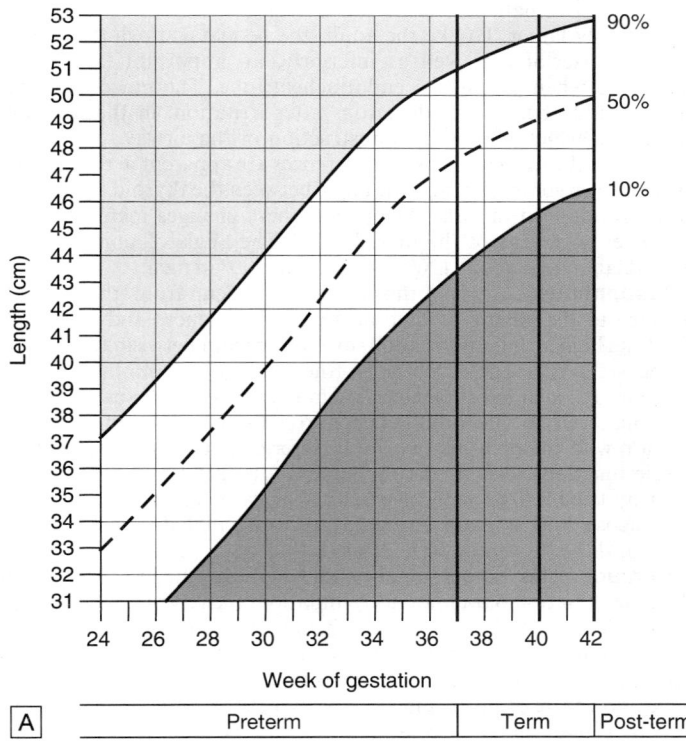

4.2 Standardized graphs of fetal length (A) and weight (B) from 24 weeks of pregnancy showing the 10th, 50th and 90th centiles.

period from birth to 7 days, and a late neonatal period from 7 to 28 days.

Neonatal measurements and gestational age

The **length** of the full-term neonate ranges from 48 to 53 cm (**4.2A**). Length of the newborn is measured from crown to heel (CHL); however, in utero length is estimated from crown–rump length (CRL), i.e. the greatest distance between the vertex of the skull and the ischial tuberosities, with the fetus in the natural curved position. Crown–rump length is very reliable for estimating gestational age between weeks 7 and 14. The **weight** of the full-term infant at parturition ranges from 2700–4000 g (**4.2B**), the average being 3400 g; 75–80% of this weight is body water with a further 15–28% composed of adipose tissue. After birth there is a general decrease in the total body water but a relative increase in intracellular fluid. Normally the newborn loses about 10% of the birth weight by 3–4 days postnatally because of loss of excess extracellular fluid and meconium. By 1 year total body water makes up 60% of the body weight.

Two populations of neonates are at particular risk:

- those with known low gestational dates, i.e. *preterm infants* (see above)
- those with a low birth weight.

Low birth weight has been defined as under 2500 g, with *very low birth weight* being under 1500 g. Infants may weigh less than 2500 g but not be premature by gestational age. Collection of the range of weights fetuses may attain before birth has led to the production of weight charts which allow babies to be described according to how appropriate their birth weight is for their gestational age, for example small for gestational age (SGA), appropriate for gestational age (AGA), and large for gestational age (LGA) (**4.3**). Small for gestational age infants are often the result of *intrauterine growth retardation* (*IUGR*); the causes of growth retardation are many and various and beyond the scope of this text.

For both premature infants and growth retarded infants an assessment of gestational age, which correlates closely with the stage of

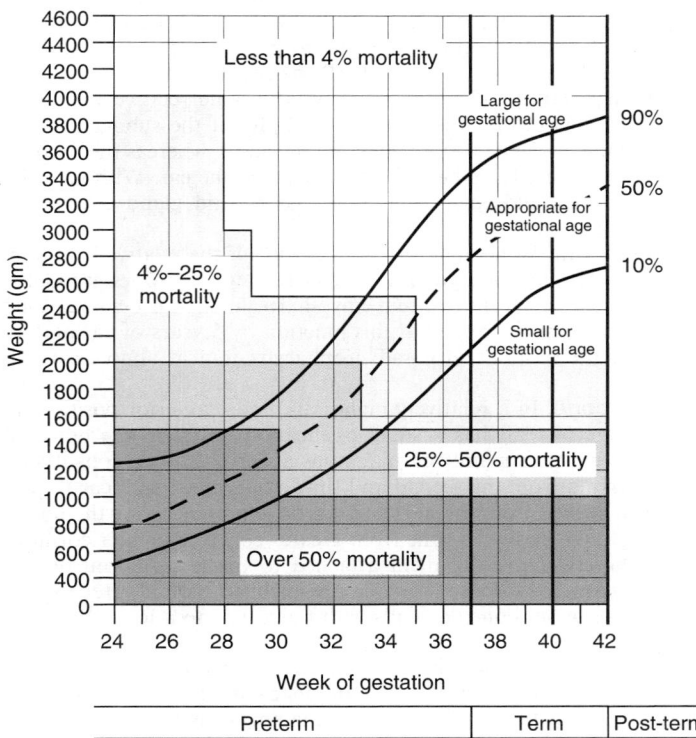

4.3 Graph showing intrauterine growth status and its appropriateness for gestational age. Gestational age is more closely related to maturity than birth weight. The mortality for the weight ranges is indicated.

maturity, is desirable. Gestational age at birth is predicted by its proximity to the estimated date of delivery and the results of the ultrasonographic examinations during pregnancy (see p. 340). It is currently assessed in the neonate by evaluation of a number of external physical and neuromuscular signs. Scoring of these signs results in a cumulative score of maturity which is usually between ±2 weeks of the infant's true age. The scoring scheme has been devised and improved over many years from gestational age assessments proposed by, inter alia, Robinson (1966), Farr et al (1966), Dubowitz et al (1970) and Dubowitz and Dubowitz (1981). For a recent account of these methods of assessing gestational age consult Gandy (1992).

DESCRIPTION OF INDIVIDUAL SYSTEMS IN THE NEONATE

GASTROINTESTINAL SYSTEM

Oral cavity. This cavity is only potential with the mouth closed. The tongue is short and broad, and its entire surface lies within the oral cavity (4.4). The posterior third of the tongue descends into the neck during the first postnatal year and by the fourth or fifth year the tongue forms part of the anterior wall of the pharynx. The hard palate is only slightly arched; it is usually corrugated by five or six irregular transverse folds which assist the newborn when suckling. The epiglottis is high and makes direct contact with the soft palate. During suckling three spaces are formed in the oral cavity. A median space between the tongue and hard palate divides into two posteriorly, forming channels each side of the approximated soft palate and epiglottis. Two lateral spaces, *lateral arcuate cavities*, are formed between the tongue medially and the cheeks laterally; the upper and lower gums situated in these spaces do not touch during suckling. Each cheek is supported by a mass of subcutaneous fat which lies between the buccinator and masseter muscles; it is sometimes termed the *suctorial pad*. As fluid passes from the oral spaces to the pharynx, the larynx is elevated so that its opening is **above** the level of the spaces which convey fluid to the pharynx. The high position of the larynx and its further elevation during suckling directs its opening into the nasopharynx enabling babies to breath while suckling. It was thought for many years that neonates preferentially breathe through the nose, resorting to mouth breathing only if the nasal passage is obstructed. Studies have shown that full-term infants are able to establish oral breathing in the presence of nasal occlusion of a mean duration of 7.8 seconds (Rodenstein 1985).

Salivary glands. These glands have the same relative weight in the neonate as in the adult. The topography of the submandibular and sublingual glands is the same as in the adult, whereas the parotid gland is rounded, lying between masseter and the ear. With growth, during infancy and early childhood, the parotid gland covers the parotid duct.

Pharynx. In the neonate this is one-third of the relative length in the adult. The nasopharynx is a narrow tube which curves gradually to join the oropharynx without any sharp junctional demarcation. An oblique angle is formed at this junction by 5 years of age and in the adult the nasopharynx and oropharynx join at almost a right angle.

Hyoid bone. In a relatively higher and more anterior position in the neonate (4.4), it has a small ossification centre in the body of the bone, which is mainly cartilaginous at birth. Its two constituent parts, derived from the second and third pharyngeal arch cartilages, can be identified from the horizontal groove present along the body. The length of the hyoid bone from greater cornu to greater cornu is 3 cm. The stylohyoid ligament attached to the lesser cornu of the hyoid passes to a more horizontally inclined styloid process. In infancy the hyoid bone descends with the larynx to a lower position in the neck.

Larynx. About one-third the size of the adult, although it is proportionately larger in the neonate, its cavity is short and funnel-shaped. At rest the upper border of the epiglottis is at the level of the second or third cervical vertebra; when the larynx is elevated it is at the level of the first cervical vertebra. The *thyroid cartilage*, which is shorter and broader than the adult, lies closer to the hyoid bone in the neonate. Neither the superior notch nor the laryngeal

prominence is as marked as in the adult. The *cricoid cartilage* is the same shape as in the adult. The *vocal folds* are 4–4.5 mm long, relatively shorter than in childhood and the adult. The ventricle of the larynx is small; however, the saccule of the larynx is often considerably larger. Unlike the adult, the neonatal subglottic cavity extends posteriorly as well as inferiorly, an important fact to be considered when passing an endotracheal tube. The mucosa of the larynx readily becomes oedematous after irritation, in the neonate and infant, which may lead to obstruction of the airway.

By about the third year sexual differences are apparent in the larynx; it becomes larger in boys and the angle between the thyroid laminae is more pronounced in girls. At puberty these changes increase, with greater enlargement of the male larynx. The angle of union of the thyroid laminae is about 120° in women and 90° in men.

Oesophagus. At birth this extends 8–10 cm from the cricoid cartilage to the gastric cardiac orifice. It commences and ends 1–2 vertebrae higher than in the adult, extending from between the fourth to the sixth cervical vertebrae to the level of the ninth thoracic vertebra. Its average diameter is 5 mm and it possesses the constrictions seen in the adult. The narrowest constriction is at its junction with the pharynx, where the inferior pharyngeal constrictor muscle functions to constrict the lumen; it is this region which may be easily traumatized with instruments or catheters. In the neonate the mucosa may contain scattered areas of ciliated columnar epithelium; these disappear soon after birth.

Stomach. This exhibits fetal characteristics until just after birth when the initiation of pulmonary ventilation, the reflexes of coughing and swallowing, and crying, cause the ingestion of large amounts of air and liquid. Once postnatal swallowing has commenced the stomach distends to four or five times its contracted state and shifts its position in relation to the state of expansion and contraction of the other abdominal viscera, and to the position of the body. Generally, in the neonate, the anterior surface of the stomach is covered by the left lobe of the liver which extends across nearly as far as the spleen (4.5, 6). Only a small portion of the greater curvature of the stomach is visible anteriorly. The capacity of the stomach is between 30–35 ml in the full-term neonate, rising to 75 ml in the second week and 100 ml by the fourth week (adult capacity is on average 1000 ml). The mucosa and submucosa are relatively thicker than in the adult; however, the muscularis is only moderately developed without co-ordinated peristalsis. At birth gastric acid secretion is low, resulting in a high gastric pH for the first 12 postnatal hours. The pH then falls rapidly with the onset of gastric acid secretion, usually after the first feed. Generally acid secretion remains low for the first 10 days postnatally. Gastric emptying and transit times are delayed in the neonate (Nagourney & Aranda 1992).

Small intestine. This forms an oval-shaped mass with a greater diameter transversely orientated in the abdomen rather than vertically as in the adult (4.6). The mass of the small intestine inferior to the umbilicus is compressed by the urinary bladder which is anterior at this point (see below). The small intestine is 300–350 cm long at birth and its width when empty is 1–1.5 cm. The ratio between the length of the small and large intestine at birth is similar to the adult. The mucosa and submucosa are fairly well developed with villi throughout the small intestine (villi are present in the large intestine earlier in development, see p. 191); however, the muscularis is very thin, particularly the longitudinal layer, and there is little elastic tissue in the wall. Generally there are few or no circular folds in the small intestine, and the jejunum and ileum have little fat in their mesentery.

Large intestine. At birth this is about 66 cm long and averages 1 cm in width. The caecum is relatively smaller than in the adult; it tapers into the vermiform appendix. The ascending colon is shorter in the neonate, due to the shorter lumbar region; the transverse colon is relatively long; the descending colon is short, but twice the length of the ascending colon (4.5). The sigmoid colon may be as long as the transverse colon; it often touches the inferior part of the anterior body wall on the left and, in approximately 50% of neonates, part of the sigmoid colon lies in the right iliac fossa. Generally in the colon the muscularis, including the taeniae coli, is poorly developed as in the small intestine. Appendices epiploicae and haustra are not present, giving a smooth external appearance to the colon. Haustra appear within the first 6 months. The rectum is relatively

1. Superior sagittal sinus
2. Falx cerebri
3. Corpus callosum
4. Septum pellucidum
5. Right interventricular foramen
6. Frontal lobe of right cerebral hemisphere
7. Optic nerve
8. Hypophysis
9. Olfactory nerve
10. Cribriform lamina
11. Sphenoid bone
12. Nasal cavity
13. Ostium of auditory tube
14. Naris
15. Hard palate
16. Foramen caecum of tongue
17. Mandible
18. Hyoid bone
19. Laryngeal ventricle
20. Vocal fold
21. Thyroid cartilage
22. Cricoid cartilage arch
23. Isthmus of thyroid gland
24. Left brachiocephalic vein
25. Thymus gland
26. Sternum
27. Auricle of right atrium
28. Aortic semilunar valves
29. Right ventricle
30. Pericardium
31. Liver
    a. left lobe
    b. caudate lobe
32. Pylorus of stomach
33. Gastrocolic ligament
34. Transverse colon
35. Transverse mesocolon
36. Greater omentum (apron)
37. Jejunum
38. Falciform ligament
39. Umbilical vein
40. Stump of umbilical cord
41. Median umbilical ligament
42. Ileum
43. Urinary bladder
44. Pubic symphysis
45. Vesico-uterine pouch
46. Clitoris
47. Urethra
48. Vagina
49. Superior cerebral veins
50. Thalamus protruding into
    3rd ventricle
51. Pineal body
52. Great cerebral vein
53. Cerebral peduncle
54. Cerebral aqueduct
55. Straight sinus
56. Pons
57. Spheno-occipital
    synchondrosis
58. 4th ventricle
59. Confluence of sinuses
60. Cerebellum
61. Medulla oblongata
62. Ligamentum nuchae
63. Median aperture of
    4th ventricle
64. Nasal part of pharynx
65. Lamina and spinous process
    of 2nd cervical vertebra
66. Oral part of pharynx
67. Soft palate
68. Epiglottis
69. Laryngeal part of pharynx
70. Arytenoid cartilage
71. Cricoid cartilage lamina
72. Subcutaneous adipose tissue
    (interscapular brown fat)
73. Trachea

74. Brachiocephalic trunk
75. Ascending aorta
76. Openings of right pulmonary
    veins in left atrium
77. Coronary sinus
78. Left ventricle
79. Oesophagus
80. Diaphragm
81. Coronary ligament
82. Spinal cord
83. Cardiac part of stomach
84. Lesser omentum
85. Omental bursa
86. Splenic artery
87. Opening of right renal artery
    in aorta
88. Left renal vein
89. Pancreas
90. Splenic vein
91. Duodenum
92. Nucleus pulposus of intervertebral
    disc between 2nd and 3rd lumbar vertebrae
93. Filum terminale among spinal nerve
    roots (cauda equina) within vertebral canal
94. Body of 5th lumbar vertebra
95. Uterus
96. Rectum
97. Sacrum
98. Median sacral artery
99. Sacral hiatus
100. Recto-uterine pouch
101. Coccyx
102. Rectovaginal septum
103. Anal canal
104. Anococcygeal ligament

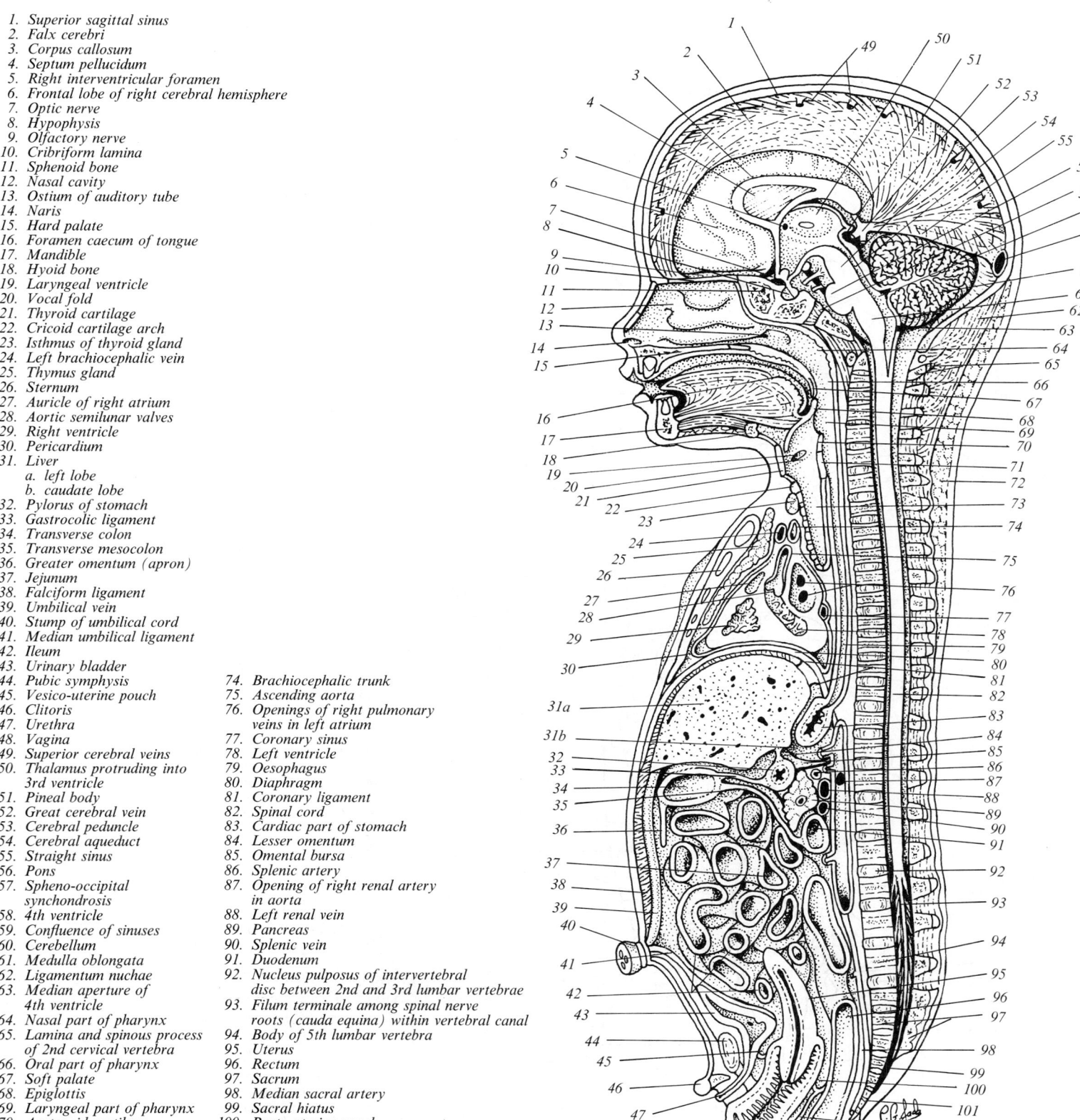

4.4 Midsagittal section through a full-term female neonate (after Crelin).

long; its junction with the anal canal forms at nearly a right angle.

Meconium. This is a dark, sticky, viscid substance formed from the passage of amniotic fluid, sloughed cells, digestive enzymes and bile salts along the fetal gut. Meconium becomes increasingly solid as gestation advances but does not usually pass out of the fetal body while in utero. Fetal distress produced by anoxia may induce the

premature defecation of meconium into the amniotic fluid, causing risk of its inhalation. At birth the colon contains 60–200 g of meconium. The majority of neonates defecate within the first 24 hours after birth.

Liver. This constitutes 4% of the body weight in neonates, compared to 2.5–3.5% in adults. It is in contact with the greater part of

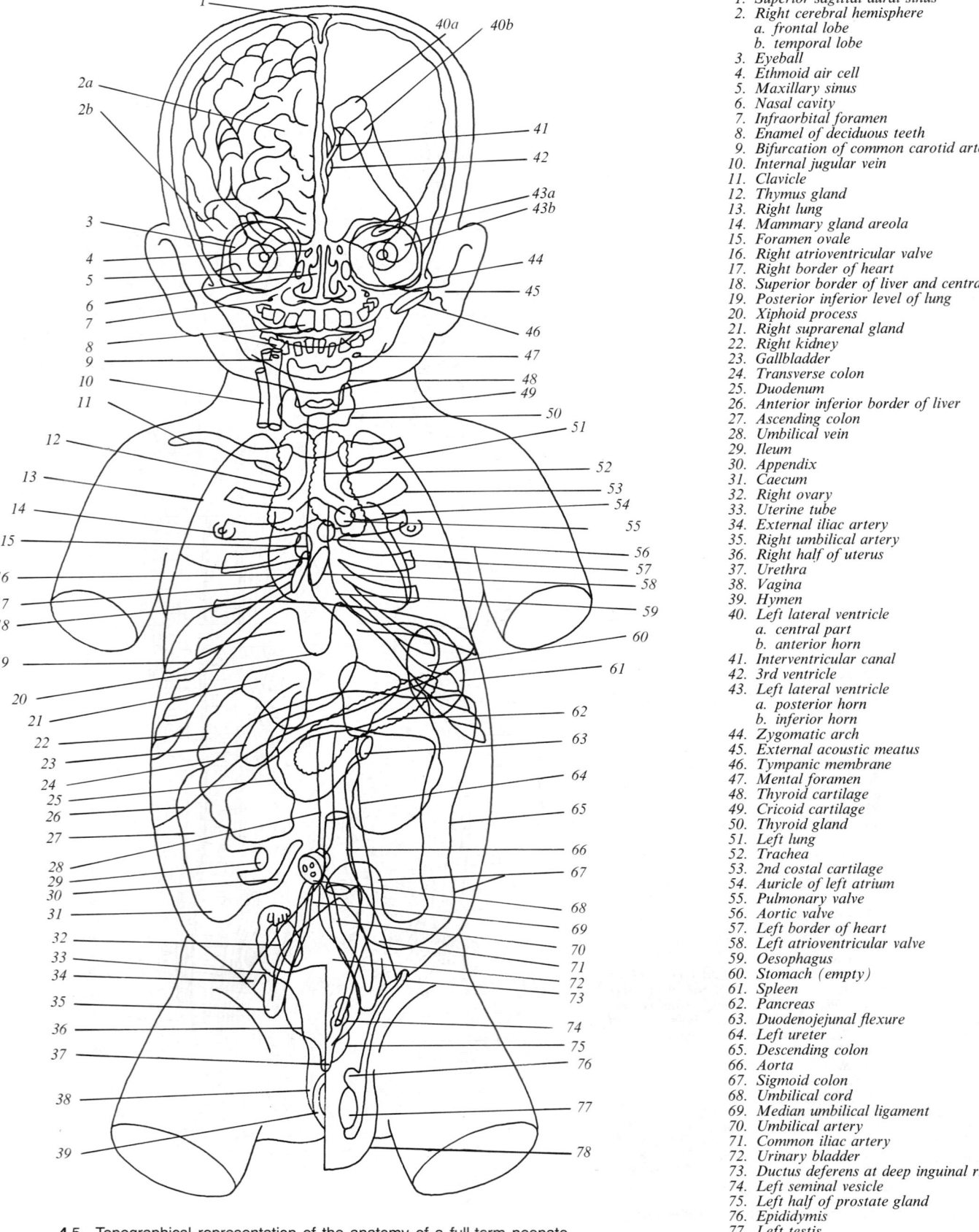

4.5 Topographical representation of the anatomy of a full-term neonate (after Crelin).

1. Superior sagittal dural sinus
2. Right cerebral hemisphere
   a. frontal lobe
   b. temporal lobe
3. Eyeball
4. Ethmoid air cell
5. Maxillary sinus
6. Nasal cavity
7. Infraorbital foramen
8. Enamel of deciduous teeth
9. Bifurcation of common carotid artery
10. Internal jugular vein
11. Clavicle
12. Thymus gland
13. Right lung
14. Mammary gland areola
15. Foramen ovale
16. Right atrioventricular valve
17. Right border of heart
18. Superior border of liver and central level of diaphragm
19. Posterior inferior level of lung
20. Xiphoid process
21. Right suprarenal gland
22. Right kidney
23. Gallbladder
24. Transverse colon
25. Duodenum
26. Anterior inferior border of liver
27. Ascending colon
28. Umbilical vein
29. Ileum
30. Appendix
31. Caecum
32. Right ovary
33. Uterine tube
34. External iliac artery
35. Right umbilical artery
36. Right half of uterus
37. Urethra
38. Vagina
39. Hymen
40. Left lateral ventricle
    a. central part
    b. anterior horn
41. Interventricular canal
42. 3rd ventricle
43. Left lateral ventricle
    a. posterior horn
    b. inferior horn
44. Zygomatic arch
45. External acoustic meatus
46. Tympanic membrane
47. Mental foramen
48. Thyroid cartilage
49. Cricoid cartilage
50. Thyroid gland
51. Left lung
52. Trachea
53. 2nd costal cartilage
54. Auricle of left atrium
55. Pulmonary valve
56. Aortic valve
57. Left border of heart
58. Left atrioventricular valve
59. Oesophagus
60. Stomach (empty)
61. Spleen
62. Pancreas
63. Duodenojejunal flexure
64. Left ureter
65. Descending colon
66. Aorta
67. Sigmoid colon
68. Umbilical cord
69. Median umbilical ligament
70. Umbilical artery
71. Common iliac artery
72. Urinary bladder
73. Ductus deferens at deep inguinal ring
74. Left seminal vesicle
75. Left half of prostate gland
76. Epididymis
77. Left testis
78. Scrotum

the diaphragm; it extends below the costal margin anteriorly, and in some cases to within 1 cm of the iliac crest posteriorly. The left lobe covers much of the anterior surface of the stomach and constitutes nearly one-third of the liver (4.5, 6). The liver is particularly large because of its precocious function as a site of haemopoiesis in the

fetus; however, although its haemopoietic functions cease before birth its enzymatic and synthetic functions are not completely mature at birth.

Gallbladder. This has a smaller peritoneal surface than in the adult, and its fundus often does not extend to the liver margin. It is

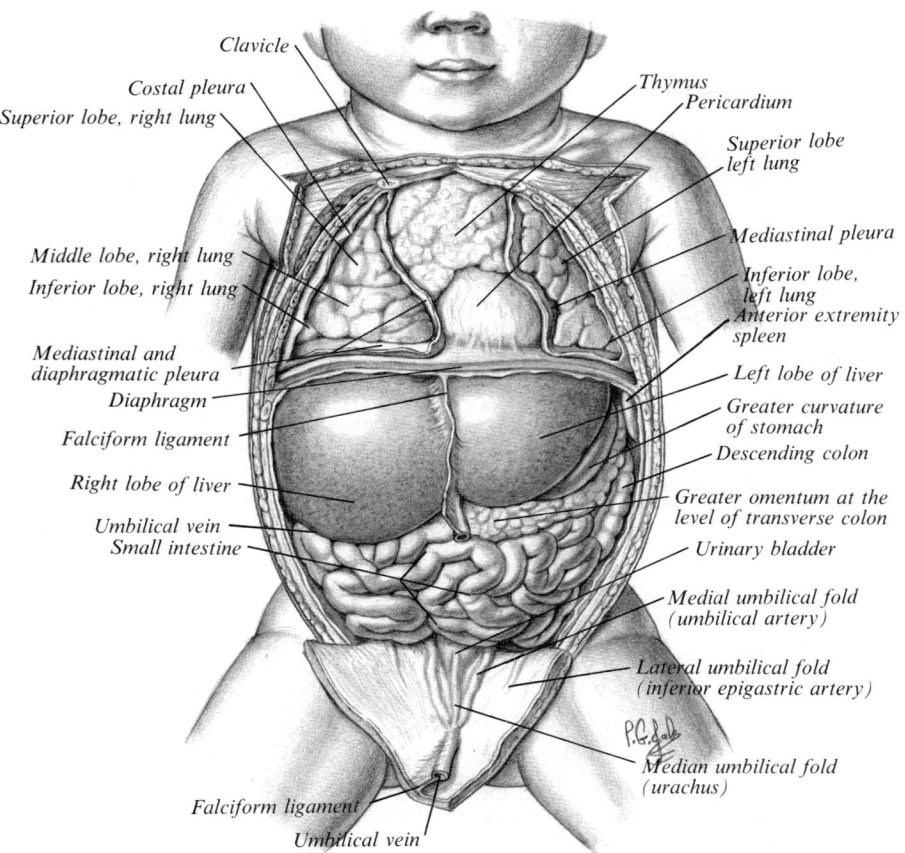

Clavicle

Costal pleura

Superior lobe, right lung

Thymus

Pericardium

Superior lobe left lung

Middle lobe, right lung

Inferior lobe, right lung

Mediastinal pleura

Inferior lobe, left lung

Anterior extremity spleen

Mediastinal and diaphragmatic pleura

Diaphragm

Left lobe of liver

Greater curvature of stomach

Falciform ligament

Descending colon

Right lobe of liver

Greater omentum at the level of transverse colon

Umbilical vein

Small intestine

Urinary bladder

Medial umbilical fold (umbilical artery)

Lateral umbilical fold (inferior epigastric artery)

Median umbilical fold (urachus)

Falciform ligament

Umbilical vein

4.6 Abdominal and thoracic viscera in situ in a full-term neonate. The anterior thoracic and abdominal wall has been removed. The lower abdominal wall has been deflected downwards.

generally embedded in the liver and in some cases may be covered by bands of liver. After the second year the gallbladder is of the relative size it is in the adult.

Pancreas (**4**.5). In the neonate this has all of the normal subdivisions of the adult. The head is proportionately larger in the newborn and there is a smooth continuation between the body and the tail. The inferior border of the head of the pancreas is found at the second lumbar vertebra; the body and tail pass cranially and to the left, and the tail is in contact with the spleen.

Peritoneal cavity (**4**.6). This is ovoid in shape in the neonate. It is fairly shallow from anterior to posterior as the bilateral posterior extensions each side of the vertebral column, which are prominent in the adult, are not present. Two factors lead to the protuberance of the anterior abdominal wall in the neonate and infant. Firstly, the diaphragm is flatter in the newborn, leading to a caudal displacement of the viscera compared to the adult. Secondly, the pelvic cavity is very small in the neonate and the organs which are normally pelvic in the adult, i.e. urinary bladder, ovaries and uterus, all extend superiorly into the abdomen (**4**.4). The pelvic cavity is joined to the abdominal cavity at less of an acute angle in the neonate as there is no lumbar vertebral curve and only a slight sacral curve.

Peritoneal attachments. These are similar to the adult; however, the greater omentum is relatively small; its constituent layers of peritoneum may not be completely fused and it does not extend much below the level of the umbilicus (**4**.4). Generally the length of the mesentery of the small intestine and of the transverse and sigmoid mesocolons are longer than in the adult, whereas the area of attachment of the ascending and descending colons is relatively smaller. The peritoneal mesenteries and omenta contain little fat.

RESPIRATORY SYSTEM

Trachea. This is relatively small in relation to the larynx in the

neonate (**4**.5). The walls of the trachea are relatively thick and the tracheal cartilages are relatively closer together than in the adult. The ability of the trachea to resist external compression is about one-third that of a one-year-old infant, a fourth that of a five-year-old child, and a sixth that of an adult (Crelin 1973). The trachea commences at the upper border of C6; a relationship conserved with growth, it bifurcates at the level of the third or fourth thoracic vertebra.

Lungs. In the neonate these are relatively shorter and broader than those in the adult (**4**.5, 6). The respiratory rate in a full-term infant is 40–44 breaths/minute (normal resting rate in an adult male is 12/min). At birth the lungs are still in the alveolar stage of development (see p. 178); this continues through the neonatal period and into childhood perhaps up to 8 years of age although the time at which this stage is complete has not yet been established.

Normal postnatal pulmonary arterial development. Immediately after birth dramatic remodelling of the pulmonary vasculature occurs to effect an abrupt reduction of pulmonary vascular resistance. This process continues at a rapid rate throughout the first 1–2 months, while the lungs adapt to extrauterine life, and then more slowly throughout childhood. Failure to remodel in the presence of an anatomically normal heart leads to persistent pulmonary hypertension (Haworth 1992).

Normal postnatal pulmonary arterial development in the full-term neonate can be divided into three stages (taken from Haworth 1992):

Stage one. Lasting from birth to about 4 postnatal days, this stage concerns the immediate adaptation to extrauterine life. At birth the endothelial cells of the precapillary arteries are squat and have narrow bases on the subendothelium, a low surface:volume ratio, and many surface projections. Five minutes after birth the endothelial cells are thinner and gradually show less cell overlap; the surface:volume ratio increases, and few cell projections are seen. The vessel wall becomes thinner and the lumen diameter increases (**4**.7).

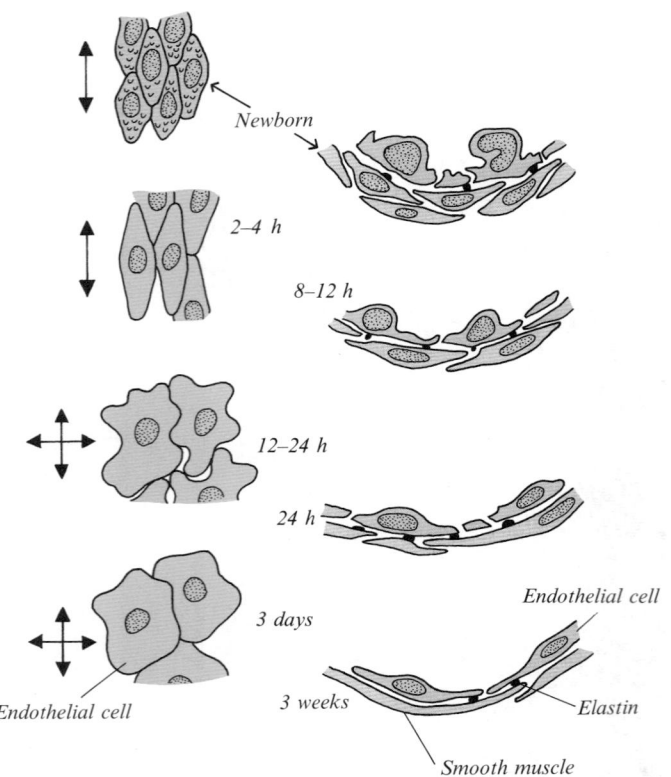

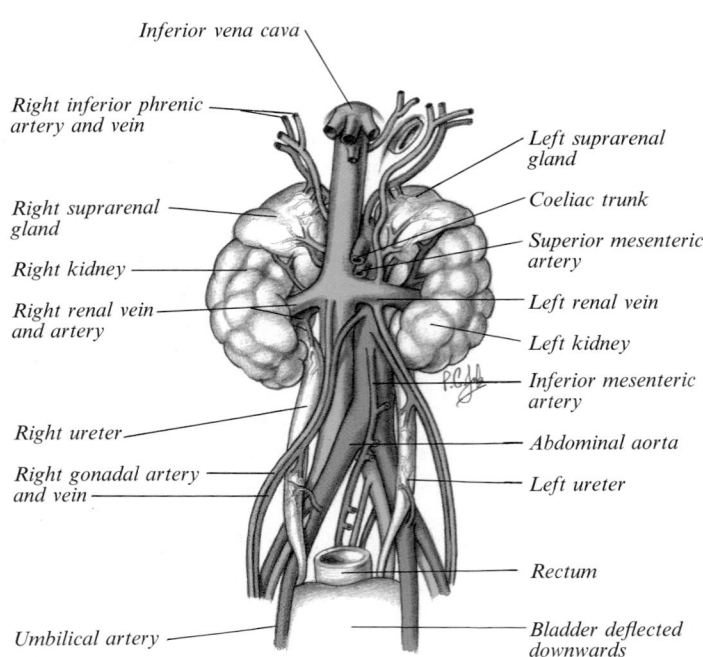

4.8 Posterior abdominal wall of a full-term neonate. Note the lobulated kidneys and relatively wide calibre of the ureters.

4.7 En face views (left) and transverse sections (right) showing the changes in the endothelial and smooth muscle cells of small muscular pulmonary arteries accompanying terminal bronchi from the neonatal period to three weeks after birth (from Haworth 1992).

The smooth muscle cells show a significant reduction in diameter during this time.

Stage two. From birth, particularly from day 4 to 3–4 weeks, the cells deposit matrix around themselves to fix their new positions. At birth the internal elastic lamina of the small muscular arteries consists only of amorphous elastin in a basal lamina-like matrix. By 3 weeks of age a definitive elastic lamina is evident; however, it is heavily fenestrated, permitting contact between the endothelial cells and the smooth muscle cells.

Stage three. This continues into adulthood. The intrapulmonary arteries increase in size and their walls increase in thickness. However, from birth all the pulmonary vascular smooth muscle cells from the hilum to the precapillary bed are immature; maturation is not advanced until 2 years.

As the distal airspaces expand there is a process of fusion of the capillary nets from one alveolus to another, forming, for a period, an extensive double capillary net. Fusion of these layers can be seen from 28 postnatal days and it becomes more extensive by 1.5 years; it is thought to be complete by 5 years.

The amount and type of connective tissue in the lung changes after birth. The neonatal lung has abundant type III and type IV collagen but little type I collagen, as seen in mature lungs. The former collagen types are not so strong, suggesting that the neonatal lung is more plastic; this would facilitate the changes in cell shape and orientation that characterize adaptation to extrauterine life. The rapid deposition of type I collagen postnatally gives structural stiffness to the blood vessel walls.

Thorax. Because it is relatively soft and flexible in the neonate, it makes the chest wall subject to collapse during negative pressure generation. The neonatal thorax has a round circumference rather than the dorsoventrally flattened profile of the adult.

At all ages during rapid eye movement (REM) sleep, there is a reduction if not a loss of tonic intercostal muscle activity. The mechanism is thought to be related to a descending spinal inhibition of the muscle spindle system. Further, there is often a destabilization of the chest wall which results in the rib cage and abdominal respiratory movements being out of phase. The neonate is at particular risk in this respect, firstly because the chest wall is flexible, and secondly, because much of the infant sleep activity is of the REM type (Woodrum 1992).

Diaphragm. To date this has not been well studied in the neonate. It is relatively flat at birth, gaining the dome shape with growth of the thorax and abdominal viscera. There is an exaggerated asymmetric movement of the neonatal diaphragm with the posterior portion showing a considerably greater excursion than the anterior portion. Thus the diaphragm after birth is potentially less effective in compressing the abdominal contents and expanding the lower thorax, having a flatter configuration and narrower zone of apposition, where the diaphragmatic fibres are parallel to the body axis and in direct contact with the lower rib cage (Woodrum 1992).

URINARY SYSTEM

Kidneys. At birth the two kidneys weigh about 23 g. They function early in development producing the amniotic fluid which surrounds the fetus. Fetal kidneys have a lobulated appearance which is still present at birth (**4.5, 8**). Addition of new cortical nephrons continues in the first few months of postnatal life after which the general growth of the glomeruli and tubules results in the disappearance of the lobulation.

The kidneys respond to the work load they are required to do; thus if one kidney is abnormal or removed, the remaining kidney becomes larger than the two kidneys combined would have done. The renal blood flow is lower in the neonate, the glomerular filtration rate at birth being approximately 30% that of the adult value; adult values for glomerular filtration are attained by 3–5 months of age and for renal blood flow by the end of the first year.

Urinary bladder. In the neonate this is egg-shaped with the larger end directed downwards and backwards (**4.4, 5, 6, 9, 10**). From the bladder neck the bladder extends anteriorly and slightly upwards in close contact with the pubis until it reaches the anterior abdominal wall. The apex of the contracted bladder is at a point midway between the pubis and the umbilicus; when the bladder is filled with urine the apex may extend up to the level of the umbilicus. There is no true fundus in the bladder as in the adult. The anterior surface is not covered with peritoneum; however, posteriorly peritoneum extends as low as the level of the urethral orifice. Although the neonatal bladder is described as abdominally placed, Symington (1887) noted that if a line is drawn from the promontory of the sacrum to the upper edge of the pubic symphysis, nearly one half of the bladder is found below that line, i.e. within the cavity of the true pelvis. However, pressure on the lower abdominal wall will express urine from an infant bladder and the bladder does not gain its adult, pelvic, position until about the sixth year. The bladder remains connected to the umbilicus by the obliterated remains of the urachus; stimulation of the umbilicus can initiate micturition in babies. Because of the elongated shape of the bladder in neonates the ureters are correspondingly reduced in length and have no pelvic portion compared to adults. In the neonate a distinct interureteric fold is present in the contracted bladder.

REPRODUCTIVE SYSTEM

Reproductive organs in the female

Ovaries. The combined weight of the ovaries at birth is about 0.3 g; they double in weight during the first 6 postnatal weeks. The ovaries are relatively large at birth and much larger than the testes (**4.5, 9**). They have surface furrows which disappear during the second and third postnatal months. In the neonate the ovaries are found in the lower part of the iliac fossae; they complete their descent into the ovarian fossae in early childhood. The long axis of the ovary is almost vertical in the neonate, becoming temporarily horizontal during descent and vertical once more in the ovarian fossa. All of the primary oöcytes for the reproductive life of the female neonate are present in the ovaries by the end of the first trimester of pregnancy. Of the 7 000 000 primary oöcytes estimated at the fifth month of gestation 1 000 000 remain at birth; this is reduced to 40 000 by puberty and only 400 are ovulated during reproductive life.

Uterus. At birth this is 2.5–5 cm long (average 3.5 cm), 2 cm wide between the uterine tubes, and about 1.3 cm thick (**4.4, 5, 9**). The body of the uterus is smaller than the uterine cervix which forms two-thirds or more of the length. The isthmus between the body and the cervix is absent. Generally the fetal female reproductive tract is affected by maternal hormones and undergoes some enlargement in the fetus. The endocervical glands are active before birth and usually

the cervical canal is filled with mucus. After birth the uterus involutes, decreasing by about one-third in length and more than a half in weight. The neonatal size and weight of the uterus is not regained until puberty. The uterine tubes are relatively short and wide. The position of the uterus in the pelvic cavity depends to a great extent on the state of the bladder anteriorly and the rectum posteriorly. If the bladder contains only a small amount of urine the uterus may be anteverted but often it is in a direct line with the vagina.

Vagina. In the neonate this is about 2.5–3.5 cm long and 1.5 cm wide at the fornices. The uterine cervix extends into the vagina about 1 cm. The posterior vaginal wall is longer than the anterior giving the vagina a distinct curve (**4.4, 9**). The cavity is filled with longitudinal columns covered with a thick layer of cornified, stratified squamous epithelium. These cells slough off after birth when the effect of the maternal hormones is removed. The orifice of the vagina is surrounded by a thick elliptical ring of connective tissue, the hymen (**4.9**). During childhood the hymen becomes a membranous fold along the posterior margin of the vaginal lumen; should the fold form a complete diaphragm across the vaginal lumen it is termed an imperforate hymenal membrane.

External genitalia. At birth these include relatively enlarged labia minora, clitoris and labia majora. The labia majora are united by a posterior labial commissure. They each contain the distal end of the round ligament of the uterus (the gubernaculum, see p. 213).

Reproductive organs in the male

Testes. These are relatively the same weight as in the adult. The long axis of the testis is almost vertical (**4.5, 10**). The testes are situated at the future deep inguinal rings by the sixth to seventh month of gestation. They descend into the scrotum before birth (see p. 212), the left testis usually migrating ahead of the right. In full-term male neonates 90% have descended testes; however, in premature babies descent may not be complete. The testes, unlike the ovaries, contain primordial germ cells which are surrounded by Sertoli cells preventing their further proliferation and meiosis until puberty. The processus vaginalis which precedes the testis in its descent into the scrotum is collapsed at birth but not necessarily obliterated. In 66% of male infants it remains patent for up to 2

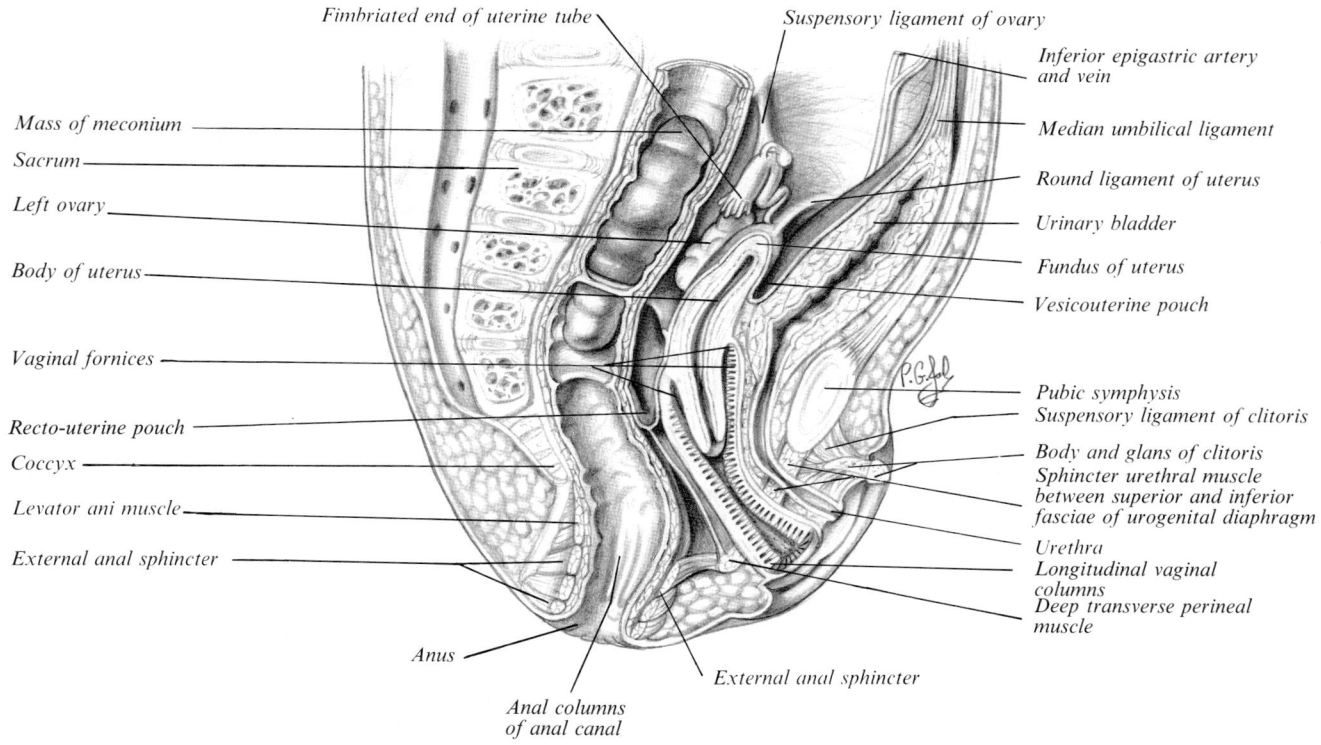

4.9 Midsagittal section through the pelvis of a full-term female neonate. Note the abdominal position of the urinary bladder and uterus.

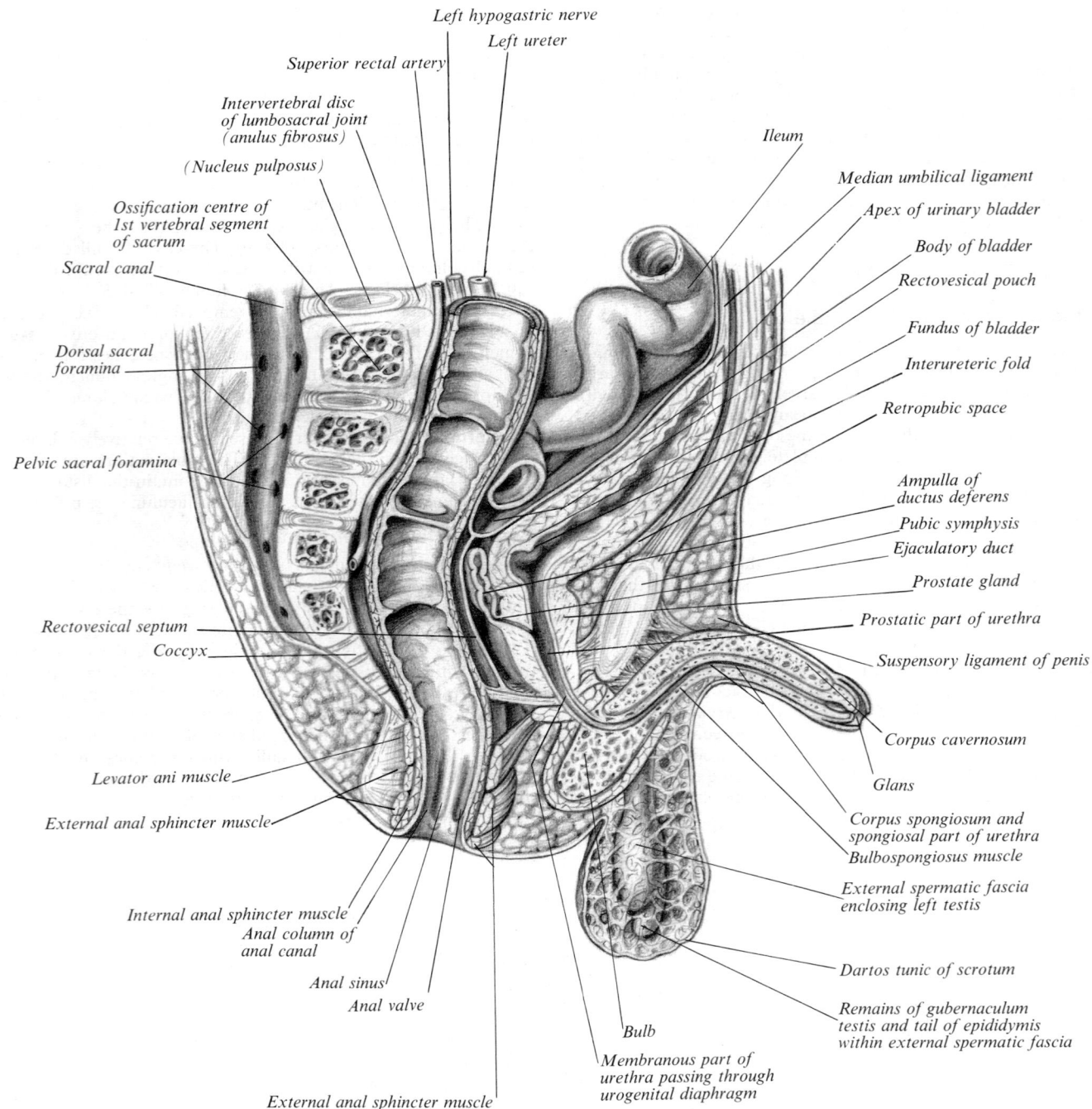

Left hypogastric nerve

Left ureter

Superior rectal artery

Intervertebral disc
of lumbosacral joint
(anulus fibrosus)

(Nucleus pulposus)

Ileum

Median umbilical ligament

Apex of urinary bladder

Ossification centre of
1st vertebral segment
of sacrum

Body of bladder

Rectovesical pouch

Sacral canal

Fundus of bladder

Interureteric fold

Dorsal sacral
foramina

Retropubic space

Pelvic sacral foramina

Ampulla of
ductus deferens

Pubic symphysis

Ejaculatory duct

Prostate gland

Rectovesical septum

Prostatic part of urethra

Coccyx

Suspensory ligament of penis

Corpus cavernosum

Glans

Levator ani muscle

Corpus spongiosum and
spongiosal part of urethra

External anal sphincter muscle

Bulbospongiosus muscle

External spermatic fascia
enclosing left testis

Internal anal sphincter muscle

Anal column of
anal canal

Dartos tunic of scrotum

Anal sinus

Remains of gubernaculum
testis and tail of epididymis
within external spermatic fascia

Anal valve

Bulb

External anal sphincter muscle

Membranous part of
urethra passing through
urogenital diaphragm

4.10   Midsagittal section through the pelvis of a full-term male neonate.
Note the abdominal position of the urinary bladder (see also **8**.183).

weeks. By between 10 and 20 days after birth the processus is
partially (or completely) obliterated in 80% of male infants, the left
side before the right. The *spermatic cord* is relatively large in the
neonate as are the seminal vesicles and adjacent ampullae of the
ductus deferens. The *prostate gland* (**4**.10) is similar to the uterine
cervix of the female in shape, size and its position; it is the only
major organ in the male neonatal pelvic cavity apart from the
rectum.

Penis and scrotum. In the neonate these are relatively large.
Although the prepuce and glans begin to separate from the fifth
month in utero they may still be joined at birth. Despite containing
less smooth muscle and elastic tissue than the adult, the neonatal
penis is capable of erection. The scrotum has a broad base which
does not narrow until after the first year. Both the septum and the
walls of the scrotum are relatively thicker than in adults.

NERVOUS SYSTEM

Brain

The brain of the full-term neonate ranges from 300–400 g with an
average of 350 g; the brains of neonatal males are slightly heavier
than those of females. Because the head is large at birth, measuring
one quarter the total body length, the brain is also proportionally
larger, and constitutes 10% of the body weight (2% in the adult).
The brain reaches 90% of its adult size by the fifth year, and 95%
by 10 years. The sulci of the cerebral hemispheres appear from the
fourth month of gestation (**3**.122) and at full term the general
arrangement of sulci and gyri are present but the insula is not
completely covered. The central sulcus is situated further rostrally
and the lateral sulcus is more oblique than in the adult. Most of the

developmental stages of sulci and gyri have been identified in the brains of premature infants.

The pons is relatively smaller in the full-term neonate; the brainstem is more oblique and has a distinct bend as it passes through the foramen magnum to become the spinal cord. Of the cranial nerves, the olfactory and the optic at the chiasma are much larger than in the adult, whereas the roots of the other nerves are relatively smaller.

Spinal cord

The spinal cord in the neonate extends to L2–L3; lumbar puncture investigations should thus never be attempted higher than the L3/L4 intervertebral space (see p. 22).

Myelination. This occurs over a protracted period beginning during the second trimester in the peripheral nervous system (PNS), with motor roots myelinating before sensory roots, and continuing in the central nervous system (CNS) where conversely the sensory nerves myelinate before the motor systems. The cranial nerves of the midbrain, pons and medulla oblongata begin myelination at about 6 months gestation. Myelination is not complete at birth; its most rapid phase occurs during the first 6 months of postnatal life, after which it continues at a slower rate up to puberty and beyond. The sequence of myelination of the motor pathways may explain, at least partially, the order of development of muscle tone and posture in the premature infant and neonate. Myelination of the various subcorticospinal pathways, i.e. vestibulospinal, reticulospinal, olivospinal and tectospinal (often grouped as bulbospinal tracts) occurs from 24–30 weeks gestation, for the medial groups, and extends to 28–34 weeks gestation for the lateral groups; lastly myelination of the corticospinal tracts occurs at term. Thus, in the preterm infant, axial extension precedes flexion, whereas finger flexion precedes extension. By term the neonate at rest has a strong flexor tone accompanied by adduction of all limbs. Neonates also display a distinct preference for a head position facing to the right, which appears to be independent of handling practices and may reflect the normal asymmetry of cerebral function at this age (Hill 1992).

The brain occupies 97.5% of the cranial cavity from birth to 6 years of age after which the space between the brain and skull increases until the adult brain occupies only 92.5% of the cranial cavity. Although the cerebral ventricles are larger in the neonate than in the adult, the newborn has a total of about 10–15 ml of cerebrospinal fluid when delivered vaginally and 30 ml when delivered by caesarian section.

Reflexes

A number of reflexes are present at birth and their demonstration is used to indicate normal development of the nervous system and responding muscles. Robinson (1966) noted that five tests of neurological development were most useful in determining gestational age. The pupillary reflex is consistently absent before 29 weeks gestation and present after 31 weeks; the glabellar tap, a blink in response to a tap on the glabella, is absent before 32 weeks and present after 34 weeks; the neck righting reflex appears between 34 and 37 weeks; the traction response, where flexion of the neck or arms occurs when the baby is pulled up by the wrists from the supine position appears after 33 weeks; head turning in response to light appears between 32 and 36 weeks. The spinal reflex arc is fully developed by the eighth week of gestation and muscle stretch reflexes at the knees and ankles may be elicited in premature infants of 19–23 weeks gestation. The Babinski response, which involves extension of the great toe with spreading of the remaining toes in response to stimulation of the lateral aspect of the sole of the foot, is elicited frequently in neonates; it reflects poor cortical control of motor function by the immature brain (Hill 1992).

The usual reflexes which can be noted in the neonate include Moro, asymmetric tonic neck response, rooting-sucking, grasp, placing (contacting the dorsum of the foot with the edge of a table produces a 'stepping over the edge' response), stepping, and trunk incurvation (elicited by stroking down the paravertebral area with the infant in the prone position). Examination of the motor system and evaluation of these reflexes allows assessment of the nervous system in relation to gestational age. The neonate also exhibits complex reflexes such as nasal reflexes and sucking and swallowing.

Nasal reflexes. These produce apnoea via the diving reflex, sneezing, sniffing, and both somatic and autonomic reflexes. Stimulation of the face or nasal cavity with water or local irritants produces apnoea in neonates. Breathing stops in expiration, with laryngeal closure, and infants exhibit bradycardia and a lowering of cardiac output. Blood flow to the skin, splanchnic areas, muscles and kidneys decreases, whereas flow to the heart and brain is protected. Different fluids produce different effects when introduced into the pharynx of preterm infants. A comparison of the effects of water and saline in the pharynx showed that apnoea, airway obstruction, and swallowing occur far more frequently with water than with saline, suggesting the presence of an upper airway chemoreflex (see Duara 1992). Reflex responses to the temperature of the face and nasopharynx are necessary for the commencement of pulmonary ventilation; local anaesthetic agents applied to the nasopharynx will prevent the onset of ventilation in newborn lambs. Midwives have for many years blown on the faces of neonates to induce the first breath.

Sucking and swallowing. This is a particularly complex set of reflexes, partly conscious and partly unconscious. As a combined reflex it requires the co-ordination of most of the 12 cranial nerves. The neonate can, within the first couple of feeds, suck at the rate of once per second, swallow approximately after five or six sucks, and breathe during every second or third suck. Air moves in and out of the lungs via the nasopharynx, and milk crosses the pharynx en route to the oesophagus without apparent interruption of breathing and swallowing, or significant misdirection of air into the stomach or fluids in the trachea (Herbst 1989).

Sucking. Although this develops, generally, slightly later than swallowing, mouthing movements have been detected in premature babies as early as 18–24 weeks gestation, and infants delivered at 29–30 weeks gestation make sucking movements a few days after birth; however, co-ordinated activities are not noted before 33–34 weeks. The concept of non-nutritive and nutritive sucking has been introduced (Wolf 1972) to account for the different rates of sucking seen in the neonate. Non-nutritive sucking, when rhythmic negative intraoral pressures are initiated which do not result in the delivery of milk, can be spontaneous or stimulated by an object in the mouth. This type of sucking tends to be twice as fast as nutritive sucking, the sucking frequency for non-nutritive sucking being 1.7 sucks/second in 37–38 week premature babies, 2 sucks/second in term neonates, and 2.7 sucks/second at 7–9 months postnatally. Corresponding times for nutritive sucking are about 1 suck/second in term neonates, increasing to 1.5 sucks/second by 7 months postnatally.

The taste of the fluid as well as nutrient content affects the efficiency of nutritive sucking in the early neonatal period. There is more sucking with milk than with 5% dextrose; however, sucking activities increased with solutions determined sweet by adult appraisal. Odour can also have some effect on sucking. If the nipples of anaesthetized female rat are washed it will cause a decrease in the number of pups attaching to nipples and an increase in the time between finding the nipple and attachment (see Herbst 1989).

Swallowing movements. First noted at about 11 weeks gestation, in utero fetuses swallow about 450 ml of amniotic fluid per day. Sucking and swallowing in premature infants (1700 g) is not associated with primary peristaltic waves in the intestine; however, in older babies and full-term neonates, at least 90% of swallows will initiate primary peristaltic waves.

In full-term neonates, the placing of a spoon or food onto the anterior part of the tongue elicits an extrusion reflex: the lips are pursed and the tongue pushes vigorously against the object. By 4–6 months the reflex changes and food deposited on the anterior part of the tongue is moved to the back of the tongue, into the pharynx, and swallowed. Rhythmic biting movements occur by 7–9 months postnatally, even in the absence of teeth.

Difficulties in suck and swallow. In infancy this may be an early indication of disturbed nervous system function. An interesting correlation between feeding styles of neonates and later eating habits has shown that children who were obese at 1 and 2 years of age, as measured by triceps skin-fold thickness, had a feeding pattern in the first month of life characterized by sucking more rapidly, producing higher pressures during prolonged bursts of sucking, and having shorter periods between bursts of sucking. Fewer feeds and higher sucking pressure were also associated with greater adiposity (Agras et al 1987).

CHROMAFFIN ORGANS

Suprarenal glands

The suprarenal glands are relatively very large at birth (**4.5, 8**) forming 0.2% of the entire body weight, compared with 0.01% in the adult. The left gland is heavier and larger than the right, as in the adult. At term each gland weighs about 4 g; the average weight of the two glands is 9 g (average in the adult is 7–12 g). The glands involute rapidly in the neonatal period with each gland losing 25% of its mass; the average weight of both glands is 5 g by the end of the second week, and 4.36 g by 3 months. The birth weight is not regained until puberty. The cortex of the suprarenal gland is thicker than in the adult and the medulla of the gland is small. Early studies on fetal suprarenal glands described extensive degeneration and necrosis within the fetal zone; however, it is believed that these studies showed disease processes rather than the normal involution of the gland. Normal involution causes the fetal zone cells of the postnatal gland to become smaller and assume the appearance and organization typical of zona fasciculata. In studies on neonatal monkeys a centripetal wave of transformation of fetal zone cells to zona fasciculata was observed, with only rare mitotic figures and no evidence of necrosis or collapse (Winter 1992).

MUSCULOSKELETAL SYSTEM

Fetal movements. These have been detected by ultrasonography in the second month of gestation (Hill 1992). Simple movements of an extremity have been observed sporadically as early as the seventh week of development (week 9 of pregnancy); combined movements of limb, trunk and head begin between weeks 12–16 of development. Fetal movements related to trunk and lower limb movements can be perceived consistently by the mother from about 16 weeks gestation (quickening). Movements of the fetus are often slow, asymmetric twisting and stretching movements of the trunk and limbs, resembling athetoid movements. Also there may be rapid, repetitive wide-amplitude limb movements, similar to myoclonus. By 32 weeks gestation symmetric flexor movements are most frequent and by term the quality of the movements has generally matured to smooth alternating movement of the limbs with medium speed and intensity. The reduced effect of gravity in utero may cause certain fetal movements to appear, on ultrasonography, more fluent than the equivalent movements observed postnatally. The number of spontaneous movements decreases after the 35th week of gestation and there is from this time an increase in the duration of fixed postures (Hill 1992). This restriction of normal fetal movements in late gestation is due to the degree of compliance of the maternal uterus; there is a slowing of growth at this time (see p. 26).

Early embryonic and fetal movements are vital to align the trabeculae within the bones, the correct attachments of the tendons, and the appropriate coiling of the constituent collagen fibres of the tendons. Movements of the fetus also encourage skin growth and flexibility indirectly as it is noted that fetuses with in utero muscular dystrophies, or other conditions resulting in small or atrophied muscles, have webs of skin, *pterygia*, passing across the flexor aspect of the joints. The condition, multiple pterygium syndrome, is characterized by webbing across the neck, the axillae and antecubital fossae. Usually the legs are maintained straight and webbing is not seen at the hip and knee.

The workload undertaken by the musculoskeletal system before birth is relatively light as the fetus is under essentially weightless conditions supported by the amniotic fluid. Thus the load on the muscles and bones is generated by the fetus itself with little gravitational effect. The reduction of gravitational force caused by the supporting fluid means that all parts of the fetus are subject to relatively equal forces and that the position assumed by the fetus relative to gravity is of little consequence. This is important to ensure the normal modelling of fetal bones especially the skull. Skulls of premature babies may become distorted due to the weight of the head on the mattress, despite regular changes in position; the application of oxygen therapy via a mask attached by a band around the head can cause dystososis of the occipital bone.

Neonatal skeleton

Generally the bones of the neonate are more spongy than the adult's because of the reduced work load undertaken by the fetus. Neonatal bones have more haemopoietic foci than adults'; haemopoiesis occurs in the red marrow of all the bones of the skeleton but later becomes limited to the red marrow of the vertebral bodies, the ribs, sternum, diploë of the skull and proximal ends of the humerus and femur (see p. 1409).

Because the adult skeleton is composed of a number of bones which fuse after birth, the neonate technically has more bones (270) than the adult (206; **4.11**).

Skull. The neurocranium is much larger than the viscerocranium in the neonate (**4.12, 15, 28**), the latter forming less than half of the length of the head, i.e. the distance from the top of the skull to the upper margin of the orbit is about 5 cm, whereas the distance from the upper margin of the orbit to the mandible is 4 cm. The ratio between the calvarial and facial portions is 8:1 at birth, changing to 2.5:1 in the adult female and 2:1 in the adult male. At birth the face is proportionally much wider than in the adult being twice as broad as its height.

Generally in the neonatal skull, the occipital condyles are elongate and flat instead of curved as in the adult. The tympanic rings are prominent features of the base of the skull; they provide attachment for the tympanic membranes (**4.14, 15**). The calvaria extends beyond the base of the skull both laterally and posteriorly. The hard palate is short (2.3 cm) and broad (2.2 cm) and the choanae are almost circular. The posterior border of the vomer at the choanae is relatively lower and more slanted than in the adult.

Fontanelles. The calvarial bones are thin at birth and ossification does not extend to the suture lines of the skull. The junctions between the calvarial bones are the sites of the fontanelles (**4.13**). Six fontanelles are present at birth; *anterior* and *posterior* fontanelles are median, paired *sphenoid* and *mastoid* are lateral, and other smaller accessory fontanelles may be present. An additional fontanelle located between the anterior and posterior fontanelles along the sagittal suture is found in some normal neonates but also in some infants with trisomy 21. The largest fontanelle is the anterior: it has an average diameter of 25 mm at birth. It overlies the superior sagittal dural venous sinus which transmits its pulsations to the overlying skin. Obliteration of the fontanelles occurs with progressive ingrowth of the edges of the bones that form their borders. The sphenoid is obliterated by 6 months as is the posterior; the anterior and mastoid are obliterated by the second year.

During parturition the calvarial bones can be displaced to the extent that they overlap each other at the sutures. Such skull 'moulding', occurring during delivery of the head, may exert tension on the great cerebral vein and be severe enough to rupture it.

Frontal bones (**4.12**). These are separated by the metopic suture at birth; this is obliterated by 6–8 years. Frontal sinuses do not develop until the second postnatal year.

Ethmoid bone (**4.16**). This has only the lateral masses containing the ethmoid air cells ossified at birth; the remainder is cartilage. The part forming the upper portion of the nasal septum ossifies during the first year, the two cribriform laminae ossify in the second year and the crista galli between the second and fourth years. These cartilaginous portions of the ethmoid fuse as they ossify, joining with the lateral masses in the sixth year.

Sphenoid bone (**4.16**). Made up of three parts, body, lesser wings, and greater wings with the pterygoid processes, these composite parts fuse during the first year. A relatively large mass of cartilage separates the body of the sphenoid from the basilar part of the occipital bone at the spheno-occipital synchondrosis; union of these bones does not begin until shortly after puberty. The optic canal in the neonate is relatively large and has a keyhole or figure of 8 shape rather than the circular profile of the adult. Sinuses do not develop in the sphenoid until the fifth year.

Temporal bones (**4.14, 15, 16**). Each consists of four parts, squamous, petrous and tympanic separated by sutures and the styloid process. The squamous part has a shallow mandibular fossa and the articular tubercle is absent. The petrous part is relatively large. The tympanic ring is thin and incomplete, with ends fused with the squamous part. The styloid process is cartilaginous except for a small ossified portion near the proximal end. The mastoid process is

1. *Anterior fontanelle*
2. *Frontal bone*
3. *Coronal suture*
4. *Sphenoid fontanelle*
5. *Roof of orbit*
6. *Fossa for lacrimal sac*
7. *Nasolacrimal canal*
8. *Floor of middle cranial fossa*
9. *Pterygoid process*
10. *Infraorbital foramen*
11. *Hard palate*
12. *Enamel of deciduous teeth*
13. *Mandibular canal*
14. *Mental foramen*
15. *Body of hyoid bone*
16. *Tympanic part of temporal bone*
17. *Clavicle*
18. *Scapula*
19. *Humerus*
    a. head
    b. body
    c. olecranon fossa
20. *Ulna*
21. *Radius*
22. *Bodies of metacarpal bones*
23. *Bodies of phalanges*
24. *Coxal bone*
    a. ilium
    b. ischium
    c. pubis
25. *Centre in talus*
26. *Centre in calcaneus*
27. *Parietal bone*
28. *Lesser wing of sphenoid bone*
29. *Posterior fontanelle*
30. *Optic canal*
31. *Squamosal suture*
32. *Hypophyseal fossa of sphenoid bone*
33. *Squamous part of temporal bone*
34. *Lambdoidal suture*
35. *Mastoid fonticulus*
36. *Subarcuate fossa*
37. *Internal acoustic meatus*
38. *Spheno-occipital synchondrosis*
39. *Petrous part of temporal bone*
40. *Occipital bone*
    a. squamous part
    b. lateral part
41. *6th cervical vertebra (3 centres)*
42. *1st rib*
43. *Centres of sternum (superimposed upon thoracic vertebrae)*
44. *12th rib*
45. *3rd lumbar vertebra (3 centres)*
46. *Centres in sacrum*
47. *Centre in coccyx*
48. *Femur*
    a. body
    b. condylar centre
49. *Tibia*
    a. condylar centre
    b. body
50. *Fibula*
51. *Bodies of metatarsal bones*
52. *Bodies of phalanges*

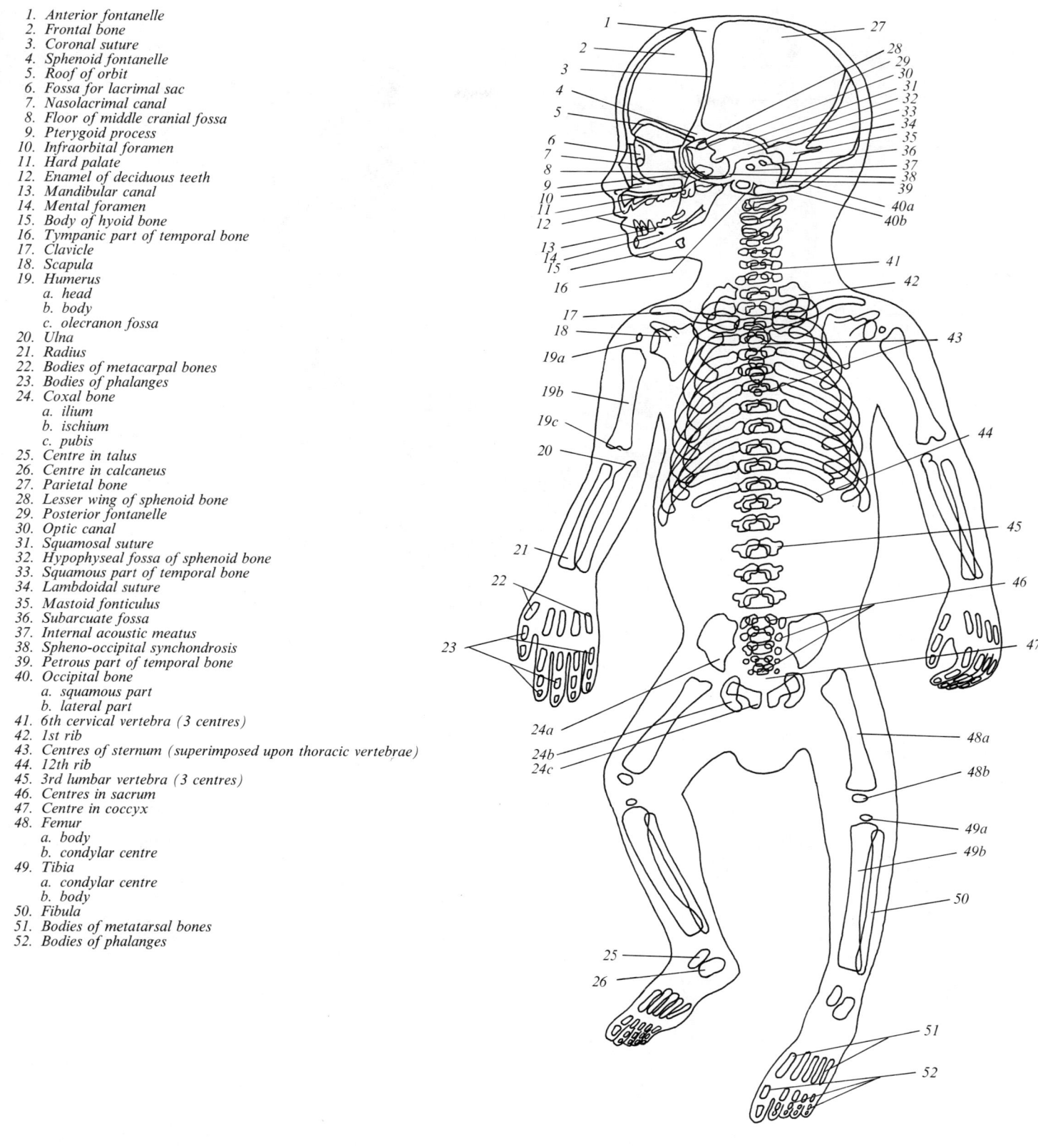

4.11   Ossified portions of the full-term neonate skeleton.

absent at birth; it develops as a small projection at the end of the first year; mastoid air cells invade it at puberty. In the neonate the petrous and squamous parts of the temporal bone are usually partially separated by the petrosquamous fissure which opens directly into the mastoid antrum of the middle ear. The fissure closes in 4% of infants during the first year but remains unclosed in 20 to 40% up to 19 years. It is a route for the spread of infection from the middle ear to the meninges.

External acoustic meatus. This is relatively long in the neonate, about two-thirds the length in the adult. It is almost straight and courses inward, downward and slightly forward. The lumen of the middle part is very narrow. The middle ear cavity is about the same size as the adult's. The epitympanic recess and the mastoid antrum are well developed. The auditory ossicles reach their adult size in the fetus by 6 months. The bony and membranous labyrinths of the inner ear are almost equal to adult size in the neonate; thus the inner

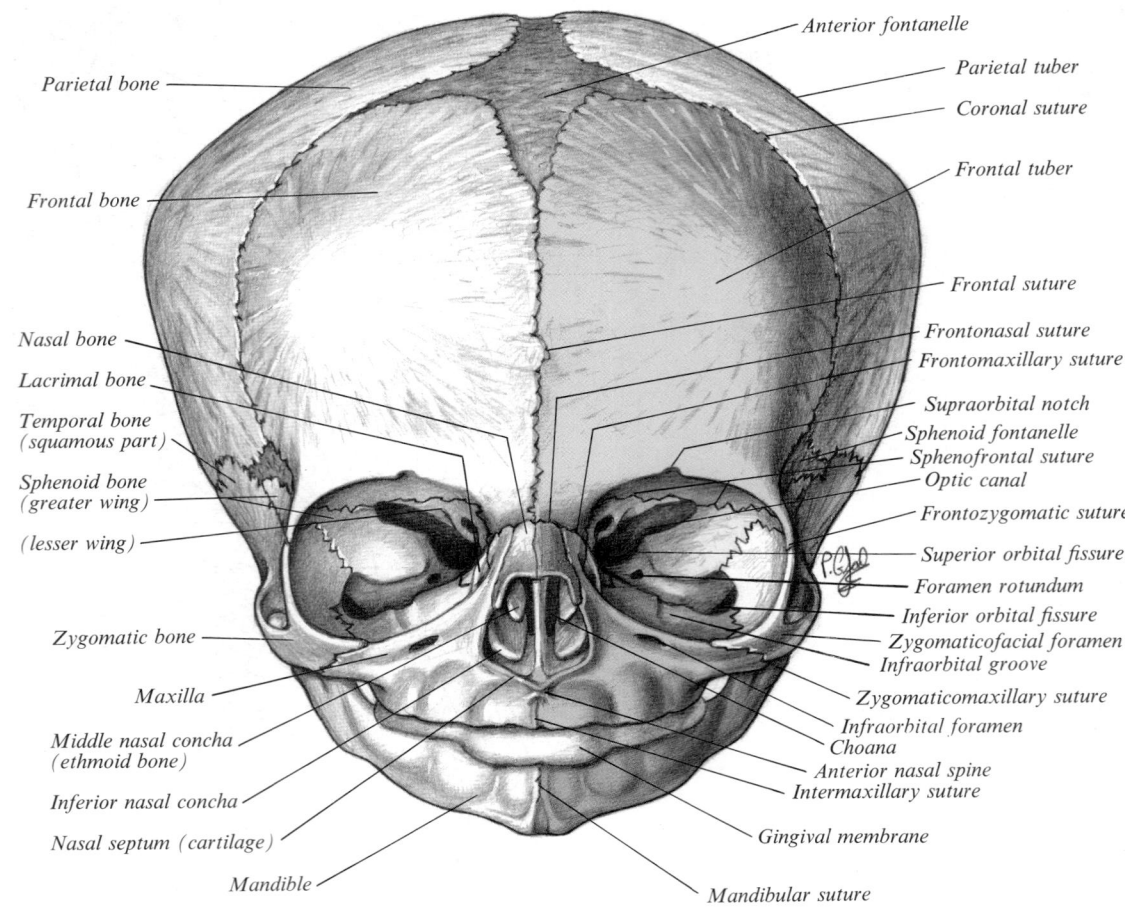

Parietal bone

Frontal bone

Nasal bone

Lacrimal bone

Temporal bone
(squamous part)

Sphenoid bone
(greater wing)

(lesser wing)

Zygomatic bone

Maxilla

Middle nasal concha
(ethmoid bone)

Inferior nasal concha

Nasal septum (cartilage)

Mandible

Anterior fontanelle

Parietal tuber

Coronal suture

Frontal tuber

Frontal suture

Frontonasal suture

Frontomaxillary suture

Supraorbital notch

Sphenoid fontanelle

Sphenofrontal suture

Optic canal

Frontozygomatic suture

Superior orbital fissure

Foramen rotundum

Inferior orbital fissure

Zygomaticofacial foramen

Infraorbital groove

Zygomaticomaxillary suture

Infraorbital foramen

Choana

Anterior nasal spine

Intermaxillary suture

Gingival membrane

Mandibular suture

4.12   Anterior aspect of the full-term neonatal skull. For a comparative view of an adult skull see **6.**135A, B.

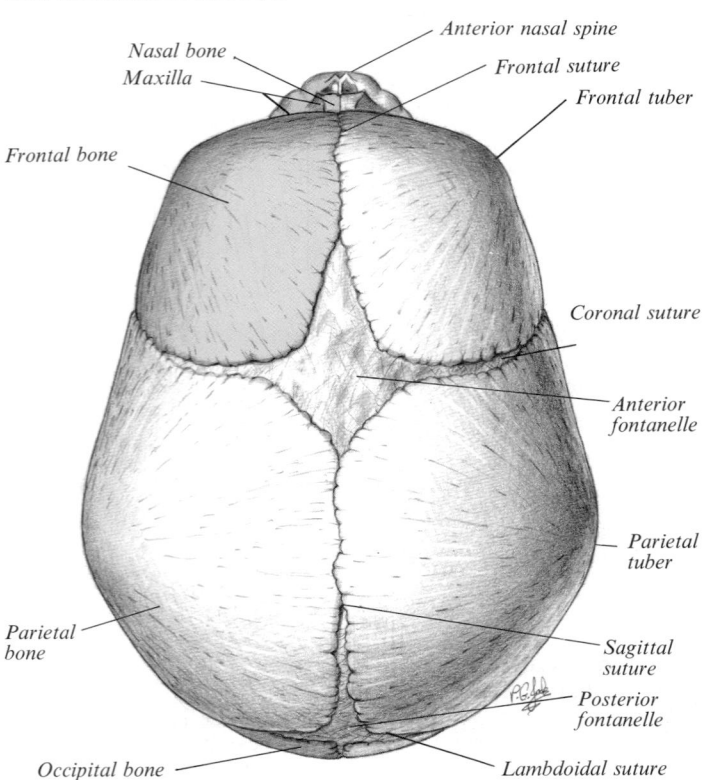

Nasal bone

Maxilla

Frontal bone

Parietal
bone

Occipital bone

Anterior nasal spine

Frontal suture

Frontal tuber

Coronal suture

Anterior
fontanelle

Parietal
tuber

Sagittal
suture

Posterior
fontanelle

Lambdoidal suture

4.13   Superior aspect of the full-term neonatal skull. For a comparative view of an adult skull see **6.**137.

ear occupies a relatively greater area of the petrous part of the temporal bone.

Internal acoustic meatus. The diameter of this in the neonate is almost as large as in the adult.

Auditory tube. In the neonate this is about half the length of the adult's; its opening from the middle ear cavity is as large as in the adult, but the pharyngeal opening in the nasal part of the pharynx is relatively smaller. The course of the auditory tube is horizontal in the newborn whereas in the adult it passes from the middle ear downward, forward and medially.

Occipital bone (**4.**11, 14, 15, 16). At birth this consists of four separate parts, a basilar part, two lateral parts and a squamous part; they are joined by cartilage and form a ring around the foramen magnum. The squamous and lateral parts fuse together from the second year; the cartilage between them is flexible at birth. The lateral parts fuse with the basilar part during years 3 and 4, but fusion may be delayed until the 7th year.

Maxillae (**4.**11, 12, 15, 16). These are low and broad with 10 large alveoli containing deciduous teeth. The bony palate is shallow at birth. Postnatal growth occurs mainly vertically. The maxillary sinus is an elongated sac in the neonate, but with eruption of the deciduous teeth it enlarges to become three times longer anteroposteriorly and five times greater in height and width. At birth the floor of the sinus is above that of the nasal cavity; in the adult it is below it.

Mandible (**4.**11, 12, 15, 16). This is formed by two halves joined by fibrous tissue at the mandibular suture which fuse after the first year. The body of the mandible is relatively large; its upper two-thirds are filled with alveoli containing the deciduous and some permanent teeth. The rami are short and broad, at an angle of 140° to the body (120° in the adult); the rami are shorter than the body (same length in the adult).

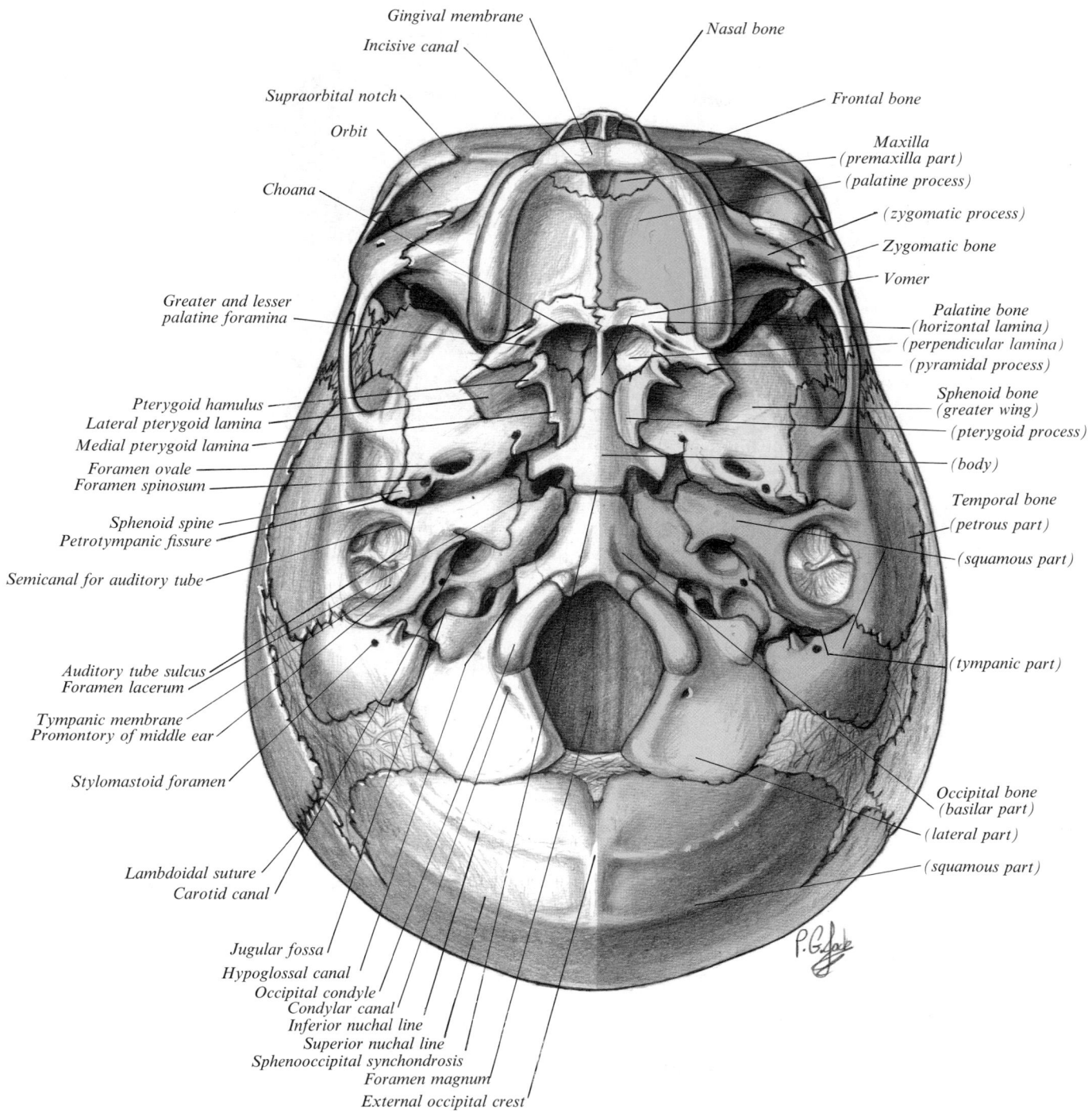

Gingival membrane
Incisive canal
Supraorbital notch
Orbit
Choana
Greater and lesser
palatine foramina
Pterygoid hamulus
Lateral pterygoid lamina
Medial pterygoid lamina
Foramen ovale
Foramen spinosum
Sphenoid spine
Petrotympanic fissure
Semicanal for auditory tube
Auditory tube sulcus
Foramen lacerum
Tympanic membrane
Promontory of middle ear
Stylomastoid foramen
Lambdoidal suture
Carotid canal
Jugular fossa
Hypoglossal canal
Occipital condyle
Condylar canal
Inferior nuchal line
Superior nuchal line
Sphenooccipital synchondrosis
Foramen magnum
External occipital crest

Nasal bone
Frontal bone
Maxilla
(premaxilla part)
(palatine process)
(zygomatic process)
Zygomatic bone
Vomer
Palatine bone
(horizontal lamina)
(perpendicular lamina)
(pyramidal process)
Sphenoid bone
(greater wing)
(pterygoid process)
(body)
Temporal bone
(petrous part)
(squamous part)
(tympanic part)
Occipital bone
(basilar part)
(lateral part)
(squamous part)

4.14 Inferior surface of the base of the full-term neonatal skull with the mandible removed. For comparative view of an adult skull see **6.**141A, 144A.

Vertebral column. This has no fixed curvatures in the neonate (**4.4**, **11**). Crelin (1973) notes that the vertebral column of the newborn is so flexible that when dissected free from the body it can easily be bent (flexed or extended) into a perfect half circle. A slight sacral curvature can be seen in the neonate; this develops as the sacral vertebrae ossify and fuse. The thoracic part of the column is the first to develop a relatively fixed curvature, concave anteriorly. The other curvatures develop later, the cervical curvature when the head can be held erect (from 3 months) and the lumbar curvature when walking starts (from 1 year). Each vertebra (excluding C1 and C2) consists of hyaline cartilage with three separate ossification centres. The atlas has only two ossification centres; it becomes a bony ring between the fifth and ninth years. The axis has four ossification centres, one for the body, two for the neural arches and one for the dens; the latter fuse between the third and sixth

years. In the neonate the intervertebral discs are composed mainly of the nucleus pulposus which becomes much reduced in the adult as the annulus fibrosus develops.

Upper limbs. Generally the upper limbs are proportionately shorter than in the adult. They are long compared to the neonatal trunk and lower limbs, extending to the upper thigh as in the adult; but the trunk is much shorter in the neonate (**4.11**). At birth the upper limbs are about the same length as the lower limbs but much more developed. When examining the proportions of parts of the upper limb, the forearm is longer than the arm in the newborn, more so in boys than girls (p. 29). Only primary centres of ossification are present in the upper limb, apart from a centre in the head of the humerus. The elbow of the newborn cannot achieve full extension, being some 10–15% short; it can flex to 145°. Crelin (1973) notes that

357

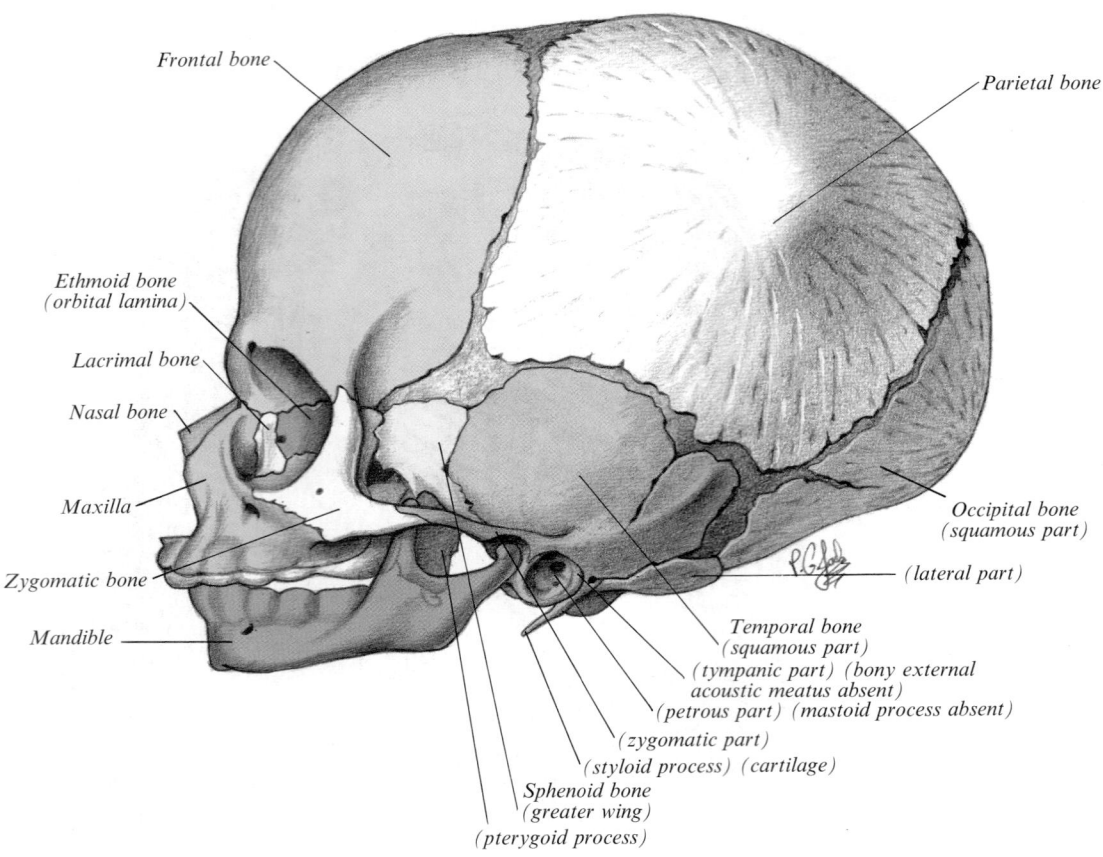

Frontal bone

Parietal bone

*Ethmoid bone
(orbital lamina)*

Lacrimal bone

Nasal bone

Maxilla

Zygomatic bone

Mandible

*Occipital bone
(squamous part)*

(lateral part)

*Temporal bone
(squamous part)*

*(tympanic part) (bony external
acoustic meatus absent)*

(petrous part) (mastoid process absent)

(zygomatic part)

(styloid process) (cartilage)

*Sphenoid bone
(greater wing)*

(pterygoid process)

4.15   Lateral view of a full-term neonatal skull. See also **6**.197. For a comparative view of an adult skull see **6**.133A, B.

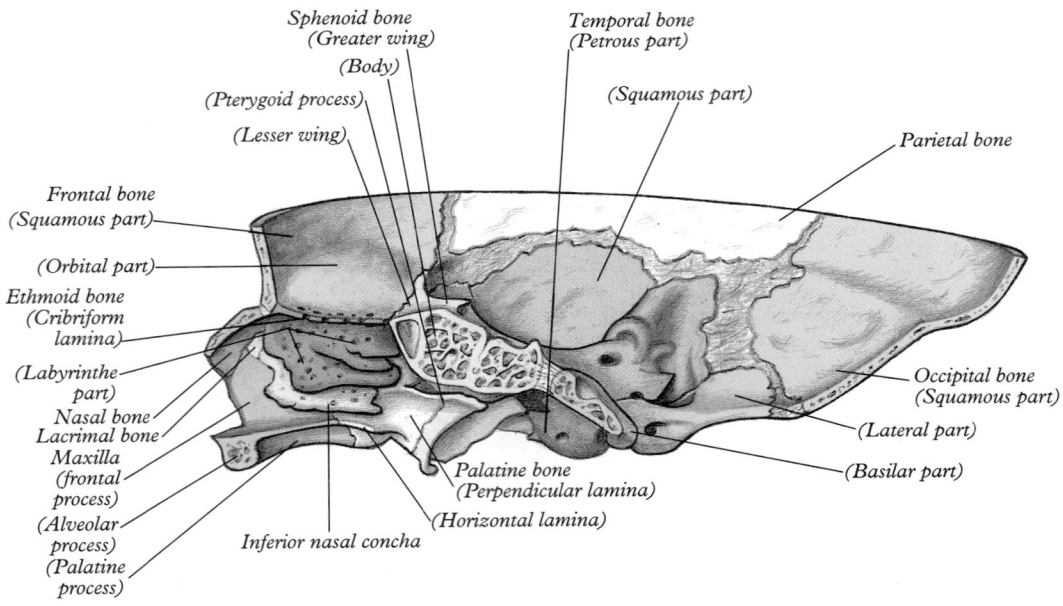

*Sphenoid bone
(Greater wing)*

(Body)

(Pterygoid process)

(Lesser wing)

*Temporal bone
(Petrous part)*

(Squamous part)

Parietal bone

*Frontal bone
(Squamous part)*

(Orbital part)

*Ethmoid bone
(Cribriform
lamina)*

*(Labyrinthe
part)*

Nasal bone

Lacrimal bone

*Maxilla
(frontal
process)*

*(Alveolar
process)*

*(Palatine
process)*

Inferior nasal concha

*Palatine bone
(Perpendicular lamina)*

(Horizontal lamina)

*Occipital bone
(Squamous part)*

(Lateral part)

(Basilar part)

4.16   Midsagittal section through a full-term neonatal skull. A sagittal section of an adult skull is presented in **6**.158.

the neonatal hand clearly shows four distinct palmar interosseous muscles, the deep head of flexor pollicis brevis being the first palmar interosseous, with a different origin and innervation to the superficial head of flexor pollicis brevis. The neonate has a relatively strong grasp, which may allow it to be pulled off a mattress within the first

few days. The fingernails of the upper limb usually extend to the finger tips or just beyond; they are soft at birth but soon dry to become quite firm and sharp.

Pelvis. In the newborn the pelvis is cone-shaped; the transverse diameter of the true pelvis is 2.2 cm, its anteroposterior diameter

2.8 cm and its length between the inlet and outlet is 2 cm. The sacrum is proportionately larger than in the adult and the sacral promontory is higher. When walking commences the sacrum descends between the ilia and the promontory develops. The bilateral ilia, ischia and pubic bones are variably ossified (see p. 669) at birth; they meet at the acetabulum which in the neonate is cartilaginous, relatively large and shallow.

Lower limbs. Compared to the upper limbs these are under-developed. They are retained in a flexed position. The leg is proportionally shorter than the thigh. In the neonate the legs appear to be bowed; however, the tibia and fibula are straight and the illusion of bow-legs is caused by the shape of the soft tissues and the slightly more advanced development of the lateral head of the gastrocnemius compared to its medial head. The femoral neck is much shorter and forms an acute angle with the shaft. The shaft of the femur is quite straight; the curvature seen in the adult is acquired with walking. The head of the femur is larger than the acetabular fossa with nearly one-third remaining external; the ligamentum teres is relatively very long. Dislocation of the hip joint is relatively easy and the femoral head can be removed from the acetabular fossa laterally, but not posteriorly; such dislocation occurs more frequently on the right side and in caucasian females. Two of the tarsal bones, the calcaneus and the talus, have an ossification centre at birth and in 50% of neonates a centre is present in the cuboid.

The muscles of the lower limb are much less developed than those in the upper limb. The fetal position, often assumed by postnatal babies, keeps the thighs in continuous abduction, stretching the adductors. The muscles which will later be used for walking are weak and the lack of gluteal development, particularly, gives the typically diminutive buttocks of the neonate.

Feet. In neonates these are usually inverted. They have a greater degree of dorsiflexion caused by the relatively greater area of the trochlea of the talus; plantar flexion on the other hand is limited, due to some extent to the shortness of the extensor muscles of the foot. At birth the footprint outlines the whole plantar surface due to deposition of subcutaneous fat beneath the longitudinal and transverse arches; thus most babies appear flat-footed.

SKIN

The surface area of the skin increases with growth. It has been estimated that the surface area of a premature neonate weighing 1505 g is about 1266 cm², whereas a neonate of 2980 g has a surface area of 2129 cm². The skin of the neonate is thinner than that of older infants and children. It cornifies over a period of 2–3 weeks providing protection; however, in the premature infant the thin epidermal layer allows absorption of a variety of substances, for example chlorhexidene and boric acid. At birth the skin is richly vascularized by a dense subepidermal plexus. The mature pattern of capillary loops and of the subpapillary venous plexus is not present at birth but develops as a result of capillary budding with migration of endothelia at some sites and the absorption of vessels from other sites (Ryan 1992). Perera et al (1970) studied the microvasculature of the skin for the first 3 months of postnatal life and noted how some regions mature faster than others. They noted, inter alia, that with the exceptions of the palms, soles and nail beds, the skin of the neonate has almost no papillary loops; the skin has a disordered capillary network which becomes more orderly from the second week when papillary loops appear; defined loops are not present until the fourth or fifth week, but all areas possess loops by 14–17 weeks postnatally.

Neonates exhibit a regional sequence of eccrine gland maturation, with the earliest sweating occurring on the forehead, followed by the chest, upper arm and, later, more caudal areas. Acceleration of maturation of the sweating response occurs in premature babies after delivery (Lane 1992).

CARDIOVASCULAR AND LYMPHATIC SYSTEMS

Heart

The heart is relatively large at birth (**4.6, 17**), and weighs about 20 g; the cardiac output is about 550 ml/minute, and the blood pressure 80/46. The fetal heart rate is approximately 150 beats a minute near term, at birth it is about 180/minute and it drops over the neonatal period to 170/minute after about 10 minutes, 120–140/minute from 15 minutes to 1 hour after birth. Obviously any signs of fetal distress will increase this general, basic level. The heart rate drops further with increasing age; thus it is normally between 113 and 127 beats/minute from 6 months to 1 year, settling to about 100/minute by the end of the first year.

At all ages the interventricular septum is considered part of the left ventricle, and the heart ratio is expressed as: weight of left ventricle and septum/weight of right ventricle. At birth the left ventricle weighs about 25% more than the right; however, the right ventricle has been working against the systemic pressure in the fetus (the pulmonary circulation being not yet active) and there is a right ventricular functional preponderance in the first 2 or 3 months after birth. With the establishment of the pulmonary circulation the work of the right side of the heart decreases; the left side of the heart, particularly the ventricle, grows rapidly to meet the demands of the active neonate and by the end of the second year it weighs twice as much as the right, a condition which continues to middle age.

Corresponding to the weight differential between the right and left ventricles, at birth the average thickness of the lateral walls of the ventricles is about equal (5 mm). By the end of the third month the left ventricle is thicker than the right, becoming twice as thick by the second year and three times as thick by puberty.

The heart is situated in the neonate midway between the crown of the head and the lower level of the buttocks (**4.5**). The anterior surface is formed mainly by the right atrium and right ventricle as in the adult; this surface is usually covered by the thymus which may extend over the base of the right ventricle.

Foramen ovale. About 4–6 mm in vertical length and 3–4 mm wide, it lies at the level of the third intercostal space with its long axis in the median plane (**4.5**). It is almost exactly in the coronal plane of the body; thus blood passes from the anteriorly placed right atrium posteriorly and upwards to reach the upper, posterior part of the left atrium. Although the foramen ovale closes functionally after pulmonary respiration is established it does not become structurally closed until some time later. It is obliterated in less than 3% of infants 2 weeks after birth, but in 87% by 4 months after birth.

Occlusion of fetal vessels after birth

Soon after birth a number of fetal vessels occlude, but the majority of vessels do not, suggesting that the walls of a population of fetal vessels are different to the remaining vessels permitting their differential constriction. In many cases the tunica media contains populations of smooth muscle, elastic fibres and connective tissue which proliferate prior to birth. Bradykinin, one of the Klinins — polypeptide hormones that induce contraction or relaxation of smooth muscle —, forms in the blood of the umbilical cord when the temperature of the cord drops at or shortly after birth. It is also formed and released by granular leucocytes in the lungs of the neonate after exposure to adequate oxygen. Bradykinin is a potent constrictor of the umbilical arteries and veins and the ductus arteriosus, while being at the same time a potent inhibitor of contraction of the pulmonary vessels (Crelin 1973). It has long been realized that intact endothelium is required for the relaxation response to bradykinin.

Ductus arteriosus. The ductus arteriosus (**4.17, 18**) shunts blood from the pulmonary trunk in the fetus to the arch of the aorta, thus bypassing the lungs. It arises as a direct continuation of the pulmonary trunk where it divides into right and left pulmonary arteries; it is 8–12 mm long. It joins the aorta at an angle of 30–35° on the left side, anterolaterally, below the origin of the left subclavian artery. The opening of the ductus arteriosus into the aorta is greatly elongated. The diameter of the ductus at its origin from the pulmonary trunk, when distended with blood, is 4–5 mm; this is nearly equal to the diameter of the adjacent ascending aorta (5–6 mm). Both arteries taper to a smaller diameter as they pass inferiorly with the aorta remaining slightly larger (4 mm; **4.18**). In the neonate the ductus arteriosus is closely related to the left primary bronchus inferiorly and the thymus gland anteriorly.

The ductus arteriosus is very different from the other great vessels arising from the heart (see p. 314). All the other great vessels develop tunicae mediae which are elastic in nature whereas the ductus has a muscular morphology (de Ruiter et al 1990). It has been proposed

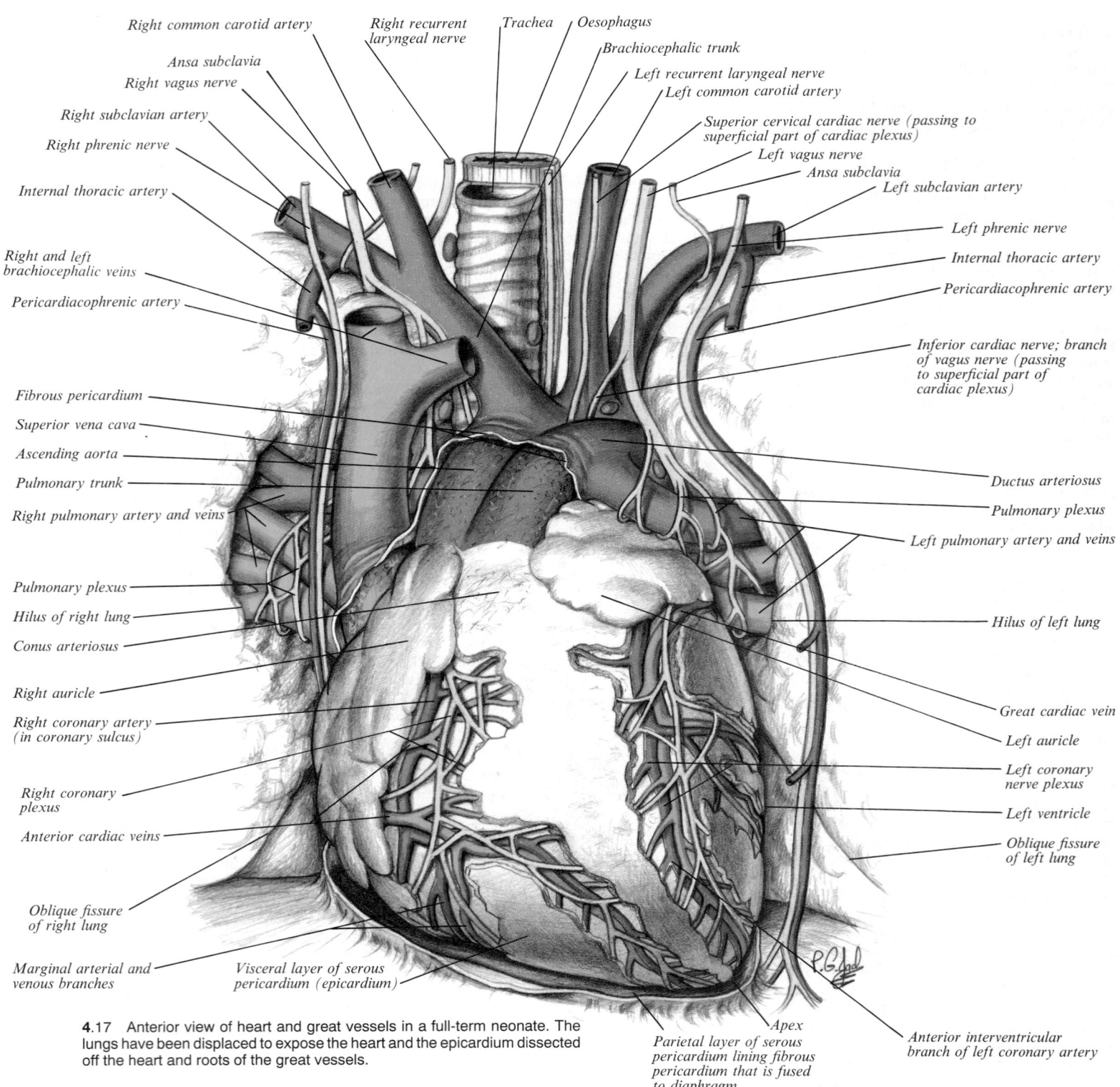

4.17 Anterior view of heart and great vessels in a full-term neonate. The lungs have been displaced to expose the heart and the epicardium dissected off the heart and roots of the great vessels.

that a relationship between the recurrent laryngeal branch of the vagus nerve and the developing ductus arteriosus could account for the histological difference in the ductus (Leonard et al 1983). The vagus nerve in the stage 16 embryo is very large in relation to the aortic arch system. The recurrent laryngeal nerve has a greater proportion of connective tissue than other nerves making it more resistant to stretch. Leonard et al (1983) suggest that tension applied by the left recurrent laryngeal nerve wrapping around the ductus arteriosus could provide a means of support which may permit the ductus to develop as a muscular artery rather than an elastic artery.

Patency of the ductus arteriosus. This is essential for fetal life. Prostaglandins appear to play a role in maintaining this patency. Fetal and neonatal ductal tissue can produce prostaglandin E_2 (PGE_2), prostaglandin I_2 (PGI_2), prostaglandin F_{2a} (PGF_{2a}). They inhibit the ability of the ductus to contract in response to oxygen.

Closure of the ductus arteriosus. Closure starts immediately after birth. The first stage is completed within 10–15 hours and the second stage takes 2–3 weeks. The first stage consists of contraction of the smooth muscle cells and development of subendothelial oedema; destruction of the endothelium and proliferation of the intima subsequently occurs, leading to permanent closure. Diverse factors have been identified which may promote ductal closure and include: increased oxygen tension; increase in the plasma catecholamine levels; suppression of PGI_2 production; switching off PGE receptors; a synergistic role of PGF_{2a} and oxygen levels; a fall in plasma adenosine level.

After birth these interrelated events together result in the closure of the ductus. It has been proposed that high oxygen tension initiates the synthesis of a hydroperoxy fatty acid which suppresses prostacyclin production, thus exposing the ductus to the contractile

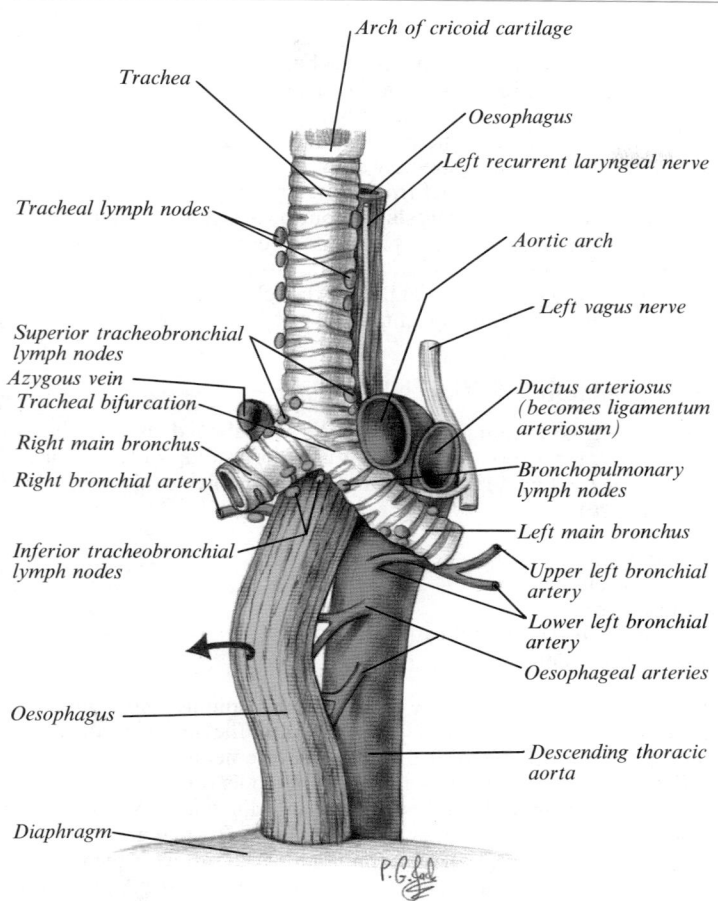

4.18 Anterior view with the heart removed to show the relationship between the left primary bronchus, the aortic arch and the ductus arteriosus in a full-term fetus.

effects of prostaglandin endoperoxide. For a discussion of the factors associated with closure of the ductus see Mathew (1992).

Umbilical vessels

Umbilical arteries (4.5). These are in direct continuation with the internal iliac arteries. Their lumen is about 2–3 mm in diameter at their origin, when distended, narrowing as they approach the umbilicus with a reciprocal thickening of the tunica media due particularly to an increase in the number of longitudinal smooth muscle fibres and elastic fibres. Before birth there is a proliferation of connective tissue within the vessel wall. After the cord is severed the umbilical arteries contract preventing significant blood loss; thrombi often form in the distal ends of the arteries. The arteries obliterate from their distal ends until by the end of the second or third month involution has occurred at the level of the superior vesical arteries. The proximal parts of the obliterated vessels remain as the medial umbilical ligaments.

Umbilical vein (4.4, 5). In the neonate this is 2–3 cm long and 4–5 mm in diameter when distended. It passes from the umbilicus, within the layers of the falciform ligament, superiorly and to the right, to the porta hepatis. Here it gives off several large intrahepatic branches to the liver and then joins the left branch of the portal vein. The umbilical vein is thin walled; it possesses a definite internal lamina of elastic fibres at the umbilical ring, but not in its intra-abdominal course. The tunica media contains smooth muscle fibres, collagen and elastic fibres. When the cord is severed the umbilical vein contracts but not so vigorously as the arteries. The rapid decrease in pressure in the vein after the cord is clamped means that the elastic tissue at the umbilical ring is sufficient to arrest any retrograde flow along the vessel. Prior to birth there is a subintimal proliferation of connective tissue around the periphery of the lumen. After birth the contraction of the collagen fibres in the tunica media and the increased connective tissue constitute the ligamentum teres, obliteration of the vessel occurring from the umbilical ring towards the hepatic end; no thrombi are formed in the obliteration process.

For up to 48 hours after birth the intra-abdominal portion of the umbilical vein can be easily dilated and in most adults the original lumen of the vein persists through the ligamentum teres and can be dilated to 5–6 mm in diameter.

Ductus venosus. This is a direct continuation of the umbilical vein arising from the left branch of the portal vein, directly opposite the termination of the umbilical vein. The ductus venosus passes for 2–3 cm within the layers of the lesser omentum, in a groove between the left lobe and caudate lobe of the liver, before terminating in the inferior vena cava, or in the left hepatic vein immediately before it joins the inferior vena cava. The tunica media of the ductus venosus contains circularly arranged smooth muscle fibres, an abundant amount of elastic fibres and some connective tissue. Obliteration of this vessel is initiated at the portal vein end and passes to the vena cava; it begins in the second postnatal week and the lumen is completely obliterated by the second or third month after birth.

Major arterial and venous vessels of the trunk. These, with their associated visceral branches, are relatively larger than those in the limbs, favouring central pooling of blood. Vessels in the periphery are nearly microscopic in the neonate and cannulation poses much more of a problem than in the adult. Large vessels are in the same relative positions as in the adult but may correspond to different vertebral levels. Thus although the bifurcation of the common carotid artery into the internal and external carotid arteries occurs at the level of the hyoid bone, as in the adult, the hyoid bone is relatively higher in the neonate neck than in the adult. The renal arteries similarly arise higher, often between T12 and L1 (in the adult upper border of L2). The abdominal aorta bifurcates into common iliac arteries at the upper border of L4 rather than at the lower border as in the adult.

Lymphoid and lymphatic tissues

Thymus (4.19). This accounts for 0.42% of the body weight at birth, compared to 0.03 to 0.05% in the adult. It weighs 10 g in the full-term neonate, increases in weight steadily until puberty, when it weighs about 30 g, and thereafter slowly decreases until old age when it may be 12.5 g. At birth the thymus is most often bilobar; it is 4–6 cm long, 2.5–5 cm wide and 1 cm thick. The gland has a cervical portion which may extend as high as the lower margin of the thyroid gland, inferiorly; the lower end of the right lobe is commonly between the right side of the ascending aorta and the right lung, anterior to the superior cava. Anterior to the gland in the neck are the sterno-hyoid and sternothyroid muscles and fascia; in the thorax the gland is covered by the manubrium, the internal thoracic vessels, the upper three costal cartilages, and laterally the pleura. Posteriorly the thymus

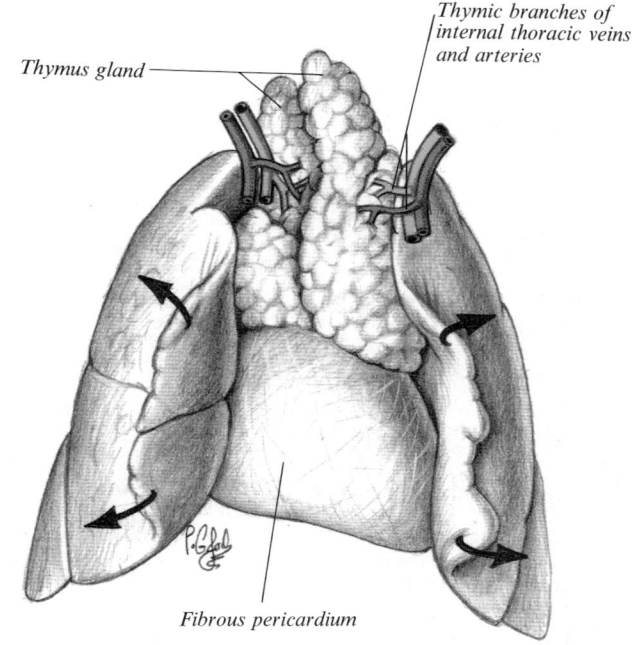

4.19 Anterior view of the thymus gland in the full-term neonate. The lungs have been displaced to show the extent of the gland.

is in contact with the vessels of the superior mediastinum, especially the left brachiocephalic vein which may be partly embedded in the gland, the upper part of the thoracic trachea, and the upper part of the anterior surface of the heart. The thickest part of the gland at birth is not at the superior thoracic aperture but lies immediately above the base of the heart. During childhood the thymus narrows and lengthens and the cervical portion becomes less noticeable. The thymus is necessary for the development of the white pulp of the spleen.

Spleen (4.5). At birth the spleen weighs, on average, 13 g. It doubles its weight in the first postnatal year and triples it by the end of the third year. Accessory spleens are very common in neonates, located in the greater omentum.

Lymph vessels and lymph nodes. The thoracic duct is the largest single lymph vessel in the body in both neonates and adults. It is about 10–11 cm long in the neonate. The right lymphatic duct that drains lymph from the right side of the head and neck is only 2–3 cm long and surrounded by lymph nodes. The total amount of lymphoid tissue in the form of lymph nodes is considerable in the neonate. Generally lymphoid tissues increase in amount during childhood because of the growth of nodes already present in the neonate. The pharyngeal tonsil (adenoid) is formed shortly before birth by infiltration of the pharyngeal bursa with masses of lymphoid cells. Definitive follicles with germinal centres are formed during the first postnatal year, and the pharyngeal tonsil reaches its maximal development at 6 years; thereafter involution is completed by puberty. The paired palatine tonsils are situated slightly higher in the tonsillar fossae in the neonate; each descends in position during the second and third postnatal year; definitive lymph nodules appear after birth. The palatine tonsils may begin to atrophy from the fifth year and involution is often complete by puberty.

ENDOCRINE GLANDS

Of the neonatal endocrine glands, the pancreas has been described under the gastrointestinal tract and the gonads under reproductive organs.

Thyroid gland (4.5). Relatively large in the neonate, it has a long narrow isthmus connecting lobes which do not yet contact the upper part of the trachea. The gland attains half the adult size by 2 years postnatally. Colloid is present in the gland from 3 months gestation and thyroxin by 4.5 months gestation.

Parathyroid glands. These are variable in size and position as in the adult. They double in size between birth and puberty. Parathyroid hormone (PTH) is produced from the 12th week of development.

Pituitary gland (hypophysis). About one-sixth the weight of the adult gland, it increases in weight to become about one-half the weight of the adult gland at 7 years, attaining adult weight at puberty. Throughout postnatal life the gland appears larger in females, in both size and weight.

EVALUATION OF THE NEONATE

The general condition of the neonate is evaluated as quickly as possible after delivery, traditionally using a grading of five clinical features devised by Virginia Apgar (1953). The five clinical features are (see 4.20):

- heart rate
- respiration
- muscle tone
- response to pharyngeal catheter
- colour of trunk.

These are each given a score from 0–2 at 1 minute and 5 minutes after delivery; evaluation is repeated until the infant's condition stabilizes. Total scores of 0–3 indicate severe neonatal distress, 4–6 indicate moderate difficulty in adjusting to extrauterine life, and scores of 7–10 indicate little difficulty in adjustment. Whereas the Apgar score alone is a poor index of asphyxia, and resuscitation may be indicated regardless of a high score, a low Apgar score invariably indicates some sort of problem. Generally the Apgar score is used alongside a narrative description of the baby at birth. The improvement in the Apgar score from 0 to 20 minutes after delivery has become an internationally understood and accepted shorthand for describing the success or otherwise of the resuscitative effort; it provides valuable information for medical practitioners examining the baby during the first years of life (Roberton 1992).

	0	1	2
Heart rate	Absent	Slow (less than 100 beats/min)	Greater than 100 beats/min
Respiratory effort	Absent	Slow or irregular	Good; crying lustily
Muscle tone	Limp	Some flexion of extremities	Active motion; well flexed
Response to pharyngeal catheter	No response	Grimace	Cough or sneeze; vigorous cry
Colour of trunk	Blue or pale	Body pink, extremities blue	Completely pink

4.20 The factors which are evaluated at birth in the Apgar scoring system. Each factor is scored from 0–2 giving a maximal score of 10. Evaluations are made at 1 minute and 5 minutes after delivery and repeated until the infant's condition is stable.

Neonatal procedures

It is estimated that 1–2% of all newborn infants in the United Kingdom receive intensive care following birth. Many of these babies are born prematurely and some require cardiorespiratory and nutritional support for one to several weeks, or even months, until functional maturity of their organ systems has occurred. Others are mature at birth but the transition to extrauterine life has been complicated by conditions such as birth asphyxia, sepsis or hypoxia, often leading to persistent pulmonary hypertension. A small number of babies require intensive care because anatomical abnormalities have occurred during their in-utero development; examples of such conditions include congenital abnormalities of the heart, obstruction to the digestive system and herniation of the abdominal contents into the chest as a consequence of congenital diaphragmatic hernia. While many of these conditions can only be corrected by operative procedures, the babies will usually require intensive care before and after their surgery.

In order to provide effective intensive care, catheterization of a central vein for pressure monitoring, placement of a 'long-line' into, or near, the heart for intra-venous feeding and insertion of an in-dwelling catheter into an artery for blood gas and arterial pressure monitoring are often required. For other infants, samples of cerebrospinal fluid, blood or urine are required to determine whether infection is present. Some of the more commonly performed procedures which are required in the newborn period are described below, with particular reference to the anatomical landmarks which are referred to to ensure safe and accurate localization.

Endotracheal intubation

The insertion of an endotracheal tube (ETT) is a procedure which is commonly performed for resuscitation of the

Table 4.1 Guidelines for endotracheal tube length*

Birth weight (kg)	Nose to mid-trachea (cm)	Lips to mid-trachea (cm)
0.5	—	6.2
0.75	—	6.5
1.0	8	6.8
1.5	9	7.3
2.0	10	7.9
2.5	11	8.5
3.0	12	9.1
3.5	13	9.7

*Hodson & Truog 1987

Table 4.2 Key anatomical points relevant to endotracheal tube positioning in the neonate*

Structure	Vertebral level
Vocal cords	C1–2
Thoracic inlet	T1
Carina	T3–4, or T4

*Blayney & Logan 1994

newborn at birth and subsequently to enable artificial ventilation. The ETT is introduced into either the nose or the mouth and guided through the vocal cords with the help of a laryngoscope. The tip of the ETT should be in the mid-trachea, well above the carina.

The required length of the tube can be estimated according to birth weight, as in Table 4.1, or, in an emergency, by measuring the distance from the tragus of the ear to the tip of the chin; the distance from the lips to the mid-trachea gives approximately the same measurement. Alternatively, a commonly used formula for the estimation of 'tip to lip' tube length is the '1-2-3 = 7-8-9 guideline'. This is based on the observation that, for a baby weighing 1 kg at birth, the distance from the lip to midtrachea is 7 cm; for a 2 kg baby it is 8 cm and for a 3 kg baby it is 9 cm (Tochen 1979). For nasotracheal tubes the formula takes into account the nasopharyngeal length needed and becomes '1-2-3 = 8-10-12'. These figure are also achieved by using the 7-8-9 figures plus the birth weight in kilograms (Kohelet et al 1982).

Confirmation of correct positioning of the ETT is obtained radiologically, either from a chest X-ray or, in order to minimize radiation exposure of the baby, from a 'coned view' of the trachea. The anatomical reference points used for the X-ray to assess the position of the ETT are the clavicles, the bodies of the vertebrae and the carina (although the latter is not always visible on X-ray). In the past it has been advised that the ETT tip should be placed just below the clavicles, at the level of the first rib (Fletcher et al 1983) or 1–2 cm above the carina (Carolene 1991). It has recently been suggested that, as positioning of the clavicles can vary according to angulation and placement of the baby and the carina cannot always be identified, the body of the first thoracic vertebra (T1) would be a more stable reference point as the target for the ETT tip (Blayney & Logan 1994). The length of the trachea in the neonate can be as short as 3.1 cm in premature infants (Coldiron 1968) and the distance from T1 to the carina ranges from 1.4 cm in babies weighing 500–1000 g to 1.8 cm in those weighing 3001–3500 g (Blayney & Logan 1994). Relevant anatomical reference points are given in Table 4.2.

UMBILICAL ARTERIAL CATHETERIZATION

Insertion of an umbilical catheter is undertaken to provide direct access to the arterial circulation. This enables arterial blood to be withdrawn repeatedly for measurement of oxygen and carbon dioxide partial pressures, pH, base excess and many other parameters of blood biochemistry and haematology; the in-dwelling catheter also provides a facility for the continuous measurement of arterial blood pressure.

The catheter is inserted directly into either the cut end or the side of one of the two umbilical arteries in the umbilical cord stump which remains attached to the baby following transection of the umbilical cord at the time of delivery. The catheter tip is then advanced along the length of the umbilical artery, through the internal iliac artery, into the common iliac artery and from there into the aorta. In order to keep the catheter patent a small volume of fluid is infused continuously through it. It is important that the tip of the catheter should be located well away from arteries branching from the aorta, to avoid potentially harmful perfusion of these arteries with the catheter fluid. Thus umbilical arterial catheter tips are placed in the descending aorta either in a 'high' position, above the coeliac artery but well below the ductus arteriosus, or in a 'low' position, below the renal and inferior mesenteric arteries but above the point where the aorta bifurcates into the two common iliac arteries. The length of catheter to be inserted can be estimated from charts relating the required catheter length to external body measurements (Dunn 1966; Rosenfeld et al 1980), or from birth weight (Shukla & Ferrara 1986). Positioning of the catheter is assessed by means of abdominal and/or chest X-rays: a 'high' catheter tip should be located in the descending aorta somewhere between the levels of the sixth and ninth thoracic vertebrae (T6–T9), while a 'low' catheter tip should be at a level between the third and fourth lumbar vertebrae (L3–L4). Relevant anatomical reference points are given in Table 4.3.

Peripheral arterial puncture

It is common practice to insert a small-bore cannula into a peripheral artery in neonates receiving intensive care when either the umbilical artery is not accessible or there are clinical reasons to avoid cannulation of the umbilical vessels. Transillumination can be used to provide an outline of the artery to be cannulated (see below) (Pearse 1978). The peripheral arteries which are most commonly used are the radial artery, just above the anterior surface of the wrist, and the posterior tibial artery, posterior to the medial malleolus. The proximity of the ulnar nerve to the ulnar artery increases the risk of nerve damage associated with arterial cannulation of the ulnar artery, and the relatively poor collateral circulation associated with the dorsalis pedis artery means that this artery is used only as a last resort. The brachial artery at the antecubital fossa also has a poor collateral circulation and the median nerve is in close proximity; it is generally considered, therefore, that cannulation of this artery is not justified.

Confirmation that an adequate col-

Table 4.3 Key anatomical reference points for umbilical arterial catheterization

Structure	Vertebral level
Ductus arteriosus	T4–5
Coeliac artery	T12
Superior mesenteric artery	T12–L1
Renal artery	L1
Inferior mesenteric artery	L3
Aortic bifurcation	L4–5

Table 4.4 Key anatomical reference points relevant to lumbar puncture

Structure	Vertebral level
End of conus medullaris	L2
Iliac crests	L3–4
End of subarachnoid space	S1–2

lateral circulation is present when cannulating the radial artery can be obtained by performing *Allen's test*, in which both the radial and ulnar arteries are compressed at the wrist following exsanguination of the hand and forearm; release of pressure on the ulnar artery while maintaining occlusion of the radial artery should result in reperfusion of the hand and lower forearm if an adequate collateral ulnar arterial supply is present. Alternatively, intact arterial flow can usually be confirmed, particularly in the preterm infant, by direct visualization of the arteries using transillumination. A cold light source is placed on the posterior aspect of the lower forearm and the shadow of the pulsating arteries can be seen on the anterior surface of the forearm.

Umbilical vein catheterization

The umbilical vein is catheterized to enable exchange and transfusion of blood, for central venous pressure measurement and, usually in an emergency, for vascular access. The catheter is inserted into the cut end of the umbilical vein and is advanced along the length of the vein, through the ductus venosus and into the inferior vena cava, the tip being placed between the ductus venosus and the right atrium. Positioning of the catheter tip is confirmed radiologically and it should be located just above the diaphragm at a point which is level with the ninth or tenth thoracic vertebrae (T9–T10). As with umbilical arterial catheters, estimation of the required catheter length can be determined from standard charts (Dunn 1966).

Percutaneous central venous catheterization

Small-bore catheters can be fed into large central veins or into the right atrium via needles or catheters inserted in the peripheral veins. Typically, the median cubital or basilic veins are used in the upper limb and the great saphenous at the medial malleolus in the lower limb. The tip of the catheter is sited at the entrance to the right atrium. The required catheter length is assessed from direct measurement of the distance between the point of surface entry in the limb to the right atrium, estimated at midsternal level.

Lumbar puncture

Cerebrospinal fluid (CSF), obtained by lumbar puncture, is often needed to determine whether meningitis is present. CSF surrounds both the spinal cord and the cauda equina; when bacterial meningitis occurs an increased inflammatory cell influx can be demonstrated by microscopical examination of CSF and pathogenic bacteria can be identified by culture and microscopy.

During gestation the relationship between the conus medullaris and the vertebral column changes such that the conus medullaris gradually ascends to lie at higher vertebral levels. By 19 weeks of gestation the conus is adjacent to the fourth lumbar vertebra (L4), and by full term (40 weeks) it is at the level of the second lumbar vertebra (L2). By 2 months postnatally the conus medullaris has usually reached its permanent position at the level of the body of the first lumbar vertebra (L1) (Barson 1970). In per-

forming a lumbar puncture it is important to enter the spinal canal below the level of the termination of the spinal cord, the tip of the conus medullaris. While this is usually at or above the level of the second lumbar vertebra (L2), in some individuals the cord may, rarely, extend as low as L3 and it is advisable, therefore, for the needle to enter the spinal canal below this level.

A lumbar puncture is performed by placing the baby in a position, either lying or 'sitting', which gives maximum convex curvature to the lumbar spine. A needle with trochar is inserted into the back between the spines of the third and fourth vertebrae and into the subarachnoid space below the level of the conus medullaris. The space between L3 and L4 is approximately level with the iliac crests and it is usual to insert the needle and trochar into the intervertebral space immediately above or below the iliac crests. The needle and trochar pass through the interspinous ligament, the ligamentum flavum, the dura mater and the arachnoid mater (see Table 4.4).

Suprapubic aspiration of the bladder

In infants under the age of two years, and particularly in neonates, urine is often collected, either as part of a general sepsis screen, when infection is suspected but neither certain nor localized, or when a specific urinary infection is suspected. In either case, there may be some urgency in initiating treatment with antibiotics and the urine must be collected before such treatment is started in order to avoid a partially treated specimen giving misleading results.

In young infants a large portion of the bladder, when it contains urine, is located above the level of the symphysis pubis, in the lower abdomen rather than in the pelvis. It is possible, therefore, to obtain urine by inserting a needle, connected to a syringe, into the bladder through the abdominal wall about 2 cm above the symphysis pubis and aspirating the contents into the sterile syringe (Nelson & Peters 1965). Since urine is obtained directly from the bladder it cannot have been contaminated by organisms around the perineum and anus, as it might be if the urine is passed into a bag or container; any growth on culture, therefore, is regarded as significant and indicative of urinary infection.

The success rate of the procedure is variable and depends upon the bladder being full. Recently, a much higher success rate has been reported by using an ultrasound scanner to locate the bladder and confirm that it contains urine prior to the insertion of the needle (Buys et al 1994).

GROWTH

Growth is a term widely used in everyday conversation and applied to both living and inanimate objects; commonly it implies an increase in mass or size. The section which follows is concerned with this general concept as it applies to the growth of cells, tissues and organs constituting a whole animal. Within this context, and indeed in others, it becomes evident that the simple definition 'increase in mass and size' is not entirely satisfactory; it becomes necessary to distinguish between different types of growth to appreciate the complex nature of the process and the exquisite control mechanisms involved.

TYPES OF GROWTH

At the cellular level distinctions can be made between protein and DNA synthesis leading to an increase in cell number by mitotic division, *cellular hyperplasia*, and synthesis of protein and cellular material without mitotic division leading to an increase in cell size, *cellular hypertrophy*. Also at this level growth may be described with reference to the amount of extracellular matrix produced by the cells (this is termed *accretionary growth*) or by the position in which cells and extracellular matrix are added, i.e. either within a tissue as in *intestinal growth* or to its surface, as in *appositional growth*.

Cellular hyperplasia

Within the normal life cycle *hyperplasia*, or *multiplicative growth*, is seen during the developmental stages of embryogenesis, organogenesis and gestational growth, and also in infancy and childhood. Generally, hyperplastic growth decreases as the individual approaches sexual maturity; however, each cell lineage normally remains in multiplicative growth for differing time periods such that whereas some cells, for example neurons, complete their mitotic proliferative phase in utero, other cells, for example type I alveolar epithelial cells, continue to divide during childhood, while still other cells, for example stem cells for blood production, divide continuously for the lifetime of the individual (see **4.21**).

Cell division is controlled at two main levels, extrinsic and intrinsic; these levels correlate to the distance effector substances travel to exert their effect. Extrinsic control of cell division depends on factors from other tissues (a hormonal effect, whereas intrinsic control depends on factors produced locally by the cells themselves (a paracrine effect.

Cellular hypertrophy

Hypertrophic or *auxetic growth* involves an increase in the size of the specific individual cells characterizing a tissue without their division. It is usually seen in cells which can no longer undergo mitosis and therefore is mainly a feature of postnatal life. It is particularly prominent in certain invertebrate tissues such as the salivary glands of Diptera, but is also well shown by some mammalian tissues. For example, there is a vast postnatal increase of both surface area and cytoplasmic volume in many neurons and glial cells; the growing striated muscle fibre, the oöcyte, the myelinating Schwann cells, and the smooth muscle cells of the pregnant uterus furnish further obvious examples. The majority of other tissues, however, show some hypertrophic growth but of limited degree, while conversely, in some sites, continued multiplicative growth is accompanied by a **reduction** in cell volume (e.g. granule cells of the cerebellar cortex, and small lymphocytes in lymphoid tissue).

It is widely held that the general nucleocytoplasmic ratio to which most of the body's cells roughly approximate reflects the fixed quantity of DNA in their diploid nuclei which, in turn, imposes a rate limitation on the replacement of cytoplasmic proteins (each of which has a characteristic turnover rate). Thus, with continuing auxetic growth of a cell, its cytoplasmic volume eventually reaches a point beyond which the structural genes cannot effectively replace the protein which is undergoing continual degradation. In some cases, growth ceases at this point, or nuclear replication with cell division occurs. The cases of hypertrophic growth cited above, however, often proceed far beyond the usual ratio of cytoplasmic

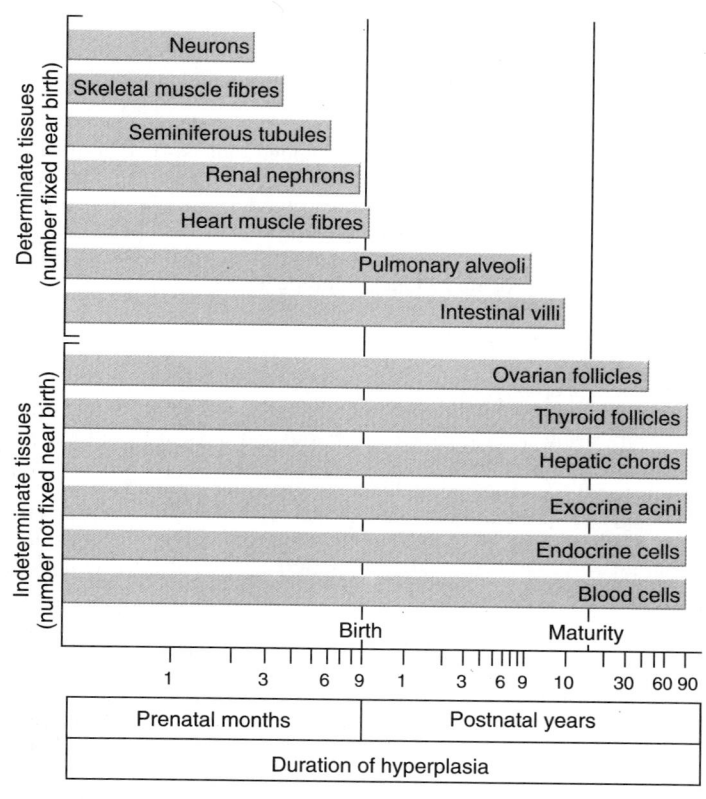

4.21 The duration of multiplicative growth for various human tissues (after Gilbert 1992).

volume to nuclear material and, in these, various methods of providing auxiliary nuclear support have emerged. The large dipteran salivary gland cells develop 'giant' polytene chromosomes containing some multiple of the diploid DNA content. The striated muscle fibre and other 'giant' cells such as megakaryocytes are, of course, multinucleate syncytia. Finally, the enlarging oöcyte and neuron (possessing but a single haploid and a single diploid nucleus, respectively) have their surfaces clothed by numerous satellite cells (follicular or glial cells). Such satellites probably provide auxiliary metabolic and nuclear support for the enlarged central cell, i.e. the two are functionally interlocked as a *cytophysiological unit*.

Hypertrophic growth can be induced; for example, muscle fibres enlarge when exercised and adipose cells enlarge with fat deposition in obesity.

Accretionary growth

Accretionary growth denotes an increase in the amount of extracellular matrix between tissue cells rather than either an increase in cell number or of cell size. Bone and cartilage are the most commonly cited examples; other less obvious examples are the other fibrous connective tissues, tendons, joint capsules, aponeuroses, fasciae, and the cornea.

Appositional growth

Appositional growth is a specific type of growth where new generations of cells and extracellular matrix are added to the surface of the tissue by the repeated division of the cells of a cambial layer which surrounds the tissue, for example periosteum and perichondrium.

Interstitial growth

Interstitial growth is seen where multiplicative and sometimes accretionary growth continues throughout the thickness of a tissue mass and it grows as a whole expanding from within.

Meristematic growth

Meristematic growth describes growth from a tip which contains populations of dividing cells. As division occurs the tip moves distally leaving populations of cells from its early divisions. An example of meristematic growth is seen in the limb buds where the progress zone produces first cells of the shoulder, then is moved distally to produce populations of the arm, and so on.

Compensatory growth

Tissue and organ growth is normally under some sort of control: a balance is achieved between loss through 'wear and tear' and the maintenance of functional tissue integrity. Large-scale loss can be compensated for either through regeneration of the tissue itself, as in the liver, or by compensatory growth elsewhere, for example following the loss of one kidney. Compensatory growth, however, appears to be strictly regulated; regenerating liver, for instance, more or less regains its original size, at which point growth ceases.

Integration of types of growth

In the later gestational months and the postnatal period all the types of growth are welded together in various patterns, with differential growth rates and directions in different parts of the system. For example, in the developing limb whereas the production of the mesenchymal populations may be an example of meristematic growth, the overlying ectoderm, in contrast, grows interstitially. Generally the differential growth patterns with either random or preferentially polarized directions of mitotic division, together with alterations in cell size, shape and surface consistency, are central features of embryonic development and are responsible for the moulding of tissues into specific shapes whether solid masses, hollow balls, tubes, sheets and so forth. Equally important in some regions, however, is a process of tissue regression, with degeneration, cell death and tissue removal.

PATTERNS OF GROWTH

When describing growth patterns of a whole body two types of growth can be considered, *isometric growth* and *allometric growth*.

Isometric growth

True isometric growth would imply a progressive proportional increase of all organs and systems with time. Clearly isometry does not occur in developing embryos where differential rates of growth obtain, a process termed allometric growth.

Allometric growth

Allometric growth describes the differences in the relative rates of growth between one part of the body and another. It is most clearly seen in the changes in body proportion between fetuses, neonates, children and adults. Between 6 and 7 weeks after fertilization the head is nearly one-half of the total embryonic length. Subsequently during gestation the head grows proportionally more slowly so that at birth it is one-quarter of the whole length. During childhood this pattern of growth continues with lengthening of the torso and limbs until, in adults, the head is one-eighth the length (**4.22**).

Allometric growth can be considered to be responsible for the variation of the vertebrate body plan, especially in, for example, skull development in mammals. It has been suggested that a basic pattern for the base of the skull is specified by the basal layer of the neural tube (see p. 274). The initial stimulus to chondrogenesis is provided by the neuroepithelial cells resulting in the arrest of migration of underlying migrating mesenchymal cells. The pattern of arrest forms the template for the base of the skull. In mammals there is some modification of the skull prior to birth but generally the mammalian skull is globular, assisting passage along the birth canal. After birth the specific skull shape for the species develops by allometric growth, resulting in either the flat, neotenous human skull, the more prognathous skulls of lower primates or the relatively extreme elongation of the skulls in horses or anteaters.

GROWTH HORMONES AND GROWTH FACTORS

Growth during the embryonic, fetal and postnatal period is controlled by a variety of processes which are as yet not understood. Postnatal growth is profoundly affected by the circulating levels of growth hormone (GH or somatotropin); growth-hormone releasing hormone (GHRH) and somatostatin; however, these hormones have not been shown to control fetal growth.

Growth hormones (GH)

Growth hormone can be detected in fetal serum by 100 days gestation (Kaplan et al 1972), the level increasing in concentration up to 30 weeks but falling in the last trimester, although the level at birth is still elevated compared to that of the mother. The level of growth hormone remains fairly constant from birth until the end of the first postnatal year.

The role of growth hormone in the fetus is unclear. Because anencephalic babies and those with genetically determined growth hormone deficiencies attain lengths within normal limits it has

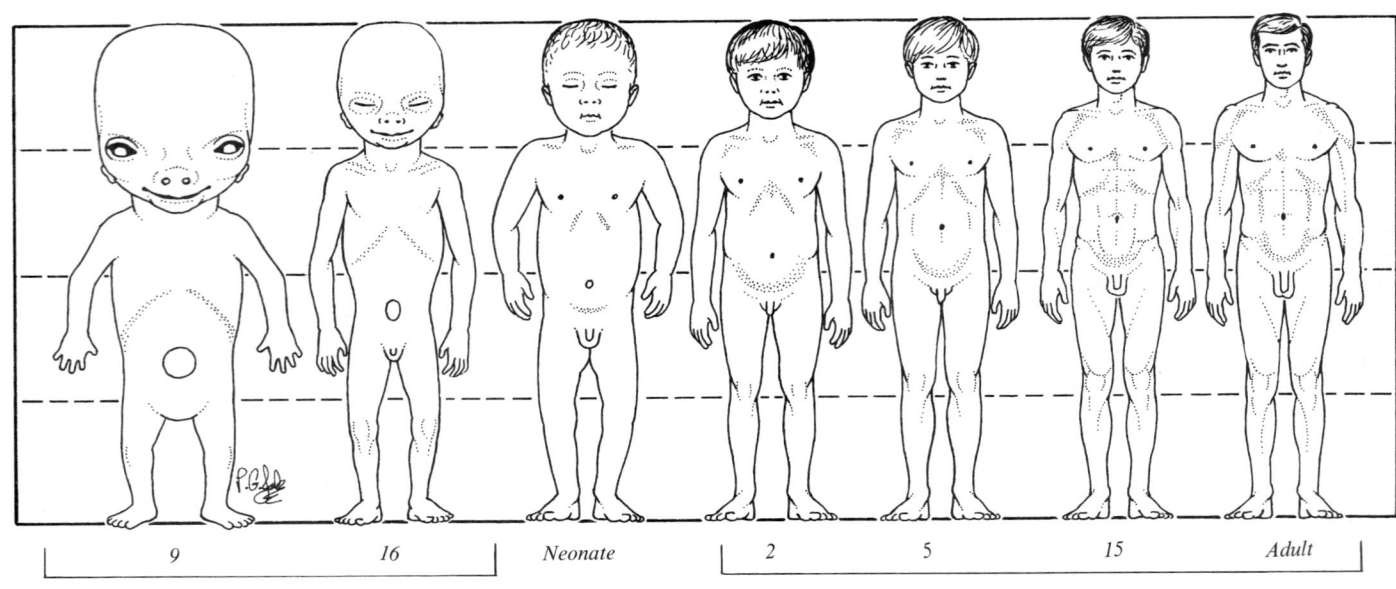

9	*16*	*Neonate*	*2*	*5*	*15*	*Adult*

Weeks of development   *Age in years*

4.22 Allometric growth in humans. The head is very large in proportion to the rest of the body during the embryonic period. After this time the head grows more slowly than the torso and limbs and by adulthood the head is only one-eighth of the body length.

been assumed that fetal growth is independent of pituitary growth hormone, a view noted as hazardous by Hindmarsh and Brook (1988).

However, the role of growth hormone in the postnatal period has been the subject of extensive study. It is clear from epidemiological studies that growth hormone is necessary after the first 2–3 months, if not before. All tissues respond to growth hormone producing a proportional body growth which slows after puberty when secretion of the hormone decreases. The effects of growth hormone are seen particularly on the epiphyseal growth plates of the long bones. Continued secretion of growth hormone will result in giantism and lack of the hormone produces proportional dwarfism. In cases of acromegaly where growth hormone is abnormally secreted (after the epiphyseal growth plates have fused), the presenting symptoms develop over many years, with enlargement of the heart and liver, thickening of the bones especially the maxilla and mandible, and thickening of the skin. Thus, in this case, all the cells and tissues which are normally responsive to growth hormone continue proliferating.

A series of complicated experiments have elucidated the specific effects of growth hormone. The gene for growth hormone was isolated in the rat and combined with a mouse gene which regulates serum zinc levels (mouse metallothionein I) to act as a promoter. The combined gene was injected into mouse pronuclei shortly after fertilization, resulting in mice with both the rat growth hormone gene and the mouse metallothionein I gene within their chromosomes. Some of the transgenic mice were then fed a diet which included zinc supplements which switched on the rat growth hormone gene inducing synthesis of rat growth hormone from the liver (the normal site of metallothionein). The transgenic mice with the zinc supplement became up to 80% larger than their littermates, with all of their organs in proportion (Palmiter et al 1982). These elegant experiments demonstrate that growth hormone controls the co-ordinated regulation of growth.

Somatomedins/insulin-like growth factors

At the cellular level growth hormone acts by stimulating somatomedin synthesis by the liver. Somatomedins are a family of insulin-like growth factors (see p. 56) including insulin-like growth factor I (IGF-I or somatomedin C) and insulin-like growth factor II (IGF-II or somatomedin A).

It has been noted that in the human embryo IGF-I levels are low and administration of growth hormone does not affect growth at this time (Hall & Sara 1983). IGF-II levels on the other hand are elevated in the fetus and their levels are not influenced by growth hormone. It has thus been suggested that the regulation of growth in the fetus is mainly regulated by IGF-II, which, in turn, may be controlled by placental lactogen (Engstrom & Heath 1988). Due to its widespread expression in the embryo and fetus IGF-II has been proposed to be the major paracrine growth factor in vivo and a major determinant of fetal growth.

There is a positive correlation between birth weight and plasma concentrations of IGFs at delivery, with decreased levels of IGFs observed in small for gestational age children. During the growth spurt of adolescence the levels of GH, IGF-I and IGF-II are increased. In pygmies the level of both GH and IGF-I is normal; however, at puberty IGF-I secretion falls to one-third compared to other adolescents, suggesting that IGF-I is necessary for the normal pubertal growth spurt (Merimee et al 1987).

Other growth factors

Various families of growth factors are discussed in the Introduction section (see p. 56) and elsewhere (see p. 112). In brief, *platelet-derived growth factor (PDGF)* stimulates division of fibroblasts, smooth muscle and glioblasts; *epidermal growth factor (EGF)* promotes division in, inter alia, epidermis, mammary gland epithelium and skeletal muscle.

Interestingly, a wide range of growth factors are secreted in breast milk. EGF is the major growth factor in human milk, unlike cow's milk which contains no EGF. Insulin is detected in low concentrations in human milk and IGF-I concentrations are 10% of those in normal human serum (Read 1988). The concentrations of these growth factors change during lactation, being maximal in day 1 colostrum and declining during the first week to reach a plateau. Despite this fall human milk still contains EGF and insulin at 10%

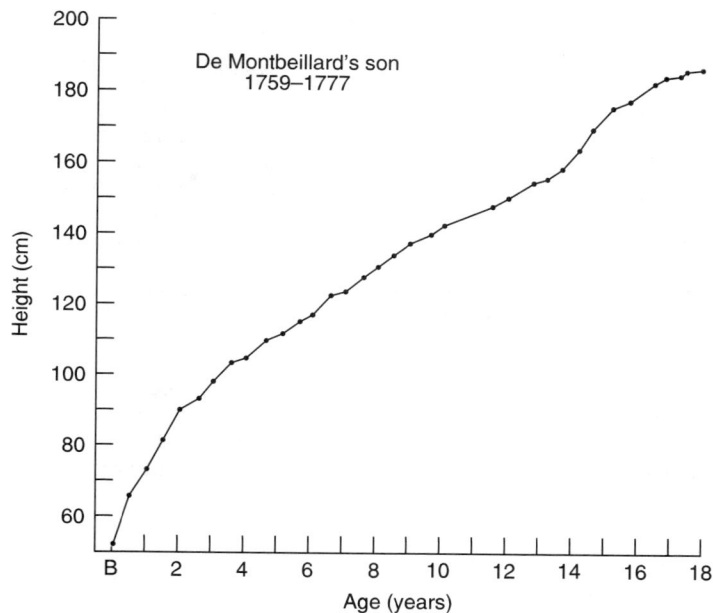

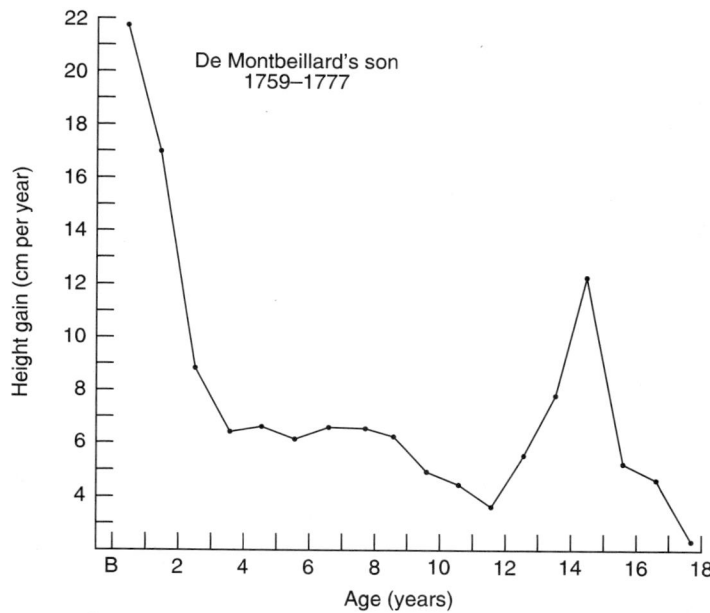

4.23 Graphs showing a longitudinal study of growth. The height of de Montbeillard's son (1759–77) from birth to 18 years is shown in the upper chart. The lower chart shows a velocity curve, plotting increments in height from year to year (from Harrison et al 1964).

of the concentrations in colostrum. Read et al (1984) have suggested that the total growth factor delivery to the baby remains nearly constant throughout lactation. As endogenous production of EGF is undetectable in the neonatal period, human milk may provide the baby's only source. However, as neonates maintained entirely on artificial formulae develop at apparently normal rates it seems unlikely that growth factors in milk are essential requirements for normal growth; Read (1988) suggests that growth factors may exist in milk as an emergency measure to improve the efficiency of neonatal growth under conditions of poor nutrition or inadequate development.

GROWTH RATES

The rate of prenatal and postnatal growth can be indicated by increments in body length or weight which when plotted form a *growth curve*. Growth curves can be plotted for individuals if accurate measurements are taken, preferably by the same person, for the entire period of growth, a *longitudinal study*. An alternate method is to collect a series of averages for each year of age obtained from different individuals; this is a *cross-sectional study*. Cross-sectional studies are valuable for the construction of standards for height and weight attained by healthy children at specific ages, and can establish percentile limits of normal growth; however, they cannot reveal individual differences in the rate of growth or in the timing of particular phases of growth. Longitudinal studies are thus of great value but laborious and time consuming to those undertaking them. The data from longitudinal and cross-sectional studies can also be used to plot the increments in height or weight from one age to the next; this forms a *velocity curve*: it reflects a child's state at any particular time much better than the growth curve in which each point is dependent on the preceding one. The oldest published longitudinal study, still of great value today, was made by Count Philibert de Montbeillard upon his son (**4.23**). It shows that the velocity of growth in height decreases from birth onwards with a

marked acceleration of growth from 13 to 15, the *adolescent growth spurt* (see below).

Cross-sectional data have provided comparison of prenatal and postnatal growth, and childhood growth charts are used to predict normal childhood development. The velocity curve for the prenatal and postnatal period (**4.24**) shows that the peak velocity for length is reached at about 4 months (note that these prenatal charts use the obstetric measurements of gestational time where fetal age is estimated from the last menstrual period, 2 weeks prior to fertilization). Growth in weight reaches its peak velocity usually after birth.

Growth has always been regarded as a regular process. Tanner (in Harrison et al 1964) stated that growth does not proceed in fits and starts, noting that the more carefully the measurements are taken, the more regular is the succession of points on a growth curve. However, a longitudinal study of growth measured weekly, semi-weekly, and daily (Lampl et al 1992) demonstrated growth in length and head circumference occurring by saltatory increments with a mean amplitude of 1.01 cm for length. Growth saltations were not periodic but episodic. This study proposes that human growth in length, during the first 2 postnatal years, occurs during intervals of less than 24 hours that punctuate a background of stasis. They suggest that stasis may be part of the normal temporal structure of growth and development. A cautionary note is provided by Wales & Gibson (1994) who, while concurring that growth in height is not a steady process but one made up of intermittent episodes of growth, add that, because of the range of factors which may affect growth, the problem of accurate measurement and the type of mathematical model used to explain growth, predictions of long-term growth from short-term observations, either of one bone or of the whole body, should not be attempted.

Effect of maternal environment

The rate of growth of fetuses slows from about 36 to 40 weeks due to the limiting influence of the maternal uterus. Birth weight thus reflects the maternal environment more than the genotype of the child. This slowing of the growth rate enables a genetically larger child developing within a small mother to be delivered successfully, after which the growth rate of the neonate picks up and in weight reaches a peak some 2 months postnatally.

This limit of prenatal growth imposed by the maternal uterus was demonstrated experimentally many years ago by the crossing of large Shire horses and Shetland ponies. A Shire mare crossed with a Shetland produces a foal of similar size to a pure-bred Shire foal, whereas a Shetland mare crossed with a Shire horse produces a foal only a third as large, similar in size to a pure-bred Shetland foal (Walton & Hammond 1938).

The predominant influence of the mother on the size at birth is steadily eroded as the infant's genotype expresses itself and by adult life the offspring bears no greater resemblance to the mother than to the father. Thus in the horses, after weaning when the foals are under the same nutritional conditions, the Shetland/Shire crosses rapidly outgrow pure-bred Shetlands; however, they do not keep up with pure-bred Shires.

Standard growth charts

Charts of height and weight correlated to age are compiled from extensive cross-sectional growth studies. Such charts show the mean height or weight attained at each age, also termed the 50th centile, and also the centile lines for the 75th, 90th and 97th centiles as well as the 25th, 9th and 2nd centile. The date shown in **4.25** are derived from United Kingdom cross-sectional references. Any comparison of an individual growth curve with these data should also take into account the ethnicity, nutritional and family history of the individual.

Adolescent growth spurt

From growth charts it can be seen that during the first year after birth body **length** increases from a neonatal range of 48–53 cm to about 75 cm, and in the second year by 12–13 cm. Thereafter 5–6 cm are added each year. In individual longitudinal growth curves an increase in the velocity of growth can be seen from 10.5–11 years in girls, and 12.5–13 years in boys. This rapid increase in growth is termed the *adolescent growth spurt* (**4.25, 26**). In both sexes this growth spurt lasts for 2–2.5 years. Girls gain about 16 cm in height during the spurt, with a peak velocity at 12 years of age; boys gain

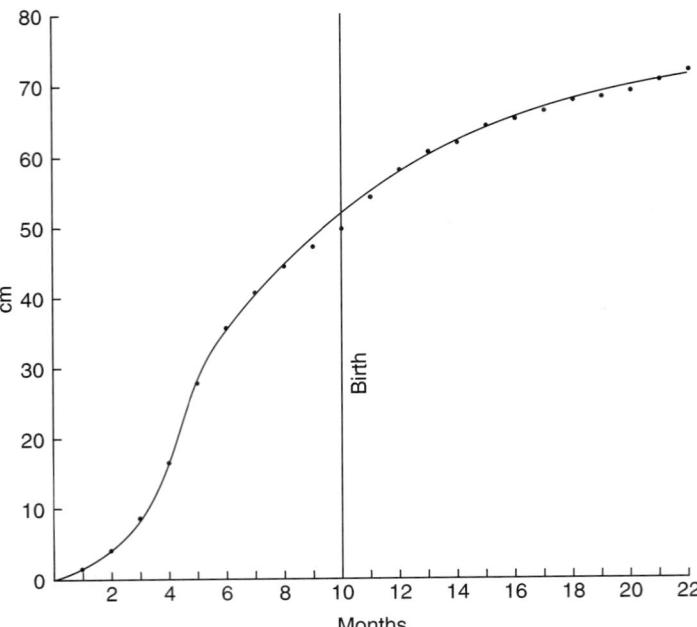

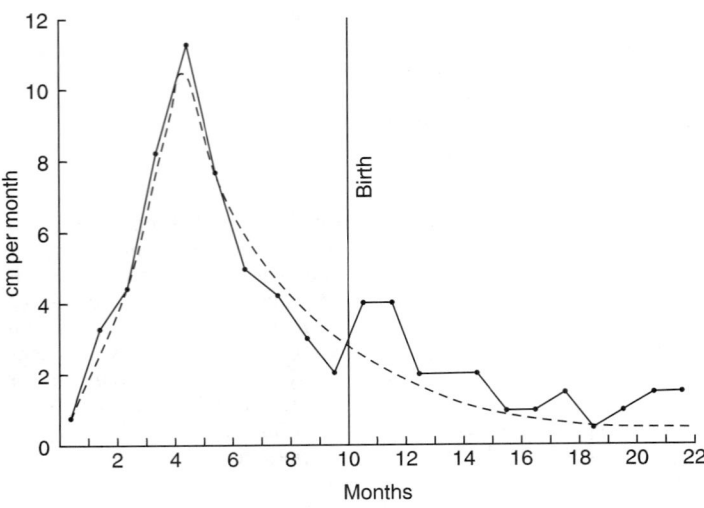

4.24 Graphs of cross-sectional data showing growth in length in the prenatal and early postnatal period, and the corresponding velocity curve for this period (from Harrison et al 1964).

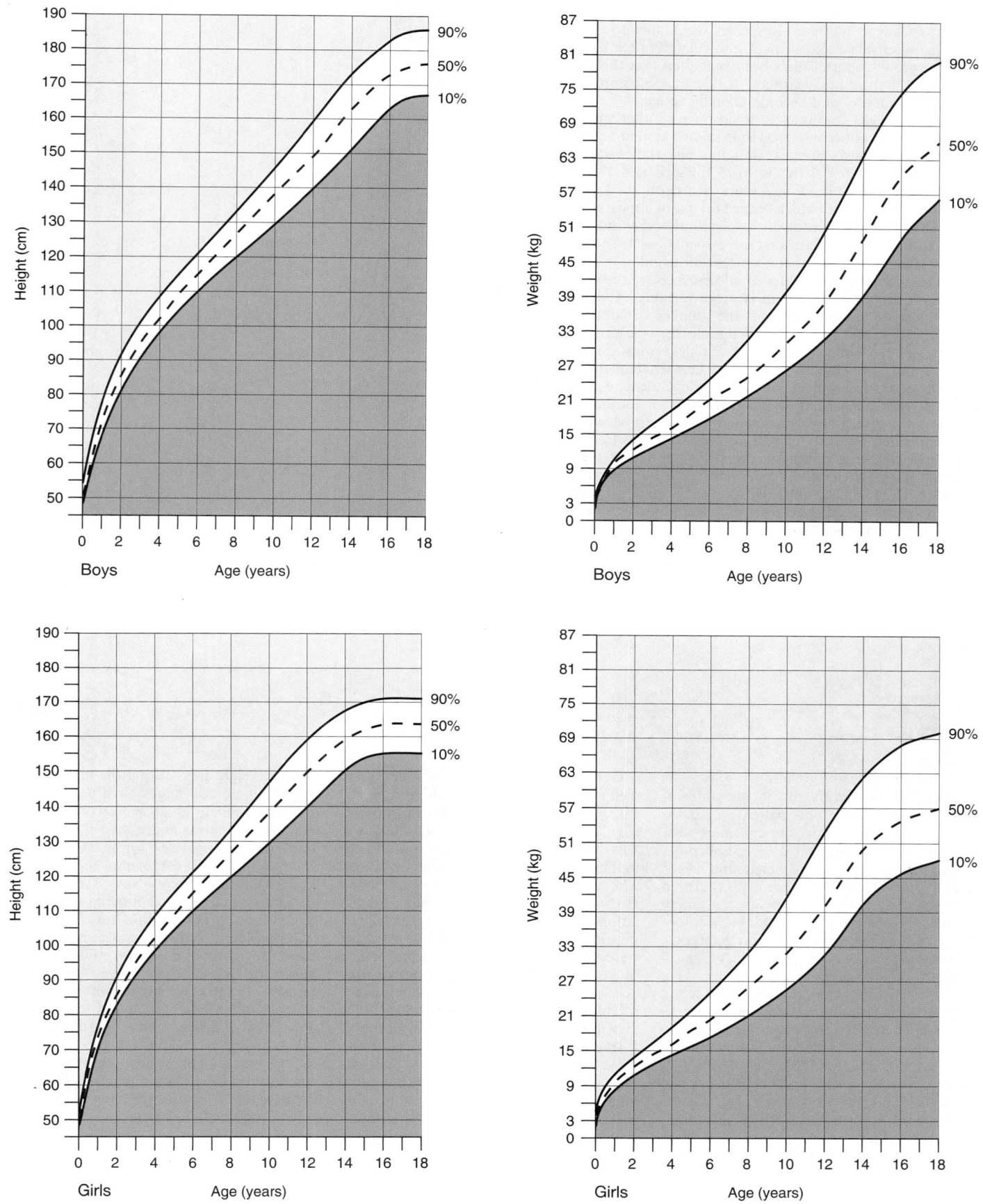

4.25 Standard growth charts of boys and girls showing the 90th, 50th and 10th centiles. (Data from Child Growth Foundation 1994/1).

about 20 cm in height (mostly by growth of the trunk), with a peak velocity at 14 years of age during which they may be growing at the rate of 10 cm a year.

Humans seem to be the only species which has a long quiescent interval between the rapid growth immediately after birth and the adolescent growth spurt. It has been suggested that this time allows the brain to mature and learning to take place before individuals pass through puberty and become sexually active.

Growth in height continues at a slower rate after the adolescent growth spurt and noticeable growth is said to stop at about 18 years in females and 20 years in males (longitudinal studies have indicated that an average figure for this is 16.25 for girls and 17.75 for boys with a normal variation of ±2 years; Harrison et al 1964). After this time any increments, which occur because of appositional growth at the cranial and caudal ends of the vertebral bodies and intervening intervertebral symphyses (discs), are so small as to be difficult to measure; after middle age there is a loss of height.

The phenomenal growth rates of adolescence are seen particularly in increased height. **Weight** gain is more variable. At birth, weight reflects the maternal environment, the number of conceptuses, the sex of the baby, and the parity of the mother. Generally full-term female babies are lighter than full-term males, twins are lighter than singletons and later children tend to be heavier than the first-born. Although the birth weight seems to be independent of the mother's diet unless there has been severe malnutrition, mothers in a low socioeconomic group have smaller babies than those with a higher rating, and small mothers tend to have small babies (see above).

The birth weight is normally tripled by the end of the first year and quadrupled by the end of the second year. Thereafter weight increases by 2.25–2.75 kg annually until the adolescent growth spurt when boys may add 20 kg to their weight and girls 16 kg. The peak velocity for weight gain lags behind the peak velocity for height by about 3 months. Body weight does not reach adult values until some time after adult height is attained.

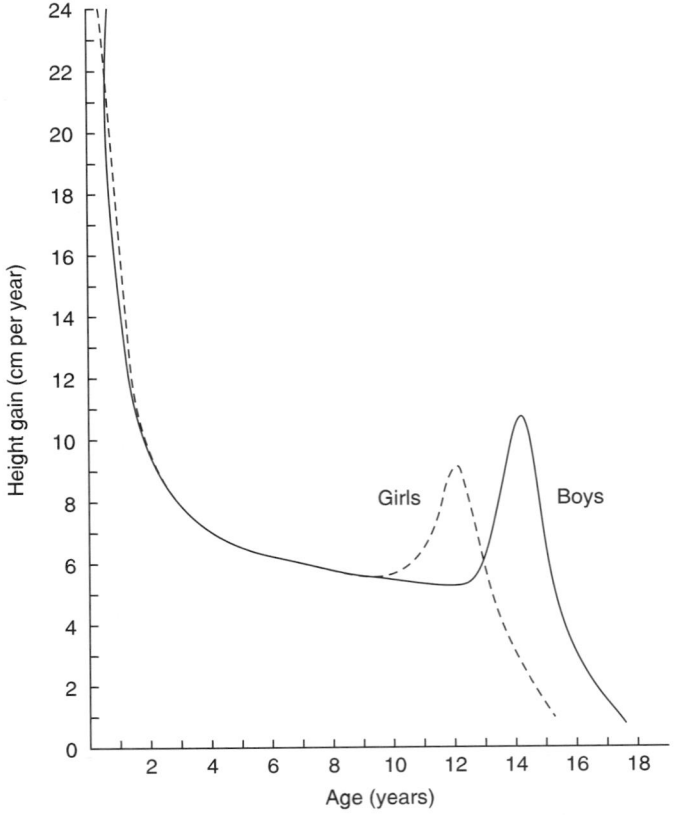

4.26 Typical individual velocity curves for height: English boys and girls (from Tanner et al 1966).

Fetal and infant growth rates and adult pathology

A very interesting relationship is now emerging between the nutritional status of the fetus in utero and patterns of pathology in late adult life. The routine assessment of weight and height of the neonate, and the re-evaluation of weight and height at 1 year of age was rigorously followed in the early years of this century in many counties in the United Kingdom. Many of these data, filed with the old birth records, remained untouched for more than 50 years, until recently when its rediscovery prompted follow up studies on as many of the original population documented as possible. Studies by Barker et al (1989, 1993a,b,c) noted the cause of death or survival health of 1586 men born in a maternity hospital in Sheffield during 1907–25, and of 5654 men born in Hertfordshire during 1911–30. Such longitudinal studies are of great value in correlating in utero status, which may be inferred by birth weight and weight at 1 year postnatally (when the peak velocity for growth in weight has occurred, see above), with childhood and adult lifestyles and with later pathology.

Generally these studies indicated that men with low birth weight and low weight at 1 year of age (on or below the 3rd centile on the standard growth chart, see **4.25**) were almost three times more likely to die of coronary heart disease than those who attained average weight at birth and at 1 year. Examination of other populations of both sexes similarly indicated that low growth rates up to 1 year of age were associated with increased prevalence of known risk factors for cardiovascular disease, including altered blood pressure, plasma concentrations of glucose, insulin, fibrinogen, factor VII, and apolipoprotein B (Barker et al 1993a). These associations were seen in babies born small for gestational age rather than in those born prematurely; however, as well as this population of infants with intrauterine growth retardation, some babies of average weight also developed later cardiovascular pathology. This latter group were small at birth in relation to the size of their placenta, were thin at birth, or, although of average weight, were short in relation to head size and had below

average weight gain during the first year.

Barker and colleagues have postulated that poor nutrition at critical stages of fetal life may permanently alter the normal developmental pattern of a range of organs and tissues, for example endocrine pancreas, liver and blood vessels, resulting in their pathological responses to certain conditions in later adult life. Such a relationship has been demonstrated experimentally in animal studies. Low birth weight in the guinea pig, caused by retardation of intrauterine growth, causes lifelong elevation of blood pressure (Persson & Jansson 1992). In the rat, a low protein diet can induce a high ratio of placental weight to birth weight. Such rats have reduced placental activity of 11-B hydroxy-steroid dehydrogenase, which may protect them from excessive maternal cortisol (the fetal blood pressure is partly regulated by cortisol), and have raised blood pressure 15 weeks after birth (Barker et al 1993b).

As different tissues and organs mature at different times in fetal life and infancy any long-term consequences of in utero malnutrition would depend on its timing and duration. Different birth phenotypes have been correlated with different pathological sequelae; for example infants who are thin at birth, with a low ponderal index (weight/length^3), tend to develop a combination of insulin resistance, hypertension, non-insulin-dependent diabetes, and lipid disorders, whereas those who are short in relation to head size tend to develop hypertension and high plasma fibrinogen concentrations (Barker et al 1993c).

Thus it is suggested that alterations in the availability of nutrients to the fetus, at particular stages of pregnancy, cause adaptive responses by the fetus which ensures fetal coping, but lead on to pathology in adult life when different conditions operate. Examples of this are as follows:

- An increase in placental size occurs in pregnancy as an adaptive response to both high altitude and mild undernutrition during midpregnancy. The larger placenta may be more able to deliver the full nutritional requirements of the fetus; however, the perfusion of a larger placenta may produce changes in fetal blood flow, changes in placental enzymes (see above), and change the normal structure of the vessel wall or of its responses to circulating trophins, for example catecholamines or angiotensin II, which will continue into adult life. Undernutrition in later pregnancy would not produce the same sequelae and placental enlargement does not occur; however, fetal growth slows and fetal wasting may occur as oxygen, glucose and amino acids are redistributed to the placenta to maintain its function.

- Maternal starvation lowers fetal insulin-like growth factor (IGF)-I concentrations which may, along with a general hypoglycaemia, impair the development of the β-cells of the pancreas; generally fetal undernutrition may induce insulin resistance in the tissues. The coexistence of both insulin resistance and impaired β-cell development in the fetus appears to be important in the pathogenesis of non-insulin-dependent diabetes. The risk of developing this type 2 diabetes is highest in those individuals with low weight at birth and at 1 year, who become obese as adults, thus challenging an already impaired glucose-insulin metabolism.

- Fetal IGF-I levels are also lower in infants who are short at birth as a result of a long period of maternal undernutrition. Such individuals have exaggerated responses to growth hormone-releasing factor (GHRF), which together with low IGF-I levels suggests a degree of growth hormone (GH) resistance. Barker et al (1993) suggest that in such individuals the normal development of their hepatic GH receptors may have been attenuated.

These studies suggest that undernutrition in pregnancy may cause fetal adaptations which permanently alter the structure and physiology of the body possibly leading to a variety of pathological conditions in adult life. The implications of these findings is that the nutritional status of pregnant women is of fundamental importance for the health of the next generation. Further studies which illuminate this hypothesis are awaited with interest.

Growth rates of tissues and organs

Although skeletal and muscular tissues generally follow the growth curves given for the whole body, as do the dimensions of organs such as the liver, spleen and kidneys, other tissues have very different growth rates. The brain and skull, lymphoid tissues, reproductive organs and subcutaneous fat show differing growth rates during childhood and adolescence (4.27).

Head. This develops early and in response to the general craniocaudal progression of embryonic development, with the brain, skull, eyes and ears developing earlier than other parts of the body. After birth, the surrounding skull thickens with age and continues ossification towards the sutures; the face, however, is relatively underdeveloped and undergoes profound changes throughout childhood and at the adolescent spurt, resulting in the eruption of the deciduous and permanent teeth, the formation of the sinuses, and the elongation of the maxilla and mandible (4.28).

Limbs. It is worth noting at this point that although the bones and muscle of the limbs contribute to the growth spurt in height, there are some changes in relative proportions within this process. The male forearm is longer relative to the upper arm than the female forearm, a difference already established at birth which increases throughout the growing period. A similar difference is noted in the sex difference in relative lengths of the second and fourth fingers. The second finger is longer than the fourth more frequently in females than in males at birth. After birth, at all ages, the dimensions of the head are in advance of those of the trunk, and the trunk is advance of the limbs. However, the more distal parts of the limb are in advance of the more proximal parts; thus the foot is nearer adult status than the calf, which is in turn more advanced than the thigh. The time at which the hands and feet are large relative to the rest of the body coincides with the adolescent growth spurt; the foot ceases growth early before almost all other parts of the skeleton.

Lymphoid tissues. These include the thymus, tonsils, appendix and intestine and show an earlier growth curve compared to other tissues. They reach their maxima before adolescence and then, probably under the influence of the sex hormones, decline to adult values (4.27). The thymus is found in the superior and anterior mediastina in childhood. In the infant it weighs on average 13 g, reaching a maximum weight of about 35 g in girls at 12 years and

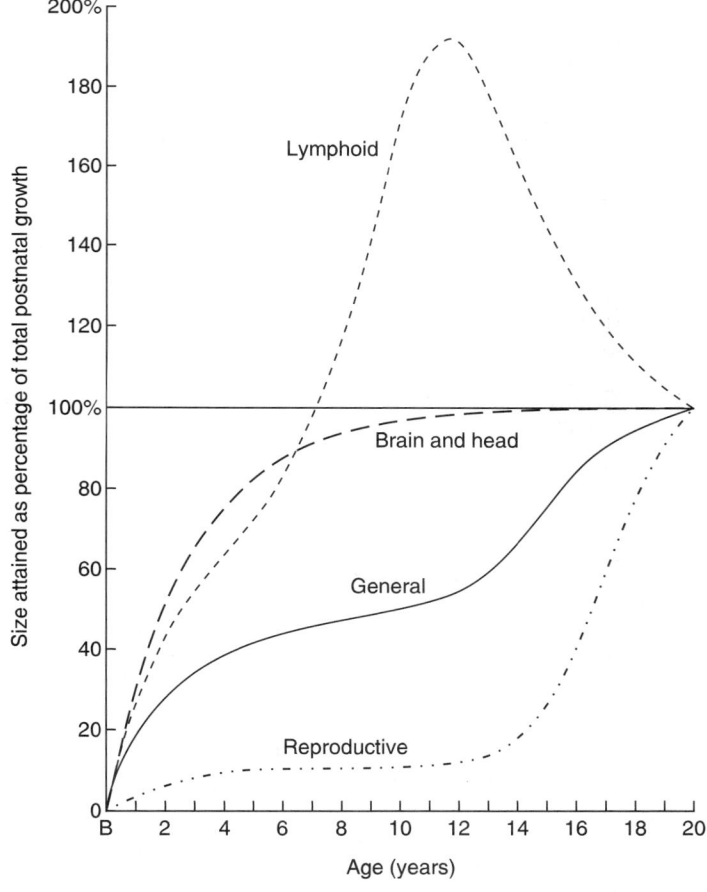

4.27 Growth curves of different tissues, regions of the body and systems. Note that the growth of lymphoid tissue, thymus, lymph nodes and intestinal lymph masses decreases after puberty (from Tanner 1962).

371

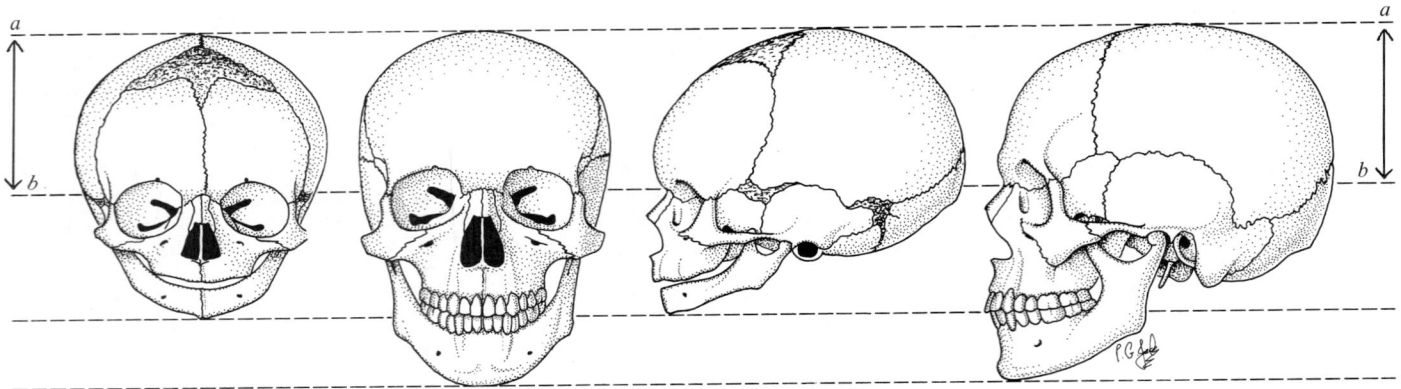

4.28 Much of the postnatal growth of the skull is concerned with development of the viscerocranium. This diagram shows that with the height of the cranial vault expressed as similar in newborn and adult skulls (lines a . . . b) the facial skeleton increases particularly during childhood and puberty.

boys at 14 years. After this time it regresses until it can no longer be found in old age. The tonsils gain their maximum size by 6 years and regress thereafter. Peyer's patches around the ileum also diminish in size towards old age.

Reproductive organs. Until the adolescent growth spurt these grow very slowly. The uterus is relatively large at birth, under the influence of maternal hormones, but it rapidly shrinks and does not regain its birth weight until adolescence. Generally the changes in the reproductive organs occur over a time period termed *puberty*. The *sequence* of these events is much less variable than the age at which they take place. **4.29A** and **4.29B** show the sequence of puberty in girls and boys.

In girls. The appearance of the breast bud is usually the first sign of puberty. The uterus and vagina develop simultaneously with the breast. Menarche occurs after the peak of the height spurt; onset is more closely related to radiological than to chronological age. It has been suggested that the menarche occurs as a critical weight of about 50 kg is attained; certainly sports and excessive restriction of diet which may reduce weight below this level can cause amenorrhoea in women who were previously menstruating normally. Tall girls reach sexual maturity earlier than short ones, but girls with a late adolescent growth spurt and later puberty are ultimately taller on the average than those passing through the menarche early, for they have longer to grow. A girl who has begun to menstruate can be predicted to grow a further 7.5 cm at most (Sinclair 1985). Menarche marks a definitive stage of uterine development but does not mean attainment of full reproductive function. Many of the early menstrual cycles may not involve ovulation.

In boys. The earliest sign of puberty is the growth of the testes and scrotum. The volume of the testes may be estimated; the average adult volume is 20 ml; a volume of 6 ml indicates that puberty has started. Later the penis, prostate and seminal vesicles begin to enlarge, and the elevation of testosterone levels from the Leydig cells of the testes promote changes in the larynx, skin and hair distribution. During puberty the enlargement of the larynx causes the vocal fold to double in length from 8 mm to 16 mm, perhaps within a year; this is associated with the voice 'breaking', the lengthening cords producing a lower pitch. Ultimately the vocal cords will reach an adult length of about 25 mm.

Subcutaneous fat. These deposits are measured by callipers applied to a fold of fat pinched up from the underlying muscles. Such measurements are taken over the triceps muscle and beneath the angle of the scapula. Fat begins to be laid down in the fetus from about 34 weeks and it increases from then to birth and from birth to 9 months. From 9 months, when the velocity is then zero, the subcutaneous fat decreases (has a negative velocity) until 6–8 years when it begins to increase again. This early decrease in fat is

less in girls than boys, so that after 1 year girls have more fat than boys.

From 7 years the increase in fat occurs in both sexes. At adolescence the fat in the limbs (triceps measurement) of boys decreases and is not gained back until the late twenties; girls show a slight slowing of the limb-fat increase, but no loss. Also at this time the

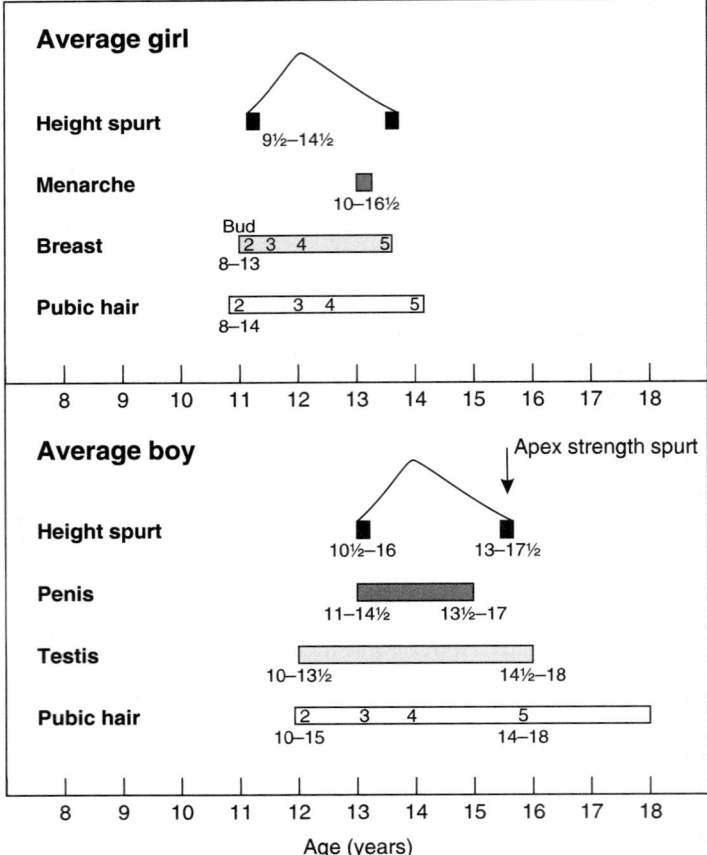

4.29 Diagram of the events which occur at adolescence in average girls and boys. The figures beneath the bars indicate the range of ages within which each event may begin and end. Figures within the bars indicate the developmental stage (from Tanner 1962).

trunk-fat (subscapular measurement) stops increasing in boys; in girls the trunk-fat shows a steady increase. Girls show fat deposits in a secondary sexual distribution, in the breasts, over the upper arms, lower abdomen and thighs. Postpubertal boys do not have this pattern of fat distribution; adult men are more likely to deposit fat around the anterior abdominal wall.

Senescence

There is a general agreement that the processes involved in aging and senescence seem to be developmentally regulated. Examination of long-term tissue culture of fibroblasts from a human embryo showed that the cells had a definite life span which could be described in three stages. Firstly, the cells acclimatize to the tissue culture conditions. Secondly, there is a rapid increase in growth with cells dividing about every 21 hours. Thirdly, after 40–50 divisions, the cells assume a larger cell volume and show longer cell cycles until they arrest in the G_1 phase of the cycle (Hayflick & Moorhead 1961). Fibroblasts retain a memory of the number of divisions they have completed and, even if suspended from division by being frozen, they will complete only the remainder of their divisions before arresting. Transplantation of the nucleus from young cells to old cells and vice versa demonstrates that the knowledge of the number of divisions a cell has passed through is contained in the nucleus (Muggleton-Harris & Hayflick 1976). The older population of fibroblasts loses the ability to respond to the normal physiological stimulators of mitosis (Phillips et al 1984) and thus cannot engage in interactions with surrounding cells and matrix molecules. Thus all processes from gastrulation to death may be driven by the same mechanisms superimposed on a time scale contained within the genome.

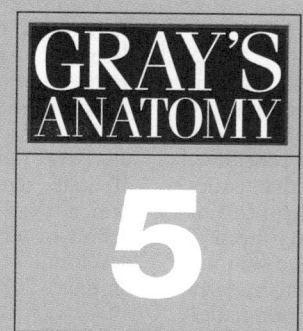

INTEGUMENTAL SYSTEM: SKIN AND BREASTS

Section Editor: Lawrence H. Bannister

Contributors: Professor Aidan Breathnach (the integument, completely rewritten and extensively illustrated); Dr Mary Dyson (dermal repair and epidermal regeneration); Mr Ian Fentiman FRCS (breast structure and function, extensively revised)

OUTLINE OF SECTION

The term *integumental system* is used here to denote the skin and its derivatives: hairs, nails, and sweat and sebaceous glands, the mucocutaneous junctions around the openings of the body orifices, and the breasts. In previous editions of *Gray's* the skin was considered in the Introductory Section with the epithelia and connective tissues, and the breasts were described with the reproductive system. In view of the importance of the skin in human biology, its nature as a composite system of tissues and the common origin of the skin and breasts from an interactive combination of ectoderm and mesoderm, it was felt appropriate to create a separate section to bring these topics together. In this account the external appearance of the integument and its variations in different parts of the body is described first, followed by the microstructure of the epidermis and dermis, and the appendages of skin including the pilosebaceous units comprising hairs, sebaceous and apocrine glands and associated smooth muscle fascicles, and the nails, and sweat glands. Concluding this part of the section, the effects of ageing on skin, and the processes of tissue repair are described briefly; the prenatal development of skin is dealt with in Embryology and Development (p. 294), and details of innervation are in Nervous System (p. 1289) although the development of cutaneous innervation is dealt with in this section on pages 398–399. In the second part of the section the topographic anatomy, microstructure and development of the breasts (female and male) are considered.

SKIN

INTRODUCTION

The skin (integument, cutis) is largely ignored by the student in the dissecting room, just being incised, reflected, and cast aside as something which hides more interesting things underneath. Yet, it is that part of the body in which, par excellence, can be demonstrated, at all levels of observation, the relation between structure and function in biological organization. Here also, a number of different body systems come together in synergy to fulfil general overall functions beyond their individual specialized capacities. In recent years, skin has increasingly become a common meeting ground for biologists with a variety of different primary interests, leading to significant cooperative basic and applied research, and the blurring of interdisciplinary boundaries.

The skin covers the entire external surface of the body, including the external auditory meatus, the lateral aspect of the tympanic membrane and the vestibule of the nose. It is continuous with the mucosae of the alimentary, respiratory, and urogenital tracts at their respective orifices, where the specialized skin of mucocutaneous junctions occurs. It also fuses with the conjunctiva at the margins of the eyelids, and with the lining of the lacrimal canaliculi at the lacrimal puncta. Skin forms about 8% of the total body mass, and its surface area varies with height and weight; in an individual of 1.8 m and weighing 90 kg, it is about 2.2 m². Its thickness ranges from about 1.5–4.0 mm, variations being due to maturation, ageing, and regional specializations.

The skin forms a self-renewing and self-repairing interface between the body and its environment, and is a major site of inter-communication in both directions between the two. Within limits, it forms an effective barrier against microbial invasion, and has proper-ties which can protect against mechanical, chemical, osmotic, thermal and photic damage. It is capable of absorption and excretion, and is selectively and regionally permeable to a variety of chemical substances. It is an important primary site of immunosurveillance against the entry of antigens, and of initiation of the primary immune response. Skin carries out many biochemical synthetic processes (Boyce 1994), including the formation of vitamin D from the pre-cursor 7-dihydrocholesterol under the influence of ultraviolet B (UVB) radiation, synthesis of cytokines and growth factors, etc., and is the target of a variety of hormones. In a sense, it can be regarded as an endocrine organ. These activities can affect the appearance and function of individual skin components, such as the sebaceous glands, the hairs and the pigment-producing cells. Control of body temperature is an important function of skin, being effected mainly by regulation of heat loss from the cutaneous circulation by vascular mechanisms which can rapidly increase or reduce the flow of blood to an extensive surface area exposed to the exterior, assisted by sweating. Skin is involved in sociosexual communication at close quarters and at a distance, and in the case of facial skin, can signal emotional states by means of muscular and vascular responses. It provides individual identification and awareness of personal identity and self-image. Herein lies the concept of 'mind and skin' in the interpretation and treatment of many dermatological disorders which can be cosmetic disasters. It is a major sense organ, richly supplied by nerve terminals and specialized receptors for touch, temperature, pain, mechanical and pleasurable stimuli. The segmental arrangement of the spinal nerves is reflected in the sensory supply of the skin, a *dermatome* being the area supplied by an individual spinal nerve (p. 1289). Knowledge of the spatial distribution of dermatomes is essential for diagnosis of local lesions of nerve roots and of the spinal cord.

Skin has good frictional properties, assisting locomotion and manipulation by its texture. It is elastic, and can be stretched and compressed within limits. The outer surface is covered by various markings, some of them large and conspicuous and others delicate to the point of being microscopic (see Millington & Wilkinson 1983), or only revealed after manipulation or incision of the skin. These are often referred to collectively as *skin lines*, and are considered in greater detail on page 381.

The colour of human skin derives from and varies with the amount of blood (and its degree of oxygenation) in the cutaneous circulation, the thickness of the stratum corneum, and the activity of specialized cells producing the pigment, *melanin*. Melanin has a protective role against ultraviolet radiation, and acts as a scavenger of harmful free radicals produced under this and other circumstances. Racial variations in colour are mainly due to differences in the amount, type and distribution of melanin, and are genetically determined.

In addition to the variations mentioned above, the appearance of skin is also affected by many other factors, for example size and shape and distribution of hairs and their follicles, and of skin glands (sudorific, sebaceous, and apocrine), changes associated with maturation, ageing, metabolic changes, pregnancy, etc. The general state of health is reflected in the appearance and condition of the skin, and the earliest signs of many systemic disorders may be observed by inspecting it. Examination of the skin, therefore, is of importance in the diagnosis of much more than purely skin diseases. Biopsy of fetal skin at amniocentesis is becoming increasingly import-ant for prenatal diagnosis of genetically determined diseases, and can involve the dermatologist in genetic counselling.

For reviews of aspects of structure and function of skin see: Millington and Wilkinson (1983), Thody and Friedmann (1986), Fitzpatrick et al (1987), Champion et al (1991), Goldsmith (1991), and special issues of the current dermatological journals. For Atlases see Breathnach (1971), and Montagna et al (1992). For special techniques related to skin, see Skerrow and Skerrow (1985).

TYPES OF SKIN

Although skin over the entire body is fundamentally of similar structure, there are many local variations in thickness, mechanical strength, softness, flexibility, degree of keratinization, sizes and numbers of hairs, frequency and types of glands, pigmentation, vascularity, innervation and other features. However, it is useful to distinguish between two major classes of skin which cover large areas of the body, but show important differences of detailed structure and functional properties; these are, *thin, hairy* (*hirsute*) *skin*, which covers the greater part of the body, and *thick, hairless* (*glabrous*)

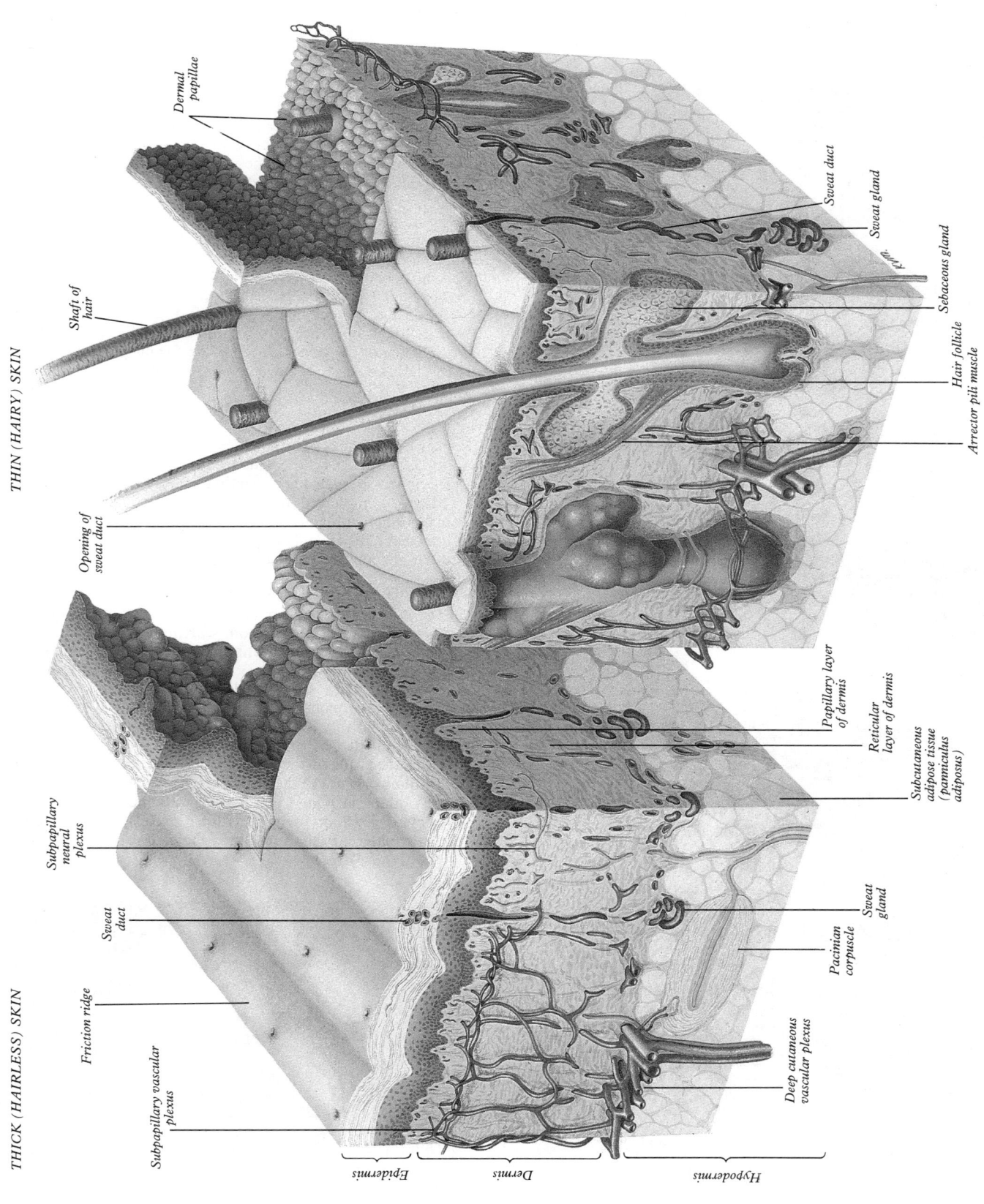

THIN (HAIRY) SKIN

THICK (HAIRLESS) SKIN

Dermal papillae

Shaft of hair

Opening of sweat duct

Sweat duct

Sweat gland

Sebaceous gland

Hair follicle

Arrector pili muscle

Papillary layer of dermis

Reticular layer of dermis

Subcutaneous adipose tissue (panniculus adiposus)

Subpapillary neural plexus

Sweat duct

Friction ridge

Subpapillary vascular plexus

Sweat gland

Pacinian corpuscle

Deep cutaneous vascular plexus

Epidermis

Dermis

Hypodermis

5.1 Schema showing the organization of skin, comparing the structures present in thick, hairless (plantar and palmar) skin and thin, hirsute skin. The epidermis has been partly peeled back in this picture, to show interdigitating dermal and epidermal papillae. For details of the innervation (yellow), see p. 962.

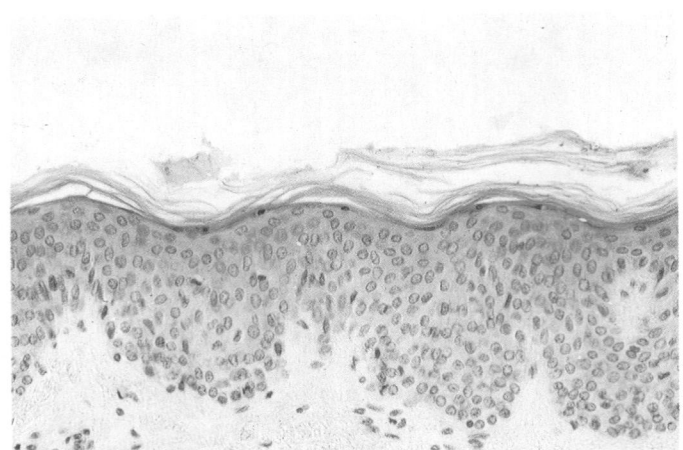

5.2 Vertical section through the epidermis of the scalp between hair follicles. Note the reduced keratinized layer (compare with **5**.3. Haematoxylin and eosin. Magnification × 200.

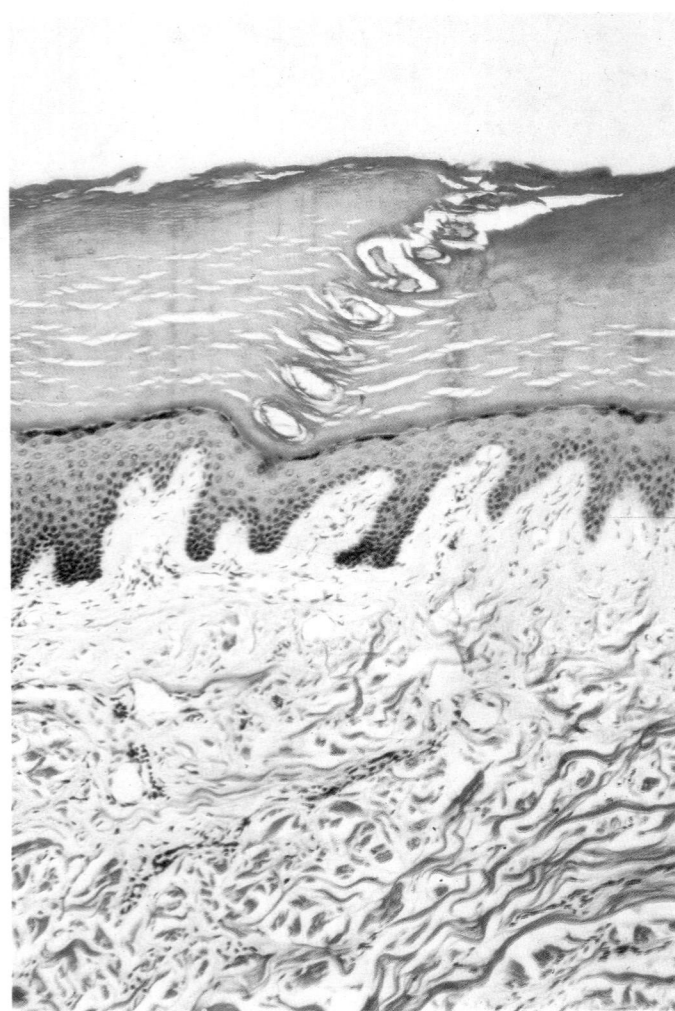

5.3 Low-power light micrograph of a vertical section through skin from the sole of the human foot: Mallory's triple stain. The finer collagen fibres of the papillary and reticular layers are stained blue and the coarser collagen of the reticular layer stains red. The epidermis is differentiated into the stratum corneum and stratum lucidum above (red-brown) and the strata basale, spinosum and granulosum, which stain blue-grey. A spiral duct from a sweat gland is also seen in vertical section. The base of the epidermis is irregularly ridged. Magnification × 150.

skin, forming the surfaces of the palms of the hands, soles of the feet, and flexor surfaces of the digits (5.1–3). These two classes differ in their surface markings, thick skin having complex patterns of friction ridges absent elsewhere on the body. As implied by their names, they also differ in the thickness of both epidermal and dermal components, and in the presence of hairs with attendant sebaceous glands and arrector pili muscles (*pilosebaceous units*). These dissimilarities reflect their distinctive functions. Thick hairless skin forms frictional surfaces for manipulation and locomotion, and requires extra strength for this purpose. It also possesses numerous sweat glands for cooling during sustained activity, and dense clusters of sensitive sensory endings with a high degree of spatial discrimination, unimpeded by the presence of hairs. Thin hairy skin is responsible for the general cutaneous functions over the remainder of the body.

Minor, specialized areas of skin also have distinctive features which do not fall into either of the major categories. The *mucocutaneous junctions* of the lips, outer rim of the anal canal, and urethral opening each have a characteristic histology: for example, the lips have a delicate epidermis lacking glands or hairs, as also do the coverings of the glans penis and glans clitoridis. Some of these regional differences are responsible for local differences in the *microclimate* of the skin surface, and in the bacterial and fungal flora that inhabits it.

SKIN LINES

The surface of the skin and its deeper structures show various linear markings. Over 35 different names, many of them synonyms, have been applied to such lines, relating to various systems of grooves, raised areas, preferred directions of stretching, lines of nervous occurrence and spread of infection. Some of these are clearly evident in intact skin, others only appear after some sort of intervention, for example pinching, while the actual existence of others is debatable.

Externally visible skin lines

Externally visible skin lines are related to various patterns of epidermal creasing, ridge formation, scarring and pigmentation.

Surface pattern lines, tension lines, skin creases (5.4–6). A simple lattice pattern of lines occurs on all major areas of the body other than the thick skin of volar and plantar surfaces. The lattice pattern typically consists of polygons (generally parallelograms) formed by relatively deep primary creases visible to the naked eye, irregularly divided by finer secondary creases into triangular areas. These, in turn, are further subdivided by tertiary creases limited to the stratum corneum of the epidermis, and, finally, at the microscopic level, by quaternary lines which are simply the outlines of individual corneocytes (Hashimoto 1974; Millington & Wilkinson 1983). Apart from the quaternary lines, all the others increase the surface area of

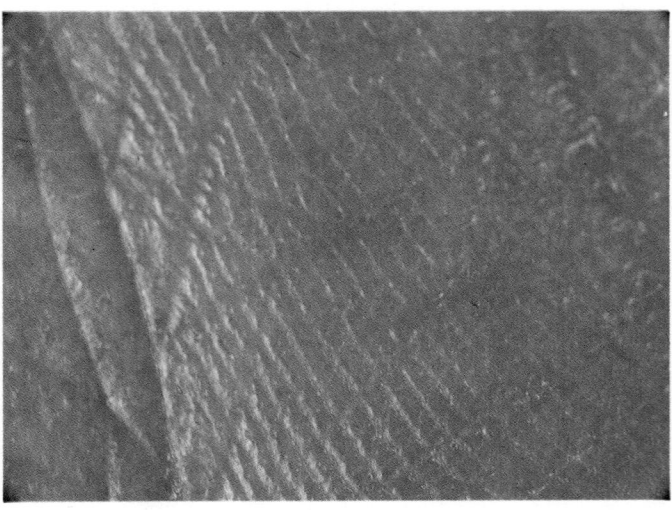

5.4 Low-power light micrograph of hairless skin, in surface view, from the palm of the hand showing epidermal friction (papillary) ridges and larger flexure lines (left). Magnification × 6.

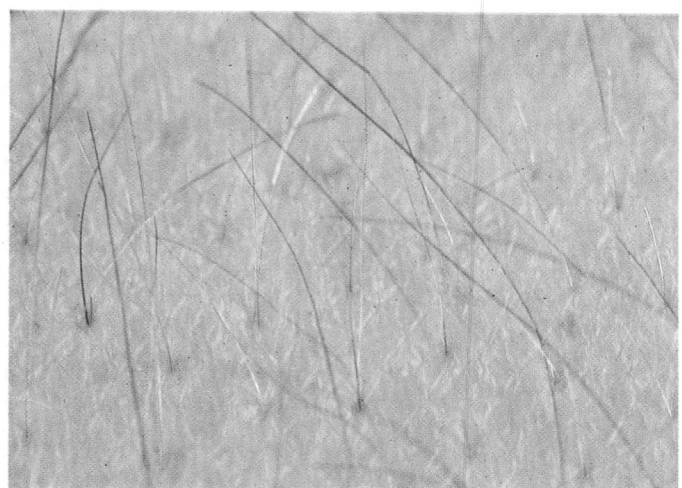

5.5 A light micrograph similar to that shown in 5.4 but taken from hairy skin on the extensor aspect of the forearm; note the pattern of surface grooves (tension lines) and hairs. The oblique direction of the emerging hair shafts points away from the pre-axial border of the limb. Magnification × 6.

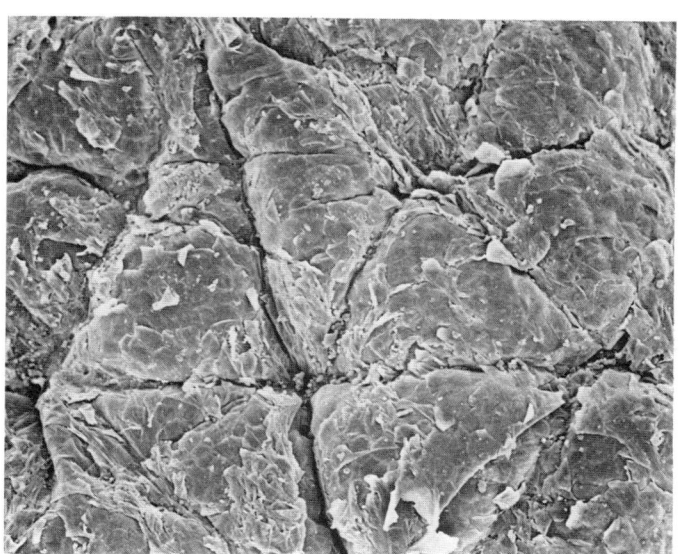

5.6 Scanning electron micrograph of the surface of thin skin (human: dorsum of thorax), showing the interlacing network of fine creases and predominantly triangular areas between them. Magnification × 400.

the skin, permitting considerable stretching and recoil and distributing stresses more evenly. Details of the pattern vary according to the region of the body; for example, on the cheek the primary creases radiate from the hair follicles, on the scalp they form hexagons, while on the calf and thigh they form parallelograms whose longer sides are inclined at about 30–40° to the vertical. There is a relationship between type of pattern and local skin extensibility (Fergus & Barbenel 1981).

Wrinkle lines. These are caused by contraction of underlying muscles and are usually disposed perpendicular to their axis of shortening. On the face they are known as *lines of expression*, and with progressive loss of skin elasticity due to ageing, they become permanent. *Occupational lines* are creases produced by repeated muscular contractions associated with particular trades or skills. *Contour lines* are lines of division at junctions of body planes, for example the cheek with the nose, and *lines of dependency* are produced by the effect of gravity on loose skin or fatty tissue in particular situations, for example the creases associated with the 'turkey-gobbler' fold beneath the chin of the aged.

Flexure (joint) lines. These are major markings found in the vicinity of synovial joints, where the skin is attached strongly to the underlying deep fascia (5.4). They are conspicuous on the flexor surfaces of the palms, soles, and digits, and in combination with

associated skin folds facilitate movement. The skin lines do not necessarily coincide with the associated underlying joint line. For example, the flexure lines demarcating the extended fingers from the palm lie approximately half an inch distal to the metacarpophalangeal joints, the positions of which are more closely related to the distal palmar crease ('heart-line'). The patterns of flexure lines on the palms and soles may vary and are to some extent genetically determined; the belief that the palmar pattern can reveal personality traits or the future of the individual underlies the practice of palmistry. In Down syndrome, the distal and middle palmar creases tend to be united into a prominent single transverse one, a sign which is of some diagnostic importance.

Papillary ridges (friction ridges). These are confined to the palms and soles and the flexor surfaces of the digits, where they form narrow parallel and often curved arrays separated by narrow furrows (5.7, 8). Along the summit of each ridge the apertures of sweat ducts open at regular intervals. The epidermal ridges correspond to an underlying interlocking pattern of dermal papillae, an arrangement which helps to anchor the two components firmly together. The pattern of dermal papillae determines the early development of the epidermal ridges, the arrangement of which is stable throughout life, unique to the individual, and, therefore, significant as a means of identification. The ridge pattern can be affected by certain abnor-

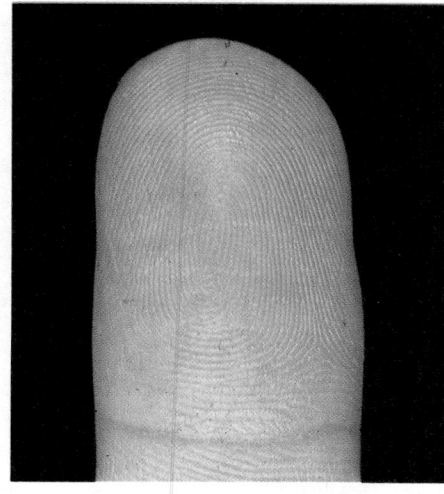

A

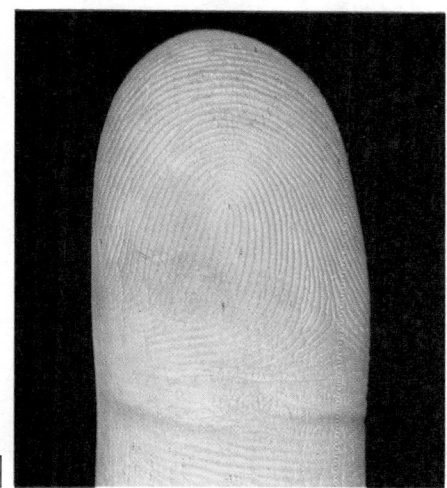

B

5.7 Photographs of the palmar aspect of a terminal phalanx in two different individuals to show the major types of pattern of the fingerprint ridges. The pattern in (A) is commonly termed a whorl; (B) is composed of loops. Note interphalangeal flexure lines.

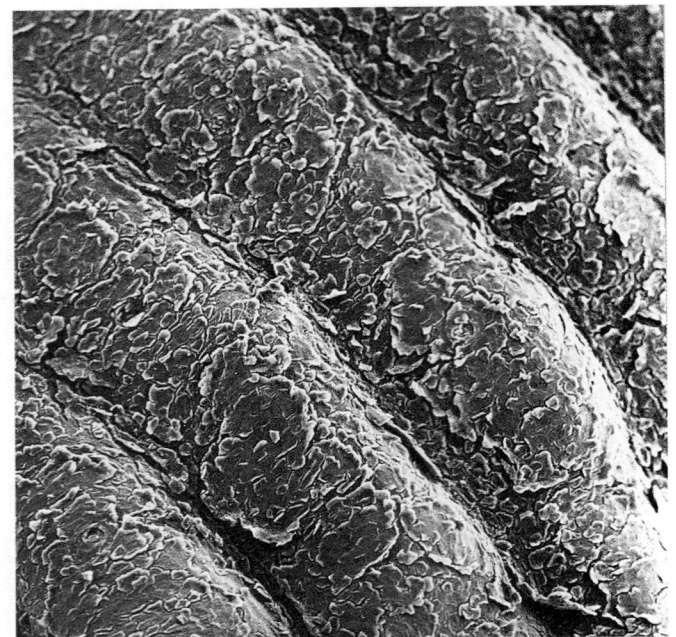

5.8 Scanning electron micrograph of the surface of thick hairless skin from the volar surface of a human digit, showing friction ridges along which open lines of sweat ducts. Magnification × 400. (Provided by Caroline Wigley, Department of Anatomy and Cell Biology, UMDS, London.)

gripping ability of hands and feet, preventing slipping, and because of the great density of tactile nerve endings beneath them they are also important sensory structures.

The analysis of ridge patterns by studying prints of them is known as *dermatoglyphics.* It has considerable forensic importance, and there are also complicated mathematical ramifications of this subject which are beyond the scope of this account (see Cummins 1926, 1964; Cummins & Midlo 1961; Penrose & Loesch 1969; Schaumann & Alter 1976). Measurable parameters include the frequency of ridges in particular patterns and the disposition of *tri-radii,* junctional areas where three sets of parallel ridges meet. Ridge configurations may differ on the terminal segments of an individual's fingers and can be separated into three major types (**5.**7): *arches* (5%), *loops* (70%), and *whorls* (25%), arches having no tri-radii, loops one, and whorls two or more. Arches may be simple or tented, loops may have a tri-radius towards the ulnar or radial side of the hand, and whorls may be symmetrical, spiral or double loop. Whorl finger patterns are more common on the right hand, and males generally have more whorls and fewer arches than females, in whom the ridges are relatively narrower. The frequency of individual patterns varies with particular fingers. Ridges within the patterns may branch or join, or may be discontinuous. Similar considerations apply to the toes. In any configuration the number of ridges may vary, the *ridge-count* being given by counting the total intersected when a line is drawn from the central point of a pattern to its nearest tri-radius. The variable features provide an astronomical number of possible combinations, so that each individual is almost certain to have a unique set of patterns.

Tri-radii also occur on the palms and soles, including the bases of each digit except the thumb; a characteristic one (the axial tri-radius) is also present on the proximal edge of the hand in the midline above the flexor retinaculum. On the palm there are six areas—interdigitals I–IV, hypothenar and thenar. The precise positions, numbers and ridge-counts associated with the tri-radii have an inherited basis and in general the genetics are multifactorial and highly complex. However, the total ridge-count of all 10 digits of the hand appears to have a simpler inheritance.

malities of early development, including genetic disorders such as Down syndrome, and skeletal malformations such as polydactyly (Thompson & Bandler 1973). Absence of epidermal ridges occurs in less than 1% of people. Functionally, epidermal ridges increase the

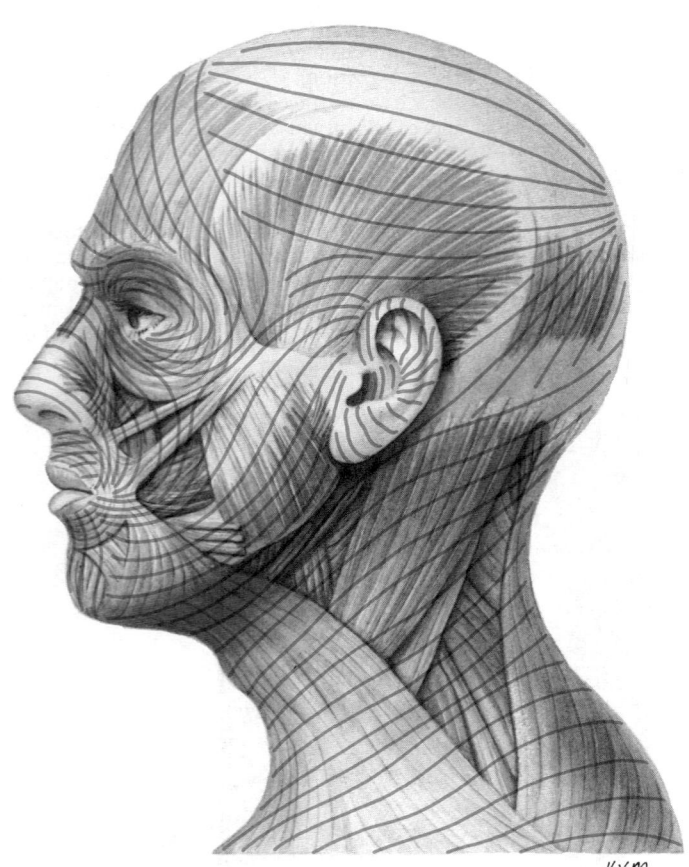

KVM

5.9A. Distribution of Langer's cleavage lines on the face. For further details see text.

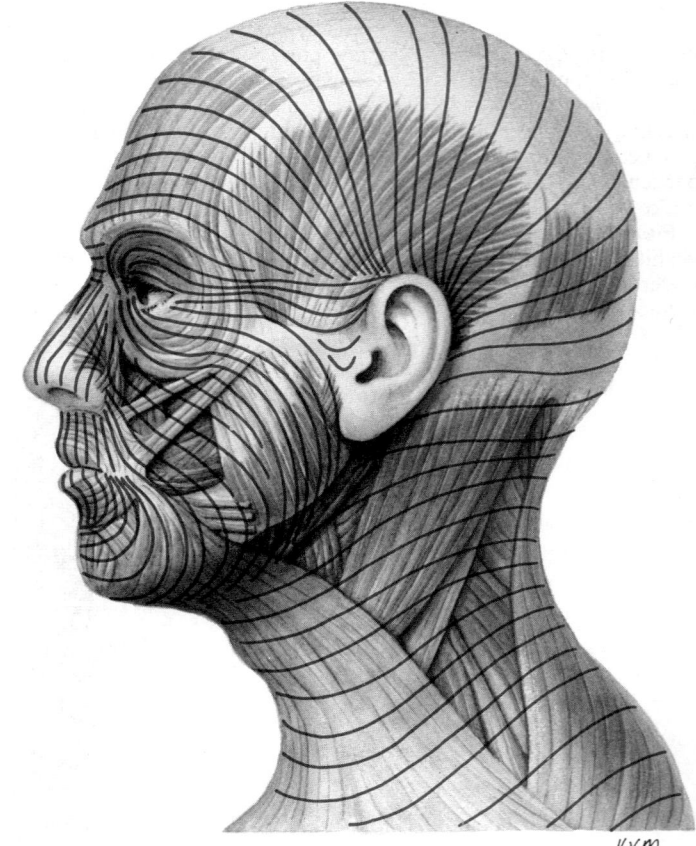

KVM

5.9B. Distribution of the lines of Kraissl's (relaxed skin tension lines) on the face. It has been reported that incisions made along these lines heal with minimum scarring (see text).

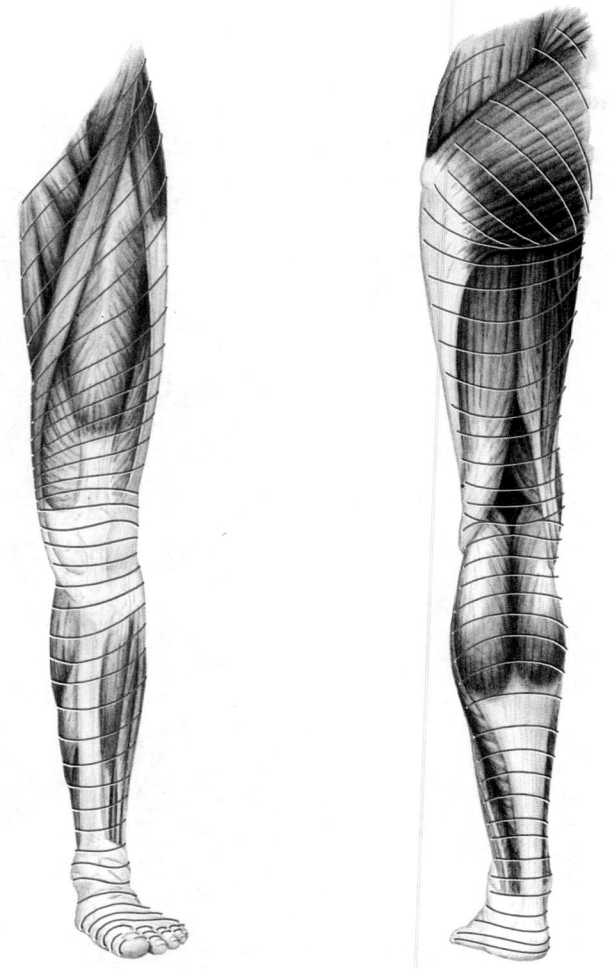

5.10 Lines of Kraissl associated with the anterior (left) and posterior (right) aspects of the lower limb.

Intrinsic scarring. If the mechanical demands placed on the skin are greater than the skin creases and the dermis can accommodate, the lateral cohesion of dermal collagen fibres is disrupted, with associated haemorrhage and cellular reaction, and eventually, formation of poorly vascularized scar tissue. Such changes can be termed *intrinsic*, to distinguish them from scars formed by external wounding (see p. 412). Sites of dermal rupture are visible externally as lines, *striae*, or stretch marks, which are initially pink in colour, but later widen and become a vivid purple or red (*striae rubrae*), and eventually fade, becoming paler than the surrounding intact skin (*striae albae*). They develop on the anterior abdominal wall of some women in pregnancy when they are termed *striae gravidarum*, associated with stretching due to the growing fetus, and in other conditions involving excessive stretching of the skin such as hypertrophy of muscle in weight-lifters and body-builders, gross obesity and rapidly growing tumours. They tend to follow Langer's lines (see below). There is thought to be a hereditary factor involved in the tendency to develop striae, and they are commoner in conditions of increased adrenal cortical activity and of excess glucocorticoids, and may be side-effects of therapeutic administration of local or systemic steroid therapy (Geschwandtner 1973; Moretti & Rebora 1976). Epidermal 'oedema' and damage to melanocytes occurs in striae rubrae; in striae albae, though melanocytes are present, they are almost totally inactive (Breathnach 1976).

Pigmentation. Variation in pigmentation can also produce externally visible lines, such as *Voigt* and *Futcher lines* on the surface of the skin. Voigt lines mark differences in pigmentation between the darker extensor and paler flexor surfaces of the arms, occurring along the anterior axial lines, extending from the sternum to the wrist. They are more common in highly pigmented races (McLaurin 1988).

Lines detectable after manipulation or incision

Lines of Langer and Kraissl (5.9, 10). Skin is normally under tension, the direction in which this is greatest varying regionally. Langer (1861) illustrated patterns of parallel cleavage lines which indicate the direction of elastic tension of skin in particular areas, and it has long been suggested that surgical incisions should be made parallel with them to minimize postoperative scarring. Unfortunately, the lines mapped out by Langer on cadavers do not always coincide with the lines of greatest tension in the living, and Kraissl's (1951) lines which often coincide with wrinkle lines are probably more appropriate lines for surgical incision. Lines of greatest tension similar to those of Kraissl have been termed 'relaxed skin tension lines' by Borges and Alexander (1962).

Blaschko lines. These refer to the way in which patterns of naevi and related dermatological pathologies are distributed or develop along certain preferred cutaneous pathways (Blaschko 1901; Rieger et al 1994). They do not appear to correspond to vascular or neural elements of the skin, and may be related to earlier developmental boundaries of a 'mosaic' nature. For more on physical properties, see Marks et al (1988).

MICROSTRUCTURE OF SKIN

EPIDERMIS

The epidermis (5.1–3, 11) is a compound tissue consisting mainly of a continuously self-replacing stratified keratinized squamous epithelium, the principal cells of which are called *keratinocytes*. Other cellular elements of different developmental origin within the mature epidermis include *melanocytes* or pigment-forming cells from the embryonic neural crest, *Langerhans cells* which are immuno-competent antigen-presenting cells derived from bone marrow, and *lymphocytes*. These disparate cells are collectively known as *non-keratinocytes* or *epidermal immigrants*. Neurally-associated *Merkel cells* are now thought to be modified keratinocytes. Sensory nerve endings are also sparsely present within the epidermis. Each component has an individual primary function, but the fact of their intimate spatial association and of functional interactions between them has led to the concept of epidermal symbionts (see p. 395). In routine sections stained with haematoxylin and eosin the non-keratinocytes and Merkel cells are poorly distinguishable, appearing as 'clear cells', due to shrinkage with a resulting clear space around them, and/or the absence of keratin filaments from the cytoplasm. However, they can be individually visualized by special light microscopic techniques or electron microscopy. The population of keratinocytes undergoes continuous renewal throughout life, a mitotic layer of cells at the base replacing those shed at the surface. As they move away from the base of the epidermis, the keratinocytes undergo progressive changes in shape and content, eventually transforming from polygonal living cells to non-viable flattened *squames* full of the protein *keratin*, a process known as keratinization.

It is usual to divide the epidermis into a number of strata from deep to superficial as follows: stratum basale, stratum spinosum, stratum granulosum, stratum lucidum (where present) and stratum corneum. The first three of these layers are metabolically active and are often grouped together as the *stratum Malpighii*. They really do not form distinct superimposed layers, and are better thought of as compartments through which cells pass, and change form as they progressively differentiate. The more superficial strata of cells achieving terminal keratinization constitute the *cornified zone*, and here, horizontal, and in some species, also vertical, layering, is evident. *Keratinization* involves not only structural changes in keratinocytes, but also alterations in their relationships with each other and with non-keratinocytes, and chemical changes within the intercellular space. The epidermal appendages (pilosebaceous units, sudoriferous glands and nails) are formed by ingrowth or other modification of the general epidermis, which is often therefore referred to as the *interfollicular epidermis*.

Keratinocyte strata of the interfollicular epidermis

Stratum basale. This includes the deepest layer of cells adjacent to the dermis, and in preparations stained by the periodic acid-Schiff (PAS) reaction or by silver impregnation, appears to rest upon a

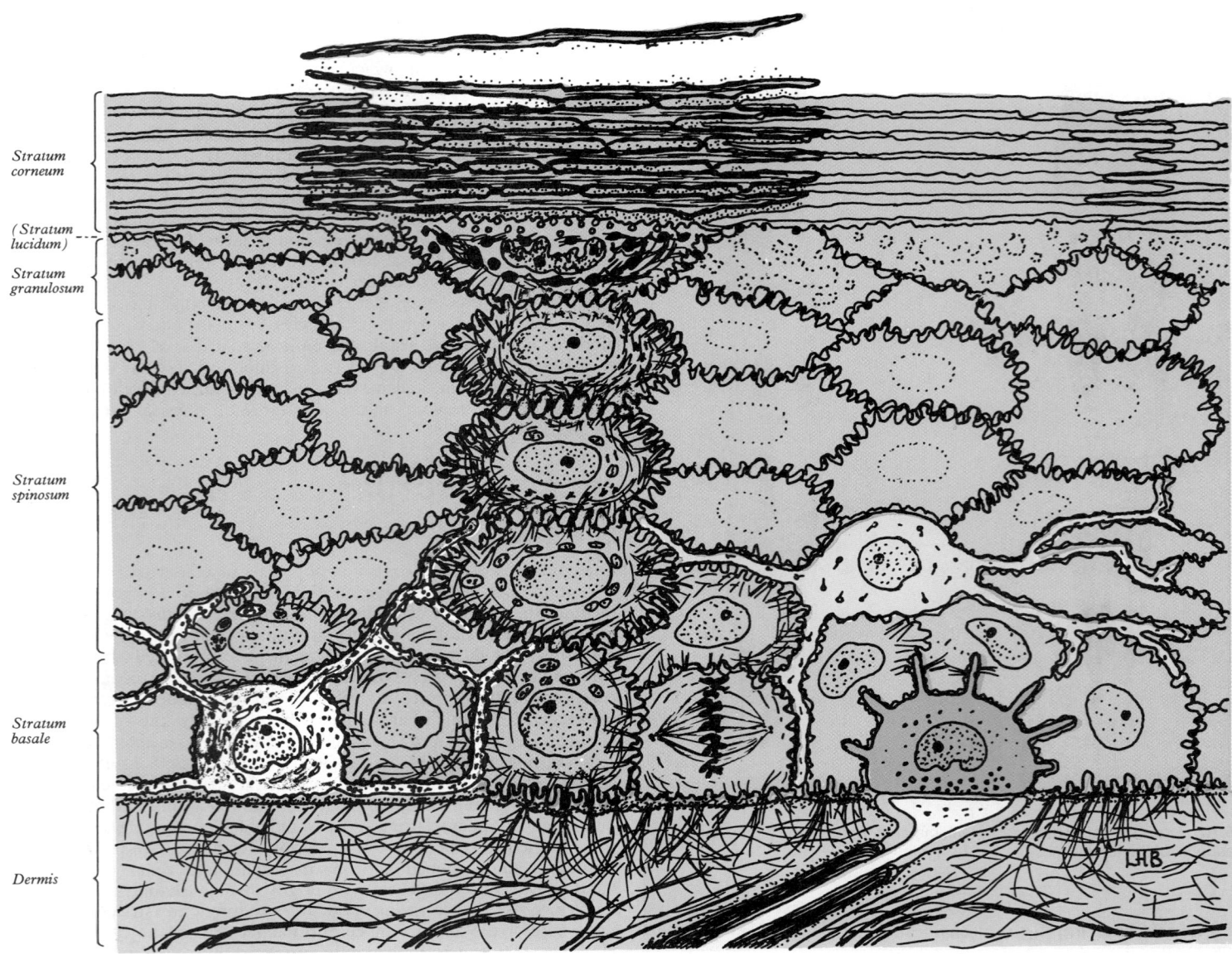

Stratum corneum

(Stratum lucidum)

Stratum granulosum

Stratum spinosum

Stratum basale

Dermis

5.11 Diagram of the main features of the epidermis, including its cell layers and different types of cell, including: keratinocytes (pink); two dendritic varieties, the melanocyte (grey) and Langerhans cell (blue); and a Merkel cell (purple). Also depicted are the dermis (green) and the sensory axon (yellow) associated with the Merkel cell. In this picture the epidermis of thin skin is shown so that the position of the stratum lucidum as it would appear in thick (hairless) skin is only indicated. For clarity only a single column of keratinocytes arising from the mitosis of a basal cell is shown in any structural detail, although desmosomal contacts are not illustrated because of the level of magnification.

continuous narrow 'basement membrane'. However, electron microscopy has shown that this is not an individual structure, and that the area apparently occupied by it, '*the basement membrane zone*' (BMZ; **5.13**, 39) includes the basal plasma membrane of the cell, a *basal lamina* consisting of lamina lucida and lamina densa, and a dermal *reticular lamina* (see p. 397). This area is also known as the *epidermal–dermal junction* (see later, p. 397). The majority of basal layer cells are columnar to cuboidal in shape, with large, mainly euchromatic nuclei and prominent nucleoli. The cytoplasm contains the common cellular organelles, variable amounts of melanosomes, and, characteristically, many cytoskeletal intermediate filaments including lower molecular-weight keratin filament bundles corresponding to the tonofilaments and tonofibrils of classical light microscopy. The plasma membranes of apposed cells are connected by desmosomes, and the basal plasma membrane has hemidesmosomes distributed along it. Occasionally, spindle-shaped 'dark cells' with more dense cytoplasm, coarser filamentous bundles and heterochromatic nuclei are seen in the basal layer. These have variably been interpreted as 'stem cells', or, more likely, older cells at a premortal stage. Melanocytes, Langerhans cells and (locally in tactile areas) Merkel cells are interspersed among the basal keratinocytes (see p. 394). Merkel cells are connected to keratinocytes

by desmosomes, but the other two lack these specialized contacts. *Intraepithelial lymphocytes* are also present in small numbers.

Stratum spinosum (prickle cell layer). This contains several layers of more mature keratinocytes packed closely and interdigitating by means of numerous projections and indentations of the cell membranes which are linked by many desmosomes (**5.11–18**), features which provide much tensile strength and coherence to the layer; gap junctions are sporadically present (**5.18A**). When skin is processed for routine histology, the cells tend to shrink away from each other except where joined by desmosomes, so giving them a spiny appearance (hence the name *spinous cells* or *prickle cells* for keratinocytes in this layer, and also the name of the stratum). Internally, spinous cells contain prominent bundles of keratin filaments, arranged concentrically around the moderately euchromatic nucleus, and attached to the dense plaques of desmosomes peripherally (for more on the general structure of desmosomes see p. 27). The cytoplasm contains the common organelles, including some lysosomes and melanosomes, the latter occurring singly or aggregated within membrane-limited organelles (compound melanosomes). Langerhans cells and the occasional associated lymphocyte are the only non-keratinocytes present in the stratum spinosum.

Stratum granulosum. In this stratum of three to four layers of

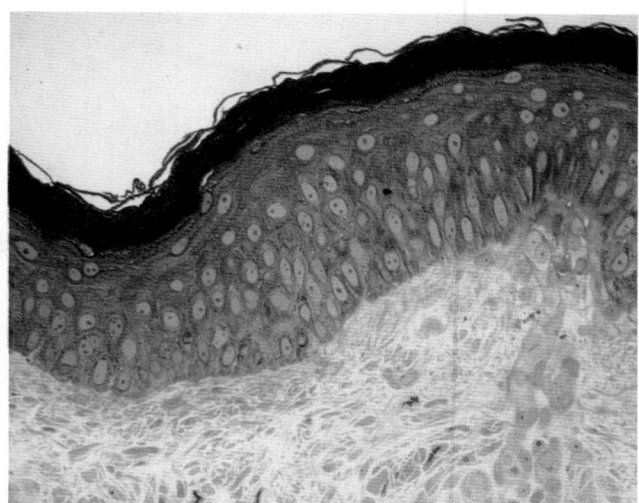

5.12   Section through epidermis and papillary dermis. Note the cellular organization of the epidermis, including the densely staining stratum corneum at the surface. Epoxy resin section stained with basic fuchsin and methyline blue. Magnification × 320. (Provided by Professor R Eady, St John's Dermatology Centre, UMDS, St Thomas' Campus, London.)

flattened cells, extensive changes in keratinocyte structure occur (Holbrook 1989). The nuclei become pycnotic and begin to disintegrate, the membranous organelles such as mitochondria, Golgi membranes and ribosomes degenerate, and keratin filament bundles become more compact and associated with, or enmeshed by, stellate or irregular densely staining *keratohyalin granules*. Small round granules (100 by 300 nm) with a lamellar internal structure (*lamellar granules*, *Odland bodies*, *membrane-coating granules*) also appear in the cytoplasm. Keratohyalin granules contain a histidine-rich, sulphur-poor protein (*profilaggrin*) which, when the cell reaches the stratum corneum, becomes modified to *filaggrin* which is thought to provide the interfilamentous matrix and to be concerned with aggregation of the keratin filaments of the corneocyte (see below under 'Epidermal keratinization'. The lamellar granules are concentrated deep to the plasma membrane of the granular cell, with which they fuse, liberating their predominantly lipid contents into the intercellular space not only of this stratum, but also into the space between it and the stratum corneum. They form an important component of the permeability barrier of the epidermis (see below, p. 386). Langerhans cells may occasionally be seen at lower levels of the stratum granulosum.

Stratum lucidum. Only found in thick glabrous palmo-plantar skin, this layer represents a poorly understood stage in keratinocyte differentiation. It stains more strongly than the stratum corneum with acidic dyes (**5**.37), is more refractile optically and often contains nuclear debris. Ultrastructurally, it resembles the *transitional cell*, an incompletely keratinized cell occasionally seen in the innermost layer of the stratum corneum of non-glabrous skin.

Stratum corneum. This stratum is the final product of epidermal differentiation, or keratinization (**5**.14, 15, 19, 22). It consists of closely-packed layers of flattened polyhedral *corneocytes*, or squames, ranging in surface area from about 800–1100 μm^2; these cells overlap at their lateral margins and interlock with cells of apposed layers by ridges, grooves and microvilli (**5**.19). In thin skin this stratum may be only a few cells deep, but in thick skin it may be more than 50 cells deep. Vertically stacked columns of corneocytes can be demonstrated with special techniques in rodents and some primates (Christophers et al 1974), but not consistently in the human stratum corneum.

The plasma membrane of the corneocyte appears thickened compared with that of keratinocytes in lower strata, but this is actually due to deposition of a dense marginal band formed by stabilization of a soluble precursor, *involucrin*, just deep to it. The outer surface is covered by a monolayer of bound lipid. In the lower layers the membrane is studded with modified desmosomes the intercellular component of which in thin sections (**5**.18B) appears as an amorphous remnant. The intercellular compartment also contains extensive lamellar sheets of glycolipid (**5**.20–22) derived from the lamellar granules of the stratum granulosum (see below, under 'permeability

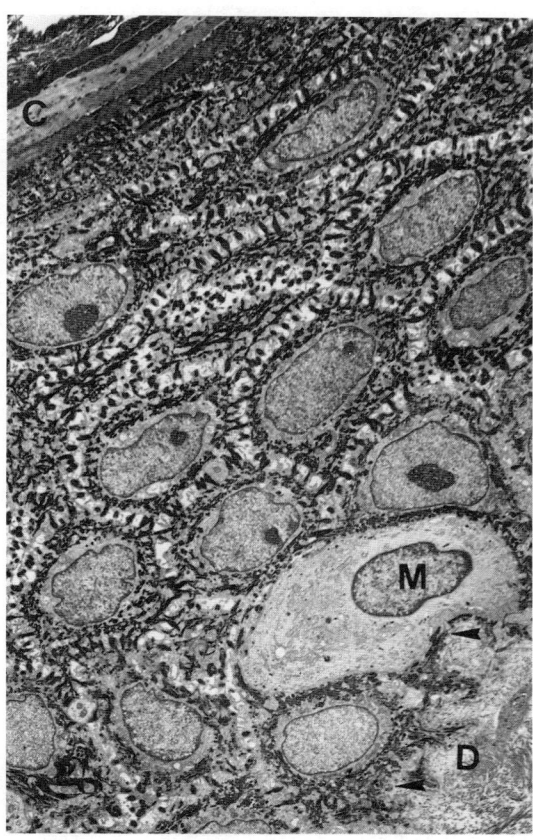

5.13   Section of full thickness of epidermis. Note melanocyte (M) in the basal layer, the characteristic 'prickle-cell' appearance of the cells of the stratum spinosum due to the arrangement of their desmosomal contacts, the flattening of the cells of the stratum granulosum, and the squames of the stratum corneum (C). D, dermis, and arrowheads indicate the epidermal–dermal junction. Magnification approx. × 2560.

barrier'). The interior of the corneocyte is devoid of nucleus and membranous organelles, consisting solely of a dense array of keratin filaments embedded in an interfilamentous matrix (**5**.15) partly composed of filaggrin derived from keratohyalin granules. In stained thin sections different 'keratin patterns' of arrangement of filaments and matrix have been described, which seem to vary with technique of processing as well as with the processor. Further consideration is given to corneocyte structure in the section dealing with the overall process of keratinization (see below).

Desquamation of the outer layers of the stratum corneum involves a poorly understood loosening of attachments (desmosomes and intercellular substances) between the cells, probably involving enzyme action, and is normally imperceptible. When excessive, it appears in hairy regions as dandruff, and more massively in certain diseases as peeling, scaling and exfoliation. Langerhans cells are not present in the stratum corneum, and, therefore, are not desquamated.

Though the stratum corneum consists of individual squames, each of which can be consecutively stripped with adhesive tape, it is important to think of it functionally also as an entity which can be separated as a single pliable sheet (Kligman 1964). The thickness of the cornified layer can be influenced by local environmental factors, particularly abrasion, which can lead to a considerable thickening of the whole epidermis including the stratum corneum, so that the soles of the feet become excessively resistant if shoes are dispensed with, and keratinized pads develop in areas of habitual pressure, for example corns from tight shoes, palmar calluses in manual workers, digital calluses in guitar players, etc. Exposure to high levels of sunshine or other stressful agents may also cause general epidermal thickening.

Epidermal keratinization

Traditionally, epidermal keratinization applied only to the final stages of keratinocyte differentiation and maturation, during which cells are converted into tough cornified squames. However, nowadays

383

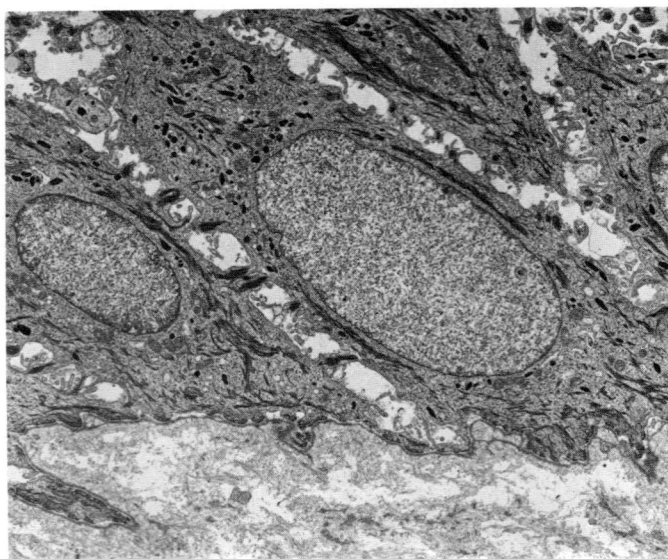

5.14A.   Electron micrograph of human epidermis showing a section through the stratum basale where it abuts the basal lamina and papillary layer of the dermis (below). Note the presence of numerous melanin granules in the epidermal cells. Magnification × 7000.

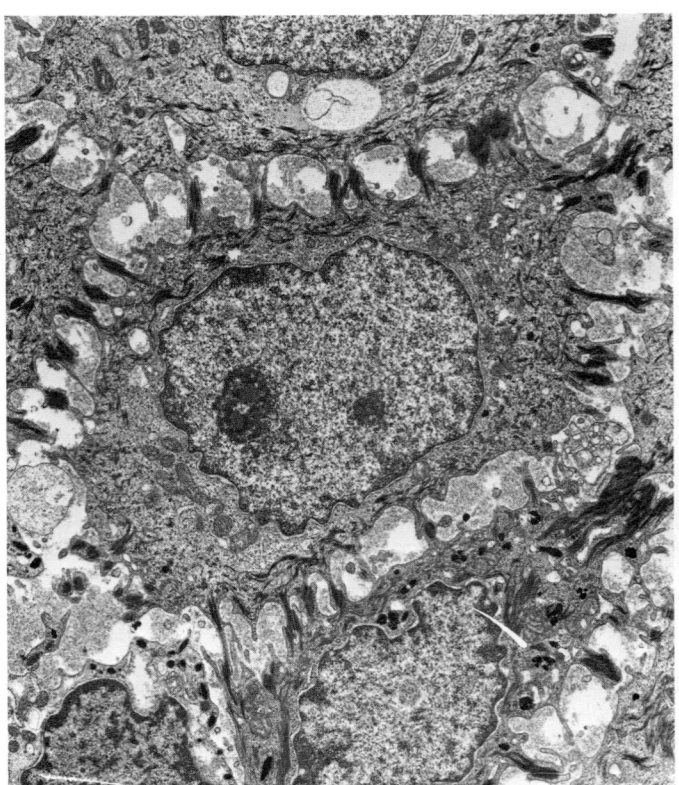

5.14B.   Electron micrograph of a keratinocyte from the stratum spinosum showing details of its cytoplasmic and nuclear structure and the desmosomal attachments between cells. Magnification × 14 000.

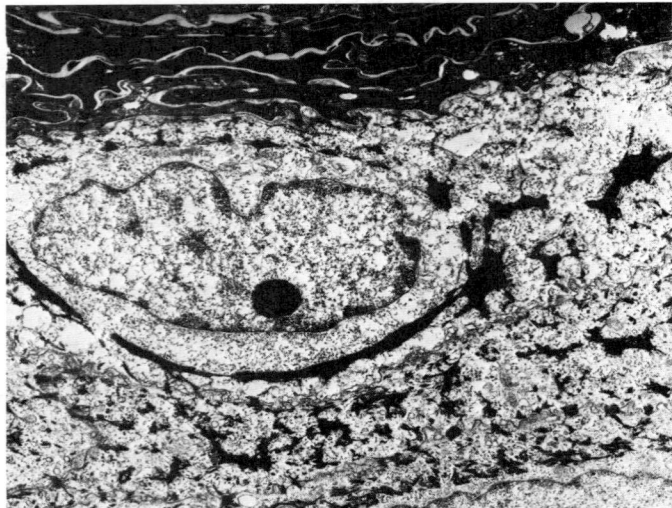

5.14C.   Electron micrograph of human skin in vertical section. This shows the transition between the stratum spinosum (below), stratum granulosum (middle) and stratum corneum (the dark laminae above). The cytokeratin bundles of the keratinocytes, below, become denser and more compact in the stratum granulosum; finally the cells flatten, becoming scale-like and electron dense. Magnification × 8000.

the term is interpreted more widely. It includes the expression and synthesis of keratin proteins in the basal layer cells, their organization into filaments, changes in their chemical composition in the upper layers, and their interaction with keratohyalin granules to form the filamentous-matrix structure of the interior of the corneocyte and strengthening of its envelope. Only a brief summary of these complicated events can be given here.

Keratins are proteins (M.W. 40 000–60 000 Da) of two types, Type I (acidic) and Type II (basic), co-expressed in pairs by epithelial cells (p. 39). Up to 30 different polypeptide chains have been recognized and numbered according to molecular weight. Chains K5 (Type II) and K14 (Type I) are expressed by basal keratinocytes and first of all assembled into two-chain coiled-coil protofilaments, then organized progressively into 4, 8 and 32 chain complexes to form the 10 nm intermediate filaments of the cytoskeleton of the basal cell (Steiner et al 1994). Filaments attach peripherally to the desmosomal plaque, and centrally may enter the nuclear pores. New keratin pairs,

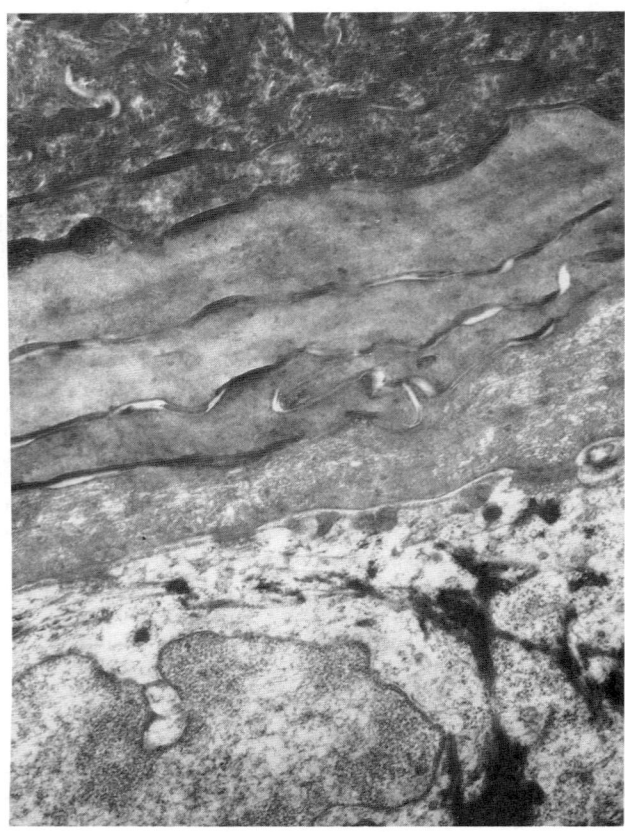

5.15   Stratum granulosum and stratum corneum. The uppermost cell of the stratum granulosum is overlain by the flattened squames of the stratum corneum. Note dense irregular keratohyalin granules in the cytoplasm of the granulosa cell. The keratinized cells of the stratum corneum are devoid of nucleus or organelles, but their internal structure is clearly not identical in all layers. Here in the five deepest layers shown, three variations of internal pattern are seen. Magnification × 20 500.

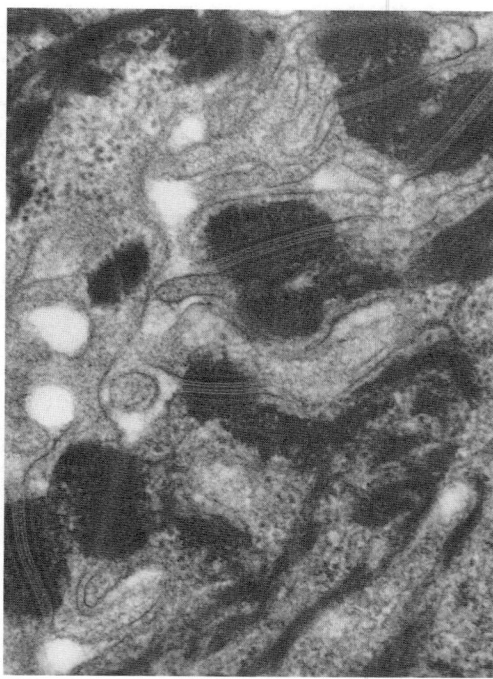

5.16 Desmosomes and cytokeratin bundles from the stratum spinosum. Magnification × 52 500.

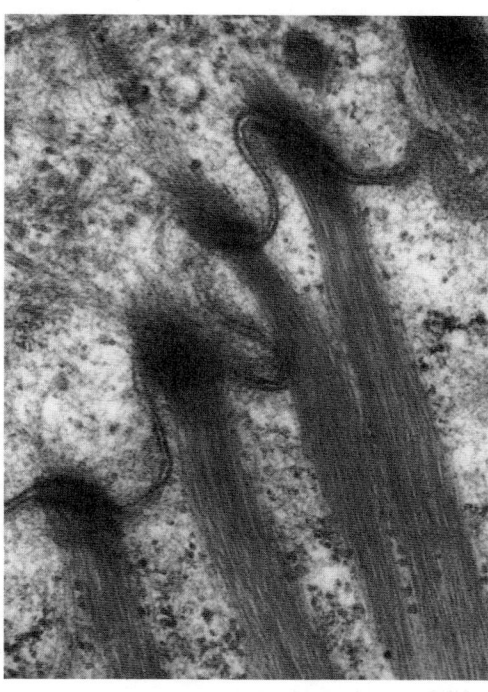

5.17 Keratin filaments attaching to the cytoplasmic aspects of desmosomes. From a keratinocyte of the outer root sheath of a hair follicle. Magnification × 47 250.

1 (Type II) and 10 (Type I), are synthesized suprabasally, and in the stratum granulosum the filaments are processed into macrofibrils and become associated with keratohyalin granules countaining profilaggrin, a histidine-rich phosphorylated protein. As the cells pass into the stratum corneum, profilaggrin is cleaved by phosphatase enzymes into filaggrin which causes aggregation of the filaments and forms the matrix in which they are embedded. As already mentioned, various patterns of filament-matrix organization within thin sections of corneocytes have been illustrated by different authors, and even in the same section different patterns may be seen in individual cells at different levels. These variations may be due to differences in processing, or to the fact that cells do not enter the stratum corneum synchronously or at exactly the same degree of terminal differentiation. This makes it difficult to define exactly what is the

final 'keratin pattern'. In freeze-fracture preparations (5.22) a picture of filaments more or less uniformly distributed within the matrix is seen.

The envelope of the corneocyte consists of a modified plasma membrane strengthened on its deeper aspect by a marginal band. Freeze-fracture (Breathnach et al 1973) reveals that intramembranous particles (IMPs) present on fracture faces of plasma membranes of cells of lower strata are generally absent from fracture faces of the corneocyte membrane, and the manner of fracture of the intramembranous component of the desmosome is also different. IMPs represent transmembrane proteins of the plasma membrane, often associated with the passage of ions and small molecules, and their absence within the corneocyte membrane could indicate that it is metabolically inert. The dense marginal band internal to the plasma

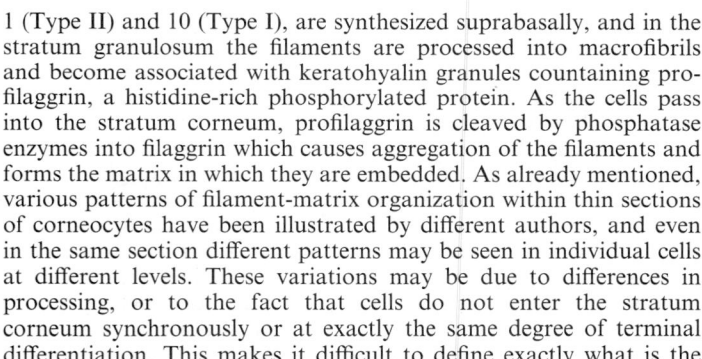

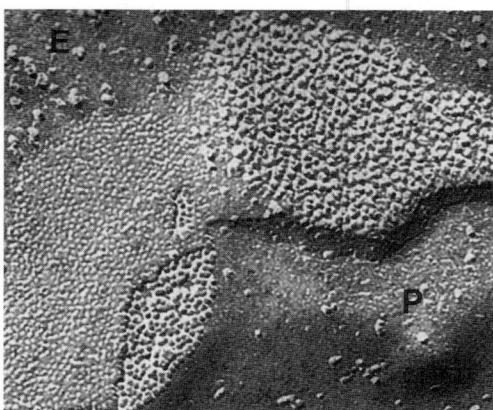

5.18A. Freeze-fracture replica of cellular contact in stratum spinosum. E and P are complementary fracture faces of the plasma membranes of the apposed cells with, on the right of the E face, aggregated particles at the site of a desmosome. Associated with it is a gap junction, defined by closely-packed particles on the P face of one cell membrane, and complementary pits on the E face of the membrane of the apposed cell. Gap junctions are not often seen in adult epidermis, and when present are nearly always closely associated with a desmosome as here. Magnification × 12 500.

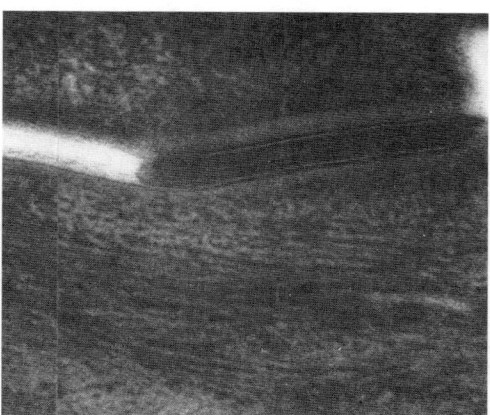

5.18B. Stratum corneum. A modified desmosome is seen between two cells with an apparent empty intercellular space on either side. However, other techniques reveal that the intervals between the corneocytes are occupied by organized lipid material derived from lamellar granules. The arrangement of internal filaments shown here is close to that commonly accepted as the typical 'keratin pattern' of the corneocyte, but in fact, it is the one least frequently seen by most observers. Magnification × 32 000.

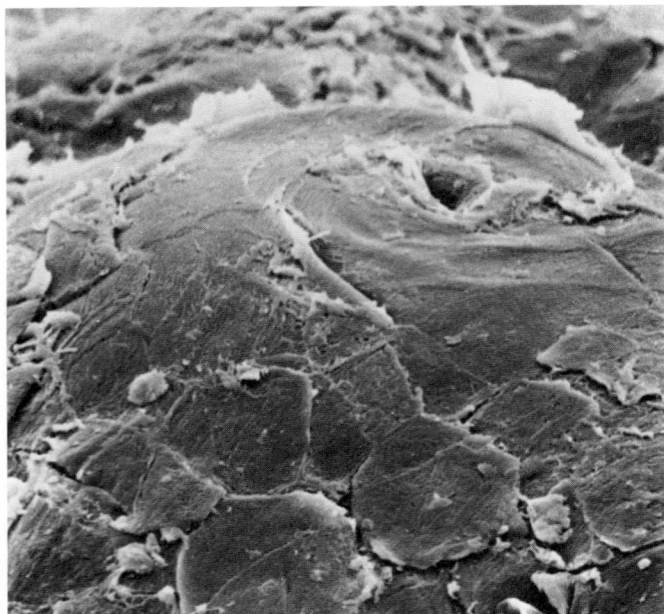

5.19 Scanning electron micrograph of a portion of the epidermal surface surrounding the aperture of a sweat duct. Several scale-like corneocytes, polygonal in form, are visible. Magnification × 2000.

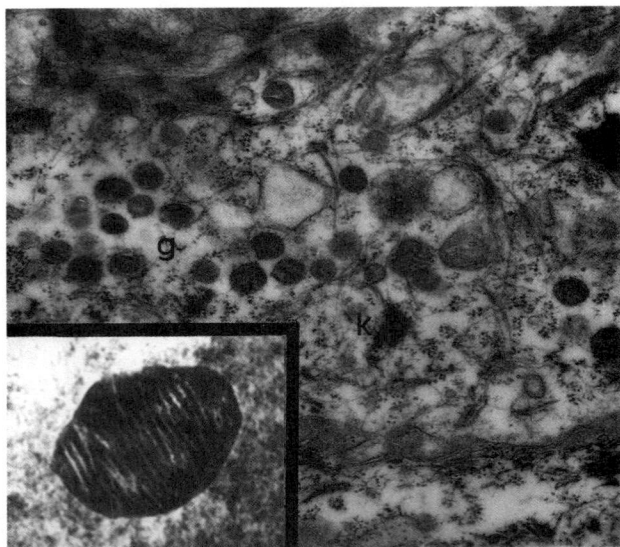

5.20 Lamellar granules (g) in cytoplasm of cell of stratum granulosum. Keratohyalin granule (k). Magnification × 23 625. Inset: granule stained by the osmium-iodide technique to show internal lamination. Magnification × 165 000. (Reproduced from Breathnach et al 1973, with permission.)

membrane results from cross-linking of a soluble precursor protein, *involucrin*, with membrane associated proteins, catalysed by a transglutaminase. It and the plasma membrane together measure 20 nm in thickness.

Other types of terminal keratinization occur elsewhere, particularly in hair and nails, where the keratin is chemically distinct and becomes much tougher than in the general epidermis ('hard keratin' as opposed to 'soft keratin'). These processes will be considered further, below (p. 402).

Extracellular compartment, permeability, barrier function and epidermal lipids

The epidermis serves as an important barrier to the loss of water and other substances through the body surface (apart from sweating and sebaceous secretion), and to their permeation from without. Theoretically, two routes of passage are available, transcellular and extracellular. In the viable strata of the epidermis the plasma membrane provides a generally effective barrier against transcellular transfer, although gap junctions provide ionic and electrical coupling between cells, important in their interactions, especially during development.

Below the stratum granulosum, the extracellular compartment appears on electron micrographs as a lucent 20 nm interval interrupted only by the intermediate components of desmosomes and the occasional gap junction. It is not, however, 'empty', but is composed of the outer glycocalices of the apposed cells containing cell surface receptors, and other molecules, and extracellular proteoglycans and ligands concerned with a variety of regulatory activities and cell–cell adhesion. Water soluble tracers, such as horseradish peroxidase (HRP), injected into the dermis can freely traverse the extracellular compartment as far as the upper levels of the stratum granulosum, but not beyond. This is the level at which lamellar granules extrude their contents and at which incomplete tight junctions are present, and it represents the deep limit of the water barrier. Experiments measuring diffusion of water from the exterior show that the entire stratum corneum provides an effective though not complete barrier. Some water soluble substances can traverse it along a polar route, probably directly through the corneocytes, and hydration makes the stratum much more permeable. Lipid-soluble substances can penetrate it more effectively, and this indicates that the water barrier must be primarily lipid in nature. It is, in fact, composed of intercellular glycolipid sheets or lamellae derived from the lamellar granules of the stratum granulosum (Breathnach et al 1973; Elias & Friend 1975; Elias 1983; Landmann 1988; Fartasch et al 1993) which are clearly seen in freeze-fracture preparations (5.22), and in thin sections of ruthenium red-fixed tissues (5.21). The contents of lamellar granules are liberated into the extracellular compartment in the form

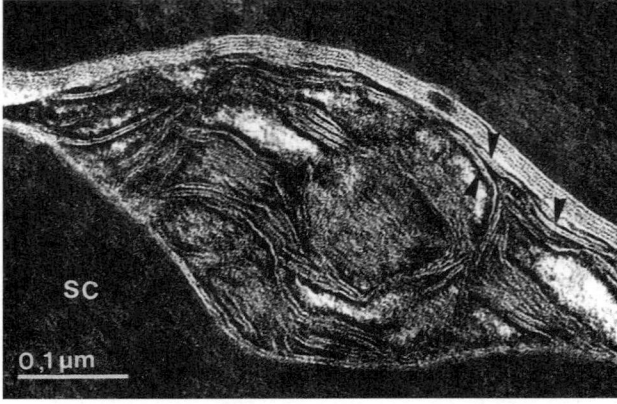

5.21A. Uncoiling prelaminar lipid sheets (arrowheads) derived from lamellar granules in the intercellular space of the stratum corneum (sc). Magnification × 73 250.

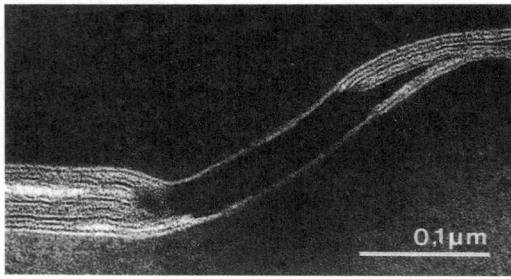

5.21B. Lipid lamellae on either side of a desmosome in the intercellular space of the stratum corneum. Magnification × 172 500. RuO₄ staining. (Reproduced from Fartasch et al 1993, with permission.)

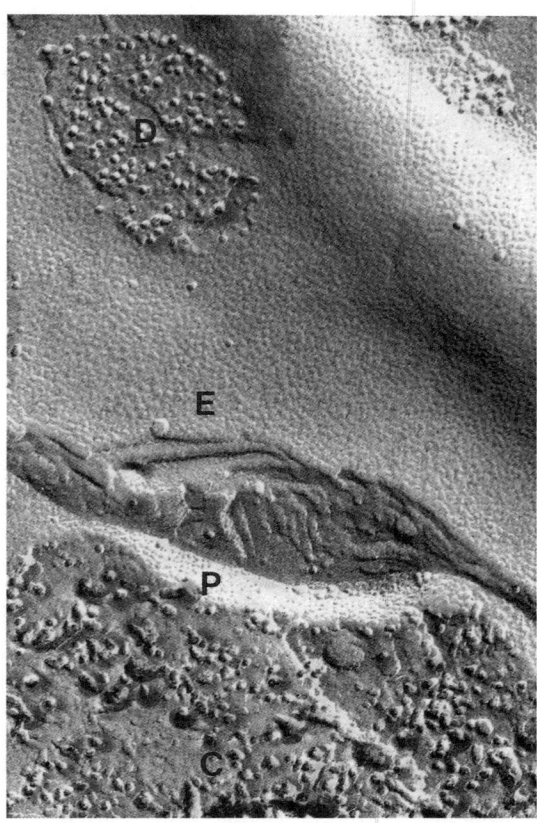

5.22 Freeze-fracture replica of stratum corneum showing lamellated material in intercellular space between fracture faces E and P of two corneocytes. In the stratum corneum, general fracture faces of the cell membranes do not exhibit intramembranous particles except at desmosomal sites (D). Fractured cytoplasm (C) of lower cell shows only filaments. Magnification × 121 500. (Reproduced from Breathnach et al 1973, with permission.)

of discs each containing two apposed lipid bilayers. After extrusion, the discs fuse edge to edge, and are chemically remodelled to form broad, multilamellar sheets throughout the extracellular compartment of the stratum corneum (**5**.20–22). The cornecytes, together with their own lipid envelopes, can, therefore, be regarded in a sense as bricks individually embedded in a lipid cement.

Epidermal lipids. A variety of lipids are present and synthesized in the epidermis, including triglycerides and fatty acids, phospholipids, cholesterol, cholesterol esters, glycosphingolipids and ceramides. Apart from their role in barrier formation, lipids, and especially phospholipids, are important components of plasma membranes and membrane-bound organelles, and serve in transmembranal signalling processes. An intermediate in the synthesis of cholesterol, 7-dehydro-cholesterol, is the precursor of vitamin D. The content and composition of epidermal lipids changes with differentiation. Phospholipids and glycolipids at first accumulate within keratinocytes above the basal layer, but higher up they are broken down and are practically absent from the stratum corneum. Cholesterol, its esters, fatty acids and ceramides also accumulate towards the surface, and are abundantly present in the stratum corneum. Whereas the lamellar arrangements of the extracellular lipids is a major factor in their barrier function, it is not clear how important the exact species composition of the sheets is. Clearly, it will be important to establish the role of individual lipids in this respect, especially in connection with delivering drugs across the barrier. Stratum corneum lipids may participate in a variety of other functions such as anti-microbial activity, antioxidant generation and xenobiote metabolism, and recognition of this is leading to a reappraisal of the stratum corneum as not just a passive, inert, selectively permeable layer, but one in which some catabolic and enzymatic activities may continue (Elias 1989). For reviews of topics referred to in this section, see Bronaugh and Maibach (1989), Maibach and Downing (1992), and Rawlings et al (1994).

Epidermal keratinocyte population dynamics

The epidermis is a cellular system undergoing continuous renewal, where, in order to maintain a constant normal thickness, the rate of cell production must equal their loss. Disturbances in division and maturation rates are common in various skin diseases, so a knowledge of the mechanisms of normal cell population dynamics (*kinetics*) is important (Davis & Wright 1991). The subject is also of importance in development wound healing and ageing of skin (see pp. 411, 412–418).

At any one time in the basal layer of the epidermis there is a variety of keratinocytes in different states of differentiation. There are *stem cells* (10%), which on division produce one of their like to maintain production, and another daughter cell, which can have a variable fate:

- it can remain for a while in the basal layer undergoing a limited number of mitoses, when it is known as a *proliferative cell* (60%) undergoing *amplification* (*transit*) divisions;
- it may remain quiescent in the basal layer for a time as a G_o cell which will resume mitosis later (see p. 23);
- it may lose the ability to divide, remaining for a time in the basal layer as a *postmitotic maturing cell* (40%).

Stem cells and proliferative cells are *recycling cells*, and postmitotic maturing cells are *non-cycling cells*; G_o cells occupy a somewhat equivocal position in this classification, since for a time they are non-cycling, but ultimately re-enter the cycle of production as proliferative cells. As a result of this activity of stem cells and proliferative cells in the basal layer, a continuous supply of non-cycling postmitotic maturing cells is passed on to the spinous layer, traversing this as *differentiating cells*, then moving into the granular layer and stratum corneum, to be finally desquamated at the surface. These layers are known as *transit compartments*, though some cell division does occur in the more basal regions of the stratum spinosum. Stem cells are thought to reside mainly at the tips of the rete pegs, and in the outer root sheath and bulge of the hair follicle, but they cannot easily be distinguished morphologically from their neighbours.

Cell proliferation kinetics can be given a degree of quantitative expression by measuring certain parameters. Techniques which have been employed include administration of colchicine to arrest mitosis, pulse-labelling with [3H]-thymidine and microradioautography, and immunocytochemical detection of 5-bromodeoxy-uridine (BUdR) incorporation. With these methods, the following can be measured: *cell cycle time*, the interval between a stem cell mitosis and the next mitosis of its daughter cell(s); *proliferative index* (mitotic index or flash-labelling index) which measures the proportion of basal cells in cycle; *turnover time*, which is the time taken to replace all cells in a compartment; *transit time*, the time it takes a cell to traverse a compartment; and *total epidermal turnover time*, the time taken for a non-cycling cell to pass from the basal layer to desquamation from the surface. Widely varying estimates of these parameters derive mainly from measurements on animals, and reliable figures for human epidermis are few. The normal total epidermal turnover time is quoted as between 52 and 75 days. Rates and times for the various parameters can vary with region, epidermal thickness, degree of skin abrasion, ambient temperature, and time of day. Circadian rhythms in the S-phase and M-phase of the mitotic cycle (p. 22) have been demonstrated. In rodents, the S-phase peaks at 3.30 a.m., and the M-phase at 8.30 a.m.; in humans, the S-phase peaks at 3.30 p.m., and the M-phase at 11.30 p.m. (Brown 1991). In some pathologies of skin, turnover rates and transit times can be exceedingly rapid; for example, in psoriasis, total epidermal turnover time may be as little as 8 days, and in such conditions differentiation of supra-basal layers is disordered, the stratum corneum does not keratinize properly and the barrier functions of the skin break down.

Potten's (1975, 1983) proposal of an *Epidermal Proliferative Unit* (EPU) seeks to unite state and rate parameters in a single concept of kinetic organization which can be demonstrated histologically. If the epidermis of some mammalian species (e.g. rats) is treated with dilute alkali before sectioning, the cells of the stratum corneum swell, and can then be seen to be stacked in regular columns (**5**.23). Beneath each column are stacked several layers of spinous and granular cells overlying a group of six to eight basal cells, each group consisting of a central stem cell with an encircling ring of what are essentially either proliferative or postmitotic maturing cells (see above). From the periphery of this ring, non-cycling cells are fed into the stratum

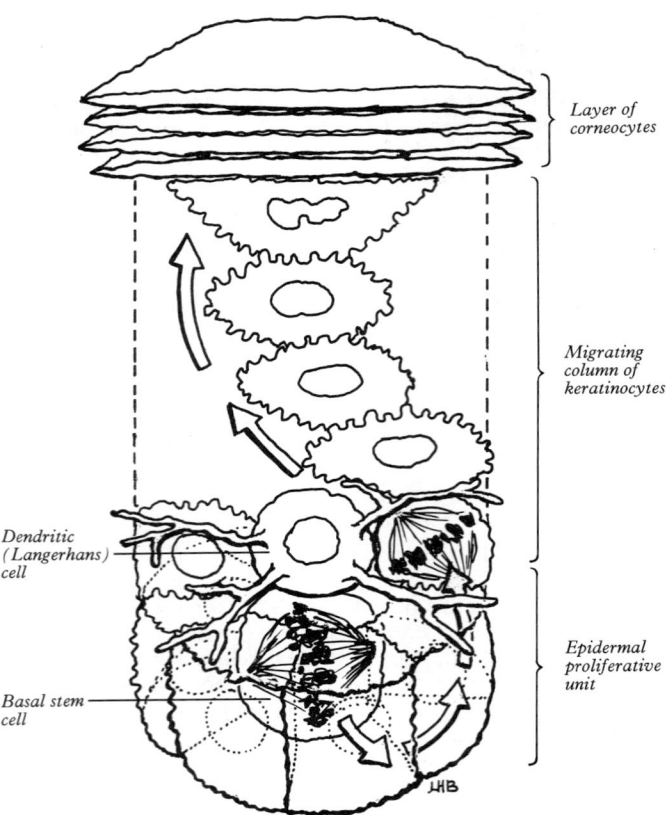

Layer of corneocytes

Migrating column of keratinocytes

Dendritic (Langerhans) cell

Epidermal proliferative unit

Basal stem cell

5.23 The concept of the epidermal proliferative unit and its relationship to the overlying column of differentiating keratinocytes, finally maturing through the stratum granulosum into the flattened corneocytes of the stratum corneum. In this model, keratinocytes arise by the repeated mitosis of a single basal stem cell, move laterally, then pass into the base of the stratum spinosum, where they may divide again one or more times before passing towards the surface. A single basal stem cell and its progeny within the stratum basale constitute the epidermal proliferative unit as initially conceived. The dendritic Langerhans cell, situated above the basal stem cell, has also been suggested as a controlling influence on cell division. For further explanation see text.

spinosum. The whole forms a cellular prism, the EPU, and each unit is a discrete entity, i.e. not feeding cells laterally into adjacent units. Whereas this arrangement seems to apply to species and sites where epidermal cell turnover is regular and not too fast, regular columns are rarely demonstrable in human epidermis, and it is questionable to what extent the concept applies here. Potten originally proposed that each unit contained a single Langerhans cell which directed mitotic activity within it, but though it can affect keratinocyte growth it is doubtful if it plays the predominant role suggested.

Under normal conditions the production of epidermal keratinocytes is matched by loss of cells from the stratum corneum, and this dynamic equilibrium is achieved by a balance of stimulating and inhibiting signals regulating proliferation of basal layer cells. Among growth- and diffusable factors which stimulate cell proliferation and differentiation are Epidermal Growth Factor (EGF), GkDa polypeptide, Transforming Growth Factor (TGF)-a, cytokines, and Basic Fibroblast Growth Factor (b-BFGF). Some of these are secreted by the basal keratinocytes themselves. Growth inhibitors include TGF-β, pentapeptide, and a- and γ-interferons. *Chalones* are substances thought to be secreted by suprabasal cells which bind to adrenaline and inhibit basal layer mitosis by a negative feedback mechanism, though evidence for their existence is mainly circumstantial. Recently, physiological cell death (*apoptosis*) has been recognized as an active regulatory mechanism in shaping and maintaining tissue size, and may play a role in normal epidermal kinetic homeostasis.

Hormones—androgens, oestrogens, corticosteroids—and vitamin A and its metabolites, the retinoids, can also affect keratinocyte turnover and differentiation, and Langerhans cells and lymphocytes are increasingly being thought of as accessory regulators in the

context of a triad of cells forming a peripheral monitoring immunological unit. Extracellular matrix components of the dermis also influence epidermal cell population dynamics, especially during development, through interactions at the basement membrane zone (BMZ) (see p. 397), and reduction of differentiating keratinocyte adhesiveness to extracellular matrix proteins, including fibronectin, facilitates their migration out of the basal layer (Nicholson & Watt 1991). Following binding of the various mediating factors to keratinocyte surface receptors, intracellular signals are triggered by 'second messengers' (see p. 24); also Elder et al 1991). Changes in keratinocyte cell to cell adhesivity during suprabasal differentiation and stratification also involves changes in the expression of adhesion molecules, such as cadherins, integrins, etc.

Clearly, separation and migration of cells to other layers involves disruption, reformation and relocation of desmosomes along the plasma membrane. Freeze-fracture replication reveals the presence of aggregated intramembranous particles composed of glycoproteins (desmogleins) within the plasma membrane at desmosomal sites (Breathnach et al 1972; Caputo & Perluchetti 1977). In fetal epidermis (Breathnach 1973), extensive areas of desmosmal particles are seen from which individual aggregates seem to bud. This suggests that certain sites on the plasma membrane may be coded for desmosome formation by lateral movement of specialized particles within the plane of the membrane, and a similar mechanism might account for their relocation and redisposition associated with asynchronous movements of previously apposed cells. Calcium could be involved as mediator in this process: addition of calcium to cultures of keratinocytes causes redistribution of desmosome-associated proteins and induces desmosome formation (Hennings & Holbrook 1983), and transmembrane desmosomal glycoproteins can bind to calcium. Calcium may also be otherwise involved in cell to cell adhesion mechanisms since it binds to the extracellular regions of the group of cell adhesion molecules known as cadherins (Farley 1991; Menon et al 1994).

Melanocytes are not involved in the movement of keratinocytes to upper levels, maintaining station along the basal lamina. This could be due partly to lack of desmosomes linking them to adjacent keratinocytes, and to the maintenance of adhesiveness to basal lamina fibronectin via integrin binding. Langerhans cells also manage to maintain position within the lower epidermal levels despite the general superficially directed current of the stream of movement, and indeed they can move against it in proceeding downward into the dermis. They might be regarded as floating or swimming in the stream, and their dendritic shape might result from, or perhaps help in, this movement.

EPIDERMAL MELANOCYTES AND SKIN PIGMENTATION (5.24–30)

Melanocytes are *melanin-pigment* forming cells derived from the neural crest and widely distributed throughout the body in vertebrates. In humans, they are present in the epidermis and its appendages, in oral epithelium, some mucous membranes, the uveal tract (choroid coat) of the eyeball, parts of the middle and internal ear and in the leptomeninges at the base of the brain. The cells of the retinal pigment epithelium, developed from the outer wall of the optic cup, also produce melanin, and neurons in different locations within the brainstem (e.g. the locus coeruleus and substantia nigra) synthesize a variety of melanin called neuromelanin.

True melanins are complicated high molecular weight polymers attached to a structural protein (to form melanoproteins), and in humans there are two classes, the brown-black *eumelanin*, and the red-yellow *phaeomelanin*, both derived from the substrate *tyrosine* by a complicated series of reactions initially catalysed by the enzyme *tyrosinase* (see p. 391). *Melanophages* are macrophages which have ingested preformed melanin, and *melanophores* are dermal melanocytes, especially common in fishes, amphibians and reptiles, though absent in humans, within which melanin can be rapidly aggregated or dispersed to change body colour in adaptation to environmental backgrounds.

Embryonic precursors of melanocytes (melanoblasts) migrate from the neural crest to enter the epidermis as melanocytes from about the eighth gestational week (Sagebiel & Odland 1972), and by the 14th week may have reached densities of 2000/mm² in some regions,

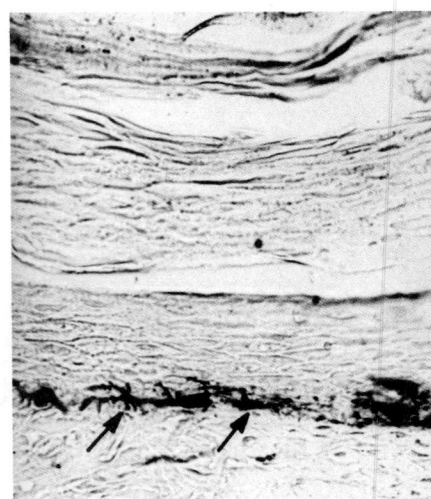

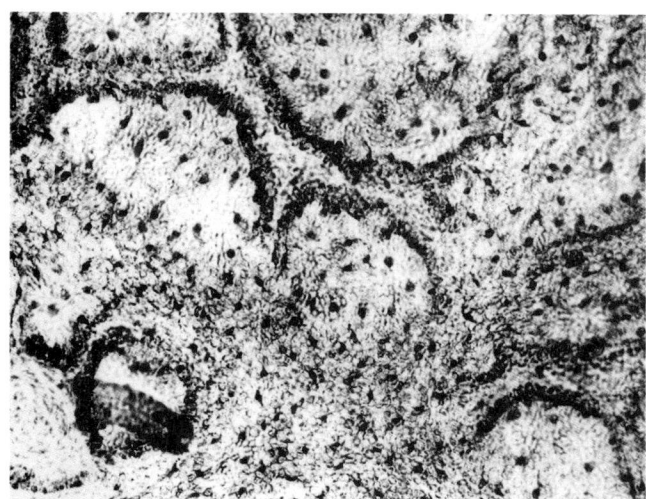

5.24 Section of skin incubated in 1 in 1000 buffered DOPA solution. Dendritic DOPA-positive melanocytes are present in the basal layer of the epidermis and stain black (arrowheads) because they contain the enzyme tyrosinase. Other cells of epidermis and dermis are DOPA-negative. The fact that faint outlines of epidermis and dermis are seen is due to non-specific staining of the solution due to auto-oxidation of DOPA during the reaction. Magnification ×320. (Reproduced from Breathnach 1960, with permission.)

5.25 'Split-skin' sheet of epidermis which was incubated in DOPA solution, viewed from the deep surface. DOPA-positive dendritic melanocytes are seen, and it is from this type of preparation that estimates of their population density per unit area of epidermis can be obtained. Not all cells are in focus because of the undulant nature of the epidermal–dermal junction, and the rete ridges of the epidermis are outlined by melanocytes superimposed at different levels along them, as well as by some melanin pigment. Magnification ×145.

partly by division of cells in situ. Shortly after their arrival, the cells engage in melanogenic activity, indicating that melanin has functions (as yet poorly understood) other than protection against solar radiation. In some oriental races, melanocytes persist for a while postnatally in the dermis of the lumbar region and buttock giving rise to bluish *Mongolian spots.* The blue colour is due to scattering of blue light by collagen bundles overlying the melanin-containing cells. In routine histological preparations stained with haematoxylin and eosin, melanocytes appear as 'clear cells' in the basal layer of the epidermis; they can be stained with Masson's ammonium silver nitrate method, but are best revealed in sections and in 'split-skin' pure epidermal sheets, by the DOPA technique (**5.24, 25**). This involves incubation in a buffered 1 in 1000 solution of DOPA (dihydroxy-phenylalanine) when the dendritic nature of the cells is well visualized. They can also be recognized in fetal epidermis by the monoclonal antibody HB-45 (Holbrook 1989). Cell counts on DOPA preparations reveal considerable regional variations in numbers of melanocytes per unit area of epidermis, ranging from 2300 per mm^2 in the cheek to 800 per mm^2 on the abdomen (Szabo 1959). It is estimated that a single melanocyte may be in functional contact via its dendrites with up to 30 keratinocytes to form an entity called the Epidermal Melanin Unit (Fitzpatrick & Breathnach 1963). In general, there are no sexual or racial differences in frequency distribution of melanocytes, and intrinsic or acquired variations in melanic pigmentation are due rather to differences in the melanizing activity of the cells than in their numbers. Melanocytes constitute a reproductive self-maintaining system of cells, although their normal turnover rate is very slow and an accurate mitotic balance sheet is lacking. They can be readily cultured in vitro (**5.28**). When locally depleted, they repopulate the epidermis, and a keratinocyte-derived growth factor, FGF-*β* (Halaban et al 1988), is probably involved as a mitogen. UV radiation also stimulates mitotic activity of melanocytes.

It should be emphasized in evaluating numerical estimates, that the DOPA reaction reveals only synthetically active melanocytes, depending as it does on the presence of the enzyme tyrosinase within the cell. In albinism, where the enzyme is either absent or blocked, melanocytes, though present, are not stained with DOPA, and relatively inactive cells in the normal epidermis may be missed through giving a weak reaction. Melanocytes decrease significantly in numbers in old age, and are absent from grey-white hair.

Ultrastructure of melanogenesis

Like the Langerhans cell, the melanocyte is a dendritic non-kera-

tinocyte (**5.25**), lacking desmosomal contacts with apposed keratinocytes, though hemidesmosomal contacts with the basal lamina are present. The nucleus is large, round, and euchromatic, and in the cytoplasm, are: intermediate filaments, a prominent Golgi complex and vesicles and associated granular endoplasmic reticulum, mitochondria, and coated vesicles, together with a characteristic marker organelle, the *melanosome* (**5.26, 27**). The melanosome is a membrane-bound structure which undergoes a sequence of four developmental stages during which melanin is synthesized and deposited within it by the tyrosine–tyrosinase reaction. The *Stage I melanosome* is a spherical vacuole, derived probably from the rough endoplasmic reticulum, and containing filamento-amorphous structural protein and vesiculoglobular bodies. Subsequent stages of eumelanosomes and phaeomelanosomes differ somewhat in morphology (**5.29A, B**). *Stage II eumelanosomes* become spherical or

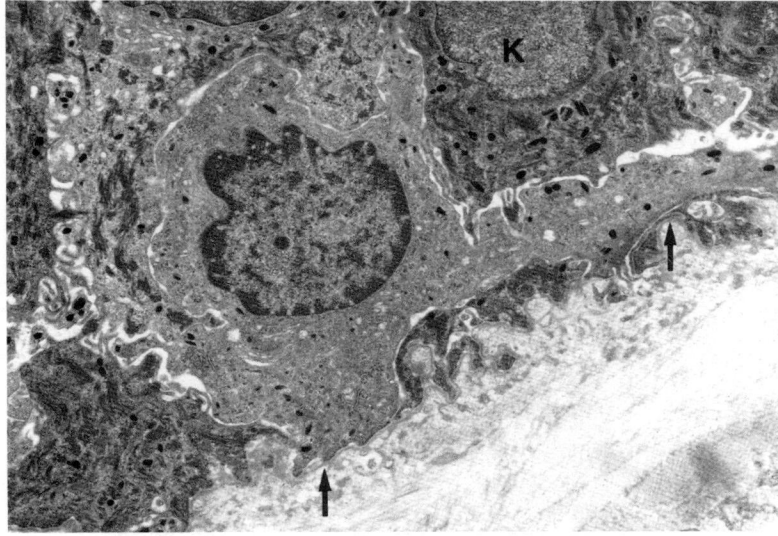

5.26 Basal epidermal melanocyte showing general ultrastructural features. There are no desmosomes connecting it with apposed keratinocytes (K), the cytoplasm contains no keratin fibrils, and melanosomes are present as individual granules in the cytoplasm. Note dendrite extending towards the right. Arrows mark the epidermal–dermal junction. Magnification ×5625.

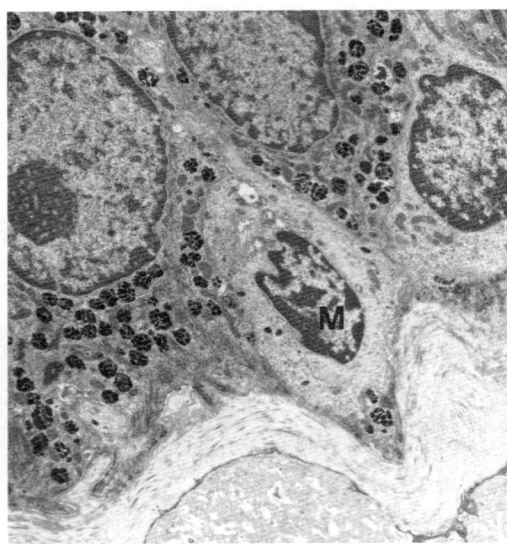

5.27　Melanosomes aggregated in groups in basal keratinocytes. Note few melanosomes in melanocyte (M). It produces the melanosomes and passes them on to the keratinocytes. Magnification × 4950.

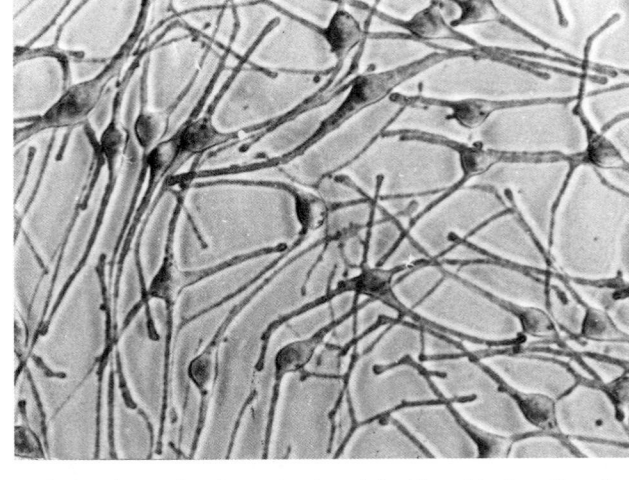

5.28　Pure culture of melanocytes from infant foreskin. In culture the cells retain their dendritic shape. Magnification × 450.

ellipsoid and the inner matrix becomes organized into filamentous sheets exhibiting a 9 nm periodicity. At *Stage III*, melanin begins to be deposited on the inner sheets, gradually obscuring their arrangement, until the final, densely-pigmented *Stage IV* is reached, exhibiting no other internal structures apart from non-melanized vesiculoglobular bodies. *Phaeomelanosomes* retain their spherical shape throughout all stages, their inner matrix is not organized into sheets, and at Stage IV a microgranular internal structure may still be apparent. In most active melanocytes, melanosomes of all stages are present; in albinos, Stages I and II are present, though the inner matrix may lack its typical organization. When mature, Stage IV melanosomes move into the dendrites along the surfaces of microtubules and are transferred to keratinocytes by a special type of phagocytosis involv-

ing the latter cell nipping off and internalizing the tip of the dendrite with the subsequent liberation of melanosomes into the keratinocyte cytoplasm (5.27). Here, they may exist as individual granules in heavily-pigmented skin, or be packaged within secondary lysosomes as melanosome complexes or compound melanosomes in lightly pigmented skin. They are often aggregated above the nucleus to form supranuclear caps. As the keratinocytes progress towards the surface, melanosomes undergo degradation, and melanin remnants in the stratum corneum are more in the form of dust-like particles.

Lipid droplets frequently occur in normal melanocytes, and in the eyelid there is a melanocyte which contains them in abundance, and which is known as the 'unicellular sebaceous gland of Wolff' (Pelfini et al 1969).

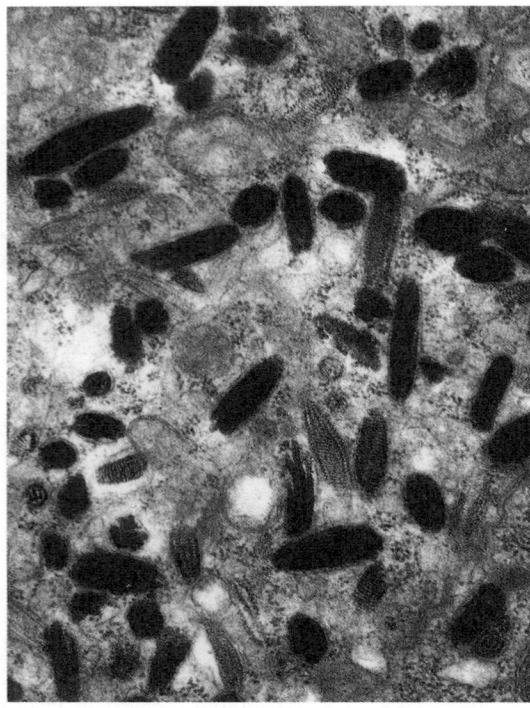

5.29A.　Cytoplasm of hair bulb melanocyte containing melanosomes at Stages II and III. From the elongated rod-shaped form, these are identified as eumelanosomes. K, keratinocyte. Magnification × 32 550.

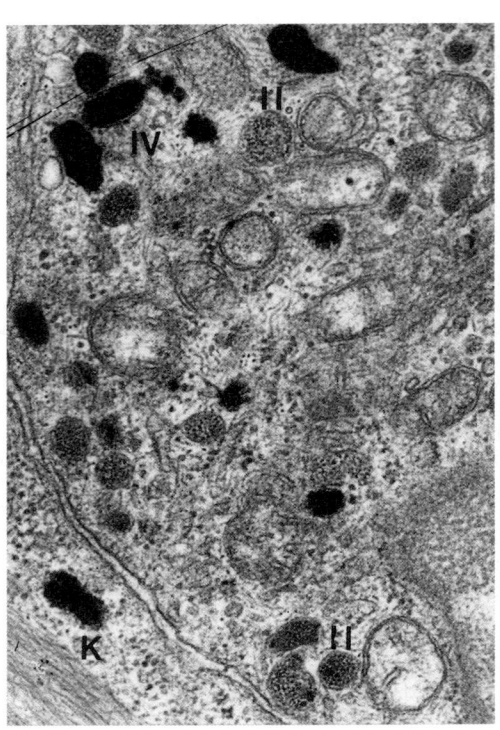

5.29B.　Cytoplasm of melanocyte containing melanosomes mainly at Stages II and IV. From the predominantly round sectional profiles and granular internal structure, these are identified as phaeomelanosomes. Magnification × 51 000.

Tyrosinase, and synthesis and properties of melanins. Tyrosinase is a copper containing metallo-enzyme, present in the form of several isozymes, which catalyses the initial stages of the synthesis of tyrosine-melanin. It is formed by ribosomes on the granular endoplasmic reticulum, conveyed to the Golgi complex, glycosylated and incorporated into coated vesicles which attach to the limiting membrane of the Stage I melanosome, liberating the active enzyme into its interior. Melanization then commences via a complicated pathway the complete details of which remain to be worked out, and which differ between eumelanin and phaeomelanin. The first two steps, oxidation of tyrosine to DOPA, and DOPA to dopaquinone, are common to both, and catalysed by tyrosinase. Next, in eumelanin synthesis, dopachrome is formed, converted into dihydroxyindoles and 5–6 dihydroxyindole-2-dicarboxylic acid by a mechanism involving a conversion factor and possibly two enzymes, dopachrome oxido-reductase, and dopachrome tautomerase, though these latter may be one and the same (Pawelek 1991). The final stages in the pathway to melanin essentially involve complex polymerizations in which tyrosinase may again be involved. In phaeomelanin synthesis, the amino-acid cysteine is added to dopaquinone to form 5-S cysteinyldopa. Evidence is increasing that most natural melanins are mixtures of eumelanin and phaeomelanin, and phaeomelanic pigments, *trichochromes*, occur in red hair.

Melanin has biophysical and biochemical properties related to its functions in skin. It protects against damaging effects of UV radiation on DNA through its spectral absorptive electron–photon coupling, and amorphous semiconductor properties, whereby it can absorb many different types of energy and dissipate them in the form of vibrational modes or heat. Its redox capacity makes it an efficient scavenger of damaging free radicals, however generated, and its ability to bind to a variety of metal ions and drugs suggests it can act as an antitoxic agent. However, if the energy input is too great, these properties can be expressed in the output of toxic activated chemical species which can be damaging (Hill 1992). Another disadvantage is that a high concentration of melanin in relation to incident solar UV may adversely affect synthesis of vitamin D.

Determination and control of melanin pigmentation

Melanin pigmentation of human skin can be analysed on two bases: *constitutive* and *facultative*. Constitutive pigmentation is the intrinsic level, genetically determined, and facultative pigmentation comprises reversible changes induced by environmental agents, for example UV and X-radiation, chemicals, and hormonal influences.

Genetics. In rodents, at least 130 genes at 50 loci are known to determine skin and coat melanization, acting not only on the melanocytes themselves, but also on their environment. Specific genes can influence differentiation of neural crest cells into melanoblasts, and also melanoblast migration to the skin, their differentiation into melanocytes, and morphological features of these latter, such as shape, size and length of dendrites, which in turn determine the size of the pool of keratinocytes to which each cell transfers its melanosomes. Other genes acting primarily within the melanocyte control the synthesis of tyrosinase, its type and activity (including inhibitors), the type of melanin synthesized, the size, shape, protein structure and number of melanosomes, their degree of melanization, and their rate of transfer to keratinocytes. Constitutive melanin pigmentation in man is probably under similar precise genetic control, though positive evidence is not easy to obtain due to co-mingling of genes. Various types of *albinism* are genetically determined.

Racial variations in pigmentation are due to differences in melanocyte morphology and activity rather than to numerical differences. In naturally heavily pigmented skins the cells tend to be larger, more dendritic, and to contain more and larger Stage III and IV melanosomes than melanocytes of paler caucasoid skins. The keratinocytes in turn contain more melanosomes, individually dispersed, whereas in caucasoids the majority are contained within secondary lysosomes to form melanosome complexes. (Melanosomes occasionally seen within Langerhans cells are always similarly enclosed.) For more on this topic, see Robins (1992).

Ultraviolet irradiation. *Photobiology* is a rapidly expanding discipline concerned with the overall effects of solar irradiation, and in particular, UV irradiation, on the skin (see Fitzpatrick et al 1974; Potten 1985; Posschier et al 1987). The response of the melanin pigmentary system to UV varies with genetic and constitutional factors. It includes *immediate tanning*, or *pigment darkening*, which can occur within a matter of minutes, probably due to photooxidation of pre-existing melanin. *Delayed tanning* occurs after about 48 hours, and involves stimulation of new melanogenesis within the melanocytes, and transfer of additional melanosomes to keratinocytes. There may also be some increase in size of active melanocytes, and in their apparent numbers, both through division, and activation of dormant cells. Keratinocytes can be directly involved in these changes through various signals. In vitro, the lower frequency end of the UV band (UVB) induces synthesis by keratinocytes of b-FGF, which is mitogenic for melanocytes, as well as Interleukin I which induces them to produce α-melanocyte stimulating hormone (α-MSH), a known stimulant of melanogenesis (see below); there is evidence that keratinocytes may also produce adrenocorticotrophic hormone (ACTH). Chronic exposure to UV results in changes dealt with below under 'Age related changes in skin' (p. 411).

Freckles in skin of red-haired individuals are usually thought to be induced by UV, though they do not appear initially until several years after birth, despite exposure. Paradoxically, melanocytes are significantly fewer in freckles than in adjacent paler epidermis, but they are larger and more active. What determines the onset of freckles, or their individual location, is not known.

Hormonal influences. In amphibians, MSH from the anterior lobe of the hypophysis, and melatonin, a skin-lightening hormone secreted by the pineal, are involved in pigmentary alterations, though their importance as normal regulatory factors in man is unclear. When administered to humans, α-MSH causes an increase in pigmentation due to a cyclic adenosine monophosphate (cAMP)-mediated increase in tyrosinase activity, and as mentioned above, UV irradiation induces MSH production by keratinocytes. ACTH is also thought to affect melanocyte activity, and is probably responsible for the hyperpigmentation associated with pituitary and adrenal disorders. The role of melatonin in the biology of human melanin pigmentation remains problematic. In pregnancy, higher levels of circulating oestrogens and progesterone are responsible for the increased melanization of the face, abdominal and genital skin, and the nipple and areola, and much of this may remain permanently. A number of other factors operating within the epidermis, such as interleukins, arachidonic acid, prostaglandins and various cytokines, also affect melanogenesis, either stimulating or inhibiting individual steps, or inhibiting natural tyrosinase inhibitors within the melanocyte. Clearly, the level of pigmentation at any given time represents a balance between a large number of competing influences, constitutive and facultative, and these must be taken into account in the analysis and diagnosis of hypo- and hyperpigmentary disorders.

Summary. Further details on all aspects of melanin pigmentation will be found in: Quevedo et al (1987), Nordlund et al (1989), Jimbow et al (1991), Prota (1992), Robins (1992), and Takeuchi and Quevedo (1992).

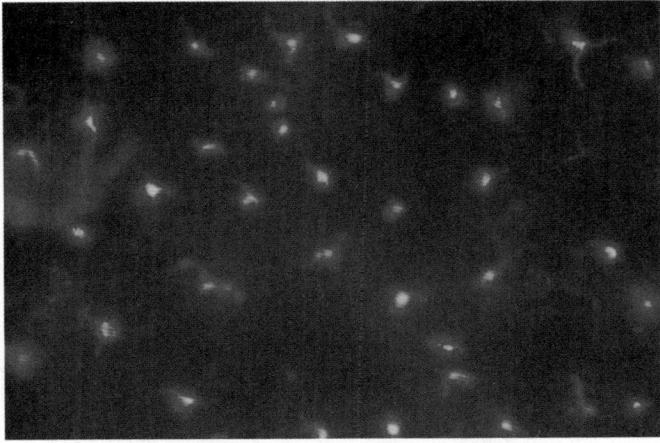

5.30 Epidermal sheet preparation. Immunofluorescence staining with Phycoerythrin anti-HLA-DR showing Langerhans cell network. Magnification ×95. (Provided by Dr S Breathnach, St John's Dermatology Centre, UMDS, St Thomas' Campus, London.)

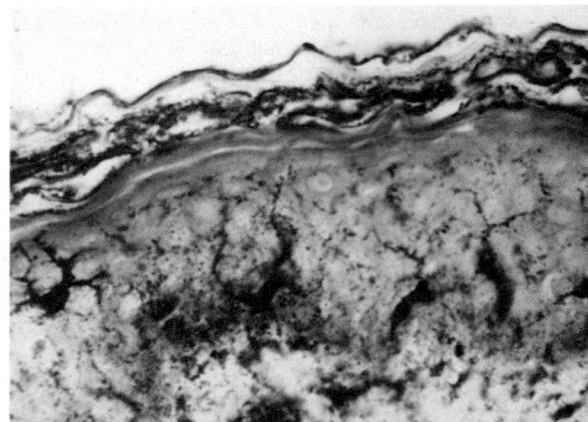

5.31 Section of skin stained with Gairn's gold chloride method. Gold-positive dendritic Langerhans cells are seen at suprabasal levels. Magnification × 315.

Langerhans cell: immunological surveillance

Langerhans cells are dendritic antigen-presenting cells regularly distributed in mammals throughout the basal and spinous layers of the epidermis (p. 381) and its appendages, apart from the sweat gland, and of other stratified squamous epithelia, including the buccal, tonsillar and oesophageal epithelia, as well as the cervical and vaginal mucosae and the transitional epithelium of the bladder. They are present in the conjunctiva, but not in the cornea. In routine H&E preparations they appear as high-level 'clear cells', and with other techniques such as staining with gold chloride or osmium-zinc iodide, their characteristic dendritic shape becomes apparent (5.31). They are also visualized in adenosine 5'-triphosphate (ATP)ase preparations and by a variety of immunofluorescence and immunocytochemical techniques (5.30). They are immunocompetent cells derived from bone marrow (Katz et al 1979), and enter the epidermis as early as the fifth to sixth week. The postnatal population (460–1000/mm², 2–3% of all epidermal cells, with regional variations) is maintained both by continual renewal from the marrow and, minimally, by division in situ. Following almost complete depletion in rodents by tape-stripping of the epidermis, or X- and UV radiation, normal numbers of Langerhans cells return by 4–15 days. Extra-epithelial Langerhans cells are present in the dermal stroma, occasionally within dermal capillaries and lymphatics, and in lymph

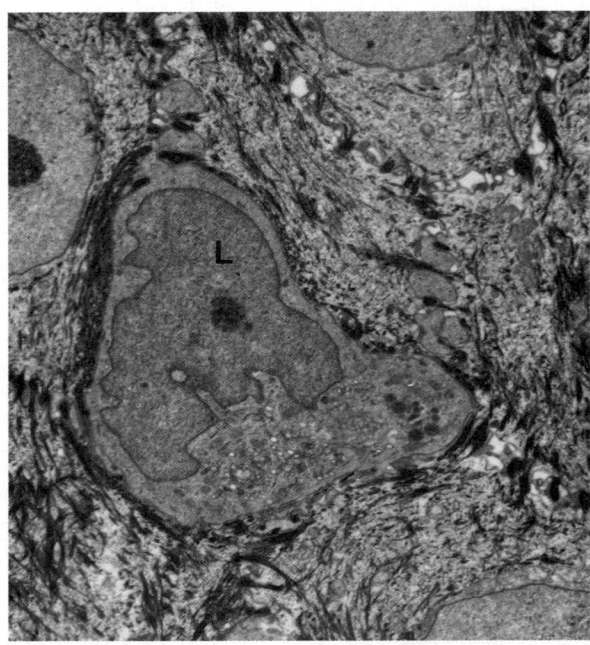

5.32 A Langerhans cell (L) in the stratum spinosum of the epidermis. Note indented nucleus, cytoplasm with no keratin filaments which are characteristic of surrounding keratinocytes, and absence of desmosomes along the plasma membrane. The characteristic granules of the cytoplasm (5.33) are too small to be clearly identified at this enlargement. Magnification × 5325.

nodes, thymus, and spleen (with, of course, a pool of precursors in the bone marrow).

Ultrastructure. Langerhans cells are non-keratinocytes in that desmosomes are absent from the plasma membrane, the cytoplasm lacks keratin filaments, they do not become keratinized and are not desquamated. The nucleus is euchromatic and markedly indented (5.32), and the cytoplasm contains a well-developed Golgi complex, lysosomes often containing ingested melanosomes, and a characteristic marker organelle, the *Birbeck granule* (Birbeck et al 1961). These structures are discoid or cup-shaped, and on section (5.33) present a variety of appearances. The commonest is that of a rod 0.5 μm long and 30 nm wide, with a linear fuzzy coat within the trilaminar limiting membrane and a central core of two linear arrays of particles with a periodicity of 9 nm. Vesiculation of the limiting membrane at either end gives an appearance similar to a tennis racket and, when sectioned obliquely, an orthogonal or lattice array of the central particles is evident. What appear to be granules may occasionally be seen continuous with the plasma membrane, and this has raised questions as to their origin, nature and function. The bulk of current evidence (Schuler et al 1991; Bartosik 1992; Bucana et al 1992) suggests that the structures attached to the plasma membrane are formed by internalization and zipping of segments of plasma membrane associated with coated vesicles, the resulting structures then undergoing unzipping, vesiculation and fusion with endosomes, to deliver molecules to the interior. There is some doubt as to the exact correspondence of classical, closed, intracytoplasmic granules with those attached to the plasma membrane, which have been referred to as 'Birbeck granule-like structures'. If they are not identical, this allows revival of the original suggestion that Birbeck granules are derived from the Golgi apparatus (see above). Hanau et al (1991) have reported the presence within ethylene diamine tetracetic acid (EDTA)-treated human blood platelets of elements ultrastructurally similar to Birbeck granules and apparently formed by collapse of the *surface-connected canalicular system*. This has led them to suggest that the granules may derive from transformation of vacuolar or canalicular structures due to ligand–receptor interactions while resident in the epidermis. Apart from this, Langerhans cells can exhibit general phagocytic activity, but not to the same extent as keratinocytes. Cells with all the features of Langerhans cells apart from the granules may be present in the basal layer, and are referred

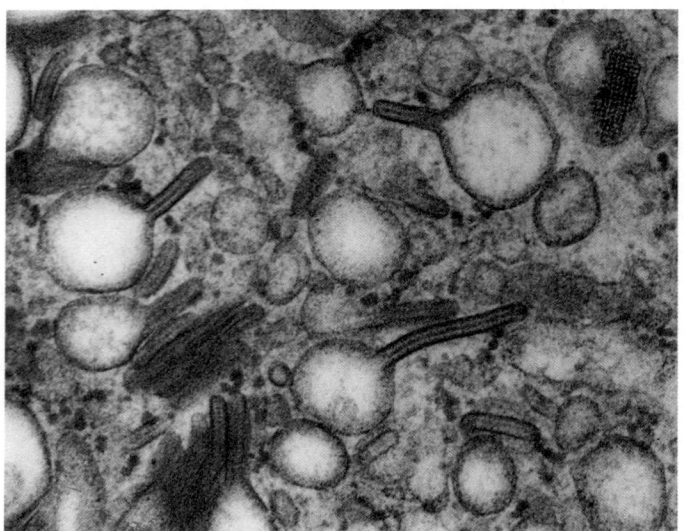

5.33 Langerhans granules. Note rod-shaped sectional profiles with central linear periodicity, and terminal blowing-out of the limiting membrane. At top right, a granule sectioned tangentially exhibits a lattice arrangement of particles. Magnification × 62 010.

to as 'indeterminate cells'; they are thought to be either immature stages, or else the most mature, about to leave the epidermis (see below). Cells with more electron-dense cytoplasm exhibiting degenerative features and present at all levels of normal epidermis except the striatum corneum (Breathnach 1981) may have been damaged by solar radiation or some other environmental insult, or, perhaps, represent a distinct phenotype or functional stage.

Another dendritic non-keratinocyte, also of bone-marrow origin, the Thy-1 + EC, is present in murine epidermis, and belongs to the T-cell lineage (see Schuler et al 1991). Any analogue of this cell type has not yet been certainly demonstrated in human epidermis.

Immunoreactivity. Langerhans cells belong to the general group of dendritic cells (DC), mononuclear phagocytic cells important in immunological reactions (see p. 1417), though their exact relationship to other members of this group, such as 'veiled cells', interdigitating reticulum cells, DC in peripheral blood and lymph, and B-cell related dendritic cells of lymphoid follicles, remains uncertain (Romani et al 1991a,b; Bergstresser et al 1992). Phenotypically, they carry receptors for the Fc portion of IgG, and for complement components (C3b–C4b and C4d), and express a variety of antigens, the number of which is being added to regularly. These include MHC Class I and Class II antigens (Ia; HLA-DR) and CDIa antigen, and the cytoplasm expresses S-100 protein. Preparation of monoclonal antibodies to these and other markers has allowed specification and visualization of Langerhans cells by immunofluorescence and immunocytochemical techniques. The phenotype of human Langerhans cells differs in some respects from that of experimental animals, and in cell culture is significantly altered, becoming more like that of dendritic cells within lymphoid tissue. The capacity of the cell to produce Birbeck granules is reduced in culture, and this, together with the change in phenotype, is regarded as a badge of 'maturity' in terms of ability to sensitize T-cells (see below). Implicit in this concept is the suggestion that the majority of resident Langerhans cells are immature from a functional point of view.

Functions. The Langerhans cell is now recognized as a key element in a Skin Associated Lymphoid Tissue (SALT) (Streilein 1983), which is the peripheral outpost of the body's immune surveillance system and involved in induction and regulation of the primary immune response. SALT comprises the Langerhans cell, T-lymphocytes and keratinocytes, together with local draining peripheral lymphatics and associated lymph nodes. In this scheme, the Langerhans cell, under appropriate conditions of normal monitoring, or in the course of a contact hypersensitivity reaction, internalizes antigen (haptens, proteins, local tumour antigens, etc.) by receptor-mediated endocytosis via 'Birbeck granule-like structures' (Bucana et al 1992), processes it, becoming 'mature' meanwhile, then migrates to the draining lymph nodes to present it to unstimulated T-cells. It initiates antigen-specific T-cell activation and proliferation, and

generation of cytotoxic T-cells (see p. 1420). These activities involve a traffic in both directions of Langerhans cells across the epidermal–dermal junction, their presence, especially in contact hypersensitivity reactions, in dermal lymphatics and nodes, and their apposition to lymphocytes within the epidermis. A positive regulatory role for the keratinocyte in SALT is becoming increasingly apparent. It also expresses Ia antigen, produces cytokines which can enhance or downregulate T-cell activation, and others which, in culture, can affect the differentiation, maturation and viability of Langerhans cells (Luger & Schwartz 1991), functions which it might well subserve in vivo. A reciprocal influence of the Langerhans cell on keratinocyte proliferation, differentiation, and keratinization is enshrined in the concept of the Epidermal Proliferative Unit (p. 387).

Langerhans cells are involved in rejection of skin grafts from histo-incompatible animals, and their absence from the cornea may be an important factor in the ease with which grafts of this tissue can be accomplished. Transplantation of bone-marrow cells from one individual to another is increasingly being used in the treatment of leukaemias and other blood discrasias, and in the process, precursor Langerhans cells will be transferred from donor to host and possibly involved, in addition to host Langerhans cells, in cutaneous manifestations of *graft-versus-host* (*GVH*) *disease* (Breathnach & Katz 1987). In acquired immunodeficiency syndrome (AIDS), epidermal Langerhans cells are greatly reduced in number, partly due to direct infection with the human immunodeficiency virus (HIV)-I, and partly due to the general state of immunosuppression.

UV light and various chemicals. Langerhans cells are adversely affected by these factors, which can inactivate them and deplete their numbers. In that they are normally involved in monitoring endogenous tumour antigens, this suppressive effect may contribute to the higher incidence of epidermal carcinomas and melanomas in caucasians habitually exposed to strong sunlight, and may play a part too in the chemical induction of neoplasms. Histiocytosis-X is a condition characterized by abnormal proliferation of cells morphologically practically identical with Langerhans cells, though differing somewhat in phenotype. Lesions occur in skin, lymph nodes, lungs and bone, and the condition is variously regarded as a tumour or a granuloma of Langerhans cells. For reviews, and citations of the voluminous literature on Langerhans cells and current unsolved problems which they present, see Schuler (1991), Bergstresser et al (1992), and Kamperdijk (1993).

Lymphocytes

Lymphocytes are occasionally seen in normal human epidermis, individually, or in apposition with Langerhans cells and melanocytes. Their presence is readily understandable in the context of SALT. Mast cells have also been reported in normal epidermis, though this raises the question of what is 'normal'. In present civilization the

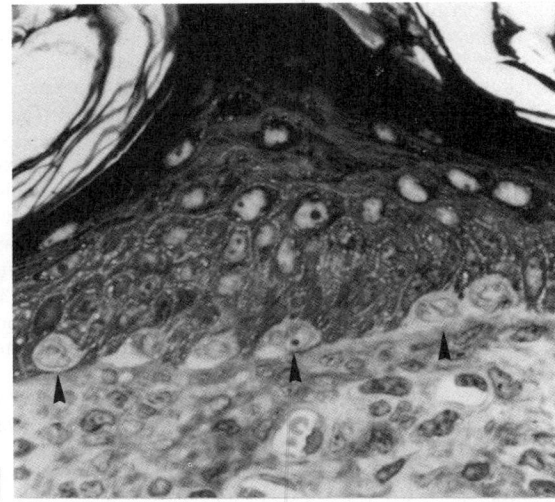

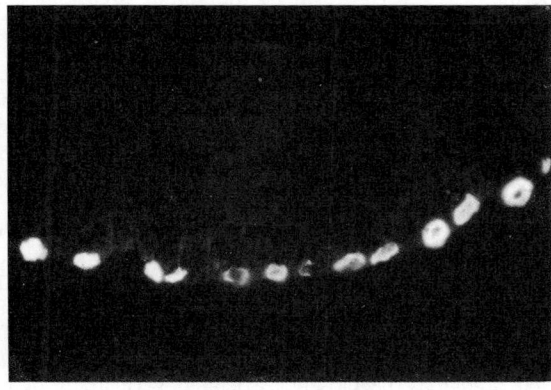

5.34 A, B. Immunolabelling of Merkel cells from rabbit lip. A shows a semi-thin section in which are 'clear cells' (arrowheads) in the basal layer of the epidermis, representing Merkel cells, as shown by later electron microscopy. B shows a similar section immunostained for the low molecular weight keratin 18 located in basally placed Merkel cells. Magnifications: A × 300, B × 280. (Provided by Professor J H Saurat, Dermatology Clinic, Cantonal Hospital of the University, Geneva, Switzerland.)

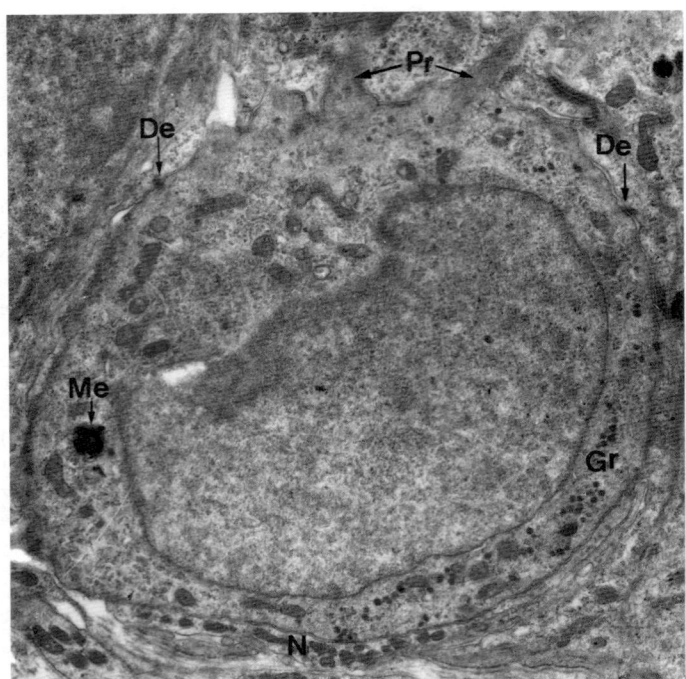

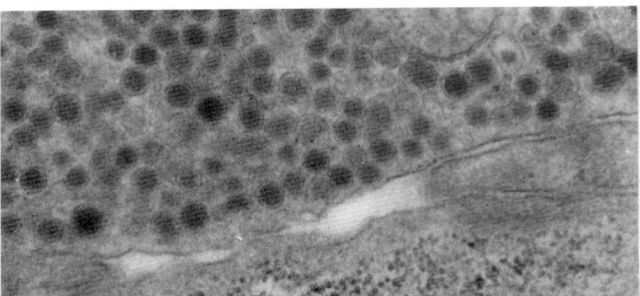

5.35B. Characteristic granules in a fetal Merkel cell, each granule consisting of a dense core separated by a lucent interval from the surrounding membrane. Magnification × 62 300. (Supplied by D Robins, Department of Anatomy, St Mary's Hospital Medical School, London. From Winkelmann and Breathnach 1973, with permission.)

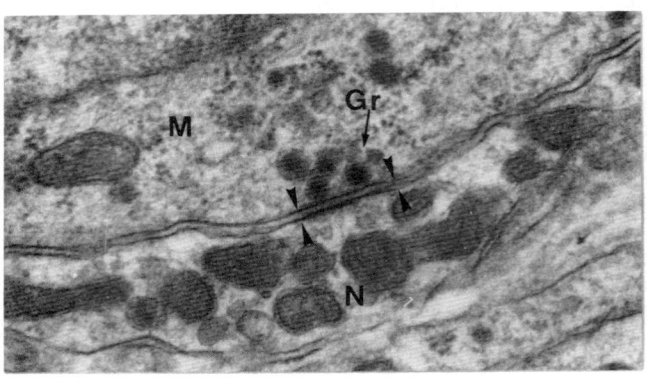

5.35 A–C. Electron microscopic appearance of Merkel cells and related structures. A is a Merkel cell in the basal epidermal layer of a human fetal finger, showing general features. Note desmosomes (De) between the Merkel cell and adjacent keratinocytes, characteristic granules (gr), phago-cytosed melanosomes (Me), nerve ending (N) in contact with the basal aspect, and spine-like processes (Pr) indenting the neighbouring kera-tinocytes. Magnification × 16 800. (From Winkelmann and Breathnach 1973, with permission.)

5.35C. A region of apposition between a fetal Merkel cell (M) and an afferent nerve terminal (N). In the segments between the arrowheads the membrane shows increased density granular vesicles (Gr) are concentrated here, resembling a type of synapse in its appearance. Magnification × 70 200. (Reproduced by permission from Breathnach 1979.)

epidermis in different cultures is submitted to so many cosmetic and environmental assaults that it is difficult to establish what might be considered as virginal normal—perhaps only the neonatal.

Merkel cell

Merkel cells are morphologically distinct cells, present in the epidermis of mammals, amphibians, and fish, and in other vertebrates. In man, they appear in routinely stained preparations as 'clear' oval cells, singly or in groups, in the basal layer of the epidermis, especially of glabrous skin, and intimately associated with a nerve terminal. They are also present in the outer root sheath of some large hair follicles. They can be distinguished from other 'clear cells' (melanocytes and Langerhans cells) by a variety of specific immunohistochemical reactions (5.34A, B). Clusters of Merkel cell–neurite complexes in glabrous skin are called *touch corpuscles* (*Tastscheiben*), and in hairy skin, *tactile hair discs* (*Haarscheiben*). Merkel cells are regarded by some as belonging to a widely-distributed system of 'neuroendocrine cells', also known as the '*amine precursor uptake and decarboxylation (APUD) system*' (Winkelmann 1977) and '*paraneurons*' (Fujita 1977).

Ultrastructure (see Halata 1975). Short, spiny processes of the plasma membrane with a cytoplasmic core of intermediate filaments insinuate between, or indent, adjacent basal keratinocytes, to which the Merkel cell is attached by small desmosomes (5.35A). The basal plasma membrane is closely apposed to the membrane of an axonal terminal packed with mitochondria and clear-cored vesicles, and areas of membrane specialization, seen as localized densities, may be present along the apposition (5.35C; see also 8.73C). The cytoplasm contains common organelles, numerous closely-packed intermediate filaments, and characteristically, 80–110 μm dense-core granules (5.35B). These are usually concentrated mainly on the side of the nucleus opposite to the Golgi apparatus, from which they are thought to be derived, and may be closely associated with areas of basal plasma membrane specialization. The nucleus may contain nuclear rodlets, also present in some nerve cells.

Immunoreactivity. Merkel cells express the low molecular-weight cytokeratins 8, 18, and 19, but not the types characteristic of

fully differentiated keratinocytes (Moll et al 1982). They also show immunoreactivity to the following antigens: neuron-specific enolase (NSE), vasoactive intestinal polypeptide (VIP), met-enkephalin, chromogranins, and bombasins (Hartschuh et al 1979; Hartschuh et al 1983; Gu et al 1981). Dense-core granule-containing neuroendocrine cells exhibit similar reactivities. Human fetal dermal Merkel cells have been reported as expressing nerve growth factor (NGF) receptors (Narisawa et al 1992).

Nature and function. The developmental lineage of Merkel cells is not yet fully established, although the view that they are modified keratinocytes (Moll et al 1986) is rapidly replacing the theory that they are immigrants which traverse the dermis along developing neurites (Breathnach 1979). In favour of the view that they are modified keratinocytes, or arise from a common ectodermal stem cell, is the observation that in development they appear in the epidermis (between weeks 8–12) earlier than in the dermis, preceding the ingrowth of nerve fibres (Moll et al 1986; Pasche et al 1990; McKenna Boot et al 1992). Human fetal skin (8–11 weeks), lacking Merkel cells and xenografted to nude mice, contained abundant epidermal Merkel cells of apparent human origin after 4–8 weeks (Moll et al 1990). This evidence suggests that fetal dermal Merkel cells are derived by migration from epidermis to dermis, and not vice versa, and that they become secondarily associated with nerve fibres. This is consistent with evidence that Merkel cells serve as targets for ingrowing axons during development, evoking directional sprouting of fibres and partially determining terminal fields (Diamond 1979).

Precise localization to Merkel cell–neurite complexes of mammals, of slowly adapting Type 1 discharges following mechanical stimulation of the skin, confirms that they are mechanoreceptors. They are capable of detecting vertical, shearing, or other directional deformations, and direction of hair movement. Morphology suggested that the Merkel cell was the prime transducer giving rise to a receptor potential activating the associated axon by a synaptic mechanism involving release of a transmitter substance from the dense-core cytoplasmic granules. However, no transmitter substance has been detected in the granules, and electrophysiological evidence of chemosynaptic transmission from Merkel cell to nerve ending is lacking. A trophic function, or a function similar to that of the Schwann cell for the neurite has also been suggested for the Merkel cell. For further details of this cell, see page 967.

Epidermal symbionts

A concept of the epidermis as a compound tissue made up of cellular elements of different developmental origins and prime functions (epidermal symbionts), existing together in biological balance and mutual dependence to perform wider collaborative functions, has grown out of early tentative ideas of Caudiere, Billingham, and Rappaport, and now includes the subconcepts of the Epidermal Melanin Unit, the Epidermal Proliferative Unit, and SALT (p. 1442). The symbionts consist of the keratinocytes, melanocytes, Langerhans cells, and lymphocytes. Whether the Merkel cell should be included is problematic. In the accounts above, many instances have been quoted of one cell type influencing proliferation, differentiation and functioning of others (sometimes facilitating, sometimes blocking activities), and being, in turn, affected similarly by these. Such interactions are of importance in development, growth, inflammation, immunology and wound-healing, and for maintaining normal homeostasis in the epidermis. They involve expression of cell-surface molecules—adhesion molecules, interleukins, various antigens, receptors—as well as growth factors, cytokines, and other factors involved in signalling, both intracellular and extracellular. For example, there is evidence that keratinocyte-derived cytokines regulate the functioning of Langerhans cells, and that Langerhans cell-derived cytokines in turn regulate the activities of keratinocytes. Identification of such substances and understanding their actions in health and disease is a major concern of current dermatological research. It has been pointed out that epidermal activities may be controlled and affected by extraepidermal influences, such as hormones, etc. and it is important to remember that substances produced within the epidermis, not only vitamin D, but also some of those mentioned above can, by diffusion or by entering the circulation, have wider local and systemic effects.

DERMIS

The dermis (5.1, 36–38) is an irregular, moderately dense, soft connective tissue, with a matrix composed of an interwoven collagenous and elastic network in an amorphous ground substance of glycosaminoglycans, glycoproteins, and bound water, which accommodates nerves, blood vessels, lymphatics, epidermal appendages and a changing population of cells. Mechanically, the dermis provides considerable strength to skin by virtue of the number and arrangement of its collagen fibres, which give it tensile strength, and it has elastic recoil because of its elastic fibres. The density of its fibre meshwork, and therefore its physical properties, varies both within an area and with different sites, and with age and sex. The dermis is vital for the survival of the epidermis, and important morphogenetic signals are exchanged at the interface between the two, the epidermal–dermal junction, or basement membrane zone (BMZ), during development and postnatally (see p. 294). The dermis can be divided into two zones, a narrow superficial *papillary layer*, and a deeper *reticular layer*, though the transition between the two is gradual.

Dermal collagen

General aspects of biosynthesis, structure, and types of collagen are dealt with elsewhere (p. 81). Types I and III form the major part of adult dermal collagen in the proportions of 80–85% and 15–20% respectively. The coarser-fibred Type I is predominant in the reticular dermis, and the finer Type III is found in the papillary dermis and around blood vessels. Type IV collagen forms the lamina densa of the basal lamina (p. 397) where it provides a scaffold for interactions between cells and amorphous matrix components such as laminin and heparan sulphate proteoglycan; it is also present in the basal laminae of Schwann cells and endothelial cells, and in anchoring plaques. Type V occurs in the lamina lucida and sparsely around cells, and Type VI forms a microfibrillar network throughout the

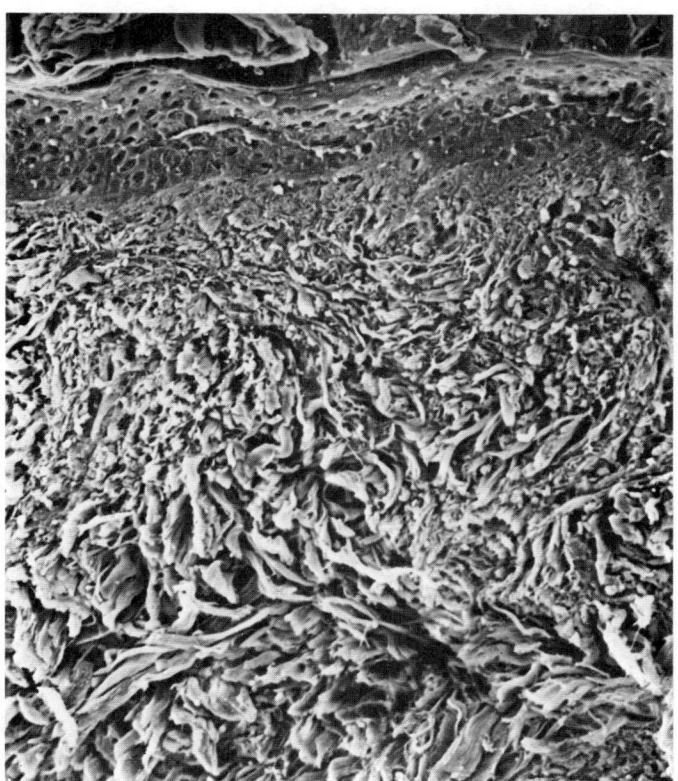

5.36 Scanning electron micrograph of the surface of a section through the skin showing the epidermis (above) and the layers of the dermis. The papillary layer close to the epidermis contains fine collagen fibres, while in the deeper reticular layer the fibres become increasingly more coarse. Magnification × 300.

dermis, enmeshing nerves and vessels. Type VII is the main component of anchoring fibrils (5.39).

Elastic fibres

For general aspects, see page 83. Elastic fibres form a fibrous network interwoven between the collagen bundles throughout the dermis (5.38). They consist of two components, amorphous elastin and 10 nm microfibrils. Close to the dermal–epidermal junction, only microfibrils known as *oxytalin* are present; somewhat deeper is *elaunin*, composed mainly of fibrils with little elastin, and deeper still are the *mature elastic fibres* with a predominance of elastin. They form a continuum extending deeper from the underside of the lamina densa.

Ground substance

For general aspects, see page 84. The ground substance of the dermis, being amorphous, can only be visualized by special techniques and consists mainly of proteoglycans (glycosaminoglycans being, predominantly, hyaluronic acid and dermatan sulphate, heparan sulphate, and some chondroitin-4 and chondroitin-6 sulphate) and fibronectins. These matrix macromolecules interact with cell surface and transmembrane molecules and maintain the cellular environment of the dermis, including its water and electrolyte composition. It is also concerned with cell movement and attachment to substratum during development and wound healing (see p. 412 et seq). For more on the extracellular matrix in general, see Hay (1981, 1982), Uitto et al (1989), and Alberts et al (1994).

Cells of the dermis

Two major categories of cells are present in postnatal dermis:

- fixed cells of organized structures such as nerves (Schwann cells, epi-, peri- and endoneurial cells), vessels (endothelial cells, pericytes, smooth muscle cells), cells of the arrector pili muscles
- a population of free cells of different origins and functions, the composition of which can vary with time and region so that it is not possible to define a normal distribution.

Among these latter cells are: fibroblasts, macrophages, mast cells, eosinophils, neutrophils, T-lymphocytes, and B-lymphocytes (including plasmacytes), and dermal Langerhans cells, all of which can be identified at light or electron microscopical level either by special staining techniques or by morphological characteristics including specific marker organelles, and whose functions are clear. Then, there are others, not easy to identify on any basis, but which have been referred to under such terms as fixed histiocytes, or monocytic cells. Headington (1986a,b) suggests the term *histiocyte* be abandoned, and identifies cells currently so described as *dermal dendrocytes* of bone-marrow derivation and capable of antigen presentation. He further suggests that many cells regarded as fibroblasts are, in fact, dermal dendrocytes. Sontheimer (1989) has described a 'dermal perivascular dendritic macrophage' expressing major histocompatibility complex (MHC) class II (HLA-DR) antigens which may engage in immunological reactions with microvascular endothelial cells, and perivascular T-lymphocytes. These observations indicate a greater participation of dermal elements in immunology than previously thought.

Layers of the dermis

Papillary layer. This is immediately deep to the epidermis (5.3, 36, 37), and is specialized to provide mechanical anchorage, metabolic support, and trophic maintenance to the overlying tissue, as well as housing rich networks of sensory nerve endings and blood vessels. Its superficial surface is marked by numerous papillae which interdigitate with recesses in the base of the epidermis and form the dermal–epidermal junction at their interface. The papillae have round or

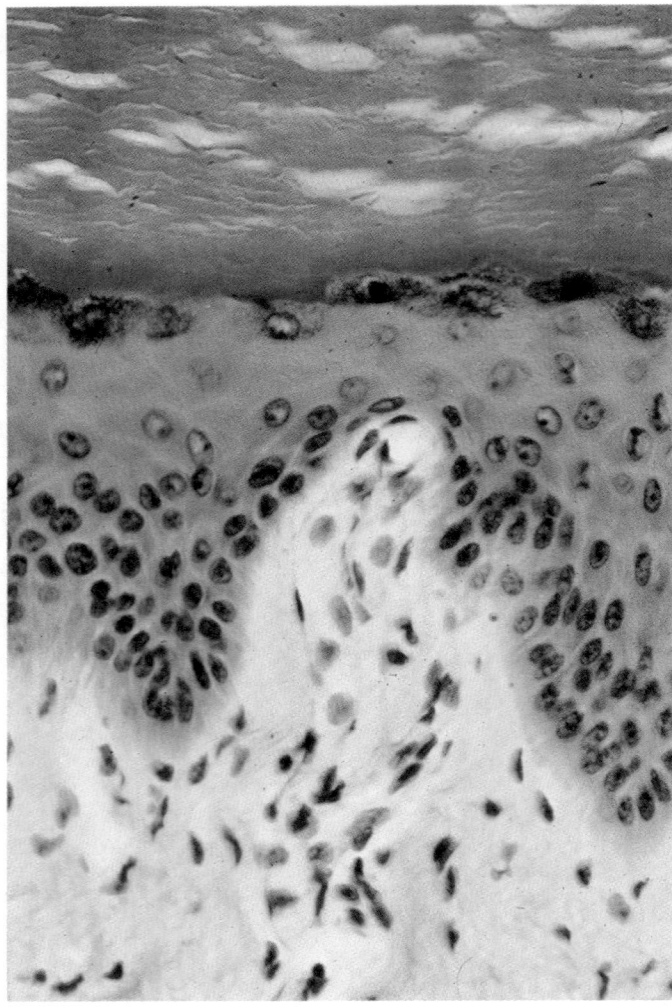

5.37 Vertical section through a dermal papilla and adjacent epidermis, showing a capillary loop. Notice the closeness of the vessel to the basal layer of the epidermis. Also visible are the layers of the epidermis, including a prominent stratum granulosum and above it the stratum lucidum stained dark orange and the paler orange stratum corneum. The section was taken from the thick skin of the foot. (Compare also 5.1 and 5.11.) Mallory's triple stain. Magnification × 800.

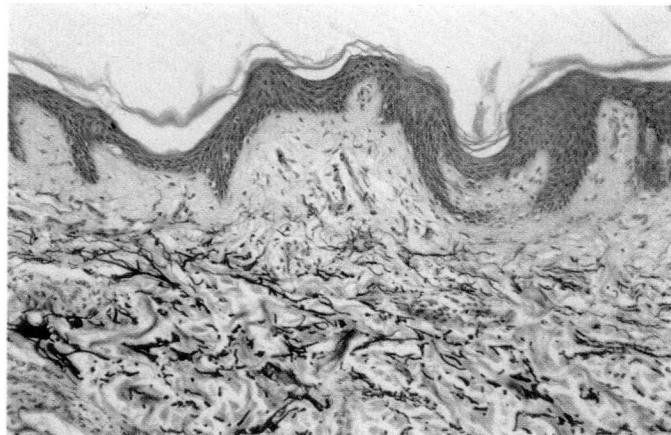

5.38 Section through thin skin, stained by the Verhoeff method to demonstrate elastin fibres. The fibres of the superficial layers of the dermis are thin while the deeper layers have more conspicuous coarser elastic fibres. Magnification × 120.

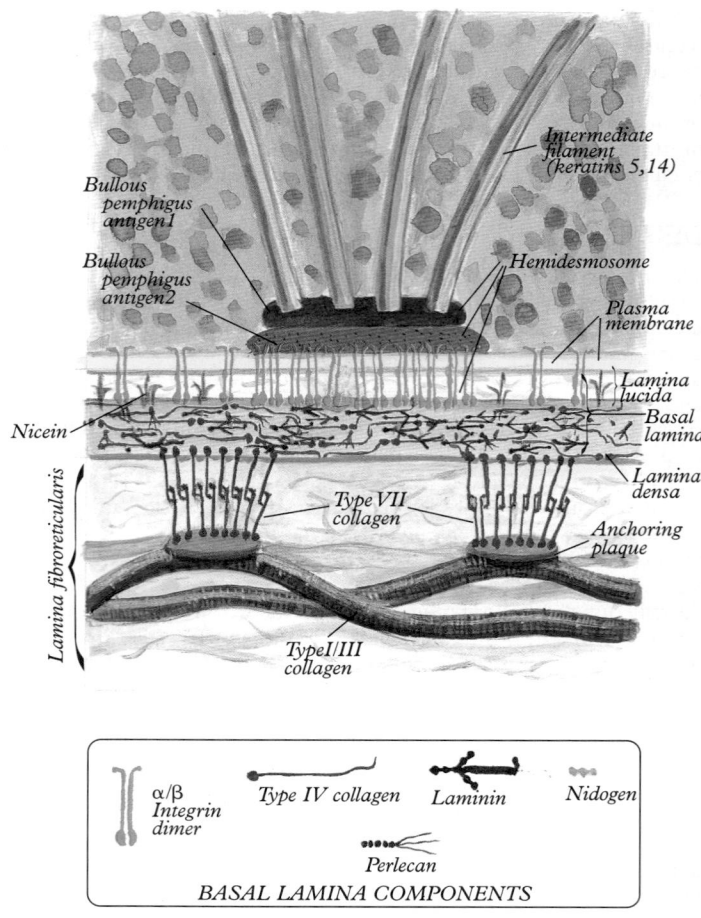

5.39 Diagram showing the major features of the basement membrane zone of skin, including some of the important molecular species involved. See text for further details.

blunt apices which may be divided into several cusps. In thin skin, especially in regions with little mechanical stress and minimal sensitivity, papillae are few and very small, while in the thick skin of the palm and sole of the foot, they are much larger, closely aggregated, and arranged in curved parallel lines following the pattern of ridges and grooves typical of these surfaces (5.1). Lying under each epidermal ridge are two longitudinal rows of papillae one on either side of epidermal *rete pegs* through which the sweat ducts pass on the way to the surface (see 5.1, 3). Each papilla contains narrow, densely interwoven bundles of fine Type I and III collagen fibres, some elastic fibrils and microfibrils, many attached to the basal lamina and extending deeper. Also present is a capillary loop, and in some sites, especially in thick hairless skin, Meissner's corpuscular nerve endings (p. 967).

Reticular layer. This merges with the deep aspect of the papillary layer (5.3, 36). Its bundles of collagen fibres are thicker than those in the papillary layer and interlace with them and with each other to form a strong yet deformable three-dimensional lattice, in which many fibres are parallel to each other, and within which lies a variable number of elastic fibres. The predominant orientation of the collagen fibres may be related to the main direction of action of the mechanical forces to which the dermis is subjected locally and thus may be involved in the development of skin surface lines (p. 378).

DERMAL–EPIDERMAL JUNCTION

In sections perpendicular to the surface, the dermal–epidermal junction exhibits various degrees and patterns of undulation related to the prominence or otherwise of dermal papillae. Staining with periodic acid-Schiff (PAS) technique reveals an apparent *basement membrane* along the junctional line, and a similar appearance occurs in other situations where cellular structures interface with the extracellular matrix (see p. 80). However, electron microscopy reveals that there is no such structural entity, and it is more correct to refer to a *basement membrane zone* (BMZ), which in the skin consists of several components (5.39–41). There is the *basal cell membrane*, studded with hemidesmosomes, beneath which is the *basal lamina* consisting of an electron-lucent *lamina lucida* of 40–50 nm traversed by *anchoring filaments* which insert into an amorphous *lamina densa* of approximately 70 nm; this may be intermittently reduplicated. Beneath the basal lamina is a shallow *reticular layer* of different fibrous elements: banded *anchoring fibrils*, attached to the lamina densa at one end, and ending freely or looping back, or being

attached to amorphous *anchoring plaques* at the other; oxytalin *microfibrils*; and small diameter *collagen fibrils*. Beneath melanocytes, anchoring filaments traverse the lamina lucida, but anchoring fibrils are practically absent beneath the lamina densa. The cytoskeleton of the epidermal keratinocyte is linked to the fibrous matrix of the dermis through the attachment of keratin filament bundles to hemidesmosomes, via anchoring filaments across the lamina lucida to the lamina densa, from which anchoring fibrils (Type VII collagen: 5.39) and oxytalin microfibrils extend deeply. This arrangement provides a mechanically stable substratum for the epidermis. Epidermis and dermis can be separated, usually in the plane of the lamina lucida, by trypsinization or immersion of skin in various chemicals. This provides '*split-skin*' preparations which are useful for examining the apposed surfaces of the two en face, providing, for example, excellent views of the pattern of dermal papillae, and detailed ultrastructure of the lamina densa (Mihara et al 1992) by scanning electron microscopy, and an opportunity to carry out counts of melanocytes in DOPA-stained epidermal sheets. In inherited bullous (blistering) diseases of the BMZ, separation can occur within the cytoplasm of the basal cell, along the plane of the lamina lucida, or just beneath the lamina densa.

Many BMZ components are precisely localized (Uitto 1992). The lamina densa is mainly composed of Type IV collagen and the anchoring fibrils of Type VII collagen (5.39). *Laminin*, a glycoprotein which binds to cells and Type IV collagen, is present in the lamina densa and lucida, and *entactin nidogen*. which binds to the other three, is present in the lamina densa. *Heparan sulphate proteoglycan* (perlecan) and *chondroitin-6-sulphate proteoglycan* are present in the lamina densa, and *bullous pemphigoid antigen* is largely localized to hemidesmosomes. Other antigens characterized by monoclonal antibodies have been recognized. These various components are synthesized by epidermal keratinocytes and/or by dermal fibroblasts, and react with one another and with fibronectins in the formation of an organized BMZ during development, in its maintenance throughout postnatal life and in its reconstitution during wound-healing and re-epithelialization. Similar interactions are involved in facilitating cell movements (Langerhans cells, lymphocytes) in either direction across the dermal–epidermal junction.

Since the epidermis is non-vascular, clearly, macromolecules and solutes essential for the nutrition of the cells must pass the barrier of the basal lamina. The permeability properties of the lamina are, therefore, of interest and significance, but it is not easy to locate definitive information in the literature.

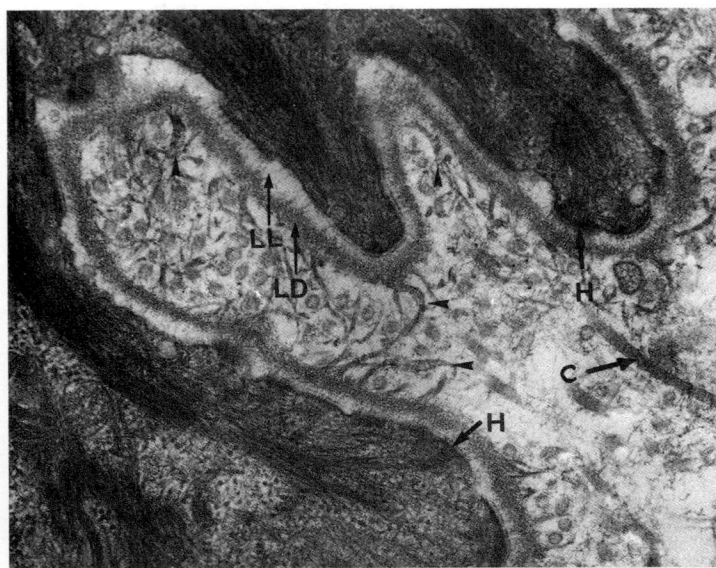

5.40   Electron micrograph of a section through the base of the epidermis showing the epidermal–dermal junction. Note the basal keratinocyte plasma membrane with hemidesmosomes (H), lamina lucida (LL), lamina densa (LD), anchoring fibrils (arrowheads) attached to its deeper aspect and adjacent collagen fibrils (C). Magnification × 45 000. (Provided by J McGrath, St John's Dermatology Centre, UMDS, St Thomas' Campus, London.)

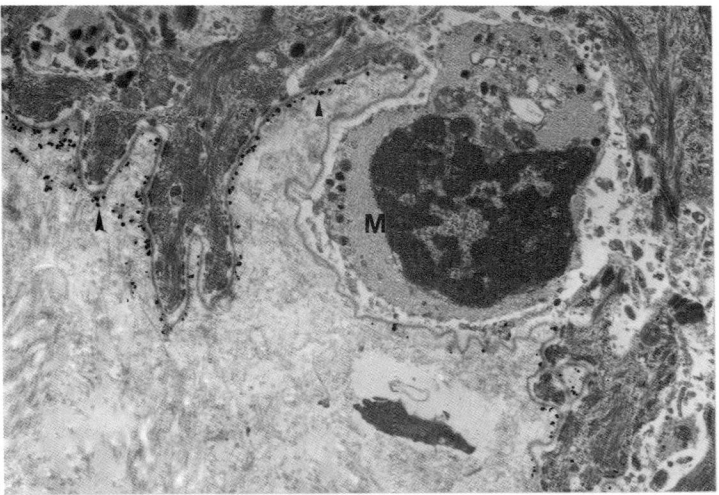

5.41   Immunogold labelling of anchoring fibrils at the epidermal–dermal junction. Gold particles (arrowheads) are seen beneath the lamina densa underlying the keratinocytes, but are virtually absent from this situation beneath a melanocyte (M). Magnification × 4680. (Provided by J McGrath, St John's Dermatology Centre, UMDS, St Thomas' Campus, London.)

INNERVATION OF SKIN

Skin is a major sensory surface, with regional variations in sensitivity to different stimuli evoking a spectrum of subjective sensations. It has a rich nerve supply, which is also concerned with autonomic functions, in particular, thermoregulation. Equating structure and distribution of fibres and receptors with function has been a major and continuing concern of neuroanatomists and neurophysiologists over the years.

Cutaneous sense provides us with a wealth of information about the external environment and its interactions with the skin, through receptors tuned to stimuli of various kinds. These latter may be classed as: mechanical (rapid or sustained touch, pressure, vibration, stretching, bending of hairs, etc.), thermal (hot and cold), and noxious (perceived as discomfort, itching and pain of various degrees of intensity). In addition, there are other stimuli evoking sensations less easy to define precisely, such as those of pleasure evoked by appropriate stroking, tickle, or wetness. All of these sensations are recorded and interpreted by a wide variety of specialized neurons distributed throughout the ascending levels of the nervous system, but the primary input is transmitted by neurons whose cell bodies lie in the spinal and cranial ganglia, and whose fibres are terminally distributed to the dermis. These may be myelinated or unmyelinated (5.42).

Efferent autonomic fibres are non-myelinated noradrenergic and cholinergic in type, innervating the arterioles, arrector pili muscles, and the myoepitheliocytes of sudorific and apocrine glands. In the scrotum, labia minora, perineal skin and nipples they also supply smooth muscle fasciculi of the dermis and adjacent connective tissue. Except in the nipples and genital area, activity of the autonomic efferent nerves is chiefly concerned with regulation of heat loss by vasodilation and vasoconstriction, sweat production, and (only incipiently in humans) pilo-erection.

Dermal plexuses, nerve terminals and receptors

On reaching the dermis, nerve fasciculi branch extensively to form a deep *reticular plexus*, which serves much of the dermis, including most sweat glands, hair follicles and the larger arterioles. Many small fasciculi pass from this plexus to ramify in another superficial *papillary plexus* at the junction between the reticular and papillary layers of the dermis. Twigs from this pass more superficially into the papillary layer, ramifying horizontally and vertically, terminating either in relation to encapsulated receptors, or as terminals reaching the level of the basal lamina, and, in some instances, entering the epidermis. As these latter fasciculi proceed superficially, the epineurial sheath merges with the general matrix collagen; the perineurium becomes reduced to a single cellular layer and eventually

terminates, leaving Schwann-cell axonal complexes, enveloped by basal lamina, in direct contact with the matrix. Perineurial cells are joined by tight junctions, so the sheath forms an effective barrier against substances or organisms entering the endoneurial compartment across it. They can, of course, gain entry and proceed proximally from below the level at which it terminates (see also p. 947).

The detailed structure, classification, and behaviour of the sensory endings are described in detail in Nervous System (p. 965).

Development of cutaneous nerves

Sensory cutaneous nerves—axons and Schwann cells—are derived by outgrowth from the neural crest (via posterior root ganglia), and motor fibres to vessels and glands arise from cells of sympathetic ganglia. As individual parts of the embryo grow, the nerves grow and lengthen with them. Small neurites are present superficially at a stage when the epidermis is bilaminar, and by 8 weeks' gestation there is already a functioning cutaneous plexus. By the fourth gestational month, the dermal plexuses are very richly developed, and by this time also, Meissner and Pacinian corpuscles appear. Whereas the overall general pattern of distribution of fibres is determined by forces intrinsic to the nervous system, the directional guidance of developing axons and the establishment of appropriate terminal connections is a very complicated matter and the subject of considerable differences of opinion amongst neuroembryologists (see p. 925). The growing tips of migrating axons have been much studied in tissue culture. The tip forms a swollen growth cone, the leading membrane of which may be flattened or ruffled, exhibiting filipodia, and it contains filaments, microtubules, and vesicles, all of which are associated with the axoplasmic transport which must accompany new membrane formation and elongation. GAP (Growth Associated Protein) 43, a protein which is a substrate for calcium-dependent and phospholipid dependent protein kinase C, influences the ability of axons to grow and is synthesized and transported to growth cones at a high concentration in extending axons. Swollen tips of axons can sometimes be observed in nerves of digital skin of human fetuses and possibly represent growth cones in vivo.

In the development of peripheral nerves, axonal outgrowth precedes migration of Schwann cells, so the latter do not serve as initial 'pathfinders'. The two soon become closely associated, however, to form the actual unit of migration, the nerve fibre whose progress is guided by local tissue conditions and influences. These are thought to include guidepost cells of other tissues, heterogeneities and gradients of matrix macromolecules along the way, and chemotropic factors released from target cells (Jessel 1991). They partly underlie the general overall processes of contact guidance and inhibition.

The ability of outgrowing neurites to adhere to cell surfaces they encounter plays a major role in directing their migration. Cell Adhesion Molecules (CAM, N-CAM) belonging to the immunoglobulin family (see p. 26) are involved, and integrins mediate adhesion between neurites and the matrix glycoproteins laminin and fibronectin. Homing of axons on to certain specific targets is thought to involve release of soluble diffusible factors, such as hormones and growth factors. Nerve Growth Factor (NGF) (Levi-Montalcini and Angeletti 1968) is produced by targets of sensitive adrenergic sympathetic neurons, such as sweat glands, and in vitro, has been shown to promote neurite outgrowth and adhesion of human sensory neurons in synergy with laminin and fibronectin (Crain et al 1980). Whether it functions in this manner in vivo has been questioned, but developing Merkel cells, which certainly serve as peripheral attractive targets for somatic terminals (Diamond 1979) have recently been reported to contain NGF (Munger 1991). It has been suggested that Epidermal Growth Factor may also be involved in directional guidance of axons during development. There is evidence that in development, terminal areas are approached by an excess of axons, and that there may be competition between them for specific targets or limited territories. Definition or limitation of final terminal distribution is governed partly by elimination of some axons, and excessive branching or extension is probably regulated by inhibitory mechanisms involving contact with neighbouring ones.

In embryos of 8–10 weeks, peripheral fascicles and their terminals consist of bundles of axons in direct contact, partially or completely enveloped by Schwann cells. Axons contain many microtubules which serve as a cytoskeleton, and are involved with axoplasmic

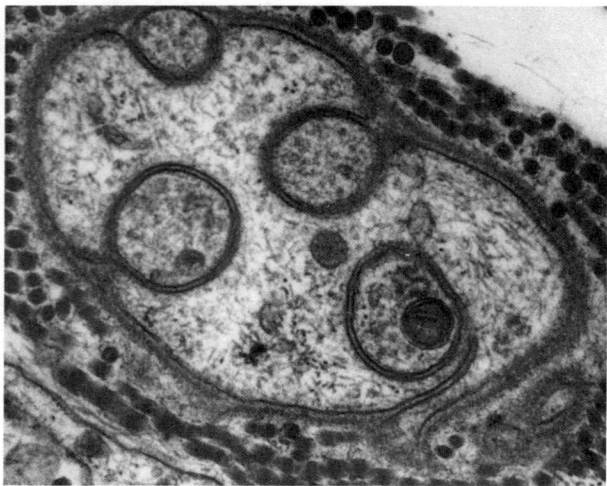

5.42 Unmyelinated neurite in papillary dermis consisting of Schwann cell process enveloping four axons. Note Schwann cell basal lamina, and sectioned collagen fibres. This is peripheral to the level at which the perineurial sheath terminates. Magnification × 39 375.

transport and motility. Schwann cells and processes soon invade the axonal bundles, separating them into progressively smaller ones, ultimately isolating them from one another, until finally a numerical relationship between cell and axon of one to one is established for myelinated fibres, and one to several for unmyelinated fibres.

These developments are associated with multiplication of Schwann cells, their migration in a transverse as well as a longitudinal direction, and degeneration of many axons. Axonal and other debris is frequently seen within fetal Schwann cells, and this potential for phagocytosis is carried forward into postnatal life.

The factors that determine myelination of an individual axon, and the final relationship between axon diameter, thickness of myelin sheath, and internodal length are matters of interest. It is generally agreed that the population of Schwann cells is uniform, and that size of axon (1 μm plus) is the trigger that signals the cell to start myelination. Axons with diameters of 1 μm undergoing myelination may be seen in human fetal cutaneous nerves as early as 12 weeks. Early during myelination, the Schwann cell expresses Myelin Associated Glycoprotein (MAG), an adhesion molecule which may be important for maintaining stability between it and the axon during initiation of the process. The total number of Schwann cells along an axon is fixed at the time of onset of myelination, as is the number of nodes of Ranvier (except in regenerating nerves).

Myelination involves the development of a multi-layered membranous sheath continuous with the Schwann cell plasma membrane. It is not a simple wrapping of pre-formed membrane around the axon, but the progressive addition of newly synthesized material at the inner and outer mesaxons, or at multiple sites. The lipid composition of myelin changes progressively during development, and is different to that of general Schwann cell plasma membrane (for further details, see p. 948).

The degree of myelination of peripheral nerves in the human fetus varies with the nerve, and the distance from the parent cell bodies at which it is examined. It is not possible therefore to give precise dates for the onset of myelination which would have general application. It can commence in the ulnar nerve as early as the twelfth week (Gamble 1966).

Early Schwann cell–axonal complexes are surrounded by and in direct contact with the general mesenchymal collagen and matrix, and there is no collagen among the axons. The first sign of the connective tissue sheaths is the appearance of single cells loosely arranged around the neurites to form a primitive *perineurium*, and collagen fibres enclosed by them can be regarded as an early *endoneurium*. The primitive perineurial cells lack a basal lamina, but acquire one as the sheath becomes multilaminar; they are thought to be modified fibroblasts, and presumably produce the perineurial collagen. Endoneurial collagen is thought to be produced by both fibroblasts and Schwann cells, and the epineurium is formed by lamination of extra-perineurial collagen around the neurites. The outer lamellar cells of Pacinian corpuscles are homologous with the perineurium, but the source of the laminar cells of the Meissner corpuscle is unclear, in view of their direct contact with terminal axons, a relationship which is never seen with perineurial cells.

VASCULARIZATION OF SKIN

Blood vessels

The metabolic demands of the skin are not generally great, and yet, under normal conditions, the blood flow exceeds by 10 times its nutritional requirements, and may amount to 5% of the cardiac output. This is because the cutaneous circulation has an additional important thermoregulatory function, and is arranged so that its capacity can be rapidly altered by as much as 20 times in either direction in response to requirements of loss or conservation of heat.

Blood enters the skin from the underlying muscles and subcutis via small perforating arterioles which form an anastomosing horizontal *reticular plexus* (5.1, 43) at the interface between cutis and dermis. From this plexus, some arterioles pass deeply to supply the adipose tissue and, where present at this level, sweat glands and hair follicles. Other arterioles pass superficially, giving off anastomotic collaterals to glands and hair follicles, and form a second major horizontal plexus, at the junction of the reticular and papillary dermis, the *papillary plexus*. Capillaries from this plexus loop into the dermal

papillae, usually one loop per papilla, and the loops drain into a *superficial venous plexus* intertwined with the arteriolar papillary plexus. This venous plexus in turn drains into a flat intermediate plexus in the reticular layer, which further drains into a deeper plexus, receiving from capillary beds surrounding glands and hair follicles, and closely associated with the arteriolar reticular plexus. This close association between arteriolar and venous plexuses permits exchange of heat between blood in vessels at different temperatures flowing in opposite directions, for example between cooler venous blood returning from the surface, and warmer arterial blood coming from the heart (counter-current heat exchange). This can allow for conservation or dissipation of heat, depending upon circumstances.

The general structure and arrangement of the microvasculature in general is dealt with in detail in another section (see p. 1452), so only features particular to skin will be considered here. In the deeper layers of the dermis, arteriovenous anastomoses are common, particularly in the extremities subject to cooling (hands, feet, ears, lips, nose), where, as *glomera* (see p. 1468) they are surrounded by thick muscular coats. Under autonomic vasomotor control, these vascular shunts, when relaxed, divert blood away from the superficial plexus and so reduce heat loss, while at the same time ensuring some deep cutaneous circulation and preventing anoxia of structures such as nerves which might otherwise be at risk. Extensive intercapillary anastomoses are also present. Generally, cutaneous blood flow is regulated and constantly adjusted according to the need for heat loss or retention, or also, in some areas of the body, according to emotional states. The normal vascular tone is a balance between neural (vasoconstrictor and vasodilator) and chemical influences affecting the musculature of the arterioles. In very cold conditions, the peripheral circulation is greatly reduced by vasoconstriction, but intermittent spontaneous intervals of vasodilatation result in recurring increases in temperature which prevent cooling to the level at which frostbite might occur (the hunting reaction). This is thought to be due to a direct effect of oxygen lack on the arteriolar constrictor muscle, rather than to a neural influence. The deeper dermal arterioles contain elastic tissue in the wall, and are surrounded by several layers of smooth muscle cells. More superficially, the muscle forms two layers, an inner longitudinal and an outer spiral one, and just before the capillary loop, individual myocytes or pericytes form an incomplete layer outside the endothelium. The postcapillary venules have one or two layers of contractile pericytes which can produce gaps between the endothelial cells and allow extravasation of fluid (Braverman 1989). Tight junctions are prominent between smooth muscle cells, pericytes, and endothelial cells, an arrangement which provides strength and stability to the vessel wall. For more on thermoregulation, see Clarke and Edholm (1993).

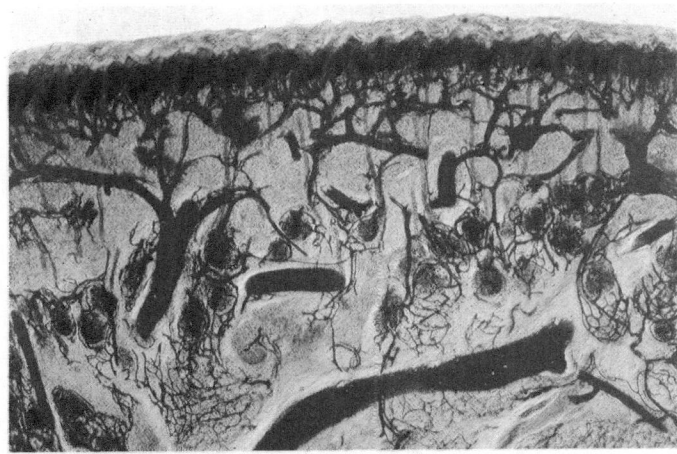

5.43   A thick vertical section through palmar skin, the arteries, arterioles and capillaries of which have been injected with red gelatin to demonstrate the pattern of dermal vascularization. At the base of the dermis a broad flat arterial plexus supplies a more superficial papillary plexus, which in turn gives off capillary loops which enter the dermal papillae. Sweat glands and their ducts are numerous in this specimen; they extend basally into the subcutaneous tissues. Magnification × 200.

Individual segments of the dermal microvasculature can be identified on the basis of level, diameter, and more precisely, the components of the vessel wall (Braverman & Yen 1977; Higgins & Eady 1981). The *capillary loop* arises from a *terminal arteriole*, and ends in a *postcapillary venule*. At the arterial end, the ascending limb consists of an endothelial tube surrounded by a homogeneous basal lamina, outside which are individual pericytes, also enveloped by basal lamina. Just beyond the apex of the loop, the basal lamina becomes duplicated, and in the postcapillary venule it is multi-laminated. Pericytes are more numerous in association with venules. Mast cells, and elongated fibroblast-like cells, or *veil cells*, are frequently seen closely associated with terminal arterioles and post-capillary venules. Sontheimer (1989) has defined a human *dermal microvascular unit* comprising the endothelial tube, pericytes, mast cells, and T-lymphocytes, and another cell, the *perivascular dendritic macrophage*, with antigen-presenting capabilities. It is probable that this cell belongs to the population of dermal dendrocytes (see p. 1415), and it may be identical with the veil cell. Sontheimer suggests the dermal microvascular unit may be a significant site of functional, immunological and other types of interaction between its cellular components.

The *endothelial cell* of the dermal microvasculature is particularly rich in microfilaments, which serve cytoskeletal and possibly contractile functions, and *Weibel-Palade bodies*, which store Factor VIII, are most numerous in the endothelium of venules. Fenestrated endothelial cells are present mainly in the capillary loops, and in association with vessels supplying the skin appendages. The endothelium must not be regarded merely as a passive, semi-permeable lining of the vessels. It has potential contractile and migratory abilities which become manifest in inflammatory and reparative processes, and expresses a large number of antigens, including Factor VIII-related antigen, and Class II major histocompatibility complex (MHC) antigens, and synthesizes cytokines, adhesion molecules and the angiotensin-converting enzyme (ACE) (Ruiter et al 1989). These synthetic properties are important in the endothelium's interactions with vasoactive amines of mast cells and nerves (Tharp 1989), in lymphocyte adhesion and migration, and in the recruitment of inflammatory cells into the skin. It is, therefore, a key cell involved in inflammatory and immunological reactions, and in wound-healing and repair.

Lymphatics

The general features and topographical arrangement of the body's lymphatic system are dealt with elsewhere (see p. 1605). The lymphatics of the skin are small terminal vessels that collect fluid and macromolecules that have leaked from the capillaries for return to the circulation via larger vessels; they also convey lymphocytes, Langerhans cells and macrophages involved in immunological reactions to and from the regional lymph nodes. They begin as blind endothelial-lined tubes or loops just below the papillary dermis, which drain into a *superficial plexus* below the subpapillary venous plexus. This plexus drains via collecting vessels into a deeper plexus at the junction of the reticular dermis and subcutis, which in turn drains into the larger subcutaneous channels.

The wall of the terminal lymphatic vessel is formed by a single layer of very flattened overlapping endothelial cells, with few cytoplasmic organelles, and a tenuous, discontinuous basal lamina (**5.44**). Gaps of varying extent are present between the cells (**5.44B**), and protrusion into the lumen of cytoplasmic processes, nuclei and the tips of the inner of two overlapping cells gives rise to the appearance of *valves*. The endothelium of the larger collecting vessels is thicker, and the cells are connected by simple specialized junctional areas (p. 1605). Cells, macromolecules and fluid enter the lymphatics through the gaps in the wall, being directed thereto by 'wringing of the tissues' through movement of limbs, contraction of muscles and pulsation of adjacent arterial vessels (Ryan 1989, 1991). Unidirectional flow within the vessels is facilitated by the valves (Daroczy 1988).

APPENDAGES OF SKIN

PILOSEBACEOUS UNIT

This comprises the hair and its follicle with associated arrector pili muscle, sebaceous gland, and sometimes an apocrine gland (**5.1, 45, 47**). Not all elements of the unit occur together in all bodily regions.

Hairs

Hairs are filamentous keratinized structures present over almost all of the body surface, though less apparent in man than in his mammalian and primate ancestors. This 'trend towards nudity' in human evolution has been explained on a number of bases by anthropologists, including selective advantage on descending from the trees and hunting in a warm climate (Ebling 1991). The phylogeny of hair has also given rise to much speculation. Hair is thought to have developed in association with scales of pro-mammals, a 'basic trio-group' of three hairs being associated with a scale. Hairs grow out of the skin at a slant, and in small mammals are streamlined mainly in a craniocaudal direction. In many species this basic arrangement is complicated by reversals of orientation, with the formation of divergent streams and whorls to form 'hair-tracts', the disposition of which is thought to be related to grooming habits,

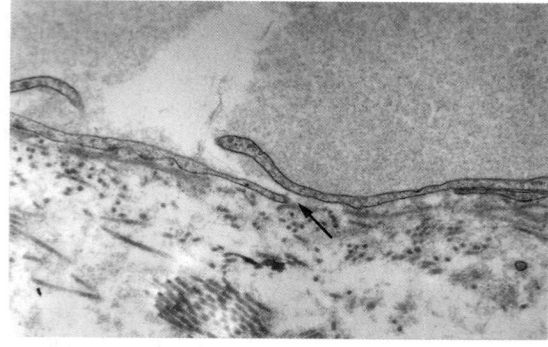

5.44A. Lymphatic from papillary dermis. The vessel is lined by a layer of flattened cytoplasm of endothelial cells the nuclei of which project into the lumen. A basal lamina is not very evident and is discontinuous. Magnification × 3840.

5.44B. Portion of wall of terminal lymphatic from papillary dermis. A gap (arrow) is present at the overlapping edges of the lining endothelial cells, and the tip of the inner cell projects into the lumen. Magnification × 10 400.

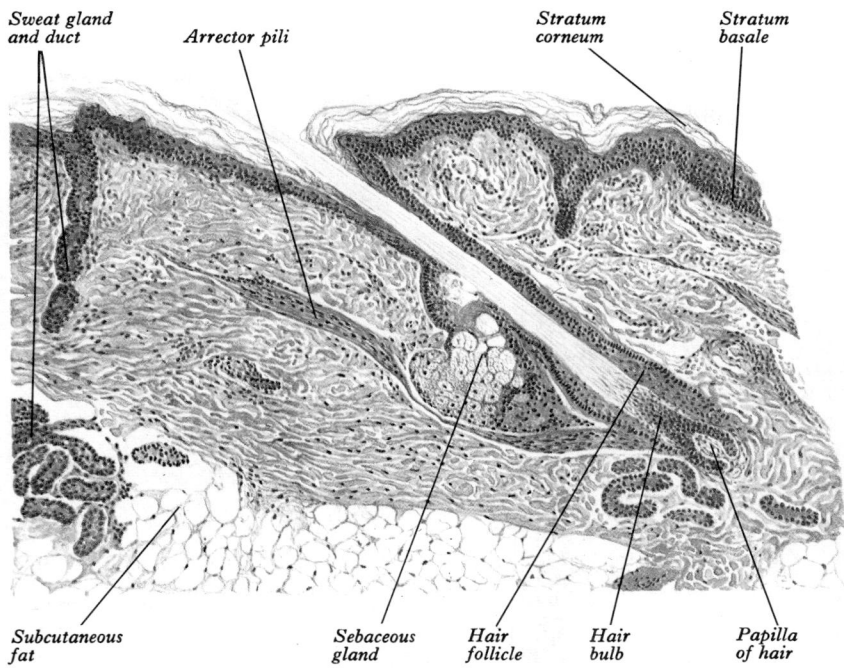

5.45 A section through the skin, showing the epidermis and dermis (corium), a hair in its follicle, an arrector pili muscle and sebaceous glands opening into the hair follicle. Magnification × 100.

posture, or movement (Clark 1939). Hair-tracts can be mapped on the skin of man (Wiedersheim 1895), and the original streamlining is still evident in the sloping of the hairs on the dorsum of forearm, hand and fingers towards the ulnar side. This feature allows an isolated middle finger to be correctly sided at first glance. Hairs are absent from a few areas of the body, including the thick skin of palms, soles and flexor surfaces of the digits and certain other regions: umbilicus, nipples, glans penis and clitoris, the labia minora and the inner aspects of the labia majora and prepuce. The presence or absence, distribution and relative abundance of hair in certain regions (face, scalp, pubis, axillae) are secondary sexual characteristics which play subtle roles in sociosexual communication, and there are also racial variations in density, form, distribution and pigmentation. Within these parameters, there are also individual variations. Hairs assist minimally in thermoregulation, on the scalp they provide some protection against injury and the harmful effects of excessive solar radiation, and generally, they have sensory functions.

Hairs vary from about 600 per cm^2 on the face to 60 per cm^2 on the rest of the body. In length they range from less than a millimetre to more than a metre, and in width from 0.005 to 0.06 mm. They vary in form, being straight, coiled, helical or wavy, and differ in colour depending on the type and degree of pigmentation. Curly hairs tend to have a flattened cross-section, and are weaker than straight hairs. In general, body hairs are longest and coarsest in caucasians and least noticeable in mongolian races. Over most of the body surface hairs are short and narrow (*vellus hairs*) and in some areas these hairs do not project beyond their follicles, for example in eyelid skin. In other regions they are longer, thicker and often heavily pigmented (*terminal hairs*); these include the hairs of the scalp, the eyelashes, eyebrows and the postpubertal skin of the axillae and pubis, and the moustache, beard and chest hairs of males.

Hair follicle

The hair follicle (**5.1**, **45–50**) is an invagination of the epidermis (see p. 377) containing a hair, which may extend deeply (3 mm) into the hypodermis, or may be more superficial (1 mm) within the dermis. Typically, the long axis of the follicle is oblique to the skin surface; with curly hairs it is also curved. There are *cycles of hair growth* and hair loss, during which the follicle presents different appearances. In the *anagen phase* the hair is actively growing and the follicle is at its maximum development; this is followed by the involuting or *catagen*

phase when hair growth ceases and the follicle shrinks; next comes the *resting* or *telogen phase*, during which the inferior segment of the follicle is absent. The next succeeding anagen phase follows. Further details of the hair growth cycle are given below, following the description of the anagen follicle and hair.

Anagen follicle. This has several regions. Deepest is the *inferior segment* including the region enclosing the *hair bulb* (**5.46**, **47**) which extends up to the level of attachment of the arrector pili muscle at the *bulge*. Between this and the site of entry of the sebaceous duct is the *isthmus*, and above this level is the *infundibulum*, or *dermal pilary canal*, which is continuous with the *intraepidermal pilary canal*. Below the sebaceous duct, hair filament and follicular wall are intimately connected, and it is only towards the upper end of the isthmus that the hair becomes free in the pilary canal. Below the infundibulum the follicle is surrounded by a thick perifollicular dermal coat containing Type III collagen, elastin, sensory nerve fibres and blood vessels, and into which blend the arrector pili muscles. Marking the interface between dermis and follicular epithelium is a broad modification of the basal lamina, the *glassy membrane*.

Hair bulb. This forms the lowermost portion of the follicular epithelium and encloses the *dermal papilla* of connective tissue cells (**5.47**). It generates the hair and its inner root sheath. A line drawn across the widest part of the hair bulb, or 'critical level', divides it into:

- a lower *germinal matrix*, of closely packed, mitotically active pluripotential keratinocytes, among which are interspersed melanocytes, and some Langerhans cells
- the '*upper bulb*' of cells arising from the matrix.

These latter move apically and differentiate along several lines. Those arising centrally form the hair *medulla*, then, radially, further out, successive concentric rings of cells will give rise to the *cortex* and *cuticle* of the hair and, outside this, the layers of the *inner root sheath*, from within out: the *cuticle of the inner root sheath*, *Huxley's layer* and *Henle's layer*. Outside Henle's layer is a layer of cells, the *outer root sheath*, which forms the wall of the follicle (**5.46**, **49**, **50**).

Differentiation and structure of the hair and its sheaths

Differentiation towards keratinization of cells of the various layers of the hair and its inner root sheath commences at the level of the

401

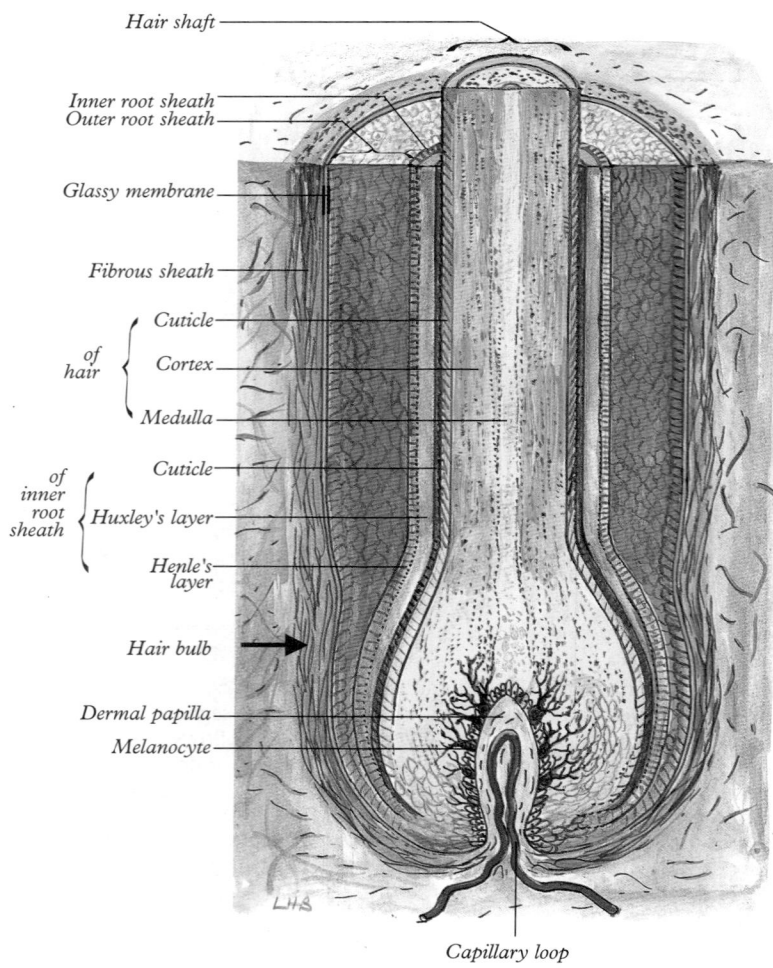

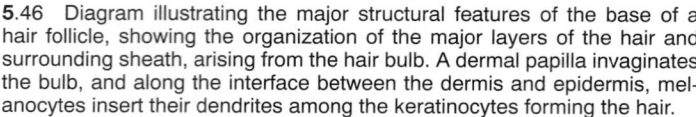

5.46 Diagram illustrating the major structural features of the base of a hair follicle, showing the organization of the major layers of the hair and surrounding sheath, arising from the hair bulb. A dermal papilla invaginates the bulb, and along the interface between the dermis and epidermis, melanocytes insert their dendrites among the keratinocytes forming the hair.

upper bulb and is asynchronous, beginning earliest in Henle's layer and Huxley's layer. It involves various morphogenetic and biochemical processes in which different cell migration patterns, cell shapes and distinct chemical forms of keratin are produced, depending upon which genes are being expressed. These processes are too extensive and complicated to be detailed here, but for morphological aspects, see Birbeck and Mercer (1957), Parakkal and Matoltsy (1964), Pucinelli et al (1967), Breathnach (1971), Montagna et al (1992), and for reviews of the biochemistry of hair keratinization see Baden (1990) and Gillespie (1991). An impression of the morphological transformations that take place is given by the illustrations in 5.46, 49, 55. Excellent reviews of fundamentals of hair biology are provided in Wuepper et al (1993).

Mature hair shaft (5.48–50). This shows three concentric zones from outwards in, the *cuticle, cortex* and *medulla*, each with different

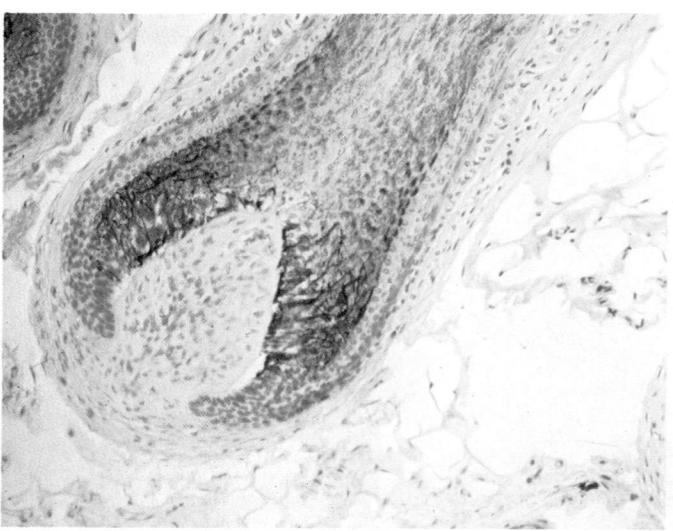

5.47 Vertical section through a hair root, showing the dermal papilla and numerous melanocyte processes extending into the matrix of the hair. Haematoxylin and eosin. Magnification × 250.

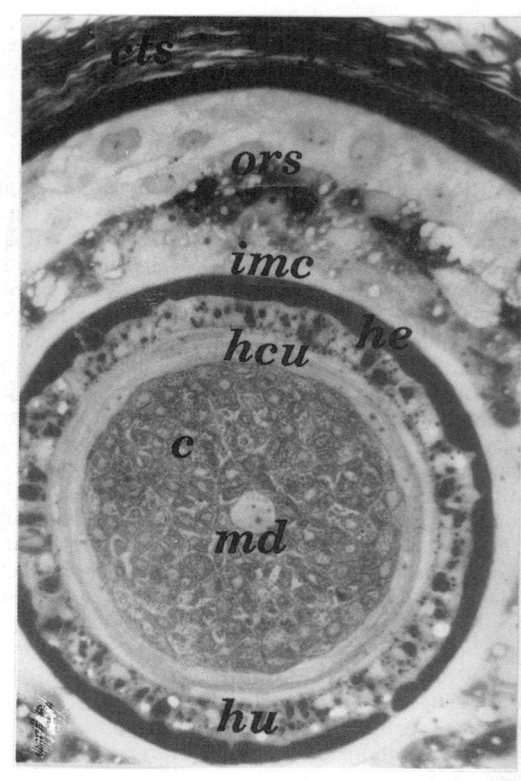

5.48 Transverse section of normal scalp anagen hair of a male aged 25, above the bulb and at a level at which only Henle's layer is keratinized. From without in are: connective tissue sheath (cts), outer root sheath (ors), innermost layer of outer root sheath (imc), keratinized Henle's layer (he), non-keratinized Huxley's layer with keratohyalin granules (hu), cuticles (hcu), outer lightly stained cuticle of inner root sheath and inner cuticle of hair, cortex (c), and medulla (md). Magnification × 525. (Reproduced from Tobin 1991, with permission.)

types of keratin. In thinner hairs the medulla is usually absent. The *cuticle* forms the hair surface and consists of several layers of overlapping keratinized squames directed apically and slightly outwards (5.51, 52). In the isthmus region cells of the outer layer interlock with those of the cuticle of the inner root sheath (5.50). Pre-keratinizing cuticle cells have dense amorphous granules aligned predominantly along the outer plasma membrane with a few fila-

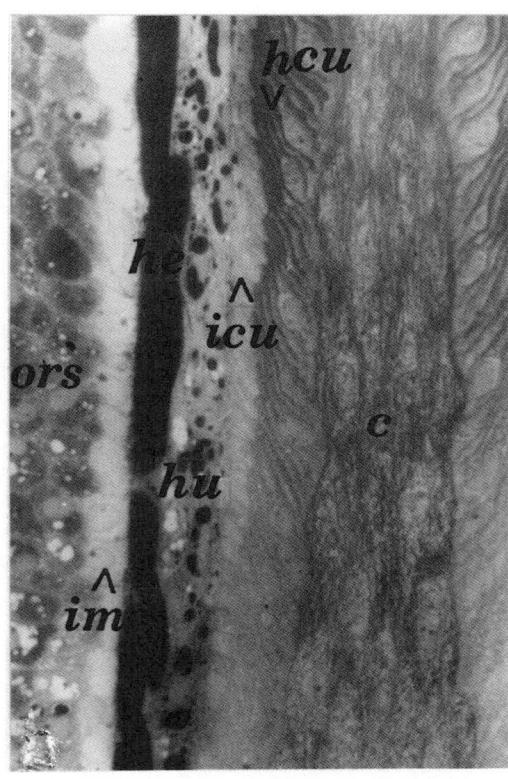

5.49 Longitudinal section of normal scalp anagen hair of a male aged 25 at a level at which only Henle's layer is keratinized. From without in are: outer root sheath (ors), innermost layer of outer root sheath (im), keratinized Henle's layer (he), non-keratinized Huxley's layer with keratohyalin granules (hu), cuticle of inner root sheath (icu) cuticle of hair (hcu), and cortex (c). Magnification × 1275. (Reproduced from Tobin 1991, with permission.)

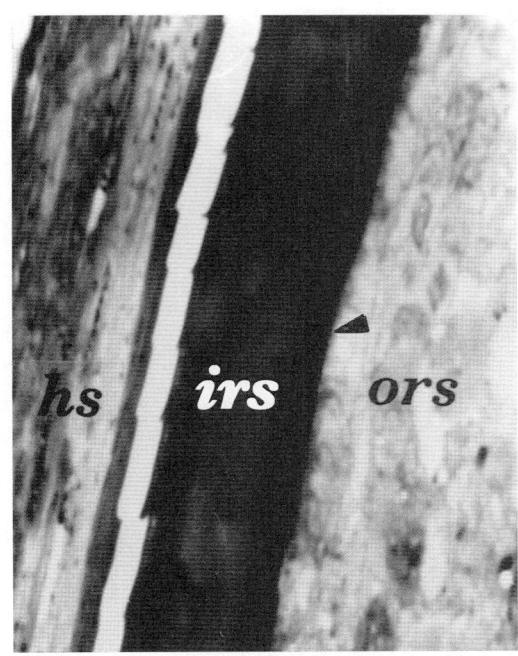

5.50 Longitudinal section of normal anagen scalp hair of a male aged 25 at a level below the entry of the sebaceous duct, and at which the hair and its inner root sheath are keratinized. From without in are: outer root sheath (ors), keratinized inner root sheath (Henle's (arrowhead) and Huxley's layers) and cuticle of inner root sheath (irs) and hair shaft (hs) consisting of narrow more deeply staining cuticle of hair and cortex. Note imbrication of apposed surfaces of cuticle of inner root sheath and cuticle of hair (bounding the artefactual space between them) which leads to interlocking. Magnification × 960. (Reproduced from Tobin 1991, with permission.)

ments, and when keratinized exhibit outer and inner zones of different densities, with a narrow dense band separating the cells (5.53). The cortex forms the greater part of the hair shaft and consists of numerous closely packed elongated keratinized cells which may contain nuclear remnants and melanosomes, and which are also separated by a narrow band of dense intercellular material. Pre-keratinizing cortical cells contain bundles of closely packed filaments but no dense granules, and when fully keratinized, exhibit a charac-

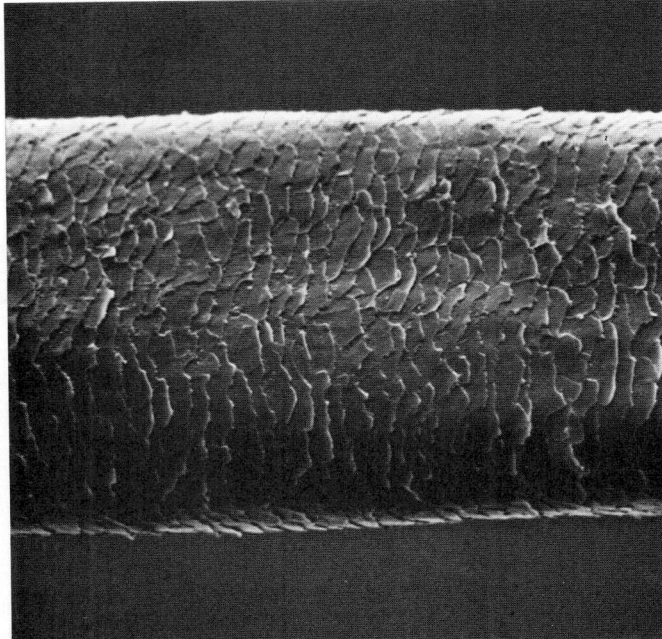

5.51 Scanning electron micrograph of a scalp hair showing details of surface structure. Note that the cuticular cells overlap each other; their free ends point towards the apex of the hair. Magnification × 370. (Specimen prepared by Michael Crowder, Guy's Hospital Medical School, London.)

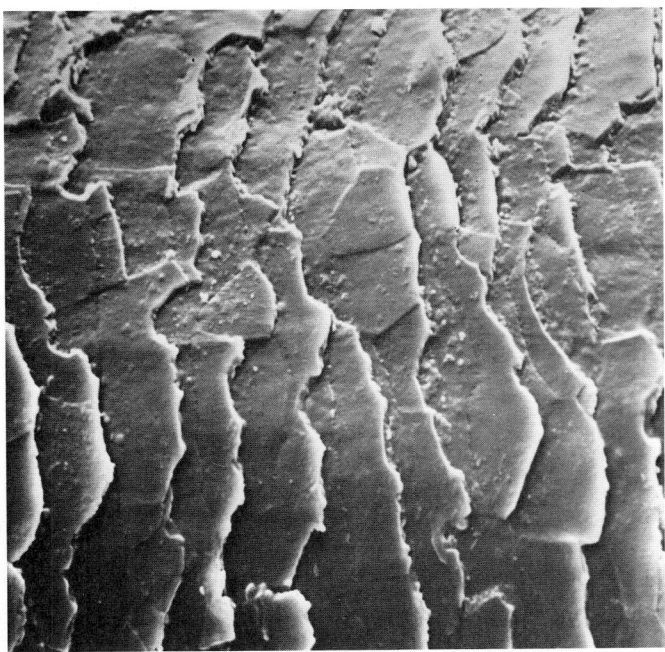

5.52 Detail of **5.51**. Magnification × 1850. (Specimen prepared by Michael Crowder, Guy's Hospital Medical School, London.)

403

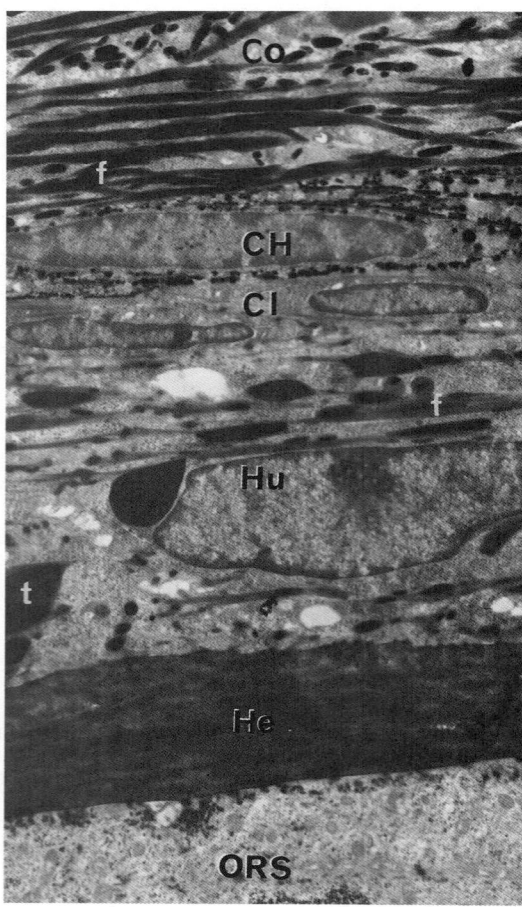

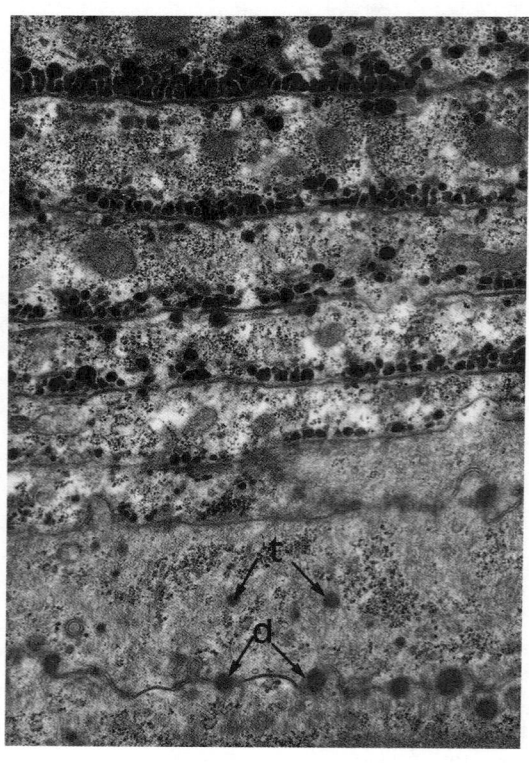

5.53　Longitudinal section of suprabulbar region of scalp hair of a 16½ week fetus. Direction of growth is towards the right. Note from without in: outer root sheath (ORS), keratinized Henle's layer (He), Huxley's layer (Hu) with trichohyalin granules (t) and filaments (f), cuticle of inner root sheath (CI), cuticle of hair (CH), and cortex (Co) with dense filamentous bundles (f). With the exception of the outer root sheath, all the layers will ultimately become keratinized from differently arranged starting materials. Magnification × 5600. (Reproduced from Breathnach 1971, with permission.)

5.54　Pre-keratinized cuticles of adult hair. Below, the cuticle of the inner root sheath contains scattered round trichohyalin granules (t) and filaments, and desmosomes (d) are prominent along apposed plasma membranes. At the upper end of the field five to six layers of cells of the cuticle of the hair show characteristic dense granules aligned predominantly along the outer plasma membranes of the flattened cells. Magnification × 17 160. (Reproduced from Breathnach 1971, with permission.)

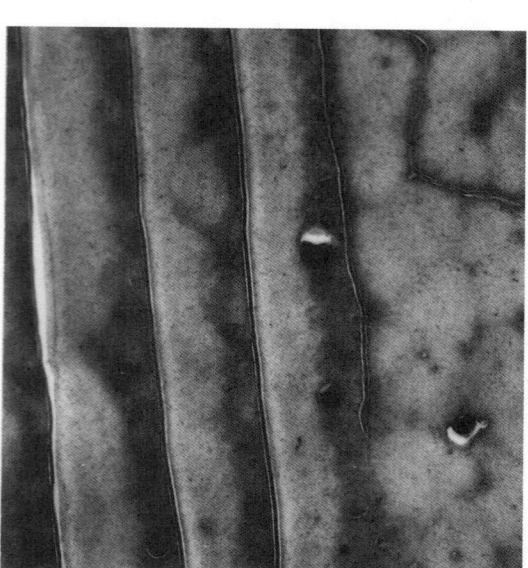

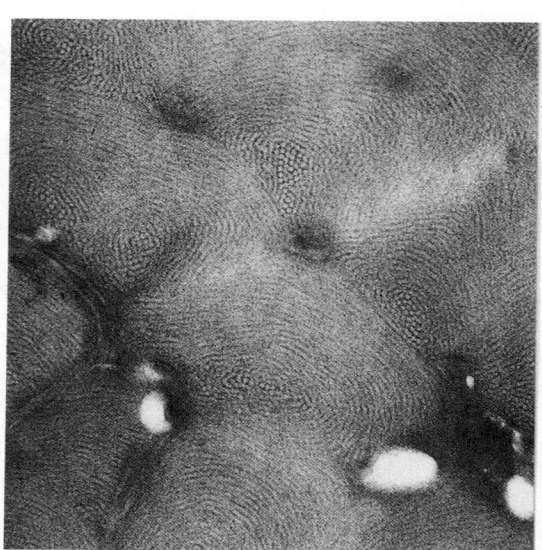

5.55A　Keratinized cuticle and cortex of adult hair. The interior of the flattened cells of the hair cuticle, on the left, exhibit two zones of amorphous material, an inner dense, and an outer more translucent one; a narrow linear dense material occupies the intercellular space. The cortex, on the right, appears to have an amorphous structure also. At higher magnification it is seen to have a filamentous substructure. Magnification × 31 200. (Reproduced from Breathnach 1971, with permission.)

5.55B.　Keratinized hair cortex, transverse section. The pattern is of axially orientated groups of electron-lucent filaments set in an amorphous matrix, and arranged in whorls to give the characteristic 'thumb-print' appearance. Dense material occupies the narrow intercellular intervals. Magnification × 8700. (Reproduced from Breathnach 1971, with permission.)

teristic 'thumb-print' appearance of electron-lucent filaments arranged axially and in whorls and set in a dense matrix (**5.55**). The medulla, when present, is composed of loosely aggregated and often discontinuous columns of partially disintegrated cells containing vacuoles, scattered filaments, granular material and melanosomes. Air cavities lie between the cells or even within them.

Inner root sheath. As already noted, this consists of three concentric layers of cells; the outermost two of which, *Henle layer*, and *Huxley's layer*, in the prekeratinized state contain irregular dense keratohyalin granules and associated filaments. At the level of the upper bulb Henle's layer begins to keratinize, as does Huxley's layer at the middle of the follicle, and when fully keratinized, cells of both have an apparently thickened envelope enclosing a filamento-amorphous matrix which undergoes some further change as they ascend. The cells of the *cuticle of the inner root sheath* have essentially the same structural components as the other two layers, though at the pre-keratinized stage the trichohyalin granules are much fewer, smaller, and rounded. Full keratinization takes place at a level lower than that of Huxley's layer, and, as with the other two layers of the sheath, before disintegration, the filamentous substructure is no longer apparent and a clear-cut pattern such as is seen in the cortical cells is not evident. As they become keratinized, the cells of the cuticles of the inner root sheath and hair become interlocked (**5.49**). Just below the level of entry of the sebaceous duct, the inner root sheath undergoes fragmentation, and the hair then lies free in the pilary canal.

Outer root sheath. Situated at the level of the upper bulb, this is a single or double layer of undifferentiated cells containing glycogen, which higher up the follicle becomes multilayered and gradually assumes the main characteristics of interfollicular epidermis, with which it is continuous. Langerhans cells and melanocytes are interspersed among its cells. At the level of entry of the sebaceous duct, it forms the wall of the pilary canal. In the fetus, the innermost cells contain keratohyalin granules and membrane-coating granules, and become keratinized, but this is less evident postnatally (Breathnach 1971). Ito (1989) describes two layers of cells in the outer root sheath with different keratin and antigen expressions during differentiation. This, and the suggestion that stem cells may reside in the sheath in the region of the bulge (see below), have directed attention towards a more active role of the outer root sheath than previously contemplated.

Dermal papilla. In the anagen follicle this consists mainly of highly cellular (fibroblastic) connective tissue continuous with the outer dermal sheath. They may be partially ensheathed by basal laminar material, and specialized contacts may be present where they are apposed (Tobin 1991). Macrophages and the occasional melanocyte may be present. During development, the dermal papilla induces formation of the hair germ, and is essential for maintenance of the follicle during ontogeny and postnatally through epidermal–dermal interactions similar to those operating at the basement membrane zone of interfollicular epidermis (see p. 294).

Pigmentation of hair. Melanocytes are present in the bulb in the region adjacent to the apex of the dermal papilla (**5.47**) and feed melanosomes to the medulla and cortex mainly. They are active only in mid-anagen, and during telogen become amelanotic, and are interspersed among the epithelial cells at the base of the club hair, where they can only be identified ultrastructurally. They are capable of producing both phaeo- and eumelanosomes, and changes in hair colour of an individual, usually in adolescence, are due to alterations in the dominant type produced. Greying of hair is due to a decline in numbers of melanocytes and their activities. In albinism, melanocytes are present in the bulb, but inactive.

Hair cycle and growth of hair

Recurrent cyclic activity of hair follicles involving growth, rest, and loss of hair (moulting) in phases are characteristic of the pelage of mammals generally, but in man the cycles are irregular, of variable duration, with regional and other variations in the length of the individual phases. In the growing or *anagen phase*, follicle and hair are as described above. This is followed by the involuting or *catagen phase* during which mitotic activity of the germinative matrix ceases, the base of the hair keratinizes into a *club* which moves upwards to the level of the arrector pili muscle, and the whole inferior segment of the follicle degenerates; the dermal papilla also ascends and

remains close to the base of the shortened follicle and its enclosed club hair. This situation persists during the resting or *telogen phase*. At the beginning of the next anagen, the epithelial cells of the base of the follicle renew mitotic activity to form a *secondary hair germ* which envelops the dermal papilla to form a new hair bulb. This grows downwards, reforming the inferior segment of the follicle, and from this a new hair grows up alongside the club hair (which is eventually shed). Cotsarelis et al (1990) have identified in mice a population of outer root sheath cells in the region of the bulb which they class as stem cells capable of regenerating the lower end of the follicle, an observation which calls into question the predominant or unique role of the matrix cells in this respect. (See also Lauer et al in Wuepper et al (1993) on this point.)

By the fifth month of fetal life the body is covered by fine, often deeply pigmented primary hairs all in anagen (collectively the *lanugo*); on the back these hairs are more frequent than those of the gorilla or chimpanzee at a similar age. Before birth some hairs may have reached catagen or telogen. Lanugal hairs are mostly shed before birth or immediately after, and are replaced by secondary *vellus hairs*, except on the scalp, eyebrows and palpebral margins. Since no further follicles are formed after birth, hairs become more widely spaced as the area of skin increases with body growth. Postnatally in man hairs exhibit regional asynchrony of cycle duration and phase leading to an irregular *mosaic pattern* of growth and replacement, as distinct from the *wave pattern* of rodents. In some regions the cycle is measured in years. Circannual variation of both scalp and thigh hair growth and loss in men occurs (Randall & Ebling 1991), with a greater number of anagen follicles on the scalp in winter, and a corresponding peak in the number shed during summer. This may represent a phylogenetic or evolutionary echo.

With puberty, hair growth and generation of much thicker hairs occurs on the pubes and axillae in both sexes, and on the face and trunk in males. The actions of hormones on hair growth are complex, and include not only sex hormones, but also those of the thyroid, adrenal cortex, pituitary and pineal (Ebling et al 1991). Androgens stimulate facial and general body hair formation and, after about the first 30 years, tend to cause the thick terminal hairs of the scalp to change to small vellus hairs, causing recession from the forehead and maybe almost complete baldness (*male pattern*). In females, oestrogens tend to maintain vellus hairs in their formation of minute hairs, and in postmenopausal life reduction of oestrogens may permit stronger facial and bodily hair growth. During midpregnancy, hair growth may be particularly active but some weeks later an unusually large number of hairs tend to enter the telogen phase and may be shed before the growth cycle recommences. In older men, growth of hairs on the eyebrows and within the nostrils and external ear canals increases, whereas elsewhere on the body growth slows and the hairs become much finer.

Figures for the rate of growth of individual hairs vary considerably, probably because of the influence of factors mentioned above. A rate of 0.2–0.44 mm per 24 hours in males is usually given, with the higher rate occurring on the scalp. Shaving does not appear to affect the growth rate, nor does hair grow after death.

Innervation of hair. Hairs are tactile organs, and are richly innervated as described on page 962. **Blood supply** is via collaterals from the reticular arteriolar plexus to the dermal papilla and from ascending branches to anastomosing networks around the bulb and the inferior segment of the follicle.

(For further details on the hair follicle see Orfanos et al 1981; Orfanos & Happle 1990.)

Sebaceous glands

Sebaceous glands are small saccular structures lying (**5.1, 46, 56**), in the dermis; these, together with the hair follicle and arrector pili muscle, constitute the major part of the pilosebaceous unit. They are present over the whole body except the thick hairless skin of the palm, soles and flexor surfaces of digits. Typically, they consist of a cluster of secretory acini opening by a short common duct into the dermal pilary canal of the hair follicle (**5.1, 45**) into which they liberate their secretory product, *sebum*. In some areas of thin skin lacking hair follicles, their ducts open instead directly onto the skin surface, for example on the lips and corners of the mouth, the buccal mucosa (Fordyce spots, p. 1688), nipples, female mammary areolae, glans penis, inner surface of the prepuce (glands of Tyson), glans

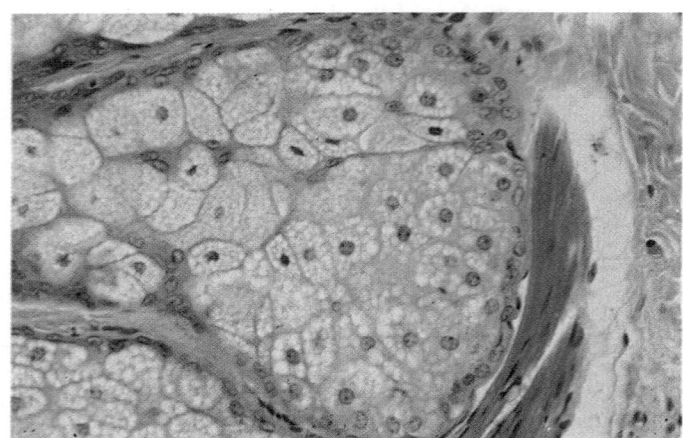

5.56 A sebaceous gland showing the progression from small polygonal cells around its margins to the large, highly vacuolated cells in the interior of a saccule. The sebum has been extracted by histological processing, leaving an empty frothy appearance in cells about to undergo holocrine secretion. Haematoxylin and eosin. Smooth myocytes of an arrector pili muscle visible on the right. Magnification × 540.

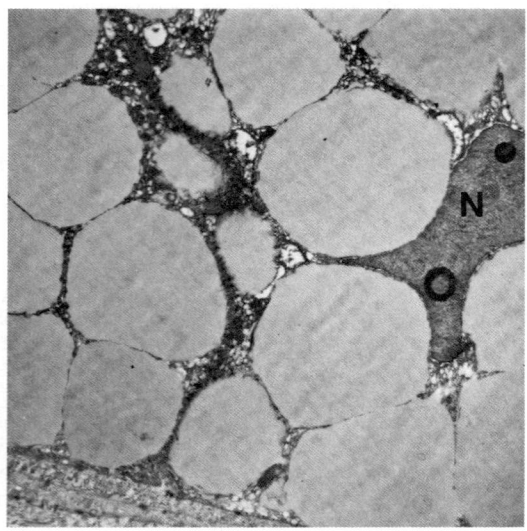

5.57 From central portion of fully differentiated sebaceous gland of an adult. The nucleus of the cell (N) is irregular due to compression by lipid droplets separated only by tenuous cytoplasmic septa. These septa will finally rupture liberating the cellular contents into the duct. Magnification × 3528. (Reproduced from Breathnach 1971, with permission.)

clitoridis and labia minora. At the margins of the eyelids, the large complex palpebral tarsal glands (Meibomian glands) are of this type, and also occurring in the eyelid is the *unicellular sebaceous gland of Wolff* (Pelfini et al 1969) which is actually a melanocyte full of lipid droplets. They are also present in the external auditory meatus.

In general, numbers of sebaceous glands in any given area reflect the distribution of hair follicles, ranging from an average of about 100/cm² over most of the body to as many as 400–900/cm² on the face and scalp. They are also numerous in the midline of the back. Individual sebaceous glands are particularly large on the face, around the external auditory meatus, chest and shoulders, and on the anogenital surfaces. Those of much of the face are related to very small vellus hairs whose investing follicles have particularly wide apertures.

Microstructure. Microscopically, the glandular acini are seen to be invested by a basal lamina supported by a thin dermal capsule and a rich capillary network. Within this, each acinus is lined by a single layer of small, flat, polygonal epithelial cells which ultrastructurally resemble undifferentiated basal keratinocytes of interfollicular epidermis. They possess euchromatic nuclei and large nucleoli, scattered keratin filaments, free ribosomes, agranular endoplasmic reticulum and rounded mitochondria, and are attached to each other by desmosomes. Functionally, they are mitotically active stem cells whose offspring move gradually towards the centre of the acinus increasing in volume, and accumulating increasingly swollen lipidic vacuoles (**5.57**), which some observers describe as membrane-limited, and others as non-limited. The nuclei become pyknotic as the cells mature, and finally the huge distended cells disintegrate, filling the central cavity and its effluent duct with a mass of fatty cellular debris. This mode of secretion, involving the total destruction of the glandular cells, is described as *holocrine* (p. 74) and takes about 2 to 3 weeks. The secretory products pass through a wide duct lined with keratinized squamous epithelium into the infundibulum of the hair follicle and thence on to the surface of the hair and the general epidermis.

The normal functions of sebum are a matter for discussion. It forms a major component of the *skin surface lipids*, the remainder being provided by the interfollicular epidermis. The lipids provide a protective coating on hairs, possibly assist waterproofing of the epidermis, discourage blood-sucking ectoparasites and contribute to characteristic body odour, a feature which in our ancestral conditions may have possessed strong positive social connotations and in the newborn could play a part in the relationship between mother and child. A general antibacterial activity has been postulated, but the presence in sebum of triglycerides which can be hydrolysed by bacteria, including *Propionobacterium acnes*, argues against this.

Sebum and sebaceous activity. When first formed, sebum is a complex mixture of which over 50% is di- and triglycerides, with smaller proportions of wax esters, squalene, cholesterol esters, cholesterol and free fatty acids, mainly of 16-carbon atom chain length; phospholipids are not present (Stewart et al 1983; Stewart 1992). At birth, sebaceous glands are quite large, regressing later until stimulated again at puberty. At that time, sebaceous gland growth and secretory activity increase greatly in both males and females, under the influence of androgens (testicular and adrenal), and possibly growth hormone from the adenohypophysis, and thyroid hormone, amongst other factors. Androgens act locally on the gland, and there is no motor innervation. Oestrogens have an effect opposite to that of androgens, and secretion is considerably lower in women, becoming greatly decreased after the age of 50 years.

Little is known of the biosynthesis of sebum because of the holocrine nature of its formation, and its expression from the duct is due to continuous pressure from behind of disintegrating cells, aided possibly by compression due to contraction of the neighbouring arrector pili muscles. Excessive amounts of sebum may become impacted within the duct, and this, associated with hyperkeratinization, may lead to it being blocked to form a 'comedone', which, becoming infected and inflamed, is the primary lesion of acne. There are now sufficient therapeutic agents available, both topical and systemic, which are largely capable of ameliorating and curing acne. What is needed in addition is an awareness of this amongst practitioners and patients, the effort to apply them and a general change in attitude towards this most distressing of skin diseases.

Apocrine glands

The apocrine glands are particularly large glands of the dermis or hypodermis, classed as a type of sweat gland, but, since they develop as outgrowths of the hair follicle and discharge secretion into the hair canal, they are appropriately considered here. They are widely distributed over the skin of mammals generally, including lower primates, in whom they serve a thermoregulatory function, but in the adult human are present in only a few areas, namely the axillae, perianal region, areolae, periumbilical skin, prepuce, scrotum, mons pubis and labia minora. Ceruminous glands of the external auditory meatus and the ciliary glands of the palpebral margins (glands of Moll) are also usually included in this category. However, their secretions are quite different and these glands should be considered as distinct, specialized subtypes (for details see p. 1369 and **8.459**, respectively).

The gland consists of a basal secretory coil and a straight duct which opens into the pilary canal above the duct of the sebaceous gland, or directly on to the skin surface if there is no associated hair.

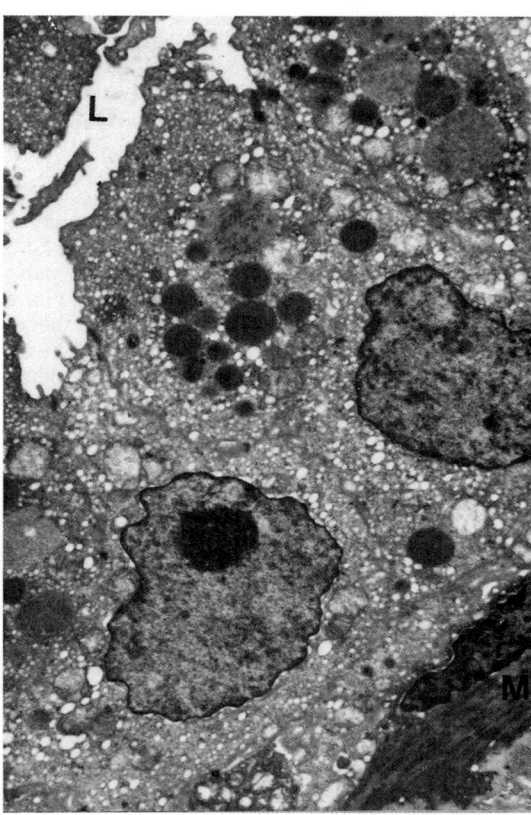

5.58 Secretory coil of axillary apocrine gland. Secretory cells containing granules project into the lumen (L), and rest upon myoepithelial cells (M). Magnification × 6000.

The secretory region may be as much as 2 mm wide and its coils often anastomose with each other to form a labyrinthine network. Each coil is lined by cuboidal secretory cells with apical caps of cytoplasm projecting into the lumen beyond terminal junctional complexes, and resting upon a layer of myoepitheliocytes (**5.58**). The whole complex of cells is limited by a thick basal lamina, and outside this is a connective tissue capsule, rich in capillaries and containing nerve terminals. The secretory cells contain vacuoles, vesicles and dense granules of varying size and internal structure, whose numbers and character vary with the cycle of synthesis and discharge. 'Clear cells' with few organelles are sporadically present basally among the myoepitheliocytes. The mechanism of secretion is still not entirely clear but may involve a number of different processes (see Hashimoto 1978), including merocrine secretion of granules, detachment or pinching off of apical caps or complete holocrine disintegration of the cells. Secretion is pulsatile, the thick, milky proteinaceous product being projected into and along the duct by contraction of the myoepitheliocytes.

Apocrine activity is minimal before puberty, after which it is androgen dependent and responsive to emotional stimuli. It is controlled by adrenergic nerves, and is sensitive to epinephrine and norepinephrine. The secretion as it emerges is sterile and odourless, but it undergoes bacterial decomposition to generate potent odorous compounds, musky or urinous in smell, including short-chain fatty acids, steroids such as 5 α-androstenone, etc. In many animals these are potent pheromonal signals important in courtship, parental and territorial behaviour, as well as in various other aspects of social life. Their role for modern humans is less certain, although there has been much speculation on the potency of, for example, axillary odours on the more subtle aspects of human interactions (see Gower et al 1987).

Arrector pili muscles

The arrector pili muscles are small fasciculi of smooth muscle cells which form diagonal links between the dermal sheaths of hair follicles and the papillary layer of the dermis (**5.1, 45, 56**). They are attached

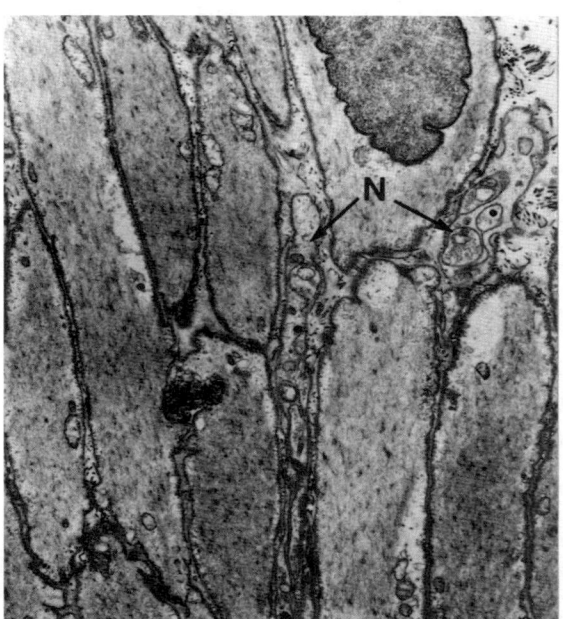

5.59A. Arrector pili muscle. Fibres are sectioned tangentially, and nerve terminals (N) and collagen fibrils are disposed among them. Magnification × 6000.

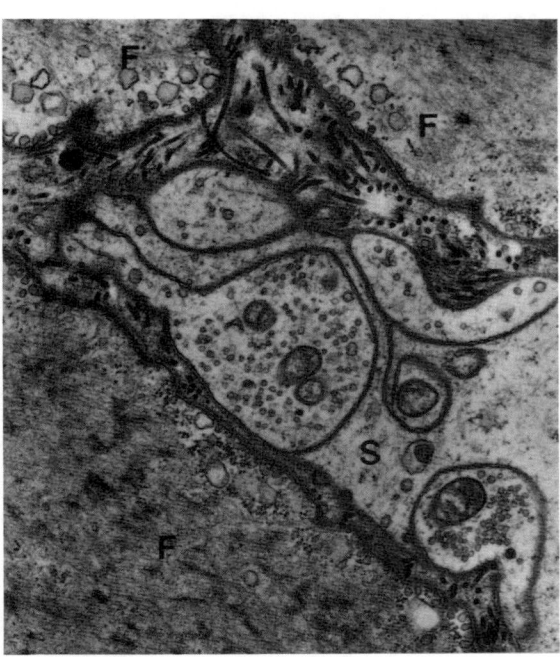

5.59B. Arrector pili muscle. Between the fibres (F) are axonal terminals enclosed in Schwann cell cytoplasm (S). The terminals contain clear-cored vesicles and mitochondria. Magnification × 15 600.

to the bulge region of the follicles by means of elastin fibrils, and are directed obliquely and superficially towards the side to which the hair slopes. The sebaceous gland occupies the angle between the muscle and the hair follicle. Contraction, therefore, tends to pull the hair into a more vertical position and to elevate the epidermis surrounding it into a small hillock, while dimpling the surface where the muscle is inserted superficially, giving the appearance of 'goose-flesh'. Arrector pili muscles are absent from facial, axillary, and pubic hairs and from eyelashes and eyebrows, and the hairs around nostrils and the external auditory meati.

The closely-packed myocytes are separated by narrow intervals containing collagen fibres and non-myelinated Schwann cell–axonal complexes (**5.59A, B**). They exhibit the typical features of smooth-

407

muscle cells—loose bundles of myofilaments associated with dense foci orientated along the long axis of the cell, with glycogen particles and pinocytotic vesicles distributed just within the plasma membrane, which has a basal lamina. The innervating axonal terminals contain mainly clear-cored vesicles (**5.59**B), and are noradrenergic sympathetic.

These muscles by virtue of their position could help to express the secretions of sebaceous glands, though it is doubtful if they act in this way. In many mammals, piloerection is a means of signalling aggression, fear, and other social responses, and can have a thermo-regulatory function by trapping an insulating layer of air within the fur.

NAIL UNIT

The nail unit has five components:

- the *nail plate*, a horny translucent plate on the extensor surface of the distal segment of each digit
- the *matrix*, the proximal extension of the nail plate underneath
- a *proximal nail fold*
- a *nail bed* on which the nail plate rests
- the *hyponychium*, which underlies the free distal edge of the nail plate, and which is separated from the adjacent volar skin of the digital tip by a shallow *distal nail groove*.

The sides of the nail plate are bordered by *lateral nail folds* continuous with the proximal fold, and *lateral* and *proximal nail grooves* marking the conjunction (**5.60**). A fold of skin, the *eponychium*, borders the proximal edge of the exposed nail.

Nail plate

The nail plate is approximately rectangular in shape (**5.60**), and is mostly convex in both longitudinal and transverse axes, though there is much variation, between both individuals and the different digits of one person. The thickness increases proximodistally from about 0.7 mm to 1.6 mm, and the terminal thickness can vary considerably from individual to individual (Johnson et al 1991). The surface of the nail plate may show fine longitudinal ridges, and its under surface is grooved by corresponding ridges of the nail bed. Disturbances of growth pattern or disease may lead to transverse ridging or grooves (Beau's lines; Meuhrcke lines), and minute trapped air-bubbles may produce white flecks. These defects move distally with growth of the plate. The colour of the nail plate is generally translucent pink, except proximally, always on the pollex, and to a varying extent on the other digits, depending upon manicuring, where a crescentic white opaque area, the *lunule*, is present, emerging from under the proximal nail fold. Its alleged greater surface area on the dominant thumb is said to be a mark of handedness.

Nails are homologous with the stratum corneum of the general epidermis, consisting of compacted, anucleate, keratin-filled squames which are variably described as being disposed in two or three horizontal layers, depending upon views as to their origins from particular parts of the nail unit (see below). Ultrastructurally, the squames contain closely-packed filaments which lie transversely to the direction of proximodistal growth, and are embedded in a dense protein matrix, which also forms a dense marginal band within the tortuous and interlocking cell membranes. Hashimoto (1971)

described the squames as being connected by desmosomes and gap junctions, but others (Parent et al 1985) observed only desmosomes. All authors, quoting Hashimoto (1971a), state that keratohyalin is not involved in keratinization of postnatal nail, which is interesting in view of the fact that it is most certainly involved in this process in fetal nail (Hashimoto et al 1966; Breathnach 1971). This point could bear re-examination. Squames are not shed from the nail plate surface, unlike the general epidermis.

The nail plate has a high content of sulphur-containing matrix proteins, but a lipid content less than that of general stratum corneum. A variety of mineral elements is present in nail, among which is calcium, though this is not responsible for the hardness of nail. This is related rather to the arrangement of the layers of squames, their mutual adhesion, and the disposition of their internal fibres (Zaias 1990). Analysis of metal elements in nail has forensic importance in diagnosing excessive ingestion, for example of arsenic, criminally administered. The water content of nail is low, but nail is 10 times as permeable to water as general epidermis (Baden 1970). Elasticity of the nail plate is related to its degree of hydration.

Proximal nail fold. Proximally, the nail plate extends under the *proximal nail fold*, forming an angle with it (Lovibond's angle), which is less than 180°. The fold is composed of two epidermal layers, superficial and deep, with a core of dermis in between. The epidermis of the superficial layer lacks hair follicles and epidermal ridges, and its stratum corneum extends over the nail plate for a little distance as the *cuticle* or *eponychium*. The ventral layer merges deeply with the *matrix* which produces the greater part of the nail plate.

Matrix. On section, the matrix is seen as a wedge of cells with its apex proximal, in which the deeper part of the nail plate is embedded (**5.61, 62**). Those cells lying dorsal to the plate are referred to as the *dorsal matrix*, and are continuous with the ventral epithelium of the proximal nail fold. Those lying ventral are known as the *ventral matrix*, which is continuous distally with the nail bed. From the apical region of the matrix fine bundles of anchoring filaments extend into the dermis. The matrix epithelium consists of typical basal and spinous layer keratinocytes with axes directed diagonally distally, among which melanocytes and Langerhans cells are intermingled. The keratinocytes produce membrane coating granules, but not keratohyalin granules (Hashimoto, 1971), although granules like those of keratinizing oral epithelia have been reported (Picardo et al 1992). Keratinized cells of dorsal and ventral matrices are steadily extruded distally to form the nail plate with the major contribution coming from the ventral matrix. This continues into the **nail bed** at the distal edge of the lunule, which is formed by the distal portion of the ventral matrix overlain by the nail plate.

Nail bed. This underlies the nail plate from the lunule to the *hyponychium*, and its surface is ridged and grooved longitudinally in correspondence with a similar pattern on the under surface of the nail plate, which results in a tight interlocking coupling of the two that prevents the invasion of microbes and the impaction of debris underneath the nail. The pattern is imposed by underlying dermal ridges, and is thought to represent the finger print pattern elsewhere. The epidermis of the nail bed consists of two to three layers of nucleated cells lacking keratohyalin granules, and a thin keratinized layer which moves distally with the growing nail plate. Until recently, the nail plate was thought to be derived entirely from the matrix, growing distally over the nail bed, and carrying the cornified cells of the latter along with it to be shed distally. In this scheme, the nail bed was regarded as providing a gliding surface for an already fully formed growing nail plate. Now, however, it is generally thought that nail bed cells differentiate towards the nail plate, contributing a significant component to it ventrally. The plate, therefore, is now thought to consist of three horizontal layers—a dorsal one from the dorsal matrix, an intermediate one from the ventral matrix and a ventral one from the nail bed. Authorities, however, are not in agreement as to the extent of contribution of the three components (Forslind & Thyresson, 1975; Parent et al 1985; Ziais 1990; Baran et al 1991; Johnson et al 1991). Beneath the epithelium of the nail bed is a dermis anchored to the periosteum of the distal phalanx without any intervening subcutis. It forms a distinct compartment and because of this, infections of the nail bed, or other local sources of rise of pressure (e.g. haematoma), may cause severe pain only relieved by excision of part or all of the nail plate. The dermis is

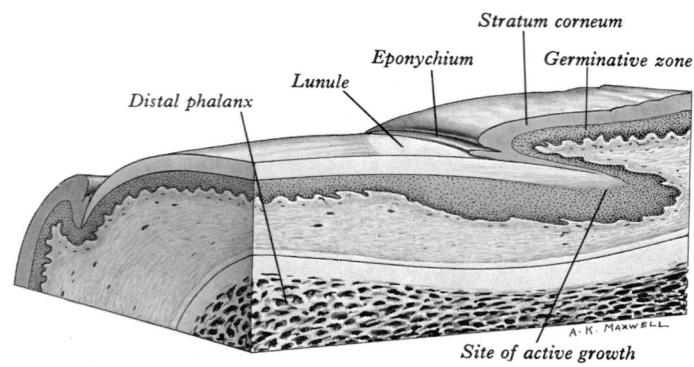

Stratum corneum

Eponychium

Germinative zone

Lunule

Distal phalanx

A·K·MAXWELL

Site of active growth

5.60   Longitudinal section through the root of a nail.

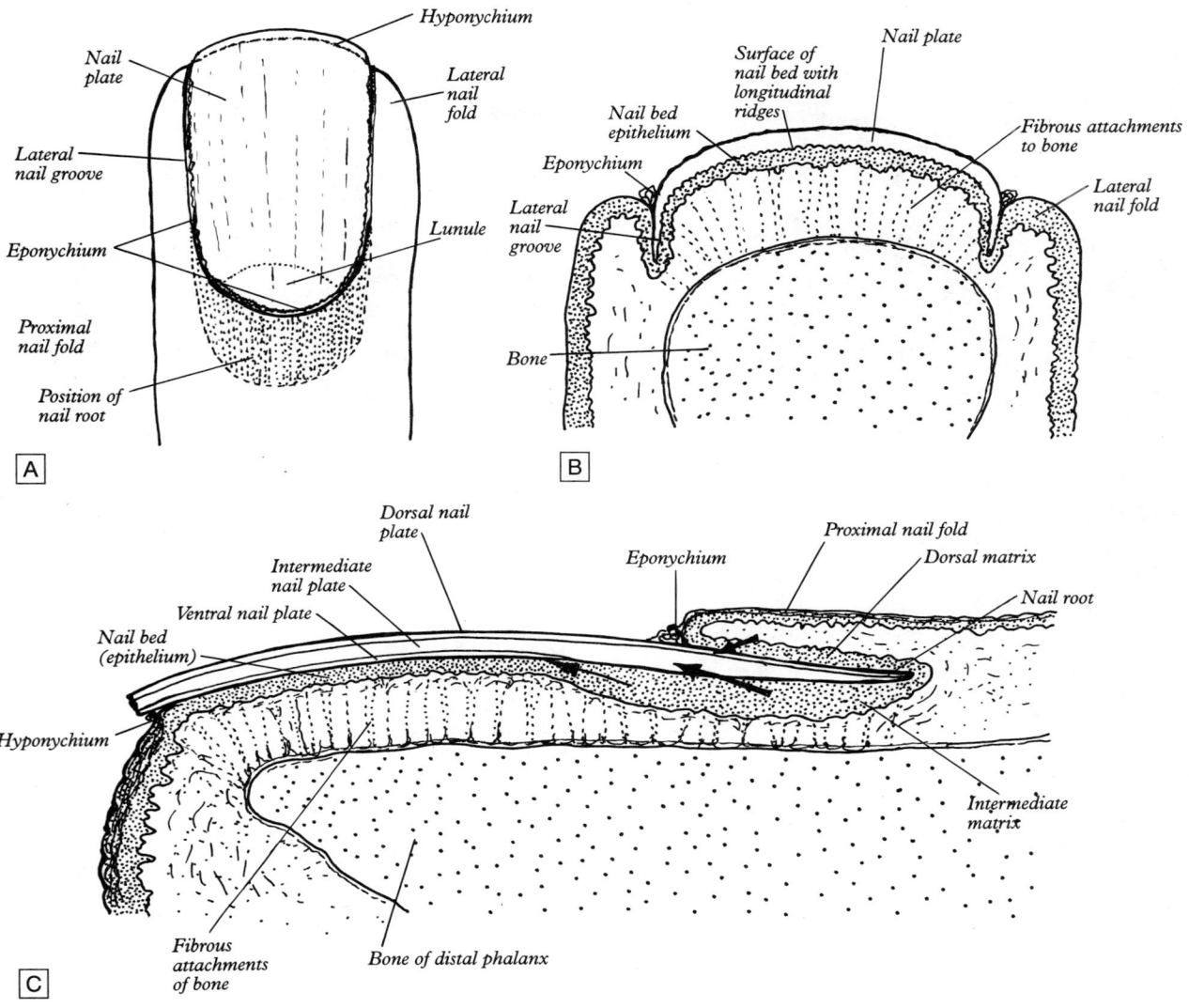

5.61 A–C. Diagram showing the organization and terminology of the structures associated with a fingernail. (A) shows the appearance of the dorsal side, indicating the extent of the hidden nail root. (B) depicts a cross section of a fingertip, and (C) a longitudinal section through a nail and its surrounding structures, indicating the areas of formation of the nail plate from the different areas of matrix.

richly vascularized, including large arteriovenous shunts (glomera), and numerous sensory nerve endings, including Merkel terminals and Meissner corpuscles. Fingernails subserve an important tactile function, providing support and counterpressure for the digital pad, thereby aiding manipulation. Spatulate (flat) nails are found in all primate species, and are an evolutionary development from sharp claws. They represent a thin superficial protective stratum of the tetrapod claw.

Hyponychium. An area of epidermis which underlies the edge of the nail plate, it extends from the nail bed to the distal groove which marks its continuation into the general epidermis of the finger tip. The basal layer cells have a semi-palisade arrangement, the granulosa cells are packed with keratohyalin granules and the stratum corneum is undulant and continually being shed. The hyponychium provides an important defence against entry of bacteria underneath the free edge of the nail plate, and may be damaged by too vigorous cleaning in this situation.

Growth of nail. The growth of nail is determined by the turnover rate of the matrix cells, which varies with digit, age, environmental temperature and season, time of day, nutritional status, trauma, such as biting, and various diseases. Generally, its speed is related to the length of the digit, being fastest (about 0.1 mm per day) in the middle finger of the hand, and slowest in the little finger. Fingernails grow up to four times faster than toenails, quicker in summer than in winter, and faster in the young than in the old. Left

unclipped and protected from erosion, nails can grow to considerable lengths, and in previous Chinese cultures they were allowed to do so by the wealthy classes as an indication that they were waited upon for everything. The long nails were protected by elaborately jewelled and decorated sheaths. Painting the toenails red was said to be a signal of menstrual status in the seraglio.

ECCRINE SWEAT GLANDS (5.63–67)

The eccrine sweat glands are long unbranched tubular structures, each with a highly coiled, wider secretory portion (the body or fundus, up to $0.4\,\mu m$ in diameter; **5.63**) situated deep in the dermis or hypodermis and a narrower, straight or slightly helical ductular portion, which in the deeper layers of the dermis is convoluted or twisted (**5.1**, **45**). The walls of the duct fuse with the base of epidermal (rete) papillae and the lumen passes between the keratinocytes often, particularly in thick hairless skin, in a tight spiral (**5.3**), to open via a rounded aperture onto the skin surface (**5.19**). In thick hairless skin, they discharge by a regular series of punctae along the centre lines of friction ridges, incidentally providing markers of fingerprint patterns for forensic purposes. Eccrine glands have an important thermoregulatory function, and their secretion enhances grip and sensitivity of the palms and soles.

Eccrine glands are absent from the tympanic membrane, margins of the lips, nail bed, nipple, inner preputial surface, labia minora,

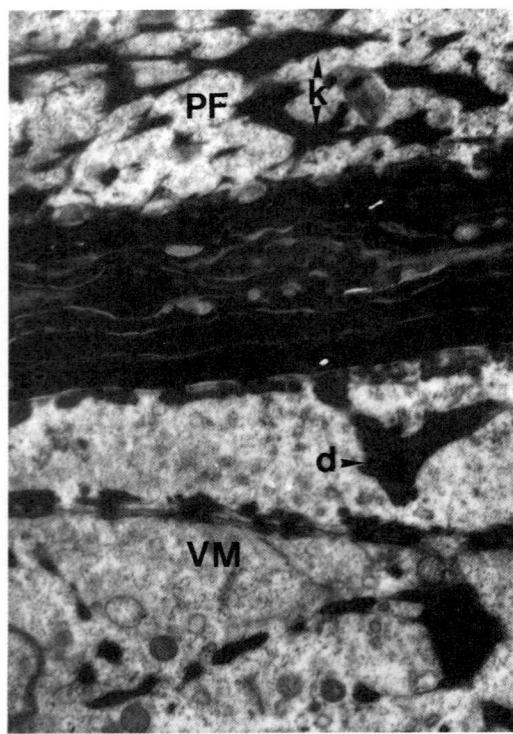

5.62 Longitudinal section of nail organ of a fetus aged 16 weeks. Dorsal to the keratinized squames of the nail plate is a cell of the proximal nail fold (PF) with typical keratohyalin granules (k) and ventral to them a cell of the ventral matrix (VM) with dense cytoplasmic granules (D) similar to those seen in areas of keratinizing oral epithelium. Magnification × 10 080. (Reproduced from Breathnach 1971, with permission.)

glans penis and glans clitoridis. Elsewhere they are numerous, their frequency ranging from 80 to over 600/cm², depending on position and genetic variation; the total number lies between 1.6 and 4.5 million (Millington & Wilkinson 1983; Ito 1988). Numbers are greatest on the plantar skin of the feet, but there are also many on the face and flexor aspects of the hands, while the surfaces of the limbs generally have the fewest. Racial groups indigenous to warmer climates tend to have more than those of cooler geographical areas. Ito (1988) has described apo-eccrine glands with features of both apocrine and eccrine glands in the human axilla.

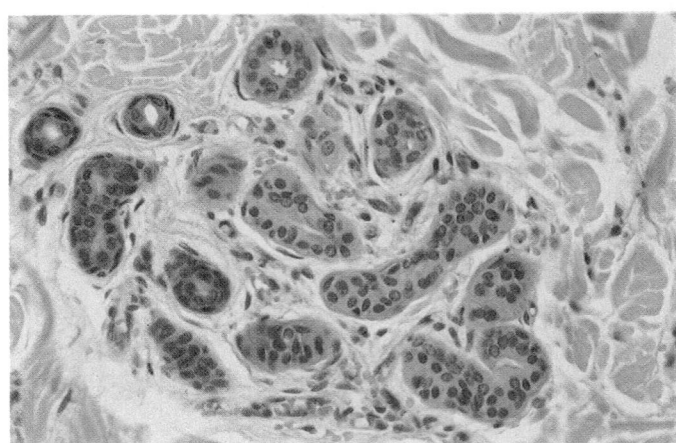

5.63 Section through the basal coil of a sweat gland showing the wider secretory portion and the narrower initial region of the sweat duct composed of two layers of small cuboidal cells. Haematoxylin and eosin. Magnification × 540.

Cell types

Microscopically the secretory coil consists of a pseudostratified epithelium enclosing a lumen with intercellular canaliculi resting on a basal lamina and enclosed by a thin fibrous dermal sheath. There are three types of cell:

- *clear* (serous) cells from which most of the secretion derives
- *dark* (mucoid) cells
- *myoepitheliocytes*.

Clear cells. These are approximately pyramidal in shape, with their bases resting on the basal lamina or myoepitheliocytes, and their microvillus-covered apical plasma membranes lining the intercellular canaliculi. The lateral plasma membrane is highly folded, inter-digitating with folds of apposed clear cells (5.66), as is also the basal plasma membrane where it abuts on the basal lamina. The cytoplasm is rich in glycogen granules and mitochondria, and granular endo-plasmic reticulum and a small Golgi complex are present, but few other formed organelles. The nucleus is rounded and moderately euchromatic.

Dark cells. These are also pyramidal, with their broad ends facing and forming the greater extent of the lining of the main lumen. The cytoplasm contains a well-developed Golgi complex, numerous

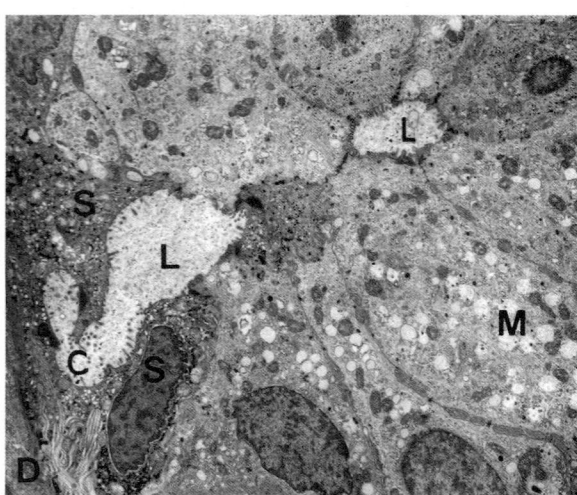

5.64 Portion of secretory coil of eccrine gland. Serous (S) and mucous (M) cells surround the lumen (L) from which an intercellular canaliculus (C) extends between serous cells. D, dermis. Magnification × 2656. (Reproduced from Breathnach 1971, with permission.)

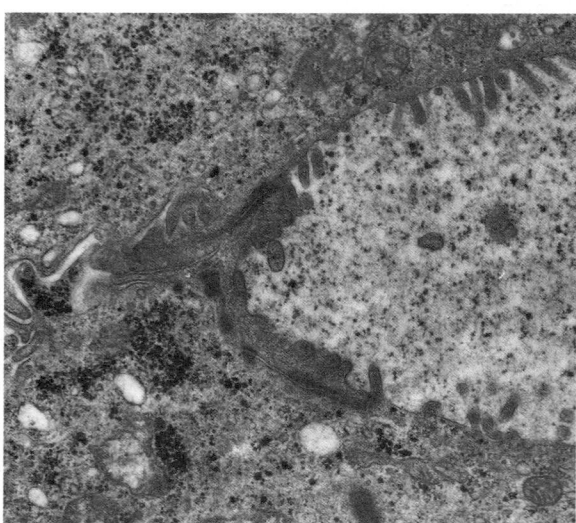

5.65 Eccrine sweat gland. Portions of two serous cells are seen bounding the lumen. Note microvilli on the luminal plasma membrane. Magnification × 14 000. (Reproduced from Breathnach 1971, with permission.)

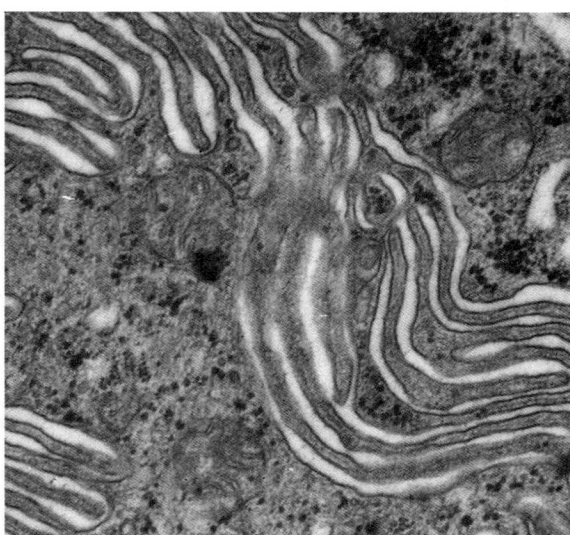

5.66   Eccrine sweat gland. This illustrates interdigitation of long villous processes of plasma membranes of apposed serous cells. Magnification × 33 440. (Reproduced from Breathnach 1971, with permission.)

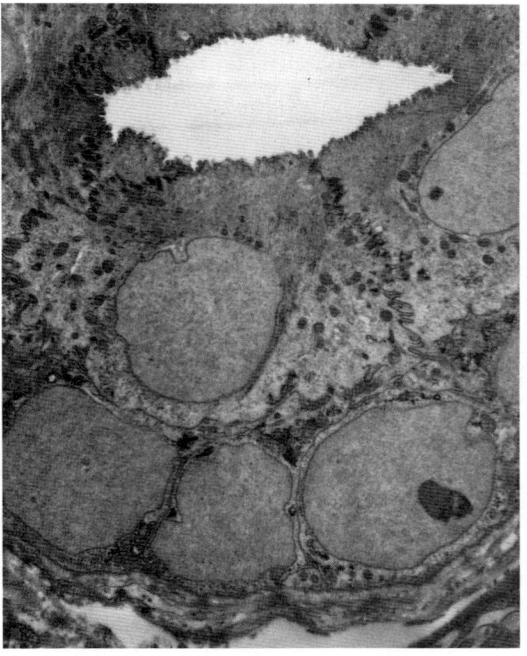

5.67   Transverse section of upper portion of intradermal sweat duct, which is composed of two cellular layers, basal and luminal. The supranuclear portions of the cells bounding the lumen appear 'clear' because the cytoplasm here contains mainly filaments, and this zone corresponds to the cuticular border of light microscopy. Magnification × 4480. (Reproduced from Breathnach 1971, with permission.)

vacuoles and vesicles and dense granules of different sizes, indicating a type of secretion different to that of the clear cells.

Myoepitheliocytes. Similar to those elsewhere (p. 780), these form an incomplete layer along the basal lamina with processes of clear cells in between. The infranuclear region of the cytoplasm is almost entirely occupied by myofilaments, the bulk of the other organelles lying superior and lateral to the nucleus.

Sweat ducts. The *intradermal sweat duct* is formed of two cell layers, an outer basal layer and an inner layer of luminal cells connected by numerous desmosomes, and with microvilli along the luminal border. The supranuclear cytoplasm is highly filamentous, corresponding to the eosinophilic 'cuticular border' of light microscopy. The *intraepidermal sweat duct* is twisted, and also consists of essentially two layers of cells which, developmentally, are different to the surrounding general keratinocytes. The outer cells near the surface contain keratohyalin granules and lamellar granules, and undergo typical keratinization. The inner cells from a mid-epidermal level contain numerous vesicles just within the microvillous luminal plasma membrane, undergo an incomplete form of keratinization, and are largely shed into the lumen at the level of the stratum corneum.

Sweat

Sweat is a clear, odourless fluid, hypotonic to tissue fluid, containing small quantities of many substances, mainly sodium and chloride ions, but also potassium, urea, lactate, amino acids, immunoglobulins and other proteins, epidermal growth factor, bicarbonate, calcium ions, etc. Heavy metals and various organic compounds are eliminated in sweat, the greater part of which is thought to be produced by the clear cells, the function of the dark cells being uncertain. The function of the myoepitheliocytes is equally obscure, but it has been suggested they provide support for the secretory cells against overdistension when large amounts of fluid are being secreted, squeeze fluid into the canaliculi and lumen, or actually separate when contracted thus exposing a greater area of the clear cell to the basal lamina and dermal extracellular fluid. When initially secreted, the fluid is similar in composition to tissue fluid, but it is modified as it passes along the duct by the action mainly of the basal cells which exhibit Na-K-adenosine 5'-triphosphate (ATP)ase activity and resorb sodium and chloride and some water too. The hormone aldosterone enhances this activity. The body's sweat glands are capable of producing up to 10 litres of sweat per day, in response to thermal, emotional, and gustatory stimuli, mediated by non-myelinated sympathetic cholinergic fibres, though the glands also respond to adrenaline (Sato et al 1991). *Thermoregulation* is a complex process involving a heat centre in the hypothalamus reacting

to changes in blood temperature and afferent stimuli from the skin, and controlling cutaneous blood supply and the rate and volume of sweat secretion for evaporation at the surface (Clerk and Edholm 1985). Excessive sweating can lead to salt depletion.

AGE-RELATED CHANGES IN SKIN

With the increase in the proportion of elderly persons in the population, interest in age-related changes in skin has greatly expanded in recent years (Montagna et al 1979; Balin & Kligman 1989; Greaves & Voorhees 1990). This interest is from both an aesthetic and a pathological point of view. Two main factors, chronological and environmental, are said to be involved in skin ageing, with the former being regarded as more physiological or intrinsic. A major environmental factor is chronic exposure to the sun, referred to as photoageing, and emphasis is laid upon differences between the two since photoageing is to some extent preventable (Gilchrest 1987; Kligman & Lavker 1988). The major features of skin are essentially formed well before birth, and during the first two to three decades of life the main changes are an expansion of its surface area and thickening of the epidermis and dermis, as well as various changes in hair and gland patterns which occur at puberty (see pp. 405, 406). The arrangement and numbers of creases and friction ridges is essentially the same from their early fetal formation onwards, although their sizes increase until cessation of growth. However, from about the third decade onwards there is a gradual change in the appearance and mechanical properties of the skin which reflect natural ageing processes, in old age becoming very marked.

Intrinsic ageing

Normal human ageing is accompanied by epidermal and dermal atrophy, which result in some changes in the appearance, microstructure and function of the skin. Alterations include wrinkling (see p. 379), dryness, loss of elasticity, thinning and a tendency towards purpura on minor injury. Epidermal atrophy is expressed by general thinning and loss of the basal rete pegs with flattening of the epidermal–dermal junction, resulting in a reduction in contact area between the two which may affect epidermal nutrition. Flattening of the junction decreases resistance to shear, leading to poor adhesion of epidermis and its separation following minor injury. The thickness of the stratum corneum is not reduced in old age, and its permeability characteristics seem little affected. Epidermal proliferative activity and rate of cell replacement decline with age, the thymidine-labelling index being reduced by up to 50%. Synthesis of vitamin D is reduced with this general decline in activity. After middle age there is a 10–20% decline in the number of melanocytes (Ortonne 1990), and Langerhans cells also become sparser, associated with a reduction in immune responsiveness (Schuler 1991). These alterations in non-keratinocytes may be aggravated by chronic exposure to UV irradiation. Depigmentation and loss of hair with some local increases—eyebrows, nose and ears in males, and face and upper lip in females—are so well known as hardly to require mention. Decrease in function of skin glands associated with degenerative changes has been described.

Dermal changes are mainly responsible for the appearance of aged skin, its stiffness, flaccidity and wrinkling, and loss of extensibility and elasticity (Lapiere 1990). Its general thickness diminishes due to a fall-off in collagen synthesis by a reduced population of fibroblasts, though the relative proportion of Type III collagen increases (Lovell et al 1987). Senile elastosis (5.68) is a degenerative condition of collagen which may be partly due to excessive exposure to sun. There is also loss and fragmentation of elastin, and alterations in matrix components, including reduction in glycosaminoglycans. The general cellularity of the dermis decreases with age, and mast cells in particular are reduced in numbers. Vascularization of the skin is also reduced, the capillary loops of the dermal papillae being particularly affected, and the tendency towards small spontaneous purpuric haemorrhages indicates a general fragility of the cutaneous microvasculature. A decrease in sensitivity of sensory perception associated with some loss of specialized receptors occurs. For further reading on this subject, see L'Evêque and Agache (1993).

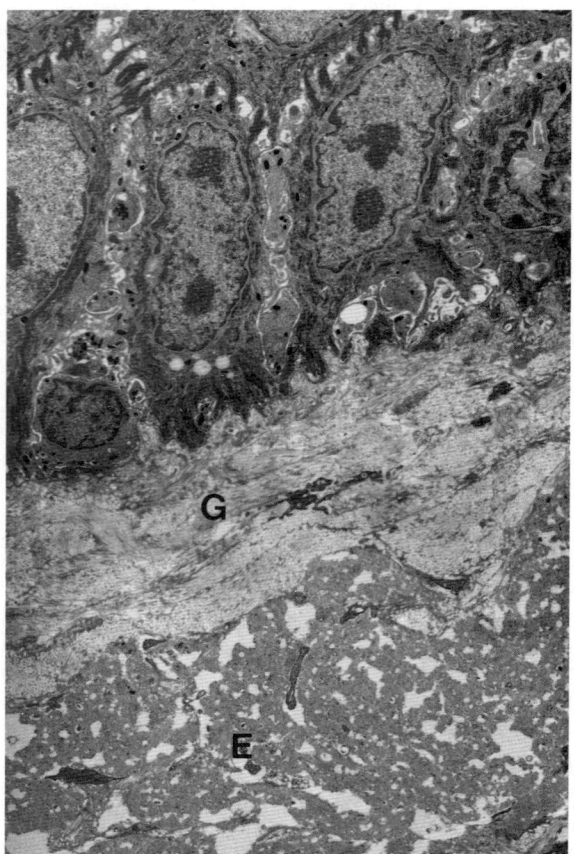

5.68 Epidermis and dermis of facial skin of woman aged over 70, to show area of solar elastosis (E), thought to result from damage to collagen due to chronic exposure to solar radiation. It is interesting that a band just beneath the epidermis, known as the Grenz zone (G), is undamaged. Magnification × 3200.

Photoageing

Reference has already been made to the developing discipline of photobiology (see p. 391), of which photoageing is a major concern because of an association with epidermal cancer, and further details may be found in the literature cited above. The effects of chronic sun exposure on melanocytes (stimulatory) and Langerhans cells (destructive) has received particular attention because of the increasing incidence of malignant melanoma among sun-worshippers, in which reduction in tumour monitoring activity of Langerhans cells may be a factor. (See Gilchrest et al 1979; Thiers et al 1984; Cruz & Bergstresser 1991; Breathnach et al 1992.)

DERMAL REPAIR

For descriptive purposes, dermal repair is divisible into three overlapping phases: *inflammation*, *proliferation* and *remodelling* (**5.69**).

Inflammation

Acute inflammation begins with the activation of platelets and mast cells as an immediate response to injury. During inflammation, haemostasis is achieved, removal of damaged tissue occurs and factors which start the formation of granulation tissue are released or deposited in the wound. Multiple interacting pathways of inflammation (**5.73**) are triggered when dermal blood vessels are injured and end automatically when the inflammatory stimuli dissipate; should these stimuli persist, then inflammation persists and wound healing is delayed.

Tissue injury and bleeding are followed by blood clotting. This involves many complex chemical interactions between components of the extravascular tissue and of blood, including activation of the Hageman factor (for intrinsic coagulation), factor VII (for extrinsic coagulation) and the activation of platelets. These are all responses to the surface adsorption and activation of specific coagulation pro-enzymes normally inhibited in intact tissues, but free to act in the protease inhibitor-free microenvironment temporarily provided by the wound. Blood clotting is a crucial part of inflammation, because activation of Hageman factor leads to bradykinin generation, initiation of the classic complement cascade (Ghebrehiwet et al 1981) and possibly also to production of anaphylatoxins C3a and C5a (Clark 1985), among many other complex and as yet poorly understood reactions. These anaphylatoxins, together with bradykinin, increase local blood vessel permeability (Williams & Jose 1981), causing leakage of plasma proteins and formation of an extravascular clot. They also stimulate release of the vasoactive mediators histamine and leukotrienes C4 and D4 from mast cells (Hugli & Müller-Eberhard 1978; Stimler et al 1982) and attract neutrophils and monocytes to the wound (Marder et al 1985). As a result of activation the platelets also liberate a host of growth factors which affect the proliferative phase of repair (see below) by stimulating the migration and proliferation of cells involved in this phase and by stimulating the synthesis of extracellular matrix components at the site of the wound. These growth factors include platelet factor-4 (Senior et al 1983), platelet-derived growth factor (PDGF) (Huang et al 1988), transforming growth factor-β (TGF-β) (Assoian 1988), epidermal growth factor (EGF) (Banks 1988), basic fibroblast growth factor (b-FGF) (Fox 1988) and platelet-derived endothelial cell growth factor (Miyazono & Heldin 1989; Pierce et al 1991).

The main function of the neutrophils while at the wound site is the phagocytosis of pathogenic bacteria. Once bacterial contamination has been controlled, neutrophil infiltration ceases and the early inflammatory phase of repair is at an end. In contrast, monocytes, which develop into macrophages on entering the wound bed, remain throughout the entire inflammatory phase. Macrophages are not only phagocytic but also release a host of biologically active materials, including growth factors essential for the initiation and propagation of granulation tissue during the next, proliferative, phase of repair.

Proliferation

During this stage, cells and intercellular substances increase greatly to form *granulation tissue*. This is a highly vascular material consisting largely of macrophages, pluripotent pericytes, fibroblasts and

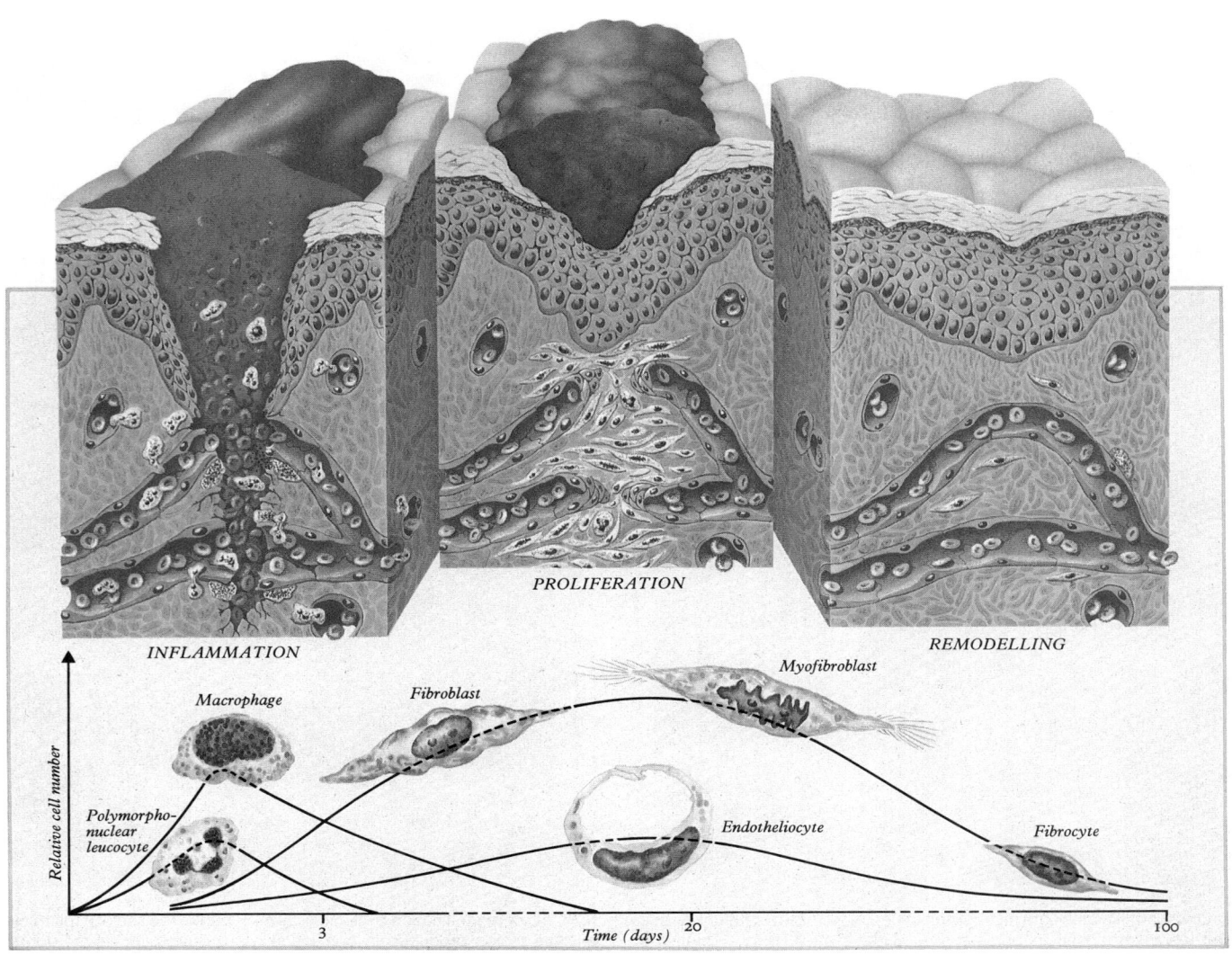

5.69 Diagrammatic representation of the normal response of skin to incision showing the changes in relative numbers of different cell types during inflammation, proliferation and remodelling. For further explanation see text.

endothelial cells lining capillaries, all embedded in a matrix of fibronectin, proteoglycans rich in hyaluronic acid, and collagen, which at first is mainly Type III, changing later to Type I. The profuse assemblies of capillaries, which are the main type of blood vessel, give this tissue its 'granular' appearance when incised, hence its name (see **5**.70, 71, 72).

Granulation tissue forms in response to various signals, which may include chemotactic and growth factors, structural molecules and proteases which digest connective tissue matrix (Clark 1985). It forms a nutritive substrate over which the regenerating epidermis can migrate and is gradually replaced by scar tissue. Apart from the absence of osteogenic cells and chondroblasts, granulation tissue resembles the blastema which develops at the site of fracture repair (p. 483).

Macrophages, fibroblasts and blood capillaries migrate into the wound bed as a mutually dependent unit termed a *wound module* (Hunt & Van Winkle 1979). In the lead are activated macrophages, followed in sequence by newly differentiated fibroblasts, dividing fibroblasts and capillaries. The macrophages release chemotactic agents which attract pericytes, fibroblasts and endothelial cells into the wound. As the fibroblasts mature they produce a matrix through which other cells can readily migrate and from which delicate new capillaries can obtain mechanical support. As each capillary loop becomes functional it brings nutrients and oxygen to nearby cells, enabling the fibroblasts to secrete materials for the matrix, through which macrophages and other cells can migrate further. The above proliferative and migratory processes are repeated sequentially until

the wound bed is filled with granulation tissue. A diagram depicting these complex processes is shown in **5**.73.

There is considerable experimental evidence to support the proposition that macrophages are key cells in dermal repair. They assist in tissue debridement, release chemotactic agents which attract fibroblasts and endothelial cells to the wound site, release growth factors which stimulate these cells to proliferate, and secrete lactate which stimulates collagen synthesis by fibroblasts (Comstock 1970), thus strengthening the tissue which develops within and adjacent to the wound (Silver 1984). Intercellular contacts between macrophages and fibroblasts (**5**.74) suggest that the cells may exert a direct effect on each other. If the migration of macrophages into the wound bed is prevented by anti-inflammatory steroids, or if they are eliminated from it by the application of antimacrophagic serum, the formation of granulation tissue is inhibited (Leibovich & Ross 1975). Inhibition due to anti-inflammatory steroids can be reversed by vitamin A administration, which permits migration of macrophages to the wound site.

During the proliferative phase of repair, fibroblasts of the granulation tissue develop into cells termed *myofibroblasts* (Majno 1979). These cells, which are responsible for wound contraction, the centripetal movement of the wound margin and the consequent reduction of the size of the wound, are immunologically similar to smooth muscle cells, contain peripherally located microfilaments and become linked together by desmosomes and other intercellular contacts (**5**.75). Links between the cells and their substrates have also been found (Ryan et al 1974). Intracytoplasmic filaments of

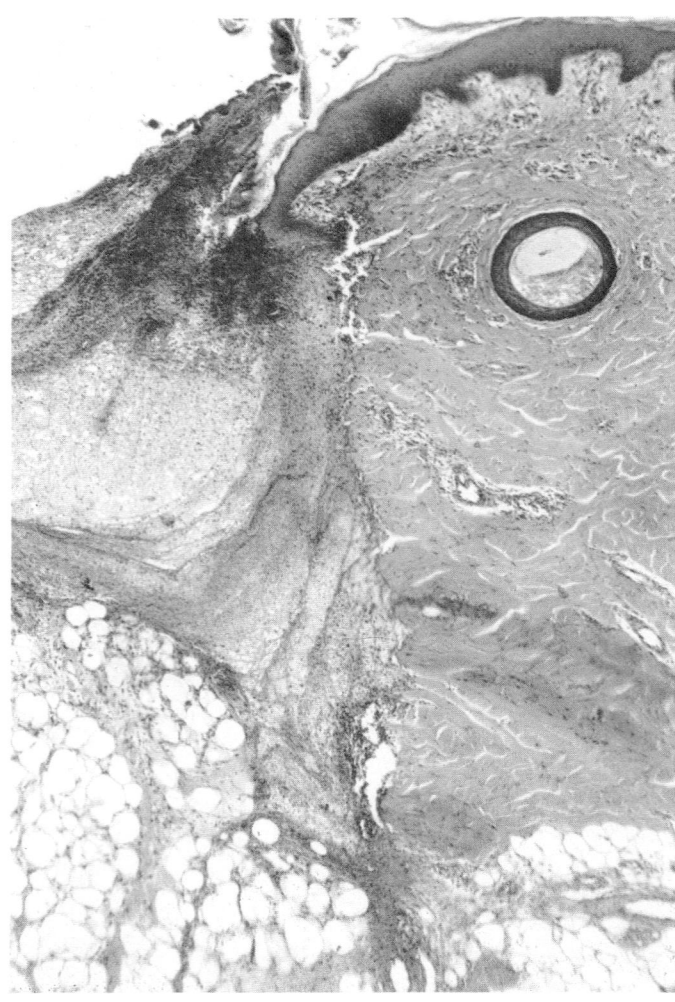

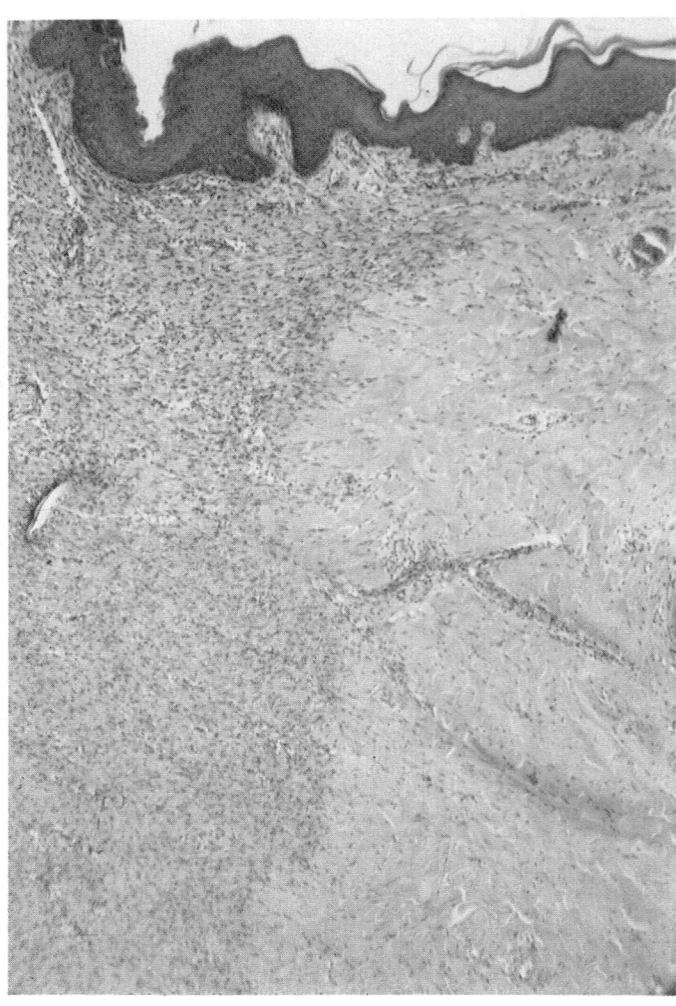

5.70 Low magnification light micrograph of part of the site of a full-thickness excised lesion produced in porcine skin, 3 days after injury, during the inflammatory phase of repair. Intact skin can be seen on the right. Poly-morphonuclear leucocytes and macrophages are present beneath the exudate covering the wound bed, and epidermal migration from the intact skin has already commenced. Stained with haematoxylin and eosin. Magnification × 135. Material supplied by S Young and photographed by Kevin Fitzpatrick, Department of Anatomy, UMDS, Guy's Campus, London.)

5.71 Low magnification light micrograph of part of the site of a full-thickness excised lesion produced in porcine skin, 10 days after injury, during the proliferative phase of repair. Granulation tissue, over which epidermal cells have migrated, fills the wound bed. Stained with haematoxylin and eosin. Magnification × 135. Material supplied by S Young and photographed by Kevin Fitzpatrick, Department of Anatomy, UMDS, Guy's Campus, London.)

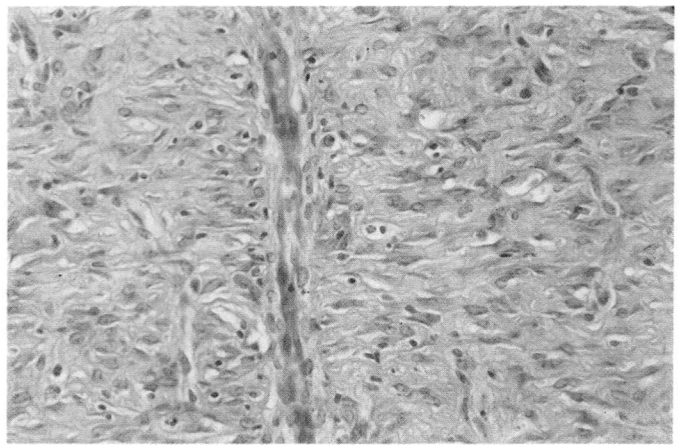

5.72 High magnification light micrograph of granulation tissue, 10 days after the production of a full-thickness excised lesion in porcine skin. The tissue is well vascularized and contains many myofibroblasts, orientated approximately parallel to the base of the wound and at right angles to the majority of the blood vessels. Magnification × 300. Material supplied by S Young and photographed by Kevin Fitzpatrick, Department of Anatomy, UMDS, Guy's Campus, London.)

actin and vinculin form co-linear assemblies, each termed a *fibronexus* (**5.75**), with extracellular matrix fibrils of fibronectin (Singer 1979) and Types I and III procollagen (Furcht et al 1980). It has been suggested (Singer et al 1984) that a fibronexus is a cohesive complex which transmits the collective forces generated by contraction of all the myofibroblasts of the granulation tissue to the wound margins, thereby effecting wound contraction.

The mechanism by which myofibroblasts or fibroblasts generate the contractile force needed for wound contraction is still unresolved. According to Gabbiani et al (1971) the contractile force is due to the muscle-like cellular contraction of myoblasts (the cell contraction-myoblast theory) whereas more recently the cell traction-fibroblast theory has been proposed (Ehrlich & Rajaratnam 1990). According to the latter, wound contraction is due to the traction-like activity of fibroblasts on the matrix of the wound bed.

Angiogenesis. This is a vital part of the proliferative phrase of dermal repair. Without it invasion of the wound bed by macrophages and fibroblasts would cease through lack of oxygen and nutrients. In vitro studies have shown that capillary endothelial cells release collagenase in response to angiogenic factors. This degrades the collagen of the basement membrane which later fragments, per-mitting migration of endothelial cells into the perivascular spaces, where they form buds which are added to by the proliferation of cells within and near the parent vessel (Kalebic et al 1983). During dermal repair these buds grow rapidly towards the free surface,

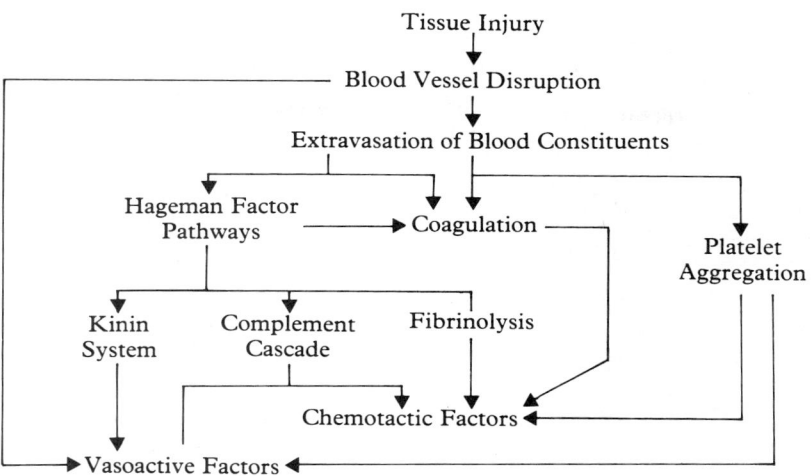

5.73   Mediator pathways of inflammation initiated by tissue injury. (After Clark 1985.)

where they branch at their tips and unite to form functional capillary loops. New buds then develop on these loops so that a superficial capillary plexus rapidly forms in the granulation tissue (**5**.76).

Although the factors responsible for angiogenesis during dermal repair remain unidentified, several candidates have been proposed. These include a macrophage-derived growth factor known to stimulate proliferation of endothelial cells in vitro (Martin et al 1981), low oxygen tension (Remensnyder & Majno 1968), lactic acid (Imre 1964), biogenic amines (Zauberman et al 1969) and hepatocyte growth factor. The last of these, also known as scatter factor, is a powerful mitogen and motility factor which acts through the tyrosine kinase receptor encoded by the metabolic equivalent (MET) proto-oncogene, stimulating endothelial cells to proliferate and migrate (Bussolino et al 1992). Endothelial migration may be more significant than proliferation during angiogenesis after injury. If so, then chemotactic factors will play a key role in vivo. Such factors include platelet-derived substances (Wall et al 1978), heparin (Azizkhan et al 1980) and fibronectin (Bowersox & Sorgente 1982). Successful angiogenesis depends not only on chemotactic and mitogenic factors, but also on the presence of a suitable substrate over which migration of endothelial cells can occur. This may be produced, at least partly, by the endothelial cells themselves, since they have been shown to synthesize fibronectin (Birdwell et al 1978) and collagen (Madri & Stenn 1982).

Remodelling

Just as the proliferative overlaps the inflammatory phase, so remodel-

ling overlaps proliferation. During remodelling the highly cellular and highly vascular granulation tissue is gradually replaced by scar tissue with few cells and blood vessels. During the process of remodelling, which may occupy months or even years, most of the fibronectin is removed from the matrix and there is a slow accumulation of large bundles of Type I collagen fibres which, as they form cross-links, increase the tensile strength of the scar tissue. Changes in the arrangement of the collagen with time after injury have been studied by scanning electron microscopy (Forrester 1973). When it first appears in the granulation tissue of the wound bed it forms randomly arranged fibrils, which gradually develop into large irregular masses without evidence of any fibrillar substructure. The absence of the characteristic pattern found in uninjured dermis may be associated with the decrease in extensibility and tensile strength which are typical of scar tissue. During subsequent remodelling, the orientation of fibres becomes less random and its strength increases. This change may be caused by the action of mechanical forces exerted on the scar during normal usage to produce orientation of the collagen fibrils in the scar tissue and improve its mechanical function, so that it resembles uninjured dermis more closely.

Such forces may also produce a piezo-electric effect which affects the arrangement of collagen fibrils and fibres. There is now convincing evidence that the pattern of collagen within granulation and scar tissue can be altered by local forces, i.e. that remodelling occurs (Forrester 1973). As long ago as 1892 Wolff noted that bone responded structurally to functional demands. It is likely that scar tissue responds in a similar manner.

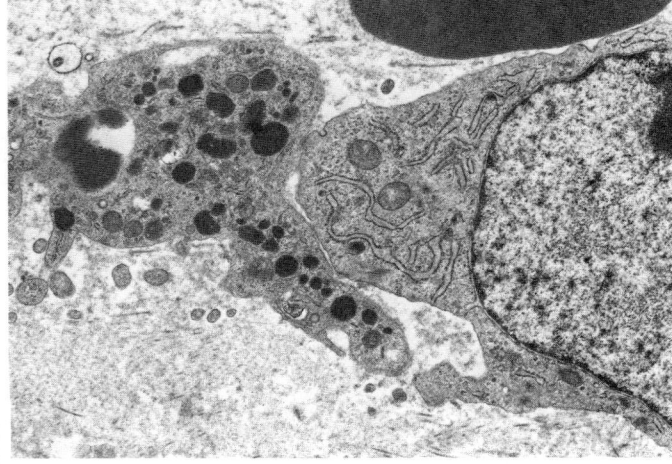

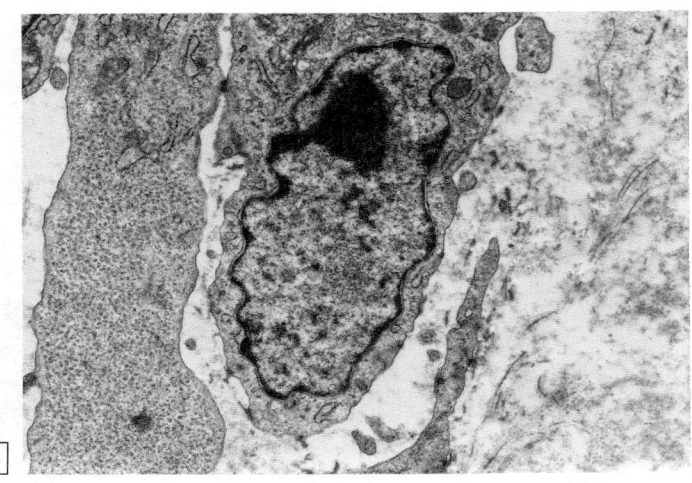

5.74   Electron micrograph showing intercellular contact between: (A) a macrophage and fibroblast in a healing, full thickness skin lesion, 3 days after trauma; (B) two myofibroblasts in a similar lesion, 7 days after trauma.

Magnification ×8000. (Provided by Rachel Hickman, Department of Anatomy, UMDS, Guy's Campus, London.)

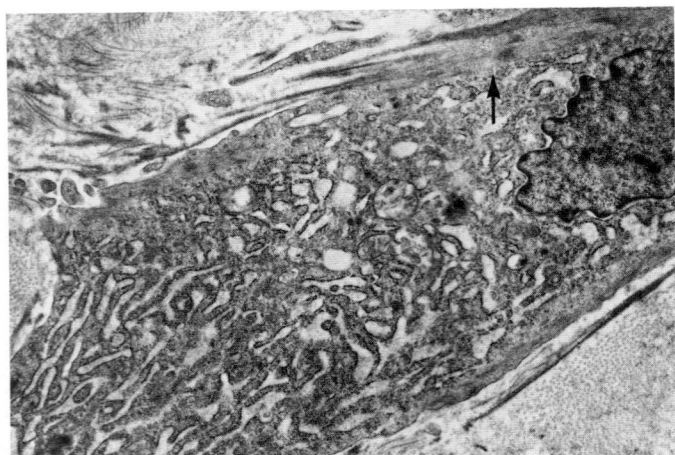

5.75 Electron micrograph showing a fibronexus, a region at the surface of a myofibroblast where there is an alignment between intracellular filaments and fibrils of the extracellular matrix (arrow). Magnification × 8000. (Provided by Rachel Hickman, Department of Anatomy, UMDS, Guy's Campus, London.)

Scar tissue is functionally inferior to the uninjured dermis, and methods of improving the quality of repair by inducing scarless healing are being sought. In the fetus, cutaneous wounds heal with either little or no scarring, whereas postnatally scar tissue develops at the wound site. Whitby and Ferguson (1991) in a comparison of fetal, neonatal and adult wound healing have found that the virtually scarless healing of fetal wounds is associated with the absence of transforming growth factor-β (TGF-β) and basic fibroblast growth factor (b-FGF), and with the early deposition of fibronectin and tenascin. This has led to attempts to decrease scarring in postnatal wounds by administering neutralizing antibodies to TGF-β, with some success (Shah et al 1992). Recently the effects of the TGF-β isoforms 1, 2 and 3 on scarring have been investigated (Levine et al 1993); TGF-β1 and TGF-β2 stimulate scarring whereas TGF-β3 appears to reduce it. The addition of mannose-6-phosphate which inhibits TGF-β activation also reduces scarring and improves the quality of wound healing (Ferguson 1994). Manipulation of the growth factor profile at the wound site by neutralizing some factors

and encouraging the synthesis of others may lead to improvement in the quality and rate of the healing response following injury.

The cellular changes involved in dermal repair can be accelerated by treatments which improve the microenvironment of the wound (Dyson et al 1988) and by application of electrotherapy modalities which increase the rate of ingress of macrophages (Dyson 1987, Dyson & Young 1986), possibly by temporarily modifying their membrane structure. The use of such techniques has considerable clinical and surgical significance.

Until recently many of the reports of the clinical effectiveness of these and other techniques designed to improve the rate and quality of repair were based either on the subjective assessment of the progress of healing or on invasive techniques which inevitably interfered with the healing process by inflicting a further injury. The need for non-invasive, painless, objective methods of assessment has led to the development of high-resolution diagnostic ultrasound scanners in which changes in the ultrasonograms of the wound bed can be quantified by means of image analysis in which fractal signatures are produced of regions of interest (ROIs) of the ultrasonograms (Whiston et al 1992). A typical ultrasonic image of an incised cutaneous wound is shown in **5.77**. Changes in fractal signatures obtained of ROIs of such images during the healing process are shown in **5.78**. As healing progresses, the fractal signatures of the wound bed approach that of intact skin. Should the wound deteriorate, this process is reversed, the fractal signature becoming less similar to that of intact skin. This technique has been used to identify adverse changes at operation sites in renal transplant patients undergoing graft rejection (Calvin et al 1994). The technique can also be used to monitor the development of scar tissue at the wound site.

EPIDERMAL REGENERATION

Changes in the epidermis leading to re-epithelialization begin within a few hours of the formation of a cutaneous wound. Intact keratinocytes at the free edge of the cut epidermis begin to migrate across the defect (Winter 1962). Migration is made possible by a change in gene expression of the cells, involving temporary dissolution of hemidesmosomes and desmosomes (p. 382), freeing the cells to move, and the formation of peripherally located actin filaments enabling them to do so (Gabbiani et al 1978). They also acquire a unique phenotype, termed the phenotype of regenerative maturation (Mansbridge & Knapp 1987), possibly as a result of exposure to low extracellular calcium concentrations (Hennings et al 1980; Clark

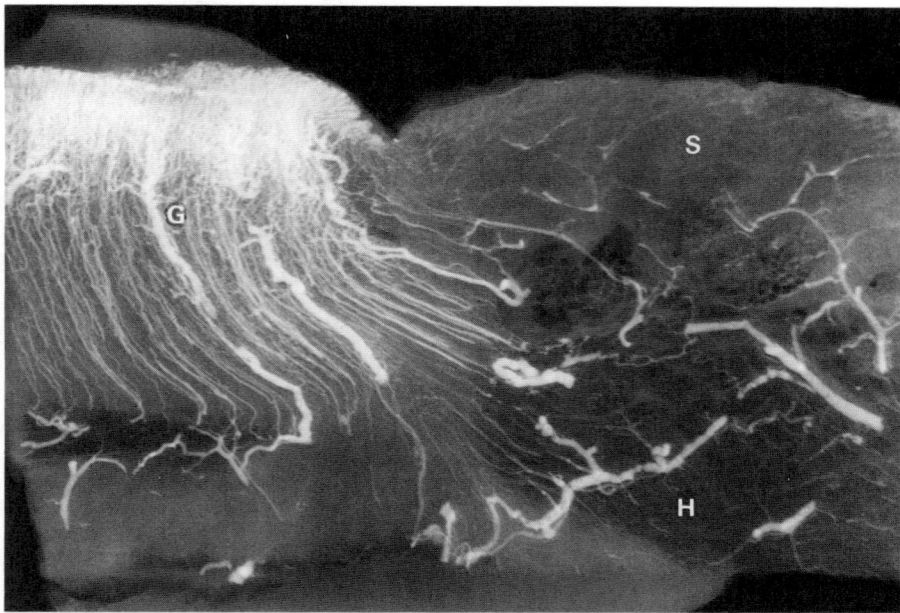

5.76 Microangiograph of a transverse section of granulation tissue (G) showing its invasion by new blood vessels; adjacent intact skin (S), and hypodermis (H) are also visible. The specimen was perfused with barium sulphate and gelatin 10 days after the production of a full-thickness excised lesion in porcine skin. The majority of the regenerating vessels lie at right angles to the surface and are linked by a superficially located capillary plexus. Magnification × 130. (Provided by S Young, Department of Anatomy, UMDS, Guy's Campus, London.)

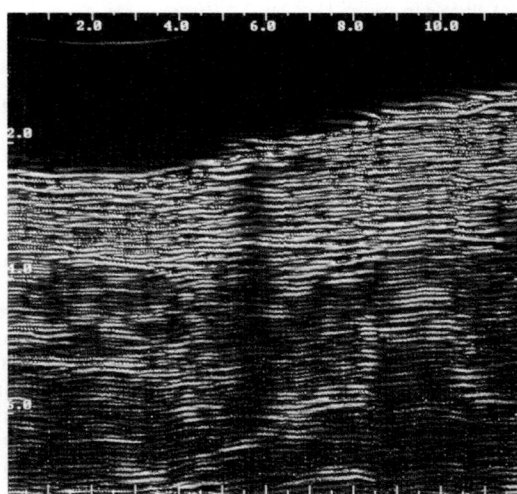

5.77 High resolution ultrasonogram of skin and subcutaneous tissue containing an incised wound identifiable by reduced echogenicity. (Provided by S Young, Department of Anatomy and Cell Biology, UMDS, Guy's Campus, London.)

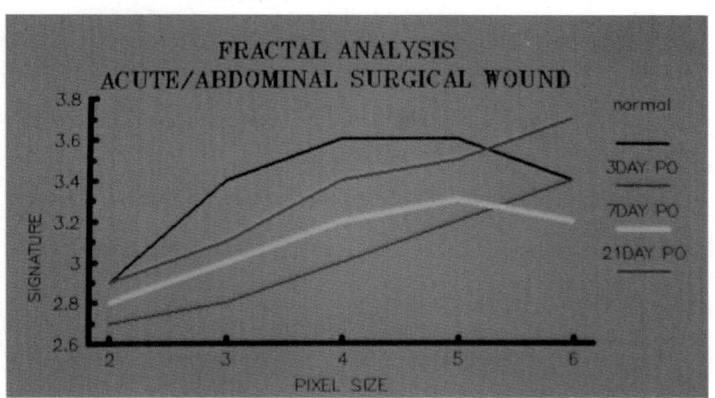

5.78 Fractal signatures obtained from high resolution ultrasonograms of an incised cutaneous wound during the inflammatory (3-day PO), proliferative (7-day PO) and remodelling (21-day PO) phases of healing, together with the signature obtained from the skin prior to injury. As healing progresses the fractal signatures of the ultrasonograms of the injured skin approach that of intact skin. PO = postoperative. (Provided by S Young, Department of Anatomy and Cell Biology, UMDS, Guy's Campus, London.)

1990). According to the 'leap-frog' hypothesis of epidermal regeneration (Winter 1962, 1964), cells superficial to the stratum basale at the edges of the wound elongate laterally and crawl over each other until they make contact with the wound bed; they then cease to move and begin to divide, producing a new supply of cells, some of which add to the thickness of the regenerating epidermis. Meanwhile other cells migrate over the first cells, reach the wound bed, divide and repeat the process in 'leap-frog' fashion until prevented from doing so by contact inhibition. According to this hypothesis no single keratinocyte moves more than about four or five cell diameters (approximately 40 μm) from its original position during epidermal regeneration. Within 48 hours of injury the basal keratinocytes of the new epidermis begin to divide, generating more cells capable of migration (Hell & Cruickshank 1963). The stimulus for epidermal proliferation after injury is still unknown. It may be the removal of an inhibitory chalone (Bullough & Laurence 1961) and/or the release of epidermal growth factors (Cohen 1965).

In shallow, partial thickness wounds of thin skin, each cut hair follicle acts as a source of reparative epidermal stem cells. These cells can be recognized by their ability to form a characteristic stem cell keratin (Type 19). After migration and division, they produce cells which manufacture other keratins (Types 9 and 16) which allow the cells to remain sufficiently flexible to migrate over the wound bed. Later products of keratinocyte division produce more rigid keratins (Types 1 and 10), typical of mature epidermis.

If the injury is sufficient to disrupt the basement membrane, the keratinocytes migrate over a temporary matrix of fibronectin, fibrin

and Type V collagen (Clark et al 1982; Repesh et al 1982; Donaldson & Mahan 1983). Keratinocytes have been shown to secrete fibronectin in vitro (Kariniemi et al 1982; O'Keefe et al 1984; Kubo et al 1984) so it is possible that they may produce at least part of the matrix over which they migrate. TGF-β encourages epithelial cell migration (Yang & Moses 1990) and stimulates fibronectin deposition (Nickoloff et al 1988). Once migration ceases, the temporary matrix is replaced by basement membrane.

Regeneration of the basement membrane zone occurs in sequential stages. Bullous pemphigoid antigen (p. 397) is always present between the basal plasma membrane of the migrating cells and the temporary matrix and can thus be considered to be the first part of the basement membrane to regenerate (Stanley et al 1981; Clark et al 1982). Once the epidermal cells cease to migrate, first Type IV collagen and then laminin become incorporated in the regenerating basal lamina (Clark et al 1982).

If the migrating keratinocytes make contact with small foreign particles of approximately 1 μm in size, the cells may remove them by phagocytosis (Odland & Ross 1968), possibly after opsonization by fibronectin (Takashima & Grinnell 1984). The keratinocytes migrate deep to any larger particles and dead tissues which lie in their path. Secretion of plasminogen activators (Isseroff et al 1982), collagenases and neutral proteases (Donoff et al 1971) by the keratinocytes may help to clear the way for their migration.

Once re-epithelialization is complete, the keratinocytes revert to their original phenotype (Clark 1985).

BREASTS (MAMMAE)

INTRODUCTION

In humans and other mammals the breasts form a secondary sexual feature of females and are the source of nutrition for the neonate, although they are also present in a rudimentary form in males. Developmentally they are derived from modified sweat glands (5.79). In females, major growth and differentiation of breast tissues occurs after puberty to give rise to a complex structure, predominantly composed (in the non-lactating breast) of adipose tissue surrounding

epithelial secretory tissue arranged in 15–20 lobes, each leading to a lactiferous duct which converges with the others upon the nipple. Connective tissue, blood vessels, lymphatics and nerves also contribute to breast structure. A specialized area of skin, the *areola*, surrounds the base of the nipple. The breasts are the site of malignant change in as many as one in ten women, and the biology of their tissues is at present the focus of much clinical research. For reviews of normal breast structure, see: Cowie (1974), Pitelka (1983), Ellis et al (1993), and Fawcett (1994).

417

FEMALE BREAST

In young adult females, each breast is a rounded eminence lying within the superficial fascia, chiefly anterior to the upper thorax but spreading laterally to a variable extent (**5.**79). Breast shape and size depend upon genetic, racial and dietary factors, together with age, parity and menopausal status of the individual, being hemispherical, conical, variably pendulous, piriform or thin and flattened. In the adult female the base of the breast (its attached surface) extends vertically from the second or third to the sixth rib, and in the transverse plane, from the sternal edge, medially, almost to the midaxillary line laterally. The superolateral quadrant is prolonged towards the axilla along the inferolateral edge of pectoralis major, from which it projects a little, and may extend through the deep fascia up to the apex of the axilla (the axillary tail of Spence).

The breast lies upon the deep pectoral fascia, which in turn overlies pectoralis major and serratus anterior, and below, obliquus externus abdominis and its aponeurosis as that forms the anterior wall of the sheath of rectus abdominis. Between the breast and the deep fascia is loose connective tissue in the retromammary (submammary) 'space', which allows the breast some degree of movement on the deep pectoral fascia. (Advanced mammary carcinoma may, by invasion, fix the breast to pectoralis major.) Occasionally, small projections of glandular tissue may pass through the deep fascia into the underlying muscle in normal subjects.

Before describing the general organization of the breast, the structure of the nipple and areola will be considered.

NIPPLE (MAMMARY PAPILLA)

The nipple (**5.**79, 80) projects centrally from the anterior aspect; its shape varies from conical to flattened, depending on nervous, hormonal, developmental and other factors. Its level in the thorax varies widely but is at the fourth intercostal space in most young women, and in the nulliparous it is pink or light brown or darker, depending on the general melanization of the body. It is covered by hairless skin; the epidermis has a deeply folded base interdigitating with dermal papillae, and scattered sebaceous glands open on to its surface. Melanocytes are quite numerous, giving the skin of the nipple a darker hue. Internally the nipple is composed mostly of collagenous dense connective tissue with numerous elastic fibres which also spread beneath the areola, wrinkling the overlying skin. Smooth muscle cells are also present in and just deep to the nipple, disposed in a predominantly circular direction and radiating out from its base into the surrounding breast; their contraction, induced by cold or tactile (e.g. in suckling), or emotional stimuli causes erection of the nipple and wrinkling of the surrounding areola. The lactiferous ducts traverse the nipple, their 15–20 minute orifices opening on to its wrinkled tip. Near its opening at the nipple each of these ducts is slightly expanded as a *lactiferous sinus* in the lactating breast by the presence of milk. Occasionally the nipple may not evert during prenatal development (p. 296), remaining permanently retracted and so causing difficulty in suckling.

AREOLA

The areola is a discoidal area of skin which encircles the base of the nipple (**5.**79, 80); its colour also varies from pink to dark brown depending on parity and race. Darkening of the nipple and areola occurs during the second month of pregnancy, and although it becomes a little paler after parturition, the change of hue is permanent. The nipple and especially the areola contains many sebaceous glands much enlarged in pregnancy and lactation as subcutaneous 'tubercles', whose oily secretion is a protective lubricant during lactation. Other glands (*areolar glands of Montgomery*) are intermediate in structure between lactiferous and sweat glands; when visible to the naked eye they are creamy in colour. At the perimeter of the areola are large sudorific and sebaceous glands, the latter not accompanied by hairs. There is no adipose tissue immediately beneath the skin of the areola and papilla.

INTERNAL ORGANIZATION OF THE BREAST

The breast (**5.**79, 81–88) contains:

- epithelial glandular tissue of the tubulo-alveolar type
- fibrous connective tissue (stroma) surrounding the glandular tissue
- interlobar adipose tissue (Cowie 1974).

Glandular tissue. This consists of branching *ducts* and terminal secretory *lobules* (**5.**81–85). The ducts converge on to the 15–20 larger lactiferous ducts which open on to the apex of the nipple. Each lactiferous duct is therefore connected to a tree-like system of ducts and lobules, enclosed and intermingled with connective tissue stroma, collectively forming a *lobe* of the mammary gland; the number of lobes is, therefore, the same as the number of lactiferous ducts. Although the lobes are usually depicted as discrete anatomical territories within the breast, they grow into one another around their edges so that they do not appear as distinct entities during surgery.

Lobules consist of the portions of the glands that are secretory (or potentially so). Their structure varies according to hormonal status (see below), but in the mature breast each lobule consists of several blind-ending branches or expansions, the *alveoli* (*acini*), converging on an *alveolar duct*, and these are the sites of milk secretion.

Breast cancers arise at the junction of the lobules and ducts, and as they increase in size they lead to fibrous tissue formation so that they are hard and irregular.

Stroma of the breast. The connective tissue *stroma* penetrates between and encloses the lobules, where it has a loose texture, allowing the rapid expansion of secretory tissue during pregnancy (**5.**79, 84). Fibrous condensations of stromal tissue extend from the ducts to the dermis, and these are often well developed in the upper part of the breast as the *suspensory ligaments* (*of Astley Cooper*), which assist in the support of the breast tissue. Pathologically, these may be contracted by fibrosis in carcinoma, causing retraction or pitting of the overlying skin. Elsewhere in the normal breast, fibrous tissue surrounding the glandular components extends to the skin and nipple, assisting in the mechanical coherence of the gland.

Adipose tissue. Highly variable in amount, this is typically present in the interlobar stroma, and not amongst the lobules.

BREAST DEVELOPMENT

Prenatal development

Prenatal development is similar in both sexes, with the epithelial mammary bud appearing at a gestational age of 35 days; by day 37 this has become a mammary line extending from the axilla through to the inguinal region (see also **5.**79). Usually invagination of the thoracic mammary bud into the mesenchyme occurs by day 49, with involution of the remaining mammary line, although accessory breast tissue may be present in adults anywhere along the milk line (polythelia), usually in the thoracic region (90%) but also occasionally in the axillary (5%) or abdominal (5%). Nipple formation begins at day 56 and primitive ducts (mammary sprouts) develop at 84 days with canalization occurring at about the 150th day. In either sex, there may be no breast development (amastia), or alternatively there may be nipple development but no breast tissue (amazia). Rarely, the nipple may not develop (athelia) although this occurs more commonly in accessory breast tissue. At birth the combination of fetal prolactin and maternal oestrogen may give rise to transient hyperplasia and secretion of 'witch's milk'. (A fuller account of prenatal development is given on p. 296.)

Postnatal development

Lobule formation occurs (exclusively in females) after puberty (**5.**79), when there is branching of ducts and development of lobules from terminal ducts. Externally recognizable breast development (thelarche) from puberty onwards can be divided into five separate phases. In *phase I* there is elevation of the nipple. In *phase II* glandular subareolar tissue is present with both nipple and breast projecting from the chest wall as a single mass. *Phase III* encompasses increase in diameter and pigmentation of the areola, with proliferation of palpable breast tissue. During *phase IV* there is further pigmentation and enlargement in the areola so that the nipple and areola form a secondary mass anterior to the main part of the breast. Finally, in *phase V* there is development of a smooth contour to the

5.79 (*opposite*) Postnatal development and structure of the female breast.

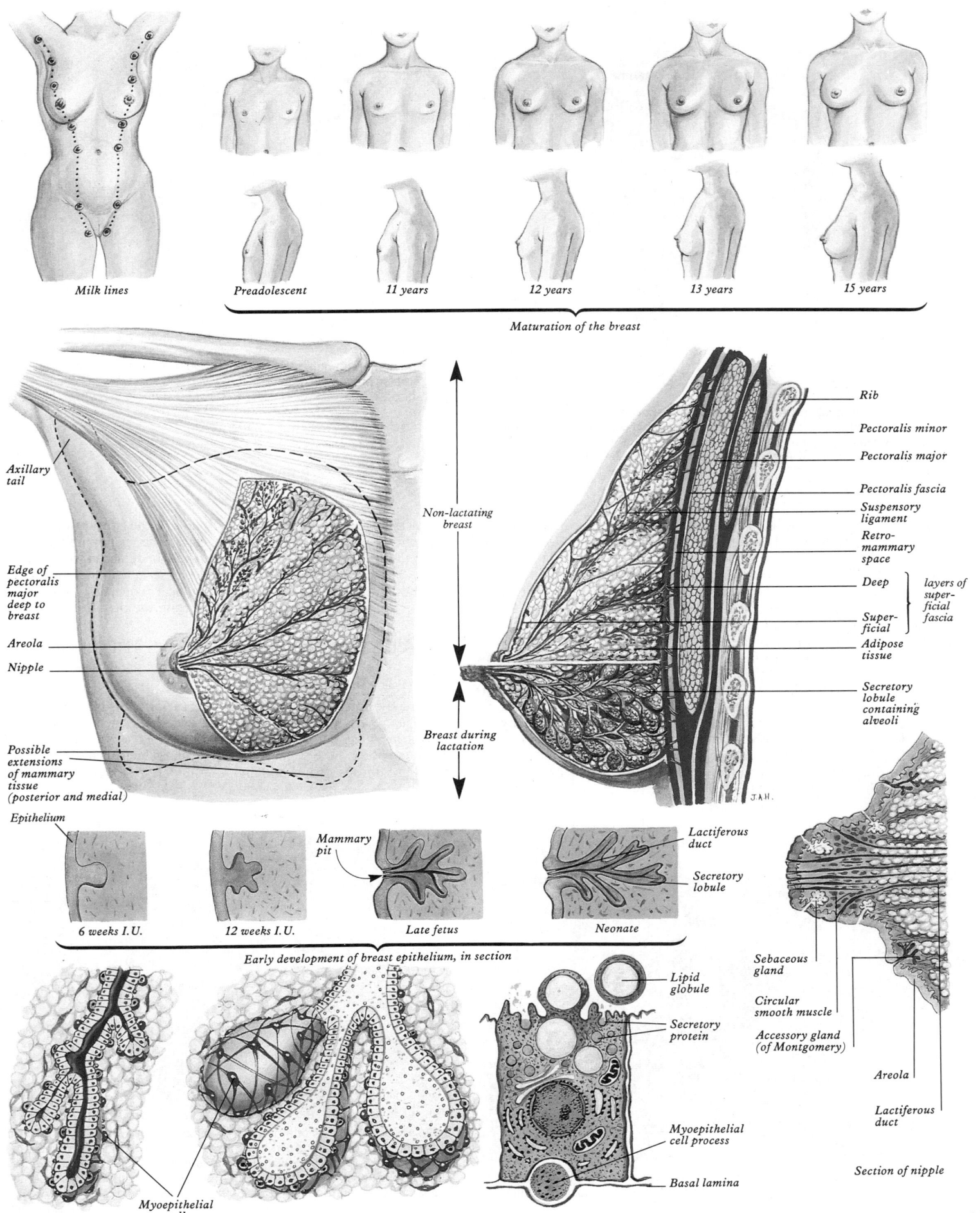

Milk lines

Preadolescent

11 years

12 years

13 years

15 years

Maturation of the breast

Axillary tail

Edge of pectoralis major deep to breast

Areola

Nipple

Possible extensions of mammary tissue (posterior and medial)

Non-lactating breast

Breast during lactation

Rib

Pectoralis minor

Pectoralis major

Pectoralis fascia

Suspensory ligament

Retro-mammary space

Deep

Super-ficial

layers of super-ficial fascia

Adipose tissue

Secretory lobule containing alveoli

Epithelium

Mammary pit

Lactiferous duct

Secretory lobule

6 weeks I.U.

12 weeks I.U.

Late fetus

Neonate

Early development of breast epithelium, in section

Sebaceous gland

Circular smooth muscle

Accessory gland (of Montgomery)

Areola

Lactiferous duct

Section of nipple

Lipid globule

Secretory protein

Myoepithelial cell process

Basal lamina

Myoepithelial cell

HISTOLOGY: Non-lactating (Nulliparous)

Lactating

Ultrastructure of secretory cell

419

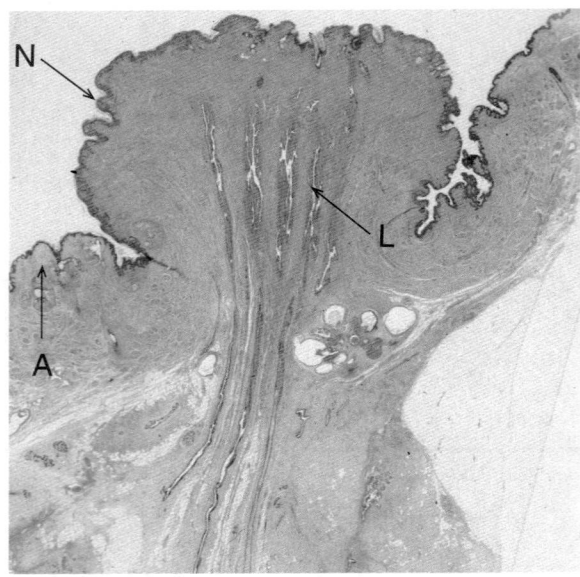

5.80 Vertical section through female nipple, showing corrugated epithelium over the nipple surface (N), the surrounding areola (A), and lactiferous ducts (L). Haematoxylin and eosin. Magnification ×6. (Photography by Sarah Smith, Department of Anatomy and Cell Biology, UMDS, Guy's Campus, London.)

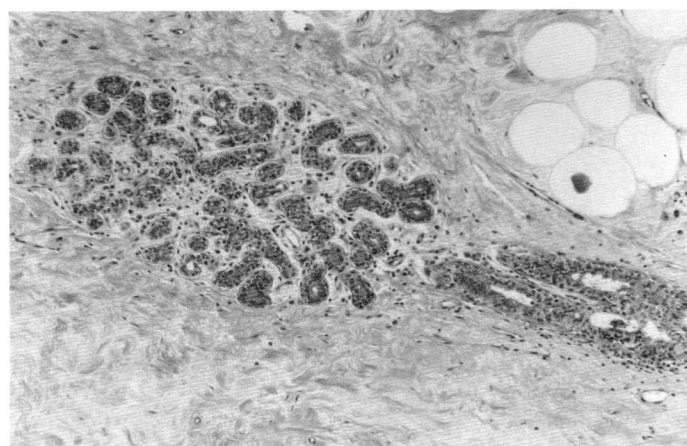

5.81 Normal non-lactating lobule with terminal duct, human breast. The duct can be seen leading to the lobule which is composed of multiple, small acini set within a loose intralobular stroma. The denser, interlobular stroma can be seen surrounding the lobule and duct. A small amount of adipose tissue is also present top right. Haematoxylin and eosin. Magnification ×450. (Provided by Dr Rosemary Millis, Consultant Pathologist, Guy's Hospital, London.)

breast. For further details of breast development, see page 296; for reviews: see Knight and Peaker (1982) and Anbazhagan et al (1991).

Pregnancy

Changes during this period are associated with further duct and lobule proliferation and epithelial growth, consisting mainly of an increase in the number of alveoli per lobule (5.84). This is completed by the sixth month of pregnancy after which the breast expands further with the increase in blood flow and secretion of colostrum (see below). Total weight gain of each breast during pregnancy is about 400 g. True lactation starts within 1–4 days after parturition and may continue for as long as $3\frac{1}{2}$ years if frequent suckling is maintained. When lactation ceases there is a progressive atrophy of the lobules and ducts, with fatty replacement of breast tissue.

Changes also occur during the menstrual cycle, with an increase in size during midcycle, mainly due to a transient increase in blood flow, with consequent greater hydration of the stromal tissue; minor changes have been reported in epithelial structure too (see below), especially during the second half (luteal phase) of the cycle. With

increasing age various changes take place in the proportions of the different components of the breast; after the menopause there is involution of the glandular tissue which may be replaced with adipose tissue, or the breast may gradually decrease in volume, and many other alterations take place in the mechanical properties, for example elasticity of the connective tissue supporting the breast.

DETAILED MICROSTRUCTURE OF THE BREAST

Before pregnancy

As already noted, mammary structure varies with age, time in the menstrual cycle, pregnancy and lactation. In the neonate there are lactiferous ducts but no alveoli, and until puberty little branching of the ducts occurs, the slight mammary enlargement being due to the growth of fibrous stroma and fat. After puberty, the ducts, stimulated

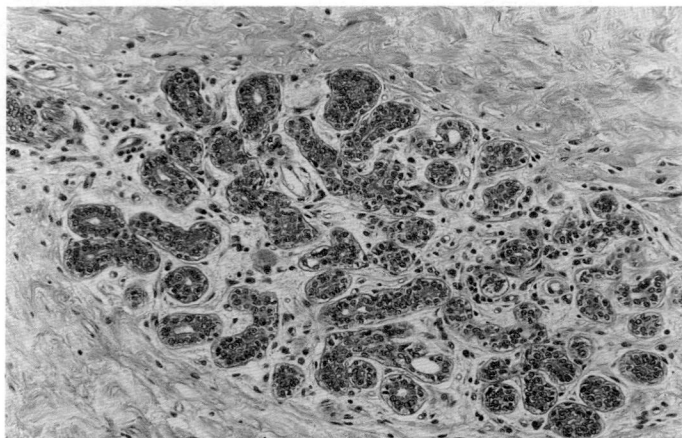

5.82 Normal non-lactating terminal duct lobular unit. The terminal duct can just be seen to the left of the picture. The lobule is composed of numerous acini. Haematoxylin and eosin. Magnification ×450. (Provided by Dr Rosemary Millis, Consultant Pathologist, Guy's Hospital, London.)

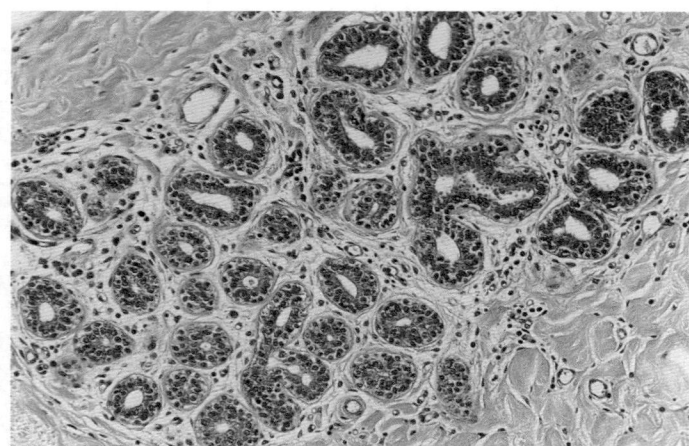

5.83 High power view of a non-lactating lobule. The two cell type lining of the acini can be clearly seen with the inner luminal epithelium and outer myoepithelial layer. The eosinophilic basement membrane can also be discerned. The loose intralobular stroma contrasts with the denser, interlobular stroma surrounding the lobule. Haematoxylin and eosin. Magnification ×800. (Provided by Dr Rosemary Millis, Consultant Pathologist, Guy's Hospital, London.)

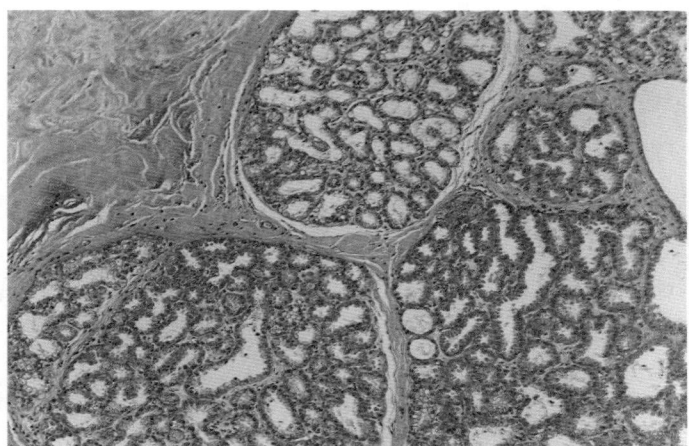

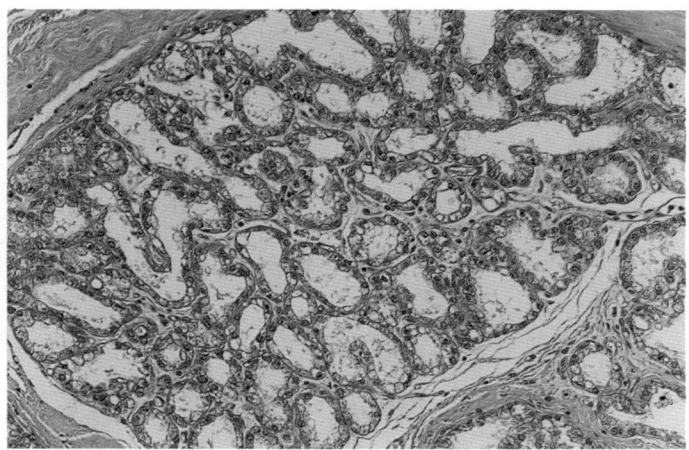

5.84 Lactating breast. The lobules are greatly expanded. Many more acini are present lined by cells showing evidence of secretory activity. The intralobular stroma has largely been displaced. Haematoxylin and eosin. Magnification × 450. (Provided by Dr Rosemary Millis, Consultant Pathologist, Guy's Hospital, London.)

5.85 High power view of lactating breast. The enlarged lobule, composed of multiple distended acini, can be seen. The vacuolated cytoplasm of the secretory epithelium is clearly visible. Myoepithelium is difficult to see. Haematoxylin and eosin. Magnification × 450. (Provided by Dr Rosemary Millis, Consultant Pathologist, Guy's Hospital, London.)

by ovarian oestrogens, develop branches whose ends form solid, spheroidal masses of granular polyhedral cells, which are potential alveoli (Stirling & Chandler 1977). In the resting state the glandular epithelium is separated from the vascular stroma by a thin avascular zone of fibroblasts (**5.83**). This 'epitheliostromal junction' may control the passage of materials to the secretory cells (Ozzello 1974) and have other important controlling influences on breast biology, mediating the actions of hormones on growth, cell division and secretion.

Ductal system. For most of their lengths, the ducts are lined by columnar epithelium (**5.81–83**); in the larger ducts these are two cells thick, but in the smaller ones only a single layer of columnar (*luminal*) cells is present. The bases of these are in close contact with numerous *myoepithelial* (*basal*) cells which invaginate their bases (**5.87**), and are so frequent that they form a distinct layer surrounding the ducts and alveoli, giving the epithelium a bilaminar appearance.

Close to the openings of the lactiferous ducts on to the nipple surface, their stratified cuboidal lining gives way to keratinized stratified squamous epithelium continuous with the epidermis; shed squames may sometimes block the duct apertures in the non-pregnant breast. External to the epithelial lining is a *basement membrane* (**5.86**)

composed of a thin *basal lamina* and a more extensive external *reticular region* blending with the stroma. The structure of the ductal complex varies with development and hormonal status, postpubertal maturation, the menstrual cycle, pregnancy and age-related regression. These factors have considerable effect on the microscopic structure of the deeper parts of the ducts (see below).

During the menstrual cycle

Demonstrable changes occur to the breast tissues in the menstrual cycle (Fanger & Ree 1974; Ferguson et al 1992); in the follicular phase (days 3–14) the stroma becomes less dense and various changes take place in the ducts, including the expansion of their lumen, with occasional mitoses but no secretion. In the luteal phase (days 15–28) there is a progressive increase in stromal density; the ducts have an open lumen containing secretion, with flattening of epithelial cells. Cell proliferation, as measured by ^{3}[H]-thymidine labelling, is maximal on day 26. Thereafter, the ductal system undergoes reduction, with epithelial cell apoptosis greatest on day 28 of the cycle. These activities have considerable clinical significance in terms of the most appropriate timing for surgery related to carcinoma of the breast (see Fentiman 1993).

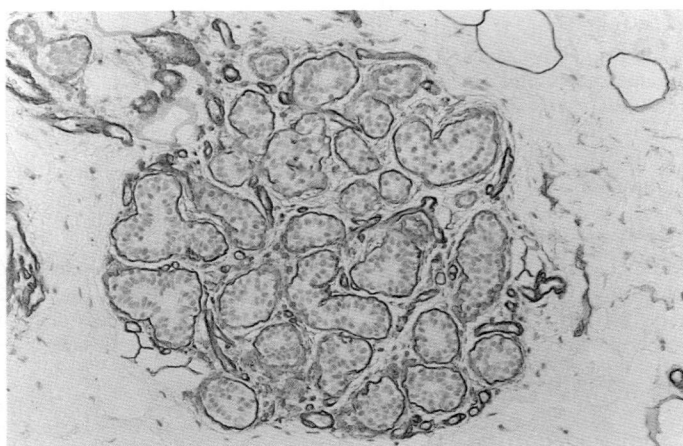

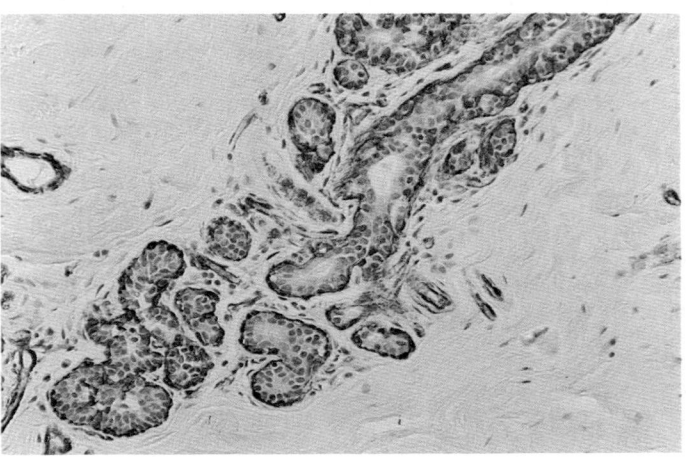

5.86 Normal non-lactating lobule stained by immunohistochemistry for collagen IV to demonstrate basement membrane. The acini of the lobule are clearly seen. Each lobule is surrounded by a well defined basement membrane. Basement membrane material can also be seen surrounding vessels and fat cells. (Immunoperoxidase method for collagen IV). Magnification × 450. (Provided by Dr Rosemary Millis, Consultant Pathologist, Guy's Hospital, London.)

5.87 Normal lobule. Stained by immunohistochemistry for actin to demonstrate myoepithelial cells. The terminal duct lobular unit can be seen. The myoepithelial cells have stained positively with the antibody to actin. A limiting ring of myoepithelial cells is seen around the ducts and acini. Staining is also demonstrated in vessel walls. (Immunohistochemistry for actin.) Magnification × 450. (Provided by Dr Rosemary Millis, Consultant Pathologist, Guy's Hospital, London.)

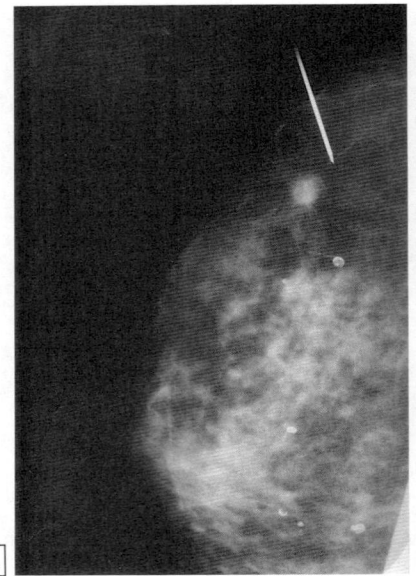 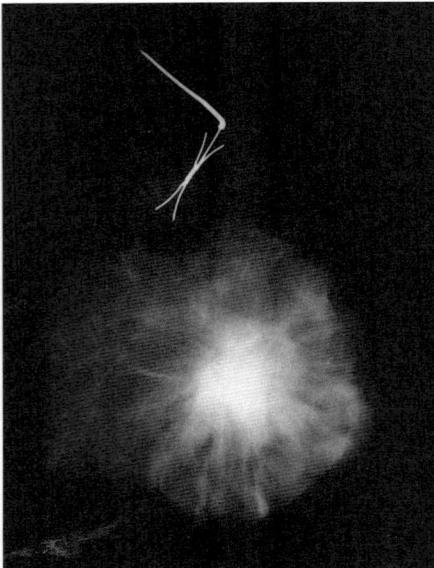 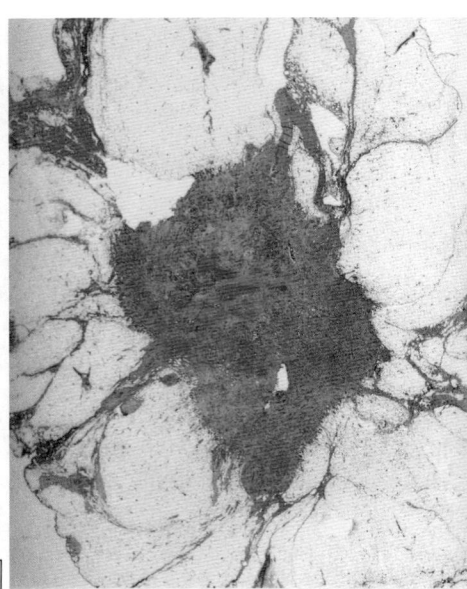

5.88 A mammogram (A), specimen radiograph (B) and histological section (C) of an infiltrating carcinoma.

A.   Mammogram of the breast with a rounded density in the upper half which has an irregular, spiculated margin. Adjacent to the density is a needle which has been inserted to localize the lesion for the surgeon prior to operation. Elsewhere in the breast foci of calcification are seen. These are large, single particles, with a smooth outline and are typical of benign calcifications.

B.   Radiograph of the surgical specimen after it has been removed from the patient. This confirms that the mammographic abnormality has been removed. Note the adjacent marker needle. The irregular margin of the rounded density can be more clearly seen in the specimen radiograph.
C.   Low power photomicrograph of the histological section showing the carcinoma in the centre with surrounding adipose tissue. The rather rounded outline of the tumour can be seen with an irregular margin which corresponds to the density seen on the radiograph. (Provided by Dr Rosemary Millis, Consultant Pathologist, Guy's Hospital, London.)

Immunolabelling shows that various antigens associated with the basal lamina of the ducts and alveoli, including laminin, Type IV collagen and fibronectin, undergo major changes during the cycle, whereas other stromal components are relatively unaffected (Ferguson et al 1992). This finding adds weight to the concept that the basal lamina is involved in the trophic control of secretory tissue behaviour.

In addition to these alterations there are changes in blood flow, which are greatest at midcycle, with a consequent increase in the water content of the stroma at that time.

In pregnancy and during suckling

As the output of placental oestrogen and progesterone rises during pregnancy, the ducts increase in the number and lengths of their branches; the secretory alveoli proliferate, and with the synthesis and secretion of milk the alveoli expand as their cells and lumen fill (5.84, 85). The myoepithelial cells, which are initially spindle-shaped, become highly branched stellate cells, especially around the alveoli. In the stroma there is a concomitant reduction in adipose tissue, but the numbers of lymphocytes including plasma cells, and of eosinophils increase greatly; blood flow through the breast also increases. The secretory activity in alveolar cells rises progressively in the latter half of pregnancy. Their product in late pregnancy and for a few days after parturition is different from the later milk and is known as *colostrum*; it contains many cytoplasmic fat globules and colostral corpuscles, which are a combination of epithelial cell membranes and macrophages, and is rich in immunoglobulins, conferring a measure of passive immunity to the neonatal alimentary tract (see also below); it also has laxative properties. True milk secretion begins a few days after parturition due to a reduction of circulating oestrogen and progesterone, a change which appears to stimulate production of prolactin by the anterior hypophysis (Wolstenholme & Knight 1972 and p. 1883). Milk distends the alveoli, at first lined by a single layer of granular, short columnar cells with stellate myoepitheliocytes near the basement membrane; the cells flatten as secretion increases. The columnar cells show accumulation of fat droplets which then undergo apocrine secretion into the lumen. After the onset of lactation there is a gradual reduction in the numbers of lymphocytes and eosinophils in the stroma, although plasma cells continue to synthesize IgA for secretion into the milk.

Postlactational breast

When lactation ceases the secretory tissue undergoes some involution, but the ducts and alveoli never return completely to the pre-pregnant state. Two major processes are responsible for the regression of the alveolar-ductal system, a reduction in epithelial cell size, and a reduction in their numbers. Size reduction appears to involve the formation of lysosomal autophagic vacuoles within the cells, reducing the numbers of their organelles and cytoplasmic volume. The loss of cells may be by apoptosis, some dead cells being shed into the lumen. At the same time, macrophages invade the stroma, and some of them also enter the alveolar/ductal lumen; in both of these sites they phagocytose dead epithelial cells, and also appear to modify or destroy the basal lamina of the epithelium, with consequent loss of epithelial cell activity which apparently depends on the integrity of this structure. Eventually, the numbers of lymphocytes and macrophages become reduced and gradually the breast tissue reverts to the resting state. If another pregnancy occurs the resting glandular tissue is reactivated, and the process outlined above recurs. Up to the age of about 50 increasing amounts of elastic tissue tend to be laid down around vessels and ducts (elastosis), and also in the stroma, although elastosis does not typically continue thereafter except in pathological changes (Martinez-Hernandez et al 1977; Farahmand & Cowan 1992).

Postmenopausal changes

After the menopause there is progressive atrophy of lobules and ducts, with fatty replacement of breast tissue, although a few ducts may remain (Ozzello 1974); the stroma becomes much less cellular and collagenous fibres decrease; the amount of adipose tissue varies widely between individuals, but the breast may return to a condition similar to the pre-pubertal state.

Cellular structure

As outlined above, the cells of the breast include:

- *epithelial cells*: alveolar, duct-lining and myoepithelial cells
- *connective tissue cells of the stroma*: fibroblasts, adipocytes, mast cells, macrophages, lymphocytes, neutrophils and eosinophils.

In addition there are cells associated with vessels and nerves.

Alveolar cells (5.79, 85, 88). As already stated, these display wide ultrastructural differences depending on the physiological state of the breast. In the resting state they are cuboidal. The apical surfaces are rich in microvilli and adjacent cells are joined around their apical ends by junctional complexes including tight junctions, adhering junctions and desmosomes; gap junctions are also present between these cells (Pitelka et al 1973). In lactation they increase in height initially to a columnar form, but as the alveoli distend with milk, stretching their epithelial linings, they may become cuboidal again. In the *secretory phase* when viewed by light microscopy, their apical cytoplasm is eosinophilic and vacuolated, and their apical surfaces often bulge into the alveolar lumen, distended by relatively huge secretory vacuoles; basally, their cytoplasm is basophilic. Ultra-structurally, the basal region possesses abundant granular endo-plasmic reticulum, mitochondria, lysosomes and free ribosomes. Apical to the basally-situated nucleus are a Golgi complex and large secretory vacuoles of two types, one proteinaceous and the other lipidic. *Protein vacuoles* contain multiple granules of micellar *casein* and other lactic proteins formed in the granular endoplasmic retic-ulum and passed to the Golgi apparatus to form larger vacuoles; these vacuoles are passed to the apical surface where they release their contents by membrane fusion (merocrine secretion). *Lipid vacuoles*, on the other hand, are formed directly in the apical cytoplasm as smaller lipid droplets which fuse with each other to create large 'milk vacuoles' up to 10 μm across, frequently protruding from the cell's surface. These are released as intact lipid droplets with a thin surround of apical plasma membrane and adjacent cytoplasm (Linzell & Peaker 1971; Saacke & Heald 1974; Hollmann 1974; Tobon & Salazar 1975; Pitelka & Hamamoto 1977; Hartmann 1991). This secretory process may be considered to be apocrine, since actual cytoplasm is lost with the secretion, although only minimally. In pregnant rats, other types of protein granule are also synthesized as precursors of normal granules; these may appear in colostrum (Murad 1970). Alveolar cells also take up IgA from adjacent plasma cells by endocytosis, and secrete it apically by a separate, merocrine mechanism.

Duct-lining (luminal) cells. The detailed structure of these varies with the diameter of the duct, but most of them are columnar to cuboidal in shape (5.81). They have relatively few organelles, and their nuclei are elliptical and euchromatic with a rim of condensed chromatin. Like other epithelial cells of the mammary gland the ductal cells are capable of cell division when hormonally stimulated, although it is not clear whether a distinctive stem cell population is responsible for this activity, or if all ductal cells can act in this capacity.

Myoepithelial cells (5.79, 87). These are similar to this type of cell in other glands (see pp. 71, 1695). In the mature mammary gland they are closely associated with the bases of alveolar and ductal cells and the long radiating, branched processes of adjacent myoepithelial cells intermesh to form a basket-like network around the alveoli and ducts, interposed between the basement membrane and the luminal cells. Internally they contain actin (5.87) and myosin filaments. Immunohistochemistry shows that they contain antigenic markers for epithelial features such as cytokeratins and also for smooth muscle (e.g. desmoplakins); a subpopulation is also positive for glial fibrillary acidic protein (GFAP) (see Viale et al 1991; Lazard et al 1993). On suitable hormonal stimulation by oxytocin they con-tract to expel the secretions into the larger ducts in readiness for suckling.

Stromal components. The cells of the stroma resemble those of other connective tissues elsewhere in the body. However, there is much evidence that they interact closely with the epithelial cells, and are an essential part of the hormonal regulatory system which controls the activity of the secretory tissue. This has been dem-onstrated for a number of stromal cell types in co-culture (including the numerous adipocytes) which are necessary for the stimulation of mammary epithelial cell growth and differentiation (Blum et al 1987). *B-* and *T-lymphocytes* are present throughout the stroma, but are particularly numerous around the ducts and alveoli, and also between the epithelial cells themselves. These cells provide immune sur-veillance of the stroma and epithelium; mature B-cells (plasmacytes) around the secretory regions are the source of immunoglobulins secreted during lactation. *Macrophages* have a distribution similar to that of lymphocytes, being both stromal and intraepithelial. In addition, some macrophages enter the lumen of the ducts, where they can phagocytose the shed epithelial cells, as noted above. Macrophages are also present in colostral milk although their sig-nificance in this respect is uncertain. Macrophages are important in regressional changes following lactation, where they dispose of degenerating epithelial cells. They are also likely to be important sources of growth factors and other chemical agents affecting the biology of the breast tissue, as they do elsewhere in the body (see p. 78).

LACTATION

The release of milk during suckling depends upon a combination of touch and negative pressure from the infant's lips on the nipple (Sala et al 1974). Stimulation of the abundant nerve terminals in the dermis of the nipple leads to oxytocin release, causing contraction of myoepithelial cells of the breast and the nipple's smooth muscle, increasing the pressure within the lactiferous ducts, and bringing about milk ejection. Cessation of suckling results in an increased intraluminal pressure which inhibits the secretory activity of the alveolar cells and subsequently the synthesis of milk.

Commonly lactation continues for 5 or 6 months after parturition, but then it progressively diminishes, according to demand, infants usually being weaned at about 9 months, although in some cultures suckling may be continued for over 3 years, during which the mother's ovulation is inhibited (see e.g. Thapa et al 1988). When lactation stops, the glandular tissue returns to the 'resting' condition, the remaining milk is absorbed and the alveoli shrink, many losing their lumina. However, due to hormonal and other disturbances, glandular tissue may fail to produce milk throughout pregnancy or secretion may cease within a few weeks of birth.

During lactation the volume of milk secretion by a mother is considerable, typically over 1100 ml/day (and nearly double this volume for twins). Amongst other nutrients, this creates a heavy demand for calcium which is obtained, as are other precursors of milk, from the circulation; interestingly, a hormone similar to parathyroid hormone has been shown to be secreted into the cir-culation from the lactating breast, assisting in the mobilization of calcium from storage sites in bones (Thiede & Rodan 1988).

Milk

Milk is a complex fluid, composed in humans of about 88% water, 7% lactose, 4% fat, 1% protein and various ions, notably calcium, sodium, potassium, phosphate and chloride. Vitamins and anti-bodies, mainly of the IgA (secretory) class, are present, the latter being largely responsible for the sterility of milk during lactation (Jenness 1974). The proteins are chiefly caseins and lactalbumin; these, with lactose and several triglycerides, are synthesized from circulating precursors by enzymes. Colostral milk is markedly differ-ent, poor in nutrients with an ionic composition like blood plasma. Table 5.1 sets out the composition of human milk. For details of lactation and human mammary structure see the review by Vorherr (1979).

Table 5.1 Major constituents of mature human milk		
Protein	total	10.6 g/l
Casein		
Lactalbumin		
Albumin		
Immunoglobulin		
Carbohydrate	total	78 g/l
Lactose		71 g/l
Oligosaccharide		6 g/l
Fucose		1 g/l
Fats	total	45.4 g/l
Water		897 g/l
Minerals		
Sodium		172 mg/l
Potassium		512 mg/l
Calcium		344 mg/l
Magnesium		35 mg/l

423

Vessels and nerves

Arteries. Supplying the female breasts are branches of the axillary artery, the internal thoracic artery, and some intercostal arteries, as follows:

- the *axillary artery* supplies blood to the breast via several branches: the supreme thoracic, the pectoral branches of the thoraco-acromial artery, the lateral thoracic and the subscapular artery;
- the *internal thoracic artery* gives perforating branches to the anteromedial part of the breast;
- the *second to fourth intercostal arteries* give perforating branches more laterally in the anterior thorax. The second perforating artery is usually the largest, supplying the upper region of the breast, and the nipple, areola and adjacent breast tissue (Bertelli & Valle Pereira 1994).

For further details, see page 1534).

Veins. Around the areola there is a circular venous plexus. From this and from the glandular tissue, blood drains in veins accompanying the arterial blood supply, i.e. to the axillary, internal thoracic and intercostal veins. Great individual variation may occur, and the axillary vein may be bifid. (See also p. 1592.)

Lymph vessels. The lymphatic drainage of the breast can be very variable (see Turner-Warwick 1959; also p. 1615). From the subareolar plexus (of Sappey) there are efferent vessels draining to the following:

- the contralateral breast
- the internal mammary lymph node chain, and thence via:

    1. the mediastinal lymph nodes to the para-aortic lymph nodes, bronchomediastinal trunks, thoracic duct and right thoracic duct

    2. inferiorly, the superior and inferior epigastric lymphatic routes to the groin

- the axillary lymph nodes, the predominant site of drainage from the breast. These number from 20–40; in the past these were named and grouped artificially as lower, central, subscapular, lateral and apical. Nowadays, a simpler nomenclature is generally adopted, based on the relation of the nodes to pectoralis minor. Those lying below pectoralis minor are the *low nodes* (level 1), those behind the muscle are the *middle group* (level 2), while the nodes between the upper border of pectoralis minor and the lower border of the clavicle are the *upper* or *apical nodes* (level 3). In addition, between pectoralis minor and major there may be one or two other nodes (*Rotter's nodes*). (See also p. 1613.)

Nerves. The nerve supply of the breast is derived from the anterior and lateral branches of the fourth to sixth intercostal nerves which carry sensory and sympathetic efferent fibres. The nipple supply is from the anterior branch of the lateral cutaneous ramus of T4; this forms an extensive nerve plexus within the nipple (see Miller & Kasahara 1959), its sensory fibres terminating close to the epithelium as free endings, Meissner corpuscles and Merkel disc endings (see p. 967). These are essential in signalling suckling to the central nervous system; however, secretory activities of the gland are largely controlled by ovarian and hypophyseal hormones rather than by efferent motor fibres.

CLINICAL ASPECTS OF THE FEMALE BREAST

Breast cancer (**5.88A–C**) is a common disease, particularly in post-menopausal women (see Wellings 1980; Fentiman 1993). Breast lumps may be classified into those with clinical signs suggesting malignancy (hard and regular, skin-tethering, muscle fixation, skin infiltration or oedema (peau d'orange)), and those which are mobile and without sinister signs. Investigations include needle aspiration which will drain cysts, or in the case of a solid lump, obtain cells for cytological evaluation. Additional investigations include mammography and ultrasonography which can distinguish cysts from solid lumps. A common problem in young women is the fibroadenoma, an overgrowth of a lobule.

If a breast lump has to be removed, incision should be based whenever possible on Langer's lines (p. 381) for best cosmetic results, although for women with larger lumps which may be malignant, the incision should be compatible with a possible subsequent mastectomy. Most women with single breast cancers up to 4 cm in diameter are treated by breast conservation rather than mastectomy. This is a combination of surgery (tumour excision and axillary lymph node sampling or clearance) together with external radiotherapy. Patients with larger tumours are treated by modified radical mastectomy with clearance of the axilla and preservation of the nerves to serratus anterior, latissumus dorsi and the lateral and medial pectoral nerves. Failure to preserve the nerve to serratus anterior will result in winging of the scapula and reduced function of the shoulder.

Patients with blood-stained nipple discharge without a palpable lump are treated by duct excision (microdochectomy) carried out through a circumareolar incision. Blood-stained nipple discharge is caused by either an intraduct papilloma, or duct extasia, and only rarely (5% of cases) is it due to malignancy.

The papillary ducts are radially orientated and incisions should hence also be radial. An obstructed lactiferous duct may distend as a galactocele. Abscesses may occur between the septa in the glandular tissue, subcutaneously near the papilla or between gland and deep fascia anterior to the pectoralis major.

Supernumerary mammae (polymastia) or papillae (polythelia) occur in males and females, usually along a line extending from the axilla to the pubic region, the milk line (**5.79**).

MALE BREAST

The male breast remains rudimentary throughout life. It is formed of small ducts (without lobules or alveoli) and a little supporting fibro-adipose tissue (see Ellis et al 1993). Sometimes the 'ducts' are largely solid cellular cords. Slight temporary enlargement may occur at puberty. The areola is well developed, although limited in area, and the nipple is relatively small (for surface anatomy, see Irstam 1962). It is usually stated that the ducts do not extend beyond the areola, but a recent survey (Cochrane et al 1992) has shown that although this is generally true, the limits of the glandular tissue may extend well beyond this boundary (35% in a sample of 40 cadavers). The male mamma may hypertrophy after puberty (gynaecomastia), usually due to imbalance between oestrogenic and androgenic hormones. (See pp. 1883, 1884, 1895 and 1905 for endocrine influences.) Male breast cancers comprise approximately 1% of all mammary malignancies (Crichlow & Galt 1990), and may include tissue beyond the areolar boundary.

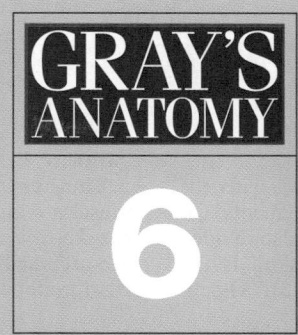

GRAY'S ANATOMY

6

SKELETAL SYSTEM

Section Editor: Roger W Soames

I am indebted to the late Professor John Pegington, friend and colleague, who, as original editor of this section provided the framework for combining osteology and arthrology into a single section: any shortcomings are mine and mine alone.

Many parts of the section have been revised and/or rewritten: histology (Professors Boyde and Jones), cervical column and craniovertebral joints (Mr Crockard and Dr Stevens), growth and development of the vertebral column (Dr Dangerfield). Essays on dating skeletal remains (Professor Day), imaging bones and joints (Dr Buckland-Wright) and arthroscopy of the knee (Mr Jackson) are included, in addition to surgically oriented essays on the major appendicular joints: shoulder (Professor Wallace and Dr Neumann), elbow (Mr Souter), wrist and hand (Mr Goddard and Mr McCullough), hip (Mr Muirhead-Allwood), knee (Mr Aichroth) and foot and ankle (Mr Helal).

MORPHOLOGY OF THE HUMAN SKELETON

INTRODUCTION

The human skeleton is bilaterally symmetrical (**6**.1, 2, 4), with the typical vertebrate pattern of an axis, divided into segments for flexibility, and of two pairs of limbs, pectoral and pelvic, also divided into jointed parts for locomotion, grasping, etc. The skull is the expanded and modified cranial end of the axis (**6**.3). Osseo-

cartilaginous sesamoid bones develop in some tendons and ligaments. All these elements are collectively termed the 'skeleton'.

The human skeleton, as in other vertebrates, is internal to the muscles with which it has evolved. It is an *endoskeleton*, unlike the *exoskeleton* of many invertebrates, such as *Insecta*, whose muscles are attached to the internal aspects of jointed elements of chitin, a rigid material also offering protection. Many features of the human

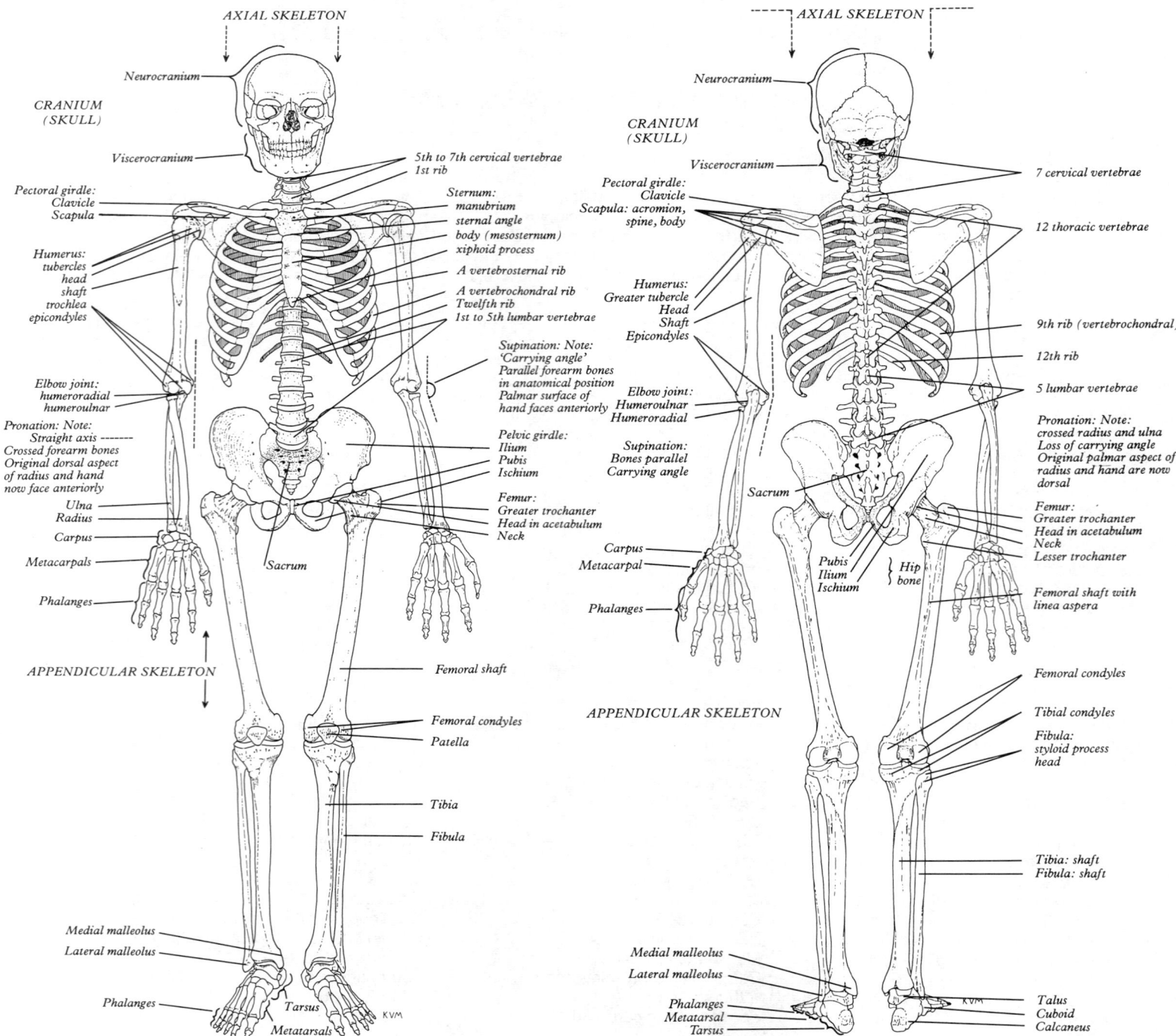

6.1   Adult male skeleton: anterior (ventral) view.

6.2   Adult male skeleton: posterior (dorsal) view.

endoskeleton are also deemed to be protective, sometimes to an extent sufficient to obscure its primary association with muscle and hence with movement. Perhaps only in the vault of the skull and spinal column is the protective role paramount, but even here there are muscle attachments. Cranially, its superficial situation reflects its evolutionary origin, as generally accepted, from the dermal bony armour of earlier vertebrates, including fish, amphibians and reptiles, both extinct and extant. The ossified dermal carapace of the tortoise is a familiar example. The maxilla, mandible, clavicle and dentine of teeth are also dermal derivatives; all are vestiges of more extensive assemblies of dermal bones from which they have been modified to form a human 'exoskeleton'.

Homologues of the branchial skeleton of fish also contribute a visceral component to the skeleton in higher vertebrates, including man. Much modified, these elements appear as ear ossicles, part of the mandible, maxilla, styloid process and hyoid bone. Some caudal branchial arches persist as the cartilaginous larynx, not usually included in the human skeleton; supportive tracheal and bronchial cartilages maintain the larger respiratory tubes, much as do the bones and cartilages of the nasal cavities. In some ungulates bone develops in cardiac connective tissue as an *os cordis*, while an *os penis* occurs in many mammals. The human skeleton is thus a complex, derived from original endoskeleton, exoskeletal dermal elements, modified branchial arches and ossification in structures such as tendons.

THE SKELETON IN LIFE

The living skeleton also includes other, non-osseous structures which are lost when bones are preserved for study since attached muscles, ligaments, periosteum and cartilages are all removed. Costal cartilages are, of course, grouped with the skeleton; but articular cartilages, functionally prominent parts of most living bones, are by custom excluded, as are ligaments, the menisci and intervertebral discs. A macerated skeleton, therefore, is completely disjointed into elements which, while convenient for examination, have lost most of their functional implications. The bone marrow also disappears, and mechanical properties such as elasticity, proper to living bone, are lost (Smith & Walmsley 1959).

The properties of living bone have been much studied (Bell 1956) at macroscopic, microscopic and ultrastructural levels, especially in relation to mechanical factors. Its intimate blend of hard inorganic and resilient organic components, almost equally resistant to compression and tension, differs from most materials used by man, which are usually better in one respect than the other. The tensile strength of bone resembles cast iron, but with only a third of its weight, breaking stresses being 2450 and 3000 kg per cm² respectively: about 15.5 and 18 metric tons per square inch (Bell et al 1941, Tables 6.1, 2 on p. 436–437). In flexibility bone resembles steel more than iron, but only has half the strength of steel. In compression it has large margins of safety for weight-bearing (Koch 1917) and for impact. Muscle contraction provides the largest proportion of pressure, even at weight-bearing joints, especially in active movement (Bell et al 1941; Williams & Svensson 1968). At the hip joint only a small part of the pressure is due to body weight (see below).

A tubular structure, typical of the shaft in many bones, is the strongest, lightest and hence most economical arrangement of material. This adaptation of form to habitual stresses is also seen in the predominant longitudinal orientation of osteons in long bones. The thickness of compact cortical bone tends to be greatest at the midshaft, where torsional and bending stresses are most severe and internal trabeculae are largely absent. In articular regions bones mainly withstand compression forces, often surprisingly large. In symmetrical standing, for example, each hip joint takes half the superincumbent body weight, with muscular activity increasing this by a factor of about six: in walking or running, full body weight (except that of the weight-bearing leg) impinges alternately on each hip joint, giving, in adult males, a total load of 270 kg (600 lb): this may double in powerful exertions. In articular regions bone structure differs from that in the shaft, being entirely trabecular, with a thin outer shell of compact bone—an arrangement also found in smaller bones, for example carpal and tarsal, and vertebral bodies, all of which are mostly stressed by compression. In joints where weight-

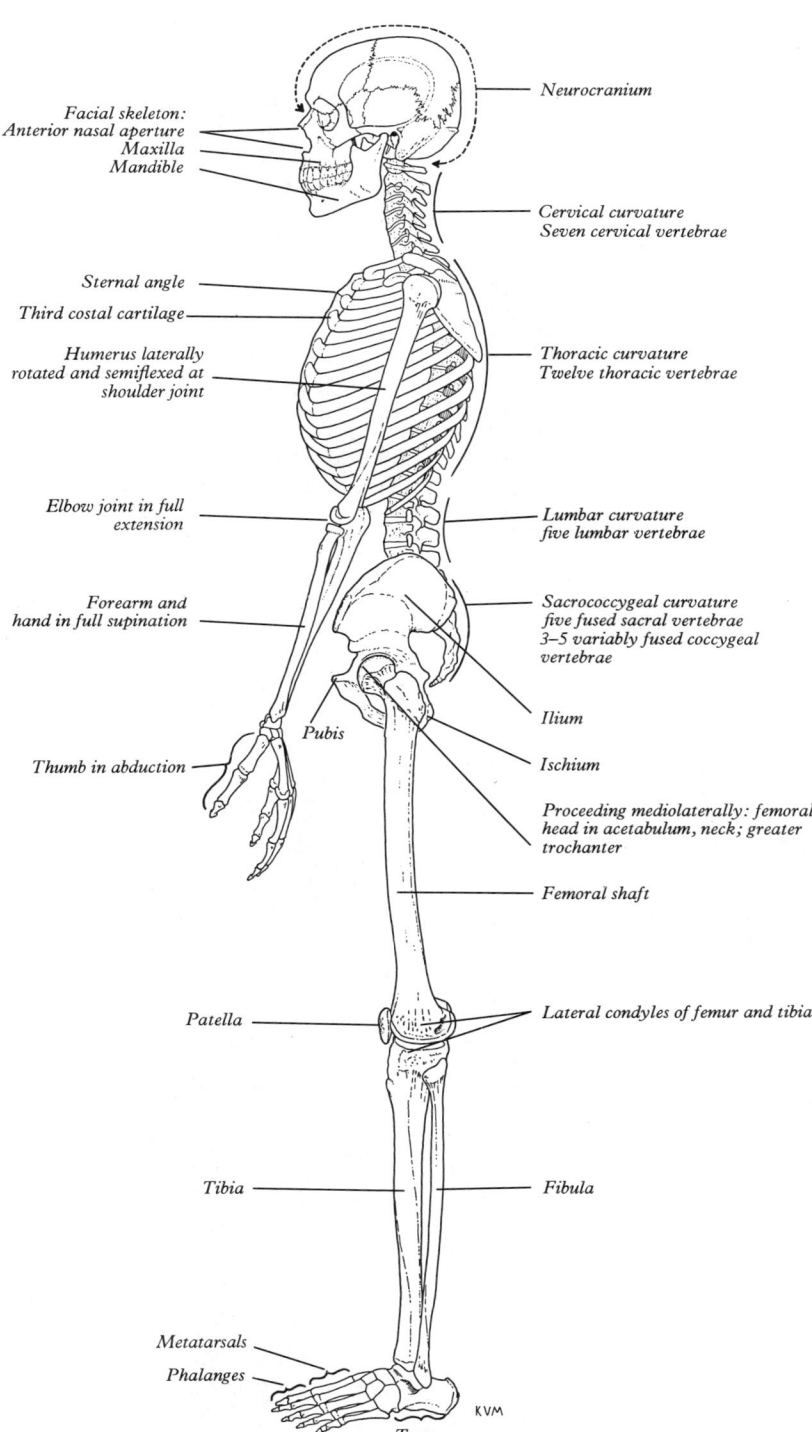

Facial skeleton:
Anterior nasal aperture
Maxilla
Mandible

Neurocranium

Cervical curvature
Seven cervical vertebrae

Sternal angle
Third costal cartilage

Humerus laterally
rotated and semiflexed at
shoulder joint

Thoracic curvature
Twelve thoracic vertebrae

Elbow joint in full
extension

Lumbar curvature
five lumbar vertebrae

Forearm and
hand in full supination

Sacrococcygeal curvature
five fused sacral vertebrae
3–5 variably fused coccygeal
vertebrae

Ilium

Pubis

Thumb in abduction

Ischium

Proceeding mediolaterally: femoral
head in acetabulum, neck; greater
trochanter

Femoral shaft

Patella

Lateral condyles of femur and tibia

Tibia

Fibula

Metatarsals
Phalanges

KVM

Tarsus

6.3 Adult male skeleton: lateral view.

bearing is slight, pressure may still be large during movement, due to muscle action.

The trabeculae of cancellous bone, though individually small, collectively provide powerful support to the thin surrounding shell of compact bone, a form of construction widespread in vertebrate skeletons, being modified only where bending, twisting and tensile forces demand a larger mass of compact bone. Many examples of both arrangements will be noted in individual bones; most larger bones show both forms, with intermediate arrays adapting to local mechanical needs. Mechanical forces influence growth and form in bones; and during protracted evolutionary time a most apt solution to mechanical demands has been reached, in accordance with nutrition, muscle power, and the best compromise between size and weight (p. 437).

Sections of trabecular bone (**6.5**, 9, 22, 23) show criss-crossing

427

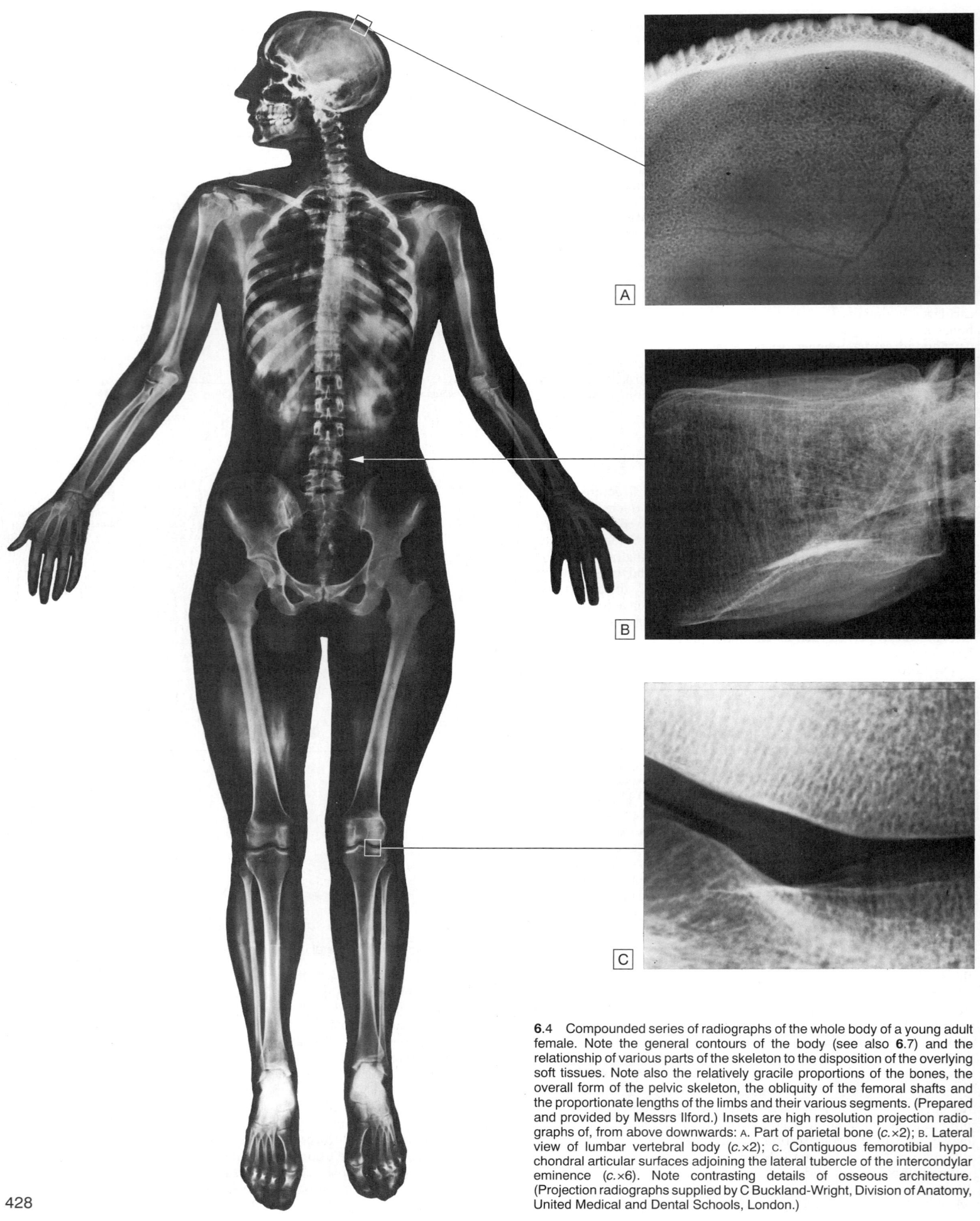

6.4 Compounded series of radiographs of the whole body of a young adult female. Note the general contours of the body (see also **6**.7) and the relationship of various parts of the skeleton to the disposition of the overlying soft tissues. Note also the relatively gracile proportions of the bones, the overall form of the pelvic skeleton, the obliquity of the femoral shafts and the proportionate lengths of the limbs and their various segments. (Prepared and provided by Messrs Ilford.) Insets are high resolution projection radiographs of, from above downwards: A. Part of parietal bone (*c.*×2); B. Lateral view of lumbar vertebral body (*c.*×2); C. Contiguous femorotibial hypochondral articular surfaces adjoining the lateral tubercle of the intercondylar eminence (*c.*×6). Note contrasting details of osseous architecture. (Projection radiographs supplied by C Buckland-Wright, Division of Anatomy, United Medical and Dental Schools, London.)

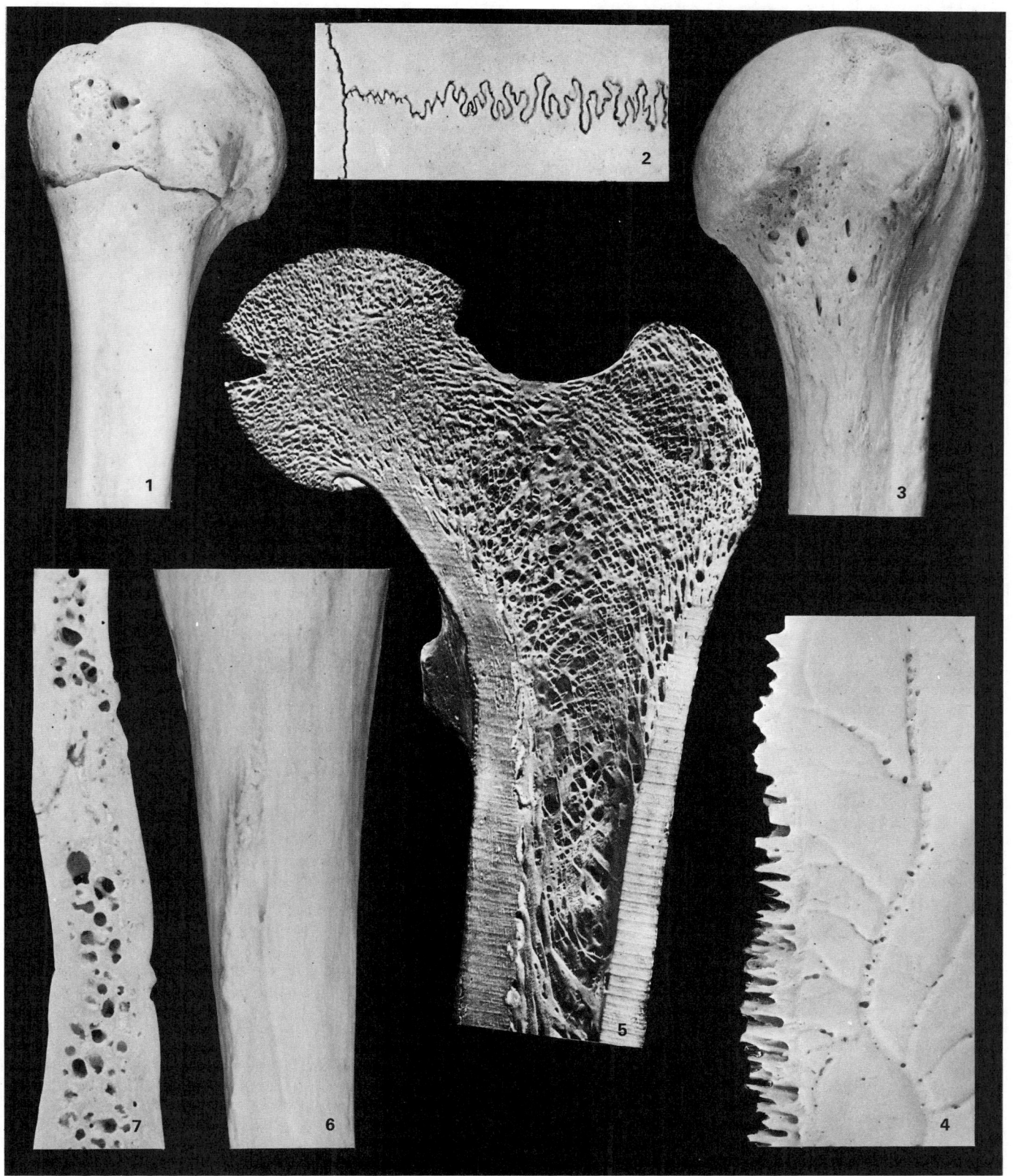

6.5 Some macroscopic features of bone structure. 1. The anterior aspect of the proximal end of an immature humerus. Note the contrasting surface characteristics of the smooth articular surface, covered in life by articular cartilage, the smooth periosteal surface of the metaphysis separating the compound epiphysis from the metaphysis—the vascular osseous fusion has not yet occurred. 2. The external aspect of part of the sagittal (horizontal) and coronal (vertical) cranial sutures. Note the variation in the form and degree of interlocking of the bones. 3. The anterior aspect of the proximal end of a mature humerus; complete osseous fusion has occurred (see 1). Note the variations in surface texture and the distribution and size of the vascular foramina. 4. The endocranial aspect of the sagittal margin of a parietal bone. Note the highly complex nature of the sutural surface, the presence of vascular grooves and multiple vascular foramina on the endo-

cranial surface. 5. A coronal section through the head, neck, greater trochanter and proximal shaft of an adult femur, clearly showing the variation in thickness of the shell of compact cortical bone, and the organization of the bony trabeculae. 6. The posterior aspect of part of the shaft of a tibia. Note the relatively smooth areas which bear 'fleshy' attachments of muscles, the ridge where dense lamellae of collagen are attached and an oblique vascular foramen which transmits the main nutrient vascular bundle to the shaft. 7. A sectioned bone of the cranial vault showing the internal and external tables of compact bone separated by the trabecular diploë, the diploic spaces of which, in life, are filled with haemopoietic red bone marrow.

The sectioned femur (5) has been reproduced using a specialized photographic technique which produced a 'bas-relief' effect. (Photographs by Kevin Fitzpatrick, United Medical and Dental Schools, London.)

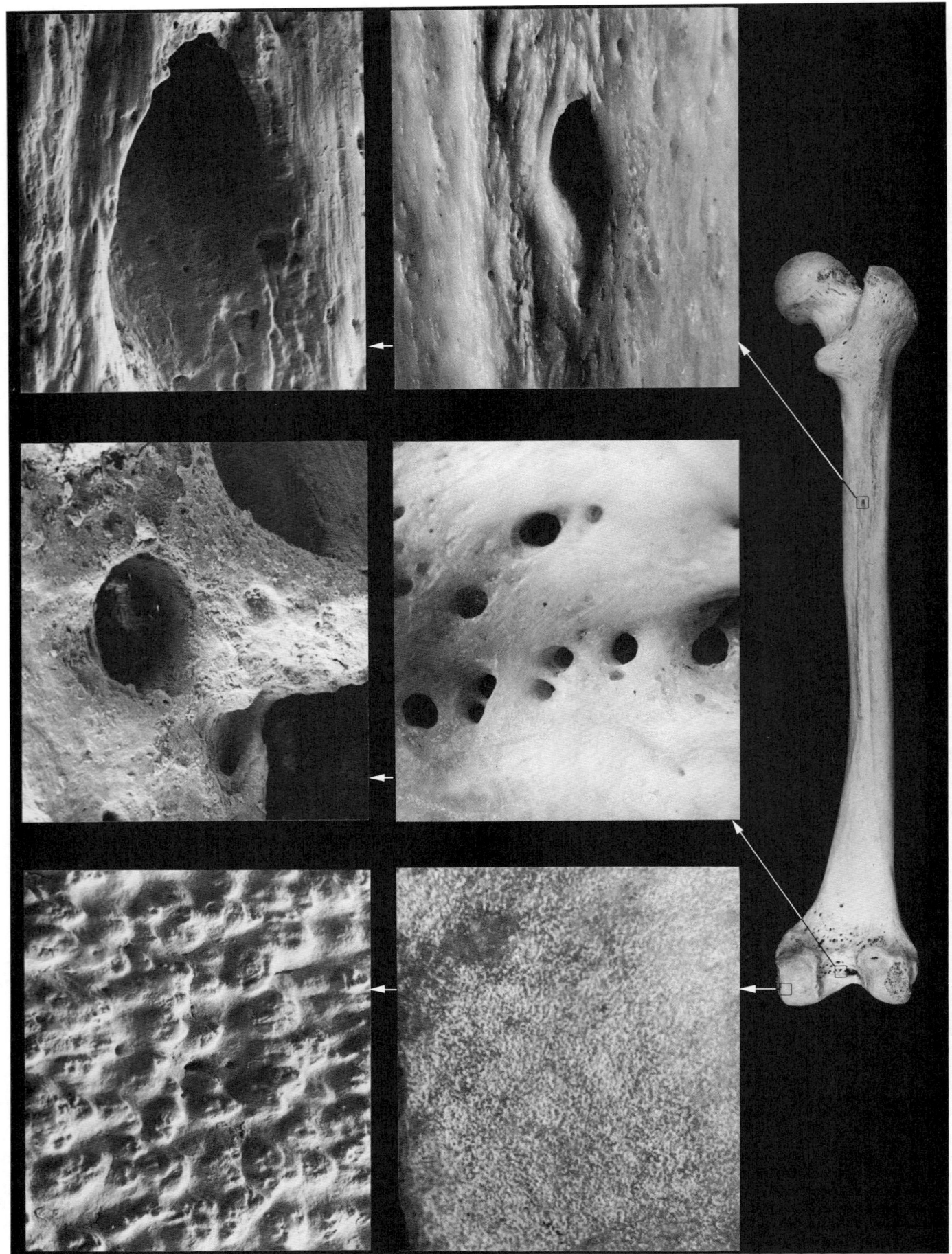

6.6 Surface details of a normal adult femur photographed at the sites indicated, by macrophotography and scanning electron microscopy, The macrophotographs which are immediately adjacent to the whole bone photo-

graphs are at a magnification of ×5, except for that showing the diaphyseal nutrient foramen which is ×4. All the scanning electron micrographs are ×80, with the exception of that showing the diaphyseal nutrient foramen, which

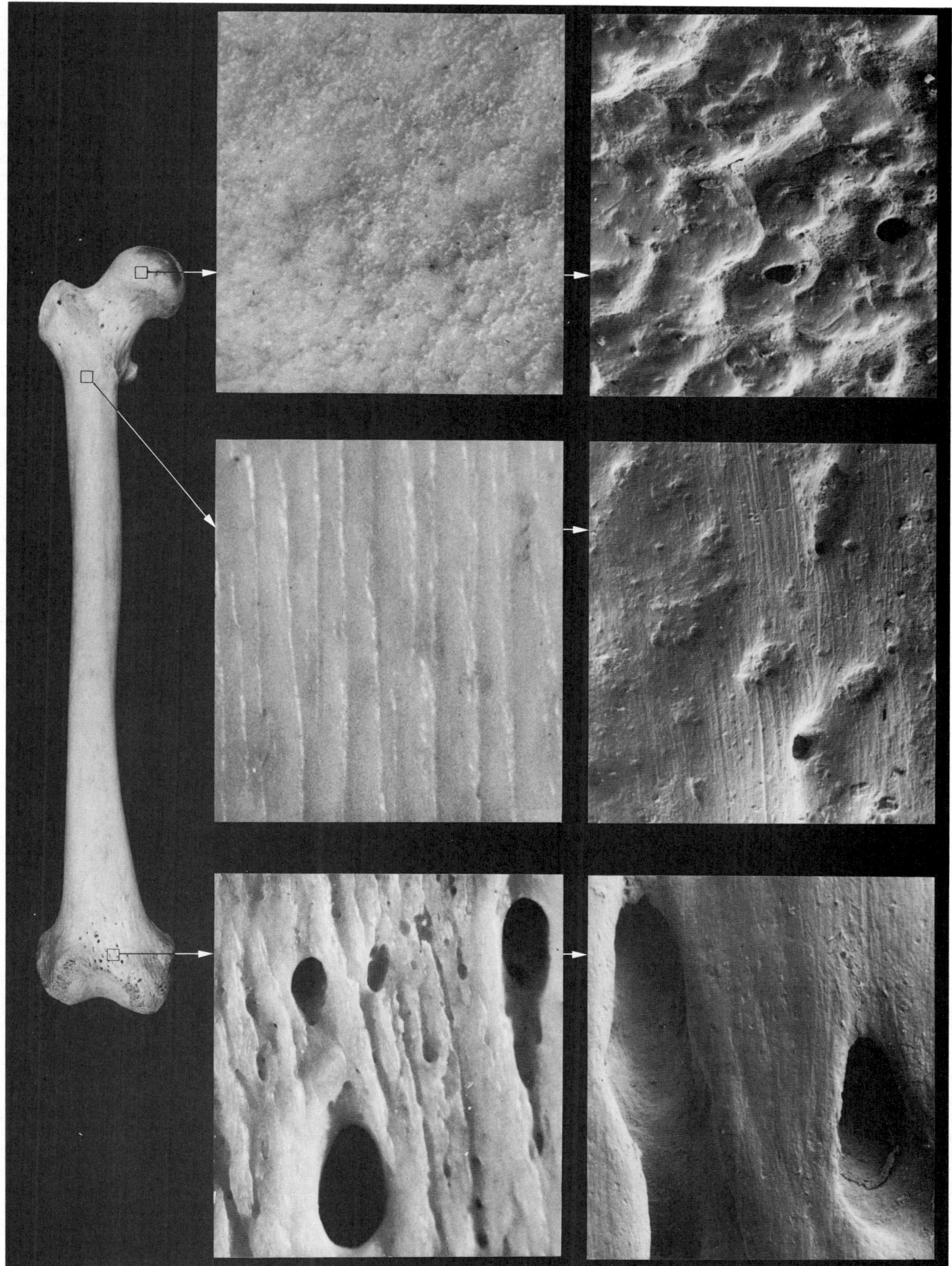

is ×15. (Prepared and provided by Kevin Fitzpatrick, Derrick Lovell and Michael Crowder, Division of Anatomy, United Medical and Dental Schools, London.)

patterns which resemble girderwork. Attempts to equate these patterns in particular bones, such as the femur and calcaneus, with lines of force in habitual stresses were made early (Ward 1838). Such architectural explanations of structure have been criticized (e.g. Murray 1936), but studies of individual bones, and the entire skeleton (Hall 1966), show an intimate correlation between stress and structure in trabecular and cortical bone. Wherever stresses are locally applied, as in tendon and ligament attachments, sections show that external features, for example ridges or facets, are not the only local changes. Compact cortical bone may also increase, together with subjacent condensations of trabeculae. It is certain that stress patterns and trabecular arrangements are related, although the precise relationship may be unclear (p. 437). Surface features of bones are clear to the naked eye (**6.5**); but much more detail and variation is revealed by a hand lens, macrophotography, incident light microscopy and scanning electron microscopy (**6.6**).

THE SHAPE AND PROPORTIONS OF BONES

Since bones vary in shape their gross appearance has led to a traditional grouping into long, short, flat and irregular bones. **Long**

bones are typical of limbs, with length reflecting both speed and power in movement. Their tubular shafts (diaphyses), with a central medullary cavity, diverge (metaphyses) towards their expanded articular ends (epiphyses), which have separate, often multiple, centres of ossification. The metacarpals, metatarsals and phalanges are smaller examples of long bones, having a proportionately greater shaft diameter and only a single epiphysis. So-called **short** bones occur in the carpus and tarsus, for example cuboid, cuneiform, trapezoid, scaphoid. Since they are generally subject to compression more than other stresses, they typically have a thin cortex of compact bone, supported by an interior which is wholly trabecular. **Flat** bones include the curved bones of the cranial vault, which have trabecular bone (*diploë*), variable in thickness, enclosed between laminae (*tables*) of compact bone (**6.5**). The scapulae, despite their irregular form, are also described as flat. **Irregular** bones include any element not easily assigned to the foregoing groups. This time-honoured classification, however, has no great merit. Bones must be studied individually, and considered in relation to the functional demands placed upon them.

In both shape and structure bones are affected by genetic, metabolic and mechanical factors, with each bone resulting from a long functional history through countless successive generations. Genetic determination of primary shape has been demonstrated by organ

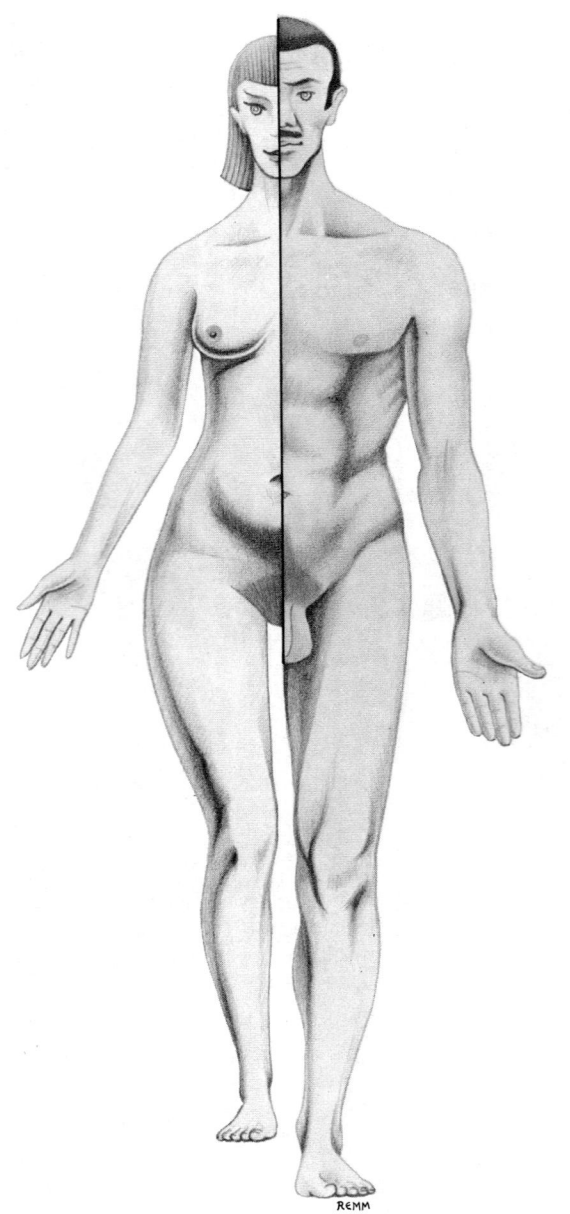
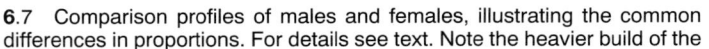
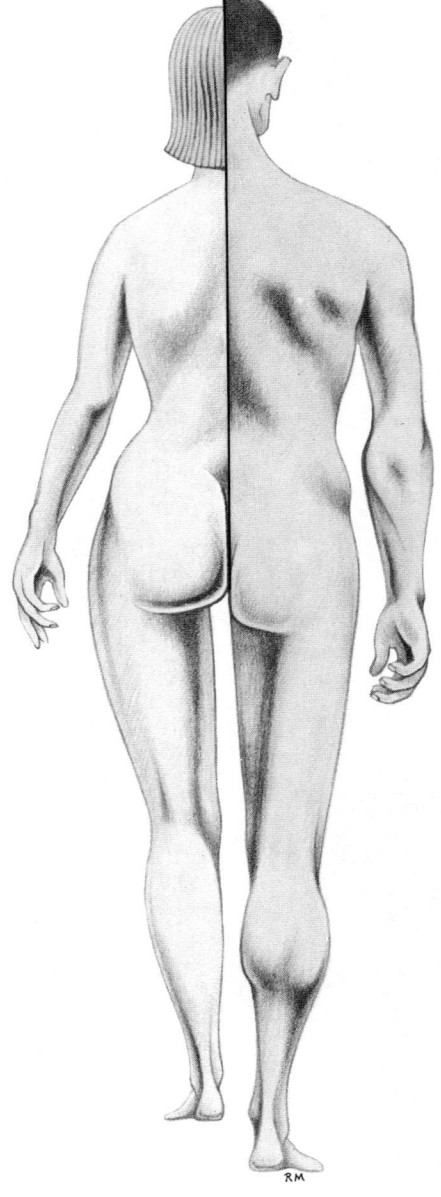

6.7 Comparison profiles of males and females, illustrating the common differences in proportions. For details see text. Note the heavier build of the male above the waist and the female below it, differences in limb proportions, carrying angle of forearm, muscularity and apparent neck length.

culture and transplantation of embryonic skeletal tissues (Murray & Huxley 1924; Fell & Canti 1934; Willis 1936); all major characteristics appear to be self-determined. Mechanical influences such as moulding by muscular activity, often regarded as of first importance, do not operate when the primary form is being established. As muscles become active during prenatal life they may influence bone growth, but to what extent is difficult to say; after birth and up to adolescence, before all the epiphyses are fused, increased activity augments growth in both length and girth. The reduced limb bone growth seen in paralyses, for example poliomyelitis, implies that muscle activity is necessary for proper skeletal development. Experimental studies involving removal of muscles point in the same direction (Appleton 1934; Washburn 1947; Wolffson 1950). Increases in strength and stature show some temporal correlation in adolescents (Jones 1949).

Metabolic influences affect bone growth at all stages of development. The availability of calcium, phosphorus, vitamins A, C and D, and secretions of the hypophysis, thyroid, parathyroid, adrenal glands and gonads, are all essential to osteogenesis (see below) and hence to skeletal form and dimensions. Disturbances in any of these factors result in recognized pathologies; however, it is often difficult to distinguish pathological from normal variation. Body height is an example: between the extremes of dwarfism and gigantism (both resulting from hormonal dysfunction), much variation in height occurs. Variations in stature and other dimensions linked with age, sex and race are in part genetically determined; but racial variations in nutrition also have profound effects (Greulich 1951; Acheson 1960; Tanner 1962).

Body proportions and absolute dimensions vary widely in respect of age and sex (**6.7**) within and between racial groups. While partly due to variability in muscularity and adiposity, such variations are chiefly skeletal; their study is *anthropometry* (Martin 1928: Hrdlička 1939). The data of anthropometry may be non-metrical, such as the presence or absence of a feature (e.g. sagittal crest in Eskimo skulls, preauricular sulcus in female innominate bones), or persistence of an entity (e.g. interfrontal suture), or degree of development (e.g. frontal ridges, projection of chin). However, most anthropometric data are measurements, by internationally agreed techniques, in living subjects or skeletal material. These may involve the whole body (e.g. stature), sections such as the limbs, or individual bones. Proportions are expressed by indices, for example breadth of the skull as a percentage of its length (the *cranial index*), which may show ethnic variation. Mongoloid people, for example, have larger cranial indices than other races; they therefore have a relatively 'broader' head, which is also absolutely wider. A Mongolian child, of course, might have a cranial width less than that of a Negro adult, and yet be proportionately broader. Ratios between length of limbs and 'sitting height', or between arm and leg, upper arm and forearm, thigh and foreleg, are all used and show differences related to age, sex and race. Details of some indices, where appropriate, are included in accounts of particular bones.

Observations and measurements suggesting age, sex, size and race of an individual skeleton, or parts of it, are not only useful in anthropology and archaeology (Brothwell 1968; Warwick 1968) but sometimes essential to identification in forensic practice (Glaister & Brash 1937; Boyd & Trevor 1953; Stewart 1954; Harrison 1957).

Estimation of skeletal age

Estimation of skeletal age involves many criteria, varying in value at different ages. Up to 25 years (including fetal life) dentition and ossification provide numerous data for assessment of age, with accuracy dependent on precision of observations, available statistics for sex and racial affinities of individuals under examination, together with their nutritional and endocrine history. The latter data are rarely forthcoming; available tables of ossification usually apply to healthy caucasian children and adolescents in Europe or America. A few studies of other racial groups exist (Todd 1931; Modi 1957): racial variations in the events of ossification would necessarily be genetic, but there is no clear evidence for this (Krogman 1962). Variations in ossification are affected by the wide divergence in nutrition between and within racial groups so far studied, in all of which data females show earlier ossification and epiphyseal fusion than males, a difference which is presumably genetic. Nevertheless, up to age 25, the age of a complete skeleton can usually be assessed to within a year, or more accurately in earlier years, especially if

dental observations are available. (For details see Teeth and individual bones.)

Above 25 years skeletal age can be estimated to within five years by the appearance of the cranial sutures and of the bony surfaces of the symphysis pubis. From midtwenties onwards, sutures exhibit progressive closure (p. 607, Todd & Lyon 1924, 1925a, b, c), which begins internally, so that without internal inspection observations may be misleading (Singer 1953; Genovese & Messmacher 1959); complications due to racial variation have been recorded (Abbie 1950). Progressive changes occur in the articular surfaces at the pubic symphysis. Features typical of ages from late teens to fifties and beyond are well-established (Todd 1920a, b, 21a, b; McKern & Stewart 1957), and this is generally considered the best method for estimation of skeletal age in maturity. Sequences of age changes have also been described in other bones (scapula, sternum and costal cartilages), but provide less accurate estimates. Lipping of the rims of vertebral bodies and at other articular surface margins, exaggerated secondary markings and ossification into tendons and ligaments all suggest advancing age, but only vaguely indicate **actual** age.

Estimation of sex

Estimation of sex in complete postpubertal human skeletons is usually easy, even without measurement. Sexual differences are marked in the pelvis (p. 673) and skull (p. 609), but not equally so in all populations. Thus 'sexing' of skeletons from one racial group is almost free from error, whereas assessment of an individual of unknown extraction is less certain. Postcranial bones other than the pelvis, especially larger limb bones, may provide clear evidence of sex, if others of like race and both sexes are available for comparison. Female bones are usually smaller and more slender than male equivalents, i.e. smaller shaft diameter relative to length. This is reflected in their comparative **weights**: in a study of Hindu femora, mean weights were 385 g in males, 279 g in females (Singh & Singh 1974).

Anatomists, anthropologists, and forensic scientists have long judged the sex of skeletal material by non-metrical observations. More recently, sexual divergence has been based upon measurements in many different bones (Montagu 1960; Krogman 1962). Discriminant analysis, for example, in which the capital dimensions of 70 humeri were analysed (Rother et al 1977), showed that sex was not easy to establish; however, approximate age could be assessed. Such studies emphasize the need for standards of sexual dimorphism in different populations. The pelvis remains, however, the most reliable region for assessing sex even before puberty, as well as in infancy (Reynolds 1947) and fetal life (Boucher 1957).

Sexual dimorphism of thoracolumbar vertebrae in Australian subjects (aged 5 to 19 years) has been observed by Taylor and Twomey (1984), with female vertebral bodies being more slender from the eighth year onwards: there being greater growth in transverse diameter in males.

Estimation of size

Estimation of size, particularly height, from measurements of limb bones has long been formulated (Rollet 1899), and with increasing accuracy as formulae have become more refined (Trotter & Gleser 1958). All such calculations depend on the fact, familiar to artists (cf. Leonardo da Vinci), that major parts, trunk and limbs, exhibit consistent ratios among themselves and relative to total height; these ratios are linked to age, sex and race. The relatively large head, long trunk, short arms and shorter legs present a familiar picture in infants which becomes grotesque in older children, and monstrous in adults. As infants grow, they change their proportions gradually towards adult shape, diverging towards one sex at puberty. The limbs become relatively longer, the shoulders broader and the pelvis narrower in adult males, as well as other differences (**6.7**). Between major races, and even smaller ethnic groups, characteristic variations in proportions appear. Negroes have comparatively long legs and arms: moreover, the calf and forearm are long relative to the thigh and arm. Consequently, formulae designed to estimate height from long bones in one population may not apply to another. Alternative formulae for the sexes must also be used, and immature bones must be recognized and suitable corrections made.

Femoral length alone has commonly been used for estimating stature by using a simple multiplier derived from comparison with known height in many individuals. Similarly, the humerus, radius, ulna, tibia and fibula have also been used; more complex formulae, using several long bone lengths, give more accurate estimates. Whatever the methods used, the estimates are merely mean values with appropriate standard deviations; hence estimated stature of unidentified remains, however careful, may be in error by several centimetres.

Since estimates of stature (and other assessments) must sometimes be made from fragments of bones, attempts have been made to establish reliable formulae (Steele 1970).

Estimation of race

Estimation of race from skeletal data has always been a central theme in anthropology, with the skull attracting most attention. An array of **non-metrical** features (Jones 1931) and of cranial, facial and mandibular indices are widely used (Martin & Saller 1961; Berry & Berry 1967; Berry 1975), with statistical analysis of **metrical** data

(Giles & Elliot 1960). In the three major racial groups, caucasian, mongoloid and negroid, perhaps 85–90% of skulls can be classified without elaborate measurement: with further racial division the error increases markedly. Worldwide mingling of races renders 'pure' races difficult to indicate. In the United States of America, large collections of skeletons, both caucasian and negroid, well attested as to origin, have stimulated comparative studies. Critical surveys (Krogman 1962) suggest that only the skull (but not the mandible) and pelvis (Todd & Lindàla 1928) have any value in estimating race. (For details of **cranial** features of racial significance see p. 609.) However, metrical peculiarities in Japanese limb bones have been claimed by Takahashi (1975, 1976). The racial significance of postcranial non-metrical characteristics has been rigorously re-examined by Finnegan (1978), who provides a summary of many findings. The value of non-metrical features in evaluating populations from skeletal data has been reviewed by Finnegan and Faust (1974).

The dating of human fossil remains

INTRODUCTION

The recovery of skeletal remains from ancient deposits is of considerable importance to human palaeontologists, since this evidence forms part of the data upon which the study of human evolution is based. It is equally important to determine the date of death of the individual, so that the remains can be placed in a chronological sequence that will assist in the interpretation of human phylogeny. In addition, it is necessary to know that the remains are contemporary with the deposit in which they have been found: the intrusive burial of recent remains into ancient deposits can cause confusion, as can the redeposition of ancient remains into younger deposits. The establishment of contemporaneity can also permit the association of human remains with faunal and floral remains in the same deposit, and thus give information concerning the palaeoenvironment that may correlate with other sites. The date in years is known as the absolute or chronometric date, while the relative date provides evidence of contemporaneity or correlation with similar sites (Oakley 1964).

RELATIVE DATING

The first consideration must be to determine the local stratigraphy and compare the fossiliferous stratum with those above and below; this ensures that no disturbances or inversions have taken place that might invalidate the normal sequence of older deposits lying below younger ones (Law of Superposition). If the sequence is normal, then account can be taken of the floral, faunal and cultural associations of the deposit; its position in other sequences can then be established. The existence of residual magnetism in rocks can help, since changes in the polarity of the earth through time have established a sequence of 'normal' and 'reversed' polarities world-

wide that is known and dated (6.8): the new deposit should fit in this sequence. These data may be sufficient to determine the stratigraphic age or the archaeological age of the deposit, for example Upper Pleistocene or Neolithic.

Laboratory tests on the human or hominid bones themselves are important, since buried bone undergoes chemical changes that relate to decomposition and to interaction with the deposit via the ground waters. Since deposits vary widely in their mineral content, such tests are principally of value in determining contemporaneity with the bones of other animals which may be extinct. The nitrogen content of buried bone, which comes from the organic fraction, diminishes with time as decomposition proceeds. Conversely, the fluorine content of buried bone tends to increase, and may reach an equilibrium with the deposit through the ground waters (Oakley 1969). A new method, Energy Dispersive X-ray Microanalysis (EDXA) can determine both qualitatively and quantitatively the spectrum of elements present in a fossil bone, and may serve to separate fossils in a mixed sample (Scott & Love 1983; Bartsiokas & Day 1993).

ABSOLUTE OR CHRONOMETRIC DATING

The determination of the time in years that has elapsed since the death of the individual is as important as an assessment of the anatomy of the bones, since both are needed in order to establish the taxonomic status and phylogenetic position of the fossil. Methods of chronometric dating can be direct, taken on the bones or teeth themselves, or indirect, taken on the deposit, or on associated remains and artefacts. The methods available vary widely in the range of years over which they are effective, and the ranges of error to which they are subject.

Radiocarbon dating (Libby 1952)

The organic and inorganic portions of bones and teeth contain carbon, part of the total carbon reservoir of the earth (biosphere, atmosphere and the seas). This reservoir consists of two stable isotopes, C^{12} and C^{13}, and the radioactive isotope C^{14}, which undergoes decay at a constant rate of about 1% per 80 years. The radioactive isotope is formed in the upper atmosphere by the bombardment of nuclei to form free secondary neutrons that collide with N^{14} to form C^{14}. This C^{14} has a half-life of 5730 ± 30 years (Mann et al 1961); $T\frac{1}{2} = 5568$ is used to calculate C^{14} dates. The C^{14} atoms do not differ chemically from the others, and are also taken up from the atmosphere, oxidized to carbon monoxide and then to carbon dioxide. A continuous supply of radioactive carbon enters the oceans and the biosphere and forms an equilibrium. This equilibrium is upset on the death of the organism, since no new radioactive carbon enters the system, and radioactive decay begins. The measurement of the C^{14} activity of organic material any time after death allows the calculation of when the organism stopped exchanging radioactive carbon with the environment, and hence the time of the death. If the quantity of radioactive carbon remaining is too small, detection will be impossible: in practice, this limits conventional radiocarbon dating to $c.40\,000$ years before the present (BP). The use since 1977 of accelerator or cyclotron radiocarbon dating has approximately doubled the range of the method (Protsch 1986).

Potassium–argon dating (Gentner & Lippolt 1969)

Naturally occurring potassic minerals contain a small proportion of an isotope of potassium that has been decaying to $Argon^{40}$ since the mineral was formed. Since the rate of decay is known, measurement of the quantity of argon present in the specimen permits the calculation of when the process began. This method is particularly useful since potassic minerals

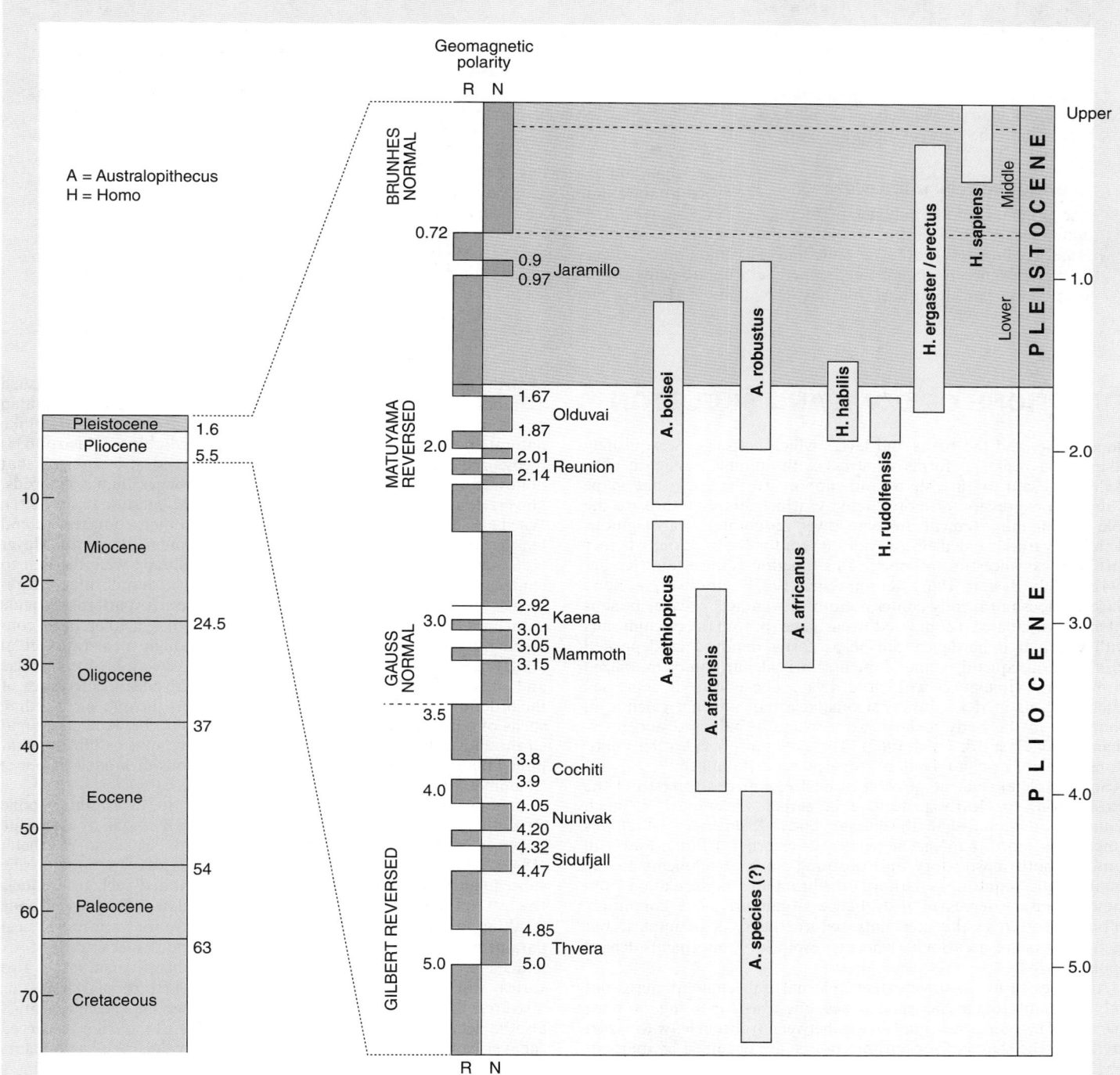

6.8 The Pliocene and Pleistocene geological periods expanded to show the geomagnetic polarity record and its correlation with the time ranges of the principal hominid, hominine and sapient human species. Dates in millions of years (BP). (Redrawn with permission after Bilsborough.)

occur widely in volcanic sediments that often preserve fossil bone. The method is indirect, and relies on other evidence of contemporaneity. It is less effective for recent material, and most effective for samples more than 400 000 years old.

Fission track dating (Fleischer et al 1975)

Naturally occurring volcanic glasses, such as obsidian, often contain radioactive uranium contaminants. When individual uranium atoms decay, they release particles that blast tracks through the glass. These tracks may be etched and counted. The sample is then put into an atomic pile and all the remaining uranium atoms decay, making fission tracks that are also counted. The difference between the naturally occurring and the induced fission track count will give the time elapsed since the formation of the glass. This method often complements potassium–argon dating, since the two methods have differ-

ing and unrelated possibilities of error.

Electron spin resonance (Ikeya 1975, 1986)

The principle of electron spin resonance dating (ESR) uses electron spins created by natural radiation resulting from the decay of uranium, thorium and potassium, in the specimen (usually tooth enamel) or in an associated deposit. Radiation ionizes atoms or molecules: thus, when an ionized electron is trapped by another atom, an electron-deficient and electron-excess atom are formed with detectable magnetic properties. The specimen is then irradiated in an atomic pile and once again a differential calculation will give the elapsed time, since the rate of natural decay is known.

Thermoluminescence (Aitken 1985)

The principle and techniques of thermoluminescence (TL) dating are much the same as those of ESR. The emission of light from experimentally heated minerals, such as archaically burnt flint, is pro-

portional to the electrons displaced since the original heating, and to the natural radiation experienced.

Amino acid racemization dating
(Bada 1985)

This technique is applicable to bones, teeth, shell and calcareous sediments. All protein-bound amino acids have a three-dimensional arrangement that is, in nature, conventionally termed the L-enantiomer (*laevo-* or *left*). Synthetic amino acids contain equal amounts of L- and D-(*dextro-*)enantiomers. The L-form

is used by animals and plants during biosynthesis of proteins as a consequence of the selectivity of the enzymes used in the synthesis. The conversion of one form into the other is termed racemization. In living forms, all amino acids are in the L-form, but after death, spontaneous racemization takes place at a rate that is temperature-dependent. The extent of racemization can be estimated, and the D/L ratio is used to calculate the elapsed time since death, provided that the average temperature is known and has been constant.

FUNCTIONS OF BONE AND SKELETON

Bone tissue, and the struts and levers which it forms, is exquisitely adapted to resist all forms of stress with suitable resilience. The skeleton is said to 'give shape and support' to the body; but shape is itself an expression of motor activity, which simply returns to the role of bone in movement. In some lower vertebrates a cartilaginous skeleton, variably calcified, provides levers for locomotion; whether cartilage was ancestral to bone in this function is uncertain (Romer 1942, 1970; Bassett 1962; Krompecher 1967). However, a bony skeleton does not merely confer a motor advantage; because bone is intensely vascularized compared to cartilage (p. 469) the calcium salts with which it is hardened can be as easily removed as deposited (p. 472). Consequently some of the osseous calcium can be mobilized into general circulation with little delay. The effects of depressed calcium levels in rickets and osteomalacia indicate that calcium in bone and in the body at large are constantly balanced and interchanged (McLean & Urist 1969). The skeleton provides the major store (97%) of calcium available for general metabolism.

Some skeletal elements protect against extraneous forces; but the exoskeleton, so clearly protective in earlier vertebrates, is much reduced and modified in the human body. Even in the skull this function is more than just a barrier to external assault. Powerful muscles, both masticatory and postural, have attachments to the cranial walls, requiring isolation of the brain and its circulation from these intrinsic sources of disturbance. Again, ribs are commonly dubbed protective: they certainly reduce the risks of impact, but such dangers are occasional, whereas respiratory movements **depend** upon the ribs.

All bones show, to some extent, internal trabeculae; patterns not only resistant to mechanical stresses but also for siting of bone marrow. The numerous small spaces between trabeculae, with larger cavities in the shafts of longer limb bones, are occupied by marrow, whether haemopoietic or adipose (p. 1409). In some cranial bones, air-filled cavities develop; these bones are termed *pneumatic*. Pneumatization may consist of large hollows, such as the maxillary *sinus*, or multiple, small, communicating *air cells*, as in the temporal mastoid process. In human skulls, the saving in weight can scarcely be as significant as it is in the pneumatized cranial vault of elephants; however, the trabecular architecture of most bones is conducive to lightness without loss of strength, with economy in use of materials. Some sinuses, particularly smaller air cells, appear to develop from trabecular tissue (diploë) in certain cranial bones, thus expressing the above principle. Larger sinuses, perhaps due merely to unusual growth patterns, may affect the timbre of the voice.

MECHANICAL PROPERTIES OF BONE

The resemblance of bones to man-made levers, supporting columns, arches, struts and girders has resulted in the concepts of mechanical engineering being applied to them. Not only are bones similar to such structures in external shape and internal architecture, but also in their uses. The apparently fragile but collectively strong lattices

of struts and trusses seen in trabecular bone and skeletal forms such as tubes, H-girders, and ridges in cortical bone, predate human invention by millennia. As human technology began to overtake natural biomechanics comparisons were inevitable. Galileo (1638) recognized the significance of trabeculation and also asserted that hollow cylinders are, weight for weight, **stronger** than solid rods. Havers described his 'systems' and their axial orientation (circa 1691); Ward (1838) likened trabecular patterns, with their compressive and tensile elements, to supporting brackets and similar structures. Meyer (1867) and his mathematical collaborator, Culman, were the first to enunciate clearly the *trajectorial* theory which, despite much argument, still survives. Basically it states that trabecular patterns coincide with lines of stress transmission; as yet this has neither been convincingly demonstrated nor disproved, although Venieratos et al (1987) report good convergence between the direction of trabeculae and stress (both compressive and tensile), with mean differences of the order of $\pm 7°$. Trabeculae must also support the thin surrounding shells of cortical bone; however, the relationship between stress and strain and trabecular pattern is often more complex than the simplified mathematical analyses applied to sections or models of bones (Kummer 1972).

In contrast to this theoretical approach to determining bone strength, direct measurement uses engineering methods to assess the response of bone samples or entire skeletal elements. Wertheim (1847), anticipating Meyer, applied physical tests to bone tissue; subsequent workers have improved and expanded such techniques. Interest in the mechanics of locomotion stimulated the study of bone resulting in the recording of a variety of values for various physical parameters of bone. Obviously bone from various species differs; sex and age are also important factors. The form of specimen tested also varies; whole bones or blocks of cortical or trabecular bone, or mixtures: all behave differently. The source of the specimens must also be defined if results are to be comparable. Bone from preserved cadavers gives misleading values, especially regarding plastic deformation (Reilly & Burstein 1974), but also in elasticity, hardness and compressive and tensile properties (Evans 1973). Dead bone, however, if kept wet, does not differ from living bone tested in vivo, whereas dried bone is harder but less deformable. Sampling from a bone also presents problems, because the varying distribution of

Table 6.1 The approximate tensile strengths of bone and a few other materials (From Gordon 1968)

Material	Tons/inch	MN/m^2
Traditional cast iron	5–10	75–150
Copper	10	150
Bone	10	150
Tendon	7	105
Wood, spruce (along grain)	7	105
Cotton	25	375

Table 6.2 Young's modulus of wet bone with the direction of load parallel to the long axis of the bone (From Reilly and Burstein 1974)

Bone species and authors	Type of loading	Young's Modulus (10×10^9 N/m^2)	Comments
Human			
Dempster & Liddicoat (1952)	Tension, low strain rate	14.1	Dry, rewetted femur, tibia, humerus, mixed data, extensometer used
Burstein *et al.* (1972)	Tension, strain rate: 0.1 sec^{-1}	14.1	Femur; extensometer used for strain
Bovine			
Burstein *et al.* (1972)	Tension, strain rate: 0.1 sec^{-1}	24.5 ± 5.10	Femur; extensometer used
Simkin & Robin (1973)	Tension, low strain rate	23.8 ± 2.21	Tibia; unreported histology; extensometer used
Other materials			
Methylmethacrylate: Plexiglass Wood: Douglas Fir Steel		8.6 13.4 210.0	(68% moisture)

Note: MN = 10^6 N   1 N = 1 kg × 1 m/s^2 = 10^5 dyn.

osteons or trabeculae may make comparisons difficult. Testing specimens or intact bones, especially to destruction, involves attachment of tension devices, often resulting in collapse at these points, especially in testing axial tension. Experimental data, therefore, present a complex picture; for example, it is almost impossible to state useful mean values for the physical properties of bone, because resistance to stress and elasticity vary in different regions of the same bone. In view of the structural complexity in any skeletal element, including variations in thickness, density, cortical modelling and internal trabeculation (**6.**9), a definition of the mechanical behaviour in any individual bone is considered by many to be improbable. Variations in the proximal end of the human femur are shown in **6.**9 (Whitehouse & Dyson 1974); similar regional variability exists in its distal end and the proximal part of the tibia (Behrens et al 1974). In the tibia strength does not appear to be directly related to trabecular pattern or total density, indicating a multifactorial relation.

Various engineering techniques have been used to assess the isolated physical properties of bone samples and whole bones, and to assess strain distribution in them under various stresses. The results of many such tests have been summarized by Ascenzi and Bell (1972), Kummer (1972) and Evans (1973). Although these values vary, there is greater disagreement regarding the transmission of forces within bone or plastic models, because of the false assumption that bone is isotropic and homogeneous. Bone is a viscoelastic, biphasic substance analogous to fibreglass, with the tropocollagen corresponding to 'fibres', and the crystalline hydroxyapatite to the 'glass'. A plastic model will therefore indicate only the **surface** behaviour of stresses in the bone it is supposedly imitating. In both bone and model, stress patterns can be studied by inspection of cracks produced in a colophonium resin (**6.**10) covering (Kuntscher 1934) or special lacquers (Gurdjian & Lissner 1945); these superficial cracks may, however, give no more than a crude picture of strains in bone. A photoelastic technique using polarized light (Hallermann 1934), later exploited by Pauwels (1965) and Kummer (1966), reveals stress patterns for bones and plastic models. However, Brekelmans et al (1972) emphasized its limitations in models as well as its oversimplified, two-dimensional mathematical analyses.

Benninghoff (1925), using the *split-line phenomenon* (**6.**10) in decalcified bones, claimed that a surface pattern of split-lines or cracks, induced by puncturing with a round awl, followed the distribution of osteons orientated about compression or tension axes. Accepting the trajectorial theory, he considered the cracks were directly related to the behaviour of cortical osteons. Tappen (1954) later made similar claims, but admitted that the patterns may follow 'immature' osteons. Isotupa (1972) considered that the cracks represent points of weakness due to vascular spaces. Subsequently Buckland-Wright (1977) has attributed them to weaker zones of bone (which may also be instrumental in fracture initiation and propagation), and included

cement-lines, interlamellar interfaces, osteocytic lacunae, and vascular canals. However, he considered the split-line technique to be unreliable in the analysis of structure and force transmission.

Strain gauges have been used to record stresses in whole bones, either during in vivo experiments or as dead, isolated elements or bone samples. Gauges cannot be attached to bone in large numbers, so the data obtained are limited; but interesting in vivo results have been obtained by Lanyon (1973) on ovine vertebrae, tibiae, and calcanei during locomotion. Although Lanyon himself criticized the method, the data confirmed the elasticity of bone and showed that its elastic modulus varied with speed of movement.

Interference holography has been applied to the study of surface strains in human mandibles (Gupta & Knoell 1973); but the technique is difficult, especially in experiments on the living.

Mathematical analysis has been developed in this field; however, since basic data are limited or are based on the oversimplification inherent in the use of models, their value is restricted (consult Koch 1917; Kummer 1966; Rybicki et al 1972).

Consequently, a combination of techniques probably offers most help in solving and understanding the mechanical properties of bone. A study by Buckland-Wright (1978) of the patterns of strain transmission in the feline skull due to biting combined radiology and projection microradiography with the use of strain gauges, colophonium resin experiments and histology, the limitations of each technique being complemented by the others. Projection microradiographs were assessed by a stereoscopic technique, permitting three-dimensional correlation between bone structure and the impressed stresses. These observations have led to the development of a modified version of the trajectorial theory.

Alexander (1984) has compared the optimum strengths of bone in terms of their habitual stresses and actual properties and has developed mathematical expressions for the balance between strength and weight of bones. He concludes that mammalian limb bones are often stronger than they need to be, but admits that the equation between stress and structure is difficult to predict with accuracy. Bacon and Griffiths (1985), using neutron diffraction patterns, have investigated texture, stress and ageing in human femora bone samples, and found a vertical orientation of hydroxyapatite crystals able to resist vertical stresses: the alignment was low at birth and maximal by about 13 years, decreasing steadily thereafter.

GROWTH OF INDIVIDUAL BONES

As in other mammals human bones are mostly preformed in hyaline cartilage; some condense in mesenchyme. Thus, a soft tissue model appears first and is gradually changed into bone by onset of osteogenesis, often at a centre from which it spreads, until the whole

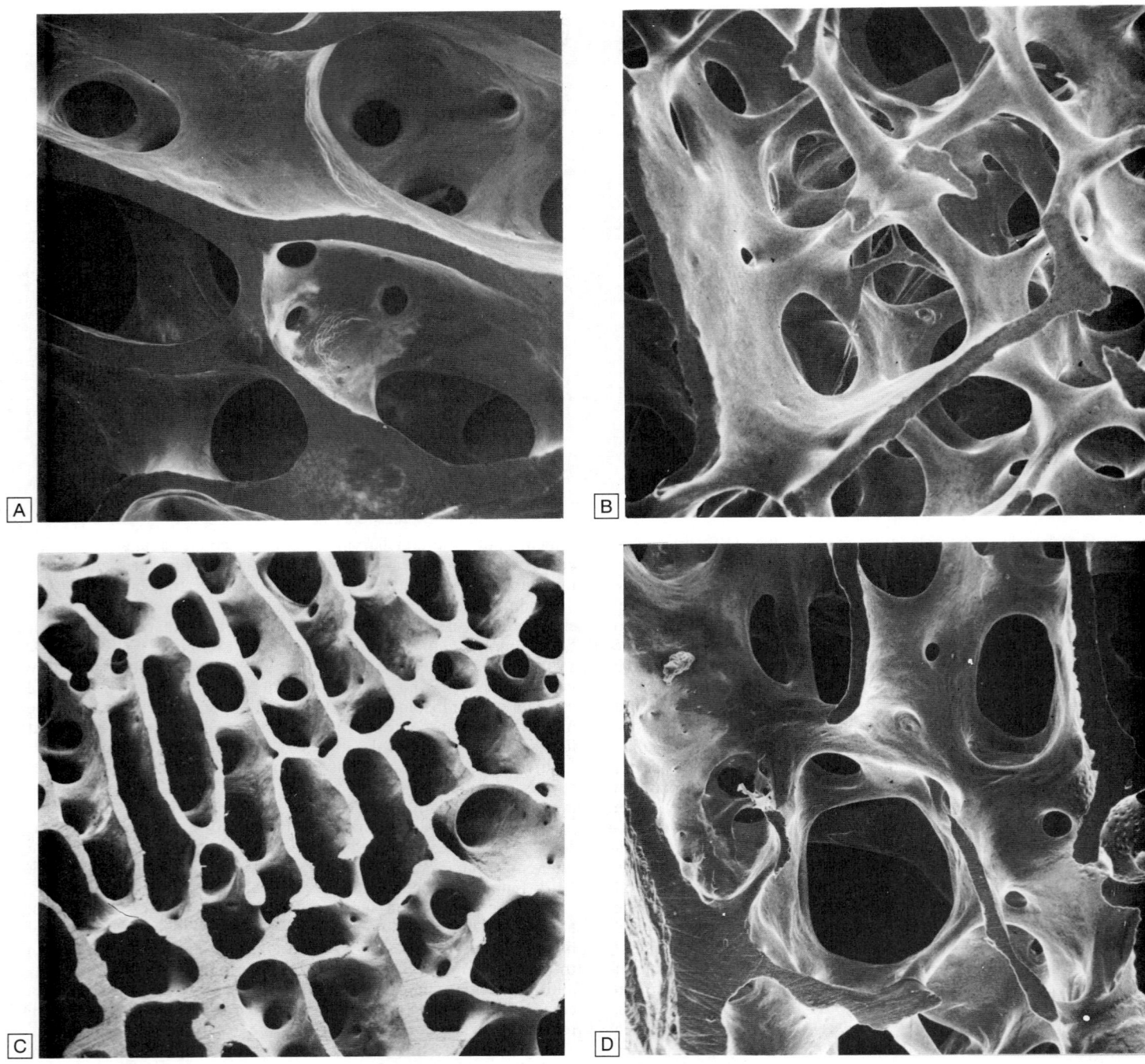

6.9 Scanning electron micrographs of trabelular bone at different sites in the proximal part of the same human femur. All fields are ×20. A is an area in the subcapital part of the neck, B and C are in the greater trochanter, and D in the rim of the articular surface of the head. Note the wide variation in the thickness, orientation and spacing of the trabeculae. (Original photographs from Whitehouse & Dyson 1974, with permission from the authors, the *Journal of Anatomy* and Cambridge University Press.)

skeletal element is transformed. Such *ossification centres* appear over a long period, many in embryonic life (**6**.11), some in prenatal life and others well into the postnatal growing period. The process is complex, and must be studied at different levels of organization. The basic phenomena of histogenesis, growth and transformation of skeletal tissues, including primitive mesenchyme and its differentiation into other forms of connective tissue, cartilage and bone at the microscopic, ultrastructural and molecular levels, are considered later (p. 473).

Initially microscopic, the ossification centres soon become macroscopic and their growth can then be followed by inspection, dissection or by using radiological and other scanning techniques. It is the latter scale of events which will be considered here.

Many bones, including carpal, tarsal, lacrimal, nasal, and zygomatic bones, inferior nasal conchae and auditory ossicles, ossify

from a single centre. Even in this limited group centres appear between the eighth intrauterine week and the tenth year, a wide sequence for studying growth or estimating age. However, most bones ossify from several centres, one of which appears in late embryonic or early fetal life (seventh week to fourth month) in the centre of the future bone (**6**.11): from here ossification progresses towards the ends, which are cartilaginous at birth (**6**.12, 13), although characteristic in shape and articular congruence. These terminal regions ossify from separate centres, sometimes multiple, appearing between birth and the late teens; they are thus *secondary* to the earlier *primary* centre from which much of the bone ossifies. This is the pattern in long bones, as well as in some shorter elements such as the metacarpals and metatarsals, and in the ribs and clavicles.

At birth a bone such as the tibia is typically ossified throughout its shaft, *diaphysis*, by a primary centre appearing in the seventh

438

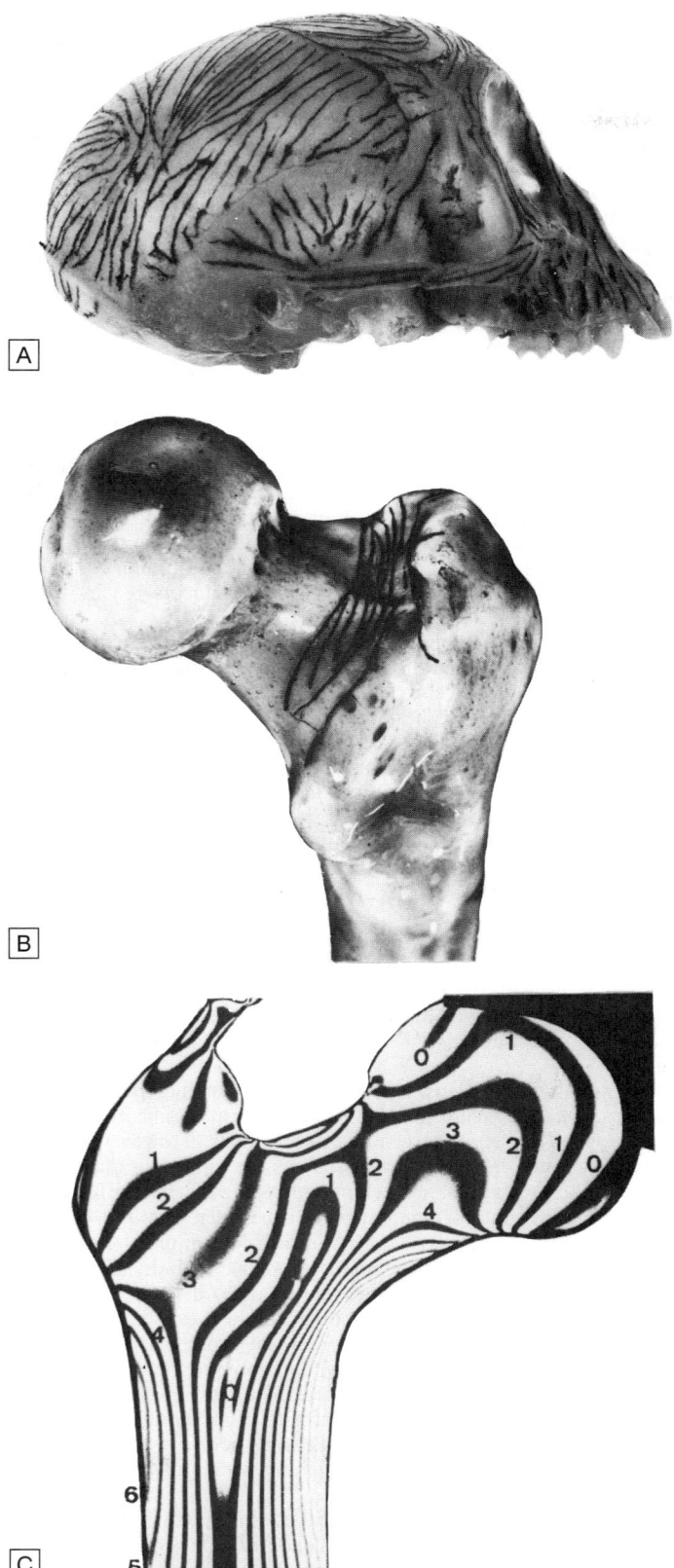

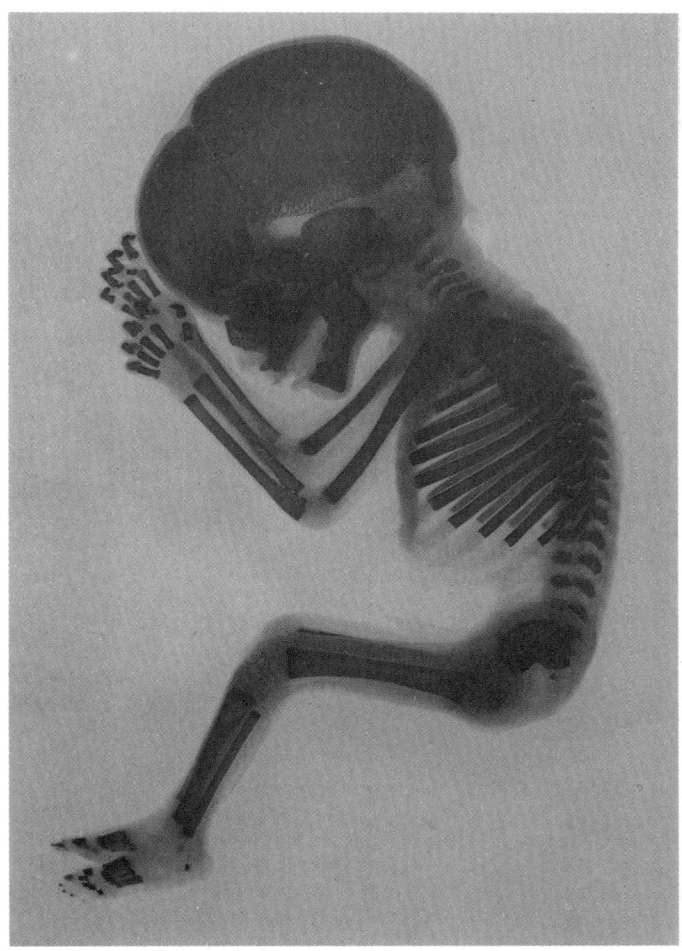

6.11 Alizarin stained and cleared human fetus of about 14 weeks in utero. Note the degree of progression of ossification from primary centres, which is endochondral in the appendicular and axial skeletons, except for the clavicles, and the intramembranous centres for the majority of the cranial bones which are visible. The carpus and tarsus are wholly cartilaginous, except for the primary centre of the calcaneus, as are the epiphyses of all the long bones. The central and neural arches of the vertebrae are separate. The sternum is still unossified. The membranous anterolateral and post-erolateral fontanelles are particularly obvious. (Photographed by Kevin Fitzpatrick, Division of Anatomy, United Medical and Dental Schools, London, from a specimen prepared by Roslyn Holthouse, formerly of the same department.)

6.10 Photographs illustrating three methods used to investigate possible interrelations between structural organization and patterns of force transmission in bone. A. Split-line patterns produced in a decalcified skull (*Macaca mulatta*) by repeated puncture with an ink-tipped needle; B. Pattern of cracks in the colophonium resin coating of a femur subjected to a compressive stress of the head, vertically applied; C. Photoelastic pattern produced in a flat plastic sheet modelled upon the proximal end of the femur. A compressive force has been applied to the femoral 'head', whilst a tensile force has been applied to its 'greater trochanter'. (C is from von Knief 1967, the others contributed by C Buckland-Wright, Division of Anatomy, United Medical and Dental Schools, London.)

intrauterine week, whereas its cartilaginous *epiphyses* ossify from secondary centres. As the epiphyses enlarge almost all the cartilage is replaced by bone, except for a specialized layer of hyaline cartilage that persists at the joint surface (p. 475) and a thicker zone between the diaphysis and epiphysis. Persistence of this *epiphyseal plate* or *disc* (*growth plate* or *growth cartilage*) allows increase in bone length until the usual dimensions are reached, by which time the epiphyseal plate has ossified. The bone has then reached maturity. Coalescence of the epiphysis and diaphysis is *fusion*, the amalgamation of separate osseous units into one.

Many bones have epiphyses at both ends, others at one end only. Long limb bones show the former, while the metacarpals, metatarsals, phalanges, clavicles and ribs have only one epiphysis, though the costal cartilages may represent epiphyses normally devoid of ossification centres. (For discussion of a *pseudoepiphysis* at the distal end of the first metacarpal see Haines 1974.) Epiphyseal ossification is sometimes more complex; for example, the proximal end of the humerus, wholly cartilaginous at birth, develops three centres during childhood, which coalesce into a single mass before fusing with the diaphysis. Only one of these centres forms an articular surface, the others forming the greater and lesser tubercles giving muscular attachments. Similar composite epiphyses occur at the distal end of the humerus and in the femur, ribs and vertebrae. Because some

439

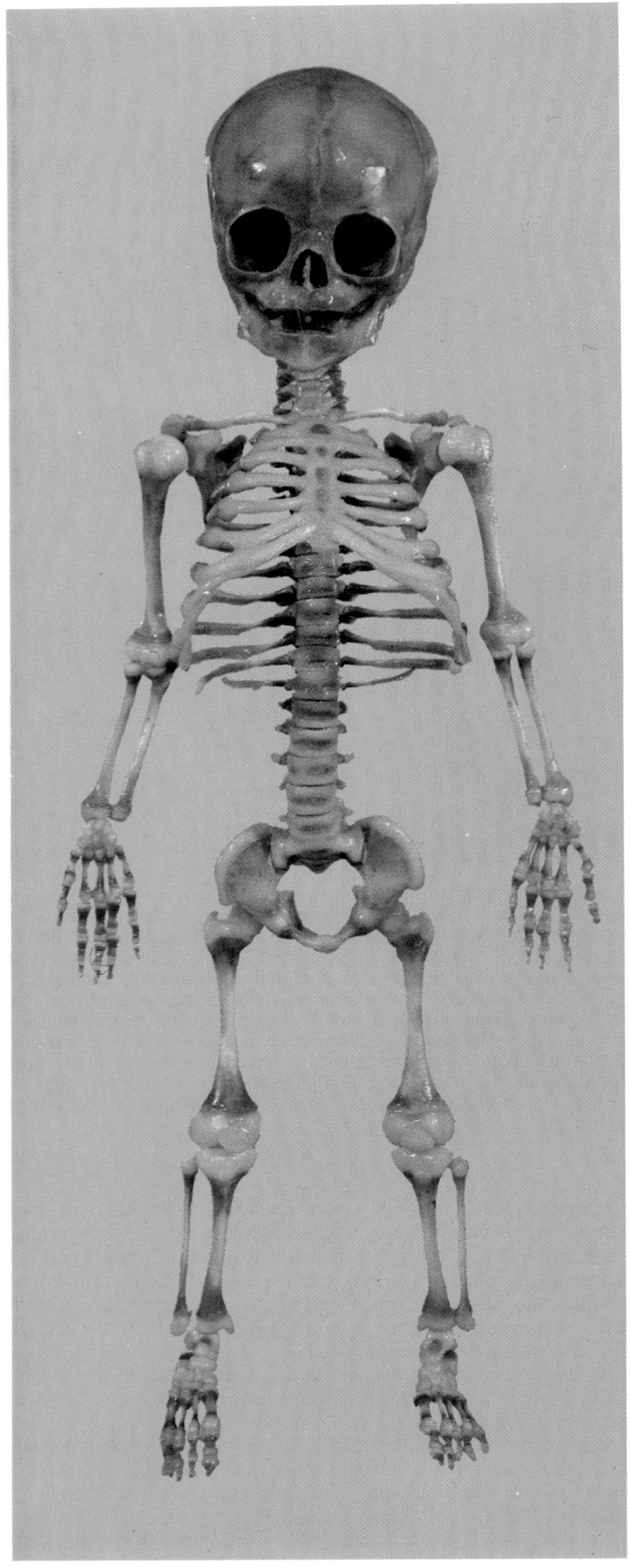

6.12 The skeleton of a neonatal infant, with all cartilages preserved. Note particularly the proportions of the neurocranium, orbital cavities and face; interfrontal (metopic) suture; sternebral ossification; extensive costal cartilages; large cartilaginous epiphyses and metaphyseal flaring of long bones, especially the humeri, femora and tibiae. (Photographed by Kevin Fitzpatrick from a preparation by Michael C E Hutchinson, of the Division of Anatomy, United Medical and Dental Schools, London.)

ossification centres appear in regions exposed to articular pressure, and others in regions subject to muscular traction, a classification into *pressure*, *traction* and *atavistic* epiphyses was proposed by Parsons (1903, 1904, 1905); the atavistic epiphyses being considered to represent skeletal elements separate at earlier evolutionary stages. Comparative morphology suggests that some mammalian bones are composites of separate reptilian or amphibian elements. The skull, clavicle, scapula and innominate bones are examples; a small centre in the human coracoid process and an epiphysis at the medial end of the clavicle may be vestiges of skeletal elements separate in earlier vertebrates, repeated during development as transient features in subsequent mammalian forms. However, the medial end of the clavicle could equally be regarded as a pressure epiphysis.

Many cranial bones ossify from multiple centres, and evidence suggests that some are atavistic. A marked reduction in the number of cranial bones in mammals, compared with older vertebrate groups, is clear. The sphenoid, temporal and occipital bones are almost certainly composites of previously multiple elements, some represented by centres which are additional evidence of fusion in dermal (membranous) and cartilaginous derivatives, at first separate but united during growth to form a complex whole (p. 588). These events in cranial development do not precisely parallel atavistic epiphyses in postcranial bones, which are always secondary. In human composite cranial bones the result is coalescence of elements, each with a primary centre.

Classification of epiphyses, of little significance per se, does, however, direct attention to matters of interest in mammalian skeletal evolution. Epiphyseal centres do not occur in other vertebrates, except sporadically in reptiles and birds (Haines 1937), and these are pressure (articular) epiphyses. Traction epiphyses are peculiar to mammals, but genetically established, for their appearance is not arrested by division of structures attached to them (Appleton 1922; Barnett & Lewis 1958). However, experimental evidence in connection with epiphyseal development is limited.

The rate of growth in ossification centres exceeds that of the cartilage in which they occur, though the latter is itself growing in concert with the increase in size and change in proportions of the skeletal element for which it is a model. Thus, the epiphyseal region, at first cartilaginous, gradually ossifies, with the exceptions noted above. The process starts at a time and continues at a rate characteristic for each bone. (Individual, sexual and racial variations must be taken into account, as far as data permit, when assessing skeletal age.)

The rate of growth also varies both in bones with epiphyseal plates and those without. Were the rate to be uniform, ossification centres would appear in a strict descending order of size. However, primary centres for bones of such different sizes as the phalanges and femora are separated by, at most, a week of embryonic life. Those for carpal and tarsal bones show some correlation between size and order of ossification, from largest (calcaneus in fifth fetal month) to smallest (pisiform in ninth to twelfth postnatal year). In individual bones, succession of centres is related to the volume of bone which each produces. The largest epiphyses, for example the adjacent ends of femur and tibia, begin to ossify the earliest (immediately before or after birth, points of forensic interest); but comparison between other bones reveals numerous inconsistencies. Masses as dissimilar as a phalangeal epiphysis and lesser tuberosity of the humerus begin to ossify about the same time, and both long before the much larger greater trochanter of the femur, indicating widely disparate rates of ossification.

Experiments in mammals show that, at epiphyseal plates, the rate of growth is initially equal at both ends of bones possessing two epiphyses, but that after birth one grows faster (Brookes 1963); since the faster-growing end also usually fuses later with the diaphysis, its contribution to length is greater. Though faster **rate** can only be presumed in human bones, **later** fusion is a radiological fact. Recurrent directions of nutrient arteries as they enter certain bones supports the above observations (cf. p. 469).

The more active end of a long limb bone is often termed the *growing end*, but this is obviously a misnomer. Variable rates of growth at epiphyses in general also show in the rate of increase of stature (Krogman 1941; Tanner 1962), which is rapid in infancy and again at puberty, but otherwise slower. The spurt at puberty, or slightly before, decreasing as epiphyses fuse in post-adolescent years, has been the subject of much study. For general reviews of fetal and postnatal growth patterns, including the skeleton, see Sinclair (1969), Tanner (1978).

Growth cartilages do not grow uniformly at all points; this accounts for changes such as the alteration in angle between the humeral shaft and its neck. On their diaphyseal surfaces epiphyses do not have a uniformly flat junction with the growth cartilages, nor indeed do the latter at their diaphyseal junction. By differential growth osseous surfaces usually become reciprocally curved, the epiphysis forming a shallow cup over the convex end of the shaft (cartilage intervening). This arrangement may resist shearing forces at this relatively weak region. Reciprocity of bone surfaces is augmented by small nodules and ridges, typical of such surfaces when denuded of cartilage. Such adaptations emphasize the formation of many immature bones from several elements held together by epiphyseal cartilages. Most human bones are such complexes, not only through the active years of childhood but also through the even more vigorous years of adolescence; the bonding of bone to bone through cartilage is thus strengthened.

Forces at growth cartilages are largely compressive, but with an element of shear. At traction epiphyses, attached by cartilage prior to fusion, attached structures create tension, perhaps promoting development of adundant collagen fibres aligned along supposed lines of stress (Smith 1962a). Interference with epiphyseal growth may occur as a result of violence, but disturbance by constitutional disease, such as fevers, is more frequent, producing visible changes in trabecular patterns of bone, visible radiographically as dense transverse *lines of arrested growth* (Harris 1933); several such lines may appear in the limb bones of children afflicted by successive illnesses.

Details of fusion are described later (p. 477). The growing part of a diaphysis adjacent to the epiphyseal cartilage, the *metaphysis*, appears to overtake the cartilage, but the epiphyseal contribution is shown by the denticulate edges of both bone elements as they bridge the cartilaginous gap. These appearances, extensively described, provide criteria for estimations of the times of fusion, by either inspection **or** radiography (Stevenson 1924). Knowledge of the sites, times of appearance, rates of growth and times of epiphyseal fusion is clinically, forensically and anthropometrically valuable. Reliable data depend upon adequate observations and standardized techniques. The variation in published figures is partly due to failure in these respects. Radiography needs to be more frequent than is usual, with the angle of view carefully controlled. Routine positions may be inadequate; for example, the centre for the lesser tubercle of the humerus is often missed, probably because its image is superimposed upon another centre.

Variation in skeletal development does, of course, occur between individuals, sexes and possibly also races. The *sequence* of events, however, shows little variation; it is their timing which varies. **Females antedate males** in all groups studied, and differences, perhaps insignificant before birth, increase thereafter, rising to two years or so in the later fusions of adolescence. Data are most reliable for caucasians, but few of their skeletal parts have been compared in sufficient detail, numbers or over adequate periods. Perhaps the best studies available are for the hand (Todd 1937; Greulich & Pyle 1959; Mathiasen 1973), knee (Pyle & Hoerr 1955) and ankle and foot (Hoerr et al 1962).

Cartilage and bone are specialized connective tissues consisting of the same three elements: *cells* embedded in a *matrix*, permeated by arrays of *fibres*; but sclerous tissues differ from soft, pliant, connective tissues, their matrix being solidified. Cartilage and bone, nevertheless, differ in structure, physical properties, vascularization and modes of growth and regeneration.

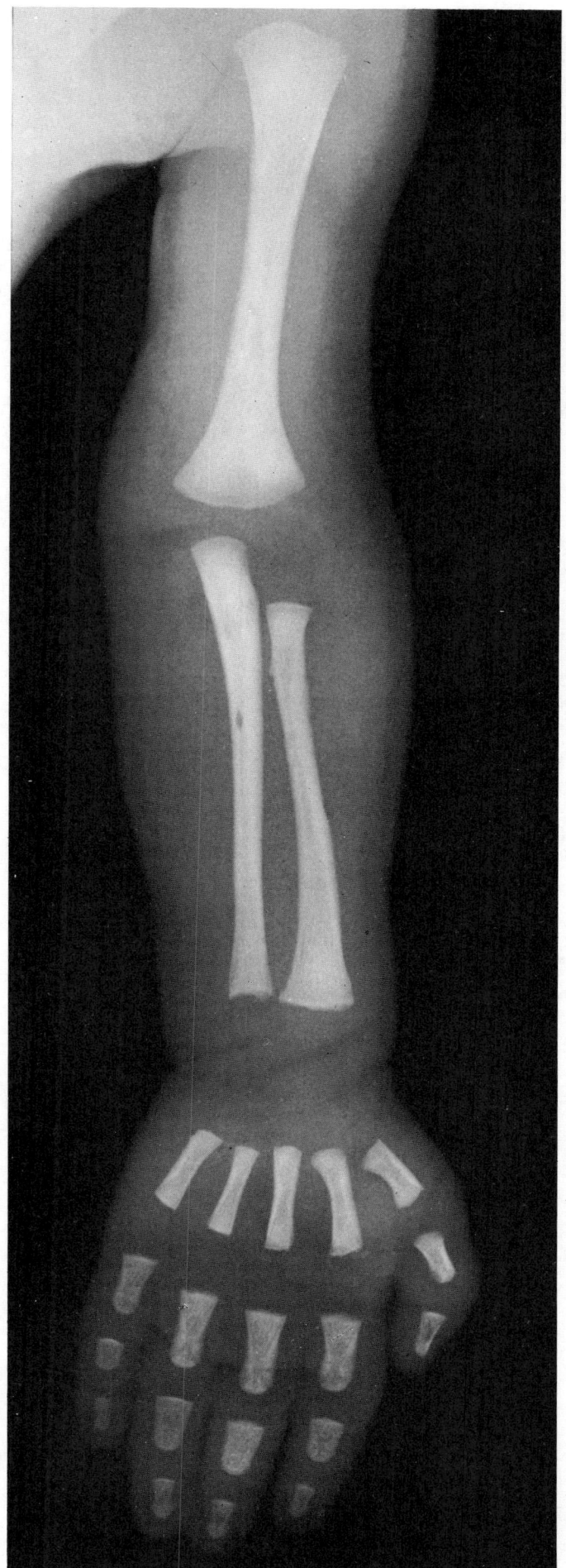

6.13A Radiograph of neonatal arm. Ossification from primary centres is well advanced in all bones except the carpals, which are still wholly cartilaginous. The gaps by which individual elements appear to be separated are filled by the radiolucent hyaline cartilage, in which epiphyseal or carpal ossification will subsequently occur. In long bones note the flaring contours, with narrow midshaft and relatively expanded metaphyses. Note also the proportions of the limb segments characteristic of this age—in particular the relatively large hand.

A

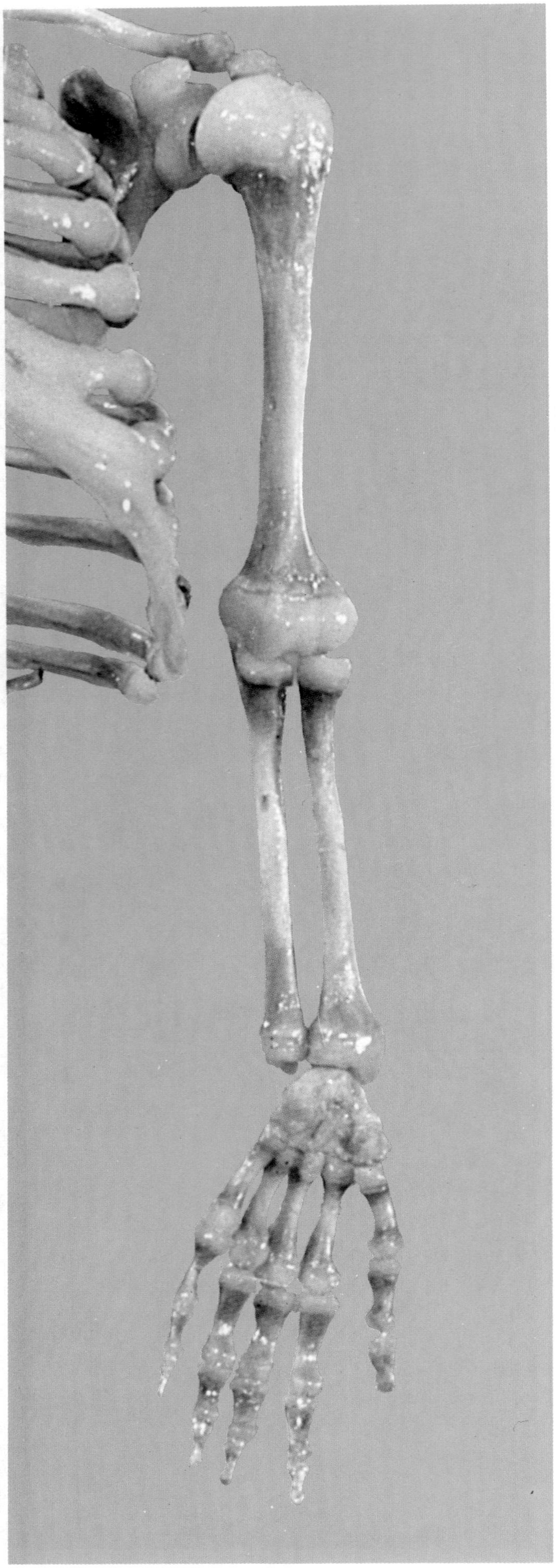

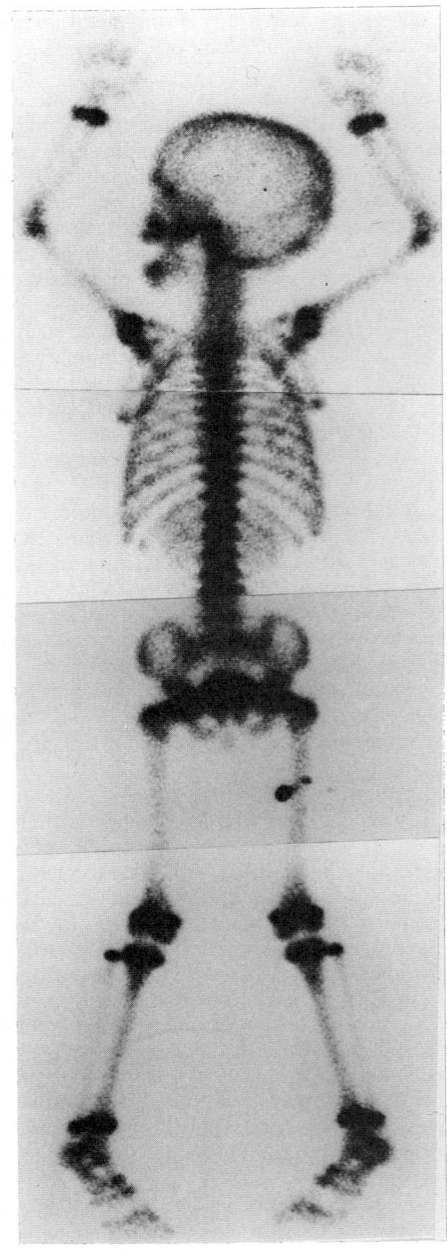

6.13B Photograph of a preparation of a neonatal left arm (from the specimen shown in 6.12). Compare the radiolucent areas in the radiograph (6.13A) with the preserved cartilaginous epiphyses and carpal elements in this specimen. (For acknowledgements see 6.12.) c Composite bone scan of a male child, aged approximately 1 year, showing sites of epiphyseal growth activity. The tracer used (technetium-99m labelled methylene diphosphonate) also shows the kidneys and bladder. (Provided by Department of Nuclear Medicine, United Medical and Dental Schools, London; photography by K Fitzpatrick and Sarah Smith.)

B

SKELETAL CONNECTIVE TISSUES

The skeletal tissues, cartilage and bone, are essentially specialized connective tissues and consist of the same components—cells embedded in a matrix permeated by a system of fibres. Physically, however, matrices of skeletal tissues differ from those of general connective tissues in being solidified. Cartilage and bone are, nevertheless, quite distinct in their structure, physical properties, vascularization and in their patterns of growth and regeneration.

STRUCTURE OF CARTILAGE

Cartilage is a phylogenetically ancient tissue, widespread in vertebrates as either a permanent or temporary skeletal component. During early fetal life the human skeleton is mostly cartilaginous, but is subsequently largely replaced by bone. In adults cartilage persists at the surfaces of synovial joints, in the walls of the larynx, trachea, bronchi, nose and external ears, in the epiglottis and as isolated small masses in the cranial base. Developmental replacement by bone is a complex process, and cartilaginous growth plates between ossifying epiphyses and diaphyses of long bones (and elsewhere) continue to proliferate, increasing the length of the bones concerned until they eventually ossify, when growth ceases (see reviews in Hall 1983).

Cartilage is essentially a type of stiff, load-bearing connective tissue. Its distinctive properties are a low metabolic rate and a vascular supply confined to its surface or to large, penetrating tunnels, a capacity for continued and often rapid interstitial and appositional growth (see below) and a high resistance to tension, compression and shearing, with some resilience and elasticity. Cartilage is covered by a fibrous *perichondrium* except at osseous junctions; at synovial surfaces, the latter are lubricated by secreted, nutrient fluid.

Cartilage matrix. This contains *chondroblasts* and *chondrocytes*, varies in appearance, composition and in the nature of its fibres. Hence there is *hyaline cartilage* (*hyalos* = glass), white *fibrocartilage* (with much collagen) or yellow *elastic cartilage* (with an elastin network). A densely *cellular cartilage*, with thin septa of matrix between its cells, is a stage in development of early *embryonic cartilage* and a permanent tissue in many mammalian pinnae. White and yellow elastic fibrocartilage are specific, relatively unvarying tissues, whereas hyaline cartilage embraces a wide range of appearances varying much in composition and properties according to age and location as well as species.

Cartilage cells (6.14A, B, 15, 16, 17). These occupy small lacunae in the matrix which conform to their shape. Young cells (*chrondroblasts*) are smaller, often flat, irregular in contour and bear many surface projections (*filopodia*) fitting complementary recesses in the matrix. Early postmitotic chondroblasts often have intercellular contacts, including gap junctions, which are necessarily transient, disappearing as matrix synthesis proceeds. As cartilage cells mature, they lose the ability to divide and become metabolically less active. Some authors reserve the name *chondrocytes* for such cells; but this term is commonly employed to denote cartilage of all degrees of activity, a practice which will largely be followed here. When appropriate, however, chondroblasts and chondrocytes are distinguished. Mature chondrocytes enlarge with age and, though rounder, still have a few filopodia and an occasional cilium. The internal structure of chondrocytes is typical of cells active in making and secreting proteins (Stockwell 1983; Kosher 1983; Sheldon 1983). Their nucleus is rounded or oval, euchromatic and possesses one or more important nucleoli. The cytoplasm is filled with granular endoplasmic reticulum, transport vesicles and Golgi complexes, and contains many mitochondria and frequent lysosomes. Also present are numerous glycogen granules, intermediate filaments (vimentin) and pigment granules. With final maturation of these cells to the relatively inactive chondrocyte stage, the nucleus becomes heterochromatic, the nucleoli smaller and the apparatus of synthesis and secretion (endoplasmic reticulum, Golgi apparatus, etc.) much reduced; often such cells accumulate lipid vacuoles, quite large in diameter.

Very little is known about the responses of chondrocytes to load bearing, or how the pericellular matrix absorbs stresses and protects the chondrocytes. Changes in shape and size of articular chondrocytes or *chondrons* of pericellular matrix encapsulating cells must occur during function but have not been described in living tissue.

Intercellular matrix. Composed of *collagen* and, in some cases, *elastin fibres*, embedded in a water-filled yet stiff ground substance (6.18, 19), these components have various chemical features which are unique to cartilage, and confer upon it unusual mechanical properties. The *ground substance* is a firm gel, rich in carbohydrates and therefore stainable with the periodic acid-Schiff (PAS) method; the carbohydrates are predominantly acidic, and are hence basophilic, strongly binding such dyes as haematoxylin, alcian blue and toluidine blue, and giving metachromatic coloration with the latter. The chemistry of the ground substance is complex, consisting mainly of water and dissolved salts, held in a meshwork of long interwoven proteoglycan molecules together with various other minor constituents, mainly proteins or glycoproteins and some lipid.

Collagen of the cartilage matrix. (6.18). Forming up to 50% of its dry weight, this is chemically distinct from that of most other tissues, being classed as Type II collagen; elsewhere this variety is only found in the notochord, the nucleus pulposus of the inter-

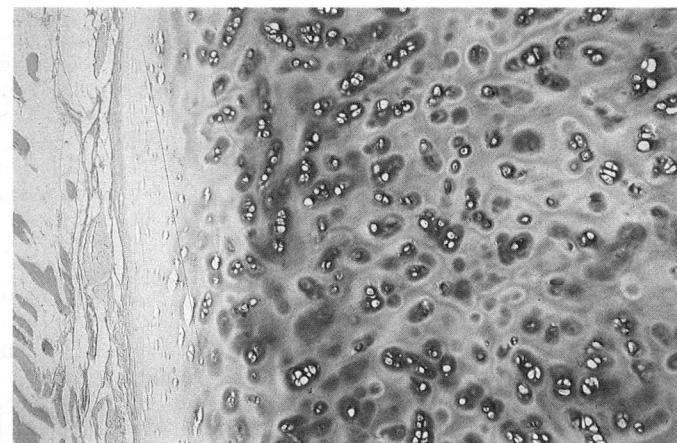

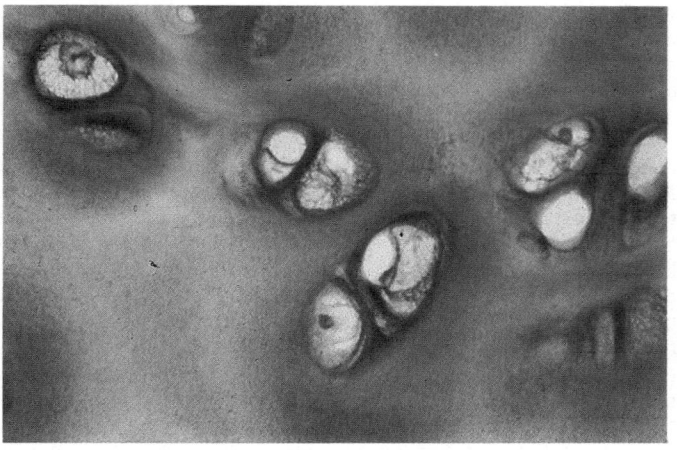

6.14 Sections through hyaline cartilage (human rib), stained with haematoxylin and eosin. A. is a low-power view, showing perichondrium, chondroblasts and mature chondrocytes embedded in the basophilic matrix.

Magnification ×150. B. Higher magnification showing groups of chondrocytes within lacunae. Note the basophilic zones (rich in proteoglycans) around the cell clusters. Magnification ×1000.

443

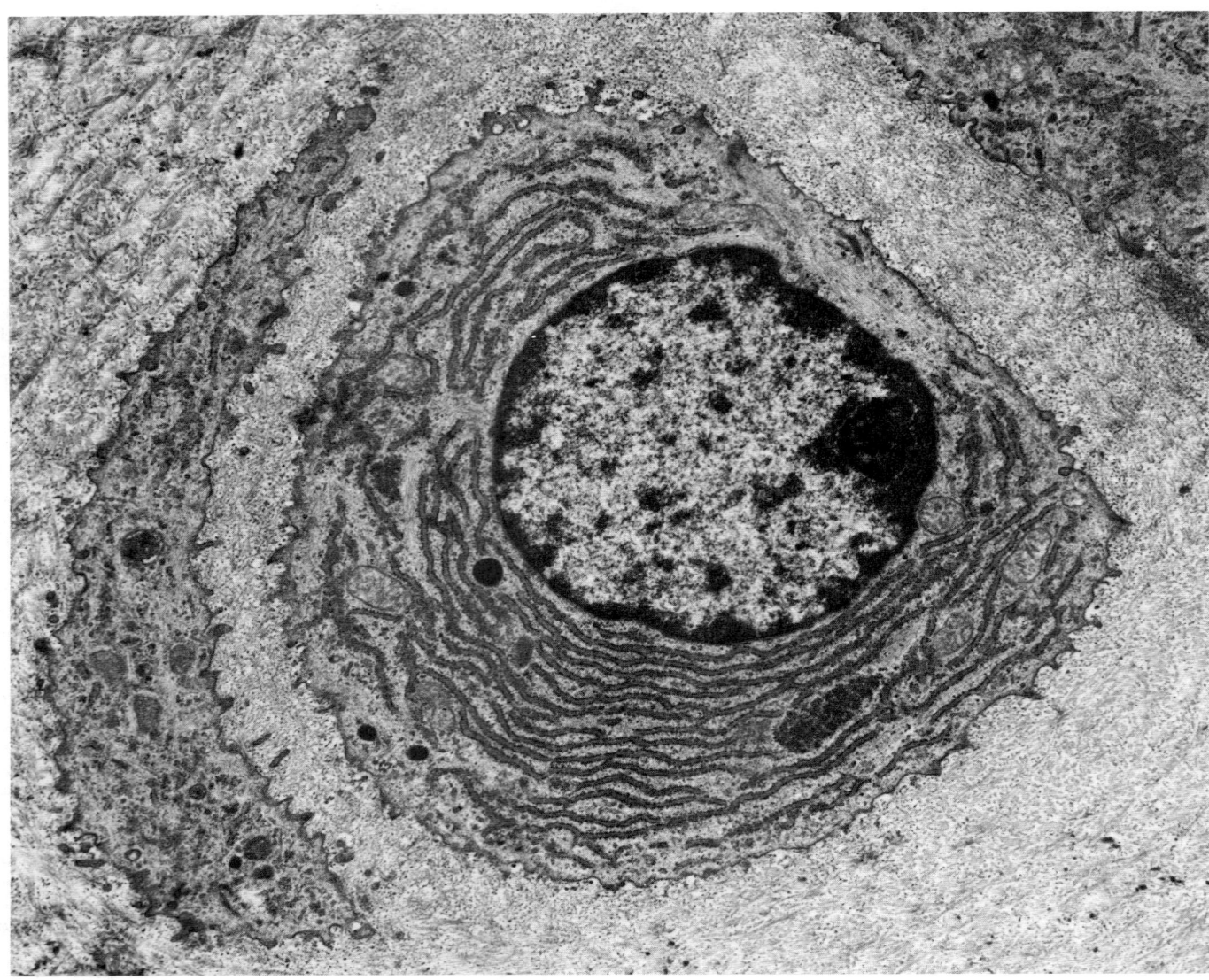

6.15 Transmission electron micrograph of an ultra-thin section of a perfusion-fixed specimen of a rabbit's femoral condylar cartilage. The centrally placed chondroblast contains an active euchromatic nucleus with a prominent nucleolus. Its cytoplasm contains a rich concentration of roughly parallel concentric flattened cisternae of rough endoplasmic reticulum, scattered mitochondria, lysosomes and aggregations of glycogen. Its plasma membrane bears numerous short filopodia which project into complementary recesses in the surrounding matrix. The latter shows a delicate fibrillary feltwork with a finely dispersed granular interfibrillary substance. No pericellular 'lacuna' is present; the matrix separates the central chondroblast from the sectioned cytoplasmic periphery of two adjacent chondroblasts. The left profile, crescentic in outline, is characteristic of chondroblasts with an almost squamous form that are sited near the articular surface. Magnification ×14 500. (Preparation by Susan Smith, Department of Anatomy, Guy's Hospital Medical School, London.)

vertebral disc, the vitreous body of the eye and in the primary corneal stroma. Its tropocollagen subunits are composed of triple helices of identical polypeptides (three α-1 chains), although collagen in the outer layers of the perichondrium and much of the collagen in white fibrocartilage belongs to the general connective tissue Type 1. The majority of the collagen fibres of cartilage are too small to be individually visible except by electron microscopy; they are relatively short, thin (mainly 10–20 nm diameter) structures with the characteristic cross-banding (67 nm, appearing as 64 nm intervals insections) and they are interwoven to create a three-dimensional meshwork linked by lateral projections of the proteoglycans associated with their surfaces. Various studies have shown that proteoglycans partially ensheath collagen fibres, and their concentrations often share the periodicity of the fibres. Proteoglycans and other organic molecules thus link collagen fibres with each other, with the interfibrillar material of the ground substance and also with the cells of cartilage. Collagen fibres vary greatly in their amounts, sizes and orientation in different types of cartilage, as also with maturity and position within the cartilage mass. In articular cartilage, collagen fibres close to the surfaces of cells are particularly narrow (4–6 nm across) and resemble fibres of Type II cartilage in non-cartilaginous sites.

In addition to Type II collagen, the principal component, minor quantities of other classes unique to cartilage are present, including Types IX, X and XI. The significance of these is as yet unclear, but they may be involved in stabilizing Type II collagen networks (Type IX) and in hypertrophic changes in some types of cartilage (Type X). Type VI collagen is also present, mainly in the vicinity of chondrocytes (Poole et al 1992; Hagiwara et al 1993) and may form a link between the chondrocyte, pericellular microenvironment and interterritorial matrix. As described below, other types of fibre are also present in some classes of cartilage; these include elastin fibres in elastic fibrocartilage and, where ligamentous structures are inserted, as in fibrocartilage, Type I collagen, derived from fibroblasts rather than chondrocytes.

Proteoglycans of cartilage. These are similar in general outline to those of general connective tissue, although with features peculiar to cartilage. They consist of various long polymers, often branched, of carbohydrates termed *glycosaminoglycans* (GAGs: Lash & Vasan 1983). These are acidic, bearing anionic sulphate and carboxyl groups which give them a net negative charge. Groups of GAGs are covalently bound to a filament of protein (the '*core protein*', with an Mr of 250 000 and a length of 300 nm) which may bear more than

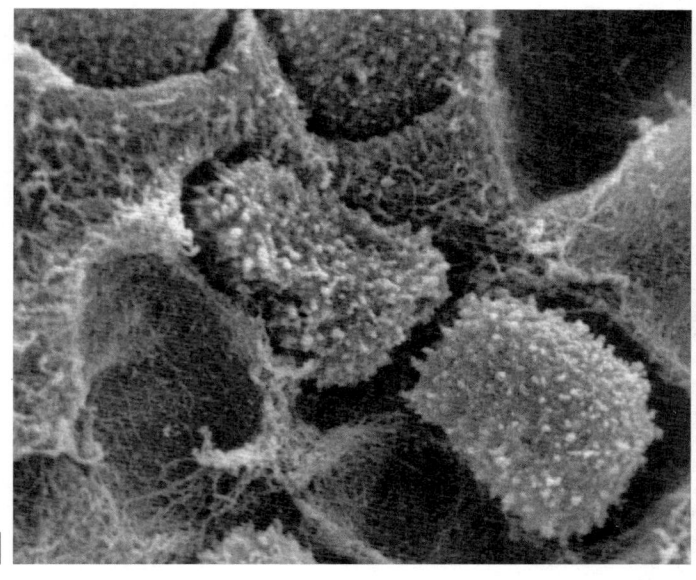

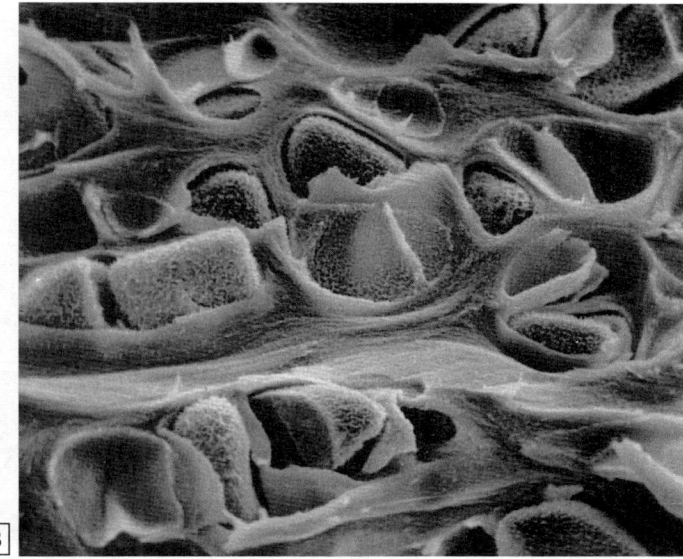

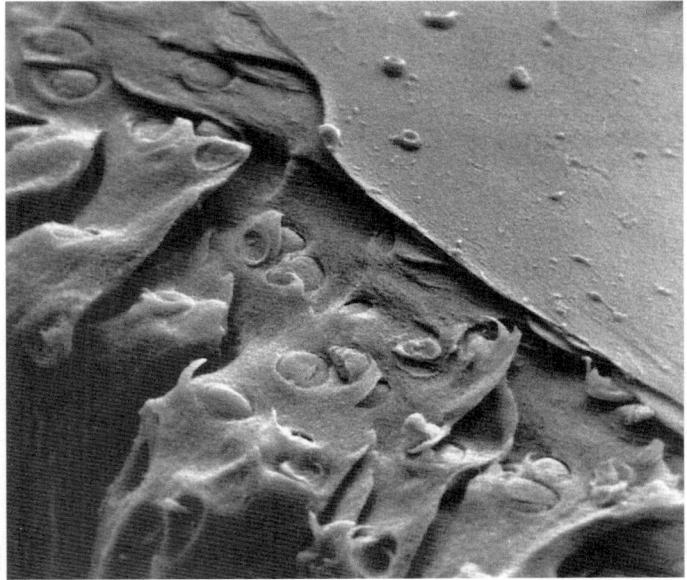

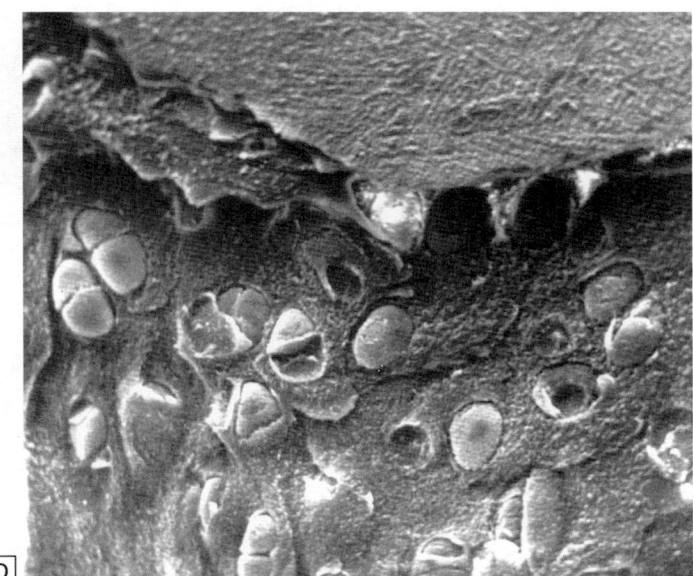

6.16A Chrondrocytes in highly cellular embryonic cartilage have many short microvilli. 17-day fetal mouse embryo phalangeal cartilage; SEM of critical point dried (cpd) tissue, field width = 43 μm. B. Isogenous chondrocytes separated only by thin septae of matrix in lacunae in chipmunk nasal septal cartilage; SEM of tissue fixed by osmic acid perfusion, cpd and fractured dry; field width = 90 μm. C. Articular surface and zones 1 and 2 of rat femur at knee joint. The joint surface is flat, and chondrocytes lie em-

bedded in a finely fibrous matrix. Fixed with glutaraldehyde and osmium, cpd and dissected dry; SEM, field width = 140 μm. D. Rat lower femoral head snap-frozen and freeze-dried showing reticulated pattern of ice crystal formation preserved in freeze-dried synovial fluid to top of figure. The cells in the immediate sub-surface zone have produced no impressions in the articular surface; SEM, field width = 127 μm.

one hundred GAGs of different types sticking out sideways like the bristles of a bottle brush (**6.19**). In turn, several such proteoglycan assemblies can be bound along the length of a relatively huge (a million or more in relative molecular mass) *hyaluronate* molecule (another type of GAG) to form highly complex, filamentous aggregates. Other, smaller '*link proteins*' are involved in this interaction. Because of the predominance of acidic groups there is a tendency for the chains to repel each other, thus standing out stiffly from the central core protein. Weak intermolecular forces hold these aggregates together as a three-dimensional network with large water-filled spaces within. This arrangement allows the ready diffusion of water and dissolved materials through the ground substance, although water and other electrolytes are also loosely bound by the electrostatic forces on the surfaces of the charged macromolecules. In the living state the molecular aggregates appear to be compressed into a smaller volume than would be expected from their shape, the length of their chains and electrical repulsions between their subunits. It has been suggested that the proteoglycans may act as minute compressed

springs, storing energy when further compacted then releasing it on recoil and so conferring elastic properties on the matrix.

In most electron microscope sections, these large molecular arrays generally collapse to small dense granules about 20 nm across as their hydration sheaths are stripped away. However, when separated by centrifugation and negatively stained or prepared by cryo-technology, their complex feathery nature is clearly visible (Hunziker & Schenk 1987).

Glycosaminoglycans (GAGs). Those in the proteoglycans of cartilage include chondroitin 4-sulphate, chondroitin 6-sulphate and dermatan sulphate, and also keratin sulphate. These are polysaccharides mainly composed of repeating disaccharides, one invariably a substituted hexosamine and the other an esterified hexuronic acid or substituted hexose. Thus chondroitin 4- and 6-sulphates comprise repeating N-acetylgalactosamine and glucuronyl sulphate disaccharides, differing only in the siting of the sulphate ester linkage. Keratin sulphate is a polymer of disaccharides composed of an N-acetylgalactosamine and a D-galactose with a sulphate ester

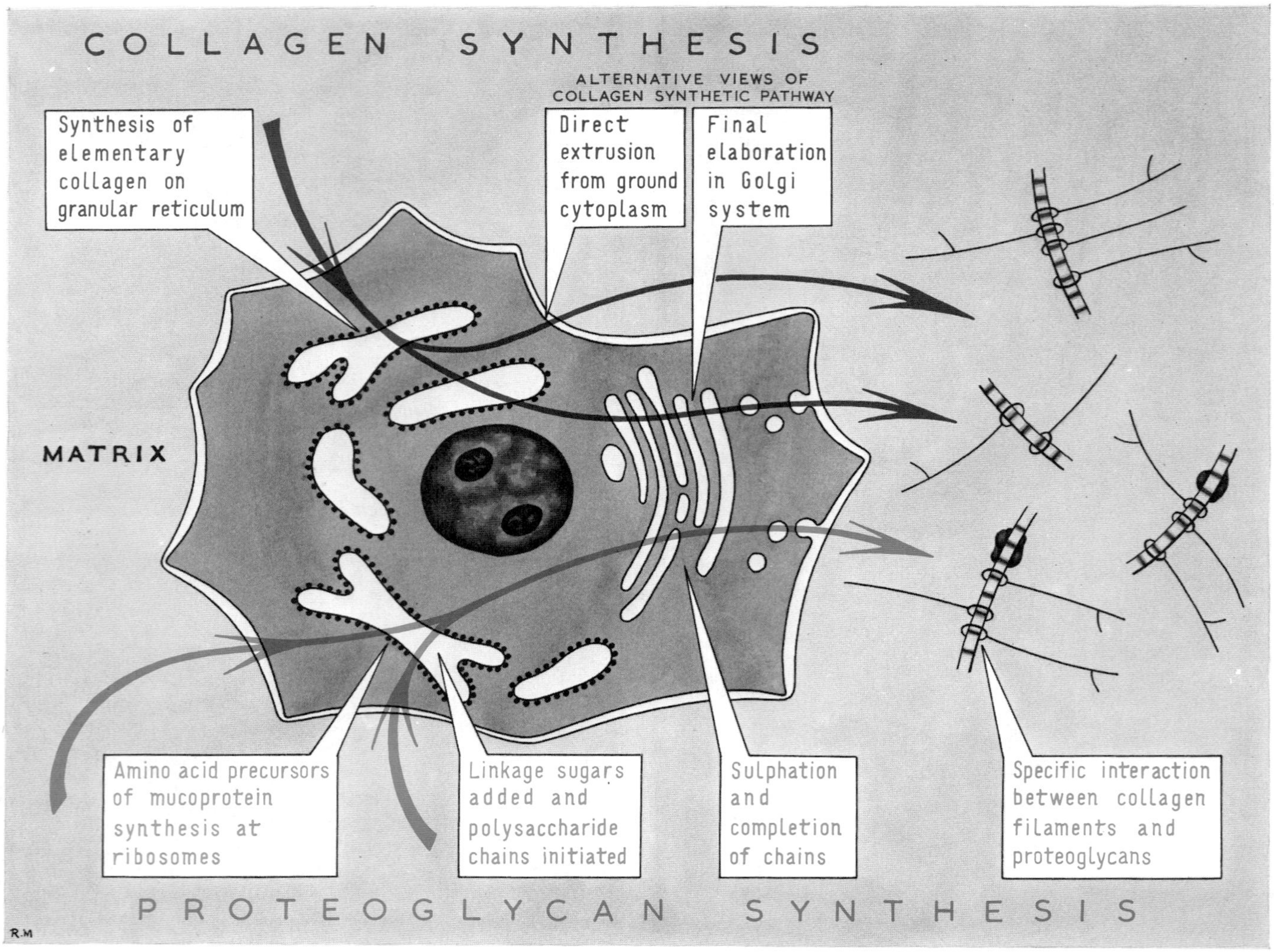

COLLAGEN SYNTHESIS

ALTERNATIVE VIEWS OF
COLLAGEN SYNTHETIC PATHWAY

Synthesis of
elementary
collagen on
granular reticulum

Direct
extrusion
from ground
cytoplasm

Final
elaboration
in Golgi
system

MATRIX

Amino acid precursors
of mucoprotein
synthesis at
ribosomes

Linkage sugars
added and
polysaccharide
chains initiated

Sulphation
and
completion
of chains

Specific interaction
between collagen
filaments and
proteoglycans

PROTEOGLYCAN SYNTHESIS

6.17 Summary of some of the important biosynthetic pathways of the chondroblast.

linkage of variable position. The relatively huge hyaluronate molecules have similar repeating disaccharides of N-acetylglucos- amine and glucuronate composition, but are not sulphated and are unbranched.

These different chemical configurations result in different numbers of electrostatic charges, different degrees of interactions between adjacent chains and other variations in bulk properties which deter- mine many of the physical and chemical properties of the matrix. The colocalization in mesenchymal cell condensations of collagen

Types II and IX and proteoglycan core protein heralds the onset of chondrogenesis.

Cell adhesion proteins. Those that include various proteins and glycoproteins have recently been shown to play an important role in the adhesion of chondrocytes to matrix components. The best known is *chondronectin*, a cartilage glycoprotein important in the adhesion of chondroblasts to Type II collagen fibres in the presence of chondroitin sulphates. It has an Mr of about 150 000 (Hewitt et al 1980); and is synthesized by chondrocytes. Another adhesion

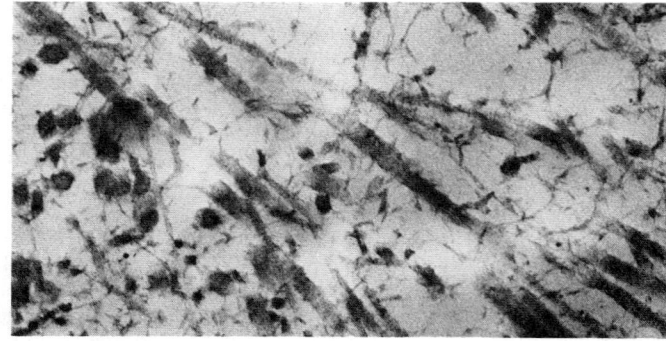

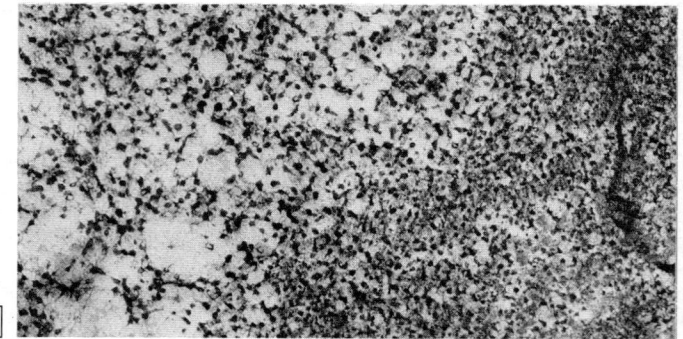

A

B

6.18 Electron micrograph of hyaline cartilage matrix. The matrix in A shows thick, banded collagen fibrils and thinner, unbanded ones. Traces of finely filamentous proteoglycan complexes can also be seen adhering to and connecting collagen fibrils. Magnification ×30 000. In B the matrix has been

fixed in the presence of ruthenium red to preserve proteoglycan complexes, which are here visible as densely staining beaded structures representing collapsed assemblies of protein and glycosaminoglycans. Magnification ×10 000. (Provided by Moya Meredith Smith.)

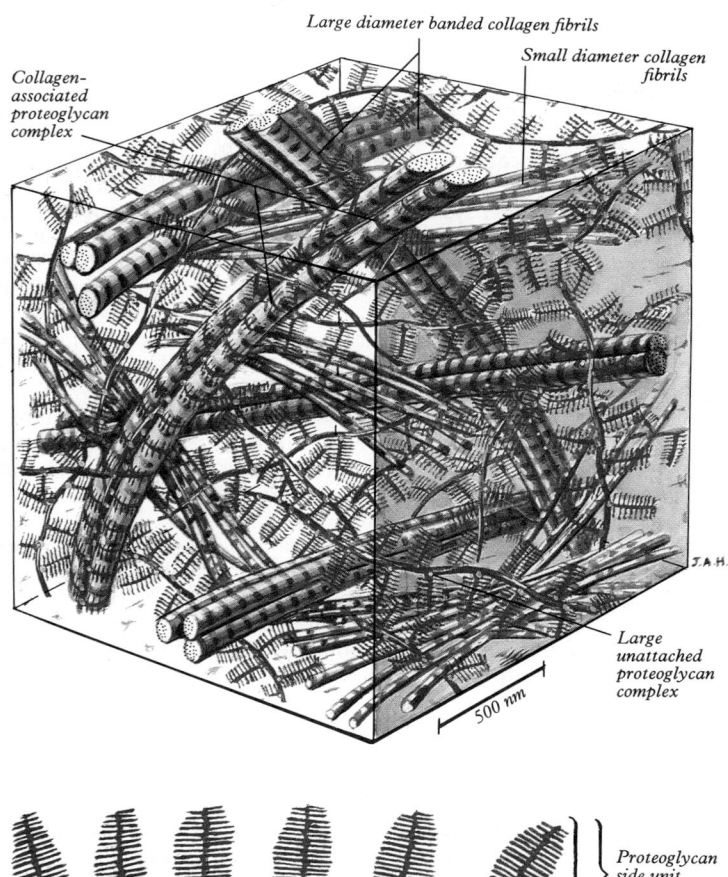

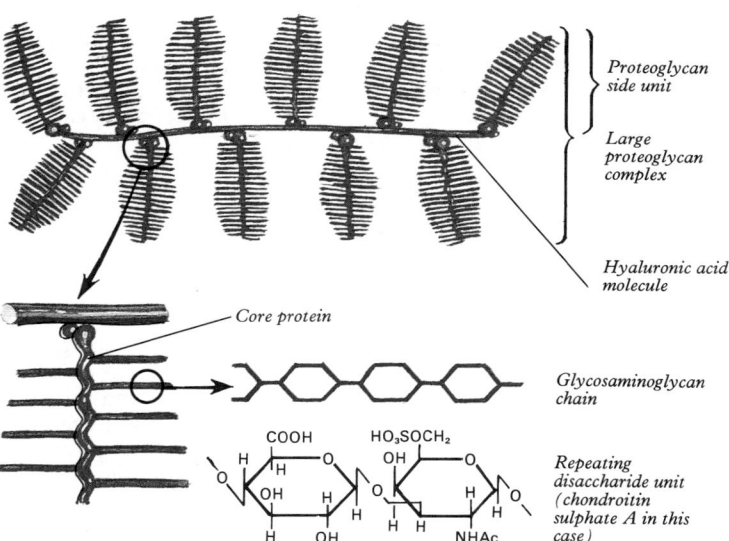

6.19 Diagram showing the fine structural organization of hyaline cartilage matrix. Depicted are large proteoglycan complexes and Type II collagen fibres of the coarser cross-banded and the narrower varieties. Proteoglycan complexes bind to the surface of these fibres and link them together. Detail shows the arrangement of glycosaminoglycans and core filaments. See text for further details.

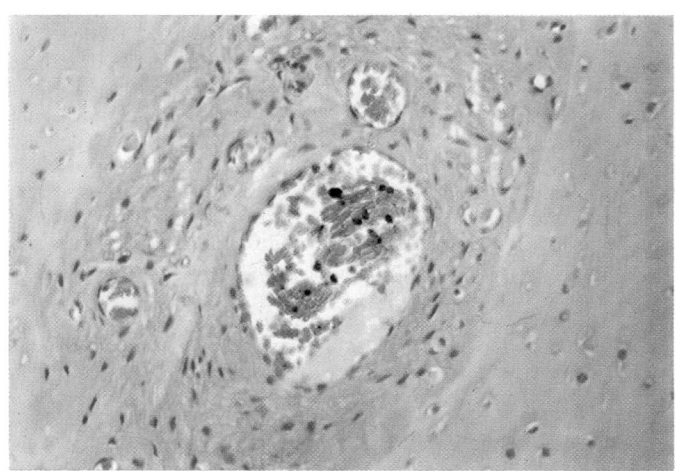

6.20 Section through the proximal cartilaginous end of the tibia of a young child showing a cartilage canal and its contained blood vessels, stained with haematoxylin and eosin.

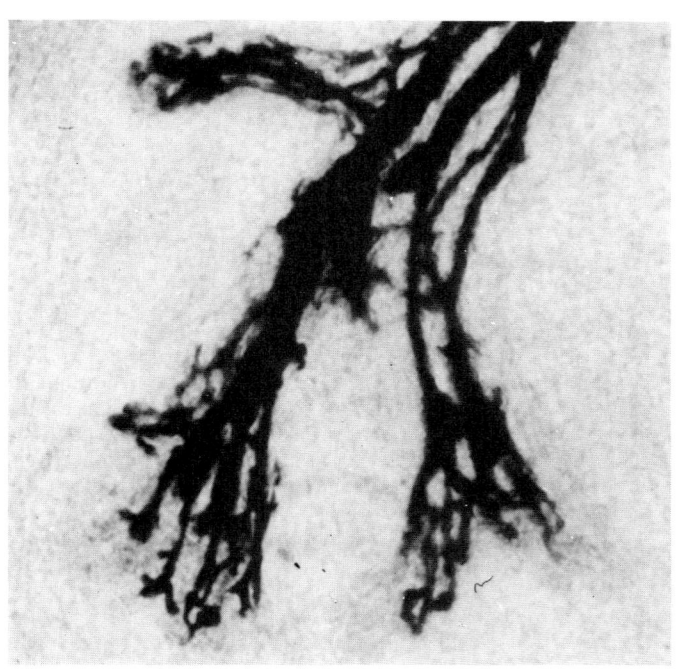

6.21 Capillary plexuses in the terminal arborization of a cartilage canal in the femoral condylar epiphysis of a seven-month human fetus. Specimen injected with Indian ink. (Provided by Murray Brookes, Department of Anatomy, Guy's Hospital Medical School, London.)

molecule is *anchorin CII* (von der Mark et al 1985), a glycoprotein with an Mr of 34 000 found at chondrocyte surfaces and binding specifically to Type II collagen. Aggregating proteoglycans, *aggrecan* and *versican*, are also produced by human chondrocytes (Grover & Roughley 1993). There may also be other similar substances which play a part in stabilizing the structural complex of cells and matrix components.

Lipid. This is also present as part of the matrix, in the form of small spheroidal masses stainable with lipid-soluble dyes for light microscopy (Meachim & Stockwell 1978). Some of this may be the result of cell disintegration, or shedding of cytoplasm, and some is membranous material or portions of cells, for example the matrix vesicles found in epiphyseal growth plates.

Summary. The matrix of cartilage is a labyrinth of protein and proteoglycan filaments, its interstices occupied by bound water, cations and various other small molecules. Reactions to mechanical stresses accordingly reflect interacting contributions from all these structural elements. The properties of the '*walls*' and '*contents*' of this molecular meshwork also affect the diffusion of nutrient and waste material throughout this remarkable tissue.

Synthesis of matrix by chondrocytes. All of the major components of the matrix are synthesized and secreted by chondrocytes (**6.**17). These processes have been studied extensively with a battery of biochemical, structural and autoradiographic methods (see the reviews by Prockop et al 1979; Mayne & von der Mark 1983). To summarize these findings briefly, collagen is synthesized within the

447

granular endoplasmic reticulum in the same way as in fibroblasts, except that Type II rather than Type I procollagen chains are made. These assemble into triple helices and some carbohydrate is added at this stage. After transport to the Golgi apparatus, where further glycosylation occurs, they are secreted as procollagen molecules into the extracellular space. Here, terminal registration peptides are cleaved from their ends, so forming tropocollagen molecules, and final assembly into collagen fibres takes place. In other regions of the granular endoplasmic reticulum, core proteins of the proteoglycan complexes are synthesized and addition of GAG chains is begun, completion of the process being carried out in the Golgi complex (Lohmander et al 1986).

The large molecules of glucuronate appear to be synthesized by enzymes inserted in the plasma membrane of the chondrocyte and are thought to be extruded directly into the matrix without passing through the endoplasmic reticulum.

NUTRITION OF CARTILAGE

Cartilage is often described as totally avascular. This is not wholly true but most cartilage cells are unusually distant from exchange vessels, which are mostly perichondrial. Between this perichondrial capillary network and chondrocytes, nutrient substances and metabolites diffuse along concentration gradients across the intervening matrix. This limitation is reflected in the restriction of most living cartilage masses to a few millimetres in thickness. Cartilage cells further than this from a nutrient vessel do not survive, and their surrounding matrix typically becomes calcified.

Cartilage contains an anti-angiogenic factor that inhibits vascular invasion (Kuettner & Pauli 1983a,b; Hall 1988) and inhibitors to many chondrolytic proteinases (Homandberg et al 1992).

Cartilage canals

Nutrition is augmented, at least in cartilaginous epiphyses of large mammals (and their analogues in birds and reptiles) by branching of cartilage canals (Brookes 1971), each containing small vessels from centripetal rami of a perichondrial artery and vein. Perfusion (Brookes 1958) and histological examination (Wilsman & Van Sickle 1972) suggest that each canal contains a central small artery or arteriole surrounded by numerous venules and perivascular capillaries (6.20, 21). The central vessel, at the blind end of the canal, forms several capillaries from which venules pass back to a parent perichondrial vein. Capillaries lined by fenestrated endothelium branch off along the canal and, with terminal capillaries, mediate metabolic exchange with the cartilage mass (Wilsman & Van Sickle 1972). The canalicular vessels lie enclosed in loose connective tissue, abundant in fibroblasts and macrophages and continuous with the perichondrium.

Various theories have been proposed for their formation. The possibility that they are derived from perichondrial vessels which have been engulfed by the appositional growth of cartilage around them is attractively simple, but does not explain many findings, for example, that cartilage canals are formed more rapidly than the growing front of cartilage moves forwards. It appears instead that canals actively invade cartilage, probably by the action of macrophages and other erosive cells (Wilsman & Van Sickle 1972); among the latter the endothelium of the central blood vessels may be important, as the ability of these cells to release chondrolytic agents has been demonstrated in tissue culture (Moscatelli et al 1981). However, chondrocytes themselves are also able to degrade cartilage matrix (*chondrocytic chondrolysis*), and may also play a part in canal formation, either subsequently dying ahead of an advancing blood vessel to present it with a series of preformed cavities or, having freed themselves from the matrix, de-differentiating to form other mesenchymally derived cells of the cartilage canals.

Cartilage canals are not random, but have a characteristic pattern in each cartilage. Canals in a fetal epiphysis form two groups, the more conspicuous passing from the non-articular surfaces towards its centre, the less prominent from vessels in the *ossification groove* (*of Ranvier*); capillary tufts at the ends of the latter are complex and glomerular, like those in postnatal subchondral circulation (Trueta & Morgan 1960). According to Brookes (1971), the pattern of arteries in some adult bony epiphyses closely resembles the canalicular pattern in corresponding fetal epiphyses, indicating that vessels in

the canals may be forerunners of main epiphyseal vessels in mature bone, and that vessels in the minor group of canals originating in Ranvier's groove are precursors of subchondral vascular networks on the epiphyseal side of growth cartilages in postnatal life.

Cartilage canals are believed to assist nutrition of large cartilages, which would depend otherwise solely on perichondrial capillaries. This process appears to be faster than formerly considered both in young and mature cartilage. Labelled ions are concentrated rapidly by chondrocytes of mature articular cartilage (Hall 1965), despite the absence of canals and perichondrium; the half-life of proteoglycans in rabbit articular cartilage is only 4 days (Mankin & Lipiello 1969). While it might be expected that large cartilages, such as fetal limb epiphyses, possess canals, it is surprising that they also occur in carpal and sesamoid cartilages in early fetal hands, and even in the epiphyses of human fetal phalanges at 11 cm crown–rump (CR) length (Gray et al 1957).

While not denying a nutritional function, most workers consider that cartilage canals are involved in forming *secondary centres of ossification* (and *primary centres* in bones without epiphyses). But puzzling anomalies remain. Distal phalangeal and proximal metacarpal epiphyses develop elaborate cartilage canals, though lacking ossification centres. There is also no clear connection between onset of chondrification, the first appearance of canals and onset of ossification; all occur at times peculiar to each skeletal element (Brookes 1971). The contents of canals appear to provide osteogenic cells and capillaries for ossification when an ossification centre appears. The control of the timing of these events remains an enigma.

In the *mandibular condylar cartilage*, canals form until the second year, when they disappear. Canals in laryngeal and nasal cartilages first form in the seventh month in utero, persisting until old age; in costal cartilages they arise in the first year, reaching the centre of the shaft about the tenth year. In long-lived canals, marrow elements may appear after the twentieth year, persisting until the sixties, when atrophy supervenes, canals retaining a mucinous material.

Cartilage canals are present in various locations apart from long bone epiphyses, occurring also, for example, in respiratory cartilages (see reviews by Kuettner & Pauli 1983a,b).

VARIETIES OF CARTILAGE

Cartilage may be *hyaline, white fibrocartilage* and *yellow elastic cartilage* and *cellular cartilage*. It may also be calcified.

Hyaline cartilage (6.16, 22A, 23A)

Hyaline cartilage has a glassy, bluish, opalescent, homogeneous appearance, firm consistency and some elasticity. Costal, nasal, some laryngeal, tracheobronchial, all temporary and most articular cartilages are hyaline, but there are marked differences in size, shape and arrangement of cells, fibres and proteoglycan composition at different sites and ages. Its cells vary in shape from quite flat near the perichondrium to rounded or bluntly angular deeper in the tissue. They are often in groups of two or more (*cell nests* or *isogenous cell groups*) which are the offspring of a common parent chondroblast; such cells have a straight outline where apposed to each other, but a rounded contour in general. The matrix is typically basophilic and metachromatic, both more pronounced where recently formed matrix bounds a lacuna. This distinctive zone is the territorial matrix or lacunar capsule, contrasting with the pale-staining interterritorial matrix between cell nests. An isogenous cell group together with the enclosing pericellular matrix is referred to as a *chondron*.

The fresh matrix is transparent and structureless, or faintly granular like ground glass when viewed by standard light microscopy. By polarized light or electron microscopy it appears permeated by fine fibrils and fibres of collagen, 10–20 nm in diameter. Electron microscopy shows that around each chondrocyte there is some zonation of the matrix. In well-fixed tissue where no cell shrinkage has occurred, the irregular surface of the chondrocyte is in direct contact with the matrix. However, there is often an encapsulating layer of proteoglycans containing fine filaments of uncertain composition, but no typical collagen, immediately surrounding the cell, probably corresponding to the limits of the lacuna seen by light microscopy. Outside this there are typical collagen fibres, often arranged in a basket-like network around one or more cells in a group, grading into the parallel fibre domain between cells, the

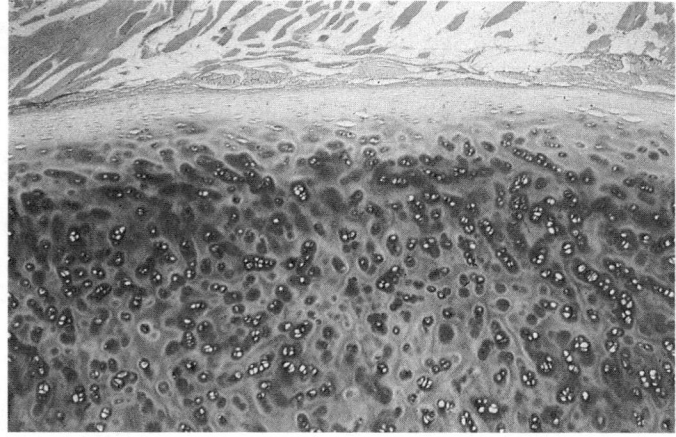

A. Hyaline cartilage (see also **6**.14 A, B) H & E. Magnification ×150.

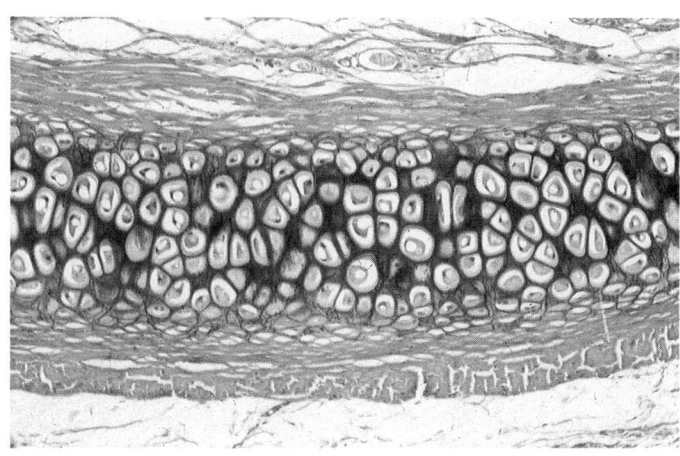

B. Elastic fibrocartilage, stained with Gomori's elastin stain (blue-black), and van Gieson's collagen stain (pink), which shows the fibrous perichondrium clearly. Pinna (rabbit). Magnification ×150.

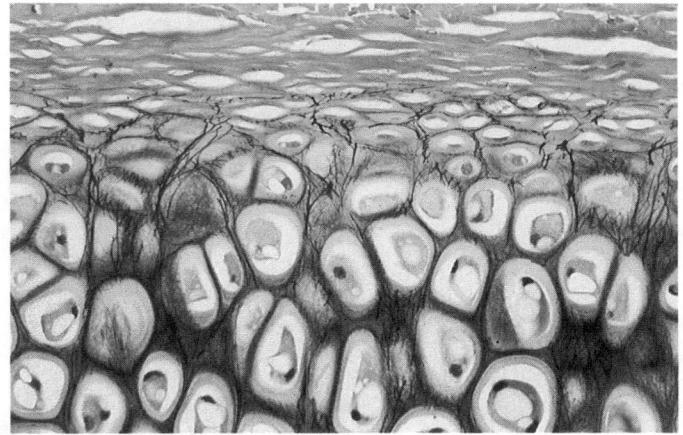

C. Higher magnification of B, showing fibrous perichondrium, chondroblasts and larger chondrocytes embedded in a matrix rich in elastin fibres. Magnification ×400.

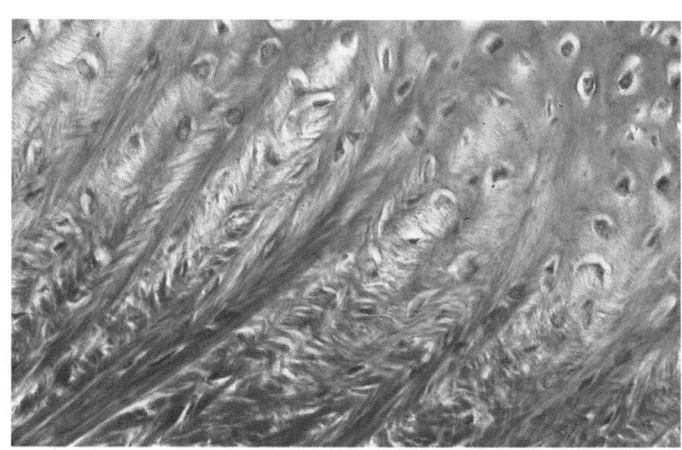

D. White fibrocartilage in late fetal intervertebral disc, showing chondroblasts between coarse collagen fibres derived from the annulus fibrosus; Mallory's triple stain. Magnification ×150.

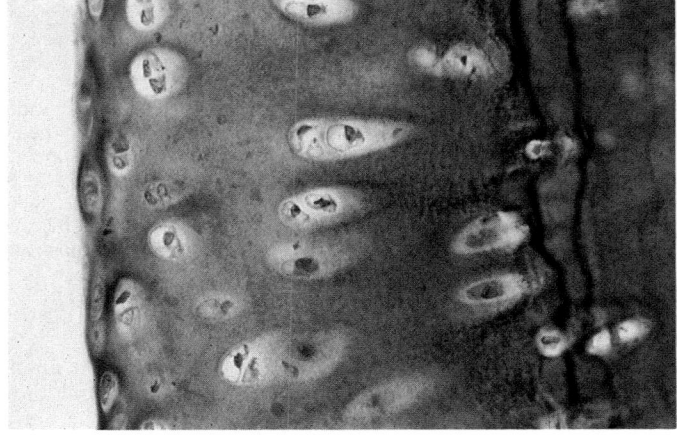

E. Articular cartilage stained with silver, showing cellular arrangement of the different layers. Note the absence of a periosteum, the superficial flattened cells of layers I and II, the more rounded chondrocytes of layer III, the lines of calcification in the deeper layer (IV) and the lamellar bone adjacent to the cartilage (see text for details). Interphalangeal joint (Rhesus monkey). Magnification ×400.

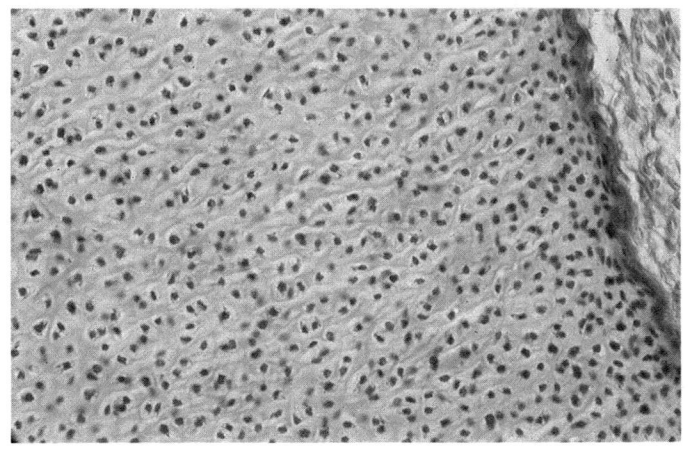

F. Fetal cartilage, human phalanx, stained with Mallory's triple stain. Note the highly cellular appearance. The cells are small and almost uniform in distribution. Magnification ×150.

6.22   Different types of cartilage

449

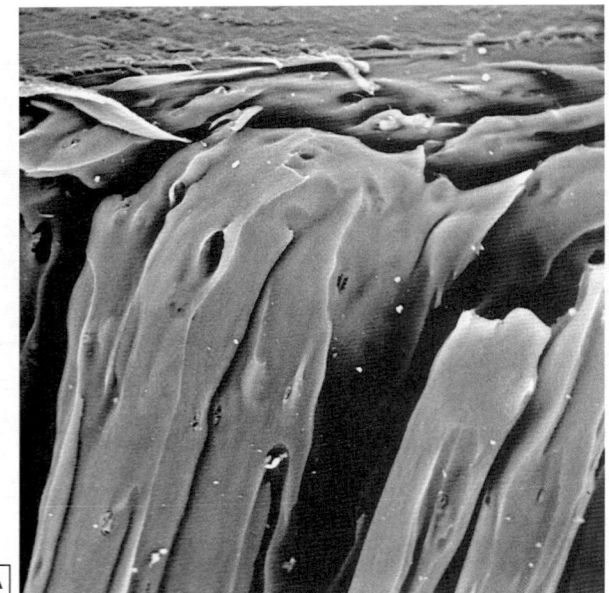

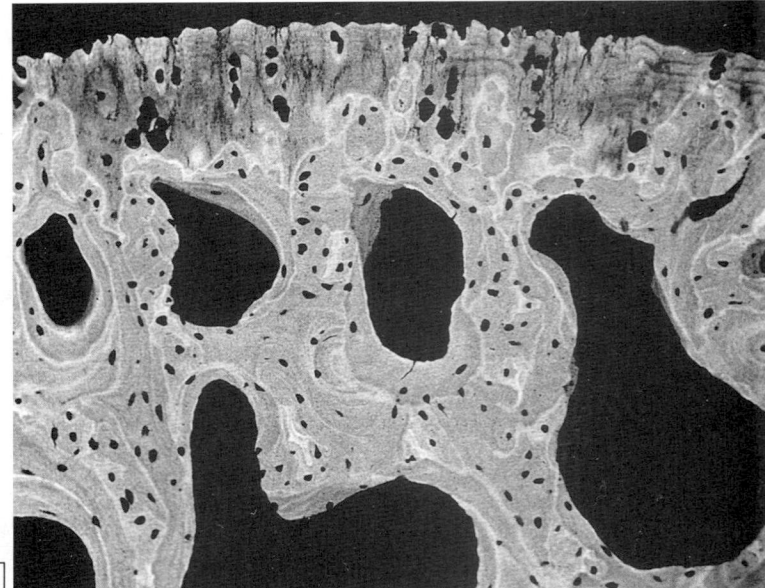

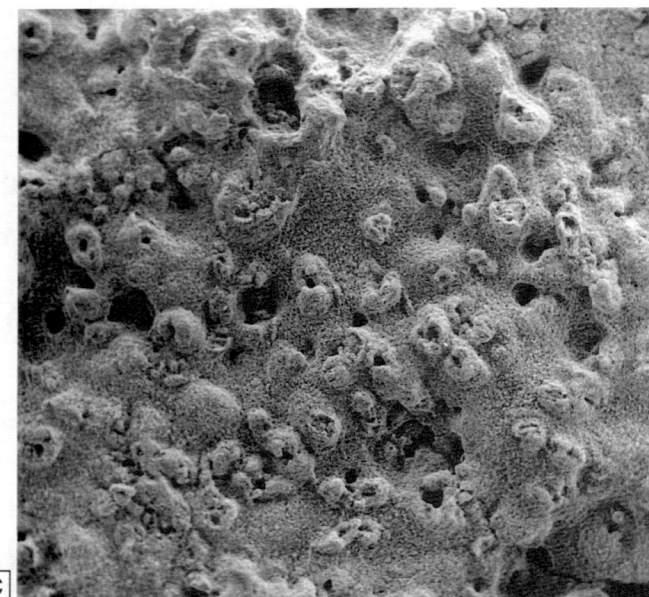

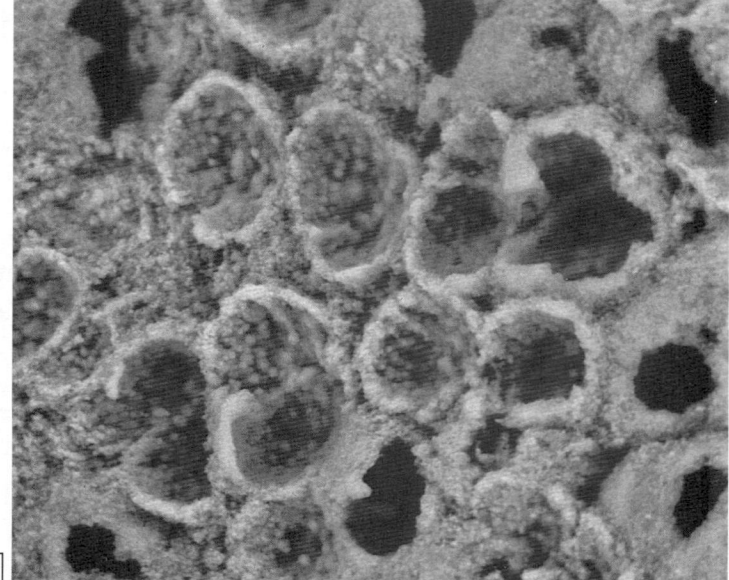

6.23A Human femoral head articular cartilage cleaved wet in ethanol and critical point dried. Vertical columns are generated in zone 3 by this wet dissection procedure; they curve over in the transitional zone 2 to become tangential in the immediate sub-articular zone 1. Backscattered electron image (BSE), field width = 820 μm. B. Calcified cartilage superficial to sub-condral bone in zone 4 of articular cartilage. Several tidemarks recording the advance of zone 4 into zone 3 can be seen. Reversal lines in the bone and at the osseochondral junction are white. Rat tibial head embedded (in PMMA, block surface polished and carbon-coated) BSE, field width = 600 μm. C. Mineralizing front of human articular cartilage (femoral head of 81 year female). The interface between zones 3 and 4 was exposed by treatment with Na_2O_2 to remove unmineralized tissue. Protuberances surround chondrocyte lacunae; SEM, field width 715 μm. D. Mineralizing front of distal tibial articular surface showing detail of pericellular mineralization. The lacunae were occupied by one or two chondrocytes. Sample made anorganic by treatment with KOH; SEM, field width = 138 μm.

interterritorial zone. Chondroitin sulphates are particularly prevalent in the vicinity of chondrocytes, whereas keratin sulphate predominates in the interterritorial zone.

Articular hyaline cartilage

Articular hyaline cartilage covers articular surfaces (**6.**16c,d, 22e, 23a) in synovial joints, providing an extremely smooth, resistant surface bathed by synovial fluid, allowing almost frictionless movement. Its elasticity, with that of other articular structures, dissipates effects of concussions, giving the whole articulation some flexibility, particularly near extremes of movement. Articular cartilage is admirably constructed to resist the large compressive forces generated by weight transmission, especially during movement.

Articular cartilage does not ossify, and varies from 1 to 7 mm in thickness; it is moulded to the shape of the underlying bone but its surface smooths, often accentuating and modifying, the surface geometry. On convex osseous surfaces it is thickest centrally, the reverse being true of concave surfaces; its thickness decreases from maturity to old age. The surface of articular cartilage is devoid of perichondrium, but around its edges the synovial membrane overlaps then grades into its structure.

Adult articular cartilage shows a zonation in structure with increasing depth from the surface (Stockwell 1979; Ghadially 1983). Except perhaps for the very surface, the matrix is pervaded by collagen fibres, those near the surface around lacunae being fine, plexiform and, at the most, faintly banded, whereas elsewhere they are coarser with the usual 64 nm banding. Their arrangement is variously described as plexiform, helical, or in the form of serial arcades radiating from the deepest zone to the surface, where they pursue a short tangential course before returning radially, as most workers confirm (Boyde & Jones 1983; Clark 1990). It has long been known (Hultkrantz 1898; Amprino 1948) that if the surface of articular cartilage is pierced by a pin a longitudinal 'split-line' shows after withdrawal and that, for any given joint, the patterns of split-lines are constant and distinctive (cf. cleavage lines of skin). Bullough and Goodfellow (1968), using polarized light and electron microscopy, demonstrated that splits follow the predominant directions of collagen bundles in tangential zones of cartilage. Such patterns probably reveal 'tension trajectories' set up in surrounding cartilage during habitual activities. Subsequent investigations have largely confirmed the views of Bullough and Goodfellow: for example, split-line analysis by transmission electron microscopy (Meachim et al 1974), polarization microscopy (Ortmann 1975) and scanning electron microscopy (Minns & Stevens 1977). The structure of the surface layer in articular cartilage is functionally important (Broom 1986; Oloyede & Broom 1993a,b) but the dynamics of articular cartilage are not well understood (Setton et al 1993; Broom & Silyn-Roberts 1989). Serafini-Fracassini and Smith (1974) propose that the basic function of articular cartilage collagen is not resistance to tensile stresses, but provision of fixation anchors for viscoelastic domains of proteoglycan molecules when subjected to deforming and displacing stresses. Clearly, no model is adequate unless it includes the dynamics of all interacting constituents of cartilage (see review by Freeman 1979 and **6.16**C,D, **22**E).

In the *superficial* or *tangential stratum* (*zone 1*) cells are small, oval or elongated, flat and parallel to the surface, and surrounded by fine tangential fibres; they have a few short projections, mainly from their lateral borders and deep surfaces, and display scattered mitochondria and small cisternae of granular endoplasmic reticulum; their Golgi apparatus is not prominent. The nature of the articular surface, the thin superficial layer, remains uncertain. The surface zone is said to be a cell-free, 3 μm thick layer containing fine collagen Type II fibrils covered superficially by a protein layer that prevents anti-Type II collagen antibody from binding to the surface (Jasin et al 1993). Deep to the superficial layer are typical banded collagen fibres, regularly tangential, their diameters and volume density increasing with depth. Mow et al (1974) described the superficial layer as sheets of tightly woven collagen fibrils parallel to the surface, from 5 to 20 nm in diameter and forming a layer from 1 to 200 μm in thickness. It is said to be poor in glycosaminoglycans but rich in hyaluronate.

The deeper cells of the *transitional* or *intermediate stratum* (*zone 2*) are larger, rounder, single or in isogenous groups. Most are largely typical active chondrocytes in ultrastructure and around them pass oblique collagen fibres.

Deeper still, in the *radiate stratum* (*zone 3*), cells are large, round, often in vertical columns, with intervening radial collagen fibres. As elsewhere, the cells, singly or in groups, are encapsulated in pericellular matrix which has fine fibrils and as well as Type II collagen contains fibronectin and Types VI and IX collagen. Hyaluron is also enriched pericellularly (Poole et al 1990). The turnover rate of the collagen in adult human cartilage is very slow (Maroudas et al 1992).

The deepest layer or *calcified stratum* (*zone 4*) adjoins the *subchondral bone* (*hypochondral osseous lamina*) of the epiphysis. These adjacent surfaces show reciprocal fine ridges, grooves and interdigitations, which, with the confluence of their fibrous arrays, resist shearing stresses due to postural changes and muscle action. The junction between zones 3 and 4 is called the *tidemark*. With age articular cartilage thins by advancement of the tidemark zone, and the replacement of calcified cartilage by bone.

Concentrations of GAGs vary according to site and species, and especially with regard to age (Stockwell 1983; Heise & Toledo 1993). The proportion of keratan sulphate increases linearly with depth; the latter is mainly in the interterritorial matrix, whereas chondroitin sulphates are largely circumlacunar. The turnover rates of glycosaminoglycans in cartilage are faster than those of collagen, and the smaller, more soluble GAGs turn over fastest. This fraction decreases with age and distance from the cells. Maroudas (1980) gives a proteoglycan turnover time of nearly 5 years for adult human articular cartilage.

The sequence of structural changes from hyaline cartilage with dispersed cells through columnar arrays of cells, a zone of calcified cartilage and eventually epiphyseal bone, is also typical of cartilaginous growth plates (**6.22**E, **23**, **24**A,B). It follows radial epiphyseal growth by the extension of endochondral ossification into overlying calcified cartilage. This ceases in maturity, but the zones persist throughout life. The same terminal mechanism also occurs in bones lacking epiphyses.

Cells of articular cartilage divide by mitosis, but mitoses are few except in young bones. Progressive loss of superficial cells from normal young joint surfaces, and their replacement by cells from deeper layers, is unconfirmed; but degenerating cells may occur in any of the four zones. This probably accounts for progressive reduction in cellularity of cartilage with advancing age, particularly in superficial layers (Stockwell 1967) and probably contributes to the variable lipid content of the matrix.

Articular cartilage may derive nutriment by diffusion from three sources: vessels of the synovial membrane, synovial fluid and hypochondral vessels of an adjacent medullary cavity, some capillaries from which penetrate and occasionally traverse the calcified cartilage (Kuettner & Pauli 1983a,b; Duncan et al 1987), and have been estimated to contact 1–7% of the osseous aspect of the cartilage. The contributions from these sources are uncertain and may change with age, but accurate determinations of permeability of articular cartilage are available (Maroudas et al 1975). Small molecules freely traverse articular cartilage, with diffusion coefficients about half those in aqueous solution. Larger molecules have diffusion coefficients inversely related to molecular size; for example, glucose, inulin and haemoglobin (relative molecular masses: 180, 5000 and 68 000) have molal distribution coefficients in the ratio 85 : 11 : 1. Permeability of cartilage to large molecules is greatly affected by variations in its glycosaminoglycan content; for example, a threefold increase multiplies the partition coefficient a hundredfold.

Costal cartilage

In costal cartilage cells and nuclei are large; the matrix is usually homogeneous and transparent, and tends to fibrous striation, especially in old age. In their thickest parts a few large vascular channels and sometimes medullary elements may appear. The xiphoid process and the cartilages of the nose, larynx and trachea (except the elastic fibrocartilaginous epiglottis and corniculate cartilages) resemble costal cartilage in microstructure. The arytenoid cartilage changes from hyaline at its base to elastic cartilage at apex. Hyaline cartilages, after adolescence, are prone to calcification, especially in costal and laryngeal sites. Quantitative studies demonstrate diminishing cellularity throughout costal cartilages with advancing age (Stockwell 1979).

White fibrocartilage

White fibrocartilage is dense, fasciculated, white fibrous tissue, with attendant fibroblasts and small interfascicular groups of chondrocytes; the cells are ovoid and surrounded by concentrically striated matrix (**6.22**D). When amassed, as in intervertebral discs, fibrocartilage has great tensile strength with appreciable elasticity. In lesser amounts, as in articular discs, glenoid and acetabular labra, the cartilaginous lining of bony grooves for tendons and some articular cartilages (see below), it is a tissue of strength and elasticity able to resist repeated pressure and friction. This tissue is unlike other types of cartilage in having much Type I (general connective tissue) collagen in its matrix; it is perhaps best regarded as a mingling of the two types of tissue, for example where a ligament or tendinous tissue inserts into hyaline cartilage, rather than a specific type of cartilage (Benjamin & Evans 1990). The fibrocartilage of joints is often altogether lacking in Type II collagen and possibly represents a quite distinctive class of connective tissue, designated cartilage only for the convenience of histologists.

The articular surfaces of bones which ossify in mesenchyme are covered by white fibrocartilage (e.g. squamous temporal, mandible and clavicle). Electron microscopy of such articular cartilages (Silva & Hart 1967) shows that *deep layers*, adjacent to hypochondral bone, resemble calcified regions of the radial zone of hyaline articular cartilage. The *superficial zone* contains dense parallel bundles of thick collagen fibres, interspersed with typical dense connective tissue fibroblasts and scanty ground substance. Fibre bundles in adjacent layers alternate in direction as in the cornea. A *transitional zone* of irregular bundles of coarse collagen and fibroblasts with prominent Golgi complexes separates the two. The fibroblasts are probably involved in elaboration of proteoglycans and collagen, and may constitute a germinal zone for deeper cartilage. Fibril diameters and types may differ at different sites according to the functional load. For permeability of white fibrocartilage in intervertebral discs consult Maroudas et al (1975).

Yellow elastic cartilage

Yellow elastic cartilage (6.22B,C) occurs in the external ear, corniculate cartilages, epiglottis and apices of the arytenoids. It contains typical chondrocytes, but its matrix is pervaded by yellow elastic fibres except around lacunae, where it resembles typical hyaline matrix with fine Type II collagen fibrils. Its elastic fibres are irregularly contoured, unaffected by acetic acid, have an affinity for orcein and show no periodic banding (Sheldon & Robinson 1958; Mecham & Heuser 1990). Cox and Peacock (1977) have reviewed the ultrastructure, histogenesis and growth of chondroblasts and matrix in the rabbit's pinna. Histogenesis of elastic fibres of cartilage (and probably other tissues) is in two stages: a glycoprotein microfibrillar framework of oxytalan first appears and then elastin. Most sites in which elastic fibrocartilage occurs have *vibrational* functions, such as laryngeal sound-wave production and their collection and transmission in the ear.

Development, growth and regeneration of cartilage

Normally cartilage is formed in embryonic mesenchyme (Glenister 1976; Serafini-Fracassini & Smith 1974; Cox & Peacock 1977). The signals that direct cellular differentiation in the first skeletal condensations are only now being discovered (Tickle 1994). Mesenchymal cells proliferate and become tightly packed, the shape of their condensation foreshadowing that of a subsequent cartilage. The cells become rounded, with prominent rotund or oval nuclei and a low cytoplasm:nucleus ratio. Gap junctions are present between the cells (Jones et al 1993). Each cell soon begins to secrete a surrounding basophilic halo of matrix, composed of a delicate network of fine type II collagen filaments, type IX collagen and cartilage proteoglycan core protein, indicating differentiation into chondroblasts (6.16A, 22F). Continued secretion of matrix further separates the cells and so typical hyaline cartilage is now recognizable. In other sites collagen synthesis predominates, many cells becoming fibroblasts and chondroblastic activity appearing only in isolated groups or rows of cells. These are soon surrounded by dense bundles of collagen fibres to form white fibrocartilage. Similarly, elsewhere, the matrix of early cellular cartilage is permeated first by anastomosing oxytalan and, later, elastin fibres. In all cases, developing cartilage is surrounded by condensed mesenchyme differentiating into a bilaminar perichondrium in which the cells of the outer layer become fibroblasts secreting a dense collagenous matrix lined externally by vascular mesenchyme; the inner layer of perichondrium contains differentiated but mainly resting chondroblasts or prechondroblasts.

The growth of cartilage is both *interstitial* and *appositional*.

Interstitial growth (i.e. from within the cartilage). This follows continued mitosis of early chondroblasts throughout the mass. When such a cell divides, its descendants temporarily occupy the same lacuna but are soon separated by thin septa of matrix, which thicken and further separate cells (6.16B). Continuing division leads to isogenous groups. Interstitial growth is obvious only in young cartilage, where presumably plasticity of matrix permits continued expansion. However, the manner of matrix expansion and reorganization and indeed the factors determining total shape of a cartilage are as yet poorly understood.

Appositional growth at the cartilage surface. This results from the proliferation of cells of the internal, chondrogenic layer of perichondrium. Some resultant superficial chondroblasts secrete matrix around themselves, thus creating superficial lacunae. This process, continuing, adds additional surface while the entrapped cells can now participate in interstitial growth. Apposition is often stated to be prevalent in more mature cartilages, but interstitial growth must persist for long periods in epiphyseal cartilages.

Regeneration and ageing. In mammals regeneration of lost hyaline cartilage is poor, defects being slowly filled by vascularized connective (granulation) tissue, which may become less vascular and persist as fibrous tissue. Occasionally, cells in such tissue become chondroblasts, but the newly made cartilage matrix does not become integrated with or properly adherent to the original tissue. Mandibular condylar cartilage is able to heal more satisfactorily and has been used to repair experimental articular defects (Girdler 1993).

Microcracks in the calcified layer of ageing articular cartilage and their extension into the subchondral bone may initiate remodelling of the tissue at the chondro–osseous junction (Mori et al 1993; Sokoloff 1993).

Interesting features of cartilage are the low antigenicity of its matrix, its relatively low vascularity and the isolation of its chondrocytes in lacunae, which permit successful homotransplantation without marked cellular or humoral immune reaction.

Normal cartilage growth depends on adequate nutrition and hormonal environment; disturbances due to these will be considered with endochondral ossification. With advancing years the matrix of many permanent cartilages becomes calcified, also an essential step in endochondral ossification during earlier development. Advancement of the tidemark zone with age leads to thinning of articular cartilage.

Mineralization patterns. The mineralization of cartilage occurs in three ways:

(1) In the process of endochondral ossification, mineralization of the growth plate is closely associated with type X collagen production in the hypertrophic zone and the incidence of matrix vesicles. Matrix vesicles originate from chondrocytes in the proliferation zone, are evident mostly in the intercolumnar regions and appear to initiate crystal formation there (6.24A).

(2) Mineralization also spreads along collagen fibres (6.24B). Collagen-based mineralization is a major feature at the tidemark (6.23B) and in fibrocartilage.

(3) A further pattern of mineralization is seen in pericellular regions enveloping the chondrocytes ahead of the general front of mineralization (6.23C,D; Boyde & Jones 1983).

Mineral clusters fuse as the rate of mineralization slows or becomes inactive. Remnants of unremodelled cartilage intercellular matrix within bone can be identified by their higher density in microradiographs or backscattered electron imaging (6.24C) and may be revealed at resorbed bone surfaces (6.24D).

Cubic calcium phosphate crystals have been detected by transmission electron microscopy in the surface zone of normal human articular cartilage from juveniles and adults (Scotchford et al 1992). The crystals have been identified as Mg whitlockite, are 50–500 nm across and are associated with lipid. They are more common in regions subject to high mechanical stress but their functional significance is not known.

BONE AS A TISSUE

Bone is essentially a highly vascular, living, constantly changing mineralized connective tissue. It is remarkable for its hardness, resilience and regenerative capacity, as well as its characteristic growth mechanisms. Like all other connective tissues, bone consists of cells and an intercellular matrix, the great majority of its cells (*osteocytes*), lying embedded within it. The matrix is composed in part (about 40% dry weight in mature bone) of organic materials, mainly collagen fibres, and the rest consists of inorganic salts rich in calcium and phosphate. Together these give bone its unique mechanical properties (see, e.g. Hancox 1972; Currey 1984a,b,c). Vascular canals ramify within bone, providing its cells with metabolic support and creating avenues of entry for other cells, including osteoclasts, capable of removing bone, and osteoblasts which can deposit it. While these features are found in all bone, their details differ widely with developmental state, site, prevailing mechanical forces and the metabolic state of the body. Bone's collagen framework, permeated with mineral salts, varies from almost randomly orientated coarse bundles (*woven bone*) when young, to a system of highly ordered, parallel-fibred sheets or lamellae (*lamellar bone*) in the mature condition. Collagen fibres and mineralized matrix together usually form minute cylinders (osteons) arranged concentrically around blood vessels both in woven and lamellar bone while, in the

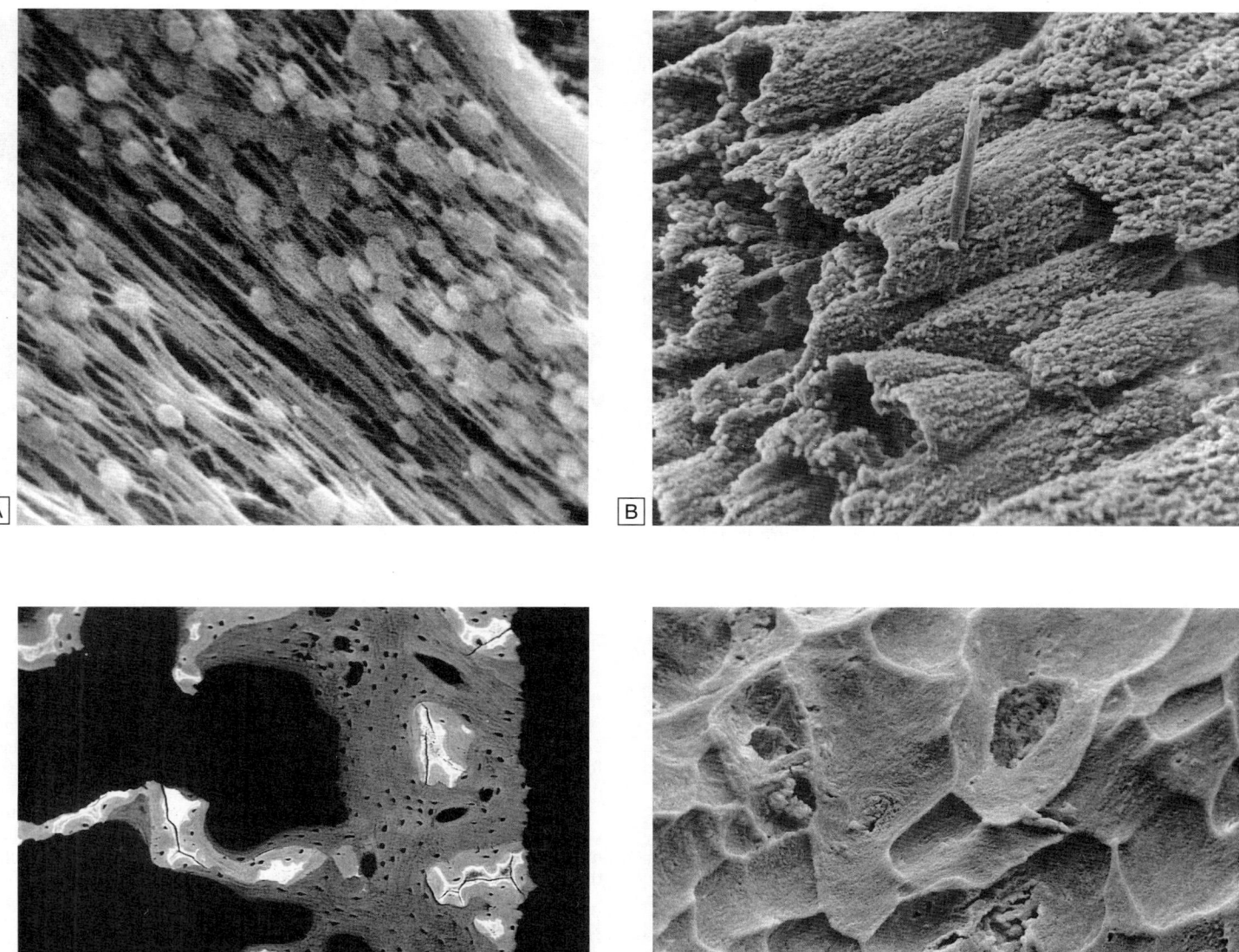

6.24A. Longitudinal freeze-fracture through rat epiphyseal growth plate cartilage showing the mineralization region. The white spherical structures are large mineral particle aggregates (microcalcospherites) believed to originate from matrix vesicles. They appear to have a special relationship with the longitudinal collagen fibres of the intercolumnar matrix; SEM, field width = 17 μm. B. Anorganic preparation of a rat femoral growth plate showing the sides of longitudinal tubes formed by mineralization in intercolumnar matrix. The mineral clusters had extended along the longitudinal collagen fibres; SEM, field width = 144 μm. C. Transverse section of human neonate rib showing calcified cartilage remnants within the bone. The centres of some of these remnants are fully mineralized. Note how the cartilage remnants (white) are surrounded by older, denser bone trabeculae (light grey), which have been incorporated endosteally in the cortical bone (dark grey) during growth and remodelling. Cortical drift is occurring from right to left; Embedded BSE, field width 823 μm. D. Endosteal surface of a human rib (7 week female) made anorganic by treatment with NaOCl. Modelling resorption has exposed regions of calcified cartilage (e.g. at centre) which may be identified by the characteristic morphology of the calcospherites. The bone is more evenly mineralized. An osteocyte lacuna is seen at top right; SEM, field width 68 μm.

mature state, the inner and outer surfaces of bones are lined by a few layers of continuous circumferential (outside) and endosteal (inside) lamellae. Bone may also incorporate bundles of collagen fibres derived from surface structures including tendons and ligaments (*bundle bone*). The outer surface of bone is always lined by a fibrocellular layer, the *periosteum*, and on the inner surface is a similar, though thinner, *endosteum*. In these layers lie osteoblasts, osteoclasts and other cells important in the biology of bone. The texture of mature bone also varies between dense (*compact*) and spongy (*cancellous*) osseous tissues which have distinctive mechanical and metabolic roles, often related to their positions within bones (**6.25**: diaphyseal, metaphyseal, epiphyseal, etc).

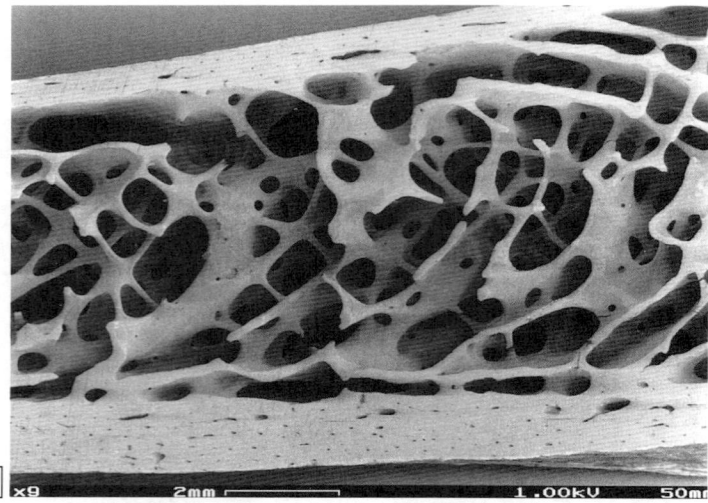

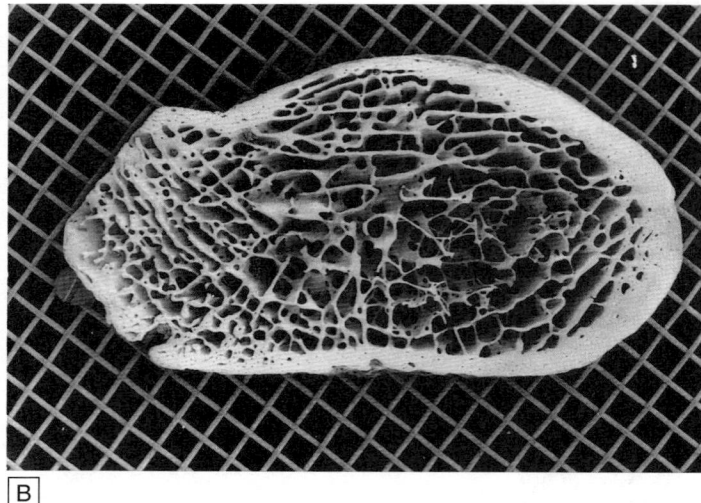

6.25A. Iliac crest of 42 year female—vertical section 2 cm below the antero-superior border which lay to the right of the field view as oriented. The cancellous bone comprises intersecting curved plates and struts. Osteonal (Haversian) canals can just be seen in the two cortices at this magnification.

Mag. bar = 2 mm. B. Transverse section of human femoral neck (45 year male) viewed from disto-lateral aspect towards the femoral head, showing the predominant pattern of curved intersecting plates in the cancellous bone. The section is 4 mm thick. Field width = 50 mm.

Classification and terminology

1. **Macroscopic appearance of cut surfaces (6.25, 26)**
   Compact bone—the ivory surface layers of mature bone.
   Trabecular bone—the interior of mature bones (also termed *cancellous* or *spongy* bone). Early embryonic bone is also spongiose—the *primary spongiosa (Os spongiosum primum)*.

2. **Developmental origin**
   Intramembranous (*mesenchymal* or *dermal* bone)—formed by direct transformation of condensed mesenchyme.
   Intracartilaginous (*cartilage* or *endochondral* bone)—replacing a preformed cartilage model.

3. **Regions of long bones**
   Diaphysis—intermediate region or shaft.
   Metaphysis—developing, juxta-epiphysical regions of shaft.
   Epiphysis—extremity with a separate centre of ossification.

4. **Organization of collagen fibres**
   Woven bone (*coarse-bundled* bone), with an irregular collagen network—includes embryonic bone, isolated patches in adult bone, and repair tissue in fractures.
   Parallel-fibred bone—includes all forms of lamellar bone and non-lamellar primary osteons.

5. **General microstructure**
   Non-lamellar bone—includes early woven bone and primary osteons.
   Lamellar bone—almost all mature bone.

6. **Disposition of lamellae**
   Circumferential lamellae (primary lamellae)—parallel to both periosteal and endosteal surfaces.
   Osteonic lamellae (secondary lamellae)—concentric lamellae around vascular canals of mature bone.
   Interstitial lamellae between osteons.

7. **Types of osteon (Haversian system)**
   Primary osteons—first formed, lamellar or non-lamellar osteons.
   Secondary osteons—concentric lamellae around vascular canals of mature bone.

8. **General terms**
   Surface bone—usually circumferential lamellae but may include woven and bundle (Sharpey or extrinsic fibre) bone.
   Interstitial bone—between osteons; often lamellar remnants of secondary osteons but may include woven or primary osteon fragments.

Developmentally, bone may form either by the direct transformation of condensed mesenchyme (*intramembranous bone*) or be preceded by a cartilage model which bone later replaces (*endochondral bone*). However, bones of different origins may show any of the features mentioned above, and can only be distinguished by a study of their genesis.

Because of these different types of classification, it may help to refer to **Classification and Terminology** set out opposite where the more commonly used terms have been grouped. The concepts which these reflect will be treated more fully in the following pages.

STRUCTURE OF MATURE BONE

MACROSCOPIC STRUCTURE

Macroscopically, living bone is white, with either a dense texture like ivory (*compact bone*), or honeycombed by large cavities, the bone being reduced to a latticework of bars and plates (*trabeculae*), in which case it is called *cancellous*, *trabecular*, or *spongy* bone (6.25, 26, 27). Compact bone is usually limited to the cortices of mature bones (cortical bone) and is of supreme importance in providing their strength. Its thickness and architecture vary for different bones, reflecting their overall shape, position and functional roles. In contrast, cancellous bone lies chiefly in their interior (6.25, 26), and particularly, in the case of long bones, within their expanded ends (metaphyses and epiphyses). Cancellous bone gives additional strength to cortices and supports the bone marrow. Bone forms a reservoir of metabolic calcium and phosphate which can be readily added to or withdrawn by cellular action under hormonal and cytokine control; this property within cancellous bone may be enhanced by its large surface area and proximity to blood vessels and marrow cells.

The proportions of compact to cancellous bone vary greatly. In the shaft of a long bone, a thick cylinder of compact bone presents only a few trabeculae and spicules on its inner surface so that a large central medullary or marrow cavity is enclosed, communicating freely with the intratrabecular spaces of the expanded bone ends. In other bones, especially flat ones such as the ribs, the interior is uniformly cancellous, compact bone forming the surface. These cavities are filled with marrow, either red, haemopoietic, or yellow, adipose, its character varying with age and site. In some bones of the skull, notably the mastoid and ethmoid, many of the cavities within are filled with air, a situation which is common in the wing-bones of most birds.

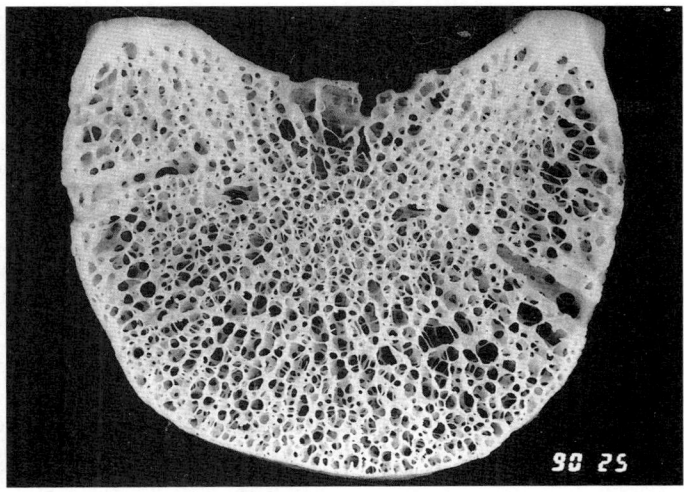

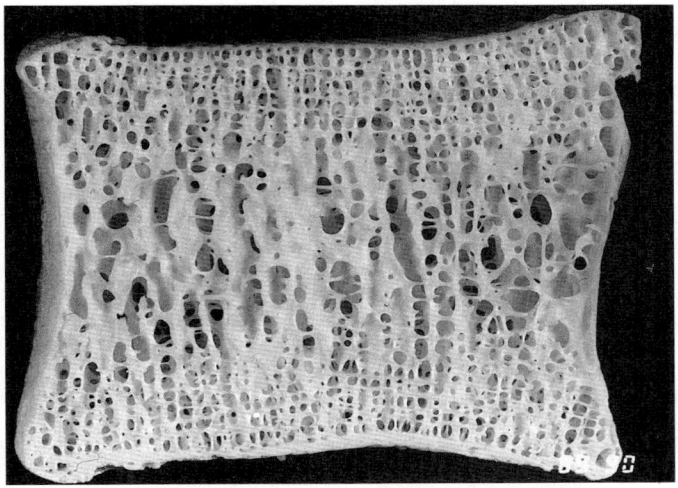

6.26A. Horizontal section through the central region of a human vertebral body (30 year female). The 4 mm thick section was photographed against a black background which is visible in many places through the honeycomb trabecular structure. Two blood vessel canals pass obliquely back from the lateral walls. Posterior is top of the illustration. Width of bone = 37 mm.

B. Human fourth lumbar vertebral body (31 year male), mid-sagittal section, superior is top of illustration. The cortical bone is very thin in vertebrae. The trabeculae in the middle zone are relatively larger and are mainly vertical plates or tubes. Photograph of 4 mm thick section, field width = 37.5 mm.

MICROSCOPIC STRUCTURE—CELLS OF BONE

As stated earlier, bone is composed of cells embedded in a stiff calcified matrix; these components will now be described in some detail, first individually and then in terms of their overall organization.

The cells of bone consist of a number of types, including:

- osteoprogenitor stromal cells which give rise to various other bone cells
- osteoblasts which lay down bone
- osteocytes within bone
- bone lining cells on its surface
- osteoclasts which erode it.

In addition to these are the cells of its vascular and nervous system and other components of the periosteum, endosteum and marrow.

Of these different cells, the first four are closely related, while the osteoclasts arise from a quite unrelated source. Vascular and nervous tissue are, of course, of external origins.

Osteoprogenitor cells

Osteoprogenitor cells are derived from pluripotential stromal stem cells present in the bone marrow and other connective tissues which can proliferate and differentiate into osteoblasts prior to bone formation. The stromal stem cells resemble young fibroblasts and are, like these, of mesenchymal origin. Such mesenchymally derived cells are responsible for all bone formation during early development. In intramembranous bone they aggregate and undergo proliferation before differentiating into osteoblasts while, during endochondral bone formation, similar cells migrate with the ingrowth of blood vessels from the perichondrium into areas of degenerating cartilage, then likewise differentiate into osteoblasts.

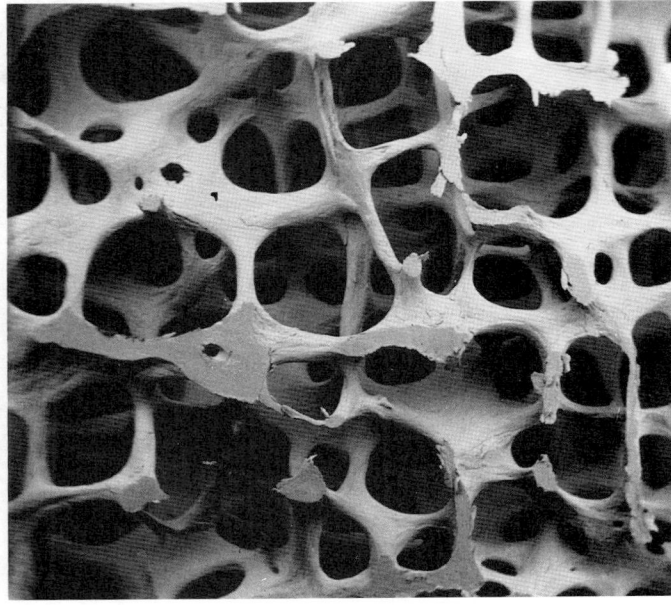

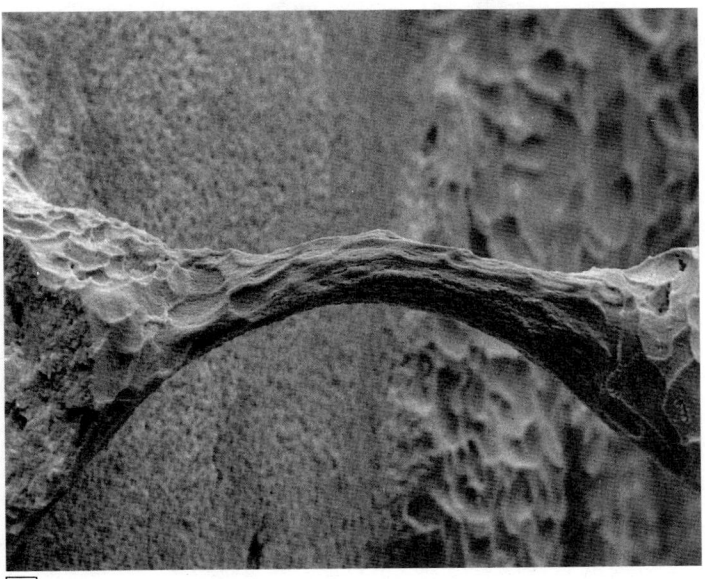

6.27A. Vertical section of cancellous bone in human second lumbar vertebra (42 year female); SEM, field width = 4 mm. B. Endosteal surface of human sixth rib (3.5 months female); showing extensive resorption of a trabeculum in the foreground and of the endosteal surface in the background at the right. The remainder of the background surface is formative; SEM of inorganic preparation, field width = 168 μm.

Cells with mesenchymal features, derived from human bone, can be grown in culture and these form cellular condensations that give rise to bone nodules in culture (Sharrard et al 1986) or new osseous tissue when implanted into animals. There is some evidence that pericytes may be osteoblast precursors as they also form mineralizing colonies in culture (Brighton et al 1992). Ectopic bone formation can also be induced experimentally in various tissues of the body, for example, skeletal muscle, by implantation of demineralized bone or dentine containing bone morphogenetic proteins, or urinary bladder epithelium; thus there may be two types or stages of osteoprogenitor cell, one totally committed to bone formation (*committed osteoprogenitors*), found associated with bones, and the other (*inducible osteoprogenitors*) widely present in connective tissue and probably able to differentiate into various connective tissue cells (e.g. fibroblasts, myoblasts, pericytes, adipose cells, chondroblasts, osteoblasts) depending on the nature of the inducer (Friedenstein 1976; Beresford et al 1992; Martin et al 1993). Cells that have differentiated in one direction may be able to revert to a proliferative phase and then differentiate into osteoblasts (Bennett et al 1991). Osteoblasts and osteoclasts were at one time thought to arise from the same progenitor cell, but it is now clear that osteoclasts have a quite separate origin (Ash et al 1981; Baron et al 1993; see 'Osteoclasts', p. 459 see also (**6.**37).

Osteoblasts (**6.**28, 29, 48, 58). Osteoblasts are basophilic, roughly cuboidal mononuclear cells about 15–30 μm across, found on the forming surfaces of growing or remodelling bone where they constitute a covering monolayer (Mårtin et al 1993). In relatively quiescent adult bones they appear to be present chiefly on the endosteal rather than periosteal surfaces, but also occur deep within compact bone where osteons are being remodelled. They are responsible for the synthesis, deposition and mineralization of bone matrix (Rodan & Rodan 1984) and a proportion of them, on becoming embedded in the matrix, finally change into osteocytes (see also **6.**47). Ultrastructurally, osteoblasts have features typical of protein-secreting cells, i.e. a pale (euchromatic) oval nucleus placed away from the secreting surface, an extensive granular endoplasmic reticulum, large Golgi complex and numerous secretory vesicles. The cells are orientated so that their secretory surface abuts on to the adjacent bone. They have prominent bundles of actin, myosin and other cytoskeletal proteins associated with the maintenance of cell shape, attachment and motility. Their plasma membranes have many extensions, some contacting neighbouring osteoblasts and osteocytes at intercellular junctions, by means of which the actions of quite large groups may be co-ordinated, as seen, for example, in their concerted action to form large domains of parallel collagen fibres. Gap junctions containing connexin-43 have been identified in bone cells (Jones et al 1993) and may integrate the response of the tissue to strain.

The surfaces of osteoblasts are rich in alkaline phosphatase activity, located at the plasma membrane. Some of this enzyme is shed and reaches the circulation where it can be detected in conditions of rapid bone formation or turnover. Osteoblasts of woven bone have protrusions which appear to bud off vesicular structures (matrix vesicles) important in mineral deposition (see below, p. 472). A major activity of osteoblasts is to synthesize and secrete the organic matrix of bone, i.e. Type I collagen, small amounts of Type V collagen, and various other macromolecules including the gamma-carboxyglutamic acid (GLA)-containing protein osteocalcin and matrix GLA-protein (of uncertain function), Sparc/osteonectin, which binds strongly to mineral and collagen, and may also be a cell adhesion factor, and some proteoglycans, latent proteases and growth factors (see the review by Delmas & Malaval 1993). Prior to its mineralization this organic matrix is called *osteoid*. An equally important osteoblast function is the mineralization of this matrix, alkaline phosphatase playing a vital but unexplained role in this process. Collagen synthesis is carried out in much the same manner as in fibroblasts, initially in the granular endoplasmic reticulum and later in the Golgi apparatus, before being secreted to the exterior.

There is also much evidence that osteoblasts may play an important though indirect role in the hormonal regulation of bone resorption, since they bear receptors for parathyroid hormone and 1,25-dihydroxy vitamin D3 and other stimulants of bone resorption. During bone deposition osteoblasts may inhibit osteoclast activity or may merely fail to stimulate them, but in the presence of bone resorption stimulators, for example parathyroid hormone (PTH), osteoblasts release various intermediaries which activate osteoclasts to remove osseous tissue. Neurohormones are also thought to regulate osteoblastic activity. This subject, and others related to bone formation

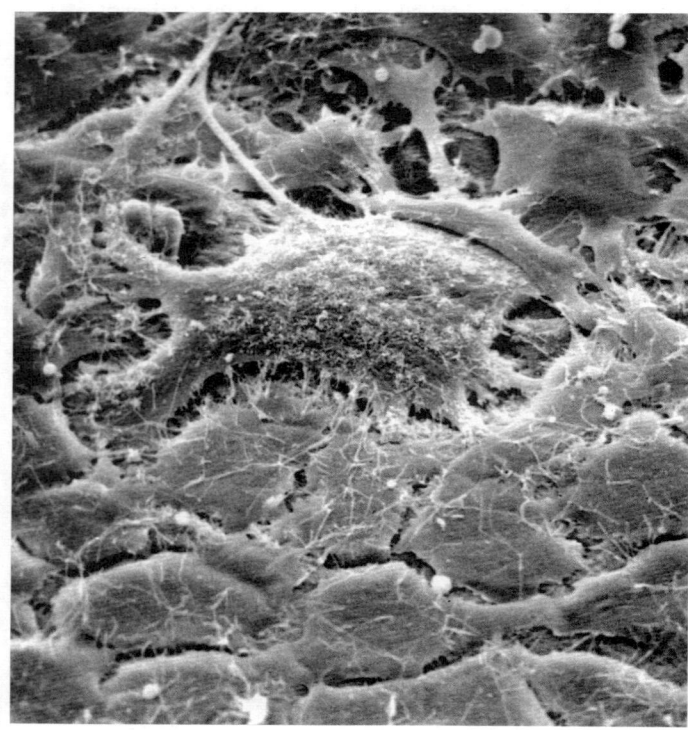

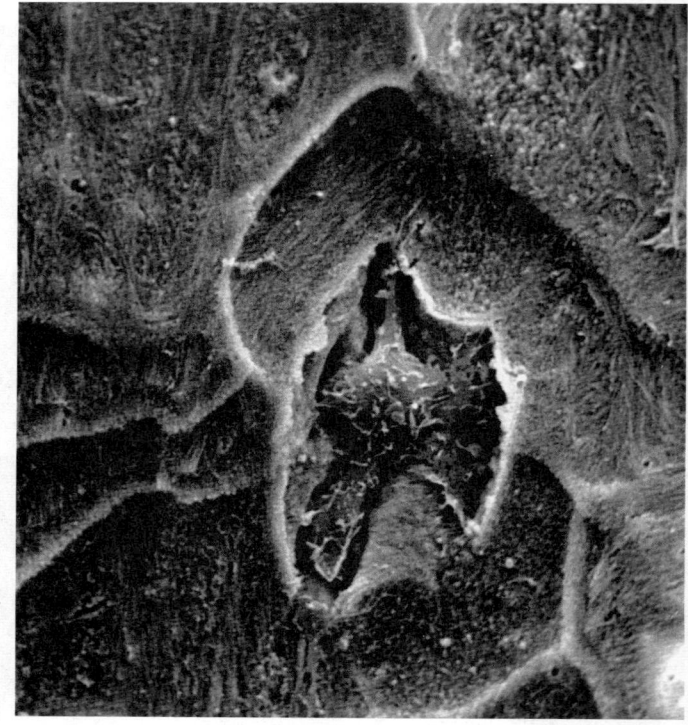

6.28A. An osteoclast (the largest cell) lies amongst osteoblasts on endocranial surface of rat calvarium. The osteoblasts form a continuous layer, one cell thick, over the bone (crevices between cells occurred during drying the specimen). Filopodia contact adjacent cells; SEM, field width = 68 μm.

B. Endosteal surface of rabbit tibia showing an osteocyte within its lacuna exposed by osteoclastic resorption of surrounding bone; SEM, field width = 34 μm.

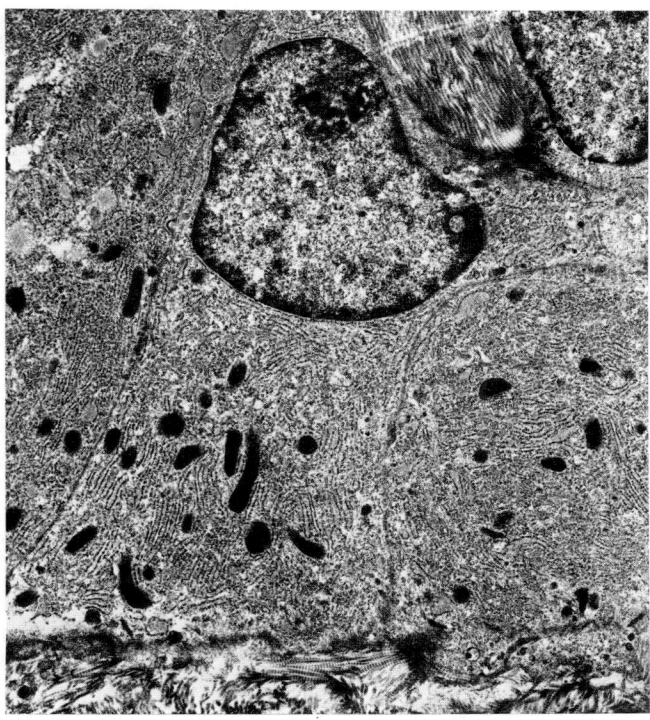

6.29   Electron micrograph of a series of osteoblasts on a bone-forming surface (below). The cytoplasm is filled with granular endoplasmic reticulum. Some banded collagen fibres are visible at the secretory front at the base of the picture. Magnification ×4000. (Provided by A Hayward.)

and turnover, will be considered more fully in the section on bone remodelling (p. 478).

Osteoblasts are differentiated, non-mitotic cells which arise from osteoprogenitor cells and also possibly by de-differentiation of osteocytes when these are released from bone during its resorption. Osteoblasts may also themselves de-differentiate into osteoprogenitor cells capable of mitosis under certain circumstances. When not active in bone formation, they may also become bone lining cells on endosteal surfaces.

Osteocytes (6.28, 30, 31, 32)

Osteocytes constitute the major cell type of mature bone, lying scattered within its matrix, but interconnected by numerous cellular extensions to form a complex cellular network. They are derived from osteoblasts which have reduced or ceased matrix formation and become enclosed in matrix, but retain contacts with each other and with cells at the surfaces of bone (i.e. osteoblasts and bone-lining cells) throughout their lifespan.

Mature, relatively inactive osteocytes possess a cell body which has the shape of a three-axis ellipsoid, the longest axis (about 25 μm) parallel to the surrounding bony lamella and its shortest axis perpendicular to the plane of the lamellae. The cytoplasm is faintly basophilic and contains relatively few organelles, including a little granular endoplasmic reticulum, a few free ribosomes and a small Golgi apparatus. The rather narrow rim of cytoplasm surrounds an oval nucleus. Younger, more active osteocytes are more rounded, with a well-developed endoplasmic reticulum and larger Golgi complexes, both signs of greater synthetic and secretory activity. Osteocytes in woven bone are large and irregular in shape (**6.31**D).

Numerous fine processes emerge from the cell body and branch a number of times to form an extensive tree. Such processes contain bundles of microfilaments and some smooth endoplasmic reticulum. At their distal tips they contact the processes of adjacent cells (other osteocytes and, at surfaces, osteoblasts and bone-lining cells), with which they form communicating gap junctions and are thus in electrical and metabolic continuity.

The bone matrix surrounds the cell bodies and processes but there appears to be a variable space between the osteocyte and its enclosing wall containing extracellular fluid. From the *lacuna* in which the cell body lies extend tens of narrow, branched tunnels (*canaliculi*) about 0.5–0.25 μm wide containing the cell processes of the osteocytes (**6.31**B). Thus the bony matrix is riddled with minute branched canals and cavities which, beside housing living cells, provide a route for the diffusion of nutrients, gases and waste products for their maintenance (Atkinson & Hallsworth 1982). Canaliculi do not usually extend through and beyond the reversal line surrounding an osteon or communicate with neighbouring systems. They may infrequently, usually at the outer limit of the osteon, loop back to their own lacuna. The walls of lacunae may be lined with a variable (0.2–2 μm) layer of unmineralized organic matrix.

The average lifespan of an osteocyte varies with the metabolic activity of the bone and the likelihood that it will be remodelled, but has been estimated as about 25 years. Old osteocytes may retract their processes from the canaliculi and, when dead, their lacunae and canaliculi may become plugged with cell debris and minerals, so hindering diffusion through the bone (**6.31**C). Dead osteocytes occur commonly in interstitial bone and the inner regions of trabecular bone which escape surface remodelling, becoming particularly noticeable by the second and third decades. Bones which experience little turnover, such as ear ossicles, are most likely to

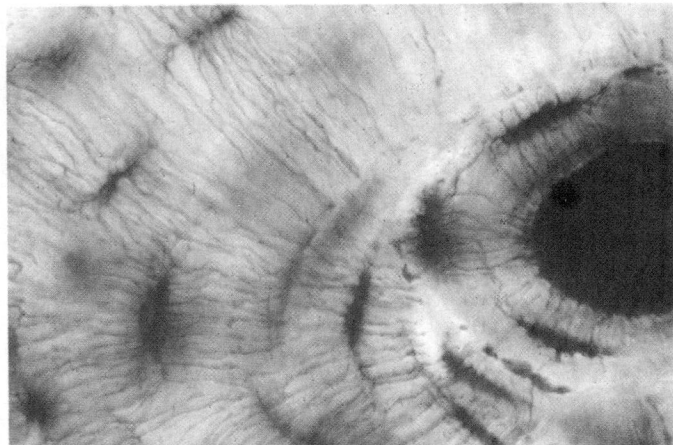

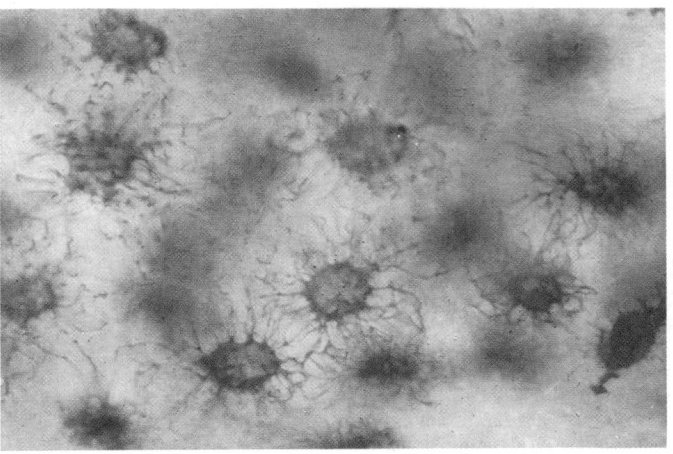

6.30A, B.   High-power view of part of an osteon in transverse section seen with transmitted light. Note the relation of the osteocyte lacunae and their canaliculi to each other, and to the central Haversian canal (black). Tangential section of oseocyte lacunae and their associated canaliculi. Contrast with their appearance in A.

457

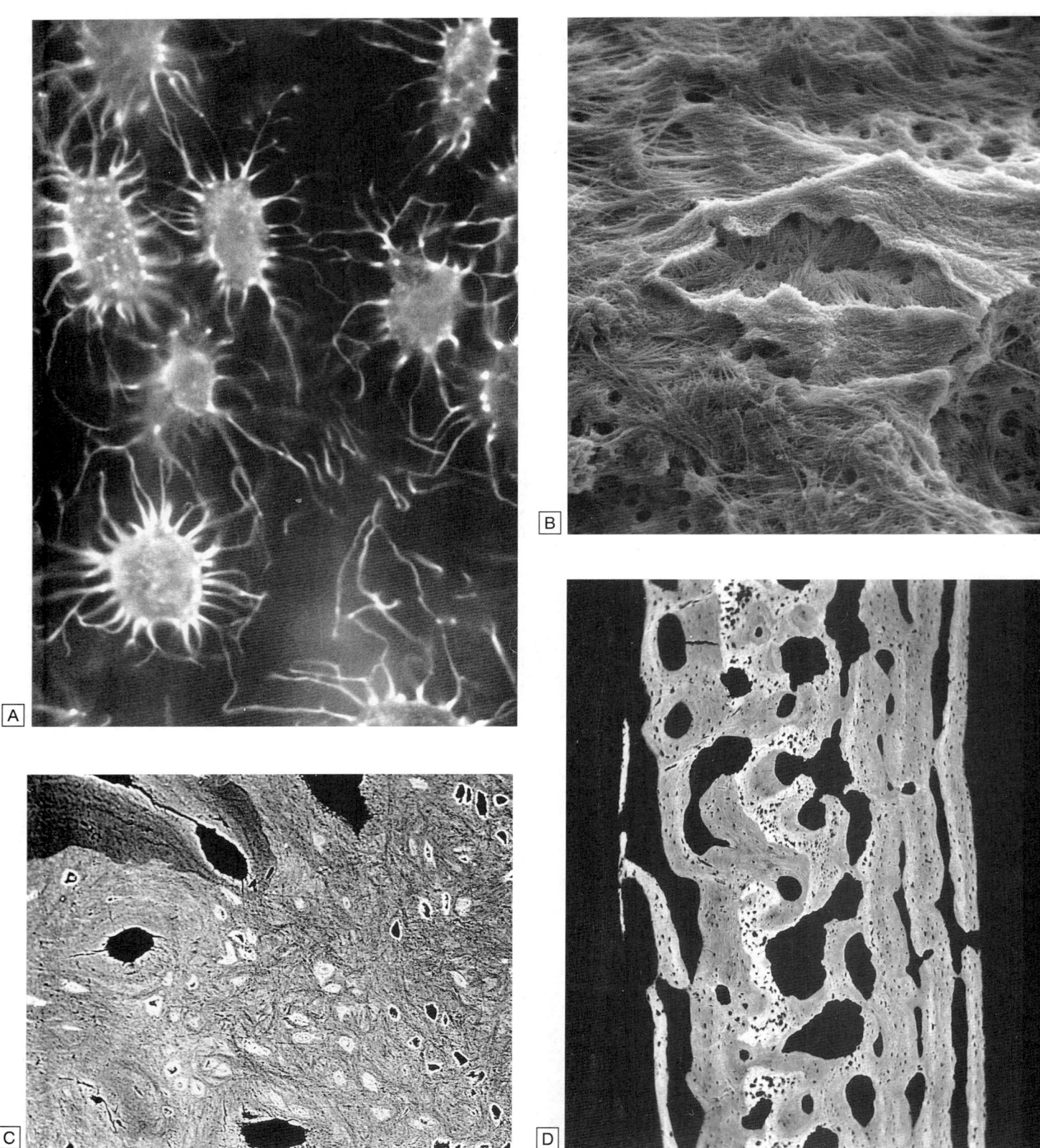

6.31A.   Osteocytes in rat parietal bone; the cell processes radiate from the soma, branching and connecting with those of other osteocytes (and osteoblasts). Fluorescence confocal scanning light micrograph, field width = 120 μm. B. Osteocyte lacuna, half-opened by osteoclastic resorption, in periosteal surface of a human rib (13 year male). Canalicular openings are seen in its wall. Surrounding this area, new intrinsic fibre matrix and the ends of Sharpey's (extrinsic) fibres can be seen. SEM, field width = 29 μm.

C. Human incus, embedded BSE, showing numerous mineralized osteocytes in their lacunae and a dense perilacuna phase in several lacunae with non-mineralized centres; field width = 330 μm. D. Human parietal bone (neonate male) showing primary osteonal bone and woven bone (white, with many large and conjoined osteocyte lacunae within, appearing black). Resorption of the bone internally is resulting in trabecularization. Embedded BSE, field width = 1335 μm.

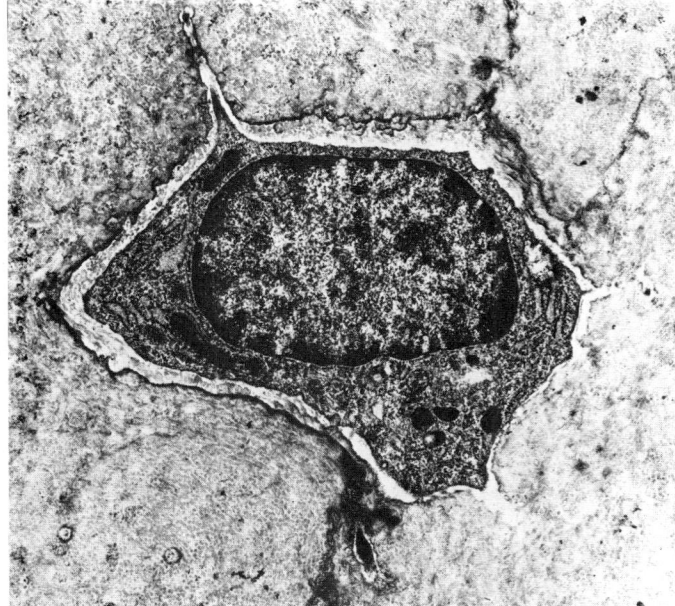

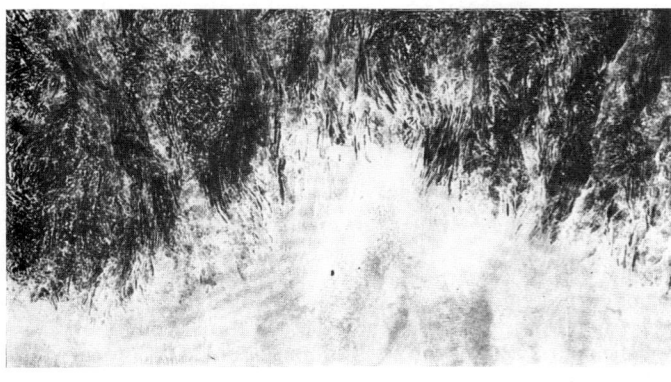

6.32 Electron micrographs A shows a young osteocyte within bone matrix (decalcified during processing for microscopy). Visible are the bases of cell processes extending within the canaliculi, the cell body containing granular endoplasmic reticulum, the lacuna with less dense matrix surrounding the cell body, and many collagen fibres in the matrix, mainly sectioned transversely in this picture. Magnification ×3000. (Provided by A Hayward.) B shows bone crystals (above) and collagen fibres at a mineralizing front on the surface of bone. Magnification × 3000. (Provided by Moya Meredith Smith.)

Bone lining cells

Bone lining cells are flattened epithelium-like cells, particularly evident in the adult skeleton, found on the resting surfaces of bone, i.e. those not undergoing deposition or resorption (Miller & Jee 1987, 1992). They form continuous layers and are in contact with each other, and with neighbouring osteocytes, through gap junctions. On the endosteal surface of narrow cavities they form the outer boundary of the marrow tissue, are present on the periosteal surface and line the system of vascular canals within osteons. Their role and lineage is not yet clear, but they may be once active osteoblasts which can revert to the active state when suitably stimulated, or be derived directly from committed osteoblast progenitors. They may play an active role in regulating the differentiation of osteoprogenitor cells, control the access of osteoclasts to the bone surface and regulate mineral homeostasis (Menton et al 1982; Miller et al 1989). It has also been suggested on the basis of in vitro experiments that bone lining cells may secrete collagenase to remove any unmineralized matrix and prepare bone surfaces for osteoclastic resorption (Chambers et al 1985).

Osteoclasts (6.33, 34, 35)

Osteoclasts are large (20 μm or more) polymorphous cells with a variable number of oval, closely packed nuclei, often 15–20 or more (see review by Baron et al 1993). They are found where there is active removal of bone and lie in close contact with the bone surface in pits termed *resorption bays* or *lacunae of Howship* (**6.36**B).

Osteoclasts contain numerous mitochondria and vacuoles, many being tartrate-resistant acid phosphatase-positive lysosomes. The granular endoplasmic reticulum is relatively sparse for the size of cell and they have extensive perinuclear Golgi complexes. Coated transport vesicles and vacuoles are numerous between the Golgi stacks and the surface of the cell at the site of bone resorption. The latter is highly folded with finger and leaf-shaped processes to form a *ruffled membrane*. Here, the bases of clefts between the irregular cell extensions may appear as vacuoles in sections. Microtubule arrays are involved in the transport of vesicles. Around the perimeter of the ruffled membrane is a well-defined zone of actin filaments, and here the osteoclast is closely attached to the bone surface, so forming a limit to the resorptive activities of the ruffled membrane zone. In tissue culture the ruffled membrane exhibits constant vigorous movement and active pinocytosis. Collagen fragments and other matrix debris have been found within its clefts. The size of the ruffled membrane varies with hormonal treatment, increasing when resorption of bone is stimulated, for example with parathyroid hormone, and disappearing in the presence of agents which directly inhibit resorption, for example calcitonin. The region surrounding the ruffled membrane and closely applied to the bone is called the *clear zone* because it has few cell organelles.

have aged osteocytes, and also low osteocyte viability (Dunstan et al 1993).

The exact functions of osteocytes are not yet clear. However, it is widely assumed that they must have an essential role in the maintenance of bone, and that their death leads to the resorption of the matrix by osteoclast activity. It is also assumed that they are involved in signalling the requirement to resorb microdamaged compact bone, and to splint fractured trabeculae with microcallus. By means of their communications with cells at the bone surface, they may act as local sensors of the mechanical and chemical state of the bone and initiate resorption or addition of matrix at the surface accordingly (Lanyon 1993a,b). Evidence that mature osteocytes are directly responsible for matrix resorption in mammals is lacking at present (Lanyon 1993a) and refuted by some (Boyde 1980). They remain responsive to parathyroid hormone and 1,25(OH)$_2$ vitamin D3 and it is possible that they are involved in mineral exchange at the adjacent, extensive lacunar and canalicular bone surface.

In some mammals, a distinct phase is found lining the walls of the osteocytic lacunae. This *perilacunar matrix* is highly mineralized, its matrix is formed within the confines of the original lacuna, and it appears to contain no collagen. In man, the osteocytes themselves are often mineralized, with the nuclear compartment still recognizable.

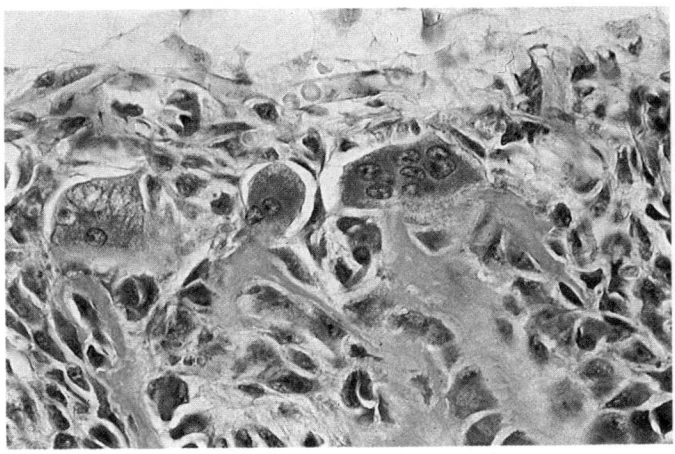

6.33 Section through developing membrane bone showing a group of large, multinucleate osteoclasts eroding spicules of bone (green). Many osteoblasts are also clustered at other surfaces of the spicules where bone is being formed. Masson's trichrome. Magnification ×1000. (Provided by Moya Meredith Smith.)

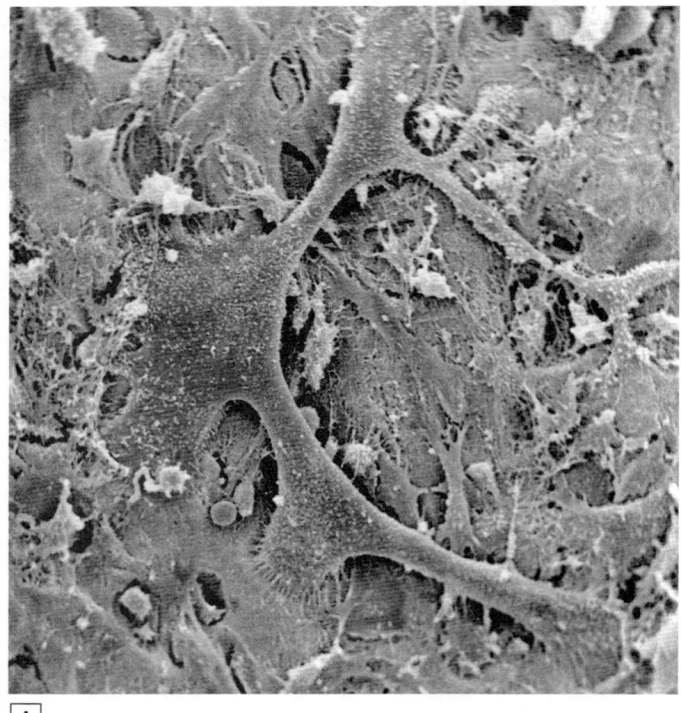

A

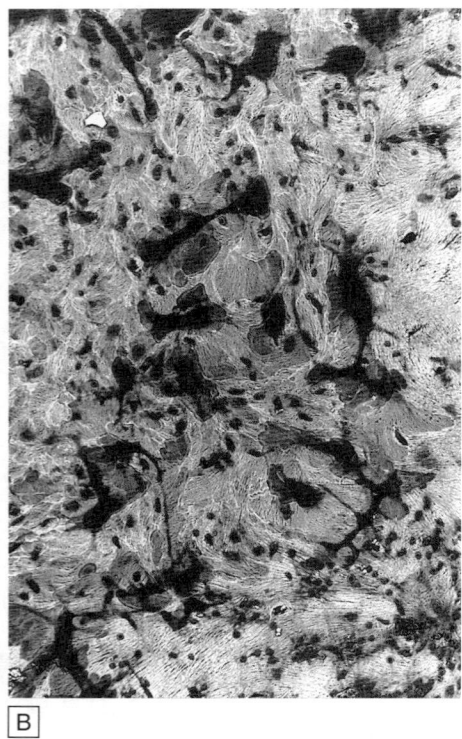

B

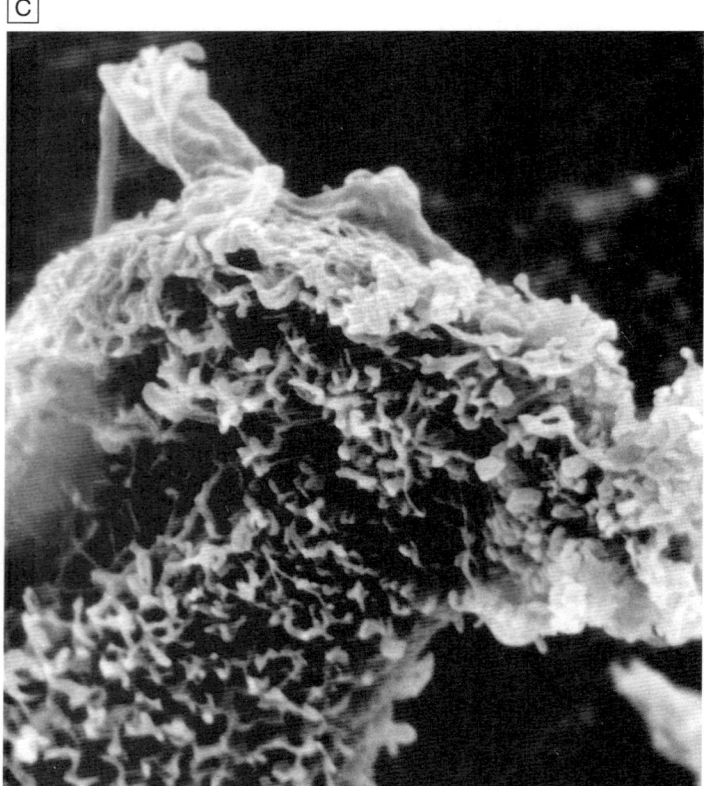

C

6.34A. A large osteoclast on the endocranial surface of rat calvarium: the cell has several resorptive sites of attachment to the bone and extends over a large area; SEM, field width = 129 μm. **B.** The varied shapes and sizes of active osteoclasts, showing as dark features against the whiter background of the more backscattering bone, on the parietal bone of a Westray mouse; BSE, field width = 266 μm. **C.** Ventral surface of an osteoclast on the endocranial surface of rat calvarium, dissected back to reveal the resorptive ruffled border zone that abutted the bone; SEM, field width 18.5 μm.

Functionally, osteoclasts are responsible for the removal of bone, although exactly how is not known. Clearly, they cause demineralization by *proton* release, and there is also structural evidence of organic matrix destruction by lysosomal and non-lysosomal enzymes (Delaisse & Vaes 1992). Demineralization of the matrix occurs locally where the osteoclast's ruffled membrane approaches the bone surface; it has been proposed that osteoclasts can only attack bone after its organic lining has been removed by osteoblasts or bone lining cells to expose the mineralized surface. However, there is also much evidence that osteoclasts can readily degrade collagen and other organic compartments of the unmineralized or demineralized matrix, perhaps by the secretion of *gelatinase/collagenase* as well as *cysteine proteases* (Delaisse et al 1993; Wucherpfennig et al 1994). Osteoclasts may also generate oxygen-derived free radicals which increase bone resorption (Baron et al 1993).

Agents responsible for stimulating osteoclasts to resorb bone appear to be multiple, including factors released by osteoblasts and probably various other cells such as macrophages and lymphocytes (see review by Mundy 1993a). A rise in intracellular calcium leads to inactivation of the osteoclast and a reduction of Ca_i to activation. Various humoral factors such as parathyroid hormone and $1,25(OH)_2$ vitamin D3 (calcitriol) are also involved in bone resorption. This subject will be discussed more fully in a later section (see bone remodelling, p. 478).

The cell lineage of osteoclasts has been much studied, and it is now established that they arise by fusion of mononuclear cells which originate in the bone marrow (Ash et al 1980; Ko & Bernard 1981) or other haemopoietic tissue (Takahashi et al 1988). Several lines of evidence point to similarities between osteoclasts and mononuclear phagocytes (macrophages) which can also fuse to form giant multi-nuclear cells with phagocytic functions. Both cell types arise from the bone marrow, have an affinity for certain supravital dyes, possess many lysosomes and are motile. However, some monoclonal antibodies specific for macrophages fail to react with osteoclasts, so it is likely that they form a distinct class of cells, although with a common precursor of the granulocyte–macrophage lineage (**6.37B**).

When bone resorption has finished, it is possible that these syncytial cells dissociate into mononuclear cells: whether these may again fuse to form active osteoclasts if suitably stimulated is unknown. The

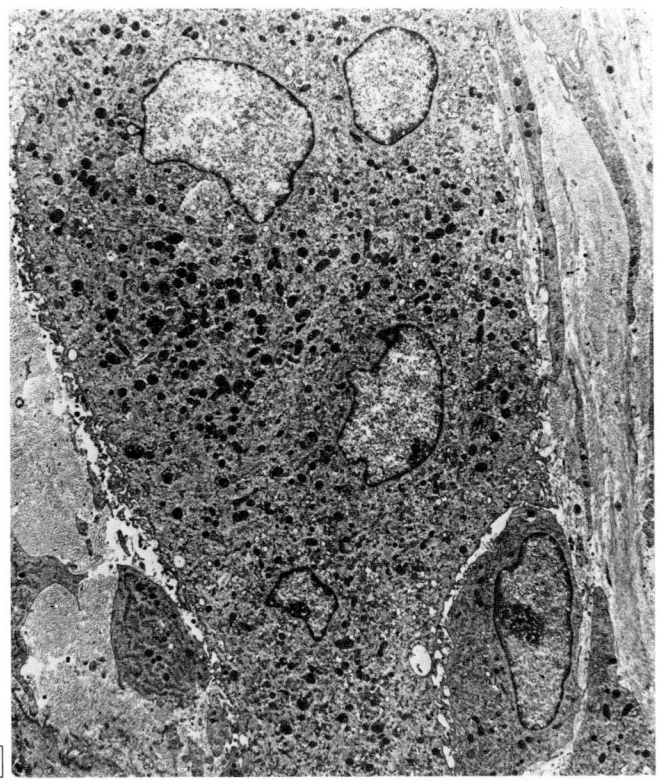

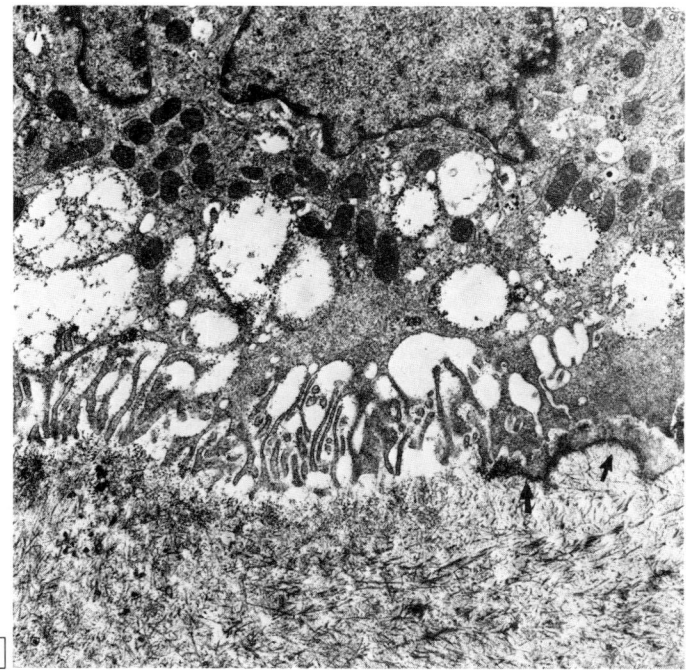

6.35 Electron micrograph of osteoclasts. A shows a large multinucleate cell close to the surface of bone, although not, in this section plane, within an erosion bay. Magnification ×2500. B is a higher magnification of an osteoclast ruffled border, where active bone resorption is occurring. The cell has been stained cytochemically for acid phosphatase activity, which is shown by the dense granular precipitate within the large (lysosomal) vacuoles in the cytoplasm. To the right arrows mark a close junction between the cell surface and the matrix below the clear zone of the osteoclast. Magnification ×6000. (Both micrographs provided by Moya Meredith Smith.)

lifespan of an osteoclast nucleus has been estimated to be about 16 days, and Jaworski et al (1981) give osteoclast survival times in vivo of over 7 weeks. However, knowledge of osteoclast longevity in humans of different ages is scant.

MICROSCOPIC STRUCTURE—BONE MATRIX

Bone matrix is the extracellular mineralized material of bone and consists of a ground substance in which are embedded numerous collagen fibres, usually ordered in parallel arrays (**6.36, 38**). In mature bone, the matrix is moderately hydrated, 10–20% of its mass being water; of its dry weight, 60–70% is made up of inorganic, mineral salts (mainly carbonate-apatite), 30–40% is collagen and the remainder (about 5%) is non-collagenous protein and carbohydrate, mainly conjugated as glycoproteins (Sparc/osteonectin, osteocalcin, decorin, bone sialoproteins, etc). The proportions of these various components vary with age, location and metabolic status. In the early stages of bone formation, before mineralization, the matrix is termed *osteoid*. In adult bones the amount of osteoid is very small, reflecting local remodelling of the bone in which mineralization follows the deposition of the organic matrix. In certain disease states where mineralization is defective, notably rickets, the amounts of osteoid are greatly increased.

Collagen

Collagen in bone closely resembles that of many other connective tissues, belonging to Type I with trace amounts of Type V which is thought to regulate fibrillogenesis. However, in some details it differs from collagen in loose connective tissue in that in bone its molecular structure is more strongly covalently cross-linked internally, and the transverse spacings within its fibrils are somewhat larger. The cross-links make it stronger and chemically more inert, and the internal gaps provide the space for deposition of the mineral phase—it has been estimated that up to two-thirds of the mineral is located within collagen fibrils (Katz & Li 1973; Katz et al 1989). It is generally believed that the crystals are initiated in the gaps between the

ends of tropocollagen subunits ('hole regions') which, in sectioned material, occur with a 64 nm repeat distance along the collagen (67 nm in hydrated tissue), emphasizing the regular banding pattern in electron microscope preparations. This opinion has recently been challenged (Arsenault 1989). Bound to the collagen structural framework are acidic phosphorylated macromolecules, also secreted by the osteoblasts, which initiate mineral deposition of a carbonate-apatite (Veis 1992).

That collagen contributes much to the mechanical strength of this tissue is clearly demonstrated in bones treated to denature or remove their collagen, when the bone becomes brittle and fragile. The precise role of collagen in bone mechanics is still not understood in detail, however, since the direction of fibres, the association of mineral crystals within and outside the fibres and other local features all modify their behaviour under stresses of different kinds, making mathematical analysis a complex matter (see e.g. Frasca et al 1981; Currey 1984a,b,c). But it is clear that besides contributing to the tensile, compressive and shearing strengths of bone, the small degree of elasticity shown by collagen imparts a measure of resilience to this tissue, helping to resist fracture when mechanically loaded.

Collagen fibres are synthesized by osteoblasts, polymerizing from tropocollagen extracellularly and becoming progressively more cross-linked as they mature. In primary bone, they form a complex interwoven meshwork (non-lamellar or *woven bone*) which is later almost entirely replaced by the regular laminar arrays of nearly parallel collagen fibres (*lamellar bone*). Partially mineralized collagen networks can be seen within osteoid on the outer and internal surfaces of bone (**6.38c, 62c**): endosteal faces and linings of vascular canal.

Collagen fibres from the periosteum are incorporated in cortical bone (*extrinsic* or *Sharpey's fibres*), anchoring this fibrocellular layer at its surface (**6.36, 38**). The terminal collagen fibres of tendons and ligaments are also included deep in the matrix of cortical bone. With cortical drift (*modelling*) and turnover (*remodelling*) they may be interrupted by new osteons and remain in islands of interstitial lamellae or even trabeculae.

461

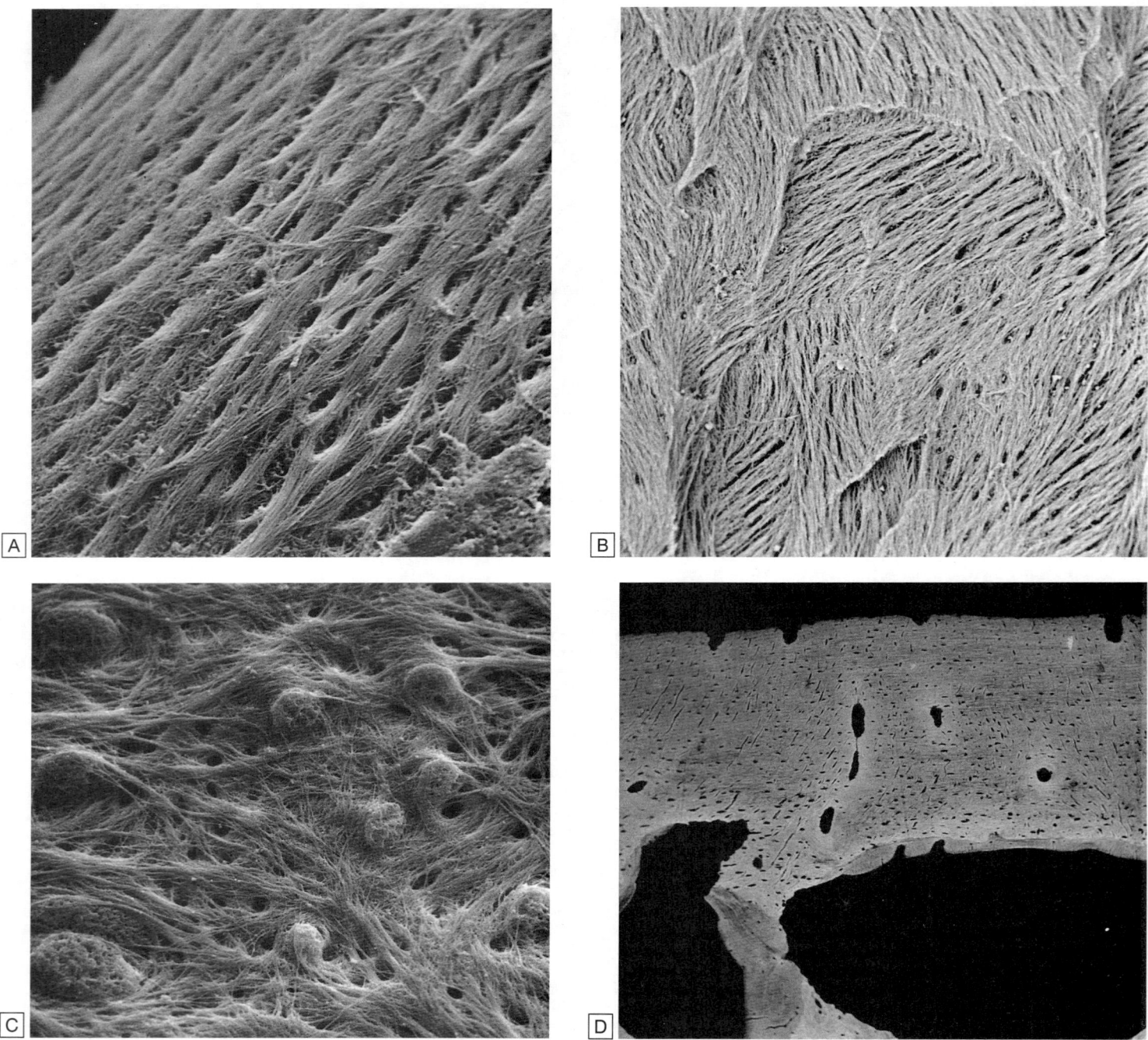

6.36A.   Collagen fibres on the surface of human trabecular bone (2 month female, sixth rib). Note the branching and rejoining of the fibres, as fibrils switch between bundles; SEM, field width = 36 μm. B. The different orientations of the collagen fibres in successive lamellae has been uncovered by osteoclastic resorption. Human sixth rib (43 year female); SEM, field width = 65 μm. C. Periosteal surface of human rib (13 year male). The ends of obliquely incorporated Sharpey's (extrinsic) fibres are seen as oval struc- tures amongst the finer intrinsic matrix fibres of the bundle bone. Canaliculi pass through the surface; SEM, field width = 32 μm. D. Polished, embedded section of human cranial bone (15 month male) showing (Sharpey's) extrinsic fibres incorporated throughout the cortex of the bone, and in the region undergoing trabecularization. The unmineralized cores of the fibres are seen as fine obliquely running black lines. Fine horizontal lines in the cortex are incremental lines. Embedded BSE, field width = 1 mm.

Other organic components of the matrix

Various complex macromolecules also exist attached to collagen fibres and surrounding bone crystals in small amounts (for review see Delmas & Malaval 1993). *Sparc/osteonectin* is a phosphorylated glycoprotein secreted by osteoblasts and bound mainly to mineral. It is involved in adhesion of cell–cell and cell–substrate interactions.

Osteocalcin is another glycoprotein, synthesized by osteoblasts, which may play a part in bone mineralization and the regulation of bone resorption. It is bound to the mineral and is used as a marker of bone formation. Matrix gamma carboxyglutamic acid (GLA)-protein is bound to collagen; its function in bone is unknown but it may inhibit mineralization.

The functions of the bone proteoglycans *biglycan* and *decorin* remain unclear, but they may regulate fibrillogenesis and cell differentiation.

Bone sialoproteins, *osteopontin* and *thrombospondin* contain the arginine-glycine-aspartic acid (RGD) sequence and are involved in cell adhesion to bone. They may also have a role in mineralization of the matrix, particularly in the nucleation of crystals and regulation of crystal size.

The bone matrix also contains many *growth factors* (Baylink et al 1993), *proteases* and *protease inhibitors* secreted by osteoblasts, often in a latent form. One, transforming growth factor-β (TGF-β), is activated in the acid conditions of the ruffled border zone of the

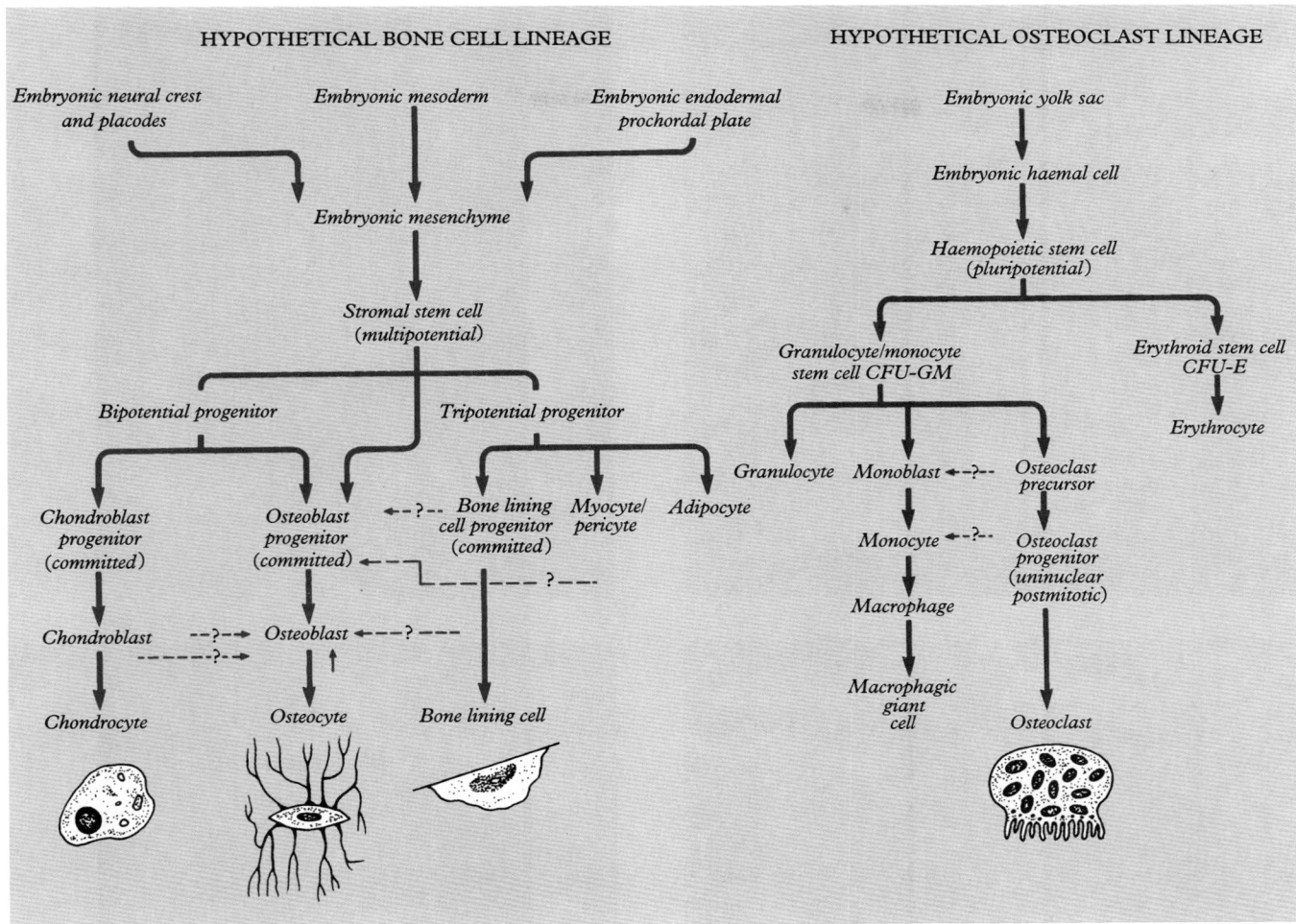

6.37 Diagram of the origins of the cells of bone, after Martin et al 1993.

osteoclast and may be a coupling factor for stimulating new bone formation at resorption sites. TGF-β is secreted by osteoclasts as well as osteoblasts (Oursler 1994).

Some plasma proteins, such as a_2HS-glycoprotein and *albumin*, are adsorbed by the bone crystals but have no proven function in bone.

Bone salts

Bone salts form the inorganic constituents of the bone matrix, conferring on bone its hardness and much of its rigidity. The mineral substances of bone are mostly soluble in dilute acids and can be removed by prolonged immersion, for example in 2% nitric acid, or in solutions of calcium chelators such as citrates or ethylene diamine tetracetic acid (EDTA). The bone then retains its shape but is highly flexible, so that a long thin bone (such as the fibula) can easily be tied in a knot. In histological sections the microstructure of the bone, including its cells, lamellae, osteons, etc. are well preserved after such gentle demineralization.

Bone crystals are small with a large surface. They take the form of thin plates or leaf-like structures ranging in size up to at least 150 nm long by 80 nm wide and 5 nm thick but mostly half that size. They are often packed quite closely together, with long axes at 3° (i.e. nearly parallel) to the collagen fibril axis, when within them, or may enshroud microfibrils. The narrow gaps between the crystals contain associated water and organic macromolecules.

The mineral portion of mature bones is composed largely of crystals made of a substance generally referred to as *hydroxyapatite*, but with an important *carbonate* content and a lower Ca/P ratio than pure hydroxyapatite ($Ca_{10}(PO_4)_6(OH)_2$), together with a small amount of non-apatitic calcium phosphate (Glimcher 1990). Thus the major ions which comprise the mineral part of bone include calcium, phosphate, hydroxyl and carbonate. Less numerous ions

are those of citrate, magnesium, sodium, potassium, fluoride, chloride, iron, zinc, copper, aluminium, lead, strontium, silicon and boron, many of these being present only in trace quantities. Fluoride ions can substitute for hydroxyl ions, and carbonate can substitute either hydroxyl or phosphate (Posner 1988). Group IIA cations such as radium, strontium and lead all readily substitute for calcium and are therefore known as bone-seeking cations; these can be either radioactive or chemically toxic and so constitute a danger to health. When present in bone, they are particularly hazardous since their position in the body close to the haemopoietic tissues of bone marrow may induce various pathologies of that tissue.

Under the electron microscope, bone crystals are electron-dense and, where packed closely together, give the matrix a solid appearance (**6.32**). Intermediate forms of calcium phosphate may occur in early stages of mineralization in developing bone. The number and size of the crystals increases in mature bone with time and the water content decreases. Autoradiographic studies using ^{45}Ca have shown that rapidly exchangeable bone calcium is found at all bone surfaces and is greatest at sites of bone formation and maturation (Parfitt 1993).

MICROSCOPIC ORGANIZATION OF BONE

While the mechanical properties of bone are dependent on the general composition of its matrix, the manner in which the different components are arranged is also of utmost importance in its strength and resilience. Two quite distinct types of organization are found: woven and lamellar bone.

Woven bone

In primary, woven bone, the most immature tissue of developing

463

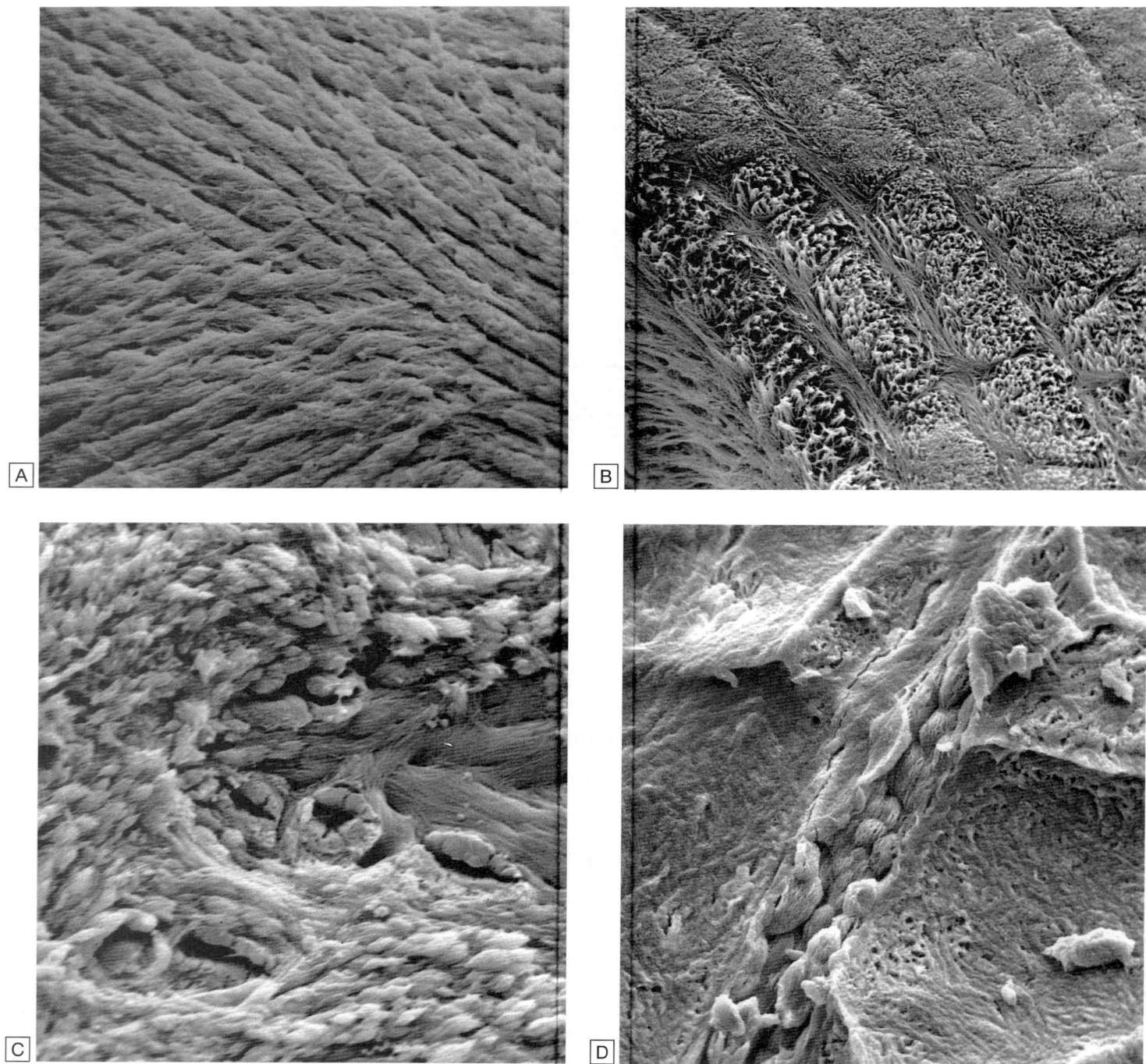

6.38A. Tapering collagen fibres border the new patch of lamellar bone and lie across those of the previous layer. Human trabecular bone in fourth lumbar vertebra (35 year male); SEM, field width = 31 μm. B. Collagen fibre orientations in the osteonal lamellae of a human femur are seen clearly in the etched region (lightly resorbed by culturing chick osteoclasts on the bone slice for 96 hours, and then removing the cells). The collagen fibres lining the osteonal canal can be seen at lower left; SEM, field width = 32 μm. C. Human bundle (Sharpey fibre) bone lining the socket of an upper first molar: unmineralized osteoid and periodontal ligament have been removed to reveal the interface with mineralized tissue. The mineralized segments of the intrinsic fibres lie in the plane of the surface; the ends of extrinsic fibres have unmineralized cores. The back wall of an osteocyte lacuna (centre right) accommodates to several extrinsic fibres, is well mineralized and shows canalicular openings. Anorganic preparation; SEM, field width = 34 μm. D. Resorbed surface of human sixth rib (5 month female); osteoclastic activity has uncovered a partly mineralized extrinsic (Sharpey's) fibre (running obliquely through the centre of the field) in the bone. Anorganic preparation; SEM, field width = 33 μm.

bones, collagen fibres (and the bone crystals within them) are irregularly arranged. The diameters of the fibres vary, fine and coarse fibres intermingling. The coarse fibres are large enough to be resolved by light microscopy and are visible in the bright (45° and 135°) sectors when a section is viewed between crossed polarizing filters, giving rise to the **appearance** of the warp and weft of a woven fabric. Woven bone is formed by very active osteoblasts in an osteogenic blastema, but its formation is stimulated in the adult by fracture, growth factors, or prostaglandin E_2 (Turner 1992). In all other situations, collagen fibres and crystals of bone salts are highly oriented within flattened lamellae.

Lamellar bone

This type of bone makes up almost all of the adult osseous skeleton. The precise arrangement of its lamellae varies from site to site, particularly between the compact cortical bone and the trabecular bone within.

Compact bone (6.30, 39, 40, 41). As already mentioned, adult

464

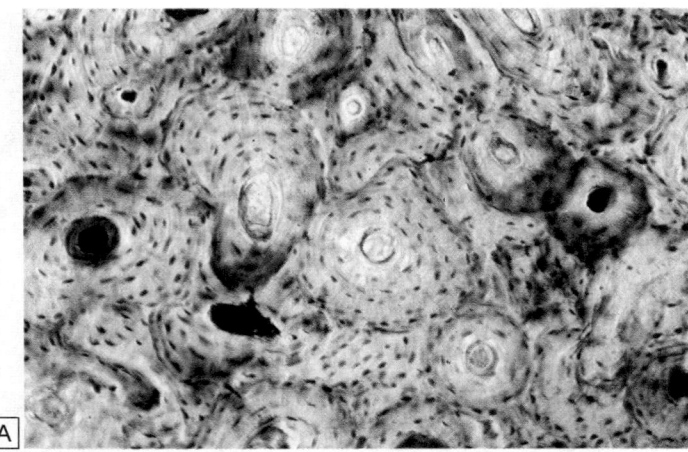

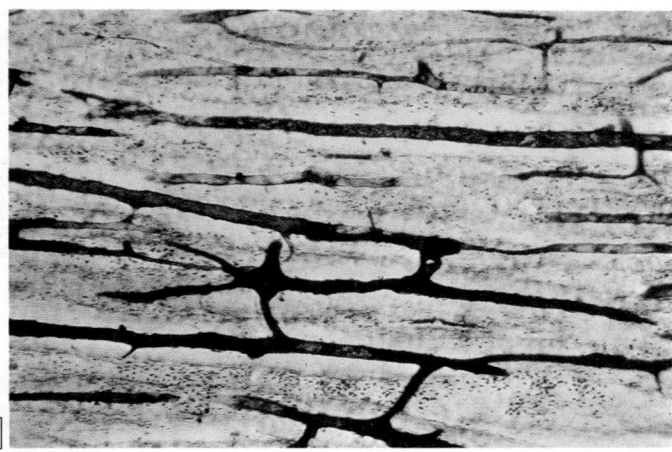

6.39   Transverse (A) and longitudinal (B) ground sections of compact bone from human femoral shaft. Note variation in shape and size of osteons and their canals and in distribution of lacunae in A. Haematoxylin staining in

B. has emphasized the osteons, predominantly longitudinal but showing intercommunications. (Material for **6**.30, **6**.39, **6**.40 prepared by David Ristow, Guy's Hospital Medical School.)

bone consists almost entirely of mineralized matrix with collagen fibres arranged in layers, embedded in which are the osteocytes. In many bones a few such lamellae form continuous layers at the surface, termed *circumferential lamellae*. By far the greatest proportion, however, are arranged in concentric cylinders around neurovascular channels (*Haversian canals*), so forming the basic units of bone construction, the *Haversian systems* or *osteons* (more correctly called *secondary osteons* to distinguish them from *primary osteons* formed during the initial generation of bone and its rapid growth, as described below). Secondary osteons usually lie parallel to each other and, in elongated bones such as those of the appendicular skeleton, with the long axis of the bone, but they frequently spiral, branch or intercommunicate and some end blindly. It has been estimated that there are about 21 million osteons in the adult skeleton (Parfitt 1983). In transverse section they are round or ellipsoidal, varying from about 100 to $400\,\mu$mm in diameter, and the number of lamellae, which are approximately $3\,\mu$mm thick, is about 30 in medium-sized osteons. Each osteon is permeated with canaliculi of its resident osteocytes which form pathways for diffusion of nutrients, gases, etc. between the vascular system and the osteons. The rather small maximum diameter ensures that no osteocyte is more than about $200\,\mu$mm from a blood vessel, a distance which may be a limiting factor in cellular survival. In the intervening spaces between secondary osteons are the fragmentary remains of osteons or circumferential lamellae of older bone which have been partially eroded before the new osteons were formed. This is termed *interstitial bone*.

The central osteonal canals vary in size, with a mean diameter of

$50\,\mu$mm; those near the marrow cavity are somewhat larger (Cohen & Harris 1958). Within each canal are one or two capillaries lined by fenestrated endothelium surrounded by a basal lamina which splits to enclose typical pericytes. Usually there are also some unmyelinated and occasional myelinated nerve fibres, $5-9\,\mu$mm in diameter (Cooper 1968). The bony surfaces of osteonic canals are perforated by the openings of myriads of canaliculi and are also lined by collagen fibres (**6**.38).

Osteonal canals communicate directly or indirectly with the medullary cavity, channels which run obliquely or transversely to the direction of the osteons now being referred to as *Volkmann's canals*. These are said not to be surrounded by concentric lamellae of bone. However, the majority of such channels appear to be simple anastomotic canals and the frequency of larger, true vascular connections with the periosteum and endosteum may be rather low (see Cohen & Harris 1958).

All secondary osteons are demarcated from their neighbours by a *cement line* which has little or no collagen and is strongly basophilic due to a high content of glycoproteins and proteoglycans; this marks the limit of bone erosion prior to the formation of an osteon and is therefore also known as a *reversal line*. Similar basophilic lines also occur in the absence of erosion, where bony growth has been interrupted and then resumed (*resting lines*). Canaliculi may sometimes pass through cement lines, so providing a route for exchange between interstitial bone and vascular channels within osteons (Atkinson & Hallsworth 1982).

Lamellation of bone (**6**.38, 40). The relative importance of different

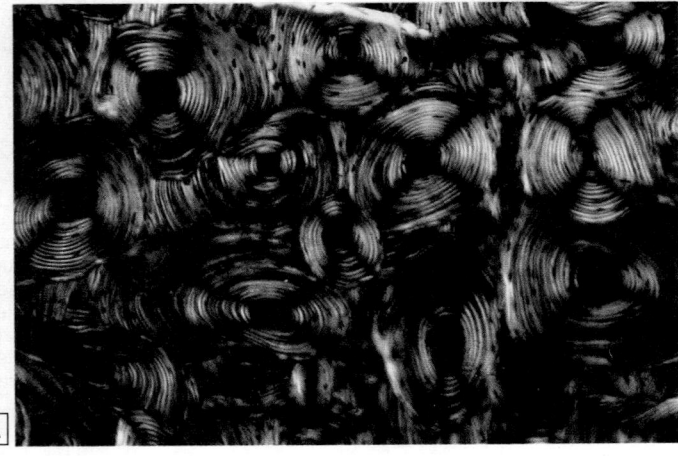

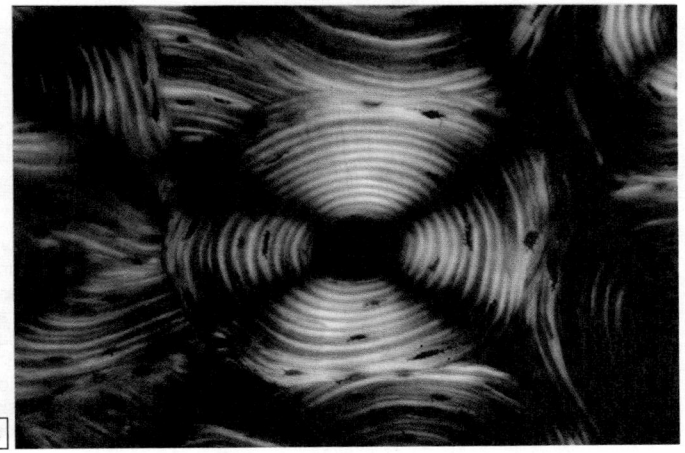

6.40A, B.   Ground transverse section of the compactum of the adult human femur photographed using polarization microscopy. Compare with **6**.39A.

B. A single secondary osteon viewed with high-power polarization optics to illustrate its lamellar architecture.

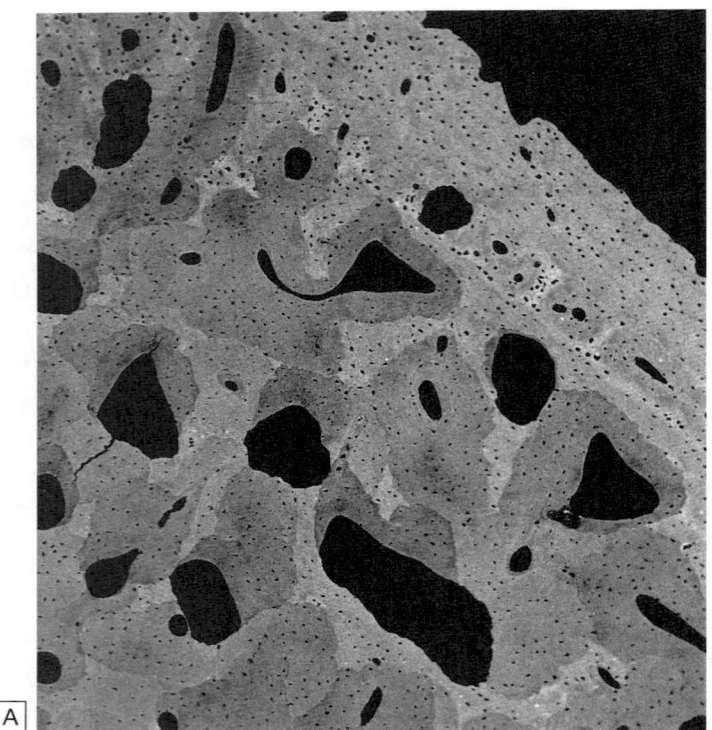

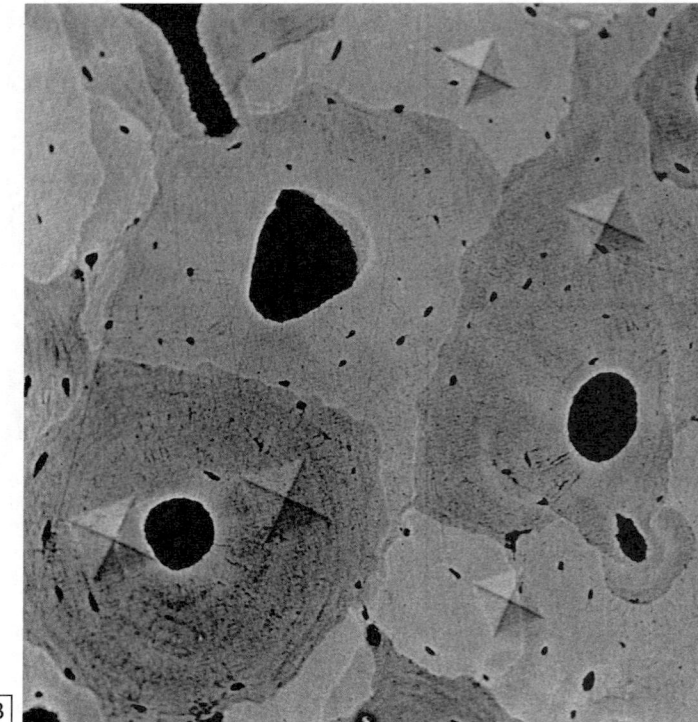

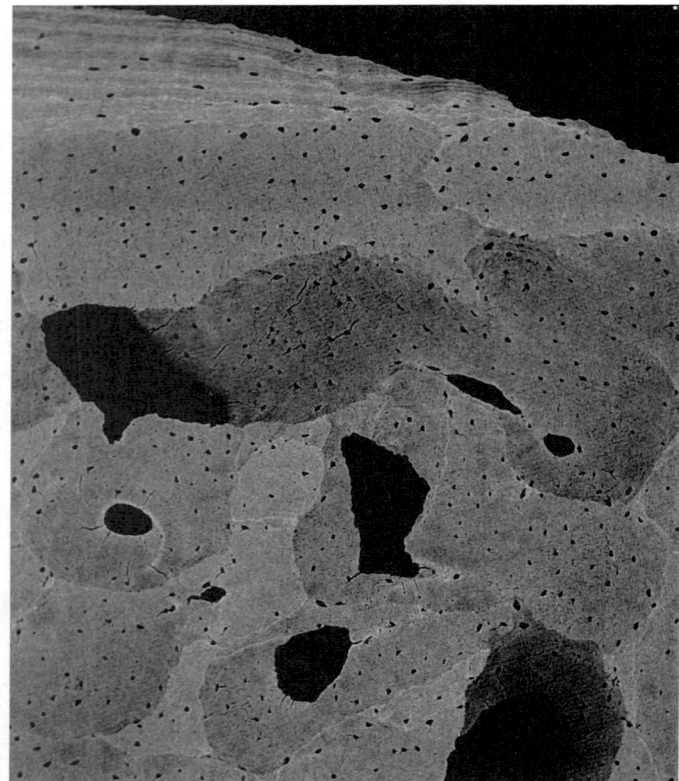

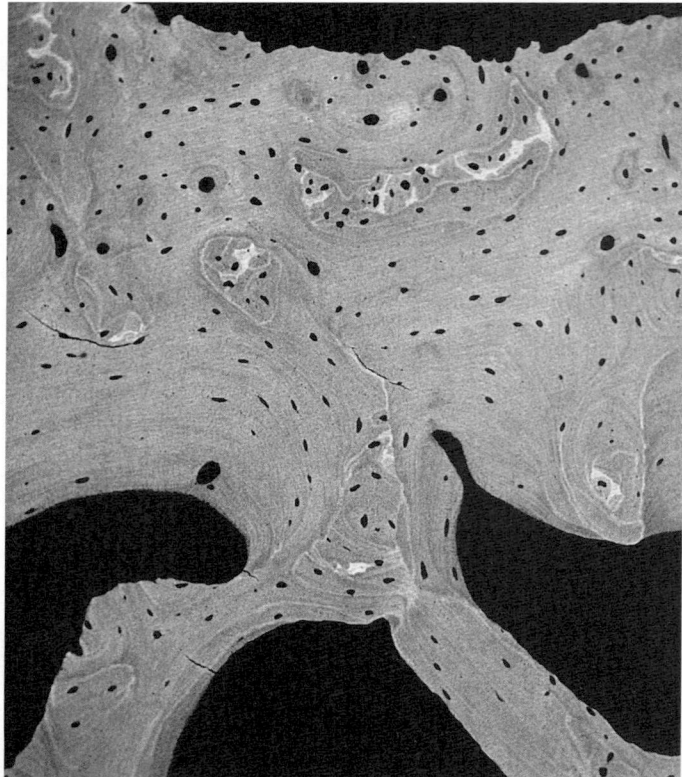

6.41 Backscattered electron images of embedded bone, coated with carbon. A. Primary osteonal bone at surface (top right) and secondary osteonal bone within. The denser (whitest) bone within the surface layer is woven bone that formed as intervascular ridges. Unremodelled primary osteonal bone is also present in the interstitial regions between secondary osteons. Eroding and infilling osteons are present. Periosteal region of human (9 year) tibia; field width = 1.55 mm. B. Adult human rib cross-section: the bone was indented with a pyramidal marker at constant load: the size of the indent indicates the hardness of the bone. Interstitial, older bone is more mineralized and harder; field width = 404 μm. C. Circumferential lamellae border the bone surface (top left) but the surface is being resorbed as modelling occurs during growth. Remodelling with generations of secondary osteons is evident within the bone. Human sixth rib (13 years); field width =780 μm. D. Calcified cartilage remnants (whitest, highly mineralized regions) within the bone of rat tibia periosteal resorption and endosteal formation are maintaining cortical width. The osteocyte lacunae demonstrate the orientation of the lamellae; field width = 600 μm.

factors which might account for the lamellar appearance are not yet entirely agreed. Each lamella consists of a sheet of mineralized matrix containing collagen fibres of similar orientation locally, which run in branching fasciculi about 2–3 μm thick, and often from one lamella to the next in depth. This interconnecting three-dimensional construction increases the strength of the bone. There is a difference in orientation between the structures (i.e. collagen fibres and bone crystals) in adjacent lamellae, varying between 0° and 90°. This alternating orientation is clearly shown by polarized light microscopy (**6**.40) and by scanning electron microscopy. A less perfect packing of collagen fibrils into bundles occurs at the borders of lamellae, with intermediate and indifferent orientations predominating. This would explain descriptions which have included a thin (0.1 μm) layer of matrix with a reduced organic content, initially a higher water content, and, in the mature condition, eventually a higher mineral content at lamellar boundaries (‘*interlamellar bone*’). Mjör (1969) supported earlier claims (Ruth 1947) that fibre-rich and fibre-poor lamellae alternate, and this view has been adopted by Marotti (1993) who proposes that (‘transverse’) collagen-rich lamellae composed of densely packed interwoven fibres alternate with (‘longitudinal’) collagen-poor lamellae with loosely packed interwoven fibres.

The earliest descriptions suggested that collagen fibres in osteons alternate between longitudinal and circumferential in successive lamellae, or that they had spiral paths of different pitches. Although a degree of spiralization has been confirmed in investigations into the structure and compressive properties of isolated osteons (Ascenzi & Bonucci 1968; Ascenzi et al 1978), scanning electron microscopy of forming or resting surfaces in osteonal canals shows only small domains or areas of nearly parallel collagen fibres visible on the bone surface. Although fibres within a domain have the same direction, domains are not parallel with each other so that variation of orientation may exist at any surface (Boyde & Hobdell 1969).

The main direction of the collagen fibres within osteons of long bone shafts varies between sites subjected predominantly to tension, where they are more longitudinal, and compression, where they are more oblique (transverse; Carando et al 1989). At any site in the diaphysis the peripheral lamellae of osteons have more ‘transverse’ fibres.

Trabecular bone (6.25, 26, 27)

The organization of trabecular bone is again basically lamellar, but the bone is in the form of branching and anastomosing curved plates, tubes and bars of various widths and lengths, limiting medullary spaces (see p. 436) and bounded by endosteal tissue. Their thickness ranges from about 50 to 400 μm (see review by Eriksen et al 1993). In general, bone lamellae are oriented parallel with the adjacent bone surface and there is the same arrangement of cells and matrix as found in circumferential and osteonic bone. Thick trabeculae may contain small osteons, but blood vessels do not otherwise lie within the bony tissue and osteocytes rely on canalicular diffusion from adjacent medullary vessels. In young bone, calcified cartilage may occur in the cores of trabeculae but this is generally replaced by bone during subsequent remodelling.

Variation in bone composition. Normal variation in composition of bone at different sites and ages is inadequately recorded, although it would be valuable in an assessment of rarefaction (porosity) due to ageing, disease or disuse. Whether *osteoporosis* is, for example, merely an actual reduction in total amount of tissue, rather than a reduction in mineralization, cannot be determined by clinical imaging methods because of problems of separation of bone from other tissues. Furthermore, measurement of sizes of vascular, lacunar and medullary spaces is still difficult even with microscopic imaging techniques. The minimization of difficulties by limiting estimates to cortical bone has been tried since trabecular is more labile than cortical bone. However, the difference in composition of trabecular and compact bone is normally considered to be slight. Overall, water content decreases and mineralization increases with age, but how the organic content varies with age is unknown.

Microradiography and backscattered electron imaging of compact bone show uneven distributions of mineral salt (**6**.41). Inner and outer circumferential and interstitial lamellae are evenly and highly mineralized. Secondary osteons exhibit variable mineralization; in a single osteon concentration varies in different areas. Young osteons have a low but increasing concentration of mineral: whilst infilling is in process, the mineralization is higher in the older, more peripheral

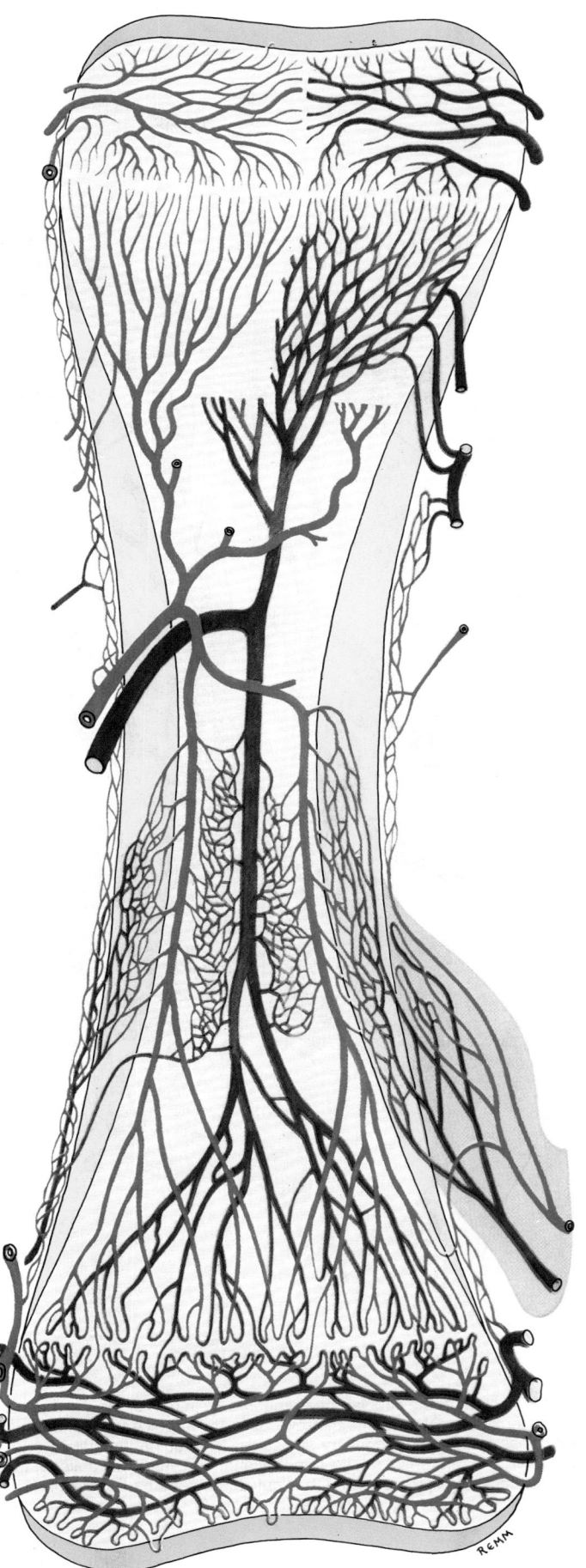

6.42 Scheme of the main features of the blood supply of a long bone based upon descriptions by M Brookes (Guy's Hospital Medical School). Note the contrasting supplies of the diaphysis, metaphysis and epiphysis, and their connections with periosteal, endosteal, muscular and periarticular vessels. Consult the text for a more extended description.

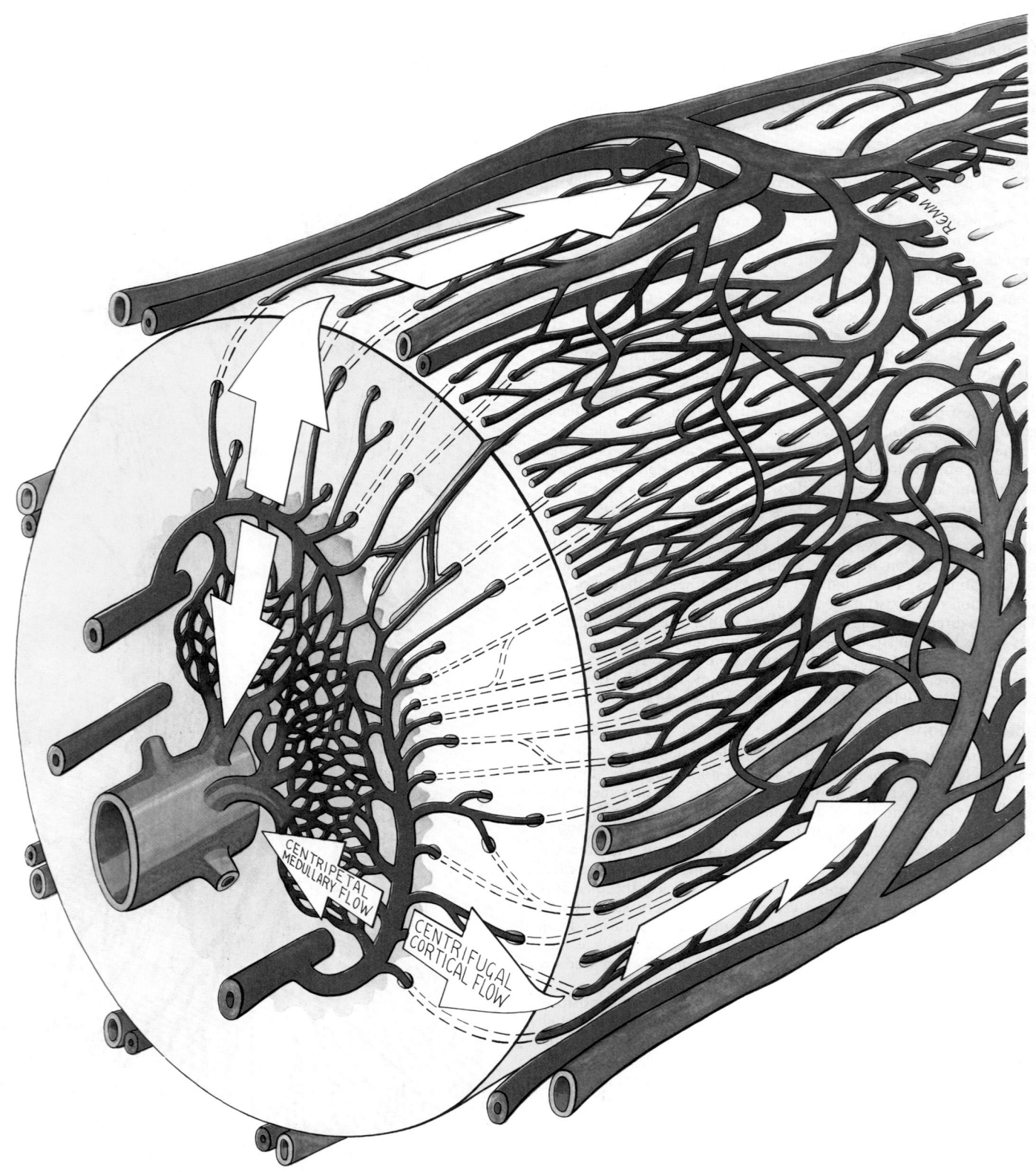

6.43 Diagram of the circulatory arrangements in part of the diaphysis of a typical long bone. Note, in the marrow cavity, the large central venous sinus, the dense network of medullary sinusoids, longitudinal medullary arteries and their circumferential rami. From the latter, longitudinally oblique, trans-cortical capillaries emerge through minute 'comet-shaped' foramina (**6.46**A) to become confluent with the periosteal capillaries and venules. Not to scale; obliquity of cortical capillaries is emphasized for clarity. (Constructed with the collaboration of M Brookes, Department of Anatomy, Guy's Hospital Medical School, London.)

bone: after the initial infill is completed, the level is higher centrally and less towards the periphery, a gradient which diminishes with age until in old, highly mineralized osteons mineral distribution is uniform. Osteons may also show one or more highly mineralized arrest lines within the wall. During remodelling, bone resorption occurs in regions of both high and low mineral concentration. In lamellar bone, mineralization reaches 70–80% in about 3 weeks, 100% much less rapidly. Woven bone mineralizes faster and can be identified from adjacent lamellar bone by its higher degree of mineralization.

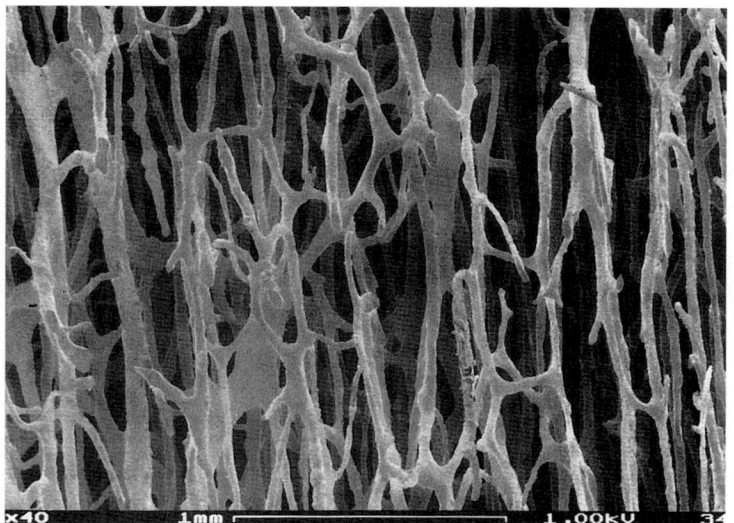

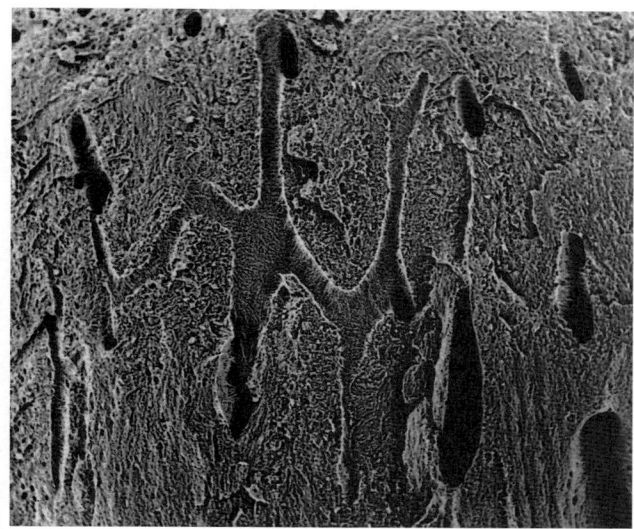

6.44A. PMMA cast of Haversian and interconnecting canals within adult human femoral cortex; SEM, scale bar = 1 mm. B. Fractured human tibial cortex (9 year male) to show arrangement of neurovascular channels; SEM, field width = 1.38 mm.

BLOOD VESSELS AND NERVES OF BONE

The osseous circulation supplies the living bone tissue, the marrow, perichondrium, epiphyseal cartilages in young bones and in part the articular cartilages. Modern researches (see review by Brookes 1993) have emphasized a *centrifugal* flow of blood through cortical bone in shafts of long bones, in contrast to an earlier concept of substantial centripetal arterial flow into the cortex from periosteal vessels. The vascular supply of a long bone depends on several points of inflow, feeding complex and regionally variable sinusoidal networks within it, which in turn drain to venous channels leaving through all surfaces not covered by articular cartilage. These vascular patterns are summarized in **6.**42, 43; see also **6.**44, 45).

One or two main *diaphyseal nutrient arteries* enter the shaft obliquely through nutrient foramina leading into nutrient canals. Long recognized (Havers 1691; Bernard 1855), their sites of entry and angulation are almost constant and characteristically directed away from the dominant growing epiphysis. This is the basis of the *growing-end hypothesis* to explain the positions and orientations of nutrient foramina and canals, but such a simple mechanism does not account for the exceptions to this pattern reported in various species and sites (Hughes 1952). However, in human long bones Mysorekar (1967) observed atypically directed canals only in the fibula, attributing this to its unique pattern of ossification. A subsequent study of metacarpal and metatarsal bones showed that, apart from a few with double or no foramina, over 90% had a single nutrient foramen in the middle third of the shaft. All foramina, single or double, slanted away from the epiphysis, supporting the above hypothesis (Patake & Mysorekar 1977). Nutrient arteries do not branch in their canals, but divide into ascending and descending branches in the medullary cavity. These approach the epiphyses, dividing repeatedly into smaller rami which pursue helical courses in the juxta-endosteal medullary zone. Near the epiphyses they are joined by terminals of numerous *metaphyseal* and *epiphyseal arteries*: the former are direct branches of neighbouring systemic vessels, the latter from periarticular vascular arcades formed on non-articular bone surfaces (**6.**43). Numerous vascular foramina penetrate bones near their ends, often at fairly specific sites; some are occupied by such arteries, but most contain thin-walled veins. Within bone these arteries are unusual in consisting of endothelium with only a thin layer of supportive connective tissue (Yoffey 1962). Epiphyseal and metaphyseal arteries quantitatively exceed the diaphyseal supply, which they can complement, for example when the latter is experimentally destroyed.

Medullary arteries of the shaft (**6.**42, 43) give off:

- centripetal branches to a hexagonal mesh of medullary sinusoids draining into a wide, thin-walled central venous sinus

- cortical branches passing through endosteal canals to feed fenestrated capillaries in Haversian systems (**6.**44).

The central sinus drains veins which retrace the paths of nutrient arteries, sometimes piercing the shaft elsewhere as independent emissary veins.

Cortical capillaries conform in their pattern to the Haversian canals, often described as longitudinal with oblique interosteonic connections (**6.**44). However, an oblique, radial pattern has been demonstrated, vessels largely radiating from the primary ossification centre (Brookes 1971). At bone surfaces cortical capillaries make capillary and venular connections with the periosteal plexuses (**6.**42, 43, 46), which are formed by arteries from neighbouring muscles contributing vascular arcades with longitudinal links to the fibrous periosteum. From this external plexus a capillary network permeates the deeper, osteogenetic periosteum. At muscular attachments periosteal and muscular plexuses are confluent and the cortical capillaries then drain into interfascicular venules.

The concept of such an almost exclusively centrifugal supply to the cortex in the shafts of long bones has received increasing support, but some (de Marneffe 1951; Morgan 1959) have described an appreciable *centripetal arterial* flow to outer cortical zones from

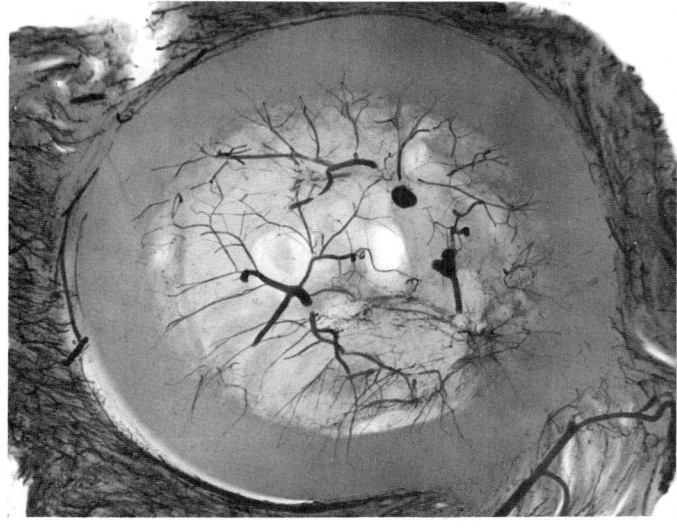

6.45 Microradiograph of long bone in which the arterial supply has been injected with a radio-opaque substance, demonstrating the centrifugal perfusion route of the blood supply. (Provided by M Brookes, Department of Anatomy, UMDS Guy's Campus, London.)

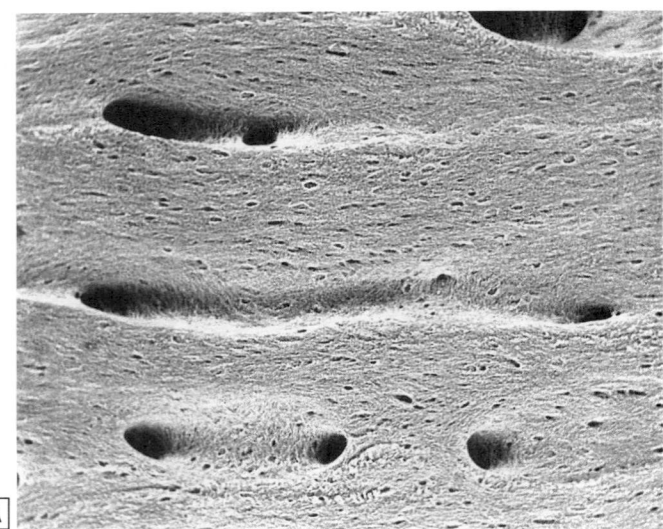

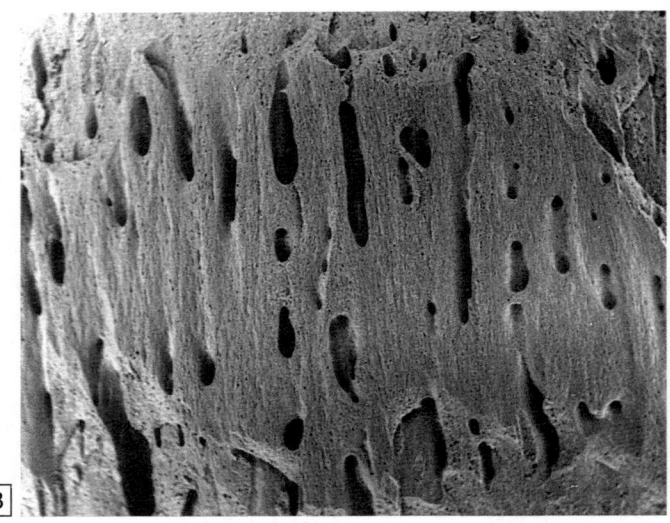

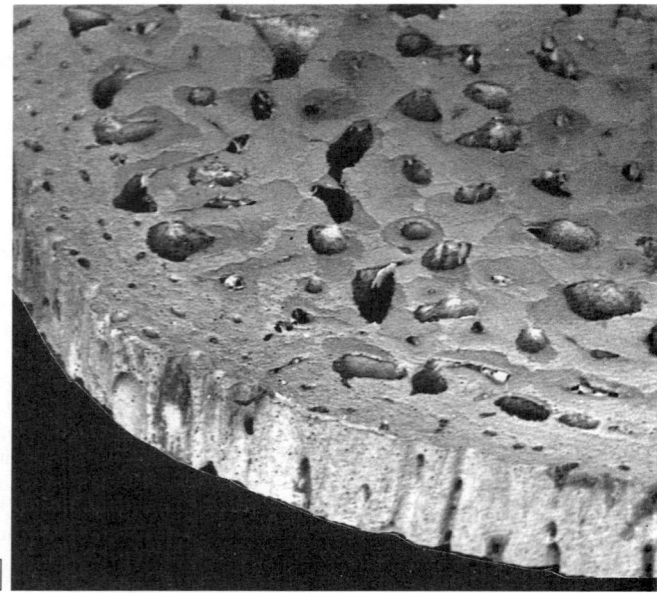

6.46A. Scanning electron micrograph of the periosteal surface of the diaphysis of an adolescent tibia. Note the oblique 'comet-shaped' groove and foramen which in life transmitted a minute neurovascular bundle; numerous foramina of this general type are scattered over the surface of the diaphysis, but their pattern, direction and degree of obliquity vary with the overall subperiosteal deposition of bone that characterizes the various growth zones of the diaphysis. B. Vascular grooves and oblique openings on the periosteal surface of human tibial shaft (9 year male): series of primary osteons develop as intervascular ridges of new bone form then close over the neurovascular tissue, incorporating it within the growing bone. C. Transverse slice of shaft showing secondary osteons which have remodelled the primary osteons deep to the surface region. Anorganic preparations; SEM, field width A = 1.11 mm, B = 2.81 mm, C = 4.39 mm.

periosteal vessels. The large nutrient arteries of epiphyses form many intraosseous anastomoses, branches passing towards the articular surfaces within trabecular spaces of the bone. Near the articular cartilages these form serial anastomotic arcades (e.g. three or four in the femoral head) from which arise end-arterial loops often piercing the thin hypochondral compact bone (**6.6**) to enter, and sometimes traverse, the calcified zone of articular cartilage before returning to the *epiphyseal venous sinusoids.*

In immature long bones the supply is similar, but the epiphysis is a discrete vascular zone; epiphyseal and metaphyseal arteries enter on both sides of the growth cartilage, anastomoses between them being few or absent. Growth cartilages probably receive a supply from both sources and also from an anastomotic collar in the adjoining periosteum, but how much from each is uncertain (Brookes 1964, 1967, 1971; Trueta & Morgan 1960; Rang 1969). Occasionally cartilage canals are incorporated into a growth plate (p. 475). Metaphyseal bone is nourished by conjoined terminal branches of metaphyseal arteries and primary nutrient arteries of the shaft. They form terminal blind ended sprouts or sinusoidal loops in the zone of advancing ossification. There may be an intimate contact between sinusoidal endothelium and cartilage, and to such vessels have been ascribed a nutritive and a chrondrolytic role (Cameron 1961; Brookes & Landon 1964). Young periosteum is more vascular; its

vessels communicate more freely with those of the shaft than in adults, and have more metaphyseal branches.

Large irregular bones, like the scapula and innominate, receive a periosteal supply and often have large nutrient arteries penetrating directly into their cancellous bone: the two systems anastomose freely.

Short bones receive numerous fine vessels from the periosteum at non-articular surfaces, supplying their compact and cancellous bone and medulla. Arteries enter vertebrae close to the bases of transverse processes; their medulla drains to two large basivertebral veins converging to a foramen on the posterior surface of the vertebral body.

Flatter cranial bones are supplied by numerous periosteal or mucoperiosteal vessels. Large veins run tortuously in diploë (cancellous bone). Being thin-walled, they gape when cut.

Lymphatic vessels accompany periosteal plexuses but have never been convincingly demonstrated in bone.

Nerves. These are most numerous in articular extremities of long bones, vertebrae and larger flat bones. Bone has a complex autonomic and sensory innervation and bone cells have receptors for several neuropeptides, for example, neuropeptide Y (NY), calcitonin gene-related peptide (CGRP), vasoactive intestinal peptide (VIP) and substance P (SP), present in nerves in bone (Bjurholm et al 1992).

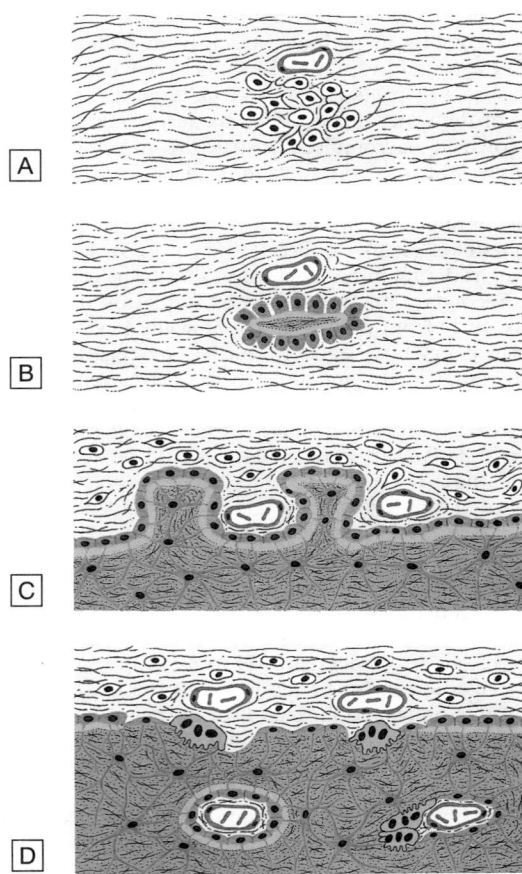

6.47 Schema of intramembraneous ossification. Different stages in the formation of intramembranous bone are shown. Colour code: osteoblasts, bone lining cells and osteocytes = blue, osteoclasts = pink, blood vessels = red, surrounding mesenchyme matrix = pale green, uncalcified bone matrix (osteoid) = dark green, and calcified bone = orange-brown.

A. Cellular condensation in mesenchyme: differentiation of Osteoprogenitor cells

B. Differentiation of cells into osteoblasts: matrix (osteoid) formation and mineralization of osteoid to form bone

c. Development of periosteal layer: osteocytes: incorporation of blood vessels

D. Consolidation of bone: remodelling by osteoclasts.

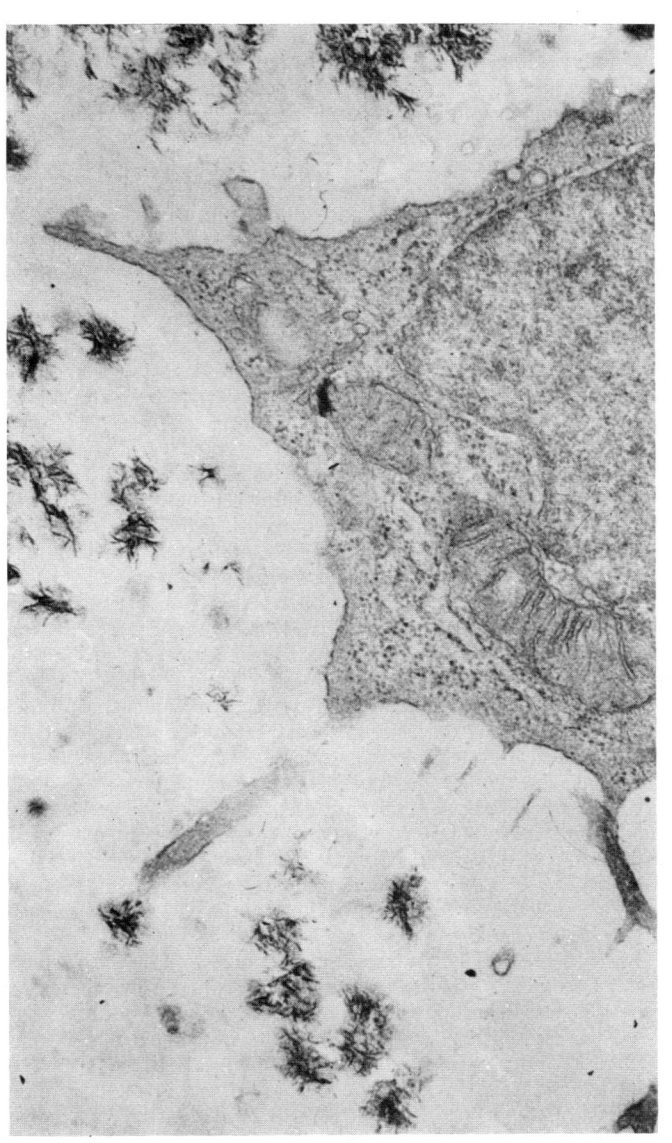

6.48 Transmission electron micrograph of part of an osteoblast, its surface bearing long filopodia which project into the surrounding intercellular matrix. Within the latter are clusters of 'matrix vesicles' which provide the initial nucleation sites for the formation of hydroxyapatite crystallites in the early mineralization of bone. The specimen is from the subperiosteal ossifying front of a chick's tibia in tissue culture.

Nerves occur widely in periosteum, and fine myelinated and non-myelinated fibres accompany nutrient vessels into bone and marrow and lie in perivascular spaces of Haversian canals.

HISTOGENESIS OF BONE

Although there is no basic difference in the deposition of bone at various sites to form the skeleton, the precursors are of two distinct classes: bones such as those in the cranial vault are preceded by a fibrocellular membrane, whereas most bones are formed in association with rods or masses of cartilage. These two types of ossification are known as intramembranous (dermal) and endochondral, respectively. They will now be considered in some detail, together with the general topic of the mineralization and subsequent fate of bone.

INTRAMEMBRANOUS (MESENCHYMAL) OSSIFICATION

Intramembranous (mesenchymal) ossification, which is essentially the direct mineralization of a highly vascular connective tissue, spreads from regular centres of ossification (**6**.47), at which differentiating mesenchymal (*osteoprogenitor*) cells (see p. 455) proliferate

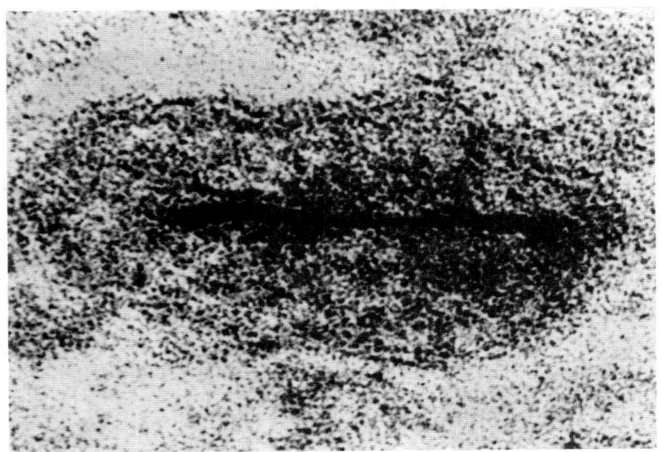

6.49 High-power transmission electron micrograph of a single 'matrix vesicle' from the specimen shown in **6**.34. The vesicle is membrane-bound, has a granular content and centrally, along its long axis, is a dense needle-shaped crystallite of hydroxyapatite. Magnification ×200 000. (Specimens provided by J J Reynolds, Strangeways Laboratory, Cambridge.)

densely around a capillary network (for review see Hansen 1993). A fine mesh of collagen fibres and ground substance appears between cells and around vessels. The central cells enlarge and fine strips of eosinophilic matrix (earliest bone) appear between. These rapidly extend and fuse into a delicate labyrinth, enclosing vessels and transforming mesenchyme, whose cells enlarge, become polygonal, cuboidal, or low columnar and form an incomplete layer of polarized *osteoblasts* (p. 456) in contact with the primitive, eosinophilic bony matrix. The secretion of osteoid constituents occurs from the osteoblast surface facing away from the blood vessel. The earliest crystals appear in association with extracellular *matrix vesicles* produced by osteoblasts (6.48, 49). Crystal formation then extends into the surrounding matrix to collagen fibrils which form increasingly widemeshed reticula in walls of an early labyrinth of *woven bone* (p. 463), the *primary spongiosa*. As layers of calcifying matrix are added to these early *trabeculae*, some osteoblasts are enclosed by matrix in primitive lacunae. Cells are sometimes incorporated in clusters to lie in conjoined lacunae. The new osteocytes retain intercellular contact by means of their surface processes and, as these elongate, matrix condenses around them to form canaliculi. Further osteoblasts are added to trabecular surfaces by differentiation of adjacent osteoprogenitor cells in the vascular mesenchyme.

As matrix secretion, calcification and enclosure of osteoblasts proceed, the trabeculae thicken and intervening vascular spaces become narrower. Where bone remains trabecular, the process slows and the spaces between them become occupied by haemopoietic tissue. Where compact bone is forming, trabeculae continue to thicken and vascular spaces to narrow. Meanwhile the collagen fibres of the matrix, secreted on the walls of narrowing spaces between trabeculae, is organized as parallel, longitudinal or spiral bundles and enclosed cells occupy concentric sequential rows. These irregular, interconnected, sometimes cylindrical masses of compact parallel-fibred bone, with a central canal, are *primary osteons* or *primary Haversian systems* (6.31D, 41A). With intervening woven bone they are later eroded and replaced by generations of lamellar *secondary osteons* (6.41) (see also pp. 465, 467, 478).

During these changes mesenchyme condenses on the surface to form a fibrovascular *periosteum*, and bone is laid down increasingly by osteoblasts differentiating from mitotic stem cells in deeper layers of the periosteum. Thus there is an advancing front of matrix deposition which entraps further periosteal vessels and also osteoblasts which then become osteocytes. Further growth is a continuation of these processes with much modelling by varying rates of resorption and deposition in different sites. Overall patterns of formation and modelling vary with the shape and structure of particular bones, and these have been studied by many techniques. Examples are considered elsewhere (p. 478); here the general processes of calcification and bone resorption will be considered in further detail.

Calcification and the osteoblast

As described above (p. 463) bone crystals have an apatitic lattice consisting of calcium, phosphate, carbonate, hydroxyl and other ion species. Traditionally calcification has been treated from the point of view of precipitation dynamics, with, initially, the only ions needed being calcium (Ca^{2+}) and phosphate (PO_4^{3-}). The extracellular fluid is supersaturated with respect to the basic calcium phosphates (Williams & Elliott 1979) yet mineralization is not a widespread phenomenon. Thus for precipitation to occur, the conditions in osteoid matrix must be in some way especially favourable to this process. Conditions that might favour calcification might be alkaline phosphatase activity in osteoblasts (raising local concentration of phosphate), or some factor raising local pH to alkaline levels, with consequent reduction in solubility of the calcium salt. However, such simple physico-chemical models are now considered inadequate (Anderson & Morris 1993).

An interesting development was the theory of *epitactic nucleation* (Neuman & Neuman 1953), based on the concept of *seeding* or *epitaxy*: a nucleus is somehow formed, probably in relation to collagen, effective in aggregating calcium and phosphate ions (Glimcher 1990). The hydroxyapatite crystal then grows spontaneously by addition of these from the saturated surrounding fluids. General acceptance of the theory of epitaxy led to many attempts

to determine the nature and distribution of nucleation sites, variously claimed to be points in periodic structure of collagen (Weiner & Traub 1989), ground substance links between collagen fibrils or structural aspects of proteoglycans. An alternative view is that the dimensions of the water-filled pore space in the matrix, particularly within the collagen macromolecular structure, are crucial in allowing both the ingress of ions, the formation of critical ion clusters and the aggregation of such clusters to form nuclei from which crystal growth can continue.

Matrix vesicles (6.49) Bonucci (1967) proposed a role for the osteoblast, considering initial nucleation sites to be cellular 'buds' or extrusions. Secondary nucleation, by the formation of critical nuclei which break away from the thermodynamically unstable surfaces of already formed crystals, leads to further aggregation of crystals around this initial locus, and thus to the formation of spherulitic mineralization nodules: these coalesce to give seams of mineralized bone, the association with collagen fibres being secondary. Such cellular '*seeds*' derived from osteoblasts would be absent in general connective tissues.

The role of the matrix vesicle has aroused intense interest and stimulated much investigation (Anderson 1990). The vesicles are membrane-bound spheres about 0.1–0.2 μm in diameter. They typically have an electron-dense core. The bone salt crystals within the matrix vesicles are often seen first in association with the inner surface of the vesicle membrane and subsequently accumulate in the vesicles (see review by Anderson & Morris 1993).

Matrix vesicles appear to be the loci of earliest crystal formation in newly forming bone, and indeed in the initial mineralization of all mineralized tissue throughout vertebrates (see review by Anderson & Morris 1993). They occur in calcifying cartilage, woven bone, dentine and subperiosteal bone. Thus matrix vesicles with similar properties can be produced by chondroblasts, odontoblasts and osteoblasts and their formation is not uniform around the cell membrane. In each case, it is thought that they are derived by polarized budding of the relevant cell. Their essential role in the initiation of calcification, however, remains disputed and it is difficult to exclude the problem of artefactual precipitation of crystals in vesicles during specimen preparation for electron microscopy. They have not always been found in mineralizing fronts in osteoid of more mature bone, and some have failed to find calcium tightly bound to matrix vesicles when using rapid freezing and freeze-substitution of tissue to preserve ultrastructure (Sumii & Inoue 1993). Being membrane-bound, vesicles separate internal and external environments, and the outer surface of the vesicle is the same as that of the cell. They show alkaline phosphatase, adenosine 5'-triphosphate (ATP)ase, inorganic pyrophosphatase, and nucleoside triphosphate pyrophosphatase activity and contain acidic phospholipids. It is possible that matrix vesicles provide the enzymes and environment to concentrate calcium and phosphate sufficiently to initiate crystallization, primarily along the inner leaflet of the membrane, which then spreads outside the vesicle. Recent studies of isolated vesicles have identified the presence of calcium-binding proteins.

While it is possible that matrix vesicles are important in beginning the process of calcification, there are also various *calcium-binding molecules* among the proteins and proteoglycans of osteoid, as mentioned above (p. 463). These might immobilize ions such that crystal nucleation occurs, and may be an important mechanism by which calcification is promoted. Alternatively, they may be inhibitory, mineralization proceeding in a controlled fashion in vivo because of the selective removal of non-collagenous calcium-binding proteins by enzymes produced by the osteoblast.

Considerable controversy concerns the shape and size of the initial crystals which are variously described as plates, rods, or needles. Most studies agree a smallest dimension of about 5 nm but estimates of length vary from 20–35 nm to values three times larger, reflecting a variety of techniques (Moradian-Oldak et al 1991). X-ray diffraction and dark-field electron microscopy give low values for length, whereas transmission electron microscopy of ion-beam thinned sections yields much larger values for mature tissue (Boyde 1974).

Calcium balance, bone resorption and the osteoclast

Many cellular activities depend on a relatively constant microenvironment (in terms of osmolality, types and concentrations of ions, pH, etc.) and finely balanced feedback systems operate to ensure this homeostasis. The level of circulating calcium ions is an example: it is preserved despite wide variation in diet, rates of bone growth and remodelling (Parfitt 1993). Involved in this process but varying quantitatively at different times are both labile and stable areas of bone salts, interacting types of cell (osteoblasts, osteocytes and osteoclasts), various hormones, including parathyroid hormone, $1,25(OH)_2$ vitamin D3 and calcitonin as well as many other factors.

Of the total body calcium, 99% is in the skeleton (Parfitt 1993). Calcium in blood and tissue fluids is constantly exchanging with calcium in bone to the extent of approximately one-quarter of ionic blood calcium each minute (Brookes 1987). The blood calcium is in equilibrium with that of tissue fluid, especially in the perivascular space in Haversian canals, and in lacunae and canaliculi—which present vast exposed areas of bone salt for such physico-chemical exchanges. The microcirculation in bone is rapid and the transport of bone fluid is probably aided by the movement of the live cells and their interconnecting processes. Markers added to the blood are detected in osteocyte lacunae within minutes. The mineral surface exposed to extracellular fluid in a 70 kg person has been estimated at between 1500 and 5000 m^2 (Robinson 1964). The calcium content of newly formed, less well mineralized bone is more labile than in older, denser tissue and provides a ready reservoir of calcium ions. However, rapid *calcium exchange* is a feature of all bone surfaces, whether quiescent or not (Parfitt 1993).

The osteonal surface area in cortical bone has been estimated to be 3.5 m^2 and the endosteal surface about 7.5 m^2: these surfaces provide activation sites for bone *remodelling*, resorption occurring at each location once every 2–5 years whilst *bone turnover* for the whole skeleton is about 10% per year (Parfitt 1983, 1993). The rate of replacement of old osteons by new ones, which continues throughout life, can also be modulated by hormones to alter blood calcium levels by increased activation or suppression of remodelling sites. Bone salt release may also be modulated by osteocytes and bone lining cells but how far direct cellular action contributes to rapid continuous turnover of calcium, or how much is simply a direct physico-chemical exchange, is uncertain. Bélanger et al (1963) proposed that osteocytes can actively resorb matrix forming the lacunar wall, a process he termed *osteocytic osteolysis*, and contribute in this way to calcium homeostasis. Criticism of the morphological evidence which led to the adoption of this view has been summarized by Boyde (1980).

The depression of circulatory ionic calcium levels increases secretion of parathyroid hormone (PTH), which raises blood calcium level by several mechanisms: direct action on bone, increased renal tubular reabsorption of calcium and increased intestinal absorption of calcium—a minor effect. The actions of PTH on bone are complex. Bone turnover is increased and the hormone stimulates osteoblasts, perhaps by the local generation of growth factors; the hormone also stimulates osteoclasts either indirectly via the osteoblasts or directly. Osteoblasts have receptors for PTH but these have not yet been unequivocally demonstrated in osteoclasts. PTH may also increase bone lining cell and osteocyte activity. Vitamin D3 modifies the action of PTH, decreasing its secretion and contributing to calcium homeostasis by increasing intestinal calcium absorption and the differentiation and activity of osteoclasts. Conversely, the rise in circulating calcium levels increases secretion of calcitonin by thyroid parafollicular cells, transiently depressing circulating calcium and suppressing the activity of osteoclasts, but this is not a significant mechanism for normal calcium homeostasis. Calcium release from bone may be altered by the stabilization of collagen, by increased osteoblastic deposition of bone and specific inhibitors thought to be released locally by bone cells (including bone-lining cells).

Osteoclasts are responsible for bone removal in both *modelling* during bone growth and later *remodelling* of osteons and surface bone, but details of osteoclastic action remain unclear (p. 460). The ruffled border compartment is acidified by the secretion of protons by the osteoclast and *bone apatite* is dissolved. The exposed matrix is then subjected to proteolytic enzyme activity. Surfaces undergoing localized resorption display large, multinuclear osteoclasts with foamy, faintly basophilic or acidophilic cytoplasm, in contact with bone in small *resorption lacunae (of Howship)*. When resorption ends osteoclasts disappear; details of this cell type are given on page 460.

INTRACARTILAGINOUS (ENDOCHONDRAL) OSSIFICATION (6.50, 51, 52)

Most human bones are preformed in cartilage: in early fetal life a 'long' bone is prefigured by a rod of hyaline cartilage (6.50, 53), replacing a similar rod of condensed mesenchyme, both foreshadowing in shape the early bone. Smaller (e.g. carpal) bones are

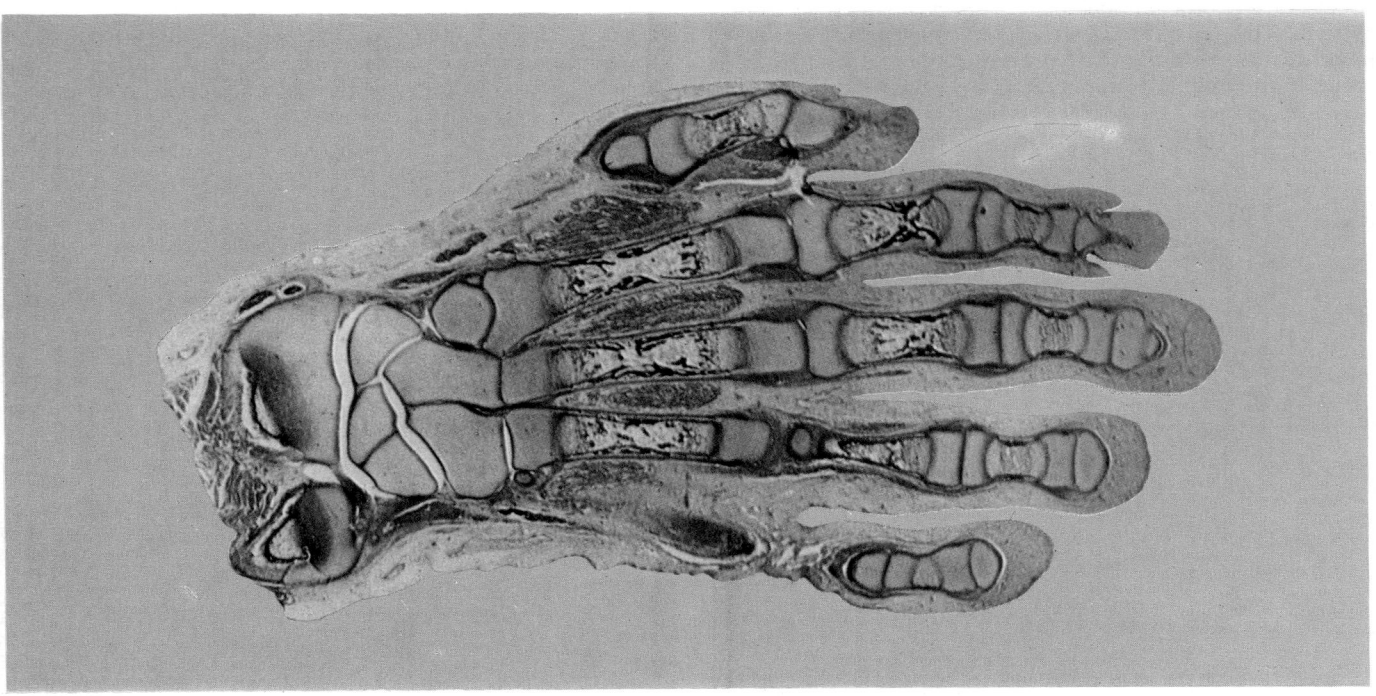

6.50 Survey photograph of a section of a fetal hand showing cartilaginous models of the carpal bones and various stages of development of primary ossification centres in the metacarpals and phalanges. Note that none of the carpal elements show any evidence of ossification. (Photography by Kevin Fitzpatrick, Guy's Hospital Medical School, London.)

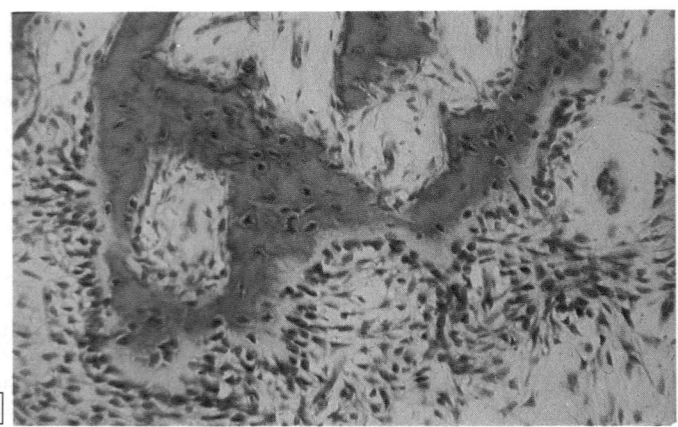

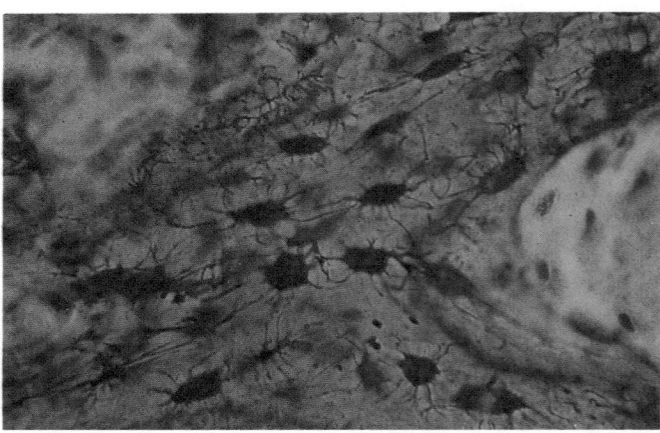

6.51 Micrographs of immature woven bone (fetal human). A is a section of part of the maxilla, stained with haematoxylin and eosin. The mineralized bone is eosinophilic, but shows a paler front of osteoid formation where many basophilic osteoblasts are clustered. Magnification ×150. Osteocytes are also visible within the bone. B is a higher magnification of woven bone stained with picrothionin to show the typically large osteocytes and their branched processes. Magnification ×800. (Both micrographs provided by Moya Meredith Smith, UMDS, Guy's Campus, London.)

also preceded by appropriately shaped cartilaginous 'models' (6.50). In such models a sequence of orderly changes signals the appearance of *centres of ossification*. The significance of these, and of growth plates, has been considered elsewhere (p. 437) and only their microscopic changes will be described here. The cartilaginous model is surrounded by vascular condensed mesenchyme or perichondrium, like that which precedes and surrounds intramembranous ossificatory centres (p. 471). Again, its deeper layers contain osteoprogenitor cells.

The first sign of a centre of primary ossification is seen when chondroblasts deep in the centre of the primitive shaft (6.53, 54) enlarge greatly, their cytoplasm becoming vacuolated and accumulating glycogen. Their intervening matrix is compressed to thin and often perforated septa. Routine histological appearances suggest that as the cells and their lacunae enlarge, the cells degenerate and may die, leaving enlarged and sometimes confluent lacunae as *primary areolae* whose thin walls have become calcified during these final stages. Simultaneously, cells in the deep layer of the perichondrium, surrounding the centre of the model, become osteoblasts and form a peripheral layer of fenestrated bone. This '*periosteal collar*', essentially formed by *intramembranous ossification* (6.53, 54), is at first a thin-walled tube enclosing the central shaft, but as it increases in diameter it also extends towards the ends of the shaft (see below).

Both the calcifying cartilage and the matrix of the calcifying perichondral bone collar contain *matrix vesicles* (see p. 472).

The periosteal collar overlying the calcified cartilage walls of chondrocyte lacunae is invaded from the deep periosteal layers by *osteogenic buds*—blind-ended capillaries and accompanying osteoprogenitor cells and osteoclasts. The latter excavate newly formed bone to pass into adjacent calcified cartilage and here continue to erode walls of primary chondrocyte lacunae, leading to fusion of these into larger, irregular, communicating spaces or *secondary areolae*. These fill with embryonic medullary tissue (vascular mesenchyme, osteoblasts and osteoclasts, haemopoietic and marrow stromal cells, etc.). Osteoblasts attach themselves to the delicate residual walls of calcified cartilage, laying down osteoid which rapidly changes firstly into patches and then continuous linings of bone. Further layers of bone are added, enclosing young osteocytes in lacunae, and narrowing the perivascular spaces. As the formation of subperiosteal bone continues, bone deposition on the more central calcified cartilage ceases. Osteoclastic erosion of the early bone spicules then creates a primitive medullary cavity in which only a few trabeculae composed of bone with central cores of calcified cartilage remain to support the developing marrow tissues. Such trabeculae soon become remodelled and replaced by more mature bone or marrow. Meanwhile cartilaginous regions near the shaft go

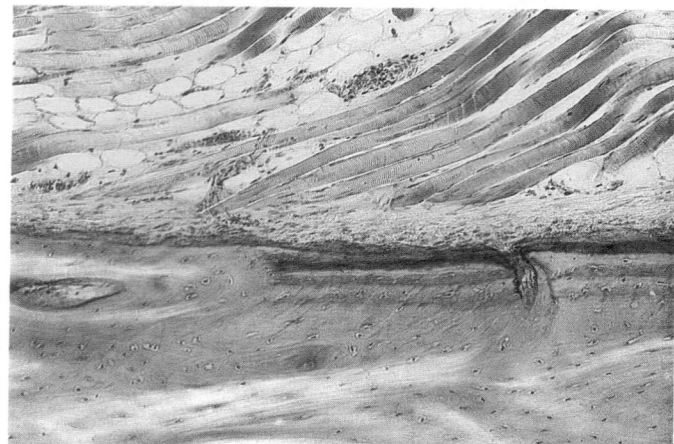

6.52 Section through the surface of a mature bone showing the periosteum into which are inserted skeletal muscle fibres. Notice both fibrous and deeper cellular components of the periosteum. Viewed by half-polarized light which demonstrates the anisotropic nature of the lamellar bone visible here; H & E. Magnification ×250. (Provided by Moya Meredith Smith.)

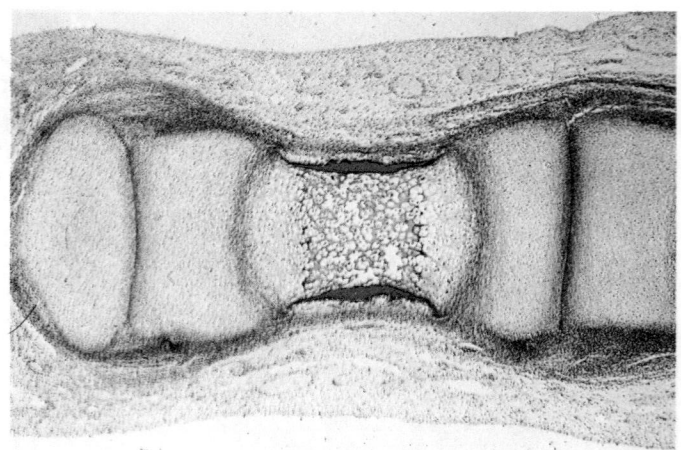

6.53 Longitudinal section of a phalanx (from the hand in 6.50) showing an early primary ossification centre. The cartilage cells in the shaft centre have hypertrophied and this region is surrounded by a delicate tube or collar of subperiosteal bone (red). Magnification ×50. (Photography by Kevin Fitzpatrick, Guy's Hospital Medical School.)

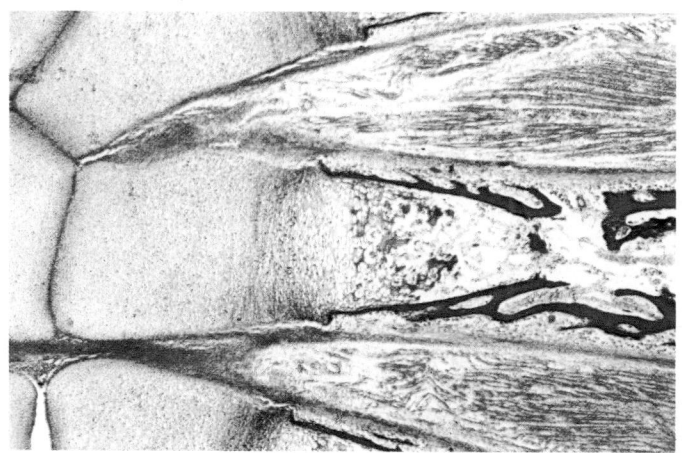

6.54 Longitudinal section of the proximal half of a fetal metacarpal bone (from **6.50**) at a more advanced stage than the phalanx in **6.53**. The periosteal collar of woven bone is thicker, contains radially disposed vascular spaces; vascular invasion of the shaft centre has occurred and is proceeding towards its extremities. Magnification ×40. (Photography by Kevin Fitzpatrick, Guy's Hospital Medical School)

through similar changes and, when covered with bone, may become incorporated in the bone of the periosteal collar. Since these are most advanced centrally and the epiphyses remain cartilaginous, the intervening zones show a sequence of changes in growing bones, when viewed in longitudinal section (**6.50**, **55**, **56**). This region, which persists until longitudinal growth of the bone ceases, is the *growth plate* or *epiphyseal plate*.

GROWTH PLATE (6.56)

Expansion of the cartilaginous extremity (usually an epiphysis) keeps pace with the rest of the bone both by appositional and interstitial growth. An organized region of rapid growth develops as the future growth plate between epiphysis and diaphysis, which grows in all dimensions. Transverse or latitudinal growth is due to occasional transverse mitoses and appositional growth due to matrix deposition by cells from the perichondrial collar (or ring) at this level. The

future growth plate thus expands in concert with the shaft and adjacent future epiphysis. On the side of the plate closest to the epiphysis is a zone of relatively quiescent chondrocytes (the *resting zone*), but further towards the shaft of the bone is an actively mitotic zone of cells. Here, the more frequent divisions in the long axis soon create numerous longitudinal columns (palisades) of discoidal or cuneiform chondrocytes, each in a flattened lacuna (**6.53**). This proliferation and column formation occupies the zone of cartilage growth (the *proliferative zone*) and continued longitudinal interstitial expansion is the basic mode of elongation of a bone. Traced centrally in the shaft, a column of cells shows increasing maturity. They increase in size and accumulate glycogen. In the proliferative zone the cells exhibit a high level of oxidative enzyme activity. Younger chondrocytes display surface projections into reciprocal recesses in lacunar walls, but projections increase greatly as they hypertrophy. The largest cells apparently withdraw their projections. In the *hypertrophic zone* there is a sharp redox change and energy metabolism is depressed at the level of the mineralizing front (**6.57**). According to most investigators, the chondrocytes degenerate and die. An alternative view (Hunziker et al 1984) is that morphological evidence of cell death may be an artefact of tissue preparation and that chondrocytes may be alive in the terminal zone. The lacunae are now separated by transverse and longitudinal walls, the longitudinal walls being impregnated with apatitic crystals (the *zone of calcified cartilage*; **6.24A,B**, **58**). The calcified partitions enter the *zone of bone formation* and are invaded by vascular mesenchyme, with its osteoblasts, osteoclasts, chondroclasts, etc. from adjacent centres of primary ossification (**6.59**). Partitions, especially the transverse ones, are next partly eroded and osteoid deposition, bone formation and osteocyte enclosure occur on surfaces of the longitudinal walls.

Chondrolysis of calcified partitions has been ascribed to osteoclastic (chondroclastic) action, aided by chondrolysis by cells associated with terminal loops or buds of a labyrinth of vascular sinusoids which occupy and come into close contact with each incomplete, columnar trabecular framework (**6.60**); Stanka et al 1991). The terminal vasculature is partly fenestrated. Longitudinal and transverse partitions of matrix differ in structure and probably chondrolytic mechanisms, the transverse being uncalcified or lightly calcified, with sparse collagen and distinctive proteoglycans susceptible to lysosomal enzymes; the more calcified, collagen-rich longitudinal septa succumb only to osteoclastic action.

Continuing cell division in the zone of growth adds to epiphyseal

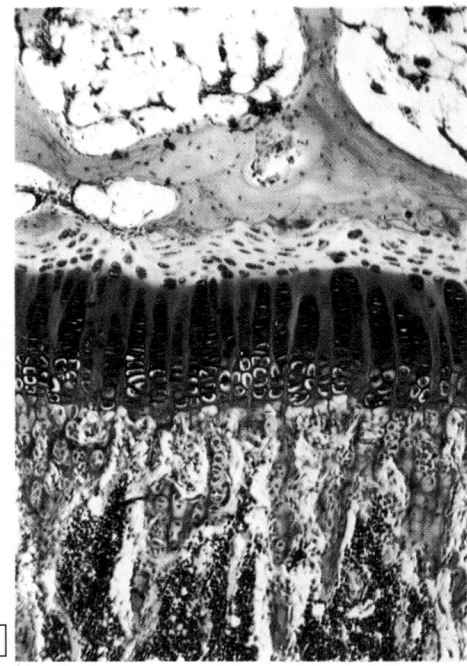

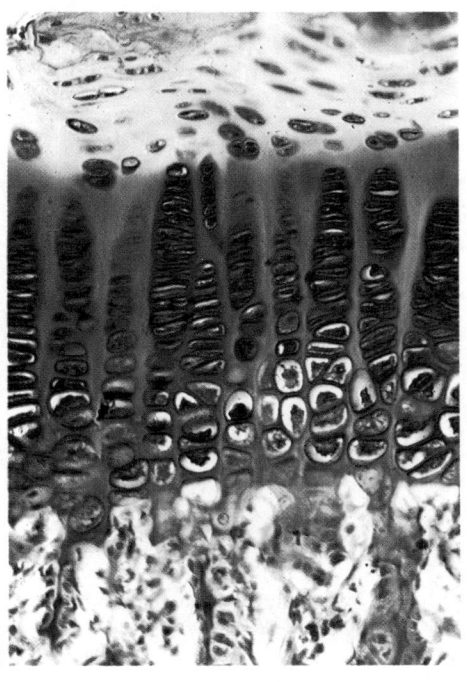

6.55 Low and intermediate magnifications of sections through the cartilaginous growth plate between the epiphysis and metaphysis (below) at the proximal end of a human tibia. Note the transition from hyaline cartilage, through zones of cell multiplication, column formation, hypertrophy, matrix calcification and partial chondrolysis to the ossifying front. Compare with **6.56** and consult text for further details.

475

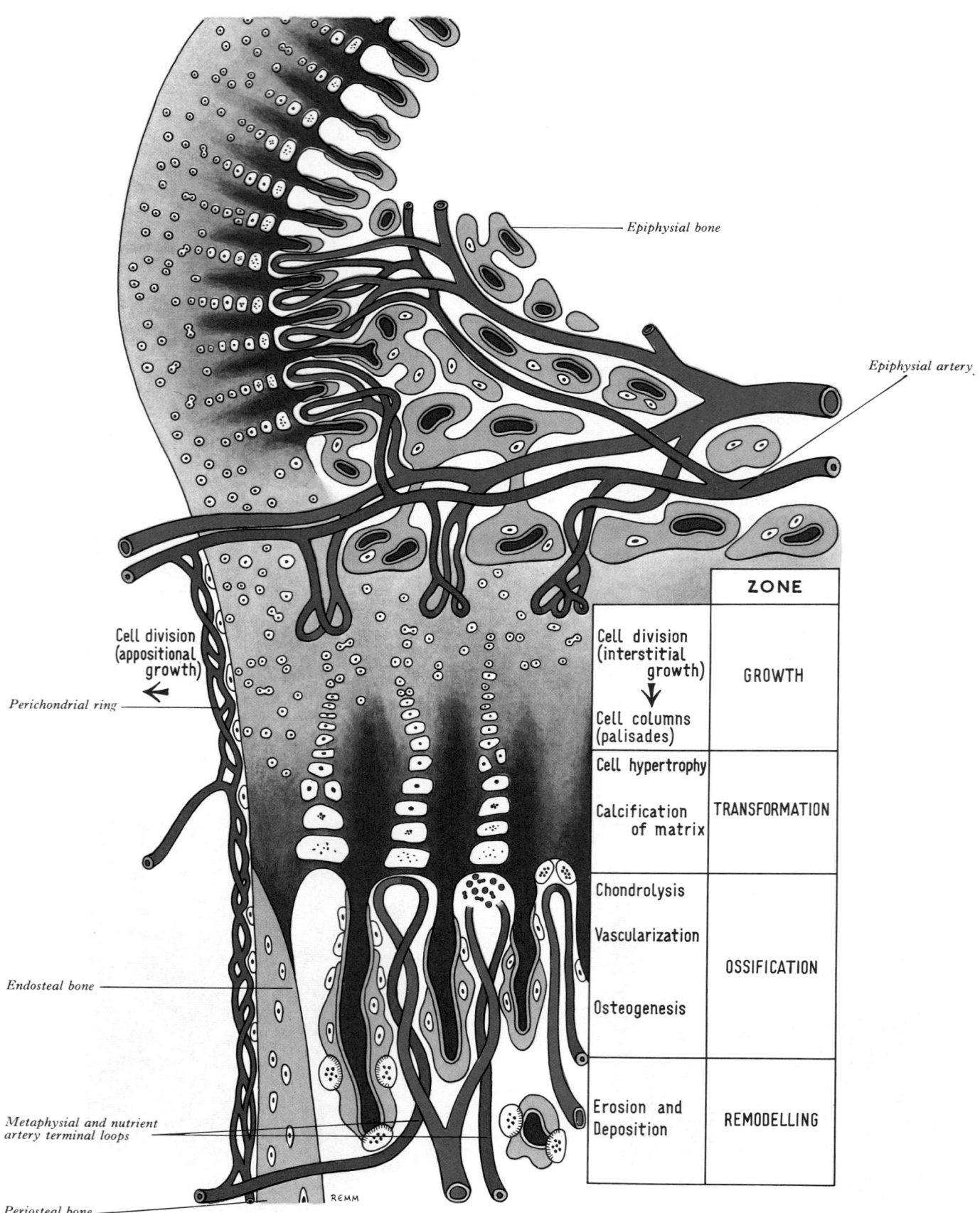

Epiphysial bone

Epiphysial artery

	ZONE
Cell division (interstitial growth) ↓ Cell columns (palisades)	GROWTH
Cell hypertrophy Calcification of matrix	TRANSFORMATION
Chondrolysis Vascularization Osteogenesis	OSSIFICATION
Erosion and Deposition	REMODELLING

Cell division (appositional growth) ←

Perichondrial ring

Endosteal bone

Metaphysial and nutrient artery terminal loops

Periosteal bone

REMM

6.56 Scheme of the main features of an active growth cartilage and the adjacent metaphysis and epiphysis. The different views concerning the mechanism of chondrolysis described in the text are indicated.

476

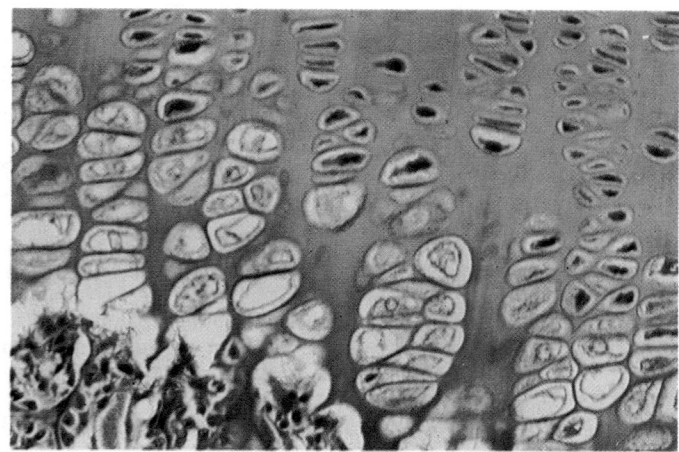

6.57 Section showing the transformation of cartilage cells and their lacunae as the ossifying front of an early primary centre of ossification is approached (below). Note the cell hypertrophy, lacunar enlargement with matrix partition reduction and increased density of the partitions following calcification. Magnification ×600.

ends of cell columns and, with the sequence of changes proceeding away from the diaphyseal centre, the bone grows in length. Meanwhile, there is continued internal erosion and remodelling of the newly formed bone tissue and, as further subperiosteal bone deposition continues towards the epiphyses, the bone also grows in diameter, its medullary cavity enlarging transversely and longitudinally.

Growth continues thus for many months or years in different bones (p. 437) but eventually one or more *secondary centres of ossification* usually appear in the cartilaginous extremities (**6.61**). Such epiphyseal centres (or ends of bones lacking epiphyses) do not at first display cell columns. Instead, isogenous cell groups hypertrophy, with matrix calcification and then invasion by osteogenic vascular mesenchyme (sometimes from cartilage canals; see

p. 448). Bone is formed on calcified cartilage, as described above for the growth plate. As an epiphysis enlarges, its cartilaginous periphery forms a zone of proliferation and its organization becomes radial, with cell columns and zones of growth, hypertrophy, calcification, erosion and ossification at increasing depths from the surface (**6.55**). The early osseous epiphysis is thus surrounded by a superficial growth cartilage; but the growth plate next to the metaphysis soon becomes the most active region, and rapidly enlarging cell columns are directed towards the metaphyseal plate, whereas elsewhere they are directed to the underlying epiphyseal ossification (Rang 1969).

As the bone reaches maturity, epiphyseal and metaphyseal ossification processes gradually encroach upon this growth plate from either side, eventually meeting, when *bony fusion of the epiphysis* occurs and longitudinal growth of the bone ceases. Events of fusion are broadly as follows (Haines 1975). As growth ceases, the cartilaginous plate becomes quiescent and gradually thins. Proliferation, palisading and hypertrophy of chondrocytes ceases; they form short, irregular conical masses. Patchy calcification is then accompanied by resorption of calcified cartilage and some adjacent metaphyseal bone. These resorption channels are invaded by vascular mesenchyme, some endothelial sprouts piercing the thin plate of cartilage, and here metaphyseal and epiphyseal vessels unite. Final bony fusion is by ossification around these vessels, spreading into the intervening zones. Such bone is visible in radiographs as a radio-dense *epiphyseal line* (a term also used for the level of the perichondrial ring around the growth cartilage of immature bones, or the surface junction between epiphysis and metaphysis in a mature bone). In smaller epiphyses, uniting earlier, there is usually one eccentric, initial area of fusion, with thinning of the residual cartilaginous plate. Subsequently the original sites of fusion are resorbed and replaced by new bone and medullary tissue extending into the whole cartilaginous plate until union is complete and no *epiphyseal 'scar'* persists. In larger epiphyses, uniting later, similar processes also involve multiple perforations in growth plates, islands of epiphyseal bone often persisting as epiphyseal scars. Calcified cartilage which, coated by bone, forms the epiphyseal scar is also found below articular cartilage, and has been called *'metaplastic' bone*, a term also applied to attachments of tendons, ligaments and other dense connective tissues (Haines & Mohuiddin 1968).

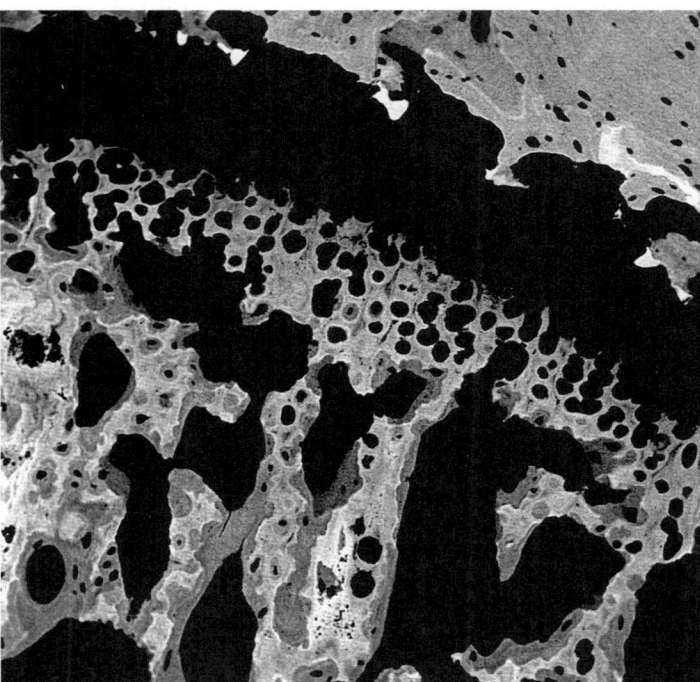

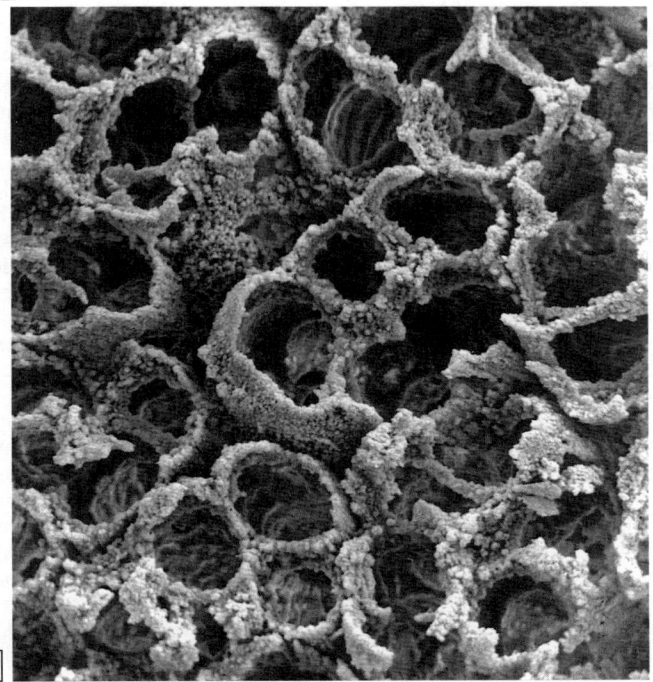

6.58A Growth plate of rat tibial epiphysis: the unmineralized zones cannot be seen in this embedded BSE image. Mineralized cartilage surrounds the hypertrophied chondrocytes (round black spaces, often appearing conjoined in lines as the partitions between cells in a column are unmineralized). Large remnants of cartilage are coated with new bone (grey) in the metaphyseal trabeculae. The epiphyseal side of the growth plate (top right) shows much less activity, with little calcified cartilage incorporated in the bone; field width = 570 μm. B. The mineralizing front of the proximal growth plate cartilage of rat femur: calcification is predominantly in the intercolumnar regions, surrounding the cells with tubes of mineralized matrix. Central regions between the tubes may or may not mineralize completely. SEM of anorganic specimen, field width = 139 μm.

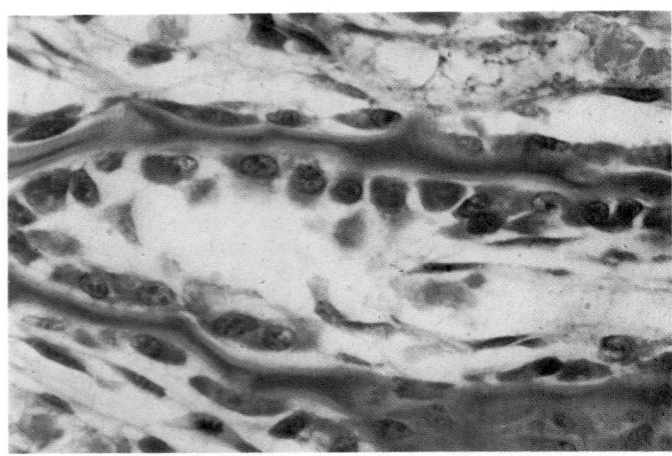

6.59 Section through the metaphysis of a fetal bone stained with haematoxylin and eosin showing developing spicules of early bone. Each spicule contains a deeply stained basophilic core of calcified cartilage, which is covered on both aspects by a lightly stained eosinophilic layer of young bone along which are ranged rows of active osteoblasts.

The cartilaginous surfaces of epiphyses involved in synovial articulations remain unossified, but the typical sequence of cartilaginous zones in them persists throughout life.

Synchondroses show a similar developmental sequence to epiphyseal growth plates, except that the proliferative rates of chondrocytes and replacement of cartilage by bone are similar, although not identical, at each side of the synchondrosis.

FURTHER DEVELOPMENT AND REMODELLING OF BONE

In both early intramembranous and endochondral ossification, bone forms the walls of a continuous labyrinth of large vascular spaces; osteocytes are irregularly scattered, there is no lamellation and collagen fascicles in the matrix form a random network. This *woven bone* is typical of young fetal bones, but occurs also in adults in excessively rapid bone remodelling and during repair of fractures. Woven bone is also found as the centres of *intervascular ridges* sprouting radially (and branching tangentially) from rapidly growing surfaces of even quite large growing bones (**6**.31D, 41A, 46). Later, concentric tracts of non-lamellar, parallel-fibred (in which collagen bundles in the matrix form parallel longitudinal spirals) or lamellar bone are deposited within the vascular spaces, dividing them by osseous bridges and narrowing them as *primary osteons* (*primary Haversian systems*) develop (**6**.41D). No bone resorption precedes formation of such osteons; hence no *cement lines* separate them from surrounding woven bone. Later again, once primary osteonal development has ceased, bone deposited circumferentially on periosteal and endosteal surfaces is mostly lamellar (**6**.36D, 41C); where lamellae are thin, lamellation is indistinct.

As bone matures, *typical Haversian systems* (*secondary osteons*) gradually replace primary osteons and woven bone. They are always preceded by resorption, usually eccentric, of the vascular channels within primary osteons or woven bone. Remodelling of the interior of bone is marked by the balanced activities of osteoclasts and osteoblasts; osteoclasts first excavate a cylindrical tunnel by concerted action (a '*cutting cone*' of about nine osteoclasts moving at about 50 μm/day: Jaworski 1992), and then they are followed by osteoblasts which fill in the space created by concentric deposition around a centrally ingrowing blood vessel (forming a '*closing cone*' with about 4000 osteoblasts/mm²: Jaworski 1992). Concentric deposition of lamellae then follows on walls of resorption cavities, narrowing the vascular channels (Polig & Jee 1990). A hypermineralized, basophilic cement line marks a site of reversal from resorption to deposition.

Formation of secondary osteons does not end with growth but continues variably throughout life; some of the earliest secondary osteons are eventually eroded (**6**.41). Remnants of woven bone,

primary osteons, circumferential lamellae and, finally, secondary osteons form interstitial bone-occupying crevices between later osteons (**6**.24C, 41D). The degree of remodelling is, in general, an indication of age, so that the number of osteons and osteon fragments have been used in attempts to estimate the age of skeletal material at death (Uberlaker 1986; Stout 1989; Castanet et al 1993).

Bone growth is solely *appositional*, i.e. new layers are added to pre-existing surfaces, osteocytes being enclosed in lacunae and not dividing. The rigidity of mineralized bone matrix prevents internal expansion, so that interstitial growth, characteristic of most tissues, is absent in bone, though essential in growth cartilages, as previously discussed.

Hence remodelling of bone, which involves either major readjustment after fracture or remodelling throughout life, depends upon delicate geometric balances between deposition and removal. Demonstrations of these main features have, with increasing refinement, spanned the last two centuries. Earlier experimenters used metal markers, such as wires encircling shafts of bones, or pellets embedded in them, to investigate modelling of growing bones. An early observation that newly formed bone is identifiably pink in growing pigs fed with the plant madder, initiated numerous studies of bone growth by alternating periods of feeding with madder and without it (Brash 1934). Intraperitoneal injection of alizarin red has been used with greater precision for the same purpose (Hoyte 1960). Such studies confirm that bone grows by accretion; later techniques have merely increased accuracy, making quantitative histological studies possible. These include administration of osseotropic isotopes followed by autoradiography, exposure to tetracyclines at intervals followed by fluorescence microscopy and microradiography. Recently, advances in techniques for the detection of autofluorescence or minimal fluorescence labelling by confocal microscopy and of changes in mineral density by backscattered electron imaging have added further precision.

Modelling, i.e. change in general shape, occurs in all growing bones (**6**.62A,B); much studied examples are cranial and long bones with expanded extremities. A bone such as the parietal thickens and expands during growth, but decreases in curvature. Accretion continues at its edges by interstitial multiplication of osteoprogenitor cells at sutures. Periosteal bone is mainly added externally and eroded internally, but not at uniform rates or at all times. The rate of formation increases with radial distance from the centre of ossification (the future parietal eminence) and formation may also occur endocranially as well as ectocranially, changing the curvature of the bone. As the skull bones thicken and grow at the sutures, the relative positions of original centres of ossification change in three dimensions, the vault of the skull expanding with growth of the brain. The development of diploë (trabeculae) and marrow space internally results in outer and inner cortical plates.

Long bones elongate mainly by extension of endochondral ossification into calcified zones of adjacent growth cartilages continually replaced by longitudinal interstitial growth of their proliferative zones, with minor additions by radial epiphyseal growth. Simultaneously diametric increases of growth cartilages and shafts occur by continuing subperiosteal deposition and endosteal erosion. In many bones, however, growth is at different rates, or even reversed, at different places. A bone initially tubular may thus become triangular in section, for example the tibia. Similarly, the waisted contours of metaphyses are preserved by differential rates of periosteal erosion and endosteal deposition, as metaphyseal bone becomes diaphyseal in position. The junction between a field of resorption and one of deposition on the surface of a bone during its growth is called a *surface reversal line*: the relative position of such a line may remain stable over long periods of cortical drift.

Tetracycline marking techniques have emphasized the mutability of even mature compact bone, where a single section may include mature quiescent osteons, and recently formed, forming or resorbing osteons. Lamellar bone forms at a variable rate; each Haversian system resorption canal being about 2 mm long forms in 1–3 months, with a new infilling osteon forming in a similar period. Internal remodelling continuously supplies young osteons with labile calcium reserves, and a malleable osseous architecture responsive to altering patterns of stress. The remodelling unit in cancellous bone equivalent to the secondary osteon is the *bone structural unit*. This has a depth (thickness) of 40–70 μm and length of about 100 μm in sections of

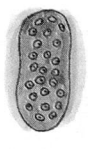

*Cartilage
model*

A

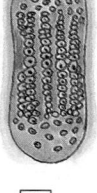

B

*Hypertrophy
of central cells*

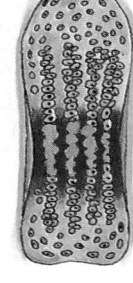

C

*Calcification of
matrix in primary
centre and
formation of
periosteal collar
of bone*

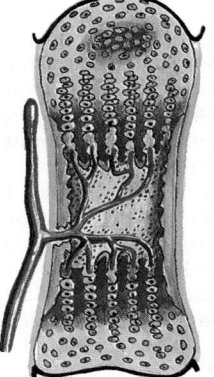

D

*Invasion of primary centre
by vascular osteogenic buds*

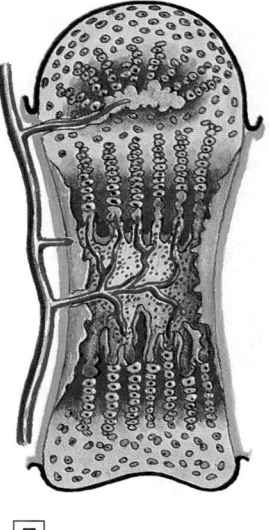

E

*Primary bone laid
down on calcified
cartilage remnants;
secondary centre of
ossification appears
and becomes
vascularised*

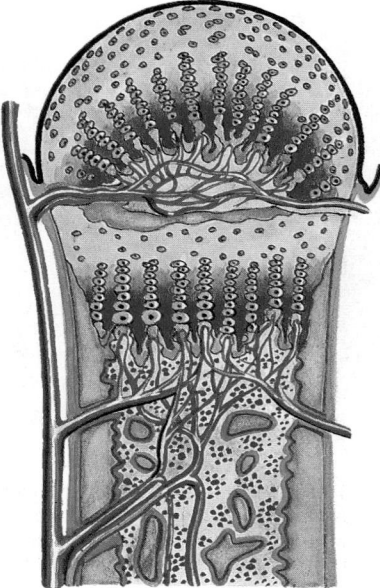

F

*Continued growth
of cartilage of
'epiphyseal' plate and
epiphysis; proliferation
of red bone marrow*

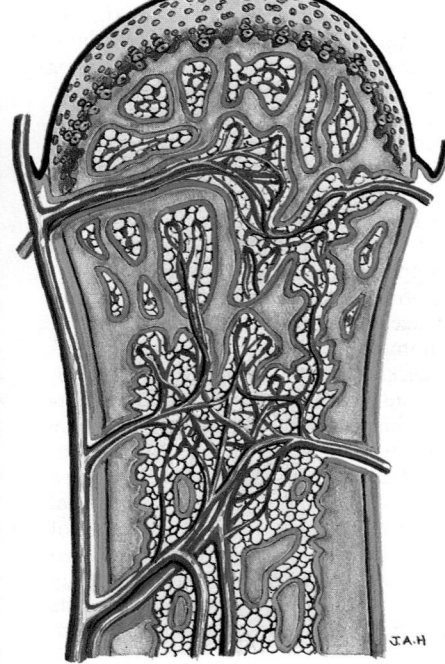

G

*Cessation of cartilage
growth and complete
ossification of
'epiphyseal' plate,
(fusion of the epiphysis).
Replacement of red
bone marrow with
yellow, adipose marrow
(as in all long bones
of the adult, except
proximal humeral
and femoral
epiphyses)*

6.60A–G Diagram depicting the stages of endochondral ossification in a long bone (e.g. a phalanx). For colour code see **6**.47; additionally, hyaline cartilage = light purple, calcified cartilage = deep purple. For further details of postnatal endochondral ossification, see **6**.56.

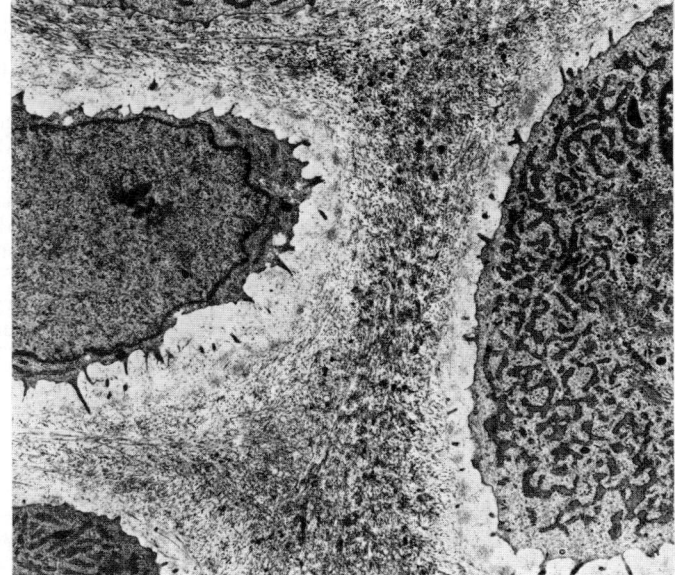

H

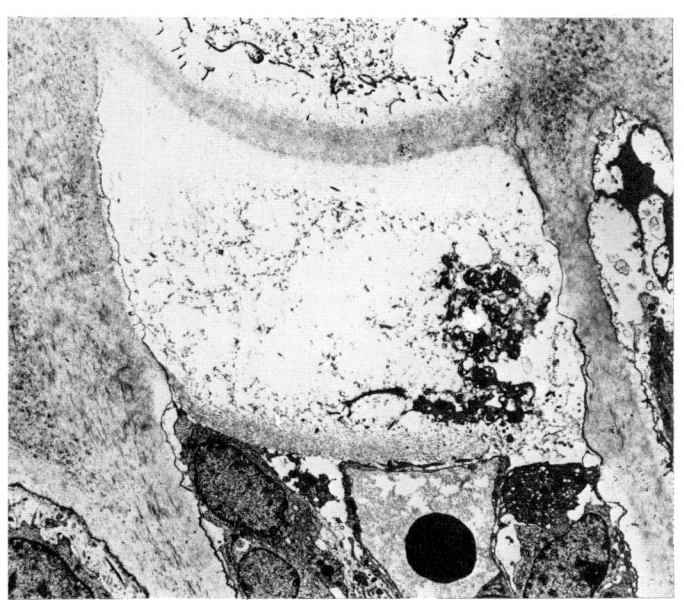

I

6.60H, I Electron micrographs showing cartilage cells in two stages of endochondral ossification in an epiphyseal plate. In G, growing chondroblasts have laid down a collagenous matrix containing numerous dense matrix vesicles. Magnification ×6000. In H the chondrocyte has hypertrophied and disintegrated, while at its base is the tip of an ingrowing capillary surrounded by osteoblasts. Magnification ×6000. (Micrographs taken by G Roberts.)

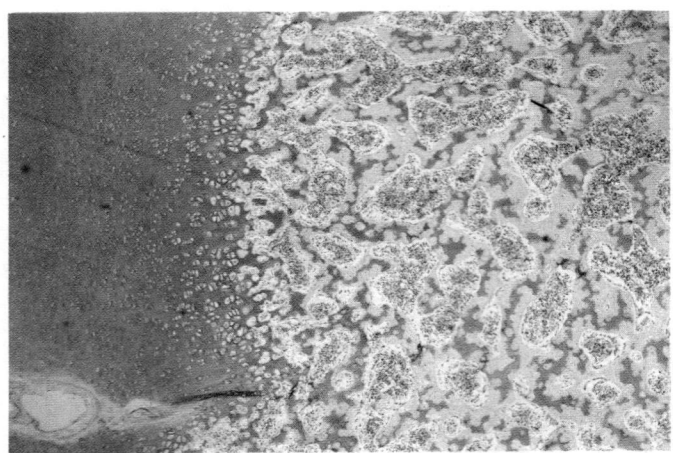

6.61 Transverse section through an epiphysis of a long bone at a more advanced stage of ossification. Note the gradation of cartilage cell lacunae (left) as the ossifying front is approached. The bony trabeculae (light pink) contain dark patches of basophilic calcified cartilage and the intertrabecular spaces are filled with red bone marrow.

bone according to Eriksen et al (1993) but many bone packets viewed en face at the surface of trabeculae are much more extensive and irregular in shape (**6**.62, 63). The morphogenetic control of shape is not clear, but suggestions largely involve responses to strain. Certainly bone resorption typically occurs when the gravitational or other mechanical stresses are reduced, as in bed rest, or in zero gravity conditions in space. Likewise bone subjected to constant pressure tends to resorb and, with constant tension, is deposited; this forms the basis of much orthodontic treatment, as teeth can be made to migrate slowly through alveolar bone by the application of steady lateral or medial pressure. However, why dermal and cartilage bones apparently respond differently to strain of a given magnitude is an enigma.

Completely dry bone is *piezo-electric*, i.e. it develops potential differences when deformed. However, there is no possibility that this phenomenon might be related to physiological effects in life. *Streaming potentials* arise when ionized fluids flow through channels with charged surfaces; they are proportional to the rate of strain; no change in the rate of fluid flow is to be expected when a deformation is simply maintained. The resulting *stress-generated electrical effects* may affect cells responsible for osteolysis and bone deposition, promoting structural remodelling (see Currey 1984a,b,c and Martin & Burr 1989 for reviews). Data concerning sources, intensities and distributions of bioelectric phenomena in stressed connective tissues in general are not yet sufficient to show causal relationships between such events and to relate them to morphogenesis. However, bone cells in culture respond to electric fields.

Metabolic and endocrine effects on bone

The roles of bone salts, PTH, 1,25-dihydroxy vitamin D3 (calcitriol) and calcitonin in regulating circulating calcium levels are considered elsewhere (p. 472). However, the normal development and maintenance of bone also require adequate intake and absorption of calcium, phosphorus, vitamins A, C and D and a balance between growth hormone, thyroid hormones, oestrogens and androgens. Various other factors, including different prostaglandins and glucocorticoids may also play important roles in the maintenance and turnover of osseous tissue (see Eriksen et al 1993; Mundy 1993b).

Prolonged deficiency of calcium causes loss of bone mineral via a loss of bone tissue and consequent bone fragility (*osteoporosis*). Vitamin D influences intestinal transport of calcium and phosphate and therefore affects circulatory calcium levels; prolonged deficiency (with or without low intake) leads, in adults, to bones which contain regions of deformable, uncalcified osteoid (*osteomalacia*). Similar deficiencies, during growth, lead to severe disturbance of growth cartilages and ossification, including reductions of regular columnar organization in growth plates and failure of cartilage calcification (although chondrocytes proliferate); growth plates also become thicker and less regular than normal (classic *rachitis* or *rickets*). In

rickets, the uncalcified or poorly calcified cartilage trabeculae are only partially eroded; osteoblasts secrete layers of osteoid, which fail to ossify in the metaphyseal regions. Ultimately gravity deforms such softened bones. (For review of the role of vitamin D, see Eisman 1993.) The local production of 1,25 dihydroxy vitamin D3 is also believed to be important in the generation of new osteoclasts from precursors.

Deficiency of vitamin C causes *scurvy*, with widespread changes in all connective tissues, particularly growth cartilages and metaphyses of long bones. Vitamin C is essential for adequate synthesis of collagen and matrix proteoglycans in connective tissues and, when deficient, growth plates become thin, ossification almost ceases and metaphyseal trabeculae and cortical bone are reduced in thickness, causing fragility and delayed healing of fractures.

Vitamin A is also necessary for normal growth and for a correct balance of deposition and removal of bone. Deficiency retards growth due to the failure of internal erosion and remodelling, particularly in the cranial base. Foramina are narrowed, sometimes causing pressure atrophy of contained nerves; the cranial cavity and spinal canal may fail to expand with the central nervous system (CNS), impairing nervous function. Conversely, excessive vitamin A stimulates vascular erosion of growth cartilages, which become thin or totally lost; as a result, longitudinal growth ceases. Retinoic acid, a vitamin A derivative, is involved in pattern formation in limb buds, and the differentiation of osteoblasts.

Balanced endocrine activities are essential to normal bone maturation, and disturbances may have profound effects. In addition to its role in calcium metabolism, parathyroid hormone in excess (*primary hyperparathyroidism*) stimulates unbridled osteoclastic erosion of bone, particularly subperiosteally and later endosteally—a condition termed *osteitis fibrosa cystica* and identified radiographically by a characteristic lacework pattern in cortical bone.

Acidophil cells of the adenohypophysis cerebri secrete *growth hormone* (GH) (*somatotropin*) necessary for normal interstitial proliferation in growth cartilages and hence increase in stature. Termination of normal growth is imperfectly understood, but may involve a fall in hormone production or in the sensitivity of chondroblasts to insulin-like growth factors regulated by GH, amongst others (Canalis et al 1993). Experimental hypophysectomy, or clinical reduction of GH in the young, leads to quiescence and thinning of growth plates and hence *pituitary dwarfism*. Conversely, continued hypersecretion in the immature leads to *gigantism*, but in maturity it results in thickening of bones by subperiosteal deposition, the mandible, hands and feet being most affected, an affliction known as *acromegaly*.

While continued longitudinal growth of bones depends on adequate levels of GH, the effective remodelling to a mature shape also requires the action of the thyroid hormones, tri-iodothyronin and tetraiodothyronin (T3 and T4); growth and skeletal maturity are also closely related to endocrine activities of the ovaries, testes and adrenal cortices. High oestrogen levels increase deposition of endosteal and trabecular bone; conversely, osteoporosis in aged women may reflect reduced ovarian function. Fluctuations in the rate of growth and the timing of skeletal maturation reflect circulating levels of adrenal and testicular androgens (p. 1853). In hypogonadism, maturation (marked by growth plate obliteration) is late and the limbs therefore elongate excessively; conversely, in hypergonadism, premature fusion of the epiphyses results in diminished stature. The normal growth and pathology of growth cartilages has a large literature, beyond the present scope, but several accounts are published (Rang 1969; Serafini-Fracassini & Smith 1974; Kember 1983).

GENERAL FEATURES OF BONES

Bones vary not only in their primary shape but also in lesser surface details, or secondary markings which appear mainly in postnatal life. Certain features—elevations and depressions, smooth areas and rough ridges—are found in many bones. For such, a repertoire of general terms is used, since the same form of marking or surface texture usually has the same functional significance wherever it occurs. For example, bones display *articular surfaces* at synovial joints with their neighbours; if small, these are *facets* or *foveae*. knuckle-shaped surfaces are *condyles*, and a *trochlea* is grooved like

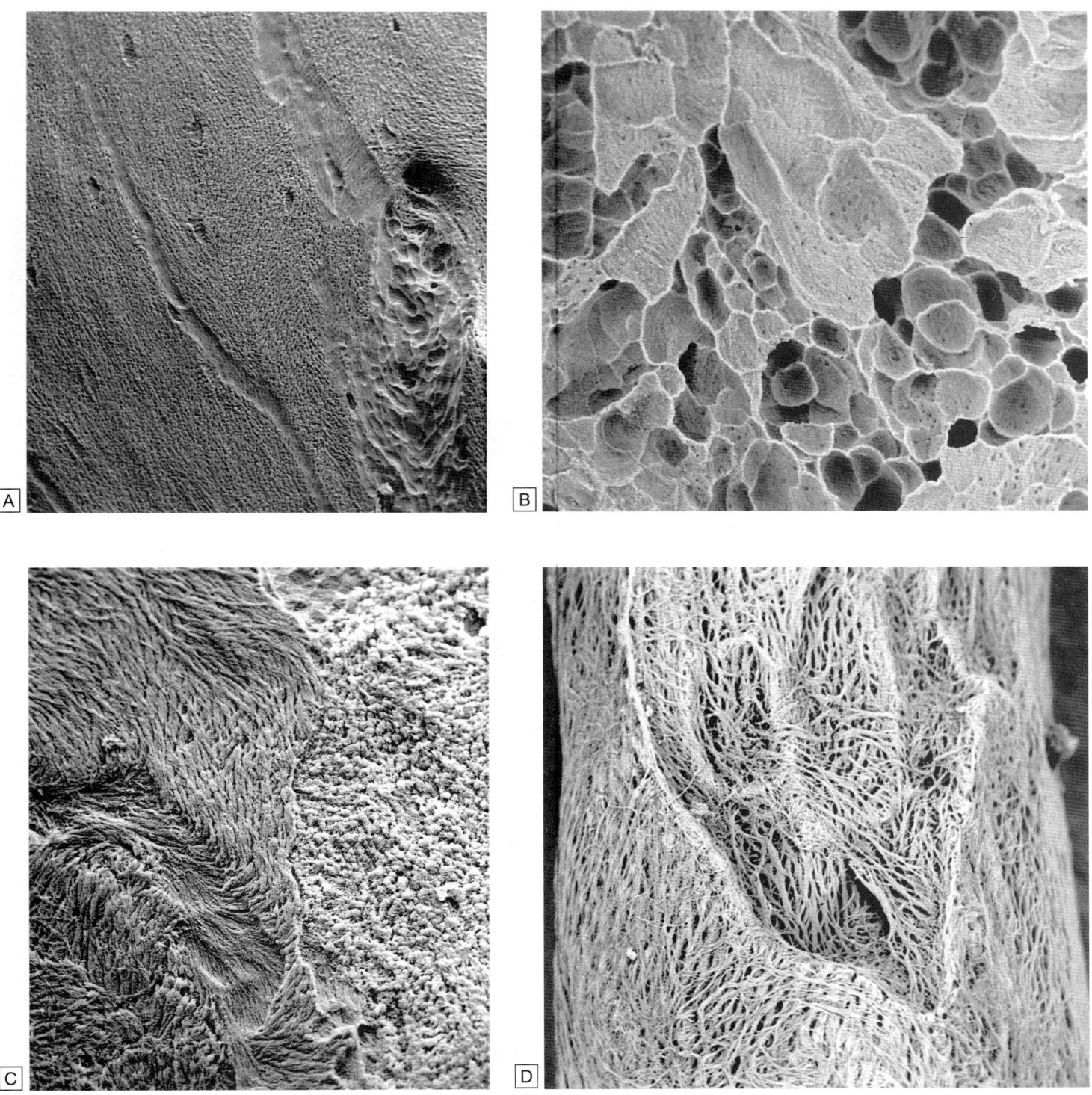

6.62A.   Endosteal surface of human sixth rib (2 year 4 month male) showing resorption trails crossing the field obliquely. The central track was made by one osteoclast migrating over the bone surface as it resorbed the bone. Note that the path of the osteoclast followed the orientation of the collagen fibres (and this would be the same as the long axes of the overlying osteoblasts).   SEM of anorganic specimen, field width = 320 μm.   B. Resorbed surface on human sixth rib (59 year male): the individual pits comprising the large Howship's lacuna vary in size and shape, but the directions taken by resorptive lobopodial extensions of osteoclasts can be identified in some places. Note also the canaliculi for osteocyte processes.

SEM, field width = 129 μm. C. Anorganic preparation of human sixth rib (70 year male). New bone formation had filled the resorbed region at the right; the mineral clusters indicate an interface with osteoid. At the upper left the collagen fibres are fully mineralized indicating a 'resting' bone surface. At the lower left corner new bone deposition had not yet extended over the whole of the resorbed area. SEM, field width = 127 μm. D. Repair with new bone of a resorbed region on a trabeculum in a human sixth rib (43 year female). The resorption pits can still be seen below the newly deposited collagen. Field width = 72 μm.

a pulley. Adapted in shape to the movement of particular joints, such surfaces are smooth, though in life they are, of course, covered by articular cartilages forming the actual surfaces of synovial joints. The texture of such osseous surfaces is due to another feature, frequently overlooked; they are devoid of the vascular foramina

typical of most other bone surfaces, articular cartilage being poorly vascularized. However, osseous articular surfaces are not completely impermeable, though the cartilage contiguous with subjacent bone is usually calcified; hence substantial interchange is improbable (the nutritive avenue to articular cartilage may be largely from synovial

481

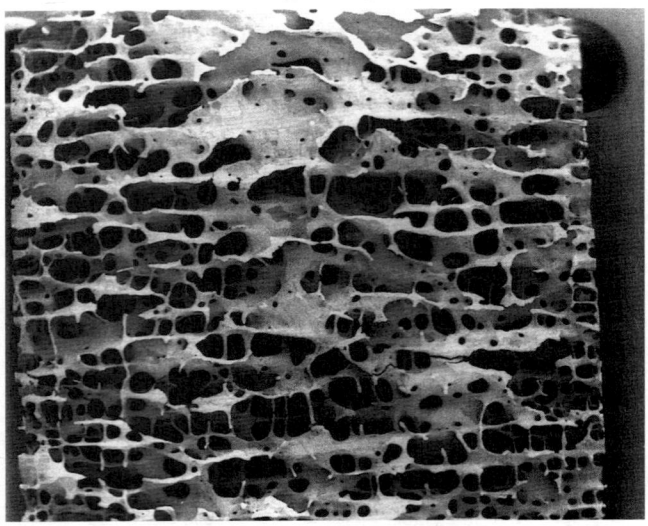

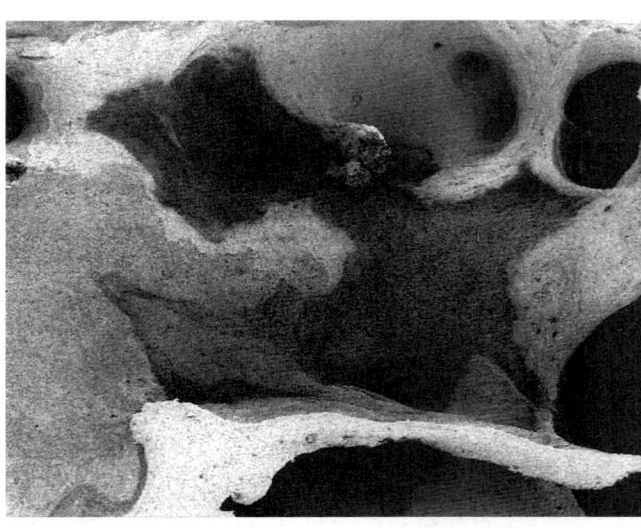

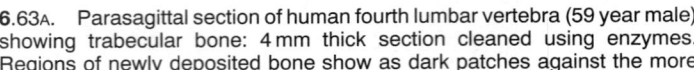

6.63A. Parasagittal section of human fourth lumbar vertebra (59 year male) showing trabecular bone: 4 mm thick section cleaned using enzymes. Regions of newly deposited bone show as dark patches against the more highly mineralized, older bone. The patch just above the centre of the field in A is shown at higher magnification in B. BSE, field widths A = 21.5 mm and B = 1.69 mm.

fluid). Scanning electron microscopy shows that all bony surfaces, including those appearing smooth to the naked eye or hand lens, display large numbers of minute foramina. The proportion of these occupied by vascular, nervous or collagenous elements is unknown.

Large tendons (e.g. adductor magnus, subscapularis) are attached to facets which lack the regular contours of articular surfaces but resemble them in texture, being poorly vascularized. Such tendon facets are sometimes depressed (the adductor 'tubercle' is often a small pit); alternatively they may surmount large elevations, for example, the humeral tuberosities.

Depressions and elevations, varying in size and shape, interrupt otherwise featureless osseous surfaces. A depression is a *fossa*, and some articular surfaces are fossae (cf. temporomandibular joint). Lengthy depressions are *grooves* or *sulci* (e.g. humeral bicipital sulcus); a notch is an *incisura*, and an actual gap is an *hiatus*. A large projection is termed a *process* or, if elongated, slender or pointed, a *spine*. A curved process is a *hamulus* or *cornu* (cf. sphenoidal pterygoid hamuli and hyoid cornua). A rounded projection is a *tuberosity* or *tubercle*, occasionally a *trochanter*. Long elevations are *crests*, or *lines* if less developed; crests are wider and present boundary edges or *lips*; however, these terms are ill-defined, and one most substantial crest is the linea aspera (cf. femur). An *epicondyle* is a projection close to a condyle and usually an attachment for the collateral ligaments of the adjacent joint or common myotendinous attachments for superficial muscle groups (cf. humerus). The terms *protuberance*, *prominence*, *eminence* and *torus* are also less often applied to certain bony projections. The expanded proximal ends of many long bones are often termed the '*head*' or *caput* (cf. humerus, femur, radius, etc.).

A hole in bone is a *foramen*; foramina are *canals* when lengthy. Large holes may be called *apertures* or, if covered largely by connective tissue, *fenestrae*. Clefts in or between bones are *fissures*. A *lamina* is a thin plate; larger laminae may be called *squamae* (e.g. the temporal squama).

Large areas on many bones are featureless and indeed often smoother than articular surfaces, but they differ from these in possessing many visible vascular foramina. Such a texture occurs where muscle is directly attached; through the foramina pass small blood vessels from bone to muscle and perhaps vice versa. Areas covered only by periosteum are similar but vessels are less numerous.

Tendons are usually attached at roughened bone surfaces; and wherever any aggregation of collagen in a muscle reaches bone, surface irregularities correspond in form and extent to the pattern of such 'tendinous fibres'. Such markings are almost always elevated above the general surface, as if ossification advanced into the collagen bundles from periosteal bone. How such secondary markings are induced is uncertain but they may result from the continued incorporation of new Sharpey's (extrinsic) fibres in the bone, necessary for minor functional adjustment. Evidence suggests that their prominence may be related to the power of muscles involved and they increase with advancing years, as if the pull of muscles and ligaments exercised an accumulative effect perhaps over a more limited area. Certainly, surface markings delineate the shape of attached connective tissue structures, whether an obvious tendon, intramuscular tendon or septum, aponeurosis, or tendinous fibres mediating otherwise direct muscular attachment. Hence markings may be facets, ridges, nodules, rough areas or complex mixtures, affording accurate data of junctions of bone with muscles, tendons, ligaments or articular capsules. Numerous examples will be described with individual bones.

Even in the so-called 'fleshy' or direct attachment of a muscle, its myocytes do not themselves adhere directly to periosteum or bone. The route of transmission of tension from contracting muscle to bone is through the connective tissue which pervades all muscles as perimysium and endomysium. These two forms of attachment of muscles, at the extremes of a range of admixtures, differ in the density of collagen fibres between muscle and bone. Where collagen is visibly concentrated, markings appear on the bone surface. In contrast, the multitude of microscopic connective tissue ties of direct attachment, necessarily over a larger area, do not visibly mark it. Here the bone appears smooth to unaided vision and touch.

RESPONSE OF BONE TO INJURY

Microdamage in bone may initiate bone remodelling; it may also precipitate bone fracture. After an injury such as a fracture, bone generally undergoes spontaneous regeneration, which in favourable conditions can result in virtually complete restoration of its anatomical structure before injury. Depending on the location of the injury, endochondral and/or intramembranous ossification (p. 471) may be involved. Exceptions to this occur in the calvarium, where fractures may be repaired permanently by fibrous union and not by regeneration of new bone, and after rigid internal fixation, where bone can form directly by primary bone healing, without the preliminary development of either fibrous tissue or cartilage.

BONE HEALING WITHOUT OPERATIVE INTERVENTION

Bone healing consists of several overlapping phases: inflammation, soft callus formation, hard callus formation and remodelling. Soft and hard callus formation are collectively equivalent to the proliferative phase of wound healing. The term 'soft callus' appears to be contradictory in that 'callus' implies hardness (Latin *callum* or *callus* = hard integument); it can be defined as the soft, collagenous, revascularizing, osteogenic blastema which unites the bone fragments and from which bone regenerates.

Inflammation

Inflammation begins immediately after fracture, overlaps with the phase of soft callus formation and typically lasts for about 4 days. It is characterized by local haemorrhage, haematoma formation, oedema and pain. Although there is some evidence that fibrin in the haematoma may stimulate the proliferation of local potentially osteogenic cells and assist in immobilizing the bone fragments, the haematoma is not generally considered to be a significant stimulator of bone healing (Heppenstall 1980).

Vascular damage causes the environment of the fracture to become hypoxic and acidic, followed by tissue necrosis at and close to the site of injury. Mast cells, polymorphonuclear leucocytes and macrophages appear at the site of injury and release cytokines, some of which may, as in the repair of skin wounds, stimulate the proliferation of reparative cells (here osteoblasts, endothelial cells and, in some circumstances, chondroblasts). Platelet-derived growth factor (PDGF), for example, is mitogenic for osteoblasts. The mast cells, some of the macrophages and the reparative cells are of local origin, while the polymorphonuclear leucocytes and the remainder of the macrophages (and osteoclast precursors) are haematogenous.

During the inflammatory phase, osteoclasts and macrophages erode necrotic and live bone and remove tissue debris from the fracture site. Osteoclasts are stimulated to resorb in an acid environment (Mundy 1993a). Recent research suggests that macrophages also secrete factors or mediators, some of which stimulate collagen synthesis and angiogenesis in wound healing, and it is conceivable that they act in a similar manner in the healing of bone.

As inflammation is overlapped by soft callus formation, cells near the fracture site are induced to develop into osteoblasts which produce new bone. Osteoprogenitor cells in the periosteum divide actively and differentiate into osteoblasts, and marrow stromal and surrounding connective tissue cells differentiate into chondroblasts. The inductive mechanism for differentiation is probably multifactorial and may involve a variety of interacting stimuli including cytokines released from mast cells, macrophages, stromal cells and endothelial cells, reduced oxygen availability and the level of bone morphogenetic proteins (Baylink et al 1993; Wozney & Rosen 1993). The notion that endothelial cells may become osteoblasts in fracture callus (Brighton & Hunt 1991) is not supported by immuno-

localization of endothelial cell proteins (Oni et al 1993), but pericytes may be osteoprogenitor cells.

Soft callus formation

During the stage of soft callus formation, which occupies approximately 3 or 4 weeks, a soft tissue blastema or soft callus develops around and between the fragments of bone, reducing their mobility (6.64A). The soft callus contains proliferating preosteoblasts, fibroblasts and often chondroblasts, embedded in a matrix, rich in glycoproteins and collagen, into which new blood vessels grow. The soft callus can be subdivided into external and internal callus, the former derived from the proliferation of osteoblast progenitors in the osteogenic layer of the periosteum, and the latter from endosteal cells. The enhanced proliferative activity of the osteogenic layer of the periosteum extends beyond the immediate fracture site, elevating the overlying fibrous component of the periosteum and producing a collar of soft external callus which unites the bone fragments. Periosteal cells located within this callus furthest from the fracture site (i.e. in a mechanically stable, well-oxygenated environment) form new osseous matrix directly, but as the more mobile and poorly oxygenated fracture site is approached the cell population becomes mixed. Although angiogenesis is in progress, proliferation is so rapid that cellularity outstrips vascularity, maintaining an oxygen gradient and keeping the fracture site relatively hypoxic (Wray 1963; Heppenstall et al 1975). Initially the periosteum supplies blood to the site of fracture, but later in the regenerative process the normal centrifugal flow of blood from the endosteal circulation is re-established.

Hard callus formation

During this stage of fracture healing the external and internal soft callus are gradually converted into woven bone (6.64B) mainly by endochondral ossification, unless the bone fragments have been surgically immobilized with a compression plate, when intramembranous ossification predominates. Both cellularity and vascularity continue to increase, but in such a manner that the oxygen gradient referred to above is maintained. The pH of the matrix of the callus gradually increases to the neutral level. While both osteogenesis and chondrogenesis are in progress, osteoclastic activity continues at the fracture site. This stage of bone healing commences at about 3 or 4 weeks after injury and continues until attainment of firm bony union, about 2 or 3 months later for most adult long bones, but sooner in the young.

Remodelling

During remodelling, which overlaps with the formation of hard callus and may continue for several years, the woven bone of the

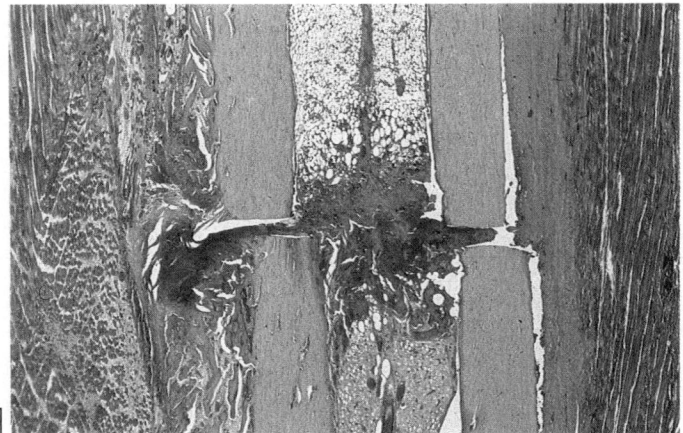

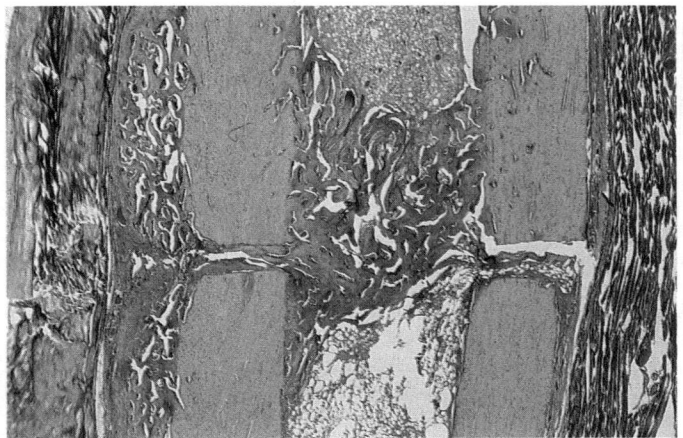

6.64 Midsagittal sections through the repairing fracture site of the lower tibia of a rabbit, held rigidly in an external fixator. Movat's hexachrome stain: undifferentiated blastemal tissue = grey; cartilage = turquoise; bone = pale green. (Sections provided by R. Brueton, Orthopaedic Research Department, Rayne Institute, St Thomas's Hospital, London; photographed by Kevin Fitzpatrick.) A. 2 weeks after injury. A distinct fracture gap separates adjacent fragments of cortex. The mainly adipose marrow contains patches

of blastemal tissue. External soft callus contains patches of cartilage; a few bone trabeculae and some cartilaginous areas are present endosteally.
B. 4 weeks after injury. A thin layer of bone lies in the fracture gap. Endosteal soft callus unites the posterior cortical fragments. Periosteal soft callus is present posteriorly, but is not yet confluent across the gap, while anteriorly only fibrous tissue is present.

hard callus is gradually converted into lamellar bone. Osteoclasts remove excess bone from the exterior of the periosteal collar and remodel its endosteal aspect so that the medullary cavity is restored across the site of the fracture (**6**.65). As a result of changes in vascularity, the oxygen supply of the fracture site returns to normal. Remodelling can be considered to be complete, a state achieved more rapidly in children than in adults, when the site of the fracture may no longer be identified either structurally or functionally. The regenerative process is, however, extremely lengthy and, until it has been completed, the injured bone is functionally less efficient than it was before damage. Attempts to accelerate the rate of regeneration have included surgical intervention and exposure to physical agents such as direct current (Friedenberg et al 1971; Brighton 1981), pulsed electromagnetic fields (Bassett et al 1974; reviewed by Barker & Lunt 1983) and ultrasound (Duarte 1983; Dyson & Brookes 1983). The bioelectrical properties of bone and its response to electrical stimuli have been reviewed by Spadaro (1991).

PRIMARY BONE HEALING

The same four overlapping stages of repair are found in fractures which are stabilized, except that no cartilage is formed in the second, soft callus phase (Brueton et al 1993; Perren et al 1969). Such 'primary bone healing' still follows an interruption of the blood supply at and near the fracture and results in local resorption, with the destruction of osteons and the generation of Haversian systems across the site of the fracture. Osteoclasts assemble at the ends of Haversian canals near to the fracture site, forming cutting cones which advance at a rate of 50–80 μm per day across the fracture, enlarging the canals as they advance; they are closely followed by osteoblasts which form new Haversian systems in the enlarged canals which now cross the fracture site and so link the fragments of bone.

The entire process only lasts about 5 or 6 weeks but has the disadvantage that the major surgical intervention required subjects the tissues to further trauma.

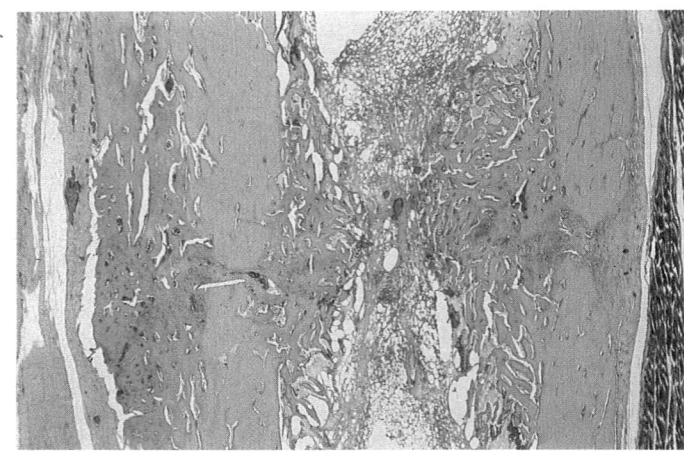

6.65 Midsagittal section through the remodelling fracture site of the lower tibia of a rabbit, held rigidly in an external fixator, 6 weeks after injury. A mass of periosteal hard callus unites the posterior cortices, while fibrous tissue is present anteriorly. Endosteal hard callus unites anterior and posterior cortices. Some soft callus lies between the fragments posteriorly. Remodelling of the marrow cavity has begun and there is a central axis of myelofibrotic material. Movat's hexachrome stain: undifferentiated blastemal tissue = grey; cartilage = turquoise; bone = pale green. (Section provided by R. Brueton, Orthopaedic Research Department, Rayne Institute, St Thomas's Hospital, London; photographed by Kevin Fitzpatrick.)

THE SCOPE OF ARTHROLOGY

The rigid nature and mode of growth of skeletal tissue requires that the skeleton consists of *multiple* osseous elements, each joined to its neighbours by a variety of structural arrangements. All such unions are grouped as *arthroses* (synonyms: *articulationes, juncturae* (classical); *joints, articulations, junctions* (Anglicized)). Arthroses are concerned with *differential growth, transmission of forces* (tensile, compressive, shear and torsion) and *movement* (from consolidation and complete rigidity at one extreme, through to relatively free but controlled movement at the other). Which of these attributes predominates varies with site and age, often changing markedly with the latter. The scientific study of the functional topography and temporal variation of arthroses is *Arthrology*. Arthroses are classified in a number of ways, with different criteria and degrees of quantitative accuracy being adopted by different groups of workers. Hence, sources limited to a single classification should be considered with respect to the intended audience, varying from a simplified introductory grouping, through a more detailed vocational grouping, to greater mensural information for orthopaedicians and finally the most comprehensive classifications—used by specialist kinesiologists. **All** these approaches to classification are given here, initially as a synopsis of principal headings and terms; in later pages and (where indicated) elsewhere, these are defined and described in greater detail. Where the morphology is mixed, or changes radically with time, and in some exceptional topographical situations (e.g. the costal cartilages and the larynx), additional classificatory groups have been included. Although unusual, this confers a more complete logic to the frameworks employed.

ARTHROSES: MAIN VARIETIES

The anlagen of all skeletal units (initially separate centres of ossification and ultimately consolidated whole bones) are derived from condensations of mesenchyme. At many sites the mesenchyme becomes increasingly fibrous and bone formation occurs directly in the tissue (*intramembranous ossification*, p. 471); elsewhere the

INTRODUCTORY CLASSIFICATION OF ARTHROSES

Either (classic nomenclature)

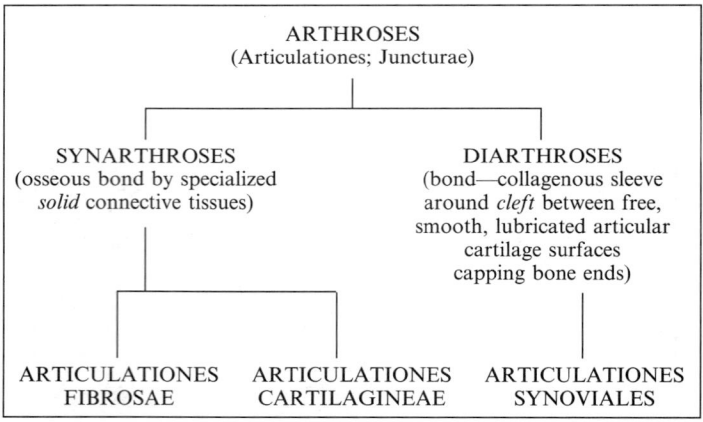

or (Anglicized nomenclature)

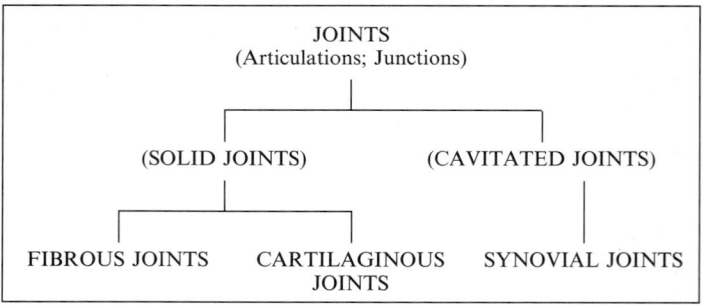

Introductory classification of arthroses (continued)

I SYNARTHROSES	bone—solid connective tissue—bone
1. FIBROUS JOINTS **(Articulationes fibrosae)**	
a. Sutures:	bone—collagenous sutural ligament—bone
b. Syndesmoses:	bone—collagenous interosseous ligament, membrane or cord—bone (elastic fibrous tissue is occasionally prominent)
c. Gomphoses:	bone—complex collagenous periodontium—dental cement
2. CARTILAGINOUS JOINTS **(Articulationes cartilagineae)**	
a. Synchondroses:	bone—hyaline cartilage—bone
(*Primary cartilaginous joints*)	
b. Symphyses:	bone—hyaline cartilage—fibrocartilaginous disc—hyaline cartilage—bone
(*Secondary cartilaginous joints*)	
SYNOSTOSES:	rigid bony union; after growth has ceased this is the normal fate of synchondroses, ultimately most sutures, and some symphyses

II DIARTHROSES	bone—cavitated connective tissue—bone
SYNOVIAL JOINTS:	bone—articular cartilage—synovial fluid in cavity—articular cartilage—bone
(*Articulationes synoviales*)	Bond: surrounding sleeve of collagenous fibrous capsule lined by synovial membrane; extrinsic and intrinsic ligaments. Occasional intracapsular ligaments, tendons, fat pads, fibrocartilaginous discs or menisci

More detailed nomenclature (see text for definitions) (A)

SYNARTHROSES

FIBROUS JOINTS (ARTICULATIONES FIBROSAE)

Sutures (Suturae)
Morphological terms:
serrate
denticulate
squamous
limbous
plane
schindylesis (wedge and groove)
Suturae cranii (33 officially recognized and systematically named)

Gomphoses
('peg and socket';
articulationes dentoalveolares)

Syndemoses
Bonding by collagenous (sometimes elastic) interosseous ligament, cord or membrane sheet. There are 12 officially recognized, named, syndemoses (see text). Criteria for inclusion (or exclusion) remain arbitrary.

SYNARTHROSES: MIXED

Many large synchondroses have localized bundles of dense collagen. Many sutures possess islands of fibrocartilage (see text).

CARTILAGINOUS JOINTS (ARTICULATIONES CARTILAGINEAE)

Synchondroses (Primary cartilaginous joints; hyaline growth cartilages)
Varieties and sites:
Synchondroses cranii (between ossific centres in the chondrocranium, within and between named bones. See text for details and names.)
Synchondroses postcranii
epiphysiodiaphyseal
epiphysiocorporeal
intra-epiphyseal
multiplex (in compound, e.g. hip, bones)
sternales (between sternebrae)
manubriosternalis (young)
xiphosternalis
sacrales (young)
costal cartilages are atypical (see text)

Symphyses (Secondary cartilaginous joints)
Bone surfaces encased in hyaline growth cartilage are bonded by fibrocartilaginous disc. All are median.
S. *manubriosternalis*
S. *intervertebrales*
S. *sacrales*
S. *pubis*
S. *menti* (atypical and temporary)

SYNARTHROSES: PERSISTENCE OR CONSOLIDATION (Synostoses)

Syndemoses, gomphoses and some symphyses grow with their surrounding tissues, the latter contributing to osseous growth; when growth ceases, however, they *persist* throughout life with only minimal age changes. Some symphyses ossify wholly or in part. Synchondroses and sutures possess both functionally important mechanical properties and are most prominently *growth mechanisms*. When growth ceases the intervening cartilage or fibrous tissue is progressively ossified, bony union occurs and they become **synostoses**. It is usually stated that 'the joint is obliterated' and uncommon to group **synostoses** with **arthroses**. Total function, however, makes it quite logical.

mesenchyme differentiates into a hyaline cartilaginous model within which an orderly sequence of transformations leads to *endochondral ossification*. The biological nature, mechanical properties, changes and fate of the specialized connective tissues interposed between adjacent osseous surfaces form the foundation for the broad classification of arthroses, firstly into two fundamentally contrasting groups. The specialized connective tissues may remain solid, often changing character with time, or they may develop a narrow but extensive, enclosed, fluid-containing cavity. *Solid* (*non-synovial*) joints are termed *synarthroses* and are commonly grouped according to the principal type of intervening connective tissue: *fibrous joints* and *cartilaginous joints*. These reflect the two modes of ossification already mentioned.

Synarthroses, of both types, characterize almost all the cranial

485

More detailed nomenclature (see text for definitions) (B)

DIARTHROSES
(ARTICULATIONES SYNOVIALES)
SYNOVIAL JOINTS
(to avoid repetition Joint or Articulation is omitted below)
General Morphology
Simple (one pair of articulating surfaces; male and female)
Compound (more than one pair of surfaces)
Complex (with intracapsular meniscus or disc)

Widely used terms
(useful approximations)
Surface shape
  plane
  spheroid (**enarthrosis**; 'ball and socket')
  ellipsoid
  ginglymus ('hinge')
  bicondylar
  trochoid ('pivot')
  sellar ('saddle-shaped')
Axes of movement
  uniaxial
  biaxial
  triaxial
  polyaxial
Types of movement
  translation
  rotation (*conjunct* or *adjunct*)
  angulation
  flexion/extension
  abduction/adduction
  circumduction
  elevation/depression
  protraction/retraction
  fixation (neuromuscular)
  fixation (mechanical: close-packing)
  During locomotion, postural adjustment and exploratory and manipulative tasks, the above analytical unitary movements are combined in complex patterned arrays at numerous joints.
Fundamental joint positions
  Loose packed—controlled free *mobility*
  Close packed—position of functional *rigidity*

Precise analytical terms
(less frequently encountered)
Surface topology
  ovoid, simple; male and female
  ovoid, compound; male and female
  sellar; male and female
Almost all synovial articular surfaces are quantitative variants of the above.
Joint mechanics
Movements are related to the concept of the *mechanical axis* of a bone (see text). Movements are all resolvable as rotations around one, two or three orthogonal axes, i.e. possessing 1–3 *degrees of freedom*.
Types of movement
Terms refer to one mobile articular surface moving relative to its fixed partner.
Spin: pure rotation of surface around its mechanical axis.
two varieties—*pure* and *impure*:
  Cardinal swing: tips of mechanical axis trace a chordal path. There is no spin.
  Arcuate swing: tips of mechanical axis trace an arcuate path. Joint topology necessitates some associated spin (i.e. conjunct rotation)

All the above terms, and others, are defined and amplified in the following pages.

junctions; their respective derivations are the desmocranium and chondrocranium; both types are also present in large numbers throughout the postcranial skeleton which, apart from the clavicle, is mainly endochondral in origin.

Cavitated (*synovial*) *joints* are formally termed *diarthroses* and, with few exceptions (the temporomandibular joint and those involving the clavicle), are between the ends or other defined surfaces of endochondral bones. Each articular surface is of specialized hyaline cartilage strongly adherent to the bone on one aspect, and presenting a free, lubricated, macroscopically smooth, wear-resistant surface on the other, which can glide over its fellow with minimal friction. The fine cleft between apposed surfaces contains lubricating and nutritive synovial fluid (*synovia*): this *synovial cavity* extends to the synovial membrane (where the fluid is produced) which lines the surrounding fibrous capsule and other non-articular joint surfaces.

SITES OF ARTHROSES

The detailed topography of individual bones including the fleshy/tendinous/aponeurotic attachments of muscles, fasciae, ligaments, articular capsules and other relationships, for example neurovascular, visceral, coelomic or bursal, together with a summary of their patterns of ossification, are considered later in this Section. Also given are the well-defined areas on the surface of a bone which are in intimate structural/functional juxtaposition with com-

plementary areas on a neighbouring bone or bones; specialized connective tissues blend strongly with the osseous surfaces, solid or cleft, and occupy all the intervening territory. Collagen, prominent in the present context, is considered in terms of varieties, dispositions, mechanical properties and biosynthesis in 'the matrix of connective tissue' in Section 1, *Introduction*, where also the less prominent elastic components are reviewed. Accounts of the development of skeletal, junctional and related locomotor structures can be found in Section 3, *Embryology and development*. (Consult tables for nomenclature of varieties of arthroses.)

FIBROUS JOINTS (ARTICULATIONES FIBROSAE)

In most instances fibrous joints consist of predominantly collagenous junctions between bones but in a minority of situations fibro-elastic tissue predominates. Three main groups of fibrous articulation are generally recognized, namely, *sutures*, *gomphoses* and *syndesmoses* (**6.66**).

SUTURES

Sutures are limited to the skull and occur wherever margins or broader surfaces of bones are separated only by connective tissue,

FIBROUS JOINTS

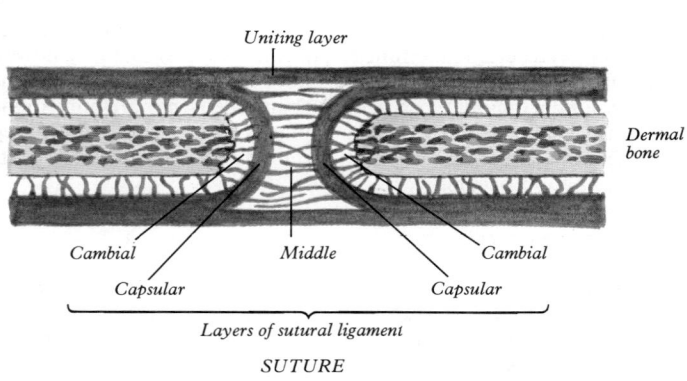

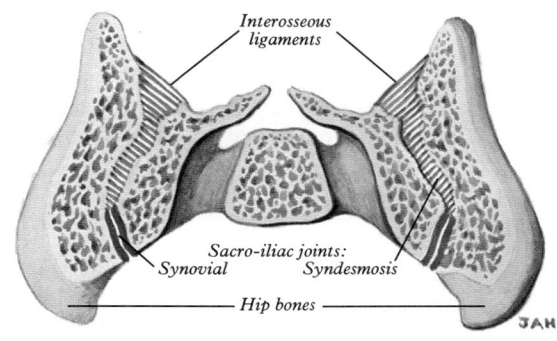

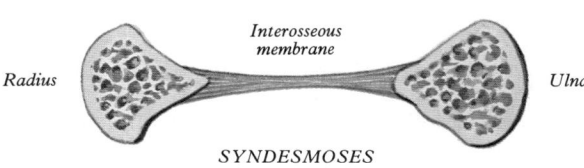

SYNDESMOSES

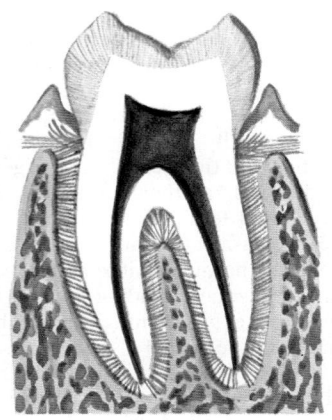

GOMPHOSIS
(Dentoalveolar joint)

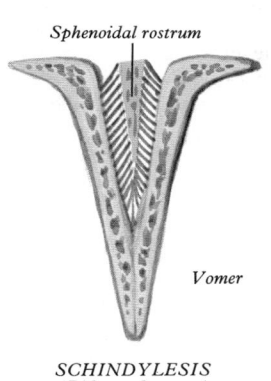

SCHINDYLESIS
(Ridge and groove)

6.66 Some examples of the principal varieties of fibrous joints (articulationes fibrosae), each shown in section. Note that schindyleses are not regarded by some as sufficiently distinct from sutures to merit a separate group. Syndesmoses are difficult to define because of the large numbers and great variety of fibrous interosseous structures. The official (internationally) recognized list has changed several times over the years, with the list increasing; however, the massive sacro-iliac ligament illustrated is not, as yet, in the official list.

the *sutural ligament* or membrane, which is a surviving unossified part of mesenchymatous sheets in which dermal bones develop (p. 548). Sutural ligaments display regions of differentiation concerned in growth and binding of apposed bone surfaces (Pritchard et al 1956). On its sutural aspect each bone is covered by a layer of osteogenic cells (the 'cambial' layer), itself overlaid by a capsular lamella of fibrous tissue (6.66), collectively corresponding to and continuous with periosteum at the margins of the sutural surfaces, both inside and outside the skull. Between these two layers of sutural periosteum is a central stratum of loose fibrous connective tissue, varying in width according to age and the interval between the bones involved. This central stratum contains thin-walled blood vessels, the veins of which communicate with diploic vessels, intracranial venous sinuses and external veins in the scalp. The fibrous periosteum adherent to the bones crosses the interval between them, as two uniting layers (external and internal) enclosing the sutural ligament and adding to its strength. During active growth the orientation of collagen fibres within sutural membranes is adaptable to several factors, particularly to the direction of growth of minute bone spicules (Koskinen et al 1976).

In view of the occurrence of fibrous tissue in synchondroses (p. 488), it is interesting that, during growth, secondary cartilage formation often occurs in sutural ligaments, suggesting a relation between fibrous and cartilaginous joints.

When cranial growth (including in its earlier stages growth at sutures) ends, osteogenic cells generally bring about complete ossification of sutural ligaments, ultimately leading to obliteration and

rigid synostosis. This is a slow process (p. 607) and does not begin until the late twenties; yet it is clearly necessary that sutures should cease to be slightly flexible joints as soon as possible after birth. Sutural ligaments may create an almost immovable bond between large areas of bone, especially where they show reciprocally adapted irregularities, even if fine as in the intermaxillary junction; but such immobility cannot be produced at narrow edges of bones in the cranial vault. Here, however, their margins develop spikes and recesses which interlock so well that the bones are difficult to separate even when denuded of all fibrous connective tissue. Where the edges are saw-like, the junction is a *serrate suture*: a *denticulate suture* has small toothlike projections, often widening towards their ends to provide even more effective interlocking. When united by sutural ligament and periosteum, such sutures are almost completely immobile: the sagittal suture is serrated as is much of the lambdoid denticulate. Where bones overlap, as at the temporoparietal suture, a *squamous suture* is formed; the adjacent bone surfaces are reciprocally bevelled and, if mutually ridged or serrated, the junction is sometimes termed a *limbous suture*. Simple apposition of contiguous surfaces, usually rough and reciprocally irregular, is inappropriately named a *plane suture*, examples being sutures between the palatine bones, between the maxillae and at the palatomaxillary sutures. Although surface demarcations between such bones show none of the interlocking evident at serrate or denticulate sutures, irregular surfaces of contact, united by wide expanses of sutural ligament, provide much resistance to shearing or torsion; like other sutures they are, for all practical purposes, immovable. In summary, sutures, although

487

in some locations providing slight perinatal flexibility, are essential structural mechanisms for sutural bone growth, providing the necessary rigidity and geometry in the upper neurocranium and in the nasofacial and palatine skeleton.

Schindylesis. This is a specialized suture where a ridged bone fits into a groove on a neighbouring element, for example the cleft between the alae of the vomer that receives the rostrum of the sphenoid.

GOMPHOSES

A *peg-and-socket joint* (*articulatio dentoalveolaris*) is a specialized fibrous articulation restricted to the fixation of teeth in alveolar sockets in the mandible and maxillae. The collagen of the periodontium connects dental cement with alveolar bone (see p. 1706, for details).

SYNDESMOSES

A syndesmosis is a fibrous articulation in which bony surfaces are bound together by an interosseous ligament, a slender fibrous cord or an aponeurotic membrane, usually allowing slight but occasionally more extensive movement between them. Long considered to be rare in mammals, the term was at one time restricted to the inferior tibiofibular joint **alone** (but see below). Clearly this was unsatisfactory since interosseous fibrous connections occur in such profusion and variety of form; nevertheless no consensus concerning a precise definition of *syndesmosis* has emerged. The following may serve to illustrate some inconsistencies and difficulties, and perhaps provide a background for the curious assortment of structures officially recognized as syndesmoses given below.

Though not usually so described, the dorsal part of the sacro-iliac junction, through its massive interosseous sacro-iliac ligaments, **is**, rather than 'closely resembles' a syndesmosis (**6.66**). The sacro-iliac joints proper, primarily synovial, are also often invaded by fibrous tissue late in life and may become entirely fibrous articulations, differing little from syndesmoses. The inferior tibiofibular joint, long accepted as a typical syndesmosis, could alternatively be considered little more than an interosseous ligament adjacent to the ankle joint, or to a synovial extension of the joint when this exists, as it occasionally does in man and regularly in other primates. If this is accepted, the term syndesmosis could be extended to many other interosseous ligaments, as in the carpus and tarsus, and also include the interosseous membranes of the forearm and calf (foreleg), especially since these are already described as 'intermediate' joints in the radioulnar and tibiofibular series (but see below). Since ligaments are almost all 'interosseous', it becomes difficult to restrict use of the term 'syndesmosis', unless only very short extrinsic ligaments close to a synovial joint are so designated. (Intrinsic and intracapsular ligaments of synovial joints must be excluded.)

In *Nomina Anatomica* (1977) the term syndesmosis was extended to include the following ligaments: pterygospinous, stylohyoid, interspinous, intertransverse, ligamenta flava and ligamentum nuchae. The *syndesmosis radioulnaris* includes the antebrachial interosseous membrane and oblique cord, the *syndesmosis tibiofibularis*, the interosseous membrane and ligament and the anterior and posterior tibiofibular ligaments. This particular choice of ligaments is, however, quite arbitrary; many others could have been included as syndesmoses: the list should be expanded within a strictly defined framework.

CARTILAGINOUS JOINTS (ARTICULATIONES CARTILAGINEAE)

As indicated earlier synarthroses, bone junctions bonded by solid connective tissue, are generally divided into two main groups: fibrous and cartilaginous joints. In most instances the distinction is quite obvious and apposite; at a number of sites, however, some admixture occurs, where a predominantly fibrous articulation contains occasional islands of cartilage or conversely a predominantly cartilaginous articulation contains aligned dense bundles of collagen (see below).

Cartilaginous joints are themselves classified into two groups: *synchondroses* (*primary cartilaginous joints*) and *symphyses* (*secondary cartilaginous joints*) (**6.67**). When fully formed each group has some distinctive structural and functional features; other features, however, although varying quantitatively, are common. The terms primary and secondary should, perhaps, be abandoned; they are only apposite in the instances of certain symphyses (see below) that, developmentally, are preceded by synchondroses within which further differentiation occurs.

SYNCHONDROSES

These articulations occur where originally separate, but adjacent, centres of ossification appear within a continuous mass of hyaline cartilage. As ossification spreads it invades the **actively growing** zone of cartilage occupying the interval between the contiguous osseous surfaces. Thus, a synchondrosis consists of two ossifying fronts closely bonded by a specialized *hyaline growth cartilage*. Structurally, passing towards an ossifying surface the growth cartilage has successive recognizable zones of: relative *quiescence*; proliferative and interstitial *growth*; *transformation* into columns, with cell hypertrophy, matrix calcification and cell death; *ossification* involving chondrolysis, vascularization and osteogenesis (see p. 471). Where the rate of ossification of both surfaces forming a synchondrosis is approximately equal (e.g. in the cranial base), the growth cartilage has a central quiescent zone equidistant from the surfaces and the zones proceed symmetrically towards **both** surfaces. Where the growth rates are unequal, the growth cartilage structure is correspondingly asymmetrical; extreme examples are synchondroses between the diaphysis and terminal epiphyses of long bones where growth and progressive ossification are mainly (but not exclusively) diaphyseal. In the latter the quiescent **zone** lies near the epiphyseal bone with the ossification zone extending towards the diaphysis. The cartilaginous growth plate grows in girth by the interstitial and subperichondrial methods described elsewhere (p. 478), with activity varying at different radial distances from its centre. In this way the overall shape of the cartilage and its associated bones are changed, sometimes profoundly. Thus, the early epiphysis of the femoral head is separated from the femoral neck, an extension of the diaphysis, by a relatively simple horizontal plate of growth cartilage. With differential growth the capitular tip of the neck becomes increasingly conical, being tightly bound to a conical growth cartilage which fits into a deep conical recess in the inferolateral part of the otherwise spheroidal ossifying femoral head.

Functionally, synchondroses are primarily *growth mechanisms* and, although contributing slightly to the more flexible skeleton of youth, their growth potential is combined with the ability to successfully resist forces, whether of compression, tension, shear or torsion. Thus they permit growth to continue, while either free but controlled, often powerful, movements can be executed at neighbouring synovial joints, or the more restricted movements at symphyses and some fibrous joints. These features are characteristic of the numerous *postcranial synchondroses*. Since, with the exception of the clavicle and areas of subperiosteal bone accretion, all postcranial centres of ossification are endochondral, synchondroses are present in all postcranial bones derived from two or more centres, i.e. the majority of postcranial bones. The carpal and most tarsal bones, however, each develop from a single endochondral centre: their ossifying surfaces advance invading *a complete encasement of growing cartilage*. Parts of the latter persist as the specialized articular surfaces of the synovial carpal and tarsal joints; elsewhere the bone approaches the perichondrium (now periosteum) providing attachment for fibrous joint capsules, tendon sheaths, interosseous ligaments, fascial septa and muscles. Clearly, these relatively small bones possess no synchondroses but their essential growth mechanisms have much in common with that of epiphyses (p. 649).

Postcranial synchondroses

Most postcranial synchondroses have not been given specific topographical names, but the general morphological group to which each belongs is given in the classification (p. 485). They may be *epiphysiodiaphyseal* (or more precisely *epimetaphyseal*, or *epicorporeal*), *intraepiphyseal* in compound epiphyses, or *multiplex* in compound bones with multiple primary centres. Examples of the

CARTILAGINOUS JOINTS

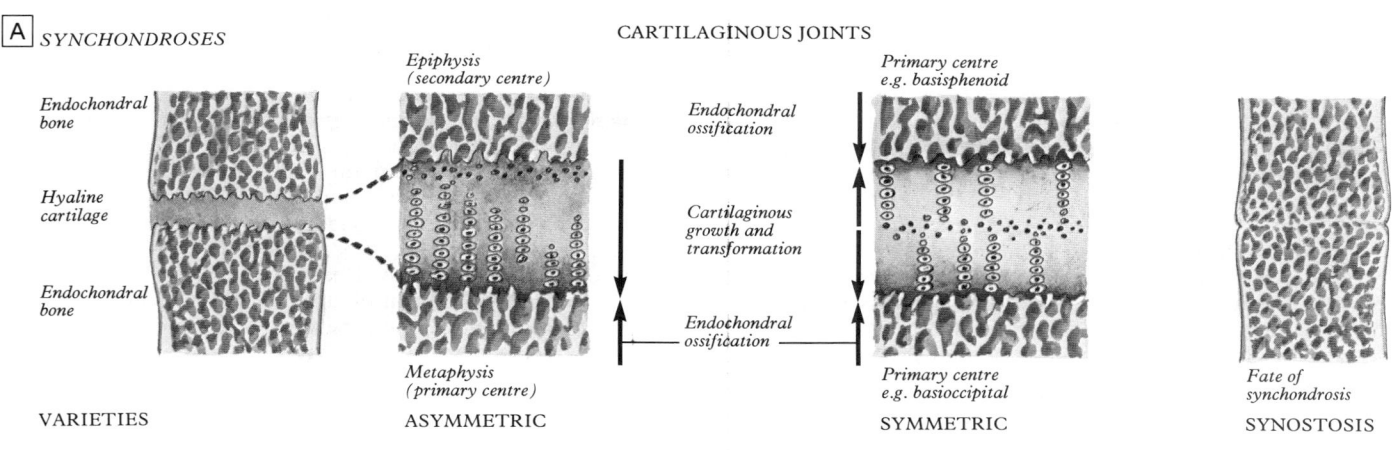

A *SYNCHONDROSES*

Endochondral bone

Hyaline cartilage

Endochondral bone

VARIETIES

Epiphysis (secondary centre)

Metaphysis (primary centre)

ASYMMETRIC

Endochondral ossification

Cartilaginous growth and transformation

Endochondral ossification

Primary centre e.g. basisphenoid

Primary centre e.g. basioccipital

SYMMETRIC

Fate of synchondrosis

SYNOSTOSIS

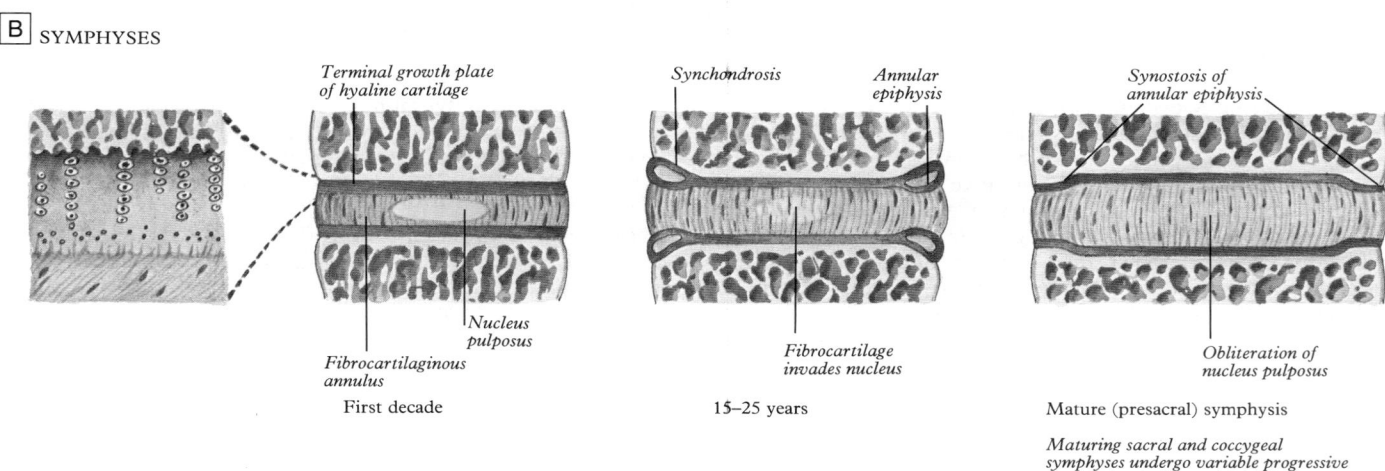

B SYMPHYSES

Terminal growth plate of hyaline cartilage

Fibrocartilaginous annulus

Nucleus pulposus

First decade

Synchondrosis

Annular epiphysis

Fibrocartilage invades nucleus

15–25 years

Synostosis of annular epiphysis

Obliteration of nucleus pulposus

Mature (presacral) symphysis

Maturing sacral and coccygeal symphyses undergo variable progressive synostosis starting peripherally

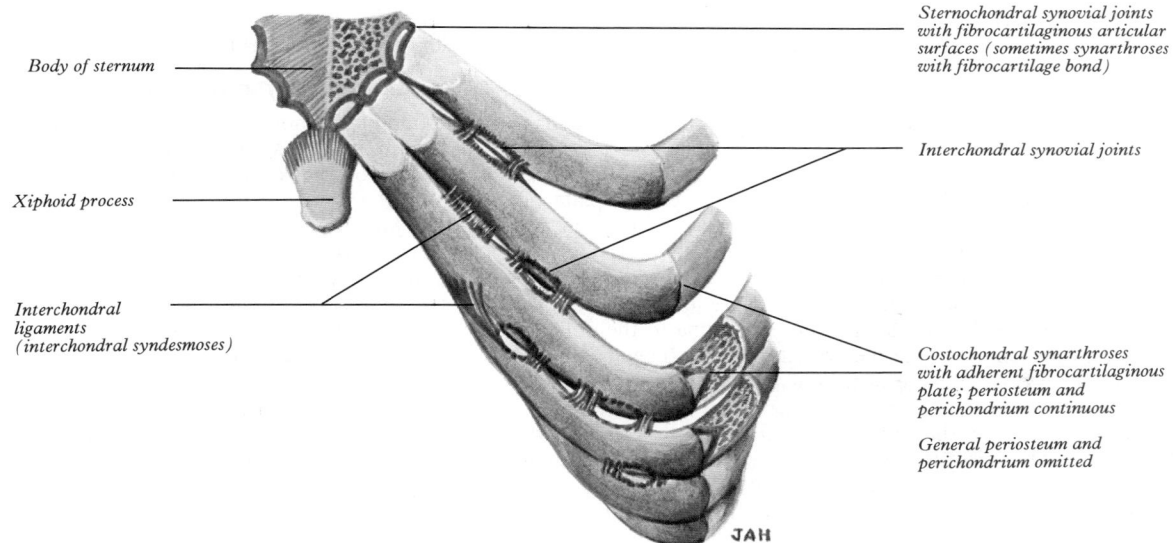

C *LESS COMMON CHONDRAL JOINTS*

Body of sternum

Xiphoid process

Interchondral ligaments (interchondral syndesmoses)

Sternochondral synovial joints with fibrocartilaginous articular surfaces (sometimes synarthroses with fibrocartilage bond)

Interchondral synovial joints

Costochondral synarthroses with adherent fibrocartilaginous plate; periosteum and perichondrium continuous

General periosteum and perichondrium omitted

JAH

6.67 Varieties of cartilaginous joints (articulationes cartilagineae). A. Synchondroses in sectional view. The principal tissues involved, more detailed architecture and main growth patterns of symmetrical and asymmetrical synchondroses. In some locations lesser degrees of asymmetry occur; synostosis is the normal fate of almost all synchondroses when *endochrondral* growth has ceased. B. Intervertebral symphyses (presacral) in sectional view, displaying changes with age. Note that partial or complete synostosis is the normal fate of sacral and coccygeal symphyses. For discussion and for manubriosternal and pubic symphyses see text and individual joints. C. Less common interchondral and osseochondral junctions; see text for other locations.

last which have topographical names are: the *triradiate acetabular cartilage* of the developing hip bone, *sternales* between growing sternebrae, *manubriosternalis* (young, before transformation to a symphysis), *xiphosternalis*, *vertebrales* confined to individual vertebrae, *sacrales centrales* (young, soon to be temporary symphyses) and *laterales* (between central, neural arches and costal processes). Structurally, the pattern of zonation mentioned above and elsewhere (p. 437) requires some amplification. Growth cartilages vary considerably with age, site and species (see Knese 1979 and Hall 1983 for reviews of the literature; Moss-Salentijn et al 1987 and Taylor et al 1987 for recent quantitative studies). Most intensively studied are certain synchondroses in small laboratory mammals (mouse, rat, rabbit), particularly the proximal tibial synchondrosis. In the embryonic stage the cartilaginous 'models' of future bones consist of generalized hyaline cartilage, its chondrocytes being randomly distributed within the matrix. With the formation and longitudinal advance of the primary centre of ossification the site of the *presumptive growth plate* of cartilage is indicated by ovoid aggregates (or clones) of chondrocytes. The full zonal pattern is only seen in the *definitive growth plate* between the advancing osseous surface of the metaphysis and that of the epiphysis. Human growth plates are relatively much thicker than those of the laboratory mammals studied, due mainly to the depth of the 'quiescent' or small cell zone adjacent to the epiphyseal bone, which accounts for 60–70% of total plate thickness. Its significance is, however, controversial, some regarding it as relatively inert while others consider it a pool of stem progenitor cells (see reviews and quantitative references). From the latter, throughout the life of the growth plate (i.e. growth of the bone), successive generations of chondrocyte columns are formed, transformed, partially eroded, then form a scaffold for advancing ossification. Thus, when fully active, a growth cartilage contains chondrocyte columns of varying length, maturity and position. Young columns extend limited distances from the small cell zone (*epiphyseal* position); mature forms are *full length* columns; old columns are again short, partly eroded and *metaphyseal* in position. (These names are purely positional, devised for quantitative analyses of growth cartilages in appendicular long bones, which as they grow and retreat all contribute to the advancing surface of metaphyseal ossification.) The dual views concerning the small cell zone may, reasonably, both be correct; the cells near the epiphyseal bone have a low growth potential while the potential to function as a pool of chondrocyte progenitor cells increases markedly as the tips of the chondrocyte columns are approached.

The chondrocytes and matrix of young growth cartilages have the three-dimensional architecture described for hyaline cartilage (p. 450) and the changes in the partitions enclosing chondrocyte columns have been mentioned (p. 476). In the latter the collagen fibrils have been termed 'ladderlike' (Eggli et al 1985). Some large growth cartilages that are habitually subjected to unusually large stresses may also develop dense bundles of collagen, the fibro-osseous disposition reflecting the stress. These *fibrous epiphyseal* (*growth*) *plates* have been studied by Smith (1962a,b). In the proximal growth plate of the human tibia the almost flat condylar parts are crossed by regularly aligned horizontal bundles lying at right angles to the long axis of the bone, which during weight bearing suffer lateral compression. Where the epiphysis descends anteriorly to form the tibial tuberosity it is subjected to shearing stress due to the oblique pull of quadriceps femoris; here the growth plate cartilage is almost completely replaced by oblique dense collagen. (Other examples of structurally mixed growth cartilages are given in the references above; for a general review of the vascularization of epiphyseal growth cartilages see Moss-Salentijn 1976.) The fates of both postcranial and cranial synchondroses are considered below, together with some unclassified or inappropriately classified junctions involving cartilage.

Cranial synchondroses

Cranial synchondroses occur between neighbouring endochondral centres of ossification that develop in the chondrocranium (for its origin, chondrification, and topographical regions, see p. 478, and Bosma 1976 for a general developmental review). Some regions of the chondrocranium remain unossified: the lateral, alar and septal nasal cartilages and remnants occupying and near the foramen lacerum. In contrast the largely endochondral auditory ossicles articulate via specialized synovial joints, while the malleus and stapes

are connected to the temporal bone by equally specialized fibrous arrangements, the fibrous stratum of the tympanic membrane (p. 1373) and the annular ligament respectively. The endochondral centres of ossification are for the inferior nasal concha (single), the ethmoid (three), the sphenoid (multiple pre- and postsphenoidal centres for the body, conchae, lesser wings and roots of greater wings, see p. 592), the temporal bones (multiple centres for each petromastoid part and styloid process), and the occipital bone (multiple centres for basilar, condylar and squamous parts up to the superior nuchal lines, see p. 585). The sites of basicranial synchondroses are numerous, some being within individual bones, others between them, with all contributing to some extent to basicranial growth. However, those that persist for limited periods, and coalesce early, are unnamed, while those that make substantial contributions to growth have official names; these are (omitting the prefix synchondrosis): *sphenoethmoidalis*, *spheno-occipitalis*, *sphenopetrosa*, *petro-occipitalis*, *intraoccipitalis anterior* and *intraoccipitalis posterior*. Although they are not officially named, presumably because of their relatively early fusion, it seems appropriate to include the main intrinsic synchondroses of the sphenoid. Suggested names are: *intrasphenoidalis transversus* between pre- and postsphenoidal parts of the body and *intrasphenoidalis lateralis*, bilaterally separating the body from the conjoined greater wings and pterygoid processes (see p. 588). The cranial synchondroses are approximately symmetrical in structure, their zones of growth and differentiation passing from the centre towards both ossifying surfaces.

The fate of synchondroses

When growth between parts of a bone or between individual bones joined by a synchondrosis nears completion, classic cartilaginous growth, transformation and endochondral ossification ceases. For a period the cartilaginous plate is relatively quiescent, but becomes irregularly thinned; complex histological changes now ensue involving the cartilage from both osseous surfaces. (For histological details and references see p. 477.) Finally, the synchondrosis is entirely replaced by complete bony union between the originally separate osseous surfaces, forming a *synostosis*, losing its cartilaginous growth potential and mechanical properties, but acquiring the maximal rigidity of bone. This enhances the effectiveness of postcranial bones in resisting a variety of powerful stresses, either in almost static postures or during movement patterns involving synovial and (to more limited degrees) median symphyseal or fibrous joints. Rigidity of the neurocranium, both during and after completion of growth, is functionally essential, providing protective support and encasement of the brain, special sense organs, their vasculature and associated fluids (blood and cerebrospinal fluid).

Terminology: some brief comments

The fate of synchondroses raises a number of points, some directly, others indirectly, which require amplification; they also provide examples of the kind of limitations inherent in many biological classifications. It is commonly stated that 'synchondroses are temporary junctions, and with cessation of growth, the joint is obliterated as bony union occurs'. Apparently useful and self-explanatory, the statement requires comment. '*Temporary junctions*': while strictly correct in relation to all true synchondroses (see below), the periods of activity and times of synostosis vary greatly in different sites. Some fuse in fetal or perinatal life, others throughout the first decade, many in the latter half of the second, while the spheno-occipital basicranial synchondrosis may continue well into the third decade (p. 588, see also 'Ossification of individual bones'). Many are, therefore, fully active for many years; consequently their essential properties are a unique combination of growth potential and strength of interosseous bonding. '*Cessation of growth*': this clearly does not refer to overall growth, for example, of the whole body, skeleton, body segment or even a whole bone. Patterns of osseous fusion are complex and extend over lengthy periods; most long bones that develop simple terminal epiphyses at each end (e.g. fibula, ulna) have asynchronous fusion times. The growth referred to is the equilibrium between endochondral ossification, cartilaginous growth plate proliferation and transformation of the specific growth plate. When fusion **has** occurred, however, subperiosteal and subendosteal bone accretion and resorption and trabecular remodelling may **continue**; at the microscopic level, osteon removal and replacement at varying rates continues throughout life. '*The joint is obliterated*': this implies acceptance of synarthroses as a major classificatory group, with synchondroses (also symphyses, sutures, syndesmoses, gomphoses) as well-defined subgroups. Osseous fusion is not included in the official nomenclature or by the majority of authors. Some authorities, however, include synostoses as extreme forms of synarthroses, especially when growth potential and rigidity are regarded as equally relevant arthrological elements as active movement.

Unusual junctions involving cartilage

Arthroses are generally defined as coaptations of osseous surfaces, with their classification stemming from the variety of specialized intervening connective tissue and its solid or cleft state. A number of junctions, however, have many arthrodial features but are not accommodated by the general classification of arthroses; these occur where substantial masses of cartilage remain unossified in normal development. (Some masses develop irregular patches of calcification in later decades.) Such junctions may be between bone (endochondral or intramembranous) and cartilage, between two adjacent cartilages, or a cartilage may join with a fibrous suture or a synchondrosis. The junctions are similar to either fibrous synarthroses or to synovial joints. Particular reference can be made to the nasal, laryngeal and costal cartilages, and to those of the auditory tube and auricle (pinna). Fibrous junctions occur between the borders of contiguous nasal cartilages; the septal cartilage is, in part, continuous with the lateral nasal cartilage but elsewhere fibrous bonds extend to the internasal suture, perpendicular plate of the ethmoid, the vomer, the nasal crest (and intermaxillary suture) and anterior nasal spine of the maxillae and the septal process of the lateral nasal cartilage. At these junctions perichondria fuse or perichondrium and periosteum (and in some sites sutural ligament) blend.

A fibrous junction joins the perichondrium of the elastic auricular fibrocartilage and the periosteum of the roughened outer rim of the external acoustic meatus. A similar fibrous union suspends the perichondrium of the superior recurved border of the cartilage of the auditory tube and the inferior perichondrium of the sphenopetrosal synchondrosis (periosteum after synostosis, the upper attachment spreading on to the petrous quadrate area). The larynx and hyoid bone are further examples of specialized and uncommon varieties of connection and junction. Most extensively the laryngeal cartilages are connected to each other, and the thyroid and epiglottic cartilages to the hyoid bone, by three-dimensional complexes of fibroelastic membranes and their ligamentous thickenings. Details of these *interchondral* and *osseochondral* structures are given on pages 485, 492; although not officially listed as synarthroses (subgroup *syndesmoses*) it seems logical to regard them as such. In addition, the cricoid cartilage bears four discrete articular surfaces, one bilateral pair on the sloping superior border of its lamina and a lateral pair at the junction of each lamina and arch. These articulate respectively with the articular surface on the base of each arytenoid cartilage and with the medial aspects of the tips of the inferior cornua of the thyroid cartilage. The crico-arytenoid and cricothyroid articulations to which these surfaces contribute (p. 1644) are *interchondral* synovial joints.

The costal cartilages are often, usefully, considered as unossified cartilaginous extensions of the ribs, with the first to seventh reaching the sternum, the eighth to tenth the cartilage above, while the eleventh and twelfth are short blunt cones with free intermuscular tips. The cartilages are, however, traditionally described as separate topographical entities (p. 544) and, depending on its level, each engages in from one to five different types of junction (p. 541). The costochondral junctions are unusual synarthroses where the convex tip of the cartilage is received by a complementary recess in the tip of the rib; perichondrium and periosteum are continuous, as are the collagenous elements of bone and cartilage. The sternochondral joints (often called sternocostal joints) vary; the second to seventh are often synovial, with *fibrocartilaginous* articular surfaces on both chondral and sternal aspects. Quite frequently synovial cavities are absent in some or all these joints, in which case a thin dense lamina of tightly adherent fibrocartilage is interposed between cartilage and bone—an unclassified variety of synarthrosis. This type of junction is usually present at the manubrial end of the first costal cartilage. (It should be noted that it is commonplace for the **whole** first costal cartilage and attached rib and sternum, or the manubriochondral junction alone, to be incorrectly classified as a synchondrosis.) The

fifth to ninth costal cartilages carry a variable number of simple interchondral synovial joints as well as irregular syndesmoses in the form of short interchondral ligaments between their borders or apices (particularly cartilages eight to ten), anchoring their tips to the superjacent border.

SYMPHYSES

A symphysis is another variety of cartilaginous synarthrosis having many features in common with other arthroses, only differing quantitatively; distinctive attributes although prominent are few. Topographically, all symphyses are median and, with one exception, are confined to the axial skeleton. The latter include the following named symphyses: the *manubriosternalis* between manubrium and sternal body; *intervertebralis* between successive vertebral bodies (regionally grouped—cervical, thoracic, lumbar, sacral and coccygeal); also axial is the *symphysis menti* between the bilateral halves of the fetal mandible, continuing only into the first postnatal year when synostosis supervenes. Histologically the mental junction is unlike other symphyses (see p. 576); however the use of its name is so widespread that retention seems inevitable. Finally the medial surfaces of the bodies of the pubes (bilateral appendicular bones) are conjoined at the *symphysis pubis*.

Ignoring regional specializations (mentioned below) the general architecture of a symphysis consists of two well-defined surface areas of articulating endochondral bones; the osseous surfaces varying from a few millimetres to over a centimetre apart being bound together by strong, tightly adherent, solid connective tissues. Each bony surface is firmly attached to a thin lamina of hyaline cartilage, which in turn blends with the surface of a thick, strong, but deformable pad (or disc) of fibrocartilage. Collagenous ligaments extend from the periostea across the symphysis and blend with the hyaline and fibrocartilaginous perichondria; they do not form a complete capsule (as in synovial joints), but are similar in containing plexuses of afferent nerve terminals, which also penetrate the periphery of the fibrocartilage. The combined strength of the ligaments and of the hyaline and fibrocartilage exceeds that of the associated bones; thus they can easily withstand the habitual range of stresses (compression, tension, shear and torsion) encountered without disruption. Tears are usually the result of sudden, massive unexpected stresses occurring with the body in an inappropriate posture. The architecture of the fibrocartilaginous tissues is such that it combines **strength** with limited degrees of elastic deformability, thus allowing a restricted but appreciable range of **movement** that characterize symphyses. Fibrocartilaginous disc compression narrows the interosseous interval, while tension increases it; when these occur simultaneously in opposite sectors of a disc it becomes cuneiform (wedge-shaped) with the attached bones becoming relatively inclined (angulated). Torsional stresses increase or decrease the spiralization of collagenous discal microarchitecture and permit slight relative rotation. Although the range of movement possible at a symphysis is not great, being primarily determined by its intrinsic anatomy, it is further limited by the additional articulations and ligaments that involve the bones but which are extrasymphyseal; for example, the numerous syndesmoses and synovial zygapophyseal joints between adjacent vertebrae, articulations of the clavicles and costal cartilages with the sternum, and the sacroiliac joints, interosseous sacroiliac, sacrotuberous and sacrospinous ligaments. All these features profoundly affect movement patterns at their related symphyses.

Further comments on symphyseal structure, functional attributes and nomenclature

Thick fibrocartilaginous pads or discs that most characterize symphyses are not simple deformable masses of feltwork, but present precise zonal variations in microstructure, particularly in their arrangement of collagenous and elastic fibres adapted to their habitual stresses. Best investigated and most complex are the intervertebral discs. (See p. 512 for their main subregions, fibre architecture, cellularity, physicochemical properties and profound age changes.)

Solid specialized connective tissues, by definition, characterize synarthroses and, while this holds for the thoracolumbar and sacrococcygeal series of intervertebral symphyses, significant proportions of the remainder develop a single central or a bilateral pair of narrow fluid-filled clefts in (or near) their fibrocartilaginous pads.   491

Over 30% of manubriosternal symphyses develop a central horizontal elongate cleft (p. 539) and over 50% of interpubic discs develop a median elongated cleft in the oblique long axis of the disc. (For variations in size and position see p. 677.) The second to sixth (occasionally seventh) cervical intervertebral discs develop laterally placed small fluid-filled cavities in the fibrous tissue between the bevelled inferolateral edge of the vertebral body above and the superolateral lip of the vertebral body below. Some regard these cavities as being in the peripheral parts of the discs and non-synovial in character; while others regard them as small synovial joints near, but external to, the discs (6.94). The synovial or non-synovial nature of all the above clefts remains controversial; they perhaps reflect a stage in the evolution of synovial joints. Caution should also prevail concerning the dogmatic assertion that no movements of translation occur between their free moist surfaces until adequate objective evidence has accumulated. Distinct possibilities seem to be translations at the cervical cavities during spinal movements and translation with distraction at the interpubic cleft, particularly during the later stages of pregnancy.

The common statement that synchondroses are temporary and concerned with growth, whereas symphyses are permanent and concerned with movement, is an oversimplification and only partly correct. **Both** are concerned with **strength** and the ability to withstand and transmit considerable stresses and with **growth**; and, in contrasting ways, both contribute either directly or indirectly to the total *movement patterns* of the parts involved. The strength and mechanical properties of cartilaginous joints need little further comment, except to re-emphasize that the rigidity of synchrondroses increases the efficiency of positive movements at related syndesmoses, symphyses and particularly synovial joints. It must be remembered that the movements at symphyses are not a simple extrapolation of the mechanical properties of a fibrocartilaginous pad or disc assessed by experimental isolation. For example, movement of a vertebra relative to its neighbour is a three-dimensional summation of the properties of **all** its intervertebral arthroses (syndesmoses and synovial joints, in addition to the complex symphysis) acting in concert, but each with its particular array of stresses. (During their growth phases the mechanical properties of the *intravertebral synchondroses* are also significant.)

The prominent role of synchondroses in skeletal **growth** is widely recognized, investigated and discussed, whereas growth of and involving symphyses is often ignored or receives but scant mention. *Symphyseal growth* may, for convenience, be considered from two aspects (although interrelated); intrinsic growth of the fibrocartilaginous disc and growth of the hyaline cartilaginous plates into which (e.g. vertebral) endochondral ossification progresses and later 'annular' epiphyses form (see below). At the manubriosternal symphysis its limiting plates of proliferative hyaline cartilage are progressively invaded by the ossifying fronts of the manubrium and first

sternebra; normally no epiphyses are formed. At the pubic symphysis, however, the growth plates of hyaline cartilage that are involved with endochondral ossification on the symphyseal aspects of the bodies of the pubes after puberty commonly develop scale-like epiphyses, usually anterosuperiorly. The occurrence of intervertebral and pubic epiphyses complicates the traditional description of symphyses. At these latter sites the epiphyses appear at (or soon after) puberty and continue slow growth for about a decade before synostosis with the main bone. During this period the epiphysis is completely encased by proliferative hyaline cartilage, its interosseous lamina being a narrow (epiphysiocorporeal) synchondrosis and its symphyseal lamina a simple extension of the terminal plate of hyaline growth cartilage: the latter being originally derived from the early embryonic cartilaginous vertebral model. These growth plates are the proliferative source of cartilage into which all endochondral ossification of the vertebral **bodies** occurs cranially and caudally, constituting about 80% of the length of the mature vertebral column (see p. 511). The remaining 20% is provided by growth of the fibrocartilaginous discs; their regional variations in thickness and their cuneiform sagittal profile (vertically thicker anteriorly) in the cervical and lumbar secondary spinal curvatures are described on page 512. Where the fibrocartilage blends with the lamina of hyaline cartilage some bundles of collagen pass without interruption from the fibrocartilage to interlace within the matrix of the hyaline cartilage, whose laminae show the zonal variation in structure previously described and common to all growth cartilages.

Terminology. Both clinically and radiologically the term intervertebral symphysis is seldom used; instead '*the intervertebral disc*', or simply '*the disc*', and radiologically '*the disc space*' are often used to indicate all tissues between the vertebral bodies. Formally, however, the fibrocartilaginous intervertebral disc, with its age-dependent nucleus pulposus (p. 513), is regarded as part of a symphysis, completed by paired laminae of terminal growth cartilages and their associated ossifying or mature osseous surfaces.

Fates of symphyses

The generalization that 'synchondroses are temporary while symphyses are permanent' is only partly correct; there are notable exceptions. Normally permanent, but exhibiting age changes, are the cervical, thoracic, lumbar and lumbosacral intervertebral symphyses, the pubic symphysis and about 90% of manubriosternal symphyses. The age changes in intervertebral discs are considered on page 514; the development of narrow fluid-filled clefts are mentioned above and under individual joints; also reference to changes in the pubic symphysis in the later stages of pregnancy are made above and on page 678. In contrast, the joints between successive sacral bodies, between sacrum and coccyx and between coccygeal segments, after preliminary stages, form well-developed symphyses; however, their normal fate is partial or complete *synostosis*; the process is slow

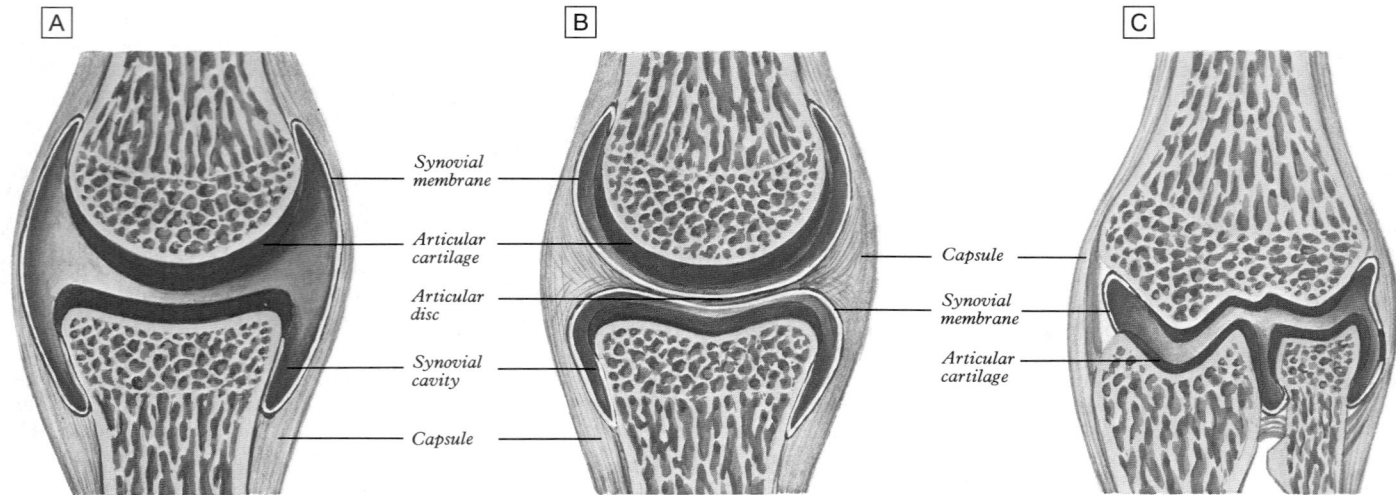

A	B	C
SIMPLE	*COMPLEX*	*COMPOUND*

6.68 Synovial joints, some main structural features and one elementary type of classification: A. simple; B. complex; C. compound joints (see text). For clarity, the articular surfaces are artificially separated. A and B are purely diagrammatic and not related to particular joints. C, however, is a simplified representation of some features of an elbow joint but the complicated contours due to the olecranon, coronoid and radial fossae and profiles of articular fat pads present in a true section have been omitted.

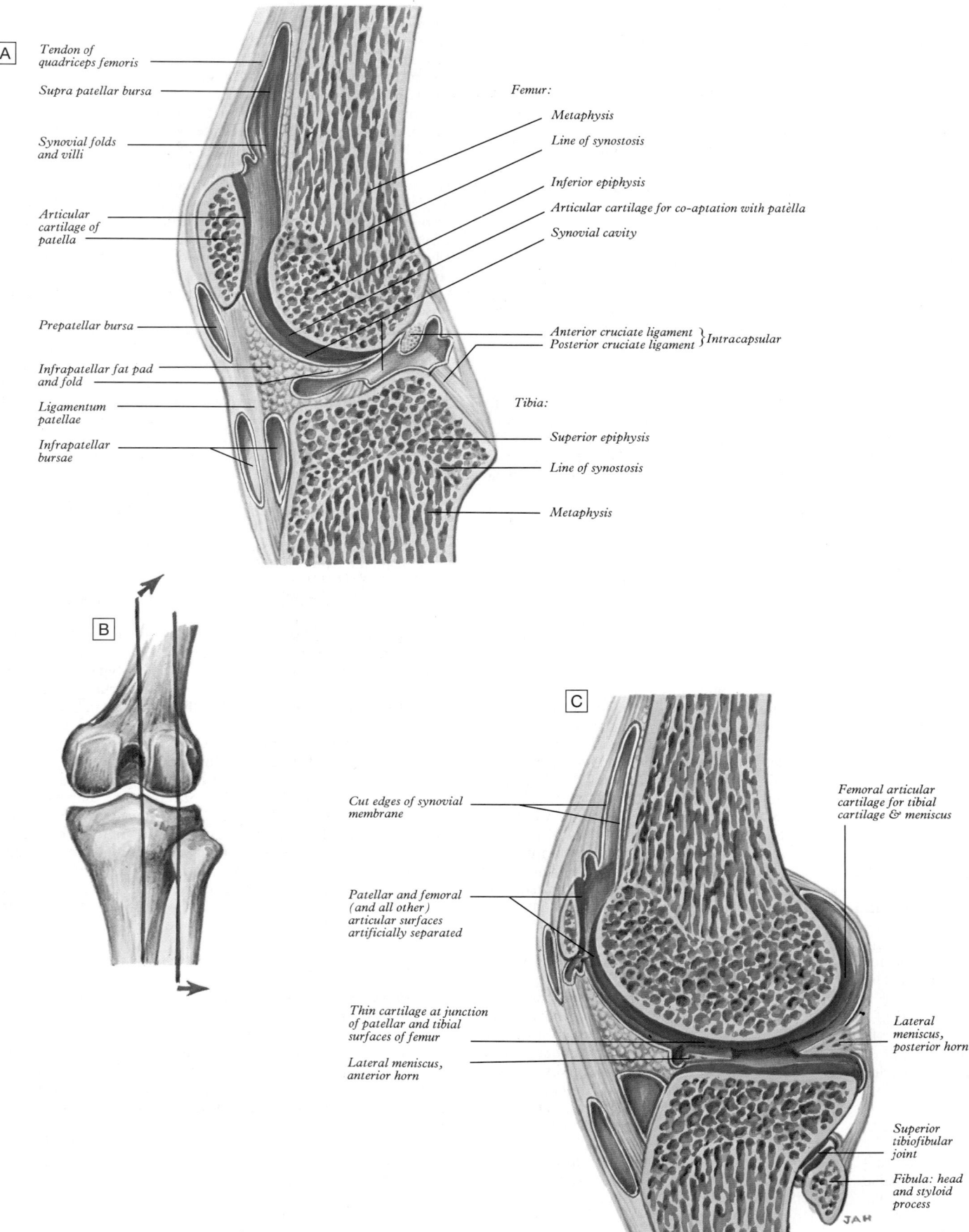

A
Tendon of
quadriceps femoris

Supra patellar bursa

Synovial folds
and villi

Articular
cartilage of
patella

Prepatellar bursa

Infrapatellar fat pad
and fold

Ligamentum
patellae

Infrapatellar
bursae

Femur:

Metaphysis

Line of synostosis

Inferior epiphysis

Articular cartilage for co-aptation with patella

Synovial cavity

Anterior cruciate ligament
Posterior cruciate ligament } Intracapsular

Tibia:

Superior epiphysis

Line of synostosis

Metaphysis

B

C

Cut edges of synovial
membrane

Patellar and femoral
(and all other)
articular surfaces
artificially separated

Thin cartilage at junction
of patellar and tibial
surfaces of femur

Lateral meniscus,
anterior horn

Femoral articular
cartilage for tibial
cartilage & meniscus

Lateral
meniscus,
posterior horn

Superior
tibiofibular
joint

Fibula: head
and styloid
process

JAH

6.69A–C   Principal structural features displayed in two parasagittal sections of the left knee joint, which is synovial and both compound and complex. B. Line diagram of the posterior aspect showing the planes of section in A and C. The synovial cavity and bursae are, for clarity, shown as slightly distended; the articular surfaces of the patella, femur and tibia and the meniscal surfaces are thus artificially separated. These illustrations should be studied both with the accompanying introductory text and also with the detailed account of the knee joint (p. 697 et seq.).

and lengthy (pp. 533, 539). After 30 years of age about 10% of manubriosternal symphyses develop partial or complete synostosis; again the phenomenon may be slow and lengthy (p. 539).

SYNOVIAL JOINTS

Synovial articulations (**6.68, 69**) operate differently from *non-synovial* fibrous and cartilaginous joints. Although the bones involved are linked by a fibrous capsule usually having intrinsic ligamentous thickenings, and often by internal or external accessory ligaments, the osseous surfaces concerned are **not** in continuity. They are covered by articular cartilage, a stratum of specialized hyaline cartilage (occasionally fibrocartilage) of varying thickness and precise topology, with contact being strictly between these cartilaginous surfaces, which have a very low coefficient of friction (Charnley 1959). Sliding contact is facilitated by viscous *synovial fluid* (synovia), like a lubricant in some respects but also concerned in the maintenance of living cells in the articular cartilages. Its properties are considered later (p. 498).

The fibrous capsule completely encloses such a joint except where it is interrupted by synovial protrusions; the exceptions are described with the individual joints. The capsule is lined by *synovial membrane*, which also covers all non-articular surfaces including non-articular osseous surfaces, tendons and ligaments partly or wholly within the fibrous capsule, as at the shoulder and knee. Where a tendon is attached inside a joint and issues from it, a prolongation of synovial membrane usually accompanies it beyond the capsule. Some extra-capsular tendons are separated from the capsule by a synovial bursa (p. 631) continuous with the joint's interior. Such protrusions are potential avenues for the spread of infection into joints.

A further intra-articular structure, **not** covered by synovial membrane, is an *articular disc* or *meniscus*, occurring between articular surfaces where congruity is low: it consists of fibrocartilage with the fibrous element usually predominant. A disc may extend across a synovial joint, dividing it structurally and functionally into **two** synovial cavities. Peripherally discs are connected to fibrous capsules, usually by vascularized connective tissue, so that they become invaded by vessels and afferent and motor (sympathetic) nerves; sometimes, however, the union is closer and stronger, as in the knee and temporomandibular joints. Their main part contains few cells, but the surfaces may have an incomplete stratum of flat cells, continuous at the periphery with adjacent synovial membrane; however, the two groups of cells are not alike (p. 497). The term *meniscus* should be reserved for incomplete discs, like those in the knee joint and occasionally the acromioclavicular joint. Complete *discs* occur in the sternoclavicular and inferior radioulnar joints, while that in the temporomandibular joint may be complete or incomplete. Discs often have small perforations; where menisci are usual, complete discs may occur or may be slightly perforated. The function of intra-articular fibrocartilages is uncertain; views advanced are deductions from structural or phylogenetic data, with the help of mechanical analogies. The plethora of suggestions is therefore not surprising and includes shock absorption, improvement of fit between surfaces, facilitation of combined movements, checking of translation at joints such as the knee, deployment of weight over larger surfaces, protection of articular margins, facilitation of rolling movements, and spread of lubricant. The temporomandibular disc has attracted particular attention because of its exceptional, perhaps unique, design and biomechanical properties. Osborn (1985) has surveyed these properties and examined some factors relating to the *stabilization* of the disc and its possible role as a *destabilizer* of the mandibular condyle, thereby permitting trauma-free complex movements (see p. 580).

In the study of the evolution of articular discs attention has concentrated on equating them with skeletal vestiges, such as the quadrate bone (jaw joint) or the os intermedium carpi (inferior radioulnar joint), and not upon comparative function. Such contentions are usually based on tenuous evidence but nodules of bone, or lunules, do occur in some primate discs but rarely in mankind (Lewis et al 1970). A more interesting comparative functional observation is that joints containing discs usually display combined translatory and other movements (p. 500). For example, in the temporomandibular joint, forward and backward translation of the condyle accompanies angulation or hinging; however, the disc (though usually thin) also occurs in carnivores where such translation is negligible. It is worth noting (Moffett 1957) that, during evolution of mammalian from primitive reptilian jaw joints, the tendon of the lateral pterygoid muscle may have been partially incorporated into the temporomandibular disc; but it is absent in earlier mammals, monotremes and marsupials. Such conflicting observations illustrate how indecisive attempts to elucidate function from morphology often prove. It is more plausible that the pliant and sometimes elastic qualities of discs and menisci provide adaptable surfaces in joints where they occur, facilitating simultaneous movements of different kinds in the compartments of a joint thus divided (p. 579), perhaps also ensuring uninterrupted lubrication (MacConaill 1932). Where translation occurs, complete congruity is impossible except in an (hypothetical) entirely plane articulation, the nearest approximation to this being some sesamoid joints. All articular surfaces exhibit some curvature and translation is always associated with some other movement (p. 500). But translation does occur and intra-articular cartilages may aid in controlling movement from one position to another, as in rolling at the knee joint (p. 707). The tapering profile of menisci enables them to fit between incongruent surfaces, obviating large collections of synovial fluid between them but preserving a filmy distribution over the articular surfaces. Advantages of this in damping turbulence and drag are in keeping with the lubrication theory.

A complete articular disc in effect creates two joints in series, comparable with concatenations of multiple joints, whose individual small ranges of movement nevertheless summate. This arrangement occurs in the carpus and tarsus but is carried further in multiplication of interphalangeal joints in flippers of extinct aquatic reptiles and extant aquatic mammals such as some whales. By such analogy one may liken the talus of some mammals to a meniscus, in terms of function; it is equally tempting to equate some menisci with degenerate skeletal elements. The various views propounded are not reciprocally exclusive; discs may have evolved by more than one route, just as they may contribute in more than one way to the smooth and efficient performance of synovial joints.

The functions of two other quite common types of intra-articular structure (*labra* and *fat pads*) are also uncertain. A labrum is a fibrocartilaginous annular *lip*, usually triangular in cross-section like a meniscus, attached to an articular margin (e.g. the glenoid fossa and acetabulum) deepening the socket and increasing the area of contact. It may act as a lubricant spreader and, like menisci, may also reduce the synovial space to capillary dimensions, thus limiting drag. However, unlike menisci, labra are not compressed between articular surfaces. Small *fibrous labra* (*connective tissue rims*) have been described along the ventral or dorsal margins of the zygapophyseal joints at lumbar levels as well as meniscus-shaped *fibro-adipose meniscoids* at the superior or inferior poles of the same joints. (For brief comments and references see p. 514.) Fat pads are closely associated with synovial membrane, with which they are therefore described (p. 497).

EVOLUTION OF SYNOVIAL JOINTS

Much speculation, observation and experiment have been directed to the mechanics of synovial joints by anatomists, orthopaedic specialists, physicists and engineers. The basic problem is to convincingly account, in terms of movement, loading and lubrication, for the efficiency by which joints preserve smoothness of action under most conditions, except when diseased. Lubrication theory has yet to explain the outstanding effectiveness of synovial joints, although progress has been made (p. 498).

What are the advantages of sliding articulations? That these are considered is shown by the increasing dominance of synovial joints in vertebrate phylogeny. Evolution of joints has attracted little attention; few joints or vertebrate groups have been systematically studied. Synovial articulation occurs as far down the scale as lungfish (Dipnoi), especially in joints of jaws (Haines 1942b). Hence, the synovial joint is not particularly novel, in general features at least. Nevertheless, most movable bony junctions in piscine ancestors of land vertebrates were simpler, as in surviving species. These simpler joints may illustrate stages in the development of synovial joints. Fibrous and cartilaginous joints may be assumed to be the simplest and probably primary form, the next step being the appearance of multiple fluid-filled cavities in the deformable tissue. A further advance is held to be union of these into a single joint cavity, surrounded by a substantial cuff of tissue uniting the skeletal components involved. This pattern resembles cavitated symphyses (p. 491). Finally, complete dissolution of continuity between bones would markedly increase range of movement. With subsequent development of a synovial stratum and a fibrous capsule, the fluid-containing cavity is confined and the fluid reduced to a mere film between surfaces approximated in smooth, sliding contact.

Examples of all such stages occur in living vertebrates; interestingly synovial joints in more primitive land animals, although they replace other arrangements in limb articulations, are in some respects inferior to piscine mandibular joints, which may have been the first vertebrate articulations refined to synovial status.

The stages considered above accord with major events in prenatal development of human synovial joints. Perhaps most significant is breakdown of interzonal mesenchyme (p. 292) to form a presumptive synovial cavity. Potentiality of mesoderm for cleavage (forming considerable cavities or clefts between surfaces in contact and hence mobilized) is clearly significant to the evolution of synovial joints. In addition to established mesodermal discontinuities, including the whole range of coelomic and synovial arrangements, fully differentiated connective tissue retains this potentiality, revealed in the occurrence of such acquired structures as adventitious bursae and pseudarthroses. It is reasonable to suppose that, once a region of pliant connective tissue is established between rigid skeletal elements, the ultimate appearance of a synovial cavity is an evolutional and mechanically significant probability.

It is considered likely that synovial joints have developed not only as discontinuities in skeletal bars but also by approximation of separate elements. Mammalian tibiofibular joints may have thus evolved, the bones being out of contact in reptiles; but these synovial arrangements are probably extensions of the knee and ankle joints and not new formations. A better example, perhaps, is the occasional synovial joint between clavicle and coracoid process (p. 622; Lewis 1959), which may consist merely of a bursa or, more frequently than either arrangement, a fibrocartilaginous junction; an excellent example of lability of joints in occurrence and structure. A synovial joint such as the sacroiliac may regress to a simpler form and may, like others such as interphalangeal, carpal and tarsal articulations, disappear entirely either by synostosis in individuals or as an evolutionary phenomenon. The avian tibiotarsus and tarsometatarsus illustrate reunion of once separate bones; the opposite tendency, towards multiplication of elements by new joint formation, is apparent in phalangeal patterns in the paddle-like extremities of some aquatic mammals and extinct reptiles.

Evolution of synovial joints at the mammalian level shows two tendencies. Firstly, their number increases by replacement of non-synovial joints, particularly in limbs, eventually reaching their smallest terminal articulations. Secondly, synovial joints increasingly specialize, particularly by limitation of movement to that habitually required. A typical non-synovial joint, such as a symphysis, is essentially multiaxial, however limited in range; its movements are basically angulation, torsion or rotation ('swing' and 'spin', see p. 505) and 'translation'; all other movements are combinations of these. From the restricted data available, the earliest synovial joints are likely to have had the same repertoire, with improvement in range and smoothness. The ancestral vertebrate limb probably had joints approximating to a 'ball-and-socket' form; palaeontological data and synovial joints in extant primitive amphibians and reptiles support this supposition. This view also entails that proximal joints have remained less specialized than those more distal; they certainly are closer to multiaxial activity. A multiaxial joint requires more complex muscular control than a biaxial, in which more reliance can be placed on ligaments, an advantage even greater in uniaxial joints. The advantage holds both in dynamic and static situations: when a multi- or biaxial articulation is moving uniaxially, muscles must be used to prevent unwanted movement about other axes. Similarly, when a joint is to be held static in a particular posture or as an adjunct to some other phase of movement, this is achieved more economically if the joint surfaces and disposition of associated ligaments limit movement in some directions. Unless this interferes with overall activity, the trend is towards uniaxial function and this

appears to be the evolutionary tendency in limbs. This is tantamount to saying that joints are adapted to motions required in the behaviour of a particular animal form. To extend the argument, a joint may even disappear if its activity ceases; examples have occurred in many mammals; in the human skeleton the process appears as synostosis of sternal and sacral segments, conferring rigidity on joints having a limited degree of mobility in some other mammals.

Refinement of a joint, in limitation of direction and range of movement to whatever is habitually required, favours skilled control and the most advantageous distribution of available muscle power. Bulky muscles around a joint may impede it; it is an advance if restraining activities can be transferred from muscles to ligaments and articular geometry. Joints may be arrested in temporary but prolonged static positions, as required of the human hip and knee in standing. If joints can be maintained in a nearly close-packed position (p. 509) by gravity, muscular effort can be reduced, for example in the usual human mechanism of standing (p. 897). This commonly cited example of joint control suggests a concept of *stability* at joints, with its associated static implications. Joints are, however, primarily *dynamic*; during movement qualities stabilizing them in one position are equally important in controlling transit from one position to another. In the medical context it is natural to view these factors as preserving articular *integrity*—a clinical approach deviating more towards factors preventing dislocation than towards functional interpretation of structure. Synovial joints of higher vertebrates are precisely engineered to accomplish habitual movements with greatest efficiency commensurate with the resources available; but, before analysis of individual joints, the intimate structure of the tissues of synovial joints must be considered.

STRUCTURE OF SYNOVIAL JOINTS

Articular surfaces

Articular surfaces are mostly formed by a special variety of *hyaline cartilage* reflecting their preformation as parts of cartilaginous models in embryonic life (Barnett et al 1961; Ghadially & Roy 1969). As exceptions to this, surfaces of the sternoclavicular and acromio-clavicular joints and both temporomandibular surfaces are of dense fibrous tissue, with isolated groups of chondrocytes and little surrounding matrix, reflecting their formation by *intramembranous* ossification. However, to regard cartilage of most articular surfaces as unmodified hyaline cartilage and merely the unossified surface sectors of growing cartilaginous models ignores its special features. In long bones articular cartilage is a specialized tissue long before the subjacent bone has ossified (Davies & Edwards 1948); the organization of mature articular cartilage is distinctly radial, with variation in cellular type and arrangement, fibrous architecture and calcification at varying levels from its surface. (Split-line phenomena in articular cartilage and their relations to structural properties are discussed on p. 451. Examples of split-line patterns in an ankle joint are shown in **6**.70.)

Articular cartilage has a wear-resistant, low-frictional, lubricated surface, slightly compressible and elastic and thus ideally constructed for easy movement over a similar surface but also able to absorb large forces of compression and shear generated by gravity and muscular power, qualities specially important at one extreme of a joint's most habitual movement, the so-called 'close-packed position' (p. 509).

The thickness of articular cartilage is said to range from 1 to 2 mm, but this is more typical of small bones in aged individuals; in youth it may reach 5–7 mm in larger joints; such young cartilages are typically white, smooth, glistening and compressible. Ageing cartilages are thinner, less cellular, firmer and more brittle, with a less regular surface and a yellowish opacity. The 'glassy' moistness of fresh, wet articular cartilage and early measurements supported the early impression of smoothness. Later, several authors emphasized the microscopic roughness of its free surface (Dowson et al 1969; Longfield et al 1969), said to be much inferior to mechanical bearings; but when covered by synovial fluid the surface has a very low coefficient of friction. Under load, 'troughs' between 'crests' in the surface have been considered to trap pools of synovial fluid. McCutchen (1959) proposed a porous nature (with a pore size of 6 nm) like a sponge, saturated at rest with synovial fluid; increasing

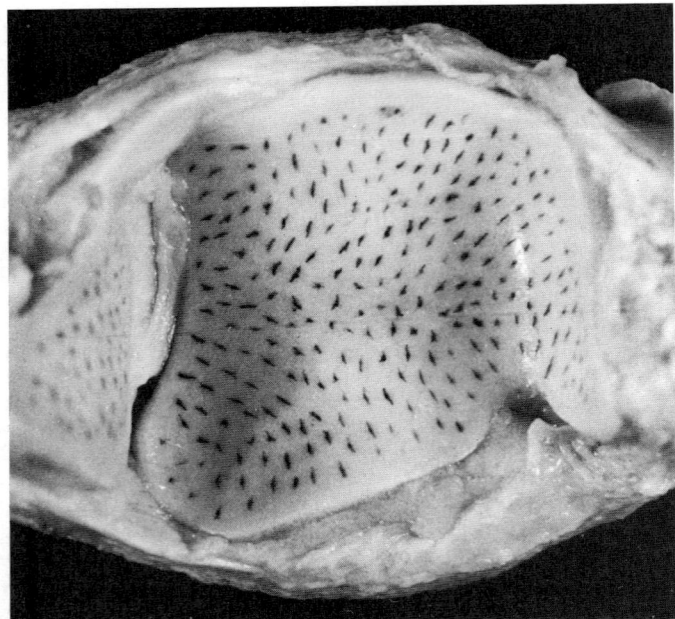

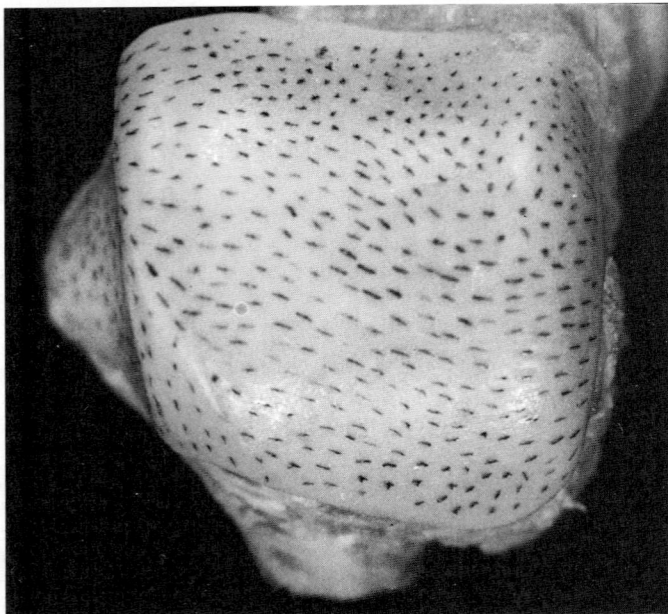

6.70 Articular surfaces of the left ankle joint demonstrating the patterns of split-lines in the articular cartilages produced by multiple insertions of a round-bodied needle, previously immersed in Indian ink. *Above*, tibiofibular mortice; note interosseous and inferior transverse tibiofibular ligaments. *Below*, superior (tibial) and lateral (fibular) surfaces of the talus. For possible significances of split-line configurations, see p. 451. (Photographs by Kevin Fitzpatrick, Guy's Hospital Medical School, London.)

load and compression was presumed to allow fluid to 'weep' from this porous surface. Using lubrication modelling, porosity has been shown to deplete rather than increase the lubricant film thickness, particularly when film thickness becomes small (Jin et al 1992). Scanning electron microscopy renewed interest in these surfaces. Although many described patterns of undulation as constant features in detached blocks of articular cartilage, undulation was not apparent in cartilage still attached to bone (Clarke 1973a; Ghadially et al 1976; Ghadially 1983), casting doubt on the 'enrichment theory' of joint lubrication. Small shallow pits, considered to overlie groups of chondrocytes in adult cartilage (Clarke 1973a,b; Ghadially et al 1976) and small 'humps' of similar size in juvenile cartilage are also likely to be artefactual due to differential shrinkage of cells and intercellular matrix during specimen preparation and examination (Boyde & Jones 1983).

Attempts have been made to circumvent such difficulties by studying fresh necropsy specimens of weight-bearing areas of lateral femoral condyles by interference fringe microscopy (Longmore 1976; Longmore & Gardner 1978). They reported primary anatomical contours, secondary undulations of 100–500 μm crest to crest; tertiary cell-related shallow hollows 20–50 μm in diameter; and quaternary ridges 1–4 μm in diameter and 130–270 nm deep. Even if this surface topography is not in part a superficial drying artefact (Bloebaum & Wilson 1980), the value of observations made on articular cartilage, the total integrity of which has been interrupted, is highly questionable.

Articular cartilages are moulded to bone, but variations in thickness often accentuate subjacent osseous surface shape. Typically, convex surfaces are thickest centrally, thinning peripherally; concave surfaces being the reverse. Precise configuration, degree of congruence in various positions and dispositions of surrounding capsule and ligaments are all related to the types and ranges of movement permitted at a joint. (For a simplified classification based on articular geometry see pp. 500, 505.)

Articular cartilage has no nerves or blood vessels (except occasional vascular loops reaching and even penetrating the calcified zone from the osseous side). Nutrition is considered to depend on a peripheral vascular plexus in synovial membrane (*circulus vasculosus articuli*), synovial fluid and blood vessels in adjacent marrow spaces; the relative importance of these is uncertain.

The zone of articular cartilage adjacent to the joint cavity is mainly a layer of collagen fibres arranged in various planes with small, oval chondrocytes lying in the matrix deep to it. Transmission electron microscopy of heavy metal stained preparations shows an interrupted electron-dense surface coat of a particulate or filamentous appearance, generally 0.03–0.1 μm thick, covering it, with a layer of proteoglycan particles and associated filaments occasionally intervening (Ghadially et al 1982). Synovial fluid and matrical lipidic debris, the product of chondrocytic necrosis, may contribute to the surface coat which is ephemeral in nature, the stable, permanent articular surface being that bounded by the most superficial collagen fibres (Ghadially 1983). The 'lamina splendens' appearing as a bright line at the free surface of articular cartilage when oblique sections are examined by negative phase contrast microscopy (MacConaill 1951) is an artefact arising at the border between regions of different refractive index and cannot be taken as evidence for an anatomically distinct surface layer (Aspden & Hukins 1979).

With advancing age, undulations of articular surfaces deepen and develop minute, ragged projections perhaps due to wear and tear. Erosion occurs in pathologically 'dry' joints and where synovial viscosity is altered; but in healthy joints changes are extremely slow. Replacement of eroded surface by proliferation of deeper layers is uncertain; mitoses are absent from adult articular cartilage.

Ultrastructural observations (Broom 1984; Broom & Marra 1986) reveal a highly complex, three-dimensional reticulum of interconnected fibrils in articular cartilage, with obvious functional implications.

Fibrous capsule of synovial joints

The fibrous capsule has parallel but interlacing bundles of white collagen fibres, forming a cuff with its ends attached continuously round the articular ends of the bones concerned, usually in small bones near the peripheries of articular surfaces, but this varies considerably in long bones; in these part or all of the attachment may be a significant distance from the surface. It is perforated by vessels and nerves and may have apertures through which synovial membrane protrudes as bursae. The capsule usually has local thickenings of parallel fibre bundles; such *capsular* (*intrinsic*) *ligaments* are named by their attachments. Some capsules are reinforced or replaced by tendons of nearby muscles or expansions from them. Accessory ligaments are separate from capsules and may be *extracapsular* or *intracapsular* in position.

All ligaments, although yielding little to tension, are pliant and do not resist normal actions, being designed to check excessive or abnormal movements. Ligaments are taut at the normal limit of a particular movement; they are, however, slightly elastic and protected from excessive tension by reflex contraction of appropriate muscles (Smith 1954).

Synovial membrane

Synovial membrane (Barnett et al 1961) derived from embryonic mesenchyme lines non-articular areas in synovial joints, bursae and tendon sheaths; all regions where movement occurs between apposed surfaces are lubricated by a fluid superficially like egg-albumin (hence named *synovia*) secreted and absorbed by the membrane. In joints it lines fibrous capsules and covers exposed osseous surfaces, intra-capsular ligaments and tendons. It is absent from *intra-articular* discs or *menisci* and ceases at the margins of articular cartilages, the peripheral few millimetres of which are a structural *transitional zone* between synovial membrane and articular cartilage.

Pink, smooth and shining, the internal synovial surface has a few small *synovial villi* (Ghadially 1983) which increase in size and number with age. Elsewhere folds and fringes may project into the joint cavity, some constant enough to be named, for example alar folds and ligamentum mucosum of the knee. Accumulations of adipose tissue (*articular fat pads*) occur in the synovial membrane in many joints. Such pads, folds and fringes are flexible, elastic and displaceable cushions occupying potential spaces and irregularities in joints which are not wholly filled by synovial fluid; during movement they accommodate to the changing shape and volume of the irregularities. They increase synovial area and may promote distribution of lubricant over articular surfaces (cf. intra-articular discs and menisci). Synovial villi are normally few but more numerous where the membrane rests on areolar tissue near articular margins and on surfaces of folds and fringes. They increase with age and become prominent in some pathological states.

Synovial membrane varies in local structure. Basically it has a cellular *intima* on a fibrovascular *subintimal lamina* (*subsynovial tissue*) often loose and areolar, but sometimes of organized lamellae of collagen and elastin fibres lying parallel to the membrane's surface, between which are fibroblasts, macrophages, mast cells and fat cells (Davies 1950; Shaw & Martin 1962). The elastic component may prevent redundant fold formation during joint movement, folds which might become compressed between articular surfaces. Sub-intimal adipose cells form compact lobules surrounded by fibro-elastic interlobular septa, which are very vascular and impart firmness, deformability and elastic recoil. Where synovial membrane covers intracapsular ligaments or tendons the subintima is scarcely a separate zone, being merged with the adjacent capsule, ligament or tendon.

The synovial intima (lamina propria synovalis or synovial lining layer)

The synovial intima consists of pleomorphic *synoviocytes* embedded in a granular, amorphous, fibre-free intercellular matrix. There is considerable regional variation in synoviocyte morphology and numbers, which appears to be dependent on the underlying sub-intimal tissue. The synoviocytes of normal human joints form an interlacing, discontinuous layer, one to three cells and 20–40 μm deep, between the subintima and the joint cavity (Castor 1962). They are not separated from the subintima by a basement membrane and are distinguished from the subintimal cells only by their association to form a superficial layer (Henderson & Pettipher 1985). In many locations, but particularly over areolar subintimal tissue, areas free from synoviocytes are commonly found, while conversely over fibrous subintimal tissue the synoviocytes may be flattened and closely packed, forming endothelioid sheets. Neighbouring cells are often separated by distinct gaps but where they approach more closely their processes may interdigitate. The latter situation is common in compact areas of rat synovial intima, where cells may be linked by tight junctions and desmosomes (Roy & Ghadially 1967), although these junctions have not been identified in human synovial tissue (Henderson & Pettipher 1985).

Human synoviocytes are generally elliptical, with numerous cytoplasmic processes (Castor 1962) but can vary considerably in form. They consist of at least two morphologically distinct populations, termed *Type A* and *Type B* (Barland et al 1962; Wynne-Roberts & Anderson 1978; Ghadially 1983).

Type A synoviocytes are macrophage-like cells characterized by surface ruffles or lamellipodia (often described as filopodia, since they resemble these when sectioned), plasma membrane invaginations and associated micropinocytotic vesicles, a prominent Golgi apparatus but little granular endoplasmic reticulum. There is immunohistochemical evidence for the presence of surface receptors characteristic of macrophages on what are believed to be Type A synoviocytes (Theofilopoulos et al 1980).

In contrast, *Type B* synoviocytes which predominate in the intima of most species (Ghadially 1983) resemble fibroblasts, have abundant granular endoplasmic reticulum but contain fewer vacuoles and vesicles and have a less ruffled and branched plasma membrane than the phagocytic Type A synoviocytes. Even when cultured, synovial fibroblasts are phenotypically distinct from ligament fibroblasts in the amount of Type III collagen and hyaluronic acid produced (Murphy et al 1993).

The possibility that precursors of Type A synoviocytes may originate in bone marrow and be part of the mononuclear phagocyte system was proposed by Fell (1978) and demonstrated by Edwards (1982), using genetic markers for tracing cell lines related to mononuclear macrophages in radiation chimeras. The derivation of Type B synoviocytes is still uncertain. Edwards and Willoughby (1982) have shown that in normal synovial membranes Type B cells are derived neither from the bone marrow nor from Type A cells. They could be of local origin from within the intima and be replaced by cell division or, as suggested by Ghadially (1983), derive from a stem cell population in the local subintima. Synoviocytes are not, however, an actively dividing cell population in normal synovial membranes (Key 1932; Coulton et al 1980), although their division rate increases dramatically in response to acute trauma and acute haemarthrosis (Ghadially 1983). In such conditions the Type B synovial fibroblasts divide in situ while the Type A cell population is increased by migration of bone marrow-derived precursors.

The *functions* of the cells of the synovial intima include the removal of debris from the joint cavity (mainly by Type A cells) and the synthesis of some of the components of the synovial fluid (by both types of cells).

Removal of debris. Once a synoviocyte has ingested particulate matter it becomes capable of migrating into the subintima (Vernon-Roberts et al 1976); it is probable that migrating synoviocytes carry ingested material to the lymphatic channels of the subintima which remove it from the joint. Fluid containing protein may be taken into the synoviocytes by micropinocytosis; there is evidence of the removal of injected peroxidase by Type A cells but not by Type B in this manner (Linck & Porte 1981).

Synthesis. It is generally assumed that some of the hyaluronic acid of synovial fluid is synthesized by the synoviocytes, although it could be manufactured by subintimal fibroblasts. There is evidence that, like most mammalian cells, synoviocytes synthesize some forms of glycosaminoglycans (GAGs), including hyaluronic acid (Henderson & Pettipher 1985; Murphy et al 1993). The presence of hyaluronic acid within the vesicles of synoviocytes could be due to micropinocytotic uptake from synovial fluid as well as synthesis by the cells. The ultrastructure of the intimal synovial cells suggests strongly that they are involved in synthesis and secretion, although the nature of the secretory products is not clear. One or both of the synoviocyte types could be involved in the secretion of the proteoglycan-like material, lubricin, which acts as an articular cartilage lubricant; it has been shown to be produced by cells isolated from the synovial membrane and is not produced by fibroblasts from other sources (Swann 1982). Synoviocytes also secrete some of the constituents of the extracellular matrix which surrounds them, for example collagen, proteoglycans and fibronectin (Henderson & Pettipher 1985). Type A synoviocytes synthesize and release lytic enzymes during the phagocytosis of joint debris, damage to joint tissues being limited by the secretion of enzyme inhibitors by Type B synovial fibroblasts.

Other functions. Some intimal synoviocytes can present antigens to lymphocytes and can, therefore, rapidly stimulate an immune response to foreign material appearing in the joint cavity (Klareskog et al 1982). They may also have some control over the functioning of chondrocytes; it is known that mononuclear cells secrete cytokines which stimulate chondrocytes to degrade their matrix (Jasin & Dingle 1981) and it is probable that Type A cells have a similar function. They may also control blood flow in the synovial membrane by the release of prostanoids such as the vasoconstrictor thromboxane A and the vasodilator prostacyclin (Blotman et al 1982; Salmon et al 1983).

Synovial fluid

Synovial fluid occupies synovial joints, bursae and tendon sheaths. In synovial joints it is clear or pale yellow, viscous, slightly alkaline at rest (diminishing in activity) and has a small mixed population of cells and metachromatic amorphous particles. Viscosity, volume and colour vary in different joints and species; it is difficult to correlate these variations with particular joints or with size, weight or exertion. In human joints volume is low; usually less than 0.5 ml can be aspirated even from a large joint such as the knee.

The *physical properties* of synovial fluid include viscous, elastic and plastic components. With low rates of shear, the fluid is highly viscous but viscosity decreases with increased rates of shear, suggesting that in slow movement weight-bearing capacity would be maximal and in fast movement impedance due to fluid drag would be reduced. However, as the product of viscosity and shear rate is almost constant so also is the weight-bearing capacity. Viscosity is very sensitive to changes in dilution and falls with increasing temperature and pH. Elasticity is similarly affected by changes in dilution, pH and temperature but it increases with higher rates of shear, unlike viscosity in similar conditions. Jay (1992) has suggested that viscosity of synovial fluid is not the basis for low friction since synovial joints have negligible sliding speeds and lubricant would therefore be expelled. He concluded that a protein, probably lubricin, rather than hyaluronic acid, is the lubricating factor but that hyaluronic acid amplifies its boundary lubricating activity (Jay et al 1992).

The *composition* of synovial fluid suggests a dialysate of blood plasma, containing protein (about 0.9 mg/100 ml) mainly derived from blood (Swann 1978), and added mucin, mostly hyaluronate, a sulphate-free glycosaminoglycan containing equimolar concentrations of glucuronic acid and N-acetylglucosamine; much evidence shows its viscoelastic and thixotropic (plastic) properties as largely due to hyaluronate content. Synovial mucin has been variously considered an attrition product of articular cartilage matrix, a secretion of subintimal mast cells, or a product of Type A or B synovial cells.

Synovial fluid protein is partly free and partly bound to GAGs, including hyaluronate. Much appears to be of haematogenous origin, the relative concentration of the individual proteins probably depending on their molecular weights and on the permeability of the synovial vessels (Swann 1978). The protein associated with hyaluronate may be either loosely or firmly bound. About 10–30% of the loosely bound protein is derived from blood plasma, as is most of that firmly bound (termed hyaluronate-protein). The remainder of the latter (some 2%) differs from plasma protein and is probably produced by synovial intimal cells. Approximately 0.5% of synovial fluid protein can be separated as a lubricating glycoprotein fraction that lubricates articular cartilage like whole synovial fluid. Although hyaluronic acid is an efficient lubricator of soft connective tissues, including synovial membrane, tests have shown that it is ineffective on articular cartilage, where the lubricating glycoprotein appears to be uniquely involved (Swann 1978, 1982).

Phosphatidylcholine, the major lipidic component of synovial fluid, has also been proposed as a boundary lubricant for articular cartilage that may also act as a protectant to the joint surface (Williams et al 1993).

The origin of non-haematogenous proteins of synovial fluid is uncertain but the ultrastructure of the Type B cells of the synovial intima is typical of that of cells manufacturing and secreting protein, suggesting that they may be sources of at least some of them.

The small tally of cells (about 60 per ml in resting human joints) includes monocytes, lymphocytes, macrophages, synovial intimal cells and polymorphonuclear leucocytes (Bauer et al 1940). Higher counts, characteristic of youth and of other species, may be due to more active movements before sampling. The amorphous, metachromatic particles and fragments of cells and fibrous tissue in synovial fluid are considered to be due to wear and tear.

Functions of synovial fluid include provision of a liquid environment with a small range of pH, and, for joint surfaces, nutrition of articular cartilages, discs and menisci, and lubrication and reduction of erosion. Its nutritive role, compared with direct diffusion from vascular plexuses, is uncertain. Despite general agreement on its lubricant value, details of its actions are still disputed.

Models proposed for *lubrication* in joints have largely paralleled current advances in engineering physics. First proposed was '*fluid film*' or '*hydrodynamic lubrication*', familiar in engineering, bearing surfaces being separated by a substantial layer of lubricant, its effectiveness depending on the rheological properties of the fluid in bulk. Later theoretical refinement included consequences of fluid elasticity, the '*elastohydrodynamic model*'; but criticism of suitability of the articular environment for simple fluid-film lubrication arose and '*boundary lubrication*' was proposed, in which properties of the solid surfaces are combined with those of extremely thin layers of lubricant molecules. '*Weeping lubrication*' followed, in which the porous, fluid-filled deformable nature of the articular surface was emphasized; it was proposed that surfaces under load were lubricated by a film of fluid expressed from the '*pores*'. Then '*boosted lubrication*' came forward suggesting that compression of articular cartilages traps fluid pools in irregularities of their surfaces; increasing compression is supposed to force a small-moleculed, mobile fraction of synovial fluid into the cartilage contact area, fluid left in the 'valleys' becoming increasingly enriched in hyaluronate and hence more viscous and thus a more effective and protective lubricant. However, ridges and valleys are probably artefacts and 'pits' and 'humps' in vivo are not proven. Considering the wide variation in joint geometry, structure and activity, it seems likely that multiple mechanisms may operate under different conditions.

Synovial membrane not only **produces** fluid but also **removes** materials from articular cavities. Small molecules of crystalloids and soluble dyes can cross it directly into subintimal capillaries and venules, the former fenestrated according to Kos (1970). Particles pass into subintimal lymphatic capillaries for transport to regional lymph nodes. Intra-articular introductions of tracers, such as thorotrast, colloidal carbon and ferritin, studied by electron microscopy, have revealed the marked phagocyte powers of Type A synovial cells, which rapidly enclose particles in phagocytic vesicles. The source of subintimal macrophages is uncertain; some may enter joints from blood but many are probably Type A cells of intimal origin which enter subintimal tissues (Ghadially & Roy 1969).

CLASSIFICATION AND MOVEMENTS OF SYNOVIAL JOINTS

Several criteria have been used in classifying synovial joints and their movements; but these differ in universality, scientific accuracy and utility. They include complexity and number of articulating surfaces, number and position of principal axes of movement, general geometry of surfaces and major movements and association of more precise geometry with analysis of movements as bases for *human kinesiology*. This can be considered only briefly here; detailed accounts are available (Steindler 1955; Barnett et al 1961; MacConaill & Basmajian 1977).

Complexity of form. Most synovial joints have two surfaces (**male** and **female**) and are *simple* articulations. In some one surface is wholly *convex* (male) and greater in area than its opposing *concave* (female) surface; in a few, both are *concavoconvex*, the larger being considered male. A joint with more than two surfaces is *compound*, for example, the elbow. (The humerus presents two male surfaces, capitulum and trochlea, which 'mate' with the radial and ulnar female surfaces. The convex (male) circumference of the radial head also 'mates' with the concave (female) radial notch of the ulna.) In all compound joints articulating territories remain distinct; male surfaces never pass on to female surfaces of an adjoining pair. When a joint contains an intra-articular disc or meniscus it is *complex*.

Degrees of freedom. Analysis of positional changes of one of a pair of articulating bones is often best effected by considering rotations around three mutually perpendicular axes, whose directions may, for convenience, vary with the joint concerned. Often they correspond to the main body planes, i.e. vertical, transverse and anteroposterior axes; but alternatives may be more appropriate; for example, many prefer to consider the movements of the humerus on the scapula around a vertical axis, an oblique transverse axis in the plane of the scapula and a third at right angles to both (**6.71**).

When movement is practically limited to rotation at one axis, a joint is termed *uniaxial*: it has *one degree of freedom*. If independent movements can occur around two axes, it is *biaxial*, with *two degrees of freedom*. Since there are three axes for independent rotation, joints

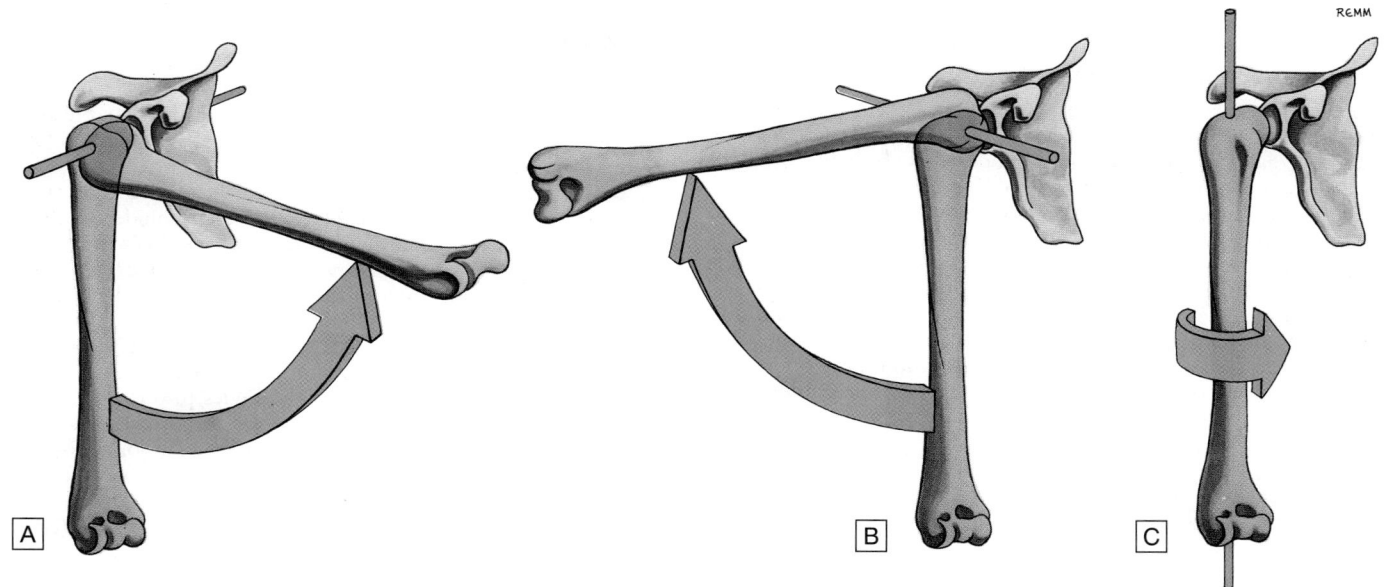

6.71   The shoulder joint is polyaxial and possesses three degrees of freedom. The three mutually perpendicular axes around which the principal movements of flexion–extension (A), abduction–adduction (B) and medial and lateral rotation (c) occur are shown. At the shoulder the axes are referred to the plane of the scapula and not to the coronal and sagittal planes of the erect body as a whole. An infinite variety of additional movements may occur at such a joint, e.g. those involving intermediate planes, or there may be movement combinations or sequences. However, these can always be resolved mathematically into components related to the three axes illustrated.

may have up to *three degrees of freedom*. This apparently simple classification requires amplification.

Firstly, a bone can rotate at a ball-and-socket joint on three main axes **and** any others in intermediate positions. Such a *multiaxial joint*, however, still has only three degrees of freedom; all intermediate rotations can be resolved into components involving **three** orthogonal axes.

Secondly, if movement in one plane is examined throughout its *full range*, a single relevant axis of movement cannot be determined in space but a succession of continuously changing axes ensues as movement progresses; because articular surfaces are not simple, their radius of curvature changes across any profile (p. 505) to a variable extent in different forms of joint. However, a *mean position* of such a moving axis is often '*the axis*' usually described. For many purposes such approximate axes are useful particularly when gross movements only are considered.

Thirdly, simple movements apparently limited to one plane are often in fact compound. For example, what appears simple angulation is often accompanied by rotation of one bone about its long axis, a direct consequence of the complex articular surfaces. When, as is usual, such rotation is not independent, i.e. never isolated, it is not considered an additional degree of freedom (e.g. movements of ulna p. 646).

Fourthly, many movements involve *translation* (which is not included in the above classification): one surface slides bodily across its partner with minimal rotation or angulation (cf. 'plane' joints, see below). Translation, however, often accompanies large angulations (e.g. shoulder joint).

General classification of synovial joints

The general shape of synovial joints has been widely used to classify them, usually into seven varieties. While this has some practical value, it affords no exclusive basis for separation because they are merely variations, sometimes extreme, of two basic forms (p. 503).

Plane joints. These are appositions of almost flat surfaces (e.g. intermetatarsal and some intercarpal joints); slight curvature is usual although often disregarded, movements being considered pure translations or sliding between bones. Nevertheless, in precise dynamics even slight curvatures cannot be ignored (see below).

Ginglymi (hinge joints). These resemble hinges and are shaped to restrict movement to one plane, i.e. they are uniaxial. They have strong collateral ligaments; interphalangeal and humeroulnar joints are examples. However, the surfaces of such biological hinges differ from regular mechanical cylinders in that their profiles are not arcs but varyingly spiral; therefore the main to-and-fro swing includes some (conjunct) rotation (see below).

Trochoid (pivot) joints. Also uniaxial, they have an osseous pivot in an osteoligamentous ring, allowing rotation only around the pivot's axis. Pivots may rotate in rings, as the head of the radius rotates within the annular ligament and ulnar radial notch; or rings may rotate, as the atlas (with its transverse ligament) rotates (carrying the head) around the dens of the axis.

Bicondylar joints. Largely uniaxial, with a main movement in one plane, they also have limited rotation about a second axis orthogonal to the first. The rotation is of two varieties: *conjunct*, an integral and inevitable accompaniment of the main movement; *adjunct* which can occur independently and may or may not accompany the principal movement. They have two *convex condyles* (knuckles) articulating with *concave surfaces* (sometimes also inappropriately named condyles). Condyles may be almost parallel (e.g. knee) with a common fibrous capsule or well apart in separate capsules (e.g. temporomandibular joints) which necessarily co-operate in all movements as a *condylar pair*.

Ellipsoid joints. These are biaxial, with an oval, *convex surface* apposed to an *elliptical concavity*, as in radiocarpal and meta-carpophalangeal joints. Primary movements are about two ortho-gonal axes (e.g. flexion–extension, abduction–adduction), which may be combined as circumduction (see below); rotation around the third axis is largely prevented by general articular shape.

Sellar (saddle) joints. Also biaxial, these have *concavoconvex surfaces*; each is most convex in a particular direction but at **right angles** to this they are maximally *concave* (p. 503). The convexity of the larger is apposed to the concavity of the smaller surface and vice versa. Primary movements occur in two orthogonal planes but articular shape causes axial rotation of the moving bone. Such *conjunct rotation*, as mentioned above, is never independent and is not simply a by-product of 'imper-fect' mechanics but is functionally significant in habitual positioning and limitation of movement (pp. 505, 510). The most familiar sellar joint is the carpometacarpal joint of the thumb; others include the ankle and calcaneocuboid joints.

Spheroidal joints ('ball-and-socket'). Formed by reception of a globoid 'head' into an opposing cup, for example hip and shoulder joints, they are multiaxial, with three degrees of freedom. Their surfaces, although resembling parts of spheres, are not strictly spherical but slightly ovoid. (*Articulatio ovoidalis* is an accepted alternative.) Consequently, in most positions congruence is not perfect, occurring only in one position, at the end of the commonest movement (see below).

Articular movements and mechanisms

Articular movement will first be considered in terms and concepts usual in standard textbooks, followed by a review of the more advanced concepts and theories of modern kinesiology. Articular movements are usually considered to be gliding and angulation, circumduction and rotation. Almost always these four are combined in a variety of ways. Where movement is slight, reciprocal surfaces are of similar size; where it is wide, the bone habitually more mobile has the larger articular surface.

Translation. The simplest motion, it involves sliding without appreciable angulation or rotation. Often combined with other movements, in some carpal and tarsal articulations it is often considered the only motion permitted; but even here cineradiography reveals considerable rotation and angulation of small carpal and tarsal bones during their movements.

Angulation. This implies change in angle between (topographical) axes of articulating bones. Two types are common, especially in limbs, around orthogonal axes:

- *flexion* or bending and *extension* or straightening
- *abduction* and *adduction*.

Flexion. A widely used term, but difficult to define. It often means approximation of two *ventral* surfaces around a *transverse* axis. But the thumb is almost at right angles to the fingers; its 'dorsal' surface faces laterally so that flexion and extension at its joints is around anteroposterior axes. At the shoulder flexion is more reasonably referred to an oblique axis through the centre of the humeral head in the plane of the scapular body, the arm moving anteromedially forwards and hence nearer to the trunk's ventral aspect. Again, flexion at the hip, which has a transverse axis, brings the thigh's morphologically *dorsal* (but topographically ventral) surface to the trunk's *ventral* aspect reflecting rotation of the hindlimb bud in early embryonic life (p. 288). Description at the ankle joint is again complicated by the foot's posture at a right angle to the leg. Elevation diminishes this angle and is sometimes termed flexion, but it is approximation of two dorsal surfaces and might equally be called extension. Flexion has also been defined as fetal posture, implying that elevation of the foot is flexion, a view supported with flexion at the knee and hip, the converse holding in crossed extensor reflexes. Definitions based on morphological and physiological grounds are

thus contradictory. To avoid confusion in this instance *dorsiflexion* and *plantarflexion* are used for ankle movements.

Throughout this section and elsewhere, therefore, it is evident that care must be exercised, when using positional terms, to indicate whether they stem from phylogenetic, ontogenetic or physiological data and how these relate to descriptions of mankind in 'the anatomical position'.

Abduction and adduction. These occur around anteroposterior axes except at the first carpometacarpal and shoulder joints for the reasons stated above. The terms generally imply lateral or medial angulation, except in digits, where arbitrary planes chosen are midlines of the middle digit of the hand and second digit of the foot, because these are least mobile in this respect. Abduction of the thumb is around a transverse axis and away from the palm. Similarly, abduction of the humerus on the scapula occurs in the scapular plane around an oblique axis at right angles to it (**6.71**).

Circumduction. This occurs when the distal end of a long bone circumscribes the base of a cone, its apex at the joint, for example shoulder and hip joints. It combines successive flexion, abduction, extension and adduction.

Rotation. Another widely, but often imprecisely, used term. Its *restricted* sense denotes movement around some notional 'longitudinal' axis, which may even be in a separate bone, for example the dens of the second cervical vertebra ('axis') on which the atlas rotates. An axis may be approximately the centre of the shaft of a long bone, as in medial and lateral humeral rotation (**6.71**). Again, it may be at an angle to the bone's topographical axis, as in movement of the radius on the ulna in pronation and supination, where it joins the centre of the radial head to the base of the ulnar styloid process, and in medial and lateral femoral rotation, where the axis joins the centre of the femoral head to the lateral femoral condyle (p. 687). In these examples rotations can be independent, as *adjunct rotations*, providing an additional degree of freedom. They must be distinguished from *conjunct rotations* which always accompany some other main movement due to articular geometry (p. 505). However, in some articulations *conjunct* may be combined with some *adjunct* rotation and the latter may either increase or nullify the former at different times. Furthermore, with the exception of slight simple translation, **all** movements are in fact rotations. For example (p. 631) medial and lateral rotation of the humerus occur around the bone's long axis (vertical, in the anatomical position); swinging, 'angular' movements (flexion–extension and abduction–adduction) are rotations around the other two axes.

The various techniques for imaging bones and joints are described in terms of their ability to detect different anatomical features: no attempt has been made to give a detailed description of the techniques themselves. A more detailed account can be found in Resnick and Niwayama (1988) or in the introductory chapters of appropriate reference works. In general, the image quality obtained by the different imaging systems depends on a number of factors, including the frequency of the electromagnetic radiation used and the sensitivity of the system employed in recording and/or generating the image. These factors also determine which features within the joint will be seen.

Standard radiography. The most widely available and well-understood method of obtaining images of joints. The

radiograph is a shadow of the X-ray beam as it passes through the joint, with the radio-opaque bony structures appearing white (**6.134, 258–261**) and the radio-translucent soft tissues dark to light grey (**6.95, 290A**). The detailed appearance of compact and cancellous bone, its shape and extent, are clearly recorded on the film with a spatial resolution of 0.1–0.2 mm. Soft tissue evaluation is limited, due to poor contrast differentiation, although in certain instances the extent of tissues such as cartilage can be determined by the configuration of adjacent bony margins in joints (**6.213, 251, 252, 305**), intervertebral spaces (**6.95, 106**) and epiphyseal growth plates (**6.212, 271**).

Arthrography. This is the introduction of either an iodine-based radio-opaque contrast medium and/or radiolucent agent such as air or carbon dioxide, into a joint

cavity to assist in visualizing and/or differentiating between soft tissues. In particular, the extent of the joint space and associated bursae can be evaluated, together with the surface of the synovial membrane, the size of the menisci (**6.317**), intra-articular ligaments and articular cartilage. Tenography is a similar method, permitting the examination of tendons and their sheaths in the hand and foot.

Soft tissue radiography. This allows particular structures in the joints of fingers, wrist, foot and ankle to be visualized by using a low kilovolt (28–35 kV) X-ray unit (Fischer 1988). This method results in a greater contrast between fat and water equivalent tissues and bone. It allows soft tissue detail, such as tendons and their sheaths, ligaments, the joint capsule, and cartilage to be imaged, as well as allowing a more precise analysis of the margins of the thinner portions of bone.

Magnification radiography. An imaging technique which provides the greatest detail of the structural organization of bone (**6.4**B, C); magnification is obtained in one of two ways (Genant & Resnick 1988): either by optical magnification of fine grain contact radiographs, or by direct radiographic magnification using X-ray equipment with a focal spot diameter of 100 μm or less. In the latter, magnification is obtained by placing the object close to the source and projecting the shadow image on to X-ray film some distance away. Of the two methods, images produced by projection radiography have greater spatial resolution and contrast range. The degree of magnification obtained is largely dependent on the size of the X-ray source; the smaller the source, the higher the magnification. With microfocal X-ray units, which have an X-ray source diameter less than 20 μm, high-resolution magnification radiographs of joints are obtained at magnifications of ×10 or more (Buckland-Wright 1989). The detail reported in these radiographs approximates to that of histology (Buckland-Wright & Bradshaw 1989). In addition, all parts of the object recorded in the film are in focus, there is minimal penumbral blurring and, because of the advantages of magnification and high spatial resolution (20–40 μm), accurate and reproducible measurements can be taken of X-ray features immeasurable by any other imaging technique (Buckland-Wright & Bradshaw 1989).

Stereoradiography. Plain film radiographs often contain overlapping structures that can hide features of interest. Stereoradiography is obtained by displacing the tube and/or object between successive exposures; this permits three-dimensional evaluation of the object when the pair of images is viewed stereoscopically. The best impression of depth is gained when the shift between object and tube equates with the parallax created by the interocular distance.

Conventional tomography. This involves the motion of two of three objects—usually the tube and film—while the third object (the patient) remains stationary. In this way the structures in the focal plane are always imaged, whereas those on either side of the plane are eliminated from the image due to blurring. Such systems are widely used in the study of the alveolar process and teeth (**12.50**) and, more recently, with the scanora, in which tomograms are obtained of the temporomandibular joint and skull base in planes perpendicular to those provided by computerized tomography (**6.72**).

Computerized tomography (CT). A radiographic technique in which X-ray images representing horizontal slices through the body are reconstructed by computer from the tissue attenuation of an X-ray beam passing at different angles through the subject (Ridyard 1986) (**6.106**, **169**); the images produced have greater

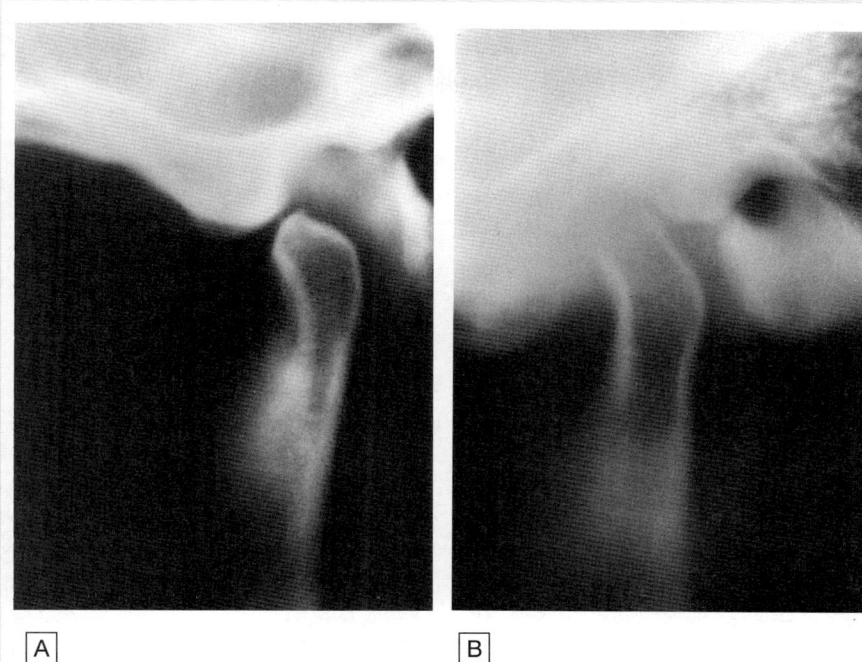

A   B

6.72   Tomogram on the temporomandibular joint showing the position of the head of the mandible with the jaw open (A) and closed (B). (Scanora tomogram prepared by Mr E J Whaites, UMDS, Guy's Hospital, London.)

contrast but poorer spatial resolution (0.4 mm) than standard radiography. The cartilage and cortex of joints such as the hip and knee are poorly imaged in horizontal sections. Three-dimensional computerized image display in sagittal and coronal planes of bones and joints are possible (**6.73**), although the quality of these images is inferior to standard radiography (Martel et al 1991). The particular advantage of CT lies in the study of complex joints, or of those that are difficult to examine by conventional techniques, such as the sacroiliac joint (**6.277**A)

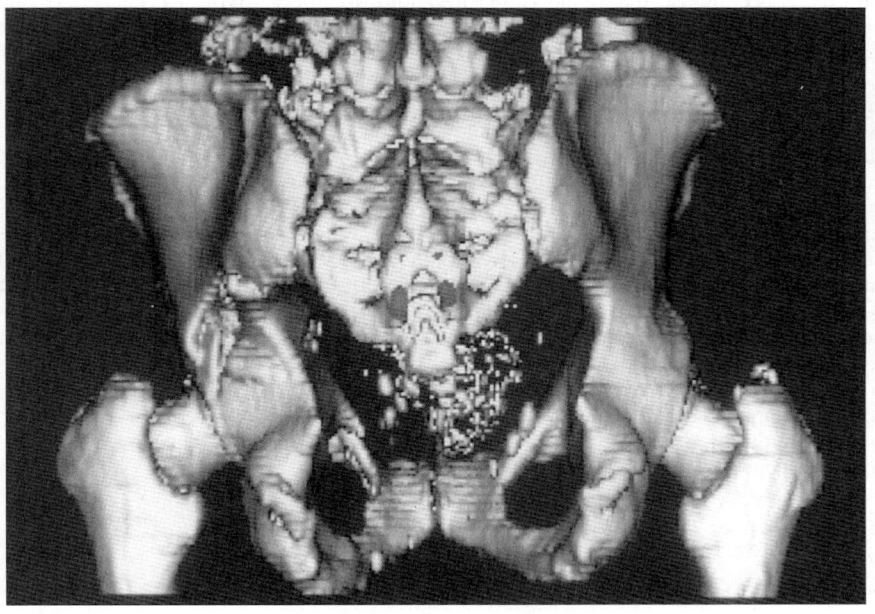

6.73   Three-dimensional computerized image reconstruction of the bones in the pelvic region obtained from serial CT scans. (Image obtained courtesy of Professor R Robb, Mayo Clinic, USA.)

or ossicles within the middle ear. Quantitative techniques have been developed for high resolution CT for assessing trabecular bone structure and mineral content (Genant et al 1987).

Ultrasonography. This is based on the detection of reflected sound waves from joint tissues. The spatial resolution within the image is between 0.2 and 0.3 mm (Martel et al 1991). Its application is mainly in the assessment of the thickness and extent of soft tissue boundaries such as the synovial membrane and bursae in the knee, the synovial sheaths of the hand, or the thickness and surface characteristics of articular cartilage.

Radionuclide imaging. Performed by injecting a radioactive tracer into the body, this process commonly uses one of two tracers: technetium pertechnate or technetium-labelled phosphate compounds. ^{99}Tc-pertechnate reflects blood flow to the synovium and picks up the highly vascular cancellous bone. ^{99}Tc-labelled phosphate compounds have similar functions to those of the pertechnate. In addition, they are absorbed into hydroxyapatite crystals associated with either bone resorption or deposition (Christensen 1985), identifying sites of bone growth (**6.13c**) and remodelling. The localization of the tracer within the tissues of the joint is more readily observed using sectional scanning, particularly in large joints. Quantitation of the radionuclide scan, expressed as the percentage uptake, can be obtained from the amount of radiation emitted from the region of interest.

Magnetic resonance imaging (MRI). A computer-generated image, it is based on the collection of the re-emission of an absorbed radio-frequency (RF) signal while the object is in a strong magnetic field (AMA 1987). The image is obtained from the signal emitted from the protons within the hydrogen nucleus. Sectional images are produced, in almost any plane, of the tissues under examination, providing a combination of both anatomical and biochemical data. Spin echo pulse sequences are generally employed, with images obtained with either T1 weighting, T2 weighting, or both. Using these sequences, hyaline cartilage appears as a grey band of tissue overlying the black line of subchondral bone (**6.74, 316**). Fat marrow appears bright on T1 weighted images, outlining the extent of the cortex and adjacent cancellous bone. Synovial

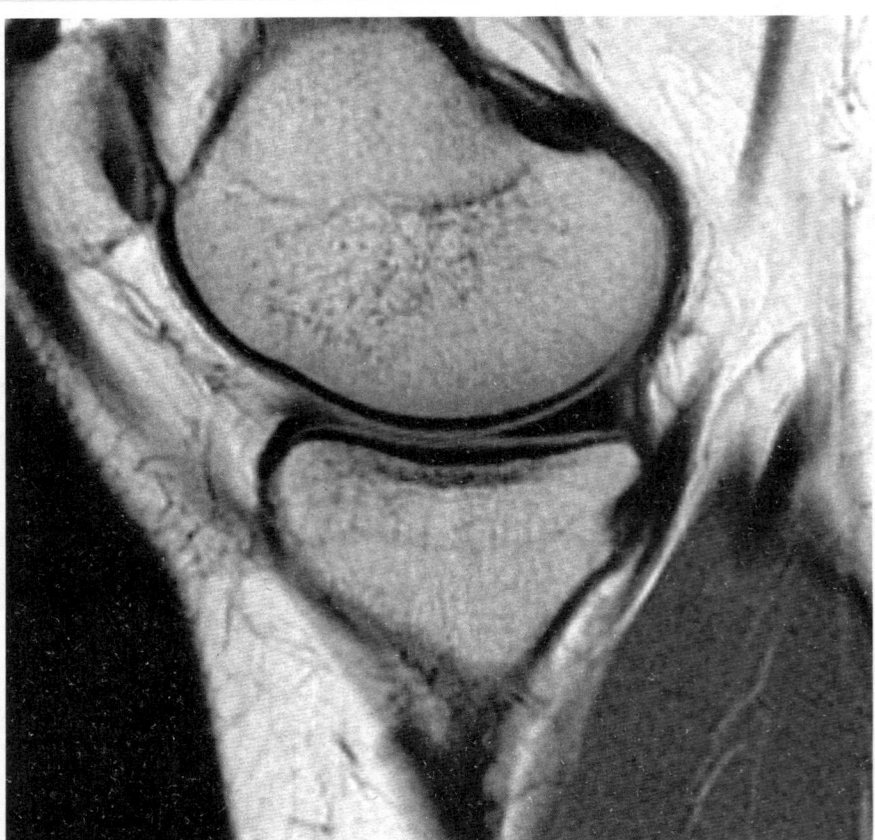

6.74 A T1 weighted MRI of a normal knee through the medial condyle. The articular cartilage appears as a grey band of tissue overlying the cortex, the latter appears black as does the medial meniscus. The fatty marrow has a high signal intensity. (Image prepared by Mr K Fitzpatrick, UMDS, Guy's Hospital, London.)

fluid will appear dark or bright on T1 and T2 weighted images, respectively, whereas menisci, collateral ligaments and tendons all appear dark on both T1 and T2 weighted images (**6.74**). The use of contrast agents allows the technique to distinguish further soft tissue detail as well as the degree of its vascularity. MRI has a spatial resolution 20–30% less than CT, and quantitative methods are still being developed; however, its superior contrast makes it a more effective technique than CT for detecting joint structures. Recent developments in small-bore magnets and RF coils have provided images at high spatial resolution (100 μm).

Multi-model imaging. In general, imaging systems fall into two broad categories: those that simply record ana-

tomical features (such as radiography), and those that detect physiological processes, as seen with radionuclide and MRI. Combining these techniques can provide additional information. With careful registration during the image acquisition process, radiographic and radionuclide images can be superimposed, using computational techniques, to provide anatomical localization of the physiological processes taking place within a joint (Hawkes et al 1991). This approach, together with new methods for quantifying cancellous bone organization (Buckland-Wright et al 1994), will provide investigators with the opportunity to study joint tissues dynamically and in even greater detail.

Kinesiology

The preceding account summarizes views and terminologies evolved over many years by simple observation of articular anatomy and obvious geometrical changes. For many purposes this is adequate. More recently closer attention has amassed more objective observations, experimental results and theory to form an emerging science of *kinesiology*, a branch of biomechanics requiring new terminology, revision of older concepts and unfamiliar mathematical treatments.

These developments are considered briefly here; useful expositions are given by MacConaill (1946, 1950, 1953, 1964, 1966, MacConaill & Basmajian 1977, Steindler (1955), Barnett et al (1961) and Kapandji (1974). Two fields of study are relevant here:

- *osteokinematics* dealing primarily with overall bone movements with little reference to joints
- *arthrokinematics*, concerned with articular mechanics.

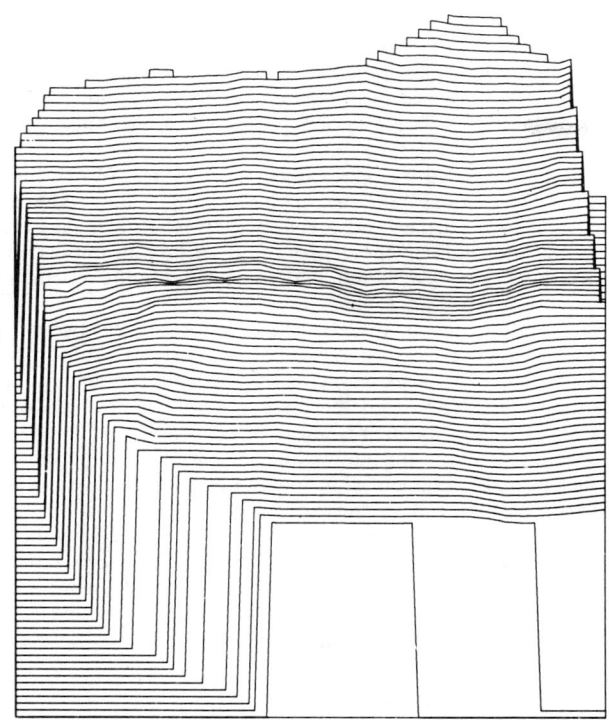

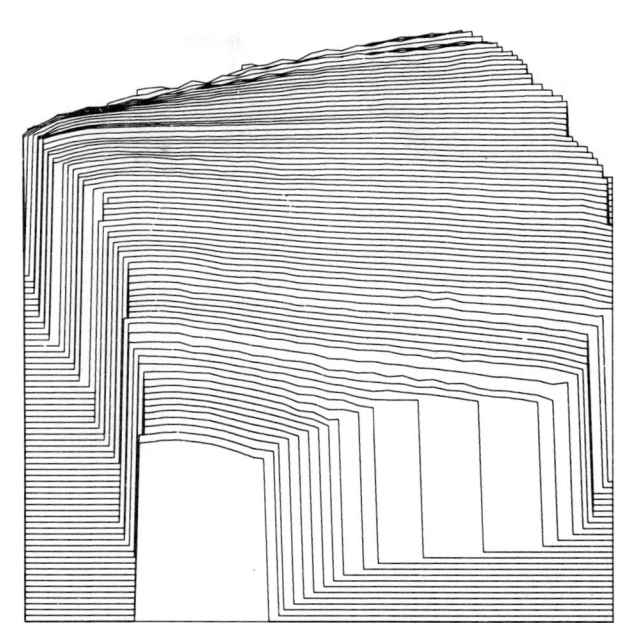

6.75A.   *Left*, a computer reconstruction of a sagitally sectioned cast of the trochlear surface of a fresh human tibia (left side, female, aged 63) viewed posteriorly. The medial malleolar surface is not included. It is a modified female sellar surface and reciprocally curved to its mating surface on the talus. Anteroposteriorly the surface is concave; lateromedially (left to right) there is a central convexity flanked by anterior and posterior concavities.

Right, a computer reconstruction of a coronally sectioned cast of the trochlear surface of a fresh human talus (left side, male, aged 62) viewed

anteriorly. The triangular facet for the 'inferior transverse ligament' part of the posterior tibiofibular ligament has been excluded. It is a modified male sellar surface, which is convex anteroposteriorly; mediolaterally (left to right) it presents a medial convexity, a central concavity and a rather flattened lateral convexity. (Reconstructions provided by A J Palfrey and Linda K Ziemer of the Department of Anatomy, Charing Cross Hospital Medical School, London.)

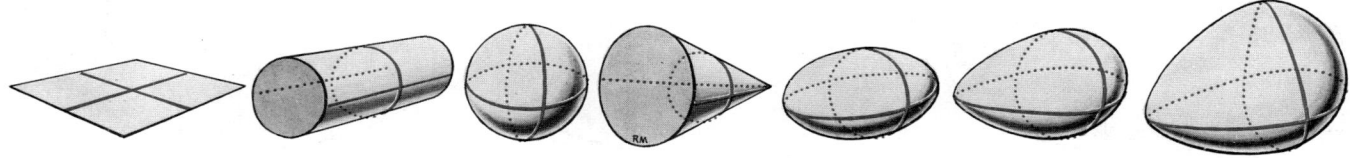

6.75B.   A variety of geometric figures to which reference is commonly made in simple classifications of synovial joints. However, such comparisons are rough approximations only—no synovial joint possesses articular surfaces

which are truly plane, cylindrical, spherical, conical or ellipsoid. Commonplace simple and compounded ovoids are included for comparison.

Certain generalizations about shapes of articular surfaces must be considered followed by replacement of an irregular bone by a single *mechanical axis*—concepts which necessarily precede study of surfaces and movements of particular joints.

The shape of articular surfaces

Although the usual classification of synovial joints into seven types is based on shape, this does **not** entail a like number of fundamentally different surface shapes. Articular surfaces are never truly flat, nor exactly parts of spheres, cylinders, cones or ellipsoids (**6**.75). They are more nearly parts of surfaces of *ovoids* (**6**.75B) or compounded of more than one such surface. When these are either convex or concave, they may be termed male or female *ovoid articular surfaces*. The other well-recognized type is *sellar*, convex in one plane and concave at approximately right angles to this; even here curvatures are convex or concave *ovoid* profiles. Articular profiles vary from nearly flat to nearly spheroidal, but evidence increasingly indicates all to be ovoid or sellar (**6**.76). However, quantitative topology of conarticular surfaces has, for

most joints (especially human), not yet been detailed. Palfrey and Ziemer 1979 (**6**.75A) have attempted such analyses on fresh ankle joints (amputation specimens); a more extensive analysis of tarsal joints has been contributed by Langelaan (1983). In the former study physical damage and desiccation were minimized (but not eliminated) and multiple casts in dental wax were made of talar and tibial trochlear surfaces; coronal and sagittal slices (3 mm or less) were prepared. Multiple points, marked along curved cartilage profiles, were assigned spatial co-ordinates determined by projection and tracing upon grid paper. Similar data were assessed for subchondral osseous surfaces. Subsequent analysis yielded two-dimensional contour maps and three-dimensional reconstructions. Much more exact data of shape, congruence, variation in thickness of cartilage, conarticular surface areas and differences between profiles of cartilage and subchondral bone were obtained.

Certain terms applied to ovoid surfaces and their properties are relevant both to movements of articular surfaces and of whole bones. Two points on an ovoid may be joined by a curved line which is the shortest distance between them, this being a *chord* distinct from any

503

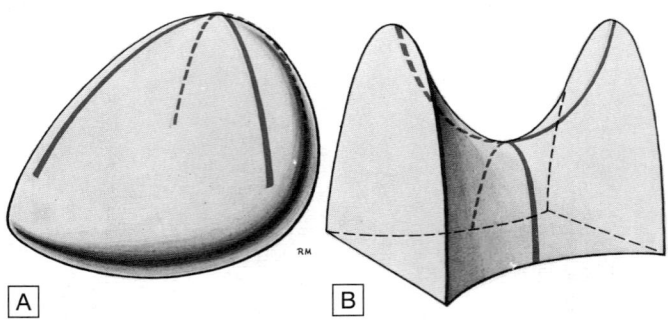

6.76 The two fundamental geometric types of articular surfaces. A. Ovoid, which may be convex (male) or concave (female). Note that the compound solid body illustrated presents different ovoid profiles in two planes at right angles and that the curvatures of the two may be different. B. Sellar or saddle-shaped surfaces, which are concavoconvex. In practice both types of surface may vary from only slightly to highly curved. Thus ovoid surfaces may be 'almost flat' or 'almost spherical' but the majority show intermediate grades of curvature and much variation in change of radius from place to place. Sellar surfaces may also be compound and have a marked asymmetry, e.g. at the ankle and patellofemoral joints.

concept imagine two points on a plane but deformable surface; these may be joined by the shortest route, a straight line, a chord (*geodesic*); **any** longer route may be called an arc (*non-geodesic*). Even if the surface is now formed into a sphere, cylinder, ovoid, sellar surface, etc., the relation between chord (geodesic) and arc (non-geodesic) is preserved.

A figure enclosed by three chords is a *triangle* (**6.77**), the sum of its angles exceeding 180° on an ovoid surface but being less than this on a sellar surface and precisely 180° when it is flat. Deviation from 180° depends on the degree of curvature, an important fact in arthrokinematics (see below). Any three-sided figure in which at least one side is an arc is a *trigone*.

Sectional profiles of ovoid surfaces (**6.78A**) reveal two properties: firstly radius of curvature varies continuously, a profile being considered a series of short segments of circles of different radius and a line joining their centres being the *evolute* of the profile. Rotation of a bone by sliding on such a profile is referrable not to one axis but to successive points on the evolute. Secondly if on a convex ovoid surface a smaller segment of a similarly curved concave surface slides (**6.78B**), the two will fit perfectly only in one position (cf. close-packed position, described below); in all other positions the surfaces are not congruent, the area of contact being much reduced and cuneiform intervals separating them elsewhere. (Theoretically, in a 'perfect', incompressible ovoid, contact would be linear; it is an area because of superficial undulations and the compressibility of cartilage.)

Mechanical axes of bones

Bones are irregular, their articular surfaces bearing no simple or symmetrical relation to their form. Hence comparison of movements of individual **bones** may be misleading in terms of **joint**

longer line joining them which is an *arc* (**6.77**) (MacConaill & Basmajian 1977). Any point moving on an ovoid surface traces a chordal or an arcuate line (or a succession of these), as will be considered further below. This usage of chord and arc is unfamiliar (they are usually applied to *circles* on plane surfaces). To clarify the

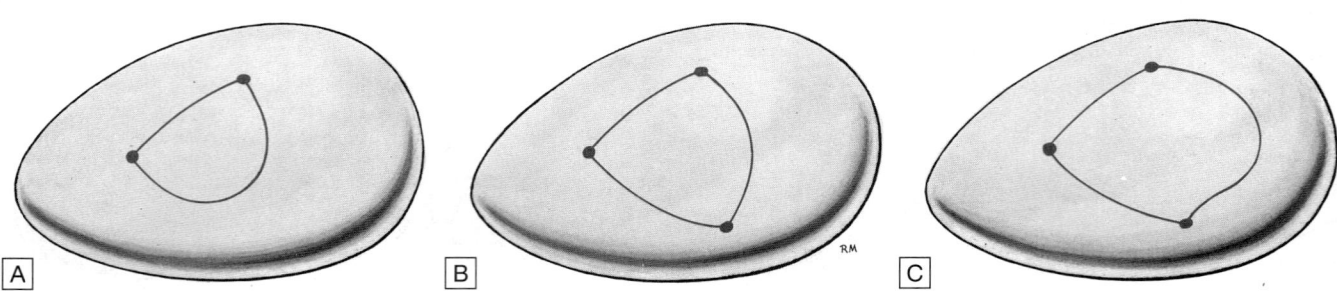

6.77 Geometric paths across ovoid surfaces, and three-sided figures enclosed by such paths. A. A chord (the shortest path between two points) and one example of an arc (any longer path between the points). B. A

triangle enclosed by three chords. C. A trigone, a three-sided figure in which one or more sides is an arc.

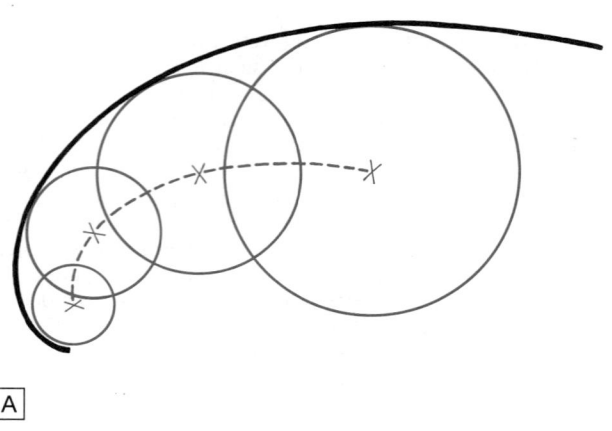

6.78A. Profile of a section through an ovoid surface showing that it may be considered as a series of segments of circles of changing radius. The (dashed) line joining the centres of the circles is the evolute of the profile.

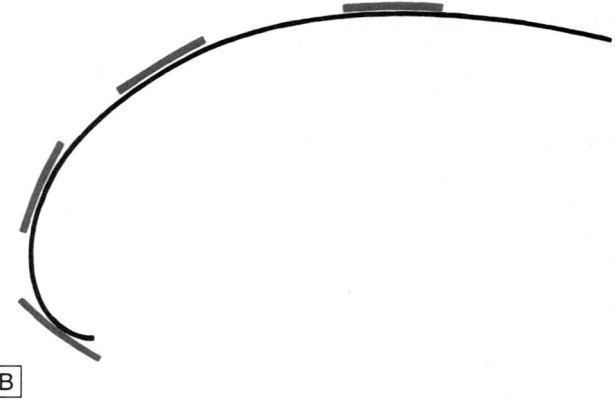

B. A small section of an ovoid profile (red) in various positions; in relation to a more extensive profile (black). The two fit perfectly (i.e. are fully congruent) in only one position.

mechanics. To aid accurate comparison the concept of the *mechanical axis* has been introduced. In **6.79**A a hypothetical, symmetrical long bone is shown with a terminal joint in the midrange of movement: a rod through the bone, ending perpendicular to the articular centre, is its mechanical axis and can represent the bone when *articular movements* are considered; in this special case of symmetry the mechanical axis coincides with shaft. In **6.79**B the joint is again in midrange but the bone is not symmetrical; consequently the mechanical axis and shaft diverge widely: *articular movements* result in similar displacements relative to the mechanical axis, but movement of the shaft is different. (See below for varieties of 'spin' and 'swing'.) Despite the usefulness of a mechanical axis in some analyses, in others it is less so because of arbitrary choice of a 'central articular point', difficult to define with precision. Mechanical axis selection might be better defined as that of *most habitual conjunct rotation*, the limit of which is the *close-packed* position of the joint concerned (see below). In spheroidal, multiaxial joints definition of a **single** mechanical axis may also be an insufficient datum for the many combinations possible.

Movements of bones

Apart from passive accessory movements due to external forces, all others are rotations; since this term is often used in a restricted sense (p. 500), new terms become necessary. Any bone solely rotating around its stationary mechanical axis is said to show pure *spin*; **any** point on the bone, outside the axis, describes an arc of a circle, with the axis as its centre (**6.79**). All other displacements of bone and axis are *swings*, which may be *pure* (**6.80**A) or *impure* when spin also occurs (**6.80**B). (In a spheroidal joint what is virtually pure spin is theoretically possible around many alternative 'mechanical axes'.)

Another useful concept is the so-called *ovoid of motion*: during any swing a point on the mechanical axis, distant from its related joint, describes a curved path in space and all such possible paths (**6.81**) are on part of an ovoid's surface (as would be expected, since they are generated from such an articular surface). Area and shape of such ovoids of motion vary for individual bones and articular surfaces. During any particular swing, therefore, a point on the mechanical axis moves from X to Y on the ovoid of motion either along a chord (a *cardinal swing*) or by a longer route from X to Y (an *arcuate swing*). Synchronously the articular end of the axis traces a reciprocal chord or arc across its opposing articular surface. A consequence of such swings is related to the presence or absence of associated spin: during a cardinal swing along a chord (an unusual movement) there is **no** *associated spin*; in an arcuate swing there must be some spin which is functionally significant (see below). Similarly, spin occurs if a movement involves two chords in series at an angle to each other (one form of *diadochal movement*), for example X to Y and Y to Z in **6.81**.

In some apparently simple swings of bones, spin was long undetected; but its occurrence can be predicted mathematically as a consequence of articular curves and is in most instances verifiable by careful inspection or cineradiography. Diagrams may assist comprehension: in **6.82**A three points, A, B and C, are on the surface of a sphere, AB, BC, and CD being the shortest distances (chords) between them. AB and AC are 'lines of longitude' meeting the equator at 90° at B and C. A model limb moves successively along chords A–B, B–C, C–A; between the initial and final positions it has 'spun' 90° (by which the sum of angles of 'triangle' ABC **exceeds** 180°. **6.82**B shows intermediate 'lines of longitude'; in each case spin equals the sum of the three angles minus 180°. This relation holds mathematically for all ovoid or sellar surfaces. Spin is imparted during the B–C movement (i.e. along a second chord at an angle to the first). An arcuate path may be analysed as a series of chords which change angle. These spins, inevitable in certain swings, are *conjunct rotations* and characteristic of sellar and most ovoid joints. Habitual movements at **all** joints always involve some demonstrable conjunct rotation; an important consequence will be best appreciated after consideration of related movements and 'fit' of articular surfaces (see below).

Beyond these basic arthrokinematics of conjunct rotations it must be added that other rotations (due to the interplay of gravity, external forces and muscle action) are *adjunct*. Adjunct

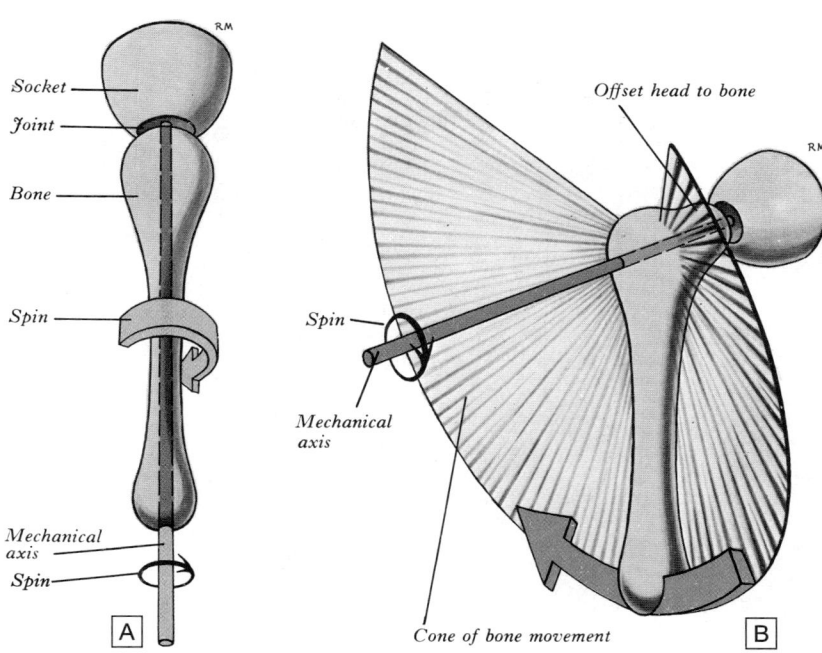

6.79 The mechanical axis: (A) in a hypothetically simple, symmetrical long bone, with a terminal joint; (B) in a bone with an offset head; a 'spin' occurs around this axis; (B) in a bone with an offset head; a similar 'spin' occurs between the articular surfaces, but the shaft of the bone traces part of the surface of a cone.

rotations occur only in joints with two or more degrees of freedom, involving either a bone undergoing **no** conjunct rotation or one in which it must be considered. In the first, factors causing adjunct rotation may generate *pure spin*; in the second, the effects of adjunct rotation may be in the *same sense* (e.g. both 'clockwise'), i.e. additive, increasing rotation and hence termed a *cospin*. Alternatively, adjunct rotations may be in *opposite sense*, reducing or nullifying the effects of conjunct rotation and hence termed *antispins*. Thus a bone starting one or a succession of arcuate swings which, if unmodified, would involve some conjunct rotation may also be subjected to *nullifying antispin*: the latter may be *gradual*, applied throughout movement or *sudden*, near its end. Therefore, while the *path* of the bone is a more or less complex *arcuate* swing, it is modified to become *quasichordal* because there is no net spin.

Movements at articular surfaces

The 'fit' of ovoid surfaces (p. 503) is precise only at one end of the joint's most common excursion, a feature of the close-packed position discussed below. In all other positions the surfaces are not fully congruent, the joint is 'loose-packed'. Changes in congruity are illustrated in the shoulder joint in **6.83**.

Where articular surfaces are not fully congruent movements can be analysed into spin, slide and roll, which must first be considered at a convex (male) surface moving on a stationary concave (female) surface, and vice versa (**6.84, 85**). In most natural movement these are combined (**6.86**). With a moving convex surface, slide and roll are simultaneous but *opposite*; with a moving concave surface they are in the *same* direction; both combinations increase possible angulation, without a comparable increase in articular surface area. The significance of these movements and variations in congruity is best considered with the basic states of 'loose-' and 'close-pack' (see below).

Joint positions

Ovoid or sellar surfaces are fully congruent in only one position, at one extreme of *most habitual articular movement* (e.g. full extension at the knee, wrist and interphalangeal joints, dorsiflexion at the ankle, abduction with lateral rotation at the shoulder). As full congruence is approached, other changes occur: attachments

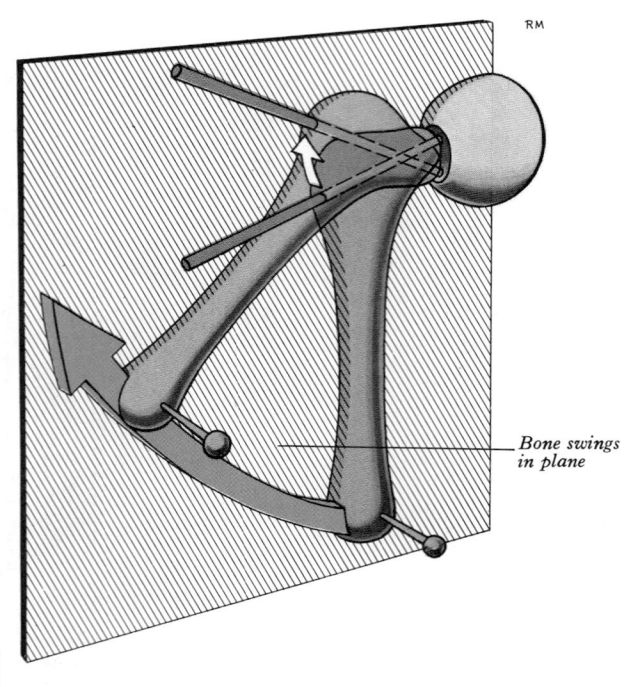

A

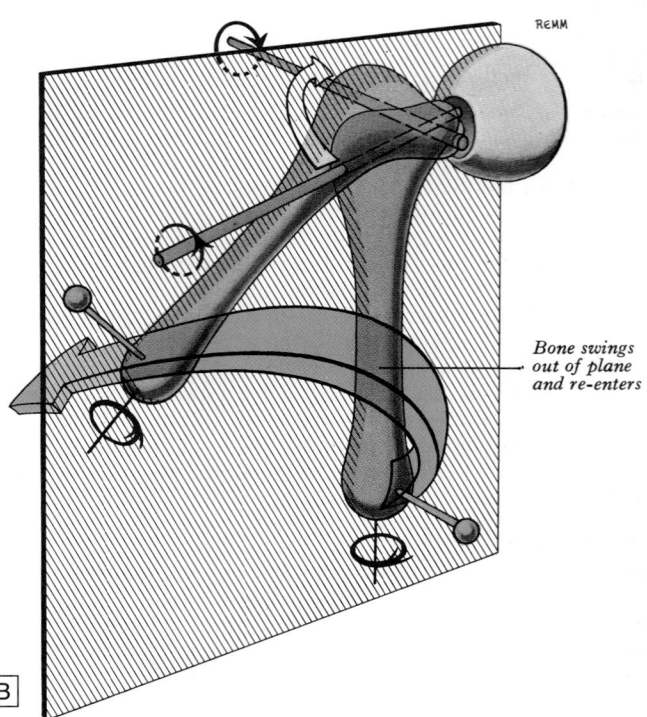

*Bone swings
in plane*

*Bone swings
out of plane
and re-enters*

B

6.80 Further movements of the bone and joint shown in **6.79**B. A. A cardinal swing. Note that the mechanical axis moves in one plane. (Its proximal end traces a chordal path at the joint and its distal end a chordal path on the ovoid of motion, see **6.81**.) There is no spin. B. An arcuate swing. Note that the bone moves out of the plane illustrated and then returns to it. The ends of the mechanical axis trace arcuate paths at the joint and on the ovoid motion. There is an associated spin or conjunct rotation around the *mechanical axis* (and a rotation around the *long axis* of the *bone shaft*).

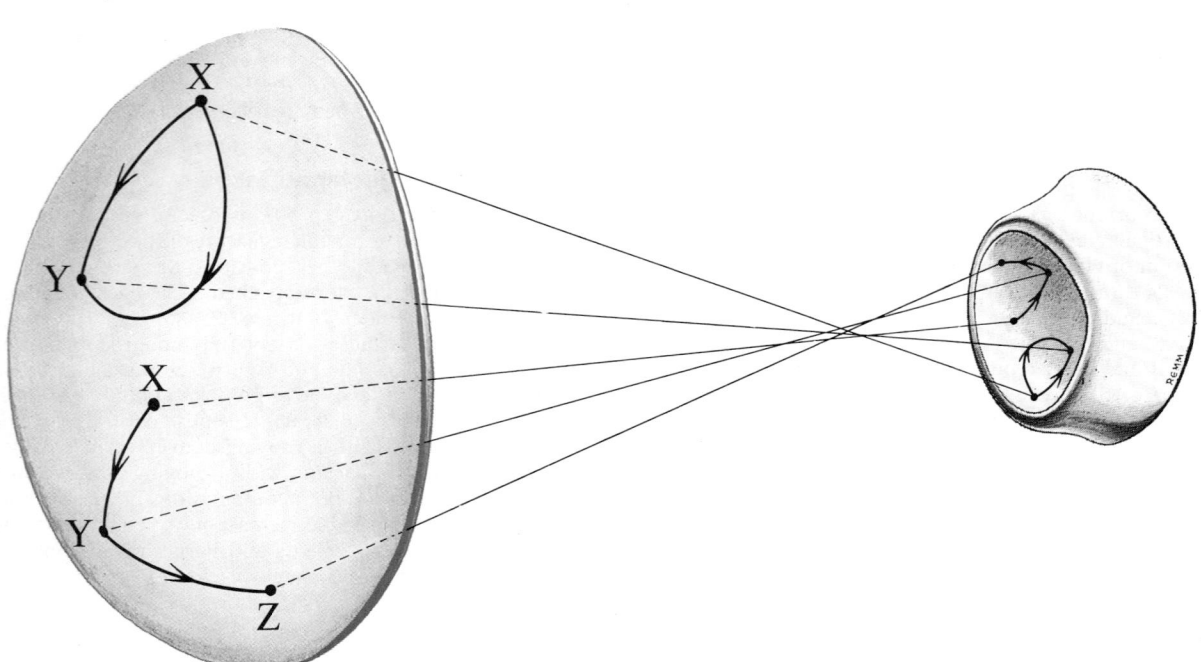

6.81 The ovoid of motion. This represents the imaginary surface which would include all possible paths of a point on the mechanical axis at some distance from its related joint. Two points on the ovoid of motion are joined by a chordal and by an arcuate path, and the reciprocal movements of the end of the axis at the joint surface are shown. A succession of two movements at an angle to each other (i.e. a diadochal movement) is also illustrated.

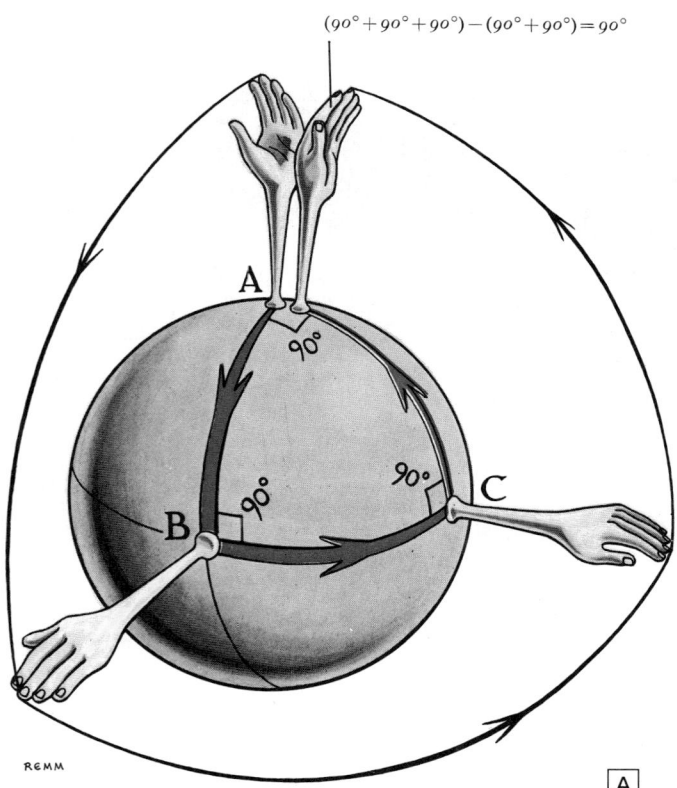

$$(90° + 90° + 90°) - (90° + 90°) = 90°$$

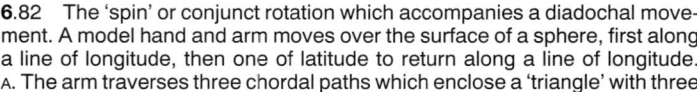

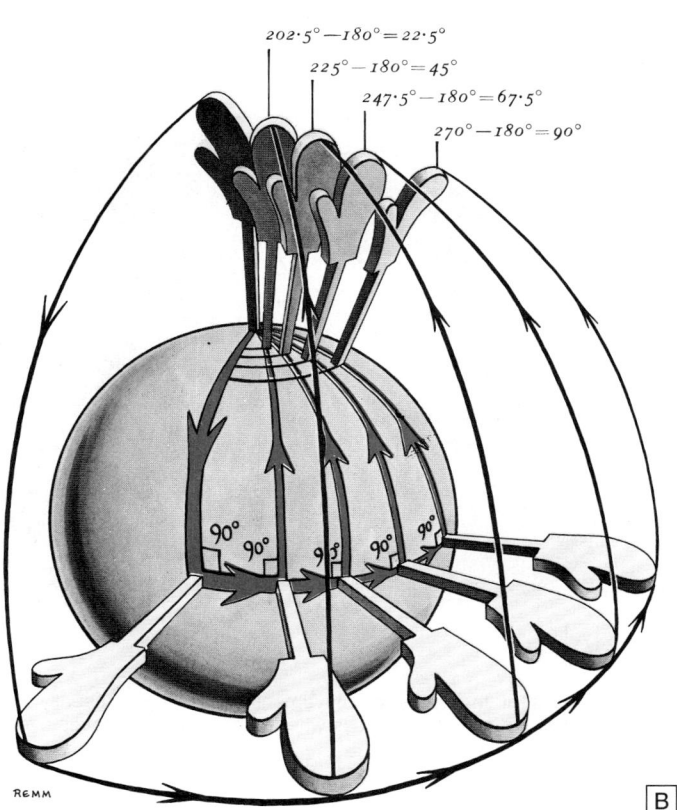

$$202·5° - 180° = 22·5°$$
$$225° - 180° = 45°$$
$$247·5° - 180° = 67·5°$$
$$270° - 180° = 90°$$

6.82 The 'spin' or conjunct rotation which accompanies a diadochal movement. A model hand and arm moves over the surface of a sphere, first along a line of longitude, then one of latitude to return along a line of longitude. A. The arm traverses three chordal paths which enclose a 'triangle' with three right angles (i.e. the sum of the angles = 270°). Note that as it passes along the line of latitude from B to C, a spin of 90° is imparted. B. This illustrates how the amount of spin imparted during a diadochal movement varies with the length and angulation of the second stage of the movement.

of fibrous capsule and ligaments increasingly separate and become taut. The conjunct rotation of all natural movements adds to this by imposing spiral twist in them. In final close-packing, therefore, surfaces are fully congruent, in maximal contact and tightly compressed or 'screwed-home', fibrous capsule and ligaments being maximally spiralized and tensed; no further movement is possible. Close-packed surfaces cannot normally be separated by external force (as they may be in other positions); bones can be regarded as temporarily locked, as if no joint existed. This extreme is only assumed when special effort is required; the rigidity and stresses generated expose articular structures maximally to trauma. Close-packing is a final, limiting position; any force which tends to

further change is resisted by reflex contraction of appropriate muscles. Movement **just short** of close-packing is physiologically most important. Ligaments and articular cartilage are to a small degree elastically deformable and in the final stages the articular position is an equilibrium between the external torque applied (often gravity) and resistance to tissue deformation by the tense, twisted capsule and compressed cartilages. In symmetrical standing, the knee and hip joints approach close-packed positions sufficiently to maintain an erect posture with minimal energy (Joseph 1960, 1975).

In all other positions the articular surfaces are not congruent and parts of the capsule are lax; the joint is *loose-packed*. Capsules are lax

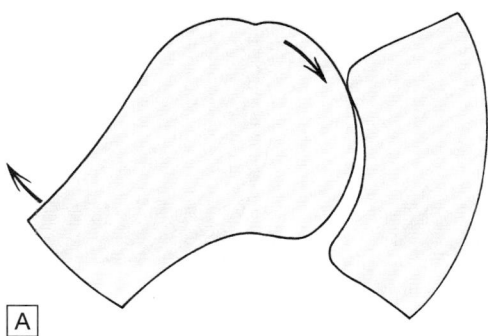

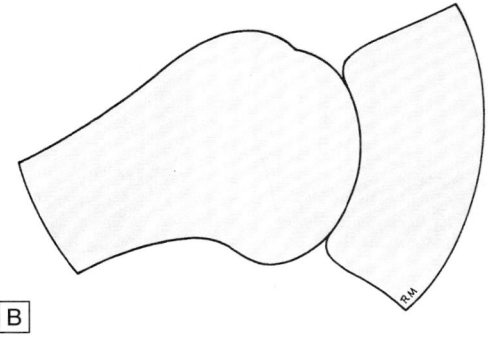

6.83 Congruence of articular surfaces. A. In loose-packed positions of a joint, e.g. the shoulder, the surfaces are not congruent (this has been over-emphasized for clarity). B. The close-packed position of the joint with close-fitting or full congruence of the surfaces.

507

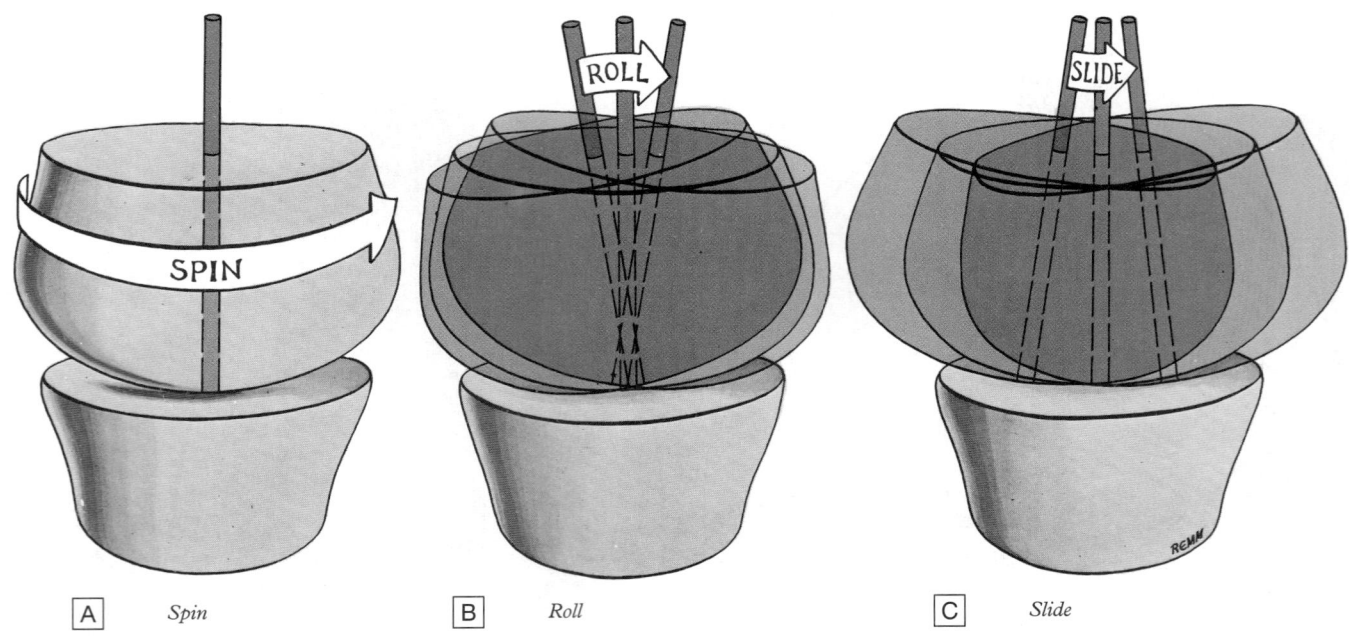

| A | *Spin* | B | *Roll* | C | *Slide* |

6.84 An analysis of the types of movement which occur (usually in combination) between articular surfaces when a male surface moves over a stationary female surface.

enough near the midrange of many movements to allow separation of surfaces by external forces. Congruence in which a convex surface has a smaller radius than a concave one is advantageous: firstly, it allows combined spin, roll and slide, a feature of such joints; secondly, contact area is greatly reduced and variable, which may diminish friction and erosion; thirdly, small cuneiform intervals between the surfaces around contact areas contain synovial fluid,

their shape perhaps a factor in maintaining efficient lubrication and nutrition of avascular articular cartilages; finally, combination of sliding and rolling increases the effective range of movement. With slide or roll alone, this could be achieved only by more extensive surfaces (**6**.86).

According to MacConaill and Basmajian (1977) the close- and loose (least)-pack positions of joints are as follows:

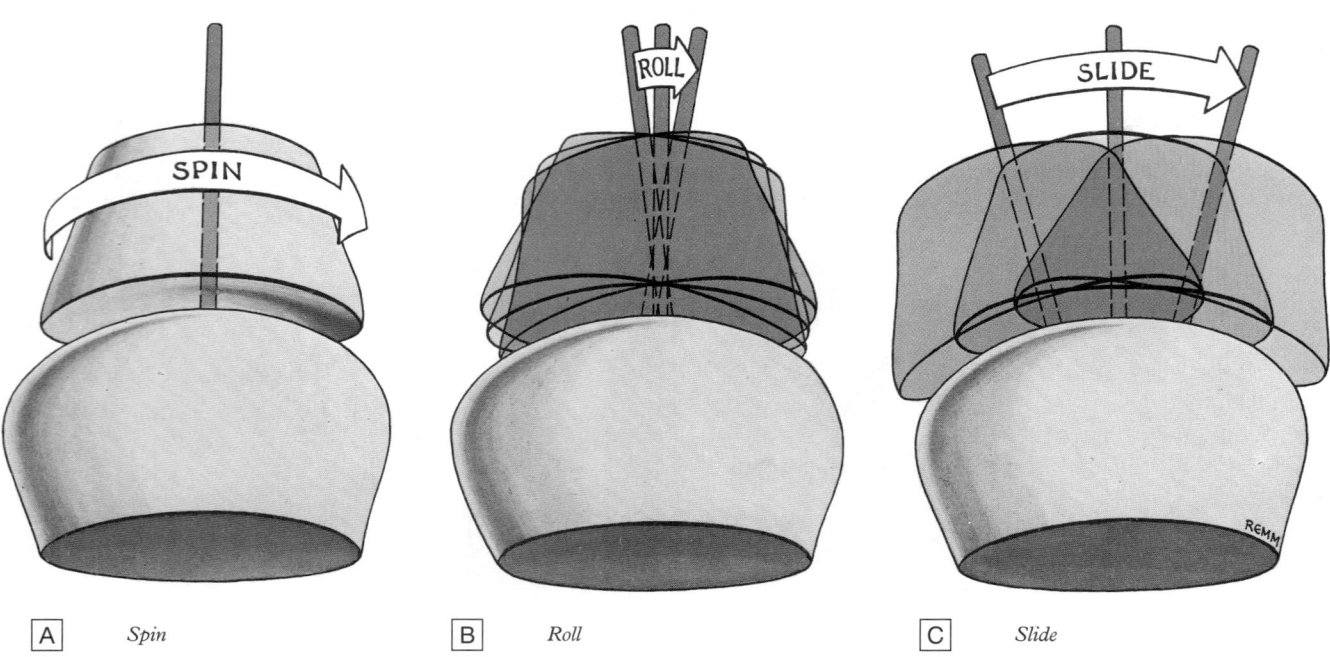

| A | *Spin* | B | *Roll* | C | *Slide* |

6.85 Articular movements. A male surface moves on a stationary male surface.

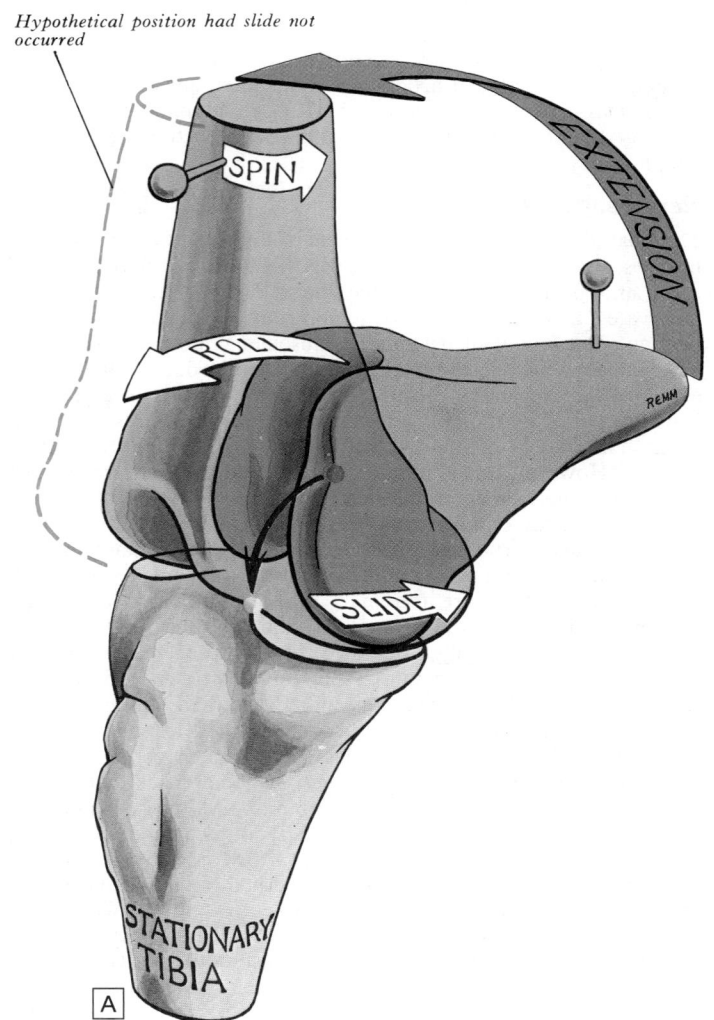

Hypothetical position had slide not occurred

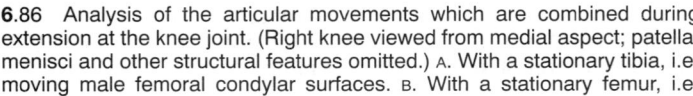

A

B

6.86 Analysis of the articular movements which are combined during extension at the knee joint. (Right knee viewed from medial aspect; patella, menisci and other structural features omitted.) A. With a stationary tibia, i.e. moving male femoral condylar surfaces. B. With a stationary femur, i.e. moving female tibial condylar surfaces. Notice that in each case elements of slide, roll and spin occur together. In A the roll and slide are in opposite directions, whereas in B they are in the same direction. See text for further description.

Joint	Close-packed position	Loose-packed position
Shoulder	Abduction + lateral rotation	Semiabduction
Ulnohumeral	Extension	Semiflexion
Radiohumeral	Semiflexion + semipronation	Extension + supination
Wrist	Dorsiflexion	Semiflexion
2nd–5th metacarpo-phalangeal	Full flexion	Semiflexion + ulnar deviation
Interphalangeal (fingers)	Extension	Semiflexion
1st carpometacarpal	Full opposition	Neutral position of thumb
Hip	Extension + medial rotation	Semiflexion
Knee	Full extension	Semiflexion
Ankle	Dorsiflexion	Neutral position
Tarsal joints	Full supination	Semipronation
Metatarsophalangeal	Dorsiflexion	Neutral position
Interphalangeal (toes)	Dorsiflexion	Semiflexion
Intervertebral	Extension	Neutral position

Opinions may vary in connection with a few of the above positions; for example a 'close-packed' position may possibly occur in occasional joints at **both** extremes of the range of movement. It is also most difficult to assess the situation in small tarsal, carpal and the first carpometacarpal joints. Intervertebral movements are, of course, the result of integrated simultaneous changes at all elements comprising the intervertebral articular complex; i.e. massive symphyses (including the discs), equally massive syndesmoses and the relatively small synovial zygapophyseal joints. Perhaps 'intervertebral' should not be included above. However, most of the positions given above do, it is true, correspond with postures adopted when maximal stress is encountered.

General concepts as set out above have much clarified joint mechanics but aspects of joint lubrication, maintenance of articular cartilage and detailed mechanics of many joints await resolution (Freeman 1973).

Accessory movements. Movements actively performed at any joint do not always include all that its structure permits. Certain movements, voluntarily impossible or limited in range, can only be produced maximally when resistance to active movements occurs (accessory movements, first type); for example, only when a solid object is grasped in the hand can the fingers be *maximally* rotated at the metacarpophalangeal joints (see p. 658). (However, a moderate degree of rotation of the *non-grasping* fingers towards the centre of the palm during flexion and its converse during extension is commonplace.) Some movements can be produced only passively (accessory movements, second type), their widest range being obtained when the muscles of a joint are relaxed; for example, when the supported arm is passively abducted at the shoulder, the humerus can be distracted from the glenoid cavity, a feature of many joints when loose-packed. Such movements are commonly termed 'passive'

509

but all movements, active or not, can be made passively when the muscles concerned are relaxed; the term 'accessory' will be used for all movements impossible in the absence of resistance (Salter 1955).

Limitation of movements. This is due to several factors, of which tension in ligaments is prominent, as is obvious in attempted hyperextension of the unfixed cadaveric knee or hip. Increasing ligamentous tension, balanced by increased compression between opposed articular surfaces, are integral factors in producing close-packing, limiting most habitual movements. But tension of antagonistic muscles is equally important, involving both *passive elastic components* of muscles (and other structures around the joint) and *reflex contraction* when stimulation of mechanoreceptors in articular and periarticular tissues reaches a critical level. Muscles as limiting factors are exemplified in flexion at the hip; with the knee extended it is much more limited in range; with the knee flexed the hamstring muscles are relaxed allowing flexion of the thigh to the abdominal wall, such *approximation of the soft parts* being a third factor in some movements, for example flexion at the elbow and knee. Contact (occlusion) of teeth obviously limits mandibular elevation.

In synovial joints, where bones are connected only by ligaments and muscles, parts of articular surfaces are in constant apposition in all positions. (Some maintain that 'apposition' implies a fine film of synovial fluid, of 10 μm or less, between adjacent surfaces.) Apposition is assisted by atmospheric pressure and cohesion between surfaces, but these are subsidiary to balanced contraction of muscle groups around the joint. When these contract, the force generated is vectorially resolvable into components (p. 787). Some maintain or alter positions of bones ('swing' and 'spin' components) and oppose internal and external resistances, including gravity. Another component is *transarticular* ('shunt' component), which increases compression between articular surfaces and helps apposition in various postures and movements (p. 786). Effects of external compressive or tensile forces, including gravity, vary with body posture and the direction of applied force. Thus gravity or load-bearing may sometimes provide a *distractive force*, tending to separate conarticular surfaces, or may exert a largely *translatory/swing force* between them. They often exert a considerable *compressive force* at surfaces.

Summary. The preceding remarks are merely an introduction to the main concepts of kinesiology. Brief references to myokinetics are on p. 785. For further analyses the references given should be consulted. (Readers with greater facility in mathematics and physics may be interested in attempts to present a 'generalized mechanics of articular swing', ranging from Aristotelian and Newtonian physics to the relativity theory and quantum mechanics; MacConaill 1978a,b,c.)

Blood supply and lymphatics of joints

Joints receive blood from periarticular arterial *plexuses* whose numerous rami pierce capsules to form subsynovial vascular plexuses. Some synovial vessels end near articular margins in an anastomotic fringe, the *circulus articularis vasculosus* (p. 470). A lymphatic plexus in the synovial subintima drains along blood vessels to the regional deep lymph nodes.

Nerve supply of joints

Movable joints are innervated in general by nerves supplying their muscles, probably establishing local reflex loops involved in movement and posture. Although the branches concerned vary, each innervates a specific capsular region but their territories freely overlap. The region made taut by muscular contraction is usually innervated by nerves supplying antagonists (Gardner 1948a,b). For example, the hip joint's capsule, on stretch inferiorly in abduction, is here supplied by the obturator nerve, tension in it thus producing reflex contraction of the adductors, usually enough to prevent damage. However, this is not so at the shoulder, where the axillary nerve innervates the anteroinferior capsular region.

Myelinated fibres in articular nerves have Ruffini endings, lamellated articular corpuscles and some like the neurotendinous organs of Golgi. Simple endings are numerous at the attachments of capsule and ligaments; they are terminals of non-myelinated and finely myelinated fibres believed to mediate pain (Gardner 1950). Ruffini end organs are variably orientated in the knee joint's capsule, principally in its flexor region, responding to stretch and adapting slowly. Lamellated corpuscles, less numerous than Ruffini endings, are sited laterally and adapt rapidly since they respond to rapid movement and vibration; both register speed and direction of movement. Golgi end organs, with the largest myelinated nerve fibres (10–15 μm diameter), are like those at neuromuscular junctions and slow to adapt (Boyd & Roberts 1953; Boyd 1954; Skoglund 1956); they mediate position sense (Stopford 1921–2; Mountcastle & Powell 1959a,b; Gardner 1967) and are concerned in stereognosis, i.e. recognition of shape in objects held (Renfrew & Melville 1960). Many non-myelinated fibres are sympathetic, ending near vascular non-striated muscle and believed to be vasomotor or vasosensory, although evidence is sparse. In synovial membrane no special end organs or even simple endings occur, except near blood vessels, the membrane being relatively insensitive to pain (Kellgren & Samuel 1950; Barnett et al 1961). For a review concerned with receptors and sensation see Wyke (1981); for histological and functional details and classification of articular nerve endings see page 969.

AXIAL SKELETON

INTRODUCTION

Dividing the skeleton into axial and appendicular sections is not merely a convention. The axial structures, cranium and vertebral column and associated ribs and sternum, are primary; the appendicular elements in fins, limbs or wings were subsequent though early additions. Both primary and secondary elements are concerned in elaboration of locomotion. An axial endoskeleton, first a notochord and then a vertebral column, is the basic feature of *Chordata* and their subphylum, the *Vertebrata*, including mankind. A stiff but flexible axis, in bilaterally symmetrical animals that show an early tendency to elongation, prevents telescoping of the body during waves of contraction in successive segmental muscles to produce the sinuous movements, especially in the tail, which are the basic mode of locomotion in aquatic vertebrates. A chain of bones, connected by discs of deformable substance, developed around and largely replaced the notochord. However, notochordal vestiges occur in vertebrae of many fish, amphibians and reptiles, and centrally in mammalian intervertebral discs. This replacement is repeated in every vertebrate embryo. These new vertebral elements are complex and variable in pattern in earlier vertebrates but from reptiles onwards the most basic part is the *centrum*, forming most of the vertebral body, ventral to the spinal cord (spinal medulla). In a typical vertebra a *neural arch*, encircling the spinal cord, fuses ventrally with the centrum and usually bears a median dorsal *spinous process* and paired lateral *transverse processes* just dorsal to the neurocentral junctions. This enclosure isolates the spinal cord from the axial musculature and protects it from external forces, thus insulating its vessels from extraneous compression.

The centrum and each half neural arch ossify from separate centres; when these extend through cartilaginous precursors to meet and fuse, the dorsolateral parts of the vertebral body are formed from the ventral ends of the neural arch. Centrum and body are therefore **not** synonyms, nor is the *vertebral arch* exactly equal to a neural arch. A centrum is somewhat less than a vertebral body, a neural somewhat more than a vertebral arch (p. 532).

Segmental muscles flexing the vertebral axis are only in part attached to vertebrae; in connective tissue septa (*myocommata*) between adjacent myotomes ribs evolve as levers for such attachments. Such costal struts first appeared **dorsally** in the axial musculature and extended ventrally into the body wall in early vertebrates. In fish **ventral** ribs also appeared, which enclosed caudal vessels in the tail. It is generally agreed that ribs of land tetrapods correspond to the dorsal piscine series (Romer 1970).

Ribs are thus intersegmental, and segmental muscles, derived basically from myotomes, bend the vertebral column; vertebrae also become intersegmental, though their embryonic pattern (p. 265) is primarily segmental. In early vertebrates dorsal ribs adjoin most vertebrae, showing little regional adaptation except in the postnatal tail. In land vertebrates, with the elaboration of appendages for locomotion, the vertebral column is adapted to new patterns of force in the distribution of weight and muscular tensions.

In hindlimbs the pelvic girdle articulates with several vertebrae, which fuse with each other and with costal elements to form a *sacrum*. Sacral vertebrae lose *individual* movement; in mammals there are three to five *fused sacral vertebrae*, and distal to these a variable number of *caudal vertebrae*, reduced to four degenerate elements fused into a *coccyx* in adult humans. Some movement persists, however, between the fused sacral mass and neighbouring vertebrae, as well as between the sacrum and pelvic girdle.

Mammalian presacral vertebrae vary in number and differentiation but can be grouped into *cervical* (neck), *thoracic* (where ribs persist) and *lumbar* vertebrae (devoid of mobile ribs) by distinguishing features. Cervical ribs are small or 'absent' (but see below); their disappearance in cervical and lumbar regions is linked to the change from breathing by gills to lungs, and to development of independent movements of the head. There is no neck in fish, the postcranial region being occupied by the branchial apparatus. Caudal shift of the respiratory apparatus in land vertebrates necessarily preceded development of a neck. Cervical vertebrae were early stabilized to seven in mammals (except tree sloths and manatees), even in such extremes as whales and giraffes. With respiratory adaptation of ribs in land animals and development of a diaphragm in mammals, well-formed ribs, articulating with but separate from vertebrae, are limited to thoracic levels. But ribs do **not** disappear completely in *cervical* and post-thoracic regions: vestigial *costal elements* are combined with transverse processes of all such vertebrae (see **3**.134, **6**.89).

The total number of vertebrae, excluding the tail, is reduced from the lemuroid and tarsloid to the anthropoid primates. Monkeys, apes and hominids (extinct and extant) show some uniformity. The cervical, thoracic, lumbar and sacral vertebrae number respectively 7, 11–15, 4 to 7, and 3–6, human values being 7, 12, 5 and 5. Caudal vertebrae vary much in number.

VERTEBRAL COLUMN

GENERAL VERTEBRAL FEATURES

A vertebra (**6**.87) essentially has a ventral *body* and a dorsal *vertebral (neural) arch*, extended by lever-like processes, together enclosing a *vertebral foramen*, occupied by the spinal cord, meninges and their vessels. Opposed surfaces of adjacent bodies are bound together by *intervertebral discs* of fibrocartilage. The complete column of bodies and discs forms a strong but flexible central axis of the body

supporting, in bipeds, the full weight of the head and trunk. It also transmits even greater forces due to muscles attached to it directly and indirectly. The foramina form a *vertebral canal* for the spinal cord, and between adjoining neural arches, near their junctions with vertebral bodies, *intervertebral foramina* transmit mixed spinal nerves, smaller recurrent nerves and blood and lymphatic vessels (see also p. 1258).

The cylindroid *vertebral body* varies in size, shape and proportions in different regions and more so in different species. Its junctional aspects vary from approximately flat (but not parallel) to sellar, with a raised peripheral smooth zone formed from the 'annular' epiphyseal disc (p. 532), within which the surface is rough. These differences in texture are due to variations in early structure of intervertebral discs (p. 265). In the horizontal plane the profiles of most bodies are convex anteriorly, but concave posteriorly where they complete the vertebral foramen. Most vertical profiles are concave anteriorly but flat posteriorly. Small vascular foramina appear on the front and sides, but posteriorly there are small arterial foramina (Willis 1949) and a large irregular orifice (sometimes double) for the exit of basivertebral veins (**6**.88). The adult vertebral **body** is **not** coextensive with the developmental **centrum** (p. 532) but includes, posterolaterally, parts of the neural arch, as already noted.

The vertebral arch has on each side a vertically narrower ventral part, the pedicle, and dorsally a broader lamina. Projecting from their junctions are paired transverse, superior and inferior articular processes; dorsally is a median spinous process.

Pedicles are short, thick, rounded dorsal projections from the superior part of the body at the junction of its lateral and dorsal surfaces, so that the concavity formed by its curved superior border is shallower than the inferior one (**6**.84). Adjacent *vertebral notches* contribute to an *intervertebral foramen* when vertebrae articulate by the intervertebral disc and zygapophyseal joints. The complete perimeter of an intervertebral foramen consists, therefore, of the notches, the dorsolateral aspects of parts of adjacent vertebral bodies and intervening disc, and the capsule of the synovial zygapophyseal joint.

Laminae, directly continuous with pedicles, are vertically flattened and curve dorsomedially to complete, with the base of the spinous process, a vertebral foramen.

The *spinous process* (*spine*) projects dorsally and often caudally from the junction of the laminae. Spines vary much in size, shape and direction. They act as levers for muscles which control posture and active movements (flexion/extension, lateral flexion and rotation) of the vertebral column.

The paired superior and inferior *articular processes* (*zygapophyses*) arise from the vertebral arch at the pediculolaminar junctions. The *superior processes* project cranially, bearing dorsal facets which may also have a lateral or medial inclination, depending on level. *Inferior processes* bulge caudally with articular facets directed ventrally, again with medial or lateral inclination depending on vertebral level. Articular processes of adjoining vertebrae thus form small synovial

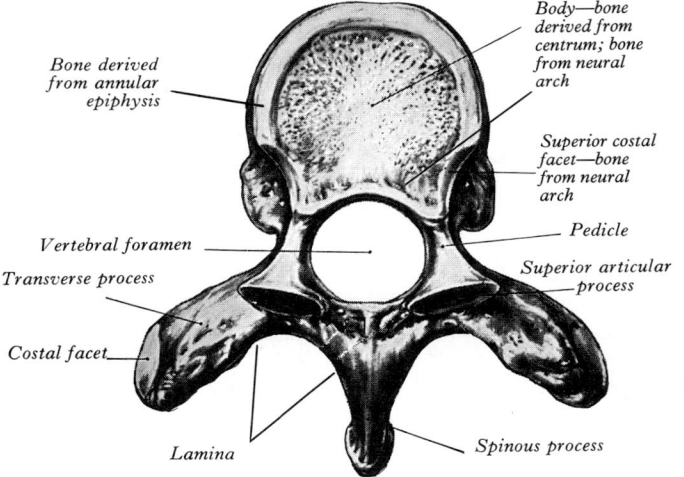

6.87 Typical thoracic vertebra: superior aspect.

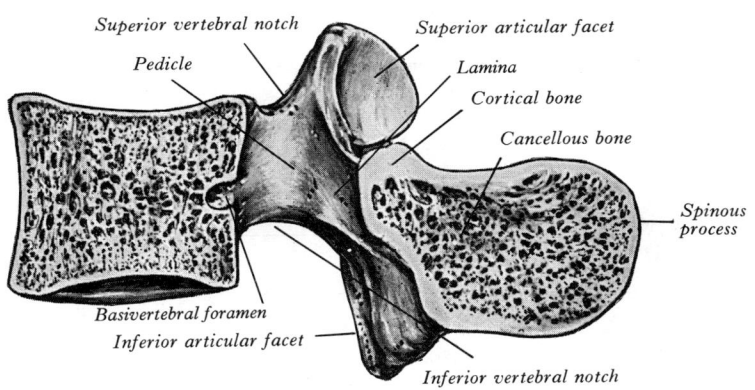

6.88 Median sagittal section through a lumbar vertebra.

zygapophyseal joints (p. 514), forming the posterior aspect of the intervertebral foramina; these joints permit limited movement between vertebrae: mobility varying considerably with vertebral level.

Transverse processes project laterally from the pediculolaminar junctions as levers for muscles and ligaments particularly concerned in rotation and lateral flexion. (The preceding comment is a simplification. In practice the activities of spinal musculature must be considered in terms of bilateral and surrounding muscle groups; weight-bearing and initial posture are also crucial.) The thoracic transverse processes articulate with ribs. At other levels the mature transverse process is a composite of 'true' transverse process (*diapophysis*) and an incorporated costal element.

Costal elements (*pleurapophyses*) develop as basic parts of neural arches in mammalian embryos, but become independent only as thoracic ribs. Elsewhere they remain less developed and fuse with the 'transverse process' of descriptive anatomy (**6.89**).

Vertebrae are internally trabecular (**6.88**), with an external shell of compact bone perforated by vascular foramina. The shell is thin on discal surfaces but thicker in the arch and its processes. The trabecular interior contains red bone marrow and one or two large ventrodorsal canals for the basivertebral veins.

A technique involving the analysis of nine dimensions of vertebral bodies and spines, from which exact anthropometric vertebral dimensions can be determined from radiographs, has been developed by Gilad and Nissan (1985).

The arterial patterns in bodies of thoracic vertebrae between ages 29th prenatal week to adulthood has been described by Ratcliffe (1980, 1981).

All vertebrae, from second cervical to first sacral, articulate by cartilaginous joints between their bodies, synovial joints between their articular processes (zygapophyses) and fibrous joints between their laminae and also between their transverse and spinous processes.

JOINTS OF VERTEBRAL BODIES

Vertebral bodies are united by anterior and posterior longitudinal ligaments and by fibrocartilaginous intervertebral discs between laminae of hyaline cartilage, together forming symphyses.

The anterior longitudinal ligament

The anterior longitudinal ligament (**6.90**) is a strong band extending along the anterior surfaces of the vertebral bodies, broader caudally, being thicker and narrower in thoracic than in cervical and lumbar regions. It is also relatively thicker and narrower opposite vertebral bodies than at the levels of intervertebral symphyses. Attached to the basilar occipital bone, it extends to the anterior tubercle of C1 (atlas), the front of the body of C2 (axis), continuing caudally to the front of the upper sacrum. Its longitudinal fibres, strongly adherent to the intervertebral discs, hyaline cartilage laminae and margins of adjacent vertebral bodies, are loosely attached at intermediate levels of the bodies, where the ligament fills their anterior concavities, flattening the vertebral profile (**6.90**). At these various levels ligamentous fibres blend with the subjacent periosteum, perichondrium and periphery of the annulus fibrosus. It has several layers, the most superficial fibres being longest extending over three or four vertebrae, intermediate between two or three, the deepest from one body to the next: laterally short fibres connect adjacent vertebrae.

The posterior longitudinal ligament

The posterior longitudinal ligament (**6.91**) on the posterior surfaces of the vertebral bodies lies in the vertebral canal, attached to the body of C2 (axis) and the sacrum; above it is continuous with the membrana tectoria (p. 522). Its smooth glistening fibres, attached to intervertebral discs, laminae of hyaline cartilage and adjacent margins of vertebral bodies, are separated between attachments by basivertebral veins and the venous rami draining them into anterior internal vertebral plexuses. At cervical and upper thoracic levels the ligament is broad and of uniform width, but in lower thoracic and lumbar regions it is denticulated, narrow over vertebral bodies and broad over discs (strictly symphyses). Its superficial fibres bridge three or four vertebrae, while deeper fibres extend between adjacent vertebrae as *perivertebral ligaments* close to and, in adults, fused with the annulus fibrosus of the intervertebral disc. The layers are more distinct in the immediate postnatal years.

Intervertebral discs

Intervertebral discs (**6.90, 92**), between adjacent surfaces of vertebral bodies from C2 (axis) to the sacrum, are the chief bonds between them. Disc outlines correspond with the adjacent bodies, thickness varying in different regions and parts of the same disc. In cervical and lumbar regions they are thicker anteriorly, contributing to the anterior convexity; in the thoracic region they are nearly uniform, the anterior concavity being largely due to the vertebral bodies. Discs are thinnest in the upper thoracic region and thickest in the lumbar regions, being adherent to thin layers of hyaline cartilage on the superior and inferior vertebral surfaces (p. 511); together the disc and hyaline cartilages form an *intervertebral symphysis*. Except for their peripheries, supplied from adjacent blood vessels, discs are avascular and supported by diffusion through the trabecular bone of adjacent vertebrae. Vascular and avascular parts differ in reaction to injury (Smith & Walmsley 1951). Connected to anterior and posterior longitudinal ligaments discs in the thoracic region are additionally tied laterally, by intra-articular ligaments, to the heads

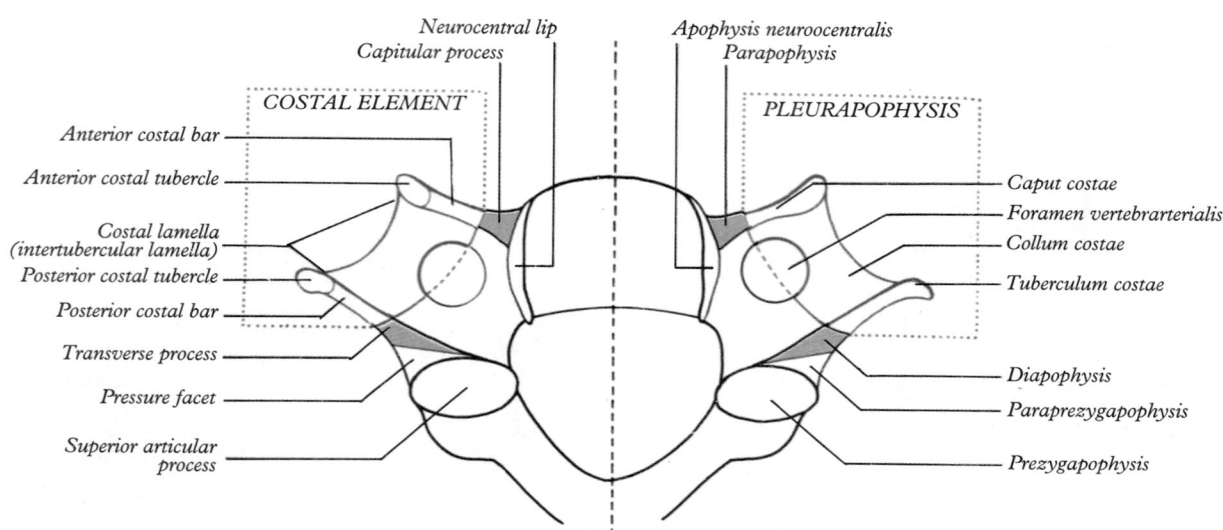

6.89 The morphology of a generalized cervical vertebra, with particular reference to the pleurapophyses. On the left the terms are zoological, on the right are alternatives for human anatomy suggested by Cave (1975).

(Reproduced with permission from the author, the *Journal of Zoology* and Cambridge University Press.)

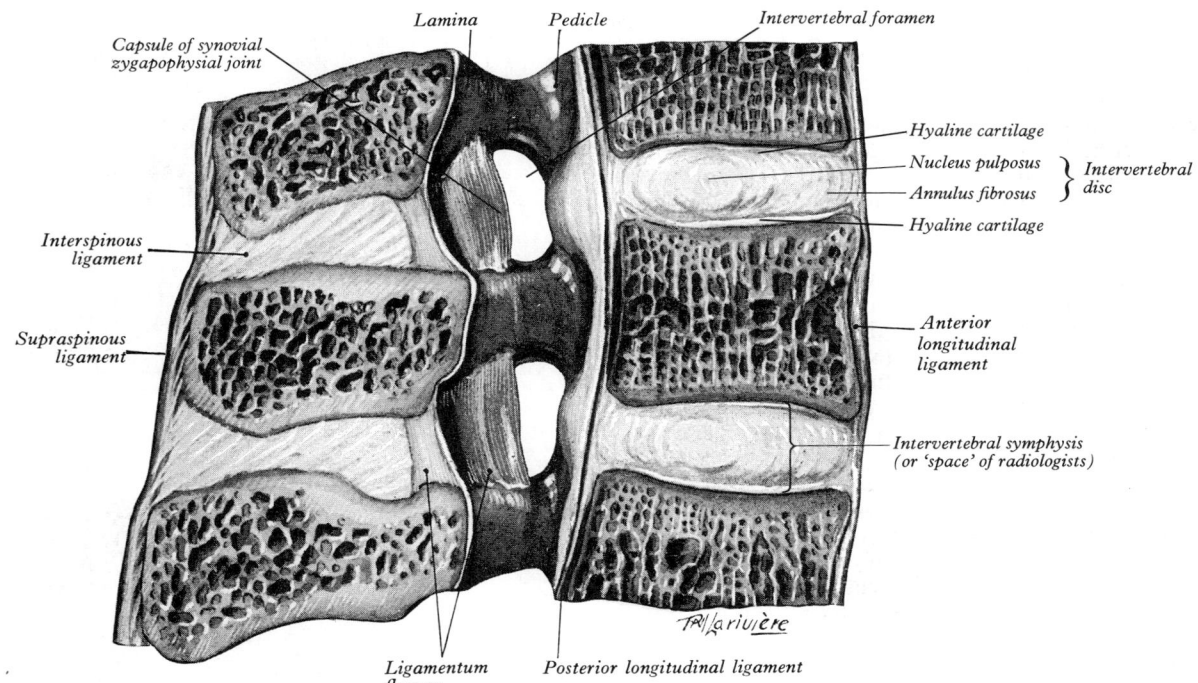

Capsule of synovial zygapophysial joint
Lamina
Pedicle
Intervertebral foramen
Interspinous ligament
Supraspinous ligament
Hyaline cartilage
Nucleus pulposus
Annulus fibrosus } *Intervertebral disc*
Hyaline cartilage
Anterior longitudinal ligament
Intervertebral symphysis (or 'space' of radiologists)
Ligamentum flavum
Posterior longitudinal ligament

6.90 Median sagittal section through part of the lumbar region of the vertebral column. Note the boundaries of intervertebral foramina. For contrasting details concerning the direction of fibre bundles in the interspinous ligaments see text and Heylings (1978).

of ribs articulating with adjacent vertebrae. Intervertebral discs (excluding the first two vertebrae) form a fifth of the postaxial vertebral column, cervical and lumbar regions having, in proportion to length, a greater contribution than the thoracic and thus being more pliant (Harris 1939). Each disc consists of an outer laminated *annulus fibrosus* and an inner *nucleus pulposus* (**6.90, 92**).

Annulus fibrosus. This has a narrow outer collagenous zone and a wider inner fibrocartilaginous zone. Its laminae, convex peripherally seen in vertical section, are incomplete collars connected by fibrous bands overlapping one another. (The internal vertical concavity of the laminae conforms to the surface profile of the nucleus pulposus.) Posteriorly, laminae join in a complex manner; fibres in the rest of each lamina are parallel and run obliquely between vertebrae; fibres in contiguous laminae criss-cross (**6.92**), thus limiting rotation in both directions. Predominantly **vertical** posterior fibres have been

described (Zaki 1973), predisposing to herniation. Obliquity of fibres in deeper zones varies in different laminae (Inoue 1973). Johnson et al (1985) have described elastic fibres in a small number of human lumbar annuli fibrosi. Hickey & Hukins (1981) have described fetal collagen fibril diameters in these structures; they also include elastic fibres.

Nucleus pulposus. Better developed in cervical and lumbar regions, this is nearer the disc's posterior surface. At birth it is large, soft, gelatinous and of mucoid material with a few multinucleated notochordal cells, invaded also by cells and fibres from the inner zone of the adjacent annulus fibrosus. Notochordal cells disappear in the first decade, followed by gradual replacement of mucoid material by fibrocartilage (Sylvén 1951), derived mainly from the annulus fibrosus and the hyaline cartilaginous plates adjoining vertebral bodies. The nucleus pulposus, hitherto distinct, now becomes

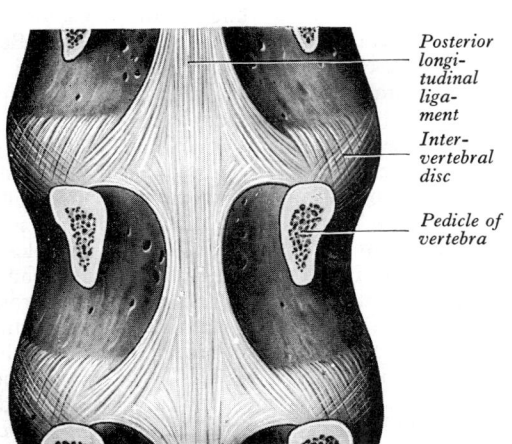

Posterior longitudinal ligament
Intervertebral disc
Pedicle of vertebra

6.91 The posterior longitudinal ligament in the lumbar region.

Annulus fibrosus
Nucleus pulposus
Laminae of fibrocartilage
Paraosseous lamina of hyaline cartilage
Vertebral body

6.92 Schematic representation of the main structural features of an intervertebral disc. The fibrocellular structure of the nucleus pulposus is omitted. For clarity the number of fibrocartilaginous laminae has been greatly reduced, since they are in fact of microscopic dimensions. Note alternating obliquity of collagen fascicles in adjacent laminae. (Modified after Inoue 1973.)

513

less differentiated from the remainder of the disc (Peacock 1952; Walmsley 1953; Töndury 1958). In lumbar discs cellularity (6000 cells/mm overall) is highest in peripheral annuli fibrosi and in hyaline cartilage nearest to the vertebral bodies, with a glucose diffusion coefficient of $2.5\,cm^2$ per second, comparable with values for cartilage elsewhere (Maroudas et al 1975). However, nutritional conditions may be more critical, especially in large lumbar discs. With these changes the nucleus pulposus becomes amorphous and sometimes discoloured. Its water-binding capacity and elasticity diminish (Püschel 1930), because these properties are due to its muco-polysaccharide and protein component (Hendry 1958). When the disc is not loaded, pressure in the nucleus pulposus is low at all ages (Nachemson 1960). Pech and Haughton (1985) have recently used cadaveric intervertebral discs to show the high correlation between radiographic and magnetic resonance (MR appearance).

For a review of the structure and function of the human inter-vertebral disc see Humzah and Soames (1988).

Clinical anatomy. In young adults intervertebral discs are so strong that violence first damages the adjacent bone. It is impossible to damage a healthy disc except by forcible flexion. After the second decade, however, degenerative changes in discs may result in necrosis, sequestration of the nucleus pulposus, softening and weakening of the annulus fibrosus. Then comparatively minor strains may cause **either** internal derangement with eccentric displacement of the nucleus pulposus **or** external derangement; the nucleus pulposus then bulges or bursts through the annulus fibrosus, usually postero-laterally. In the former unequal tension in the joint causes muscle spasm and sudden violent pain, acute *lumbago*; in the latter a herniated nucleus pulposus may press on adjacent nerve roots with resultant referred pain, *sciatica*. Such derangements are usually in the lower lumbar region, especially at the lumbosacral joint, and sometimes at the levels of C5–7. Motor effects, with loss of power and reflexes, may ensue.

The nerve supply to the outer part of the annulus fibrosus, which is frequently torn, may be an underlying cause of 'idiopathic backpain'. For a review of the various mechanisms of spinal pain see O'Brien (1984).

JOINTS OF VERTEBRAL ARCHES

Joints between vertebral articular processes (zygapophyses) are syn-ovial and vary in shape with vertebral level (p. 511); the laminae, spines and transverse processes are connected through syndesmoses constituted by ligamenta flava, interspinous, supraspinous and inter-transverse ligaments and the ligamentum nuchae. Some authorities group these various fibrous structures as accessory ligaments of the zygapophyseal joints, while others, as here, classify them as officially recognized, named syndesmoses.

Zygapophyseal joints

Zygapophyseal joints are of the simple (cervical and thoracic) or complex (lumbar) synovial variety: the hyaline covered articular cartilage mating surfaces are carried on mutually adapted articular processes. Their size, shape and topology vary with spinal level and are described with individual vertebrae.

Articular capsules. These are thin and loose and attached peri-pherally to the articular facets of adjacent zygapophyses; they are longer and looser in the cervical region.

Zygapophyseal lumbar specializations. Three types of lumbar intracapsular structure have been identified by Engel and Bogduk (1982):

- *adipose tissue fat pads* either anterosuperior, posteroinferior or both
- *fibroadipose 'menisci'* (*meniscoids*) at the superior or inferior pole, or both
- *connective tissue rims* either anterior, posterior or both.

The rims are inflections of fibrous capsule; the fat pads are similar to those in many other joints; the meniscoids have an expanded, vascularized, fibroadipose base attached to and sometimes per-forating the capsule, a poorly vascularized adipose core and a firm flattened fibrous apex. They project into the crevices between non-congruent articular surfaces but their function is conjectural; they are possibly significant clinically. **All** of the 82 specimens in the

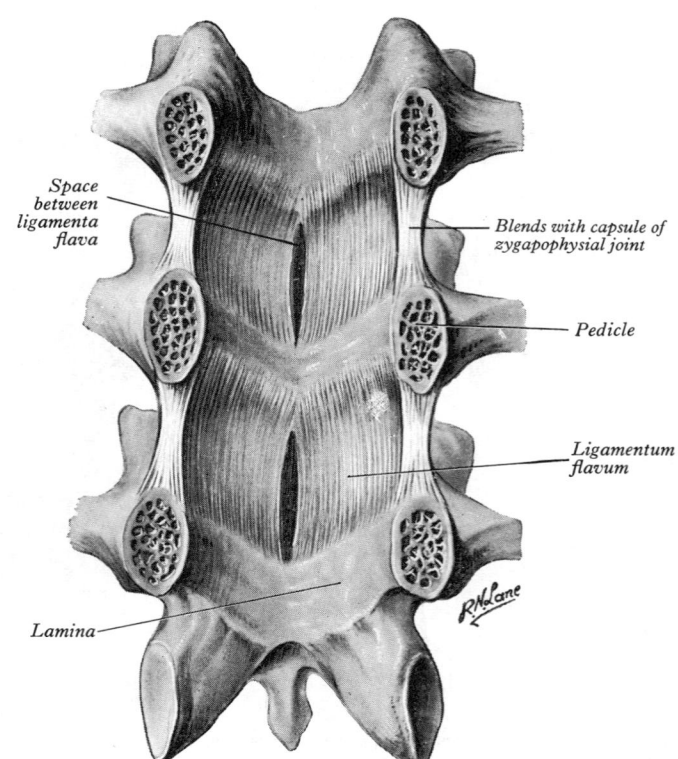

6.93 Ligamenta flava (anterior aspect in the lumbar region).

above study presented at least one of these features, with more than 50% presenting two or more features.

Intervertebral syndesmoses

Ligamenta flava (6.90, 93). They connect laminae of adjacent ver-tebrae in the vertebral canal. Their attachments extend from zyga-pophyseal capsules to where laminae fuse to form spines; here their posterior margins meet and are partially united, intervals being left for veins connecting internal to posterior external vertebral venous plexuses. Their predominant tissue is yellow elastic tissue, whose almost perpendicular fibres descend from the lower anterior surface of one lamina to the posterior surface and upper margin of the lamina below. The ligaments are thin, broad and long in the cervical region, thicker in the thoracic and thickest at lumbar levels. They arrest separation of the laminae in spinal flexion, preventing abrupt limitation, and also assist restoration to an erect posture after flexion, perhaps protecting discs from injury.

Supraspinous ligament (6.90). A strong fibrous cord connecting the tips of spinous process from C7 to the sacrum, it is thicker and broader at lumbar levels and intimately blended with neighbouring fascia. The most superficial fibres extend over three or four vertebrae, the deeper span two or three, while the deepest connect adjacent spines being continuous with interspinous ligaments. Between the spine of C7 and the external occipital protuberance it is expanded as the ligamentum nuchae. Heylings (1978) considers supraspinous ligaments to cease at the fifth lumbar spine.

Ligamentum nuchae. This is a bilaminar fibroelastic inter-muscular septum often considered homologous with, but structurally distinct from, supraspinous and interspinous ligaments in the neck. In structure, its dense bilateral fibroelastic laminae are separated by a tenuous layer of areolar tissue; the laminae are blended at its posterior free border. The latter is superficial and extends from the external occipital protuberance to the spine of C7. From this the fibroelastic laminae are attached to the median part of the external occipital crest, the posterior tubercle of C1 and the medial aspects of the bifid spines of cervical vertebrae, as a septum for bilateral attachment of cervical mucles and their sheaths. In bipeds it is the reduced representative of a much thicker, complex elastic ligament which, in quadrupedal mammals, aids suspension of the head and modifies its flexion, functioning like ligamenta flava.

Interspinous ligaments (6.90). These are thin and almost membranous, and connect adjoining spines, their attachments extending from the root to the apex of each. They meet the ligamenta flava in front of the supraspinous ligament behind. Narrow and elongated in the thoracic region, broader, thicker and quadrilateral at lumbar levels, they are poorly developed in the neck. (Some observers allocate all cervical bundles as part of the ligamentum nuchae; others regard them, although tenuous, as distinct interspinous fasicles.) Their fibres are usually described as obliquely *posteroinferior*; Heylings (1978), however, observed them to be obliquely *posterosuperior* at lumbar levels.

Intertransverse ligaments. Found between transverse processes these consist at cervical levels of a few, irregular fibres, largely replaced by intertransverse muscles; in the thoracic region they are cords intimately blended with adjacent muscles; in the lumbar region they are thin and membranous.

Nerves of the joints

Intervertebral joints (symphyses, syndesmoses and synovial) are all innervated by adjoining spinal (and sympathetic) nerves, particularly by their dorsal divisions.

INTERVERTEBRAL FORAMINA

Closely related to some of the main intervertebral articulations are the principal routes of entry and exit to and from the vertebral canal, the intervertebral foramina. (Minor routes occur between the median, often partly fused, margins of the ligamenta flava.) Between the axis and sacrum, despite some quantitative and structural regional variations, essentially they conform to the same general plan; because of their construction, contents and susceptibilities to multiple disorders, they are loci of great biomechanical, functional and clinical significance. The specializations cranial to the axis and at sacral levels are described with the individual bones and articulations. The **boundaries** of a generalized intervertebral foramen are: **anteriorly**, from above downwards, periosteum of the posterolateral aspect of the superior vertebral body (thin compact osseous shell over red bone marrow containing cancellous bone); posterolateral aspect of the intervertebral symphysis (including the disc)—the curved collagen fascicles here may be regarded as either the outer lamina of the annulus fibrosus or as extensions of perivertebral ligaments (distinctions of little importance)—finally a small (variable) periosteum-covered posterolateral part of the body of the inferior vertebra (structure as above); **superiorly**, the compact bone of the deep arched inferior vertebral notch of the vertebra above; **inferiorly**, the compact bone of the shallow superior vertebral notch of the vertebra below; **posteriorly** a part of the ventral aspect of the fibrous capsule of the zygapophyseal synovial joint. Cervical intervertebral foramina are distinct in having superior and inferior vertebral notches of almost equal depth which, in accord with the direction of the pedicles, face **anterolaterally**; external to them, and in the same direction, is the complex transverse process and foramen transversarium (p. 516). The thoracic and lumbar intervertebral foramina face **laterally** and their transverse processes are posterior. The first to tenth thoracic foramina have additionally as anteroinferior boundaries the articulations of the head of a rib, the capsules of double synovial joints with the demifacets on adjacent vertebrae and the intra-articular ligament between the costocapitular ridge and the intervertebral symphysis. Note that the lumbar foramina lie **between** the two principal lines of vertebral attachment of the psoas major muscle. The walls of each foramen are, as noted, covered throughout by collagen, either periosteal, perichondrial, annular or capsular. *Contents* are: a segmental mixed spinal nerve and its sheaths, from two to four recurrent meningeal (sinu-vertebral) nerves (pp. 1259, 1261), variable spinal arteries (for origins, branches and distribution see p. 1546), and plexiform venous connections between internal and external vertebral venous plexuses (p. 1595). These structures, particularly the nerves, may be affected by trauma or one of the many disorders of the tissues bordering the foramen: i.e. fibrocartilage of the annulus fibrosus; in earlier decades the nucleus pulposus; the highly vascular red bone marrow occupying the cancellous bone of the vertebral bodies; the compact bone of the pedicles; the capsules, synovial membranes, articular cartilages (and at lumbar levels fibroadipose meniscoids, fat pads, fibrous labra, p. 514) of the synovial

zygapophyseal joints; and additionally at thoracic levels tissues of the complex synovial costocapitular joints.

MOVEMENTS OF THE VERTEBRAL COLUMN

Movement between vertebrae is restricted by the limited deformation of intervertebral symphyses (particularly the discs), whose greater thickness at cervical and lumbar levels increases individual ranges. It is also limited by the topography of the zygapophyseal joints and by concomitant changes in tension of the ligamentous syndesmoses. Although movements between individual vertebrae are small, their summation gives a large total range to the vertebral column in flexion, extension, lateral flexion, rotation and circumduction.

In *flexion* the anterior longitudinal ligament becomes relaxed as the anterior parts of intervertebral discs are compressed; at its limit the posterior longitudinal ligament, ligamenta flava, interspinous and supraspinous ligaments and posterior fibres of intervertebral discs are tensed; interlaminar intervals widen, inferior articular processes glide on superior processes of subjacent vertebrae and their capsules become taut. Tension of extensor muscles is also important in limiting flexion, for example when carrying a load on the shoulders. Flexion is most extensive in the cervical region.

In *extension* the opposite events occur with compression of posterior discal fibres; it is limited by tension of the anterior longitudinal ligament, anterior discal fibres and approximation of spines and zygapophyses. Marked in cervical and lumbar regions, extension is much less at thoracic levels, partly because of thinner discs but also because of the presence of the thoracic skeleton and musculature. In full extension the axis of movement has been described as behind the articular processes, moving forwards as the column straightens and passes into flexion, reaching the centre of the vertebral bodies in full flexion (Wiles 1935).

In *lateral flexion*, which is always combined with rotation, intervertebral discs are laterally compressed and contralaterally tensed and lengthened, motion being limited by tension of antagonist muscles and ligaments. Lateral movements occur in all parts of the column but are greatest in cervical and lumbar regions.

Rotation involves twisting of vertebrae relative to each other with accompanying torsional deformation of intervening discs. Although slight between individual vertebrae, it summates along the column. Movement is slight at cervical level, greater in the upper thoracic and least in the lumbar region.

Circumduction is limited and merely a succession of preceding movements.

The extent and direction of vertebral movements are guided by the articular facets. Although often described as *plane*, they are never truly flat but *ovoid*, with opposing surfaces being reciprocally concave and convex. In the *cervical* region the upward inclination of the superior articular facets allows free flexion and extension; the latter usually being greater and checked above by locking of the posterior edges of the superior facets of C1 in the occipital condylar fossae and below by slipping of the inferior processes of C7 into grooves inferoposterior to the first thoracic superior articular processes. Flexion stops where the cervical convexity is straightened, checked by apposition of the projecting lower lips of vertebral bodies on subjacent bodies. Cervical lateral flexion and rotation are always combined; superomedial inclination of superior articular facets imparts rotation during lateral flexion. In the *thoracic* region, especially above, all movements are limited, reducing interference with respiration; lack of upward inclination of superior articular facets prohibits much flexion, extension being checked by contact of the inferior articular margins with laminae and of spines with each other. Thoracic rotation is freer; its axis is in the vertebral bodies in the midthoracic region, in front of them elsewhere, so that rotation involves some lateral displacement (Davis 1959; Davis et al 1965). The direction of articular facets would allow free lateral flexion but this is limited in the upper thoracic region by resistance of the ribs and sternum. Rotation is usually combined with slight lateral flexion to the same side. *Lumbar* extension is wider in range than flexion and some lateral flexion and rotation can also occur: rotation being limited by the absence of a common centre of curvature for right and left articular facets (Putz 1976). Functional transition between thoracic and lumbar regions is usually between the eleventh and twelfth thoracic vertebrae (p. 525), where zygapophyseal joints of the

515

vertebral arches usually fit tightly, slight compression locking them, preventing all but flexion.

Muscles producing vertebral movements. The spinal column is moved both by intrinsic muscles attached to it and by muscles attached to other bones, acting indirectly. Gravity also always plays a part.

Flexion: longus cervicis, scaleni, sternocleidomastoid and rectus abdominis of both sides.

Extension: the erector spinae complex, splenius and semispinalis capitis and trapezius of both sides.

Lateral flexion: longissimus and iliocostocervicalis, oblique abdominal muscles and flexors on the side of lateral flexion.

Rotation: rotatores, multifidus, splenius cervicis and oblique abdominal muscles.

Extension, principally lumbar, occurs commonly from a stooping position. Initial extension is mainly at the hips and knees; continuous lumbar extension is delayed, with little or no activity in erector spinae. In lifting heavy weights there is considerable initial compression of lumbar intervertebral discs, with large rises in thoracic and abdominal pressure, which may resist flexion (Davis 1963; Davis et al 1965). Pal and Routal (1986) have studied the mechanics of weight transmission via the vertebral arches. In contrast with the usual view, that the major, almost only, factor is contributed by vertebral bodies and intervertebral discs, they find that, on the basis of areal and other measurements, the vertebral arches and their zygapophyseal joints are, at cervical levels, also a considerable factor in weight transmission. For an extensive view of lumbar backache see Wyke (1980).

CERVICAL VERTEBRAE

The seven cervical vertebrae (**6.94–96**), the smallest of the movable vertebrae, are typified by a foramen in each transverse process. The first, second and seventh have special features and will be considered separately. The third, fourth and fifth cervical are almost identical; the sixth, while typical in its general features, has minor differences which usually enable its distinction from others.

Typical cervical vertebra

The typical cervical vertebra (**6.97**) has a small, relatively broad vertebral *body*. The *pedicles* project posterolaterally and the longer laminae posteromedially, enclosing a large, roughly triangular *vertebral foramen*; the vertebral canal here accommodates the cervical enlargement of the spinal cord. The pedicles are inserted midway between the discal surfaces of the vertebral body, so the superior and inferior vertebral notches are of similar depth. The *laminae* are thin and slightly curved, with a thin superior and slightly thicker inferior border. The *spinous process* (spine) is short and bifid, with two tubercles which are often unequal in size. The junction between lamina and pedicle bulges laterally between the superior and inferior *articular processes* to form, when articulated, an articular pillar on each side. The *transverse process* is morphologically composite around the *foramen transversarium*. Its dorsal and ventral *roots* or *bars* terminate laterally as corresponding *tubercles*. The tubercles are connected, lateral to the foramen, by the *costal* (or intertubercular) *lamella*: these three elements represent morphologically the capitellum, tubercle and neck of a cervical costal element, sometimes referred to as the *pleurapophysis*. The attachment of the posterior root to the pediculolaminar junction represents the morphological transverse process (*diapophysis*) and the attachment of the ventral root to the ventral body the capitellar process (*parapophysis*; **6.89**).

The vertebral body has a convex anterior surface. The discal margin gives attachment to the anterior longitudinal ligament, and shallow anterolateral depressions lodge the vertical parts of longus colli. The posterior surface is flat or minimally concave, and its discal margins give attachment to the posterior longitudinal ligament. The central area displays several vascular foramina, of which two are commonly relatively larger and known as the *basivertebral foramina*: these transmit basivertebral veins to the anterior internal vertebral veins. The superior surface is saddle-shaped, formed by flange-like lips which arise from most of the lateral circumference of the upper margin of the vertebral body; these are sometimes referred

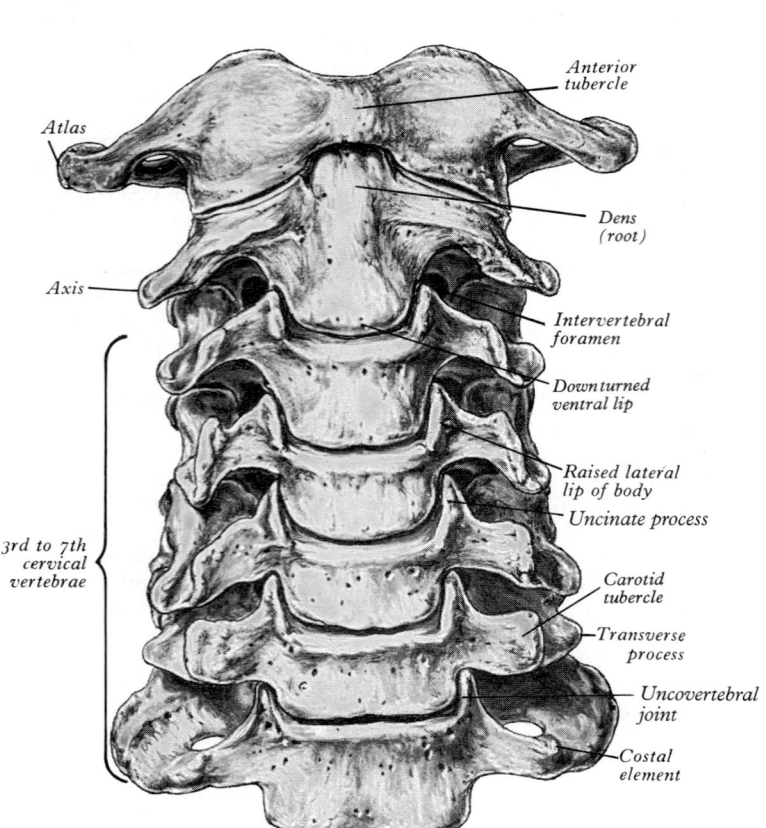

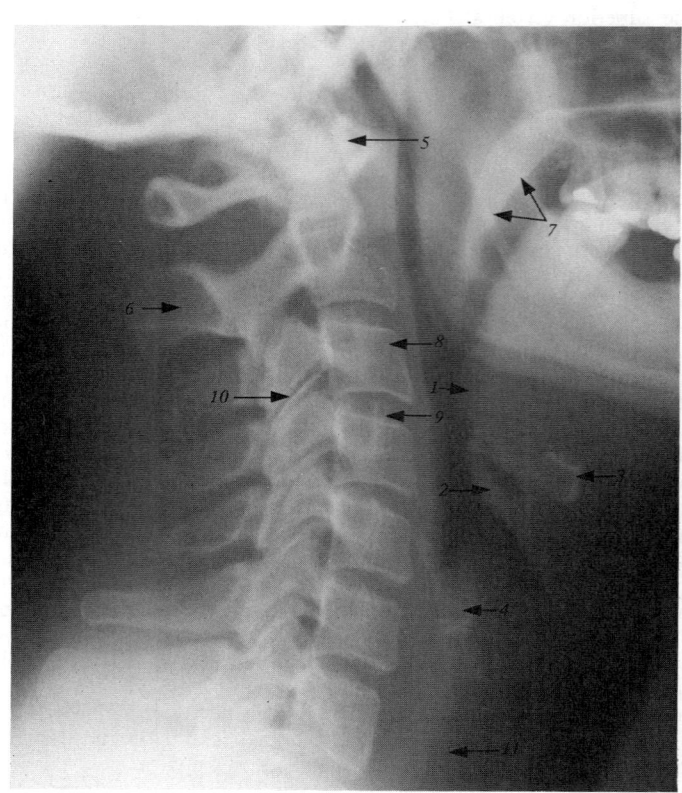

6.95 Lateral radiograph of the neck. The cervical curve of the vertebral column is well shown. The arrows point to 1. the pharyngeal part of the tongue; 2. the epiglottis; 3. the body of the hyoid bone; 4. the thyroid cartilage which is undergoing calcification; 5. the anterior tubercle of the atlas; 6. the spinous process of the axis; 7. the soft palate; 8. characteristic cervical body; 9. intervertebral disc; 10. zygapophysial joint; 11. air in trachea. (Provided by Shaun Gallagher; photography by Sarah Smith.)

6.94   The cervical vertebrae: anterior aspect.

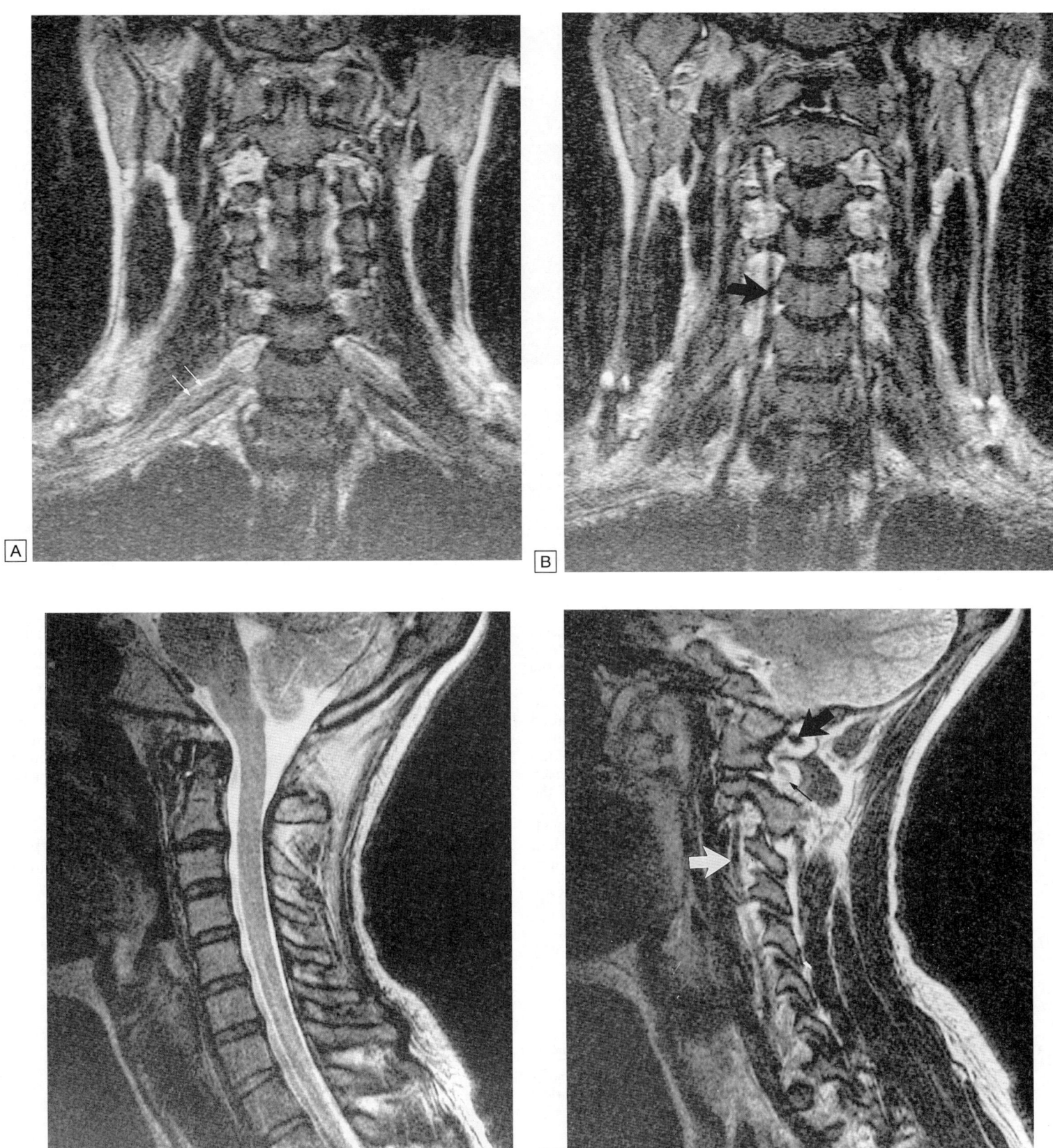

6.96 Magnetic resonance images (MRI) of the cervical spine in a 26-year-old man. (A) and (B) are in the coronal plane passing through the cervical vertebral bodies, (A) being centred 3.5 mm anterior to (B). (C) and (D) are in the sagittal plane, (C) centred to the midpoints of the vertebral bodies, (D) centred to the articular pillars. Large arrow in (B) and (D) is the vertebral artery; small arrows in (A) are the trunks of the brachial plexus; small arrow in (D) is the dorsal root ganglion of the second cervical nerve. There is an appearance suggestive of midsagittal clefting of the upper cervical centra, perhaps indicating that they formed from right and left ossification centres like the centrum of the atlas. It is a relatively common appearance on computed images in the appropriate plane. (Images supplied by J M Stevens and H A Crockard.)

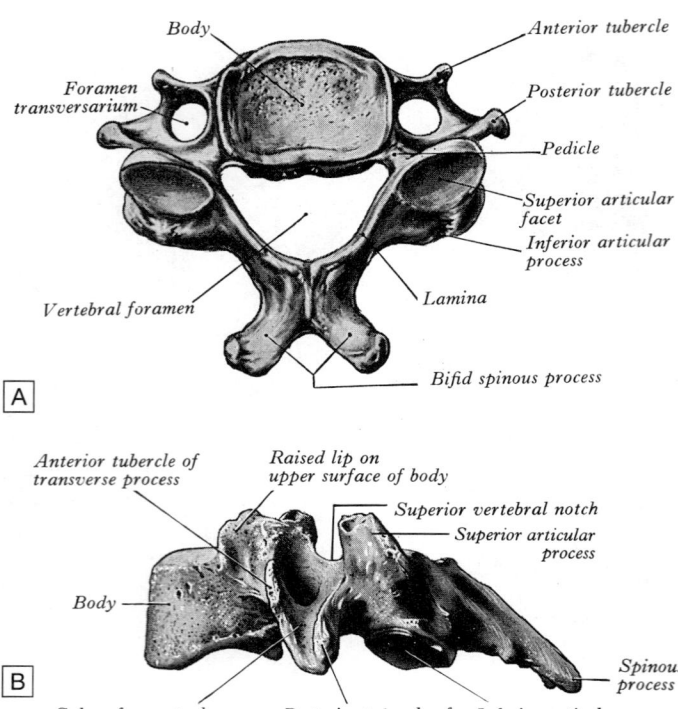

6.97 Typical cervical vertebra: A. Superior aspect. B. Left lateral aspect.

to as *uncinate* or *neurocentral* lips or processes. The inferior discal surface is also concave, the convexity being produced mainly by a broad projection from the anterior margin which partly overlaps the anterior surface of the intervertebral disc. The discal surfaces of cervical vertebrae are so shaped in order to restrict both lateral and anteroposterior gliding movements during articulation. The paired ligamenta flava extend from the superior border of each lamina below to the roughened inferior half of the anterior surfaces of the lamina above. The superior part of the anterior surface of each lamina is smooth, like the immediately adjacent surfaces of the pedicles: these are usually in direct contact with the dura mater and cervical root sheaths, to which they may become loosely attached. To the spinous processes are attached the ligamentum nuchae and numerous deep extensors, including semispinalis thoracis and cer-

vicis, multifidus, spinales and interspinales. The spinous process of the sixth cervical vertebra is larger, and is often not bifid.

The superior articular facets, flat and ovoid, are directed supero-posteriorly, whereas the corresponding inferior facets are directed mainly anteriorly, and lie nearer the coronal plane than the superior facets. The dorsal rami of the cervical spinal nerves curve posteriorly close to the anterolateral aspects of the articular pillars, and may actually lie in shallow grooves, especially on the third and fourth pair. A small, functionless tubercle, lateral to a small pressure facet, is often present close to the superior articular facet, and is regarded by morphologists as a paraprezygapophysis (Cave 1975). The dorsal root ganglion of each cervical spinal nerve lies between the superior and inferior vertebral notches of adjacent vertebrae; the large anterior ramus passing posterior to the vertebral artery, which lies on the concave upper surface of the costal lamella: the concavity of the lamellae increasing from the fourth to the sixth vertebra. The fourth to sixth anterior tubercles are elongated and rough for tendinous slips of salenus anterior, longus capitis and longus colli; the sixth is the longest and is often called the *carotid tubercle*. The carotid artery can be immobilized and compressed in the groove formed by the vertebral bodies and the larger anterior tubercles, especially the sixth—hence its name. The posterior tubercles are rounded and more laterally placed than the anterior, and all but the sixth are also more caudal, with the sixth being at about the same level as the anterior. Attached to the posterior tubercles are the splenius, longissimus and ilio-costalis cervicis, levator scapulae and scalenus posterior and medius.

Seventh cervical vertebra

The seventh cervical vertebra (**6**.98), or vertebra prominens, has a long spinous process visible at the lower end of the nuchal furrow. It ends in a prominent tubercle for the attachment of the ligamentum nuchae, along with the following muscles: trapezius, spinalis capitis, semispinalis thoracis, multifidus and interspinales. The thick and prominent transverse processes are behind and lateral to the transverse foramina; the latter transmits vertebral veins, not the artery, and is often divided by a bony spicule. The costal lamella is relatively thin and may be partly deficient, or it may be separate as a *cervical rib*. It is grooved superiorly for the anterior ramus of the seventh cervical nerve, and usually carries a small and inconspicuous anterior tubercle. The posterior tubercle, by contrast, is prominent. The anterior border of the transverse process receives the attachment of scalenus minimus (pleuralis), when present, and also the suprapleural membrane (p. 1663). The first pair of levatores costarum is also attached to the transverse processes.

Atlas

The atlas, the first cervical vertebra (**6**.99), supports the head. It is unique in that it fails to incorporate a centrum, the expected position

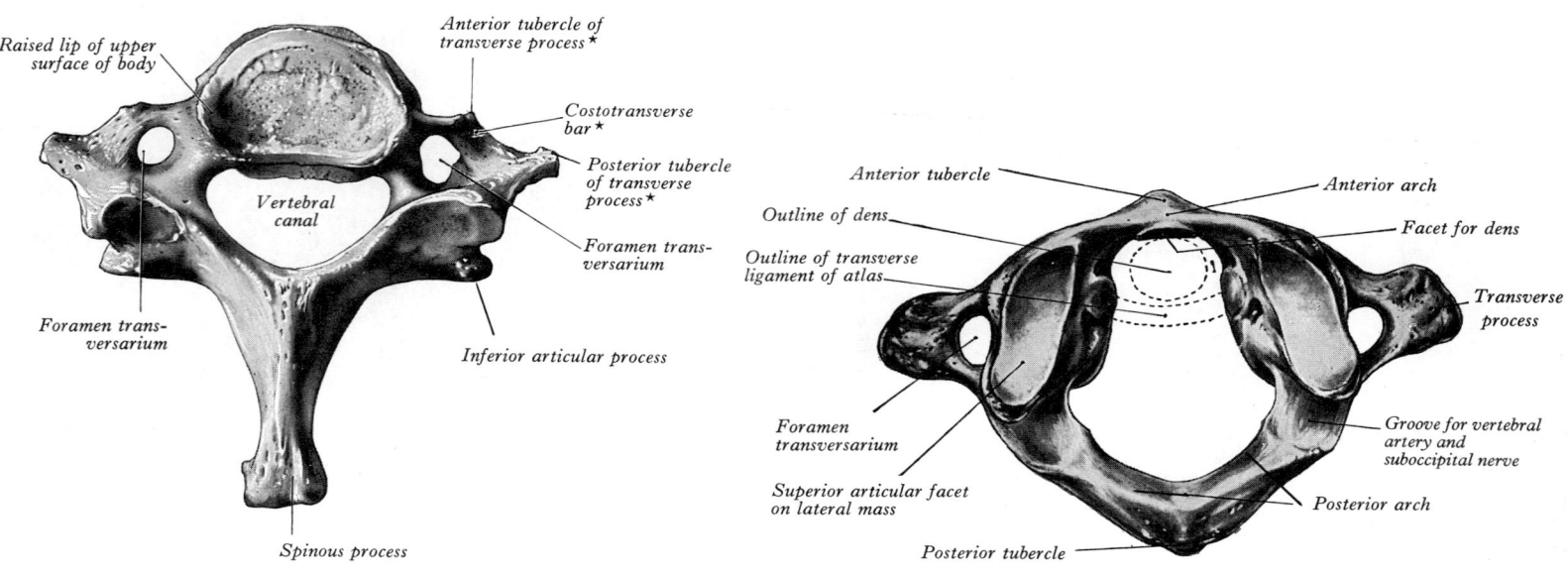

6.98   The seventh cervical vertebra: superior aspect. See text and **6**.89 for alternative terms.

6.99   The first cervical vertebra, or atlas: superior aspect.

of which is occupied by a cranial protuberance of the axis known as the *dens*. The atlas consists of two *lateral masses* connected by a short *anterior* and a longer *posterior* arch. The *transverse ligament* retains the dens against the anterior arch. Jenkins (1969) has shown that the dens in this location is not homologous with the centrum of the atlas, as often stated, but evolved as an addition to the postdens ossification, which is the true atlas body and has become fused to the body of the axis. The anterior arch of the atlas is morphologically a hypocentrum, ossifying in fibrocartilage formed from the embryonic hypochordal bow. Both the anterior arch and transverse ligament can be regarded as a modified intervertebral disc into which an anterior protuberance of the atlas centrum, the dens, is invaginated (Jenkins 1969; O'Rahilly et al 1983).

The *anterior arch* is slightly convex anteriorly, and carries a roughened *anterior tubercle*, to which is attached the anterior longitudinal ligament (cord-like at this level) and the superior oblique part of longus colli on each side. Its upper and lower borders provide attachment to the anterior atlanto-ocipital membrane and diverging lateral parts of the anterior longitudinal ligament. The posterior surface of the anterior arch carries a concave, almost circular facet for the dens.

The *lateral masses* are ovoid, their long axes converging anteriorly. Each bears a reniform superior articular facet for the respective occipital condyle; sometimes it is completely divided into a larger anterior and a smaller posterior part (Singh 1965; Lang 1986). The inferior articular facet of the lateral mass is almost circular, and is flat or slightly concave. It is orientated more obliquely to the transverse plane than the superior facet, facing more medially and very slightly backwards. On the medial surface of each lateral mass is a roughened area bearing vascular foramina and a tubercle for attachment of the transverse ligament (**6.99**). In adults the distance between these tubercles, shorter than the transverse ligament itself, has a mean value of 16.34 mm (range 12.0–19.0 mm; Lang 1986). The anterior surface of the lateral mass gives attachment to rectus capitis anterior.

The *posterior arch* forms three-fifths of the circumference of the atlantal ring. The superior surface bears a wide groove for the vertebral artery and venous plexus immediately behind and variably overhung by the lateral mass: the first cervical nerve intervenes. Frequently a bony spur arises from the anterior and posterior margins of this groove, sometimes referred to as *ponticles*, which convert the groove into a foramen in about 14% of individuals: more frequently, however, the foramen is incomplete superiorly (Lamberty & Zivanovic 1973; Lang 1986). The flange-like superior border gives attachment to the posterior atlantoaxial membrane, and the flatter inferior border to the highest pair of ligamenta flava. The posterior tubercle is a rudimentary spinous process, roughened for attachment of the ligamentum nuchae, and lateral to this the rectus capitis posterior minor.

The *transverse processes* are longer than those of all cervical vertebrae except the seventh (**6.94**). They act as strong levers for the muscles making fine adjustments for keeping the head balanced. Maximum atlantal width varies from 74–95 mm in males and 65–76 mm in females, affording a useful criterion for assessing sex in human remains. The apex of the transverse process, which is usually broad, flat and palpable between the mastoid process and ramus of the mandible, is homologous with the posterior tubercle of typical cervical vertebrae: the remaining part of the transverse process consists of the costal lamella. A small anterior tubercle is sometimes visible on the anterior aspect of the lateral mass. The costal lamella is sometimes deficient, leaving the foramen transversarium open anteriorly. Superiorly is rectus capitis lateralis with superior oblique located more posteriorly: laterally, on the apex, is inferior oblique below which are slips of levator scapulae, splenius cervicis and scalenus medius.

Axis

The axis, the second cervical vertebra (**6.100**), is an axle for rotation of the atlas and head around the strong *dens* (odontoid process), which projects cranially from the superior surface of the body. The dens is conical in shape, with a mean length of 15.0 mm (range 9–21 mm) in adults (McManners 1983; Lang 1986). It may be tilted a little, up to 14°, posteriorly, or, less often, anteriorly, on the axis body: it may also tilt laterally up to 10° (Lang 1986). The posterior

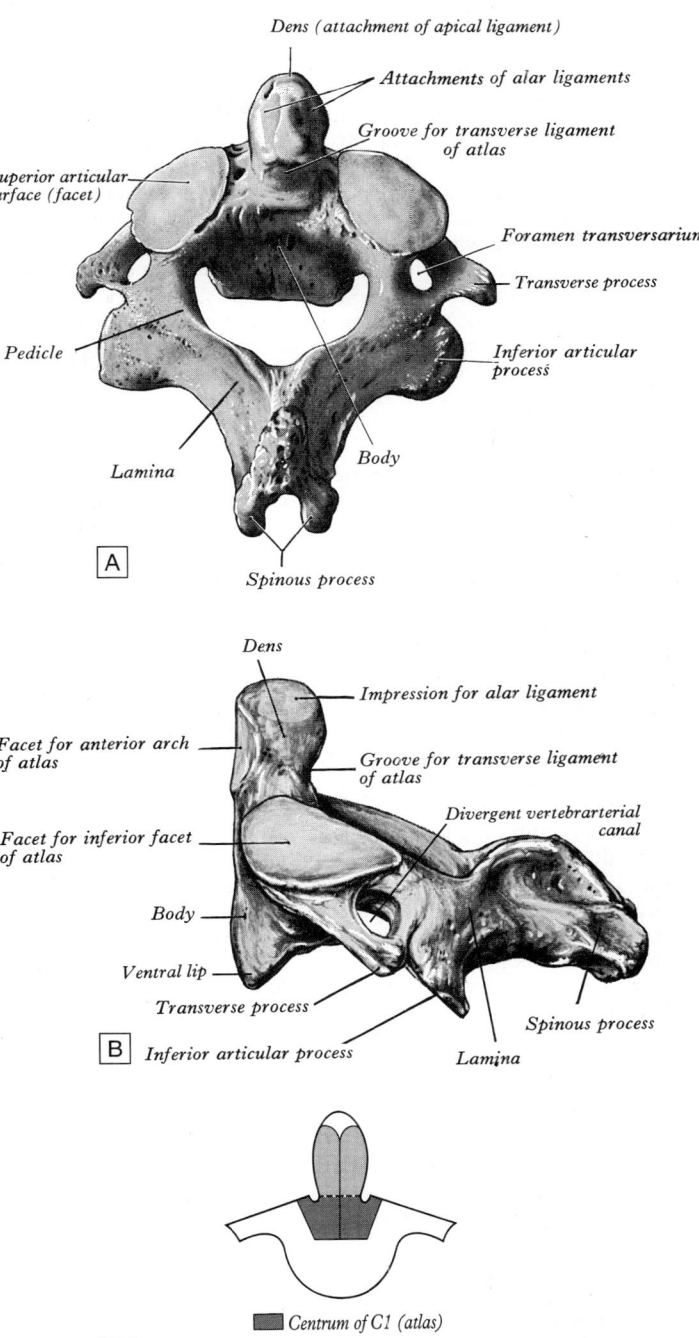

6.100 The second cervical vertebra (axis), posterosuperior (A) and left lateral (B) aspects. C. Morphology of the axis with particular reference to the centrum of the atlas and its derivatives (modified from Jenkins 1969).

surface bears a broad groove for the cartilage-covered transverse ligament. The apex is pointed, and from this point arises the apical ligament; the alar ligaments are attached to the somewhat flattened posterolateral surfaces above the groove for the transverse ligament. The anterior surface bears an ovoid articular facet for the anterior arch of the atlas, and the surface is pitted by many vascular foramina, which are most numerous near the apex. Schiff and Parke (1973) studied the arterial blood supply of the dens and found that small twigs arose mainly from the vertebral artery at the level of the intervertebral foramen for the third cervical nerve, which formed paired anterior and posterior longitudinal channels, branches entering the dens near the base and more distally near the apex. However, the anterior also received numerous twigs from nearby branches of the external carotid via branches to the longus colli and ligaments

519

of the apex. Hence vascular necrosis does not occur after fracture of the base of the dens. The *body* consists of less compact bone than the dens. It is, in fact, composite, consisting of the partly fused centra of atlas and axis, and a rudimentary disc (synchondrosis) between: this usually remains detectable deep within the axis body throughout life (**6**.100c). Large ovoid articular facets are present on either side of the dens at the junction of the body and neural arch, which are flat or slightly convex for articulation with the masses of the atlas. They lie in a plane anterior to the plane of the intercentral articulations, with which they are, in part, homologous (Jenkins 1969; Cave 1975). The anterior surface of the body carries a deep depression on each side for the attachment of the vertical part of longus colli. The somewhat triangular downward projecting anterior border gives attachment to the anterior longitudinal ligament. Posteriorly, the lower border receives the posterior longitudinal ligament and the membrana tectoria (p. 512, 522).

The *pedicles* are stout, with the superior surface carrying part of the superior articular facet, which also projects laterally and downwards on to the transverse process. The anterolateral surface is deeply grooved by the vertebral artery, and the lateral part of the inferior surface of the superior articular facet, which can become quite thin. The inferior surface of each pedicle bears a deep, smooth inferior intervertebral notch, in which lies the large root sheath of the third cervical nerve. Here is a short interarticular part of the pedicle, between the relatively small posterior articular process located at the pediculolaminar junction, with its equally small anteriorly facing facet, and the superior articular surface.

The *transverse process* is pointed and projects inferiorly and laterally, arising from the pediculolaminar junction and the lateral aspect of the interarticular area of the pedicle. The rounded tip is homologous with the posterior tubercle of typical cervical vertebrae. The foramen transversarium is directed laterally as the vertebral artery turns abruptly laterally under the superior articular facet. Small anterior tubercles may be present near the junction of the costal lamella with the body. To the tips of the transverse processes are attached the levator scapulae, between scalenus medius and splenius cervicis, and to their upper and lower surfaces the intertransverse muscles (p. 812).

The *laminae* are thick, affording attachment to the ligamenta flava. The *spinous process* is large, with a bifid tip and a broad base, concave inferiorly. The lateral surfaces of the spinous process give

origin to the inferior obliques, with the rectus posterior major a little more posteriorly. The inferior concavity receives the semispinalis and spinalis cervicis, and, deeper, the multifidus: near the apex it receives interspinales. The ligamentum nuchae is attached to the apical notch.

Clinical anatomy. Abnormalities of the dens of the axis are common, and often result in atlantoaxial subluxation. Most are acquired, but many result from fractures through the base of the dens which do not unite due to interposition of the transverse ligament (Crockard et al 1993). Others, occurring particularly in some skeletal dysplasias, represent an abnormal ossification pattern in which the dens ossifies separately and much later than the atlantal centrum (of which it is part): this is probably a result of abnormal mobility in the cartilaginous anlage, and may be restored to normal if motion is prevented by surgical arthrodesis (Stevens et al 1991). Hypoplasia of the dens is usually accompanied by atlanto-occipital assimilation and basilar invagination. Incomplete segmentation is common in the cervical spine, and most commonly involves the axis and third cervical vertebra. The costal element of the seventh cervical vertebra may articulate with the transverse process as an independent rib of variable size.

CRANIOVERTEBRAL JOINTS

The articulation between the cranium and vertebral column is specialized to provide a wider range of movement than in the rest of the axial skeletal. It consists of the occipital condyles, atlas and axis, and functions like a universal joint, permitting horizontal and vertical scanning movements of the head, which is superbly adapted for eye-head co-ordination (Rabischong 1992).

Atlanto-axial joints

Articulation of atlas to axis is at three synovial joints, a pair between lateral masses, and a median complex between the dens of the axis and the anterior arch and transverse ligament of the atlas.

The lateral atlantoaxial joints. These are often classified as planar but the bony *articular surfaces* are more complex in shape, usually reciprocally concave in the coronal plane, with the medial parts being somewhat convex in the sagittal plane, especially that of the axis. The cartilaginous articular surfaces are usually less concave. Fibrous capsules attached to their margins are thin, loose and lined by synovial membrane. Each has a posteromedial *accessory ligament* attached below to the axial body near the base of its dens, and above to the lateral atlantal mass near the lateral ligament.

Anteriorly, the vertebral bodies are connected by the anterior longitudinal ligament (**6**.101): here a strong, thickened band attaches above to the lower border of the anterior tubercle of the anterior arch of the atlas and below to the front of the axial body. Posteriorly the vertebral bodies are joined by the ligamenta flava (**6**.102), attaching to the lower border of the atlantal arch above, and to the upper borders of the axial laminae. At this level these ligaments are a thin membrane, pierced laterally by the second cervical nerves.

The median atlantoaxial joint. A pivot between the dens and a ring formed by the anterior arch and transverse ligament of the atlas, it has two synovial cavities which sometimes communicate (Cave 1975). A vertically ovoid facet on the anterior dens articulates with one on the posterior aspect of the anterior atlantal arch. The fibrous capsule, which is lined by synovial membrane, is relatively weak and loose, especially superiorly. The synovial cavity of the posterior component of the median joint complex is larger, lying between the horizontally orientated ovoid facet, grooving the posterior surface of the dens and the *cartilaginous* anterior surface of the transverse ligament (**6**.103): communication often exists with one or both of the atlanto-occipital joint cavities.

The transverse atlantal ligament (**6**.99, 103, 104). This is a broad, strong band arching across the atlantal ring behind the dens: it is variable in length (mean 20.1 mm) (Dvorak et al 1988b). It is attached laterally to a small but prominent tubercle on the medial side of each atlantal lateral mass, and broadens medially where it is covered anteriorly by a thin layer of articular cartilage. It consists almost entirely of collagen fibres, which, in the central part of the ligament, cross one another at an angle to form an interlacing mesh (Dvorak et al 1988b). From its upper margin a strong median longitudinal band arises which inserts into the basilar part of the occipital bone

Anterior atlanto-occipital membrane

Basilar part of occipital bone

Jugular foramen

Mastoid process

Articular capsule of atlanto-occipital joint

Transverse process of atlas

Articular capsule of atlanto-axial joint

Anterior longitudinal ligament at attachment to anterior tubercle of atlas

Anterior longitudinal ligament

Cleft between vertebral bodies

6.101 Atlanto-occipital and atlanto-axial joints: anterior aspect. On each side a small cleft has been opened between the lateral part of the upper surface of the body of the third cervical vertebra and the bevelled, inferior surface of the body of the axis.

between the apical ligament of the dens and membrana tectoria, and from its inferior surface a weaker and less consistent longitudinal band passes to the posterior surface of the axis. These transverse and longitudinal components together constitute the *cruciform ligament*.

The transverse ligament divides the ring of the atlas into unequal parts (**6**.99); the posterior and larger surrounds the spinal cord and meninges, the anterior contains the dens, which is retained in position even when all other ligaments are divided.

Movements at the atlantoaxial joints. These are simultaneous at all three joints and consist almost exclusively of rotation of the axis. The shape of the articular surfaces determines that, when rotation occurs, the axis ascends slightly into the atlantal ring (Kapandji 1974; Lang 1986), which limits stretch on the lateral atlantoaxial joint capsules. Rotation is limited mainly by the alar ligaments, with a minor contribution from the accessory atlantoaxial ligament. The normal range of atlantoaxial rotation has been measured as being 41.5° (range 29–54°) (Dvorak et al 1988a).

Muscles producing atlantoaxial rotation. These act on the cranium, transverse processes of the atlas and spinous process of the axis. They are mainly obliquus capitis inferior, rectus capitis posterior major and splenius capitis of one side, and the contralateral sterno-cleidomastoid.

Atlanto-occipital joints

Each joint consists of two reciprocally curved *articular surfaces*, one on the occipital condyle the other on the lateral mass of the atlas; the atlantal facets are concave and tilted medially. The bones are connected by articular capsules and the anterior and posterior atlanto-occipital membranes.

Fibrous capsules. The capsules surround the occipital condyles and superior atlantal articular facets. They are thicker posteriorly and laterally, where the capsule is sometimes deficient, and may communicate with the joint cavity between the dens and the transverse ligament of the atlas (Cave 1934; Lang 1986).

The anterior atlanto-occipital membrane (**6**.101). Broad, and of densely woven fibres, it connects the anterior margin of the foramen magnum to the upper border of the anterior arch of the atlas. Laterally, it blends with the capsular ligaments, and medially

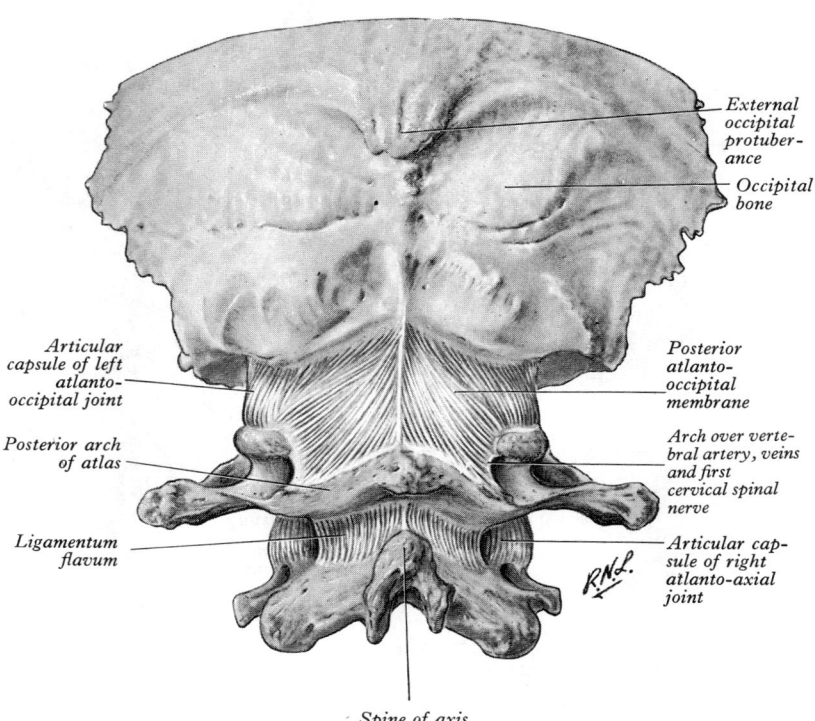

6.102   Atlanto-occipital and atlantoaxial joints: posterior aspect.

it is strengthened by a median cord which is the anterior longitudinal ligament stretching between the basilar occipital bone and anterior atlantal tubercle.

The posterior atlanto-occipital membrane (**6**.102). This is also broad, but relatively thin, connecting the posterior margin of the foramen magnum to the upper border of the posterior atlantal arch,

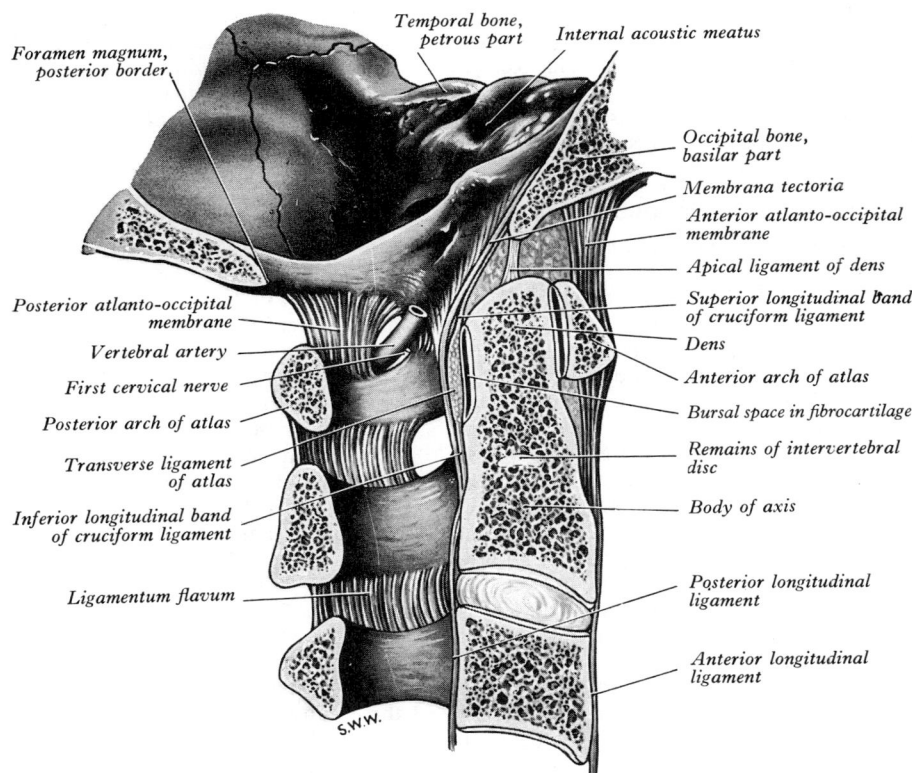

6.103   Median sagittal section through the occipital bone and the first to third cervical vertebrae.

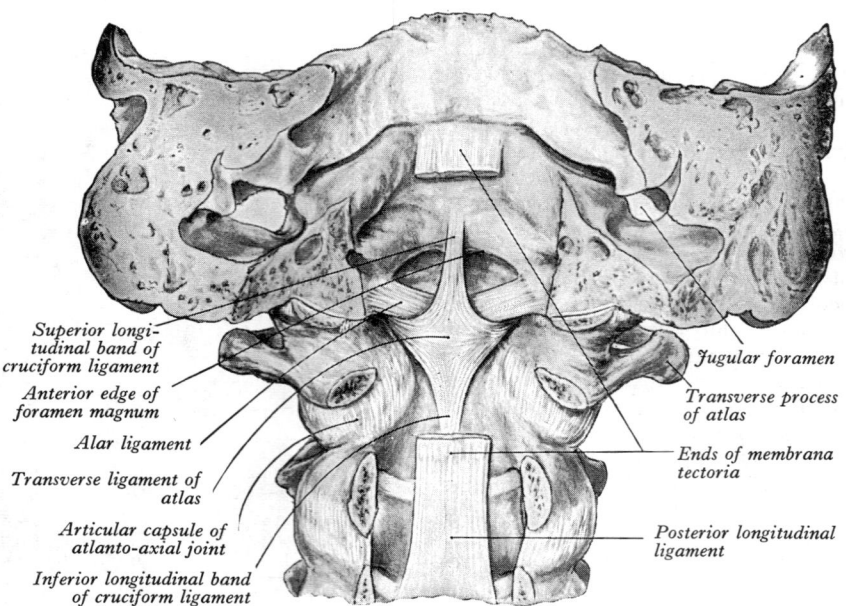

Superior longi-
tudinal band of
cruciform ligament

Anterior edge of
foramen magnum

Alar ligament

Transverse ligament of
atlas

Articular capsule of
atlanto-axial joint

Inferior longitudinal band
of cruciform ligament

Jugular foramen

Transverse process
of atlas

Ends of membrana
tectoria

Posterior longitudinal
ligament

6.104   Posterior aspect of the atlanto-occipital and atlantoaxial joints, after removal of the posterior part of the occipital bone and the laminae of the upper cervical vertebra. The atlanto-occipital joint cavities have been opened.

blending laterally with the joint capsules. It arches over the grooves for the vertebral arteries, venous plexuses and first cervical nerve: the ligamentous border of the arch is sometimes ossified.

Movements at the atlanto-occipital joints. The long (topographical) axes run anteromedially; because of this and their articular curvatures, the joints act as one around transverse and anteroposterior axes of movement but **not** about a vertical axis. The main movement is flexion, with a little lateral flexion and rotation. In young individuals the flexion range has been measured at 16.8–20.8° (Johnson et al 1977), lateral flexion at 3° and rotation at 5.7° (Dvorak et al 1988a).

Muscles producing movements at the atlanto-occipital joints. These are for *flexion*: longus capitis and rectus capitis anterior; *extension*: recti capitis posteriores major and minor, obliquus capitis superior, semispinalis capitis, splenius capitis and trapezius (cervical part); *lateral flexion*: rectus capitis lateralis, semispinalis capitis, splenius capitis, sternocleidomastoid and trapezius (cervical part); *rotation*: obliquus capitis superior, rectus capitis posterior minor, splenius capitis and sternocleidomastoid.

Ligaments connecting axis and occipital bone

These consist of the membrana tectoria, and paired alar and median apical ligaments.

Membrana tectoria (**6**.103, 104). Inside the vertebral canal, this is a broad strong band representing the upward continuation of the posterior longitudinal ligament (p. 512). Its superficial and deep laminae are both attached to the posterior surface of the axial body, the superficial lamina expanding as it ascends to the **upper** surface of the basilar occipital bone, attaching above the foramen magnum, where it blends with the cranial dura mater. The deep lamina has a strong median band ascending to the foramen magnum, and two lateral bands which pass and blend with the capsules of the atlanto-occipital joints as they reach the foramen magnum. The membrane is separated from the cruciform ligament of the atlas by a thin layer of loose areolar tissue, and sometimes by a bursa.

Alar ligaments (**6**.104). Thick cords about 11 mm long, they extend from the longitudinally ovoid flattenings on the posterolateral aspect of the apex of the dens horizontally and laterally to the roughened areas on the medial side of the occipital condyles. In most individuals there is also an anteroinferior band about 3 mm long which inserts into the lateral mass of the *atlas* in front of the transverse ligament; a few fibres are occasionally found passing from the dens to the anterior arch of the atlas (Dvorak and Panjabi 1987). In addition, in about 10% of cases a continuous transverse band of fibres passes between the occipital condyles immediately above the transverse

ligament, the *transverse occipital ligament* (Dvorak et al 1988b). These ligaments consist mainly of collagen fibres arranged in parallel. The main function of the alar ligaments is now considered to be limitation of atlantoaxial rotation, the left becoming taut on rotation to the right and vice versa. The slightly upward movement of the axis during rotation helps permit a wider range of movement by reducing tension in the alar ligaments, as it does also in the capsules and accessory ligaments of the lateral atlanto-occipital joint.

Apical ligament of the dens (**6**.103). It fans out from the apex of the dens into the anterior margin of the foramen magnum between the alar ligaments. It represents the cranial continuation of the notochord and its sheath (Ganguly & Roy 1964; O'Rahilly et al 1974). It is separated for most of its extent from the anterior atlanto-occipital membrane and cruciform ligament by pads of fatty tissue, though it blends with their attachments at the foramen magnum, and with the alar ligaments at the apex of the dens.

Ligamentum nuchae (p. 514). This also connects cervical vertebrae with the cranium.

Clinical anatomy. The transverse ligament is stronger than the dens, which usually fractures before rupture of the ligament. The alar ligaments are weaker, and combined head flexion and rotation may avulse one or both alar ligaments: rupture of one side results in an increase in the range of rotation of about 30% to the opposite side (Dvorak et al 1987). Pathological softening of the transverse and adjacent ligaments, usually due to connective tissue disorders, or of the lateral atlantoaxial joints results in atlantoaxial subluxation (Bogduk & Macintosh 1984), which may cause spinal cord injury. An interesting syndrome has been described in which atlantoaxial rotation causes entrapment of the second cervical spinal nerve, resulting in unilateral cervico-occipital pain, and, because afferent fibres pass from the lingual nerve via the hypoglossal nerve to the second cervical nerve, pain and numbness in the ipsilateral side of the tongue (Lance & Anthony 1980).

THORACIC VERTEBRAE

The twelve thoracic vertebrae (**6**.87, 105, 106) increase in size caudally, like other vertebrae, due to increased loading from above. All their bodies display lateral costal facets and all but the lowest two or three transverse processes also have facets, articulating with the head of the rib or its tubercle respectively. The first and ninth to twelfth vertebrae also have atypical features; except for relatively minor details the rest are alike.

The *body* is typically a waisted cylinder except where the vertebral foramen encroaches, transverse and anteroposterior dimensions

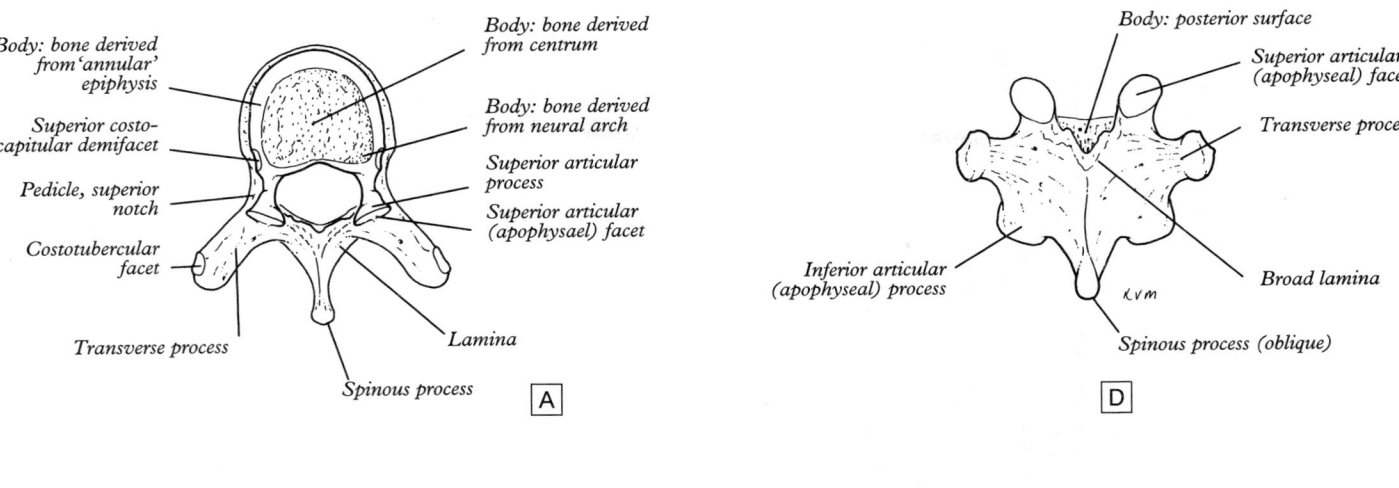

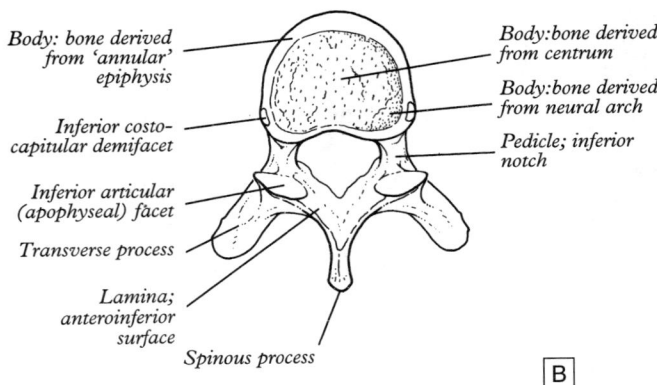

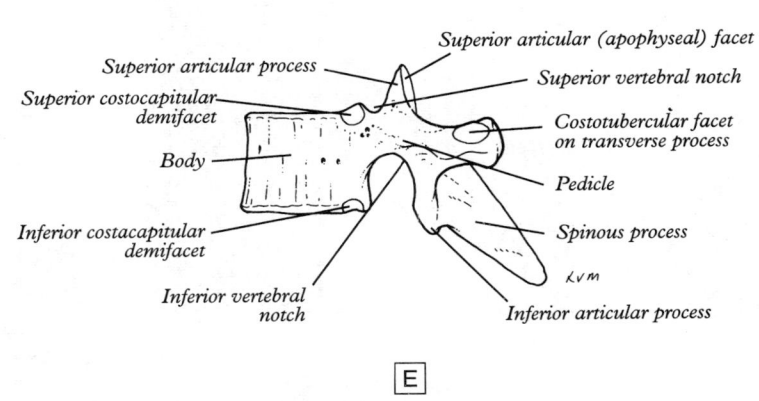

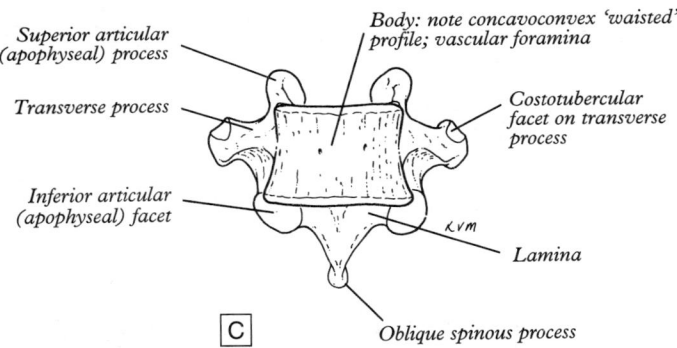

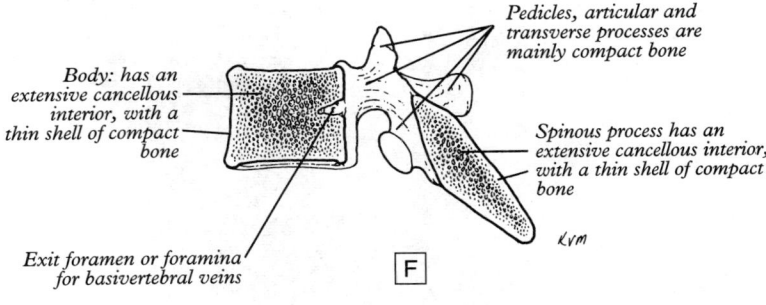

6.105   Typical thoracic vertebra. A. Superior aspect B. Inferior aspect C. Anterior aspect D. Posterior aspect E. Lateral aspect F. Longitudinal section.

being almost equal. One each side are *two costal facets* (really *demifacets*), the superior pair (usually larger) at the upper border anterior to the pedicles, the inferior at the lower border anterior to the vertebral notches (6.105D). The *vertebral foramen* is small and circular; thus the *pedicles* do not diverge as in cervical vertebrae; also the thoracic spinal cord is smaller and more circular. The *laminae* are short, thick and broad overlapping from above downwards. The *spinous process* slants downward. The thin and almost flat *superior articular processes* project from the pediculolaminar junctions and face posteriorly, a little superolaterally. The *inferior processes* project down from the laminae with their facets directed forwards, a little superomedially. The large, club-like *transverse processes* also project from the vertebral arch at the pediculolaminar junctions. Each passes posterolaterally and has, near its tip, anterior oval facets for articulation with the tubercle of the corresponding rib.

First thoracic vertebra (6.107). This has circular upper costal facets for articulation with the whole facet on the head of the first

rib; the smaller, semilunar inferior facets articulate, as do most thoracic vertebrae, with a demifacet on the rib head. The long, thick spine is horizontal and commonly as prominent as the seventh cervical.

Ninth thoracic vertebra (6.107). Otherwise typical, it often fails to articulate with the tenth ribs in which case the inferior demifacets are absent.

Tenth thoracic vertebra (6.107). This only articulates with the tenth pair of ribs. Consequently superior facets only appear on the body; these are usually large and semilunar, or oval when the tenth ribs fail to articulate with the ninth vertebrae and intervening disc. The transverse process may or may not bear a facet for the tenth rib tubercle.

Eleventh thoracic vertebra (6.107). This articulates only with heads of the eleventh ribs. The circular costal facets are close to the upper border of the body extending on to the pedicles. The small transverse processes lack articular facets.

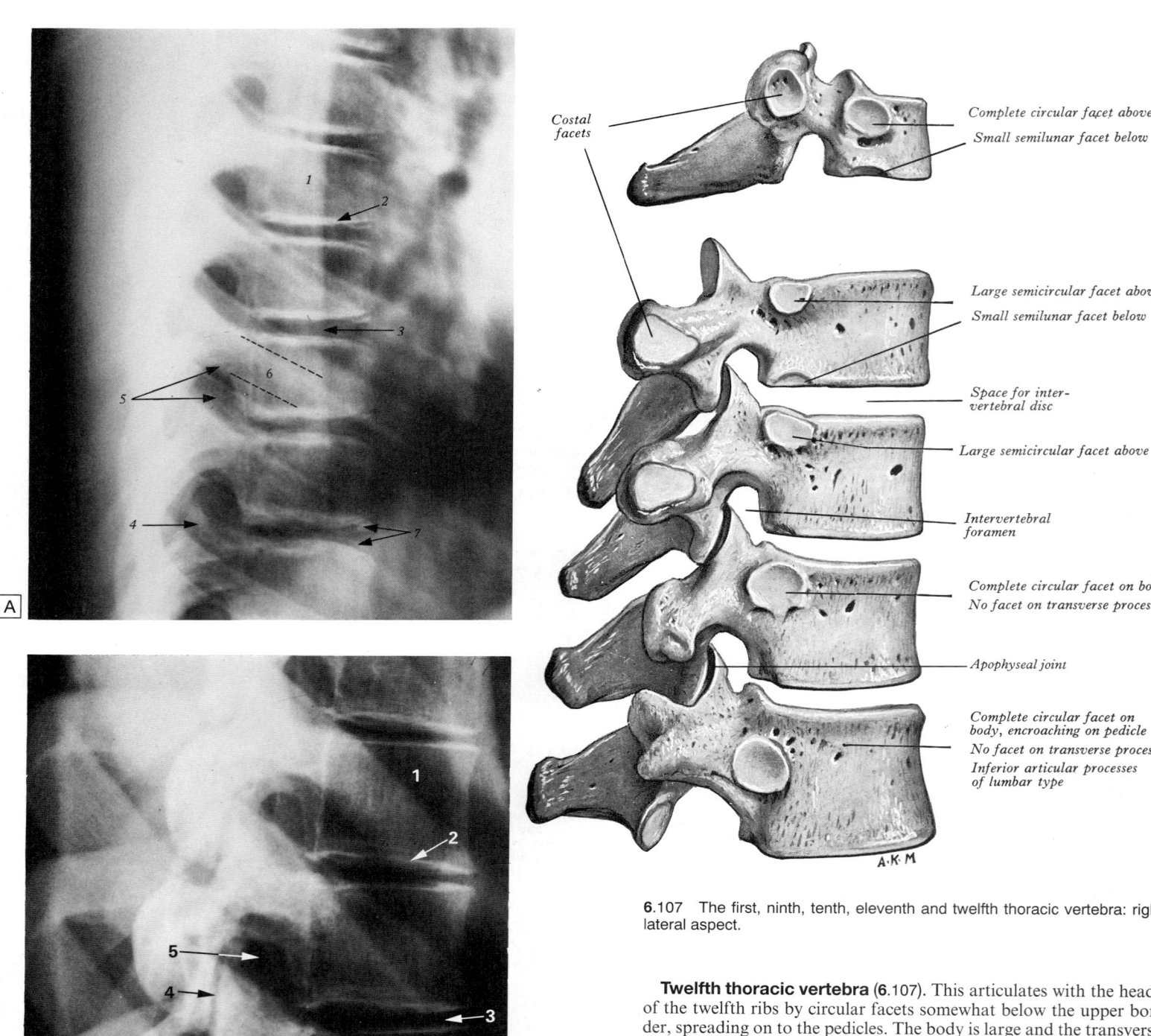

6.107 The first, ninth, tenth, eleventh and twelfth thoracic vertebra: right lateral aspect.

Labels on illustration: Costal facets; Complete circular facet above; Small semilunar facet below; Large semicircular facet above; Small semilunar facet below; Space for inter-vertebral disc; Large semicircular facet above; Intervertebral foramen; Complete circular facet on body; No facet on transverse process; Apophyseal joint; Complete circular facet on body, encroaching on pedicle; No facet on transverse process; Inferior articular processes of lumbar type

A·K·M

Twelfth thoracic vertebra (6.107). This articulates with the heads of the twelfth ribs by circular facets somewhat below the upper border, spreading on to the pedicles. The body is large and the transverse processes small; the vertebra has some lumbar features (see below).

Changes in thoracic vertebrae

The *bodies* of upper thoracic vertebrae gradually change from cervical to thoracic in type, while the lower change from thoracic to lumbar. The body of the first is typically cervical, its transverse diameter being almost twice the anteroposterior; the second retains a cervical shape, but its two diameters differ less. The third body is the smallest having a convex anterior aspect unlike the flattened first and second. The remaining bodies increase in size and, owing to its increased anteroposterior diameter, the fourth is typically 'heart-shaped' (cordate). The fifth to eighth increase their anteroposterior dimension but change little transversely. These four, in transverse section, are asymmetrical, their left sides being flattened by pressure of the thoracic aorta. The rest increase more rapidly in all measurements, so that the twelfth body resembles that of a typical lumbar vertebra. Geometrical analysis suggests that these modifications are also adaptations to a greater range of flexion-extension at the cervical and lumbar ends of the thoracic vertebral column (Veleanu et al 1972). To borders of the bodies are attached the anterior and posterior longitudinal ligaments, and around the margins of costal facets are

6.106 Lateral radiographs of midthoracic vertebral column in a child of 14 years (A) and an adult female of 22 years (B).
1. Cancellous bone of vertebral body. 2. Shell of compact bone. 3. Site of intervertebral disc. 4. Synovial joint between articular processes. 5. Intervertebral foramen. 6. Superimposed shadow of rib. 7. Ossification occurring in unfused annular epiphyses of vertebral bodies. (A supplied by Shan Gallagher, Guy's Hospital; photography by Sarah Smith.)

capsular and radiate ligaments of the costovertebral joints. Longus colli arises from the upper three thoracic vertebral bodies, lateral to the anterior longitudinal ligament, and psoas major and minor from the side of the twelfth near its lower border.

Thoracic *pedicles* show a successive caudal increase in thickness. The superior vertebral notch is recognizable only in the first thoracic, but the inferior notch is deep in all. Ligamenta flava are attached at the upper borders and lower anterior surfaces of laminae, and rotatores to their posterior aspects.

Thoracic *transverse processes* shorten in caudal succession. In the upper six (or five), the costal facets are concave and face antero-laterally; at lower levels the facets are flatter and face superolaterally and slightly forwards. To the anterior surface medial to the facet is attached the costotransverse ligament, to its tuberculated apex the lateral costotransverse ligament and to its lower border the superior costotransverse ligament. Upper and lower borders also provide attachment for intertransverse muscles or fibrous vestiges and the posterior surface for deep dorsal muscles; posteriorly on the apex is the levator costae.

Thoracic *spines* overlap from the fifth to eighth, which is the longest and most oblique. (In quadrupeds most thoracic spines slope caudally and lumbar spines cranially, the change in inclination occurring at a lower thoracic *anticlinal* vertebra; its human equivalent is the eleventh.) Supraspinous and interspinous ligaments, trapezius, rhomboid major and minor, latissimus dorsi, serratus posterior

superior and inferior and many deep dorsal muscles are attached to thoracic spines.

The first thoracic vertebra resembles a cervical vertebra in its body, both in shape and posterolateral lipping, the latter forming the anterior border of the superior vertebral notch, a distinctive feature. The upper costal facet is often incomplete, the first rib then articulating with the seventh cervical and intervening disc. Below the facet a small, deep depression often occurs.

The eleventh and twelfth thoracic spinous processes are triangular, with blunt apices, a horizontal lower and an oblique upper border. The twelfth thoracic transverse process is replaced by three small tubercles; the superior is largest, projects upwards and corresponds to a lumbar mamillary process, though not so close to the superior articular process. The lateral tubercle is the homologue of a transverse process, the inferior the homologue of a lumbar accessory process. These two vertebrae can be distinguished by the size and shape of the transverse process and the distance between the costal facet and upper border (see above).

A change in orientation of articular processes from thoracic to lumbar type usually occurs at the eleventh thoracic vertebra, some-times the twelfth or tenth. In the transitional vertebra the superior articular processes are thoracic, facing posterolaterally, while the inferior are transversely convex and face anterolaterally. This vertebra marks the site of a sudden change in degree from rotational to non-rotational function (p. 515; Davis 1955).

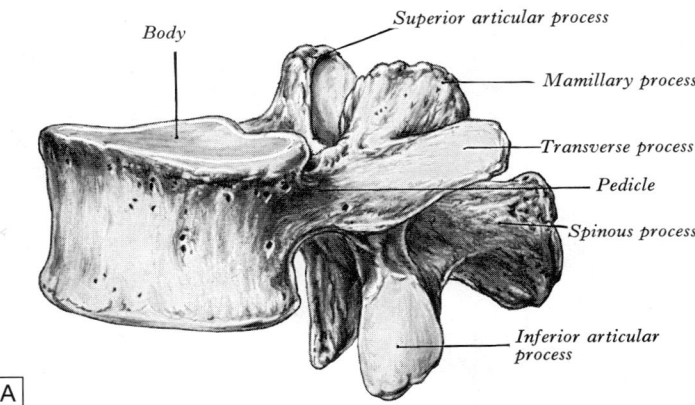

6.108A.   Lumbar vertebra: left lateral aspect.

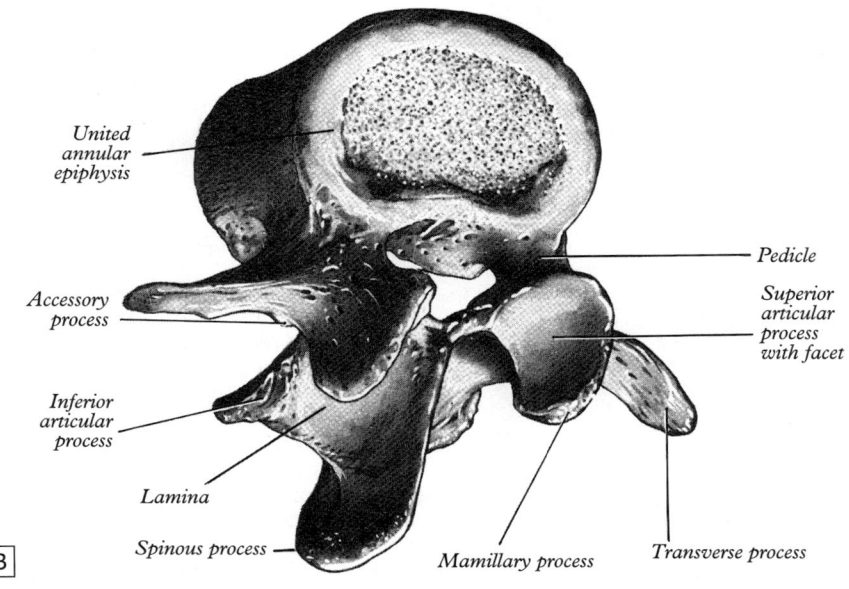

6.108B.   Lumbar vertebra: posterosuperior aspect, viewed obliquely from the left side.

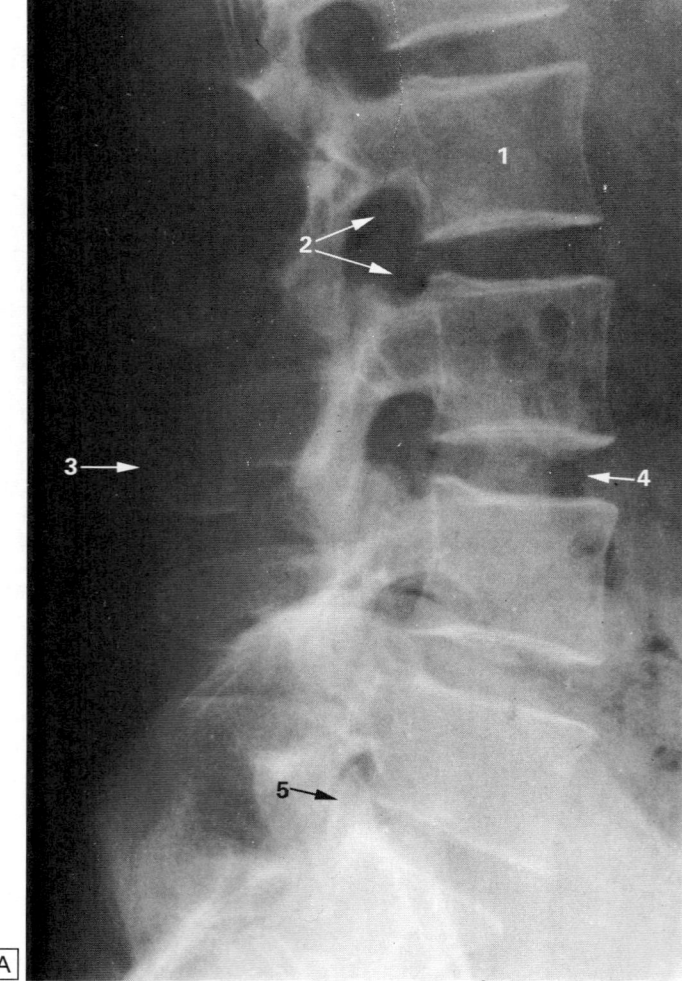

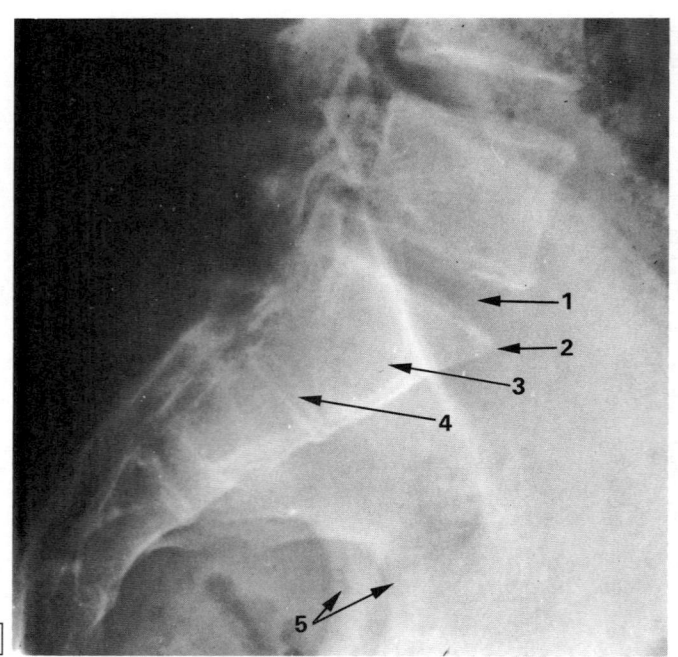

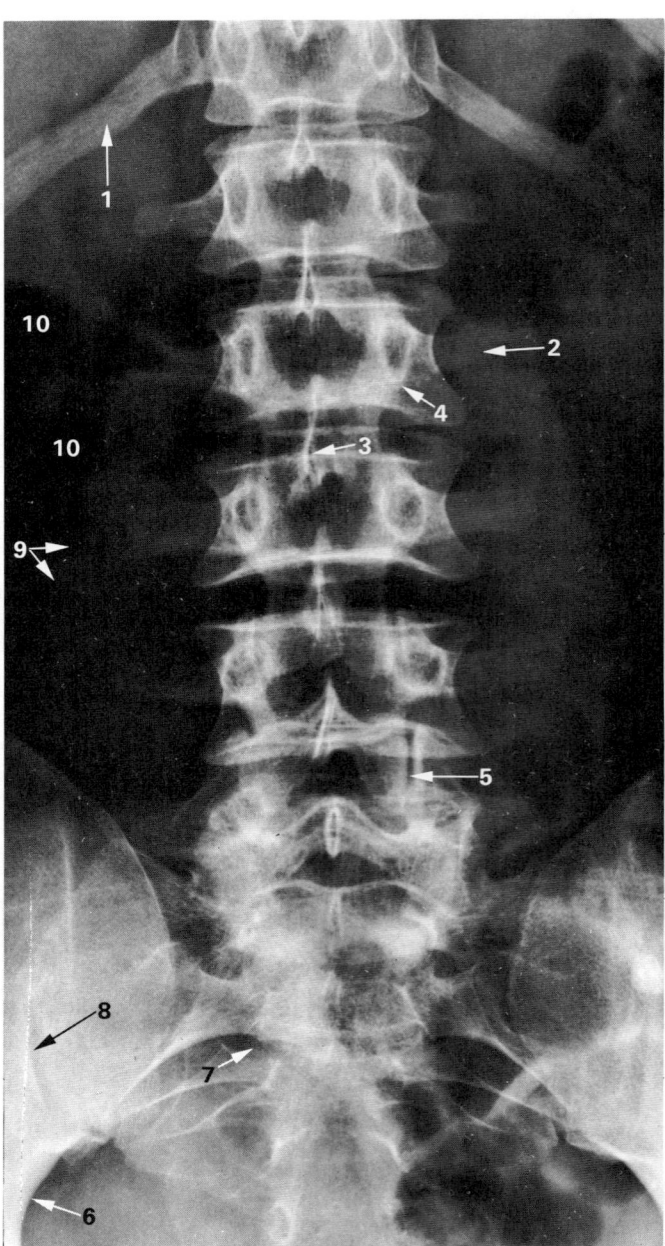

6.109   c. Anterosuperior radiograph of lumbosacral vertebral column in a young adult male aged 22 years. 1. Twelfth rib. 2. Transverse process. 3. Spinous process (2nd lumbar). 4. Compact bony shell of pedicle (2nd lumbar). 5. Joint between articular processes (4th and 5th lumbar). 6. Pelvic brim. 7. Anterior sacral foramen. 8. Sacro-iliac joint. 9. Lateral border of psoas major. 10. Gas in colon.

6.109A, B.   Lateral radiographs of lumbosacral vertebral column in an adult male aged 26 years.

A 1. Lumbar vertebral body. 2. Intervertebral foramen. 3. Spinous process. 4. Site of intervertebral disc. 5. Synovial joint between articular processes. Note slightly cuneiform profile of fifth lumbar vertebral body. B 1. Site of lumbosacral disc. Note cuneiform shape. 2. Sacral promontory. 3. First sacral segment. 4. Remains of sacral intervertebral disc. 5. Profiles of greater sciatic notches.

LUMBAR VERTEBRAE

The five lumbar vertebrae (**6**.108, 109) are distinguished by their large size and absence of costal facets and transverse foramina. The *body* is wider transversely and deeper in front. The *vertebral foramen* is triangular, larger than at thoracic but smaller than at cervical levels. The *pedicles* are short. The *spinous process* is almost horizontal, quadrangular and thickened along its posterior and inferior borders. The *superior articular processes* bear vertical concave articular facets facing posteromedially, with a rough mamillary process on their posterior borders. The *inferior articular processes* have vertical convex articular facets facing anterolaterally. The *transverse processes* are thin and long, except the more substantial fifth pair. A small accessory process marks the posteroinferior aspect of the root of each transverse process. Measurement of 338 third and fourth lumbar vertebrae, from both sexes aged 20–90 years, showed that breadth of the body increases with age; in males, posterior height decreases

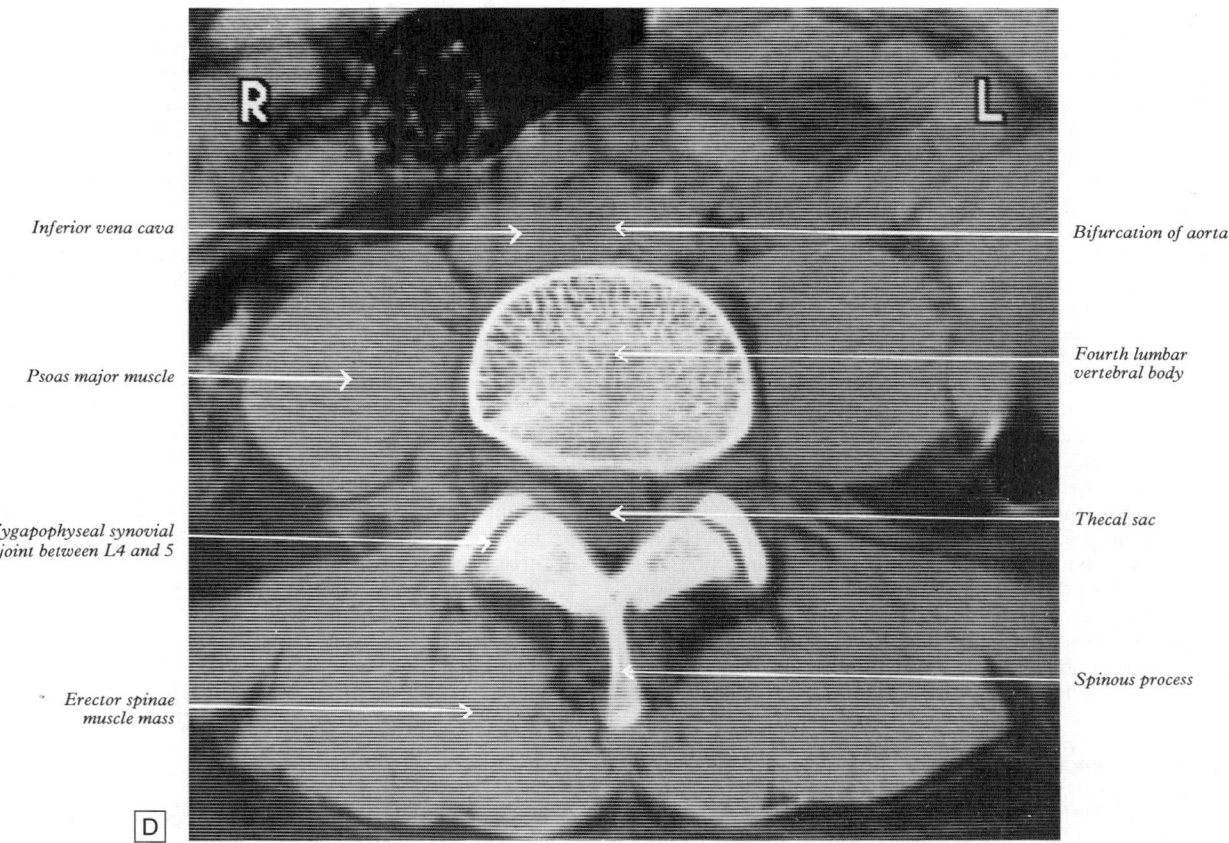

Inferior vena cava

Psoas major muscle

Zygapophyseal synovial joint between L4 and 5

Erector spinae muscle mass

Bifurcation of aorta

Fourth lumbar vertebral body

Thecal sac

Spinous process

R   L

D

6.109D.   High resolution computed tomogram through posterior abdominal wall at the level of the body of the fourth lumbar vertebra, showing zyga- pophyseal joints between fourth and fifth lumbar vertebrae. (Supplied by Shaun Gallagher, Guy's Hospital; photography by Sarah Smith.)

relatively; in both sexes anterior height of the body decreases relative to breadth (Ericksen 1976). Twomey et al (1983), in a study of 93 adult vertebral columns, observed a reduction in bone density of lumbar vertebral bodies, principally due to a reduction in transverse trabeculae (more marked in females), associated with increased diameter and increasing concavity in their juxtadiscal surfaces. Amonoo-Kuofi (1982, 1985) compared lumbar interpedicular distances in 150 males and 140 females by radiography, expressing these as a ratio of vertebral body width. Values varied much, but the ratio (in Nigerians) was most constant: racial variation was discussed.

A recent study has shown significant sex difference in the angle of inclination and depth of curvature of the superior articular facets of all lumbar vertebrae, in addition to which considerable asymmetry was also observed, being greatest at L1 and least at L5 (Tulsi & Hermanis 1992).

Fifth lumbar vertebra (6.110). This has a massive *transverse process* continuous with the **whole of the pedicle and encroaching on**

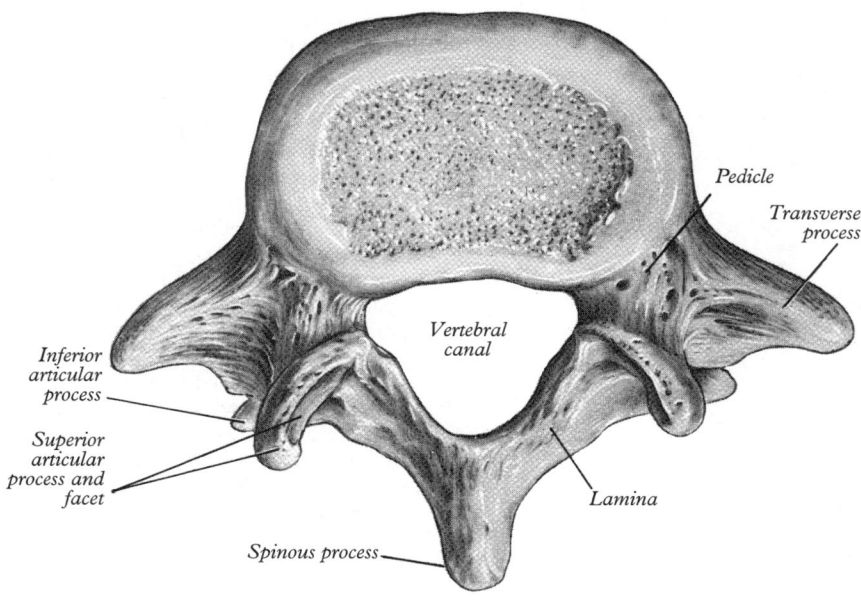

Pedicle

Transverse process

Inferior articular process

Superior articular process and facet

Vertebral canal

Lamina

Spinous process

6.110   The fifth lumbar vertebra: superior aspect.

the body. The body is usually the largest and markedly deeper in front, thus contributing to the lumbosacral angle.

Attachments of lumbar vertebrae. Upper and lower borders of lumbar *bodies* give attachment to the anterior and posterior longitudinal ligaments (p. 512). Lateral to the anterior ligament the upper bodies (three on the right, two on the left) give attachments to the crura of the diaphragm. Posterolaterally, psoas major is attached to the upper and lower margins of all lumbar bodies; between these, tendinous arches carry its attachments across their concave sides. The first lumbar *vertebral foramen* contains the conus medullaris of the spinal cord, the lower foramina the cauda equina and spinal meninges. Strong paired pedicles arise posterolaterally from each body near its upper border. Superior vertebral notches are shallow, inferior ones deep. The laminae are broad and short but do not overlap as much as do the thoracic. To spinous processes are attached the posterior lamella of the thoracolumbar fascia, erectores spinae, spinales thoracis, multifidi, interspinal muscles and ligaments, and supraspinous ligaments. The fifth spine is smallest, its apex often rounded and down-turned. Upper lumbar superior articular processes are further apart than inferior ones, but the difference is slight in the fourth and negligible in the fifth. The articular facets are reciprocally concave (superior) and convex (inferior), allowing flexion, extension, lateral bending and some degree of rotation. Transverse processes, except the fifth, are anteroposteriorly compressed and project posterolaterally. The lower border of the fifth transverse process is angulated, passing laterally and then superolaterally to a blunt tip, the whole process presenting greater upward

---

inclination than the fourth. The angle on the inferior border may represent the tip of the costal element and the lateral end the tip of the true transverse process. The lumbar transverse processes increase in length from first to third and then shorten. Thus, as noted, the fifth pair incline both **upwards** and posterolaterally. All lumbar transverse processes present a vertical ridge on the anterior surface, nearer the tip, which marks the attachment of the anterior layer of the thoracolumbar fascia, and separates the surface into medial and lateral areas for psoas major and quadratus lumborum respectively. The middle layer of the fascia is attached to the apices of the transverse processes; to the first pair the medial and lateral arcuate ligaments (lumbocostal arches) also attach, and to the fifth the iliolumbar ligament. Posteriorly the transverse processes are covered by deep dorsal muscles; fibres of longissimus thoracis are attached to them. To their upper and lower borders the lateral intertransverse muscles are attached. The mamillary process, homologous with the superior tubercle of the twelfth thoracic vertebra, gives attachment to multifidus and the medial intertransverse muscle. To the accessory process, which is sometimes difficult to identify, is attached the medial intertransverse muscle. The costal element is incorporated in the mature transverse process. (For a discussion of homologies of all three processes consult Jones 1912.)

Clinical anatomy. The various methods of estimating the diameter of the lumbar vertebral canal, which is sometimes subject to stenosis, have been reviewed by Amonoo-Kuofi (1982), who considers radiographic estimation of interpedicular dimensions to be a reliable technique: racial variation has been found to occur in the sagittal dimension of the canal (Amonoo-Kuofi 1985).

SACRUM

The sacrum (**6.**111–113) is a large, triangular fusion of five vertebrae and forms the posterosuperior wall of the pelvic cavity, wedged between the two innominate bones. Its blunted, caudal *apex* articulates with the coccyx and its superior, wide *base* with the fifth lumbar vertebra at the *lumbosacral angle.* It is set obliquely and curved longitudinally, its dorsal surface being convex, the pelvic concave (**6.**111c). This ventral curvature increases pelvic capacity. Between base and apex are *dorsal, pelvic* and *lateral* surfaces and a *sacral canal.* In childhood, individual sacral vertebrae are connected by cartilage and separable by maceration; the adult bone also retains many vertebral features.

Base (**6.**112). This is the upper surface of the *first sacral vertebra,* the least modified from the typical vertebral plan. The *body* is large and wider transversely, its anterior projecting edge is the *sacral promontory.* The vertebral foramen is triangular, its *pedicles* being short and divergent posterolaterally. The *laminae* are oblique, inclining down posteromedially to meet at a *spinous tubercle.* The *superior articular processes* project cranially, with concave articular facets directed posteromedially to articulate with inferior articular processes of the fifth lumbar vertebra. The posterior part of each process projects, bearing laterally a rough area homologous with a lumbar mamillary process. The *transverse process* is much modified; a broad, sloping mass projects laterally from the body, pedicle and superior articular process (**6.**112)—a unique feature, although foreshadowed in the fifth lumbar. It consists of transverse process and costal element fused together and to the rest of the vertebra, forming the superior part of the sacral *lateral mass* or *ala.*

Pelvic surface (**6.**111A). Anteroinferior, it is vertically and transversely concave, but the second sacral body may produce a convexity. Four pairs of *pelvic sacral foramina* communicate through intervertebral foramina with the sacral canal, transmitting ventral rami of the upper four sacral spinal nerves. The large area between right and left foramina, formed by flat pelvic aspects of the sacral bodies, shows their fusion by four *transverse ridges.* The bars between foramina are *costal elements,* fused to the vertebrae. Lateral to the foramina the costal elements unite together and posteriorly with transverse processes to form the *lateral part* of the sacrum (which expands basally as the ala).

The pelvic surface gives attachment to the piriformes (**6.**111A). Emerging from the pelvic sacral foramina the first three sacral ventral rami pass anterior to piriformis. Medial to the foramina the sympathetic trunks descend in contact with bone, as do the median sacral vessels in the midline. Lateral to the foramina lateral sacral

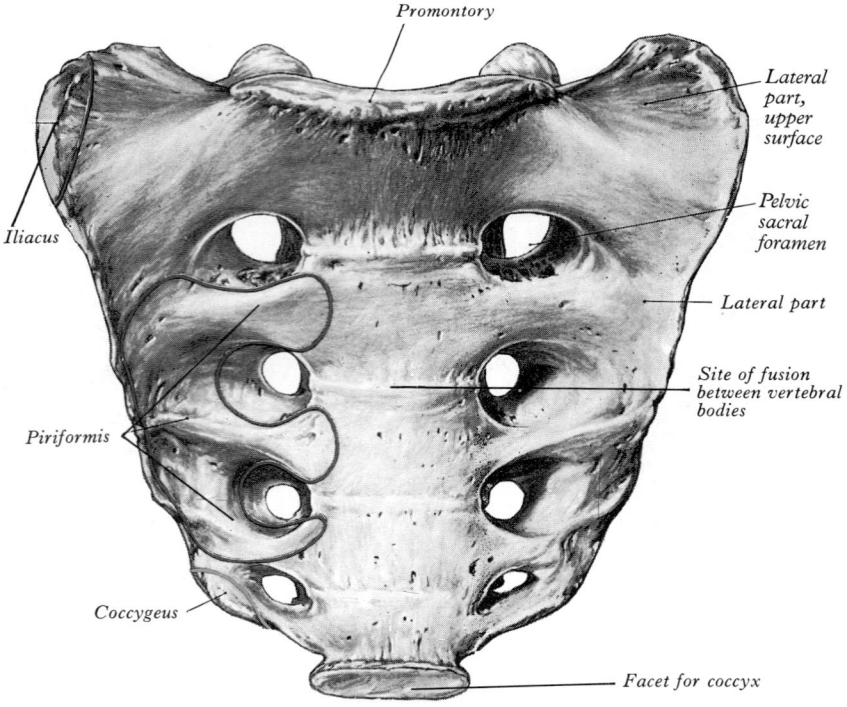

Promontory

Lateral part, upper surface

Pelvic sacral foramen

Lateral part

Site of fusion between vertebral bodies

Facet for coccyx

Iliacus

Piriformis

Coccygeus

528   6.111A.   Pelvic surface.

Colour coding of muscle attachments. The structural/functional ideas implicit in the traditional terms 'origin' and 'insertion' applied to muscle attachments do not accord with modern myokinetics; the latter envisages many more complex and flexible responses (p. 788). Nevertheless, some introductory and practical courses retain the terms, and the delineation of *all* muscle attachments by a single colour has proved an impediment to occasional groups of students. Some trunk muscles and those of the girdles and free limbs have, in this edition, a dual colour code; this facilitates their separate recognition. The axial, paraxial, or medial attachments of free limb muscles are delineated in *blue* (the historical 'insertion'). In contrast, on a series of diagrams of the skull, multiple colour coding is used to group muscles in terms of their embryological origin and nerve supply. Above comments on red and blue lines apply in most instances; occasional exceptions may be noted in a minority of individual muscles and bones.

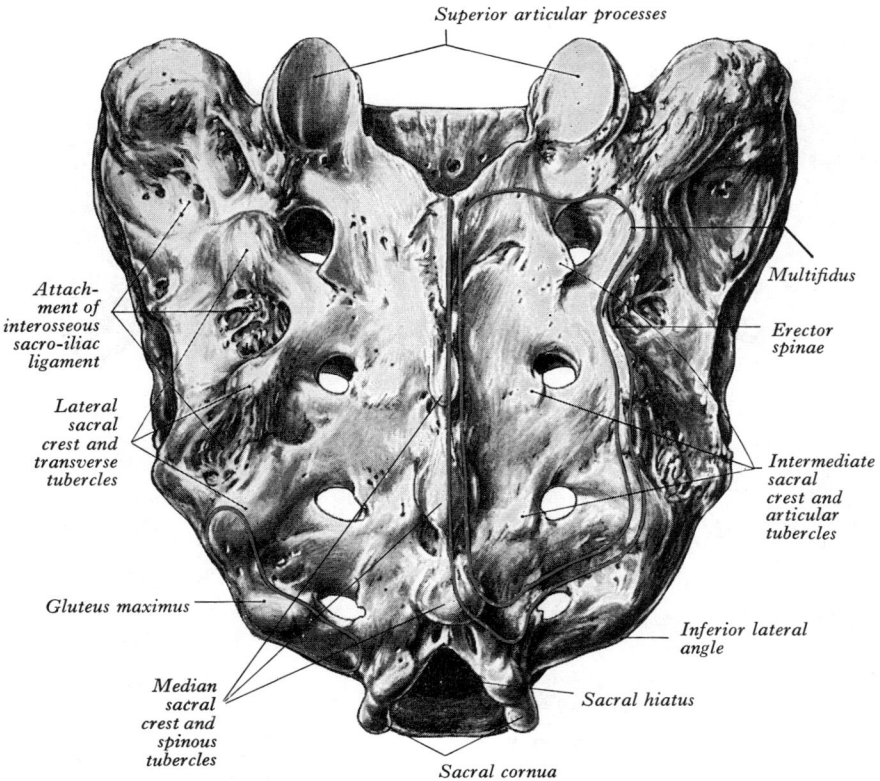

6.111B.   Dorsal surface of the sacrum.

vessels are related to bone. Ventral surfaces of the first, second and partly third sacral bodies are covered by parietal peritoneum and crossed obliquely, left of the midline, by the attachment of the sigmoid mesocolon. The rectum is in contact with the pelvic surfaces of the third to fifth sacral vertebrae and with the superior rectal artery's bifurcation between the rectum and third sacral vertebra.

Dorsal surface (6.111B). Convex and posterosuperior, it has a raised, interrupted, *median sacral crest* with four (sometimes three) spinous tubercles representing fused sacral spines. Below the fourth (or third) an arched *sacral hiatus* in the posterior wall of the sacral canal, due to failure of the fifth pair of laminae to meet, exposes the dorsal surface of the fifth body. Flanking the median crest the posterior surface is formed by fused laminae and lateral to this are four pairs of *dorsal sacral foramina*. Like the pelvic foramina they lead into the sacral canal through intervertebral foramina; each transmits the dorsal ramus of a sacral spinal nerve. **Medial** to the foramina, and vertically below each articular process of the first sacral, is a row of four small tubercles, collectively the *intermediate sacral crest*; these, sometimes termed *articular*, represent fused articular processes. The fifth inferior articular processes project caudally and flank the sacral hiatus as *sacral cornua*, connected to coccygeal cornua by intercornual ligaments. **Lateral** to the dorsal sacral foramina is a *lateral sacral crest* formed by fused transverse processes, whose apices appear as a row of *transverse tubercles*.

The dorsal surface gives attachment to erector spinae by an elongated U-shaped area of spinous and transverse tubercles, covering multifidus which occupies the enclosed area (6.111B). The upper three sacral spinal dorsal rami pierce these muscles as they emerge via dorsal foramina.

Lateral surface (6.111C). This is a fusion of transverse processes and costal elements: wide above, it rapidly narrows in its lower part. The broad, upper part bears an *auricular surface* for articulation with the ilium, the area posterior to this being rough and deeply pitted by attachment of ligaments. The auricular surface, borne by costal elements, is like an inverted letter L. The shorter, cranial limb is restricted to the first sacral vertebra, the caudal descending to the middle of the third. Beyond this the lateral surface is non-articular and reduced in breadth. Caudally it curves medially to the body of

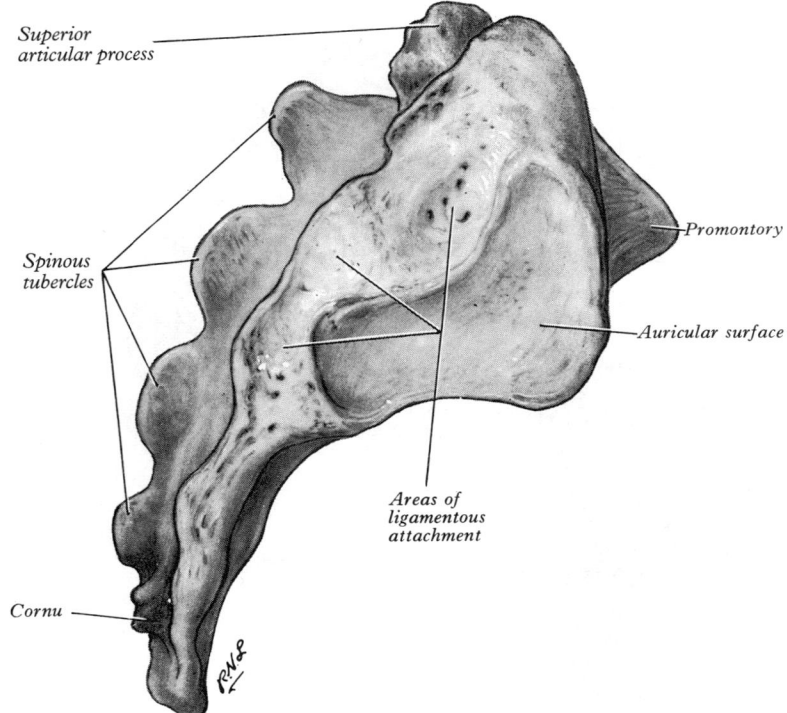

6.111C.   Right lateral aspect of the sacrum.

the fifth sacral vertebra at the *inferior lateral angle*, beyond which the surface becomes a thin lateral border. A variable *accessory* sacral articular facet sometimes occurs.

The auricular surface is covered by hyaline cartilage, and formed entirely by costal elements. It shows cranial and caudal elevations and an intermediate depression, posterior to which, in the elderly, is

529

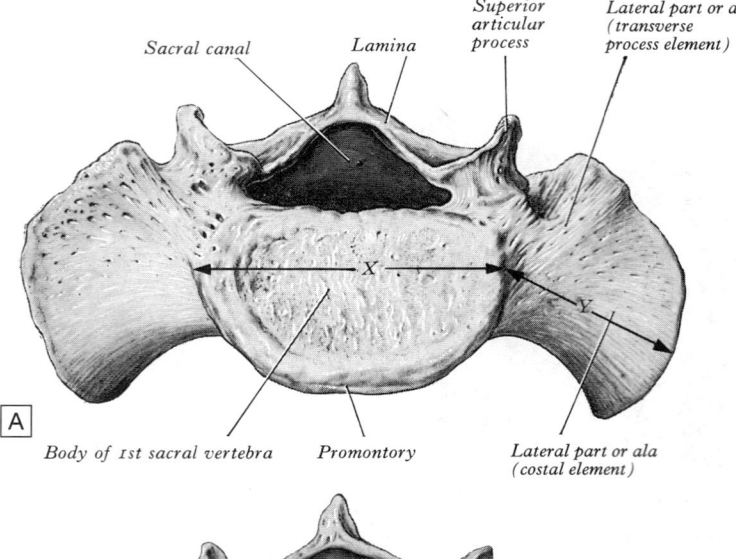

Sacral canal Lamina Superior articular process Lateral part or ala (transverse process element)

A

Body of 1st sacral vertebra   Promontory   Lateral part or ala (costal element)

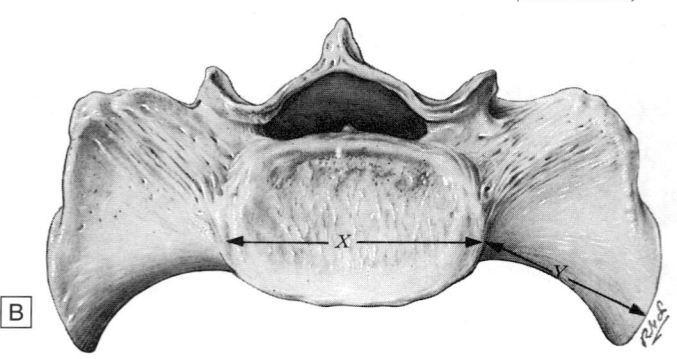

B

6.112 Base of the sacrum in the male (A) and in the female (B). The body of the first segment (*x*) forms a larger part of the breadth of the base in the male than it does in the female. In the latter the body is relatively smaller and the lateral, costal part (*y*), the ala, is relatively broader.

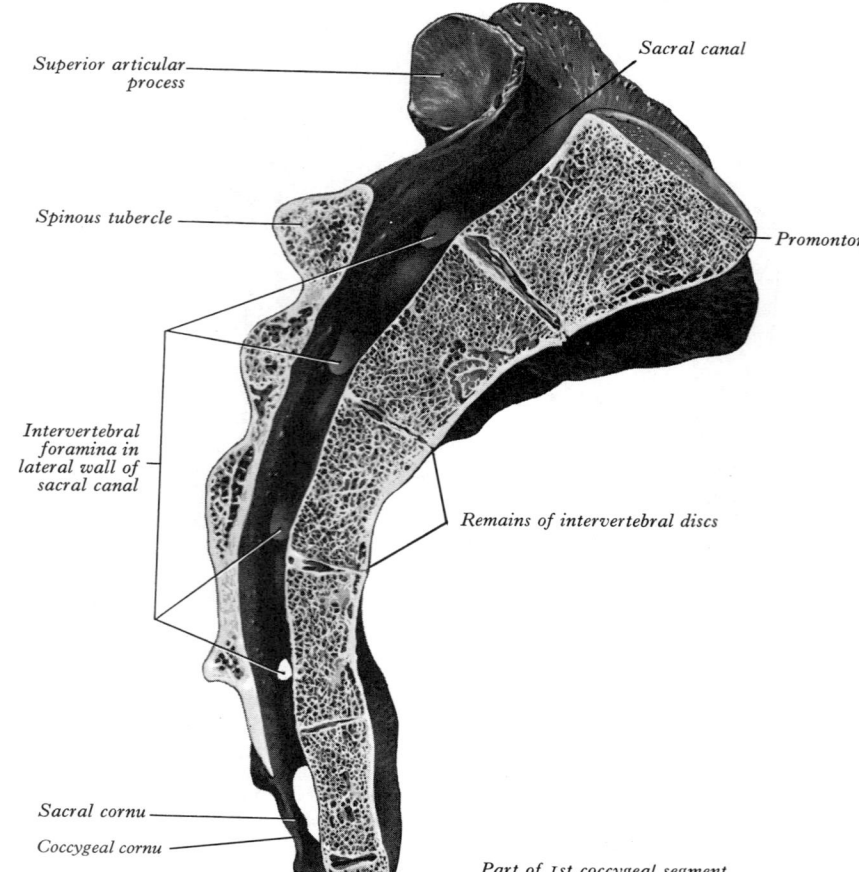

Superior articular process   Sacral canal

Spinous tubercle

Promontory

Intervertebral foramina in lateral wall of sacral canal

Remains of intervertebral discs

Sacral cornu

Coccygeal cornu

Part of 1st coccygeal segment recently united to sacrum

530   6.113 Median sagittal section through the sacrum.

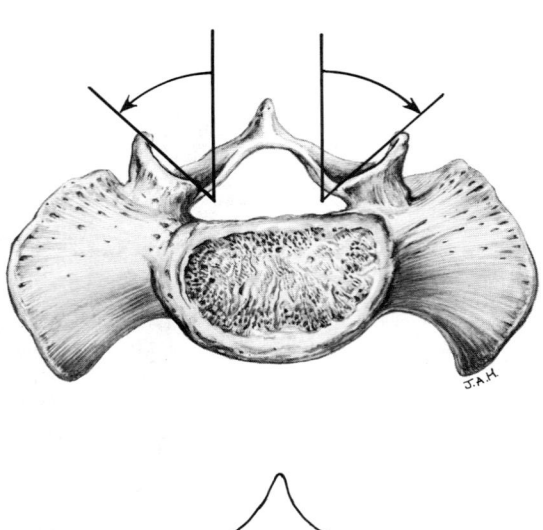

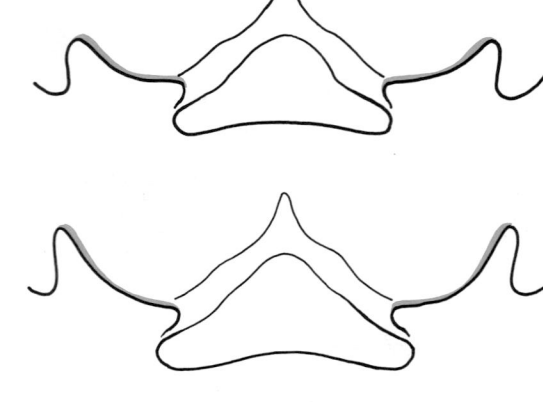

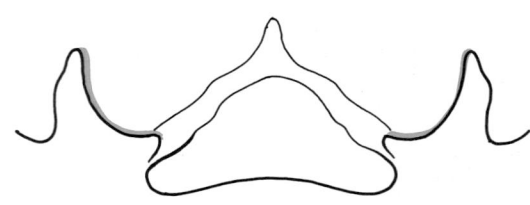

6.114 The method employed by Čihák (1970) to measure the inclinations of articular surfaces of the lumbosacral zygapophyseal joints (above). The lower profiles depict three degrees of increasing curvature and inclination. For quantitative data derived from 132 human sacra consult the original paper.

a third elevation. The rough area behind the auricular surface shows two or three marked depressions for attachment of strong interosseous sacroiliac ligaments. Below the auricular surface are attached gluteus maximus, the sacrotuberous and sacrospinous ligaments and coccygeus, from behind forwards.

Sacral apex. The inferior aspect of the fifth sacral vertebral body, it bears an oval facet for articulation with the coccyx.

Sacral canal (6.113). Formed by sacral vertebral foramina, it is triangular in section. Its upper, basal opening is oblique but, owing to sacral inclination, is directed cranially in the standing position. Each lateral wall presents four intervertebral foramina, through which it is continuous with pelvic and dorsal sacral foramina. Its caudal opening is the *sacral hiatus*.

The sacral canal. This contains the cauda equina (including its filum terminale) and spinal meninges. Near its midlevel subarachnoid and subdural spaces cease and lower sacral spinal roots and filum terminale pierce the arachnoid and dura maters. The filum terminale emerges at the sacral hiatus and traverses the dorsal surface of the fifth sacral vertebra and sacrococcygeal joint to reach the coccyx. The fifth sacral spinal nerves also emerge through the hiatus medial to the sacral cornua, grooving the lateral aspects of the fifth sacral vertebra.

Attachments of the first sacral body. To the ventral and dorsal surfaces of the first sacral body are attached terminal fibres of the anterior and posterior longitudinal ligaments. Its upper laminar borders receive the lowest pair of ligamenta flava. Superiorly the ala is smooth, medially concave and laterally rough. It is covered almost entirely by psoas major. The smooth area is obliquely grooved by the lumbosacral trunk. The rough area is for the lower band of the iliolumbar ligament, lateral to the fifth lumbar spinal nerve and to the anterior sacroiliac ligament. Iliacus reaches the anterolateral part of this area (**6**.111A).

Sex differences in sacra. Typical male or female sacra are easily identified but sexual differences are not always marked; identification is sometimes difficult. The female sacrum is shorter and wider, producing a wider pelvic cavity. Sacral width, as a percentage of length, yields a *sacral index*. The loci used in making these measurements are discussed on p. 671. The ventral concavity is deeper in females and its deepest point is usually higher than in males; curvature above this point is greater in the female. The dorsal protrusion of the second sacral vertebra (p. 674) is therefore usually less prominent in males. In females the pelvic surface faces downwards more than in males, increasing the pelvic cavity and making the lumbosacral angle more prominent. The female auricular surface is shorter but in both sexes usually extends along the first three sacral vertebrae. Owing to the great size of the fifth **lumbar** body, the first **sacral** body occupies a larger proportion of the sacral base in the male, its transverse diameter exceeding the length of an ala; the female dimensions are roughly equal.

Structure. The sacrum consists of trabecular bone enveloped by a shell of compact bone of variable thickness.

Variations. The sacrum may contain six vertebrae, by development of an additional sacral element or by incorporation of the fifth lumbar or first coccygeal vertebrae. Inclusion of the fifth lumbar (*sacralization*) is usually incomplete and limited to one side. In the most minor degree of the abnormality a fifth lumbar transverse process is large and articulates, sometimes by a synovial joint, with the sacrum at the posterolateral angle of its base. Reduction of sacral constituents is less common but *lumbarization* of the first sacral vertebra occurs; it remains partially or completely separate. The dorsal wall of the sacral canal may be variably deficient, due to imperfect development of laminae and spines. Orientation of the superior sacral articular facets (and hence the relation between the planes of the two zygapophyseal lumbosacral joints) displays wide variation according to Čihák (1970): the chords of the concave sacral facets formed an angle with the sagittal plane varying from 20° to 90° in 132 sacra, the majority between 40° and 60° (**6**.114). Curvatures of the facets and their degree of asymmetry also varied.

LUMBOSACRAL JOINTS

Articulations between the fifth lumbar and first sacral vertebrae resemble those of others. Their bodies are united by a symphysis including a large intervertebral disc, deeper anteriorly at the lumbosacral angle with anterior and posterior longitudinal ligaments adherent to it. Their zygapophyseal joints are separated by a wider interval than those above. They have ligamenta flava, interspinous and supraspinous ligaments. The fifth lumbar vertebra is attached to the ilium and sacrum by the iliolumbar ligament. These joints vary much in geometry (p. 528; **6**.114).

Iliolumbar ligament (**6**.278). It is attached to the tip and antero-inferior aspect of the fifth lumbar transverse process, and sometimes has a weak attachment to the fourth. It radiates laterally and is attached by main bands to the pelvis: a lower one, the *lumbosacral ligament*, from the inferior aspect of the fifth lumbar transverse process to the anterosuperior lateral surface of the sacrum, blending with the anterior sacroiliac ligament; and an upper, partial attachment of quadratus lumborum, passing to the iliac crest anterior to the sacroiliac joint, continuous above with the thoracolumbar fascia. Innervation is from dorsal divisions of spinal nerves.

COCCYX

The coccyx (**6**.115), a small triangular bone, usually consists of four fused rudimentary vertebrae but the number varies from five to three, the first sometimes being separate. It descends ventrally from the sacral apex, its pelvic surface being tilted upwards and forwards, its dorsum downwards and backwards. Orientation varies, of course, with its mobility.

The *base*, or upper surface of the *first coccygeal vertebral body*, has an oval, articular facet for the sacral apex. Posterolateral to this, two *coccygeal cornua* project upwards to articulate with sacral cornua; they are homologues of pedicles and superior articular processes of other vertebrae. A rudimentary *transverse process* projects superolaterally from each side of the first coccygeal body and may articulate or fuse with the inferolateral sacral angle, completing the fifth sacral foramina.

The *second* to *fourth coccygeal vertebrae* diminish in size and are usually mere fused nodules, representing rudimentary vertebral bodies, though the second may show traces of transverse processes and pedicles.

Laterally on the *pelvic surface* and including the rudimentary transverse processes, the levatores ani and coccygei are attached, as is the anterior sacrococcygeal ligament, to the front of the first and sometimes second coccygeal vertebral bodies (**6**.278), and to the *cornua* the intercornual ligaments. The gap between fifth sacral body and articulating cornua represents, on each side, an intervertebral foramen, transmitting the fifth sacral spinal nerve, whose dorsal ramus descends behind the rudimentary transverse process, its ventral ramus passing anterolaterally between the transverse process and sacrum with, laterally, the lateral sacrococcygeal ligament which connects the process to the inferolateral sacral angle. To the *dorsal surface* are attached the glutei maximi, at its tip the sphincter ani externus, and in its median area the deep and superficial posterior sacrococcygeal ligaments, the superficial descending from the margins of the sacral hiatus and sometimes closing the sacral canal. The filum terminale, between the two ligaments, blends with them on the dorsum of the first coccygeal vertebra.

SACROCOCCYGEAL JOINT

The sacrococcygeal joint is a symphysis between the sacral apex and

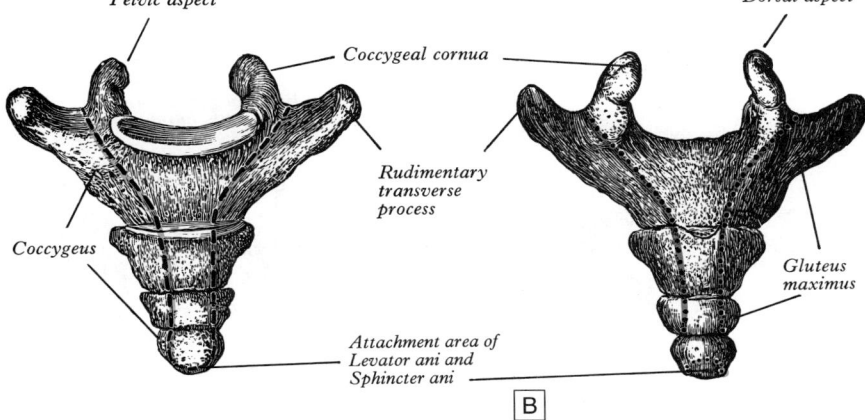

Pelvic aspect

Coccygeal cornua

Rudimentary transverse process

Coccygeus

Attachment area of Levator ani and Sphincter ani

Dorsal aspect

Gluteus maximus

A   B

6.115   The coccyx: A. Pelvic aspect; B. Dorsal aspect.

coccygeal base, united by a fibrocartilaginous disc, remnants of hyaline cartilage and anterior, posterior and lateral ligaments.

Fibrocartilage disc. A thin disc between contiguous surfaces of the sacrum and coccyx, somewhat thicker in front and behind than laterally. Its surfaces carry hyaline cartilage varying from thin veils to small islands. Occasionally the coccyx is more mobile, the joint being synovial.

The anterior sacrococcygeal ligament (6.278). Consisting of irregular fibres descending on the pelvic surfaces of both sacrum and coccyx, it is attached like the anterior longitudinal ligament.

The superior posterior sacrococcygeal ligament. It is flat and passes from the margin of the sacral hiatus to the dorsal coccygeal surface (6.265), roofing the lower sacral canal.

The deep dorsal sacrococcygeal ligament. Passing from the back of the fifth sacral vertebral body to the dorsum of the coccyx, it corresponds to the posterior longitudinal ligament.

A lateral sacrococcygeal ligament. This is on each side, like an intertransverse ligament. It connects a coccygeal transverse process to an inferolateral sacral angle, completing a foramen for the fifth sacral spinal nerve.

The intercornual ligaments. These connect sacral and coccygeal cornua on each side. A fasciculus also connects the sacral cornua to the coccygeal transverse processes.

INTERCOCCYGEAL JOINTS

The intercoccygeal joints are symphyses, with thin discs of fibrocartilage, between coccygeal segments in the young. Segments are also connected by extension of the anterior and posterior sacrococcygeal ligaments. In adult males all segments are united comparatively early but in females union is later. In advanced age the sacrococcygeal joint is obliterated. Occasionally the joint between the first and second segments is synovial; the apex of the terminal segment is connected to overlying skin by white fibrous tissue.

OSSIFICATION OF THE VERTEBRAL COLUMN

For earlier stages of vertebral development consult page 265 and 3.134. A typical vertebra is ossified from three primary centres (6.116A), one in each half vertebral arch and one in the centrum. Centres in arches appear at the roots of the transverse processes, ossification spreading backwards into laminae and spines, forwards into pedicles and posterolateral parts of the body, laterally into transverse processes and upwards and downwards into articular processes. Classically centres in *vertebral arches* are said to appear first in upper cervical vertebrae in the ninth to tenth week, and then in successively lower vertebrae, reaching lower lumbar levels in the twelfth week. However, in a radiographic study of unsexed human fetuses, of which 33 were of appropriate age (Bagnall et al 1977), a pattern was noted differing from such a simple craniocaudal sequence. A regular cervical progression was not observed. Centres

first appeared in the lower cervical/upper thoracic region, quickly followed by others in the upper cervical region. After a short interval a third group appeared in the lower thoracolumbar region and remaining centres then appeared, spreading regularly and rapidly in craniocaudal directions. The body's major part, the *centrum*, ossifies from a primary centre dorsal to the notochord. (Centra are occasionally ossified from *bilateral* centres which may fail to unite. Suppression of one of these produces a *cuneiform vertebra*, a recognized cause of lateral spinal curvature (scoliosis). The condition is frequently multiple.) This centre first appears at lower thoracic levels in the ninth to tenth week, spreading craniocaudally and reaching the second cervical vertebra in the twelfth week. In the study by Bagnall et al (1977) these events were largely confirmed, but the earliest centres were in lower thoracic **and** upper lumbar regions; cranial progression was rather faster than caudal, the last centre being in the fifth sacral vertebra. (For the later and erratic ossification of the coccyx see below.) During early postnatal years the centrum is connected to each half neural arch by a synchondrosis or *neurocentral joint*. In thoracic vertebrae costal facets on bodies are **posterior** to neurocentral joints. At birth a vertebra consists of three ossifying elements, a centrum and two half arches, united by cartilage. During the first year the arches unite behind, first in the lumbar region and then through thoracic and cervical regions. In upper cervical vertebrae centra unite with arches about the third year, but in lower lumbar vertebrae union is not complete until the sixth. Until puberty the upper and lower surfaces of bodies and apices of transverse and spinous processes are cartilaginous but now *five secondary centres* appear, one in the apex of each transverse and spinous process and two annular epiphyseal 'rings' for circumferential parts of upper and lower surfaces of the body (6.116B, C). Costal articular facets are extensions of the annular epiphyses (Dixon 1920). These epiphyses fuse with the rest of the bone at about 25 years. In bifid cervical spinous processes there are two secondary centres. The annular 'epiphyses' of vertebrae probably cannot be equated with epiphyses of long bones. In most mammals they are complete osseous discs. For discussion consult François and Dhem (1974).

Sexual dimorphism in vertebrae has received little attention, but Taylor and Twomey (1984) have described radiological differences in adolescent humans, female vertebral bodies having a lower ratio of width to depth.

Exceptions to this pattern of ossification occur in the first, second and seventh cervical and in lumbar vertebrae.

Atlas. This is commonly ossified from three centres (6.116D): one in each lateral mass at about the seventh week, gradually extending into the posterior arch where they unite between the third and fourth years, directly or occasionally through a separate centre. At birth, the anterior arch is fibrocartilaginous; here a separate centre appears about the end of the first year, uniting with the lateral masses between the sixth and eighth, the lines of union extending across anterior parts of the superior articular facets. Occasionally the

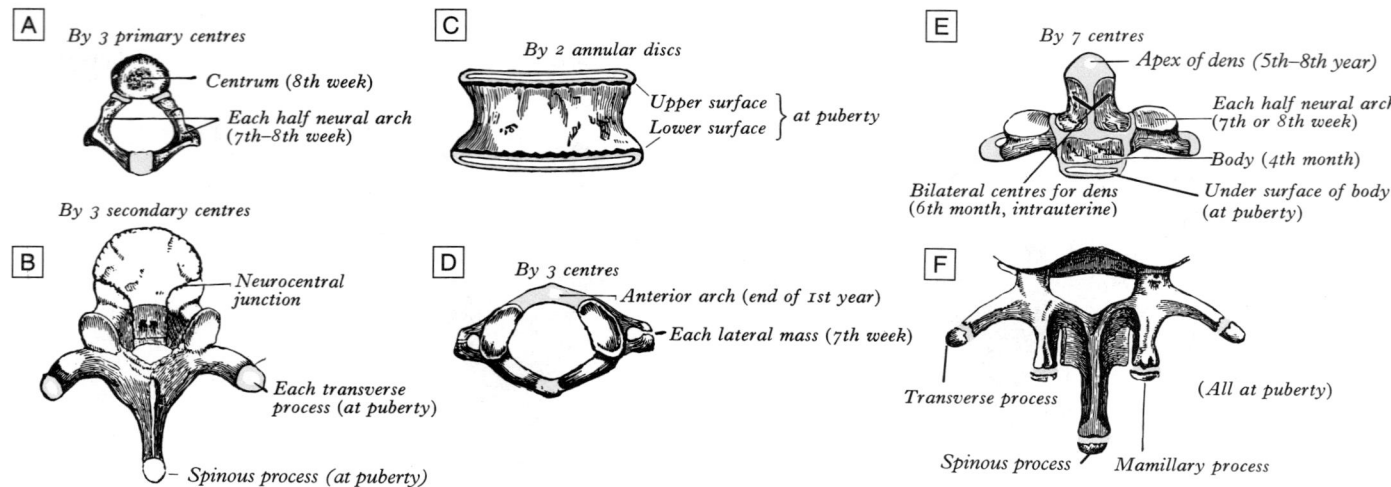

6.116 Ossification of the vertebral column. A. Typical vertebra. B. Typical vertebra at puberty. C. Body of a typical vertebra at puberty. D. The atlas. E. The axis. F. Lumbar vertebra. For further details consult text.

anterior arch is formed by extension and ultimate union of centres in the lateral masses, sometimes from two lateral centres in the arch itself.

Axis. This is ossified from five primary and two secondary centres (6.116E), the vertebral arch from two primary, the centrum from one, as in a typical vertebra. The former appear about the seventh or eighth week, that for the centrum about the fourth or fifth month. The dens is largely ossified from bilateral centres, appearing about the sixth month and joining before birth to form a conical mass, deeply cleft above by cartilage. This cuneiform cartilage forms the apex of the odontoid process and in it a centre appears, which shows considerable individual variation in both time of appearance and time of fusion to the rest of the dens: it most often appears between five and eight years, but sometimes even later (Ogden 1984), fusing with the main mass about the twelfth year. It has been widely regarded as a part of the cranial sclerotomal half of the first cervical segment or pro-atlas (Gadow 1933), but see below. The dens is separated from the body by a cartilaginous disc, the circumference of which ossifies while its centre remains cartilaginous until old age; in the disc possible rudiments of adjacent epiphyses of atlas and axis may occur. A thin epiphyseal plate is formed inferior to the body around puberty. The dens has long been considered the atlantal centrum, secondarily fused with the axis. This view was undermined by studies in a variety of mammals by Jenkins (1969), who regarded the dens as a new formation. Ganguly and Singh-Roy (1965) consider the apical centre for the dens as derived from the pro-atlas, which may also contribute to lateral atlantal masses.

Some observers regard the dens as the centrum of the pro-atlas.

Seventh cervical vertebra. In this vertebra separate centres for its costal processes appear about the sixth month and join the body and transverse processes between the fifth and sixth years; they may remain separate and grow anterolaterally as cervical ribs (p. 518). Separate ossific centres may, on occasion, also occur in the costal processes of the fourth to sixth cervical vertebrae.

Lumbar vertebrae (6.116F). These have two additional centres for mamillary processes. In the fifth lumbar a pair of scale-like epiphyses usually appear on the tips of costal elements.

Sacrum (6.117). This resembles typical vertebrae in the ossification of its segments. Primary centres for the centrum and each half vertebral arch appear between the tenth and twentieth weeks. Primary centres for costal elements of the upper three or more segments appear superolateral to the pelvic sacral foramina, between the sixth and eighth prenatal months. Each costal element unites with its half vertebral arch between the second and fifth years, and the conjoined element so formed unites anteriorly with the centrum and posteriorly with its opposite fellow at about the eighth year. Thereafter the upper and lower surfaces of each sacral body are covered by an epiphyseal plate of hyaline cartilage separated by a fibrocartilaginous precursor of an intervertebral disc. Laterally, successive conjoined vertebral arches and costal elements are separated by hyaline cartilage; a cartilaginous epiphysis, sometimes divided into upper and lower parts, develops on each auricular and adjacent lateral surface. Soon after puberty the fused vertebral arches and costal elements of adjacent vertebrae begin to coalesce from below upwards. At the same time epiphyseal centres develop for:

- upper and lower surfaces of bodies
- spinous tubercles
- transverse tubercles and
- costal elements.

The costal epiphyseal centres appear at the lateral extremities of the hyaline cartilages **between** adjacent costal elements; two anterior and two posterior appear in each interval between first, second and third segments. Ossification spreads from these into the auricular epiphyseal plates. One costal epiphyseal centre appears anteriorly in each remaining interval; from these ossification spreads to the epiphyseal plate covering the lower lateral surface. Sacral bodies unite at their adjacent margins after the twentieth year, but the central mass and most of each intervertebral disc remain unossified up to or beyond middle life. Available information is based on few specimens (McKern & Stewart 1957; Fawcett 1907).

Coccyx. Each segment is ossified from one primary centre but the incidence and timing are uncertain. A centre in the first segment appears about birth and its cornua may soon ossify from separate centres. Remaining segments ossify at wide intervals up to the

twentieth year or later. Segments slowly unite; union between the first and second is frequently delayed until 30 years. The coccyx often fuses with the sacrum in later decades, especially in females.

VERTEBRAL COLUMN AS A WHOLE

The structure of the vertebral column undergoes progressive change in the postnatal period, affecting its growth and morphology. This process continues in adulthood and leads eventually to decline in senescence. Vertebral column morphology is influenced **externally** by mechanical and environmental factors and **internally** by genetic, metabolic and hormonal factors. These all affect its ability to react to the dynamic forces of everyday life, such as compression, traction and shear. These dynamic forces can vary in magnitude and are much influenced by occupation, locomotion and posture (Nachemson 1963; Gracovetsky 1988).

The vertebral column comprises some 33 vertebral segments, each separated by a fibrocartilaginous intervertebral disc. Its function is to support the trunk and to protect the spinal cord. It lies in the general vertebrate plane, and is median and posterior in the body. Its total length in males is about 70 cm and in females about 60 cm. Individual regions of the column account for approximately 8% of overall body length for the cervical, 20% for the thoracic, 12% for the lumbar and 8% for the sacrococcygeal. Although the usual number of vertebrae is 7 cervical, 12 thoracic, 5 lumbar, 5 sacral and 4 coccygeal, this total is subject to frequent variability, with reports of a variation between 32 and 35 bones (Bergman et al 1988). The demarcation of groups by their morphological characteristics may be blurred: for example, there may be thoracic costal facets on the seventh cervical, giving it the appearance of an extra thoracic vertebra; lumbarlike articular processes may be found on the lowest thoracic vertebra; and the fifth lumbar vertebra may be wholly or partially incorporated into the sacrum. Thus, due to these changes

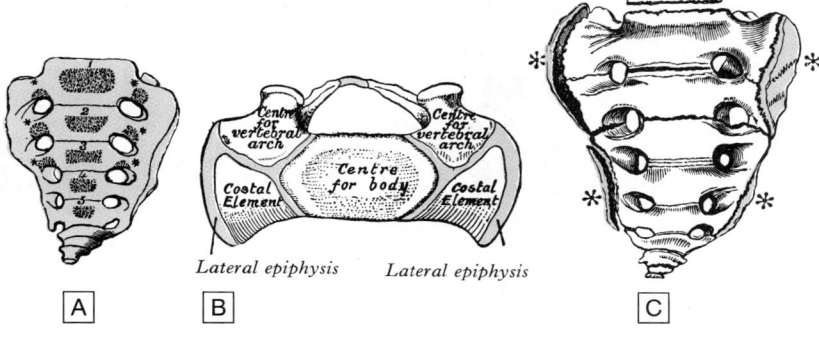

Lateral epiphysis   *Lateral epiphysis*

A   B   C

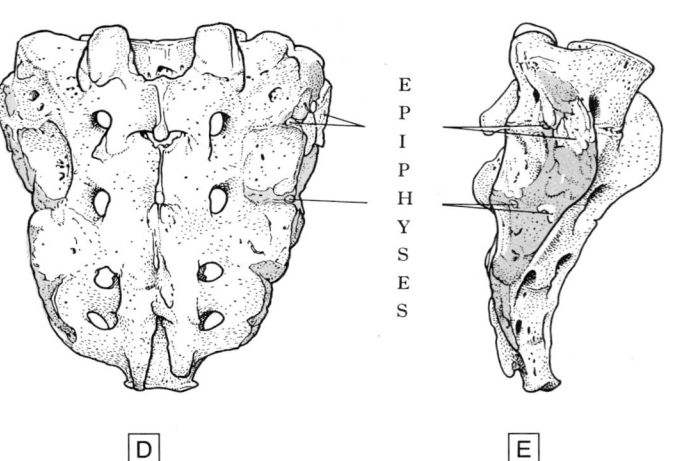

E
P
I
P
H
Y
S
E
S

D   E

6.117 Ossification of the sacrum and coccyx: A. At birth; B. The base of the sacrum of a child of about four years of age; C. At the twenty-fifth year. In C The epiphyseal plates for each lateral surface are marked by asterisks. D, E. The epiphyses of the costal and transverse process of the sacrum at the eighteenth year.

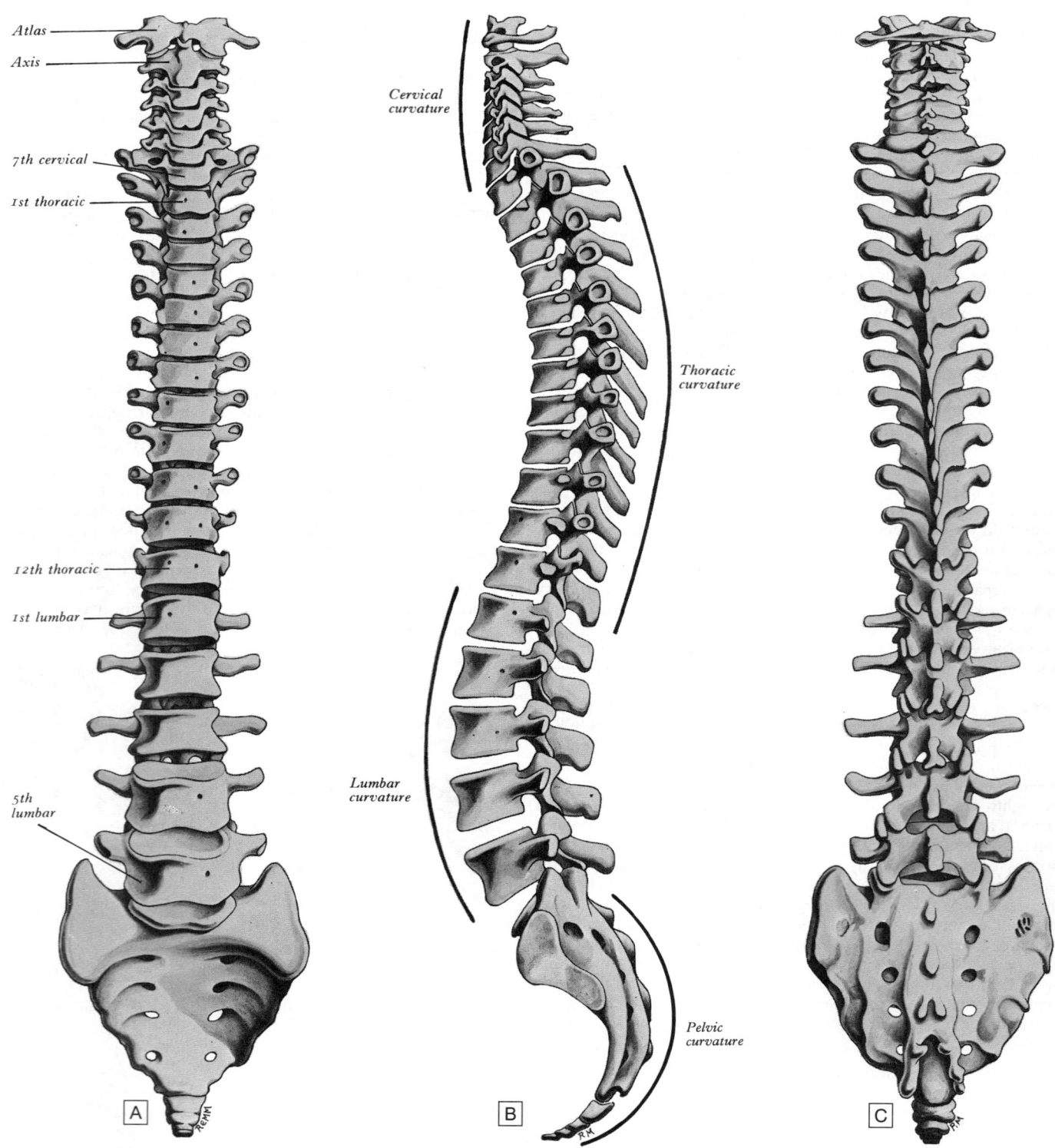

Atlas

Axis

7th cervical

1st thoracic

12th thoracic

1st lumbar

5th lumbar

Cervical curvature

Thoracic curvature

Lumbar curvature

Pelvic curvature

A

B

C

6.118 The vertebral column: A. Anterior aspect; B. Lateral aspect (note curvatures); C. Dorsal aspect. Note slight sinuous, lateral, thoracolumbar curvature visible from both dorsal and anterior aspects.

in transition between vertebral types, there may be 23–25 mobile presacral vertebrae.

The line of gravity of the vertebral column

The well-balanced, erect body has a line of gravity which extends from the level of the external auditory meatus, through the dens of the atlas, just anterior to the body of the second thoracic vertebra, through the centre of the body of the twelfth thoracic vertebra and through the rear of the body of the fifth lumbar vertebra to lie anterior to the sacrum.

Curvatures of the vertebral column

In the normal vertebral column, there are no lateral curvatures, but there are well-marked curvatures in the sagittal plane. However, in the upper thoracic region there is often a slight lateral curvature, convex to the right in right-handed persons, and left in left-handed. The sagittal curvatures are present in the cervical, thoracic, lumbar and pelvic regions (**6.118, 119**). Such curvatures are the result of three million years of evolution, in which rounding of the thorax and pelvis have developed as an adaptation to bipedal gait. Curvatures appear as a response to *fetal movements* as early as 7 weeks in utero,

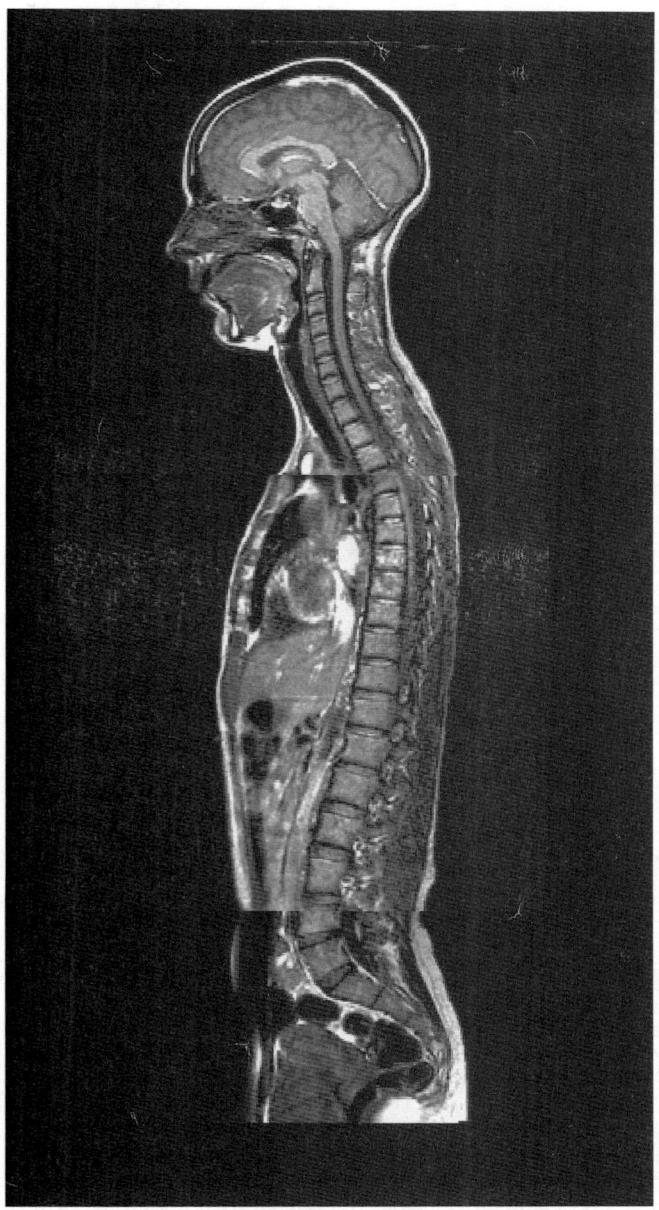

6.119 A composite T1-weighted midline sagittal magnetic resonance image of the vertebral column of a 27-year-old female. The subject had no history of back pain at the time of imaging but one year later suffered acute pain following the prolapse of the L4/5 intervertebral disc which had been identified as degenerate on a T2-weighted image obtained as part of a research study. (Image provided by Dr N Roberts, Magnetic Resonance Centre, University of Liverpool.)

and become more pronounced after birth when the baby begins to hold up his or her head. Although the embryo develops in flexion, resulting in *primary* thoracic and pelvic curves which are concave anteriorly, functional muscle development leads to the early appearance of *secondary* cervical and lumbar spinal curvatures in the sagittal plane.

The *cervical curvature* appears before birth, probably as early as the seventh week in utero, in response to fetal development of the muscles responsible for head extension, an important component of the 'gasp reflex' (Bagnall et al 1977). Radiographic study of 195 human fetuses aged from 8 to 23 weeks demonstrated the presence of secondary cervical curvature in 83% of the sample. Ultrasound investigations support the role of movement in the development of these curvatures. *Lumbar flattening* has also been identified as early as the eighth week (O'Rahilly et al 1980). However, the early appearance of these secondary curves is probably accentuated by postnatal muscular and nervous system development when the ver-

tebral column is highly flexible and when it may assume almost any curvature (Wood-Jones 1946). An infant can support its head at about 3 or 4 months, sit upright at about 9 months, and will commence walking between 12 and 15 months. Such functional changes exert a major influence on the development of the secondary curvatures in the vertebral column and changes in the proportional size of the vertebrae, in particular in the lumbar region. The secondary *lumbar curvature* becomes important to maintain the centre of gravity of the trunk over the legs when walking commences, and thus changes in body proportions exert a major influence on the subsequent shape of curvatures in the vertebral column. Support for this view comes from recent research which has demonstrated that long-term training of monkeys aimed at stable upright posture resulted in marked lumbar lordosis, a feature which is comparable to the human condition both morphologically and functionally. The induced lordosis was retained even in normal pronograde posture of the monkeys: bone remodelling occurred in the postcranial skeleton, attributable to functional adaptation to stresses induced by sustained bipedalism.

In adults, the *cervical curve* is convex forwards and the least marked: this is a *lordosis*. It extends from the atlas to the second thoracic vertebra, with its apex between the fourth and fifth cervical vertebrae. Sexual dimorphism in the cervical curvatures has also been found (Knussman & Finke 1977).

The *thoracic curve* is *kyphotic*, i.e. concave forwards. It extends between the second and the eleventh and twelfth thoracic vertebrae, with its apex lying between the sixth and ninth thoracic vertebrae. This curvature is caused by the increased posterior depth of the thoracic vertebral bodies.

The *lumbar curve* is *lordotic*, i.e. convex forwards. It has a greater magnitude in females and extends from the twelfth thoracic vertebra to the lumbosacral angle, with an increased convexity of the last three segments due to greater anterior depth of intervertebral discs and some anterior wedging of the vertebral bodies. Its apex is at the level of the third lumbar vertebra.

The *pelvic curve* is concave anteroinferiorly and involves the sacrum and coccygeal vertebrae, extending from the lumbosacral junction to the apex of the coccyx.

Vertebral bodies

Viewed anteriorly there is a cephalocaudal **increase** in vertebral body width from the second cervical to the third lumbar vertebra, associated with increased weight-bearing. The increase is linear in the neck but not in the thoracic and lumbar regions. There is some variation in size of the last two lumbar bodies, but thereafter width diminishes rapidly to the coccygeal apex. In the two lowest lumbar vertebrae there is an inverse relation between the areas of the upper and lower surfaces of bodies and size of the pedicles and transverse processes, suggesting that the latter transmit some of the vertebral compressive forces from spine to pelvis (Davis 1961). They are also transitional towards the sacral region (Panjabi et al 1992). Vertebral diameter may be used as a basis for sex prediction as the posterior aspect of the body is less dimorphic than the anterior region (MacLaughlin & Oldale 1992).

Spinous processes

The spinous processes lie approximately in the median plane and project posteriorly, although in some individuals a minor deflection of the processes to one side may be seen. This deviation also occurs in fractures and dislocations and can be associated with congenital abnormalities of the vertebra. The third thoracic spinous process is level with the spine of the scapula, and the seventh with the inferior scapular angle when the arm is by the side. The fourth lumbar spine is level with the summits of the iliac crests (a point useful in lumbar puncture), and the second sacral spine with the posterior superior iliac spines.

Lateral to the vertebral spines, vertebral grooves contain the deep dorsal muscles: at cervical and lumbar levels these grooves are shallow and mainly formed by laminae; in the thoracic region they are deeper, broader and formed by both laminae and transverse processes. The laminae are broad for the first thoracic vertebra, narrower for the second to seventh, broadening again from the eighth to eleventh, but become narrow thereafter down to the third lumbar vertebra.

Transverse processes

Lateral to the laminae are articular processes, and, still more lateral, transverse processes. Cervical transverse processes are anterior to articular processes, lateral to pedicles and between the intervertebral foramina. In the thoracic region, they are posterior to the pedicles, considerably behind those of the cervical and lumbar processes. In the lumbar region, the processes are anterior to articular processes, but posterior to intervertebral foramina. There is considerable regional variation in structure and length of the transverse processes. In the cervical region, the atlantal transverse process is long and broad, allowing the rotator muscles maximum mechanical advantage. Breadth varies little from second to sixth cervical, but increases in the seventh. In thoracic vertebrae the first is widest, and breadth decreases to the twelfth, whose transverse elements are usually vestigial. In the upper three lumbar vertebrae, the transverse processes become broader, diminishing in the fourth and fifth. The transverse process of the fifth is the most robust and arises directly from the body and pedicle to allow for weight transference to the pelvis through the iliopelvic ligament.

Lateral aspect of the vertebral column

The lateral aspect of the vertebral column is arbitrarily separated from the posterior by articular processes in the cervical and lumbar regions and transverse processes in the thoracic. Anteriorly it is formed by the sides of vertebral bodies, with costal facets at thoracic levels. The intervertebral foramina, behind bodies and between pedicles, are oval, and smallest at cervical and upper thoracic levels increasing progressively in size in the thoracic and lumbar regions: they contain spinal and other nerves and various vessels.

Vertebral canal

The vertebral canal follows the vertebral curves. In the cervical and lumbar regions, which exhibit free mobility, it is large and triangular, but where movement is less, in the thoracic region, it is small and circular. These differences are matched by variations in the diameter of the spinal cord and its enlargements. In the lumbar region, the spinal canal has a gradual decrease in measurement between L1 and L5, with a greater relative width in the female. The lumbar canal/vertebral body ratio ranges between 1:2 and 1:5; any ratio greater than 1:5 would constitute lumbar vertebral canal stenosis.

Diurnal variation

In 1852, Bishop reported that body height was affected by changes from recumbency to upright posture. These diurnal variations appear to be due to changes that occur within the cervical, thoracic and lumbar spine. Recent investigations using stereophotogrammetry have demonstrated that 40% of diurnal changes occur in the thoracic spine, affecting the degree of kyphosis, and a further 40% in the lumbar spine, without affecting the lordosis (Wing et al 1992). The greatest change in vertebral column length has been found in adolescents and young adults (De Puky 1935). The height loss occurs within 3 hours of rising in the morning (Reilly et al 1984), with the overall loss being approximately 16 mm (Fitzgerald 1972; Krag et al 1990). Although the curvatures within the vertebral column contribute to these changes in height, the intervertebral disc is also likely to account for observed height loss. Recent magnetic resonance imaging (MRI) investigations reveal a dynamic movement of fluid into and out of both the intervertebral disc (6.120) and adjacent vertebral body over a 24-hour period (Roberts et al 1991, 1994). This is related to body position and could have profound implications for the biomechanics of the column when it is under axial compression (Dangerfield et al 1994).

Growth of the vertebral column

At birth, the column is approximately 24 cm in length (Scammon & Calkins 1929). Its growth through childhood and adolescence to adulthood is influenced by sexual, hormonal, genetic, biomechanical and other factors, with variation in absolute and relative size of the individual component vertebrae (Falkner & Tanner 1986; Roche 1992).

The size of component parts of the vertebral column varies with age, with relatively smaller lumbar and sacral components in the neonate compared to the adult: this is due to cephalocaudal devel-

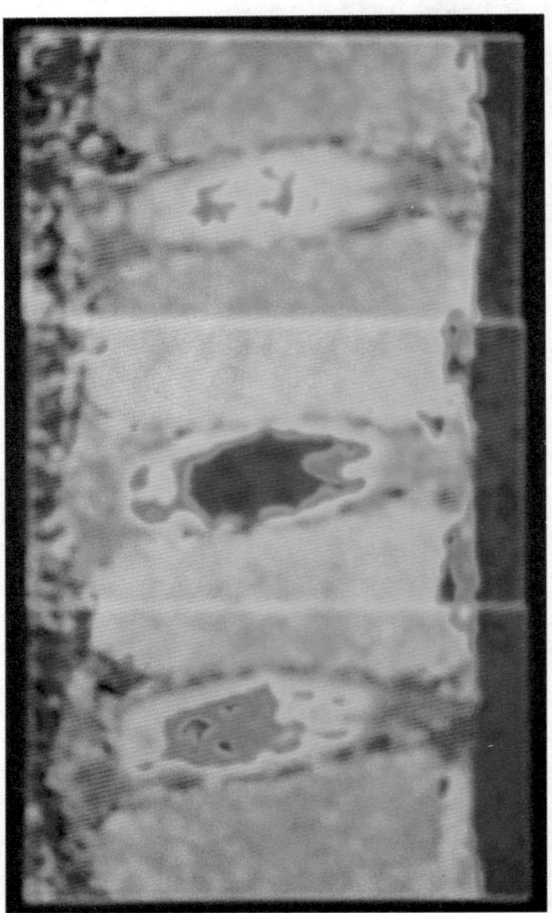

6.120 Three MR images, enhanced after image processing, of intervertebral discs showing, from top to bottom, low water content at midnight = pale green, high water content in the morning after a night recumbent = dark blue, and an intermediate state in the afternoon. (Images provided by Dr N Roberts, Magnetic Resonance Research Centre, University of Liverpool.)

opmental gradients. These vertebrae, therefore, grow more to attain adult size. Different velocities of skeletal maturation (heterochrony) may also be determined by intrinsic bony mechanisms (Burwell et al 1980). The lumbar vertebrae have a threefold increase in body width and a fourfold increase in body height. These changes are determined genetically and display sexual dimorphism, with discrete and constant differences between the sexes being identified in anthropometric studies based on computerized tomography (CT) (Cooper et al 1992).

Changes in the mechanics of the lumbar region are potent factors in influencing growth changes in the proportions of vertebral bodies and intervertebral discs, especially in the fifth lumbar and the disc below it, and the shape of the lumbar curvature (Taylor 1975).

Vertebral column growth is due to the summation of growth of individual vertebrae; the length of the spine being a major component of overall stature. At birth the ossified component of the vertebra has the same height as the intervertebral cartilaginous component (Brandner 1970), becoming 75% of the total by adulthood. Growth in the vertebral column is due to *proliferative* changes in the cartilaginous end plates, similar to the epiphyseal cartilages of long bones. *Growth in height* occurs at the upper end after puberty and can still be identified in subjects in their midtwenties (Bernick & Caillet 1982). The annular tension apophysis takes no part in the growth of the body, with its ossification status having no relationship with vertebral growth, although its diameter keeps pace with the body. This is because it lies outside the plane of the epiphyseal growth plate.

The *neural arch processes* grow from *primary* centres by subperiosteal bone deposition and extension into the adjacent cartilage. At the tips of the transverse processes and spinous processes, traction epiphyses appear. The *facet joints* grow as a result of extension into the extra-articular zone of cartilage and subarticular growth. Changes in posture and body proportions alter the orientation of each articular surface (Roaf 1971).

Adolescent growth spurts within the vertebral column occur in both males and females, with sexual difference for the time of onset and the achievement of adulthood. The spurt occurs in males between ages 13 and 15 years, and in females between 9 and 13 years (Anderson et al 1965; Taylor & Twomey 1984). The female growth increment is 65% greater than the male between 9.5 and 12.5 years. Female vertebrae are also more slender than male.

Although growth in standing height is usually complete by 18 years in Caucasian girls and 20 years in males, evidence has been found to suggest that vertebral growth may continue well into adulthood: changes in the cartilaginous endplates of the vertebrae have been demonstrated in subjects in the midtwenties (Tanner et al 1966; Bernick & Caillet 1982). In male East Africans, changes in height of the lumbar vertebrae have been found at up to 45 years of age (Allbrook 1956).

Vertebral column in the elderly

In older people, age-related changes in the structure of bone lead to broadening and loss of height of the vertebral bodies, these changes being more severe in females. The bony changes in the vertebral column are accompanied by changes in the collagen content of the discs and by decline in the activity of spinal muscle dynamics. This leads to progressive decline in vertebral column mobility, particularly in the lumbar spine. Lumbar lordosis decreases as a result of increased loading, due to an increase in body weight. The development of a 'dowager's hump' in the midthoracic region in females, due to age-related osteoporosis, increases the thoracic kyphosis and cervical lordosis. Overall, these changes in the vertebral column lead directly to loss of total height in the individual.

Other changes affect the vertebral bodies. Osteophyte activity on the anterior and lateral surfaces of the bodies leads to spurs arising from the compact cortical bone. Although individual variations occur, these changes appear in most individuals from about 20 years onwards. They are most common on the anterior aspect of the body and appear to be related to movement, especially as their incidence is highest at C5, T8 and L3/4, regions where spinal movement is greatest (Nathan 1962). They never involve the ring epiphysis. Osteophytic spurs are frequently asymptomatic, but may result in diminished movements within the spine.

Movement of the vertebral column

Normal movements between adjacent vertebrae are limited, but they have a cumulative effect over the whole column, allowing a considerable degree of bending or rotation (p. 515). Although bony deformation in the subchondral bone and articular cartilage may contribute, the vertebral discs both tie vertebrae together and are the principal sites of vertebral column movement. By elastic deformability, they permit tilting and torsion between vertebral bodies, and they also add compressibility to the column. This ability to absorb stresses is augmented by the column's sinuous curvature: forces transmitted with little loss by a straight column are largely expended against the pliability of the spinal curves. Effects of weight, muscle activity and thrust from the feet, whether trivial (as in walking) or large (as in running and jumping), are smoothed out by the discs and curvatures.

Despite the prominent role of intervertebral discs in spinal dynamics, regional variations in mobility also depend on the disposition, properties and geometry of intervertebral synovial joints and ligamentous complexes attached to all parts of each vertebra (p. 515).

Articular trophism or asymmetrical orientation of the apophyseal joints results in the orientation of one joint becoming more inclined in the frontal or sagittal plane than the orientation of the contralateral joint. Trophism is present in up to 25% of human spines (Grieve 1989), occurring frequently in L4 and L5, and leads to imbalanced movement between the facets (Kraft & Levinthal 1951). This, in turn, may hasten degenerative damage.

Abnormalities of the vertebral column

Scoliosis is a term applied to abnormal lateral curvature of the spine, frequently accompanied by severe rotation of the vertebral bodies and torsions within the laminae and pedicles. Such abnormal curvatures may be postural or structural. Postural curvatures may result from the lower limbs being unequal in length: since these curves are non-structural, they should disappear when the inequality is corrected. Fixed structural curvatures can be due to congenital abnormalities of the vertebrae (e.g. hemivertebrae); they may be secondary to disease (such as poliomyelitis or muscular dystrophies), or they may be idiopathic. The causes of the latter have been attributed to growth and nervous system factors (Burwell & Dangerfield 1992).

In spondylolisthesis (present in 5% of skeletons) the spine, laminae and inferior articular processes of the fifth (and sometimes the fourth) lumbar vertebra are joined together but separate from the rest of the bone. The condition is probably congenital, the suggestion being that each half vertebral arch ossifies from two primary centres which fail to fuse. There is, however, no clear evidence for this.

Fractures to the column

Injury to the vertebral column may result from **five** different mechanisms: flexion, extension, rotation, shear and axial load. In forced flexion injury, such as a violent blow on the back, fractures usually occur at the fifth or sixth cervical vertebra. If the violence is transmitted axially, for example by a fall on to the feet or head, the injury is also a flexion fracture (because of the normal spinal curvature), often between the ninth thoracic and second lumbar. Vertebral stability is maintained by the disc-body complex and does not require an intact posterior ligament complex (Bedbrook 1971). This clinical observation has led to the biomechanical concept of the three-column theory for spinal stability (Dennis 1983). The anterior column is formed by the anterior longitudinal ligament, the anterior part of the vertebral body and the anterior annulus fibrosus. The middle column is made up of the posterior longitudinal ligament, the posterior wall of the vertebral body and the posterior annulus fibrosus; and the posterior column consists of the posterior body arch complex and the posterior ligamentous complex. This concept forms the basis of classification of vertebral column fractures (Dennis 1983).

STERNUM

The sternum is confined to land vertebrates, and aquatic mammals such as seals; it is absent in fish. The elongate human form is typical of mammals, the sternum being a plate, often composite, in amphibians and reptiles. Though associated with shoulder girdles and ribs from its earliest appearance, it is often considered axial. Its embryonic development and ossification indicate an origin separate from ribs. The human sternum (**6**.121, 122) consists of a cranial *manubrium* (prosternum), an intermediate *body* or mesosternum and a caudal *xiphoid process* (metasternum). Its total length in males is about 17 cm, less in females (Jit & Bakshi 1984). The ratio between manubrial and mesosternal lengths differs in the sexes, but racial differences have not been established. Such data are complicated by possible continuation of growth beyond the third decade and even throughout life (Ashley 1956; Rother et al 1975). In addition to the three major sections, the mesosternum in early life consists of four *sternebrae*, which from costal relations appear to be intersegmental. In natural stance the sternum slopes down and slightly forwards. It is convex in front, concave behind and broadest at the junction with the first costal cartilages, narrow at the manubriosternal joint, below which it widens to its articulation with the fifth cartilages, narrowing again below this.

Manubrium sterni. Broad and thick above, it narrows to its junction with the mesosternum. Its *anterior surface* is smooth, convex transversely, vertically concave. Its *posterior surface* is concave and smooth. The *superior border* is thick, with a central *jugular* (*suprasternal*) *notch* between two oval fossae directed up and posterolaterally for articulation with the sternal ends of the clavicles (*clavicular notches*). The *inferior border*, oval and rough, carries a thin layer of cartilage for articulation with the mesosternum. The *lateral borders* are marked above by a depression for the first costal cartilage and below by a small articular demifacet, which, with one on each superior mesosternal angle, articulates with part of the second costal cartilage. Between these facets the narrow curved edge descends medially.

Mesosternum (body). Longer, narrower and thinner than the manubrium, it is broadest near its lower end. Its *anterior surface*,

537

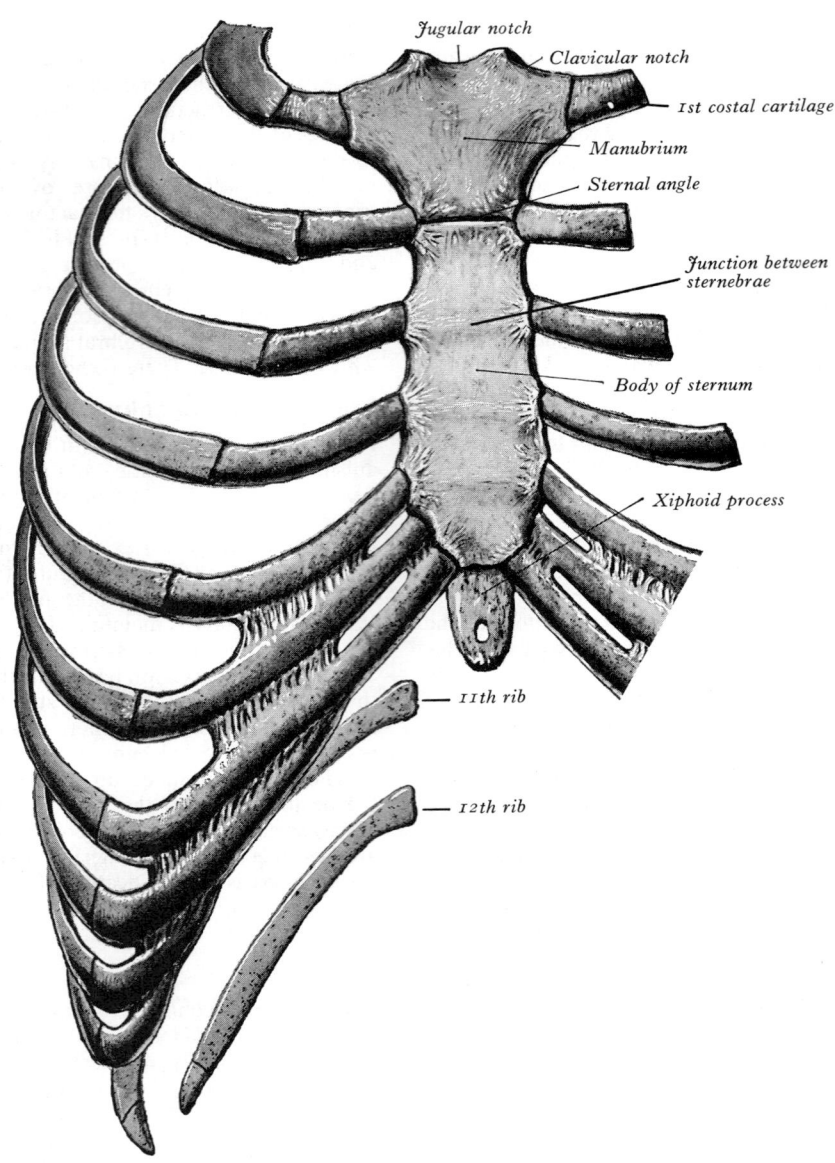

Jugular notch
Clavicular notch
1st costal cartilage
Manubrium
Sternal angle
Junction between sternebrae
Body of sternum
Xiphoid process
11th rib
12th rib

6.121   The sternum and costal cartilages: anterior aspect.

nearly flat, faces slightly upwards and has three variable transverse ridges at levels of fusion of its four *sternebrae* (see below). A *sternal foramen*, of varying size and form, may occur between the third and fourth sternebrae (p. 539). The *posterior surface*, slightly concave, also displays three less distinct transverse lines. The *oval upper end* articulates with the manubrium (*manubriosternal joint*) at the level of the *sternal angle*, an anterior ridge usually being palpable. A posterior transverse groove also marks the manubriosternal joint (**6**.122A). The *lower end* is narrow and continuous with the xiphoid process. On each *lateral border* (**6**.122B), at its superior angle, a small notch receives in part the second costal cartilage; below this, four *costal notches* articulate with the third to sixth costal cartilages; the inferior angle has a small facet, which, with the xiphoid process, receives the seventh costal cartilage. Between these articular depressions a series of curved edges diminish in length downwards, forming the anterior limits of the intercostal spaces.

Xiphoid process (xiphisternum). The smallest and most variable sternal element, it may be broad and thin, pointed, bifid, perforated, curved or deflected. It is cartilaginous in youth, but more or less ossified in adults. It is continuous with the mesosternum's lower end at the *xiphisternal joint.* Anterior to its superolateral angles are demifacets for parts of the seventh costal cartilages (**6**.122).

The manubrium is level with the third and fourth thoracic vertebrae; the *sternal angle* is opposite the inferior border of the fourth

vertebral body. To the manubrial *anterior surface* the sternal ends of the pectoralis major and sternocleidomastoid muscles are attached and to its *posterior surface* the sternothyroids, opposite the first costal cartilages; above are the most medial fibres of the sternohyoids. This surface is the anterior wall of the superior mediastinum; inferiorly (approximately the vertical lower half) it is related to the aortic arch, above this to the left brachiocephalic vein and brachiocephalic, left common carotid and left subclavian arteries; laterally it is related to lungs and pleurae. To the *jugular notch* are attached fibres of the interclavicular ligament. On the *lateral border* the manubriocostal joint (first costal cartilage) is a synchondrosis, unlike other sternocostal joints.

The mesosternum is level with the fifth to ninth thoracic vertebrae. To its *anterior surface* articular capsules of sternocostal joints and sternal fibres of pectoralis major are attached, and to its *posterior surface* the transversus thoracis (sternocostalis). Right of the median plane it is related to pleura and the thin, anterior border of the right lung, projecting between sternum and pericardium. The left half of the upper two sternebrae is related to left pleura and lung, the lower two directly to pericardium. To the *borders* the external intercostal membranes are attached between costal facets. Except for the first and sixth, the cartilages of 'true' ribs articulate with the sternum at junctions of its segments.

The xiphoid process is in the epigastrium. To its *anterior surface* are attached the most medial fibres of rectus abdominis and aponeuroses of external and internal obliques, to its *lower end* the linea alba, and to its *borders* the aponeuroses of internal oblique and transversus abdominis. To its *posterior aspect* slips of diaphragm are attached and it is here related to the liver.

The sternum contains highly vascular trabecular bone enclosed by a compact layer thickest in the manubrium between clavicular notches. The medulla contains *red bone marrow*. The internal trabecular pattern has been examined intensively by scanning electron microscopy and by computer analysis of metrical parameters (Whitehouse 1975). Centrally the bone is lightly constructed, the trabeculae being thicker and wider apart in lateral regions. No completely satisfactory explanation of these variations, or of those already noted in ribs and lumbar vertebrae, has been formulated. Pismenov and Zapetski (1977) have described the vascular supply of the sternum in detail.

Little has been recorded of racial or sexual variation in the sternum. Jit et al (1980), and Jit and Harjeet (1982) stated that, except in combined length of manubrium and mesosternum, sexing is not possible, the sternal angle being unreliable.

Ossification (6.123)

The sternum is formed by fusion of two cartilaginous *sternal plates* (p. 268) flanking the median plane. Arrangement and number of ossificatory centres vary in relation to completeness and time of fusion of the sternal plates and to the width of the adult bone (Ashley 1956). Incomplete fusion leaves a *sternal foramen*. (For incidence in Indian sterna, see Jit & Bakshi 1984.) The manubrium is ossified from one to three centres appearing in the fifth fetal month, and the first and second sternebrae usually from single centres about the same time. Centres in the third and fourth sternebrae are commonly paired and appear in the fifth and sixth months respectively, but one of either pair may be delayed until the seventh or even eighth month; the fourth sternebral centre may be absent (Paterson 1904). The xiphoid process begins to ossify in the third year or later. In some sterna all centres are single and median, in others the manubrial centre is single and the sternebral all paired, symmetrical or asymmetrical. Union between mesosternal centres begins at puberty and proceeds from below upwards; by 25 all are united.

Suprasternal ossicles, paired or single, occur in about 7% of sterna. They may fuse to the manubrium or articulate posteriorly at the lateral border of the jugular notch. When well formed they are pyramidal, the base being articular. Cartilaginous at birth, they ossify during adolescence.

STERNAL JOINTS

Manubriosternal joint

Lying between the manubrium and sternal body, it is usually a symphysis, the bony surfaces covered by hyaline cartilage and connected by a fibrocartilage which may ossify in the aged. In more than 30% the central part of the disc is absorbed and the joint **appears** synovial; similar cavitation may occur in the symphysis pubis (see pp. 491, 677). The two are also connected by a fibrous membrane enveloping the whole bone. In 10% of all over 30 years the manubrium is joined to the sternal body by bone but the intervening cartilage may be only superficially ossified; it is in the aged that this is complete. Early synostosis has been attributed to a persistent synchondrosis in place of a symphysis (Ashley 1954). In the newborn union is by collagenous and elastic fibres without chondrocytes.

Movements. The symphysis permits a small range of angulation between longitudinal axes of the manubrium and body of the sternum and also limited anteroposterior displacement. A study of these movements in 62 male athletes yielded (standing position) mean values of 162.7° (full inspiration) and 164.7° (full expiration) for the manubriosternal angle (Constantinescu 1974). Both movements contribute to respiratory excursions of the sternum.

Xiphisternal joint

This is between xiphoid process and corpus sterni and is also a symphysis. Usually transformed to a synostosis by the fortieth year, it sometimes remains unchanged even in old age.

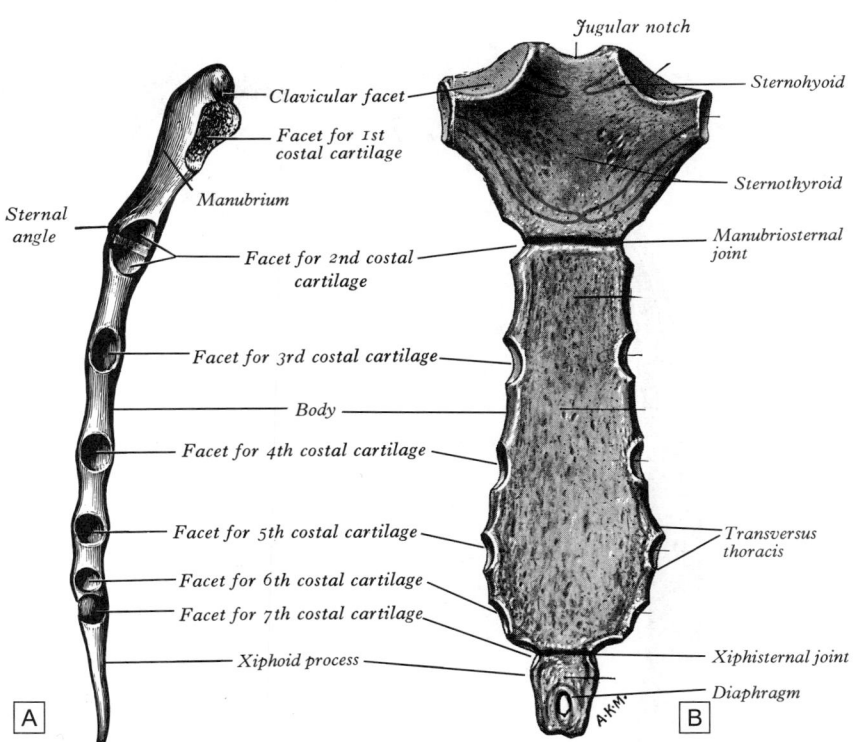

6.122   The sternum: A. Lateral aspect; B. Posterior aspect.

RIBS

The ribs are elastic arches, connected posteriorly with the vertebral column, forming much of the thoracic skeleton. The 12 pairs may be increased by cervical or lumbar ribs or reduced to 11 by absence of the twelfth pair. The superior seven pairs are connected by costal cartilages to the sternum (**6**.121), as *true* ribs. The remaining five are so-called *false* ribs, cartilages of the eighth to tenth joining the superjacent costal cartilage; the eleventh and twelfth, being free at their anterior ends, are sometimes termed *floating* ribs. (The tenth rib is also **usually** 'floating' in the Japanese, also recorded in other races, see p. 542.)

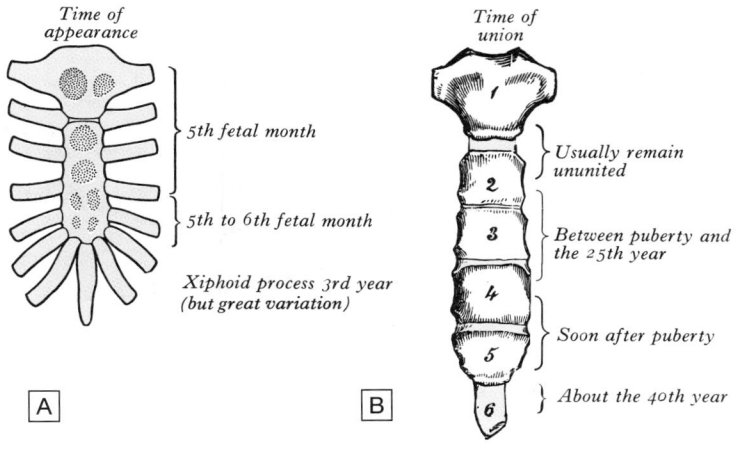

6.123   The ossification of the sternum: A. Before birth; B. At puberty.

Between ribs are *intercostal spaces*, which are deeper in front and between the upper ribs. Upper ribs are less oblique than the lower, obliquity being maximal at the ninth and decreasing to the twelfth. They increase in length from first to seventh, diminishing to the twelfth. In breadth they decrease downwards; in the upper 10 the greatest breadth is anterior. The first two and last three present special features, the rest conforming to a common plan.

A typical rib

It has a shaft with anterior and posterior ends (**6**.124). The *anterior, costal end* has a small concave depression for its cartilage's lateral end. The *shaft* has an external convexity and is grooved internally near its lower border, which is sharp, in contrast to its rounded upper border. The *posterior, vertebral end* has a head, neck and tubercle. The *head* presents two facets, separated by a transverse *crest*. The lower and larger facet articulates with the body of the corresponding vertebra, its crest attaching to the intervertebral disc above it. The *neck* is the flat part beyond the head, anterior to the corresponding transverse process. It is oblique, facing antero-superiorly. Its posteroinferior surface is rough and pierced by foramina. Its upper border is the sharp *crest of the neck*, its lower border rounded. The *tubercle* is posteroexternal at the junction of neck with shaft; more prominent in upper ribs, it is divided into medial articular and lateral non-articular areas. The articular part bears a small, oval facet for the transverse process of the corresponding vertebra; the non-articular area is roughened by ligaments. The shaft is thin and flat with external and internal surfaces, superior and inferior borders. It is curved, bent at the *posterior angle* 5–6 cm from the tubercle, and also twisted about its long axis: the part behind the angle inclines superomedially, its *external surface* hence posteroinferior; in front of the angle it faces slightly up; it is convex and smooth, and crossed near the tubercle by a rough line, directed inferolaterally, at the *posterior angle*. The *internal surface* is smooth and marked by the *costal groove*, bounded below by the inferior border. The superior border of the groove continues behind the lower border of the neck, but terminates anteriorly at the junction of middle and anterior thirds of the shaft, anterior to which the groove is absent. (See below concerning an *anterior angle*.)

Ribs consist of highly vascular trabecular bone, enclosed in a thin layer of compact bone and containing large amounts of red marrow.

The first rib (6.125A)

Most acutely curved and usually shortest, it is broad and flat, its surfaces superior and inferior, its borders internal and external. It slopes obliquely down and forwards to its sternal end. The *head* is small, round and bears an almost circular facet, articulating with the first thoracic vertebral body. The *neck* is rounded and ascends posterolaterally. The *tubercle*, wide and prominent, is directed up and backwards; medially an oval facet articulates with the first thoracic transverse process. At the tubercle the rib is bent, its head turned slightly down; angle and tubercle therefore coincide. The *superior surface* of the flattened shaft is crossed obliquely by two shallow grooves, separated by a slight ridge which ends at the internal border as a usually small, pointed projection, the *scalene*

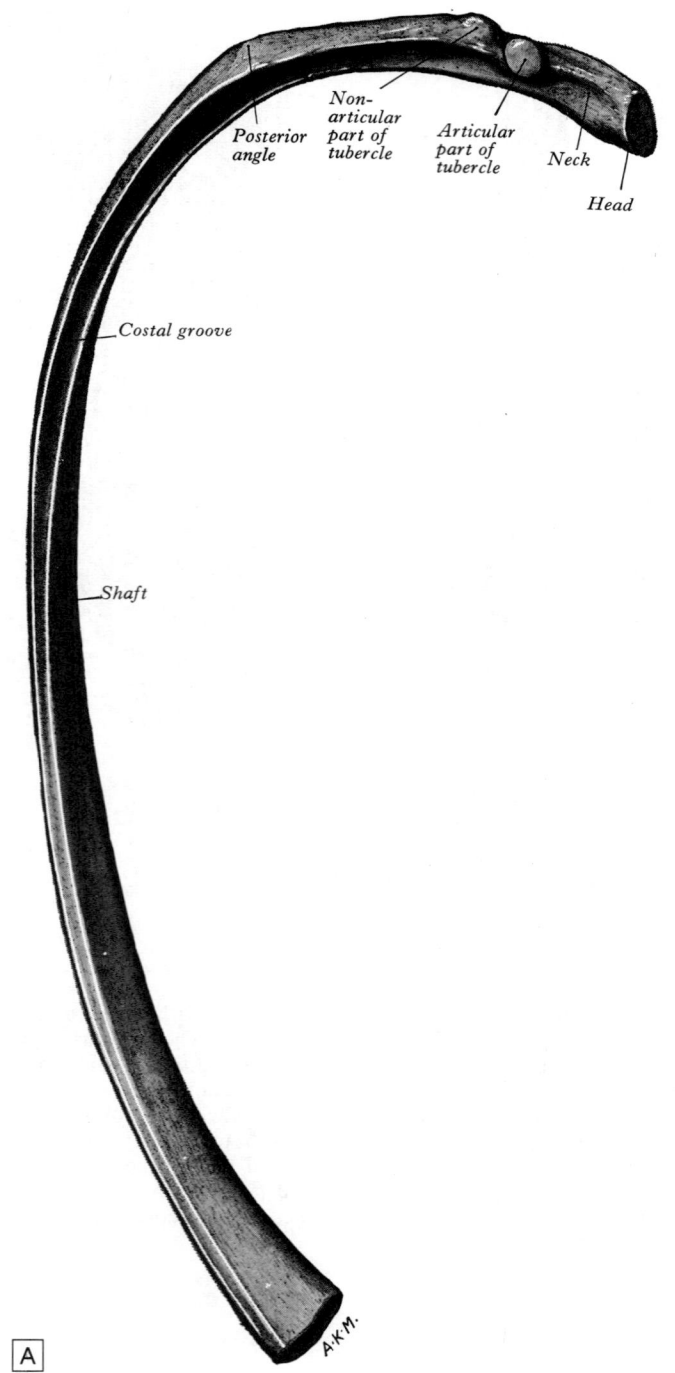

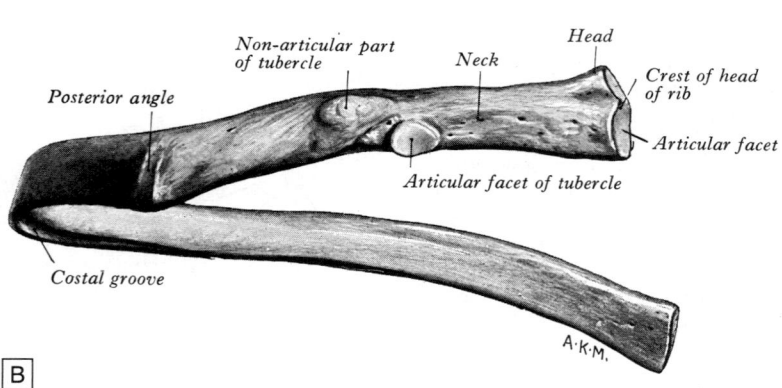

6.124 A typical rib of the left side: A. Inferior; B. Posterior aspects.

tubercle. The *inferior surface* is smooth and ungrooved. The *external border* is convex, thick behind, thin in front. The *internal border* is concave and thin, with a scalene tubercle near its midpoint. The *anterior end* is larger than in any other rib.

The second rib (6.125B)

It is twice the length of the first, with a similar curvature. The non-articular area of the *tubercle* is small. The *angle* is slight and near the tubercle. The *shaft* is not twisted, but at the tubercle is convex upwards, as in the first rib but less so. The *external surface* of the shaft is convex and superolaterally marked centrally by a rough, muscular impression; the latter continues posteromedially towards the tubercle as a narrow roughened ridge. The *internal surface*, smooth and concave, faces inferomedially with posteriorly a short costal groove.

The tenth rib

This has a single facet on its head which may articulate with the intervertebral disc above as well as the upper border of the tenth thoracic vertebra near its pedicle.

The eleventh and twelfth ribs (6.126)

Each has one large, articular facet on the head, but no neck or tubercle; their pointed anterior ends are tipped with cartilage. The eleventh has a slight angle and shallow costal groove. The twelfth has neither, being much shorter and sloping cranially at its vertebral end. The internal surfaces of both ribs face slightly **upwards**, more so in the twelfth.

Ossification

Each rib, except the first and last two, is ossified from a primary centre for the shaft and secondary centres for the head and articular and non-articular parts of the tubercle (Fawcett 1911a,b) but not for non-articular parts of tubercles below the sixth or seventh. The primary centre appears near the angle, late in the second month, first in the sixth and seventh ribs. Secondary centres for the head and tubercle appear about puberty, uniting to the shaft soon after 20. The first rib has a primary centre for the shaft, a secondary for the head but only one for the tubercle; the eleventh and twelfth, without tubercles, have two centres each.

COSTAL CARTILAGES

The costal cartilages (**6**.121), flat bars of hyaline cartilage, extend from the anterior ends of ribs, contributing much to thoracic mobility

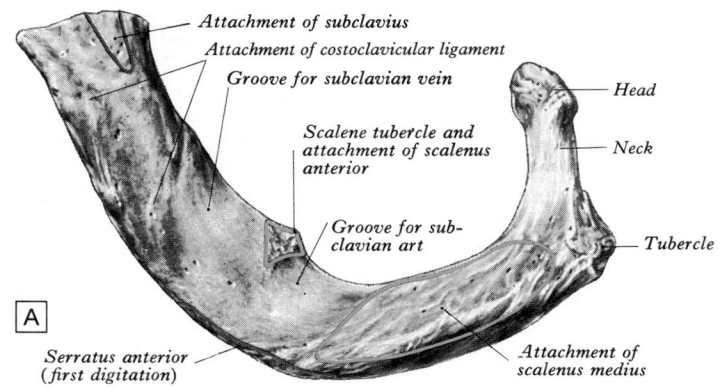

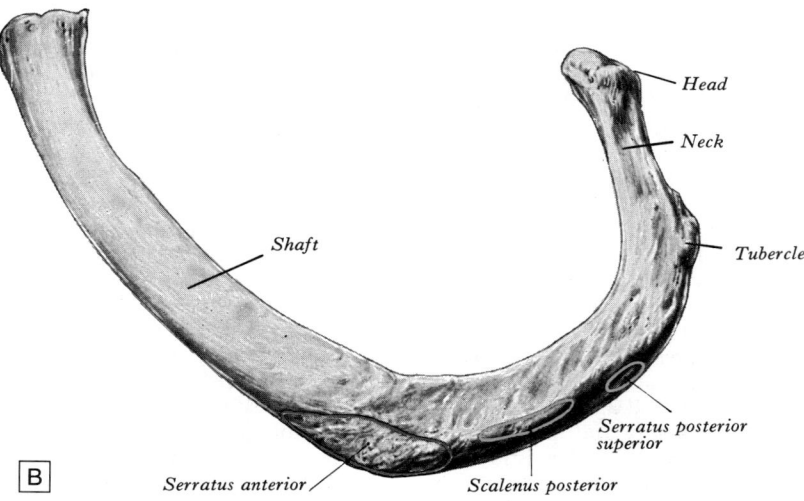

6.125   The superior aspects of the first (A) and second (B) left ribs.

and elasticity. The upper seven pairs join the sternum; the eighth to tenth articulate with the lower border of the cartilage above; the lowest two have free pointed ends in the abdominal wall. They increase in length from first to seventh, decreasing again to the

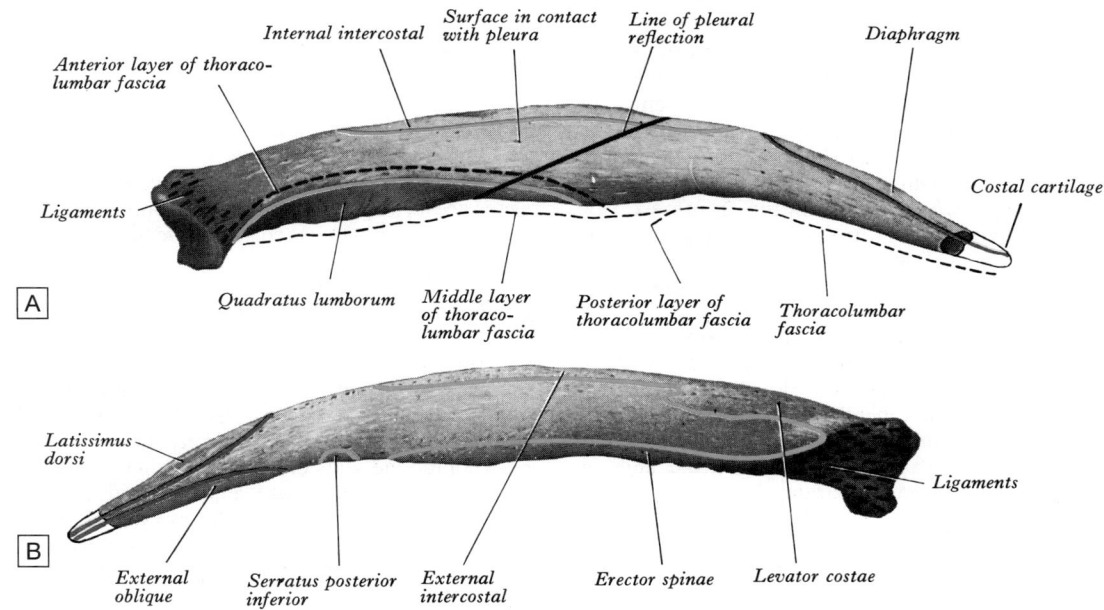

6.126   The twelfth rib of the left side. A. Anterior aspect; B. Posterior aspect.

twelfth. They diminish in breadth from first to last, like the intercostal spaces. They are broad at their costal continuity and taper as they pass forward; but the first and second are of even breadth and the sixth to eighth enlarge where their margins are in contact. The first descends a little, the second is horizontal and the third ascends slightly, the others being angulated and inclining up towards the sternum or cartilage above, a little anterior to their ribs.

Each costal cartilage has two surfaces, borders and ends. The *anterior surface* is convex, facing anterosuperior; to the first cartilage are attached the sternoclavicular articular disc, costoclavicular ligament and subclavius and to the first six of seven medially is pectoralis major. The others are covered by the partial attachments of the anterior abdominal muscles. The *posterior surface* is concave, and really posteroinferior; attached to the first cartilage is sternothyroid, to the second to sixth, transversus thoracis, and to the six lower transversus abdominis. To the concave *superior* and convex *inferior* borders are attached the internal intercostal muscles and external intercostal membranes. The inferior borders of the fifth (sometimes), and sixth to ninth cartilages project at points of greatest convexity. Oblong facets on these projections articulate with facets on slight projections from the superior borders of subjacent cartilages. The *lateral end* of each cartilage is continuous with its rib; the *medial end* of the first is continuous with the sternum; those of the six succeeding cartilages are round and articulate with shallow costal notches on the lateral margins of the sternum; those of the eighth to tenth are pointed, each connected with the cartilage above; those of the eleventh and twelfth are pointed and free. Excepting the synchondrosis of the first rib and sternum, all these articulations are synovial (p. 544).

The tenth rib is usually united anteriorly with the ninth by a fibrous joint (p. 545); but frequently it is free and pointed like the eleventh and twelfth. The incidence of a 'floating' tenth rib varies from 35% to 70% in different races (Shimaguchi 1974).

In old age the costal cartilages tend to ossify superficially, losing pliability and becoming brittle. The histology (Amprino & Bairati 1933), histochemistry (Quintarelli & Dellovo 1966), and ultrastructure of such senile changes have been reviewed by Stockwell (1967) (and see p. 451). An increase in keratan sulphate is noted maximally in the subperichondrial zone.

ATTACHMENTS AND RELATIONS OF RIBS

To the *head of a typical rib* the radiate ligament is attached along its anterior border, and the intra-articular ligament to its crest. Its anterior surface is related to costal pleura and in lower ribs the sympathetic trunk. The *neck's anterior surface* is divided by a faint transverse ridge for the internal intercostal membrane and is continuous with the *inner* lip of the superior border of the shaft. The area above the ridge, more or less triangular, is separated from the membrane by fatty tissue; the lower, smooth area is covered by costal pleura. The *neck's posterior surface* receives the costotransverse ligament and is pierced by vascular foramina. The *crest of the neck* is for attachment of the superior costotransverse ligament and extends laterally into the *outer* lip of the shaft's superior border. The neck's rounded inferior border continues laterally into the upper border of the costal groove, receiving the internal intercostal membrane. The *articular area of the tubercle* in the upper six ribs is convex and faces posteromedially; in the succeeding three or four it is almost flat and faces down, back and slightly medially. The lateral costotransverse ligament is attached to the *non-articular area*.

The ridge on the shaft's *external surface* (near its posterior angle) in a typical rib receives an upward continuation of thoracolumbar fascia and lateral fibres of iliocostalis thoracis. From second to tenth ribs the distance between angle and tubercle increases. Medial to the angle the external surface gives attachment to a levator costae and is covered by erector spinae. Near this surface's sternal end an indistinct, oblique line (anterior 'angle') separates the attachments of external oblique and serratus anterior (or latissimus dorsi, in ninth and tenth ribs). To the *costal groove* (internal surface) is attached the internal intercostal muscle, separating bone from the intercostal vessels and nerve. At the vertebral end the groove faces down, its borders in the same plane. Near the posterior angle the shaft broadens and the groove reaches its internal surface; to the groove's

superior rim innermost intercostal is attached, rarely extending to the rib's anterior quarter. Posteriorly this rim meets the neck's lower border. To the sharp inferior costal border is attached an external intercostal muscle. The superior border has two lips posteriorly: to the inner are attached both the external intercostal, to the outer only the internal and innermost intercostal.

The *first rib* (**6**.125A) has a *tubercle for scalenus anterior*, which is also attached to adjoining parts of the *upper surface*. The groove anterior to this forms a bed for the subclavian vein; and the rough area between this and the first costal cartilage receives the costoclavicular ligament and, more anteriorly, subclavius. Passing in the groove behind the tubercle is the subclavian artery and usually the lower trunk of the brachial plexus. Behind this, as far as the costal tubercle, scalenus medius is attached. The obliquity of the first ribs accounts for the appearance of pulmonary and pleural apices in the neck.

The first rib's external border is covered behind by scalenus posterior descending to the second; the first digitation of serratus anterior is, in part, attached to it, behind the subclavian (arterial) groove. To the internal border is attached the suprapleural membrane, covering the pleura's cervical dome.

The *second rib* (**6**.125B) is marked by *serratus anterior*, its rough prominence extending from just behind the midpoint of its external surface; to this tubercle the lower part of the first and the second digitation are attached. The second intercostal nerve is between the rib and pleura for most of its course. The distinct lips of the upper border are widely separated behind; in front of the angle the outer lip receives scalenus posterior and, below this, serratus posterior superior.

The *twelfth rib* (**6**.126) has numerous attached muscles and ligaments. To the lower part of its *anterior surface*, in its medial half to two-thirds, quadratus lumborum and its anterior covering layer of thoracolumbar fascia are attached, the upper part being related to the costodiaphragmatic pleural recess. At or near the *upper border* are attachments of the internal intercostal medially and laterally the diaphragm. The *lower border* gives attachment to the middle lamella of the thoracolumbar fascia and, lateral to quadratus lumborum, the lateral arcuate ligament (p. 816) and posterior lamella of the thoracolumbar fascia. Posteriorly, close to the head, is attached the lumbocostal ligament (p. 543), connecting it to the first lumbar transverse process. To the *external surface* are attached the lowest levator costae, longissimus thoracis and iliocostalis in its medial half and laterally serratus posterior inferior, latissimus dorsi and external oblique. Along the *upper border* the external intercostal is attached. These attachments vary; those of the internal intercostal, levator costae and erector spinae merge and those of latissimus dorsi, diaphragm and external oblique may reach the costal cartilage. The lower limit of the pleural sac crosses in front of the rib, approximately where it is crossed by the lateral border of iliocostalis. Its lateral end is usually below the line of costodiaphragmatic pleural reflection and therefore not covered by pleura.

COSTOVERTEBRAL JOINTS

Articulations of the ribs with the vertebral column connect their heads to vertebral bodies (costocorporeal) and necks and tubercles to transverse processes (costotransverse).

Joints of costal heads

Heads of typical ribs articulate with facets (often termed demifacets) on the margins of adjacent thoracic vertebral bodies and with intervertebral discs between them (**6**.127). The first and tenth to twelfth ribs articulate with a single vertebra by a simple synovial joint; in the others an intra-articular ligament bisects the joint. Double synovial compartments result, the joint being classified as both compound and complex. Often inaccurately described as plane, their articular surfaces are slightly ovoid and the upper and lower synovial articulations are obtusely angled to each other (**6**.127). Ligaments are capsular, radiate and intra-articular.

Fibrous capsules. They connect costal heads to the circumference of articular surfaces formed by intervertebral discs and demifacets of adjacent vertebrae; some of their upper fibres traverse their intervertebral foramina to blend with the posterior aspects of intervertebral discs (strictly symphyses); posterior fibres are continuous with costotransverse ligaments.

Radiate ligaments. These connect the anterior parts of each costal head to the bodies of two vertebrae and their intervening intervertebral disc. Each is attached to the head just beyond its articular surface. Superior fibres ascend to the vertebral body above, inferior to the body below; intermediate fibres, shortest and least distinct, are horizontal and attached to the disc. In the first rib's joint the radiate ligament is attached to the seventh cervical and first thoracic vertebrae. In joints of the tenth to twelfth ribs, articulating with single vertebrae, the ligament is attached to this and the one above.

Intra-articular ligament. A short, flat band, it is attached laterally to the crest between the costal articular facets and medially to the intervertebral disc, dividing the joint; from the first and tenth to twelfth joints the ligament is absent.

Costotransverse joints

The facet of a costal tubercle articulates reciprocally with the transverse process of its corresponding vertebra (**6**.128). The eleventh and twelfth ribs lack this articulation; in the upper five or six joints articular surfaces are reciprocally curved but below this are flatter (**6**.129). Their ligaments are capsular, costotransverse, superior and lateral costotransverse. The *fibrous capsule* is thin and attached to articular peripheries; it has a synovial lining.

The superior costotransverse ligament. This has an anterior layer attached between the crest of the costal neck and lower aspect of the transverse process above (**6**.127); laterally it blends with the internal intercostal membrane and it is crossed by intercostal vessels and nerve; its posterior layer is attached posteriorly on the costal neck, ascending posteromedially to the transverse process above; laterally it blends with the external intercostal muscle. The first rib has no such ligament; the shaft of the twelfth, near its head, is connected to the base of the first lumbar transverse process by a *lumbocostal ligament* in series with the superior costotransverse ligaments.

Accessory ligament. This is usually present and medial to the superior costotransverse ligament, being separated from it by the dorsal ramus of a thoracic spinal nerve and accompanying vessels (**6**.127). Variable in attachments, such bands usually pass from a depression medial to a costal tubercle to the inferior articular process immediately above; some fibres also pass to the base of the transverse process.

The costotransverse ligament. This fills the *costotransverse foramen* between the rib neck and its adjacent corresponding transverse process. Its numerous short fibres extend back from the posterior rough surface on the neck to the anterior surface of the transverse process. In the eleventh and twelfth ribs it is rudimentary or absent.

The lateral costotransverse ligament. Short, thick and strong, it passes obliquely from the apex of the transverse process to the rough non-articular part of the adjacent costal tubercle. The ligaments of upper ribs **ascend** from their transverse processes; they are shorter and more oblique than those of the lower ribs, which descend.

Movements at costotransverse joints. Costal heads are so firmly tied to vertebral bodies by radiate and intra-articular ligaments that only slight gliding can occur; strong ligaments binding costal necks and tubercles to transverse processes also limit movements at costotransverse joints to slight gliding, guided by the shape and direction of articular surfaces (**6**.129); those on tubercles of the upper six ribs are oval and vertically convex, fitting corresponding concavities on the anterior surfaces of transverse processes; hence up and down movements of tubercles involve rotation of costal necks about their long axes. Articular surfaces of the seventh to tenth tubercles are almost flat, facing down, medially and backwards; opposing surfaces are on the upper aspects of transverse processes. Hence when these tubercles ascend they also move posteromedially. Both sets of joints move simultaneously and in the same directions; the costal neck moves as if at a single joint, the two articulations forming its ends. In the upper six ribs the neck moves slightly up and down but its chief movement is one of rotation about its long axis, downward rotation of its anterior aspect being associated with depression and upward rotation with elevation of the shaft and anterior end of the rib. In the seventh to tenth ribs the neck ascends posteromedially or descends anterolaterally, increasing or

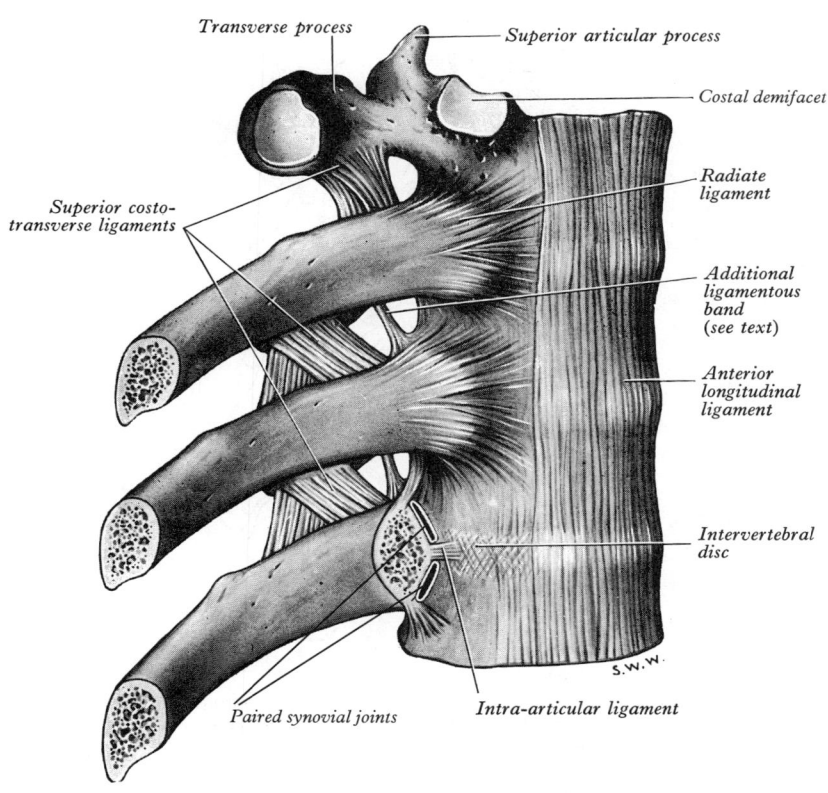

6.127 Costovertebral joints: right anterolateral aspect. In the lowest joint shown most of the radiate ligament and the anterior part of the head of the rib have been excised to show the two joint cavities and the intra-articular ligament between them.

diminishing the infrasternal angle; slight rotation accompanies these movements. The muscles involved in respiration are considered on page 818.

STERNOCOSTAL JOINTS

Costal cartilages join small concavities on the lateral sternal borders (*chondrosternal articulations*, **6**.130). Perichondrium and periosteum are continuous. The first costal cartilage joins by an unusual variety

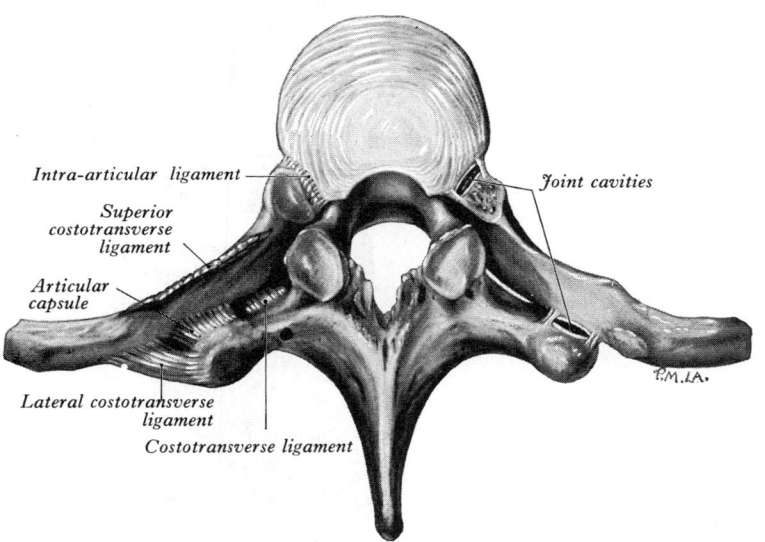

6.128 Costovertebral joints: superior aspect. On the left the free demifacet superior to the intra-articular ligament is apparent on the rib's head. On the right the inferior costovertebral and costotransverse synovial cavities have been opened.

543

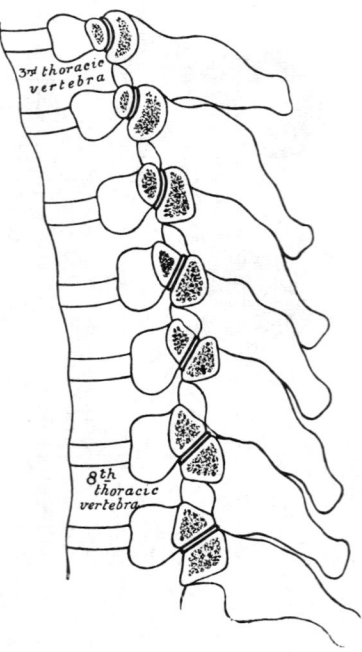

6.129 Section through the costotransverse joints from the third to the ninth inclusive. Contrast the concave facets on the upper with less curved facets on the lower transverse processes.

of synarthrosis (see p. 491; this is often inaccurately called a synchondrosis) while the second to seventh articulate by synovial joints; articular cavities are often absent, particularly in lower joints. Articular surfaces are *fibrocartilaginous* and this tissue also unites costal cartilages to the sternum where cavities are absent (Gray & Gardner 1943). Ligaments involved are capsular, radiate sternocostal, intra-articular and costoxiphoid. According to Sick and Koritke (1976) the seventh costosternal joint may be synovial or 'symphyseal'.

Fibrous capsules. These surround the second to seventh sternocostal joints. They are thin, blended with the sternocostal ligaments and are strengthened above and below by fibres connecting the costal cartilages to the sternum.

Radiate sternocostal ligaments. Broad, thin bands, they radiate from the front and back of the sternal ends of the costal cartilages of true ribs to corresponding sternal surfaces. Their superficial fibres intermingle with adjacent ligaments above and below, with those of the opposite side and with tendinous fibres of pectoralis major, forming a thick fibrous membrane around the sternum, more markedly in its lower part.

Intra-articular ligaments. These are constant only between the second costal cartilages and sternum. The second costal cartilage's ligament extends from the costal cartilage to the fibrocartilage uniting the manubrium and sternal body and is therefore intra-articular. Occasionally the third sternal cartilage is connected with the first and second sternal segments by a similar ligament. Fibrocartilaginous strands may occur in the third and lower joints. Articular cavities may be absent at all ages.

Costoxiphoid ligaments. Connecting anterior and posterior surfaces of the seventh costal cartilage (and sometimes sixth) to the same surfaces of the xiphoid process; they vary in length and breadth, the posterior being less distinct.

Movements. Slight gliding movements occur at sternocostal joints, sufficient for respiration (p. 818).

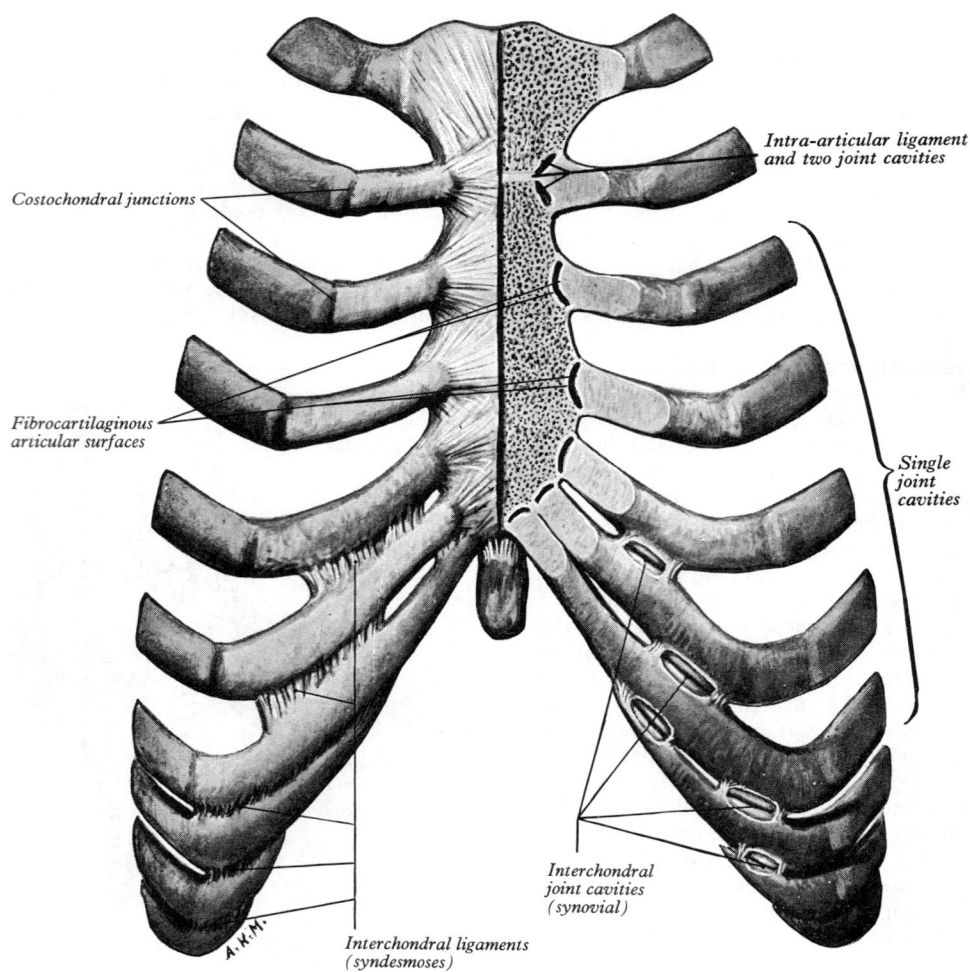

Costochondral junctions

Fibrocartilaginous articular surfaces

Intra-articular ligament and two joint cavities

Single joint cavities

Interchondral joint cavities (synovial)

Interchondral ligaments (syndesmoses)

6.130 Sternocostal and interchondral joints: anterior aspect.

INTERCHONDRAL JOINTS

Contiguous borders of the sixth to ninth costal cartilages articulate by apposition of small oblong facets, each articulation being enclosed in a thin *fibrous capsule*, lined by synovial membrane with lateral and medial *interchondral ligaments* (**6**.130). Sometimes the fifth cartilage, more rarely the ninth, articulate at their inferior borders with adjoining cartilages, this connection being more often by ligamentous fibres. Articulation between the ninth and tenth cartilages is never synovial and sometimes absent (p. 491). For further comments on chondral arthroses see page 542.

COSTOCHONDRAL JUNCTIONS

The costal cartilages are persistent, unossified anterior parts of cartilaginous models preceding fully developed ribs. Artificially separated from its rib a costal cartilage has a rounded end, the rib a depression. Across junctions periosteum and perichondrium are continuous and the collagen of the osseous and cartilaginous matrices blend. No movement occurs there.

THORAX

The thoracic skeleton (**6**.131) is an osteocartilaginous frame around the principal organs of respiration and circulation. It is narrow above, broad below, flattened anteroposteriorly and longer behind.

It is reniform in horizontal section due to the forward projection of vertebral bodies.

Posteriorly the thorax includes thoracic vertebrae and posterior parts of the ribs. On both sides of the vertebral column is a large groove due to the posterolateral curvature of the ribs from their vertebral ends to their angles. **Anteriorly** are the sternum, anterior parts of ribs and costal cartilages; this aspect is slightly convex. **Laterally** the thorax is convex and formed by ribs alone. Ribs and costal cartilages are separated by 11 intercostal spaces, occupied by intercostal muscles and membranes, neurovascular bundles and lymphatic channels.

The *thoracic inlet* is reniform, about 5 cm anteroposteriorly, and about 10 cm transversely. Its plane slopes down and forwards, bounded by the first thoracic vertebral body behind, the superior border of the manubrium sterni in front and first rib on each side. The *outlet* is limited behind by the twelfth thoracic vertebral body, the twelfth and eleventh ribs laterally, and in front by the tenth to seventh ribs, which ascend to form the *infrasternal angle*. The outlet is wider transversely and oblique, sloping down towards the back, and is closed by the diaphragm which forms a floor to the thoracic cavity.

Thoracic variations in dimensions and proportions are partly individual and also linked to age, sex and race. At birth the transverse diameter is relatively less but adult proportions develop as walking begins. In females capacity is less, absolutely and proportionately, the sternum being shorter, the thoracic inlet more oblique and the suprasternal notch level with the third thoracic vertebra (second in males). The upper ribs are more mobile in females, allowing greater upper thoracic expansion. In tall thin individuals the thorax usually

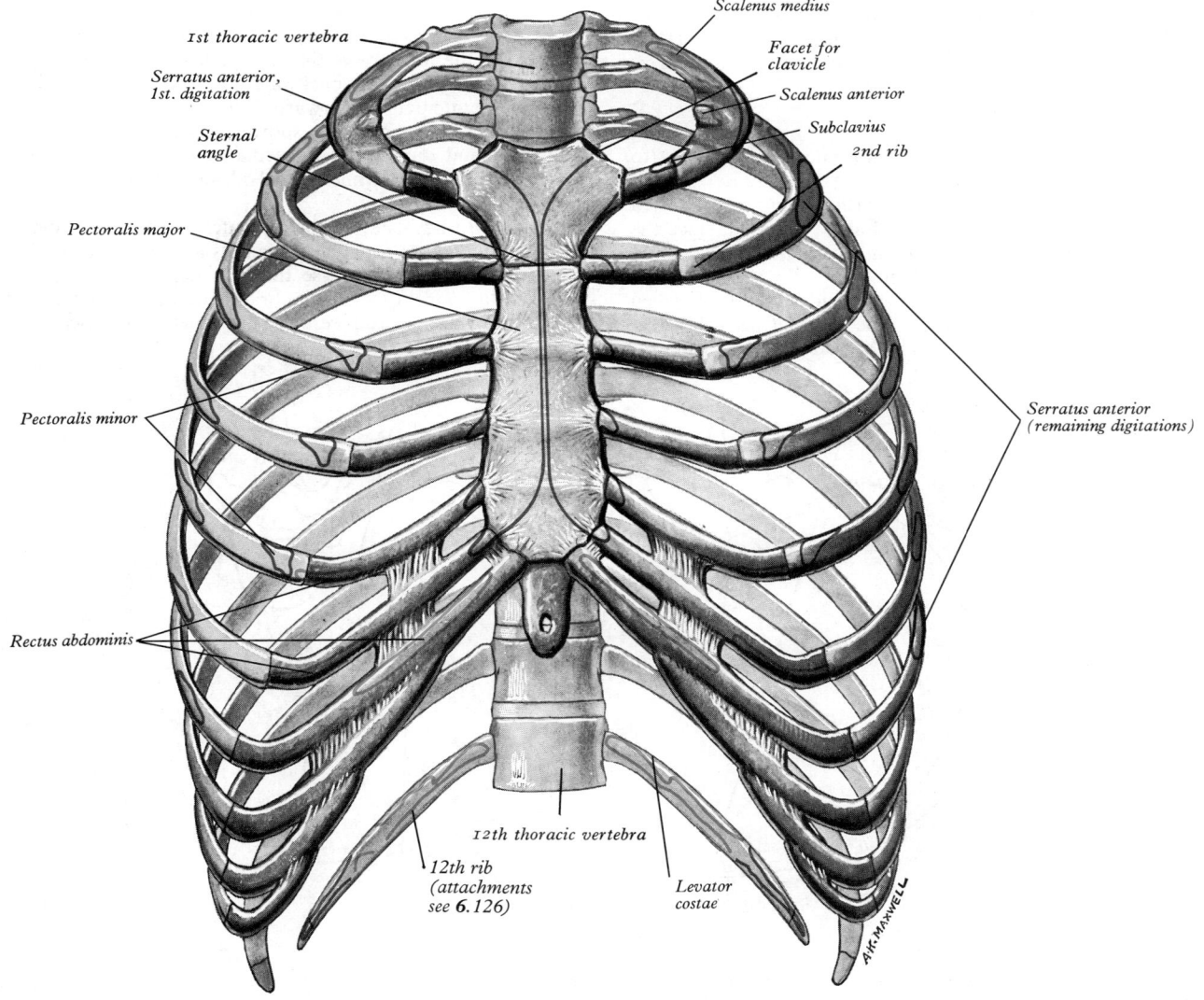

1st thoracic vertebra

Serratus anterior,
1st. digitation

Sternal
angle

Pectoralis major

Pectoralis minor

Rectus abdominis

Scalenus medius

Facet for
clavicle

Scalenus anterior

Subclavius

2nd rib

Serratus anterior
(remaining digitations)

12th thoracic vertebra

12th rib
(attachments
see **6**.126)

Levator
costae

A.K.MAXWELL

6.131   The skeleton of the thorax: anterior aspect.

shows corresponding proportions, and a similar correspondence also occurs in the short and broad individuals. Racial variations are also linked to stature and proportions in a like manner.

The prime function of the thorax is respiration. The obvious protection afforded is fortuitous but many muscles are attached to it, not all primarily concerned with respiration, although they may assist it. Muscles of the arm, especially those acting on the pectoral girdle and humerus, those of the abdominal wall and spinal column, all have widespread thoracic attachments.

Elastic recoil of ribs, which suspend the sternum, may explain the rarity of sternal fractures. Despite their pliability, the ribs are much more frequently broken, middle ribs being the most vulnerable. Since traumatic stress is usually due to compression of the thorax, the usual site of fracture is the rib's weakest point, just in front of the angle. Direct impact may fracture a rib anywhere and the broken ends of bone may be driven inwards, with possible injury to thoracic or upper abdominal viscera.

A *cervical rib*, the costal element of the seventh cervical vertebra, may be a mere epiphysis on its transverse process but more often has a head, neck and tubercle, with or without a shaft which, varying in length, extends anterolaterally into the posterior triangle of the neck, where it may end freely or join the first rib or costal cartilage, or even the sternum. It may be partly fibrous, but its effects are not related to the size of its osseous part. If it is long enough its relations are those of a first thoracic rib: the brachial plexus (usually lower trunk) and subclavian vessels are *superior* and apt to suffer compression in a narrow angle between rib and scalenus anterior. Hence cervical ribs may first be revealed by nervous and vascular symptoms, particularly due to pressure on the eighth cervical and first thoracic spinal nerves, with motor and sensory effects in structures supplied. According to Cave (1975) a cervical rib or pleurapophysis may show synostosis or diarthrosis with either the anterior (parapophyseal) or posterior (diapophyseal) 'roots' of the so-called seventh cervical transverse process or, more usually, with both (**6.89**).

MECHANISM OF THE THORAX

Each rib has its range and direction of movement contributing to thoracic respiratory excursions. Each acts as a lever, its fulcrum immediately lateral to its costotransverse articulation; hence, when the shaft is elevated, the neck is depressed and vice versa; since the lever's arms differ much in length, slight movement at the vertebral end is much magnified at the anterior end.

Anterior costal ends are lower than posterior; therefore, when shafts are raised they move forwards. The midshaft is below the ends so that when the shaft is raised it also spreads laterally. Further,

each rib is part of a curve greater than that of the rib above; therefore, costal elevation increases transverse thoracic diameter at higher levels. (Modifications of rib movements at vertebral ends are described on p. 544.) Modifications also result from attachments of anterior costal ends with different movements of vertebrosternal, vertebrochondral and vertebral ribs.

Vertebrosternal ribs (6.132A). The first moves little, except in deep respiration about an oblique axis through the neck; the shaft rises laterally in inspiration, its inferomedial surface becoming more directly inferior, an impossible movement if the cartilage is calcified, as it may be; first ribs and manubrium then move as a unit about a transverse axis through their costotransverse joints. The second rib also moves little in quiet respiration; elevation of third to sixth ribs thrusts their anterior ends upwards and forwards, mostly by backward rotation at their necks; this also moves the sternum similarly at the manubriosternal joint, increasing the anteroposterior thoracic diameter. As this action ceases, an elevating force raises the middle parts of their shafts, everting their lower borders, opening the costochondral angle and increasing the transverse thoracic diameter. Measurements of sternal respiratory movements reveal large excursions, especially in fit adult males (Constantinescu 1974). Between full inspiration and expiration the suprasternal notch may move 31 mm, excursions at the superior (34 mm) and inferior (37 mm) ends of the sternal body being increased by changes in the sternal angle.

Vertebrochondral ribs (6.132B). These ribs, including the seventh, assist thoracic respiratory enlargement and they also increase upper abdominal space for the viscera displaced by diaphragmatic descent, although abdominal relaxation accounts in part for this. Costal cartilages, through their joints, push each other up, the final thrust forcing the lower sternum upwards and forwards. Elevation of their anterior ends is limited by the very slight rotation possible at their necks. Elevation of shafts is accompanied by outward and backward movement, the former everting their anterior ends and opening the infrasternal angle, while backward movement retracts the anterior ends and counteracts the forward thrust of elevation, most noticeably in the lower ribs which are shortest. The result is an increase in transverse and diminution in median anteroposterior diameters of the upper abdomen, while its lateral anteroposterior diameters are increased.

Vertebral ribs. They have free anterior ends and costovertebral joints without intra-articular ligaments and may move a little in all directions. As other ribs rise they are depressed and fixed by the quadrati lumborum to aid diaphragmatic action of the diaphragm. The muscles which produce these movements are discussed on page 818.

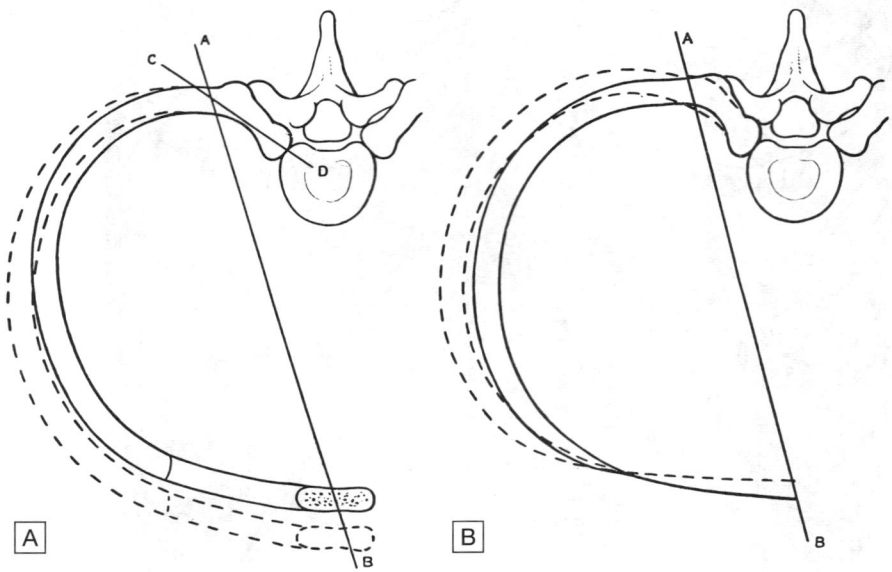

6.132A. Diagram showing the axes of movement (AB and CD) of a vertebrosternal rib. The interrupted lines indicate the position of the rib in inspiration. B. Diagram showing the axis of movement (AB) of a vertebrochondral rib. The interrupted lines indicate the position of the rib in inspiration.

SKULL

INTRODUCTION

The vertebrate skull is the most modified part of the axial skeleton. Whatever truth may reside in the hypothesis that it is partly derived from metameric elements such as modified vertebrae, palaeontology and comparative anatomy clearly indicate that from earliest times it has been a skeletal complex adapted to support the brain and organs

magnum, displaceable in either direction. Even the brainstem can be displaced through the foramen magnum by raised intracranial pressure. Variability in volume of fluid in the cerebral ventricular system and numerous connections between intra- and extracranial veins add to the complexity of the situation. Nevertheless, it appears undeniable that enclosure of the brain in an otherwise invariable space must be a factor in the control of cerebral circulation. This peculiar location of the brain entails some penalties, however well-adapted to ordinary circumstances: lesions which occupy space can

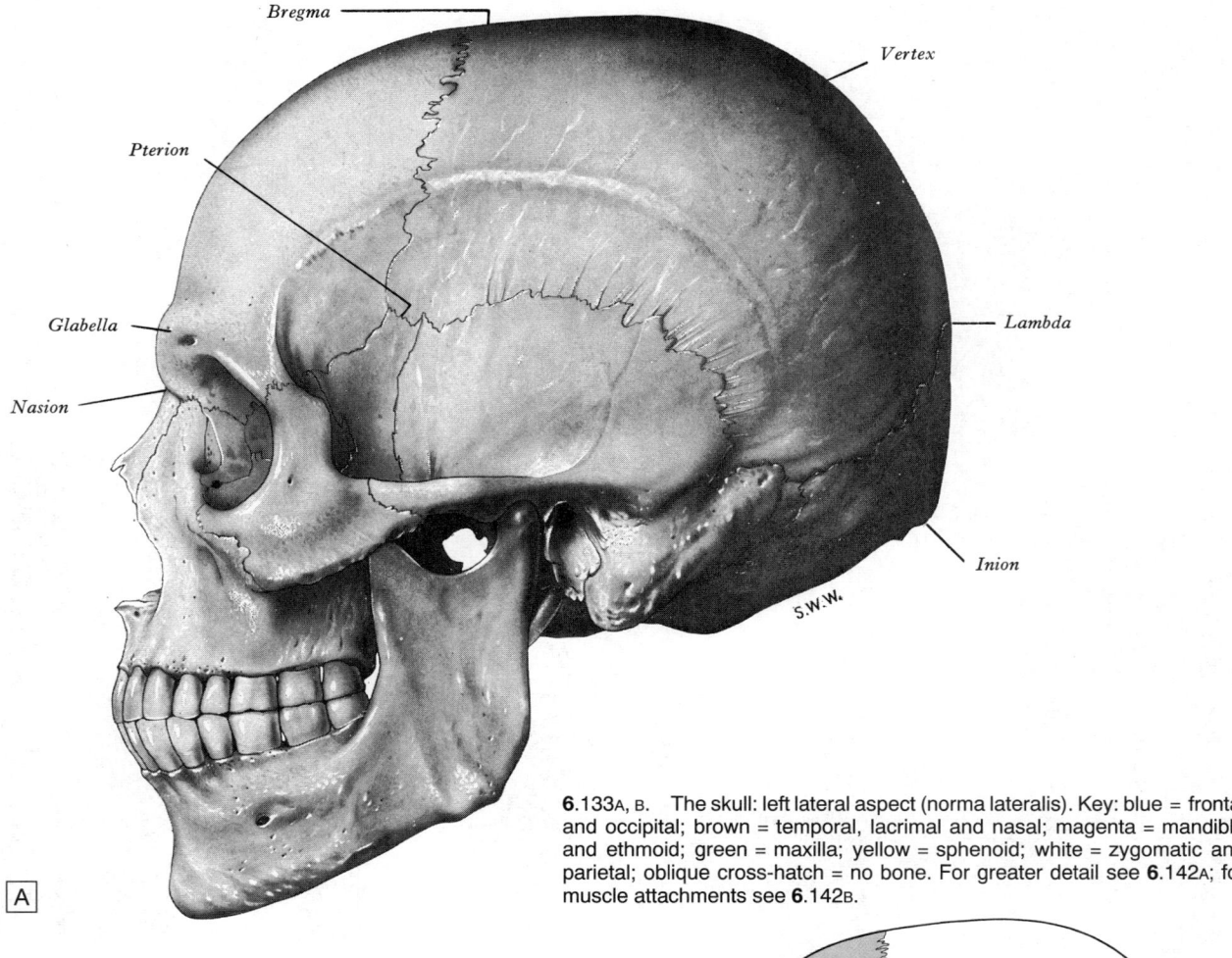

[A]

6.133A, B.   The skull: left lateral aspect (norma lateralis). Key: blue = frontal and occipital; brown = temporal, lacrimal and nasal; magenta = mandible and ethmoid; green = maxilla; yellow = sphenoid; white = zygomatic and parietal; oblique cross-hatch = no bone. For greater detail see **6**.142A; for muscle attachments see **6**.142B.

of special sense and to secure food. Siting of special receptors, tactile, chemical and visual, and a feeding orifice at the leading end of an elongate creature, such as a vertebrate, have advantages so obvious as to be overlooked. This concentration of functions is linked with elaboration of the fore end of the nervous system into a brain, whose size and dominance have increased throughout vertebrate evolution. The very size of the human brain emphasizes the skull's **cerebral** function, overshadowing others. Even in this limited role the cranium cannot be considered merely protective. Sporadic protection of brain from external impacts is of undoubted value; need of a barrier against stresses from powerful masticatory and axial musculature is less obvious but nevertheless continual. In addition to these extraneous forces, the rigid cranial walls provide continuous isolation for cerebral circulation. Moreover, the reputed buffering by meninges, the subarachnoid space and contained fluid could only be effective within a rigid container.

The brain's extreme dependence on an uninterrupted blood flow is well known; independence of cerebral arterial pressure from extra-cranial variations, due to some form of autoregulation as yet unidentified, is also established. It appears likely that siting of a brain in a rigidly maintained space is a factor in such mechanisms, despite lack of exact evidence. Of course, the cranial cavity is not closed: cerebrospinal fluid passes freely through the foramen

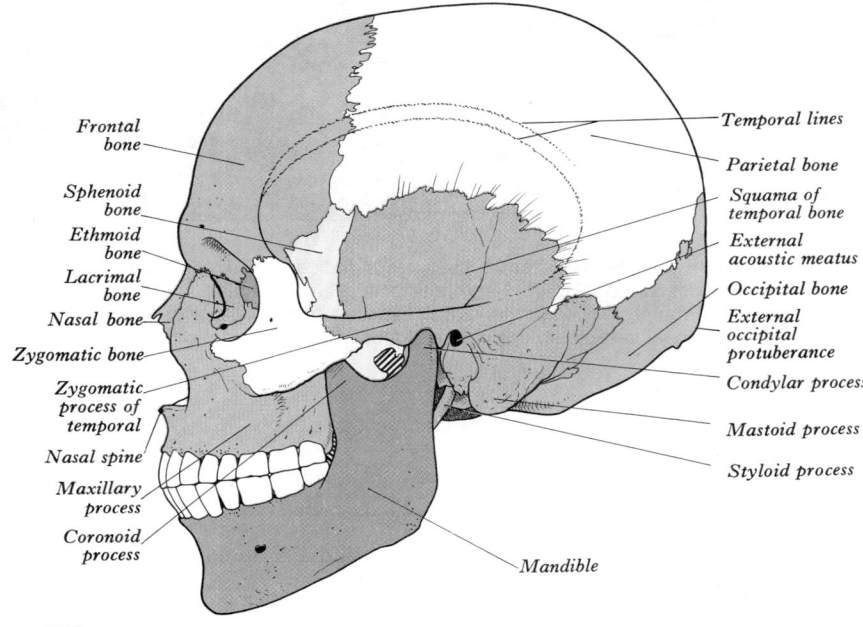

[B]

547

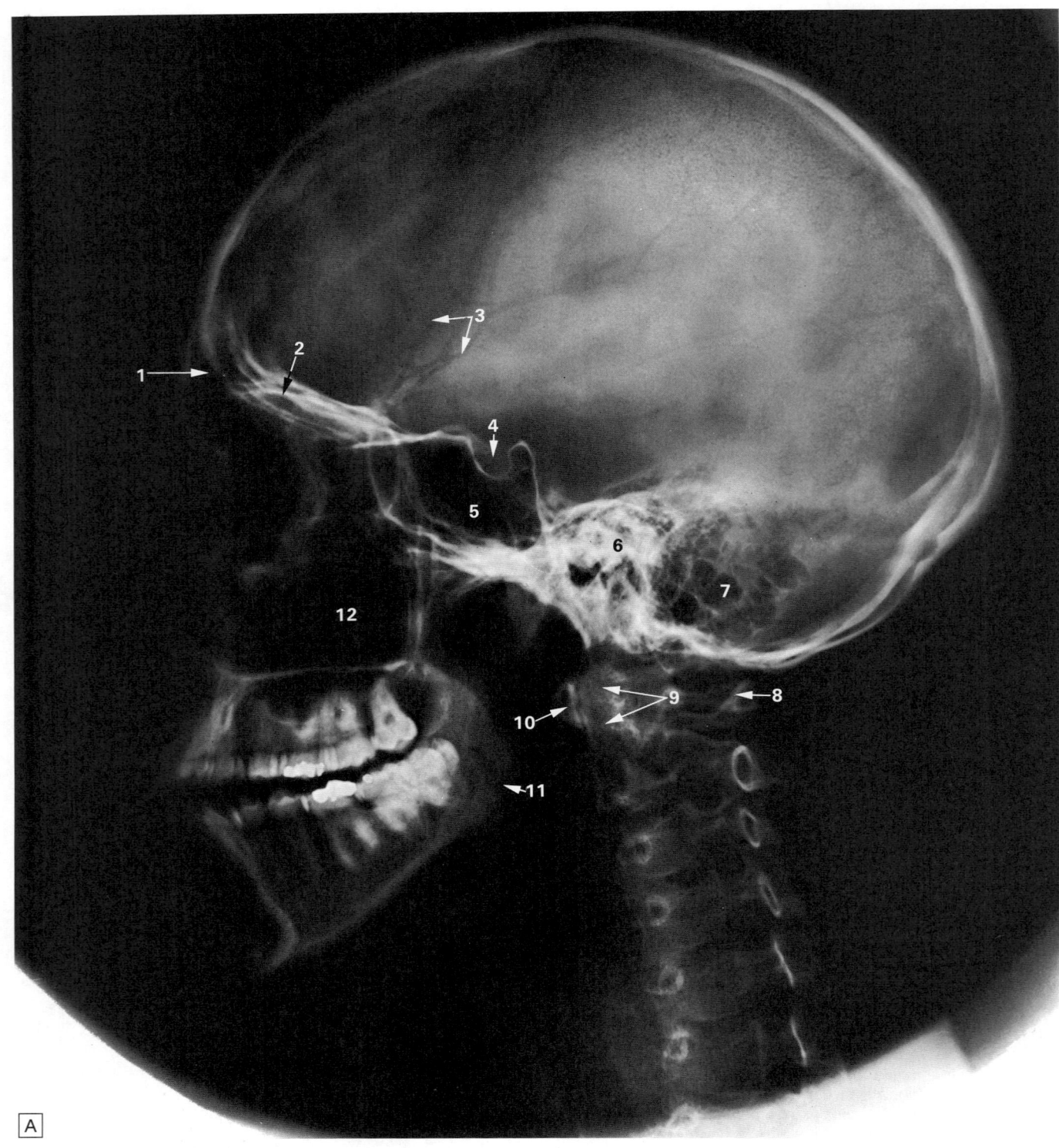

A

6.134   Lateral (A) and anteroposterior (B) radiographs of adult female skull. (Provided by R D Hoare, Neuroradiologist, Guy's Hospital.)
A. 1. Frontal sinus. 2. Orbital roof. 3. Grooves for anterior branches of middle meningeal vessels. 4. Hypophyseal fossa. 5. Sphenoidal sinus. 6. Dense shadow of petrous part of temporal bone. 7. Mastoid air cells. 8. Posterior arch of atlas. 9. Dens of axis. 10. Anterior arch of atlas. 11. Angle of mandible. 12. Maxillary sinus.

raise pressure within the cranium far more easily than elsewhere and with far more devastating effects.

Even in primitive vertebrates the *neurocranium*, derived from cartilages ventral to the brain, as in human embryos (p. 271), has been joined by cartilaginous supports for external nares and olfactory receptors, eyeballs and labyrinths. With the addition of jaws, of branchial origin, and dermal or 'membrane' bones, arising in subcutaneous mesenchyme over the head and jaws and in the buccal roof, the vertebrate skull is defined in all its complexity. Cartilaginous elements are usually ossified, except in minor groups such as sharks,

where cartilage is considered degenerate rather than primitive. Moreover, some dermal elements are as ancient, judging by fossil records, as 'cartilage' bones, and may even have preceded them. It is misleading to regard cartilage as the primeval substance in this respect. Bone may arise by two major routes: by direct ossification in mesenchyme or indirectly in cartilage, itself derived from mesenchyme. The roof and sides of the neurocranium are developed in mesenchymal sheets, or membranes, in or subjacent to dermis; hence the terms 'membrane' or 'dermal' bone, the latter perhaps being more informative. Dermal parts of the cranium box are currently

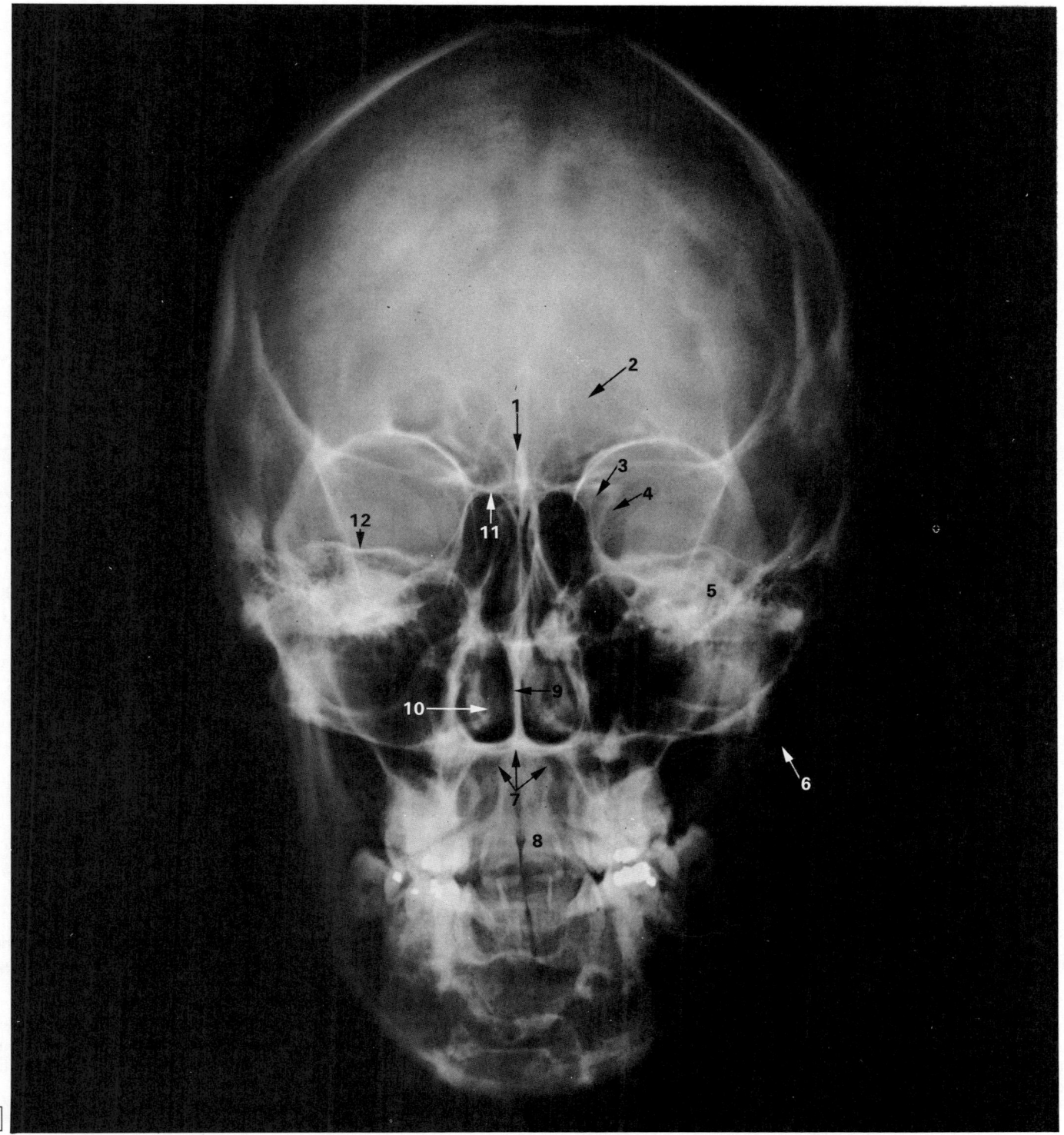

B

1. Crista galli. 2. Frontal sinus. 3. Optic canal. 4. Superior orbital fissure. 5. Dense shadow of petrous part of temporal bone. 6. Apex of mastoid process. 7. Dens of axis. 8. Upper central incisor tooth. 9. Nasal septum. 10. Inferior concha. 11. Cribriform plate. 12. Superior border of petrous part of temporal bone.

considered at least as primitive in origin as its chondrocranial base. In jaws, events appear more certain: primary cartilaginous elements, derived from the branchial apparatus, have been replaced by dermal bone.

The 'capsules', enclosing special sensory organs and integrated into the skull, are obviously protective but also confer less obvious but more basic advantages. Primitive nostrils in lower vertebrates are gustatory and olfactory; even when they lead to nasal cavities after development of a secondary palate in land vertebrates, olfactory function persists with new respiratory arrangements and both functions require open airways, whatever sphincteric mechanisms are

added. Circumocular skeletal elements have long provided sockets, more or less complete, containing not only eyeballs but also their muscles. The latter, in attachments to this optic 'capsule', have varied only in minor details since their appearance in earliest vertebrates— judging from extant forms. Their effects are largely rotatory, and it is difficult to envisage how such actions could be effective without a socket, which not only aids ocular location during rotation but also ensures stability of interocular distance, a necessary prelude to binocular vision.

The siting of labyrinths deep in cartilage or bone entails a fixed relationship between the three semicircular canals; fusion of otic

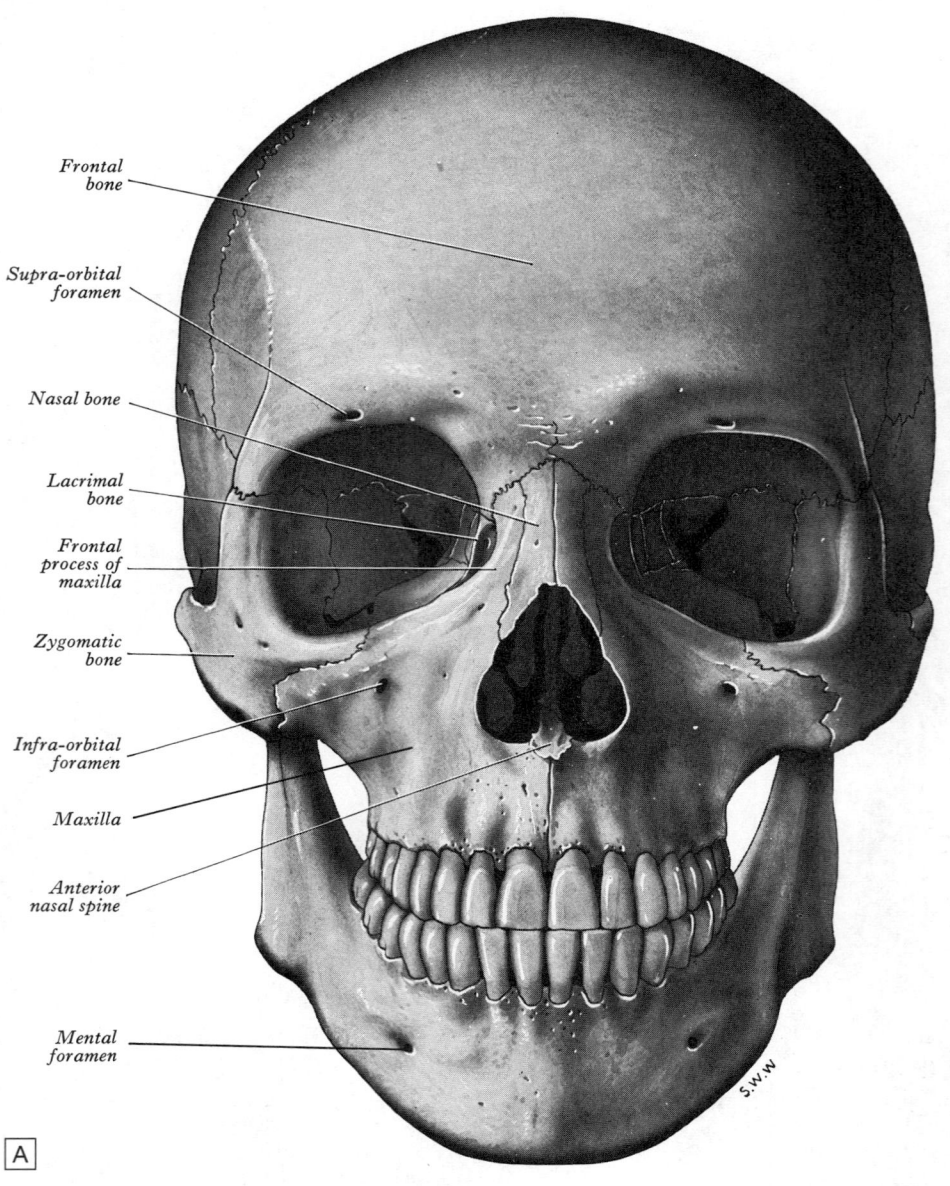

Frontal
bone

Supra-orbital
foramen

Nasal bone

Lacrimal
bone

Frontal
process of
maxilla

Zygomatic
bone

Infra-orbital
foramen

Maxilla

Anterior
nasal spine

Mental
foramen

A

6.135A, B The skull: anterior aspect (norma frontalis). Key: blue = frontal; yellow = sphenoid; green = maxillae; brown = lacrimal, nasal, temporal and vomer; magenta = mandible; uncoloured = parietal, zygomatic and ethmoid bones. Compare with **6.136**.

capsules into the cranial base determines the strict relation of all six canals both to each other and to the head itself, and without this no orderly correlation could evolve between these receptors and central nervous connections.

Axial muscles extending from the vertebral column to caudal aspects of the cranium have become more elaborate and massive in land animals with the development of necks and increasing problems of cranial suspension in quadrupeds. In all but jawless fishes (*Agnatha*, such as lampreys, a numerically insignificant class) the primitive skull is invaded by the ligamentous and muscular apparatus of the jaws, the maxillae being integrated into the skull at an early stage. These large muscles, both axial and mandibular, transmit strains to the skull which are sometimes very great and associated with extensive cranial modifications to resist and absorb stress. Even in humans, with modest masticatory and neck musculatures, the whole body can be suspended from the bite of the teeth. In other mammals, especially quadrupeds, greater relative size of the jaws and weight of the head led to the development of large plates, bars and buttresses, which owe little in origin to the protection which they fortuitously offer. A perfect example is the high cranial dome of elephants, which is associated with providing a large attachment for the massive extensor muscles necessary for suspension of so heavy a head. Perhaps enough has now been said to emphasize

the diversity of cranial function beyond its obvious protectiveness; exclusive emphasis upon protection, characteristic of anatomical texts, is purblind and belittles the skull's multifunctional adaptations.

GENERAL CRANIAL FEATURES

The term *cranium* is sometimes reserved for the skull without its mandible but this strict usage is not adhered to here. Its upper part is a box enclosing the brain, often termed the *calvaria*, the remainder being the *facial skeleton*; its upper part is immovably fixed to the calvaria, the lower being the mobile mandible. The skull is clearly of greater practical interest, viewed as a whole, than its constituent bones. Nevertheless, the general positioning of these must first be considered (**6.**133–135). The skull may be viewed from above (*norma verticalis*), below (*norma basalis*), behind (*norma occipitalis*), the front (*norma frontalis*) and the side (*norma lateralis*). The calvarial roof or *calva* (skull cap) must be removed to examine its interior. In the erect attitude the lower margins of the orbital openings and upper margins of the external acoustic meatuses are near the same horizontal (Frankfurt) plane, an important convention of orientation in description.

The forehead is formed by the *frontal bone* (**6.**133, 135), passing back in the vault of the skull to the *coronal suture* to meet the

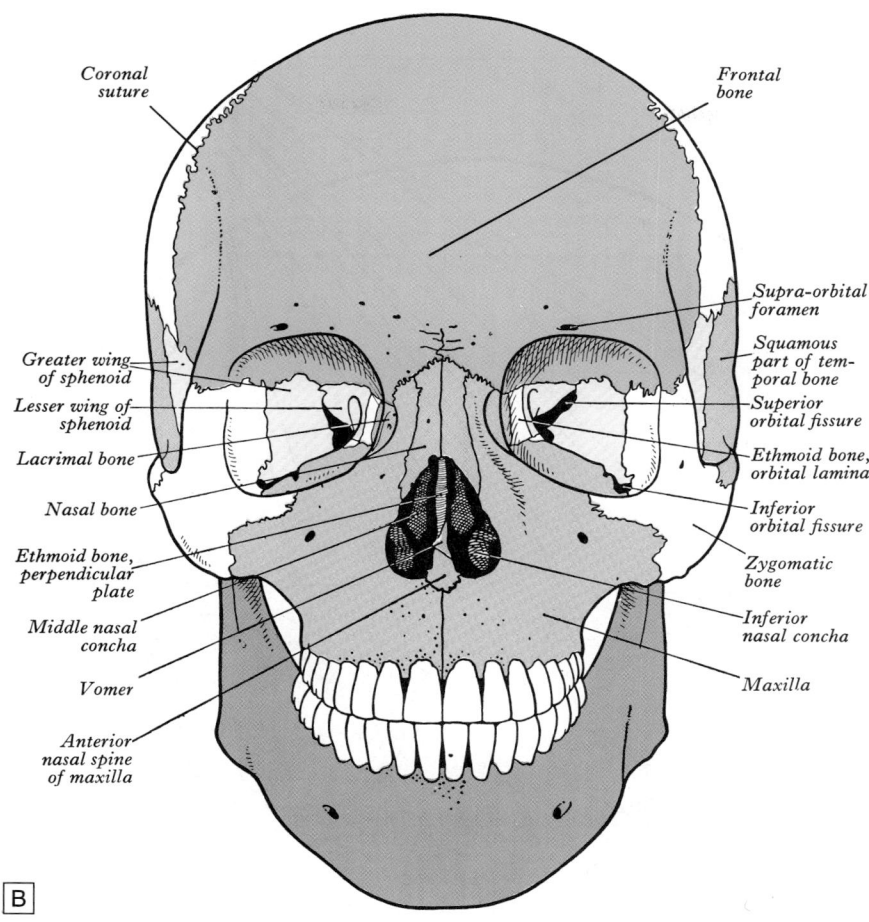

Coronal suture

Frontal bone

Greater wing of sphenoid

Lesser wing of sphenoid

Lacrimal bone

Nasal bone

Ethmoid bone, perpendicular plate

Middle nasal concha

Vomer

Anterior nasal spine of maxilla

Supra-orbital foramen

Squamous part of temporal bone

Superior orbital fissure

Ethmoid bone, orbital lamina

Inferior orbital fissure

Zygomatic bone

Inferior nasal concha

Maxilla

B

anterior borders of the *parietal bones*, right and left, which form most of the cranial vault, articulating together at the median, serrated, *sagittal suture*. Posteriorly they meet the *occipital bone*, which forms the back of the skull (occiput). The suture between parietal and occipital bones is called the *lambdoid suture*, after the Greek capital letter lambda, Λ, which it resembles in shape. Each parietal bone curves down as the side of the vault to the upper limit of the *greater wing* of the *sphenoid bone* in front, and the *squamous part* of the *temporal bone* behind. When the calva is removed, saw cut passes through the frontal and usually across the lower part of the parietal bones, but may also involve the temporal squamae; posteriorly the section cuts the occipital bone. The calva thus consists of a large part of the frontal bone, most of the two parietals, possibly small parts of temporal squamae and part of the occipital. When it is removed, the *calvarial floor* or *base of the skull* is revealed. It shows natural subdivision into three regions: anterior, middle and posterior *cranial fossae*. These are considered in detail on pages 568, 570, 572; here, as a preliminary, is a brief synopsis of their principal osseous boundaries.

The anterior cranial fossa (see **6**.151). A little less than the base's anterior third, it is limited behind by a sharp edge on each side. Note that it roofs the orbits and between them the nasal cavity. On each side an *orbital part* projects back from the *frontal bone* forming most of the orbital roof, these two plates being separated by a narrow interval occupied by a perforated strip, the *cribriform plate* of the *ethmoid bone*, forming much of the nasal roof; the rest of the ethmoid is in the lateral walls and septum of the nasal cavity. The cribriform plate bears a median *crista galli* on its upper surface. Posteriorly the floor of the anterior fossa is formed by parts of the *sphenoid bone*, the front of whose *body* meets the cribriform plate; on each side a narrow *lesser wing* projects laterally from it to the posterior margin of the orbital plate of the frontal bone, forming a sharp posterior border, the posterior limit of the floor of the anterior cranial fossa. These borders are adapted to the lateral cerebral fissures (p. 1108).

The middle cranial fossa (see **6**.151). Immediately behind the

anterior it is of small median extent but expanded posterolaterally on both sides. The narrow median region is formed by the sphenoid body and its cranial aspect presents a hollow for the hypophysis cerebri (pituitary gland). The lateral parts are formed by the *greater wings* of the *sphenoid* in front and the *petrous temporal bones* behind. Each greater wing curves from the side of the body in the base, then the side of the skull to the parietal's anteroinferior angle. Posterior to this the anterior surface of the petrous temporal bone continues laterally into the squama.

The posterior cranial fossa (see **6**.151). Almost circular and occupying about two-fifths of the cranial base, it is largely *occipital bone*. Through its large *foramen magnum* the brainstem and spinal cord are continuous. The anterior region is the *basilar part* of the *occipital bone*, fused in front with the body of the sphenoid. On each side the fossa is formed by the posterior surface of the petrous temporal bone above and *lateral (condylar) part* of the *occipital bone* below. The temporal's mastoid part, posterolateral to the petrous, joins the occipital squama to complete the fossa.

Further details

In frontal view (*norma frontalis*; **6**.135, 136) the *orbits* and *anterior nasal aperture* are apparent. Inferiorly is the *mandibular body*; above this are the *maxillae*, or upper jaws, separated by the teeth. The maxillae form much of the buccal roof and the inferolateral margin of the anterior nasal aperture; each forms the inferomedial orbital margin (completed laterally by the zygomatic bone) and a *frontal process* ascends to the frontal bone in the medial orbital margin. Between the bilateral maxillary frontal processes are two *nasal bones*, the upper boundary of the nasal aperture.

In lateral view (*norma lateralis*; **6**.133, 134) the *mandibular ramus* ascends from the posterior end of its body to the cranial base. The *mandibular head*, surmounting the posterior border of the ramus, fits the *articular fossa* on the inferior aspect of the temporal squama. It is separated from the *external acoustic meatus* by the temporal *tympanic plate*. Anterosuperior to the meatus the temporal *zygomatic process* reaches to the zygomatic bone, forming the *zygomatic arch*, 551

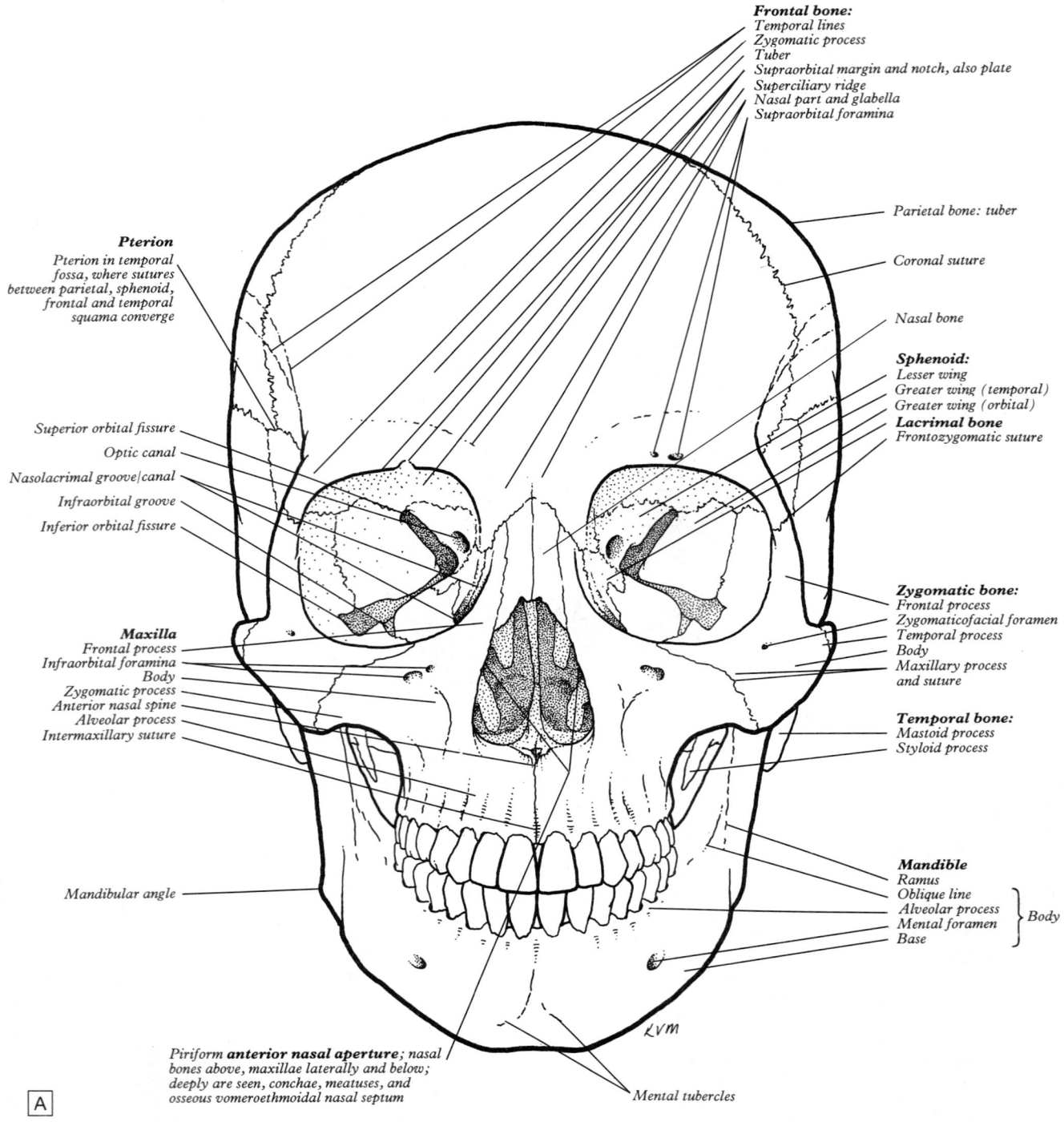

Frontal bone:
Temporal lines
Zygomatic process
Tuber
Supraorbital margin and notch, also plate
Superciliary ridge
Nasal part and glabella
Supraorbital foramina

Parietal bone: tuber

Coronal suture

Nasal bone

Sphenoid:
Lesser wing
Greater wing (temporal)
Greater wing (orbital)
Lacrimal bone
Frontozygomatic suture

Pterion
Pterion in temporal fossa, where sutures between parietal, sphenoid, frontal and temporal squama converge

Superior orbital fissure
Optic canal
Nasolacrimal groove/canal
Infraorbital groove
Inferior orbital fissure

Zygomatic bone:
Frontal process
Zygomaticofacial foramen
Temporal process
Body
Maxillary process and suture

Maxilla
Frontal process
Infraorbital foramina
Body
Zygomatic process
Anterior nasal spine
Alveolar process
Intermaxillary suture

Temporal bone:
Mastoid process
Styloid process

Mandible
Ramus
Oblique line
Alveolar process ⎫
Mental foramen ⎬ *Body*
Base ⎭

Mandibular angle

Piriform **anterior nasal aperture***; nasal bones above, maxillae laterally and below; deeply are seen, conchae, meatuses, and osseous vomeroethmoidal nasal septum*

Mental tubercles

ℓvm

A

6.136A.   The skull: anterior aspect (norma frontalis).

or *zygoma*, separated from the side of the skull. The *zygomatic bone* forms the prominence of the cheek and inferolateral orbital margin, ascending in the lateral orbital margin to the frontal bone.

With mandible removed (see **6.**145) it is easier to see behind the maxilla, the *pterygoid process* projecting down from the sphenoid at the root of its greater wing as a large *lateral pterygoid plate* reaching alveolar level, and a smaller *medial plate* ending as a hamulus. The plates are walls of the *pterygoid fossa*.

The inferior cranial aspect (*norma basalis*; see **6.**145, 146), the exterior of its base, shows posteriorly the *occipital bone* and foramen magnum, lateral to which the occipital bone articulates with the *mastoid parts* of the temporal bones and anterolaterally with their *petrous parts*, extending forwards almost to the roots of the pterygoid processes. Anteriorly the *osseous palate*, part of the buccal roof, lies within the maxillary alveolar arch; both maxillae and palatine bones

contribute to it, its anterior three-fourths formed by maxillary *palatine processes*, meeting in the midline, the posterior fourth by palatine *horizontal plates*. The *perpendicular palatine* plates ascend from the horizontal plates as parts of the lateral nasal walls.

The *lacrimal bones*, anterior in the medial orbital walls, the *vomer*, a large part of the nasal septum, and the *inferior conchae*, in the lateral nasal walls, can be seen effectively when the orbits and nose are examined (pp. 555, 574).

EXTERIOR OF THE SKULL

NORMA VERTICALIS

Seen from above (**6.**137), cranial contour varies greatly but is usually

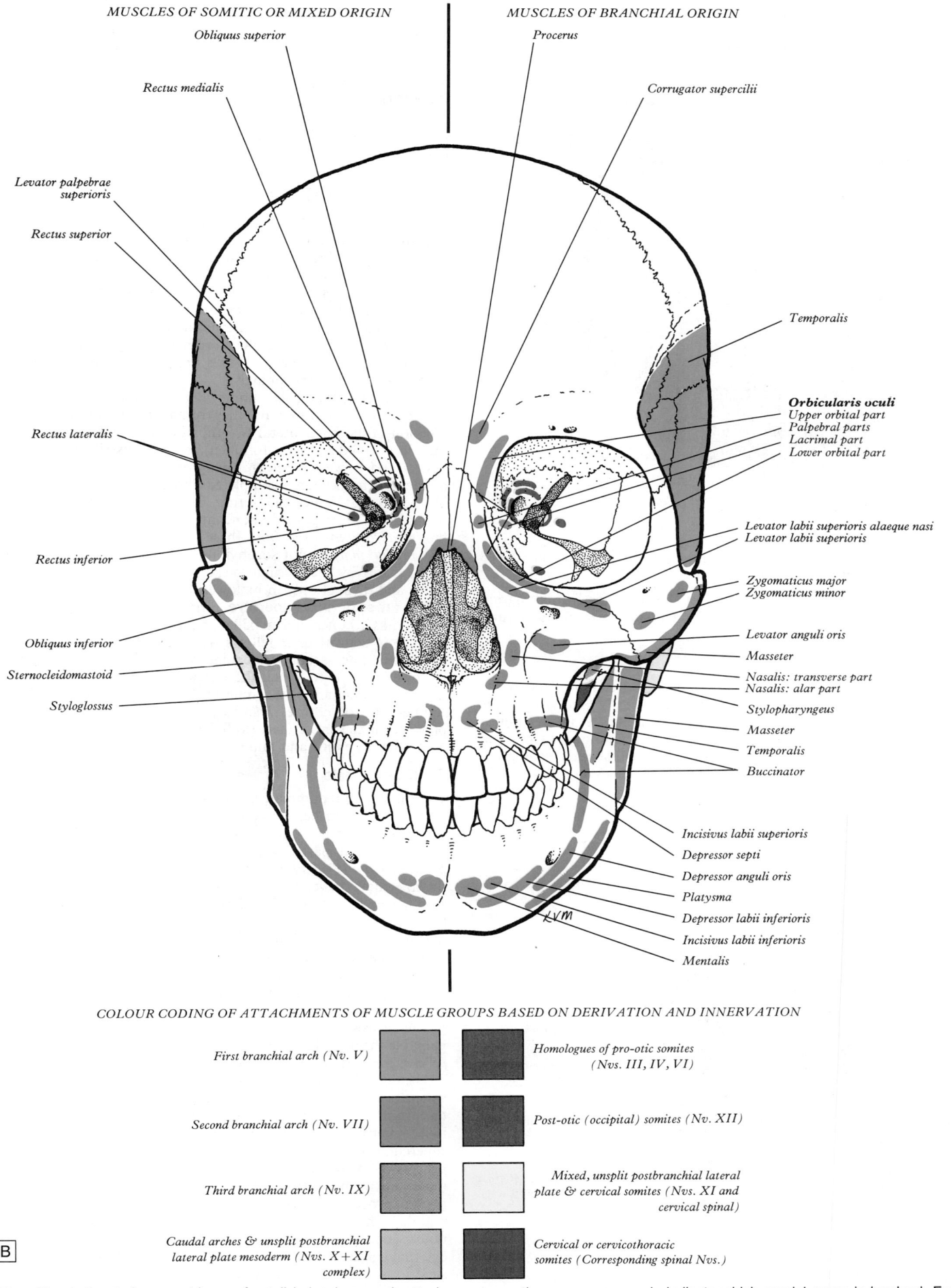

MUSCLES OF SOMITIC OR MIXED ORIGIN

MUSCLES OF BRANCHIAL ORIGIN

Obliquus superior

Rectus medialis

Levator palpebrae superioris

Rectus superior

Rectus lateralis

Rectus inferior

Obliquus inferior

Sternocleidomastoid

Styloglossus

Procerus

Corrugator supercilii

Temporalis

Orbicularis oculi
Upper orbital part
Palpebral parts
Lacrimal part
Lower orbital part

Levator labii superioris alaeque nasi
Levator labii superioris

Zygomaticus major
Zygomaticus minor

Levator anguli oris

Masseter

Nasalis: transverse part
Nasalis: alar part

Stylopharyngeus

Masseter

Temporalis

Buccinator

Incisivus labii superioris

Depressor septi

Depressor anguli oris

Platysma

Depressor labii inferioris

Incisivus labii inferioris

Mentalis

COLOUR CODING OF ATTACHMENTS OF MUSCLE GROUPS BASED ON DERIVATION AND INNERVATION

First branchial arch (Nv. V)

Homologues of pro-otic somites (Nvs. III, IV, VI)

Second branchial arch (Nv. VII)

Post-otic (occipital) somites (Nv. XII)

Third branchial arch (Nv. IX)

Mixed, unsplit postbranchial lateral plate & cervical somites (Nvs. XI and cervical spinal)

Caudal arches & unsplit postbranchial lateral plate mesoderm (Nvs. X + XI complex)

Cervical or cervicothoracic somites (Corresponding spinal Nvs.)

B

6.136B. The skull: anterior aspect (norma frontalis) showing muscle attachments, colour coded to indicate embryological origin and innervation. Refer to caption; roman numerals indicate which cranial nerve is involved. For spinal nerve sources consult individual muscles and peripheral nerves.

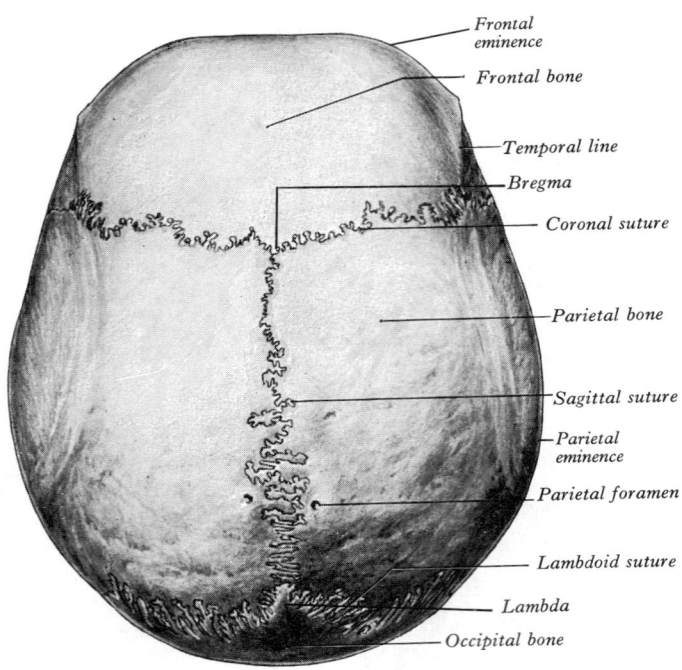

6.137   The skull: superior aspect (norma verticalis).

ellipsoid (strictly, a modified ovoid), its greatest width nearer to its occipital pole; it displays three sutures:

- the *coronal suture* is the junction of the posterior frontal margin with anterior borders of the parietal bones, descending around and forwards across the cranial vault.
- The *sagittal suture* is median between the interlocking medial parietal borders.
- The *lambdoid suture* joins the posterior parietal borders to the superior occipital margin, descending laterally and across the cranial vault. The coronal and sagittal sutures meet at the *bregma* and in the fetal skull (together with the temporary interfrontal suture) they form the boundaries of a diamond-shaped membrane-filled *anterior fontanelle* (p. 607). The latter persists until about 18 months after birth. The *lambda* is at the junction of the sagittal and lambdoid sutures, the site of a similar *posterior fontanelle* (p. 607) which closes more rapidly.

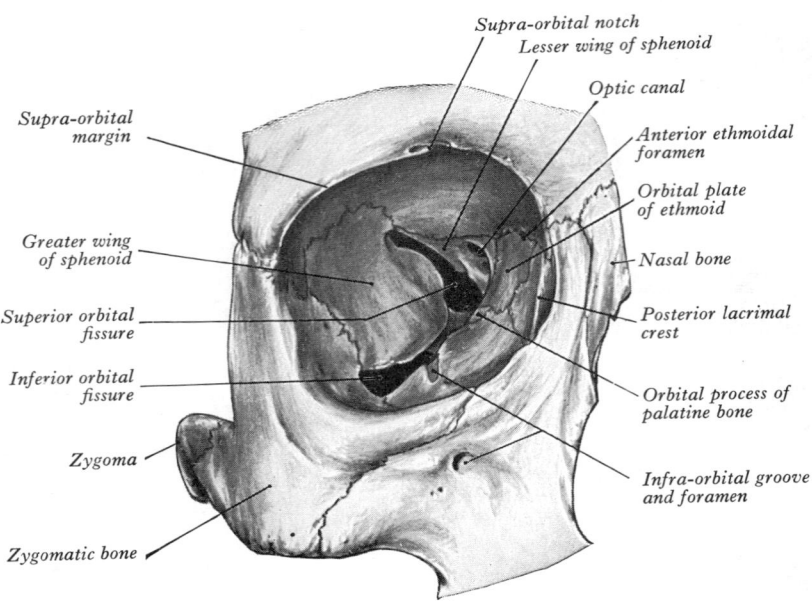

Maximal parietal convexity is the palpable *parietal tuber* (*eminence*), on each side, where the norma verticalis passes into the norma lateralis and occipitalis without distinct demarcation. A *parietal foramen*, often absent, pierces each parietal bone near the sagittal suture about 3.5 cm anterior to the lambda. It transmits a small emissary vein from the superior sagittal sinus. An incidence of about 40–60% (in different races) is ascribed to this foramen (p. 609). Anteriorly the norma verticalis slopes into the norma frontalis.

NORMA FRONTALIS

From the front (6.135–137) the skull appears roughly oval, wider and smooth above in its frontal region, but below this is irregular and interrupted by the orbits and anterior nasal aperture. Supero-medial to each orbit is a rounded *superciliary arch*, better marked in males, between is a median elevation, the *glabella*, below which, where the nasal bones meet the frontal, is a depression at the root of the nose. The junction of internasal and frontonasal sutures is the *nasion*. Above each superciliary arch is a slightly elevated *frontal tuber* or *tuberosity*. These features are palpable and useful to both the surgeon and anthropologist.

Orbital opening. This is somewhat quadrangular, its *supraorbital margin* formed entirely by the frontal bone, interrupted at the junction of its sharp lateral two-thirds and rounded medial third by the supraorbital notch (or foramen), which transmits the supraorbital vessels and nerve. The *lateral margin* is largely the frontal process of the zygomatic bone, completed above by the zygomatic process of the frontal bone: the suture between them being a palpable depression. The zygomatic bone laterally and maxilla medially form the *infraorbital margin*. Both these margins are sharp and palpable. The *medial margin*, not so obvious, is formed above by the frontal bone, below by the lacrimal crest of the maxillary frontal process, sharp and distinct only in its lower half.

The anterior nasal aperture. Piriform, wider below, and bounded by the nasal bones and maxillae, which articulate with each other, with their contralateral fellows and with the frontal bone above. Each nasal bone articulates behind with a maxillary frontal process; its lower border, to which the lateral nasal cartilage is attached, is the upper boundary of the anterior nasal aperture (6.135). The nasal cavities are, of course, *bilateral*; a **single** anterior nasal aperture presents in the macerated skull because various cartilages (septal, lateral nasal, major and minor alar) are lost during preparation.

Further details

The maxillae predominate in the facial skeleton, and their growth elongates the face between 6 and 12 years. Only the anterior surface is visible in norma frontalis, with a medial well-marked *nasal notch* (the lower and partly lateral border of the nasal aperture). The prominent *anterior nasal spine* marks the intermaxillary junction in the aperture's lower boundary. It is palpable in the nasal septum. About 1 cm below the infraorbital margin is the *infraorbital foramen*, for infraorbital vessels and nerve; it is on or near a vertical passing through the supraorbital notch. The maxillary *alveolar process* contains sockets for the upper teeth, best seen in basal view (p. 600). The short, thick *zygomatic process* from the superolateral region of the anterior surface has an oblique upper surface forming, with the zygomatic bone, a zygomaticomaxillary suture. The inferior border of the process meets the body above the first molar tooth and is palpable through the cheek or buccal vestibule. The maxillary *frontal process* ascends posterolateral to the nasal bone to reach the frontal.

The *glabella* may show the remains of the interfrontal suture, which ascends in about 9% of skulls to the coronal suture, indicating the frontal bone's formation by fusion of two halves, ossifying independently. To the medial part of the *superciliary arch* corrugator supercilii is attached; to the nasal part of the frontal bone and frontal process of the maxilla, the orbital part of orbicularis oculi. Between these the medial palpebral ligament is attached to the maxillary frontal process (6.136B), and procerus to the nasal bone near the midline. The lower margin of the nasal bone usually bears a small notch, converted by the lateral nasal cartilage into a foramen for the external nasal nerve. In front of orbicularis oculi the levator labii superioris alaeque nasi is attached to the maxillary frontal process and, more laterally, levator labii superioris to the maxilla between the infraorbital margin and foramen.

A *canine eminence*, due to the tooth's large root, appears between the lateral *canine* and medial *incisive fossae*. Levator anguli oris is attached in the canine fossa whilst, to the surface bordering the nasal notch, nasalis and depressor septi and below them the incisive muscle gain attachment.

In the zygomatic bone, near the junction of inferior and lateral orbital margins, is a small *zygomaticofacial foramen* (see **6.141B**, **196B**), sometimes duplicated, for the so-named nerve and artery; below the foramen are attached zygomaticus minor and, more laterally, zygomaticus major. The foramen was absent in 12–30% of different populations in a series of 580 crania (p. 609).

ORBITAL CAVITY

The orbits (**6.138, 139**) contain the eyes, associated muscles, vessels and nerves, lacrimal apparatus, fascial strata and soft fat. Each is pyramidal, with a base at the orbital opening and a long, postero-medially directed axis. It has a roof, floor, medial and lateral walls, a base and apex.

The superior wall or roof. This is a thin, frontal plate, gently concave on its orbital aspect, which lies largely between the orbital contents and brain in the anterior cranial fossa. Anteromedially it is bilaminated by the frontal sinus; here it presents the *trochlear fovea* or *spine* where the annular pulley for superior oblique is attached (pp. 595, 1355). Anterolaterally is a deep *lacrimal fossa* for the lacrimal gland's orbital part. Posteriorly, at the junction of its roof and medial wall, the *optic canal* or *foramen* connects the orbit to the middle cranial fossa and transmits the optic nerve and ophthalmic artery. Near the superior, medial and lower margins of the orbital opening of the canal the *common tendinous ring* of the four recti is attached to bone (p. 455).

The medial wall (6.140). This is extremely thin except posteriorly and curves inferolaterally into the floor. Anterior is the vertical *lacrimal groove* for the lacrimal sac, opening below into the nasal cavity via the laterally inclining *nasolacrimal canal*, little more than 1 cm long. The floor of the groove separates the orbital and nasal cavities, but more posteriorly the ethmoidal sinuses intervene. The medial wall is related most posteriorly to the anterior region of the sphenoidal sinus, forming its lateral wall.

The inferior wall or floor (6.139). This is thin and largely roofs the maxillary sinus (**6.140**). Not quite horizontal, it ascends a little laterally. Anteriorly it curves into the lateral wall; posteriorly it is separated by the *inferior orbital fissure*, connecting the orbit posteriorly to the pterygopalatine fossa, and more anteriorly to the infratemporal fossa. The maxillary nerve traverses the fissure, whose medial lip is notched by the *infraorbital groove*, passing forwards and sinking into the floor to become the *infraorbital canal*, opening at the *infraorbital foramen*. Groove, canal and foramen contain the infraorbital nerve. The inferior orbital fissure transmits a connection between the inferior ophthalmic vein and pterygoid plexus in the infratemporal fossa. The infraorbital foramen is sometimes double, even multiple (Harris 1933), *accessory* foramina being usually smaller and recorded at incidences of 2–18% in various populations (p. 609).

The lateral wall (6.140). The thickest wall, especially posteriorly where it separates the orbit from the middle cranial fossa; anteriorly it separates the orbit and temporal fossa. The lateral wall and roof are continuous anteriorly but separated posteriorly by the *superior orbital fissure*, tapering laterally but widened at its medial end (**6.138**), its long axis descending posteromedially. It communicates with the middle cranial fossa and transmits the oculomotor, trochlear and abducent nerves, branches of the ophthalmic nerve and the oph-thalmic veins. Where the fissure begins to widen, its inferolateral edges shows a projection, often a spine, for the lateral attachment of the annular tendon (**8.455**). Royle (1973) has described an '*infra-orbital*' sulcus, in 22 of 64 orbits, from the superolateral end of the superior orbital fissure towards the orbital floor, associated some-

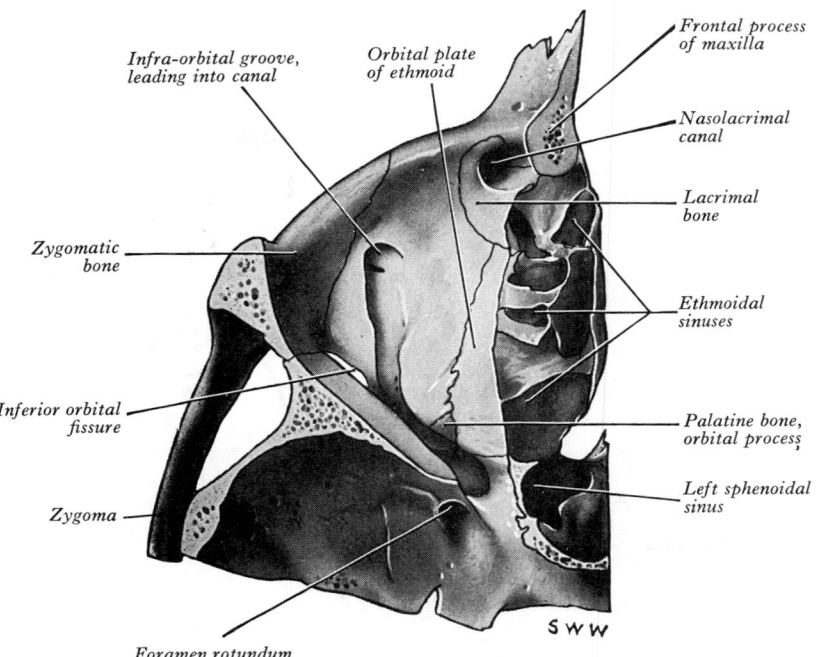

6.139 Horizontal section through the left orbit and nasal cavity viewed from above.

Infra-orbital groove, leading into canal
Orbital plate of ethmoid
Frontal process of maxilla
Nasolacrimal canal
Lacrimal bone
Zygomatic bone
Ethmoidal sinuses
Inferior orbital fissure
Palatine bone, orbital process
Zygoma
Left sphenoidal sinus
Foramen rotundum

Anterior ethmoidal foramen
Orbital plate of ethmoid
Posterior ethmoidal foramen
Left frontal sinus
Supra-orbital foramen
Lacrimo-maxillary suture
Nasal bone
Lesser wing of sphenoid
Orbital process of palatine bone
Uncinate pro-cess of ethmoid
Inferior concha, maxillary process
Pterygomaxillary fissure
Anterior nasal spine
Perpendicular plate of pala-tine bone
Lateral pterygoid lamina
Maxillary sinus
Pyramidal process of palatine bone
Alveolar process of maxilla
Pterygoid hamulus
Maxillary tuberosity

A

Lesser wing of sphenoid
Frontal sinus
Orbital plate of frontal bone
Superior orbital fissure, lateral part
Orbital surface of zygomatic bone
Foramen for zygomatico-facial nerve
Orbital surface of greater wing of sphenoid
Inferior orbital fissure, lateral end
Orbital surface of maxilla
Maxillary sinus
Wire in infra-orbital groove, canal, and foramen.

B

6.140A. Oblique parasagittal section through the anterior part of the skull, showing the medial wall of the left orbit and the medial wall of the left maxillary sinus. B. The lateral wall of the left orbit, viewed from the medial side. Compare with **6.137A**, which represents the opposite part of the same section of the skull.

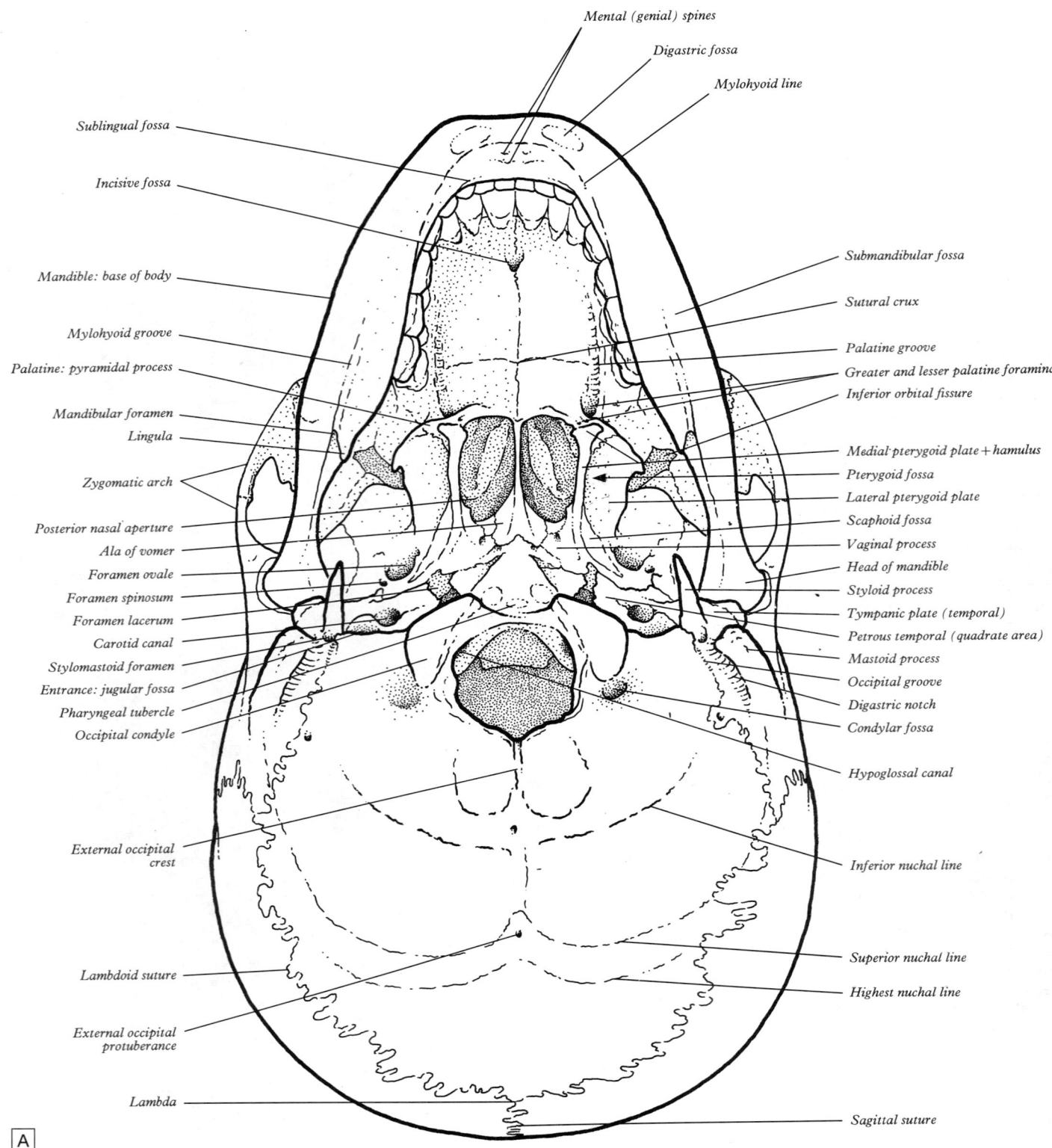

Mental (genial) spines
Digastric fossa
Mylohyoid line
Sublingual fossa
Incisive fossa
Mandible: base of body
Mylohyoid groove
Palatine: pyramidal process
Mandibular foramen
Lingula
Zygomatic arch
Posterior nasal aperture
Ala of vomer
Foramen ovale
Foramen spinosum
Foramen lacerum
Carotid canal
Stylomastoid foramen
Entrance: jugular fossa
Pharyngeal tubercle
Occipital condyle
External occipital crest
Lambdoid suture
External occipital protuberance
Lambda

Submandibular fossa
Sutural crux
Palatine groove
Greater and lesser palatine foramina
Inferior orbital fissure
Medial pterygoid plate + hamulus
Pterygoid fossa
Lateral pterygoid plate
Scaphoid fossa
Vaginal process
Head of mandible
Styloid process
Tympanic plate (temporal)
Petrous temporal (quadrate area)
Mastoid process
Occipital groove
Digastric notch
Condylar fossa
Hypoglossal canal
Inferior nuchal line
Superior nuchal line
Highest nuchal line
Sagittal suture

A

6.141A.   The skull: norma occipitalis and norma basalis with the mandible in situ.

times with an anastomosis between the middle meningeal and infra-orbital arteries; this feature has been confirmed in 45% of 100 orbits by Santo Neto et al (1984).

Further details

The boundaries of the *orbital opening* have already been described (p. 554). The *apex* of the orbit is near the medial end of the superior orbital fissure.

The *roof*, almost entirely frontal orbital plate, includes posteriorly a part of the inferior aspect of the lesser sphenoidal wing. The suture between these being almost horizontal. The *optic canal* is between the roots of the lesser wing, bounded medially by the sphenoid body. As noted, near the junction of the roof and medial wall, close to the orbital opening, a *trochlear fovea* or *spine* marks attachment of the fibrous loop for the superior oblique's tendon.

To the *medial wall* (**6**.140), limited in front by the *anterior lacrimal*

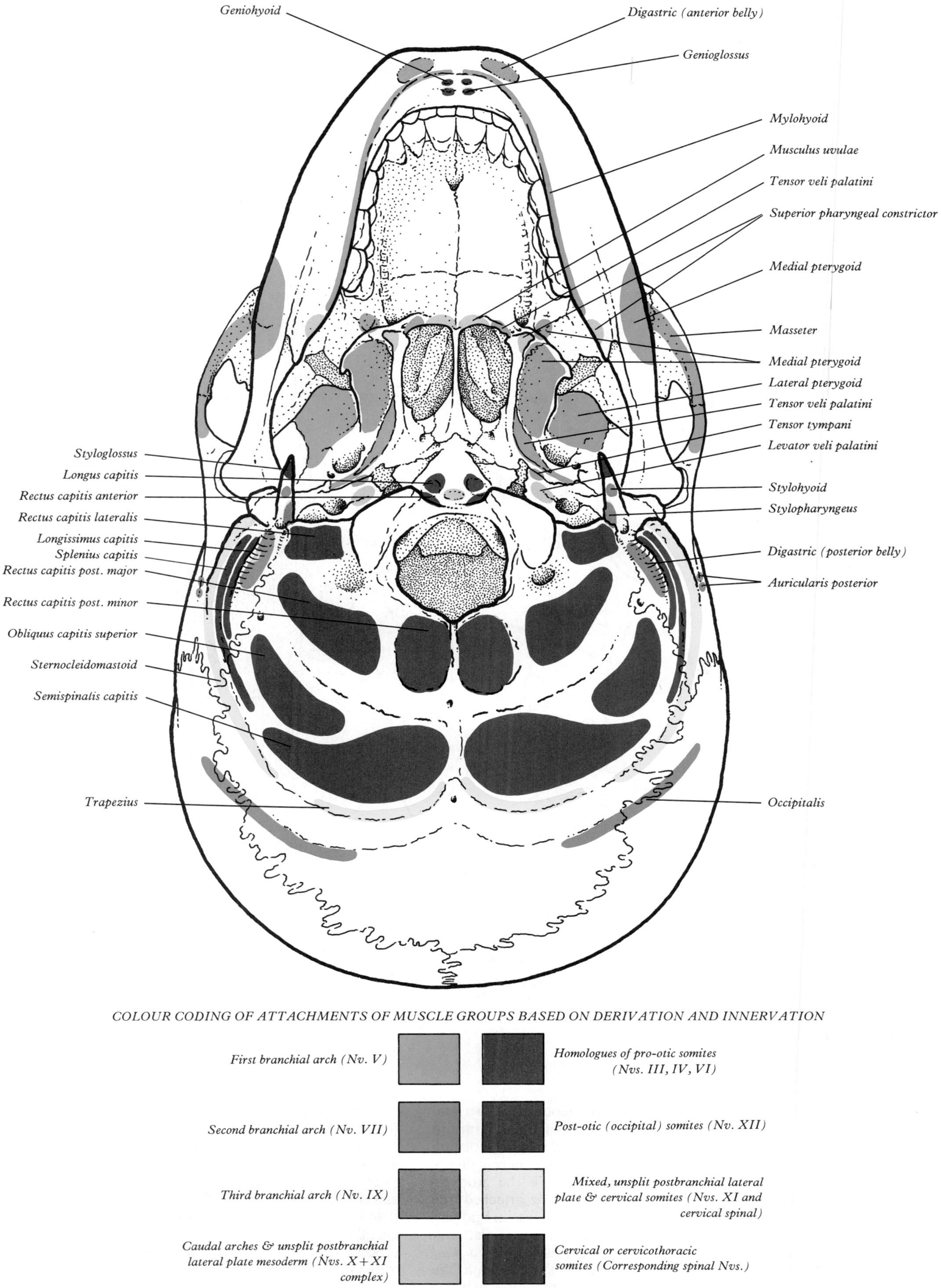

Geniohyoid

Digastric (anterior belly)

Genioglossus

Mylohyoid

Musculus uvulae

Tensor veli palatini

Superior pharyngeal constrictor

Medial pterygoid

Masseter

Medial pterygoid

Lateral pterygoid

Tensor veli palatini

Tensor tympani

Levator veli palatini

Styloglossus

Longus capitis

Rectus capitis anterior

Rectus capitis lateralis

Longissimus capitis

Splenius capitis

Rectus capitis post. major

Rectus capitis post. minor

Obliquus capitis superior

Sternocleidomastoid

Semispinalis capitis

Stylohyoid

Stylopharyngeus

Digastric (posterior belly)

Auricularis posterior

Trapezius

Occipitalis

COLOUR CODING OF ATTACHMENTS OF MUSCLE GROUPS BASED ON DERIVATION AND INNERVATION

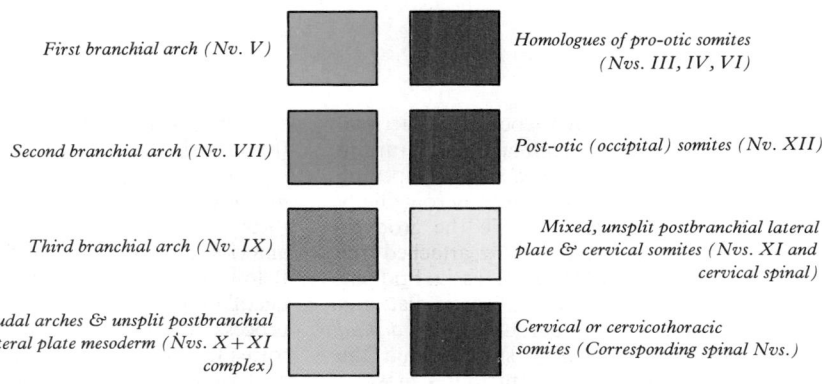

First branchial arch (Nv. V)			Homologues of pro-otic somites (Nvs. III, IV, VI)
Second branchial arch (Nv. VII)			Post-otic (occipital) somites (Nv. XII)
Third branchial arch (Nv. IX)			Mixed, unsplit postbranchial lateral plate & cervical somites (Nvs. XI and cervical spinal)
Caudal arches & unsplit postbranchial lateral plate mesoderm (Nvs. X + XI complex)			Cervical or cervicothoracic somites (Corresponding spinal Nvs.)

B

6.141B. The skull: norma occipitalis and norma basalis with the mandible in situ showing muscle attachments.

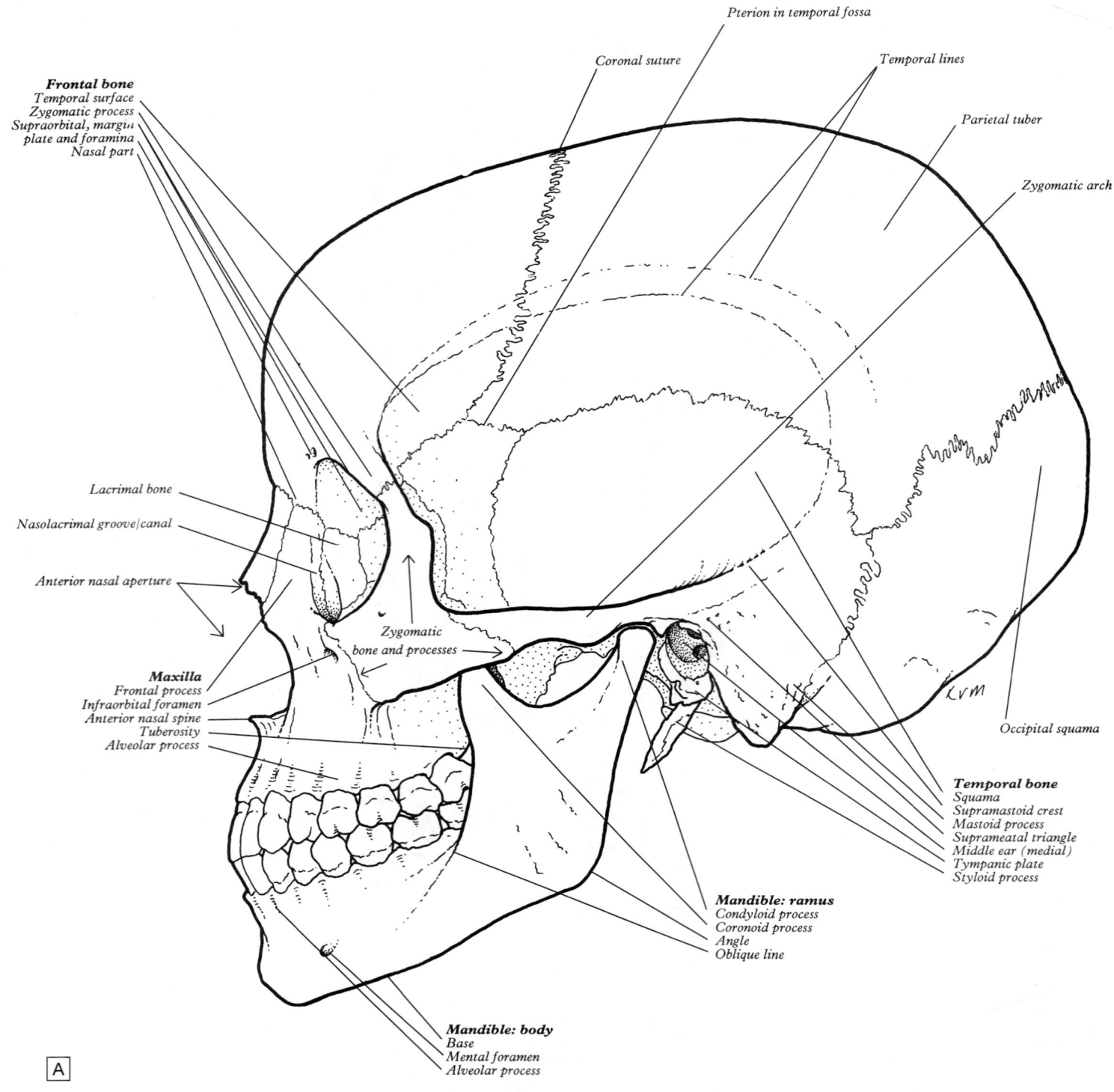

Frontal bone
Temporal surface
Zygomatic process
Supraorbital, margin
plate and foramina
Nasal part

Coronal suture

Pterion in temporal fossa

Temporal lines

Parietal tuber

Zygomatic arch

Lacrimal bone

Nasolacrimal groove/canal

Anterior nasal aperture

Zygomatic
bone and processes

Maxilla
Frontal process
Infraorbital foramen
Anterior nasal spine
Tuberosity
Alveolar process

Occipital squama

Temporal bone
Squama
Supramastoid crest
Mastoid process
Suprameatal triangle
Middle ear (medial)
Tympanic plate
Styloid process

Mandible: ramus
Condyloid process
Coronoid process
Angle
Oblique line

Mandible: body
Base
Mental foramen
Alveolar process

A

6.142A. The skull: norma lateralis.

crest on the maxilla's frontal process, orbicularis oculi and lacrimal fascia are attached. Behind this crest is a maxillolacrimal suture in the *lacrimal groove's* floor. The *nasolacrimal canal's* upper opening is completed laterally by the *lacrimal hamulus*, curving anteromedially to the lower part of the anterior lacrimal crest. To the groove's *posterior lacrimal crest* (mostly lacrimal bone) are attached the lacrimal part of orbicularis oculi (p. 791) and lacrimal fascia, bridging the groove. Posteriorly the lacrimal's orbital surface is flat and articulates by a vertical suture with the ethmoid labyrinth's *orbital plate*. The frontolacrimal and lacrimomaxillary sutures limit the medial wall in front; the ethmoid *orbital plate* contributes most to it. Almost rectangular, it is very thin, forming the lateral walls to

ethmoidal sinuses. Above, it articulates with the medial edge of the frontal orbital plate at a suture interrupted by *anterior* and *posterior ethmoidal foramina*, and occasionally (28% of skulls examined) a *middle* ethmoidal foramen (Downie et al 1995). These canals transmit their vessels and nerves (the posterior is often absent) into the anterior cranial fossa at the lateral edge of the cribriform plate. Below, the ethmoid plate articulates with the medial edge of the maxilla's orbital surface and posteriorly with the palatine orbital process. Posteriorly it articulates with the sphenoid's body which forms the orbit's medial wall posteriorly, separated from the orbital roof by the optic canal. Analysis of racial and sexual variation in position and incidence of ethmoidal canals in 580 crania from several

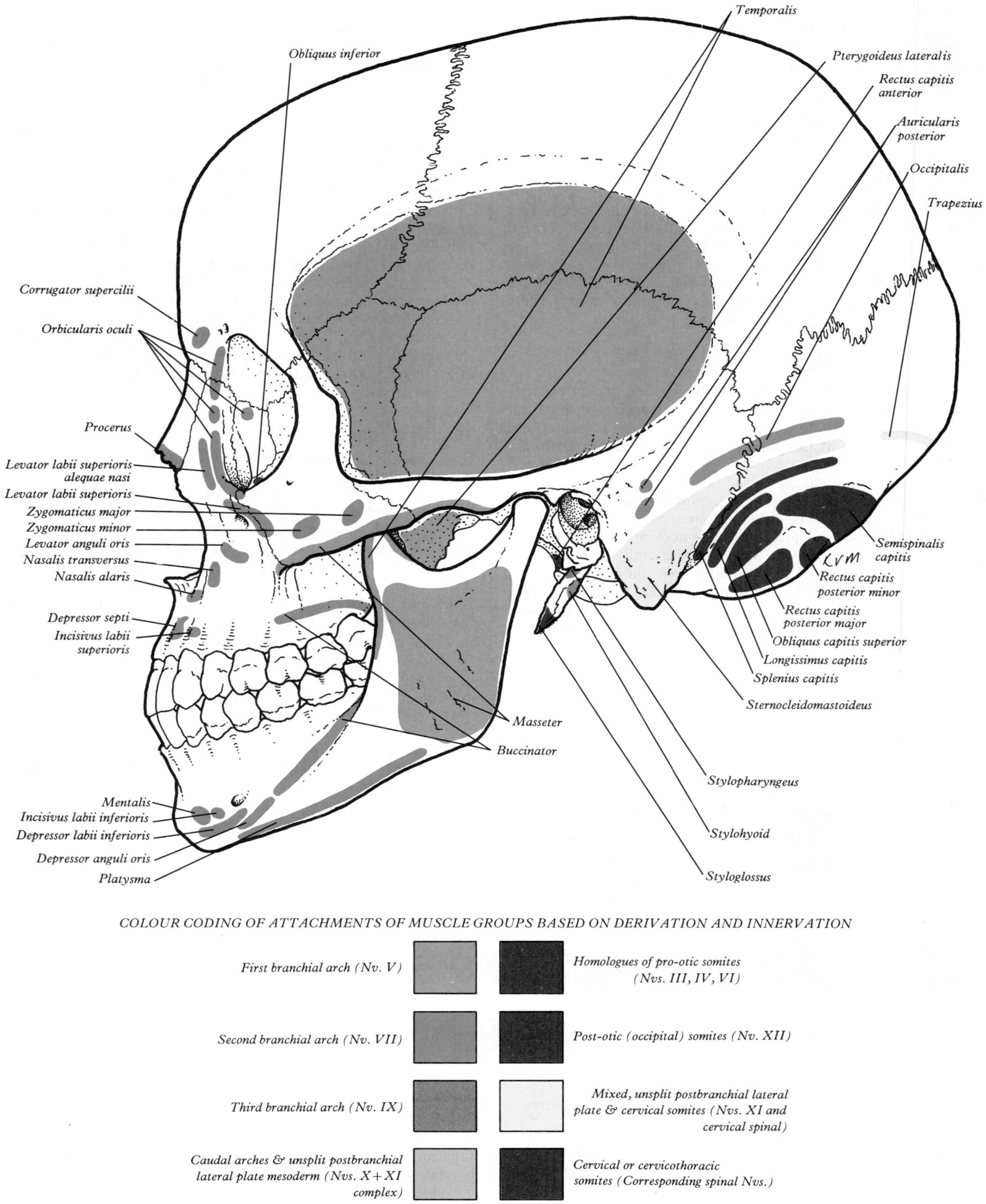

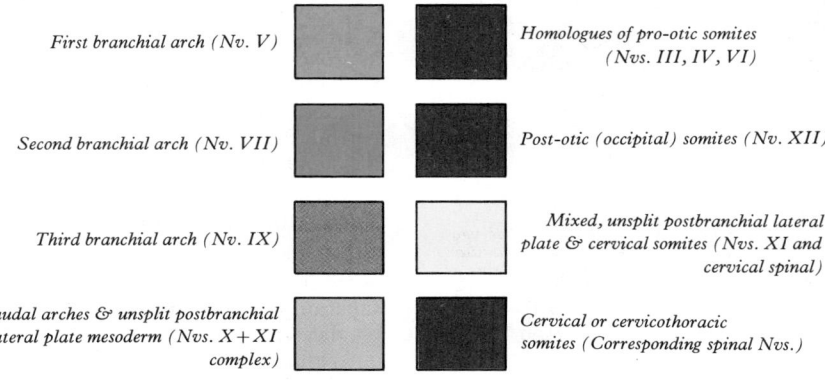

Obliquus inferior

Temporalis

Pterygoideus lateralis

Rectus capitis anterior

Auricularis posterior

Occipitalis

Trapezius

Corrugator supercilii

Orbicularis oculi

Procerus

Levator labii superioris aleguae nasi

Levator labii superioris

Zygomaticus major

Zygomaticus minor

Levator anguli oris

Nasalis transversus

Nasalis alaris

Depressor septi

Incisivus labii superioris

Semispinalis capitis

Rectus capitis posterior minor

Rectus capitis posterior major

Obliquus capitis superior

Longissimus capitis

Splenius capitis

Sternocleidomastoideus

Masseter

Buccinator

Stylopharyngeus

Mentalis

Incisivus labii inferioris

Depressor labii inferioris

Depressor anguli oris

Platysma

Stylohyoid

Styloglossus

COLOUR CODING OF ATTACHMENTS OF MUSCLE GROUPS BASED ON DERIVATION AND INNERVATION

First branchial arch (Nv. V)

Homologues of pro-otic somites (Nvs. III, IV, VI)

Second branchial arch (Nv. VII)

Post-otic (occipital) somites (Nv. XII)

Third branchial arch (Nv. IX)

Mixed, unsplit postbranchial lateral plate & cervical somites (Nvs. XI and cervical spinal)

Caudal arches & unsplit postbranchial lateral plate mesoderm (Nvs. X + XI complex)

Cervical or cervicothoracic somites (Corresponding spinal Nvs.)

B

6.142B.   The skull: norma lateralis showing muscle attachments.

populations (p. 609), showed the anterior foramen to lie outside the frontoethmoidal suture in 10–20% of several modern races and 62% out of 53 Peruvian crania.

The floor of the orbit (**6**.139), mostly formed by maxilla and zygomatic bone anterolaterally, contains posteromedially, adjoining the medial wall, a triangular area from the palatine orbital process.

559

The *inferior orbital fissure* transmits the maxillary nerve, infraorbital vessels, zygomatic nerve and rami of the pterygopalatine ganglion; it is bounded above by the greater wing of the sphenoid, below by the maxilla and the palatine orbital process and laterally by the zygomatic bone or zygomaticomaxillary suture. In 35–40% of skulls, maxilla and sphenoid meet at the fissure's anterior end, excluding the zygomatic. Anteromedially, lateral to the lacrimal hamulus, a small maxillary depression may mark the attachment of the inferior oblique muscle.

The lateral wall (**6.**140B) is formed by the orbital surfaces of the greater wing of the sphenoid and anteriorly by the zygomatic bone's frontal process, meeting at the sphenozygomatic suture. This zygomatic surface has openings of minute canals for zygomaticofacial and zygomaticotemporal nerves, the former near the junction of the floor and lateral wall, the latter at a slightly higher level, sometimes near the suture. The *superior orbital fissure* lies between the greater wing (below) and lesser wing (above) of the sphenoid, its body being medial. For contents see p. 555 and **8.**455.

NORMA OCCIPITALIS

The skull's posterior aspect is convex above and laterally flatter below. The *lambdoid suture*, entirely visible, is deeply serrated but less so inferolaterally. Inferiorly it meets the *occipitomastoid* and *parietomastoid sutures* at the postero-inferior parietal angle (**6.**133). Sutural bones are common at the *lambda* (meeting of lambdoid and sagittal sutures) and along the lambdoid suture (pp. 583, 606). The main feature is the median *external occipital protuberance* (**6.**141A) and associated ridges. The protuberance may overhang, being easily palpable at the upper end of the median posterior nuchal furrow. The *superior nuchal lines*, often sharp, pass laterally from the protuberance at the junction of the scalp and neck; the occipital region below them appears foreshortened and is seen better in norma basalis. The *highest nuchal lines*, when present, curve laterally from the protuberance, about 1 cm above the superior, and are more arched. In various ethnic groups their incidence varies from 3.6 to 40% (p. 609).

The *inion* is the summit of the external occipital protuberance, to whose lower part are attached the ligamentum nuchae and to its

upper part, fibres of trapezius. The latter fibres spread to the superior nuchal line, to which laterally (see **6.**146B, 166B) are attached posterior fibres of sternocleidomastoid and, below this, splenius capitis. To the highest nuchal line are attached the galea aponeurotica and laterally the occipital belly of occipitofrontalis.

NORMA LATERALIS

Much of the side of the skull (**6.**133, 142, 143) has already been described from other aspects, but not its central features. Above is the *temporal line*, arching up and back from the frontal's zygomatic process across the coronal suture to the parietal bone. Salient and palpable in front, it is less distinct on the parietal and usually becomes **two curved ridges**, enclosing a smooth strip. Posteriorly the superior line fades away, but the inferior again becomes more prominent as it curves down across the temporal squama above the mastoid process, where, as the *supramastoid crest*, it continues into the processes forming the zygomatic arch. The temporal line marks the periphery of the temporalis muscle and its fascia, the muscle attachment being limited by its inferior ridge, the temporal fascia by the superior ridge.

Temporal fossa

It is delineated by the zygomatic arch, temporal line, frontozygomatic processes and supramastoid crest; to its floor temporalis is attached. An irregularly H-shaped meeting of sutures in the fossa has as a horizontal limb the suture between the antero-inferior parietal angle and the apical border of the greater sphenoid wing. The frontal, sphenoid, parietal and temporal squama are here all close together (**6.**133A, 139A): a small circular area includes parts of all four and is termed the *pterion*, whose centre, an important surgical landmark, is on average 4.0 cm above the zygomatic arch and 3.5 cm behind the frontozygomatic suture (**6.**133A, 139A). It marks the anterior middle meningeal arterial ramus and the axial position of the lesser wing of the sphenoid; the latter is lodged in the stem of the lateral (Sylvian) cerebral fissure. Hence the term *Sylvian point*. The fossa's anterior wall is the temporal surface of the zygomatic bone, adjoining part of the greater wing of the sphenoid and a small area of frontal bone. These structures separate the fossa from the orbit; inferiorly the fossa merges with the infratemporal fossa between zygomatic arch and cranial wall; here the tendon and some fibres of temporalis descend to the mandible (p. 577).

Zygomatic arch

Formed by temporal and zygomatic processes, it is palpable and visible where cheek and temple meet. Its sharp upper border is obscured by attachment of temporal fascia, the lower by masseter; the latter is also attached to its medial aspect. The gap between arch and temple is deeper anteriorly; here the arch is crossed obliquely down and back by the zygomaticotemporal suture.

The *zygomatic process* of the temporal bone widens as it approaches the squama, dividing into: an *anterior root* passing medially in front of the *mandibular fossa* to the smooth *articular tubercle*, the anterior boundary of the fossa; and a *posterior root* passing back, lateral to the fossa, its upper border continuing into the supramastoid crest.

The external acoustic meatus

Below the posterior zygomatic root, it has rough margins, especially anteroinferiorly, for attachment of meatal cartilage. Posterosuperiorly the margin is formed by the temporal squama, the rest by the temporal's *tympanic plate*. The squamotympanic suture is anterosuperior, the posterior meatal (tympanomastoid) suture usually obliterated in adults, except for a canaliculus for the auricular branch of the vagus. Below the meatus the tympanic plate projects as a rough triangular area. Posterosuperior is often a small depression with a *suprameatal spine* in its anterior margin; within is a *suprameatal triangle*, bounded above by the supramastoid crest, in front by the posterosuperior meatal margin and behind by a posterior vertical tangent to the meatal margin. This triangle is the lateral wall of the mastoid (tympanic) antrum (p. 589) and is hence of surgical interest.

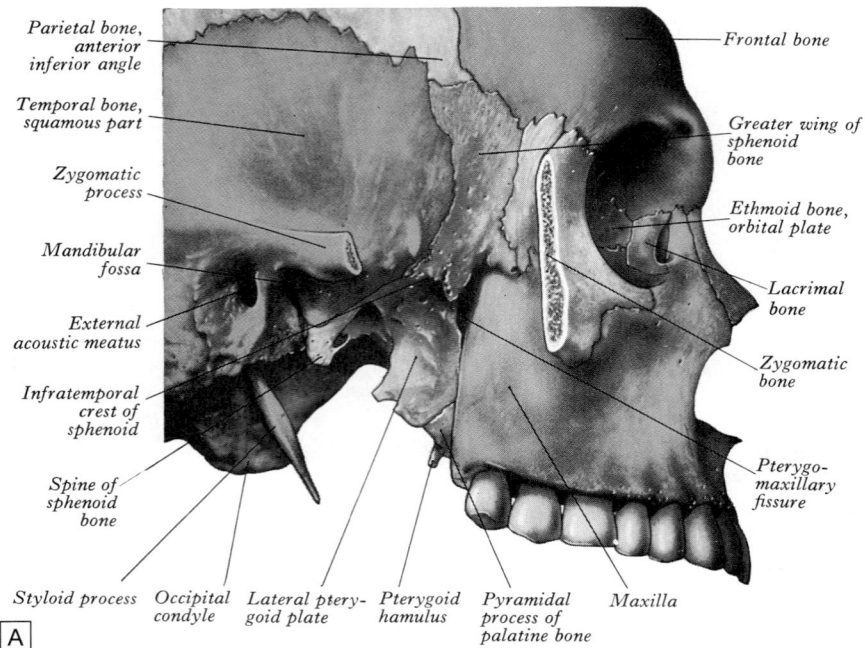

Parietal bone, anterior inferior angle

Temporal bone, squamous part

Zygomatic process

Mandibular fossa

External acoustic meatus

Infratemporal crest of sphenoid

Spine of sphenoid bone

Styloid process

Occipital condyle

Lateral pterygoid plate

Pterygoid hamulus

Pyramidal process of palatine bone

Maxilla

Frontal bone

Greater wing of sphenoid bone

Ethmoid bone, orbital plate

Lacrimal bone

Zygomatic bone

Pterygomaxillary fissure

A

6.143A. The right infratemporal fossa: seen in norma lateralis after detachment of mandible and removal of zygomatic arch. Blue = frontal bone; yellow = sphenoid and lacrimal bones; brown = temporal and nasal bones; green = maxilla. The parts shown of the parietal, zygomatic, ethmoid and palatine bones are uncoloured.

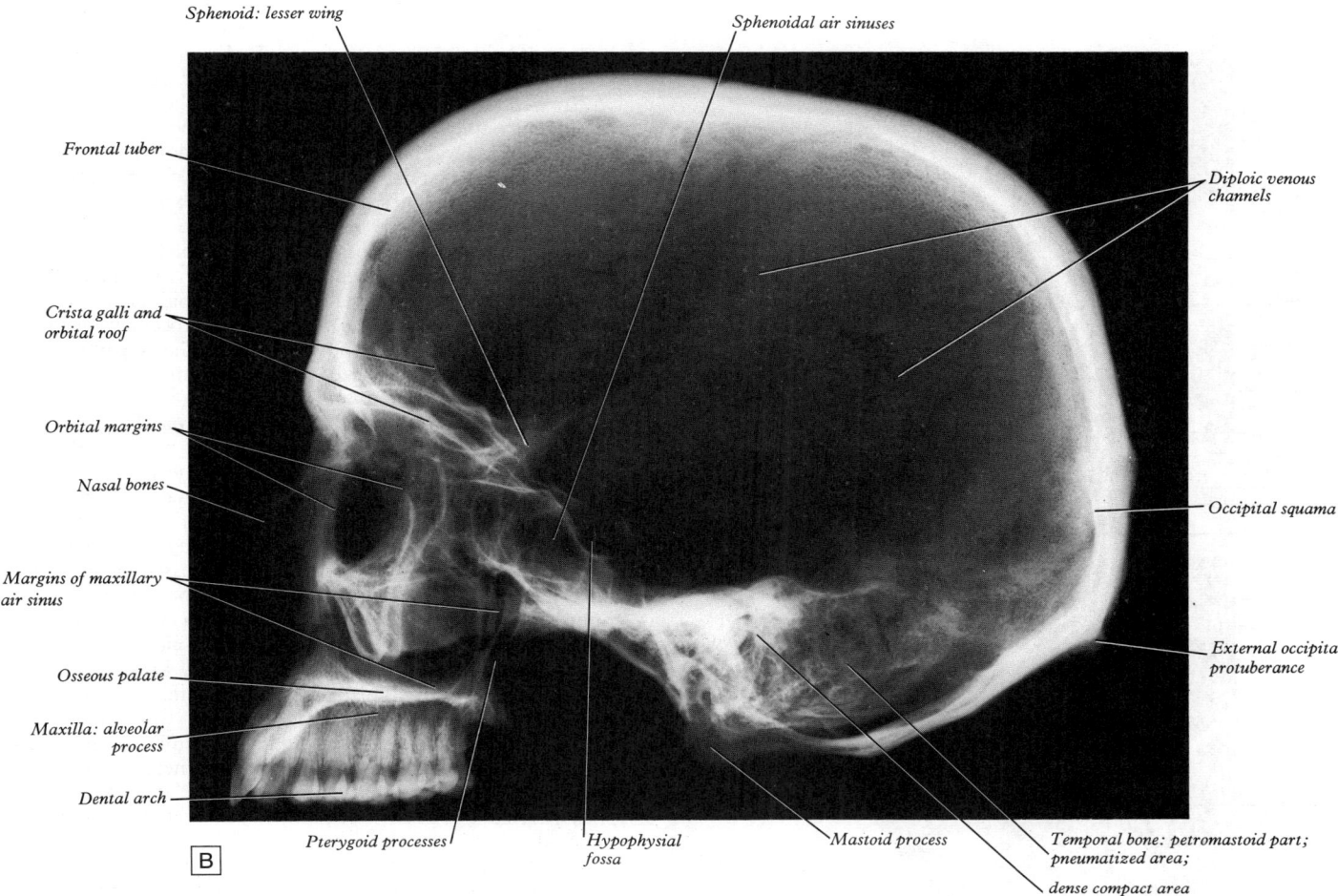

Sphenoid: lesser wing

Sphenoidal air sinuses

Frontal tuber

Diploic venous channels

Crista galli and orbital roof

Orbital margins

Nasal bones

Margins of maxillary air sinus

Occipital squama

Osseous palate

External occipital protuberance

Maxilla: alveolar process

Dental arch

B

Pterygoid processes

Hypophysial fossa

Mastoid process

Temporal bone: petromastoid part; pneumatized area;

dense compact area

6.143B. Lateral radiograph of adult female skull, with mandible omitted. (Supplied by P J Liepins; photography by Sarah Smith.)

Mastoid part of the temporal bone

Posterior to the meatus, it is continuous above with the squama in front. Its upper border forms behind this with the posteroinferior parietal angle a *parietomastoid suture* and, by its posterior border with the occipital squama, an *occipitomastoid suture*. These two meet the lateral end of the lambdoid suture at the *asterion*. The *mastoid process* (**6.142A**), a breast-like inferior projection from the mastoid temporal bone, is posteroinferior to the external acoustic meatus and palpable under the ear's lobule. The *mastoid foramen* is near or in the occipitomastoid suture; it transmits an emissary vein from the sigmoid sinus. Sutural ossicles may appear in the parietomastoid suture, often at or near the asterion, the site of a *posterolateral fontanelle* (Le Double 1903), but also elsewhere along the suture.

Styloid process (6.142A)

A slender spike attached to the skull's base, is best viewed in norma lateralis. Anterior and medial to the mastoid process, its base partly ensheathed by the tympanic plate, it descends anteromedially, its tip usually reaching a point medial to the posterior margin of the mandibular ramus. The styloid process is, however, very variably developed, ranging in length from a few millimetres to a few centimetres, often approximately straight, but on occasion curved; an anteromedial concavity is more common, a posterior concavity is infrequent. From its apex the stylohyoid ligament descends forward to the hyoid's lesser cornu (p. 582) as a cranial suspension.

Infratemporal fossa (6.144A)

An irregular, postmaxillary space, it communicates with the temporal fossa between the zygomatic arch and lower temple. Medially its roof is the infratemporal surface of the sphenoid's greater wing and

part of the temporal squama. Here the greater wing displays the foramina ovale and spinosum. Medial is the lateral pterygoid plate, described in norma basalis (p. 566). Behind, below and laterally the fossa is open. Its anterior and medial walls converge below but are separated above by the *pterygomaxillary fissure*, through which the infratemporal and pterygopalatine fossae connect. The fissure is continuous above with the *inferior orbital fissure*'s posterior end, by which route the infratemporal and pterygopalatine fossae connect with the orbit (p. 560).

Pterygopalatine fossa

A small pyramidal space below the orbital apex, it communicates with the infratemporal fossa via the pterygomaxillary fissure, with the nasal cavity by the sphenopalatine foramen and the orbit by the medial end of the inferior orbital fissure. The foramen rotundum, in its posterior wall, is traversed by the maxillary nerve.

Further details

The floor of the *temporal fossa* bears a few vascular furrows, the most constant being above the external acoustic meatus produced by middle temporal vessels. In its anterior wall the *zygomaticotemporal foramen* passes up and backwards from the zygomatic bone's posterior surface, transmitting the *zygomaticotemporal* nerve and a minute artery. The tendon of temporalis descends and the deep temporal vessels and nerves ascend, deep to the muscle, between the zygomatic arch and cranial wall. The temporal bone's zygomatic process bears a small *tubercle of the anterior root of the zygoma*, to which the lateral temporomandibular ligament is partly attached (see **6.162C**). It is palpable in front of the mandibular head. Behind the

561

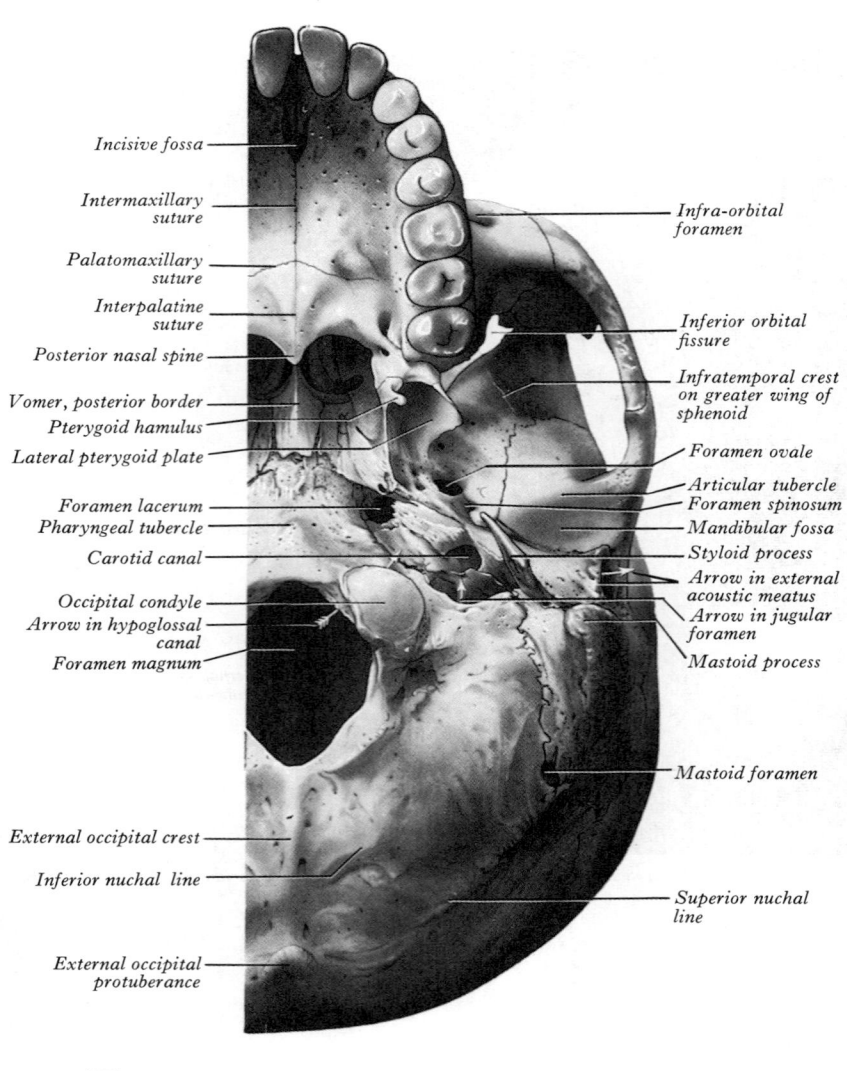

Incisive fossa
Intermaxillary suture
Palatomaxillary suture
Interpalatine suture
Posterior nasal spine
Vomer, posterior border
Pterygoid hamulus
Lateral pterygoid plate
Foramen lacerum
Pharyngeal tubercle
Carotid canal
Occipital condyle
Arrow in hypoglossal canal
Foramen magnum
External occipital crest
Inferior nuchal line
External occipital protuberance

Infra-orbital foramen
Inferior orbital fissure
Infratemporal crest on greater wing of sphenoid
Foramen ovale
Articular tubercle
Foramen spinosum
Mandibular fossa
Styloid process
Arrow in external acoustic meatus
Arrow in jugular foramen
Mastoid process
Mastoid foramen
Superior nuchal line

A

6.144A. The inferior of the left half of the base of the skull (norma basalis) with the mandible removed, see **6**.144B (blue = occipital bone; yellow = sphenoid bone; green = maxilla).

mandibular fossa the postglenoid tubercle descends from the zygoma's posterior root to meet the tympanic plate anterosuperiorly at the external acoustic meatus (see **6**.173); its anterior aspect is a small part of the mandibular fossa.

The posterolateral surface of the *mastoid process* and its apex give attachment to sternocleidomastoid, splenius capitis and longissimus capitis, from before backwards (**6**.143, 144B). Anterior and parallel to this area partially obliterated remains of the squamomastoid suture may be visible. Hence the suprameatal triangle's floor, and therefore the lateral wall of the mastoid antrum, is formed by temporal squama. The tympanomastoid fissure is on the base of the process; the mastoid canaliculus (see **6**.177), which transmits the vagal auricular branch, opens in the fissure.

The *styloid process* is related laterally to the parotid gland, medially to the internal jugular vein. Stylohyoid is attached by a slender tendon to its posterior aspect near the base, styloglossus to the tip and adjacent anterior aspect, stylopharyngeus medially to its base and the stylomandibular ligament laterally near its tip. Behind its base the facial nerve emerges from the stylomastoid foramen crossing lateral to the process in the parotid gland.

The *infratemporal fossa* (**6**.144A) contains temporalis as it reaches the mandibular coronoid process and adjacent ramus; the maxillary artery and its rami, and the pterygoid venous plexus lie medial

562

to the muscle and usually lateral to the lateral pterygoid. Deepest are the medial pterygoid, mandibular nerve and chorda tympani, the mandibular nerve entering the fossa through the foramen ovale in its roof to divide into terminal rami medial to the lateral pterygoid; these leave the fossa for other regions. The chorda tympani enters the fossa medial to the sphenoidal spine to join the lingual nerve. The maxillary nerve appears in its upper part between the pterygopalatine fossa and inferior orbital fissure. The anterior wall is pierced by small foramina for posterior superior alveolar vessels and nerves and is limited below by the maxilla's alveolar part behind the molar teeth. Here a strip of maxilla is covered by gingival mucosa and above this are attached upper fibres of buccinator, extending back on to the maxillary tuberosity. The fossa's medial wall, the lateral pterygoid plate, is completed below by the palatine bone's pyramidal process wedged between the maxillary tuberosity and the plate. The superficial head of medial pterygoid is attached to the pyramidal process but also spreads onto the maxillary tuberosity.

The *pterygomaxillary fissure*, between maxilla and pterygoid process, admits the maxillary artery to the pterygopalatine fossa; its uppermost part contains the maxillary nerve.

The *pterygopalatine fossa* (**6**.144A) is bounded **behind** by the root of the pterygoid process and adjoining anterior surface greater wing of the sphenoid, **medially** by the palatine bone's perpendicular plate with its orbital and sphenoidal processes, **anteriorly** by the superomedial part of the maxilla's posterior surface. **Laterally** it connects with the infratemporal fossa via the pterygomaxillary fissure. Its main contents are the maxillary nerve, pterygopalatine ganglion and terminal rami of the maxillary artery. The pterygoid canal inferomedial to the foramen rotundum transmits the pterygoid nerve and artery from the anterior wall of the foramen lacerum to the pterygopalatine ganglion; inferomedially the palatovaginal canal transmits the pharyngeal nerve and artery from the ganglion to the pharyngeal roof. In the medial wall the *sphenopalatine foramen* (see **6**.157A) is bounded above by the sphenoid's body, elsewhere by parts of the palatine bone, in front by its orbital process, behind by its sphenoidal process, and below by the upper border of the palatine bone's perpendicular plate. It carries into the nasal cavity the nasopalatine nerve and vessels. A fifth foramen, placed inferiorly at the junction of the anterior and posterior walls, leads into the *greater palatine canal* and descends between the maxilla and palatine perpendicular plate. This canal transmits anterior, middle and posterior palatine nerves and greater and lesser palatine vessels, which emerge onto the bony palate.

NORMA BASALIS

The inferior cranial aspect is complex, extending from upper incisor teeth to the superior nuchal lines of the occiput. Laterally are the postincisor teeth, zygomatic arches and their posterior roots and mastoid processes (which reach the lateral limits of the superior nuchal lines). It is conveniently divided into anterior, middle and posterior parts, the anterior being the hard palate and alveolar arches, on a lower level than the rest, the rest being arbitrarily divided into middle and posterior parts by a transverse plane through the anterior margin of the foramen magnum.

Anterior part of norma basalis

The *bony palate* (**6**.145), within the superior alveolar arch, is formed by the maxillary palatine processes and palatine horizontal plates, meeting at a *cruciform suture* formed of intermaxillary, interpalatine and palatomaxillary sutures. The palate is arched sagittally and transversely, its depth and breadth variable but is always greatest in the molar region. The *incisive fossa* is anterior and median; the *lateral incisive foramina*, via which incisive canals pass to the nasal cavity (p. 574), are in its lateral walls and the median incisive foramina, present in some skulls, open on its anterior and posterior walls. The *greater palatine foramen* is near the lateral palatal border behind the palatomaxillary suture (**6**.145), and a vascular groove, deep posteriorly, leads forwards from it. The *lesser palatine foramina*, usually two, behind the greater, pierce the *palatine pyramidal process* wedged between the lower ends of the medial and lateral pterygoid plates. (Accessory lesser foramina have a high incidence, with racial and sexual variation from 30–70%; see p. 609.) The palate is pierced by many other small foramina and marked by pits for palatine glands. Near its sharp, gently arched bilaterally posterior border, also slightly curved, variably prominent *palatine crests* extend medially from behind the greater palatine foramina. The posterior border projects back as a median *posterior nasal spine*. The alveolar arch has 16 sockets or *alveoli* for teeth, varying in size and depth, some single, some divided by septa in adaptation to tooth roots. The lateral incisive foramen transmits terminal rami of the greater palatine vessels and nasopalatine nerve. When median incisive foramina occur, the left nasopalatine nerve traverses the anterior and the right posterior foramen. The lateral foramina are, some claim, in the line of fusion of an os incisivum (premaxilla) with the maxilla proper, as a primitive bucconasal communication. In young skulls a dubious bilateral suture between os incisivum and maxilla may extend from the posterior part of the incisive fossa to septa between the roots of the lateral incisor and canine teeth (but see p. 577).

The greater palatine nerve and vessels traverse their foramina, the vessels grooving the palate towards the incisive fossa. The lesser palatine foramina, usually two but sometimes three, contain lesser palatine nerves and vessels. To the palatine crest is attached part of the tendon of tensor veli palatini, to the posterior border the palatine aponeurosis and to the posterior nasal spine musculus uvulae. These collagenous elements, although often described separately, are in fact blended as the osseous surfaces are approached. Margins of the median palatal intermaxillary suture are sometimes raised into a *palatine torus*, variably smooth, pitted or rough. A similar longitudinal *maxillary torus* may appear on the alveolar process, palatal to the upper molar roots.

Middle part of norma basalis

The middle part of norma basalis (**6.146**) extends posteriorly from the osseous palate to an arbitrary line through the anterior margin of the foramen magnum. Anteriorly the *posterior border* of the *vomer* separates two *posterior nasal apertures*, behind which a posterior area of interior sphenoid surface is continuous with that of the *basioccipital bone*, forming a broad bar sloping down to the foramen magnum. Convex transversely, wider behind, it bears, in front of the foramen, a small midline *pharyngeal tubercle*, the highest attachment of the superior pharyngeal constrictor.

Pterygoid process. Descending behind the third molar tooth from the junction of the sphenoid's greater wing and its body, it has medial and lateral pterygoid plates, separated by a cuneiform *pterygoid fossa*, facing posterolaterally. Anteriorly the plates are fused, except below, where they are separated by the *pyramidal process* of the *palatine*; sutures are usually discernible. Anteromedially the processes articulate with the posterior border of the palatine's perpendicular plate, forming a flat area in the posterior nasal aperture's lateral wall and nasopharynx. Laterally they are separated from the posterior maxillary surface by the pterygomaxillary fissure (**6.144A**). The *medial pterygoid plate* is narrower and projects directly backwards, its medial surface covered by mucous membrane of the posterior nasal aperture's lateral rim and part of the nasopharynx. Its posterior border is sharp, with a small projection near the midpoint, above which it is curved and attached to the pharyngeal end of the auditory tube; superiorly it divides to enclose the *scaphoid fossa* (**6.147**, **168B**); below, it projects as a slender *pterygoid hamulus* which curves laterally and is grooved anteriorly by the tendon of tensor veli palatini. The *lateral pterygoid plate* projects posterolaterally; its lateral surface is the medial wall of the infratemporal fossa. Superiorly it is continuous with the *infratemporal surface* of the *sphenoid's greater wing*, anterior in the roof of the infratemporal fossa. This surface, inferolateral, is almost pentagonal; anterior is the posterolateral border of the inferior orbital fissure, anterolateral the infratemporal crest. Laterally it articulates with the temporal squama; medially it is continuous with the pterygoid process and side of the sphenoid's body; posteromedially it articulates with the petrous part of the temporal bone.

The medial pterygoid plate. At the root of its posterior border the *scaphoid fossa* receives anterior fibres of tensor veli

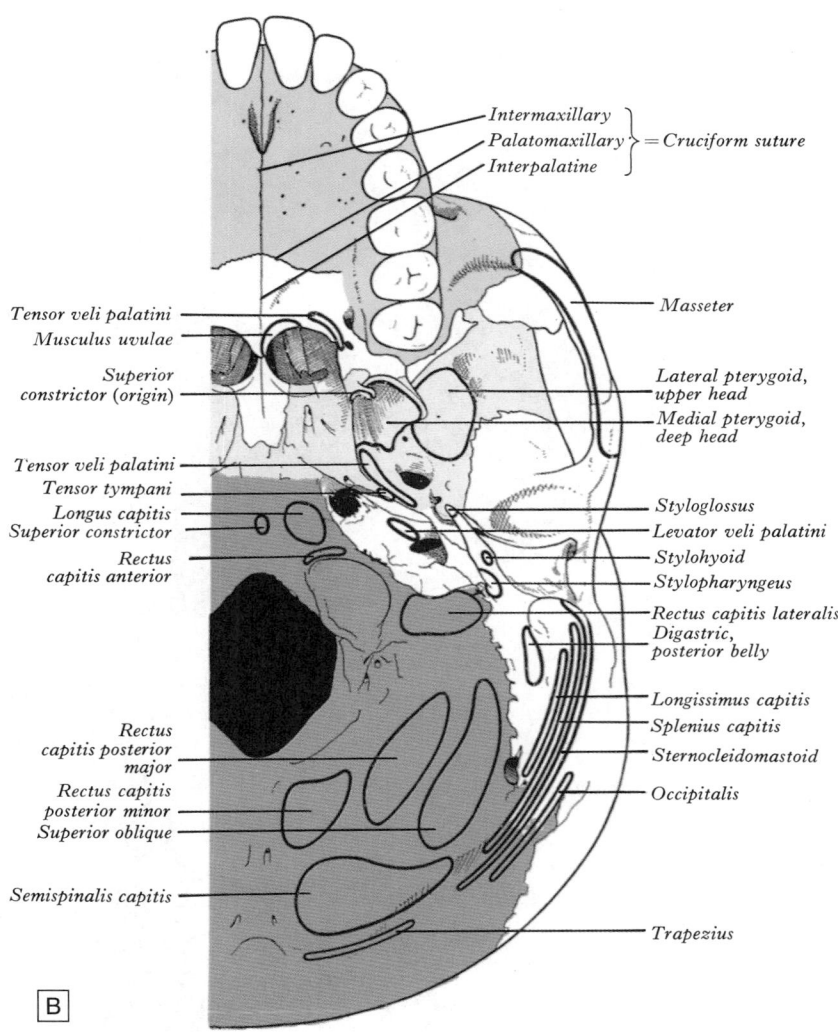

6.144B. Outline drawing showing the attachments of named but unclassified muscles (blue = occipital; yellow = sphenoid; green = maxilla).

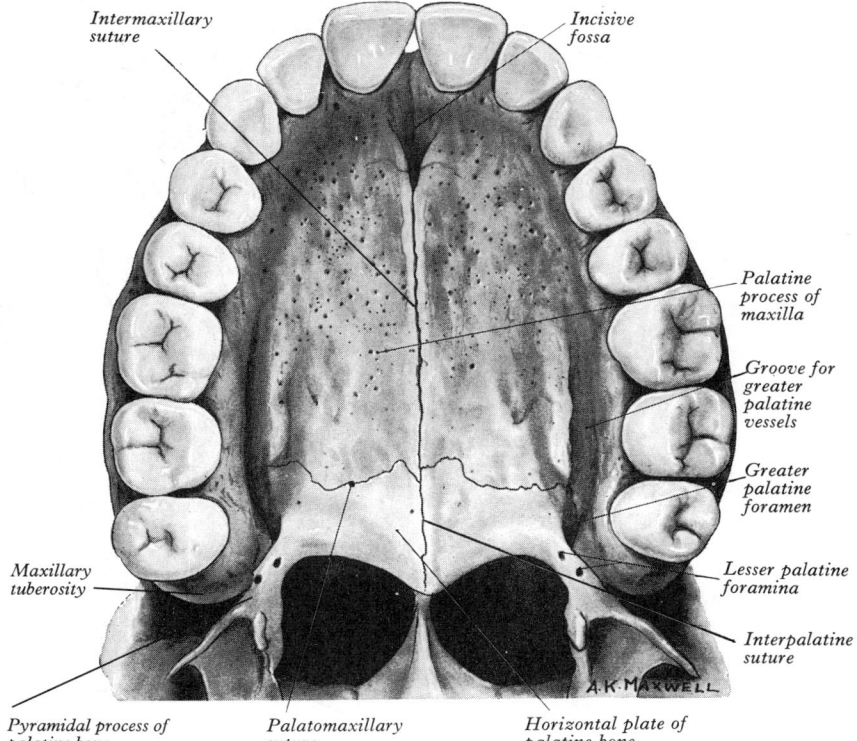

6.145 The bony palate and the alveolar arch: inferior aspect.

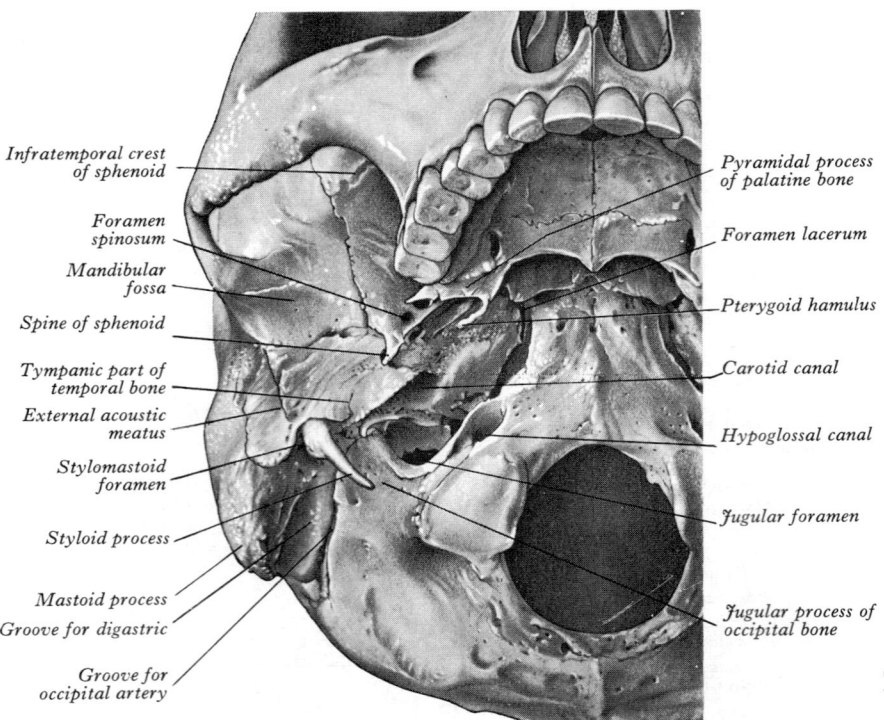

Infratemporal crest of sphenoid

Foramen spinosum

Mandibular fossa

Spine of sphenoid

Tympanic part of temporal bone

External acoustic meatus

Stylomastoid foramen

Styloid process

Mastoid process

Groove for digastric

Groove for occipital artery

Pyramidal process of palatine bone

Foramen lacerum

Pterygoid hamulus

Carotid canal

Hypoglossal canal

Jugular foramen

Jugular process of occipital bone

6.146 The right and part of the left side of the norma basalis of the skull. To show some features to better advantage, the anterior end of the skull has been elevated so that the Frankfurt plane is tilted to an angle of about 45° to the horizontal.

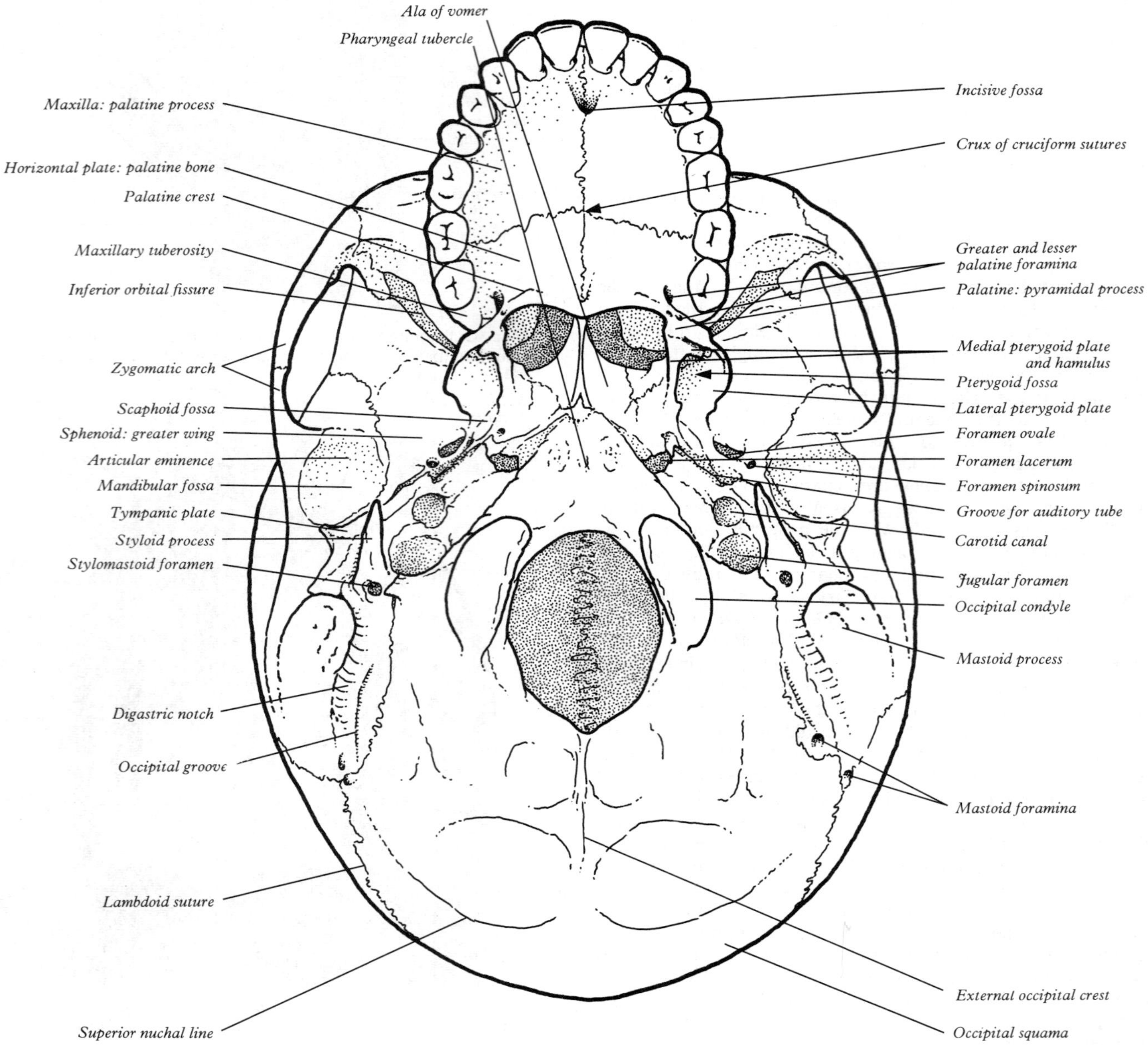

Ala of vomer

Pharyngeal tubercle

Maxilla: palatine process

Horizontal plate: palatine bone

Palatine crest

Maxillary tuberosity

Inferior orbital fissure

Zygomatic arch

Scaphoid fossa

Sphenoid: greater wing

Articular eminence

Mandibular fossa

Tympanic plate

Styloid process

Stylomastoid foramen

Digastric notch

Occipital groove

Lambdoid suture

Superior nuchal line

Incisive fossa

Crux of cruciform sutures

Greater and lesser palatine foramina

Palatine: pyramidal process

Medial pterygoid plate and hamulus

Pterygoid fossa

Lateral pterygoid plate

Foramen ovale

Foramen lacerum

Foramen spinosum

Groove for auditory tube

Carotid canal

Jugular foramen

Occipital condyle

Mastoid process

Mastoid foramina

External occipital crest

Occipital squama

A

564   **6.**147A.   The skull: norma basalis without mandible.

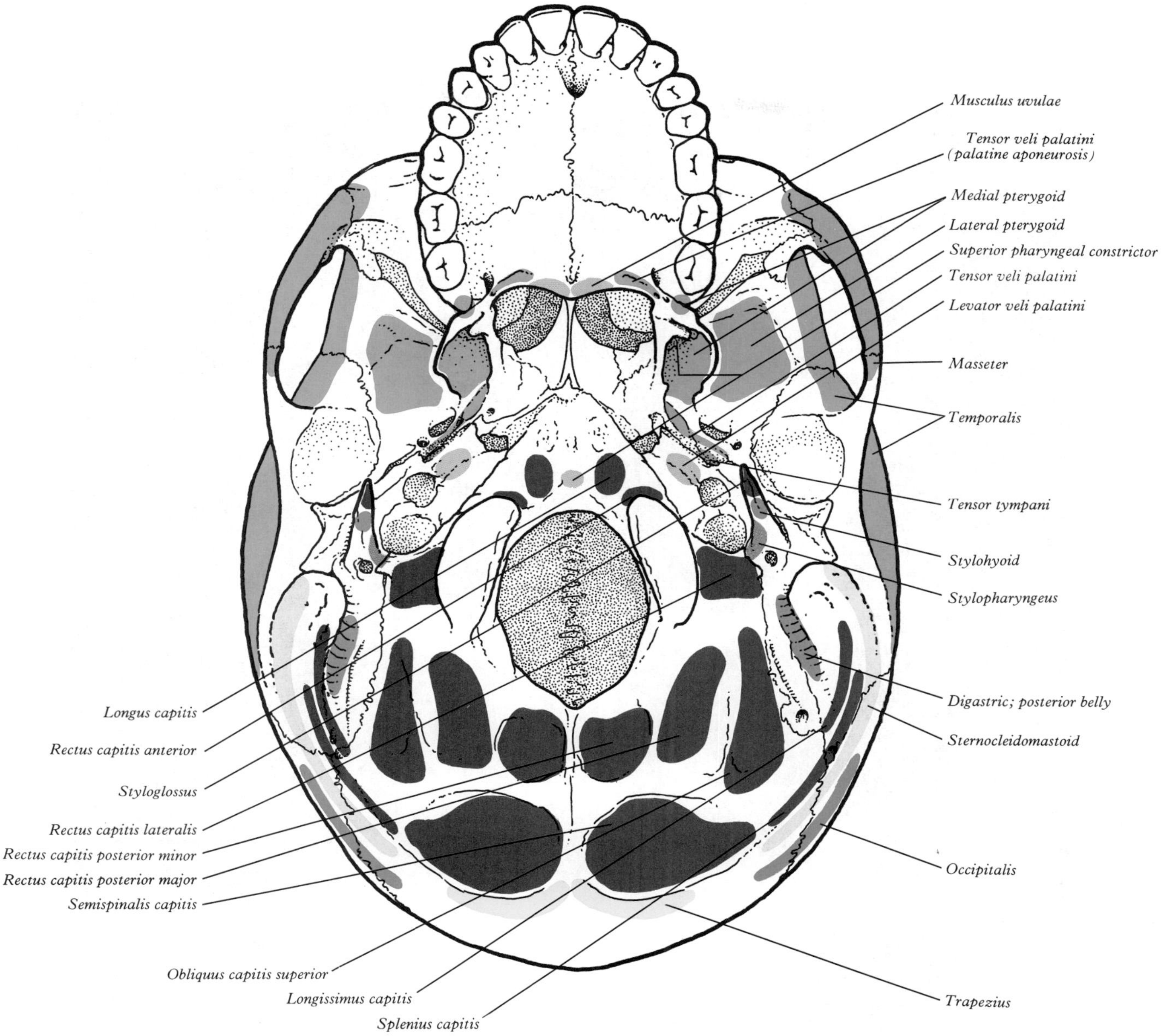

Musculus uvulae

Tensor veli palatini
(palatine aponeurosis)

Medial pterygoid

Lateral pterygoid

Superior pharyngeal constrictor

Tensor veli palatini

Levator veli palatini

Masseter

Temporalis

Tensor tympani

Stylohyoid

Stylopharyngeus

Digastric; posterior belly

Sternocleidomastoid

Occipitalis

Trapezius

Longus capitis

Rectus capitis anterior

Styloglossus

Rectus capitis lateralis

Rectus capitis posterior minor

Rectus capitis posterior major

Semispinalis capitis

Obliquus capitis superior

Longissimus capitis

Splenius capitis

COLOUR CODING OF ATTACHMENTS OF MUSCLE GROUPS BASED ON DERIVATION AND INNERVATION

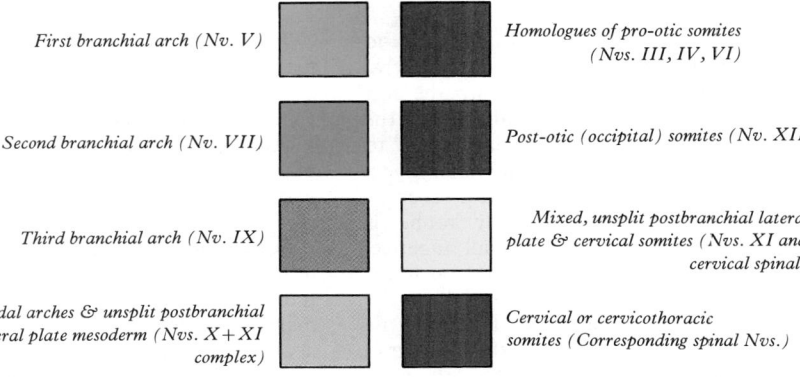

First branchial arch (Nv. V)

*Homologues of pro-otic somites
(Nvs. III, IV, VI)*

Second branchial arch (Nv. VII)

Post-otic (occipital) somites (Nv. XII)

Third branchial arch (Nv. IX)

*Mixed, unsplit postbranchial lateral
plate & cervical somites (Nvs. XI and
cervical spinal)*

*Caudal arches & unsplit postbranchial
lateral plate mesoderm (Nvs. X + XI
complex)*

*Cervical or cervicothoracic
somites (Corresponding spinal Nvs.)*

6.147B.   The skull: norma basalis without mandible, showing muscle attachments.

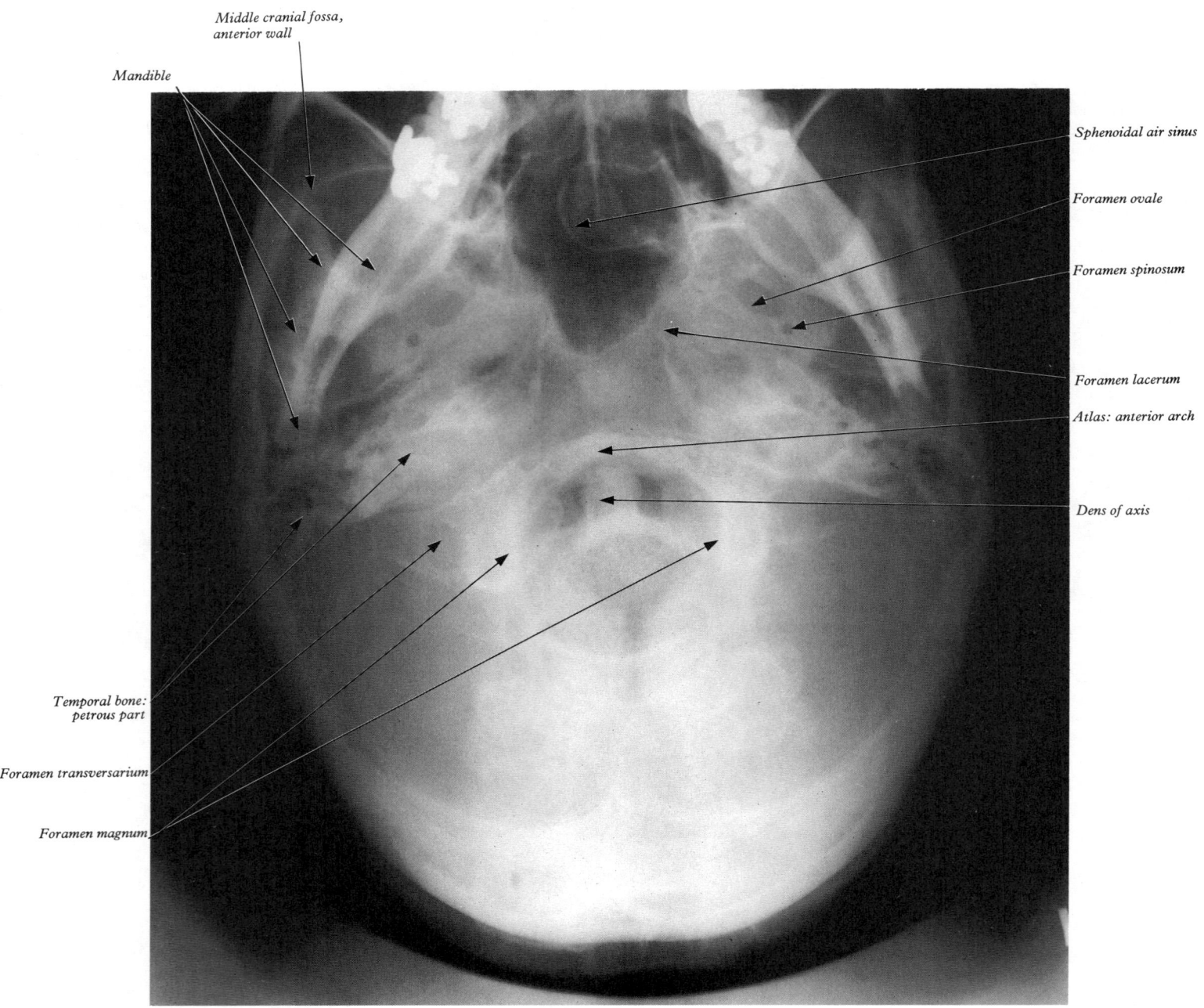

Middle cranial fossa,
anterior wall

Mandible

Sphenoidal air sinus

Foramen ovale

Foramen spinosum

Foramen lacerum

Atlas: anterior arch

Dens of axis

Temporal bone:
petrous part

Foramen transversarium

Foramen magnum

6.148 Radiograph of base of skull (submento-vertical view) to show foramina. (Supplied by Shaun Gallagher, Guy's Hospital; photography by Kevin Fitzpatrick.)

palatini, which descend along the plate's lateral surface and posterior border to reach the *hamulus,* around the anterolateral aspect of which the muscle's tendon twists medially into the soft palate. To the plate's posterior border, notched above by the auditory tube (p. 588), is attached the pharyngobasilar fascia, to its lower part the anterior highest fibres of the superior pharyngeal constrictor; these curve up and medially to the pharyngeal tubercle. To the tip of the hamulus the pterygomandibular raphe is attached. High on the plate's posterior border a small tubercle, medial to the scaphoid fossa, projects back below the posterior opening of the *pterygoid canal,* which opens anteriorly on the pterygopalatine fossa's posterior wall. The canal transmits its nerve and vessels and is in the line of fusion of the pterygoid process and greater wing with the sphenoidal body. The *pterygoid fossa,* between the pterygoid plates, is completed anteroinferiorly by the palatal pyramidal process.

The lateral pterygoid plate (6.144). This is wider than the medial. A variable *pterygospinous process* on its irregular posterior border is connected by a ligament (sometimes ossified) to the sphenoid spine. To its rougher, lateral surface is attached the lower head of lateral pterygoid and to the medial surface most of medial pterygoid. Attached to the lateral aspect of the *palatine pyramidal process* are some fibres of the superficial slip of medial pterygoid.

Foramina ovale and spinosum. Sited on the greater wing's infratemporal surface (6.148), they transmit some large structures: the *foramen ovale,* near the lateral pterygoid plate's posterior margin, transmits the trigeminal mandibular division and the accessory meningeal artery (if present). To its sharp posterior border fibres of tensor veli palatini are attached between the nerve and auditory tube. Posterolaterally is the *foramen spinosum* which transmits the middle meningeal artery and meningeal branch of the mandibular nerve to the middle cranial fossa; it is much the smaller and circular. Posterolateral to the foramen spinosum projects the irregular *spine of the sphenoid* whose medial surface is flat and forms, with the adjoining posterior border of the greater wing, the anterolateral wall of a groove, completed posteromedially by part of the petrous temporal bone. This groove contains the cartilaginous *pharyngotympanic (auditory) tube* and leads posterolaterally into an osseous canal for the tube in the petrous temporal bone and also anteromedially to the medial pterygoid plate's superior border. In the roof of the groove the posterior border of the greater wing and the anterior border of the petrous temporal meet at a petrosphenoidal suture. Occasionally the foramina ovale and spinosum are confluent, frequency varying from 0.7–10.4% in modern populations. Similarly, the foramen spinosum's posterior edge may be defective, with an incidence of 2–17% (p. 609). Posteromedial to this groove is the *inferior surface* of the *petrous temporal* between the sphenoid's greater wing and the basioccipital bone. Anteriorly the surface is rough, its apex separated from the posterolateral aspect of the sphenoid's body by an irregular *foramen lacerum*. Behind this rough area and posterolateral to the foramen lacerum, a large, almost circular foramen opens into the *carotid canal*, which ascends then turns anteromedially to reach the posterior wall of the foramen lacerum. Emerging from the canal the internal carotid artery turns up into the cranial cavity. Inferiorly the foramen lacerum is filled by fibrocartilage; this is not traversed by large structures.

The temporal bone's tympanic part (6.146). It is separated from the temporomandibular joint by the parotid gland, usually containing the auriculotemporal nerve. It is thinnest centrally and occasionally deficient (p. 592). Its grooved upper aspect forms the anterior wall, floor and lower posterior wall of the external acoustic meatus. Except where it ensheathes the styloid process, its posterior surface is fused with the petromastoid bone.

Further details. From the base of the spine of the sphenoid the *squamotympanic fissure* runs posterolaterally between the tympanic plate and mandibular fossa, usually reaching the anterior margin of the external acoustic meatus but sometimes obliterated near its lateral end. The *mandibular fossa*, deeply concave sagitally, and transversely gently concave, is wider laterally. It contains the head of the mandible when the jaw is elevated. Anteriorly the articular surface invades a transverse rounded *articular tubercle*, continuous laterally with the zygoma's anterior root. In front is the part of the temporal squama in the roof of the infratemporal fossa. Behind the squamotympanic fissure the *temporal tympanic plate*, separating mandibular fossa and external acoustic meatus, is roughly triangular, its apex at the medial end of the fissure near the root of the spine of the sphenoid. Its lower border skirts the anterolateral margin of the inferior opening of the carotid canal, extending posterolaterally to the root of the styloid process. There it forms a *sheath of the styloid process*, longer and prominent laterally where the tympanic plate is fused with the rest of the temporal bone below and behind; it is free above, forming the anterior border of the external acoustic meatus.

The upper border of the *vomer*, applied to the inferior aspect of the sphenoid's body, expands into an *ala* on each side (6.147A, 188), a median groove between them fitting the sphenoid's rostrum. The lateral border of each ala reaches a thin *vaginal process* projecting medially from the medial pterygoid plate. The two may merely touch or the alar edge may be overlapped inferiorly by the vaginal process, whose inferior surface bears an anteroposterior groove, converted into a canal anteriorly by the superior aspect of the sphenoidal process of the palatine bone. This *palatovaginal canal*, opening anteriorly on the pterygopalatine fossa's anterior wall, transmits a pharyngeal branch of the pterygopalatine ganglion and a pharyngeal branch from the third part of the maxillary artery. A second, *vomerovaginal canal*, medial to the palatovaginal, may exist between ala and vaginal process, leading into the anterior end of the palatovaginal canal.

Anterior to the pharyngeal tubercle the basioccipital bone is related to the roof of the nasal part of the pharynx and the pharyngeal tonsil. Anterolateral to the tubercle, longus capitis is attached and posterior to this rectus capitis anterior, immediately anterior to the occipital condyle and medial to the hypoglossal canal.

The greater wing's infratemporal surface is an attachment of the

upper head of lateral pterygoid and is crossed by the deep temporal and masseteric nerves, between muscle and bone. Between the foramen ovale and scaphoid fossa a small *sphenoidal emissary foramen* may contain an emissary vein from the cavernous sinus. Attached to the *spine* of the *sphenoid*, variably sharp or blunt, is the sphenomandibular ligament. The spine is related laterally to the auriculotemporal nerve, medial to chorda tympani, by which it may be grooved, and to the auditory tube. Posterior fibres of tensor veli palatini are attached posterior to it. The groove for the tube varies in width and depth, its roof occasionally completed by fibrous tissue; its lateral sphenoidal wall gives attachment posteriorly to fibres of tensor tympani. Laterally on the petrous temporal bone's posterior surface levator veli palatini is attached.

The *foramen lacerum* is bounded in front by the sphenoid body and adjoining roots of the pterygoid process and greater wing, posterolaterally by the apex of the petrous temporal and medially by the basioccipital; it is nearly 1 cm long, but no large structure completely traverses it. The carotid canal's orifice opens posteriorly; this artery and its venous and sympathetic plexuses ascend through its upper end. In the foramen the deep and the greater petrosal nerves join to form the nerve of the pterygoid canal, which opens low in the anterior wall. Meningeal branches of the ascending pharyngeal artery, and emissary veins from the cavernous sinus traverse the foramen. Cartilage in its lower part is a remnant of the chondrocranium.

The *mandibular fossa*'s thin floor is below the most lateral part of the middle cranial fossa and covered by white fibrocartilage (p. 579). To the *tubercle of the root of the zygoma* is attached the lateral temporomandibular ligament. A thin edge of bone may appear at the medial end of the *squamotympanic fissure*; it is the lower border of the down-curved lateral edge of the tegmen tympani, a part of the petrous temporal. It partly divides the squamotympanic into *petrotympanic* and *petrosquamous* fissures. Through the former the chorda tympani, in its anterior canaliculus, escapes anteroinferiorly from the tympanic cavity; the anterior tympanic branch of the maxillary artery traverses the same fissure.

Posterior part of norma basalis

Anteromedian in this region (6.144, 147, 148) is the *foramen magnum*, which is oval, wider behind, its greatest diameter being anteroposterior. It contains the medulla oblongata's lower end. Anteriorly its margin is slightly overlapped by the *occipital condyles*, projecting down to articulate with the superior articular facets on the lateral masses of the atlas. Oval in outline, each condyle is oblique, its anterior end nearer the midline, markedly convex anteroposteriorly, less so transversely. Its medial aspect is roughened by ligamentous attachments. Above each condyle, anteriorly, is an *hypoglossal (anterior condylar) canal*, directed laterally and slightly forwards from the posterior cranial fossa and containing the hypoglossal nerve.

The *hypoglossal canal* also contains a meningeal branch of the ascending pharyngeal artery and an emissary vein from the basilar plexus. Sometimes it is divided by a spicule of bone (p. 584). A *condylar fossa* of variable depth, posterior to the condyle, is sometimes pierced by a *condylar canal* for an emissary vein from the sigmoid sinus. Incidence of condylar canals shows racial variation from 13.3% in modern Palestinians to 70% in Peruvian crania; it also illustrates sexual variation, occurring in 58% of male Burmese, but only 31% of females (p. 609). Lateral to each condyle a *jugular process* joins the petrous temporal; its anterior border is the posterior boundary of the *jugular foramen*.

Jugular foramen. A large irregular hiatus **between** occipital and petrous temporal bones, it is at the posterior end of the petro-occipital suture. Anteriorly it is separated from the inferior carotid opening by a ridge, related laterally to the medial aspect of the styloid sheath and separated from the hypoglossal canal by a thin osseous bar. Its long axis is directed anteromedially, the right foramen usually being larger. Its anterior part contains the inferior petrosal sinus, its intermediate part the glossopharyngeal, vagus and accessory nerves and its posterior part the internal jugular vein. When the vein's superior bulb is well developed the jugular fossa of the petrous temporal is expanded superolaterally.

Foramen magnum. This is a wide communication between the posterior cranial fossa and the vertebral canal. Anteriorly the apical ligament of the dens and membrana tectoria are in it, both attached to the upper surface of the basioccipital bone. Its wider, posterior part contains the medulla oblongata and meninges. In the subarachnoid space spinal rami of the accessory nerves and vertebral arteries, with their sympathetic plexuses, ascend into the cranium; the posterior spinal arteries descend, posterolateral to the brainstem, as does the anterior spinal artery anteromedian to it. The cerebellar tonsils may project into the foramen. To its *anterior margin* is attached the anterior atlanto-occipital membrane, continuous on each side with capsular ligaments of the atlanto-occipital joints, to its *posterior margin* the posterior atlanto-occipital membrane, and to rough medial condylar areas, the alar ligaments.

Stylomastoid foramen. This is posterior to the styloid root at the anterior end of the mastoid notch, and the facial nerve emerges from the stylomastoid foramen near the digastric's posterior belly, supplying it before entering the parotid gland. The foramen also contains the stylomastoid artery. A groove across the inferior aspect of the temporal bone, medial to the mastoid notch, is related to the occipital artery; it is absent when the vessel is lower than usual, between splenius and longissimus capitis instead of medial to both. To the area **below** the inferior nuchal line are attached medially rectus capitis posterior minor, laterally rectus capitis posterior major (**6.**147B). In the interval **between** the inferior and superior nuchal lines is attached, medially, semispinalis capitis and, laterally, the superior oblique. **Medially** to the superior nuchal line the highest fibres of trapezius are attached, laterally fibres of sternocleidomastoid and, more anteriorly, splenius capitis.

Further details. The jugular foramen (**6.**148B) ascends posteromedially; externally its apparent size is increased laterally by the jugular fossa, its floor separating the superior jugular bulb from the tympanic cavity. A minute *mastoid canaliculus* on the fossa's lateral wall transmits the vagal auricular branch. Passing laterally, this nerve is very near the facial canal, finally emerging in the tympanomastoid suture; it is extracranial at birth but surrounded by bone as the tympanic plate and mastoid process develop. On or near the ridge between the jugular fossa and carotid canal is the *tympanic canaliculus*, transmitting to the middle ear the tympanic branch of the glossopharyngeal nerve. Medial on the upper boundary of the jugular foramen a small notch, more easily identified internally, contains the inferior glossopharyngeal ganglion. The orifice of the *cochlear canaliculus* (p. 592) is at the notch's apex; its projecting edges may reach the occipital bone to trisect the foramen. To the inferior surface of the occipital jugular process rectus capitis lateralis is attached.

Posterior to the styloid process a *stylomastoid foramen* contains the facial nerve. Posterolateral to the foramen the *mastoid process* projects down and forwards as the lateral wall of the *mastoid notch*, in which the posterior belly of digastric is attached. Medial to the notch the temporal bone may be grooved by the occipital artery (**6.**146).

In the midline, posterior to the foramen magnum, the occipital squama has a median *external occipital crest* to which is attached the ligamentum nuchae. The crest ends in the external occipital protuberance; *inferior nuchal lines* curve posterolaterally from its midpoint, almost parallel to the *superior nuchal lines*, which also extend from the protuberance and may form a distinct crest medially.

INTERIOR OF THE CRANIUM

The cranial cavity contains the brain, pineal and hypophysis cerebri, parts of cranial and spinal nerves, blood vessels, meninges and cerebrospinal fluid. It is contained by the frontal, parietal, sphenoid, temporal and occipital bones, and, in part, the ethmoid, all lined by fibrous *endocranium*, the external zone of the dura mater, which traverses various foramina to join the external periosteum, the *pericranium*. Both membranes are blended with sutural ligaments or cartilages in the narrow interosseous intervals.

The cavity's walls vary in thickness in different regions and individuals, but tend to be thinner where covered by muscles, for example in the temporal and posterior cranial fossae. Most cranial bones display *outer* and *inner tables* of compact bone, separated by *diploë*, trabecular bone containing red bone marrow. The inner table

is thinner and more brittle, the outer generally very resilient. Many bones are so thin that the tables are fused, for example the vomer and pterygoid plates. The skull is thicker in some races and individuals, but no relation exists between this and cranial capacity; in all races, it is thinner in women and children. The interior may be described in two parts: the internal surface of the skull 'cap' or calva and that of the cranial base.

Internal surface of cranial vault (calva)

The calva (**6.**149) includes most of the frontal and parietal bones and the upper occipital squama and hence the coronal, sagittal and lambdoid sutures unless fusion, which begins internally, has obliterated them. The cranial vault, deeply concave, presents numerous vascular furrows and cerebral grooves.

The anteromedian *frontal crest* projects back for attachment of the falx cerebri, grooved by the beginning of the *sagittal sulcus*, accommodating the superior sagittal sinus, the groove widening as it progresses back below the sagittal suture. On each side of it are irregular depressions, *granular foveolae*, which become larger and more numerous as skulls age; they are adapted to arachnoid granulations.

The frontal branch of the middle meningeal vein, and sometimes the artery, groove bone deeply just behind the coronal suture, corresponding to the precentral cerebral sulcus. Branches of both and their parietal branches ascend backwards, grooving the internal parietal surface. Smaller grooves may mark the frontal and occipital bones. *Parietal foramina* may occur near the sagittal sulcus, about 3.5 cm anterior to the lambdoid suture, for emissary veins of the superior sagittal sinus. *Impressions for cerebral gyri* are less distinct on the vault than the cranial base, and most obvious near the latter.

Internal surface of cranial base

The internal surface of the cranial base shows clear division into anterior, middle and posterior cranial fossae. It is irregular, partly due to impressions for cerebral gyri, especially conspicuous in the anterior and middle fossae, reflecting the pattern of corresponding cerebral surfaces. Dura mater is firmly adherent to the whole area and through all foramina and fissures its outer layer, endocranium, is continuous with the external periosteum.

ANTERIOR CRANIAL FOSSA

The anterior cranial fossa (**6.**150, 151) is formed at the front and sides by the frontal bone, its floor by the frontal's orbital plate, the

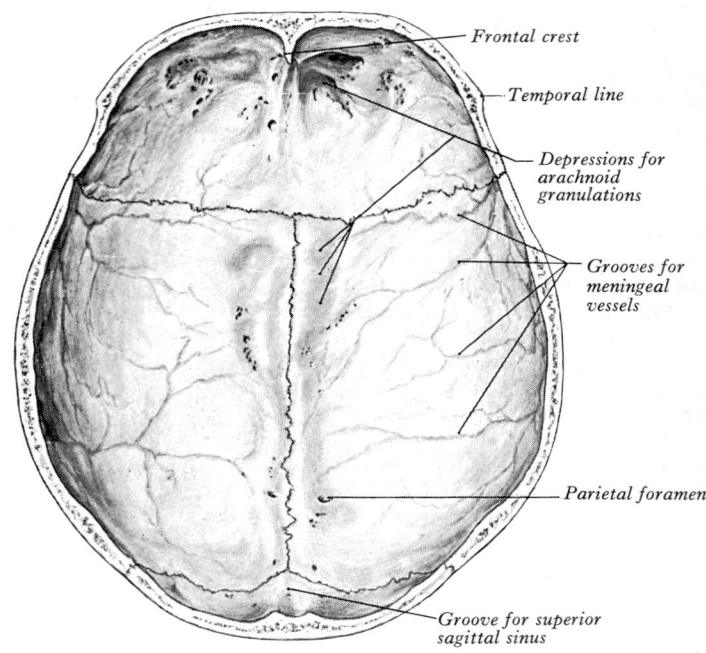

Frontal crest

Temporal line

Depressions for arachnoid granulations

Grooves for meningeal vessels

Parietal foramen

Groove for superior sagittal sinus

6.149 The internal (endocranial) surface of the skull cap or calva.

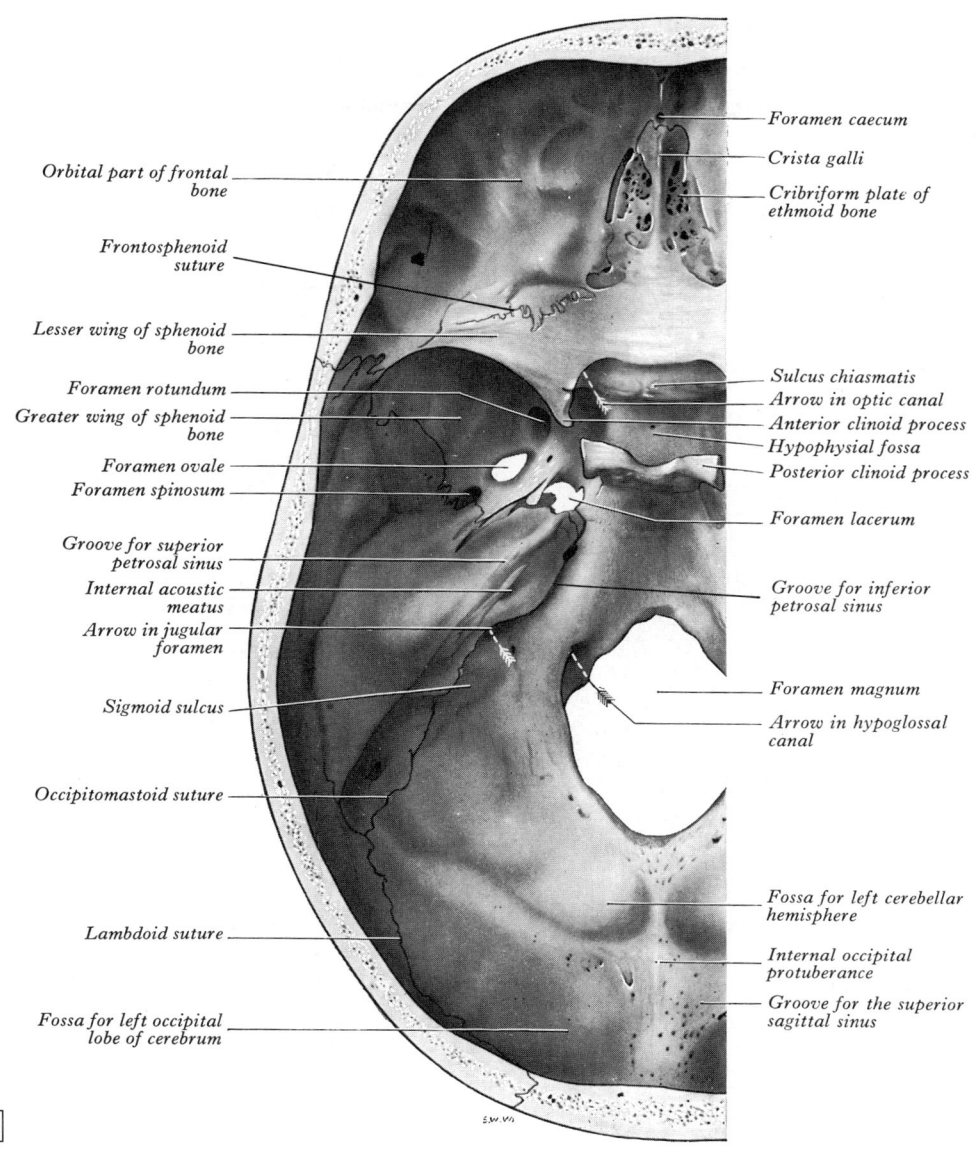

Orbital part of frontal bone

Frontosphenoid suture

Lesser wing of sphenoid bone

Foramen rotundum

Greater wing of sphenoid bone

Foramen ovale

Foramen spinosum

Groove for superior petrosal sinus

Internal acoustic meatus

Arrow in jugular foramen

Sigmoid sulcus

Occipitomastoid suture

Lambdoid suture

Fossa for left occipital lobe of cerebrum

Foramen caecum

Crista galli

Cribriform plate of ethmoid bone

Sulcus chiasmatis

Arrow in optic canal

Anterior clinoid process

Hypophysial fossa

Posterior clinoid process

Foramen lacerum

Groove for inferior petrosal sinus

Foramen magnum

Arrow in hypoglossal canal

Fossa for left cerebellar hemisphere

Internal occipital protuberance

Groove for the superior sagittal sinus

A

6.150A.   The internal (endocranial) surface of the left half of the base of the skull. Compare with Key, **6**.150B.

ethmoid's cribriform plate, and the sphenoid's lesser wings and anterior part of its body.

Cribriform plate of the ethmoid. This spreads across the midline between the frontal orbital plates, but depressed below them, separating the anterior cranial fossa from the nasal cavity, whose roof it helps to form (see **6**.182A). Anteriorly its median *crista galli* projects up between the cerebral hemispheres. A depression between the crista galli and *crest* of the *frontal bone* is crossed by the frontoethmoidal suture and displays the *foramen caecum*. On each side the crista galli is separated from the frontal bone by a narrow region with numerous small foramina transmitting olfactory nerves from the nasal mucosa to the olfactory bulb. Posteriorly each cribriform plate articulates with the sphenoid's body.

Orbital plates of the frontal. These form most of the fossa's floor on each side of the ethmoid, separating the orbital contents from the cerebral frontal lobe. Its convex cranial surface shows impressions for cerebral gyri and small grooves for meningeal vessels. Anteromedially it is split to contain part of the *frontal sinus*. Medially each orbital plate excludes the ethmoidal labyrinth from the anterior cranial fossa. Posteriorly it joins the anterior border of the lesser wing of the sphenoid. The frontal bone bears a median *frontal crest*, which projects between the cerebral hemispheres and narrows upwards on the bone's internal surface.

Sphenoid bone. This completes the fossa's floor posteriorly, centrally by the anterior part of its upper surface, the *jugum sphenoidale*; this separates the fossa from paired sphenoidal sinuses in the sphenoid body (see **6**.156, 157A). Anteriorly the jugum articulates with the cribiform plate; posteriorly it is the anterior bank of the *sulcus chiasmatis* crossing the sphenoid body centrally in the middle cranial fossa and connecting the optic canals. Lateral to the jugum, the anterior fossa is floored by the *lesser wings* of the sphenoid, whose posterior margins overhang the middle fossa. Laterally each lesser wing tapers to a point, meeting the suture between the frontal bone and greater wing at or near the superolateral end of the superior orbital fissure. The medial end of its posterior border is the *anterior clinoid process*. Medially each lesser wing joins the sphenoid body by two roots, separated by the *optic canal*; the anterior, broad and flat, is continuous with the jugum sphenoidale, the posterior, smaller and thicker, joins the sphenoid body near the posterior bank of the chiasmal sulcus.

Further details

To the crista galli and frontal crest the falx cerebri is attached. The foramen caecum between them, usually blind, occasionally accommodates a vein from nasal mucosa to the superior sagittal sinus. Lateral to the crista is the gyrus rectus; the olfactory bulb lies

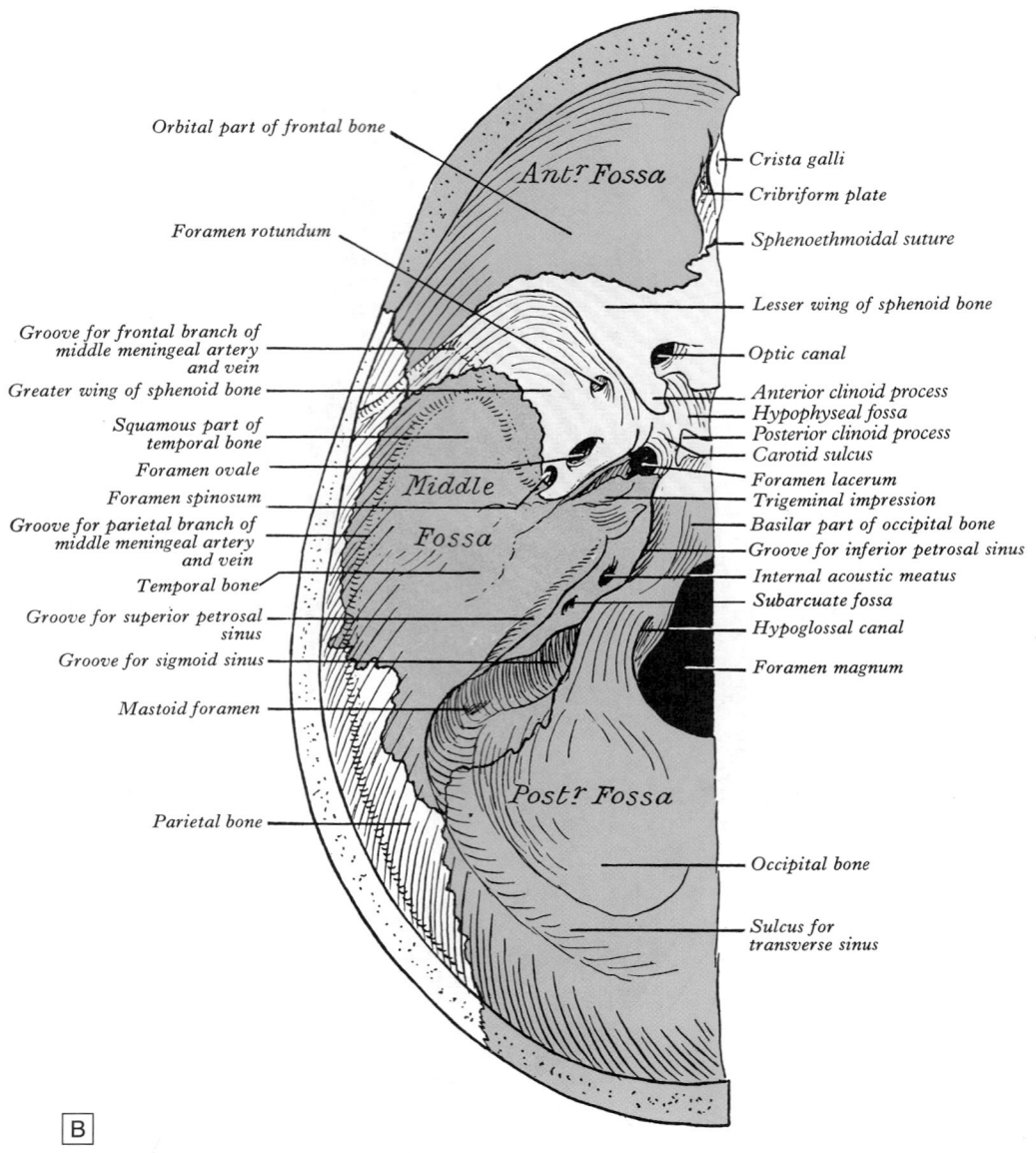

Orbital part of frontal bone

Foramen rotundum

Groove for frontal branch of
middle meningeal artery
and vein

Greater wing of sphenoid bone

Squamous part of
temporal bone

Foramen ovale

Foramen spinosum

Groove for parietal branch of
middle meningeal artery
and vein

Temporal bone

Groove for superior petrosal
sinus

Groove for sigmoid sinus

Mastoid foramen

Parietal bone

Ant.r Fossa

Middle

Fossa

Post.r Fossa

Crista galli

Cribriform plate

Sphenoethmoidal suture

Lesser wing of sphenoid bone

Optic canal

Anterior clinoid process

Hypophyseal fossa

Posterior clinoid process

Carotid sulcus

Foramen lacerum

Trigeminal impression

Basilar part of occipital bone

Groove for inferior petrosal sinus

Internal acoustic meatus

Subarcuate fossa

Hypoglossal canal

Foramen magnum

Occipital bone

Sulcus for
transverse sinus

B

6.150B. The internal surface of the left half of the base of the skull. Key: blue = frontal and occipital; yellow = sphenoid; brown = temporal; white = parietal and ethmoid bones.

on the medial edge of the frontal orbital plate. The *anterior ethmoidal canal* opens in the *cribrofrontal suture* (**6.**152A, 182A) behind the crista galli and is difficult to identify, being overlapped by the orbital plate. It transmits the anterior ethmoidal nerve and vessels, which then run forward under the dura mater to descend through a slit-like foramen at the side of the crista galli into the nasal cavity. The *posterior ethmoidal canal* opens at the posterolateral corner of the cribriform plate and is overhung by the sphenoid. It transmits the posterior ethmoidal vessels.

The posterior border of each lesser wing fits the stem of the lateral cerebral sulcus and may be grooved by the sphenoparietal sinus. Above is the inferior surface of the frontal lobe, and medially, the anterior perforated substance. Inferiorly, it bounds the superior orbital fissure, completing the orbital roof. Each anterior clinoid process receives the free border of the tentorium cerebelli and is grooved medially by the internal carotid artery leaving the cavernous sinus. It may be connected to the middle clinoid process by a thin osseous bar, completing a *caroticoclinoid foramen* around the artery. Parts of gyri recti and olfactory tracts are above the jugum sphenoidale.

MIDDLE CRANIAL FOSSA

The middle cranial fossa (**6.**150, 153), deeper and more extensive than the anterior, particularly laterally, is bounded in front by the posterior borders of the lesser wings, anterior clinoid processes and

sulcus chiasmatis, behind by the superior borders of the petrous temporal bones and sphenoid's dorsum sellae, laterally by the temporal squamae, parietal bones and greater wings of the sphenoid.

Centrally the floor is narrower and formed by the sphenoid body. The chiasmal sulcus, connecting the optic canals, is rarely in contact with the optic chiasma, which is usually posterosuperior. Each *optic canal*, between the roots of a lesser wing and, medially, the sphenoid body, descends a little anterolaterally, containing the optic nerve, ophthalmic artery and meninges. Behind the sulcus the upper sphenoid surface is the *sella turcica*, whose anterior slope bears a median *tuberculum sellae*, behind which is the *hypophyseal fossa* (**6.**150A). The fossa's floor is part of the roof of the sphenoidal sinuses (**6.**134, 156, 157A); posterior to it the *dorsum sellae* projects up and forwards. The superolateral angles of the dorsum are expanded as the *posterior clinoid processes*. Lateral to the sella turcica the sphenoid has a shallow *groove for the internal carotid artery*, here turning anteriorly from the foramen lacerum. A small elevation on the groove's medial edge is the *middle clinoid process*; it may be joined to the anterior process, as noted above. Posterolaterally the groove may be deepened by a small projecting *lingula* (see **6.**168A).

Laterally the middle fossa is deep and supports the temporal lobes. In front are the cerebral surfaces of the greater wings of the sphenoid, behind are the anterior surfaces of the petrous temporal bones and, laterally, the cerebral surfaces of the temporal squamae between the former two. Anteriorly are the orbits, laterally the temporal fossae, inferiorly the infratemporal fossae. The middle cranial fossa com-

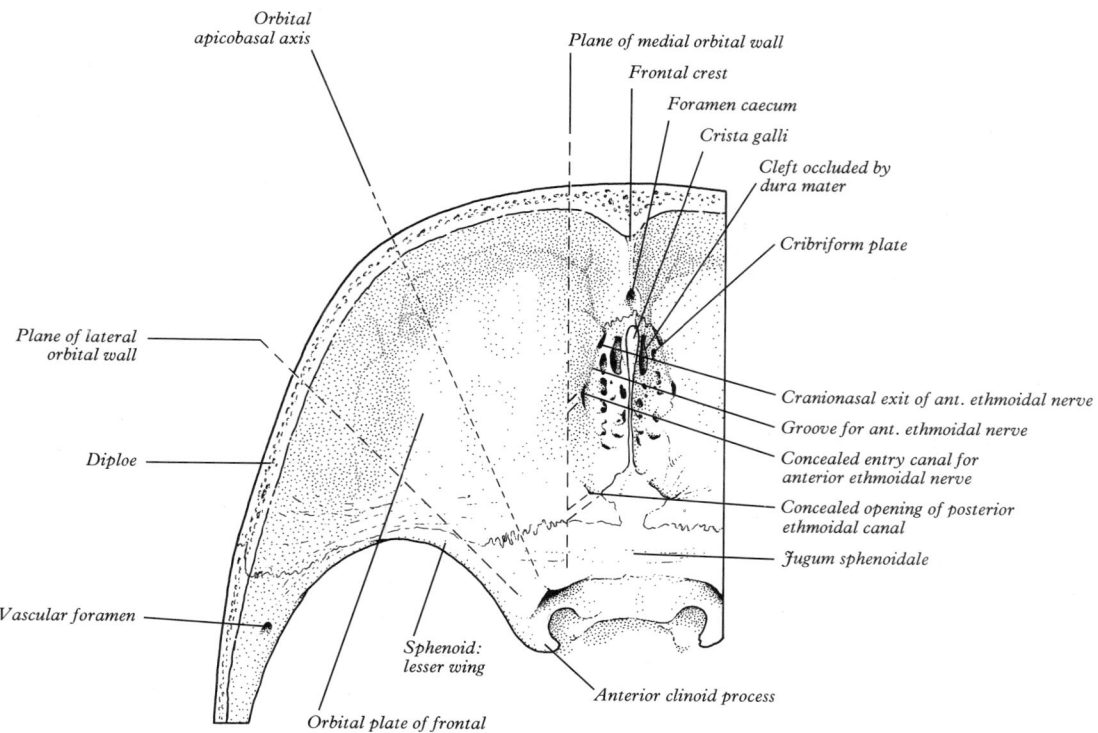

6.151   Anterior cranial fossa.

municates with the orbits by the *superior orbital fissures*, each bounded above by a lesser wing, below by a greater wing, and medially by the sphenoidal body; each fissure is wider medially, with a long axis sloping inferomedially and forwards. Each transmits the terminal branches of the ophthalmic nerve, the ophthalmic veins, the oculomotor, trochlear and abducent nerves and smaller vessels (see below).

Foramen rotundum. This is in the greater sphenoidal wing just below and behind the medial end of the superior orbital fissure. It leads forwards into the pterygopalatine fossa, to which it conducts the maxillary nerve.

Foramen ovale. Is posterior to the foramen rotundum, lateral to the lingula and posterior end of the carotid groove. It opens into the infratemporal fossa and transmits the mandibular nerve.

Foramen spinosum. Posterolateral to foramen ovale, transmits the middle meningeal artery which, with companion veins, ascends lateral to the temporal squama, turns anterolaterally across the sphenosquamosal suture to the greater wing to divide into frontal and parietal branches. The frontal ascending across the pterion (p. 560) to the anterior part of the parietal bone; at or near the pterion it is often in a bony canal. The parietal branch runs back and up on to the temporal squama, crossing the squamosal suture to gain the parietal bone. These arteries and veins groove the floor and lateral wall of the middle cranial fossa.

Foramen lacerum. This is at the posterior end of the carotid groove, posteromedial to the foramen ovale, bounded behind by the petrous apex, in front by the body and posterior border of the sphenoid's greater wing, where it contains the internal carotid artery and accompanying sympathetic and venous plexuses. Posterior to the foramen the anterior surface of the petrous temporal has near its apex a shallow *trigeminal impression* adapted to the trigeminal ganglion. Posterolateral to this is a shallow pit, limited posteriorly by a rounded *arcuate eminence*, and produced by the anterior semicircular canal, where it is closely related to the floor of the fossa. Lateral to the impression a narrow groove passes posterolaterally into the *hiatus for the greater petrosal nerve*, lateral to which is the *hiatus for the lesser petrosal nerve*. Anterolateral to the arcuate eminence the anterior petrous surface is formed by the *tegmen tympani*, a thin osseous lamina in the roof of the tympanic cavity, extending anteromedially above the auditory tube. Lateral to the eminence the posterior part of the tegmen tympani roofs the mastoid

antrum (which is continuously anteriorly with the tympanic cavity). The superior border of the petrous temporal separates middle from posterior cranial fossae. Behind the trigeminal impression it is grooved by the superior petrosal sinus.

Further details

The *superior orbital fissure* (**6**.138) is between the orbit's roof and lateral wall. To its lower border is attached the common tendinous ring. At its superolateral end the greater wing articulates with the

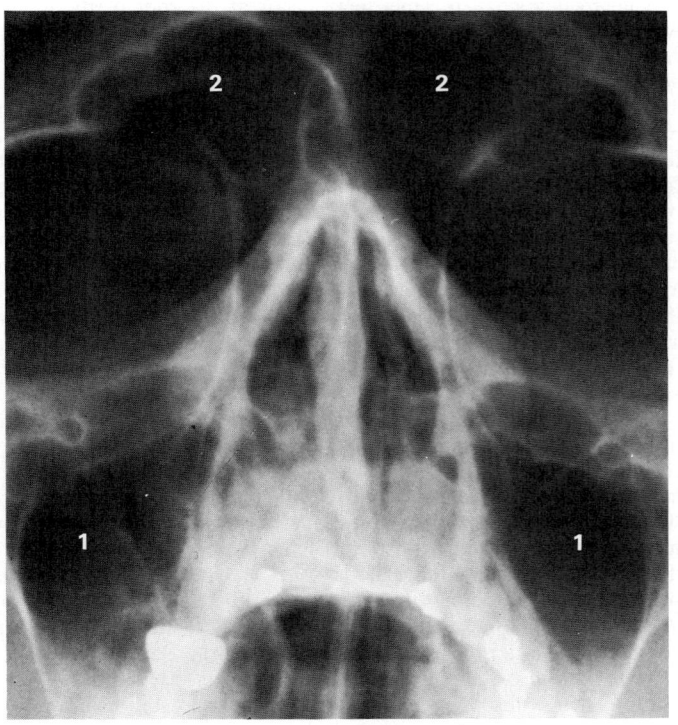

6.152   Radiograph of adult skull: frontal view. 1. Maxillary sinus. 2. Frontal sinus. Both infra-orbital canals are shown.

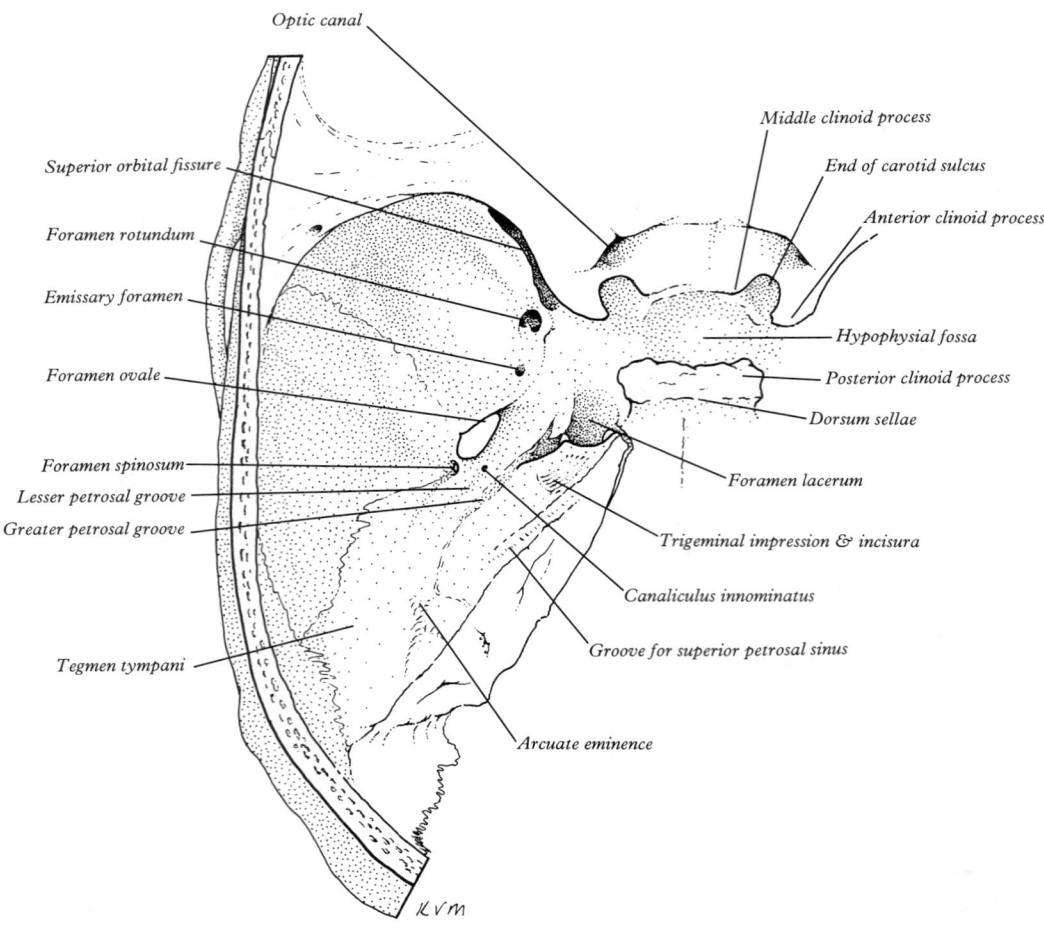

Optic canal

Superior orbital fissure

Foramen rotundum

Emissary foramen

Foramen ovale

Foramen spinosum
Lesser petrosal groove
Greater petrosal groove

Tegmen tympani

Middle clinoid process

End of carotid sulcus

Anterior clinoid process

Hypophysial fossa

Posterior clinoid process

Dorsum sellae

Foramen lacerum

Trigeminal impression & incisura

Canaliculus innominatus

Groove for superior petrosal sinus

Arcuate eminence

6.153   Middle cranial fossa.

frontal orbital plate (p. 595). The *foramen rotundum*, like the superior orbital fissure's medial end, is near the lateral wall of the sphenoidal sinus. Originally part of the fissure, the latter is secondarily separated. Medial to it a small foramen may occur at the root of the greater wing; this *emissary sphenoidal foramen* transmits a vein from the cavernous sinus. The *foramen ovale* transmits the mandibular nerve, accessory meningeal artery and, sometimes, the lesser petrosal nerve. The *foramen spinosum* contains the middle meningeal artery and meningeal branch of the mandibular nerve. Both foramina are at first notches on the greater wing's margin and later converted into foramina. The *foramen lacerum* is a short canal completely **traversed** only by meningeal branches of the ascending pharyngeal artery and small veins. The internal carotid artery pierces its posterior wall and curves to ascend through its upper end. The greater petrosal nerve, leaving its hiatus, runs in its groove on the petrous temporal bone, then turns down to partly traverse the foramen lateral to the artery and joins the deep petrosal nerve. The nerve of the pterygoid canal, thus formed, leaves the foramen lacerum by a *pterygoid canal* in its anterior wall.

On each side of the sphenoid body a cavernous sinus extends from the superior orbital fissure to the apex of petrous temporal bone. It contains the internal carotid artery, its sympathetic plexus, oculomotor, trochlear, abducent and ophthalmic nerves, but only the artery contacts bone. An anterior intercavernous sinus crosses the tuberculum sellae and a posterior sinus crosses the dorsum sellae; they connect the two cavernous sinuses. The diaphragma sellae surrounds the infundibulum, spreading from the tuberculum in front to the dorsum sellae behind. To the posterior clinoid process are attached the anterior limit of the fixed margin of the tentorium cerebelli and also the petrosphenoidal ligament (p. 1240).

In young skulls a petrosquamous suture may be visible at the lateral limit of the *tegmen tympani* but is obliterated in adults; the tegmen then turns down as a lateral wall of the osseous auditory tube; its lower border may appear in the squamotympanic fissure

(p. 590). Lateral to the tegmen's anterior part, the temporal squama is thin over a small area near the mandibular fossa's deepest part.

Anteromedial to the groove for the superior petrosal sinus, on the upper border of the petrous temporal, a smooth *trigeminal notch* leads into the *trigeminal impression*; here the trigeminal nerve separates sinus from bone. To a tiny spicule, directed anteromedially at the notch's anterior end, is attached the petrosphenoidal ligament; anterior to it the abducent nerve bends sharply across the upper petrous border between this ligament and the dorsum sellae.

POSTERIOR CRANIAL FOSSA

The posterior cranial fossa (**6**.150A, 154), the largest and deepest of the cranial fossae, is bounded in front by the dorsum sellae and posterior aspects of the sphenoidal body and basioccipital bone, behind by the lower part of the occipital squama, laterally by petrous and mastoid parts of the temporal bone and lateral parts of the occipital and, above and behind, by the mastoid angles of the parietal bones. It contains the cerebellum, pons and medulla oblongata.

Internal acoustic meatus. This is separated at its *lateral fundus* from the internal ear by a vertical plate divided unequally by a *transverse crest* (**6**.155), above which anteriorly is a *facial canal* conducting its nerve through the petrous temporal to the stylomastoid foramen. Posterior to this a small, depressed *superior vestibular area* presents openings for nerves to the utricle and anterior and lateral semicircular ducts. Below the crest is an anterior *cochlear area* in which a spiral of small holes, the *tractus spiralis foraminosus*, encircles the central cochlear canal. Behind this the *inferior vestibular area* bears openings for saccular nerves. Most posteroinferior is a *foramen singulare* for the nerve to the posterior semicircular duct.

Foramen magnum (p. 567). This is in the fossa's floor, surrounded by the basilar part of the occipital bone in front, its lateral parts on each side and a small part of its squama behind. Anterior to its transverse diameter it is narrowed by the two occipital condyles,

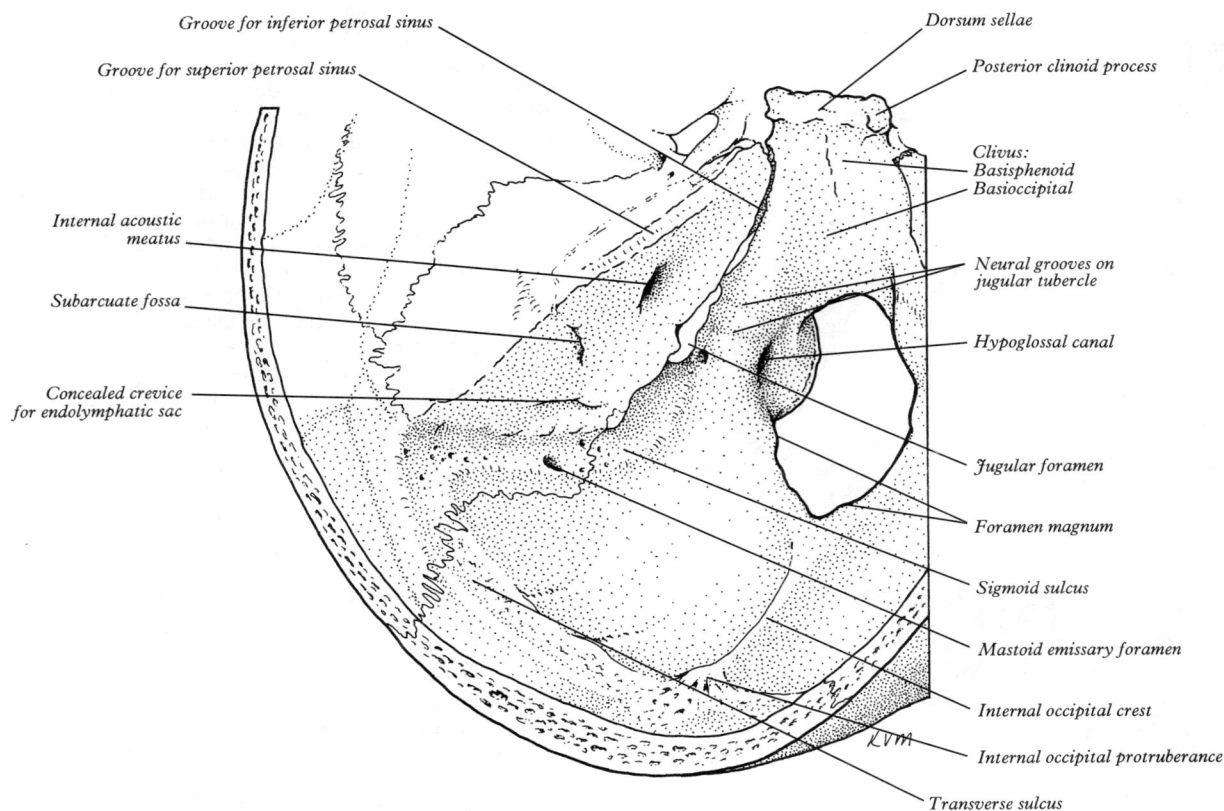

Groove for inferior petrosal sinus

Groove for superior petrosal sinus

Internal acoustic meatus

Subarcuate fossa

Concealed crevice for endolymphatic sac

Dorsum sellae

Posterior clinoid process

Clivus: Basisphenoid Basioccipital

Neural grooves on jugular tubercle

Hypoglossal canal

Jugular foramen

Foramen magnum

Sigmoid sulcus

Mastoid emissary foramen

Internal occipital crest

Internal occipital protruberance

Transverse sulcus

6.154 Left posterior cranial fossa. Viewed obliquely from a position above, slightly behind, and to the right.

being hence somewhat ovoid and wider behind. Its anterior part is above the dens of the axis; its posterior part communicates with the vertebral canal and here the medulla oblongata and spinal cord become continuous.

Anterior to the foramen, in sequence, are the basioccipital, the posterior part of the sphenoid's body and then the dorsum sellae forming a sloping *clivus*, which is concave transversely and placed antero-inferior to the pons and medulla oblongata. On each side the clivus is separated from the petrous temporal bone by a petro-occipital fissure, filled by a thin plate of cartilage and limited behind by the jugular foramen. Its margins are grooved by the inferior petrosal sinus.

Jugular foramen (p. 567). Sited at the posterior end of the petro-occipital fissure, it descends anterolaterally to the exterior. Its upper border is sharp and irregular, with a *notch for the glossopharyngeal nerve*; its lower border is smooth. Posteriorly is the sigmoid sinus, continuous below with the internal jugular vein, and anteriorly the accessory, vagus and glossopharyngeal nerves from behind forwards. Medial to its lower border is the rounded *jugular tubercle*, antero-superior to the internal opening of the *hypoglossal canal*, at the junction of the basilar and lateral parts of the occipital bone.

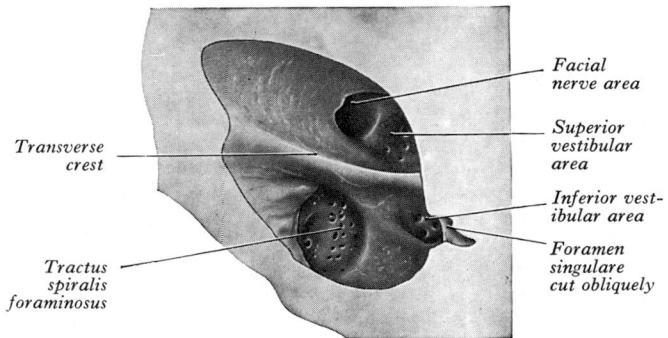

Transverse crest

Tractus spiralis foraminosus

Facial nerve area

Superior vestibular area

Inferior vest-ibular area

Foramen singulare cut obliquely

6.155 The fundus of the right internal acoustic meatus, exposed by a section through the petrous part of the right temporal bone nearly parallel to the line of its superior border.

Further details

The petrous temporal bone's posterior surface forms much of the posterior cranial fossa's anterolateral wall. Anterosuperior to the jugular foramen the *internal acoustic meatus* (6.150, 153, 154) runs laterally. It is about 1 cm long, closed laterally by a plate of bone separating it from the internal ear and perforated by facial and vestibulocochlear nerves, nervus intermedius and labyrinthine vessels.

Behind the petrous temporal (the posterior fossa's lateral wall) is the mastoid part of the temporal bone. Anteriorly is a wide *sigmoid sulcus* running forwards and downwards, then downwards and medially and finally forwards to the jugular foramen. It contains the sigmoid sinus (6.150, 174). Superiorly, where it touches the parietal bone's mastoid angle, the groove is continuous with one for the transverse sinus, and crosses the parietomastoid suture. It descends **behind** the *mastoid antrum* and here is sited a *mastoid foramen* for an emissary vein from the sinus. The lowest part of the sulcus crosses the occipitomastoid suture and grooves the occipital bone's jugular process. The right sulcus is usually larger.

Posterior to the foramen magnum the occipital squama has a median *internal occipital crest*, ending above in an *internal occipital protuberance*, on each side of which a wide sulcus curves laterally with an upward convexity, to the parietal bone's mastoid angle. Produced by the transverse sinus, it is usually deeper on the right and, on both sides, continuous with its sigmoid sulcus. Below this *transverse sulcus* the internal occipital crest separates two shallow fossae, adapted to the cerebellar hemispheres.

When a *condylar canal* is present, its internal orifice is postero-lateral to that of the hypoglossal canal. It contains a sigmoid emissary vein.

The clivus (anterior wall of the posterior fossa) is related to the plexus of basilar sinuses connecting the inferior petrosal sinuses and joining below the internal vertebral venous plexus. Anterior to the foramen magnum the membrana tectoria is attached to the basi-occipital (6.104), behind attachment of the apical ligament. The jugular tubercle is often grooved by the glossopharyngeal, vagus and accessory nerves as they enter the jugular foramen. In addition to its nerve the hypoglossal canal, often subdivided (p. 584), transmits a meningeal branch of the ascending pharyngeal artery. To the rough

573

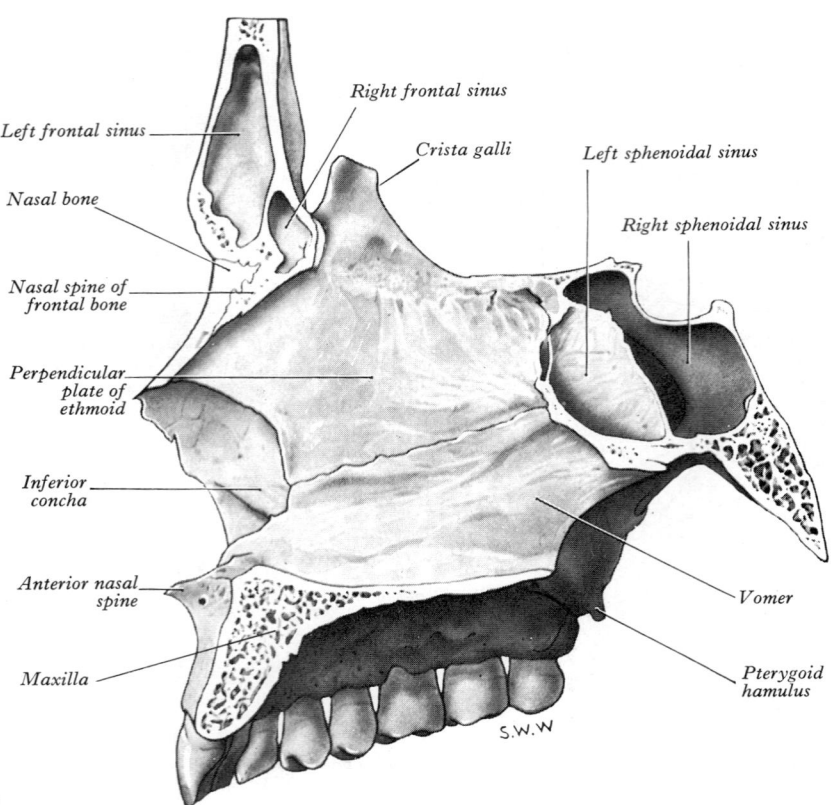

Left frontal sinus

Nasal bone

Nasal spine of frontal bone

Perpendicular plate of ethmoid

Inferior concha

Anterior nasal spine

Maxilla

Right frontal sinus

Crista galli

Left sphenoidal sinus

Right sphenoidal sinus

Vomer

Pterygoid hamulus

S.W.W.

6.156   The bony nasal septum: left side. An enlarged part of **6**.158.

medial aspect of the occipital condyle (see **6**.166B) the alar ligament is attached.

The lower, posterior borders of the jugular foramen (pp. 567, 572) are smooth, its upper border being sharp and notched; sometimes the margins of the notch extend to divide the foramen into two or three compartments. In the deepest part of the notch appears the *cochlear canaliculus*, containing the perilymphatic 'duct' (p. 1379).

Behind the internal acoustic meatus a thin plate with an irregularly curved margin projects back, bounding a slit containing the *vestibular*

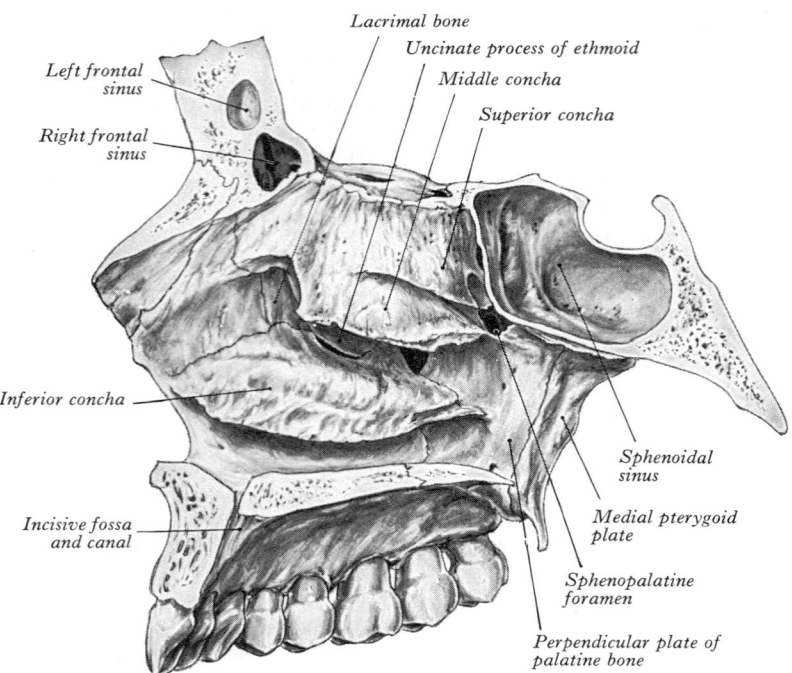

Lacrimal bone

Uncinate process of ethmoid

Middle concha

Superior concha

Left frontal sinus

Right frontal sinus

Inferior concha

Sphenoidal sinus

Medial pterygoid plate

Incisive fossa and canal

Sphenopalatine foramen

Perpendicular plate of palatine bone

6.157A.   The roof, floor and lateral wall of the right nasal cavity.

aqueduct's opening (see **6**.174); within, it carries the saccus and ductus endolymphaticus (p. 1384) and a small artery and vein. Between the internal acoustic meatus and aqueductal opening is a small *subarcuate fossa* (**6**.150B, 174), containing dura mater; near the superior petrous border the fossa is pierced by a small vein. In infants the fossa is a relatively large blind tunnel under the anterior semicircular duct; it corresponds to the floccular fossa of some animals.

In addition to its emissary vein the *mastoid foramen* transmits a meningeal branch of the occipital artery, sometimes large enough to groove the occipital squama. The internal occipital crest, to which the falx cerebelli is attached, may be grooved by the occipital sinus. Its lower end adjoins the inferior vermis. The internal occipital protuberance is close to the confluence of sinuses and bilaterally grooved by the transverse sinuses, to the margins of which are attached the two layers of the tentorium cerebelli. Bone flanking the internal occipital crest is thin, even translucent, contrasting with the occipital's thick crest and protuberance.

NASAL CAVITY

The nasal cavity, an irregular space between buccal roof and cranial base, is divided by a vertical *septum* (**6**.156), approximately median. In macerated skulls the septum is deficient anteriorly, leaving a single *anterior nasal aperture* in norma frontalis, but it reaches the posterior limit of the cavity, leading into the nasopharynx through a pair of *posterior nasal apertures*, above the posterior osseous (hard) palatal border. The cavity is wider below than above, but widest and vertically deepest in its central region. It communicates with the frontal, ethmoidal, maxillary and sphenoidal paranasal sinuses. Each half cavity has a roof, floor, lateral and medial walls, the medial being the nasal septum.

The posterior nasal apertures, or choanae. These are separated by the posterior vomerine border, each being limited below by the posterior border of the palatine bone's horizontal plate, above by the sphenoid and laterally, on each side, by its medial pterygoid plates.

The anterior nasal aperture. This is described on page 554.

Roof

The roof (**6**.156, 157) is centrally horizontal but descends in front and behind. The anterior slope is formed by the frontal's nasal spine and nasal bones, contributing to the external nose. The horizontal region is the ethmoid's cribriform plate separating the nasal cavity and median region of anterior cranial fossa's floor, and has a separate anterior foramen for the anterior ethmoidal nerve and vessels. Its numerous small perforations contain the olfactory nerves. The posterior slope is formed by the anterior aspect of the body of the sphenoid (interrupted on each side by an opening of a sphenoidal sinus), with which the sphenoidal conchae are fused; below this are the vomerine alae and palatine bones' sphenoidal processes.

Floor

The floor is smooth, concave transversely, and slopes up from anterior to posterior apertures. It is the upper surface of the osseous palate. Anteriorly the maxillary palatine processes and, behind them, the palatine horizontal plates articulate in the midline and with each other. Anteriorly, near the septum, a small infundibular opening in the nasal floor leads into the *incisive canals* (p. 602).

The nasal floor (**6**.157A) is crossed at the junction of its middle and posterior thirds by the palatomaxillary suture. Anteromedian are the incisive canals, descending to the palatine incisive fossa; they may traverse the union of the os incisivum (premaxilla) with the maxillae; they represent a primitive bucconasal communication (p. 602).

The medial wall

The medial wall or *nasal septum* (**6**.156, 158), between the roof and floor, is a thin sheet of bone with a wide anterior deficiency occupied by septal cartilage; its bony part is largely vomer and perpendicular plate of the ethmoid. The *vomer* extends from the sphenoidal body to the bony palate, forming the posteroinferior region, including the posterior border; it is furrowed by vessels and nerves. The *perpendicular plate* of the *ethmoid* forms the septum's anterosuperior part (**6**.156), continuous above with cribriform plate (p. 597). The septum is often deviated, most commonly at the vomero-ethmoidal suture.

At the upper and lower limits of the medial wall (**6**.157B) other bones make minor contributions to the septum: anterosuperior are the nasal bones and frontal's nasal spine, posterosuperior are the sphenoid's rostrum and crest, and inferiorly, the maxillary and palatine nasal crests. The vomer is grooved by the nasopalatine nerves and vessels.

The lateral wall

The lateral wall (**6**.157, 183) is irregular, due to three projections: the inferior, middle and superior nasal *conchae*. It is formed largely by the maxilla anteroinferiorly, by the palatine's perpendicular plate posteriorly, and superiorly by the ethmoidal labyrinth, separating the nasal cavity from the orbit. The conchae curve inferomedially, each roofing a groove, or meatus, open to the nasal cavity.

The inferior concha. This is a thin, curved and independent bone and articulates with the nasal surface of the maxilla and palatine perpendicular plate; its free lower border is gently curved; the subjacent *inferior meatus* reaches the nasal floor. It is the largest meatus, extending along almost all the lateral nasal wall. It is deepest at the junction of its anterior and middle thirds, where the inferior opening of the nasolacrimal canal appears.

The middle concha. Much the larger, it extends back to articulate with the palatine bone's perpendicular plate above the *middle meatus*, whose lateral wall can be examined only after the removal of the concha (**6**.157B); its upper part is the rounded *ethmoidal bulla*, which contains middle ethmoidal air cells; anteroinferior to this a thin, curved *uncinate process* of the *ethmoid* descends back across the large opening of the maxillary sinus. The curved gap (**6**.157B) between process and bulla is the *hiatus semilunaris*; at its upper end it is continuous with the *ethmoidal infundibulum*, a short canal receiving anterior ethmoidal air cells and then ascending in the labyrinth to the frontal sinus. However, the infundibulum often ends blindly; the frontal sinus then opens directly into the middle meatus. The middle ethmoidal air cells open above, or near, the bulla.

The superior concha. A small curved lamina, posterosuperior to the middle concha, it roofs the *superior meatus*. It is the shortest and shallowest of the three conchae and receives into it open the posterior ethmoidal air cells. Posterior to it the sphenopalatine foramen (occluded by mucosa) leads into the pterygopalatine fossa. A narrow *sphenoethmoidal recess* separates the superior concha and anterior aspect of the sphenoid's body, through which the sphenoidal sinus connects with the nasal cavity. The *middle* and *superior conchae* are medial processes of the ethmoidal labyrinth.

Further details. The lateral wall (**6**.157, 183), additionally, is formed anterosuperiorly by the nasal bone and maxillary's frontal process. Behind the latter, and articulating with its posterior border, lies the lacrimal bone which reaches the middle meatus to articulate with the lacrimal process of the inferior concha, thus forming the nasolacrimal canal's medial wall (**6**.157B, 186), which conveys the nasolacrimal duct to the inferior meatus. Posteriorly the lacrimal bone articulates with the ethmoidal labyrinth to complete some of the ethmoidal air cells. The *uncinate process* from this part of the labyrinth curves posteroinferiorly in the lateral middle meatal wall. It is thin, fragile, about 3 mm wide, and curves across the maxillary hiatus to the inferior conchal ethmoidal process. Its concave, posterior border forms the medial edge of the hiatus semilunaris and helps to form a medial wall of the maxillary sinus; its convex anterior border is free only above. The *maxillary hiatus*, a wide defect in the maxillary's nasal surface (see **6**.194A), is much reduced by neighbouring bones; being covered below by the inferior concha and its maxillary process, above by ethmoid's uncinate process, behind by palatine's perpendicular plate and anterosuperiorly by small parts of ethmoidal labyrinth and lacrimal bone (**6**.157B). Thus the hiatus is sometimes reduced to a single orifice in the floor of the posterior part of the hiatus semilunaris, but usually additional openings exist both between the inferior concha and the uncinate process and also behind the uncinate process. The *ethmoidal bulla*, variable in size and shape, may be fused with the uncinate process, and then the duct of the frontal sinus opens into the middle meatus medial to the blind end of the infundibulum. A *concha suprema* often exists on the medial surface of the ethmoidal labyrinth posterosuperior to the superior concha's posterior end (sphenoethmoidal recess); it is merely a ridge, separated from the superior concha by a depression. The *sphenopalatine foramen* (**6**.157A) is posterior to the superior meatus and transmits the sphenopalatine artery and nasopalatine and

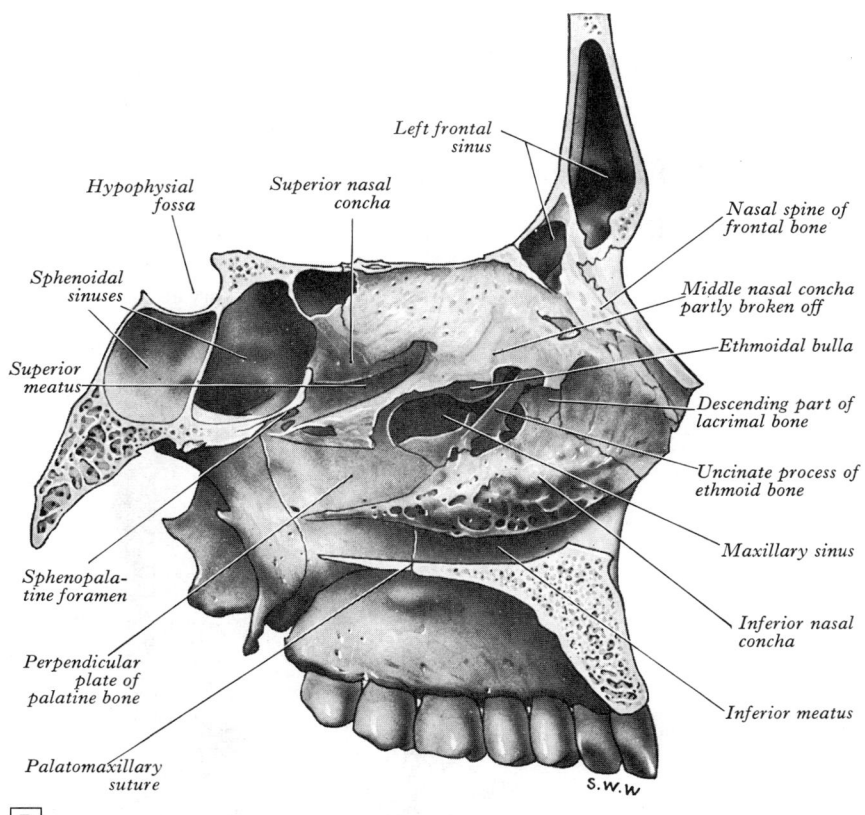

Left frontal sinus

Hypophysial fossa

Superior nasal concha

Nasal spine of frontal bone

Sphenoidal sinuses

Middle nasal concha partly broken off

Ethmoidal bulla

Superior meatus

Descending part of lacrimal bone

Uncinate process of ethmoid bone

Sphenopala- tine foramen

Maxillary sinus

Inferior nasal concha

Perpendicular plate of palatine bone

Palatomaxillary suture

Inferior meatus

S.W.W

B

6.157B. The lateral wall of the left nasal cavity with part of the middle concha removed to expose some of the middle meatus.

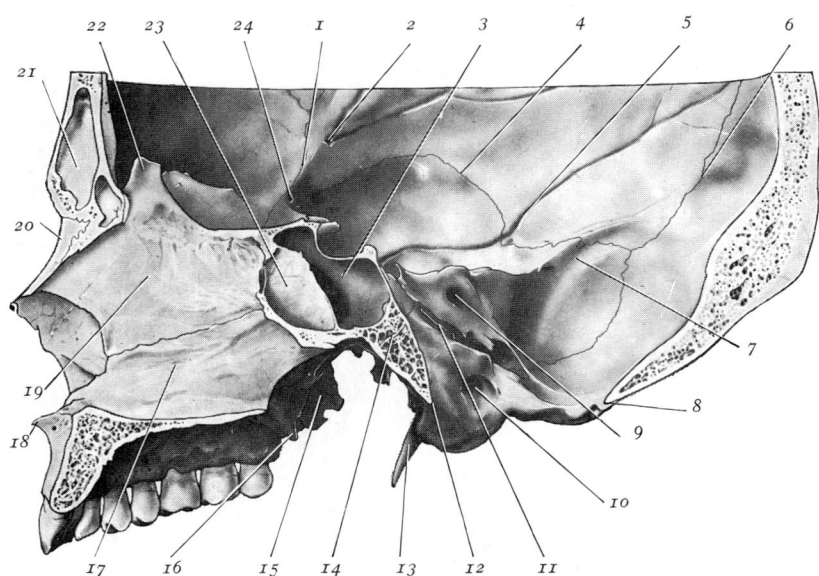

6.158 Sagittal section through the lower part of the skull, slightly to the left of the median plane. 1. Frontosphenoidal suture. 2. Bony canal for middle meningeal vessels, frontal branches, upper orifice. 3. Right sphenoidal sinus. 4. Squamosal suture. 5. Groove for parietal branches of middle meningeal vessels. 6. Lambdoid suture. 7. Groove for transverse sinus. 8. Posterior margin of foramen magnum. 9. Internal acoustic meatus. 10. Hypoglossal canal. 11. Petro-occipital suture in floor of groove for inferior petrosal sinus. 12. Anterior margin of foramen magnum. 13. Styloid process. 14. Line of occipitosphenoidal junction. 15. Lateral pterygoid plate. 16. Pterygoid hamulus. 17. Vomer. 18. Anterior nasal spine. 19. Perpendicular plate of ethmoid. 20. Nasal bone. 21. Frontal sinus. 22. Crista galli. 23. Left sphenoidal sinus. 24. Bony canal for frontal divisions of middle meningeal vessels, lower orifice.

superior nasal nerves from the pterygopalatine fossa. The foramen is bounded above by the sphenoidal body and concha, below by the superior border of palatine perpendicular plate, in front and behind by the palatine's orbital and sphenoidal processes (see **6.194, 195**).

INDIVIDUAL CRANIAL BONES

MANDIBLE

The mandible (**6.159**), the largest, strongest and lowest bone in the face, has a horizontally curved *body*, convex forwards, and two broad *rami*, ascending posteriorly.

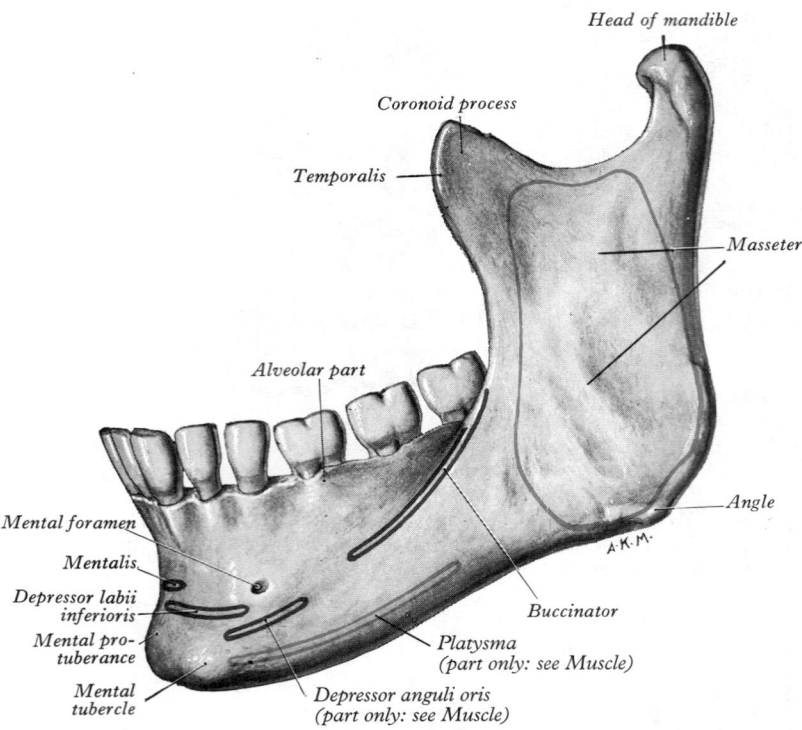

6.159A.   The left half of the mandible: lateral (external) aspect.

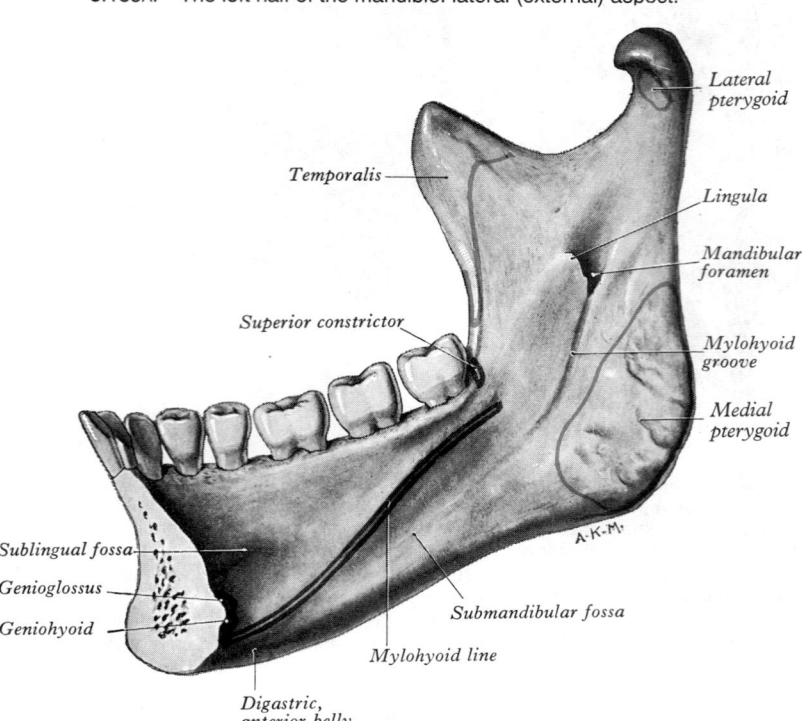

576   **6.159B.**   The right half of the mandible: medial (internal) aspect.

Mandibular body

The mandibular body, somewhat U-shaped, has external and internal surfaces, separated by upper and lower borders. Anteriorly, the upper *external surface* shows a faint median ridge, often absent, indicating fusion of the halves of the fetal bone (*symphysis menti*); inferiorly this ridge divides to enclose a *triangular mental protuberance*, its base centrally depressed but raised on each side as a *mental tubercle*. Below the interval between the premolar teeth, or the second premolar, is the *mental foramen*, from which emerge the mental nerve and vessels; its posterior border is smooth accommodating the posterolaterally emerging nerve (Warwick 1950a). A faint *oblique line* ascends backwards from each mental tubercle, sweeping below the foramen, becoming more marked as it continues into the anterior border of the ramus.

The body's lower border, the *base*, extends posterolaterally from the symphysis into that of the ramus behind the third molar tooth. Near the midline, on each side, is a rough *digastric fossa*, behind which the base is thick and rounded, with a slight anteroposterior convexity. As the ramus is approached, this changes to a gentle concavity; thus, in profile, the whole base is sinuous.

The upper border, the *alveolar part*, contains 16 *alveoli* for roots of teeth, varying in size and depth, some being multiple.

The *internal surface* is divided by an oblique *mylohyoid line*, sharp and distinct near the molars, faint in front and extending from behind the third molar, a centimetre from the upper border, to the mental symphysis between the digastric fossae. Below this line is the slightly concave *submandibular fossa*; the area above it widens anteriorly into a triangular *sublingual fossa*. Above the latter and extending back to the third molar, the bone is covered by oral mucosa. Above the anterior ends of the mylohyoid lines, the posterior symphyseal aspect has a small elevation, often divided into upper and lower parts, the *mental spines* (genial tubercles). Posteriorly the *mylohyoid groove* extends down and forwards from the ramus below the mylohyoid line's posterior part. Superior to the mental spines most mandibles display a *lingual (genial) foramen* opening into a canal, which traverses the bone to approximately 50% of the buccomandibular dimension of the mandible (McDonnell et al 1994): it contains a branch of the lingual artery. As yet its development is uncertain; however, it is a useful radiological landmark see also *accessory mandibular foramina*, p. 577.) Above the mylohyoid line, medial to the molar roots, a rounded torus mandibularis sometimes appears: for its incidence consult Mayhall et al (1970) and Berry (1975).

Mandibular ramus

The mandibular ramus (**6.159**) is quadrilateral, with two surfaces, four borders and two processes. The flat *lateral surface* has oblique ridges in its lower part; the medial presents, a little above centre, an irregular *mandibular foramen*, leading into the *mandibular canal*, curving downwards and forwards into the body to its mental foramen (but see below and p. 577). Anteromedially the foramen is overlapped by a thin, triangular *lingula*. The *mylohyoid groove* descends forwards from behind the lingula; the surface behind it being marked by short ridges. The *inferior border*, continuous with the mandibular base, meets the posterior border at the *angle*. This is typically everted, but in females frequently inverted. The thin *upper border* bounds the *mandibular incisure*, surmounted in front by the somewhat triangular, flat, *coronoid process*, behind by a strong *condylar process*. The *posterior border*, thick and rounded, extends from the condyle to the angle, being gently convex backwards above, and concave below; it is in contact with the parotid gland. The *anterior border* is thin above and continuous with that of the coronoid process, and thicker below and continuous with the oblique line.

The ramus and its processes provide attachment for muscles of mastication, much of its *lateral surface* to masseter, except posterosuperiorly, where it is covered by the parotid gland; the *medial surface* receives the medial pterygoid on the roughened area posteroinferior to the mylohyoid groove. To the *lingula* the sphenomandibular ligament is attached, posterior to which the mylohyoid nerve and vessels enter the *mylohyoid groove*, reaching the mandibular body below the mylohyoid line; they then pass superficial to mylohyoid. Below the lingula, but above the roughened attachment mentioned above, the medial surface of the ramus is related to the medial pterygoid, the lingual nerve being between the muscle and bone. The lowest attachment of temporalis descends beyond the coronoid process to the anterior ramal border and particularly its adjoining medial surface. To the area posterosuperior to the mandibular foramen the maxillary artery and its inferior alveolar branch are related, and lateral pterygoid to the area near the mandibular incisure. The mandibular incisure transmits the masseteric nerve and vessels from the infratemporal fossa.

Coronoid process. This projects upwards and slightly forwards. Its posterior border bounds the mandibular incisure; its anterior continues into that of the ramus. Its margins and medial surface are attachments for most of temporalis. It is covered laterally by the anterior part of masseter descending to its attachment on the ramus. The *anterior border* is palpable below the zygoma, most evident when opening the mouth.

Condylar process. Apically enlarged as the fibrocartilage covered *head* or *condyle*, it projects more at its medial pole to articulate with the temporal bone's mandibular fossa via an intermediate articular disc. It is convex in all directions, with the transverse dimension being greater. Its lateral aspect is a blunt projection, palpable in front of the auricular tragus. As the mouth opens the condyle descends forwards, admitting a finger-tip towards its vacated fossa. Below the head is the narrower *neck*, slightly flattened from before backwards, its anterior aspect overlapped laterally by the mandibular incisure's margin, medial to which the neck's anterior surface bears a rough *pterygoid fovea*.

Further details. The *articular surface* descends only a little on its anterior surface, but covers the whole of its superior aspect and descends 5 mm posteriorly. Its projecting lateral part is separated from the cartilaginous external acoustic meatus by the parotid gland. Laterally on its neck the lateral ligament of the temporomandibular joint is attached (see **6.162A**), covered by the parotid gland. The pterygoid fovea, anterior on the neck, receives the lateral pterygoid. The neck's medial surface is related to the auriculotemporal nerve above and maxillary artery below.

The *parotid gland* is below the external acoustic meatus and lies between the ramus and mastoid process, with the styloid process medial; but it extends forwards lateral to the temporomandibular joint and to the exposed ramus behind the masseter. It also curls round the posterior border to the medial aspect of the ramus above the attachment of medial pterygoid.

Mandibular canal. This descends obliquely forwards in the ramus from the mandibular foramen, then horizontally forwards in the body below the alveoli, with which it communicates by small canals. It contains the inferior alveolar nerve and vessels, from which branches enter tooth roots, periodontal sockets and septa. Between the roots of the first and second premolars, or below the second, the canal divides into *mental* and *incisive* parts; the mental canal swerves up, back and laterally to the mental foramen; the incisive canal continues below the incisor teeth. (See p. 1700 for variations.)

Mandibular body. This bears a small shallow *incisive fossa* below the incisors, an attachment for mentalis and part of orbicularis oris. To the anterior ends of the oblique lines are attached depressors labii inferioris and anguli oris, and platysma to bone below and backwards beyond them. Adjoining the alveolar border, bone is covered by oral mucosa and, below this in the molar region, the buccinator has a linear attachment extending medially behind the last molar to the pterygomandibular raphe.

Mylohyoid line. It gives attachment to the mylohyoid muscle and, above its posterior end, the superior pharyngeal constrictor, some retromolar fasicles of the buccinator, and the *pterygomandibular raphe* behind the third molar. Although usually described separately, here the constrictor, buccinator and the raphe are blended and jointly attach to the mandibular periosteum. The lingual nerve reaches the tongue above the mylohyoid line, closely related to bone near its posterior end (p. 1239); often the nerve is accommodated in a shallow, curved groove. To the superior mental spines are attached the genioglossi, to the inferior the geniohyoids. The *submandibular fossa* adjoins submandibular lymph nodes as well as the salivary gland; the facial artery usually descends here to curl round the base of the mandible, sometimes making a shallow groove. The *digastric fossa* is for attachment of the anterior belly of digastric.

Accessory foramina of the mandible. These are usually unnamed and infrequently described. Yet a study of 300 mandibles yielded a count of 2449 accessory foramina (Sutton 1974). Since many transmit auxiliary nerves to teeth (from facial, mylohyoid, buccal, transverse cervical cutaneous and other nerves), their occurrence is significant in dental blocking techniques.

Further mandibular variants. These include *lingual depressions*, molar or canine, *variable position of mental foramen, multiple mental foramina, lingual fenestrations* of molar sockets, *retromolar foramina* and *condylar defects*. For incidences in 125 mandibles see Azaz and Lustmann (1973).

Aspects of mandibular structure

In addition to variable mandibular canals (Fawcett 1895; Carter & Keen 1971), numerous analyses have been made of the structure of surface tables and buttresses of compact bone and the geometry of trabeculation in attempts to relate these to habitual functional stresses (Beltrani 1946; Seipel 1948; Dal Pont 1960; Scott & Symons 1977; Mercier et al 1970a,b). Holographic interferometry has been used to study surface strains induced by orthodontic forces (Hewitt 1977).

Ossification

The mandible forms in dense fibromembranous tissue lateral to the inferior alveolar nerve and its incisive branch and also in the lower parts of Meckel's cartilage (**6.160**). Each half is ossified from a centre appearing near the mental foramen about the sixth week, i.e. just after the clavicle's primary centre (p. 620). From this, ossification spreads medially and posterocranially to form the body and ramus, first below, then around the inferior alveolar nerve and incisive branch and upwards, initially forming a trough and later crypts for developing teeth. By the tenth week Meckel's cartilage below the incisor rudiments is surrounded and invaded by bone (p. 277. Secondary cartilages appear later (**6.160**): a conical mass, the *condylar cartilage*, extends from the mandibular head downwards and forwards in the ramus, contributing to its growth in height; though it is largely replaced by bone by midfetal life, its proximal end persists as proliferating cartilage under articular fibrocartilage until the third decade. The orientation and growth patterns in the condylar cartilage are one (of many) important determinants of co-ordinated craniofacial growth. Another secondary cartilage, which soon ossifies,

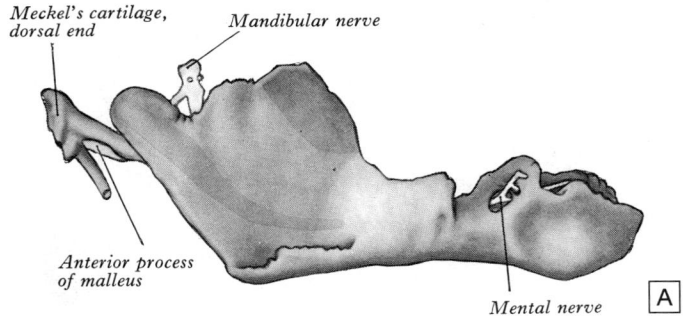

Meckel's cartilage, dorsal end
Mandibular nerve
Anterior process of malleus
Mental nerve
A

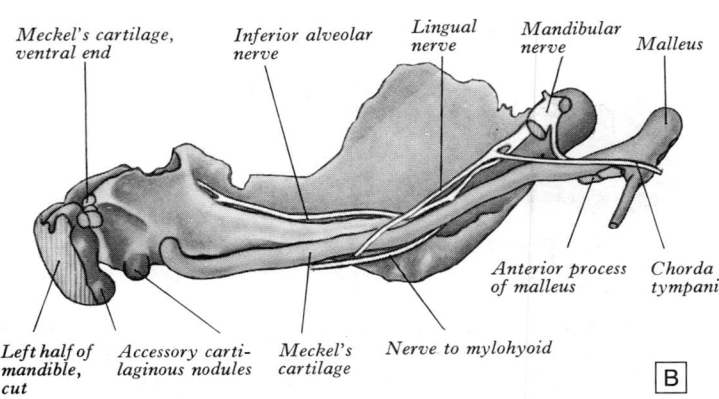

Meckel's cartilage, ventral end
Inferior alveolar nerve
Lingual nerve
Mandibular nerve
Malleus
Anterior process of malleus
Chorda tympani
Left half of mandible, cut
Accessory cartilaginous nodules
Meckel's cartilage
Nerve to mylohyoid
B

6.160 The right half of the mandible of a human embryo, 95 mm long; A. lateral aspect; B. medial aspect. Blue = cartilage; yellow = bone. (Reconstruction by A Low.)

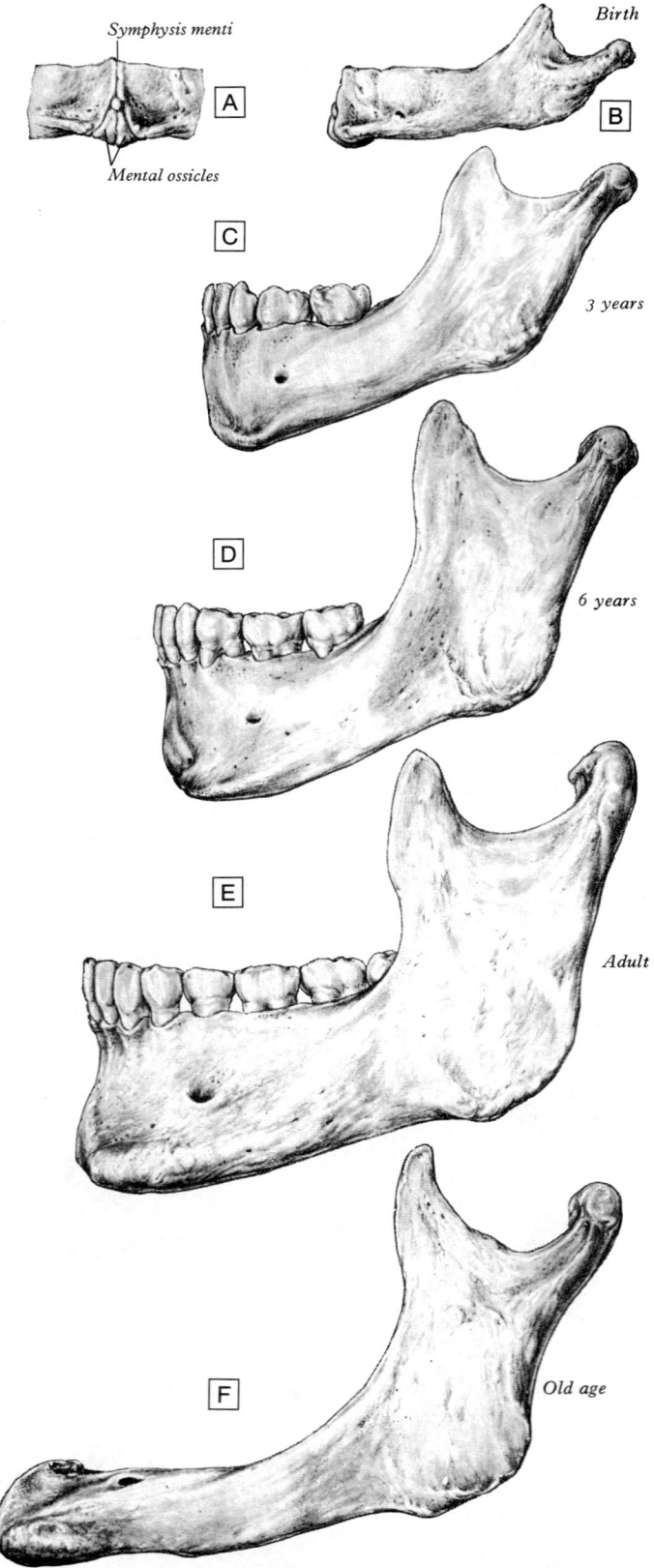

Symphysis menti

A

B *Birth*

Mental ossicles

C *3 years*

D *6 years*

E *Adult*

F *Old age*

6.161   The mandible at different periods of life.

growth in condylar cartilage, which expanded by surface accretion only (Kvinnsland & Kvinnsland 1975).

Age changes in the mandible

At birth (**6**.161) the two halves of the mandible are united by a fibrous *symphysis menti*. Anterior ends of both rudiments are covered by cartilage, separated only by a symphysis. Until fusion occurs new cells are added to each cartilage from symphyseal fibrous tissue, ossification on its mandibular side proceeding towards the midline; when the latter process overtakes the former, extending into median fibrous tissue, the symphysis fuses but details are uncertain. At this stage the body is a mere shell, enclosing imperfectly separated sockets of deciduous teeth. The mandibular canal is near the lower border; the mental foramen opens below the first deciduous molar and is directed forwards (Warwick 1950a). The coronoid process projects above the condyle.

In the first to third postnatal years (**6**.161) the two halves join at their symphysis from below upwards; separation near the alveolar margin may persist into the second year. The body elongates, especially behind the mental foramen, providing space for three additional teeth (pp. 1712–1718). During the first and second years, as a chin develops, the mental foramen alters direction from anterior to posterosuperior, and then almost horizontally posterior, as in adults (Warwick 1950), accommodating a changing direction of the emerging mental nerve. The proximal zone of the conical condylar cartilage persists as an epiphyseal plate. Its proliferation contributes to the vertical increase in the ramus and to general mandibular growth which is essentially **downwards** and **forwards**. With its antimere it also adapts the intercondylar distance to the widening cranial base. The condylar cartilage is covered on its articular aspect by self-perpetuating fibrous tissue, deep to which a proliferating intermediate zone is responsible for ramal growth and thus displacement of the whole mandible. Beneath this are hypertrophic chondrocytes and then bone (Blackwood 1959). As the depth of the body increases, alveolar growth makes room for the roots of the teeth, the subalveolar region becoming thicker and deeper. After eruption of permanent teeth (**6**.161D,E) the mandibular canal is a little above the mylohyoid line, and the mental foramen occupies its adult position. As the mandible increases in size, bone is added at the posterior borders of the ramus and coronoid process, absorption occurring at their anterior borders. This remodelling is continuous until adult size is reached, allowing alveolar parts to accommodate the permanent molar teeth (Enlow & Harris 1964). Organ culture of condylar cartilage in rats shows no growth potential, but in vivo all mandibular growth cartilages respond to mechanical forces (Petrovic 1972).

In adults (**6**.161E) alveolar and subalveolar regions are about equal in depth, with the mental foramen midway between the upper and lower borders; the mandibular canal nearly parallels the mylohyoid line. The *angle* between the lower border of the body and a plane touching the posterior surface of condyle above, and ramus below, diminishes as ramal height increases with age; but radiographs at different ages (Brodie 1941) show that its (*genial*) *contour* remains unaltered.

In old age (**6**.161F) the bone is reduced in size as teeth are lost and the alveolar region absorbed; the mandibular canal and mental foramen are nearer the superior border. Both may even disappear, exposing the inferior alveolar nerve (Gabriel 1958). The ramus becomes oblique, the angle about 140°, and the neck inclined backwards (Fawcett et al 1924). Absorption affects chiefly the thinner alveolar wall (lingual or labial) and, after completion, a linear *alveolar ridge* is left at the superior border of the mandible (and inferior border of the maxilla). In the mandible the labial wall is thinner in incisor and canine regions, the lingual wall in the molar. The mandibular alveolar ridge hence is within the line of teeth in the former but outside it in molar regions, forming a curve wider posteriorly than that of the line of the teeth, but intersecting it near the premolars. In the maxilla, however, the labial wall is everywhere thinner and after absorption its maxillary alveolar ridge is entirely within the line of the teeth.

TEMPOROMANDIBULAR JOINTS

Each joint involves the temporal articular tubercle and anterior part of the mandibular fossa above and mandibular condyle below.

appears along the anterior coronoid border, disappearing before birth. One or two cartilaginous nodules also occur at the symphysis menti; about the seventh month these may ossify as variable *mental ossicles* in symphyseal fibrous tissue, uniting to adjacent bone before the end of the first postnatal year (Lebourg & Champagne 1951; Sicher 1962; Scott & Symons 1977; and **6**.161A). It may be mentioned here that H-thymidine labelling in the *rat* showed no interstitial

Articular surfaces are covered by white fibrocartilage in which collagen fibres predominate and cartilage cells are few. An articular disc divides the joint, usually completely, into upper and lower parts. (Sometimes, however, the disc is perforated.) Commonly described as 'condylar', they are preferably termed *ellipsoid*, right and left joints forming a *bicondylar* articulation.

Fibrous capsule

Each part of the joint can be considered to be surrounded by short capsular fibres which stretch from the condyle to the disc, and from the disc to the temporal bone forming two joint capsules (Fennol et al 1992). Longer bands extending from the condyle to the temporal bone may be regarded as reinforcing fibres. However, true capsular fibres passing between the mandible and temporal bone are present only on the lateral side of the joint: posteriorly, anteriorly and medially the upper and lower laminae of the articular disc are attached separately either to the temporal bone or mandibular condyle (Schmolke 1994). The 'capsule' is attached **above** anteriorly to the articular tubercle, posteriorly to the lips of the squamo-tympanic fissure and between these to the edges of the mandibular fossa; **below** to the mandibular neck. Above the articular disc it is loose; below it is taut.

Synovial membrane. This lines the capsule, above and below the disc (but does not cover the disc); thus, on each side it lines the non-articular surfaces of both superior and inferior synovial compartments. Below the disc the capsular synovial membrane is reflected upwards along the mandible's neck and lateral pterygoid tendon to reach the condylar articular cartilage.

The lateral temporomandibular ligament

The lateral temporomandibular ligament (**6**.162A), close to the capsule, is attached above to the tubercle on the zygoma's root, below to the lateral surface and posterior border of the mandibular neck, its fibres sloping **downwards** and **backwards** deep to the parotid gland. Variations (macroscopic and microscopic) in the ligament have been reported (Nell et al 1994).

Sphenomandibular ligament

The sphenomandibular ligament (**6**.162B), medial to and separate from the capsule, is a flat, thin band descending from the spine of the sphenoid and widening to reach the lingula of the mandibular foramen. Superolateral to it are the lateral pterygoid muscle and auriculotemporal nerve; inferior to this it is separated from the mandibular neck by maxillary vessels, below which the inferior alveolar vessels and nerve and a parotid lobule separate it from the mandibular ramus; here the vessels and nerve to the mylohyoid pierce the ligament with the medial pterygoid muscle inferomedial. It is separated from the pharynx by fat and pharyngeal veins and, near its upper end, is crossed by the chorda tympani. Some fibres traverse the medial end of the petrotympanic fissure to the anterior malleolar process as a vestige (the anterior ligament of the malleus) of the dorsal end of Meckel's cartilage (p. 277). The role of this vestigial ligament in mandibular mechanics is negligible.

Stylomandibular ligament

The stylomandibular ligament (**6**.162A), a specialized band of deep cervical fascia (p. 802), stretches from the apex and adjacent anterior aspect of the styloid process to the mandible's angle and posterior border. It can be considered only accessory to the joint and of uncertain function.

Articular disc

The articular disc (**6**.162C, 163), an oval plate of fibrous tissue shaped like a peaked cap, completely divides the joint. Its upper surface is sagittally concavoconvex to fit the articular tubercle and fossa,

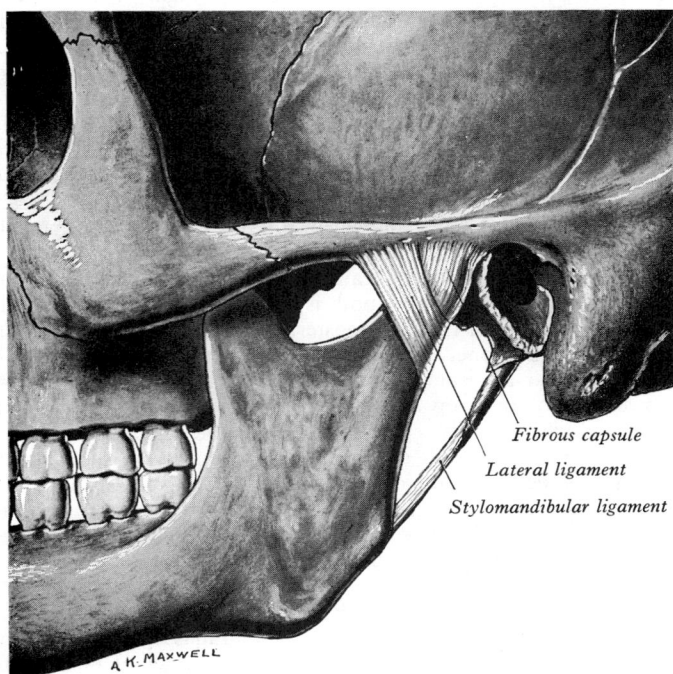

Fibrous capsule
Lateral ligament
Stylomandibular ligament

A

A.K.MAXWELL

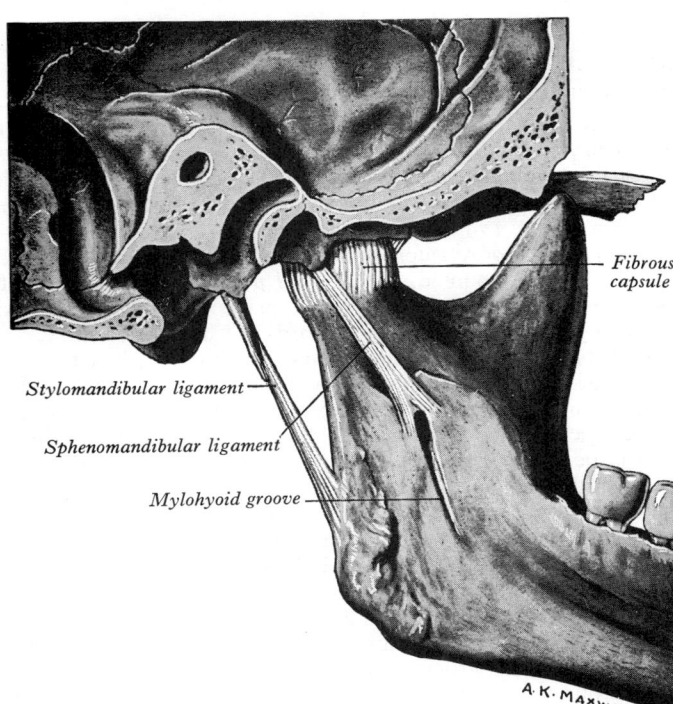

Fibrous capsule

Stylomandibular ligament
Sphenomandibular ligament
Mylohyoid groove

B

A.K.MAXWELL

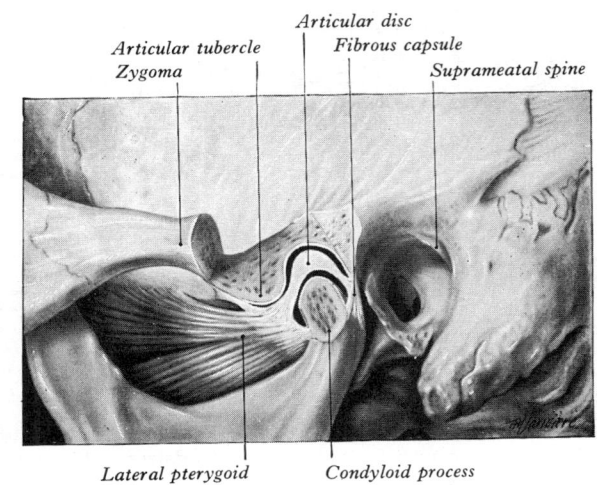

Articular tubercle   *Articular disc*
Zygoma   *Fibrous capsule*
    Suprameatal spine

C

Lateral pterygoid   *Condyloid process*

6.162   The left temporomandibular joint; A. lateral aspect; B. medial aspect; C. sagittal section.

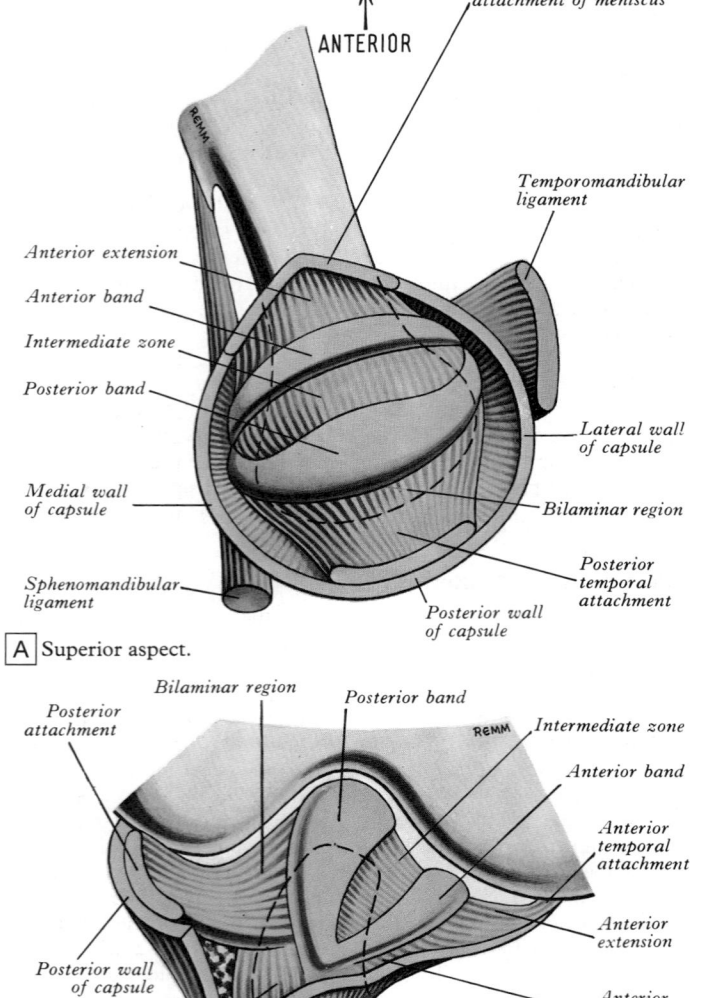

A | Superior aspect.

B | Lateral aspect.

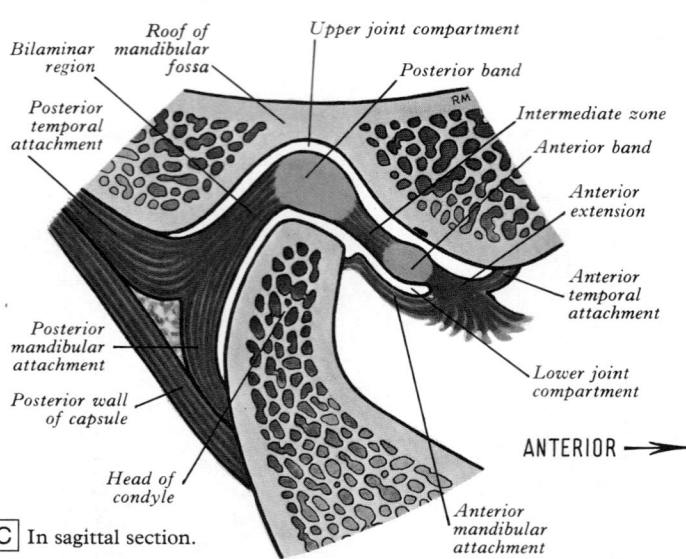

C | In sagittal section.

6.163 Form, subdivisions and thickness variations of the intra-articular disc in the temporomandibular joint. See text for details and for alternative interpretations. Based upon Rees (1954) and with permission from the *British Dental Journal*.

its inferior concave surface adapted to the mandibular head. Its circumference blends with the fibrous capsule and, anteromedially, the tendon of lateral pterygoid (p. 801). Medial and lateral, short, strong bands pass from its margins to the medial and lateral condylar poles, ensuring that the disc and condyle move together in protraction and retraction. Posteriorly in the disc a venous plexus separates upper and lower layers, the **upper** of fibroelastic tissue attaches to the fossa's posterior margin, the **lower** of non-elastic fibrous tissue attaches to the back of the condyle. Though variable, the disc is thickest behind its centre, in the deepest part of the mandibular fossa where Rees (1954) has described two thick regions (anterior and posterior bands) with thinner zones between. Mediolateral variations are equally relevant. An interesting analysis with some alternative proposals concerning the design, formation, possible functional roles and derangements of the disc have been provided by Osborn (1985). He emphasizes the largely fibrous nature of the highly non-congruent articular surfaces and views the interposed disc as a viscoelastically deformable pad coextensive with the cranial articular surface (i.e. much more extensive than the mandibular condyle). Compression forces (increased during chewing, biting, grinding) **thin** an area of disc between the condyle and the posterior slope of the articular eminence, thereby 'squeezing out' material to form a thickened zone, the *annulus* of Osborn, which surrounds the thin area—a recess for the mandibular condyle. (It should be noted that the anterior and posterior thickened bands shown in **6.163** are continuous medially and laterally with the mandibular condyle.) The question of whether the shape of the disc is genetically determined, produced mainly by biomechanical constraints or both is also discussed. The supposedly non-elastic nature of the inferoposterior (mandibular) lamina of the disc is also questioned (see also below). Postnatal development of the disc up to 21 years, described by Wright and Moffet (1974), showed at no stage any chondrocytes in the disc, which is flat at birth and develops its sigmoid profile as the articular eminence enlarges. From the fifth decade it also often shows macroscopic evidence of degeneration (fraying, thinning and perforation) that this can be regarded as 'normal' ageing. Weisengreen (1975) found such degeneration in 40% of 183 individuals between 40 and 90 years. The disc, often incomplete, is variably perforated.

Vessels and nerve supply to the joint

Innervation is from the auriculotemporal and masseteric branches of the mandibular nerve, **arteries** are from the superficial temporal and maxillary arteries. Klineberg and Wyke (1975) have detailed the distribution of mechanoreceptors in the joint and suggested their role in mastication.

Movements

The mandible can be depressed or elevated, protruded or retracted and, since both joints always act together but may differ in actual movement, some rotation (around a vertical axis, see below) may occur. These actions involve gliding, spin, roll and angulation. (The last is another variety of rotation around a dynamic transverse axis, see below.)

In the *position of rest* upper and lower teeth are slightly apart; in closure they are apposed, the *occlusal position*. When the mouth **opens** the mandibular 'condyles' rotate on a common horizontal axis and also glide forwards and downwards on the inferior surfaces of their articular discs, which slide in the same direction on the temporal bones due to their attachments to the mandibular heads and to contraction of the lateral pterygoids drawing the heads and discs on to the articular tubercles. Discal sliding ceases when their posterior fibroelastic attachments to the temporal bones are stretched to their limit. Further hinging and gliding of the condyles brings them into articulation with the most anterior parts of the discs as the mouth opens fully. In **closure** the movements are reversed: each head glides back and hinges on its disc, still held by the lateral pterygoid, which relaxes to allow the disc to glide back and up into the mandibular fossa. The full cycle is shown in **6.164**, derived from observations by Rees (1954). Osborn (1985) presents alternative interpretations; he regards the fibrous articular surfaces as particularly susceptible to trauma during the arthrokinematic roll, spin and glide executed when the joint is maximally loaded. The deformable viscoelastic articular disc's primary function is to permit these activities while reducing the risk of trauma. The *disc* is thought to be stabilized by

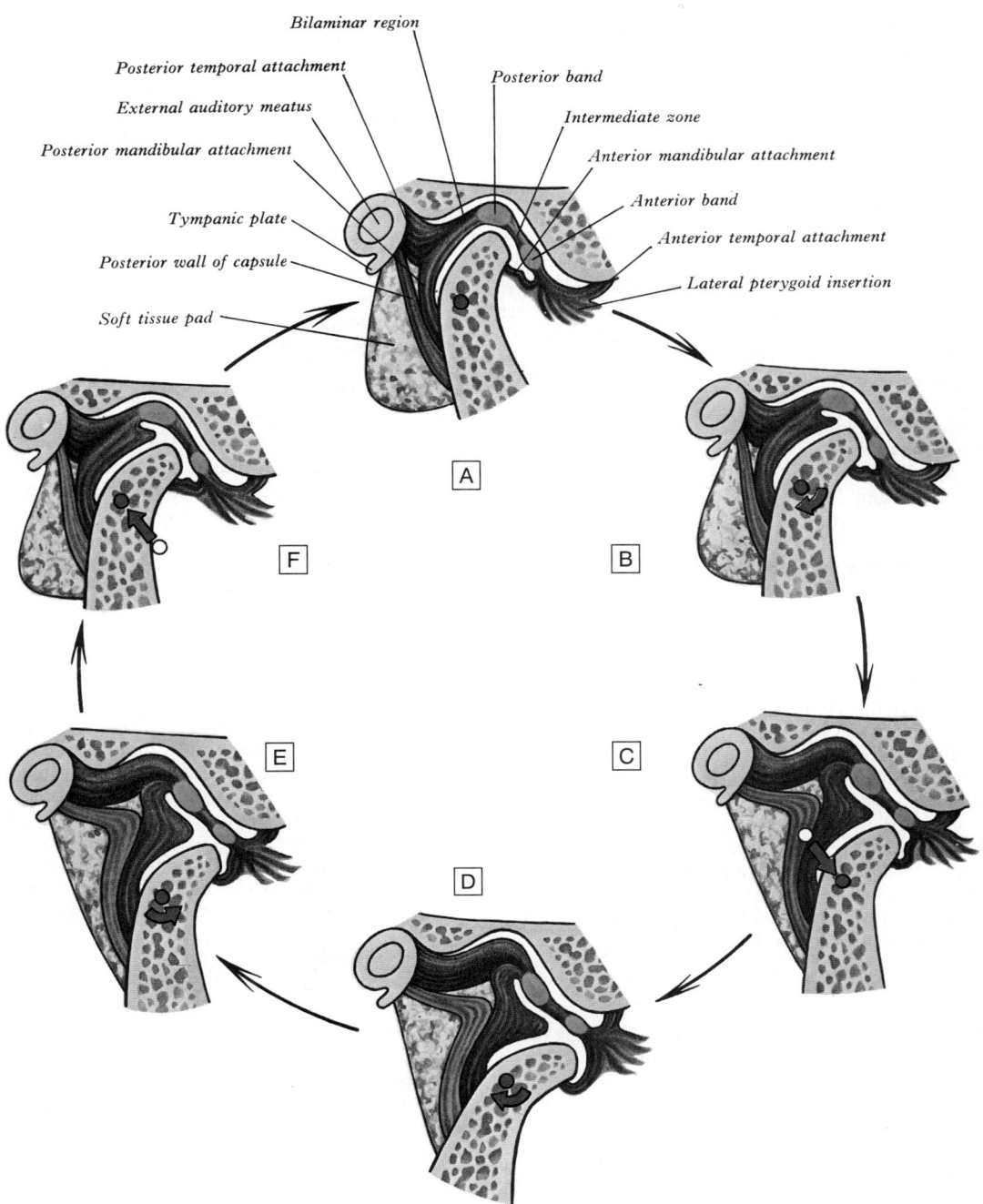

Bilaminar region
Posterior temporal attachment
External auditory meatus
Posterior mandibular attachment
Tympanic plate
Posterior wall of capsule
Soft tissue pad
Posterior band
Intermediate zone
Anterior mandibular attachment
Anterior band
Anterior temporal attachment
Lateral pterygoid insertion

A B C D E F

6.164 Changing relationships of the condyle of the mandible, the articular disc and the articular surface of the temporal bone during one complete opening (A→D) and closing (D→A) cycle of the mouth. Based upon Rees (1954) with permission of the late Professor J J Pritchard, on behalf of the late Leonard A Rees and the *British Dental Journal*. See also alternative hypotheses proposed by Osborn (1985).

its inherent viscoelasticity; increasing loads thicken its annulus (see above) and prolapse is prevented. Activity of the lateral pterygoid and presence of elastic tissue in the posterior bilaminar zone are regarded as secondary features in disc stabilization. An unusual proposition is that while the disc is *self-stabilizing* its other principal role is to *destabilize* the mandibular condyle and allow complex free movement under load. The elastic tissues may act to withdraw tissues and thus prevent entrapment between the articular surfaces during mouth closure. In *protrusion* the teeth are parallel to the occlusal plane but variably separated, the lower carried forwards by both lateral pterygoid muscles. In *retraction* the mandible is returned to the position of rest. In rotatory movements of mastication (in the *occlusal plane*, but clearly not in *occlusion*), one head with its disc glides forwards, rotating around a vertical axis immediately behind the opposite head, then glides backwards rotating in the opposite direction, as the opposite head comes forward in turn. This alternation swings the mandible from side to side (Sarnat 1951).

Measurement of mandibular movements is of clinical interest; in adults incisors may separate by 50–60 mm, maximal lateral displacement and protrusion being about 10 mm, with much individual variation. Adult range is reached earlier in females (*c.* 10 years) than in males (*c.* 15 years) in accord with postnatal development of the articular profiles (Wright & Moffet 1974), adult form being reached between 6 and 12 years.

Muscles producing movements

Protrusion: lateral and medial pterygoid muscles.
Retraction: temporales (posterior fibres), assisted by middle and deep parts of the masseters, digastric and geniohyoid muscles.
Elevation: temporalis, masseter, medial pterygoid, of both sides. In closure each mandibular head is retracted by the posterior fibres of the temporalis before elevation. The temporales maintain the position of rest (Latif 1957).
Depression: lateral pterygoids, aided when the mouth is open widely

581

or against resistance, by digastric, geniohyoid and mylohyoid muscles.

Lateral movements: medial and lateral pterygoid of each side, acting alternately.

Such a list, though useful, obscures the complex integrations of simultaneous contraction and lengthening of many muscles.

Alternative descriptions of mandibular movements have been proposed, with a detailed analysis of biting, chewing and deglutition being given by Kraus et al (1969). For a mathematical model relating patterns of human mandibular movement to biomechanical constraints see Baragar and Osborn (1984).

An unresolved controversy concerning forces transmitted at temporomandibular joints must be noted. A proposal that they carry no load, or are subject to little transarticular compression, has been supported by Wilson (1920), Scott (1955), Steinhardt (1958) and others; while later views (e.g. Smith & Savage 1959; Turnbull 1970) oppose this. Most observations involve vertebrates other than mammals; few reliable experimental data are available for man according to Gingerich (1971). Analysis, both theoretical and involving electromyography (integrated and quantitative), in man, however, favours a force-transmitting function (Barbenel 1972, 1974), supported by observations by Crompton & Hiemae (opossum, 1969) and by Buckland-Wright (cat, 1978). In view of the complex activities at these joints, both views may be correct at times. It is only in 'hinge' movements of limited extent, as in biting, that controversy need exist.

Clinical anatomy

The mandible is dislocated only forwards. With the mouth open, the condyles are on the articular eminences and sudden violence, even muscular spasm (a convulsive yawn), may displace one or both into the infratemporal fossa. Reduction involves depressing the jaw posteriorly, at the same time elevating the chin. Downward pressure overcomes spasm in the masseter, temporalis and pterygoid muscles; elevation of the chin forces the condyles backwards. Derangement of a disc may follow trauma, by overclosure with backward displacement of a condyle or malocclusion; clicking and pain on movement result. In operations, rami of the facial nerve overlying the joint must be preserved. Changes in occlusion may lead to remodelling of the temporomandibular articular surfaces (Moffet et al 1964).

HYOID BONE

The U-shaped hyoid bone (**6**.165) is suspended from the tips of the (bilateral) styloid processes by the stylohyoid ligaments. It has a body, two greater and two lesser cornua.

Body

This is irregular, elongated and quadrilateral. Its *anterior surface* is convex, facing anterosuperiorly, and is crossed by a transverse ridge with a slight downward convexity; often a vertical median ridge bisects the body; the upper part of this vertical ridge is usually present, the lower part is rare. The *posterior surface* is smooth, concave, faces posteroinferiorly, and is separated from the epiglottis by the thyrohyoid membrane and loose areolar tissue, with a bursa between the bone and the membrane.

The greater cornua

These are connected to the body in early life by cartilage, but after middle age they are usually united by bone. They project backwards (curving posterolaterally) from the lateral ends of the body; horizontally flattened, they taper posteriorly, each ending in a tubercle. When the throat is gripped between finger and thumb above the thyroid cartilage, the greater cornua can be identified and the bone can be moved from side to side.

The lesser cornua

They are two small, conical projections at the junctions of the body and greater cornua, connected at their base to the body by fibrous tissue and occasionally to the greater cornua by synovial joints, which occasionally become ankylosed (see below).

Further details

Attached to most of the body's *anterior surface* is geniohyoid, above and below the transverse ridge; but the medial part of hyoglossus invades the lateral geniohyoid area (**6**.165B). The lower anterior surface gives attachment to mylohyoid, above the sternohyoid medially and omohyoid laterally. To the rounded *superior border* the lowest fibres of the genioglossi, the hyoepiglottic ligament and (most posteriorly) the thyrohyoid membrane are attached; to the *inferior border* are attached sternohyoid medially and omohyoid laterally, sometimes with the medial fibres of thyrohyoid and levator glandulae thyroideae, when present.

To the *upper surface* of each *greater cornu* the middle pharyngeal constrictor and, more laterally (superficially), hyoglossus, are attached along its whole length. Near the junction of the cornu with the body stylohyoid is attached, lateral to hyoglossus, and a little posterior to this, is the fibrous loop for the digastric tendon. To the *medial border* is attached the thyrohyoid membrane, to the *lateral border* anteriorly the thyrohyoid. The oblique *inferior surface* is separated from the thyrohyoid membrane by fibroareolar tissue.

At the *posterior* and *lateral aspects of the lesser cornua* are the attachments of the middle pharyngeal constrictors. To their apices are attached the stylohyoid ligaments, often partly ossified, and to the medial aspects of their bases, the chondroglossi.

Ossification

The hyoid bone evolves from cartilages of the second and third visceral arches, the lesser cornua from the second, the greater from the third and the body from the fused ventral ends of both (p. 277). Chondrification begins in the fifth fetal week in these elements, completed in the third and fourth months. Ossification proceeds from six centres—a pair for the body, one for each cornu—commencing in the greater cornua towards the end of intrauterine life, in the body shortly before or after birth, and in lesser cornua around puberty. The greater cornual apices remain cartilaginous until the third decade and epiphyses may occur here. They fuse with the body. Synovial joints between the greater and lesser cornua may be obliterated by ossification in later decades.

OCCIPITAL BONE

The occipital bone (**6**.166), forming much of the back and base of the cranium, is trapezoid and internally concave. It encloses the *foramen magnum*; the expanded plate posterosuperior to this is the *squama* (*squamous part*), the massive quadrilateral part anterior to it being the *basilar part* (*basioccipital*); on each side of the foramen is a *lateral part* (*exoccipital*).

Squama

The squama is convex externally and concave internally. The *external surface* presents, midway between its summit and the foramen magnum, the *external occipital protuberance*. On each side two curved lines extend laterally from this; the upper, faintly marked and often almost imperceptible, is the *highest nuchal line* to which the epicranial aponeurosis is attached; the lower is the *superior nuchal line*. The surface above the highest nuchal lines is smooth and covered by the occipital part of occipitofrontalis; below this it is rough and irregular for the attachment of muscles. From the external occipital protuberance the median *external occipital crest*, often faint, descends

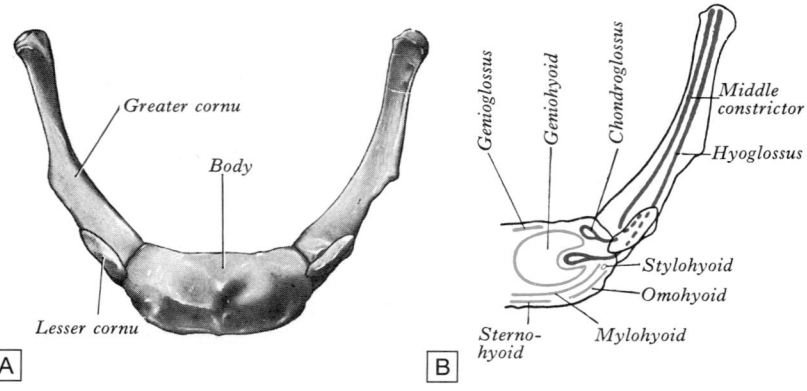

6.165A. The hyoid bone: anterosuperior aspect. B. Drawing of the left half of the hyoid bone to show the muscular attachments: superior aspect.

to the foramen magnum and is an attachment of the ligamentum nuchae; on each side an *inferior nuchal line* spreads laterally from the crest's midpoint. Areas of muscular attachment are shown in **6.141, 147, 166B**. The posterior atlanto-occipital membrane is attached posterolaterally just outside the foramen magnum's margin.

The squama's *internal surface* is divided into four deep fossae by an irregular *internal occipital protuberance* and by ridged sagittal and horizontal extensions from it. The two superior fossae are triangular and adapted to the cerebral occipital poles, the inferior are quadrilateral and shaped to accommodate the cerebellar hemispheres. A wide groove, with raised banks, ascends from the protuberance to the squama's superior angle—the *superior sagittal sulcus*. The posterior part of the falx cerebri is attached to its margins. A prominent *internal occipital crest* descends from the protuberance, for attachment of the falx cerebelli, and bifurcates near the foramen magnum; the occipital sinus, sometimes double, lies in this attachment. At the crest's lower end a small *vermian fossa* may exist, occupied by part of the inferior cerebellar vermis. On each side a wide *sulcus for the transverse sinus* extends laterally from the protuberance; to the margins of these sulci the tentorium cerebelli is attached. The right sulcus is usually larger, passing into the sulcus for the superior sagittal sinus, but the left may be larger or both almost equal in size. The position of this *confluence of sinuses* is indicated by a depression on one side of the protuberance.

The *superior angle* at the squama's summit meets the occipital angles of the parietal bones, the position of the fetal *posterior fontanelle*. The *lateral angles* of the squama', marked internally by the ends of the transverse sulci, project between the parietal and temporal bones. The *lambdoid borders* extend from superior to lateral angles, serrated for articulation with the occipital borders of the parietals at the *lambdoid suture*. The *mastoid borders* extend from the lateral angles to the jugular processes, articulating with the mastoid parts of the temporal bone. A variety of ossicles may occur at or near the lambda (p. 606 and Srivastava 1977), for example the 'interparietal' (Inca bone or ossicle of Goethe).

Basilar part

The basilar part extends anterosuperiorly from the foramen magnum, fusing with the sphenoid in adults. In young skulls a rough and uneven surface is joined to the body of the sphenoid by a growth cartilage. By the twenty-fifth year this plate has ossified and occipital and sphenoid bones are fused.

The *inferior surface* of the basioccipital, about 1 cm anterior to the foramen magnum, bears a small *pharyngeal tubercle* for attachment of the fibrous pharyngeal raphe. Longus capitis is attached anterolateral to the tubercle and rectus capitis anterior to a small depression immediately anterior to the occipital condyle which, on occasion, may be replaced by a small *precondylar tubercle*, of low incidence, but relatively frequent in Mexican and Burmese crania (p. 609). To the anterior margin of the foramen magnum the anterior atlanto-occipital membrane is attached.

The *superior basioccipital surface* is a broad groove, part of the *clivus*, which ascends anteriorly from the foramen magnum; above it are the medulla oblongata and lower pons. Near the foramen the membrana tectoria and axial apical ligament are attached to the clivus. On its lateral margins are *sulci of the inferior petrosal sinuses*, below which the lateral margins articulate with the petrous temporal bones.

Lateral (condylar) parts

The lateral (condylar) parts of the occipital bone flank the foramen magnum; on their *inferior surfaces* are *occipital condyles* for articulation with the superior atlantal facets. They are oval or reniform, their long axes converging anteromedially. Their anterior ends invade the basioccipital, level with the foramen's centre. The articular surfaces, wholly convex, face inferolaterally; they are occasionally constricted and a condyle may be in two parts (p. 610). The atlantal superior articular facets are also frequently constricted and occasionally 'double' (Singh 1965). Medial to each facet a tubercle gives attachment to an alar ligament. Anteriorly above each condyle is a

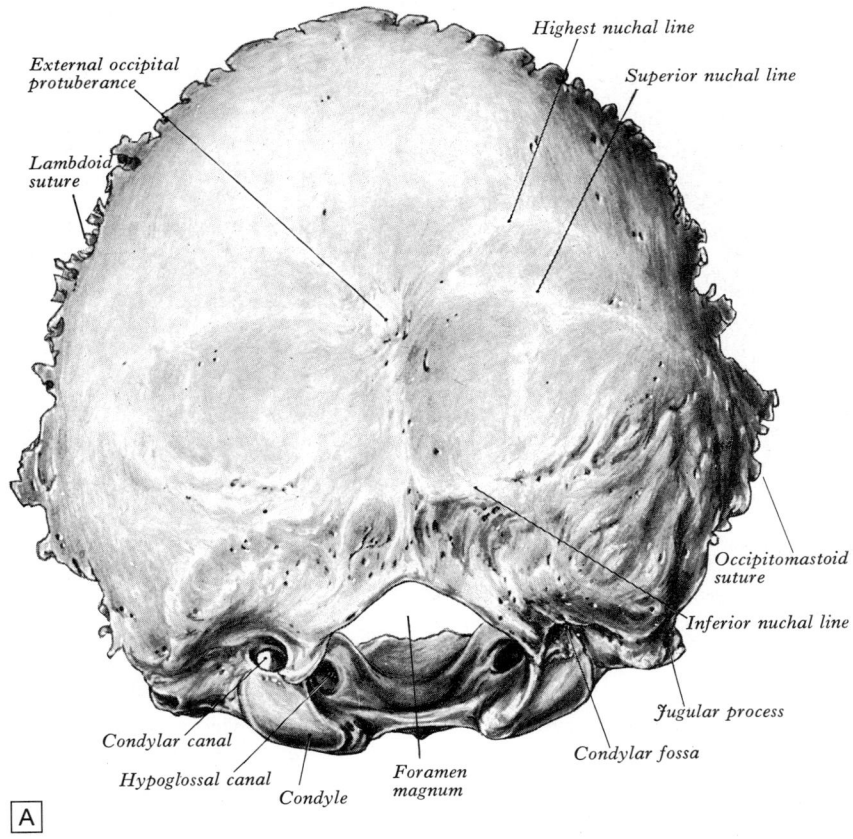

External occipital protuberance

Lambdoid suture

Highest nuchal line

Superior nuchal line

Occipitomastoid suture

Inferior nuchal line

Jugular process

Condylar fossa

Condylar canal

Hypoglossal canal

Condyle

Foramen magnum

A

6.166 The occipital bone; A. Posterior (external) aspect; B. Inferior aspect; C. Internal aspect. The condylar canal was only present on the left side in this specimen. (B. and C. overleaf).

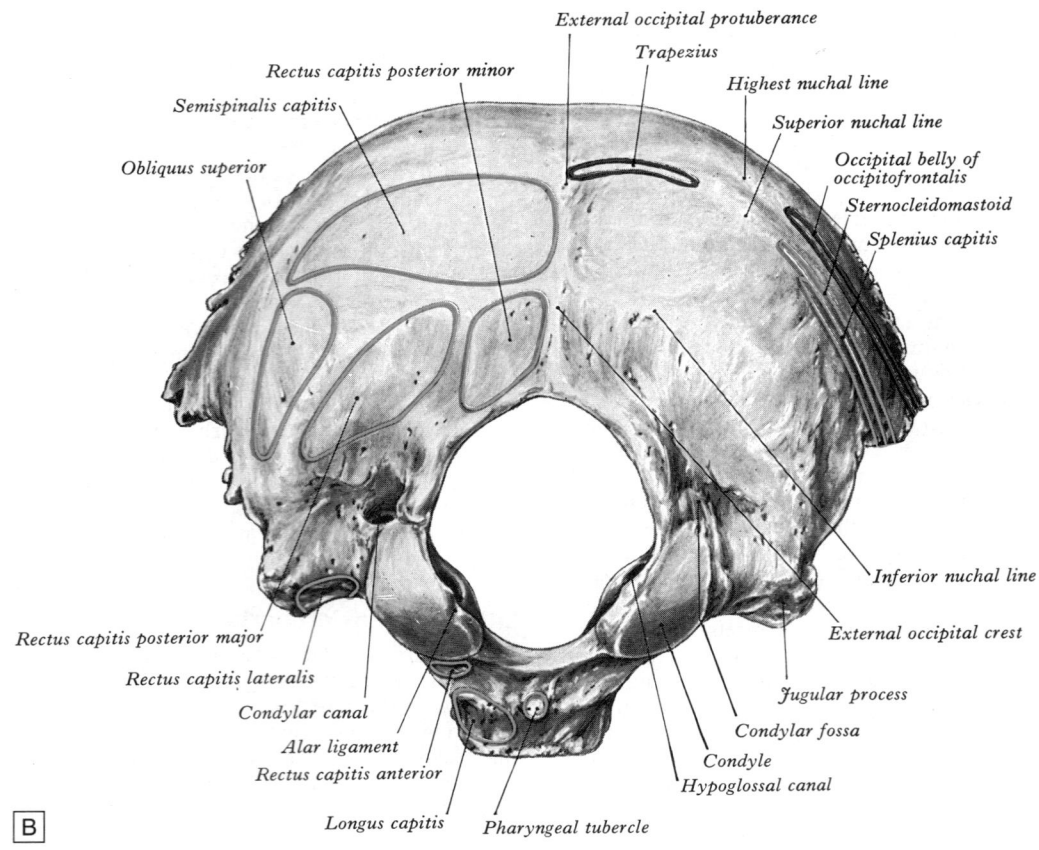

External occipital protuberance

Rectus capitis posterior minor

Trapezius

Semispinalis capitis

Highest nuchal line

Superior nuchal line

Obliquus superior

Occipital belly of occipitofrontalis

Sternocleidomastoid

Splenius capitis

Inferior nuchal line

External occipital crest

Rectus capitis posterior major

Jugular process

Rectus capitis lateralis

Condylar fossa

Condylar canal

Condyle

Alar ligament

Hypoglossal canal

Rectus capitis anterior

Longus capitis

Pharyngeal tubercle

B

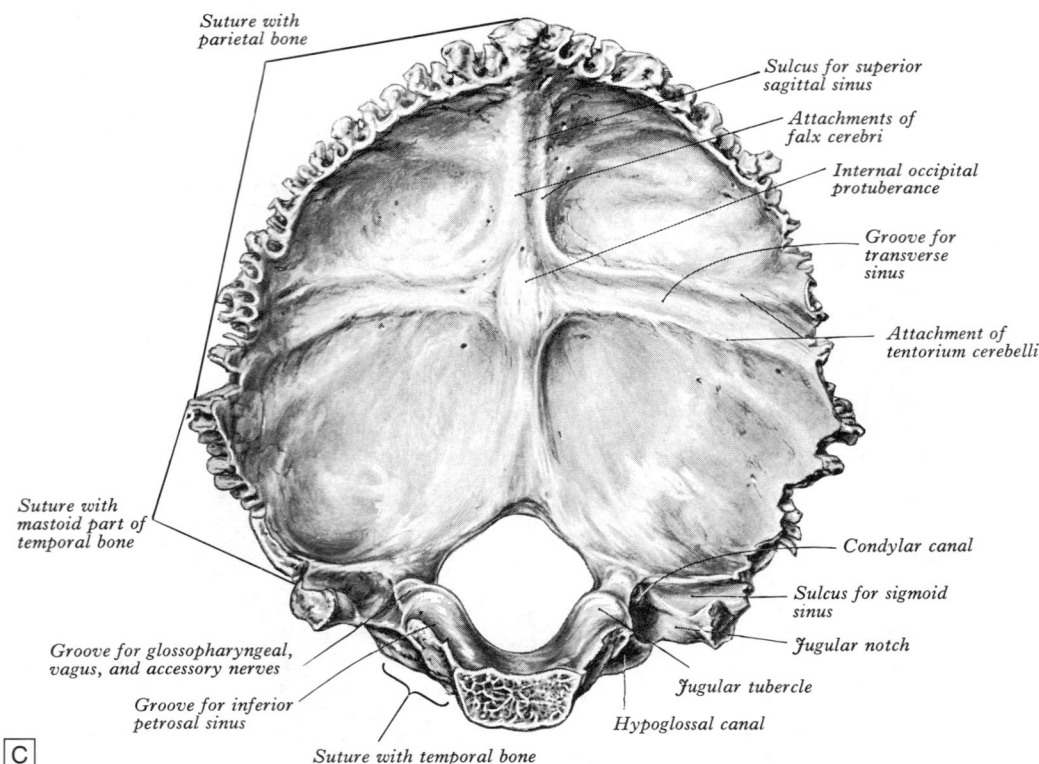

Suture with parietal bone

Sulcus for superior sagittal sinus

Attachments of falx cerebri

Internal occipital protuberance

Groove for transverse sinus

Attachment of tentorium cerebelli

Suture with mastoid part of temporal bone

Condylar canal

Sulcus for sigmoid sinus

Groove for glossopharyngeal, vagus, and accessory nerves

Jugular notch

Jugular tubercle

Groove for inferior petrosal sinus

Hypoglossal canal

Suture with temporal bone

C

hypoglossal canal, which starts internally a little above the anterolateral part of the foramen magnum and continues anterolaterally. It may be partly or wholly divided by a spicule of bone and transmits the hypoglossal nerve and a meningeal branch of the ascending pharyngeal artery. A *condylar fossa*, behind each condyle, fits the posterior margin of the superior atlantal facet in full extension; its floor is sometimes perforated by a *condylar canal* for a sigmoid emissary vein. The *jugular process*, jutting laterally from the posterior

half of each condyle, is a quadrilateral plate, indented in front by a *jugular notch*, the posterior part of the jugular foramen. This notch is sometimes partly divided by a small *intrajugular process*, projecting anterolaterally. The jugular process' inferior surface is roughened by attachment of rectus capitis lateralis; a *paramastoid process* sometimes projects down and may even articulate with the atlantal transverse process. Laterally the jugular process has a rough quadrilateral or triangular area joined to the jugular surface of the temporal bone by a cartilaginous growth plate, which begins to ossify at about 25 years. For variations of jugular foramen, processes, etc., consult Solter and Paljan (1973). Though rare or absent in many populations, a paramastoid process was recorded in 44% of 149 male and 31% of 137 female American Indians (Finnegan 1972).

On the superior condylar surface an oval *jugular tubercle* overlies the hypoglossal canal, its posterior part often bearing a shallow furrow for the glossopharyngeal, vagus and accessory nerves. On the jugular process' superior surface a deep groove, curving antero-medially around a hook-shaped process, ends at the jugular notch; it contains the end of the sigmoid sinus. Near the groove's medial end the condylar canal opens into the posterior cranial fossa.

Foramen magnum

The foramen magnum is described on page 572.

Structure

The occipital, in common with many parts of other cranial bones, consists of two compact lamellae, *outer* and *inner plates*, enclosing trabecular bone or *diploë*; the bone is thick at ridges, protuberances and condyles, and in the anterior basioccipital; in lower parts of cerebellar fossae, however, it is thin, semitransparent and devoid of diploë. As noted earlier, the intertrabecular spaces (cancelli) of the diploë are occupied by haemopoetic red bone marrow (p. 568), the latter being drained by radicles of the wide diploic veins (p. 1581), of which the occipital diploic vein is usually the largest.

Ossification

A common but **oversimplified** account of occipital ossification states that above the highest nuchal lines the squama is developed in a fibrous membrane and ossified from two centres, one on each side from about the second fetal month; this part may remain separate as the *interparietal bone*; the rest is preformed in cartilage. Below the highest nuchal lines, the squama ossifies from two centres, appearing in about the seventh week and soon uniting. These two regions of the squama unite in the third postnatal month but the line of union is recognizable at birth (6.167).

An occasional centre appears in the posterior margin of the foramen magnum in about the sixteenth week (Kerckring 1970); it unites with the rest of the squama before birth. From a survey of literature and examination of 620 human skulls for anomalies of the occipital squama, however, Srivastava (1977) has proposed a more complex developmental history. He regards the *membranous* (*dermal*) part above the nuchal lines as compounded of *interparietal* and *pre-interparietal* parts, the interparietal consisting of two *lateral plates* and a *central piece*. The intramembranous centres proposed for these are a pair for each lateral plate and two for the central piece of the interparietal, additionally a pair of centres for the pre-interparietal. Pal et al (1984) have criticized the views of Srivastava (1977); they consider the so-called pre-interparietal elements as probably sutural; but it has to be stated that much uncertainty persists regarding the

status of these accessory ossicles. Fusion may fail, partly or completely, between any of these elements. To the *cartilaginous supra-occipital* Srivastava allots five endochondral centres, a pair each for right and left *lateral segments* and one for the *central segment* (the latter may correspond to Kerckring's centre). Each lateral (condylar or exoccipital) part ossifies from one centre, appearing during the eighth prenatal week. The basioccipital is ossified from one centre appearing about the sixth week. Near the end of the second year the squama unites with condylar parts and by the sixth year the bone is one entity. Between the eighteenth and twenty-fifth years the occipital and sphenoid bones unite. Metrical study of the occipital bone (Olivier 1975) suggests that squamous and basilar parts have independent parameters of growth, and that sexual differences are chiefly evident in condylar regions. Routal et al (1984) have described sexual dimorphism, chiefly difference in size, in the foramen magnum.

SPHENOID BONE

The sphenoid bone is in the base of the skull, 'wedged' (as its name implies) between the frontal temporal and occipital bones. It has a central *body*, paired *greater* and *lesser wings* spreading laterally from it and two *pterygoid processes*, descending from the junctions of the body and greater wings.

Body

The body is cuboidal and contains two large air sinuses, separated by a septum. The *cerebral* or *superior surface* (6.153, 168A) articulates in front with the ethmoidal cribriform plates; anteriorly it is the smooth jugum sphenoidale, related to gyri recti and olfactory tracts. The jugum is bounded behind by the anterior border of the *sulcus*

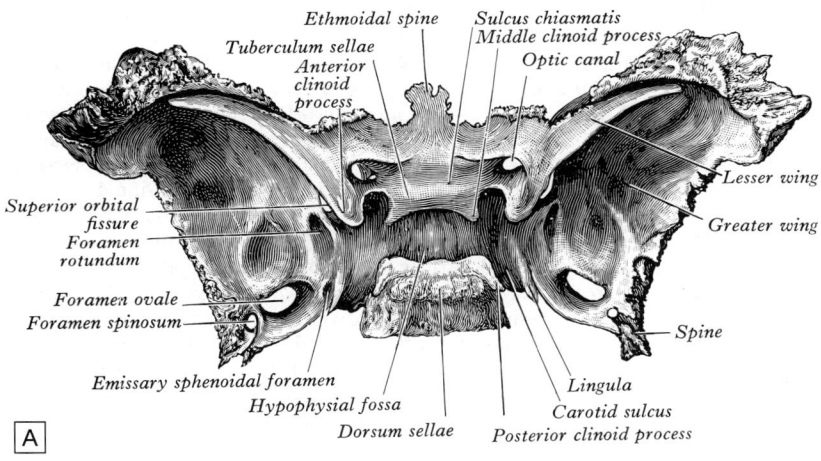

Ethmoidal spine · Sulcus chiasmatis · Middle clinoid process · Tuberculum sellae · Anterior clinoid process · Optic canal · Lesser wing · Greater wing · Superior orbital fissure · Foramen rotundum · Foramen ovale · Foramen spinosum · Spine · Emissary sphenoidal foramen · Hypophysial fossa · Dorsum sellae · Lingula · Carotid sulcus · Posterior clinoid process

A

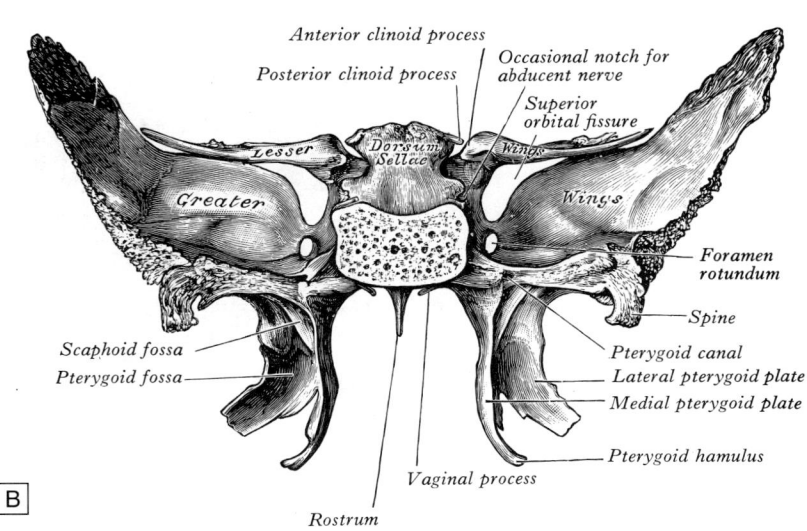

Anterior clinoid process · Posterior clinoid process · Occasional notch for abducent nerve · Superior orbital fissure · Lesser · Dorsum Sellae · Wings · Greater · Wings · Foramen rotundum · Spine · Scaphoid fossa · Pterygoid fossa · Pterygoid canal · Lateral pterygoid plate · Medial pterygoid plate · Pterygoid hamulus · Vaginal process · Rostrum

B

Upper part of squama

Line of union between upper and lower parts of squama

Lower part of squama

Kerckring's centre

Lateral part

Basilar part

S.W.W

6.167   The occipital bone of a newborn child: external surface. Parts of the chondrocranium still unossified are shown in blue.

6.168   The sphenoid bone; A. superior aspect; B. posterior aspect.

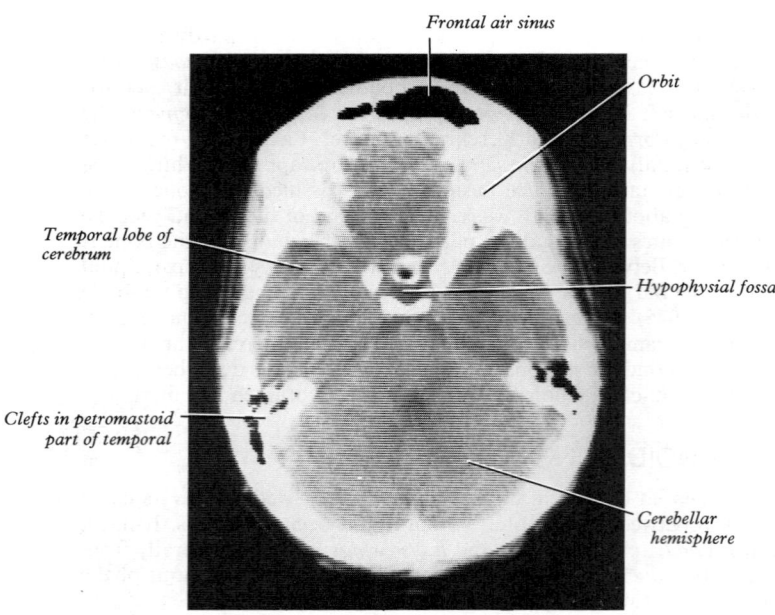

Frontal air sinus

Orbit

Temporal lobe of
cerebrum

Hypophysial fossa

Clefts in petromastoid
part of temporal

Cerebellar
hemisphere

6.169   Computed tomogram through the head at the level of the pituitary fossa of the sphenoid. (Supplied by Shaun Gallagher, Guy's Hospital; photography by Sarah Smith.)

chiasmatis, leading laterally to the *optic canals*. Posterior to this is the *tuberculum sellae*, behind which the deeply concave *sella turcica* contains the hypophysis cerebri in the *hypophyseal fossa* (**6**.169). The sella's anterior edge is completed laterally by two *middle clinoid processes* (**6**.168A), posteriorly by a square *dorsum sellae*, the superior angles of which bear variable *posterior clinoid processes*, for attachment of the tentorium cerebelli. On each side, below the dorsum sellae, a small *petrosal process* articulates with the apex of the petrous temporal bone. (For variations in sella turcica see Kinman 1977; Lang 1977.) Posterior to the dorsum sellae the sphenoid body slopes directly into basioccipital bone in adults, together forming the *clivus*. The latter's sphenoidal part lies beneath the upper pons.

The *lateral surfaces* are united both with the greater wings and the medial pterygoid plates. Above the root of each wing a broad *carotid sulcus* accommodates the internal carotid artery and cavernous sinus and a series of closely related nerves. It is deepest posteriorly, overhung medially by the petrosal process and has a sharp lateral margin, the *lingula*, which continues back over the posterior opening of the pterygoid canal.

On the *anterior surface* (**6**.170) a median triangular, structurally bilaminar *sphenoidal crest* forms a small part of the nasal septum; its anterior border joins the ethmoid's perpendicular plate; on each

side of it opens a *sphenoidal sinus*. The sphenoidal sinuses (p. 1637), two large, irregular cavities within the body, are usually separated by an asymmetrical septum. Varying in form and size, each sinus is partially divided by bony laminae. A lateral recess may extend into the greater wing and lingula (Cope 1917) and may even invade the basioccipital bone almost to the foramen magnum. Trans-sphenoidal surgical approach to the hypophysis cerebri has prompted classification into types: *conchal*—a small sinus separated from the sella turcica by about 10 mm of trabecular bone; *presellar*—a sinus not extended posteriorly to the tuberculum sellae; and *sellar*—the sinus extended, as described above, at variable distances beyond the tuberculum (Hammer & Råadberg 1961; Kinman 1977; Lang 1977). In the articulated state they are closed anteroinferiorly by the *sphenoidal conchae* (p. 588), leaving openings by which each communicates with its sphenoethmoidal recess. Each half anterior surface of the body consists of:

- a superolateral depressed area joined to the ethmoid labyrinth, completing the posterior ethmoidal sinuses
- its lateral margin articulates with the ethmoid's orbital plate above and palatine's orbital process below
- an inferomedial, smooth, triangular area, forming the posterior nasal roof; near its superior angle is the orifice of a sphenoidal sinus.

The *inferior surface* bears a median triangular *sphenoidal rostrum*, embraced above by the diverging lower margins of the crest, its narrow antero end fitting into a fissure between the anterior parts of the vomerine alae. Posterior ends of the sphenoidal conchae flank the rostrum, articulating with vomerine alae. On each side of the posterior part of the rostrum, behind the sphenoidal concha's apex, a thin *vaginal process* projects medially from the base of the medial pterygoid plate (**6**.170).

Greater wings

The greater wings, strong processes, curve broadly superolaterally from the body. Posteriorly each is triangular, fitting the angle between petrous and squamous parts of the temporal bone (**6**.144A) at a sphenosquamosal suture. The *cerebral surface* (**6**.168A) is an anterior part of the middle cranial fossa. Deeply concave, its undulating surface is adapted to the anterior gyri of the temporal lobe. Anteromedial is the *foramen rotundum* for the maxillary nerve, posterolateral to this the *foramen ovale* for the mandibular nerve, accessory meningeal artery and sometimes the lesser petrosal nerve, which may have a special *canaliculus innominatus* medial to the foramen spinosum. A small *emissary sphenoidal foramen* exists on one or both sides in 40% of skulls; it opens below, lateral to the scaphoid fossa, and transmits a small vein from the cavernous sinus. Anteromedial to the sphenoidal spine the *foramen spinosum* transmits the middle meningeal artery and meningeal branch of the mandibular nerve.

The *lateral surface* (**6**.144A) is vertically convex and divided by a transverse *infratemporal crest* into temporal (upper) and infra-

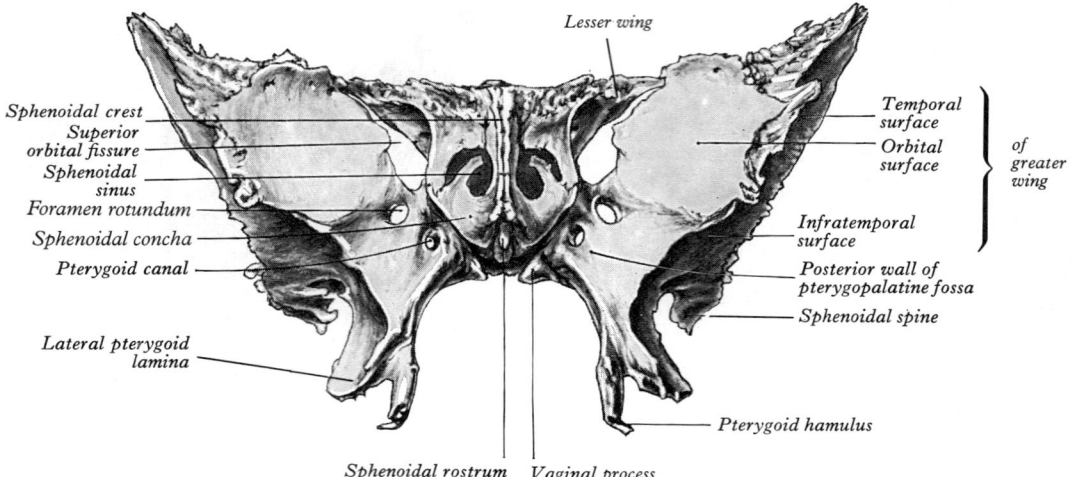

Lesser wing

Sphenoidal crest
Superior
orbital fissure
Sphenoidal
sinus
Foramen rotundum
Sphenoidal concha
Pterygoid canal

Lateral pterygoid
lamina

Temporal
surface
Orbital
surface

of
greater
wing

Infratemporal
surface

Posterior wall of
pterygopalatine fossa

Sphenoidal spine

Pterygoid hamulus

Sphenoidal rostrum   Vaginal process

6.170   The sphenoid bone of an eight-year-old child: anterior aspect.

temporal (lower) surfaces; to the upper surface temporalis is attached; the lower is directed downwards and, with the infratemporal crest, it is the attachment of the upper fibres of lateral pterygoid. It presents the foramen ovale and foramen spinosum. Posteriorly is the small downward projecting *spine of the sphenoid*; its medial side shows a faint anteroinferior groove for the chorda tympani and also appears in the lateral wall of the sulcus for the auditory tube (p. 1374): to its tip is attached the sphenomandibular ligament. Medial to the anterior end of the infratemporal crest a triangular process is part of the lateral pterygoid's attachment; a ridge, descending medially from this to the front of the lateral pterygoid plate, is a posterior boundary of the pterygomaxillary fissure.

The quadrilateral *orbital surface* (**6**.170) faces anteromedially as a posterior part of the lateral orbital wall. Its serrated upper edge articulates with the frontal's orbital plate, its serrated lateral margin with the zygomatic bone. Its smooth inferior border is the postero-lateral edge of the inferior orbital fissure. Its sharp medial margin is the inferolateral edge of the superior orbital fissure; on it a small tubercle gives partial attachment of the common annular ocular tendon (p. 1355). Below the superior fissure's medial end a grooved area forms the posterior wall of the pterygopalatine fossa, pierced by the foramen rotundum.

The irregular *margin of the greater wing* (**6**.168B), from sphenoid body to spine, is in its medial half an anterior limit of the *foramen lacerum* and displays the posterior aperture of the pterygoid canal. Its lateral half articulates with the petrous temporal bone at a *sphenopetrosal synchrondrosis*. Inferior to this the *sulcus tubae* contains the cartilaginous auditory tube. Anterior to the sphenoidal spine the concave *squamosal margin* is serrated (bevelled internally below, externally above) for articulation with the temporal squama. The tip of the greater wing, bevelled internally, articulates with the parietal's sphenoidal angle at the *pterion*. Medial to this, a triangular

rough area articulates with the frontal bone, its medial angle continuous with the inferior boundary of the superior orbital fissure, its anterior angle by a serrated articulation with the zygomatic bone.

Lesser wings

The lesser wings are triangular, pointed plates protruding laterally from the anterosuperior regions of the body (**6**.168). The *superior surface* of each is smooth and related to the cerebral frontal lobe. The *inferior surface* is a posterior part of the orbital roof and upper boundary of the *superior orbital fissure*; it overhangs the middle cranial fossa. The posterior border projects into the lateral cerebral fissure; its medial end is the *anterior clinoid process*, for attachment of the anterior end of the free tentorial border. The anterior and middle clinoid processes are sometimes united to form a *caroticoclinoid foramen*. The lesser wing is connected to the body by an anterior root, thin and flat, and a posterior, thick and triangular root; between them the *optic canal* contains the optic nerve and ophthalmic artery. Growth of the posterior root is closely associated with variations in the canal (Kier 1966), whose cranial opening may be duplicated (Warwick 1951). More often the division is incomplete.

Superior orbital fissure

The superior orbital fissure, triangular and connecting the cranial cavity and orbit, is bounded medially by the sphenoid body, above by the lesser wing, below by the medial margin of the orbital surface of the greater wing; it is completed laterally, between greater and lesser wings, by the frontal bone. For its contents see page 1355 and **8**.455.

Pterygoid processes

The pterygoid processes (**6**.168B, 170, 171) descend perpendicularly from the junctions of the greater wings and body. Each consists of

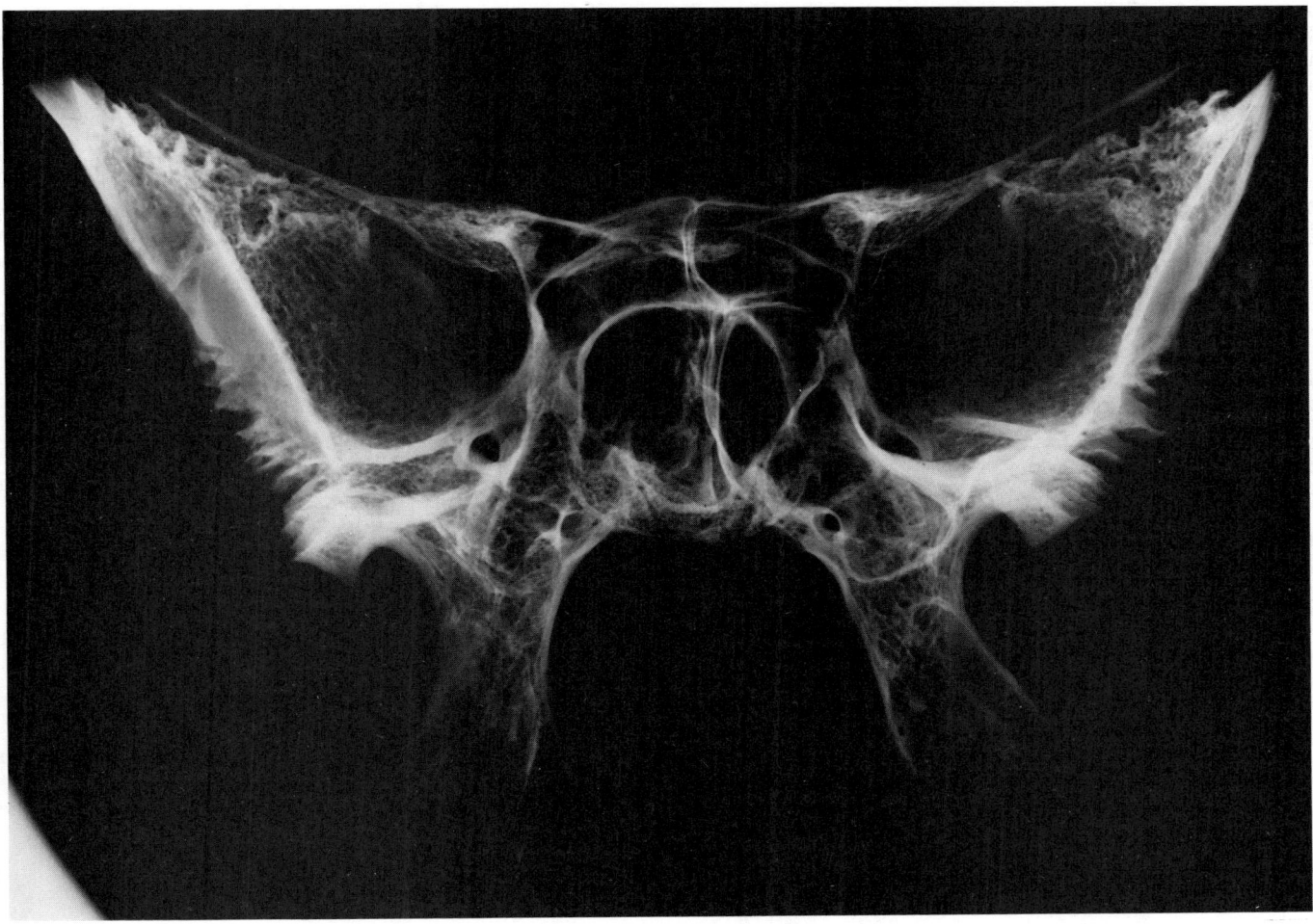

6.171   High resolution projection microradiograph of the sphenoid bone (anteroposterior projection). Note in particular the sphenoidal body and its contained sinuses, the architecture of the greater and lesser wings, and pterygoid processes and the disposition of the optic canal, superior orbital fissure, foramen rotundum and pterygoid canal. (Contributed by C Buckland-Wright, Department of Anatomy, Guy's Hospital Medical School, London.)

a medial and lateral plate, their upper parts fused anteriorly. They are separated below by the angular *pterygoid fissure*, whose margins articulate with the palatine's pyramidal process. They diverge behind and the cuneiform *pterygoid fossa* between them contains the medial pterygoid and tensor veli palatini. Above is the small, oval, shallow *scaphoid fossa*, formed by division of the upper posterior border of the medial plate; to it part of the tensor veli palatini is attached. The anterior surface of the root of the pterygoid process is broad and triangular and is the pterygopalatine fossa's posterior wall, pierced by the anterior opening of the *pterygoid canal*.

Lateral pterygoid plate

The lateral pterygoid plate is broad, thin and everted, its *lateral surface*, being part of the medial wall of the infratemporal fossa, gives attachment of the lower part of the lateral pterygoid; its *medial surface* is the lateral wall of the pterygoid fossa and to it most of the medial pterygoid is attached. The upper part of its *anterior border* is a posterior boundary of the pterygomaxillary fissure; the lower part articulates with the palatine bone. Its *posterior border* is free.

Medial pterygoid plate

The medial pterygoid plate is narrower and longer than the lateral; its lower end curves into the lateral, unciform *pterygoid hamulus*, which deflects the tendon of the tensor veli palatini, and the pterygo-mandibular raphe attached to it. The *lateral surface* is the medial wall of the pterygoid fossa; the tensor veli palatini adjoins it; the *medial surface* is a lateral boundary of the posterior nasal aperture. The medial plate is prolonged above on the sphenoid body's inferior aspect as the thin *vaginal process*, articulating anteriorly with the palatine's sphenoidal process and medially with the vomerine ala. Inferiorly it has a furrow, anteriorly made into a canal by the palatine sphenoidal process; this *palatovaginal canal* transmits pharyngeal branches of the maxillary artery and pterygopalatine ganglion. To the whole of the medial plate's posterior margin the pharyngobasilar fascia is attached and to its lower end the superior pharyngeal constrictor. At its upper end is a small *pterygoid tubercle*, just below the pterygoid canal's posterior opening. Projecting back near the margin's midpoint is the *processus tubarius*, supporting the auditory tube's pharyngeal end. The plate's anterior margin, in its lower part, articulates with the posterior border of the palatine's perpendicular plate.

Sphenoidal conchae

The sphenoidal conchae (**6**.170) are two thin, curved platelets, attached anteroinferiorly to the sphenoid body; the superior concave surface of each is the anterior wall and part of the floor of a sphenoidal sinus. They are largely destroyed in disarticulating a skull; in situ each has anterior vertical, quadrilateral and posterior horizontal, triangular parts. The anterior part consists of:

- a superolateral depressed area, completing the posterior ethmoidal sinuses and joining below with the orbital process of a palatine bone
- an inferomedial area, smooth and triangular and part of the nasal roof, perforated above by the round opening connecting the sphenoidal sinus and sphenoethmoidal recess.

Anterior parts of the two bones meet in the midline, protruding as the sphenoidal crest. The horizontal part appears in the nasal roof and completes the sphenopalatine foramen; its medial edge articulates with the sphenoid's rostrum and vomerine ala; its apex, directed posteriorly, is superomedial to the vaginal process of the medial pterygoid plate and joins the posterior part of the ala. A small conchal part sometimes appears in the medial orbital wall between the ethmoid's orbital plate in front, the palatine's orbital process below and the frontal bone above.

Ossification

Until the seventh or eighth month in utero the sphenoid body has a *presphenoidal part*, anterior to the tuberculum sellae, with which the lesser wings are continuous, and a *postsphenoidal part*, comprising the sella turcica and dorsum sellae, and integral with the greater wings and pterygoid processes. Much of the bone is preformed in cartilage. There are six ossificatory centres for the presphenoidal and

eight for postsphenoidal parts. This multiplicity accords with the sphenoid's evolution from a number of elements, such as the median presphenoid and basisphenoid homologous with the human parts defined above. The lesser wings, primitively separate orbitosphenoids, show a tendency to fusion with the body in mammals.

Presphenoidal part. About the ninth fetal week a centre appears in each wing, lateral to the optic canal; a little later two bilateral centres appear in the presphenoidal body. Each sphenoidal concha has a centre, appearing superoposteriorly in the nasal capsule in the fifth month in utero; as this enlarges it partly surrounds a posterosuperior expansion of the nasal cavity, which becomes the sphenoidal sinus. The posterior conchal wall is absorbed and the sinus invades the presphenoid. In the fourth year the concha fuses with the ethmoidal labyrinth and before puberty with the sphenoid and palatine bones. Its anterior deficiency persists as an opening for the sphenoidal sinus.

Postsphenoidal part. First centres appear in the greater wings about the eighth fetal week, one in each below the foramen rotundum in the wing's basal cartilage; this centre forms only the wing's root, near the foramen rotundum and pterygoid canal; the remainder is ossified in mesenchyme, spreading also into the lateral pterygoid plate. About the fourth fetal month two centres appear, flanking the sella turcica, and soon fuse. The medial pterygoid plates are also ossified in 'membrane', a centre in each probably appearing about the ninth or tenth week; the hamulus is *chondrified* during the third fetal month and at once begins to ossify (Fawcett 1905). Medial and lateral pterygoid plates join about the sixth fetal month; during the fourth a centre appears for each lingula, soon joining the body.

Further details. Presphenoidal and postsphenoidal parts fuse about the eighth month in utero, but an unciform cartilage persists after birth in lower parts of the junction. At birth the bone is tripartite (**6**.172): a central part, body and lesser wings, and lateral parts each comprising a greater wing and pterygoid process. During the first year the greater wings and body unite around the pterygoid canals and the lesser wings extend medially above the body's anterior part, meeting to form the smooth, elevated *jugum sphenoidale*. By the twenty-fifth year sphenoid and occipital bones are completely fused. Anterior in the hypophyseal fossa is an occasional vascular foramen, often erroneously termed the *craniopharyngeal canal* (p. 258). (For discussion of cartilage canals in fetal spheno-occipital synchondrosis consult Moss-Salentijn 1975.)

The sphenoidal sinus before birth is an extension of the nasal cavity into the sphenoidal concha. In the second or third year it spreads into the presphenoid and later invades the postsphenoid, reaching full size in adolescence. As age advances it often enlarges further by absorption of its walls.

Certain sphenoidal parts are connected by ligaments which occasionally ossify, such as the *pterygospinous*, between the sphenoid spine and upper part of lateral pterygoid plate; the *interclinoid*, joining the anterior to the posterior clinoid process; and the *caroticoclinoid*, connecting the anterior to the middle clinoid process. For details of fetal and perinatal development of the optic foramen and canal consult Kier (1966). Lang (1977) has surveyed ossificatory variations of the sella turcica.

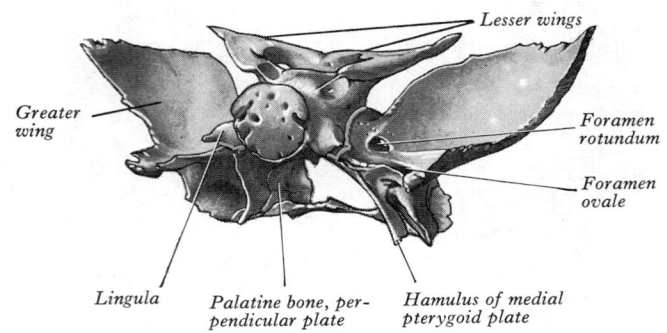

6.172 The sphenoid bone at birth, viewed from behind and from the right side. The blue strip indicates the cartilage between the central and the lateral parts on the right side; this is only partly visible on the left. Note that the two palatine bones are in situ.

Premature synostosis of the junction between pre- and post-sphenoidal parts, or of the spheno-occipital suture, produces a characteristic appearance, obvious in profile, of an abnormal depression of the nasal bridge (*hypertelorism*).

TEMPORAL BONES

The temporal bones in the sides and base of the skull are developmentally divisible into *squamous, petromastoid, tympanic* and *styloid* parts. These morphologically distinct elements have fused during the evolution of higher vertebrates. The squamous part is a dermal bone evolved to help enclosure of the brain. The petromastoid part is preformed in cartilage; it preserves precise orientation of the membranous labyrinth. The tympanic part, formed in mesenchyme, is homologous with the os angulare, part of the composite lower jaw of many reptiles and osseous fishes, integrated into the skull and adapted to form part of the tympanic cavity and external acoustic meatus and to support the tympanic membrane, all concerned in sound transmission. The styloid process is the dorsal element of the hyoid arch. Fusion of these parts and inclusion of the tympanic cavity and auditory ossicles are discussed on page 263.

In structure the temporal squama is like other cranial bones: the mastoid part is trabecular and variably pneumatized, the petrous part compact.

Squamous part

The squamous part or squama, anterosuperior in the bone, is thin and partly translucent. Its *temporal surface* (**6**.173) is smooth, slightly convex, and part of the temporal fossa for attachment of temporalis; above the external acoustic meatus it is grooved vertically by the middle temporal artery. The *supramastoid crest* curves backwards and upwards across its posterior part; it is an attachment of temporal fascia and muscle. The junction between squamous and mastoid parts is about 1.5 cm below this crest; traces of the squamomastoid suture may persist. Between the anterior end of the crest and posterosuperior quadrant of the external acoustic meatus is the *suprameatal triangle*, a depression marking the mastoid antrum, medial to it at a depth of about 1.25 cm (p. 610); anteriorly it usually contains a small *suprameatal spine*.

The *cerebral surface* (**6**.174) is concave; its depressions correspond to convolutions of the temporal lobe, its grooves to middle meningeal vessels; its lower border is fused to the anterior petrous surface, but traces of a petrosquamosal suture often appear in adult bones. The *superior border* is thin, bevelled internally and overlaps the parietal's inferior border at the squamosal suture. Posteriorly it forms an angle with the mastoid element. The *antero-inferior border*, thin above and thick below, joints with the greater wing; above it is bevelled internally, below externally.

Zygomatic process. This part of the *zygoma*, juts forwards from the squama's lower region. Its triangular posterior part has a broad base directed laterally, its surfaces superior and inferior. The process then twists anteromedially, so that its surfaces become medial and lateral. The posterior part's superior surface is concave and continuous with that of the squama; the inferior surface is bounded by *anterior* and *posterior roots*, converging into the anterior part of the process. At the junction of the roots the *tubercle of the zygomatic root* gives attachment to the lateral temporomandibular ligament. The posterior root is prolonged forwards above the external acoustic meatus, its upper border continuing into the supramastoid crest. The anterior root juts almost horizontally from the squama; its inferior surface, with an anteroposterior convexity covered by cartilage, contacts the joint's articular disc, forming a short semicylindrical *articular tubercle*, the anterior limit of the mandibular fossa. Very rarely the squama is perforated above the posterior root by a *squamosal foramen*, transmitting the petrosquamous sinus (p. 1584).

The zygomatic process' anterior part is thin and flat. To its superior border the temporal fascia is attached, to the inferior, short and arched, some fibres of masseter. The convex lateral surface is subcutaneous; the medial is concave and provides an attachment for part of masseter. The anterior end is deeply serrated and slopes obliquely posteroinferiorly to articulate with the zygomatic bone's temporal process. Anterior to the articular tubercle a small triangular area forms part of the roof of the infratemporal fossa, separated from the squama's temporal surface by a ridge, continuous behind with the zygomatic process' anterior root, in front with the infratemporal crest of the sphenoid's greater wing.

Mandibular fossa. The fossa, limited in front by the articular tubercle, has an anterior articular area, formed by temporal squama,

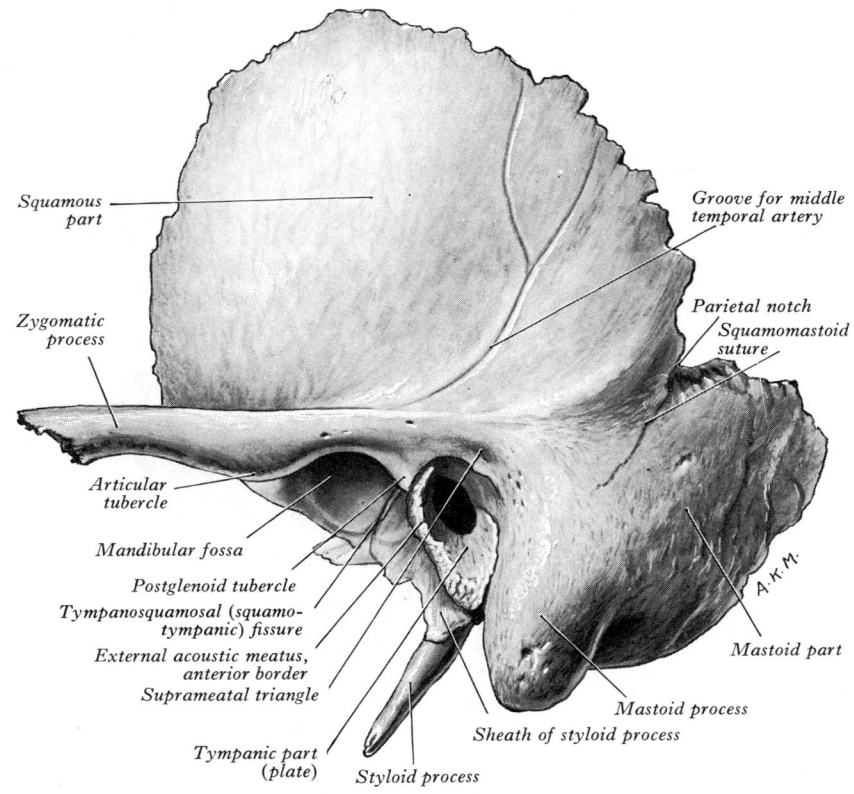

Squamous part

Zygomatic process

Articular tubercle

Mandibular fossa

Postglenoid tubercle

Tympanosquamosal (squamo-tympanic) fissure

External acoustic meatus, anterior border

Suprameatal triangle

Tympanic part (plate)

Styloid process

Groove for middle temporal artery

Parietal notch

Squamomastoid suture

A.K.M.

Mastoid part

Mastoid process

Sheath of styloid process

6.173   The left temporal bone: external aspect.

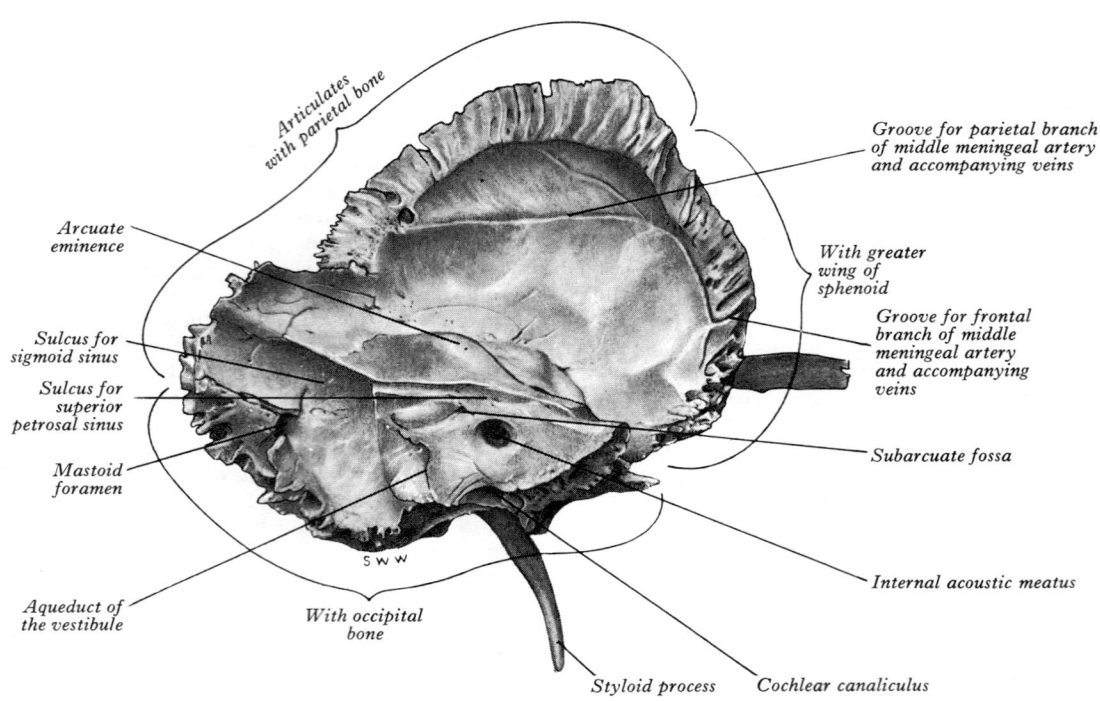

6.174   The left temporal bone: internal aspect. Note **6**.173 and **6**.174 were painted at different times by different artists and from different specimens. Contrast curvatures of the styloid processes (see text).

and a posterior non-articular area, formed by the tympanic element. The *articular surface*, smooth, oval and deeply hollow, articulates with the temporomandibular disc; the non-articular area sometimes contains part of the parotid gland. A small, conical *postglenoid tubercle* separates the articular surface laterally from the tympanic plate; it is prominent in some mammals, descending behind the mandibular condyle to prevent backward displacement; it is sometimes described as a third root of the zygomatic process. (For a multivariate analysis of this articular surface (and many other cranial parameters) in modern and fossil mankind and apes, and an evaluation of functional deductions, consult Ashton et al 1976, Ashton &

Moore 1980.) Between the medial part of the articular fossa and the tympanic plate is the *squamotympanic fissure*, into which the anterolateral edge of the tegmen tympani turns down; the *petro-tympanic fissure* is between this plate and the tympanic part; it leads into the tympanic cavity and contains an anterior malleolar ligament and anterior tympanic branch of the maxillary artery. At the fissure's medial end is the anterior opening of the *anterior canaliculus for the chorda tympani*. Rarely, a *postglenoid foramen* exists anterior to the external acoustic meatus in the line of fusion of the squama and tympanic part; it replaces the squamosal foramen noted above and transmits the petrosquamous sinus (p. 1584).

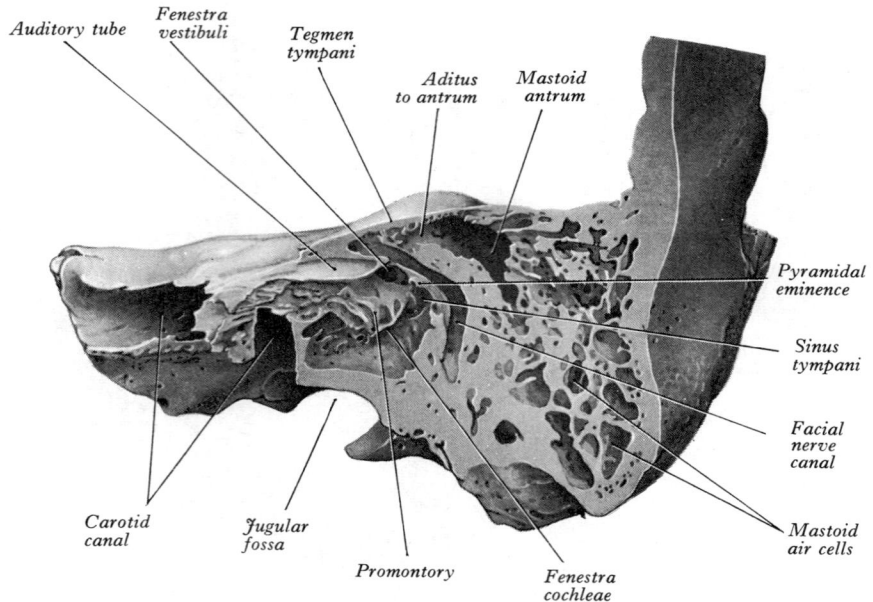

6.175   Oblique vertical section through the left temporal bone in the long axis of the tympanic cavity. The lateral surface of the medial half of the bone is shown.

Petromastoid part

The petromastoid part of the temporal bone, morphologically one element (p. 593), is conveniently described in mastoid and petrous parts.

Mastoid part. This is the posterior region of the temporal bone, and has an *outer surface* (**6**.173) roughened by attachments of the occipital belly of occipitofrontalis and auricularis posterior. Frequently near its posterior border is a *mastoid foramen*, traversed by a vein from the sigmoid sinus and a small dural branch of the occipital artery. Its position and size vary; it may be in the occipital or occipitotemporal suture. It is parasutural in 40–50% of crania (p. 609) but may be absent. The mastoid part projects down as the conical *mastoid process*, larger in adult males. To its lateral surface sternocleidomastoid, splenius capitis and longissimus capitis are attached and, medially, in a deep *mastoid notch*, the posterior belly of digastric. Medial to this a shallow *occipital groove* contains the occipital artery. The *internal mastoid surface* (**6**.174) bears a deep, curved *sigmoid sulcus* for the sigmoid venous sinus and posteriorly the mastoid foramen. The sulcus is separated from the innermost mastoid air cells merely by a thin lamina of bone. The air cells (**6**.175, 176) and *mastoid antrum* are described on page 1374. The mastoid's *superior border* is thick and serrated for articulation with the mastoid angle of the parietal bone. Its serrated *posterior border* articulates with the inferior border of the occipital between its lateral angle and jugular process. The mastoid element is fused with the descending process of the squamous part: below, it appears in the posterior wall of the tympanic cavity.

Petrous part. This is wedged between the sphenoid and occipital bones in the cranial base (**6**.150), and inclined superiorly and antero-medially; it has a base, apex, three surfaces and margins. The acoustic labyrinth is within it.

The *base*, an artificial concept, corresponds to the suture between the petrous and squamous elements, though this disappears soon after birth. Since a mastoid process is a postnatal petrous development, the base is arbitrary but indicated by partial separation due to the mastoid antrum.

The *apex*, blunt and irregular, is angled between the posterior border of the greater wing of the sphenoid and the basioccipital bone; it contains the carotid canal's anterior opening and limits posterolaterally the foramen lacerum.

The *anterior surface* partly floors the middle cranial fossa and is continuous with the cerebral surface of the squamous part, although the petrosquamosal suture often persists late in life. The whole surface is adapted to the inferior temporal gyri. Behind the apex is a *trigeminal impression* for the trigeminal ganglion. Bone antero-lateral to this roofs the anterior part of the carotid canal, but is often deficient. A ridge separates the trigeminal impression from another hollow behind, which partly roofs the internal acoustic meatus and cochlea. This in turn is limited behind by the *arcuate eminence* (**6**.174) and raised by the anterior semicircular canal. Laterally it roofs the vestibule and, partly, the facial canal. Between the squamous part laterally and the arcuate eminence and the hollows just described medially, the surface is formed by the *tegmen tympani*. This thin plate of bone, roof of the mastoid antrum, extends forwards above the tympanic cavity (**6**.175) and the canal for the tensor tympani. Its lateral margin meets the squama at the petrosquamosal suture, turning down in front as the lateral wall of the canal for the tensor tympani and the osseous part of the auditory tube; its lower edge is in the squamotympanic fissure (p. 567). Anteriorly the tegmen bears a narrow groove, passing posterolaterally to enter bone anterior to the arcuate eminence by a hiatus for the greater petrosal nerve, passing forwards to the foramen lacerum. A smaller, more lateral hiatus transmits the lesser petrosal nerve from the tympanic plexus; the bone in front of this hiatus may be grooved. The posterior slope of the arcuate eminence overlies the posterior and lateral semicircular canals; lateral to it the posterior part of the tegmen tympani roofs the mastoid antrum.

The *posterior surface* (**6**.174) is an anterior part of the posterior cranial fossa, continuous with the internal mastoid surface. Near its centre is the *internal acoustic meatus* (p. 572), behind which a small slit, almost hidden by a thin plate of bone, leads to the *vestibular aqueduct*, containing the saccus and ductus endolymphaticus together with a small artery and vein. The terminal half of the saccus

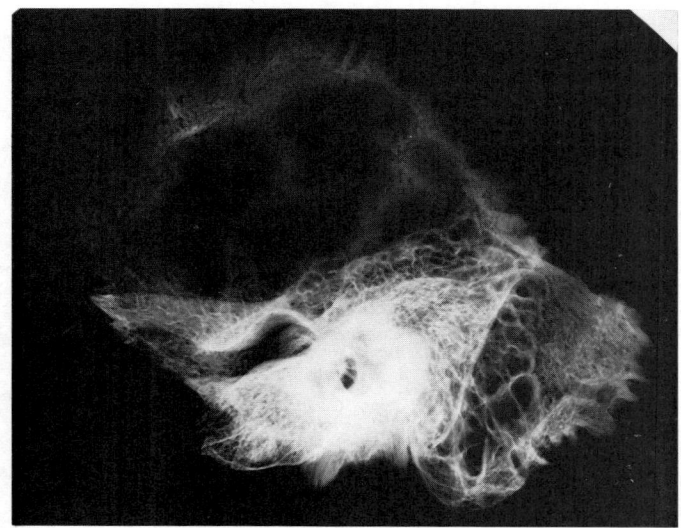

A

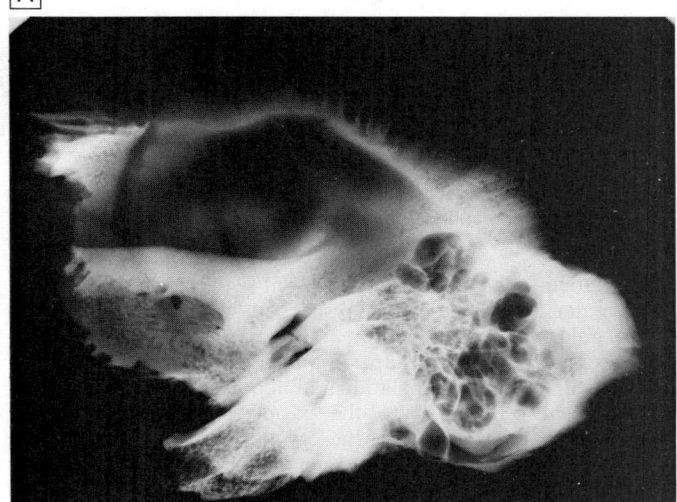

B

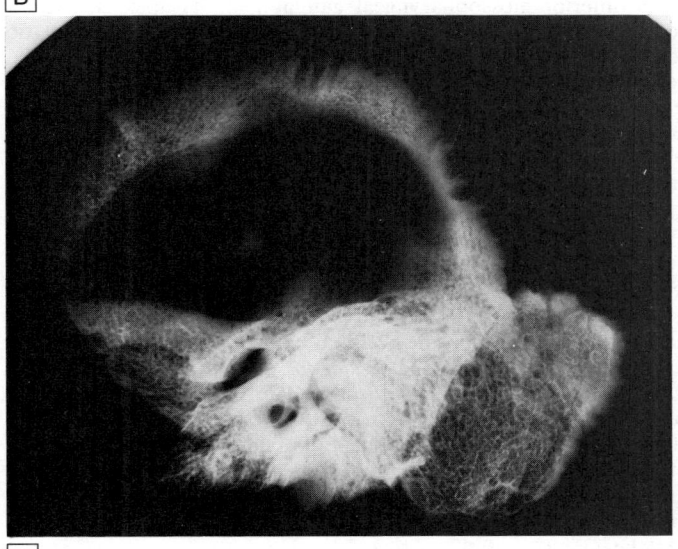

C

6.176 High resolution projection microradiographs of the petromastoid, tympanic and squamous parts of three temporal bones (mediolateral projection), showing marked variation in extent and mode of pneumatization. A. The air-cells are comparatively large and extend beyond the mastoid process as far as the mandibular fossa. B. The cells are large but restricted to the post-otic and mastoid regions of the bone. C. Obvious pneumatization is absent; a fine meshwork of trabecular bone occupies the core of the mastoid process. (Prepared and contributed by C Buckland-Wright, Department of Anatomy, Guy's Hospital Medical School, London.)

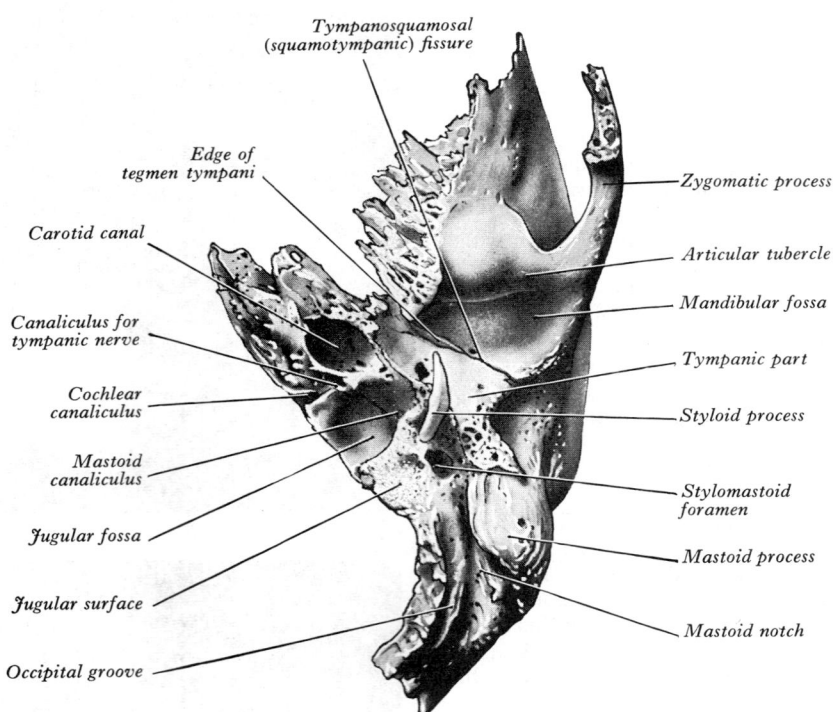

Tympanosquamosal (squamotympanic) fissure

Edge of tegmen tympani

Carotid canal

Canaliculus for tympanic nerve

Cochlear canaliculus

Mastoid canaliculus

Jugular fossa

Jugular surface

Occipital groove

Zygomatic process

Articular tubercle

Mandibular fossa

Tympanic part

Styloid process

Stylomastoid foramen

Mastoid process

Mastoid notch

6.177   The left temporal bone: inferior aspect.

endolymphaticus protrudes through the slit between the periosteum and dura mater. Above these openings is the *subarcuate fossa* (p. 572).

The irregular *inferior surface* (**6**.177) is part of the exterior of the cranial base. Near the petrous apex a quadrilateral area is partly for attachment of levator veli palatini and the cartilaginous auditory tube, and partly connected to the basioccipital bone by dense fibrocartilage. Behind this is the large, circular opening of the *carotid canal* (p. 567), behind which is the *jugular fossa* of variable depth and size and containing the superior jugular bulb. Anteromedial to this, below the internal acoustic meatus, is a triangular depression for the inferior glossopharyngeal ganglion; at its apex is a small opening into the *cochlear canaliculus*, occupied by the perilymphatic duct, a tube of dura mater and a vein from the cochlea to the internal jugular vein. On the ridge between the carotid canal and jugular fossa is a *canaliculus for the tympanic nerve* from the glosso-pharyngeal. Lateral in the jugular fossa is the *mastoid canaliculus* for the vagal auricular branch. Behind the fossa the *jugular surface*, a rough quadrilateral, is covered by cartilage joining it to the jugular process of the occipital bone.

The *superior border*, the longest, is grooved by the superior petrosal sinus, the tentorium cerebelli being attached to the groove's edges except at its medial end, where it is crossed by the trigeminal roots. The *posterior border*, intermediate in length, bears medially a sulcus which forms, with one on the occipital bone, a gutter for the inferior petrosal sinus. Behind this the *jugular fossa* forms, with the occipital jugular notch and the jugular foramen, and is also notched by the glossopharyngeal nerve. Bone on either or both sides of the jugular notch may meet the occipital bone and divide the foramen into two or three parts. The *anterior border* is joined laterally to the temporal squama at the *petrosquamosal suture*; medially it articulates with the sphenoid's greater wing.

At the junction of the petrous and squamous parts two canals exist, one above the other, separated by a thin osseous plate. Both lead to the tympanic cavity, the upper containing the tensor tympani, the lower the auditory tube.

Tympanic part

The tympanic part of the temporal bone (**6**.177) is a curved plate below the squama, anterior to the mastoid process. Internally it fuses with the petrous part and appears between this and the squama, where it is inferolateral to the auditory orifice. Behind, it fuses with the squama and mastoid process and is the anterior limit of the

tympanomastoid fissure. Its concave *posterior surface* forms the anterior wall, floor and part of the posterior wall of the external acoustic meatus. (Its posteroinferior wall may display a longitudinal *auditory torus*.) Medially on this surface is a narrow *tympanic sulcus* for attachment of the tympanic membrane. The quadrilateral and concave *anterior surface* is the posterior wall of the mandibular fossa and may contact the parotid gland. Its rough *lateral border* forms most of the margin of the external acoustic meatus and is continuous with its cartilaginous part. Laterally the *upper border* is fused with the back of the postglenoid tubercle; medially it is the posterior edge of the petrotympanic fissure. The *inferior border* is sharp, splitting laterally to form, at its root, a *sheath of the styloid process* (vaginal process). Centrally the tympanic part is thin, often perforated. Between the styloid and mastoid processes the *stylomastoid foramen*, the external end of the facial canal, transmits the facial nerve and stylomastoid artery.

Styloid process

The styloid process, slender, pointed, about 2.5 cm in length, projects anteroinferiorly from the temporal bone's inferior aspect. Its curvature is somewhat variable (**6**.176). Its proximal part (*tympanohyal*) is ensheathed by the tympanic plate, especially anterolaterally; to its distal part (*stylohyal*) are attached muscles and ligaments (p. 561). The process is covered laterally by the parotid gland; the facial nerve crosses its base, the external carotid artery its tip, embedded in the gland. Medially the process is separated from the beginning of the internal jugular vein by the attachment of stylopharyngeus.

External acoustic meatus

The external acoustic meatus, about 16 mm long, slopes down anteromedially; its floor is convex upwards. In sagittal section it is oval or elliptical with a long axis directed down and slightly back. Its anterior wall, floor and lower posterior wall are formed by the tympanic plate, its roof and upper posterior wall by the temporal squama. Its medial end is closed by tympanic membrane, the outer bounded above by the posterior zygomatic root, below which a *suprameatal spine* may exist.

Ossification

The four temporal components ossify independently (**6**.178). The *squama* is ossified in a sheet of condensed mesenchyme from a single centre near the zygomatic roots, appearing in the seventh or eighth

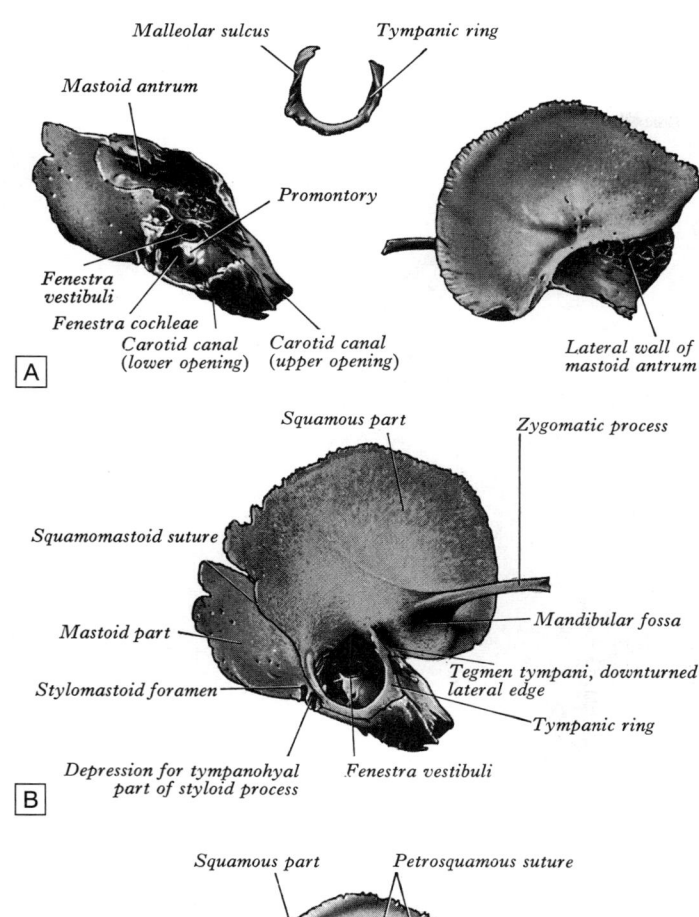

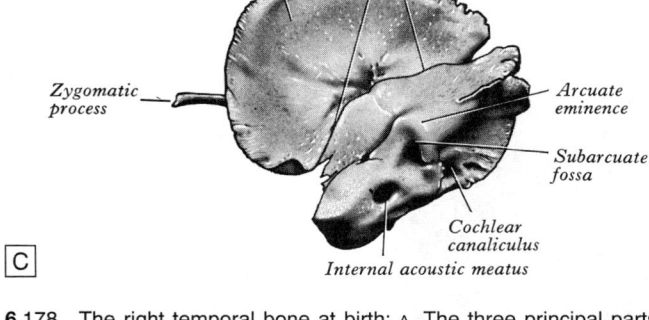

6.178 The right temporal bone at birth; A. The three principal parts are, from left to right, petromastoid part (lateral aspect), tympanic ring (medial aspect) and squama (medial aspect); B. Lateral aspect with the rudimentary styloid process removed (yellow = tympanic part, brown = squamous part, petromastoid part = uncoloured); c. Medial aspect.

week in utero. The *petromastoid part* has several centres appearing in the cartilaginous otic capsule (p. 263) during the fifth month. As many as 14 have been described, variable in order of appearance. Several are small and inconstant, soon fusing with others. This multiplicity accords with numerous otic bones in earlier forms. The otic capsule is almost fully ossified by the end of the sixth month. The *tympanic part* is also ossified in mesenchyme from a centre identifiable about the third month; at birth it is an incomplete *tympanic ring*, deficient above (6.178), its concavity grooved by a tympanic sulcus for the tympanic membrane. Inclined obliquely downwards and forwards across the medial aspect of the anterior part of the ring is the *malleolar sulcus* (6.178A) for the anterior malleolar process, chorda tympani and anterior tympanic artery. The *styloid process* is developed at the cranial end of cartilage in the second visceral or hyoid arch (p. 277) by two centres: a proximal, for the tympanohyal, appearing before birth; the other, for the distal stylohyal, after birth. The tympanic ring unites with the squama shortly before birth, the petromastoid fusing with it and the tympanohyal during the first year. The stylohyal does not unite with the rest of the process until after puberty and may never do so.

During ossification, the tympanic cavity, mastoid antrum and posterior end of the auditory tube are all in bone. The petrous part forms the roof, floor and medial wall of the cavity; the squama and tympanic part, with the membrana tympani, form its lateral wall. **At birth** the middle and inner ears are **adult size** (Dahm et al 1993), with the tympanic cavity, mastoid antrum, tympanic membrane and auditory ossicles all almost adult size. The anterior process does not join the malleus until 6 months later. The internal acoustic meatus is about 6 mm in horizontal diameter, 4 mm vertically and 7 mm in length at birth, adult diameters being 7.7 mm and 11 mm.

After birth and apart from general growth, changes in the temporal bone are:

- The tympanic *ring* extends posterolaterally to become cylindrical, growing into a fibrocartilaginous *tympanic plate*, which forms the adjacent part of the external acoustic meatus at this stage. This growth is not equal but is rapid in the anterior and posterior regions, which meet and blend; thus, for a time, there is in the floor an opening (*foramen of Huschke*), usually closed at about the fifth year, but sometimes permanent (in 5–46% of adult crania from ancient and modern populations, p. 609); in Burmese crania a marked sexual difference occurs (25% in males, 40% in females). By posterior extension the tympanic plate ensheathes the styloid process and extends medially over the petrous bone to the carotid canal.
- The mandibular fossa is first shallow, facing more laterally, then deepening and ultimately facing downwards. Posteroinferiorly the squama grows down behind the tympanic ring to form the lateral wall of the mastoid antrum.
- The mastoid part is at first flat, the stylomastoid foramen and rudimentary styloid process being immediately behind the tympanic ring. As mastoid air cells develop the lateral mastoid region grows down and forwards to form the mastoid process, styloid process and stylomastoid foramen, becoming inferior. Descent of the foramen lengthens the facial canal. Not until late in the second year is the mastoid process perceptible.
- The subarcuate fossa is gradually filled and almost obliterated.

For a discussion of postnatal growth of the temporal bone see Dahm et al (1993).

The external acoustic meatus is relatively as long in children as in adults, but the canal is fibrocartilaginous, whereas its medial two-thirds are osseous in adults. Surgical access to the tympanic cavity is via the mastoid antrum; in children only a thin scale of bone must be removed in the suprameatal triangle to reach the antrum (p. 1374).

PARIETAL BONES

Parietal bones (6.179) form most of the cranial roof and sides. Irregularly quadrilateral, each has two surfaces, four borders and four angles.

The *external surface* (6.179A) is convex and smooth, with a central *parietal tuber (tuberosity)*. Curved *superior* and *inferior temporal lines* cross it, forming posterosuperior arches; to the superior arch is attached the temporal fascia; the inferior indicates the upper limit of attachment of temporalis. Above these lines is the *epicranial aponeurosis* (galea aponeurotica), below them part of the temporal fossa. Posteriorly, close to the sagittal (superior) border, a *parietal foramen* transmits a vein from the superior sagittal sinus and sometimes a branch of occipital artery; the foramen is sometimes absent.

The *internal surface* (6.179B) is concave and marked by cerebral gyri and grooves for the middle meningeal vessels which ascend, inclining backwards, from the *sphenoidal (anteroinferior) angle* and posterior half or more of its inferior border. Along the sagittal border is a *groove for the superior sagittal sinus*, completed by the opposite parietal; the falx cerebri is attached to its edges. *Granular foveolae* for arachnoid granulations flank the sagittal sulcus, being most pronounced in old age.

The dentated *sagittal border*, longest and thickest, articulates with the opposite parietal at the sagittal suture. In the *squamosal (inferior)* border the anterior part is short, thin and truncated, bevelled externally and overlapped by the greater wing of the sphenoid; the middle is arched, bevelled externally and overlapped by the temporal squama; the posterior part is short, thick and serrated for articulation with the mastoid bone. The *frontal border* is deeply serrated, bevelled

593

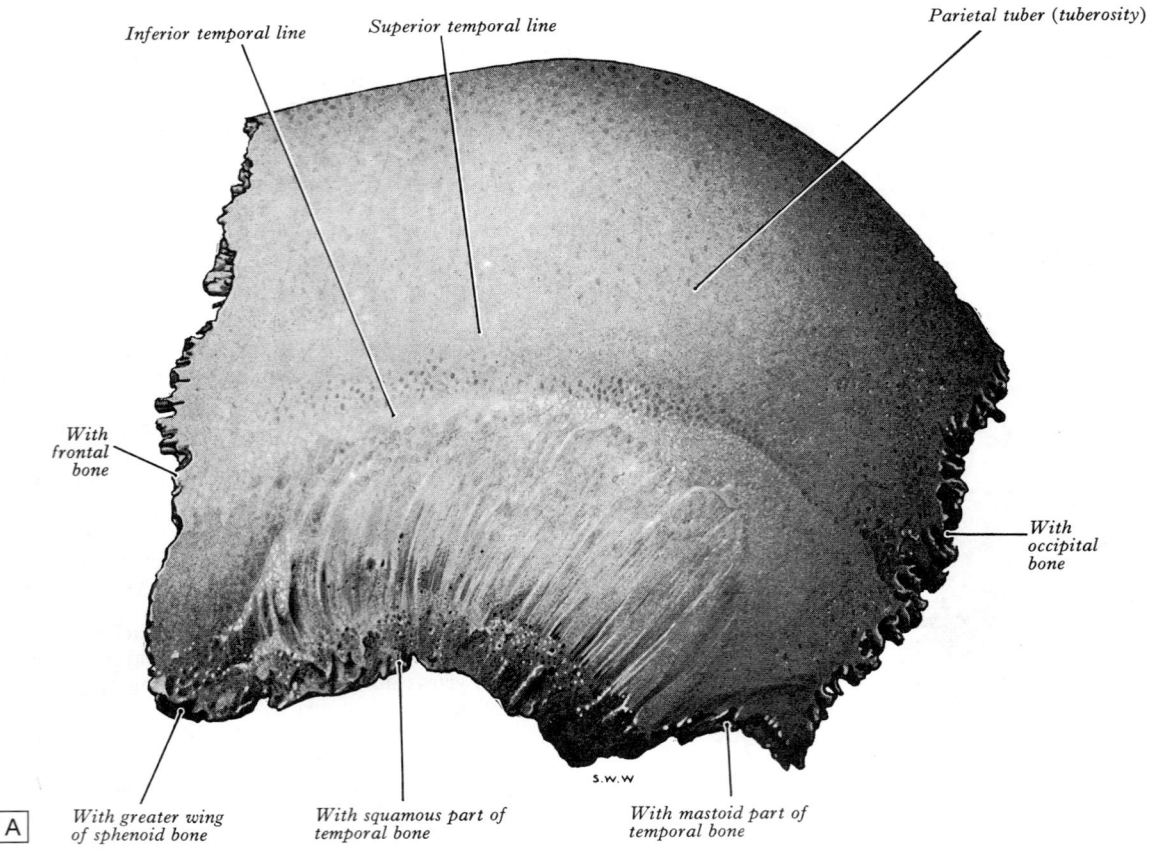

Inferior temporal line

Superior temporal line

Parietal tuber (tuberosity)

With
frontal
bone

With
occipital
bone

S.W.W

A

With greater wing
of sphenoid bone

With squamous part of
temporal bone

With mastoid part of
temporal bone

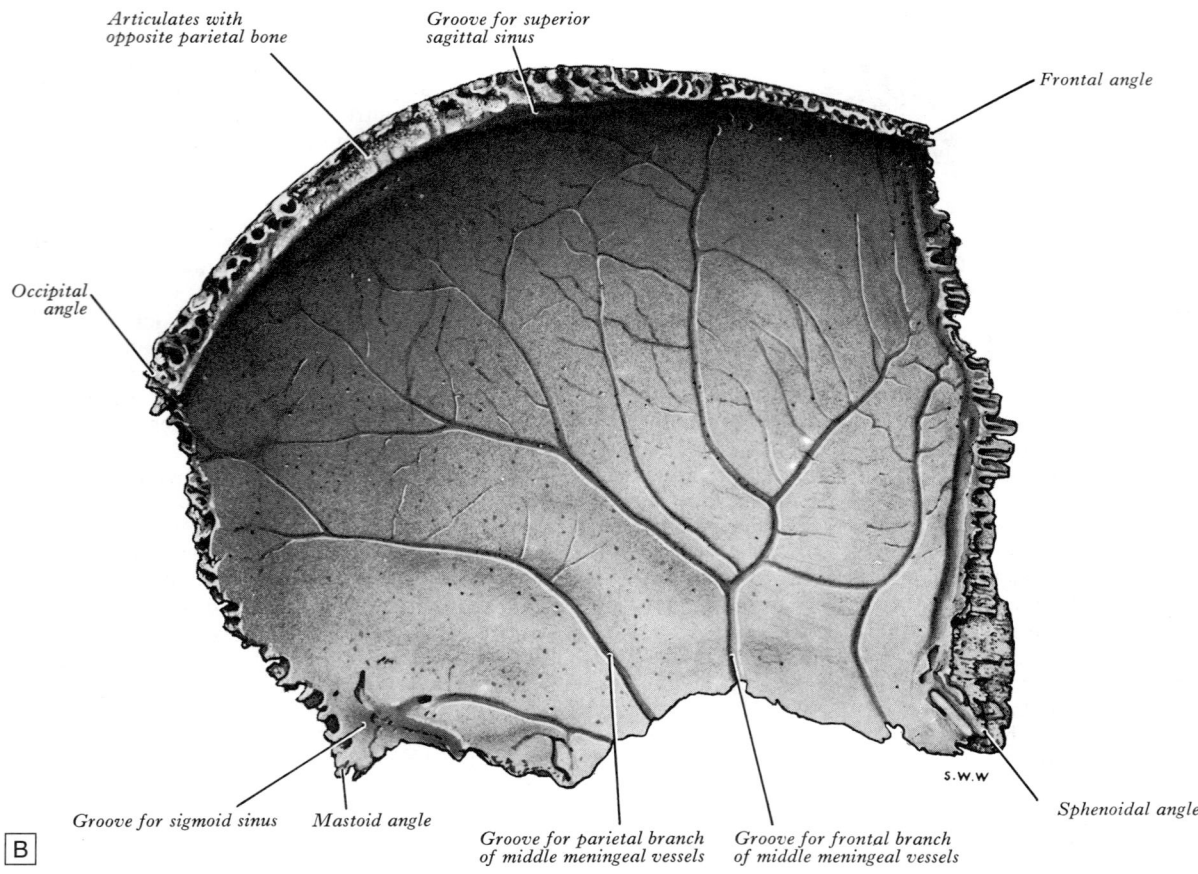

Articulates with
opposite parietal bone

Groove for superior
sagittal sinus

Frontal angle

Occipital
angle

Sphenoidal angle

S.W.W

B

Groove for sigmoid sinus

Mastoid angle

Groove for parietal branch
of middle meningeal vessels

Groove for frontal branch
of middle meningeal vessels

6.179   The left parietal bone; A. external surface; B. internal surface.

externally above, internally below, and articulates with the frontal bone to form half the coronal suture. The *occipital border*, deeply dentated, articulates with the occipital, forming half the lambdoid suture.

The *frontal (anterosuperior) angle*, almost 90°, is at the *bregma* (meeting of the sagittal and coronal sutures). The *sphenoidal (antero-inferior) angle* is between the frontal bone and greater wing of the sphenoid, its internal surface marked by a deep groove, sometimes a canal, for the frontal branches of the middle meningeal vessels. The frontal sometimes meets the temporal squama, the parietal then failing to reach the greater wing. Where these four bones meet is the *pterion* (p. 560). (Frontotemporal articulation shows racial variation, probably epigenetic; its incidence varies from almost zero in a British seventeenth century cemetery to 9.8% in Nigerian crania.) The rounded *occipital (posterosuperior) angle* is at the *lambda*, the meeting of the sagittal and lambdoid sutures. The blunt *mastoid (posteroinferior) angle* articulates with the occipital and mastoid temporal bones. Internally it bears a broad, shallow groove for the junction of transverse and sigmoid sinuses.

Ossification

Each parietal is ossified from two centres, appearing one above the other near its tuberosity at about the seventh week in utero in dense mesenchyme. These unite early; ossification radiates towards the margins; the angles are consequently the last to be ossified and hence fontanelles occur at these sites (p. 607). At birth the temporal lines are low down, reaching their final position after the eruption of the molar teeth. Occasionally the parietal is divided by an anteroposterior suture.

FRONTAL BONE

The frontal bone is like half a shallow, irregular cap forming the forehead or *frons*; on each side a horizontal *orbital part* roofs most of an orbital cavity.

The *external surface* (**6.**180A) has a rounded *frontal tuber* (*tuberosity*) about 3 cm above the midpoint of each supraorbital margin. These tubera vary, but are especially prominent in young skulls and more so in adult females than males. Below them, separated by a shallow groove, are two curved *superciliary arches*, medially prominent and joined by a smooth median elevated *glabella*; they are more prominent in males, depending partly on the size of the frontal sinuses; but prominence is occasionally associated with small sinuses. Inferior to the arches are curved *supraorbital margins* of the orbital openings, their lateral two-thirds sharp, the medial third rounded, and at each junction is a *supraorbital notch* (or *foramen*) containing supraorbital vessels and nerve. Medial to it a small *frontal notch* or *foramen* occurs in 50% of skulls. Berry (1975) has recorded incidences of frontal and supraorbital *foramina* and *notches* (incisures). A supraorbital notch or foramen occurs equally in some populations (e.g. 51% of Mexican crania). A frontal foramen occurs in 15–87% in various ethnic groups. Both features show sexual dimorphism (Kimura 1977).

The supraorbital margin ends laterally in a *zygomatic process*, strong, prominent and meeting the zygomatic bone. From this a line curves posterosuperiorly, dividing into *superior* and *inferior temporal lines*, continued on the temporal squama.

The region between supraorbital margins is the *nasal part*. Inferiorly a serrated *nasal notch* articulates with the nasal bones and, laterally, with the maxillary frontal processes and lacrimal bones. From the centre of the notch posteriorly the bone projects antero-inferiorly behind the nasal bones (**6.**156) and maxillary frontal processes, supporting the nasal bridge. The region ends in a sharp *nasal spine*, on each side of which a small grooved surface partly roofs the ipsilateral nasal cavity. The nasal spine also contributes slightly to the nasal septum; in front it articulates with the crest of the nasal bones and behind with the perpendicular ethmoidal plate (**6.**156).

The *temporal surface*, posteroinferior to the temporal lines, forms the anterior part of the temporal fossa and an attachment of temporalis (**6.**142B). The *internal surface* (**6.**180B) is concave. Its upper, median part has a vertical *sulcus for the sagittal sinus*, the edges of which unite below as the *frontal crest*; the sulcus contains the superior sagittal sinus (anterior part); to its margins and frontal

crest part of the falx cerebri is attached. The crest ends in a small notch, completed to form a *foramen caecum* (p. 569) by the ethmoid bone. The internal surface shows impressions of cerebral gyri and small furrows for meningeal vessels. Several *granular foveolae* usually exist near the sagittal sulcus, for arachnoid granulations.

The *parietal (posterior) margin* is thick, deeply serrated, bevelled internally above and externally below; inferiorly it becomes a rough, triangular surface for the greater wing of the sphenoid.

Orbital parts of the frontal bone

The orbital parts of the frontal bone are two thin, curved, triangular laminae, largely forming the orbital roofs and separated by a wide *ethmoidal notch*.

The *orbital surface* (**6.**180B) of each plate is smooth and concave, with a shallow anterolateral *fossa for the lacrimal gland*. Below and behind the medial end of the supraorbital margin, midway between the supraorbital notch and frontolacrimal suture, is the *trochlear fovea* (or *spine*) for attachment of a fibrocartilaginous trochlea for the superior oblique muscle. The convex *cerebral surface* is marked by frontal gyri and faint grooves for meningeal vessels.

The quadrilateral *ethmoidal notch* (**6.**180B) is occupied by the ethmoid's cribriform plate. Inferior to its lateral margins parts of several ethmoidal air cells are visible, completed when the ethmoid is in position. Two transverse grooves across each margin are converted into *anterior* and *posterior ethmoidal canals* by the ethmoid; these open on the medial orbital wall, transmitting anterior and posterior ethmoidal nerves and vessels.

Openings of the *frontal sinuses* (**6.**180B) are anterior to the eth-moidal notch, lateral to the nasal spine. These two irregular cavities ascend posterolaterally for a variable distance between the frontal laminae, separated by a thin septum, usually deflected from the median plane; the sinuses are hence rarely symmetrical. Rudimentary at birth, usually well-developed by the seventh or eighth year, they reach full size after puberty, being most variable in size and larger in males. Each communicates with the middle meatus in the ipsilateral nasal cavity by a *frontonasal canal*. The degree of development is linked to prominence of the superciliary arches, which are a response to masticatory stresses (Weinmann & Sicher 1955). The sinuses show a primary expansion with eruption of the first deciduous molars and again when the permanent molars begin to appear in the sixth year. With advancing age osseous absorption may lead to further enlargement.

The posterior borders of the orbital plates are thin and serrated to articulate with the lesser wings of the sphenoid; their lateral parts usually appear in the middle cranial fossa between greater and lesser wings.

Structure

The frontal bone is thick with trabecular tissue between two compact laminae, trabeculae being absent near the frontal sinuses. The orbital plates, entirely of compact bone, are thin and often translucent posteriorly; they may be partly absorbed in old age.

Ossification

The frontal bone is ossified in fibrous mesenchyme from two primary centres appearing in the eighth week in utero, one near each frontal tuber. Ossification extends superiorly to form half the main part of the bone, posteriorly to form orbital and inferiorly to form nasal parts (**6.**181). No secondary centres occur, except two for the nasal spine described as appearing about the tenth year (Inman & Saunders 1937). At birth the bone consists of two halves which may remain separate, a *metopic suture* persisting (Montagu 1951; Tongerson 1951; Linc & Fleischmann 1968). Such *metopism* has been assessed at 0–7.4% of individuals in various ethnic groups (Berry 1975). In a group of 206 Nigerian skulls (Ajmani et al 1983) incidence was 3.4%. It is high in mongoloids—10% according to Woo (1949).

ETHMOID BONE

The ethmoid bone, cuboidal and fragile, lies anteriorly in the cranial base, and is involved in the structure of the medial orbital walls, nasal septum, the roof and lateral walls of the nasal cavity. It is described as having a horizontal, perforated *cribriform plate*, a median *perpendicular plate* and two lateral *labyrinths*.

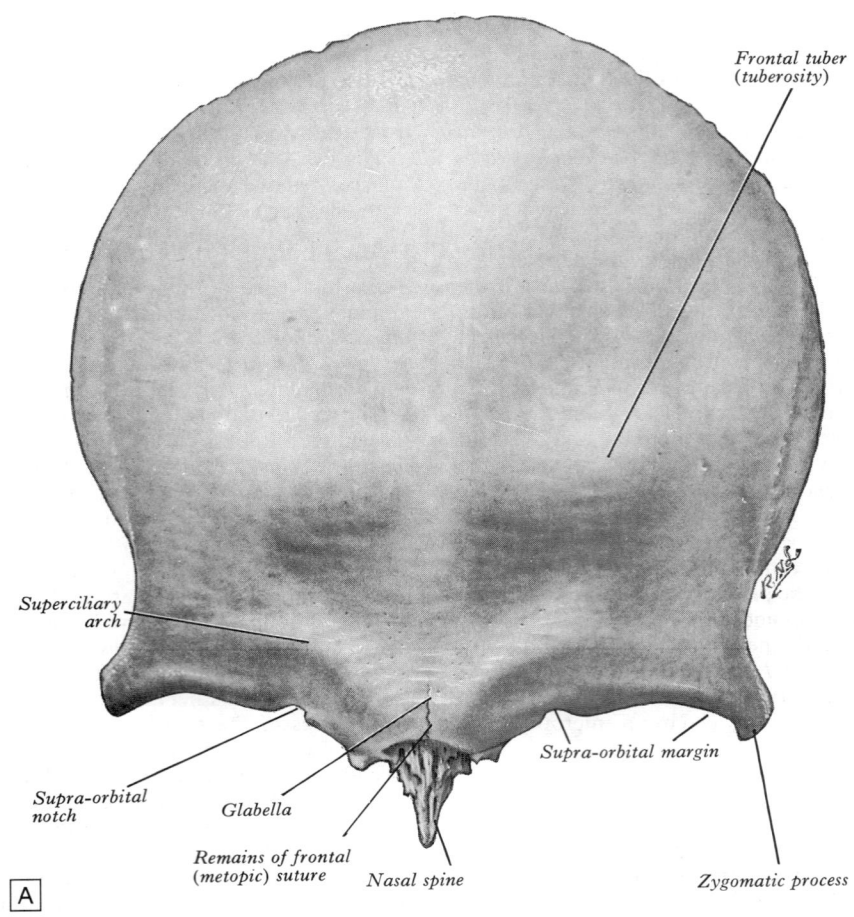

Frontal tuber (tuberosity)

Superciliary arch

Supra-orbital notch

Glabella

Remains of frontal (metopic) suture

Nasal spine

Supra-orbital margin

Zygomatic process

A

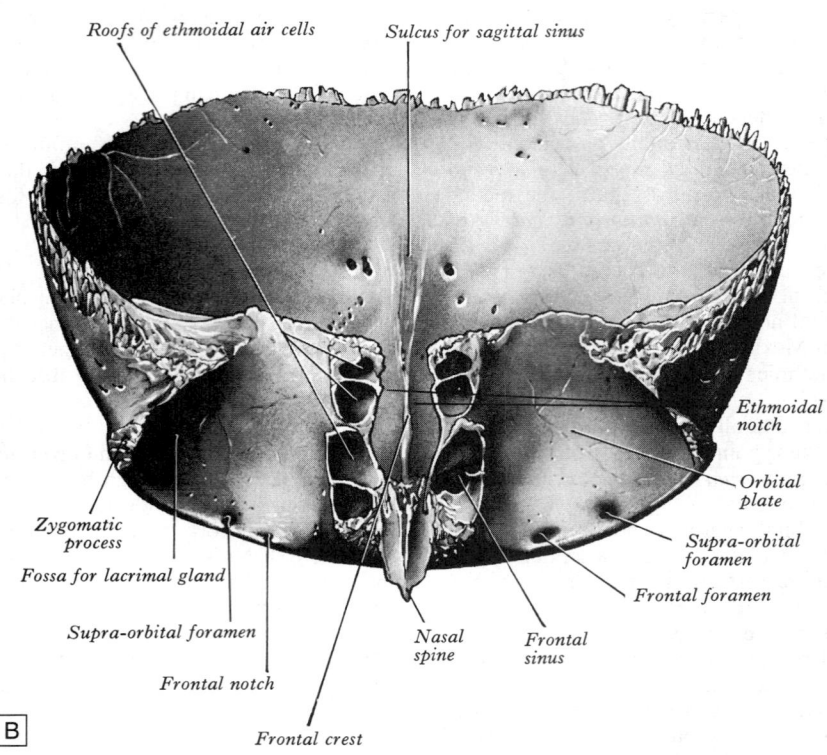

Roofs of ethmoidal air cells

Sulcus for sagittal sinus

Ethmoidal notch

Orbital plate

Supra-orbital foramen

Frontal foramen

Zygomatic process

Fossa for lacrimal gland

Supra-orbital foramen

Frontal notch

Nasal spine

Frontal sinus

Frontal crest

B

6.180   The frontal bone; A. External aspect; B. Inferior aspect.

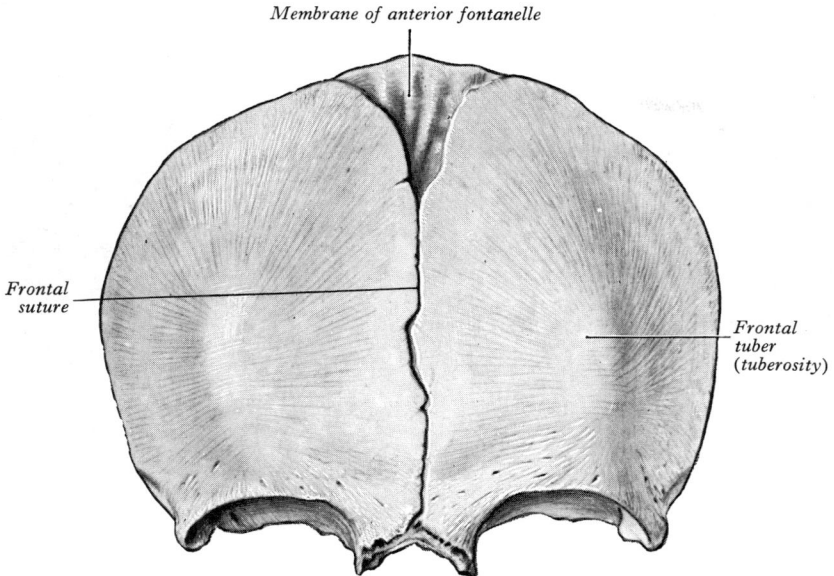

Membrane of anterior fontanelle

Frontal
suture

Frontal
tuber
(tuberosity)

6.181   The frontal bone at birth: anterior aspect. Note that at this stage the bone consists of right and left halves connected by the frontal suture.

Cribriform plate

The cribriform plate (**6**.182A) fills the frontal ethmoidal notch as a large part of the nasal roof. A thick, smooth, triangular, median *crista galli* projects up from this lamina; to its thin and curved posterior border the falx cerebri is attached. Its shorter, thick, anterior border joins with the frontal bone by two small *alae*, completing the *foramen caecum* (p. 569). Its sides are smooth but sometimes bulged by air cells. On both sides of the crista galli the cribriform plate is narrow, depressed and related to the gyrus rectus and olfactory bulb above it; its numerous foramina transmit olfactory nerves. Anteriorly on each side of the crista is a small slit occupied by dura mater. A foramen carrying anterior ethmoidal nerve and vessels to the nasal cavity is anterolateral to this slit; a groove runs forwards to it from the anterior ethmoidal canal.

Perpendicular plate

The perpendicular plate (**6**.182B, D), thin, flat, quadrilateral and median, descends from the cribriform plate to form the upper part of the nasal septum, usually a little deflected. Its *anterior border* meets the frontal's nasal spine and crest of the nasal bones, its *posterior border* joining the sphenoidal crest above and vomer below. The thick *inferior border* is attached to the nasal septal cartilage. Its surfaces are smooth, except above, where numerous grooves and canals lead to medial foramina in the cribriform plate for filaments of the olfactory nerves.

Ethmoidal labyrinths

The ethmoidal labyrinths consist of thin-walled ethmoidal air cells, in *anterior, middle* and *posterior groups* between two vertical plates (p. 1636); the lateral, *orbital plate* is part of the medial orbital wall, the medial being part of lateral nasal wall. In the disarticulated bone many air cells are open, but closed when articulated with adjoining bones, except where they open into the nasal cavity. The *superior surface* (**6**.182A) shows open air cells, completed by edges of the frontal ethmoidal notch (**6**.180B). It is crossed by two grooves completing *anterior* and *posterior ethmoidal canals* with the frontal. On the *posterior surface* (**6**.182B) large air cells are completed by sphenoidal conchae and the palatine's orbital process. The *lateral surface* (**6**.182C), thin, smooth and oblong, is the *orbital plate*, which covers the middle and posterior ethmoidal air cells. It articulates superiorly with the frontal's orbital plate, inferiorly with the maxilla and palatine's orbital process, anteriorly with the lacrimal and posteriorly with the sphenoid bone (**6**.152).

A few air cells lie anterior to the orbital plate, their walls completed by the lacrimal bone and frontal process of the maxilla. A thin,

curved *uncinate process*, variable in size, projects posteroinferiorly from the labyrinth, appearing in the medial wall of the maxillary sinus (**6**.152) as it crosses the hiatus maxillaris to join the inferior nasal concha's ethmoidal process. The upper edge of this process is a medial boundary of the hiatus semilunaris in the middle meatus.

The *medial surface* of the labyrinth (**6**.183) forms part of the lateral nasal wall as a thin lamella descending from the inferior surface of the cribriform plate to end as the convoluted *middle nasal concha*. Above this the surface shows many vertical grooves for olfactory nerves. Posteriorly it is divided by the narrow, oblique *superior meatus*, bounded above by the thin, curved *superior nasal concha*; posterior ethmoidal air cells open into this meatus. Antero-inferior to the superior meatus the middle concha's convex surface extends along all the medial surface of the labyrinth, its lower edge thick, its lateral surface concave and part of the *middle meatus*. Middle ethmoidal air cells produce a swelling (*bulla ethmoidalis*) on the lateral wall of the middle meatus (**6**.157B); on the bulla, or above it, these cells open into the meatus. A curved *infundibulum* extends up and forwards from the middle meatus, communicating with anterior ethmoidal sinuses; in more than 50% of crania it continues up as the frontonasal duct.

Ossification

The ethmoid bone ossifies in the cartilaginous nasal capsule from three centres: one in the perpendicular plate, and one in each labyrinth. The latter two appear in the orbital plates between the fourth and fifth months in utero, extending into the ethmoid conchae. At birth, the labyrinths, although ill-developed, are partially ossified, the remainder cartilaginous. During the first year the perpendicular plate and crista galli begin to ossify from the median centre, fusing with the labyrinths early in the second year. The cribriform plate is ossified partly from the perpendicular plate, partly from the labyrinths. Ethmoidal air cells begin to develop in utero; in the newborn they are narrow pouches.

INFERIOR NASAL CONCHAE

The inferior nasal conchae are curved horizontal laminae in the lateral nasal walls (**6**.184A). Each has two surfaces, borders and ends. The *medial surface* (**6**.184A) is convex, much perforated, and longitudinally grooved by vessels. The *lateral surface* is concave (**6**.184B) and part of the inferior meatus. The *superior border*, thin and irregular, may be divided into three regions: an anterior articulating with the maxillary conchal crest, a posterior with the palatine conchal crest and a middle with three *processes*, variable in size and form. Of these the *lacrimal process*, small and pointed, at

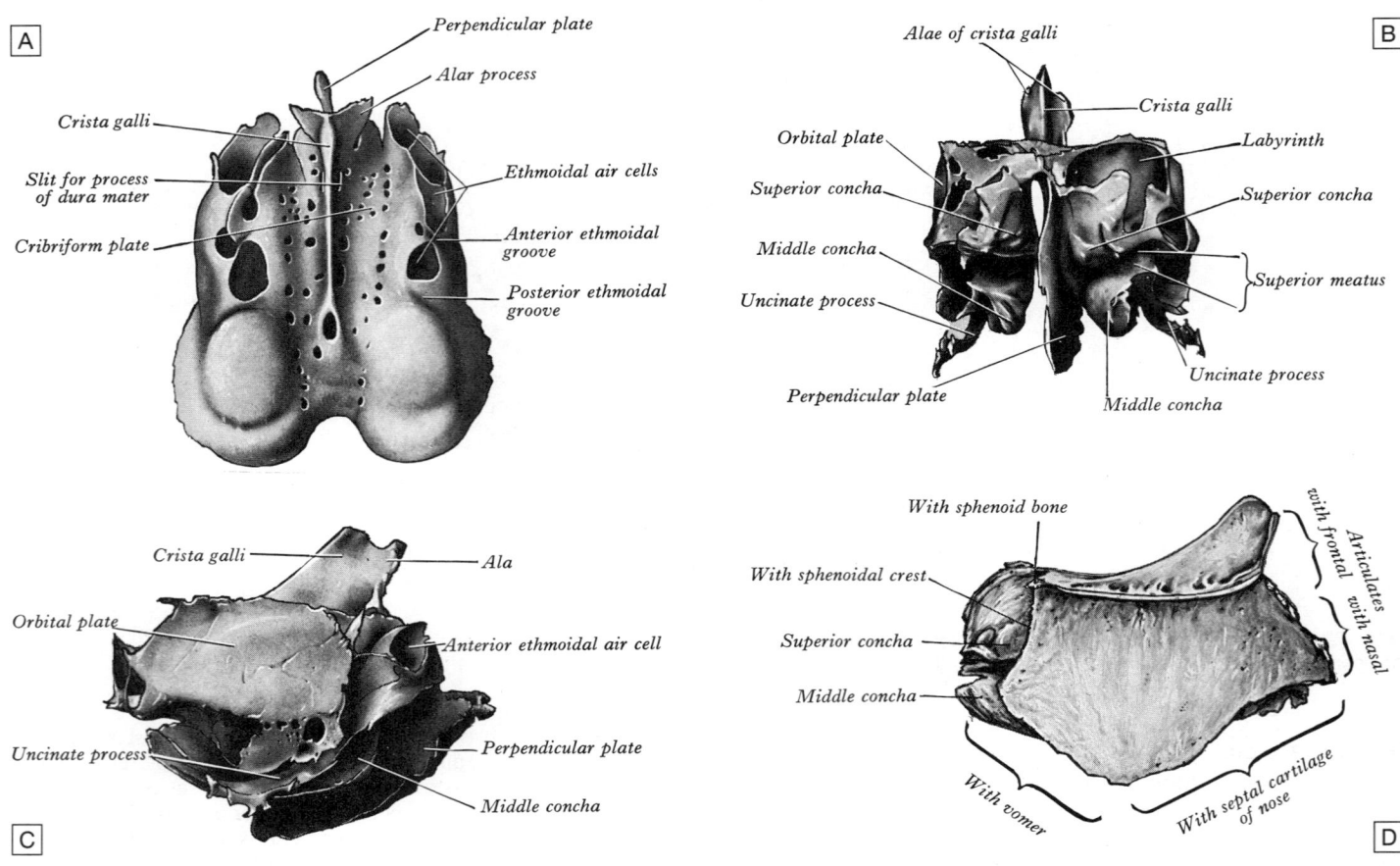

6.182   The ethmoid bone: A. Superior aspect; B. Posterior aspect; C. Right lateral aspect; D. The perpendicular plate viewed from the right side with the right ethmoidal labyrinth removed.

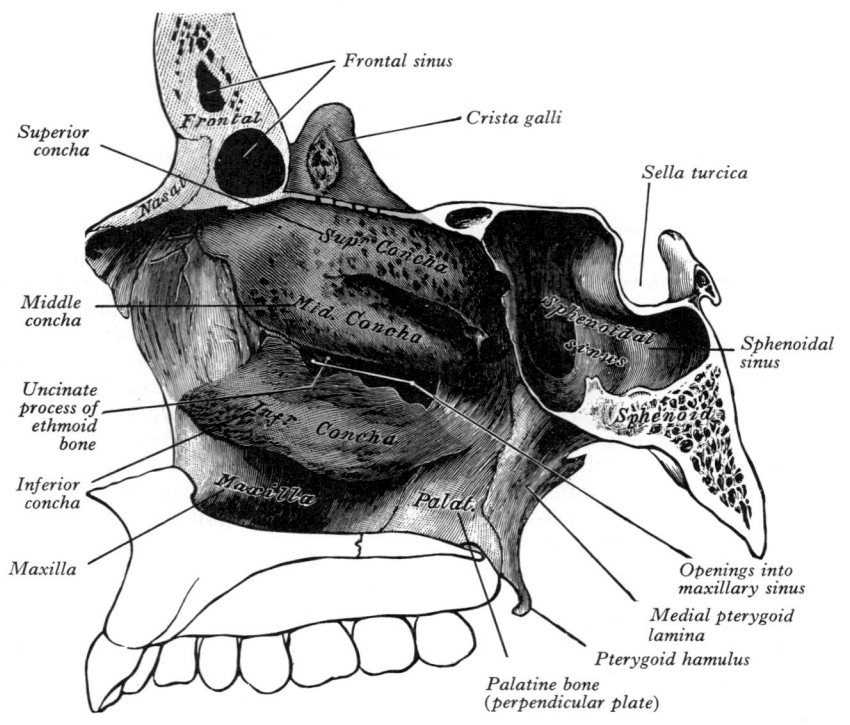

6.183   The lateral wall of the right half of the nasal cavity, showing the ethmoid bone (coloured brown) and the inferior nasal concha (coloured blue) in position.

the junction of the anterior with the posterior three-fourths of the border, articulates apically with a descending lacrimal process (**6.185**) and, by its margins, with the edges of the nasolacrimal groove on the medial maxillary surface, thus completing the nasolacrimal canal. Most posteriorly, a thin *ethmoidal process* ascends to the ethmoid uncinate process (**6.157B**). An intermediate thin *maxillary process* curves inferolaterally to articulate with the maxilla and maxillary process of the bone as part of the maxillary sinus' medial wall. The *inferior conchal border* is thick and spongiose, especially in its midpart. Both *conchal ends* are more or less tapered, the posterior more so.

Ossification

Ossification is from one centre, appearing at about the fifth month in utero in the incurved lower border of the cartilaginous nasal capsule's lateral wall. It loses continuity with the capsule during ossification.

MAXILLAE

The maxillae, largest of the facial bones excepting the mandible, jointly form the whole upper jaw (**6.135, 137**), most of the buccal roof, floor and lateral wall of nasal cavity, orbital floors, in part the infratemporal and pterygopalatine fossae and inferior orbital and pterygomaxillary fissures. Each has a body and zygomatic, frontal, alveolar and palatine processes.

Maxillary body

The maxillary body, roughly pyramidal, has anterior, infratemporal (posterior), orbital and nasal surfaces, enclosing the maxillary sinus.

Anterior surface. This (**6.136B, 185**), faces anterolaterally and displays inferior elevations overlying the roots of teeth. Above the incisors is a shallow *incisive fossa* in which is attached the depressor septi; to the alveolar border below this a slip of orbicularis oris is attached, and superolateral to it is the nasalis. Lateral to this fossa is a larger, deeper *canine fossa*, separated from it by the *canine eminence*, over the canine socket. In the canine fossa the levator anguli oris is attached. Above it is the *infraorbital foramen*, the anterior end of its canal, transmitting infraorbital vessels and nerve. Above the foramen a sharp border, dividing the anterior and orbital surfaces, is part of the orbital opening's rim; attached nearby is the levator labii superioris. Medially the anterior surface ends at a deeply concave *nasal notch*, ending in a pointed process which, with its fellow, forms the *anterior nasal spine*. To the anterior surface near the notch, the nasalis and depressor septi are attached.

Infratemporal surface. This (**6.185**) is concave and faces posterolaterally, forming the anterior wall of the infratemporal fossa and is separated from the anterior surface by the maxilla's zygomatic process and a ridge ascending to it from the first molar socket. Near its centre are apertures of two or three *alveolar canals*, containing posterior superior alveolar vessels and nerves. Posteroinferior is the *maxillary tuberosity*, rough superomedially where it meets the palatine bone's pyramidal process (**6.185A, 186**); a few fibres of medial pterygoid are attached to it, and sometimes it articulates with the lateral pterygoid plate. Above this is the smooth anterior boundary of the pterygopalatine fossa, grooved by the maxillary nerve as it passes laterally and slightly upwards into the infraorbital groove on the orbital surface.

Orbital surface. This (**6.139, 185**) is smooth and triangular, forming most of the orbital floor. Anteriorly its *medial border* bears a *lacrimal notch*, behind which it joints with the lacrimal bone, the ethmoid's orbital plate and, posteriorly, the palatine's orbital process (**6.186**). Its *posterior border* is smoothly rounded, forming most of the anterior edge of the inferior orbital fissure; central is the infraorbital groove. The *anterior border* is part of the orbital margin, continuous medially with the lacrimal crest of the maxilla's frontal process (p. 600). The *infraorbital groove*, for similarly named vessels and nerve, begins midway on the posterior border, continuous with a groove on the posterior surface, and passes forwards into the *infraorbital canal*, which opens on the anterior surface below the infraorbital margin. Near its midpoint the canal has a small lateral branch for the anterior superior alveolar nerve and vessels; this *canalis sinuosus* (Wood Jones; see Jones 1939a) descends in the orbital floor lateral to the infraorbital canal and curves medially in the

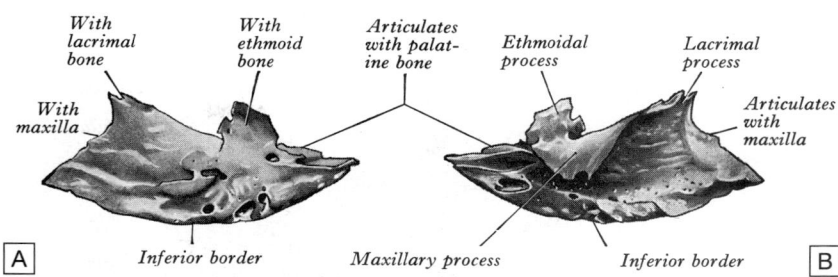

6.184   The right inferior nasal concha. A. Medial aspect; B. Lateral aspect.

anterior wall of the maxillary sinus. It passes below the infraorbital foramen to the margin of the anterior nasal aperture in front of the anterior end of the inferior concha; it then follows the aperture's lower margin to open near the nasal septum in front of the incisive canal. Anteromedial in the orbital surface and lateral to the lacrimal groove, the attachment of inferior oblique may make a small depression.

Nasal surface. This (**6.186**) displays posterosuperiorly the large, irregular *maxillary hiatus* leading into the sinus. At the upper hiatal border are parts of air sinuses completed by the ethmoid and lacrimal bones; the smooth concave surface below the hiatus is part of the inferior meatus, and behind it a rough surface meets the palatine's perpendicular plate; this surface is traversed by a groove, descending forwards from the midposterior border; it is converted into a *greater palatine canal* by the palatine's perpendicular plate. Anterior to the hiatus a deep groove, continuous above with the lacrimal groove (p. 605), makes about two-thirds of the circumference of the naso-lacrimal canal, the rest being the lacrimal's descending part, and the lacrimal process of the inferior nasal concha (see **6.193**). This canal leads the nasolacrimal duct to the inferior meatus (**6.157B**). More anterior is an oblique *conchal crest* for the inferior nasal concha; the concavity below it being part of the inferior meatus; above it the surface is part of the atrium of the middle meatus.

Maxillary sinus

The maxillary sinus (**6.185, 187**), a large pyramidal cavity, has thin walls corresponding to orbital, alveolar, facial and infratemporal aspects of the maxilla. Its lateral, truncated *apex* extends into the zygomatic process, sometimes into the zygomatic bone; its *base* is medial and is the lateral wall of the nasal cavity, appearing in the maxillary hiatus in a disarticulated bone. This hiatal aperture is reduced by the ethmoidal uncinate process and descending part of the lacrimal bone above, the maxillary process of the inferior nasal concha below, and the palatine's perpendicular plate behind (**6.157B, 186**). The maxillary sinus hence connects only with the middle meatus, usually by two small holes, one of which is usually closed by mucous membrane. Its *posterior wall* contains *alveolar canals*, conducting posterior superior alveolar vessels and nerves to molar teeth; these canals may ridge the sinus, whose *floor* is formed by the alveolar process, its lowest part being about 1.25 cm below the nasal floor. Radiating septa of varying size usually spring from the sinual floor between adjacent dental roots; sometimes it is perforated by molar roots (p. 1637). The infraorbital canal usually ridges the sinus from *roof* to *anterior wall*. The cavity's size varies, even between sides of a single skull (p. 1637).

Clinical anatomy. Because of the extreme thinness of the sinual walls, a tumour may push up the orbital floor and displace the eyeball, project into the nasal cavity, protrude onto the cheek or spread back into the infratemporal fossa or down into the mouth. Extraction of molar teeth may damage the floor, and impact may fracture its walls.

Zygomatic process

The zygomatic process is a pyramidal projection where anterior, infratemporal and orbital surfaces converge. **In front** it merges into the maxillary body's facial surface; **behind** it is concave and continuous with the infratemporal surface; **above** it is roughly serrated for articulation with the zygomatic bone; **below** an arched border separates facial (anterior) and infratemporal surfaces.

599

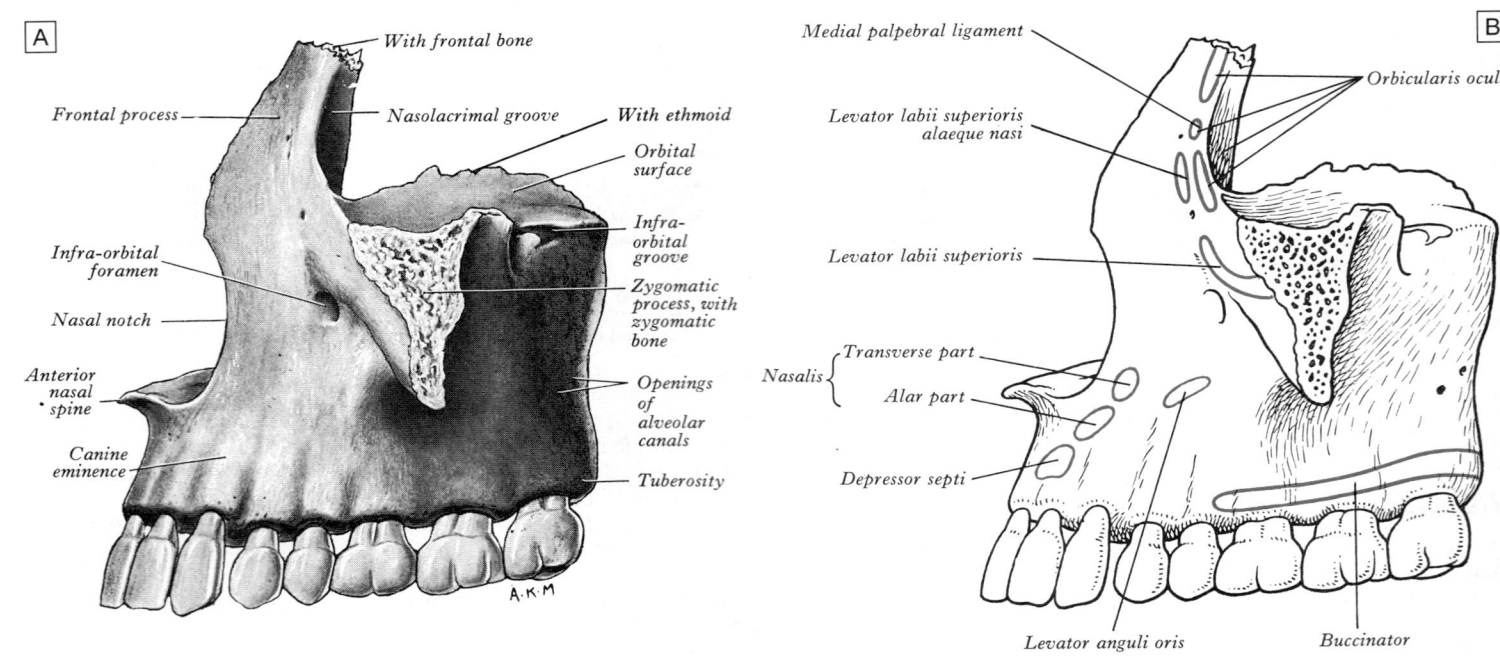

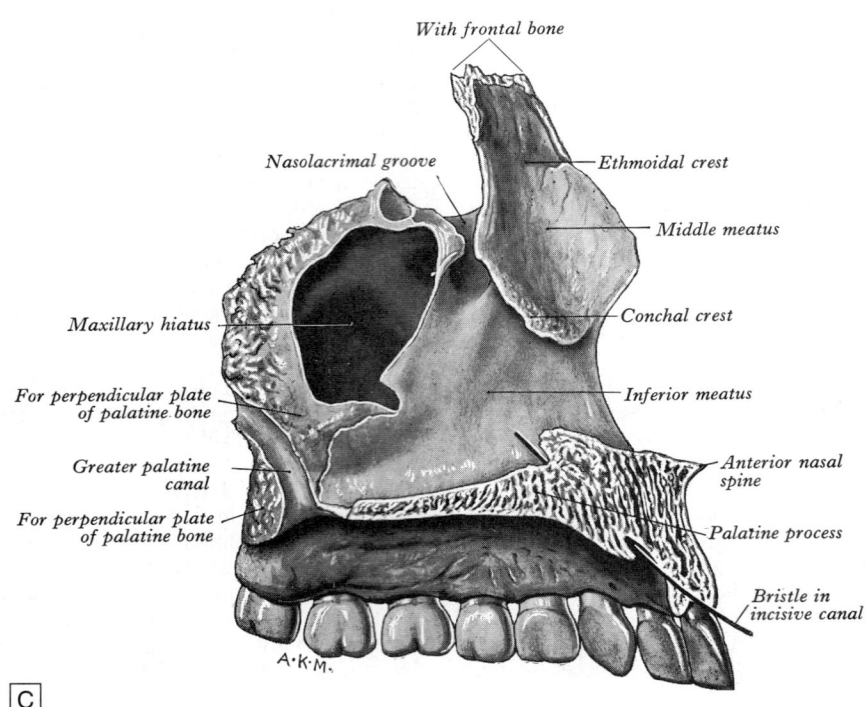

6.185   The left maxilla; A. Lateral aspect; B. Outline showing muscle attachments; C. Medial aspect.

Frontal process

The frontal process projects posterosuperiorly between the nasal and lacrimal bones (**6.133**A, **186**). Its *lateral surface* (**6.142**A, **186**) is divided by a vertical *anterior lacrimal crest* for attachment of the medial palpebral ligament and is continuous below with the infraorbital margin. At the junction of the crest and orbital surface a small palpable tubercle is a guide to the lacrimal sac. The smooth area anterior to the lacrimal crest merges below with the body's anterior surface; part of orbicularis oculi and levator labii superioris alaeque nasi are attached here (**6.136**B, **143**). Behind the crest a vertical groove combines with one on the lacrimal bone to complete the lacrimal fossa. The *medial surface* (**6.185**) is part of the lateral nasal wall. A rough subapical area joints with the ethmoid and closes anterior ethmoidal air cells. Below this an oblique *ethmoidal crest* articulates posteriorly with the middle nasal concha and anteriorly underlies

the *agger nasi*, a ridge anterior to the concha on the lateral nasal wall; the crest is the upper limit of the atrium of the middle meatus. The frontal process joints apically with the frontal's nasal part, its *anterior border* with the nasal bone, its *posterior* with the lacrimal.

Alveolar process

The alveolar process is thick and arched, wide behind, and socketed for tooth roots. The eight sockets on each side vary according to contained teeth. That for the canine is deepest, those for molars widest and subdivided into three by septa, those for incisors and second premolar single, that for the first premolar sometimes double. The buccinator is attached to the external alveolar aspect, as far forwards as the first molar. In articulated maxillae the processes form the *alveolar arch*. Occasionally a longitudinal *maxillary torus* variably prominent, appears on the palatal aspect of the process near the molar sockets.

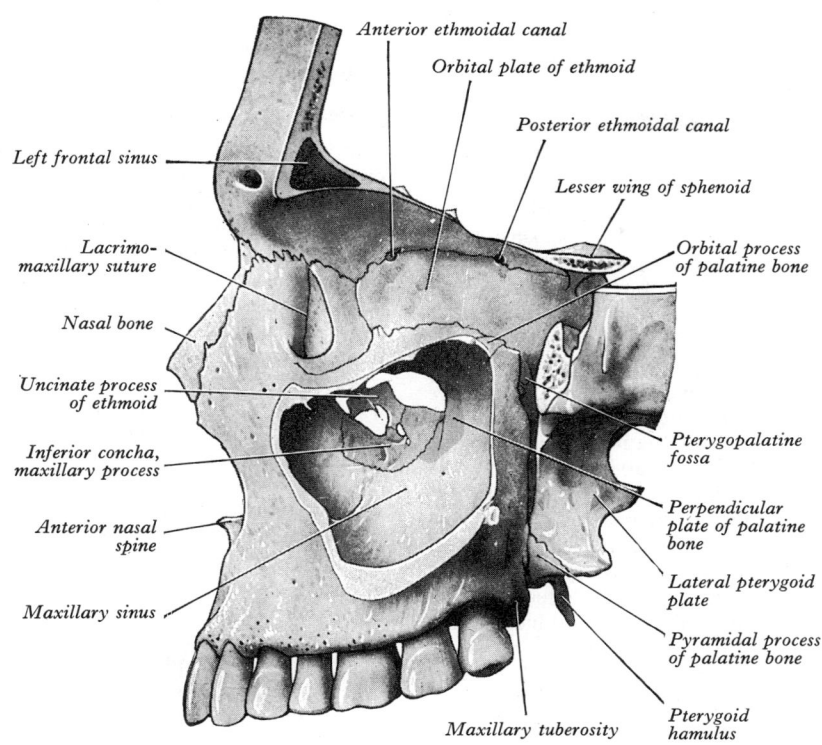

Anterior ethmoidal canal

Orbital plate of ethmoid

Posterior ethmoidal canal

Left frontal sinus

Lesser wing of sphenoid

*Lacrimo-
maxillary suture*

*Orbital process
of palatine bone*

Nasal bone

*Uncinate process
of ethmoid*

*Pterygopalatine
fossa*

*Inferior concha,
maxillary process*

*Perpendicular
plate of palatine
bone*

*Anterior nasal
spine*

*Lateral pterygoid
plate*

Maxillary sinus

*Pyramidal process
of palatine bone*

Maxillary tuberosity

*Pterygoid
hamulus*

6.186 Oblique sagittal section through the anterior part of the skull, showing the medial wall of the left orbit and the medial wall of the left maxillary sinus. The inferior concha is shown in yellow and the perpendicular plate of the palatine bone in blue.

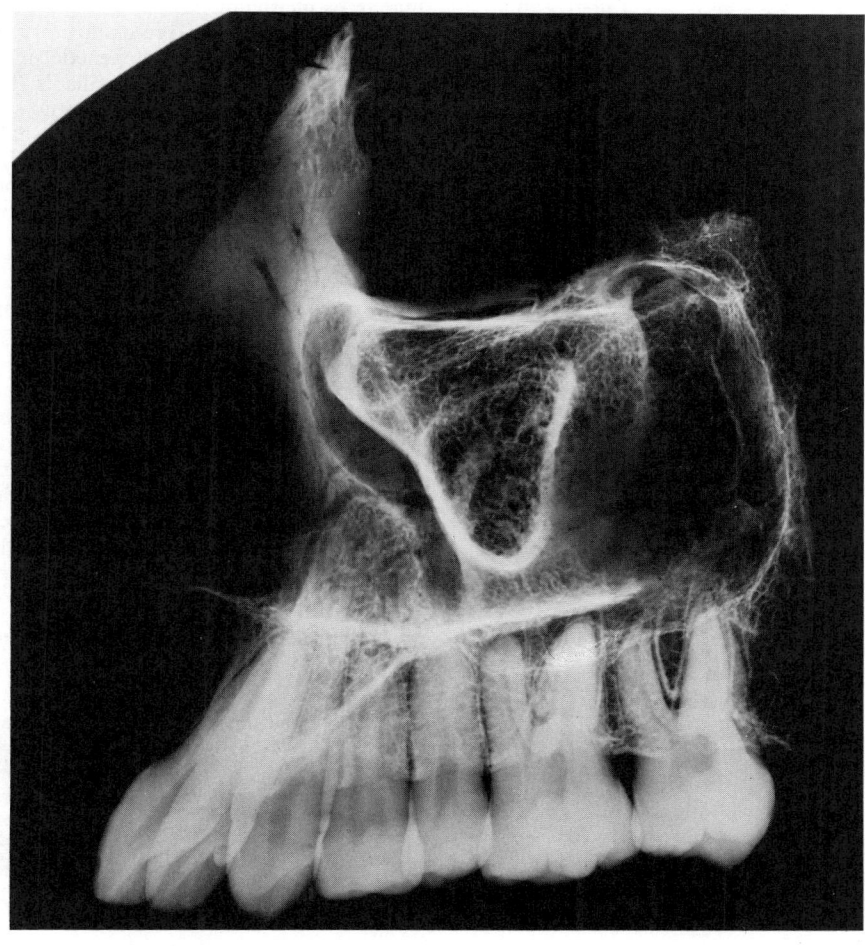

6.187   High resolution projection microradiograph of a maxilla (mediolateral view). Note particularly the distribution of compact and trabecular bone, the extent of the profile of the maxillary sinus and its relation to the dental alveoli, the compact bone of the *laminae durae* of the latter, the hard tissues, pulp cavities, root canals and foramina of the teeth. Contrast the dense shells of compact bone in the frontal, zygomatic and palatine processes with the fine filigree of trabecular bone in much of the alveolar process, interior of the zygomatic process and the posterior wall of the sinus. (Contributed by C Buckland-Wright, Guy's Hospital Medical School, London.)

Palatine process

The palatine process, thick, strong and horizontal, projects medially from the lowest part of the medial maxillary aspect, forming a large part of the nasal floor and palate; it is much thicker in front. Its *inferior surface* (6.145) is concave, uneven and forms with its fellow about the anterior three-fourths of the osseous palate. It displays numerous vascular foramina and depressions for palatine glands and, posterolaterally, two grooves containing greater palatine vessels and nerves. Between the maxillae the infundibular *incisive fossa* appears behind the incisor teeth, posterior to which is the median intermaxillary palatal suture—a little uneven but relatively flat on its oral aspect. However, its bony margins are sometimes raised into a prominent longitudinal *palatine torus* (p. 563), incidence of which varies (p. 609); for example, it is rare in Burmese, but frequent in English crania (29% in males, 48% in females among nineteenth-century Londoners). In the *incisive fossa* are openings of two lateral *incisive canals*; each ascends into its half of the nasal cavity, transmitting terminations of the greater palatine artery and nasopalatine nerve. Occasionally two additional median openings exist: *anterior* and *posterior incisive foramina*, transmitting the nasopalatine nerves, the left passing anterior. On the inferior palatine surface a fine groove, sometimes termed the *incisive suture* and prominent in young skulls, may be observed in adults where it extends anterolaterally from the incisive fossa to the interval between the lateral incisor and canine teeth. Anterior to this supposed suture is the *os incisivum*, long considered to represent the premaxilla, a separate element in most vertebrates including primates. This view has been criticized (see below). The *superior surface* of the palatine process is concave transversely, smooth and forms most of the nasal floor; anteriorly, near its median margin, is the incisive canal. The *lateral border* is continuous with the maxillary body. The *medial border*, thicker in front, is raised into a *nasal crest* which, with its fellow, forms a groove for the vomer. The front of this ridge rises higher as an *incisor crest*, prolonged forwards into a sharp process which, with its fellow, forms an *anterior nasal spine*. The *posterior border* is serrated for the palatine's horizontal plate.

Ossification

The maxilla ossifies in a sheet of mesenchyme superficial to the nasal capsule. Three centres are described: one for the main maxillary mass appears above the canine fossa at about the sixth week in uterine; two others are ascribed to the *premaxillary* region, the so-called *os incisivum*, which corresponds in position with a true premaxilla. Of these two 'premaxillary' centres, reputed to occur in human embryonic upper jaw (Woo 1949; Noback & Moss 1953), the principal one is said to appear above the incisor tooth germs in the seventh week; a second, sometimes called *paraseptal* or *prevomerine*, is considered to begin in the medial wall of a paraseptal cartilage at the ventral margin of the nasal septum, fusing almost at once with the maxilla's palatine process. Bone formed by the principal premaxillary centre is reputedly overgrown by bone from the main maxillary mass, fusing along its anterior limit with the maxilla's alveolar process. (This junction may be discernible as the *interalveolar*

suture of Farmer.) This would explain the absence, after the third month in utero, of any *facial* indication of a premaxilla (*os incisivum*). However a suture, or what appears to be one, may occur on the nasal floor behind its anterior margin. When identifiable postnatally, this suture passes medially on each side to the incisive canal. Moreover, a suture or cleft is always visible at birth anterior in the palate; diverging on each side from the incisive fossa it runs to the septum between the lateral incisor and canine teeth (rarely between the canine and first premolar). This *palatal* sign of separation between the os incisivum and the rest of the maxilla may persist until the middle decades. Considered together, these features delineate a separate element, anterior to the incisive fossa and canals, forming parts of the incisor alveoli. Being fused anteriorly with an overlap from the maxillary centre, this 'os incisivum' has no facial representation.

Regular occurrence of a premaxilla in other primates, as a separate bone, has naturally prompted attempts to identify a human homologue. Despite early disagreements (Fawcett 1911a), the above description of maxillary development has become standard, conveniently equating the os incisivum with the mammalian premaxilla. This argument depends primarily on supposed ossificatory centres in the os incisivum. One study of serial sections in human embryos strongly suggested that ossification in it is merely an extension from the maxillary centre (Wood et al 1969). The osseous lamina developing from this centre, as in the mandible, is complex, appearing in more than one place in some sections and suggesting multiple centres. It was claimed that their continuity is clear in serial sections, providing a welcome simplification for complexities of maxillary development. Extension from a supposed initial 'premaxillary' centre to form the frontal and palatine processes can thus be ascribed instead to the main maxillary centre. But this simplification does not explain various sutures, clefts and grooves held to delineate the human os incisivum.

Whether patterns of pre-ossificatory mesenchymal condensation in the region have any phylogenetic significance remains uncertain; the status of a human premaxilla is thus problematical. There is strong evidence, at least, that it has no specific centre of ossification.

The maxillary sinus appears as a shallow groove (6.188) on the nasal aspect at about the fourth month in utero. Infraorbital vessels and nerve are for a time in an open groove in the orbital floor; its anterior part being converted into a canal by a lamina growing in from the lateral side.

Age changes in the maxilla

At birth the transverse and sagittal maxillary dimensions are greater than the vertical. The frontal process is prominent, but the body little more than an alveolar process, its alveoli reaching almost to the orbital floor, the maxillary sinus is a mere furrow on the lateral nasal wall. In adults the vertical dimension is greatest, owing to development of the alveolar process and enlargement of the sinus. If all teeth are lost, in old age or earlier, the bone reverts towards infantile shape: its height diminishes, the alveolar process is absorbed (p. 607) and lower parts of the bone contracted and reduced in thickness at the expense of the labial wall (p. 578). Differences in the

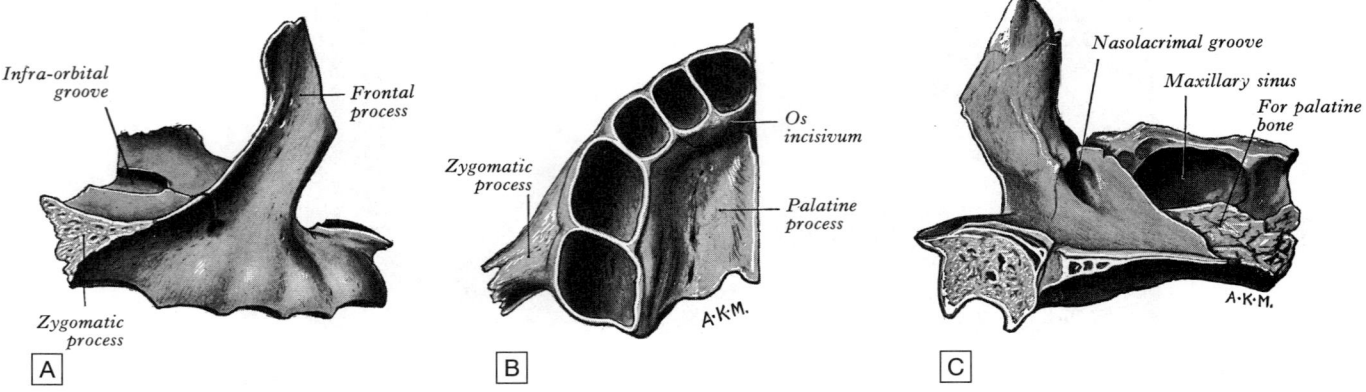

6.188   The right maxilla at birth. A. Lateral aspect; B. Inferior aspect; C. Medial aspect. Note alveoli for deciduous teeth (B) and rough articular area for opposite maxilla (C).

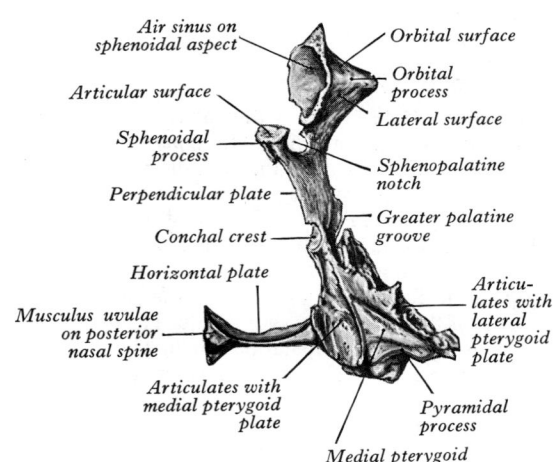

6.189   The right palatine bone: posterior aspect.

mode of alveolar absorption in maxilla and mandible are of practical importance in fitting dentures.

PALATINE BONES

The palatine bones are posteriorly placed in the nasal cavity between the maxillae and sphenoid's pterygoid processes (**6**.157B); they contribute to the nasal floor and lateral walls, to the palate and orbital floors, and to the pterygopalatine and pterygoid fossae and inferior orbital fissures. Each resembles a letter L in its *horizontal* and *perpendicular plates*, with three processes: *pyramidal*, inclining down and posterolaterally from the junction of these plates, *orbital* and *sphenoidal*, surmounting each perpendicular plate and separated by the deep sphenopalatine notch.

Horizontal plate

The horizontal plate (**6**.145, 189) is quadrilateral, with two surfaces and four borders. The *nasal surface*, transversely concave, forms the posterior nasal floor; the *palatine surface* forms, with its fellow, a posterior quarter of the bony palate; near its posterior margin a curved *palatine crest* often exists. The *posterior border* is thin and concave; to it and its adjacent surface behind the palatine crest the expanded tendon of tensor veli palatini is attached. Medially the posterior border forms, with its fellow, a median *posterior nasal spine* for attachment of the uvular muscle. The serrated *anterior border* articulates with the maxillary palatine process. The *lateral border* is

continuous with the perpendicular plate and marked by a *greater palatine groove*. The *medial border*, thick and serrated, articulates with its fellow in the midline, forming the posterior part of the *nasal crest*, which articulates with the posterior part of the vomer's lower edge; and the latter is continuous anteriorly with the maxillary nasal crest.

Perpendicular plate

The perpendicular plate (**6**.189, 190), thin and oblong, has two surfaces and four borders. The *nasal surface* bears inferiorly a broad depression, part of the inferior meatus. Above this the horizontal *conchal crest* articulates with the inferior concha; above this again a shallow depression forms part of the middle meatus. This last depression is limited above by an *ethmoidal crest* for the middle nasal concha, above which a narrow, horizontal groove forms part of the superior meatus. The *maxillary surface*, largely rough and irregular, articulates with the maxillary's nasal surface; posterosuperiorly it is a smooth medial wall to the pterygopalatine fossa; its anterior area, also smooth, overlaps the maxillary hiatus from behind to form a posterior part of the medial wall of the maxillary sinus (**6**.186). Posteriorly on this maxillary surface is the deep, obliquely descending *greater palatine groove*, converted into a canal by the maxilla; it transmits the greater palatine vessels and nerve.

The *anterior border* is thin and irregular; level with the conchal crest a pointed lamina projects below and behind the maxillary process of the inferior concha, articulating with it and so appearing in the medial wall of the maxillary sinus (**6**.186). The *posterior border* (**6**.189) has a serrated suture with the medial pterygoid plate and is continuous above with the palatine's sphenoidal process, and expanding below into its pyramidal process. From the *superior border* project both the *orbital* and *sphenoidal processes* separated by the *sphenopalatine notch* (made into a *foramen* by the sphenoid body). This foramen connects the pterygopalatine fossa to the posterior part of the superior meatus, transmitting sphenopalatine vessels and the posterior superior nasal nerves. The *inferior border*, continuous with the lateral border of the horizontal plate, bears the lower end of the greater palatine groove in front of the pyramidal process.

Pyramidal process

The pyramidal process slopes down posterolaterally from the junction of the horizontal and perpendicular palatine plates into the angle between the pterygoid plates. On its *posterior surface* a smooth, grooved triangular area, limited on each side by rough articular furrows articulating with the pterygoid plates, completes the lower part of the pterygoid fossa, and is a partial attachment of the medial pterygoid muscle. Anteriorly the *lateral surface* articulates with the maxillary tuberosity; posteriorly a smooth triangular area appears low in the infratemporal fossa between the tuberosity and lateral

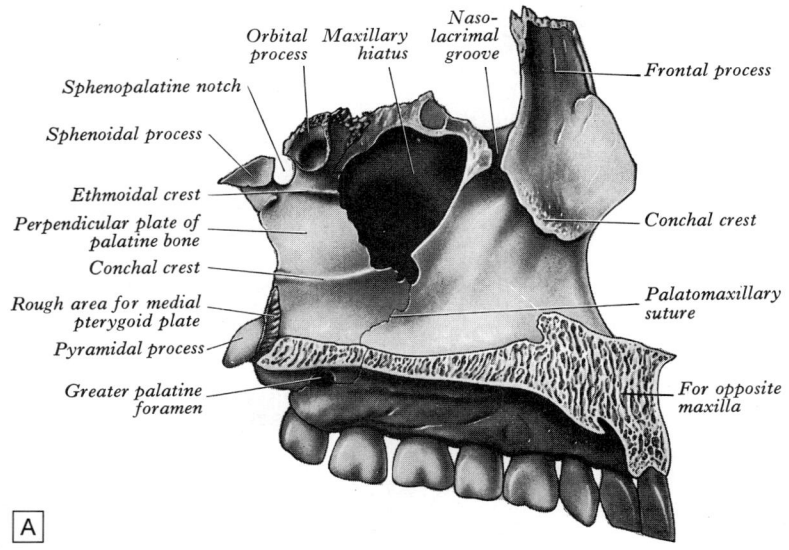

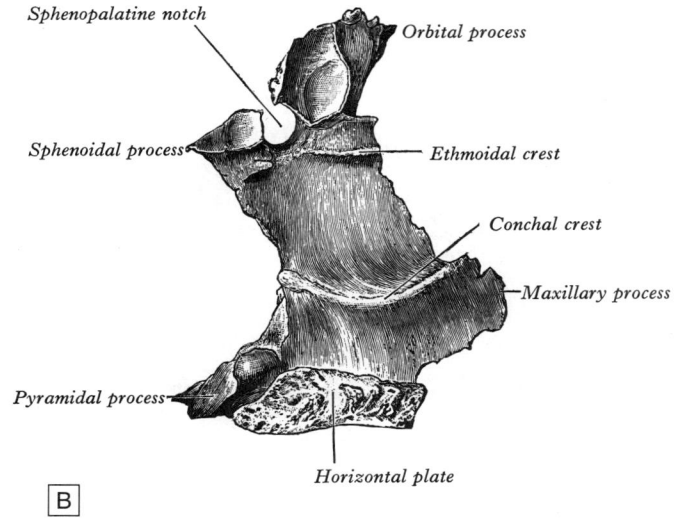

6.190   The medial aspect of the left palatine bone; A. In articulation with the left maxilla; B. Enlarged.

pterygoid plate (**6.144A**). The *inferior surface*, near its union with the horizontal plate, shows the *lesser palatine foramina* for the corresponding nerves and arteries (**6.145**).

Orbital process

The orbital process (**6.189, 190**), directed superolaterally from in front of the perpendicular plate with a constricted 'neck', encloses an air sinus and presents three articular and two non-articular surfaces. Of the articular surfaces:

- the oblong *anterior* or *maxillary* faces down and anterolaterally to articulate with the maxilla;
- the *posterior* or *sphenoidal*, directed up and posteromedially, bears the opening of an air sinus, usually communicating with the sphenoidal sinus and completed by a sphenoidal concha;
- he *medial* or *ethmoidal*, facing anteromedially, articulates with the ethmoid's labyrinth.

The sinus sometimes opens on the surface, communicating with the posterior ethmoidal air cells; more rarely it opens on the ethmoidal **and** sphenoidal surfaces, communicating with posterior ethmoidal air cells **and** the sphenoidal sinus. Of the non-articular surfaces:

- the triangular *superior* or *orbital* is directed superolaterally to the posterior part of the orbital floor (**6.139**);
- the *lateral* is oblong, faces the pterygopalatine fossa and is separated from the orbital surface by a rounded border, a medial part of the lower margin of the inferior orbital fissure; this surface may present a groove, directed superolaterally, for the maxillary nerve and is continuous with the groove on the upper maxilla's posterior surface (p. 602).

The border between the lateral and posterior surfaces descends anterior to the sphenopalatine notch.

Sphenoidal process

The sphenoidal process (**6.189, 190**), a thin plate smaller and lower than the orbital, directed superomedially. Its *superior surface* articulates with the sphenoidal concha and, above it, the root of the medial pterygoid plate; it carries a groove helping to form the palatovaginal canal. The concave *inferomedial surface* is part of the nasal roof and lateral wall. Posteriorly the *lateral surface* articulates with the medial pterygoid plate; its smooth anterior region is part of the medial wall of the pterygopalatine fossa. The *posterior border* articulates with the vaginal process of the medial pterygoid plate. The *anterior border* is the posterior edge of the sphenopalatine notch. The *medial border* articulates with the vomerine ala. The *sphenopalatine notch*, between the two processes, becomes a foramen by articulation with the sphenoidal body. Sometimes the processes themselves unite.

Ossification

Ossification is in mesenchyme from one centre, appearing during the eighth week in the perpendicular plate. From this, ossification spreads into all parts. At birth the height of the perpendicular plate equals the width of the horizontal, but in adults it is almost twice as great, a change in proportions according with those in the maxilla.

ZYGOMATIC BONES

Each zygomatic bone forms the prominence of a cheek, contributes to the lateral orbital wall and floor, parts of the walls of temporal

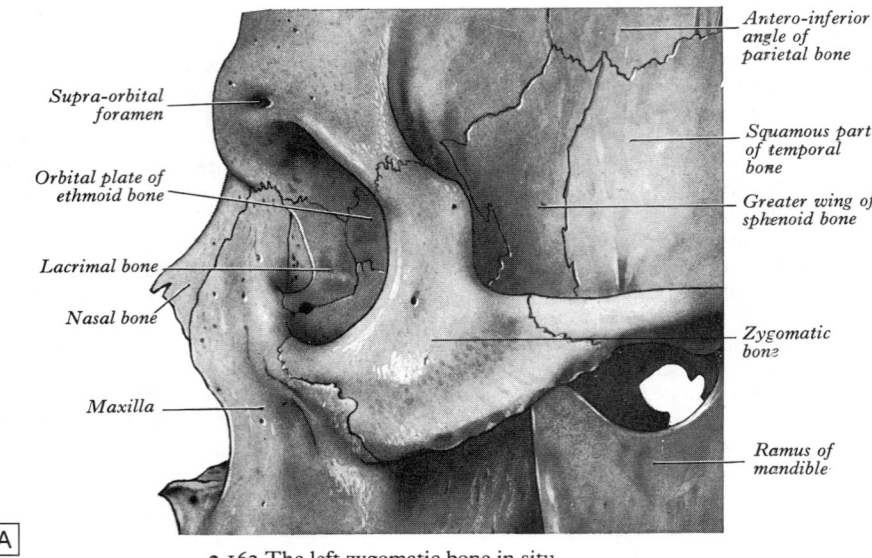

3.163 The left zygomatic bone in situ.

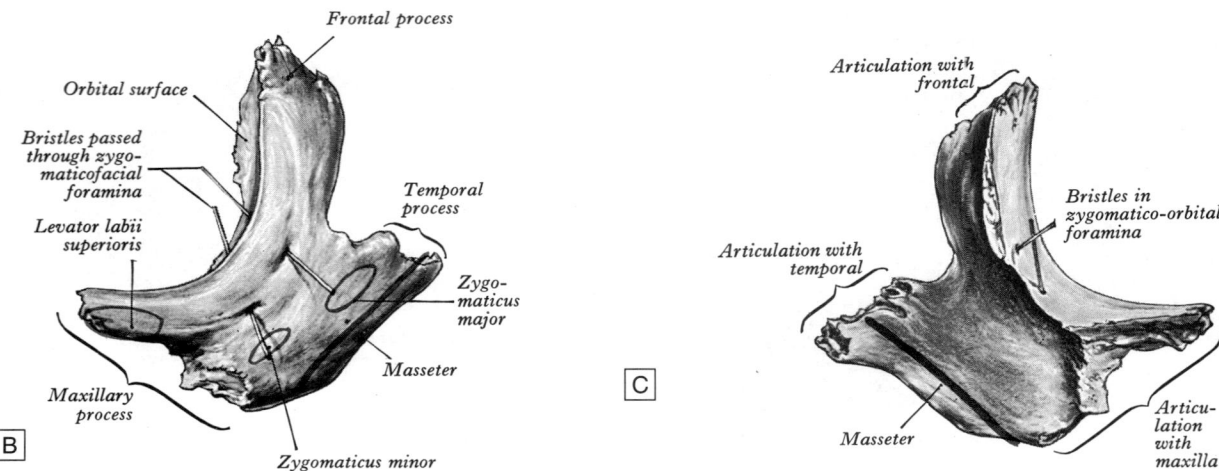

6.191 The left zygomatic bone; A. In situ; B. Lateral aspect showing muscle attachments; C. Medial aspect.

and infratemporal fossae and completes the zygomatic arch (**6.191**A). It is roughly quadrangular with anteromedial and frontal processes. It can be described as having three surfaces, five borders and two processes.

The *lateral surface* (**6.191**), really anterolateral, is convex and pierced near its orbital border by the *zygomaticofacial foramen* (often double) for the zygomaticofacial nerve and vessels; below this zygomaticus minor and, posteriorly, zygomaticus major are attached. The zygomaticofacial foramen is sometimes absent (p. 609). The posteromedial *temporal surface* (**6.191**) has a rough anterior area for articulation with the maxilla and a smooth, concave posterior area extending up posteriorly on its frontal process as the anterior aspect of the temporal fossa. It also extends back on the medial aspect of the temporal process as an incomplete lateral wall for the infratemporal fossa. The *zygomaticotemporal foramen* pierces this surface near the base of the frontal process. The *orbital surface* (**6.191**B, C), smooth and concave, is the anterolateral part of the orbital floor and adjoining lateral wall, extending up on the medial aspect of its frontal process. It usually bears *zygomatico-orbital foramina*, openings of canals leading to zygomaticofacial and temporal foramina.

The smoothly concave *anterosuperior* or *orbital border* forms the inferolateral circumference of the orbital opening, separating the orbital and lateral surfaces. The *anteroinferior* or *maxillary border* articulates with the maxilla; its medial end tapers to a point above the infraorbital foramen; near the orbital margin a part of the levator labii superioris is attached. The *posterosuperior* or *temporal border* is sinuous, convex above, concave below and continuous with the posterior border of the frontal process and upper border of the zygomatic arch; attached to it is the temporal fascia. Below the frontozygomatic suture is often a small *marginal tubercle*, easily palpable. The *posteroinferior border* is roughened by attachment of masseter. The serrated *posteromedial border* articulates with the sphenoid's greater wing above, and orbital surface of the maxilla below. Between these serrated regions a short, concave, non-articular part usually forms the lateral edge of the inferior orbital fissure; it is sometimes absent, the fissure then being completed by junction of the maxilla and sphenoid or a small sutural bone between them.

The *frontal process*, thick and serrated, articulates above with the frontal's zygomatic process and behind with sphenoid's greater wing. On its orbital aspect, within the orbital opening and about 1 cm below the frontozygomatic suture, a tubercle of varying size and form, observed in 95% of skulls (Whitnall 1932), is the attachment of the lateral palpebrae ligament (p. 1361), suspensory ligament and part of the aponeurosis of levator palpebrae superioris (p. 1353). The *temporal process*, directed backwards, has an oblique, serrated end articulating with the temporal zygomatic process to complete the zygomatic arch.

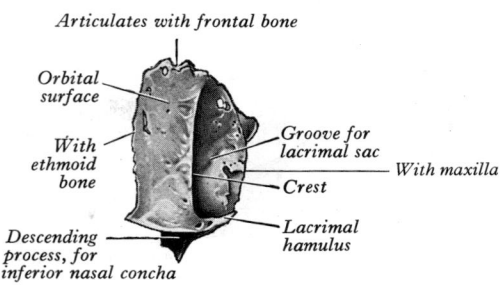

6.192   The right lacrimal bone: lateral aspect.

Ossification

Ossification is from one centre, appearing in fibrous tissue about the eighth week. The bone is sometimes divided by a horizontal suture into a larger upper and smaller lower divisions.

LACRIMAL BONES

The lacrimal bones, the smallest and most fragile of cranial bones, lie anteriorly in the medial orbital walls (**6.152**). Each has two surfaces and four borders. The *lateral, orbital surface* (**6.192**) is divided by a vertical *posterior lacrimal crest*, anterior to which is a vertical groove, its anterior edge meeting the posterior border of the frontal process of the maxilla to complete the *fossa for the lacrimal sac*. The groove's medial wall is prolonged by a descending process (**6.193**) helping to form the nasolacrimal canal by joining the lips of the maxillary nasolacrimal groove and lacrimal process of the inferior nasal concha. Behind the crest is a smooth part of the medial orbital wall. To this surface and crest the lacrimal part of orbicularis oculi is attached; the surface ends below in the *lacrimal hamulus* which, with the maxilla, completes the upper opening of the nasolacrimal canal (**6.139**); the hamulus may be a separate *lesser lacrimal bone*. The anteroinferior region of the *medial (nasal) surface* is part of the middle meatus; its posterosuperior part meets the ethmoid to complete some anterior ethmoidal air cells. The *anterior lacrimal border* articulates with the frontal process of the maxilla, the *posterior* with the ethmoid's orbital plate, the *superior* with the frontal bone, and the *inferior* with the maxillary orbital surface (**6.139**).

Ossification

Ossification is from a centre appearing at about the twelfth week in mesenchyme around the nasal capsule. In later life the lacrimal is subject to patchy erosion.

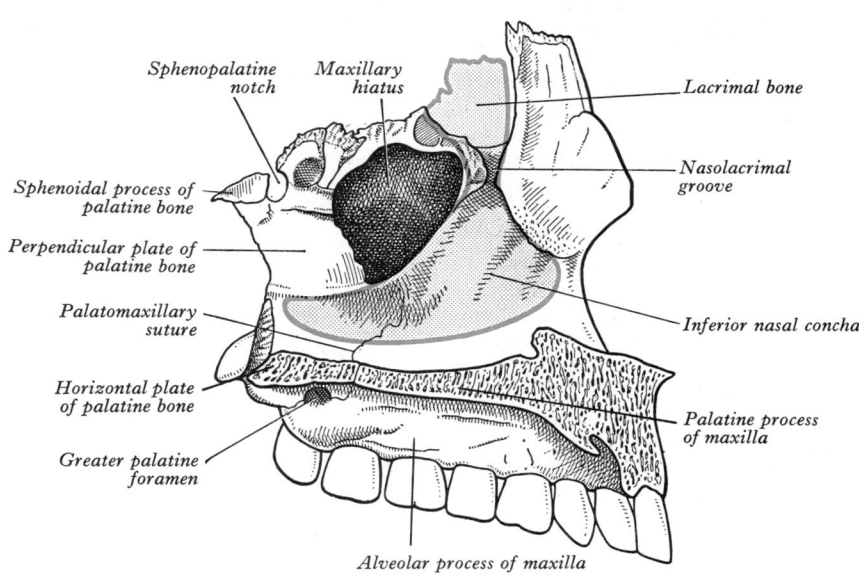

6.193   Drawing to show how the medial wall of the nasolacrimal canal is formed by the articulation of the descending process of the lacrimal bone with the lacrimal process of the inferior nasal concha.

605

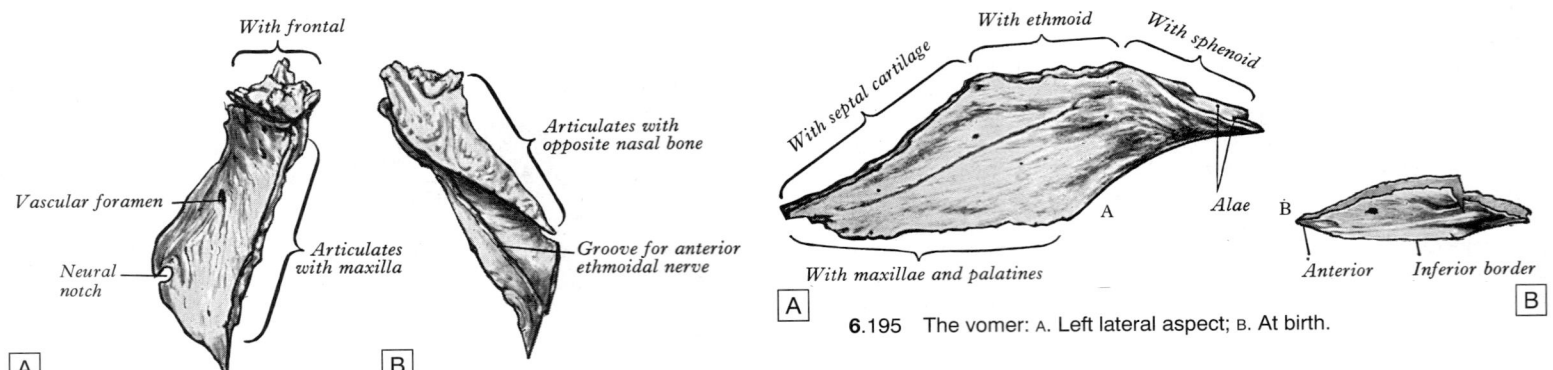

6.194   The left nasal bone: A. External aspect; B. Internal aspect.

6.195   The vomer: A. Left lateral aspect; B. At birth.

NASAL BONES

Nasal bones are small, oblong, variable in size and form, and placed side by side between the frontal processes of the maxillae; they jointly form the nasal bridge (**6.134, 157B**).

Each has two surfaces and four borders. The *external surface* (**6.194A**) has a descending concavoconvex profile and is transversely convex. It is covered by the procerus and nasalis muscles and perforated centrally by a small venous foramen. The *internal surface* (**6.194B**), transversely concave, is traversed by a longitudinal groove for the anterior ethmoidal nerve. The *superior border*, thick and serrated, articulates with the frontal. The *inferior border*, thin and notched, is continuous with the lateral nasal cartilage. The *lateral border* joins the frontal process of the maxilla. The *medial border*, thicker above, meets its fellow and projects behind as a vertical crest, a small part of the nasal septum, articulating from above with the nasal spine of the frontal, the ethmoid's perpendicular plate and the nasal septal cartilage.

Ossification

Ossification is from a centre which appears early in the third month in mesenchyme overlying the cartilaginous anterior part of the nasal capsule.

VOMER

The vomer is thin, flat, and almost trapezoid, forming the postero-inferior part of the nasal septum (**6.156**); it has lateral surfaces and four borders. Both *surfaces* (**6.195**) are marked by grooves for nerves and vessels, one obliquely anteroinferior for the nasopalatine nerve and vessels. The *superior border* is thickest, with a deep furrow between projecting alae which fits the sphenoidal rostrum; the alae articulate with the sphenoidal conchae, sphenoidal processes of the palatine bones and vaginal processes of the medial pterygoid plates. Where each ala is between the sphenoid's body and the vaginal process its inferior surface helps to form the vomerovaginal canal (p. 567). The *inferior border* articulates with the median maxillary and palatine nasal crests. The *anterior border*, the longest, articulates in its upper half with the ethmoid's perpendicular plate; the lower half is cleft to receive the inferior margin of the nasal septal cartilage. The *posterior border* is concave, separating the posterior nasal apertures; it is thick and bifid above, thin below. The anterior end articulates with the posterior margin of the maxillary incisor crest and descends between the incisive canals.

Ossification

The nasal septum is at first a plate of cartilage, part of which is ossified above to form the ethmoid's perpendicular plate; its antero-inferior region persists as septal cartilage, the vomer being ossified in strata of connective tissue covering it on each aspect in its postero-inferior part. About the eighth week two centres appear flanking the midline and in the twelfth week these unite below the cartilage, forming a deep groove (**6.195B**) for the nasal septal cartilage. Union of the bony lamellae progresses anterosuperiorly, while intervening

cartilage is absorbed; by puberty they are almost united, but the bilaminar origin remains in the everted alae and anterior marginal groove (**6.195A**).

SUTURAL BONES

Additional ossificatory centres may occur in or near sutures, giving rise to isolated *sutural bones* (**6.196**). Usually irregular in size and shape, and most frequent in the lambdoid suture, they sometimes occur at fontanelles, especially the posterior, perhaps representing a *pre-interparietal* element, a true *interparietal* or some composite. An isolated bone at the lambda is sometimes dubbed the *Inca bone* or *Goethe's ossicle* (p. 583). One or more *pterion ossicles* or *epipteric bones* may appear between the parietal's sphenoidal angle and sphenoid's greater wing, varying much in size, but more or less symmetrical. Sutural bones usually have little morphological significance, with notable exceptions (p. 591). There are often only two or three, but they appear in great numbers in hydrocephalic skulls. They have therefore been linked with rapid cranial expansion, but this is unproven. For a detailed analysis of these and other *epigenetic variations* in 585 adult crania, consult Berry and Berry (1967), who discuss genetic identification of populations by such criteria, subsequently providing further data (Berry 1975). A report of their occurrence in fetal skulls (El-Najjar & Dawson 1977) supports a genetic factor.

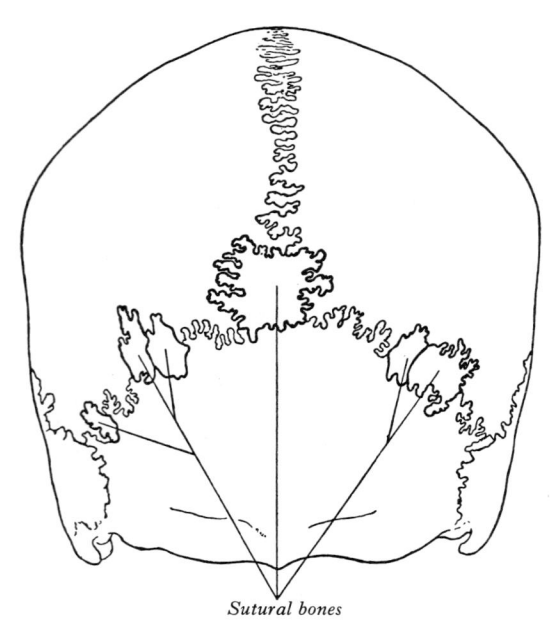

Sutural bones

6.196   Sutural bones in the lambdoid and sagittal sutures.

CRANIAL CHARACTERISTICS AT DIFFERENT AGES

THE SKULL AT BIRTH

At birth the skull is large in proportion to other skeletal parts, but the facial region is relatively small, only about one-eighth of the neonatal cranium, compared with half in adult life. Smallness of the face at birth is due to the rudimentary stage of the mandible and maxillae, non-eruption of the teeth and the small size of maxillary sinuses and the nasal cavity. The latter is almost entirely between the orbits, the lower border of the piriform nasal aperture being only slightly below the orbital floors. The large size of the calvaria, especially the cranial vault, is related to precocious cerebral growth. The cranial base is relatively short and narrow and, although the middle and internal auditory parts are almost adult in size, the petrous temporal bones are generally far from adult dimensions. Bones of the cranial vault are unilaminar and without diploë. Frontal and parietal tuberosities are prominent and in norma verticalis the greatest width is between the parietal tuberosities (p. 609). The glabella, superciliary arches and mastoid processes are not developed.

Ossification is incomplete, many bones being still in several elements united by fibrous tissue or cartilage. The 'os incisivum' is continuous with the maxilla (p. 602); pre- and postsphenoids have just united, but the halves of frontal bone and mandible, and squamous, lateral and basilar parts of occipital bone are all separate. A second styloid centre (*stylohyal*) has not appeared and parts of the temporal bones are separate except for the commencing fusion of the tympanic with the petrous and squamous parts. The fibrous membrane, forming the cranial vault before ossification, is unossified at the angles of the parietal bones, leaving six *fonticuli* (*fontanelles*), two median (anterior and posterior) and two lateral pairs (sphenoidal and mastoid). The *anterior fontanelle* (**6.197**), the largest, is at the junction of the sagittal, coronal and frontal sutures, hence rhomboid, and about 4 cm in anteroposterior and 2.5 cm in transverse dimensions. The *posterior fontanelle* (**6.197**), at the junction of the sagittal and lambdoid sutures, is hence triangular. The *sphenoidal* (anterolateral) and *mastoid* (posterolateral) fontanelles (**6.197**) are small, irregular and at sphenoidal and mastoid angles of the parietal bones.

At birth the orbits are large and the germs of developing teeth are near their orbital floors. Temporal bones differ greatly from their adult form. The internal ear, tympanic cavity, auditory ossicles and mastoid antrum are almost adult, the tympanic plate is an incomplete ring and the mastoid process absent. Hence the external acoustic meatus is short, straight, unossified and wholly fibrocartilaginous. The external aspect of the tympanic membrane faces **down** rather than laterally, in accord with the basal cranial contour. The stylomastoid foramen is exposed on the lateral surface of the skull; the styloid process has not fused with the temporal bone; the mandibular fossa is flat and more lateral and its articular tubercle undeveloped. Paranasal sinuses are rudimentary or absent; only the maxillary sinuses are usually identifiable.

During birth the skull is moulded by slow compression; that part of the scalp which is more central in the birth canal is often temporarily oedematous due to interference with venous return and is called the *caput succedaneum*. Fontanelles and the width of the sutures allow bones of the cranial vault some overlap. The skull is compressed in one plane with compensatory elongation orthogonal to this. These effects disappear within a week.

POSTNATAL GROWTH

Co-ordinated postnatal growth of the calvarial and facial skeleton proceeds at different rates and periods, the cranial cavity being related to cerebral growth, the facial skeleton to the development of the teeth, muscles of mastication and tongue; but growth of the cranial base is not at the same rate as that of the vault. Therefore the three regions must be considered separately. The anterior part of the cranial base is a *zone of interaction* between facial and cerebral growth (Brash 1924; Scott 1967).

Growth of the vault

This is rapid during the first year and slower to the seventh, by which time it has reached almost adult dimensions. For most of this period expansion is largely concentric; form is determined early in the first year, remaining thereafter largely unaltered (Brodie 1941; Weinmann & Sicher 1955; Hoyte 1966; Scott & Symons 1977). That **shape** of the vault is not directly related to cerebral growth but to genetic factors is supported by the great range of cranial indices and shapes in racial groups. During the first and early second years growth of the vault is mainly by ossification at apposed margins of bones, which possess an osteogenic layer (p. 487), accompanied by some accretion and absorption of bone at surfaces to adapt to continually altering curvatures. Growth in **breadth** occurs at the sagittal, sphenofrontal, sphenotemporal and occipitomastoid sutures and petro-occipital cartilaginous joints, while growth in **height** occurs at the frontozygomatic and squamosal sutures, pterion (p. 560) and asterion (p. 561). During this period fontanelles are closed by ossification of the bones around them, but separate centres may convert them into sutural bones. The sphenoidal and posterior fontanelles 'fill in' within 2 or 3 months of birth, mastoid fontanelles usually near the end of the first year and the anterior fontanelle at about the middle of the second, by which time calvarial bones have interlocked at sutures, commencing early in the first year. Further expansion is chiefly by accretion and absorption on external and internal surfaces respectively (Ford 1956). Meanwhile the bones thicken, but not uniformly. At birth the vault is unilaminar, tables and intervening diploë appearing about the fourth year, with maximal differentiation at about 35 years, when diploic veins are prominent in radiograms. Thickening of the vault and development of external muscular markings are related to the development of the masticatory and neck muscles. The mastoid process is a visible bulge in the second year and invaded by air cells in the sixth; Galli et al (1976) have recorded metrical studies of it.

Growth of the base

This is responsible for much of the cranial **lengthening**, mostly at cartilaginous joints between the sphenoid and ethmoid, and especially between the sphenoid and occipital bones. Largely independent of cerebral growth, it continues at the occipitosphenoid synchondrosis until the eighteenth to twenty-fifth year, a period prolonged by continued expansion of the jaws to accommodate erupting teeth, and by growth in the muscles of mastication and those of the nasopharynx. However, there is some evidence that growth may cease at about 15 years (Latham 1966). A pubertal growth spurt has been ascribed to both sexes, about two years earlier in females; considerable postpubertal growth, up to 17.5 years in males (Roche & Lewis 1974), has been described. For a review of studies on basal growth consult Hoyte (1975), and for labelling studies of growth in craniofacial cartilages (in rats) see Kvinnsland and Kvinnsland (1975). Buranarugsa and Houghton (1981) have applied multivariate analysis to Cartesian co-ordinates of cranial landmarks in Polynesian crania; they claim considerable independence in the growth and positioning of the segments noted above. Trenouth (1984) has contributed an extensive study of 60 fetal cranial profiles and draws attention to the effects of disproportionate growth of the brain and face, and the result of this in changing the developing cranial base. It is to be hoped that this series of observations can be linked with pre- and postnatal changes.

Growth of the face

This occupies a longer period than the calvaria. Much information is derived from serial radiography (Salzmann 1961). The ethmoid and the orbital and upper nasal cavities have almost completed growth by the seventh year (**6.198**). Orbital and upper nasal growth is achieved by sutural accretion with deposition of bone on the facial aspects of the margins. The maxilla is carried **downwards** and **forwards** by expansion of the orbits and nasal septum and sutural growth, especially at the fontanelles and zygomaticomaxillary and pterygomaxillary sutures. In the first year growth in width occurs at the symphysis menti and midpalatal, internasal and frontal sutures; but such growth is diminished or even ended when the symphysis menti and frontal suture close during the first few years, even though the midpalatal suture persists until mature years. Facial growth in this

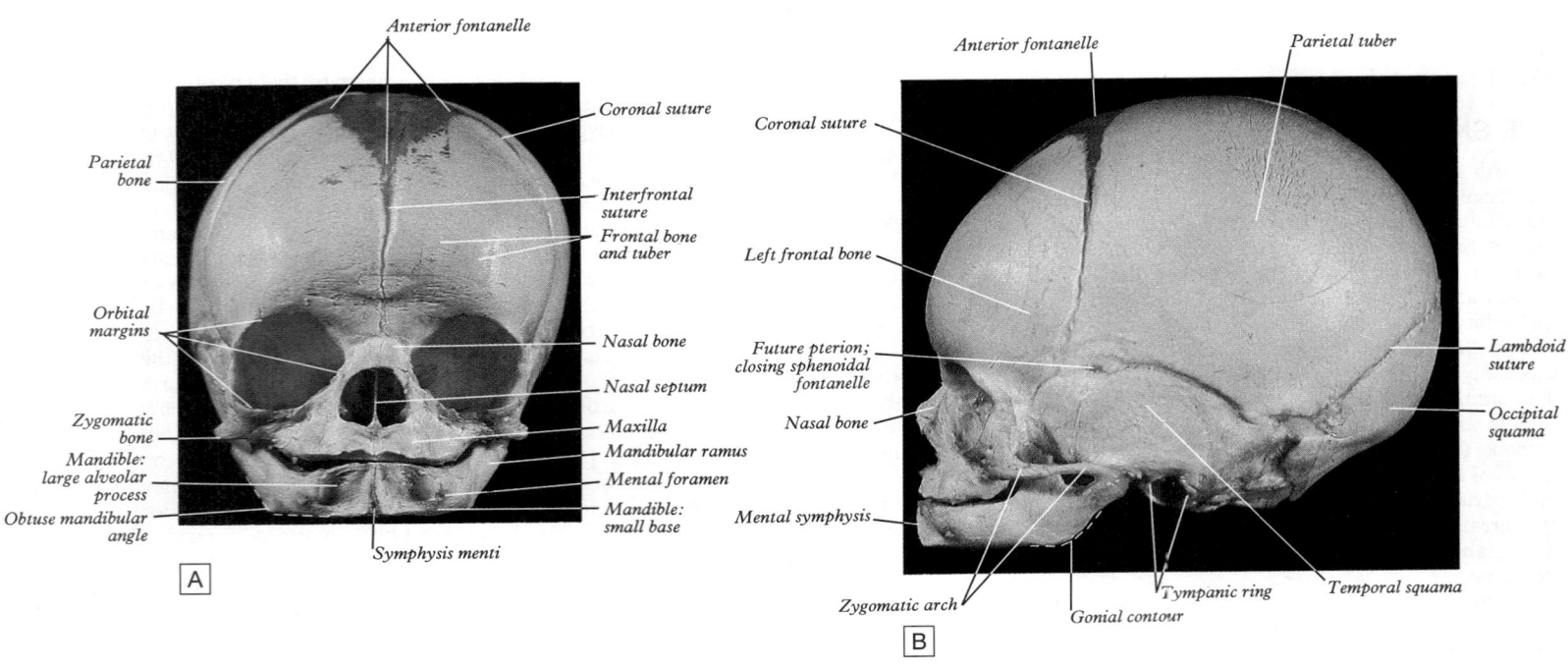

A.
Anterior fontanelle
Coronal suture
Parietal bone
Interfrontal suture
Frontal bone and tuber
Orbital margins
Nasal bone
Nasal septum
Zygomatic bone
Maxilla
Mandible: large alveolar process
Mandibular ramus
Mental foramen
Obtuse mandibular angle
Mandible: small base
Symphysis menti

B.
Anterior fontanelle
Parietal tuber
Coronal suture
Left frontal bone
Future pterion; closing sphenoidal fontanelle
Nasal bone
Lambdoid suture
Occipital squama
Mental symphysis
Zygomatic arch
Gonial contour
Tympanic ring
Temporal squama

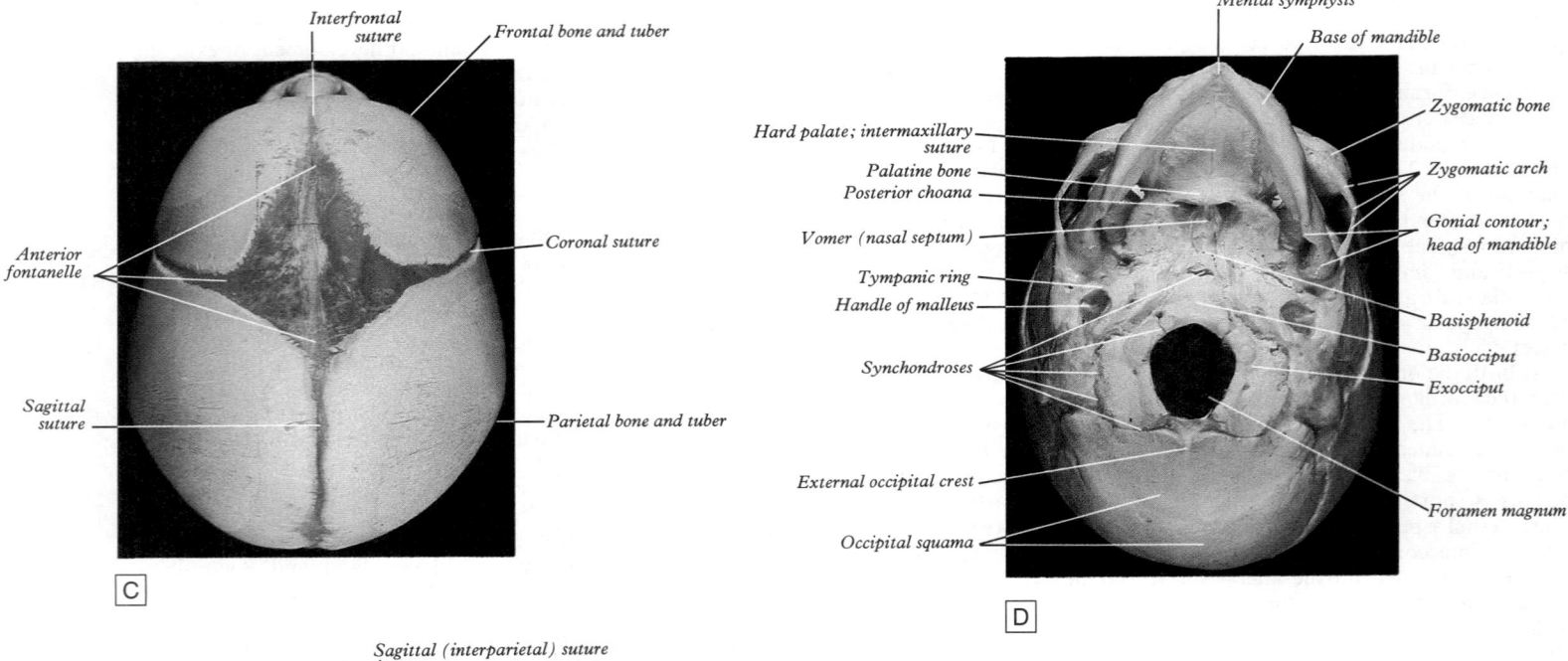

C.
Interfrontal suture
Frontal bone and tuber
Anterior fontanelle
Coronal suture
Sagittal suture
Parietal bone and tuber

D.
Mental symphysis
Base of mandible
Hard palate; intermaxillary suture
Zygomatic bone
Palatine bone
Posterior choana
Zygomatic arch
Vomer (nasal septum)
Gonial contour; head of mandible
Tympanic ring
Handle of malleus
Basisphenoid
Synchondroses
Basiocciput
Exocciput
External occipital crest
Foramen magnum
Occipital squama

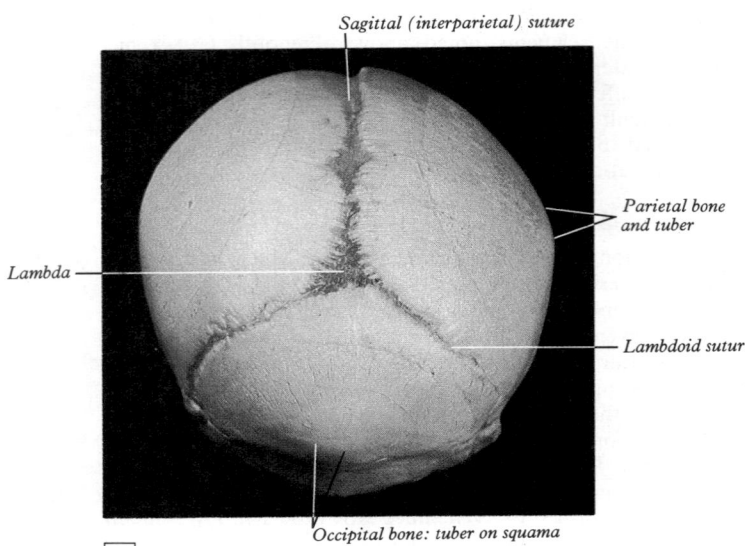

E.
Sagittal (interparietal) suture
Parietal bone and tuber
Anterior fontanelle
Lambda
Lambdoid suture
Occipital bone: tuber on squama

6.197 Skull of newborn infant: A. Anterior aspect; B. Lateral aspect; C. Superior aspect; D. Basal aspect; E. Posterior occipital aspect. (Photograph by K Fitzpatrick.)

period continues to puberty and later, linked with the eruption of the permanent teeth. After sutural growth, near the end of the second year, expansion of the facial skeleton is by surface accretion on the face, alveolar processes and palate, with resorption in the walls of the maxillary sinuses, the upper surface of the hard palate and the labial aspect of the alveolar process. Co-ordinated growth and divergence of the pterygoid processes is due to deposition and resorption of bone on appropriate surfaces. Mandibular growth is described on page 576.

Obliteration of the calvarial sutures progresses with age, commencing between 30 and 40 years internally, about 10 years later on the exterior, but closure times vary greatly (Todd & Lyon 1924, 1925a,b; Abbie 1950; Singer 1953). Obliteration usually begins at the bregma, extending into the sagittal, coronal and lambdoid sutures, in that order. In old age the skull becomes thinner and lighter, but occasionally the reverse. The most striking senile feature is diminution in size of the mandible and maxillae following the loss of teeth and absorption of alveolar bone. This reduces the vertical depth of the face and increases the mandibular angles (**6**.198; p. 578).

SEXUAL AND RACIAL DIFFERENCES IN THE CRANIUM

Until puberty there is little sexual difference in skulls; the adult female's is a little lighter and smaller, its capacity about 10% less; its walls are thinner and muscular ridges less marked; the glabella, superciliary arches and mastoid processes are less prominent; air sinuses are smaller; tympanic plates are smaller and their margins less rough; the upper orbital margins are sharper, the forehead vertical, the frontal and parietal tuberosities prominent and the vault somewhat flattened; the facial contour is rounder, facial bones

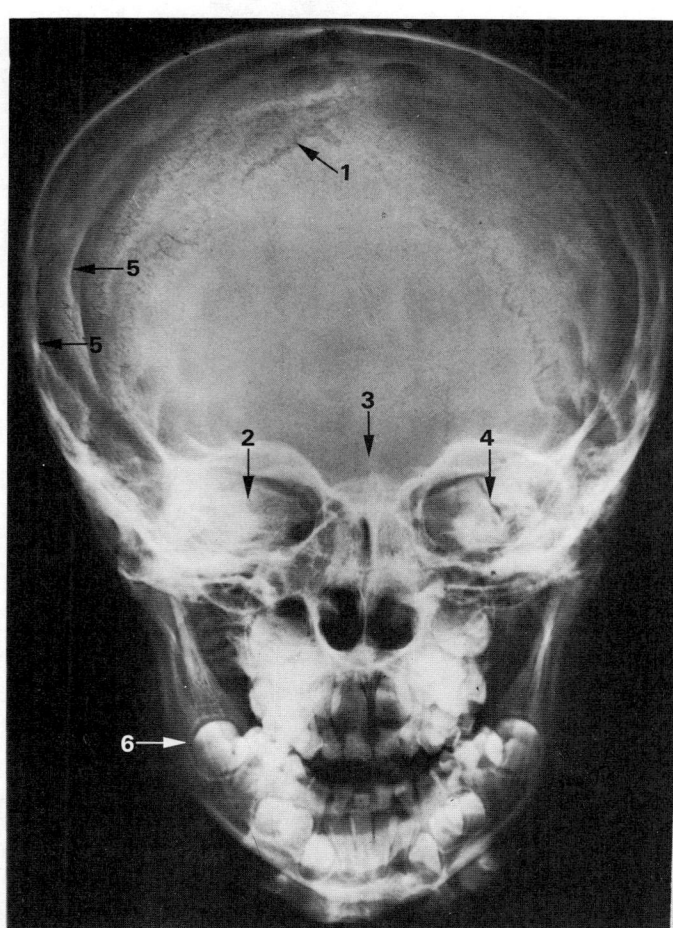

6.198 Radiograph of child's skull, aged seven: occipitofrontal view. 1. Lambdoid suture. 2. Petrous portion of right temporal bone, seen through the cavity of the orbit. 3. Crista galli of the ethmoid bone. 4. Fracture through petrous portion of left temporal bone, seen through the cavity of the orbit. 5. Impressions for cerebral gyri. 6. Second permanent molar tooth, not yet erupted.

smoother and the mandible and maxillae and contained teeth are smaller. Thus, more childhood characteristics are retained in females. Typical male or female skulls are easily recognized, but in some characteristics are so indeterminate that diagnosis of sex is difficult or impossible.

Sexual dimorphism

Generally less marked in humans than other primates, this is associated with the *paedomorphic* tendency of human stock, females and even males being less divergent in adult development from their own juvenile form, a tendency less apparent in other primates, especially in males (Abbie 1952; Schultze 1956). Exaggerated sexual differences occur in most anthropoid apes and some monkeys in the form of enlarged canines in males, with associated jaw development, accentuated muscular ridges and total size of the skull. These excesses are typified in the gorilla, orang-utan, and many species of baboon, in which males also much exceed females in stature and physique. Even in extinct human forms sexual dimorphism, on available fossil evidence, appears to have been less than in other primates. In modern humans differences are further reduced but the degree of sexual divergence in cranial size and proportions varies in racial groups. Such sexual differences have been less exactly assessed than general ethnic differences. In both, assessment depends on observation of two kinds of feature:

- those which cannot be measured, for which no satisfactory quantitative technique has, as yet, been devised (e.g. size of mastoid process, prominence of chin);
- those expressed as actual measurements or indices (e.g. cranial capacity, orbital index).

Examples of the former category in distinguishing sex have been cited above; more exhaustive lists exist (Keen 1950). Use of such features in judging sex or race in isolated crania is dependent on the observers' experience but, where many are available from a single ethnic group, both types of assessment are more certain. Distinction of three major races by non-metrical traits can be effected with some confidence (Todd & Tracy 1930). Incidences of many variations have been observed on a racial basis, for example metopism and other sutural variants (Berry & Berry 1967), and are of considerable ethnic but lesser forensic interest. Berry (1975) made a special study of *non-metrical* human cranial variations; these include:

- Highest nuchal line (p. 560).
- Os suturale at lambda (p. 606).
- Ossa suturalia in lambdoid suture (p. 506).
- Parietal foramen (p. 554).
- Os suturale at bregma (p. 607).
- Frontal suture (metopism) (p. 595).
- Ossa suturalia in coronal suture (p. 606).
- Epipteric os suturale (p. 606).
- Frontotemporal articulation (p. 595).
- Parietomastoid os suturale (p. 561).
- Os suturale at asterion (p. 561).
- Tympanic foramen of Huschke (p. 593).
- Extrasutural mastoid foramen (p. 591).
- Absence of mastoid foramen (p. 591).
- Patent condylar canal (p. 567).
- Double condylar facet (p. 583).
- Precondylar tubercle (p. 583).
- Double hypoglossal canal (p. 584).
- Incomplete foramen ovale (p. 567).
- Incomplete foramen spinosum (p. 567).
- Accessory palatine foramina (p. 563).
- Maxillary torus (p. 602).
- Palatine torus (pp. 563, 602).
- Occurrence of zygomaticofacial foramen (pp. 555, 605).
- Supraorbital foramen or incisure (p. 595).
- Frontal foramen or incisure (p. 595).
- Extrasutural anterior ethmoid foramen (p. 559).
- Absence of posterior ethmoid foramen (p. 558).
- Accessory infraorbital foramen (p. 585).
- Interparietal bone (p. 585).
- Paramastoid process (p. 584).
- Auditory torus (p. 592).

Although many have studied these and other cranial variants (e.g. the mandibular torus, p. 576), few studies have been quantitative. These authors have been reviewed by Berry and Berry (1967) and Berry (1975), with extensive statistical data; they have assessed which cranial variations exhibit racial (and sometimes sexual) correlation. The interested reader should also consult Czarnetzki (1971) and Hjarnø et al (1974).

To achieve a more objective racial assessment, metrical studies have long been practised; internationally accepted techniques of *craniometry* have promoted a large corpus of comparable ethnic data for males and, to a lesser extent, females. Many standard measurements are used; only major dimensions and examples of indices derived from them are included here (**6.199, 200**). The calvarial part of the skull is measured as follows:

A. Maximal cranial length	summit of glabella to furthest occipital point
B. Maximal cranial breadth	greatest breadth, at right angles to median plane
C. Cranial height	from basion (median point on anterior rim of foramen magnum) to bregma

All measurements are to the nearest millimetre. From these three dimensions, three indices are calculated: *B/A, C/A* and *C/B* and expressed as percentages.

The breadth/length ratio is the *cranial index* (*cephalic index* in the

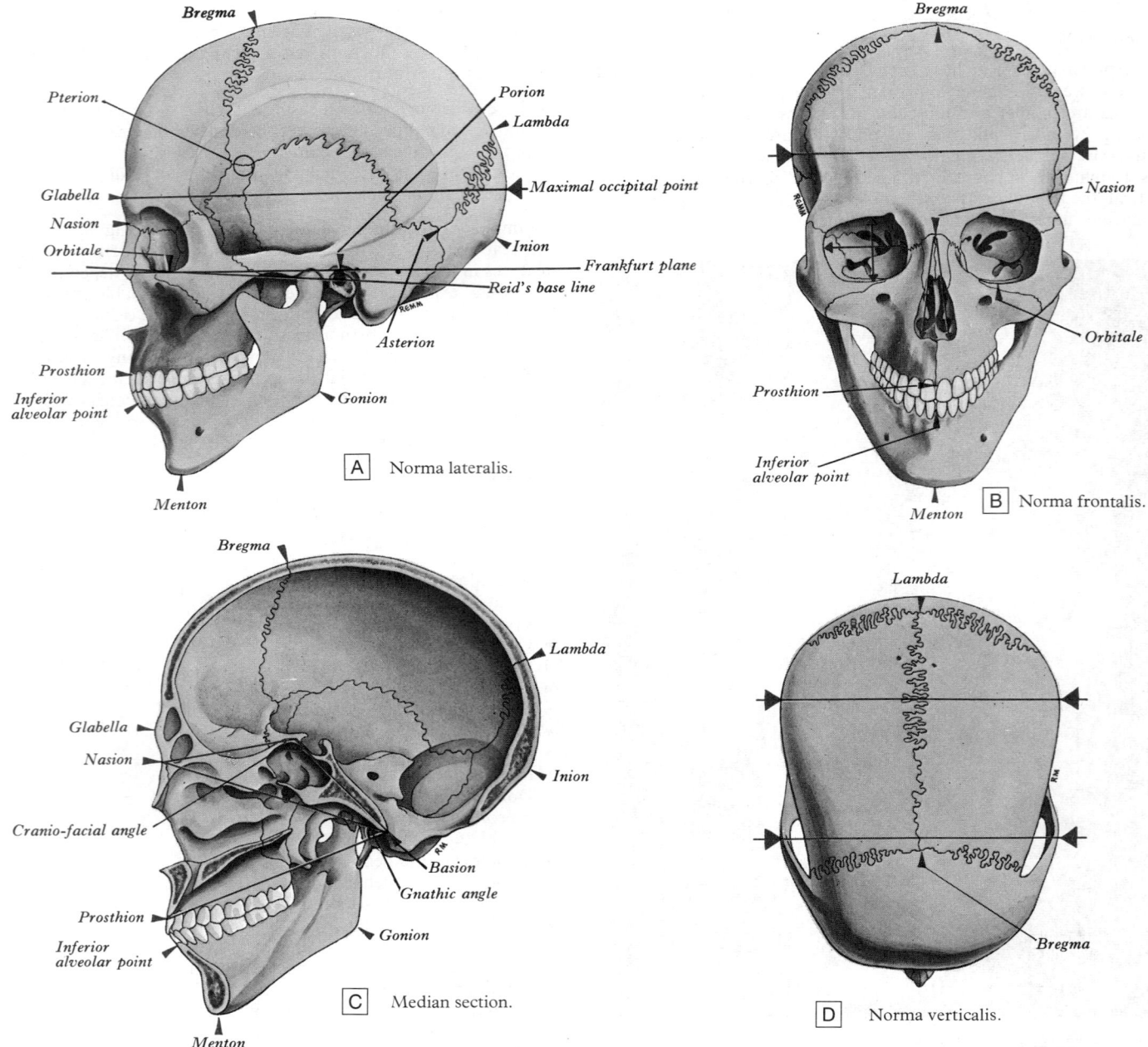

A Norma lateralis.

B Norma frontalis.

C Median section.

D Norma verticalis.

6.199 These diagrams illustrate the cranial points used, by international agreement, in making linear and certain angular measurements in anthropometry. In all four views the skull is in the standard orientation, that is, with the Frankfurt plane as a horizontal. The point at which the craniofacial angle is measured is not named; it corresponds to the midpoint of the chiasmal groove.

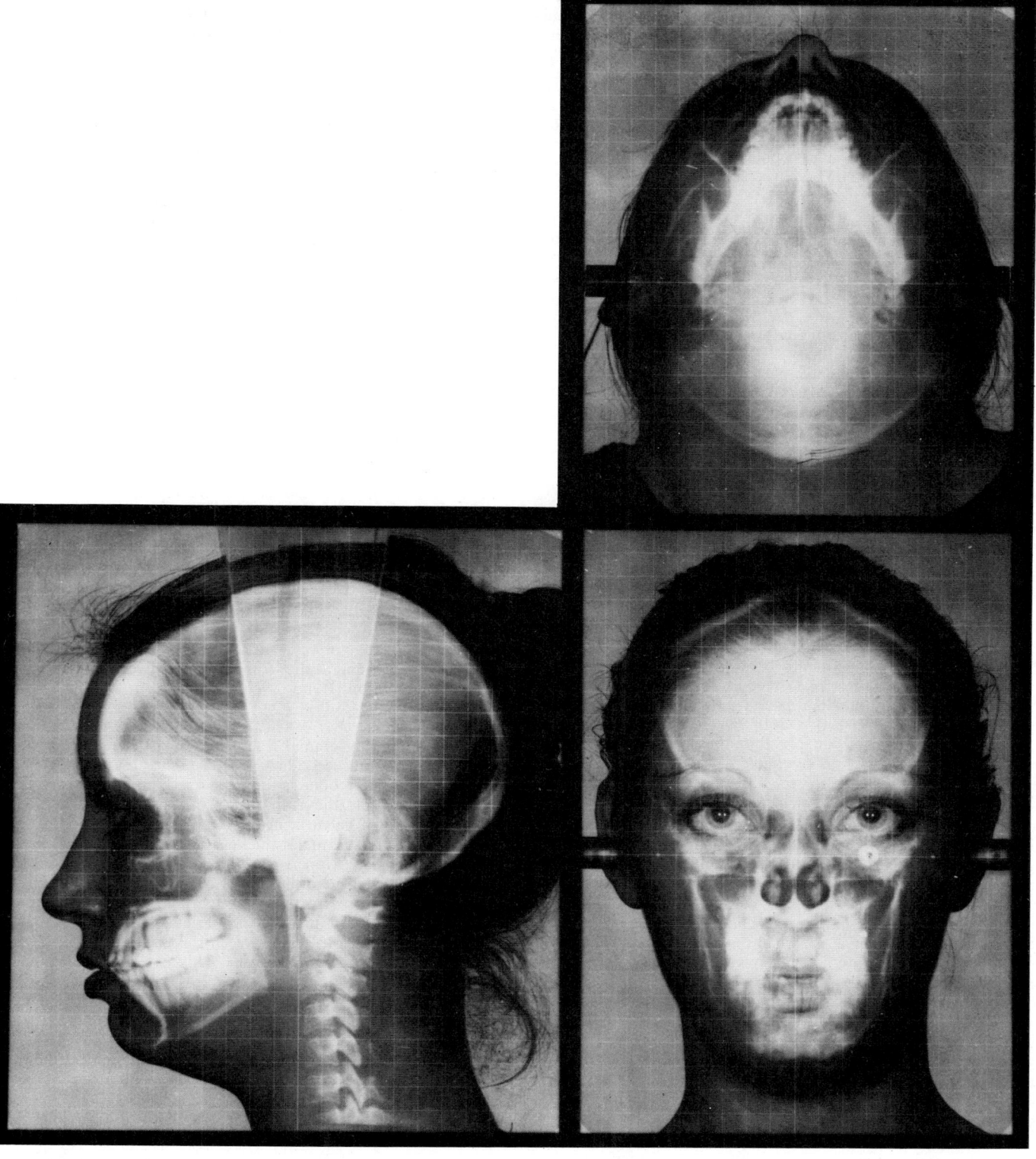

6.200 Combined, accurately superimposed photographs and radiographs of the kind shown here are currently being used to produce a computerized analysis of metrical relations between a selection of datum points in the skeletal and soft tissue components of human heads and faces. The technique, known as morphanalysis, has been elaborated by Dr G P Rabey, to whom we are indebted for these records. Both photographs and radiographs are produced in the three primary planes and hence the morphometric analysis is three-dimensional. For further information see Rabey (1968, 1971, 1980).

living). Its recorded range of variation is high, as with other skull or head indices. All ranges are arbitrarily divided into steps, usually covering 5% sections of the total range; to each step a specific term is applied. For example:

(*Maximal breadth/maximal length*) × 100 = cranial or cephalic index

Up to 74.9 = dolichocranic or dolichocephalic
75.0 to 79.9 = mesocranic or mesocephalic
80.0 to 84.9 = brachycranic or brachycephalic

Distinction between measurement of dried crania and living heads, by the two sets of terms, is not rigidly applied. The 'cephalic' terms are more common, often used for both purposes. Other indices in common use are:

(*a*) *Total facial index* = (nasion–gnathion height/bizygomatic breadth) × 100. The nasion is the point where the internasal suture meets the frontal bone. The gnathion is the midpoint of the lower mandibular border

(*b*) *Upper facial index* = (nasion–prosthion length/bizygomatic breadth) × 100. The prosthion is the midpoint of the maxillary alveolar rim, between the central incisors. The bizygomatic breadth is the greatest distance measured by trial between zygomatic arches on external aspects

(*c*) *Nasal index* = (nasal breadth/nasal height) × 100. Breadth is the horizontal maximum across the nasal aperture, and height is from nasion to the mean between the two lowest points on the aperture's lower border

(*d*) *Orbital index* = (maximal orbital height/maximal orbital breadth) × 100

(*e*) *Palatal index* = (maximal palatal breadth/maximal palatal length) × 100

(*f*) *Gnathic index* = (basion–prosthion/basion–nasion) × 100.

Indices provide a system for *metrical* recording of sizes and proportions of cranial features in place of subjective impressions. If a group is said to be dolichocephalic, this does not (or should not) imply a vague comparison, but that the index is within known numerical limits. It can be observed that the orbital opening appears rounder in females, but this statement can be quantified and is then far more valuable. Again, jaws project more in some races, a fact determinable by inspection alone when the condition is pronounced; the gnathic index yields a numerical expression and comparisons are then permissible.

The following measurements are applied to mandibles: (*a*) height of symphysis, (*b*) length of body, (*c*) length of ramus, (*d*) bigonial width (between angles), (*e*) bicondylar width, and so on. The angle between the body and ramus is also often estimated. Since the mandible is often missing from skulls and moreover is considered less reliable in assessing racial affinity (Morant 1936), its measurements are less widely used.

Other forms of cranial measurement are employed. Horizontal circumference and various arcs and contours are sometimes measured. Radiographic studies make it possible to extend classic craniometry and to measure directly certain angles, for example the gnathic angle, between basion–nasion and basion–prosthion lines. The *craniofacial* or *cranial base angle* is of special interest, representing the degree of cranial flexure. The human angle has a value of about 130°, probably achieved by birth, little further change occurring. Its

high human value has been linked with translation of the tongue towards pharynx, a change sometimes regarded as essential to speech (Schulter 1976). Radiographic techniques for the estimation of endocranial volume has been evolved (Haas 1952). *Cranial capacity*, an indication of brain volume, can be assessed directly by filling the cavity with lead shot, millet seed or other particulate materials suitable for volumetric measurement when poured out again. Several formulae have also been constructed to give cranial capacity from the length, breadth and height of the cranium. Examples are:

Males: 0.000337 (L-11) (B-11) (H-11) + 406.01 cc
Females: 0.000400 (L-11) (B-11) (H-11) + 206.60 cc

In these formulae, L and B are length and breadth, and H is the *auricular height*, measured to the vertex from the external acoustic meatus. All measurements are in millimetres, but such methods involve some inaccuracy, and various corrections do not entirely remove this (Hrdlička 1939; Montagu 1960).

Attempts to establish reliable craniometric differentiation between races are as old as craniometry. Though mandibular data and cranial capacity are less dependable, satisfactory differentiation is possible in some groups, especially between Caucasians and Negroes. When several measurements are treated by discriminant analysis, an accuracy of over 90% can be expected (Giles & Elliot 1960). Multivariate analysis may also elucidate cranial growth. Cranio-metric methods are useful in forensic identification when cranial remains can be compared with existing photographic and radiographic records (Glaister & Brash 1937), and in attempts to reconstruct appearance in life of individuals represented only by skeletal remains (Stewart 1954). Cephalometry has also been applied in plastic and oral surgery concerned with craniofacial deformity. A development in this field is *morphanalysis*, which uses gridded radiographs and photographs universally related in three dimensions (**6.200**). Such standardized records enable diagnostic comparison between patients and the normal population (Rabey 1968, 1971).

Clinical anatomy

Factors preventing cranial fracture are elasticity, round shape and construction from secondary elastic arches, each derived from a single bone. Where bone is thin, the overlying muscles may cushion blows, for example the temporal squama and inferior occipital fossa. The thickness of calvaria in 28 Caucasians (from 15 to 82 years) averaged 5.8 mm. In males thickness increased with age, in females the reverse is true (Lippert & Kafer 1974).

The commonest site of basal fracture is through the middle cranial fossa; fracture starts from the point struck, usually near the parietal tuberosity, descends through the parietal and temporal squamata and across the petrous region, often traversing the internal acoustic meatus, to the foramen lacerum. This explains various sequelae: thus, if the internal acoustic meatus is damaged, injury to the facial and vestibulocochlear nerves may result, with consequent facial paralysis and deafness; if it extends through the semicircular ducts, vertigo ensues; if the arachnoid around these nerves in the meatus is torn and when the internal ear and tympanic cavity communicate and the tympanic membrane is torn, as it often is, cerebrospinal fluid may escape.

Facial bones are sometimes fractured by direct violence, most commonly the nasal bones and mandible. Nasal fracture is usually transverse, about 1.25 cm from the free margin, the broken edges being displaced backwards or more often to one side by direct blows. The commonest site of mandibular fracture is near the canine tooth, whose deep socket weakens the bone; next most frequent is the angle. Occasionally a double fracture may occur, in both halves of the bone, and is usually compound, with laceration of the oral mucosa.

APPENDICULAR SKELETON

PHYLOGENY AND FUNCTIONS

The ancestral vertebrates, *Agnatha*, were not only jawless but limbless, like surviving representatives such as lampreys (Young 1962; Romer 1970). Two continuous ventrolateral finfolds probably preceded the separated fins which appear in fossil remains of the earliest fish possessing jaws, the *Placoderms*. These sometimes displayed more than two pairs of appendages, but in their descendant bony and cartilaginous classes, the *Osteicthyes* and *Chondricthyes*, the vertebrate pattern of two pairs, pectoral and pelvic, was stabilized, except in such forms as snakes, which have subsequently lost their limbs. Appendicular skeletons of fossils and extant fish vary but show a common plan of 'girdle' bones, embedded in body musculature, and rodlike elements radiating into the mobile fin, with an intermediate joint of the ball and socket type. In many orders of *Osteicthyes* homologues of the pectoral and pelvic components of terrestrial limbs can be identified, as well as those of the proximal segments, arm and forearm or thigh and foreleg (Bolk et al 1931–9). Distal equivalence is less clear; but the multiplicity of small bony units in fins at least resembles the extremities, hand and foot, of land tetrapods.

Terrestrial vertebrates are grouped as *tetrapods* because their four limbs are an outstanding common feature, although the pectoral pair may be modified for flight. They are probably derived from a primitive order, the *Crossopterygii* ('fringe-finned'), related to another ancient group, *Dipnoi* or lungfish, species of which still survive. The crossopterygians were known only as fossils until 1938, when a living specimen of a suborder, *Coelacanthus*, was captured off the coast of South Africa; further coelacanths have been secured near the Comoro Islands and elsewhere in the Indian Ocean. These possess lobed fins with a narrowed attachment, and from such appendages tetrapod limbs can most plausibly be derived.

In the change to terrestrial environment, during evolution of primitive amphibians from crossopterygians, two major adaptations began. The first, already foreshadowed in fins, was a repositioning of these limb-like paddles for more effective support and propulsion on land. The *forelimbs* rotated **laterally** at joints with the pectoral girdle so that the hinging of the elbow, at first pointing away from the body as it still does in amphibians and reptiles, finally projected backwards. In contrast, the *hindlimbs* rotated **medially** at their pelvic joints into opposite positions, so that the knees projected forwards. These opposite changes rotated the *preaxial* or leading *border*, corresponding with the 'first' digit, pollex or hallux, from an anterior to lateral position in the pectoral limb. This changed orientation of the forelimb necessitates a complementary *pronation* of its radio-ulnar segment to achieve a plantigrade appendage, a compensation unnecessary in the hindlimb. Coupled with these growing distinctions between fore and hind extremities was a second modification— articulation of pelvic girdles with the spinal column, unknown in fish but uniform in tetrapods, except some fossil amphibians.

With the evolution of amphibians, a general skeletal pattern of tetrapod limb was defined and, apart from minor modifications, has persisted through subsequent vertebrates. This *primitive pentadactyl limb* typically terminates in five digits, reduction of which is frequent, especially in mammals. But the primates, including humans, have retained the full number and are in this respect unspecialized.

Of the girdles the *pectoral* always comprises a dorsal *scapula*, but varies in ventral components, commonly a mixture of endochondral and dermal bones. Of these the *coracoid* and *clavicle* persist in mammals, the former reduced in size and fused to the scapula. The clavicle, sole mammalian survivor of a variety of dermal elements in lower vertebrates (e.g. the *cleithrum* and *interclavicle*), is also often reduced and even lost in some mammals, especially fast-running or bounding types of quadruped. Its persistence in primates is linked with the development of forelimbs for grasping and climbing; the clavicle acts as a mobile strut, at the lateral end of which the rest of the limb can be variably positioned (Watson 1917). The *pelvic girdle*, in contrast, contains only endochondral elements; the primitive dermal armour only extended far enough caudally to permit incorporation of dermal elements into the pectoral but not the pelvic

girdle. The latter developed a ventral *symphysis* in fish, which in tetrapods contains distinguishable pubic and ischial elements. The dorsal ilium, though present in some fish, is not well developed. In land animals the need for larger muscles to support the body's weight and to impart thrust through the hindlimbs, leads to greater iliac size and articulation with the sacral spinal column. Throughout tetrapods these pelvic entities, *pubis, ischium* and *ilium*, are more uniformly arranged than in fish. They also show an increasing tendency to fuse into an *innominate* bone, especially in adult mammals. The two innominate bones are joined ventrally at a symphysis pubis and to the sacrum dorsally at sacroiliac articulations. Thus is established a *pelvis*, primarily locomotor, conducting stresses between the axial skeleton and the limbs. The term pelvis, a basin, is misleading; it is more of an irregular ring which, being at the caudal end of the body cavity, inevitably surrounds certain viscera, a relation which in human anatomy obscures its essentially appendicular origin and function. Since the cloaca is immediately caudal to it, not only the hindgut but other tubes, urinary and genital, must traverse the pelvis, even though separate external openings evolve in mammals. During birth, the offspring must also traverse the pelvis, and their comparatively large size in human females entails obstetric considerations (p. 673), which again may temporarily overshadow the somatic locomotor nature of the hindlimb girdles.

In mammals functional differences between fore- and hindlimbs, accentuated in the human primate, are associated with structural divergence in their girdles. Major differences (ignoring the possible status of e.g. the coracoid complex) are as follows:

Pectoral girdle	Pelvic girdle
(1) Dermal and endochondral	Entirely endochondral
(2) Two principal components, clavicle and scapula, which remain separate. (However, see above and p. 620)	Three components, pubis, ischium and ilium, which fuse into a single innominate bone
(3) No articulation with the vertebral column	Articulates with sacral vertebrae
(4) No direct ventral articulation (clavicles connected only by interclavicular ligament)	Direct ventral articulation at symphysis pubis
(5) Articulations of clavicles with axial skeleton (sternum) are relatively small, mobile and ventral	Articulations of innominate bones with axial skeleton (sacrum) are relatively large, capable of limited movement only, and dorsal
(6) Comparatively lightly built for mobility	Massively constructed for resistance to stress, rather than for mobility
(7) Resilient to thrust	Transmits thrust between vertebral column and hindlimb
(8) Shallow joint with limb, allowing wide range of movement	Deep joint with limb, limiting range of movement

Both girdles articulate with the distal, freely movable parts of the limbs by 'ball and socket' joints, the first segment of each limb containing a single *humerus* or *femur*. Shoulder and hip joints are the same in mechanism, allowing some movement in all directions, though more limited in the hip. Even in quadrupedal mammals, where limbs are walking props mainly adapted to fore and aft movement, greater mobility is usual at the shoulder, particularly in abduction, permitting splaying of the forelimbs. Throughout tetrapods the shoulder region shows a greater range of structural adaptation to changing function. Scapular orientation in relation to the thorax and humerus varies far more than hindlimb equivalents, even in quadrupeds, but the difference is most extreme in bipedal primates (Ashton et al 1976), whose adoption of an arboreal habitat, in which they climb, walk, run and swing, accords with the development of highly mobile and prehensile forelimbs and similar but lesser changes

613

in hindlimbs. Equally to be emphasized is the habit of **sitting** upright, even in primates such as baboons which have returned to a predominantly quadrupedal life on the ground; forelimbs are thus released for manipulative use, activities of the profoundest significance to human evolution.

In modern mammals, *Eutheria*, the articular head of the humerus is usually directed dorsocaudally and the scapular glenoid socket ventrocranially. While this may favour quadrupedal use, it prevents movement of the humerus into the vertical position so easily assumed by primates in reaching up above the head. This entails reorientation of the humeral head relative to its shaft, the head being directed **medially** rather than caudally. Coincident with reorganization of the shoulder is a change in maximal thoracic diameter from dorsoventral to transverse, the former being typical of quadrupeds, the latter of bipedal primates. This is coupled with the retention of clavicles in primate mammals and altered scapular orientation. The scapulae come to face ventrally, rather than medially, and their glenoid fossae more laterally. These changes and correlated muscular alterations are linked with a wider range of movement at the shoulder.

The tubercles and bicipital groove of the humerus partly share in the rotation of its head, but the distal end retains its transverse orientation (Martin 1932). Hence a radial axis through the centre of the head is approximately at right angles to the axis of the lower end in most *Eutheria*, because the head is directed caudally. As it becomes more medial this angle increases above 90°. It is still 95° in Carnivora, rises to about 100° in monkeys, 120° in apes, and from 135° to 165° or more in man. This change in the primate humerus has been considered torsional and the angle termed *angle of torsion*. The term is misleading; there is no evidence of any true 'twisting' of the humeral shaft; spiralling of the radial nerve and its groove predates this change. Nor is there anything specially human in the torsion angle. It reaches 180° (where the axes are parallel) in birds and was apparently nearly as high in mammal-like reptiles, returning to about 90° in *Metatheria* (marsupials). A word of caution is needed concerning methods of recording angles of humeral torsion. As defined here, the angle is measured between articular 'axes' of the shoulder and elbow joints. However, Krahl (1944, 1976), sometimes quoted in textbooks, measured the angle between the axis of the elbow joint and a line orthogonal to the axis of the shoulder joint; his values, therefore, differ by 90° from those cited here. Neither method is conceptually satisfactory, but very similar figures are obtained (*mutatis mutandis*). Krahl's work thus supports the view put forward here, that change in orientation of the humeral head has involved alterations at the proximal end of the bone and has not been accomplished by an evolutionary twisting of the shaft. Racial and sexual differences have been recorded (Kate 1968).

In the lower limb the state is like that of mammal-like reptiles (and birds), with the two axes almost parallel. (The human femoral head and long axis of its neck are anteverted about 16° relative to the transcondylar femoral axis.) This condition is said not to have varied in the lower limbs, unlike the upper. Lability of the humeral 'torsion' angle may be coupled with greater variability in forelimb activity, especially in bipedal forms, with the consequent release of the forelimbs.

Intermediate segments of limbs, and their joints with the humerus and femur, show similarities and differences. The differences are greater in bipeds; in quadrupeds similarities are more evident. Both segments initially contained **parallel** elements, radius and ulna, tibia and fibula (but see below). Primitively both pairs articulate with the single proximal element but in most mammals, as in man, the fibula withdraws from the knee joint, leaving a *preaxial* tibia as the major lever and prop. In the forearm the ulna, a *postaxial* bone, becomes the main force-transmitting strut at the elbow.

Both elbow and knee are hinge joints in quadrupedal mammals; but, while this was the primitive tetrapod state in knees, elbows had an initial potentiality for *rotation*. The hindlimb turns medially, bringing its extensor surface forwards, so that the foot, hinged at the ankle, projects forwards with its plantar surface on the ground. This typical *plantigrade* habit of many quadrupeds brings the hindlimbs under the body as serially hinged levers adapted for propulsion and support. Note that the tibia and fibula remain **parallel**; but the **lateral** rotation of the forelimbs which turns the extensor aspects backwards, entails *pronation* at the elbow to bring the 'hand' forwards, palm downwards, for plantigrade locomotion. This brings

the *preaxial* radius anteromedially across the ulna, and both are stabilized in this relation in a large majority of quadrupeds, including **all** four-footed mammals. Both forearm and foreleg bones tend to fuse in such mammals, particularly in those with a reduced number of digits and usually *digitigrade* in habit (e.g. Carnivora), contact with the ground being restricted to flexor aspects of the remaining digits.

A rotatory potential at the elbow, retained and refined in primates, allows free *pronation* and *supination*, essential to the development of manual skills. These movements are impossible in legs. At primate elbows, the ulna forms a massive hinge with the humerus but tapers to a small distal end; the radius being reciprocal: its upper end is small and adapted for rotation, the lower enlarged to carry the hand. Thus, when the radius revolves it takes the hand with it, turning round the distal end of the ulna.

Both wrist and ankle joints are hinges, but wrists can also *adduct* and *abduct*. The *carpus* and *tarsus* contain small bones between the forearm or foreleg and digits. They are much modified throughout tetrapods, and the two groups show some divergence. But, however modified, both are derivable from the same primary arrangement in the primitive pentadactyl limb. This consisted of a proximal row of three, a distal row of five, articulating with five digits, and a central intermediate group, probably four, wedged between these rows. By fusion, loss and modification in size, shape and articulation, carpal and tarsal bones display much variation (particularly reduction). Tracing homologies between primitive elements and subsequent transformations (structural and functional) has aroused much controversy (Broom 1901; Jones 1949; Lewis 1964a), but agreement has largely been reached. Authorities disagree in minor details, but generally accepted homologies are shown in Table **6**.3.

Main divergences between mammalian carpus and tarsus, apart from the latter's greater size in primates, are threefold. Firstly, the carpus usually remains more primitive, retaining a full proximal row, all articulating with the forearm bones; in the tarsus only one (the talus) retains this role in most mammals, including the primates. Secondly, a single proximal tarsal bone (the calcaneus) projects back as a lever behind the tibia and fibula; this does not occur in the carpus. Thirdly, tarsal bones at intermediate joints permit some rotation (inversion/eversion and pronation/supination), an adaptation to uneven surfaces, which may be met in some forelimbs by pronation and supination between the **forearm** bones and some abduction and adduction at the wrist and intercarpal joints. In all three modifications the tarsus is more advanced. Evolution of the calcanean lever is a **mammalian**, not a solely primitive or human modification. Its high development in the human foot and the resemblance of other primate feet to hands, may superficially suggest that it is a **human** characteristic. (Consult Lewis 1983 for a detailed account, with extensive bibliography, of the evolution of the architecture of the mammalian foot.)

Occurrence of small supernumerary bones, pre- or postaxial in position in both carpus and tarsus, has been taken as evidence of additional digits (Jones 1941) suggesting an ancestral pattern of more than five digits, but all known tetrapods show the orthodox five and often less. The five metacarpal and metatarsal bones originally articulated each with a separate carpal or tarsal, which are reduced to four by fusion of the fourth and fifth even in the pentadactyl primates. In mammals with reduced or lost digits, metacarpals and metatarsals as well as phalanges are involved. An example exists in Carnivora, whose first digit, pollex or hallux, is degenerate and useless, though often still clawed; another more extreme example is the horse, which retains only the middle digit, with a greatly enlarged metapodial bone.

The *metapodial* (metacarpal or metatarsal) *formula* puts these bones in order of length and number. In humans it is usually 2>3>4>5>1 in hands, and 1>2>3>4>5 in feet. The *phalangeal formula*, starting from the preaxial digit, pollex or hallux, numbers the phalanges in each digit. In many primitive reptiles it is 2.3.4.5.3. in primitive mammals 2.3.3.3.3. for hand and foot, as in humans. In horses it is 0.0.3.0.0. A *digital formula* denoting relative lengths of digits is sometimes used, especially in comparing primate extremities.

In all tetrapods pollex and hallux tend to diverge from other digits, perhaps as a prop. Some early mammals were probably arboreal, using hands as primates do, with a grasp between the preaxial digit and the remainder. Primate prehension is developed in hands and feet, though absent from human feet and not always

Table 6.3 Homologization of the primitive tetrapod and human carpus and tarsus

	Tetrapod carpus	Human carpus		Human tarsus		Tetrapod tarsus	
Proximal row	Os Radiale	Scaphoid	Scaphoid minus tubercle	Talus	Navicular minus tubercle	Os Tibiale	Pre-axial
	Os Intermedium	Lunate			Talus	Os Intermedium	
	Os Ulnare	Triquetral		Calcaneus		Os Fibulare	Postaxial
Central elements	Os Centrale	Absent	Tubercle of Scaphoid	Navicular	Tubercle of Navicular	Os Centrale	
Distal row	Os Carpale 1	Trapezium		Medial Cuneiform		Os Tarsale 1	Pre-axial
	Os Carpale 2	Trapezoid		Intermediate Cuneiform		Os Tarsale 2	
	Os Carpale 3	Capitate		Lateral Cuneiform		Os Tarsale 3	
	Ossa Carpalia 4 and 5	Hamate		Cuboid		Ossa Tarsalia 4 and 5	Postaxial

N.B. Alternative views have been stated for the carpal scaphoid and the tarsal navicular. In each case the most widely accepted view is on the left. In the case of the talus the anomalous persistence of its posterior process as a separate element, an *os trigonum*, may have influenced the orthodox view of the talus as an amalgam of ossa tibiale and intermedium. If it becomes accepted that the talus is merely the os intermedium, the main residual controversies concern the scaphoid and navicular, centred on the possible derivation of each bone's tubercle from the corresponding os centrale. It should be added that the *centrale* element has been shown as singular in this table, though there were probably a variable number of centralia in the ancestral forms.

effective in primate hands. In gibbons the hands are used as hooks in brachiating from branch to branch; thumbs are not effectively opposable to the other digits, although the feet have an excellent grasp. In most primates the distal end of the first metatarsal is not tied by ligaments to the second, allowing the hallux marked freedom. But the human first and second metatarsals are so connected, all five metatarsal heads being tied by ligaments. In contrast, human thumbs are even better developed for *opposition* than in other primates, in which the joint between the pollicial metacarpal and trapezium (*os carpale I* of the primitive tetrapod carpus) permits the thumb to flex and rotate towards the fingers, either in a 'power' grip, when the thumb and fingers wrap around opposite sides of an object such as a branch, weapon or tool, or in a 'precision' grip, in which the thumb is opposed to a single finger, often the index, in more accurate manipulations (Napier 1966).

Bones in human limbs, when compared functionally, are excellent examples of adaptation. In the lower limb, the massive, almost immobile pelvic girdle directly articulates with the vertebral column; the limited ball-and-socket mechanism at the hip is adapted for fore and aft swinging but allows some abduction to effect a steady stance in bipeds; the hinging knee and ankle joints give resilient propulsion in walking, running and springing; and the powerful lever of the foot is arched for resilience in the final thrust of take-off and impact of landing. All these features produce a limb highly developed for *locomotion*.

The upper limb presents different adaptations, divisible into various components, but integrated in action. The scapula is suspended by muscles, strutted by a slender mobile clavicle, its only axial connection. A **shallow** ball-and-socket joint allows a far wider range for the reaching, grasping, 'inquisitive' hand. Flexion at the elbow and rotation of the forearm bring the hands within the arena of vision, providing a steady but adjustable carpal base for fine movements of an opposable thumb and highly mobile fingers. Endlessly variable manipulations, entailing delicate muscular adjustments, are thus developed; with the constant feedback of stereoscopic vision and tactile sensation, a limitless horizon for manual dexterity in invention and cerebral development has been opened.

In ourselves we see the arm and hand at the end of several hundred million years of evolution. Perhaps it is not the 'end' but, even were the human upper limb to evolve no further, it has, with growing excellence of cerebral control, accomplished such a mastery over the environment as to deflect the whole course of evolution into a new channel (Huxley 1942).

UPPER LIMB

INTRODUCTION

The human upper limb has almost no locomotor function; instead it has acquired a great degree of freedom of movement, being adapted essentially for grasping and manipulation. Nevertheless, it still retains the ability to act as a locomotor prop, as when grasping an immobile object and pulling the body towards the hand or when used in conjunction with a walking aid to support the body during gait. The bones of the upper limb are not as robust as their counterparts in the lower limb.

The pectoral girdle serves to attach the limb to the trunk; the only point of articulation being at the sternoclavicular joint. Between the trunk and hand are a series of highly mobile joints and a system of levers, which allow the hand to be brought to any point in space to be held steadily and securely while it performs its task. In this respect the importance of the opposability of the thumb is paramount in permitting effective grasping and manipulation of objects of varying shapes and sizes. In grasping the thumb is of equal value to the remaining four digits; loss of the thumb is almost as disabling as loss of all the other digits.

Since the human upper limb is largely concerned with load carriage and manipulation, stability at its various joints often has to be maintained in usual postures, depending to a large extent on ligamentous and muscular action to counteract the constant gravitational tendency to cause distraction. In addition, because the limb itself is heavy every movement is accompanied by postural adjustments to compensate for shifts in the body's centre of gravity.

The upper limit of the upper limb is not as easily defined as in the lower limb because of muscle attachments to the head, neck and thorax; the free upper limits can be considered as the superior surfaces of the clavicle and scapula. Between the shoulder and elbow joints is the arm; between elbow and wrist the forearm; beyond the wrist the hand. Because of its many motor and sensory functions, the hand has an extensive vascular network to support its metabolic requirements.

SCAPULA

The scapula (**6**.201, 202), a large, flat, triangular bone, overlaps in part the second to seventh ribs on the posterolateral thoracic aspect. It has costal and dorsal surfaces, superior, lateral and medial borders, inferior, superior and lateral angles, and three processes—spinous, acromial and coracoid. The lateral angle is truncated by the glenoid cavity for articulation with the humerus, sometimes regarded as the *head*, connected to the body by an inconspicuous neck. The long axis of the scapula (from 'head' to inferior angle) is nearly vertical and much thickened. The relatively featureless costal surface contrasts with the dorsal, which is divided by the spine (**6**.201).

The costal surface (**6**.201A). Anteromedial when the arm is pendent it is slightly hollow especially above, and presents near the lateral border a rounded ridge, prominent near the neck, less so below and separated from the border by a narrow groove.

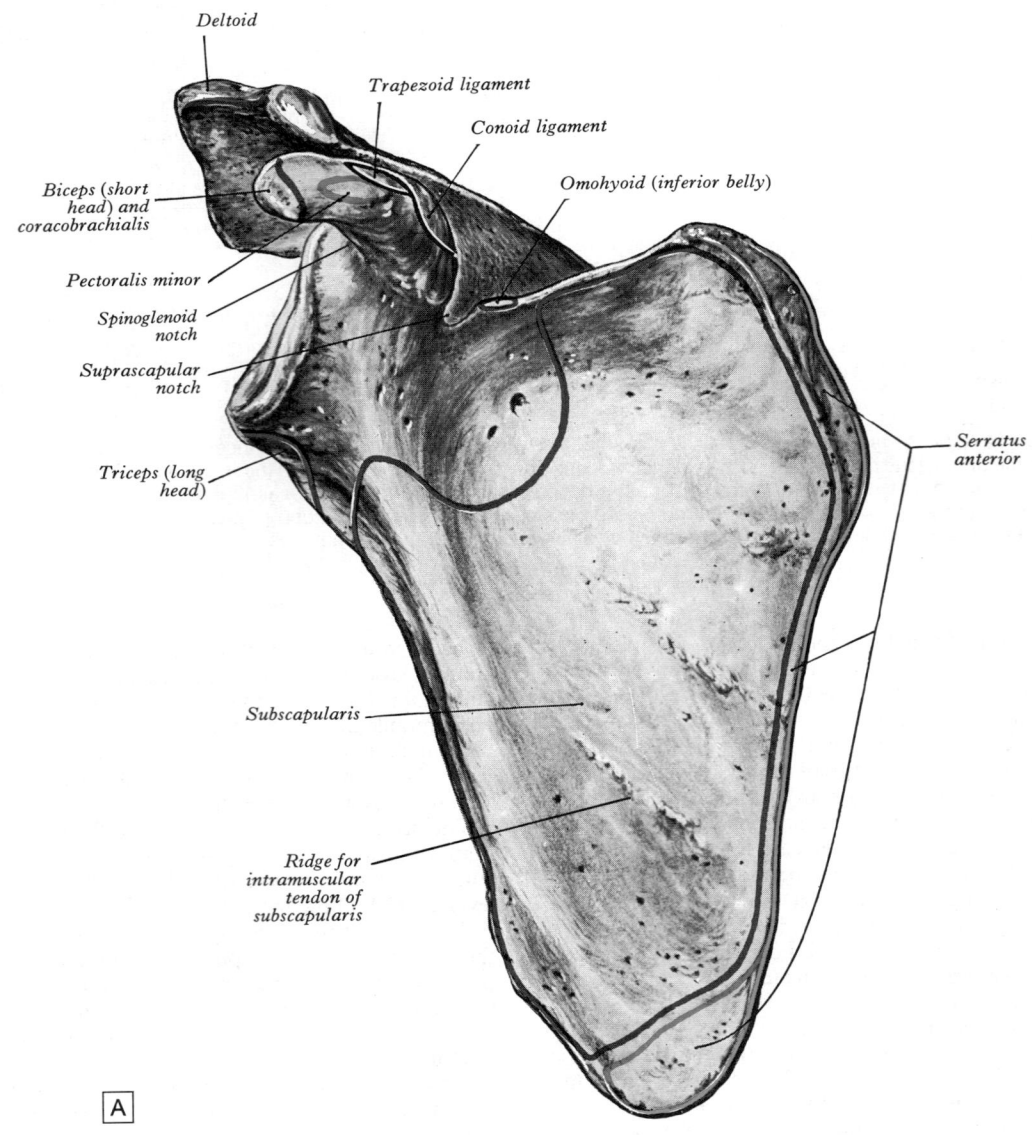

Deltoid

Trapezoid ligament

Conoid ligament

Biceps (short
head) and
coracobrachialis

Omohyoid (inferior belly)

Pectoralis minor

Spinoglenoid
notch

Suprascapular
notch

Triceps (long
head)

Serratus
anterior

Subscapularis

Ridge for
intramuscular
tendon of
subscapularis

A

6.201   The right scapula: A. Anterior (costal) surface; B. Posterior (dorsal) surface.

The dorsal surface (**6**.201B). Divided by the shelf-like *spine of the scapula* into a small upper and a large lower area, they are confluent at a *spinoglenoid notch* between the spine's lateral border and the neck's dorsal aspect.

The lateral border. A sharp, rough and sinuous ridge, it has an adjoining flat dorsal strip, for muscular attachments, from the inferior angle to the glenoid cavity. Superiorly it widens into a rough, triangular *infraglenoid tubercle* (**6**.201). It is covered by muscles and cannot clearly be palpated. It is described as thick because the grooved part of the costal surface, the narrow flat lateral strip of the dorsal surface and adjacent thickened ridge (**6**.201A), are often included in it during clinical examination.

The medial border. From the inferior to the superior angle, it is easily felt in its inferior two-thirds but its upper third is too deep.

The superior border. Thin, sharp and shortest, it is separated laterally from the coracoid process by the *suprascapular notch*.

The scapular angles. The *inferior angle* overlies the seventh rib or intercostal space. Palpable through the skin and covering muscles, it is also visible as it advances round the thoracic wall when the arm is raised. The *superior angle*, at the junction of the superior and medial borders, is obscured by muscles. The *lateral angle*, truncated and broad, is the 'head', bearing the *glenoid cavity* and forming a glenohumeral joint with the humerus. It provides a shallow, and a limited, socket for the humeral head; its outline is piriform, narrower above (**6**.202). Just above it a small rough *supraglenoid tubercle*

encroaches on the root of the coracoid process. The *anatomical neck*, the constriction adjoining the rim of the glenoid cavity, is most distinct at its inferior and dorsal aspects. Anteriorly and posteriorly it extends between the infraglenoid and supraglenoid tubercles, passing lateral to the root of the coracoid process. Some authorities describe a *surgical neck*, best distinguished posteriorly. Commencing inferiorly, near the glenoidal rim, it passes upwards and laterally through the deepest part of the spinoglenoid (greater scapular) notch continuing to the anterior border of the suprascapular notch, thence medial to the coracoid, and is completed by an ill-defined, but corresponding ventral line.

Spine of the scapular (**6**.201B). This projects from the upper dorsal surface and is triangular. Its lateral border, thick and rounded, helps to form the *spinoglenoid (great scapular) notch*, between it and the neck's dorsal aspect. Anteriorly it joins the dorsal surface along a line running laterally and slightly up from the junction of the upper and middle thirds of the medial border. The fairly flat scapular body is, however, bent along this junction, accentuating the concavity of the upper costal surface. The dorsal border is the *crest of the spine*, mainly subcutaneous expanding medially into a smoother, triangular area. Elsewhere its upper and lower borders and surface are roughened by muscular attachments. The concave superior surface of the spine widens laterally, forming with the dorsal surface of the upper body the *supraspinous fossa*. The spine's inferior surface is overhung by the crest's medial, narrow end, but is gently convex in

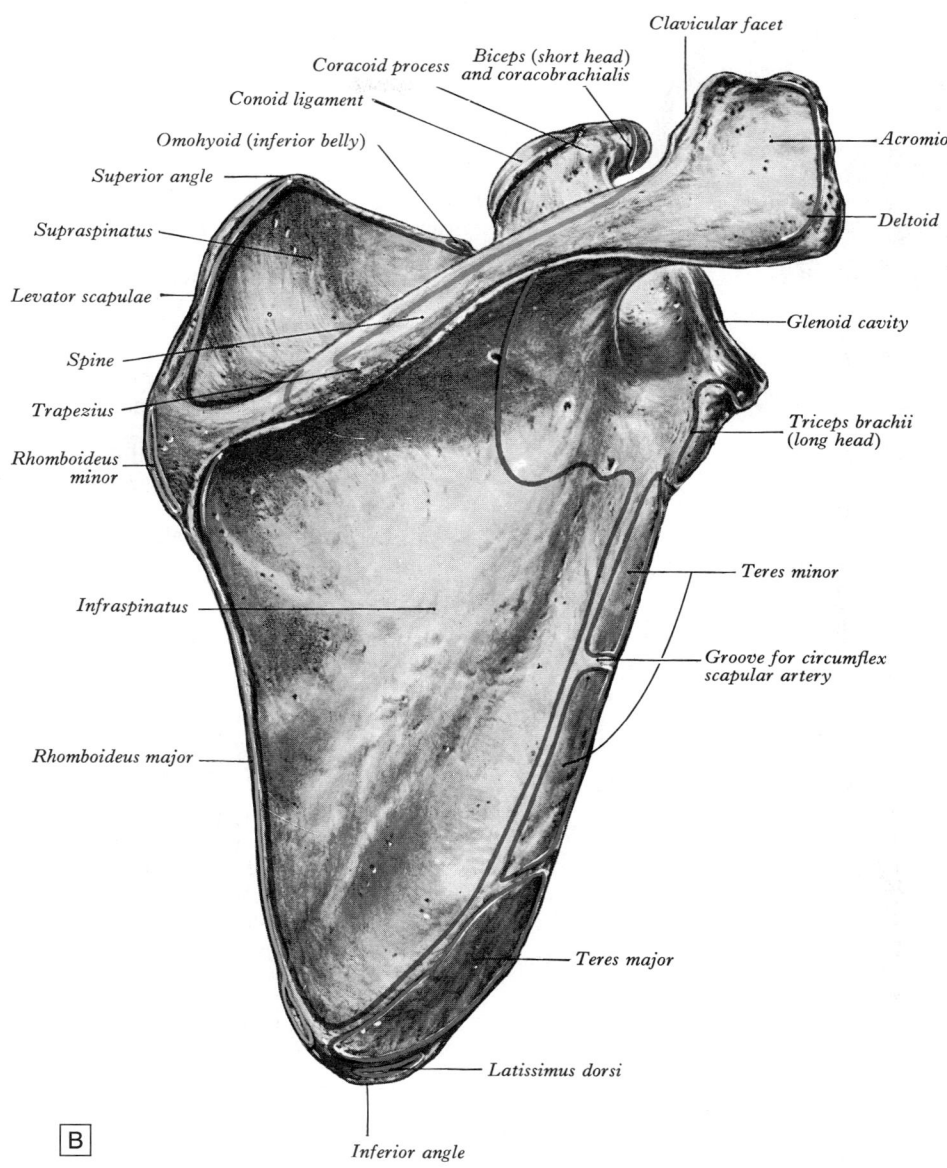

Clavicular facet

Biceps (short head)
and coracobrachialis

Coracoid process

Conoid ligament

Omohyoid (inferior belly)

Superior angle

Supraspinatus

Levator scapulae

Spine

Trapezius

Rhomboideus
minor

Infraspinatus

Rhomboideus major

Acromion

Deltoid

Glenoid cavity

Triceps brachii
(long head)

Teres minor

Groove for circumflex
scapular artery

Teres major

Latissimus dorsi

B

Inferior angle

its wider lateral part; with the lower dorsal surface it forms the *infraspinous fossa*, continuous with the supraspinous at the spinoglenoid notch.

Acromion. Projecting forwards, almost at right angles, from the lateral end of the spine, the inferior border of the crest and lateral border of the acromion are continuous at the *acromial angle*, a visible, subcutaneous landmark. The medial acromial border is short, bearing anteriorly a small, oval facet directed superomedially for articulation with the clavicle's lateral end. The lateral border, tip and superior surface are easily palpable. An accessory articular facet may occur on the acromion's inferior surface.

A recent study, which examined 270 scapulae, reported an incidence of *os acromiale* of 8.2%, with the free fragment being approximately one-third the length of the acromion; it included the acromioclavicular facet and principal areas of attachment of the coracoacromial ligament (Edelson et al 1993).

Coracoid process (6.201). This arises from the summit of the scapular head and hooks slightly laterally and forwards. With the arm pendent, it points almost straight forwards. Its enlarged tip is palpable, though covered by the anterior part of deltoid. It is about 2.5 cm below the junction of lateral fourth and the rest of the clavicle. The supraglenoid tubercle at the root of the process adjoins the upper part of the glenoid cavity. On the coracoid's dorsal aspect, where it changes direction, is an impression for the conoid part of the coracoclavicular ligament.

Further details

On the *costal surface* subscapularis (6.201A) attaches to almost the whole area, including much of the lateral groove but excluding the region of the neck. Intramuscular tendons are attached to radiating rough ridges dividing this surface incompletely into smooth areas. The neck's anterior aspect is separated from the tendon of subscapularis by a synovial protrusion of the joint (subscapular 'bursa'). To an almost oval area near the inferior angle, the lower five or six digitations of serratus anterior are attached. The upper fibres are attached to a narrow ventral strip along the medial border, which is wider above for the large first digitation. Longitudinal thickening near the lateral border provides a lever to withstand the pull of serratus anterior on the inferior angle during lateral scapular rotation, by which the glenoid cavity is turned up as the arm is raised against gravity.

On the *dorsal surface*, to the medial two-thirds of the supraspinous fossa, is attached supraspinatus, the covering fascia attaching to the fossa's margins. The flat strip near the lateral border has teres minor attached to it in its upper two-thirds, grooved near the midpoint by the circumflex scapular vessels, which pass between muscle and bone into the infraspinous fossa. The lower limit of the muscle's attachment is an oblique ridge, which runs from the lateral border towards the inferior angle, separating the attachment of teres minor from a somewhat oval area for teres major. Except for the area near the neck, the remaining infraspinous fossa gives attachment to

617

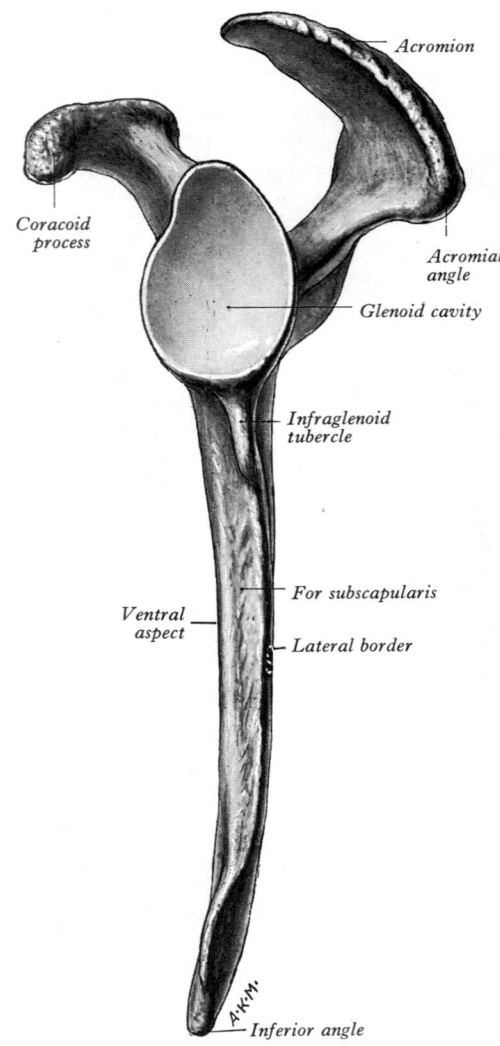

Acromion

Coracoid
process

Acromial
angle

Glenoid cavity

Infraglenoid
tubercle

Ventral
aspect

For subscapularis

Lateral border

Inferior angle

6.202   The left scapula: lateral aspect.

infraspinatus, the aponeurosis of which passes on to teres minor and major sending the fascial septa between them marking the bone at the limits of their attachments.

The *lateral border* separates the attachments of subscapularis and teres minor and major. These muscles project beyond the bone and, with latissimus dorsi, make the border impalpable. To the infraglenoid tubercle the long head of the triceps brachii is attached.

The *medial border* is thin and angled opposite the spine; to a narrow strip, from the superior angle to this point, is attached levator scapulae and, below this, opposite the spine, rhomboid minor. The rest of the border is taken up by rhomboid major (p. 843).

The *superior border* is thin; near the suprascapular notch the inferior belly of omohyoid is attached. Crossing the notch is the superior transverse ligament, attached laterally to the root of the coracoid process, medially to the notch; it is sometimes ossified. The foramen, thus completed, conducts the suprascapular nerve to the supraspinous fossa, the suprascapular vessels passing above the ligament.

The *inferior angle* is covered dorsally by the upper border of latissimus dorsi, which frequently receives a small slip from it. The *superior angle* is covered by the upper part of trapezius. The *lateral angle* bears the *glenoid cavity* covered by hyaline articular cartilage; to its anterior margin are attached glenohumeral ligaments (p. 628), to the *supraglenoid tubercle* the long head of biceps brachii, to the *infraglenoid tubercle* the long head of triceps brachii.

To the *scapular spine's* upper and lower surfaces the supra- and infraspinatus muscles are attached. The triangular area at its root, opposite the third thoracic spine, is played over by the tendon of trapezius, a bursa intervening. The crest's lower border is occupied by the posterior fibres of the deltoid, its upper border by the middle

fibres of trapezius, the lowest part of which ends as a flat triangular tendon gliding over the area noted above and attached to the so-called *deltoid tubercle* on the spine's dorsum lateral to the area.

The *acromion* is subcutaneous posteriorly, covered only by skin and superficial fascia. Its lateral border, thick and irregular, and its tip as far round as the clavicular facet are the attachment of the middle part of deltoid. To its summit medially, and below deltoid, the lateral end of the coracoacromial ligament is attached. The articular capsule of the acromioclavicular joint is attached to the rim of the clavicular facet. Behind the facet, the acromion's medial border receives the horizontal fibres of trapezius. The smooth inferior aspect of the acromion, together with the coracoacromial ligament and coracoid process, forms a *coracoacromial arch* over the shoulder joint. The tendon of supraspinatus, below the overhanging acromion, is separated from both it and deltoid by the subacromial bursa.

The *coracoid process*, below the junction of the lateral fourth with the rest of the clavicle, is connected to it by the coracoclavicular ligament (p. 622; **6**.201A), which also receives the pectoralis minor. To its lateral border is attached the wider, medial end of the coraco-acromial ligament and, below this, the coracohumeral ligament. To the coracoid apex is attached the coracobrachialis medially and the short head of biceps laterally. The apex is covered by the anterior edge of deltoid and is palpable under the lateral border of the infraclavicular fossa.

The human coracoacromial ligament is a trait shared only with other hominoid primates, according to Ciochon and Corruccini (1977), who devised a *coracoacromial projection index*: *projection height* (i.e. vertical distance from supraglenoid tubercle to a line between the most lateral points on the acromial and coracoid apices) divided by the *height of the glenoid cavity*. They claim that their observations reflect specialized locomotor and feeding adaptations in *Hominoidea*.

Detailed geometric anatomy, based on data from 28 scapulae, has been presented by Mallon et al (1992), giving precise dimensions (distances, angles, radii of curvature) which are discussed in terms of their clinical relevance to the pathomechanics of rotator cuff disease, total shoulder arthroplasty and recurrent shoulder dislocation. An earlier study of 200 scapulae observed that the slope and length of the acromion and the height of the coracoacromial arch were closely related to degenerative change on the acromion (osteophyte formation and spurs on the anterior margin) (Edelson & Taitz 1992).

Ligaments of the scapula

The main scapular ligaments (see **6**.217A) are the coracoacromial and superior transverse scapular; there may also be a weaker, variable inferior transverse (spinoglenoid) ligament.

Coracoacromial ligament. A strong triangular band between the coracoid process and acromion, it is attached apically to the acromion anterior to its clavicular articular surface and by its base on the whole lateral coracoid border. With the coracoid process and acromion it completes an *arch* above the humeral head. It may have two strong marginal bands with a thinner centre; when occasionally the pectoralis minor is inserted into the humeral capsule instead of the coracoid process, its tendon passes between the bands (p. 839). The subacromial bursa (p. 631 and **6**.214) facilitates movement between the coracoacromial arch and the subjacent supraspinatus muscle and shoulder joint, functioning as a secondary synovial articulation.

The superior transverse scapular (suprascapular) ligament. It converts the scapular notch into a foramen and is sometimes ossified. A flat fasciculus, it narrows towards its ends, attached to the base of the coracoid process and medial side of the scapular notch. The suprascapular nerve traverses the foramen; suprascapular vessels cross above the ligament.

Inferior transverse (spinoglenoid) ligament. This membranous ligament may stretch from the scapular spine's lateral border to the glenoid margin forming an arch over the suprascapular nerve and vessels entering the infraspinous fossa; it is often absent.

Structure

The main processes, and thicker parts of the scapula, contain trabecular bone; the rest consists of a thin compact layer. The central supraspinous fossa and most of the infraspinous fossa are thin and

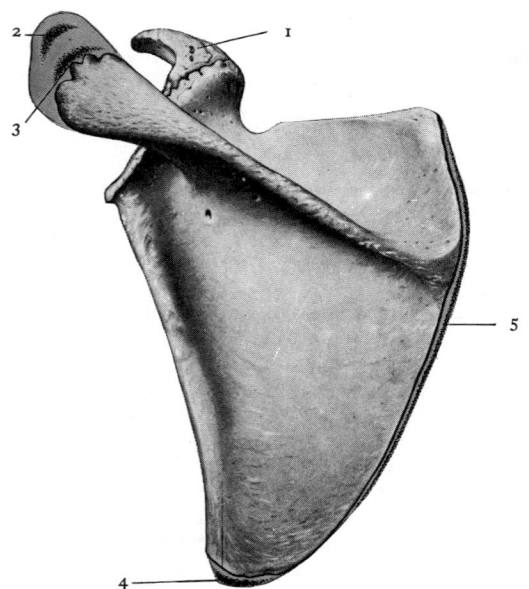

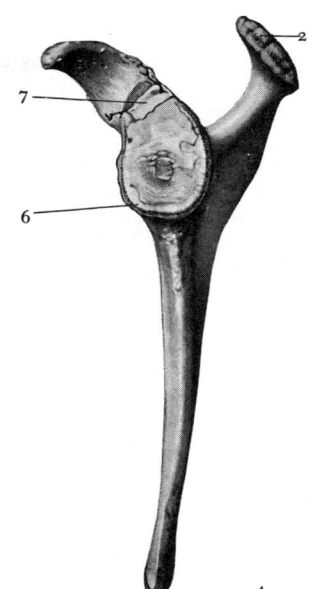

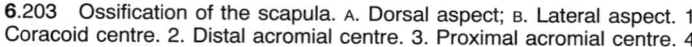

6.203 Ossification of the scapula. A. Dorsal aspect; B. Lateral aspect. 1. Coracoid centre. 2. Distal acromial centre. 3. Proximal acromial centre. 4. Centre at inferior angle. 5. Centre for medial border. 6. Glenoid centre. 7. Subcoracoid centre.

even translucent; occasionally the bone in them is deficient, gaps being filled by aponeurotic tissue.

Ossification

The cartilaginous scapula is ossified from eight or more centres: one in the body, two each in the coracoid process and the acromion, one each in the medial border, inferior angle and lower glenoid rim (**6.203**). The centre for the body appears in the eighth intrauterine week. Ossification begins centrally in the coracoid process in the first year, occasionally before birth; it joins the rest of the bone in about the fifteenth year. At or soon after puberty, centres appear in the coracoid root (subcoracoid centre), in the lower glenoid rim, often in the coracoid apex, in the acromion, inferior angle and contiguous medial border and in the medial border. A variable part of the glenoid cavity, usually the upper third, is ossified from the subcoracoid centre, uniting in the fourteenth (females) to seventeenth (males) year. A crescentic epiphysis for the lower glenoid rim, thicker peripherally, converts the child's flat cavity into the gently concave adult fossa.

The acromial base is an extension from the spine; the remaining acromion is ossified from two centres which unite and join the spinous extension. The various scapular epiphyses have all fused by about the twentieth year.

CLAVICLE

The clavicle (**6.204**) extends laterally and almost horizontally across the neck from the manubrium to the acromion, being wholly subcutaneous. It struts the shoulder and enables the limb to swing clear of the trunk, transmitting part of its weight to the axial skeleton. Its flat *lateral, acromial end* articulates with the medial aspect of the acromion; the enlarged *medial, sternal end* articulates with the manubrial clavicular facet and first costal cartilage. The shaft is sinuous, being convex forwards in its medial two-thirds, and concave forwards lateral to this. The *inferior* aspect of its intermediate part is grooved in its long axis.

The lateral third. This is flat, with superior and inferior surfaces,

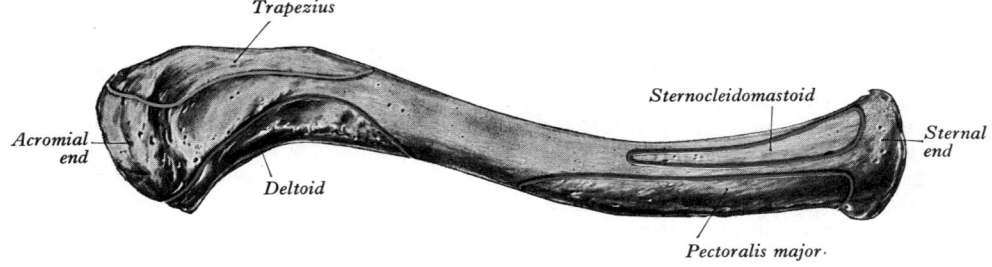

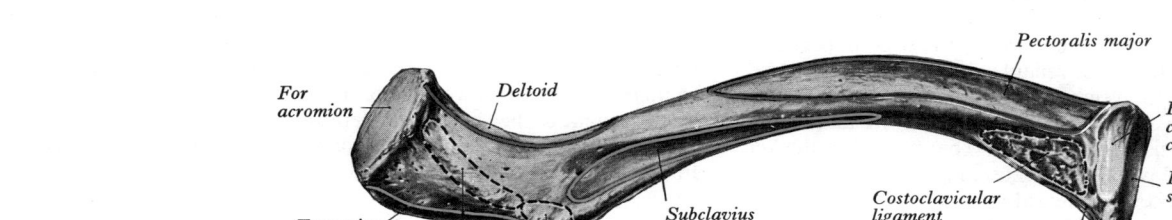

6.204 The right clavicle: A. Superior surface; B. Inferior surface.

and anterior and posterior borders. A small oval articular facet, for articulation with the medial aspect of the acromion, faces laterally and slightly downwards. The *anterior border* is concave, thin, rough and may show a small deltoid tubercle; the *posterior border*, also roughened by muscular attachments, is convex. The palpable *superior surface* is rough near its margins but otherwise smooth. The *inferior surface* presents, near its posterior border and at the junction of the lateral fourth with the rest of the shaft, a prominent *conoid tubercle* for the conoid part of the coracoclavicular ligament; from the lateral side of this a narrow, rough strip (*trapezoid line*) runs anterolaterally, almost to the acromial apex (6.204B), for the ligament's trapezoid part.

Attached to the lateral third is deltoid anteriorly, trapezius posteriorly, both reaching the superior surface. The coracoclavicular ligament, attached to the conoid tubercle and trapezoid line (6.204B), transmits the weight of the upper limb to the clavicle, counteracted by trapezius supporting its lateral part (p. 835). From the conoid tubercle weight is transmitted medially by the shaft to the axial skeleton; a fracture medial to it interrupts this transmission, almost all weight then being supported by trapezius which is unable to meet the demand, and the limb therefore droops.

The medial two-thirds. Roughly cylindrical or prismatic with four surfaces; the inferior is often a mere ridge. *Anterior* and *superior surfaces* are largely rough but laterally smooth and rounded above the infraclavicular fossa (p. 838). The *posterior surface* is smooth, the *inferior* marked near its sternal end by a rough oval area, often depressed, for the costoclavicular ligament. Rarely, this area is smooth or even raised and may form a synovial joint with the first rib (Cave 1961) on the lateral half of the inferior surface is a groove for the attachment of subclavius.

The sternal end. Directed medially slightly downwards and forwards, it articulates with the clavicular notch of the manubrium: its sternal surface, usually irregular and pitted, is quadrangular (sometimes triangular) and slightly rough above for attachment of the interclavicular ligament, sternoclavicular capsule and articular disc. The articular surface is otherwise smooth and extends on to the inferior surface to articulate with the first costal cartilage. The sternal end projects above the manubrium and can be felt and usually seen (a prominent clinical landmark) in the lateral wall of the jugular fossa.

Further details

The medial two-thirds provides attachment, anteriorly, for the clavicular part of pectoralis major, the area being usually visibly marked. The clavicular part of sternocleidomastoid is attached to the medial half of the superior surface but marks it little. The smooth posterior surface is devoid of attachments except near its sternal end, where part of sternohyoid is attached. Medially this surface is related to the lower end of the internal jugular vein (separated by sternohyoid), the end of the subclavian and beginning of the brachiocephalic vein. More laterally, the clavicle curves in front of the trunks of the brachial plexus and the third part of the subclavian artery. The suprascapular vessels are related to the upper part of this surface. On the inferior surface is subclavius in its groove (6.204B). To the edges of this groove is attached the clavipectoral fascia, which encloses the muscle; the posterior edge of the groove runs to the conoid tubercle, where fascia and conoid ligament merge. A nutrient foramen, lateral in the groove, is inclined laterally. Medially an impression for the costoclavicular ligament varies greatly in texture and outline (see above and Cave 1961).

The female clavicle is shorter, thinner, less curved and smoother, its acromial end carried lower than the sternal; in males it is level with, or slightly above, the sternal end when the arm is pendent. Midshaft circumference is the most reliable single indicator of sex, but a combination of this with weight and length yields better results (Olivier 1951; Jit & Singh 1966); however, consult Jit and Sahni (1983) for statistical analysis and literature. The clavicle is thicker and more curved in manual workers, its muscular attachments being marked. The clavicle is trabecular internally, with a shell of compact bone much thicker in its shaft. Although elongate, the clavicle is unlike typical long bones; it usually has no medullary cavity.

Ossification

The clavicle begins to ossify before any other bone, the shaft

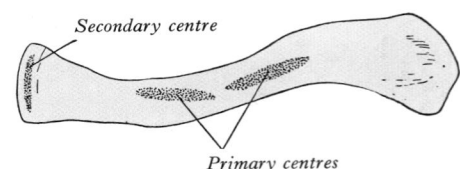

6.205 Diagram showing the three constant centres of ossification of the clavicle.

from medial and lateral primary centres appearing in condensed mesenchyme between the fifth and sixth weeks and fusing approximately 1 week later; cartilage at both ends of the clavicle then develops (Ogata & Uhthoff 1990; 6.205). The medial cartilaginous mass contributes more to growth in length than does the lateral mass: the junction of these two ossification centres being between the middle and lateral thirds of the clavicle. A secondary centre for the sternal end appears in late teens, or even early twenties, usually 2 years earlier in females. Fusion is probably rapid but reliable data are lacking. An acromial secondary centre sometimes develops at about 18 to 20, but this epiphysis is always small and rapidly joins the shaft (Todd & D'Erico 1928). In a study of the sternal epiphysis in 684 Punjabis, ossification occurred from 11 to 19 years (both sexes) and fusion at 18 to 25 years (Jit & Kulkaria 1976). Comparison suggests racial differences. Such assessment by radiological appearances is, of course, not devoid of fallacy.

However, clavicular development is not only by intramembranous ossification. In 14-mm embryos the clavicle is a band of condensed mesenchyme between the acromion and apex of the first rib, and continuous with the sternal rudiment. In this band medial and lateral zones of early cartilage transformation ('precartilage') occur, and in mesenchyme between them intramembranous centres of ossification appear and soon fuse. Sternal and acromial zones soon become true cartilage, into which ossification extends from the shaft. Length increases by interstitial growth of these terminal cartilages, which develop zones of hypertrophy, calcification and advancing endochondral ossification as in other growth cartilages. Diameter is increased by subperichondral deposition in the extremities and subperiosteal deposition in the shaft. Epiphyses are endochondral and probably fuse as in long bones which are **primarily** cartilaginous. Defects of ossification in the clavicle and primarily intramembranous cranial bones occasionally coincide as the condition of cleidocranial dysostosis.

The primitive reptilian pectoral girdle comprises a dorsal scapula and two ventral elements, an anterior (cranial) precoracoid and posterior (caudal) coracoid. Of the three pelvic elements, the ilium is homologous with the scapula, the pubis with the precoracoid, the ischium with the coracoid. The clavicle, dermal in origin and therefore morphologically distinct, is an addition to the pectoral girdle with no pelvic equivalent. It is doubtful whether any trace of precoracoid persists in the human skeleton, but the double primary clavicular ossification centre may indicate that human clavicles contain reptilian precoracoid and clavicle. Some believe that the first coracoid centre represents the precoracoid element and the subcoracoid centre the caudal ventral element of reptilian girdles. The clavicle is absent from forelimbs used principally or entirely for progression, for example in ungulates and carnivores; but it is present and well-developed in prehensile limbs, for example in many rodents, primates and man.

The clavicle is often fractured, commonly by indirect forces, due to violent impacts to hand or shoulder, the break being at the junction of lateral and intermediate thirds, where its curvature changes, for this is its weakest part. Consequent deformity is caused by the weight of the arm, which depresses the lateral fragment, forces being transmitted through the coracoclavicular ligament; the medial fragment is usually little displaced.

STERNOCLAVICULAR JOINT

Involved in the sternoclavicular joint are the sternal end of the clavicle and the sternal clavicular notch, together with the adjacent superior surface of the first costal cartilage (6.206). The larger

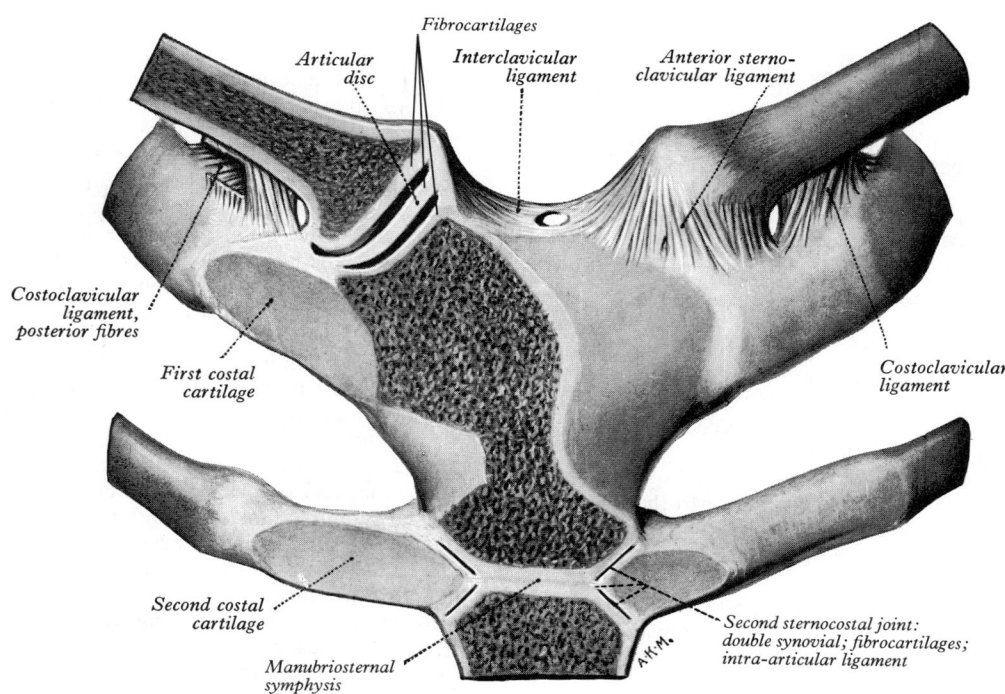

6.206   Sternoclavicular joints: anterior aspect; left joint intact and right in coronal section.

clavicular *articular surface* is covered by fibrocartilage, thicker than the fibrocartilaginous lamina on the sternum. Convex vertically but slightly concave anteroposteriorly, it is therefore sellar; the sternal clavicular notch is reciprocally curved but the two surfaces are not fully congruent. (For their variations see p. 620.) An articular disc completely divides the joint. Its ligaments are *capsular, anterior and posterior sternoclavicular, interclavicular* and *costoclavicular.*

Fibrous capsule

This is thickened in front and behind; but above and especially below it is little more than loose areolar tissue.

The anterior sternoclavicular ligament

Broad and attached above to the anterosuperior aspect of the clavicle's sternal end, it passes inferomedially to the upper anterior aspect of the manubrium, spreading onto the first costal cartilage.

The posterior sternoclavicular ligament

A weaker band posterior to the joint, it descends inferomedially from the back of the clavicle's sternal end to the back of the upper manubrium.

Interclavicular ligament

Continuous above with deep cervical fascia, it unites the superior aspect of the sternal ends of both clavicles; some fibres are attached to the superior manubrial margin. When present, *suprasternal ossicles* (p. 539) are in this ligament.

Costoclavicular ligament

Like an inverted cone but short and flattened, with anterior and posterior laminae attached to the upper surface of the first rib and costal cartilage, it ascends to the margins of an impression on the inferior clavicular surface at its medial end. Fibres of the anterior lamina ascend laterally and shorter fibres of the posterior lamina ascend medially (**6**.206); they fuse laterally and merge medially with the capsule. Between them a bursa suggests separate functions (Cave 1961). Probably each is tensed at opposite extremes of clavicular axial rotation.

Articular disc

Flat and almost circular, between the sternal and clavicular surfaces, it is attached above to the superoposterior border of the clavicular articular surface, below the first costal cartilage near its sternal junction and by the rest of its circumference to the capsule. It is thicker peripherally, especially in its superoposterior part and a smaller inferomedial one. The capsule around the former is more lax, movements between the clavicle and the disc being more extensive than those between the discs and sternum. The sellar shape of the articular surfaces permits **movement** in approximately anteroposterior and vertical planes, about the long axis of the clavicle, (30° according to Kapandji 1974), which is conjunct. Close-packing probably coincides with maximum posterior rotation associated with full scapular rotation. Some anteroposterior translation also occurs.

Vessels and nerve supply to the joint

Arteries are branches from the internal thoracic and suprascapular arteries; **nerves** are from the anterior supraclavicular nerve and the nerve to subclavius. For details of vascularization consult Sick and Ring (1976).

Clinical anatomy

The joint's strength depends on ligaments, especially its disc. This and the usual transmission of forces along the clavicle make dislocation rare and fracture far more common.

ACROMIOCLAVICULAR JOINT

The acromioclavicular joint is between the clavicle's acromial end and the medial acromial margin (see **6**.215, 218), and is approximately plane; but either surface may be slightly convex, the other reciprocally concave. **Both** are covered by *fibrocartilage*, the clavicular being a narrow, oval area facing inferolaterally and overlapping a corresponding facet on the medial acromial border. The long axis is anteroposterior. Ligaments are *capsular, acromioclavicular* and *coracoclavicular.*

Fibrous capsule

This completely surrounds the articular margins and is strengthened above by the acromioclavicular ligament.

Acromioclavicular ligament

Quadrilateral and above the joint, it extends between the upper aspects of the lateral end of the clavicle and the adjoining acromion.

621

Its parallel fibres interlace with the aponeuroses of trapezius and deltoid.

Articular disc

This often occurs in the joint's upper part, partially separating the articular surfaces (de Palma 1957): rarely it completely divides the joint.

Coracoclavicular ligament (see 6.217A)

This connects the clavicle and coracoid process of the scapula. Though separate from the acromioclavicular joint it is a most efficient accessory ligament, maintaining apposition of the clavicle to the acromion. Its *trapezoid* and *conoid parts*, usually separated by fat or, frequently, a bursa, connect the medial horizontal part of the coracoid process and lateral end of the subclavian groove of the clavicle; these adjacent areas may even be covered by cartilage to form a *coracoclavicular joint* (Lewis 1959).

Trapezoid part. Anterolateral, it is broad, thin and quadrilateral, ascending slightly from the upper coracoid surface to the trapezoid line on the inferior clavicular surface. It is almost **horizontal**, its anterior border free, its posterior joined to the conoid part, forming an angle projecting backwards.

Conoid part. Posteromedial, it is a dense almost **vertical** triangular band. It has its base attached to the conoid tubercle of the clavicle and its inferior apex attached posteromedially to the root of the coracoid process in front of the scapular notch.

Movements

Movements at the joint are like those of the sternoclavicular joint. Axial rotation of the clavicle is said to be about 30° (Kapandji 1974), the two joints together, therefore, permitting about 60° of scapular rotation. Angulation with the scapula occurs in any direction. Rotation and angulation both tense the coracoclavicular ligament at their extremes; rotation tightens the capsule by spiralization. According to MacConaill and Basmajian (1977) close-packing occurs when the angle between the superior scapular border and clavicular shaft reaches about 90°. This 'opening' (*ouverture*) of the angles tenses the conoid part of the coracoclavicular ligament (Kapandji 1970); further scapular rotation is due to rotation at the sternoclavicular joint.

Vessels and nerve supply to the joint

The **arterial supply** is from branches from the suprascapular and thoracoacromial arteries, the **nerve supply** is from suprascapular and lateral pectoral nerves.

Clinical anatomy

In acromioclavicular dislocation the coracoclavicular ligament is torn and the scapula falls away from the clavicle. Owing to the flatness and orientation of the joint surfaces, dislocation readily recurs.

MOVEMENTS OF THE PECTORAL (SHOULDER) GIRDLE

Clavicular movements at their sternoclavicular and acromioclavicular joints are always associated with those of the scapula, which, in turn, are usually accompanied by humeral movements. Therefore, this account should be amplified by reference to pages 631 and 632. The acromioclavicular joint allows the acromion, and hence the scapula, anteroposterior gliding and rotation on the clavicle; but scapular range is increased by movements at the sternoclavicular joint. Analysis is clarified by considering *scapular movements*, primarily analysed as (1) elevation and depression, (2) protraction and retraction round the thorax, (3) rotation laterally (glenoid fossa faces upwards) and medially (glenoid fossa faces downwards), with the inferior angle as the reference point.

(1) *Scapular elevation* and *depression*, as in 'shrugging the shoulders', do not necessarily imply movement at the shoulder joint. In elevation slight angulation or swing occurs at the acromioclavicular joint but the clavicle's sternal end, rotating about an anteroposterior axis through the bone above the medial attachment of the costoclavicular ligament, slides down over the articular disc (*translation*);

this is checked by antagonist muscles and tension in the costoclavicular ligament and lower capsule. It is produced by trapezius (upper part) and levator scapulae; since these tend to rotate the scapula in opposite directions, pure elevation can occur.

In the reverse movement (depression) slight angulation occurs at the acromioclavicular joint, but at the sternoclavicular joint the clavicle slides up on the disc, the movements being checked by antagonist muscles, the interclavicular and sternoclavicular ligaments and articular disc. This role of the interclavicular ligament, suspension of the depressed clavicle, has been confirmed by experiment (Bearn 1967). Usually gravity alone is sufficient, but serratus anterior (lower part) and pectoralis minor are, when necessary, active depressors.

(2) *Protraction* (*forward movement*) round the thoracic wall occurs in pushing, thrusting and reaching movements, usually with some lateral rotation. The acromion advances over the clavicular facet to the limit and the shoulder is simultaneously advanced by forward movement of the lateral end of the clavicle and posterior translation of its sternal end over the sternal facet, carrying the disc with it. Antagonist muscles and the anterior sternoclavicular and costoclavicular (posterior lamina) ligaments check backward slide of the sternal end. Serratus anterior and pectoralis minor are prime movers and maintain continuous apposition of the scapula, especially its medial border, in smooth gliding on the thoracic wall. The upper part of latissimus dorsi also acts like a strap across the inferior scapular angle in protraction and lateral rotation.

In scapular *retraction*, bracing back the shoulders, movements are reversed and checked at the sternoclavicular joint by the posterior sternoclavicular and costoclavicular (anterior lamina) ligaments. Trapezius and the rhomboids are prime movers, but gravity may also produce retraction when the weight of the trunk is taken by the arms in leaning forwards, to a degree controlled by protractive musculature.

When force is applied at the end of an outstretched arm, for example in a fall on the hand, pressure transmitted to the glenoid fossa tends to drive the sloping acromial facet below the clavicle's acromial end but also tenses the trapezoid ligament, which resists the displacement; and, unless the fall is unexpected, even greater forces are available to resist dislocation.

(3) *Lateral rotation of the scapula* increases the range of *humeral elevation* by turning the glenoid cavity to face almost directly up (as in raising an arm above the head), a movement always associated with some humeral elevation and with protraction of the scapula. Scapular rotation requires movement at the sternoclavicular and the acromioclavicular joints: the sternoclavicular permitting elevation of the lateral end of the clavicle, a movement almost complete when the arm is abducted to 90°. The acromioclavicular joint moves in the first 30° of abduction when the conoid ligament becomes taut and thereafter is accompanied by clavicular rotation at the sternoclavicular joint around the bone's longitudinal axis, also with further depression of its medial end as the lateral end continues to rise. Some acromioclavicular movement also occurs in the final stages of humeral abduction (Inman et al 1944). Trapezius (upper part) and the serratus anterior (lower part) are prime movers.

Medial rotation is usually by gravity, gradual active lengthening of trapezius and serratus anterior being sufficient to control it. When more force is needed the levator scapulae, rhomboids and in the initial stages pectoralis minor are prime movers in returning the scapula to a position of rest.

Muscles which are antagonists in one movement may combine as prime movers in another. Movements, not muscles, are represented in cerebral motor areas; muscles are not grouped unalterably in nervous control but can be variably combined as demands dictate. Thus serratus anterior and trapezius are opposed in scapular movement round the thorax but combine as prime movers in its lateral rotation.

In all scapular movements subclavius probably steadies the clavicle by drawing it medially and downwards, although its inaccessibility makes its role uncertain. Scapular movements on the thoracic wall are facilitated by areolar tissue between subscapularis and serratus anterior and the chest wall. With the arm pendent the shoulder girdle's normal posture relative to the trunk involves moderate activity in trapezius and serratus anterior (Basmajian 1967), which obviously must increase when the limb is loaded.

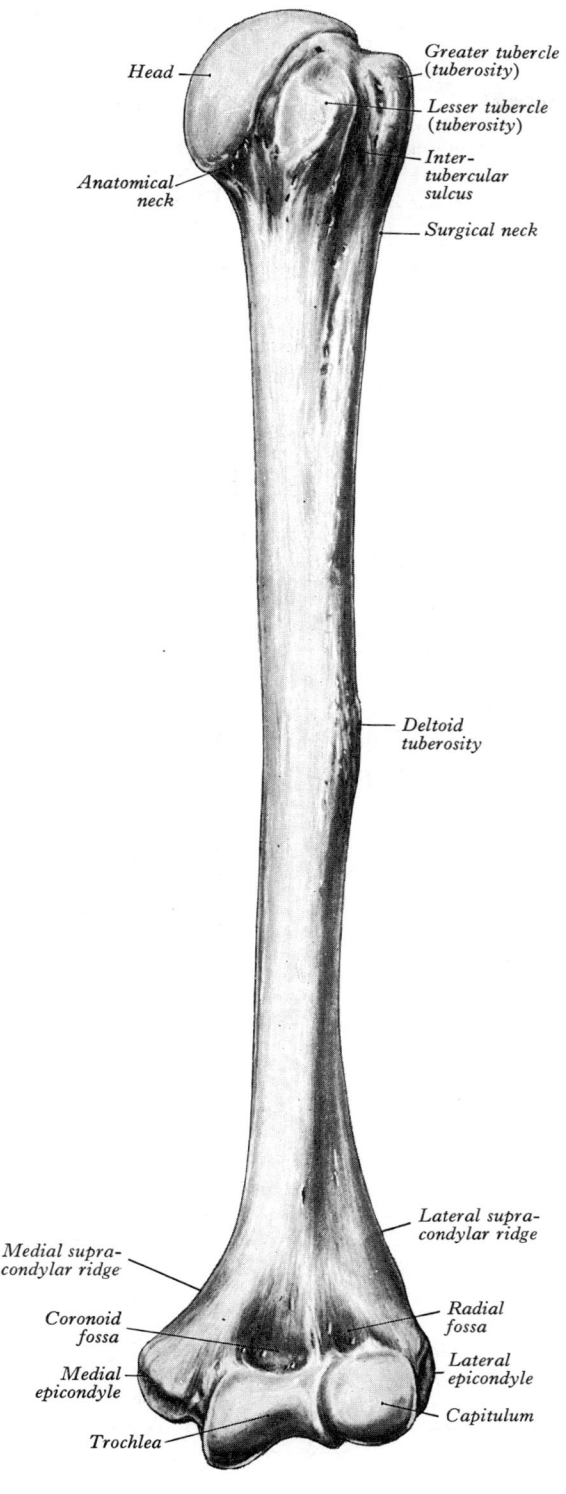

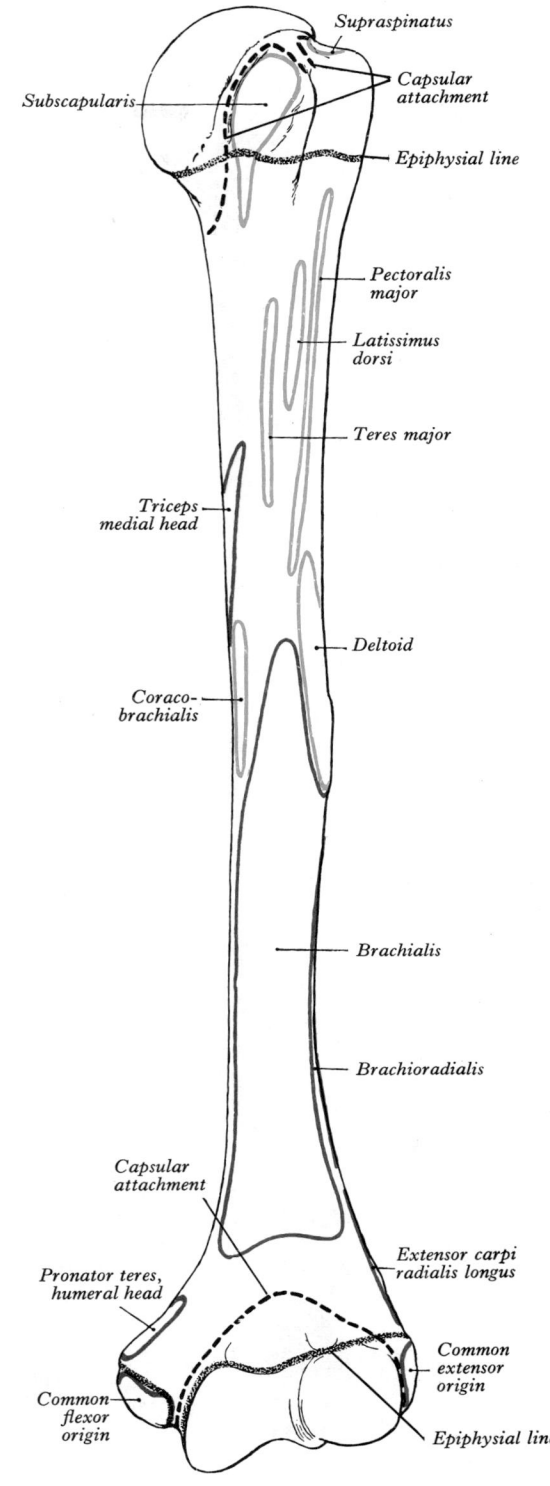

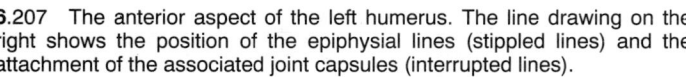

6.207   The anterior aspect of the left humerus. The line drawing on the right shows the position of the epiphysial lines (stippled lines) and the attachment of the associated joint capsules (interrupted lines).

HUMERUS

The humerus (**6**.207, 208), the longest and largest bone in the upper limb, has expanded ends and a shaft. Proximally a round 'head' forms with the scapular glenoid cavity an enarthrodial articulation. The distal end, loosely termed 'condylar', is adapted to the forearm bones at the elbow joint.

The proximal end

This includes a head, neck and greater and lesser tubercles (tuberosities).

Head (**6**.207, 208). At the proximal end, it is slightly less than half a spheroid; in sectional profile it is spheroidal (strictly ovoidal, see p. 627). The articular surface is covered by hyaline cartilage, thicker centrally, and is directed posteromedially and upwards towards the glenoid cavity in the pendent arm. The humeral articular surface exceeds that of the glenoid cavity, only part of it being in glenoid contact in any position of the joint.

The anatomical neck. Directly adjoining the articular head's margin, it is a slight constriction, least apparent near the greater tubercle, and superiorly, and for some distance continuing anteriorly and posteriorly, indicates the line of capsular attachment of the   **623**

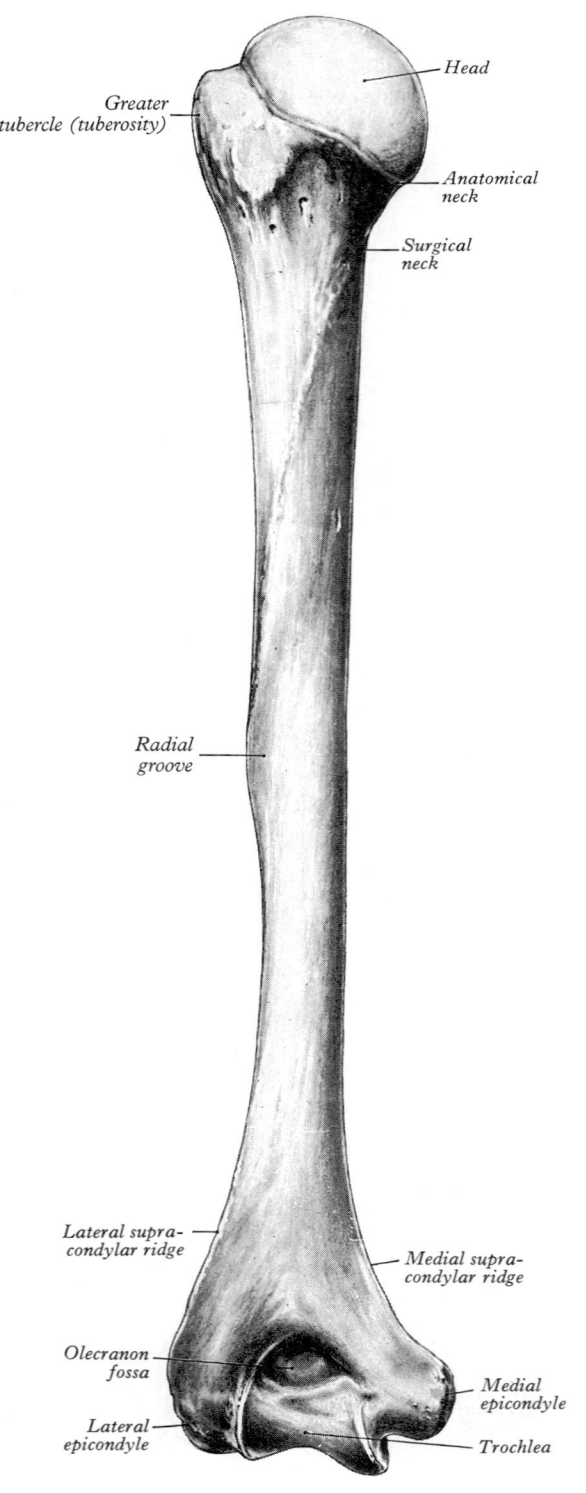

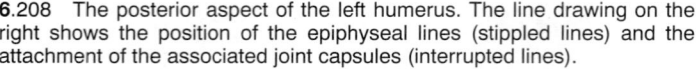

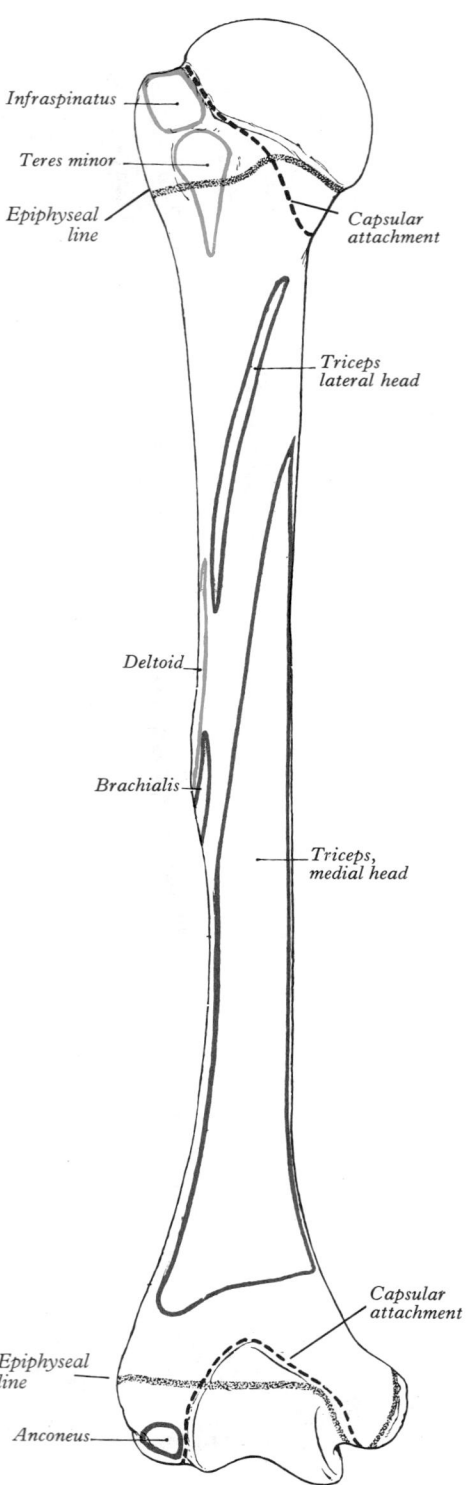

6.208 The posterior aspect of the left humerus. The line drawing on the right shows the position of the epiphyseal lines (stippled lines) and the attachment of the associated joint capsules (interrupted lines).

shoulder joint (**6**.207, 208), except at the intertubercular sulcus, where the long tendon of biceps emerges. However, medially, the capsular attachment diverges from the anatomical neck descending 1 cm or more onto the shaft.

The lesser tubercle (tuberosity). This is anterior and just beyond the anatomical neck; it has a smooth, muscular impression palpable through the deltoid 3 cm below the acromial apex, moving when the humerus rotates. Its sharp lateral edge is part of the medial border of the intertubercular sulcus. Subscapularis attaches to the lesser tubercle (**6**.207), and to the lateral margin the transverse ligament of the shoulder joint.

The greater tubercle (tuberosity). This is the most lateral part of the proximal end of the humerus and in the shoulder region projects beyond the acromion and, covered by deltoid, produces the shoulder's round contour. Its posterosuperior aspect, near the anatomical neck, bears three smooth impressions for tendons. Between the tubercles is the *intertubercular sulcus*. The humeral proximal end tapers into the shaft as an ill-defined 'surgical neck', medial to which are the axillary nerve and posterior humeral circumflex artery (**6**.208).

The three impressions on the greater tubercle are for the tendons, the supraspinatus (uppermost), infraspinatus (middle) and teres minor (lowest) (**6.208B**). Its projecting lateral surface has many vascular foramina and is covered by the deltoid; a subacromial bursa may separate deltoid from the tubercle. The attachments of subscapularis and teres minor are not confined to their respective tubercles, but extend for varying distances on to the adjacent metaphysis.

Shaft

Almost cylindrical proximally, it is prismatic (in section) distally and anteroposteriorly compressed. It is not directly palpable due to the large muscles around it. Its three surfaces and borders are not equally obvious.

The anterior border. It descends from the front of the greater tubercle almost to the distal end of the bone. Its proximal third is the lateral edge of the intertubercular sulcus, marked by muscular attachments. Beyond this, as the anterior edge of the deltoid tuberosity, it is also rough but smoothly rounded in its distal half.

The lateral border. Distally sharp and rough along its anterior aspect, its proximal two-thirds are barely discernible, although sometimes traceable to the posterior aspect of the greater tubercle. Centrally it is interrupted by a wide, shallow groove (*radial* or *spiral groove*), descending obliquely laterally and forwards.

The medial border. Rounded in its distal half, it bears a roughened strip just below its midpoint; proximal to this it is indistinct but reappears as the medial lip of the intertubercular sulcus, where it is again rough and reaches the lesser tubercle.

Surfaces. *The anterolateral surface* is between the anterior and lateral borders; just proximal to its midpoint is the rough *deltoid tuberosity*, tapering to a distal apex. Behind this the radial groove descends, fading distally when it reaches the lateral border a little beyond the tuberosity. The *anteromedial surface*, between the anterior and medial borders, forms in its proximal third the rough floor of the intertubercular sulcus, but the rest is smooth. Near its midpoint a nutrient foramen opens, its canal directed distally. The *posterior surface*, between medial and lateral borders, is the most extensive. A ridge, sometimes rough, descends laterally across its proximal third. The middle third is crossed by the beginning of the radial groove. The distal third is an extensive, flat surface, which widens distally.

The distal end of the humerus (6.207, 209)

Basically a modified *condyle*, it is wider transversely and has articular and non-articular parts. The articular part joints with the radius and ulna at the elbow and is divided into a lateral, convex *capitulum* and a medial, pulley-shaped *trochlea*. The non-articular condyle includes *medial* and *lateral epicondyles*, olecranon, coronoid and *radial fossae*.

Capitulum. Less than half a sphere, it includes anterior and inferior surfaces of the condyle laterally, but not its posterior surface. It articulates with the discoid radial head, which abuts the inferior surface in full extension but slides on to the anterior surface during flexion.

Trochlea. This is like part of a pulley, occupying anterior, inferior and posterior surfaces of the humeral condyle medially; it is separated laterally from the capitulum by a faint groove; all aspects of its

medial margin project. It articulates with the trochlear notch of the ulna. In extension the inferoposterior trochlear circumference contacts the ulna, but in flexion the trochlear notch slides on to the anterior aspect, the posterior being uncovered. The projecting medial trochlear edge is a main determinant of the angulation between the long axes of the humerus and ulna when the forearm is extended and supinated (p. 642).

The medial epicondyle. A blunt medial projection on the medial condyle, it is subcutaneous and usually visible in passive flexion. Its smooth posterior surface is crossed by the ulnar nerve in a shallow sulcus as it enters the forearm, and here the nerve can be rolled against the bone. If it is jarred against the epicondyle, characteristic tingling sensations result. Distally the anterior epicondylar surface is marked by the attachment of the superficial forearm flexors. The medial humeral border ends at the medial epicondyle and is distally the *medial supracondylar ridge*.

The lateral epicondyle. The lateral non-articular part of the condyle, it does not project beyond the lateral border. It has an anterolateral impression for the superficial forearm extensors. Its posterior surface, slightly convex, is easily felt in a depression visible behind the extended elbow. The lateral humeral border ends at the lateral epicondyle, from which, extending proximally, is its distal part, the *lateral supracondylar ridge*.

Further details

A deep hollow, the *olecranon fossa*, on the condyle's posterior surface, proximal to the trochlea, contains the apex of the olecranon in the extended elbow. Its floor is always thin and may be deficient. A smaller *coronoid fossa*, immediately proximal to the trochlea on the anterior surface, accommodates the margin of the ulnar coronoid process in full flexion. A shallow *radial fossa*, proximal to the capitulum and lateral to the coronoid fossa, is related to the margin of the radial head in full flexion.

In lower mammals the longest axes of the proximal and distal humeral articular surfaces make an angle with each other of a little more than 90°. But the proximal human humerus appears to have rotated laterally, so that the angle has been increased to about 164°

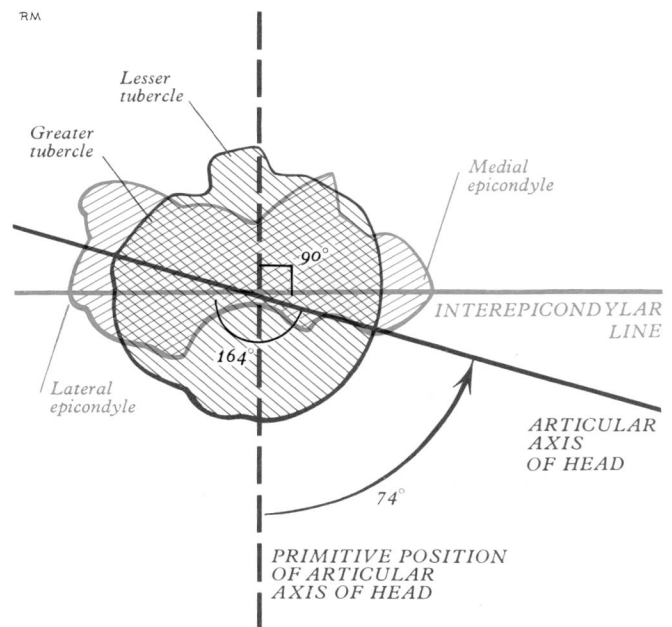

6.210   This diagram illustrates the concept of humeral 'torsion'. The left humerus is viewed distally along its length, with its proximal end (magenta) superimposed upon the distal (blue). The 'axes' of the two extremities are shown at right angles, as in early tetrapods and most quadrupedal mammals. In primates, including mankind, the axis of the head is directed medially, and the angle which this now makes with the 'primitive' anteroposterior position of the axis is the so-called angle of torsion. This is on average 74° in man: some authorities add to this the original angle of 90°, giving a total of 164°. See text for more detailed explanation.

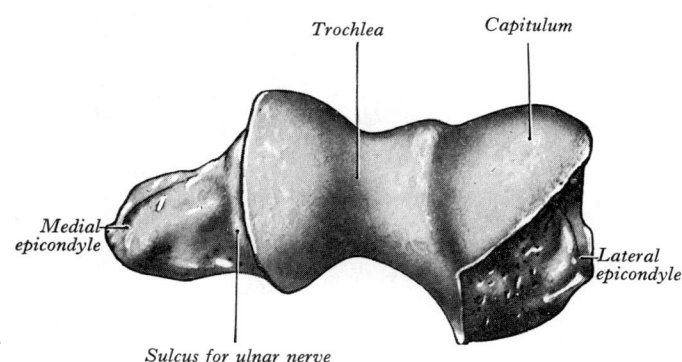

6.209   The inferior aspect of the distal end of the left humerus.

(6.210), the angle of 'humeral torsion'. It is greater in males and adults, and less in anthropoid apes. Krahl (1976) claims that the angle increases with age until fusion of the epiphysis (p. 614).

The *intertubercular sulcus* (bicipital groove) contains the long tendon of biceps, its synovial sheath, and an ascending branch from the anterior circumflex humeral artery. The groove's lateral lip is marked by the tendon of pectoralis major, its floor by that of latissimus dorsi and its medial lip by that of teres major. The attachment of pectoralis major extends beyond teres major's, that of latissimus dorsi being least extensive. Distal to the sulcus a small area of anteromedial surface is devoid of muscular attachment, but its distal half is occupied by the medial part of the brachialis (6.207). The rough strip on the medial border is for the coracobrachialis. Near its distal end the medial supracondylar ridge has a narrow area for the humeral part of pronator teres, and the ridge itself for the medial intermuscular septum.

To the oblique ridge across the *posterior surface* the lateral head of triceps is attached; proximal to this the axillary (circumflex) nerve and posterior circumflex humeral vessels curve round the 'surgical neck' deep to deltoid; distally the radial groove, containing the nerve and profunda vessels, descends laterally to the anterolateral surface. The medial head of triceps occupies much of the posterior surface in a long triangular area, its apex medial on this surface and **proximal** to the distal limit of teres major, widening distally over the whole dorsal surface almost to its distal end (6.208).

Proximally the *anterolateral surface* is smooth and covered by deltoid, which is attached to its tuberosity; distally it is occupied by part of brachialis, ascending into the floor of the radial groove (6.208). The lateral supracondylar ridge, in its proximal two-thirds, gives attachment to brachioradialis and in its distal third extensor carpi radialis longus. Behind these, the lateral intermuscular septum is attached to the ridge.

The articular region of the humeral condyle is so curved that the anterior and posterior surfaces are anterior in plane to corresponding surfaces of the shaft. The trochlear groove spirals posterolaterally from the anterior to the posterior surface; posteriorly it is wider, deeper and more symmetrical; anteriorly its medial flange is longer and the convex surface adjoining its projecting medial margin is adapted to the medial arc of the coronoid articular surface. These asymmetries entail varying angulation between the humeral and ulnar axes, together with some conjunct rotation (p. 631).

The elbow joint capsule (6.207, 208) is attached to the proximal limits of the radial and coronoid fossae, which are therefore intra-capsular and lined by synovial membrane, and also to the medial aspect of the trochlear rim and root of the medial epicondyle. Posteriorly it ascends almost to the upper margin of the olecranon fossa, which is also intracapsular and covered by synovial membrane. Laterally it skirts the borders of the trochlea and capitulum, lying medial to the lateral epicondyle.

The common superficial flexor tendon arises from the medial epicondylar epiphysis, which is wholly extracapsular. The common superficial extensor tendon is attached to the lateral epicondyle, also outside the articular capsule; to its posterior surface anconeus is attached (6.208). The medial epicondyle turns slightly backwards, the lateral slightly forwards.

With the upper limb pendent, the medial epicondyle is **posterior** in plane to the lateral; the humeral head is directed almost equally **backwards** and **medially**, the posterior surface of the shaft facing posterolaterally. Since the glenoid fossa of the scapula faces antero-laterally, the humerus is not rotated medially *relative to the scapula* in this position of rest; but it *is* so rotated relative to the *conventional anatomical position*. This must be remembered when movements of the arm and forearm are considered (pp. 631 and 642).

A hook-shaped *supracondylar process*, from 2 to 20 mm in length, occasionally projects from the anteromedial surface of the shaft, about 5 cm proximal to the medial epicondyle. It curves distally and forwards, its apex connected to the medial border, proximal to the epicondyle, by a fibrous band, to which part of pronator teres is attached. The foramen so formed usually encloses the median nerve and brachial artery, but sometimes only the nerve or perhaps nerve plus the ulnar artery in a high division of the brachial artery. A groove for the artery and nerve usually exists behind the process. It is the homologue of the *entepicondylar foramen* of many animals and may protect the nerve and artery from compression by muscles. These skeletal features may aid in assessing racial affinities (p. 434).

Ossification

The humerus is ossified from eight centres, in shaft, head, greater and lesser tubercles, capitulum and lateral trochlea, medial trochlea and both epicondyles (6.211A). The shaft begins to ossify centrally in the eighth week with gradual extension to its ends, and the humeral head usually during the first 6 months after birth, but just before it in 20% of individuals. The greater and lesser tubercles begin to ossify in the second and fifth years in males, about a year earlier in females. By the sixth year the head and tubercles have become a single epiphysis, **hollow** inferiorly (6.211B) to fit the conical end of the diaphysis and fusing with it about the twentieth year in males, 2 years earlier in females. Some deny a centre in the lesser tubercle, perhaps because it is often obscured in the usual anteroposterior radiological views (6.212). In the distal end, during the first year, ossification begins in the capitulum and extends to form most of its articular surface; a centre for the medial region of the trochlea appears in the ninth year in females and tenth in males. Ossification begins in the medial epicondyle in the fourth year in females, sixth in males, and in the lateral epicondyle about the twelfth year. Centres for the lateral epicondyle, capitulum and trochlea fuse around puberty and the composite epiphysis unites with the shaft in the fourteenth year in females, sixteenth in males. The medial epicondyle is a separate epiphysis, entirely extracapsular (6.207, 208), from a centre posteromedial in it. It is separated from the distal epiphysis by a downgrowth of shaft, with which it unites in about the twentieth year.

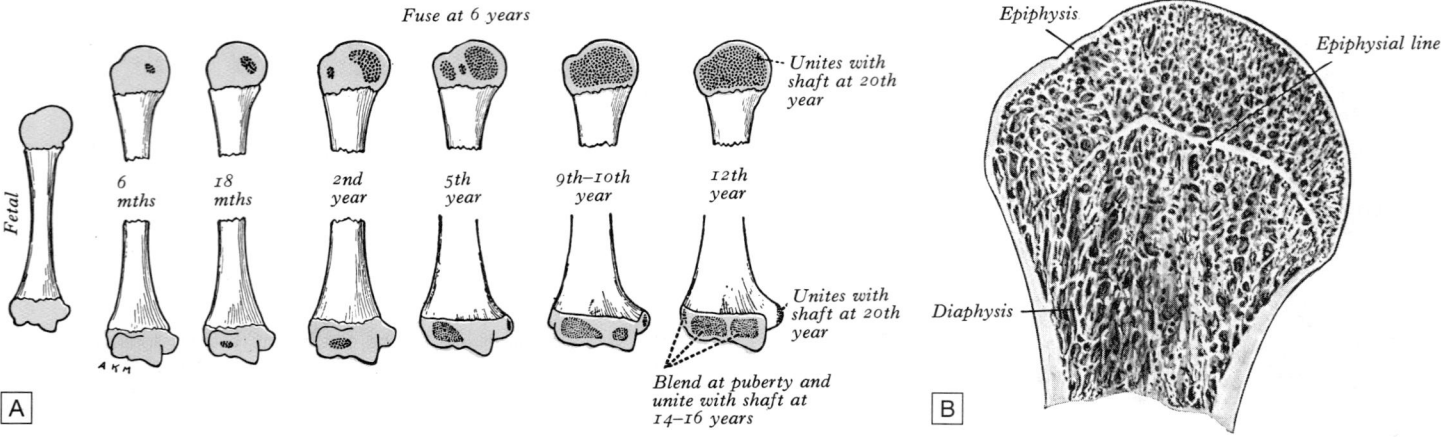

Fuse at 6 years

Unites with shaft at 20th year

Fetal · 6 mths · 18 mths · 2nd year · 5th year · 9th–10th year · 12th year

Unites with shaft at 20th year

Blend at puberty and unite with shaft at 14–16 years

Epiphysis

Epiphysial line

Diaphysis

A   B

6.211A. The stages in ossification of the humerus (not to scale); B. Longi-tudinal section through the head of the right humerus.

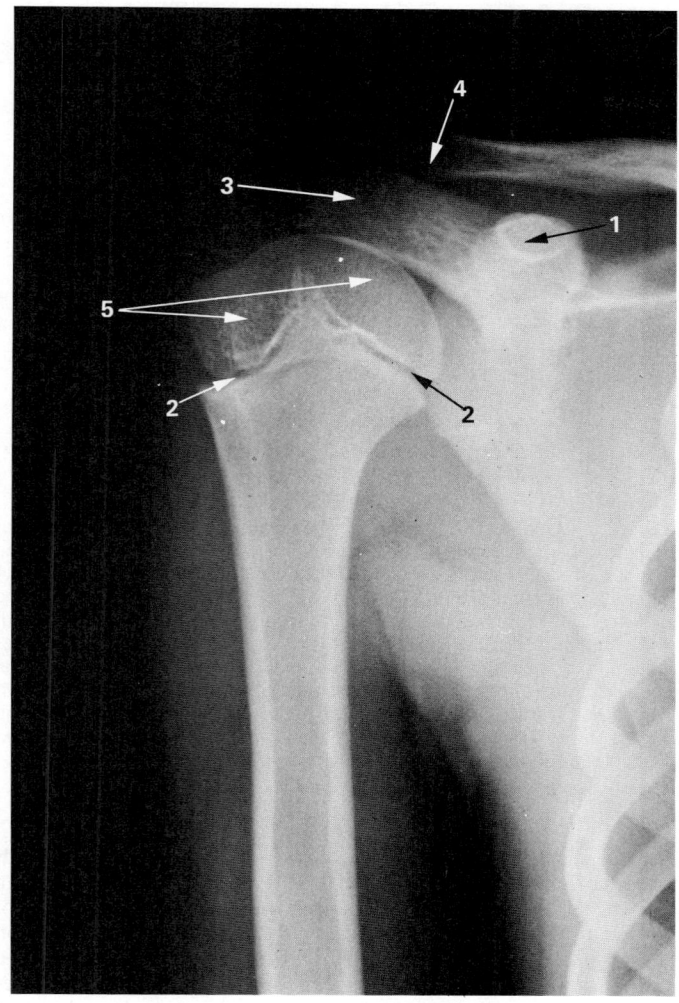

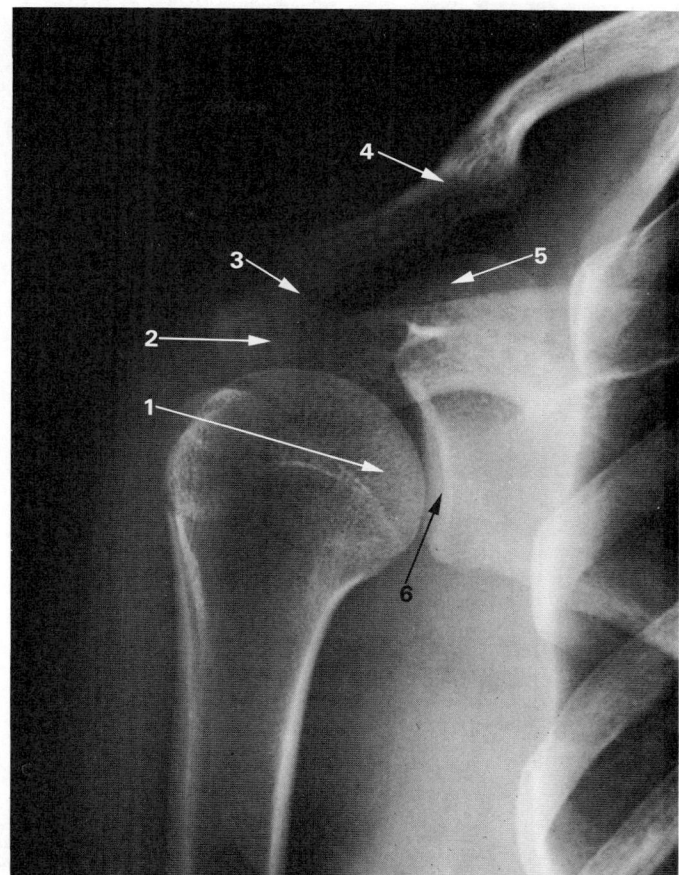

6.212   Anteroposterior radiograph of the right shoulder in a boy aged 11.
1. Coracoid process. 2. Growth plate of cartilage at upper end of humeral
diaphysis. 3. Acromion. 4. Lateral end of clavicle, not yet completely ossified.
5. Proximal humeral epiphysis. Note its conical junction with the diaphysis.

Clinical anatomy

The proximal epiphysis joins the shaft later than the distal, and
growth in length is predominantly due to the proximal growth
cartilage. Hence, after amputation through the arm in youth, the
humerus continues to grow, its lower end progressively moulding
the soft tissues and making the stump conical. Fractures are comparatively common and at almost any level. Muscular action is more
often the cause than in any other long bone; it is usually the shaft,
below the attachment of deltoid, which is broken. Hence the radial
nerve may be injured in its groove and is sometimes involved later
in the growth of callus. Non-union is commoner than in any other
bone except the tibia. Fractures at the proximal end may damage
the axillary nerve, and at the medial epicondyle the ulnar nerve.
Late fusion of this epicondyle may be misdiagnosed as a fracture.

SHOULDER (GLENOHUMERAL) JOINT

The shoulder is a multiaxial spheroidal joint (**6**.213) possessing three
degrees of freedom between the roughly hemispherical humeral head
and shallow scapular glenoid fossa, an arrangement allowing much
movement but reducing security. Skeletally the joint is weak, and
depends for support on the surrounding muscles more than on its
shape and ligaments. However, the coracoacromial arch overhangs
it.

The *articular surfaces*, reciprocally curved, are really *ovoids* (see
p. 503). Here, as in the hip, where ovoid surfaces are almost spherical
they are often termed *spheroidal*; small deviations from sphericity of
less than 1% of the radius have been recorded (Soslowsky et al
1992a). The humeral convexity exceeds in area that of the glenoid

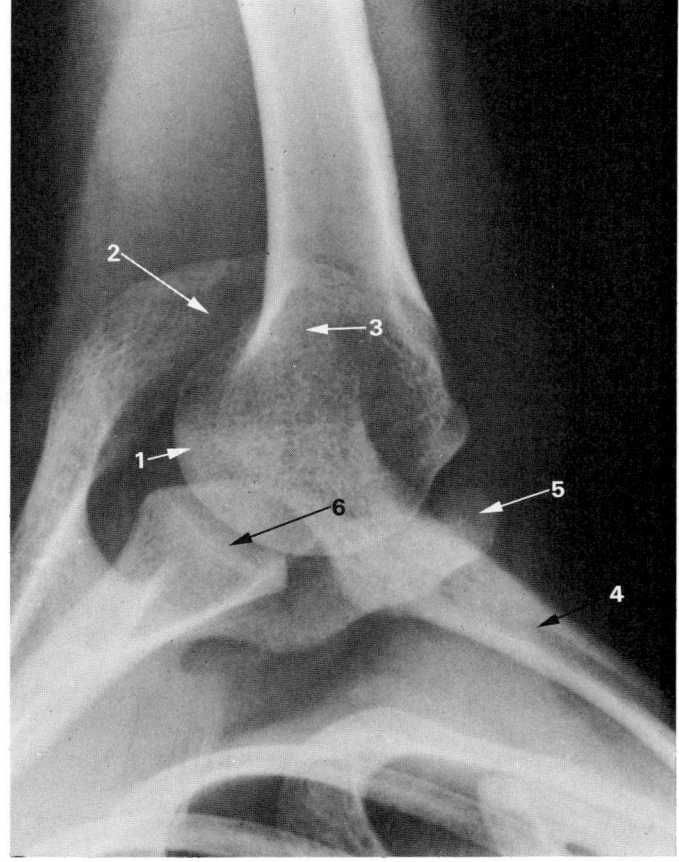

6.213   Radiograph of shoulder in a young female of 18 years in anteroposterior view (A) and axillary view with the arm abducted (B). 1. Head of
humerus. 2. Acromion. 3. Acromioclavicular joint. 4. Clavicle. 5. Coracoid
process. 6. Glenoid (osseous, subchondral) articular surface.

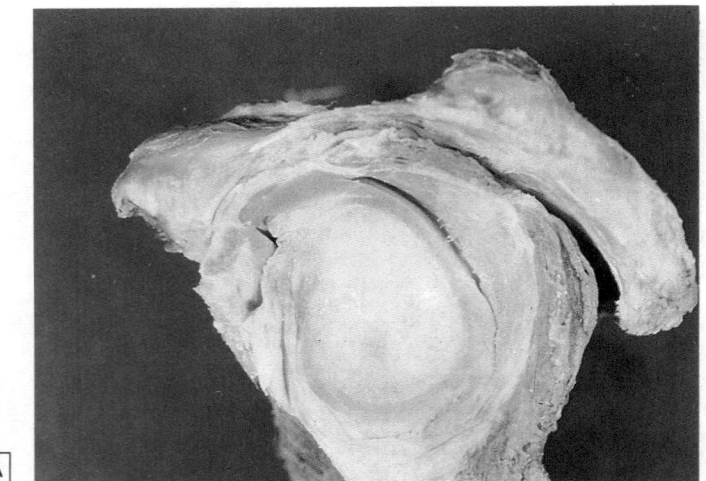

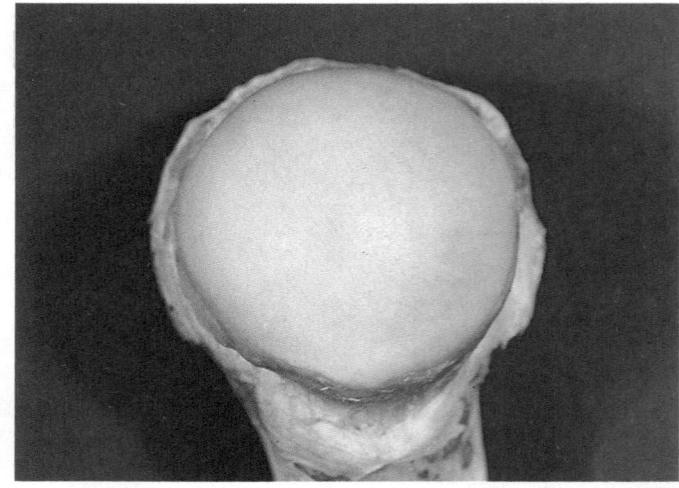

6.214A, B. Dissections from a preserved cadaver showing the articular surfaces and periarticular structures of the shoulder joint. A shows the glenoid cavity covered by articular cartilage and the glenoidal labrum; note the intracapsular part of the tendon of the long head of the biceps sectioned near the supraglenoid tubercle, the fibrous capsule intimately blended with 'rotator cuff' musculature, the subacromial bursa, and the superjacent cora-coacromial arch complex. B displays the much more extensive spheroidal articular surface of the head of the humerus and the pendant inferior part of the fibrous articular capsule. (Preparation by M C E Hutchinson and photography by Kevin Fitzpatrick, Guy's Hospital Medical School, London.) C. Section through the shoulder joint. The synovial membrane is in blue.

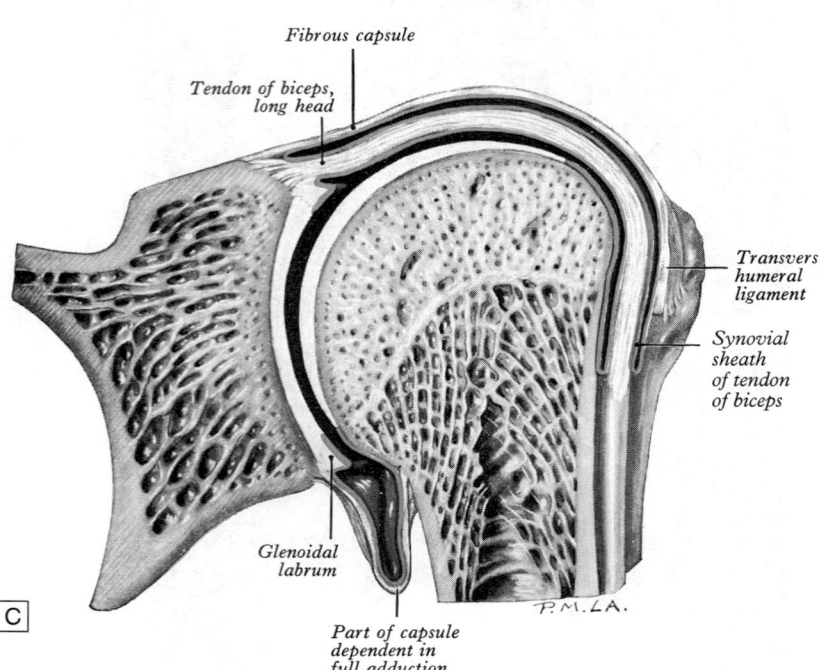

Fibrous capsule

Tendon of biceps, long head

Transverse humeral ligament

Synovial sheath of tendon of biceps

Glenoidal labrum

P.M.LA.

Part of capsule dependent in full adduction

concavity (**6.214**) such that only a small portion opposes the glenoid in any position, the remaining capitular articular surface being in contact with the capsule; contact on the glenoid is much more uniformly distributed over its entire articular surface (Soslowsky et al 1992b). The radius of curvature of the glenoid cavity (**6.214, 215, 216**) in the coronal plane is greater than that of the humeral head (Iannotti et al 1992); consequently it is deepened by a fibro-cartilaginous rim, the *glenoid labrum*. Both articular surfaces are covered by hyaline cartilage: on the humerus it is thickest centrally, thinner peripherally; the reverse in the glenoid cavity. In most positions, their curvatures are not fully congruent, the joint being loose-packed (Saha 1961). Full congruence (close-packing) is reached with the humerus abducted and laterally rotated (see pp. 509, 631; and **6.71, 83**). When the arm is dependent, the anterior glenoid edge can be represented by a laterally concave line descending 3 cm from a point just lateral to the coracoid apex; it lies over the joint's lower half. Ligaments are *capsular, glenohumeral, coracohumeral* and *transverse humeral*.

Fibrous capsule

A fibrous capsule (**6.214, 217A**) envelops the joint, attaching medially to the glenoid margin outside the glenoid labrum, and encroaching on the coracoid process to include the attachment of the long head of biceps. Laterally, it is attached to the humeral anatomical neck,

i.e. near the articular margin, except inferomedially where it descends more than 1 cm on the humeral shaft. It is so lax that the bones can be distracted for 2 or 3 cm. This accords with a very wide range of movement. However, such unnatural separation requires relaxation of the upper capsule by abduction. The fibrous capsule is supported by the tendons of supraspinatus (above), infraspinatus and teres minor (behind), subscapularis (in front) and by the long head of triceps (below). All but triceps blend with the capsule as the *rotator cuff* which reinforces the capsule and actively supports it unless the muscles are fully relaxed. Triceps is separated from the capsule by the axillary nerve and posterior circumflex humeral vessels as they pass back from the axilla (**6.217B**). Inferiorly the capsule is therefore least supported and also subjected to the greatest strain, being stretched tightly across the humeral head in full abduction. The capsule is also strengthened in front by extensions from the tendons of pectoralis major and teres major.

The capsule usually has two or three openings: an anterior, below the coracoid process, connects the joint to a bursa behind the subscapular tendon; another, between the humeral tubercles (tuberosities), transmits the long tendon of biceps and its synovial sheath; a third, inconstant and posterior, connects the joint to a bursa under the infraspinatous tendon.

Glenohumeral ligaments. Anteriorly three *glenohumeral ligaments*, best visible from within the joint (**6.216, 218**), reinforce the capsule. The *superior glenohumeral ligament* passes from the upper part of the glenoid labrum and base of the coracoid process (deep to the coracoacromial ligament) to the upper part of the neck of the humerus, between the lesser tubercle and the articular margin. The *middle glenohumeral ligament* arises from a wide attachment, below the superior glenohumeral ligament, along the anterior glenoid margin as far as the inferior third of the rim (Shahan 1983), and passes obliquely inferolaterally, enlarging as it does, to attach to the lesser tuberosity deep to the tendon of subscapularis, with which it blends. The thicker and longer *inferior glenohumeral ligament* arises from the anterior, middle and posterior margins of the glenoid labrum, below the epiphyseal line, and passes anteroinferiorly to attach to the inferior and medial aspects of the neck of the humerus. The anterior, superior edge of the inferior ligament is thickened as the *superior band* (Spencer & Turkel 1981; Bigliani et al 1992), the diffuse thickening of the anterior part of the capsule to which it attaches being known as the *axillary pouch* (Spencer & Turkel 1981).

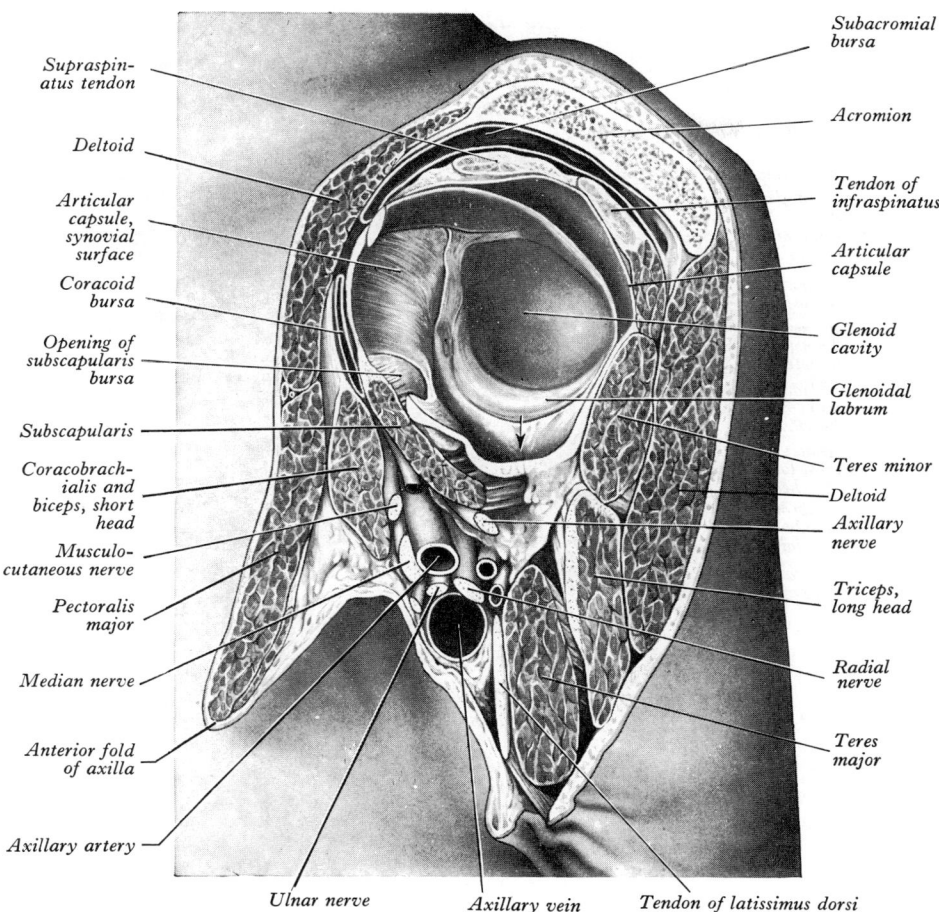

Supraspin-
atus tendon

Deltoid

Articular
capsule,
synovial
surface

Coracoid
bursa

Opening of
subscapularis
bursa

Subscapularis

Coracobrach-
ialis and
biceps, short
head

Musculo-
cutaneous nerve

Pectoralis
major

Median nerve

Anterior fold
of axilla

Axillary artery

Subacromial
bursa

Acromion

Tendon of
infraspinatus

Articular
capsule

Glenoid
cavity

Glenoidal
labrum

Teres minor

Deltoid

Axillary
nerve

Triceps,
long head

Radial
nerve

Teres
major

Ulnar nerve   Axillary vein   Tendon of latissimus dorsi

6.215   An obliquely coronal section through the left shoulder and shoulder joint, in the plane of the glenoidal labrum, dissected after removal of the upper limb. The arrow points into the dependent part of the articular capsule. Note: the relations of the axillary vessels to each other and to the branches of the brachial plexus as displayed in this dissected section may appear unfamiliar and the reader is referred to **6.92** for a more usual view. Compare, also, with **6.216**.

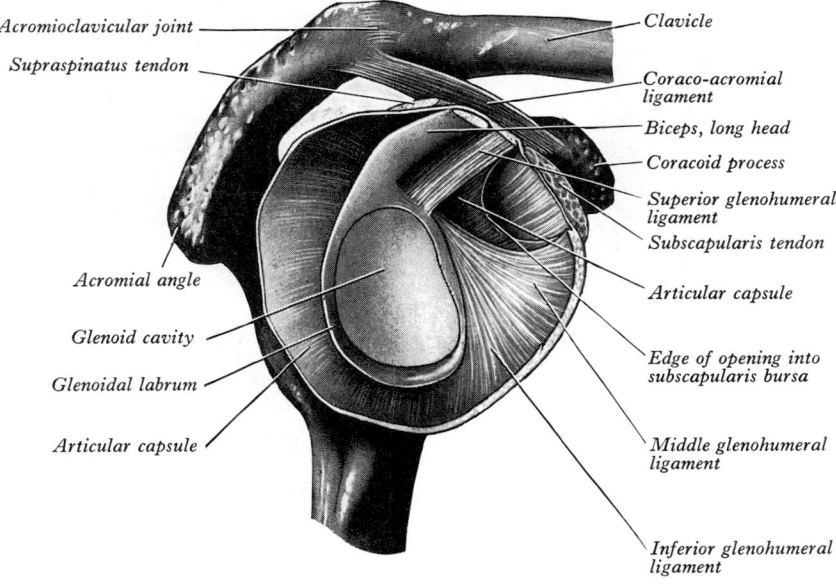

Acromioclavicular joint

Supraspinatus tendon

Acromial angle

Glenoid cavity

Glenoidal labrum

Articular capsule

Clavicle

Coraco-acromial
ligament

Biceps, long head

Coracoid process

Superior glenohumeral
ligament

Subscapularis tendon

Articular capsule

Edge of opening into
subscapularis bursa

Middle glenohumeral
ligament

Inferior glenohumeral
ligament

6.216   Interior of the right shoulder joint: anterolateral aspect.

Synovial membrane. This lines the capsule and covers parts of the anatomical neck. The long tendon of biceps traverses the joint in a synovial sheath which continues into the intertubercular sulcus as far as the humeral surgical neck (**6.214, 217A**).

Coracohumeral ligament

The coracohumeral ligament (**6.217A**), a broad thickening of the upper capsular region, passes from the lateral border of the root of the coracoid process to the front of the greater tubercle, blending with the supraspinatous tendon; its inferoposterior border blends with the capsule.

The transverse humeral ligament

The transverse humeral ligament (**6.217A**) is a broad band passing

629

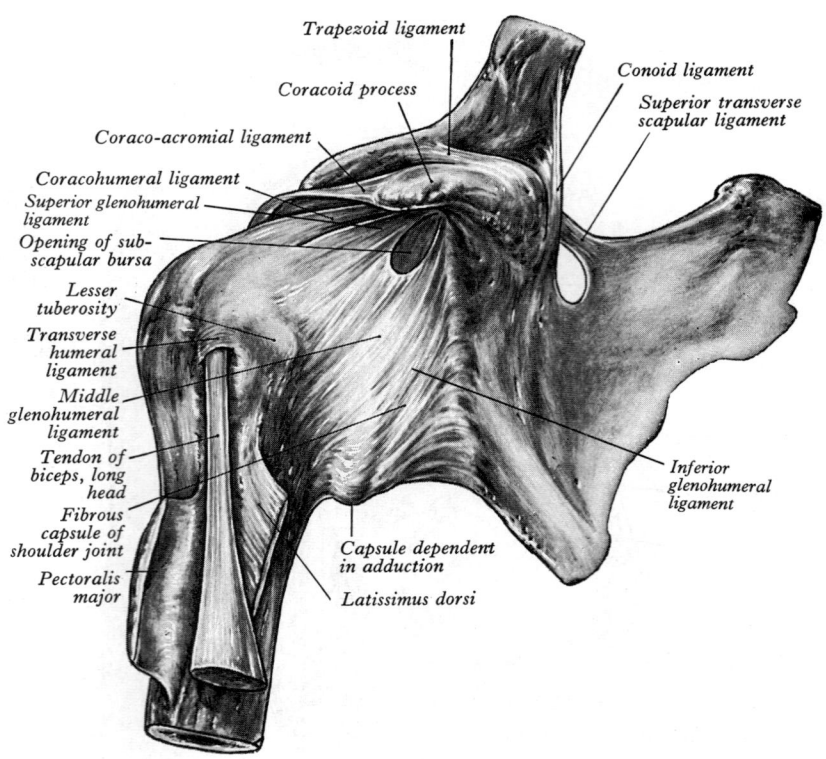

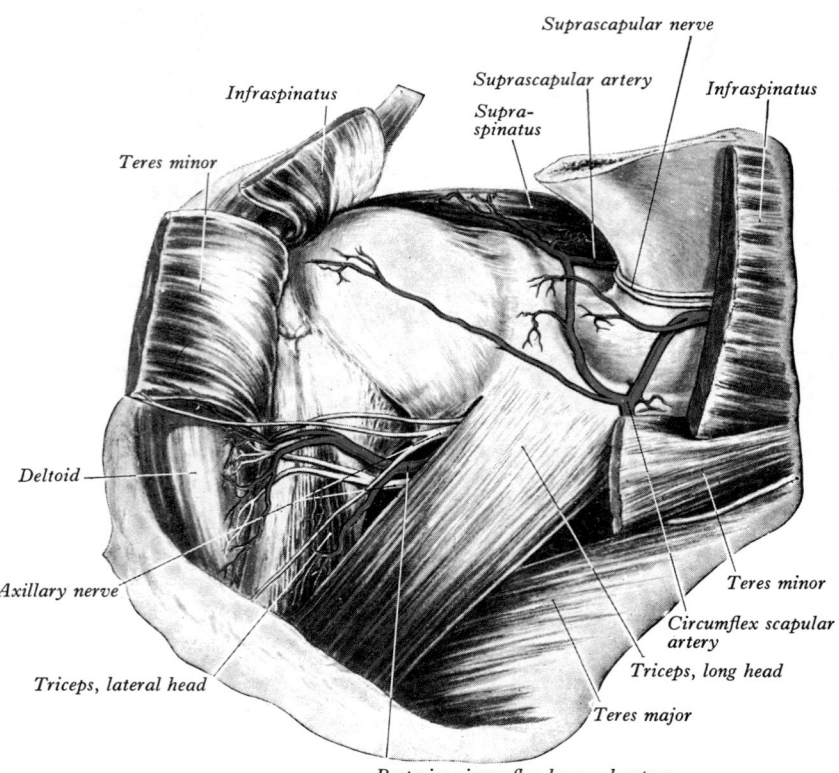

6.217A. The anterior aspect of the right shoulder; B. posterior aspect of the left shoulder joint with the acromion removed. Parts of infraspinatus and teres minor have been excised and their tendons turned forwards.

between the humeral tubercles, attaching superior to the epiphyseal line. It converts the intertubercular sulcus into a canal, and acts as a retinaculum for the long tendon of biceps.

Glenoid labrum

630   The glenoid labrum (**6.215**), a fibrocartilaginous rim round the

glenoid fossa, is triangular in section, its base attached to the fossa's margin, its thin margin projecting as a continuation of the curve of the glenoid. It blends above with two fasciculi from the long tendon of biceps. It deepens the cavity, may protect bone and probably assists lubrication (p. 594). Its attachment is sometimes partly deficient; synovial membrane may protrude through such gaps.

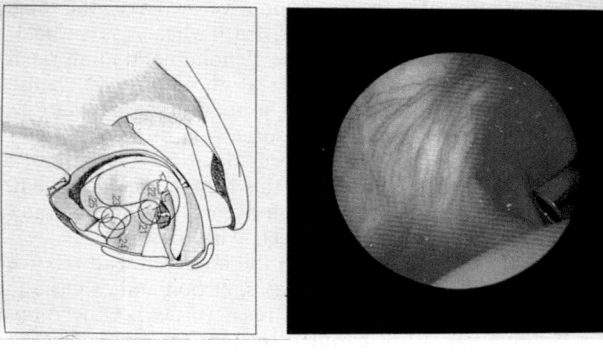

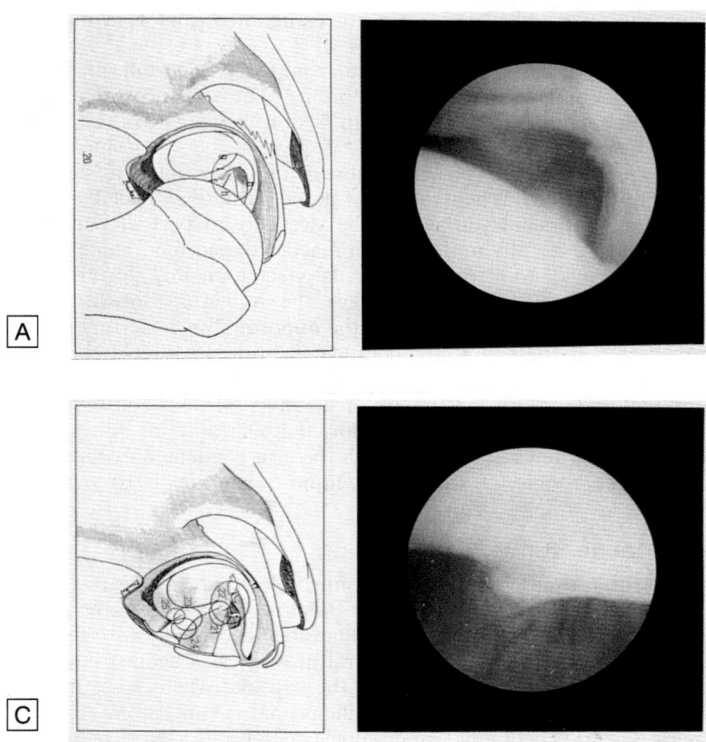

6.218 The superior (A), middle (B) and inferior (C) glenohumeral ligaments viewed arthroscopically. The line drawings illustrate the orientation of each view. (Supplied by Dr K Zyto, Department of Orthopaedics and Accident Surgery, Queen's Medical Centre, Nottingham)

Bursae

Many bursae adjoin the shoulder joint:

- between the subscapular tendon and articular capsule (6.216), communicating with the joint between the superior and middle glenohumeral ligaments;
- sometimes between the infraspinatous tendon and capsule, occasionally opening into the joint;
- the *subacromial bursa* (6.215) between deltoid and the capsule, non-communicating but prolonged under the acromion and coracoacromial ligament, and between them and supraspinatus: it appears to be attached, together with the subdeltoid fascia, to the acromion (Birnbaum & Lierse 1992);
- on the superior acromial aspect;
- frequently between the coracoid process and capsule;
- sometimes behind coracobrachialis;
- between teres major and the long head of triceps;
- anterior and posterior to the tendon of latissimus dorsi.

Related muscles

These are: supraspinatus (above), long head of triceps (below), subscapularis (in front), infraspinatus and teres minor (behind), long tendon of biceps (intracapsular). Deltoid covers the joint in front, behind and laterally (6.215).

Vessels and nerve supply to the joint

Arteries are from the anterior and posterior circumflex humeral as well as the suprascapular and circumflex scapular vessels (Cooper et al 1992; de la Garcia et al 1992). **Nerves** are mainly from the posterior brachial cord and from the suprascapular, axillary and the lateral pectoral nerves. The suprascapular supplies the posterior and superior, axillary anteroinferior and the lateral pectoral antero-superior parts of the capsule (Gardner 1948b).

Movements

The shoulder, as a multiaxial spheroidal joint, is capable of any combination of swing and spin over a very wide range (p. 507), all movements analysable as rotations around three orthogonal axes, i.e. it has three degrees of freedom (p. 498). Classically, *flexion–extension*, *abduction–adduction*, *circumduction* and *medial* and *lateral rotation* (p. 500) are assigned to it. Laxity of the capsule, and a humeral head which is large relative to the shallow glenoid fossa,

afford a wider range of movement than at any other joint. However, with the arm dependent, even when moderately loaded, supraspinatus and tension in the upper capsule prevent downward displacement of the humerus (Basmajian 1967).

In analysis of shoulder movements it is preferable to refer humeral movement to the scapula, rather than to conventional anatomical planes, the relevant axes being shown in 6.71. When the arm hangs at rest the glenoid fossa faces almost equally forwards and laterally, and the humeral capitular and scapular (topographical) axes correspond, although the humerus, relative to the anatomical position, is medially rotated (p. 500). *Flexion* carries the arm anteromedially on an axis through the humeral head orthogonal to the glenoid fossa at its centre. *Abduction* and *adduction* occur in a vertical plane orthogonal to that of flexion–extension, the axis being horizontal, through the humeral head, parallel to the glenoid plane (Flecker 1929). Pure abduction raises the arm **anterolaterally in the plane of the scapula**. However, when referred to the *trunk*, flexion and extension are in the paramedian plane, abduction and adduction in the coronal plane. Raising the arm vertically from flexion (in this sense) or raising it from abduction (in this sense) are both accompanied by humeral rotation in opposite directions. Whether 'scapular' or any other plane of abduction is described, these are selections from an infinite series. In scapular abduction points on the humeral surface pursue vertical chords but in rotation they are horizontal. In 'pure' flexion–extension, in a plane orthogonal to the scapular, the axis of movement (and the notional 'mechanical axis', p. 505) are regarded as projected from the centre of the glenoid cavity.

Glenohumeral abduction is about 90° (Kapandji 1974) but angles up to 120° have been stated (Inman et al 1944). About 60° further abduction occurs at the sterno- and acromioclavicular articulations. Contralateral vertebral flexion also aids in bringing the arm vertical. However, during active elevation movements at the glenohumeral and acromioclavicular joints are simultaneous, except in the initial 25°–30°, when most and often all movement is glenohumeral. For every 15° of elevation, glenohumeral movement is said to be 10° and scapular 5°.

In flexion, however, the humerus swings at right angles to the scapular plane and scapular rotation cannot increase elevation (120°) obtainable in full flexion. If the fully flexed humerus is also abducted, elevation increases pro rata until, when the humerus reaches the scapular plane, i.e. when true abduction is reached, 180° of elevation becomes possible. In *rotation*, medial or lateral, the humerus revolves about one-quarter of a circle around a vertical axis; the range being greatest when the arm is pendent, least when it is vertical. When assessing the rotational range at the glenohumeral joint, the forearm should be flexed to a right angle at the elbow, preventing mis-interpretation due to superadded pronation or supination in the pendent limb. In *circumduction*, a succession of the foregoing move-ments, the distal end of the humerus describes the base of a cone, its apex at the humeral head, but this glenohumeral movement can be much increased by scapular movements; the combination is exemplified in acts of slinging objects with force.

Because of the offset position of the humeral head relative to the shaft's longitudinal topographical axis, flexion and extension involve almost pure 'spins' in the glenoid fossa (p. 505). Other movements are an infinite variety of cardinal or arcuate swings or successions of these (pp. 503, 505).

The peculiar relation of the long head of biceps to the shoulder joint may serve several purposes. By its connection with both the shoulder and elbow the muscle harmonizes their actions as an elastic ligament during all their movements. It helps to prevent the humeral head impinging on the acromion when deltoid contracts and to steady it in movements of the arm. In paralysis of supraspinatus it may also help initiate abduction of the arm, particularly when the humerus is laterally rotated.

Accessory movements. A wide range of accessory movements (p. 509) occurs at the shoulder joint. The humeral head can be translated in any direction relative to the glenoid fossa and, in abduction when accessory movements are most free, the articular surface can be separated by traction.

Muscles producing movement

The muscles producing movement may be divided into those acting on the pectoral girdle and those acting on the glenohumeral joint.

Muscles acting on the pectoral girdle. These are considered on page 622.

Muscles acting at the glenohumeral joint. Principally deltoid, pectoralis major, latissimus dorsi and teres major. All converge on the humerus, acting at mechanical advantage on a joint which, owing to glenoid shallowness and capsular laxity, is relatively unstable, a condition counteracted by the short muscles attached nearer to it, viz. the 'rotator cuff' (subscapularis, supraspinatus, infraspinatus and teres minor), which function as postural muscles retaining the

humeral head and glenoid in correct alignment and resisting skid during active movements.

Flexion: pectoralis major (clavicular part), deltoid (anterior fibres) and coracobrachialis assisted by biceps. The sternocostal part of pectoralis major is a major force in flexion forwards to the coronal plane from *full extension*.

Extension: deltoid (posterior fibres) and teres major, from the pendent position. When the fully flexed arm is extended against resistance, latissimus dorsi and the sternocostal part of pectoralis major act powerfully until the arm reaches the coronal plane.

Abduction: deltoid, but initially its effect is mainly upward and, unless opposed, would so displace the humerus. Subscapularis, infraspinatus and teres minor are the opposing force exerting down-ward traction; these three and deltoid constitute a 'couple' to produce abduction in the scapular plane. Supraspinatus assists in effecting and maintaining this movement but its precise role is controversial.

Medial rotation: pectoralis major, deltoid (anterior fibres), lat-issimus dorsi, teres major and, with the arm pendent, subscapularis.

Lateral rotation: infraspinatus, deltoid (posterior fibres) and teres minor.

Clinical anatomy

Good rotator muscle strength and intact glenohumeral ligaments are both required for normal shoulder stability, but owing to the joint's shallowness it is the most frequently dislocated, usually with the arm abducted. In such cases the humeral head presses against and may tear the antero-inferior aspect of the capsule, where it is thinnest and least supported; dislocation being primarily subglenoid. (Further degrees are subcoracoid and subclavicular.) If, after reduction, abduction is prevented, dislocation cannot recur. In cases of trau-matic anterior dislocation of the shoulder it is common for the inferior glenohumeral ligament to be stretched (Spencer & Turkel 1981) or rendered dysfunctional by avulsion of its glenoid attachment (Bigliani et al 1992), occurring as a consequence of detachment of the anterior and inferior glenoid labrum, thereby creating the typical Blankart lesion.

If the shoulder joint ankyloses, loss of movement is partly com-pensated by increased scapular mobility. When ankylosis is likely the humerus should be positioned as if the palm were to be placed on the back of the neck, i.e. abducted, to make full use of scapular mobility.

Shoulder joint replacement

Surgical replacement of the glenohumeral joint has become a routine procedure: results are improving as new designs of prosthesis are introduced. Good results can be achieved when care is taken to restore the anatomy of the joint during the procedure. Shoulder replacement can be carried out as a hemiarthroplasty in which the joint surface of the humerus only is replaced, or as a total arthroplasty in which the glenoid surface is also replaced.

The metal humeral prosthesis usually consists of a stem placed inside the med-ullary cavity and is either a one-piece or modular (separate head and stem) pros-thesis: the stem may either be cemented to the bone or left uncemented, depending on its design. Solid fixation of the glenoid component can be a problem due to the limited bone stock available, and conse-quently numerous designs are available. The prosthetic articular surface is ultra

high molecular weight polyethylene, either fixed directly to bone with cement, or if backed with metal, fixed with cement, or with screws (uncemented).

The commonest indications for total shoulder replacement are rheumatoid arthritis (**6.219**) and osteoarthritis (**6.220**). A hemiarthroplasty is usually preferred for comminuted fractures of the neck and head of the humerus, and as secondary procedures in mal-union and non-union of fractures.

Shoulder replacement is performed with the patient half-sitting: the 'deckchair pos-ition'. The skin incision extends from the junction of the middle and lateral third of the clavicle to lateral and just distal to the anterior axillary fold. The deltopectoral groove is exposed and the cephalic vein is isolated; branches from deltoid are cau-terized to allow the vein to be preserved and retracted medially. Deltoid is then either retracted or reflected laterally, using

a longitudinal osteotomy of the lateral third of the clavicle (less than a third of the width of the clavicle is detached; **6.221**) with the insertion of the anterior third of deltoid. Retraction of deltoid must be done carefully because of the close prox-imity of the axillary nerve to its deep surface: denervation of the anterior third of deltoid results in severely impaired function and weak shoulder flexion.

The deep anterior part of the shoulder is now exposed. Medially the conjoined tendons (coracobrachialis and short head of biceps) are left untouched, giving pro-tection to the musculocutaneous nerve. The interval between the lesser and greater tuberosities is identified by locating the tendon of the long head of biceps. The shoulder joint is approached either by performing a tenotomy of the sub-scapularis tendon or by osteotomizing the lesser tuberosity together with the sub-scapularis tendon.

The rotator cuff is now divided longi-tudinally from the superior border of the bicipital groove towards the base of the coracoid process, in the rotator interval

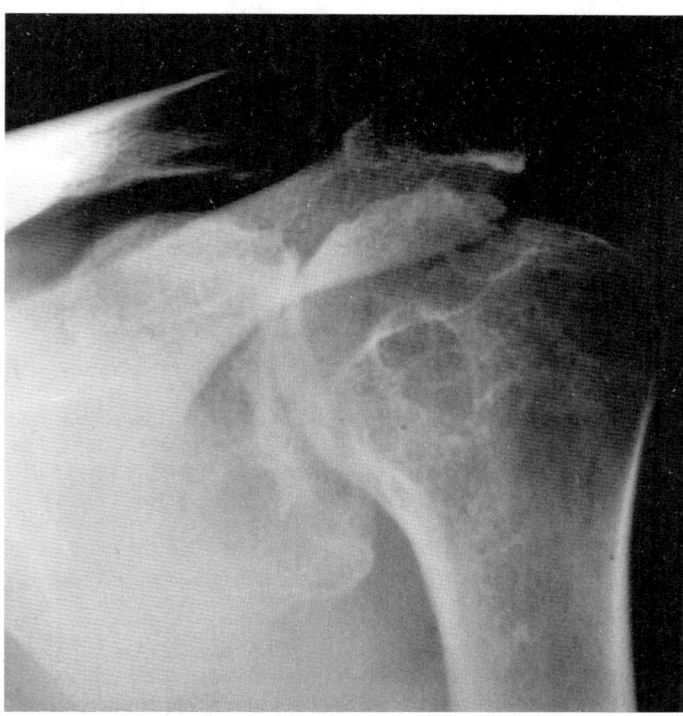

6.219 Shoulder with rheumatoid arthritis. Typical degenerated bone tissue with cysts and wear is apparent. The humeral head has moved medially, and due to proximal wear of the glenoid, has also subluxed upwards, causing impingement. The rotator cuff is in severe danger.

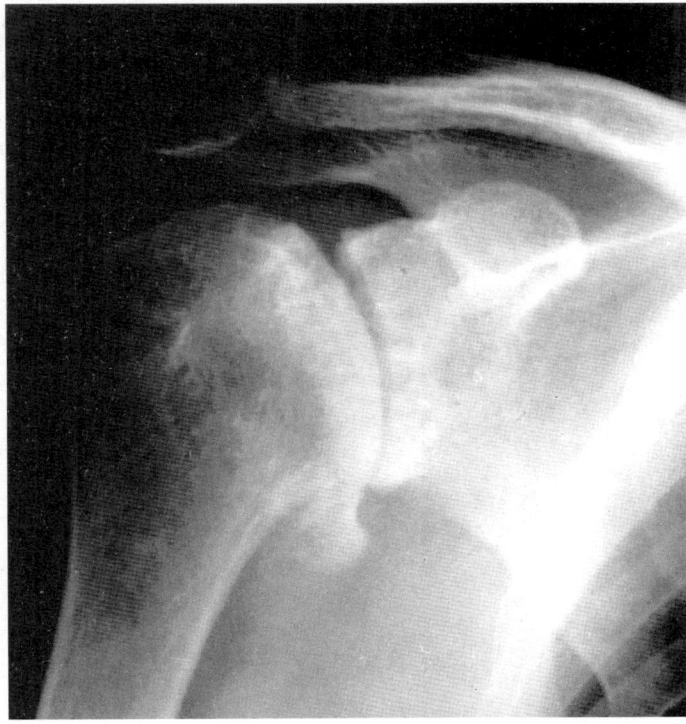

6.220 Shoulder with osteoarthritis. Inferior osteophytes on the head are typical, as is the loss of cartilage indicated by the direct bony contact between the head of the humerus and the glenoid. The bone quality is good, as is usually the condition of the soft tissues.

(junction between the supraspinatus and subscapular tendons). The subscapularis tendon is reflected medially, the joint exposed and dislocated anteriorly: in the osteoarthritic shoulder the presence of osteophytes, mainly on the inferior, but also on the posterior border of the humeral joint surface, as well as on the glenoid, may cause difficulties in dislocating the joint. The humeral head is cut in the anteroposterior plane using the angles devised for the prosthesis: anatomically the humeral head is retroverted some 30° with respect to the intercondylar plane of the elbow, to allow optimal rotational movement of the joint depends on this retroversion.

For total joint replacement, the glenoid surface, which is often severely worn and has formed osteophytes, is then prepared. In refacing the glenoid, its normal plane (at a right angle to the plane of the blade of the scapula and facing laterally) must be recreated. When removing inferior osteophytes from the humeral head or lower pole of the glenoid, the axillary nerve should, as a routine, be protected by a retractor inserted between the joint capsule and the muscles. Having prepared the glenoid surface the prosthesis is inserted using the technique applicable to the type of prosthesis used.

Due to the restricted movement usually present prior to surgery, the rotator cuff tendons are usually found to be retracted and shortened. To restore movement they need to be mobilized: the subscapularis tendon, in particular, should be mobilized from the anterior surface of the scapula.

The medullary canal of the humerus is now reamed, and the prosthetic stem inserted, with or without cement. The cut surface of the humerus should be well covered by the head of the prosthesis; however, the prosthesis head should not extend beyond the cut surface of the humeral head, as this will cause anterior and posterior impingement on the rotator cuff tendons. Proximally, the head should be flush with the superior margin of the greater tuberosity: if it is lower then impingement of the tuberosity against the acromion will occur; if it is higher, the rotator cuff tents over the rim of the head and will wear against the acromion.

As the shoulder is an unconstrained joint stability is predominantly dependent on the soft tissues, which should be tight and in balance: if too tight, movement will be reduced; if too loose, the shoulder can become unstable. As well as selecting and inserting appropriate components, additional soft tissue releases may be needed to achieve a satisfactory result. Insertion of the glenoid component with the correct inferior tilt creates a good subacromial space, preventing impingement under the acromion during elevation of the arm.

When closing wounds the subscapularis

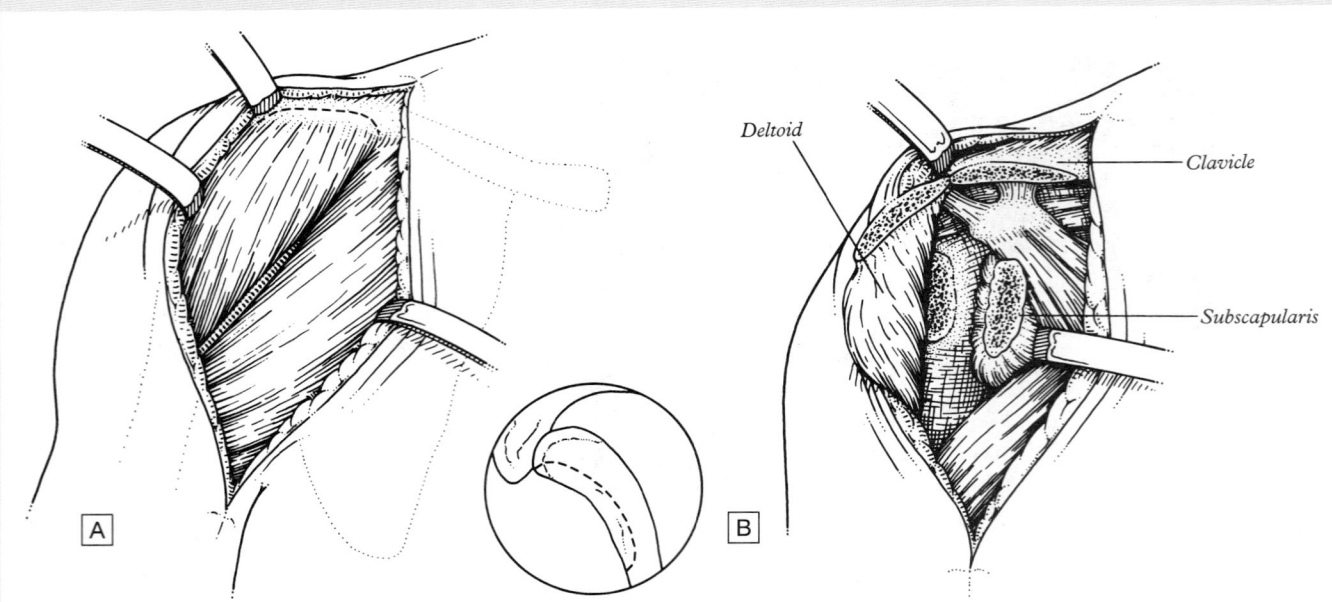

6.221A, B.   Clavicular osteotomy. Osteotomy of a bony bar, together with the insertion of the anterior third of deltoid, gives easy access to the shoulder joint and allows solid reattachment of the muscle.

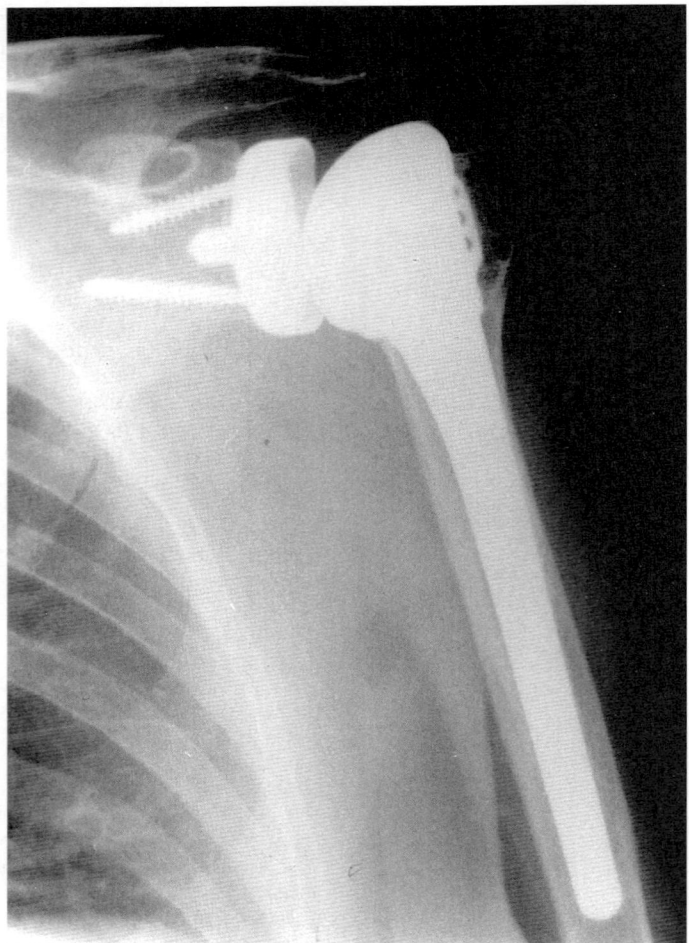

tendon is repaired with non-absorbable heavy sutures: if osteotomy has been performed transosseous sutures are used. The rotator interval is closed, and the prosthesis is completely covered by the repaired rotator cuff. If a clavicular osteotomy has been used, deltoid and the bar of bone are reattached with resorbable sutures using a cerclage-technique around the clavicle. The deltopectoral groove is closed with a few interrupted sutures to avoid a permanent gap; the subcuticular tissues and skin are closed in the usual manner.

The joint replacement (**6.222**) so performed should allow immediate rehabilitation to take place. Shoulder immobilization, even for short periods of time, is a well-known cause of restriction of movement, particularly in the recently operated shoulder where the different layers of tissues may unite and the necessary sliding movement in the subacromial space is lost.

6.222   X-ray after total shoulder replacement. A biomodular, total shoulder prosthesis (Biomet Inc.) in a previously osteoarthritic shoulder. A wide subacromial gap is recreated: the overall alignment of the components resembles that of the original joint surfaces.

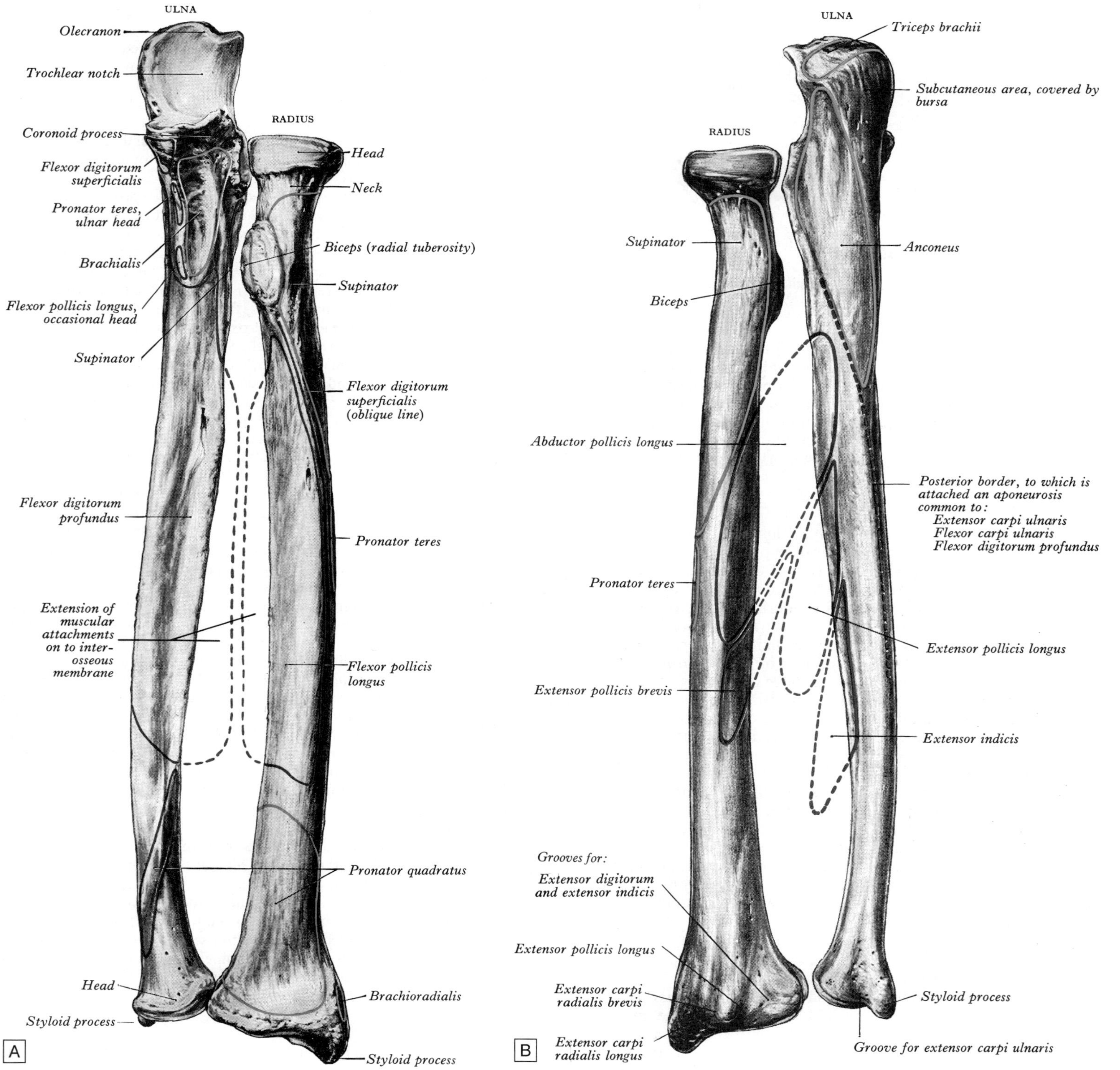

A

ULNA
Olecranon
Trochlear notch
Coronoid process
Flexor digitorum
superficialis
Pronator teres,
ulnar head
Brachialis
Flexor pollicis longus,
occasional head
Supinator
Flexor digitorum
profundus
Extension of
muscular
attachments
on to inter-
osseous
membrane
Head
Styloid process

RADIUS
Head
Neck
Biceps (radial tuberosity)
Supinator
Flexor digitorum
superficialis
(oblique line)
Pronator teres
Flexor pollicis
longus
Pronator quadratus
Brachioradialis
Styloid process

B

ULNA
Triceps brachii
Subcutaneous area, covered by
bursa
Anconeus

RADIUS
Supinator
Biceps
Abductor pollicis longus
Posterior border, to which is
attached an aponeurosis
common to:
    Extensor carpi ulnaris
    Flexor carpi ulnaris
    Flexor digitorum profundus
Pronator teres
Extensor pollicis longus
Extensor pollicis brevis
Extensor indicis
Grooves for:
Extensor digitorum
and extensor indicis
Extensor pollicis longus
Extensor carpi
radialis brevis
Extensor carpi
radialis longus
Styloid process
Groove for extensor carpi ulnaris

6.223 The left radius and ulna: A. Anterior aspect; B. Posterior aspect;
C. Transverse section viewed from above showing the attachment of the
interosseous membrane.

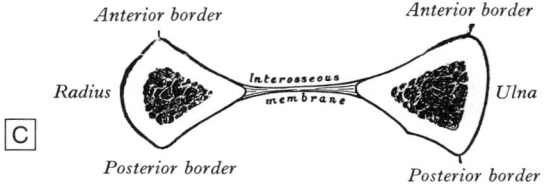

Anterior border   Anterior border
Radius   Interosseous membrane   Ulna
Posterior border   Posterior border

C

RADIUS

The radius (**6**.223), lateral in the forearm, has expanded proximal
and distal ends, the distal much the broader. The shaft widens
rapidly towards its distal end, is convex laterally and concave
anteriorly in its distal part.

The proximal end

It includes a head, neck and tuberosity. The *head* is discoid, its

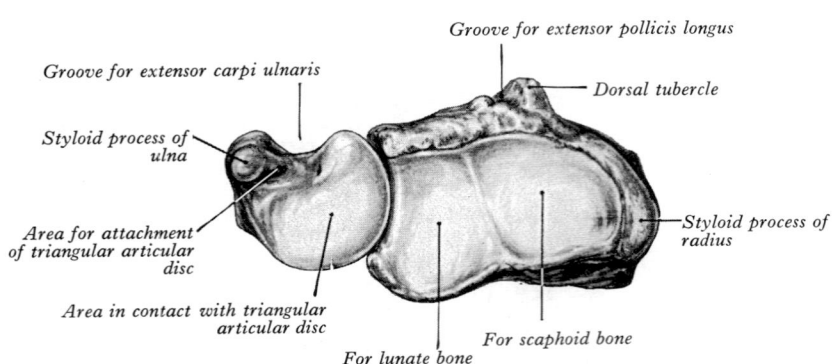

Groove for extensor carpi ulnaris

Groove for extensor pollicis longus

Dorsal tubercle

Styloid process of ulna

Area for attachment of triangular articular disc

Styloid process of radius

Area in contact with triangular articular disc

For scaphoid bone

For lunate bone

6.224 The inferior aspect of the distal ends of the right radius and ulna.

proximal surface a shallow cup for the humeral capitulum. Its smooth *articular periphery* is vertically deepest medially, where it contracts the ulnar radial notch. Its posterior surface is palpable in a small depression on the lateral side of the back of the extended elbow. The *neck* is the constriction distal to the head, which overhangs it, especially on the lateral side. The *tuberosity* is distal to the medial part of the neck; it is posteriorly rough but anteriorly usually smooth.

Shaft

This has a lateral convexity, in section triangular (**6.223c**), but only its *interosseous border* is sharp, except proximally, near the tuberosity; distally it is the posterior margin of a small, elongated, triangular area, proximal to the *ulnar notch*, the two areas forming a so-called *medial surface*. To its distal three-fourths the interosseous membrane is attached, connecting radius to ulna. The *anterior border* is obvious at both ends but rounded and indefinite between them. It descends laterally from the anterolateral part of the tuberosity as the *anterior oblique line*, distally a sharp, palpable crest along the lateral margin of the anterior surface. The *posterior border* is well defined only in its middle third; proximally it ascends medially towards the posteroinferior part of the tuberosity; distally it is merely a rounded ridge. The *anterior surface*, between anterior and interosseous borders, is concave transversely and shows a distal forward curvature. Near its midpoint is a proximally directed nutrient foramen and canal. The *posterior surface*, between interosseous and posterior borders, is largely flat but may be slightly hollow in the proximal area. The *lateral surface* is gently convex; proximally, due to the obliquity of the anterior and posterior borders, it encroaches on the anterior and posterior aspects and is here slightly rough. A finely irregular oval area occurs near the midshaft; beyond this the surface is smooth.

The distal end

The widest part, it is four-sided in section. Its *lateral surface* is slightly rough, projecting distally as a *styloid process* palpable when tendons around it are slack. Distal (**6.224**) is the smooth *carpal articular surface*, divided by a ridge into medial and lateral areas, the medial quadrangular, the lateral triangular and curving on to the styloid process. The *anterior surface* is a thick, prominent ridge, palpable even through overlying tendons, 2 cm proximal to the thenar eminence. The *medial surface* is the *ulnar notch*, smooth, anteroposteriorly concave for articulation with the ulna's head. The *posterior surface* displays a palpable *dorsal tubercle*, limited medially by an oblique groove and in line with the cleft between the index and middle fingers. A wide, shallow groove, lateral to it, is divided by a faint vertical ridge. A similar but undivided groove is medial to the tubercle.

Further details

The *proximal articular surface* of the radial head and its *circumference* are covered by hyaline cartilage, the upper rim (margin) of the latter fitting the groove between the capitulum and trochlea and invading the radial fossa in flexion. The articular circumference joints with the ulnar radial notch and annular ligament, within which it rotates in pronation and supination. The radial neck is enclosed by the

ligament's narrower, distal part, separated by a synovial protrusion from the superior radioulnar joint.

The posterior area of the *tuberosity* is marked by the biceps tendon, but the latter is separated from a smooth anterior area by a bursa, distal to which the oblique cord is attached.

Proximally on the *anterior border* the thin, wide radial head of flexor digitorum superficialis is attached, and to its conspicuous distal part the lateral edge of the extensor retinaculum. The small, triangular area proximal to the ulnar notch is for the deepest part of pronator quadratus.

The proximal two-thirds of the *anterior surface* provides an extensive area for flexor pollicis longus, which conceals the nutrient foramen; the distal quarter is for pronator quadratus. A rough area on the *lateral surface*, midway at its maximal curvature, is for pronator teres. Proximally, the *lateral surface* widens, encroaching on the anterior and posterior, into a long V-shaped area (**6.223**) for supinator. Distal to pronator teres, the lateral surface is covered by tendons of the radial extensors. Proximally on the *posterior surface* abductor pollicis longus is attached and, more distally, extensor pollicis brevis. The remaining surface is devoid of attachments but covered by the long and short extensors of the thumb.

The radial *styloid process* projects beyond that of the ulna, its apex concealed by the tendons of abductor pollicis longus and extensor pollicis brevis. The carpal lateral ligament is attached to its tip. The *lateral surface*, near the styloid, receives brachioradialis and is crossed obliquely, downwards and forwards, by the tendons of abductor pollicis longus and extensor pollicis brevis. The terminal ridge on the *anterior surface* of the lower end is an attachment for the palmar radiocarpal ligament. To a smooth ridge distal to the ulnar notch the base of the triangular articular disc of the inferior radioulnar joint is attached. From the latter, a narrow protrusion of synovial membrane extends proximally anterior to the lower end of the interosseous membrane (p. 646). The lateral part of the *carpal articular surface* articulates with the scaphoid and the medial part with the lateral part of the lunate; in full adduction the latter's proximal surface is wholly in contact with the radius.

The radial *dorsal tubercle* receives a slip from the extensor retinaculum and is grooved medially by the tendon of extensor pollicis longus. The wide groove lateral to the tubercle contains the tendons of extensor carpi radialis longus laterally, extensor carpi radialis brevis medially and their synovial sheaths. Medially the dorsal surface is grooved by the tendons of extensor digitorum, but extensor indicis and the posterior interosseous nerve separate these from the bone. Attached to the distal margin of this surface is the dorsal radiocarpal ligament.

Ossification. The radius ossifies from three centres, in the shaft, appearing centrally in the eighth week, and in each end (**6.225, 226**). Near the end of the first postnatal year ossification begins in the distal epiphysis, and in the proximal at the fourth year in females, fifth in males. The proximal fuses in the fourteenth year in females, seventeenth in males, the distal in the seventeenth and nineteenth years respectively. A fourth centre sometimes appears in the tuberosity about the fourteenth or fifteenth year.

ULNA

The ulna (**6.223, 224**) is medial to the radius in the supinated forearm. Its proximal end is a massive hook (**6.227**), concave forwards. The shaft's lateral border is a sharp (interosseous) crest. The bone diminishes progressively from its proximal mass throughout almost its whole length, but at its distal end expands into a small rounded head and styloid process. The shaft is triangular in section but has no appreciable double curve. In its whole length it is slightly convex posteriorly; but mediolaterally its profile is sinuous; the proximal half has a slight laterally concave curvature, the distal half a medially concave curvature.

The proximal end

The proximal end (**6.227**) has large olecranon and coronoid processes and trochlear and radial notches articulating with the humerus and radius. The *olecranon*, more proximal, is bent forwards at its summit like a beak, which enters the humeral olecranon fossa in extension. Its posterior surface is smooth, triangular and subcutaneous, its proximal border being the elbow's 'point'. In extension it can be felt

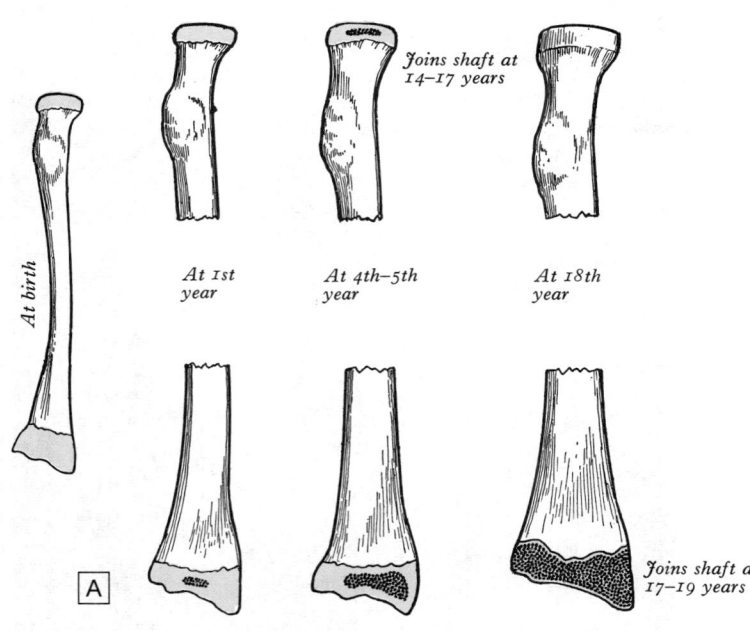

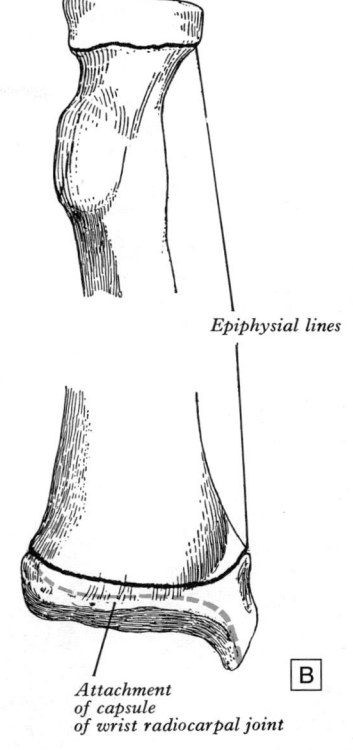

6.225A. Stages in the ossification of the radius (not to scale); B. The epiphyseal lines of the adolescent left radius, anterior aspect. The attachment of the wrist joint capsule is in blue.

near a line joining the humeral epicondyles, but in flexion it descends, the three osseous points forming an isosceles triangle. Its anterior, articular surface forms the proximal area of the trochlear notch. Its base is slightly constricted where it joins the shaft and narrowest part of the proximal ulna. The *coronoid process* projects anteriorly distal to the olecranon, its proximal aspect forming the distal part of the trochlear notch, distal to which, on the lateral surface, is a shallow smooth, oval *radial notch* for articulation with the radial head. Distal to this the surface is hollow to accommodate the radial tuberosity during pronation and supination. The coronoid's anterior surface is triangular, its distal part being the *tuberosity of the ulna*. Its medial border is sharp and bears a small tubercle proximally.

The *trochlear notch* articulates with the trochlea of the humerus. It is constricted at the junction of the olecranon and coronoid processes, where their articular surfaces may be separated by a narrow rough non-articular strip. A smooth ridge, adapted to the humeral trochlea's groove, divides the notch into medial and lateral parts, the medial fitting to the trochlear flange. The *radial notch* (6.227), an oval or oblong proximal depression on the lateral aspect of the coronoid, articulates with the periphery of the radial head, separated from the trochlear notch by a smooth ridge.

The shaft

The shaft is triangular in section (6.223C) in its proximal three-fourths, but distally almost cylindrical. It has anterior, posterior and medial surfaces and interosseous, posterior and anterior borders. The *interosseous border* is a conspicuous lateral crest in its middle two-fourths. Proximally continuous with the posterior border of a depression distal to the radial notch as the *supinator crest*, it disappears distally. The rounded *anterior border* commences medial to the ulnar tuberosity, descending backwards and usually traceable to the base of the styloid process. The *posterior border*, also rounded, descends from the apex of the olecranon's posterior aspect, curving laterally to reach the styloid process. It is *palpable throughout* in a longitudinal furrow most obvious with the elbow in full flexion.

The *anterior surface* (6.223A), between the interosseous and anterior borders, is longitudinally grooved, sometimes deeply. Proximal to its midpoint is a nutrient foramen, directed proximally and containing a branch of the anterior interosseous artery. Distally, it is crossed obliquely by a rough, variable prominence, descending from the interosseous to the anterior border. The *medial surface*, between the anterior and posterior borders, is transversely convex and smooth.

The *posterior surface* (6.223B), between the posterior and interosseous borders, is divided into three areas, the most proximal limited by a sometimes faint oblique line ascending laterally from the junction of the middle and upper thirds of the posterior border to the posterior end of the radial notch (6.227). The region distal to this line is divided into a larger medial and narrower lateral strip by a vertical ridge, usually distinct only in its proximal three-fourths.

The distal end

The distal end, a little expanded, has a head and styloid process. The *head* is visible in pronation on the posteromedial carpal aspect and can be gripped when the supinated hand is flexed. Its lateral convex articular surface fits the radial ulnar notch. Its smooth distal surface (6.224) is separated from the carpus by an articular disc, the apex of which is attached to a rough area between the articular surface and *styloid process*. The latter, a short, round, posterolateral projection of the ulna's distal end, is palpable (most readily in supination) about 1 cm proximal to the plane of the radial styloid. A posterior vertical groove is present between the head and styloid process.

Further details

To the proximal *olecranon* surface, anteriorly, is attached the elbow joint capsule, and to its rough posterior two-thirds the tendon of triceps; these may be separated by a smooth bursal area. Its medial surface is marked proximally by attachment of the posterior and oblique bands of the ulnar collateral ligament and ulnar part of flexor carpi ulnaris. The smooth area distal to this is the most proximal attachment of flexor digitorum profundus. To the lateral olecranon surface, and the adjoining posterior surface of the ulnar shaft as far as its oblique line (6.223B, 227), anconeus is attached. Its posterior surface is separated from the skin by a subcutaneous bursa.

To the anterior surface of the *coronoid process*, including the ulnar tuberosity, brachialis is attached. To a small tubercle at the proximal end of the medial border are attached the oblique and anterior bands of the ulnar collateral ligament and the distal part of the humero-ulnar slip of flexor digitorum superficialis. Distal to this the margin provides attachment for the ulnar part of pronator teres. An ulnar part of flexor pollicis longus may be attached to the lateral or, more rarely, the medial border of the coronoid process (Martin 1958); to its medial surface are attached fibres of flexor digitorum profundus. To the anterior rim of the radial notch the annular ligament is

637

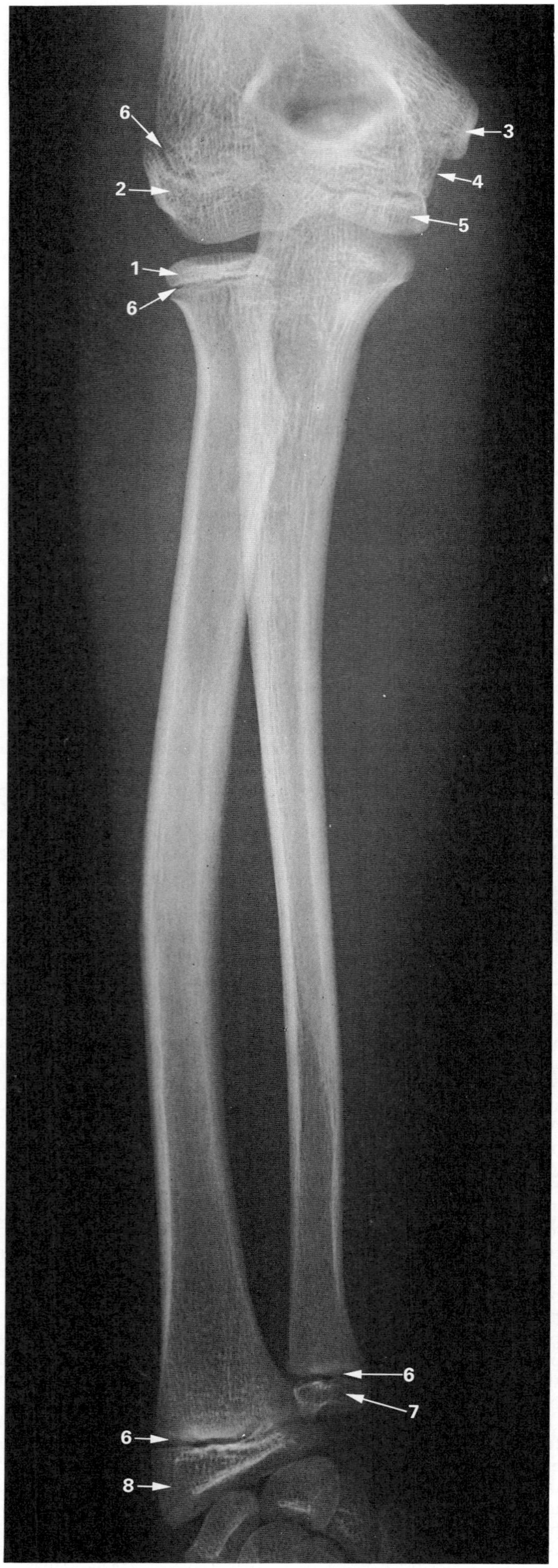

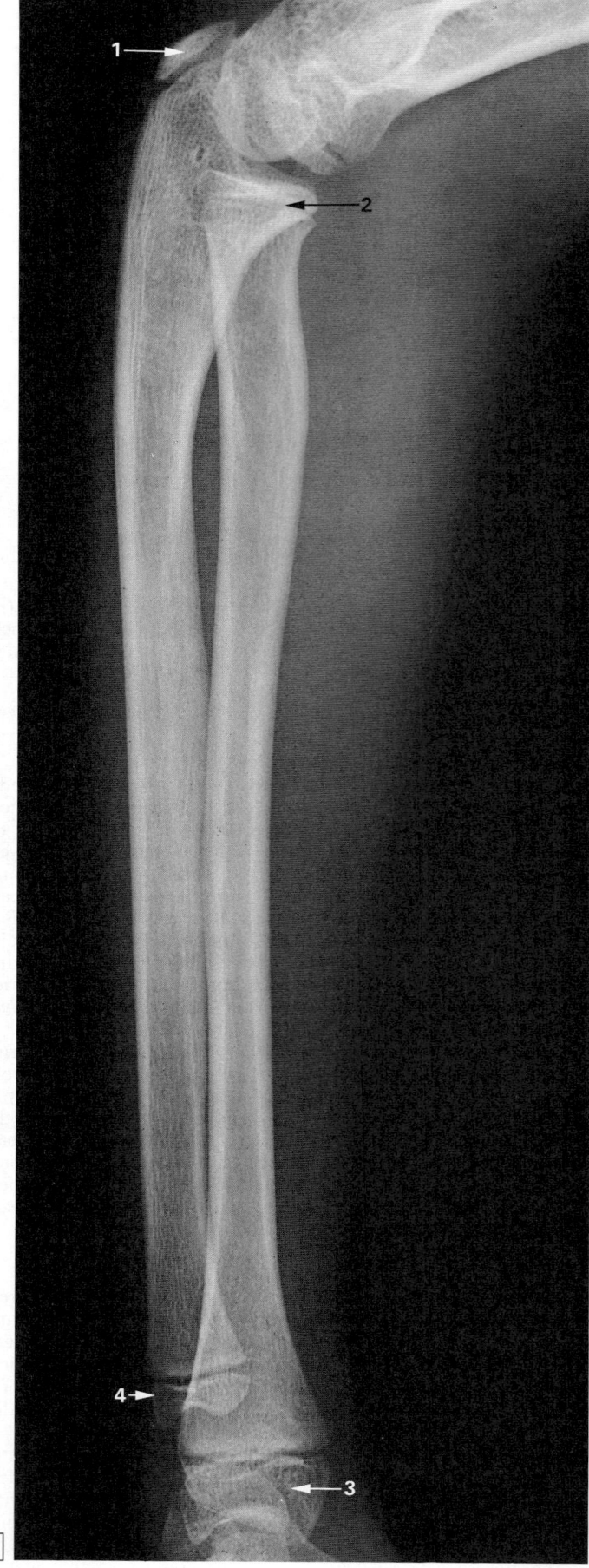

6.226A. Anteroposterior radiograph of the forearm of a girl aged 11.
1. Proximal radial epiphysis. 2. Conjoined epiphyses of capitulum and
lateral epicondyle. 3. Epiphysis of medial epicondyle. 4. Diaphysial bone.
5. Trochlear epiphysis. 6. Cartilaginous growth plates. 7. Distal ulnar
epiphysis. 8. Distal radial epiphysis. B. Lateral radiograph of forearm of a
girl of 11 years, semiflexed at the elbow. Note following epiphyses and
adjacent radiotranslucent growth cartilages: 1. Olecranon. 2. Proximal radial.
3. Distal radial. 4. Distal ulnar.

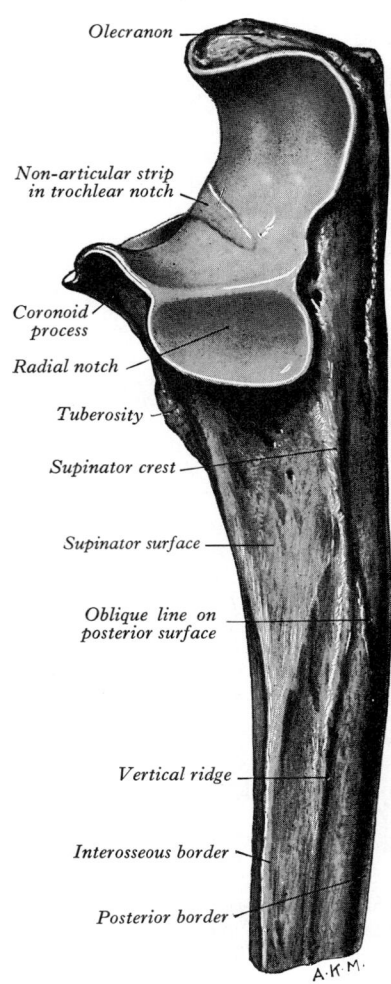

6.227 The proximal end of the left ulna: lateral aspect.

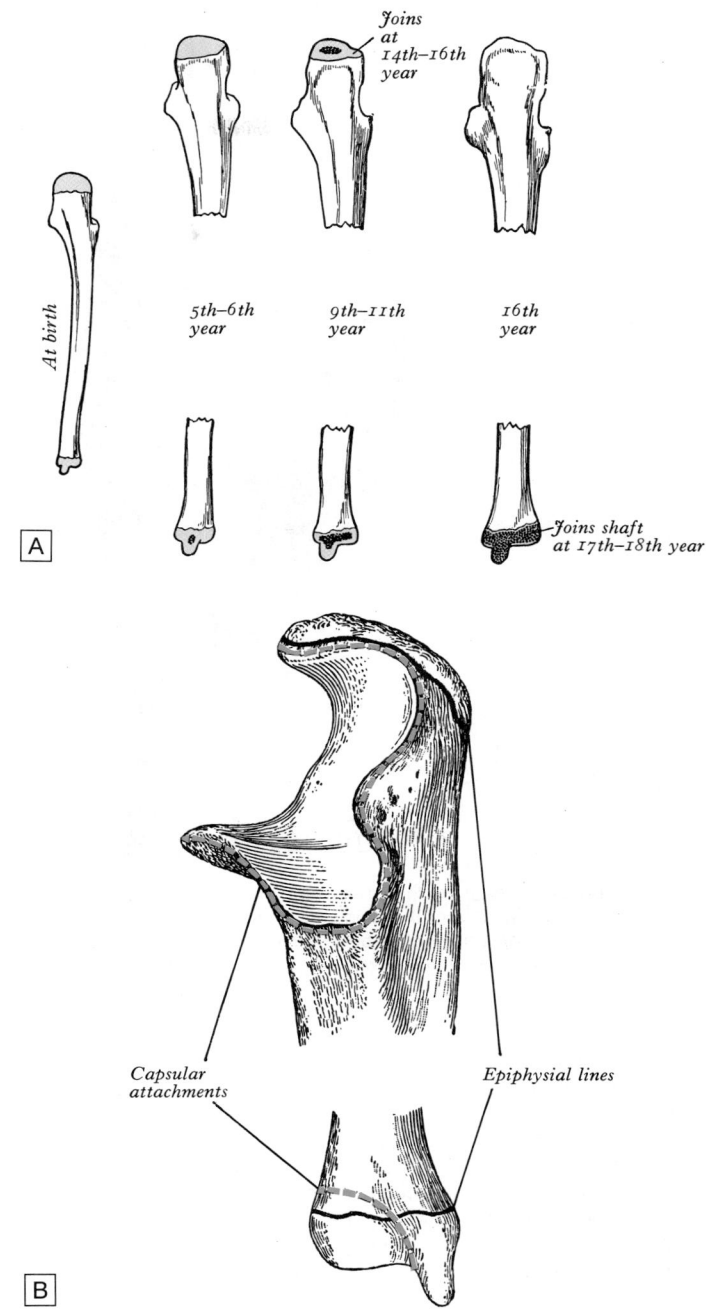

6.228A. Stages in the ossification of the ulna. The diagram is simplified in relation to the ossification of the olecranon epiphysis, which is said to have two centres (see Porteous 1960 and the text); B. The epiphyseal lines of the adolescent left ulna, lateral aspect. The attachment of the joint capsules is in blue.

attached and posteriorly to a ridge at or just behind the notch's posterior margin. The depressed area distal to the notch is limited behind by the *supinator crest*, both providing attachment for supinator.

The olecranonic area of the *trochlear notch* is usually divided into three areas: the most medial faces anteromedially, and is grooved to fit the medial flange of the humeral trochlea with which it makes increasing contact during flexion; a flat intermediate area fits the lateral flange and the most lateral, a narrow strip, abuts the trochlea but only in extension (p. 625). The articular surface is narrower than the olecranon's base; resulting non-articular parts are related to the synovial processes (see 6.230). The coronoid area of the trochlear notch is also divided, its medial and lateral areas corresponding to medial and intermediate olecranonic areas. The medial is hollower, conforming to the convex medial trochlear flange (p. 625); to its medial and anterior borders, the medial and anterior parts of the capsular ligament are attached.

To the subcutaneous *posterior border* is attached the deep fascia of the forearm, which is also, in its proximal three-quarters, an aponeurotic attachment for flexor digitorum profundus; in its proximal half it is another attachment for flexor carpi ulnaris and, in its middle third, for extensor carpi ulnaris. These muscles thus connect with the posterior border through a common blended aponeurosis. To the *interosseous border*, except proximally, is attached the interosseous membrane. To the proximal three-fourths of the *anterior border* flexor digitorum profundus is attached.

The *anterior surface*, in its proximal three-fourths, is for flexor digitorum profundus, as are the anterior border and *medial surface*, ascending medial to the coronoid process and olecranon. The rough strip across the distal fourth of the anterior surface is an attachment of pronator quadratus. Anconeus is attached to the *posterior surface* proximal to the oblique line and lateral to the olecranon. The narrow strip between the interosseous border and vertical ridge is for three deep muscles: abductor pollicis longus from the proximal fourth, and (with a ridge sometimes interposed) from the succeeding fourth for extensor pollicis longus; extensor indicis is attached to the third quarter. The broad strip medial to the vertical ridge is merely covered by extensor carpi ulnaris, whose tendon grooves the posterior aspect of the ulna's distal end. The ulnar collateral ligament is attached to the apex of the *styloid process*.

For an account of ulnar vascularization consult Fischer et al (1974).

Ossification

The ulna ossifies from four main centres, one each in the shaft and distal end and two in the olecranon (6.228). Ossification begins in the midshaft about the eighth fetal week, extending rapidly. In the

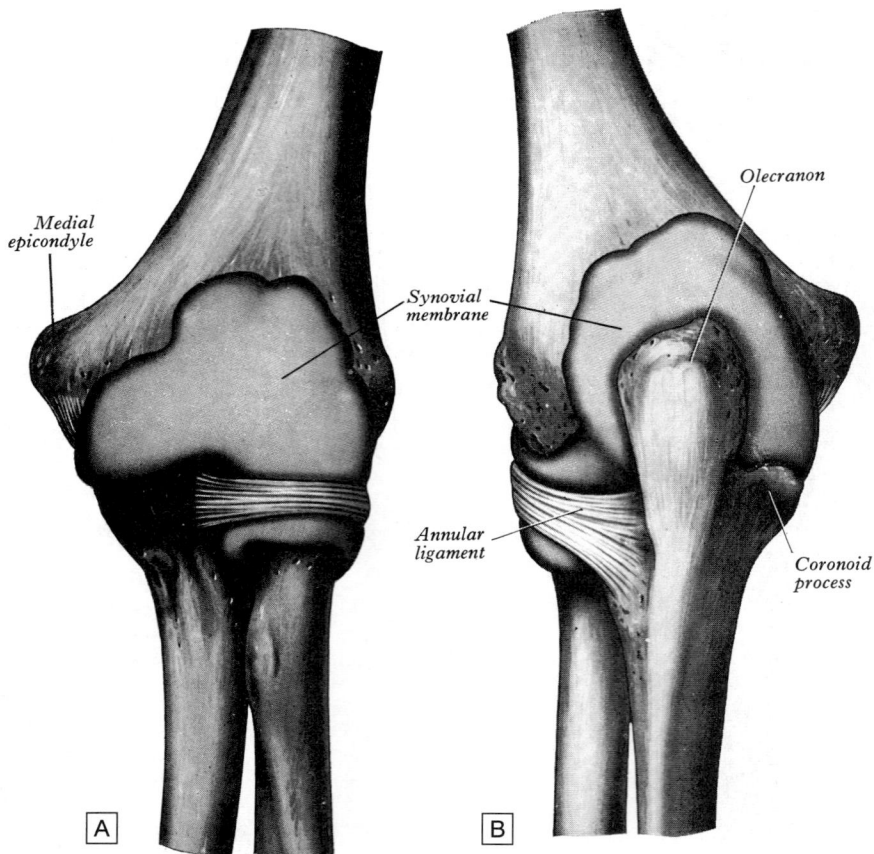

Medial epicondyle

Synovial membrane

Annular ligament

Olecranon

Coronoid process

A

B

6.229A. Synovial cavity of the left elbow joint, partially distended: anterior aspect. The fibrous capsule of the elbow joint has been removed but the thick part of the annular ligament has been left in situ. Note that the synovial membrane descends below the lower border of the annular ligament.

B. Synovial cavity of the left elbow joint, partially distended: posterior aspect of the specimen represented in A. In A and B a small part of the ulnar (medial) collateral ligament may be seen. (Originally drawn from a specimen prepared by J C B Grant.)

fifth (females) and sixth (males) years a centre appears in the distal end, extending into the styloid process. The distal olecranon is ossified as an extension from the shaft, the remainder from two centres, one for the proximal trochlear surface, and a thin scale-like proximal epiphysis on its summit (Porteous 1960). The latter appears in the ninth year in females, eleventh in males; the whole proximal epiphysis has joined the shaft by the fourteenth year in females, sixteenth in males. The distal epiphysis unites with the shaft in the seventeenth year in females, eighteenth in males.

ELBOW JOINT

The elbow joint (**6.229, 230**) includes two articulations:

* *humeroulnar*, between the trochlea of the humerus and the ulnar trochlear notch
* *humeroradial*, between the capitulum of the humerus and the radial head.

It is hence a *compound* synovial joint. Its complexity is increased by continuity with the superior radioulnar joint.

The *articular surfaces* are the humeral trochlea and capitulum, and the ulnar trochlear notch and radial head. The trochlea is not a simple pulley as its medial flange exceeds its lateral, thus projecting to a lower level so that the plane of the joint, about 2 cm distal to the interepicondylar line, is tilted inferomedially; the trochlea is also widest posteriorly and here its lateral edge is sharp. The trochlear notch is not wholly congruent with it; in full extension the medial part of its upper (olecranon) half is not in contact with the trochlea and a corresponding lateral strip loses contact in flexion. The trochlea has an asymmetrical sellar surface, largely concave transversely, convex anteroposteriorly; sections show that these profiles are compounded spirals. Consequently swing is accompanied (as in all hinge joints) by screwing and conjunct rotation (p. 505). Olecranon and

coronoid parts of the trochlear notch are usually separated by a rough strip, devoid of articular cartilage and covered by fibro-adipose tissue and synovial membrane. The capitulum and the radial head are reciprocally curved; closest contact occurs with a semiflexed radius in midpronation. The rim of the head, more prominent medially, fits the groove between humeral capitulum and trochlea.

Since the humeroulnar and humeroradial articulations form a largely uniaxial joint, ligaments are *capsular* and *ulnar* and *radial collateral*.

Fibrous capsule

The fibrous capsule (**6.231, 232**) is anteriorly broad and thin, attaches proximally to the front of the medial epicondyle and humerus above the coronoid and radial fossae, and distally to the edge of the ulnar coronoid process and annular ligament (p. 645), being continuous at its sides with the ulnar and radial collateral ligaments. Anteriorly it receives numerous fibres from brachialis. Posteriorly the capsule is thin and attached to the humerus behind its capitulum and near its lateral trochlear margin, to all but the lower part of the olecranon fossa's edge and to the back of the medial epicondyle. Inferomedially it reaches the olecranon's superior and lateral margins and is laterally continuous with the superior radioulnar capsule deep to the annular ligament (p. 645). It is related posteriorly to the tendon of triceps and to anconeus.

The synovial membrane (**6.229, 231**). It extends from the humeral articular margins, lines the coronoid, radial and olecranon fossae, the flat medial trochlear surface, the capsule's deep surface and the lower part of the annular ligament. Projecting between the radius and ulna from behind is a crescentic synovial fold, partly dividing the joint into humeroradial and humeroulnar parts; irregularly triangular, it contains extra synovial fat (**6.233**). Between the capsule and synovial membrane are three other pads of fat: the largest, at the olecranon fossa, is pressed into it by triceps during flexion; the

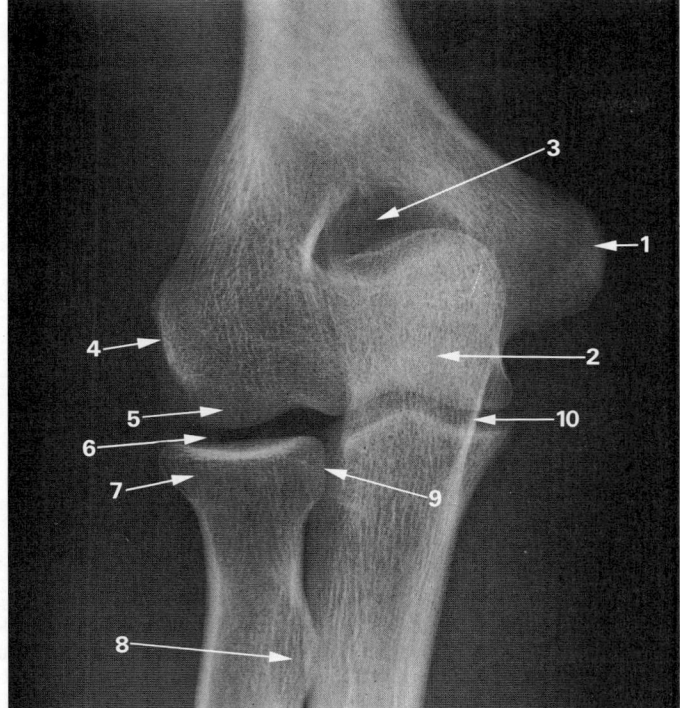

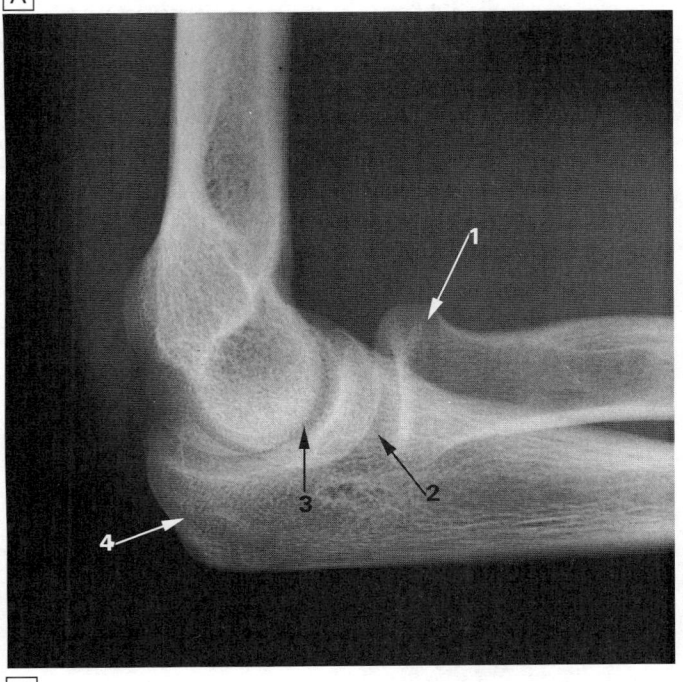

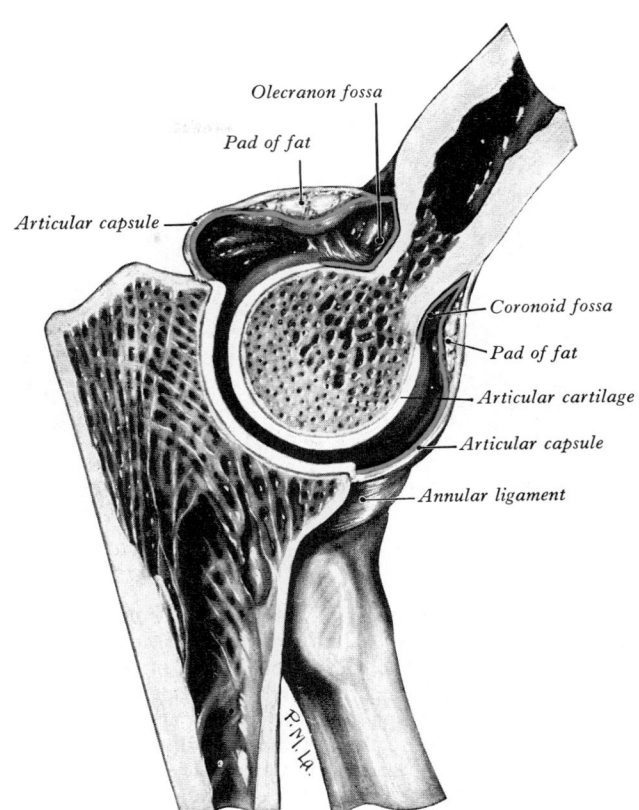

6.231 Sagittal section through the left elbow joint: medial aspect. The synovial membrane is shown in blue.

6.230 Anteroposterior (A) and lateral (B) radiographs of an adult elbow joint. The joint is semiflexed in B.

A. 1. Medial humeral epicondyle. 2. Shadow of olecranon superimposed on trochlea. 3. Olecranon fossa. 4. Lateral epicondyle. 5. Capitulum. 6. Humeroradial joint. 7. Head of radius. 8. Radial tuberosity. 9. Radial head articulating with radial notch of ulna. 10. Humeroulnar joint.

B. 1. Head of radius. 2. Profile of capitulum. 3. Profile of trochlea. 4. Olecranon.

Ulnar collateral ligament

The ulnar collateral ligament is a triangular band, with thick anterior, posterior and inferior parts united by a thin region (**6.232**A). The strongest and stiffest *anterior part* is attached by its apex to the front of the medial epicondyle and by its broad distal base to a proximal tubercle on the medial coronoid margin. The *posterior part*, also triangular, is attached low on the back of the medial epicondyle and to the olecranon's medial margin. Between these two bands intermediate fibres descend from the medial epicondyle to an inferior, *oblique band*, often weak, between the olecranon and coronoid processes, converting a depression on the medial margin of the trochlear notch into a foramen, by which the intracapsular fat pad is continuous with extracapsular fat medial to the joint. The anterior band is taught throughout most of the range of flexion, while the posterior band becomes taut between half and full flexion (Regan et al 1991).

The ulnar collateral ligament is related to triceps, flexor carpi ulnaris and the *ulnar nerve*. Along it, anteriorly, the attachment of flexor digitorum superficialis extends from the medial epicondyle to the medial coronoid border.

Radial collateral ligament

The radial collateral ligament (**6.232**B) is attached low on the lateral epicondyle and to the annular ligament, some of its posterior fibres crossing the ligament to the proximal end of the ulna's supinator crest. It is intimately blended with attachments of supinator and extensor carpi radialis brevis. It is taut throughout most of the range of flexion (Regan et al 1991).

Muscles related to the joint

Muscles related to the joint are: (in front) brachialis, (behind) triceps and anconeus, (laterally) supinator and the common extensor tendon, and (medially) the common flexor tendon and flexor carpi ulnaris.

Vessels and nerve supply to the joint

Articular arteries are from the numerous periarticular anastomoses

other two, at the coronoid and radial fossae, are pressed in by brachialis during extension. They are all slightly displaced in contrary movements. Smaller synovial-covered tags of fat project into the joint near constrictions flanking the trochlear notch (p. 637), covering small non-articular areas of bone.

641

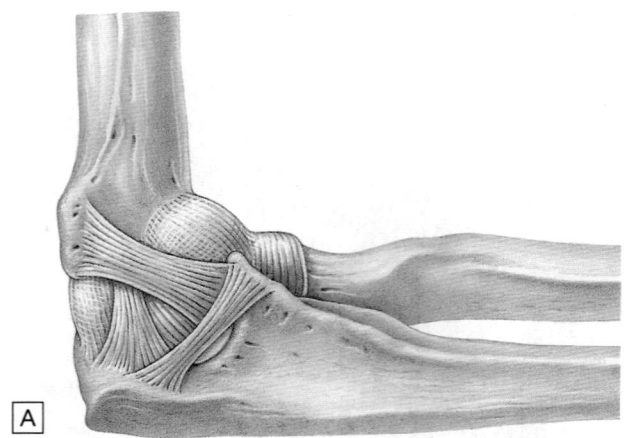

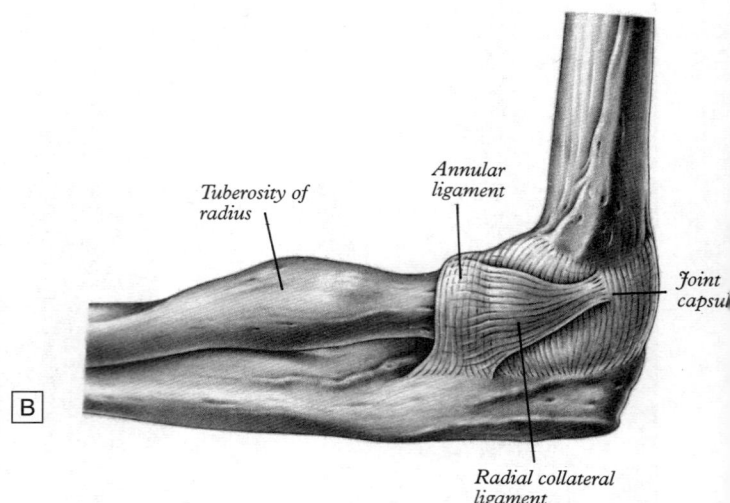

6.232   The left elbow joint; A. Medial aspect; B. Lateral aspect.

(**10**.102). **Articular nerves** are mainly from the musculocutaneous and radial, but the ulnar, median and sometimes anterior interosseous nerves also contribute. The musculocutaneous branch is from the nerve to brachialis and innervates an anterior part of the capsule; branches of the radial supply its posterior and anterolateral regions and come from the nerve to anconeus and the ulnar collateral branch to the medial head of triceps. The ulnar nerve supplies the ulnar collateral ligament behind the medial epicondyle (Gardner 1948b). These articular nerves accompany blood vessels supplying the synovial membrane, fat pads and epiphyses; they presumably contain vasomotor fibres as well as afferent fibres serving pain and proprioception.

Movements

Being a uniaxial joint the elbow allows flexion and extension, ulna moving on the trochlea, radial head on the capitulum. However, ulnar flexion–extension is not a pure swing but accompanied by slight conjunct rotation, the ulna being slightly pronated in extension, supinated in flexion. Since the capitulum is smaller than the radial facet, the head of the radius can be felt at the back of the joint in full extension, which is limited by tension in the capsule and muscles anterior to the joint (extension being the close-packed position) and the entry of the tip of the olecranon into the olecranon fossa; flexion is limited chiefly by apposition of soft parts; in full flexion the rim of the radial head and the tip of the ulnar coronoid process enter the radial and coronoid fossae of the humerus respectively.

When the forearm is fully extended and supinated, it diverges laterally forming with the upper arm a 'carrying angle' of about 163° (Steel & Tomlinson 1958); its ulnar border cannot contact the lateral surface of the thigh. The 'carrying angle' is caused partly by projection of the medial trochlear edge about 6 mm beyond its lateral edge and partly by obliquity of the coronoid's superior articular surface, which is not orthogonal to the ulna's shaft. Tilt of the humeral and ulnar articular surfaces is approximately equal; hence the carrying angle disappears in full flexion, the two bones reaching the same plane. When the adducted arm is flexed the little finger meets the clavicle, due to the position of the resting humerus (p. 631); with the humerus rotated laterally, the hand reaches the front of the

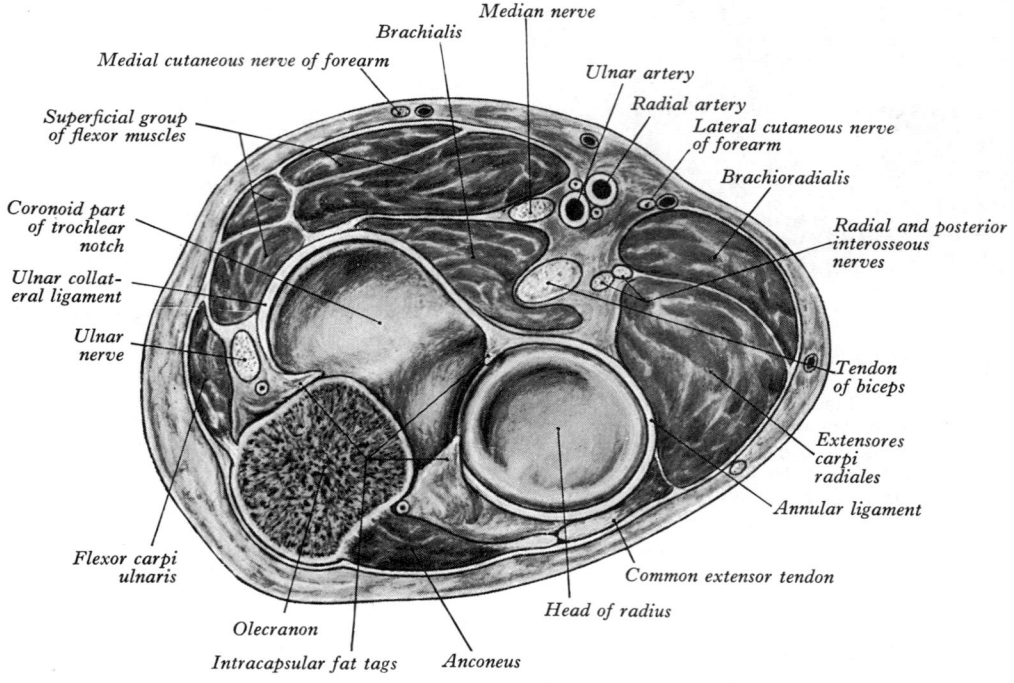

6.233   Transverse section of the right elbow joint to show the relations of the joint: superior aspect. Note the intracapsular fat 'tags' with meniscoid transverse-sectional profiles.

shoulder. The carrying angle is also masked by pronation of the extended forearm, which brings the upper arm, semipronated forearm and hand into line, increasing manual precision in full extension of the elbow or during extension.

Accessory movements. These are limited to slight ulnar screwing, abduction and adduction, and anteroposterior translation of the radial head on the humeral capitulum. In translation the radial head moves on the ulnar radial notch and the annular ligaments are slewed backwards and forwards, more so when the elbow is semiflexed.

Muscles producing movement

Flexion: brachialis, biceps and brachioradialis. In slow flexion or its maintenance against gravity, brachialis and biceps are principally involved, even for light loads. With increasing speed, activity in brachioradialis is increasingly prominent (MacConaill 1949; Basmajian 1959); due to its attachments it acts most effectively in midpronation. Against resistance pronator teres and flexor carpi radialis may also act.

Extension: triceps, anconeus and gravity. In rapid extension brachioradialis may again be active.

Elbow arthroplasty

Excision arthroplasty—current practice and status

Excision arthroplasty of the elbow was first successfully performed in 1797 by Moreau in Paris. During the following century the technique became well established in the surgical repertoire, being discussed in great detail by Ollier in 1988. Today excision arthroplasty remains the preferred option in many centres.

Over the years the original radical excision has been modified to a more anatomical re-contouring of the joint, frequently supplemented by the introduction of an interpositional membrane. Historically a variety of materials have been tried; currently the most frequently used are fascia lata, dura mater or skin.

Evidence from the literature suggests that provided excision arthroplasties are performed on patients younger than 50 with good musculature, satisfactory pain relief and a useful range of movement can be achieved in 50–70% of cases (Knight & van Zandt 1952). The largest clientele for arthroplasty, at present, are patients suffering from rheumatoid arthritis. For them, however, excision arthroplasty has serious limitations: although marked pain relief and a useful range of movement can be achieved, joint stability is often poor due to a lack of muscle power to stabilize the pseudarthrosis. Moreover, such patients appear to be liable to develop further bone resorption such that an initially satisfactory arthroplasty may become completely dislocated (Hurri et al 1964; Souter 1990; 6.234). Because of these problems the development of total replacement arthroplasty of the elbow has been of considerable interest over the last 25 years.

Metallic hinge arthroplasty—early failures

The first total elbow replacement (a metallic hinge) was reported by Boerema and de Waard (1942), following which hemi- and total arthroplasty for individual patients were developed. Real interest, however, developed in the late 1960s with the advent of cemented metallic hinge prostheses. Early results were successful but soon unacceptably high levels of humeral loosening, with the accompany-

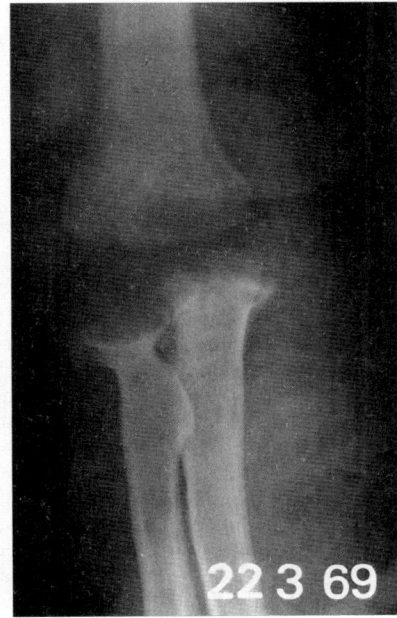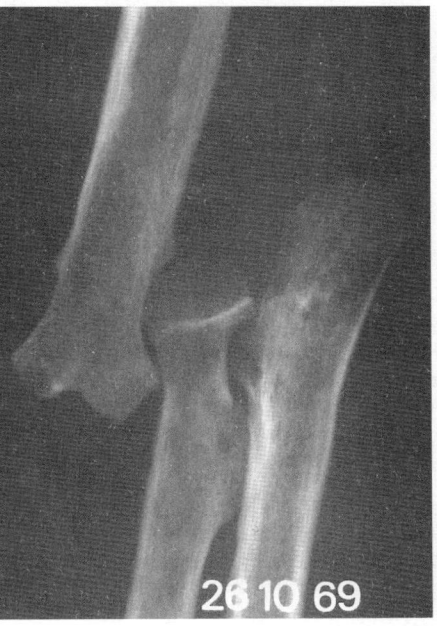

6.234 Radiographs of excision arthroplasty immediately after surgery and 18 months later. Note the degree of bone resorption which has occurred leading to complete dislocation of the pseudarthrosis.

ing danger of grossly comminuted fractures of the thinned and ballooned distal humeral shaft, became apparent, especially in the event of a fall (Dee 1977; Souter 1977).

Reasons for failure

Surprisingly high forces are transmitted across the elbow; however, it is not the compressive loads which are most likely to cause loosening of any constrained implant, but rather a combination of the torsional forces generated during ordinary daily activities and the anteroposterior force vectors, which are constantly reversing during any cycle of elbow movement (Nicol et al 1977; Amis et al 1981; Morrey & Brian 1985).

Development and classification of current prostheses

During the last two decades prosthetic designs and methods of fixation which successfully resist displacing forces have been developed. The resulting variety of prostheses can be classified into two main groups:

(1) Linked prostheses, based on a hinge mechanism, conferring great stability. Hinge design has improved through the use of longer stems, the introduction of high density polyethylene (HDP) bushing, and the incorporation of flanges or metal shells to resist torsional and anteroposterior forces. Several degrees of freedom of movement have been introduced into the hinge mechanism with regard to valgus/varus and axial movements to allow the ligaments to resist some of the stresses. Such prostheses (Inglis & Pellicci 1980; Gschwend et al 1988; Morrey & Adams 1992) appear to be achieving good success (6.235).

(2) Unlinked prostheses use designs approaching the normal anatomy of the humeroulnar joint and rely to a large degree on the collateral ligaments and other soft tissues for stability (Souter 1990; Kudo & Iwano 1990; Ewald et al 1993; 6.236). Preservation of the collateral ligaments is therefore of great importance for the success of most types of unlinked elbow arthroplasty.

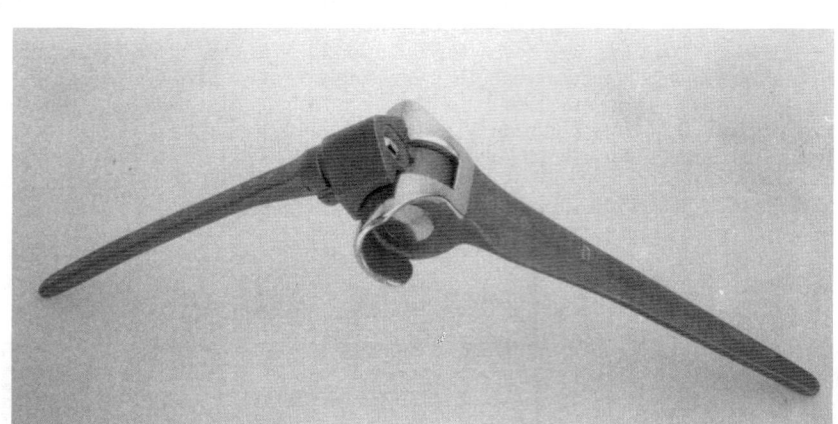

6.235 GSB III linked prosthesis incorporating a sloppy hinge mechanism and projecting metal shells to fit over the residual humeral condyles to provide resistance to torsional and anteroposterior forces.

during closure may produce puckering and tightness in the ligament inducing an Osborne lesion: routine release of the arcuate ligament greatly diminishes the incidence of ulnar neuritis.

Other significant problems accompanying total elbow replacement are dislocation or disassembly of the joint mechanism, infection and aseptic loosening. However, these problems can each be contained within an incidence of 3–4%: such complications often overlap so that revision rates as low as 5–6% are currently reported. This appears to be an acceptable level of performance to establish total joint replacement as the treatment of choice for grade 4 erosions of the elbow or even perhaps for late grade 3.

Conclusions with regard to current status and applications of total elbow replacement

Following the improved results of elbow replacement in the management of rheumatoid disease, the operation is now increasingly used in the management of trauma, juvenile chronic arthritis, and some skeletal dysplasias. With many of the post-traumatic problems collateral ligament support has been lost and linked prostheses become essential: this is also the case for much revision surgery.

No single implant can provide an ideal solution for all problems; however, with a variety of endoprostheses or a graduated system of implants comprising both linked and unlinked joints, the entire spectrum of elbow pathology, including tumours, are now amenable to reconstructive surgery.

Results

For both the newer linked and unlinked prostheses survivorship at 10 years is similar to that of hip and knee replacement. Relief of pain and the recovery of movement especially flexion, pronation and supination has been very satisfactory; the recovery of extension, however, has been less satisfactory (Inglis & Pellicci 1980; Gschwend et al 1988; Souter 1990; Kudo & Iwano 1990; Morrey & Adams 1992; Ewald et al 1993).

Complications

Ulnar neuritis can be an annoying postoperative complication, especially with

unlinked techniques aiming to restore the normal anatomy of the humeroulnar joint. Such operations result in a reversal of the proximal migration of the ulna which inevitably follows severe erosion of the trochlea. Thus in the immediate postoperative period the ulnar nerve may be subjected to significant stretch, the effect of which may be increased by pressure from the arcuate ligament between the two heads of flexor carpi ulnaris, which itself will have been made tighter by the distal displacement of the ulna. Moreover, during exposure, the arcuate ligament and ulnar head of flexor carpi ulnaris are detached from the coronoid. Resuture

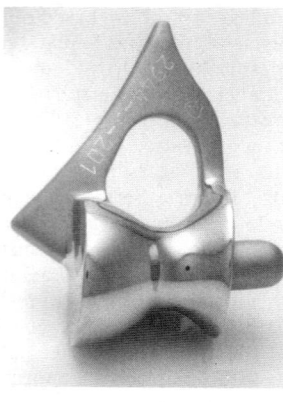
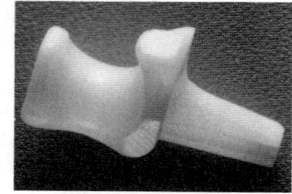
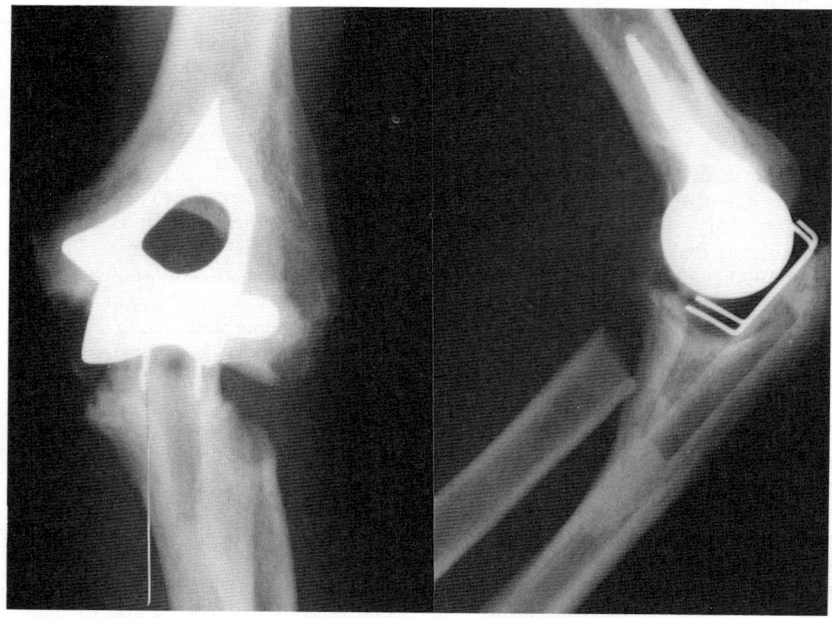

6.236 Souter-Strathclyde unlinked prosthesis with radiographs components cemented in position. Note the anatomically contoured articular surfaces of the trochlea and the stirrup fixation within the humeral condyles and supracondylar ridges.

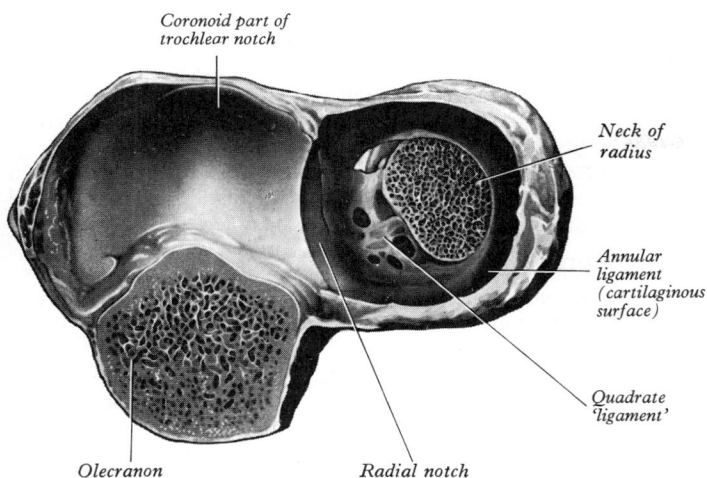

*Coronoid part of
trochlear notch*

*Neck of
radius*

*Annular
ligament
(cartilaginous
surface)*

*Quadrate
'ligament'*

Olecranon

Radial notch

6.237   Distal socket of the superior radioulnar joint. The radial neck is transected and its head withdrawn. The socket consists of the chondrified aspect of the annular ligament, the articular cartilage of the radial notch of the ulna and the lax almost retiform quadrate 'ligament'. Section at the olecranon's base reveals, anteriorly, the sellar articular surface of the coronoid part of the trochlear notch (humeroulnar joint).

RADIOULNAR JOINTS

The radius and ulna articulate by synovial *superior* (*proximal*) and *inferior* (*distal*) *radioulnar joints* and by an intermediate interosseous membrane and ligament, a non-synovial *middle radioulnar union*.

The superior (proximal) radioulnar joint

The superior radioulnar joint is a uniaxial pivot between the circumference of the radial head and the fibro-osseous ring made by the ulnar radial notch and annular ligament.

Annular ligament (6.232, 237). A strong band, it encircles the radial head, holding it against the ulna's radial notch. Forming about four-fifths of the ring, it is attached to the notch's anterior margin, broadens posteriorly and may divide into several bands and is attached to a rough ridge at or behind the notch's posterior margin; diverging bands may also reach the lateral margin of the trochlear notch above and proximal end of the supinator crest below. The proximal annular border blends with the elbow joint capsule, except posteriorly where the capsule passes deep to the ligament to reach the posterior and inferior margins of the radial notch. From the distal annular border a few fibres pass over reflected synovial membrane to attach loosely on the radial neck. A thin, fibrous quadrate ligament covers the synovial membrane on the joint's distal surface (Martin 1958). The annular ligament's external surface blends with the radial collateral ligament and is an attachment of part of supinator. Posterior to it are anconeus and the interosseous recurrent artery. Internally the ligament is thinly covered by cartilage where it is in contact with the radial head; distally it is covered by synovial membrane, reflected up onto the radial neck.

The middle radioulnar union

The radial and ulnar shafts are connected by syndesmoses—an oblique cord and an interosseous membrane.

Oblique cord (6.238). This is a small, inconstant, flat fascial band on the deep head of supinator, extending from the lateral side of the ulnar tuberosity to the radius a little distal to its tuberosity. Its fibres are at right angles to those in the interosseous membrane. Its functional significance is dubious.

Interosseous membrane (6.238). A broad, thin, collagenous sheet, its fibres slant distomedially between the radial and ulnar interosseous borders, and its distal part is attached to the posterior division of the radial border. Two or three posterior bands occasionally descend distolaterally across the other fibres. The membrane is deficient proximally, starting about 2 or 3 cm distal to the radial tuberosity. It is broader at midlevel and has an oval aperture near its distal margin conducting the anterior interosseous vessels to the back of the forearm. Between its proximal border and the oblique

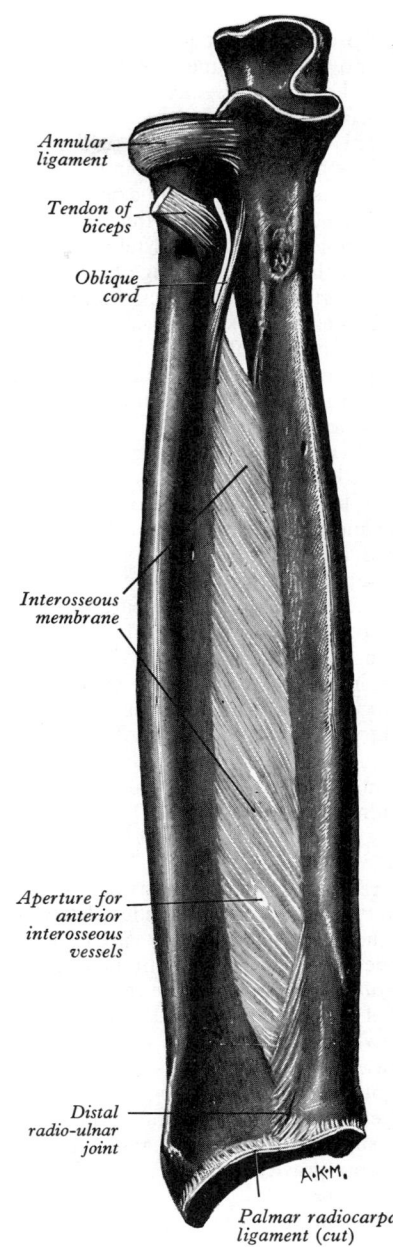

*Annular
ligament*

*Tendon of
biceps*

*Oblique
cord*

*Interosseous
membrane*

*Aperture for
anterior
interosseous
vessels*

*Distal
radio-ulnar
joint*

A·K·M.

*Palmar radiocarpal
ligament (cut)*

6.238   Interosseous membrane and oblique cord of the forearm: anterior aspect. Membrane and cord are syndesmoses.

cord is a gap for the posterior interosseous vessels. The membrane provides attachments of the deep forearm muscles and connects the two bones. Its fibres appear to transmit to the ulna and humerus forces acting proximally from the hand to the radius; however, it is only tense when the hand is midway between prone and supine positions and is relaxed in complete pronation and supination; the hand is usually pronated when subject to such forces. Moreover, the radius can transmit substantial forces directly to the humerus (Travill 1964). **Anteriorly** the membrane is related, in its proximal three-quarters, laterally to flexor pollicis longus and medially to flexor digitorum profundus, between them to the anterior interosseous vessels and nerve, and in its distal quarter to pronator quadratus; **posteriorly** are supinator, abductor pollicis longus, extensores pollicis brevis, longus and indicis and, near the carpus, the anterior interosseous artery and posterior interosseous nerve.

The inferior (distal) radioulnar joint

The inferior radioulnar joint is a uniaxial pivot between the convex distal head of the ulna and the concave ulnar notch of the radius; these surfaces are enclosed by a capsule and connected by an articular disc. The fibrous capsule is thicker in front and behind, proximally lax and lined by synovial membrane projecting proximally between the radius and ulna as a *recessus sacciformis* in front of the distal part of the interosseous membrane (see **6.250**).

Articular disc. This is fibrocartilaginous (collagen with few elastic fibres in the young) and is triangular, binding the distal ends of the ulna and radius. Its periphery is thicker, its centre sometimes perforated. It is attached by a blunt, thick apex to a depression between the ulnar styloid process and distal articular surface and by its wider thin base to the prominent edge between the ulnar notch and carpal articular surface of the radius. Its margins are united to adjacent carpal ligaments, its surfaces smooth and concave; the proximal articulates with the ulnar head, the distal is part of the radiocarpal joint, articulating with the lunate and, when the hand is adducted, the triquetral. Mikić (1978) and Mikić et al (1992) have observed, in studies on 237 wrists and articular discs ranging from fetuses to 94 years, that the discs show age-dependent degeneration: progressively reduced cellularity, loss of elastic fibres, mucoid degeneration, exposure of collagen fibres, fibrillation, ulceration, abnormal thinning and ultimate perforation. The structure of various parts of the disc is adapted to the functional stresses exerted on them; in central parts the tissue is more cartilaginous while the peripheral margins have a ligament-like pattern (Mikić et al 1992). No perforations appeared in the first two decades, 7.6% in the third, 18.1% in the fourth, 40% in the fifth, 42.8% in the sixth and 53.1% in those over 60. Comparable degenerative changes frequently occur in the 'discal' surfaces of the ulna and lunate.

Vessels and nerve supply to the joint. The **arterial supply** to the joint and disc is mainly from the palmar and dorsal branches of the anterior interosseous artery, reinforced by the posterior interosseous and ulnar arteries (Mikić 1992).

Movements

Movements at the radioulnar joint complex pronate and supinate the hand. In *pronation* the radius carrying the hand turns anteromedially obliquely across the ulna, its proximal end remaining lateral, its distal becoming medial. During this action the interosseous membrane becomes *spiralled*. In *supination* the radius returns to a position lateral and parallel to the ulna (and the interosseous membrane becomes *unspiralled*). The hand can be turned thus through 140°–150° and, with the elbow extended, this can be increased to nearly 360° by humeral rotation and scapular movements. Power is greater in supination, affecting the design of nuts, bolts and screws, which are tightened by supination in right-handed persons. Moreover, supination is an **anti gravity** movement (with a pendent upper arm, and semiflexed forearm); in seizing objects for examination or manipulation, pronation is merely a preliminary and is **aided** by gravity.

The axis for pronation and supination is often represented as a line through the centre of the radial head (proximal) and the ulnar attachment of the articular disc (distal). More correctly this is the axis of movement of the **radius relative to the ulna** and it **does not remain stationary**. The radial head rotates in the fibro-osseous ring: its distal lower end and articular disc swing round the ulnar head. During rotation of the radial head in this ring its proximal surface spins on the humeral capitulum. The distal end of the ulna is **not stationary** during this movement; it moves a variable amount along a curved course, posterolaterally in pronation, anteromedially in supination. This entails that the axis, as defined above, is displaced laterally in pronation, medially in supination. Hence **the axis for supination and pronation of the whole forearm and hand** passes **between** the bones at both the superior and inferior radioulnar joints, when ulnar movement is marked, but through the centres of the radial head and ulnar styloid when it is minimal. The axis may be prolonged through any digit, depending on medial or lateral displacement of the distal end of the ulna (Ray et al 1951). Note that this displacement is not conjunct rotation; it can be varied at will. For example, the index finger and thumb, in a precision grip (p. 867), can describe arcs of varying radius according to functional demands. Greatest radius of arc involves minimal ulnar deviation, whereas rotation of opposed digits around a virtually fixed point (often necessary in manipulation of tools and instruments) involves marked and even maximal ulnar displacement. Ulnar movements are possible because of the incongruence of the trochlea and trochlear notch, therefore

occurring **without** humeral rotation, whether the elbow is flexed, semiflexed or extended. Since this incongruence persists in all elbow positions, the 'close-packed position' of the humeroulnar articulation at terminal elbow extension depends on ligaments rather than articular geometry.

Accessory movements. These include backward and forward translation of the radial head on the ulnar radial notch (p. 637) and the ulnar head likewise on the radial ulnar notch.

Muscles producing movement

Pronation: pronator quadratus, aided in rapid movement and against resistance by pronator teres (Basmajian & Travill 1961). Gravity also assists.

Supination: supinator, in slow unresisted movement and extension, assisted by biceps in fast movements in flexion, especially when resisted.

Electromyographic studies have not confirmed activity in brachioradialis during pronation and supination.

Clinical anatomy

At the elbow joint backward dislocation with ulnar abduction are commonest, the former often complicated by fracture of the coronoid process. Owing to the strength of collateral ligaments, the medial epicondyle is frequently torn off in lateral dislocations.

In acute synovitis the joint cavity becomes distended, bulging most around the olecranon, due to capsular laxity here. There is often some swelling above the radial head or the whole elbow may become fusiform.

Dislocation of the radial head alone is not uncommon, most frequently in youth from falls on the hand with the forearm extended and supinated, the head being displaced forwards, with rupture of the annular ligament. Occasionally a peculiar injury, supposedly a subluxation, occurs in children. The radial head appears to be displaced distally in the annular ligament; its upper border is folded over the head between it and the capitulum; the small size of the head in children predisposes to this. The forearm becomes fixed in semiflexion, midway between supination and pronation.

WRIST AND HAND

The hand's skeleton has three regions:

- the carpus
- the metacarpus
- the phalanges.

In the following description *proximal* and *distal* are used in preference to *superior* and *inferior*, and *palmar* and *dorsal*, which are self-explanatory, rather than *anterior* and *posterior*.

CARPUS

General features

The carpus (**6.239, 240**) contains eight bones in proximal and distal rows of four. Proximally, in lateral to medial order, are the *scaphoid*, *lunate*, *triquetral* and *pisiform*; in the distal row are the *trapezium*, *trapezoid*, *capitate* and *hamate*. The pisiform articulates with the palmar surface of the triquetral, thus separated from the other carpal bones, all of which articulate with their neighbours. The other three proximal bones form an arch proximally convex, articulating with the radius and articular disc of the inferior radioulnar joint. The arch's concavity is a distal recess embracing, proximally, the projecting aspects of the capitate and hamate; the two rows are thus mutually and firmly adapted without any loss of movement.

The dorsal carpal surface is convex and the palmar forms a deeply concave *carpal groove*, accentuated by the palmar projection of the lateral and medial borders. The medial projection is formed by the *pisiform* and the *hamulus* (*hook*), an unciform palmar process of the *hamate*. The pisiform is at the proximal border of the hypothenar eminence, medial in the palm; it is easily felt in front of the triquetral. The hamulus is concave laterally, its tip palpable 2.5 cm distal to the pisiform, in line with the radial border of the ring finger. The ulnar nerve's superficial division can be rolled on it. The lateral border of the carpal groove is formed by the *tubercles* of the *scaphoid* and

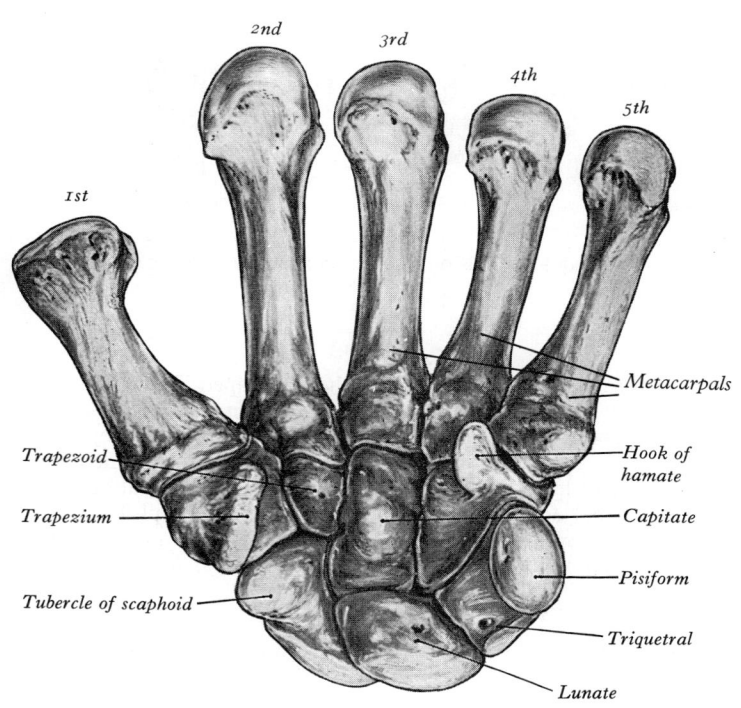

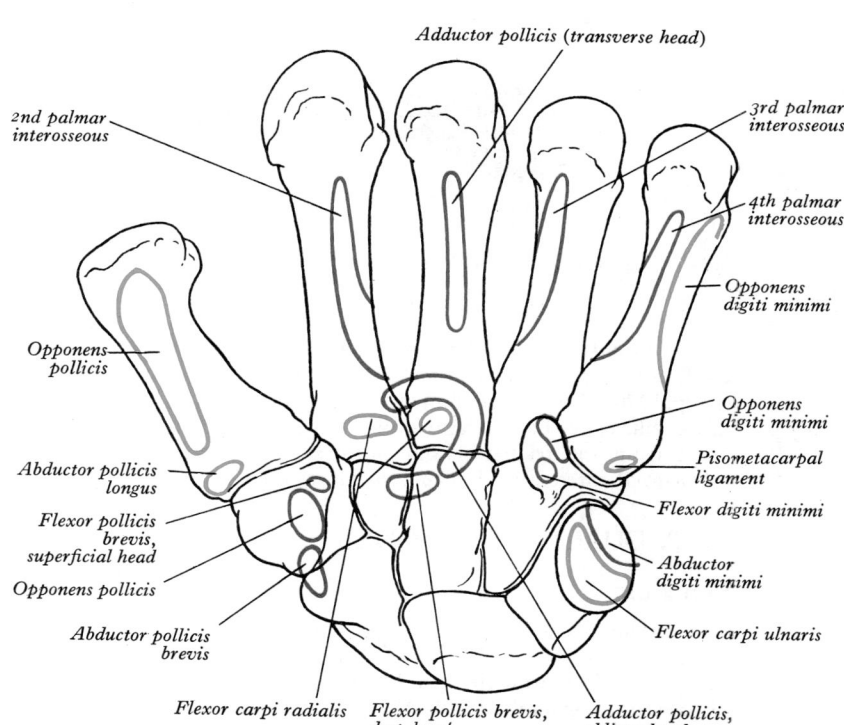

6.239 The palmar aspect of the carpal and metacarpal bones of the left hand. Muscle attachments, except for the dorsal interossei, are shown on the line drawing on the right.

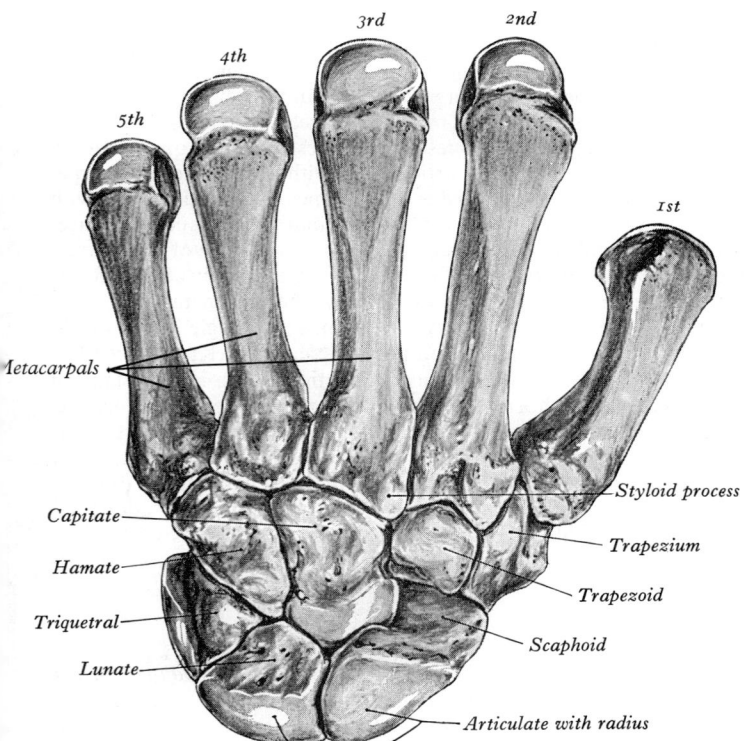

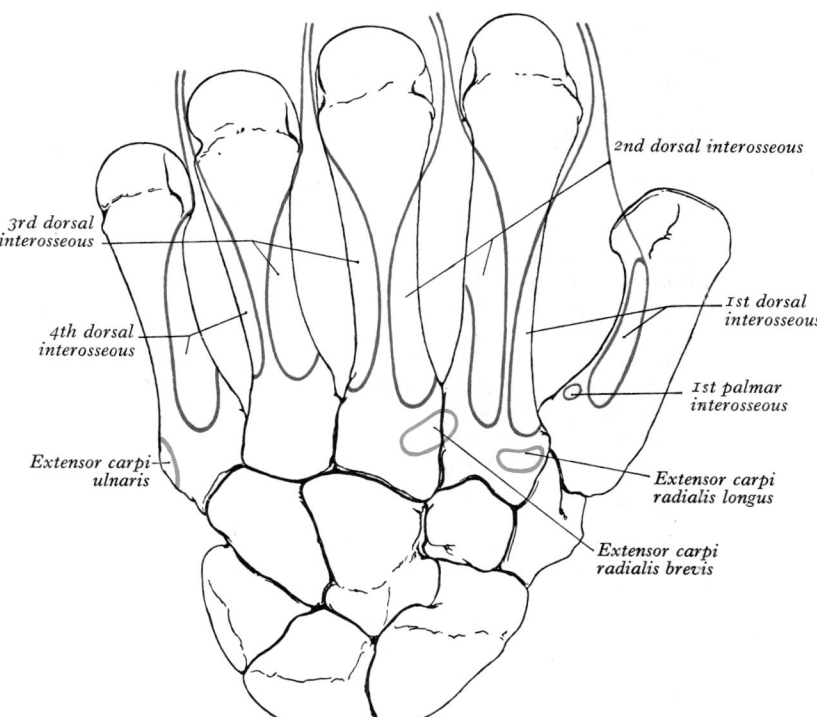

6.240 The dorsal aspect of the carpal and metacarpal bones of the left hand. Muscle attachments are shown on the line drawing on the right.

trapezium. The former is distal on the anterior scaphoid surface and palpable, sometimes also visible, as a small medial knob at the proximal border of the palmar thenar eminence, lateral to the tendon of flexor carpi radialis. The tubercle of the trapezium is a vertically rounded ridge on the bone's anterior surface, slightly hollow medially and just distal and lateral to the scaphoid tubercle; it is difficult to palpate. (Both the scaphoid and trapezium may be grasped individually and moved passively, by firm pressure between an opposed index finger and thumb applied to the palmar surface and anatomical snuff-box simultaneously.) The carpal groove is made into an osseo-

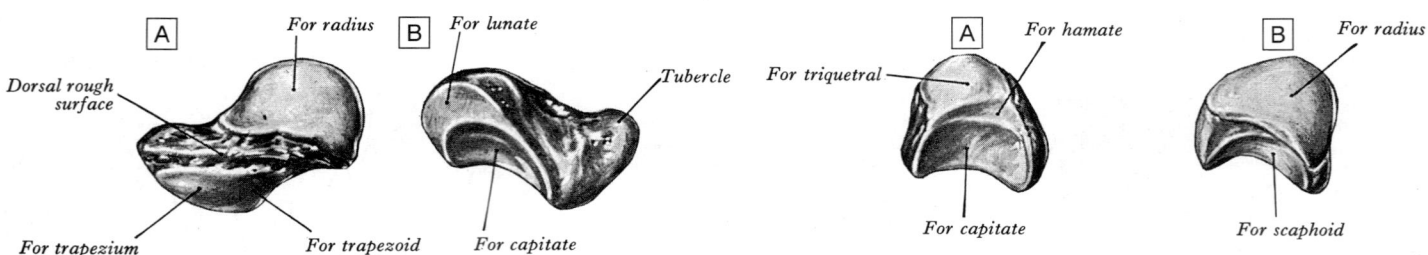

6.241   The left scaphoid: A. Dorsal, B. Palmar aspects.

6.242   The left lunate: A. Distomedial; B. Proximolateral aspects.

fibrous *carpal tunnel* by a fibrous retinaculum attached to its margins; the tunnel carries flexor tendons and the median nerve into the hand (see p. 1270). The retinaculum strengthens the carpus and augments flexor efficiency. Palmar and dorsal surfaces of the carpal bones, apart from the triquetral and pisiform, are attachments of the *radiocarpal, intercarpal* and *carpometacarpal* ligaments.

INDIVIDUAL CARPAL BONES

Scaphoid

The scaphoid (**6.241**), largest element in the proximal carpal row, has a long axis which is distal, lateral and slightly palmar in direction. Its round tubercle on the distolateral part of its *palmar surface* is directed anterolaterally (**6.239A**), and is an attachment of the flexor retinaculum and abductor pollicis brevis; it is crossed by the tendon of flexor carpi radialis. The rough *dorsal surface* is slightly grooved, narrower than the palmar, and pierced by small nutrient foramina, often restricted to the distal half (13%) (Obletz & Halbstein 1938), an observation of clinical significance. The *lateral surface*, also narrow and rough, has the radial collateral ligament attached to it. The remaining surfaces are all articular: the *radial surface* is convex, proximal and directed proximolaterally; the *lunate surface* is flat, semilunar, facing medially; the *capitate surface* is large, concave and distal, directed distomedially. The *surface* for the *trapezium* and *trapezoid* is continuous, convex and distal.

Lunate

The lunate (**6.242**), approximately semilunar, articulates between the scaphoid and triquetal in the proximal carpal row. Its rough *palmar surface*, almost triangular, is larger and wider than the rough *dorsal surface*. Its smooth convex *proximal surface* articulates with the radius and articular disc of the inferior radioulnar joint. Its narrow *lateral surface* bears a flat semilunar facet for the scaphoid. The *medial surface*, almost square, articulates with the triquetral and is separated from the distal surface by a curved ridge, usually somewhat concave (**6.242A**) for articulation with the edge of the hamate in adduction. The *distal surface* is deeply concave to fit the medial part of the head of the capitate.

Triquetral

The triquetral (**6.243**), somewhat pyramidal, bears an oval isolated facet for articulation with the pisiform on its distal *palmar surface*. Its *medial* and *dorsal surfaces* are confluent, marked distally by attachment of the ulnar collateral ligament but smooth proximally for the articular disc of the inferior radioulnar joint in full adduction. The *hamate surface*, lateral and distal, is concavoconvex, broad proximally, narrow distally. The *lunate surface*, almost square, is proximal and lateral.

Pisiform

The pisiform (**6.244**), as its name implies, is shaped like a pea, with a *dorsal* flat *articular facet* for the triquetral; it has a distolateral long axis. The palmar non-articular area, surrounding and projecting distal to the articular surface, has the tendon of the flexor carpi ulnaris attached to it and also the tendon's distal continuations, the pisometacarpal and pisohamate ligaments. Hence the pisiform has attributes of a sesamoid bone (see p. 735), which it almost certainly is, being unrepresented in primitive carpalia (p. 616).

Trapezium

The trapezium (**6.245**) has a tubercle and groove on its rough palmar surface. The groove is medial and contains the tendon of flexor carpi radialis; to its margins are attached two layers of the flexor retinaculum **7.106** and page 852. The *tubercle* is obscured by attached thenar muscles, opponens pollicis between flexor pollicis brevis distally and abductor pollicis brevis proximally (**6.239B**). The elongate, rough *dorsal surface* is related to the radial artery. The large *lateral surface* is rough for attachment of the radial collateral ligament and capsular ligament of the pollicial carpometacarpal joint. A large *sellar surface* faces distolaterally for the base of the first metacarpal, its surface area being significantly smaller in females, as well as having a fundamentally different shape from that in males (Ateshian et al 1992). Most distally it projects between the bases of the first and second metacarpal bones and carries a small, quadrilateral, distomedially directed facet articulating with the second metacarpal base. The large *medial surface* is gently concave for articulation with the trapezoid. The *proximal surface* is a small, slightly concave facet for the scaphoid. Due to its contribution to mobility of the thumb, the metacarpal articular surface has attracted much attention. Its ridge or 'summit', fitting the concavity of the first metacarpal base, extends in a palmar and lateral direction, at an angle of about 60° with the plane of the second and third metacarpals (Kuczynski 1974, pp. 657 and 865). Abduction and adduction occur in the plane of the ridge, which is shorter than the corresponding metacarpal groove; contours of both vary reciprocally, being more curved near the second metacarpal base, with a longer radius of curvature away from this. The two surfaces are not completely congruent, the area of close contact probably moving towards the palm in adduction and dorsally in abduction (see p. 657). While the axis of flexion–extension passes through the trapezium, that for adduction–abduction is in the metacarpal base (Hollister et al 1992).

Trapezoid

The trapezoid (**6.246**), small and irregular, has a rough *palmar surface* narrower and smaller than its rough *dorsal surface*, the former invading the lateral aspect. The *distal surface*, articulating with the grooved second metacarpal base, is triangular, convex transversely

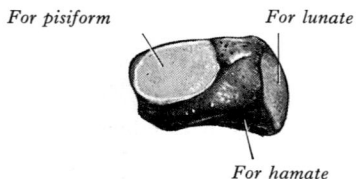

6.243   The left triquetral: palmar aspect.

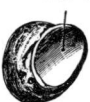

6.244   The left pisiform: dorsal aspect.

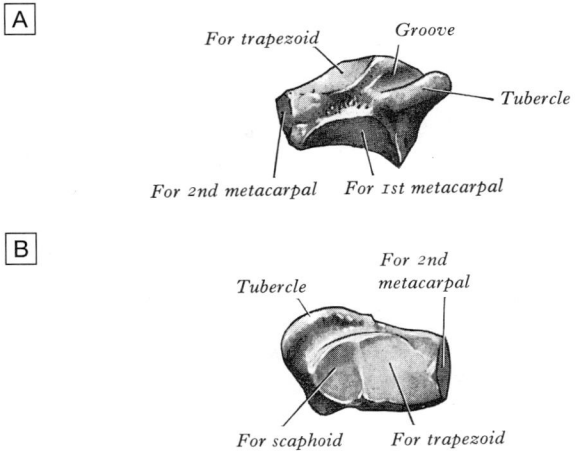

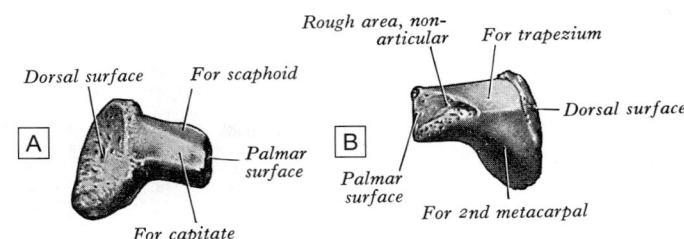

6.246   The left trapezoid: A. Proximomedial; B. Distolateral aspects.

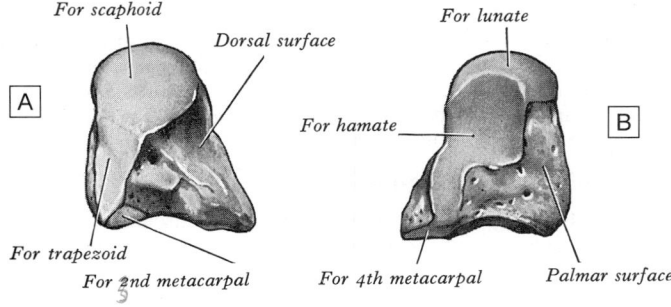

6.245   The left trapezium: A. Palmar; B. Proximomedial aspect.

and concave at right angles to this. The *medial surface* articulates, by a concave facet, with the distal part of the capitate, the lateral surface with the trapezium and the proximal with the scaphoid bone.

Capitate

The capitate (**6.**247), the central and largest carpal bone, articulates with the third metacarpal base, its triangular *distal surface* concavoconvex for this. Its *lateral border* is a concave strip for the medial side of the second metacarpal base; its *dorsomedial angle* usually bears a facet for the fourth metacarpal base. The *head* projects into the concavity formed by the lunate and scaphoid, its *proximal surface* articulating with the lunate and the lateral with the scaphoid. The facets for the scaphoid and trapezoid, usually continuous on the *distolateral surface*, may be separated by a rough interval. The *medial surface* has a large facet for the hamate, deeper proximally where it is partly non-articular. *Palmar* and *dorsal surfaces* are roughened for carpal ligaments, the dorsal being the larger.

Hamate

The hamate (**6.**248) is cuneiform with an unciform *hamulus* (hook) projecting from the distal part of its rough *palmar surface*; the hamulus is curved with a lateral concavity and its tip inclines laterally contributing to the medial wall of the carpal tunnel. To the hamular apex is attached the flexor retinaculum. Distally, on the hamular base, a slight transverse groove may be in contact with the ulnar nerve's terminal deep branch. The remaining *palmar surface*, like the dorsal, is rough for ligaments. A faint ridge divides the *distal surface* into a smaller lateral facet articulating with the fourth metacarpal base and a medial facet for the fifth. The *proximal surface*, the thin margin of the wedge, usually bears a narrow facet contacting the lunate in adduction. The *medial surface* is a broad strip, convex proximally, concave distally, articulating with the triquetral; distally a narrow medial strip is non-articular. The *lateral surface* articulates

with the capitate by a facet covering all but its distal palmar angle.

Ossification

Carpal bones (see **6.**258–261) are cartilaginous at birth, but ossification may have started by then in the capitate and hamate. Each carpal is ossified from one centre, capitate first, pisiform last; but the order in the others varies. The capitate begins to ossify in the second **month**, the hamate at the end of the third, triquetral in the third **year**, lunate during the fourth and scaphoid, trapezium and trapezoid in the fourth in females, fifth in males; the pisiform begins to ossify in the ninth or tenth year in females, twelfth in males. The order varies according to sex (Garn & Rohmann 1960), nutrition and, possibly, race (Shakir & Zaini 1974; Wingerd et al 1974). Occasionally an *os centrale* (p. 616) occurs between the scaphoid, trapezoid and capitate bones; during the second prenatal month it is a cartilaginous nodule usually fusing with the scaphoid. Occasionally, lunate and triquetral elements may fuse; other fusions and accessory ossicles have also been described (O'Rahilly 1953, 1956).

Clinical anatomy

The scaphoid is the most frequently fractured carpal bone, the fracture usually crossing the long axis. Fractures of its proximal part or its 'waist' may fail to unite, possibly because the proximal fragment, devoid of nutrient foramina in about 13% (p. 648), has lost its blood supply. Palmar dislocation of the lunate is often associated with scaphoid fracture. The displaced lunate may compress the median nerve against the flexor retinaculum.

RADIOCARPAL (WRIST) JOINT

The radiocarpal joint (**6.**249, 250), biaxial and ellipsoid, is formed by articulation of the distal end of the radius and the triangular articular disc with the scaphoid, lunate and triquetral. The radial articular surface and distal discal surface form an almost elliptical, concave surface with a transverse long axis; but the radial surface is bisected by a low ridge into two concavities. A similar ridge usually appears between the medial radial concavity and the concave distal discal surface. Proximal articular surfaces of the scaphoid, lunate and triquetral and their interosseous ligaments form a smooth convex surface, received into the proximal concavity. The surface projection of the joint is a line, convex upwards, joining the radial and ulnar styloid processes (**6.**250).

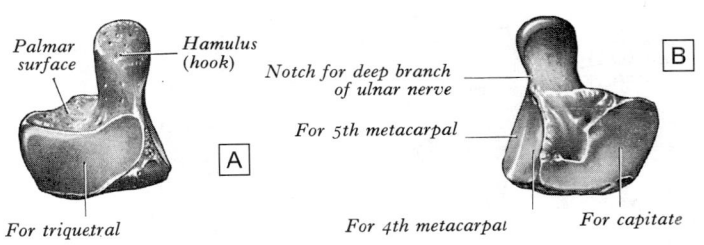

6.247   The left capitate: A. Lateral; B. Medial aspects.

6.248   The left hamate: A. Medial; B. Lateral aspects.

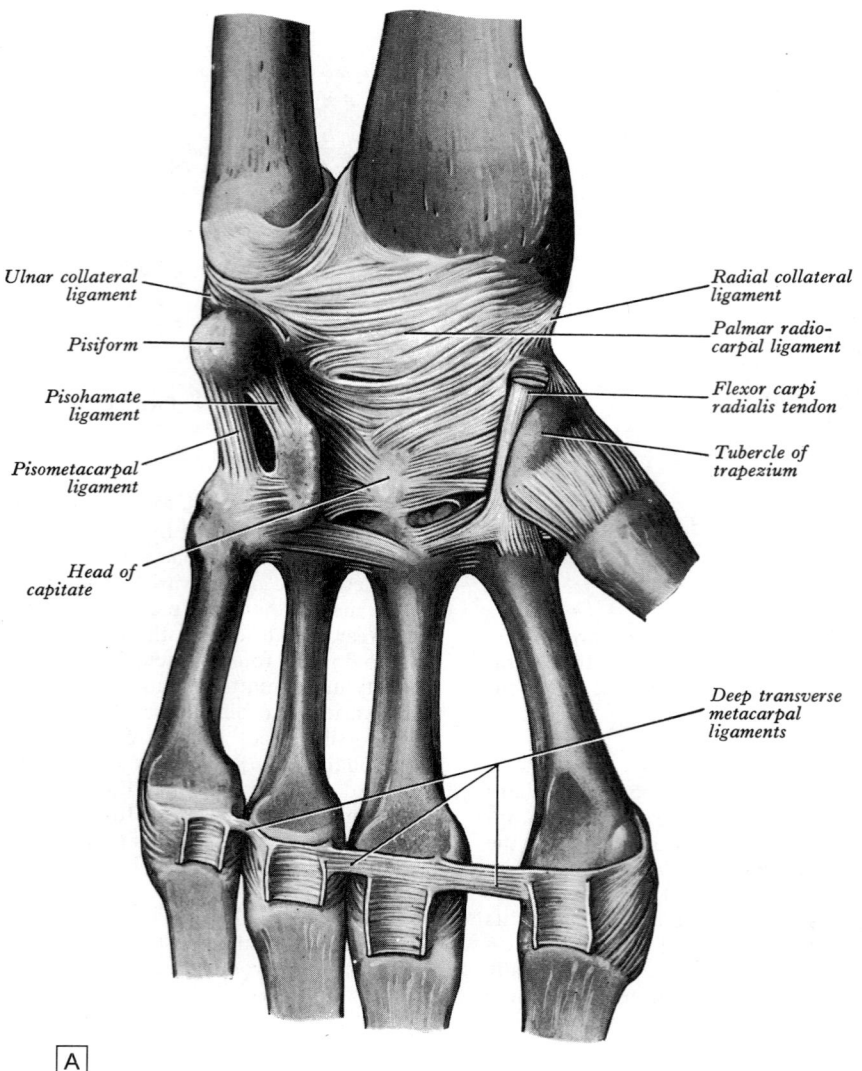

Ulnar collateral ligament

Pisiform

Pisohamate ligament

Pisometacarpal ligament

Head of capitate

Radial collateral ligament

Palmar radio-carpal ligament

Flexor carpi radialis tendon

Tubercle of trapezium

Deep transverse metacarpal ligaments

A

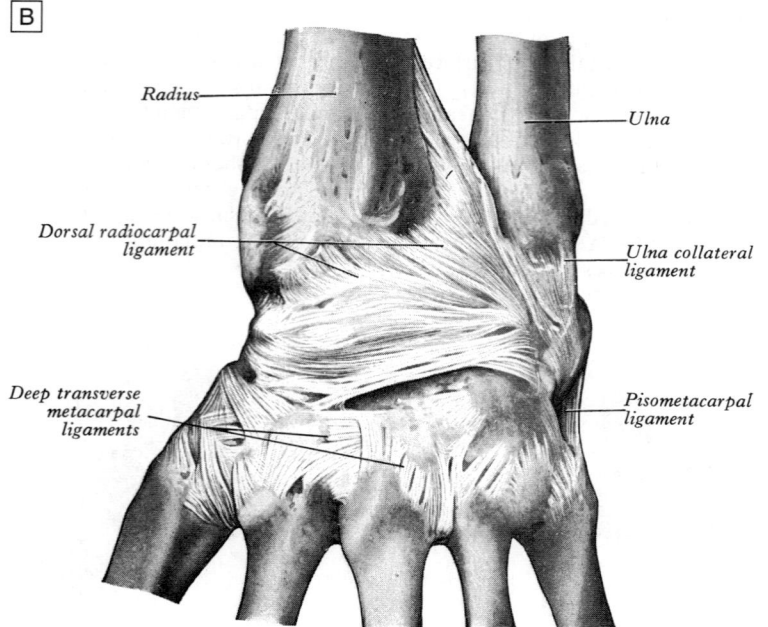

Radius

Dorsal radiocarpal ligament

Deep transverse metacarpal ligaments

Ulna

Ulna collateral ligament

Pisometacarpal ligament

B

6.249 Ligaments of the left wrist: A. Palmar aspect also showing the deep transverse metacarpal ligaments; B. Dorsal aspect.

Fibrous capsule

The fibrous capsule is lined by *synovial membrane* which is usually separate from that of the inferior radioulnar and intercarpal joints; but a protruding *prestyloid recess* (*recessus sacciformis*), anterior to the articular disc, is present and ascends close to the styloid process. The recess is bounded distally by a fibrocartilaginous meniscus, projecting from the ulnar collateral ligament between the tip of the ulnar styloid process and the triquetral (**6.250**); both are clothed with hyaline articular cartilage. The meniscus may ossify (Lewis et al 1970). The capsule is strengthened by *palmar radiocarpal* and *ulnocarpal*, *dorsal radiocarpal* and *radial* and *ulnar collateral* ligaments.

Palmar radiocarpal ligament

The palmar radiocarpal ligament (**6.249**A), a broad membranous band, is attached to the anterior margin of the distal end of the radius and its styloid process, its fibres passing distomedially to the anterior surfaces of the scaphoid, lunate and triquetral, some reaching the capitate. It is partly intracapsular.

Palmar ulnocarpal ligament

The palmar ulnocarpal ligament is a rounded fasciculus from the base of the ulnar styloid process and anterior margin of the articular disc to the lunate and triquetral. Lewis et al (1970) and Mayfield et al (1976) regard both palmar carpal ligaments as intracapsular; the latter also divide the radiocarpal ligament into three and the ulnocarpal ligament into two parts, each named by its attachments, for

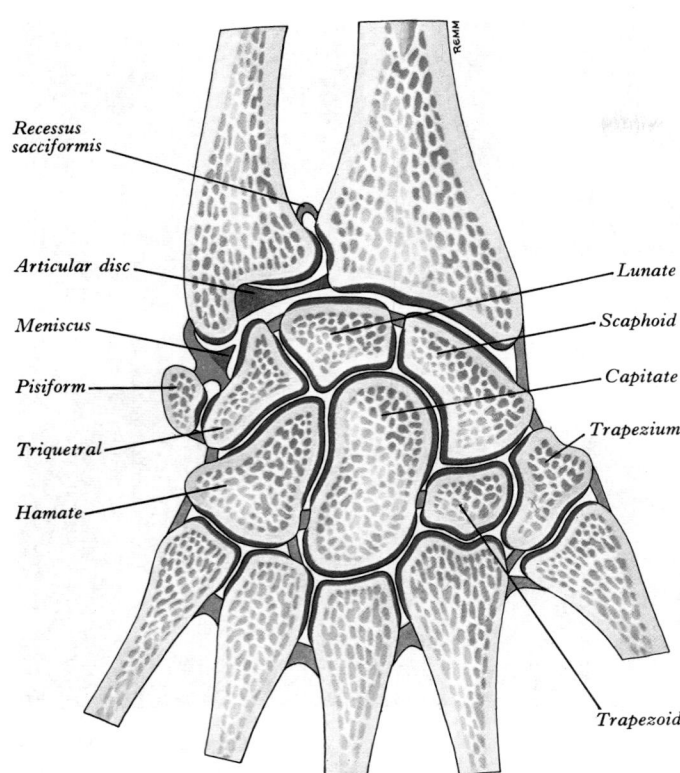

6.250 Coronal section through the distal ends of the radius and ulna, the carpus and the proximal ends of the metacarpals, showing the general form of the articular surfaces (blue), synovial cavities, interosseous ligaments (green) and fibrocartilages (purple). Partly after Lewis et al (1970).

example radiocapitate, ulnolunate, etc. It is not clear whether the ligaments are totally intracapsular, i.e. separate from the overlying articular capsule. (See also p. 494.) The palmar carpal ligaments are perforated by vessels and are related anteriorly to the tendons of flexor digitorum profundus and flexor pollicis longus.

Dorsal radiocarpal ligament

The dorsal radiocarpal ligament (**6.249B**), thinner than the palmar, is attached to the posterior border of the distal end of the radius, its fibres descending distomedially to the dorsal surfaces of the scaphoid, lunate and triquetral and continuing into the dorsal intercarpal ligaments. It is related posteriorly to the carpal and digital extensor tendons, their synovial sheaths and the posterior interosseous nerve; anteriorly it is blended with the disc of the inferior radioulnar articulation.

Ulnar collateral carpal ligament

The ulnar collateral carpal ligament (**6.249**) is attached to the apex of the ulnar styloid process, it divides into two fasciculi, one attached to the medial side of the triquetral, the other to the pisiform. Attached to the ligament's deep (lateral) aspect is a small fibrocartilaginous *meniscus* which is the distal boundary of the synovial *prestyloid recess* (**6.250**).

Radial collateral carpal ligament

The radial collateral carpal ligament (**6.249**) extends from the tip of the radial styloid process to the radial side of the scaphoid; some fibres are prolonged to the trapezium. It is related to the radial artery, curving round laterally between the ligament and tendons of abductor pollicis longus and extensor pollicis brevis. Both collateral ligaments are relatively weak.

Vessels and nerve supply to the joint

Arteries supplying the joint are the anterior interosseous, anterior and posterior carpal branches of the radial and ulnar, palmar and dorsal metacarpals and recurrent rami of the deep palmar arch. **Nerves** are from the anterior and posterior interosseous.

Movements

Movements accompany those of the intercarpal and midcarpal joints and are described together on page 652. The close-packed position is in full extension.

INTERCARPAL JOINTS

The intercarpal joints interconnect the carpal bones and may be summarized as:

- joints between the proximal row of carpal bones
- joints between the distal row of carpal bones
- a complex joint between the rows, the midcarpal joint.

Carpal bones are connected by an extensive array of ligaments, not all specifically named. In addition to those described, the flexor retinaculum (p. 852) is an accessory intercarpal ligament. Articular surfaces are either sellar, ellipsoid or spheroidal.

Joints of the proximal carpal row

(a) The scaphoid, lunate and triquetral are connected by *dorsal*, *palmar* and *interosseous* ligaments.
Dorsal and palmar ligaments. These are transverse, connecting scaphoid to lunate and lunate to triquetral. The palmar ligaments are weaker. Mayfield et al (1976) described a distinct ligament (in 28 dissections) between the palmar aspects of the capitate and triquetral which crosses the hamate.
Interosseous ligaments (6.250). Two narrow bundles, one connecting the lunate and scaphoid, the other the lunate and triquetral, they are attached near their proximal surfaces, forming part of the convex articular radiocarpal surface.
(b) The pisiform articulates with the palmar surface of the triquetral at a small, oval, almost flat, synovial *pisotriquetral joint*; ligaments are the *capsular*, *pisohamate* and *pisometacarpal*. A thin capsule surrounds the joint; the synovial cavity is usually separate but may communicate with that of the radiocarpal joint.
Pisohamate and pisometacarpal ligaments. These connect the pisiform to the hook of the hamate and the base of the fifth metacarpal respectively (**6.249A**). Both are continuations of the tendon of flexor carpi ulnaris and are misnamed.

Joints of the distal carpal row

Bones of the distal carpal row are connected by *dorsal*, *palmar* and *interosseous* ligaments.
Dorsal and palmar ligaments. These extend transversely between trapezium and trapezoid, trapezoid and capitate, and capitate and hamate.
Interosseous ligaments. Usually thicker than in the proximal row, three unite the four bones, that between the capitate and hamate being strongest; one or both of the other two are often absent.

Midcarpal joint

The midcarpal joint, between the scaphoid, lunate and triquetral (proximally) and trapezium, trapezoid, capitate and hamate (distally) is a compound articulation divided descriptively into medial and lateral parts. Throughout most of the *medial compartment* the convexity of the head of the capitate and hamate articulate with a reciprocal concavity formed by the scaphoid, lunate and much of the triquetral; however, most medially the curvatures are reversed, thus forming a compound sellar joint. In the *lateral compartment* the trapezium and trapezoid articulate with the scaphoid, forming a second compound articulation, often said to be plane but which is also sellar. The ligaments are *dorsal*, *palmar* and *collateral*.
Carpal synovial membrane. This is most extensive (**6.250**), lining an irregular articular cavity, its proximal part being between the distal surfaces of the scaphoid, lunate and triquetral and the proximal surfaces of the second carpal row. It has proximal prolongations between scaphoid and lunate, lunate and triquetral and three distal prolongations between the four bones of the second row. The prolongation between trapezium and trapezoid or between trapezoid and capitate is, due to the absence of an interosseous ligament, often continuous with corresponding carpometacarpal joints, variably from the second to fifth or often second and third only. If the latter, the joint between the hamate and fourth and fifth metacarpal bones has

651

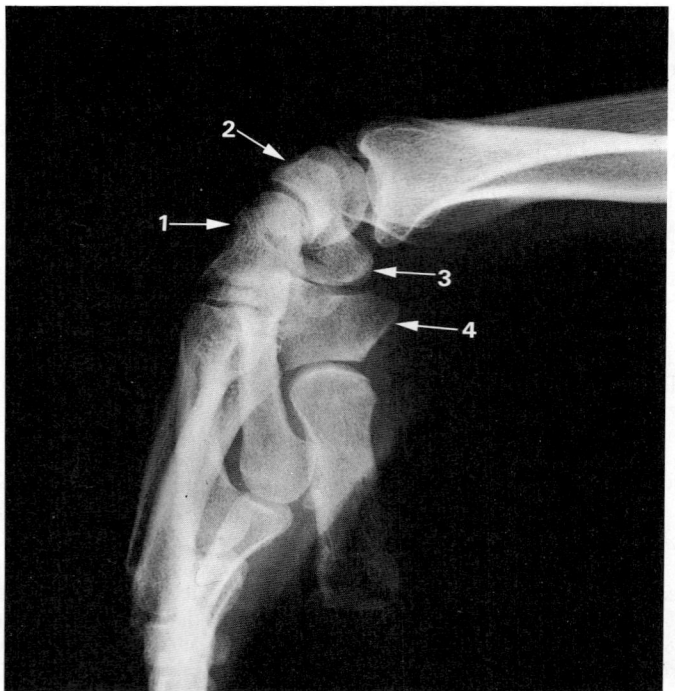

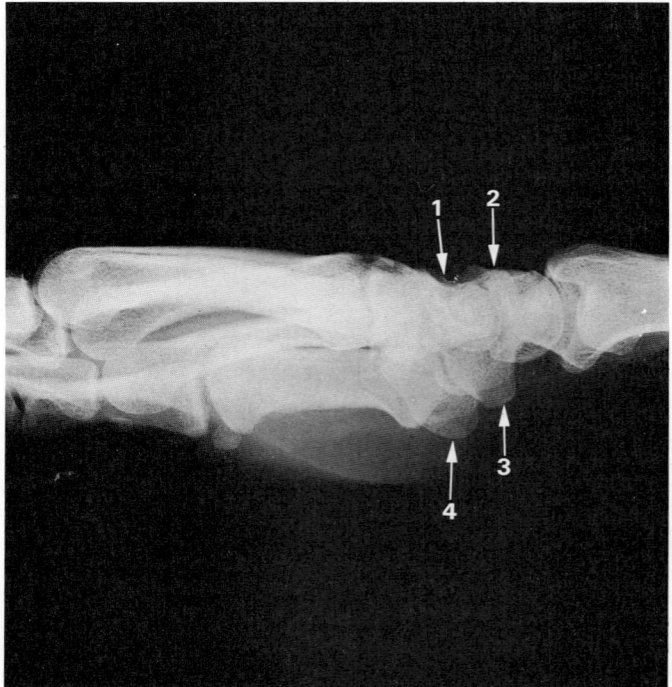

6.251A. Radiograph of the hand and wrist in full flexion: lateral aspect. The arrows point to: (1) the capitate; (2) the lunate; (3) the tubercle of the scaphoid; (4) the tubercle of the trapezium. Compare with **6.251B** and note the relative positions of the capitate and lunate, and the lunate and radius.

6.251B. Radiograph of the hand and wrist: lateral aspect. The long axes of the third metacarpal, the capitate and the lunate are, approximately, in line with the long axis of the radius. The arrows point to the same structures as in **6.251A**. Note the relative positions of the capitate and lunate, and the lunate and radius.

a separate synovial membrane; interposed (**6.250**) is the carpometacarpal interosseous ligament. Synovial cavities of carpometacarpal joints are prolonged slightly between the metacarpal bases. The synovial joint between the pisiform and triquetral is usually isolated.

Dorsal and palmar ligaments. Short, irregular bundles, they are found between the bones of the first and second carpal rows. Palmar fascicles radiate from the head of the capitate to surrounding bones as the *radiate carpal ligament*.

Radial and ulnar collateral ligaments. These are very short. The stronger and more distinct radial connects the scaphoid and trapezium, while the ulnar connects the triquetral and hamate; they are continuous with corresponding collateral ligaments of the wrist joint. A slender interosseous band sometimes connects the capitate and scaphoid but does not completely divide the midcarpal synovial cavity.

Radiocarpal and intercarpal movements

The movements at the radiocarpal and intercarpal joints are considered together since they are both involved in **all** movements as well as being acted upon by the same muscles. Active movements are flexion (*c.* 85°), extension (*c.* 85°), adduction (ulnar deviation) (*c.* 45°), abduction (radial deviation) (*c.* 15°) and circumduction.

The range of flexion is greater at the radiocarpal joint, while in *extension* there is more movement at the midcarpal joint (**6.251**). Hence the proximal surfaces extend further posteriorly on the lunate and scaphoid bones. These movements are limited chiefly by antagonistic muscles; therefore, the range of flexion is perceptibly diminished when the fingers are flexed, due to increased tension in the extensors. Only when the joints are forced to the limits of flexion or extension are the dorsal or palmar ligaments fully stretched (but see below).

Adduction of the hand is considerably greater than *abduction*, perhaps due to the more proximal site of the ulnar styloid process. Most adduction occurs at the radiocarpal joint; the lunate articulates with both the radius and articular disc when the hand is in the midposition (**6.250**) but in adduction it articulates solely with the radius (**6.252A**). Much of the proximal articular surface of the scaphoid becomes subcapsular beneath the radial collateral ligament

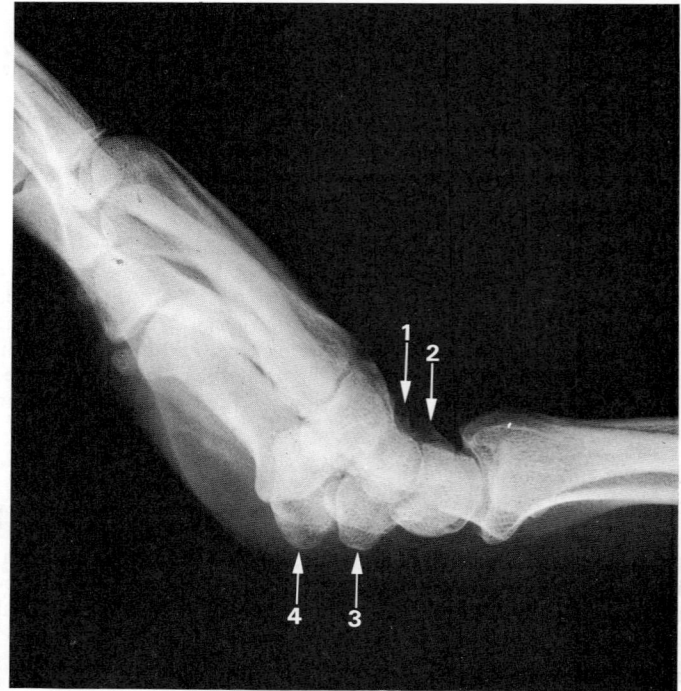

6.251C. Radiograph of the hand and wrist in full extension: lateral aspect. The arrows point to the same structures as in **6.251A**. Compare with **6.251B** and note the alterations in the relative positions of the capitate and lunate, and the lunate and the radius.

and forms a smooth, convex, palpable prominence in the floor of the anatomical 'snuff box'.

Abduction from the neutral position occurs at the midcarpal joint, the proximal carpal not moving (Youm & Flatt 1980); radiographs of abducted hands show that the capitate rotates round an antero-

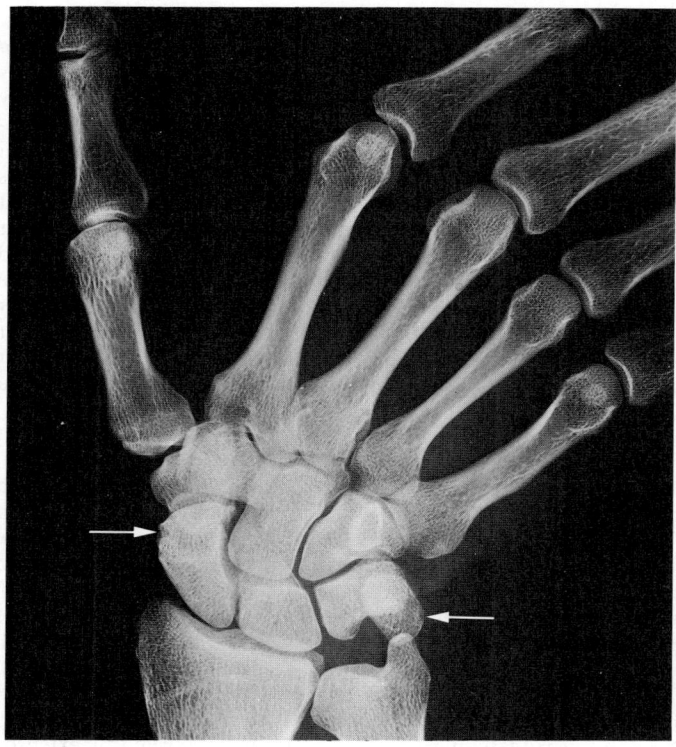

A

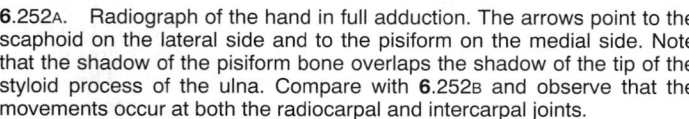

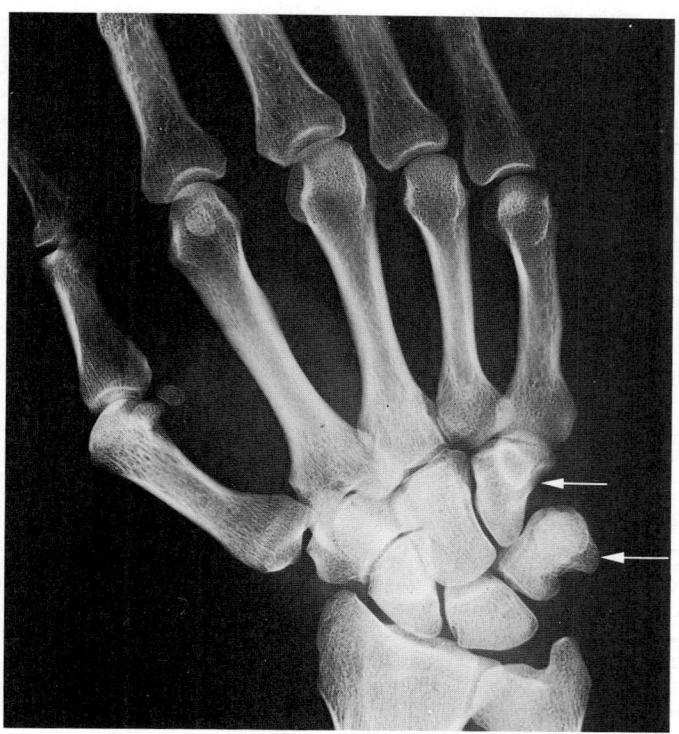

B

6.252A. Radiograph of the hand in full adduction. The arrows point to the scaphoid on the lateral side and to the pisiform on the medial side. Note that the shadow of the pisiform bone overlaps the shadow of the tip of the styloid process of the ulna. Compare with **6.252B** and observe that the movements occur at both the radiocarpal and intercarpal joints.

6.252B. Radiograph of the same hand in full abduction. The arrows point to the hamate and pisiform. Compare with **6.252A** and note that: (1) the scaphoid and lunate have passed medially so that the latter articulates to a large extent with the articular disc of the inferior radioulnar joint; (2) the pisiform is now widely separated from the styloid process of the ulna; (3) the scaphoid, having rotated round a transverse axis, is much foreshortened; (4) the apex of the hamate has been thrust away from the lunate by the rotation of the capitate around an anteroposterior axis; (5) a gap has opened up between the distal portions of the hamate and triquetral; and (6) the long axes of the capitate and lunate are now almost in the same straight line.

posterior axis so that its head passes medially and the hamate conforms to this, the distance between the lunate and the apex of the hamate being increased (**6.252B**). The scaphoid rotates around a transverse axis; its proximal articular surface moves away from the capsule to articulate solely with the radius. Movements are limited by antagonistic muscles and, at extremes, by the carpal collateral ligaments.

Circumduction of the hand is not rotatory but successive flexion, adduction, extension and abduction or vice versa.

Abduction–adduction movements are of special functional value. The hand is commonly used with the carpus slightly extended and the forearm in midposition. Skilled abduction–adduction movements manipulate a large variety of precision tools, from fine needles to hammers.

Accessory movements. Largely radiocarpal, these are more easily observed in flexion than extension. The carpus can be moved backwards and forwards on the radius and articular disc as well as being axially rotated to a considerable extent. Some side-to-side movement is also possible.

Additional analysis of radiocarpal and intercarpal movements

A 'link' joint has been suggested as the mechanical equivalent of the radiocarpal and medial midcarpal complex, in simple form illustrated by a bicycle chain. This is stable only when under tension and 'on centre' with the links in line; unless strengthened by a 'stop' device it buckles under longitudinal compression, especially when 'off centre'. But some advantages are inherent: since the range of movement at each unit is less than the total, articular surfaces can be flatter than in a single joint of the same total range and are better adapted to pressure. Further, overlying tissues are less disturbed by squeezing at the extremes of movement.

Other views contrast sharply with the foregoing (MacConaill 1941). In most manual positions the carpal bones are loose-packed and relatively mobile, becoming a rigid block (close-packed) only in full extension; close-packing is achieved in **two** stages. The carpus is envisaged in four functional units:

(1) trapezium
(2) scaphoid
(3) hamate, capitate and trapezoid
(4) triquetral and lunate.

From full flexion to full extension the stages considered to occur are: firstly the distal row (3) moves on the proximal (2 and 4) until the hand and forearm are in line; hamate, capitate, trapezoid and scaphoid coming into mutual close-pack to form a rigid mass (i.e. 2 + 3). Secondly this mass moves upon the triquetral and lunate, which move at the radiocarpal joint until full extension is reached, with close-packing of the radiocarpal and most carpal joints (i.e. except articulations of the pisiform and trapezium). In this position, adopted only for special effort, very large forces can be transmitted through the articular structures. A similar position is often adopted to resist falls on the outstretched hand, and commonly results in damage, for example a 'supination' (Colles') fracture of the radius, fracture of the scaphoid or dislocation of the lunate. Mayfield et al (1976), studying the behaviour of carpal ligaments in experimental carpal fractures, have corroborated this dorsal 'locking' of the carpus and made further analysis of the roles of the carpal ligaments in progressive intercarpal slides ending in close-packing. During the initial stages of the movement, the scaphoid acts with the proximal carpal row but in later stages with the distal row. The trapezio-scaphoid joint is not considered to be involved in general close-packing of the carpus, perhaps due to the thumb's functional independence when the remainder of the carpus becomes a rigid mass.

Further analysis by Kauer (1974) continues the concept of articular links but emphasizes *rotations* of the lunate and scaphoid relative to the radius and disc; during flexion–extension both rotate relative to each other and to the capitate. The proximal curvatures of the lunate and scaphoid are different, thus dictating some independence of movement, although this is limited, their independence being determined by the biomechanical properties of their interosseous ligament.

Muscles producing carpal movement

Flexion: flexors carpi radialis and ulnaris and palmaris longus, assisted by flexors digitorum superficialis and profundus, flexor pollicis longus and abductor pollicis longus.

Extension: extensors carpi radialis longus, brevis and ulnaris, assisted by extensors digitorum, digiti minimi, indicis and pollicis longus.

Adduction: flexor and extensor carpi ulnaris.

Abduction: flexor carpi radialis, extensors carpi radialis longus and brevis, with abductor pollicis longus and extensor pollicis brevis.

METACARPUS

The metacarpus (Singh 1959) consists of five metacarpal bones, conventionally numbered in lateromedial order. These are miniature long bones, with a distal head, shaft and expanded base. The rounded *heads* articulate with the proximal phalanges. Their articular surfaces are convex, less so transversely, and extend further on the palmar surfaces, especially at their margins. The familiar knuckles are produced by the metacarpal heads. The metacarpal bases articulate with the distal carpal row and with each other, except the first and second. The *shafts* have longitudinally concave palmar surfaces, forming hollows for the palmar muscles. Their dorsal surfaces have a distal triangular area, continued proximally as a round ridge. These flat areas are palpable proximal to the knuckles.

The *medial four metacarpals* are sometimes described as parallel; strictly they diverge somewhat, radiating gently proximodistally. However, the *first metacarpal*, relative to the others, is more anterior and **rotated medially** on its axis through 90°, so that its morphologically **dorsal** surface is **lateral**, its radial border palmar, its palmar surface medial and its ulnar border dorsal. Hence the thumb flexes medially across the palm and can be rotated into opposition with each finger. Such opposition depends on medial rotation and is the prime factor in manual dexterity; when an object is grasped, fingers and thumb encircle it from opposite sides, greatly increasing the power and skill of the grip. Lewis (1977) has made an extended study of human metacarpals and their articulations with the carpus and phalanges, in an explanation of evolving human skills.

INDIVIDUAL METACARPAL BONES

The first metacarpal (6.253)

It is short and thick. (Caution should be exercised when considering descriptions of this bone; here, morphological terms are used supplemented, in places, by their topographical equivalents.) Its *dorsal* (*lateral*) *surface* can be felt to face laterally; its long axis diverges distolaterally from its neighbour. The *shaft* is flattened, dorsally broad and transversely convex. The *palmar* (*medial*) *surface* is longitudinally concave and divided by a ridge into a larger lateral (anterior) and smaller medial (posterior) part. Opponens pollicis is attached to the radial border and adjoining palmar surface; the first dorsal interosseous muscle (radial head) is attached to its ulnar border and adjacent palmar surface. The *base* is concavoconvex and articulates with the trapezium (p. 648). On its lateral (palmar) side abductor pollicis longus is attached, to its ulnar side the first palmar interosseous muscle (p. 860). The *head* is less convex than in other metacarpals and contrasts in being transversely broad. On its palmar aspect ulnar and radial angles form two articular eminences, on which glide sesamoid bones.

The second metacarpal (6.254)

This has the longest shaft and largest *base*, which is grooved in a dorsopalmar direction for the trapezoid; medial to the groove a deep ridge articulates with the capitate; laterally, nearer the base's dorsal surface, is a quadrilateral facet for the trapezium, and just dorsal to this a rough impression marks the attachment of extensor carpi radialis longus. On the *palmar surface* a small tubercle or ridge receives flexor carpi radialis. The base's medial side articulates with the third metacarpal base by a long facet, centrally narrowed. The *shaft* is prismatic in section and longitudinally curved, convex dorsally, concave towards the palm. Its *dorsal surface* is distally broad but proximally narrows to a ridge and is covered by extensor tendons of the index finger; its converging borders begin at the tubercles, one on each side of its head for the attachment of collateral ligaments (p. 659). Proximally the *lateral surface* inclines dorsally for the ulnar head of the first dorsal interosseous muscle. The *medial surface*, inclining similarly, is divided by a faint ridge into a palmar strip for the second palmar interosseous and a dorsal for the radial head of the second dorsal interosseous muscle.

The third metacarpal (6.255)

It has a short *styloid process*, projecting proximally from the radial side of the dorsal surface. Its *base* articulates with the capitate by a facet anteriorly convex but dorsally concave where it invades the styloid process on the lateral aspect of its base. A strip-like facet, constricted centrally, articulates with the second metacarpal base (laterally) and the fourth metacarpal base (medially), the latter by two oval facets. The palmar facet may be absent; less frequently the

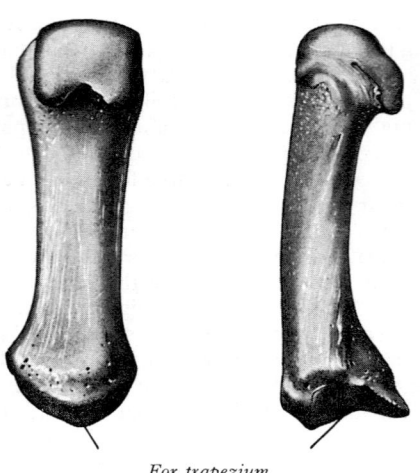

For trapezium

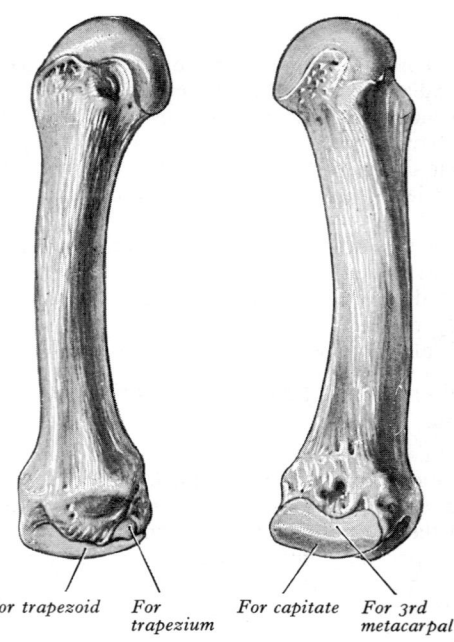

For trapezoid   *For trapezium*   *For capitate*   *For 3rd metacarpal*

6.253 The first right metacarpal bone: palmar and lateral aspects.

6.254 The left second metacarpal bone: dorsolateral and medial aspects.

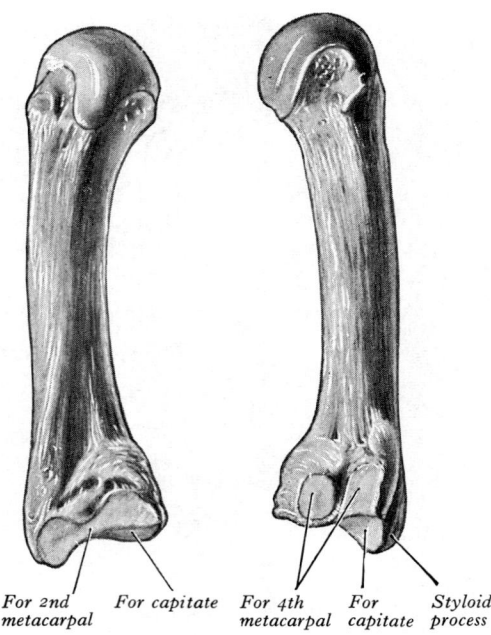

For 2nd   For capitate   For 4th   For   Styloid
metacarpal   metacarpal   capitate process

6.255   The left third metacarpal bone: lateral and medial aspects.

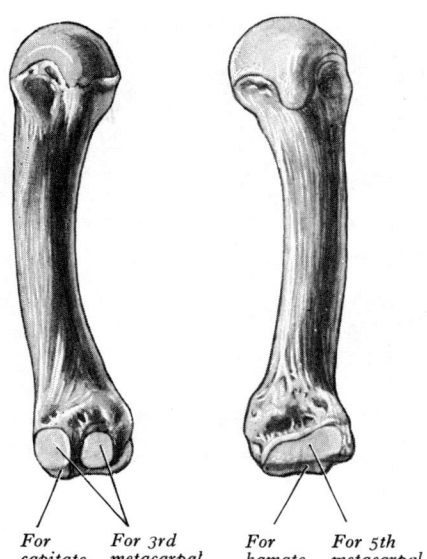

For   For 3rd   For   For 5th
capitate   metacarpal   hamate   metacarpal

6.256   The left fourth metacarpal: lateral and medial aspects.

facets are connected proximally by a narrow bridge. The base's palmar surface receives a slip from the flexor carpi radialis tendon; to its dorsal surface, beyond the styloid process, extensor carpi radialis brevis is attached. The *shaft* resembles that of the second metacarpal. To its lateral surface the ulnar head of the second dorsal interosseous muscle is attached, to its medial surface the radial head of the third dorsal interosseous and to the intervening palmar ridge in its distal two-thirds the transverse head of adductor pollicis. Its dorsal surface is covered by the extensor tendon.

The fourth metacarpal (6.256).

Shorter and thinner than the second and third, it displays on its *base* two lateral oval facets for the third metacarpal base (see above), the dorsal usually larger and proximally in contact with the capitate. A single medial elongate facet is for the fifth metacarpal base. The quadrangular *proximal surface* articulates with the hamate, being anteriorly convex, dorsally concave. The *shaft* is like the second, but a faint ridge on its lateral surface separates the attachments of the third palmar interosseous and the ulnar head of the third dorsal interosseous muscles. To the medial surface the radial head of the fourth dorsal interosseous is attached.

The fifth metacarpal (6.257).

This differs in its medial basal surface, which is non-articular and bears a tubercle for extensor carpi ulnaris. The lateral basal surface is a facet, transversely concave, convex from palm to dorsum, for articulation with the hamate. A lateral strip articulates with the fourth metacarpal base. The *shaft* has a triangular dorsal area almost reaching the base; the lateral surface inclines dorsally only at its proximal end. To the medial surface opponens digiti minimi is attached; the lateral is divided by a ridge, sometimes sharp, into a palmar strip for the fourth palmar interosseous and a dorsal strip for the ulnar part of the fourth dorsal interosseous.

Ossification

Each metacarpal ossifies from a primary centre for the shaft and a secondary in the *base* of the first and *heads* of the other four. Ossification begins in the midshaft about the ninth week. Centres for the second to fifth metacarpal heads appear in that order in the second year in females, and between $1\frac{1}{2}$ to $2\frac{1}{2}$ years in males. They unite with the shafts about the fifteenth or sixteenth year in females, eighteenth or nineteenth in males. The first metacarpal base begins late in the second year in females, early in the third year in males, uniting before the fifteenth year in females and seventeenth in males

(Joseph 1951). Sometimes the styloid process of the third metacarpal is a separate ossicle. For wider assessments of range of variability consult Modi (1957) and Krogman (1962) (6.258–261).

The thumb metacarpal ossifies like a phalanx; some, therefore, consider the thumb skeleton to consist of three phalanges; others believe the distal phalanx represents fused middle and distal phalanges, a condition occasionally observed in the fifth toe (Broom 1930). (When the thumb has **three** phalanges, the metacarpal has a distal and a proximal epiphysis. It occasionally bifurcates distally, the medial branch, with no distal epiphysis, bearing **two** phalanges, the lateral showing a distal epiphysis, and **three** phalanges (Nicholson 1937). The existence of only a *distal* metacarpal epiphysis may be associated with a greater range of movement at the metacarpophalangeal joint. In the thumb, it is the carpometacarpal joint which has the wider range, and a *basal* epiphysis in the first metacarpal may be attributable to this. However, a distal epiphysis may appear in the first, and a proximal in the second metacarpal.

Growth studies of 1700 children, aged one to 18 years, favour the

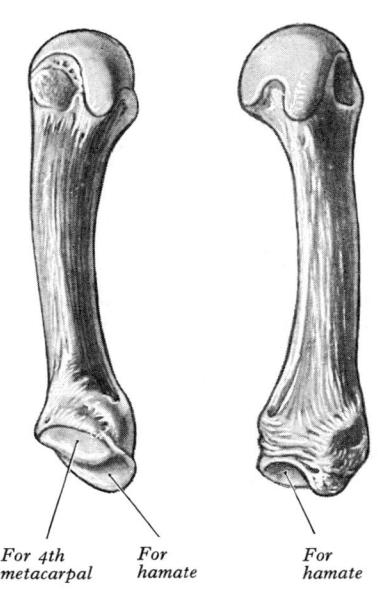

For 4th   For   For
metacarpal   hamate   hamate

6.257   The left fifth metacarpal: lateral and medial aspects.

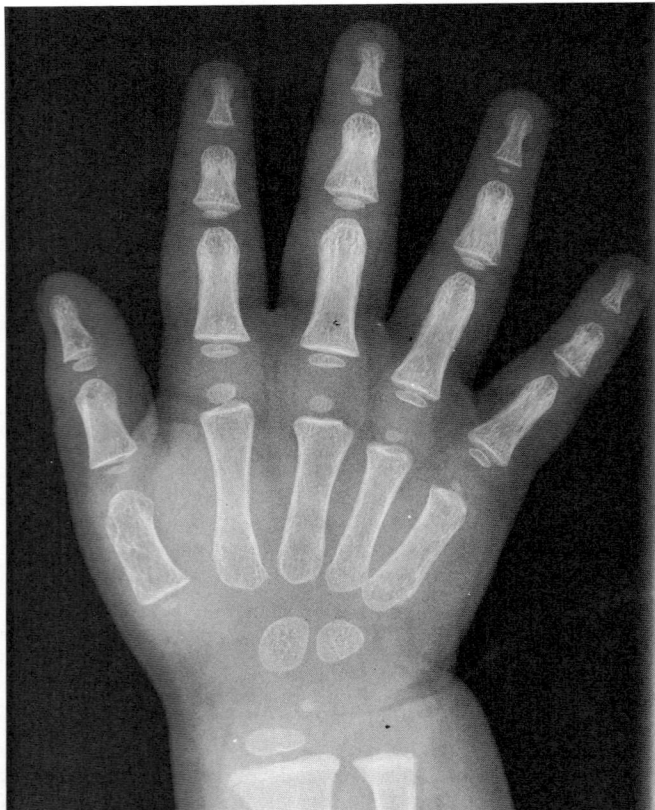

6.258 Radiograph of a hand at 2½ years (male). Note early stages of ossification in epiphyses at proximal ends of phalanges and first metacarpal, at distal ends of remaining metacarpals and radius and in the capitate, hamate and lunate. The last is more usually preceded by the centre for the triquetral. Compare with **6.259** and **6.260**.

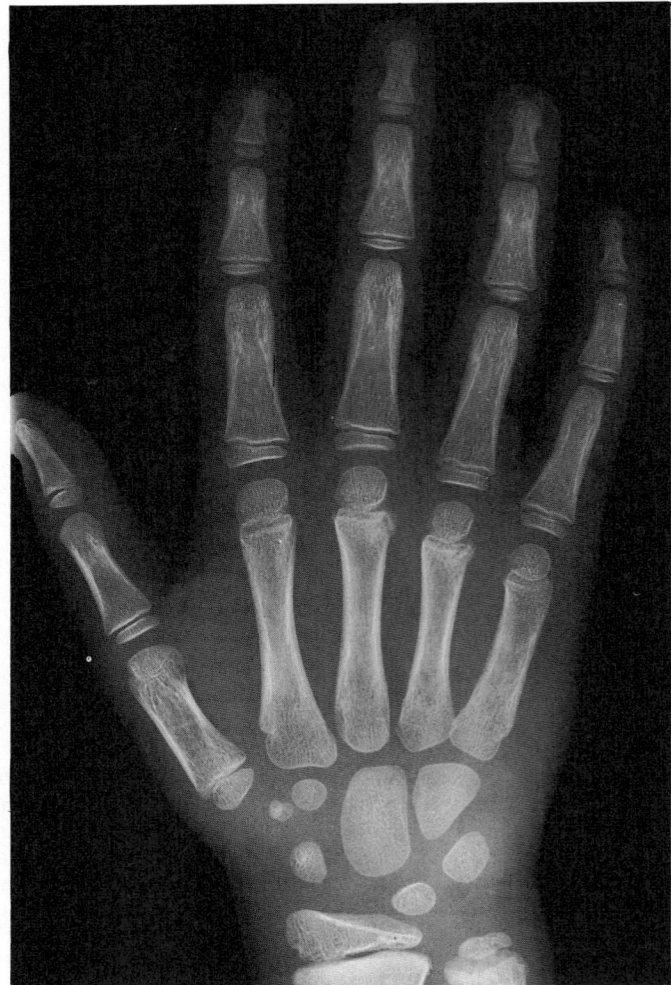

6.259 Radiograph of a hand at 6½ years (male). Note the more advanced state of the centres of ossification already visible in **6.258**, and additional centres in the distal ulnar epiphysis and in the triquetral, scaphoid, trapezium and trapezoid.

view of the thumb metacarpal as a proximal phalanx (as first suggested by Vesalius in 1543). But this ignores the observations that the so-called distal epiphysis of the first metacarpal is usually (if not always) a diaphyseal prolongation into terminal cartilage, rather than a separate centre. A review of the data concerning such 'pseudo-epiphyses' corroborates this description (Haines 1974).

CARPOMETACARPAL JOINT OF THE THUMB (POLLEX)

The carpometacarpal joint of the thumb is a *sellar* joint between the first metacarpal base and trapezium, and enjoys wide mobility due to its extensive articular surfaces and their topology. It has a fibrous capsule, thick but loose, extending from the circumference of the metacarpal base to the rough rim of the distal trapezial articular facet; it is thickest laterally and dorsally. The synovial membrane is separate (**6.250**). The first metacarpal and trapezium are connected by *lateral*, *anterior* and *posterior* ligaments and the capsule.

Lateral ligament. This broad ligament runs from the lateral surface of the trapezium to the radial side of the metacarpal base.

Palmar and dorsal ligaments. These are oblique bands converging to the ulnar side of the metacarpal base from the palmar and dorsal surfaces of the trapezium respectively.

Relations

The joint's *palmar surface* is covered by the thenar muscles, its *dorsal surface* by the long and short extensors. **Medial** is the first dorsal interosseous space, and the tendon of flexor pollicis longus; **lateral** are the tendons of abductor pollicis longus and extensor pollicis brevis.

Movements

Active movements are flexion–extension, abduction–adduction,

rotation, and circumduction. In the resting position of the first metacarpal (p. 865) flexion and extension are parallel to the palmar plane, abduction and adduction at right angles to this. Except at initiation, flexion is accompanied by medial rotation; conversely, medial rotation involves flexion. Linkage of movements is largely due to the shape of the articular surfaces, imposing some conjunct rotation, and to the obliquity of the dorsal ligament, which when taut anchors the ulnar side of the metacarpal base while its radial side continues to move. Contraction of flexor pollicis brevis, assisted by opponens pollicis, thus produces medial rotation with flexion (Napier 1955); combined with abduction this brings the thumb pulp into contact with those of the slightly flexed fingers, a movement termed *opposition*. (The flexed fingers have varying degrees of *lateral metacarpophalangeal rotation*, minimal in the index but maximal in minimus.) Conversely, full extension of the pollicial metacarpal entails slight lateral rotation (Kuczynski 1974), attributable also to the sellar form of the joint and to the action of the *palmar* ligament, similar to the dorsal ligament in flexion.

These rotations are conjunct, inevitably accompanying flexion–extension, with spiralling and tightening of the joint capsule and balanced conarticular compression at the extremes of these movements. Close-packing is said to occur in powerful opposition, when greatest forces are transmitted to the joint. (For analysis consult Haines 1944; Kapandji 1963, 1970; Kuczynski 1974; MacConaill & Basmajian 1977.)

Accessory movements. These are axial rotation in the position of rest, and distraction.

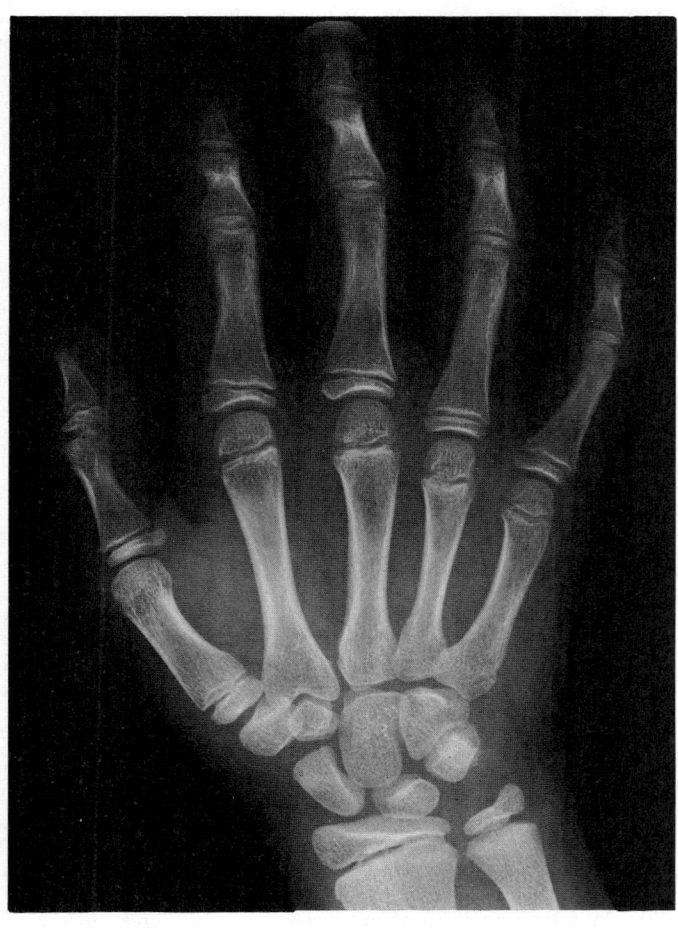

6.260 Radiograph of a hand at 11 years (female). Note the maturing shapes of all the ossifications previously seen in **6.258** and **6.259**, with the addition of the pisiform.

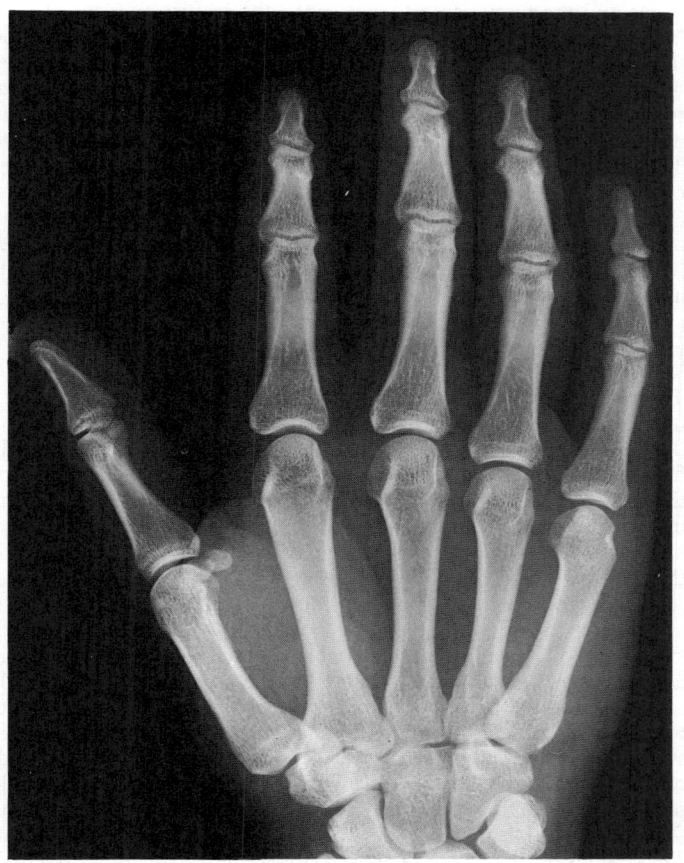

6.261 Radiograph of adult hand for comparison (male of 19 years). Note additional ossification in the sesamoid bones of the thumb.

Muscles producing movement

Flexion: flexor pollicis brevis and opponens pollicis, aided by flexor pollicis longus when the other joints of the thumb are flexed. Flexion entails medial rotation.

Extension: abductor pollicis longus and extensors pollicis brevis and longus. In full extension extensor pollicis longus, owing to its oblique pull and the disposition of the palmar ligament, rotates the thumb laterally and draws it dorsally, i.e. slightly adducts it.

Abduction: abductors pollicis brevis and longus. When abduction is maximal the digit and metacarpal are not in line, the thumb being abducted at both metacarpophalangeal and carpometacarpal joints.

Adduction: adductor pollicis alone.

Opposition: opponens pollicis and flexor brevis pollicis simultaneously flex and medially rotate the abducted thumb. Interpulpal pressure, or that generated by digital grasping, is increased by adductor pollicis and flexor pollicis longus.

Circumduction: the above muscle groups acting consecutively, extensors, abductors, flexors and adductors in this or reverse order.

THE SECOND TO FIFTH CARPOMETACARPAL JOINTS

The joints between the carpus and second to fifth metacarpals, although widely classed as plane, have curved articular surfaces often of complex sellar shape (pp. 503–505). The bones are united by articular capsules, *dorsal*, *palmar* and *interosseous* ligaments.

Synovial membranes. These are often continuous with those of the intercarpal joints. Occasionally, the joint between the hamate and fourth and fifth metacarpal bones has a separate synovial cavity, bounded laterally by the medial interosseous ligament and its extensions to the palmar and dorsal parts of the capsule (**6**.250).

Dorsal ligaments. These are the strongest, connecting the dorsal surfaces of the carpal and metacarpal bones. The second metacarpal has two, from the trapezium and trapezoid; the third also has two, from the trapezoid and capitate; the fourth two, from the capitate and hamate; the fifth a single band from the hamate continuous with a similar palmar ligament, forming an incomplete capsule.

Palmar ligaments. These are similar, except for the third metacarpal, which has three: a lateral from the trapezium, superficial to the tendon sheath of flexor carpi radialis, an intermediate from the capitate and a medial from the hamate.

Interosseous ligaments. Two short, thick, fibrous bands, they are limited to one part of the carpometacarpal articulation; they connect contiguous distal margins of the capitate and hamate with adjacent surfaces of the third and fourth metacarpal bones: they may be united proximally.

INTERMETACARPAL JOINTS

The second to fifth metacarpal bases articulate reciprocally by small cartilage-covered facets connected by *dorsal*, *palmar* and *interosseous* ligaments.

Dorsal and palmar ligaments. These pass transversely from bone to bone.

Interosseous ligaments. These connect contiguous surfaces just distal to their articular facets.

Synovial membranes. These are continuous with those of the carpometacarpal articulations.

Movements

Movements at the carpometacarpal and intermetacarpal articulations are limited to slight gliding, sufficient, however, to permit some flexion–extension and adjunct rotation, ranges varying in different joints. They are **partly** accessory movements occurring when the palm is 'cupped', as in grasping an object. Active movements also

657

occur and are familiar, for example, to the pianist or violinist. The fifth metacarpal is most movable, then the fourth, the second and third being least mobile. These variations are easily demonstrated by opposing each digit to the thumb over the palmar centre. About two-thirds of the movements are pollicial, as described above, but during opposition to minimus, the latter is flexed, abducted and laterally rotated, accounting for the remaining third. These actions occur at both the carpometacarpal and metacarpophalangeal joints. (For a more extensive description of digital, including pollicial, movement see below.) The close-packed position probably coincides with carpal extension, as in gripping. Further accessory movements are spiral twisting of the whole metacarpus on the carpus.

PHALANGES OF THE HAND

There are 14 phalanges, three in each finger, two in the thumb. Each has a head, shaft and proximal base. The *shaft* tapers distally, its dorsal surface transversely convex. The palmar surface is transversely flat but gently concave anteriorly in its long axis. The *bases* of the *proximal phalanges* carry concave, oval facets adapted to the metacarpal heads, their own heads smoothly grooved like pulleys and encroaching more on to the palmar surfaces. Conforming to this, the *bases* of the *middle phalanges* carry two concave facets separated by a smooth ridge. Middle phalangeal *heads* are also pulley-like, to which the bases of the distal phalanges are adapted; the latter's own heads are non-articular but carry a rough, crescentic *palmar tuberosity* to which the pulps of the finger tips are attached.

In addition to articular ligaments, the phalanges give attachments to numerous muscles: to the base of the distal phalanx on its palmar surface a corresponding tendon of flexor digitorum profundus and, on its dorsal surface, extensor digitorum; to the sides of a middle phalanx a tendon of flexor digitorum superficialis (p. 847) and its fibrous sheath; to the base dorsally, a part of extensor digitorum. To the sides of a proximal phalanx a fibrous flexor sheath is attached; to its base, laterally, part of the corresponding dorsal interosseous, and, medially, another dorsal interosseous muscle are attached (p. 860).

The phalanges of minimus and the thumb differ: attached to the medial side of the base of the former's proximal phalanx are abductor and flexor digiti minimi; to the base of the proximal pollicial phalanx are attached, dorsally, the tendon of extensor pollicis brevis and the oblique head of adductor pollicis and, medially, oblique and transverse heads of adductor pollicis, sometimes conjoined with the first palmar interosseous (p. 860).

The margins of the proximal pollicial phalanx are not sharp, the fibrous sheath being less strongly developed than in the other digits.

Ossification

Phalanges are ossified from a primary centre for the shaft and a proximal epiphyseal centre. Ossification begins prenatally in shafts as follows: distal phalanges in the eighth or ninth week, proximal phalanges in the tenth, middle phalanges in the eleventh week or later. Epiphyseal centres appear in proximal phalanges early in the second year (females), and in its later months (males); in middle and distal phalanges in the second year (females), third or fourth (males). All epiphyses unite about the fifteenth to sixteenth year in females, seventeenth to eighteenth in males (6.258–261, 262).

METACARPOPHALANGEAL JOINTS

The metacarpophalangeal joints (6.263) are usually considered ellipsoid, but the metacarpal heads, adapted to shallow concavities on the phalangeal bases, are not regularly convex but partially divided on their palmar aspects and thus almost bicondylar (p. 654). Each joint has a *palmar* and **two** *collateral ligaments*.

Palmar ligaments. These are unusual, being thick, dense and fibrocartilaginous, sited between and connected to the collateral ligaments. They are attached loosely to the metacarpals but firmly to the phalangeal bases. Their palmar aspects are blended with the deep transverse palmar ligaments and are grooved for the flexor tendons, whose fibrous sheaths connect with the sides of the grooves. Their deep surfaces increase articular areas for the metacarpal heads.

The deep transverse metacarpal ligaments. Three short, wide, flat bands, they connect the palmar ligaments of the second to fifth

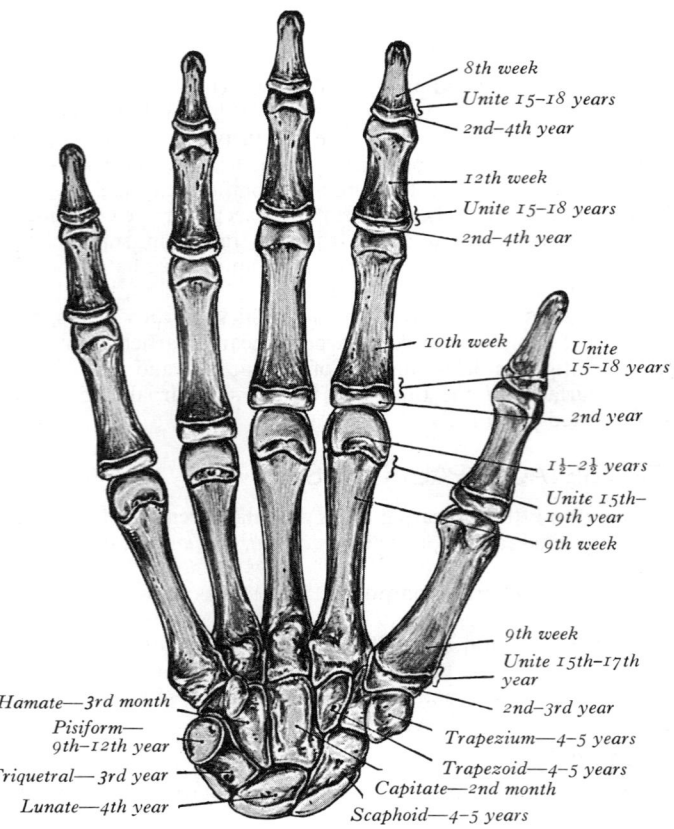

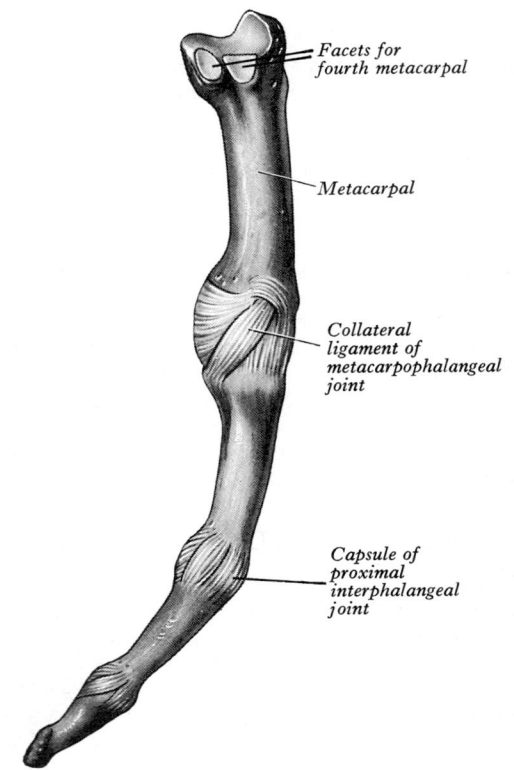

6.262 The bones of the hand of a child, indicating the general plan of ossification.

6.263 Metacarpophalangeal and digital joints of the right third finger: medial aspect.

metacarpophalangeal joints (**6.**249A, 263) and are related anteriorly to the lumbricals and digital vessels and nerves, posteriorly to the interossei. Bands from the digital slips of the central palmar aponeurosis join their palmar surfaces (p. 854). On both sides of the third and fourth metacarpophalangeal joints (but only the ulnar side of the second and radial side of the fifth) transverse bands of the dorsal digital expansions (p. 858) join the deep transverse metacarpal ligaments; **anterior** to this band are the lumbricals and phalangeal attachments of dorsal interossei and **dorsal** to it are the remaining attachments of dorsal interossei and palmar interossei (p. 858 and **7.**113).

Collateral ligaments. Strong, round cords, they flank the joints, each attached to the posterior tubercle and adjacent pit on the side of its metacarpal head and each passing distoanteriorly to the side of the anterior aspect of its phalangeal base (**6.**263B).

Further details

Extensions from the extensor expansion, each collateral ligament and the palmar ligament pass into the joint cavity (Fisher et al 1985), providing a significant increase to the articular surface area of the phalangeal base; their deformable nature improving joint congruence.

On the dorsal surfaces of these joints the fibrous capsules are thin and often separated from the extensor tendons by bursae. In a proportion of instances, however, part of the long extensor tendon is intercalated into the dorsal capsule and some authorities then regard the tendon as forming the capsule on this aspect. Their sensory nerve supply has been detailed by Sathian and Devanandan (1983), who found abundant Paciniform corpuscles but few Ruffini endings and no Golgi type receptors in association with these joints.

Movements

Movements are flexion, extension, adduction, abduction, circumduction and limited rotation, the last of which cannot occur in isolation but may accompany flexion–extension; this, however, can be initiated voluntarily in the free hand (e.g. each finger flexing and rotating to place its tip near the palmar centre); the range of rotation is frequently increased due to the resistance of a grasped object.

Flexion is almost 90°, *extension* just a few degrees; both are limited chiefly by antagonistic muscles but flexion is commonly terminated by resistance of a grasped object. *Abduction* and *adduction* are also relatively small and in flexion negligible. The metacarpophalangeal joint of the thumb has a flexion–extension range of about 60° (almost entirely flexion); other movements are adduction–abduction (maximal range 25°) which invariably accompanies the corresponding carpometacarpal movements and increases their combined range; also some slight conjunct rotation, but greater adjunct rotation, accompanying flexion–extension. Of the other metacarpophalangeal joints the second is most mobile in adduction–abduction (*c.* 30°), followed by the fifth, fourth, and third. (For further analyses of these movements see p. 865.)

Accessory movements. These are further rotation (marked in the thumb), anteroposterior and lateral translation of a phalanx or metacarpal, and distraction.

Muscles producing movement

Flexion: flexors digitorum superficialis and profundus, assisted by the lumbricals and interossei (Long et al 1961) and, in the minimus, the flexor digiti minimi brevis; in the thumb, by flexors pollicis longus and brevis and the first palmar interosseous. Slight lateral rotation accompanies digital flexion of digits 3–5. Flexion of the index may be accompanied by minimal lateral or no rotation; frequently a small degree of **medial** rotation can be observed.

Extension: in the third and fourth digits extensor digitorum, assisted respectively in the second and fifth digits by extensor indicis and extensor digiti minimi; in the thumb, by extensors pollicis longus and brevis.

Adduction: in extended fingers, palmar interossei; during flexion the long flexors are predominant. In the thumb the limited metacarpophalangeal adduction possible is slightly attributable to adductor pollicis and the first palmar interosseous.

Abduction: in extended fingers, dorsal interossei assisted by the long extensors except in the middle finger; in minimus the abductor digiti minimi. In the thumb, abductor pollicis brevis produces the slight abduction possible, most often one factor contributing to opposition. When the fingers are flexed, active abduction is impossible; but, if the long digital flexors are inactive, passive abduction is free. Inability to abduct actively in this position may be due to shortening of the dorsal interossei and abductor digiti minimi by flexion, but the altered line of pull of the interossei relative to the axis of movement is probably the determining factor; while in digital extension the axis of lateral movements is anteroposterior, in flexion it is proximodistal, the line of pull of the interossei being then nearly *parallel* to the axis.

INTERPHALANGEAL JOINTS

The interphalangeal joints are uniaxial hinge joints (**6.**263), each with a fibrous capsule, *palmar* and **two** *collateral* ligaments, arranged as in the metacarpophalangeal joints. Long extensor tendons take the place of the dorsal capsular ligaments.

Again extensions from the extensor expansion, each collateral ligament and the palmar ligament pass into the joint cavity (Fisher et al 1985), providing a significant increase to the articular surface area of the phalangeal base; their deformable nature improving joint congruence.

Movements

Movements (active) at interphalangeal joints are flexion and extension, greater in range at proximal joints. *Flexion* is considerable, *extension* limited by tension of the digital flexors and terminated by tension in the palmar ligaments and conarticular compression. Full extension is the close-packed position, assumed whenever the fingers are used as props to transmit body weight or powerful thrust. (In contrast, alternatively, the fully clenched fist may be used.) Flexion and extension are accompanied by slight conjunct rotation; during flexion this turns the digital pulps slightly laterally, i.e. to face the opposed thumb. An opposite rotation occurs during extension.

Accessory movements. These are limited rotation, abduction, adduction and anteroposterior translation, and permit the fingers to adapt to the shapes of objects gripped and provide against stresses and strains.

Muscles producing movement

Flexion: at proximal interphalangeal joints, flexors digitorum superficialis and profundus; at the distal, flexor digitorum profundus; at the thumb interphalangeal joint, flexor pollicis longus.

Extension: extensors digitorum, digiti minimi and pollicis longus, in association with abductor pollicis longus and extensor pollicis brevis. Extension occurs simultaneously in both joints in digits 2–5.

Simultaneous *flexion* at the metacarpophalangeal and *extension* at the interphalangeal joints of a digit are essential in the fine movements of writing, drawing, threading a needle, etc. The lumbricals and interossei have long been accepted as not only primary agents in flexing the metacarpophalangeal joints but also in extending the interphalangeal joints via their attachments to the dorsal digital expansions (p. 858). Also, when the lumbricals and interossei flex the metacarpophalangeal joints, it has been claimed that the balance between the tension of the digital flexors and extensors alters in favour of the extensors and that this alone is responsible for the extension of interphalangeal joints (Braithwaite et al 1948). However, the lumbricals and interossei alone can both extend these joints (Sunderland 1945b see also pp. 861, 862).

Replacement arthroplasty in the wrist and hand

Introduction

The joints of the wrist and hand may be damaged by injury or progressively destroyed by degenerative or inflammatory disease, resulting in pain, stiffness, instability and deformity. Reconstructive surgery, either arthrodesis or arthroplasty, may then be required, the nature of which will depend on the degree of destruction and the joint involved.

Arthrodesis involves stiffening the joint in a functional position by fusing the adjacent bones. Normal joint motion is therefore lost, the resulting deficit being dependent on the joint involved. Pain-free stability is of prime importance at the wrist, the metacarpophalangeal and interphalangeal joints of the thumb, the proximal interphalangeal joint of the index finger and the distal interphalangeal joints of all fingers. In addition, mobility at the carpometacarpal joint of the thumb is advisable so that the thumb can be used for prehensile activities. Similarly, mobility is also essential at the metacarpophalangeal joints of the fingers and at the proximal interphalangeal joints of the middle, ring and little fingers for power gripping. If objects are to be placed into the palm of the hand, extension of the fingers at the metacarpophalangeal joints is essential. If one wrist is stiff, as may occur in patients with rheumatoid arthritis, mobility should be maintained at the other wrist.

Replacement arthroplasty, in which the diseased joint is excised and replaced with a prosthesis, is therefore of value at the wrist, at the base of the thumb, the metacarpophalangeal joints of the fingers and the proximal interphalangeal joints of the middle, ring and little fingers.

Wrist joint

The carpal region is unique in that there are no tendon attachments to any of the individual bones; stability, therefore, depends on the nature of the opposed articulating surfaces, the integrity of both the extrinsic and intrinsic ligaments and the normal functioning of muscles crossing the region. In general, some or all of these components are lacking in patients requiring wrist replacement; an unbalanced wrist, frequently with ulnar deviation, being the end result.

Patients with post-traumatic osteoarthritis, and often those with degenerative osteoarthritis, usually have single wrist joint involvement. Frequently these patients are involved in heavy work, and a replacement arthroplasty is contraindicated, since the stresses across the wrist joint from heavy lifting, for example, lead to prosthetic loosening or fracture: arthrodesis is usually performed in such

patients. However, patients with rheumatoid arthritis often have bilateral involvement; a replacement arthroplasty of one wrist will allow useful movement, particularly if the other wrist is to undergo arthrodesis or is stiff as a result of the disease. Other contraindications for arthroplasty include previous infection, ruptured extensor tendons and a non-functioning hand.

The prostheses currently available are designed to restore function and not necessarily to reproduce the original anatomy, nor do they attempt to reproduce the range and complexity of movements of the normal wrist: they aim to enable 20° each of flexion and extension. The ideal prosthesis should be non-constrained, require minimal bone resection (because of the possible need for salvage), and have the facility to restore carpal height, provide support for the first and fifth rays, as well as to restore the anatomical centre of rotation within the head of the capitate.

The most commonly used prosthesis is a flexible hinge made from silicone rubber (silastic), which fits snugly into the bone and around which a strong 'capsule' of fibrous tissue forms within a few weeks of insertion, thus providing stability: 10-year follow-up studies have shown good pain relief. More complicated designs are essentially adaptations of a 'ball-and-socket' type of joint following flexion and extension, and abduction and adduction with a small degree of rotation. The bearing surfaces are metal and high density polyethylene in a variety of combinations, with fixation achieved by medullary stems with or without the use of cement: such implants, however, frequently loosen in the porotic bone. The major problems associated with wrist replacement are alignment of the prosthesis, restoration of the anatomic centre of rotation and balancing the soft tissues crossing the joint: fixation and wear of the prosthesis are less of a challenge.

Historically the silastic interposition arthroplasty has played an important supplementary role especially in the low-demand patient with rheumatoid disease. While not a 'total' replacement the combination of a flexible implant, synovectomy and resection arthroplasty maintains the alignment of the bony skeleton, but is not capable of correcting a deformity or of ensuring long-lasting stability of the joint. Pain relief is generally excellent with functional, although limited, mobility: complications include wear, breakage, dislocation, bone resorption and silicone synovitis.

Wrist arthroplasty is rarely performed in isolation, usually being combined with synovectomy, tendon reconstruction, sta-

bilization or resection of the inferior radio-ulnar joint and intercarpal fusion.

Alternatives to replacement include synovectomy, proximal row carpectomy, flexible implant arthroplasty, partial or total wrist fusion. Fusion provides a strong, stable, pain-free wrist and can be achieved relatively easily in most cases, especially in rheumatoid disease. However, given the current relatively high failure rate of arthroplasties total wrist replacement can provide a viable alternative, particularly when other reconstructive procedures are unsuitable.

Salvage options in the case of failure include revision and reimplantation, resection/excision arthroplasty, arthrodesis and soft tissue reconstruction and rebalancing, but tend to leave the patient with a weaker grip due to the absence of extension together with a potential deleterious effect on the joints of the hand.

Although total wrist replacements are becoming increasingly available, they have as yet to become commonplace; they demand precise surgical techniques especially with regard to soft tissue balancing. Currently available implants still have a relatively high early failure and complication rate, as high as 35% at five years' follow up. Both prostheses and techniques are still evolving.

Surgical approach

A midline longitudinal incision is made on the dorsum of the wrist, avoiding the superficial veins, and the extensor retinaculum is reflected from the ulnar side of the wrist as far as its insertion onto the radius. The extensor tendons to the fingers are retracted towards the ulna while extensors pollicis longus and carpi radialis longus and brevis are retracted towards the radius. A distally based capsular flap is raised from the posterior rim of the radius and reflected from the underlying carpus. The articular surface and subchondral bone are excised from the radius, resection being perpendicular to the long axis. The triquetrum, scaphoid and lunate are removed and the proximal half of the capitate resected. A track is made across the capitate and along the shaft of the third metacarpal for the distal stem of the prosthesis, while the proximal stem fits into the medullary cavity of the radius (**6.264**). The capsule is then secured to the posterior rim of the distal radius. The wrist is supported in plaster for 3 weeks, following which gentle movements are started.

Metacarpophalangeal and interphalangeal joints

Rarely, single joints may require replacement in patients with post-traumatic or degenerative osteoarthrosis. However, in

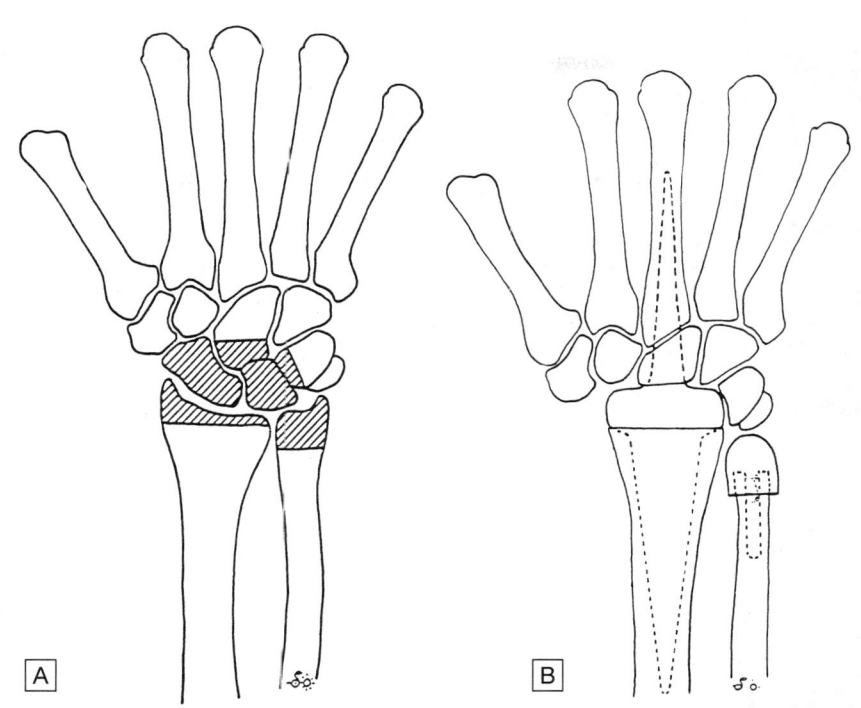

6.264 Silastic radiocarpal arthroplasty. A. the bone to be resected; B. the implant seated with stems in the middle metacarpal and radial shafts. Also shown is a replacement of the head of the ulna.

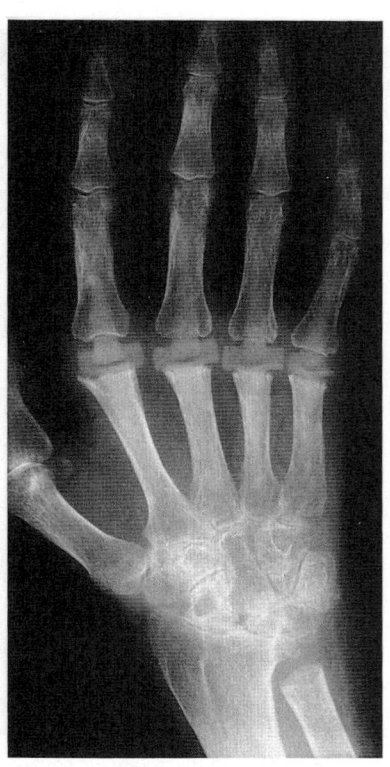

6.265 Postoperative radiograph showing metacarpophalangeal joint replacement in all fingers, using a silastic flexible hinge prosthesis, in a patient with rheumatoid arthritis. The distal ulna has also been excised (excision arthroplasty).

rheumatoid arthritis all metacarpophalangeal joints are often diseased, resulting in the classic deformity of fixed flexion and ulnar deviation of the fingers; secondary deformities may develop at the interphalangeal joints. The fingers cannot then be moved out of the palm to enable objects to be grasped; grip strength is reduced. Replacement of the damaged joints, together with soft tissue realignment, corrects the clinical deformity and allows approximately 50° of movement. Hand function is therefore improved, both by enabling the fingers to be cleared from the palm to permit objects to be held and by increasing the strength of power grip. Flexible silicone rubber hinge prostheses are frequently used.

Similar hinge prostheses can be used at the proximal interphalangeal joints of the middle, ring and little fingers, where flexion is important in power gripping.

Surgical approach. A curved longitudinal or transverse undulation incision is made over the metacarpophalangeal joint; the ulnar side of the extensor hood is incised to release the intrinsic insertions and free the ulnar deforming force: in the little finger the tendon of abductor digiti minimi is divided. The joint capsule is incised longitudinally and diseased synovium removed; the metacarpal head is resected at the level of the flare. The medullary canals of both the metacarpal and proximal phalanx are reamed and the prosthetic stems inserted (**6.265**). The radial capsule is reefed to realign the extensor tendon and, for the index finger, the radial collateral ligament is advanced proximally to increase stability and enhance thumb : index pinch.

Carpometacarpal joint of the thumb

The indication for replacement arthroplasty at this joint is usually degenerative osteoarthrosis, and almost never rheumatoid arthritis. Both thumbs may be involved and there is often a characteristic deformity of fixed abduction of the thumb with hyperextension laxity of the metacarpophalangeal joint. Soft tissue procedures are required to release the adductor contracture and to stabilize the metacarpophalangeal joint. Carpometacarpal joint arthritis can be treated by excising the trapezium (excision arthroplasty) and reconstructing the inter-

metacarpal ligament between the first and second metacarpals. Alternatively, the trapezium can be replaced with a silastic prosthesis which has a peg inserted into the first metacarpal shaft (**6.266** see over). A strip of flexor carpi radialis tendon is used to supplement the capsular repair and provide stability for the prosthesis.

Many surgeons no longer use the silastic prosthesis at this site as silicone synovitis, a giant cell foreign body reaction to silicone particles, may occur leading to erosion of adjacent bone. Silicone rubber prostheses may cause this reaction at other sites in the hand, but to a much lesser extent.

Surgical approach. A curved longitudinal incision is made over the dorsoulnar aspect of the carpometacarpal joint, taking care to protect the fine branches of the superficial radial nerve. The radial artery is exposed at the proximal border of the joint and a small branch supplying the joint is ligated. A longitudinal incision is made in the capsule and it is dissected from the trapezium, which is then bisected and removed. The base of the metacarpal is broached and the shaft reamed to receive the stem of the prosthesis. The

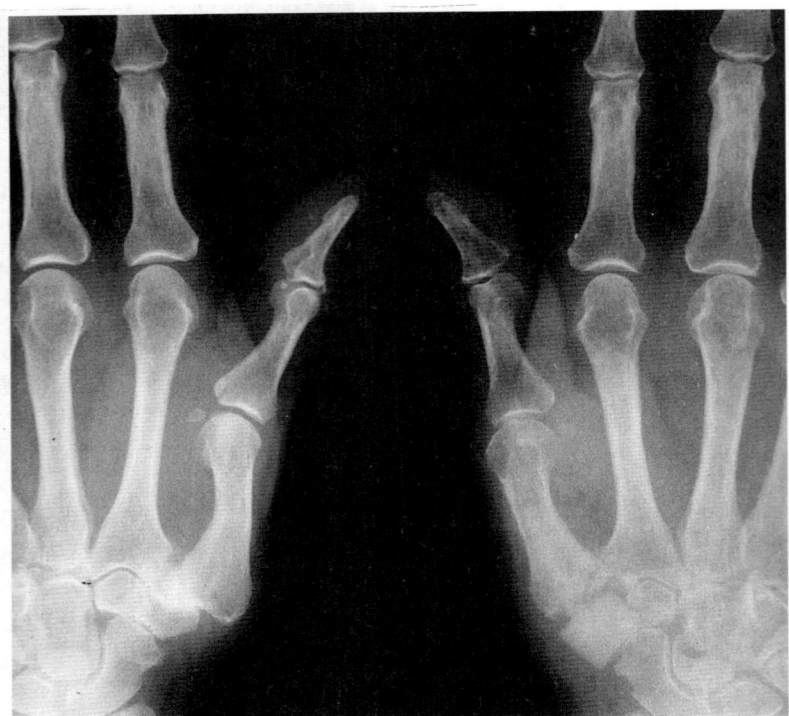

capsule is repaired and strengthened with a strip of the flexor carpi radialis tendon. (For further details see Swanson 1973; Swanson & de Groot Swanson 1974; Volz 1976; Meuli 1980; Beckenbaugh & Linscheid 1982; Stanley 1991.)

6.266   The left thumb shows severe pantrapezial osteoarthrosis with subluxation of the carpometacarpal joint: the classic deformity is demonstrated with metacarpal abduction and hyperextension at the metacarpophalangeal joint. In the right the trapezium has been excised and replaced with a silastic prosthesis; the soft tissues have been rebalanced correcting the pre-operative deformity.

FLEXURE LINES OF WRIST AND HAND

Flexure lines commonly crease the skin across the flexor surfaces of wrist and hand (10.110). Though not all directly over their functionally related subjacent skeletal joints they result from adhesion of the skin to subjacent deep fascia and are sites of folding of the skin during movement: such flexures have often been termed 'skin joints'. Nevertheless, they are useful landmarks. Less often mentioned, but quite prominent, although less regular, there are crease-line complexes, mainly transverse but with varying curvatures, which are centred over the dorsal (extensor) aspects of the radiocarpal, carpal, metacarpophalangeal and interphalangeal joints. During flexion the dorsal skin is stretched and the lines become less prominent (but can still be identified). During extension the now redundant skin becomes increasingly puckered and the lines are finally maximally prominent. (For a general review of 'skin lines' see p. 378.)

Near the junction of the carpus and forearm there are usually three *anterior* transverse lines; the proximal marks the proximal limit of flexor synovial sheaths, an intermediate line overlies the wrist joint and a distal line is at the proximal border of the flexor retinaculum.

In the palm a curved *radial longitudinal line* encircles the thenar eminence, ending at the palm's lateral margin; medial and roughly parallel to it are several less constant longitudinal lines. *Proximal* and *distal transverse lines* ascend medially across the palm. The proximal begins at the distal end of the radial longitudinal line and runs obliquely to the middle of the hypothenar eminence across the shafts of the metacarpals; the distal begins at or near the cleft between the index and middle finger and traverses the palm with a proximal convexity over the second to fourth metacarpal heads, near the proximal ends of the fibrous flexor sheaths. For further details see Bugbee and Botte (1993).

The second to fifth digits show proximal, middle and distal sets of transverse lines. The **proximal**, often double, are at the digital roots, about 2 cm **distal** to the metacarpophalangeal joints; the **middle** are typically double, proximal members being **directly over** the proximal interphalangeal joints; the **distal lines**, usually single, are **proximal** to the distal interphalangeal joints, their levels are sometimes marked by a fainter, more distal line. The free pollicial base is partly encircled by a line starting on the radial side and crossing distally over the metacarpophalangeal joint to end between the thumb and index finger level with the base of the proximal pollicial phalanx. A second, shorter crease is about 1 cm distal to this. At the interphalangeal joint of the thumb are two lines comparable to the middle digital lines in other digits.

LOWER LIMB

INTRODUCTION

The lower limb is primarily adapted for weight-bearing and locomotion, which together with the attainment of an habitual erect bipedal posture has resulted in a change in both the functional and mechanical requirements of all skeletal structures. Consequently more strength and stability are required than in the upper limb: the bones are larger and more robust, their form and structure being adapted to provide support and resist mechanical stresses; the internal architecture (trabecular systems) has specific arrangements in relation to these functions. Many bones, particularly the innominate and to a lesser extent the femur, also show sexual differences in line with the requirement for childbirth in the female.

An important consequence of the bipedal posture is that the centre of gravity of the body has been brought closer towards the vertebral column, to lie slightly behind and at the same level as the hip joint (anterior to the second sacral segment), reducing the tendency of gravity to pull the trunk forwards. From here the line of weight transmission passes anterior to both the knee and ankle joints: at the knee it passes towards the outside, at the ankle it passes through the navicular. Because of the angulation of the femur the foot, the tibia and knee of each limb remain close to the path followed by the centre of gravity, and the energy expenditure required to maintain the centre of gravity above the supporting limb during walking is therefore minimal. Balance is thus improved and there is more time for the free leg to swing forward promoting an increase in stride length. The alternation of the line of gravity is carried into the foot where it passes to the inner side. However, weight is also transmitted to the outside of the foot thus bringing the whole of the foot into use as a stabilizing element.

To reduce the possibility of collapse or dislocation, due to the higher forces to which they are subjected, the joints of the lower limb are structurally more stable than their upper limb counterparts. The increased stability is due to the shape of the articular surfaces (compare the shoulder and hip joints); the size, number and strength of associated ligaments (compare the elbow and knee joints); and the size and strength of the muscles related to the joint.

The pelvic girdle connects the lower limb to the axial skeleton via the posterior articulation with the sacrum. This articulation, the sacroiliac joint, has sacrificed mobility for stability and strength for weight transmission from the trunk to the lower limb; the area of contact between sacrum and ilium relative to ilial area has increased during evolution. Similarly the acetabulum and femoral head have also increased in relative size. The knee too has undergone change in that it has become closer to the midline as part of the strategy of centring the body mass, thereby reinforcing skeletal rather than muscular equilibrium.

The foot has perhaps undergone the greatest evolutionary change within the lower limb, with a reduction in its original primate function of being a grasping tactile organ to becoming a locomotor prop; the joints within the human foot are much less mobile, an adaptation to ground walking. During walking the foot acts as a lever adding propulsive force to that of the leg, with the point of pivot being the subtalar joint. The forefoot has been relatively shortened accentuating the power capabilities of the foot as a whole. The arches convert the foot into a complex spring, held in tension by ligaments and tendons, able to transmit the stresses involved in walking, both when body momentum is checked at heel strike and in propelling the body forwards at toe off. The lateral arch steadies the foot on the ground, while the medial transmits the main propulsive thrust. It is the arched form of the foot which helps to minimize energy expenditure and therefore increase the efficiency of walking.

INNOMINATE

The innominate or hip bone (**6.267, 268**) is large, irregular, constricted centrally and expanded above and below. Its *lateral surface* has a deep, cup-shaped *acetabulum*, articulating with the femoral head, anteroinferior to which is the large, oval or triangular *obturator foramen*. Above the acetabulum the bone widens into a plate with a sinuously curved *iliac crest*.

The bone articulates in front with its fellow, to form the pelvic girdle (p. 613). Each has three parts, *ilium*, *ischium* and *pubis*, connected by cartilage in youth but united as one bone in adults, the principal union being in the acetabulum (**6.267**B, **268**B). The ilium includes the upper acetabulum and expanded area above it; the ischium includes the lower acetabulum and bone posteroinferior to it; the pubis forms the anterior acetabulum, separating the ilium from ischium, and the anterior median region where the pubes meet.

ILIUM

The ilium, so named because it supports the *flank*, may be described as having upper and lower parts and three surfaces. The smaller, lower part forms a little less than the upper two-fifths of the acetabulum, the upper part being much expanded, with gluteal, sacropelvic and iliac (internal) surfaces. The posterolateral *gluteal surface* is an extensive rough area; the anteromedial *iliac fossa* is

smooth and concave; the *sacropelvic surface* is medial and posteroinferior to the fossa, separated from it by the *medial border*.

Iliac borders

Iliac crest. This is the ilium's superior border, convex upwards but sinuously curved, internally concave in front, the reverse behind. Its ends project as anterior and posterior superior iliac spines. The *anterior superior iliac spine* is palpable at the lateral end of the inguinal fold; the *posterior superior iliac spine* is not palpable but often indicated by a dimple, about 4 cm lateral to the second sacral spine above the medial gluteal region (buttock). The crest has ventral and dorsal segments: the ventral is slightly more than the anterior two-thirds of the crest and its prominence is associated with changes in iliac form due to the emergence of the upright posture; the dorsal segment, about the posterior third in mankind, exists in all land vertebrates. The iliac crest's ventral segment has internal and external lips, the rough intermediate zone being narrowest centrally. The *tubercle of the crest* (**6.267**A) projects onto the outer lip about 5 cm posterosuperior to the anterior superior spine. The dorsal segment has two sloping surfaces separated by a longitudinal ridge ending at the posterior superior spine. The crest's *summit*, a little behind its midpoint, is level with the interval between the third and fourth lumbar spines. The lower part of the ilium will be described with the acetabulum (p. 668).

Anterior border. This descends to the acetabulum from the anterior superior spine. Superiorly it is concave forwards; inferiorly is a rough *anterior inferior iliac spine*, immediately above the acetabulum.

Posterior border. This is irregularly curved (**6.268**), descending from the posterior superior spine at first forwards, with a posterior concavity forming a small notch. At the lower end of the notch is a wide, low projection, the *posterior inferior iliac spine*; here the border turns almost horizontally forwards for about 3 cm and finally down and back to join the posterior ischial border. Together they form a deep *greater sciatic notch*, bounded above by the ilium, below by the ilium and ischium (**6.268**B).

Medial border. Separating the iliac fossa and the sacropelvic surface, this is indistinct near the crest, rough in its upper part, then sharp where it bounds an articular surface for the sacrum, and finally rounded. The latter part is the *arcuate line*, which inferiorly reaches the posterior part of the *iliopubic (iliopectineal) eminence*, marking the union of the ilium and pubis.

Gluteal surface

The *gluteal surface* (**6.267**), facing inferiorly in its posterior part, laterally and slightly downwards in front, is bounded above by the iliac crest, below by the upper acetabular border and by the anterior and posterior borders. It is rough and curved, convex in front, concave behind, and marked by three gluteal lines. The *posterior gluteal line* is shortest, descending from the external lip of the crest about 5 cm in front of its posterior limit and ending in front of the posterior inferior iliac spine. Above, it is usually distinct, but inferiorly it is ill-defined and frequently absent. The *anterior gluteal line*, the longest, begins near the midpoint of the superior margin of the greater sciatic notch and ascends forwards into the crest's outer lip, a little anterior to its tubercle. The *inferior gluteal line*, rarely well-marked, begins posterosuperior to the anterior inferior iliac spine, curving posteroinferiorly to end near the apex of the greater sciatic notch. Between the inferior gluteal line and the acetabular margin is a rough, shallow groove. Behind the acetabulum the lower gluteal surface is continuous with the posterior ischial surface, the union marked by a low elevation.

Iliac fossa

The *iliac fossa*, the internal concavity of the ilium, faces anterosuperior being limited above by the iliac crest, in front by the anterior border and behind by the medial border, separating it from the sacropelvic surface. It forms the smooth and gently concave posterolateral wall of the greater pelvis. Below it is continuous with a wide shallow groove (**6.268**A), which is bounded laterally by the anterior inferior iliac spine and medially by the iliopubic eminence.

Sacropelvic surface

The *sacropelvic surface* (**6.268**A), the posteroinferior part of the medial   **663**

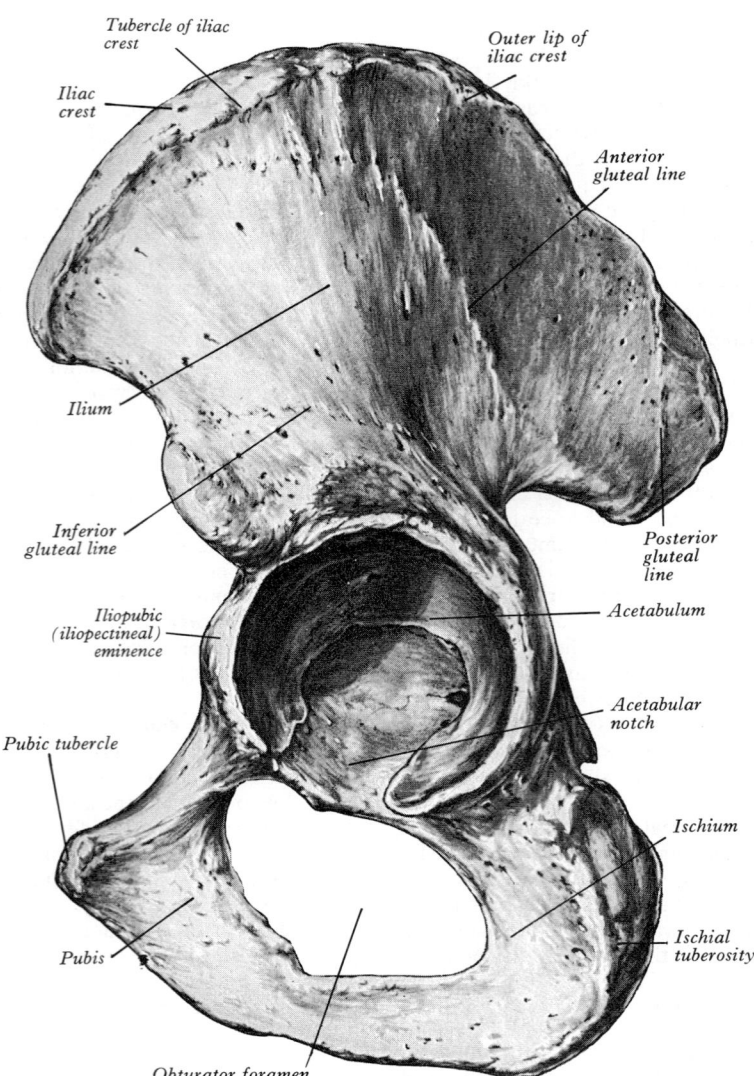

Tubercle of iliac crest

Iliac crest

Outer lip of iliac crest

Anterior gluteal line

Ilium

Inferior gluteal line

Iliopubic (iliopectineal) eminence

Pubic tubercle

Pubis

Posterior gluteal line

Acetabulum

Acetabular notch

Ischium

Ischial tuberosity

A

Obturator foramen

6.267 The left innominate bone; A. Lateral (external) aspect: B. Line drawing showing muscle attachments; the epiphyseal lines are stippled.

iliac surface, is bounded posteroinferiorly by the posterior border, anterosuperiorly by the medial border, posterosuperiorly by the iliac crest and anteroinferiorly by the line of fusion of the ilium and ischium. It is divided into iliac tuberosity, auricular and pelvic surfaces. The *iliac tuberosity*, a large, rough area below the dorsal segment of the iliac crest, shows cranial and caudal areas separated by an oblique ridge and connected to the sacrum by the interosseous sacroiliac ligament. The *auricular surface* (**6.268B**), immediately anteroinferior to the tuberosity, articulates with the lateral sacral mass. Shaped like an ear, its widest part is anterosuperior, its 'lobule' posteroinferior and on the medial aspect of the posterior inferior spine. Its edges are well-defined, but the surface, though articular, is rough and irregular. The *pelvic surface* is anteroinferior to the acutely recurved part of the auricular surface, contributing to the lateral wall of the lesser pelvis. Its upper part, facing down, is between the auricular surface and the upper limb of the greater sciatic notch; its lower region faces medially and is separated from iliac fossa by the arcuate line. Anteroinferiorly it extends to the line of union of the ilium and ischium; this is usually obliterated, but passes from the depth of the acetabulum to, roughly, the middle of the inferior limb of the greater sciatic notch.

Further details

Iliac crest. Approximating to the lower limit of the waist, it is an attachment for lateral abdominal and dorsal muscles, fasciae and muscles of the lower limb (**6.267B, 268B**). To the *outer lip* and *tubercle*

of its ventral segment (p. 663) the fascia lata and iliotibial tract are attached, anterior to its tubercle tensor fasciae latae; to its anterior two-thirds, the lower fibres of the external oblique and, just behind its summit, the lowest fibres of latissimus dorsi. A variable interval exists between the most posterior attachment of external oblique and the most anterior attachment of latissimus dorsi, and here the crest is the base of the lumbar triangle. The crest's *intermediate area* receives internal oblique. To the anterior two-thirds of its *inner lip* transversus abdominis is attached, and behind this the thoracolumbar fascia and quadratus lumborum. To the crest's dorsal segment (p. 663), on its lateral slope, the highest fibres of gluteus maximus are attached; from its medial slope erector spinae and, along its medial margin, the interosseous and posterior sacroiliac ligaments arise.

The anterior superior spine. To this is attached the lateral end of the inguinal ligament below which the attachment of sartorius extends down the *anterior border*.

The anterior inferior spine. This is divided indistinctly into an upper area for the straight part of rectus femoris and a lower area extending laterally along the upper acetabular margin to form a triangular impression for the iliofemoral ligament.

The posterior border. To the upper part the upper fibres of the sacrotuberous ligament are attached and in front of the posterior inferior spine (i.e. on the upper border of the greater sciatic notch) fibres of piriformis. The superior rim of the notch is related to the superior gluteal vessels and nerve. The lower part of the border (i.e.

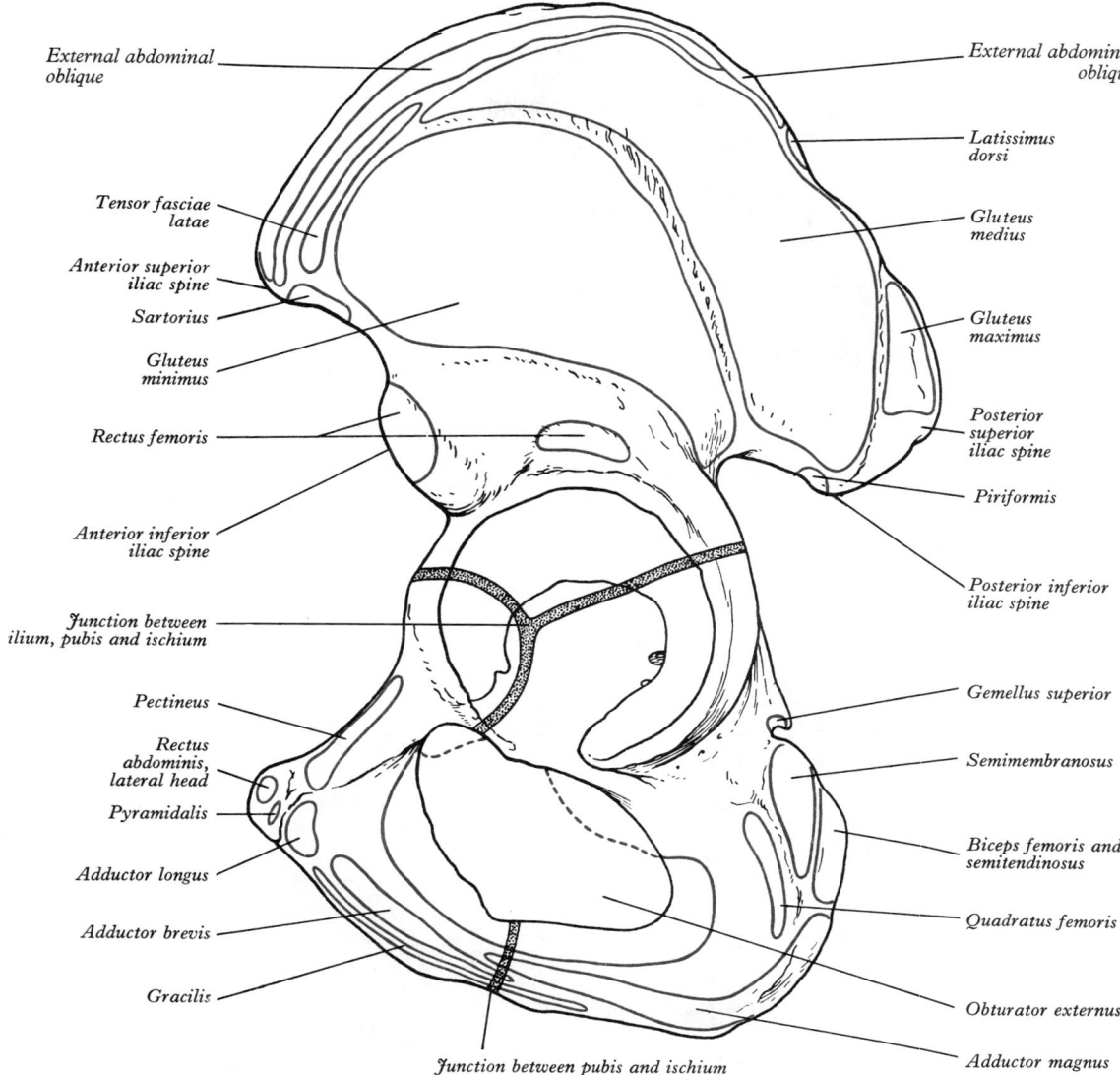

External abdominal
oblique

External abdominal
oblique

Latissimus
dorsi

Tensor fasciae
latae

Gluteus
medius

Anterior superior
iliac spine

Sartorius

Gluteus
maximus

Gluteus
minimus

Rectus femoris

Posterior
superior
iliac spine

Piriformis

Anterior inferior
iliac spine

Posterior inferior
iliac spine

Junction between
ilium, pubis and ischium

Gemellus superior

Pectineus

Semimembranosus

Rectus
abdominis,
lateral head

Pyramidalis

Biceps femoris and
semitendinosus

Adductor longus

Quadratus femoris

Adductor brevis

Gracilis

Obturator externus

Adductor magnus

B

Junction between pubis and ischium

the lower margin of the greater sciatic notch) is covered by piriformis and related to the sciatic nerve, which, however, largely adjoins the ischium.

Gluteal surface. This is divided by the three gluteal lines into four areas (**6.267**):

- behind the posterior line, its upper rough part being for the upper fibres of the gluteus maximus and its lower, smooth region for part of the sacrotuberous ligament and iliac head of piriformis;
- between the posterior and anterior lines, below the iliac crest, for gluteus medius;
- between the anterior and inferior lines for gluteus minimus;
- below the inferior line, where there are many vascular foramina.

Attached to a curved groove above the acetabulum is the reflected head of rectus femoris and to an area adjoining the acetabular rim is the articular capsule; most of this area is covered by gluteus minimus. Posteroinferiorly, near the union of the ilium and ischium, the bone is related to piriformis. The vascular foramina on the iliac gluteal aspect may lead into large vascular canals in the bone (Sirang 1973).

Iliac fossa. In its upper two-thirds, it provides attachment for the iliacus (**6.268B**), also related to the lower third; branches of the iliolumbar artery run between the muscle and bone, one entering a large nutrient foramen often posteroinferior in the fossa. The wide groove between the anterior inferior iliac spine and the iliopubic eminence is occupied by the converging fibres of iliacus laterally and the tendon of psoas major medially, the tendon separated from bone

by a bursa. The right iliac fossa contains the caecum, and often the vermiform appendix and terminal ileum; the left one houses the end of the descending colon.

Iliac tuberosity. This (sacropelvic surface) gives attachment to the posterior sacroiliac ligaments and, behind the auricular surface, the interosseous sacroiliac ligament. To its anterior part is attached the iliolumbar ligament and above this is the medial part of quadratus lumborum.

Auricular surface. This articulates with the sacrum and is reciprocally shaped (p. 674). To its sharp anterior and inferior borders the anterior sacroiliac ligament is attached. The narrow part of the **pelvic surface**, between the auricular surface and the upper rim of the greater sciatic notch, often shows a rough *preauricular sulcus* for the lower fibres of the anterior sacroiliac ligament, more apparent in females. However, its unreliability in sex determination was shown in a study of 237 Indian pelves (Jit & Gandhi 1966), but also consult Finnegan and Faust (1974) and Finnegan (1978). Lateral to the sulcus, piriformis is sometimes, in part, attached, and to the more extensive remainder of the pelvic surface is attached part of the obturator internus (**6.268B**).

PUBIS

The pubis is the ventral part of the innominate bone and forms a median cartilaginous *pubic symphysis* with its fellow. From its anteromedial body a superior ramus passes up and back to the

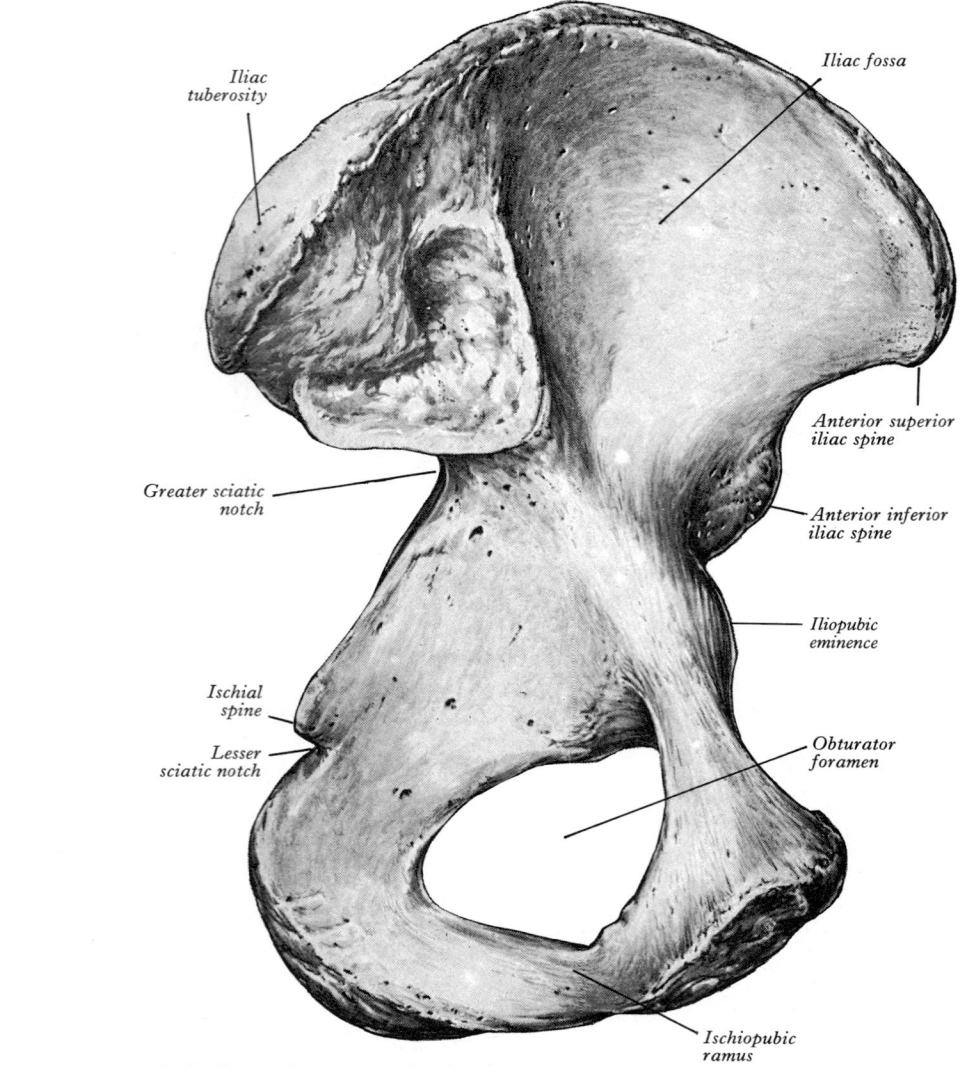

Iliac tuberosity

Iliac fossa

Anterior superior iliac spine

Greater sciatic notch

Anterior inferior iliac spine

Iliopubic eminence

Ischial spine

Lesser sciatic notch

Obturator foramen

A

Ischiopubic ramus

6.268 The left innominate bone. A. Medial (internal) aspect: B. Line drawing showing muscle attachments; the epiphyseal lines are stippled.

acetabulum and an inferior ramus passes back, down and laterally to join the ischial ramus inferomedial to the obturator foramen.

Body

The *body*, anteroposteriorly compressed, has anterior, posterior and symphyseal (medial) surfaces and an upper border, the *pubic crest*. The *anterior surface* also faces inferolaterally; it is rough supero-medially and elsewhere smooth, affording attachment for medial femoral muscles. The smooth *posterior surface* faces upwards and backwards as the oblique anterior wall of the lesser pelvis and is related to the urinary bladder. The *symphyseal surface* is elongate and oval, united by cartilage to its fellow at the pubic symphysis. Denuded of cartilage it has, in the elderly, an irregular surface of small ridges and furrows or nodular elevations, varying much with age (Todd 1920a,b, 1921a,b; Brooks 1955; McKern & Stewart 1957; Suchey et al 1979), features of obvious forensic value. Pal and Tamankar (1983), in a series of 60 male and 60 female pubes of Northern Indians, aged from 14 to 60 years, found that accepted data gave inaccurate values, some 'over-ageing' their specimens, some the reverse. The *pubic crest* is the rounded upper border of the body, which overhangs the anterior surface (**6.267**A), its lateral end being the rounded *pubic tubercle*. Both crest and tubercle are pal-pable, the latter partly obscured in males by the spermatic cord, crossing above it from the scrotum to the abdomen. The *pubic rami* diverge posterolaterally from the lateral corners of the body.

The *anterior surface* of the pubic body faces the femoral adductor region; on its medial part and to a rough strip, which is wider in females, attaches the anterior pubic ligament. In the angle between

its upper end and the pubic crest the tendon of adductor longus is attached and below this, to a line near the medial border extending down to the inferior ramus, gracilis attaches. Lateral to gracilis adductor brevis is attached to the body and inferior ramus. Obturator externus is attached laterally to the anterior surface, spreading onto both rami (**6.267**B).

The *posterior surface* is separated from the urinary bladder by retropubic fat; near its centre anterior fibres of levator ani are attached, more laterally obturator internus, and this extends to both rami. Medial to levator ani the puboprostatic ligaments are attached.

The superior pubic ramus

The superior pubic ramus passes upwards, backwards and laterally from the body, superolateral to the obturator foramen to reach the acetabulum. Triangular in section, it has three surfaces and borders. Its anterior, *pectineal surface*, tilted slightly up, is triangular in outline and extends from the pubic tubercle to the iliopubic eminence (**6.268**B). It is bounded in front by the rounded *obturator crest* and behind by the sharp *pecten pubis* (*pectineal line*) which, with the crest, is the pubic part of the *linea terminalis* (i.e. anterior part of the pelvic brim). The posterosuperior, *pelvic surface*, medially inclined, is smooth and narrows into the posterior surface of the body, bounded above by the pecten pubis and below by a sharp *inferior border*. The *obturator surface*, directed down and back, is crossed by the *obturator groove* sloping down and forwards; its limit in front is the *obturator crest* and, behind, the inferior border.

To the *pectineal surface* of the superior ramus along its upper part pectineus is attached, covering the rest of the surface (**6.267**B).

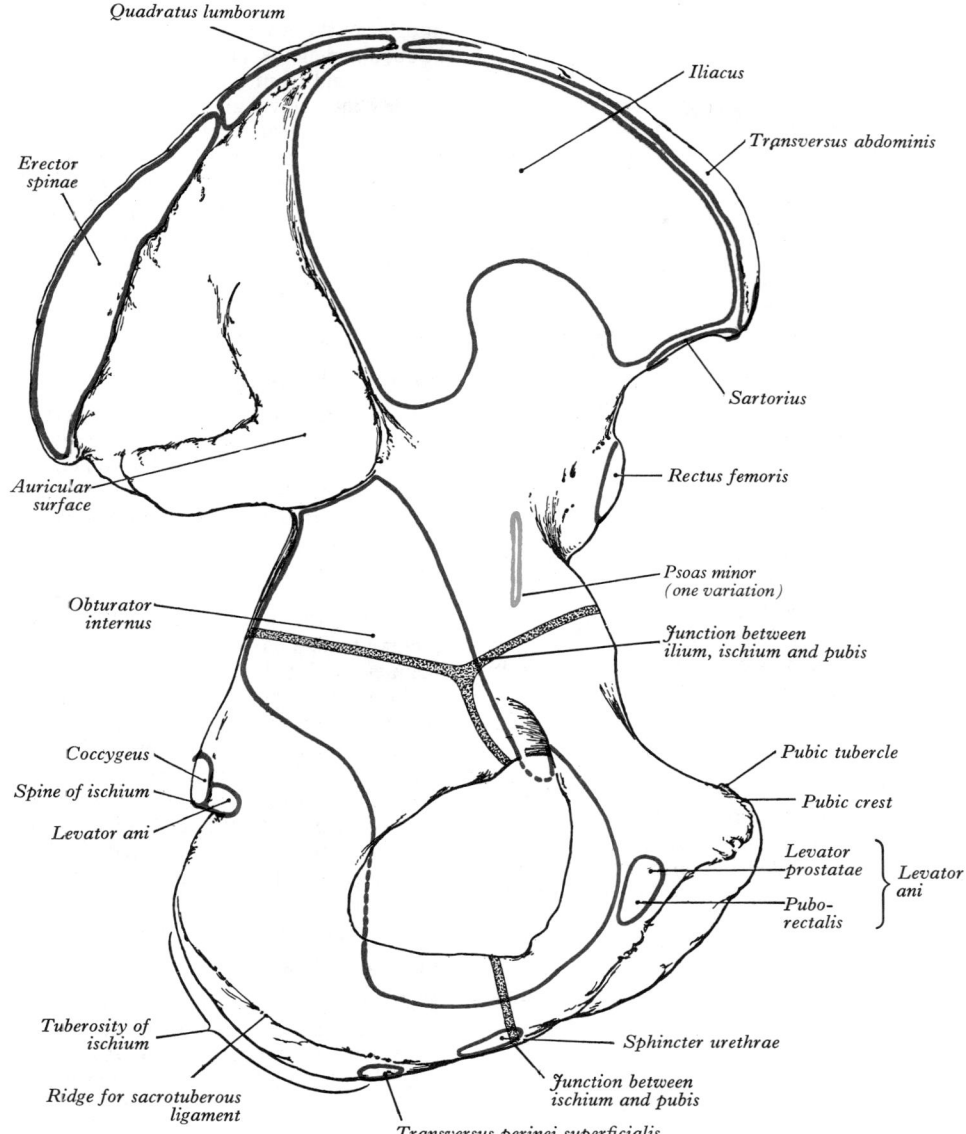

The inferior pubic ramus

The inferior pubic ramus, an inferolateral process of the body, descends inferolaterally to join the ischial ramus medial to, and below, the obturator foramen. The union may be locally thickened, but not obviously so in adults. The ramus has two surface and borders. The *anteroexternal surface*, continuous above with that of the pubic body, faces the thigh and is marked by muscles, its lateral limit being the margin of the obturator foramen and, medially, the rough anterior border. The *posterointernal surface* is continuous above with that of the body and transversely convex, its medial part is often everted in males (see **6.274B**) and connected to the crus penis. This surface faces the perineum medially, its smooth lateral part tilted up towards the pelvic cavity.

To the *external surface* of the inferior ramus are attached gracilis, adductor brevis and obturator externus, in mediolateral order. In addition, the adductor magnus usually extends from the ischial ramus on to the lower part of the inferior pubic ramus between adductor brevis and obturator externus. The *internal surface* is indistinctly divided into medial, intermediate and lateral areas. The medial area faces inferomedially in direct contact with the crus penis, limited above and behind by an indistinct ridge for attachment of the inferior fascia of the urogenital diaphragm (p. 832). To the intermediate area, related to the dorsal penile nerve, internal pudendal vessels and their fascial sheath, may be attached some inner fibres of sphincter urethrae, and to the lateral area, fibres of

obturator internus. The *medial margin* of the ramus, strongly everted in males, is an attachment of the fascia lata and the membranous layer of the superficial perineal fascia.

Pubic tubercle

The pubic tubercle is a medial attachment of the inguinal ligament in the floor of the superficial inguinal ring and is crossed by the spermatic cord; ascending loops of cremaster are also attached to it. Laterally on the *pubic crest* are attached the lateral part of rectus abdominis and, below it, pyramidalis. Medially the crest is crossed by the medial part of rectus abdominis, ascending from ligamentous fibres interlacing in front of the pubic symphysis.

Pecten pubis

The pecten pubis is the sharp, superior edge of the pectineal surface. Attached at its medial end are the conjoint tendon and lacunar ligament, along the rest of it a strong fibrous *pectineal ligament* (p. 822) and, near its centre, psoas minor when present. The smooth *pelvic surface* is separated from parietal peritoneum only by areolar tissue, in which the lateral umbilical ligament descends forwards across the ramus and, laterally, the ductus deferens passes backwards. The *obturator groove*, converted to a canal by the upper borders of the obturator membrane and obturator muscles, transmits the obturator vessels and nerve from the pelvis to the thigh. To the lateral end of the *obturator crest* (**6.268B**) some fibres of the pubofemoral ligament are attached.

667

ISCHIUM

The ischium, the inferoposterior part of the innominate bone, has a body and ramus, the body having upper and lower ends and femoral, posterior and pelvic surfaces (**6**.267, 268, 269). Above, it forms the inferoposterior part of the acetabulum; below, its ramus ascends anteromedially at an acute angle to meet the descending pubic ramus, completing the obturator foramen.

The *femoral surface*, facing down, forwards and laterally towards the thigh, is bounded in front by the margin of the obturator foramen and a lateral border, indistinct above but well-defined below, forming the lateral limit of the ischial tuberosity. The *posterior surface*, facing superolaterally, is continuous above with the iliac gluteal surface, and here a low convexity follows the acetabular curvature. This surface is inferiorly the upper part of the ischial tuberosity, above which is a wide, shallow groove on its lateral and medial aspects. The *ischial tuberosity* (**6**.269) is a large, rough area on the ischium's lower posterior surface and inferior extremity. Though obscured by gluteus maximus in extension, it is palpable in flexion. It is 5 cm from the midline and about the same distance above the gluteal fold (p. 878). Elongate, widest above, tapering inferiorly, it is the attachment of the posterior femoral muscles. The ischial posterior aspect is between the lateral and posterior borders. The *posterior border* blends above with that of the ilium, helping to complete the inferior rim of the *greater sciatic notch*, the posterior end of which has a conspicuous *ischial spine*. Below this, the rounded border is the floor of the *lesser sciatic notch*, between the ischial spine and tuberosity. The *pelvic surface* is smooth and faces the pelvic cavity; below this is part of the lateral wall of the ischiorectal fossa.

Ischial ramus

This has anterior and posterior surfaces continuous with those of the inferior pubic ramus; the former is really antero-inferior and roughened by the attachment of the medial femoral muscles. The smooth *posterior surface* is partly divided into perineal and pelvic areas, like the inferior pubic ramus. The *upper border* completes the obturator foramen; the rough *lower border*, together with the medial border of the inferior pubic ramus, bounds the subpubic angle and pubic arch.

The *anterior surface* and *ischial ramus* faces the adductor region.

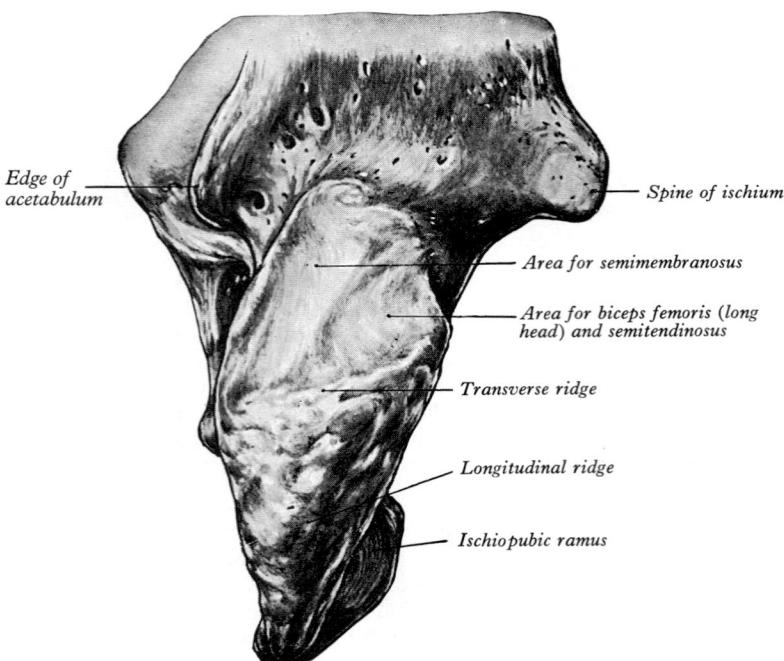

Edge of acetabulum

Spine of ischium

Area for semimembranosus

Area for biceps femoris (long head) and semitendinosus

Transverse ridge

Longitudinal ridge

Ischiopubic ramus

6.269 The left ischial tuberosity: posterior aspect. The *transverse ridge* forms the lower boundary of the area for the hamstring muscles and separates it from the lower half of the tuberosity, which is divided into lateral and medial areas by the *longitudinal ridge*. To the lateral area is attached the adductor magnus; the medial area is covered with fibro-adipose tissue and supports the body in the sitting posture.

The obturator externus above, anterior fibres of adductor magnus and, near the lower border, gracilis are all attached here. Between adductor magnus and gracilis the attachment of adductor brevis may descend from the inferior pubic ramus. The *posterior surface* is divided into pelvic and perineal areas; the former, facing back, has part of obturator internus attached to it; the perineal area faces medially, its upper part related to the crus penis or clitoridis, with the sphincter urethrae attached to it, and below this ischiocavernosus and the transverse superficial perineal muscle. The inferior fascia of the urogenital diaphragm is attached below the ridge between the perineal and pelvic areas and above the areas for the crus of the penis and sphincter urethrae. The *lower border* of the ramus is an attachment of fascia lata and a membranous layer of the superficial perineal fascia.

Ischial tuberosity

Divided nearly transversely into upper and lower areas (**6**.269), the upper is subdivided by an oblique line into a superolateral part for semimembranosus and an inferomedial part for the long head of biceps femoris and semitendinosus; the lower region, narrowing as it curves on to the inferior ischial aspect, is subdivided by an irregular vertical ridge into lateral and medial areas. The larger lateral area is for part of adductor magnus, the medial is covered by fibro-adipose tissue, usually containing the ischial bursa of gluteus maximus and supporting the body in sitting. Medially the tuberosity is limited by a curved ridge passing on to the ramus, to which the sacrotuberous ligament and its falciform process are attached (**6**.268B). Many fibres of biceps femoris pass into the ligament, an interesting fact, since the sacrum and posterior part of the ilium are primitive mammalian attachments of biceps femoris—the tuberosity being a secondary attachment, the ligament representing, at least in part, remains of primitive tendon.

Superomedial to the tuberosity the posterior surface has a wide, shallow groove, usually covered by hyaline cartilage, with a bursa between it and the tendon of obturator internus. To the lower margin of the groove, near the tuberosity, gemellus inferior is attached, and to the upper margin, near the ischial spine, gemellus superior.

Ischial spine

This projects downwards and a little medially. To its margins is attached the sacrospinous ligament, separating the greater from the lesser sciatic foramen (see **6**.278). It is crossed posteriorly by the internal pudendal vessels and the nerve to obturator internus. Its pelvic surface is an attachment of coccygeus (coextensive with the sacrospinous ligament) and the most posterior fibres of levator ani. Various structures traverse these foramina (p. 677).

To the smooth *pelvic ischial surface*, in its upper part, is attached obturator internus, converging on the lesser sciatic notch (foramen) and covering the rest of this surface, except the pelvic aspect of the ischial spine. The muscle and its fascia separate the bone from the ischiorectal fossa.

Acetabulum (6.267A)

An approximately hemispherical cavity central on the lateral aspect of the innominate bone, it faces anteroinferiorly; it is surrounded by an irregular margin deficient **inferiorly** at the *acetabular notch*. The *acetabular fossa* is the cavity's central floor, which is rough and non-articular and has an articular *lunate surface*, widest above, where weight is transmitted to the femur. On this crescentic surface, covered with cartilage, the head of the femur slides. All three innominate elements contribute to the acetabulum in man, but unequally. The pubis forms the anterosuperior fifth of the articular surface, the ischium forms the fossa's floor and rather more than the postero-inferior two-fifths of the articular surface, and the ilium the remainder. A linear defect may cross the acetabular surface from the *superior border* to the acetabular fossa, but does not follow any junction between the main morphologic parts of the innominate bone.

Obturator foramen

Below and slightly anterior to the acetabulum, it is between the pubis and ischium. It is rimmed above by the grooved obturator surface of the superior pubic ramus, medially by the pubic body and its inferior ramus, below by the ischial ramus, laterally by the anterior border of the ischial body, including the margin of the acetabular notch. The foramen is almost closed by the *obturator membrane* which is attached to its margins, except above, where a communication remains between the pelvis and thigh; this free edge is attached to an *anterior obturator tubercle* at the anterior end of the inferior border of the superior pubic ramus, and a *posterior obturator tubercle* on the anterior border of the acetabular notch; these tubercles are sometimes indistinct. Since the tubercles lie in different planes and the obturator groove crosses the foramen's upper border, the acetabular rim is in fact a spiral. The foramen is large and oval in males, but smaller and nearly triangular in females.

Further details

Attached below to the *femoral surface* of the *ischial body* is part of obturator externus (**6.267**B) and along the upper part of the lateral border of the ischial tuberosity is quadratus femoris. Below the acetabulum, to the lateral border, the ischiofemoral ligament is attached. Above the ischial tuberosity the *posterior surface* is crossed by the tendon of obturator internus and the gemelli; between them and bone is the nerve to quadratus femoris. At a higher level the femoral surface is covered by piriformis, partially separated by the sciatic nerve and the nerve to quadratus femoris.

Structure

The thicker parts of the innominate are trabecular, encased by two layers of compact bone; the thinner parts, for example in the acetabulum and central iliac fossa, are often translucent, consisting of one lamina of compact bone. In the upper acetabulum and along the arcuate line, i.e. the route of weight transmission from the sacrum to the femur, compact bone is increased and subjacent trabecular bone displays two sets of pressure lamellae. They start together near the upper auricular surface and diverge to impinge on two strong buttresses of compact bone, from which two similar sets of lamellar arches start and converge on the acetabulum (Wakeley 1929). Because of frequent use for biopsy puncture the anterior iliac crest has been much studied as regards distribution of cortical and trabecular bone. Whitehouse (1977) has surveyed these studies; his own observations, by scanning electron micrography, indicate that the cortical bone is very porous, being only 75% bone, decreasing to 35% near the anterior superior iliac spine; denser cortical bone commences at the margins of the crest, thickening rapidly below it on both aspects of the iliac squama.

Studies of the internal stresses within the innominate have revealed a systemic pattern of trabeculae that corresponds well with the expected patterns of theoretical stress trajectories (Holm 1980); however, the patterns are much more complicated than in any other major bone. Stresses are higher in the acetabular than the iliac region (Goel et al 1978), the ilium being an area subjected to insignificant stresses on the pelvic side with stress lower than those on the lateral side. Venieratos et al (1987) have observed a good correlation (convergence) between the direction of the trabeculae and both compressive and tensile stresses, the convergence being better in those parts of the bone where the stresses are greatest, the mean difference being ± 7°.

Ossification

Ossification is by three primary centres, for the ilium, ischium and pubis; the iliac appears above the greater sciatic notch prenatally about the ninth week (Laurenson 1964), the ischial in its body in the fourth month, and the pubic in its superior ramus between the fourth and fifth months. At birth some parts are still cartilaginous: the whole iliac crest, the acetabular floor and inferior margin (**6.270**A); the acetabulum is still a cartilaginous cup with a triradiate stem extending medially to the pelvic surface as a Y-shaped epiphyseal plate between the ilium, ischium and pubis (Harrison 1957), including also the anterior inferior iliac spine. Cartilage along the inferior margin also covers the ischial tuberosity, forms (temporarily) conjoined ischial and pubic rami and continues to the pubic symphyseal surface and along the pubic crest to its tubercle.

The ossifying ischium and pubis fuse to form a continuous ramus at the seventh or eighth year (**6.271**). Secondary centres, other than for the acetabulum, appear about puberty and join between the fifteenth and twenty-fifth years (**6.270**B); there are usually two for the iliac crest (which rapidly fuse), and single centres for the ischial tuberosity (in cartilage close to the inferior acetabular margin and spreading forwards), anterior inferior iliac spine (although it may ossify from the triradiate cartilage) and symphyseal surface of the pubis (the pubic tubercle and crest may have separate centres).

Between age eight and nine years three major centres of ossification appear in the acetabular cartilage (Ponseti 1978a); the largest appears in the anterior wall of the acetabulum and fuses with the pubis, one in the iliac acetabular cartilage superiorly and fuses with the ilium and one in the ischial acetabular cartilage posteriorly and fuses with the ischium. At puberty these epiphyses expand towards the periphery of the acetabulum contributing to its depth (Ponseti 1978a). Fusion between the three bones within the acetabulum occurs between the sixteenth and eighteenth years. Delaere et al (1992) have suggested that ossification of the ilium is similar to that of a long bone, possessing three cartilaginous epiphyses and one cartilaginous process; however, it tends to undergo osteoclastic resorption comparable with that of cranial bones. During development the acetabulum increases in breadth at a faster rate than it does in depth (Meszaros & Kery 1980).

SKELETAL PELVIS

The term *pelvis*, 'a basin', is vaguely applied to the skeletal ring formed by the innominate bones and the sacrum, the cavity within them and even the entire region where the trunk and lower limbs meet. It is used here in the skeletal sense, for the irregular osseous girdle between the femoral heads and fifth lumbar vertebra. It is massive, because its primary function is to withstand compression and other forces due to body weight and powerful musculature, mechanisms considered elsewhere (p. 678). Here, we are concerned with metrical and other features of sexual significance, and hence of obstetric, forensic and anthropological application.

The pelvis can be regarded as having greater and lesser segments, the true and false pelves, arbitrarily divided by an oblique plane, passing through the sacral promontory behind and *lineae terminales* elsewhere. Each linea terminalis includes the iliac arcuate line (p. 663), pecten (iliopectineal line) and pubic crest. But the segments are continuous, and parts of the body cavity which they enclose are also continuous through the superior pelvic aperture or pelvic inlet (**6.272**).

The greater pelvis

This consists of iliac flanges above the lineae terminales and the sacral base. This junctional zone is structurally massive, forming powerful arches from the acetabular fossae to the vertebral column around the visceral cavity which is, of course, part of the abdomen; because of the pelvic inclination it has little anterior wall.

The lesser pelvis

This encloses a true basin when soft tissues of the pelvic floor are in

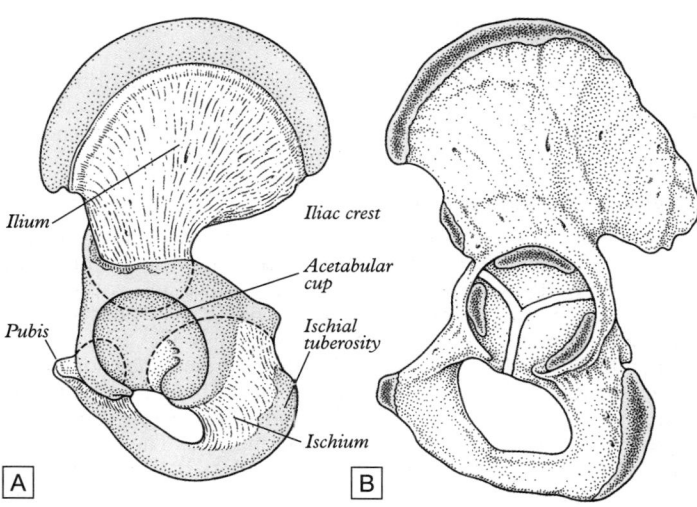

6.270A. The innominate bone at birth; B. The adolescent innominate, more heavily stippled areas indicate the secondary centres of ossification. See text for dates of appearance of the various secondary centres.

Ilium

Iliac crest

Acetabular cup

Pubis

Ischial tuberosity

Ischium

A

B

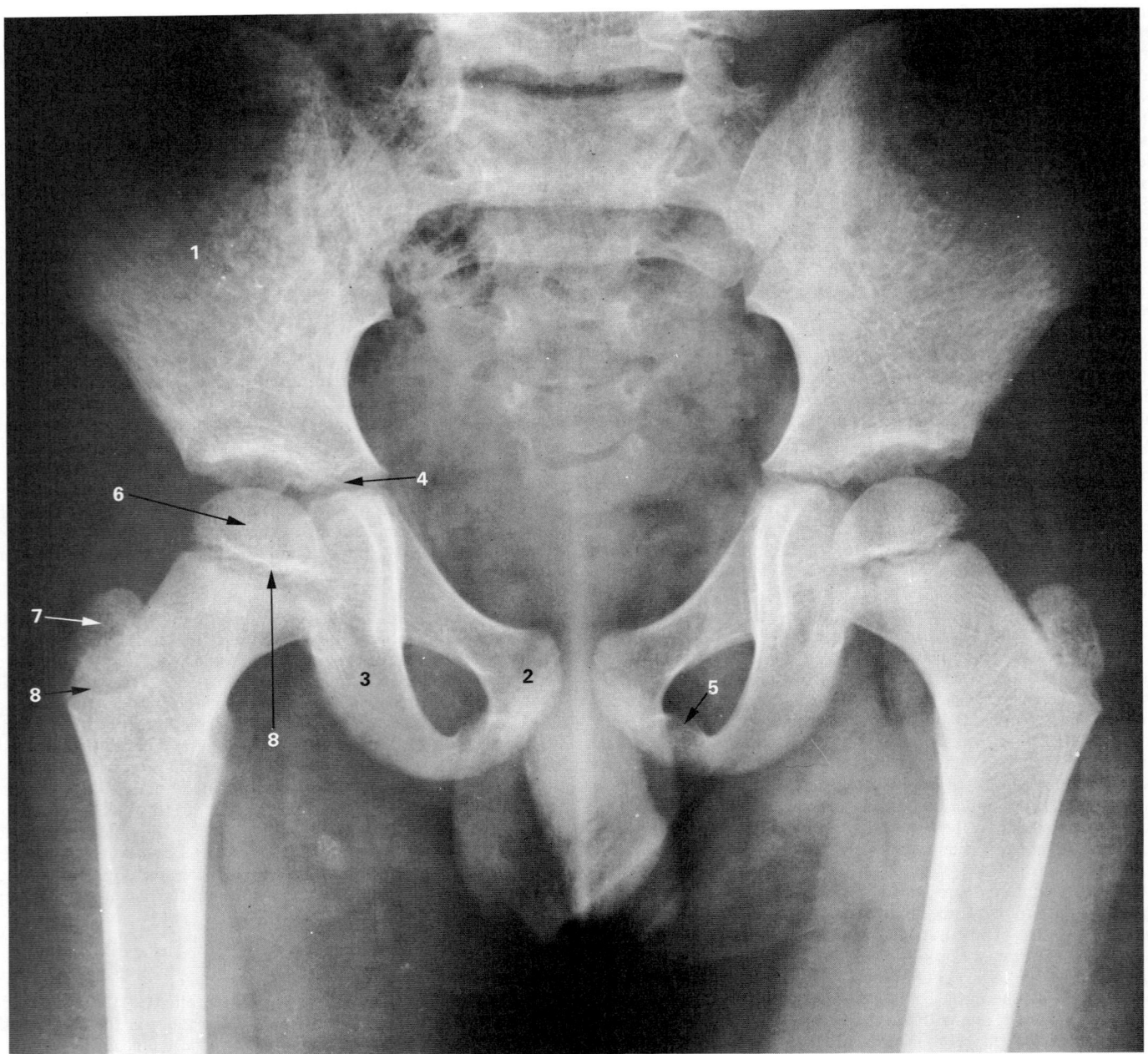

6.271 Anteroposterior radiograph of the pelvis of a boy aged seven. 1. Ilium. 2. Pubis. 3. Ischium. 4. Part of triradiate growth cartilage. 5. Cartilage between pubic and ischial rami. 6. Superior femoral epiphysis. 7. Ossifying greater trochanter. 8. Cartilaginous growth plates.

place. Skeletally it is a narrower continuation of the greater pelvis, with irregular but more complete walls around its cavity. Naturally of great obstetric importance, it has a *median curved axis*. It has superior and inferior openings, the superior occupied in life by viscera, the inferior largely closed by the pelvic floor and its sphincters.

The superior pelvic aperture (pelvic inlet)

Variable in contour—round or oval—it is encroached upon by the sacral promontory. Its boundary, described as *pelvic brim*, is obstetrically important (6.272A) and has also long been measured for anthropological reasons, as has the pelvic cavity; much information is available, especially for females. Data of different observers vary, being founded on differing racial and economic groups. Data cited here are merely approximate samples of values in Europeans (Martin 1928). Three dimensions of the pelvic inlet have become conventional:

A. *Anteroposterior diameter* (true conjugate) is measured between the midpoints of the sacral promontory and upper border of the symphysis pubis (male 100 mm, female 112 mm).

B. *Transverse diameter* is the maximum distance between similar points (assessed by eye) on opposite sides of the pelvic brim (male 125 mm, female 131 mm).

C. *Oblique diameter* is measured from the iliopubic eminence to the opposite sacroiliac joint (male 120 mm, female 125 mm).

Cavity of the lesser pelvis

Short and curved, it is markedly longer in its posterior wall. Anteroinferiorly it is bounded by pubic bones, their rami and symphysis; posteriorly by the concave anterior sacral surface and coccyx; and on each side by the smooth quadrangular pelvic aspect of the fused ilium and ischium. The region thus enclosed is the pelvic cavity proper, through which pass, in all land vertebrates, the ends of the alimentary canal and urogenital ducts. Thus in humans its contents are rectum, bladder and parts of the reproductive organs. The rectum is posterior, bladder anterior, uterus intermediate. The cavity must also permit passage of the fetal head.

Pelvic diameters are often measured and while this can be done at many levels, measurements are usually chosen at approximately midlevel:

A. *Anteroposterior diameter* is measured between the midpoints of the third sacral segment and posterior surface of the symphysis pubis (male 105 mm, female 130 mm).

B. *Transverse diameter* is the widest transverse distance between the side walls of the cavity, and often the greatest transverse dimension in the whole cavity (male 120 mm, female 125 mm).

C. *Oblique diameter* is the distance from the lowest point of one sacroiliac joint to the midpoint of the contralateral obturator membrane (male 110 mm, female 131 mm).

The inferior pelvic aperture (pelvic outlet) (6.272B)

Less regular in outline than the superior, it is indented behind by the coccyx and sacrum and bilaterally by the ischial tuberosities. Its perimeter thus consists of three wide arcs; anterior is the *pubic arch*, between the converging ischiopubic rami; between the sacrum and coccyx posteriorly and the ischial tuberosities laterally are two large sciatic notches, divided, on both sides, by the sacrotuberous and sacrospinous ligaments into *greater* and *lesser sciatic foramina* (p. 677). With ligaments included, the inferior aperture is rhomboidal, its anterior limbs being the ischiopubic rami (joined by the inferior pubic ligament), its posterior the sacrotuberous ligaments, with the coccyx median. The outlet is thus not rigid in its posterior half, being limited by ligaments and the coccyx, all slightly yielding. Even with the sacrum taken as the posterior midline limit (more reliable for measurement), there remains slight mobility at the sacroiliac joints. Note also that a plane of the inferior aperture is merely conceptual: the anterior, ischiopubic part has a plane inclined down and back to a transverse line between the lower limits of the ischial tuberosities, and the posterior half has a plane approximating to the sacrotuberous ligaments, sloping down and forwards to the same line. Dimensions of the inferior aperture are measured as follows:

A. *Anteroposterior diameter* is usually measured from the coccygeal apex to the midpoint of the lower rim of the symphysis. The lowest sacral point may also be used (male 80 mm, female 125 mm).

B. *Transverse diameter* is measured between the ischial tuberosities at the lower borders of their medial surfaces. Hence the term *bituberous diameter* (male 85 mm, female 118 mm).

C. *Oblique diameter* extends from the midpoint of the sacrotuberous ligament on one side to the contralateral ischiopubic junction (male 100 mm, female 118 mm).

Further details

Apart from these main measurements, by consensus the basis of pelvic osteometry, other planes and measurements are used in obstetric practice. The *plane of greatest pelvic dimensions*, an obstetrical concept, represents the most capacious pelvic level, between the pelvic brim and midlevel plane, corresponding with the latter anteriorly (midsymphysis) but ascending slightly to the disc between the second and third sacral segments. The *plane of least pelvic dimensions* is said to be at about midpelvic level; its transverse diameter is between the apices of the ischial spines; most difficulty in parturition occurs here. The *posterior median diameter* is the part of any anteroposterior diameter behind its intersection with the transverse diameter, and thus assessable at any level or plane as an indicator of capacity of the posterior pelvic segment. Because the direct measurement of osseous dimensions is impracticable in living patients, except by radiological methods, indirect measurements may be used.

The *diagonal* (*oblique*) *conjugate* is the distance from the sacral promontory to the lower symphyseal border, measured per vaginam, and a guide to the 'true' conjugate. This, like all pelvic diameters described anatomically, largely disregards soft tissues. The *intercristal* and *interspinous diameters*, respectively the greatest widths between the iliac crests and the anterior superior iliac spines, are sometimes compared in females. Average values are 250 mm (intercristal) and 275 mm (interspinous), the difference between them being an indication of the width of the pelvic cavity; the iliac crests do not turn medially at their anterior ends to the same extent in females as in males. The method's value is dubious and correlation between such sexual characteristics in the pelvis is uncertain.

MORPHOLOGICAL CLASSIFICATION OF PELVES

Interest in the above dimensions is primarily obstetric and, less frequently, forensic. All pelvic measurements display, as others elsewhere, individual variation; values quoted are means from limited

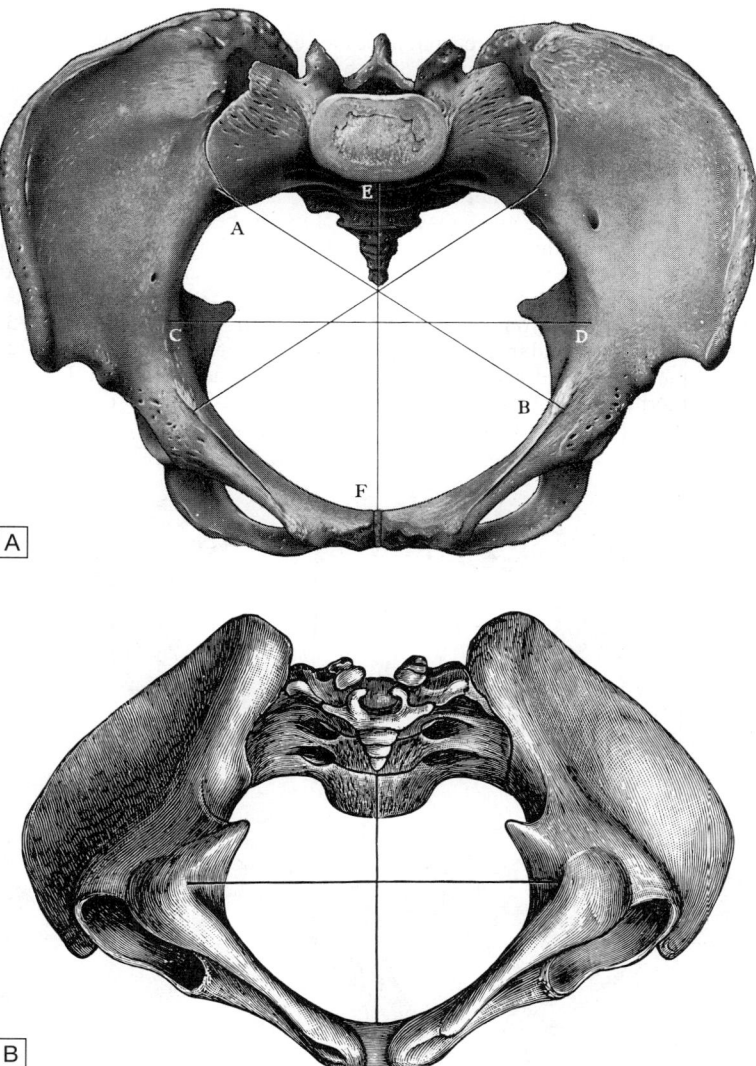

6.272 The diameters of the female lesser pelvis: A. Superior aperture; B. Inferior aperture (oblique diameter not shown). A. sacroiliac joint; B. iliopubic eminence; C, D. middle of pelvic brim; E. sacral promontory; F. pubic symphysis.

surveys. Sexual and racial differences also occur. The range in any group, for both sexes, is large when adequately assessed. Measurements are on skeletonized pelves in the most extensive studies; such data are not only of anthropological interest but also the basis of attempts to define clinically identifiable forms of the pelvis without resort to the full range of measurements, which are not all possible in the living, although radiological pelvimetry has become a refined technique (Borell & Fernström 1960). In the female patient it is *her* measurements which are significant, not average values; comparison between her dimensions and a fetal head are the principal concern. These values can satisfactorily be assessed only by radiographic techniques. Hence modern pelvimetry and fetal cephalometry have replaced obstetric measurement by calipers whenever requisite expertise is available (Lewis 1964a).

Pelvic measurements, however obtained, have been analysed by many anatomists, anthropologists, obstetricians and radiologists in attempts to classify human pelves, especially the female. *Pelvic brim index*—(ant-post./trans. diameters) × 100—was an early attempt to define the shape of the pelvic cavity (Turner 1886). Like the cephalic index (p. 610) its range is divided into steps, by which pelves are classified as *platypellic* (transversely flat), *mesatipellic* (intermediate) and *dolichopellic* (anteroposteriorly long); on anatomical and radiological data a *brachypellic* form is added, also known as *android* and responsible for most cases of severe obstruction in childbirth (Greulich & Thomas 1938, 1939; Thoms 1940). Such classification is equally applicable to both sexes and various ages; for example, in one large series, children and males were predominantly dolichopellic, females mostly mesatipellic and brachypellic. Platypellic pelves are comparatively rare in all series. Another classification depends jointly on anatomical and radiological data, the latter including qualitative and metrical observations (Caldwell & Moloy 1933; Caldwell et al 1940). This divides the superior pelvic aperture by its transverse diameter into an anterior *forepelvis* and a *hindpelvis*, the latter more variable in shape and capacity. The slope of the pelvic walls, whether radiographically straight, convergent or divergent, pelvic depth and shape and size of the greater sciatic notch (lateral radiographs) and shape of the subpubic arch are all considered. This study led to wide acceptance of four pelvic types (shown in Table **6**.4 and **6**.273) depending fundamentally on skeletal measurement, although frequently applied somewhat subjectively in clinical practice. Though intermediate forms exist, the classification is claimed to embrace all but a very small percentage.

Table 6.4   Pelvic types, their mean diameter values and incidence (based on data by Caldwell et al)

Pelvic type	Conjugate diameter (mm)	Transverse diameter (mm)	White females (%)	Negro females (%)
Gynaecoid (= mesatipellic)	108.5	137.6	41.4	42.1
Android (= brachypellic)	105.9	135.6	32.5	15.7
Anthropoid (= dolichopellic)	117.5	129.4	23.5	40.5
Platypelloid (= platypellic)	85.5	144.5	2.6	1.7

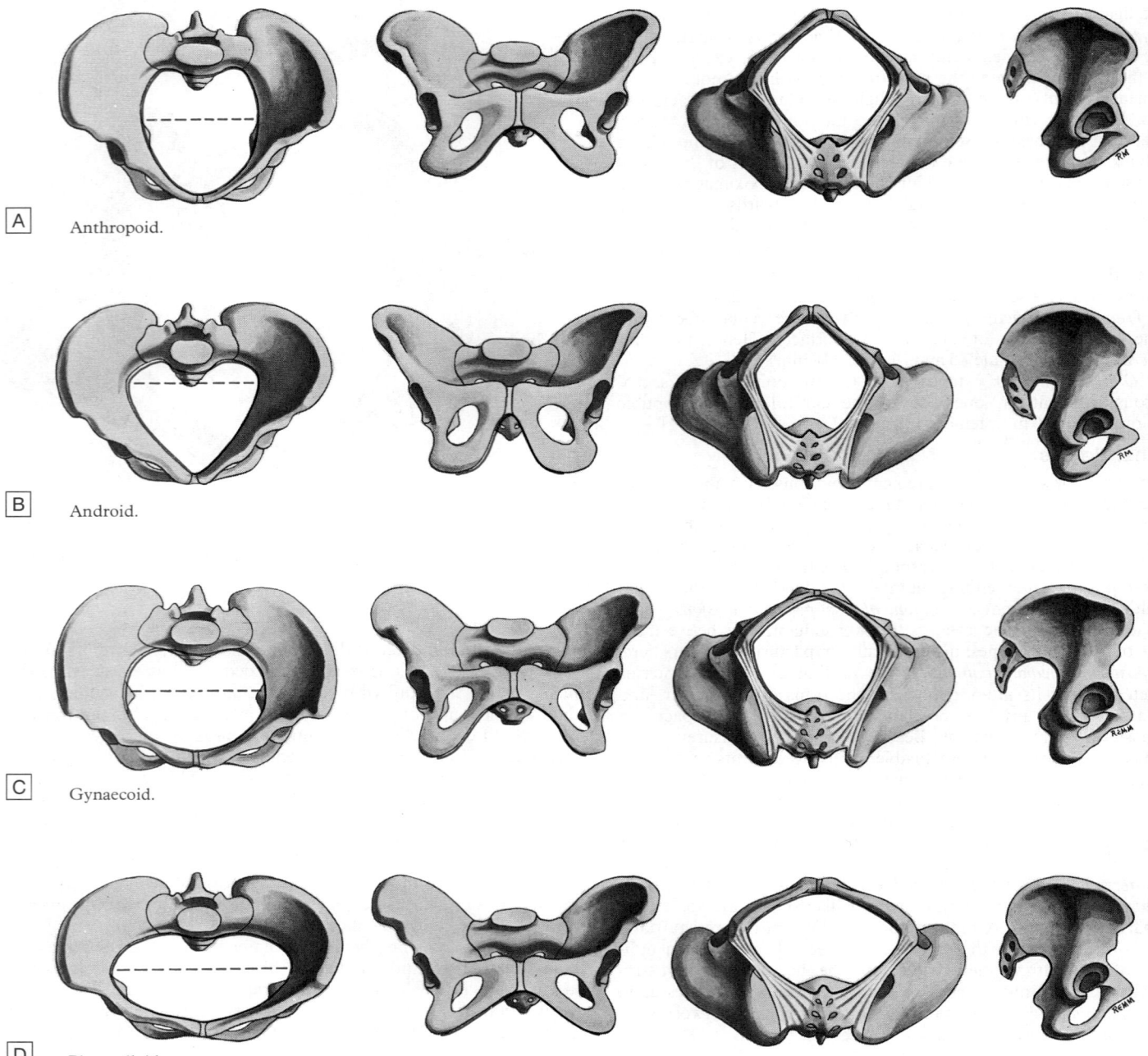

A   Anthropoid.

B   Android.

C   Gynaecoid.

D   Platypelloid.

6.273   The major differences between the four types of pelvis in the most widely accepted classification. Types shown in A and B are commonest in males, B and C in females, while D is rare, even in females. Note the variations in superior and inferior apertures, greater sciatic notch, and subpubic arch. Note varying proportion between fore- and hind-pelvis, anterior and posterior to transverse diameter of the inlet. (Caldwell and Moloy's Classification, after Clyne 1933.)

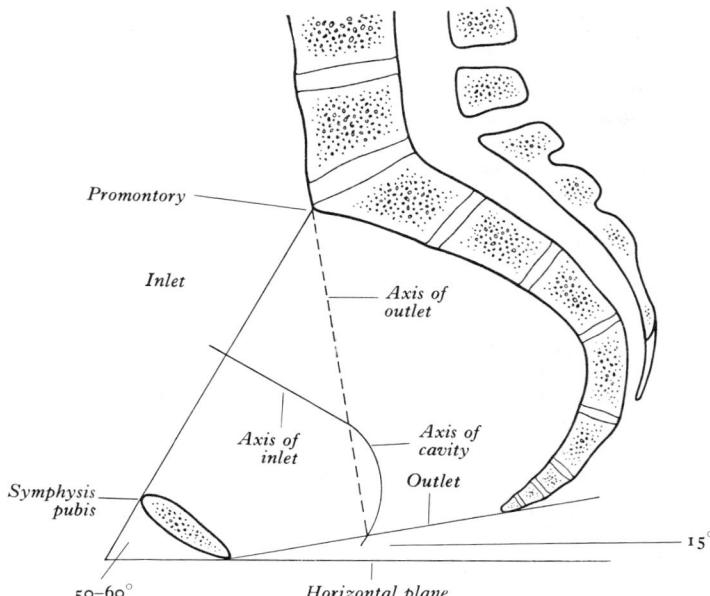

6.274 Median sagittal section through the female pelvis to show the planes of inlet and outlet and their relation to each other and the horizontal plane. The curved axis of the pelvic cavity is also shown. It should be noted that, as depicted in this section, the curve of the sacrum affects the lower part of the third and the upper part of the fourth sacral vertebrae. In many cases the curve is restricted to the fourth vertebra only. Difficulties in defining the plane of the outlet are mentioned in the text.

Apart from racial differences (e.g. high rate of anthropoid pelves in Negro women), such observations emphasize the low incidence of the platypelloid form. Children (under 9 years) and adult males show a high incidence of dolichopelly, perhaps indicating a paedomorphic trait in males. The platypelloid pelvis has been described as 'ultra-human'.

Correlation of pelvic type with general bodily physique is uncertain (Smout et al 1969). It has been claimed, for example, that women with the dangerous android pelvis are stout, short-necked and broad-shouldered (Kenny 1944), views regarded as unreliable by others (Ince & Young 1940).

Pelvic axes and inclination

The *axis* of the superior pelvic aperture traverses its centre at right angles to its plane, directed down and backwards; when prolonged (projected) it passes through the *umbilicus* and *midcoccyx*. An axis is similarly established for the inferior aperture; projected up it impinges on the *sacral promontory*. Axes can likewise be constructed for any plane, and one for the whole cavity is a concatenation of an infinite series of such lines. It follows the cavity's curvature, indicated by the profile of the sacrum and coccyx in lateral views (**6**.274). The form of this *pelvic axis* and disparity in depth between the anterior and posterior contours of the cavity are prime factors in the mechanism of fetal transit in the *pelvic canal*.

In the standing position the pelvic canal curves obliquely back relative to the trunk and abdominal cavity (**6**.274). The whole pelvis is tilted forwards, the plane of the pelvic brim making an angle of 50° to 60° with the horizontal. The plane of the inferior aperture is tilted likewise to about 15°, posterior parts of both planes being thus above the anterior. Strictly, the pelvic outlet has two planes, an anterior passing back from the pubic symphysis and a posterior passing forwards from the coccyx, both descending to meet at the intertuberous line. In standing, the pelvic aspect of the symphysis pubis faces as much upwards as backwards and the sacral concavity is directed anteroinferiorly. The front of the symphysis and anterior superior iliac spines are in the same vertical plane. In sitting, body weight is transmitted through inferomedial parts of the ischial tuberosities, with variable soft tissues intervening, and anterior superior iliac spines are in a vertical plane through the acetabular centres, the whole pelvis being tilted back and the lumbosacral angle somewhat diminished at the sacral promontory.

Sexual differences in the pelvis

The pelvis obviously provides the most marked skeletal differences between male and female (**6**.275, 276); surprisingly, distinction can be made even during fetal life, particularly in the subpubic arch (Boucher 1957). Radiographic pelvic studies in American children during their first postnatal year show that male infants exceed females in dimensions of the whole pelvis, but usually females exceed males in the size of pelvic cavity (Reynolds 1945). From 2 to 9 years a similar distinction prevails; but the difference is said to be maximal at 22 months, decreasing in later childhood (Reynolds 1947). Sexual differences in adults, which have been much assessed (Genovese 1959), are divisible into metrical and non-metrical features, the range of most overlapping between the sexes.

Differences are inevitably linked to function. While primary pelvic function in **both** sexes is locomotor, the pelvis is adapted to parturition in females, particularly the lesser pelvis, changes in which variably affect proportions and dimensions of the greater pelvis. Since males are distinctly more muscular and therefore more heavily built, overall pelvic dimensions, such as intercristal measurement, are greater, markings for muscles and ligaments more pronounced

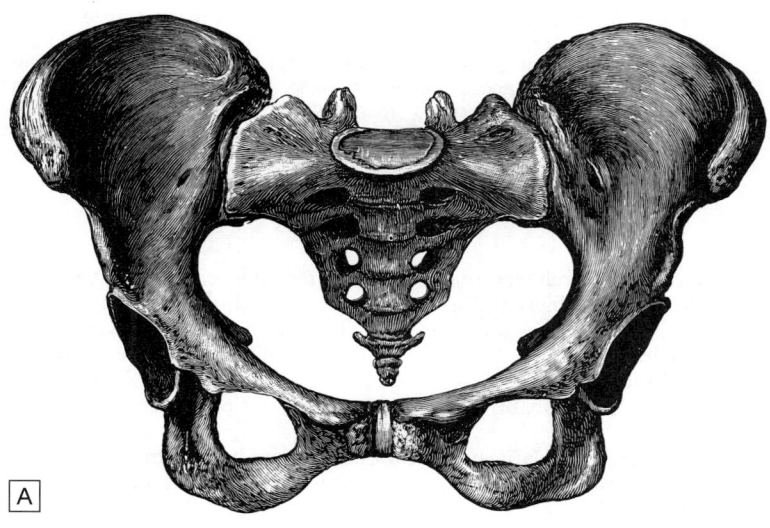

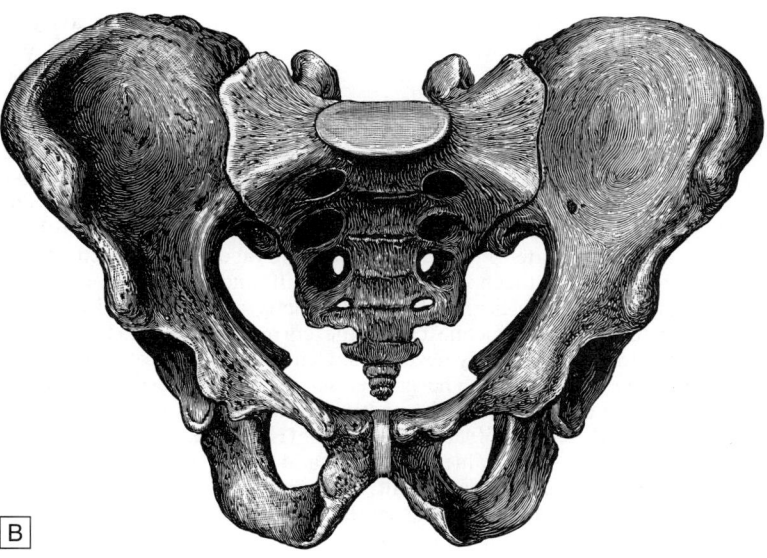

6.275 The anterior aspect of the female (A) and male (B) pelves.

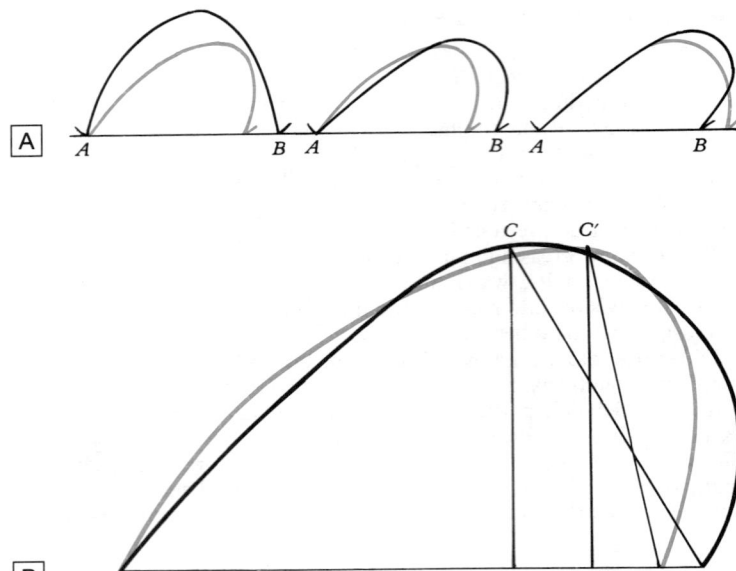

6.276A. Three common profiles of the greater sciatic notch in males (blue) and females (black). B. Points, axes and angles utilized in mensuration of the greater sciatic notch. AB = *maximal width*, i.e. distance between the tip of the ischial spine and a tubercle marking attachment of the piriformis muscle. OC = *maximal depth* (perpendicular to AB). OB = *posterior segment* of width. Index I = OC × 100/AB. Index II = OB × 100/AB. ACB = *total angle*. BCO = *posterior angle*. (Modified, with permission, from Singh & Potturi 1978.)

and general architecture heavier. The male iliac crest is more rugged and more medially inclined at its anterior end; in females the crests are less curved in all parts. The iliac blades are more vertical in females, but do not ascend so far; the iliac fossae are therefore shallower and each iliopectineal line more vertical. These iliac peculiarities probably account for the greater prominence of female hips.

The male is relatively and absolutely more heavily built above the pelvis, with consequent differences at the lumbosacral and hip joints. The sacral basal articular facet for the fifth lumbar vertebra and intervening disc is more than a third of the total sacral basal width in males but less than a third in females, whose sacrum is also relatively broader, accentuating this difference. Thus the female has relatively broader sacral alae. The male acetabulum is absolutely larger and its diameter about equal to the distance between its anterior rim and symphysis pubis. But in females acetabular diameter is usually less than this distance, not only because it is absolutely smaller but also because the anterolateral wall of the cavity is comparatively and often absolutely wider. The female symphysis and adjoining parts of the pubis and ischium, forming the anterior pelvic wall, are also absolutely less in height, producing a somewhat triangular obturator foramen, which is more ovoid in males. Differing pubic growth is also expressed in the subpubic arch below the symphysis and between the inferior pubic rami. It is more angular in males, being 50° to 60°; in females it is rounded, less easy to measure and usually 80° to 85°. Associated with pubic width in females is a greater separation of the pubic tubercles. The ischiopubic rami are also much more lightly built and narrowed near the symphysis; in males they bear a distinctly rough, everted area for attachment of the penile crura, the corresponding attachment for the clitoris being poorly developed. Ischial spines are closer in males, being more inturned. The greater sciatic notch is usually wider in females; comparisons of its width and angle yield mean values for males and females of 50.4° and 74.4° (Hanna & Washburn 1953); the greater female values for angle and width are associated with increased backward sacral tilt and greater anteroposterior pelvic diameter, especially at lower levels. A method for comparing **depth** of the notch is reported by Jovanovic and Zivanovic (1965). More recently, detailed analysis of dimensions and derived indices in relation to sex determination at the greater sciatic notch has been

made by Singh and Potturi (1978), based on a study of 200 adult hip bones (120 males and 80 females). Using defined points (Jit & Singh 1966) they assessed maximal width and depth, posterior segment of width, total angle and posterior angle. Two indices were also assessed (**6.276**). Width and depth of the notch per se were found valueless for determining sex: the posterior angle was the best single parameter, while the length of the posterior segment and index II were also highly effective, especially in females.

The sacrum displays metrical sexual differences, in addition to orientation. Female sacra are less curved, the curvature being most marked between the first and second segments and the third and fifth, with an intervening flatter region. Male sacra are more evenly curved, relatively long and narrow and more often exceeding five segments (by addition of a lumbar or coccygeal vertebra). The *sacral index* compares sacral breadth (between the most anterior points on the auricular surfaces) with length (between midpoints on the anterior margins of the promontory and apex); average values for males and females are 105 and 115%. Auricular surfaces are relatively smaller and more oblique in females; contrary to a common statement, they extend on the upper **three** sacral vertebrae in **both** sexes. The dorsal auricular border is more concave in females (Weisl 1954a). Many differences are summarized in the generalization that the pelvic cavity is longer and more conical in males, shorter and more cylindrical in females; but in both the axis is curved. Differences are greater at the inferior aperture than the brim, where in absolute measurements males are not as different from females as sometimes stated. But the superior aperture is more likely to be anthropoid or android in males, gynaecoid or android in females, the sexes overlapping to this extent.

In forensic practice identification of human skeletal remains (sometimes fragmentary) usually involves diagnosis of sex, and this is most certainly established from the pelvis. Even parts of the pelvis may be useful. Several studies of metrical characteristics in various pelvic regions have been made, leading to various indices. The ilium has received particular attention; for example, one index essentially compares the pelvic and sacroiliac parts of the bone (Derry 1923). A line is extended back from the iliopectineal eminence to the nearest point on the anterior auricular margin and thence to the iliac crest. The auricular point divides this *chilotic line* into anterior (pelvic) and posterior (sacral) segments, each expressed as a percentage of the other. Such *chilotic indices* display reciprocal values in the sexes, the pelvic part of the chilotic line being predominant in females, the sacral part in males. The most detailed metrical study of the ilium, involving several indices, indicates its limited reliability in 'sexing' pelves (Straus 1927). However, the higher incidence and definition of the female preauricular sulcus was confirmed (p. 665). A *pubo-ischial index*, based on maximum lengths of the ischium and pubis, measured from their acetabular junction, produced values of 83.7% and 100.0% for American males and females (Washburn 1949); when this was correlated with the angle of the sciatic notch, it was claimed that the sex of 98% of pelves could be deduced. The desirability of correlation of all available metrical data is to be emphasized; when a range of pelvic data can be combined, especially if they are metrical, 95% accuracy should be achieved. Complete accuracy has been claimed when the rest of the skeleton is available. Nevertheless, assessment of sex in isolated and often incomplete human remains cannot always be absolutely certain.

SACROILIAC JOINT

The sacroiliac joint, a synovial articulation between the sacral and iliac auricular surfaces (**6.277A**), although often termed plane, is nearly flat only in infants; in adults the surfaces are irregular, often markedly so, and sometimes sinuous. Their curvatures and irregularities, greater in males, are reciprocal; they restrict movements and contribute to the joint's considerable strength in transmitting weight from the vertebral column to the lower limbs. According to Putschar (1931) and Schunke (1938) the sacral surface is covered by hyaline cartilage and the iliac by fibrocartilage. The sacral cartilage is indeed typically hyaline (Bowen & Cassidy 1981), being thicker anteriorly than posteriorly in adults; the thinner iliac cartilage is also hyaline as confirmed by the presence of Type II collagen (Paquin et al 1983). Fibrous adhesions and gradual obliteration occur in both sexes, earlier in males, after the menopause in females. A radiological

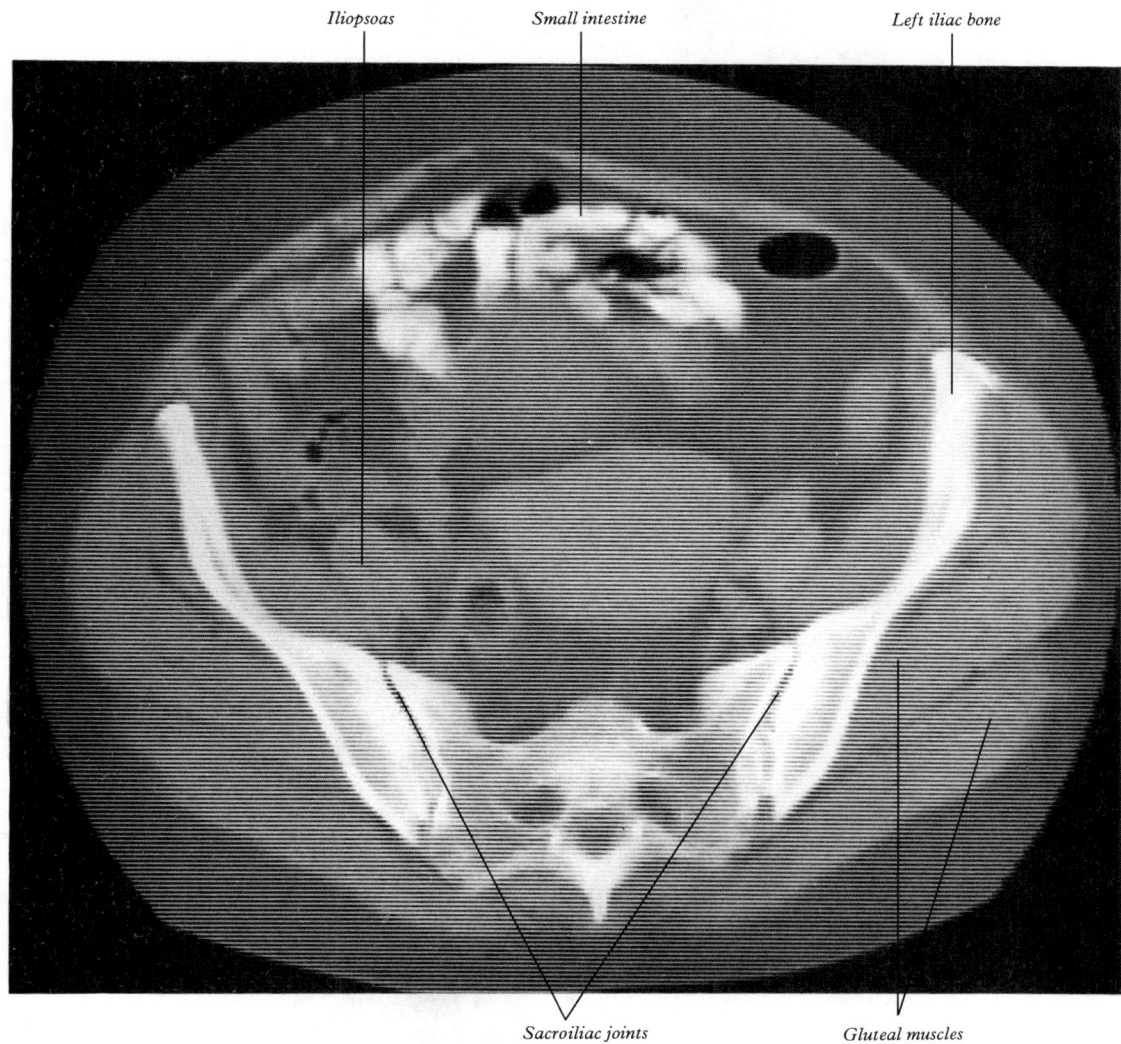

Iliopsoas   *Small intestine*   *Left iliac bone*

A

Sacroiliac joints   *Gluteal muscles*

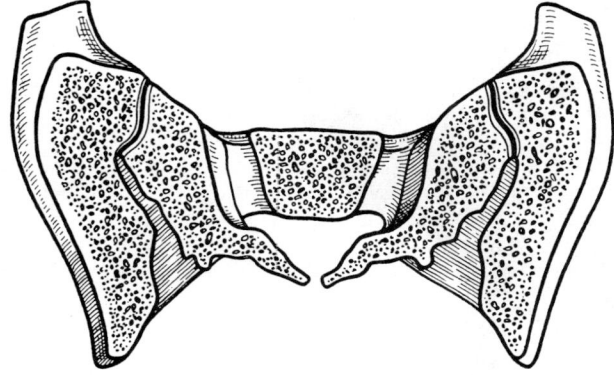

B

6.277A. Computed tomogram in the transverse plane showing the sacro-iliac joints. (Supplied by Shaun Gallagher; photography by Sarah Smith). B. Coronal section through the middle segment (see text) of the sacroiliac joints: the sacrum and pelvis are in the anatomical position.

study of 94 healthy individuals (Cohen et al 1967) showed such changes in 6% before 50 years, in 24% thereafter. In old age the joint may be completely fibrosed and occasionally even ossified. The articular capsule is attached close to both articular margins. Ligaments are *anterior*, *interosseous* and *posterior sacroiliac*.

Accessory sacroiliac articulations are not uncommon and are thought to represent acquired fibrocartilaginous joints resulting from the stresses of weight bearing (Ehara et al 1988), developing behind the articular surface between the lateral sacral crest and posterior superior iliac spine and iliac tuberosity (Trotter 1937). They may be single, double, unilateral or bilateral (Weisl 1954a), and have a joint

capsule and are saddle-shaped, occurring more frequently in some races than in others (Trotter 1937).

The anterior sacroiliac ligament (6.278)

An anteroinferior capsular thickening, it is particularly well-developed near the arcuate line and the posterior inferior iliac spine, where it connects the third sacral segment to the lateral side of the preauricular sulcus. It is thin elsewhere.

Interosseous sacroiliac ligament

Not officially recognized but the largest typical *syndesmosis* (p. 488), it is the major bond between the bones filling the irregular space posterosuperior to the joint (6.277B); it is covered superficially by the posterior sacroiliac ligament. Its deeper part has superior and inferior bands passing from depressions posterior to the sacral auricular surface to those on the iliac tuberosity. These bands are covered by, and blend with, a more superficial fibrous sheet connecting the posterosuperior margin of a rough area posterior to the sacral auricular surface to the corresponding margins of the iliac tuberosity. This sheet is often partially divided into superior and inferior parts, the former uniting the superior articular process and lateral crest on the first two sacral segments to the neighbouring ilium as a *short posterior iliac ligament* (6.279).

The posterior sacroiliac ligament

This lies over the interosseous ligament, but intervening are the dorsal rami of the sacral spinal nerves and vessels. It has several weak fasciculi connecting the intermediate and, below this, the lateral sacral crests to the posterior superior iliac spine and internal lip of the iliac crest at its posterior end. Inferior fibres, from the third and fourth sacral segments, ascend to the posterior superior iliac spine

675

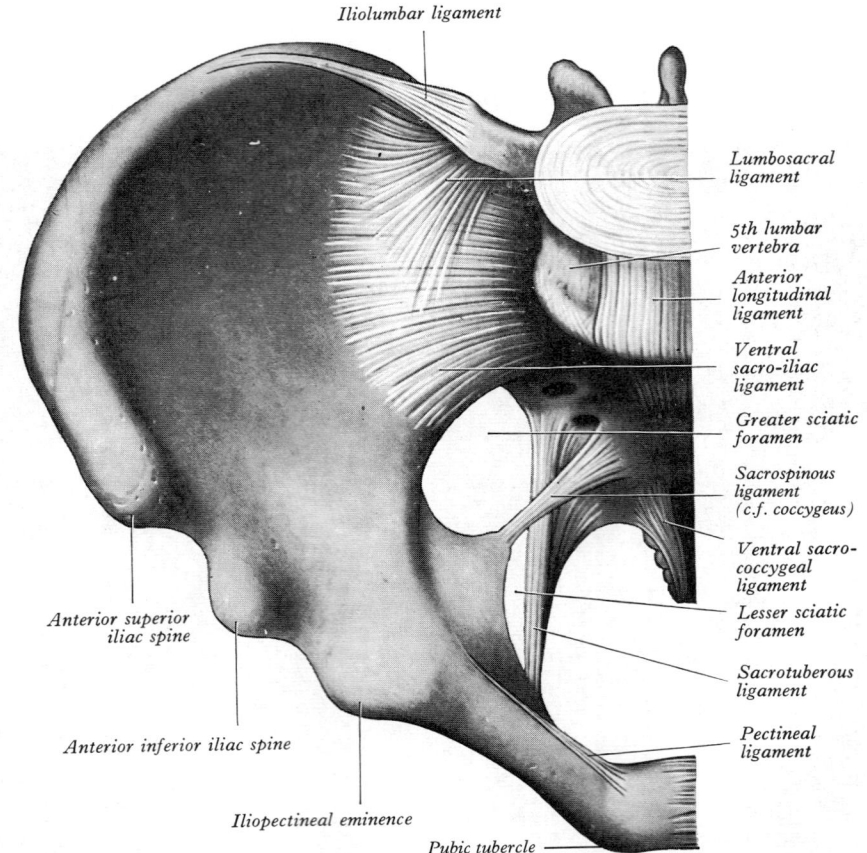

Iliolumbar ligament

Lumbosacral ligament

5th lumbar vertebra

Anterior longitudinal ligament

Ventral sacro-iliac ligament

Greater sciatic foramen

Sacrospinous ligament (c.f. coccygeus)

Ventral sacro-coccygeal ligament

Lesser sciatic foramen

Sacrotuberous ligament

Pectineal ligament

Anterior superior iliac spine

Anterior inferior iliac spine

Iliopectineal eminence

Pubic tubercle

6.278   Joints and ligaments of the right half of the pelvis: anterior aspect. Anterior superior iliac spine and pubic tubercle are in the same coronal plane. Note the inclination of the 'brim' (inlet) of the lesser (true) pelvis, the boundaries of the sciatic foramina and the (partly obscured) pelvic outlet.

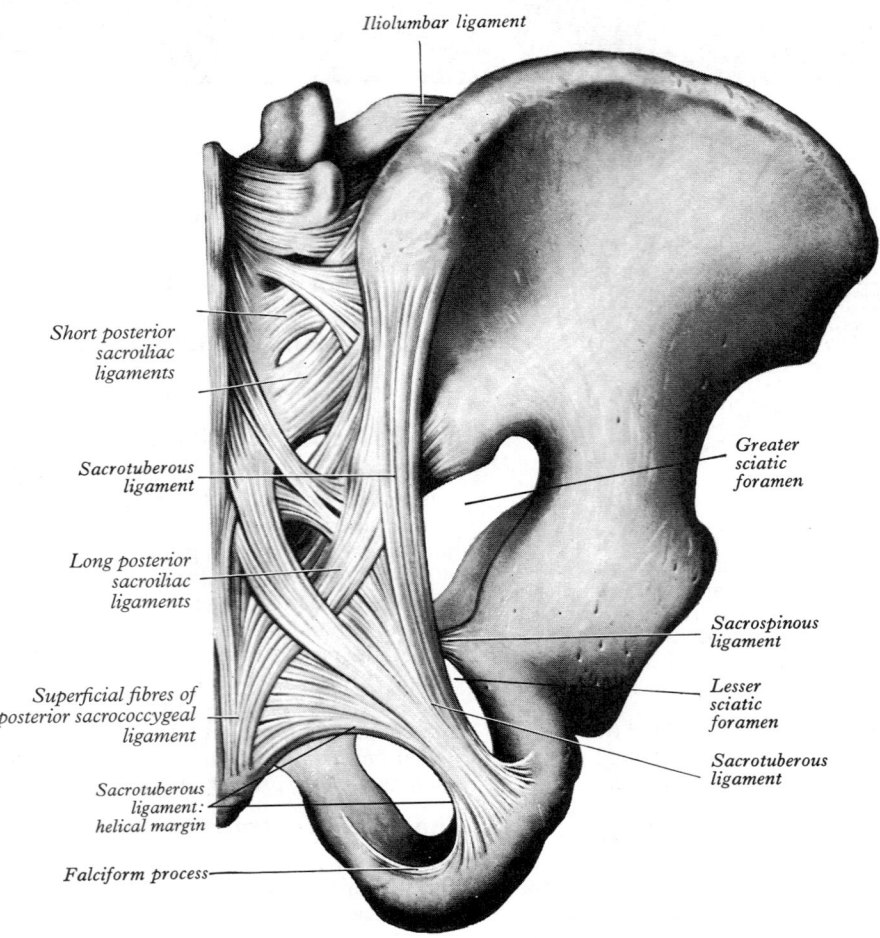

Iliolumbar ligament

Short posterior sacroiliac ligaments

Sacrotuberous ligament

Long posterior sacroiliac ligaments

Superficial fibres of posterior sacrococcygeal ligament

Sacrotuberous ligament: helical margin

Falciform process

Greater sciatic foramen

Sacrospinous ligament

Lesser sciatic foramen

Sacrotuberous ligament

6.279   Joints and ligaments on the posterior aspect of the right half of the pelvis and fifth lumbar vertebra.

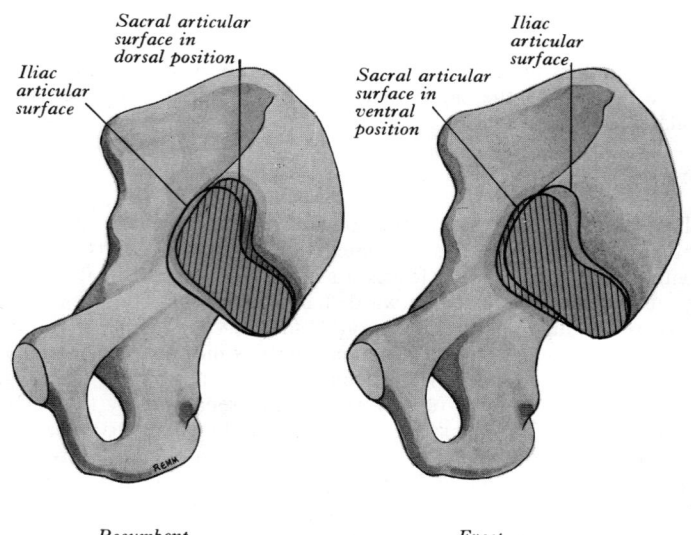

Recumbent   Erect

6.280 The changing relation (rotation) of the auricular surface of the sacrum and that of the ilium when changing from a recumbent to an erect posture. (Based upon work by H Weisl 1953, with permission of the author.)

and internal lip of the iliac crest at its posterior end. Inferior fibres, from the third and fourth sacral segments, ascending to the posterior superior iliac spine, may form a separate *long posterior sacroiliac ligament* (**6**.279); the latter is continuous laterally with part of the sacrotuberous ligament and medially with the thoracolumbar fascia's posterior lamina (Weisl 1954a).

Movements

A little anteroposterior rotation occurs around a transverse axis about 5–10 cm vertically below the sacral promontory (Weisl 1955). This accompanies flexion and extension of the trunk; its range is the same in males and non-pregnant females; it is increased in pregnancy. The greatest sacral movement relative to the iliac bones is in rising from a recumbent to a standing position (**6**.280). The sacral promontory advances as much as 5–6 mm as body weight impinges on the sacrum; backward movement of the lower end of the sacrum is less. Movement is not simple rotation, the axis being dynamic (Weisl 1953); some translation is associated with it.

Accessory movements. When lying prone a small degree of rotation of the sacrum with respect to the pelvis is possible when downward pressure is applied to the sacral apex.

Vertebropelvic ligaments

Each ilium is connected to the fifth lumbar vertebra by an *iliolumbar ligament* (p. 531, **6**.278) and the sacrum to the ischium by *sacrotuberous* and *sacrospinous* ligaments. (Further attachments are detailed below.)

Sacrotuberous ligament (**6**.278, 279). Broadly attached by its base to the posterior superior iliac spine, it is partly blended with the posterior sacroiliac ligaments, to the lower transverse sacral tubercles and the lateral margins of the lower sacrum and upper coccyx. Its oblique fibres descend laterally, converging to form a thick, narrow band which widens again below and is attached to the ischial tuberosity's medial margin. It then spreads along the ischial ramus as the *falciform process*, whose concave edge blends with the fascial sheath of the internal pudendal vessels (p. 1561) and pudendal nerve. To the sacrotuberous ligament's posterior surface are attached the lowest fibres of gluteus maximus; superficial fibres of the ligament's lower part continue into the tendon of biceps femoris. The ligament is pierced by the coccygeal branches of the inferior gluteal artery, the perforating cutaneous nerve and filaments of the coccygeal plexus.

Sacrospinous ligament (**6**.278). Thin and triangular, it extends from the ischial spine to the lateral margins of the sacrum and coccyx anterior to the sacrotuberous ligament with which it blends. Its anterior surface is **muscular** and constitutes the coccygeus; the ligament is often regarded as a degenerate part of the muscle. (When

pelvic and gluteal topographical relations are under consideration, it must be emphasized that muscle and ligament are coextensive and are the anterior and posterior aspects of the **same structure**.)

Further details. The sacrotuberous and sacrospinous ligaments oppose upward tilting of the lower part of the sacrum under downward thrust at its upper end. They also convert the sciatic notches into foramina.

The greater sciatic foramen. This is bounded anterosuperiorly by the greater sciatic notch, posteriorly by the sacrotuberous and inferiorly by the sacrospinous ligament and ischial spine. It is partly filled by the emerging piriformis, above which the superior gluteal vessels and nerve leave the pelvis; below it, the inferior gluteal vessels and nerve, internal pudendal vessels and pudendal nerve, sciatic and posterior femoral cutaneous nerves and nerves to obturator internus and quadratus femoris also leave the pelvis.

The lesser sciatic foramen. This is bounded anteriorly by the ischial body, superiorly by its spine and sacrospinous ligament, posteriorly by the sacrotuberous ligament. It transmits the tendon of obturator internus, the muscle's nerve and the internal pudendal vessels and pudendal nerve.

PUBIC SYMPHYSIS

The pubic bones meet in the midline at a fibrocartilaginous *pubic symphysis* (**6**.281), connected by *superior* and *arcuate pubic* ligaments.

The superior pubic ligament

This connects the bones above, extending to the pubic tubercles.

Arcuate pubic ligament

A thick arch of fibres, it connects the lower borders of the symphyseal pubic surfaces, bounding the pubic arch. Superiorly it blends with the *interpubic disc* and extends laterally attached to the inferior pubic rami; its base is separated from the anterior border of the urogenital diaphragm by an opening for the deep dorsal vein of the penis or clitoris.

Interpubic disc

It connects the medial pubic surfaces, each covered by a thin layer of tightly adherent hyaline cartilage (surface growth cartilage in the young). The junction is not flat (p. 666) but marked by reciprocal

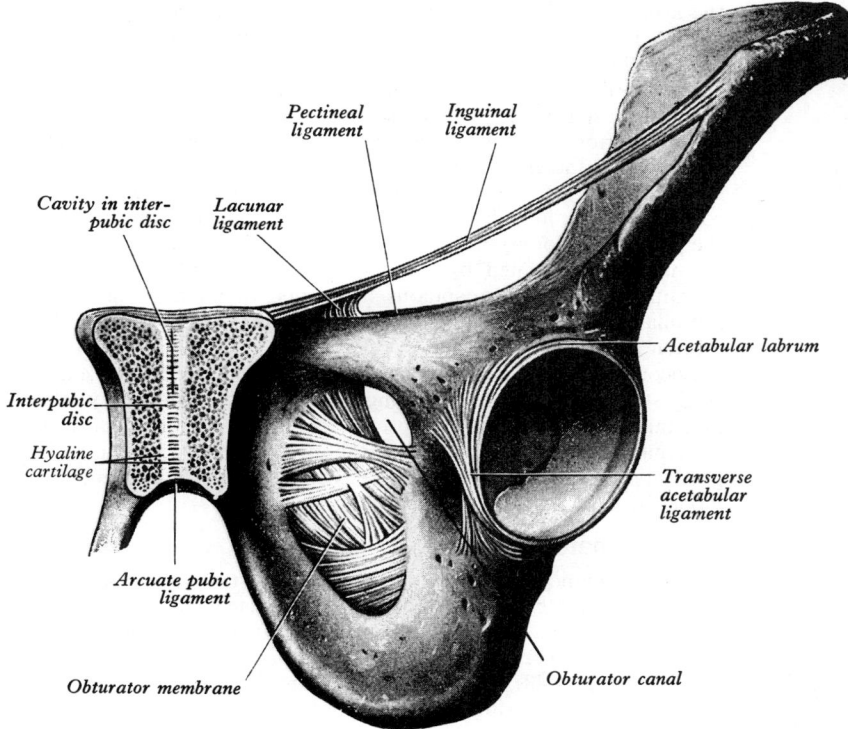

6.281 An obliquely coronal section through the pubic symphysis: antero-inferior aspect.

crests and papillae. Theoretically this would resist shearing. The surfaces of hyaline cartilage are connected by fibrocartilage, varying in thickness. It often contains a cavity, probably due to absorption, rarely appearing before the tenth year and non-synovial. Better developed in females, it is usually posterosuperior but may reach the front or even occupy most of the cartilage (**6**.281). The disc is strengthened anteriorly by several interlacing collagenous fibrous layers, passing obliquely from bone to bone, decussating and interweaving with fibres of the external oblique aponeuroses and the medial tendons of the recti abdominis.

Movements

Movements have been little described. Angulation, rotation and displacement are possible but slight and are likely in activities at the sacroiliac and hip joints. Some separation is held to occur late in gestation and during childbirth.

PELVIC MECHANISM

The skeletal pelvis undoubtedly supports and protects the contained viscera, but is primarily part of the lower limbs, affording wide attachment for leg and trunk muscles. It is the major mechanism in transmitting the weight of the head, trunk and upper limbs to the lower limbs. It may be considered as two arches divided by a vertical transacetabular plane. The posterior arch, chiefly concerned in transmitting weight, consists of the upper three sacral vertebrae and strong pillars of bone from the sacroiliac joints to the acetabular fossae (p. 668). The anterior arch, formed by the pubic bones and their superior rami, connects these lateral pillars as a tie-beam preventing separation; it also acts as a compression strut against medial femoral thrust. The sacrum, as summit of the posterior arch, is loaded at the lumbosacral joint; theoretically this force has two components, one thrusting the sacrum downwards and backwards between the iliac bones, the other thrusting its upper end downwards and forwards. Sacral movements are regulated by osseous shape and massive ligaments. The first component therefore acts against the wedge, its tendency to separate iliac bones resisted by the sacroiliac and iliolumbar ligaments and symphysis pubis.

Vertical coronal sections through the sacroiliac joints suggest division of the (synovial) articular region of the sacrum into three segments. In the *anterosuperior segment*, involving the first sacral vertebra, the articular surfaces are slightly sinuous and almost parallel. In the *middle segment* (**6**.279A) the posterior width between the articular markings is greater than the anterior, and centrally a sacral concavity fits a corresponding iliac convexity, an interlocking mechanism relieving the strain on the ligaments due to body weight. In the *posteroinferior segment* the anterior sacral width is greater than the posterior and here its sacral surfaces are slightly concave. Anteroinferior sacral dislocation by the second component (of force) is prevented, therefore, mainly by the middle segment, owing to its cuneiform shape and interlocking mechanism. However, some rotation occurs, in which the anterosuperior segment tilts down and the posteroinferior segment up. 'Superior' segmental movement is to a small degree limited by wedging but chiefly by tension in the sacrotuberous and sacrospinous ligaments. In all movements the sacroiliac and iliolumbar ligaments and symphysis pubis resist separation of the iliac bones.

Locomotor significance of structural data has been more extensively studied on primate, including human, pelves than on any other skeletal element, except perhaps the femur. As an introduction to such metrical analysis consult Zuckerman et al (1973). Muscular, gravitational and inertial forces have been analysed in a mathematical model by Goel and Svensson (1977).

Clinical anatomy

During pregnancy the pelvic joints and ligaments relax, while movements increase. Relaxation renders the sacro-iliac locking mechanism less effective, permitting greater rotation and perhaps allowing alterations in pelvic diameters at childbirth, although the effect is probably small (Young 1940). The impaired locking mechanism diverts the strain of weight-bearing to the ligaments, with frequent sacroiliac strain after pregnancy. After childbirth the ligaments tighten and the locking mechanism improves; but this may occur in a position adopted during pregnancy. Such sacroiliac 'subluxation' causes pain

by unusual ligamentous tension; reduction by forcible manipulation may be attempted. The most common position in this condition of subluxation is believed to be backward rotation of the innominate bone relative to the sacrum; usually unilateral, it is on occasion bilateral.

FEMUR

The femur (**6**.282, 283) is the longest and strongest bone in the human body. Its length is associated with a striding gait, its strength with weight and muscular forces. Its *shaft*, almost cylindrical in most of its length and bowed forward, has a proximal round, *articular head* projecting mainly medially on its short *neck*, a medial curvature of the proximal shaft. The distal extremity is more massive, being a double 'knuckle' or *condyle* articulating with the tibia. In standing, the femora are oblique (**6**.1–3), their heads separated by the pelvic width, their shafts converging downwards and medially to where the knees almost touch. Since the tibia and fibula descend vertically from the knees, the femoral obliquity approximates the feet, bringing them under the line of body weight in standing or walking. The narrowness of this base detracts from stability but facilitates forward movement by increasing speed and smoothness. Femoral obliquity varies but is greater in women, due to the relatively greater pelvic breadth and shorter femora. Proximally the femur (**6**.284, 285) comprises a head, neck and greater and lesser trochanters.

Proximal end. Slightly more than half a 'sphere' (but see pp. 503, 684), it faces anterosuperomedially to articulate with the acetabulum. (More precisely, the head is not part of a true sphere, but rather it is sphenoidal and part of the surface of an ovoid.) Its smoothness is interrupted posteroinferior to its centre by a small, rough *fovea*.

Femoral neck. About 5 cm long, it connects the head to the shaft at an angle of about 125° (*angle of inclination*): this facilitates movement at the hip joint, enabling the limb to swing clear of the pelvis. The neck is also laterally rotated with respect to the shaft (*angle of anteversion*) some 10°–15° (Reikeras et al 1983), although values as low as 7° have been reported (Yoshioka & Cooke 1987): there also appears to be some racial variation in anteversion (Eckhoff et al 1994a). (Methodology for measuring anteversion has been reviewed by Kirby et al (1993), while Ruwe et al (1992) present a method for its clinical determination.) Narrowest in its midpart, widest laterally, the contours of the neck are rounded, the upper almost horizontal and slightly concave above, the lower straighter but oblique, directed inferolaterally and backwards to the shaft near the lesser trochanter. On all aspects the neck expands as the articular surface of the head is approached. The neck's anterior surface is flat and marked at the junction with the shaft by a rough *intertrochanteric line* (**6**.282A). The posterior surface, facing back and up, is transversely convex, and concave in its long axis; its junction with the shaft is marked by the rounded *intertrochanteric crest* (**6**.283A, 284).

Greater trochanter. Large and quadrangular, it projects up from the junction of the neck and shaft. Its posterosuperior region projects superomedially (**6**.283A, 284) to overhang the adjacent posterior surface of the neck and here its medial surface presents the rough *trochanteric fossa*. The trochanter's proximal border is a hand's breadth below the iliac tubercle, level with the centre of the femoral head. It has an anterior rough impression, its lateral surface being divided by an oblique, flat strip, wider above, crossing it down and forwards; this aspect is palpable and, with the muscles (**6**.285) relaxed, can be gripped. The trochanteric fossa occasionally presents a tubercle or exostosis, a useful non-metrical racial characteristic (p. 434).

Lesser trochanter (**6**.284). A conical posteromedial projection of shaft at the posteroinferior aspect of its junction with the neck, its summit and anterior surface are rough, but its posterior surface, at the distal end of the intertrochanteric crest, is smooth. It is not palpable.

Intertrochanteric line. At the junction of the anterior surfaces of neck and shaft (**6**.282), it is a prominent ridge, descending medially from a tubercle, superomedial on the anterior aspect of the greater trochanter to the neck's lower border, level with but in front of the lesser trochanter, often ending in a second tubercle. Distally it is continuous with the *spiral line* (see below).

Intertrochanteric crest (**6**.283A, 284). At the junction of the posterior surface of the neck with the shaft, it is a smooth ridge,

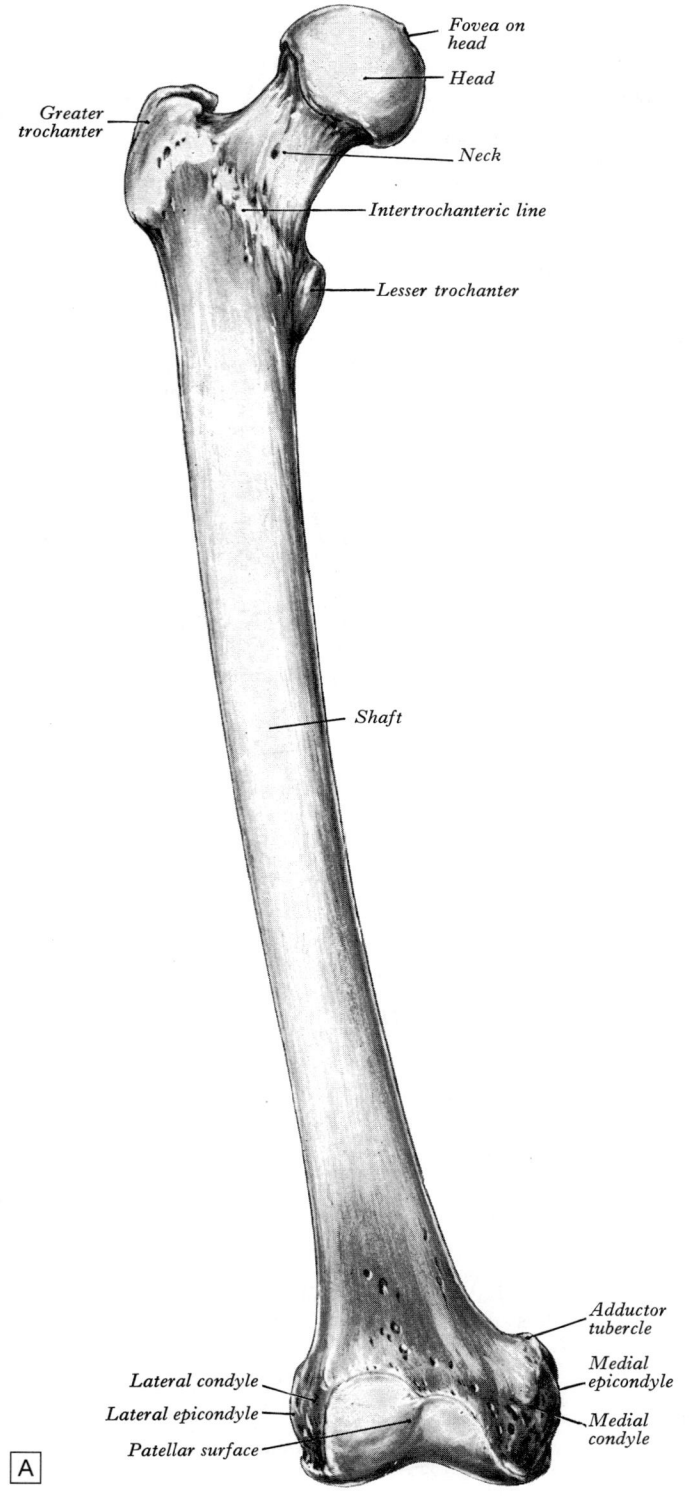

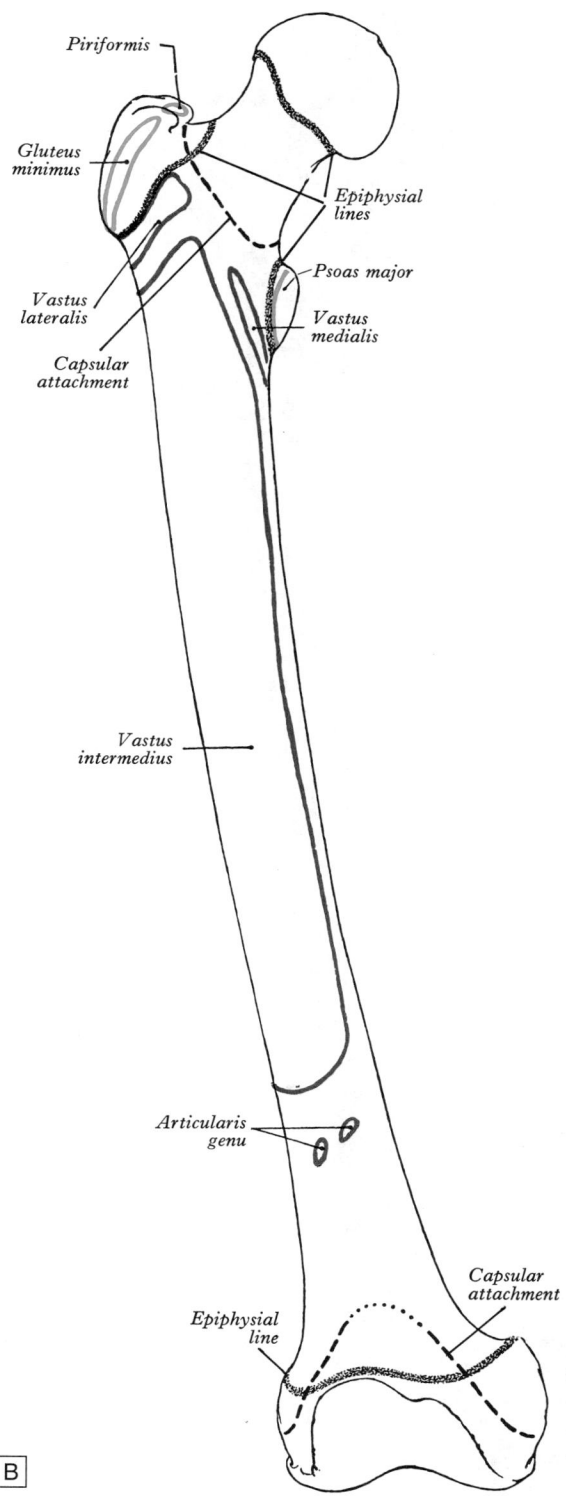

6.282A. Anterior aspect of the right femur; B. Line drawing showing muscle attachments. The epiphyseal lines are stippled; the interrupted lines are the capsular attachments, with the dotted part of the interrupted line indicating the site of communication between the knee joint and the suprapatellar bursa.

descending medially from the posterosuperior angle of the greater to the lesser trochanter. A little above its centre is a low, rounded *quadrate tubercle*.

Shaft (6.282, 283)

Narrowest centrally, it expands a little upwards, but more so towards its distal end. Its long axis makes an angle of some 7° with the vertical, and diverges about 10° from the long axis of the tibia. Its *middle third* has three surfaces and borders. The extensive *anterior surface*, smooth and gently convex, is between the lateral and medial borders, both round and indistinct. The *lateral surface*, really posterolateral, is bounded behind by the posterior border, the broad, rough *linea aspera*, usually a crest with lateral and medial edges; its subjacent compact bone is augmented to withstand compressive forces concentrated here by the shaft's anterior curvature. The *medial surface* is posteromedial, smooth like the others, bounded in front by the indistinct medial border and behind by the linea aspera. In its *proximal third* the shaft has a fourth, *posterior surface*, bounded medially by a narrow, rough *spiral line*, continuous proximally with the intertrochanteric line, distally with the medial edge of linea

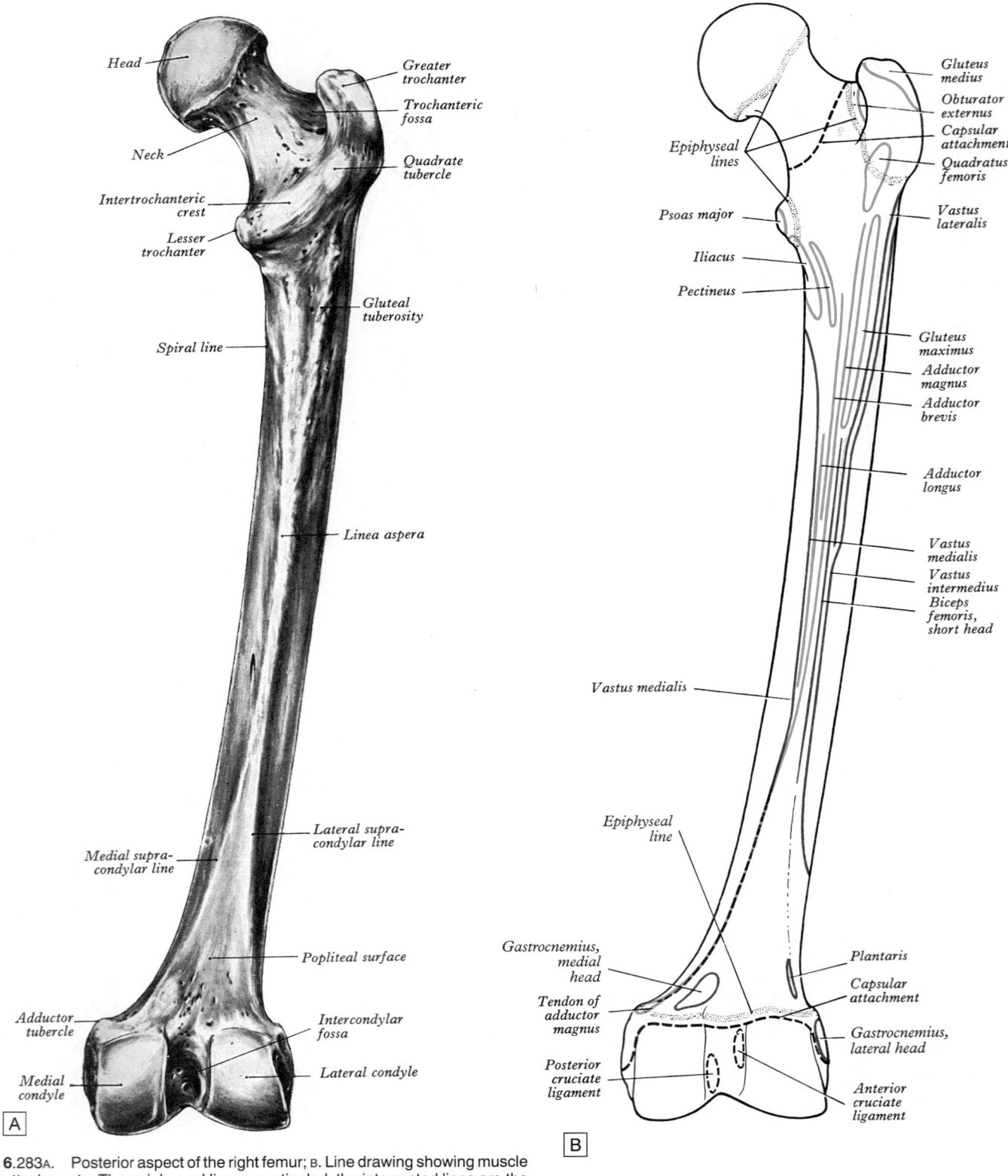

6.283A. Posterior aspect of the right femur; B. Line drawing showing muscle attachments. The epiphyseal lines are stippled; the interrupted lines are the capsular attachments.

aspera. Laterally this surface is limited by the broad, rough, *gluteal tuberosity*, ascending a little laterally to the greater trochanter and descending to the lateral edge of the linea aspera; this surface is triangular. In its *distal third* the shaft also has a fourth, *posterior surface*, between the *medial* and *lateral supracondylar ridges*, continuous above with the corresponding edges of the linea aspera; the lateral is the more distinct. Proximally the medial ridge is partly obliterated where the femoral artery is close to bone, slanting back to the popliteal fossa. This *popliteal surface* (6.283A) is also triangular, in its distal medial part rough and slightly elevated.

Distal end

Widely expanded as a bearing surface for transmission of weight to the tibia, it has two massive *condyles*, which are partly *articular*. Anteriorly the condyles unite and continue into the shaft, posteriorly separated by a deep *intercondylar fossa* and projecting beyond the plane of the popliteal surface. The *articular surface* is a broad area, like an inverted U, for the patella above and the tibia (6.286). The *patellar surface* extends anteriorly on both condyles, but largely the lateral; transversely concave, it is vertically convex and grooved for the posterior patellar surface. The *tibial surface* is divided by the intercondylar fossa but is anteriorly continuous with the patellar surface; its medial part is a broad strip on the convex inferoposterior surface of the medial condyle, gently curved with a medial convexity; its lateral part covers similar aspects of the lateral condyle but is broader and passes straight back. Heiple and Lovejoy (1971) regarded a deep patellar groove as a hominid feature, concerned with bipedal gait; others disagreed. The role of the groove in preventing lateral patellar subluxation is often repeated, but remains uncertain.

Lateral condyle (6.286, 287). Laterally flat and less prominent than the medial, it is more massive and more directly in line with the femoral shaft, and hence transmits more weight to the tibia. Its most prominent point is the *lateral epicondyle*; its whole lateral aspect is palpable. A short groove, deeper in front, separates the lateral epicondyle posteriorly from the articular margin. The medial surface is the lateral wall of the intercondylar fossa. Its lateral surface projects beyond the shaft. To its lateral epicondyle is attached the fibular collateral ligament and, to an impression posterosuperior to this, part of the lateral head of gastrocnemius. Attached anteriorly in the groove is popliteus (6.287), whose tendon is in it in full flexion; in extension it crosses the articular margin and may groove it. Adjoining the margin a strip of condyle, 1 cm broad, is intracapsular, covered by synovial membrane except for the attachment of popliteus.

Medial condyle. This has a bulging, convex medial aspect, easily palpable. Proximally its *adductor tubercle* (6.283A) receives the tendon of adductor magnus, an important surgical landmark most readily identified from above, but often a facet. The condyle's summit, the *medial epicondyle*, is anteroinferior to the tubercle. The medial condyle's lateral surface is the medial wall of the intercondylar fossa. The condyle projects distally so that, despite the shaft's obliquity, the profile of the distal end is almost horizontal. A curved strip, about 1 cm wide, adjoining the medial articular margin, is covered by synovial membrane and is inside the joint's capsule. The medial epicondyle, proximal to this, receives the tibial collateral ligament.

Further details

Femoral head. This is intracapsular, encircled lateral to its equator by the acetabular labrum. Its periphery is distinct, except anteriorly, where the articular surface extends to the neck. To its fovea (6.284) is attached the ligament of the head; the head's anterior surface is separated inferomedially by the tendon of psoas major, the psoas bursa, and the articular capsule from the femoral artery. Its blood supply is from a vascular circle around the neck, near the attachment of the fibrous capsule, supplied by medial and lateral circumflex arteries; from this rami pierce the capsule (under its zona orbicularis, (p. 684) to ascend the neck beneath the reflected synovial membrane. These divide into metaphyseal branches entering the neck and epiphyseal rami to peripheral non-articular parts of the head to supply the epiphysis. During growth, territories of the two groups are separated by the epiphyseal plate; after osseous union of the head and neck, they anastomose freely. A small supply reaches the head along its ligament (pp. 1566 and 444) by the acetabular branches of the obturator and medial femoral circumflex arteries; these anastomose with the epiphyseal vessels (Crock 1965, 1980). Observations on developmental patterns of this supply in late fetal and early postnatal periods modify the above description: though medial and lateral circumflex arteries at first contribute equally, two major branches of the medial are the final supply, both related posterior to the neck (Ogden 1974). The supply from the lateral circumflex diminishes and the arterial circle is interrupted. As the femoral neck elongates, the extracapsular circle becomes more distant from the epiphyseal part of the head.

Neck. With numerous vascular foramina, especially anterior and posterosuperior, its angle with the shaft is widest at birth and diminishes until adolescence; it is less in females. Its *anterior surface* is intracapsular; the capsular ligament extends laterally attaching to the intertrochanteric line. Facets, often covered by extensions of articular cartilage, and various imprints frequently occur here; though attributed to squatting habits, they are not always so associated; their cause is uncertain (Kostick 1963). One such feature, the *cervical fossa* (of Allen), may be racial (p. 434). On the *posterior surface* the capsule does not reach the intertrochanteric crest (6.283); little more than the medial half of the neck is intracapsular. The

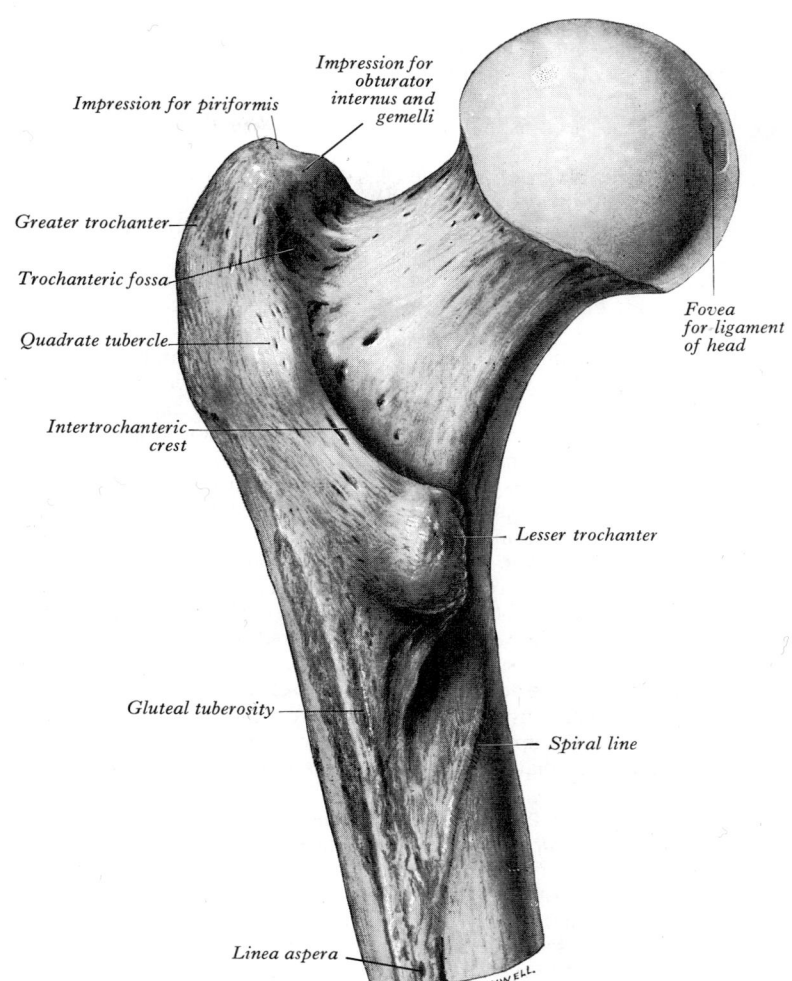

6.284 The proximal part of the left femur: posterior aspect.

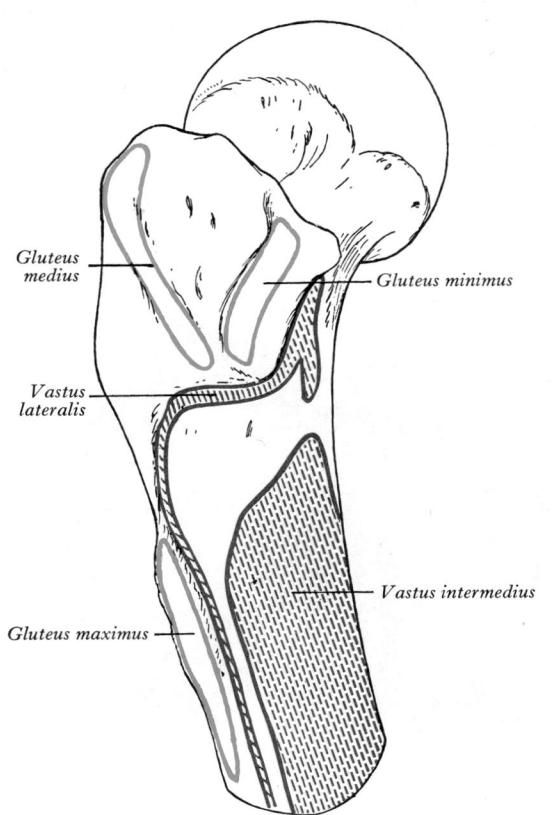

6.285 The proximal part of the right femur: lateral aspect.

681

anterior surface adjoining the head and covered by cartilage is related to the iliofemoral ligament. A groove spirals across the neck's posterior surface in a proximolateral direction, produced by the tendon of obturator externus approaching the trochanteric fossa. The neck is **not** in the plane of the shaft, but inclined forwards.

The greater trochanter (6.282B, 283B, 285). This provides attachment for most of the gluteal muscles: gluteus minimus to its rough anterior impression, gluteus medius to its lateral oblique strip, the area anterior to this separated from its tendon by a trochanteric bursa; the area behind is covered by deep fibres of gluteus maximus, with part of its trochanteric bursa interposed. To the trochanter's upper border is attached the tendon of piriformis, to its medial surface the common tendon of obturator internus and the gemelli; at their attachment these two tendons are often variably fused. The trochanteric fossa receives the tendon of obturator externus.

The lesser trochanter. This has psoas major attached to its summit and anteromedial surface. To the medial or anterior surface of its base iliacus is attached, descending a little behind the spiral line. Adductor magnus (upper part) plays over its posterior surface, with sometimes an interposed bursa.

Intertrochanteric line. This is the lateral limit of the hip joint capsule, and at its proximal and distal parts with their tubercles are attached the upper and lower bands of the iliofemoral ligament. The most proximal fibres of vastus lateralis are attached to its proximal end, those of vastus medialis distally.

Intertrochanteric crest. Above the *quadrate tubercle*, it is covered by gluteus maximus, separated distally from the muscle by quadratus femoris and the upper border of adductor magnus. To the tubercle and the immediately distal bone quadratus femoris is attached (6.283B).

Shaft (6.282B, 283B). This is surrounded by muscles and is impalpable. Its *anterior* and *lateral surfaces* are attachments in its proximal three-fourths for vastus intermedius and distal to this for slips of articularis genus. The distal anterior surface, for 5 to 6 cm above the patellar articular surface, is covered by a suprapatellar bursa, between bone and muscle. The distal lateral surface is covered by vastus intermedius. The *medial surface*, devoid of attachments, is covered by vastus medialis.

Gluteal tuberosity. This may be an elongate depression or a ridge. It may in part be prominent enough to be dubbed a *third trochanter*. It receives the deeper fibres of the distal half of gluteus maximus and, at its medial edge, pubic fibres of adductor magnus, distal to which adductor magnus is attached to the linea aspera and aponeurotically to the proximal part of the medial supracondylar ridge, remaining fibres forming a large tendon attached to the adductor tubercle (p. 681), with an aponeurotic expansion to the distal part of the medial supracondylar ridge. Lozanoff et al (1985) have devised a metrical technique associating various femoral dimen-

sions with the incidence of a third trochanter in human femora, finding that increased incidence is associated with short femora bearing large epiphyses. Though this series is limited, the metrical technique applied is commendable.

Vastus lateralis has a linear attachment from in front of the greater trochanter's base to the proximal end of the gluteal tuberosity, and along the latter's lateral margin to the proximal half of the lateral edge of the linea aspera. Similarly, vastus medialis is attached from the distal end of the intertrochanteric line along the spiral line to the medial edge of the linea aspera and thence to the medial supracondylar line; it receives many fibres from the aponeurotic attachments of adductor magnus.

Between the gluteal tuberosity and spiral line, the posterior femoral surface receives pectineus and adductor brevis, the former at a line, sometimes slightly rough, from the lesser trochanter's base to the linea aspera. The adductor brevis is attached lateral to the pectineus and beyond this to the proximal part of the linea aspera, medial to adductor magnus.

Linea aspera. This receives adductor longus, intermuscular septa and the short head of biceps femoris, inseparably blended at their attachment. The perforating arteries cross the linea laterally under tendinous arches in adductor magnus and biceps. Nutrient foramina appear in the linea aspera, varying in number and site, one usually near its proximal end, usually a second near its distal end. They are directed proximally.

Popliteal surface. The proximal floor of the popliteal fossa, it is covered by variable amounts of fat separating the popliteal artery from bone. The superior medial genicular artery, from the popliteal artery, arches medially above the medial condyle. It is separated from bone by the medial head of gastrocnemius, attached a little above the condyle, distal to which may be a smooth facet underlying a bursa for the medial head of the gastrocnemius. More medially, proximal to the articular surface, is often an imprint which in flexion is close to a rough tubercle on the medial tibial condyle for the attachment of semimembranosus (Kostick 1963). The superior lateral genicular artery arches up laterally proximal to the lateral condyle but is separated from bone by the attachment of plantaris to the distal part of the lateral supracondylar line.

The lateral supracondylar line. Most distinct in its proximal two-thirds, where the short head of biceps femoris and lateral intermuscular septum are attached, its distal third has a small rough area for plantaris, often encroaching on the popliteal surface.

The medial supracondylar line. Indistinct in its proximal two-thirds, where there is the attachment of vastus medialis, proximally it is crossed by femoral vessels entering the popliteal fossa from the adductor canal. It is often sharp for 3 or 4 cm proximal to the adductor tubercle, and here the lower membranous expansion from the tendon of adductor magnus is attached.

Intercondylar fossa. This separates the two condyles distally and

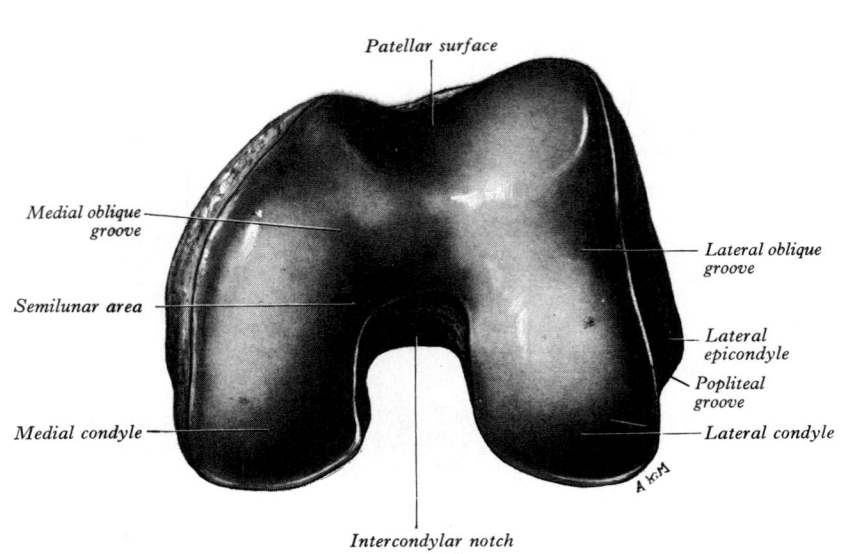

Patellar surface

Medial oblique groove

Semilunar area

Medial condyle

Lateral oblique groove

Lateral epicondyle

Popliteal groove

Lateral condyle

Intercondylar notch

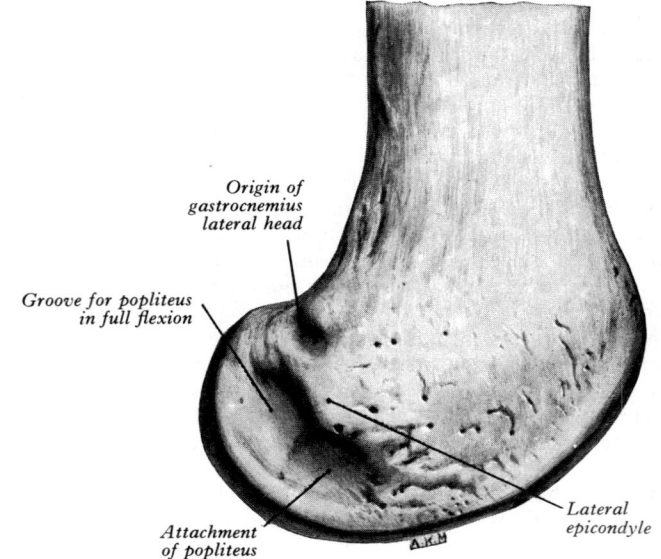

Origin of gastrocnemius lateral head

Groove for popliteus in full flexion

Attachment of popliteus

Lateral epicondyle

6.286 Inferior aspect of the distal end of the left femur.

6.287 Lateral aspect of the distal end of the right femur.

behind. In front it is limited by the distal border of the patellar surface, behind by an *intercondylar line*, separating it from the popliteal surface. It is intracapsular but largely extrasynovial. Its lateral wall, the medial surface of the lateral condyle, has a flat, posterosuperior impression spreading to the fossa's floor near the intercondylar line for the proximal attachment of the anterior cruciate ligament. The fossa's medial wall, lateral surface of the medial condyle, bears a similar larger area for the proximal attachment of the posterior cruciate ligament, sited anteriorly and extending to the fossa's anterior floor. Both impressions are smooth, and largely devoid of vascular foramina like most attachments of tendons or ligaments; the rest of the fossa is rough and pitted by vascular foramina, but a bursal recess between the ligaments may ascend to it. To the intercondylar line is attached the capsular ligament and, laterally, the oblique popliteal ligament, and to the fossa's anterior border, the infrapatellar synovial fold (p. 699).

Patellar surface. This extends proximally more on the lateral side; its proximal border is hence oblique and runs distally and medially (**6.282**A, 286), separated from the tibial surfaces by two faint grooves, which cross the condyles obliquely. The lateral groove is more distinct (**6.286**); it runs laterally and slightly forwards from the front of the intercondylar fossa and expands to form a faint triangular depression, resting on the anterior edge of the lateral meniscus with the knee fully extended. The medial groove is restricted to the medial part of the medial condyle and rests on the anterior edge of the medial meniscus in full extension; where it ceases, the patellar surface continues back to the lateral part of the medial condyle as a semilunar area adjoining the anterior region of the intercondylar fossa; this area articulates with the patella's medial vertical facet in full flexion; it is not distinct in outline in most femora. In habitual squatters articular cartilage may extend to the lateral aspect of the lateral condyle under vastus lateralis. The tibial surfaces are transversely convex in all directions. Anteroposterior curvature of both surfaces is not uniform, with a shorter radius posteriorly; the medial surface is longer anteroposteriorly, and has a slight laterally concave profile. These differences are important determinants of rotatory movements, both adjunct and conjunct (p. 505), at the knee joint (p. 707).

Structure

The femoral shaft is a cylinder of compact bone, with a large medullary cavity. The wall is thick in its middle third, where the femur is narrowest and the medullary cavity most capacious; but proximally and distally the compact wall becomes progressively thinner, the cavity gradually filling with trabecular bone; the extremities, especially where articular, consist of trabecular bone within a thin shell of compact bone; their trabeculae being disposed along lines of greatest stress (p. 688). In the proximal end (**6.288**A) the main trabeculae form a series of plates orthogonal to the articular surface, converging to a central dense wedge, which is supported by strong trabeculae passing to the sides of the neck, especially along its upper and lower profiles. Force applied to the femoral head is hence transmitted to the wedge and thence to the junction of the neck and shaft. This junction is strengthened by dense trabeculae extending laterally from the lesser trochanter to the end of the neck's superior aspect, thus resisting tensile or shearing forces applied to the neck through the head. A smaller bar across the junction of the greater trochanter with the neck and shaft resists shearing due to muscles attached to it. These two bars are proximal layers of arches between the sides of the shaft, transmitting to it forces applied to the proximal end. A thin vertical plate, *calcar femorale* (**6.288**B), ascends from the compact wall near the linea aspera into the trabeculae of the neck. Medially it joins the posterior wall of the neck; laterally it continues into the greater trochanter, dispersing into general trabecular bone. It is thus in a plane anterior to the trochanteric crest and base of the lesser trochanter. Scanning electron microscopy of the proximal femoral end, in a small series of specimens, has partly confirmed these details (Whitehouse & Dyson 1974). Wide variation in metrical parameters of trabecular pattern in the femoral head and neck was nevertheless observed. Tensile and compressive tests of 40 human femora also indicate that axial trabecular tissue of the femoral head withstands much greater stresses than do peripheral trabeculae. In the distal femoral end trabeculae spring from the entire internal surface of compact bone, descending perpendicular to the articular surface; proximal to the condyles these are strongest and most accurately perpendicular. Horizontal planes of trabecular bone, arranged like crossed girders, form a series of cubical compartments.

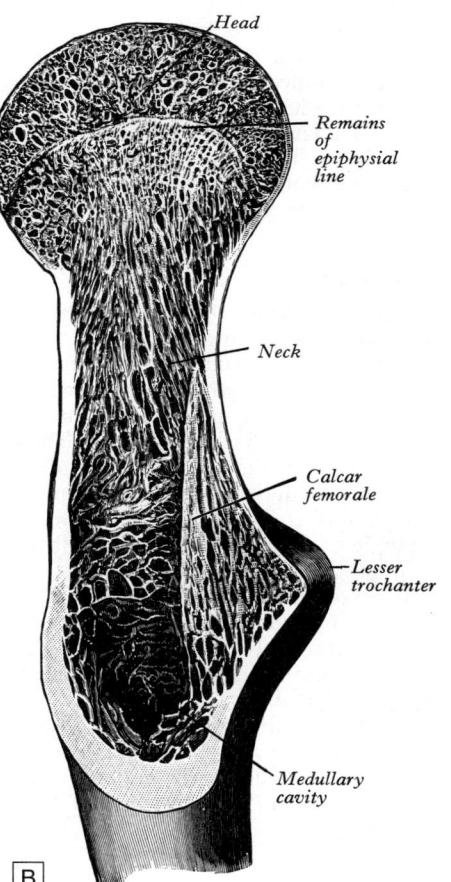

Head

Remains of epiphysial line

Acetabular labrum

Capsular ligament

Zona orbicularis

Ligament of head of femur

Pad of fat

Transverse ligament of acetabulum

Capsular ligament

Zona orbicularis

Neck

Calcar femorale

Lesser trochanter

Medullary cavity

A   B

6.288A. Section through the hip joint. B. Oblique section through the proximal end of the left femur showing the trabecular architecture, calcar femorale, medullary cavity and variations in cortical thickness. Compare with **6.5** and **6.292**A.

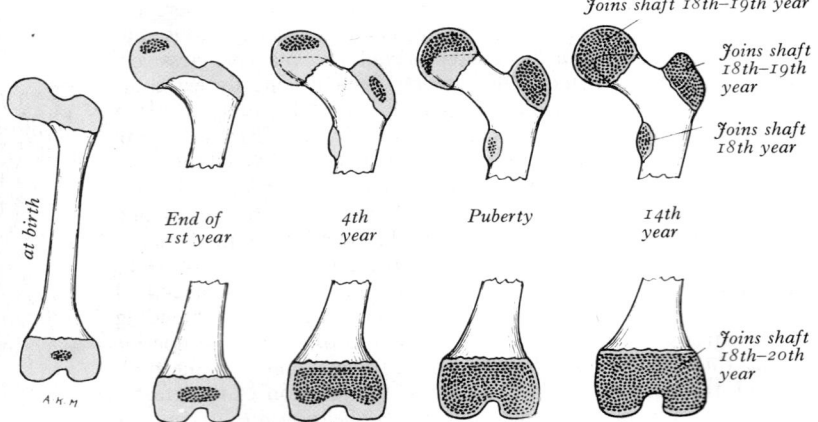

Joins shaft 18th–19th year

Joins shaft 18th–19th year

Joins shaft 18th year

Joins shaft 18th–20th year

at birth

End of 1st year

4th year

Puberty

14th year

A K M

6.289 Stages in the ossification of the femur. Note how the neck, which is ossified as an extension from the shaft, invades, and is partly enclosed by, the cartilaginous head (not to scale).

Ossification

Ossification (6.282B, 283B, 289) of the femur is from five centres: in the shaft, head, greater and lesser trochanters and the distal end. Excepting the clavicle, it is the first long bone to ossify, this beginning in the midshaft in the seventh prenatal week and extending to produce a miniature shaft largely ossified at birth. Secondary centres appear in the distal end during the ninth month (from which the condyles and epicondyles are formed) (see 6.303), in the head during the first six months after birth, in the greater trochanter during the fourth year and in the lesser between the twelfth and fourteenth year. Note that the centre in the cartilaginous head is restricted to it until the tenth year, so that the epiphyseal line (6.271) is horizontal and the inferomedial part of the articular surface is on the neck (6.289). The medial epiphyseal margin later grows over this part of the articular surface. Thus, the mature epiphysis is a **hollow cup** on the neck's summit. The epiphyseal line follows the articular margin except where separated superiorly from the articular surface by a non-articular area; here blood vessels enter the head (Trueta 1957; Smith 1962a). The epiphyses fuse independently, the lesser trochanter soon after puberty, then the greater, the head at the fourteenth year in females, seventeenth in males and the distal end at the sixteenth year in females, eighteenth in males. Note that the distal epiphyseal plate traverses the adductor tubercle (6.282B).

Clinical anatomy

The distal end of the femur is the only epiphysis in which ossification constantly starts just before birth, a most reliable indicator that a dead newborn child was viable. Since the epiphyseal plate is level with the adductor tubercle, the epiphysis does not form all the distal end covered by synovial membrane; hence operations here may damage the distal epiphyseal cartilage in children and entail subsequent shortening of the leg. Fractures of the femoral neck are usually due to transmitted stress, as in tripping over obstructions. The trunk continues to advance and, overbalancing, twists and imposes excessive medial rotation on the thigh and leg. Before 16 years the usual injury is a spiral fracture of the shaft, but between 16 and 40 a crescentic tear of the medial meniscus is frequent. Between 40 and 60, a common result is fracture of the tibia, but over 60, fracture of the femoral neck is common, because of osteoporotic changes in ageing bones. Women are more liable, their bones being lightly built.

Normally, with the lower limb aligned with the trunk, the greater trochanter's apex is on the line joining the anterior superior iliac spine and the most prominent part of the ischial tuberosity (Nelaton's line). In displacements due to fracture of the neck the trochanter may be above this line.

HIP JOINT

The hip joint is a multiaxial joint of ball-and-socket (spheroidal, cotyloid) type. The femoral head articulates with the cup-shaped

(cotyloid) acetabulum, its centre lying a little below the middle third of the inguinal ligament (6.290). (The profile of the joint's ventral margin is also **parallel** to the middle third of the inguinal ligament.) The articular surfaces are reciprocally curved but neither coextensive nor completely congruent. The close-packed position is in full extension, with slight abduction and medial rotation. As in the shoulder joint, the surfaces are considered ovoid or spheroid rather than spherical but this is controversial (Hammond & Charnley 1967; Bullough & Goodfellow 1968; Greenwald & Haynes 1972). Evidence favours spheroid and slightly ovoid (p. 503) surfaces, becoming almost spherical with advancing age. The femoral head is covered by articular cartilage, except for a rough pit for the *ligament of the head* (6.284); in front the cartilage extends laterally over a small area on the adjoining neck; it is thickest centrally. Kurrat and Oberländer (1978) measured acetabular and femoral articular cartilages in 10 human joints, finding maximal thickness in the acetabulum's anterosuperior quadrant and anterolateral on the femoral head (6.291). Meachim and Allibone (1984) have described topographical variation in a calcified zone in this cartilage. The acetabular articular surface is an incomplete ring, the *lunate surface*, broadest above where the pressure of body weight falls in the erect posture, narrowest in its pubic region. It is deficient below opposite the acetabular notch and covered by articular cartilage, thickest where the surface is broadest. The acetabular fossa within it is devoid of cartilage but contains fibroelastic fat largely covered by synovial membrane. Acetabular depth is increased by a fibrocartilaginous *acetabular labrum*, which bridges the acetabular notch via the *transverse acetabular ligament*. Ligaments include the *iliofemoral, ischiofemoral, pubofemoral* and the *ligament of the head of the femur*.

Acetabular labrum (6.281, 292). A fibrocartilaginous rim attached to the acetabular margin, deepening the cup, it bridges the acetabular notch as the *transverse acetabular ligament*, completing the circle. Triangular in section, it is attached by its base to the acetabular rim, the apex being its free margin. The acetabular cavity is constricted by the labral rim which embraces the femoral head.

The transverse acetabular ligament (6.281). This is part of the labrum but has no cartilage cells. Its strong, flat fibres cross the notch forming a foramen through which vessels and nerves enter the joint.

Fibrous capsule (6.293)

Strong and dense, it is attached above to the acetabular margin 5–6 mm beyond its labrum, in front to the outer labral aspect and, near the acetabular notch, to its transverse acetabular ligament and the adjacent rim of the obturator foramen. It surrounds the femoral neck and is attached **in front** to the intertrochanteric line; **above** to the base of the femoral neck; **behind** about 1 cm above the intertrochanteric crest; **below** to the femoral neck near the lesser trochanter (6.293A). Anteriorly many fibres ascend along the neck as longitudinal *retinacula*, containing blood vessels for both the femoral head and neck (p. 1567). The capsule is thicker anterosuperiorly, where maximal stress occurs, particularly in standing; posteroinferior it is thin and loosely attached. It has two sets of fibres, circular and longitudinal. The circular fibres (*zona orbicularis*) are internal (6.292), forming a collar round the femoral neck; though partly blended with the pubofemoral and ischiofemoral ligaments, these fibres are not directly attached to bone. Externally, longitudinal fibres are most numerous in the anterosuperior region, reinforced by the *iliofemoral ligament*. The capsule is also strengthened by the *pubofemoral* and *ischiofemoral* ligaments; externally it is rough, covered by muscles and separated from psoas major and iliacus by a bursa.

Synovial membrane. Starting from the femoral articular margin, it covers the intracapsular part of the femoral neck, then passes to the capsule's internal surface to cover the acetabular labrum, ligament of the head and fat in the acetabular fossa. It is thin on the deep surface of the iliofemoral ligament where it is compressed against the femoral head and sometimes is even absent here. The joint may communicate with the subtendinous iliac (psoas) bursa (p. 872) by a circular aperture between the pubofemoral and the vertical band of the iliofemoral ligament.

Iliofemoral ligament

Triangular and very strong, it is anterior and intimately blended with the capsule; its apex is attached between the anterior inferior

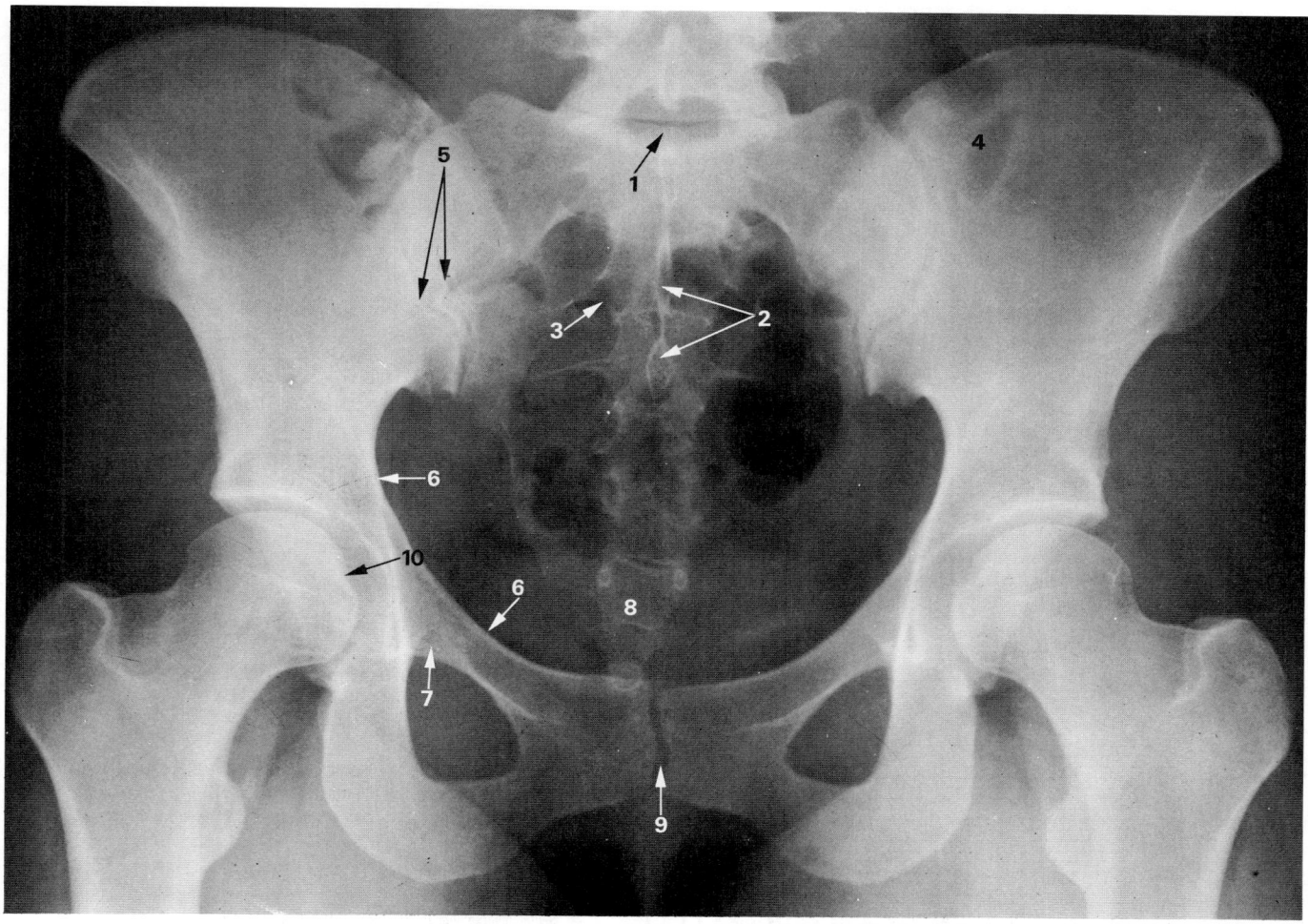

6.290 Anteroposterior radiograph of adult female pelvis. 1. Sacral prom-ontory. 2. Sacral spinous crest. 3. Margin of anterior sacral foramen. 4. Gas in pelvic colon. 5. Sacroiliac joint. 6. Pelvic brim. 7. Obturator groove. 8. Coccyx. 9. Symphysis pubis. 10. Fovea of femoral head.

iliac spine and acetabular rim, its base to the intertrochanter line: it is often referred to as the Y-shaped ligament (6.293A). Fuss and Bacher (1991) distinguish a weaker central section, referred to as the *greater iliofemoral ligament*, with thicker, more dense margins, the *lateral* and *medial iliofemoral ligaments*. The oblique lateral ligament attaches to a tubercle at the superolateral end of the intertrochanteric line; the vertical medial ligament reaches the inferomedial end.

Pubofemoral ligament

Also triangular, it has a base attached to the iliopubic eminence, superior pubic ramus, obturator crest and membrane; it blends distally with the capsule and deep surface of the medial iliofemoral ligament (6.293A). However, Fuss and Bacher (1991) consider this ligament to consist of four crura.

Ischiofemoral ligament

This thickens the back of the capsule (6.293B) and consists of three distinct parts (Fuss & Bacher 1991). From the ischium, postero-inferior to the acetabulum, the central part, the *superior ischiofemoral ligament* spirals superolaterally behind the femoral neck, some fibres blending with the zona orbicularis, to attach to the greater trochanter deep to the iliofemoral ligament. *Lateral* and *medial inferior ischi-ofemoral ligaments* embrace the posterior circumference of the femoral neck.

Ligament of the head of the femur

A triangular flat band, its apex is attached anterosuperiorly in the pit on the femoral head; its base is principally attached on both sides of the acetabular notch, between which it blends with the transverse ligament (6.294). (However, it receives weaker contributions from the margins of the acetabular fossa.) Ensheathed by flattened tubular synovial membrane, it varies in strength; occasionally its synovial sheath alone exists, without a core; rarely both ligament and sheath are absent. The ligament appears to tense when the thigh is semiflexed and adducted and to relax in abduction.

Relations

The joint capsule is surrounded by muscles (6.295). *Anteriorly*, lateral fibres of pectineus separate its most medial part from the femoral vein; lateral to this the tendon of psoas major, with iliacus lateral to it, descends across it, partly separated by a bursa. The femoral artery is anterior to the tendon; the femoral nerve deep in a groove between tendon and iliacus. More laterally the straight head of rectus femoris crosses the joint with a deep layer of the fascial iliotibial tract, which blends with the capsule under the muscle's lateral border. *Superiorly*, the reflected head of rectus femoris contacts the capsule medially, while gluteus minimus covers it laterally, being closely adherent. *Inferiorly*, lateral fibres of pectineus adjoin the capsule and, more posteriorly, obturator externus spirals obliquely to its posterior aspect. *Posteriorly*, the lower capsule is covered by the tendon of obturator externus, separating it from quadratus femoris and accompanied by an ascending branch of the medial circumflex femoral artery; above this the tendon of obturator internus and the gemelli contact the joint, separating it from the sciatic nerve; the nerve to quadratus femoris is deep to the obturator internus tendon, the nerve descending most medially on the capsule. Above this, the joint's posterior surface is crossed by piriformis.

Vessels and nerve supply to joint

Articular arteries are branches from the obturator, medial circumflex femoral, and superior and inferior gluteal arteries. **Nerves** are from the femoral or its muscular branches, the obturator, accessory

685

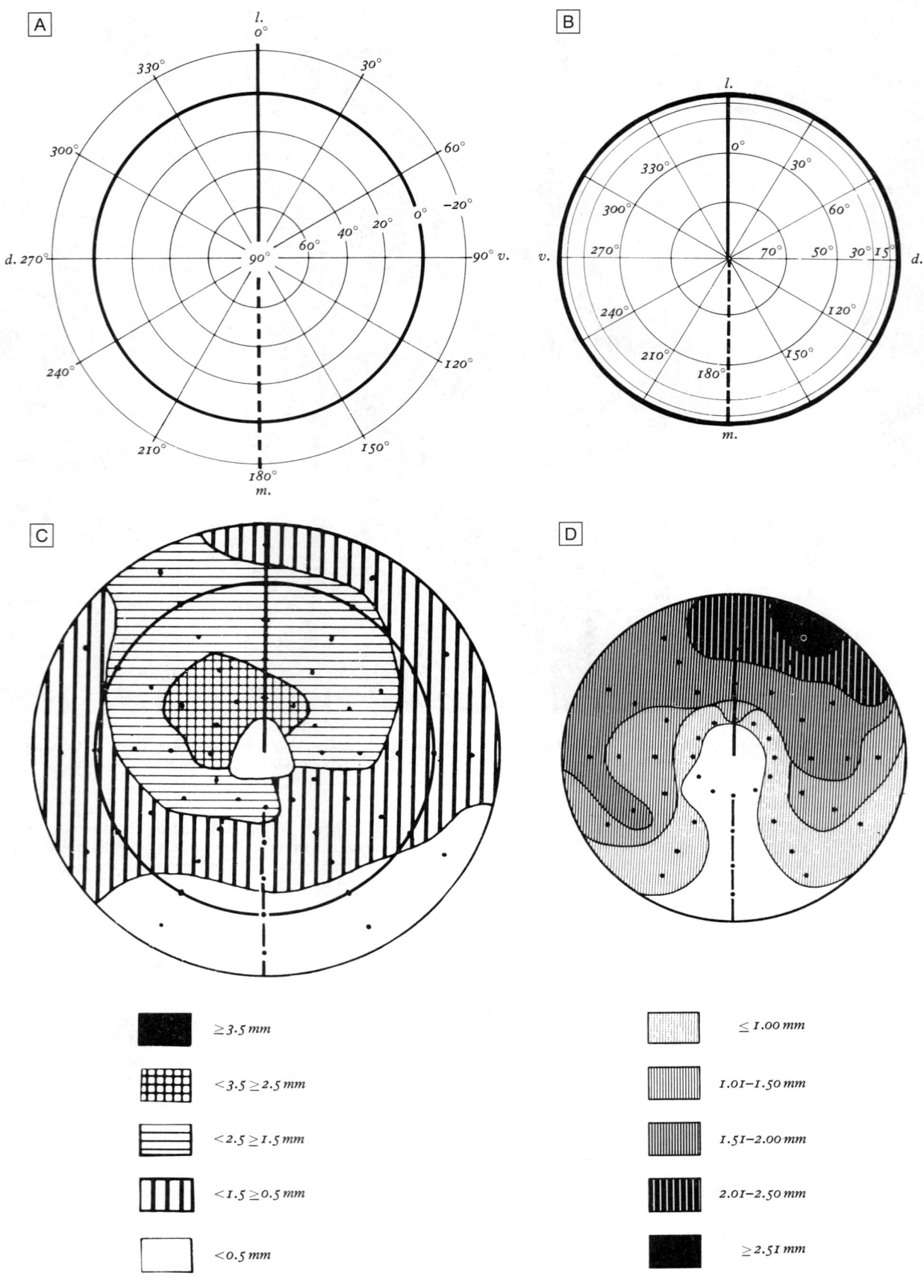

6.291 Variations in the thickness of the articular cartilages of the femoral head (A and C) and the lunate surface of the acetabulum (B and D). Diagrams A and B are reference grids by which the distance and angular direction of sampling points are measured from the centres of the femoral head and of the acetabulum. Diagrams C and D show the average contours of the thickness ranges indicated in the shading codes included below. Anterior and posterior aspects are denoted as 'a' and 'p'; 'l' and 'm' denote super-olateral and inferomedial points on the circumference of the femoral articular surface. The black dots indicate the intersections of lines of 'longitude' and 'latitude' and also represent sampling points. It is immediately apparent that this method does not provide a detailed representation of the graded topology of the articular surfaces. (See p. 504 for an alternative methodology, more recently introduced.) (Provided from the paper by H J Kurrat & W Oberländer, 1978 by courtesy of Cambridge University Press.)

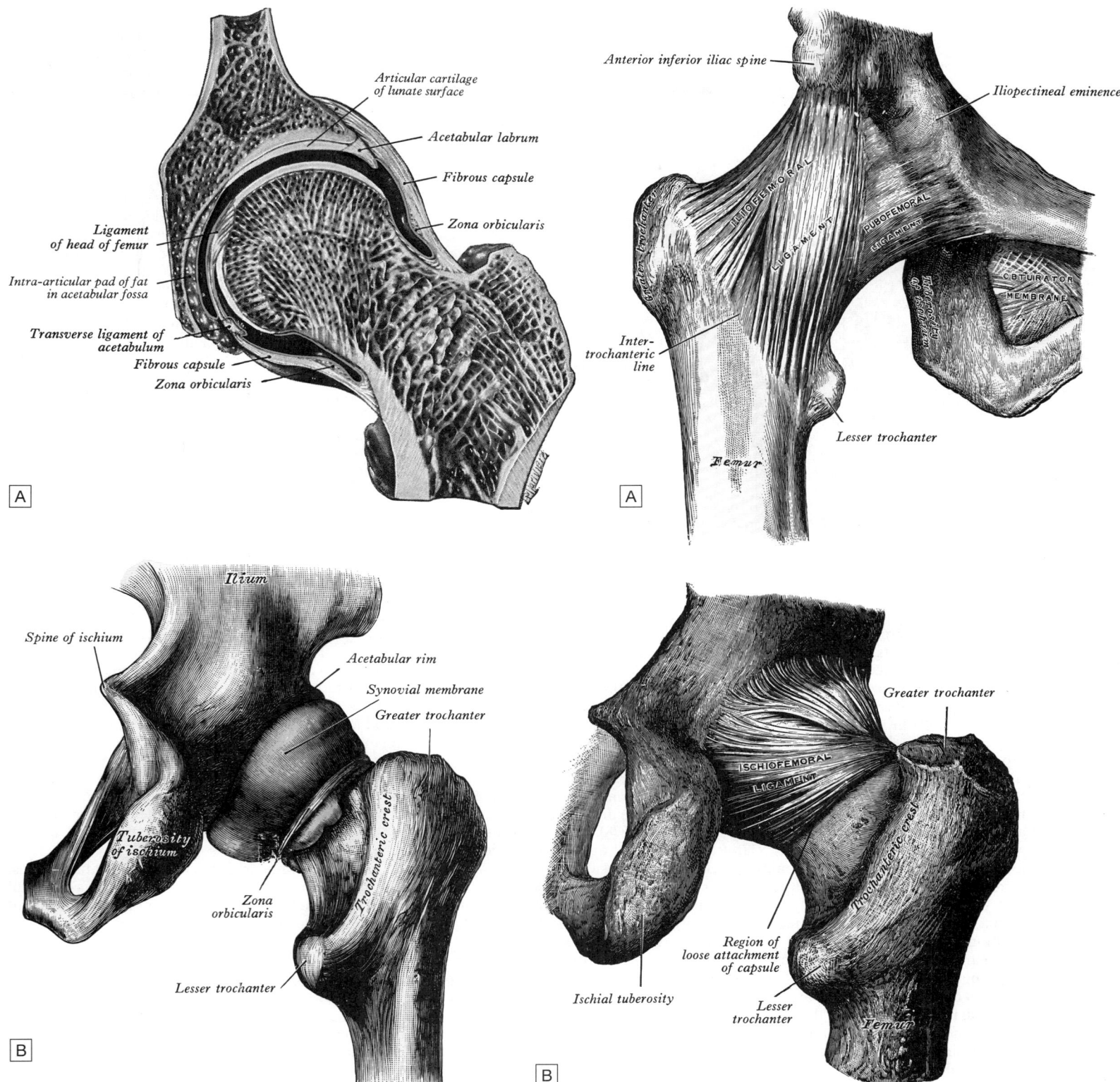

6.292A.   Section through the hip joint. The synovial membrane is shown in blue. B. Synovial cavity of the right hip joint (distended); posterior aspect.

6.293   The right hip joint; A. Anterior aspect: B. Posterior aspect.

obturator, the nerve to quadratus femoris and the superior gluteal nerves (Gardner 1948a).

Movements

Movements can be categorized as *flexion–extension, adduction–abduction, circumduction, medial* and *lateral rotation,* conveniently considered as rotations around three orthogonal axes, but when femoral movements are considered in relation to the articular surfaces, the length and angulation of the neck in relation to shaft must be remembered. When the thigh is flexed or extended, the femoral head

'spins' in the acetabulum on an approximately transverse axis; conversely, the acetabula rotate around similar axes in flexion and extension of the trunk on stationary femoral heads. Medial and lateral femoral rotation have a vertical axis through the centre of the femoral head and lateral condyle, with the foot **stationary** on the ground. Such rotations are the inevitable conjunct rotations accompanying terminal extension or initial flexion at the knee joint (pp. 707–708). Because of the relation of this axis to the whole femur (with its angulated neck and oblique shaft), during medial rotation the medial condyle moves in an arc **backwards** on the medial tibial

687

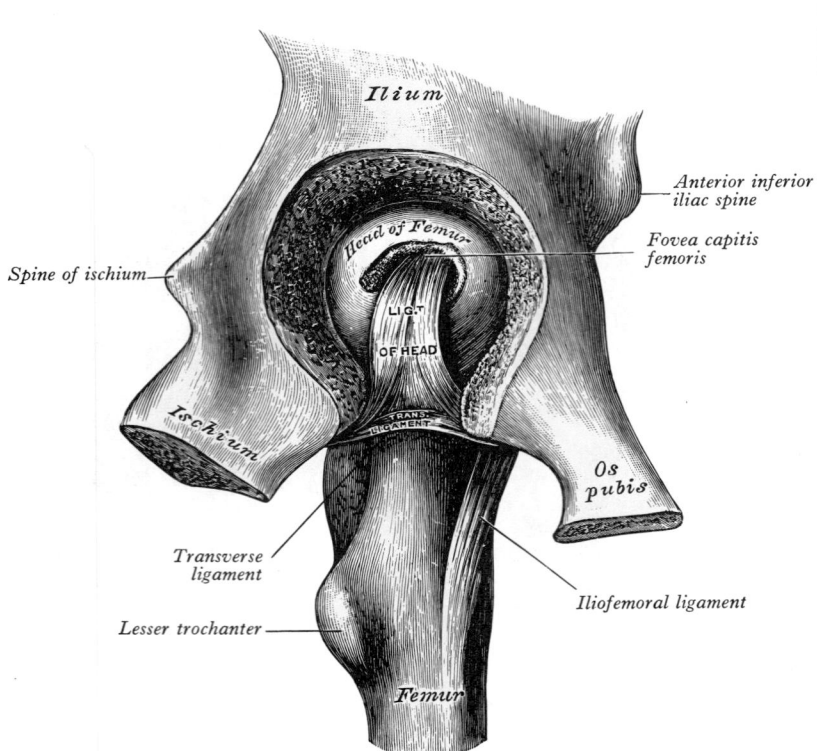

Anterior inferior
iliac spine

Fovea capitis
femoris

Spine of ischium

Transverse
ligament

Lesser trochanter

Iliofemoral ligament

6.294 Left hip joint, opened by the removal of the floor of the acetabulum from within the pelvis.

condyle and the greater trochanter simultaneously in a **forward** arc: converse movements occur during lateral rotation. With the foot in loose contact or free, medial and lateral adjunct rotation of the whole lower limb occurs around variable axes, all through the femoral head and any part of the foot. Conversely, with one foot stationary and the other free, the whole trunk may rotate on one femoral head—as in cross-kicking. Abduction and adduction are around an anteroposterior axis through the femoral head; but since this is not truly spherical no axis is satisfactory (Walmsley 1928). Some kinesiologists refer to a *mechanical axis* coincident with the topographical long axis of the femoral neck, impinging on the approximate centre of its head's articular surface (p. 678), making extension and flexion of the thigh relatively pure 'spins' at the hip joint and most effective in tightening or relaxing the capsular ligaments. All other movements are regarded as pure or impure swings (p. 505). While this permits analysis closer to actual articular function than a cardinal triaxial system, related arbitrarily to the 'anatomical' position, the mechanical axis is itself (incorrectly) regarded by some as dynamic, because forms of apparent dynamic 'spin' may occur in many positions; this view stems from an imprecise definition of the varieties of axes employed in arthrokinematics. The mechanical axis is not dynamic relative to the femur. It is stationary during pure spins; it moves relative to its coarticular surface in chordal or arcuate paths during pure or impure swings respectively.

Simple flexion is possible to 90°–100° from the **vertical**; extension beyond the **vertical** is limited (perhaps 10°–20°). Both movements are augmented by adjustments of the spinal column and pelvis, flexion of the knee and concomitant medial or lateral hip rotation. For example, knee flexion (lessening tension in the posterior femoral muscles) increases hip flexion to 120°; the thigh can be drawn passively to the trunk, though with some spinal flexion. Extension in walking, running, etc., is increased by forward inclination of the body, pelvic tilting and rotation and lateral hip rotation. (For analyses consult Kapandji 1963, 1974; Joseph 1975.) Abduction and adduction can be similarly increased.

The hip joint differs much from the shoulder joint in limitation of its movements. The articular surface of the humeral head much exceeds that of the glenoid cavity and movements are little restrained by the capsule. In the hip, in contrast, the femoral head is closely fitted to the acetabulum in an area of almost half a sphere, embraced

more closely by its labrum, being held in place even when the capsule is divided. The iliofemoral is the strongest of all ligaments and is progressively tightened when the femur extends to the line of the trunk. The pubofemoral and ischiofemoral ligaments also tighten and, as the joint approaches close-packing, resistance to an extending torque rapidly increases.

No accessory movements occur, except for very slight separation effected by strong traction.

Muscles producing movement

Flexion: psoas major and iliacus, assisted by pectineus, rectus femoris and sartorius. The adductors, particularly adductor longus, also assist, especially in early flexion from full extension.

Extension: gluteus maximus and the hamstring (posterior femoral) muscles. In the fully erect posture with pendent arms a vertical through the body's centre of gravity is behind a line joining the centres of the femoral heads; therefore the body tends to incline backwards but is counterbalanced by ligamentous tension and congruence and compression of the articular surfaces with the hip joints in the close-packed position. Under increased loading of the trunk or leaning backwards, these resistive but passive factors are assisted by active contraction of the joint's flexors. In swaying forwards at the ankles, or when the arms are stretched forward, and also in forward bending at the hip, the line of body weight moves in front of the transverse axis and the posture adopted, or the rate of change of posture, is largely controlled by the hamstrings which, although powerful **flexors** of the knee, are equally strong **extensors** of the hip. Gluteus maximus only becomes active when the thigh is extended against resistance, as in rising from a bending position or climbing.

Abduction: gluteus medius and minimus (p. 878), assisted by tensor fascia lata and sartorius. Abduction is limited by adductor tension, the pubofemoral ligament and medial band of the iliofemoral ligament. These muscles are consistently involved in walking or running (p. 897), contracting periodically at precise phases of the walking or running cycle.

Adduction: adductors longus, brevis and magnus, assisted by pectineus and gracilis. Adduction is limited by contact with the opposite limb but its range is wider with the thigh flexed when it is limited by the abductor muscles, the lateral band of the iliofemoral ligament and ligament of the femoral head.

Medial rotation: tensor fascia lata and the anterior fibres of gluteus minimus and medius. It is relatively weak and is limited by the lateral rotators, ischiofemoral ligament and posterior part of the capsule. Electromyographic data suggests that the adductors usually assist in medial rather than lateral rotation but this is, of course, dependent on the primary position.

Lateral rotation: obturator muscles, gemelli and quadratus femoris, assisted by piriformis, gluteus maximus and sartorius. It is a powerful action and limited by tension in the medial rotators and the lateral band of the iliofemoral ligament.

Clinical anatomy

The iliofemoral ligament is rarely torn during dislocation, an advantage in reduction because it can act as the fulcrum to a lever, its long arm the femoral shaft, the short arm being the femoral neck. Congenital dislocation is more common at the hip than elsewhere and is often associated with a cartilaginous ridge, formed almost exclusively by a bulge of acetabular cartilage sometimes covered by an inverted labrum (Ponseti 1978b). Displacement is usually to the gluteal surface of the ilium, the acetabular rim being deficient above. In a study of 280 hips in 140 normal fetuses, 65 of 92 hips (46 fetuses between 12 weeks and term) showed morphological variants involving the acetabular labrum, ligament of the head and capsule, but none were subluxated or dislocated (Walker 1980). There was, however, a significant relationship with age in the frequency of these variants. The suggestion is that they are subclinical manifestations of congenital hip disease.

In manipulation of the sacroiliac joints the surgeon takes advantage of the tautness of the iliofemoral and ischiofemoral ligaments in hip extension. So strong are they that forcible hyperextension with forward pressure on the iliac crest produces sacroiliac movement.

The forces transmitted across the hip joint vary according to activity; during single limb stance forces of 2.1 times body weight

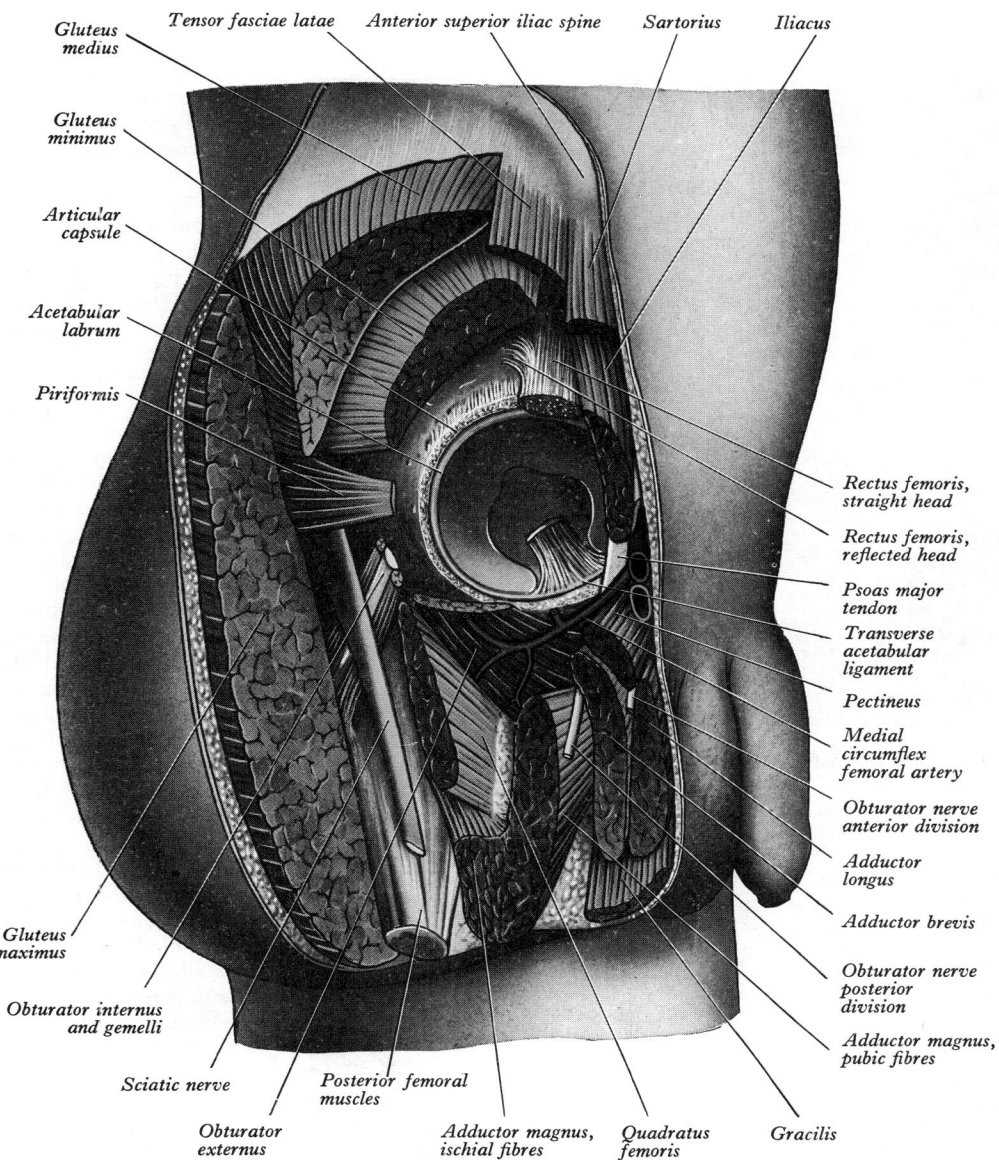

6.295   Dissection to display the structures surrounding the right hip joint. The head of the femur has been disarticulated and removed.

have been recorded, while in the stance phase of gait forces are 2.6–2.8 times body weight (Davy et al 1988). The highest hip contact pressures, recorded over a 36-month period, were consistently found to be localized to the superior and posterior regions of the acetabulum, corresponding to observed sites of degenerative change (Hodge et al 1989).

Total hip replacement

Total hip replacement has, over the last 25 years, become one of the most successful surgical operations, with over 35 000 performed annually in the United Kingdom alone.

The indications for total hip replacement are pain and loss of function: hip pain is classically felt over the greater trochanteric region, in the groin and radiating down the front of the thigh to the knee, this distribution reflecting the innervation of the joint from branches of the sciatic, femoral and obturator nerves. Loss of function presents as stiffness, fixed deformity, limb shortening and a limp. The conditions most commonly requiring hip replacement are osteoarthritis and rheumatoid arthritis (6.296); other conditions include psoriatic arthritis, ankylosing spondylitis, avascular necrosis, trauma and tumours.

The standard present-day hip replacement consists of an ultra-high molecular weight polyethylene hemispherical socket fixed into the acetabulum and a spherical metallic head supported by a metal stem (either of stainless steel, titanium alloy or chrome cobalt alloy) fixed into the medullary cavity of the femur: both the socket and stem are fixed using methylmethacrylate cement (6.297).

Hip replacement requires surgical access to the upper femur, femoral head and acetabulum. Charnley used a true lateral approach in which, after making a longitudinal skin incision over the lateral aspect of the hip, the fascia lata is then divided to expose the greater trochanter. The

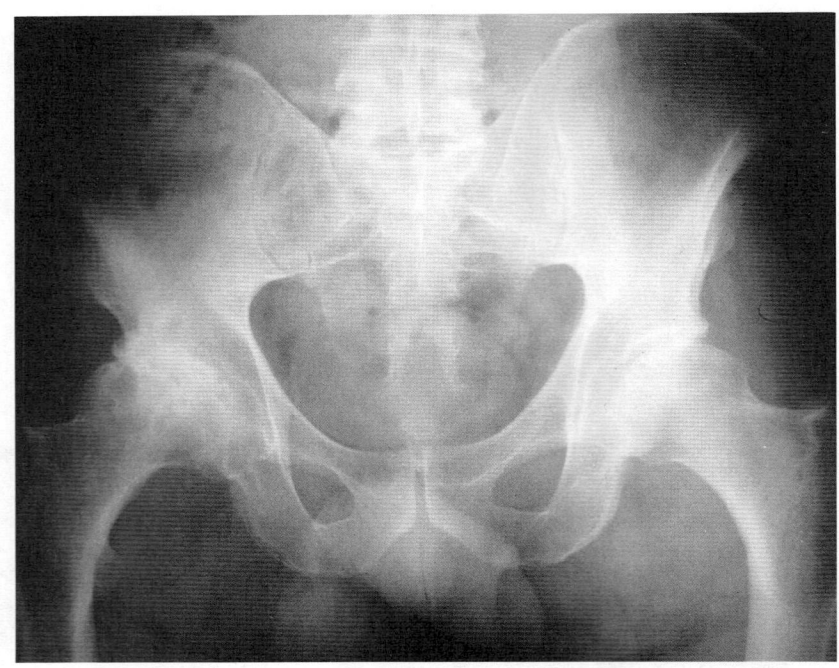

6.296   X-ray of pelvis showing osteoarthritic right hip with loss of joint space, osteophytes, sclerosis and cysts.

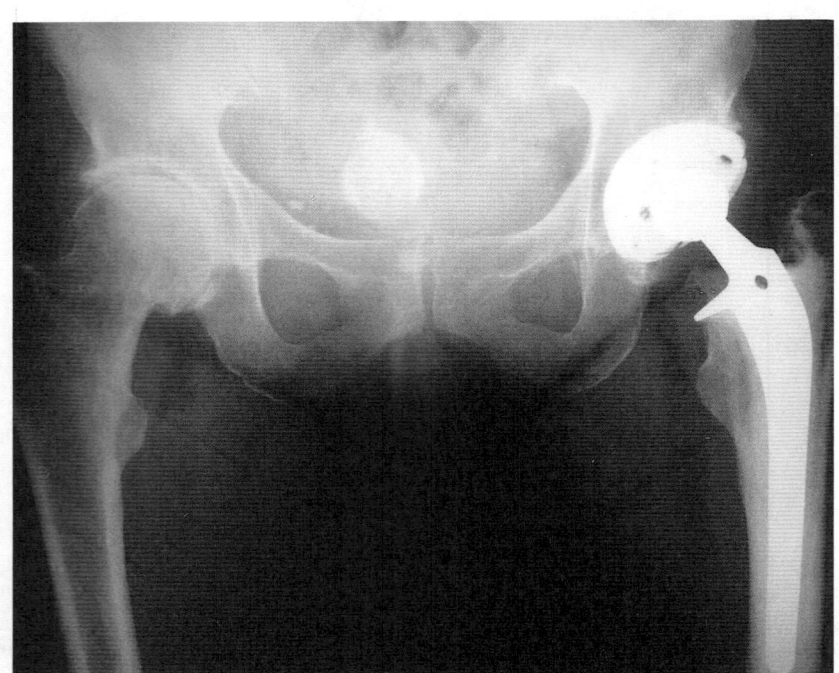

6.297   X-ray showing a left hybrid total hip replacement using an uncemented cup and cemented stem.

medius and tensor fasciae latae is incised. Each approach has its advantages, with all allowing the femoral neck to be resected giving access to both the acetabulum and the femoral intramedullary canal.

In an ideal hip replacement the stresses transmitted across the joint would exactly reproduce the natural pattern and magnitude. The forces on the hip, which can be as high as 20 times body weight, are transmitted via the cancellous bone of the pelvis to the acetabular subchondral bone, and hence across the hip joint to the complex architecture of cancellous bone of the femoral head and neck to the femoral shaft. Hip replacement is mechanically crude in comparison. In the acetabulum, the complex horseshoe-shaped subchondral bone plate is replaced by material with a constant stiffness. In the femur, the constraints of strength (to prevent fatigue fractures) and the difficulty of providing a strong bone–prosthesis interface means that large, stiff pieces of metal are implanted into the femoral shaft, generally with stems longer than 120 mm. Stems of this length considerably alter the overall stiffness of the proximal femur, leading to proximal stress shielding and subsequent remodelling of the upper femur, with a loss of cortical thickness.

Nevertheless, a technically well-performed cemented total hip replacement, in a patient who pursues limited activities, has a 95% chance of surviving 10 years. Total hip failure is, in part, accounted for by infection and dislocation, but by far the largest failure occurs from prosthetic loosening, either because the cemented interface is not sufficiently strong to bear the loads, or because the interface was weak originally, or because the applied loads have been excessive. Particulate debris causes bone resorption and, if a fibrous layer exists between the cement and bone, the debris can be transported into the membrane, setting up a giant cell reaction and producing substances such as interleukins, osteoclast-activating factor and tumour necrosis factor, all of which cause bone resorption. The source of the particulate debris can be the polyethylene cup, the metal stem or the polymethacrylate cement, which can abrade on either bone or metal. The particulate size may be less than 1 μm; it is estimated that a polyethylene bearing surface can produce billions of these particles each year.

Attempts to improve the longevity of hip replacement have focused on improving the bond at the prosthesis–bone interface; one effective way of doing this is to improve the cementing technique. Much time and effort have been expended on developing cementless prostheses. The advantages of such prostheses are that the structural weakness of the cement, and one source of particulate debris, are avoided: uncemented replacements rely on an inter-

trochanter is then divided, allowing it to be proximally retracted, together with its attached muscles—thereby creating access to the joint capsule. Alternative approaches are: a posterior approach in which the short external rotator muscles (piriformis and the gemelli) are divided, allowing access to the posterior joint capsule; or an anterolateral approach in which the interval between the gluteus

ference fit. The metal surfaces are rough or porous and bone can be encouraged to grow into the surface, thereby fixing the prosthesis. This technique is probably of value for the acetabulum, but has not yet produced superior results for the femur. More recently, prostheses with a hydroxyapatite ceramic coating have been used: the hydroxyapatite has a similar chemical composition to the bone's apatite, attracting bone to grow directly onto its surface without any fibrous interposition. The long-term performance of these prostheses has yet to be evaluated, but early results are encouraging.

The actual bearing surfaces, commonly of metal on ultra-high molecular weight polyethylene, are another weak area of the prosthetic hip joint: titanium heads increase polyethylene particulate debris; consequently metal heads should be of chrome cobalt or stainless steel. Part of the poor performance of metal on polyethylene bearing surfaces in the past may have been due to poor manufacturing quality control. Ceramic heads coupled with polyethylene sockets, ceramic on ceramic, and metal on metal bearing surfaces are being evaluated.

As a surgical procedure, hip replacement has been extremely successful with the standard hip, i.e. an ultra-high molecular weight polyethylene socket and a metal stem, both cemented into the bone with methylmethacrylate cement. To produce a hip with the performance in sport and longevity to match the normal hip is proving more problematical.

PATELLA

The patella (**6.**298, 303, 304), the largest sesamoid bone, is embedded in the tendon of quadriceps femoris anterior to the knee joint. Flat, distally triangular, proximally curved, it has anterior and posterior surfaces, three borders and an apex. In the living, when standing, its distal apex is a little proximal to the line of the knee joint.

The subcutaneous, convex *anterior surface* is perforated by nutrient vessels. It is longitudinally striated, separated from skin by a prepatellar *bursa* and covered by an expansion from the tendon of quadriceps femoris, which blends distally with superficial fibres of the so-called patellar *ligament*, strictly the continued *tendon* of quadriceps. The *posterior surface* has a proximal smooth, oval, articular area, crossed by a smooth vertical ridge, which fits the groove on the femoral patellar surface and divides the patellar articular area into medial and lateral facets, the lateral being larger. The 'ridge' and flanking facets are, of course, continuously covered by articular cartilage. (Degenerative changes in this cartilage, associated with ageing, have been reported by Meachim 1982.) A narrow strip, proximally broader, is marked off medially from the medial facet; this contacts the medial femoral condyle in extreme flexion. Distal to the articular surface the *apex* is roughened by attachment of the patella ligament and, proximal to this, the area between the roughened apex and articular surface is covered by an infrapatellar pad of fat.

The thick *superior border* slopes down and forwards; except near its posterior margin, it is an attachment for quadriceps femoris (rectus femoris and vastus intermedius). The *medial* and *lateral borders* are thinner and converge distally, and to them are attached expansions of the tendons of vastus medialis and lateralis termed the *medial* and *lateral patellar retinacula* (p. 698). The lateral retinaculum receives contributions from the iliotibial tract. Near the superolateral angle is a shallow, circular depression for a distinct part of the tendon of vastus lateralis (vasti medialis and lateralis).

Structure

The patella consists of almost uniformly dense trabecular bone, covered by a thin compact lamina. Trabeculae beneath the anterior surface are parallel with it; elsewhere they radiate from the articular surface to other parts.

Ossification

Several centres appear during the third to sixth years and quickly coalesce. Accessory marginal centres appear later and fuse with the central mass (Hellmer 1935; Prakash et al 1979).

TIBIA

The tibia (**6.**299, 300), medial to and much stronger than the fibula, is exceeded in length only by the femur. Its shaft is prismoid in section, with expanded ends, the smaller distal end having a strong *medial malleolus* projecting distally. The anterior border is sharp, curving medially towards this malleolus; the anterior, together with medial and lateral borders, defines three surfaces.

Proximal end

The proximal end, expanded especially transversely, is a bearing surface for body weight transmitted through the femur; it has massive *medial* and *lateral condyles*, an intercondylar area and tibial tuberosity. The condyles overhang the shaft's proximal posterior surface, and both have proximal articular surfaces separated by an irregular intercondylar area. The condyles are visible and palpable at the sides of the patella ligament, the lateral being more prominent. In the passively flexed knee the anterior *margins* of the condyles are palpable in fossae flanking the patellar ligament. The proximal tibial surface slopes posteriorly and downwards relative to the shaft's long axis; the tilt, maximal at birth, decreases with age; it is more marked in habitual squatters (Kate & Robert 1965). The *medial articular surface* is **oval** (long axis anteroposterior) and perceptibly longer in conformity with differences between the femoral condyles (p. 681). Around its anterior, medial and posterior margins it is related to the medial meniscus, the area of contact being flat. The meniscal imprint, wider behind, narrower anteromedially, is often discernible. The surface is otherwise concave; its raised lateral margin partly invades the medial intercondylar tubercle. The *lateral articular surface* is more **circular**; like the medial it is adapted to its meniscus. Elsewhere the surface, slightly concave to fit the femoral condyle, has a raised medial margin spreading to the lateral intercondylar tubercle. Its articular margins are sharp, except posterolaterally, where the edge is round and smooth; here the tendon of popliteus is in contact with bone.

Medial condyle. The medial condyle is larger but projects less. Its **oval** articular surface (**6.**301) is concave and its lateral border, deepening the concavity, extends on to a *medial intercondylar tubercle*. Its posterior surface, distal to the articular margin, has a horizontal, rough groove; its anteromedial surface is a rough strip, separated from the shaft's medial surface by an inconspicuous ridge.

Lateral condyle. The lateral condyle overhangs the shaft posterolaterally above a small circular facet for articulation with the

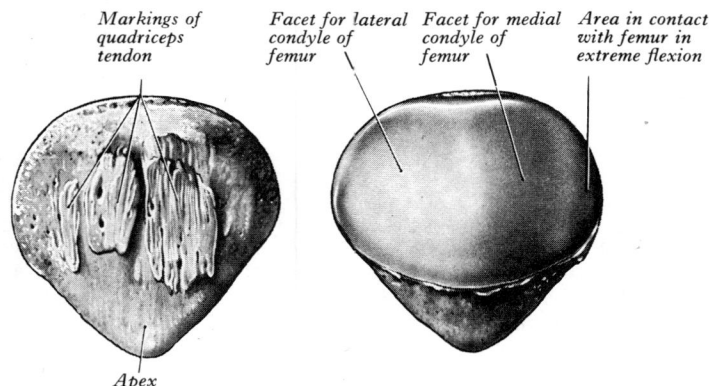

Markings of quadriceps tendon   *Facet for lateral condyle of femur*   *Facet for medial condyle of femur*   *Area in contact with femur in extreme flexion*

Apex

6.298   The left patella: anterior and posterior aspects, drawn from a fresh, unmacerated specimen, with the articular cartilage preserved.

691

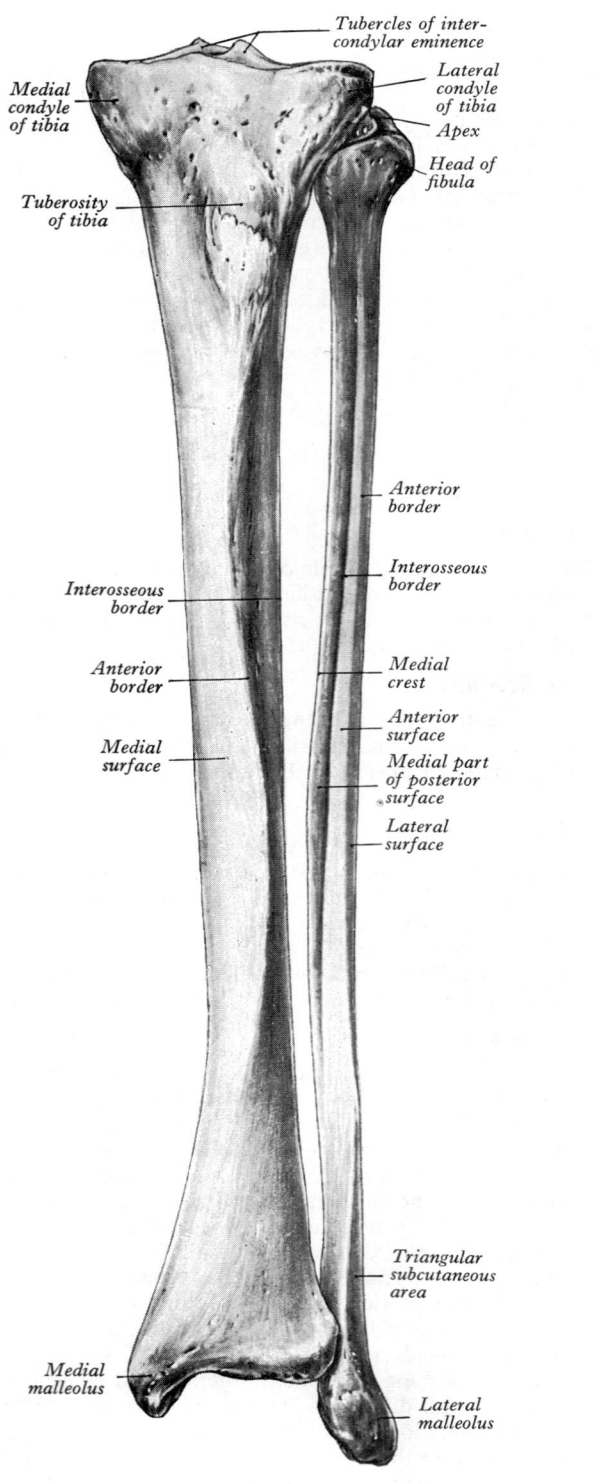

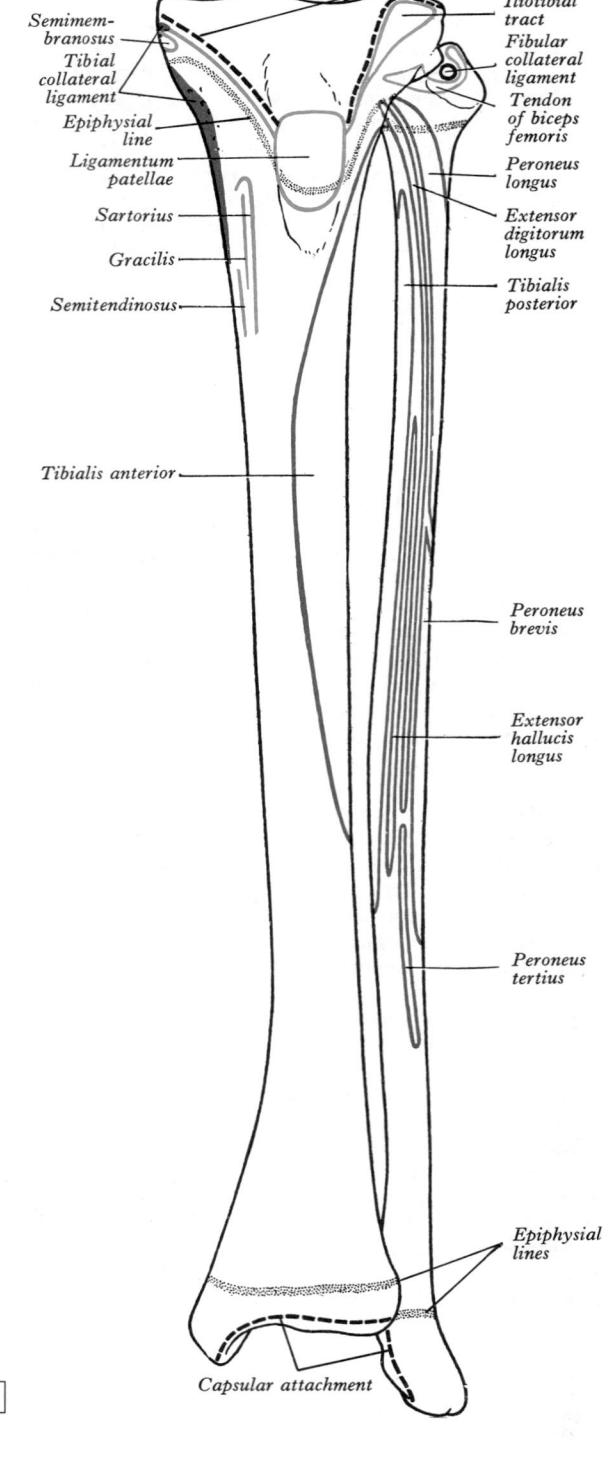

6.299A. Anterior aspect of the left tibia and fibula; B. Line drawing showing muscle attachments. The epiphyseal lines are stippled; the interrupted lines are the capsular attachments.

fibula. The proximal, articular surface (6.301) for the lateral femoral condyle is almost **circular**, centrally concave, its medial border extending onto a *lateral intercondylar tubercle*. Its posterior, lateral and anterior edges are rough.

The anterior condylar surfaces are continuous with a large triangular area; its apex is distal and formed by the tibial tuberosity, whose lateral edge is a sharp ridge between the lateral condyle and lateral surface of the shaft.

The tibial tuberosity. At the proximal end of the anterior border,

this is the truncated apex of a triangular area, where the anterior condylar surfaces merge. It projects little, and is divided into a distal rough and a proximal smooth region. The former is palpable, separated from skin merely by a subcutaneous *infrapatellar bursa*; to the proximal part the patella ligament is attached.

Intercondylar area. The intercondylar area (6.301), between the condylar articular surfaces, is rough, narrowest centrally and here forms an *intercondylar eminence*, edges of which project slightly proximally as *lateral* and *medial intercondylar tubercles*. At the back

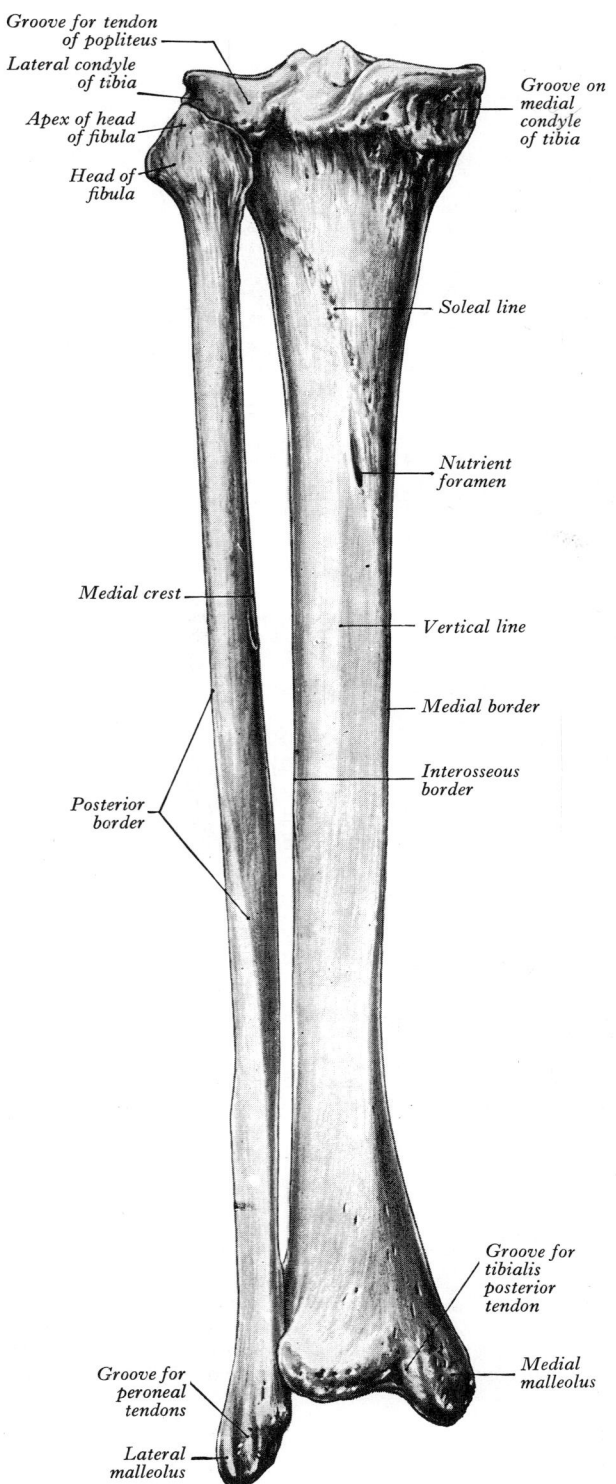

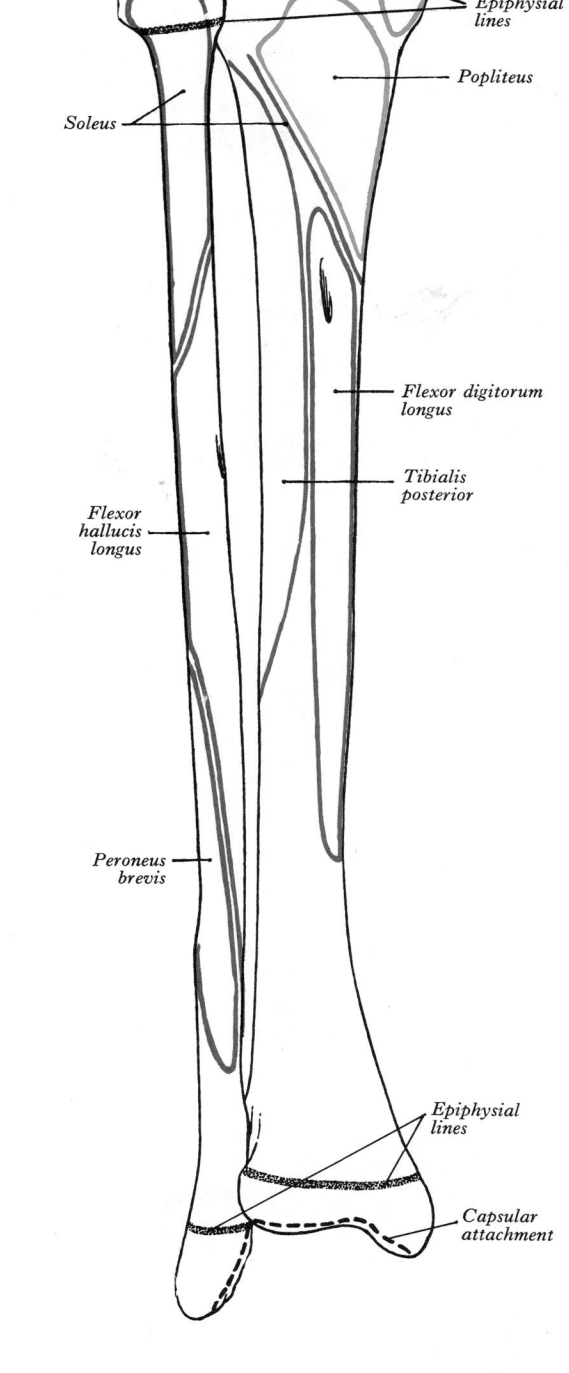

6.300 A. Posterior aspect of the left tibia and fibula; B. Line drawing showing muscle attachments. The epiphyseal lines are stippled; the interrupted lines are the capsular attachments.

and front of the eminence the intercondylar area widens as the articular surfaces diverge.

The anterior intercondylar area (6.301). Widest anteriorly, it bears on its anteromedial area, anterior to the medial articular surface, a depression in which the anterior horn of the medial meniscus is attached. Behind this a smooth area receives the anterior cruciate ligament. The anterior horn of the lateral meniscus is attached anterior to the intercondylar eminence, lateral to the anterior cruciate ligament. The eminence, with medial and lateral

tubercles, is the narrow, central part of the area. To its posterior slope the posterior horn of the lateral meniscus is attached.

The posterior intercondylar area. Behind the posterior horn of the lateral meniscus the posterior intercondylar area inclines down and back. A depression behind the base of the medial intercondylar tubercle is for the posterior cornu of the medial meniscus. The rest of the area is smooth and for attachment of the posterior cruciate ligament, spreading back to a ridge for the capsular ligament.

Further details. To the proximal edge of the groove on the medial

693

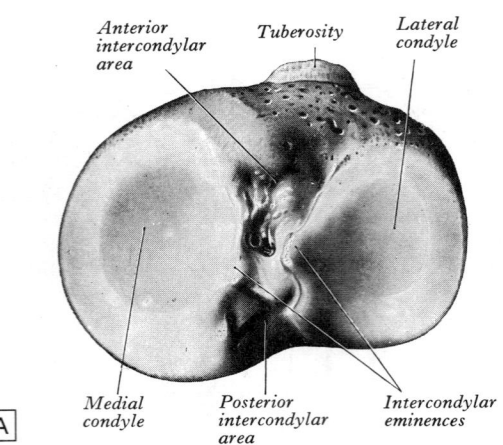

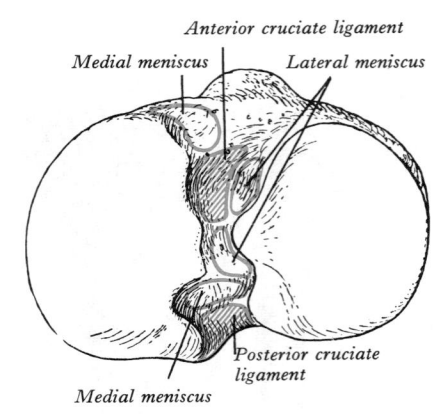

6.301A. The proximal articular surface of the right tibia. The imprints of the menisci were very conspicuous in this specimen.

6.301B. Outline of A showing the attachments of the menisci and cruciate ligaments.

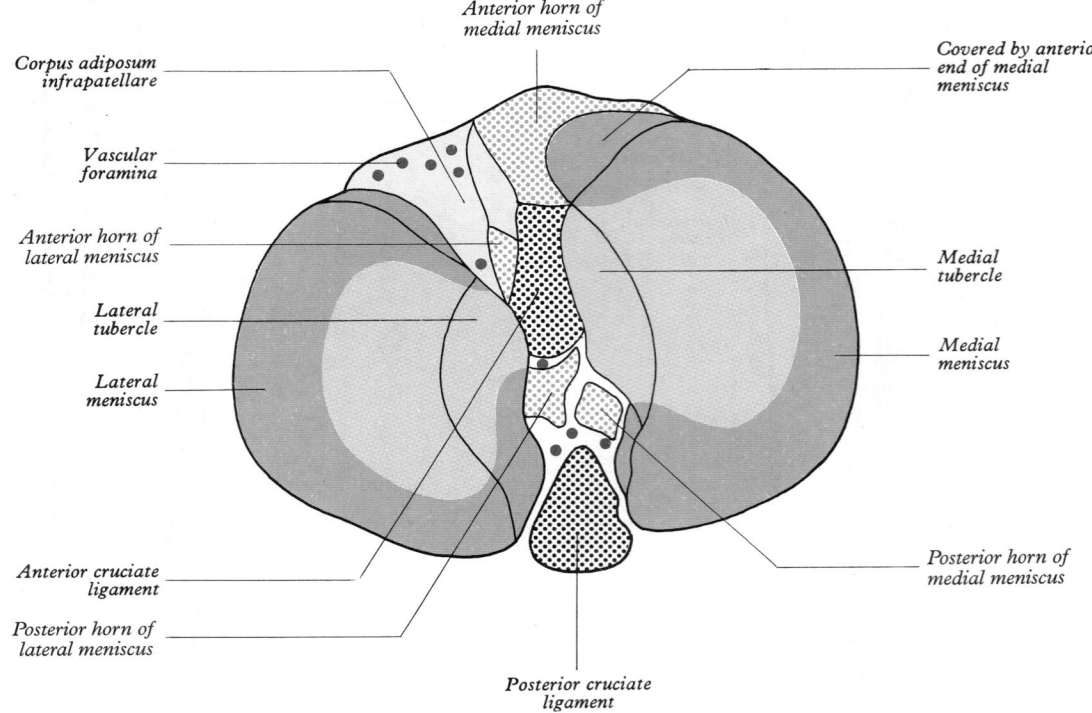

6.301C. Detailed analysis of the surface features of the proximal aspect of the human tibia (left). The condylar areas are shown in full blue, the parts in contact with the menisci being in deep blue, while the remaining condylar regions are in light blue. The attachments of the meniscal horns are in blue stipple, and those of the cruciate ligaments are in black stipple. The yellow area indicates the extent of contact with the corpus adiposum and the red dots signify vascular foramina. (Adapted with permission from Klaus Jacobsen, Department of Orthopaedic Surgery, The Gentofte Hospital, Copenhagen, *Journal of Anatomy* and Cambridge University Press.)

condyle's posterior surface are attached the capsular and posterior part of the tibial collateral ligaments; its distal edge receives semimembranosus. At the lateral end of the groove a tubercle is the main attachment of the tendon of semimembranosus (Cave & Porteous 1958). To medial and anterior condylar surfaces, marked by vascular foramina, the medial patellar retinaculum is attached.

Measurement of 13 healthy knee joints, with observations on 75 macerated specimens, yielded a highly detailed plan of ligamentous and other attachments (Jacobsen 1974 and **6.**301C); much variation was noted; dense fibrous attachments produced facets, separated by more porous areas.

The tibia has been investigated stereometrically by Ljungren (1976); analysis confirmed functional adaptation of curvatures and inclinations of tibial condyles and the tuberosity, and these were correlated with habits of locomotion in different racial groups.

The *fibular facet* on the lateral condyle faces distally and posterolaterally. Superomedial to it the condyle is grooved posteriorly by the tendon of popliteus, with a synovial recess between the tendon and bone. The condyle's anterolateral aspect is separated from the shaft's lateral surface by a sharp margin for attachment of deep fascia. The iliotibial tract makes a flat but definite marking (triangular and facet-like) on its anterior aspect. Slips from the tendon of biceps femoris are attached anteroproximal to the fibular facet, distal to which proximal fibres of extensor digitorum longus and occasionally peroneus longus are attached.

A line across the tibial tuberosity marks the distal limit of the epiphyseal line (**6.**299B and p. 697); the patellar ligament is attached to the smooth bone proximal to this, its superficial fibres reaching a rough area distal to the line; the attachment may be marked distally by a slight ridge (Lewis 1958a). Distally the tuberosity is subcutaneous; proximal to it bone is related to the deep aspect of the patellar ligament, but a *deep infrapatellar bursa* and fibro-adipose tissue intervene. In habitual squatters a vertical groove on the anterior surface of the lateral condyle is occupied by the ligament's edge in flexion.

Shaft

The shaft (**6.299, 300**), triangular in section, has medial, lateral and posterior surfaces, separated by anterior, lateral (interosseous) and medial borders. It is thinnest at the junction of the middle and distal thirds, expanding towards both ends.

The *anterior border* descends from the tuberosity to the anterior margin of the medial malleolus and is subcutaneous throughout; except in its distal fourth, where it is indistinct, it is a sharp crest, slightly sinuous and turning medially in its distal fourth. The *interosseous border* begins distal and anterior to the fibular facet and descends to the anterior border of the fibular notch; to most of it is attached the interosseous membrane, connecting tibia to fibula; above it is indistinct. The *medial border* descends from the anterior end of the groove on the medial condyle to the posterior margin of the medial malleolus. Its proximal and distal fourths are ill-defined, its middle region sharp.

The *medial surface* (really **antero**medial), between the anterior and medial borders, is broad, smooth and almost entirely subcutaneous. The broad, smooth *lateral surface*, between the anterior and inter-osseous borders, faces laterally in its proximal three-fourths and is transversely concave. Its distal quarter swerves anteriorly, due to the medial deviation of the anterior and distal interosseous borders. This part of the surface is somewhat convex. The *posterior surface*, between the interosseous and medial borders, is widest above, where it is crossed distomedially by an oblique, rough *soleal line* (**6.300A**), from the centre of which a faint vertical line descends but soon fades. A large vascular groove adjoins the line's end, descending distally into bone; it may be lateral or medial to the vertical line. To the *anterior border* is attached deep fascia and, proximal to the medial malleolus, the medial end of the superior extensor reti-naculum. Proximal to the soleal line the *medial border* is an attach-ment of popliteal fascia, the posterior fibres of the tibial collateral ligament and slips of semimembranous; distal to it some fibres of soleus and the fascia covering deep calf muscles are attached. The distal medial border merges into the medial lip of a groove for the tendon of tibialis posterior. To the *lateral border* the interosseous membrane is attached, except at its extremes. It is proximally indistinct where a large gap in the membrane transmits the anterior tibial vessels; distally the border is the anterior boundary of the fibular notch; the anterior tibiofibular ligament is attached to it.

The *medial surface* bears proximally, near the medial border, an area about 5 cm long and 1 cm wide for the anterior part of the tibial collateral ligament and, behind this, semimembranosus; anterior to this are from before, backwards, linear attachments of the tendons of sartorius, gracilis and semitendinosus, which rarely mark the bone (**6.299B**). The remaining surface is subcutaneous but crossed obliquely by the great saphenous vein ascending from **in front** of the medial malleolus.

The *lateral surface* is, in its proximal two-thirds, an attachment for the tibialis anterior. Its distal third, devoid of attachments, is crossed by the tendon of tibialis anterior (lateral to the anterior border), extensor hallucis longus, the anterior tibial vessels and nerve, extensor digitorum longus and peroneus tertius, in medio-lateral order.

To the *posterior surface* popliteus is attached in a triangular area proximal to the soleal line, except near the fibular facet, and to the *soleal line* the popliteal aponeurosis, soleus and its fascia and deep transverse fascia. Proximally the line does not reach the interosseous border and has a tubercle for the medial end of the tendinous soleal arch; lateral to it the posterior tibial vessels and nerve descend on tibialis posterior. Distal to the soleal line, the *vertical line* separates the attachments of flexor digitorum longus (medial) and tibialis posterior (**6.300B**). The surface's distal quarter has no attachments, but is crossed medially by the tendon of tibialis posterior travelling to a posterior groove on the medial malleolus. Flexor digitorum longus crosses obliquely behind tibialis posterior; but the posterior tibial vessels and nerve and flexor hallucis longus contact only the lateral part of the distal posterior surface.

Distal end

The distal end of the tibia, slightly expanded, has anterior, medial, posterior, lateral and distal surfaces. It projects inferomedially as the *medial malleolus*. The distal end of the tibia, when compared to the proximal end, is laterally rotated (*tibial torsion*), the torsion beginning in utero and progressing throughout childhood and adolescence to skeletal maturity (Staheli & Engel 1972). Tibial torsion is about 30° in Caucasian and Oriental populations (Yoshioka et al 1989; Yagi & Sasaki 1986), but is significantly greater in Africans (Eckhoff et al 1994b).

Its smooth *anterior surface* bulges beyond the distal surface, separated from it by a narrow groove, continuing the shaft's lateral surface. The *medial surface*, smooth and continuous above and below with the medial surfaces of the shaft and malleolus, is subcutaneous and visible. The *posterior surface* is crossed near its medial end by a nearly vertical, but slightly oblique groove, usually conspicuous, extending to the posterior surface of the malleolus; elsewhere it is smooth and continuous with the shaft's posterior surface. The *lateral surface* is the triangular *fibular notch*, bound by ligaments to the

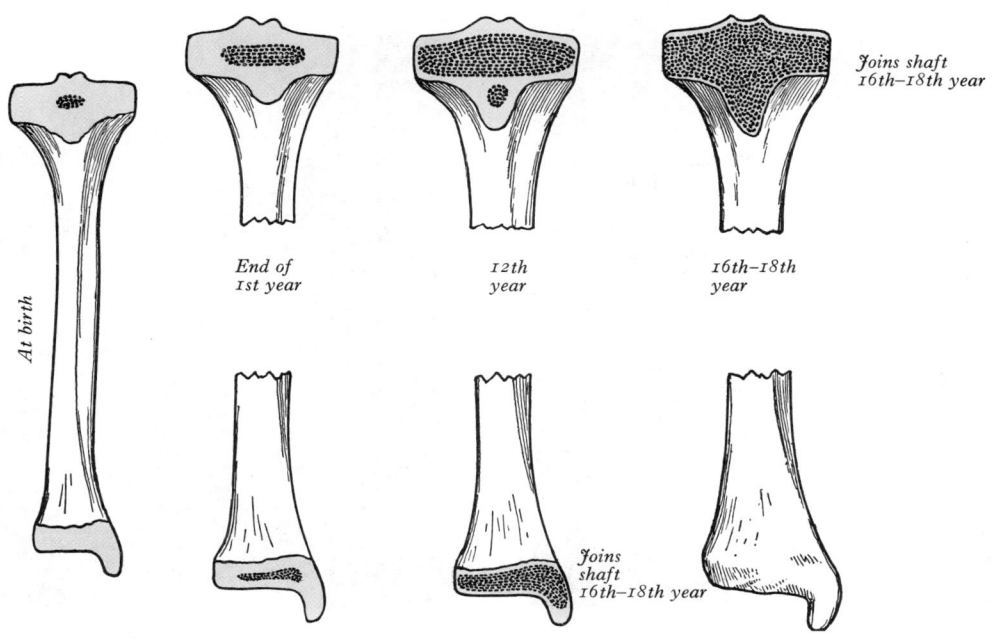

End of
1st year

12th
year

16th–18th
year

Joins shaft
16th–18th year

At birth

Joins
shaft
16th–18th year

6.302   Stages in the ossification of the tibia (not to scale).

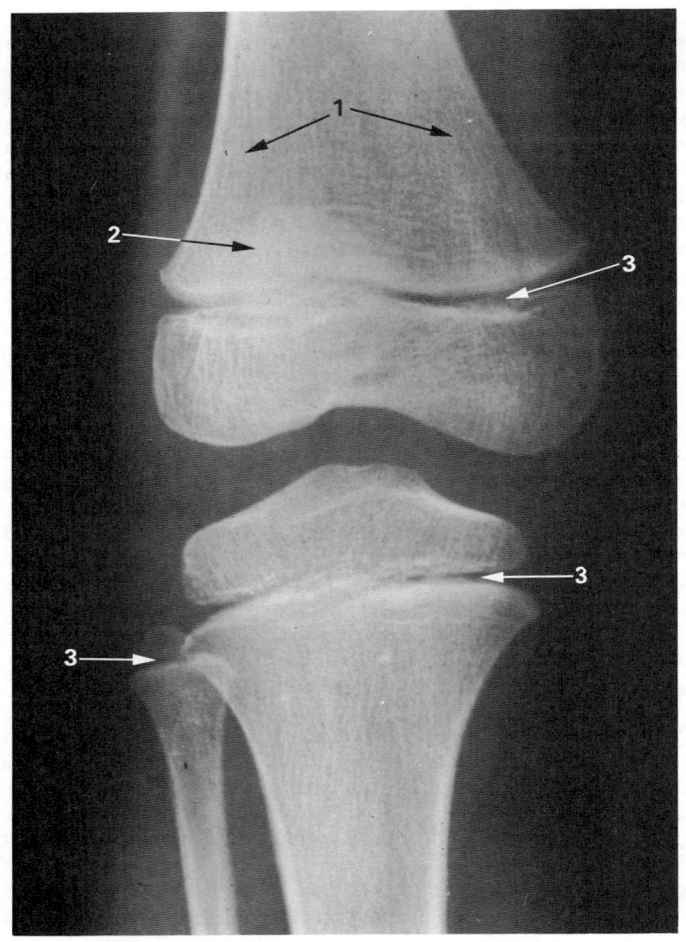

A

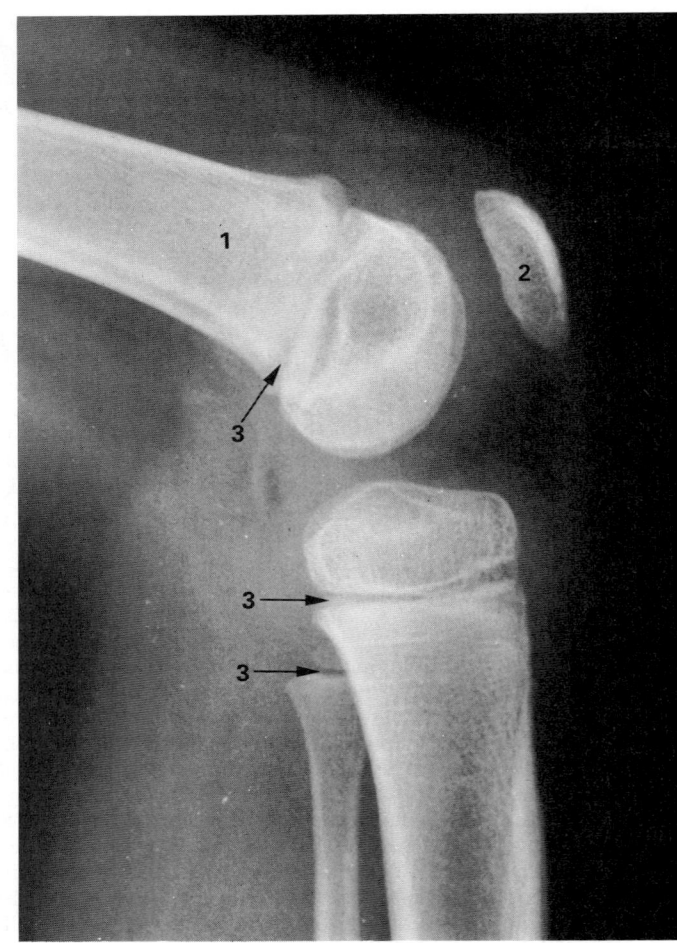

B

6.303 Anteroposterior (A) and lateral (B) radiographs of the knee in a girl aged six. 1. Flared femoral metaphysis. 2. Patella. 3. Cartilaginous growth plates with adjacent epiphyses. Note early stage of ossification in fibular epiphysis.

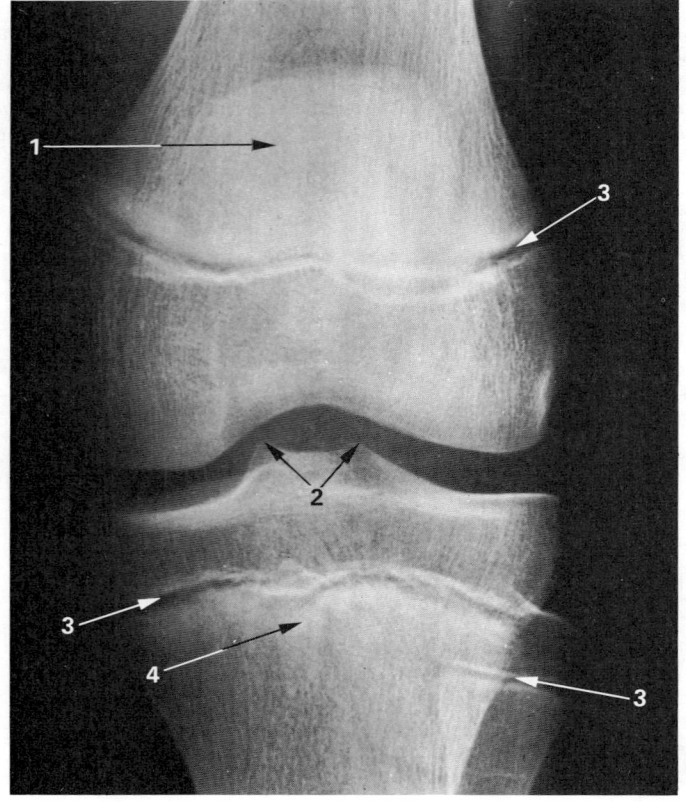

A

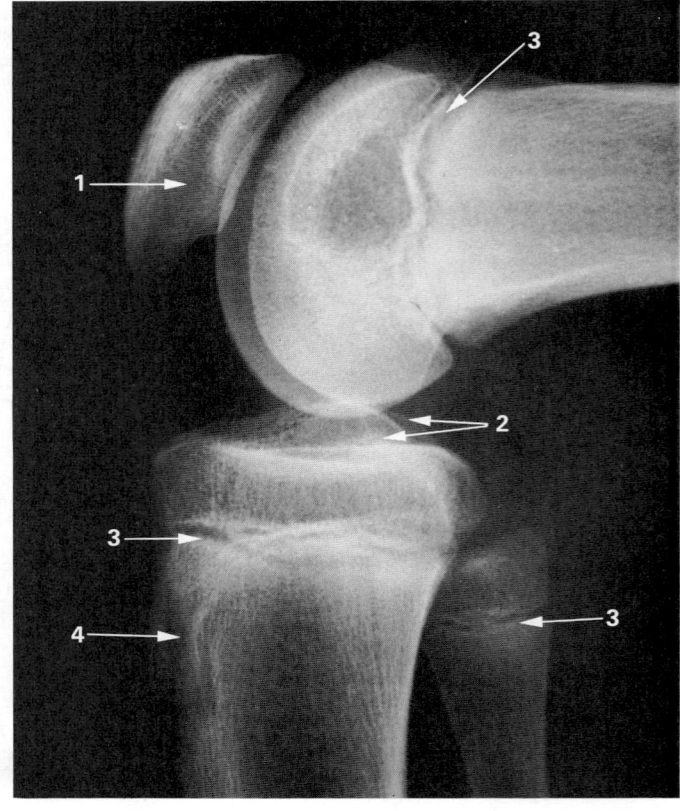

B

6.304 Anteroposterior (A) and lateral (B) radiographs of the knee in a boy aged 14. 1. Patella. 2. Intercondylar eminences. 3. Cartilaginous growth plates with adjacent epiphyses. 4. Prolongation of proximal tibial epiphysis and growth plate forming the tibial tuberosity.

fibula; its anterior and posterior edges project and converge proximally to the interosseous border. The floor of the notch is roughened proximally by a substantial interosseous ligament, but is smooth distally and sometimes covered by articular cartilage. The *distal surface*, articulating with the talus, is wider in front, concave sagittally and transversely slightly convex (i.e. it is **sellar**). Medially it continues into the malleolar articular surface. This articular surface may extend into the groove (see above), separating it from the shaft's anterior surface. Such extensions, medial or lateral or both, are *squatting facets*, articulating with reciprocal talar facets (p. 714) in extreme dorsiflexion. These features have been used in racial evaluation (p. 434).

Medial malleolus. The medial malleolus, short and thick, has a smooth lateral surface with a crescentic facet articulating with the medial talar surface. Its anterior aspect is rough and its posterior continues the groove on the shaft's posterior surface. The distal border is pointed anteriorly, posteriorly depressed.

Further details. The distal end is related anteriorly to tendons, vessels and nerves lateral to the tibial shaft. To an anterior groove near the articular surface, the capsule of the ankle joint is attached. The posterior groove is adapted to the tendon of tibialis posterior, which usually separates that of flexor digitorum longus from bone. More laterally, the posterior tibial vessels and nerve and flexor hallucis longus are in contact with this surface. To the edges of the *fibular notch* are attached anterior and posterior tibiofibular ligaments. The *medial malleolus* ends proximal to the lateral malleolus, which is also more posterior in plane. To its anterior surface is attached the ankle joint's capsule. To the groove for the posterior tibial tendon, on its prominent medial border, the flexor retinaculum is attached. The deltoid ligament, proximal to the distal malleolar border, is attached to its apex and depression.

Ossification

Ossification of the tibia is by three centres (**6.299**B, 300B, 302, 303,

304) in the shaft and both epiphyses. It begins in midshaft about the seventh intrauterine week. The proximal epiphyseal centre is usually present at birth; at about 10 years a thin anterior process from it descends to form the smooth part of the tibial tuberosity (**6.302**), but a separate centre for this may appear about the twelfth year, soon fusing with the epiphysis. Distal strata of the epiphyseal plate are of dense collagenous tissue, the fibres of which are aligned with the patellar ligament. This peculiar structure is attributed to large tensile stresses transmitted via the ligament (Lewis 1958a; Smith 1962b). The distal epiphyseal centre appears early in the first year, joining the shaft about the fifteenth in females, seventeenth in males. The proximal epiphysis fuses in the sixteenth year in females, eighteenth in males. The medial malleolus is an extension from the distal epiphysis, commencing to ossify in the seventh year; it may have a separate centre.

KNEE JOINT

The knee, largest of human joints, is *compound* and sometimes derived from a primitive double condylar articulation, although contrary evidence exists (Haines 1942a). Despite its single cavity in man, it is convenient to describe it as two condylar joints between the femur and tibia and a sellar joint between the patella and femur. The former are partly divided by menisci between corresponding articular surfaces. (Strictly, the joint is therefore also classified as *complex*.) The level of the joint is at the (palpable) proximal margins of the tibial condyles (**6.305**).

Articular surfaces

The articular surfaces (pp. 681, 691) are most incongruent. The femoral condyles, bearing articular cartilage, are almost wholly convex; in lateral profile both are spiral with a curvature increasing posteriorly, the lateral condyle more rapidly. The tibial surfaces are also cartilage-covered areas, separated by the intercondylar region;

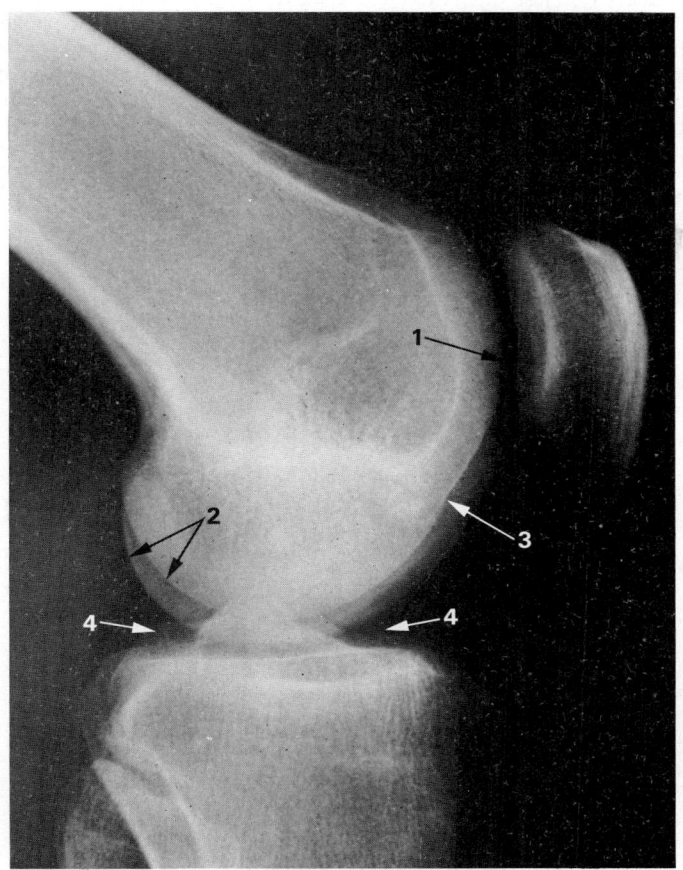

6.305A. Anteroposterior radiograph of an adult knee (male aged 22 years). 1. Shadow of patella superimposed on femur. 2. Adductor tubercle. 3. Medial femoral condyle. 4. Radiotranslucent space occupied by medial meniscus and articular cartilages. 5. Medial tibial condyle. 6. Intercondylar eminences.

7. Head of fibula. B. Lateral radiograph of the partly flexed adult knee (same as in A). 1. Patellar surface of femur. 2. Spiral profiles of femoral condyles. 3. Groove impinging on anterior end of meniscus in full extension. 4. Note marked incongruity of femorotibial joint surfaces.

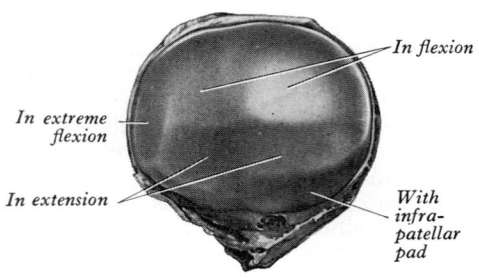

6.306 Posterior surface of the right patella, showing areas of contact with the femur and infrapatellar fat pad in different positions of the knee joint as indicated.

each is gently hollow centrally and flattened peripherally where a meniscus rests. The lateral tibial articular surface is almost circular and smaller, the medial oval with a longer anteroposterior axis. Both tibial surfaces slope up near the intercondylar area on to its eminences; posteriorly the lateral is prolonged onto the back of its condyle, in relation to the popliteal tendon; anteriorly, near the anterior horn of the lateral meniscus, it descends on to the anterior sloping condylar surface. Femorotibial congruence is improved by the menisci, shaped to increase the concavity of tibial surfaces, the combined lateral tibiomeniscal surface being deeper. The lateral femoral condyle has in front a faint groove, resting on the peripheral edge of the lateral meniscus in full extension. A similar groove appears on the medial condyle but does not reach its lateral border, where a narrow strip contacts the medial patellar articular surface in full flexion. These grooves demarcate the femoral patellar and condylar surfaces, the latter articulating only with the tibia and menisci. The distal outlines of the femoral surfaces conform to the tibiomeniscal articular surfaces. The lateral femoral surface is almost circular, the medial is larger, somewhat oval but curved with a lateral concavity. These differences correlate with movements of the joint. The surfaces approach congruence in full extension, the close-packed position, as confirmed by casting techniques and radiological studies of excised human joints. (See below for a detailed discussion of close-packing and consult Kettlekamp & Jacobs 1972 for relevant bibliography.)

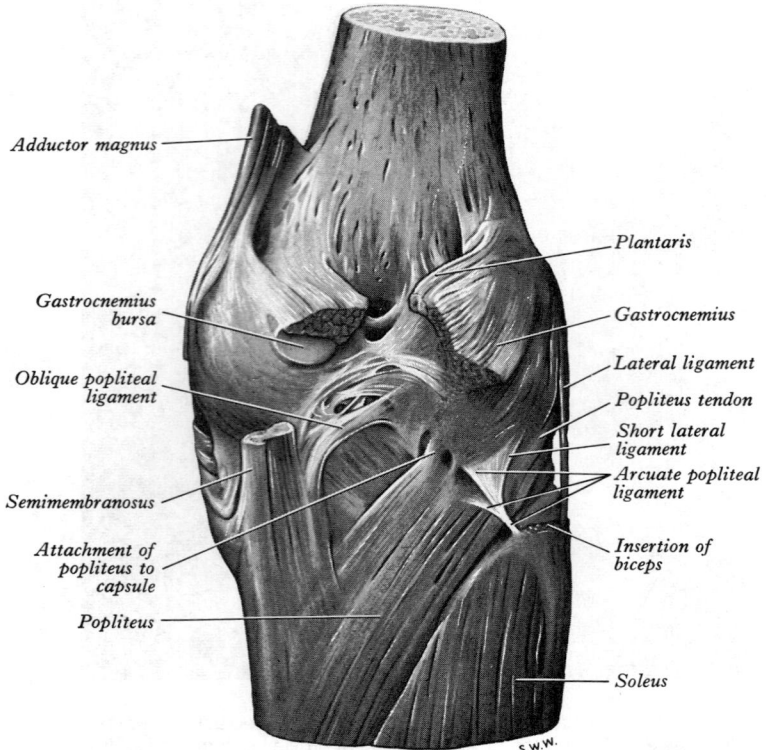

Adductor magnus

Gastrocnemius bursa

Oblique popliteal ligament

Semimembranosus

Attachment of popliteus to capsule

Popliteus

Plantaris

Gastrocnemius

Lateral ligament

Popliteus tendon

Short lateral ligament

Arcuate popliteal ligament

Insertion of biceps

Soleus

S.W.W.

6.307 Posterior aspect of right knee joint.

The patella's articular surface is adapted to the femoral surface (p. 691), which extends onto the anterior surfaces of both condyles like an inverted U. An oblique groove, descending a little laterally, divides the femoral patellar surface into a larger lateral and smaller medial area; the lateral is wider, passes more steeply on to the prominent anterior boss of the lateral condyle and ascends higher on its anterior surface. Since the whole area is concave transversely and parasagittally convex, it is an asymmetrical sellar surface (p. 503). A rounded, almost vertical ridge, dividing the articular surface of the patella also into larger lateral and medial areas, fits the corresponding femoral groove; but the two areas are not fully congruent with those of the femur. The patellar surface may be subdivided by two faint, horizontal ridges which, with the vertical ridge, map out three pairs of facets. But in many patellae there is only **one** horizontal ridge, better marked laterally, and the upper lateral facet is more deeply hollowed. Medially, a second vertical ridge separates a narrow semilunar strip from the medial border which contacts the lateral anterior end of the medial femoral condyle in full flexion, when the highest lateral patellar facet contacts the anterior part of the lateral condyle. As the knee extends, the middle patellar facets contact the lower half of the femoral surface; in full extension only the lowest patellar facets are in contact with the femur (**6.306**). Seedhom and Tsubuku (1977) have applied a special technique for study of contact areas between viscoelastic bodies to the patella. They emphasize temporal factors in compressive contacts.

Ligaments of the joint are the patellar ligament (*ligamentum* (*tendo*) *patellae*), *tibial* and *fibular collateral*, *oblique* and *arcuate popliteal*, *anterior* and *posterior cruciate* and *transverse* ligaments.

Fibrous capsule

The fibrous capsule is complex, partly deficient and partly augmented by expansions from adjacent tendons. Its *posterior, vertical fibres* are attached proximally to the posterior margins of the femoral condyles and intercondylar fossa and distally to the posterior margins of the tibial condyles and intercondylar area; proximally on each side it blends with the attachments of gastrocnemius and is centrally strengthened by the oblique popliteal ligament. *Medial capsular fibres* are attached to the femoral and tibial condyles just beyond their articular margins; here the capsule blends with the tibial collateral ligament. Between the medial epicondyle and the convex border of the medial meniscus is a capsular thickening, a deep component of the tibial collateral ligament (Last 1948). *Lateral capsular fibres*, attached to the femur above popliteus, descend over its tendon to the tibial condyle and fibular head. The fibular collateral ligament is separated from the capsule by fat and the inferior lateral genicular vessels and nerve. **Anteriorly** the capsule does not pass proximal to the patella or over the patellar area; elsewhere it blends with expansions from the vasti medialis and lateralis; these are attached to the patellar margins and patellar ligament, extending back to the corresponding collateral ligaments and distally to the tibial condyles. They form *medial* and *lateral patellar retinacula*, the lateral being augmented by the iliotibial tract. Proximal to the patella an absence of capsule allows continuity of the suprapatellar bursa (p. 875) with the joint. The posterior capsular attachment to the lateral tibial condyle is interrupted where popliteus emerges (**6.307**) but elsewhere the oblique popliteal ligament, derived from the tendon of semimembranosus, thickens the posterior capsule. A prolongation of the iliotibial tract fills the interval between the oblique popliteal and fibular collateral ligaments, partly covering the latter; its expansions also reach the lateral patellar retinaculum and patellar ligament. Medially, expansions from sartorius and semimembranosus ascend to the tibial collateral ligament. Internally the capsule is attached to the meniscal rims, connecting them to the tibia by short *coronary ligaments*.

Synovial membrane. The synovial membrane of the knee is the most extensive and complex in the body. At the proximal patellar border, it forms a large *suprapatellar* bursa between quadriceps femoris and the lower femoral shaft (**6.308, 309**). This is, in practice, an extension of the joint cavity, sustained by articularis genus which is attached to it. Alongside the patella the membrane extends beneath the aponeuroses of the vasti, more extensively under the medial. Distal to the patella the synovial membrane is separated from the patellar ligament by the *infrapatellar fat pad*, covering which the membrane projects into the joint as two fringes, or *alar folds*; these

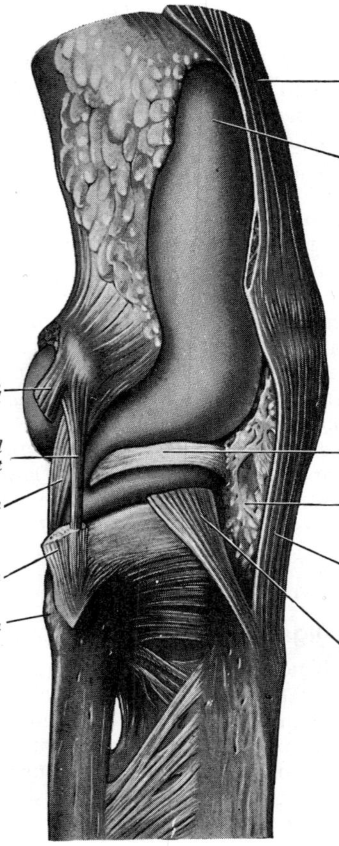

Tendon of
quadriceps femoris

Suprapatellar bursa

Gastrocnemius,
lateral head

Fibular collateral
ligament

Popliteus tendon

Biceps tendon

Head of fibula

Lateral meniscus

Infrapatellar pad
of fat

Ligamentum patellae

Lateral patellar
retinaculum,
cut and drawn
backwards

6.308   Dissection of the right knee joint: lateral aspect. The joint cavity has been injected and the synovial membrane is coloured blue.

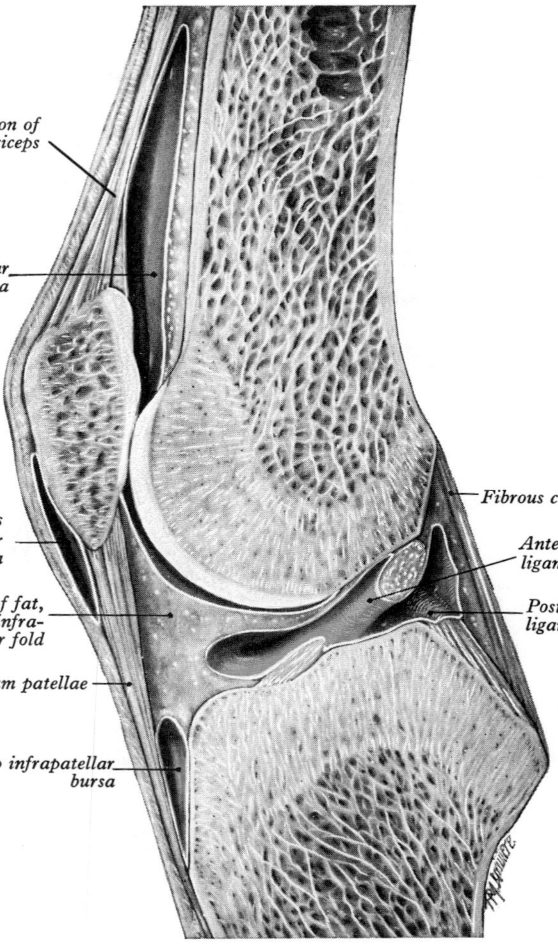

Tendon of
quadriceps

Suprapatellar
bursa

Subcutaneous
prepatellar
bursa

Infrapatellar pad of fat,
extending into infra-
patellar fold

Ligamentum patellae

Deep infrapatellar
bursa

Fibrous capsule

Anterior cruciate
ligament

Posterior cruciate
ligament

6.309   Sagittal section through the left knee joint: lateral aspect. The synovial membrane is shown in colour. See also **6**.69, 70.

bear villi and then converge posteriorly to form the single *infrapatellar fold* (*ligamentum mucosum*) which curves posteriorly to its attachment in the femoral intercondylar fossa (**6**.310); this may be a vestige of the inferior boundary of an originally separate femoropatellar joint (p. 697). At the sides of the joint the synovial membrane descends from the femur, lining the capsule as far as the menisci whose surfaces have no synovial covering. Posterior to the lateral meniscus the membrane forms a *subpopliteal recess* between a groove on the meniscal surface and the tendon of popliteus (**6**.311); this may connect with the superior tibiofibular joint (p. 711). The relation of the synovial membrane to the cruciate ligaments is described on page 703.

Bursae

Bursae associated with the knee are numerous.

Anteriorly there are:

(1) a large *subcutaneous prepatellar bursa* between the lower patella and skin;
(2) a small *deep infrapatellar bursa* between the tibia and patellar ligament;
(3) a *subcutaneous infrapatellar bursa* between the distal part of the tibial tuberosity and skin;
(4) a large *suprapatellar bursa* between the femur and quadriceps femoris (**6**.309); although developing separately it is later continuous with the joint and best regarded as part of it.

Laterally there are:

(1) a bursa between the *lateral head of gastrocnemius* and *joint capsule* (sometimes continuous with the joint);

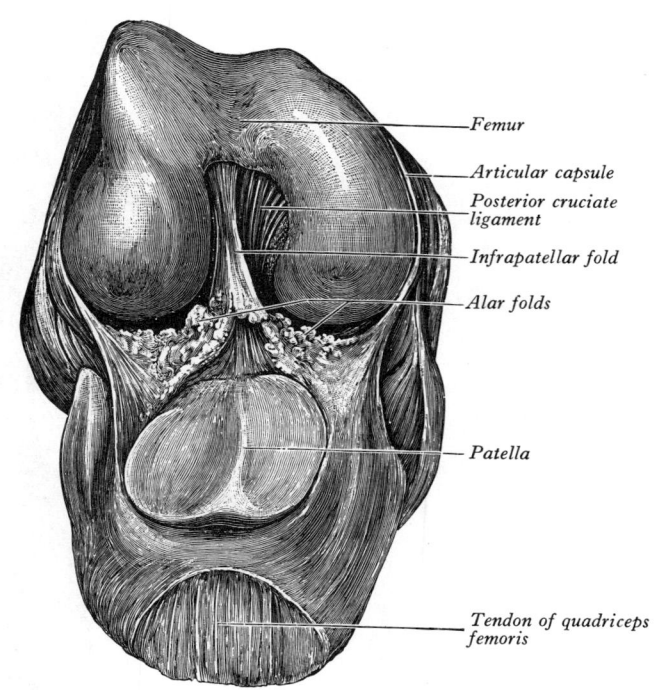

Femur

Articular capsule

Posterior cruciate
ligament

Infrapatellar fold

Alar folds

Patella

Tendon of quadriceps
femoris

6.310   Right knee joint in flexion: anterior exposure.

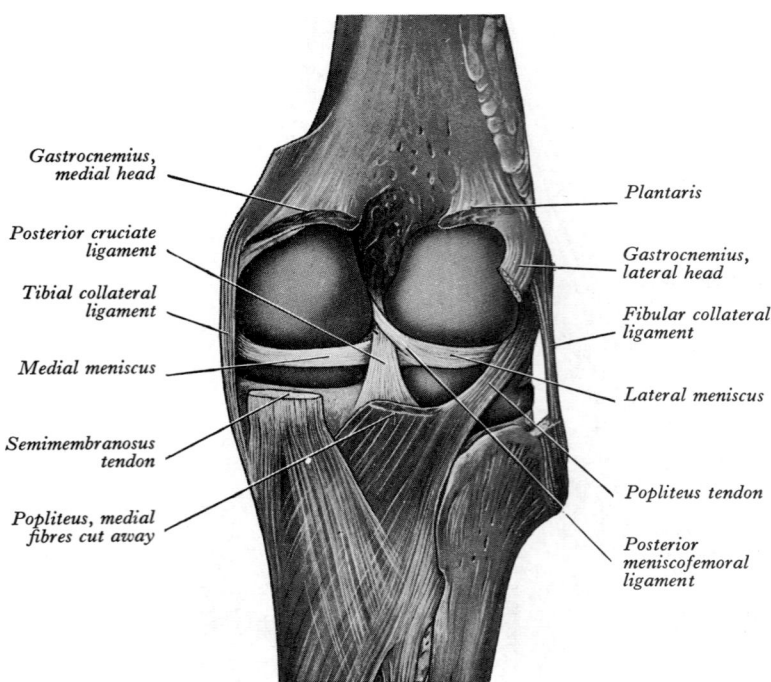

Gastrocnemius,
medial head

Posterior cruciate
ligament

Tibial collateral
ligament

Medial meniscus

Semimembranosus
tendon

Popliteus, medial
fibres cut away

Plantaris

Gastrocnemius,
lateral head

Fibular collateral
ligament

Lateral meniscus

Popliteus tendon

Posterior
meniscofemoral
ligament

6.311 Posterior dissection of the right knee joint. The fibrous capsule has been removed, exposing the unopened synovial membrane which is coloured blue. The cavity of the joint has been partially distended by injection.

(2) one between the *fibular collateral ligament* and the *tendon of biceps femoris*;

(3) one also between the *fibular collateral ligament* and the *tendon of popliteus* (sometimes an expansion from (4) below);

(4) one between the *tendon of popliteus* and the *lateral femoral condyle*, usually an extension from the joint.

Medially there are:

(1) a bursa between the *medial head of gastrocnemius* and *fibrous capsule*, with a prolongation between the medial tendon of gastrocnemius and the tendon of semimembranosus, often communicating with the joint;

(2) a bursa between the *tibial collateral ligament* and the *tendons of sartorius, gracilis* and *semitendinosus*;

(3) variable bursae, in number and position, deep to the *tibial collateral ligament* between the *capsule, femur, medial meniscus, tibia* or *tendon of semimembranosus*;

(4) a bursa between the *tendon of semimembranosus* and the *medial tibial condyle* and also the *medial head of gastrocnemius* (the *semimembranosus bursa*) which may communicate with (1) above;

(5) an occasional bursa between the *tendons of semimembranosus* and *semitendinosus*.

Posteriorly, bursae are variable.

Patellar ligament (ligamentum patella, 6.312)

This is the central band of the tendon of quadriceps femoris, continued distally from the patella to the tibial tuberosity. It is strong, flat, about 8 cm in length, attached proximally to the apex, adjoining margins and to rough areas on the anterior surface and on the depression on the distal posterior patellar surface, and distally to the superior smooth area of the tibial tuberosity. Its superficial fibres are continuous over the patella with the tendon of quadriceps

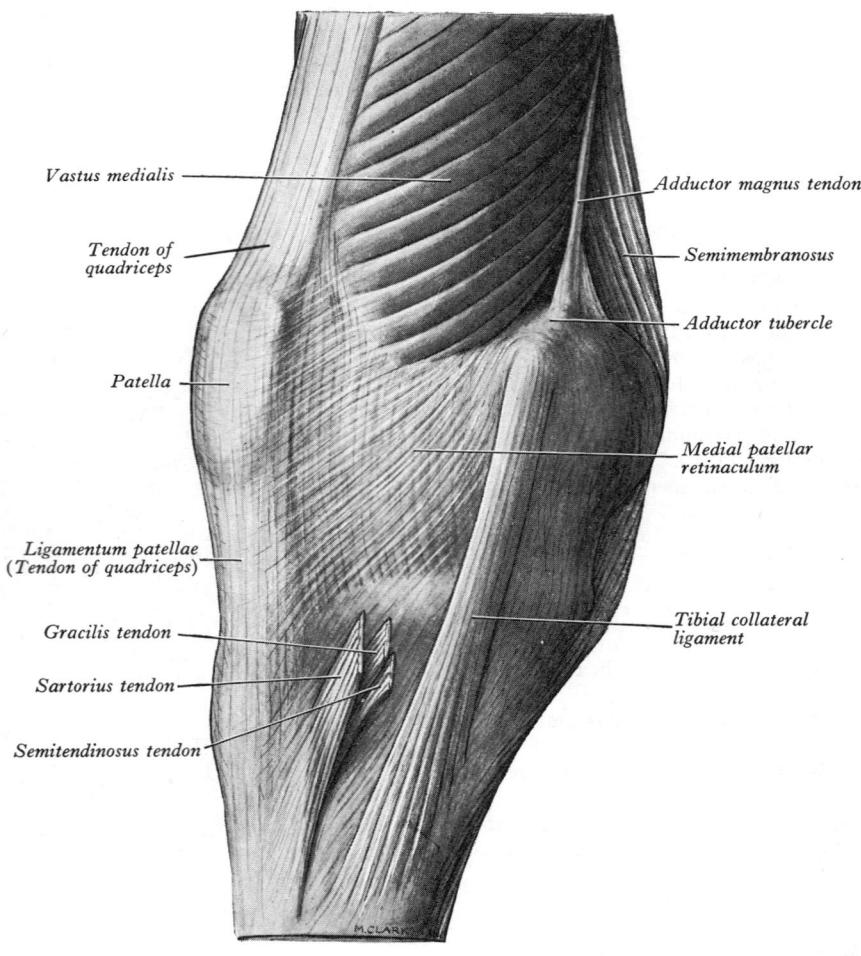

Vastus medialis

Tendon of
quadriceps

Patella

Ligamentum patellae
(Tendon of quadriceps)

Gracilis tendon

Sartorius tendon

Semitendinosus tendon

Adductor magnus tendon

Semimembranosus

Adductor tubercle

Medial patellar
retinaculum

Tibial collateral
ligament

6.312 Anteromedial aspect of right knee joint.

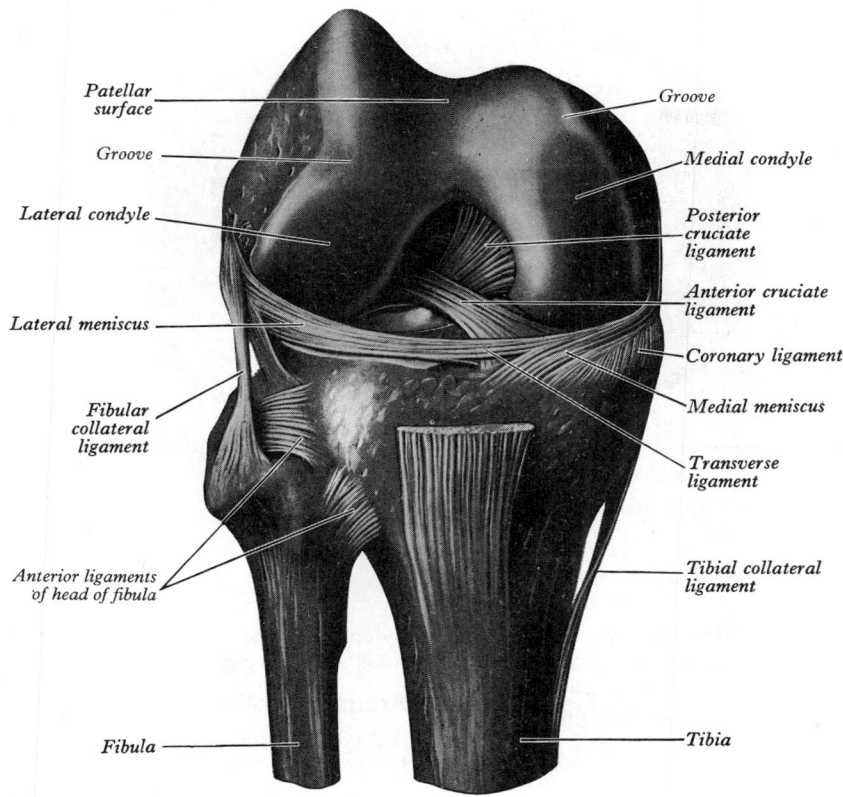

Patellar surface

Groove

Lateral condyle

Lateral meniscus

Fibular collateral ligament

Anterior ligaments of head of fibula

Fibula

Groove

Medial condyle

Posterior cruciate ligament

Anterior cruciate ligament

Coronary ligament

Medial meniscus

Transverse ligament

Tibial collateral ligament

Tibia

6.313 Right knee joint in full flexion: dissection from anterior aspect.

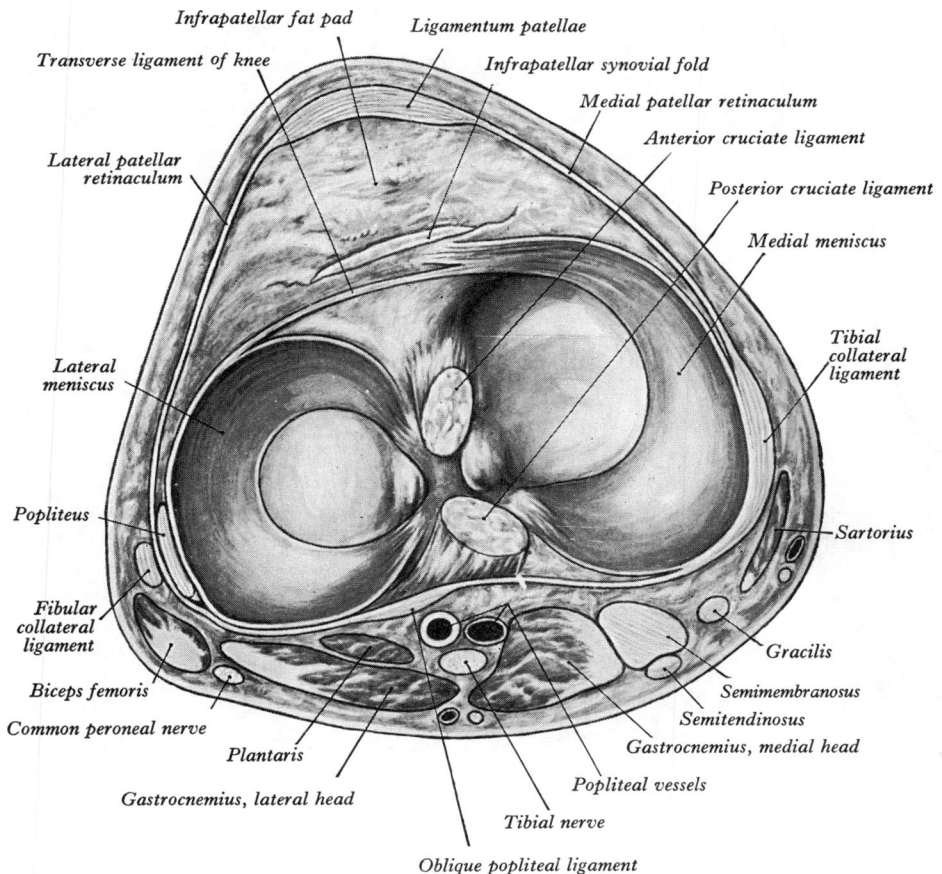

Infrapatellar fat pad

Transverse ligament of knee

Ligamentum patellae

Infrapatellar synovial fold

Medial patellar retinaculum

Lateral patellar retinaculum

Anterior cruciate ligament

Posterior cruciate ligament

Medial meniscus

Lateral meniscus

Tibial collateral ligament

Popliteus

Sartorius

Fibular collateral ligament

Gracilis

Biceps femoris

Semimembranosus

Common peroneal nerve

Semitendinosus

Plantaris

Gastrocnemius, medial head

Gastrocnemius, lateral head

Popliteal vessels

Tibial nerve

Oblique popliteal ligament

6.314 Transverse section of the left knee joint; superior aspect, to show the relations of the joint.

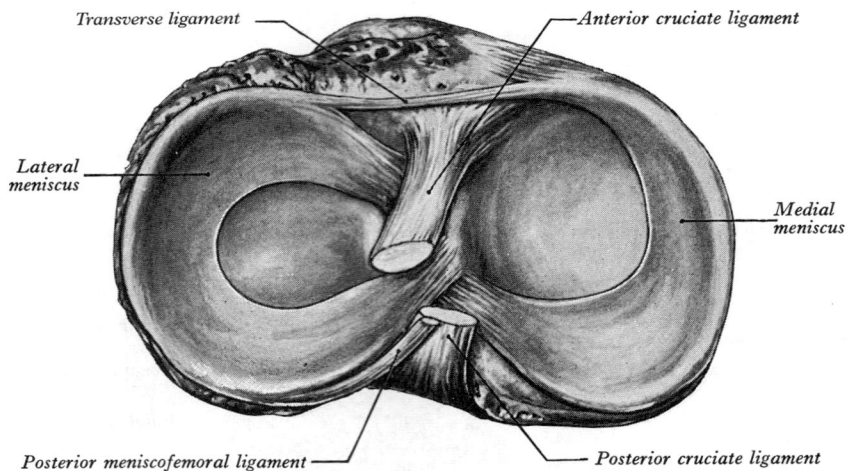

Transverse ligament — — *Anterior cruciate ligament*

Lateral meniscus

Medial meniscus

Posterior meniscofemoral ligament — — *Posterior cruciate ligament*

6.315 Superior aspect of the left tibia, showing the menisci and the tibial attachments of the cruciate ligaments.

femoris, medial and lateral parts of which descend, flanking the patella, to the sides of the tibial tuberosity, merging into the fibrous capsule as *medial* and *lateral patellar retinacula*. The patellar ligament is separated from the synovial membrane by a large infrapatellar fat pad and from the tibia by a bursa (**6.296**).

Oblique popliteal ligament (6.307)

It expands from the tendon of semimembranosus, blends partly with the capsule and ascends laterally to the lateral part of the intercondylar line and lateral femoral condyle. Its fasciculi are separated

by apertures for vessels and nerves; it is in the floor of the popliteal fossa with the popliteal artery in contact.

Arcuate popliteal ligament (6.307)

A Y-shaped mass of capsular fibres, it has a stem attached to the head of the fibula; its posterior limb arches medially over the emerging tendon of popliteus to the posterior border of the tibial intercondylar area; the anterior limb, sometimes absent, extends to the lateral femoral epicondyle, being connected with the lateral head of gastrocnemius and is often termed the *short lateral genual ligament*.

Adductor tubercle   *Epiphyseal line*

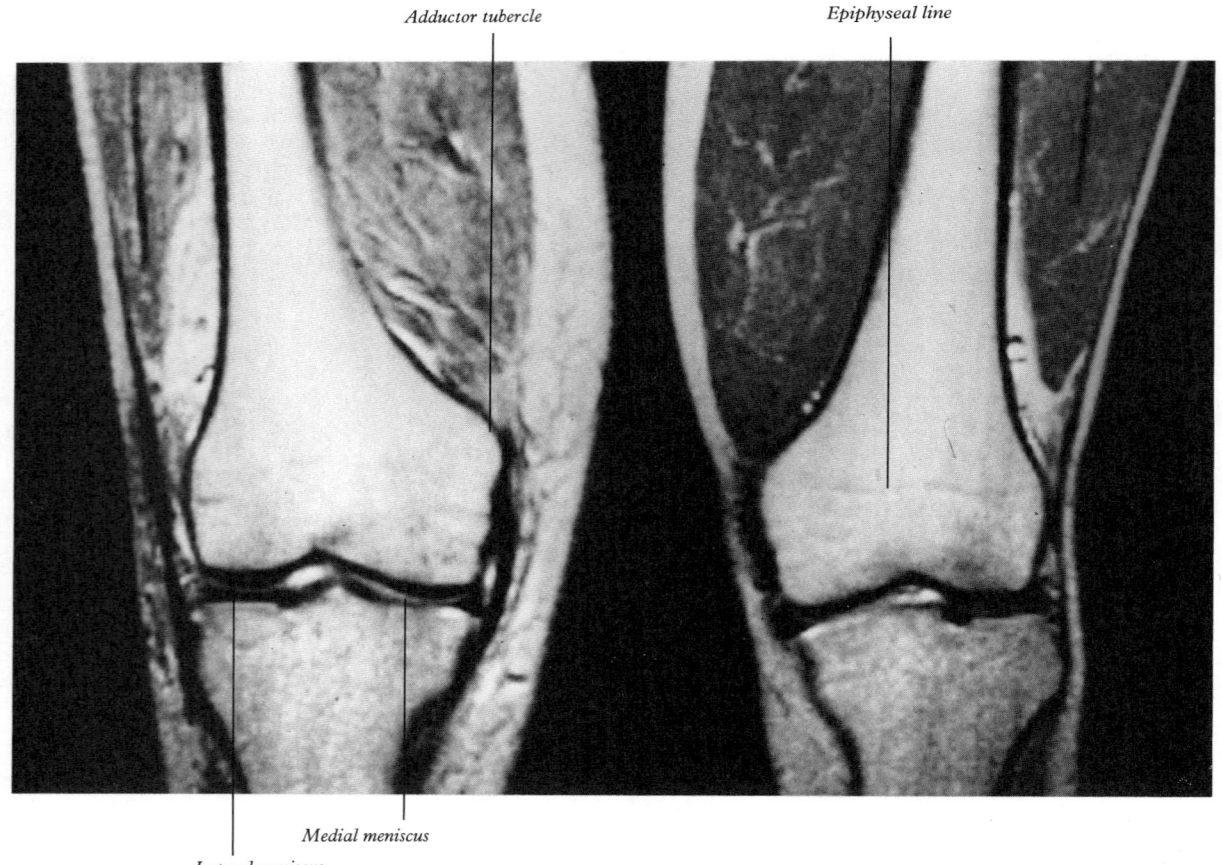

Medial meniscus

Lateral meniscus

6.316 Magnetic resonance imaging scan of the knee joints of an adult male, showing the menisci. (Supplied by Philips Medical Systems; photographed by Sarah Smith.)

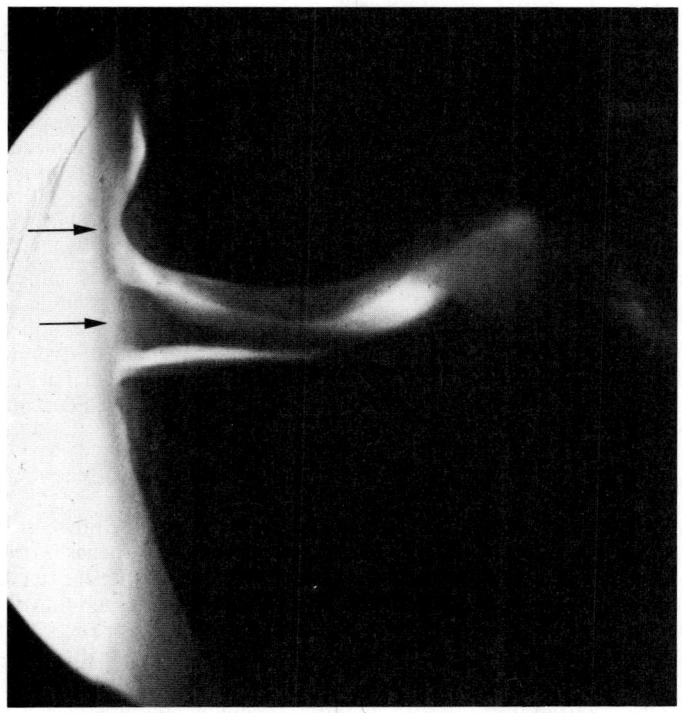

6.317 Radiograph taken after injection of air into the knee joint, showing the shadow thrown by the medial meniscus. The upper arrow points to the medial ligament and the lower to the medial meniscus. (Aerogram by A A Butler, RAF.)

Tibial collateral ligament (6.305, 311, 312)

A broad flat band nearer the back of the joint, it extends from the medial femoral epicondyle, immediately distal to the adductor tubercle, to the medial meniscus, tibial condyle and adjacent shaft. Its *anterior part* is flat, about 10 cm long, and may be separated from the capsule and medial meniscus by one or more bursae (Brantigan & Voshell 1943). It slopes anteriorly as it descends to the medial margin and posterior medial surface of the tibial shaft where it is crossed by the tendons of sartorius, gracilis and semitendinosus, with a bursa interposed. It lies over the medial inferior genicular vessels and nerve and anterior part of the tendon of semimembranosus, and may have tenuous connections with the latter. Its *posterior part* fans out to blend with the back of the capsule; it is short and descends posteriorly to the medial tibial condyle proximal to the groove for semimembranosus.

Fibular collateral ligament (6.313, 314).

A strong cord, it is attached to the lateral femoral epicondyle, proximal to the popliteal groove, and extends to the fibular head in front of its apex. It is largely overlapped by the tendon of biceps femoris, which embraces and partly blends with it; deep to the ligament are the tendon of popliteus and the inferior lateral genicular vessels and nerve. The ligament is **not** attached to the lateral meniscus.

Cruciate ligaments

They are very strong and sited a little posterior to the articular centre. They are termed *cruciate* because they cross, *anterior* and *posterior* from their *tibial* attachments. Their disposition suggests identification with collateral ligaments of originally separate medial and lateral femorotibial joints (p. 697).

Synovial membrane. This almost surrounds the ligaments but is reflected posteriorly from the posterior cruciate to adjoining parts of the capsule. Thus the intercondylar part of the posterior region of the fibrous capsule has no synovial covering. A synovial bursal recess intrudes between the ligaments from their lateral aspect (6.309) and may reach the medial wall of the femoral intercondylar fossa.

The anterior cruciate ligament (6.315). It is attached medially to the anterior intercondylar area of the tibia partly blending with the anterior horn of the lateral meniscus; it ascends **posterolaterally**, twisting on itself and fanning out to attach to the posteromedial aspect of the lateral femoral condyle (Last 1951). It is anterolateral to the posterior cruciate.

The posterior cruciate ligament (6.313, 315). Stronger, less oblique with some shorter fibres, it is attached to the **posterior** intercondylar area and posterior horn of the lateral meniscus; it ascends **anteromedially**, broadening out to its attachment on the lateral surface of the medial femoral condyle.

Mensuration. Observations on 24 fresh joints (Girgis et al 1975) suggested that each ligament has a main posterolateral and a smaller anteromedial band, which behave differently in movement. Spiralization is apparent and more pronounced in certain positions. Average dimensions were: anterior cruciate 38 mm, width 11 mm; posterior cruciate length 38 mm, width 13 mm. Odensten & Gillquist (1985) in a functional and surgical study gave a mean length of 31.3 mm in 33 adult cadavers (Swedish).

It should be noted that these ligaments have substantial cross-sectional areas and attachments that are not only in orthogonal planes but also displaced anteroposteriorly; all these factors introduce difficulties during mensuration, particularly determinations of 'length'.

Menisci

The menisci (semilunar cartilages) (6.315) are crescentic laminae deepening the articulation of the tibia which receives the femur. Their peripheral attached borders are thick and convex; their free borders are thin and concave. Their peripheral zone is vascularized by capillary loops from the fibrous capsule and synovial membrane; their inner regions are avascular (Davies & Edwards 1948). The meniscal horns are richly innervated compared with the remainder, with the central thirds being devoid of innervation (Gronblad et al 1985). The proximal surfaces are smooth and concave, in contact with the articular cartilage on the femoral condyles, while their distal surfaces are smooth and flat, resting on the tibial articular cartilage. Each covers about two-thirds of its tibial articular surface. Canal-like structures have been observed opening onto the surface of menisci in infants and young children (Bird & Sweet 1987), which are thought to transport nutrients to deeper avascular areas.

Two structurally different regions of the menisci have been identified, the medial two-thirds consisting of radially organized collagen bundles and the peripheral third consisting of larger circumferentially arranged bundles (Beaupre et al 1986). The articular surfaces of the medial part are lined by thinner collagen bundles parallel to the surface, while the outer portion is covered by synovium. Such a structural arrangement suggests specific biomechanical functions; mainly compression medially and tension peripherally: with ageing and degeneration compositional changes occur within the menisci reducing the ability to resist tensional forces (Ghosh & Taylor 1987). Outward displacement of the menisci by the femoral condyles is resisted by firm anchorage of the peripheral circumferential fibres to the intercondylar bone. Ghadially et al (1983) have detailed meniscal ultrastructure.

Menisci probably assist lubrication, facilitate combined sliding, rolling and spinning, and may cushion extremes of flexion and extension (p. 707). Seedhom et al (1974, 1979) and Voloshin & Wosk (1983) have demonstrated their role in cushioning compression forces.

The menisci meet a functional need as shown by their reformation after full excision, regeneration being from peripheral vascular tissue. Prior to such reformation the knee joint shows no instability, but if it is subjected to continued violent exercise, subsequent history indicates that articular cartilage suffers permanent damage, perhaps due to inefficient lubrication.

Medial meniscus. Broader behind, it is almost a **semicircle** (6.315), attached by its *anterior horn* to the anterior tibial intercondylar area in front of the anterior cruciate ligament, its posterior fibres being continuous with the transverse ligament. The anterior horn is in the floor of a depression medial to the upper part of the patellar ligament. The *posterior horn* is fixed to the posterior tibial intercondylar area, between the attachments of the lateral meniscus and posterior cruciate ligament. Its peripheral border is attached to the fibrous capsule and the deep surface of the tibial collateral ligament (6.316, 317).

703

Lateral meniscus. About four-fifths of a circle (**6.315**), it covers a larger area than the medial meniscus. Its breadth is uniform, except that of the short tapering horns; it is grooved posterolaterally by the popliteal tendon, separating it from the fibular collateral ligament. Its *anterior horn* is attached in front of the intercondylar eminence, posterolateral to the anterior cruciate ligament, with which it partly blends. Its *posterior horn* is attached behind this eminence, in front of the posterior horn of the medial meniscus. Its anterior attachment is twisted, its free margin facing posterosuperiorly, the anterior horn resting on the anterior slope of the lateral intercondylar tubercle. Near its posterior attachment it commonly sends a *posterior meniscofemoral ligament* (**6.315**) superomedially behind the posterior cruciate ligament to the medial femoral condyle. An *anterior meniscofemoral ligament* may also connect the posterior horn to the medial femoral condyle anterior to the posterior cruciate ligament. The meniscofemoral ligaments are often the sole attachments of the posterior horn of the lateral meniscus. More medially, however, part of the popliteal tendon is attached to the lateral meniscus and mobility of its posterior horn may thus be controlled by the meniscofemoral ligaments and popliteus (Last 1948). A *meniscofibular ligament* has been described in about 80% of knee joints (Živanović 1973).

Transverse ligament (**6.315**). It connects the anterior convex margin of the lateral to the anterior horn of the medial meniscus; it varies in thickness and may be absent. According to Živanović (1974) this *meniscomeniscal ligament* varies much and is absent in about 40% of joints. A *posterior meniscomeniscal ligament* was observed in 20% of 300 knee joints; other inconstant ligaments have been described.

Relations

Anterior are the tendon or quadriceps femoris enclosing and attached to non-articular surfaces of the patella, the tendon's continuation, the patellar ligament and tendinous expansions from vastus medialis and lateralis extending over the **anteromedial** and **anterolateral** aspects of the capsule respectively, as patellar retinacula. **Posteromedial** is sartorius, with the tendon of gracilis along its posterior border, both descending across the joint. **Posterolaterally** the biceps tendon, with the common peroneal nerve medial to it, is in contact with the capsule, separating it from popliteus (**6.314**). **Posteriorly** the popliteal artery and associated lymph nodes are on the oblique popliteal ligament, with the popliteal vein posteromedial or medial and the tibial nerve posterior to both. The nerve and vessels are overlapped by both heads of gastrocnemius and laterally by plantaris. Around the vessels gastrocnemius contacts the capsules and medial to its medial head semimembranosus is between the capsule and semitendinosus.

Vessels and nerve supply to the joint

Arteries supplying the joint are the descending genicular branches of the femoral; superior, middle and inferior genicular branches of the popliteal; anterior and posterior recurrent branches of anterior tibial; the circumflex fibular artery and the descending branch of the lateral circumflex femoral. (For genicular anastomoses see p. 1570.) Scapinelli (1968) and Wladmirow (1968) showed a penetrative ligamentous supply, even the cruciate ligaments receiving small vessels. **Nerves** are from the obturator, femoral, tibial and common peroneal nerves (Gardner 1948a; Freeman & Wyke 1967).

Arthroscopy of the knee

The modern arthroscope was pioneered some 35 years ago. Subsequent improvements in fibre optics, video systems and instruments allowed first the growth of diagnostic arthroscopy and then an ever-increasing repertoire of arthroscopic procedures. The knee, being a large and superficial joint devoid of important neurovascular structures on three sides, lent itself to these developments. Open arthrotomy is now unusual for the treatment of internal derangements of the knee: 'arthroscopic-assisted' procedures are appropriate for the treatment of cruciate ligament injuries and some intra-articular fractures. The increased accuracy of diagnosis, low morbidity and rapid recovery, matched by the financial attractions of day case surgery, have made arthroscopy the commonest type of orthopaedic procedure currently undertaken in Western countries.

While general anaesthesia is preferable, knee arthroscopy can be performed using local or regional anaesthesia. Examination of the fully relaxed knee for ligament stability should be undertaken before commencing the arthroscopy. Individual techniques vary, but a tourniquet is commonly used and sometimes combined with a thigh holder, which supports the leg while valgus and varus stress are employed to open up the medial and lateral joint compartments respectively.

ARTHROSCOPIC PORTALS
(**6.318**)

The conventional starting point for arthroscopy is the anterolateral portal, adjacent to the lateral margin of the patellar tendon about 2 centimetres above the tibial plateau, avoiding damage to the meniscus. When inserting instruments into the joint, care should also be taken to avoid damaging the articular cartilage, which has minimal capacity for repair. The 30° arthroscope is the instrument chosen for most surgical procedures, and for making the first inspection sweep of the knee. A 70° arthroscope is useful for

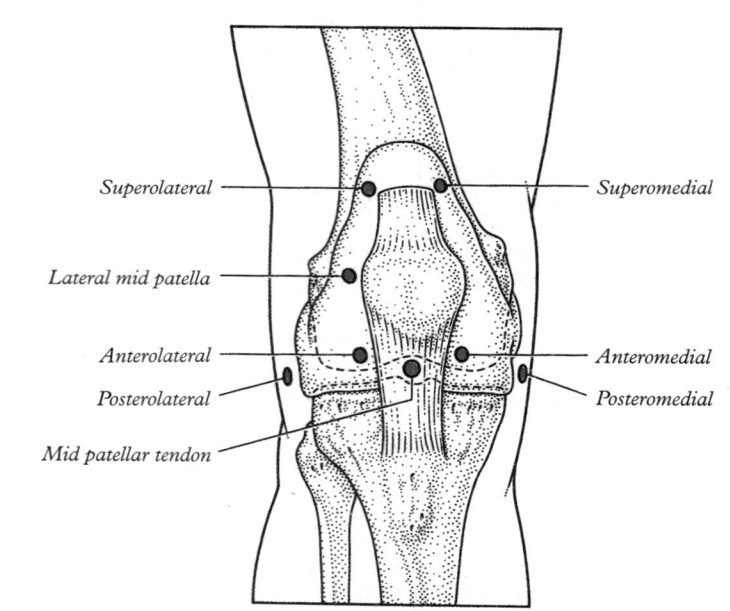

Superolateral

Superomedial

Lateral mid patella

Anterolateral

Anteromedial

Posterolateral

Posteromedial

Mid patellar tendon

6.318 The standard arthroscopy portals.

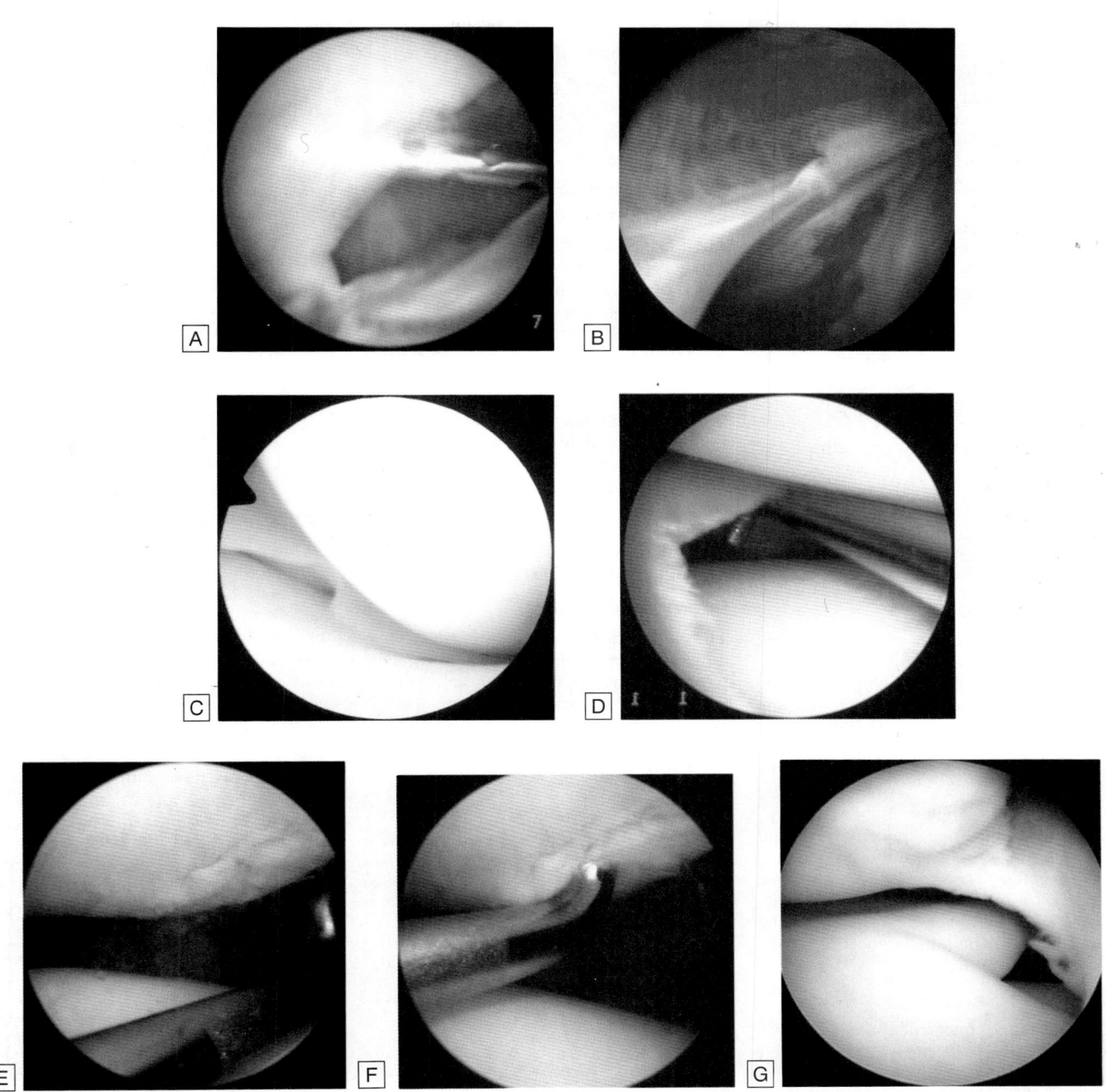

6.319 All photographs are of the right knee, taken through the anterolateral portal. A. Looking upwards into the suprapatellar pouch; the medial suprapatellar plica is seen with the irrigation cannula behind it: B. Medial plica with haemorrhagic synovium adjacent: c. Normal medial meniscus with a wavy free margin: D. Hook being used to view underside of meniscus: E. Irregular undersurface of patella: F. Probe showing deep fissures in patellar articular cartilage: G. Complete type discoid meniscus: there is no attachment of the posterior horn to the tibia. (Some of the above photographs were provided by Mr Malcolm Glasgow.)

looking round corners, and particularly when inspecting the posterior compartments from the front of the knee via the intercondylar notch. The irrigation system which distends and washes out the joint is set up at the time of the initial arthroscope insertion. The cannula is usually inserted via a superolateral or superomedial portal.

The anteromedial portal is generally the second to be placed, a similar height above the tibial plateau on the opposite side of the patellar tendon. The first instrument through this portal is the inspection hook, which is used to probe the articular surface, pull on the menisci and retract the synovium. Graduations on the hook help the surgeon appreciate size and magnification. The art of working an arthroscope through one portal and an instrument through another is known as 'triangulation'.

A central or transpatellar tendon portal gives good access to the intercondylar notch area and posterior compartments; however, its use damages the central fibres of the patellar tendon, which itself might be needed as a graft in an anterior cruciate-deficient knee. The superolateral and superomedial portals, which enter the suprapatellar pouch, should be sited 2 centimetres above the upper pole of the patella. As well as being used for irrigation, these portals can provide an excellent view of the patellofemoral joint from above: patellofemoral tracking can be observed during passive flexion and extension of the knee. The posterolateral and posteromedial portals may be required for the removal of loose bodies, for synovectomy of the knee, or for posteriorcruciate reconstruction. Entry should be made with the knee flexed and the joint distended. Illumination of the posterior corner of the knee from within, and the preliminary passage of a needle into the posterior compartment are useful guides for the precise placement of these portals. The midlateral portal is useful for viewing the front of the knee.

NORMAL ARTHROSCOPIC FINDINGS

A systematic arthroscopic inspection of the joint is necessary before any operative procedure is undertaken, and begins via the anterolateral portal.

Suprapatellar pouch

With the knee in extension and distended with fluid the pouch is easy to inspect. The fibres of vastus intermedius can often be seen through the filmy synovium lining the roof. In 80% of knees medial and lateral crescentic folds of synovium, *plicae*, project into the joint at the junction of the pouch and knee joint proper; a further fold of synovium, the *medial plica* or *shelf*, may be present in 50% of knees, and if large, may be intermittently pinched between patella and condyle and become a source of anterior knee pain. A medial plica is best seen by looking between the medial facet of the patella and the medial femoral condyle (6.319A, B).

Patellofemoral joint

The deep surface of the patella can be seen with the arthroscope rotated so that the operator is looking upwards. A combination of side-to-side movement of the arthroscope within the knee and manipulation of the patella from outside allows all of the articular surface to be scanned. The trochlear groove should also be inspected and the patellofemoral articulation viewed during extension and flexion of the joint (6.319C, D).

Lateral recess

The lateral recess is a space between the cheek of the lateral femoral condyle and the lateral side of the joint. It is inspected from above downwards until the popliteal tunnel is clearly seen. The opening of the tunnel is bounded laterally by synovium and medially by the lateral meniscus, and transmits the popliteal tendon. It is a favourite hiding place for loose bodies and, if suspected, the tunnel should be

massaged from outside the knee while its entrance is viewed through the arthroscope. Anterior to the tunnel, the meniscosynovial junction can be inspected.

Medial femoral condyle

The condyle is inspected as the knee is flexed and extended, looking particularly at the 'osteochondritis dissecans' area on the lateral aspect adjacent to the notch.

Medial compartment

The medial compartment is opened up if a valgus force is applied to the knee when in 15° of flexion. The medial meniscus can be clearly seen; the free margin has a wavy edge in a healthy meniscus. The probe can be used to view the superior and tibial surface of the meniscus and, by applying traction with a hook, the meniscus can be tested for stability (6.319E, F): in a tight knee it may be difficult to see the posterior third of the medial meniscus. The articular surface of the femur and tibia should be probed, since fissures not obvious at first sight may be revealed; softening of articular cartilage should be regarded as the first sign of chondromalacia.

Intercondylar notch

The margins are first inspected. Invariably, a ligamentum mucosum extends from the fat pad to the apex of the notch. Within the notch the anterior cruciate ligament is clearly seen arising from the intercondylar area between the tibial spines, merging anteriorly with the anterior horn of the lateral meniscus. The anterior draw test, or Lachman test, can be performed with the ligament visualized; it should also be probed to determine its integrity. Occasionally, distinct anterolateral and posteromedial bands can be recognized. The femoral origin of the posterior cruciate can sometimes be seen through the synovium, and can always be felt with the probe.

Lateral compartment

Inspection is performed with the leg in the sartorial ('Figure 4') position. Again the hook is essential for inspection. When pulled forwards, the lateral meniscus is more mobile than the medial.

Posterior compartment

The posteromedial compartment can be inspected from the anterolateral portal via the intercondylar notch; the meniscosynovial junction of the posterior horn of the medial meniscus can readily be seen. By moving the arthroscope to the anteromedial side, it is usually possible to enter the posterolateral compartment. This portal (anteromedial) is also well-placed for inspecting the medial gutter and for viewing the articular surface of the lateral femoral condyle. If a discoid meniscus is suspected of filling the lateral compartment, diagnostic arthroscopy can be started from the anteromedial portal.

ANATOMICAL VARIATIONS

Plicae

The plicae show great anatomical variation (Hardaker et al 1980). The suprapatellar plicae are remnants of an embryonic septum which completely separates the suprapatellar pouch from the knee joint: rarely, a complete septum persists. If it does, it will interfere with irrigation at the start of the arthroscopy, in which case the septum needs to be broken down or resected. Occasionally, an almost complete septum is seen with a small central opening.

The ligamentum mucosum running from the fat pad to the apex of the intercondylar notch may be enlarged, forming a complete curtain separating medial and lateral compartments. Such a curtain, or infrapatellar plica, can be extremely troublesome since, until resected, it prevents vision across the front of the knee.

Discoid lateral meniscus

The discoid lateral meniscus occurs in 5% of the population: often bilateral, it is nevertheless unusual to see this abnormality on the medial side of the joint. The distinguishing features of a discoid lateral meniscus are its shape and posterior ligamentous attachments. A classification of the abnormality, based on Watanabe et al (1979), is proposed:

(1) In its mildest form, the incomplete discoid meniscus is simply a wider form of the normal lateral meniscus. The tapered free margin is interposed between femoral and tibial condyles, but it does not completely cover the tibial plateau.

(2) A complete discoid meniscus appears as a biconcave disc with a rolled medial edge and totally covers the lateral tibial plateau, completely cushioning the lateral femoral condyle (6.319G). Often the only posterior attachment is to the femur by the anterior or posterior meniscofemoral ligaments passing in front of and/or behind the posterior cruciate ligament.

(3) The Wrisberg type of meniscus has the same shape as a complete discoid meniscus, but its posterior ligamentous attachment is by the meniscofemoral ligaments. The normal tibial attachment of the posterior horn of the lateral meniscus is missing, but the posterior meniscofemoral ligament persists. As a result, this type of meniscus is attached anteriorly to the tibia and posteriorly to the femur. This renders the posterior horn unstable and liable to attrition. As the knee extends from the flexed position, the poorly anchored meniscus may sublux into the intercondylar area with a jolt: this being one explanation of the classical presenting symptom of the 'clunking knee' in some patients.

Smillie (1948) tried to explain these abnormalities on the basis of arrested embryological development. However, subsequent studies have shown that the lateral meniscus does not assume a discoid shape during normal development, and other explanations have been sought. Kaplan (1957) proposed that the primary pathology was the abnormal posterior attachment, and that mechanical factors related to the habitual subluxation of the hypermobile cartilage helped to alter its shape towards a discoid configuration. This does not explain the origin of discoid menisci with stable and more posterior attachments. Some forms of discoid menisci, at least, would appear to be true congenital anomalies, and rare fetal discoid menisci have been reported.

Recognition of the different types of meniscus can be difficult in arthroscopy, particularly when the lateral compartment is completely filled by a bulky and torn structure. The rolled edge can usually be viewed via the anteromedial portal and mobility tested with the hook. If the posterior horn is rounded and can be elevated from the tibia, then the Wrisberg configuration is confirmed. A discoid meniscus should not be removed simply because it

exists: treatment of the symptomatic discoid meniscus depends upon its type (Dickhaut & Delee 1982). If the posterior attachment is solely of the Wrisberg type, lateral menisectomy is advocated. If the posterior horn is stable, it may be possible to trim the meniscus down to a more normal configuration. In difficult cases, distinction of stable and 'Wrisberg ligament only' types of discoid menisci may not be possible until trimming has started.

Absent anterior cruciate ligament

Congenital absence of the anterior cruciate ligament is rare, and usually seen only in association with lower limb dysplasia (Thomas et al 1985). Unlike traumatic rupture of the anterior cruciate ligament, the instability that can be revealed by clinical examination does not usually lead to significant symptoms of instability during physical activity.

COMPLICATIONS OF ARTHROSCOPY

There are relatively few complications of arthroscopic surgery. A prospective series

of over 10 000 operations revealed two complications in particular that have an anatomical basis (Small 1992):

- First, postoperative haemarthrosis sufficient to require aspiration or evacuation is the commonest complication, occurring in 1% of the series. This complication is most likely the result of lateral retinacular release: division of the lateral superior genicular artery being the cause of the bleeding. This complication can be avoided if the vessel is properly secured under vision at the time of surgery.
- Secondly, the advent of meniscal repair, which is appropriate for some peripheral tears in younger patients, brought a dramatic increase in neurovascular complications. The common peroneal nerve is particularly vulnerable when suturing the posterior horn of the lateral meniscus using long needles passed from within the knee joint outwards. Experience and improved operating techniques have greatly reduced these complications (Bach & Bush–Joseph 1992).

Movements

Movements are customarily described as *flexion*, *extension*, *medial* and *lateral rotation*. Flexion and extension differ from true hinging: firstly, the spiral profiles of the femoral condyles shift the axis upwards and forwards during extension, backwards and downwards during flexion; secondly, with the foot fixed, the last 30° of extension involves conjunct medial femoral rotation and early flexion entails corresponding lateral rotation. These conjunct rotations are due to the geometry of the articular surfaces and the disposition of ligaments. Conversely, with the foot free to move, extension involves lateral rotation of tibia and flexion a medial rotation. In full flexion posterior parts of the tibial surfaces contact posterior parts of the femoral articular surfaces. During extension the tibia and menisci glide forward on the femoral condyles, the area of contact increasing and also moving forwards. As movement progresses flatter parts of the femoral condyles contact the tibia, and the menisci are opened out, their anterior ends moving forwards, the posterior moving little. In flexion the reverse occurs so that the menisci, moving with the tibia, adapt to the curves of the femoral condyles where contact occurs.

Rotations have a smaller range than flexion and extension, and involve translation of the menisci **with** the femoral condyles on the tibia. These rotations are *conjunct*, integral with flexion and extension, but can be *adjunct* and independent, best demonstrated with the knee semiflexed.

The range of extension is about 5°–10° beyond a vertical femorotibial axis, flexion about 120° with the hip extended, or 140° when it is flexed, and 160° when a passive element such as sitting on the heels aids it. *Passive* rotation is about 60°–70° but conjunct rotation only about 20°.

Conjunct medial rotation of the femur on the tibia in later stage of extension is part of a 'locking' mechanism, an asset when the fully extended knees are subjected to strain. Full extension is the close-packed position, with maximal spiralization and tightening of the ligaments. The roles of the articular surfaces, musculature and ligaments in generating conjunct rotations have been much disputed (Barnett 1952; Kapandji 1974; Girgis et al 1975; Rajendran 1985) but the following points can be made. The **lateral** combined meniscotibial 'receiving surface' is smaller, more circular and more deeply concave.

The lateral femoral articular surface is also smaller, rounder and flattens more rapidly. Consequently, the lateral femoral condyle approaches full congruence with the opposed surface about 30° before full extension (well before the medial condyle). Simple extension cannot continue but medial rotation of the femur occurs on a vertical axis through its head and lateral condyle, the medial femoral condyle moving backwards in an arc, while rotation of the lateral femoral condyle and meniscus brings the latter's anterior horn on to the anterior slope of the lateral tibial condyle. Full congruence of the lateral condyle is thus delayed by this deformation of its 'receiving surface' and extension continues. Rotation and extension follow simultaneously and smoothly until final close-packing of both condyles coincides. At the beginning of flexion from full extension (with the foot fixed) lateral femoral rotation occurs, 'unlocking' the joint. While joint surfaces and many ligaments are again similarly involved, electromyographic evidence shows that contraction of popliteus is important, pulling down and backwards on the lateral femoral condyle, **lateral** to the axis of femoral rotation. Through its attachment to the lateral meniscus, it also retracts its posterior horn during lateral rotation and continuing flexion, preventing traumatic compression (Last 1950).

During extension femoral rotation is observable about 30° before full extension; it first progresses slowly, but more rapidly in the last 5°, when there is a progressive increase in passive mechanisms resisting further extension, i.e. spiralizing and tightening of ligaments, increasing congruence and compression of the articular surfaces and gradually increasing tension in all extra-articular tissues crossing the joint's posterior aspect (Smith 1956). Any actual position of extension adopted is a balance between forces (torque) extending the joint and passive mechanisms resisting this. The range **near** to close-packing is functionally important. In symmetrical standing, the line of body weight is anterior to the transverse axes of the knee joints but the **passive** mechanisms noted above preserve posture with minimal muscular effort (Joseph 1960). Active contraction of the extensors and a close-packed position only occur in asymmetrical postures, in leaning forward, heavy loading or when powerful thrust is needed.

In extension parts of both cruciate ligaments, the tibial and fibular collateral ligaments, the posterior capsular region, the oblique posterior ligament, skin and fasciae are all taut; passive and sometimes active tension exists in the hamstrings and gastrocnemius, and the anterior parts of the menisci are compressed between femoral and tibial condyles. (Kaplan 1958 and Evans 1973 have suggested the iliotibial tract as a strong tibial collateral ligament, see p. 703.) During extension the patellar ligament is tightened by quadriceps femoris but is relaxed in the erect attitude. When the knee flexes the fibular collateral and **posterior** part of the tibial collateral ligament relax but the cruciate ligaments and **anterior** part of the tibial collateral remain taut; posterior parts of the menisci are compressed between the femoral and tibial condyles. Flexion is checked by quadriceps femoris, anterior parts of the capsule, posterior cruciate ligament and compression of soft tissues behind the knee. In extreme **passive** flexion, contact of the calf with the thigh may be the limiting factor; parts of both cruciate ligaments also tense. In addition to conjunct rotation with terminal extension or initial flexion, relaxed collateral ligaments allow independent medial and lateral rotation (adjunct rotation) when the joint is flexed. One cruciate ligament at least is taut in all positions; it acts as a direct bond between the tibia and femur, limiting the former's translation back or forwards. In extension the collateral ligaments assist the cruciate ligaments in this role. Forward gliding of the tibia on the femur is prevented by the anterior cruciate, backward gliding of tibia on femur by the posterior cruciate ligament.

During femoral extension on a fixed tibia, the femoral articular surfaces simultaneously roll forward, slide back and spin medially. However, tibial extension on a relatively fixed femur involves simultaneous forward tibial roll, slide and lateral spin. For geometrical analysis consult (1977).

Accessory movements. Wider rotation can be obtained by passive movements when the knee is semiflexed; the tibia can also, to a limited extent, be translated back and forwards on the femur. Abduction and adduction are prevented in full extension by the collateral and cruciate ligaments. With the knee slightly flexed limited adduction and abduction are possible, both passive and active. Slight separation of the femur and tibia results from strong traction.

Muscles producing movement

Flexion: biceps femoris, semitendinosus and semimembranosus, assisted by gracilis, sartorius and popliteus. With the foot stationary, gastrocnemius and plantaris also assist.

Extension: quadriceps femoris, assisted by tensor fascia lata.

Medial rotation of flexed leg: popliteus, semimembranosus and semitendinosus, assisted by sartorius and gracilis.

Lateral rotation of flexed leg: popliteus, biceps femoris.

Clinical anatomy

The knee appears to be an insecure joint. Between the two longest bones, it is subject to much leverage; the articular surfaces are poorly congruent and the range of motion is great. Nevertheless, the powerful ligaments and strong muscles concerned make it one of the strongest joints in the body. Many muscles have direct attachments to the fibrous capsule. Traumatic dislocation is rare. Injuries of a meniscus are, however, common, resulting from twisting strains applied to the slightly or fully flexed knee. Damage may be a complete tear across the full width, a partial split extending from the free border or a longitudinal tear within the cartilage; occasionally its periphery is detached from the capsule. The torn or detached part may be displaced centrally and jam between the femoral and tibial, arresting all movement. Menisci are largely avascular; a tear cannot heal unless close to the capsule (p. 703). The medial meniscus is more commonly injured, probably because it is more securely attached to the medial capsule and ligaments and less adaptable to sudden change of position. During rotation of a flexed or partially flexed knee the medial cartilage moves more than the lateral. On the other hand, the medial fibres of popliteus may draw the posterior part of the lateral meniscus back on to the groove behind the lateral tibial condyle, preventing trapping between the articular surfaces.

Injuries to the cruciate ligaments are also common, ranging from sprain to rupture. The anterior is more commonly affected. Damage to the tibial collateral ligament is less common, since excessive strain is likely only in full extension.

Osteoligamentous preparations have aided analysis of excessive movements due to ligamentous injuries. In a flexed knee the fibular collateral and posterior part of the tibial collateral ligaments relax. If either cruciate ligament is cut, tibial gliding is increased. Rotation is increased if either cruciate or the tibial collateral ligaments are cut. Division of both collateral ligaments allows excessive lateral rotation but medial rotation is unchanged. Abduction and adduction are excessive if both cruciate ligaments are cut.

Acute traumatic synovitis is frequent in the knee. When its cavity is distended with fluid, the swelling shows above and alongside the patella, 5 cm or more above the femur's patellar surface, and extends a little more under vastus medialis than under lateralis; the synovial membrane descends just below the tibial plateau.

Bursae sometimes become distended: distension of the subcutaneous prepatellar or infrapatellar bursae is frequently caused by excessive kneeling. The semimembranosus bursa is occasionally enlarged, forming a fluctuant swelling at the back of the knee. During extension it is tense but in flexion soft, if it communicates with the joint.

During level walking the force across the femorotibial joint can reach five times body weight (Johnson & Waugh 1979), although for most of the cycle it is between two and four times body weight (Morrison 1970): in contrast the force across the patellofemoral joint is no more than 50% body weight. Not surprisingly peak force transmission across the joint increases sequentially as the menisci, articular cartilage and subchondral bone are damaged and/or removed (Hoshino & Wallace 1987). Ascending and descending stairs have little influence on femorotibial forces but significantly increase patellofemoral forces to two (ascending) and three (descending) times body weight as a result of the change in angle of the quadriceps tendon and patellar ligament during flexion (van Eijden et al 1987). However, the patella has two complex mechanisms for ameliorating forces transmitted across it: the extensor lever arm is lengthened as the axis of rotation moves posteriorly during flexion, particularly between 30° and 70° (Nisell et al 1986); and that between 30° and 90°, the contact area between the patella and femur, almost triples (Hungerford & Barry 1979).

Total knee replacement arthroplasty

Surgical replacement of the knee is required in severe destructive arthritis of the joint: the patient suffers from pain, stiffness and loss of function. The joint may also be contracted and deformed by articular erosion and derangement, most commonly due to osteoarthritis or rheumatoid disease.

Over the past 25 years the development of knee joint arthroplasty has progressed from simple hinge devices to sophisticated surface replacement of the femur, tibia and usually the patella: it is now very successful. The materials used are similar to those in total hip replacement; the main articulation is either metal (a cobalt/chrome alloy) or ultra-high density polyethylene, producing a low friction bearing surface. The tibial tray is titanium and encloses polyethylene spacers of various thicknesses (**6.320**). When necessary, the patellar surface is usually replaced with an inlaid button (**6.321**).

Technique

A vertical midline incision is made over the anterior aspect of the joint; the capsule is opened by a medial parapatellar incision extending from the quadriceps tendon above to the tibial tubercle below. The

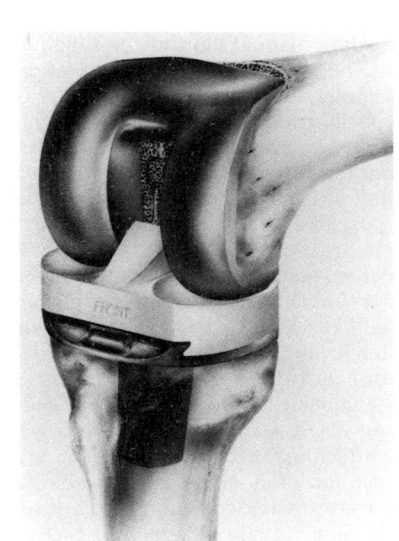

6.320 Total condylar replacement arthroplasty of the knee.

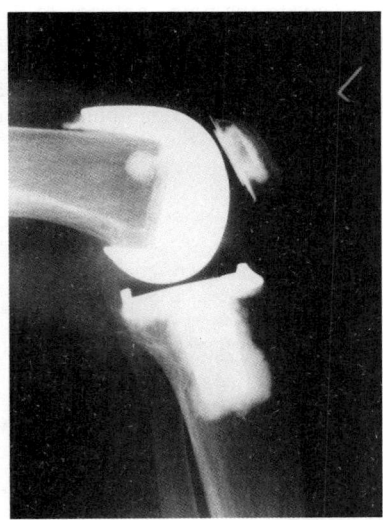

6.321 Lateral view of the condylar prosthesis with patellar replacement and metal-backed tibial component.

The cement hardens in about 8 minutes. The patella may require realignment, achieved by lateral capsular release, if it has undergone lateral subluxation.

Cementless prostheses (**6.323**) are also used, in which the metal surfaces are coated with hydroxyapatite. This thin ceramic layer allows bony ingrowth to bond the prosthetic components to the femoral condyles and tibial plateau.

For the grossly destroyed knee joint, a modular system of condylar replacement is also available, consisting of long stems, inserts and a semiconstrained adaptation to maintain alignment and stability.

Postoperative rehabilitation

Within a few hours postoperatively, the patient's knee is moved using a constant passive motion machine. The knee is then exercised to ensure early return of quadriceps and hamstring function: weight-bearing is allowed within 2 to 3 days; crutch supports are dispensed with as soon as there is good muscle control and adequate comfort. A satisfactory range of movement following this type of condylar replacement arthroplasty is from full extension to 110–120° flexion.

Results

This type of condylar prosthetic replacement produces good results, with a survival rate of 90% at 15 years follow-up (Insall 1994). Newer models, with a metal-backed tibial polyethylene component,

have a 98% survival rate at 7 years, being better than that achieved in total hip replacement anthroplasty.

The development of new prosthetic components continues, which, together with cementless coatings (including ceramics), will provide additional benefit for disabled patients affected by a destructive arthropathy.

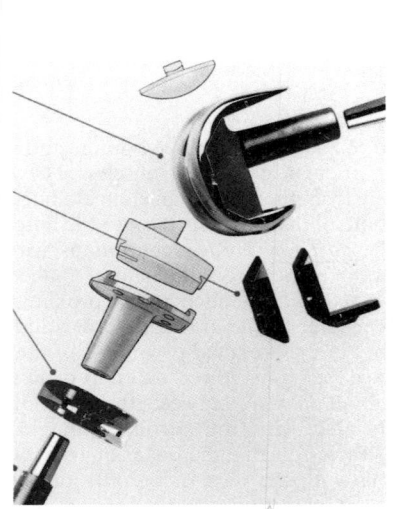

6.322 Modular prosthetic components for total knee replacement arthroplasty.

joint surface replacement maintains the capsular structures and collateral ligaments; however, appropriate soft tissue releases may be required to realign the knee. In osteoarthritis the knee is usually in varus alignment: consequently the medial capsule and collateral ligament and the pes anserinus (sartorius, gracilis, semitendinosus) are all released to allow satisfactory realignment before bone cuts are made. Various jigs and guides are used to cut the surface accurately ready to receive the prosthetic components (**6.322**), which are set in polymethyl methacrylate.

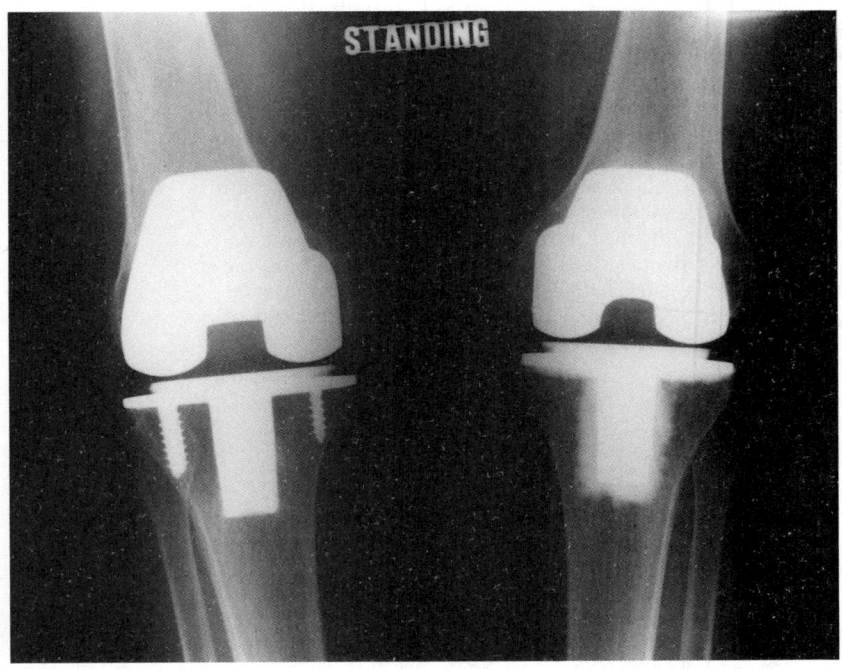

6.323 Radiological appearance (anteroposterior) of a cemented (on the right) and uncemented (on the left) prosthesis.

FIBULA

The fibula (**6.299, 300**) is much more slender than the tibia, not being directly involved in transmission of weight. It has a proximal *head*, a long *shaft* and a distal *lateral malleolus*. A thinner part near the head is the *neck*. The shaft varies in form, being variably moulded by attached muscles; these variations may be confusing.

Head

The head, slightly expanded, projects in front, behind and laterally. A round facet, on its proximomedial aspect, articulates with a facet on the inferolateral surface of the lateral tibial condyle; it faces proximally and anteromedially. A blunt *apex* (*styloid process*) projects proximally from its posterolateral aspect, palpable about 2 cm distal to the knee joint. The common peroneal nerve crosses posterolateral to the neck and can be rolled against bone, causing tingling sensations on the dorsum of the foot and toes, especially on the medial side of the hallux.

Shaft

The shaft (**6.299, 300**) has three borders and surfaces, each associated with a particular group of muscles. The *anterior border* ascends proximally from the apex of an elongated, triangular area continuous with the lateral malleolar surface, to the anterior aspect of the fibular head. The *posterior border*, continuous with the medial margin of the posterior groove on the lateral malleolus, is usually distinct distally, but often rounded in its proximal half. The *interosseous border* is medial to the anterior border and usually more posterior (**6.324**), but in the proximal two-thirds of the bone they approximate, the 'surface' being narrowed to 1 mm or less.

The *lateral surface*, between the anterior and posterior borders and associated with the peroneal muscles, faces laterally in its proximal three-fourths; the distal quarter twists (spirals) to become continuous with the *posterior groove* of the lateral malleolus. The *anteromedial* (sometimes simply termed *anterior*, or *medial*) *surface*, between the anterior and interosseous borders, usually faces anteromedially but often forwards. Distally wide, it narrows in its proximal half and may be a mere ridge; it is associated with the extensor muscles. The *posterior surface*, the largest, between the interosseous and posterior borders, is associated with the flexor muscles. Its proximal two-thirds is divided by a longitudinal *medial crest*, separated from the interosseous border by a grooved surface, directed medially; the rest of the surface faces back in its proximal half, but its distal half curves on to the medial aspect; distally this area occupies the tibia's fibular notch, roughened by the attachment of the principal interosseous tibiofibular ligament.

The triangular area proximal to the lateral surface of the lateral malleolus (**6.299A**) is **subcutaneous**; the rest of the shaft is obscured by muscles. To the *fibular head* are attached extensor digitorum longus in front, peroneus longus anterolaterally and soleus behind; the fibular collateral ligament is attached in front of its apex and embraced by the main attachments of biceps femoris. To the margins of the articular facet is attached the tibiofibular capsular ligament.

The *anterior border* divides distally into two ridges enclosing the subcutaneous triangular surface (**6.299A**). The anterior intermuscular septum is attached to its proximal three-fourths, the lateral end of

the superior extensor retinaculum distally on the anterior border of the triangular area. Distally on the triangular area's posterior margin is attached the lateral end of the superior peroneal retinaculum. The *interosseous border* ends at the proximal limit of the rough area for the interosseous ligament. The interosseous membrane attached to it does not reach the fibular head, leaving space for the anterior tibial vessels. The *posterior border* is proximally indistinct, the posterior intermuscular septum attached to all but its distal end. The *medial crest* is related to the peroneal artery, with a nutrient foramen on or near it close to the midshaft. Also attached to it is a layer of deep fascia separating tibialis posterior from flexor hallucis longus and flexor digitorum longus.

The *anteromedial* (*extensor*) *surface* has attached to it extensor digitorum longus, extensor hallucis longus and peroneus tertius (pp. 884–885). To the *lateral* (*peroneal*) *surface* peroneus longus is attached to its whole width in its proximal third but in its middle third only from its posterior part, behind peroneus brevis (p. 885). The latter continues its attachment almost to the distal end of the fibula's shaft. The *posterior surface*, divided longitudinally by the medial crest, has complex attachments: between the crest and interosseous border it is concave and often crossed by an oblique ridge for an intramuscular tendon of tibialis posterior, which is attached throughout much of this region—usually confined to the proximal three-fourths. Between the crest and posterior border in the proximal fourth of the posterior surface the soleus is attached, its tendinous arch being attached to it proximally. Distal to soleus on this surface flexor hallucis longus is attached, almost to the bone's distal end. A little proximal to its midpoint it is pierced by a nutrient foramen, directed distally, for a branch of the peroneal artery.

To the anterior surface of the *lateral malleolus* the anterior talofibular ligament is attached and, to the notch anterior to its apex, the calcaneofibular ligament. The tendons of peroneus brevis and longus groove its posterior aspect, the latter superficial and covered by the superior peroneal retinaculum. In the *malleolar fossa* (**6.325**), pitted by vascular foramina, the posterior tibiofibular ligament is attached posteriorly and, distal to this, the posterior talofibular ligament.

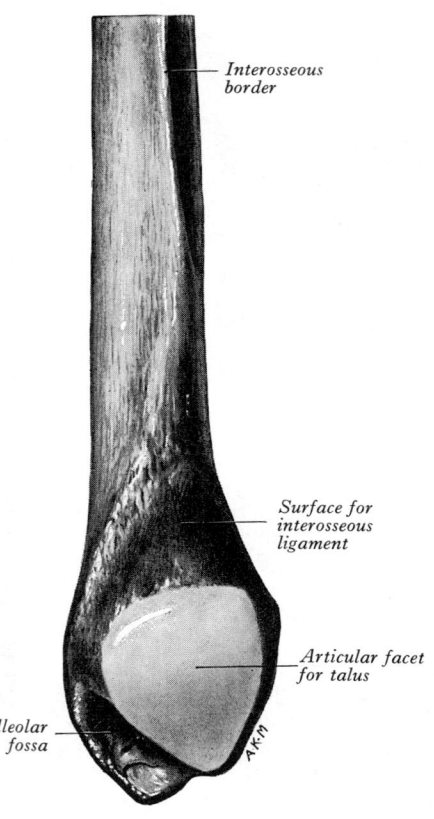

6.325   Medial aspect of the distal end of the left fibula.

6.324   Transverse section through the right tibia and fibula, showing the attachment of the interosseous membrane: proximal aspect.

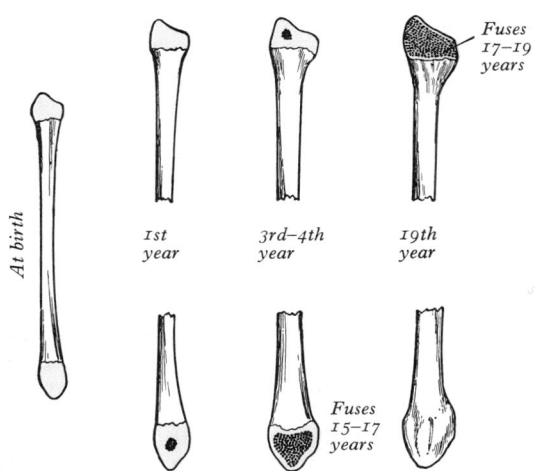

6.326   Stages in the ossification of the fibula.

Distal end

The distal end or lateral malleolus projects distally and posteriorly. Its *lateral aspect* is subcutaneous; its *posterior aspect* has a broad groove with a prominent lateral border. Its *anterior aspect* is rough, round and continuous with the tibial inferior border. The *medial surface* has a triangular articular facet, vertically convex, its apex distal (**6.325**); it articulates with the lateral talar surface. Behind the facet is a rough *malleolar fossa*.

Ossification

Ossification of the fibula is by three centres (**6.326, 327**) in the shaft

and extremities. It begins in the shaft about the eighth intra-uterine week, in its distal end in the first year and in its proximal about the third in females and fourth in males. The distal epiphysis unites with the shaft about the fifteenth year in females, seventeenth in males, whereas the proximal does not unite until about the seventeenth year in females, nineteenth in males. In this respect the fibula reverses the ossificatory pattern in other long bones.

TIBIOFIBULAR ARTICULATIONS

The tibia and fibula are connected by a proximal synovial and distal fibrous joint; their shafts are also united by an interosseous membrane. The fibrous joint and interosseous membrane are syndesmoses.

Proximal tibiofibular joint

The proximal tibiofibular joint (**6.328**) is an almost plane joint between the lateral tibial condyle and fibular head. The *articular surfaces* vary in size, form and inclination. The fibular facet is usually elliptical or circular, almost flat or slightly grooved. The surfaces are covered with hyaline cartilage, with *anterior* and *posterior* ligaments.

Fibrous capsule. This is attached to the margins of rims of facets on the tibia and fibula and are anteriorly and posteriorly thickened. In about 10% the synovial membrane is continuous with that of the knee joint via the subpopliteal recess (p. 699). The *anterior ligament* has two or three flat bands, passing obliquely up from the fibular head to the front of the lateral tibial condyle. The *posterior ligament*, a thick band, ascends obliquely between the posterior aspects of the fibular head and the lateral tibial condyle, covered by the popliteal tendon. These ligaments are not entirely separate from the capsule.

Vessels and nerve supply to the joint. Arteries are from the anterior and posterior tibial recurrent rami of the anterior tibial artery, **nerves** from the common peroneal and nerve to popliteus.

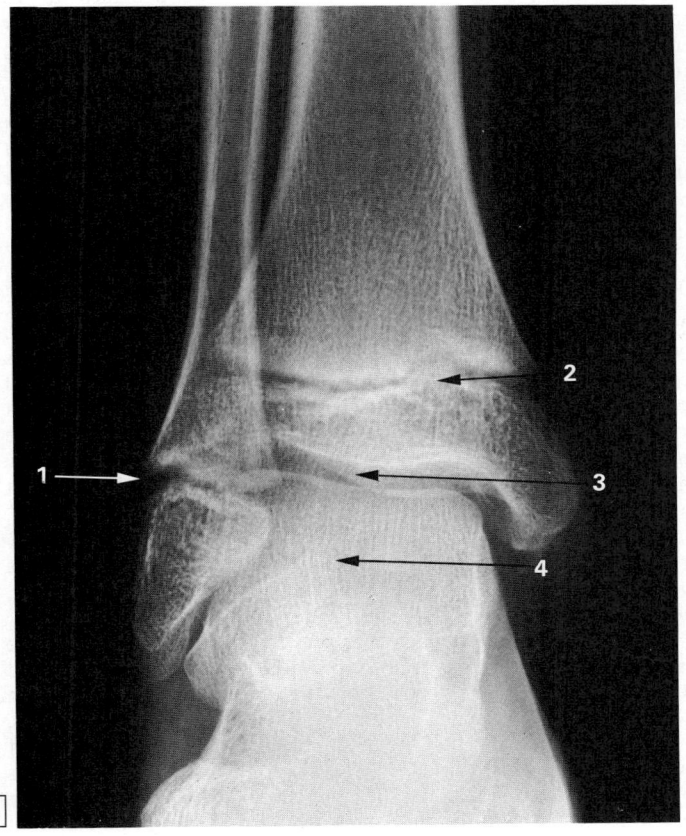

A

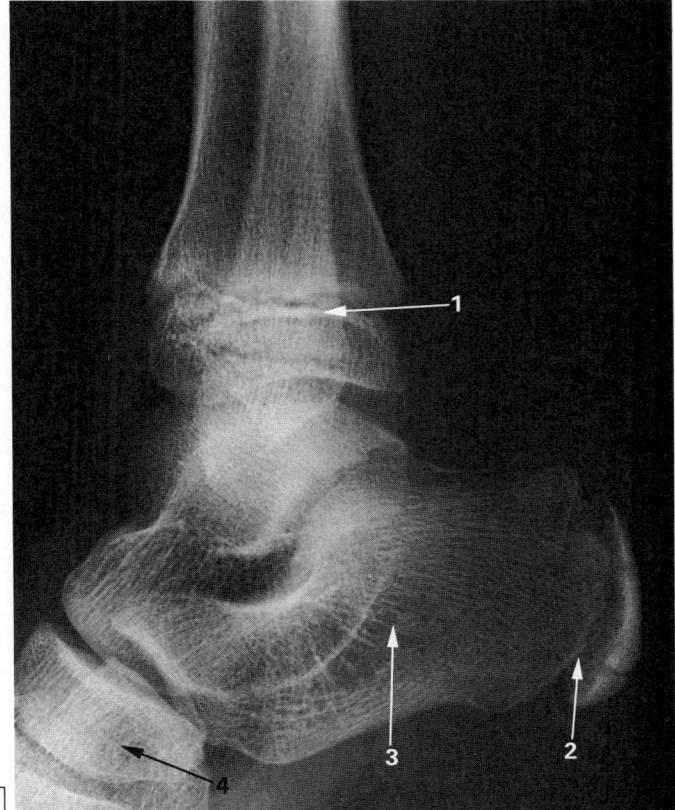

B

6.327   Ankle region of a child of 10 in plantarflexion. A. Obliquely antero-posterior. B. Lateral.

A. 1. Inferior growth cartilage of fibula. 2. Inferior growth cartilage of tibia. 3. Ankle joint. 4. Talus. Note that the fibular growth cartilage is approximately at the level of the ankle joint.

B. 1. Tibial growth cartilage. 2. Growth cartilage of epiphysis of posterior surface of calcaneous. 3. Note trabecular pattern in calcaneus. 4. Shadow of navicular bone superimposed on that of cuboid.

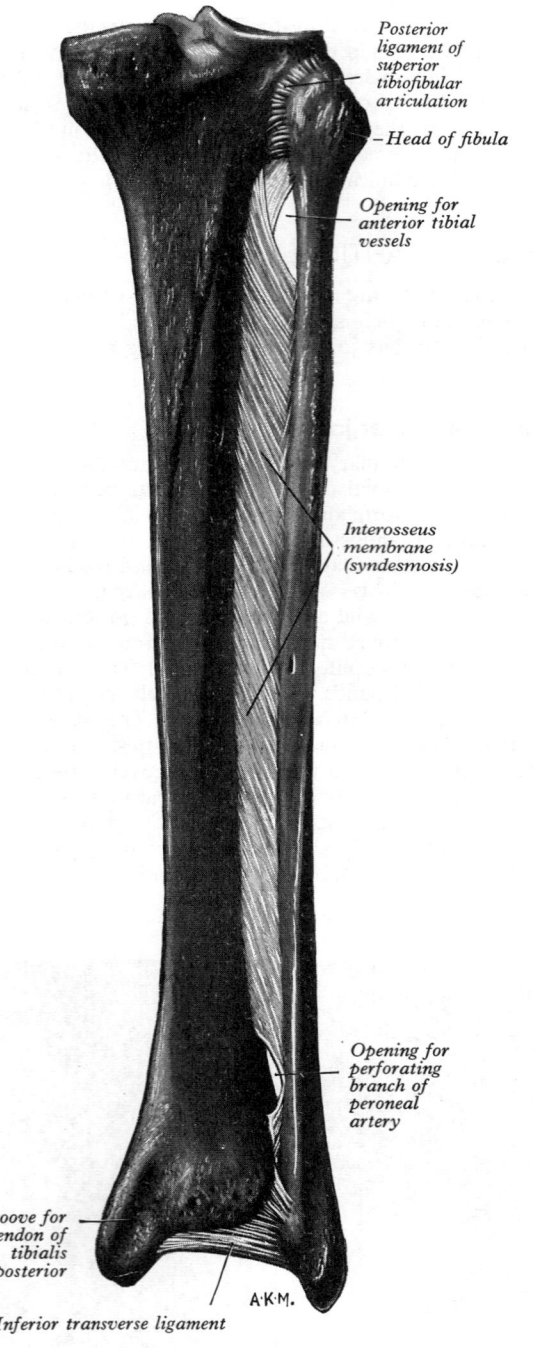

Posterior ligament of superior tibiofibular articulation

— Head of fibula

Opening for anterior tibial vessels

Interosseus membrane (syndesmosis)

Opening for perforating branch of peroneal artery

Groove for tendon of tibialis posterior

A·K·M.

Inferior transverse ligament

6.328 Posterior aspect of the interosseous membrane. Note the contrasting directions of fibre bundles around both vascular openings.

Interosseous membrane

The interosseous membrane (**6.328**) connects the interosseous borders of the tibia and fibula, separating the anterior and posterior muscles in the leg, some being attached to it. The anterior tibial artery passes forwards through a large oval opening near the membrane's proximal ends; distally the perforating branch of the peroneal artery pierces it. Its fibres, largely oblique, mainly descend laterally but a few descend medially including a bundle at the proximal border of the proximal opening. The membrane is continuous distally with the interosseous ligament of the distal tibiofibular joint. Anterior to it are tibialis anterior, extensors digitorum longus and hallucis longus, peroneus tertius, the anterior tibial vessels and deep peroneal nerve; posterior to it, tibialis posterior and flexor hallucis longus.

Distal tibiofibular joint

The distal tibiofibular joint is between the rough, medial **convex** surface on the distal end of the fibula and the rough **concave** surface of the fibular notch of the tibia, which are separated distally for about 4 mm by a synovial prolongation from the ankle joint and may be covered by articular cartilage in its lowest part. The joint is usually considered a syndesmosis (p. 488).

The anterior tibiofibular ligament (see **6.343**). A flat band, it descends laterally between the adjacent margins of the tibia and fibula, anterior to the syndesmosis.

The posterior tibiofibular ligament (see **6.340**). Stronger and disposed similarly on the posterior aspect of the syndesmosis, its distal, deep part is the *inferior transverse ligament*, a thick band of yellow fibres crossing from the proximal end of the lateral malleolar fossa to the posterior border of the tibial articular surface almost to the medial malleolus. The ligament projects distal to the bones, in contact with the talus. Its colour reflects its content of yellow elastic fibres.

Interosseous ligament. Continuous with the interosseous membrane, it contains many short bands between the rough adjacent tibial and fibular surfaces and is the strongest bond between the bones.

Vessels and nerve supply to the joint. Arteries are from the peroneal perforating branch and medial malleolar rami of the anterior and posterior tibial arteries. **Nerves** are from the deep peroneal, tibial and saphenous nerves.

Movements

The tibiofibular joints permit only slight movement. Due to the varying slope of the talar lateral malleolar surface, the fibula rotates laterally a little during dorsiflexion at the ankle (Barnett & Napier 1952), the bones being also slightly separated. Although slight bending or torsion of the fibular shaft might permit movements at the distal tibiofibular joint, the proximal probably also helps (p. 722).

ANKLE AND FOOT

Functionally the skeleton of the foot may be divided into tarsus, metatarsus and phalanges or digital bones. In this description the terms *plantar* and *dorsal*, which are self-explanatory, are used, anterior and posterior being inappropriate. The terms proximal and distal are also usually employed, with the same significance as in limbs generally. Rotation occurring in the early stages of development of the limbs (p. 613) explains that, whereas the thumb is the most lateral in the hand, the hallux (great toe) is the most medial in the foot. **Note**. These remarks are only valid with reference to the widely adopted descriptive Standard Anatomical Position.

TARSUS

The seven tarsal bones occupy the proximal half of the foot (**6.329, 330, 331**). The tarsus and carpus are homologous, but tarsal elements are larger to support and distribute weight. As in the carpus, tarsal bones are arranged in proximal and distal rows, but medially is a single intermediate tarsal element. The proximal row comprises the *talus* and *calcaneus*, the former's long axis inclined anteromedially and down, its distal head being medial to the calcaneus and at a higher level. The distal row contains, mediolaterally, *medial*, *intermediate* and *lateral cuneiforms* and the *cuboid*, which are roughly in parallel and form a transverse arch dorsally convex. Medially, the *navicular* is interposed between the talus and cuneiforms. Laterally, the calcaneus articulates with the cuboid.

The foot is at right angles to the leg in standing, with the tarsus and metatarsus arranged to form intersecting longitudinal and transverse arches. Hence thrust and weight are not transmitted from the tibia to the ground (or vice versa) directly through the tarsus, but are distributed through the tarsal and metatarsals to the ends of the longitudinal arches (p. 733). In this connection, the cancellous structure of tarsal bones has been reviewed by Sinha (1985). For description each tarsal bone is arbitrarily considered to be cuboidal in form with six surfaces.

STRUCTURE OF TARSAL BONES

The internal structure of tarsal bones has attracted relatively little

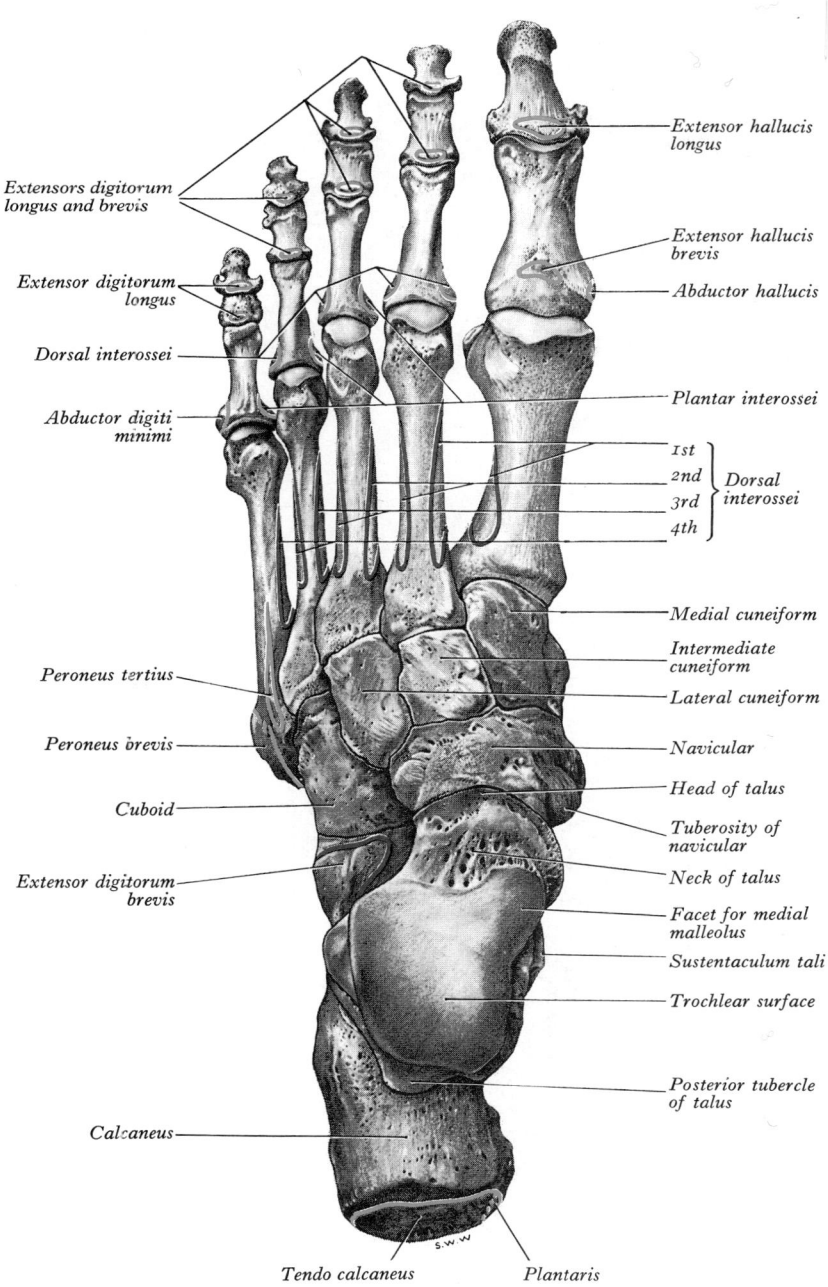

Extensors digitorum
longus and brevis

Extensor digitorum
longus

Dorsal interossei

Abductor digiti
minimi

Peroneus tertius

Peroneus brevis

Cuboid

Extensor digitorum
brevis

Calcaneus

Tendo calcaneus

Plantaris

Extensor hallucis
longus

Extensor hallucis
brevis

Abductor hallucis

Plantar interossei

1st
2nd Dorsal
3rd interossei
4th

Medial cuneiform

Intermediate
cuneiform

Lateral cuneiform

Navicular

Head of talus

Tuberosity of
navicular

Neck of talus

Facet for medial
malleolus

Sustentaculum tali

Trochlear surface

Posterior tubercle
of talus

6.329 Dorsal aspect of the skeleton of the left foot.

attention (Jones 1949). Sinha (1985), in a small series of 10 cadavers, has described the cancellous architecture of all seven bones. His observations emphasize the variation, from the mixed fine and coarse pattern of lamellae in the calcaneus, to the more widely spaced, thicker lamellae of the navicular, and he attempts to equate these appearances with functional stresses acting on these bones. The subject is of considerable kinematic and clinical interest and deserves further study. One such investigation (Bacon et al 1984), using a neutron beam technique on thin sections, shows how the orientation of hydroxyapatite crystals may be used to analyse the cancellous architecture and to associate this pattern with the effects of non-osseous structures, such as the plantar aponeurosis.

INDIVIDUAL TARSAL BONES

Talus

The talus (**6.332**) is the link between the foot and leg, through the ankle joint. Its rounded distal head, proximal trochlear surface for

the tibia, facet for the lateral malleolus, and its neck and body are its main features.

Head. Directed distally and somewhat inferomedially, it has a *distal surface*, oval and convex, with its long axis also inclined inferomedially to articulate with the proximal navicular surface. The *plantar surface* of the head has three articular areas, separated by smooth ridges; the most posterior and largest is oval, slightly convex and rests on a shelf-like medial calcanean projection, the *sustentaculum tali*. Anterolateral to this and usually continuous with it, a flat articular facet rests on the anteromedial part of the dorsal (proximal) calcanean surface; distally it continues into the navicular surface. Medial to these two calcanean facets a part of the talar head is covered with articular cartilage, continuous with the calcanean navicular areas (**6.332B**) and in contact with the *plantar cal-caneonavicular ligament* (p. 725) which is covered here, superiorly, by fibrocartilage. When the foot is inverted passively, the dorsolateral aspect of the head is visible and palpable about 3 cm distal to the tibia, but is hidden by extensor tendons when the toes are dorsiflexed.

Neck. This is the narrow region between the head and body, it is

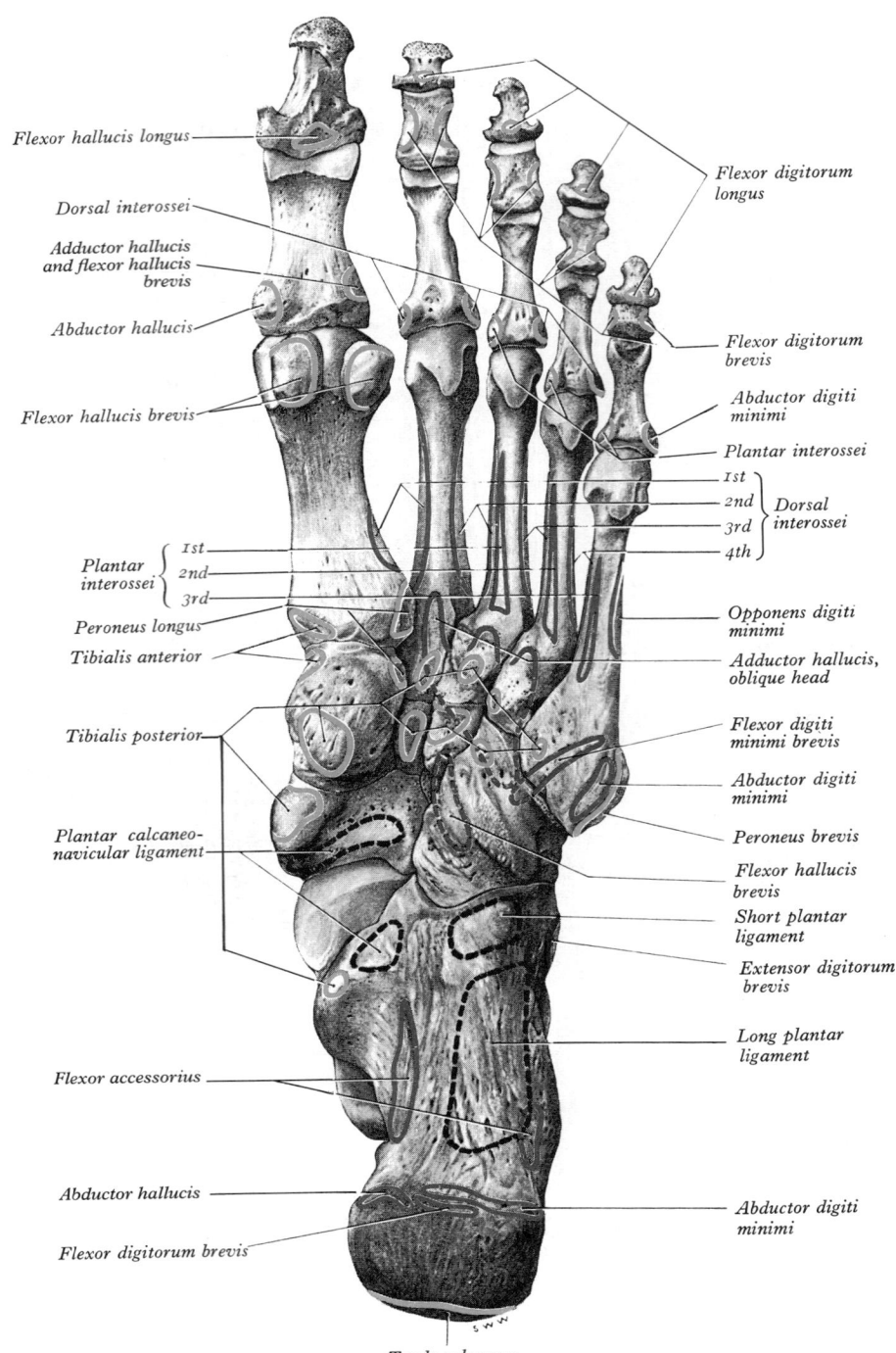

Flexor hallucis longus

Dorsal interossei

Adductor hallucis and flexor hallucis brevis

Abductor hallucis

Flexor hallucis brevis

Flexor digitorum longus

Flexor digitorum brevis

Abductor digiti minimi

Plantar interossei

1st
2nd } *Dorsal interossei*
3rd
4th

Plantar interossei { 1st 2nd 3rd

Peroneus longus

Tibialis anterior

Opponens digiti minimi

Adductor hallucis, oblique head

Flexor digiti minimi brevis

Abductor digiti minimi

Peroneus brevis

Flexor hallucis brevis

Short plantar ligament

Extensor digitorum brevis

Long plantar ligament

Tibialis posterior

Plantar calcaneo-navicular ligament

Flexor accessorius

Abductor hallucis

Flexor digitorum brevis

Abductor digiti minimi

Tendo calcaneus

6.330 Plantar aspect of the skeleton of the left foot. The attachments of tibialis posterior to the metatarsals vary, with those to the third and fifth sometimes being absent. The interrupted lines are the attachments of adductor hallucis (oblique head) and flexor hallucis brevis from ligamentous and tendinous extensions in the sole of the foot and not directly from the bone.

medially inclined. Its rough surfaces are for ligaments; the medial plantar surface has a deep *sulcus tali* which, when the talus and calcaneus are articulated, roofs the *sinus tarsi*, occupied by interosseous talocalcanean and cervical ligaments.

The *long axis of the neck*, inclined downwards, distally and medially, makes an angle of about 150° with that of the body; it is smaller (130°–140°) at birth (**6.333**), accounting in part for the inverted foot in young children. To its dorsal surface the dorsal talonavicular ligament and ankle articular capsule are attached distally, leaving its proximal part intracapsular. The medial articular facet and part of the trochlear surface may extend onto the neck, especially in childhood (**6.333**). A dorsolateral *squatting facet* commonly occurs on the neck in Indians, but seldom in adult Europeans, articulating with the anterior tibial margin in extreme dorsiflexion

(Barnett 1954; Singh 1959); the facet may be double. Laterally on the neck is attached the anterior talofibular ligament, spreading along the adjacent anterior border of the lateral surface. To the neck's inferior surface the interosseous talocalcanean and cervical ligaments are attached (p. 723).

Body. This is cuboidal, covered dorsally by a *trochlear surface* articulating with the tibia's distal end. It is anteroposteriorly convex, transversely gently concave, widest anteriorly and, therefore, sellar. The triangular *lateral surface* is smooth and vertically concave for articulation with the lateral malleolus. Superiorly it is continuous with the trochlear surface; inferiorly its apex is a *lateral process*. The *medial surface* is proximally (posterosuperiorly) covered by a comma-shaped facet, deeper in front and articulating with the medial malleolus, distal to which the surface is rough with numerous

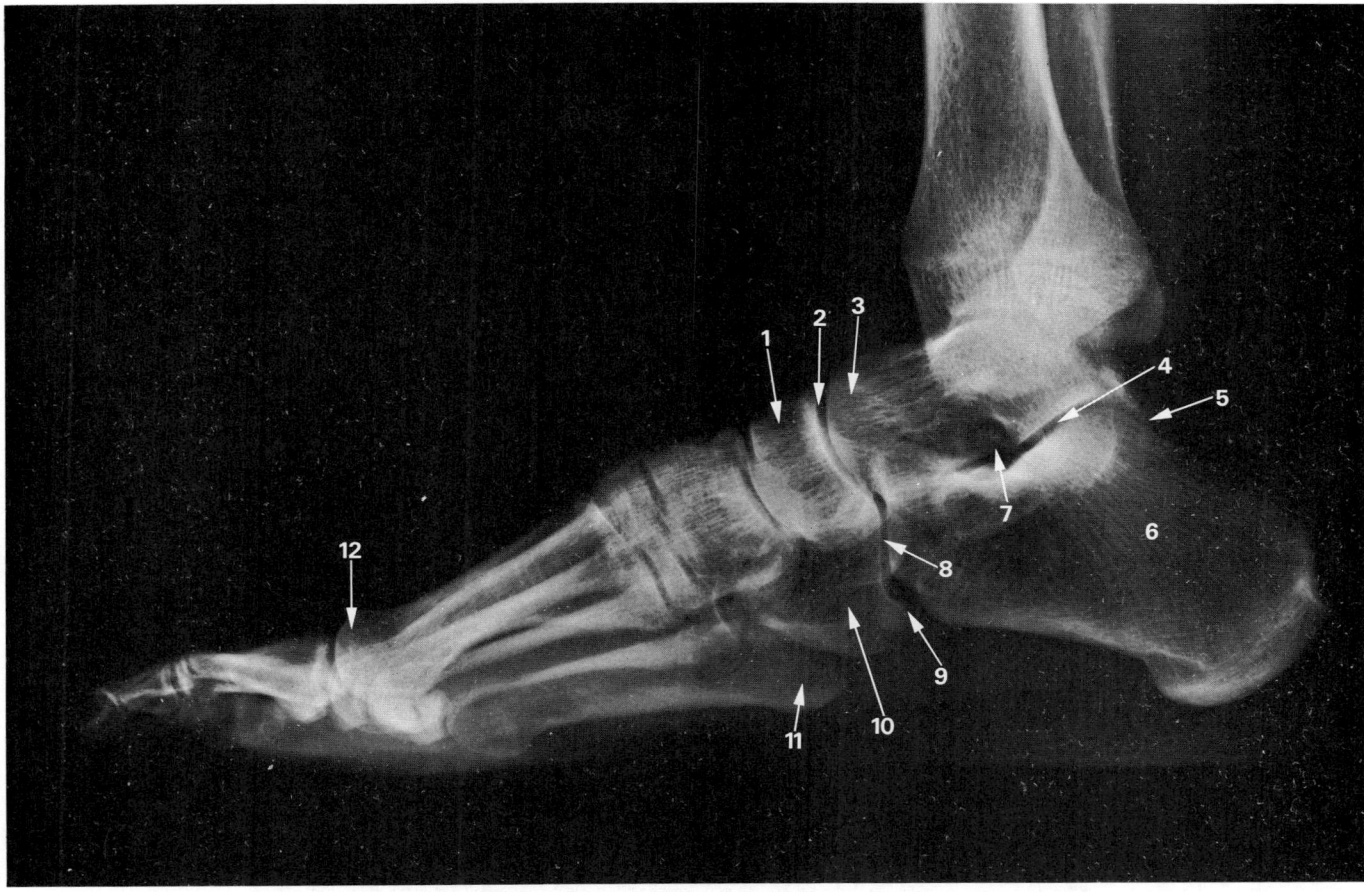

6.331A.   Lateral radiograph of ankle and foot in full plantigrade contact with the ground, during symmetrical standing, of a man aged 44 years. 1. Navicular. 2. Talonavicular joint. 3. Head of talus. 4. Subtalar joint. 5. Os trigonum. 6. Calcaneus. Note trabecular pattern. 7. Sinus tarsi. 8. Calcaneocuboid joint. 9. Sesamoid in tendon of peroneus longus. 10. Cuboid. 11. Tuberosity on base of fifth metatarsal. 12. Head of first metatarsal.

vascular foramina. The small *posterior surface* is the rough projecting *posterior process*, marked by an oblique groove between two tubercles; the *lateral tubercle* is usually larger, the *medial* less prominent and immediately behind the sustentaculum tali (see **6.334**). The plantar surface articulates with the middle third of the dorsal calcanean surface by an oval concave facet, its long axis directed distolaterally at an angle of about 45° with the median plane.

The *medial edge* of the trochlear surface is straight but its lateral edge inclines medially in its posterior part, often broadened into a small elongated triangular area, in contact with the posterior tibiofibular ligament in dorsiflexion.

To the posterior process is attached the posterior talofibular ligament, which extends up to the groove, or depression, between the process and posterior trochlear border. To its plantar border the posterior talocalcanean ligament is attached. The *groove* between the tubercles of the process contains the tendon of flexor hallucis longus, continuing distally into the groove on the plantar aspect of the sustentaculum tali. To the medial tubercle the medial talocalcanean ligament is attached below, whilst above the tubercle are attached the most posterior superficial fibres of the deltoid ligament; its deep fibres are attached still higher to the rough area immediately below the comma-shaped articular facet on the medial surface (**6.332c**).

No muscles but many ligaments (see **6.340, 342, 343**) are attached to the talus, since it is involved in ankle, subtalar and talocalcaneonavicular joints.

Mensuration. Sex differences in talar dry weight have been recorded (Singh & Singh 1975); the ranges in adult Indian males and females were 15.1 to 36.8 and 6.0 to 20.5 g, respective means being 23.50 and 15.32 g. Estimation of sex by dimensions has been claimed by Steele (1976).

Calcaneus

The calcaneus (**6.334**), the largest tarsal bone, projects posterior to the tibia and fibula as a short lever for muscles of the calf attached to its posterior surface. It is irregularly cuboidal, its long axis inclined distally upwards and laterally. Its smooth, articular anterior end contrasts with its larger, rough posterior aspect. The dorsal surface bears centrally a large articular facet and the plantar is rough; the lateral surface is flat, the medial hollowed.

The superior or proximal surface. This is divisible into three: the posterior third is rough, concavoconvex, the convexity transverse; it supports fibroadipose tissue between the calcanean tendon and ankle joint; the middle third carries the *posterior talar facet*, oval and convex anteroposteriorly; the anterior third is partly articular; distal (anterior) to the posterior articular facet a rough depression narrows into a groove on the medial side, the *sulcus calcanei*, which completes the sinus tarsi with the talus. Distal and medial to this groove an elongated articular area covers the sustentaculum tali, extending distolaterally on the bone's body. This facet is often divided by a non-articular interval at the anterior limit of the sustentaculum tali, forming *middle* and *anterior talar facets*, the incidence of which varies with sex and race. Rarely, all three facets on the upper surface of the calcaneus are fused into one irregular area (Bunning & Barnett 1963, 1965). A detailed analysis of patterns of **anterior** talar articular facets in a series of 401 Indian calcanei revealed four types. Type 1 (67%) showed one continuous facet on the sustentaculum extending to the distomedial calcanean corner; Type II (26%) presented two facets, one sustentacular, one distal calcanean; Type III (5%) possessed only a single sustentacular facet; and Type IV (2%) showed all anterior and posterior facets confluent.

The anterior surface. The smallest, it is an obliquely set concavoconvex articular facet for the cuboid.

The posterior surface. It is divided into three: a smooth proximal (superior) area separated from the tendo calcaneus by a bursa and adipose tissue; a middle area, the largest, limited above by a groove, below by a rough ridge, for the calcanean tendon; and a distal

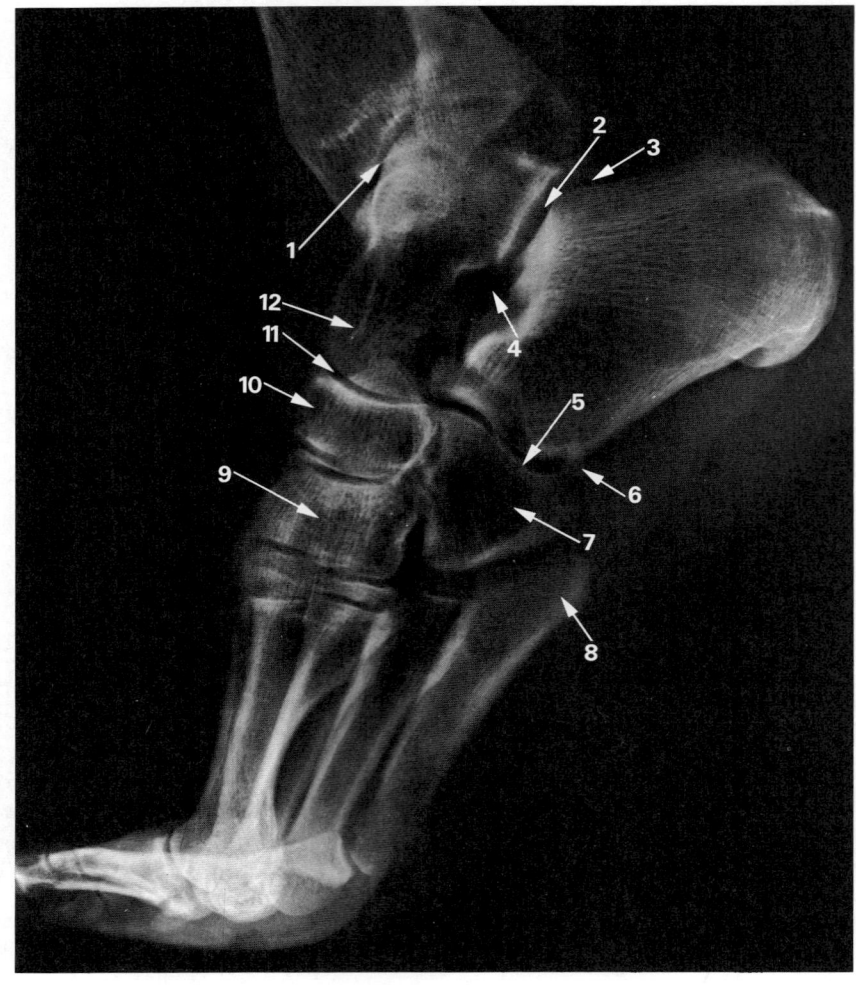

B

6.331B. The same foot as in A with heel raised from the ground, as near the end of the 'stance phase' in walking. Note the forward angulation of the leg bones, plantar flexion at the ankle joint and the position of the metatarsals and phalanges. 1. Ankle joint. 2. Subtalar joint. 3. Os trigonum. 4. Sinus tarsi. 5. Calcaneocuboid joint. 6. Sesamoid in peroneus longus tendon. 7. Cuboid. 8. Tuberosity on base of fifth metatarsal. 9. Cuneiforms. 10. Navicular. 11. Talonavicular joint. 12. Head of talus.

(inferior) area inclined downwards and forwards, vertically striated, which is the subcutaneous weight-bearing surface.

The plantar surface. This is rough, especially proximally, as the *calcanean tuberosity*, the *lateral* and *medial processes* of which extend distally, separated by a notch. The medial is longer and broader (**6.334B**). Further distally, an *anterior tubercle* marks the distal limit of the attachment of the long plantar ligament.

The lateral surface. Almost flat, it is proximally deeper and palpable on the lateral aspect of the heel distal to the lateral malleolus. Distally it presents the *peroneal trochlea* (*tubercle* **6.334C**), exceedingly variable in size and, when well developed, palpable 2 cm distal to the lateral malleolus. It has an oblique groove for the tendon of peroneus longus and a shallower proximal one for the tendon of peroneus brevis. About 1 cm or more behind and above the peroneal trochlea a second elevation may exist for attachment of the calcaneofibular part of the lateral ligament.

The medial surface. Vertically concave, its concavity is accentuated by the *sustentaculum tali* projecting medially from the distal part of its upper border (**6.334D**). Superiorly the process bears the middle talar facets and inferiorly a groove continuous with that on the talar posterior surface for the tendon of flexor hallucis longus (**6.334B**). The medial aspect of the sustentaculum tali can be felt immediately distal to the tip of the medial malleolus; occasionally it is also grooved by the tendon of flexor digitorum longus.

Further details. In the *calcanean sulcus* are attached the interosseous talocalcanean and cervical ligaments (p. 723) and the medial root of the inferior extensor retinaculum; the non-articular area distal to the posterior talar facet is the attachment of extensor

digitorum brevis (in part), the principal band of the inferior extensor retinaculum and the stem of the bifurcated ligament.

To the *medial process of the tuberosity*, at its prominent medial margin, abductor hallucis and the superficial part of the flexor retinaculum and, distally, the plantar aponeurosis and flexor digitorum brevis are all attached. To the *lateral process* is attached abductor digiti minimi, extending medially to the medial process. The rough region between the process proximally and extending to the anterior tubercle distally is the attachment of the long plantar ligament, whilst the tubercle and area distal to it is the attachment of the short plantar ligament. The lateral tendinous head of flexor accessorius is attached distal to the lateral process near the lateral margin of the long plantar ligament. To the *posterior surface*, which is wider below, and near the medial side of the tendo calcaneus, plantaris is attached. The anterior part of the *lateral surface* is crossed by the peroneal tendons, but is largely subcutaneous (p. 891). The calcaneofibular ligament is attached about 1–2 cm proximal to the peroneal trochlea, usually to a low rounded elevation.

The *sustentaculum tali* is dorsally part of the talocalcaneonavicular joint; its plantar surface is grooved by the tendon of flexor hallucis longus, margins of the groove giving attachment to the deep part of the flexor retinaculum. To the medial margin of the sustentaculum, which is narrow, rough and convex, the plantar calcaneonavicular ligament is attached distally (p. 725); proximally are attached a slip from the tendon of tibialis posterior, and superficial fibres of the deltoid and medial talocalcanean ligament. Distal to the attachment of the deltoid ligament the tendon of flexor digitorum longus is related to the margin of the sustentaculum and may groove it. Distal

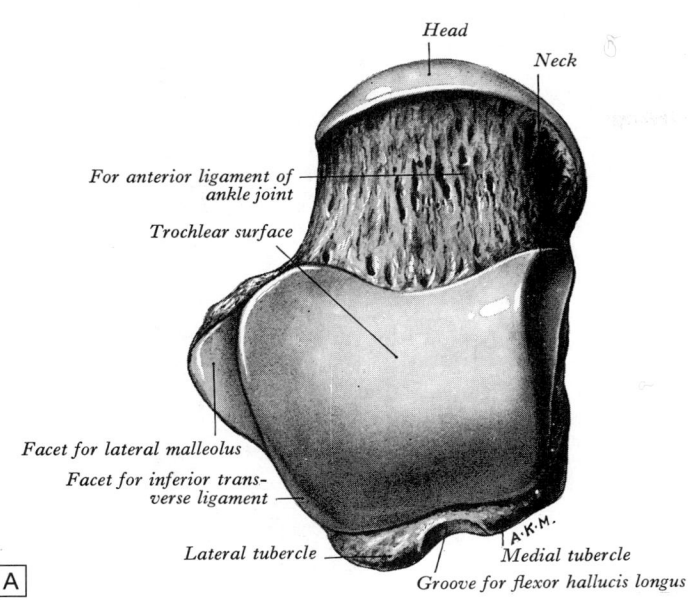

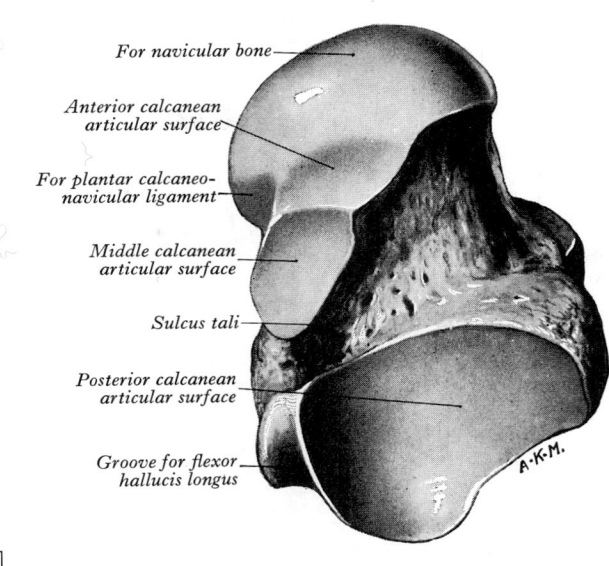

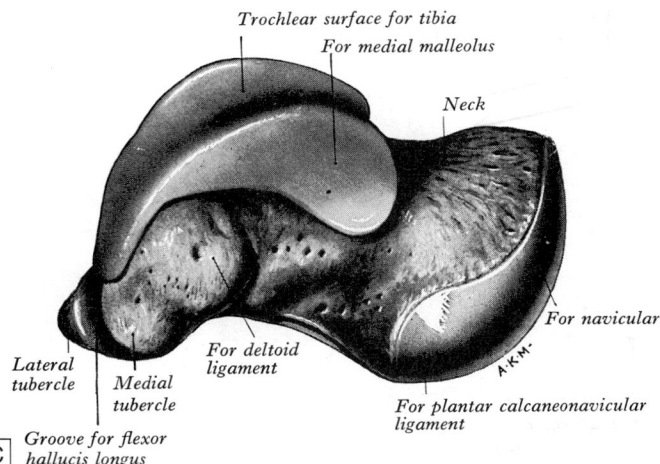

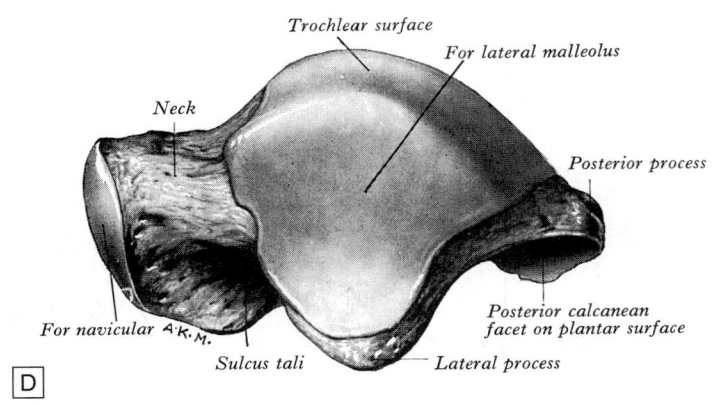

6.332 The left talus: A. Dorsal (superior) aspect; B. Plantar (inferior) aspect; C. Medial aspect; D. Lateral aspect.

to the groove for flexor hallucis longus the large medial head of flexor accessorius is attached.

Mensuration. Singh and Singh (1975) studied variations in calcanean dry weight in both sexes in adult Indians. The male range was 23.3 to 56.8 g (mean 36.64), and 13.0 to 33.0 g (mean 24.75) in females. Steele (1976) has claimed sex differentiation on dimensional data. Comparison of right and left calcanei in 52 adults (Webber & Garnett 1976) showed greater density on the side of hand preference; the evidence suggested that the concordance was determined before birth.

Navicular

The navicular (**6.335**) articulates between the talar head proximally and cuneiform bones distally. Its *distal surface* is transversely convex and divided into three facets (the medial being the largest) for articulation with the cuneiforms. The *proximal surface*, oval and concave, articulates with the talar head. The *dorsal surface* is rough and convex; the *medial*, also rough, continues into a prominent *tuberosity*, palpable about 2.5 cm distal and plantar to the medial malleolus. The *plantar surface*, rough and concave, is separated from the tuberosity medially by a groove. The *lateral surface* is rough, irregular and often bears a facet for articulation with the cuboid.

The facet for the medial cuneiform is roughly triangular, its rounded apex is medial and its 'base' often markedly curved; those for the intermediate and lateral cuneiforms are also triangular with plantar apices. The facet for the lateral cuneiform may approach a

wide crescent or a semicircle rather than a triangle (**6.335**A). To the dorsal navicular surface are attached dorsal talonavicular, cuneonavicular and cubonavicular ligaments. The tuberosity is the main attachment of tibialis posterior; a groove lateral to it transmits part of the tendon distally to the cuneiforms and middle three metatarsal bases. To a slight projection lateral to the groove and adjacent to the proximal surface the plantar calcaneonavicular ligament is

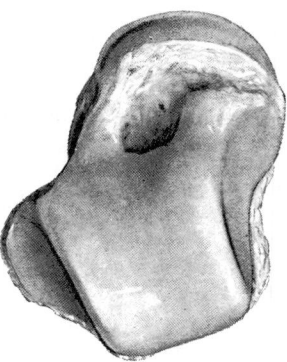

6.333 The left talus of a newborn infant: superior aspect. Compare with **6.332**A, and note the angle which the axis of the neck makes with the long axis of the body of the bone.

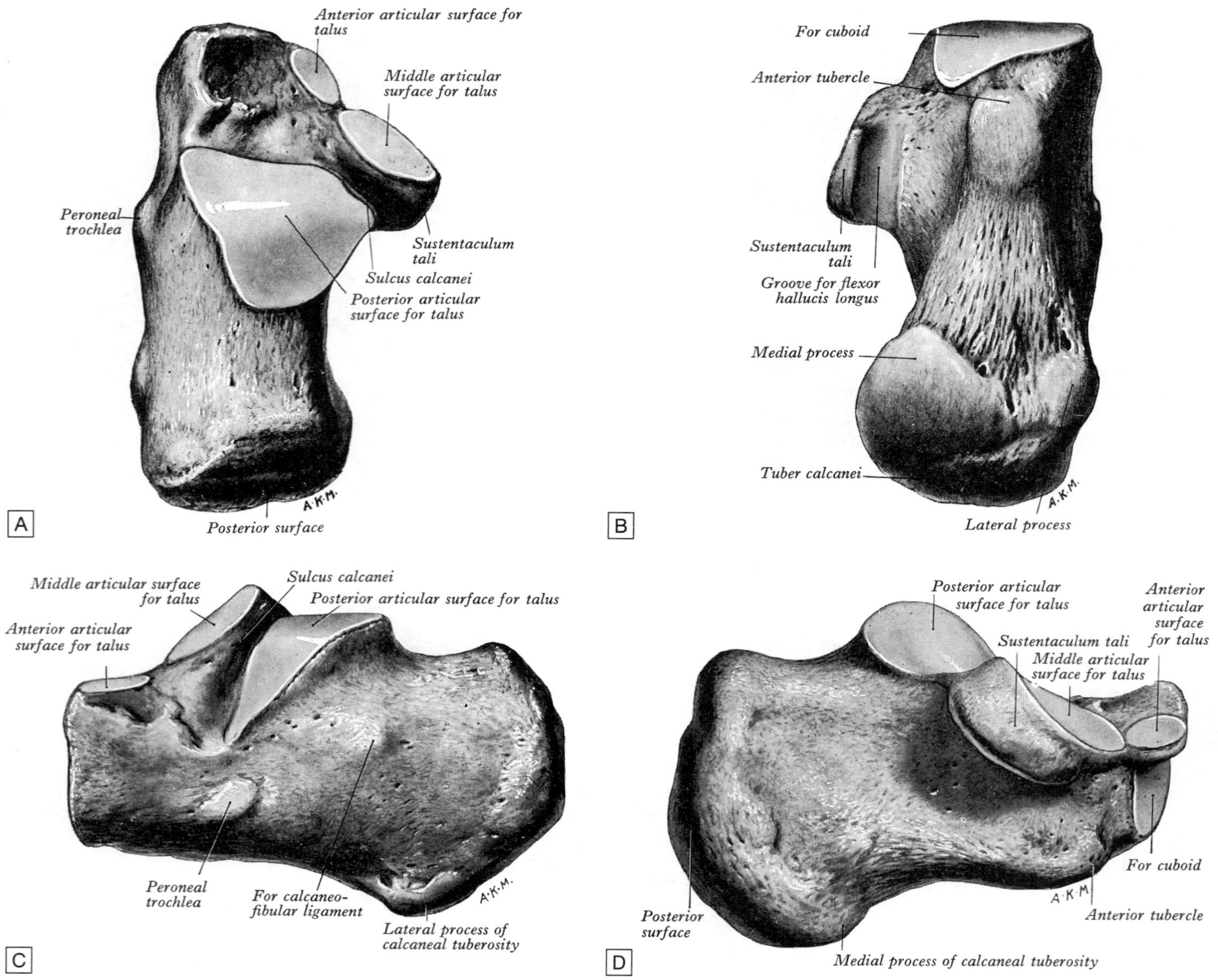

A

Anterior articular surface for talus

Middle articular surface for talus

Peroneal trochlea

Sustentaculum tali

Sulcus calcanei

Posterior articular surface for talus

Posterior surface

B

For cuboid

Anterior tubercle

Sustentaculum tali

Groove for flexor hallucis longus

Medial process

Tuber calcanei

Lateral process

C

Middle articular surface for talus

Sulcus calcanei

Posterior articular surface for talus

Anterior articular surface for talus

Peroneal trochlea

For calcaneo-fibular ligament

Lateral process of calcaneal tuberosity

D

Posterior articular surface for talus

Anterior articular surface for talus

Sustentaculum tali

Middle articular surface for talus

For cuboid

Anterior tubercle

Posterior surface

Medial process of calcaneal tuberosity

6.334 The left calcaneus: A. Dorsal aspect; B. Plantar aspect; C. Lateral aspect; D. Medial aspect.

attached. To the rough part of the lateral surface is attached the calcaneonavicular part of the bifurcated ligament.

Cuneiforms

The wedge-like cuneiform bones articulate with the navicular proximally and the bases of the first to third metatarsals distally; the medial is the largest, the intermediate smallest. In the intermediate and lateral cuneiforms the dorsal surface is the base of the wedge but in the medial the wedge is reversed, a prime factor in shaping the transverse arch. The proximal surfaces of all three form a concavity for the navicular, medial and lateral cuneiforms project distally beyond the intermediate, forming a recess for the second metatarsal base.

Medial cuneiform (6.336). Articulating with the navicular and first metatarsal base, it has a rough, narrow *dorsal surface*. The *plantar surface* receives a slip from the tendon of tibialis posterior. The *distal surface* is a reniform facet for the first metatarsal base, its 'hilum' being lateral. The *proximal surface* bears a piriform facet for the navicular, concave vertically, dorsally narrowed. The *medial surface*, rough and subcutaneous, is vertically convex; its distal–plantar angle carries a large impression for most of the tendon of tibialis anterior (6.336A). The *lateral surface* is partly non-articular; along its proximal and dorsal margins is a smooth right-angled strip for the intermediate cuneiform; its distal dorsal area is separated by

a vertical ridge from a small, almost square facet for the dorsal part of the medial surface of the second metatarsal base. Plantar to this the medial cuneiform is attached to the medial side of the second metatarsal base by a strong ligament. Proximally an interosseous intercuneiform ligament connects this surface to the intermediate cuneiform. The surface's distal and plantar area is roughened by attachment of part of the peroneus longus tendon (6.336B).

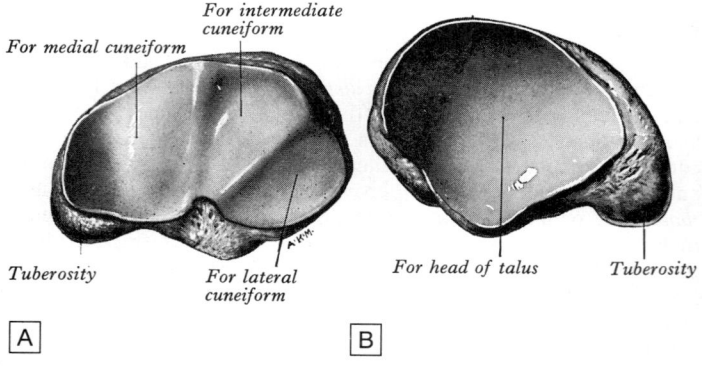

For medial cuneiform

For intermediate cuneiform

Tuberosity

For lateral cuneiform

For head of talus

Tuberosity

A

B

6.335 The left navicular: A. Distal aspect; B. Proximal aspect.

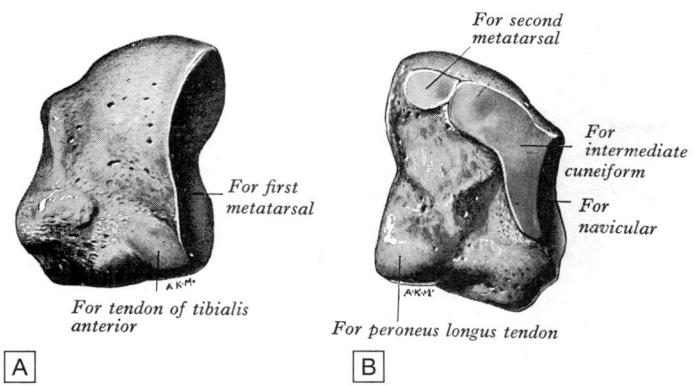

6.336 The left medial cuneiform: A. Medial aspect; B. Lateral aspect.

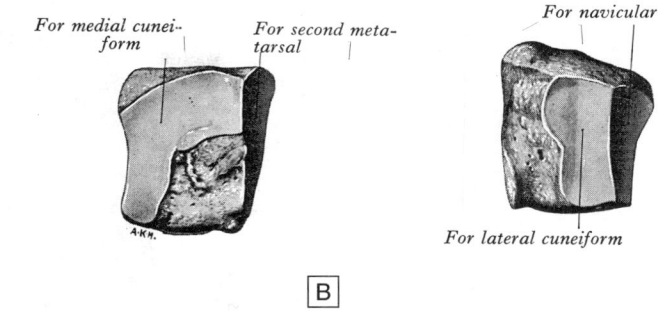

6.337 The left intermediate cuneiform: A. Distal and medial aspect; B. Proximal and lateral aspect.

Intermediate cuneiform (6.337). Articulating with the navicular and distally with the second metatarsal base, it has a narrow, *plantar surface* receiving a slip from the tendon of tibialis posterior. The *distal* and *proximal surfaces*, both triangular articular facets, articulate with the second metatarsal base and navicular respectively. The *medial surface* is partly articular; along its proximal and dorsal margins a smooth, angled strip, occasionally double, articulates with the medial cuneiform. The *lateral surface* also is partly articular; along its proximal margin a vertical strip, usually indented, abuts with the lateral cuneiform. Strong interosseous ligaments connect non-articular parts of both surfaces to adjacent cuneiforms.

Lateral cuneiform (6.338). This is between the intermediate cuneiform and cuboid, articulating also with the navicular and, distally, the third metatarsal base. Like the intermediate, its *dorsal surface*, rough and almost rectangular, is the base of the wedge. Its narrow *plantar surface* receives a slip from the tibialis posterior and sometimes part of the flexor hallucis brevis. The *distal surface* is a triangular articular facet for the third metatarsal base. The *proximal surface* is rough on its plantar aspect, but its dorsal two-thirds articulates with the navicular by a triangular facet. The *medial surface*, partly non-articular, has on its proximal margin a vertical strip, indented for the intermediate cuneiform; on its distal margin a narrower strip (often two small facets) articulates with the lateral side of the second metatarsal base. The *lateral surface*, also partly non-articular, has a triangular or oval proximal facet for the cuboid; a semilunar facet on its dorsal and distal margin articulates with the dorsal part of the medial side of the fourth metatarsal base. Non-articular areas of the medial and lateral surfaces receive intercuneiform and cuneocuboid ligaments, important in the transverse arch.

Cuboid

The cuboid (6.339), most lateral in the distal tarsal row, is between the calcaneus proximally and the fourth and fifth metatarsals distally. Its *dorsal surface*, really dorsolateral, is rough for the attachment of ligaments. The *plantar surface* is crossed distally by an oblique *groove* for the tendon of peroneus longus, bounded proximally by a ridge ending laterally in the *tuberosity of the cuboid*, the lateral aspect of which is faceted for a sesamoid bone or cartilage frequent in the

peroneal tendon. Proximal to its ridge the rough plantar surface, due to the obliquity of the calcaneocuboid joint, extends proximally and medially, making its medial border much longer than the lateral. The *lateral surface* is rough; from a deep notch on its plantar edge extends the groove for peroneus longus. The *medial surface*, much more extensive and partly non-articular, bears an oval facet for the lateral cuneiform and proximal to this another (sometimes absent) for the navicular, the two forming a continuous surface separated by a smooth vertical ridge. The *distal surface* is divided vertically into a medial quadrilateral articular area for the fourth metatarsal base and a lateral triangular area, its apex lateral, for the fifth metatarsal base. The *proximal surface*, triangular and concavoconvex, articulates with the distal calcanean surface; its medial–plantar angle projects proximally and inferior to the distal end of the calcaneus.

To the dorsal surface are attached dorsal calcaneocuboid, cubonavicular, cuneocuboid and cubometatarsal ligaments, and, to the proximal edge of the plantar ridge, deep fibres of the long plantar ligament. To the projecting proximomedial part of the plantar surface are attached a slip of the tendon of tibialis posterior and flexor hallucis brevis. To the rough part of the medial cuboidal surface are attached interosseous, cuneocuboid and cubonavicular ligaments, and proximally the medial calcaneocuboid, which is the lateral limb of the bifurcated ligament.

ANKLE (TALOCRURAL) JOINT

The joint is approximately uniaxial. The lower end of the tibia and its medial malleolus, with the lateral malleolus of the fibula and inferior transverse tibiofibular ligament, form a deep recess for the body of the talus. Its line is judged by the anterior margin of the tibia's distal end, which is palpable when the overlying tendons are relaxed. Although it appears a simple hinge, usually styled 'uniaxial',

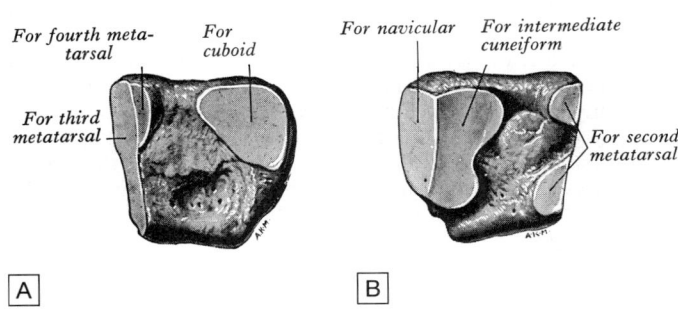

6.338 The left lateral cuneiform: A. Distal and lateral aspect; B. Proximal and medial aspect.

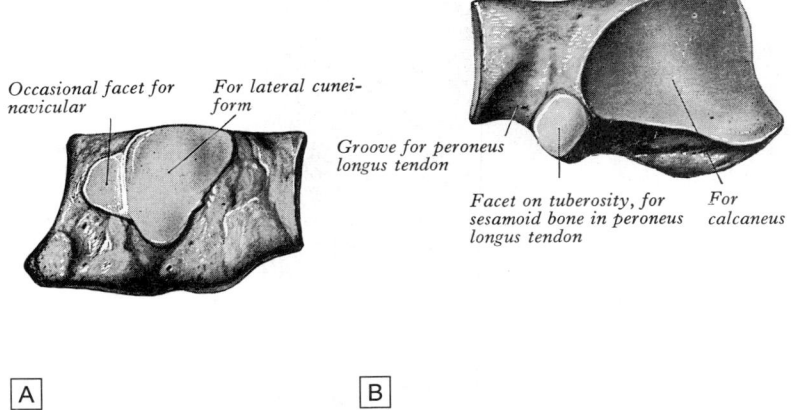

6.339 The left cuboid: A. Medial aspect; B. Proximal and lateral aspect.

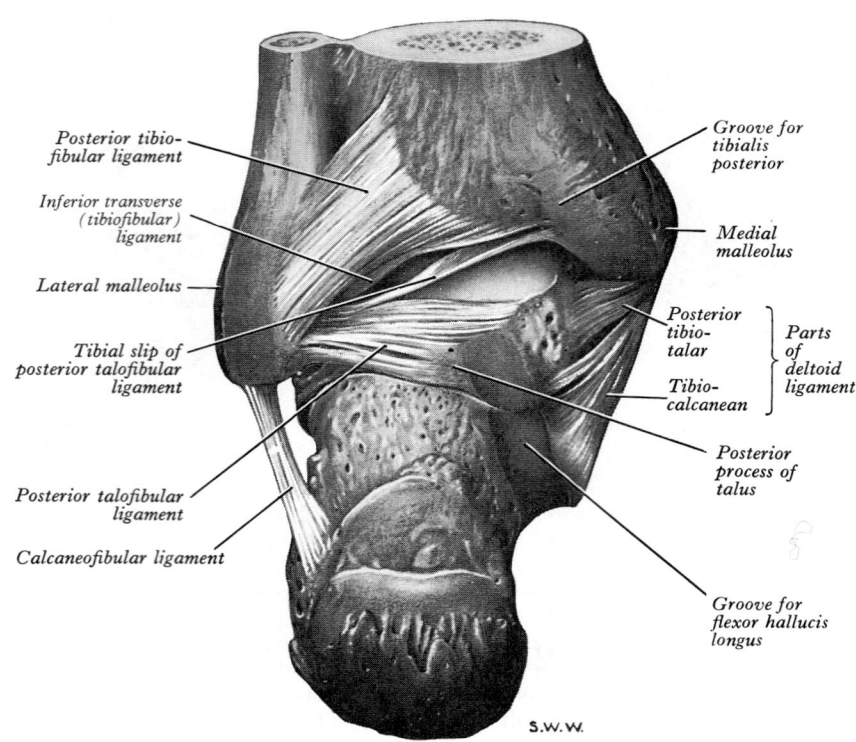

Posterior tibio-
fibular ligament

Inferior transverse
(tibiofibular)
ligament

Lateral malleolus

Tibial slip of
posterior talofibular
ligament

Posterior talofibular
ligament

Calcaneofibular ligament

Groove for
tibialis
posterior

Medial
malleolus

Posterior
tibio-
talar

Tibio-
calcanean

} Parts
of
deltoid
ligament

Posterior
process of
talus

Groove for
flexor hallucis
longus

S.W.W.

6.340   Posterior aspect of the left ankle joint. (Drawn from a specimen in
the Museum of the Royal College of Surgeons of England, with permission
from the Council.)

its axis of rotation is dynamic, shifting during dorsi- and plantar
flexion (Sammarco 1977; Jend et al 1985; Lundberg et al 1989).

Articular surfaces are covered by hyaline cartilage. The talar
trochlear surface, convex parasagittally, transversely gently concave,
is wider in front; the distal tibial articular surface is reciprocally
curved. The talar articular surface for the medial malleolus is a
proximal area on the medial talar surface, being fairly flat, comma-

shaped and anteriorly deeper. The larger lateral talar articular surface
is triangular and vertically concave, that on the lateral malleolus is
reciprocally curved. Posteriorly the edge between the trochlear and
fibular articular surfaces of the talus is bevelled to a narrow, flat
triangular area articulating with the inferior transverse tibiofibular
ligament (**6.**340): all surfaces are continuous. The bones are connected
by a fibrous capsule, *medial* (*deltoid*), *anterior* and *posterior talofibular*
and *calcaneofibular* ligaments.

Fibrous capsule

Around the joint this is thin in front and behind, attached proximally
to the borders of the tibial and malleolar articular surfaces and
distally to the talus near the margins of its trochlear surface,
except in front where it reaches the dorsum of the talar neck. It is
strengthened by strong collateral ligaments. Its posterior part is
mainly of transverse fibres. It blends with the inferior transverse
ligament and is thickened laterally where it reaches the fibular
malleolar fossa.

Synovial membrane. Lining the capsule, it ascends as a short
vertical recess between the tibia and fibula (**6.**341).

Medial ligament (deltoid collateral) (6.342)

This is a strong, triangular band, attached to the apex and the
anterior and posterior borders of the medial malleolus. Of its
superficial fibres the anterior (*tibionavicular*) pass forwards to the
navicular tuberosity and behind this blend with the medial margin of
the plantar calcaneonavicular ligament; intermediate (*tibiocalcaneal*)
fibres descend almost vertically to the whole length of the sustentaculum tali; posterior fibres (*posterior tibiotalar*) pass posterolaterally to the medial side of the talus and its medial tubercle.
The *deep fibres* (*anterior tibiotalar*) pass from the tip of the medial
malleolus to the non-articular part of the medial talar surface. The
ligament is crossed by the tendons of tibialis posterior and flexor
digitorum longus.

Lateral ligament

This comprises discrete parts. The *anterior talofibular ligament* (**6.**343)
extends anteromedially from the anterior margin of the fibular
malleolus to the talus, attached in front of its lateral articular facet

Interosseous ligament of
inferior tibiofibular
syndesmosis

Medial malleolus

Body of talus

Deltoid ligament

Tendon of tibialis
posterior

Sustentaculum tali

Tendon of flexor digit-
orum longus

Tendon of flexor hallucis
longus

Lateral malleolus

Posterior talofibular
ligament

Interosseous talo-
calcanean ligament

Body of calcaneus

Tendon of peroneus brevis

Tendon of peroneus longus

720   **6.**341   Coronal section through the left ankle and talocalcaneal joints.

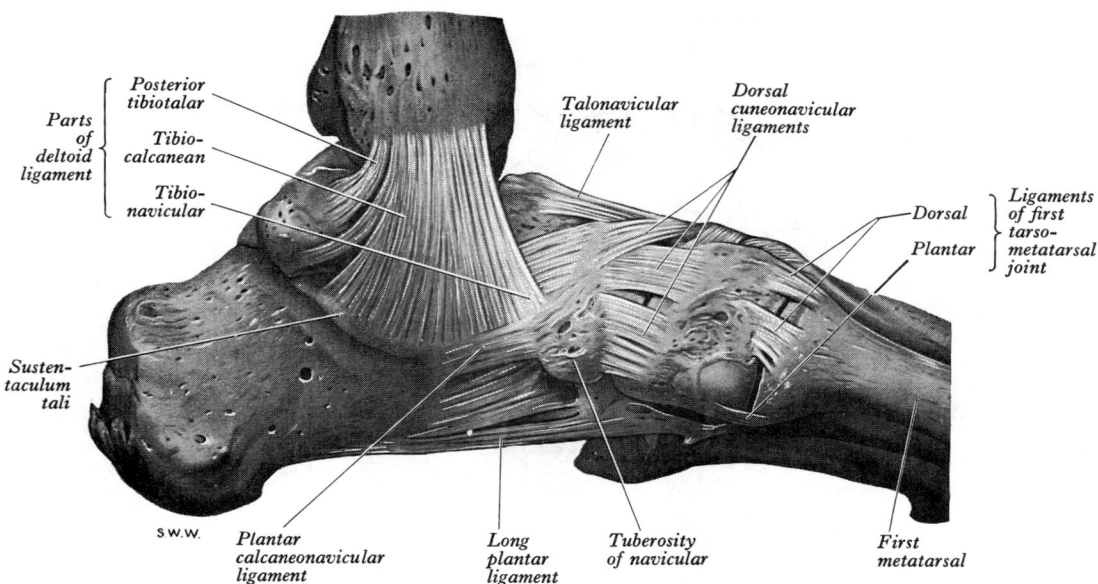

6.342 Medial aspect of the left ankle and tarsal joints. (Drawn from a specimen in the Museum of the Royal College of Surgeons of England, with permission from the Council.)

and to the lateral aspect of its neck. The *posterior talofibular ligament* (**6.340**) runs almost horizontally from the distal part of the lateral malleolar fossa to the lateral tubercle of the posterior talar process. A 'tibial slip' of fibres connects it to the medial malleolus. The *calcaneofibular ligament* (**6.343**), a long cord, runs from a depression anterior to the apex of the fibular malleolus to a tubercle on the lateral calcaneal surface and is crossed by the tendons of peroneus longus and brevis.

Relations

Anteriorly, from the medial side, are tibialis anterior, extensor hallucis longus, the anterior tibial vessels, deep peroneal nerve, extensor digitorum longus and peroneus tertius; **posteriorly** from the medial side, are tibialis posterior, flexor digitorum longus, the posterior tibial vessels, tibial nerve, flexor hallucis longus; in the groove behind

the lateral malleolus are the tendons of peroneus longus and brevis (**6.344**).

Vessels and nerve supply to the joint

Arteries are from malleolar rami of the anterior tibial and peroneal arteries. **Nerves** are from the deep peroneal and tibial nerves.

Movements

When the body is upright and the foot at right angles to the leg, *active movements* of the joint are dorsiflexion (*c.* 10°) and plantar flexion (*c.* 20°), the former moving the dorsum of the foot towards the anterior calf thereby decreasing the angle between the leg and foot, the latter moving the dorsum away from the anterior calf. Dorsiflexion is the 'close-packed' position, with maximal congruence and ligamentous tension; from this position all major thrusting

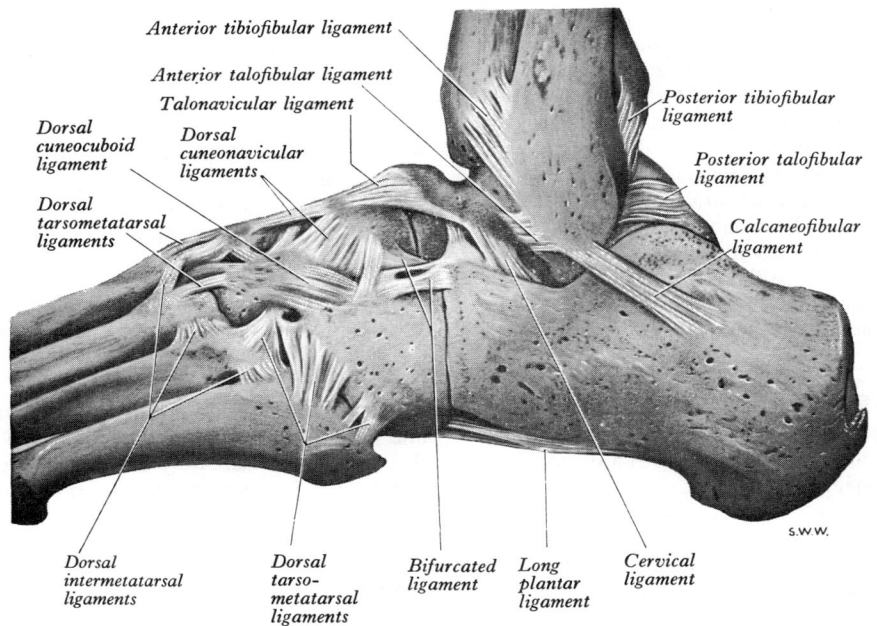

6.343 Lateral aspect of the left ankle and tarsal joints. (Drawn from a specimen in the Museum of the Royal College of Surgeons of England, with permission from the Council.)

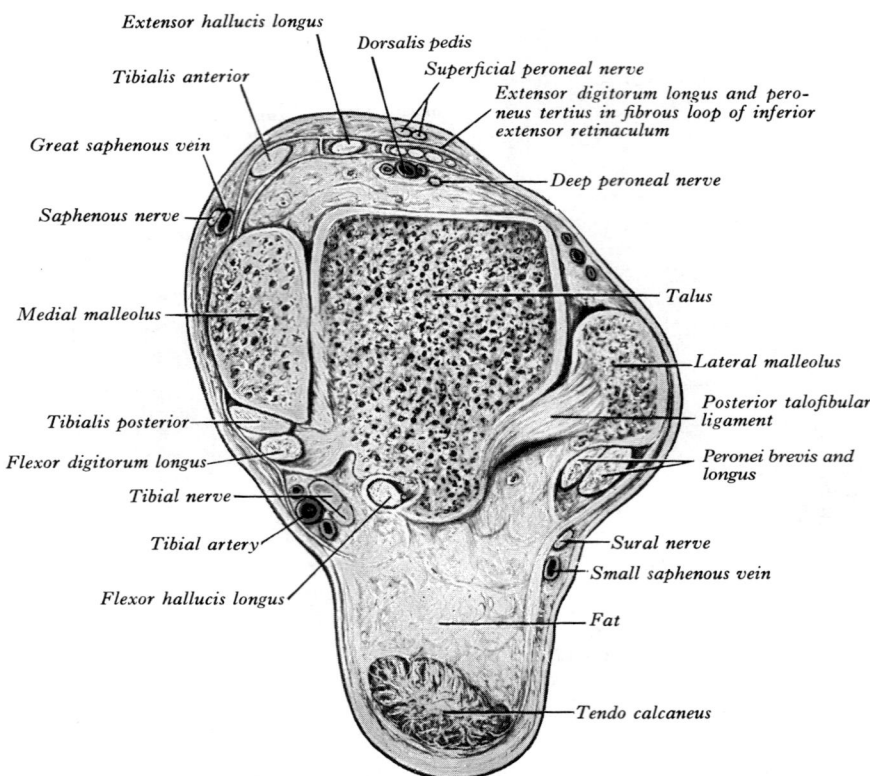

Extensor hallucis longus

Dorsalis pedis

Tibialis anterior

Superficial peroneal nerve

*Extensor digitorum longus and pero-
neus tertius in fibrous loop of inferior
extensor retinaculum*

Great saphenous vein

Deep peroneal nerve

Saphenous nerve

Talus

Medial malleolus

Lateral malleolus

*Posterior talofibular
ligament*

Tibialis posterior

Flexor digitorum longus

*Peronei brevis and
longus*

Tibial nerve

Tibial artery

Sural nerve

Small saphenous vein

Flexor hallucis longus

Fat

Tendo calcaneus

6.344   Transverse section through the lower part of the right ankle joint:
superior aspect.

movements are exerted, in walking, running and jumping. The
malleoli embrace the talus; even in relaxation no appreciable lateral
movement can occur without stretch of the inferior tibiofibular
syndesmosis and slight bending of the fibula. The superior talar
surface is broader in front, and in dorsiflexion the malleolar gap is
increased by slight lateral rotation of the fibula by 'give' at the inferior
tibiofibular syndesmosis and gliding at the superior tibiofibular joint.
The medial (deltoid) ligament is very strong and is even able to resist
forces which tear the bone to which it is attached. Its middle part,
with the calcaneofibular ligament, binds the leg firmly to the foot,
resisting displacement in all directions. The posterior talofibular
ligament assists the calcaneofibular in resisting posterior displacement, deepening the joint for the talus. The anterior talofibular
ligament limits anterior displacement. Plantarflexion is limited by
the opposing muscles, the anterior fibres of the medial (deltoid) and
the anterior talofibular ligaments. Dorsiflexion is limited by the
tendocalcaneus and contraction of triceps surae, the posterior fibres
of the medial (deltoid) and the calcaneofibular ligaments (**6**.344).
Dorsi- and plantarflexion are increased by intertarsal movements,
adding about 10° to the former, 20° to the latter.

Accessory movements. Slight amounts of side-to-side gliding,
rotation, abduction and adduction are permitted, when the foot is
plantarflexed.

Muscles producing movement

(see also pp. 883–890, 897–900.)
Dorsiflexion: tibialis anterior, assisted by extensors digitorum longus
and hallucis longus, and peroneus tertius.
Plantarflexion: gastrocnemius and soleus, assisted by plantaris,
tibialis posterior, flexors hallucis longus and digitorum longus.

In symmetrical standing the line of body weight is anterior to the
ankle joints, which are not even near their close-packed position.
Stability requires continuous action by soleus, increasing (often
involving gastrocnemius) with leaning forward and vice versa. If
backward sway takes the projection of the centre gravity ('weight
line') posterior to the transverse axes of the ankle joints, the plantar
flexors relax and the dorsiflexors contract.

Clinical anatomy

Owing to its depth the ankle joint is rarely dislocated without
malleolar fracture. So-called sprains of the joint are almost always
abduction sprains of *subtalar joints*, although some medial (deltoid)
fibres may also be torn. True sprains are usually due to forcible
plantarflexion, resulting in capsular tears in front (most commonly
of the anterior talofibular ligament) and bruising by impaction of
structures behind the joint. In ankylosis the optimal position is slight
plantarflexion.

Compressive forces transmitted across the joint during gait reach
five times body weight while tangential shear forces, the result of
internally rotating muscle forces and externally rotating inertial
forces associated with the body moving over the foot, may reach
80% body weight (Stauffer et al 1977). For most of the stance
phase the tangential shear is directed forwards. The load distributed
through the fibula with the ankle in the neutral position has been
reported as 7% of the total force transmitted across the joint (Goh
et al 1992); fibula resection will therefore markedly increase the load
borne by the tibia.

INTERTARSAL JOINTS

Subtalar (talocalcaneal) joint

There are anterior and posterior articulations between the calcaneus
and talus, forming a functional unit often termed the 'subtalar joint';
this term is used here only for the posterior articulation, the anterior
being treated as part of the talocalcaneonavicular joint.

The subtalar joint proper involves the **concave** posterior calcaneal
facet on the posterior part of the inferior surface of the talus and
the **convex** posterior facet on the superior surface of the calcaneus
(**6**.345). The joint is modified multiaxial and its permitted movements
are considered together with those at other tarsal joints. The bones
are connected by a fibrous capsule, *lateral, medial, interosseous
talocalcaneal* and *cervical* ligaments.

Fibrous capsule. It envelops the joint, its fibres being short
and attached to its articular margins; it is split into slips, between

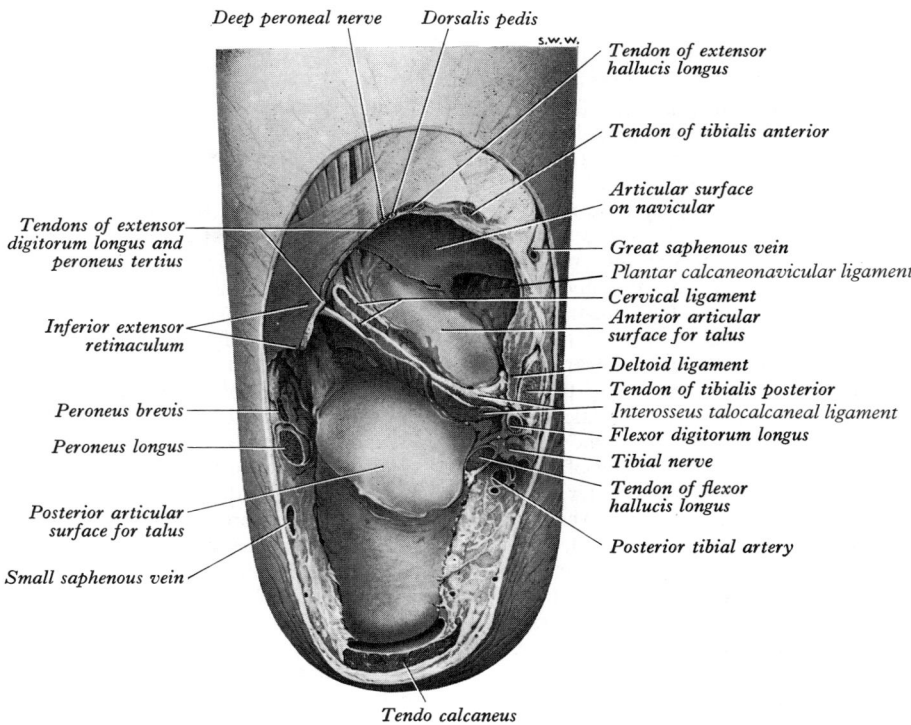

Deep peroneal nerve   Dorsalis pedis
s.w.w.
Tendon of extensor
hallucis longus

Tendon of tibialis anterior

Articular surface
on navicular

Tendons of extensor
digitorum longus and
peroneus tertius

Great saphenous vein
Plantar calcaneonavicular ligament
Cervical ligament
Anterior articular
surface for talus

Inferior extensor
retinaculum

Deltoid ligament
Tendon of tibialis posterior
Interosseus talocalcaneal ligament
Flexor digitorum longus
Tibial nerve
Tendon of flexor
hallucis longus

Peroneus brevis

Peroneus longus

Posterior articular
surface for talus

Posterior tibial artery

Small saphenous vein

Tendo calcaneus

6.345 Left talocalcaneal and talocalcaneonavicular joints. Exposed from above by removal of the talus.

which it is thin; its synovial membrane is separate from other tarsal joints.

Lateral talocalcaneal ligament. A short flat fasciculus, it descends obliquely back from the lateral talar process to the lateral calcaneal surface and is attached anterosuperior to the calcaneofibular ligament.

Medial talocalcaneal ligament. This connects the medial talar tubercle to the back of the sustentaculum tali and adjacent medial surface of the calcaneus. Its fibres blend with the medial (deltoid) ligament, the most posterior fibres lining the groove for flexor hallucis longus between the talus and calcaneus.

Interosseous talocalcaneal ligament (6.341, 345). A broad, flat, bilaminar transverse band in the sinus tarsi, it descends obliquely and laterally from the sulcus tali to sulcus calcanei. Its medial fibres are taut in eversion. The ligament's posterior lamina is associated with the talocalcanean joint, its anterior lamina with the talocalcaneonavicular joint (see below).

Cervical ligament (6.343). Just lateral to the sinus tarsi and attached to the superior calcaneal surface, it is medial to the attachment of extensor digitorum brevis, whence it ascends medially to an inferolateral tubercle on the talar neck (Barclay-Smith 1896; Smith 1958). It is considered to be taut in inversion.

Movements. Between the talus and calcaneus movements accompany those at the talocalcaneonavicular joint and will be described with that joint.

Talocalcaneonavicular joint

The talocalcaneonavicular joint, a compound articulation, is multiaxial; the ovoid talar head is continuous with the triple-faceted anterior area of its inferior surface (p. 714) and the whole fits the concavity formed by the posterior surface of the navicular, the middle and anterior talar facets of the calcaneus and the superior fibrocartilaginous surface of the plantar calcaneonavicular ligament. The reverse of the subtalar joint, the proximal talocalcaneonavicular surface is **convex**. The joint's position is judged by the talar head, visible and palpable about 3 cm anterior to the lower end of the tibia, with the foot passively inverted. The bones are connected by a fibrous capsule and three ligaments: *talonavicular*, *plantar calcaneonavicular* and the *calcaneonavicular part* of the *bifurcated ligaments*.

Fibrous capsule. This is poorly developed, except posteriorly, where it is thick and is the anterior part of the interosseous ligament filling the sinus tarsi.

Talonavicular ligament (6.342, 343). A broad, thin band, it connects the dorsal surfaces of the neck of the talus and the navicular; it is covered by extensor tendons. The plantar calcaneonavicular ligament (p. 725) and the calcaneonavicular part of the bifurcated ligament (6.343) are the joint's plantar and lateral ligaments respectively.

Movements

Gliding and rotation occur at the subtalar and talocalcaneonavicular joints, by which the calcaneus and navicular, carrying the **non-weight-bearing** foot, rotate medially on the talus, thus elevating the medial and depressing the lateral border of the foot, bringing its plantar aspect medial. This is *inversion*, occurring mainly at the subtalar joint and the complex articulation between the talar head, with its plantar extensions, and the sustentaculum tali, calcaneus, plantar calcaneonavicular ligament and posterior navicular surface. The joint surfaces are reciprocally curved but in opposite directions in the two joints, and movements at them have been likened to those between the radius and ulna at the superior and inferior radio-ulnar joints. This axis joins their approximate centres of curvature, ascending anteromedially from the back of the calcaneus, crossing the sinus tarsi obliquely to reach the superomedial aspect of the talar neck (Shepard 1951). Axial obliquity explains, in part, the adduction and slight plantarflexion of the foot (but to a greater degree the forefoot) in inversion. Movement of the calcaneus around the talus, however, also involves movement at the *transverse tarsal articulation* (talonavicular and calcaneocuboid joints); forefoot range is thereby increased. These joints are almost in one transverse plane; during inversion the navicular rotates on the talar head, while the cuboid glides down and rotates at the sellar calcaneocuboid joint. The range of inversion is further increased in plantar flexion; the narrow part of the talar trochlear surface now occupies the tibiofibular mortice and slight talar movement increases adduction with inversion. The opposite movement, more limited in range, is *eversion*.

Inversion is chiefly checked by the peroneal muscles and the lateral part of the interosseous talocalcaneal ligament. The other tarsal interosseous ligaments and the calcaneofibular ligament are less powerful factors. Eversion is arrested by tibialis anterior and the posterior and medial (deltoid) ligament.

The complex actions of inversion and eversion described above refer to changes in the whole foot (with minor movements of the talus), when it is **off the ground**. The fully inverted foot is also plantarflexed; conversely, eversion is linked with dorsiflexion. When the foot is **transmitting weight** or thrust these movements are modified to maintain plantigrade contact. The distal tarsus and metatarsus are *pronated* or *supinated* relative to the talus, pronation involving a downward rotation of the medial border and hallux; supination being the reverse, both bring the lateral border into plantigrade contact. Further, when there is *angulation* of the tibia and fibula in the coronal plane, either laterally but particularly medially, these bones and their distal mortice carry the talus with them in their movements. The talus tilts (rotates) around the oblique transarticular intercentroid axis (described above) at first, relative to the rest of the subtalar foot and moving at the subtalar and talocalcaneonavicular joints. When close-packing occurs between the talus and calcaneus, further angulation is accompanied by tilting of the functional unit of the combined talus **and** calcaneus, the latter involving the calcaneocuboid joint. Unfortunately, the terms inversion and eversion are often confused with pronation and supination, the latter being **components** of the former, like the slight adduction and abduction which may accompany inversion and eversion. Supination and pronation can be dissociated from inversion and eversion in adaptation of the forefoot in plantigrade stance or progression (pp. 733–735, 897–900).

Terminology of foot movements is somewhat confused amongst orthopaedists, kinesiologists and others. The above account represents widely accepted usage (MacConaill 1950; Kapandji 1970; MacConaill & Basmajian 1977). According to Kapandji (1970), inversion is a combination of adduction and supination, with eversion involving abduction and pronation.

Muscles producing movement. *Inversion*: tibialis anterior and posterior.

Eversion: peroneus longus and brevis.

Calcaneocuboid joint

The articular surfaces of the calcaneocuboid joint, which is 2 cm proximal to the tubercle, on the fifth metatarsal base, are sellar. Its ligaments are: the fibrous capsule, *calcaneocuboid part* of the *bifurcated ligament*, the *long plantar* and *plantar calcaneocuboid* ligaments.

Fibrous capsule. This is thickened dorsally as the *dorsal calcaneocuboid ligament*. The synovial membrane is distinct from other tarsal articulations (6.346).

Bifurcate ligament (6.343). A strong Y-shaped band, it is attached by its stem proximally to the anterior part of the upper calcaneal surface; distally it divides into calcaneocuboid and calcaneonavicular parts. The (*medial*) *calcaneocuboid ligament* extends to the dorsomedial aspect of the cuboid, forming a main bond between the two rows of tarsal bones; the (*lateral*) *calcaneonavicular ligament* is attached to the dorsolateral aspect of the navicular.

The long plantar ligament (6.343, 347, 348). The longest ligament associated with the tarsus, it extends from the plantar surface of the calcaneus (anterior to its tuberosity's processes) and from its anterior tubercle, to the ridge and tuberosity on the cuboid's plantar surface, to which deep fibres are attached, more superficial fibres continuing to the bases of the second to fourth and sometimes fifth metatarsals. This ligament, with the groove on the cuboid's plantar surface, makes a tunnel for the tendon of peroneus longus. It is a most powerful factor limiting depression of the lateral longitudinal arch (p. 734).

Plantar calcaneocuboid ligament. This *short plantar ligament* (6.348) is deeper than the long plantar ligament, from which it is separated by areolar tissue. It is a short, wide band of great strength, stretching from the anterior calcaneal tubercle and the depression anterior to it to the adjoining part of the plantar surface of the cuboid; it also sustains the lateral longitudinal arch.

Movements. Movements between the calcaneus and cuboid are gliding with conjunct rotation upon each other during inversion and eversion of the whole foot and during pronative or supinative changes between the fore- and hindfoot (pp. 733–735).

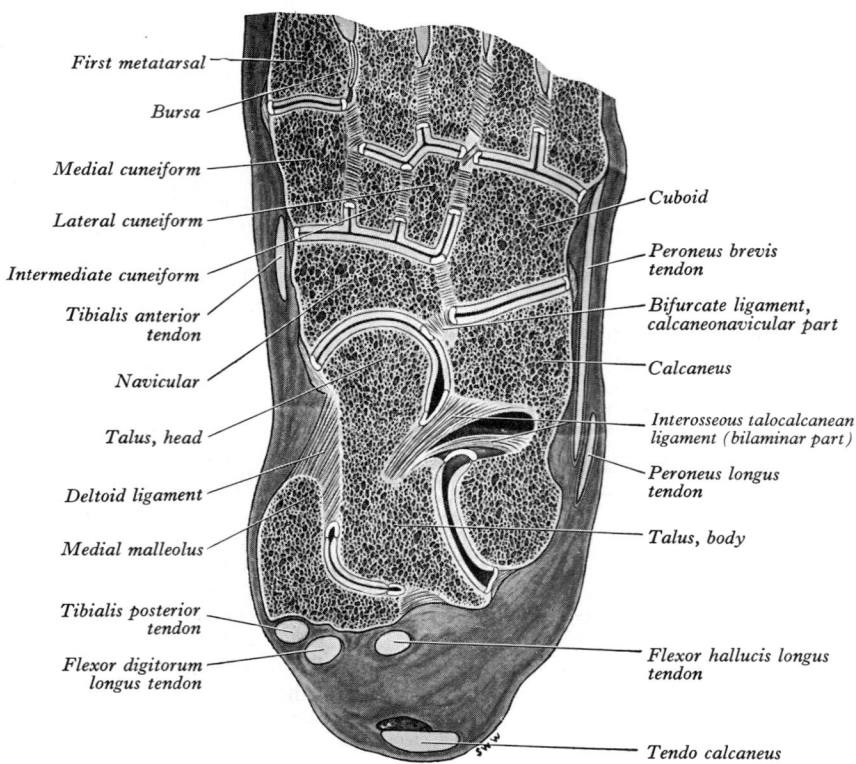

First metatarsal
Bursa
Medial cuneiform
Lateral cuneiform
Intermediate cuneiform
Tibialis anterior tendon
Navicular
Talus, head
Deltoid ligament
Medial malleolus
Tibialis posterior tendon
Flexor digitorum longus tendon

Cuboid
Peroneus brevis tendon
Bifurcate ligament, calcaneonavicular part
Calcaneus
Interosseous talocalcanean ligament (bilaminar part)
Peroneus longus tendon
Talus, body
Flexor hallucis longus tendon
Tendo calcaneus

6.346 Oblique section that descends mediolaterally through the right foot, showing the synovial cavities of the intertarsal and tarsometatarsal joints; also the medial malleolar part of the ankle joint: superior aspect. Note: the section passed below the joint between the medial cuneiform and the base of the second metatarsal; no synovial joint was present between the navicular and cuboid. The laminae of the interosseous talocalcaneal ligament form accessory ligaments to the fibrous capsules of the talocalcaneonavicular and subtalar (posterior talocalcaneal) joints. The (diagrammatic) apparently uniform thickness of the articular cartilages obscures the variations in thickness and curvature that obtain in life.

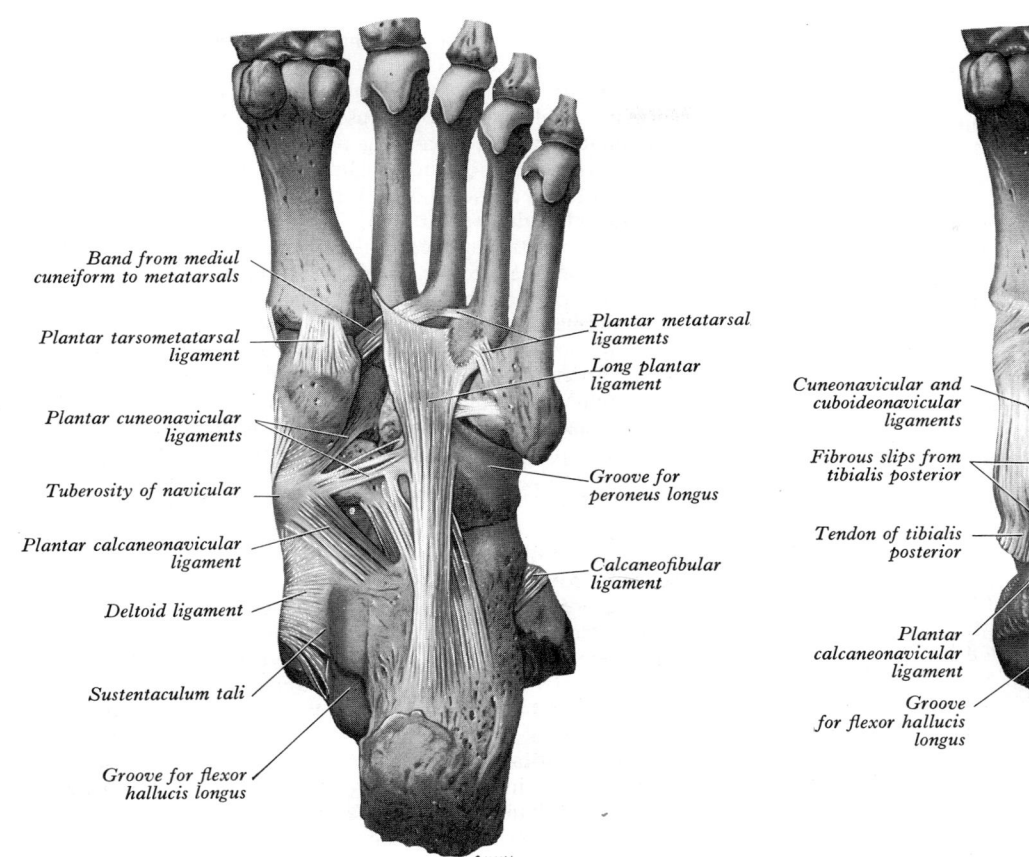

6.347 Ligaments of the plantar surface of the left foot. Some of the fibres of the long plantar ligament which arise in front of the medial tubercle of the calcaneus have been removed. (Drawn from a specimen in the Museum of the Royal College of Surgeons of England, by permission of the Council.)

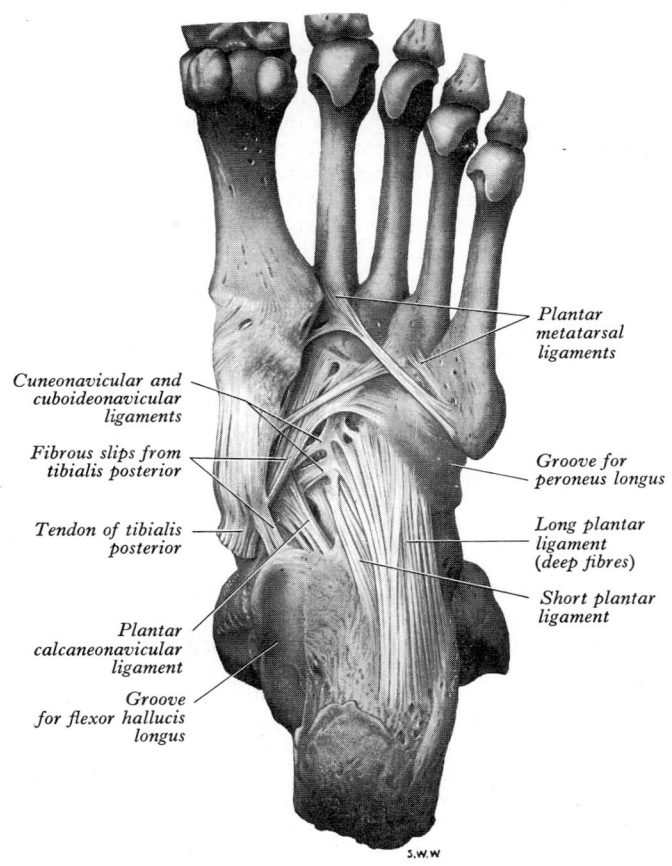

6.348 Ligaments on the plantar surface of the left foot. The long plantar ligament has been removed. (Drawn from a specimen in the Museum of the Royal College of Surgeons of England, with permission from the Council.)

Ligaments connecting the calcaneus and navicular

Though the calcaneus and navicular do not articulate directly, they are connected by *calcaneonavicular* and *plantar calcaneonavicular ligaments*. The calcaneonavicular ligament has been described above as the medial band of the bifurcated ligament.

Plantar calcaneonavicular (spring) ligament (6.342, 345, 348). A broad, thick band, it connects the anterior margin of the sustentaculum tali to the navicular's plantar surface. It ties the calcaneus to the navicular below the head of the talus as part of its articular cavity; it sustains the foot's medial longitudinal arch (p. 733). The ligament's *dorsal surface* has a triangular fibrocartilaginous facet on which part of the talar head rests (6.345). Its *plantar surface* is supported medially by the tendon of tibialis posterior and laterally by the tendons of flexors hallucis longus and digitorum longus; its *medial border* is blended with the anterior superficial fibres of the medial (deltoid) ligament. There is no real evidence that the 'spring' ligament is particularly resilient.

Cuneonavicular joint

The navicular articulates distally with the cuneiform bones at a compound joint often described as plane although the distal navicular surface is transversely convex and divided into three facets by low ridges, adapted to the proximal, slightly curved cuneiform surfaces. Its capsule is continuous with those of the intercuneiform and cuneocuboid joints, as is its synovial cavity, and it is connected also to the second and third cuneometatarsal joints and intermetatarsal joints between the second to fourth metatarsal bones (p. 728).

Dorsal and plantar ligaments. These connect the navicular to each cuneiform; of the three dorsal ligaments, one is attached to each cuneiform. The fasciculus from the navicular to the medial cuneiform is continued as the joint's capsule around its medial aspect, and then blends medially with the plantar ligament. Plantar ligaments have similar attachments and receive slips from the tendon of tibialis posterior.

Cuboideonavicular joint

The cuboideonavicular joint is usually a fibrous joint, the bones being connected by *dorsal, plantar* and *interosseous* ligaments. This syndesmosis is often replaced by a synovial joint, almost plane, its articular capsule and synovial lining continuous with that of the cuneonavicular joint. The dorsal ligament extends distolaterally, the plantar nearly transversely from the cuboid to the navicular. The interosseous ligament, of strong transverse fibres, connects non-articular parts of adjacent surfaces to the two bones (6.346).

Intercuneiform and cuneocuboid joints

The intercuneiform and cuneocuboid joints are all synovial and approximately plane or slightly curved. Their articular capsules and synovial linings are continuous with the cuneonavicular joint. The bones are connected by *dorsal, plantar* and *interosseous* ligaments.

Dorsal and plantar ligaments. Each have three transverse bands, between the medial and intermediate cuneiform, intermediate and lateral cuneiform and between the lateral cuneiform and cuboid. The plantar ligaments receive slips from the tendon of tibialis posterior.

Interosseous ligaments. These connect non-articular areas of adjacent surfaces and are strong agents in maintaining the transverse arch (p. 734).

Movements

Movements at the cuneonavicular, cuboideonavicular, inter-cuneiform and cuneocuboid joints are merely slight gliding and rotation during pronation or supination of the foot (p. 733), i.e. in alterations of a loaded foot in contact with the ground. For example, they increase suppleness when the forefoot is stressed, as in the initial thrust of running and jumping.

Ossification

Each of these has a single centre (see **6**.354), except the calcaneus, which has a scale-like posterior epiphysis (but see below). Centres for the calcaneus and talus appear prenatally in the third and sixth month respectively. A detailed study of the calcaneus in 177 human fetuses between 49 and 150 mm (crown-rump length) showed 16% with a lateral perichondral mesenchymatous centre and 11% with an endochondral centre, while only 2% possessed both (Meyer & O'Rahilly 1976). The cuboid frequently begins to ossify before birth; its centre has usually appeared by 6 months after birth. The medial cuneiform may have two centres and begins in the second year, the intermediate cuneiform and navicular in the third and lateral cuneiform in the first. The calcanean epiphysis covers most of the posterior and a little of the plantar surface; it begins to ossify in the sixth year in females, eighth in males, uniting in the fourteenth or sixteenth respectively. The posterior talar process sometimes has its own centre, and may remain separate or connected to the rest of the bone by cartilage as an os trigonum. Other accessory bones occur and may lead to radiological misinterpretation (Trolle 1947).

METATARSUS

The five metatarsal bones, distal in the foot, connect the tarsus and phalanges. Like metacarpals, they are miniature long bones, with a shaft, proximal base and distal head. Excepting the first and fifth, the *shafts* are long and slender, longitudinally convex on the dorsal, concave on the plantar aspects. Prismatic in section, they taper distally. Their *bases* articulate with the distal tarsal row and with each other. The line of each tarsometatarsal joint, except the first, inclines proximally and laterally, metatarsal bases being oblique relative to their shafts. The *heads* articulate with the proximal phalanges, each by a convex surface passing farther on to its plantar aspect, where it ends on the summits of two eminences. The sides of the heads are flat, with a depression surmounted by a dorsal tubercle for a collateral ligament of the metatarsophalangeal joint.

INDIVIDUAL METATARSALS

The first metatarsal (**6**.349). Shortest and thickest, it has a strong *shaft*, of marked prismatic form. The *base* sometimes has a lateral facet or ill-defined smooth area due to contact with the second metatarsal. Its large proximal surface, usually indented on the medial and lateral margins, articulates with the medial cuneiform;

its circumference is grooved for tarsometatarsal ligaments and, medially, part of the tendon of tibialis anterior is attached; its plantar angle has a rough, oval, lateral prominence for the tendon of peroneus longus. To the shaft's flat lateral surface the medial head of the first dorsal interosseous muscle is attached. The large *head* has a plantar elevation separating two grooved facets, the medial larger, on which sesamoid bones glide. (For the arterial supply of the first metatarsal consult Jaworek 1973.)

The second metatarsal (**6**.350). This is the longest. Its cuneiform *base* bears four articular facets: a proximal one, concave and triangular, for the intermediate cuneiform; a dorsomedial one for the medial cuneiform, variable in size and usually continuous with that for the intermediate cuneiform; two lateral, dorsal and plantar, separated by non-articular bone, each divided by a ridge into distal demifacets articulating with the third metatarsal base and a proximal pair (sometimes continuous) for the lateral cuneiform; these areas vary, particularly the plantar facet, which may be absent (Singh 1960). An oval pressure facet, due to contact with the first metatarsal, may appear on the medial side of the base, plantar to that for the medial cuneiform. To the shaft's medial and lateral surfaces are respectively attached the lateral head of the first dorsal interosseous and medial head of the second.

The third metatarsal (**6**.351). This has a flat triangular *base*, articulating proximally with the lateral cuneiform; medially, dorsal and plantar facets articulate with the second metatarsal and, laterally, a single facet with the dorsal angle of the fourth. The medial plantar facet is frequently absent. To the shaft's medial surface the lateral head of the second dorsal interosseous and first plantar are attached, to its lateral surface the medial head of the third dorsal interosseous.

The fourth metatarsal (**6**.352). This is smaller than the third. Proximally its base has an oblique quadrilateral facet for articulation with the cuboid, laterally a single facet for the fifth metatarsal and medially an oval facet for the third, sometimes divided by a ridge, the proximal part then articulating with the lateral cuneiform. To the medial surface the lateral head of the third dorsal and second plantar interossei are attached; to the lateral surface is the medial head of the fourth dorsal interosseous.

The fifth metatarsal (**6**.353). This has a *tuberosity* (*styloid process*) on the lateral side of its base. The base articulates proximally with the cuboid by a triangular, oblique surface, medially with the fourth metatarsal. The tendon of peroneus tertius is attached to the medial part of the dorsal surface and medial border of the shaft, that of peroneus brevis to the dorsal surface of the tuberosity. A strong band of the plantar aponeurosis, sometimes containing muscle,

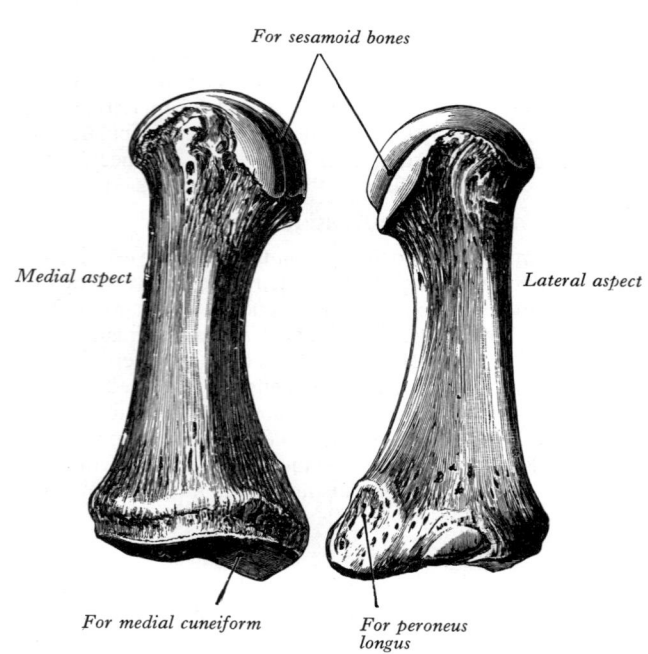

For sesamoid bones

Medial aspect

Lateral aspect

For medial cuneiform

For peroneus longus

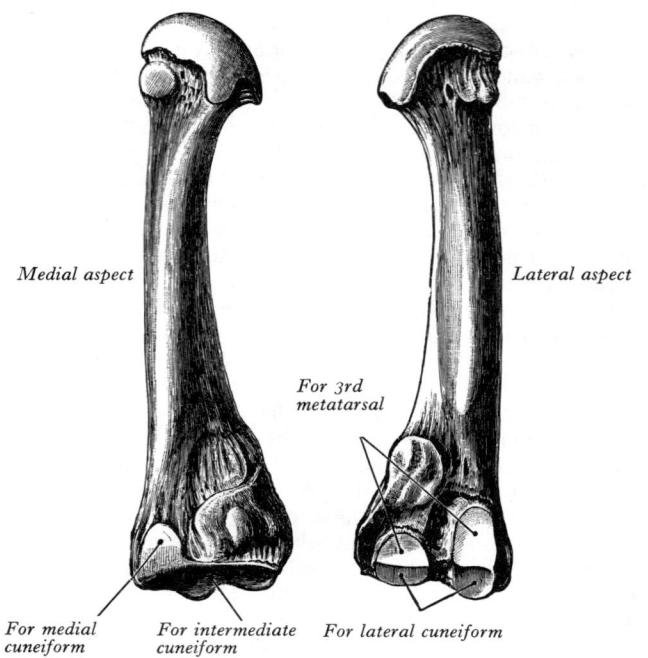

Medial aspect

Lateral aspect

For 3rd metatarsal

For medial cuneiform

For intermediate cuneiform

For lateral cuneiform

6.349   Medial and lateral aspects of the left first metatarsal.

6.350   Medial and lateral aspects of the left second metatarsal.

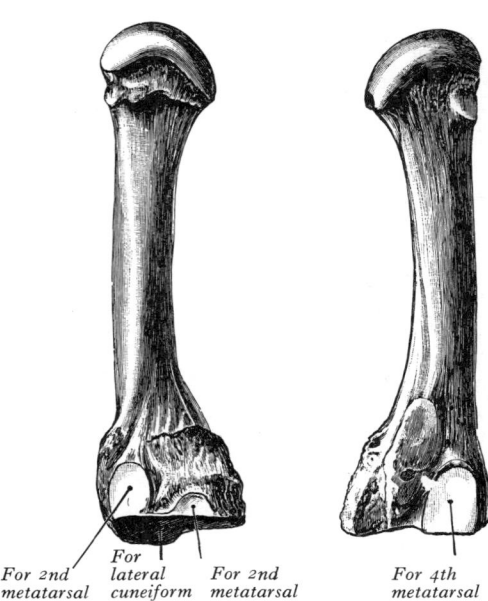

6.351   Medial and lateral aspects of the left third metatarsal.

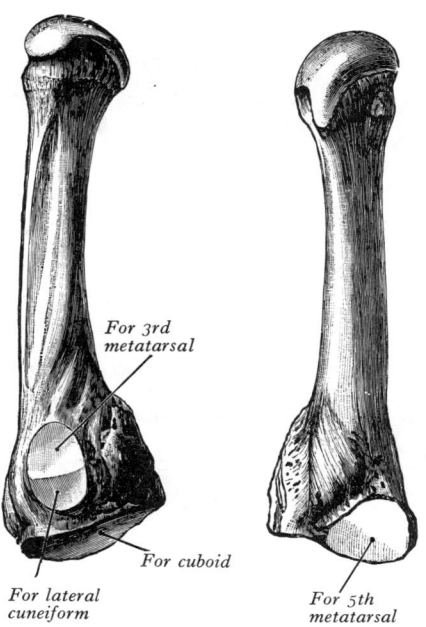

6.352   Medial and lateral aspects of the left fourth metatarsal.

connects the apex of the tuberosity to the lateral process of the calcanean tuberosity. The plantar surface of the base is grooved by the tendon of abductor digiti minimi and the flexor digiti minimi brevis is attached here. To the shaft's medial side are attached the lateral head of the fourth dorsal and the third plantar interossei. The tuberosity can be seen and felt midway along the foot's lateral border; in acute inversion it may be fractured.

Ossification

The metatarsals ossify from a primary centre for the shaft and a secondary epiphysis for the base of the first and for the head in the other four (**6.354**). In the second to fourth ossification begins in the midshaft in the ninth prenatal week, in the first and fifth about the tenth week. The centre in the first *base* appears about the third year, those for second to fifth metatarsal *heads* between the third and fourth years; all unite between the seventeenth and twentieth years. Like the first *metacarpal* (p. 654), the first metatarsal may also have an epiphysis for its head. The basal tubercle of the fifth metatarsal bone is often an epiphysis.

TARSOMETATARSAL ARTICULATIONS

Tarsometatarsal articulations are approximately plane synovial joints. The first metatarsal articulates with the medial cuneiform; the second is recessed between the medial and lateral, articulating with the intermediate cuneiform; the third articulates with lateral cuneiform; the fourth with the lateral cuneiform and cuboid; and the fifth with the cuboid. The joints are approximately on a line from the fifth metatarsal's tubercle to the tarsometatarsal joint of the hallux, except for that between the second metatarsal and intermediate cuneiform, which is 2–3 mm proximal (**6.346**). The hallucial joint has its own capsule; articular capsules and cavities of the second and third are continuous with intercuneiform and cuneonavicular joints but separated from the fourth and fifth joints by an interosseous ligament between the lateral cuneiform and fourth metatarsal base. The bones are connected by *dorsal* and *plantar tarsometatarsal* and *interosseous cuneometatarsal* ligaments.

Dorsal ligaments

Strong and flat, the first metatarsal is joined to the medial cuneiform by an articular capsule; the other tarsometatarsal capsules blend with the dorsal and plantar ligaments. The second metatarsal receives a band from each cuneiform, the third from the lateral cuneiform, fourth from lateral cuneiform and cuboid, fifth from the cuboid alone.

Plantar ligaments

These are longitudinal and oblique bands, less regular than the dorsal. Those for the first and second metatarsals are strongest; the second and third metatarsals are joined by oblique bands to the medial cuneiform, the fourth and fifth by a few fibres to the cuboid.

Interosseous cuneometatarsal ligaments

These comprise:

- one (the strongest) from the lateral surface of the medial cuneiform to the adjacent angle of second metatarsal (**6.346**);
- one connecting the lateral cuneiform to the adjacent angle of second metatarsal; it does not divide the joint between the second metatarsal and lateral cuneiform and is inconstant;
- one connecting the lateral angle of the lateral cuneiform to the adjacent fourth metatarsal base.

Movements

Movements between the tarsal and metatarsal bones are limited to

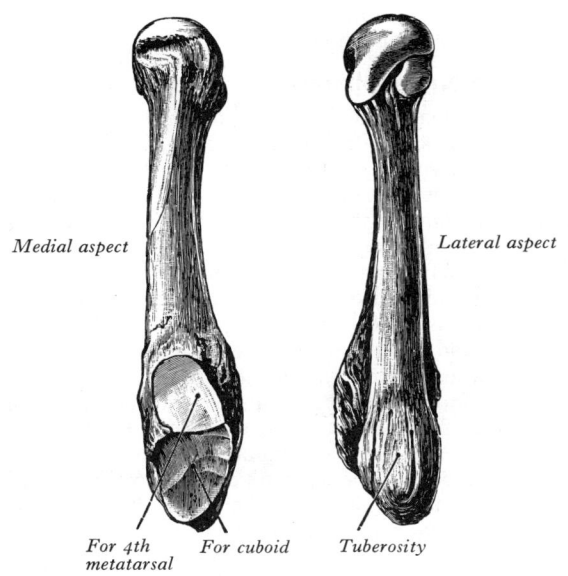

6.353   Medial and lateral aspects of the left fifth metatarsal.

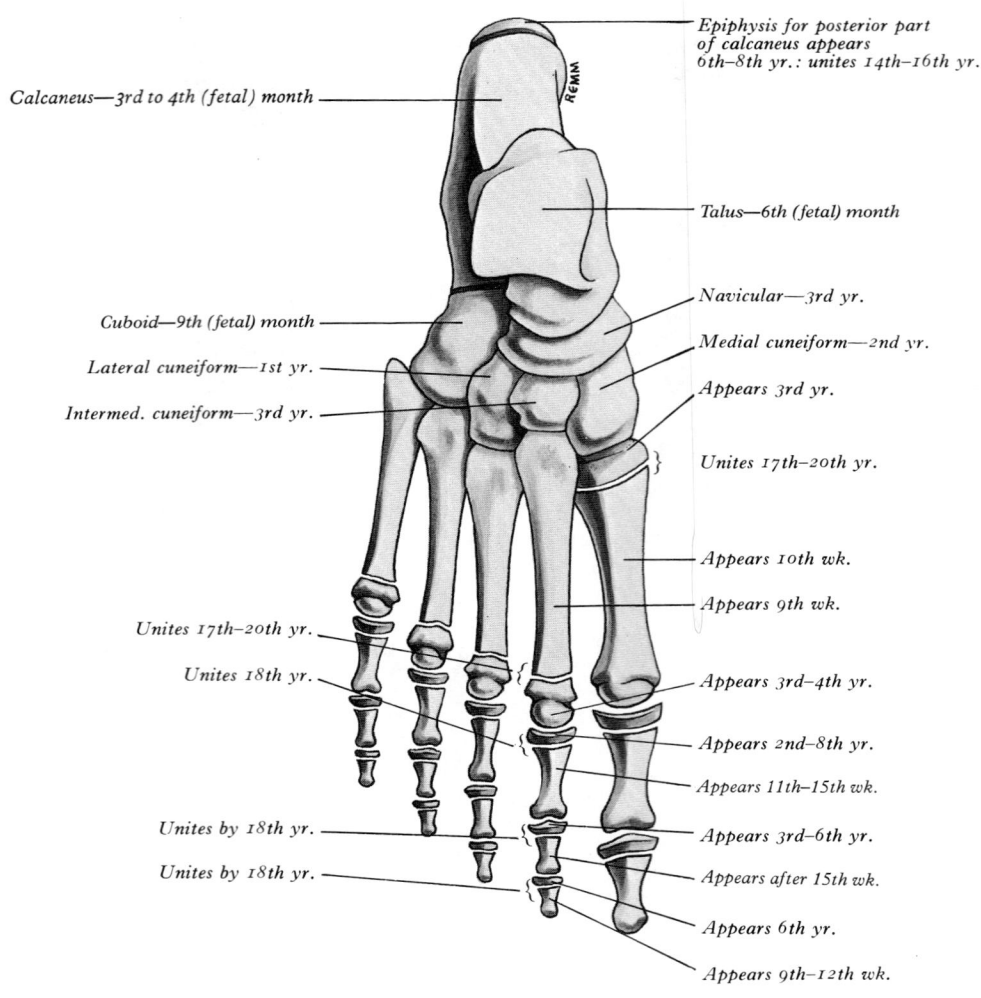

*Epiphysis for posterior part
of calcaneus appears
6th–8th yr.: unites 14th–16th yr.*

Calcaneus—3rd to 4th (fetal) month

Talus—6th (fetal) month

Navicular—3rd yr.

Cuboid—9th (fetal) month

Medial cuneiform—2nd yr.

Lateral cuneiform—1st yr.

Appears 3rd yr.

Intermed. cuneiform—3rd yr.

Unites 17th–20th yr.

Appears 10th wk.

Appears 9th wk.

Unites 17th–20th yr.

Unites 18th yr.

Appears 3rd–4th yr.

Appears 2nd–8th yr.

Appears 11th–15th wk.

Unites by 18th yr.

Appears 3rd–6th yr.

Unites by 18th yr.

Appears after 15th wk.

Appears 6th yr.

Appears 9th–12th wk.

6.354   Ossification of the bones of the foot.

gliding, very limited in range except between the medial cuneiform and first metatarsal, where appreciable **passive** metatarsal flexion, extension and rotation are possible with the muscles relaxed but all occurring **actively** in standing and walking to maintain plantigrade contact. Being recessed between the medial and lateral cuneiforms, the second is the least mobile metatarsal. Proximal articular profiles of the cuneiforms bring them into a close-packed state in plantarflexion, splaying them out in dorsiflexion.

Pronation and supination

Pronation and supination keep the feet in plantigrade apposition in a range of stances, from wide straddling to crossed legs. This is usually but inaccurately attributed to inversion or eversion, because these involve the whole unsupported foot beyond the talus and even including the talus, if the slight adduction and abduction possible at the plantarflexed ankle are added.

Feet planted far apart are wholly 'inverted' but relative positions of the forefoot and hindfoot must also change to maintain plantigrade contact, because each talus tilts medially with the tibiofibular extremities and its inferior mortice and talar tilt is followed by the calcaneus when limited movement between them is used up. If the rest of the foot followed this tilting (inversion), weight would be largely taken from the lateral to the medial border. To correct this and distribute weight by plantigrade contact, the **forefoot rotates** in the opposite sense, i.e. it **supinates** or **untwists**. This largely occurs at the transverse tarsal joint but others contribute, especially the hallucial cuneometatarsal. Conversely, when the feet are together or even crossed, contact with the ground can only be maintained by maximal **pronation** of the forefoot relative to the calcaneus and talus (pp. 733–735).

Intermetatarsal joints

The first metatarsal *base* is not connected to the second by ligaments; in this respect the hallux resembles the pollex (but differs in being distally connected). A small bursa often occurs between first and second metatarsal bases (**6**.346). Second to fifth metatarsal bases are connected by *dorsal, plantar* and *interosseous* ligaments. All metatarsal *heads* are connected indirectly by *deep transverse metatarsal ligaments* (p. 729). *Dorsal* and *plantar* ligaments pass transversely between adjacent *bases. Interosseous* ligaments are strong transverse bands connecting non-articular parts of the adjacent surfaces (**6**.346).

Movements

Movements between the tarsal ends of metatarsal bones are slight gliding when the forefoot is working under load (cf. intercuneiform joints, p. 725).

SYNOVIAL ARRANGEMENTS OF TARSUS AND METATARSUS

Synovial cavities (**6**.346) between the tarsus and metatarsus are:

- subtalar
- talocalcaneonavicular
- calcaneocuboid
- a complex of cuneonavicular, intercuneiform, cuneocuboid
- intermediate and lateral cuneiform respectively with the second and third metatarsals
- second to fourth metatarsals
- medial cuneiform with first metatarsal
- cuboid with fourth and fifth metatarsals.

A small synovial cavity sometimes occurs between the navicular and cuboid, usually communicating with that between the cuboid and lateral cuneiform.

PHALANGES OF THE FOOT

The phalanges (**6.329, 330**) in general resemble those in the hand; there are two in the hallux, and three in each of the other toes. They are, however, much shorter and their shafts, especially those of the proximal set, are compressed from side to side. In proximal phalanges the compressed *shaft* is convex dorsally, with a plantar concavity. The *base* is concave for articulation with a metatarsal *head* and the head is a trochlea for a middle phalanx. Middle phalanges are small and short, but broader than the proximal. Distal phalanges resemble those in the fingers, but are smaller and flatter; each has a broad base for a middle phalanx and an expanded distal end; a rough *tuberosity* on the plantar aspect of the latter is an attachment for the pulp, and a wider area for weight-bearing.

Tendons of the long digital flexor and extensors are attached to the plantar and dorsal aspects of the bases of the lateral four distal phalanges. In the hallux, flexor hallucis longus and extensor hallucis are likewise attached. The bases of the middle phalanges also receive the tendons of flexor digitorum brevis and extensors digitorum. The second, third and fourth proximal phalanges each receive a lumbrical on the medial side and an interosseous on each side (Jones 1949). For further details of muscular, capsular and ligamentous arrangements in the toes see **6.329, 330** and pages 892–893. The terminal phalanx of the hallux normally shows a small degree of valgus (lateral) deviation, as may the proximal, even in persons who have never worn shoes (Barnett 1962). Comparison of the angulation in 30 students (18–21 years) and 35 aged individuals showed no increase in the latter. The deviation has also been observed in fetal specimens (Wilkinson 1954).

Ossification

Phalanges (**6.354**) are ossified from a primary centre for shaft and a basal epiphysis. Primary centres for the distal phalanges appear between the ninth and twelfth prenatal weeks, and even later in the fifth digit; those for the proximal phalanges appear between the eleventh and fifteenth weeks, and later for intermediate phalanges, with wide variation. Basal centres appear between the second and eighth years (usually second or third in the hallux), uniting by the eighteenth year (Venning 1956a,b). Much variation appears in different reports; racial differences probably exist (Kraus 1961).

METATARSOPHALANGEAL ARTICULATIONS

Metatarsophalangeal articulations are ovoid or ellipsoid joints between the rounded metatarsal heads and shallow cavities on the proximal phalangeal bases. They are 2.5 cm proximal to the webs of the toes.

Articular surfaces cover the distal and plantar aspects of the metatarsal heads but not the dorsal. The plantar aspect of the first metatarsal head has two longitudinal grooves separated by a ridge; each articulates with a sesamoid bone embedded in the joint's capsule, formed here by tendons of intrinsic hallucial muscles. Articular areas on the proximal phalangeal bases are concave. Ligaments are *capsular, plantar, deep transverse metatarsal* and *collateral*.

Fibrous capsules

These are attached to their articular margins. Thin dorsally, they may be separated from the long extensor tendons by small bursae or they may be replaced by the tendons: they are inseparable from the plantar and collateral ligaments.

Plantar ligaments

Thick and dense, they are between and blend with the collateral ligaments; their attachment to the metatarsals is loose but firm to phalangeal bases. Their margins blend with the deep transverse metatarsal ligaments. Their plantar surfaces are grooved for the flexor tendons, whose fibrous sheaths connect with the edges of the grooves. Their deep surfaces extend the articular areas for metatarsal heads.

The deep transverse metatarsal ligaments

These are four short, wide, flat bands uniting the plantar ligaments of adjoining metatarsophalangeal joints. Dorsal to them are the interosseous muscles, whereas the lumbricals and digital vessels and nerves are plantar. They resemble the deep transverse metacarpal ligaments (p. 658) **but** connect with the plantar ligament of the hallucial metatarsophalangeal joint.

Collateral ligaments

Strong cords flanking each joint they are attached to the dorsal tubercles on the metatarsal heads and the corresponding side of the phalangeal bases; they slope downwards and forwards.

Movements

Movements are like those at the hand's corresponding joints but differ in range. Unlike that of the hand, the range of active extension (50°–60°) is greater than flexion (30°–40°), an adaptation to the needs of walking and a difference even more marked in the hallucial joint where flexion is a few degrees while extension may reach 90°. When the foot is on the ground metatarsophalangeal joints are already extended to at least 25°, because the metatarsals slope up in the foot's longitudinal arches (**6.355**). **Passive** range in these joints is 90° (extension) and 45° (flexion), according to Kapandji (1974). Adduction is linked to flexion, abduction to extension; but abduction of the fifth toe is always linked with slight flexion.

Accessory movements. As in the hand, these are gliding and rotation of the phalanges about their long axes.

Muscles producing movement

Flexion: flexor digitorum brevis, the lumbricals and interossei, assisted by flexors digitorum longus and accessorius. In the fifth toe flexor digiti minimi brevis assists; in the hallux flexors hallucis longus and brevis are the only flexors.

Extension: extensors digitorum longus and brevis, extensor hallucis longus.

Adduction: adductor hallucis; in the third to fifth toes, the first, second and third plantar interossei respectively.

Abduction: abductor hallucis; in the second toe, first and second

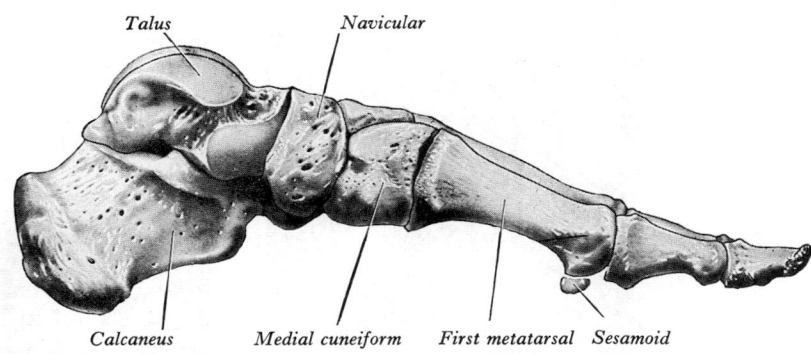

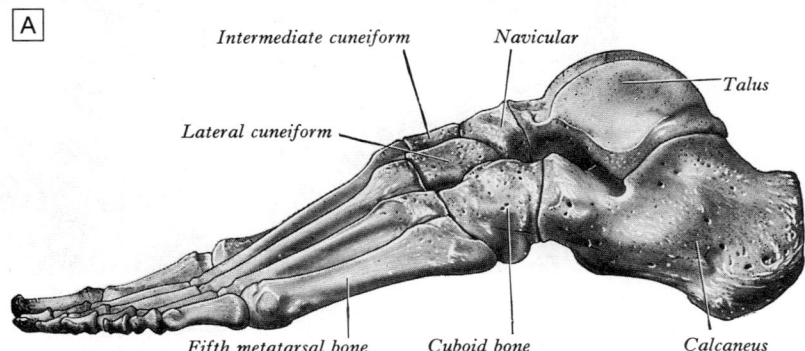

6.355   Medial (A) and lateral (B) aspects of the skeleton of the left foot. Note the height and number of bones in both the medial and lateral longitudinal arches.

dorsal interossei; in the third and fourth, corresponding dorsal interossei; in the fifth, abductor digiti minimi.

    Note. The line of reference for adduction and abduction is along the **second digit**, whose metatarsal is least mobile. This is hence 'abducted' by both its interossei medially or laterally.

INTERPHALANGEAL ARTICULATIONS

Interphalangeal articulations are almost pure hinge joints in which the trochlear surfaces on the phalangeal heads articulate with reciprocally curved surfaces on adjacent phalangeal bases. Each has an articular capsule and two collateral ligaments, as in the metatarsophalangeal joints (see above). The capsule's plantar surface is a thickened fibrous plate, like the plantar metatarsophalangeal ligaments, and is often termed the plantar ligament.

Movements

Movements are flexion and extension, greater in amplitude between the proximal and middle phalanges than the middle and distal. Flexion is marked, but extension is limited by tension of the flexor muscles and plantar ligaments. Flexion and extension are accompanied by slight conjunct rotation.

    Accessory movements. These are abduction, adduction and rotation.

Muscles producing movement

Flexion: flexors digitorum longus, brevis and accessorius, flexor hallucis longus.

    Extension: extensors digitorum longus and brevis, extensor hallucis longus.

Prosthetic replacement in the ankle and foot

Joint replacements in the ankle and foot have a limited application; consequently indications and selection criteria need to be carefully assessed in order to achieve a reasonable success rate: ankle prostheses have, on the whole, proved disappointing.

Indications

Insertion of prostheses in the foot and ankle should only be undertaken following careful consideration of the patient as a whole, in particular their expectations and essential physical requirements, and after an assessment of the biomechanical state of the more proximal parts of the limb and adjacent joints, as well as of the contralateral limb.

    Replacements are confined to the severely crippled polyarthritic, with most prostheses being implanted in the rheumatoid arthritic in whom joint destruction and ankylosis of other joints has made walking virtually impossible. In such patients a small range of motion may allow a degree of independence not otherwise possible.

Ankle joint

Ankle prostheses used in solitary joint involvement following severe trauma or joint degeneration, or after osteochondritic damage to the articular surface and other similar conditions, leads to early breakdown of the prosthesis and subsequent conversion to an arthrodesis (the procedure of choice). Such prostheses will not tolerate a normal degree of activity, even in those leading relatively sedentary lives. Early loosening is the usual cause of failure, with a small percentage (5%) failing due to infection. Only one design of prosthesis is currently available: the Kirkup prosthesis (**6.356**). A new design with a polythene meniscus separating the metal tibial and talar components may prove more satisfactory, given time (**6.357**) (Buechal & Pappas 1992).

Subtalar joint

A number of devices are available, mainly to control severe valgus of the hindfoot, both in connective tissue disorders, where the fibro-fatty pad is destroyed, and in disorders of the adjoining bone, which tend to limit excursion of the joint in eversion—the so-called 'valgus stop' mechanism (Freeman et al 1977). Such devices are usually introduced into the lateral side of the tarsal tunnel thus opening the lateral side of the subtalar joint, thereby correcting hindfoot valgus: indications are the valgus hindfoot of rheumatoid arthritis. Some surgeons, especially in Spain and Italy, use these devices to treat the severe mobile planovalgus foot in childhood; however, if the child's foot is mobile and painless orthoses should suffice to correct the condition, which often resolves spontaneously in ado-

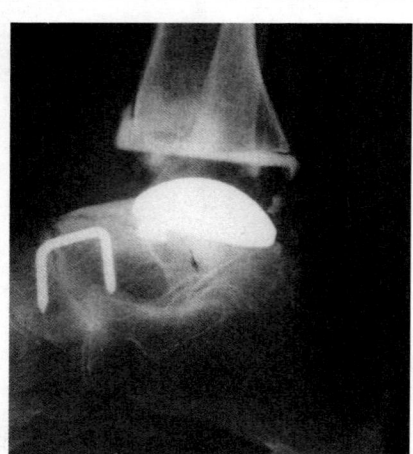

6.356 The metal talar dome and polythene tibial component of the Kirkup prosthesis (1990) (A), and shown in situ (B).

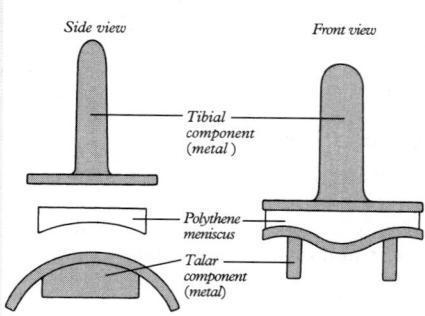

6.357 A new design of prosthesis (Buechal Pappas) coated with hydroxyapatite for direct union of metal to bone.

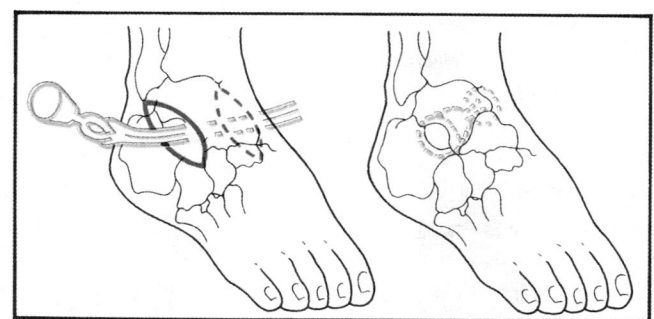

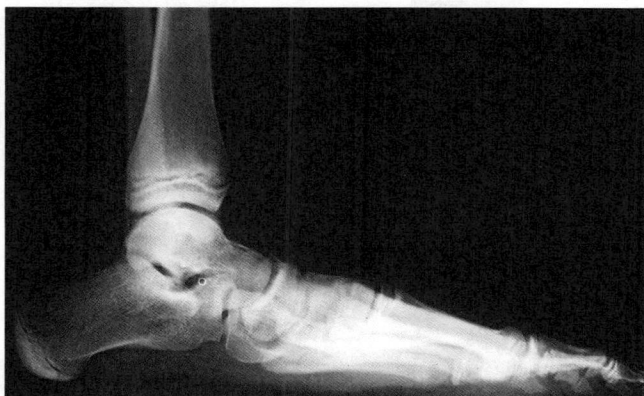

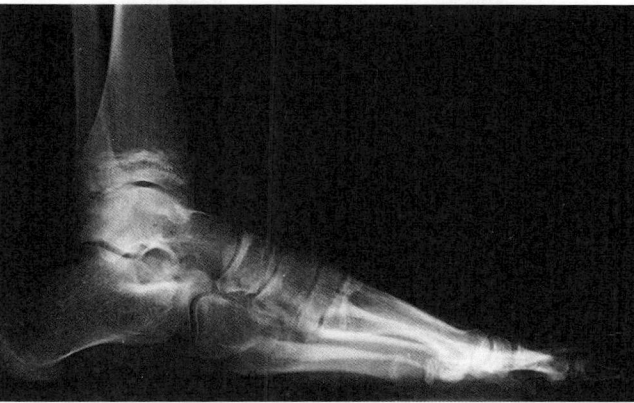

6.358   A silicone wine glass-shaped prosthesis introduced into the lateral side of the subtalar tunnel (A); in situ with the foot weight-bearing and flat (B). (C) shows that the arch is lifted as the heel valgus is corrected.

lescence. An early design was a metal and polythene device (Freeman et al 1977): two types are currently available, the silicone rubber Viladot prosthesis (**6**.358) and the absorbable polymer Giannini prosthesis, which can be expanded to the required size by a polymer screw (**6**.359). The talonavicular joint tends to be involved very early in polyarthritis: the original Freeman device attempted to preserve mobility at this joint, thereby sparing the remaining tarsal joints from the additional stresses produced by an arthrodesis (the surgery of choice in most instances). Subtalar and midtarsal joint problems often occur simultaneously and both these joints can be replaced (**6**.360).

The first metatarsophalangeal joint

The first metatarsophalangeal joint is an important joint in the forefoot which can be destroyed by connective tissue disorders such as rheumatoid disease, or by metabolic conditions such as gout. Sesamometatarsal diseases such as chondromalacia may progress to severe degeneration resulting in damage to the articular cartilage with shedding of debris into the metatarsophalangeal joint. In 20% of cases early hallux limitans can result from a tight band of plantar fascia which produces severe articular cartilage compression in the sesamoids resulting in degeneration: division of the band at an early stage restores movement and arrests the progress of osteoarthritis. Frequently articular damage can occur from an area of osteochondritis in the first metatarsal head.

A stiff joint can be treated in a number of ways. The initial limitation is in dorsiflexion: a dorsal wedge osteotomy of the proximal phalanx brings the arc of movement into extension to allow more dorsiflexion and relieve symptoms. Arthrodesis is not favoured because of the increased stresses imposed on the interphalangeal joints as well as the difficulty of securing the correct angle of fixation. Arthroplasty may be suitable when sporting activity such as running is not important and may simply involve excision of the joint, part of the metatarsal head or the base of the proximal phalanx: it may be enhanced by the insertion of a silicone spacer (**6**.361).

Despite the large forces generated, even in level walking, these devices are often long lasting, probably due to the protection afforded by the pseudocapsule of condensed fibrous tissue which forms around them, which also serves to maintain the length and mobility of the great toe if the prosthesis has to be removed. Other designs of metal on polythene, which require fixation, have not proved successful.

The lesser metatarsophalangeal joints

The lesser metatarsophalangeal joints sometimes have to be excised for severe deformity with metatarsalgia, usually in rheumatoid disease, and sometimes after deformity or arthritis of the joint in Freiberg's infraction (**6**.362). Several designs of joint have been tried to enhance the simple excision, but there is, as yet, no evidence that these improve the long-term results. In Freiberg's infraction with only one or two joints involved a small silicone spacer, combined with osteotomy of the remaining lesser metatarsals to 'level' the tread, has proved effective and worthwhile. Where sesamoids have been destroyed by injury or arthritis artificial silicone sesamoids can be inserted (**6**.363). For general information see Helal (1988, 1992).

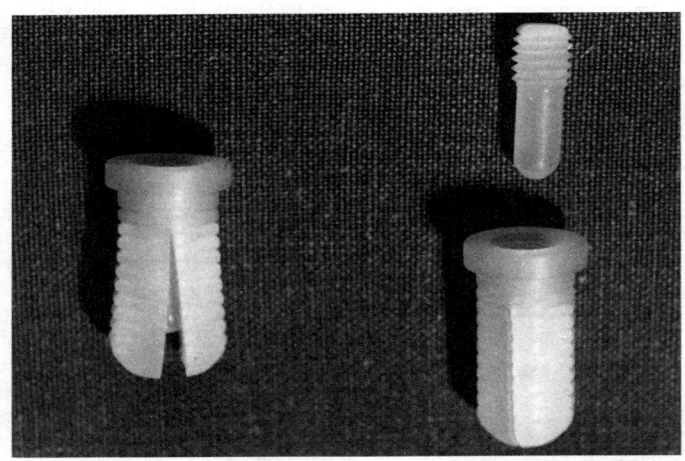

6.359   The Giannini device which slowly and completely absorbs as the screw section is inserted expanding the outer side of the subtalar tunnel.

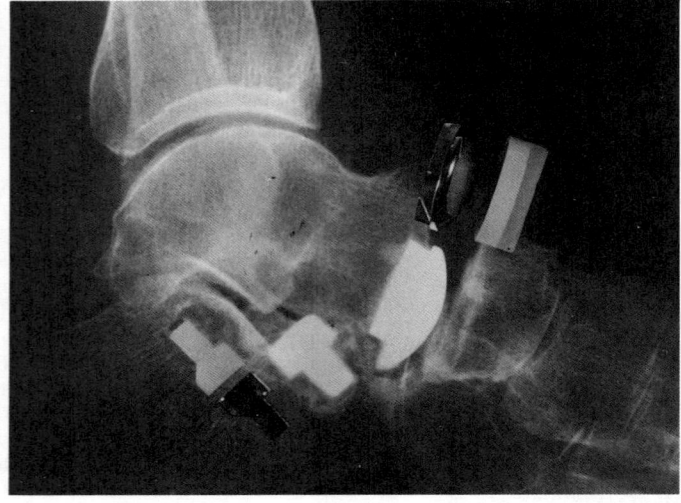

6.360   Combined subtalar and midtarsal or talonavicular prosthesis.

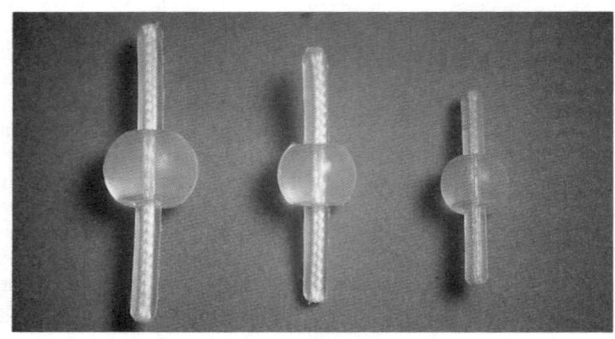

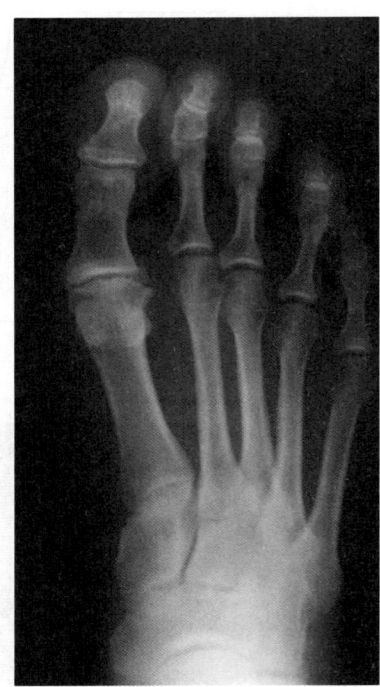

B

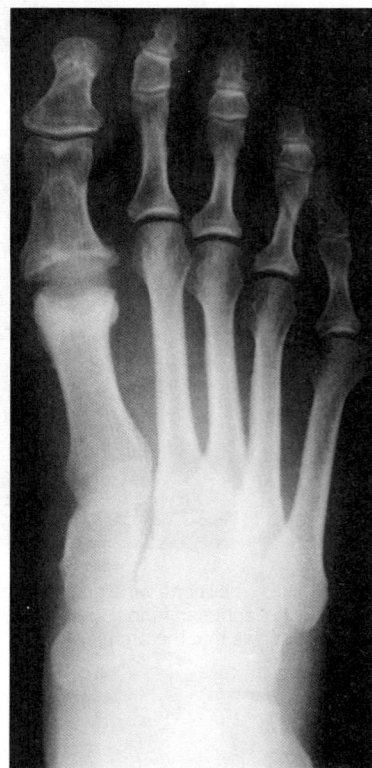

C

6.361   The silicone rubber Universal Small Joint Spacer (A). An osteoarthritic first metatarsophalangeal joint (hallux rigidus) (B) with the joint replaced by a small spacer (C) giving an almost full range of movement.

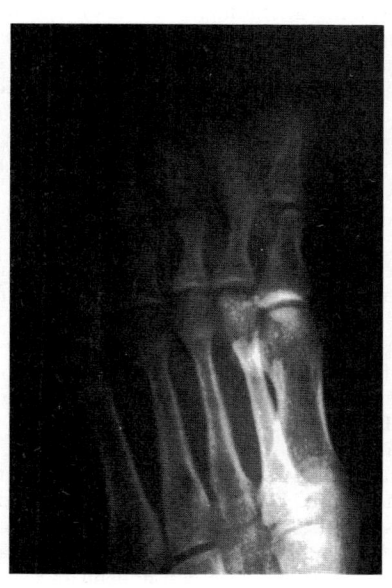
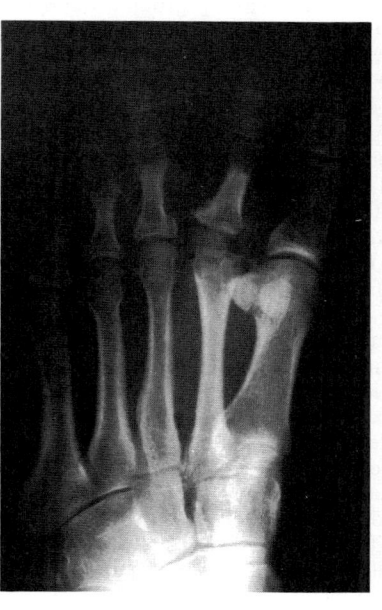

A   B

6.362   An osteoarthritic (Freiberg's infraction) of the second metatarsal head (A) which has been replaced by a silicone rubber ball spacer (B) giving pain relief and restoring movement.

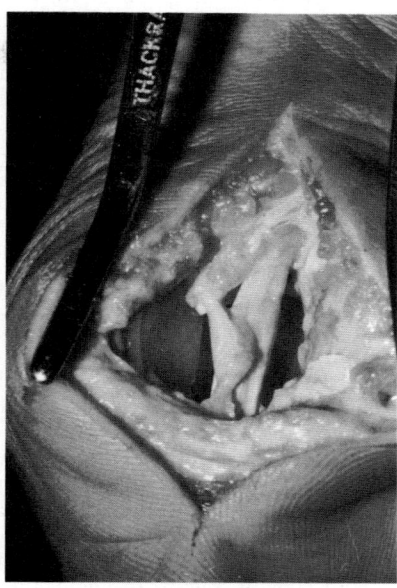

6.363   Badly damaged (fractured) sesamoids have been removed and replaced by silicone rubber sesamoids, restoring the smooth sesamometatarsal articulation and maintaining the height of the metatarsal head preventing lateral metatarsalgia.

MOVEMENTS OF THE FOOT

The foot may move both **off the ground**, freely and relatively only to the leg, or while **on the ground**, bearing weights or transmitting thrust. The latter movements are more limited and partly imposed from the leg by body weight but are also the result of muscular contraction (pp. 897–900).

Active movements occur at the ankle, talocalcaneonavicular and subtalar joints. At the ankle joint movements are almost restricted to dorsi- and plantarflexion, but slight rotation may occur in plantar flexion; at the talocalcaneonavicular and subtalar joint the ranges of movement are greater and here inversion and eversion largely occur.

With the foot on the ground, body weight causes some supination, with flattening of the longitudinal arches; about one-third of the weight borne by the forefoot is taken by the first metatarsal's head. When a resting position becomes active, on starting to walk, the foot is *pronated* by muscular effort; the first metatarsal (the second less so) is *depressed*, accentuating the longitudinal arch to its maximum height (Hicks 1953a,b). Similar changes can be imposed on a weight-bearing foot by active lateral femoral rotation, which is transmitted through the tibia to the talus. This entails passive inversion of the foot at the subtalar joints. Medial femoral rotation has an opposite effect. When the foot is grounded and immobile, muscles which move it when freely suspended may exert effects **on the leg**; for example, the dorsiflexors can then pull the **leg forwards** at the ankle joint.

The foot has two major functions:

(1) to support the body in standing and progression;
(2) to lever it forwards in walking, running and jumping.

To fulfil the first the pedal platform must be able to spread the stresses of standing and moving and be pliable enough for uneven and sloping surfaces. To fulfil its second function it must be transformable into a strong adjustable lever to resist inertia and powerful thrust. A segmented lever can best meet such stresses if arched in form.

In infants and young children plantar amassed, fatty, connective tissue may give the foot a flat appearance; soft tissues variably modify its appearance at all ages. But the human foot, alone among primates, is normally arched in its **skeletal** basis, usually with visible concavity in the sole. The word 'arch' so applied has perhaps become too architectural, imposing rigidity on classical descriptions of curved pedal form and differences of interpretation more linguistic than factual. The word has several meanings and doubtless 'arches of the foot' has various implications. As a start, at simplest, the term implies little more than a curved form, concave on the plantar aspect. Such an arch should not be compared with static masonry, with pediments on terra firma and an intermediate keystone structure. The pedal arch is dynamic; muscles and ligaments are functionally inseparable. Moreover, its heel is often **off** the ground. In this account, therefore, 'arch' denotes no more than curved form, just as the back is merely curved when 'arched'.

This curvature is customarily analysed into longitudinal and transverse arches, of some value in initial analysis. They vary individually in height, especially the longitudinal in its medial part, and, being dynamic, in different phases of activity. Arches are often said to be mainly dependent on osseous shapes and ligamentous ties, the associated muscles playing a secondary role (Jones 1941; Hicks 1955). But clinical experience points to muscular insufficiency as the commonest cause of flat foot, in which ligaments elongate and bones in consequence alter in shape. It is perhaps unwise to give any factor major emphasis; all function together in the living foot. Loading experiments, on amputated legs and by electromyography in the living, show that in **standing** ligaments play a major role; but as soon as movement occurs muscles predominate. Longitudinal curvature is usually described as composed of medial and lateral arches, a division partly justified by differences in osseous arrangement and function in the foot's medial and lateral regions.

The *medial arch* contains the calcaneus, talus, navicular, cuneiform

733

and medial three metatarsal bones. Its summit is at the superior talar articular surface, taking the full thrust from the tibia and passing it backwards to the calcaneus, forwards through the navicular and cuneiforms to the metatarsals. When the foot is grounded these forces are transmitted through the three metatarsal heads and calcaneus (especially its tuberosity). This arch is higher, more mobile and resilient than the lateral; its flattening progressively tightens the plantar calcaneonavicular ligament (p. 725) and plantar fascia. Tibialis posterior, flexor digitorum longus, flexor hallucis longus and intrinsic muscles all act on the curvature of the medial arch; they are adjustable, unlike ligaments. Nevertheless, they are often considered secondary and claimed to be usually inactive in standing but markedly active in any movement elevating the arch. This view, as regarded static posture, does not accord with clinical experience in the aetiology of flat foot.

The *lateral arch* contains the calcaneus, cuboid and lateral two metatarsals; its summit is considered to be the subtalar articulation. It is hence skeletally lower than the medial. Its main joint is the calcaneocuboid part of the 'transverse tarsal joint' (p. 723), of very limited range. The lateral arch, being lower and less mobile, is adapted to transmit weight and thrust rather than to absorb such forces. As it flattens, the long plantar and plantar calcaneocuboid ligaments tighten; its special muscles are peroneus longus and the intrinsic muscles of the fifth toe. It makes contact with the ground more extensively than the medial arch. With the foot flat its anterior and posterior ends or 'pillars' (heads of the lateral two metatarsals and calcanean tuberosity) of course transmit forces; but, as it flattens,

an increasing fraction of load traverses soft tissues inferior to the whole arch. In fact the whole lateral border usually touches the ground; the medial border does not but is visibly concave, usually even in standing. This explains the familiar outline of human footprints (though this varies with the position of the feet, apart or together (6.364), development of soft tissues and the nature of the surface). As soon as the heel rises, in any activity, the toes are extended and muscular structures (including the plantar aponeurosis) tighten up in the sole, accentuating the longitudinal arches. (It is suggested by Hicks 1955 that in this phase tension diminishes in deeper plantar ligaments.)

Since the sole is transversely concave, both in skeletal form and usually in external appearance, serial transverse arches, most developed inferior to the metatarsus and adjoining tarsus, are usually described. Apart from the metatarsal heads and to some degree along the lateral border, the transverse arches cannot transmit forces though subjacent soft tissues do; medially, only the metatarsal heads can do so. Hence the foot has been likened to a half-dome, its plantar concavity directed medially, a complete dome forming when feet are close together. Peroneus longus is a strong agent in maintaining the transverse curvature.

The foregoing structural analysis is a necessary prelude to the study of activities in the living. Direct observation, coupled with electromyography, kinesiology and clinical data, all contribute to understanding the dynamic events in the foot during natural use. Unfortunately, disagreements persist with consequent uncertainties. The following remarks are hence not to be taken as dogmatic.

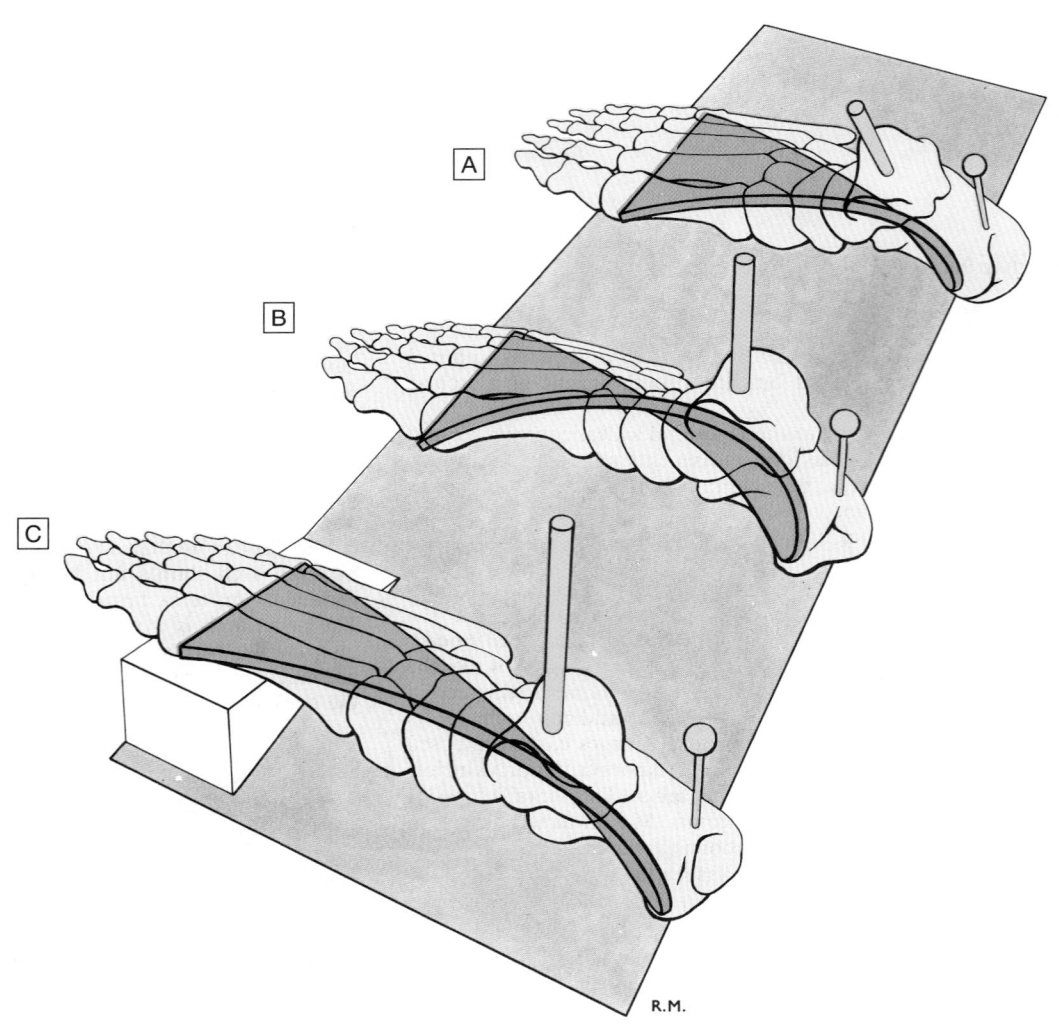

R.M.

6.364 The concept of the foot skeleton as a twisted plate which may be untwisted (supination) or further twisted (pronation) during the maintenance of a plantigrade stance in various positions of the foot. (Based upon MacConaill 1945, 1950.) A. The foot skeleton in supination, as in standing with the feet widely separated. Note the marked medial tilting of the talus and, to a lesser degree, of the calcaneus and the depression of the medial longitudinal arch. B. Relative pronation of the foot, as in standing with the feet close together. C. Supination of the foot when standing on an inclined surface; if the position of the wedge had been reversed, the foot skeleton would, of course, approach maximal pronation.

In standing, with only body weight to support, both the intrinsic and extrinsic muscles appear to relax, the plantar ligaments being relied on to tie the bones into an arched form. This they can do only if the longitudinal arches are allowed to sink by muscular relaxation. The medial arch is more elevated when the feet are together than when they are apart; i.e. inversion with supination increases as the feet are separated. This medial sag can be countered by voluntary contraction of muscles such as the anterior tibial. Pronation and supination ensure that in standing, whatever the position of the feet, a maximal weight-bearing area is grounded, from the metatarsal heads along the lateral border to the calcaneus. Twist imparted by pronation (partly undone in supination) prompted MacConaill (1945, 1950) to liken the foot to a twisted but resilient plate (**6.364**); this would ensure adequate ground contact whatever the angle between the foot and leg, also imparting adaptable resilience in standing and progression. Such a form would strengthen the foot in leverage, perhaps by spiralization of the ligaments.

In walking, the suspended foot, arches accentuated by muscles, is swung forward until the heel meets the ground. As it plantarflexes, the lateral border, from the heel to the metatarsal heads, rolls into contact, the foot supinated for maximum contact. As it now rises, heel first, pronation (with elevation of the medial arch) transfers the thrust largely to the 'ball' of the hallux. The dorsiflexed ankle and elevated metatarsus, being now near their 'close-packed' position, are adapted to the stresses of maximum thrust. As in repetitive actions at the hip and knee joints, a cycle from a position of near close-pack coupled with maximal effort and return to a mobile range of joints prepares re-entry into a phase of thrust. Kapandji (1970) has analysed foot movements in extension. For a scholarly discussion of the evolution of the mammalian foot, in structure and function, see Lewis (1983).

COMPARISON OF BONES OF HAND AND FOOT

The origin of skeletal elements in the hand and foot from terminal segments of primitive pentadactyl limbs has already been considered (p. 615); similarities and differences can now be further examined. Both hand and foot consist of proximal, intermediate and distal components, i.e carpus/tarsus, metacarpus/metatarsus and phalanges. Carpus and tarsus both contain seven elements (omitting the sesamoid pisiform); although more or less cubical, they vary much in shape and size. The carpal bones are smaller, are concerned in the transmission of smaller forces and have retained primitive alignment in rows more than the tarsal bones. Articulation of the tarsus with the foreleg is reduced to one bone (talus); the whole tarsus is divisible into two groups, corresponding to their location in the principal longitudinal arches, with a degree of independent movement absent from the carpus. The calcaneal lever has no equivalent in the *primate* carpus, although similar *carpal* arrangements exist in some quadrupedal mammals.

Digital components, metacarpus/metatarsus and phalanges, are more alike. Metacarpals and metatarsals are similar in form, both bound by soft parts into a structural entity. Mobility is very limited at their bases, where they articulate with the carpals or tarsals and with each other. Between both are interosseous muscles, and first and fifth digits also have short intrinsic muscles. On the flexor aspects in hand and foot are large arterial anastomotic arches, superficial and deep to the long flexor tendons crossing them to enter the free parts of the digits. The distal ends of the metacarpals and metatarsals are slightly more mobile than the bases; but the third metacarpal and second metatarsal are relatively fixed as axes about which neighbouring elements exercise limited movements concerned with adaptation of the hand's grip to uneven objects and the plantigrade foot to inequalities of surface. The digits can flex and extend through considerable arcs at metacarpo- and metatarsophalangeal joints, with a lesser range of abduction and adduction, all better developed in the hand. Phalanges of the foot are much shorter; and though the phalangeal formula is usually the same, reduction of the phalanges by fusion or loss, especially in the fifth digit, is more frequent in the foot.

The functions of the human hand and foot differ greatly and general skeletal similarity is much modified in detail. Greater length and mobility of the fingers, and especially preservation of a free-ranging opposable thumb, are essential to the grasping habit of a prehensile limb. Divergence of the pollicial metacarpal and its specialized joint with the trapezium contrast with arrangements in the hallux. The pollex is rotated about 90° on its long axis relative to the fingers so that, in the resting position, it is halfway to opposition with them. But the hallux is in the same plane as the other toes, its flexor surface also facing the ground. Moreover, it is tied by a transverse metatarsal ligament to the second metatarsal, thus integrated with its fellows and adapted for propulsion. This has led to a different digital formula in the foot: in the hand the middle digit projects most, in the foot it is the hallux, taking the major stress transmitted through the lever of the foot in locomotion. Dorsiflexion of the foot to a right angle with the leg, an obvious adaptation to plantigrade habit, is sometimes said to be peculiar to man; but it is the primitive plantigrade adaptation in ancestral mammal-like reptiles. While most mammals become varyingly digitigrade, bringing the foot and hand into line with the rest of their limbs, most primates and some carnivores, such as bears, retain plantigrade adaptation in the foot. The outstanding human peculiarity is loss of opposition in the hallux, distinguishing man even from other primates. The foot is, indeed, in general far more specialized for the bipedal habit in man than in any other primate animal. The strong build of the hallux in its metatarsals and phalanges, and the elongation and strength of tarsal bones, together make a powerful lever, on which the whole body can be elevated to add impetus and spring in running and jumping. The arched foot, with a lateral arch to steady it on the ground and a medial arch for thrust in propulsion, are specializations absent from the hand (pp. 863–870, **6.252**, **6.365**). The rotational element in the foot, movements of inversion and eversion and pedal pronation and supination (p. 615), are also absent from the hand, which rotates with the forearm in supination and pronation. Lewis (1983) has extensively surveyed the evolution of the mammalian foot.

SESAMOID BONES

Sesamoid bones, like the seeds of sesame, are usually ovoid nodules a few millimetres in diameter, but vary in shape and size, some being large, for example the patella (Bizarro 1921). They are not always fully ossified and may be dense fibrous tissue, cartilage and bone in varying proportions, but most are partly ossified. They are usually embedded in tendons closely related to articular surfaces or where tendons angle sharply round bony surfaces. In both sites the sesamoid surface related to another bone is covered by articular cartilage and slides over it, itself often part of an articular surface, as in the pollicial metacarpophalangeal joint. This entails that the tendons involved are partly fused with an articular capsule, as is exemplified by the relation between the patella, quadriceps femoris tendon and knee joint (p. 697). In other sites, for example the tendon of peroneus longus (p. 883), the sesamoid articular aspect glides over a cartilage-covered osseous surface, here a facet on the cuboid's tuberosity, all enclosed within a so-called bursa, which could well be termed a joint capsule, for the arrangement has all the essentials of a synovial joint. Some consider the sesamoids as **primarily** articular, i.e. embedded in articular capsules, their association with tendons being **secondary** (Patterson 1946). Despite their association with articulations, the precise functions of sesamoids are not clear. They may modify pressure, diminish friction and sometimes alter a tendon's direction of pull, for example the patella. Where a tendon is acutely deflected close to bone, a sesamoid, if ossified, may aid local circulation, bone being able to resist pressures which could compress the vessels in a tendon; these are, however, sparse and prolonged pressure is unlikely, except perhaps in the foot.

Since sesamoid elements appear during fetal life and in greater numbers than later, they are phylogenetic parts of the skeleton, not merely results of local physical factors; but this possibility cannot be dismissed in every instance. They are much more numerous in the extremities of many other mammals. In reptiles, intratendinous ossification near the ends of some limb bones produces nodules like sesamoids, but some fuse later and may be traction epiphyses (Haines 1942a). The proximal epiphysis of the olecranon is an example. Experiments on the patella suggest that phylogenetic and other factors act in the formation of sesamoid bones. Transplantation of limb bud fragments from chick embryos to chorioallantoic membrane has led to the development of a patella, indicating a self-differentiating mechanism (Murray & Huxley 1924). Conversely, removal of the patella in young dogs has been followed by regeneration, provided that normal activity of quadriceps femoris was allowed (Carey et al 1927), suggesting that local mechanical factors are necessary to the formation of sesamoids and perhaps also a parallel between sesamoids and bursae, since the latter also appear regularly before birth in certain sites, but can develop in others as adventitious structures, apparently in response to local conditions.

The incidence of sesamoid bones has received much attention, but numerical data for individual sites are not always available, and onset and progress of ossification has been little studied.

In the upper limb, sesamoid nodules associated with joints are limited to the palm, two being almost constant in the tendons of adductor pollicis and flexor pollicis brevis, the medial being larger. They articulate with the palmar facets on the joint surface of the first metacarpal head; since they are firmly attached in the articular capsule, and in the tendons involved they probably conduct some muscular pull to articular ligaments. A sesamoid is embedded in tendons anterior to the metacarpophalangeal joint of the index digit (35% of hands) and of the fifth (70%), where it is occasionally double. Less frequently, similar sesamoids occur in the third and fourth digits and, in a majority of hands (73%), one exists on the palmar aspect of the pollicial interphalangeal joint (Gray et al 1957). Sesamoid elements in non-articular sites are rare in the upper limb, but one occasionally appears in the biceps tendon near the radial tuberosity.

In the lower limb, the patella is the largest articular sesamoid bone; its relation to the tendon of quadriceps femoris and the capsule of the knee joint exemplifies the arrangements around all sesamoids integrated into synovial articulations. In the foot, sesamoid distribution is like that in the hand. Two, both sometimes double (prompting fallacious diagnosis of fracture), always exist in the tendons of flexor hallucis brevis, plantar to the hallucial metatarsophalangeal joint; they are bound to adjacent ligamentous structures, including the medial part of the plantar aponeurosis. Single sesamoids may occur in the plantar capsule of this joint in all the toes and in interphalangeal joints (**6**.365).

Non-articular sesamoid bones or cartilages are more frequent in the lower limb; that in peroneus longus has been mentioned above. Another, usually appearing later and therefore perhaps adventitious, occurs in the tendon of tibialis anterior where it contacts the distal part of the medial surface of the medial cuneiform bone; the tendon of tibialis posterior may contain a sesamoid gliding on the medial side of the talar head. Sesamoids may also occur in the lateral part of gastrocnemius, behind the lateral femoral condyle, in the tendon of psoas major where it is in contact with the ilium, in the tendon of gluteus maximus as it passes over the greater trochanter and in tendons deflected by the malleoli. In many such sites bursal arrangements occur, and opposing bony surfaces are covered by articular cartilage, as in a synovial articulation. The sesamoid occurring in the gastrocnemius is a *fabella*, articulating with the lateral femoral condyle, and is hence an 'articular' sesamoid.

Sesamoid bones ossify relatively late, except the patella (p. 691), for example the hand in early teens. In a group of Caucasians, those sesamoids associated with the thumb began to ossify in males between 12 and 15 years, and in other digits between 15 and 18 years, dates for females being three years earlier (Joseph 1951). No such data appear available for large mixed or other racial groups. Figures for the lower limb are scant and vague.

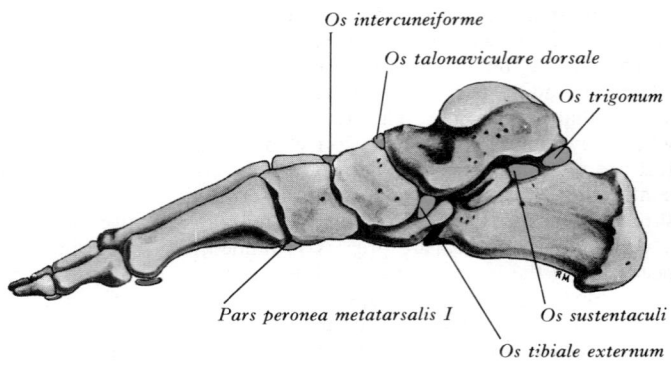

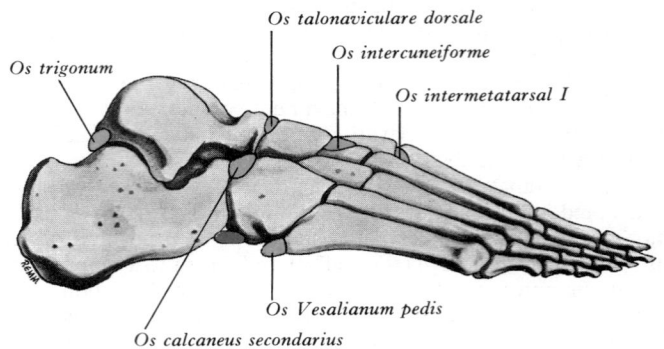

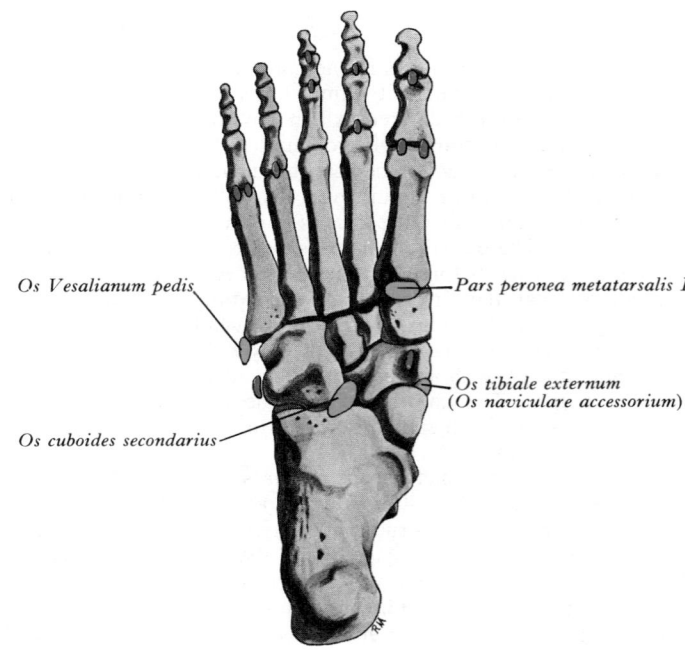

6.365 The sites of sesamoid (red) and accessory bones (blue) in the human foot.

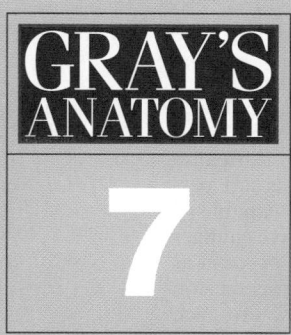

GRAY'S ANATOMY

7

MUSCLE

Section Editor: Stanley Salmons

The Section includes essays by: R McN Alexander (*Standing, walking, and running*); R H Crompton (*Mastication*); M Cullen (*Dystrophin*); D M Denison (*The movements of respiration*); Y H Edwards (*Myogenic determination factors*); L E Klenerman (*Actions of the intrinsic muscles of the foot*); D A McGrouther (*Co-ordinated movements of the upper limb*); T A Partridge (*Regeneration and genetic modification of skeletal muscle*). The remaining essays were contributed by the Section Editor.

The following made expert contributions in the topic areas indicated: P J R Barton (development of cardiac muscle), Y H Edwards and T A Partridge (development of skeletal muscle), G Gabella (excitation, innervation, development and hypertrophy of smooth muscle), T R Helliwell (response of skeletal muscle to denervation and disuse), L E Klenerman (gross anatomy of the foot), D A McGrouther (gross anatomy of the upper limb), P S Rudland (myoepithelial cells and myofibroblasts), B R Russell (non-myofibrillar structures of skeletal muscle), J V Small (subcellular structure of smooth muscle), J Trinick (contractile and structural proteins of skeletal muscle), C P Wendell-Smith (muscles and fasciae of the pelvis and perineum), the late P L Williams (blood supplies to muscles of the upper and lower limb and trunk).

New figures were realized through the skills of Robert Britton, Patrick Elliott, Jenny Halstead, Lesley J. Skeates and Philip Wilson.

In thanking these contributors, and the colleagues who contributed photographic illustrations, the Section Editor also wishes to express his appreciation of the help and advice he has received from V. Baltzopoulos, D A Eisner, M Gunther, J C Jarvis, R E Major, R L Moss, S C O'Neill, and M D O'Brien.

INTRODUCTION

If cells were mere bags of cytoplasm they would, like soap bubbles, assume a spherical shape. In most cases cells are not spherical, even when they are separated from adjacent structures, and this is because they possess an internal skeleton (p. 21). This structure is not permanent, however: some elements of the cytoskeleton are capable of lengthening or shortening, enabling the cell to undergo active changes of shape. Such a capacity is important in a variety of cellular functions, for example: locomotion, phagocytosis, mitosis, extension of processes and withdrawal from noxious stimuli. How are such changes accomplished? Some filamentous proteins—actin and tubulin, for example—can vary their length by adding and subtracting subunits through a finely regulated process of polymerization and depolymerization. Other combinations of proteins—now referred to as molecular motors—can effect changes of length much more rapidly by using energy from the hydrolysis of adenosine 5'-triphosphate (ATP) to drive them past one another. Of these systems, one of the most widespread is based on the combination of actin with myosin.

In muscle cells the filaments of actin and myosin and their associated proteins are so abundant that they almost fill the interior of the cell. Furthermore they align predominantly in one direction, so that interactions at the molecular level are translated into linear contraction of the whole cell. The ability of these specialized cells to change shape has thus become their most important property. Assemblages of muscle cells—the muscles—are, in effect, machines for converting chemical energy into mechanical work. The forces so generated move limbs, inflate the lungs, pump blood, close and open tubes and so on. In man, muscle tissue constitutes 40–50% of the body mass.

BRIEF SURVEY OF THE MAJOR TYPES OF MUSCLE

Muscle cells are also known as *myocytes* (the prefixes *myo-* and *sarco-* are frequently used in naming structures associated with muscle). Myocytes differentiate along one of three main pathways to form *skeletal, cardiac* and *smooth muscle*. Other contractile cells—*myofibroblasts* and *myoepithelial cells*—are different in character and origin, but contain smooth-muscle-related contractile proteins; they are found singly or in small groups. Both skeletal and cardiac muscle may be referred to as *striated* muscle, because in these types of muscle the myosin and actin filaments are organized into repeating elements that give the cells a finely cross-striated appearance when they are viewed in a light microscope.

Skeletal muscle

Skeletal muscle consists of parallel bundles of long, multinucleate fibres. By virtue of the regular organization of its contractile proteins, this type of muscle is capable of powerful contractions, around 100 watts per kilogram for human skeletal muscle. The price paid for this organization is a limited range of contraction, but wherever a larger range of movement is required it is achieved through the amplification provided by the lever systems of the skeleton. These characteristic attachments give skeletal muscle its name. It is sometimes referred to as *voluntary muscle*, because the movements in which it participates are often initiated under conscious control. This is, however, an unsatisfactory term, since it is involved in many movements—breathing, blinking, swallowing, and the actions of muscles of the perineum and the middle ear are examples—that are usually or exclusively driven at an unconscious level. Skeletal muscle is innervated by somatic motor nerves. It has its embryological origin in mesenchymal condensations in the somites and in equivalent areas of mesenchyme in the head and branchial pouches. It forms the bulk of the muscular tissue of the body.

Cardiac muscle

Cardiac muscle consists of a branching network of individual cells that are linked electrically and mechanically to function as a unit. Compared to skeletal muscle, cardiac muscle is much less powerful (about 3–5 watts per kilogram) but far more resistant to fatigue.

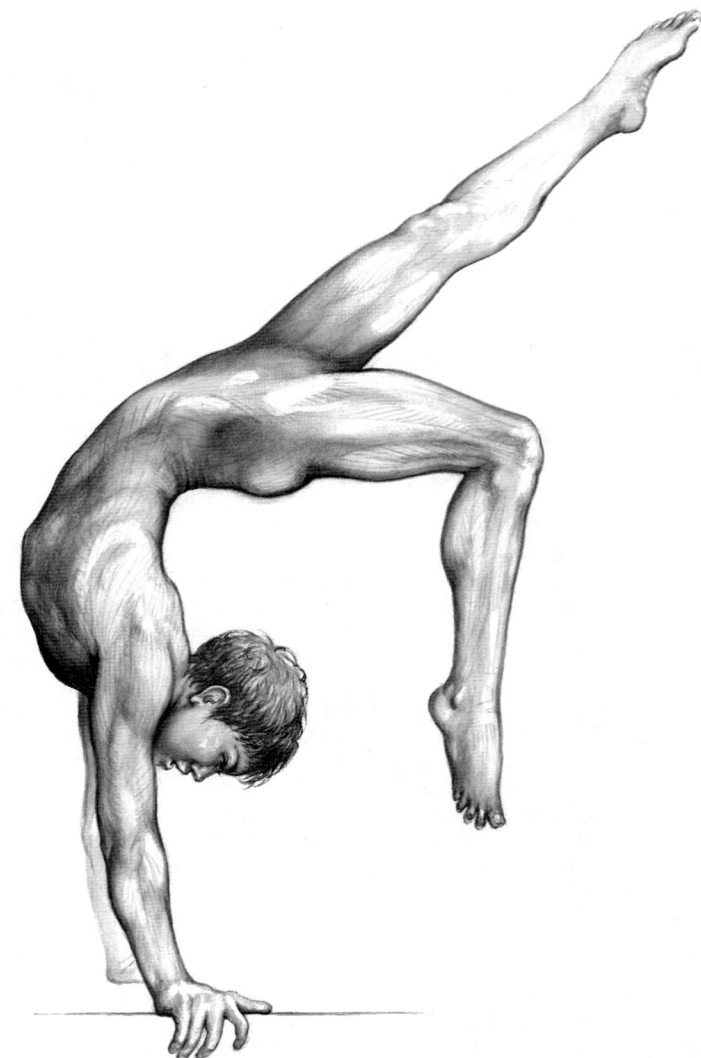

7.1 Molecular motors convert chemical energy into mechanical work in muscle—the most efficient and adaptable machine known to man.

These differences are not unconnected: in cardiac muscle, space that could otherwise have been filled with contractile machinery is occupied by the blood vessels around the fibres and the mitochondria within them, specializations that are essential for the continuous supply of energy. This type of muscle is found only in the heart, but extends into the walls of large veins where they enter the heart. It differs structurally and functionally from skeletal muscle in some important respects: it is, for example, intrinsically capable of rhythmic contraction, with a rate and strength that is nevertheless responsive to hormonal and autonomic nervous control. During embryological development, cardiac muscle arises from a continuous sheet of cuboid cells that line the ventral splanchnic wall of the pericardial cavity.

Smooth muscle

Smooth muscle contains actin and myosin, but these are not organized into repeating units and its microscopic appearance is therefore unstriated or 'smooth'. The elongated cells are smaller than those of striated muscle, and taper at the ends. They are capable of slow but sustained contractions, and although this type of muscle is less powerful than striated muscle, the amount of shortening can be much greater. These functional attributes are well illustrated by its role in the walls of tubes and sacs, where its action regulates the size of the enclosed lumen. A smooth muscle cell may be excited in several ways, most commonly by an autonomic nerve fibre, a blood-borne transmitter substance or conduction from a neighbouring smooth muscle cell. Since none of these routes are under conscious control, smooth muscle is sometimes referred to as *involuntary muscle*. It is found in all systems of the body: in the walls of the viscera, including most of the gastrointestinal, respiratory, urinary and reproductive tracts; in the tunica media of blood vessels; in the dermis (as the arrector pili muscles); in the intrinsic muscles of the eye; and the dartos muscular layer of the scrotum. In some places, smooth muscle fasciculi are associated with those of skeletal muscle. Examples of these sites are: the sphincters of the anus and the urinary bladder; the tarsal muscles of the upper and lower eyelids; the suspensory muscle of the duodenum; a transitional zone in the oesophagus; and fasciae and ligaments on the pelvic aspect of the pelvic diaphragm. Smooth muscle develops from mesenchymal cells in many parts of the embryo.

SKELETAL MUSCLE

LIGHT MICROSCOPIC APPEARANCE OF SKELETAL MUSCLE

The cellular units of skeletal muscle are the muscle fibres (7.2). These long, cylindrical structures tend to be consistent in size within a given muscle, but in different muscles may range from 10–100 μm in diameter and from millimetres to many centimetres in length. Some typical skeletal muscle fibres are seen in longitudinal section in 7.3. Their staining characteristics are dominated by the contractile apparatus, which constitutes much of the cytoplasm or *sarcoplasm*. The contractile proteins are organized into cylindrical *myofibrils*. These are too tightly packed to be visible under these conditions, although occasional separation (usually artefactual) can give the appearance of longitudinal striations or streaks. Of greater significance are transverse striations, which are the result of alignment across the fibre of repeating elements, the *sarcomeres*, within the myofibrils. These cross-striations are usually evident in sections stained by the conventional haematoxylin and eosin technique, but are demonstrated more effectively with the use of special stains (7.3).

Even more striking is the appearance of such muscle in the polarization microscope (7.4), in which the striations are seen as a pattern of alternating dark and light bands. The darker bands rotate the plane of polarized light strongly and are known as Anisotropic or *A-bands*; the lighter bands rotate the plane of polarized light only slightly and are known as Isotropic or *I-bands*. The structures responsible for this appearance will be better appreciated when we examine them at the ultrastructural level (see below).

In mammalian muscle, the multiple nuclei are oval and located at the periphery of the fibres, under the plasma membrane or *sarcolemma*. They are especially numerous in the region of the neuro-muscular junction (p. 752). The nuclei are moderately euchromatic and usually have one or more nucleoli. They occupy a thin transparent rim of sarcoplasm between the myofibrillar material and the sarcolemma (7.3). Other nuclei belonging to vascular endothelial cells, Schwann cells, fibroblasts, etc., may be present in the spaces between the fibres, where blood vessels and nerve fibres course through layers of fine connective tissue.

In transverse section, the profiles of the fibres are usually polygonal (7.5); this is because the bounding connective tissue enforces tight apposition of the fibres as they grow. Some muscles, such as the extrinsic muscles of the larynx, tend to be less tightly packed; in such situations, as well as in conditions of generalized wasting or muscle damage, the fibres adopt a more rounded profile. The sarcoplasm has a stippled appearance, because the myofibrils are resolved as dots (7.6). (The tendency for these dots to aggregate in small groups—the so-called fields of Cohnheim—is now known to be an artefact of preparation.) In this view, the peripheral, subsarcolemmal location of the nuclei may be confirmed; the nuclei often appear flattened in cross-section. Capillaries on the surface of the fibres frequently lie in gutters, and the unwary may confuse the endothelial cell nuclei with muscle nuclei.

BASIC ULTRASTRUCTURE OF THE CONTRACTILE APPARATUS

Skeletal muscle fibres are large, and electron micrographs, unless they are taken at very low magnification, seldom reveal more than

part of the interior of a fibre (7.7). *Myofibrils* are the dominant ultrastructural feature of such micrographs. They are cylindrical structures of about 1 μm diameter, which appear as ribbons in longitudinal section. At regular intervals along these ribbons are thin, very densely stained transverse lines, which correspond to discs in the parent cylindrical structure. They are called *Z-lines*, *Z-bands* or *Z-discs* (German: *Zwischenscheibe* = literally, 'between-disc'). These Z-discs divide the myofibril into a linear series of identical contractile units, *sarcomeres*, each of which is about 2.2 μm long in resting muscle (7.7).

At higher power, sarcomeres are seen to consist of two types of filament, thick and thin, organized into regular arrays (7.8, 10). The thick filaments, which are approximately 15 nm in diameter, are composed mainly of *myosin*. The thin filaments, which are 9 nm in diameter, are composed mainly of *actin*. The interpenetrating arrays of thick and thin filaments form a partially overlapping structure in which the electron density varies according to the amount of protein present. The A-band, which was identified with the polarization microscope (7.4), actually consists of the thick filaments, together with the portions of the thin filaments that overlap with the thick filaments at either end (7.8, 10). The central, paler region of the A-band, into which the thin filaments have not penetrated, is called the *H-zone* (from the earlier term, *Henson's line*). At their centres, the thick filaments are linked together transversely by material that constitutes the *M-line*. The *I-band*, also identified with the polarization microscope, consists of the adjacent portions of two neighbouring sarcomeres in which the thin filaments are not overlapped by thick filaments. (The term 'I-band' was applied to what appeared under the polarization microscope to be a continuous structure; the electron microscope shows that the I-band is actually bisected by the Z-disc, in which the thin filaments of adjacent sarcomeres are anchored.) In addition to the thick and thin filaments, there is now strong evidence for filaments of a third type, which join the ends of thick filaments to the Z-disc; these filaments are elastic and are composed of *titin* (see below). The high degree of organization of the filament arrays is equally evident in electron micrographs of transverse sections (7.9). The thick myosin filaments form a hexagonal lattice, and in the regions where they overlap with the thin filaments each myosin filament is surrounded by six actin filaments at the trigonal points of the lattice (7.10). In the I-band, the thin filament pattern changes from hexagonal to square as the filaments approach the Z-disc, where they are incorporated into a square lattice structure.

The banded appearance of individual myofibrils is thus attributable to the regular alternation of the thick and thin filament arrays. However, myofibrils are at the limit of resolution of optical microscopy, and the fact that cross-striations are also visible at that level is the result of alignment in register of the bands in adjacent myofibrils across the breadth of the fibre. In suitably stained, relaxed material (see, for example, 7.3) the A-, I- and H-bands are quite distinct, but the Z-discs, which are such a prominent feature of electron micrographs, are thin and much less conspicuous in the light microscope, and M-lines cannot be seen at all.

SLIDING FILAMENT MECHANISM OF CONTRACTION

Electron microscopy shows that the lengths of the thick and thin filaments do not change during muscle contraction; instead the sarcomere shortens by the sliding of thick and thin filaments past one another (Huxley A F & Niedergerke 1954; Huxley H E & Hanson 1954). This draws the Z-discs towards the middle of each sarcomere (7.10). As the overlap increases, the I- and H-bands narrow to extinction, while the width of the A-bands remains constant. Since the overlapping arrays of thick and thin filaments have an almost crystalline regularity, it has been possible to use X-ray diffraction not only to confirm the main features of this sliding filament mechanism in single fibres of living muscle, but also to adduce further detail about the underlying molecular changes (Squire 1981).

The head portions of the myosin molecules from which a thick filament is assembled project from its surface at regular intervals (7.2, 12; see p. 742 for a more detailed description of myosin). The projections are present throughout the thick filaments except in a region 150 nm long around the M-line, called the *bare* or *pseudo-H*

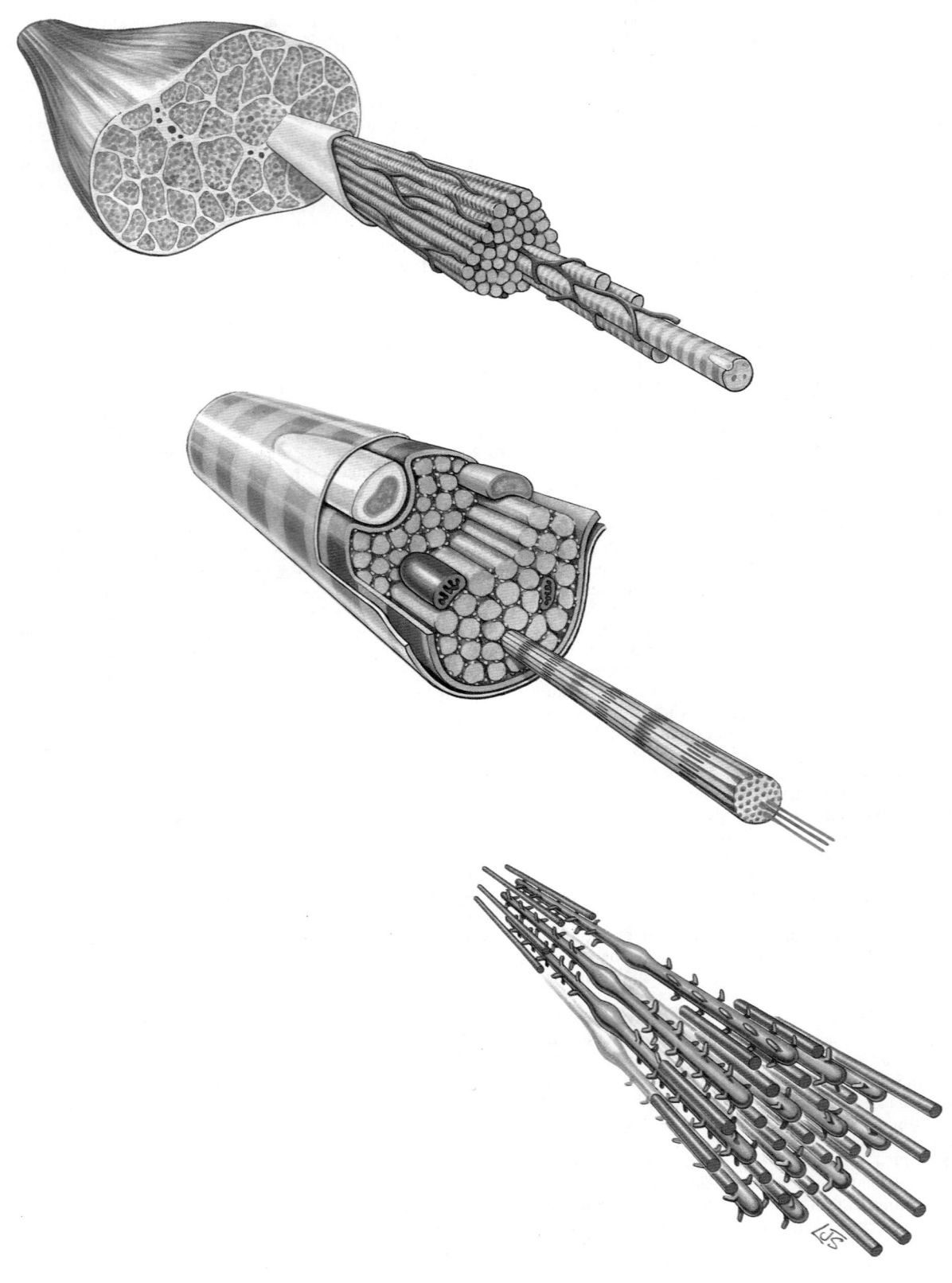

7.2 Diagram illustrating the levels of organization within a skeletal muscle, from whole muscle to fasciculi, single fibres, myofibrils and myofilaments. A satellite cell is depicted lying beneath the basement membrane of the muscle fibre. (Artist: Lesley Skeates.)

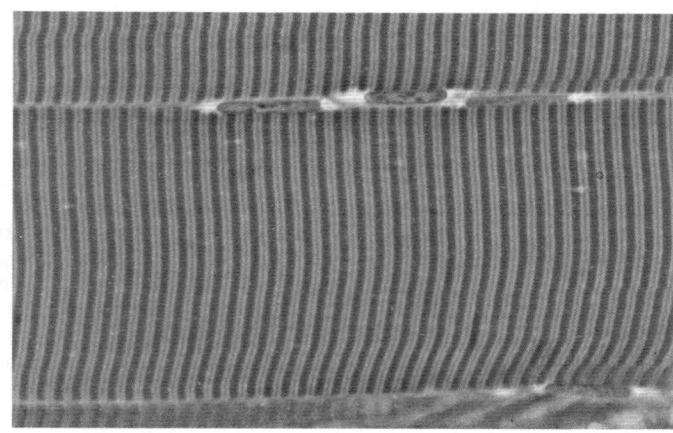

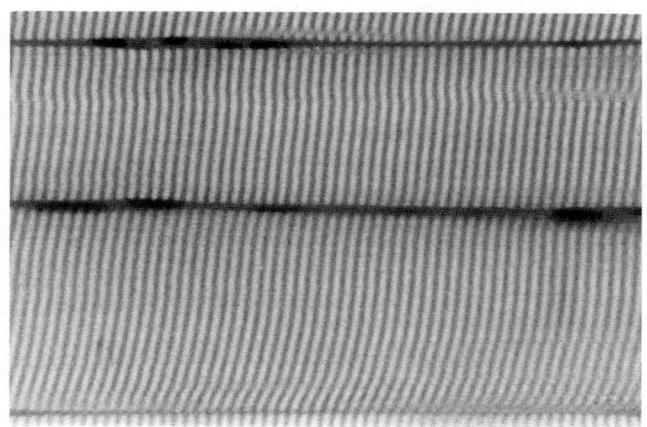

7.3 Light micrograph of a longitudinal section of relaxed rabbit skeletal muscle. The 3 μm-thick resin section has been stained with PTAH and shows the characteristic striations formed by alternation of A-bands (dark-stained) with I-bands (light-stained). These correspond to the dark and light bands in **7.4**. Each I-band is transected by a thin Z-disc. Muscle nuclei are seen occupying peripheral positions. (Photograph by Stanley Salmons.)

7.4 Longitudinal section of uncontracted rabbit skeletal muscle viewed in a polarization microscope to reveal the transverse striations. The birefringent A-bands are darker than the I-bands, but finer structure is not seen. Longitudinal streaks are due to slight separation or loss of register between myofibrils. The 3 μm-thick resin section had been stained lightly with haematoxylin and eosin, but similar pictures could be generated from unstained or even living tissue. Magnification × 800. (Photograph by Stanley Salmons.)

zone, where the myosin molecules assemble tail-to-tail (**7.2, 10, 11**). The projections can form *cross-bridges* by interacting with sites on the adjacent thin filaments. This interaction is the key to the contractile process. It consists of a sequence of mechanical events linked with a corresponding sequence of chemical events. The energy for contraction comes from hydrolysis of ATP to adenosine diphosphate (ADP) and inorganic phosphate, and the necessary enzyme, an ATPase, is an inherent part of the cross-bridge. After ATP has been split, the products of hydrolysis remain bound to the cross-bridge, and in this state the cross-bridge binds weakly (and reversibly) to an actin monomer in the thin filament (**7.13A**). When the muscle is activated (see below, Proteins of the thin filament) there follows a series of intermediate reaction steps (**7.13B–E**), in the course of which the cross-bridge first binds strongly (**7.13B**) and then undergoes a conformational change (**7.13C–D**) that produces a relative movement of 5 to 10 nm between the filaments. During this 'power stroke' at least part of the free energy released by ATP hydrolysis is stored as elastic energy, either in the head or in its attachment to the tail. By the end of this sequence, the products of hydrolysis—ADP and inorganic phosphate—have been released and the cross-bridge is attached at an angle of about 45° to the thin filament (the so-called 'rigor' condition, **7.13E**). In the absence of ATP (as in death) this state is maintained, and is responsible for the muscle stiffness known as *rigor mortis*. In the living muscle, however, a fresh molecule of ATP is available to bind (**7.13F**); the cross-bridge then detaches from the actin and resets to its initial state (**7.13A**). If the muscle remains activated this process can repeat, at a rate of 1–3 per second. The main features of this 'tilting cross-bridge model of force generation' were outlined by H. E. Huxley (1969), although the concept has evolved towards a sequence of attachment configurations rather than a single conformational change, in order to account for the observed chemical kinetics (Lymn & Taylor 1971) and single-fibre mechanical properties (Huxley A. F. & Simmons 1971).

Large-scale sliding movement between the thick and thin filaments is the result of repeated cycles of cross-bridge attachment and detachment, involving a succession of binding sites along the thin filament. Many such cross-bridges are working asynchronously when the muscle is active, and the net effect is therefore to exert a continuous pull on the thin filaments. Because of the cyclical nature of the process, cross-bridges can exert a tractive force even when the muscle is not actually shortening, for example, when it is contracting against a load that it cannot move, or when it is being extended by the action of opposing muscles or gravity.

Measurements of the contractile force exerted by a muscle under conditions in which it is not allowed to shorten (isometric contraction) have shown that the tension developed varies with the

degree of initial stretch. Highly extended muscles can produce little active force; at progressively shorter lengths tension rises, reaches a maximum, and then falls again. This behaviour is readily explained in terms of the sliding filament model (Gordon et al 1966). The force developed by the muscle is directly proportional to the number of attached cross-bridges, which depends in turn on the extent of overlap between the thick and thin filaments. Little tension is developed when the sarcomeres are stretched to more than about 3.5 μm because there is little overlap between the myofilaments. Tension is maximal when the filament overlap is greatest, at a sarcomere length of 2.25 μm in mammalian muscle. Tension falls at shorter sarcomere lengths, because thin filaments cross the M-line from both sides and begin to interfere with cross-bridge formation in the other half of the sarcomere. This double overlap appears as *contraction bands*, which can be seen in the light microscope. There is a further drop in tension as the thick filaments abut the Z-discs on either side. Although such extreme changes in sarcomere length, over a range say from 1.0 to 5.0 μm, are explored in order to test hypotheses, they bear little relationship to the way that muscles actually work. In the body, skeletal muscles are arranged to be used

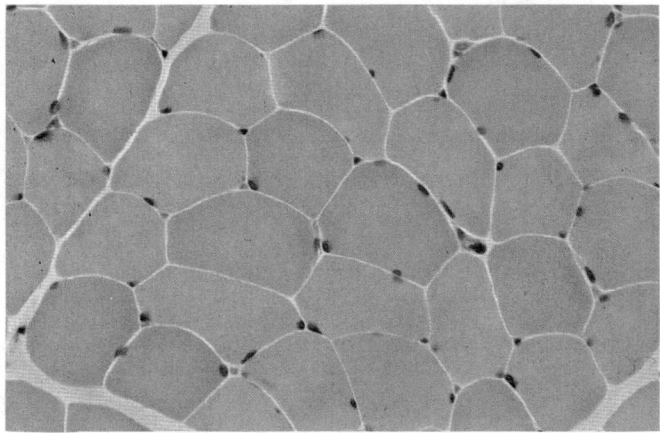

7.5 Transverse cryostat section of adult human skeletal muscle, stained with haematoxylin and eosin. Note the tight packing of the fibres and the peripheral location of the nuclei. Magnification × 250. (Photograph by Stanley Salmons, from a specimen supplied by Tim Helliwell, Department of Pathology, University of Liverpool.)

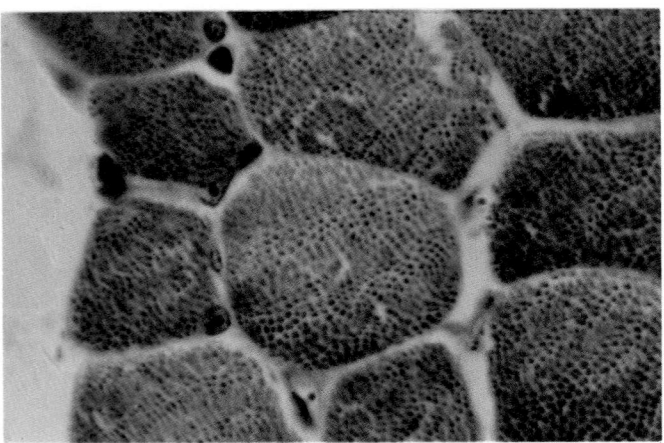

7.6   Transverse section of skeletal muscle. Myofibrils are seen within the muscle fibres, giving them a stippled appearance. Silver stain. Magnification × 800.

efficiently, so the orientation of fibres within muscles and the bony levers through which they act usually constrain the working range to allow near-maximum filament overlap at all times.

MYOFIBRILLAR PROTEINS

In the following account, the myofibrillar proteins will be considered in three groups:
- proteins of the thick filament
- proteins of the thin filament
- scaffold proteins.

Proteins of the thick filament

Myosin, the protein of the thick filament, is the most abundant contractile protein, comprising 60% of the total myofibrillar protein. The thick filaments of skeletal and cardiac muscle are 1.6 μm long and contain an estimated 274 myosin molecules. Each myosin molecule (M_r 520 000) is about 180 nm long. It is composed of six polypeptide chains: two heavy chains (M_r 222 000) and four light chains ($M_r \sim 20\,000$).

The C-terminal portions of the *myosin heavy chains* are largely *α*-helical, and they wind together along part of their length to form a two-chain coiled-coil structure: the rod-like tail of the myosin molecule. The remaining portions of the heavy chains fold separately, each forming a globular head that has both ATPase and actin-binding activity. When myosin molecules assemble to form thick filaments, the tails self-associate to form the backbone of the filament, from which the head portions project as the cross-bridges. The thick filaments are bipolar, the myosin molecules facing outward from a central region, where they are assembled tail-to-tail. The absence of

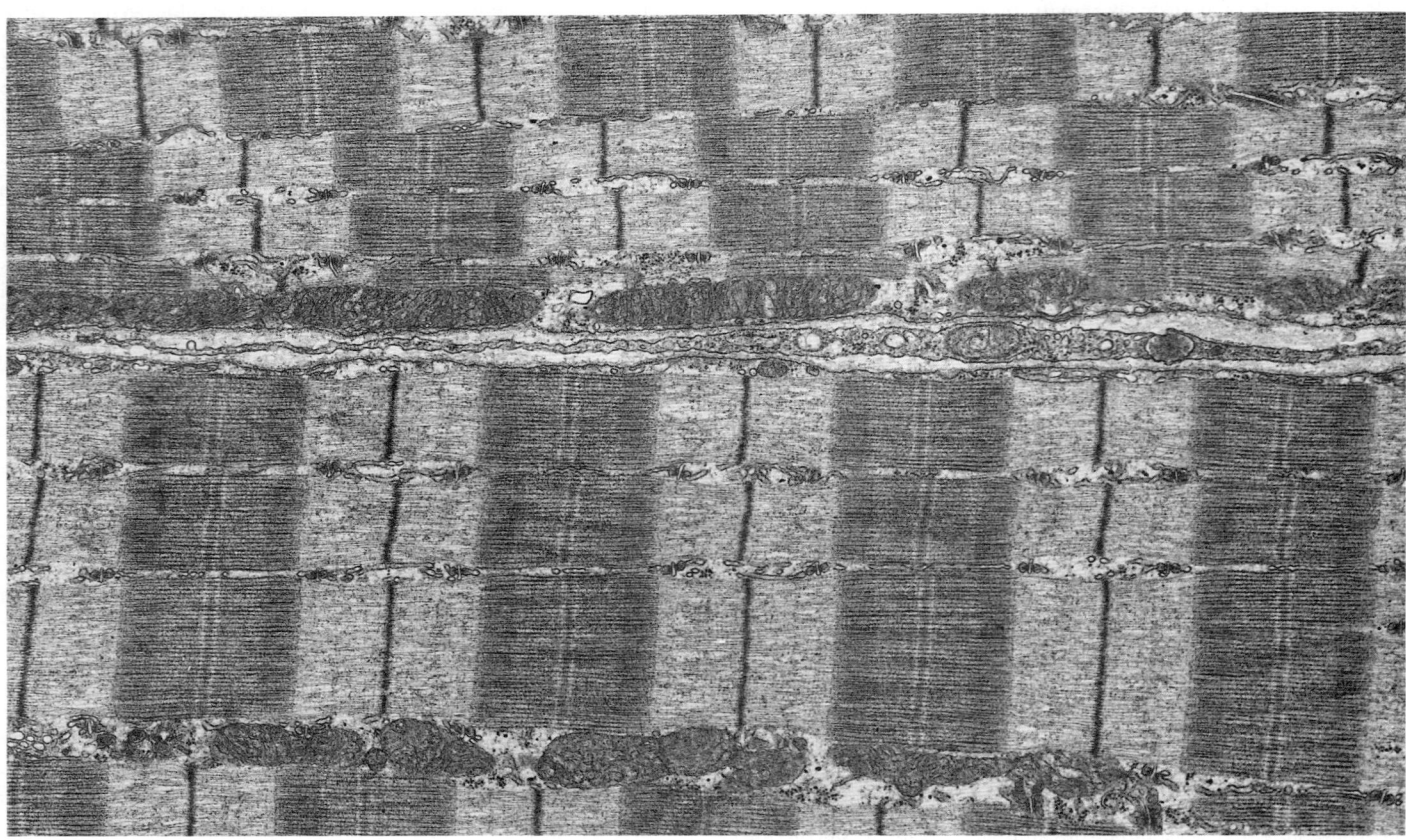

7.7   Low-power electron micrograph of skeletal muscle in longitudinal section, showing myofibrils. (Photograph by Brenda Russell, Department of Physiology and Biophysics, University of Illinois at Chicago.)

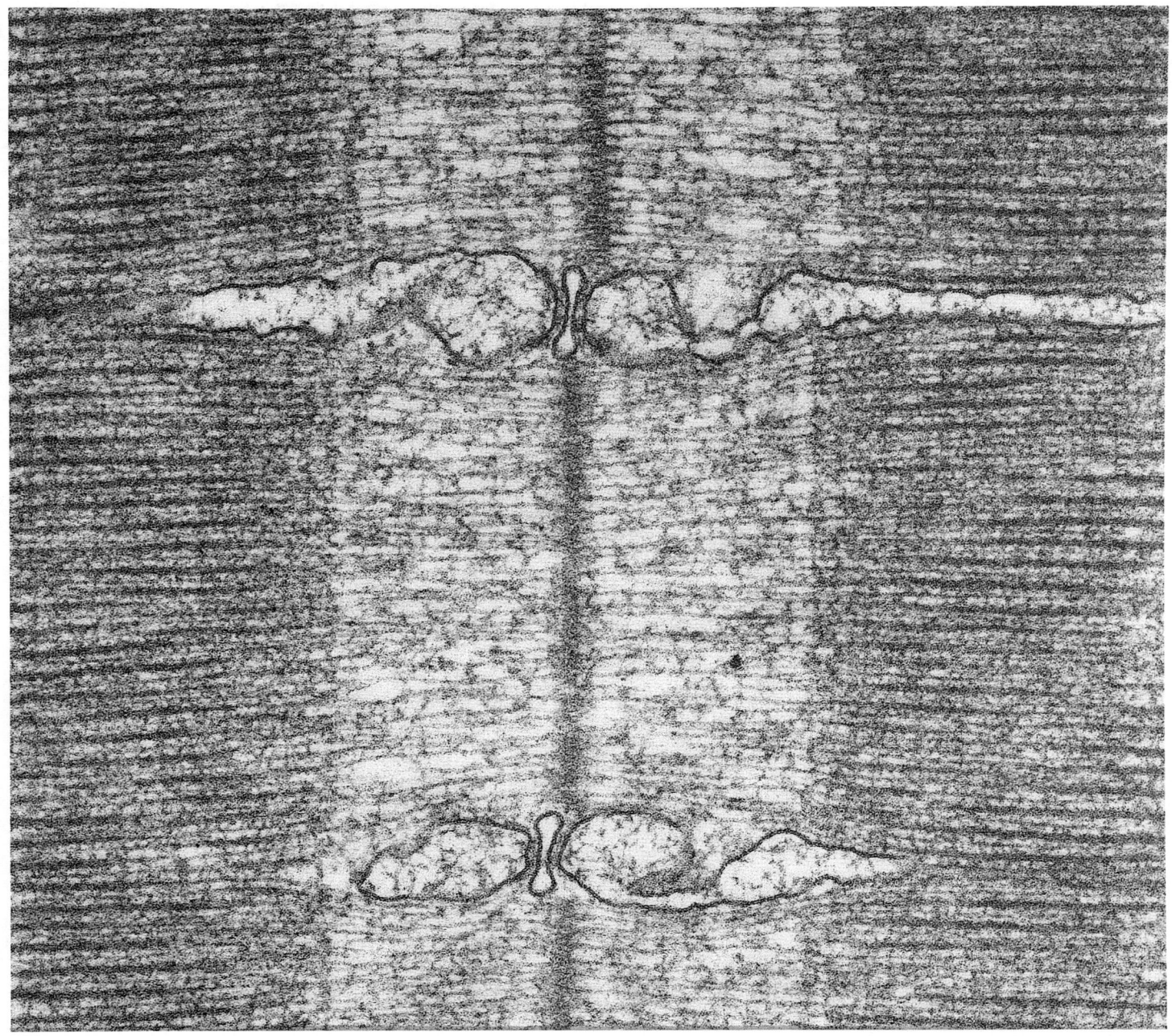

7.8 High-power electron micrograph of frog skeletal muscle in longitudinal section, showing triads, thick and thin filaments and cross-bridges bridging the spaces between them. Note the overlap of thin filaments within the Z-disc at the top of the micrograph. (Photograph by Brenda Russell, Department of Physiology and Biophysics, University of Illinois at Chicago.)

cross-bridges from this region accounts for the electronlucent pseudo-H-zone referred to above.

It appears that the two heads of a myosin molecule can act fairly independently; they may even bind to different actin filaments. This freedom results from a flexible point of attachment between the heads and the tail: each head can both swing and rotate about a point near the head–tail junction. Cleavage by proteolytic enzymes at this point divides the molecule into two subfragments: light meromyosin (LMM), which represents most of the tail, and heavy meromyosin (HMM), which contains the rest of the tail and the two globular heads. Heavy meromyosin can be cleaved further to yield the two heads separately (HMM subfragment-1 or S1), leaving behind a short segment of the tail (HMM subfragment-2 or S2). HMM S1, a folded chain of about 900 amino acids, retains all the enzymic and actin-binding properties of the parent molecule, and therefore all the elements needed for the production of force and movement.

In the presence of ATP and magnesium ions, HMM S1 can bind to actin filaments, which are then 'decorated' in a helical pattern, giving the appearance of arrowheads in electron micrographs. This property has been used as a specific labelling technique for demonstrating the presence of actin; it has also provided important insights into the structure of the actomyosin complex (Moore et al 1970).

After suitable chemical modification, HMM S1 produces crystals of sufficient quality for X-ray crystallographic analysis, and this approach has provided the most detailed description to date of the three-dimensional molecular structure of myosin (Rayment et al 1993b). A particularly interesting feature is a prominent cleft in the heavy chain which carries components of the actin-binding site on either side. Combining the crystallographic data with image reconstruction of S1-decorated actin filaments (Schröder et al 1993) provides insight into the docking of the two proteins. It is suggested that the actin filament lies quite deeply in this cleft, and that the

743

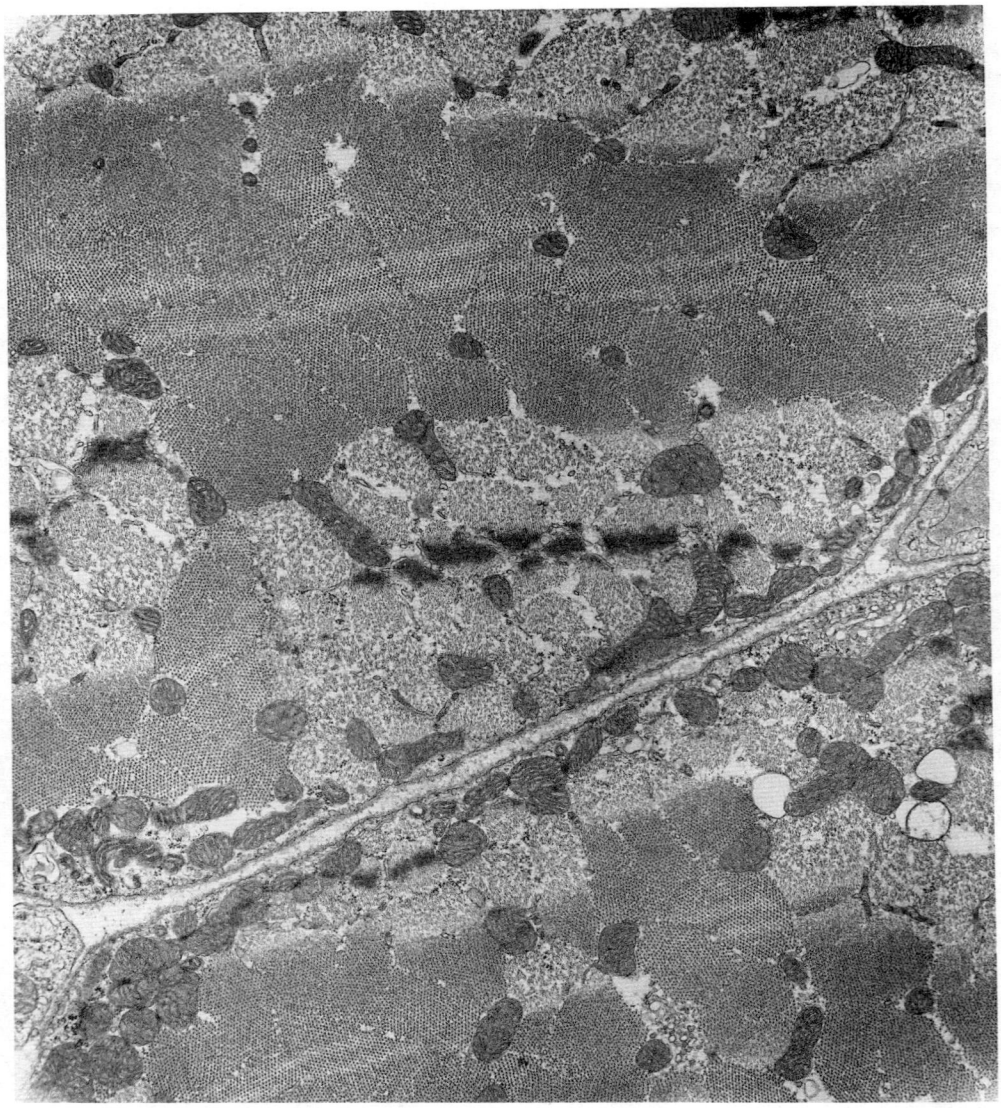

7.9   Low-power survey electron micrograph of skeletal muscle in transverse section, showing parts of two muscle fibres with their myofibrils and mitochondria. A capillary is seen in transverse section in the endomysial space. The variation in the appearance of myofibrils in cross-section is explained in **7**.10. (Photograph by Brenda Russell, Department of Physiology and Biophysics, University of Illinois at Chicago.)

cleft opens and closes in response to the state of the nucleotide bound at the ATP site, thus modifying the actin-S1 interaction (Rayment et al 1993a). At the end of the cross-bridge cycle, for example, the binding of the terminal phosphate of ATP at this site would open the cleft and release the myosin from the actin. The power stroke itself would involve a change in the curvature of the neck region of the myosin head, with most of the S1 remaining in the same orientation to the actin. This is consistent with earlier proposals (Cooke 1986) and explains why it has not proved possible to demonstrate cross-bridge configurations intermediate between the relaxed condition (cross-bridges detached) and the so-called rigor condition (cross-bridges at 45°).

The *myosin light chains* are of two chemically and structurally distinct types, and each myosin head contains one of each type. Their amino acid sequences bear strong similarities to the Ca^{2+}-binding proteins calmodulin and troponin-C, and in some species they mediate the Ca^{2+}-sensitive regulation of the ATPase activity of myosin (Kawasaki & Kretsinger 1994). In vertebrate striated muscle, evolutionary divergence has reduced their ability to bind divalent cations (Collins 1991), and although some involvement of the light chains in ATPase activity has been suggested, their major role appears to be structural: one of them appears to stabilize an α-helical portion of the heavy chain that runs through the globular head and may serve to amplify the working stroke (Rayment et al 1993b;

Lowey et al 1993). Note that in smooth muscle the light chains do regulate the myosin ATPase activity, although the Ca^{2+}-sensitive steps have been removed to other proteins (p. 778).

Both heavy and light chains exist as families of molecules which are strongly related but differ to some extent in their amino acid sequences. These myosin *isoforms* appear either at different stages of development or in functionally distinct muscle fibres in the adult. The fibres may be distinguished by histochemical techniques that exploit differences in the pH lability of the ATPase activity (**7**.20B) or by antibodies specific to the different myosin heavy chains (**7**.20C, D; see also p. 754).

Proteins of the thin filament

After myosin, actin is the next most abundant contractile protein, comprising 20% of the total myofibrillar protein. In its filamentous form (F-actin) it is the principal protein of the thin filaments; the other components, the proteins tropomyosin and troponin, play a major part in the control of contraction, a process referred to as *regulation*.

Actin filaments are about 1.0 μm long and consist of chains of globular actin (G-actin) subunits (M_r 41 700). These subunits (or monomers) are more highly conserved than myosin. They can be thought of as lying on two helical tracks wound around each other and repeating every 79 nm (**7**.12; see for example, Holmes et al 1990).

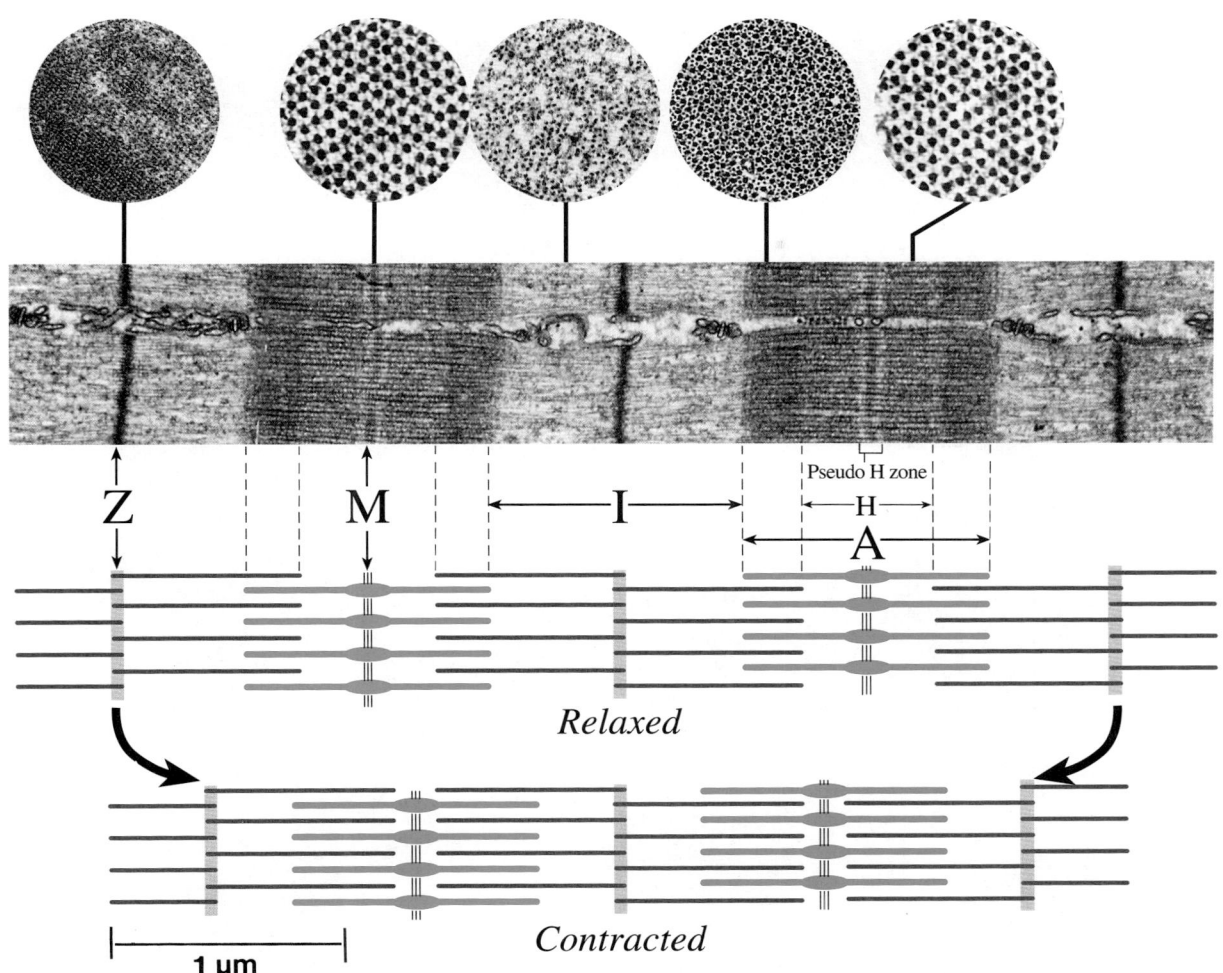

Z M I Pseudo H zone H A

Relaxed

Contracted

1 µm

7.10 Sarcomeric structures. In the centre is an electron micrograph of a myofibril sectioned longitudinally. The drawings below the micrograph indicate the corresponding disposition of the thick and thin filaments. Relaxed and contracted states are shown to illustrate the changes that occur during shortening. Insets at the top show the electron micrographic appearance of transverse sections through the sarcomere at the levels shown. Note that the packing geometry of the thin filaments changes from a square array at the Z-disc to a hexagonal array where they interdigitate with thick filaments in the A-band. (Photographs by Brenda Russell, Department of Physiology and Biophysics, University of Illinois at Chicago; artwork by Lesley Skeates.)

The number of subunits in this distance is not integral but is about 27. Actin has an orientation, or polarity, which may be determined by observing the direction of the arrowheads in S1-decorated filaments. In the sarcomere, the actin filaments are orientated in opposite directions on either side of the Z-disc. This, together with the bipolar construction of the adjacent thick filaments, ensures that active sliding always takes place in such a direction as to shorten the sarcomeres.

Arranged at regular intervals along both sides of the actin filament are the regulatory proteins, *tropomyosin* and *troponin*, such that for every 7 actin subunits there is one molecule each of tropomyosin and troponin (**7**.12). *Tropomyosin* ($M_r \sim 68\,000$) is a rod-like molecule consisting of a two-chain α-helical coiled coil. It is about 41 nm long and follows the long-pitch grooves in the thin filament, spanning 7 actin monomers and overlapping slightly with the next tropomyosin molecule. Troponin is a complex of three subunits arranged as a globular head and tail with an overall length of 27 nm. The three subunits are named after their principal properties: troponin-I (M_r 20 900; *I*nhibitory), troponin-C (M_r 17 800; *C*alcium-binding), and troponin-T (M_r 30 500; *T*ropomyosin-binding). Like myosin, tropomyosin and the troponin subunits exist in different isoforms.

Together these molecules form a calcium-sensitive switch that is believed to control the interaction between actin and myosin in the following way (Ebashi et al 1969). In the resting muscle, the presence of the tropomyosin on the actin filaments prevents them from interacting strongly with myosin, presumably by obstructing access to the S1 contact sites on one or more actin monomers. When muscle is activated, there is a sudden increase in the concentration of free Ca^{2+} in the cytoplasm. Calcium ions bind to four Ca^{2+}-binding sites on the troponin and induce a conformational change. This causes tropomyosin to roll deeper into the groove formed by the two helical rows of actin monomers, relieving the steric block and allowing a more complete actin–myosin interaction to take place.

Scaffold proteins

Grouped under this heading are proteins that are neither contractile nor regulatory but are responsible for the structural integrity of the myofibrils, particularly their regular internal arrangement. We also consider here an intermediate filament protein (desmin) that connects myofibrils together within the muscle fibre.

Z-discs provide anchorage for the thin filaments. Because of their electron density, they are the most prominent feature in longitudinal electron micrographs, in which they appear as dark bands. The thickness of these bands varies with the type of striated muscle and the species from which it is derived (Rowe 1973). The simplest Z-discs are found in fish (Franzini-Armstrong 1973; Luther 1991) and have a zig-zag appearance, from which the thin filaments emerge at the points. Although this is the appearance denoted in countless texts, the mammalian Z-disc has greater thickness, and appears to correspond to multiple layers of the fish type. Such a structure can be generated if it is assumed that each actin filament is connected by fine bridging strands to actin filaments from the adjacent sarcomere. If the actin filaments overlap within the Z-disc, another layer of strands can bind to the actin 38.5 nm further down, a distance that corresponds to the helix cross-over repeat. Further overlap would allow yet another layer of bridges to form (Squire

745

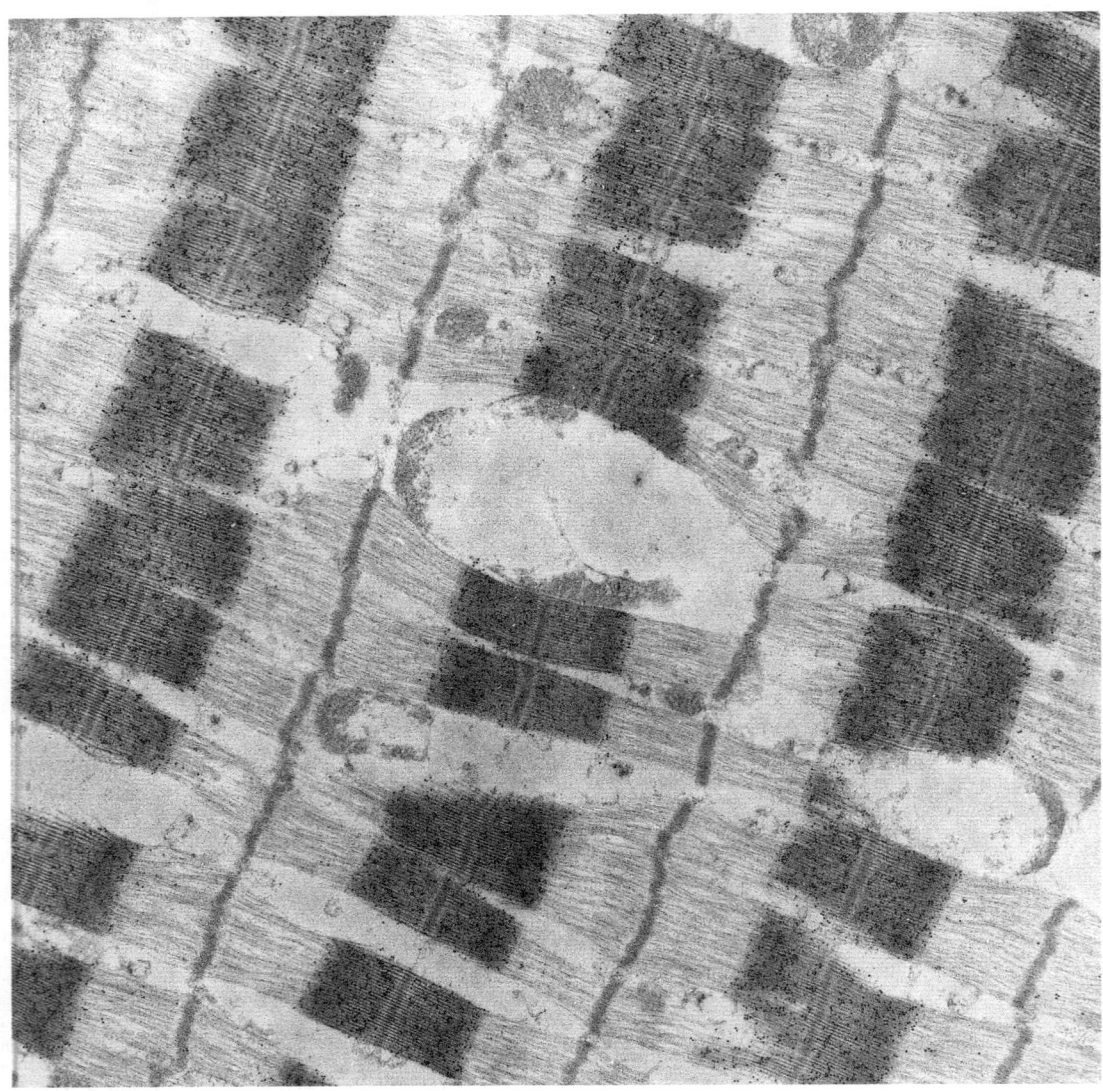

7.11 Low-power electron micrograph of a longitudinal section through rabbit skeletal muscle. The lightly fixed section has been stained by a gold-conjugated monoclonal antibody to myosin. The distribution of colloidal gold particles corresponds to the presence of myosin in the A-bands. The antibody is specific to a site in the cross-bridge portion of the myosin; hence particles are not found in the central, pseudo-H zone of the A-band, where the myosin molecules are assembled tail-to-tail. (Photograph by Leslie L Franchi, Department of Anatomy, University of Birmingham. See also Franchi et al 1990.)

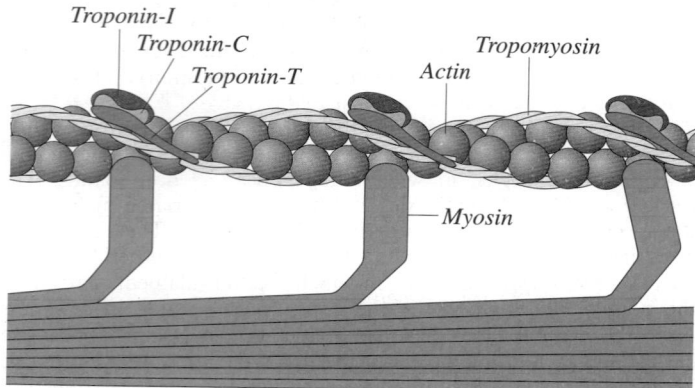

7.12 Schematic illustration of the relationship between actin, myosin and the regulatory proteins tropomyosin, troponin-I, troponin-C and troponin-T. (Artwork by Lesley Skeates, based on an illustration by Richard L Moss, Department of Physiology, University of Wisconsin-Madison.)

1981). These distances correspond closely to measurements of the apparent overlap of actin filaments in fast (39 nm) and slow (78 nm) skeletal muscle (Salmons et al 1978; see p. 755 for fast and slow types of skeletal muscle). The presence of the bridging strands is confirmed when the Z-disc structure is viewed face-on: in transverse sections close to the Z-discs, the thin filaments lie in a square array, but within the Z-disc itself a finer square lattice is formed by strands that bridge between the thin filaments (**7**.10). The most likely candidate for the bridging protein is *a-actinin*, a rod-shaped molecule composed of two similar chains, each of M_r 95 000, which has been localized in the Z-disc. Several other proteins have been identified as probable constituents of the Z-disc, including *CapZ*, *Z-nin* and *zeugmatin*, but the arrangement of these is not known.

At the centre of the A-band is the *M-line* (**7**.10). This is not one line but several, the actual number varying according to the muscle type and the species (Sjöström & Squire 1977). The M-*line* structure is formed by sets of *M-bridges*, which interconnect adjacent thick filaments at their centres and probably maintain them in their regular hexagonal array. The three strongest sets of M-bridges are connected together by short *M-filaments*, which run parallel to the thick filaments. In addition, there are finer connections joining the

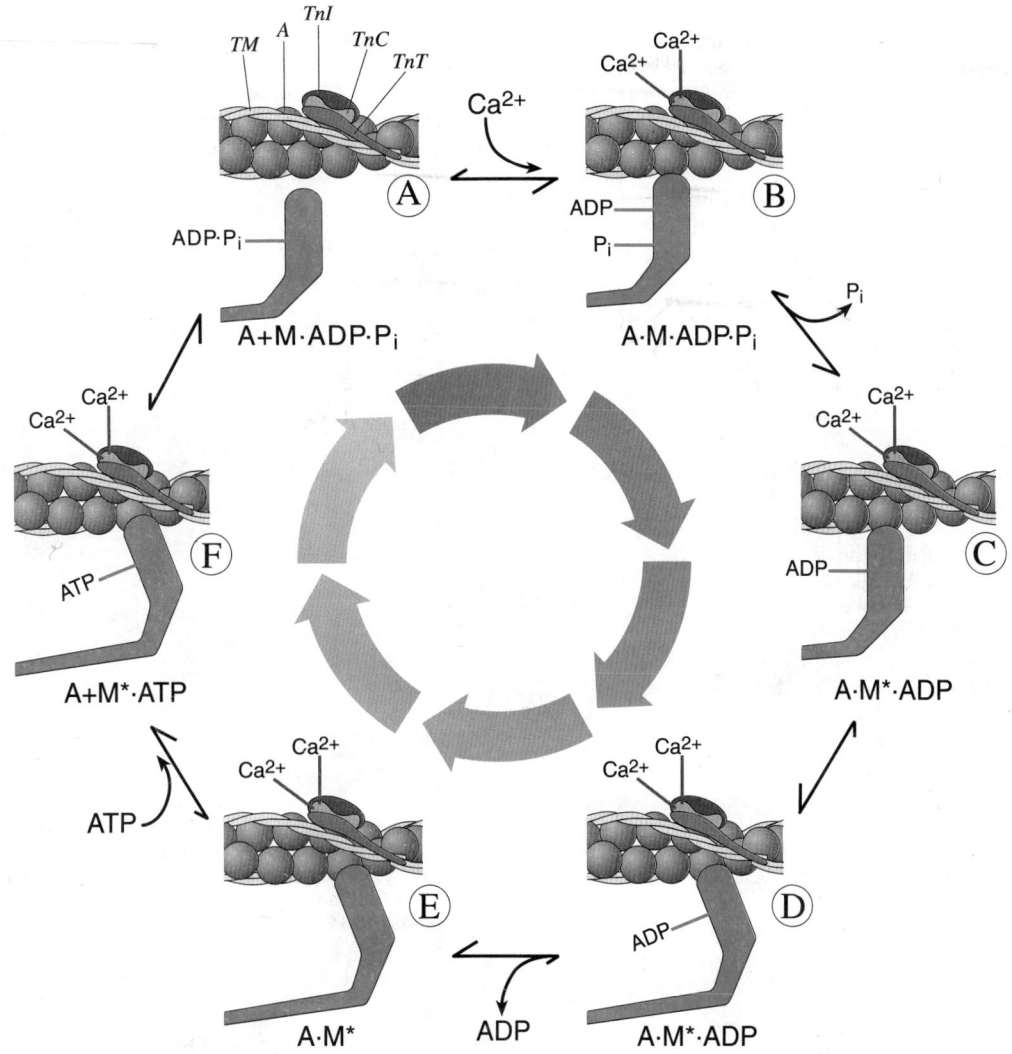

7.13 The mechanochemical cycle of muscle contraction. One of the cross-bridges of **7.**12 is shown at different stages of the contraction cycle. TM = tropomyosin, A = actin, TnI = troponin-I, TnC = troponin-C, TnT = troponin-T, M = myosin, M* = myosin (force-generating state). A. Weak binding. B. Strong binding. C–D. Conformational change. E. 'Rigor' condition. F. ATP-binding, followed by detachment. (See text for more detail.) (Artwork by Lesley Skeates, based on an illustration by Richard L Moss, Department of Physiology, University of Wisconsin-Madison.)

M-filaments at sites between the M-bridges (Luther & Squire 1978). Which proteins form each of these structural elements is not yet well established, but proteins of chain molecular weight 185 000 (*myomesin*), 165 000, 215 000 (*skelemin*) and 43 000 are known to be located in this region. The 43 000 M-protein is an isoform of the enzyme *creative kinase*.

Note that the Z-disc and the M-line impose different packing symmetries on the filaments: the thin filaments, which are arranged in a square array close to the Z-disc, adopt a hexagonal pattern when they interdigitate with the thick filaments in the A-band.

In many skeletal muscles, the length of the thin filament is specified exactly, but in other cases—such as cardiac muscle—there is more variation in length. A possible mechanism for length regulation involves the giant protein *nebulin* ($M_r \sim 800\,000$). Single molecules of nebulin appear to span entire thin filaments (Wright et al 1993) and are thought to act as templates for precise thin filament assembly.

In addition to the thick and thin filaments, there are long sarcomeric filaments of a third type which connect the ends of the thick filaments to the Z-disc. These filaments are formed by the giant protein, *titin* ($M_r \sim 3\,000\,000$; Wang et al 1979), also found in the literature as *connectin* (Maruyama et al 1977), which is the largest known polypeptide. Single titin molecules span the half-sarcomere between the M-lines and the Z-discs, with a bound portion in the A-band and an elastic portion in the I-band (see, for example, Trinick 1992). In the A-band, titin is thought to be attached to the outside of the thick filament shaft. In the I-band, the elastic sections of titin molecules centre the A-band between adjacent Z-discs. These filaments also provide the main route for mechanical continuity through relaxed myofibrils.

The titin molecule appears to be composed mainly of a linear series of 100-amino-acid-residue domains that are similar to domains in immunoglobulins (type C-2) and fibronectin (type III). These types of domain were once thought to belong exclusively to extracellular proteins, but several myofibrillar proteins are now known to have them. The feature uniting this sub-group of muscle proteins is that they all bind to myosin. The 165 000 M-protein, already mentioned in the context of the M-line, belongs to this group formed from domains. *C-protein* ($M_r\ 128\,000$) is a thick filament component of unknown function consisting of 11 such domains. When myofibrils are labelled with antibodies to pure C-protein, they show a pattern of stripes in the middle of each half of the A-band. These studies show that C-protein is bound at 7 or 8 sites, 43 nm apart in each half of the thick filament. *X-protein*, a C-protein isoform, occupies similar positions in slow muscle fibres. Other components, some so far unidentified, also contribute to a pattern that numbers some 11 equally-spaced, accessory protein stripes in each half-A-band.

The I-band, too, contains accessory stripes, referred to as the *N-lines* (see, for example, Locker & Wild 1984). Their visibility varies, reflecting perhaps variability in the binding of the proteins that form them. The N_1 line is located 110 nm from the Z-disc and may be the site at which the thin filament lattice changes from square to hexagonal. There are up to four N_2 lines in the middle of the I-band and two N_3 lines near the ends of the thin filaments. The distance from the Z-disc to the N_2 and N_3 lines varies with sarcomere length, suggesting that these lines may be associated with titin. The proteins responsible for the N-lines have yet to be identified, with the possible exception of the N_3 line, which may be formed by AMP-deaminase.

A skeletal muscle fibre appears cross-striated in the light microscope because the bands in adjacent myofibrils are aligned across the breadth of the fibre. The protein responsible for this alignment is *desmin* (M_r 55 000, also found in the literature as *skeletin*), which is a muscle-specific member of the class of intermediate filament proteins (Lazarides 1980). Desmin filaments cross-link adjacent myofibrils at the level of the Z-disc, maintaining the sarcomeres in register.

Dystrophin

Dystrophin is the product of the gene for Duchenne muscular dystrophy, a fatal disorder that develops when mutation of the gene leads to the absence of this protein. A milder form of the disease, Becker muscular dystrophy, is associated with a reduced size and/or abundance of dystrophin. Dystrophin, first described in 1987 (Hoffman et al 1987), was identified by reverse genetics: its gene and cDNA were isolated and its amino acid sequence was then deduced from the DNA sequence. At approximately 2500 kb, the gene is the largest yet discovered and this may account for the high mutation rate of Duchenne muscular dystrophy (roughly 35% of new cases).

Dystrophin (M_r 427 000) shares some structural features with spectrin and *α*-actinin. On the basis of these structural homologies it can be divided into four domains:

- the N-terminal, with sequence homologies to the F-actin binding domain of *α*-actinin
- a major rod-like domain, comprising 25 repeating elements similar to those in spectrin
- a cysteine-rich domain, with a weak homology to *α*-actinin
- a unique and highly conserved C-terminal domain that has some similarity to an autosomal analogue of dystrophin (Dystrophin-Related Protein or utrophin, Love et al 1989).

Dystrophin is confined to the periphery of the muscle fibre, close to the cytoplasmic face of the plasma membrane. It is associated with a large oligomeric complex of glycoproteins which span the membrane and link specifically with laminin in the extracellular matrix (7.14; Ibraghimov-Beskrovnaya et al 1992). The glycoprotein-binding site of dystrophin is confined to the cysteine-rich domain and the first half of the C-terminal domain. At the opposite end of the molecule, the N-terminal domain, dystrophin binds to F-actin.

The precise cellular function of dystrophin is not yet clear, but the roles that have been proposed fall roughly into three categories:

- it may contribute mechanical strength to the membrane

- it may anchor an integral membrane protein (part of the glycoprotein complex) to the cytoskeleton
- it may act as a link between the cell cytoskeleton and the extracellular matrix.

There is evidence for each of these functions. Lack of dystrophin, together with the loss of the associated glycoproteins, may leave the membrane more permeable or more susceptible to mechanical damage (Gorospe & Hoffman 1992; Matsumura & Campbell 1994). Because of its importance in understanding the structural and functional deterioration that takes place in muscular dystrophy, this is an extremely active and ongoing area of research.

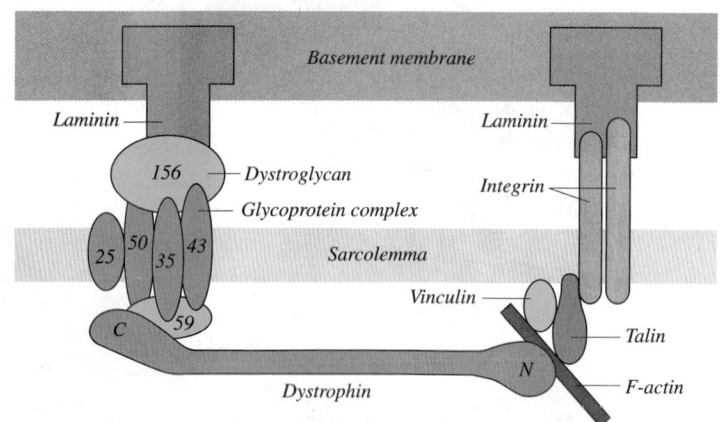

7.14 Schematic model, speculative in places, of the proteins that bridge between the subsarcolemmal cytoskeleton and the basement membrane. (Artwork by Stanley Salmons and Lesley Skeates, based loosely on Gorospe & Hoffman 1992; Isenberg & Goldmann 1992; Matsumura & Campbell 1994).

NON-MYOFIBRILLAR STRUCTURES OF THE SARCOPLASM

Although myofibrils are the dominant feature in electron micrographs of muscle, the fibres contain other organelles essential to cellular function, such as ribosomes, Golgi apparatus and mitochondria, most of which are located around the nuclei between the myofibrillar material and the sarcolemma and, to a lesser extent, between the myofibrils (Eisenberg 1983). Mitochondria, lipid droplets and glycogen provide the metabolic support needed by active muscle.

The *mitochondria* are elongated and their cristae are closely packed. Their profiles are usually seen in longitudinal orientation between the myofibrils (7.7) or in transverse orientation in the I-band (7.9); a small proportion are found at the periphery of the fibre, where their presence may help to maximize the extraction of oxygen from adjacent capillaries. The number of mitochondria in an adult muscle fibre is not fixed, but can increase or decrease quite readily in response to sustained changes in activity (Eisenberg & Salmons 1981; Salmons & Henriksson 1981; Eisenberg et al 1984). This explains the wide variation in the mitochondrial content of fibres whose roles in movement and posture pose different functional demands (see p. 754). Spherical *lipid droplets*, of about 0.25 μm diameter, are distributed uniformly throughout the non-myofibrillar spaces. They represent a rich source of energy which can, however, be tapped only by oxidative metabolic pathways; they are therefore more common in fibres that have a high mitochondrial content and good capillary blood supply. *Glycogen* is distributed in small clusters of granules between myofibrils and among the thin filaments. In brief bursts of activity it provides an important source of energy that is immediately available, and not dependent on nutrient blood flow to the muscle fibre, because it is stored close to where it is needed and because it can be partially metabolized in the absence of oxygen.

The *sarcolemma* has the ultrastructural appearance of a typical plasma membrane, including an external basal lamina, to which collagen fibres and other connective tissue components adhere. At the ends of the muscle fibre, where force is transmitted to adjacent connective tissue structures, the sarcolemma is folded into numerous finger-like projections; these strengthen the junctional region by increasing the area of attachment (Eisenberg & Milton 1984).

The *tubular system* consists of tubular invaginations of the sarcolemma, which penetrate between the myofibrils in a transverse plane at the limit of each A-band (**7.15**). The lumina of these *T-*, or *transverse*, *tubules* can be shown to remain in continuity with the extracellular space: tracer substances infused extracellularly can be found subsequently in the T-tubules, within which they can diffuse into the depths of a muscle fibre (Peachey & Franzini-Armstrong 1983).

The *sarcoplasmic reticulum* is a specialized form of agranular endoplasmic reticulum: markers that are found in the endoplasmic reticular membrane of other cell types are also found in sarcoplasmic reticulum. It consists of a plexus of anastomosing membranous passages filling much of the space between myofibrils and expanding into larger sacs—*junctional sarcoplasmic reticulum* or *terminal cisternae*—where it comes into close contact with the T-system (**7.8, 16**). At this point, electron micrographs show a structure called a *triad*, comprising a central T-tubule flanked on either side by two terminal cisternae, the latter filled with dense, granular material (**7.16**). (The functional significance of this structure will be outlined in the next section.) The membranes of the sarcoplasmic reticulum contain calcium–ATPase pumps, which transport calcium ions into the terminal cisternae. There the ions are bound to *calsequestrin*, a protein that has a high affinity for calcium, in the dense storage granules. In this way calcium can be accumulated and retained in the terminal cisternae at a much higher level than anywhere else in the sarcoplasm.

Excitation–contraction coupling

The sarcolemma is an excitable membrane, and action potentials generated at the neuromuscular junction (see p. 752) propagate rapidly over the entire surface of the muscle fibre. The action potentials are conducted radially into the interior of the fibre via the T-tubules, an arrangement which ensures that all parts of the muscle fibre are activated rapidly and almost synchronously. *Excitation–contraction coupling* is the process whereby the action potential triggers the release of calcium from the storage granules of the terminal cisternae into the cytosol, activating the calcium-sensitive switch in the thin filaments and so initiating contraction. This process depends on the apposition of two sets of proteins, one belonging to the T-tubule and the other to the sarcoplasmic reticulum, that span the 15-nm gap between the two membranes where they come together in the triad (Block et al 1988). The protein complex in the T-membrane consists of groups of four particles, or tetrads, that correspond to the *dihydropyridine* (*DHP*) *receptors* (Rios & Pizarro 1991); these are believed to act as voltage-sensors, responsive to the change in electrical field produced by the action potential. The corresponding structures on the membrane of the sarcoplasmic reticulum protrude from its junctional face, typically in two rows, like the feet of a caterpillar (Peachey & Franzini-Armstrong 1983). These junctional 'feet' are composed of the large cytoplasmic domain of four *calcium-release channels*, often referred to as the *ryanodine receptor* because the plant alkaloid ryanodine binds specifically to the channel complex. It is believed that the arrival of an action potential induces a conformational change in the DHP receptor in

the T-tubule (Schneider & Chandler 1973) which is coupled to the release of stored calcium ions through the foot protein complexes in the junctional face of the terminal cisternae (Fleischer & Inui 1989; Rios & Pizarro 1991). At the end of excitation, the T-tubular membrane repolarizes, calcium release through the junctional feet ceases, calcium ions are actively transported back to the calsequestrin stores by the calcium–ATPase pumps, and the muscle relaxes.

THE INTERFACE BETWEEN MUSCLE AND CONNECTIVE TISSUE

The delicate networks of connective tissue that surround the muscle fibres are referred to collectively as the *endomysium*. This forms the immediate external environment of the muscle fibres. It is the site of metabolic exchange between muscle and blood, and capillaries run, together with small nerve branches, in this layer. Ion fluxes associated with the electrical excitation of muscle fibres take place through its proteoglycan matrix. The endomysium is continuous with more substantial septa of connective tissue which constitute the *perimysium*; this ensheathes groups of muscle fibres to form parallel bundles or *fasciculi*. The perimysium carries larger blood vessels and nerves and also accommodates neuromuscular spindles (p. 969). The perimysial septa are themselves the inward extensions of a collagenous sheath, the *epimysium*. This develops some thickness and forms part of the fascia which invests whole muscle groups.

Collagen types I, III, IV and V may be demonstrated in these layers by fluorescent antibody techniques. Epimysium consists mainly of type I collagen, perimysium contains type I and type III collagen, and endomysium contains collagen types III, IV and V, the latter two associated particularly with the basement membrane that invests each muscle fibre (Duance et al 1980).

The epimysial, perimysial, and endomysial sheaths coalesce where the muscles connect to adjacent structures: tendons, aponeuroses, and fasciae. The result is to give such attachments great strength, since the tensile forces are distributed in the form of shear stresses, which are more easily resisted. This principle extends to the submicroscopic level at the ends of the muscle fibres, which divide into finger-like processes, allowing collagen fibres to penetrate into the intervening spaces (Trotter et al 1981; Eisenberg & Milton 1984; **7.17**). Although there are no desmosomal attachments at these *myotendinous junctions*, there are other specializations that assist in the transmission of force from the interior of the fibre to the extracellular matrix. Actin filaments from the adjacent sarcomeres, which would normally insert into a Z-disc at this point, penetrate instead into a dense subsarcolemmal matrix that provides attachment to the plasma membrane. This matrix is similar in character to the cytoplasmic face of an adherens junction (Geiger & Ginsberg 1991). Although its composition has still to be defined in detail, the major structural components are likely to be actin, *a*-actinin and vinculin, interacting with each other and with additional components, such as talin and the transmembrane protein integrin (Isenberg & Goldmann 1992). The structure is homologous to the intercalated discs of cardiac muscle and the adherens junctions of smooth muscle, which also provide anchorage for actin filaments (Jockusch et al 1993; and see below). Beyond the surface of the sarcolemma, fine junctional microfibrils, about 5–10 nm thick and of unknown composition, bridge across the lamina lucida to the prominent lamina densa of the junctional basement membrane, which in turn adheres closely to collagen and reticulin fibres of the adjacent tendon or other connective tissue structure (Law & Lightner 1993). Cell–substratum connections are not confined to the junctional region of the fibre. The Z-discs of peripheral myofibrils are each linked to the plasma membrane by vinculin-containing elements, which have been termed *costameres* (Pardo et al 1983a). These form part of another system of intracellular, transmembrane and extracellular proteins involved in transmitting force from the myofibrils laterally to the sarcolemma and beyond to the extracellular matrix (Law & Lightner 1993).

When a relaxed muscle is extended, the tension rises in a way that is determined by the hierarchy of connective tissue sheaths, by the systems of membrane-associated proteins, and by the titin filaments which provide mechanical continuity through the myofibrils. These passive elastic properties are also important in active muscle because they influence the rapidity with which force is transmitted from the

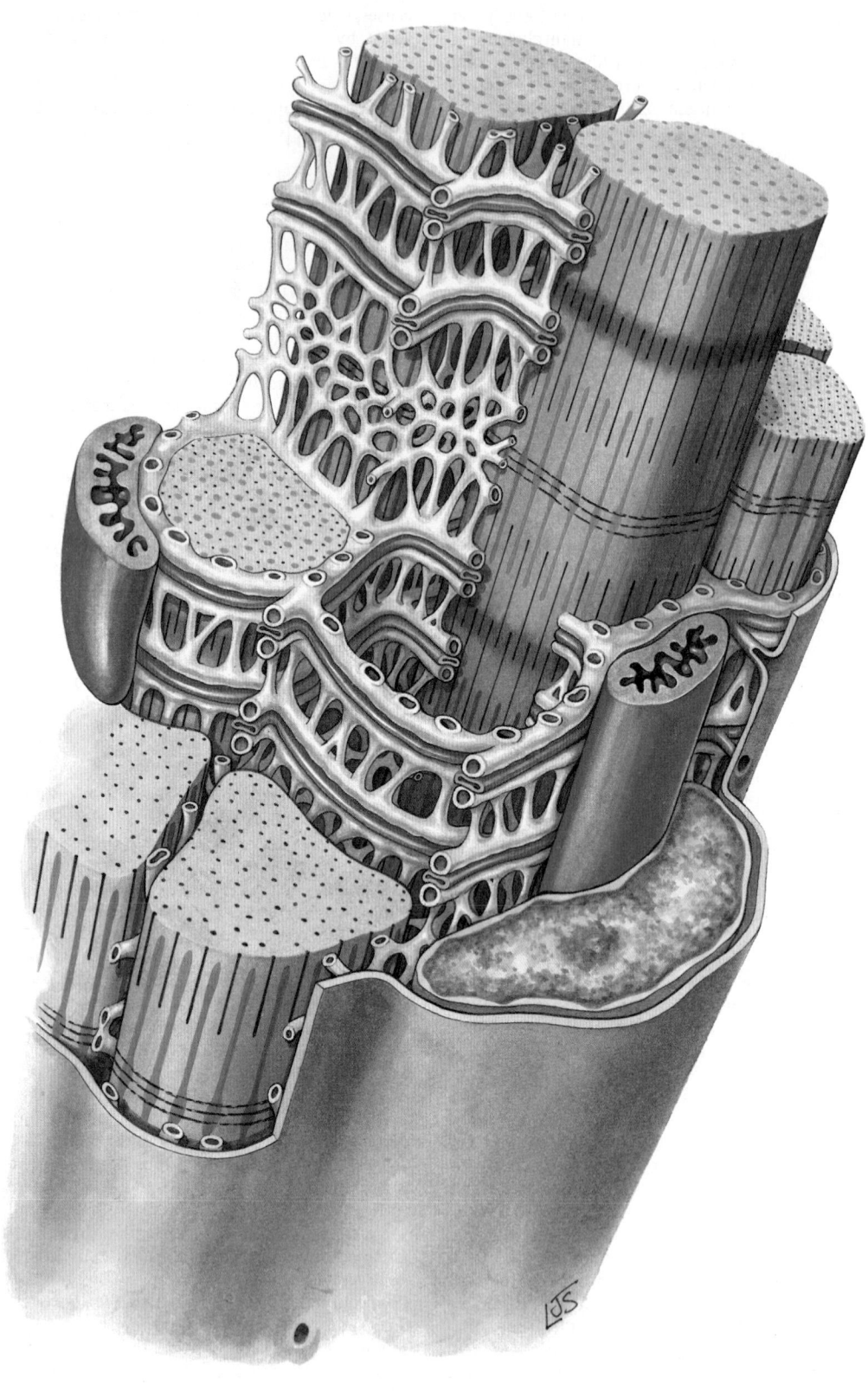

7.15 Three-dimensional reconstruction of a fibre of mammalian skeletal muscle, showing in particular the organization of the transverse tubules (orange) and sarcoplasmic reticulum (yellow). Mitochondria (blue) lie between the myofibrils and a muscle nucleus (green) at the periphery. Note that transverse tubules are found at the level of the A/I junctions, where they form triads with the terminal cisternae of the sarcoplasmic reticulum. (Artist: Lesley Skeates.)

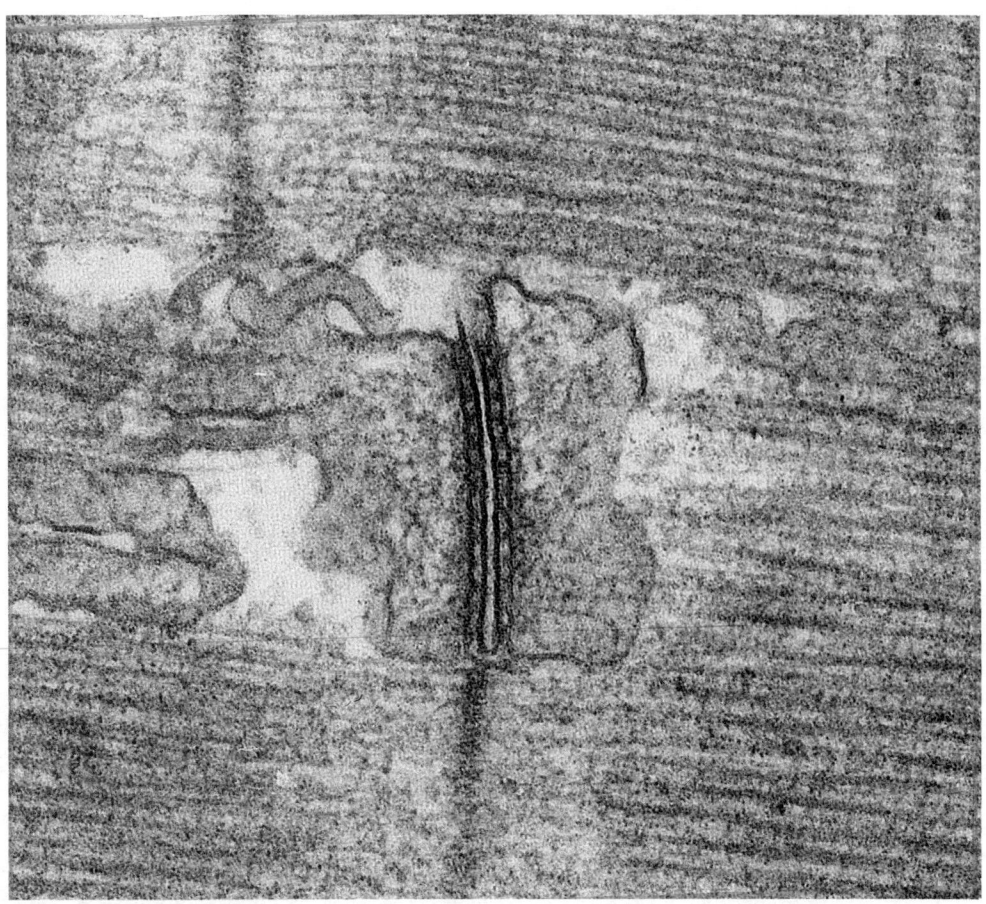

7.16 High-power electron micrograph of a portion of a triad of frog skeletal muscle in longitudinal section. The central T-tubule is flanked on each side by a terminal cisterna of the sarcoplasmic reticulum. Just visible are structures that bridge the 15-nm gap between the membranes; these are formed by the proteins responsible for excitation-contraction coupling (see text). In lower vertebrates, unlike mammals, it is usual for triads to be located, as here, at the level of the Z-discs. (Photograph by Brenda Russell, Department of Physiology and Biophysics, University of Illinois at Chicago.)

contractile components to adjacent structures (Hill 1970). Finally, elastic energy stored in these elements may be returned, particularly during cyclic movements, effecting worthwhile gains in efficiency (see p. 897).

GENERAL FEATURES OF THE BLOOD SUPPLY TO SKELETAL MUSCLES

In most muscles the major source artery enters on the deep surface, frequently in close association with the principal vein and nerve, which together form a neurovascular hilum. The vessels course and branch within the connective tissue framework of the muscle, with the smaller arteries and arterioles ramifying in the perimysial septa and giving off capillaries that run in the endomysium. While the smaller vessels lie mainly parallel to the muscle fibres, they also branch and anastomose around the fibres, forming an elongated mesh (**7.18A, B**).

In muscle cross-sections, the number of capillary profiles found adjacent to fibres usually varies from 0 to 3. Fibres that are involved in sustained activities—such as posture—are served by a denser capillary network than fibres which are recruited only infrequently (see Fibre types of adult skeletal muscle, p. 753). It is common for muscles to receive their arterial supply via more than one route. The accessory arteries penetrate the muscle at places other than the hilum and ramify in the same way as the principal artery, forming vascular territories (**7.18A**). The boundaries of adjacent territories are spanned by anastomotic vessels, sometimes at constant calibre but more commonly through reduced-calibre arteries or arterioles referred to as 'choke vessels'; these arterial arcades link the territories into a continuous network (Taylor & Palmer 1987).

Veins branch in a similar way, forming venous territories that correspond closely to the arterial territories. In the zones where the arterial territories are linked by choke vessels, the venous territories are linked by anastomosing veins, in this case without change of calibre. On either side of these venous bridges, the valves in the adjacent territories direct flow in opposite directions towards their respective pedicles, but the connecting veins themselves lack valves and would therefore permit flow in either direction (Watterson et al 1988).

Because of the potential for relative movement within muscle groups, vessels tend not to cross between muscles; rather, they radiate to them from more stable sites or cross at points of fusion. Where a muscle underlies the integument, vessels bridge between the two. These may be primarily skin vessels, supplying the skin directly but contributing small branches to the muscle as they pass through it, or they may be the terminal branches of intramuscular vessels, which leave the muscle to supplement the blood supply to the skin; the latter are less frequent where the muscle is mobile under the deep fascia (Taylor & Palmer 1987). The correspondence between the vascular territories in the skin and underlying tissues has given rise to the notion of *angiosomes*, composite blocks of tissue supplied by named distributing arteries and drained by their companion veins (Taylor & Palmer 1987; Watterson et al 1988).

The pressure exerted on valved intramuscular veins during contraction enables them to function as a 'muscle pump', promoting venous return to the heart. In some cases this role appears to be amplified by veins that pass through the muscle after originating elsewhere in superficial or deep tissues (Watterson et al 1988).

Various experiments, including the use of isotopic sodium as a tracer (Barlow et al 1961) and microscopic techniques (Grant & Wright 1968), provide evidence for the existence in muscle of arteriovenous anastomoses, through which blood can be returned directly to the venous system without having traversed the capillaries. The extent to which the muscle capillary bed is perfused can thus be varied in accordance with functional demand (see also p. 1467).

The lymphatic drainage of muscles commences as capillaries in

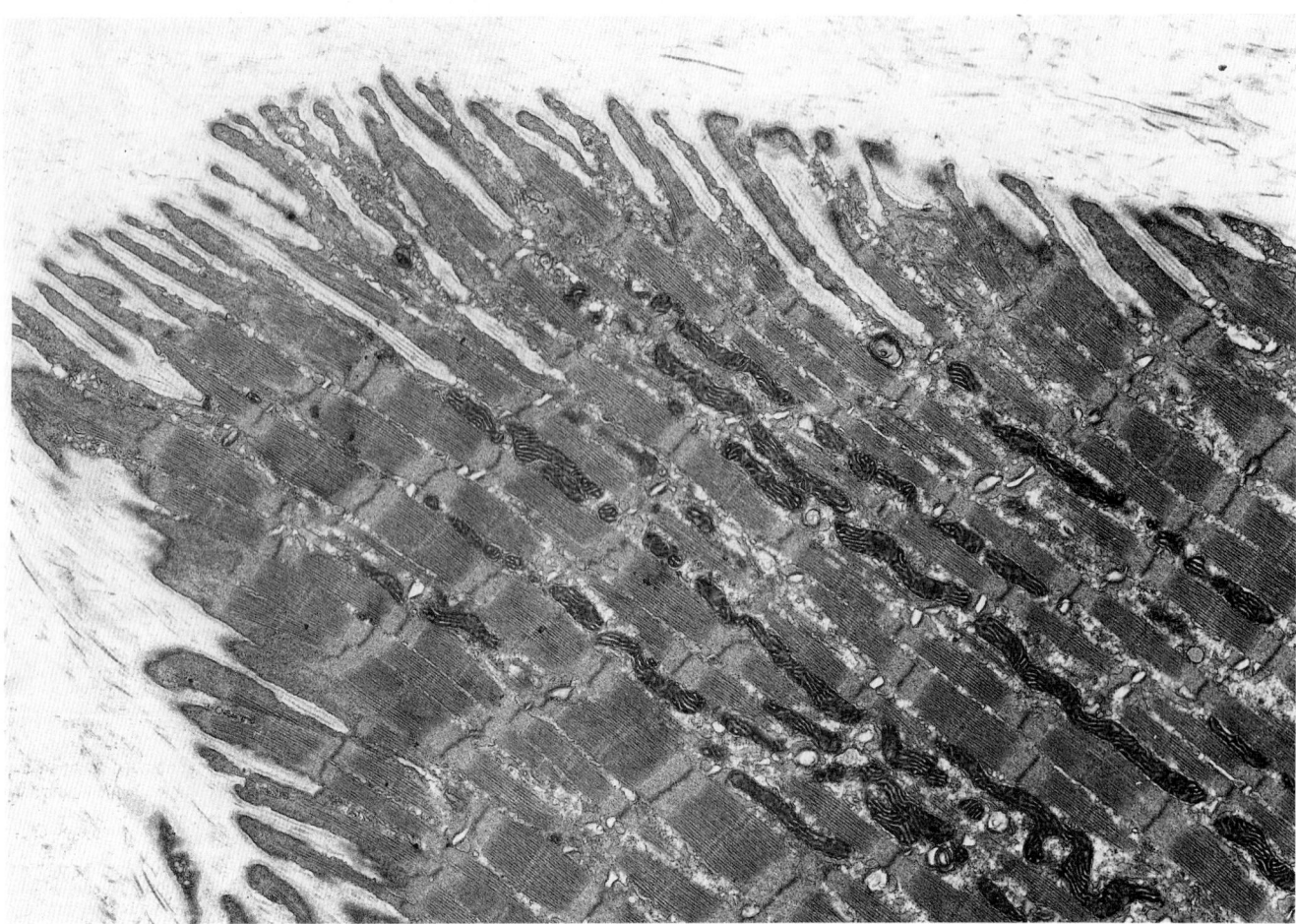

7.17 Electron micrograph of the terminal portion of a frog skeletal muscle fibre in longitudinal section, showing the myotendinous junction. Magnification × 12 000. (Photograph by Brenda Russell, Department of Physiology and Biophysics, University of Illinois at Chicago.)

epimyseal and perimysial, but not endomysial, sheaths. These converge to form larger lymphatic vessels which accompany the veins, draining to the regional lymph nodes.

INNERVATION OF SKELETAL MUSCLE

Every skeletal muscle is supplied by one or more nerves. In the limbs, face and neck there is usually a single nerve, although its axons may correspond to several spinal cord segments. Muscles such as those of the abdominal wall, which originate from several embryonic segments, are supplied by more than one nerve. In most cases the nerve travels with the principal blood vessels as a neurovascular bundle, approaches the muscle near to its least mobile attachment and enters the deep surface, at a position which is more or less constant for each muscle (see Brash 1955; Coers & Woolf 1959).

Muscle nerves are frequently referred to as 'motor nerves', but they contain both motor and sensory components. The major *motor* component consists of the large, myelinated axons that supply the muscle fibres; these α-efferents, or α-motor axons are among the fastest-conducting nerve fibres in the body. In addition, the nerve carries small, myelinated γ-efferents, or fusimotor fibres, which innervate the intrafusal muscle fibres of neuromuscular spindles, and fine, non-myelinated autonomic efferents (C fibres), which innervate vascular smooth muscle. The *sensory* component consists of the large, myelinated 2A afferents from the neuromuscular spindles, the slightly smaller myelinated 2B afferents from the Golgi tendon organs and fine myelinated and non-myelinated fibres conveying pain and other sensations from free terminals in the connective tissue sheaths

of the muscle. For a fuller consideration of this topic, see pages 948, 971.

Within muscles, nerves follow the connective tissue sheaths, coursing in the epimysial and perimysial septa before entering the fine endomysial tissue around the muscle fibres. α-motor axons branch repeatedly before they lose their myelinated sheaths and terminate near the middle of muscle fibres. These terminals tend to cluster in a narrow zone towards the centre of the muscle belly known as the *motor point*. Clinically, this is the place on the muscle from which it is easiest to elicit a contraction with stimulating electrodes.

A specialized synapse, the *neuromuscular junction*, is formed where the terminal branch of an α-motor axon contacts the muscle fibre. The axon terminal gives off several short, curling branches over an elliptical area, the *motor end plate*. Within the underlying discoidal patch of sarcolemma, the *sole plate* or *subneural apparatus*, the sarcolemma is thrown into deep synaptic folds. This discrete type of neuromuscular junction is an example of an *en plaque* ending and is found on muscle fibres that are capable of propagating action potentials. A different type of ending is found on slow tonic muscle fibres, which do not have this capability. This type of fibre is more common in birds and reptiles but is present in the extrinsic ocular muscles and the stapedius muscle of the middle ear in man. In this case the propagation of excitation is taken over by the nerve terminals, which branch over an extended distance to form a number of small neuromuscular junctions (*en grappe* endings). Some muscle fibres of this type receive the terminal branches of more than one motor neuron. The terminals of the γ-efferents that innervate the intrafusal muscle fibres of the neuromuscular spindle also take a variety of different forms, including *en plaque* endings and long trail

752

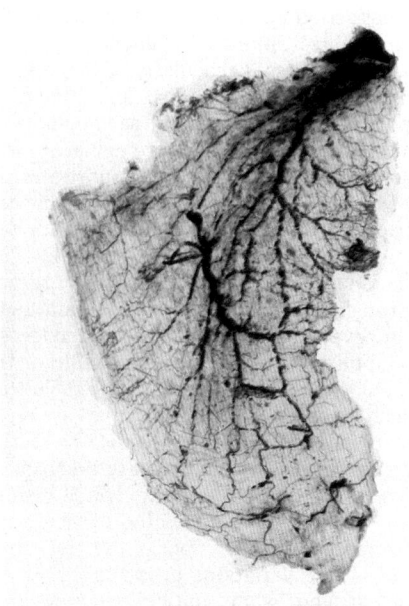

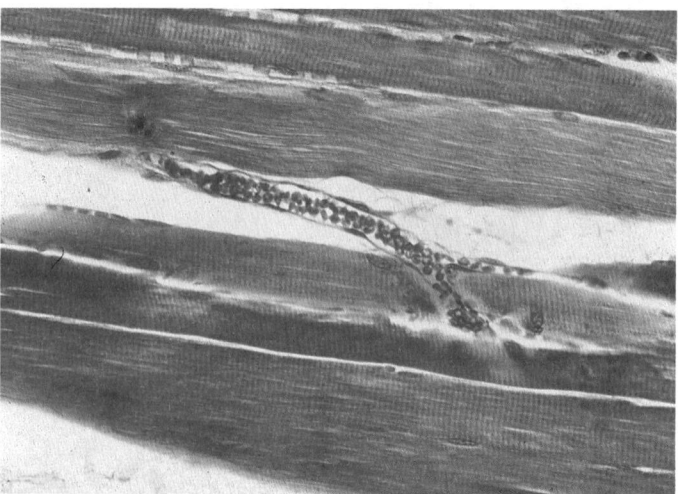

territories of these two arteries (see text). The blood supply of the human latissimus dorsi differs in detail (p. 1536), but shows the same broad features. (Photograph by Amanda J Craven, Department of Human Anatomy and Cell Biology, University of Liverpool.) B. A capillary in rabbit tibialis anterior muscle, stained with Heidenheim's haematoxylin. (Photograph by Stanley Salmons.)

7.18A, B. Blood supply of skeletal muscle. A. Vascular cast of the right latissimus dorsi muscle of a rat, viewed from the dorsal surface. The muscle was removed after systemic injection of blue resin, and air-dried to render it transparent. Two sources of blood supply are demonstrated: the thoracodorsal artery, entering below the tendinous humeral attachment of the muscle (top right), and a dorsal perforating artery, entering on the deep surface (centre). Anastomotic channels may be traced between the vascular

endings. Neuromuscular junctions are considered in more detail elsewhere (p. 957).

The arrival of an action potential at the motor end plate causes *acetylcholine* (ACh) to be released from storage vesicles into the 30–50 nm synaptic cleft that separates the nerve ending from the sarcolemma. The ACh is rapidly bound by receptor molecules located in the junctional folds, triggering an almost instantaneous increase in the permeability, and hence conductance, of the postsynaptic membrane. This generates a local depolarization (the *end-plate potential*) whose duration is self-limited by voltage dependent conformational changes in the membrane. The activity of the neurotransmitter is rapidly terminated by the enzyme *acetylcholinesterase* (AChE), which is bound to the basement membrane in the junctional folds. Because of the extended geometry of the neuromuscular junction, the end-plate potential is normally several times larger than is needed to initiate an action potential in the surrounding sarcolemma. This ensures that excitation is passed with high security to the muscle so that, except under conditions of extreme fatigue, a muscle action potential is generated for each nervous impulse. The action potential propagates along the length of the muscle fibre at about 5 metres per second (Arendt-Nielson & Zwarts 1989) and spreads into its interior along the T-tubules, initiating contraction (p. 749).

MOTOR UNITS AND MOTOR CONTROL

Motor units and their recruitment

The terminal branches of *a*-motor axons are normally in a 'one-to-one' relationship with their muscle fibres: a muscle fibre receives only one branch, and any one branch innervates only one muscle fibre. When a motor neuron is excited, an action potential is propagated along the axon and its branches to all of the muscle fibres that it supplies. The motor neuron and the muscle fibres that it innervates can therefore be regarded as a functional unit, the *motor unit*, which accounts for the more or less simultaneous contraction of a number of fibres within the muscle. The actual size of the motor units varies considerably: in muscles that are employed for precision tasks, such as extraocular muscles, interossei and extralaryngeal muscles, each motor neuron innervates only about 10 muscle fibres, whereas in a large limb muscle the ratio may exceed 1000. Within a

muscle, the fibres belonging to one motor unit are distributed over a wide territory, without regard to fascicular boundaries, and intermingle with the fibres of other motor units (Edström & Kugelberg 1968; Burke et al 1973). The motor units become larger in cases of muscle nerve damage, because denervated fibres induce collateral or ultraterminal sprouting of the remaining axons, and each new branch can reinnervate a fibre (Edström & Kugelberg 1969). Mapping of motor unit territories is therefore of clinical interest, and may be achieved by electrophysiological techniques (see Electromyography, p. 785).

The passage of a single action potential through a motor unit elicits a twitch contraction that lasts 25–75 ms. However, the motor neuron can deliver a second nervous impulse in less time than it takes for the muscle fibres to relax. When this happens, the muscle fibres contract again, building the tension to a higher level. Because of this *mechanical summation*, a sequence of impulses can evoke a larger force than a single impulse, and—within certain limits—the higher the impulse frequency, the more force is produced. This force–frequency relationship is one of the strategies used by the nervous system to gradate the contraction it elicits from the muscle. The other strategy is to recruit more motor units. In practice, the two mechanisms appear to operate in parallel, but their relative importance may depend on the size of the muscle: in large muscles with many motor units, recruitment is probably the more important mechanism (Jones & Round 1990).

Recruitment is not a random process; neither is there an alternation (or 'rotation') of active motor units, as was once thought. Low-level contractions are associated with low levels of excitation within the spinal cord, and—with only very minor exceptions—these conditions always produce regular firing of the same population of small motor neurons. As the force increases, motor neurons of larger size become involved, and the largest motor neurons are activated only when the highest forces have to be generated (7.19). Since large motor neurons have axons of large diameter, which divide into more numerous branches, the order of recruitment of motor units is in every sense one of increasing size. This 'size principle' was formulated by E. Henneman in a series of papers notable for their experimental elegance and rigour (Henneman et al 1965a; Henneman et al 1965b; Henneman et al 1974). Although it now seems likely that this principle is actually based on some property related to motor neuron size, rather than to size per se (Stuart & Enoka 1983), the important concept is that motor units contribute to movement and posture in an orderly and predictable way.

Fibre types of adult skeletal muscle

Tonic muscle fibres, which are slow-contracting and cannot propagate

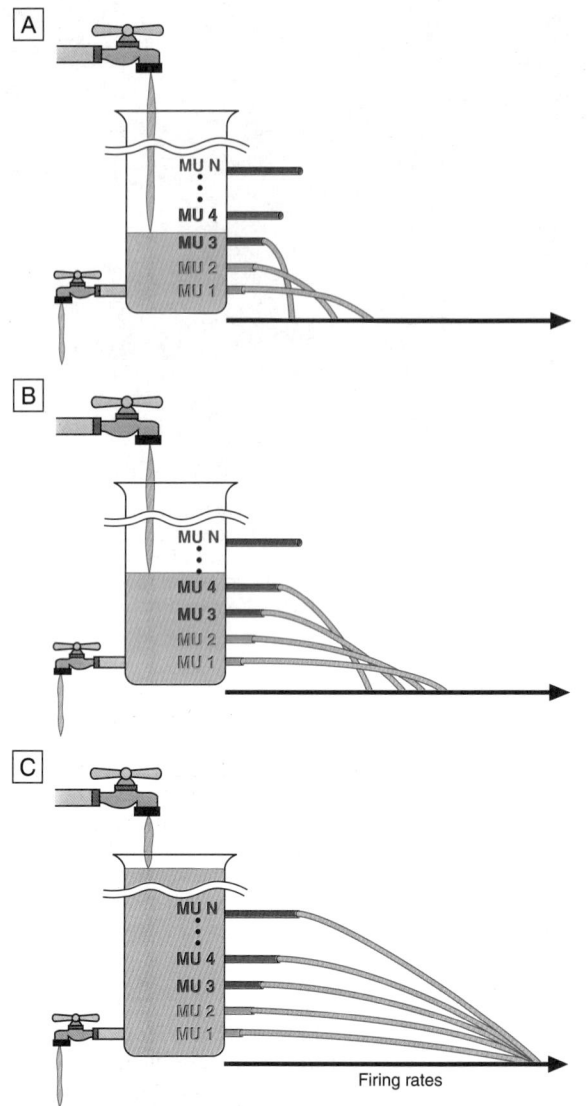

7.19 This simplified hydraulic analogy illustrates the main features of motor unit firing behaviour. The model is based on the concept of common drive, which refers to the tendency of motor units to change their firing rates together as if modulated by a common controlling factor. The water flowing into and out of the tank corresponds to excitation and inhibition impinging on the motor neurone pool; the level of water in the tank thus corresponds to the net excitation, or drive, to the motor neurone pool. The spouts represent motor units (MU 1, 2, ... N), which become active in a fixed order as the excitation level rises. The distance the outflow travels from the tank signifies firing rate, whose value at first recruitment is determined by the length of the spout. Thus, the higher the recruitment threshold, the higher the initial firing rate. As the water level rises (net excitation increases) the distance of the outflow (firing rate) increases; this embodies the observation that, at any one time, motor units recruited earlier tend to have higher firing rates than those recruited later. In (A), the drive is sufficient to recruit only three motor units; in (B), the drive to the pool has increased, resulting in the recruitment of a new motor unit and increases in the firing rates of motor units already active; in (C), drive is maximum: all motor units have been recruited and the firing rates are converging towards similar maximal values. (Modified, with permission, from De Luca & Erim 1994.)

action potentials over their membranes, are found in birds and reptiles, where they have a postural role: for example, the anterior latissimus dorsi muscle of the chicken maintains the folded position of the wing. Such fibres are uncommon in man and other mammals, where they are restricted to the extrinsic ocular muscles, the stapedius muscle of the middle ear and the intrafusal muscle fibres of the neuromuscular spindle. (For a review of slow tonic muscle, see Morgan & Proske 1984.)

With the exception of these rare tonic fibres, mammalian skeletal muscles are composed entirely of fibres of the *twitch* type. These

fibres can all conduct action potentials but they are not the same in other respects. Some fibres obtain their energy very efficiently by aerobic oxidation of substrates, particularly of fats and fatty acids. They have a high content of mitochondria and contain *myoglobin*, an oxygen-transport pigment related to haemoglobin. They are supported by a well-developed network of capillaries, which maintains a steady nutrient supply of oxygen and substrates. Such fibres are well suited to functions such as postural maintenance, in which moderate forces need to be sustained for prolonged periods. At the other extreme are fibres that have few mitochondria, little myoglobin, and a sparse capillary network. Their immediate energy requirements are met largely through anaerobic glycolysis, a route that provides prompt access to energy stores but is less efficient and less sustainable than oxidative metabolism. Such fibres are capable of brief bursts of intense activity, but these must be separated by extended quiescent periods during which glycogen and other reserves are replenished.

In many mammals these types of fibre tend to be segregated into different muscles: some muscles therefore have a conspicuously red appearance, derived from the rich blood supply and high myoglobin content associated with a predominantly aerobic metabolism, whereas others have a much paler appearance, reflecting a more anaerobic character. These variations in colour have been known for centuries, and 'red' and 'white' muscles were described clearly more than a hundred years ago by Ranvier (1874).

In man, all muscles are of the mixed variety, in which fibres that are specialized for aerobic working conditions intermingle with fibres of a more anaerobic or intermediate metabolic character. These different types of fibre are not readily distinguished in sections stained by conventional histological techniques, but they emerge quite clearly when more specialized *histochemical* techniques are used. An example is seen in **7.**20A. This section has been treated for the demonstration of an enzyme associated mainly with mitochondria, so that the colour develops most strongly in fibres that are rich in mitochondria.

On the basis of the metabolic differences that such a technique reveals, it is possible to classify the individual fibres as *red* (or *oxidative*), *white* (or *glycolytic*), and *intermediate* (or *oxidative-glycolytic*). (The terms 'red' and 'white' here refer to the appearance of whole muscles that are composed predominantly or exclusively of these types of fibre, such as the animal muscles described by Ranvier.)

Ranvier also noted that the 'red' muscles contracted and relaxed more slowly than the 'white' muscles. This difference in contractile speed is now known to be due in large part to molecular differences between the myosin heavy chains of these types of muscle, differences which affect the rate of cycling of the propulsive cross-bridges (Bárány 1967; p. 741). The different molecular isoforms of myosin (p. 744) may be demonstrated by histochemical techniques that link the enzymatic, ATP-splitting, properties of the molecule to a visualization reaction (Guth & Samaha 1970; Brook & Kaiser 1970). Although differences in the ATPase activity have been utilized directly in some techniques (Mabuchi & Sréter 1980), the methods in common use depend on the stability of this part of the molecule to changes in pH and formaldehyde treatment. These characteristics provide a more dependable basis for fibre type classification than oxidative activity, as seen in **7.**20B, which shows an example of a muscle section that has been stained for ATPase activity after being exposed to formaldehyde and alkaline pH (Tunell & Hart 1977). The dark fibres, which are termed Type 2B, contain a myosin heavy chain isoform that confers a fast contractile speed. Fibres of intermediate density are classified as Type 2A, and contain a slightly different 'fast' heavy chain. The lightly stained fibres are classified as Type 1; they contain a myosin heavy chain isoform that confers a slow contractile speed.

There are sufficient structural differences between the isoforms of myosin that antibodies can be made which distinguish between them: these antibodies can then be used to label the fibres in a muscle section by attaching fluorescent or enzymic markers to them (**7.**20C, D). The particular value of these immunocytochemical techniques, and their advantage over histochemical techniques, lies in their ability to probe the myosin composition of fibres in which more than one isoform is present: such fibres are quite usual in human jaw muscle (Thornell et al 1984) and may not be uncommon in human limb muscle (Larsson & Moss 1993; Sant' Ana Pereira et al 1995). Moreover, immunocytochemical techniques lend themselves to the

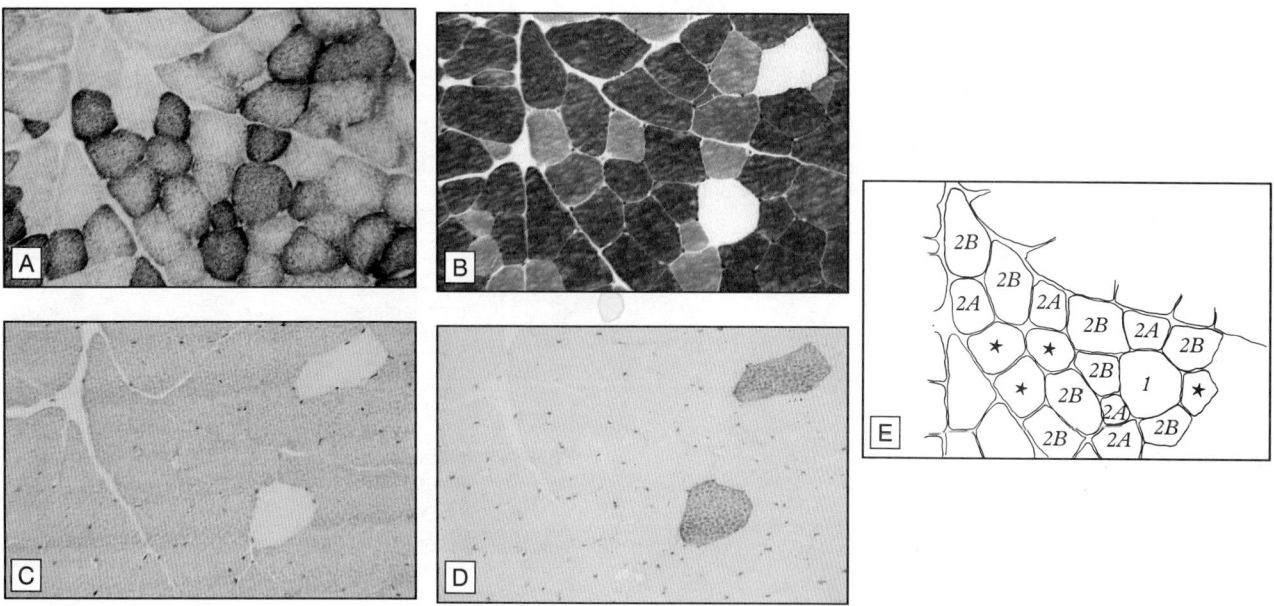

7.20 Light micrographs of serial transverse sections of rabbit tibialis anterior muscle, stained histochemically and by the immunoperoxidase technique to demonstrate differences between skeletal muscle fibre types. A. NADH tetrazolium reductase, an enzyme associated with oxidative metabolism. B. Myofibrillar ATPase after alkali and formaldehyde pre-incubation (method of Tunell and Hart 1977). C. Monoclonal antibody to fast muscle myosin heavy chains. This antibody reacts with both 2A and 2B subtypes. D. Monoclonal antibody to slow muscle myosin heavy chain. This antibody reacts only with Type 1 myosin. E. Key to fibre types. Fibres indicated by asterisks are more strongly oxidative in A, than might be expected from their ATPase reaction in B; this illustrates the metabolic overlap referred to in Table 7.1 and in the text. (Specimens prepared by Hazel Sutherland, Department of Human Anatomy and Cell Biology, University of Liverpool. Photographs by Stanley Salmons.)

detection of other proteins, such as the troponins, that also exist in fast and slow isoforms but are not suited to histochemical demonstration.

In many muscles, a classification of fibres into Types 1, 2A, and 2B is reasonably robust, based as it is on **qualitative** differences in myosin. Correspondence between this classification and more **quantitative** schemes based on metabolism is considerably less secure because of the amount of metabolic variation within fibres of a given type (Pette & Staron 1990). In broad terms, however, Type 1 and Type 2A fibres tend to be predominantly oxidative in character, whereas Type 2B fibres rely more heavily on anaerobic glycolysis. This tells us something more about the physiological properties of these fibre types:

- Type 2B fibres are fast-contracting and susceptible to fatigue
- Type 2A fibres are fast-contracting and fatigue-resistant
- Type 1 fibres are slow-contracting and fatigue-resistant.

Some fibre type characteristics lead to recognizable differences at the level of the electron microscope, particularly if quantitative, stereological techniques are employed (Eisenberg & Kuda 1976). Oxidative fibres are characterized by a larger volume fraction of mitochondria and lipid droplets. The Z-disc is wider in slow fibres than in fast fibres, and the fine structure of the M-line differs in a fibre-type-specific, muscle-specific and species-specific way (Sjöström & Squire 1977). The internal membrane systems of the

muscle fibre, the T-tubules and the sarcoplasmic reticulum, are much more elaborate in fast than in slow fibres. In relation to a given volume of sarcoplasm there are more nuclei in slow than in fast fibres, reflecting the fact that these metabolically more active fibres also synthesize and break down their proteins more rapidly.

Table 1 summarizes some of the major physiological, structural and biochemical properties of these basic fibre types. All classification schemes tend to be oversimplified, for they disregard the considerable gradation of properties shown by the fibres of a given muscle. They are, however, convenient for directing attention to particular fibre populations in a muscle and as a means of describing—and to some extent quantitating—compositional differences between muscles. Such studies reveal, for example, that a named muscle may vary in terms of fibre type proportions between individuals of different age or athletic ability. It will also vary in composition from one species to another, especially where the normal posture of the limb requires it to perform a different functional role. Even the properties of a given fibre type vary between species: broadly, all fibre types tend to be faster-contracting but more oxidative in small animals and slower-contracting but more glycolytic in large animals (Davies & Gunn 1972). On such a scale, man is, of course, one of the larger animals. (The muscles of dogs are somewhat exceptional, being unusually oxidative in relation to the body size of the animal: this feature may have evolved in relation to pack-hunting.)

Within a given muscle, deeper portions tend to have a higher

Table 7.1 Physiological, structural and biochemical characteristics of the major histochemical fibre types.

Characteristics	Fibre types		
	Type 1	Type 2A	Type 2B
Physiological			
Function	sustained forces, as in posture	—powerful, phasic movements—	
Motor neuron firing threshold	low	intermediate	high
Motor unit size	small	large	large
Firing pattern	tonic, low-frequency	—phasic, high-frequency—	
Maximum shortening velocity	slow	fast	fast
Rate of relaxation	slow	fast	fast
Resistance to fatigue	fatigue-resistant	fatigue-resistant	fatigue-susceptible
Power output	low	intermediate	high
Structural			
Capillary density	high		low
Mitochondrial volume	high	intermediate*	low
Z-band	broad	narrow	narrow
T and SR systems	sparse		extensive
Biochemical			
Myosin ATPase activity	low		high
Oxidative metabolism	high	intermediate*	low
Anaerobic glycolysis	low	intermediate*	high
Calcium transport ATPase	low		high

*Metabolic characteristics vary between species, and may show considerable overlap between fibre types. (See text for further detail and references.)

proportion of slow, red (Type 1) fibres (Narusawa et al 1987). Recent work suggests that proximity to the bone, rather than depth per se, may be responsible for these gradients (Lexell et al 1994). During embryological development, the muscle blocks of the limb form and divide in relation to skeletal elements, and the fibres formed during the primary wave of myogenesis express adult Type 1 myosin (see p. 754). More superficial parts of the muscle are populated by subsequent waves of myogenesis, so this gradient may be retained. Similar arguments may be advanced to explain the subtle gradients in fibre type proportion that can be detected within single fascicles (Sjöström et al 1986; Salmons 1987; Pernus & Erzen 1991). Major vessels usually enter a muscle on its deep aspect, so the greater development of the vascular supply in this part of the muscle may also be a factor in supporting a locally enhanced oxidative metabolism. Of course the presence in a developing muscle of spatial cues of a molecular nature cannot be ruled out.

Although it is often feasible and convenient to classify fibres according to their content of Type 1, 2A or 2B myosin heavy chains, it is also necessary to recognize the limitations of such a simple scheme. The nomenclature can be modified to accommodate fibres that express a mixture of these isoforms, but it must be elaborated still further if it is to cope with the other isoforms of myosin whose existence has emerged in recent years. For example, another 'fast' myosin isoform, 2X or 2D, has been found in some mammalian muscles: the corresponding fibres appear to be metabolically intermediate between Type 2B and 2A (Bär & Pette 1988; Schiaffino et al 1989). It now seems that a closely related isoform is expressed in Type 2B fibres from human limb muscle, so it may prove necessary to redesignate the human Type 2B fibre as Type 2X (Ennion et al 1995; Smerdu et al 1995). Muscles of cranial origin express a distinctive complement of myosin isoforms, often within the same fibres. For example, human adult jaw muscles contain a specific 'superfast' myosin, described originally in the jaw muscles of carnivores but found in every primate examined so far (Rowlerson et al 1983; J F Y Hoh, personal communication). These muscles also express a 'cardiac' α-myosin heavy chain isoform (Bredman et al 1991) and continue to express embryonic or fetal isoforms that are normally confined to the developmental period (p. 770; Butler-Browne et al 1988). Extraocular muscles also contain a great diversity of myosin isoforms: these are now known to include the 'cardiac' α-myosin heavy chain isoform (Rushbrook et al 1994), embryonic and fetal isoforms, and isoforms that appear to be unique to these muscles (Wieczorek et al 1985; Sartore et al 1987). These features may be related to differences in embryological derivation and development.

Fibres that belong to one motor unit resemble one another much more closely than fibres derived from different motor units (Edström & Kugelberg 1968; Burke et al 1973; Nemeth et al 1986). This is an important generality, but in sections of normal muscle, such as that of **7.20B**, it tends to be obscured by the overlap between different motor territories. It emerges much more clearly in muscles that have been partially denervated: the surviving axons reinnervate adjacent fibres (p. 753), producing local aggregations of fibres with very similar histochemical staining characteristics. This phenomenon is referred to by muscle pathologists as *fibre type grouping*. The increased fibre type grouping that occurs with advancing age is probably due to a neurogenic process that results in a progressive reduction in the number of functioning motor units (Lexell 1993).

Fatigue and the functional significance of motor unit organization

Diversity of muscle fibre properties is an important element in the organization of the motor system. Motor units that are active for much of the time are composed of slow, Type 1 fibres—the type of fibre that is best suited for sustaining tension without fatigue for long periods. Motor units that are active only infrequently are composed of fast, Type 2B fibres—the type of fibre that is best suited to generating powerful contractions on an intermittent basis. Between these extremes, the Type 2A motor units cope with routine activity against a background of more continuous postural tension provided by the Type 1 motor units.

This organization minimizes the possibility of muscle fatigue. The units that are recruited most frequently have the metabolic capability for sustained use. The units that are recruited only infrequently have time to replenish their anaerobic reserves between bouts of activity.

Fatigue can also be deferred if the muscle is activated in an economical way. Muscle fibres consume energy to reaccumulate the calcium ions released with each nerve impulse: energy would therefore be conserved if the required force could be developed and maintained with fewer impulses. In practice this is achieved in three ways. First, motor units discharge at a rate that correlates closely with the contractile speed of the muscle fibres: thus, motor neurons innervating slow muscle fibres fire at lower frequencies than those innervating fast fibres (Kernell 1986). Second, motor units discharge asynchronously, and as a consequence tension at the whole muscle level can develop smoothly at lower average impulse frequencies (Rack & Westbury 1969). Third, individual motor units do not fire at a constant frequency. Fast motor units, in particular, tend to commence firing at a high frequency, usually in the form of a double pulse, which produces a rapid rise of tension. The impulse frequency then declines, but tension is sustained, a phenomenon sometimes referred to as the 'catch' property of skeletal muscle (Marsden et al 1983).

DEVELOPMENT AND DIFFERENTIATION OF SKELETAL MUSCLE

Myogenesis

Modern understanding of the origins and movements of muscle-forming cells has come largely from the analysis and localization of muscle-specific proteins and their mRNAs. Among these, the multiple isoforms of the myosin heavy chain (Buckingham 1985) and the myogenic determination factors (see Myogenic determination factors, p. 757) have been particularly important. Most of our information about the early development of the skeletal musculature in man has been derived from other vertebrate species, principally chick, mouse, rat and sheep. However, where direct comparisons with the developing human embryo have been made, the patterns and mechanisms of muscle formation have been found to be the same, and the animal studies may therefore be assumed to provide an appropriate model. In the following account, the time course refers to human development.

Skeletal muscle originates from a pool of premyoblastic cells which arise in the *dermamyotome* of the maturing somite and begin to differentiate into *myoblasts* at *4 to 5 weeks* of gestation. By *6 weeks*, cells have migrated from the dermamyotomal compartment to form the *myotome* in the centre of the somite (**7.21**; Keynes & Stern 1988; Jones & Round 1990; see also p. 265). These myotomal precursor cells are identified by the expression of myogenic determination factors; they will eventually differentiate within the somite to form the axial (or *epaxial*) musculature (erector spinae). A distinct cohort of precursor cells migrates away from the somite to invade the lateral regions of the embryo; there they form the muscle of the limbs, limb girdles and body wall (*hypaxial* musculature; **7.21**). Virtually all cells in the lateral half of the newly formed somite are destined to migrate in this way. Myogenic determination factors are not expressed in these cells until the muscle masses coalesce. The appearance of myotomal myoblasts, and migration of myoblasts to the prospective limb region, occurs first in the cranial somites; thereafter these processes follow the general craniocaudal progression of growth, differentiation and development of the embryo (Buckingham 1992; see also p. 265). It needs to be emphasized that the myoblastic cells from which the limb muscles develop do not arise in situ from local limb bud mesenchyme, as was once thought, but migrate from the lateral half of the somite.

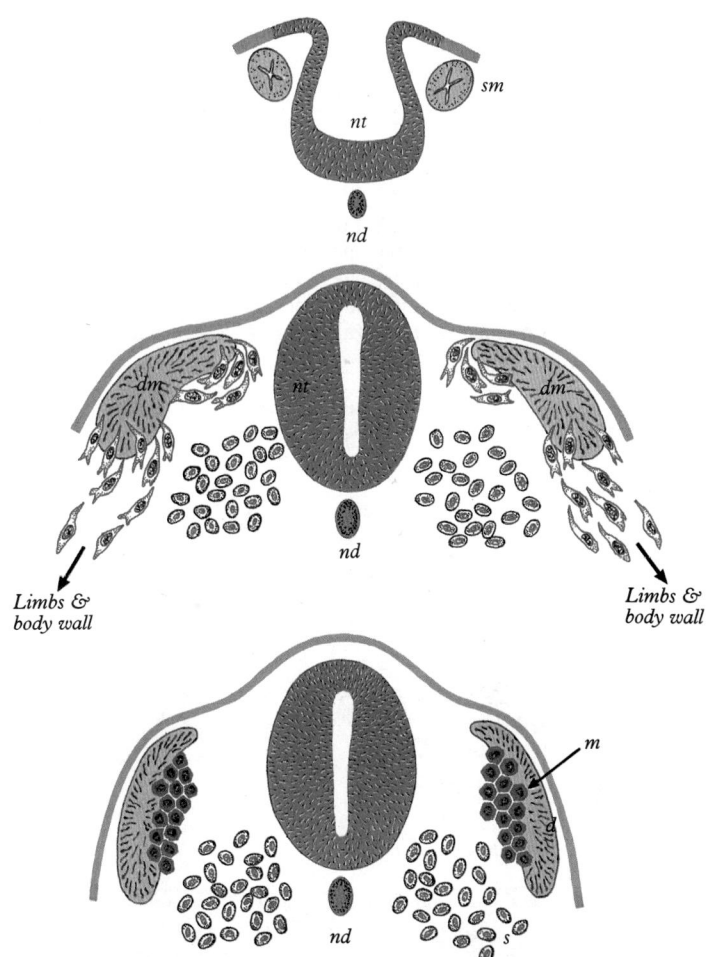

7.21 Diagram showing in three stages the early events of myogenesis which take place between 4 weeks and 6 weeks of gestation. Premyoblast stem cells arise in the dermamyotomal compartment of the early somite and migrate to form the myotome and the limb and body wall muscle. nt = neural tube; nd = notochord; sm = early somite; dm = dermamyotome; s = sclerotome; d = dermatome. (Terry Partridge, Department of Histology, Charing Cross Hospital Medical School and Yvonne Edwards, MRC Human Biochemical Genetics Unit, University College London.)

Myogenic Determination Factors

The myogenic determination factors—Myf-5, myogenin, MyoD and Myf-6 (herculin)—are a family of nuclear phosphoproteins. They have in common a 70-amino-acid, basic helix-loop-helix (bHLH) domain that is essential for protein–protein interactions and DNA binding. Outside the bHLH domain there are sequence differences between the factors which probably confer some functional specificity. The myogenic bHLH factors play a crucial role in myogenesis. Forced expression of any of them diverts non-muscle cells to the myogenic lineage (Weintraub et al 1991; Buckingham 1992). They activate transcription of a wide variety of muscle-specific genes by binding directly to conserved DNA sequence motifs (–CANNTG–, known as E-boxes) that occur in the regulatory regions (promoters and enhancers) of these genes. Their effect may be achieved co-operatively, and can be repressed (by some proto-oncogene products, for example). Some of the bHLH proteins can activate their own expression (Braun et al 1989). Accessory regulatory factors, whose expression is induced by the bHLH factors, provide an additional tier of control.

The myogenic factors do not all appear at the same stage of myogenesis (Braun et al 1989; Lyons & Buckingham 1992). The following account is based on studies in the mouse (numbers in parentheses refer to days post coitum in the mouse embryo).

In the somites Myf-5 is expressed early (8 d)—before myotome formation—followed by myogenin (8.5 d). MyoD is expressed relatively late (10.5 d) together with the contractile protein genes. Myf-6 is expressed transitorily (9–10 d) in the myotome and becomes the major transcript postnatally. Whether this specific timing is important for muscle development is not yet clear. The creation of mutant mice deficient in the bHLH proteins (gene 'knock-out') has shown that myogenin is crucial for the development of functional skeletal muscle, and that while neither Myf-5 nor MyoD are essential to myogenic differentiation on their own, lack of both results in a failure to form skeletal muscle (Buckingham 1994; Olsen & Klein 1994). In the limb bud the pattern of expression of the bHLH genes is generally later than in the somite: Myf-5 is expressed first but transitorily (10.5–

11 d), followed by myogenin and MyoD (11 d), and eventually Myf-6 (14.5 d). These differences provide evidence at the molecular level for the existence of distinct muscle cell populations in the limb and somites. It may be that the myogenic cells which migrate to the limb differ at the outset from those that form the myotome, or their properties may diverge subsequently under the influence of local epigenetic factors.

In both myotomes and limb buds, myogenesis proceeds in the following way. Myoblasts become spindle-shaped and begin to express muscle-specific proteins. The mononucleate myoblasts aggregate and fuse to form multinucleate cylindrical syncytia, or *myotubes*, with the nuclei aligned in a central chain (**7.22, 23**). These *primary myotubes* attach at each end to the tendons and developing skeleton. Note that the initiation of fusion does not depend on the presence of nerve fibres, which do not penetrate muscle primordia until after the formation of primary myotubes.

Fusion of myoblasts is not prerequisite for the synthesis of contractile machinery, but this proceeds much more rapidly after fusion. Sarcomere formation begins at the Z-disc, which binds actin filaments to form I–Z–I complexes. The myosin filaments assemble on the I–Z–I complexes to form A-bands. Nebulin and titin are among the first myofibrillar proteins to be incorporated into the sarcomere, and may well determine the length and position of the contractile filaments. Intermediate filaments connect the Z-discs to the sarcolemma at an early stage, and these connections are retained.

Myogenic cells continue to migrate and to divide, and during *weeks 7 to 9* there is extensive de novo myotube formation. Myoblasts aggregate near the midpoint of the primary myotubes and fuse with each other to form *secondary myotubes* (Jones & Round 1990; Draeger et al 1987; Maier et al 1992). Several of these smaller-diameter myotubes may be aligned in parallel with each of the primary myotubes (**7.24**). Each develops a separate basement membrane and makes independent contact with the tendon. Initially, the primary myotube provides a scaffold for the longitudinal growth of the secondary myotubes, but eventually they separate. At the time of their formation, the secondary myotubes express an 'embryonic' isoform of the myosin heavy chains, whereas the primary myotubes express a 'slow' muscle isoform apparently identical to that found in adult slow muscle fibres. In both primary and secondary myotubes sarcomere assembly begins at the periphery of the myotube and progresses inwards towards its centre. There is constant addition of myofibrils, which lengthen by adding sarcomeres to their ends. T-tubules are formed, growing initially in a longitudinal direction. Since they contain specific proteins that are not found in plasma membranes, they are probably assembled via a different pathway to that which supports the growth of the sarcolemma. The sarcoplasmic reticulum wraps around the myofibrils at the level of the I-bands.

By *9 weeks*, the primordia of most muscle groups are well defined, contractile proteins have been synthesized and the primitive beginnings of neuromuscular junctions can be observed, confined initially to the primary myotubes. Although some secondary fibre formation can take place in the absence of the nerve, most is initiated at sites of innervation of the primary myotubes. The pioneering axons

Immigration of myoblasts

Proliferation of myoblasts

Fusion of myoblasts

Primary myotube formation

Secondary myotube formation

Secondary myoblasts

Primary muscle fibre

Secondary myotubes

Axon

Neuromuscular junction

Maturing muscle fibre

Satellite cell

7.22 Stages in formation of skeletal muscle. Mononucleate myoblasts fuse to form multinucleate primary myotubes, characterized initially by central nuclei. Midway along the primary myotubes other myoblasts begin to fuse, forming secondary myotubes. As the contractile apparatus is assembled, the nuclei move to the periphery, cross-striations become visible and primitive features of the neuromuscular junction emerge. Later, small adult-type myoblasts—satellite cells—can be seen lying between the basement membrane and the plasmalemma of the muscle fibre. (Terry Partridge, Dept of Histology, Charing Cross Hospital Medical School and Yvonne Edwards, MRC Human Biochemical Genetics Unit, University College London.)

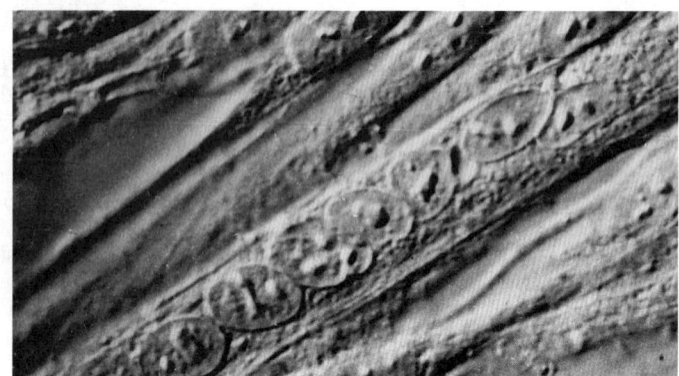

7.23 Light micrograph of cultured muscle cells, showing the fusion of myoblasts to form myotubes. Note the chain of centrally placed nuclei. (Photograph by Yvonne Edwards, MRC Human Biochemical Genetics Unit, University College London.)

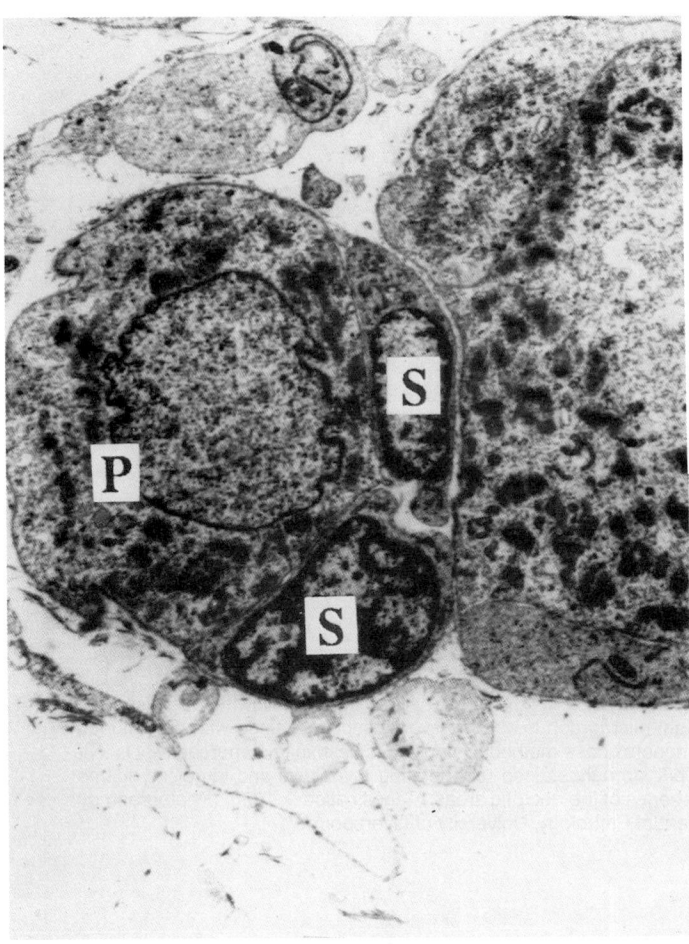

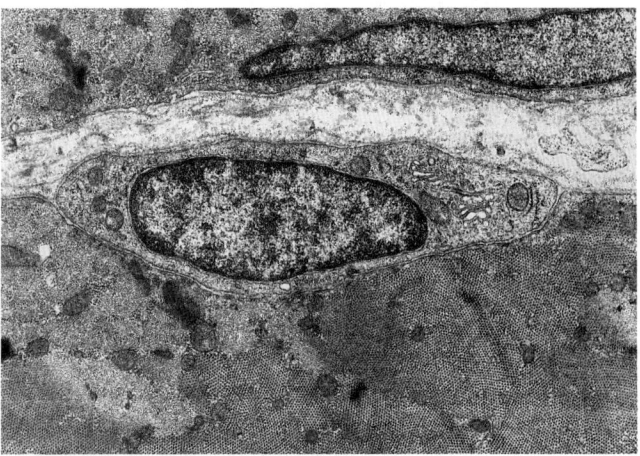

7.25 Electron micrograph of a satellite cell. Note the two plasma membranes that separate the cytoplasm of the satellite cell from that of the muscle fibre, and the basement membrane of the muscle fibre, which continues over the satellite cell (see also **7.2**). Compare this appearance with the normal muscle nucleus which is seen in the adjacent fibre. (Photograph by Terry Partridge, Department of Histology, Charing Cross Hospital Medical School, London.)

7.24 Electron micrograph of developing muscle. Closely apposed to a primary myotube (P) are two myoblasts forming secondary myotubes (S). At this stage the primary and secondary myotubes are enclosed within the same basement membrane. (Photograph by Yvonne Edwards, MRC Human Biochemical Genetics Unit, University College London.)

subsequently branch and establish contact with the secondary myotubes. By *10 weeks* the nerve-muscle contacts have become functional neuromuscular junctions and the fibres are contracting in response to impulse activity in the motor nerves. Under this new influence the secondary fibres express 'fetal' (sometimes referred to as 'neonatal') isoforms of the myosin heavy chains. At this stage several crucial

events take place which may be dependent on, or facilitated by, contractile activity. As the myofibrils encroach on the centre of the myotube, the nuclei move to the periphery, and the characteristic morphology of the adult skeletal muscle myofibre is established. The myofibrils become aligned laterally, and cross-striations are visible at the light microscopic level. T-tubules change from a longitudinal to a transverse orientation and adopt their adult positions; in this process they may be guided by the sarcoplasmic reticulum, which is more strongly bound to the myofibrils.

The myotubes and myofibres are grouped into fascicles by growing connective tissue sheaths, and the fascicles are assembled to build up entire muscles. As development proceeds, remodelling of the connective tissue matrix takes place to accommodate the increase in intramuscular volume.

At *14 to 15 weeks*, primary myotubes are still in the majority, but by *20 weeks* the secondary myotubes predominate. During *weeks 16 to 17* a new type of myotube may be seen; these are small and adhere to the secondary myotubes, with which they share a basement membrane (Draeger et al 1987; Maier et al 1992). These *tertiary myotubes* become independent by *18–23 weeks*, their central nuclei move to the periphery and they contribute a further generation of myofibres. The secondary and tertiary myofibres are always smaller and more numerous than the primaries. In some large muscles, higher order generations of myotubes may be formed (Maier et al 1992).

Late in fetal life, a final population of myoblasts arises; these cells are destined to become the *satellite cells* of adult muscle (Mauro 1961). These normally quiescent cells are associated so closely with muscle fibres that their nuclei were originally mistaken for muscle nuclei. With the electron microscope it is possible to see that the satellite cells lie outside the sarcolemma but beneath the basement membrane (**7.2, 25**). A cell adhesion protein of possible regulatory significance, *M-cadherin*, can be demonstrated at the site of contact between the quiescent satellite cell and the parent fibre (Irintchev et al 1994).

In a young individual, there is one satellite cell for every 5–10 myonuclei. Myonuclei themselves are incapable of DNA synthesis and mitosis, and satellite cells are therefore important as the sole source of additional myonuclei during postnatal growth of muscle (**7.26**). Following division, one of the daughter cells fuses with the growing myofibres, leaving behind a daughter satellite cell that is capable of further rounds of division (Moss & Leblond 1971). Similar events may take place to support exercise-induced hypertrophy of adult skeletal muscle. Satellite cells also provide a reservoir of myoblasts capable of initiating regeneration of an adult muscle after damage (see Regeneration and genetic modification of skeletal muscle, p. 760).

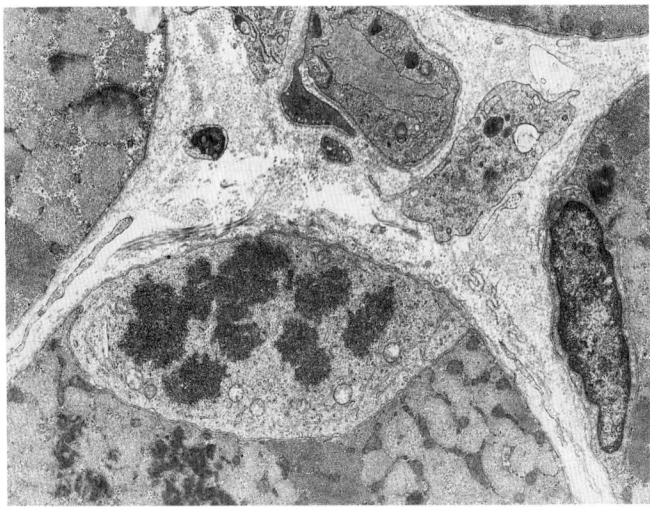

7.26 Electron micrograph of a satellite cell in mitosis. Normal skeletal muscle nuclei are incapable of division. A second, non-mitotic satellite cell is seen in the adjacent fibre on the right. (Photograph by Terry Partridge, Department of Histology, Charing Cross Hospital Medical School, London.)

759

Regeneration and Genetic Modification of Skeletal Muscle

In normal adult skeletal muscle, satellite cells are quiescent: their nuclear chromatin is less activated than that of sub-sarcolemmal nuclei, and they express neither muscle-specific proteins nor myogenic determination factors. Certain challenges to the muscle, such as injury or denervation, activate the satellite cells: they then proliferate and fuse, either with one another or with existing fibres. Evidence from cultured cells indicates that they express myogenin and MyoD prior to the appearance in the cytoplasm of mRNAs encoding myofibrillar proteins (Montarras et al 1991). Satellite cells appear to be more resistant than mature skeletal muscle fibres to chemical, mechanical or ischaemic insult. Thus conditions severe enough to produce necrosis of muscle fibres may activate, rather than kill, satellite cells, which go on to repair the muscle by replacing damaged segments or even whole fibres (Mauro 1979; **7**.27).

This regenerative capability raises the possibility of introducing new or missing genes into muscle fibres by grafting satellite cells containing those genes into damaged muscles, the normal repair process being used to integrate the grafted cells into the defective muscle fibres (**7**.28).

An opportunity for testing this approach was provided by the discovery of the *mdx* mouse, an animal model which has the genetic defect responsible for Duchenne and Becker muscular dystrophies in man (see p. 748). Grafts of satellite cells obtained from normal mice were shown to restore production of dystrophin in the muscle of *mdx* dystrophic mice (Karpati et al 1989; Partridge et al 1989). More recently the dystrophin gene has been introduced into muscle fibres by direct transfection with naked DNA encoding dystrophin (Acsadi et al 1991) and by infection with retrovirus (Dunkley et al 1992) or adenovirus (Ragot et al 1993) engineered to carry 'mini' versions of the dystrophin gene. Even when the introduced gene is not integrated into the genomic DNA it appears to be extremely stable and continues to be expressed as mRNA and protein for many months.

These developments have led to the idea of using muscle as a factory to supply systemic proteins, such as hormones and clotting factors, in which an individual may be deficient or absent (Dhawan et al 1991; Barr & Leiden 1991; Dai et al 1992).

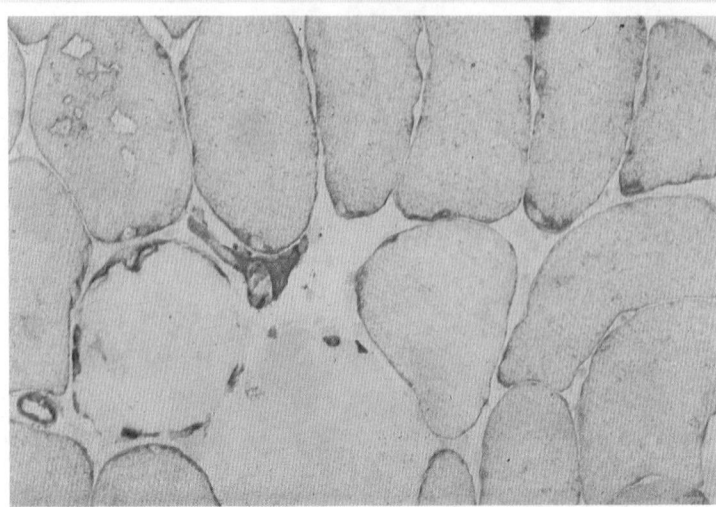

7.27   Skeletal muscle regeneration in human quadriceps muscle following an episode of rhabdomyolysis. The light micrograph is of a transverse section stained with an antibody to desmin by the immunoperoxidase method. Cytoplasmic desmin immunoreactivity is lost in two necrotic fibres, but strongly stained regenerating myoblasts and larger myotubes are present at the peripheries of the necrotic areas. Magnification × 1030. (Photograph by Tim Helliwell, Department of Pathology, University of Liverpool.)

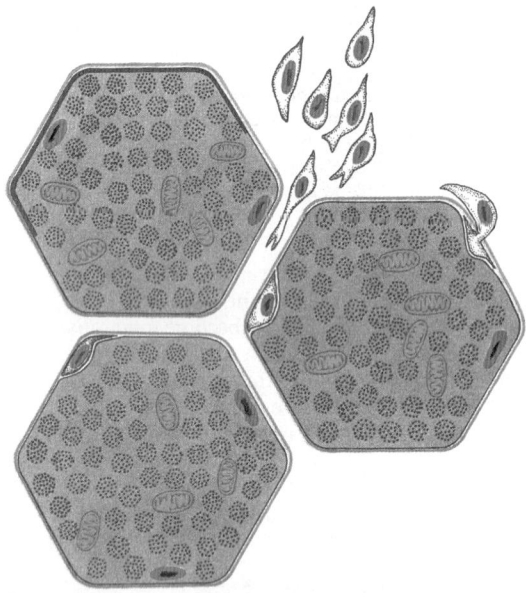

7.28   The principle of myoblast transplantation as a treatment for muscular dystrophy relies on the natural mobility of injected myogenic cells that carry copies of the normal dystrophin gene (red) within their nuclei. These cells spread from the injection site, migrating through endomysial and perimysial connective tissue, penetrating the basement membranes, and fusing with surviving portions of damaged muscle fibres. Once inside the muscle fibres, the normal dystrophin genes are expressed, compensating for the defective genes in the recipient's nuclei (brown). Injected myogenic cells can also form satellite cells within muscle fibres of the recipient. (Artwork by Terry Partridge, Department of Histology, Charing Cross Hospital Medical School, London.)

The emergence of fibre types

As already stated, the fibres of developing muscle do not express adult isoforms of myosin immediately. The type of myosin synthesized by myotubes at the time of their formation is an embryonic isoform, which is subsequently replaced by fetal and adult myosin isoforms (Whalen et al 1981). The major isoform of sarcomeric actin in fetal skeletal muscle is cardiac α-actin (Ordahl 1986; Vandekerckhove et al 1986); only later is this replaced by skeletal α-actin. The significance of these developmental sequences is not known: they may be needed for the assembly of filaments and filament arrays, they may reflect changes in functional requirements, or they may recapitulate a phylogenetic sequence.

The pattern of expression is fibre-specific as well as stage-specific. In primary myotubes, embryonic myosin is replaced by adult slow myosin from about 9 weeks onwards. In secondary and higher order myotubes the embryonic myosin isoform is superseded first by fetal and then by adult fast myosin, and a proportion go on to express adult slow myosin. Other fibre-specific, tissue-specific and species-specific patterns of myosin expression have been described in mammalian limb muscles (Hoh et al 1988a; Hughes et al 1993) and jaw muscles (Butler-Browne et al 1988; Hoh et al 1988b; Bredman et al 1992).

The origin of this diversity in the temporal patterns of expression of different fibres—even within the same muscle—is far from clear. It has been suggested that intrinsically different lineages of myoblast emerge at different stages of myogenesis or in response to different extracellular cues (Stockdale 1992). If this is the case, their internal programmes may be retained or overridden when they fuse with other myoblasts or with fibres that have already formed (Stockdale 1992; Hughes & Blau 1992). The fibres that emerge from this process go on to acquire a phenotype that will depend on the further influence of hormones and neural activity.

In man, unlike many smaller mammals, the muscles are histologically mature at birth, but fibre type differentiation is far from complete at this stage. The expression of Type 1 myosin in postural muscles, such as the soleus, increases significantly over the first few years of life, and during this period the fibre type proportions in other adult muscles become somewhat more divergent (Johnson et al 1973). The presence in adult muscles of a small proportion of fibres with an apparently transitional combination of protein isoforms suggests that changes in fibre type continue to some extent in all muscles and throughout adult life (see below, Fibre type transformation and the adaptive capacity of skeletal muscle). This dynamic element must contribute to interindividual variation in the fibre type composition of named muscles. Fibre type transitions also occur in relation to damage or neuromuscular disease, and under these conditions the developmental sequence of myosins may be recapitulated in fibres that are undergoing regeneration (see Regeneration and genetic modification, p. 760).

Fibre type transformation and the adaptive capacity of skeletal muscle

Mammalian skeletal muscle is a highly differentiated tissue, and it acquires a further level of specialization through divergence of fibre type characteristics (Table 7.1), yet it has a remarkable capacity for changing these characteristics, even in adult life. This 'plasticity' was discovered by Buller, Eccles and Eccles (1960) in the course of experiments in which they cut and cross-anastomosed the nerves to a fast, white and a slow, red muscle so that each muscle would be reinnervated by the other's nerve. Under these conditions a remarkable change in contractile speed took place, the fast muscle becoming slower-contracting and the slow muscle faster-contracting. In order to explain these effects, the authors suggested that the muscles had responded to the influence of 'quickening' and 'slowing' chemical trophic factors transported to them along the motor nerves. This explanation was widely accepted, despite a lack of direct evidence for the existence of these factors. There was, however, an alternative possibility. The nerves to fast muscles carry brief, high-frequency bursts of impulses, whereas those supplying slow muscles conduct prolonged, low-frequency trains (Eccles et al 1958; Vrbová 1963). The neural influence could therefore have something to do with these different patterns of impulse traffic in the nerves. Salmons (1967) developed an implantable miniature electronic stimulator, and for the first time it became possible to impose an artificial pattern of activity on the nerve supplying a fast muscle and to maintain it for long periods. This led to the discovery that fast muscles which were stimulated continuously for several weeks at 10 Hz—a pattern similar to that normally experienced by slow muscles—developed slow contractile characteristics (Salmons & Vrbová 1969). Later it was shown that changes in the pattern of impulse activity could account fully for the cross-reinnervation experiments of Buller and his colleagues: on the one hand, chronic stimulation of a fast muscle via its own nerve made the muscle even slower than reinnervating it with a slow muscle nerve; on the other hand, chronic stimulation of

a slow muscle could reverse completely the increase in contractile speed that normally took place when it was cross-reinnervated with a fast muscle nerve (Salmons & Sréter 1976). Chronically stimulated fast muscles resembled slow muscles in more than their speed of contraction; they acquired a red appearance and a resistance to fatigue that was even greater than that of slow muscles (Salmons & Sréter 1976).

Since the early 1970s, histochemical and biochemical studies have been providing an increasingly detailed account of the phenotypic changes responsible for these stimulation-induced changes in contractile speed and fatigue resistance (Salmons & Henriksson 1981; Pette & Vrbová 1992). The initial phase of slowing can be explained by less rapid cycling of calcium, the result of a reduction in the extent of the sarcoplasmic reticulum (Eisenberg & Salmons 1981) and changes in the amount and molecular type of proteins involved in calcium transport and binding (Heilmann & Pette 1979; Lederer et al 1986). Chronic stimulation also triggers the synthesis of myosin heavy and light chain isoforms of the slow muscle type (Brown et al 1983), and the associated changes in cross-bridge kinetics result in a lower intrinsic speed of shortening (Jarvis 1993). The muscle becomes more resistant to fatigue through changes in the metabolic pathways responsible for the generation of ATP. These consist of a reduced dependence on anaerobic glycolysis and a switch to oxidative pathways, particularly those involved in the breakdown of fat and fatty acids (Heilig & Pette 1980; Henriksson et al 1986). There is an associated increase in capillary density (Hudlicka 1991) and in the fraction of the intracellular volume occupied by mitochondria (Eisenberg & Salmons 1981).

These changes take place in an orderly sequence and bring about a complete transformation of fibre type. If stimulation is discontinued, the sequence of events is reversed and the muscle regains, over a period of weeks, all of its original characteristics (Brown et al 1989; Salmons 1990). The reversibility of transformation is one of several lines of evidence that the changes take place within existing fibres, and not by a process of degeneration and regeneration (Lexell et al 1992).

Many of the changes in the protein profile of a muscle that are induced by stimulation are now known to be the result of regulatory events taking place at a pretranslational stage. For example, analysis of the messenger RNA species encoding myosin heavy chain isoforms shows that the fast myosin heavy chain mRNA is substantially suppressed within a few days of the onset of chronic stimulation, while the slow myosin heavy chain mRNA undergoes a corresponding increase (Brownson et al 1992a,b). At this stage nothing is known about the sequence of intracellular events that underlies these changes in gene expression.

Although myosin expression is responsive to the radical increase in use brought about by chronic stimulation, it tends to be stable under physiological conditions unless these involve a sustained departure from normal postural or locomotor behaviour. Other protein systems can change more easily: increases in enzymes of oxidative metabolism, for example, may be induced not only by chronic stimulation but also by exercise programmes, such as endurance training (Holloszy & Booth 1976). These observations suggest that some muscle properties are continuously regulated by contractile activity, whereas myosin isoform transitions tend not to occur unless certain threshold levels of activity are crossed. Such a concept could help to explain how the influence of a parameter as variable as the pattern of activity reaching a muscle fibre can be reconciled with the existence of histochemically distinct classes of fibre (Salmons 1994).

The transformation of type induced by increased contractile activity may be interpreted as evidence of a natural adaptive capacity of skeletal muscle fibres (Salmons & Henriksson 1981). According to this hypothesis, fibres subjected to sustained high levels of use tend to develop properties at the slow, fatigue-resistant end of the spectrum. These properties are suited to postural activity that involves maintenance of tension but little change of muscle length: the slow type of myosin is more energy-efficient under these conditions (Barclay et al 1993), and a well-developed aerobic metabolism provides the capacity for generating ATP on a continuous basis. Fibres that are less active retain, or revert to, a native fast state. Their properties are suited to dynamic activity, for which instantaneous power is more important than endurance. The concept emerges of a machine that can optimize its properties to suit the type of work most often demanded of it (Salmons 1980). The functional matching of the neural and muscular elements of a motor unit (p. 753) may have its origins in connectivities set up during development, but there seems little doubt that it is finely tuned throughout adult life by the ability of the muscle fibres to adapt continuously to changes in their pattern of use.

Cardiac Assistance from Skeletal Muscle

Cardiac disease is the major cause of death in the industrialized world. Those that survive an ischaemic attack, or suffer from conditions that weaken the heart, often face the debilitating consequences of progressive cardiac failure. For some years the surgical treatment of heart failure has been restricted to cardiac transplantation. The procedure is not without its problems. Many patients cannot have transplant surgery, and of those who are placed on a transplant list 25–30% die while awaiting a suitable donor. Transplanted hearts often fail through rejection or accelerated restenosis of the coronary arteries. There is therefore a need for a viable surgical alternative.

More than 60 years ago, surgeons had the idea of using the patient's own skeletal muscle as a source of contractile tissue for assisting or repairing a failing heart. Their attempts failed because they could not persuade skeletal muscle to perform cardiac work without fatiguing. The discovery of the adaptive capabilities of skeletal muscle (see p. 761) has now made this approach feasible. Skeletal muscle that has been transformed (or 'conditioned') by stimulation is so fatigue-resistant that it can perform cardiac levels of work on a continuous basis (Acker et al 1987).

In the surgical procedure known as cardiomyoplasty (Chagas et al 1989; Hagege et al 1990), the latissimus dorsi muscle is mobilized with its neurovascular pedicle intact, transferred into the chest and wrapped around the heart. After a delay to allow for revascularization, the grafted muscle is conditioned and finally stimulated in synchrony with the heart (7.29). The clinical benefits of this procedure, which has now been carried out on several hundred patients worldwide, are due mainly to the reinforcing effect of the wrap, which reduces ventricular wall stress and restricts enlargement (Hooper & Salmons 1993, Chiu 1994).

Other, less conservative, configurations are being investigated that could harness more effectively the power available from skeletal muscle (Salmons & Jarvis 1992). A separate skeletal muscle ventricle can be made by winding the latissimus dorsi muscle around a former, which is subsequently removed (7.30). The device may be used either in counterpulsation or in parallel with the left ventricle. In one experimental dog such a ventricle pumped

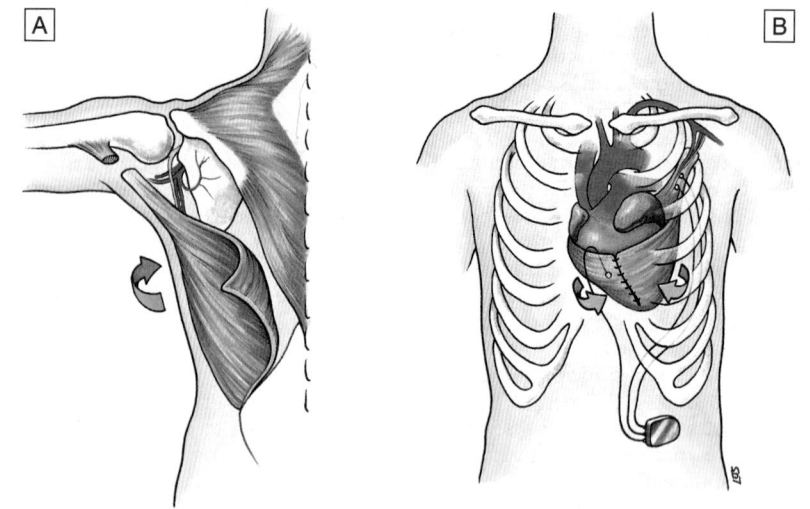

7.29 In cardiomyoplasty the latissimus dorsi muscle is mobilized (leaving the neurovascular pedicle intact), transferred into the chest and wrapped around the heart. Electrical pulses from the implantable stimulator are conveyed to branches of the thoracodorsal nerve by two stimulating electrodes which are woven into the proximal portion of the muscle. The pulse trains are triggered via the electrocardiographic lead so that contraction is appropriately synchronized with systole. (Artist: Lesley Skeates.)

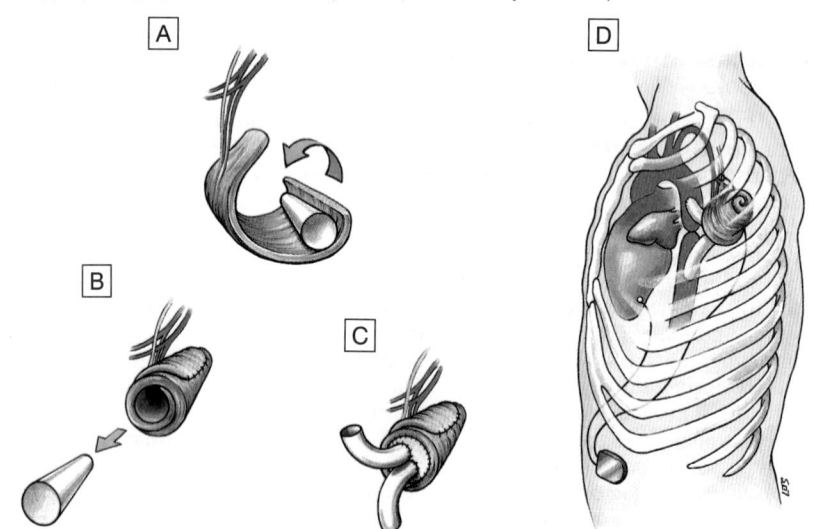

7.30 A skeletal muscle ventricle is a separate auxiliary blood pump formed by winding the latissimus dorsi muscle to form a tube or pouch. In the configuration shown, the skeletal muscle ventricle is stimulated to contract during diastole. Note again the cardiac sensing lead. In this example, a bipolar lead has been used to convey stimulating pulses to a cuff placed around the thoracodorsal nerve. (Artist: Lesley Skeates.)

in circulation for over 2 years (Mocek et al 1992). In terms of pumping power, skeletal muscle ventricles could rival the best mechanical artificial ventricles, but— unlike those devices—every component can be implanted, so they offer no psychological challenge to the patient (Salmons & Salmons 1992).

GROWTH AND REGULATION OF SKELETAL MUSCLE SIZE

Growth and regulation of fibre diameter

In man, the number of fibres in each muscle does not increase after about 24 weeks of gestation (Jones & Round 1990). Thereafter, growth in the size of the muscle takes place through an increase in the cross-sectional area of individual fibres (i.e. by *hypertrophy*, not *hyperplasia*). Within the fibres, existing myofibrils enlarge initially by accretion of myofilaments. There seems to be an upper limit to myofibril diameter, however, for at a certain point they appear to split longitudinally. It has been suggested that this is due to disruption of the Z-disc by radial stresses (Goldspink 1971).

Growth of fibres continues into postnatal life, and there is an associated increase in the number of myonuclei. Since myonuclei themselves cannot divide, these additional nuclei must come from fusion of satellite cells with established fibres. Fibres will undergo further hypertrophy in response to periodic bouts of intense exercise, of the type performed by weight-lifters. An increase in fibre number may occur under these conditions (Gonyea 1980), but the mechanism is unclear: histological appearances suggestive of fibre splitting could also be interpreted as de novo fibre formation at the surface of existing fibres. Muscle fibres can also undergo hypertrophy in response to increased loading when this is caused by pathological conditions involving a partial loss of functional motor units from a muscle or its synergists; in these cases the deficit may be compensated to some extent by hypertrophy of the remaining muscle fibres.

After the age of about 25, the total number of fibres in a muscle declines progressively, although there is no change in the relative numbers of fast and slow fibre types. This loss of fibres is one reason for the decline in motor function that occurs with advancing age (Lexell et al 1988). The other reason is a reduction in size (*atrophy*) of the fast fibres (see below).

In man, as in many other vertebrates, muscle development is greater in the male, and since the divergence from females occurs during puberty it is generally attributed to an anabolic action of testosterone. Attempts to synthesize substances that could offer this anabolic effect in isolation led to the development of anabolic steroids (see Anabolic steroids, below). Postnatal growth of skeletal muscle is also affected by thyroid hormones and growth hormone, the latter acting particularly through local production of insulin-like growth factor 1 (Jones & Round 1990). Adrenal corticosteroids reduce muscle bulk, and this is a serious and well-recognized side-effect of corticosteroid therapy.

Anabolic Steroids

In the 1950s the need for an effective pharmacological treatment of wasting diseases stimulated a search for synthetic compounds that had the anabolic properties of testosterone without the virilizing side-effects (Kochakian 1976). Evidence of myotrophic (muscle-growth-promoting) actions was based on the sensitivity of two highly atypical muscles: the so-called 'levator ani' muscle (more correctly, the sphincter ani externus muscle) of the castrated male rat and the temporal muscle of the female (or castrated male) guinea-pig. Candidate substances were normally assayed by comparing the weight gain of the levator ani muscle (myogenic effect) with the weight gain of secondary sexual organs such as seminal vesicles (androgenic effect) in a gonadectomized male animal (Eisenberg & Gordan 1950; Hershberger et al 1953). Measured in this way, myogenic:androgenic ratios were, at best, about 11:1. It has been widely assumed that these effects extend to the general skeletal musculature; in fact there is a good deal of evidence that they do not (Ryan 1981; Crist et al 1983; Kuhn & Max 1985). In man, there have been few adequately controlled studies, and observations have been complicated by other effects, such as an increase in overall body weight due to retention of salt and water or the reported increase in exercise tolerance, which may have very little to do with muscle. In animals, the problem is again to distinguish a specific muscle response from a generalized growth response that could, for example, be due to secondary changes in appetite, the levels of growth hormone, insulin, corticosteroids or thyroxine (Heitzmann 1979). For this reason, studies in which the increase in muscle weight occurs in direct proportion to body weight cannot be taken as adequate evidence of a direct myotrophic action.

A direct myotrophic response has been demonstrated in one limb muscle of the rabbit (Salmons 1992). The effect did not appear to be species-specific, but it was highly muscle-specific. It is possible that expression of anabolic/androgenic receptors in muscle tissue is global at the time of puberty but is withdrawn, except in a few muscles, thereafter. If the response were similarly selective in man, hypertrophy of individual muscles could unbalance the action of the muscles around a joint, with risk of joint damage and tendon rupture.

While there is serious doubt about any generalized influence of anabolic steroids on muscle power, there is no such doubt about their side-effects. Inappropriate androgenic effects cause behavioural changes in men, masculinizing changes in women, and growth abnormalities in children. A catalogue of further changes includes compromised reproductive function, fluid retention, toxic effects on the liver, and the possibility of accelerated coronary artery disease.

The notorious abuse of anabolic steroids by athletes continues, despite the pressures of legislation and informed public opinion, and these substances are still widely used in the meat industry.

Growth and regulation of fibre length

Muscle fibres grow in length by addition of sarcomeres to the ends of the myofibrils (Williams & Goldspink 1971). It is important throughout life for the number of sarcomeres to be regulated so that the mean sarcomere length, and hence filament overlap, is optimized for maximum force (Herring et al 1984). This is achieved by addition or removal of sarcomeres in response to any prolonged change of length (Tabary et al 1972). For example, if a limb is immobilized in a plaster cast, the fibres of muscles that have been fixed in a shortened position lose sarcomeres, and those that have been fixed in a lengthened position add sarcomeres; the reverse process occurs after the cast has been removed.

Denervation and disuse atrophy

Denervation leads to atrophy of muscle fibres. Because motor unit territories overlap, and the corresponding muscle fibres intermingle, the atrophic fibres may occur singly or in small groups, and are compressed into angular shapes by the adjacent normal fibres (Jennekens 1982). Denervation is accompanied by the spread of neuromuscular junction-associated proteins along the sarcolemma and by the re-expression of developmental proteins, such as fetal myosin heavy chains (Sawchak et al 1989).

In man, disuse of muscles for 1–4 months leads to the atrophy of fast and slow muscle fibres (Sargeant et al 1977; Hikida et al 1989). Longer term disuse caused by disease or injury results in the preferential atrophy of fast fibres (Budschu et al 1973). The selective Type 2 atrophy that occurs in the muscles of older people may likewise be attributed to disuse resulting from restricted physical activity, for this component of ageing atrophy can be reversed by appropriate training, even in the very elderly (Lexell et al 1988; Lexell 1993).

CARDIAC MUSCLE

In cardiac muscle, as in skeletal muscle, the contractile proteins are organized into sarcomeres; these are aligned in register across the fibres, producing fine cross-striations that are visible in the light microscope. The term *striated muscle* therefore applies to cardiac as well as skeletal muscle. The same contractile proteins are present (although many are synthesized as cardiac isoforms), they are assembled in a similar way, and the molecular basis for contraction is believed to be the same. To restate this briefly, energy from the hydrolysis of ATP is coupled to cyclic conformational changes in the myosin cross-bridges that propel the arrays of thick and thin filaments past each other (p. 741). The interaction between actin and myosin is regulated by a calcium-sensitive switch formed by a complex of proteins associated with the thin filaments: troponin-C, troponin-I, troponin-T and tropomyosin (p. 745). Release of Ca^{2+} into the cytosol triggers contraction, corresponding to cardiac systole, the pumping phase of the heart cycle; reuptake of Ca^{2+} produces relaxation, corresponding to cardiac diastole, the filling phase of the cycle.

Despite the similarities, there are major functional, morphological and developmental differences between cardiac and skeletal muscle. It will be helpful to describe first some of the ways in which cardiac muscle differs morphologically from skeletal muscle, before going on to consider other aspects of form and function that are unique to cardiac muscle.

DISTINCTIVE MORPHOLOGICAL FEATURES OF CARDIAC MUSCLE

The *myocardium*, the muscular component of the heart, constitutes the bulk of that organ. It consists of cardiac muscle cells, usually up to $100\,\mu m$ long and $10–15\,\mu m$ in diameter in a normal adult. Each cell has one large nucleus, occasionally two, occupying the central part of the cell; this contrasts sharply with the multiple, peripherally placed nuclei of skeletal muscle. The cells are branched at their ends, and the branches of adjacent cells are so tightly associated that the light microscopic appearance is that of a network of branching and anastomosing fibres (7.31).

The syncytial appearance is, however, misleading: electron microscopy clearly reveals the elaborate junctions that bind the cells

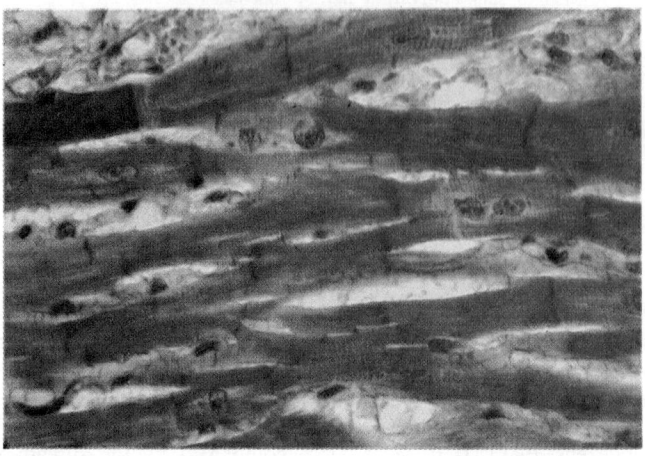

7.31 A longitudinal section through cardiac muscle reveals a network of fibres made up of branched cardiac cells. The cells have cross-striations and one or two centrally placed nuclei. The specialized junctions between the cells are visible as darkly staining transverse lines, the intercalated discs. Magnification × 800.

together (7.32, and see p. 768, Intercalated discs), and individual cardiac myocytes can be isolated from the tissue by chemical treatments that weaken the binding. Thus the 'fibres' of cardiac muscle are not single cells, as they are in skeletal muscle.

Fine fibrocollagenous connective tissue is found between the cardiac muscle fibres. Although this is the approximate equivalent of the endomysium of skeletal muscle, it is less regularly organized because of the complex three-dimensional geometry set up by the branching cardiac cells. Numerous capillaries and some nerve fibres are found within this layer. Coarser connective tissue, equivalent to the perimysium of skeletal muscle, separates the larger bundles of muscle fibres, and is particularly well developed near to the condensations of dense fibrous connective tissue that form the 'skeleton' of the heart (p. 1493). At the gross anatomical level, the ventricles of the heart are composed of spiralling layers of fibres running in different directions; as a consequence, histological sections of ventricular muscle inevitably contain the profiles of cells cut in a variety of orientations. A linear arrangement of cardiac muscle fibres is found only in the papillary muscles.

Electron micrographs of cardiac cells in longitudinal section show that the myofibrillar material separates before it courses around the nucleus, leaving a zone that is occupied by organelles, including sarcoplasmic reticulum, Golgi complex, mitochondria, lipid droplets, and glycogen. At the light microscopic level, these zones appear as unstained—or at best lightly stained—areas at the poles of each nucleus (7.31). In transverse section, they may give the appearance of central holes in fibre profiles that have been sectioned close to a nucleus (7.33) These zones often contain lipofuscin granules, which accumulate there in individuals over the age of 10; the reddish-brown pigment may be visible even in unstained longitudinal sections.

The cross-striations of cardiac muscle are less conspicuous than those of skeletal muscle. The reason for this may be found in electron micrographs such as 7.34, which show the contractile apparatus of cardiac muscle to be embedded in an abundant sarcoplasm that is especially rich in mitochondria. The myofibrils are also less well delineated than in skeletal muscle, and in transverse sections they often fuse into a continuous array of myofilaments, irregularly bounded by mitochondria and longitudinal elements of sarcoplasmic reticulum.

The large and numerous mitochondria, with their closely spaced cristae, reflect the highly developed oxidative metabolism of a tissue that has to work hard and unceasingly. Accumulations of mitochondria are found beneath the sarcolemma, adjacent to the nucleus, and between the myofibrils (7.34). The proportion of the cell volume occupied by mitochondria is even greater in cardiac muscle than it is in slow, red skeletal muscle. The high demand for oxygen is also reflected in high levels of myoglobin and an exceptionally rich network of capillaries around the fibres.

The force of contraction is transferred through the ends of the cardiac muscle cells by virtue of the junctional strength provided by the intercalated discs (see below). As in skeletal muscle, force is also transmitted laterally to the sarcolemma and extracellular matrix via *costameres*, vinculin-containing elements bridging between the Z-discs of peripheral myofibrils and the plasma membrane (Pardo et al 1983b).

With some qualification, the above description applies to both ventricular and atrial muscle. Atrial muscle cells are smaller and have few or no T-tubules. However, their most striking ultrastructural feature is the presence, in the region of the Golgi complexes at the poles of the nuclei, of dense, membrane-bounded granules. These atrial granules contain the precursor of *atrial natriuretic factor*, a hormone whose action is to promote loss of sodium, potassium and water in the kidneys, reducing body fluid volume and thereby lowering blood pressure. The hormone is released in response to stretch of the atrial wall. Its actions are normally balanced by the opposing effects of aldosterone and vasopressin.

EXCITATION OF CARDIAC MUSCLE

The molecular interaction between actin and myosin that underlies the generation of force is initiated in the same way in cardiac and skeletal muscle. Contraction is activated by raising the concentration of cytosolic free Ca^{2+}, thus promoting the binding of Ca^{2+} to the calcium-sensitive protein complex on the thin filaments. Relaxation

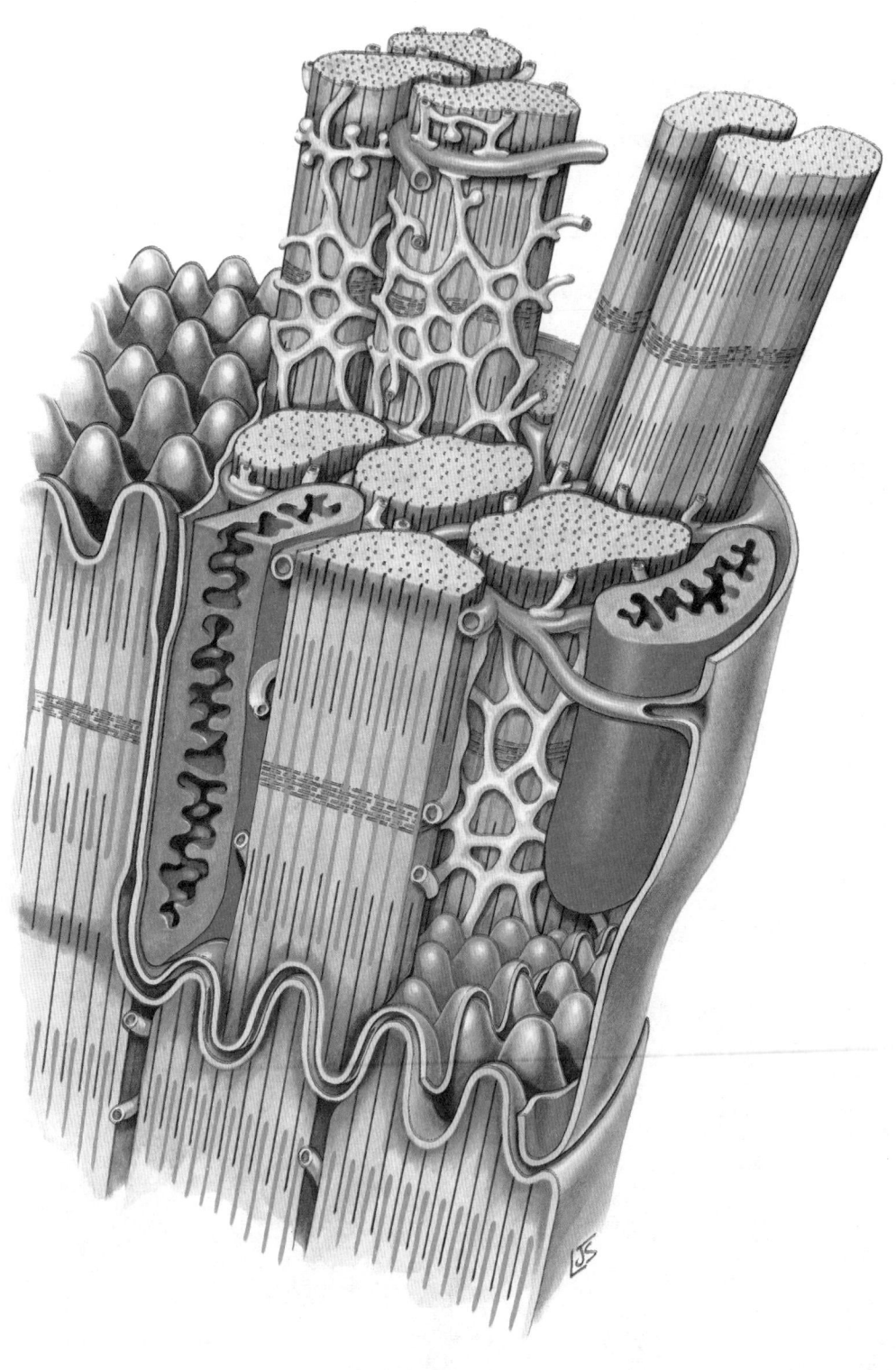

7.32 Three-dimensional reconstruction of cardiac muscle cells, showing in particular the organization of the transverse tubules (orange) and sarcoplasmic reticulum (yellow). The colour scheme is the same as in 7.15, to facilitate comparison with skeletal muscle. Note the large diameter of the transverse tubules, their location at the level of the Z-discs, and the formation of diads with the junctional sarcoplasmic reticulum. An intercalated disc, with desmosomes and a gap junction, is depicted at the bottom and left. (Artist: Lesley Skeates.)

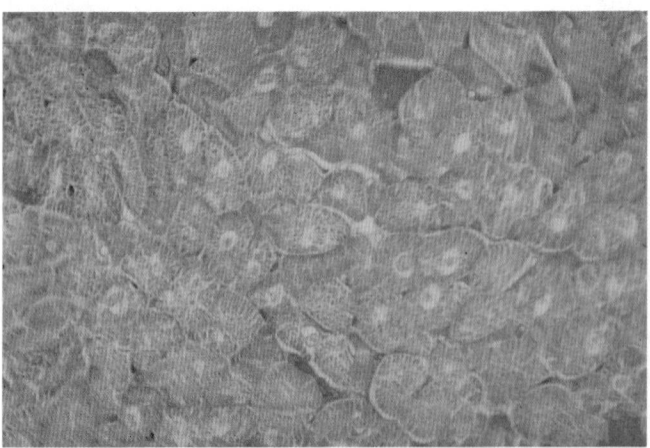

7.33 Transverse section through cardiac muscle. The cardiac cells have centrally placed nuclei surrounded by myofibrils. Note the spaces around the nuclei, which may give the appearance of holes when the nucleus is out of the plane of section. Blue strands of connective tissue form incomplete septa. Magnification × 300.

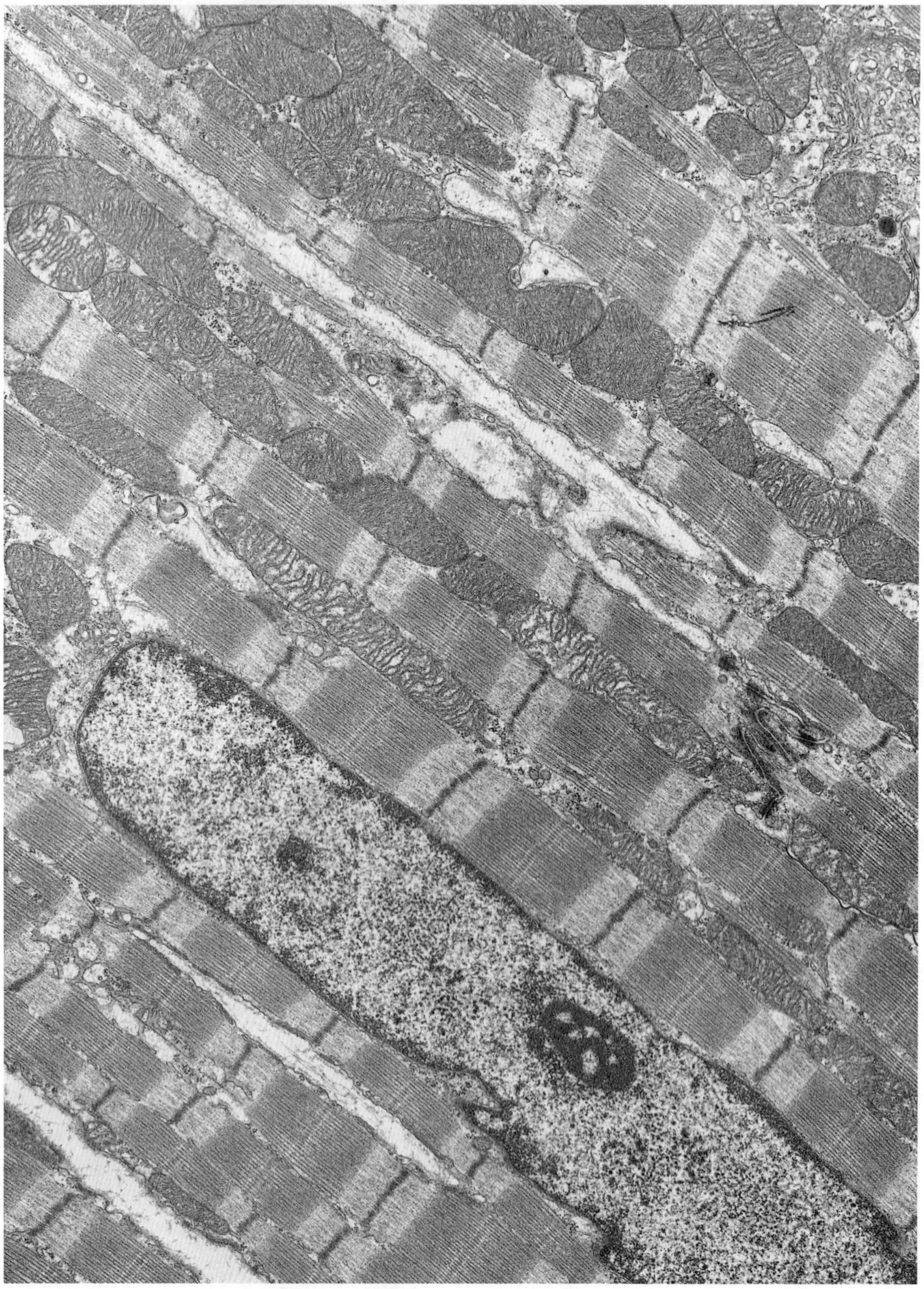

7.34 Electron micrograph of cardiac muscle in longitudinal section. Note the centrally placed nucleus, the abundant mitochondria, sarcoplasmic reticulum (lower left) and an intercalated disc (middle, right). Magnification × 10 000. (Photograph by Brenda Russell, Department of Physiology and Biophysics, University of Illinois at Chicago.)

is initiated by lowering free Ca^{2+} to its original level by active uptake into membrane-bound stores. The basic elements responsible for the Ca^{2+} transient in cardiac muscle—the sarcolemma, the transverse (or T-) tubules, and the sarcoplasmic reticulum—have been encountered before in the context of skeletal muscle. There are, however, differences in the physical arrangement and molecular composition of these elements in cardiac muscle that have a profound influence on contractile function in this tissue.

Membrane systems of cardiac muscle

The sarcolemma of cardiac muscle cells invaginates to form T-tubules, which penetrate the sarcoplasm at the level of the Z-discs (**7.32**). This location differs from that found in mammalian skeletal muscle (cf. **7.15**), although it is usual in the skeletal muscle of lower vertebrates. The T-tubules are interconnected at intervals by longitudinal branches. In skeletal muscle, the T-tubules serve to conduct the action potential into the depths of the cell. Their function is probably similar in cardiac muscle but may be less crucial, as T-tubules do not appear to be a feature of cardiac muscle in non-mammalian vertebrates. The T-tubules of cardiac muscle have a much wider lumen than those of skeletal muscle.

The *sarcoplasmic reticulum* is a membrane-bound tubular plexus which surrounds groups of myofilaments, defining, sometimes incompletely, the outlines of individual myofibrils. Its main role is the storage, release and re-accumulation of calcium ions. It comes into close contact with the T-tubules, leaving a 15-nm gap which is spanned by structures termed *junctional processes*. These processes appear to be very similar—biochemically, structurally and functionally—to the ryanodine receptor–calcium release channels found in skeletal muscle at the junctional surface of the terminal cisternae (p. 749 and see Wier 1993). Sarcoplasmic reticulum that bears junctional processes has been termed *junctional sarcoplasmic reticulum*, to distinguish it from the *free sarcoplasmic reticulum* that forms a longitudinal network of smooth-surfaced tubules (Sommer & Jennings 1986). Junctional sarcoplasmic reticulum makes contact with both the T-tubules and the sarcolemma (of which the T-tubules are, of course, an extension). *Corbular sarcoplasmic reticulum* is a component of sarcoplasmic reticulum that forms small globular extensions (French: *corbeille* = basket) in the vicinity of the Z-discs, but not in immediate relation to T-tubules or the sarcolemma. Since the junctions between T-tubules and sarcoplasmic reticulum usually involve only one structure of each type, the corresponding profiles in electron micrographs are referred to as *diads*, rather than *triads* as in skeletal muscle (compare **7.32** and **7.15**).

Excitation–contraction coupling in cardiac muscle

The calcium release channels of the sarcoplasmic reticulum are sensitive to the concentration of free Ca^{2+} in the cytoplasm. This is the basis of 'calcium-induced calcium release' (Fabiato 1985), which is believed to be the principal—and possibly the sole—mechanism involved in the liberation of Ca^{2+} from the sarcoplasmic reticulum during physiological activation. The passage of an action potential depolarizes the sarcolemma, opening membrane channels that allow some Ca^{2+} to enter from the extracellular space. This produces a small rise in the intracellular free Ca^{2+} concentration which opens the calcium release channels, allowing Ca^{2+} ions to flow down the concentration gradient from the sarcoplasmic reticulum into the cytoplasm. Calcium-induced calcium release may also involve calcium release channels located in non-junctional parts of the sarcoplasmic reticulum. (There must also be a process—as yet undiscovered—for turning the Ca^{2+} release off, else the mechanism described would result in the regenerative release of all the Ca^{2+} in the sarcoplasmic reticulum.)

Systolic activation is terminated by uptake of Ca^{2+} from the cytosol. Although both the sarcolemma and the mitochondrial membrane have some capacity for Ca^{2+} transport, the main route of uptake is into the sarcoplasmic reticulum, via a high-affinity, Ca^{2+}-transporting ATPase. The activity of this ATPase controls the rate of decay of the Ca^{2+} transient and is therefore a determinant of the rate of relaxation of the heart. The sarcoplasmic reticulum, in particular the corbular and junctional sarcoplasmic reticulum, contains *calsequestrin*, a somewhat distant cousin of the protein found in skeletal muscle. This calcium-binding protein lowers the free Ca^{2+} concentration inside the sarcoplasmic reticulum, allowing it to store considerable amounts of total calcium without increasing the gradient against which the Ca^{2+}-ATPase must pump. It may also facilitate subsequent release by interacting with proteins in the junctional sarcoplasmic reticulum (Ikemoto et al 1989).

Regulation of contraction in cardiac muscle

One of the major functional differences between cardiac and skeletal muscle is the way in which contractile force is regulated. Smoothness and gradation of contraction in a skeletal muscle depend in the first instance on the recruitment and asynchronous firing of different numbers of motor units. This mechanism is not available to the heart, in which the entire mass of muscle must be activated almost simultaneously. In skeletal muscle, gradation is possible even within individual motor units, which can build up a contraction through a brief series of re-excitations. Mechanical summation of this type is not possible in cardiac muscle, because the cells are electrically refractory until mechanical relaxation has taken place. How, then, does mammalian cardiac muscle regulate the force of contraction?

In cardiac muscle cells, as in skeletal muscle cells, contraction is initiated when Ca^{2+} binds to troponin-C, a component of the regulatory protein complex on the thin filaments. During basal activity of the heart, the amount of Ca^{2+} bound to troponin-C during each systole induces less than half-maximal activation of the contractile apparatus (see Ruegg & Solaro 1993). There is therefore scope for producing more force by increasing the Ca^{2+} bound to troponin-C. This can be achieved by controlling the amount of free Ca^{2+} released into the cytosol during systole.

A special feature of the cardiac cell is the prolonged duration of its action potential (Reiter 1988). The long-lasting plateau of depolarization allows a slow inward flux of Ca^{2+} to take place via so-called L-type Ca^{2+} channels in the sarcolemma. The Ca^{2+} is then actively pumped into the sarcoplasmic reticulum—indeed the extent to which the sarcoplasmic reticulum is loaded is crucially dependent on this entry of extracellular Ca^{2+}. The greater the amount of Ca^{2+} stored in the sarcoplasmic reticulum, the more is available for release during subsequent contractions. In man and many other species these Ca^{2+} movements provide an automatic mechanism for matching any increase in heart rate with a progressive increase in contractile force: the so-called *Bowditch staircase* or *treppe phenomenon*. At higher heart rates, more Ca^{2+} enters in unit time and is pumped into the sarcoplasmic reticulum; each systole is then more forceful, because the amount of Ca^{2+} that can be delivered into the cytosol is greater.

The most potent physiological means of enhancing cardiac contractility is through the action of β-adrenergic agents, such as adrenaline and noradrenaline. These increase Ca^{2+} taken up by the sarcoplasmic reticulum in two ways. Firstly, β-adrenergic stimulation increases the amount of Ca^{2+} that enters during depolarization by keeping the L-type Ca^{2+} channels open for longer (for references, see Reiter 1988). Secondly, β-adrenergic stimulation can enhance the activity of the Ca^{2+}-pumping ATPase by phosphorylating an associated protein, *phospholamban* ($M_r 27000$) (for references, see Movsesian 1993). The second of these two effects also enables the Ca^{2+} pump to lower the cytosolic free Ca^{2+} more rapidly, contributing to the accelerated relaxation produced by β-adrenergic agonists. Phosphorylation of phospholamban is brought about by a cyclic AMP-dependent protein kinase, and phosphodiesterase inhibitors (which raise the intracellular concentration of cyclic AMP) exert some of their effects through the same pathway. (Phospholamban is also found in slow—although not in fast—skeletal muscle (Pette & Staron 1990), so it is possible that this protein also contributes to the regulation of Ca^{2+} uptake in slow fibres.)

Because of the clinical importance of *positive inotropic* agents (substances that increase the strength of cardiac contraction) in conditions such as heart failure, there is great interest in the multiple control sites that might provide targets for pharmacological intervention. Some of these are related to another important set of ionic fluxes through the sarcolemma via the Na^+/K^+ and the bidirectional Na^+/Ca^{2+} exchange channels (Lederer et al 1986; **7.35**). The drugs in current clinical use all work on the principle of enhancing Ca^{2+} entry, Ca^{2+} uptake, or Ca^{2+} flow to the myofilaments, but there is interest in a new class of drugs that acts by increasing the affinity of the troponin complex for Ca^{2+}, thus sensitizing the myofilaments to calcium (Ruegg & Solaro 1993).

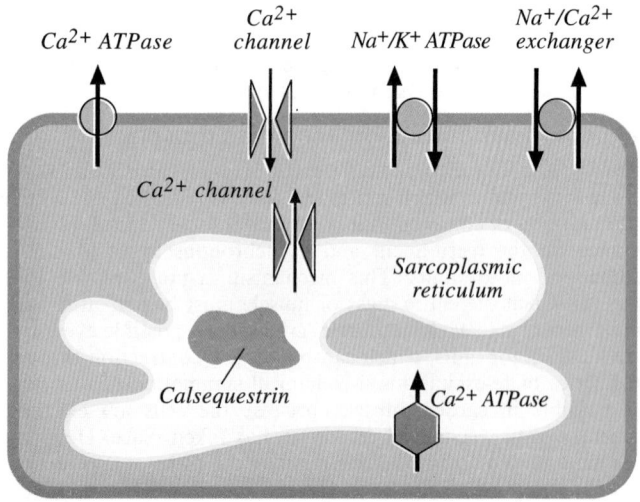

7.35 Schematic illustration of the major ion channels, pumps and exchangers in the sarcolemma and sarcoplasmic reticulum of a cardiac muscle cell. (Artwork by Stanley Salmons and Lesley Skeates.)

Intercalated discs

Intercalated discs are unique to cardiac muscle. In the light microscope they are seen as dark, transverse lines crossing the tracts of cardiac cells (**7**.31). They may step irregularly within or between adjacent tracts, and may appear to jump to a new position as the plane of focus is altered. At the ultrastructural level these structures are seen to correspond to elaborate junctions between the cardiac muscle cells (**7**.32, 34, 36). The junctions have transverse and lateral portions. A *transverse portion* is found wherever myofibrils abut the end of the cell, taking the place of the last Z-disc. At this point the actin filaments of the terminal sarcomere insert into a dense subsarcolemmal matrix which anchors them, together with other cytoplasmic elements such as intermediate filaments, to the plasma membrane. This structure is homologous, and probably similar in composition, to that found on the cytoplasmic face of the myotendinous junction (p. 749; Jockusch et al 1993). It is a focal type of adherens junction (Geiger & Ginsberg 1991). Prominent desmosomes, often with a dense line in the intercellular space, are seen at intervals along the transverse portion. The net effect is to provide firm adhesion and a route for the transmission of contractile force from one cell to the next.

The *lateral portion* of the intercalated disc runs parallel to the myofilaments for a distance that corresponds to one or two sar-

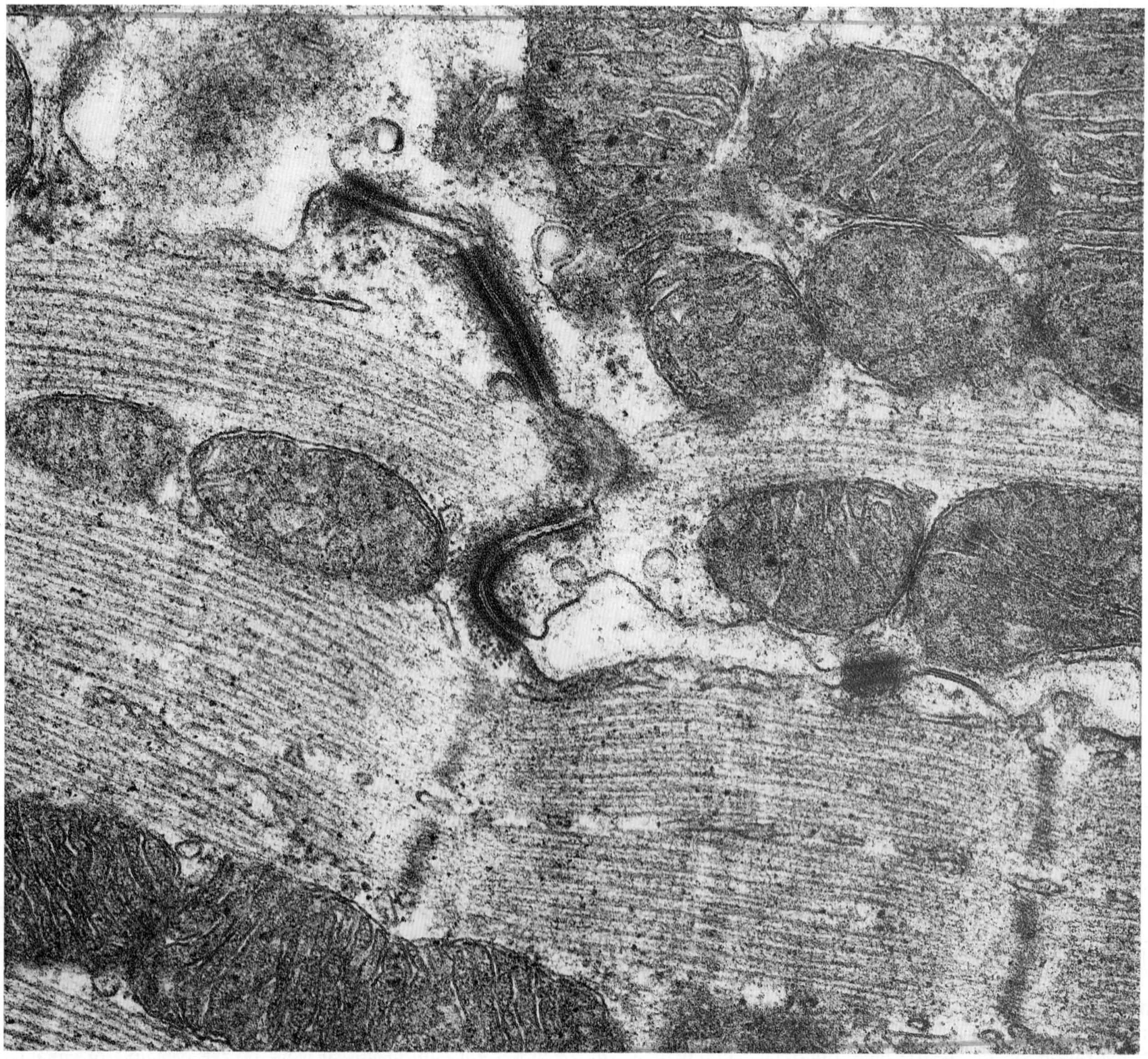

7.36 High-power electron micrograph of cardiac muscle at an intercalated disc, which shows several zones of fascia adherens and a gap junction.

Magnification × 57 100. (Photograph by Brenda Russell, Department of Physiology and Biophysics, University of Illinois at Chicago.)

comeres before the junction turns again to form another transverse portion. Thus it is responsible for the stepwise progression of the intercalated disc that can be seen in the light, as well as the electron, microscope. The important feature of the lateral portion is the presence of gap junctions (**7.36**, p. 768), which are the structures responsible for electrical coupling between the adjacent cells (Spray & Burt 1990; Severs 1990). Conductance channels within these junctions enable the electrical impulse to propagate from one cell to the next, spreading excitation and contraction rapidly along the branching tracts of interconnected cells. In this way the activity of the individual cells of the heart is co-ordinated so that they function as a syncytium.

Impulse-conducting tissues of the heart

The cells of cardiac muscle differ further from those of skeletal muscle in having the inherent ability to contract and relax spontaneously. This myogenic rhythm is shown by small pieces of cardiac tissue, and even isolated myocytes. The underlying mechanism appears to be based on a further specialization of the sarcolemma which permits a slow inward leakage of sodium ions. Ventricular cells contract and relax at a lower frequency than atrial cells, but in the intact heart both are synchronized to a more rapid rhythm generated by pacemaker tissue and conveyed to them by a system of fibres specialized for conduction. The anatomical arrangement of these tissues will be described in the context of the heart (p. 1495); here consideration is restricted to the cells that make up the impulse-generating and conducting system. All are modified cardiac cells. Three types may be distinguished morphologically from normal working cardiac cells (James 1978; James & Sherf 1978):

- *P (= Pale-staining = Primitive = Pacemaker) cells*
- *transitional cells*
- *Purkinje fibres*

Although these terms will be used in the following account, it may be equally important to emphasize the extent to which there is a continuum of morphology between P cells, transitional cells, Purkinje fibres, and working cardiac muscle cells.

Overview of the conducting system. Of all the cells in the heart, those of the *sinoatrial node* generate the most rapid rhythm, and therefore function as the pacemaker of the heart. The impulse, believed to be generated in the P cells, is transmitted over preferentially conducting pathways to right and left atria and to the *atrioventricular node*. At the atrioventricular node the impulse is delayed by about 40 ms. This delay allows the atria to eject their contents fully before contraction of the ventricles begins; it also places an upper limit on the frequency of signals that can be transmitted on to the ventricles. Slender transitional cells, closer in morphology to normal cardiac cells, extend from the node into the stem and principal branches of the atrioventricular bundle (*of His*). Here they become continuous with cells of more distinctive appearance, the Purkinje fibres. Conduction of the impulse is rapid in the bundle and its branches (about 2–3 metres per second, as opposed to 0.6 metres per second in normal myocardium). The cardiac impulse therefore arrives at the apex of the heart before spreading through the ventricular walls, producing a properly co-ordinated ventricular ejection.

Sinoatrial node. The sinoatrial node is an elliptical structure, about 10–20 mm long, a consistent feature of which is a surprisingly large central artery. *Nodal cells* are grouped circumferentially around this artery, interwoven into its dense collagenous adventitia; the functional implications of this relationship are not fully understood. Many nerve fibres are present, although none appears to terminate on cells; there are no ganglia within the node, although many border it anteriorly and posteriorly. P cells are most abundant in the central region. They are small, empty-looking cells, about 5–10 μm in greatest diameter, with a large central nucleus. The pale appearance is due to sparsity of organelles: myofibrils are few and irregularly arranged, there is no proper sarcotubular system and little glycogen. P cells are less abundant in the periphery of the node, where they mix with slender, fusiform transitional cells. The latter are part of a heterogeneous group intermediate in appearance between P cells and normal working cardiac cells. They link P cells to other cells.

Atrioventricular node. Internodal conduction pathways converge on the atrioventricular node. This is similar in general appearance to the sinoatrial node, although the collagenous component is less dense. The majority of cells are of the transitional type, but P cells resembling those of the sinoatrial node are found in a more fibrous central region. Autonomic ganglia are present between the node and the coronary sinus. In both sinoatrial and atrioventricular nodes, the intercellular contacts between P cells, and between P cells and transitional cells, are much less specialized than the intercalated discs between normal cardiac cells. A sparsity of gap junctions is consistent with the absence from these areas of *connexin-43*, which is a major protein component of mammalian gap junctions (Yancey et al 1989; Oosthoek et al 1990). This probably accounts for the observed difficulty in exciting these cells from adjacent cells (Merideth et al 1968). The atrioventricular delay may owe much to this relative inexcitability of the P cells, which appears to disturb the spread of potential in a manner that delays propagation (LeBlanc & Dubé 1993). The narrow diameter of the transitional cells may account for part of the conduction delay.

Purkinje fibres. In many species, such as ungulates, the Purkinje fibres are quite conspicuous, but in man the differences are more subtle. As in other parts of the myocardium, the 'fibres' are actually tracts of single cells. These cells are larger in diameter (30 μm) and shorter (20–25 μm) than normal cardiac myocytes and often contain more than one nucleus. The sparse myofibrils are very thin, but, unlike those in the P cells, they tend to be longitudinally orientated. They skirt the nucleus, leaving a clear zone that may contain many mitochondria; other mitochondria are scattered between the myofibrils. The cytoplasm contains abundant glycogen and also acetylcholinesterase. There is a well-developed internal membrane system which is, however, lacking in T-tubules. Intercellular contacts are made via fully developed intercalated discs, which incorporate extensive gap junctions at both the ends and the sides. Purkinje fibres are the main type of cell in the bundle of His, where they are found in longitudinal strands separated by collagen fibres. In the peripheral branches, the strands may be interspersed with cardiac cells of normal appearance. As the branches of the conducting bundle spread and subdivide, the Purkinje fibres undergo a transition, losing their distinctive character and blending into the cardiac fibres of the ventricular walls.

Although Purkinje fibres attain their largest development in the bundle branches, cells with similar morphology—and therefore included in this category—are found interspersed with other cells at the margins of the nodes and in the internodal pathways.

Rapid conduction in the Purkinje fibres of the atrioventricular bundle is probably the product of several factors: the low resistance pathway provided by the short, large-diameter cells; the extensive development of gap junctions between the cells; and the absence of a fully developed T-system, which would be expected to result in a lower membrane capacitance. This said, it is a mistake to assume the converse: that all cells involved in rapid conduction must look like Purkinje fibres (James 1978). Such an assumption may account for continuing reluctance, despite electrophysiological evidence, to recognize the existence of preferentially conducting pathways in the atria.

INNERVATION OF CARDIAC MUSCLE

Although the impulse-generating and conducting system of the heart establishes an endogenous rhythm, the rate and force of contraction are under neural influence. Both divisions of the autonomic nervous system supply non-myelinated postganglionic fibres to the heart. Although this innervation is derived bilaterally, it is functionally asymmetric. In the case of the sympathetic component, stimulation of the left stellate ganglion has little effect on heart rate but increases ventricular contractility, whereas stimulation of the right stellate ganglion influences both rate and contractility. In the case of the parasympathetic component, the action of the right vagus nerve in slowing heart rate is exerted mainly through its influence on the sinoatrial node, whereas that of the left vagus is exerted mainly by slowing propagation of the impulse through the atrioventricular node.

Sympathetic nerve fibres from the cervical sympathetic ganglia reach the heart via the cardiac nerves; parasympathetic fibres in the heart originate in ganglion cells which are innervated by efferent fibres of the vagus nerve. Adrenergic, cholinergic and peptidergic endings have been demonstrated in the myocardium by light and electron microscopy (Kyösola et al 1976; Rechardt et al 1986). Fibres often end close to myocytes and blood vessels but junctional specializations are not seen, and a gap of at least 110 nm remains. It is assumed that neurotransmitters diffuse across this gap to the adjacent cells. Some of the endings represent efferent nerve terminals; others function as pain, mechano- or chemoreceptors; still others, which are found in close apposition, may represent sites of peripheral modulation. The full range of autonomic control possibilities suggested by these structures has yet to be worked out.

BLOOD SUPPLY OF CARDIAC MUSCLE

The heart's incessant activity is equivalent to a constant power expenditure of about 1.3 watts under basal conditions, escalating to 3 watts or more during physical exertion. The cardiac muscle cells contain glycogen, which may be called upon as a reserve during intermittent peaks of activity, but the great bulk of their energy requirement is continuous in nature and can be supplied only through a highly developed oxidative metabolism. This is clearly evident from the high proportion of the cell volume given over to mitochondria, which are large and have closely spaced cristae (7.34). Such a metabolism has to be supported by a blood supply of commensurate oxygen-carrying capacity. Myocardium has a very high perfusion rate: 0.5 ml/min/g of tissue (about 5 times that of liver and 15 times that of skeletal muscle). No cardiac muscle cell is more than about 8 μm from a capillary (Wearn 1941), and measurements in rabbit myocardium show that vascular channels occupy about 60% of the total interstitial space (Frank & Langer 1974).

The heart is supplied by the coronary vessels (p. 1505). Although there is some variability in the detailed distribution of the arterial branches, the left ventricle, which has the highest workload, consistently receives the highest arterial blood flow. Branches run in the myocardium along the coarser aggregations of connective tissue and ramify extensively in the endomysial layer, creating a rich plexus of anastomosing vessels. This plexus includes lymphatic as well as blood capillaries, differing in this respect from skeletal muscle.

The high oxygen requirement of the myocardium also renders it vulnerable to ischaemic damage arising from atheroma or embolism in the coronary arteries. Arterial anastomoses, often more than 100 μm in diameter, are found throughout the heart (James 1961). They are clearly an important factor in determining whether an adequate collateral circulation can develop after a coronary occlusion. Recent experiments involving the local application of angiogenetic growth factors may encourage attempts to revascularize ischaemic myocardium from exogenous tissues or vessels (Schlaudraff et al 1993).

DEVELOPMENT OF CARDIAC MUSCLE

The early development of the heart is described in detail elsewhere (p. 299). Here we focus on the embryological origin of cardiac muscle.

Formation of cardiac muscle is an early event in embryonic life, for cells capable of forming myocardial tissue can be detected in the pregastrulation embryo (Icardo & Manasek 1992). In the late presomite and early somite embryo, presumptive myocardial cells are found as a continuous sheet of cuboidal cells that line the ventral splanchnic wall of the pericardial cavity, the *myocardial plate* (Kaufman & Navaratnam 1981). At about the 1–2 somite stage of development, paired tubular spaces form within the primitive endocardial tissue subjacent to the myocardial plate. The developing endocardial tubes begin to be surrounded by cells of the myocardial plate. During the 3–4 somite stage, the endocardial tubes fuse in the midline to form a single endocardial tube, by which time they are invested in a nearly complete layer of presumptive myocardial cells, the *myocardial mantle*. The myocardial mantle is separated from the endocardial lining of the primitive heart tube by an acellular matrix, formerly referred to as *cardiac jelly*, which is secreted by the myocardial cells; this matrix has the composition of a basement membrane and contains inductive signals, also secreted by the myocardial cells, that transform competent cells of the endocardial epithelium into free mesenchymal cells (p. 299). Thus during cardiac development, presumptive myocardial cells engage in several processes at once: they divide and differentiate to form a functional myocardium; they secrete matrix and inductive factors that will modify the differ-

entiation of other cells; and they participate in the bending and rotation of the primitive heart tube, and differential growth within its walls, which will ultimately produce the four-chambered adult heart.

Overt differentiation of the primitive myocardial cells begins at about the time of fusion of the endocardial tubes (Icardo 1988). As the primitive heart tube is formed, the presumptive myocytes start to express genes that encode constituents characteristic of the myocardial cell, including myosin, actin, troponin and other components of the contractile apparatus. Myofibrils begin to appear in the developing myocytes, and the first functional heart beats start soon afterwards.

The regulatory mechanisms underlying differentiation of cardiac muscle appear to be distinct from those of skeletal muscle. Although it is anticipated that counterparts will be found for the transcriptional factors Myf-5, myogenin, MyoD and Myf-6 that are responsible for inducing differentiation of skeletal muscle (p. 757), the corresponding factors for cardiac myogenesis have yet to be identified (Bishopric et al 1992). During fetal maturation, successive changes in gene expression (Lyons et al 1990) give rise to the characteristics of fetal, neonatal and adult myocardium (Schiaffino et al 1993; Nadal-Ginard & Mahdavi 1989) and are responsible for divergence of the properties of atrial and ventricular myocytes.

As has been seen, the committed cardiac myoblasts do not fuse to form multinucleated myotubes as in skeletal muscle, but remain as single cells coupled physically and electrically through intercellular junctions (Severs 1990). Moreover, differentiated cardiac myocytes continue to divide during fetal development, withdrawing from the cell cycle only after birth (Litvin et al 1992). This is markedly different to skeletal muscle development, in which differentiation (including the activation of muscle-specific genes) coincides with withdrawal from the cell cycle.

Contractile protein isoforms of cardiac muscle

As in skeletal muscle, the contractile proteins of cardiac muscle exist in a number of tissue- and stage-specific forms. The cardiac isoform of a-actin is not identical to the skeletal muscle form, and is encoded by a different gene, although the two are so similar as to be functionally interchangeable (Bishopric et al 1992). Both skeletal and cardiac isoforms of sarcomeric actin are expressed in fetal ventricular muscle (Gunning et al 1983; Vandekerckhove et al 1986). In the rat, the skeletal a-actin is down-regulated after birth, but in man the mRNA for this isoform increases postnatally and exceeds that of cardiac actin in the adult (Boheler et al 1991).

The myosin heavy chain of human cardiac muscle exists in two isoforms, a and β, both of which are present in the fetal heart. The a-form persists as the adult isoform of atrial muscle, whereas the β-form predominates in ventricular muscle (Emerson & Bernstein 1987). Interestingly, the β-form of myosin heavy chain in cardiac muscle is identical to the isoform in slow skeletal muscle. This identity between cardiac and slow skeletal protein isoforms is true of several proteins, including ventricular myosin light chains and cardiac troponin-C; other proteins, such as troponin-I and -T, exist in cardiac specific forms (Bishopric et al 1992).

Under some experimental conditions the contractile protein isoforms expressed by mature cardiac muscle may change in the adult mammal. Two established influences in this respect are thyroid hormone (Izumo et al 1986), and mechanical stretch induced by pressure overload (Swynghedauw 1986). Transitions in both the heavy chains and light chains of myosin have been shown to take place in the human heart under conditions of pathological overload (Schaub et al 1984; Cummins 1982), but it is not known whether these changes have any functional significance.

Development of the impulse-conducting tissues

The impulse-generating and conducting system of the heart is formed from myocytes that differ in their morphology from the working cardiac cells which make up the bulk of the myocardium (p. 308; Icardo & Manasek 1992). Myocytes of the mature conduction system retain some similarities to the myocardium of the early heart tube, and share with that embryonic tissue a distinctive pattern of expression of many genes, including those encoding contractile proteins and acetylcholinesterase. This suggests that divergence of conducting tissues and working myocardium takes place at an early embryonic stage. Efforts have been made to trace the development of the conduction tissue in the chick (Vassall-Adams 1982; Lamers et al 1991), the mouse (Viragh & Challice 1977a,b) and man (Wenink 1976; Wessels et al 1992). There are clearly difficulties in carrying out such studies based on histological criteria alone, and the results have been controversial. An important recent development is the use of cytological marker specific for the conduction system: the sulphate-3-glucuronyl carbohydrate moiety of glycoproteins that is recognized by monoclonal antibodies Leu-7 (Ikeda et al 1990), GlN2 (Wessels et al 1992) and HNK-1 (Nakagawa et al 1993). This is expressed by 32 days of development and is downregulated during the later stages of cardiac septation. Its distribution strongly suggests that the conduction tissue in man originates in a ring of specialized myocytes located at the interventricular foramen of the early heart (Wessels et al 1992; and see p. 308).

Lack of regeneration of cardiac muscle

In skeletal muscle development a population of precursor cells—satellite cells—is retained in adult life, and constitutes a pool of myoblasts capable of dividing, fusing with existing muscle fibres, and initiating regeneration after damage. Cardiac muscle contains no equivalent of these cells: it therefore has no capacity for regeneration. Temporary ischaemia (of up to 15 min duration in the dog) injures cardiac cells in a reversible manner (Jennings et al 1960); longer periods of ischaemia produce irreversible damage, the unavoidable outcome of which is necrosis of contractile cardiac tissue and its replacement by scar tissue.

GROWTH AND HYPERTROPHY OF CARDIAC MUSCLE

Although differentiated cardiac myocytes continue to divide during fetal development, this process generally ceases after birth. A further increase in the number of cells can take place if the heart is pathologically stressed in the first few months of life, but postnatal growth of cardiac muscle, like that of skeletal muscle, is normally brought about by hypertrophy of the myocytes.

In addition to the normal processes of growth, conditions that chronically increase the mechanical stress on the myocardium result in a compensatory hypertrophy of the cells, and a consequent thickening of the cardiac walls. There are two common causes of such stress: increased resistance to ventricular emptying, and increased ventricular filling (Schlant 1978). In the case of the left ventricle, increased resistance to ventricular emptying (increased afterload, or 'pressure overload') is often the result of a rise in peripheral vascular resistance, or of narrowing of the aorta or aortic valve. It produces *concentric hypertrophy*, in which there is marked thickening of the left ventricular walls, including the interventricular septum, but the left ventricular cavity is of normal, or in some instances less than normal, size. There is an increase in contractile cardiac mass, which is a reflection of changes at the subcellular level that involve parallel accretion of myofilaments. Increased ventricular filling (increased preload or 'volume overload') is commonly the result of regurgitation

through the aortic or mitral valves or a ventricular septal defect. It produces *eccentric hypertrophy*, characterized by an increase in both the thickness of the left ventricular wall and the size of the ventricular chamber. The subcellular changes that bring about ventricular dilatation consist of an increase in individual sarcomere length, addition of sarcomeres in series as well as in parallel, and slippage between and within myofibrils. There is also slippage between fibres and between fibre bundles. The right ventricle responds similarly to overload conditions: for example, left ventricular changes that produce a rise in diastolic pressure can elevate the pressure in pulmonary vessels, resulting in right ventricular hypertrophy.

Although it may be assumed that the basic stimulus for hypertrophy is an increase in wall stress, the underlying mechanisms remain unknown.

SMOOTH MUSCLE

DISTINGUISHING FEATURES OF SMOOTH MUSCLE

The ability of muscle tissues to contract is based in all cases on the interaction between the contractile proteins, actin and myosin. In skeletal and cardiac muscle, these proteins assemble to form sarcomeres—repeating elements whose precise alignment across the cells produces a striated appearance in the light microscope. In the third major type of muscle tissue the contractile proteins are not organized into sarcomeres, and the cytoplasm has a smooth, unstriated appearance from which the tissue derives its usual name. Smooth muscle is also referred to as *non-striated*, or *involuntary muscle*, the latter term referring to the fact that its activity is neither initiated nor monitored consciously. It is more variable, in both form and function, than either of the other major types of muscle tissue, a reflection of its varied roles in different systems of the body.

The myocytes of smooth muscle are smaller than those of striated muscle (**7.37**). Their length can range from 15 μm in small blood vessels to 200 μm, and even to 500 μm or more in the uterus during pregnancy (Csapo 1962; Huddart & Hunt 1975). The cells are spindle-shaped, tapering towards the ends from a central diameter of 3 to 8 μm. The single nucleus is located at the midpoint, and is often distorted or folded by the contraction of the cell. Smooth muscle cells aggregate with their long axes parallel and staggered longitudinally, so that the wide central portion of one cell lies next to the tapered end of another (**7.38**). Such an arrangement achieves both close packing and a more efficient transfer of force from cell to cell. The effect in transverse section is to present an array of circular or slightly polygonal profiles of very varied size, with nuclei present only in the centres of the largest profiles (**7.39**). This appearance contrasts markedly with that of skeletal muscle cells, which show a consistent diameter and peripherally placed nuclei in cross-sections throughout their length.

Smooth muscle is typically found in the walls of tubular structures and hollow viscera, where it serves to regulate diameter (for example, in blood vessels, and branches of the bronchial tree), to propel

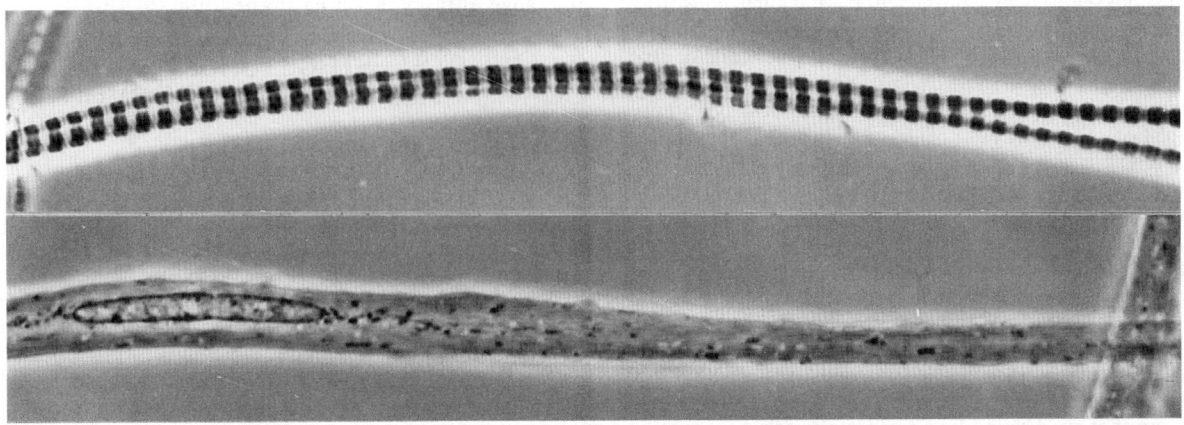

7.37 Part of a smooth muscle cell (lower panel) and two skeletal muscle myofibrils (upper panel). The two micrographs, reproduced at the same magnification, illustrate the difference in size between skeletal and smooth muscle cells, since a complete skeletal muscle fibre would contain many thousands of myofibrils. (Photographs by Vic Small, Institute of Molecular Biology, Austrian Academy of Sciences.)

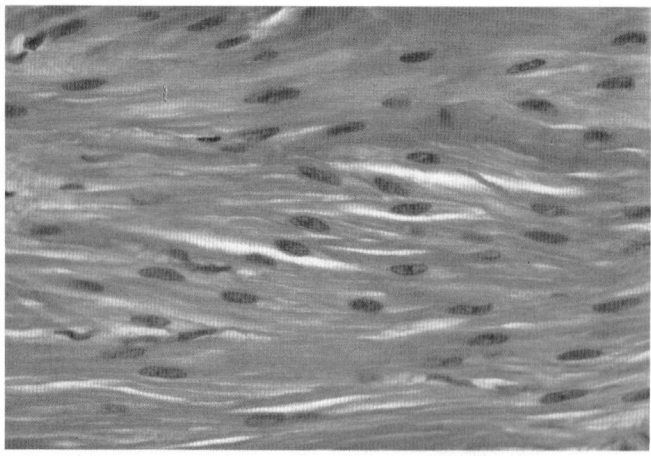

7.38 Longitudinal section of smooth muscle, stained with haematoxylin and eosin. Magnification × 410.

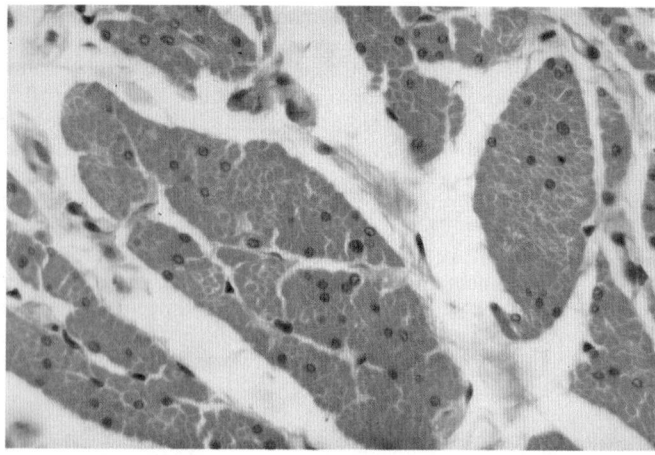

7.39 Transverse section of smooth muscle, stained with haematoxylin and eosin. The fascicles, appearing here as islands of tissue, contain numerous profiles of smooth muscle cells, only a small proportion of which contain nuclei. Note that where a nucleus is present it almost fills the cross-section of the cell (cf. skeletal muscle, **7.**5 and cardiac muscle, **7.**33). Magnification × 410.

liquids or solids (for example, in ureter, hepatic duct, and intestines) or to expel the contents (for example, in urinary bladder and uterus). The actual arrangement of the cells varies with the tissue. In respiratory bronchioles and the efferent ductules to the epididymis, the smooth muscle layer may be only two cells thick; in the tunica media of muscular arteries the cells are arranged circularly or spirally in multiple layers, packing so closely together that no capillaries penetrate between them. In the walls of the intestines, as for most of the alimentary tract, the smooth muscle is organized into well-orientated inner circular and outer longitudinal layers; in the wall of the urinary bladder, fascicles of smooth muscle interlace in several directions. Still different arrangements are found in the arrectores pilorum muscles of the skin and the iris of the eye. Because of this variation, the account that follows will be concerned, for the most part, with properties that are common to all forms of smooth muscle, leaving the implications of more specialized morphology and behaviour to be dealt with in the anatomical contexts in which they are encountered.

The blood supply of smooth muscle is less extensive than that of striated muscle. Where the tissue is not too densely packed, afferent and efferent vessels gain access via connective tissue septa, and capillaries run in the connective tissue between small fascicles. Capillaries are not found in relation to individual cells, as they are in striated muscle.

Smooth muscle has no attachment structures equivalent to the fasciae, tendons and aponeuroses associated with skeletal muscle, and individual cells start and finish within the body of the tissue. There is therefore a special arrangement for transmitting force from cell to cell and, where necessary, to other soft tissue structures. Within a fascicle, the cells are separated by a gap of 40–80 nm. Each cell is covered almost entirely by a prominent basal lamina, consisting of filamentous proteins embedded in a glycosaminoglycan matrix. This merges with a reticular layer consisting of a network of fine elastin, reticulin and collagen fibres (**7.**40). These elements bridge the gaps between adjacent cells, providing mechanical continuity throughout the fascicle. At the boundaries of fascicles, the connective tissue fibres become interwoven with those of interfascicular septa, so that the contraction of different fascicles is communicated through the tissue and to neighbouring structures.

The reticular network around each cell can be seen in the light microscope in sections stained by silver or trichrome techniques. The glycosaminoglycan matrix itself is weakly positive for the periodic acid–Schiff stain, which outlines the cells in pink. The extracellular matrix has also been strikingly demonstrated in electron micrographs of deeply etched specimens (Somlyo & Franzini-Armstrong 1985a). The components—the ground substance and the collagenous and elastic fibres—are not synthesized by fibroblasts or other connective tissue cells (which are rarely found within fasciculi) but by the smooth muscle cells themselves. This ability can be demonstrated in vitro (Scott et al 1977) and is one of several respects in which

affinities can be found between smooth muscle cells and fibroblasts.

Electron micrographs reveal places in which the basal laminae disappear from adjacent cells, and the membranes approach to 2–4 nm of one another to form a *gap junction* or *nexus* (Cobb & Bennett 1969). These junctions are believed to be structurally similar to their counterparts in cardiac muscle. They provide a low-resistance pathway through which electrical excitation can pass between cells, producing a wave of contraction. The incidence of gap junctions varies with the anatomical site of the tissue, and they appear to be more abundant in the type of smooth muscle that generates rhythmic activity (see p. 779, Innervation of smooth muscle).

Although some smooth muscles can generate as much force per unit cross-sectional area as skeletal muscle, the force always develops much more slowly than in striated muscle. On the other hand, smooth muscles from different sites in the body show specializations that are more relevant to function than mere contractile power. Smooth muscle can contract by more than 80%, a much greater range of shortening than the 30% or so to which a sarcomeric muscle is limited. The significance of this property is usefully illustrated by the urinary bladder, which must be capable of emptying completely from an internal volume of 300 ml or more. Smooth muscles can maintain tension for long periods with very little expenditure of energy. As an example, the muscular coat of an artery can maintain vascular tone despite the complete absence of a capillary supply. Many smooth muscle structures are capable of generating spontaneous contractions: examples are found in the walls of the intestines, ureter and fallopian tube. Thus, although it is easy to view smooth muscle as a primitive tissue, whose contractile mechanism is reminiscent of the contractility of non-muscle cells, there is a sense in which this versatile type of muscle is especially well adapted to the range of tasks that it has to perform.

FILAMENTOUS STRUCTURES AND THE CONTRACTILE MECHANISM OF SMOOTH MUSCLE

Although electron microscopy revealed the presence of filaments in smooth muscle some years ago (**7.**42), this observation alone has provided little insight into their possible functional organization because of the lack of any obvious filament order. Recent work, in which specific proteins were localized by high-resolution immunocytochemistry, has now revealed enough of the internal architecture of the cell to suggest a structural basis for contractile function (North et al 1994b). The model, which is illustrated in **7.**40, depends on the mutual interaction of two systems of filaments, one forming the cytoskeleton and the other the contractile apparatus.

Cytoskeleton

Excluding the perinuclear region, the cytoplasm of the smooth muscle cell effectively consists of two structural domains: the contractile

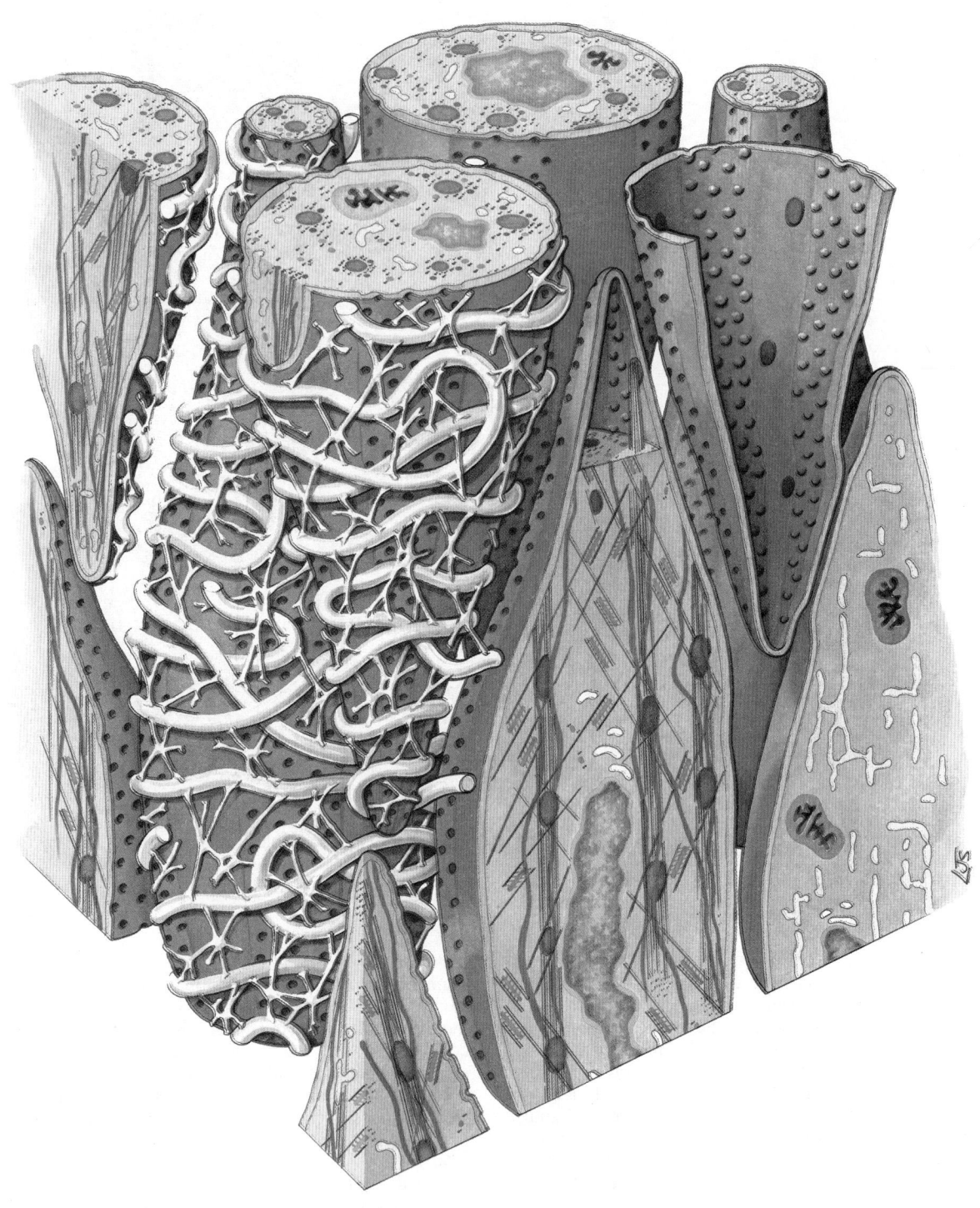

7.40 Three-dimensional reconstruction of smooth muscle cells. In the interests of clarity, some structural features have been separated for illustration in different cells. The spindle-shaped cells interdigitate with their long axes parallel; mechanical continuity between the cells is provided by a reticular layer (left). Internally, the structure of the cell is dominated by two systems of filaments (front). The cytoskeletal framework consists of intermediate filaments (brown) and thin filaments of cytoplasmic actin (black) organized into longitudinal bundles in association with dense bodies. The contractile apparatus consists of oblique filaments of myosin (green) and actin, which interact with the cytoskeleton to produce contraction of the cell. The sarcolemma contains alternating domains of anchoring adherens junctions and caveolae (top right). There is a sparse sarcoplasmic reticulum (yellow, bottom right). (Artist: Lesley Skeates.)

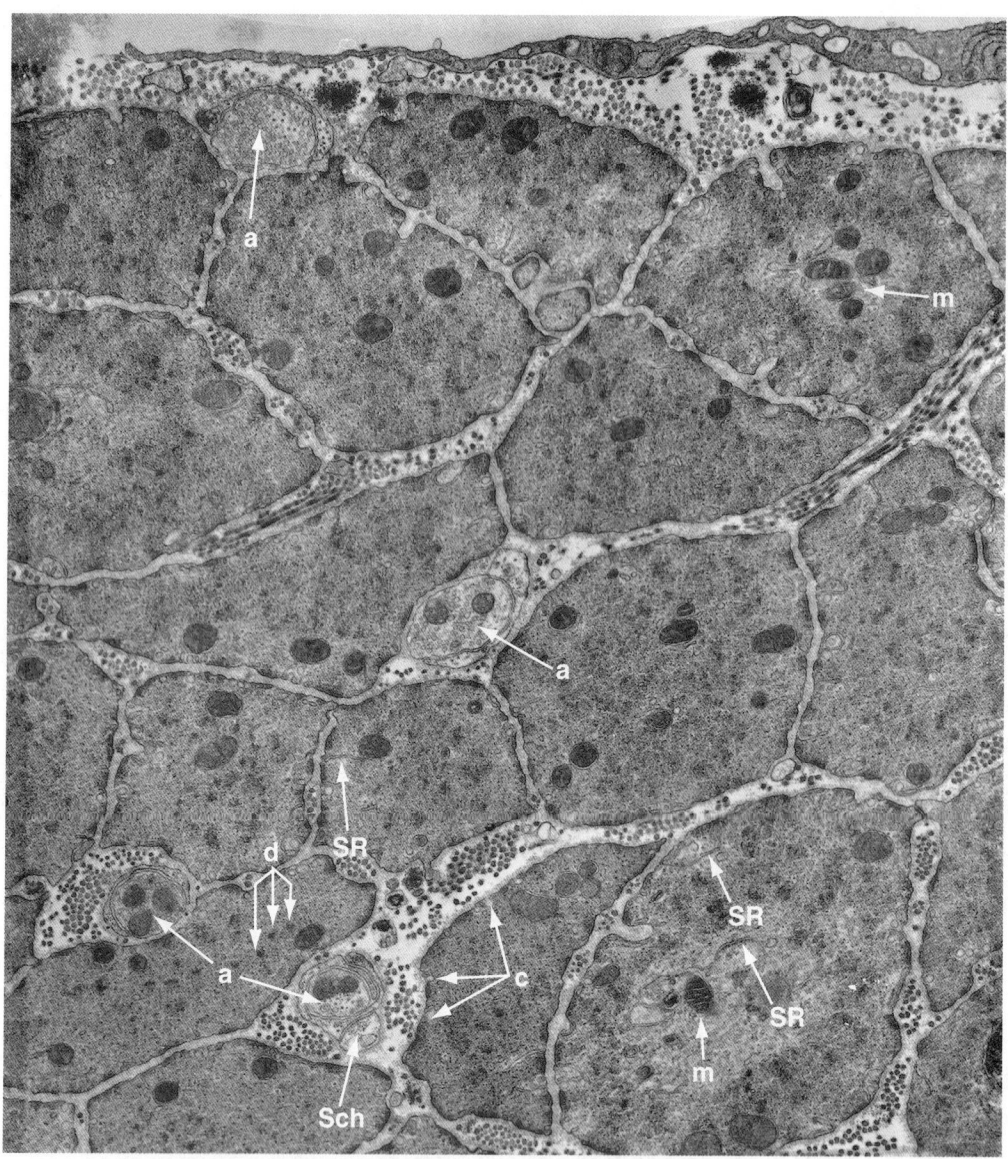

7.41 Low-power electron micrograph of smooth muscle cells from the rat detrusor muscle in transverse section. This muscle is well innervated, and four axonal profiles (a) are seen, all accompanied by Schwann cell expansions (Sch). Gap junctions are not seen. Note mitochondria (m), dense bodies (d), caveolae (c), and the flattened tubular profiles of sarcoplasmic reticulum (SR). Magnification × 6940. (Photograph by Georgio Gabella, Department of Anatomy, University College London.)

apparatus and the cytoskeleton. The cytoskeleton is a structural framework that maintains the spindle-like form of the cell and provides an internal scaffold with which other elements can interact. Its major structural component is the *intermediate filament*, composed in this case of *desmin*, with the addition of *vimentin* in vascular smooth muscle. The intermediate filaments are arranged mainly in longitudinal bundles, but some filaments interconnect the bundles with each other and with the sarcolemma to form a three-dimensional network (**7**.40). The cytoskeleton also contains filaments composed of a non-muscle isoform of *actin*, *β*-cytoplasmic actin, together with proteins, such as *filamin*, that associate specifically with actin. The bundles of intermediate filaments are associated with electron-dense, ovoid structures, about 0.1 μm in diameter, which are distributed uniformly throughout the cytoplasm (Draeger et al 1990); these are commonly referred to as *cytoplasmic dense bodies* (**7**.40, 43). Like the Z-discs of striated myocytes, the dense bodies contain the actin-binding protein *α-actinin*. They provide anchorage for the non-muscle actin filaments of the cytoskeleton, and also for the actin filaments of the contractile apparatus, a point to which we will return.

Contractile apparatus

774   The precise three-dimensional arrangement of *actin* and *myosin*

filaments in the contractile apparatus has not been completely resolved. However, several lines of evidence (see Small et al 1990) indicate that the myofilaments are arranged in fibrils that form connections with the longitudinally-orientated cytoskeleton at a shallow angle; this angle increases as the cell shortens (**7**.40, 42). Electron micrographs of transverse sections (**7**.43) show thick filament profiles surrounded by rosettes containing up to 15 thin filaments, but the spatial arrangement is often quite irregular (Rice et al 1970).

The myosin filaments are about 1.5 to 2 μm long (Small et al 1990). Smooth muscle myosin filaments have a unique structure, which differs from that of the thick filaments of the striated myocyte. Whereas the latter is bipolar (see p. 742), smooth muscle myosin filaments are 'face polar'—that is, the ribbon-like filaments are built in such a way that myosin molecules on the two sides point in opposite directions (Trybus 1991). With this type of polarity, actin filaments can slide along the whole length of a myosin filament during contraction. This difference underpins the ability of smooth muscle to undergo much greater changes in length than sarcomeric muscle.

The actin filaments are about 5 μm in length (Small et al 1990); in cross-sections this would give a somewhat exaggerated impression of their number relative to the shorter myosin filaments. Ultrastructural

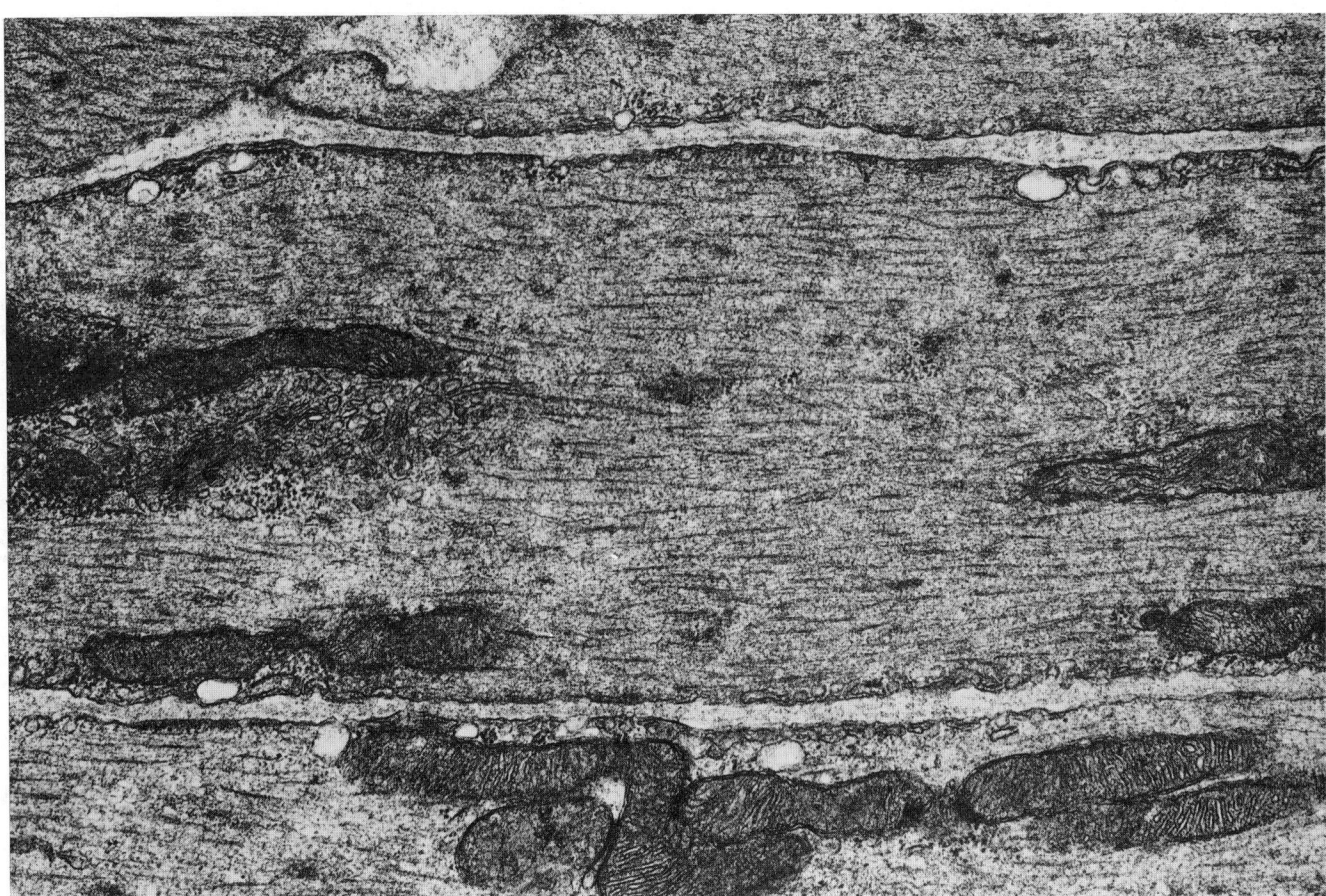

7.42 High-power electron micrograph of a smooth muscle showing myosin filaments surrounded by thin actin filaments, dense bodies and adherens junctions. (Photograph by Vic Small, Institute of Molecular Biology, Austrian Academy of Sciences.)

evidence clearly shows that actin filaments of the contractile apparatus insert into dense bodies and, importantly, they insert with a polarity that is opposite on either side of the dense body (Bond & Somlyo 1982; Tsukita et al 1983).

Contractile mechanism

The possible nature of the contractile unit may now be envisaged (**7.40**). The dense body is analogous to the Z-disc of skeletal muscle (p. 739), creating an I-band-like structure with a reversal of actin polarity at its centre. By virtue of its face–polar construction, a myosin filament can interact with the oppositely polarized actin filaments from two dense bodies, drawing together the cytoskeletal structures to which they are attached (Small 1977). The sliding of these obliquely orientated actin–myosin complexes makes the cell shorter and fatter, while their angle relative to the axis of the cell becomes steeper.

One of the key elements of this model is the interaction between the contractile apparatus and the cytoskeleton, which removes the need for a given contractile unit to span the cell from membrane to membrane. Indeed, actin filaments of the contractile apparatus do not actually have to be attached directly to the sarcolemma, although such attachments are possible (see below). There is no good evidence that the short myosin filaments are tethered to form A-band-like groupings, and the model does not require them to be: their role is to produce **relative** motion between oppositely directed actin filaments.

Membrane skeleton

From the nature of the contractile process it is clear that tension produced within the smooth muscle cell is not concentrated at the ends of the cell, as in the striated myocyte, but is distributed over much of the surface. The sarcolemma shows corresponding specializations. Electron microscopy reveals dense submembranous patches or plaques at more or less regular intervals around the periphery (**7.41, 43, 47**). These have the structural and immunocytochemical character of *adherens junctions*, which are involved in linking actin filaments to the cell membrane (Geiger & Ginsberg 1991). This justifies the earlier term 'attachment plaques', and indicates homology with the similar junctional specializations at the myotendinous junction in skeletal muscle and the intercalated disc in cardiac muscle. However, it is not certain that adherens junctions provide direct anchorage for actin filaments of the contractile apparatus, although cytoskeletal actin filaments of the non-muscle type, as well as intermediate filaments, have been located at these sites.

Between the adherens junctions are uncoated membrane regions of similar size that bear many vesicular invaginations or *caveolae* (Gabella 1984; **7.40, 41, 42, 45**). Filament anchorage does not occur in these domains. Fluorescent antibody labelling shows that the adherens junctions and caveolar domains are arranged in alternating longitudinal strips at the cell surface (**7.44A–D**).

Transmission of mechanical tension to the surrounding connective tissue is mediated by a chain of molecules at the adherens junctions which connects actin filaments on the cytoplasmic side of the membrane via transmembrane molecules, *integrins*, to extracellular matrix molecules, such as *fibronectin* and *laminin*, in the surrounding basal lamina. The sarcolemma in the intervening caveolar domains is the site of localization of the membrane-skeleton protein *dystrophin* (North et al 1993), which may have a stabilizing role similar to that suggested for skeletal muscle (see Dystrophin p. 748).

Isoforms of filamentous proteins

Smooth muscle contains several isoforms of actin and myosin. These are not segregated into different cells, so smooth muscle does not have the equivalent of the distinctive fibre types of skeletal muscle. Nevertheless, the balance between the isoforms changes with the stage of development, the tissue of origin, and the species, and is responsive to conditions such as hypertrophy and regeneration (Somlyo 1993; Malmqvist et al 1991; Eddinger & Wolf 1993).

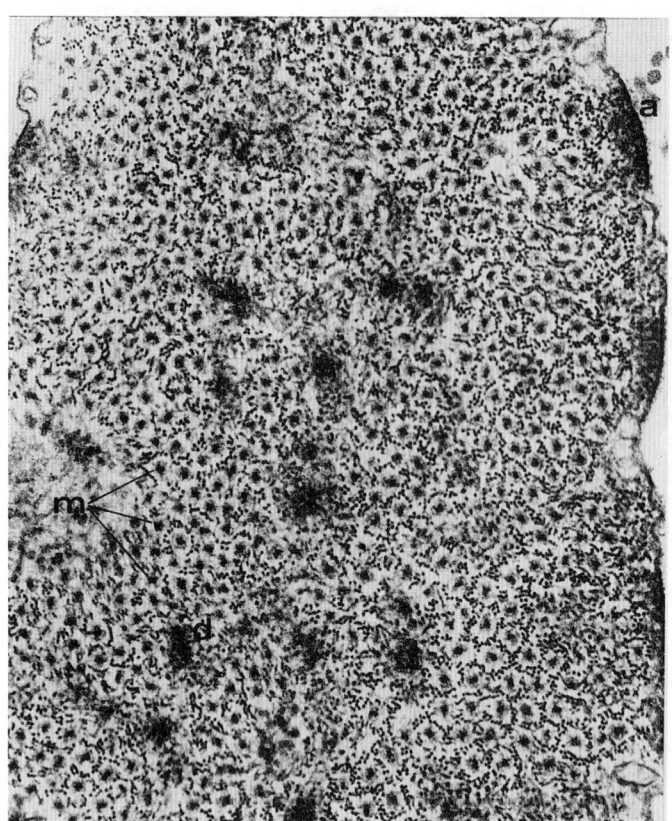

7.43 Electron micrograph of a transverse section through part of a smooth muscle cell, showing filamentous structures. The profiles of myosin filaments (m) are surrounded by an irregular pattern of thin filaments (contrast **7.10**). Also present are cytoplasmic dense bodies (d) and, at the surface membrane, adherens junctions (a). (Photograph by Vic Small, Institute of Molecular Biology, Austrian Academy of Sciences. Reproduced from Journal of Cell Science 1977 with permission of Company of Biologists Ltd.)

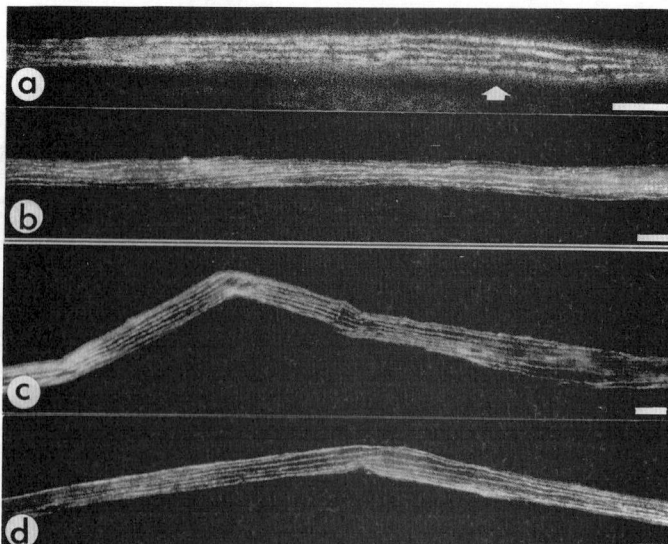

7.44 Light micrographs of isolated smooth muscle cells from guinea pig taenia coli labelled with a monoclonal antibody to vinculin and a fluorescent second antibody. The label reveals the presence of longitudinal, largely continuous (but see arrow), vinculin-containing strips on the cell surface, corresponding to the anchorage sites for actin filaments. Bars = 5 μm. (Reproduced with permission from Small 1985.)

There are two major isoforms of smooth muscle myosin heavy chain, referred to as SM-1 and SM-2 (Rovner et al 1986). They differ only in a terminal 43-residue sequence that is present on SM-1 but not SM-2, and in fact are the products of a single gene, from which they are produced by alternative RNA splicing. In most tissues and species, the ratio of SM-1 to SM-2 is about 60:40, although in human urinary bladder SM-2 is slightly predominant. Other heavy chain isoforms have been recognized, and some smooth muscles also contain non-muscle heavy and light chain isoforms (Somlyo 1993). It is not known whether these differences in myosin isoform composition have any functional significance.

Actin is present in α, β and γ isoforms, and the γ isoforms include both smooth muscle and non-muscle actins (Malmqvist et al 1991 and work cited therein). Recent evidence suggests that the non-muscle actin isoforms may be restricted to the cytoskeleton (North et al 1994b). Differences in the actin isoform composition of smooth muscle are of interest and potential importance as markers of development and change.

NON-FILAMENTOUS STRUCTURES OF SMOOTH MUSCLE

Although small groups of mitochondria may be found at any point in the cytoplasm of a smooth muscle cell, these and other organelles—such as a Golgi complex, free ribosomes, cisternae of rough and smooth endoplasmic reticulum, glycogen granules, lysosomes and lipid droplets—tend to be gathered in a filament-free perinuclear zone, particularly at the poles of the nucleus (Gabella 1973; Huddart & Hunt 1975; Gabella 1981; **7.45**).

A sparse, irregular sarcoplasmic reticulum ramifies between the myofilaments, its terminal sacs lying under the plasma membrane (**7.46**; Popescu & Diculescu 1975). It sequesters calcium ions via a

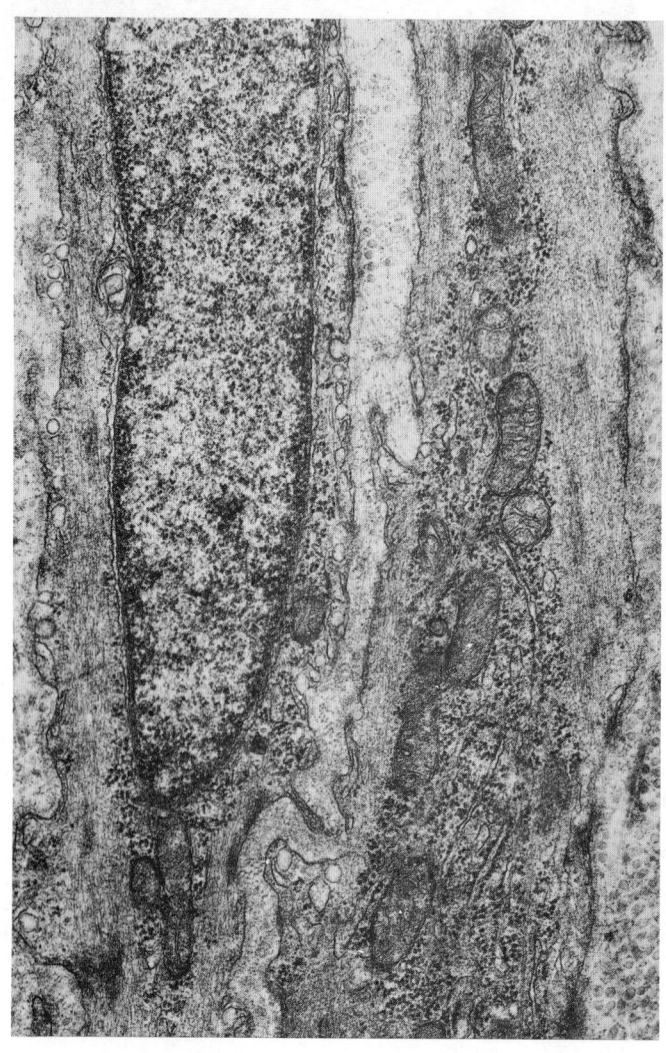

7.45 Low-power electron micrograph of a longitudinal section through two smooth muscle cells from the wall of the ileum. Note their irregular outline. The cell on the left shows a nucleus and numerous caveolae; that on the right contains mitochondria and several tubular profiles of sarcoplasmic reticulum. Fine collagen fibrils lie in the intercellular spaces. Magnification × 8000.

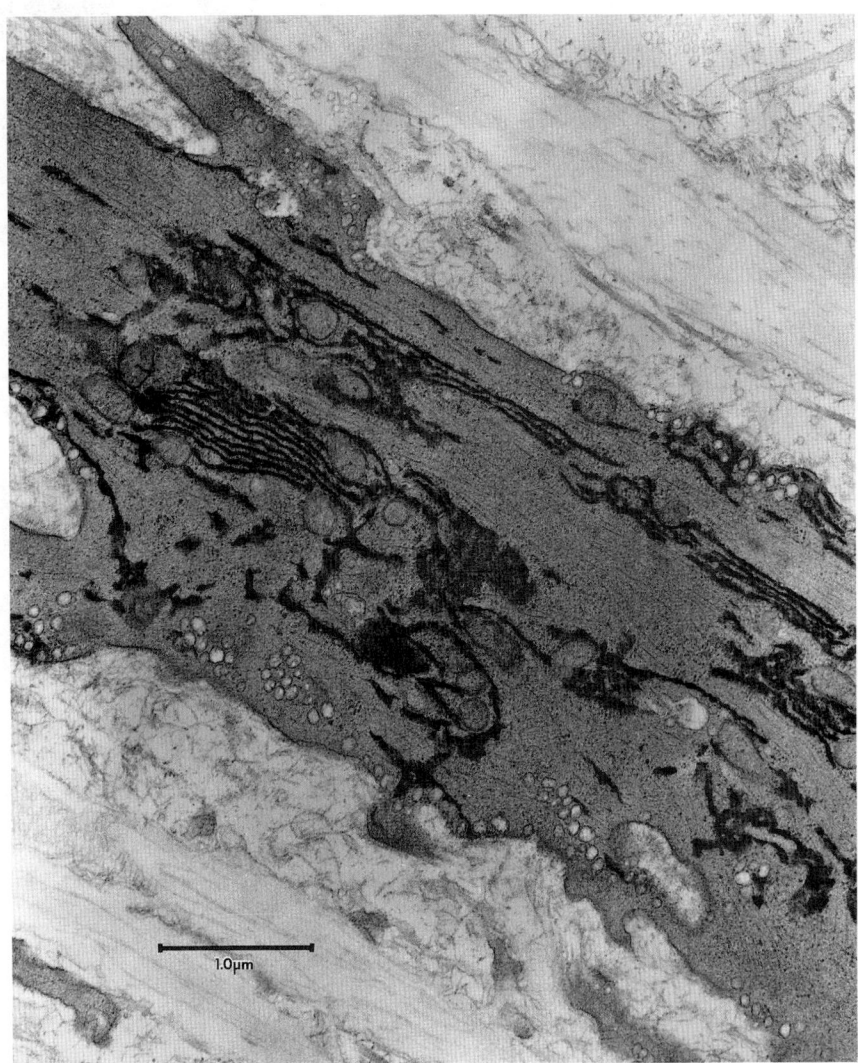

7.46 Electron micrograph of a longitudinal section through a rabbit arterial smooth muscle cell. The sarcoplasmic reticulum has been stained selectively with osmium ferrocyanide. This tonic type of smooth muscle has a particularly extensive sarcoplasmic reticulum, comprising both tubules and fenestrated sheets. (Reproduced with permission from Somlyo & Somlyo 1993.)

Ca^{2+}-transport ATPase that is antigenically related to the ATPase in the sarcoplasmic reticulum of cardiac and slow, but not fast, skeletal muscle (Raeymaekers & Wuytack 1993). The maximum rate of Ca^{2+} uptake is about 100 times slower than that of skeletal muscle sarcoplasmic reticulum, and this seems to be due mainly to the comparative paucity of transport sites in the membrane (Raeymaekers & Wuytack 1993).

The plasma membrane also contains a Ca^{2+} pump, which differs somewhat from that of the sarcoplasmic reticulum in its molecular structure and mode of activation (reviewed by Raeymaekers & Wuytack 1993).

Mention has already been made of *caveolae*, the characteristic cup-like invaginations of the plasma membrane; these have a superficial resemblance to endocytotic vesicles but do not appear to be engaged in uptake of extracellular material. Their function is not fully understood. Among other things they may provide the cell with a reservoir of additional plasma membrane that accommodates changes in surface area during shortening and lengthening. It has also been suggested that caveolae are involved in the transfer of electrical excitation or ions into the cell. Their definitive role, and that of the protein *caveolin* specifically associated with them (North et al 1993) remains to be established. The surface also shows occasional projections of unknown function (**7.47**).

EXCITATION OF SMOOTH MUSCLE

Excitation–contraction coupling in smooth muscle

In smooth muscle, as in all types of muscle, the primary trigger for contraction is a rise in the free Ca^{2+} concentration in the cytosol. This increase in Ca^{2+} is brought about by mobilization of intracellular Ca^{2+} stores (in the sarcoplasmic reticulum and bound to the cell membrane) and/or influx of Ca^{2+} from the extracellular fluid. Increase of cytosolic Ca^{2+} promotes further release from intracellular stores, probably by a mechanism similar to calcium-induced calcium release in cardiac muscle (Itoh et al 1983).

Excitation–contraction coupling in smooth muscle takes two forms: *electromechanical coupling*, and *pharmacomechanical coupling*.

Electromechanical coupling. This involves depolarization of the cell membrane by an action potential. It may be generated when a membrane receptor—usually linked with an ion channel—is occupied by a neurotransmitter, hormone or other blood-borne substance. Alternatively, it may be initiated by direct transmission of electrical excitation from an adjacent cell via a gap junction. In some types of smooth muscle, depolarization may be the consequence of other stimuli, such as cooling, stretching, and even light.

Pharmacomechanical coupling. This is a receptor-mediated process whereby transmitters or drugs can bring about release of Ca^{2+}

777

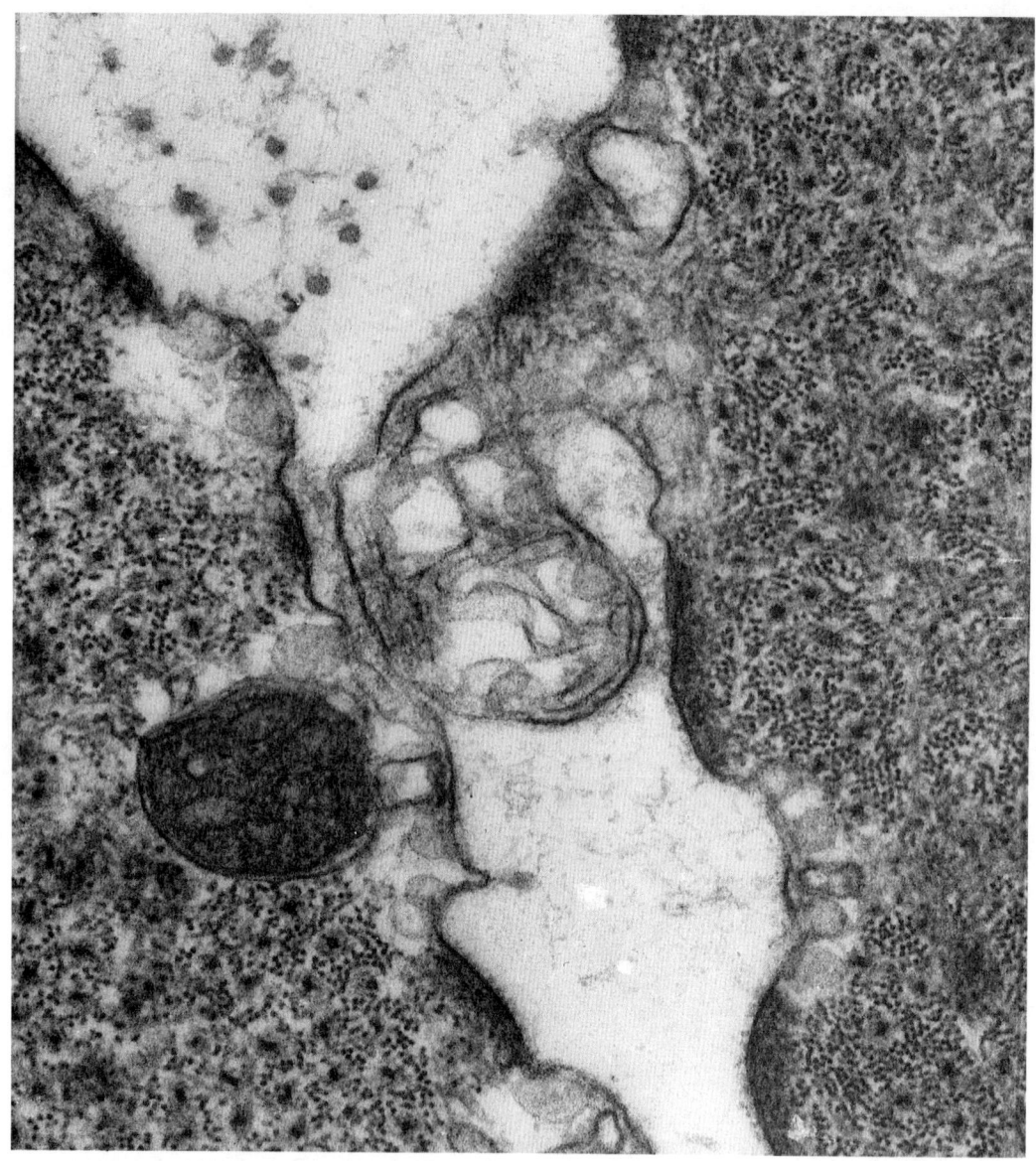

7.47 High-power electron micrograph of a transverse section through two adjacent smooth muscle cells, showing actin and myosin filaments, adherens junctions and a surface projection of unknown function.

(Photograph by Vic Small, Institute of Molecular Biology, Austrian Academy of Sciences.)

from intracellular stores without depolarization of the membrane. In pharmacomechanical coupling, receptor-binding may open Ca^{2+} channels in the sarcolemma, or trigger the formation of inositol triphosphate, which acts as a signal for intracellular Ca^{2+} release (Somlyo et al 1985a).

Thick filament regulation in smooth muscle

The way in which a rise in cytosolic Ca^{2+} concentration activates the contractile apparatus of smooth muscle differs in major respects from the mechanism that has been described for striated muscle. In vertebrate striated muscle, contraction is regulated, that is to say, actin–myosin interaction is prevented, by the tropomyosin/troponin complex on the thin filament. Ca^{2+} acts by binding to troponin-C, triggering a fast conformational change that releases the inhibition. Smooth muscle has a different regulatory mechanism, based on the thick filaments (Sobieszek & Small 1977; Adelstein 1982).

In smooth muscle, two of the myosin light chains have a regulatory function: myosin will bind to actin only if one or both of these light chains is phosphorylated (Ebashi 1983). Although the light chains themselves possess Ca^{2+} binding sites, they do not seem to bind Ca^{2+} under physiological conditions. Instead, the primary Ca^{2+}-receptor is a structurally related protein called *calmodulin* (M_r 17 000),

which has a variety of Ca^{2+}-dependent signalling roles. The Ca^{2+}–calmodulin complex can activate a specific protein kinase, *myosin light-chain kinase*. This phosphorylates the regulatory myosin light chain, and actin–myosin interaction—and contraction—can then take place. On the simplest view, there is an equilibrium between phosphorylation of myosin, mediated by light-chain kinase activity, and dephosphorylation of myosin, mediated by the activity of one or more light-chain phosphatases. When the cytosolic free Ca^{2+} concentration is lowered, by re-uptake of Ca^{2+} into the sarcoplasmic reticulum and/or extrusion across the sarcolemma, the Ca^{2+}–calmodulin complex dissociates. This renders the myosin light-chain kinase inactive again, shifting the equilibrium in favour of phosphatase activity; the myosin becomes dephosphorylated, and relaxation follows.

The problem with this basic scheme is that it does not explain all the phenomena of smooth muscle contraction. It appears that dephosphorylation of myosin does not lead to immediate detachment of the myosin cross-bridges. Under these conditions force can be maintained with the cross-bridges cycling slowly, or perhaps not at all, so that the energy expenditure is very low; this condition is referred to as the '*latch state*' (Hai & Murphy 1989). Such a condition is clearly important, for example, in relation to the control of tone in vascular smooth muscle, but the underlying mechanism is still a matter of debate (Schaub & Kunz 1986; Word & Stull 1993; and see below).

Thin filament regulation in smooth muscle

Phosphorylation of myosin appears to be essential for contraction, but it may not be the only control mechanism. In recent years there has been considerable interest in a potential regulatory process centred on the thin filaments. The thin filaments of smooth muscle do not contain troponin; they do, however, contain tropomyosin, together with a protein called *caldesmon* (M_r 87 000). In the presence of tropomyosin and caldesmon, actin–myosin interaction is markedly inhibited, and the inhibition is removed by Ca^{2+}. The concept therefore emerges of a caldesmon–tropomyosin complex which functions in a manner analogous to the troponin–tropomyosin complex of striated muscle (Marston & Smith 1985). In this complex, caldesmon appears to behave as the equivalent of both troponin-I and troponin-T, and an additional Ca^{2+}-binding protein adds the Ca^{2+}-sensitivity that would, in striated muscle, be conferred by troponin-C (Marston & Smith 1985; Pritchard & Marston 1989). Although it is necessary to confirm these phenomena in the intact tissue, it now seems likely that this constitutes a second regulatory system. There are thus two switches: a slow switch working by covalent modification through the thick filaments, and a fast switch working by conformational change through the thin filaments. Phosphorylation of caldesmon removes the inhibitory effect, providing an additional potential for slow regulation via the thin filament, but it is not certain that this occurs in vivo. A further possibility is that caldesmon is involved in producing the 'latch state' by direct cross-linking of the thick and thin filaments (Sobue & Sellers 1991; Marston et al 1992).

Calponin (M_r 34 000) is another actin-binding protein associated with the thin filaments of smooth muscle. It is more abundant than caldesmon, but resembles it in several respects. It has recently been shown to inhibit actin–myosin interaction, the inhibition being relieved by phosphorylation (Winder & Walsh 1990). Its physiological significance has yet to be established. Whereas caldesmon is found only in the contractile apparatus of smooth muscle, calponin resides in both the contractile apparatus and the cytoskeleton (North et al 1994a).

Modulation of smooth muscle contraction

Regulation of smooth muscle contraction is evidently an intricate process, which is susceptible to modulation at a number of points. Several hormones influence contraction by enhancing or depressing the sensitivity of the contractile apparatus to Ca^{2+}, achieving these effects via the thin-filament-based regulatory system in some cases and the thick-filament-based system in others. For example, the action of β-adrenergic agonists on the thick filament system promotes myosin dephosphorylation, and hence relaxation, an outcome that contrasts sharply with the increased force of contraction produced by these agents in cardiac muscle. β-agonists also promote relaxation of smooth muscle through an increase in the uptake of Ca^{2+} by the sarcoplasmic reticulum—recalling, in this case, a similar action in cardiac muscle (see Regulation of contraction in cardiac muscle, p. 767). The stimulation of Ca^{2+} uptake is, however, much weaker in the sarcoplasmic reticulum of smooth muscle, possibly because the predominant Ca^{2+} pump isoform is different and phospholamban is not the major phosphorylatable protein present (Raeymaekers & Wuytack 1993).

Control of contraction at a multiplicity of sites, by the regulatory systems and by ion transport across the membranes of the sarcoplasmic reticulum or sarcolemma, provides opportunities for the development of new, more selectively targeted, drugs for the treatment of conditions such as hypertension (Schaub & Kunz 1986; Raeymaekers & Wuytack 1993).

INNERVATION OF SMOOTH MUSCLE

Contraction of smooth muscle may be excited by nerves, hormones or electrical depolarization transferred from neighbouring cells. The importance of these different routes varies with the location of the tissue. Some muscles receive a dense innervation that tightly defines their contractile activity. In the case of the iris, for example, specific

nervous control can produce either pupillary constriction or dilatation. Such muscles have been referred to as *multi-unit smooth muscles* (Burnstock 1970). Other muscles are more sparsely innervated; they tend to display *myogenic* activity, initiated spontaneously or in response to stretch, which spreads from cell to cell via gap junctions and may be markedly influenced by hormones. In these muscles, which include those in the walls of the gastrointestinal tract, urinary bladder, ureter, uterus and fallopian tube, innervation tends to exert a more global influence on the rate and force of intrinsically generated contractions. Such muscles have been referred to as *unitary smooth muscles*. These terms are mentioned here because they are widely encountered; in practice, such distinctions are better regarded as the extremes of a continuous spectrum.

The efferent nerve fibres to smooth muscles are the non-myelinated processes of neurons whose cell bodies are located in autonomic ganglia, either in the sympathetic chain or, in the case of parasympathetic fibres, closer to the point of innervation. They ramify extensively, spreading over a large area of the muscle and sending branches into the muscle fasciculi (7.41). The neuromuscular terminals of these autonomic efferents are considered in more detail elsewhere (p. 959), and a brief description will suffice here. Along its terminal portion, each axonal branch has a beaded structure, which consists of expanded portions, or *varicosities*, packed with vesicles and mitochondria, separated by thin, intervaricose portions. Each varicosity is regarded as a transmitter release site, and hence a 'nerve ending' in the functional sense, although only the last varicosity along a branch is an ending in the anatomical sense. This pattern allows a very large number of nerve endings (up to tens of thousands) to be present in the axonal arborization of a single autonomic neuron, as opposed to a maximum of a few hundred in somatic motor neurons.

The neuromuscular junctions in smooth muscles do not show the consistent appearance seen in skeletal muscles. The neurotransmitter diffuses across a gap that can vary from 10 to 100 nm; even separations up to 1 μm may still allow neuromuscular transmission to take place, albeit more slowly. The nerve ending is packed with vesicles, but the adjacent area of the muscle cell is not structurally differentiated from that of non-junctional regions and it is not known whether it has a higher concentration of receptors.

Intramuscular afferent fibres are the peripheral processes of small neurons in the dorsal root ganglia. Since they are also unmyelinated, contain axonal vesicles and have a beaded appearance, they are difficult to distinguish from efferent fibres.

SITE-SPECIFIC VARIATION IN SMOOTH MUSCLE

It is worth emphasizing that differences between smooth muscle cells from different sites in the body extend beyond general architecture and degree of innervation to actual contractile behaviour. The smooth muscle of large arteries and the trachea, for example, is slow-contracting and tonic in nature, sustaining force for long periods. That of the intestines and bladder is faster-contracting and more phasic in its activity. Some of this variability may be generated by differences in the nature and relative importance of the regulatory systems on the thin and thick filaments. It may also reflect variations in myosin isoform composition (Somlyo 1993).

It is possible for the same stimuli to produce contrasting responses in different smooth muscles. In the smooth muscle of resistance vessels, for example, the usual consequence of a fall in intracellular pH is relaxation, but in the vascular bed of the rabbit ear and in human ureteral muscle the same stimulus results in increased force (Wray 1988).

In view of these and other individual variations, it is wise to resist the temptation to generalize when an observation has been made in smooth muscle from a single location.

DEVELOPMENT OF SMOOTH MUSCLE

Smooth muscle cells develop from mesenchymal cells in the walls of the anlagen of the viscera and around the endothelium of blood vessels. An exception is the smooth muscle of the iris, which is derived from ectodermal cells near the margin of the optic cup.

The following account of the differentiation of precursor cells into smooth muscle cells is taken from studies of the chick embryo gizzard

(Gabella 1989; Chou et al 1992). Following a period of proliferation, clusters of myoblasts become elongated in the same orientation. Dense bodies, associated with actin and cytoskeletal filaments, appear in the cytoplasm, and the surface membrane starts to acquire its specialized features—caveolae, adherens junctions and intercellular junctions. Cytoskeletal filaments extend to insert into the submembranous densities. Thick filaments are seen a few days after the first appearance of thin filaments and intermediate filaments, and from this time the cells are able to contract. During development, dense bodies increase in number and further elements of the cytoskeleton are added. In addition to synthesizing the cytoskeleton and contractile apparatus, the differentiating cells express and secrete components of the extracellular matrix.

In a developing smooth muscle all the cells express characteristics indicative of the same stage of differentiation; there are no successive waves of differentiation. From its earliest appearance to maturity, a smooth muscle increases several hundredfold in mass, by a 2–4-fold increase in the size of individual cells, but mainly by a very large increase in cell number. Growth occurs by division of cells in every part of the muscle, not just at its surface or ends. Mitoses occur in cells in which differentiation is already well advanced, as evidenced by the presence of myofilaments and membrane specializations. Mitotic smooth muscle cells may be found at any stage of life, but their numbers peak before birth, at a time that differs for different muscles, and become rare in the adult unless the tissue is stimulated to hypertrophy or to repair. (The ability of mature cells to undergo mitosis is therefore gradated between the three major types of muscle: skeletal muscle cells cannot divide at all after differentiation; cardiac muscle cells can divide, but only before birth; and smooth muscle cells appear to remain capable of division throughout life.)

During the early stages, smooth muscle expresses embryonic and non-muscle isoforms of myosin. The proportions of these isoforms decrease during development (see Somlyo 1993, and references therein). Initially, SM-1 is the dominant or exclusive smooth muscle heavy chain isoform; the SM-2 isoform becomes more established as development progresses (Borrione et al 1989; Kuro-O et al 1989; Eddinger & Wolf 1993; Woodcock-Mitchell et al 1993).

HYPERTROPHY OF SMOOTH MUSCLE

Hollow viscera can become distended when there is a chronic, partial obstruction that impairs flow or voiding of the luminal contents. Under these conditions, the smooth muscle component of the wall is placed under increased stretch, and it responds adaptively by undergoing hypertrophy. This situation may be encountered in growing subjects, especially in the presence of congenital malformation. It is also found in adult and ageing subjects when there is obstruction—for example, in the urinary bladder when the prostate gland is enlarged, or in an intestine partly blocked by a tumorous growth. A special case of hypertrophy is the increase in myometrial mass associated with the enlargement of the uterus during gestation.

Smooth muscle hypertrophy involves an increase in cell number, or *hyperplasia*, brought about by mitotic division of pre-existing muscle cells, combined with a 2–4-fold increase in the size of individual muscle cells (Owens 1989; Gabella 1990). Although the net result is an increase in force-generating capacity, there is often a reduction in the force per unit cross-sectional area. During cell growth, the fraction of the cell volume occupied by some organelles, such as sarcoplasmic reticulum, increases; that of others, such as mitochondria, decreases. Both actin and myosin increase in amount, but the increase in actin exceeds that of myosin. There is a major increase in intermediate filaments (Berner et al 1981) which outweighs that of the myofilaments; this is reflected in an increase in the desmin:actin ratio (Malmqvist et al 1991). The hypertrophic muscle has many new blood vessels and an increased collagen content. Its innervation is more sparse, and the neurons that supply it also hypertrophy.

In vitro experiments show that stretch alone is a sufficient stimulus for smooth muscle hypertrophy (Karim et al 1992). Nevertheless, hypertrophy often occurs in response to stretch combined with hormonal or other influences. A case in point is the enlargement of the myometrium during pregnancy, in which hormonal influences play a major role.

Chronic hypertension produces an adaptive hypertrophy of the smooth muscle in the larger resistance vessels, which results in thickening of the arterial walls. There is evidence that this response involves vasoconstrictor peptides such as angiotensin II and arginine vasopressin, which promote a generalized increase in protein synthesis and a larger, selective increase in the synthesis of muscle-specific proteins (Owens 1991). Inappropriate—that is to say, non-adaptive—proliferation and hypertrophy of vascular smooth muscle cells is the hallmark of a number of vascular diseases, and is the focus of considerable research interest. According to one view, mature smooth muscle cells de-differentiate to a 'fetal' phenotype that exhibits proliferative behaviour. An alternative view is that cells of this phenotype are a clonally selected subpopulation whose expansion is supported by an autocrine growth factor (Benditt 1974). A variety of agents have been implicated in the proliferative response, including: the vasoconstrictor peptides, such as angiotensin II; cytokines, such as Interleukin-1; growth factor peptides, such as Fibroblast Growth Factor, Platelet-Derived Growth Factor, and Insulin-like Growth Factor-1; lipoproteins; and extracellular matrix components. An opposing influence has also been described: under in vitro conditions, human vascular smooth muscle cells synthesize Transforming Growth Factor-β, which inhibits proliferation (Kirschenlohr et al 1993).

For atheromatous changes in the muscular walls of arteries, see p. 1458.

REGENERATION OF SMOOTH MUSCLE

Smooth muscle has a capacity for self-renewal following damage. The extent of this capability varies with the site, from limited repair with connective tissue replacement in the walls of the alimentary tract, to complete regeneration in blood vessels. This variation may depend on the source of mitotic cells. In general, regenerative activity does not depend upon the presence of a pool of undifferentiated precursor cells analogous to the satellite cells of skeletal muscle. Nonetheless, it seems that fully mature smooth muscle cells are not able to re-enter the cell cycle, for the cells that undergo proliferation after injury are less differentiated, lacking expression of smooth muscle myosin isoforms. This 'fetal' phenotype may be reached either by de-differentiation of mature cells or by clonal expansion of pre-existing immature cells (Benditt 1974; Pauly et al 1992; Woodcock-Mitchell et al 1993).

In some cases, the proliferative response of the smooth muscle goes beyond what is necessary to repair the injury. For example, inappropriate proliferation of vascular smooth muscle cells following the endothelial injury caused by balloon angioplasty can result in re-stenosis of the vessel. The obvious clinical importance of this response has stimulated much interest in the underlying mechanisms. The factors believed to be responsible for triggering proliferation in the uninjured tissue, listed above in the context of hypertrophy, are probably equally active in the response to injury (Reidy 1992). To these must be added factors to which the smooth muscle cells are exposed as a result of damage to adjacent tissues, including platelet-derived mitogens and thrombin (Wilcox 1993). Some of these factors may act synergistically (Hahn et al 1993).

MYOEPITHELIAL CELLS

Myoepithelial cells are found in association with a number of secretory glands, including salivary, lacrimal, sweat, mammary and possibly prostate glands. They contain smooth-muscle-like contractile elements but are of ectodermal origin. Thus they may be identified by the presence of myofilament proteins that are related to those of smooth muscle in conjunction with intermediate filaments that contain *cytokeratin*, the latter expressing their affinity with epithelia (Rudland 1987).

The cells are located between the glandular epithelial cells and the basement membrane. In the secretory part of the gland they may take a stellate or basket-like form, depending on the physiological state, with long dendritic extensions clasping an adjacent glandular acinus; examples are found in salivary and lacrimal glands, mammary acini and the secretory portions of sweat glands. They may also be found in relation to secretory ducts, such as the intralobular ducts of salivary glands, where they have a more cuboidal or fusiform appearance and are arranged longitudinally (p. 1695). The cells are rich in alkaline phosphatase, ATPase and adenyl cyclase (Han et al 1976). They show extensive desmosomal attachments to surrounding tissues and may be connected to one another via gap junctions. In many cases they are innervated by the autonomic nervous system, which can stimulate them to contract, expressing the secretion and helping to propel it along the glandular ducts. In the mammary gland, this control function is performed partly by the hormone oxytocin (Hamperl 1970). By virtue of their position, sandwiched between the glandular epithelial cells and the stroma containing the blood vessels, they may also have a role in transport processes and/or control of glandular metabolism (Ellis 1965). Indeed they produce much of the basement membrane, and synthesize growth factors that maintain the health of the glandular epithelium and support its growth (Fernig et al 1991).

MYOFIBROBLASTS

The ability to synthesize and to secrete components of the extra-cellular matrix is one respect in which smooth muscle cells show strong affinities to fibroblasts. Another strong homology is found between the adherens junctions of smooth muscle cells and the focal adhesions of fibroblasts, in which similar assemblages of proteins anchor cytoplasmic actin filaments to the cell membrane (North et al 1993). Conversely, some fibroblastic cells show pronounced contractile behaviour. These so-called myofibroblasts contain vari-able amounts of smooth-muscle-like contractile elements, and may develop from interstitial fat cells or fibroblasts. They are identifiable as containing smooth-muscle-related actin, and intermediate fila-ments that are composed of vimentin (Skalli et al 1989). The mesangial cells of the kidney express a-smooth muscle actin, and may be best characterized as myofibroblasts (Waldherr et al 1992). Myofibroblasts are also observed in various fibrotic conditions, where they are responsible for tissue contraction and for synthesizing much of the extracellular matrix (Oda et al 1990), together with growth factors that support the formation of vascular capillaries (Sato et al 1990).

ATTACHMENTS OF SKELETAL MUSCLES

The forces developed by skeletal muscles are transferred to bones by connective tissue structures: tendons, aponeuroses and fasciae. The nature of the junction between the tissues has already been considered (p. 749, The interface between muscle and connective tissue). Here the connective tissue structures themselves are considered in more detail.

TENDONS

Tendons take the form of cords or straps of round or oval cross-section. They consist of fascicles of Type I collagen, orientated mainly parallel to the long axis but to some extent interwoven. The fasciculi may be conspicuous enough to give tendons a longitudinally striated appearance to the unaided eye; they may coalesce to form two or more distinct cords in the tendon, or bridge between two adjacent tendons. Tendons have smooth surfaces but large tendons may be ridged longitudinally by coarse fasciculi (for example, the osseous aspect of the angulated tendon of obturator internus, p. 878). Loose connective tissue between fascicles provides a pathway for small vessels and nerves, and condenses on the surface as a sheath or *epitendineum*, which may contain elastic and irregularly arranged collagen fibres. The loose attachments between this sheath and the surrounding tissue present little resistance to movements of the tendon, but in situations where greater freedom of movement is called for, a tendon is separated from adjacent structures by a synovial sheath (see below). Tendons are strongly attached to bones, both at the periosteum and through fasciculi (Sharpey's fibres) that continue deep into the cortex. Sections of fresh bone show that at sites of tendinous attachment there is often a smooth plate of white fibrocartilage, which may cushion and reinforce the attachment zone (Benjamin et al 1986; p. 451).

The tensile strength of tendons is similar to that of bone, namely, half that of steel: a tendon with a circular cross-section of diameter 10 mm would support 600–1000 kg. The forces that tendons are required to withstand in use are normally deduced from force plate measurements, but direct measurement in vivo is possible with the use of a buckle transducer (Barnes & Pinder 1974; Salmons 1975; Walmsley et al 1978). (See p. 902 for forces on the Achilles tendon during running.)

Tendons are slightly elastic and may be stretched by up to 6% of their length without damage. Recovery of the elastic energy stored in tendons can make movement more economical (p. 902). Although they resist extension they are flexible and can, therefore, be diverted around osseous surfaces or deflected under retinacula to redirect the angle of pull.

Since tendons are composed of collagen and their vascular supply is sparse, they appear white. The blood supply to tendons is not, however, unimportant; small arterioles from adjacent muscle tissue pass longitudinally between the fascicles, branching and ana-stomosing freely, accompanied by venae comitantes and lymphatic vessels. This longitudinal plexus is augmented by small vessels from adjacent loose connective tissue or synovial sheaths (Edwards 1946). No vessels pass between bone and tendon at osseous attachments: the junctional surfaces are usually devoid of foramina (p. 427). The metabolic rate of tendons is very low but increases during infection or injury. Repair involves the initial proliferation of fibroblasts followed by interstitial deposition of new fibres (Potenza 1963).

During postnatal development, tendons enlarge by interstitial growth, particularly at myotendinous junctions, where there are high concentrations of fibroblasts. Growth decreases along the tendon from the muscle to the osseous attachments. The thickness finally attained by a tendon depends on the size and strength of the associated muscle, but appears to be influenced by additional factors, including the degree of pennation of the muscle (Elliott & Crawford 1965).

The nerve supply to tendons is largely—perhaps solely—sensory; there is no evidence of any capacity for vasomotor control. Spe-cialized endings that are sensitive to force (Golgi tendon organs, p. 964) may be found near myotendinous junctions; their large myelinated afferent fibres course centrally within branches of mus-cular nerves or in small rami of adjacent peripheral nerves (Stillwell 1957; Matthews 1972).

SYNOVIAL SHEATHS AND BURSAE

Synovial sheaths and bursae are found where there is a need to minimize friction between moving structures that are in tight appo-sition. Such a need is frequently encountered in relation to tendons—particularly near joints, where they may be deflected around bone or under retinacula.

Typically a bursa (Latin: *bursa* = purse) takes the form of a flattened sac of synovial membrane, in which the opposed walls are separated by a mere film of fluid. The outer surfaces are tethered to the adjacent tissues, and the inner surfaces slide over each other as relative movement takes place. The capillary film of lubricant syn-ovial fluid also nourishes the lining of synovial cells.

Synovial bursae

Most *synovial bursae* are found where movement occurs between a tendon and a bone or ligament, or between two tendons (*subtendinous*). Others occur where a muscle moves in relation to a bone, tendon or ligament (*submuscular*), between aponeuroses and bone (*subfascial*), between ligaments, and between the skin and subcutaneous structures—bony prominences, muscles or tendons (*subcutaneous*). During adult life, *adventitious* bursae may appear subcutaneously in places where the skin undergoes frequent dis-placement and pressure. This suggests that mechanical factors may be important in the evolution of bursae. However, the constant bursae develop in utero and must therefore be determined genetically.

Where a bursa occurs near to a joint, its synovial membranes and fluid may be continuous with those of the articular cavity. Such *communicating* bursae may arise separately during development, and connect with the joint only at a later stage. In some cases they ensheath tendons as they emerge from attachments within the capsule.

Some tendons contain osseous or cartilaginous sesamoids, closely applied to the osseous surface. In such places, the apposed surfaces are cartilage-covered and enveloped within a localized bursa, forming in effect a synovial joint; an example is the sesamoid in the tendon of peroneus longus where it articulates with the cuboid bone (p. 883).

Synovial tendon sheaths

Synovial tendon sheaths are found where tendons pass under ligamentous bands and retinacula or through fascial slings and osseofibrous tunnels. Their precise shape varies with the shape of the enclosed tendon and the surrounding tissues and with other mechanical factors. A synovial tendon sheath can be thought of as a bursa that extends around the tendon to envelop it. The internal (*visceral*) layer is attached by loose connective tissue to the tendon; the external (*parietal*) layer is similarly tethered to adjacent periosteum or other connective tissue structures; the two are separated by a thin film of synovial fluid. The inner and outer layers are in continuity at each end of the sheath, but in some cases they are also connected, continuously or at intervals along the length of the sheath, by a *mesotendon*. The mesotendon provides a degree of mechanical stability and a route whereby nerves and blood vessels can gain access to the tendon other than at the ends of the sheath. Some mesotendons have become reduced to one or more cords, e.g. the vincula tendinum of the digital tendon sheaths (p. 858).

APONEUROSES

When a tendon is distributed over a larger area, it becomes a broad, thin sheet of connective tissue referred to as an *aponeurosis*. Aponeuroses often have a longitudinally-striated appearance, imparted by large fascicles separated by loose connective tissue. The fascicles consist of compact, well-orientated bundles of collagen fibres, a structural characteristic that they share with tendons. The fibres are usually arranged in several layers, fasciculi in a given layer lying parallel to each other but at an angle to those in adjacent layers. The parallel arrays of fibres at the surface may impart a general iridescence to an aponeurosis in the fresh state, since they diffract light like an optical grating.

The term 'aponeurosis' was originally employed to denote a sheet of connective tissue extending from the sides of a tendon (the term *neuron* used to be applied indiscriminately to tendons and nerves) and providing additional attachment; examples may be found in relation to the levator palpebri superioris and the retinacula of the quadriceps extensor tendon. The term now embraces any sheet of dense connective tissue that carries tensile forces directly or indirectly from skeletal muscles to fasciae, other muscles, cartilage or bone. In some instances, a whole attachment is aponeurotic (e.g. obliquus externus abdominis); in others, aponeuroses provide large auxiliary areas of attachment for muscle fibres (e.g. supra- and infraspinous aponeuroses). Some major aponeuroses interlace at linear, sometimes multiple, decussations or raphes (e.g. ventrolateral abdominal aponeuroses, p. 825).

FASCIA

Fascia is a term so vague in use that it signifies little more than assemblages of connective tissue large enough to be visible to the unaided eye. (The practice of attaching a name to any aggregation that is large enough to dissect is of dubious value.) Its structure is highly variable, but the collagen fibres tend to be interwoven and seldom show the compact, parallel orientation seen in tendons and aponeuroses.

Fascia takes many forms. In dissection it appears as condensations on the surfaces of muscles and other tissues. Although it is termed *investing fascia*, this may not be its sole function. Between muscles that move extensively it takes the form of loose areolar connective tissue, and provides a degree of mechanical isolation. It constitutes the loose packing of connective tissue around peripheral nerves, blood and lymph vessels as they pass between other structures, often linking them together as neurovascular bundles. It forms a dense connective tissue layer investing some large vessels, such as the common carotid and femoral arteries; its presence here could be functionally significant, aiding venous return by approximating large veins to pulsating arteries, or it could simply represent a primary tissue response to the pulsatile forces created by neighbouring arteries.

Superficial fascia

Superficial fascia is a layer of loose connective tissue of variable thickness which merges with the deep aspect of the dermis. It is often adipose, particularly between muscle and skin (for *adipose tissue*, see p. 76). It provides for increased mobility of skin, and the adipose component both contributes to thermal insulation and constitutes a store of energy for metabolic use. Subcutaneous nerves, vessels and lymphatics travel in the superficial fascia, their main trunks lying in its deepest part, where adipose tissue is scant. Superficial fascia also contains skin muscles, such as *platysma*, a remnant of more extensive sheets of skin-associated musculature found in other mammals. The quantity and distribution of subcutaneous fat differs in the sexes. It is generally more abundant and widely distributed in females; in males it diminishes from the trunk to the extremities, and this distribution is more obvious in middle age, when the total amount increases in both sexes. There is an association with climate (rather than race), superficial fat being more abundant in colder geographical regions. The superficial fascia is most distinct on the lower anterior abdominal wall, where it contains much elastic tissue and appears many-layered as it passes through inguinal regions into the thighs. It is similarly differentiated in limbs and the perineum but is thin where it passes over the dorsal aspects of the hands and feet, the sides of the neck and face, around the anus, and over the penis and scrotum. It is almost absent from the external ears but is particularly dense in the scalp, palms and soles, permeated in these regions by numerous strong connective tissue bands binding the superficial fascia and skin to underlying structures; these come under the general heading of *deep fascia*, but are known regionally as aponeuroses of the scalp, palm and sole.

Deep fascia

Deep fascia is also composed mainly of collagenous fibres but these are compacted and in many cases arranged so regularly that the deep fascia may be indistinguishable from aponeurotic tissue. In limbs, where deep fascia is well developed, the collagen fibres are longitudinal or transverse, condensing into a tough, inelastic sheath around the musculature. In both upper and lower limbs some muscles are attached to the internal aspects of deep fascia, which then functions as an aponeurosis. Wherever deep fascia contacts a bone it fuses with the periosteum and thus transmits the pull of any attached muscles. The iliotibial tract is a powerful band of deep femoral fascia that transmits the pull of tensor fasciae latae and most of gluteus maximus to the femur and tibia (p. 871). Biceps brachii is partly attached to deep forearm fascia; the palmar aponeurosis is the deep fascia of the palm, receiving the pull of a number of muscles—palmaris longus (when present), and to some extent the intrinsic muscles of the thumb and little finger.

In the neck and limbs, laminae of the deep fascia pass between groups of muscles and connect extensively with bone. Such *intermuscular septa* may incidentally compartmentalize muscles or muscle groups that have different actions, developmental histories and innervations. Clinically, they may be significant in restricting the space available to muscles, causing pain syndromes when the volume of a muscle expands, for example as a result of oedema; an example is the anterior (tibial) compartment syndrome, also called anterior or lateral 'shin-splints', suffered by sportsmen when an inappropriate running activity or unsuitable shoe results in overload and inflammation of the dorsiflexors of the ankle. Functionally, septa often connect rather than separate muscles, which may be attached to both aspects of what is, in effect, an *intermuscular aponeurosis*.

In some sites, prime examples being found near the wrist and ankle, localized transverse thickenings of the deep fascia are attached at both ends to local osseous prominences. These are *retinacula*, so termed because they **retain** tendons deep to them, preventing them from springing out of position during activity. Tendons are deflected through such osseofibrous channels to pull effectively in a different direction, freedom of action being aided by synovial sheaths. Similar tunnels of deep fascia and bone form the fibrous sheaths in which digital flexor tendons of the hand and foot are retained, again surrounded by synovial sheaths (pp. 857, 892). In the lower limb particularly, deep fascia contributes to the efficiency of venous return, limiting the distension of deeper veins.

FORM AND FUNCTION IN SKELETAL MUSCLES

SHAPE AND FIBRE ARCHITECTURE

It is possible to attempt a classification of muscles based on their general shape and the predominant orientation of their fibres relative to the direction of pull (**7.48**). Muscles with fibres that are largely **parallel** to the line of pull vary in form from flat, short and *quadrilateral* (e.g. thyrohyoid) to long and *straplike* (e.g. sternohyoid, sartorius). In such muscles, individual fibres may run for the entire length of the muscle, or over shorter segments when there are transverse, *tendinous intersections* at intervals (e.g. rectus abdominis). In a *fusiform* muscle, the fibres may be close to parallel in the 'belly', but converge to a tendon at one or both ends. Where fibres are **oblique** to the line of pull, muscles may be *triangular* (e.g. temporalis, adductor longus) or *pennate* (= 'feather-like') in construction. The latter vary in complexity (see **7.48**) from *unipennate* (e.g. flexor pollicis longus), and *bipennate* (e.g. rectus femoris, dorsal interossei) to *multipennate* (e.g. deltoid). In some muscles the fibres pass obliquely between deep and superficial aponeuroses, in a kind of 'unipennate' form (e.g. soleus). In other sites muscle fibres start from the walls of osteofascial compartments, and converge obliquely on a central tendon in *circumpennate* fashion (e.g. tibialis anterior). Some muscles have a *spiral* or twisted arrangement (e.g. sternocostal fibres of pectoralis major and latissimus dorsi, which undergo a 180° twist between their median and lateral attachments). Some muscles spiral around a bone (e.g. supinator, which winds obliquely around the proximal radial shaft). Another type of spiral arrangement is shown by muscles, sometimes referred to as *cruciate*, that have two or more planes of fibres arranged in differing directions (**7.48**);

sternocleidomastoid, masseter and adductor magnus are all partially spiral and cruciate. Many muscles have more than one of these major types of arrangement, and show regional variations that correspond to contrasting, and in some cases independent, actions.

FUNCTIONAL IMPLICATIONS

Consideration will now be given to how such variations in the size, shape, fascicular architecture and form of attachment of a muscle relate to its functional role.

Direction of action

Although muscles differ in their internal architecture, the resultant force is directed along the line of the tendon; any forces transverse to this direction must therefore be in balance. In the strap-like forms of **7.48**, the transverse component is negligible. In the fusiform, bipennate and multipennate forms of **7.48**, symmetry in the arrangement of the fibres produces a balanced opposition between transverse components. In asymmetrical muscles, such as the unipennate forms of **7.48**, the fibres generate an unopposed lateral component of force which is balanced by intramuscular pressure (van Leeuwen & Spoor 1993).

Muscles that incorporate a twist in their geometry unwind it as they contract, so that they tend not only to approximate their attachments but also to bring them into the same plane (**7.49**). Similarly, muscles that spiral around a bone tend to reduce the spiral on contraction, imparting rotational force.

Force and range of contraction

The force developed by an active muscle is the summation of the tractive forces exerted by millions of cross-bridges as they work asynchronously in repeated cycles of attachment and detachment

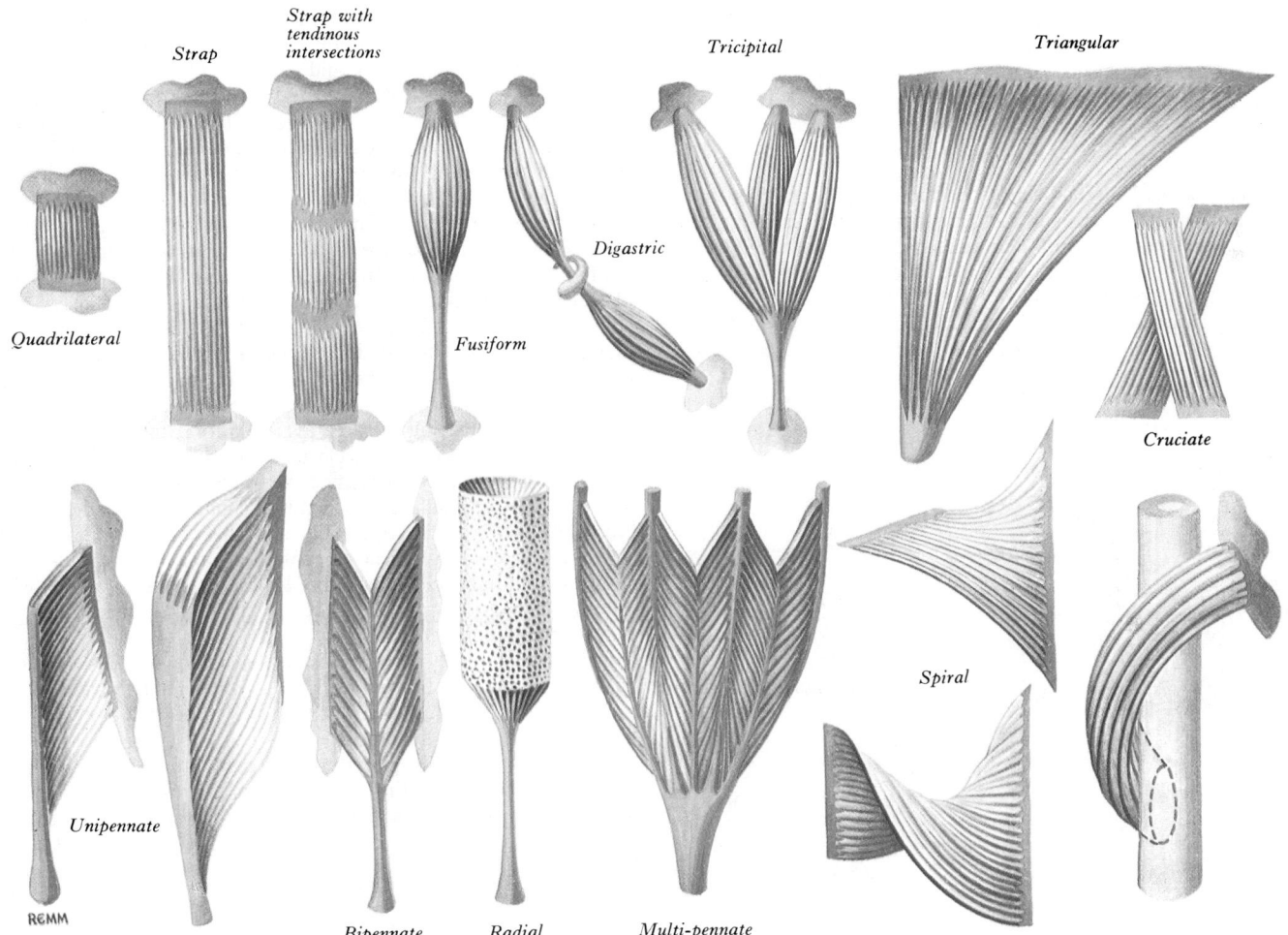

7.48 Morphological 'types' of muscle based on their general form and fascicular architecture.

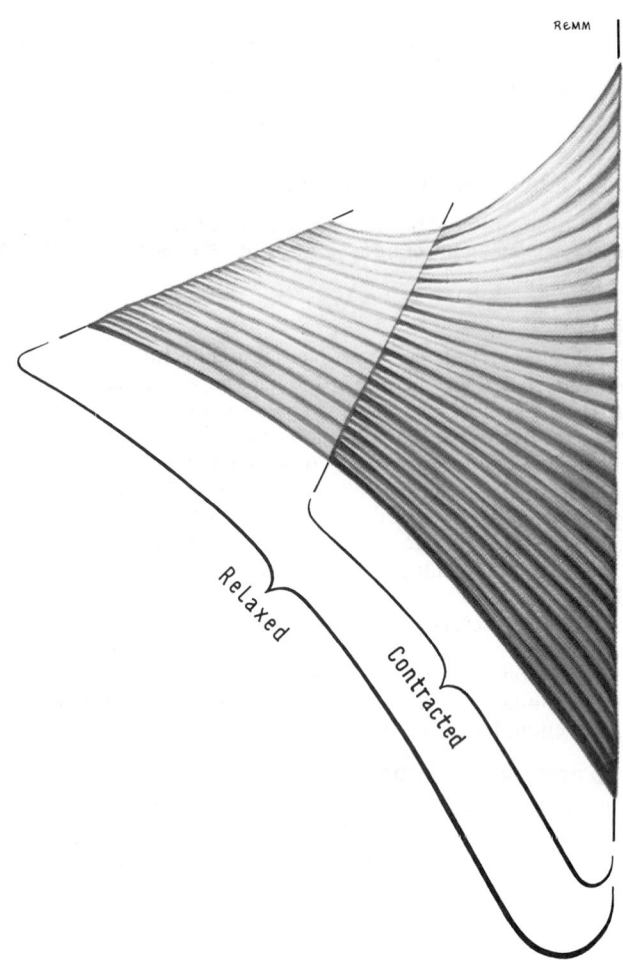

REMM

Relaxed

Contracted

7.49 Drawing to illustrate the 'detorsion' or untwisting that results from the contraction of a spirally arranged muscle.

(see Sliding filament mechanism of contraction, p. 739). This force depends on the amount of contractile machinery that is assembled in parallel, and therefore on the cross-sectional area of the muscle. The phrase 'contractile machinery' has been deliberately chosen here: from the mechanical point of view it matters little that the myofilaments are assembled into myofibrils, the myofibrils into fibres, and the fibres into fascicles (**7.2**); it is the total area occupied by

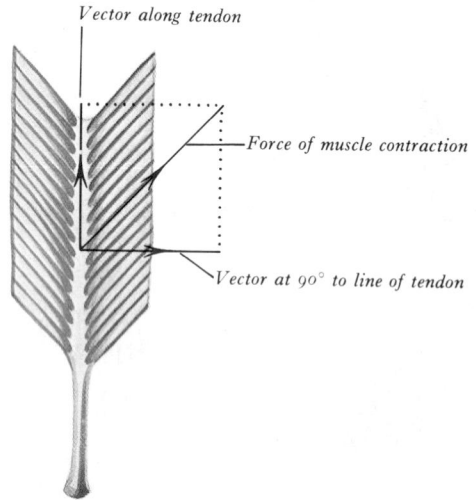

Vector along tendon

Force of muscle contraction

Vector at 90° to line of tendon

7.50 Force vectors in an idealized pennate muscle. The increase in effective cross-sectional area made possible by this architecture outweighs the small reduction in the component of force acting in the direction of the tendon. (See text for a more detailed explanation.)

myofilamentous arrays that determines force. If the fibres are small, the force will be influenced only to the extent that more of the cross-sectional area will be occupied by non-contractile elements, such as endomysial connective tissue; similarly, if there are many small fascicles this will increase the amount of perimysial connective tissue in the cross-section.

The range of contraction generated by an active muscle depends on the relative motion that can take place between the overlapping arrays of thick and thin filaments in each sarcomere (see Sliding filament mechanism of contraction, p. 739). In vertebrate muscle, the construction of the sarcomere sets a natural limit to the amount of shortening that can take place: from the minimum overlap to the maximum overlap of the thick and thin filaments represents a shortening of about 30%. Since the sarcomeres are arranged in series, the muscle fibres shorten by the same percentage. The actual movement that takes place at the ends of the fibres will depend on the number of sarcomeres in series, i.e. it will be proportional to fibre length. By way of illustration, if one takes two muscles, fixed at one end, with fibres parallel to the line of pull and the same cross-sectional area, and one muscle is twice as long as the other, then the force developed by each muscle will be the same, but the maximum movement produced at the free ends will be twice as much for the longer muscle.

Muscles in which the fibres are predominantly parallel to the line of pull are often long and thin, exemplified by the straplike form in **7.48** (e.g. sartorius). Such muscles develop rather low forces, but are capable of a long range of contraction. Where greater force is required the cross-sectional area must be increased, and the pennate type of construction is a way of achieving this in a compact way. **7.50** illustrates the principle for an idealized bipennate muscle. The fibres are set at an angle to the axis of the tendon (the angle of pennation). The range of contraction produced by such a muscle will be less than that of a straplike muscle of the same mass, because the fibres are short and because a smaller fraction of the shortening takes place in the direction of the tendon. The obliquely directed force can be resolved vectorially into two components, one acting along the axis of the tendon, and one at 90° to this. In symmetrical forms, such as that illustrated, the transverse force is balanced by fibres on the opposite side of the tendon. The functionally significant component is the one that acts along the tendon axis and, as the lengths of the vectors show, less force is available in this direction than is developed by the fibres themselves. In practice this loss is not very great: angles of pennation are usually less than 30°, so the force in the direction of the tendon may be 90% or more of that in the fascicles (cos 30° = 0.87). Nonetheless we can see that angulation of a set of fibres does not, of itself, confer any advantages: on the contrary, it reduces both the force and the range of contraction along the axis of the tendon. These negative consequences are, however, outweighed by the design advantage conferred by pennation, which is the opportunity it affords to extend the tendinous aponeurosis, increasing the area available for attachment of muscle fibres. A given mass of muscle can then be deployed as a large number of short fibres, increasing the total cross-sectional area, and hence the force, available. In a multipennate muscle, the effective cross-sectional area is larger still, and the fibres tend to be even shorter. The 'gearing' effect of pennation on a muscle thus results from the internal exchange of fibre length for total fibre area, which allows much greater forces to be developed, at the expense of a reduced range of contraction.

Of course muscle geometry is not dictated entirely by biomechanical considerations such as these. A muscle may have a pennate architecture simply because it is formed by fibres that converge from multiple sources of attachment.

Although the terms **power** and **strength** are often used interchangeably with **force**, they are not synonymous. **Power** is the rate at which a muscle can perform external work and is equal to force × velocity. Since force depends on the total cross-sectional area of fibres, and velocity—the rate of shortening—depends on their length, power is related to the total mass of a muscle. **Strength** is usually measured on intact subjects in tasks that require the participation of several muscles; it is then as much an expression of the skilful activation and co-ordination of these muscles as it is a measure of the forces that they contribute individually. Thus it is possible for strength to increase without a concomitant increase in the true force-generating capacities of the muscles involved, especially during the early stages of training (Jones & Round 1990).

MUSCLES AND MOVEMENT

The study of muscle action

Historically, attempts were made to elucidate the actions of muscles by gross observation. The attachments were identified by dissection, and the probable action deduced from the line of pull. With the use of localized electrical stimulation it became possible to study systematically the actions of selected muscles in the living subject. This approach was pioneered above all by Duchenne de Boulogne (1867). Such knowledge is necessarily incomplete: a study of isolated muscles, whether by dissection post mortem or stimulation in vivo, cannot reveal the way in which those muscles behave in voluntary movements, in which several muscles may participate in a variety of synergistic and stabilizing roles. Duchenne appreciated this, and supplemented his use of the

induction coil with clinical observations on patients with partial paralysis to make more accurate deductions about the way in which muscles acted together in normal movement (see account in Rowbottom & Susskind 1984). Manual palpation can be used to detect contraction of muscles during the performance of a movement, but tends to be restricted to superficially placed muscles, with examination taking place under quasi-static conditions. Modern knowledge of muscle action has been acquired almost entirely by recording the electrical activity that accompanies mechanical contraction, a technique known as electromyography (EMG) (see Electromyography, below). This technique can be used to study voluntary activation of deep as well as superficial muscles, under static or dynamic conditions. Multiple channels of EMG can be used to examine co-ordination between the different muscles that participate in a movement. These data can be further supplemented by adding transducers such as goniometers and force plates to monitor joint angle and ground reaction, and by recording the movement simultaneously on videotape or with a full three-dimensional motion analysis system.

Electromyography (EMG)

In normal subjects, the unit of contractile activity is the motor unit (p. 753). The nearly simultaneous depolarization of all the muscle fibres that make up a motor unit generate a signal that is readily detectable via electrodes placed in or suitably near the muscle. These *motor unit potentials* have an amplitude of 0.3–2 mV, between 10 and 100 times larger than the action potentials recorded from a single muscle fibre. Their duration, 4–10 ms, is longer than the 1 ms typical of a single-fibre action potential. This is because of the temporal dispersion introduced by conduction along axon branches of different length; the distance of the recording electrodes from the active fibres, and inhomogeneities in the conductive medium between them, have important effects on amplitude (Veen et al 1994) but little influence on duration. The distinction between single-fibre action potentials and motor unit potentials is clinically important. Damage to the motor nerve results in a loss of motor unit activity, followed by the spontaneous firing of individual muscle fibres known as *fibrillation*. When such signals are played through a loudspeaker they are audibly different, the motor unit potentials making a 'plopping'

sound, and the fibrillation potentials a sharp 'crack'. EMG can therefore be used to diagnose denervation and to follow the progress of reinnervation.

Normal, relaxed muscles are electrically silent (Joseph et al 1955). This raises the question as to what is meant by muscle *tone* or *tonus*. Tone is **not** a basal level of contractile activity: it is the ability of the muscle to respond to disturbance, including stretch and palpation, with an opposing force. It is absolutely dependent on intact connections to the central nervous system (CNS). If any part of the stretch reflex arc—motor or sensory—is destroyed, tone is abolished; the muscle becomes flaccid and presents no resistance to stretch. Conversely, damage that affects descending influences on the motor neuron can result in a pathological increase in tone.

As a voluntary muscle contraction is increased in intensity, the motor unit potentials of asynchronously firing units normally combine to form a continuous, multiphasic waveform, the so-called *interference pattern*. Efforts have been made to quantify such activity, both to provide objective diagnosis of myopathic conditions in which it is deficient and to

explore the relationship between the EMG and mechanical activity of the muscle (reviewed by Lenman 1974). Integration of the rectified electromyographic waveform provides a measure of electrical excitation which is proportional to force under isometric conditions (Lippold 1952) and to shortening velocity if force is held constant (Bigland & Lippold 1954). The normal voluntary movements of an unrestrained subject are not tightly defined in this way, and it should not be assumed that the integrated EMG will be correlated with either force or shortening velocity under these conditions. This is particularly true in fatigue, when a given level of force is associated with heightened electrical activity (Edwards & Lippold 1956).

Multichannel instruments can be used to record EMG activity in all of the muscles associated with a movement, providing accurate timing of the onset and cessation of contractile activity in each muscle. When the channels are connected to multiple electrodes within the same muscle, time-locked signal-averaging techniques can be used to map the territory of single motor units, or to look for pathological variation in the neuromuscular conduction delays between single fibres belonging to the same motor unit (Stålberg & Trontelj 1994; Bertorini et al 1994).

Actions of muscles

Classically, the action of a muscle is defined as the movement that takes place when it contracts. This should be treated as an operational definition, because a view that equates 'contraction' with shortening, 'relaxation' with lengthening, is simplistic in the context of whole muscles and real movements. Contraction can be considered as an attempt on the part of the muscle to approximate its attachments.

Whether it actually does so depends on the degree to which it is activated and the forces against which it has to act. These opposing forces are: gravitational and inertial forces; forces generated by any external contact or impact; forces generated actively by opposing muscles; and forces generated passively by the elastic and viscous resistance of all the structures that undergo extension and deformation, some within the muscle itself, others in joints, inactive muscles and soft tissues. Depending on the conditions, therefore, an active muscle may maintain its original length, shorten or lengthen, and during this time its tension may increase, decrease or stay the same. Movements that involve shortening of the active muscle are termed *concentric*; movements in which the active muscle undergoes lengthening are termed *eccentric*.

Natural movements are accomplished by groups of muscles. Each muscle may be classified, according to its role in the movement, as a:

- prime mover
- antagonist
- fixator
- synergist.

These roles will now be examined in a little more detail.

It is usually possible to identify one or more muscles that are consistently active in initiating and maintaining a movement: they are its *prime movers*. Muscles that wholly oppose the movement, or initiate and maintain the opposite movement, are *antagonists*. As an example, brachialis has the role of prime mover in elbow flexion; triceps is the antagonist. To initiate a movement, a prime mover must overcome passive and active resistance and impart an angular acceleration to a limb segment until the required angular velocity is reached; it must then maintain a level of activity sufficient to complete the movement. Antagonists may be transiently active at the beginning of the movement; thereafter they remain electrically quiescent until the deceleration phase, when units are activated to arrest motion. During the movement, the active prime movers are not completely unrestrained, being balanced against the passive, inertial and gravitational forces already mentioned.

When prime movers and antagonists contract together they behave as *fixators*, stabilizing the corresponding joint by increased transarticular compression, and creating an immobile base on which other prime movers may act. As an example, flexors and extensors of the wrist co-contract to stabilize the wrist when an object is grasped tightly in the fingers. In some cases, sufficient joint stability can be afforded by gravity, acting either on its own (e.g. knee and hip joints when they are in or near the close-packed position in erect posture, p. 507), or in conjunction with a single prime mover (e.g. shoulder joint when it is stabilized by supraspinatus with the arm pendent, p. 628). In other cases, and whenever strong external forces are encountered, prime movers and antagonists contract together, holding the joint in any required position.

A prime mover, acting across a uniaxial joint, produces a simple movement. Prime movers that act at multiaxial joints or across more than one joint may produce more complex movements, containing elements that have to be eliminated by contraction of other muscles. Those muscles, which assist in accomplishing the movement, are considered to be *synergists*, although they may act as fixators, or even as partial antagonists of the prime mover. As an example, flexion of the fingers at the interphalangeal and metacarpophalangeal joints is brought about primarily by the long flexors, superficial and deep. These also cross intercarpal and radiocarpal joints, and if movement there were unrestrained, finger flexion would be less efficient. Synergistic contraction of the carpal extensors eliminates this movement, and even produces some carpal extension, increasing the efficiency of the desired movement at the fingers.

In the context of different movements, a given muscle may act as a prime mover, antagonist, fixator or synergist. Even the same movement may involve a muscle in different ways if it is assisted or opposed by gravity. For example, under normal conditions (e.g. when thrusting out the hand), triceps is the prime mover responsible for extending the forearm at the elbow, and the flexor antagonists are largely inactive. However, when the hand lowers a heavy object the extensor action of the triceps is replaced by gravity, and the movement is controlled by active lengthening of the flexors. This example should remind us that all movements take place against the background of gravity, and its influence must not be overlooked.

Attachments and levers: the biomechanics of movement

Skeletal muscles have a limited range of contraction, for two reasons. Firstly, the fibres themselves must work within inherent limits imposed by their sarcomeric construction. Secondly, the internal design of many muscles can reduce the excursion at the tendon still further if short, oblique fibres have been used to deliver force at the expense of range of contraction. Where it is necessary to produce a greater range of movement, this is achieved through the action of the muscles on the bony levers of the skeleton.

To produce a large range of movement, force has to be applied close to the axis of the joint. An example of this is given in **7.51A**, based on the action of the triceps on the olecranon, which produces extension at the elbow. The closeness of the muscle attachment to the joint produces a large arc of motion at the hand. However, the motion could be prevented by applying to the hand a force very much less than that developed by the muscle. In fact, the **force** available at any point along the forearm, wrist and hand is **reduced** by the same factor as the **range of motion** there is **increased**. The same see-saw type of lever is found in the action of the triceps surae on the calcaneus when it produces plantar flexion of the non-weight-bearing foot. This type of lever, in which force is applied on one side of the joint axis, and loads that resist motion appear on the other, is known as a *lever of the first class*. (If the lengths of the lever arms on either side of the joint were interchanged, it would be possible to use this type of lever to produce an increased force and a reduced range of motion—the principle of the crow-bar—but this configuration is not found in the body.)

In *levers of the second class*, the load appears between the force and the joint axis. This is illustrated in **7.51B**, where plantar flexion of the weight-bearing foot raises the body. The principle involved is similar to raising the handles of a loaded wheel-barrow. In contrast to the previous example, the range of motion of the load is actually **less** than that produced by the muscle, and the force is **multiplied** by the same factor. The nutcracker action of molar teeth is obtained in a similar way.

In *levers of the third class*, the force is applied between the load and the joint axis. This is illustrated in **7.51C**, based on the contribution to flexion at the elbow produced by the action of the biceps brachii. The effect is similar to that in the first example: an **increase** in the range of motion, but a **decrease** in the available force.

Most of the levers of the body are of the first and third class: in each case they are arranged to produce a magnified version of the movement at the muscle tendon, either in the opposite sense (first class) or in the same sense (third class), and in each case this is achieved at the expense of a reduction in usable force. This effect is greater when the moving muscle attachment is closer to the joint. At first sight it seems paradoxical that the fibre architecture of so many muscles should be designed to maximize force at the expense of overall shortening, when their force has then to be scaled down by levers in order to achieve the desired range of motion. There are, however, biological advantages to such an arrangement. It is, for example, far more compact, enabling the limbs to be lighter and more slender. This trend is most obvious in fast-moving animals, such as horses, in which lever lengths are increased by running on the toes, and the powerful muscle masses lie close to the body, where they do not add significantly to the inertia of the extremities.

In **7.51A–C** the force is shown acting approximately at right-angles (90°, or **normal**) to the lever in each case. A force in this direction produces the greatest turning effect. It is, however, more usual for only part of the force exerted by a muscle to be directed in this way. The general case is illustrated in **7.52**; a muscle is shown crossing the joint between the two bones, one fixed and one mobile. The force exerted by the muscle has two main consequences:

Turning effect. The tendency of the *force* (*F*) to turn the bones about the joint is measured in terms of the *turning moment* (*M*). This is simply the product:

$$M = F \times L$$

where L is the moment arm (**7.52A**). Note that the latter is **not** the distance between the muscle attachment and the joint: it is the **perpendicular** distance between the line of pull of the muscle and the instantaneous centre of rotation. Thus the turning moment takes account of the magnitude of the force exerted by the muscle, the positions of the muscle attachments relative to the joint, the degree of angulation of the joint and the shape of the articulating surfaces. The turning effect of the force (F) can be regarded as that of a smaller force directed at right-angles to the axis of the mobile bone

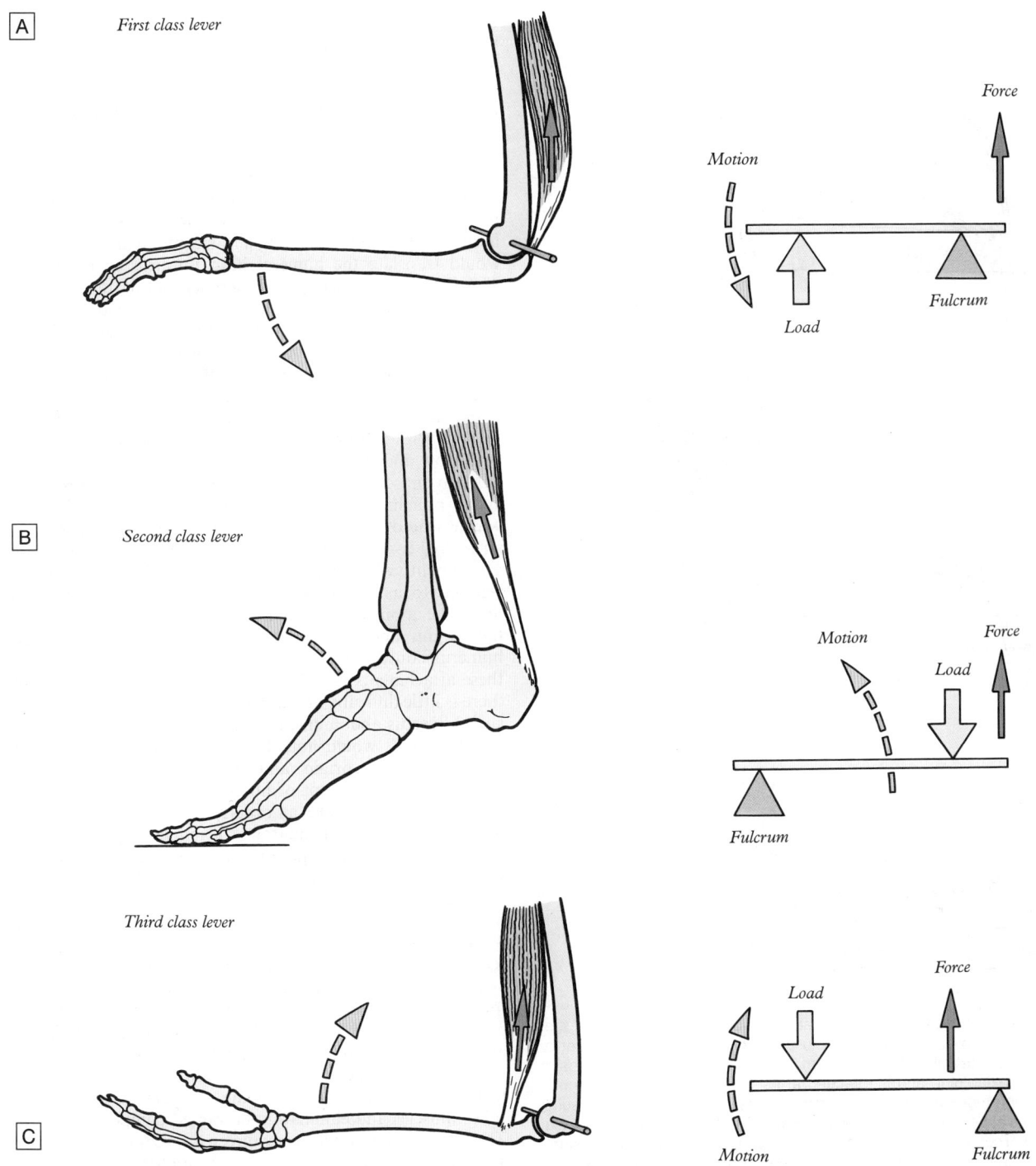

7.51 Drawings to illustrate the types of lever found in the body. A. Levers of the first class. B. Levers of the second class. C. Levers of the third class.

(blue arrow in **7.52B**), referred to in some analyses as the *transaxial, swing*, or *spurt* component (Williams et al 1989).

This description of the turning effect of a single muscle is complete only when movement takes place in one plane. The muscle may be attached to the mobile bone at a point that lies to one side or other of this plane. In this case contraction will introduce an additional turning effect, sometimes referred to as the *spin* component. In **7.52B** this component will tend to rotate the shaft of the bone about its axis.

Reaction at the joint. Newton's Third Law demands that the force on the bone is balanced by an equal and opposite reactive force generated at the joint. The reactive force can be resolved into components normal and tangential to the surfaces at the principal point of contact (**7.52C**).

The *normal* component (F_c) results from **compression** of the art-

iculating surfaces. The presence of this component contributes to the stability of the joint by helping to maintain articular contact, particularly during rapid swings, when an unresisted centrifugal force would tend to separate the joint surfaces (MacConaill & Basmajian 1977). It is referred to in some analyses as the *transarticular, paraxial,* or *shunt* component (Williams et al 1989).

The *tangential* component (F_s) represents the reaction to a shear force. If this shear force were unopposed, it would tend to produce **translation** of the articulating surfaces. A degree of translational movement is, of course, a normal feature of movement at some joints (p. 500), but ultimately it must be resisted or disarticulation would occur. The *tangential* component supplies the required balancing force. In practice, it is a composite generated by: gravitational and inertial forces; the elastic and viscous resistance of structures in and around the joint—including ligaments, the articular capsule and

787

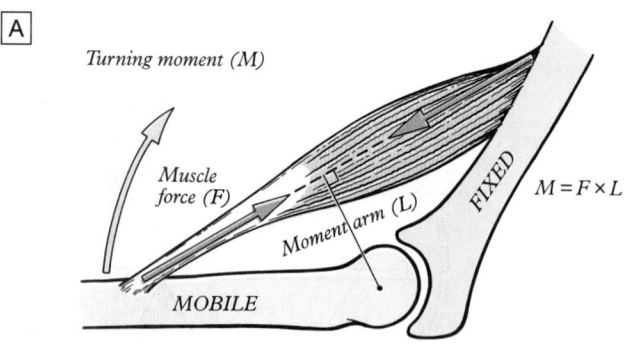

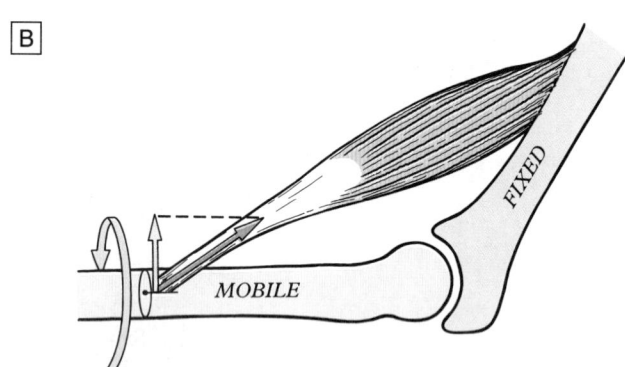

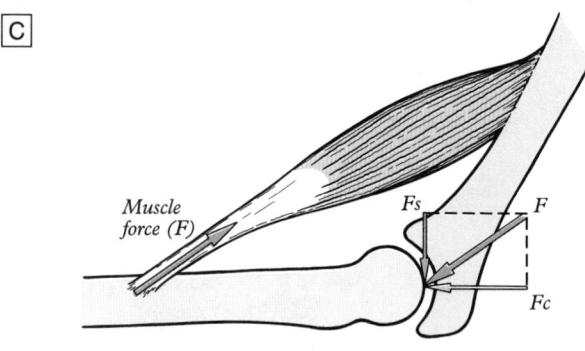

7.52 A generalized example to illustrate the biomechanical effects of the force generated by a muscle. The muscle (which does *not* represent a specific anatomical muscle) arises from a fixed base or 'origin', crosses a single multi-axial joint, and is attached at its 'insertion' to a mobile bone. A. The turning moment about the joint. B. The spin component that results from off-axis attachment. C. The reactive force (F) at the joint can be resolved into a normal component (F_c), which represents the reaction to compression, and a tangential component (F_s), which represents the reaction to shear. (See text for a fuller explanation.)

surrounding soft tissues—that are translated, stretched or compressed by the movement; and last, but by no means least, the restraining action of other muscles.

Normally there is more than one muscle acting at the joint. Each contributes a turning moment, and these turning moments can be added arithmetically. The resultant moment may impart angular acceleration to the mobile bone in either a clockwise direction (flexion in **7.52A**) or an anti-clockwise direction (extension in **7.52A**). Similarly, summation of the spin components yields a resultant moment that

may maintain the position of the shaft or rotate it about its axis in either direction. Each muscle also generates a reactive force at the joint, and these have to be added vectorially (using the polygon of forces, for example). Stability of the joint demands that when this resultant force is taken together with the gravitational and passive components already mentioned, and with the forces generated by any external contact or impact, the overall effect is neutral.

As an example, many of these elements may be seen in the actions of muscles around the shoulder joint when the arm is raised. During the initial stages of abduction, the force exerted by the acromial fibres of deltoid has a strong shear component which, if unresisted, would translate the humeral head upwards in the glenoid cavity. This is counteracted in part by gravity, but more importantly by the downward pull of subscapularis, infraspinatus and teres minor. The turning moment exerted by deltoid on the humeral shaft then adds to the moment exerted by supraspinatus to abduct the arm. The value of the analytical approach outlined briefly here is that it enables one to progress from such a verbal description to a quantitative understanding of the biomechanics of movement. Further detail may be sought in a number of modern texts, including Cochran (1982) and Mow and Hayes (1991).

Many muscles work in the manner indicated in **7.52**, from a more stable attachment to a more mobile one. The stable attachment, which would normally be part of a heavier and more proximal structure, is commonly referred to as the *origin*; the more mobile attachment, which would typically be lighter and more distal, is referred to as the *insertion*. Thus, in a muscle such as latissimus dorsi, the aponeurotic attachments to spine, pelvis and ribs constitute the origin, and the tendinous attachment to the highly mobile humerus constitutes the insertion. Although the relative mobility of these attachments can be reversed—during climbing, for example—there is little difficulty about defining habitual use. For other muscles, such as rectus abdominis, it is less easy to identify the more mobile attachment. It would not, therefore, be functionally meaningful to try to define an 'origin' and 'insertion' for every muscle. On the other hand, the concept of fibres arising, coursing, and converging on an insertion provides an orderly way of describing, and a helpful way of visualizing, the anatomy of individual muscles. No attempt will therefore be made here to abandon this terminology, which is widely accepted and, on the whole, well understood.

An interesting, and puzzling, feature of the mechanics of joint movement is the sheer number of muscles that are involved, even in quite simple movements. It is fairly clear that there is little actual redundancy in the system, and this is well illustrated by attempts to synthesize gait in paraplegic patients by electrical stimulation of the intact motor nerves (Kralj & Bajd 1989). Early attempts produced a gait that was jerky and robotic; at least 30 channels of stimulation appear to be needed to achieve a more co-ordinated and fluid motion (Marsolais & Kobetic 1987). Certainly some of these muscles act as fixators and synergists, providing a stable base for the action of other muscles and eliminating unwanted components of movement. The combination of variously directed forces may also provide more scope for achieving a balanced reaction at the joint, so that stability is less heavily dependent on passive connective tissue elements, such as ligaments and the articular capsule. The limited range over which muscles can operate effectively may mean that a sequence of contraction, involving several muscles that work optimally at different joint angles, is the only way to deliver adequate force over the full arc of movement. However, any comprehensive explanation needs to take into account the dynamic, as well as the static, aspects of movement at a joint. Stern (1974) integrated mechanics and physiology in a mathematical model that simulated the dynamic movement of a limb under the action of a muscle. The model predicted the different sets of attachment sites needed to maximize, say, velocity or power. It suggests that a joint acted upon by multiple muscles, each with different attachment sites, will be more versatile in terms of the available movement strategies.

Naming of Muscles

The names given to individual muscles are usually descriptive, based on their shape, size, number of heads or bellies, position, depth, attachments, or actions. It can be helpful to know the meaning of some of the terms used.

Shape

- deltoid (= triangular)
- quadratus (= square)
- rhomboid (= diamond-shaped)
- teres (= round)
- gracilis (= slender)
- rectus (= straight)
- lumbrical (= worm-like)

Size

- major, minor, longus (= long)
- brevis (= short)
- latissimus (= broadest)
- longissimus (= longest)

Number of heads or bellies

- biceps (= 2 heads)
- triceps (= 3 heads)
- quadriceps (= 4 heads)
- digastric (= 2 bellies)
- biventer (= 2 bellies)

Position

- anterior, posterior, interosseus (= between bones)
- supraspinatus (= above spine of scapula)
- infraspinatus (= below spine of scapula)
- dorsi (= of the back)
- abdominis (= of the abdomen)
- pectoralis (= of the chest)
- brachii (= of the arm)
- femoris (= of the thigh)
- oris (= of the mouth)

Depth

- superficialis (= superficial)
- profundus (= deep)
- externus (or externi)
- internus (or interni)

Attachment

- sternocleidomastoid (from sternum and clavicle to mastoid process)
- coracobrachialis (from the coracoid process to the arm)

Action

- extensor, flexor
- abductor, adductor
- levator (= lifter), depressor
- supinator, pronator
- constrictor, dilator

These terms are often used in combination: thus, *flexor digitorum longus* (= long flexor of the digits), *latissimus dorsi* (= broadest muscle of the back).

The names given to individual muscles or muscle groups are often oversimplified. Terms denoting action, in particular, emphasize only one of a number of habitual actions. A given muscle may play different roles in different movements, and these roles may change if the movements are assisted or opposed by gravity. The functional roles implied by names should therefore be interpreted with caution.

MUSCLES AND FASCIAE OF THE HEAD

Muscles of the head are customarily divided into two groups.

- *Craniofacial muscles* are related mainly to the orbital margins and eyelids, the external nose and nostrils, the lips, cheeks and mouth, the pinna, scalp and cervical skin. (Collectively these are often referred to, not very accurately, as 'muscles of facial expression'.)
- *Masticatory muscles* are concerned primarily with movements of the temporomandibular joint.

This division of head musculature reflects differences in embryonic origin and innervation. In functional terms, however, activities such as mastication, deglutition, vocalization, communicative and emotional expression, respiration, ocular, aural and nasal action are brought about by close co-operation and interdependence between muscles of the two groups.

Other muscle groups of the head are described elsewhere: these include *ocular* and *extraocular* muscles (pp. 1328, 1331, 1353), *auricular* and *tympanic* muscles (pp. 1368, 1376), *lingual, palatal* and *upper pharyngeal* muscles (pp. 1689, 1723, 1729).

CRANIOFACIAL MUSCLES

The craniofacial muscles all receive their innervation from branches of the facial nerve. Those described here are grouped (topographically and functionally) as:

- *epicranial*
- *circumorbital* and *palpebral*
- *nasal*
- *buccolabial*.

Most muscles can easily be assigned to one of the major groups named above; for some, however, the allocation is more arbitrary. Craniofacial myology is structurally and functionally complex, and a synthesis of the literature is not always easy to achieve because of individual variations, including some pronounced world differences, and differences in terminology. What follows is an account of widely accepted features; for further details consult the references with bibliographies cited below (see also Anatomy of speech, p. 1651).

EPICRANIAL MUSCLES

Superficial fascia of the scalp. The *superficial fascia* of the scalp is firm, dense and fibro-adipose, and adheres closely to both skin and the underlying epicranius, including its *epicranial aponeurosis*, the *galea aponeurotica* (see below). Posteriorly it is continuous with the superficial fascia of the back of the neck. Laterally, it is prolonged into the temporal region, where it is looser in texture.

Epicranius

Epicranius consists of two main parts: occipitofrontalis and temporoparietalis.

Occipitofrontalis

Occipitofrontalis covers the dome of the skull from the highest nuchal lines to the eyebrows. It is a broad, musculofibrous layer consisting of four thin, quadrilateral parts—two occipital and two frontal—connected by the epicranial aponeurosis. Each occipital part (*occipitalis*) arises by tendinous fibres from the lateral two-thirds of the highest nuchal line of the occipital bone and the mastoid part of the temporal bone, and ends in the aponeurosis. Each frontal part (*frontalis*; **7.53**) is adherent to the superficial fascia, particularly of the eyebrows, is broader than the occipital part and has fibres that are longer and paler. Although frontalis has no bony attachments of its own, the medial fibres are continuous with those of procerus, the intermediate fibres blend with corrugator supercilii and orbicularis oculi, and the lateral fibres also blend with orbicularis over the zygomatic process of the frontal bone. From these attachments the fibres ascend to join the epicranial aponeurosis in front of the coronal suture. The medial margins of the frontal bellies are joined together for some distance above the root of the nose, but between the occipital bellies there is a considerable, though variable gap, occupied by an extension of the epicranial aponeurosis.

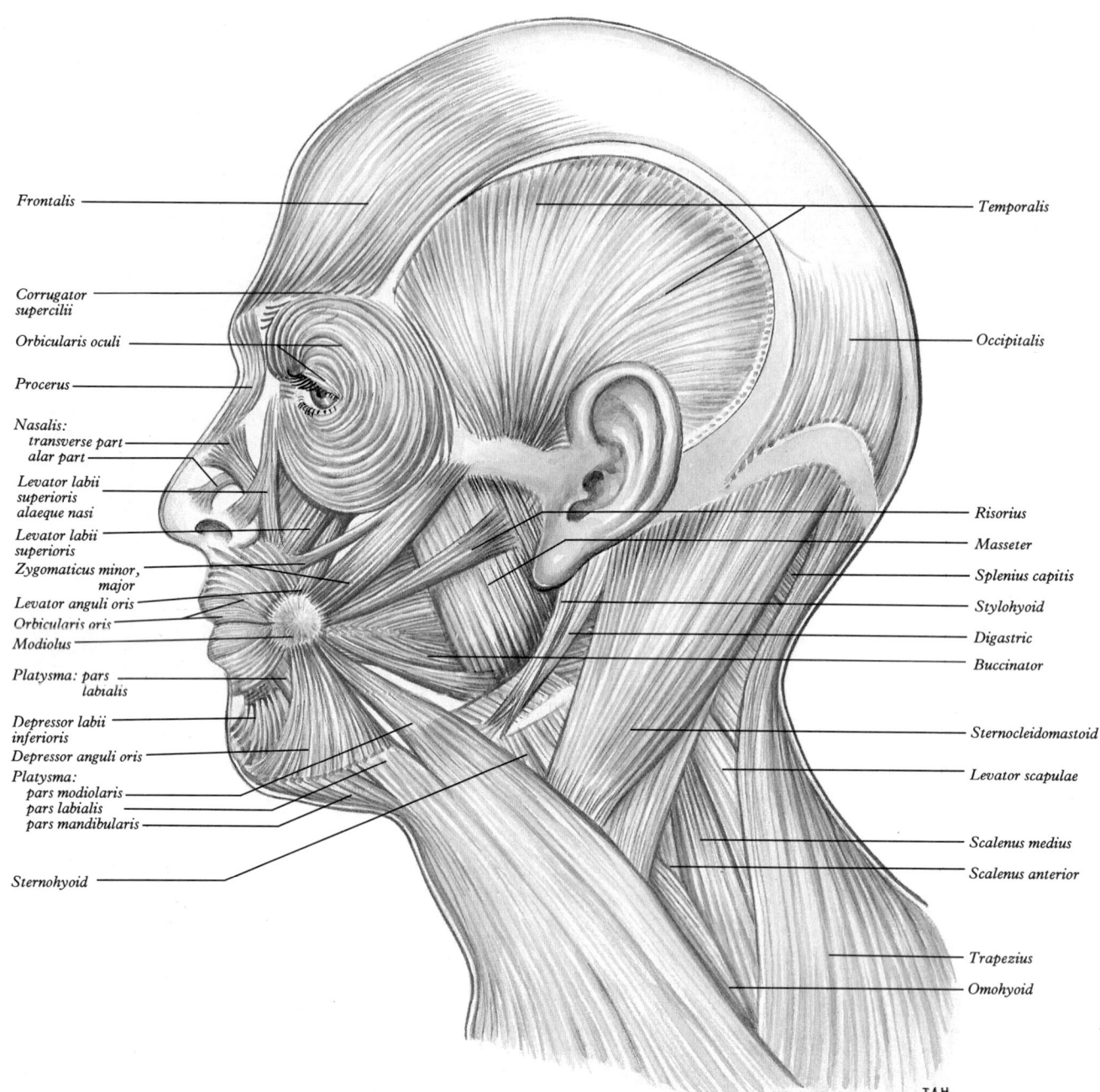

7.53 Muscles of the head and neck (superficial lateral view) including circumorbital, buccolabial, nasal, epicranial, masticatory and cervical groups. The articular muscles are omitted. Risorius, a variable muscle, here has two fasciculi, of which the lower one is unlabelled. The nature of the modiolus; the modiolar muscles and their co-operation in facial movement is described in the text. The laminae of the direct labial tractors to both upper and lower lips have been transected to reveal orbicularis oris underneath.

Temporoparietalis

Temporoparietalis is a variably developed sheet of muscle that lies between the frontal parts of occipitofrontalis and the anterior and superior auricular muscles.

The epicranial aponeurosis

The epicranial aponeurosis covers the upper part of the cranium and with the epicranial muscle forms a continuous fibromuscular sheet extending from the occiput to the eyebrows. Posteriorly, between the occipital parts of occipitofrontalis, it is attached to the external protuberance and highest nuchal line of the occipital bone. Anteriorly it splits to enclose the frontal parts and sends a short narrow prolongation between them. On each side the anterior and superior auricular muscles are attached to it; here it is thinner, and continues over the temporal fascia to the zygomatic arch. Over the cranial vault it is united to the skin by the fibrous superficial fascia, but it is connected more loosely to the pericranium by areolar tissue and

this allows it to move freely, carrying with it the skin of the scalp (7.54). Chayen and Nathan (1974) have subdivided this 'loose' subaponeurotic tissue into three layers, the middle one being dense and similar to the aponeurosis in its attachments.

Variations. A thin muscular slip, *transversus nuchae*, is present in about 25% of people. It arises from the external occipital protuberance or from the superior nuchal line, either superficial or deep to trapezius; it is frequently inserted with auricularis posterior, but may blend with the posterior edge of sternocleidomastoid.

Nerve supply. The occipital part is supplied by the posterior auricular branch, and the frontal part by the temporal branches of the facial nerve.

Actions. Acting from above, the frontal parts raise the eyebrows and the skin over the root of the nose: elevation of the eyebrows is a common accompaniment of glancing upwards, and is also part of expressions of surprise, horror, or fright, etc. Acting from below, the frontal parts draw the scalp forwards, throwing the forehead into transverse wrinkles. There are five to ten major transverse creases and variable intermediate minor ones. The 'transverse' lines form a series of roughly concentric arches above the orbits and parallel to the superior orbital margins, i.e. convex upwards. The medial ends of many of the arches are continuous across a median strip about 2 cm wide, but here the curvature is reversed, i.e. convex downwards. The occipital parts draw the scalp backwards. Acting alternately, the occipital and frontal parts can move the entire scalp backwards and forwards.

Clinical relevance. The scalp consists of five layers—skin, subcutaneous tissue, epicranius and its aponeurosis, subaponeurotic areolar tissue and pericranium (7.54). It is best to regard the first three as a single layer, since when torn off in accidents, or turned down surgically, they remain firmly connected to each other. Because the subcutaneous tissue is so dense any inflammatory swelling is slight, and a wound that does not involve epicranius or its aponeurosis does not gape. The dense nature of this tissue impedes contraction and retraction of arteries and therefore haemorrhage from scalp wounds is often copious. Subaponeurotic areolar tissue is surgically important. It is loose and lax, and is easily torn; hence, it is this tissue that is avulsed when surgical exposures are made. The vessels are in the avulsed tissue, and since they anastomose freely, necrosis is unusual.

CIRCUMORBITAL AND PALPEBRAL MUSCLES

The circumorbital and palpebral group of muscles are orbicularis oculi, corrugator supercilii and levator palpebrae superioris. The first two will be described here; the last is dealt with in the context of the eye (p. 1353).

Orbicularis oculi

Orbicularis oculi (7.53, 55) is a broad, flat elliptical muscle which surrounds the circumference of the orbit and spreads into the eyelids, anterior temporal region, infraorbital cheek and superciliary region. It has orbital, palpebral and lacrimal parts.

The *orbital part* arises from the nasal part of the frontal bone, the frontal process of the maxilla (7.56), and the medial palpebral ligament (see below) between them. Its fibres form complete ellipses, without interruption on the lateral side, where there is no bony attachment. The upper orbital fibres blend with the frontal part of occipitofrontalis and corrugator supercilii. Many of them are inserted into the skin and subcutaneous tissue of the eyebrow, constituting a

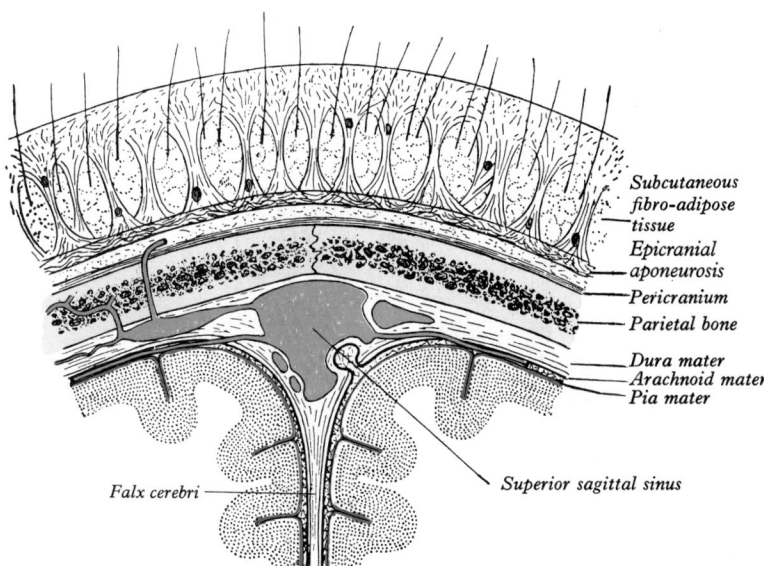

Subcutaneous fibro-adipose tissue
Epicranial aponeurosis
Pericranium
Parietal bone
Dura mater
Arachnoid mater
Pia mater
Falx cerebri
Superior sagittal sinus

7.54 Coronal section through the scalp, skull and brain. Note: loculated fat between fibrous septa blending with dermis and epicranial aponeurosis (galea aponeurotica); loose subaponeurotic areolar tissue; emissary, diploic, dural and neuropial veins. The superior sagittal sinus and lateral lacunae are more complex than depicted (see p. 1582).

depressor supercilii. Inferiorly, the ellipses overlap or blend to some extent with the attachments of levator labii superioris alaeque nasi, levator labii superioris and zygomaticus minor. Medially some ellipses may reach the upper lateral fibres of procerus. At the extreme periphery, sectors of complete, and sometimes incomplete, ellipses have a loose areolar connection with the temporal extension of the epicranial aponeurosis. The inferomedial margins of the orbital part may be continuous with the variable muscle malaris (see below).

The *palpebral part* is thinner and paler than the orbital part. It arises from the medial palpebral ligament, chiefly from its superficial, but also from its deep, surface (although not from its lower margin). It also arises from the bone immediately above and below the

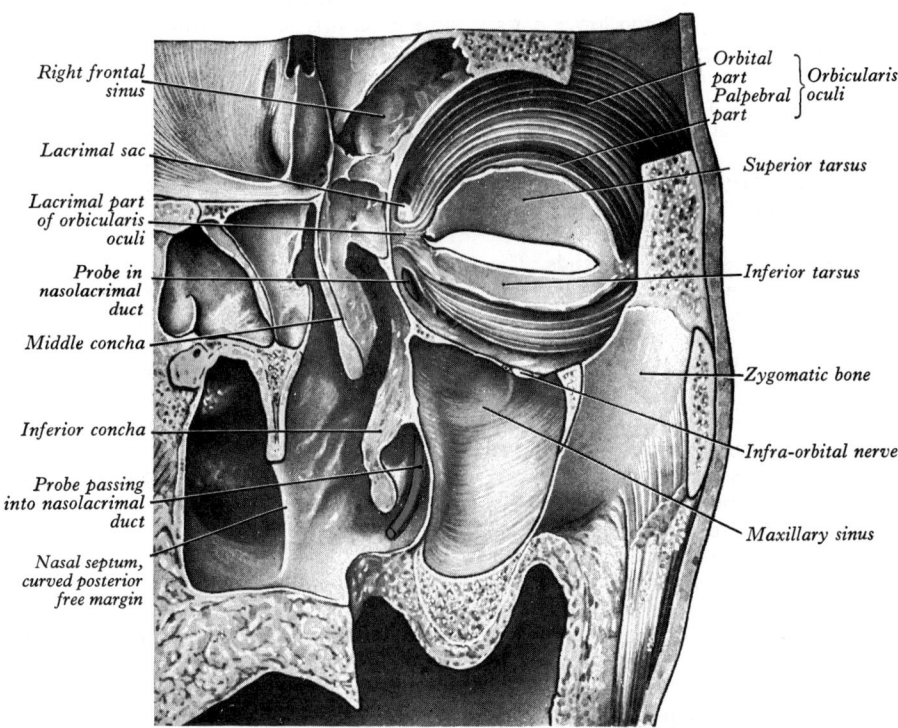

Right frontal sinus
Lacrimal sac
Lacrimal part of orbicularis oculi
Probe in nasolacrimal duct
Middle concha
Inferior concha
Probe passing into nasolacrimal duct
Nasal septum, curved posterior free margin
Orbital part / Palpebral part } Orbicularis oculi
Superior tarsus
Inferior tarsus
Zygomatic bone
Infra-orbital nerve
Maxillary sinus

7.55 Dissection to expose the right orbicularis oculi from behind.

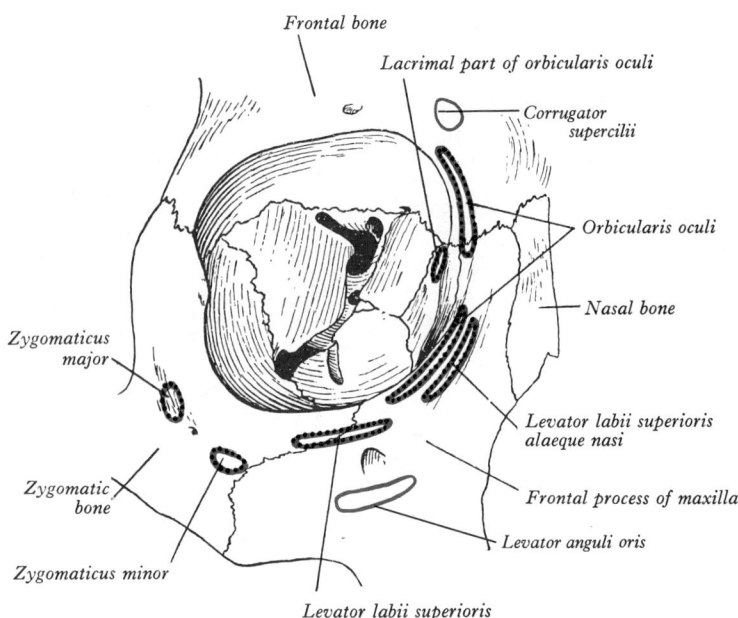

Frontal bone

Lacrimal part of orbicularis oculi

Corrugator supercilii

Orbicularis oculi

Nasal bone

Zygomaticus major

Levator labii superioris alaeque nasi

Zygomatic bone

Frontal process of maxilla

Levator anguli oris

Zygomaticus minor

Levator labii superioris

7.56 Frontal view of attachments of muscles around the right orbital opening.

ligament. The fibres sweep across the eyelids anterior to the orbital septum (p. 1361) interlacing at the lateral commissure to form the *lateral palpebral raphe*. A small group of fine fibres, close to the margin of each eyelid behind the eyelashes, is called the *ciliary bundle*.

The *lacrimal part* lies behind the lacrimal sac, separated from it by the lacrimal fascia. It is attached to the lacrimal fascia, to the upper part of the crest of the lacrimal bone and the adjacent lateral surface of the lacrimal bone (**7.56**). Passing laterally behind the lacrimal sac the muscle divides into upper and lower slips. Some fibres are inserted into the tarsi of the eyelids close to the lacrimal canaliculi, but most continue across in front of the tarsi and interlace in the lateral palpebral raphe.

The *medial palpebral ligament* is about 4 mm long and 2 mm broad. It is attached to the frontal process of the maxilla anterior to the nasolacrimal groove. Crossing the lacrimal sac, from which it is separated by lacrimal fascia, it divides into upper and lower parts, each attached to the medial end of the corresponding tarsus.

The *lateral palpebral raphe* is a much weaker structure, formed by the interlacing lateral ends of the palpebral fibres of orbicularis oculi, strengthened on its deep surface by the orbital septum. A few lobules of the lacrimal gland or, more frequently, a small lobule of fat may lie between it and the more deeply placed lateral palpebral ligament.

Nerve supply. Orbicularis oculi is supplied by temporal and zygomatic branches of the facial nerve.

Actions. Orbicularis is the sphincter muscle of the eyelids. The palpebral portion can be contracted voluntarily, closing the lids gently as in sleep, or reflexly, closing the lids protectively in blinking. The orbital portion is usually activated under voluntary control. Although the major factor in eye closure is lowering of the upper eyelid, there is also considerable elevation of the lower lid. Thus the palpebral part has upper *depressor* and lower *elevator* fascicles. Since levator palpebrae superioris raises the upper eyelid, it is the antagonist for the depressor action of the superior palpebral fibres. When the entire orbicularis oculi muscle contracts, the skin of the forehead, temple and cheek is drawn towards the **medial** angle of the orbit, and the eyelids are not only firmly closed but also displaced a little medially. The skin is thrown into folds which radiate from the lateral angle of the eyelids; in the middle decades these wrinkles often become permanent—the so-called 'crow's feet'. Orbicularis oculi is important in tear transport. The lacrimal part of the muscle draws the eyelids and the lacrimal papillae medially; this exerts traction on the lacrimal fascia and may aid drainage of tears by dilating the lacrimal sac (p. 1366). It may also influence pressure gradients within the lacrimal gland and ducts; assist in the sinuous

flow of tears across the cornea; direct the puncta lacrimalia into the lacus lacrimalis; and express secretions of the ciliary and tarsal glands. The muscle is an important element in facial expression and various ocular reflexes. Narrowing of the palpebral fissure together with bunching and protrusion of the eyebrows reduces the amount of light entering the eyes. This action of the upper orbital fibres produces vertical furrowing above the bridge of the nose—a feature that is markedly developed in people habitually exposed to strong sunlight.

Corrugator supercilii

Corrugator supercilii is a small pyramidal muscle located at the medial end of each eyebrow, deep to the frontal part of occipitofrontalis and orbicularis oculi, with which it is partially blended. Its fibres arise from bone at the medial end of the superciliary arch and pass laterally and slightly upwards to exert traction on the skin above the middle of the supraorbital margin.

Nerve supply. Temporal branches of the facial nerve.

Actions. The muscle co-operates with orbicularis oculi in drawing the eyebrows medially and downwards to shield the eyes in bright sunlight. It is also involved in frowning. The combined action of the two muscles produces mainly vertical wrinkles on the supranasal strip of the forehead. The most common pattern is a bilateral pair of major vertical wrinkles, 2–4 cm long and about 1 cm apart; these are above eyebrow level but their lower ends curve laterally around or through the medial end of the eyebrows. A variable number of lesser vertical wrinkles occurs, mainly lateral to the major ones.

NASAL MUSCLES

The nasal muscle group comprises procerus, nasalis and depressor septi (**7.53**). (Nerve supply is given at the end of the group.)

Procerus

Procerus is a small pyramidal slip close to, and often partially blended with, the medial side of the frontal part of occipitofrontalis. It arises from a fascial aponeurosis covering the lower part of the nasal bone and the upper part of the lateral nasal cartilage. It is inserted into the skin over the lower part of the forehead between the eyebrows. Normally its lower aponeurosis blends with that of the transverse part of nasalis; occasionally, however, a few muscle fascicles of procerus continue to the nasal ala, some even reaching the upper lip.

Actions. Procerus draws down the medial angle of the eyebrow and incidentally produces the transverse wrinkles over the bridge of the nose. It is active in frowning and 'concentration'. It also aids in reducing the glare of bright sunlight.

Nasalis

Nasalis consists of transverse and alar parts which may be continuous at their origins. The *transverse* part (*compressor naris*) arises from the maxilla just lateral to the nasal notch. Its fibres pass upwards and medially and expand into a thin aponeurosis. At the bridge of the nose, the aponeuroses of the paired muscles merge with each other and with the aponeurosis of procerus. The *alar* part (*dilatator naris*) arises from the maxilla below and medial to the transverse part, with which it partly merges. It is attached to the cartilaginous ala nasi. (See also depressor septi, below.)

Actions. The transverse part of nasalis compresses the nasal aperture at the junction of the vestibule with the nasal cavity. The alar part draws the ala downwards and laterally and so assists in widening the anterior nasal aperture. These actions accompany deep inspiration, and are thus associated with exertion but also with some emotional states.

Depressor septi

Depressor septi is often regarded as part of dilatator naris. It arises from the maxilla above the central incisor tooth and ascends to attach to the mobile part of the nasal septum. It is immediately deep to the mucous membrane of the upper lip.

Actions. Depressor septi co-operates with the alar part of nasalis to widen the nasal aperture.

Nerve supply. All the muscles of this group are supplied by the superior buccal branches of the facial nerve.

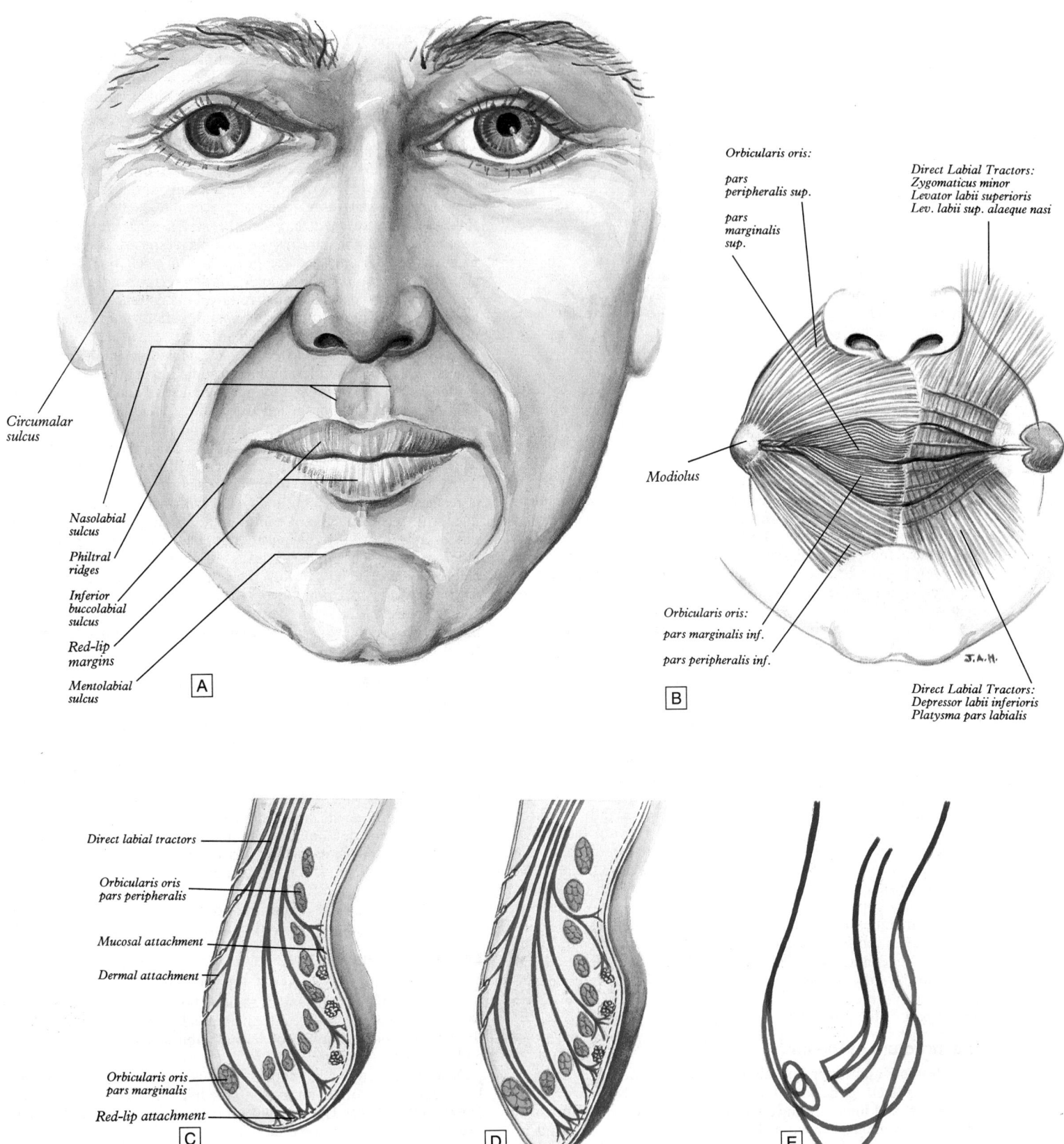

Circumalar
sulcus

Nasolabial
sulcus

Philtral
ridges

Inferior
buccolabial
sulcus

Red-lip
margins

Mentolabial
sulcus

A

Orbicularis oris:

pars
peripheralis sup.

pars
marginalis
sup.

Direct Labial Tractors:
Zygomaticus minor
Levator labii superioris
Lev. labii sup. alaeque nasi

Modiolus

Orbicularis oris:

pars marginalis inf.

pars peripheralis inf.

J.A.H.

B

Direct Labial Tractors:
Depressor labii inferioris
Platysma pars labialis

Direct labial tractors

Orbicularis oris
pars peripheralis

Mucosal attachment

Dermal attachment

Orbicularis oris
pars marginalis

Red-lip attachment

C   D   E

7.57 A. The principal sulci, creases and ridges of the face referred to at various points in the text. Note particularly those defining the 'labial hexagon' (see text). B. The disposition of the modiolus and orbicularis oris pars peripheralis and pars marginalis (on the left); the successively transected laminae of the direct labial tractors of both upper and lower lips (on the right). C. is a parasagittal section of the upper lip in repose. On the left is thin skin with oblique hair follicles; on the right is thick mucosa with mucous glands and mucosal shelf; between them is the red-lip margin. D as C but slightly contracted, forming a narrowed profile (labial cord). E. Superimposed outlines of C (magenta) and D (blue).

793

BUCCOLABIAL MUSCLES

The shape of the buccal orifice and the posture of the lips are controlled by a complex three-dimensional assembly of muscular slips (7.53). These include:

- *elevators*, *retractors* and *evertors of the upper lip*: levator labii superioris alaeque nasi, levator labii superioris, zygomaticus major and minor, levator anguli oris and risorius
- *depressors*, *retractors* and *evertors of the lower lip*: depressor labii inferioris, depressor anguli oris, and mentalis
- a *compound sphincter*: orbicularis oris, incisivus superior and inferior
- buccinator.

(Nerve supply will be given for groups of muscles.)

Before describing the buccolabial musculature, it will be convenient to have to hand an account of the limits of the labial area and the structure of the lips (7.53, 57A–E).

The labial area

When the face is in repose, the lips in gentle contact and the teeth slightly apart, the labial area is approximately hexagonal. The *superior border* of this area is between the attached lower margin of the external nose and the upper lips, and includes both *circumalar sulci* (7.57A). The *superolateral boundaries* correspond to the *nasolabial sulcus* (*groove* or *furrow*, 7.57A) on each side. They slope downwards and laterally from the upper end of the circumalar sulcus to the *modiolus*, a fibromuscular condensation located about 12 mm lateral to the buccal angle (7.53, 57A, B and see The modiolus and its role in facial movements, p. 796). The *inferolateral boundaries* extend downwards and medially from the lateral angles of the hexagon to the lateral ends of the *mentolabial sulcus* (7.53A), which itself forms the transverse *inferior boundary*. A horizontal line between the two external angles divides the labial area into a larger superior area and an inferior area of about half the size, and runs along the line of contact between the lips.

As is well known, the size and curvature of the exposed red-lip surfaces is subject to considerable individual, male–female and world variation. The junction between the external, hair-bearing skin and the red, hairless surface in the upper lip almost invariably takes the form of a double-curved Cupid's bow. From the centre it rises rapidly on each side to an apex that corresponds to the lower end of each ridge of the philtrum; it then slopes gently downwards and usually ends horizontally but sometimes curves slightly upwards (infrequently downwards). The line of contact between the red-lip surfaces is often almost horizontal but quite frequently takes the form of a much less wavy Cupid's bow. In the lower lip the junction between the skin and the red-lip varies greatly between individuals in its vertical depth at the centre; in all individuals, however, the lateral extremities descend medially for a few millimetres. With shallow lower red-lips the line of junction runs almost parallel to the line of lip contact; with the deepest lower red-lips, the junctional line is downwardly convex all along its length; lips of intermediate depth may have a flat section or even a reverse curvature in the central part of the junctional line.

The structure of the lips

In both upper and lower lips, about the central three-fifths consists mainly of a thick epithelialized fold of tissue, which has free external (cutaneous) and internal (mucous) surfaces. Where labial mucosa is reflected into gingival mucosa the upper lip has a narrow band of smooth tissue related to the subnasal maxillae. The corresponding reflexion in the lower lip coincides approximately with the mentolabial sulcus; here the lip is continuous with mental tissues. From the lateral extremities of the lips, the labial epithelia and internal tissues radiate over the boundaries of the labial hexagon to become continuous with those of the cheek. The upper and lower lips differ in cross-sectional profile: neither is a simple fold of uniform thickness. The upper lip has a bulbous asymmetrical profile, the skin and red-lip having a slight external convexity, and the adjoining red-lip and mucosa a pronounced internal convexity, creating a mucosal ridge or 'shelf' that can be wrapped around the incisal edges of the parted teeth. The lower lip is on a more posterior plane than the upper and, in the position of neutral lip contact, its external surface is concave; internally, elevation of the mucosal surface is minimal or absent. The profile of the lips can be modified by muscular activity (7.57C–E, and see Movements of the lips, p. 799).

Approximately in the centre of each lip is a thick fibrous strand, consisting of parallel bundles of skeletal muscle fibres and their attachments to skin, mucosa or other muscle fibres. The muscles concerned are the elements grouped collectively as orbicularis oris, together with incisivus superior and inferior, and the direct labial tractors; their disposition will be described in more detail later. The external surfaces are covered by a thin, fully keratinized epidermis; the dermis is well vascularized and accommodates numerous hair follicles (many of them large in the male), sebaceous glands and sweat glands. Subcutaneous panniculus adiposus is scanty. The mucous internal surfaces are lined with a thick non-keratinizing stratified squamous epithelium. Its cells are replaced continuously by mitosis in the deep germinative layer; the flattened dying or dead surface cells contain some eleidin and keratohyalin, retain their nuclei and are continuously shed into the saliva. The substantial submucosa is well vascularized and accommodates numerous labial mucous glands, up to a few millimetres in diameter, the largest being palpable with the tip of the tongue. Because of the thickness of its semi-opaque epithelium the mucosa of the everted lip appears moist, glistening and pink. Between the skin and mucosa, the free red-lip margin is covered with a specialized stratified squamous epithelium which is thin near the skin, increases in thickness slightly as the mucosa is approached, and then thickens abruptly when true mucosa is reached. The epithelium is covered with dead squames that are filled with eleidin and are transparent; its deep surface is deeply pitted and grooved, receiving abundant long dermal papillae. The latter carry a rich capillary plexus, responsible for the dusky red colour of these labial surfaces. Their rich innervation is consistent with their high discriminative sensitivity. These surfaces are, of course, hairless and their dermis carries no sebaceous, sweat or mucous glands; they are intermittently moistened with saliva by the tip of the tongue.

Levator labii superioris alaeque nasi

Levator labii superioris alaeque nasi arises from the upper part of the frontal process of the maxilla and, passing obliquely downwards and laterally, divides into medial and lateral slips. The medial slip is inserted into the greater alar cartilage of the nose and the skin over it. The lateral slip is prolonged into the lateral part of the upper lip, where it blends with levator labii superioris and orbicularis oris. Superficial fibres of the lateral slip curve laterally across the front of levator labii superioris and attach along the floor of the dermis at the upper part of the nasolabial furrow and ridge.

Actions. The lateral slip raises and everts the upper lip and raises, deepens and increases the curvature of the top of the nasolabial furrow. The medial slip dilates the nostril, displaces the circumalar furrow laterally, and modifies its curvature.

Levator labii superioris

Levator labii superioris starts from the inferior orbital margin, where it arises from the maxilla and zygomatic bone above the infraorbital foramen. Its fibres converge into the muscular substance of the upper lip between the lateral slip of levator labii superioris alaeque nasi and zygomaticus minor.

Actions. Levator labii superioris raises and everts the upper lip. Acting with other muscles, it modifies the nasolabial furrow (7.57A, B) that descends laterally from the side of the nose to fade out over the modiolus. In some faces this furrow is a highly characteristic feature; it is often deepened in expressions of sadness or seriousness. The prominent superolateral rim of the furrow, the *nasolabial ridge*, delimits the *infraorbital cheek*; the flatter, deeper inferomedial rim bounds the *superior labial area*. The buccal panniculus adiposus is thickest in the nasolabial ridge, and vanishingly thin in the labial area. The disposition of the furrow is affected by the posture of the lips and nasal ala. These indirect influences are supplemented directly by the state of contraction of levator labii superioris alaeque nasi (lateral slip), zygomaticus minor, levator anguli oris and, when present, malaris.

Zygomaticus minor

Zygomaticus minor arises from the lateral surface of the zygomatic bone immediately behind the zygomaticomaxillary suture, and passes downwards and medially into the muscular substance of the upper lip. Superiorly it is separated from levator labii superioris by a narrow triangular interval (7.53); inferiorly it blends with this muscle.

Actions. Zygomaticus minor elevates the upper lip, exposing maxillary teeth. As mentioned above, it also assists in deepening and elevating the nasolabial furrow (7.57A, B). Acting together, the main elevators—levator labii superioris alaeque nasi, levator labii superioris and zygomaticus minor—curl the upper lip in smiling, and in expressing smugness, contempt or disdain. (Some earlier investigators regarded these three muscles as individual 'heads'—named angularis, infraorbitalis and zygomaticus, respectively—of one compound *musculus quadratus labii superioris*.)

Levator anguli oris (*caninus*)

Levator anguli oris (caninus) arises from the canine fossa, just below the infraorbital foramen (7.56), and inserts into the modiolus, lateral to the angle of the mouth (7.53). Its fibres mingle there with the fibres of zygomaticus major, depressor anguli oris and other muscular bands, including orbicularis oris; some superficial fibres curve anteriorly and attach to the dermal floor of the lower part of the nasolabial furrow. Between levator anguli oris and levator labii superioris are the infraorbital vessels and nervous plexus.

Actions. Levator anguli oris raises the angle of the mouth, incidentally displaying the teeth in smiling, and contributes to the depth and contour of the nasolabial furrow.

Zygomaticus major

Zygomaticus major (7.53, 56) extends from the zygomatic bone, in front of the zygomaticotemporal suture, to the modiolus, where it blends with the fibres of levator anguli oris, orbicularis oris and more deeply placed muscular bands.

Actions. Zygomaticus major draws the angle of the mouth upwards and laterally as in laughing.

Malaris

Malaris is a thin sheet of muscle that is sometimes found covering zygomaticus major and minor levator labii superioris. It is subject to much individual and world variation, ranging from absence, or a few superficial fascicles, to a partial or complete (but rarely substantial) sheet. When present it is continuous with the inferior limit of orbicularis oculi, from which it is possibly derived (Lightoller 1925). Its fibres incline medially and downwards, covering zygomaticus major and minor and levator labii superioris. Its deep fascicles blend and distribute with those muscles. Some of its superficial fascicles have a dermal attachment to the nasolabial ridge and sulcus; others pass directly to the modiolus; the remainder enter the outer third of the upper lip and intersect with bundles of orbicularis oris.

Nerve supply. All six preceding muscles are supplied by the buccal branches of the facial nerve.

Mentalis

Mentalis is a conical fasciculus lying at the side of the frenulum of the lower lip. The fibres arise from the incisive fossa of the mandible and descend to attach to the skin of the chin.

Actions. Mentalis raises the lower lip, mental tissues and mentolabial sulcus (7.57A), wrinkling the skin of the chin. Since it raises the base of the lower lip, it helps in protruding and everting it in drinking and also in expressing doubt or disdain. Electromyography is said to show fairly continuous activity in mentalis, even to some extent during sleep, a finding that is unexplained.

Depressor labii inferioris

Depressor labii inferioris (7.53, 57B) is a quadrilateral muscle that arises from the oblique line of the mandible, between the symphysis menti and the mental foramen. It passes upwards and medially into the skin and mucosa of the lower lip, blending with the paired muscle from the opposite side and with orbicularis oris. Below and laterally it is continuous with platysma (pars labialis). Fat cells mingle with the superficial fibres of this muscle but the panniculus adiposus overlying it is very thin.

Actions. Depressor labii inferioris draws the lower lip downwards

and a little laterally in masticatory activity, and may assist in its eversion. It contributes to the expression of irony, sorrow, melancholy, and doubt.

Depressor anguli oris

Depressor anguli oris has a long, linear origin from the mental tubercle of the mandible and its continuation, the oblique line, below and lateral to depressor labii inferioris (7.53). It converges into a narrow fasciculus that blends at the modiolus with orbicularis oris and risorius; some fibres continue into levator anguli oris. Depressor anguli oris is continuous below with platysma and cervical fasciae. Some of its fibres may pass below the mental tubercle and cross the midline to interlace with their contralateral fellows; these constitute the *transversus menti* muscle (the 'mental sling').

Actions. Depressor anguli oris draws the angle of the mouth downwards and laterally in opening the mouth and in expressing sadness. During opening of the mouth the *buccolabial sulci* (7.57A) are stretched and flattened; the mentolabial sulcus becomes more horizontal and its central part deeper.

Nerve supply. Mentalis, depressor labii inferioris and depressor

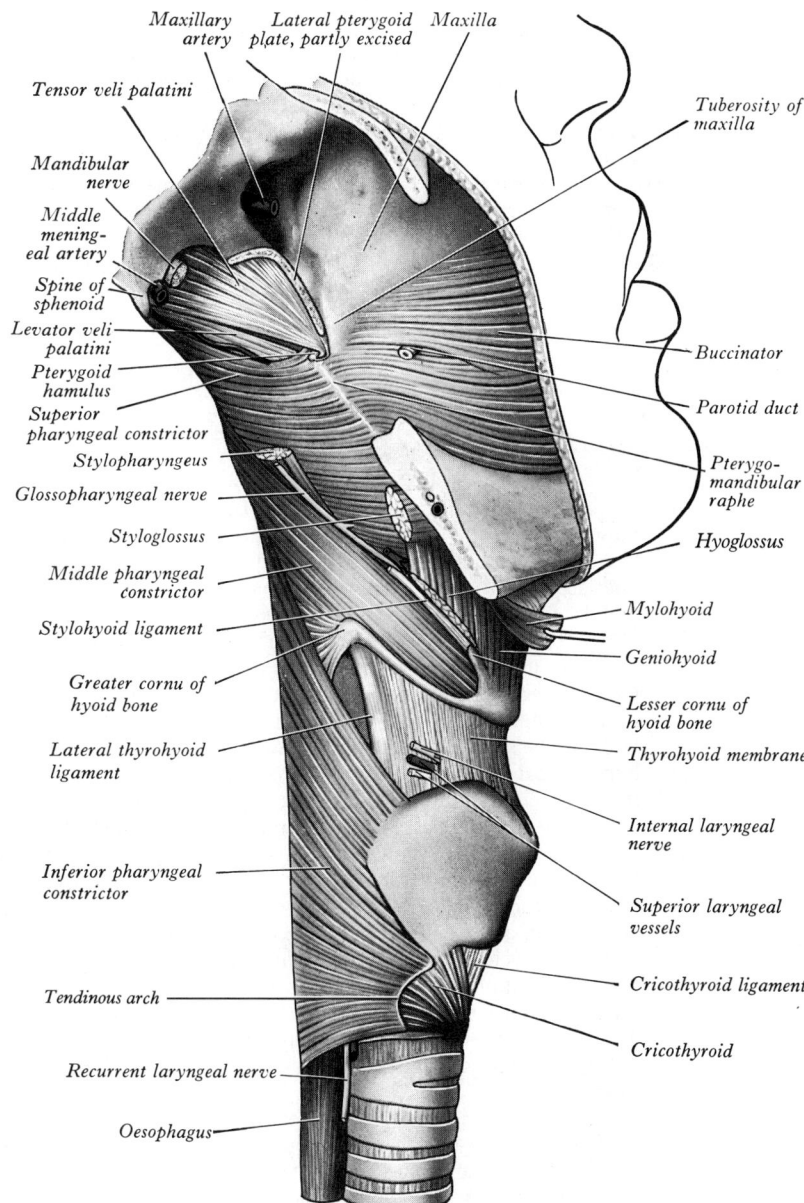

7.58 Buccinator and the muscles of the pharynx. The zygomatic arch, masseter, the ramus of the mandible, temporalis and a large part of the lateral pterygoid plate and the pterygoids have all been removed. In addition, the upper parts of stylopharyngeus and styloglossus have been excised, together with the posteroinferior part of hyoglossus and all the infrahyoid muscles.

anguli oris are all supplied by the mandibular marginal branch of the facial nerve.

Buccinator

Buccinator (7.58) is a thin quadrilateral muscle that occupies the interval between the maxilla and the mandible in the cheek. It is attached to the outer surfaces of the alveolar processes of the maxilla and mandible opposite the molar teeth, and, behind, to the anterior border of the pterygomandibular raphe (see below), which separates the muscle from the superior constrictor of the pharynx. Between the tuberosity of the maxilla and the upper end of the pterygomandibular raphe a few fibres spring from a fine tendinous band that bridges between the maxilla and the pterygoid hamulus. On its way to the soft palate the tendon of tensor veli palatini pierces the pharyngeal wall in the small gap that lies behind this tendinous band (7.58). Thus the posterior part of buccinator is deeply placed, internal to the mandibular ramus and its attachments and in the plane of the medial pterygoid plate; its anterior part curves out behind the third molar tooth to lie in the submucosa of the cheek and lips. The fibres of buccinator converge towards the modiolus, near the angle of the mouth, where the central (pterygomandibular) fibres intersect each other, those from below crossing to the upper part of orbicularis oris, those from above crossing to the lower part; the highest (maxillary) and lowest (mandibular) fibres continue forward to enter their corresponding lips without decussation. There is good evidence that as buccinator courses through the cheek and modiolar base substantial numbers of its fibres are diverted internally to attach to submucosa.

Relations. **Posteriorly**, buccinator lies in the same plane as the superior pharyngeal constrictor and is covered there by the buccopharyngeal fascia.

Superficially, a large mass of fat separates its posterior part from the ramus of the mandible, masseter and part of temporalis; this fat was originally named the suctorial pad, although its association with suckling is far from obvious.

Anteriorly, the **superficial surface** of buccinator is related to zygomaticus major, risorius, levator and depressor anguli oris, and the parotid duct, which pierces it opposite the third upper molar tooth; it is crossed by the facial artery, facial vein and branches of the facial and buccal nerves. Its **deep surface** is related to the buccal glands and mucous membrane of the mouth.

Nerve supply. Buccinator is supplied by lower buccal branches of the facial nerve.

Actions. The buccinators compress the cheeks against the teeth and gums; during mastication they assist the tongue in directing food between the grinding molar teeth. As the mouth closes, the teeth glide over the buccolabial mucosa, which must be retracted progressively from their occlusal surfaces by buccinator (and other submucosally attached muscles). When the cheeks have been distended with air, the buccinators expel it between the lips, a traditional method of blowing that accounts for the name (Latin *buccinator* = trumpeter): in modern wind instrumental technique, these muscles would be used to create pressure **without** distension of the cheeks. The labial extensions of the muscle are mentioned below.

The pterygomandibular raphe

The pterygomandibular raphe is a strand of tendinous fibres that stretches from the hamulus of the medial pterygoid plate down to the posterior end of the mylohyoid line of the mandible. It is easily palpated **medially**, where it is covered by the mucous membrane of the mouth; **laterally** it is separated from the ramus of the mandible by a quantity of adipose tissue. It gives attachment **posteriorly** to the superior constrictor of the pharynx, and **anteriorly** to the central part of buccinator (7.58).

The Modiolus and its role in Facial Movements

On each side of the face a number of muscles converge towards a focus just lateral to the buccal angle, where they interlace to form a dense, compact, mobile, fibromuscular mass: the *modiolus* (7.53). This can be palpated most effectively by using the opposed thumb and index finger to compress the mucosa and skin simultaneously. The name modiolus refers to the superficial resemblance to the hub of a cartwheel, the muscles radiating from a central point. However, the muscles lie in different planes, their modiolar stems are often spiralized, and most divide into two bundles, some into three or four, each of them interlacing and attaching in a distinctive way. Since there are nine muscles (or more, depending on the classification employed) attached to each modiolus, the structure has a high degree of three-dimensional complexity and has proved correspondingly difficult to analyse.

The shape and dimensions of the modiolus have to be given approximately because they are subject to individual, age, sexual and world variation; furthermore there are no precise histological boundaries but rather an irregular zone where dense, compact interlacing tissue grades into the stems of individually recognizable muscles. The modiolus has the rough form of a blunt cone. The base of the cone (*basis moduli*) is adjacent and adherent to the mucosa; it is roughly elliptical in outline and extends vertically about 20 mm above and 20 mm below a horizontal line through the buccal angle; it also extends laterally a similar distance from the angle. The blunt apex of the cone (*apex moduli*) is about 4 mm across, and is centred about 12 mm lateral to the buccal angle. From mucosa to dermis the thickness of the mass is about 10 mm, divided approximately equally into basal, central and apical parts. The central body has an oblique fibrous cleft or channel that transmits the facial artery, an arrangement that may limit the extent to which it is compressed by contraction of the buccolabial musculature. The cone shape is modified by two round-edged flanges (or *cornua*) that extend into the lateral free lip tissues above and below the corner of the mouth. The tip of the *superior cornu* extends 5–15 mm medial to the buccal angle, the tip of the *inferior cornu* only 3–5 mm. With these additions, the modiolar base becomes kidney-shaped, with the buccal angle projecting towards the hilum.

The apex of the modiolus is deep and adherent to the panniculus fibrosus, which extends posteromedially as a thin sloping sheet down to the buccal angle. There its free border forms a crescentic, narrow, flexible, subcutaneous fibro-elastic cord that accommodates the varying postures of the modioli, lips, mouth and jaws.

Modiolar muscles

Muscles radiate from the modiolus like an array of fans, some almost closed and strap-like, others widely open, their planes varying from sagittal through different degrees of obliquity almost to coronal. In some, the rays of the fan do not remain in a single plane but curve in conformity with buccal and labial tissue planes. Some muscles may be considered to form a large compound fan: thus, when well developed, zygomaticus major, risorius, platysma pars modiolaris and depressor anguli oris together have been likened to a wide hemicircular fan centred on the modiolus and extending peripherally from the zygomatic bone to the mental tubercle. Most of the muscle stems rotate as they approach the modiolus, and depressor anguli oris and the quadrants of orbicularis oris provide particularly clear examples of this. Peripherally the attachment of the depressor lies in the plane of the body of the mandible, whereas at the modiolus it lies in an apicobasal direction. Similarly the orbicular bundles in the free lip lie in a roughly coronal plane, but the stem thickens dorsoventrally and attaches at the modiolus from apex to base. Thus both muscles spiral through at least 90° between their attachments. This general pattern is further complicated by mutual spiralization of adjacent individual muscle bundles.

Some investigators have found it helpful to group the muscles in terms of their general geometrical relationship to the modiolus when the face is in repose, the teeth just apart, the lips in light contact and the modiolus in its 'resting' or neutral position.

Cruciate modiolar muscles: zygomaticus major, levator anguli oris, depressor anguli oris, platysma pars modiolaris. When viewed from the apex, these muscles resemble a compound X.

Transverse modiolar muscles: buccinator, risorius, the various parts of orbicularis oris, incisivus superior and inferior.

Attachment at the modiolus consists of interdigitation, partly with neighbouring bundles but mainly with direct physiological antagonists. A few muscles (risorius, platysma pars modiolaris, occasionally malaris and pars marginalis orbicularis oris) may be regarded as each possessing a single zone of attachment; the rest have superficial and deep (or multiple) zones. Most fibres terminate after attachment within the modiolus; occasional bundles escape and may be traced from one muscle to another.

Zygomaticus major slopes down to the modiolus and is separated into superficial and deep parts by the converging fibres of levator anguli oris. Many of the latter interlace with ascending bundles of depressor anguli oris at the 'angular complex' (the *caninotriangular complex* of earlier anatomists). The **superficial** fibres of zygomaticus major spread into the modiolar apex, where they interlace with the attachments of risorius, modiolar parts of platysma and malaris and with the underlying angular complex. Any or all of these muscles may interchange scattered fascicles. The **deep** fibres of zygomaticus attach to the centre of the modiolar body and to the superior cornu of its base. The central fibres interlace with corresponding fibres of buccinator and with the overlying angular fibres; interchange may occur with depressor anguli oris. Both the superficial and deep parts of zygomaticus major may send extensions into the peripheral part of orbicularis oris.

Levator anguli oris, as already stated, enters the modiolus between the superficial and deep parts of zygomaticus major, and is closely adherent to the superficial part. Thereafter its fibres radiate in many planes and intermesh with adjacent bundles. Many pass superficially and blend with depressor anguli oris. Deep bundles attach to the modiolar base inferior to the buccal angle. Some fascicles of levator anguli oris are continuous with orbicularis oris pars peripheralis inferior, others with buccinator. Most of its fibres end blindly in the modiolus. Depressor anguli oris, too,

has superficial and deep bundles: the superficial bundles interlace with the muscles converging on the modiolar apex; both superficial and deeper bundles interweave with levator anguli oris; basal fibres attach near the deep fibres of zygomaticus major. Some continuous fascicles pass into the territories of buccinator and the superior and inferior peripheral parts of orbicularis oris. Buccinator blends with the whole lateral aspect of the modiolar base and continues to interlace with many of the muscles attached to the base. The modiolar attachments of orbicularis oris (marginal and peripheral parts), incisivus superior and incisivus inferior are described in the relevant paragraphs of the main text.

Modiolar movements

Controlled three-dimensional mobility of the modioli enables them to integrate the activities of the cheeks, lips and oral fissure, the oral vestibule and the jaws. Such activities include: biting, chewing, drinking, sucking, swallowing, changes in vestibular contents and pressure, the innumerable subtle variations involved in speech, the modulation (and occasional generation) of musical tones, production of harsher sounds in shouting and screaming, crying, and all the permutations of facial expression, ranging from mere hints to gross distortion, symmetrical or asymmetrical. Major modiolar movements appear to involve many, if not all, of its associated muscles, and there is little value in considering the actions of the individual muscles in isolation. While the most obvious determinant of modiolar position and mobility is the balance between the forces exerted by muscles that are directly attached to it, another influential factor is the degree of separation or 'gape' between the upper and lower teeth. Starting from the occlusal position, and with the lips maintained in contact, the teeth can be separated by about 1.25 cm near the midline, and the mentolabial sulcus descends by a similar distance. With further separation the lips part, and as gape increases to its maximum, interlabial and interdental distances approach 4 cm, at which point the mentolabial sulcus has descended a further 2 cm. In this posture the modiolus has descended about 1 cm to lie over the interdental space, into which its basal and surrounding buccal mucosa projects a few millimetres, and its cornua diverge into their respective lips at an obtuse angle to each other, the dispositions of the modiolar muscles being correspondingly modified. The general hexagonal shape of the labial area changes as the mouth and jaws open progressively. In maximal opening, the distance between the superior and inferior boundaries has increased by 3–3.5 cm at the centre; the transverse distance between its lateral angles has decreased by about 1 cm and

the angles are obtuse; the nasolabial sulci are longer, straighter and more vertical; and the inferior buccolabial sulci are less deep and curved. These soft tissue changes radiate from the bilateral modioli.

With the lips in contact and the teeth in tight occlusion, the modiolus can move a few millimetres in all directions. However, mobility is maximal when there is 2–3 mm clearance between the teeth: the apex of the modiolus may then move vertically upwards about 10 mm, downwards 5 mm, posterolaterally 10 mm, and anteromedially 10 mm, these movements occurring in the curved planes of the cheek and lips. Specific movements of the modiolus may occur to any point, and along any path, within the boundaries of the envelope of movement thus defined. When the mouth is opened wide, the modiolus becomes immobile. From the neutral position the modiolus may be displaced superficially along its apicobasal axis for up to 5–10 mm by liquids or solids in the vestibule, or by an increase in air pressure that 'balloons' the cheeks and lips.

In all movements (elevation, depression, retraction, protraction, or any combination of these) the modiolus with its cornua, the buccal angle and the lip margins bordering the ends of the oral fissure, maintain the same fundamental relationships. A line that bisects the buccal angle can be projected through the centre of the modiolus, intersecting its apicobasal axis at a right angle. During elevation of the modiolus (and buccal angle), the line of intersection inclines upwards and laterally, accompanied by medial rotation of the modiolus around its apicobasal axis. Lowering of the modiolus is combined, similarly but to a lesser extent, with lateral rotation.

Many activities take place in three phases.

(1) A particular modiolar muscle group becomes dominant over its antagonists and the modiolus is rapidly relocated.

(2) The modiolus is transiently fixed in this new site by simultaneous contraction of modiolar muscles, principally the cruciate muscles.

(3) Acting from this fixed base the main physiological effectors, buccinator and orbicularis oris, carry out their specific actions.

These actions are usually integrated with partial separation or closure of the jaws and with varying degrees of activity in the direct labial tractors. All these factors combine to determine the positions of the lips and oral fissure from moment to moment. Modiolar movements may be bilaterally symmetrical, unilateral or asymmetrical. With both modioli at their posterolateral limits, and the oral fissure at its greatest horizontal length, activity in orbicularis oris causes compression between 'thin', stretched, smooth lips.

With both modioli at their anteromedial limits, and the oral fissure at its minimum length, orbicularis compresses 'thick' pursed, wrinkled lips. The most extreme modiolar excursions are achieved during horizontal asymmetrical movements, for example with the modioli moving either in succession or simultaneously to the right. This produces a markedly eccentric oral fissure: the ridges of the philtrum and the paired vertical sulci of the lower lip curve sharply to the right of the midline, and compression of the lips is most effective in the (original) left quadrants and less so in the right quadrants. Other asymmetric combinations are possible: one modiolus may remain static or slightly lowered while the other is raised. It is worth noting that in many facial expressions the **movement** (modiolar translocation) is often more significant than the final position.

Orbicularis oris

Orbicularis oris (**7.53, 57**) is so named because for long it was assumed that the oral fissure was surrounded by a series of complete ellipses of striated muscle that acted together in the manner of a sphincter. A variety of techniques (observations of normal function, the effects of neurological deficits, electrical stimulation and electromyographic recording) clearly demonstrate that the muscle actually consists of four substantially independent quadrants (upper, lower, left and right) each of which contains a larger *pars peripheralis* and a *pars marginalis*. (A pars peripheralis is found in many mammals; the pars marginalis is absent in non-primate mammals, marginally different in non-human primates and uniquely developed with speech in the human.) Marginal and peripheral parts are apposed along lines that correspond externally to the lines of junction between the red-lip and the skin. Thus orbicularis oris is composed of eight segments, each of which is named systematically according to its location. As with most modiolar muscles, each segment resembles a fan with its stem at the modiolus (see The modiolus and its role in facial movements, p. 796). Each fan is open in peripheral segments and almost closed in marginal segments.

Pars peripheralis. Pars peripheralis has, in each quadrant, a lateral stem attached to the labial side of the modiolus over its full thickness, from apex to base, including the corresponding upper or lower cornu. Most of these stem fibres are thought to originate within the modiolus, although it is possible that some are direct continuations from the other modiolar muscles. The usual view is that these fibres are reinforced directly by fibres from the following muscles:

- *in the upper lip*: from buccinator (upper fibres and decussating lower central fibres) and depressor anguli oris
- *in the lower lip*: from buccinator (lower fibres and decussating upper central fibres), levator anguli oris and the superficial part of zygomaticus major.

The fibres of orbicularis oris enter their respective superior and inferior labial areas and diverge to form triangular muscular sheets (**7.57B**). These are thickest at the junctions between skin and red-lip and become progressively thinner as they reach the limits of the labial region (as defined above). The greater part of each sheet enters the free lip, where its fibres aggregate into cylindrical bundles orientated parallel to the red-lip margin. Fibres of the direct labial tractors (see below) pass to their submucosal attachments between these cylindrical bundles and between pars peripheralis and pars marginalis (**7.57C**). In the upper lip, the highest fibres run near the nasolabial sulcus; a few fibres attach to the sulcus, and a few to the nasal ala and septum. In the lower lip, the lowest fibres reach and attach to the mentolabial sulcus. Of the main body of fibres, it is often said that a small proportion ends in the labial connective tissue, dermis or submucosa as it traverses its quadrant of free lip; this has not been satisfactorily demonstrated. Most fibres continue towards the median plane and cross some 5 mm into the opposite half-lip; at this point the fibres from the two sides interlace on their way to their dermal insertions, creating the ridges of the philtrum of the upper lip and the less marked corresponding depression in the lower lip (Latham & Deaton 1976).

Pars marginalis. Pars marginalis of the orbicularis oris is developed to a unique extent in human lips and is closely associated with speech and the production of some kinds of musical tone. In each quadrant the pars marginalis consists of a single (or in some cases double) band of narrow diameter muscle fibres lodged within the tissues of each red-lip margin. At their medial end, the marginal fibres meet and interlace with their contralateral fellows and then attach to the red-lip dermis a few millimetres beyond the median plane in a manner similar to pars peripheralis. At their lateral ends, the fibres converge and attach to the deepest part of the modiolar base along a horizontal strip level with the buccal angle.

The relations between pars marginalis and pars peripheralis are not simple. In a full thickness section of an upper lip at right angles to the red-lip margin, the cylindrical bundles of peripheralis fibres form an S-shape, with an external convexity above and an internal convexity below—the classical analogy is to the shank and initial curved part of a hook. Beyond peripheralis, the hook-shape is completed by the blunted triangular profile of marginalis, which occupies the core of the red-lip with its base adjacent to peripheralis and its apex reaching upwards and anteriorly towards the junction between red-lip and skin. In a similar section through the lower lip, peripheralis bundles form a continuous curve that is concave towards the external surface. This is surmounted by the flattened triangular profile of marginalis, which curves anteriorly, its apex again nearing the red-lip/cutaneous junction. Thus, throughout the red zones of both lips, marginalis lies substantially anterior to the adjacent bundles of peripheralis. However, as the muscles are traced laterally beyond the red-lip and across the buccal angle, this relationship alters: marginalis becomes inverted as it wraps progressively around the adjacent edge of peripheralis to reach its deep (submucosal) surface, and maintains this position up to its attachment at the modiolar base. The functional implications of this arrangement are mentioned below (see Lightoller 1925; Burkitt & Lightoller 1926; Duckworth 1947).

Nerve supply. Orbicularis oris is supplied by the lower buccal and mandibular marginal branches of the facial nerve.

Incisivus labii superioris

Incisivus labii superioris, an accessory muscle of the oral orbicular complex, has a bony origin from the floor of the incisive fossa of the maxilla above the eminence of the lateral incisor tooth. Initially it lies deep to orbicularis oris pars peripheralis superior. Arching laterally, its fibre bundles become intercalated between and parallel to the orbicular bundles. Approaching the modiolus, it segregates into superficial and deep parts: the former blends partially with levator anguli oris and attaches to the body and apex of the modiolus; the latter attaches to the superior cornu and base of the modiolus.

Incisivus labii inferioris

Incisivus labii inferioris, also an accessory orbicular muscle, has many features in common with incisivus labii superioris. Its osseous attachment is to the floor of the incisive fossa of the mandible, lateral to mentalis and below the eminence of the lateral incisor tooth. Curving laterally and upwards, it blends to some extent with orbicularis oris pars peripheralis inferior before reaching the modiolus, where superficial bundles attach to the apex and body and deep bundles attach to the base and inferior cornu.

Platysma

Platysma (**7.53**) is described on page 804, but also needs to be considered here. Its *pars mandibularis* attaches to the lower border of the body of the mandible. Posterior to this a substantial flattened bundle separates and passes superomedially to the lateral border of depressor anguli oris, where a few fibres join this muscle. The remainder continue deep to depressor anguli oris and reappear at its medial border. Here they continue within the tissue of the lateral half of the lower lip, as a direct labial tractor, platysma *pars labialis*. Pars labialis occupies the interval between depressor anguli oris and depressor labii inferioris; it is in the same plane as the latter and their adjacent margins blend. They have similar labial attachments. Platysma *pars modiolaris* constitutes all the remaining bundles posterior to pars labialis except for a few fine fascicles that end directly in buccal dermis or submucosa. Pars modiolaris is posterolateral to depressor anguli oris; it passes superomedially, deep to risorius, to apical and subapical modiolar attachments.

Risorius

Risorius (7.53) is a highly variable muscle that ranges from one or more slender fascicles to a wide, thin superficial fan. Its peripheral attachments may include some or all of the following: the zygomatic arch, parotid fascia, fascia over the masseter anterior to the parotid, fascia enclosing pars modiolaris of platysma, and fascia over the mastoid process. Its fibres converge to apical and subapical attachments at the modiolus. It is inappropriately named: it is not more associated with laughter than any other modiolar muscle; conversely, it participates in numerous facial activities other than laughter. (Some earlier investigators recognized a single large compound *musculus triangularis* with the following 'heads' or *capita* of peripheral attachment: *c. menti*—cf. transversus menti; *c. longum*—from the mental tubercle; *c. latum*—from fascia and the oblique line, cf. depressor anguli oris; *c. buccale*—usually called risorius.)

Nerve supply. Risorius is supplied by buccal branches of the facial nerve.

Direct labial tractors

Direct labial tractors, as their name suggests, pass directly into the tissues of the lips and not via the modioli. In broad terms, the force exerted by tractors is directed vertically at an approximate right angle to the oral fissure. Their action will therefore elevate and/or evert the whole or part of the upper lip, and depress and/or evert the whole or part of the lower lip. The tractors are, from medial to lateral:

- *in the upper lip*: the labial part of levator labii superioris alaeque nasi, levator labii superioris and zygomaticus minor
- *in the lower lip*: depressor labii inferioris and platysma pars labialis.

In both upper and lower lips the tractors blend into a continuous sheet that, as it enters the free lip, divides into a series of superimposed coronal sheets anterior to the muscle bundles of pars peripheralis orbicularis oris (7.57B, C). The sheets may be divided into three groups at increasing depths from the skin surface, each with a distinct zone of attachment. The *superficial group* comprises a succession of fine fibre bundles that curve anteriorly a short distance before attaching in a series of horizontal rows to the dermis between the hair follicles, sebaceous glands and sweat glands. The *intermediate group* attaches to the dermis of the modified skin of the red lip, which they reach by two routes: the more superficial bundles continue past the skin/red-lip junction, then curve posteriorly over pars marginalis orbicularis oris to punctate attachments on the ventral half of the red-lip dermis; the deeper bundles first pass posteriorly between pars peripheralis and pars marginalis, then curve anteriorly to punctate attachments on the dorsal half of the red-lip dermis. The *deep group* is closely applied to the anterior surface of pars peripheralis orbicularis oris, between the parallel bundles of which it sends fine tractor fibres posteriorly to attachments on the submucosa and periglandular connective tissue.

Movements of the lips

The various groups of direct labial tractors may act together or individually and their effects may involve a complete labial quadrant or be restricted to a short segment. For example, partial contraction of the superior labial tractors can result in localized elevation of a segment of the upper lip, in a postural expression reminiscent of the 'canine snarl'. Normally, however, the activity of the tractors is modified by the superimposed activity of orbicularis oris and the modiolar muscles. The resultant actions range from delicate adjustments of the tension and profile of the lip margins to large increases of the oral fissure with eversion of the lips.

Lip protrusion is passive in its initial stages; it may be suppressed by powerful contraction of the whole of orbicularis or enhanced by selective activation of parts of the direct labial tractors. However lip movements must accommodate separation of the teeth brought about by mandibular depression at the temporomandibular joints. Beyond a certain range of mouth opening, labial movements are almost completely dominated by mandibular movements. Thus over the last 2.5–3 cm interincisal distance of wide jaw separation, strong contraction of orbicularis oris cannot effect lip contact; instead it causes full-thickness inflection of upper and lower lips—including the red-lip margins—towards the oral cavity, wrapping them around the incisal edges, canine cusps and premolar occlusal surfaces. The involvement of the lips in speech, intonation and the production of less patterned sounds is mentioned elsewhere (p. 1651) but some aspects relevant to the actions of orbicularis oris pars marginalis deserve comment here. The main features of pars marginalis have already been described: its cross-sectional configuration as a sharply recurved hook in the upper lip and a gently curved 'half-hook' in the lower lip; the spiralling of marginalis over the adjacent edge of peripheralis; and their linear attachment to the basis modioli. Contraction of marginalis is considered to alter the cross-sectional profile of the red-lip rim: both the gentle bulbous profile of the upper lip and the smooth posterosuperior convexity of the lower lip change to a narrow, symmetrical triangular profile. The transformed rims, whose length and tension can be delicately controlled, have been evocatively named *labial cords*. They are known to be involved in the production of some consonantal (labial) sounds. A labial cord may also function as the so-called 'lip' of a closed organ pipe or as a vibrating 'reed' in whistling or playing a wind instrument such as the trumpet.

MASTICATORY MUSCLES

The muscles most immediately concerned with the movements of the mandible in mastication (and speech) are masseter, temporalis and the pterygoid muscles.

Parotid fascia

The parotid fascia is a strong layer of fascia, derived from the deep cervical fascia, that covers masseter and is firmly connected to it. It is attached to the lower border of the zygomatic arch, and invests the parotid gland (p. 1691).

Masseter

Masseter (7.67) is a quadrilateral muscle consisting of three layers which blend anteriorly. The *superficial layer* is the largest: it arises by a thick aponeurosis from the maxillary process of the zygomatic bone, and from the anterior two-thirds of the inferior border of the zygomatic arch. Its fibres pass downwards and backwards, to insert into the angle and lower posterior half of the lateral surface of the mandibular ramus. Intramuscular tendinous septa in this layer are responsible for the ridges on the bone. The *middle layer* arises from the medial aspect of the anterior two-thirds of the zygomatic arch and from the lower border of the posterior third and inserts into the central part of the mandibular ramus. The *deep layer* arises from the deep surface of the zygomatic arch and inserts into the upper part of the mandibular ramus and into its coronoid process. The middle and deep layers together constitute the deep part of the masseter referred to in the Nomina Anatomica (MacDougall 1955); they form a *cruciate* muscle (7.48). Because it is so close to the skin, the masseter is easily palpated when it contracts, as in clenching the teeth. MacConaill (1975) has stated that the most superficial fibres of masseter are continuous at the lower border of the mandible with the attachment of the medial pterygoid muscle. Schumacher (1961) and Yoshikawa and Suzuki (1969) have published more complex accounts of the lamination.

Relations. **Superficial** are skin, platysma, risorius, zygomaticus major, and parotid gland; the muscle is crossed by the parotid duct, branches of the facial nerve, and the transverse facial vessels. **Deep** are temporalis and the mandibular ramus. A mass of fat separates it in front from buccinator and the buccal nerve. The masseteric nerve and artery reach the deep surface of the muscle by passing through the dorsal part of the mandibular incisure. The **posterior**

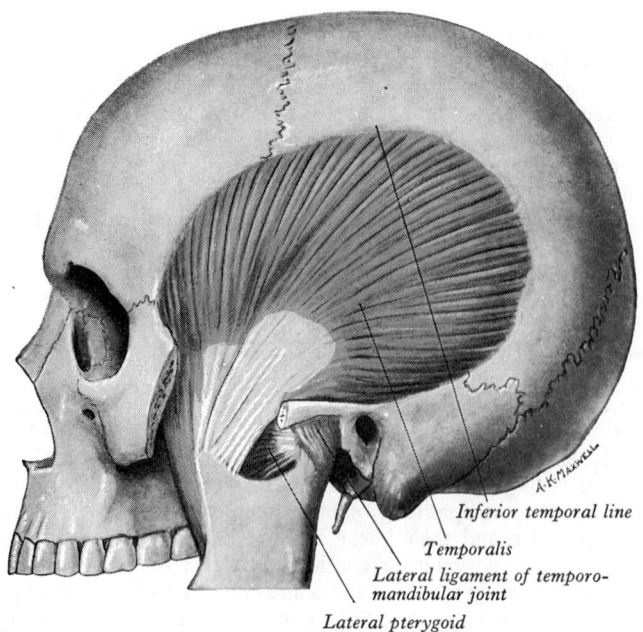

7.59 Left temporalis: the zygomatic arch and masseter have been removed. Note the changing orientations of the muscle fibres, from vertical anteriorly to horizontal posteriorly.

margin is overlapped by the parotid gland; the **anterior margin** projects over buccinator and is crossed below by the facial vein.

Nerve supply. Masseter is supplied by a branch of the anterior trunk of the mandibular nerve.

Actions. Masseter elevates the mandible to occlude the teeth in mastication. Its electrical activity in the resting position of the mandible is minimal. Masseter has a small effect in side-to-side movements, protraction and retraction. Rinqvist (1974) has analysed

numbers and diameter distribution of muscle fibres in relation to dental occlusive forces.

Temporal fascia

The temporal fascia that covers temporalis is a strong aponeurosis overlapped by auriculares anterior and superior, the epicranial aponeurosis and part of orbicularis oculi. The superficial temporal vessels and the auriculotemporal nerve ascend over it. **Above**, it is a single layer, attached to the whole of the superior temporal line; **below**, it has two layers, one attached to the lateral and the other to the medial margin of the upper border of the zygomatic arch. Between these layers are the zygomatic branch of the superficial temporal artery, the zygomaticotemporal branch of the maxillary nerve and a small quantity of fat. The deep surface of the fascia affords attachment to the superficial fibres of temporalis.

Temporalis

Temporalis (**7.59**) arises from the whole of the temporal fossa (except the part formed by the zygomatic bone) and from the deep surface of the temporal fascia. Its fibres converge and descend into a tendon which passes through the gap between the zygomatic arch and the side of the skull, and attaches to the medial surface, apex, anterior and posterior borders of the coronoid process and the anterior border of the mandibular ramus almost to the last molar tooth. The anterior fibres of temporalis are orientated vertically, the most posterior fibres almost horizontally, and the intervening fibres with intermediate degrees of obliquity, in the manner of a fan. Because of the tough temporal fascia, the muscle is not easy to palpate, but its contraction is easily felt. Its upper limit can be made out along the inferior temporal line when the teeth are firmly clenched.

Relations. **Superficial** are skin, auriculares anterior and superior, the temporal fascia, the superficial temporal vessels, the auriculotemporal nerve, the temporal branches of the facial nerve, the zygomaticotemporal nerve, the epicranial aponeurosis, the zygomatic arch and masseter. **Deep** are the temporal fossa, lateral pterygoid, the superficial head of medial pterygoid, a small part of buccinator, the maxillary artery and its deep temporal branches, the deep temporal nerves and the buccal nerve and vessels. Behind the tendon

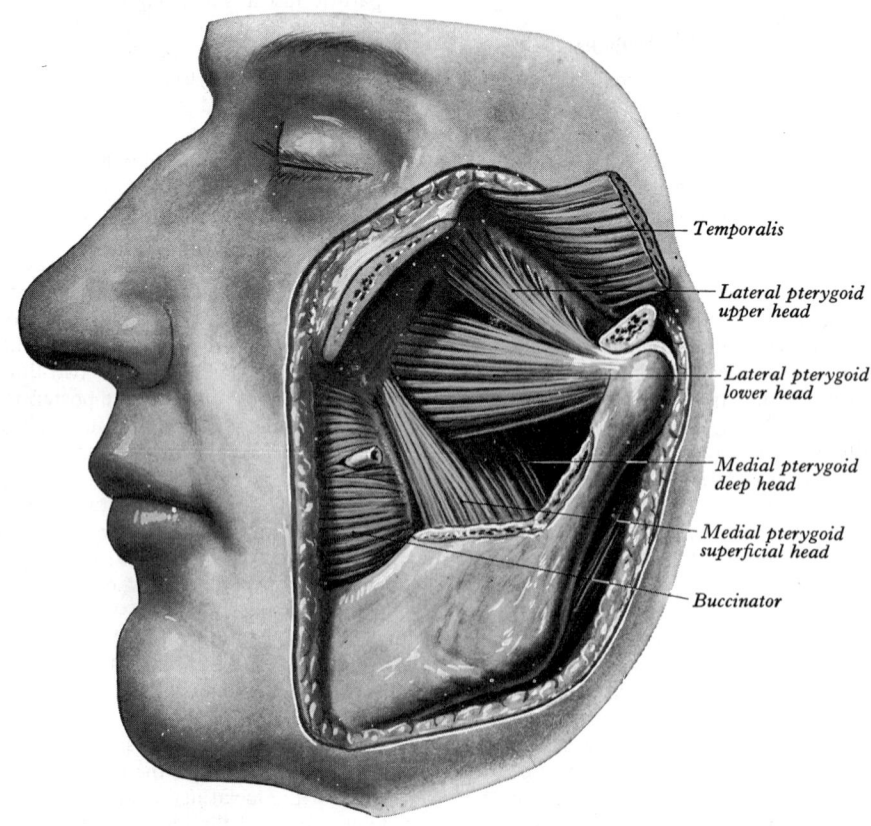

7.60 Left pterygoid muscles: the zygomatic arch and part of the ramus of the mandible have been removed.

of the muscle the vessels and masseteric nerve traverse the mandibular incisure. The anterior border is separated from the zygomatic bone by a mass of fat.

Nerve supply. Temporalis is supplied by the deep temporal branches of the anterior trunk of the mandibular nerve.

Actions. Temporalis elevates the mandible and so closes the mouth and approximates the teeth. This movement requires both the upward pull of the anterior fibres and the backward pull of the posterior fibres, because the head of the mandibular condyle rests on the articular eminence when the mouth is open. The muscle is also a contributor to side-to-side grinding movements. The posterior fibres retract the mandible after it has been protruded. Electromyographic studies have added little to this analysis: Vitti and Basmajian (1977) suggest that the temporalis is active in forcible elevation, but not in slow elevation without occlusion: otherwise their study confirms the above description.

Lateral pterygoid

Lateral pterygoid (7.60) is a short, thick muscle with two parts or heads: an *upper head* arising from the infratemporal surface and infratemporal crest of the greater wing of the sphenoid bone, and a *lower head* from the lateral surface of the lateral pterygoid plate. Its fibres pass backwards and laterally, to be inserted into a depression on the front of the neck of the mandible, and into the articular capsule and disc of the temporomandibular joint.

Early in the third month of intrauterine life the muscle inserts into mesenchyme that condenses around the developing condyle of the mandible, but part of its tendon sweeps backwards above the condyle and inserts into the portion of Meckel's cartilage that later forms the head of the malleus (Harpman & Woollard 1938). This part of the tendon becomes incorporated into the articular disc of the temporomandibular joint; its attachment to the malleus does not persist (Rees 1954).

Relations. **Superficial** are the mandibular ramus, the maxillary artery, which crosses either deep or superficial to the muscle, the tendon of temporalis, and masseter. **Deep** are the upper part of medial pterygoid, the sphenomandibular ligament, the middle meningeal artery, and the mandibular nerve. The **upper border** is related to the temporal and masseteric branches of the mandibular nerve; the **lower border** to the lingual and inferior alveolar nerves. The buccal nerve and the maxillary artery pass between the two heads of the muscles (7.61).

Nerve supply. The lateral pterygoid is supplied by a branch from the anterior trunk of the mandibular nerve.

Actions. Lateral pterygoid assists in opening the mouth by pulling forward the condylar process of the mandible and the articular disc, while the head of the mandible rotates on the articular disc (Posselt 1952). During closure of the mouth, the backward gliding of the articular disc and mandibular condyle is controlled by slow elongation of lateral pterygoid, while the masseter and temporalis restore the jaw to the occlusal position. Acting with the ipsilateral medial pterygoid, lateral pterygoid advances the condyle of that side so that the jaw rotates about a vertical axis through the opposite condyle. When medial and lateral pterygoids of the two sides act together they protrude the mandible, so that the lower incisors project in front of the upper. It has been said that the upper head is involved mainly in chewing, the lower head in protrusion. See Grant (1973) for a review and a mechanical assessment.

Medial pterygoid

Medial pterygoid (7.60) is a thick, quadrilateral muscle with a deep origin from the medial surface of the lateral pterygoid plate and the grooved surface of the pyramidal process of the palatine bone; a more superficial slip arises from the lateral surfaces of the pyramidal process and maxillary tuberosity, and lies at first on the inferior aspect of the lower head of the lateral pterygoid. Its fibres descend

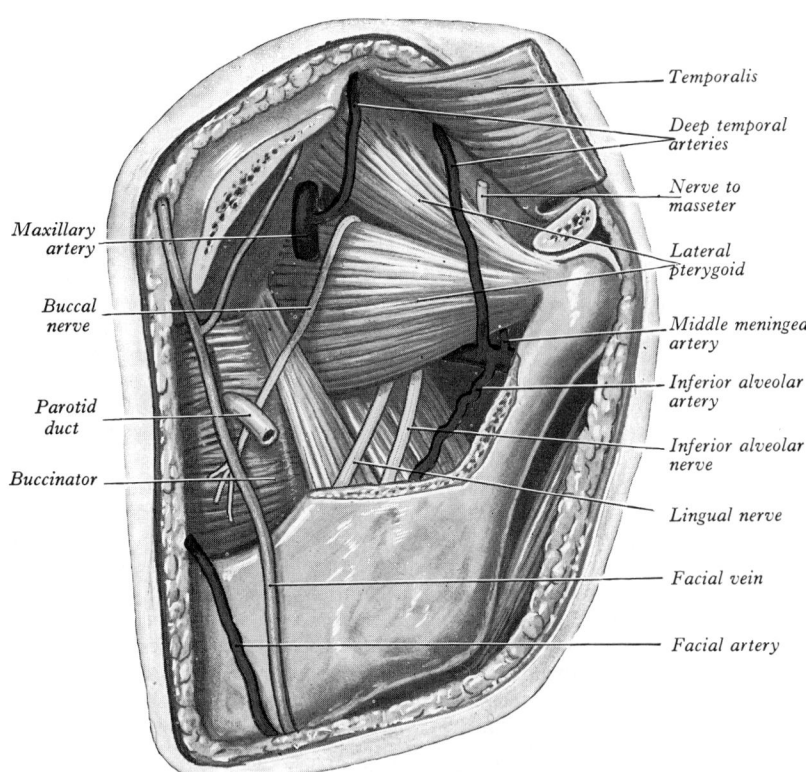

7.61 Structures related to the left pterygoid muscles.

Maxillary artery
Buccal nerve
Parotid duct
Buccinator
Temporalis
Deep temporal arteries
Nerve to masseter
Lateral pterygoid
Middle meningeal artery
Inferior alveolar artery
Inferior alveolar nerve
Lingual nerve
Facial vein
Facial artery

posterolaterally and are attached by a strong tendinous lamina to the postero-inferior part of the medial surfaces of the mandibular ramus and angle, as high as the mandibular foramen and almost as far forwards as the mylohyoid groove (6.122). This area is often rugged, because of tendinous fasciculi in the attachment.

Relations. The **lateral surface** is related to the mandibular ramus, from which it is separated above its insertion by lateral pterygoid, the sphenomandibular ligament, the maxillary artery, the inferior alveolar vessels and nerve, the lingual nerve and a process of the parotid gland. The **medial surface** is related to tensor veli palatini, and separated from the superior constrictor by styloglossus, stylopharyngeus and some areolar tissue.

Nerve supply. The medial pterygoid is supplied by a branch from the mandibular nerve. In a detailed study, Schumacher et al (1976) found that the nerves followed a very similar pattern of branching in all the masticatory muscles.

Actions. The medial pterygoids assist in elevating the mandible. Acting with the lateral pterygoids they protrude it. When the medial and lateral pterygoid muscles of one side act together, the corresponding side of the mandible is rotated forwards and to the opposite side, with the opposite mandibular head as a vertical axis (p. 580). Alternating activity in the left and right sets of muscles produces side-to-side movements, which are used to triturate food. (For further analysis see pp. 581–582 and Mastication.)

Pterygospinous ligament

The pterygospinous ligament, which is occasionally replaced by muscle fibres, stretches between the spine of the sphenoid bone and the posterior border of the lateral pterygoid plate near its upper end. It is sometimes ossified, and then completes a foramen which transmits the branches of the mandibular nerve going to temporalis, masseter and lateral pterygoid.

Mastication

Mastication is the process in which food items are held, chewed, and moved within the oral cavity, in preparation for swallowing (*deglutition*). The masticatory apparatus consists primarily of the teeth, the upper and lower jaws, and the muscles that act on them; however, the tongue, together with the hyoid and its musculature, the buccinator muscles and the rugosities of the palate, all play ancillary roles in placing and holding food items for chewing. The function of chewing is to increase the surface area of food items available to the action of the digestive juices by inducing fractures in the food. When these fractures are complete the food particles are also reduced in size and can be transported more easily. In humans, food is fractured primarily by the postcanine teeth; these compress items until they crack, cut them between paired blades, and tear them until they fail under tension. The pattern of fracture depends on the mechanical properties of the food: hard or soft, brittle or elastic. The form of the upper and lower postcanine teeth accommodates these variations by providing points (or cusps) to fracture brittle foods and to tear elastic foods, blades or crests to cut soft foods, and basins to retain food particles while they are reduced (Lucas 1979). Thus chewing consists of tooth–food–tooth interactions, rather than direct occlusal contact between teeth.

Compressive or tensile loads are applied to the food by movements of the jaws. Adduction of the mandible is brought about by the action of the masseter, medial pterygoid and temporalis muscles and the superior head of the lateral pterygoid. Secondary movements of the whole head, brought about by the prevertebral musculature, may contribute by depressing the maxillary teeth against food items, particularly when large chunks of food are bitten off for ingestion into the oral cavity (Möller 1966; DuBrul 1980; McDevitt 1989). When large food items are chewed bilaterally the mandible may act without a fulcrum, supported entirely in 'slings' formed by the masticatory muscles. At all other times the mandible functions as a bent second- or third-class lever, whose fulcrum or pivot is the articular eminence of the temporomandibular joint (Hylander 1975).

In non-mammals, opening and closing movements of the mandible are brought about symmetrically and bilaterally by rotation of both condyles against the articular disc, in combination with anterior or posterior translation of the disc–mandible complex against the articular eminence. In mammals the situation is different: although gross opening and closing of the jaws—during incisal biting, for example—is achieved in the same way, most chewing is asymmetric and unilateral. On the **working** side, where the food item is being chewed, by far the greatest proportion of the adductor force acts on the food item, and the articular eminence is not subjected to substantial loads; on the contralateral or **balancing** side, the mandibular condyle will apply large loads to the articular eminence if there are no food items between the upper and lower teeth. The reactive forces on the mandible load it asymmetrically, particularly in the later stages of chewing, when tooth–tooth or firm tooth–food–tooth contacts occur (Walker 1978).

The *chewing cycle* comprises an opening stroke, a closing stroke in which the jaws close towards the food, and a power stroke in which the food is reduced. In primates and ungulates the power stroke is conventionally divided into two phases:

- Buccal or Phase I, in which the lower teeth move upward and medially into maximal intercuspation
- Lingual or Phase II, in which the buccal cusps of the lower teeth slide downwards and medially against the palatal cusps of the upper teeth (Hiiemae & Crompton 1985).

During the power stroke, the working side condyle moves laterally by about 1.5 mm (Bennett's movement) and slightly posteriorly against the resistance of the deep part of the temporomandibular ligament and the lateral pterygoid of the same side; the contralateral condyle remains protruded by the action of both heads of the lateral pterygoid muscle of the balancing side. Activity of the adductor muscles fades shortly after the first tooth–tooth contact, but food reduction may continue to occur through intercuspation and the movements of Phase II. The action of the adductor muscles and the lateral pterygoids, together with the reaction forces from the bite point and balancing side condyle, create stresses which tend to pull the two condyles together, so that the mandibular symphysis is subjected to twisting, shearing and bending. In many mammals these stresses produce rotation at the symphysis but in humans, monkeys and apes such movement is resisted by the bony union of the symphysis, which also allows muscular force to be transferred from the balancing side adductors to the bite point.

ANTEROLATERAL MUSCLES AND FASCIAE OF THE NECK

Anterolateral muscles of the neck will be considered in the following groups:

- Superficial and lateral cervical muscles
- Suprahyoid muscles
- Infrahyoid muscles
- Anterior vertebral muscles
- Lateral vertebral muscles.

Anterior and posterior triangles of the neck

Sternocleidomastoid divides the side of the neck into two main triangles, anterior and posterior (**7.62, 63**). The boundaries of the *anterior cervical triangle* are: in front, the median ventral line; above, a line running along the base of the mandible and continuing from the mandibular angle to the mastoid process; behind, the anterior border of the sternocleidomastoid. The apex of the triangle is at the upper border of the sternum. The boundaries of the *posterior cervical triangle* are: in front, the posterior border of the sternocleidomastoid; below, the middle third of the superior surface of the clavicle; behind, the anterior margin of trapezius. The apex is at the convergence of sternocleidomastoid and trapezius on the occipital bone. (The subdivisions and contents of these major triangles are given on pp. 1521–1523.)

Superficial cervical fascia

The superficial cervical fascia is usually a thin lamina covering platysma and is hardly demonstrable as a separate layer. It may, however, contain considerable amounts of adipose tissue, especially in females. Like all superficial fascia it is not a separate stratum, but merely a zone of loose connective tissue between dermis and deep fascia, and joined to both.

Deep cervical fascia

The deep cervical fascia (**7.64**) consists of fibro-areolar tissue lying internal to platysma and investing the muscles and other structures of the neck. In certain situations it forms well-defined fibrous sheets; elsewhere it is loosely arranged. It condenses around the blood vessels as fibrous sheaths which—here, as elsewhere in the body—bind the arteries and their accompanying veins closely together. The

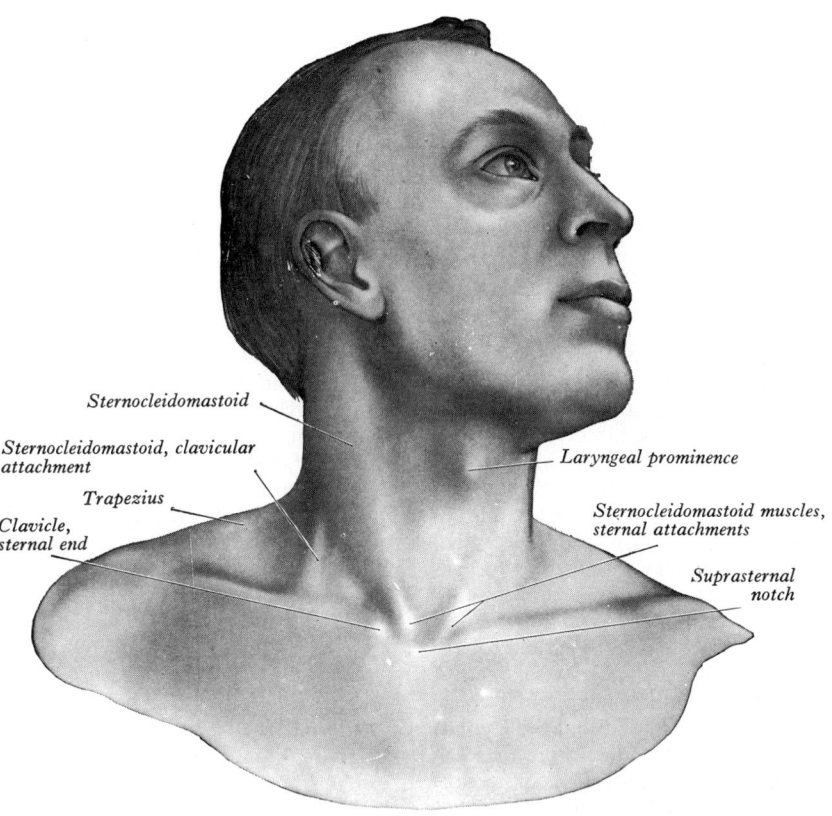

7.62   Surface landmarks of the neck.

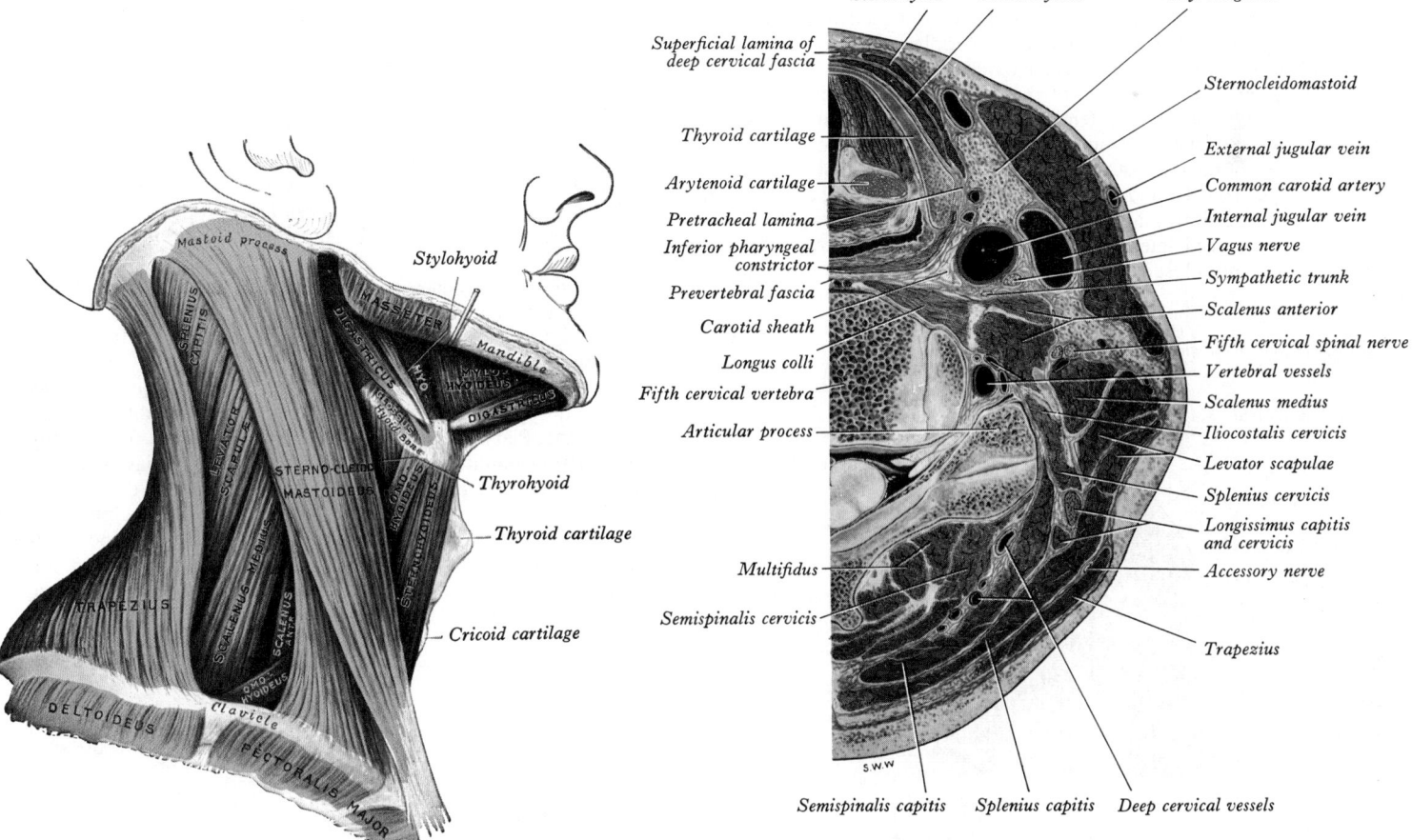

7.63   Muscles of the neck: right lateral aspect.

7.64   Transverse section through the left half of the neck to show the arrangement of the deep cervical fascia. (Specimen provided by R E M Bowden, Royal Free Hospital School of Medicine.)

superficial (investing) lamina of the deep cervical fascia is continuous behind with the ligamentum nuchae and the periosteum covering the spine of the seventh cervical vertebra. It forms a thin covering for trapezius, and continues forwards from the anterior border of this muscle as a loose areolar layer over the posterior triangle of the neck to the posterior border of sternocleidomastoid, where it becomes denser. It divides around sternocleidomastoid, enclosing it, and reunites at the anterior margin as a single lamina, which covers the anterior triangle of the neck and reaches forwards to the midline. Here it meets the corresponding lamina from the opposite side and adheres to the symphysis menti and the body of the hyoid bone. **Above**, deep fascia fuses with periosteum along the superior nuchal line of the occipital bone, over the mastoid process and along the entire base of the mandible. Between the mandibular angle and the anterior edge of sternocleidomastoid it is particularly strong. Between the mandible and the mastoid process it ensheathes the parotid gland. The layer superficial to the gland extends upwards as the *parotid fascia* and is attached to the zygomatic arch. From the layer deep to the gland, the strong *stylomandibular ligament* ascends to the styloid process (p. 579). **Below**, deep fascia is attached to the acromion, clavicle and manubrium sterni, fusing with their periostea. A short distance above the manubrium it splits into superficial and deep layers. The superficial layer is attached to the anterior border of the manubrium, the deep layer to its posterior border and to the interclavicular ligament. Between these two layers is a slit-like interval, the *suprasternal space*, which contains a small amount of areolar tissue, the lower parts of the anterior jugular veins and the jugular venous arch, the sternal heads of the sternocleidomastoid muscles and sometimes a lymph node. Over the lower part of the posterior triangle, between trapezius and sternocleidomastoid, the deep fascia again divides into superficial and deep layers. The superficial layer is attached below to the superior border of the clavicle. The deep layer surrounds the inferior belly of omohyoid and, deep to sternocleidomastoid, its intermediate tendon; it blends below with the fascia around subclavius and the periosteum on the posterior surface of both the clavicle and anterior end of the first rib.

The *carotid sheath* is a condensation of cervical fascia around the common and internal carotid arteries, the internal jugular vein, the vagus nerve and the constituents of the ansa cervicalis. It is thicker around the arteries than the vein. Peripherally it is connected to adjacent layers by loose areolar tissue (**7.65**).

The *prevertebral lamina* of the cervical fascia covers the anterior vertebral muscles and extends laterally on scalenus anterior, scalenus medius and levator scapulae, forming a fascial floor for the posterior triangle of the neck. As the subclavian artery and the brachial nerves emerge from behind scalenus anterior they carry the prevertebral fascia downwards and laterally behind the clavicle as the *axillary sheath*. Traced laterally, the prevertebral fascia becomes thin and areolar and is lost as a definite fibrous layer under cover of trapezius.

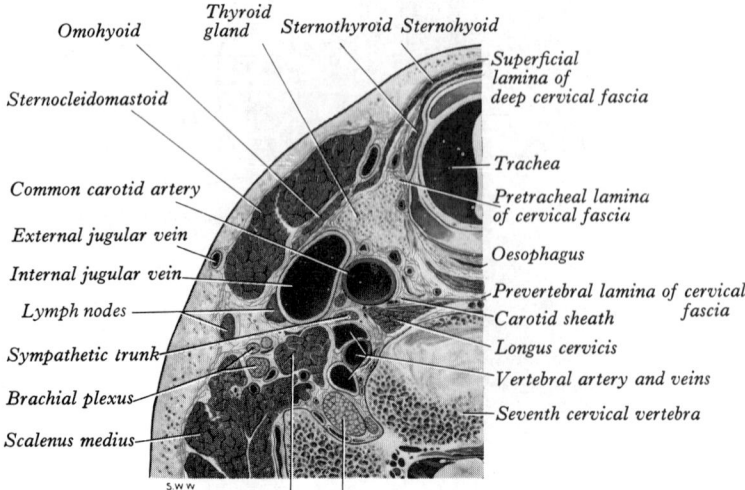

7.65 Part of a transverse section through the lower part of the neck at the level of the seventh cervical vertebra, showing the arrangement of the deep cervical fascia. (Specimen provided by R E M Bowden.)

Superiorly it is attached to the base of the skull; inferiorly it descends in front of longus colli into the superior mediastinum, where it blends with the anterior longitudinal ligament. Anteriorly the prevertebral lamina is separated from the pharynx and its covering buccopharyngeal fascia by a loose areolar zone, which is termed the *retropharyngeal space*; laterally this loose tissue connects the prevertebral lamina to the carotid sheath and the fascia on the deep surface of sternocleidomastoid. All the ventral rami of the cervical nerves are initially behind the prevertebral lamina. The nerves to the rhomboids and serratus anterior and the phrenic nerve retain this position throughout their course in the neck but the accessory nerve lies superficial to the prevertebral fascia (p. 1253).

The *pretracheal lamina* of the cervical fascia is very thin, but provides a fine fascial sheath for the thyroid gland. Above, it attaches to the arch of the cricoid cartilage; below it continues into the superior mediastinum with the inferior thyroid veins.

Clinical relevance. The superficial lamina of deep cervical fascia opposes the spread of abscesses towards the surface, and pus beneath it tends to migrate laterally. If the pus is in the anterior triangle, it may find its way into the mediastinum, anterior to the pretracheal lamina, but because the fascia here is so thin it more often approaches the surface and 'points' above the sternum. Pus behind the prevertebral lamina may extend laterally and point in the posterior triangle, or it may perforate the lamina and the buccopharyngeal fascia to bulge into the pharynx as a retropharyngeal abscess.

SUPERFICIAL AND LATERAL CERVICAL MUSCLES

The superficial and lateral cervical muscles include platysma, trapezius, and sternocleidomastoid.

Platysma

Platysma (**7.53**) is a broad sheet of muscle that arises from the fascia covering the upper parts of pectoralis major and deltoid. Its fibres cross the clavicle and ascend medially in the side of the neck. **Anterior** fibres interlace across the midline with the fibres of the contralateral muscle, below and behind the symphysis menti. **Intermediate** fibres attach to the lower border of the mandibular body (*pars mandibularis*) or pass upwards and medially, deep to depressor anguli oris, to attachments in the lateral half of the lower lip (*pars labialis*, see p. 799). **Posterior** fibres cross the mandible and the anterolateral part of masseter to attach to the skin and subcutaneous tissue of the lower face, many of them blending with modiolar muscles near the buccal angle (*pars modiolaris*, p. 799). Deep to platysma the external jugular vein descends from the angle of the mandible to the middle of the clavicle.

Variations. Platysma varies considerably in extent, and may even be absent on one side or both. It may be joined by slips from the mastoid process, the occipital bone or the fascia over the upper part of trapezius (occipitalis minor).

Nerve supply. Cervical branch of the facial nerve, which descends on the deep surface of the muscle close to the mandibular angle.

Actions. Platysma does not seem to be important functionally. Its contraction diminishes the concavity between the jaw and the side of the neck and produces tense oblique ridges in the skin of the neck. Its anterior portion, the thickest part of the muscle, may assist in depressing the mandible. Through its labial and modiolar attachments it can draw down the lower lip and corners of the mouth in expressions of horror or surprise. Electromyographic studies show the muscle to be active in sudden deep inspiration (de Sousa 1964). It often contracts vigorously during sudden, violent effort.

Trapezius

Trapezius is described on page 835 in the context of scapular musculature.

Sternocleidomastoid

Sternocleidomastoid (**7.63**) descends obliquely across the side of the neck and forms a prominent surface landmark (**7.62**), especially when contracted. It is thick and narrow centrally, and broader and

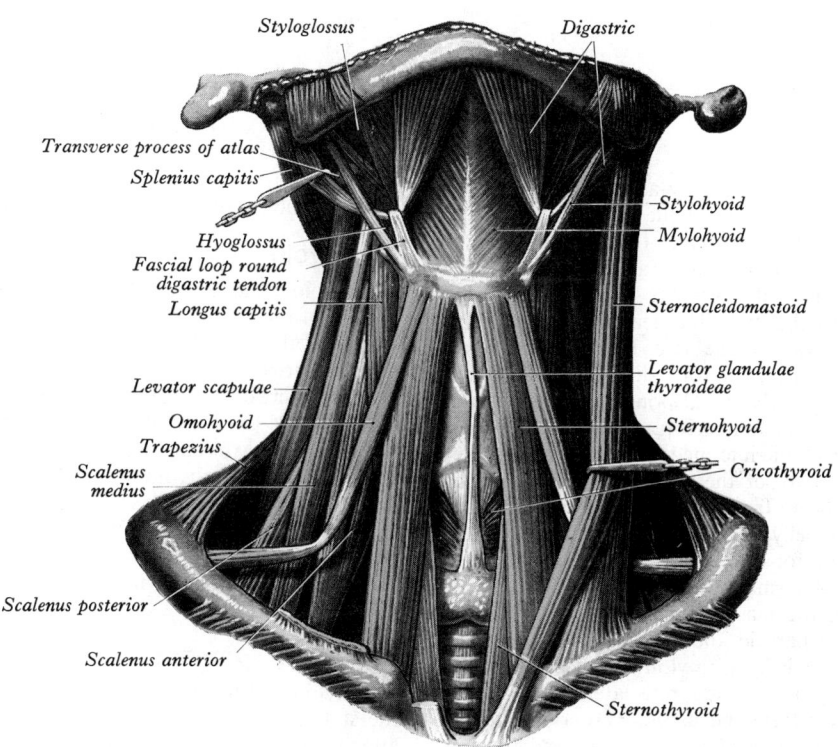

Styloglossus   *Digastric*

Transverse process of atlas

Splenius capitis

Stylohyoid

Mylohyoid

Hyoglossus

Fascial loop round digastric tendon

Longus capitis

Sternocleidomastoid

Levator glandulae thyroideae

Levator scapulae

Omohyoid

Sternohyoid

Trapezius

Scalenus medius

Cricothyroid

Scalenus posterior

Scalenus anterior

Sternothyroid

7.66 Muscles of the front of the neck. Sternocleidomastoid has been removed on the subject's right side. In this subject, the origin of the scalenus medius extended up to the transverse process of the atlas.

thinner at each end. It is attached inferiorly by two heads. The *medial* or *sternal head*, a rounded tendinous fasciculus, arises from the upper part of the anterior surface of the manubrium sterni and ascends posterolaterally (**7.62, 66**). The *lateral* or *clavicular head*, which is variable in width and contains muscular and fibrous fasciculi, ascends almost vertically from the superior surface of the medial third of the clavicle (**7.62, 63, 66**). The two heads are separated near their attachments by a triangular interval which corresponds to a surface depression, the *lesser supraclavicular fossa*. As they ascend, the clavicular head spirals behind the sternal head and blends with its deep surface below the middle of the neck, forming a thick, rounded belly. The muscle inserts superiorly by a strong tendon into the lateral surface of the mastoid process from its apex to its superior border, and by a thin aponeurosis into the lateral half of the superior nuchal line. The clavicular fibres are directed mainly to the mastoid process; the sternal fibres are more oblique and superficial, and extend to the occiput. The direction of pull of the two heads is therefore different, and the muscle may be classed as 'cruciate' and slightly 'spiralized' (**7.48**).

Relations. The **superficial** surface of the muscle is related to skin and platysma; between the surface and platysma lie the external jugular vein, the great auricular and transverse cervical nerves and the superficial lamina of the deep cervical fascia. Near its insertion the muscle is overlapped by a small part of the parotid gland. The **deep** surface of the muscle is, near its origin, related to the sternoclavicular joint, sternohyoid, sternothyroid and omohyoid. The anterior jugular vein crosses deep to it, but superficial to the infrahyoid muscles, immediately above the clavicle. The carotid sheath and the subclavian artery are deep to these muscles. Between omohyoid and the posterior belly of digastric, the **anterior** part of sternocleidomastoid lies superficial to the common, internal and external carotid arteries, the internal jugular, facial and lingual veins, the deep cervical lymph nodes, the vagus nerve and the rami of the ansa cervicalis. The sternocleidomastoid branch of the superior thyroid artery crosses deep to the muscle at the upper border of omohyoid. The **posterior** part of sternocleidomastoid is related on its internal surface to splenius, levator scapulae and the scaleni, the cervical plexus, the upper part of the brachial plexus, the phrenic

nerve and the transverse cervical and suprascapular arteries. The occipital artery crosses deep to the muscle at, or under cover of, the lower border of the posterior belly of digastric. At this point the accessory nerve passes deep to sternocleidomastoid; it pierces (and supplies) the muscle, and reappears just above the middle of the posterior border. At its insertion the muscle lies superficial to the mastoid process, splenius, longissimus capitis and the posterior belly of digastric.

Nerve supply. Accessory nerve and branches from the ventral rami of the second, third and sometimes fourth cervical spinal nerves. For some time these cervical rami were believed to be solely proprioceptive, but clinical evidence suggests that some of their fibres are motor (see Fitzgerald et al 1982).

Actions. Acting alone, one sternocleidomastoid will tilt the head towards the ipsilateral shoulder, simultaneously rotating the head so as to turn the face towards the opposite side. This movement occurs in an upward, sideways glance, but a much more common visual movement is a more or less level rotation from side to side, and this probably represents the most frequent use of the sternocleidomastoids. Acting together from below, the muscles draw the head forwards and so help the longi colli to flex the cervical part of the vertebral column. This movement is common in feeding. The two muscles are also used to raise the head when the body is supine. With the head fixed, they help to elevate the thorax in forced inspiration. Electromyographic observations (e.g. de Sousa 1973) suggest that the sternal fibres are more active in contralateral rotation, but that both parts of the muscle are involved to some extent in all of the above movements. This study also indicates that the muscle is involved in extension as well as flexion of the neck.

Clinical relevance. Torticollis (or *wryneck*), a postural deformity of the neck, is due to a permanent contracture of the sternocleidomastoid. Spasmodic torticollis, a condition that can develop in adult life, begins with tonic or clonic spasm of one sternocleidomastoid muscle, followed by a spasm of trapezius, particularly its clavicular portion. Such abnormal conditions illustrate the action of the muscle in isolation, but this is a caricature of its ordinary activities, which are invariably modified by synergists and antagonists, such as splenius capitis (p. 809).

SUPRAHYOID MUSCLES

The suprahyoid muscles include digastric, stylohyoid, mylohyoid and geniohyoid.

Digastric

Digastric (**7.66, 67**) has two bellies joined by a rounded tendon. It lies below the mandible, and extends from the mastoid process to the chin. The posterior belly, which is longer than the anterior, is attached in the mastoid notch of the temporal bone, and slopes downwards and forwards. The anterior belly is attached to the digastric fossa on the base of the mandible near the midline, and slopes downwards and backwards. The two bellies meet in an intermediate tendon, which runs in a fibrous sling that is attached to the body and greater cornu of the hyoid bone and is sometimes lined by a synovial sheath. The tendon perforates stylohyoid (**7.66**).

Variations. Digastric may lack the intermediate tendon and is then attached midway along the body of the mandible. The posterior belly may be augmented by a slip from the styloid process or arise wholly from it. The anterior belly may cross the midline to some extent and it is not uncommon for it to fuse with mylohyoid.

Relations. **Superficial** are platysma, sternocleidomastoid, part of splenius, longissimus capitis, the mastoid process, stylohyoid, the retromandibular vein and the parotid and submandibular salivary glands. **Medial to the anterior belly** is mylohyoid; **medial to the posterior belly** are superior oblique, rectus capitis lateralis, the transverse process of the atlas vertebra, the accessory nerve, internal jugular vein, occipital artery, hypoglossal nerve, internal and external carotid, facial and lingual arteries and hyoglossus (**7.67**).

Nerve supply. Anterior belly: mylohyoid branch of the inferior alveolar nerve. *Posterior belly*: facial nerve. These different nerve supplies to the two parts are associated with their separate deri-vations from the mesenchyme of the first and second branchial arch (p. 284).

Actions. Digastric depresses the mandible and can elevate the hyoid bone. Electromyography indicates that the paired digastric muscles always act together and are secondary to the lateral ptery-goids in mandibular depression, coming into play especially when depression is maximal (Moyers 1950). The posterior bellies are especially active during swallowing and chewing.

Stylohyoid

Stylohyoid (**7.66, 67**) arises by a small tendon from the posterior surface of the styloid process, near its base. Passing downwards and forwards, it inserts into the body of the hyoid bone at its junction with the greater cornu and just above omohyoid. It is perforated, near its insertion, by the intermediate tendon of digastric.

Variations. Occasionally the muscle is absent or double. It may lie medial to the external carotid artery. It may end in digastric or in suprahyoid or infrahyoid muscles.

Nerve supply. Facial nerve.

Actions. Stylohyoid elevates the hyoid bone and draws it back-wards, elongating the floor of the mouth. Its precise roles in speech, mastication and swallowing remain to be fully analysed, although some radiographic data are available (Delmas & Senecail 1977).

Stylohyoid ligament

The stylohyoid ligament is a fibrous cord extending from the tip of the styloid process to the lesser cornu of the hyoid bone. It gives attachment to the highest fibres of the middle pharyngeal constrictor and is intimately related to the lateral wall of the oral pharynx (**7.58**). Below, it is overlapped by hyoglossus. The ligament is derived from the cartilage of the second branchial arch (p. 284). It may be partially ossified and in many mammals it forms a distinct bone, the *epihyal*.

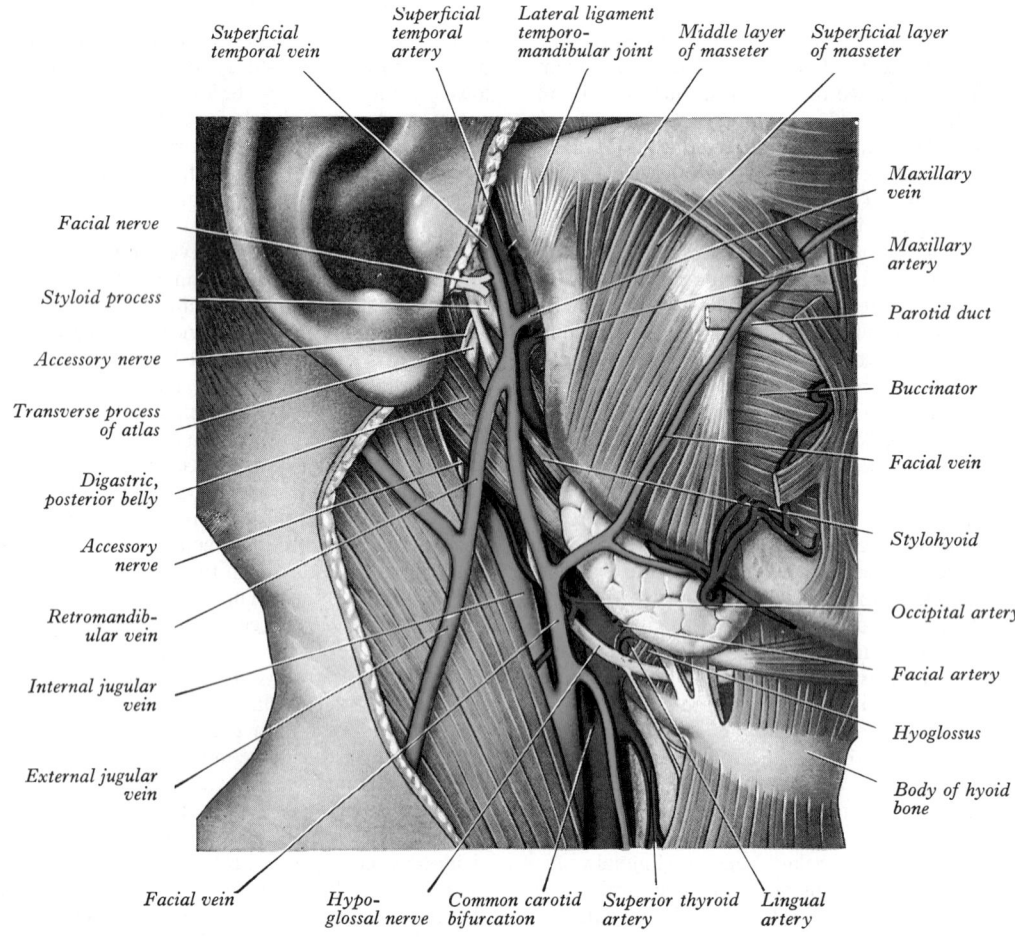

7.67 Relations of the posterior belly of digastric, exposed by the removal of only skin, fasciae, parotid gland and cutaneous branches of the cervical plexus.

Mylohyoid

Mylohyoid (**7.58, 63, 66**) lies superior to the anterior belly of digastric and, with its contralateral fellow, forms a muscular floor for the oral cavity. It is a flat, triangular sheet attached to the whole length of the mylohyoid line of the mandible. The posterior fibres pass medially and slightly downwards to the front of the body of the hyoid bone near its lower border. The middle and anterior fibres from each side decussate in a median fibrous raphe which stretches from the symphysis menti to the hyoid bone.

Variations. The median raphe is sometimes absent, in which case the two muscles form a continuous sheet. Sometimes mylohyoid is fused with the anterior belly of digastric. In about one-third of subjects there is a hiatus in the muscle through which a process of the sublingual gland protrudes (Gaughran 1963).

Relations. The **inferior (external) surface** is related to platysma, the anterior belly of digastric, the superficial part of the submandibular gland, the facial and submental vessels, and the mylohyoid vessels and nerve. The **superior (internal) surface** is related to geniohyoid, part of hyoglossus, styloglossus, the hypoglossal and lingual nerves, the submandibular ganglion, the sublingual gland, the deep part of the submandibular gland and its duct, the lingual and sublingual vessels and, posteriorly, with the mucous membrane of the mouth.

Nerve supply. The mylohyoid branch of the inferior alveolar nerve.

Actions. The muscle elevates the floor of the mouth in the first stage of deglutition (Whillis 1946). It may also elevate the hyoid bone or depress the mandible.

Geniohyoid

Geniohyoid (**7.58**) is a narrow muscle lying above the medial part of mylohyoid. It arises from the inferior mental spine on the back of the symphysis menti, runs backwards and slightly downwards, and attaches to the anterior surface of the body of the hyoid bone. The paired muscles are contiguous and may occasionally fuse with each other or with genioglossus.

Nerve supply. First cervical spinal nerve, through the hypoglossal nerve (p. 1256).

Actions. Geniohyoid elevates the hyoid bone and draws it forwards; it therefore acts partly as an antagonist to stylohyoid. When the hyoid is fixed, it depresses the mandible.

INFRAHYOID MUSCLES

The infrahyoid muscles are sternohyoid, sternothyroid, thyrohyoid and omohyoid. As a group they may be regarded as antagonists to the suprahyoid group, since they depress the hyoid bone. However, the suprahyoid and infrahyoid muscles also act together to stabilize the hyoid bone, which then serves as a fixed base for the action of muscles of the tongue attached to it. In addition the two groups may co-operate in cyclic movements of the hyoid. The actions of these muscles in deglutition are described on page 1732.

Sternohyoid

Sternohyoid (**7.63, 66**), a thin, narrow strap muscle, arises from the posterior surface of the medial end of the clavicle, the posterior sternoclavicular ligament and the upper posterior aspect of the manubrium sterni. It ascends medially and is attached to the inferior border of the body of the hyoid bone. Below, there is a considerable gap between the muscle and its contralateral fellow, but the two usually come together in the middle of their course, and are contiguous above this.

Variations. Sternohyoid may be absent or double, augmented by a clavicular slip (*cleidohyoid*), or interrupted by a tendinous intersection.

Nerve supply. Branches from the ansa cervicalis (C1, 2, 3).

Action. Sternohyoid depresses the hyoid bone after it has been elevated in deglutition. It would also be expected to play a part in speech and mastication.

Sternothyroid

Sternothyroid (**7.66**) is shorter and wider than sternohyoid, and lies deep and partly medial to it. It arises from the posterior surface of the manubrium sterni, inferior to the origin of sternohyoid, and from the posterior edge of the cartilage of the first rib. It is attached above to the oblique line on the lamina of the thyroid cartilage. In the lower part of the neck the muscle is in contact with its contralateral fellow, but the two diverge as they ascend. It is applied to the anterolateral surface of the thyroid gland.

Nerve supply. Branches from the ansa cervicalis (C1, 2, 3).

Action. Sternothyroid draws the larynx downwards after it has been elevated by, for example, swallowing or vocal movements. In the singing of low notes, this downward traction would be exerted with the hyoid bone relatively fixed.

Thyrohyoid

Thyrohyoid, a small, quadrilateral muscle, may be regarded as an upward continuation of sternothyroid. From the oblique line on the lamina of the thyroid cartilage it passes upwards and is attached to the lower border of the greater cornu and adjacent part of the body of the hyoid bone.

Nerve supply. A branch of the hypoglossal nerve. Like the nerve to geniohyoid, this branch contains fibres of the first cervical spinal nerve.

Actions. Thyrohyoid depresses the hyoid bone. With the hyoid bone stabilized, it pulls the larynx upwards—for example, when high notes are sung. These actions can be produced in varying combinations.

Omohyoid

Omohyoid (**7.63, 66**) consists of two bellies united at an angle by an intermediate tendon. It arises from the upper border of the scapula, near the scapular notch, and occasionally from the superior transverse scapular ligament (p. 618). The *inferior belly* is a flat, narrow band, which inclines forwards and slightly upwards across the lower part of the neck; it then passes behind sternocleidomastoid and ends there in the intermediate tendon. The inferior belly divides the posterior triangle of the neck into upper (occipital) and lower (supraclavicular) triangles (p. 1521). The *superior belly* begins at the intermediate tendon, passes almost vertically upwards near the lateral border of sternohyoid, and is attached to the lower border of the body of the hyoid bone, lateral to the insertion of sternohyoid. The intermediate tendon varies in length and form; it usually lies adjacent to the internal jugular vein, opposite the arch of the cricoid cartilage. The angulated course of the muscle is maintained by a band of deep cervical fascia, attached below to the clavicle and the first rib, which ensheathes the tendon.

Variations. A variable amount of skeletal muscle may be present in the fascial band. Either belly may be absent or double. The inferior belly may be attached directly to the clavicle; the superior is sometimes fused with sternohyoid. These variations have been confirmed by Buntine (1970).

Nerve supply. Superior belly: branches from the ramus superior of the ansa cervicalis (C1). *Inferior belly*: the ansa cervicalis itself (C2, 3).

Actions. Omohyoid depresses the hyoid bone after it has been elevated. It has been speculated that the muscle tenses the lower part of the deep cervical fascia in prolonged inspiratory efforts, reducing the tendency for soft parts to be sucked inward. Electromyographic data for the hyoid musculature as a whole have been sparse.

ANTERIOR VERTEBRAL MUSCLES

The anterior vertebral group of muscles includes longi colli and capitis and recti capitis anterior and lateralis, all to some extent flexors of the head and neck (**7.68**).

Longus colli

Longus colli is applied to the anterior surface of the vertebral column, between the atlas and the third thoracic vertebra. It can be divided into three parts: inferior oblique, superior oblique and vertical; all are attached by tendinous slips. The *inferior oblique part* is the smallest; it runs upwards and laterally from the fronts of the bodies of the first two or three thoracic vertebrae to the anterior tubercles of the transverse processes of the fifth and sixth cervical vertebrae. The *superior oblique part* passes upwards and medially

807

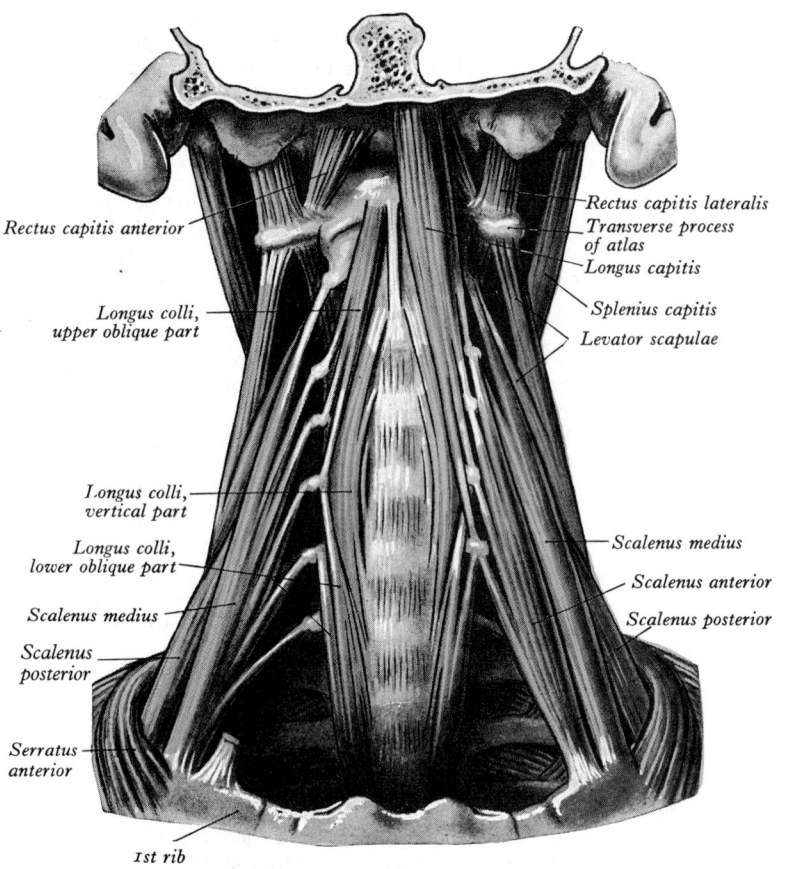

7.68 The anterior and lateral vertebral muscles. Scalenus anterior and longus capitis have been removed on the subject's right side.

Labels on figure:
Rectus capitis anterior
Longus colli, upper oblique part
Longus colli, vertical part
Longus colli, lower oblique part
Scalenus medius
Scalenus posterior
Serratus anterior
1st rib
Rectus capitis lateralis
Transverse process of atlas
Longus capitis
Splenius capitis
Levator scapulae
Scalenus medius
Scalenus anterior
Scalenus posterior

from the anterior tubercles of the transverse processes of the third, fourth and fifth cervical vertebrae to be attached by a narrow tendon to the anterolateral surface of the tubercle on the anterior arch of the atlas. The *vertical intermediate part* ascends from the fronts of the bodies of the upper three thoracic and lower three cervical vertebrae to the fronts of the bodies of the second, third and fourth cervical vertebrae.

Nerve supply. Branches from the ventral rami of the second, third, fourth, fifth and sixth cervical spinal nerves.

Actions. Longus colli flexes the neck forwards; in addition, the oblique parts flex it laterally, and the inferior oblique part rotates it to the opposite side. Despite its deep situation the muscle has been studied electromyographically (Fountain et al 1966); the findings confirmed much of the above, but called into question the role of longus colli in lateral flexion. Its main antagonist is longissimus cervicis.

Longus capitis

Longus capitis is broad and thick above, where it is attached to the inferior surface of the basilar part of the occipital bone, and narrow below, where it is attached by tendinous slips to the anterior tubercules of the transverse processes of the third, fourth, fifth and sixth cervical vertebrae.

Variations. Both longus capitis and longus colli vary chiefly in the number of their vertebral slips.

Nerve supply. Branches from the ventral rami of the first, second and third cervical spinal nerves.

Actions. Longus capitis flexes the head.

Rectus capitis anterior

Rectus capitis anterior is a short, flat muscle situated behind the upper part of longus capitis. It arises from the anterior surface of the lateral mass of the atlas and the root of its transverse process, and ascends almost vertically to the inferior surface of the basilar part of the occipital bone immediately anterior to the occipital condyle.

Nerve supply. Branches from the loop between the ventral rami of the first and second cervical spinal nerves.

Action. Rectus capitis anterior flexes the head at the atlanto-occipital joints.

Rectus capitis lateralis

Rectus capitis lateralis is a short, flat muscle which arises from the upper surface of the transverse process of the atlas and inserts into the inferior surface of the jugular process of the occipital bone. In view of its attachments and its relation to the ventral ramus of the first spinal nerve. rectus capitis lateralis is regarded as homologous with the posterior intertransverse muscles.

Nerve supply. Branches from the loop between the ventral rami of the first and second cervical spinal nerves.

Action. Rectus capitis lateralis flexes the head laterally to the same side.

The actions of these deep-seated muscles can only be deduced, and their precise roles in normal activity remain to be demonstrated in a technically satisfactory way.

LATERAL VERTEBRAL MUSCLES

The scaleni—anterior, medius and posterior—extend obliquely like ladders (Latin *scala* = ladder) between the upper two ribs and the cervical transverse processes (**7**.68).

Scalenus anterior

Scalenus anterior lies at the side of the neck deep (posteromedial) to sternocleidomastoid. Above, it is attached by musculotendinous fascicles to the anterior tubercles of the transverse processes of the third, fourth, fifth and sixth cervical vertebrae. These converge, blend and descend almost vertically, to be attached by a narrow, flat tendon to the scalene tubercle on the inner border of the first rib, and to a ridge on the upper surface of the rib anterior to the groove for the subclavian artery.

Relations. **Anterior** are the clavicle, subclavius, sternocleido-mastoid, omohyoid, the lateral part of the carotid sheath, the transverse cervical, suprascapular and ascending cervical arteries, the subclavian vein, the prevertebral fascia and the phrenic nerve. **Posterior** are the suprapleural membrane (p. 1663), the pleura, the roots of the brachial plexus and the subclavian artery; the latter two separate the muscle from scalenus medius. Below its attachment to the sixth cervical vertebra, the medial border of the muscle is separated from longus colli by an *angular interval* (**7**.68) in which the vertebral artery and vein ascend to reach the foramen transversarium of the sixth cervical vertebra. The inferior thyroid artery crosses the interval from the lateral to the medial side near its apex. The sympathetic trunk and its cervicothoracic ganglion are closely related to the posteromedial side of this part of the vertebral artery (**10**.68). On the left side the thoracic duct crosses this triangular interval at the level of the seventh cervical vertebra and usually comes into contact with the medial edge of scalenus anterior. The musculotendinous attachments of scalenus anterior to anterior tubercles are separated from those of longus capitis by the ascending cervical branch of the inferior thyroid artery.

Nerve supply. Branches from the ventral rami of the fourth, fifth and sixth cervical spinal nerves.

Actions. Acting from below, scalenus anterior bends the cervical portion of the vertebral column forwards and laterally and rotates it towards the opposite side. Acting from above, the muscle helps to elevate the first rib.

Clinical relevance. The proximity of the muscle to the lower brachial plexus, subclavian artery and vein can give rise to compression syndromes (Katirji & Hardy 1995).

Scalenus medius

Scalenus medius, the largest and longest of the scaleni, is attached above to the transverse process of the axis and the front of the posterior tubercles of the transverse processes of the lower five cervical vertebrae, and frequently extends upwards to the transverse process of the atlas (**7**.66). Below it is attached to the upper surface of the first rib, between the tubercle of the rib and the groove for the subclavian artery.

Relations. The anterolateral surface of the muscle is related to sternocleidomastoid; it is crossed by the clavicle and omohyoid; anteriorly, it is separated from scalenus anterior by the subclavian artery and ventral rami of the cervical spinal nerves. Levator scapulae and scalenus posterior are posterolateral to it. The upper two roots of the nerve to serratus anterior and the dorsal scapular nerve (to the rhomboids) pierce the muscle and appear on its lateral surface.

Nerve supply. Branches from the ventral rami of the third to eighth cervical spinal nerves.

Actions. Acting from below, scalenus medius bends the cervical part of the vertebral column to the same side; acting from above, it helps to raise the first rib. The scalene muscles, particularly scalenus medius, are active during inspiration, even during quiet breathing in the erect attitude (Campbell 1955).

Scalenus posterior

Scalenus posterior, the smallest and most deeply situated of the scaleni, passes from the posterior tubercles of the transverse processes of the fourth, fifth, and sixth cervical vertebrae to the outer surface of the second rib, behind the tubercle for serratus anterior, where it is attached by a thin tendon.

Variations. Scalenus posterior is occasionally blended with scalenus medius. The scalene muscles vary a little in the number of vertebrae to which they are attached, in their degree of separation, and their segmental innervation.

Nerve supply. Branches from the ventral rami of the lower three cervical spinal nerves.

Actions. When the second rib is fixed, scalenus posterior bends the lower end of the cervical part of the vertebral column to the same side. When its upper attachment is fixed, it helps to elevate the second rib.

Scalenus minimus (*pleuralis*)

Scalenus minimus (pleuralis) is associated with the suprapleural membrane and cervical pleura, and is considered in that context (p. 1663).

MUSCLES AND FASCIAE OF THE TRUNK

For purposes of description it is convenient to consider the muscles of the trunk in six groups:

- Deep muscles of the back
- Suboccipital muscles
- Muscles of the thorax
- Muscles of the abdomen
- Muscles of the pelvis
- Muscles of the perineum.

These will be discussed together with the associated fasciae.

DEEP MUSCLES OF THE BACK

The deep or intrinsic muscles of the back are a complex group extending from the pelvis to the skull. They include extensors and rotators of the head and neck (splenius capitis and cervicis), short segmental muscles (interspinales and intertransversarii), and extensors and rotators of the spine (erector spinae and transversospinalis, the latter comprising semispinales, rotatores and multifidus). Collectively these muscles control the vertebral column (7.69).

Superficial and *deep fasciae* of the neck are described on page 802.

A note on blood supply. The deep muscles of the back receive their blood supply from the following arteries: vertebral artery (p. 1530); deep cervical artery (p. 1536); superficial and deep descending branches of the occipital artery (p. 1519); deep branch of the transverse cervical artery, when present; superior intercostal artery via dorsal rami of upper two posterior intercostal arteries (p. 1535); posterior intercostal arteries of lower nine spaces via dorsal rami (p. 1546); dorsal branches of the subcostal arteries (p. 1546); dorsal branches of the lumbar arteries (p. 1558); dorsal branch of arteria lumbalis ima (p. 1558); dorsal branches of the lateral sacral arteries (p. 1562).

Thoracolumbar (lumbar) fascia

The thoracolumbar (lumbar) fascia covers the deep muscles of the back and the trunk. **Above**, it passes anterior to the serratus posterior superior and is continuous with the superficial lamina of the deep cervical fascia on the back of the neck. In the **thoracic region** the thoracolumbar fascia provides a thin fibrous covering for the extensor muscles of the vertebral column and separates them from the muscles connecting the vertebral column to the upper extremity. **Medially**, it is attached to the spines of the thoracic vertebrae; **laterally**, to the angles of the ribs. In the **lumbar region** the thoracolumbar fascia is in three layers (7.70). The *posterior layer* is attached to the spines of the lumbar and sacral vertebrae and to the supraspinous ligaments. The *middle layer* is attached **medially** to the tips of the transverse processes of the lumbar vertebrae and the intertransverse ligaments, **below** to the iliac crest, and **above** to the lower border of the twelfth rib and the lumbocostal ligament (p. 543). The *anterior layer* covers the quadratus lumborum and is attached **medially** to the anterior surfaces of the transverse processes of the lumbar vertebrae behind the lateral part of psoas major; **below**, it is attached to the iliolumbar ligament and the adjoining part of the iliac crest; **above**, it forms the lateral arcuate ligament (p. 816). The posterior and middle layers unite at the lateral margin of erector spinae, and at the lateral border of quadratus lumborum they are joined by the anterior layer to form the aponeurotic origin of transversus abdominis.

Splenius capitis

Splenius capitis (7.91) arises from the dorsal edge of the lower half of the ligamentum nuchae, the spines of the seventh cervical and upper 3–4 thoracic vertebrae, and their supraspinous ligaments (deep to rhomboids and trapezius). The muscle passes upwards and laterally under cover of sternocleidomastoid to be attached to the mastoid process and the rough surface on the occipital bone just below the lateral third of the superior nuchal line. The muscle forms part of the floor of the posterior triangle of the neck, above and behind levator scapulae.

Nerve supply. Lateral branches of the dorsal rami of the middle cervical spinal nerves.

Splenius cervicis

Splenius cervicis ascends from the spines of the third to the sixth thoracic vertebrae to the posterior tubercles of the transverse processes of the upper 2–3 cervical vertebrae immediately anterior to the attachment of levator scapulae.

Variations. The splenii may be absent or vary in their vertebral attachments. Accessory slips also occur.

Nerve supply. Lateral branches of the dorsal rami of the lower cervical spinal nerves.

Actions. Acting together, the splenii of the two sides draw the head directly backwards. Acting separately, they draw the head to one side, and rotate it slightly, turning the face to the same side. Each is therefore synergistic with the contralateral sternocleidomastoid.

ERECTOR SPINAE (SACROSPINALIS)

The erector spinae muscle complex, and its prolongations into thoracic and cervical levels, lies in a groove on the side of the vertebral column (7.69), covered in the lumbar and thoracic regions by the thoracolumbar fascia, serratus posterior inferior below and rhomboids and splenii above. It forms a large musculotendinous mass, which varies in size and composition at different levels of the vertebral column. In the sacral region it is narrow and U-shaped, and becomes increasingly tendinous—and very strong—as it

809

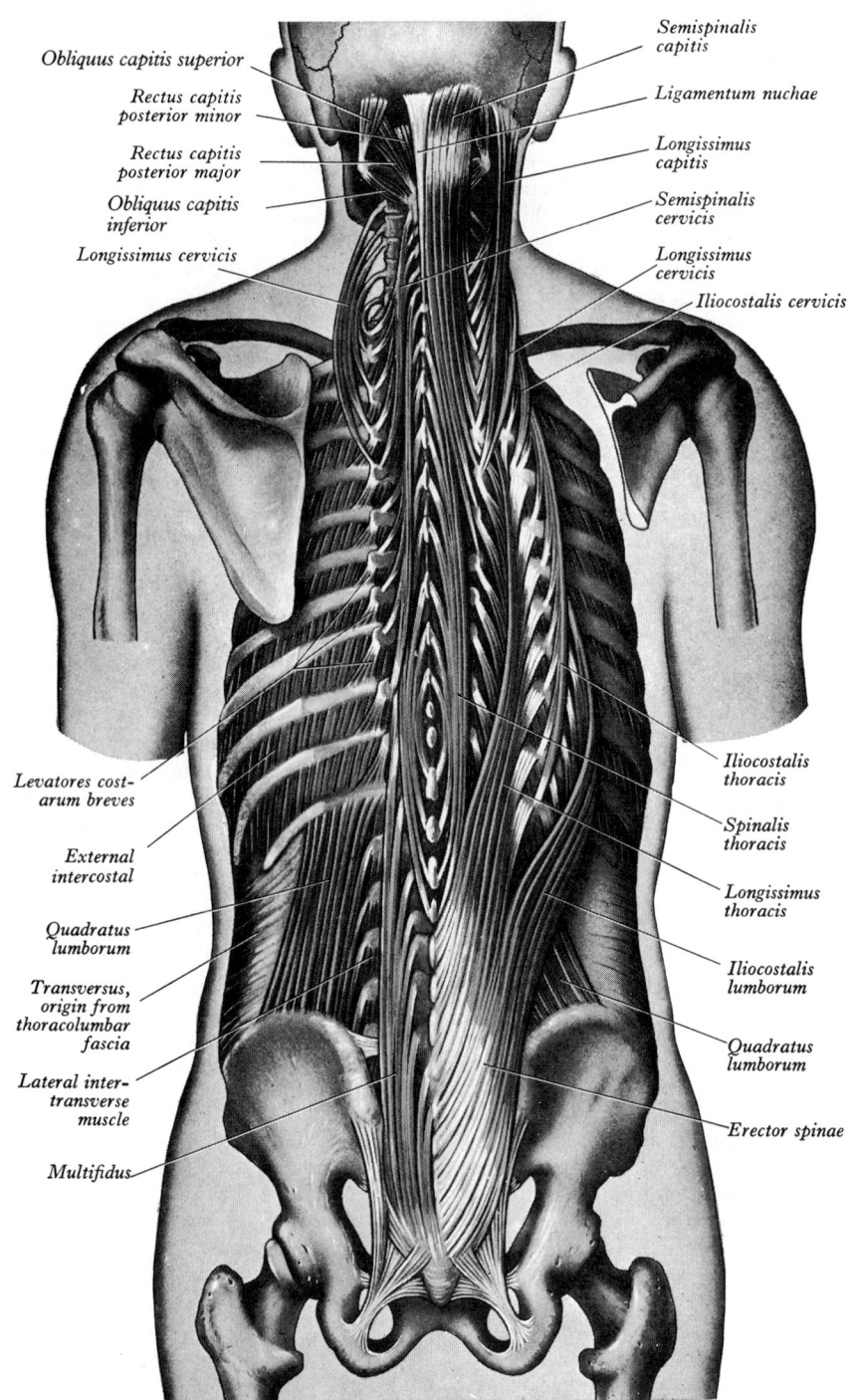

Obliquus capitis superior

Rectus capitis posterior minor

Rectus capitis posterior major

Obliquus capitis inferior

Longissimus cervicis

Semispinalis capitis

Ligamentum nuchae

Longissimus capitis

Semispinalis cervicis

Longissimus cervicis

Iliocostalis cervicis

Levatores cost- arum breves

External intercostal

Quadratus lumborum

Transversus, origin from thoracolumbar fascia

Lateral inter- transverse muscle

Multifidus

Iliocostalis thoracis

Spinalis thoracis

Longissimus thoracis

Iliocostalis lumborum

Quadratus lumborum

Erector spinae

7.69 The deep muscles of the back. On the left side erector spinae and its upward continuations (with the exception of longissimus cervicis, which has been displaced laterally) and semispinalis capitis have been removed.

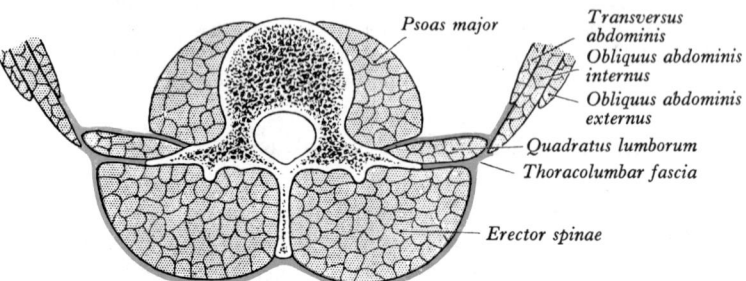

Psoas major

Transversus abdominis

Obliquus abdominis internus

Obliquus abdominis externus

Quadratus lumborum

Thoracolumbar fascia

Erector spinae

7.70 Transverse section through the posterior abdominal wall, showing the disposition of the thoracolumbar fascia. All other connective tissue strata have been omitted.

approaches its attachments. In the lumbar region it expands to form a thick fleshy mass which can readily be felt in the living subject. Its lateral border is flanked by a visible groove (**7.71**), which ascends over the back of the thorax, traversing the ribs at their angles and running first laterally, then vertically, and finally medially until it is obscured by the scapula.

Erector spinae arises from the anterior surface of a broad, thick tendon, which is attached (on the medial limb of the U) to the median sacral crest, the spines of the lumbar and the eleventh and twelfth thoracic vertebrae, their supraspinous ligaments, and (on the lateral limb of the U) the medial aspect of the dorsal part of the iliac crest (p. 664), and the lateral sacral crests (p. 529), where it blends with the sacrotuberous and dorsal sacro-iliac ligaments. Some of its fibres are continuous with gluteus maximus and multifidus. Muscle fibres arise from all aspects of the tendon and form a large fleshy mass which divides in the upper lumbar region into three columns: lateral, *iliocostocervicalis*; intermediate, *longissimus*; and medial, *spinalis*. Each of these is regionally subdivided into three parts as follows:

Iliocostocervicalis	Longissimus	Spinalis
Iliocostalis lumborum	Longissimus thoracis	Spinalis thoracis
Iliocostalis thoracis	Longissimus cervicis	Spinalis cervicis
Iliocostalis cervicis	Longissimus capitis	Spinalis capitis

Iliocostalis lumborum

Iliocostalis lumborum is attached, by flattened tendons, to the inferior borders of the angles of the lower six or seven ribs.

Iliocostalis thoracis

Iliocostalis thoracis starts from the upper borders of the angles of the lower six ribs medial to the tendons of insertion of iliocostalis lumborum; it ascends to the superior borders of the angles of the upper six ribs and the back of the transverse process of the seventh cervical vertebra.

Iliocostalis cervicis

Iliocostalis cervicis ascends from the angles of the third to the sixth ribs, medial to the tendons of insertion of iliocostalis thoracis, to the posterior tubercles of the transverse processes of the fourth, fifth and sixth cervical vertebrae.

Nerve supply. Dorsal rami of the lower cervical, thoracic and upper lumbar spinal nerves.

Actions. Extension and also lateral flexion of the vertebral column (p. 812).

Longissimus thoracis

Longissimus thoracis is the largest of the continuations of the erector spinae. In the lumbar region, where it blends with the iliocostalis lumborum, some of its fibres are attached to the whole length of the posterior surfaces of the transverse processes and the accessory processes of the lumbar vertebrae, and to the middle layer of the thoracolumbar fascia. In the thoracic region it is attached, by rounded tendons, to the tips of the transverse processes of all the thoracic vertebrae, and by fleshy slips to the lower nine or ten ribs between their tubercles and angles.

Longissimus cervicis

Longissimus cervicis lies medial to longissimus thoracis. It is attached by long thin tendons to the transverse processes of the upper four or five thoracic vertebrae, and again by tendons to the posterior tubercles of the transverse processes of the second to the sixth cervical vertebrae.

Longissimus capitis

Longissimus capitis lies between longissimus cervicis and semispinalis capitis. It arises by tendons from the transverse processes of the upper four or five thoracic vertebrae, and the articular processes of the lower three or four cervical vertebrae, and inserts into the posterior margin of the mastoid process, deep to splenius capitis and sternocleidomastoid. It is usually traversed by a tendinous intersection near its upper end.

Nerve supply. Dorsal rami of the lower cervical, thoracic and lumbar spinal nerves.

Actions. Longissimi thoracis and cervicis bend the vertebral column backwards and laterally; longissimus capitis extends the head, and turns the face towards the same side as the muscle.

Spinalis thoracis

Spinalis thoracis, the medial continuation of erector spinae, is barely separable as a distinct muscle. It lies medial to longissimus thoracis, and blends intimately with it. It arises below by three or four tendons from the eleventh thoracic to the second lumbar vertebral spines; these unite in a small muscle which is attached above by separate tendons to the spines of the upper thoracic vertebrae, the number varying from four to eight. It blends closely with semispinalis thoracis, which lies anterior to it.

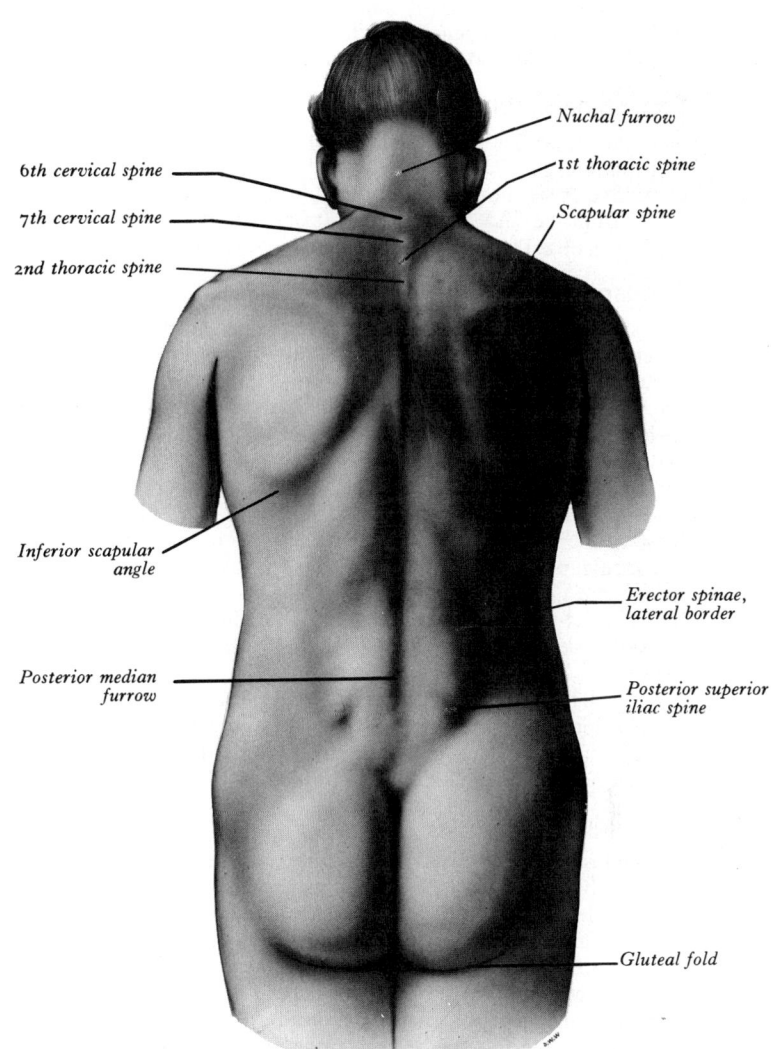

7.71 Dorsal view of the trunk, showing principal surface landmarks.

Spinalis cervicis

Spinalis cervicis, when it is present, ascends from the lower part of the ligamentum nuchae and the spine of the seventh cervical vertebra (and sometimes the first and second thoracic vertebrae) to the spine of the axis, and occasionally to the spines of the two vertebrae immediately below it. It is often absent.

Spinalis capitis

Spinalis capitis usually blends to some extent with semispinalis capitis (see below), but can be morphologically separate (Martin 1994).

Nerve supply. Dorsal rami of the lower cervical and thoracic spinal nerves.

Actions. Extension of the vertebral column.

TRANSVERSOSPINALIS

The transversospinalis muscular group consists of the following:

Semispinalis thoracis	Multifidus	Rotatores thoracis
Semispinalis cervicis		Rotatores cervicis
Semispinalis capitis		Rotatores lumborum

These muscles run obliquely upwards and medially from transverse processes to adjacent, and sometimes more distant, spinous processes.

Semispinalis thoracis

Semispinalis thoracis consists of thin, fleshy fasciculi interposed between long tendons. It arises below by a series of tendons from the transverse processes of the sixth to the tenth thoracic vertebrae,

811

and inserts above, again by tendons, into the spines of the upper four thoracic and lower two cervical vertebrae.

Semispinalis cervicis

Semispinalis cervicis (7.69), a thicker muscle, arises below by a series of tendinous and fleshy fibres from the transverse processes of the upper five or six thoracic vertebrae; it inserts above into the cervical spines from the fifth to the second (axis). The fasciculus connected with the axis is the largest, and is composed chiefly of muscle.

Semispinalis capitis

Semispinalis capitis (7.69) is situated at the back of the neck, under cover of the splenius and medial to longissimi cervicis and capitis. It arises by a series of tendons from the tips of the transverse processes of the upper six or seven thoracic and seventh cervical vertebrae, from the articular processes of the fourth, fifth, and sixth cervical vertebrae and, occasionally, from the spine of the seventh cervical or first thoracic vertebra. The tendons come together in a broad muscle, which passes upwards to the medial part of the area between the superior and inferior nuchal lines of the occipital bone. The medial part of the muscle, which is usually more or less distinct from the rest, is called *spinalis capitis*, and sometimes *biventer cervicis*, because it is traversed by an incomplete tendinous intersection.

Nerve supply. Dorsal rami of the cervical and thoracic spinal nerves.

Actions. Semispinales thoracis and cervicis extend the thoracic and cervical regions of the vertebral column, and rotate them towards the opposite side; semispinalis capitis extends the head, and turns the face slightly towards the opposite side.

Multifidus

Multifidus (7.69) consists of a number of fleshy and tendinous fasciculi lying deep to the foregoing muscles and filling the groove at the side of the spines of the vertebrae from the sacrum to the axis. Its fasciculi arise as follows: most caudally, from the back of the sacrum as low as the fourth sacral foramen, from the aponeurosis of the erector spinae, the posterior superior iliac spine and dorsal sacro-iliac ligaments; in the lumbar region, from all the mamillary processes; in the thoracic region, from all the transverse processes; in the cervical region, from the articular processes of the lower four vertebrae. Each fasciculus passes obliquely upwards and medially, and is attached to the whole length of the spine of one of the vertebrae above. The fasciculi vary in length: the most superficial pass from one vertebra to the third or fourth above; those next in depth run from one vertebra to the second or third above; the deepest connect contiguous vertebrae.

Nerve supply. Dorsal rami of the spinal nerves.

The *rotatores* lie deep to multifidus and are fully developed only in the thoracic region.

Rotatores thoracis

Rotatores thoracis consists of eleven pairs of small, roughly quadri-lateral muscles. Each connects the upper and posterior part of the transverse process of one vertebra to the lower border and lateral surface of the lamina of the vertebra immediately above. The first is found between the first and second thoracic vertebrae; the last between the eleventh and twelfth. One or more may be absent from the upper or lower ends of the series.

Rotatores cervicis and lumborum

Rotatores cervicis and lumborum are represented only by irregular and variable muscle bundles, whose attachments are similar to those of rotatores thoracis.

Nerve supply. Dorsal rami of the spinal nerves.

Interspinales

Interspinales are short paired muscular fasciculi attached above and below to the apices of the spines of contiguous vertebrae, one on either side of the interspinous ligament. They are most distinct in the cervical region, where they consist of six pairs, the first between the axis and third vertebra, and the last between the seventh cervical and first thoracic vertebrae. In the thoracic region they occur between the first and second vertebrae—sometimes between the second and

third—and the eleventh and twelfth vertebrae. In the lumbar region there are four pairs between the five lumbar vertebrae. A pair is occasionally found between the last thoracic and first lumbar vertebrae, and another between the fifth lumbar vertebra and the sacrum. Sometimes cervical interspinales span more than two vertebrae.

Nerve supply. Dorsal rami of the spinal nerves.

Intertransversarii

Intertransversarii are small muscles between the transverse processes of the vertebrae. They are best developed in the **cervical** region, where they consist of posterior and anterior sets of muscles separated by the ventral rami of spinal nerves. *Posterior intertransverse muscles* are divisible into medial and lateral slips, which are supplied by the dorsal and ventral rami of the spinal nerves, respectively. Each **medial** slip, the intertransverse muscle 'proper', is often further subdivided into medial and lateral parts by the passage through it of a dorsal spinal nerve ramus. *Anterior intertransverse muscles* and **lateral** parts of the posterior muscles connect the costal processes of contiguous vertebrae; **medial** parts of the posterior muscles connect true transverse processes. There are seven pairs of these muscles, the highest between the atlas and axis, and the lowest between the seventh cervical vertebra and the first thoracic, but the anterior muscles between atlas and axis are often absent. In the **thoracic** region they consist of single muscles, which are present between the transverse processes of only the last three thoracic and first lumbar vertebrae. In the **lumbar** region they again consist of two sets of muscles. One set, *intertransversarii mediales*, connect the accessory process of one vertebra with the mamillary process of the next. The other set, *intertransversarii laterales*, can be divided into ventral and dorsal parts (Cave 1937; Morrison 1954): ventral parts connect the transverse processes (costal elements) of the lumbar vertebrae; dorsal parts connect the accessory processes to the transverse processes of succeeding vertebrae.

Thoracic intertransverse muscles and ligaments are homologous with the medial slips of the 'proper' posterior intertransverse muscles of the cervical region; *levatores costarum* (see p. 815) are homologous with their lateral slips. The lateral branch of a dorsal spinal nerve ramus separates thoracic intertransverse from levator costae muscles. The lumbar levatores costarum are represented by the medial intertransverse muscles; the lateral intertransverse are homologous with the intercostal muscles. For other views on the homologies and classification of transversospinal musculature consult Sato (1973a).

Nerve supply. Lumbar intertransversarii mediales, thoracic intertransversarii and medial parts of cervical posterior intertransversarii are supplied by dorsal rami of the spinal nerves; the others are supplied by ventral rami.

Actions. The short muscles of the back probably function, for the most part, as postural muscles. The vertebral column consists, in effect, of a series of short, jointed levers. A mechanical arrangement of this type is unstable under compression and will tend to buckle unless movement at the individual joints is controlled. The short muscles may serve to stabilize adjoining vertebrae, controlling their movement during motion of the vertebral column as a whole, and providing for more effective action of the long muscles. In theory, the short muscles could produce extension (multifidus, spinales), lateral flexion (multifidus, intertransversarii) and rotation (multifidus and rotatores), but their detailed patterns of activity are not known. The deep muscles of the back are certainly involved in the control of posture: they contract intermittently during the swaying movements that take place from an upright position. Contraction of the erectores spinae extends the trunk, a movement controlled largely by opposing activity of the rectus abdominis muscles. Conversely, flexion of the trunk is initiated by flexor muscles such as the recti abdominis, and as the centre of gravity moves forward control is transferred to the erectores spinae. Lateral flexion is controlled by the contralateral erector spinae. When the trunk is fully flexed the erectores spinae are relaxed and electromyographically quiet; in this position, flexion may be limited by passive forces generated by tension in the spinal ligaments and resistance to deformation of the intervertebral discs (Floyd & Silver 1955; Joseph 1960). As would be expected, electromyographic activity in the erector spinae group is greater when work is carried out on a low surface from a standing position (Jonsson 1974).

SUBOCCIPITAL MUSCLES

Small suboccipital muscles (**7.72**) are involved in extension of the head at the atlanto-occipital joints (recti capitis posteriores major and minor) and rotation of the head and atlas on the axis (obliqui capitis superior and inferior).

Blood supply. The suboccipital muscles receive their blood supply from the vertebral artery (pp. 1530, 1532) and deep descending branches of the occipital artery (p. 1517).

Rectus capitis posterior major

Rectus capitis posterior major originates in a pointed tendon on the spine of the axis, becomes broader as it ascends, and attaches to the lateral part of the inferior nuchal line and the occipital bone immediately below it. As the muscles of the two sides pass upwards and laterally, they leave between them a triangular space in which parts of the recti capitis posteriores minores are visible.

Actions. Extension of the head, with rotation of the face towards the same side as the muscle.

Rectus capitis posterior minor

Rectus capitis posterior minor arises by a narrow pointed tendon from the tubercle on the posterior arch of the atlas. As it ascends it broadens before attaching to the medial part of the inferior nuchal line and also the occipital bone between the line and the foramen magnum (p. 582). Either muscle may be doubled longitudinally. An unsuspected connective tissue extension to the dura mater has been demonstrated recently for this muscle (see Thompson 1995).

Action. Extension of the head.

Obliquus capitis inferior

Obliquus capitis inferior, the larger of two oblique muscles, passes laterally and slightly upwards from the lateral surface of the spine and the adjacent upper part of the lamina of the axis to the inferoposterior aspect of the transverse process of the atlas.

Action. Rotation of the face towards the same side. By virtue of the length of the transverse process of the atlas, and the near-horizontal line of action, the muscle works with considerable mechanical advantage.

Obliquus capitis superior

Obliquus capitis superior arises by tendinous fibres from the upper surface of the transverse process of the atlas. It expands in width as it ascends dorsally, and attaches to the occipital bone between the superior and inferior nuchal lines, lateral to semispinalis capitis and overlapping the insertion of rectus capitis posterior major.

Actions. Flexion of the head backwards and to the same side. Obliquus capitis superior and the two recti are probably more important as postural muscles than as prime movers, but this is difficult to confirm by direct observation.

Nerve supply. All the suboccipital muscles are supplied by the dorsal ramus of the first cervical spinal nerve.

The suboccipital triangle

The boundaries of the suboccipital triangle are: **above** and **medially**, rectus capitis posterior major; **above** and **laterally**, obliquus capitis superior; **below** and **laterally**, obliquus capitis inferior (**7.72**). **Medially**, it is covered by a layer of dense adipose tissue, deep to semispinalis capitis; **laterally**, it lies under longissimus capitis and sometimes splenius capitis, both of which overlap obliquus capitis superior. The *'floor'* of the triangle is formed by the posterior atlanto-occipital membrane and the posterior arch of the atlas; the vertebral artery and the dorsal ramus of the first cervical nerve (**7.72**) lie in a groove on the upper surface of the posterior arch of the atlas.

MUSCLES OF THE THORAX

The thoracic group (**7.73, 74, 75**) consists of muscles that connect adjacent ribs (intercostales—externi, interni, and intimi), span several ribs between their attachments (subcostales), connect the ribs to the sternum (transversus thoracis) or to vertebrae (levatores costarum, serratus posterior superior and inferior) and the diaphragm. All are involved in producing movements of the ribs and therefore have a potential role in respiration.

A note on blood supply. Muscles of the thoracic wall receive their blood supply from the following arteries: internal thoracic artery, direct rami (p. 1534); anterior intercostal arteries, **two** to each

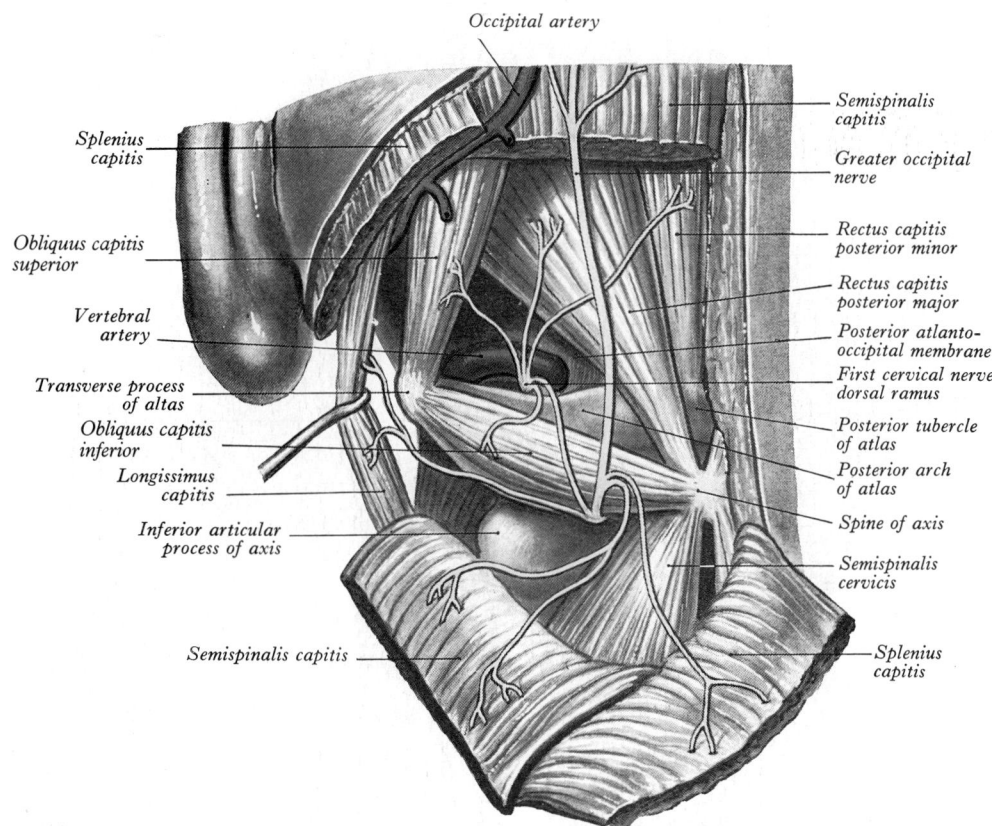

7.72 Posterior view of the left suboccipital triangle and its contents.

Occipital artery

Splenius capitis

Obliquus capitis superior

Vertebral artery

Transverse process of atlas

Obliquus capitis inferior

Longissimus capitis

Inferior articular process of axis

Semispinalis capitis

Semispinalis capitis

Greater occipital nerve

Rectus capitis posterior minor

Rectus capitis posterior major

Posterior atlanto-occipital membrane

First cervical nerve dorsal ramus

Posterior tubercle of atlas

Posterior arch of atlas

Spine of axis

Semispinalis cervicis

Splenius capitis

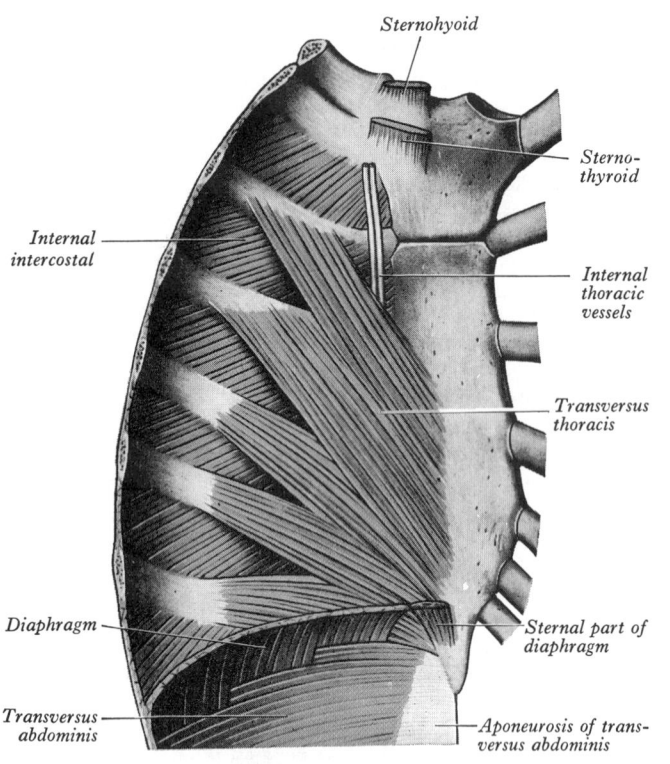

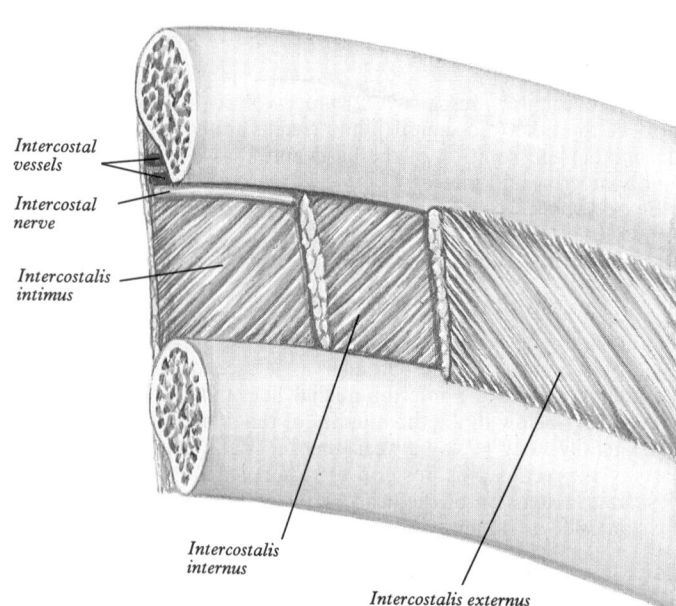

7.74   Dissection of a part of the thoracic wall, showing the position of the intercostal vessels and nerve relative to the intercostal muscles.

7.73   The left transversus thoracis, exposed and viewed from its posterior aspect. Note that, in the interval between the sternal and costal origins of the diaphragm, the lower border of transversus thoracis is in contact with the upper border of transversus abdominis.

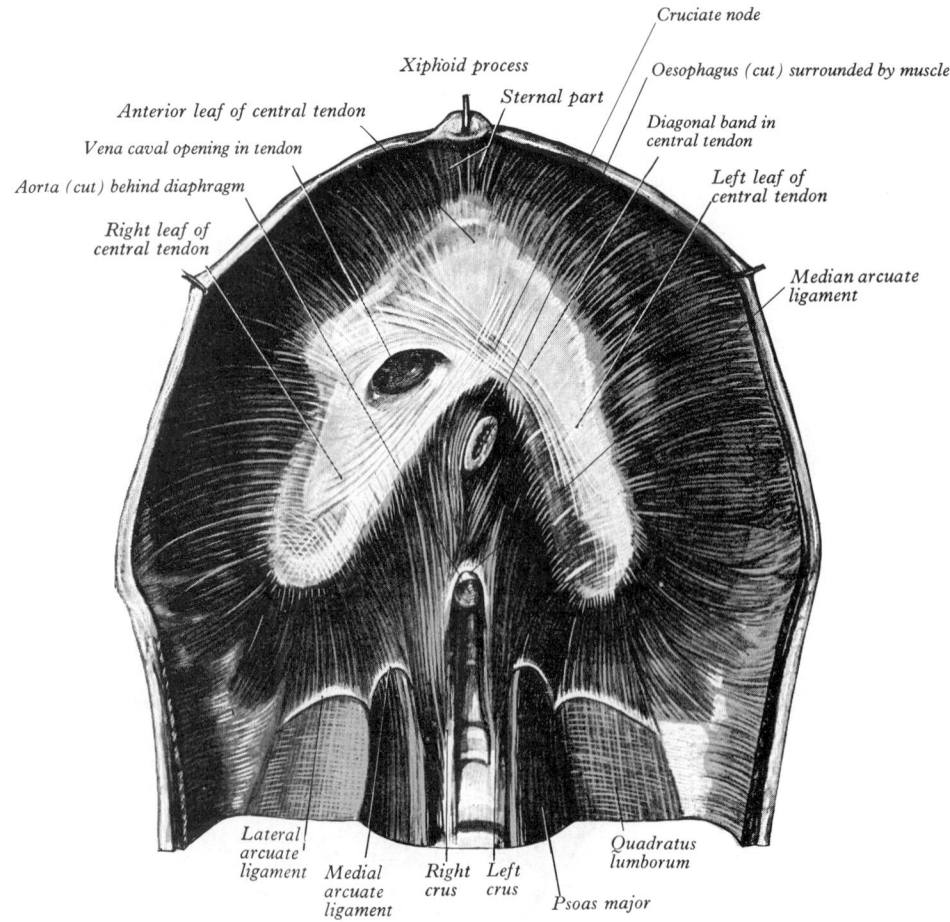

7.75   Abdominal aspect of the diaphragm. Note that the fibres descend from their relatively 'high' anterior sternocostal attachments steeply and obliquely to their complex 'low' posterior attachments.

intercostal space, upper six spaces from the internal thoracic artery (p. 1534), remaining spaces from the musculophrenic artery (p. 1534); posterior intercostal arteries, upper two spaces from superior intercostal artery (p. 1535), lower nine spaces from descending thoracic aorta (p. 1546); subcostal arteries (p. 1546); superior thoracic arteries (p. 1537). Additional contributions come from vessels noted in the context of muscles of the upper limb, namely: suprascapular artery (p. 1535); superficial cervical artery (p. 1535); thoracoacromial artery (p. 1537); lateral thoracic artery (p. 1538); subscapular artery (p. 1538). The blood supply to the diaphragm is dealt with separately (p. 1538).

Intercostales

The intercostales (7.73, 74, 81, 82) are thin multiple layers of muscular and tendinous fibres that occupy the intercostal spaces. Their names are derived from their spatial relationship—intercostales externi, interni and intimi.

Intercostales externi. Eleven pairs of these muscles extend from the tubercles of the ribs, where they blend with the posterior fibres of the superior costotransverse ligaments, almost to the costal cartilages, where each continues forwards to the sternum as an aponeurotic layer called the *external intercostal membrane*. Each muscle passes from the lower border of one rib to the upper border of the rib below. In the lower two spaces they extend to the free ends of the costal cartilages; in the upper two or three spaces they do not quite reach the ends of the ribs. They are thicker than intercostales interni. Their fibres are directed obliquely downwards and laterally at the back of the thorax, and downwards, forwards and medially at the front.

Intercostales interni. Also consisting of eleven pairs of muscles, intercostales interni begin anteriorly at the sternum, in the interspaces between the cartilages of the true ribs, and at the anterior extremities of the cartilages of the 'false' ribs. The muscles have their greatest thickness in this intercartilaginous or *parasternal* part. They continue back as far as the posterior costal angles, where each is replaced by an aponeurotic layer called the *internal intercostal membrane*. This aponeurotic membrane is continuous posteriorly with the anterior fibres of a superior costotransverse ligament, and anteriorly with the fascia between the internal and external intercostal muscles. Each of these muscles descends from the floor of a costal groove and adjacent costal cartilage, and inserts into the upper border of the rib below. Their fibres are directed obliquely nearly at right angles to those of the external intercostal muscles.

Actions. See The movements of respiration (p. 818).

Intercostales intimi. These muscles were once regarded as internal laminae of the internal intercostal muscles, and fibres in the two layers do coincide in direction. Each muscle is attached to the internal aspects of two adjoining ribs. They are insignificant, and sometimes absent, at highest thoracic levels, but become progressively more substantial below this, extending through about the middle two quarters of the lower intercostal spaces. Walmsley (1915) considered them to be in the plane of the transversus abdominis and suggested the term musculi intracostales, a view supported by Davies et al (1932). Posteriorly the intercostales intimi, in those spaces where they are well developed, may come together with the corresponding subcostales, which Davies et al regarded as a fourth layer; however, general opinion favours Walmsley's three-layered arrangement. The intercostales intimi are related internally to the endothoracic fascia and parietal pleura, and externally to the intercostal nerves and vessels.

Actions. In the absence of reliable information, these muscles are presumed to act with the internal intercostal muscles.

Subcostales

Subcostales consist of muscular and aponeurotic fasciculi, and are usually well developed only in the lower part of the thorax. Each descends from the internal surface of one rib, near its angle, to the internal surface of the second or third rib below. Their fibres run parallel to those of the internal intercostals. Like intercostales intimi they lie between the intercostal vessels and nerves and the pleura. Their incidence and distribution have been recorded by Sato (1974).

Actions. The subcostales probably depress the ribs.

Transversus thoracis

Transversus thoracis (also called *triangularis sternae* and *sternocostalis*) spreads over the internal surface of the anterior thoracic wall (7.73). It arises from the lower third of the posterior surface of the sternum, the xiphoid process, and the costal cartilages of the lower three or four true ribs near their sternal ends. Its fibres diverge and ascend laterally as slips which pass into the lower borders and inner surfaces of the costal cartilages of the second, third, fourth, fifth and sixth ribs. The lowest fibres of this muscle are horizontal, and are contiguous with the highest fibres of transversus abdominis; the intermediate fibres are oblique; the highest are almost vertical. This muscle varies in its attachments, not only between individuals but even on opposite sides of the same individual. Like intercostales intimi and subcostales, transversus thoracis separates the intercostal nerves from the pleura.

Actions. The muscle draws down the costal cartilages to which it is attached.

Nerve supply. All the above muscles are supplied by the adjacent intercostal nerves.

Levatores costarum

Levatores costarum (7.69) are strong bundles, twelve on each side, which arise from the tips of the transverse processes of the seventh cervical and 1st to 11th thoracic vertebrae. They pass obliquely downwards and laterally, parallel with the posterior borders of the external intercostals, and each is attached to the upper edge and external surface of the rib immediately below the vertebra from which it takes origin, between the tubercle and the angle (*levatores costarum breves*). Each of the four lower muscles divides into two fasciculi: one is attached as already described; the other descends to the second rib below its origin (*levatores costarum longi*).

Nerve supply. Lateral branches of the dorsal rami of the corresponding thoracic spinal nerves (Morrison 1954; Sato 1973b).

Actions. The levatores costarum elevate the ribs but their importance in respiration is disputed (Primrose 1952); they are also said to act from their costal attachments as rotators and lateral flexors of the vertebral column.

Serratus posterior superior

Serratus posterior superior is a thin, quadrilateral muscle, external to the upper posterior part of the thorax. It arises by a thin aponeurosis from the lower part of the ligamentum nuchae, the spines of the seventh cervical and upper two or three thoracic vertebrae and their supraspinous ligaments. It descends laterally, ending in four digitations attached to the upper borders and external surfaces of the second, third, fourth and fifth ribs, just lateral to their angles. It is superficial to the thoracic part of the thoracolumbar fascia and deep to the rhomboids. The number of digitations can vary from three to six, and the muscle may even be absent.

Nerve supply. Second, third, fourth and fifth intercostal nerves.

Actions. Its attachments clearly indicate that this muscle could elevate the ribs, but experiments in dogs do not support a respiratory function (Ogawa et al 1960). Its role in man is uncertain.

Serratus posterior inferior

Serratus posterior inferior (7.91) is a thin irregularly quadrilateral muscle at the junction of the thoracic and lumbar regions. It arises by a thin aponeurosis from the spines of the lower two thoracic and upper two or three lumbar vertebrae and their supraspinous ligaments; this aponeurosis blends with the lumbar part of the thoracolumbar fascia. It ascends laterally, and its four digitations pass into the inferior borders and outer surfaces of the lower four ribs, a little lateral to their angles. There may be fewer digitations and in rare cases the whole muscle may be absent.

Nerve supply. Ventral rami of the ninth, tenth, eleventh and twelfth thoracic spinal nerves.

Actions. The muscle draws the lower ribs downwards and backwards, although possibly not in respiration.

DIAPHRAGM

The diaphragm (7.75, 121) is a curved musculofibrous sheet that separates the thorax from the abdominal cavity, its mainly convex upper surface facing the former, and its concave inferior surface directed towards the latter. Its muscle fibres arise from the highly oblique circumference of the thoracic outlet, the attachments being low posteriorly and laterally, but high anteriorly. Although it is a continuous sheet the muscle can be considered to form three parts—sternal, costal and lumbar—based on the regions of peripheral attachment. The *sternal part* arises by two fleshy slips from the back of the xiphoid process; it is not always present. The *costal part* arises from the internal surfaces of the lower six costal cartilages and their adjoining ribs on each side, interdigitating with transversus abdominis (**7.73**). The *lumbar part* arises from two aponeurotic arches, the medial and lateral arcuate ligaments (sometimes termed *lumbocostal arches*) and from the lumbar vertebrae by two pillars or *crura* (sing. *crus*).

The *lateral arcuate ligament*, a thickened band in the fascia that covers quadratus lumborum, arches across the upper part of that muscle. It is attached **medially** to the front of the transverse process of the first lumbar vertebra, and **laterally** to the lower margin of the twelfth rib near its midpoint.

The *medial arcuate ligament* is a tendinous arch in the fascia that covers the upper part of psoas major. **Medially**, it is continuous with the lateral tendinous margin of the corresponding crus, and is thus attached to the side of the body of the first or second lumbar vertebra; **laterally**, it is fixed to the front of the transverse process of the first lumbar vertebra.

The *crura* are tendinous at their attachments, and blend with the anterior longitudinal ligament of the vertebral column. The *right crus* is broader and longer than the left. It arises from the antero-lateral surfaces of the bodies and intervertebral discs of the upper **three** lumbar vertebrae. The *left crus* arises from the corresponding parts of the upper **two** lumbar vertebrae. The medial tendinous margins of the crura meet in the midline to form an arch across the front of the aorta at the level of the thoracolumbar disc; this *median arcuate ligament* is often poorly defined.

From these circumferential attachments the fibres of the diaphragm converge into a central tendon. Fibres from the xiphoid process are short, and run almost horizontally; they are occasionally aponeurotic. Fibres from the medial and lateral arcuate ligaments, and more especially those from the ribs and their cartilages, are longer; they rise almost vertically at first and then curve towards their central attachment. Fibres from the crura diverge, the most lateral becoming more lateral as they ascend to the central tendon. Medial fibres of the right crus embrace the oesophagus where it passes through the diaphragm, the more superficial fibres ascending on the left and deeper fibres covering the right margin. This important structure will be returned to again (see Oesophageal aperture, below). Sometimes a fleshy fasciculus from the medial side of the left crus crosses the aorta and runs obliquely through the fibres of the right crus towards the vena caval opening, but this fasciculus does not continue upwards around the oesophageal passage on the right side (Low 1907).

The *central tendon* of the diaphragm is a thin but strong apo-neurosis of closely interwoven fibres situated near the centre of the muscle, but closer to the front of the thorax, so that the posterior muscular fibres are longer. In the centre it lies immediately below the pericardium, with which it is partially blended. Its shape is trifoliate. The middle, or anterior, leaf has the form of an equilateral triangle with the apex directed towards the xiphoid process. The right and left folia are tongue-shaped and curve laterally and back-wards, the left being a little narrower. The central area of the tendon consists of four well-marked *diagonal bands* fanning out from a thick central *node* where compressed tendinous strands decussate in front of the oesophagus and to the left of the vena cava.

The diaphragmatic apertures

Structures pass between the thorax and abdomen through apertures in the diaphragm. There are three large openings—for the aorta, the oesophagus and the vena cava (**7.75**)—and a number of smaller ones.

The *aortic aperture* is the lowest and most posterior of the large openings; it is at the level of the lower border of the twelfth thoracic vertebra and the thoracolumbar intervertebral disc, slightly to the left of the midline. It is an osseo-aponeurotic opening defined by the diaphragmatic crura laterally, the vertebral column posteriorly and the diaphragm anteriorly. Strictly speaking, therefore, it lies behind the diaphragm and its median arcuate ligament (when present).

Occasionally some tendinous fibres from the medial parts of the crura also pass **behind** the aorta, converting the opening into a fibrous ring. The aortic opening transmits the aorta and the thoracic duct and sometimes the azygos and hemiazygos veins (p. 1593); some lymphatic trunks also descend through it from the lower posterior thoracic wall.

The *oesophageal aperture* is located at the level of the tenth thoracic vertebra, above, in front, and a little to the left of the aortic opening. It transmits the oesophagus, gastric nerves, oesophageal branches of the left gastric vessels and some lymphatic vessels. The elliptical opening, whose long axis is slightly oblique, is bounded by muscle fibres that originate in the medial part of the right crus and cross the midline (Low 1907). These fibres form a chimney about 2.5 cm long, which accommodates the terminal portions of the oesophagus. The outermost fibres run in a craniocaudal direction, and the innermost fibres are arranged circumferentially (Mittal 1990). There is no direct continuity between the oesophageal wall and the muscle around the oesophageal opening. The fascia on the inferior surface of the diaphragm, which is continuous with the transversalis fascia (p. 829) and is rich in elastic fibres, extends upwards into the opening as a flattened cone to blend with the wall of the oesophagus 2 to 3 cm above the oesophagogastric (squamocolumnar) junction. Some of its elastic fibres penetrate to the submucosa of the oeso-phagus. This peri-oesophageal areolar tissue is referred to as the *phreno-oesophageal ligament*; it connects the oesophagus flexibly to the diaphragm, permitting some freedom of movement during swallowing and respiration and at the same time limiting upward displacement of the oesophagus (Allison 1951; Hayward 1961).

The *vena caval aperture*, the highest of the three large openings, lies at about the level of the disc between the eighth and ninth thoracic vertebrae. It is quadrilateral, and located at the junction of the right leaf with the central area of the tendon, so its margins are aponeurotic. It is traversed by the inferior vena cava, which adheres to the margin of the opening, and some branches of the right phrenic nerve.

There are two lesser apertures in each crus; one transmits the greater and the other the lesser splanchnic nerve. The ganglionated trunks of the sympathetic usually enter the abdominal cavity behind the diaphragm, deep to the medial arcuate ligament. Openings for minute veins frequently occur in the central tendon.

On each side of the diaphragm are small areas where the muscle fibres are replaced by areolar tissue. One, between the sternal and costal parts, contains the superior epigastric branch of the internal thoracic artery and some lymph vessels from the abdominal wall and convex surface of the liver. The other, between the costal part and the fibres springing from the lateral arcuate ligament, is less constant; when it is present, the posterosuperior surface of the kidney is separated from the pleura only by areolar tissue.

Shape and relations of the diaphragm

The upper surface of the diaphragm lies in relation to three serous membranes: on each side, the pleura separates it from the base of the corresponding lung, and over the middle folium of the central tendon the pericardium is interposed between it and the heart. The latter area, which is almost flat, is referred to as the *cardiac plateau*; it extends more to the left than the right. In anteroposterior view the superior profile of the diaphragm rises on either side of the cardiac plateau to a smooth convex dome or *cupola*, the cupola on the right being higher and slightly broader. Most of the inferior surface is covered by peritoneum. The right side is accurately moulded over the convex surface of the right lobe of the liver, the right kidney and right suprarenal gland; the left side conforms to the left lobe of the liver, the fundus of the stomach, the spleen, the left kidney and the left suprarenal gland. (In view of these differences in the profile and anatomical relationships of the right and left diaphragm, the side should always be specified in clinical descriptions.)

Blood supply. Musculophrenic arteries (p. 1534); superior epi-gastric arteries (p. 1535); pericardiacophrenic arteries (p. 1535); inferior phrenic arteries (p. 1558); upper three right lumbar arteries (p. 1558); upper two left lumbar arteries (p. 1558); superior phrenic branches of lower descending thoracic aorta (p. 1545); right and left lower three posterior intercostal arteries (p. 1546).

Nerve supply. The diaphragm receives its motor supply via the phrenic nerves. Sensory fibres are distributed to the peripheral part of the muscle by the lower six or seven intercostal nerves. It has been suggested that the motor innervation of the crural fibres comes from intercostal nerves, but Shehata (1966) has confirmed that the phrenic nerves are the source of supply. The right crus of the diaphragm, whose fibres divide to the right and left of the oesophageal opening, is innervated by both right and left phrenic nerves. Although the crural fibres are not innervated separately from the rest of the diaphragm, there is some evidence that this part of the diaphragm contracts slightly before the costal part (Mittal 1990), and this may be functionally significant (see below).

Actions. During inspiration the lowest ribs are fixed, and contraction of the diaphragm draws the central tendon downwards. In this movement the curvature of the diaphragm is scarcely altered; the cupolae move downwards and a little forwards almost parallel to their original positions. The associated downward displacement of the abdominal viscera is permitted by the extensibility of the abdominal wall, but the limit of this is soon reached. The central tendon, its motion arrested by the abdominal viscera, then becomes a fixed point from which the fibres of the diaphragm continue to contract, elevating the lower ribs and through this action pushing forwards the body of the sternum and the upper ribs. The right cupola of the diaphragm, which lies on the liver, has a greater resistance to overcome than the left, which lies over the stomach, but in compensation for this the right crus and the fibres of the right side are more substantial than those of the left. The balance between descent of the diaphragm and protrusion of the abdominal wall ('abdominal' breathing) and elevation of the ribs ('thoracic' breathing) varies in different individuals and with the depth of respiration. The thoracic element is usually more marked in females, but increases in both sexes during deep inspiration. The essential role of the diaphragm in breathing is considered further in The movements of respiration (p. 818).

The diaphragm lends additional power to all expulsive efforts. Thus, sneezing, coughing, laughing, crying, urinating, defaecating, and expelling the fetus from the uterus, are all preceded by a deep inspiration. A deep inspiration, followed by closure of the glottis, is a common preliminary to powerful recruitment of the trunk muscles, as in lifting heavy weights, the raised intra-abdominal pressure providing pneumatic bracing of the vertebral column. Any of these activities could cause gastric contents to reflux into the oesophagus, with risk of inhalation into the lungs. This is normally prevented by a physiological *antireflux barrier* located at the gastro-oesophageal junction (reviewed by Mittal 1990; see also p. 1753). The major components of this barrier are the specialized smooth muscle of the wall of the lower oesophagus and the encircling fibres of the crural diaphragm. These structures exert a radial pressure that can be measured by a sensing device as it is withdrawn from the stomach into the oesophagus. If reflux is to be prevented, this pressure must always exceed the difference between the pressures on either side of the junction, i.e. the difference between intra-abdominal pressure (transferred to the stomach, and augmented by any contraction of the stomach wall itself) and intrathoracic pressure (transferred to the oesophagus). During *expiration*, pressure exerted by tonic contraction of the smooth muscle of the lower oesophagus is normally sufficient to oppose the gastro-oesophageal pressure gradient. During *inspiration*, intra-abdominal pressure rises and intrathoracic pressure becomes more negative, increasing the risk of reflux. This tendency is opposed by additional pressure exerted by contraction of the crural fibres of the diaphragm. (Activation of the crural diaphragm slightly before the costal diaphragm would ensure that contraction of peri-oesophageal fibres preceded the increase in gastro-oesophageal pressure gradient.) The antireflux barrier must of course be lowered for swallowing and vomiting. Swallowing is followed immediately by expiration, which relaxes the crural fibres and allows the oesophageal contents to be transferred to the stomach by peristaltic movement (Whillis 1931). Vomiting is produced by bursts of activity involving co-contraction of the diaphragm, intercostal and abdominal muscles

in a pattern distinct from that of respiration; this activity is coordinated with relaxation of the crural fibres around the oesophagus (see Miller 1990).

Diaphragmatic excursion is about 1.5 cm in quiet breathing; during deep respiration the maximum movement ranges from 6 to 10 cm (Campbell 1958). After a forced inspiration, as when breathing is partially obstructed, the right cupola of the diaphragm can descend to about the level of the eleventh thoracic vertebra, while the left cupola may reach the level of the body of the twelfth. After a forced expiration the right cupola of the diaphragm is level anteriorly with the fourth costal cartilage, laterally with the fifth, sixth and seventh ribs, and posteriorly with the eighth; the left cupola is a little lower.

The level of the diaphragm is affected not only by the phase and depth of respiration but also by the degree of distension of the stomach and intestines and the size of the liver. Radiographs show that the height of the diaphragm within the thorax also varies considerably with posture. It is highest when the body is supine, and in this position it performs the largest respiratory excursions with normal breathing. When the body is erect the diaphragm is lower, and its respiratory movements become smaller. The diaphragmatic profile is still lower in the sitting posture, and respiratory excursions are smallest under these conditions. When the body is horizontal and on one side, the two halves of the diaphragm do not behave in the same way. The uppermost half sinks to a lower level even than in sitting, and moves little with respiration; the lower half rises higher in the thorax than it does even in the supine position, and its respiratory excursions are considerably greater.

Clinical relevance. Changes in the level of the diaphragm with alterations in posture explain why patients with severe dyspnoea are most comfortable and least short of breath when sitting up (see also The movements of respiration, p. 818). Paradoxical movements of the diaphragm can result from unilateral disease of the pleura or lungs, and (more commonly) from viral or surgical damage to one phrenic nerve. This is best observed fluoroscopically, with the patient first in the upright position (diaphragm unloaded) and then supine with a small weight on the abdomen (diaphragm loaded). Electrical stimulation of the diaphragm, by 'pacing' of one or both phrenic nerves, has been used with some success in infants with central alveolar hypoventilatory syndrome ('Ondine's Curse'; Ibawi et al 1985) and in patients with high cervical lesions of the spinal cord, in whom the diaphragm is paralysed but the lower motor neurons are intact (Glenn et al 1984). Electrodes are placed adjacent to the nerves, sometimes in the neck but more usually in the chest, and a respiratory rhythm is established by trains of stimuli delivered by an implanted device (Glenn et al 1984; Elefteriades et al 1992). Because this is an unphysiological way of recruiting the muscle, the fibres must be 'conditioned' during the initial period of stimulation so that they acquire the necessary resistance to fatigue (Glenn et al 1984; Salmons 1989; Elefteriades et al 1992; see also Cardiac assistance from skeletal muscle, p. 762).

Abdominal organs, usually the stomach, may herniate through the diaphragm into the thorax. There are three sites at which such hernias can occur: posterolateral (Bochdalek's), subcostosternal (Morgagni's) and oesophageal. The *posterolateral hernia* occurs as a result of a defect in the posterior diaphragm in the region of the 10th or 11th ribs. It is more common on the left and presents with abdominal contents in the left hemithorax at birth. Respiratory distress often results and the condition is life-threatening. *Subcostosternal hernias*, first described by Morgagni, are uncommon and occur through a defect in the anterior diaphragm just lateral to the xiphoid process. They are frequently asymptomatic. *Oesophageal hernias*, known as *hiatal hernias*, are common: when the oesophagogastric junction slides into the thorax, it is termed a *sliding hernia*; when the stomach herniates into the thorax alongside the oesophagus, it is termed a *para-oesophageal hernia*.

Because of common nerve root origins in the neck, diaphragmatic pain is frequently felt at the tip of the scapula (see Referred pain, p. 1005).

The movements of respiration

Introduction

In both mammalian evolution and embryological development the thoraco-abdominal wall begins as a roughly ovoid musculotendinous sheet running from the pelvic bowl at the caudal end to the clavicles and scapulae at the cranial end. It is penetrated by urogenital and alimentary tubes that are guarded by sphincters. The wall has certain primary roles: protecting the viscera; bracing, flexing, extending, and rotating the thoracolumbar spine; and permitting the passage of materials into and out of the cavity. Only later does the cavity develop lungs and eventually a transecting diaphragm. With this developmental history it is not surprising that individual muscles that make up the wall fulfil several functions, and that there is much redundancy, so that similar effects can be achieved in different ways.

A model of the basic mechanics of breathing

Consider any musculotendinous bag, filled with an almost incompressible fluid (e.g. water) and perforated by a single tube guarded by a valve. If the bag is spherical and tense it already contains the maximum volume of fluid for its surface area. Until the valve opens, any contraction of the wall will be isometric, and pressure in the bag will rise according to Laplace's Law. When the valve opens, the emergent flow will be determined by the geometry of the tube, the length–tension characteristics of the wall, and the flow properties of the fluid. So long as contraction of the wall is uniform the wall will continue to be spherical: it will alter in size but not shape. If the bag is initially slack, or contractions of the wall are not uniform, the more active parts of the wall will force the more yielding parts to move paradoxically (i.e. outwards), and the bag will change shape—but not volume—until the valve opens. The pressure developed within the container will depend mainly on the length–tension characteristics of the slacker elements of the wall. Now if the bag, spherical or otherwise, is filled with gas, which is compressible, contractions will never be isometric, and the pressures developed before the valve opens will be determined by the interactions of Boyle's and Laplace's Laws.

Let the wall of the bag be reinforced by roughly semi-circular stiffeners. If the apices of these half-hoops are maximally displaced from the axis of the bag, any movements of the hoops are bound to decrease its volume; if they are not, they may also increase its volume. Finally let the half-hoops be connected along one margin of the bag by a flexible but incompressible rod while their centres are joined along the opposite margin of the bag by an inflexible plate. Flexion of the middle of the rod away from the plate now increases the volume of the bag; flexion towards the plate decreases the volume of the bag.

These basic biomechanical principles will be recognized in the account that follows.

Observations in man

Just before birth the thoraco-abdominal cavity is divided by a domed diaphragm into two gas-free compartments: the poorly filled thorax above and the fuller abdomen below. Some (mainly phrenic) respiratory movements flush amniotic fluid in and out of the lungs. The work of moving the viscous fluid is high, despite its surfactant content, and this work may contribute to the training of the respiratory muscles for the task to come. During natural birth the infant's chest is squeezed into an expiratory position by the birth canal, expelling some fluid from the lungs. After the first breath or two of air, the lungs expand and the ribs move outwards maximally.

The caudal end of the cavity is closed by the pelvic bowl, which can be thought of as the fixed, rigid element of the wall. The ribs are at right-angles to the spinal axis, so their movements can only be expiratory. Respiration is entirely diaphragmatic. When the diaphragm descends, the anterolateral abdominal wall must relax and distend, because the abdominal contents are virtually incompressible. If excursion of the abdominal wall is prevented, for example by pain or tight strapping, the baby will suffocate. For the same reason it will also breathe with more difficulty in the prone than in the supine position. Because the infant's ribs are slender arcs of cartilage, the thoracic wall is compliant and may move paradoxically inwards and downwards on inspiration (see Watchko et al 1991). Contraction of the opposed intercostals and of the scalenes stiffen the chest wall and limit this paradoxical motion. On expiration, the elastic recoil of the lungs, the weight of the abdominal viscera, and some contraction of the abdominal wall drive the dome of the diaphragm back into the thorax, and also return the ribs to their initial, maximally displaced, positions.

Over the next few years, as the child develops, sits up and walks, the direct action of gravity on the abdominal wall pulls the ribs downwards and inwards. Now active upward movements of the ribs can be inspiratory. Maximal inspirations are achieved by relaxing the anterolateral abdominal wall, descending the diaphragm, raising the ribs, and flexing the spine backward. Maximal expirations are made by contracting the abdomen, relaxing the diaphragm, depressing the ribs and flexing the spine forward.

The actions of the respiratory muscles in man and other mammals can be studied in several ways, none of which is complete in itself. Morphological analysis of the cross-sectional area and fibre type composition of respiratory muscles gives some idea of their power and capacity for sustained or intermittent action (Mizuno 1991). Non-invasive optical techniques permit the motion of the thoracic and abdominal walls to be studied in great detail in healthy subjects and in patients with various neuromuscular disorders (see Morgan et al 1984, 1985; Peacock et al 1984; Goldman et al 1986a,b). Such studies describe the motions but do not explain how they are achieved. Action potentials recorded from thoracic, abdominal and phrenic muscles and their nerves signal the intention to contract but do not reveal whether there were actual changes in muscle length or respiratory consequences (see DiMarco et al 1989, 1990a,b,c, 1992, 1993). Artificial stimulation of specific nerves or nerve roots demonstrates what individual muscles can do when other muscles are relaxed but does not show what the target muscles actually do in concert with other muscles in natural breathing (Budzinka et al 1989; Decramer 1990; Han et al 1993). After section of specific nerves to eliminate the actions of individual muscles it is possible to imply by subtraction the function of those muscles before section. However, this requires careful interpretation of changes in the pattern of movement that may have taken place to compensate for the loss. The patterns of breathing after various surgical procedures on the thorax and abdomen and after spinal injury provide similar information and present similar interpretive difficulties (Bolton & Weiman 1993; Ford et al 1993).

Taken together, the evidence from these various approaches leads to the following current beliefs about the actions of the respiratory muscles in man. Respiration is a highly co-ordinated abdominal and thoracic process in which the diaphragm is the major muscle of inspiration, responsible for some two-thirds of the vital capacity. The external intercostal muscles are most active in inspiration and the internal intercostals, which are not as strong, are most active in expiration, but their primary roles are to act together to stiffen the chest wall, preventing paradoxical motion during descent of the diaphragm in inspiration. This becomes most obvious immediately after high spinal injury, when there is flaccid paralysis of the entire trunk and only the diaphragm is left functioning. In a healthy adult with a vital capacity of 4.5 litres or thereabouts, some 3 litres is accounted for by diaphragmatic excursion; immediately after high spinal injury the vital capacity falls to about 300 ml, although the diaphragm is moving maximally, because some 2.7 litres is lost by paradoxical incursion of the flaccid chest wall as the diaphragm descends. With time (usually several weeks) the paralysis becomes spastic, stiffening the chest wall, and the vital capacity rises towards its phrenic limit of about 3 litres (see Morgan & De Troyer 1984; Morgan et al 1984, 1985).

In the same way, high spinal injury reveals the role of the abdomen in inspiration and expiration. The abdomen is the major muscle of active expiration in man. During the flaccid stage of high spinal paralysis the only mechanisms available for returning the relaxed diaphragm into the thorax on expiration are passive recoil of the lungs and chest wall, and the weight of the abdominal viscera. The latter is the most important, and operates only when patients are lying down. If they are sat up or raised upright they are unable to breathe out. Such patients can be helped by trussing the abdomen with an elastic binder. Conversely, when paralysis becomes spastic, the stiff abdominal wall opposes inspiration (see Goldman et al 1986a,b, 1988; De Troyer & Estenne 1991).

The role of the abdomen in breathing is often underestimated. If, for example, the anterolateral wall were made of steel, linking the pelvic rim rigidly to the costal margins, inspiration would be impossible: the diaphragm could not descend, because the abdominal contents are incompressible, and the ribs could not rise, because the links to the pelvis would be inextensible. During normal breathing the abdomen relaxes as the diaphragm contracts. It is possible to oppose this motion by tensing the abdomen, as in the 'beach posture' adopted to exaggerate the size of the chest. In this case the abdominal contents fix the central tendon of the diaphragm, so that it raises the rib cage as it contracts, but it is a condition of that manoeuvre that the gap between the ribs and the pelvic rim widens.

During maximal respiratory movements, and particularly when breathing encounters resistance, the muscles already mentioned become more active and additional muscles are brought into play. In forced inspiration, the first rib is elevated by the scalene muscles, anterior and medius, and by the sternocleidomastoid indirectly through the clavicle and costoclavicular ligament and directly through the manubrium sterni. The twelfth rib is fixed by quadratus lumborum so that the diaphragm can exert a more powerful downward thrust on the abdominal viscera (Boyd et al 1965). Activity in the erectores spinae increases appreciably, and muscles connecting the upper limb to the trunk, such as pectoralis major, may be partially recruited. In forced expiration (and also during expulsive efforts such as coughing and sneezing), muscles of the abdominal wall, particularly the oblique and transverse muscles, and both latissimi dorsi, contract strongly, pushing the diaphragm upwards and drawing the lower ribs downwards and inwards.

The respiratory muscles must also work during sleep, when the pharyngeal muscles relax and upper airway resistance rises (see Henke et al 1992). It is now appreciated that in some people, particularly the obese, this relaxation can lead to periodic apnoea and marked hypoxia during sleep. This implies that the pharyngeal muscles have an important respiratory role in waking life. It is also clear that although respiratory muscles rarely tire in normal life (Fitting 1990, 1991) they do fatigue when placed under abnormal loads, as in obstructive lung disease (Goldberg & Roussos 1990; Hill 1991) or in poisoning by malnutrition (Fiaccadori & Borghetti 1991; Heijerman 1993), by some common drugs (Aldrich & Prezant 1990; Dekhuijzen & Decramer 1992), or by the metabolic consequences of organ failures that lead to the need for intensive care (Rochester 1993; Aubier 1993).

In summary, breathing is a complex and highly orchestrated neuromuscular activity, about which there is still much to be learned. That knowledge is unlikely to be acquired by the study of individual muscles in isolation.

MUSCLES OF THE ABDOMEN

It is convenient to consider the muscles of the abdomen in anterolateral and posterior groups.

ANTEROLATERAL MUSCLES OF THE ABDOMEN

The anterolateral group consists of four large flat muscular sheets that form the abdominal wall (obliqui externus and internus, transversus and rectus abdominis), and two smaller elements (cremaster and pyramidalis). The traditional account of the larger muscles and their aponeuroses that follows is adequate as an introduction, and indeed for most practical purposes. This description may be elaborated by referring to newer observations on the arrangement of the aponeuroses, the rectus sheath and the linea alba (see A more recent view of structures of the anterolateral abdominal wall). The actions of the larger muscles will be dealt with, together with pyramidalis, after they have been described individually.

Blood supply. Muscles of the anterolateral abdominal wall are supplied by the following arteries: lower two or three posterior intercostal arteries (p. 1546); subcostal artery (p. 1546); musculophrenic artery (p. 1534); superior epigastric artery (p. 1535); inferior epigastric artery, including its pubic branch and the cremasteric artery (p. 1563); superficial epigastric artery (p. 1566); superficial circumflex iliac artery (p. 1566); deep circumflex artery, particularly its ascending branch (p. 1563); continuation of four lumbar arteries (p. 1558); continuation of arteria lumbalis ima (p. 1559); rami from lumbar branch of iliolumbar artery (p. 1562). Additional contributions come from anastomoses between many of the above arteries.

Superficial fascia

The superficial fascia of the abdominal wall consists, for the most part, of a single layer that contains a variable amount of fat. In the lower part, however, particularly in obese individuals, the fascia differentiates into a superficial and a deep layer, between which are superficial vessels, nerves and the superficial inguinal lymph nodes. Either of these layers may be multiple, but the extent and significance of subdivision is disputed.

The *superficial layer* is thick, areolar in texture and contains a variable amount of fat in its meshes. Inferiorly it passes over the inguinal ligament to merge with the superficial fascia of the thighs. In the male this layer continues over the penis and outer surface of the spermatic cord into the scrotum, where it changes its character, becoming thin, devoid of adipose tissue and pale reddish in colour. In the scrotum it also contains smooth muscle fibres, which form the dartos muscle. From the scrotum it may be traced backwards into continuity with the superficial fascia of the perineum. In the female it continues from the abdomen into the labia majora and perineum.

The *deep layer* of the fascia is more membranous than the superficial, and contains elastic fibres. It is loosely connected by areolar tissue to the aponeurosis of external oblique, but in the midline it is intimately adherent to the linea alba and symphysis pubis. In the male it is prolonged on the dorsum of the penis, contributing to its *fundiform ligament* (7.77). Above, it is continuous with the superficial fascia over the rest of the trunk; below and laterally, it passes over the inguinal ligament and fuses with the overlying superficial layer and the underlying fascia lata in the inguinal flexure line or skin crease of the thigh (7.77). In the male its inferomedial continuation is over the penis and spermatic cord to the scrotum, where it becomes

819

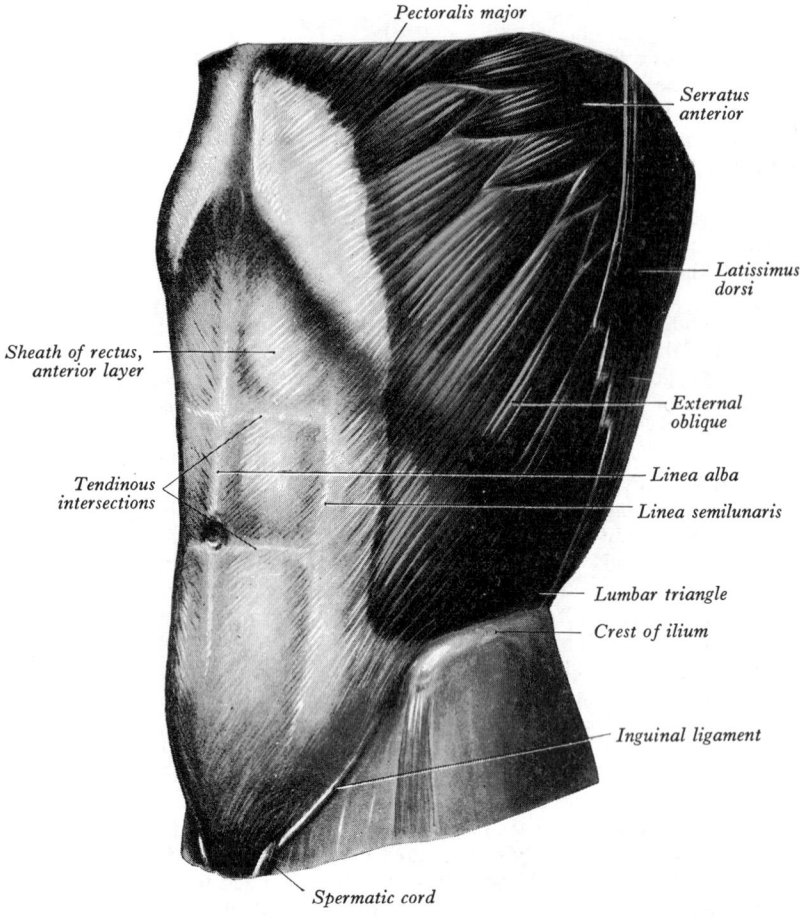

Pectoralis major

Serratus anterior

Latissimus dorsi

Sheath of rectus, anterior layer

External oblique

Linea alba

Tendinous intersections

Linea semilunaris

Lumbar triangle

Crest of ilium

Inguinal ligament

Spermatic cord

7.76 The left obliquus externus abdominis.

continuous with the membranous layer of the superficial fascia of the perineum (p. 832). In the female it continues into the labia majora and thence to the fascia of the perineum.

In the child the testis can frequently be retracted out of the scrotum into the interval occupied by loose areolar tissue between external oblique and the deep layer of superficial fascia over the inguinal canal. This interval is sometimes called the *superficial inguinal pouch* (Browne 1938).

Obliquus externus abdominis

Obliquus externus abdominis (**7.76**) curves around the lateral and anterior parts of the abdomen. It is the largest and the most superficial of the three flat muscles in this region. It arises by eight fleshy slips from the external surfaces and inferior borders of the lower eight ribs; these slips interdigitate with serratus anterior and latissimus dorsi, along an oblique line which extends downwards and backwards, the upper ones being attached close to the cartilages of the corresponding ribs, the middle ones to the ribs at some distance from their cartilages, and the lowest to the apex of the cartilage of the last rib. The fibres diverge as they pass to their insertions. Those from the lower two ribs pass nearly vertically downwards, and are attached to the anterior half or more of the outer lip of the ventral segment of the iliac crest (p. 664); the middle and upper fibres pass downwards and forwards, and end in an aponeurosis along a line drawn vertically from the ninth costal cartilage to a little below the level of the umbilicus; they then turn laterally towards the anterior superior iliac spine. The muscle fibres rarely descend beyond a line from the anterior superior iliac spine to the umbilicus. The posterior border of the muscle is free (**7.91**).

The *aponeurosis* of external oblique is a strong tendinous sheet that descends medially and meets the aponeurosis of the opposite muscle in the midline in a tendinous raphe which stretches from the xiphoid process to the symphysis pubis, the *linea alba* (**7.76**, and see p. 827). Below and medially each aponeurosis is attached to the upper border of the pubic symphysis and the pubic crest as far as the pubic tubercle. The margin of the part of the aponeurosis between

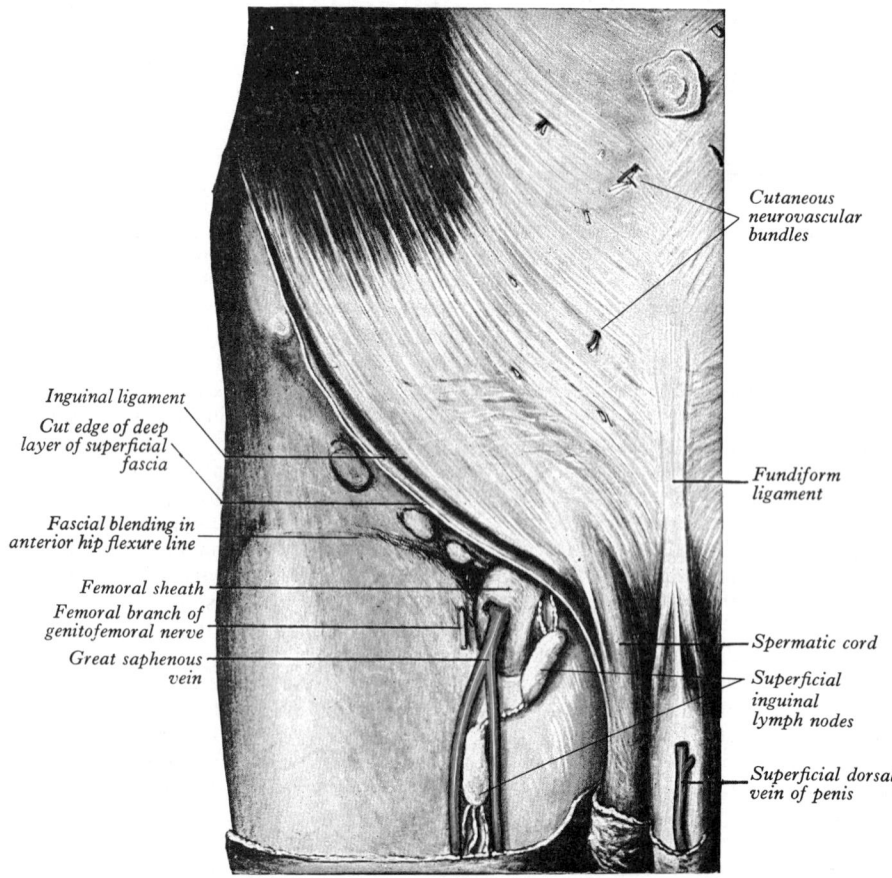

Cutaneous neurovascular bundles

Inguinal ligament

Cut edge of deep layer of superficial fascia

Fascial blending in anterior hip flexure line

Fundiform ligament

Femoral sheath

Femoral branch of genitofemoral nerve

Great saphenous vein

Spermatic cord

Superficial inguinal lymph nodes

Superficial dorsal vein of penis

7.77 Superficial structures of the inguinal region and lower part of the anterior abdominal wall on the right side.

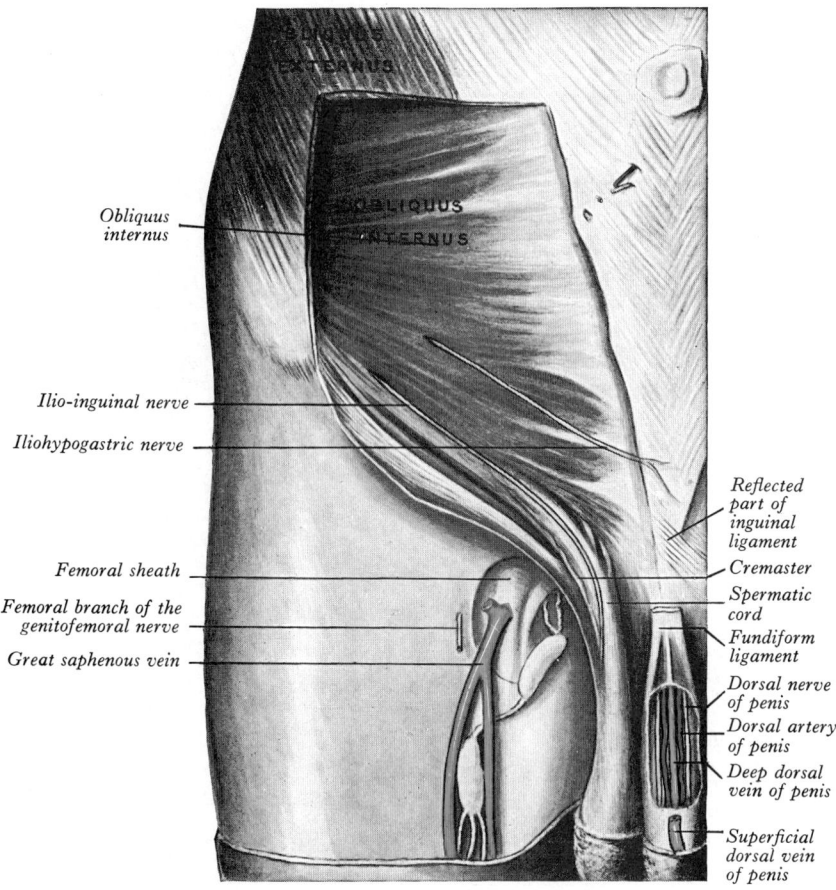

7.78 Dissection of the regions shown in **7.77**, with part of obliquus externus removed.

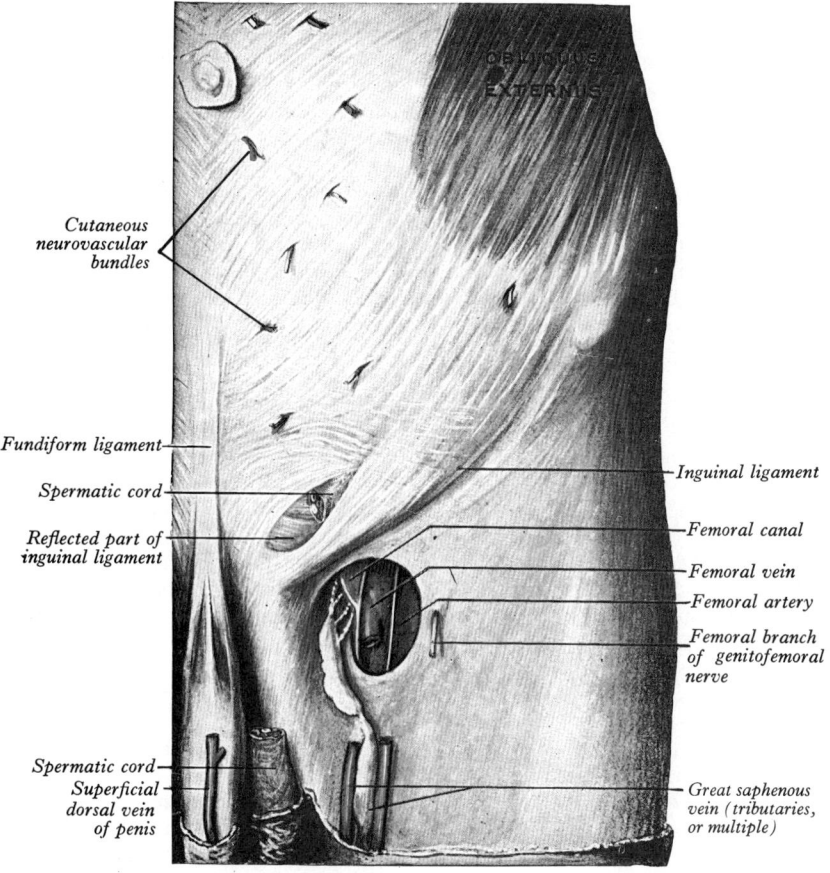

7.79 Superficial structures of the inguinal region and lower part of the anterior abdominal wall on the left side with the superficial aponeurotic layer removed.

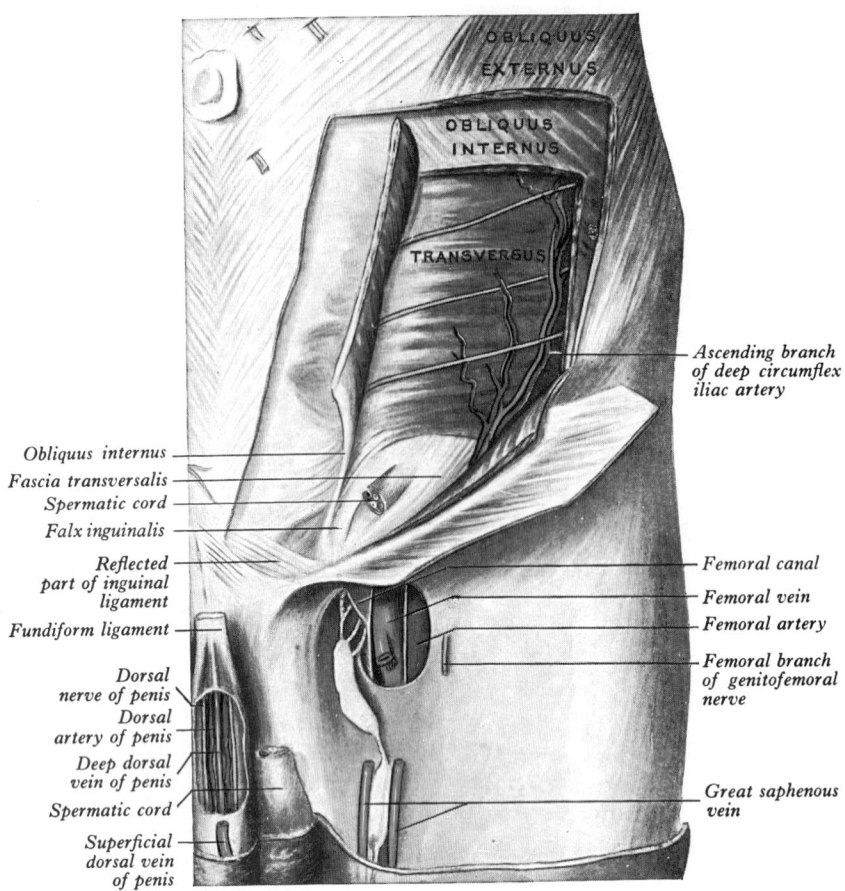

7.80 Dissection of the regions shown in **7.79**, with parts of the external and internal oblique muscles removed.

the anterior superior iliac spine and the pubic tubercle is a thick band, infolded so as to present a grooved upper surface; this is the *inguinal ligament* (see below). The deep fibres of the external oblique aponeurosis are not initially parallel to the long axis of the inguinal ligament: they approach the latter obliquely at an angle of 10–20°. On reaching the ligament, each fibre turns **medially**, most running along the ligament to reach the pubic tubercle. Fibres that are still deeper splay out posteromedially to the pecten pubis (Lytle 1974).

Variations. The upper and lower digitations may be absent; digitations or even the whole muscle may be reduplicated. Digitations may also be continuous with pectoralis major or serratus anterior.

Nerve supply. Ventral rami of the lower six thoracic spinal nerves.

Inguinal ligament

The inguinal ligament (**7.77, 79**) is, as already noted, the thick, inrolled lower border of the aponeurosis of external oblique, and stretches from the anterior superior iliac spine to the pubic tubercle; its grooved abdominal surface forms the 'floor' of the inguinal canal. (It has also been called the *crural arch*, the *superficial crural arch*, and *Poupart's ligament*.) The ligament is curved along its length, the convexity pointing towards the thigh, where it is continuous with the fascia lata. In adults it is 12–14 cm in length and inclined at 35–40° to the horizontal. Its lateral half is rounded and more oblique; its medial half gradually widens towards its attachment to the pubis, where it becomes more horizontal and supports the spermatic cord. At the medial end, fibres that do not attach to the pubic tubercle extend in two directions. An expansion posteriorly and laterally to the pecten pubis is known as the *lacunar ligament complex*. Fibres also pass upwards and medially to join the rectus sheath and the linea alba; these constitute the *reflected part of the inguinal ligament* (**7.80**).

Lacunar ligament

The lacunar ligament (*pectineal part of the inguinal ligament*) (**6.281**, p. 677) has been described as composite (Lytle 1974). Its abdominal, 'deep' part (the classic lacunar ligament) extends posteriorly and laterally from the medial part of the inguinal ligament to the medial end of the pecten pubis. It is triangular, and aligned almost horizontally when the body is upright; it is a little larger in the male, and measures about 2 cm from base to apex. Its thin base, directed laterally, is concave and forms the medial boundary of the femoral ring; its apex is attached to the pubic tubercle. Its posterior margin is attached to the pecten pubis, and is continuous with the pectineal fascia; its anterior margin continues into the inguinal ligament. It has superior and inferior surfaces. A strong fibrous band, the *pectineal ligament* (of *Astley Cooper*), extends laterally from its base (**6.281**, p. 677) along the pecten pubis. It is augmented by the pectineal fascia and by a lateral expansion from the lower end of the linea alba (*adminiculum lineae albae*, p. 827). The lacunar formation as described here is best seen from its abdominal aspect. In the living subject, however, a second, distinct lacunar fibrous sheet is distinguishable when approached from the thigh. This is derived from an inflexion of the *fascia lata* which joins the posterior border of the inguinal ligament, receives reinforcement from the transversalis fascia, fuses with pectineal fascia for a distance of about 1 cm, and then ascends to fuse with the thickened periosteum of the pecten pubis. This *fascial lacunar ligament* also presents a thickened curved lateral border which fits closely around the medial wall of the femoral sheath; because of its pectineal fascial attachment it is about 1 cm below and anterior to the pecten pubis, and some 3 cm lateral to the pubic tubercle.

Reflected part of the inguinal ligament

The reflected part of the inguinal ligament (**7.77, 80**) is an expansion from the lateral crus of the superficial inguinal ring. It passes upwards and medially behind the medial end of the superficial inguinal ring, behind external oblique and in front of the falx inguinalis; fibres of the right and left ligaments decussate in the linea alba.

Superficial inguinal ring

The superficial inguinal ring (**7.77, 79**) is a hiatus in the aponeurosis, just above and lateral to the crest of the pubis. It transmits the spermatic cord in the male, the round ligament of the uterus in the female and the ilio-inguinal nerve in both. The aperture is somewhat triangular, its long axis aligned with the deep fibres of the aponeurosis. Although it varies in size it does not usually extend laterally beyond the medial third of the inguinal ligament. Its base is the crest of the pubis, and its sides are the margins of the opening in the aponeurosis, the crura of the ring. The lateral crus is the stronger, and is formed by fibres of the inguinal ligament inserted into the pubic tubercle. The medial crus is a thin, flat band attached to the front of the symphysis pubis and interlacing with the opposite crus. In the external layer of the investing fascia of external oblique are bands of fibres of variable development and distribution which course at right angles to the fibres of the aponeurosis of the muscle. Some of these bands may arch above the apex of the superficial inguinal ring as *intercrural fibres*.

In the male the lateral crus is curved so as to form a kind of groove, in which the spermatic cord rests. If the skin of the scrotum is invaginated upwards and laterally the spermatic cord can be followed up to the superficial inguinal ring. If the examining finger is then directed backwards, the crura of the ring can be recognized and the size of the ring explored. From the margins of the ring the external oblique aponeurosis and overlying fascia continue downwards, forming a delicate tubular prolongation of fibrous tissue around the spermatic cord and testis. They form the outermost

covering, the *external spermatic fascia*. The superficial inguinal ring is only a distinct aperture when the continuity of this fascia with the aponeurosis is interrupted (Anson et al 1960). The ring is smaller in the female.

Obliquus internus abdominis

Obliquus internus abdominis (**7.81, 85**) lies beneath the external oblique for much of its extent, and is thinner and less bulky. Its muscle fibres arise from the lateral two-thirds of the grooved upper surface of the inguinal ligament, from the anterior two-thirds of the intermediate line of the ventral segment of the iliac crest and from the thoracolumbar fascia (**7.70**). It has been described as attached to the iliac fascia and not directly to the inguinal ligament (McVay & Anson 1940a) but the fascia and ligament are adherent at this point (p. 822). The posterior (iliac) fibres pass upwards and laterally to the inferior borders and tips of the lower three or four ribs and their cartilages, where they are continuous with the internal intercostals. The uppermost fibres form a short, free superomedial border. The lowest fibres, which originate from the inguinal ligament, are paler in colour; they arch downwards and medially across the spermatic cord in the male and the round ligament of the uterus in the female. They become tendinous and attach to the corresponding part of the aponeurosis of transversus abdominis to the crest and medial part of the pecten pubis, forming the *falx inguinalis* (*conjoint tendon*).

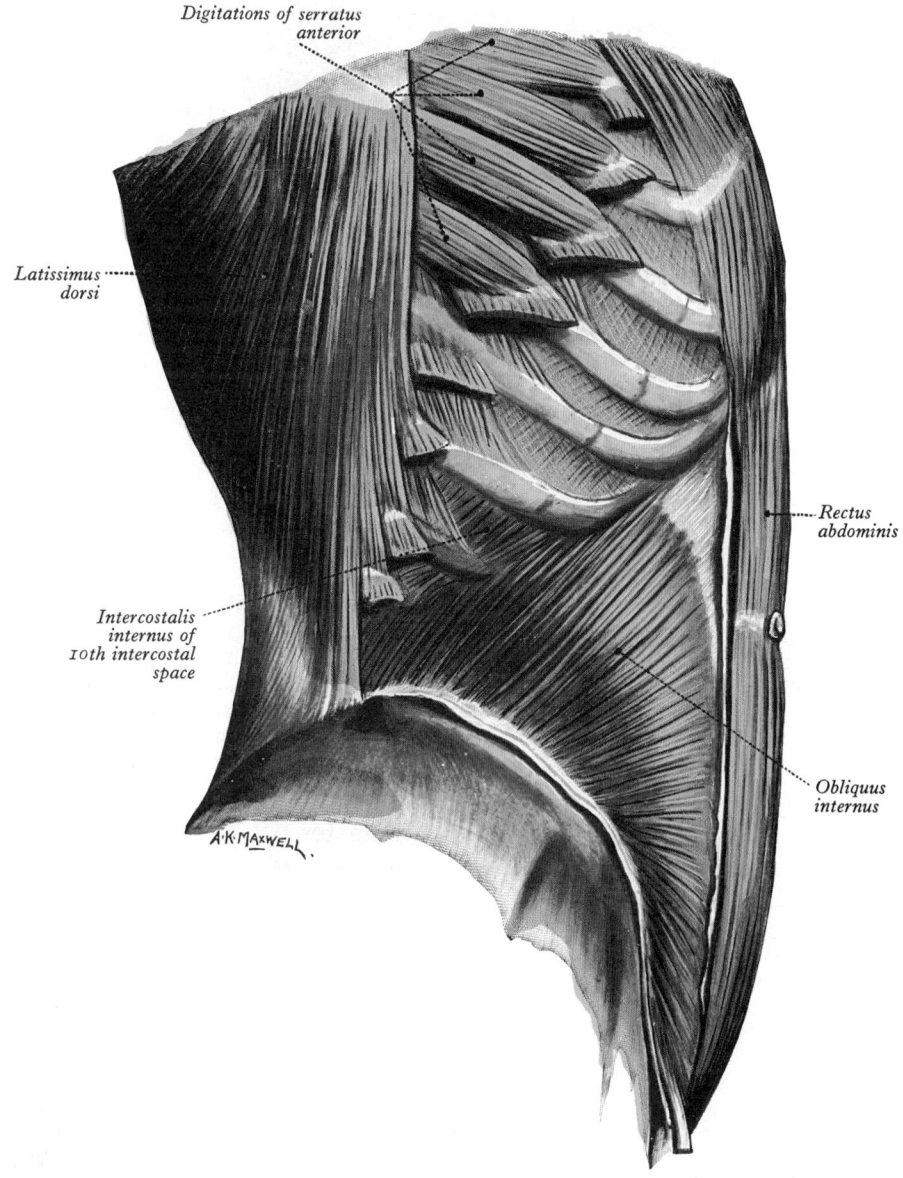

7.81 Muscles of the right side of the trunk. The external oblique has been removed to show the internal oblique, but its digitations from the ribs have been preserved. The sheath of rectus abdominis has been opened and its anterior lamina removed.

823

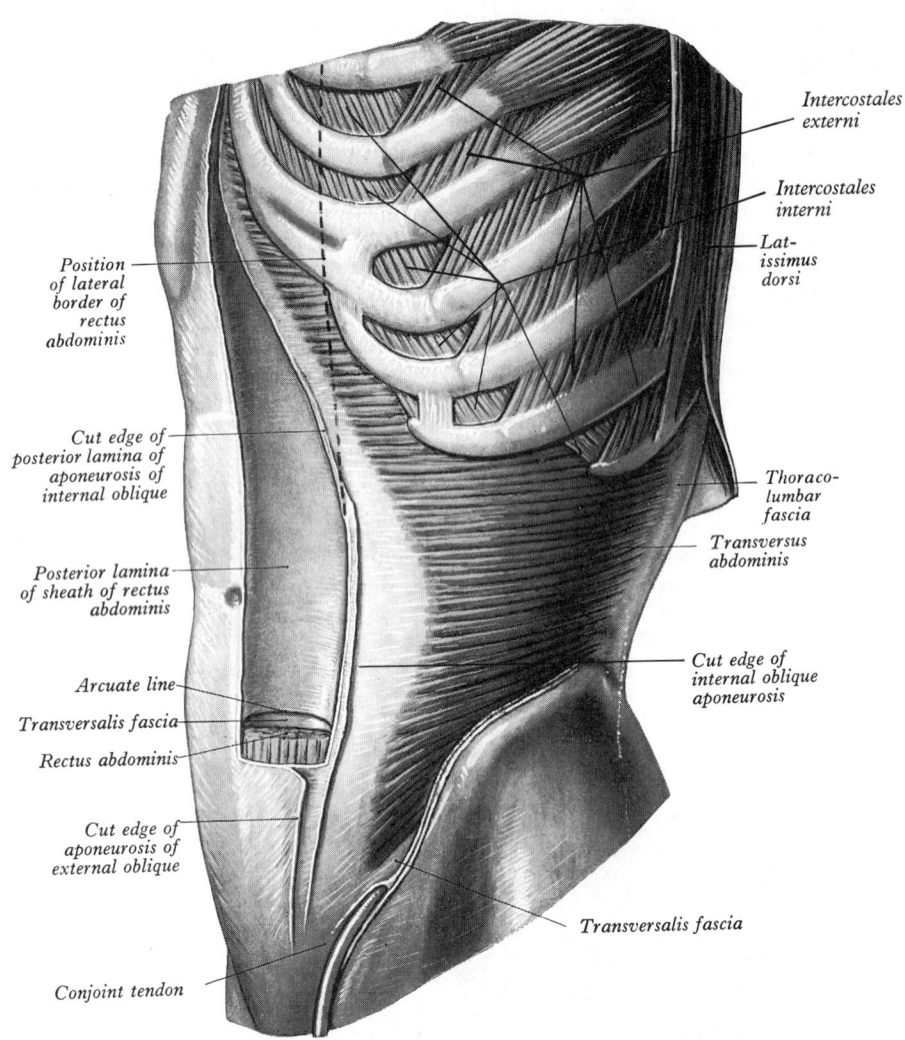

Intercostales externi

Intercostales interni

Latissimus dorsi

Position of lateral border of rectus abdominis

Cut edge of posterior lamina of aponeurosis of internal oblique

Thoracolumbar fascia

Transversus abdominis

Posterior lamina of sheath of rectus abdominis

Arcuate line

Transversalis fascia

Rectus abdominis

Cut edge of internal oblique aponeurosis

Cut edge of aponeurosis of external oblique

Transversalis fascia

Conjoint tendon

7.82 The left transversus abdominis. This diagram incorporates the traditional features of an aponeurosis of transversus (for an alternative analysis, see p. 828).

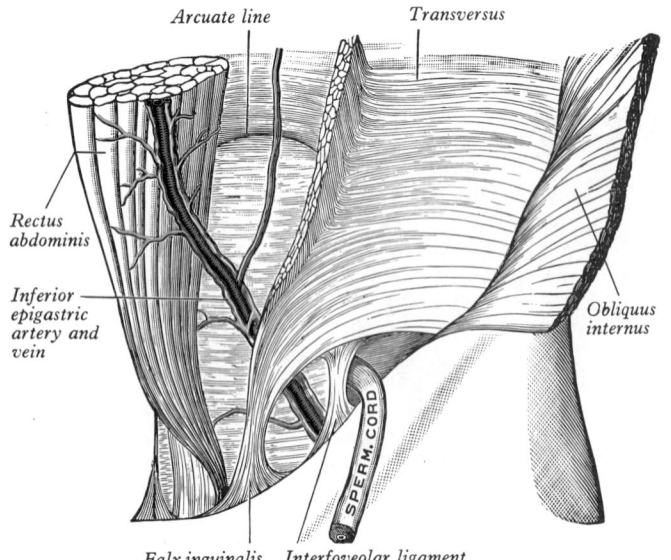

Arcuate line

Transversus

Rectus abdominis

Inferior epigastric artery and vein

Obliquus internus

SPERM. CORD

Falx inguinalis   Interfoveolar ligament

7.83 The lower part of the anterior abdominal wall on the left side, showing the relations of the spermatic cord at the deep inguinal ring. (Modified from Braune.) The posterior wall of the rectus sheath is depicted as terminating abruptly at the arcuate line; according to more recent views, this transition would be more gradual (see p. 828).

The intermediate fibres of internal oblique diverge and end in an aponeurosis which gradually broadens from below upwards. In its upper two-thirds this aponeurosis splits at the lateral border of rectus abdominis into two laminae which pass around it and reunite in the linea alba, which they help to form. The uppermost part is attached to the cartilages of the seventh, eighth and ninth ribs.

Nerve supply. Ventral rami of the lower six thoracic and the first lumbar spinal nerves.

Cremaster

Cremaster (**7.78**) consists of loosely arranged muscle fasciculi lying along the spermatic cord and united by areolar tissue to form the sac-like *cremasteric fascia* around the cord and testis within the external spermatic fascia. The *lateral part* of the muscle, arising from the inguinal ligament, has been variously described as: in continuity with the medial edge of the internal oblique; deep to the internal oblique, extending as far as the anterior superior iliac spine and in continuity with either the internal oblique or transversus; a pointed tendon from the middle of the inguinal ligament, piercing the internal oblique near its medial margin. In one extensive study, all sixty subjects had both a tendinous attachment and cremasteric fibres derived from obliquus internus and transversus (Blunt 1951). The fibres pass along the lateral aspect of the spermatic cord through the superficial inguinal ring and then spread out in loops of increasing length along its anterolateral aspect. The shortest and most superior fasciculi turn inwards in front of the cord to join the medial part;

longer fasciculi blend with the fascia over the cord and upper part of the tunica vaginalis. (In the female a few fibres descending on the round ligament of the uterus represent the lateral part of cremaster.) The *medial part* of the muscle is variably developed and may be absent. It arises from the pubic tubercle and possibly from the pubic crest, falx inguinalis and lower border of transversus. Its fasciculi loop on the posteromedial aspect of the cord, interlacing with those of the lateral part. The whole muscle may be described as forming continuous loops from the middle of the inguinal ligament as far as the tunica vaginalis and then returning to attach to the pubic tubercle. Shafik (1977) divides the muscle into two distinct parts—*cremaster internus* and *externus*—separated by the internal spermatic fascia.

Nerve supply. Genital branch of the genitofemoral nerve, derived from the first and second lumbar spinal nerves.

Action. The cremaster pulls the testis up towards the superficial inguinal ring. Although its fibres are striated, it is not usually under voluntary control. Stroking the skin of the medial side of the thigh evokes a reflex contraction of the muscle and this *cremasteric reflex* is much more active in children. This may be a protective response, but the cremaster appears to have a more significant role in testicular thermoregulation. Shafik (1977) considers that the position of the testis is adjusted by combined action of cremaster and dartos, the latter being attached to the testis by a 'scrotal ligament' (p. 1856).

Transversus abdominis

Transversus abdominis (**7.82, 85**) is the innermost of the flat muscles of the abdominal wall. Its muscle fibres arise from the lateral third of the inguinal ligament. The anterior two-thirds of the inner lip of the ventral segment of the iliac crest, the thoracolumbar fascia between the iliac crest and the twelfth rib, and the internal aspects of the lower six costal cartilages, where it interdigitates with the diaphragm (**7.73**). There is some disagreement as to whether the fibres arise directly from the inguinal ligament or from adjacent iliac fascia (McVay & Anson 1940). The muscle ends in an aponeurosis of variable extent, the lower fibres of which curve downwards and medially together with those of the aponeurosis of internal oblique to the crest and pecten of the pubis, to form the *falx inguinalis* (**7.83**). The rest of the aponeurosis passes medially, and the fibres decussate at and blend with the linea alba. The upper costal and anterior iliac fibres of transversus are short, the lower costal and posterior iliac fibres are longer, and the thoracolumbar fibres are longest. Near the xiphoid process the aponeurosis is formed only 2–3 cm from the linea alba, so the muscular part of transversus extends behind rectus, to an extent that decreases down to the level of the tip of the eleventh rib. The lateral limit of the aponeurosis, from above, curves first downwards and laterally and is widest (5–6 cm lateral to rectus) at umbilical levels; it then recurves downwards and medially towards (but not reaching) the middle of the superior crus of the superficial inguinal ring.

Variations. Fusiform defects filled with fascia occur in the lower muscular and aponeurotic parts of both internal oblique and transversus abdominis. The two muscles are sometimes fused; transversus may be absent.

Nerve supply. Ventral rami of the lower six thoracic and the first lumbar spinal nerves.

Falx inguinalis

The falx inguinalis (conjoint tendon) of internal oblique and transversus (**7.80, 83**) is formed mainly by the lower part of the aponeurosis of transversus, and inserts into the crest and pecten of the pubis. It descends behind the superficial inguinal ring, thus serving to protect from behind what would otherwise be a weak point in the abdominal wall. The attachment to the pecten pubis is frequently absent. Medially the falx inguinalis fuses with the anterior wall of the sheath of rectus abdominis. Laterally, it may blend with an inconstant ligamentous band, the *interfoveolar ligament* (**7.83**), which sometimes connects the lower margin of transversus to the superior ramus of the pubis and occasionally contains a few muscular fibres. Muscular fasciculi attached to the pecten pubis behind the falx inguinalis may reach the transversalis fascia, the aponeurosis of the muscle, or even the lateral end of the arcuate line.

Clinical relevance. The falx inguinalis may be parted or distended

by intestinal protrusion in a common type of direct inguinal hernia (see p. 1788).

Rectus abdominis

Rectus abdominis (**7.84**) is a long strap-like muscle that extends along the whole length of the front of the abdomen, widening as it ascends. The paired recti are separated in the midline by the linea alba. Each arises by two tendons: the larger lateral one is attached to the crest of the pubis and may extend beyond the pubic tubercle to the pecten pubis; the medial tendon interlaces with the contralateral muscle and blends with the ligamentous fibres covering the front of the symphysis pubis. Additional fibres may spring from the lower part of the linea alba. Above, each muscle is attached by three slips of unequal size to the fifth, sixth and seventh costal cartilages. The most lateral fibres are usually attached to the anterior end of the fifth rib; in some cases this slip is absent, in others it may extend to the fourth and third ribs. The most medial fibres are occasionally connected to the costoxiphoid ligaments and the side of the xiphoid process.

The muscle fibres of rectus are interrupted by three fibrous bands or *tendinous intersections*: one is usually situated at the level of the umbilicus, another opposite the free end of the xiphoid process, and a third about midway between the other two. These intersections pass transversely or obliquely across the muscle in a zigzag manner; they are rarely full-thickness and may only extend half-way through. They adhere closely to the anterior lamina of the sheath of the muscle. Sometimes one or two incomplete intersections are present below the umbilicus. The intersections may occur secondarily during development, but one controversial suggestion is that they represent the myosepta delineating the myotomes that form the muscle.

The medial border of rectus is closely related to the linea alba; its lateral border may show on the surface of the anterior abdominal wall as a curved groove, the *linea semilunaris*, which extends from the tip of the ninth costal cartilage to the pubic tubercle. In a muscular subject it is readily visible, even when the muscle is not actively contracting, but in a corpulent individual it may be completely obscured.

Nerve supply. Rectus abdominis is supplied by the ventral rami of the lower six or seven thoracic spinal nerves.

Rectus sheath

(The traditional description that follows may be elaborated by reference to A more recent view of structures of the anterolateral abdominal wall, p. 828.) Rectus abdominis is enclosed between the aponeuroses of the oblique and transverse muscles, which form the so-called *rectus sheath* (**7.76, 82, 85**). At the lateral margin of rectus abdominis the aponeurosis of the internal oblique divides: one lamina passes anterior to rectus and blends there with the aponeurosis of the external oblique; one passes behind it and blends there with the aponeurosis of transversus. These laminae come together again at the medial border of rectus and contribute to the linea alba (**7.85**). This is the arrangement from the costal margin down to about halfway between the umbilicus and symphysis pubis, at which point the posterior wall of the sheath ends in a curved margin, called the *arcuate line* (**7.82, 83**), whose concavity points downwards or downwards and laterally. The aponeuroses of the internal oblique and transversus extend only to the costal margin, so above that level the rectus rests directly on the costal cartilages; the anterior layer of the sheath here is formed only by the aponeurosis of the external oblique. Below the costal margin, but still in the upper part of the sheath, the muscular fibres of transversus abdominis continue behind rectus abdominis nearly to the linea alba, as described earlier; thus the posterior layer of the sheath is to some extent muscular at this point. Below the arcuate line the aponeuroses of the internal oblique and transversus pass into the anterior layer, so that all three muscles are in front of the rectus. The aponeuroses of the transversus and internal oblique fuse intimately, but that of the external oblique is bound to them only by loose connective tissue until it approaches the midline. The posterior layer of the sheath is again lacking at this level, and only transversalis fascia separates rectus from the peritoneum (**7.85B**).

In addition to rectus abdominis, the rectus sheath also contains pyramidalis (see over), the superior and inferior epigastric vessels, and the terminal portions of the lower intercostal nerves.

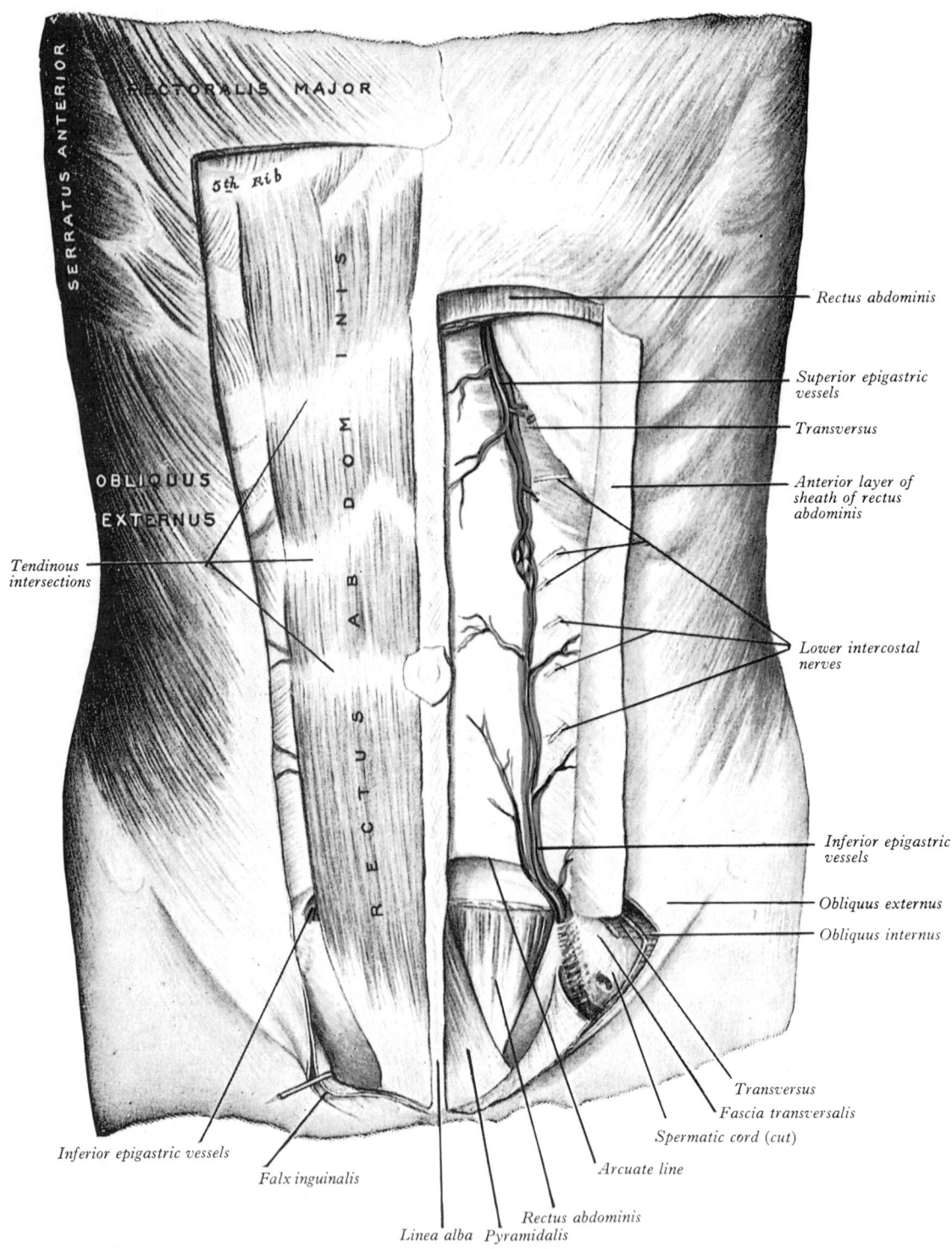

7.84 The right rectus abdominis and the left pyramidalis. The greater part of the left rectus abdominis has been removed to show the superior and inferior epigastric vessels.

Pyramidalis

Pyramidalis (**7.84**) is a triangular muscle that lies in front of the lower part of rectus abdominis within the rectus sheath. It is attached by tendinous fibres to the front of the pubis and to the ligamentous fibres in front of the symphysis. The muscle diminishes in size as it passes upwards, and ends in a pointed extremity which is attached to the linea alba, usually midway between the umbilicus and pubis but sometimes higher. The muscle varies considerably in size; it may be larger on one side than on the other, absent on one or both sides, or even doubled.

Nerve supply. The subcostal nerve, which is the ventral ramus of the twelfth thoracic spinal nerve.

Actions of the anterolateral abdominal muscles

The major muscles of the anterolateral abdominal group provide a firm but elastic wall that retains the abdominal viscera in position and opposes the action of gravity on them in both erect and sitting postures. This function depends principally on the oblique muscles, especially internal oblique. When the thorax and pelvis are fixed, the active contraction of these muscles exercises a compressive force on

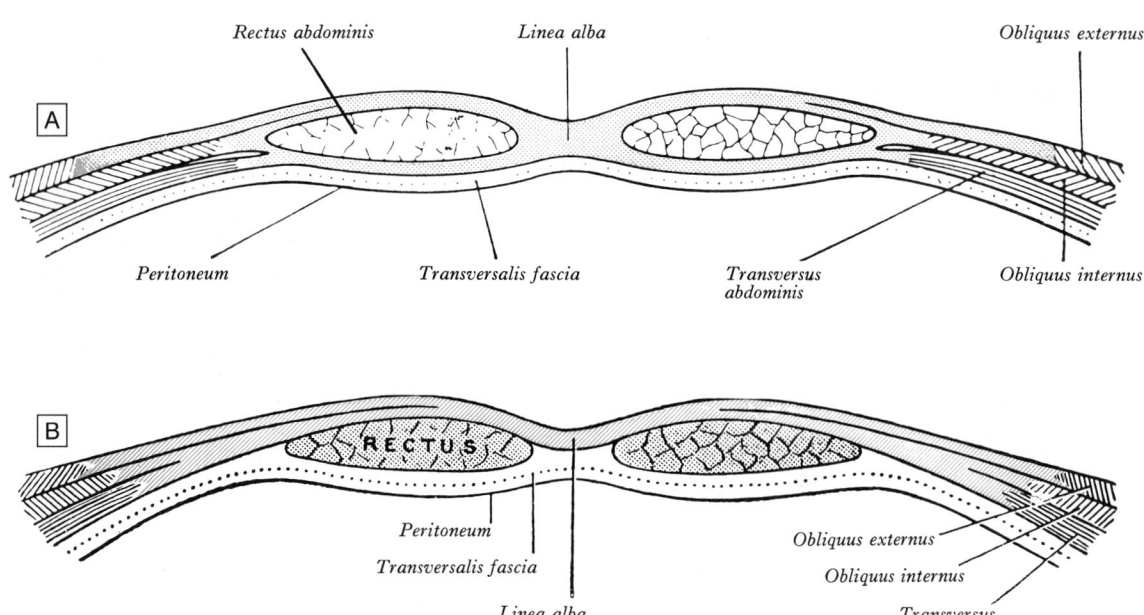

7.85   Transverse sections through the anterior abdominal wall, according to the traditional view: A. immediately above the umbilicus; B. below the arcuate line. Note the extent to which the external oblique aponeurosis remains as a separate entity, passing medially, ventral to the rectus, before blending with the other aponeuroses; these have already fused lateral to rectus. (The traditional view is retained here to maintain historical perspective and will suffice for many readers. For a modern analysis, see the essay entitled 'A more recent view of structures of the anterolateral abdominal wall', p. 828.)

the abdominal viscera. This plays an important part during expiration (see Movements of respiration, p. 818), and in the expulsion of faeces from the rectum, urine from the bladder, the gastric contents in vomiting and the fetus from the uterus. The action is mainly that of the oblique muscles, which tense the rectus sheath and lineae alba and semilunaris; rectus abdominis itself plays a minor role. If the pelvis and vertebral column are fixed, the external oblique muscles aid expiration further by depressing and compressing the lower thorax. With the pelvis fixed, the recti of the two sides, aided to some extent by the obliqui, flex the lumbar part of the vertebral column, bending the trunk forwards; with the thorax fixed, they draw the front of the pelvis upwards, also flexing the vertebral column (Floyd & Silver 1950). If the muscles are active only on one side, the trunk is bent towards that side. In addition, external oblique turns the front of the abdomen towards the opposite side, and internal oblique turns it to the same side. Electromyographic studies suggest that the abdominal musculature is little involved in most movements of the trunk, whether they take place in the sitting or the standing position, unless considerable resistance is applied. Extension of the trunk produces heightened activity in these muscles; flexion does not. All activity ceases in the supine position, but the recti, in particular, spring into action at once even when it is only the head that is raised. Further flexion brings the obliques into action, but less forcibly. In general the obliques appear to be concerned mainly in compressive and forcible twisting movements, the recti in flexion when gravitational or other resistance has to be overcome. In normal standing there is little postural activity in the entire musculature, except for the lower part of internal oblique, which can be accessed by electromyographic electrodes through the aponeurosis of external oblique (see Inguinal canal, p. 822).

Transversus is difficult to study with electromyographic techniques.

It acts to compress the abdominal contents and probably has no appreciable effect on the vertebral column.

Pyramidalis tenses the linea alba. The fact that the muscle is absent in about 1 out of 6 individuals studied (Anson et al 1938) suggests that this action is not highly significant.

Linea alba

The linea alba (**7.76, 85**) is a tendinous raphe extending from the xiphoid process to the symphysis pubis and pubic crest. It lies between the recti, and is formed by the interlacing aponeurotic fibres of the oblique and transverse muscles (for more detail see A more recent view of structures of the anterolateral abdominal wall, p. 828). A little below its midpoint is a fibrous cicatrix, covered by a puckered adherent area of skin—the *umbilicus*. Below the umbilicus the linea alba is narrow, corresponding to the linear interval between the recti, and visible only in the lean and muscular as a slight groove. Above the umbilicus the recti diverge from one other; the linea alba is correspondingly broader, and can be recognized on the surface as a shallow groove. The linea alba is doubly attached at its lower end: its superficial fibres pass **in front of** the recti to the symphysis pubis; its deeper fibres form a triangular lamella, attached **behind** the recti to the posterior surface of the pubic crest on each side and named the *adminiculum lineae albae*. The linea alba is traversed by a few minute vessels. In the fetus the umbilicus transmits the umbilical vessels, urachus and, up to the third month, the vitelline or yolk stalk. It closes a few days after birth, but the vestiges of the vessels and urachus remain attached to its deep surface. The remnant of the fetal left umbilical vein is the *ligamentum teres* of the liver; the obliterated umbilical arteries form the medial umbilical ligaments, enclosed in peritoneal folds of the same name; and the partially obliterated remains of the urachus persist as the median umbilical ligament.

A more recent view of structures of the anterolateral abdominal wall

The traditional view of the anterolateral abdominal musculature is that the oblique and transverse muscles each form a single, unilaminar aponeurosis that divides or passes around the rectus and ends in the midline at the linea alba. This is a simple and adequate description for all practical (including surgical) purposes and has accordingly formed the basis for the main account in this text. It can, however, be elaborated in the light of a detailed and extensive study of human cadaveric and other mammalian material by Rizk (1980). That paper should be consulted for further information, but the revised view that it offers is summarized briefly here in a simplified way.

The main departures from the traditional account are as follows:

- Obliquus externus, obliquus internus and transversus abdominis each have a *bilaminar* aponeurosis.
- Of the six laminae formed in this way, three pass anterior to rectus and three posterior.
- A given aponeurotic lamina does not stop at the midline but decussates there with other aponeuroses and continues as an aponeurotic layer of the contralateral muscle or of another muscle. Thus sheets of collagenous fibres cross each other at the midline, and the linea alba is formed by compaction of these linear decussations.
- The continuation of aponeurotic laminae across the midline effectively combines the bilateral oblique and transverse muscles in pairs, so that these could be regarded as digastric muscles, albeit with their central tendon firmly anchored in the linea alba.

The bilaminar aponeuroses of the obliquus externus are illustrated in (7.86). They consist of deep and superficial layers, their fibres approximately at right angles to each other. The deep layer forms a sheet of parallel, straight fibres, over the top of which the superficial layer forms a series of parallel, wide S-shaped curves. At the midline the fibres from the deep layer on each side decussate to continue as the superficial layer in the contralateral half of the abdominal wall.

From these and similar observations a more detailed picture emerges of the structure of the rectus sheath. From the costoxiphoid margin to the umbilical level the anterior wall of the rectus sheath is trilaminar. It consists (externally to internally) of:

- the anterior lamina of the external oblique aponeurosis
- the posterior lamina of the external oblique aponeurosis
- the anterior lamina of the internal oblique aponeurosis.

In the first and third of these layers the fibres are parallel, and course obliquely upwards and medially as they approach the midline. The fibres in the second layer, sandwiched between them, are at right angles to this. This construction is similar to the cross-grain of plywood. In most individuals the same arrangement is present in the posterior wall of the sheath which (continuing in the same direction) consists of:

- the posterior lamina of the internal oblique aponeurosis (fibres directed upwards and medially)
- the anterior lamina of the transversus abdominis aponeurosis (fibres directed downwards and medially)
- the posterior lamina of the transversus abdominis aponeurosis (fibres directed upwards and medially).

Between the level of the umbilicus and the iliac crest the layers change in their superficial-to-deep sequence and near the pubis they are modified by the formation of the falx inguinalis. Note that in this newer account the posterior layer of the sheath does not undergo a sudden transition at an arcuate line; instead it is slowly attenuated, with fibres transferring progressively to the anterior layer and to the falx inguinalis, and the transversalis fascia thickening posteriorly to compensate.

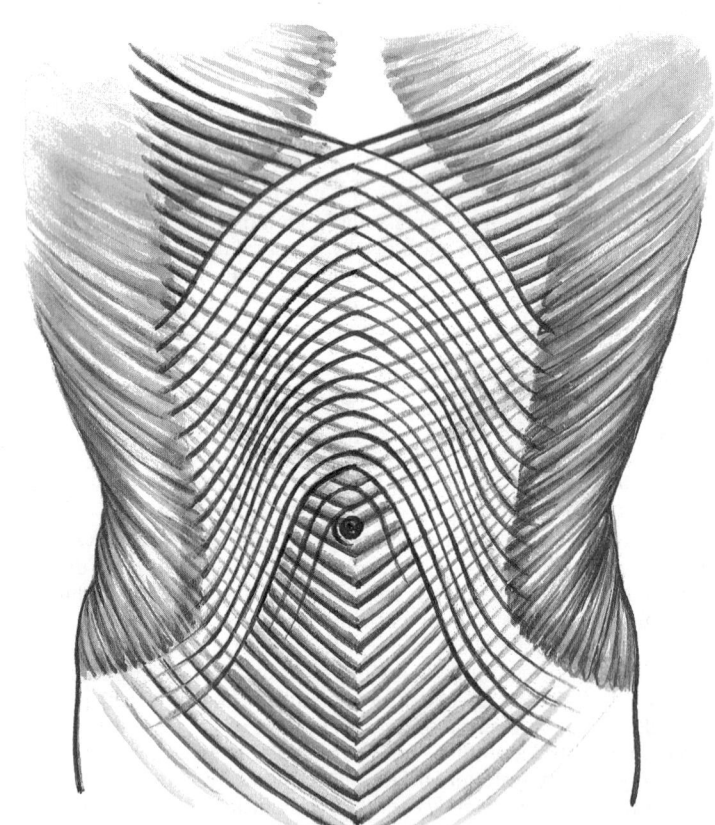

7.86 The concept of bilaminar aponeuroses of the external oblique muscles. Note that the fibres of the superficial and deep layers are approximately at right angles; decussations occur as part of the linea alba (modified from Rizk 1980).

Transversalis fascia

The transversalis fascia (7.82) is a thin stratum of connective tissue lying between the internal surface of transversus and the extra-peritoneal fat. It is part of the general layer of fascia between the peritoneum and the abdominal walls, and is continuous with the iliac and pelvic fasciae. In the inguinal region it is thick and dense, and augmented by the aponeurosis of the transversus, but it thins as it ascends to the diaphragm and blends with the fascial covering of its inferior surface. Behind, it fuses with the anterior lamina of the thoracolumbar fascia. Below, it is attached posteriorly to the whole length of the iliac crest between the origins of transversus and iliacus and to the posterior margin of the inguinal ligament between the anterior superior iliac spine and the femoral vessels, blending there with the iliac fascia. Medial to the femoral vessels it is thin and fused to the pecten pubis behind the falx inguinalis, with which it is united. It descends in front of the femoral vessels to form the anterior part of the femoral sheath (p. 1564) and the fascia is strengthened here by transversely arched fibres which spread laterally towards the anterior superior iliac spine and diverge medially behind rectus abdominis; some descend to the pecten pubis behind the falx inguinalis. These arched fibres constitute the *deep crural arch*. The spermatic cord in the male, or the round ligament of the uterus in the female, pass through the transversalis fascia at the deep inguinal ring (see below). This opening is not visible externally since the transversalis fascia is prolonged on these structures as the *internal spermatic fascia*. Around the testis this blends with the areolar tissue on the parietal layer of the tunica vaginalis (p. 1848); it sometimes contains smooth muscle fibres (Barrett 1951). The curved fibres of the deep crural arch thicken the inferomedial part of the rim of the deep inguinal ring.

The deep inguinal ring

The deep inguinal ring (7.83) is situated in the transversalis fascia, midway between the anterior superior iliac spine and the symphysis pubis and about 1.25 cm above the inguinal ligament. It is oval, with the long axis vertical. Its size varies between individuals but it is always much larger in the male. It is related above to the arched lower margin of transversus abdominis, and medially to the inferior epigastric vessels and the interfoveolar ligament, when present. Traction on the fascial ring exerted by the internal oblique muscle may constitute a valve-like safety mechanism when intra-abdominal pressure is raised (Lytle 1970).

Inguinal canal

The inguinal canal contains the spermatic cord in the male, the round ligament of the uterus in the female, and the ilio-inguinal nerve in both sexes. It is oblique and about 4 cm long, and slants downwards and medially, parallel with and a little above the inguinal ligament; it extends from the deep to the superficial inguinal rings. It is bounded: **in front**, by the skin, superficial fascia and aponeurosis of external oblique, and in its lateral one-third by the muscular fibres of the internal oblique; **behind**, by the reflected inguinal ligament, the falx inguinalis and the transversalis fascia, which separate it from extraperitoneal connective tissue and peritoneum; **above**, by the arched fibres of the internal oblique and transversus abdominis; **below**, by the union of the transversalis fascia with the inguinal ligament and, at its medial end, by the lacunar ligament.

The presence of the canal would appear to weaken the lower part of the anterior abdominal wall, but this is compensated in part by the obliquity of the canal and the arrangement of the structures in its walls. Owing to the oblique direction of the canal the two inguinal rings do not coincide, and increases in intra-abdominal pressure exercise their effect not only at the deep inguinal ring but also on the posterior wall of the canal, thus pressing it to the anterior. The posterior wall is strengthened by the falx inguinalis and the reflected inguinal ligament that lie directly behind the superficial inguinal ring, and internal oblique contributes to the formation of the anterior wall, where it overlaps the deep inguinal ring (see p. 823). The parts of internal oblique and transversus that are attached to the inguinal ligament (i.e. the muscle fibres that 'arch' over the oblique canal) are constantly active in standing; their activity is augmented by any increase in intra-abdominal pressure (for example, during coughing or straining).

Clinical relevance. Protrusion of the intestine into the inguinal canal is known as an oblique or indirect inguinal hernia (see p. 1788).

Extraperitoneal connective tissue

The extraperitoneal connective tissue is a stratum of areolar connective tissue lying between the peritoneum and the general fascial lining of the abdominal and pelvic cavities. The amount of this extraperitoneal tissue varies. It is especially abundant on the posterior wall of the abdomen, particularly around the kidneys, where it contains much fat. It is scanty on the anterolateral wall, except in the pubic region, above the iliac crest and in the pelvis.

Such fasciae are usually no more than the general connective tissue that is found between differentiated structures. In some regions, however, there may be aligned bundles of collagen, elastic fibres and (particularly in the pelvis) bundles or sheets of smooth muscle. Extraperitoneal tissue is continuous with the epimysium of muscles of the abdominal wall and its extensions into those muscles.

POSTERIOR MUSCLES OF THE ABDOMEN

Although psoas major and minor, and iliacus, with the fasciae covering them, form part of the abdominal parietes, they are also muscles of the lower limb and are described with them. Only quadratus lumborum will be considered here.

The *fascia* covering quadratus lumborum is the anterior layer of the thoracolumbar fascia (p. 809). Its attachments are as follows; **medially**, to the anterior surfaces of the transverse processes of the lumbar vertebrae; **below**, to the iliolumbar ligament; **above**, to the apex and lower border of the twelfth rib. **Laterally**, it blends with the fused posterior and middle layers of the thoracolumbar fascia (7.70). Its upper margin, which extends from the transverse process of the first lumbar vertebra to the apex and lower border of this rib, is the lateral arcuate ligament (p. 816).

Quadratus lumborum

Quadratus lumborum (7.69, 75) has an irregularly quadrilateral shape .which is broader inferiorly. It is attached below by aponeurotic fibres to the iliolumbar ligament and the adjacent portion of the iliac crest for about 5 cm, and above to the medial half of the lower border of the twelfth rib, and by four small tendons to the apices of the transverse processes of the upper four lumbar vertebrae, and sometimes to the transverse process or body of the twelfth thoracic.

Variations. Occasionally a second layer of this muscle is found in front of the first: it passes from the upper borders of the transverse processes of the lower three or four lumbar vertebrae to the lower margin and the lower part of the anterior surface of the last rib.

Relations. Anterior to quadratus lumborum are the colon, kidney, psoas major and minor, and diaphragm; the subcostal, iliohypogastric and ilio-inguinal nerves are anterior to the fascia over the muscle, but are bound down to it by the medial continuation of the transversalis fascia.

Blood supply. Lumbar arteries (p. 1558); arteria lumbalis ima (p. 1558); the lumbar branch of the iliolumbar artery (p. 1562); subcostal artery (p. 1546).

Nerve supply. Ventral rami of the twelfth thoracic and upper three or four lumbar spinal nerves.

Actions. Quadratus lumborum fixes the last rib, and acts as a muscle of inspiration by helping to stabilize the lower attachments of the diaphragm. It has been suggested that this action might also provide a fixed base for controlled relaxation of the diaphragm in the precise adjustment of expiration needed for speech and singing (Taylor 1960). With the pelvis fixed, quadratus acts upon the vertebral column, flexing it to the same side. When both muscles contract they probably help to extend the lumbar part of the vertebral column.

MUSCLES AND FASCIAE OF THE PELVIS

The muscles arising within the pelvis form two groups:

- piriformis and obturator internus, described with muscles of the lower limb (pp. 879, 880)
- levator ani and coccygeus which, with the corresponding muscles of the opposite side, form the *pelvic diaphragm*.

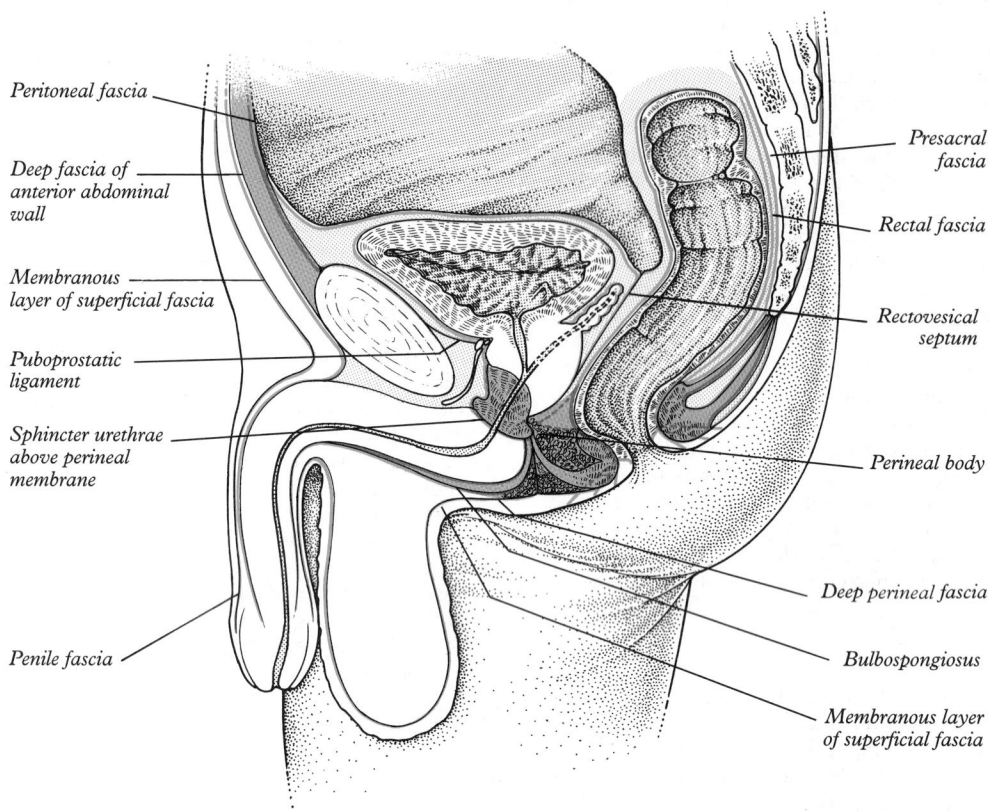

Peritoneal fascia

Deep fascia of anterior abdominal wall

Membranous layer of superficial fascia

Puboprostatic ligament

Sphincter urethrae above perineal membrane

Penile fascia

Presacral fascia

Rectal fascia

Rectovesical septum

Perineal body

Deep perineal fascia

Bulbospongiosus

Membranous layer of superficial fascia

7.87 Median sagittal section through the pelvis, showing the arrangement of the fasciae, depicted in green.

The fasciae investing the muscles (**7.87**) are continuous with visceral pelvic fascia above, perineal fascia below and obturator fascia laterally. (For perineal muscles and fasciae see pp. 832–834.)

FASCIAE OF THE PELVIS

Pelvic fascia (**7.87**) may be resolved for description into:

- *parietal pelvic fascia*, mainly sheaths of pelvic muscles
- *visceral pelvic fascia*, sheaths of pelvic viscera and their vessels and nerves (for which see individual organs).

Parietal pelvic fascia

The parietal pelvic fascia on the pelvic surface of obturator internus is well differentiated as *obturator fascia*. Above, it is connected to the posterior part of the arcuate line of the ilium, and is there continuous with iliac fascia. Anterior to this, as it follows the line of origin of obturator internus, it gradually separates from iliac fascia, continuity between the two being retained only via periosteum. It arches below the obturator vessels and nerve, completing the obturator canal, and is attached anteriorly to the back of the pubis. Behind the obturator canal the fascia is markedly aponeurotic and gives origin to levator ani (p. 831); below this origin it is thin and forms part of the lateral wall of the ischiorectal fossa (p. 832). It has indirectly continuity, via periosteum, with the fascia on piriformis.

Fascia of piriformis

The fascia of piriformis is very thin, and fuses with periosteum on the front of the sacrum at the margins of the anterior sacral foramina, where it ensheathes the sacral anterior primary rami emerging from these foramina (hence these nerves are often described as lying **behind**

the fascia). Internal iliac vessels are, however, **in front of** piriform fascia, and their branches take sheaths of extraperitoneal tissue into the gluteal region, above and below piriformis.

Fascia of the pelvic diaphragm

The fascia of the pelvic diaphragm covers both of the surfaces of the pelvic diaphragm. On the **lower** surface is the thin *inferior fascia of the pelvic diaphragm*, which is continuous with the obturator fascia laterally, covers the medial wall of the ischiorectal fossa, and blends below with fasciae on sphincter urethrae and sphincter ani externus. On the **upper** surface is the *superior fascia of the pelvic diaphragm*, which is attached anteriorly to the back of the body of the pubis, about 2 cm above its lower border, and extends laterally across the superior ramus of the pubis, blending with obturator fascia and continuing along an irregular line to the spine of the ischium. It is continuous behind with piriform fascia and the anterior sacro-coccygeal ligament. In lower mammals the levator ani springs dorsally (posteriorly) from the pelvic brim but in the human its attachment is lower (more caudal, or inferior), leaving its aponeurosis as a thickened upper part of the obturator fascia. Tendinous fibres of the attachment may reach the pelvic brim. Medially, the superior fascia of the pelvic diaphragm blends with the visceral pelvic fascia. The 'fascia' on obturator internus above the attachment of levator ani is therefore composed of:

- the obturator fascia
- the superior and inferior pelvic diaphragmatic fasciae
- the degenerated aponeurosis of levator ani.

The thickening where these structures fuse is the *tendinous arch of levator ani*. Below it, within the superior fascia, is the *tendinous arch of the pelvic fascia*, a thick white band extending from the lower part

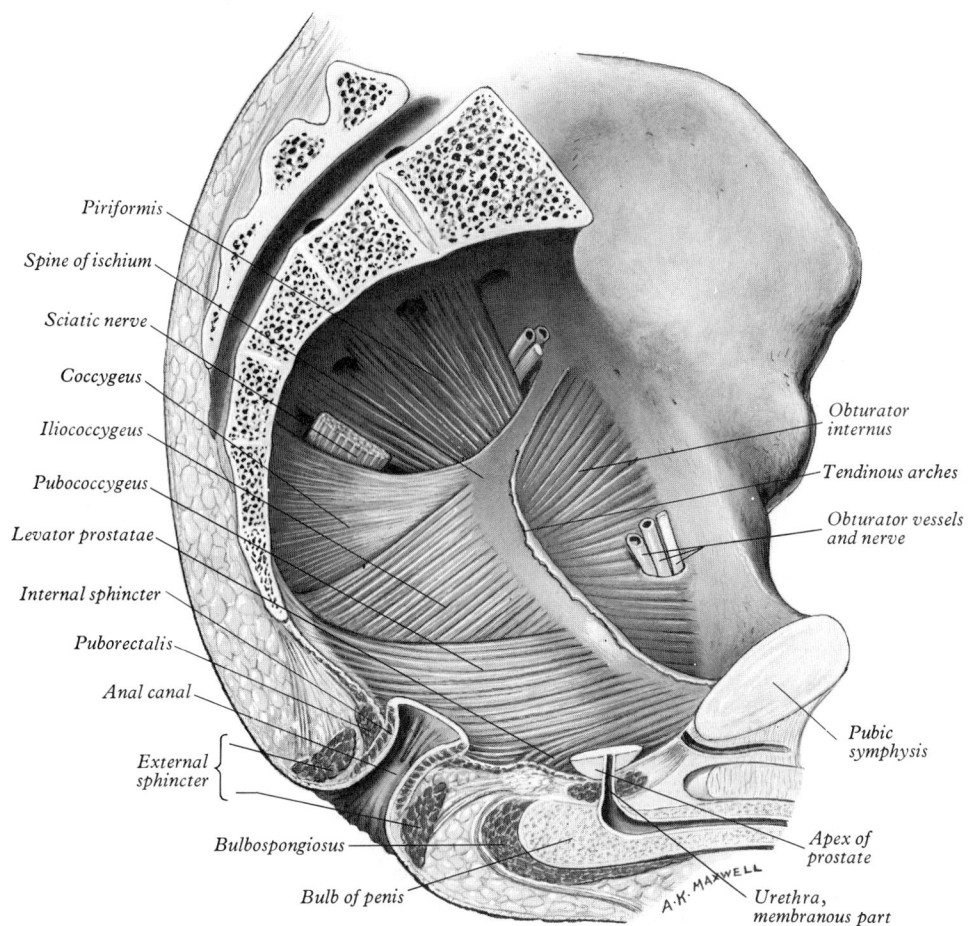

Piriformis

Spine of ischium

Sciatic nerve

Coccygeus

Iliococcygeus

Pubococcygeus

Levator prostatae

Internal sphincter

Puborectalis

Anal canal

External sphincter

Bulbospongiosus

Bulb of penis

Obturator internus

Tendinous arches

Obturator vessels and nerve

Pubic symphysis

Apex of prostate

Urethra, membranous part

A.K. MAXWELL

7.88 Pelvic aspect of the left levator ani and coccygeus. The superior gluteal vessels and nerve have been cut close to the upper border of piriformis; the anal canal has been divided below the anorectal flexure and the greater part of the prostate has been removed. The constituent parts of levator ani are shown. Note: coccygeus is fused and coextensive with the sacrospinous ligament; the latter is viewed from the gluteal aspect.

of the symphysis pubis to the inferior margin of the spine of the ischium. This is the attachment of the lateral, 'true' ligament of the urinary bladder. Anteriorly the same fascia forms two thick bands, the paired *puboprostatic* (*pubovesical*) *ligaments.*

Presacral fascia

The presacral fascia lies between the fascial sheath of the rectum and the superior pelvic diaphragmatic fascia. It is a hammock-like sheet extending between the tendinous arches of the pelvic fascia on either side. Below, it extends to the anorectal junction, where it fuses with the sheath of the rectum; above, it can be traced to the origin of the superior hypogastric plexus which, with right and left hypogastric nerves and inferior hypogastric (pelvic) plexuses, is embedded in it (Roberts et al 1964).

MUSCLES OF THE PELVIS

Levator ani

Levator ani (**7.88**) is a broad muscular sheet of variable thickness attached to the internal surface of the true pelvis; it unites with its contralateral counterpart to form most of the pelvic floor. A *pubococcygeal part* arises from the back of the body of the pubis and passes back almost horizontally: the most medial fibres relate to sphincter urethrae (and in the male to the prostate as the so-called *levator prostatae*) forming part of the periurethral musculature; further back some fibres insert into the walls of the vagina in the female (*pubovaginalis*) and the perineal body (p. 833) and rectum in both sexes. These latter fibres, *puboanalis*, decussate and blend with the longitudinal rectal muscle and fascial elements to form the conjoint longitudinal coat of the anal canal (p. 1370). Behind the rectum most pubococcygeal fibres form a tendinous plate which

attaches to the anterior surface of the coccyx. A thick *puborectal part* is inseparable from pubococcygeus at its origin but subsequently passes below it and joins its fellow from the opposite side, and sphincter ani externus, to form a sling behind the anorectal junction. A thin or aponeurotic *iliococcygeal part* arises from obturator fascia between the obturator canal and the ischial spine. Its fibres contribute to the anococcygeal ligament, forming a raphe and attaching to the sides of the last two segments of the coccyx. An accessory slip at its posterior part is *iliosacralis.* Complete homologies are controversial (Wendell-Smith 1967) but in tailed mammals pubococcygeus, iliococcygeus and ischiococcygeus (coccygeus) are attached only to caudal vertebrae; iliococcygeus and ischiococcygeus effect lateral movements of the tail and pubococcygeus draws the tail between the hind limbs. In man, loss of the tail has freed these muscles to make a more complete pelvic floor, a particular necessity in bipeds. Levator and depressor caudae of tailed mammals may be represented in the human by the rudimentary anterior and posterior sacrococcygeal muscles, which run from the sacrum to the coccyx anterior and posterior to the sacrococcygeal joint.

Relations. The *superior* (*pelvic*) *surface* of levator ani is separated only by fascia (superior pelvic diaphragmatic, visceral and extraperitoneal) from the urinary bladder, prostate or uterus and vagina, rectum and peritoneum. Its *inferior* (*perineal*) *surface* is the medial wall of the ischiorectal fossa and the superior wall of its anterior recess (p. 832), both being covered by inferior pelvic diaphragmatic fascia. The *posterior border* is separated from coccygeus by areolar tissue. The *medial borders* of the two levator muscles are separated by the visceral outlet, through which pass the urethra, vagina, and anorectum.

Nerve supply. Fibres originating mainly in the second and third sacral spinal segments reach the levatores from below and above, respectively, by a variety of routes (Wendell-Smith & Wilson 1991). Most commonly the anteromedial part is supplied by the pudendal nerve (p. 1287) and the posterolateral part by direct branches from the sacral plexus.

Actions. All the medial fibres are lateral compressors of visceral canals; puborectalis also reinforces sphincter ani externus, helps to create the anorectal angle, and reduces the anteroposterior dimension of the ano-urogenital hiatus. Thus all medial fibres contribute to continence and must relax to permit expulsion. The levatores form much of the basin-shaped muscular *pelvic diaphragm*, which supports pelvic viscera and contracts with abdominal muscles and the abdominothoracic diaphragm to raise intra-abdominal pressure. Like the abdominothoracic diaphragm, but unlike abdominal muscles, they are active in the inspiratory phase of quiet respiration. These observations are supported by scanning techniques, but complete analysis is elusive (Wendell-Smith & Wilson 1991). In the gravid female, the pelvic floor directs the fetal head into the anteroposterior diameter of the pelvic outlet. Injuries to muscles and/or nerves of the pelvic floor often occur in parturition. A tear involving the perineal body (p. 833) may permit divarication of the levatores and contribute to uterovaginal prolapse. This may be prevented by incising the perineum (*episiotomy*) in order to provide a clean, easily reparable wound.

Coccygeus

Coccygeus (7.88) is posterosuperior to, and in the morphological plane of, the levator ani. It is a triangular musculotendinous sheet that arises by its apex from the pelvic surface and tip of the ischial spine and is fused with the sacrospinous ligament; it is attached at its base to the lateral margins of the coccyx and the fifth sacral segment. It is occasionally absent, but more often varies in the proportions of its muscular and fibrous tissue content. It lies on the pelvic aspect of the sacrospinous ligament, which is commonly regarded as a degenerate part or an aponeurosis of the muscle. The muscle and ligament are coextensive, the former being visible from the pelvic aspect and the latter from the gluteal aspect. The muscle is well developed, and the ligament often absent, in mammals with a mobile tail.

Nerve supply. Third and fourth sacral spinal nerves.

Actions. The coccygei act with the levatores (see above).

MUSCLES AND FASCIAE OF THE PERINEUM

The perineum is the region below the pelvic diaphragm and has the same skeletal boundaries as the pelvic outlet: **anteriorly**, the pubic arch and its arcuate ligament; **posteriorly** the tip of the coccyx; and **on each side** the inferior pubic and ischial rami, ischial tuberosities and sacrotuberous ligaments. It extends superficially to the skin and its lateral limits are reached at the buttocks and the medial sides of the thighs. The perineum is trapezoidal, but not planar. On the surface of the body the perineum in the male is defined by the scrotum in front, the buttocks behind and the medial sides of the thighs laterally. A transverse line in front of the ischial tuberosities divides the region into two triangular parts: a posterior *anal triangle*, with its apex at the coccyx, contains the anal canal; an anterior *urogenital triangle*, with its apex at the pubic symphysis, contains external urogenital structures. The urogenital triangle slopes downwards and backwards, whereas the anal triangle slopes downwards and forwards. Clinically, the term perineum may be used in a more restricted way to apply to the perineal body and overlying skin (see below).

MUSCLES AND FASCIAE OF THE ANAL TRIANGLE

Superficial fascia

The superficial fascia of the region is thick, areolar and contains many fat cells. A pad of fatty tissue extends deeply into the *ischiorectal fossa* between levator ani and obturator internus on each side.

Deep fascia

The deep fascia lines each ischiorectal fossa; it comprises the inferior fascia of the pelvic diaphragm and that part of the obturator fascia below the attachment of levator ani.

Ischiorectal fossa

The ischiorectal fossa is wedge-shaped, with its base on perineal skin and its thin edge at the junction of obturator internus and levator ani, covered by the obturator and inferior pelvic diaphragmatic fasciae. **Medially** are sphincter ani externus and the pelvic diaphragmatic fascia; **laterally** are the ischial tuberosity and the obturator fascia. **Posteriorly**, the fossa is partly limited by the lower border of gluteus maximus but extends deep to it as far as the sacrotuberous ligament. **Anteriorly**, the fossa is partly bounded by the posterior aspect of the muscles of the urogenital triangle, but it is prolonged above them as a narrow recess, sometimes reaching as far as the retropubic space. This *anterior recess* retains the same relation to obturator internus and levator, but is deep (superior) to the urogenital muscles and fascia.

In the lateral wall of the ischiorectal fossa are the internal pudendal vessels and accompanying nerves, enclosed in fascia that forms the *pudendal canal*. This fascia fuses with the lower part of the obturator fascia, which ascends to blend with the inferior pelvic diaphragmatic fascia and descends to fuse with the falciform process of the sacrotuberous ligament (p. 677). It is sometimes termed the *lunate fascia*, and is regarded as forming the roof and lateral wall of the fossa. It passes forwards above the urogenital muscles and fasciae, blending with their lateral margin where they attach to the inner surface of the inferior pubic ramus.

Sphincter ani externus

Sphincter ani externus (7.89) surrounds the lowest part of the anal canal and is intimately adherent to skin; above, it overlaps the internal anal sphincter. It is described in detail on page 1780, and therefore only briefly here. It has deep, superficial and subcutaneous parts. The deep part exchanges fibres with the puborectal sling above it (p. 833) and, via the perineal body (see p. 833), with deep perineal muscles anterior to it. The superficial part exchanges fibres with superficial perineal muscles; this part, and to a lesser extent the other parts, is attached to both the coccyx and the anococcygeal ligament. Above this attachment a retrosphincteric space connects the ischiorectal fossae of the two sides.

Nerve supply. Perineal branch of the fourth sacral spinal nerve and rami of the inferior rectal branch of the pudendal nerve (second and third sacral spinal nerves).

Anococcygeal ligament

The anococcygeal ligament is a layered musculotendinous structure in the midline between anorectum and coccyx. With the overlying presacral fascia it forms the *postnatal plate* (Wendell-Smith & Wilson 1977), on which sits the terminal rectum. From above downwards its layers are the presacral fascia, the tendinous plate of pubococcygeus, the muscular raphe of iliococcygeus and the posterior attachments of puborectalis and sphincter ani externus. Elevation of the postanal plate reduces the anteroposterior length of the ano-urogenital hiatus.

MUSCLES AND FASCIAE OF THE MALE UROGENITAL TRIANGLE

The muscles of the urogenital region (7.89) are involved in urination, copulation and general support of the pelvic contents. They may be considered to form two groups:

- a *superficial* group, occupying the *superficial perineal space*
- a *deep* group, occupying the *deep perineal space*:

Superficial urogenital muscles	Deep perineal muscles
A median bulbospongiosus	A sphincter urethrae
Right and left ischiocavernosi	Right and left transversi perinei
Right and left transversi perinei superficiales	profundi

They do not form a diaphragmatic sheet, but extend through the visceral outlet into the lower reaches of the pelvic cavity; thus there is no *urogenital diaphragm* as such (Oelrich 1980).

Superficial fascia

The superficial fascia of this region has a superficial adipose and a deeper membranous layer.

The *adipose layer* is thick and areolar, and contains variable amounts of fat. It is continuous with the thin dartos muscle of the scrotum, with thicker circumanal subcutaneous areolar tissue, and laterally with the superficial femoral fascia. In the midline it is adherent to skin and the membranous layer.

The *membranous layer* (**7.87**) is thin, aponeurotic and strong. It, too, is continuous with the dartos muscle, and with the fascia penis and the membranous layer of the superficial fascia of the anterior abdominal wall. **Laterally** it is attached to the margins of the rami of the pubis and ischium, lateral to the crura penis and as far back as the ischial tuberosities; **posteriorly** it curves round the superficial transversi perinei to join the posterior margin of the perineal membrane (see below) and perineal body. Abcesses and extravasations deep to the membranous layer may track down into the scrotum, along the penis and up into the abdominal wall.

Perineal body

The perineal body (the Latin term, *centrum tendineum perinei*, is inappropriate, since the body is neither tendinous nor restricted to the centre) is a pyramidal fibromuscular node located in the midline in the angle between the anal canal and the urogenital apparatus, with the *rectovesical* (*rectovaginal*) *septum* at its apex. Below this, muscles and their fasciae converge and interlace (cf. the *facial modiolus*, p. 796). Described from above downwards they are:

- the smooth muscle of internal sphincter ani and the conjoint longitudinal coat of the rectum
- the two levatores prostatae (pubovaginales)
- the deep and some superficial perineal muscles.

The deep muscles comprise sphincter urethrae, the two deep transversi perinei and the deep part of sphincter ani externus. The superficial muscles comprise bulbospongiosus, the two superficial transversi perinei and the superficial part of sphincter ani externus. The attachments of these muscles to the pubes, ischia and coccyx determine the position of the perineal body and hence of the visceral canals in the pelvic outlet. Electrical stimulation of the perineal body causes the pelvic floor as a whole to contract; intermittent application of such stimulation has been employed to try to correct weakness in this musculature. The *perineal raphe* is a median ridge in the skin and fasciae overlying the perineal body that runs forwards from the anus; in the male it is continuous with the raphe of the scrotum.

Deep perineal fascia

The deep perineal fascia (Roberts et al 1964) is attached to the ischiopubic rami and to the posterior margin of the perineal membrane and perineal body above the membranous layer. In front it fuses with the suspensory ligament of the phallus and the fasciae of external oblique and the rectus sheath, so that extravasations deep to it are limited to the superficial perineal space.

Superficial perineal space

The superficial perineal space lies between the deep perineal fascia and the perineal membrane. It contains the root of the phallus and the muscles associated with it, branches of the internal pudendal vessels and the pudendal nerves. The associated muscles are superficial transversi perinei, bulbospongiosus and ischiocavernosi.

Transversus perinei superficialis

Transversus perinei superficialis is a narrow muscular strip which passes more or less transversely across the superficial perineal space anterior to the anus. It is very variable, often feebly developed and sometimes absent. It arises by tendinous fibres from the medial and anterior aspects of the ischial tuberosity and runs medially to its insertion, which is mainly into the perineal body but sometimes also into the ipsilateral bulbospongiosus or sphincter ani externus. In the perineal body its fibres decussate and pass into the contralateral bulbospongiosus or transversus perinei or sphincter ani externus.

Action. Considered with transversus perinei profundus (see below).

Bulbospongiosus

Bulbospongiosus (*bulbocavernosus*) is a midline muscle anterior to the anus. It consists of two symmetrical parts united by a median fibrous raphe. The fibres arise from the perineal body, in which they decussate and continue as the contralateral transversi and sphincter

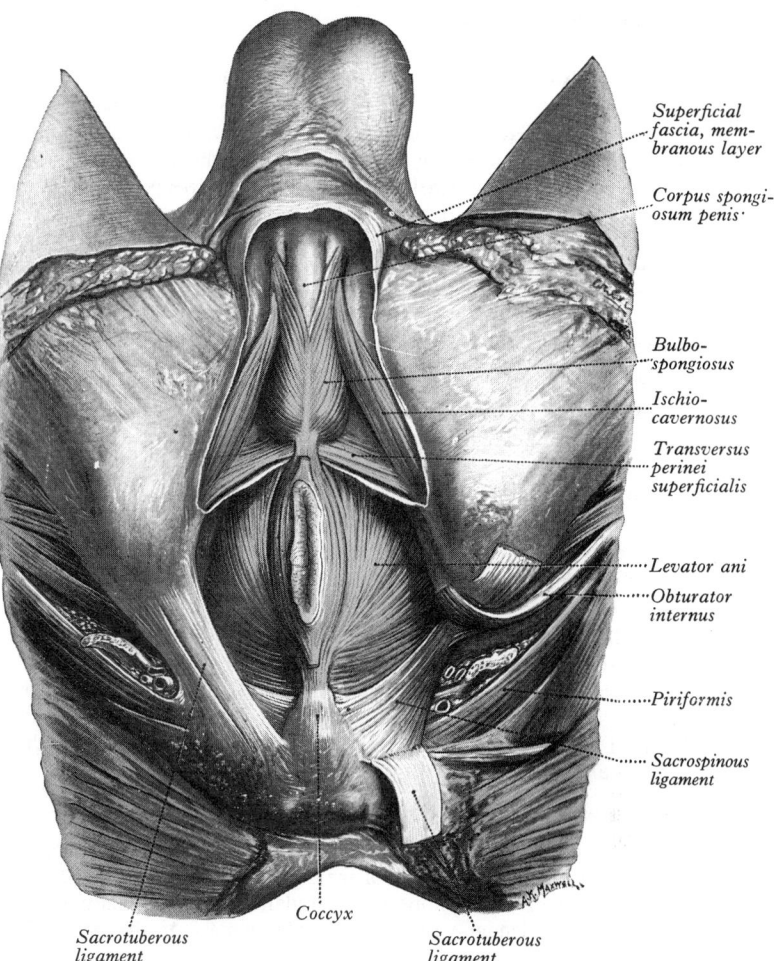

7.89 Muscles of the male perineum. (Modified from Quain's *Anatomy*, 11th edn.)

ani externus, and from the median raphe itself. The fibres diverge like the halves of a feather: a thin layer of posterior fibres disperses on the perineal membrane; the middle fibres encircle the penile bulb and adjacent corpus spongiosum and attach to an aponeurosis on the dorsal surfaces; the anterior fibres spread out over the sides of the corpora cavernosa, ending partly in them, anterior to ischiocavernosus, and partly in a tendinous expansion which covers the dorsal vessels of the penis.

Actions. Bulbospongiosus helps to empty the urethra, after the bladder has emptied; it is relaxed during micturition, usually contracting only at the end of the process, but able to arrest it. It assists in erection: the middle fibres probably compress the erectile tissue of the bulb, and the anterior fibres contribute by compressing the deep dorsal vein of the penis (p. 1858). Like other perineal muscles it has not been investigated extensively with electromyography, but the results suggest that—with sphincter urethrae—it contracts repeatedly in ejaculation.

Ischiocavernosus

Ischiocavernosus covers the crus penis. It is attached by tendinous and muscular fibres to the medial aspect of the ischial tuberosity behind the crus and to the ischial ramus on both sides of the crus. The muscle fibres end in an aponeurosis attached to the sides and under surface of the crus penis.

Action. Compression of the crus penis, maintaining penile erection. These muscles form a triangle on each side, with bulbospongiosus medially, ischiocavernosus laterally, transversus perinei superficialis posteriorly and the perineal membrane in its floor. Posterior scrotal vessels and nerves travel forwards across it in the roof of deep perineal fascia, while the perineal branch of the posterior femoral cutaneous nerve travels between superficial and deep perineal fasciae (Roberts et al 1964). The transverse perineal artery follows the posterior boundary of the triangle.

833

Perineal membrane

The perineal membrane (*inferior fascia of the urogenital diaphragm*) forms a base for superficial and deep perineal muscles and is sandwiched between them. The triangular membrane stretches almost horizontally across the pubic arch. Its base, directed backwards, is fused with the perineal body and is continuous above with the fascia over deep transversi perinei and below with the deep perineal and membranous layer of superficial fasciae, behind the transversi perinei superficiales. Its lateral margins are attached to the inferior ramus of the pubis and the ramus of the ischium, above the crura penis. Its apex, directed forwards, is thickened as the *transverse perineal ligament*; between this ligament and the pubic arcuate ligament the deep dorsal vein of the penis enters the pelvis and the dorsal nerve of the penis leaves it. The membrane is perforated by:

- urethra, 2–3 cm behind the inferior border of the symphysis, the aperture being circular and about 6 mm in diameter
- arteries and nerves to the bulb
- ducts of the bulbo-urethral glands, near the urethra
- deep arteries of the penis, near the pubic arch and halfway along its attached margin
- dorsal arteries of the penis, near its apex
- posterior scrotal vessels and nerves, near its base.

The fascia on the upper surface of the deep transversi perinei and sphincter urethrae is poorly defined but covers them and is continuous laterally with obturator fascia. Behind, it blends with inferior pelvic diaphragmatic fascia, perineal body and deep and membranous layer of superficial fasciae of the perineum. It is pierced by the urethra and continuous with prostatic fascia.

Deep perineal space

The deep perineal space lies deep to the perineal membrane and contains the membranous part of the urethra, deep transversi perinei and sphincter urethrae, bulbo-urethral glands and proximal parts of their ducts, pudendal vessels and dorsal nerves of the penis (in forward continuations of the pudendal canals), arteries and nerves of the bulb of the penis and a plexus of veins.

Transversus perinei profundus

Transversus perinei profundus extends from the medial aspect of the ischial ramus to the perineal body. Here its fibres decussate with those of its contralateral counterpart, the deep part of sphincter ani externus behind and sphincter urethrae.

Action. The superficial and deep transversi perinei tether the perineal body, and hence the visceral canals, in the median plane.

Sphincter urethrae surrounds not only the lower urethra but also the bladder neck and, between the two, has elements within the prostate (see p.1860). Its *inferior fibres* encircle the membranous urethra; some attach to the inner surface of the inferior pubic ramus; ventral fibres continue into the prostate. Its *superior fibres* form a horseshoe whose dorsal ends merge into the smooth muscle of the bladder; again ventral fibres continue into the prostate (Oelrich 1980).

Actions. Compression of the urethra, particularly when the bladder contains fluid. Like bulbospongiosus, it is relaxed during micturition, but it contracts to expel final drops of urine, or of semen, from the membranous urethra.

Nerve supply. The axons that supply the perineal muscles originate from cell bodies in the pudendal nerve nucleus (Onuf's nucleus) and those that supply the pelvic diaphragm from cell bodies related to that nucleus. From those origins, axons reach their destinations by different routes. Muscles of the pelvic floor are supplied from below by the perineal branch of the pudendal nerve (second, third and fourth sacral spinal nerves from anterior to posterior) and from above by branches from the sacral plexus and the pelvic splanchnic nerves. Muscles that lie at the interface between pelvic diaphragm and perineal muscles, such as the deep sphincters, may be supplied from above, from below, or from both above and below; those at the somatic-visceral interface, which often contain a mixture of skeletal and smooth muscle fibres, may receive both somatic and

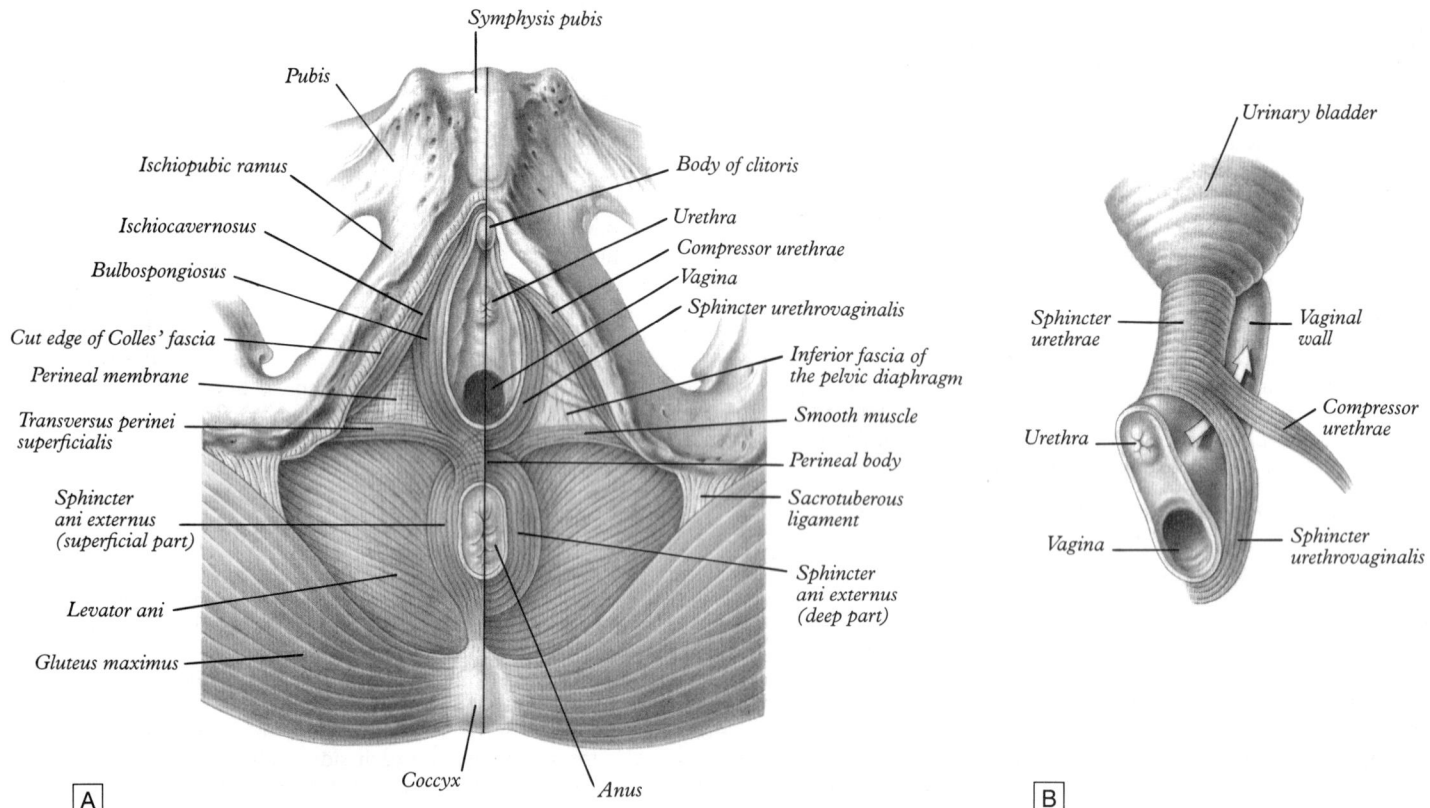

7.90 Muscles of the female perineum. On the subject's right side, the membranous layer of superficial fascia has been removed (note the cut edge). On the subject's left side, the symphysis pubis, pubis, part of the ischiopubic ramus, superficial perineal muscles and inferior fascia of the urogenital diaphragm have been removed to show the deep perineal muscles. The smaller figure illustrates the continuity of the deep perineal muscles with sphincter urethrae.

visceral innervation via pelvic splanchnic nerves. Sphincter urethrae, extending as it does from the perineum through the urogenital hiatus into the pelvic cavity, may receive innervation via the pudendal nerve, a branch of the sacral plexus and the pelvic splanchnic nerves. For further details see Wendell-Smith & Wilson (1991).

MUSCLES AND FASCIAE OF THE FEMALE UROGENITAL TRIANGLE

The female urogenital triangle includes muscles, fasciae and spaces similar to those in the male, with some differences in size and disposition due to the presence of the vagina and female external genitalia (**7.90**).

Transversus perinei superficialis

Transversus perinei superficialis is a narrow muscular slip which differs little from the corresponding muscle in the male.

Bulbospongiosus

Bulbospongiosus covers the superficial parts of the vestibular bulbs and greater vestibular glands and passes forwards on each side of the vagina to attach to the corpora cavernosa clitoridis; a fascicle crosses over the dorsum of the body of the clitoris. It is attached posteriorly to the perineal body, where its fibres decussate with those of sphincter ani externus and the contralateral transversi perinei.

Actions. Constriction of the vaginal orifice and expression of the secretions of the greater vestibular glands. Anterior fibres contribute to erection of the clitoris by compressing its deep dorsal vein.

Ischiocavernosus

Ischiocavernosus, being related to a smaller crus clitoris, is smaller than, but otherwise similar to, the corresponding muscle in the male.

Actions. Compression of the crus clitoridis, retarding venous return and thus serving to erect the clitoris.

Perineal membrane

The perineal membrane, being divided into two halves by the vagina and urethra, is less well defined and less tense than in the male. It forms a triangle on each side, between the urogenital outlets and the ischiopubic ramus, but is perforated by structures corresponding to those listed for the male (p. 834). On each side it is continuous anteriorly with a pubo-urethral ligament, there being no transverse perineal ligament as such in the female (Milley & Nichols 1971). Above the membrane, three muscles lie edge to edge along the urethra: sphincter urethrae, compressor urethrae and sphincter urethrovaginalis (Oelrich 1983, **7.90**). Their actions will be considered together below.

Sphincter urethrae

Sphincter urethrae surrounds more than the middle third of the urethra. It blends above with the smooth muscle of the bladder neck and below with the smooth muscle of the lower urethra and vagina.

Compressor urethrae

Compressor urethrae arises from the ischiopubic rami of each side by a small tendon, from which fibres pass forwards to meet their fellows of the opposite side in a flat band, ventral to the urethra, below sphincter urethrae. A variable number of fibres from the same origin fan medially to reach the vagina. Rarely do they reach the perineal body and form a deep transversus perinei; instead the posterior edge of the perineal membrane is occupied by a mass of smooth muscle.

Sphincter urethrovaginalis

Sphincter urethrovaginalis arises from the perineal body and its fibres pass forwards on either side of the vagina and urethra to meet their contralateral counterparts in a flat band, ventral to the urethra, below compressor urethrae.

Actions. The location of sphincter urethrae around the region of highest urethral closing pressure suggests that it plays an important role in the continence of urine. It may be stimulated via a vaginal tampon electrode, and this approach has been used effectively in the treatment of stress incontinence of urine. The direction of the fibres of compressor urethrae and sphincter urethrovaginalis suggests that they produce elongation as well as compression and thus aid continence.

MUSCLES AND FASCIAE OF THE UPPER LIMB

Muscles of the upper limb may be grouped as follows:

- Muscles connecting the upper limb with the vertebral column
- Muscles connecting the upper limb with the thoracic wall
- Muscles of the scapula
- Muscles of the upper arm
- Muscles of the forearm
- Muscles of the hand.

See pages 868–869 for notes and further information on the segmental innervation of muscles of the upper limb.

MUSCLES CONNECTING THE UPPER LIMB WITH THE VERTEBRAL COLUMN

Trapezius, rhomboid major and minor, and levator scapulae extend from the cervico-dorsal vertebral column to the pectoral girdle; latissimus dorsi reaches beyond this to the humerus.

Superficial fascia

The superficial fascia is thick, strong, and adipose in the cervicodorsal region, and is continuous with the general superficial fascia. In the upper neck it is tough, with much white connective tissue attaching it to skin.

Deep fascia

The deep fascia of the region is a thin, fibrous membrane, which thickens to a dense fibrous layer where it is attached to the superior nuchal lines and ligamentum nuchae, and to the spines and supraspinous ligaments of all the vertebrae below the seventh cervical. It is attached laterally to the spine and acromion of the scapula and continues downwards over the deltoid into the arm; on the thorax it is continuous with the deep fasciae of the axilla and chest; on the abdomen it merges with fascia covering the abdominal muscles; below, it is attached to the iliac crest.

Trapezius

Trapezius (**7.91**) is a flat, triangular muscle that extends over the back of the neck and upper thorax. The paired trapezius muscles form a diamond shape, from which the name is derived: lateral angles at the shoulder tips, superior angle at the occipital protuberance and superior nuchal lines, inferior angle at the spine of the twelfth thoracic vertebra. Each muscle is attached to the medial third of the superior nuchal line, external occipital protuberance, ligamentum nuchae, and apices of the spinous processes and their supraspinous ligaments from C7 all the way down to T12. Superior fibres descend, inferior fibres ascend, and the fibres between them proceed horizontally, all converging laterally on the shoulder. Here the superior fibres are attached to the posterior border of the lateral third of the clavicle; the middle fibres are attached to the medial acromial margin and superior lip of the crest of the scapular spine; the inferior fibres pass into an aponeurosis, which glides over a smooth triangular surface at the medial end of the scapular spine and is attached to a tubercle at its lateral apex. Occipital attachment is by a fibrous lamina, which is also adherent to the skin; from the sixth cervical to

835

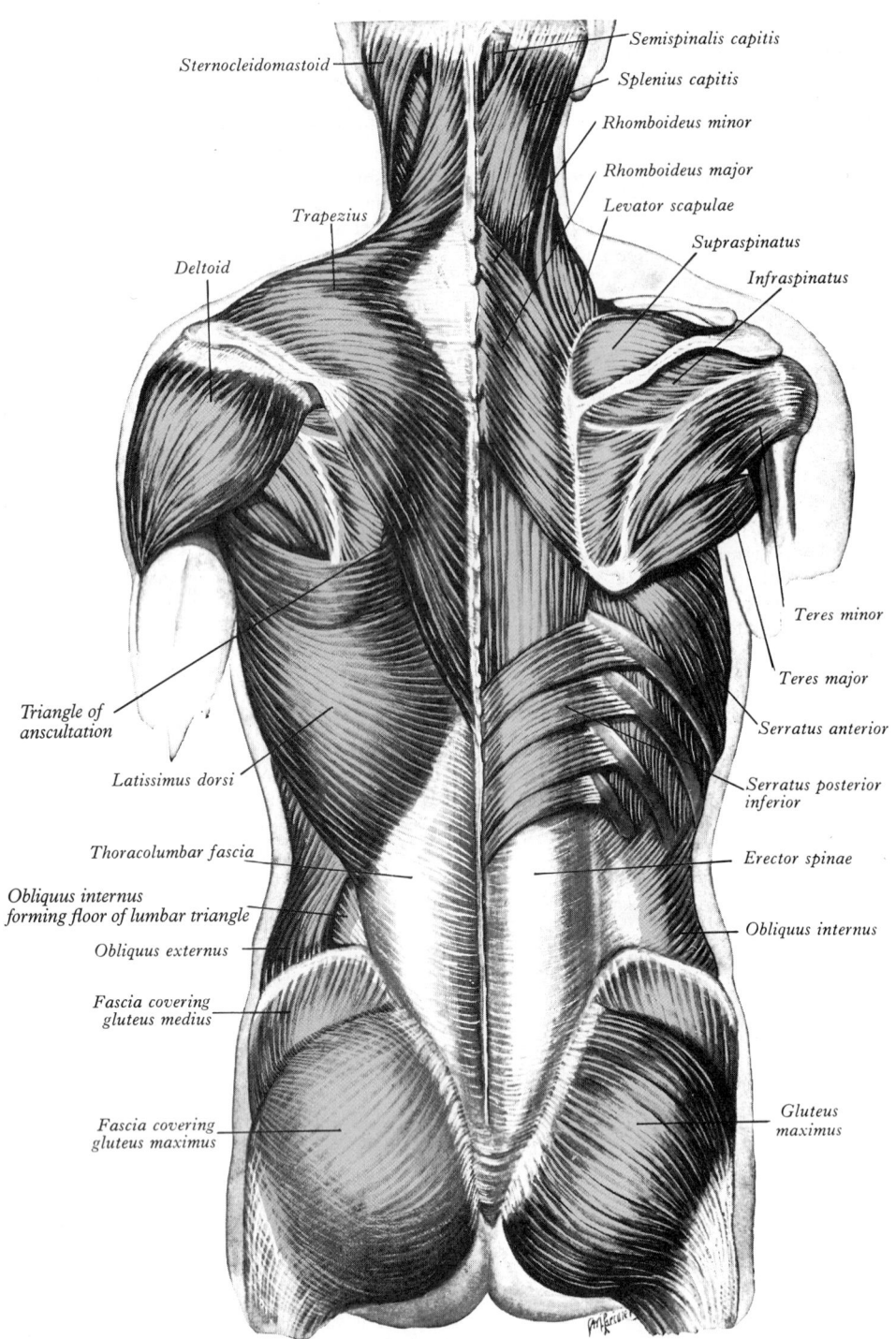

7.91 Superficial muscles of the back of the neck and trunk. On the left only the skin, superficial and deep fasciae (other than gluteofemoral) have been removed; on the right, sternocleidomastoid, trapezius, latissimus dorsi, deltoid and obliquus externus abdominis have been dissected away.

the third thoracic vertebra, spinal attachment is by a broad triangular aponeurosis; below this, attachment is by short tendinous fibres.

Variations. The clavicular attachment of trapezius varies in extent, sometimes reaching mid-clavicle and occasionally blending with sternocleidomastoid. The vertebral attachment sometimes ceases at the eighth thoracic spine. The occipital attachment may be absent. Cervical and dorsal parts are occasionally separate.

Blood supply. Superficial cervical artery or superficial branch of the transverse cervical artery (pp. 1535–1536); acromial branch of suprascapular artery (p. 1535); dorsal perforating branches of posterior intercostal arteries (p. 1546).

Nerve supply. The accessory nerve (spinal part) is the dominant motor supply, and contains sensory (proprioceptive) branches from the ventral rami of C3 and C4 (Fitzgerald et al 1982).

Actions. Trapezius co-operates with other muscles in **steadying the scapula**, controlling it during movements of the arm and maintaining

the level and poise of the shoulder. In the unloaded arm, electromyographic activity is minimal; heavy loads can be suspended with a small contribution from its upper part (Bearn 1961). With levator scapulae, its upper fibres **elevate** the scapula and with it the point of the shoulder; with serratus anterior it **rotates the scapula forward** so that the arm can be raised above the head; with the rhomboids it **retracts** the scapula, bracing back the shoulder. With the shoulder fixed, trapezius may bend the head and neck backwards and laterally. Trapezius, levator scapulae, rhomboids and serratus anterior combine in producing a variety of scapular rotations (p. 841).

Latissimus dorsi

Latissimus dorsi (**7.91**) is a large, flat, triangular muscle that sweeps over the lumbar region and lower thorax and converges to a narrow tendon. It arises by tendinous fibres from the spines of the lower six thoracic vertebrae anterior to the trapezius and from the posterior layer of thoracolumbar fascia (p. 809), by which it is attached to the spines and supraspinous ligaments of the lumbar and sacral vertebrae, and the posterior part of the iliac crest. It also springs by muscular fibres from the posterior part (outer lip) of the iliac crest lateral to the erector spinae, and by fleshy slips from the three or four lower ribs, interdigitating with obliquus abdominis externus (7.76). From this extensive attachment, fibres pass laterally with different degrees of obliquity (the upper fibres near horizontal, the middle oblique, and the lower almost vertical) to form a sheet about 12 or 13 mm thick that overlaps the inferior scapular angle. The muscle curves around the inferolateral border of teres major to its anterior surface. Here it ends as a flattened tendon, about 7 cm long, in front of the tendon of teres major, and is attached to the floor of the intertubercular sulcus of the humerus, with an expansion to the deep fascia; this attachment extends higher on the humerus than that of teres major. A bursa sometimes occurs between the muscle and the inferior scapular angle. As the muscle curves round teres major the fasciculi rotate around each other, so that fibres that originate **lowest** at the midline insert **highest** on the humerus, and fibres that originate **highest** at the midline insert **lowest** on the humerus. The tendons of latissimus and teres major are united at their lower borders, with a bursa between them near their humeral attachments.

Latissimus dorsi and teres major together form the *posterior axillary fold*. When the arm is adducted against resistance, this fold is accentuated; the whole inferolateral border of latissimus dorsi can then be traced to its attachment to the iliac crest.

The lower, lateral margin of the muscle is usually separated from the posterior border of the external oblique by a small *lumbar triangle*; the base of the triangle is the iliac crest and its floor the internal oblique (7.91). This is not to be confused with the *triangle of auscultation*, which is medial to the scapula, and is bounded above by the trapezius, below by latissimus dorsi and laterally by the medial scapular border; part of rhomboideus major is exposed in the triangle. If the scapulae are drawn forwards, by folding the arms across the chest, and the trunk is bent forwards, parts of the sixth and seventh ribs and the interspace between them (overlying the apex of the lower pulmonary lobe) become subcutaneous.

Variations. The muscle commonly receives some additional fibres from the scapula as it traverses the inferior scapular angle. A muscular axillary arch, 7–10 cm in length and 5–15 mm in breadth, may cross from the edge of latissimus dorsi, midway in the posterior fold, over the front of the axillary vessels and nerves to join the tendon of pectoralis major, coracobrachialis or fascia over the biceps. It is present in about 7% of cases and may be multiple (Kasai & Chiba 1977). The vertebral and costal attachments of latissimus dorsi may be reduced or, in rare cases, increased. A fibrous slip usually passes from the tendon, near its humeral insertion, to the long head of triceps; occasionally muscular, it is the homologue of the dorso-epitrochlearis brachii of apes.

Blood supply. The blood supply of the latissimus dorsi is particularly important because of its applications in plastic reconstructive surgery and cardiac assistance (see Cardiac assistance from skeletal muscle, p. 762). After the subscapular artery has branched to give off the circumflex scapular artery, it continues as the *thoracodorsal artery* (p. 1538). This is joined by one (rarely, two) veins and the thoracodorsal nerve, to form a neurovascular pedicle, which enters the muscle at a single neurovascular hilum on its internal (costal) surface 6 to 12 cm from the subscapular artery and 1 to 4 cm medial to the lateral border of the muscle. The artery gives off one to three large branches to the serratus anterior muscle before dividing at—or even before—the hilum to supply latissimus dorsi itself. The basic pattern of branching is a bifurcation, the larger, lateral branch following a course parallel to, and 1 to 4 cm from, the upper border of the muscle, the smaller branch diverging at an angle of 45° and travelling medially (Bartlett et al 1981; Tobin et al 1981). In two-thirds of cases there is a trifurcation: this usually yields a small recurrent branch that returns to supply the proximal part of the muscle, but in 20% of cases it provides a third major branch to the distal part of the muscle (Radermecker et al 1992). Occasionally the lateral branch gives off a further collateral to the serratus anterior muscle. This branching pattern does not appear to differ significantly between sexes (Tobin et al 1981). The two or three major branches give off 5 to 9 longitudinal branches which travel distally, parallel

to the muscle fibres. This blood supply is preserved when the muscle is moved as a pedicle graft. The distal portion of the muscle, adjacent to its costal, spinal and pelvic attachments, is supplied by dorsal perforating arteries derived from the 9th, 10th and 11th posterior intercostal and 1st, 2nd and 3rd lumbar arteries, which enter the muscle on its deep surface. There are usually two major perforating vessels, and there may be several smaller ones; these have to be ligated and divided at the time that the muscle is mobilized. The contribution from the perforating vessels used to be regarded as minor, but it is now recognized that in some mammals, including man, it may extend over as much as two-thirds of the muscle area. The basis for the survival of the distal part of the mobilized flap appears to be a series of small anastomotic channels that bridge between the territories of the thoracodorsal artery and perforating arteries (Tobin et al 1981; Taylor & Palmer 1987; Radermecker et al 1992; Craven et al 1994; see also 7.18A).

Nerve supply. The muscle is supplied by the thoracodorsal nerve from the posterior cord of the brachial plexus, C6, **7** and 8. This runs in the neurovascular pedicle and divides about 1.3 cm proximally to the point of bifurcation or trifurcation of the thoracodorsal artery. The pattern of branching follows closely that of the artery, and the neural and vascular branches travel together (Tobin et al 1981; Radermecker et al 1992).

Actions. Latissimus dorsi is active in adduction, extension and especially medial rotation of the humerus. Humeral adduction and extension are most powerful when the initial position of the arm is one of partial abduction, flexion or a combination of the two. With the sternocostal part of pectoralis major and teres major it adducts the raised arm against resistance. It assists backward swinging of the arm, as in walking and many athletic pursuits. When the arms are raised above the head, as in climbing, it pulls the trunk upwards and forwards. It takes part in all violent expiratory efforts, such as coughing or sneezing; this is readily confirmed by palpation. Electromyography (EMG) suggests that it aids deep inspiration, but the muscle is also active towards the end of forcible expiration, for example when blowing a sustained note on a musical instrument. When the arm is elevated, the stretched fibres of latissimus dorsi press on the inferior scapular angle, keeping it in contact with the chest wall. Despite this range of actions, surgical transposition of the muscle does not produce any serious restriction of normal activity.

Rhomboideus major

Rhomboideus major (7.91) is a quadrilateral sheet of muscle that arises by tendinous fibres from the spines and supraspinous ligaments of the second to fifth thoracic vertebrae, and descends laterally to the medial scapular border between the root of the spine and the inferior angle. Most of its fibres usually end in a tendinous band between these two points, joined to the medial border by a thin membrane; occasionally this is incomplete and some muscular fibres then insert directly into the scapula. The attachments of rhomboideus major (and also those of rhomboideus minor, levator scapulae and serratus anterior) can be more extensive, with 'folds' or extensions passing to both dorsal and costal aspects of the scapula adjacent to its medial margin (Bharihoke & Gupta 1986).

Rhomboideus minor

Rhomboideus minor (7.91) is a small, cylindrical muscle that runs from the lower ligamentum nuchae and the spines of the seventh cervical and first thoracic vertebrae to the base of the smooth triangular surface at the medial end of the scapular spine. Here, dorsal and ventral layers enclose the inferior border of levator scapulae (Bharihoke & Gupta 1986). The dorsal layer of rhomboideus minor is attached to the rim of the triangular surface, dorsolateral to and below levator scapulae. The ventral layer is strong and wide, extending 2–3 cm medial to and below the levator; here the fasciae of rhomboideus minor and serratus anterior are tightly fused. Rhomboideus minor is usually separate from rhomboideus major but the muscles overlap and are occasionally united.

Variations. There is some variability in the vertebral and scapular attachments of the rhomboids, and a slip of muscle may extend from the upper border of rhomboideus minor to reach the occipital bone (*rhomboideus occipitalis*).

Blood supply. Dorsal scapular artery or deep branch of the transverse cervical artery (p. 1535); dorsal perforating branches of the upper 5–6 posterior intercostal arteries (p. 1546).

Nerve supply. The rhomboids are supplied by a branch of the dorsal scapular nerve, C4, 5.

Actions. Considered together with levator scapulae (see below).

Levator scapulae

Levator scapulae (**7.68, 91**) is a slender muscle attached by tendinous slips to the transverse processes of the atlas and axis, and the posterior tubercles of the transverse processes of the third and fourth cervical posterior vertebrae. It descends diagonally to approach the medial scapular border between its superior angle and the triangular smooth surface at the medial end of the scapular spine. Bharihoke and Gupta (1986) described the scapular end of the muscle as consisting of two 'flaps' or 'folds' that are partly fused just above the superior scapular angle. The posterior fold had an aponeurotic attachment to the dorsal aspect of the medial margin, opposite the supraspinous fossa. The anterior fold had a fascial attachment 2–3 cm wide to the fascial sheath of serratus anterior, below the muscular attachment of the latter, enclosing the superior scapular angle. Below, the anterior fold tapered to a narrow tendon attached to the costal surface of the medial border at the level of the root of the scapular spine.

Variations. Levator scapulae varies considerably in its vertebral attachments and the extent to which it separates into slips. Accessory attachments may be found to the mastoid process, occipital bone, first or second rib, scaleni, trapezius, and serrate muscles.

Blood supply. The blood supply is chiefly from the transverse cervical and ascending cervical arteries. The vertebral extremity of the muscle is supplied by rami of the vertebral artery, an important consideration in transposition of the muscle (Smith et al 1974).

Nerve supply. C3, 4 and 5, by direct branches of the third and fourth cervical spinal nerves and from the fifth cervical via the dorsal scapular nerve.

Actions. The rhomboids and levator scapulae assist other scapular muscles in controlling the position and movement of the scapula. Acting with trapezius, rhomboids retract the scapula, bracing back the shoulder; with levator scapulae and pectoralis minor they rotate the scapula, depressing the point of the shoulder. With the cervical vertebral column fixed, levator scapulae acts with the trapezius to elevate the scapula or to sustain a weight carried on the shoulder; with the shoulder fixed, the muscle inclines the neck to the same side.

MUSCLES CONNECTING THE UPPER LIMB WITH THE THORACIC WALL

Serratus anterior and pectoralis minor connect the ribs to the scapula, pectoralis major extends from the upper thorax and abdomen to act on the humerus, and the small subclavius attaches only to the first rib and the clavicle.

Superficial fascia

The superficial fascia of the anterior thoracic region is continuous with that of the neck and upper limb above, and abdomen below. It contains the mammary gland, sends numerous septa between its lobes and connects it, by fibrous *mammary suspensory ligaments*, to the skin and nipple.

Pectoral fascia

The pectoral fascia is a thin (deep fascial) lamina that covers pectoralis major and extends between its fasciculi. It is attached medially to the sternum, above to the clavicle and is continuous inferolaterally with the fascia of the shoulder, axilla and thorax. Although thin over pectoralis major, it is thicker between this muscle and latissimus dorsi, to which it crosses, forming the floor of the axilla. This *axillary fascia* divides at the lateral margin of latissimus dorsi into two layers, which ensheathe the muscle and are attached behind to the spines of the thoracic vertebrae. As the fascia leaves the lower edge of pectoralis major to cross the axilla, a layer from it ascends under cover of the muscle; this layer splits to envelop pectoralis minor, at whose upper edge it becomes the *clavipectoral*

fascia (see below). The hollow of the armpit is produced mainly by the action of this fascia in tethering the skin to the floor of the axilla; it is sometimes referred to as the *suspensory ligament of the axilla.* Axillary fascia is pierced by the tail of the mammary gland (p. 417). In the lower thoracic region the deep fascia is well developed and continuous with the fibrous sheath of rectus abdominis.

Pectoralis major

Pectoralis major (**7.92**) is a thick, fan-shaped muscle, arising from the anterior surface of the sternal half of the clavicle, from half the breadth of the anterior surface of the sternum down to the level of the sixth or seventh costal cartilage, from the first to the seventh costal cartilages (first and seventh often omitted), from the sternal end of the sixth rib, and from the aponeurosis of obliquus externus abdominis. The clavicular fibres are usually separated from the sternal fibres by a slight cleft. The muscle converges to a flat tendon, about 5 cm across, which is attached to the lateral lip of the intertubercular sulcus of the humerus. The tendon is bilaminar. The thicker *anterior lamina* is formed by fibres from the manubrium, which are joined superficially by clavicular fibres and deeply by fibres from the sternal margin and second to fifth costal cartilages. Clavicular fibres may be prolonged into the deltoid tendon. The *posterior lamina* receives fibres from the sixth (and often seventh) costal cartilages, sixth rib, sternum, and aponeurosis of the obliquus abdominis externus. Costal fibres join the lamina without twisting; fibres from the sternum and aponeurosis curve around the lower border, turning successively behind those above them, this part of the muscle being so twisted that the fibres that are lowest at their medial origin are highest at their insertion on the humerus (Ashley 1952). The posterior lamina reaches higher on the humerus than the anterior, and gives off an expansion that covers the intertubercular sulcus and blends with the capsular ligament of the shoulder joint. An expansion from the deepest part of the lamina, at its linear insertion, lines the intertubercular sulcus; from its lower border another expansion descends into the deep fascia of the upper arm.

The rounded lower border of the muscle forms the anterior axillary fold, and becomes conspicuous in abduction against resistance.

Variations. The abdominal slip from the aponeurosis of the external oblique is sometimes absent. There is variation in the number of costal attachments and in the extent to which the clavicular and costal parts are separated. Right and left muscles may decussate across the sternum. A superficial vertical slip, or slips, may ascend from the lower costal cartilages and rectus sheath to blend with sternocleidomastoid or to attach to the upper sternum or costal cartilages. This is the *sternalis (rectus sternalis)*. Agenesis can result in the partial or complete absence of the muscle. For this and other variations consult Čihák and Popelka (1961) and Kasai and Chiba (1977).

Relations. **Anterior** are skin, superficial fascia, platysma, anterior and middle supraclavicular nerves, mammary gland, and deep fascia. **Posterior** are sternum, ribs and costal cartilages, clavipectoral fascia, subclavius, pectoralis minor, serratus anterior, and external intercostal muscles and membranes. Pectoralis major forms the superficial stratum of the anterior axillary wall, and hence lies anterior to axillary vessels and nerves and the upper parts of biceps and coracobrachialis. Its **upper border** is separated from the deltoid by the infraclavicular fossa, in which are the cephalic vein and deltoid branch of the thoraco-acromial artery. Its **lower border** forms the anterior axillary fold. On the medial axillary wall, pectoralis major is well separated from latissimus dorsi but the two muscles converge as they approach the lateral axillary wall (the floor of the intertubercular sulcus, between their attachments).

Blood supply. Pectoral and deltoid branches of the thoraco-acromial artery (p. 1537), and a minor contribution from perforating branches of the internal thoracic arteries (p. 1534); superior and lateral thoracic arteries (p. 1538).

Nerve supply. Pectoralis major is supplied through the medial and lateral pectoral nerves. Fibres for the clavicular part are from **C5** and 6; those for the sternocostal part are from C6, **7**, 8, and T1.

Actions. The two parts of the muscle can act separately or together. The whole muscle assists adduction and medial rotation of the humerus against resistance. It swings the extended arm forwards and medially, its clavicular part (*portio attollens*) acting with the anterior fibres of deltoid and coracobrachialis; in this movement the sterno-

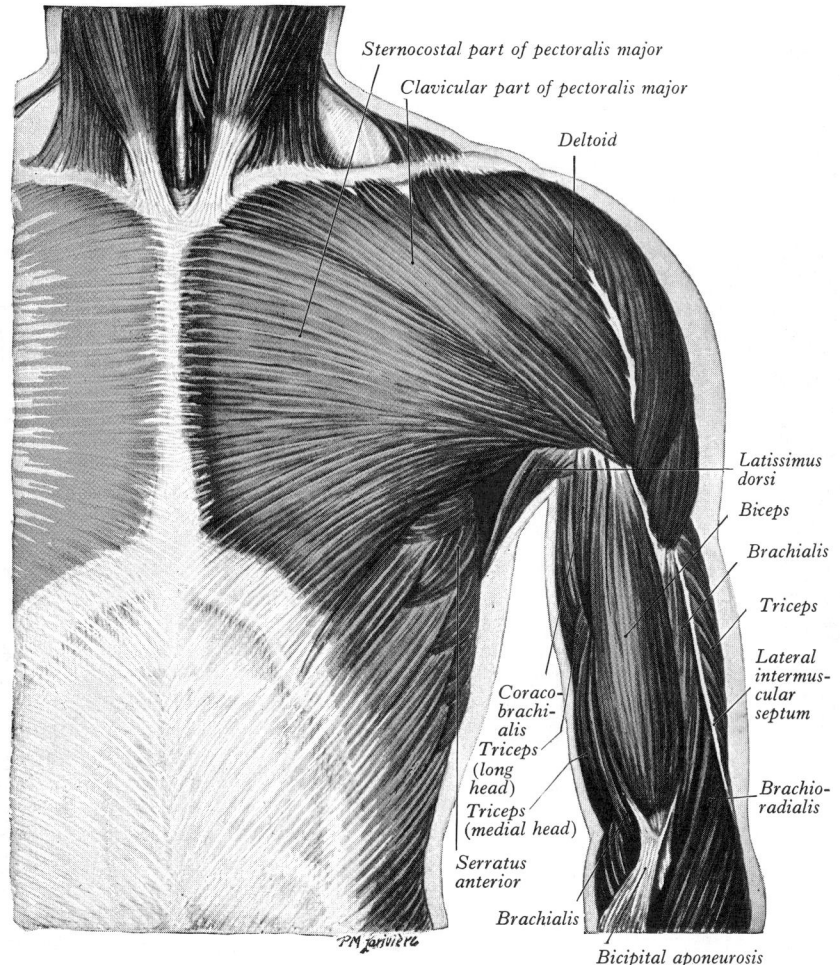

Sternocostal part of pectoralis major

Clavicular part of pectoralis major

Deltoid

Latissimus dorsi

Biceps

Brachialis

Triceps

Lateral intermus-cular septum

Coraco-brachi-alis

Triceps (long head)

Triceps (medial head)

Brachio-radialis

Serratus anterior

Brachialis

Bicipital aponeurosis

7.92 Superficial muscles of the front of the chest and left upper arm.

costal part is relaxed. The opposite movement is usually aided by gravity; when it is resisted the sternocostal part (*portio deprimens*) acts together with latissimus dorsi, teres major and the posterior fibres of deltoid, and the clavicular part is relaxed. With the raised arms fixed, e.g. gripping a branch, the same combination of muscles draws the trunk up and forwards in climbing. Pectoralis major is active in deep inspiration. Electromyography suggests that the clavicular part acts alone in medial rotation.

Clavipectoral fascia

Clavipectoral fascia is a strong fibrous sheet behind the clavicular part of pectoralis major. It fills the gap between pectoralis minor and subclavius, and covers the axillary vessels and nerves. It splits around subclavius and is attached to the clavicle both anterior and posterior to the groove for subclavius; the posterior layer fuses with the deep cervical fascia that connects the omohyoid to the clavicle (p. 807) and with the sheath of the axillary vessels. Medially it blends with fascia over the first two intercostal spaces and is attached to the first rib, medial to subclavius. Laterally, it is thick and dense, and is attached to the coracoid process, blending with the coraco-clavicular ligament. Between the first rib and coracoid process the fascia often thickens to form a band, the *costocoracoid ligament*; below this it becomes thin, splits around pectoralis minor and descends to blend with the axillary fascia and laterally with the fascia over the short head of biceps. The cephalic vein, thoraco-acromial artery and vein, and lateral pectoral nerve pass through the fascia.

Pectoralis minor

Pectoralis minor (**7.93**) is a thin, triangular muscle lying posterior (deep) to pectoralis major. It arises from the upper margins and outer surfaces of the third to fifth ribs (frequently second to fourth),

near their cartilages, and from the fascia over adjoining external intercostals. Its fibres ascend laterally under cover of pectoralis major, converging in a flat tendon attached to the medial border and upper surface of the coracoid process of the scapula. Part or all of the tendon may cross the process into the coraco-acromial ligament, or even beyond to the coracohumeral ligament, whereby it is attached to the humerus.

Variations. Slips of the muscle are sometimes separated and vary in number and level. In rare cases, one passes from the first rib to the coracoid (*pectoralis minimus*). Anson et al (1953) recorded the costal attachments of 1000 muscles as: 2nd to 5th ribs—337; 3rd to 5th—334; 2nd to 4th—193; 3rd to 4th—67. The muscle was never absent in this study, but it can be present or absent when the pectoralis major is absent.

Relations. **Anterior** are pectoralis major, the lateral pectoral nerve and pectoral branches of the thoraco-acromial artery. **Posterior** are ribs, external intercostals, serratus anterior, the axilla, axillary vessels, lymphatics and brachial plexus. The **upper border** of pectoralis minor is separated from the clavicle by a triangular gap filled by the clavipectoral fascia, posterior to which are the axillary vessels, lymphatics and nerves. The lateral thoracic artery follows the **lower border**. The medial pectoral nerves pierce and partly supply the muscle.

Blood supply. Pectoral and deltoid branches of the thoraco-acromial artery (p. 1537); superior and lateral thoracic arteries (p. 1538).

Nerve supply. Through the medial and lateral pectoral nerves, C5, 6, **7**, **8** and T1.

Actions. The muscle assists serratus anterior in drawing the scapula forwards around the chest wall. With levator scapulae and the rhomboids it rotates the scapula, depressing the point of the shoulder. Both pectoral muscles are electromyographically quiescent in normal inspiration, but are active in forced inspiration.

839

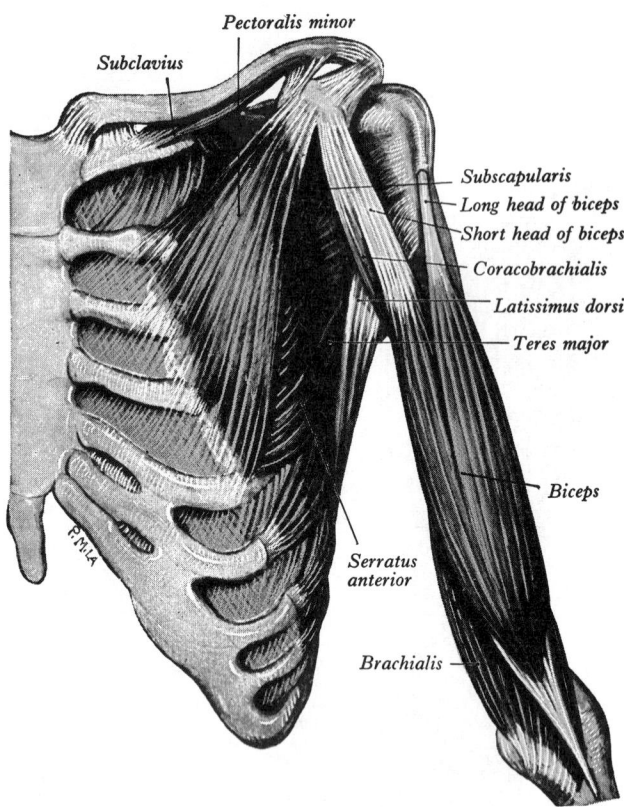

7.93 Deep muscles of the front of the chest and left arm.

Subclavius

Subclavius (**7.93**) is a small, triangular muscle tucked between the clavicle and the first rib. It arises from the junction of the first rib and its costal cartilage, anterior to the costoclavicular ligament, by a thick tendon, which is prolonged at its inferior margin (Cave & Brown 1952). It passes upwards and laterally to the groove on the under surface of the middle third of the clavicle, where it is attached by muscular fibres.

Variations. Subclavius may reach the coracoid process or the upper border of the scapula in addition to, or instead of, the clavicle.

Relations. **Posteriorly** it is separated from the first rib by the subclavian vessels and brachial plexus, **anteriorly** from pectoralis major by the anterior lamina of the clavipectoral fascia.

Blood supply. Clavicular branch of the thoraco-acromial artery (p. 1537); suprascapular artery (p. 1535).

Nerve supply. The subclavian branch of the brachial plexus, containing fibres from C5 and 6 (p. 1266).

Action. Subclavius probably pulls the point of the shoulder down and forwards and braces the clavicle against the articular disc of the sternoclavicular joint, but it is inaccessible to palpation and difficult to investigate by electromyography.

Serratus anterior

Serratus anterior (**7.92, 93**) is a large muscular sheet that curves around the thorax, arising from an extensive costal attachment and inserting on the scapula. Fleshy digitations spring anteriorly from the outer surfaces and superior borders of the upper eight, nine or even ten ribs, and from fasciae covering the intervening intercostals; these attachments lie on a long, slightly curved, line that passes inferolaterally across the thorax. The first springs from the first and second ribs and intercostal fascia, the others from a single rib; the lower four interdigitate with the upper five slips of obliquus externus abdominis. The muscle follows closely the contour of the chest wall, passes ventral to the scapula and reaches the medial border of the scapula in the following way. The first digitation encloses, and is attached to, a triangular area of both costal and dorsal surfaces of the superior scapular angle. The next two or three digitations form a triangular sheet attached to the costal surface along almost the entire medial border. The lower four or five digitations converge to

be attached by musculotendinous fibres to a triangular impression on the costal surface of the inferior angle; however, they enclose the inferior angle and are also attached to a smaller triangular part of its dorsal surface near its tip (Bharihoke & Gupta 1986).

Variations. Digitations may be absent, particularly the first and eighth but also sometimes the intermediate part. The muscle may be partly fused with levator scapulae, adjacent external intercostals or obliquus externus abdominis.

Blood supply. Superior and lateral thoracic arteries, and branches given off by the thoracodorsal artery before (and occasionally after) it divides in the latissimus dorsi muscle.

Nerve supply. The long thoracic nerve (C5, 6 and 7), which descends on the external surface of the muscle.

Actions. With pectoralis minor it protracts (draws forward) the scapula, as a prime mover in all reaching and pushing movements. The upper part, with levator scapulae and upper fibres of the trapezius, suspends the scapula, but slight activity is sufficient to support the unloaded arm. The heavier insertion lower down pulls the inferior scapular angle forwards around the thorax, assisting the trapezius in upward rotation of the bone, an action that is essential to raising the arm above the head (p. 841). In the initial stages of abduction serratus anterior helps other muscles to fix the scapula, so that deltoid acts effectively on the humerus, and not the scapula. While the deltoid is raising the arm to a right-angle with the scapula, serratus anterior and trapezius are simultaneously rotating the scapula, and the combination allows the arm to be raised to the vertical. To effect this upward rotation of the scapula, forward pull on the inferior angle by the lower digitations of the serratus anterior is coupled with an upward and medial pull on the lateral end of the clavicle and acromion by the trapezius (upper fibres) and a downward pull on the base of the scapular spine by the trapezius (lower fibres). Conversely, slow downward scapular rotation assisted by gravity is achieved by controlled lengthening of these muscles; more powerful downward rotation requires balanced contraction of the upper fibres of serratus anterior, levator scapulae, rhomboids, pectoralis minor and the middle part of trapezius. When weights are carried in front of the body, serratus anterior prevents backward rotation of the scapula. Electromyography shows that serratus anterior is not active in normal human respiration (Catton & Gray 1951); but this may not apply to laboured respiration, in which asthmatics and athletes may be observed to fix the scapula by grasping a rail!

Clinical relevance. When serratus anterior is paralysed, the medial border of the scapula, and especially its lower angle, stand out prominently. The patient cannot raise the arm fully or push effectively; attempts to do so produce further projection, known as 'winging' of the scapula.

MUSCLES OF THE SCAPULA

The shoulder joint is closely surrounded by six muscles: deltoid, supraspinatus and infraspinatus, subscapularis, and teres major and minor, all extending from scapula to humerus. These muscles are attached close to the joint, which they can manoeuvre so that articular contact is maintained under all static and dynamic conditions. This arrangement allows considerable freedom of movement in every direction while preserving the stability of this shallow joint.

Deep fascia

Deep fascia over the deltoid sends numerous septa between its fasciculi and is continuous with pectoral fascia in front and infraspinous fascia behind, the latter being thick and strong. Above it is attached to the clavicle, acromion and crest of the scapular spine; below it is continuous with the brachial fascia.

Deltoid

Deltoid (**7.92**), a thick, curved triangle of muscle, arises from the anterior border and superior surface of the lateral third of the clavicle, the lateral margin and superior surface of the acromion and the lower edge of the crest of the scapular spine (but not its smooth medial triangular surface). The fibres converge inferiorly to a short, substantial tendon attached to the deltoid tuberosity, on the lateral aspect of the humeral midshaft. Anterior and posterior fibres converge directly to the humeral tendon. The intermediate part is multipennate, four intramuscular septa descending from the acromion to interdigitate with three ascending from the deltoid tuberosity; these septa are connected by short muscle fibres, providing powerful traction. The fasciculi are large, producing a coarse longitudinal striation. The muscle surrounds the humeral articulation on all sides except inferomedially, lending the shoulder its rounded profile. In contraction its borders are easily seen and felt. The tendon gives off an expansion into the brachial deep fascia which may reach the forearm.

Variations. The muscle may be partitioned into the three parts described, may fuse with pectoralis major and may receive additional slips from trapezius, infraspinous fascia or lateral scapular border.

Relations. **Superficial** are skin, superficial and deep fasciae, platysma, lateral supraclavicular and upper lateral brachial cutaneous nerves. **Deep** are the coracoid process, coraco-acromial ligament, subacromial bursa, tendons of pectoralis minor, coracobrachialis, both heads of biceps, pectoralis major, subscapularis, supraspinatus, infraspinatus, teres minor, long and lateral heads of triceps, circumflex humeral vessels, axillary nerve, and humeral surgical neck and upper shaft of the humerus, including both tuberosities. The **anterior border** of the deltoid is separated proximally from pectoralis major by the infraclavicular fossa, in which the cephalic vein and deltoid branches of the thoraco-acromial artery lie; distally the muscles are in contact, their tendons usually united. Its **posterior border** overlies infraspinatus and triceps.

Blood supply. Acromial and deltoid branches of the thoraco-acromial artery (pp. 1537–1538); posterior and anterior circumflex humeral arteries (p. 1538); subscapular artery (p. 1538); and profunda brachii (deltoid branch) (p. 1539).

Nerve supply. The axillary nerve, **C5** and 6.

Actions. The parts of the muscle can act independently as well as together. Anterior fibres assist pectoralis major in drawing the arm forwards and rotating it medially. Posterior fibres act with latissimus dorsi and teres major in drawing the arm backwards and rotating it laterally. The multipennate, acromial part of deltoid is a strong abductor: aided by supraspinatus it abducts the arm until the joint capsule is tense below, movement taking place in the plane of the body of the scapula; this is the only way that scapular rotation can be fully effective in raising the arm above the head (p. 621). In true abduction (**6.71B**), acromial fibres contract strongly, clavicular and posterior fibres preventing departure from the plane of motion. In the early stages of abduction, traction by the deltoid is upward, but the humeral head is prevented from translating upward by the synergistic downward pull of subscapularis, infraspinatus and teres minor. Electromyography suggests that deltoid contributes little to medial or lateral rotation but confirms that it takes part in most other shoulder movements. It may also aid supraspinatus in resisting the downward drag of a loaded arm (see below). A common action of the deltoid is arm-swinging while walking. Ergonomic study of its clavicular part by Jonsson and Hagberg (1974) shows that it adjusts the hand to various heights in manual tasks.

Clinical relevance. Lesions affecting the axillary nerve cause atrophy of the deltoid; the acromion then appears to be more prominent, simulating dislocation of the shoulder joint. The distance between the acromion and the humeral head is increased, to the extent that the fingertips can be inserted between them.

Subscapular fascia

Subscapular fascia is a thin aponeurosis attached to the entire circumference of the subscapular fossa; subscapularis itself is partly attached to its deep surface.

Subscapularis

Subscapularis (**7.93**) is a bulky, triangular muscle that fills the subscapular fossa. In its medial two-thirds, the fibres are attached to the periosteum of the costal surface of the scapula; other fibres arise from tendinous intramuscular septa, which are attached to ridges on the bone, and from the aponeurosis that covers the muscle and separates it from teres major and the long head of triceps. The fibres converge laterally into a broad tendon that is attached to the lesser tubercle of the humerus and the front of the articular capsule. The tendon is separated from the neck of the scapula by the large subscapular bursa, which communicates with the shoulder joint.

Variations. Variation is unusual. A separate slip may pass from

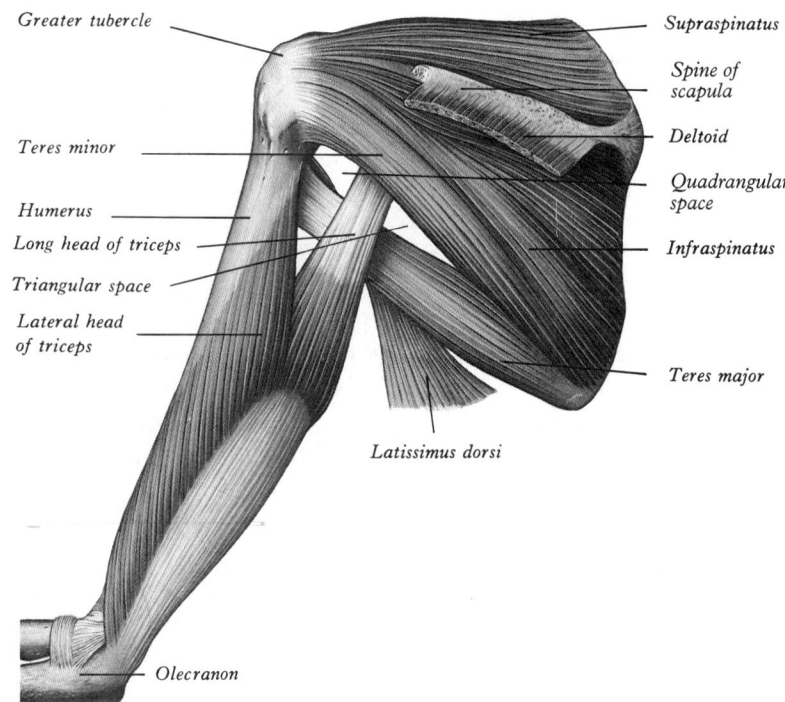

7.94 The dorsal scapular muscles and triceps of the left side. The spine of the scapula has been divided near its lateral end and the acromion has been removed together with a large part of deltoid. The humerus is laterally rotated and the forearm pronated.

the medial scapular border to the glenohumeral capsule or to periosteum medial to the intertubercular sulcus of the humerus.

Relations. The muscle forms much of the *posterior axillary wall.* Its **anterior surface** is apposed inferomedially to serratus anterior, and superolaterally to coracobrachialis and biceps, the axillary vessels, brachial plexus and subscapular vessels and nerves. Its **posterior surface** is attached to the scapula and glenohumeral capsule. Its **lower border** contacts teres major and latissimus dorsi.

Blood supply. Small rami from the suprascapular, axillary and subscapular arteries (pp. 1535–1538).

Nerve supply. The upper and lower subscapular nerves, C5, **6**.

Actions. These are considered below with supraspinatus, infraspinatus, and teres minor.

Supraspinous fascia

Supraspinous fascia completes the osseofibrous compartment in which supraspinatus is attached. It is thick medially, but thinner laterally under the coraco-acromial ligament. It is attached to the scapula around the boundaries of the attachment of supraspinatus.

Supraspinatus

Supraspinatus (**7.94**) arises from the medial two-thirds of the supraspinous fossa and from the supraspinous fascia. The fibres converge, under the acromion, into a tendon that crosses above the shoulder joint to attach to the highest facet of the greater tubercle of the humerus; the tendon blends into the articular capsule. A slip may pass from it to the tendon of pectoralis major. Fibrocartilage has been described at the tendinous insertion (Evans & Benjamin 1984), as in other tendons attached to epiphyseal bone.

Blood supply. Suprascapular artery (p. 1535); dorsal scapular artery (p. 1536).

Nerve supply. The suprascapular nerve, C5 and 6.

Actions. These are considered below with subscapularis, infraspinatus and teres minor.

Clinical relevance. The tendon of supraspinatus is separated from the coraco-acromial ligament, acromion and deltoid by the large subacromial bursa; when this is infected, abduction of the shoulder joint is painful. The tendon is the most frequently ruptured element of the musculotendinous cuff around the shoulder joint.

841

Infraspinous fascia

Infraspinous fascia covers the infraspinatus and is attached to the margins of the infraspinous fossa. The fascia is continuous with the deltoid fascia along the overlapping posterior border of deltoid.

Infraspinatus

Infraspinatus (**7.94**) is a thick triangular muscle occupying most of the infraspinous fossa. It arises by muscular fibres from the medial two-thirds of the fossa and by tendinous fibres from ridges on its surface; it also arises from the deep surface of the infraspinous fascia, which separates it from teres major and minor. Its fibres converge to a tendon, which glides over the lateral border of the scapular spine and passes across the posterior aspect of the capsule of the shoulder joint to the middle facet on the greater tubercle of the humerus.

Variations. The tendon is sometimes separated from the capsule by a bursa, which may communicate with the joint cavity. The muscle is sometimes fused with teres minor.

Blood supply. The suprascapular artery and the circumflex scapular artery (p. 1538).

Nerve supply. The suprascapular nerve, C**5** and 6.

Actions. These are considered below with subscapularis, supraspinatus, and teres minor.

Teres minor

Teres minor (**7.94**) is a narrow, elongate muscle, which springs from the upper two-thirds of a flattened strip on the dorsal surface of the scapula, adjoining its lateral border, and from two aponeurotic laminae that separate it from infraspinatus and teres major. It runs upwards and laterally; its upper fibres end in a tendon attached to the lowest facet on the greater tubercle of the humerus; its lower fibres insert directly into the humerus distal to this facet and above the origin of the lateral head of triceps. The tendon passes across, and blends with, the lower posterior surface of the capsule of the shoulder joint.

Variations. The muscle may be fused with infraspinatus.

Blood supply. The circumflex scapular artery, which pierces the origin of the muscle as it turns upward in the infraspinous fossa (p. 1538), and the posterior circumflex humeral artery (p. 1538).

Nerve supply. The axillary nerve C**5** and 6.

Actions. Swings of the humerus (p. 623) involve complex movements of the articular surfaces of the glenohumeral joint which contain elements of rolling, sliding and spinning. Excessive translation can easily occur at such a shallow articulation. While actual movement of the humerus is achieved by muscles with greater leverage, the muscles that insert close to the shoulder joint—subscapularis, supraspinatus, infraspinatus and teres minor—form a musculotendinous cuff, the 'rotator cuff', with the important function of steadying the head of the humerus, maintaining it in suitable apposition to the glenoid cavity and checking excessive translation (p. 622). During the initial stages of abduction, subscapularis, infraspinatus and teres minor counteract the strong **upward** component of pull of the deltoid, which would otherwise cause the humeral head to slide up; the additive turning moments exerted by deltoid and supraspinatus about the shoulder joint can then abduct the arm. When the loaded or unloaded upper limb is pendent, there is a tendency for the humeral head to be translated downwards in the glenoid cavity; electromyographic data and simple palpation show that this is resisted by supraspinatus, rather than deltoid. In contrast, forward and backward traction on the humerus are resisted by the posterior and anterior parts of the deltoid, respectively. Infraspinatus and teres minor, acting with the posterior fibres of the deltoid, are lateral rotators of the humerus. Subscapularis assists in medial rotation when the arm is by the side.

Teres major

Teres major (**7.94**) is a thick, flat muscle which arises from the oval area on the dorsal surface of the inferior scapular angle and from the fibrous septa interposed between the muscle and teres minor and infraspinatus. The fibres ascend laterally and end in a flat tendon, about 5 cm long, which is attached to the medial lip of the intertubercular sulcus of the humerus. The tendon lies behind that of latissimus dorsi, from which it is separated by a bursa; the tendons

are, however, united along their lower borders for a short distance.

Variations. The muscle may be fused with the scapular part of latissimus dorsi. A slip from it may join the long head of triceps or the brachial fascia.

Blood supply. The thoracodorsal branch of the subscapular artery on its way to latissimus dorsi (q.v.) and the posterior circumflex humeral artery (p. 1538).

Nerve supply. The lower subscapular nerve, C5, 6 and 7.

Actions. Despite its name, teres major has a nerve supply and action that is distinct from teres minor. Teres major draws the humerus backwards and rotates it medially. Electromyographic studies disagree about its major role in movement, but its involvement as a contributor to static posture and arm-swinging is not contested.

MUSCLES OF THE UPPER ARM

This group comprises coracobrachialis, which acts only on the shoulder joint; biceps and triceps, which cross both shoulder and elbow joints; and brachialis, which acts only at the elbow joint.

Brachial fascia

Brachial fascia, the deep fascia of the upper arm, is continuous with the fascia covering deltoid and pectoralis major; it forms a thin, loose sheath for muscles of the upper arm, and sends septa between them. It is thin over biceps, but thicker over triceps and the humeral epicondyles; it is strengthened by fibrous aponeuroses from pectoralis major and latissimus dorsi medially and from deltoid laterally. Extending from it on each side are strong *medial* and *lateral intermuscular septa*.

The *lateral intermuscular septum* extends distally from the lateral lip of the intertubercular sulcus along the lateral supracondylar ridge to the lateral epicondyle, and blends with the tendon of deltoid. It gives attachment to triceps behind, and brachialis, brachioradialis and extensor carpi radialis longus in front. It is perforated near the junction of its upper and middle thirds by the radial nerve and the radial collateral branch of arteria profunda brachii. The thicker *medial intermuscular septum* extends from the medial lip of the intertubercular sulcus, distal to teres major, along the medial supracondylar ridge to the medial epicondyle, and blends with the tendon of coracobrachialis. It gives attachment to triceps behind, and brachialis in front. It is perforated by the ulnar nerve, superior ulnar collateral artery, and the posterior branch of the inferior ulnar collateral artery. At the elbow, the brachial fascia is attached to the epicondyles of the humerus and the olecranon of the ulna, and is continuous with the antebrachial fascia. Medially, just below the middle of the upper arm, it is traversed by the basilic vein and lymphatic vessels and, at various levels, branches of the brachial cutaneous nerves.

Coracobrachialis

Coracobrachialis (**7.93, 95**) arises from the apex of the coracoid process, together with the tendon of the short head of the biceps, and also by muscular fibres from the proximal 10 cm of this tendon; it ends on an impression, 3–5 cm in length, midway along the medial border of the humeral shaft between the attachments of triceps and brachialis. The muscle forms an inconspicuous rounded ridge on the upper medial side of the arm; pulsation of the brachial artery can be felt and often seen in the depression behind it. Accessory slips may be attached to the lesser tubercle, medial epicondyle or medial intermuscular septum.

Relations. Coracobrachialis is perforated by the musculocutaneous nerve. **Anteriorly** it is related to pectoralis major above and, at its humeral insertion, to the brachial vessels and median nerve, which cross it. **Posterior** are the tendons of subscapularis, latissimus dorsi, and teres major, the medial head of triceps, the humerus and the anterior circumflex humeral vessels. **Medial** are the axillary artery (third part) and proximal parts of the median and musculocutaneous nerves. **Lateral** are biceps and brachialis.

Blood supply. Brachial artery; anterior circumflex humeral artery (p. 1538).

Nerve supply. The musculocutaneous nerve, C5, 6 and 7.

Actions. Coracobrachialis flexes the arm forward and medially, especially from a position of brachial extension. In abduction it acts

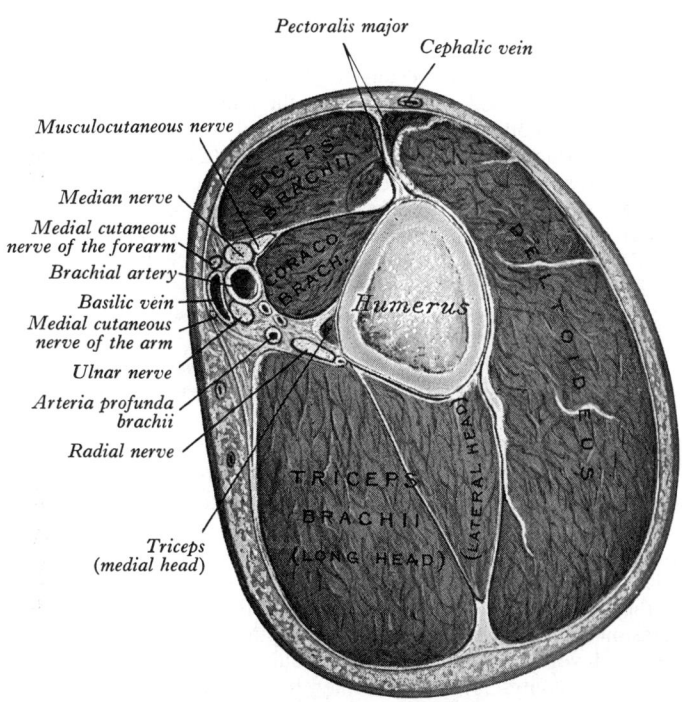

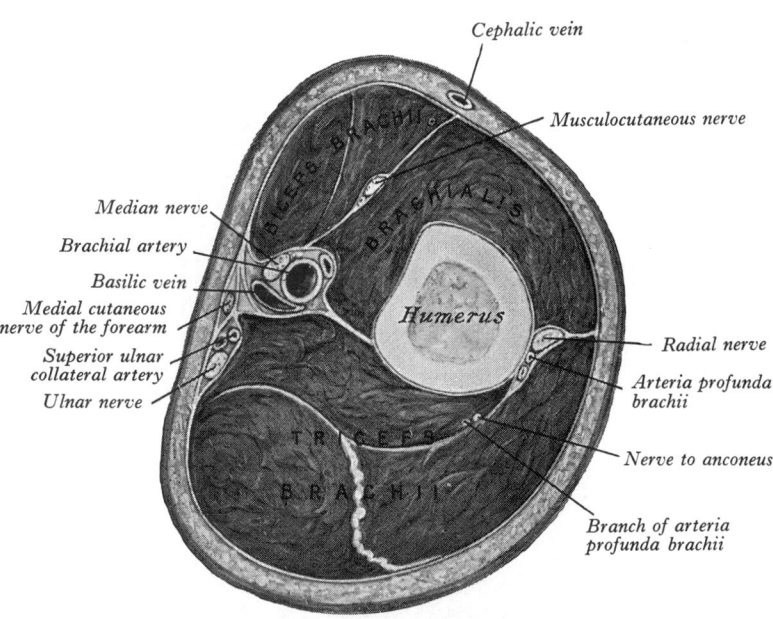

7.96 Transverse section through the right arm, a little below the middle of the shaft of the humerus: superior (proximal) aspect.

7.95 Transverse section through the right arm at the junction of the proximal and middle thirds of the humerus: superior (proximal) aspect.

with anterior fibres of the deltoid to resist departure from the plane of motion.

Biceps brachii

Biceps brachii (**7.93, 95, 96**), a large, fusiform muscle in the flexor compartment of the upper arm, derives its name from its two proximally attached parts or 'heads'. The *short head* arises by a thick flattened tendon from the coracoid apex, together with coracobrachialis. The *long head* starts within the capsule of the shoulder joint as a long narrow tendon, running from the supraglenoid tubercle at the apex of the glenoidal cavity, and continuous here with the glenoidal labrum (p. 623). The tendon of the long head, enclosed in a double tubular sheath (an extension of the synovial membrane of the joint capsule), arches over the humeral head, emerges from the joint behind the transverse humeral ligament, and descends in the intertubercular sulcus, where it is retained by the transverse humeral ligament and a fibrous expansion from the tendon of pectoralis major. The two tendons lead into elongated bellies which, although closely applied, can be separated to within 7 cm or so of the elbow joint. At the joint they end in a flattened tendon which is attached to the rough posterior area of the radial tuberosity; a bursa separates the tendon from the smooth anterior area of the tuberosity. As it approaches the radius, the tendon twists (spirals), its anterior surface becoming lateral before being applied to the tuberosity. The tendon has a broad medial expansion, the *bicipital aponeurosis*, which descends medially across the brachial artery to fuse with deep fascia over the origins of the flexor muscles of the forearm (**7.98, 10.98**). The tendon can be split without difficulty as far as the tuberosity, whence it can be confirmed that its anterior and posterior layers receive fibres from the short and long heads, respectively.

Variations. In 10% of cases, a third head arises from the superomedial part of brachialis and is attached to the bicipital aponeurosis and medial side of the tendon of insertion. It usually lies behind the brachial artery, but it may consist of two slips which descend in front of and behind the artery. Less often, other slips may spring from the lateral aspect of the humerus or intertubercular sulcus.

Relations. Biceps is overlapped proximally by pectoralis major and the deltoid; distally it is covered only by fasciae and skin, and it forms a conspicuous elevation on the front of the arm. Its long head passes through the shoulder joint; its short head is anterior to the joint. Distally it lies anterior to brachialis, the musculocutaneous nerve and supinator. Its **medial border** touches coracobrachialis, and

overlaps the brachial vessels and median nerve; its **lateral border** is related to deltoid and brachioradialis.

Blood supply. Brachial artery; anterior circumflex humoral artery (p. 1538).

Nerve supply. The musculocutaneous nerve, C5 and 6, with separate branches passing to each belly.

Actions. Biceps is a powerful supinator, especially in rapid or resisted movements. It flexes the elbow, most effectively with the forearm supinated, and acts to a slight extent as a flexor of the shoulder joint. It is attached, via the bicipital aponeurosis, to the posterior border of the ulna, the distal end of which is drawn medially in supination. The long head helps to check upward translation of the humeral head during contraction of deltoid. When the elbow is flexed against resistance, the tendon of insertion and bicipital aponeurosis become conspicuous.

Lowering the hand under the influence of gravity by extension at the elbow calls for controlled lengthening of biceps. This is an example of a habitual movement in which muscle tension increases despite increasing length. As the hand descends and the elbow extends, the vertical through the centre of gravity of the forearm is carried further from the fulcrum of movement; the turning moment exerted by the load therefore increases and must be matched by an increase in the moment exerted by the muscle.

Brachialis

Brachialis (**7.93, 96, 97**) arises from the lower half of the front of the humerus, starting on either side of the insertion of deltoid, and extending distally to within 2.5 cm of the cubital articular surface. It also arises from the intermuscular septa, more from the medial than the lateral, since it is separated distally from the lateral intermuscular septum by brachioradialis and extensor carpi radialis longus. Its fibres converge to a thick, broad tendon, which is attached to the ulnar tuberosity and to a rough impression on the anterior aspect of the coronoid process.

Variation. Brachialis may be divided into two or more parts. It may be fused with brachioradialis, pronator teres or biceps. In some cases it sends a tendinous slip to the radius or bicipital aponeurosis.

Relations. **Anterior** are biceps, the brachial vessels, musculocutaneous and median nerves. **Posterior** are the humerus and capsule of the elbow joint. **Medial** are pronator teres, and the medial intermuscular septum, which separates it from triceps and the ulnar nerve. **Lateral** are the radial nerve, radial recurrent and radial collateral arteries, brachioradialis and extensor carpi radialis longus.

Blood supply. Brachial artery, directly and via the ulnar artery (p. 1542); superior and inferior ulnar collateral arteries (p. 1539); anterior ulnar recurrent artery (p. 1543); radial collateral branch of profunda brachii (p. 1539); and radial recurrent artery (p. 1541).

843

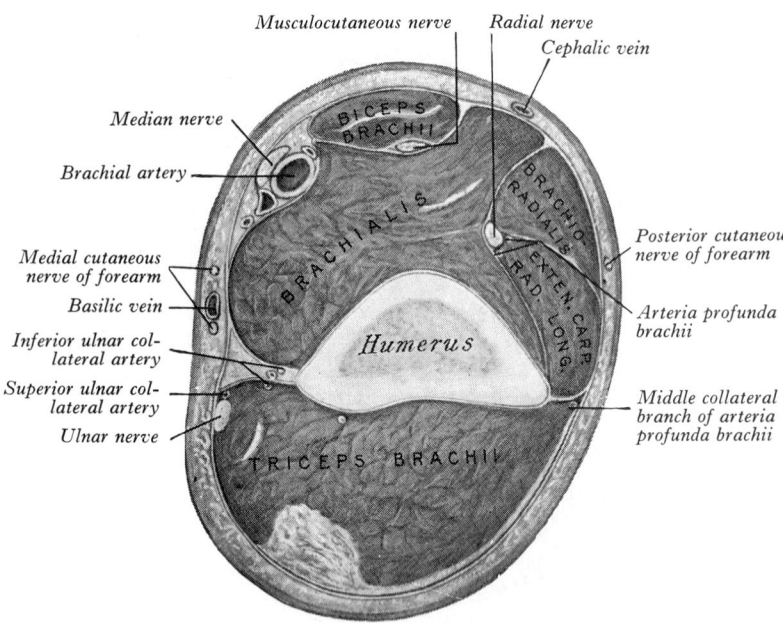

7.97 Transverse section through the right arm, a little proximal to the medial epicondyle of the humerus: superior (proximal) aspect.

Nerve supply. The musculocutaneous nerve (C5 and **6**), and radial nerve (C7) to a small lateral part of the muscle (Ip & Chang 1968).

Action. Brachialis is a flexor of the elbow joint with the forearm either prone or supine, whether or not the movement is resisted.

Triceps

Triceps (**7.94, 97**) fills most of the extensor compartment of the upper arm. It arises by **three** heads (long, lateral and medial), from which it takes its name.

The *long head* arises by a flattened tendon from the infraglenoid tubercle of the scapula, blending above with the glenohumeral capsule; its muscular fibres descend medial to the lateral head and superficial to the medial head, and join them to form a common tendon.

The *lateral head* arises by a flattened tendon from a narrow, linear, oblique ridge on the posterior surface of the humeral shaft, and from the lateral intermuscular septum. The origin on the humerus ascends with varying obliquity from its lateral border above the radial groove and behind the deltoid tuberosity to the surgical neck medial to the insertion of teres minor. These fibres also converge to the common tendon.

The *medial head*, which is overlapped posteriorly by the lateral and long heads, has a particularly extensive origin, from the entire posterior surface of the humeral shaft, below the radial groove from the insertion of teres major to within 2.5 cm of the trochlea, from the medial border of the humerus, the medial intermuscular septum and the lower part of the lateral intermuscular septum. Some muscular fibres reach the olecranon directly, the rest converge to the common tendon.

The tendon of triceps begins near the middle of the muscle. It has two laminae, one superficial in the lower half of the muscle, the other in its substance. After receiving the muscle fibres, the two layers unite above the elbow and are attached, for the most part, to the upper surface of the olecranon; on the lateral side a band of fibres continues down over anconeus to blend with antebrachial fascia.

The long head descends between teres minor and major, dividing the wedge-shaped interval between them and the humerus into triangular and quadrangular parts (**7.94**). The triangular space contains the circumflex scapular vessels; it is bounded above by teres minor, below by teres major, laterally by the long head of triceps. The quadrangular space transmits the posterior circumflex humeral vessels and the axillary nerve; it is bounded above by subscapularis, teres minor and the articular capsule, below by teres major, medially by the long head of triceps, and laterally by the humerus.

The lateral head of triceps forms an elevation, parallel and medial to the posterior border of the deltoid; it stands out prominently when the elbow is actively extended. The mass which lies medial to it, and disappears under the deltoid, is the long head.

Articularis cubiti (subanconeus) is formed by a few fibres from the deep surface of the lower part of triceps (medial head) which blend posteriorly with the fibrous capsule of the elbow joint.

Blood supply. Posterior circumflex humeral artery (p. 1538); numerous branches of profundus brachii—deltoid, middle collateral and direct (p. 1539); superior and inferior ulnar collateral artery (p. 1539); interosseous recurrent artery (p. 1543).

Nerve supply. The radial nerve, C6, **7** and 8, with separate branches for each head (p. 1274).

Actions. Triceps is the major extensor of the forearm at the elbow joint. The medial head is active in all forms of extension. The lateral and long heads are minimally active except in extension against resistance (Basmajian 1967), as in thrusting or pushing or supporting body weight on the hands with the elbows semiflexed. When the flexed arm is extended at the shoulder joint, the long head may assist in drawing back and adducting the humerus to the thorax. The long head supports the lower part of the capsule of the shoulder joint, especially when the arm is raised. Articularis cubiti probably draws up the posterior part of the capsule of the elbow joint during extension of the forearm. In forceful supination of the semiflexed forearm, involving contraction of both supinator and biceps brachii, the triceps contracts synergistically to maintain the semiflexed position. The human triceps brachii is the subject of an interesting comparison of geometric and dynamic parameters by Cnockaert and Pertuzon (1974).

MUSCLES OF THE FOREARM

The antebrachial (forearm) muscles consist of *anterior* and *posterior* groups; these are morphologically flexors and extensors, but their actions are often combined in more complex activities.

The *anterior group* of forearm muscles consists of two layers:

- superficial flexors (having origins mainly on the humerus)
- deep flexors (arising from the radius and ulna)

(Note that the superficial 'flexors' include pronator teres, while the deep 'flexors' include pronator quadratus.)

The *posterior group* of forearm muscles can also be described conveniently in terms of two layers:

- superficial extensors
- deep extensors

Following a note on the antebrachial fascia, each of these layers will be described in turn.

Antebrachial fascia

The antebrachial fascia (deep fascia of the forearm), which is continuous above with the brachial fascia, is a dense general sheath for muscles, collectively and individually, in this region. It is attached to the olecranon and posterior border of the ulna, and from its deep surface septa pass between muscles, providing partial attachment; some of these septa reach bone. Muscles also arise from its internal aspect, especially in the upper forearm. Transverse septa, anterior and posterior, separate deep from superficial muscles. The fascia is much thicker posteriorly and in the lower forearm. It is strengthened above by tendinous fibres from biceps and triceps. Near the wrist, two localized thickenings, the *flexor* and *extensor retinacula* (pp. 852–854), retain the digital tendons in position. Vessels and nerves pass through apertures in the fascia; one large aperture anterior to the elbow transmits a venous communication between superficial and deep veins.

SUPERFICIAL FLEXORS OF THE FOREARM

Muscles of this group arise from the medial epicondyle of the humerus by a common tendon. They are pronator teres, flexor carpi radialis, palmaris longus, flexor carpi ulnaris, and flexor digitorum superficialis (**7.98, 99**). They have additional attachments to the

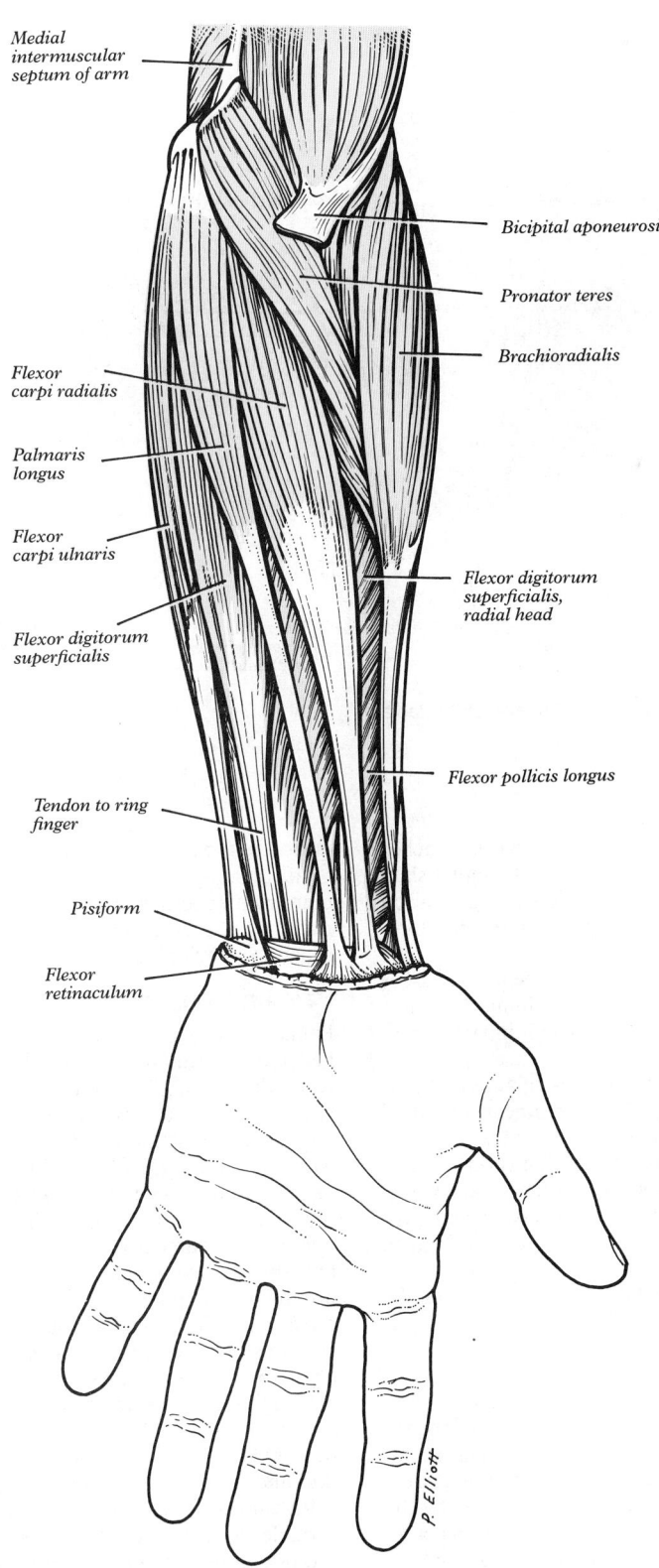

7.98 Superficial flexor muscles of the left forearm.

Medial
intermuscular
septum of arm

Bicipital aponeurosis

Pronator teres

Brachioradialis

Flexor
carpi radialis

Palmaris
longus

Flexor
carpi ulnaris

Flexor digitorum
superficialis

Flexor digitorum
superficialis,
radial head

Flexor pollicis longus

Tendon to ring
finger

Pisiform

Flexor
retinaculum

antebrachial fascia near the elbow and to the septa that pass from this fascia between individual muscles.

Pronator teres

Pronator teres (7.98, 99) has humeral and ulnar attachments. The *humeral head*, the larger and more superficial of the two, arises just proximal to the medial epicondyle, from the common tendon of

origin of the flexor muscles, from the intermuscular septum between it and flexor carpi radialis and from antebrachial fascia. The smaller *ulnar head* springs from the medial side of the coronoid process of the ulna, distal to the attachment of flexor digitorum superficialis, and joins the humeral head at an acute angle. In 83% of cases, the median nerve enters the forearm between the two heads, and is separated from the ulnar artery by the ulnar head. The muscle passes

845

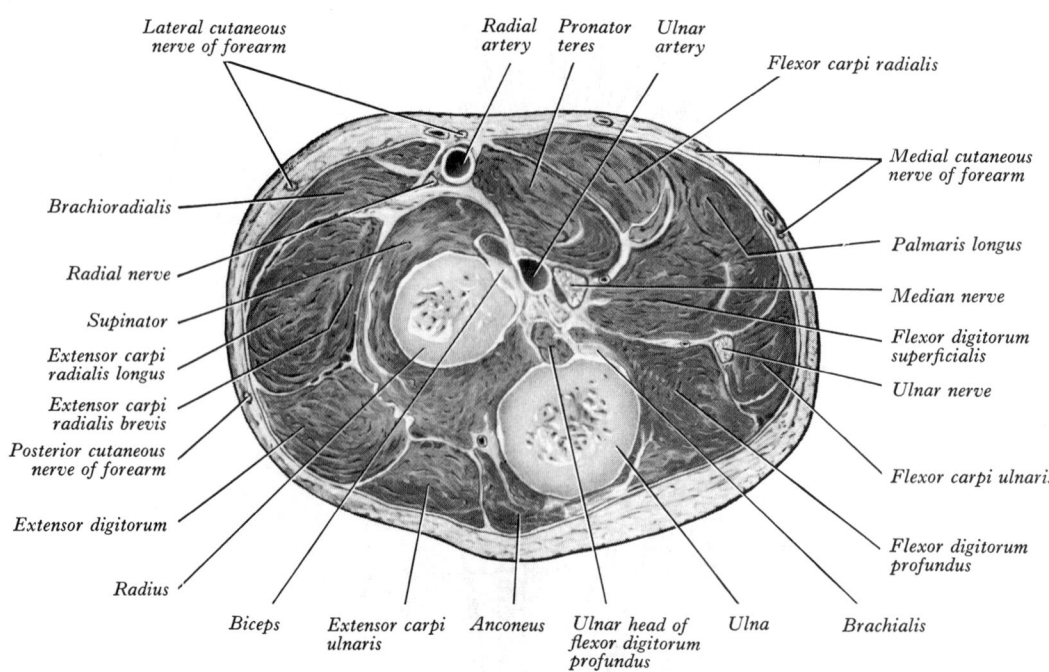

Lateral cutaneous nerve of forearm

Radial artery

Pronator teres

Ulnar artery

Flexor carpi radialis

Brachioradialis

Medial cutaneous nerve of forearm

Radial nerve

Palmaris longus

Supinator

Median nerve

Extensor carpi radialis longus

Flexor digitorum superficialis

Extensor carpi radialis brevis

Ulnar nerve

Posterior cutaneous nerve of forearm

Extensor digitorum

Flexor carpi ulnaris

Radius

Flexor digitorum profundus

Biceps

Extensor carpi ulnaris

Anconeus

Ulnar head of flexor digitorum profundus

Ulna

Brachialis

7.99   Transverse section through the left forearm at the level of the radial tuberosity: superior (proximal) aspect.

obliquely across the forearm to end in a flat tendon that is attached to a rough area midway along the lateral surface of the radial shaft (at the 'summit' of its lateral curve). The lateral border of the muscle is the medial limit of the triangular hollow anterior to the elbow joint, the *cubital fossa*.

Variations. The coronoid attachment may be absent. Accessory slips may arise from a supracondylar process of the humerus, if it is present, or from biceps, brachialis or the medial intermuscular septum.

Blood supply. Ulnar artery by direct rami (p. 1542); anterior ulnar recurrent artery (p. 1543); radial artery (radial attachment) (p. 1540).

Nerve supply. The median nerve, C6 and 7.

Actions. The muscle rotates the radius on the ulna (pronation of the forearm), turning the palm medially so that it faces backwards. It acts with pronator quadratus—which is always active in pronation—only in rapid or forcible pronation, but its activity is said always to be less (Basmajian & Travill 1961). Like all of the muscles arising from the medial epicondyle, it acts as a weak flexor of the elbow joint.

Flexor carpi radialis

Flexor carpi radialis (**7**.98, 99, 100) lies medial to pronator teres, and arises from the medial epicondyle via the common flexor tendon, from the antebrachial fascia and from adjacent intermuscular septa. Its belly is fusiform and ends, rather more than halfway to the wrist, in a long tendon. This passes through a lateral canal, formed by the flexor retinaculum above and a groove on the trapezium beneath, within a synovial sheath. It inserts on the palmar surface of the base of the second metacarpal, sending a slip to the third metacarpal. These distal attachments are hidden by the oblique head of adductor pollicis (**7**.114, 115). In the lower part of the forearm the radial artery lies between the tendon of this muscle and that of brachioradialis. The surface groove for the radial pulse is well known to all physicians.

Variations. The muscle may be absent. It may have accessory slips from the biceps tendon, bicipital aponeurosis, coronoid process or radius. Distally it may also be attached to the flexor retinaculum, trapezium or fourth metacarpal.

Blood supply. Ulnar artery by direct rami (p. 1542); superior and inferior ulnar collateral arteries (p. 1539); (variable) anterior and posterior ulnar recurrent arteries (p. 1543). In the flexor retinaculum, superficial palmar branch of the radial artery (p. 1544); at the insertion, palmar metacarpal arteries and perforating branches from the deep palmar arch (p. 1544).

Nerve supply. The median nerve, C6 and 7.

Actions. Acting with flexor carpi ulnaris, and sometimes flexor digitorum superficialis, flexor carpi radialis flexes the wrist; it helps radial extensors of the wrist in abducting the hand. (See also its function in gripping, p. 869.)

Palmaris longus

Palmaris longus (**7**.98, 99) is a slender, fusiform muscle medial to flexor carpi radialis. It springs from the medial epicondyle by the common tendon, from adjacent intermuscular septa and deep fascia. It converges on a long tendon, which passes **anterior** (superficial) to the flexor retinaculum. A few fibres leave the tendon and interweave with the transverse fibres of the retinaculum; most of the tendon passes distally. As the tendon crosses the retinaculum it broadens out to become a flat sheet, which then splits longitudinally to send bundles of ligamentous fibres to the 4 digital rays, with a variable fibre bundle extending towards the thumb. The diverging bundles occupy a triangular area in the midpalm with its apex pointing proximally. The ligamentous structures in this area have been described as the *palmar fascia* or *aponeurosis*, a terminology that tends to disguise the precise organization of the fibres into 5 groups of longitudinally orientated fibres. (In clinical practice the term *pretendinous fibres* is used.) The precise distal insertions of the fibres will be described later, but palmaris longus has wide insertions into skin and fascia in the distal palm and digital webs.

Variations. Often absent on one or both sides, the muscle is very variable (Machado & DiDio 1967; Stack 1973).

Blood supply. Ulnar artery (p. 1542); superior and inferior ulnar collateral arteries (p. 1539); (variable) anterior and posterior ulnar recurrent arteries (p. 1543); rami from the ends of the superficial palmar arch (p. 1544).

Nerve supply. The median nerve, C7 and 8.

Actions. Palmaris longus has been suggested to be a phylogenetically degenerate metacarpophalangeal joint flexor (Wood Jones 1941). Although consideration of the line of action would suggest an action in carpal flexion, the main function appears to be as an anchor for the skin and fascia of the hand, resisting horizontal shearing forces in a distal direction (as in holding a golf club) which would tend to deglove the skin of the palm.

Flexor carpi ulnaris

Flexor carpi ulnaris (**7**.98, 99, 100) is the most medial of the superficial forearm flexors. It arises by two heads, humeral and ulnar, connected

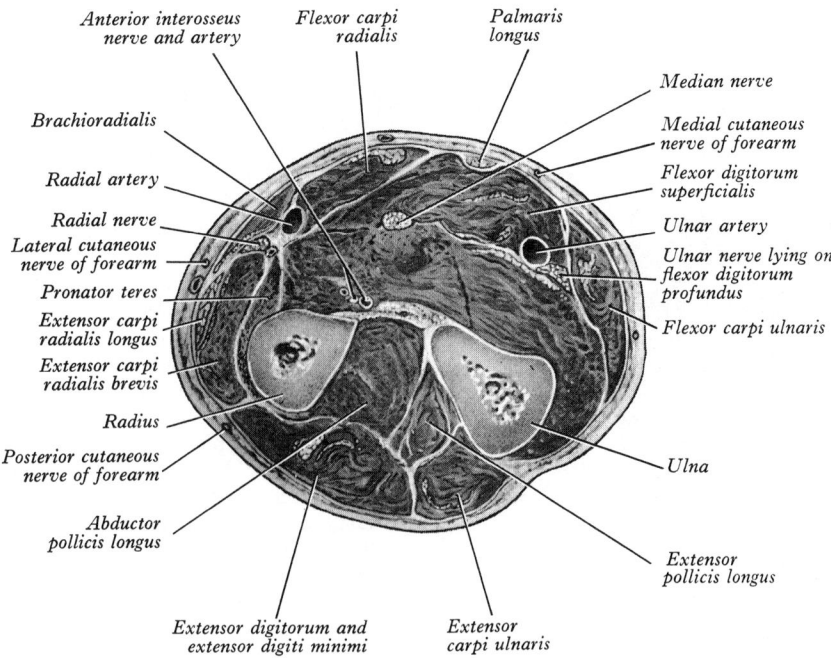

7.100 Transverse section through the middle of the left forearm: superior (proximal) aspect.

by a tendinous arch, under which the ulnar nerve and posterior ulnar recurrent artery pass. The small *humeral head* arises from the medial epicondyle via the common tendon; the ulnar head has an extensive origin from the medial margin of the olecranon and proximal two-thirds of the posterior border of the ulna by an aponeurosis shared with extensor carpi ulnaris and flexor digitorum profundus, and from the intermuscular septum between it and flexor digitorum superficialis. A thick tendon forms along the anterolateral border of the muscle in its distal half and is attached to the pisiform bone, a sesamoid, thence prolonged to the hamate and fifth metacarpal bones by so-called pisohamate and pisometacarpal ligaments (**6.249A**); a few fibres blend with the flexor retinaculum. Ulnar vessels and nerve lie lateral to the tendon of insertion.

Variations. A coronoid slip may occur, and distally there may be a more substantial attachment to the flexor retinaculum and to the fourth or fifth metacarpal bones.

Blood supply. Ulnar artery (p. 1542); superior and inferior ulnar collateral arteries (p. 1539); anterior and posterior ulnar recurrent arteries (p. 1543); ulnar end of superficial palmar arch (p. 1544).

Nerve supply. The ulnar nerve, C7 and **8** and T1.

Actions. With flexor carpi radialis it flexes the wrist; with extensor carpi ulnaris it adducts (ulnar deviates) the hand. (See also Hand function in Co-ordinated movements of the upper limb, p. 862.)

Flexor digitorum superficialis

Flexor digitorum superficialis (or *sublimis*, **7.98, 99, 100**) lies deep to the preceding muscles. It is the largest of the superficial flexors, and arises by two heads. The *humero-ulnar head* arises from the medial epicondyle of the humerus via the common tendon, from the anterior band of the ulnar collateral ligament, from adjacent intermuscular septa, and from the medial side of the coronoid process proximal to the ulnar origin of pronator teres. The *radial head*, a thin sheet of muscle, arises from the anterior radial border extending from the radial tuberosity to the insertion of pronator teres. The median nerve and ulnar artery descend between the heads. The muscle usually separates into two strata, directed to digits 2–5 as follows: the superficial stratum, joined laterally by the radial head, divides into two tendons for the middle and ring finger; the deep stratum gives off a muscular slip to join the superficial fibres directed to the ring finger, and then ends in two tendons for the index and little finger. As the tendons pass behind the flexor retinaculum they are arranged in pairs: the superficial pair going to the middle and ring fingers, the deep to the index and little finger. The student can remember this relative positioning in the carpal tunnel by forming the appropriate pattern with their own hand, touching the index and little finger under the middle and ring fingers. Distal to the carpal tunnel the four tendons diverge, each passing towards a finger superficial to the corresponding flexor digitorum profundus tendon. The two tendons for each finger enter the digital flexor sheath (which commences over the metacarpophalangeal joint) in this relationship, and thereafter there is a curious arrangement: the superficialis splits into two bundles which pass around the profundus to lie posteriorly. In this position they reunite and some fibres interchange from one bundle to another to form the *Chiasma of Camper*. The two slips then insert into the anterior surface of the middle phalanx. (See Flexor tendon sheaths, p. 892.) A detailed description has been provided by Shrewsbury and Kuczynski (1974).

Variations. The radial head may be absent. The muscular slip from the deep stratum may provide most or all of the fibres acting on the index finger. The part of the muscle associated with the little finger may be absent, replaced by a separate slip from the ulna, flexor retinaculum or palmar fascia. Variations also occur in the tendons. Dylevský (1968) and Chaplin and Greenlee (1975) have discussed these variations in relation to development.

Blood supply. Ulnar artery (p. 1542); superior and inferior ulnar collateral arteries (p. 1539); anterior and posterior ulnar recurrent arteries (p. 1543); superficial palmar arch (p. 1544); common and proper palmar digital arteries (p. 1542).

Nerve supply. The median nerve, C8 and T1.

Actions. Flexor digitorum superficialis is potentially a flexor of all the joints over which it passes; proximal interphalangeal, metacarpophalangeal and wrist joints. Its precise action depends on which other muscles are acting (see Co-ordinated movements of the upper limb, p. 862).

It has independent muscle slips to all four fingers, unlike flexor digitorum profundus, which has a muscle group common to the middle, ring and little fingers. Flexor digitorum superficialis is therefore able to flex one proximal interphalangeal joint at a time, a useful test in assessing a hand laceration.

DEEP FLEXORS OF THE FOREARM

This group comprises flexor digitorum profundus, flexor pollicis longus and pronator quadratus.

Flexor digitorum profundus

Flexor digitorum profundus (**7.99, 100, 101**) arises deep to the superficial flexors from about the upper three-quarters of the anterior and

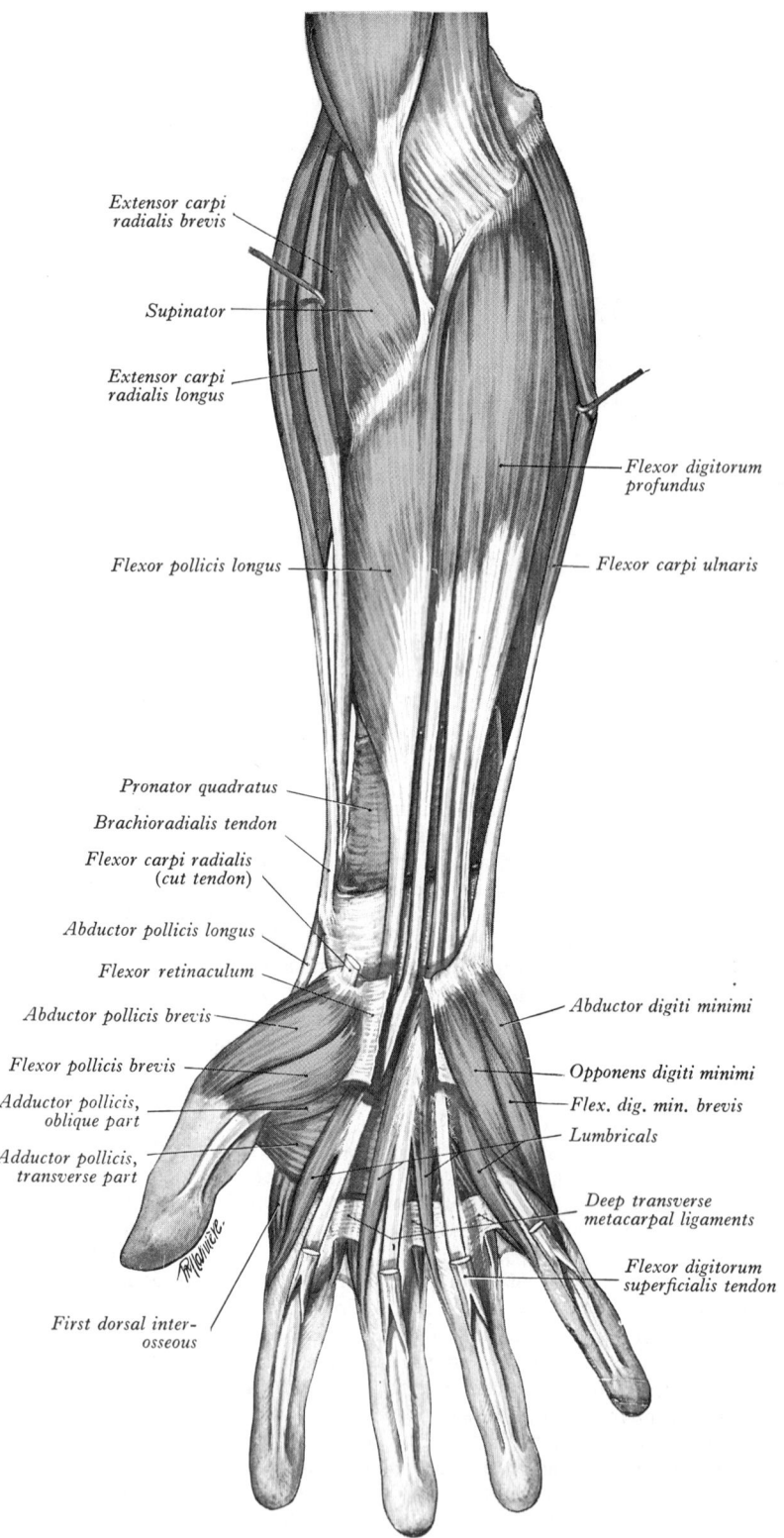

Extensor carpi
radialis brevis

Supinator

Extensor carpi
radialis longus

Flexor pollicis longus

Flexor digitorum
profundus

Flexor carpi ulnaris

Pronator quadratus

Brachioradialis tendon

Flexor carpi radialis
(cut tendon)

Abductor pollicis longus

Flexor retinaculum

Abductor pollicis brevis

Flexor pollicis brevis

Adductor pollicis,
oblique part

Adductor pollicis,
transverse part

First dorsal inter-
osseous

Abductor digiti minimi

Opponens digiti minimi

Flex. dig. min. brevis

Lumbricals

Deep transverse
metacarpal ligaments

Flexor digitorum
superficialis tendon

7.101 The deep flexor muscles of the right forearm.

medial surfaces of the ulna, embracing the attachment of brachialis above and extending distally almost to pronator quadratus. It also arises from a depression on the medial side of the coronoid process, from the upper three-quarters of the posterior ulnar border by an aponeurosis shared with flexor and extensor carpi ulnaris, and from the anterior surface of the ulnar half of the interosseous membrane. The muscle ends in four tendons, which run initially posterior (deep) to the tendons of flexor digitorum superficialis and the flexor retinaculum. The part of the muscle acting on the index finger is usually distinct throughout, but the tendons for other fingers are

interconnected by areolar tissue and tendinous slips as far as the palm. Anterior to their proximal phalanges, the tendons pass through the tendons of flexor digitorum superficialis (see above) to insert on the palmar surfaces of the bases of the distal phalanges. The tendons of the profundus undergo fascicular rearrangement as they pass through those of superficialis (Wilkinson 1953; Martin 1958). The muscle forms most of the surface elevation medial to the palpable posterior ulnar border.

Variations. The muscle may be joined by accessory slips from the radius (acting on the index finger), from flexor superficialis, flexor pollicis longus, the medial epicondyle or the coronoid process.

Blood supply. Posterior ulnar recurrent artery (p. 1543); posterior and anterior interosseous arteries (p. 1543); palmar 'carpal' arch (p. 1544); palmar metacarpal, common and proper digital palmar arteries (p. 1542). In addition, the **lateral** part is supplied by ulnar collaterals (p. 1539) and the deep palmar arch (p. 1544) and the **medial** part is supplied by the ulnar artery (p. 1542).

Nerve supply. Medial part by the ulnar nerve, lateral part by the anterior interosseous branch of the median nerve, **C8** and T1.

Actions. Like superficialis, flexor digitorum profundus is capable of flexing any or all of the joints over which it passes. It therefore has a role in coordinated finger flexion (p. 860), but it is the only muscle capable of flexing the distal interphalangeal joints. The index finger tendon is usually capable of independent function, whereas the other three work together. Electromyographically (Long 1968) flexor digitorum profundus acts alone in gentle digital flexion and is reinforced by superficialis for greater force and/or velocity.

Lumbrical muscles are attached to the tendons of flexor digitorum profundus in the palm (p. 860).

Flexor pollicis longus

Flexor pollicis longus (**7.**101, 106) is lateral to flexor digitorum profundus. It arises from the grooved anterior surface of the radius extending from below its tuberosity to the upper attachment of pronator quadratus. It also arises from the adjacent interosseous membrane, and frequently by a variable slip from the lateral, or more rarely medial, border of the coronoid process, or from the medial epicondyle of the humerus (Martin 1958). The muscle ends in a flattened tendon, which passes behind the flexor retinaculum, between opponens pollicis and the oblique head of adductor pollicis, to enter a synovial sheath, and finally to insert on the palmar surface of the base of the distal phalanx of the thumb. The anterior interosseous nerve and vessels descend on the interosseous membrane between flexor pollicis longus and flexor digitorum profundus.

Variations. Flexor pollicis longus is sometimes connected to flexor digitorum superficialis, or profundus, or pronator teres. The interosseous attachment, and indeed the whole muscle, may be absent.

Blood supply. Radial artery by direct rami (p. 1540); anterior interosseous artery (p. 1543); arteria princeps pollicis (p. 1544); palmar carpal arch (p. 1544).

Nerve supply. The anterior interosseous branch of the median nerve, C7 and **8**.

Action. The muscle flexes the phalanges of the thumb (p. 860).

Pronator quadratus

Pronator quadratus (**7.**101) is a flat, quadrilateral muscle extending across the front of the lower parts of the radius and ulna. It arises from the oblique ridge on the anterior surface of the shaft of the ulna (**6.**223A), from the medial part of this surface, and from a strong aponeurosis which covers the medial third of the muscle. The fibres pass laterally and slightly downwards to the distal quarter of the anterior border and surface of the shaft of the radius; deeper fibres insert into the triangular area above the ulnar notch of the radius.

Blood supply. Radial artery (p. 1540); anterior interosseous, anterior descending branch (p. 1543); recurrent branches of palmar 'carpal' arch (p. 1544).

Nerve supply. The anterior interosseous branch of the median nerve, C7 and **8**.

Action. The muscle is the principal pronator of the forearm, assisted by pronator teres only in rapid or forceful pronation. The deeper fibres oppose separation of the distal ends of the radius and ulna when upward thrusts are transmitted through the carpus.

SUPERFICIAL EXTENSORS OF THE FOREARM

Brachioradialis

Brachioradialis (**7.**98, 99, 100, 102) is the most superficial muscle along the radial side of the forearm, and forms the lateral border of the cubital fossa. It arises from the proximal two-thirds of the lateral supracondylar ridge of the humerus and from the anterior surface of the lateral intermuscular septum. The radial nerve and the anastomosis between arteria profunda brachii and the radial recurrent artery lie between the septum and brachialis. The muscle fibres end above midforearm level in a flat tendon which inserts on the lateral side of the distal end of the radius, just proximal to its styloid process. The tendon is crossed near its distal termination by the tendons of abductor pollicis longus and extensor pollicis brevis; the radial artery is on its ulnar (medial) side.

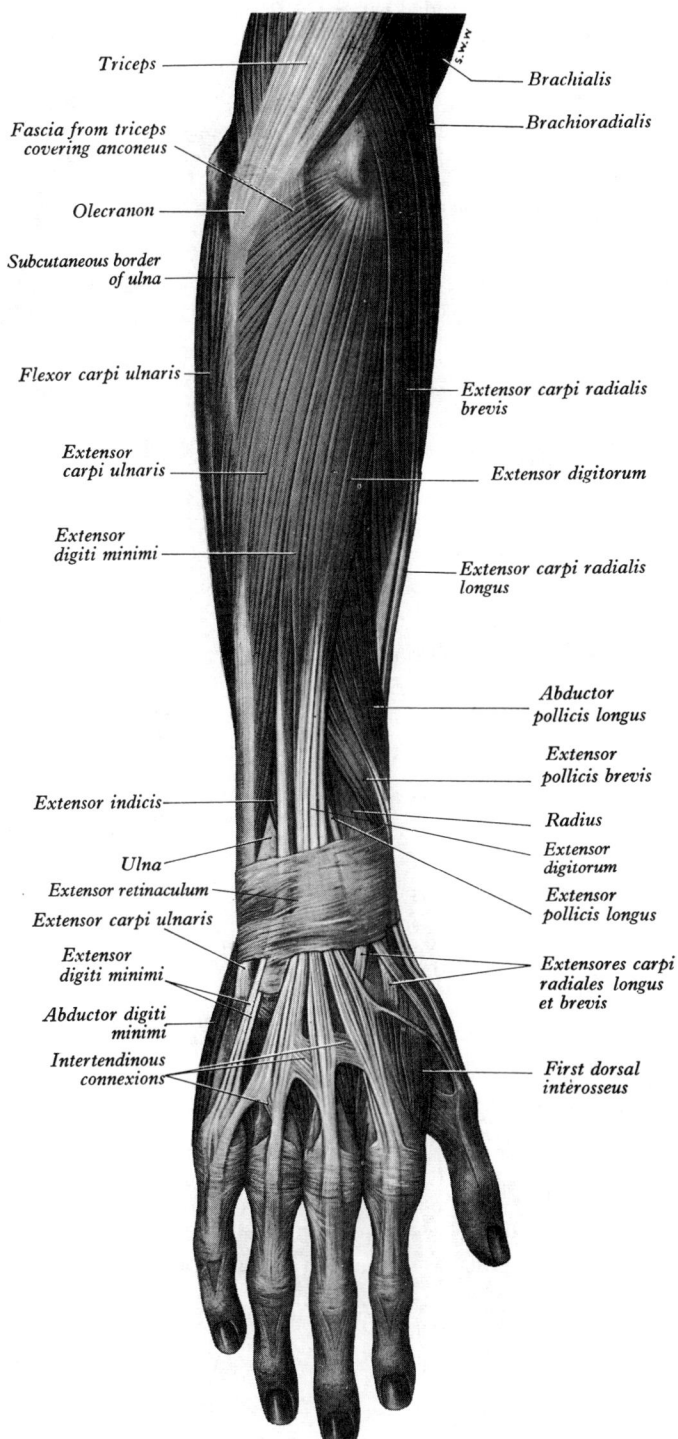

Triceps

Fascia from triceps covering anconeus

Olecranon

Subcutaneous border of ulna

Flexor carpi ulnaris

Extensor carpi ulnaris

Extensor digiti minimi

Extensor indicis

Ulna

Extensor retinaculum

Extensor carpi ulnaris

Extensor digiti minimi

Abductor digiti minimi

Intertendinous connexions

Brachialis

Brachioradialis

Extensor carpi radialis brevis

Extensor digitorum

Extensor carpi radialis longus

Abductor pollicis longus

Extensor pollicis brevis

Radius

Extensor digitorum

Extensor pollicis longus

Extensores carpi radiales longus et brevis

First dorsal interosseus

7.102 The superficial extensor muscles of the right forearm.

Variations. The muscle is often fused proximally with brachialis. Its tendon may divide into two or three separately attached slips. In rare instances it is double or absent. Its radial attachment may be much more proximal than the base of the styloid process.

Blood supply. Radial collateral branch of profunda brachii (p. 1539); inferior ulnar recurrent artery (p. 1539); the radial artery, directly and via the radial recurrent artery (p. 1541).

Nerve supply. The radial nerve, C5, **6**.

Action. Brachioradialis is a flexor of the elbow (despite being supplied by an 'extensor' nerve). It acts most effectively with the forearm in mid-pronation, and it stands out prominently, when the semi-pronated forearm is flexed against resistance. It is minimally active in slow, easy flexions, or with the forearm supine, but generates a powerful burst of activity in **both flexion and extension** when movement is rapid. Under these conditions it develops a pronounced transarticular component of its force which helps to stabilize the elbow joint by balancing the centrifugal force of rapid swings in either direction (p. 785; MacConaill & Basmajian 1977).

Extensor carpi radialis longus

Extensor carpi radialis longus (**7.**100, 102) is partly overlapped by brachioradialis. It arises mainly from the distal third of the lateral supracondylar ridge of the humerus and from the front of the lateral intermuscular septum, but some fibres come from the common tendon of origin of the forearm extensors. The belly ends at the junction of the proximal and middle thirds of the forearm in a flat tendon, which runs along the lateral surface of the radius, deep to abductor pollicis longus and extensor pollicis brevis; the tendon then passes under the extensor retinaculum where it lies in a groove on the back of the radius just behind the styloid process. It inserts on the radial side of the dorsal surface of the base of the second metacarpal. It may send slips to the first or third metacarpal bones, and it contributes to intermetacarpal ligaments.

Blood supply. Radial collateral continuation of profunda brachii (p. 1539); radial recurrent artery (p. 1541); interosseous recurrent artery (p. 1543); posterior interosseous artery (p. 1543).

Nerve supply. The radial nerve, C6 and 7.

Action. Considered with extensor carpi radialis brevis, below.

Extensor carpi radialis brevis

Extensor carpi radialis brevis (**7.**100, 102, 106) is shorter than extensor carpi radialis longus and is covered by it. It arises from the lateral epicondyle of the humerus by a tendon of origin which it shares with other forearm extensors (see below), and also from the radial collateral ligament of the elbow joint, from a strong aponeurosis which covers its surface, and from adjacent intermuscular septa. Its belly ends at about midforearm in a flat tendon that closely accompanies that of the longer carpal extensor to the wrist. The tendon passes deep to abductor pollicis longus and extensor pollicis brevis, then under the extensor retinaculum to be attached to the dorsal surface of the base of the third metacarpal on its radial side, distal to its styloid process, and on adjoining parts of the second metacarpal base. Under the extensor retinaculum the tendon lies in a shallow groove on the back of the radius, medial to the tendon of extensor carpi radialis longus, and separated from it by a low ridge.

Blood supply. As extensor carpi radialis longus.

Nerve supply. The posterior interosseous nerve, C7 and 8.

The tendons of the two radial carpal extensors pass under the extensor retinaculum in a single, common synovial sheath. They are easily palpated as the fist is clenched and relaxed. They may split into slips, variably attached to the second and third metacarpal bones. The muscles themselves may be united or may exchange muscular slips.

Actions. Acting with extensor carpi ulnaris the two muscles extend the wrist; with flexor carpi radialis they abduct it.

Extensor digitorum

Extensor digitorum (**7.**100, 102, 106) springs from the lateral epicondyle of the humerus via the common extensor tendon, from the adjacent intermuscular septa and from the antebrachial fascia. It divides distally into four tendons, which pass, together with the tendon of extensor indicis, through a separate tunnel under the extensor retinaculum in a common synovial sheath. The tendons then diverge on the dorsum of the hand, one to each finger. The tendon to the index is accompanied by extensor indicis, which lies medial to it. On the dorsum, adjacent tendons are linked by three variable *intertendinous connections*, which are inclined downwards and laterally. The medial connection is strong and pulls the tendon of the little finger towards that of the ring finger; the connection between the middle two tendons is weak and may be absent (Leslie 1954). The function of these bands is not clear; they **may** affect independent extension of digits.

The digital attachments enter a fibrous expansion on the dorsum of the proximal phalanges in which lumbrical, interosseous and digital extensor tendons all participate (see Dorsal digital expansion, p. 858).

Variations. The tendons of extensor digitorum may be variably deficient, but more often they are doubled or even tripled in one or more digits, most often the index finger or the middle finger. Occasionally a slip of tendon passes to the thumb.

Blood supply. Posterior interosseous artery (p. 1543); interosseous recurrent artery and its anastomosing vessels (p. 1543); continuation of the anterior interosseous artery after it pierces the interosseous membrane (p. 1543); dorsal carpal arch (p. 1544); dorsal metacarpal, digital and perforating arteries (p. 1541).

Nerve supply. The posterior interosseous nerve, C7 and 8.

Actions. Extensor digitorum can extend any or all of the joints over which it passes: wrist, metacarpophalangeal and, through the extensor expansion of the digits, the proximal and distal interphalangeal joints. Its role in coordinated finger movements is described below (p. 863). When acting on the metacarpophalangeal joints, extensor digitorum tends to spread the digits apart, an action that is due principally to the different axes of the individual joints because of the transverse arch of the hand. This is a 'trick' movement used by patients with interosseous muscle paralysis.

Extensor digiti minimi

Extensor digiti minimi (**7**.102) is a slender muscle medial to, and usually connected with, extensor digitorum. It arises from the common extensor tendon by a thin tendinous slip and from adjacent intermuscular septa. Its long tendon slides in a separate compartment of the extensor retinaculum just behind the inferior radio-ulnar joint. Distal to this, it divides into two, the lateral slip being joined by a tendon of extensor digitorum (**7**.102). All three tendons are attached to the dorsal digital expansion of the fifth digit.

Variations. The muscle usually has an additional origin from antebrachial fascia. Its tendon does not always divide and it may send a slip to the fourth digit. It is rarely absent, but sometimes is fused with extensor digitorum.

Blood supply. Posterior interosseous artery (p. 1543); interosseous recurrent artery and its anastomosing vessels (p. 1543); continuation of the anterior interosseous artery after it pierces the interosseous membrane (p. 1543); dorsal carpal arch (p. 1544); dorsal metacarpal, digital and perforating arteries (p. 1541).

Nerve supply. The posterior interosseous nerve, C7 and 8.

Actions. Extensor digiti minimi can extend any of the joints of the little finger, or contribute to wrist extension. It is not entirely clear why there should be an independent muscle for little finger extension, as there is for the index, but the reader will note that it is possible to extend either the little finger or the index finger independently of the other digits even in extremes of ulnar or radial wrist deviation.

Extensor carpi ulnaris

Extensor carpi ulnaris (**7**.100, 102) arises from the lateral epicondyle via the common extensor tendon, from the posterior border of the ulna by an aponeurosis shared with flexor carpi ulnaris and flexor digitorum profundus, and from overlying fascia. It can be felt lateral to the groove that overlies the posterior subcutaneous border of the ulna. It ends in a tendon that slides in a groove between the head and the styloid process of the ulna, in a separate compartment of the extensor retinaculum. It is attached to a tubercle on the medial side of the fifth metacarpal base.

Blood supply. Posterior interosseous artery (p. 1543); interosseous recurrent artery (p. 1543).

Nerve supply. The posterior interosseous nerve, C7 and 8.

Actions. Together with extensores carpi radiales longus and brevis, it acts synergistically with digital flexors to extend and to fix the

wrist when objects are being gripped or when the fist is clenched. Observation shows that it is impossible to grip strongly unless the wrist is extended. Acting with flexor carpi ulnaris, it adducts the hand.

Anconeus

Anconeus (**7**.102, 103) is a small, triangular muscle behind the cubital joint. It is partially blended with triceps, of which it is an integral part in some primates. It arises by a separate tendon from the posterior surface of the lateral epicondyle of the humerus. Its fibres diverge medially towards the ulna, covering the posterior aspect of the annular ligament, and are attached to the lateral aspect of the olecranon and proximal quarter of the posterior surface of the shaft of the ulna.

Variations. The muscle varies in the extent of fusion with triceps or extensor carpi ulnaris.

Blood supply. Interosseous recurrent artery (p. 1543); middle collateral (posterior descending) branch of profunda brachii (p. 1539).

Nerve supply. The radial nerve, C6, 7 and 8.

Action. Anconeus assists triceps in extending the elbow joint. Its

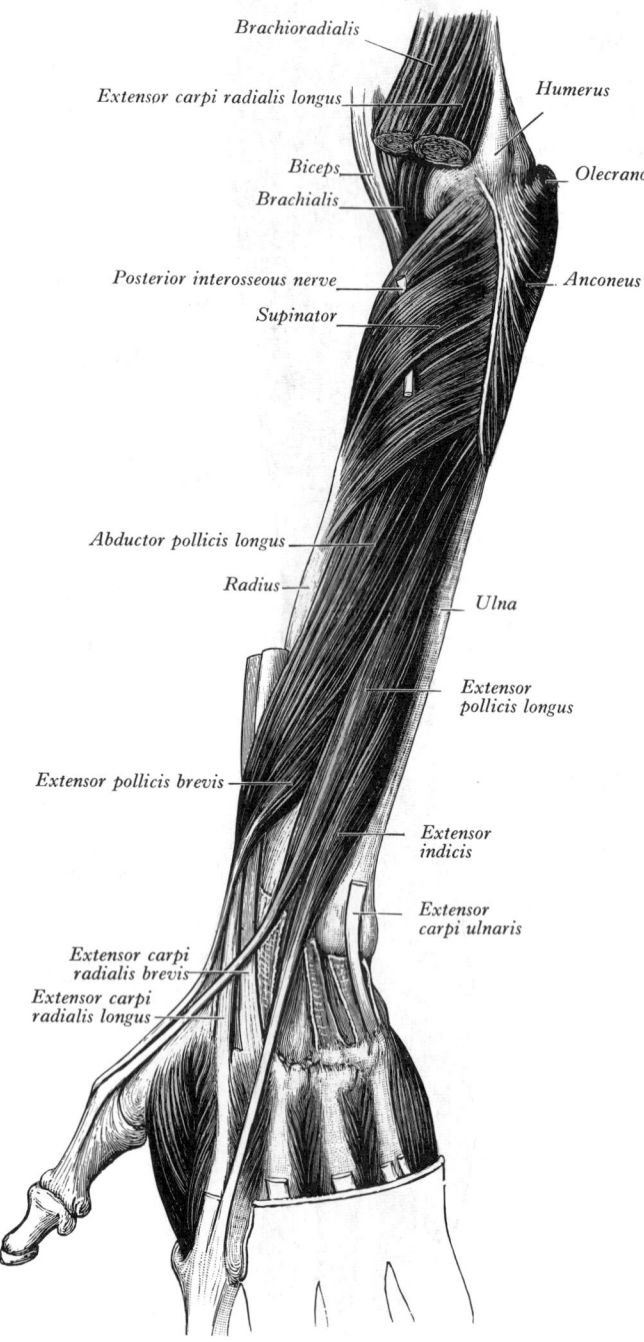

Brachioradialis

Extensor carpi radialis longus

Humerus

Biceps

Brachialis

Olecranon

Posterior interosseous nerve

Anconeus

Supinator

Abductor pollicis longus

Radius

Ulna

Extensor pollicis longus

Extensor pollicis brevis

Extensor indicis

Extensor carpi ulnaris

Extensor carpi radialis brevis

Extensor carpi radialis longus

7.103   The deep extensor muscles of the left forearm.

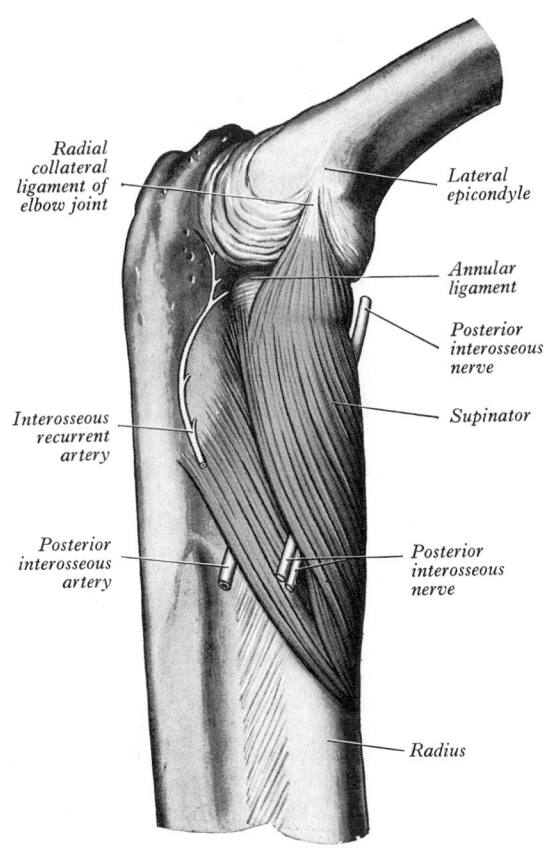

7.104   The right supinator muscle: posterolateral aspect.

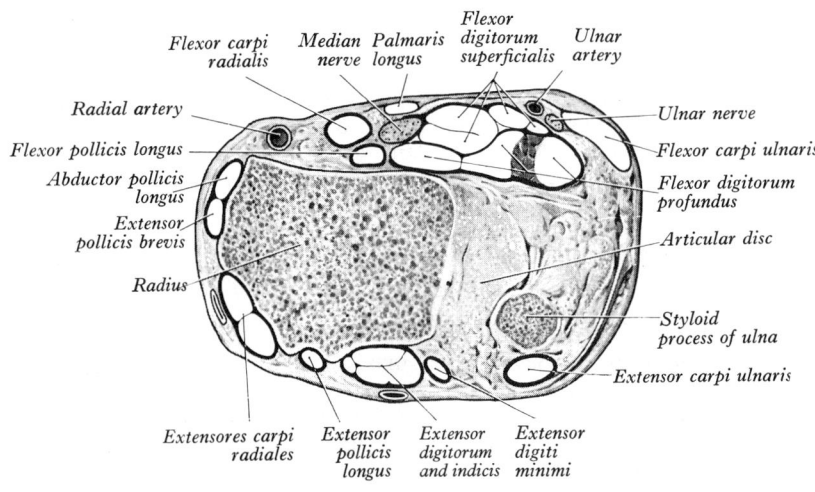

7.105   Transverse section through the right forearm, passing through the distal end of the radius and the styloid process of the ulna, with the hand and forearm in full supination: distal (inferior) aspect.

major function is not clear but it may be the control of ulnar abduction in pronation, which is necessary if the forearm is to turn over the hand without translating it medially. In this way a tool can be revolved 'on the spot' or it can be swept through an arc.

DEEP EXTENSORS OF THE FOREARM

The deep forearm extensor muscles (7.103, 105) consist of three that act on the thumb (abductor pollicis longus, extensor pollicis longus and extensor pollicis brevis), extensor indicis and supinator. Apart from supinator, all are attached proximally only to the forearm bones.

Supinator

Supinator (7.101, 103, 104) surrounds the proximal third of the radius and has superficial and deep layers, between which the posterior interosseous nerve passes (7.103). The two parts arise together—the superficial by tendinous and the deep by muscular fibres—from the lateral epicondyle of the humerus, from the radial collateral ligament of the elbow joint and the annular ligament of the superior radio-ulnar joint, from the supinator crest of the ulna and the posterior part of the triangular depression in front of it, and from an aponeurosis covering the muscle. The muscle attaches distally to the lateral surface of the proximal third of the radius, down to the insertion of pronator teres. The radial attachment extends on to the anterior and posterior surfaces (p. 636, 6.223B), between the anterior oblique line and the fainter posterior oblique 'ridge'.

Variations. The muscle is subject to frequent variation, small parts of it often receiving individual names, e.g. lateral and medial tensors of the annular ligament (Hast & Perkins 1984).

Blood supply. Radial artery (p. 1540); posterior interosseous artery (p. 1543); radial recurrent artery (p. 1541); interosseous recurrent artery (p. 1543); middle collateral artery (p. 1539).

Nerve supply. The posterior interosseous nerve, C6 and 7.

Action. Supinator rotates the radius so as to bring the palm anterior. It acts alone in slow, unopposed supination and together with biceps brachii in fast or forceful supination. An object, which may be heavy, is often picked up with the forearm initially pronated.

The more powerful supinators lift it against gravity, and rotation is often combined with increasing elbow flexion to bring the object towards the eyes.

Abductor pollicis longus

Abductor pollicis longus (7.100, 102, 103) arises, distal to the supinator and close to extensor pollicis brevis, from the posterior surface of the shaft of the ulna distal to anconeus, from the adjoining interosseous membrane, and from the middle third of the posterior surface of the radius distal to the attachment of supinator. It descends laterally, becoming superficial in the distal forearm, where it is visible as an oblique elevation (7.102). The muscle fibres end in a tendon just proximal to the wrist; this runs in a groove on the lateral side of the distal end of the radius accompanied by the tendon of extensor pollicis brevis. The tendon usually splits into two slips, one being attached to the radial side of the first metacarpal base, and one to the trapezium.

Variations. Fasciculi of the tendon may continue into opponens pollicis or abductor pollicis brevis. Occasionally the muscle itself may be wholly or partially divided.

Blood supply. Posterior interosseous artery (p. 1543); continuation and perforating rami of anterior interosseous artery (p. 1543). **Tendon:** radial artery in the 'anatomical snuff-box' (p. 1540); 1st dorsal metacarpal artery (p. 1541); dorsal carpal arch (p. 1541).

Nerve supply. The posterior interosseous nerve, C7 and 8.

Actions. Acting with abductor pollicis brevis, the muscle abducts the thumb radially (i.e. in the plane of the palm); with the pollicial extensors it extends the thumb at its carpometacarpal joint (p. 858).

Extensor pollicis brevis

Extensor pollicis brevis (7.102, 103) is medial to, and closely connected with, abductor pollicis longus; it arises from the posterior surface of the radius distal to the abductor, and from the adjacent interosseous membrane. Its tendon turns around a bony fulcrum, *Lister's tubercle* (palpable on the posterior surface of the lower radius) which changes the line of pull from that of the forearm to that of the thumb.

In the distal forearm, abductor pollicis longus and extensor pollicis brevis emerge between extensor carpi radialis brevis and extensor digitorum. They pass obliquely across the tendons of the radial extensors of the wrist, cover the distal part of brachioradialis, and pass through the most lateral compartment of the extensor retinaculum in a single synovial sheath, sharing a groove in the distal radius. Finally they cross, superficial to the radial styloid process and radial artery, to reach the dorsolateral base of the proximal phalanx of the thumb.

Variations. Extensor pollicis brevis commonly has an additional attachment to the base of the **distal** phalanx, usually through a fasciculus which joins the tendon of extensor pollicis longus (Muller

1959). The muscle may be absent or fused completely with abductor longus. Its tendon sometimes unites with that of the long pollicial extensor.

Blood supply. Posterior interosseous artery (p. 1543); continuation and perforating rami of anterior interosseous artery (p. 1543). **Tendon:** radial artery in the 'anatomical snuff-box' (branches to radial side of pollex, p. 1540); 1st dorsal metacarpal artery (p. 1541); dorsal carpal arch (p. 1541).

Nerve supply. The posterior interosseous nerve, C7 and 8.

Actions. The muscle extends the proximal phalanx and metacarpal of the thumb.

Extensor pollicis longus

Extensor pollicis longus (**7.102, 103**) is larger than extensor pollicis brevis, whose proximal attachment it partly covers. It arises from the lateral part of the middle third of the posterior surface of the shaft of the ulna below abductor pollicis longus, and from the adjacent interosseous membrane. It ends in a tendon which passes through a separate compartment of the extensor retinaculum, in a narrow, oblique groove on the back of the distal end of the radius. It then crosses obliquely the tendons of extensores carpi radiales longus and brevis (**7.103**), and is separated from extensor pollicis brevis, when the thumb is fully extended, by a triangular depression or fossa, still termed the 'anatomical snuff-box'. Bony structures can be felt in the floor of this fossa by deep palpation. In proximal to distal order they are: the radial styloid, the smooth convex articular surface of the scaphoid, the trapezium and the base of the first metacarpal. The latter are more easily felt during metacarpal movement and the scaphoid during adduction and abduction of the hand. The scaphoid can be palpated bidigitally between the examining index finger and thumb, one in the fossa, the other on the palmar tubercle. The tendon is attached to the base of the distal phalanx of the thumb. On the dorsum of the proximal phalanx the sides of the tendon are joined by expansions from the tendon of the abductor pollicis brevis laterally, and that of the first palmar interosseous and adductor pollicis medially.

Blood supply. As for extensor pollicis brevis.

Nerve supply. The posterior interosseous nerve, C7 and 8.

Actions. The muscle extends the distal phalanx of the thumb and, acting in association with extensor pollicis brevis and abductor pollicis longus, it extends the proximal phalanx and the metacarpal. In continued action, owing to the obliquity of its tendon, extensor pollicis longus adducts the extended thumb and rotates it laterally (p. 494).

Extensor indicis

Extensor indicis (**7.103**) is a narrow, elongated muscle, medial and parallel to extensor pollicis longus. It arises from the posterior surface of the ulna distal to extensor pollicis longus, and from the adjacent interosseous membrane. Its tendon passes under the extensor retinaculum in the compartment containing the tendons of extensor digitorum; opposite the head of the second metacarpal bone it joins the ulnar side of the tendon of the extensor digitorum for the index finger.

Variations. The muscle occasionally sends accessory slips to the extensor tendons of other digits. Rarely its tendon may be interrupted on the dorsum of the hand by an additional muscle belly (*extensor indicis brevis manus*).

Blood supply. Posterior interosseous artery (p. 1543); interosseous recurrent artery and its anastomosing vessels (p. 1543); continuation of the anterior interosseous artery after it pierces the interosseous membrane (p. 1543); dorsal carpal arch (p. 1541); dorsal metacarpal, digital and perforating arteries (p. 1541).

Nerve supply. The posterior interosseous nerve, C7 and 8. The distribution of neuromuscular spindles in this muscle has been studied by Gorp and Kennedy (1974); they tend to be concentrated near the motor point.

Actions. The muscle helps to extend the index finger and the wrist.

RETINACULA, FASCIAE, AND SYNOVIAL SHEATHS OF THE WRIST AND HAND

To provide an overview of muscle function in the hand, it is first necessary to describe the fascial framework and the part it plays in function. This will be followed by an account of the hand's own muscles (the clinical term 'intrinsic' is often used). By synthesizing this knowledge with the function of the forearm ('extrinsic') muscles, it is possible to gain an understanding of the way in which the many functions of the hand are co-ordinated.

FLEXOR ASPECT OF THE WRIST

Flexor retinaculum

This strong, fibrous band (**7.106, 107**) crosses the front of the carpus and converts its anterior concavity into the *carpal tunnel*, through which pass the flexor tendons of the digits and the median nerve (p. 1271). The retinaculum is short and broad, about 2.5–3 cm both transversely and proximodistally. It is attached medially to the pisiform and the hook of the hamate; laterally, it splits into two laminae, one superficial, attached to the tubercles of the scaphoid and trapezium, and one deep, attached to the medial lip of the groove on the trapezium (**7.106**). With this groove the two laminae form a tunnel, lined by a synovial sheath containing the tendon of flexor carpi radialis. The retinaculum is crossed superficially by the ulnar vessels and nerve, and the palmar cutaneous branches of the median and ulnar nerves. The tendons of palmaris longus and flexor carpi ulnaris are partly attached to its anterior surface; distally some intrinsic muscles of the thumb and little finger are attached to it.

Synovial sheaths of the carpal flexor tendons

Two synovial sheaths envelop the digital flexor tendons as they traverse the carpal tunnel, one for the flexores digitorum superficialis and profundus, the other for flexor pollicis longus (**7.106**). These sheaths extend into the forearm for about 2.5 cm proximal to the flexor retinaculum, and occasionally communicate with each other deep to it. The sheath of the flexores digitorum tendons reaches about halfway along the metacarpal bones, where it ends in blind diverticula around the tendons to the index, middle and ring fingers (**7.107**). It is prolonged around the tendons to the little finger and is

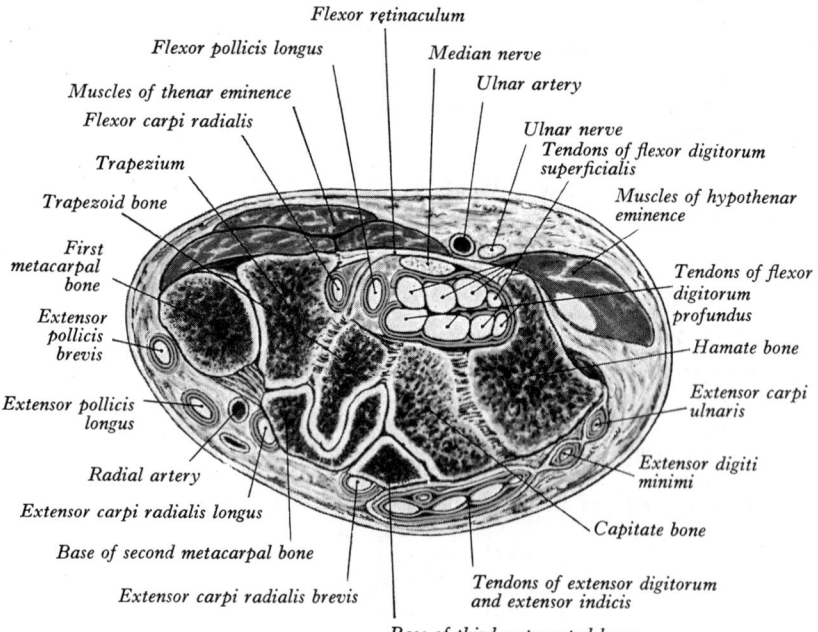

Flexor retinaculum
Flexor pollicis longus
Median nerve
Muscles of thenar eminence
Ulnar artery
Flexor carpi radialis
Ulnar nerve
Tendons of flexor digitorum superficialis
Trapezium
Muscles of hypothenar eminence
Trapezoid bone
First metacarpal bone
Tendons of flexor digitorum profundus
Extensor pollicis brevis
Hamate bone
Extensor pollicis longus
Extensor carpi ulnaris
Radial artery
Extensor digiti minimi
Extensor carpi radialis longus
Capitate bone
Base of second metacarpal bone
Extensor carpi radialis brevis
Tendons of extensor digitorum and extensor indicis
Base of third metacarpal bone

7.106 Transverse section through the left wrist, showing the tendons and their synovial sheaths: proximal (superior) aspect. The section is slightly oblique and passes through the distal row of the carpus and the bases of the first, second and third metacarpal bones. The arrangement of the tendons of the flexors of the fingers shown in the figure is not diagrammatic but represents the actual condition at this level. Observe that the carpometacarpal joint of the thumb is separate from the joint between the trapezium and the base of the second metacarpal bone.

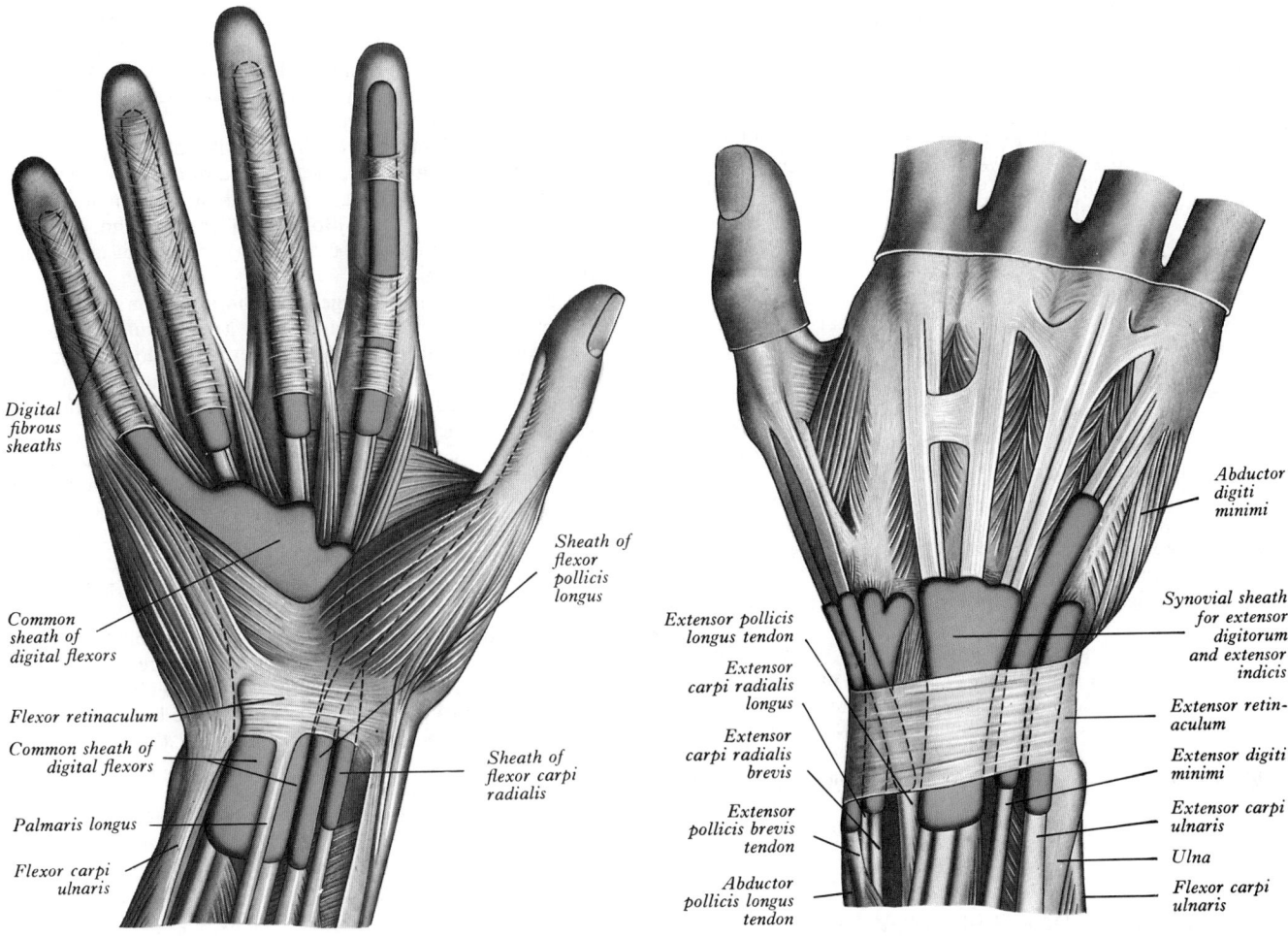

Digital fibrous sheaths

Common sheath of digital flexors

Flexor retinaculum

Common sheath of digital flexors

Palmaris longus

Flexor carpi ulnaris

Sheath of flexor pollicis longus

Sheath of flexor carpi radialis

Extensor pollicis longus tendon

Extensor carpi radialis longus

Extensor carpi radialis brevis

Extensor pollicis brevis tendon

Abductor pollicis longus tendon

Abductor digiti minimi

Synovial sheath for extensor digitorum and extensor indicis

Extensor retinaculum

Extensor digiti minimi

Extensor carpi ulnaris

Ulna

Flexor carpi ulnaris

7.107 The synovial sheaths of the tendons on the flexor aspect of the right wrist and hand (preparation by Professor J C B Grant). Where they are exposed, the synovial sheaths are shown in blue; where they are hidden by overlying structures, their margins are indicated by interrupted black lines. For simplicity and clarity the digital synovial sheaths are represented as smooth cylinders; they are described more fully under Flexor tendon sheaths, (p. 857).

7.108 A simplified representation of the synovial sheaths of the tendons on the extensor aspect of the right wrist (preparation by Professor J C B Grant). The synovial sheaths are shown in blue, but they have not been coloured where they lie deep to the extensor retinaculum. In this situation, and where one sheath lies deep to another, the margins of the sheaths are indicated by broken lines.

usually continuous with their digital synovial sheath. A transverse section through the carpus (**7.106**) shows that the tendons are invaginated into the sheath from the lateral side. The parietal layer lines the flexor retinaculum and the floor of the carpal tunnel and is reflected laterally as the visceral layer over the tendons of flexor digitorum superficialis on the ventral side and over those of flexor digitorum profundus on the dorsal side. Medially a recess formed by the visceral layer of the sheath is insinuated between the two groups of tendons and passes laterally for a variable distance. The sheath of flexor pollicis longus, which is usually separate, is continued along the thumb as far as the insertion of the tendon. The fibrous sheaths enveloping the terminal parts of the tendons of the flexores digitorum will be described below.

Clinical relevance. The anterior aspect of the wrist is not a traditional anatomical 'region'. It is neither a fossa nor a triangle with clear boundaries. Nevertheless knowledge of this area is important for all who would feel a pulse! It is frequently injured and a knowledge of the order of structures allows a mental picture to form of how deep the cut has penetrated (Lister 1985). It is an area of great importance not only to surgeons but also to physicians, for injections into the carpal tunnel, or to anaesthetists, for regional nerve anaesthesia.

There are surface landmarks that every student of anatomy should know. Looking at the wrist one can see that flexion produces transverse skin creases at the wrist, usually two or three. The dominant one overlies the proximal edge of the flexor retinaculum

and the carpal tunnel therefore lies distal to this under palmar skin. At the ulnar end of the skin crease the pisiform can be palpated and, distally, the hook of the hamate. Just distal to the radial end of the skin crease is the tubercle of the scaphoid.

Proximal to the wrist crease, the prominent tendon of flexor carpi radialis can be seen and palpated, with the radial artery to its lateral side. By palpating on the lateral side of the flexor carpi radialis 3 or 4 cm proximal to the wrist crease, it is possible to palpate flexor pollicis longus: bending and straightening the thumb will confirm that the examining finger is in the correct place. However it is the area on the ulnar side of flexor carpi radialis that is packed most densely with functionally important structures. The median nerve is very close to the skin surface and therefore often injured in lacerations. It is covered by palmaris longus, when that muscle is present (best confirmed by pinching thumb and ring finger together, when the muscle will be seen to stand out). When the muscle is absent there is only a thin covering of subcutaneous fat and deep fascia between skin and nerve. Deep to the median nerve are the four tendons of flexor digitorum superficialis, the middle and ring finger tendons in front of index and little finger tendons as they pass deep to the retinaculum. Deeper still are the tendons of flexor digitorum profundus. On the ulnar (medial) side of the front of the wrist the large and robust tendon of flexor carpi ulnaris is easily palpated and the ulnar nerve, artery and venae comitantes lie in the shelter of its radial edge. Any sharp injury powerful enough to cut through this strong tendon usually has enough energy left to cut nerve and vessel as well.

EXTENSOR ASPECT OF THE WRIST

Extensor retinaculum

The extensor retinaculum (7.108) is a strong, fibrous band which extends obliquely across the back of the wrist. It is attached laterally to the anterior border of the radius, medially to the triquetral and pisiform bones, and, in passing across the wrist, to the ridges on the dorsal aspect of the distal end of the radius.

Synovial sheaths of the carpal extensor tendons

Deep to the extensor retinaculum there are six tunnels for the passage of the extensor tendons, each containing a synovial sheath (7.108). They are:

(1) on the lateral side of the styloid process of the radius, for the tendons of abductor pollicis longus and extensor pollicis brevis

(2) behind the styloid process, for the tendons of extensores carpi radiales longus and brevis

(3) on the medial side of the dorsal tubercle of the radius, for the tendon of extensor pollicis longus

(4) on the medial side of the latter, for the tendons of extensor digitorum and extensor indicis

(5) opposite the interval between the radius and ulna, for extensor digiti minimi

(6) between the head and the styloid process of the ulna, for the tendon of extensor carpi ulnaris.

The tendon sheaths of abductor pollicis longus, extensores pollicis brevis and longus, extensores carpi radiales and extensor carpi ulnaris stop immediately proximal to the bases of the metacarpal bones; those of extensor digitorum, extensor indicis and extensor digiti minimi are sometimes prolonged a little more distally along the metacarpus.

FASCIAL CONTINUUM OR FRAMEWORK

The hand has many fascial and connective tissue structures; some can be identified as separate structures but others appear to be part of a three-dimensional network of connective tissue. Taken together this fascial continuum can be considered as a fibrous skeleton or framework designed to assist in the hand's mechanical role. The most defined connective tissue structures, tendons and ligaments, are well known and named individually, but the more delicate structures also have important functional roles; they are more than mere packing material. What is more, they have very different special-izations on the palmar and dorsal surfaces. The palm is adapted for padding and anchorage whereas the dorsum is particularly developed for gliding. The terms 'palmar fascia' or 'palmar aponeurosis' deserve special mention as they have often been used clinically as a generic term for fascia in the hand. These terms are best reserved for the well-developed planes of longitudinal and transverse fibres in the central part of the palm (7.109). The longitudinal fibres represent the distal fascial bundles of palmaris longus when it is present (the fibres are present even when the muscle is absent). These fibres (the clinical term 'pretendinous' is often used) are arranged in bundles corresponding to the four digital rays; in addition there is a variable bundle crossing the thenar eminence towards the radial side of the thumb. This structural arrangement was well known to early anatomists and surgeons (Albinus 1734; Weitbrecht 1742; Dupuytren 1831; early works have been carefully translated by Stack 1973).

The thin fascial coverings over the thenar and hypothenar muscles have sometimes been termed lateral and medial parts of the palmar aponeurosis, but these are much thinner and more flexible than the central part. Much has been written about palmar spaces, particularly in relation to the accumulation of pus in infections (Kanavel 1925), but there are many potential spaces and it is difficult to define their margins. Pus can certainly spread proximally within flexor tendon sheaths, but from a clinical point of view it is almost as disastrous in those digits whose sheaths do not communicate with the carpal tunnel sheaths (index, middle, ring) as in those that do (thumb, little finger). It is preferable to know the structures rather than the potential spaces between them.

Detailed descriptions of fascial structure have been reported by Wood Jones (1941), Kaplan (1965), Stack (1973), McFarlane (1974), Landsmeer (1976), McGrouther (1982) and Zancolli (1992).

It is possible to define a number of different functions of the fascial continuum of the hand.

Channelling of structures in transit between forearm and digits, principally tendons, nerves and neurovascular bundles. Examples of this function are provided by the longitudinal septa described and illustrated by Bojsen-Møller and Schmidt (7.110A–C) which act as spacers between the tendons and neurovascular bundles of the individual digital rays.

Where tendons must change direction around a concave surface the channels are thickened and have a retinacular role, forming sheaths with specialized pulleys to prevent tendon springing away from the underlying skeleton (see Flexor tendon sheaths, below). The term 'retinaculum' (meaning that which retains or keeps in place) is not restricted to sheaths but is also used in relation to the fingers for various retaining ligaments of the extensor apparatus which keep it in place over convex surfaces. In this instance the retinacular ligaments form not pulleys but guy-ropes, sufficiently long to allow the extensor apparatus to glide backwards and forwards.

Where pulleys exist, i.e. on concave surfaces, these allow the direction of pull in a tendon to change as it rounds a corner, and in so doing the pulley must itself apply a considerable lateral load on the tendon. It must therefore have considerable strength and a system of lubrication to prevent frictional resistance to gliding.

Transmission of loads. Where compressive loading is applied to the hand there is a shock absorber system; this has the general pattern of loculi of fat contained within defined fibrous boundaries, such that the shape of each loculus can change but not its volume. Thus the compliance or deformability of the boundaries determines the amount of shock absorption. The clinical term 'turgor' means deformability and is a measure of this anatomical property together with the vascular supply, since the local blood volume also has a major influence on tissue compliance. The finger pulp is designed in this way, as is the subcutaneous fat on the palmar area. The palm has a second dimension of shock absorber function: in addition to the subcutaneous fat loculi, there are much larger fibrous compartments between skin and skeleton containing muscles, tendons and other structures. The honeycomb pattern of these, elegantly illustrated by Bojsen-Møller and Schmidt (7.110c) forms a total palmar shock absorption system. No plane of fascia therefore has a simple mech-anical role; all are involved in pushing, and distortion of the tissues and the many fibre orientations in the fascia reflect this function. The soft padded parts of the hand are able to conform to the contours of objects being grasped, allowing better interpretation of sensation and better grip.

The other type of loading that the hand must resist is tensile loading. Tendons and ligaments are particularly suitable for resisting such forces but there are many parts of the fascial continuum that must also have a major function in resisting 'pulling' forces. The anchorage system of the palm is an example and will be discussed next.

Anchorage. Skin is retained by fascial ligaments in an ingenious system that allows the hand to flex while retaining the skin in position. The skin folds at palmar and digital creases which themselves have few deep anchoring fibres; it is the skin on either side of the crease lines that has the best developed deep anchorage ligaments, allowing the unanchored skin between to fold in a repetitive pattern; the palmar creases have been described as skin 'joints'. Fascial anchors may be vertical (perpendicular to the palm), as in the midpalm where scattered fibres run from the dermis down into the depths of the hand, or horizontal (in the plane of the palm), or oblique to the skin surface.

A well-developed horizontal anchorage system is the insertion of the longitudinal (pretendinous) fibres of the palmar aponeurosis, which represents the distal part of palmaris longus, when that muscle is present. These fibres are, however, well developed even when the tendon is absent, in which case the fibres may merge with other fascial systems in the region of the flexor retinaculum or receive an insertion from flexor carpi ulnaris (Fahrer 1980). The most superficial longitudinal fibres insert into the dermis of the distal palm. This arrangement resists horizontal shearing force in such gripping tasks

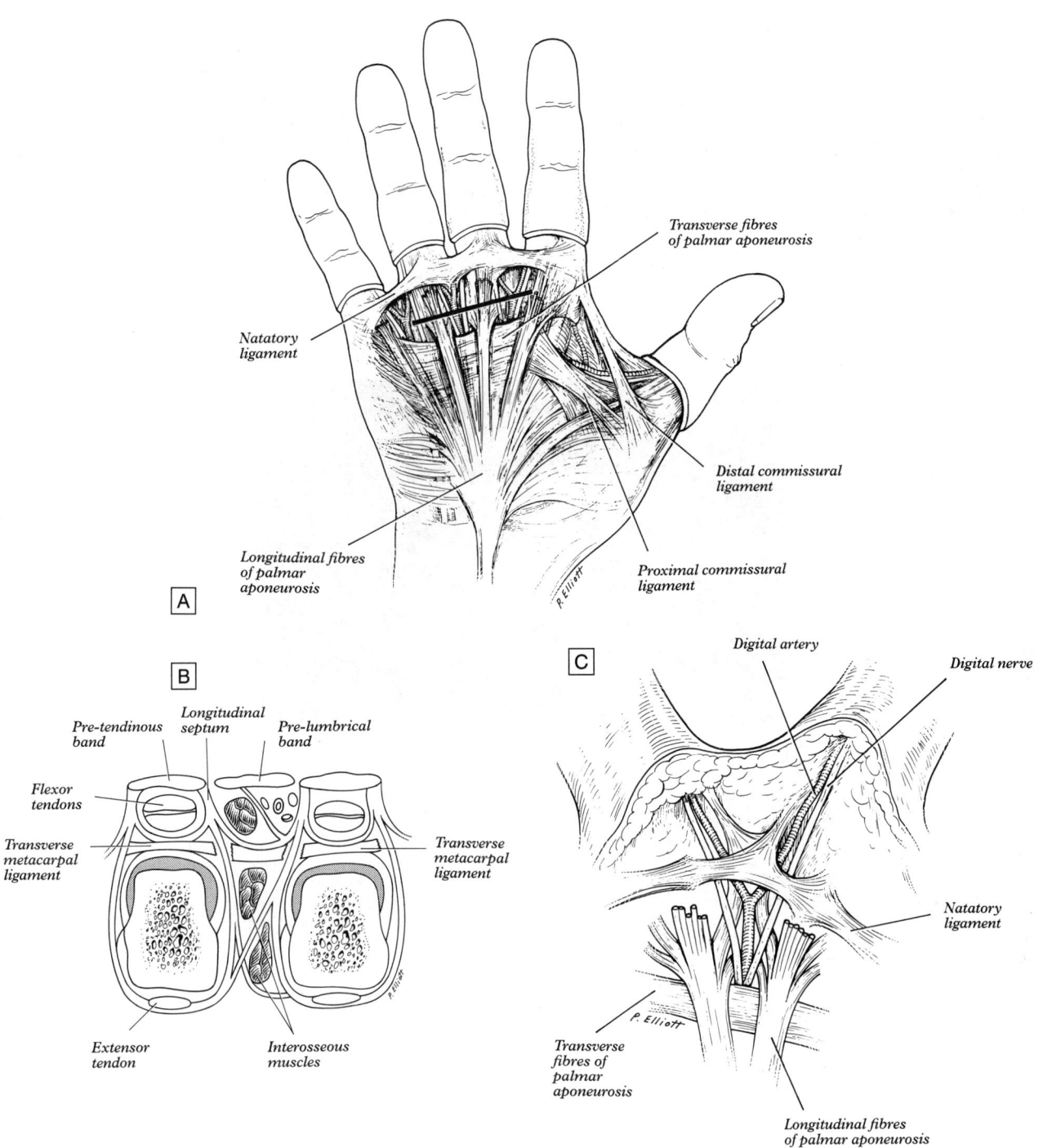

7.109 A. The right palmar aponeurosis, dissected to demonstrate transverse fascial structures in the palm and first web space. B. A cross-section of the hand at the level of the heads of the metacarpal bones, as indicated in A. C. More detailed view of structures at the level indicated in A.

as holding a golf club, in which it prevents distal skin slippage or degloving of the palm on striking the golf ball. The characteristic blisters on the palms of those unaccustomed to such sports map out the sites of the skin anchorage points. The reader can demonstrate this anchorage system on his own hand by flexing the palm until the skin of the distal palm folds loosely. This loose skin can then be pinched by the thumb and forefinger of the other hand. An attempt to pull the skin distally will reveal the anchoring longitudinal fibres of the palmar aponeurosis.

There are two deeper types of anchorage of the longitudinal fibres (7.110). The first is a layer that passes underneath a transverse fibre system named the *superficial transverse metacarpal ligament* (*natatory ligament*) and deep to the neurovascular bundles towards the digits.

When this fascial system becomes involved in Dupuytren's Contracture, an idiopathic contracture of the fascia of the hand, the neurovascular bundle can be displaced, making it vulnerable to surgical injury. The deepest layer of longitudinal fibres passes around the sides of the flexor sheath and metacarpophalangeal joint to merge with various deep fascial structures (McGrouther 1990). Thus the longitudinal fibres of the palmar fascia have wide insertions into skin and fascia in the distal hand.

Oblique anchors occur in the fingers where *Cleland's ligaments* tether the skin of proximal and middle segments of the digits to the region of the proximal interphalangeal joints. Cleland's ligaments lie anterior to the neurovascular bundles, whereas *Grayson's ligaments* are transversely orientated skin-retaining ligaments anterior to the

855

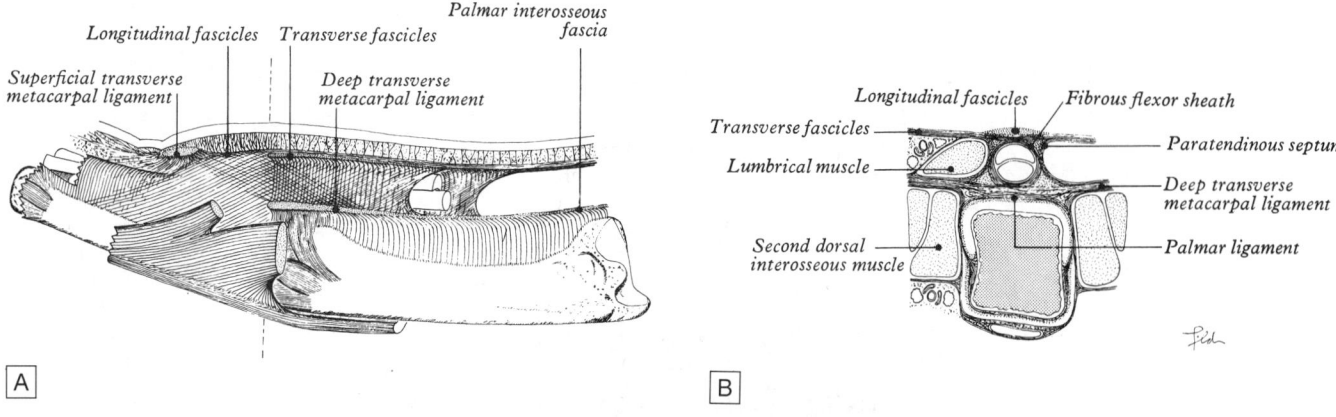

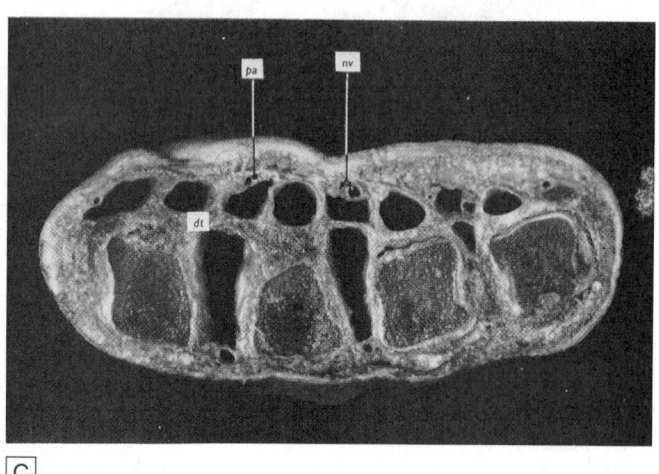

7.110 A. Drawing of the course of the fibres of the fasciae around the left third metacarpal bone and proximal phalanx viewed from the radial side. The deep transverse metacarpal ligament connects both with the metacarpal bone and with the longitudinal and transverse fibres of the palmar aponeurosis and, via their retinacula, with the skin. The palmar interosseous fascia is connected by means of a sagittal septum to the shaft of the third metacarpal bone. B. Transverse section through the head of the third metacarpal bone showing the course of the fibres between the palmar aponeurosis and the deep transverse metacarpal ligament, and their attach-ments to the metacarpal bone. C. Section through the hand at the level of the heads of the 2nd to 5th metacarpal bones, demonstrating the subdivision of the distal part of the central compartment into eight narrow compartments. The interdigital nerves and vessels (nv) have been left to show their relation to the lumbrical compartments. The deep transverse metacarpal ligaments (dt) and palmar aponeurosis (pa) are also shown (from Bojsen-Møller & Schmidt 1974, by courtesy of the authors and the Cambridge University Press). For a recent description of the flexor tendon sheaths, see pages 857–858.

bundles (Cleland 1878; Grayson 1941; Milford 1968; McFarlane 1974).

'Binding role'. The transversely orientated fascial structures have a role in maintaining the transverse arch of the hand by 'binding' the skeletal structures or the tendon sheaths. The deepest is the transverse structure extending across the four digital metacarpals, the *deep transverse metacarpal ligament*, which runs from one metacarpophalangeal joint volar plate to another thus crossing the hand (Weitbrecht 1742; Zancolli 1979). The next more superficial layer is that of the transverse fibres of the palmar aponeurosis, which lie immediately deep (posterior) to the longitudinal fibres, and form tunnels over the neurovascular bundles and flexor tendons (Legueu & Juvara 1892; Skoog 1967). They have been considered to form part of the flexor tendon pulley system (Manske & Lesker 1983). The most superficial transverse fibres have the name *superficial transverse metacarpal ligaments*, but the German description *Schwimmband* (Grapow 1887), or *natatory ligament*, better describes their position at the margins of the interdigital webs. This system has two components: transverse fibres, and fibres curving around the webs. They seem to limit web abduction and are described below.

Limiting or tethering role. Joint motion is limited by joint ligamentous action, but also in some cases by skin tightness. In the interdigital webs the skin is generally reinforced by fascial liga-mentous fibres running just beneath the dermis and in a direction so as to resist the stretch. They are well developed in the thumb web (Defrenne 1977).

Lubricating role. Flexor tendon sheaths have low friction and a system of lubrication by synovial fluid. There are many other gliding planes. On the dorsum of the digits there is a gliding plane between periosteum and extensor apparatus and between the latter and skin.

Vascular protection and pumping action. The delicate blood vessels of the hand must be protected from pressure by surrounding them with a cuff of tough fascia or a fatty pad. When the hand is compressed, as in gripping, the relatively incompressible fascial structures act as a venous pumping mechanism to assist return of blood from the limb. On the dorsum, in contrast, there are large capacitance veins in gliding skin. The fascia around these veins is loose areolar tissue, which allows venous dilatation.

Framework for muscle origins and insertions. Many of the small muscles of the hand arise from the fascial skeleton, at least in part (e.g. abductor pollicis brevis from the flexor retinaculum). Other muscles insert into it (palmaris longus). The fascial framework can also be visualized as a harness by which the muscles act on the underlying skeleton. For example, the metacarpophalangeal joint is surrounded by a ring of fascial and ligamentous structures by which the joint is moved, there being no insertions of long flexor or extensor muscles into the proximal phalanx.

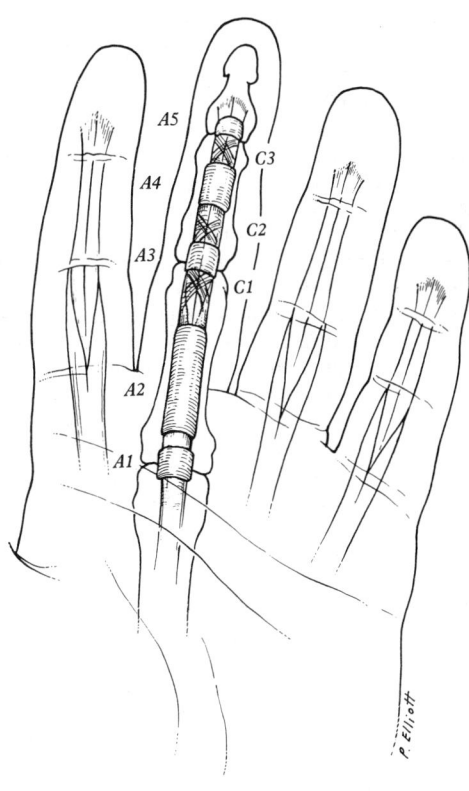

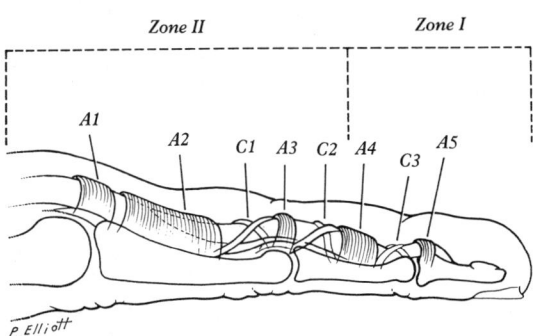

7.111 The arrangement of the annular and cruciate pulleys of the flexor tendon sheath. A. Palmar aspect of left hand. B. Lateral view.

Flexor tendon sheaths

The fibrous sheaths of the flexor tendons are specialized parts of the palmar fascial continuum. Each finger has an osseo-aponeurotic tunnel extending from midpalm to the distal phalanx, and there is a tunnel for flexor pollicis longus from the metacarpal to distal phalanx. The proximal border is to some extent a matter of definition, as the transverse fibres of the palmar aponeurosis may be considered to be a part of the pulley system. The structure of the sheath consists basically of arcuate fibres arching anteriorly over the tendons where the sheath is required to be stiff, overlying bone or at the centres of joints, where a bucket-handle of arcuate fibres is a mechanically favourable arrangement. In contrast, where the sheath is required to fold to permit joint flexion there is an arrangement of cruciate fibres supporting a thin synovial membrane to provide a sealed lubrication system containing synovial fluid. Within the fibrous sheath, the synovial membrane forms a continuous lining from the distal phalanx to midpalm in the case of the index, middle and ring fingers, but further proximally in the case of the little finger (**7.107**). This digit has a continuity with the flexor sheath in front of the wrist. The thumb has a similar arrangement. The parietal synovial membrane is reflected onto the surface of the flexor tendon, forming a visceral synovium.

A standard nomenclature for the arcuate and cruciform pulleys that comprise the sheath has been adopted by the American Society for Surgery of the Hand: the letters A and C are used respectively (Doyle & Blythe 1975). The usual pattern is as follows (**7.111**).

The A1 pulley is situated anterior to the palmar cartilaginous plate of the metacarpophalangeal joint and may extend over the proximal part of the proximal phalanx. The A2 overlies the middle third of the proximal phalanx. It is the strongest pulley and arises from well-defined longitudinal ridges on the palmar aspect of the phalanx. Its distal edge is well developed and in sagittal cross-section it is seen that there is a pouch or recess of synovium superficial to the free edge of the pulley fibres so that the free edge forms a lip protruding into the synovial space (Lundborg & Myrhage 1977; Jones & Amis 1988). A3 is a narrow pulley lying palmar to the proximal interphalangeal joint. A4 overlies the middle third of the middle phalanx, and A5 the distal interphalangeal joint. The cruciate fibres are numbered in a slightly different manner, there being a single system, C0, palmar to the metacarpophalangeal joint to allow flexion. In contrast, there are two cruciate zones, C1 and C2, at the proximal interphalangeal joint just proximal and distal respectively to A3. At the distal interphalangeal joint there is one pronounced cruciate system C3, between A4 and A5. Variations occur frequently. During flexion, the cruciate fibres become orientated more transversely in the digits and the edges of adjacent annular pulleys

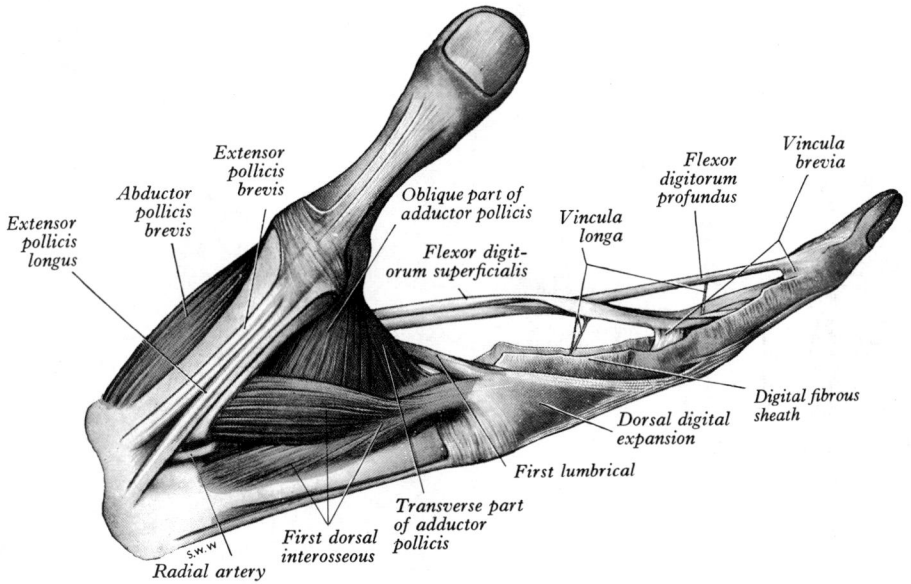

7.112 Lateral part of the right hand showing the tendons and vincula tendinum of the index finger and the muscles in the first intermetacarpal space.

approximate to form, in full flexion, a continuous tunnel of transversely orientated fibres.

The phenomenon of tendon gliding within a fibrous sheath requires a very specialized arrangement of vascular supply. Folds of synovial membrane, containing a loose plexus of fascial fibres, carry blood vessels to the tendons at certain defined points (7.112). These folds, termed *vincula tendinum* (singular: *vinculum tendinum*) are of two kinds. *Vincula brevia* (singular: *vinculum brevium*), of which there are two in each finger, are attached to the deep surfaces of the tendons near to their insertions. There is thus one vinculum brevium attaching flexor digitorum profundus to the region of the distal interphalangeal joint, and a more proximal vinculum deep to flexor digitorum superficialis at the proximal interphalangeal joint. The *vincula longa* are filiform, and usually two are attached to each superficial tendon, one to each deep tendon (Leffert et al 1974; Armenta & Fisher 1984).

MUSCLES OF THE HAND

The intrinsic muscles of the hand may be described in three groups:

- Muscles that act on the thumb: these include abductor pollicis brevis, opponens pollicis, and flexor pollicis brevis, within the thenar eminence, and adductor pollicis
- Muscles of the hypothenar eminence: these consist of muscles acting on the little finger—abductor digiti minimi, flexor digiti minimi and opponens digiti minimi—together with palmaris brevis
- Muscles acting on the fingers: the interossei and the lumbricals.

Dorsal digital expansion

In describing these muscles, reference will be made to the *dorsal digital* or *extensor expansion*. This is a fibrous expansion on the dorsum of the proximal phalanx of each digit. It can be regarded as an aponeurotic extension of the tendon of extensor digitorum (p. 849), but its location and its involvement in the attachment of the lumbrical and interosseous muscles make it convenient to consider it in the context of the hand. The expansion is triangular, and the base of the triangle, which is proximal, wraps around the dorsal and collateral aspects of the metacarpophalangeal joint. A tendon of extensor digitorum blends with the expansion along its central axis, and is separated from the metacarpophalangeal joint by a small bursa. The base of the expansion, which connects this tendon to the adjoining interosseous muscles on each side, is stabilized by numerous transverse fibres and by links that extend to the deep transverse metacarpal ligaments. It separates the *phalangeal* attachment of the dorsal interosseus from the rest of the muscle, and also the palmar interosseus from the lumbrical muscle (7.113A–C).

The margins of these expansions are thickened laterally by the tendons of lumbrical and interosseous muscles and medially by the tendon of an interosseous alone or, in the case of the fifth digit, by abductor digiti minimi. In clinical practice these attachments of the intrinsic muscles are referred to as 'wing tendons'. Proximal and distal 'wings' can be identified in the fingers (7.113A–C) usually on both sides of each expansion. The attachments of the interossei to these wings has led some to classify these muscles as 'distal' and 'proximal' in place of the more usual 'palmar' and 'dorsal'. The expansion is almost translucent between its margins and the extensor digitorum tendon. As that tendon approaches the proximal interphalangeal joint, it divides into an axial part and two collateral slips. The former, which receives some fibres from the lumbrical and interosseous tendons (Landsmeer 1949), passes over the dorsal aspect of the joint to insert on the base of a middle phalanx. Each collateral slip is joined by the corresponding thickened border of the digital expansion and the two unite to be attached to the dorsal aspect of the base of the distal phalanx. The distal 'wing tendon' is just proximal to this attachment.

Each expansion forms a movable hood (Bunnell 1949), which moves distally when the metacarpophalangeal joint is flexed and proximally when it is extended, in which position it is most closely applied to the joint. Landsmeer (1949) and Haines (1951) have described *retinacular* ('*link*') ligaments, which correlate movements at interphalangeal joints: from a proximal attachment to the side of

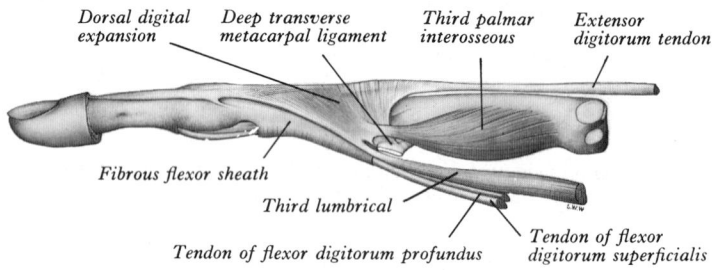

7.113B   The dorsal digital expansion of the ring finger in extension (lateral aspect). Compare the position of the proximal edge of the expansion with that in 7.113C.

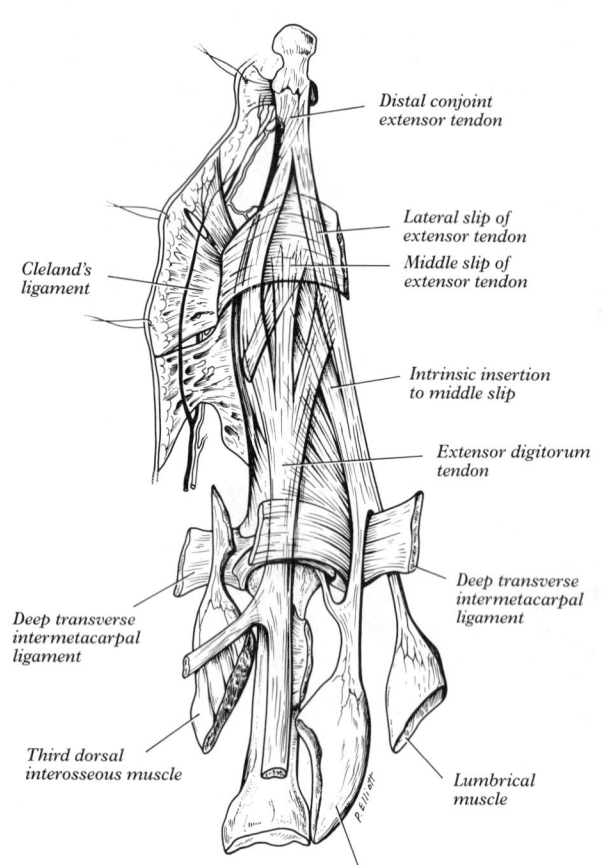

7.113A   Dorsal digital expansion, represented here by the middle finger of the left hand. (After Zancolli 1979.)

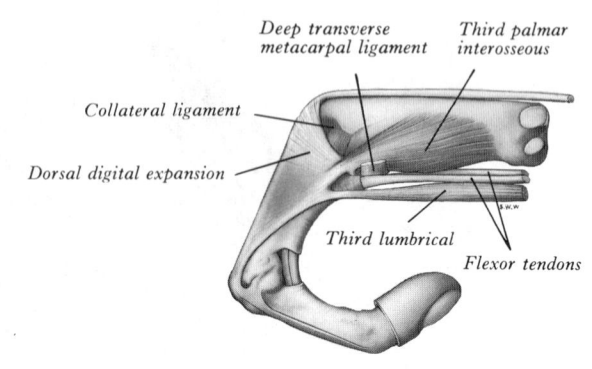

7.113C   The dorsal digital expansion of the ring finger in flexion (lateral aspect). Note the movement of the proximal edge of the expansion compared to 7.113B. (Preparations in 7.113B and C by James Whillis.)

the proximal phalanx where the fibrous sheath reaches bone, and from the sheath itself, they extend distally to blend with the margin of the dorsal extensor expansion. In this way two retinacular ligaments reach the base of the terminal phalanx in each digit.

THENAR MUSCLES AND ADDUCTOR POLLICIS

Abductor pollicis brevis

Abductor pollicis brevis (7.114) is a thin, subcutaneous muscle in the lateral part of the thenar eminence. It arises mainly from the flexor retinaculum, but a few fibres spring from the tubercles of the scaphoid bone and trapezium, and from the tendon of abductor pollicis longus (p. 851). Its medial fibres are attached by a thin, flat tendon to the radial side of the base of the proximal phalanx of the thumb; its lateral fibres join the dorsal digital expansion of the thumb.

Variations. The muscle may receive accessory slips from the long and short extensors of the thumb, opponens pollicis or from the styloid process of the radius.

Blood supply. Radial artery, superficial palmar branch (p. 1544); often an independent branch direct from radial artery to radial aspect of thumb.

Nerve supply. The lateral terminal branch of the median nerve, C8 and T1.

Actions. Abductor pollicis brevis draws the thumb ventrally in a plane at right angles to the palm of the hand (abduction); see Thumb function (p. 865).

Opponens pollicis

Opponens pollicis (7.114) lies deep to abductor pollicis brevis. It arises from the tubercle of the trapezium and the flexor retinaculum, and is attached to the whole length of the lateral border, and the adjoining lateral half of the palmar surface, of the metacarpal bone of the thumb.

Blood supply. Radial artery, superficial palmar branch (p. 1544); (when present) first palmar metacarpal artery (p. 1542); arteria princeps pollicis (p. 1541); arteria radialis indicis (p. 1541); deep palmar arch (p. 1544).

Nerve supply. The lateral terminal branch of the median nerve, C8 and T1 and commonly a ramus of the deep terminal branch of the ulnar nerve. Dissections by Day and Napier (1961) and Forrest (1967), and electromyographic tests by Harness et al (1974) indicate

double innervation in 92 out of 120 hands, and this must therefore be regarded as the usual arrangement.

Actions. Opponens pollicis flexes the metacarpal bone of the thumb (see Thumb function p. 865).

Flexor pollicis brevis

Flexor pollicis brevis (7.114) lies medial to abductor pollicis brevis. It has superficial and deep parts. The superficial head arises from the distal border of the flexor retinaculum and the distal part of the tubercle of the trapezium; it passes along the radial side of the tendon of flexor pollicis longus, and is attached, by a tendon containing a sesamoid bone, to the **radial** side of the base of the proximal phalanx of the thumb. The deep part arises from the trapezoid and capitate bones and from the palmar ligaments of the distal row of carpal bones; it passes deep to the tendon of flexor pollicis longus and unites with the superficial head on the sesamoid bone and base of the first phalanx.

Variations. The superficial head is frequently blended with opponens pollicis. The deep head varies considerably in size and may even be absent.

Blood supply. Radial artery, superficial palmar branch (p. 1544); rami from arteria princeps pollicis (p. 1541) and radialis indicis (p. 1541).

Nerve supply. The superficial head is usually supplied by the lateral terminal branch of the median nerve and the deep head by the deep branch of the ulnar nerve, C8 and T1. Some variation is not uncommon (Day & Napier 1961).

Actions. Flexor pollicis brevis flexes the metacarpophalangeal joint.

Adductor pollicis

Adductor pollicis (7.109, 114) arises by oblique and transverse heads. The *oblique head* is attached to the capitate bone, the bases of the second and third metacarpal bones, the palmar ligaments of the carpus and the sheath of the tendon of flexor carpi radialis. Most of the fibres converge into a tendon, which contains a sesamoid bone, unites with the tendon of the transverse head, and is attached to the **ulnar** side of the base of the proximal phalanx of the thumb. The deepest fibres may pass into the medial side of the dorsal digital expansion of the thumb. On the lateral side of the oblique head a considerable fasciculus passes deep to the tendon of flexor pollicis longus to join flexor pollicis brevis; this has been described as the 'deep head' of flexor pollicis brevis (Day & Napier 1961). The *transverse head* (7.109, 114) is the deepest of the pollicial muscles. It is triangular, and arises from the distal two-thirds of the palmar surface of the third metacarpal; the fibres converge to be attached, with the oblique head of the muscle and the first palmar interosseous muscle, to the base of the proximal phalanx of the thumb.

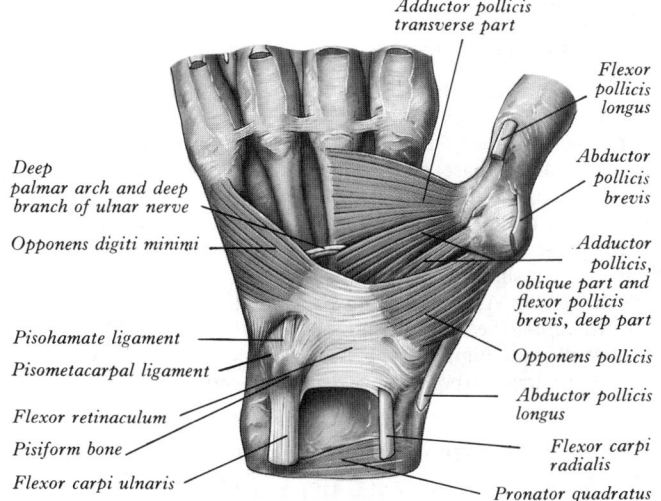

Adductor pollicis transverse part

Adductor pollicis, oblique part

2nd palmar interosseous

2nd dorsal interosseous

3rd dorsal interosseous

1st dorsal interosseous

1st palmar interosseous

Opponens pollicis

Abductor pollicis brevis

Flexor pollicis brevis   *Tendon of flexor carpi radialis*   *Flexor retinaculum*

Adductor pollicis transverse part

Flexor pollicis longus

Abductor pollicis brevis

Deep palmar arch and deep branch of ulnar nerve

Opponens digiti minimi

Adductor pollicis, oblique part and flexor pollicis brevis, deep part

Opponens pollicis

Pisohamate ligament

Pisometacarpal ligament

Abductor pollicis longus

Flexor retinaculum

Pisiform bone

Flexor carpi radialis

Flexor carpi ulnaris

Pronator quadratus

7.114 Dissection of the left thenar eminence and palm over the two lateral intermetacarpal spaces. The parts of adductor pollicis, including that sometimes designated the 'deep head' of flexor pollicis brevis, have been transected.

7.115 Deep dissection of the right palm, showing opponens pollicis and opponens digiti minimi and the two parts of adductor pollicis including the 'deep head' of flexor pollicis brevis. The superficial thenar and hypothenar muscles and palmaris longus have been removed.

Variations. The two parts of the adductor vary in relative size and degree of connection.

Blood supply. Arteria princeps pollicis (p. 1541); arteria radialis indicis (p. 1541); these two arteries are sometimes combined as the first palmar metacarpal artery (p. 1542); deep palmar arch (p. 1544).

Nerve supply. The deep branch of the ulnar nerve, C8 and **T1**.

Action. Adductor pollicis approximates the thumb to the palm of the hand, acting to greatest advantage when the abducted, rotated and flexed thumb is opposed to the fingers in gripping (see Thumb function p. 865).

HYPOTHENAR MUSCLES

Apart from palmaris brevis, a superficial muscle, this group of muscles flexes, abducts and opposes the fifth digit.

Palmaris brevis

Palmaris brevis (**7.109**) is a thin, quadrilateral muscle, lying beneath the skin of the ulnar side of the palm. It arises from the flexor retinaculum and the medial border of the central part of the palmar aponeurosis; it is attached to the dermis on the ulnar border of the hand. It is superficial to the ulnar artery and the superficial terminal branch of the ulnar nerve.

Blood supply. Ulnar end of superficial palmar arch (p. 1544).

Nerve supply. The superficial branch of the ulnar nerve, C8 and T1.

Action. Palmaris brevis wrinkles the skin on the ulnar side of the palm of the hand and deepens the hollow of the palm by accentuating the hypothenar eminence. In this way it may contribute to the security of the palmar grip.

Abductor digiti minimi

Abductor digiti minimi (**7.108**) arises from the pisiform bone, the tendon of flexor carpi ulnaris and the pisohamate ligament. It ends in a flat tendon which divides into two slips, one attached to the ulnar side of the base of the proximal phalanx of the little finger, the other to the ulnar border of the dorsal digital expansion of extensor digiti minimi.

Variations. This muscle may have two or three slips. It may be fused with flexor brevis. An additional slip may arise from the flexor retinaculum, antebrachial fascia, or tendons of palmaris longus or flexor carpi ulnaris. The muscle may be partly attached to the fifth metacarpal by a slip from the pisiform.

Blood supply. Ulnar artery, deep palmar branch (p. 1544); ulnar end of superficial palmar arch (p. 1544); palmar digital artery for medial border of little finger.

Nerve supply. See below.

Action. Abductor digiti minimi abducts the little finger away from the fourth, e.g. in the habitual spreading of the digits when they are extended. Abduction is also possible when digits 2–4 are tightly adducted in flexion or extension.

Flexor digiti minimi brevis

Flexor digiti minimi brevis (**7.116**) lies lateral to the abductor. It arises from the convex surface of the hook of the hamate bone and the palmar surface of the flexor retinaculum, and inserts into the ulnar side of the base of the proximal phalanx of the little finger with abductor digiti minimi. Its origin is separated from that of the abductor by the deep branches of the ulnar artery and nerve.

Variations. This muscle may be missing, or fused with the abductor. It may have a slip attached to the distal end of the fifth metacarpal.

Blood supply. As for abductor digiti minimi.

Nerve supply. See below.

Action. Flexor digiti minimi brevis produces flexion of the little finger at its metacarpophalangeal joint, together with some lateral rotation.

Opponens digiti minimi

Opponens digiti minimi (**7.115, 116**) is a triangular muscle, lying under cover of the flexor and abductor. It arises from the convexity of the hook of the hamate bone, and the contiguous portion of the flexor retinaculum; it inserts along the whole length of the ulnar margin of the fifth metacarpal bone, and the adjacent palmar surface.

Variations. The muscle is often divided into two lamellae by the deep branches of the ulnar artery and nerve. It blends to a variable degree with its neighbours.

Blood supply. Ulnar artery, deep palmar branch (p. 1544); medial end of the deep palmar arch (p. 1544).

Action. Opponens digiti minimi flexes the fifth metacarpal bone, drawing it forwards and rotating it laterally at the carpometacarpal joint; this deepens the hollow of the palm. These actions, together with flexion and some lateral rotation at the metacarpophalangeal and interphalangeal joints, bring the digit into opposition with the thumb.

Nerve supply. All the muscles of the little finger are supplied by the deep branch of the ulnar nerve, C8 and T1.

INTEROSSEOUS AND LUMBRICAL MUSCLES

The *interossei* occupy the intervals between the metacarpal bones, and are divided into a dorsal and a palmar set.

Dorsal interossei

The dorsal interossei (**7.117**) consist of four bipennate muscles, each arising from the adjacent sides of two metacarpal bones, but more extensively from the metacarpal bone of the finger into which the muscle passes. They insert on the bases of the proximal phalanges and separately into the dorsal digital expansions (p. 858). Between the double origin of each of these muscles there is a narrow triangular interval; the radial artery passes through the first of these intervals, and a perforating branch from the deep palmar arch passes through each of the others. The *first* and largest muscle is sometimes named *abductor indicis*; it is attached to the radial side of the proximal phalanx of the index finger and to the capsule of the adjoining metacarpophalangeal joint. The *second* and *third* are attached to the radial and ulnar sides of the middle finger, respectively. Whereas the second generally reaches the digital expansion and the proximal phalanx, the third usually extends only to the digital expansion (**7.113A**). The *fourth*, too, may be wholly attached to the digital expansion but it often sends an additional slip to the proximal phalanx.

Palmar interossei

The palmar interossei (**7.118**) are smaller than the dorsal interossei and are on the palmar surfaces of the metacarpal bones rather than between them. With the exception of the first, each of the four arises from the entire length of the metacarpal bone of one finger, and passes to the appropriate (adductor) side of the dorsal digital expansion (Salsbury 1937; Landsmeer 1949).

The middle finger has no palmar interosseus; the remaining digits have palmar interossei on their aspects facing the middle finger. The *first* arises from the ulnar side of the palmar surface of the base of the first metacarpal bone and is inserted into a sesamoid bone on the ulnar side of the proximal phalanx and thence to the phalanx and usually also into the dorsal digital expansion (Lewis 1965). It lies in front of the lateral head of the first dorsal interosseous muscle, and is overlapped anteriorly by the oblique head of adductor pollicis (**7.114**). The *second* arises from the ulnar side of the second metacarpal bone, and is inserted into the same side of the digital expansion of the index finger. The *third* arises from the radial side of the fourth metacarpal bone, and is inserted together with the third lumbrical (**7.113B, C**). The *fourth* arises from the radial side of the fifth metacarpal bone, and is attached with the fourth lumbrical and also to the base of the proximal phalanx. The attachment of these muscles to the dorsal digital expansions (**7.113B, C**) stabilizes the extensor tendons on the convex heads of the metacarpal bones during flexion and extension at the metacarpophalangeal joints.

Variations. The interossei do not vary a great deal; they are occasionally reduplicated, a condition perhaps associated with the origin of palmar interossei from paired short flexors (Lewis 1965).

Blood supply. Dorsal interossei: 1st–4th dorsal metacarpal arteries (p. 1541); 2nd–4th palmar metacarpal arteries (p. 1541); radial (1st) (p. 1540); 1st arteria princeps pollicis (p. 1541); arteria radialis indicis (p. 1541); three perforating branches from the deep palmar arch (proximal perforating arteries) (p. 1541); three distal perforating branches (p. 1541). **Tendons:** common and proper palmar digital arteries (p. 1542); dorsal digital arteries (p. 1541).

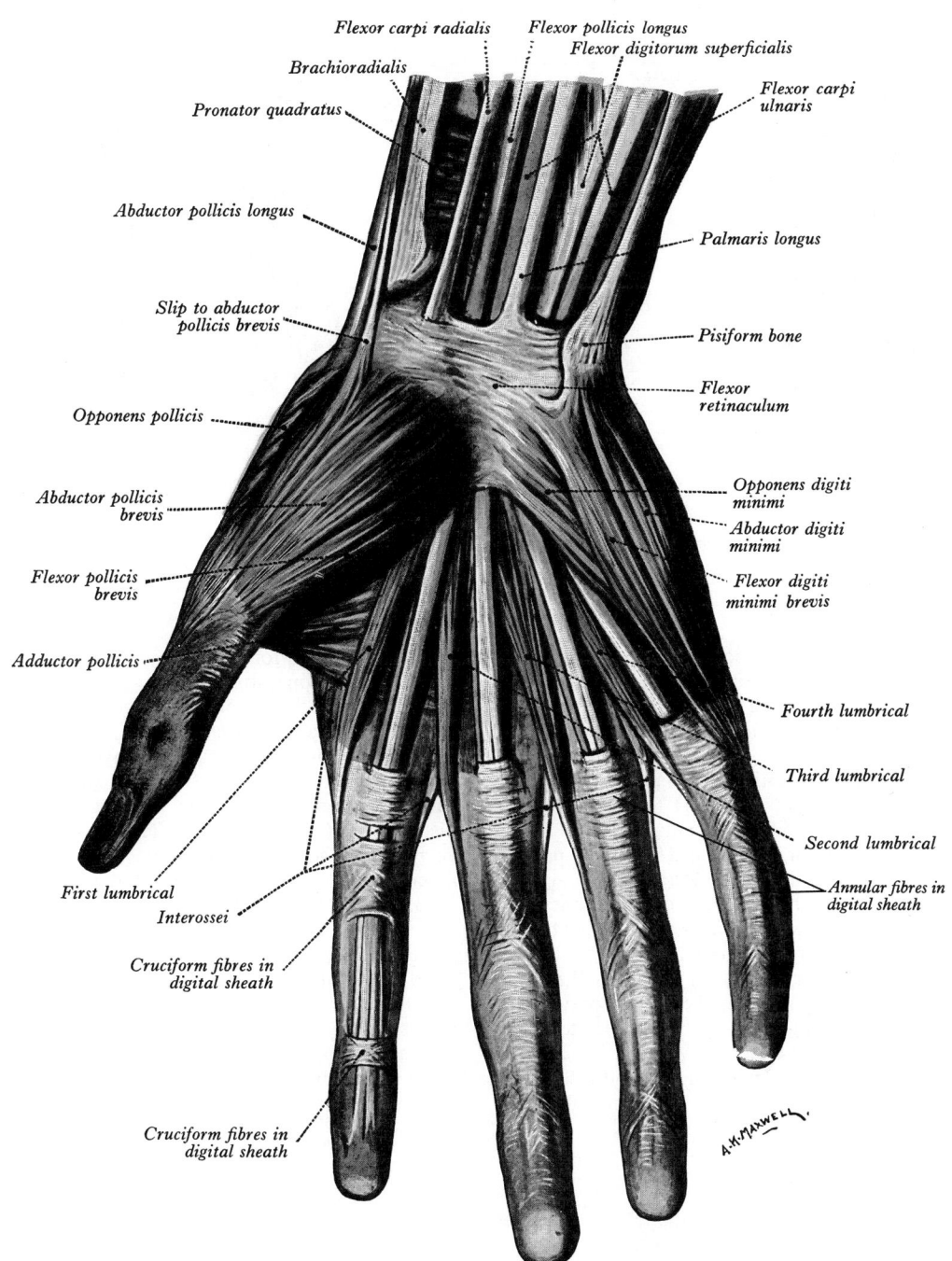

Flexor carpi radialis
Brachioradialis
Pronator quadratus
Flexor pollicis longus
Flexor digitorum superficialis
Flexor carpi ulnaris
Abductor pollicis longus
Palmaris longus
Slip to abductor pollicis brevis
Pisiform bone
Opponens pollicis
Flexor retinaculum
Abductor pollicis brevis
Opponens digiti minimi
Abductor digiti minimi
Flexor pollicis brevis
Flexor digiti minimi brevis
Adductor pollicis
Fourth lumbrical
Third lumbrical
Second lumbrical
First lumbrical
Annular fibres in digital sheath
Interossei
Cruciform fibres in digital sheath
Cruciform fibres in digital sheath

7.116 Superficial dissection of muscles of the palm of the right hand. Refer to **7.111A, B** for a more detailed description and classification of the annular and cruciate pulleys of the flexor tendon sheath.

Palmar interossei: deep palmar arch (p. 1544); arteria princeps pollicis (p. 1541); arteria radialis indicis (p. 1541); palmar metacarpal arteries (p. 1542); proximal and distal perforating arteries (p. 1541); common and proper digital (palmar) arteries (p. 1542). **Tendons:** as dorsal interossei.

Nerve supply. All the interossei are supplied by the deep branch of the ulnar nerve, C8 and **T1**.

Actions. Dorsal interossei abduct the fingers from an imaginary longitudinal axis through the centre of the middle finger; palmar interossei adduct the fingers to this axis (see also p. 863). The interossei have a considerable cross-sectional area and therefore contribute strongly to metacarpophalangeal joint flexion and interphalangeal extension. When paralysed, as in ulnar nerve paralysis, the grip strength of the hand is severely impaired and the arc of finger motion is abnormal, with a tendency for the fingers to claw. Their role in digital extension is explained below (see p. 864, Opening the hand), but it must not be forgotten that each one has a

considerable ability to rotate the digit at the metacarpophalangeal joint; generally this is not apparent, as they act in pairs, but it may occur where one interosseus is deficient as a result of injury or congenital deformity.

Lumbrical muscles

The lumbricals (**7.116**) are four small fasciculi which arise from the tendons of flexor digitorum profundus—the first and second from the radial sides and palmar surfaces of the tendons of the index and middle fingers respectively, the third, from the adjacent sides of the tendons of the middle and ring fingers, and the fourth, from the adjoining sides of the tendons of the ring and little fingers. Each passes to the **radial** side of the corresponding finger, and is attached to the lateral margin of the dorsal digital expansion of extensor digitorum that covers the dorsal surface of the finger.

Variations. Variations in the attachments of the lumbricals are common. Any of them may be unipennate or bipennate: when

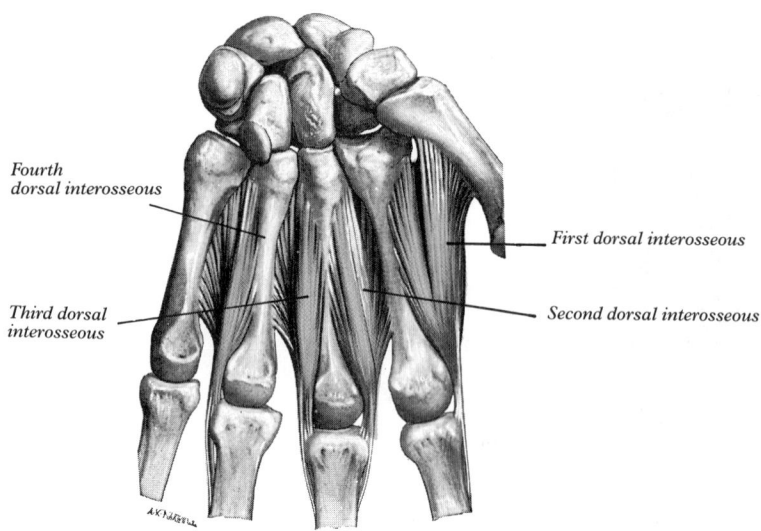

7.117 The dorsal interosseous muscles of the left hand: palmar aspect.

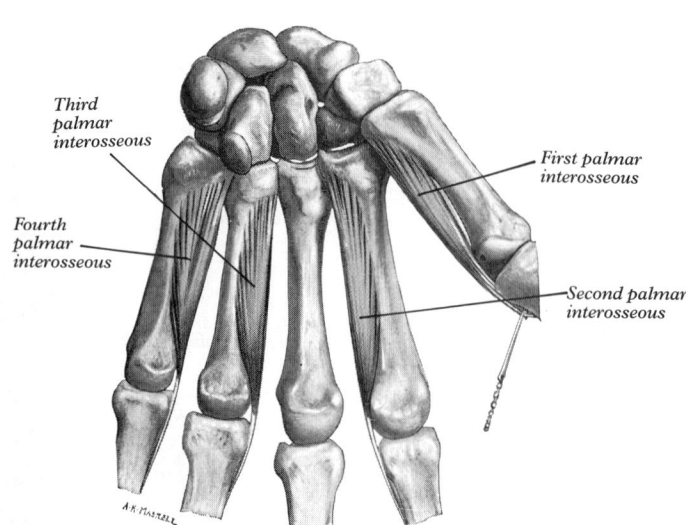

7.118 The palmar interosseous muscles of the left hand: palmar aspect.

bipennate, the two heads arise from adjoining tendons of flexor digitorum profundus, and from the tendon of flexor pollicis longus in the case of the first lumbrical (Goldberg 1970). Accessory lumbrical slips may be attached to an adjacent tendon of flexor digitorum superficialis.

Blood supply. First and second lumbricals: first and second dorsal metacarpal and dorsal digital arteries (p. 1541) (tendons); arteria radialis indicis (p. 1541); first common palmar digital artery (p. 1542). Third and fourth lumbricals: second and third common palmar digital arteries (p. 1542); third and fourth dorsal digital arteries (p. 1544) and their anastomoses with the palmar digital arteries.

Nerve supply. The first and second lumbricals are supplied by the median nerve, C8 and T1; the third and fourth lumbricals by the deep terminal branch of the ulnar nerve, C8 and T1. The third lumbrical frequently receives a supply from the median nerve. The first and second are also occasionally supplied by the deep terminal branch of the ulnar nerve (Mehta & Gardner 1961).

Actions. The lumbricals arise from flexor tendons and insert into the extensor apparatus. Since both attachments are mobile, they have the potential for producing movement at either. The action on the extensor apparatus is easier to understand and consists of extension of both interphalangeal joints in a co-ordinated manner. (The co-ordination mechanism is explained below: see p. 864, Opening the hand.) Detailed electromyographic studies by Backhouse and Catton (1952) and by Long and Brown (1964) have confirmed this action, and have shown that the lumbricals are functionally distinct from the interossei. The mode of action at the metacarpophalangeal joints is disputed but if there is a flexor action it is very weak. The effect on the flexor digitorum profundus attachment is to pull the tendon distally. The combined action on both origin and insertion is therefore to alter the posture of the finger to allow more interphalangeal extension. Pinching the index finger against the thumb without a lumbrical would result in a nail-to-nail contact; the addition of the lumbrical increases the interphalangeal joint extension, resulting in pulp-to-pulp pinch. In addition to their mechanical role, the lumbricals contain many muscle spindles and have a long fibre length; they therefore appear to have a significant role in proprioception.

Co-ordinated movements of the upper limb

PROXIMAL UPPER LIMB FUNCTION

The muscles of the shoulder girdle and elbow act together to position the hand accurately for manipulative function. It would be wrong to attribute precision and delicacy to the hand alone, as the more proximal upper limb has sufficient proprioception and muscle control to allow neat writing even when the hand has been amputated and replaced by a prosthesis. The major function of the shoulder is, however, to position the hand as a terminal working tool. The combined range of upper limb joint motion available is such that it is possible to touch the spinous process of T4 either by raising the arm, flexing the elbow and passing the hand over the shoulder, or by extending the shoulder, internally rotating the humerus, flexing the elbow and passing the hand behind the back—a range of movement that allows you to scratch any part of your own back!

The whole upper limb may be stiffened for transmitting thrust or supporting weight, yet it can offer controlled resilient flexion when it is absorbing forces. In other primates the upper limb has an important role in locomotion: grasp can be used as an aid to propulsion when pulling on branches, and loads can be transmitted to the ground through any one of several surfaces (e.g. palm, knuckles). In man the role in locomotion remains only in certain sports, but the arm is used as a pendulum in walking and running.

Although this function is imperfectly understood (see p. 899, **Standing, walking and running**) it has been observed that the loss of an upper limb, or even joint stiffness, may affect the loading of the axial skeleton and even the pattern of gait.

Man is said to be distinguished from other primates by his opposable thumb and 'prehension', a term that, while difficult to define precisely, denotes an ability to reach out and grasp objects. The prehensile role has been classified by Napier (1956) in terms of various forms of grip, which will be discussed later, but overall limb movement also contributes to prehension and can be analysed by considering the key actions of reaching out and pulling back.

Reaching out

The three major components of reaching out are: scapular movement and stabilization; glenohumeral abduction; and elbow motion. All of these functions involve a variety of muscle activities, which depend on the exact starting configuration of the limb, the position to be achieved, the effect of gravity, and also whether the movement takes place in air or in water! During abduction of the arm from the anatomical position, trapezius and serratus anterior are the major muscles involved in rotating the scapula forward, around the chest wall. The fixing of the scapula, in which many muscles participate, allows deltoid to act on the humerus; this muscle, together with supraspinatus, then abducts the arm. Although these muscles are the main players, many others are involved in moving and fixing the scapula or stabilizing the glenohumeral joint. For a fuller account the reader is referred to pages 104 et seq. In everyday activities, reaching out will often commence from a position in which the elbow is flexed and, depending on the height of the object reached for, the position of the elbow will be determined by interplay between the elbow flexors (biceps, brachialis and brachio-radialis) and extensors (triceps).

Pulling back

The activity involved in returning the arm to the side from a position of shoulder elevation or flexion depends upon whether the arm is simply falling under the force of gravity and having its trajectory controlled precisely by muscular forces, or whether the limb is being pulled back towards the trunk against a resisting force, as in climbing. For a gentle gravitational return, the muscles concerned are mainly those that contracted during abduction, and which now undergo controlled lengthening. For a forceful return, the shoulder girdle is equipped with strong adductors: pectoralis major and latissimus dorsi.

Limb posture has a major influence on the force that can be exerted in pulling back. A particularly strong pull can be achieved by keeping the arm partly abducted and using the elbow flexors to approximate the hand to the trunk. A strong hand grip is achieved in mid-pronation and wrist extension. Such factors explain in part the difficulty of defining prehension in precise anatomical terms.

HAND FUNCTION

The apparently simple human functions of closing the hand to grasp an object, or opening the palm to release it, are in reality tasks of considerable mechanical complexity, requiring the simultaneous contraction of many individual muscles. As a basis for understanding such integrated activities it is helpful to consider first the mechanical actions of individual muscles (for a more detailed treatment of muscle action see pp. 785–788). The isolated action of a single muscle may be inferred from the positions of its origin and insertion, and the estimated line of action (usually the centre line of the muscle) in relation to the axes of all the joints traversed by the muscle and its tendon. The limb can be regarded as a chain of joints crossed by muscles and, provided that we know which muscles are active, the reason why one joint moves and others do not is a matter of simple mechanical relationships. For example, flexor pollicis longus is considered to have a major role as a flexor of the interphalangeal joint of the thumb, but the position of its tendon relative to more proximal joints in the limb gives it the potential for producing flexion at the metacarpophalangeal joint and also at the trapezio-metacarpal and wrist joints. In the living subject the actual motion that takes place depends on which other muscle groups are acting, so the potential for movement must be considered for each joint in the chain in turn. Motion at the wrist is generally balanced by wrist extensors. Motion at the trapezio-metacarpal joint is balanced by abductor pollicis longus. Flexor pollicis longus will then have an action as a flexor of the metacarpophalangeal and interphalangeal joints only.

The factor that determines whether one or both of two joints will move is the turning moment at each (for a consideration of turning moment, see pp. 786–787). The greater the perpendicular distance from the line of muscle or tendon pull to the axis of the joint, the stronger is the turning effect of the muscle at the joint, but the smaller the range of joint motion that can be produced. In the case of flexor pollicis longus, the tendon is situated further from the axis of the metacarpophalangeal joint than from the axis of the interphalangeal joint: it will therefore tend to produce flexion preferentially at the metacarpophalangeal joint unless that joint is restrained by extensor pollicis brevis. In this way different postures of the thumb can be produced by the interplay of flexor and extensor forces. Although there is scope for more elaborate biomechanical analysis, these simple guiding principles will provide an understanding of muscle action in the hand that is sufficient for most purposes.

In considering the role of a particular muscle, we tend to concentrate especially on motion. Indeed, many muscles are named on the basis of the movements that they generate, although others (often those whose actions are the most difficult to interpret) are described according to their morphology or situation (see Naming of muscles, p. 789). A more important function may be the nature of the force generated. We have considered, for example, the potential of flexor pollicis longus for flexing the thumb. A large range of flexion is actually required only in a few activities, such as certain ripping tasks; in most pinch and manipulative tasks the role of the thumb is to apply isometric force, which it does with such precision that it is possible to pick up an egg and neither crush nor drop it. Thus for much of the time flexor pollicis longus behaves as an extremely sophisticated mechanism for the application of force, in which contraction and proprioception are equally important. ('Gripper pollicis longus' might be a more appropriate description.)

The anatomical position of the hand (palm flat and pointing anteriorly, forearm supinated) is a convenient standard for studying structural relationships. The hand in the relaxed (anaesthetized) position adopts a posture of partial flexion and mid-supination/pronation (the reader can verify this by relaxing completely and observing forearm and hand position). The surgeon must therefore be prepared to encounter structures in rather different relationships from those in anatomical descriptions. Hand surgeons tend to describe the position of structures as lying on the radial or ulnar sides of the hand, or on the palmar or dorsal surfaces, rather than lateral and medial, or anterior and posterior. During cadaveric fixation, some degree of digital flexion is usual and this must be taken into account during dissection.

With these general points in mind we can now go on to analyse the special functions of the hand:

- *Closing the hand*
- *Opening the hand*
- *Thumb function*
- *Grips.*

Closing the hand

It is clear that the fingers and palm of the hand flex in gripping, grasping or making a fist, but there are subtle differences in hand posture in these various activities. Initially the basic mechanisms of hand closure will be described; special grips will be considered later.

As the digits flex, the wrist usually extends (dorsiflexes) at the same time. The involvement of the long digital flexors in this movement will be considered first, followed by an analysis of the role of the wrist.

The role of the long digital flexors. Flexor digitorum superficialis acts to flex principally the proximal interphalangeal joints, through its insertions into the middle phalanges. In each digit there is also an action on the metacarpophalangeal joint, because the tendon passes anterior to that joint; for the same reason there is the potential for producing flexion at the wrist. The fact that each tendon arises from an individual muscle slip allows the clinician to test one finger at a time. The reader can verify this by attempting to flex one digit at a time while using the other hand to keep the distal interphalangeal joints of the remaining fingers in extension. This test is frequently used in clinical practice and is useful for the middle and ring fingers, where flexion of one finger alone must be attributed to flexor digitorum superficialis. The index finger, however, has its own profundus musculo-tendinous unit and may therefore move independently under the action of this tendon. Many individuals cannot flex the proximal interphalangeal joint of the little finger alone, probably because superficialis is deficient, although most can flex the metacarpophalangeal joint of the little finger using flexor digiti minimi.

Flexor digitorum profundus has similarities to superficialis but because it reaches further (to the distal phalanx) it is the only muscle available for flexion of the distal interphalangeal joint. It also contributes, together with superficialis, to flexion at the proximal interphalangeal and metacarpophalangeal joints. These two long flexors (sometimes called extrinsic flexors, because the muscle bellies are outside the hand) can be considered to act together to flex the finger. However, their action alone would wind up the interphalangeal before the metacarpophalangeal joints and the finger would not move in a normal arc of flexion. This is precisely what happens in an ulnar nerve paralysis, in which the interossei and lumbrical muscles are not functioning. These small (intrinsic) muscles have been discussed before in terms of their individual actions; for their role in co-ordinated activity it is sufficient to appreciate that their contribution changes the arc produced by the long flexors, increasing flexion at the metacarpophalangeal joint and reducing flexion at the proximal interphalangeal joint. All three joints are then angulated to the same degree and the fingers form a normal arc of flexion.

As the finger flexes, the long extensor tendons (extensor digitorum, extensor indicis and extensor digiti minimi) aid the process by relaxing and allowing the extensor apparatus to glide distally on the dorsum of the phalanges.

The role of the wrist. As the fingers wind up to make a fist, the wrist tends to extend, particularly when force is applied. This extension has a marked effect on the excursion of the long flexor tendons. On its own, digital flexion would require the long tendons to move proximally in their sheaths and the flexor muscles in the forearm would shorten. Dorsiflexion of the wrist tends to produce a lengthening of the same muscles, which in normal use is almost enough to balance the shortening due to finger flexion; the net effect is a very slight shortening (approximately 1 cm) of the long flexors in the forearm. The wrist can therefore be seen as a mechanism for maximizing force, for it allows the fingers to flex while maintaining the resting length of the extrinsic muscles near to the peak of the force–length curve. It is, of course, possible to wind up the fingers with the wrist held in a neutral position, but the grip is somewhat weaker. With the wrist in full flexion it is not possible to flex the fingers fully.

If we now turn our attention to the extensor surface of the wrist, the flexion of the fingers on gripping tends to result in a distal excursion of the long extensors. This tendency is, however, counteracted by dorsiflexion of the wrist. The net effect is a very small proximal excursion of the long extensor tendons on gripping, mirroring the effect on the flexor surface. If the movement of the wrist is exaggerated so that the wrist is a little flexed on opening the hand, and fully dorsiflexed on closing it, the net excursion of long flexors and extensors is zero, i.e., this whole movement sequence can be completed with the forearm flexor and extensor muscles contracting isometrically.

The reader can observe the relationship between digits and wrist by performing the following manoeuvre. The wrist is held in a relaxed, mid-supinated position, with the elbow flexed at 90°. If the forearm is now rotated into pronation, the wrist will fall into flexion and the fingers will automatically extend. If the forearm is rotated into supination, the wrist will extend and the fingers flex. The finger movements compensate for the wrist movements and are entirely automatic; they are made without the need for any excursion of forearm flexor or extensor tendons. This test, the *wrist tenodesis test*, is a useful way of examining the limb for tendon injury. The pointing finger (which does not move with wrist motion) 'points to' a tendon injury.

Wrist motion is controlled principally by two wrist flexors (flexor carpi radialis and flexor carpi ulnaris) and three extensors (extensors carpi radialis longus and brevis, and extensor carpi ulnaris). Although the radio-carpal joint has some functional similarity to a ball and socket joint, it is possible to conceive of the wrist as a variable hinge joint, the axis of which may be set in a number of inclinations. For example, in using a hammer it is useful to rotate the wrist backwards and forwards about an axis that permits not only wrist flexion but also ulnar deviation. It would be very restricting to have a pure hinge joint with collateral ligaments of fixed length. In this context, the wrist flexors and extensors may be regarded as variable collateral ligaments, which allow the joint to be set about a number of different axes.

For movement about major axes, the wrist tendons can be considered to act in pairs:

Wrist flexion:	flexor carpi radialis and flexor carpi ulnaris
Wrist extension:	extensor carpi radialis longus and brevis, and extensor carpi ulnaris
Ulnar deviation:	extensor carpi ulnaris and flexor carpi ulnaris
Radial deviation:	flexor carpi radialis and extensor carpi radialis longus and brevis

Making a tight fist. It is possible to observe and to palpate the muscle groups that are active in making a tight fist. The flexor compartment of the forearm is contracted tightly and EMG evidence confirms that flexor digitorum profundus and flexor digitorum superficialis are active. Flexor carpi ulnaris may be seen and felt to contract strongly. The extensor compartment is also tightly contracted and the wrist extensors would certainly be expected to be active. Palpation of the long digital extensors on the back of the wrist will show these to be contracting as well. It seems that when the fingers are held tightly closed, the long digital extensors are unable to move the extensor apparatus: they have acquired a new fixed point on which to act, namely the proximal limit of the extensor apparatus over the metacarpophalangeal joint. They therefore perform the only task available to them and act together as an additional wrist extensor.

In the thumb web, palpation confirms that the first dorsal interosseous is contracting, as are all the other interossei and the thenar and hypothenar muscles. As the firm fist is swung forward in anger the brachioradialis stands out, and at the moment of impact virtually every muscle in the limb is in a state of contraction, with the exception of the lumbricals.

Opening the hand

The hand is opened from its relaxed balanced posture, for example, when we stretch out to reach an object. This motion comprises extension of distal interphalangeal, proximal interphalangeal and metacarpophalangeal joints. The hand is provided with an ingenious mechanism that allows this to happen. The laws of mechanics would suggest that one motor would be required for every joint in a chain, together with some sort of controlling mechanism to ensure that the chain of joints moved together in a co-ordinated fashion. These requirements are achieved in the hand through an extensor apparatus, which economizes on the number of motors required for movement by allowing the muscles to act on more than one joint and by linking different levels in the mechanism so that the arc of motion is controlled. We can now look at the parts played by the various muscles involved.

The tendons of extensor digitorum run distally over the metacarpal heads, forming the major component of the extensor apparatus. Extensor digitorum has no insertion into the proximal phalanx and therefore exerts its extensor action on the metacarpophalangeal joint indirectly through more distal insertions. The first point of insertion is at the base of the middle phalanx (in clinical practice the term *central slip* has been adopted). If one considers the action of extensor digitorum at this insertion alone, the muscle can extend both metacarpophalangeal and proximal interphalangeal joints together. The interossei are also active in hand-opening: they will tend to increase extension of the proximal interphalangeal joint. There is therefore a range of possibilities. At one extreme, with no interosseous contribution, the long extensor will exert all of its action at the metacarpophalangeal joint: this leads to full extension, and even hyperextension, while the proximal interphalangeal joint remains flexed (the typical claw hand of ulnar nerve paralysis, or '*intrinsic minus*' hand). At the other extreme, when the intrinsics act strongly together with extensor digitorum, the proximal interphalangeal joint will extend completely while the metacarpophalangeal joint remains flexed ('*intrinsic plus*' hand). Thus the hand possesses in the proximal part of the extensor apparatus a variable mechanism that allows different amounts of relative metacarpophalangeal or proximal interphalangeal joint motion.

In contrast, the more distal part of the extensor apparatus acts as an automatic or fixed mechanism which determines that the two interphalangeal joints, proximal and distal, will move together. The lateral slips of the extensor apparatus arise from extensor digitorum; they pass distally on either side of the central slip and thus over the proximal interphalangeal joint. Being further lateral they are nearer the joint axis, because the dorsal surface curves away on each side. A helpful analogy that has been suggested for this arrangement is to consider it as two pulleys of different size on one axle (Brand et al 1987). The central slip can be regarded as a cord that passes over the larger wheel. Each lateral slip is a cord that passes over a smaller wheel; because these pulleys are smaller there is less longitudinal excursion for a given rotation of the wheel, and this allows some of the excursion to be used for another function, namely extension at the distal joint. There is an additional mechanism by which the lateral slips move laterally during flexion of the proximal interphalangeal joint. This was described by Winslow (1752) and has been reviewed extensively by Zancolli (1979). The effect of this lateral movement is to reduce further the distance between the lateral slips and the joint axis, thereby reducing the amount of excursion at the proximal

interphalangeal joint still more and allowing more excursion at the distal joint. When the hand flexes, this mechanical linkage system allows both interphalangeal joints to flex together in a co-ordinated way.

The extensor expansion also receives contributions from the interossei and lumbrical muscles, which approach the digits from the webs and join the corresponding expansion in the proximal segment of the digit. These small muscles can therefore act on the extensor apparatus at two levels: they can extend the proximal interphalangeal joint through fibres that radiate towards the central slip, and they can act on the distal interphalangeal joint through fibres that join the lateral slip.

Apart from the components of the extensor expansion that are concerned with joint function, the whole structure requires additional anchorage. This must be arranged in such a way that it is not displaced from the underlying skeleton, yet it must not restrict longitudinal movement. These difficult requirements are met by transverse retinacular ligaments at the level of the joints, the transverse ligaments running to relatively fixed attachment points in the region of the joint axis. As the expansion glides backwards and forwards the transverse fibres move like bucket handles. Smooth gliding layers are required under the expansion and retinacular ligaments to allow motion to occur without friction.

One final component of the extensor apparatus provides an additional automatic function. This is a fibrous anchorage system, *Landsmeer's oblique retinacular ligament* (Landsmeer 1976) which anchors the distal expansion to the middle phalanx.

Thumb function

An opposable thumb requires a different system of control from the other digits. Since the metacarpal is much more mobile than in the digits, muscles are needed to control the extra freedom of movement. Were the thumb to have three phalanges (which happens in rare cases as a congenital anomaly) an extremely complex anatomical arrangement would be required to incorporate all of the digital complexity already described above on the end of a mobile metacarpal!

The thumb does not easily assume the classical anatomical position. Therefore the normal descriptive anatomical terms—anterior, posterior, medial and lateral—do not readily apply. The terms 'palmar, dorsal, ulnar and radial' have been adopted in clinical practice.

Movements of the thumb. For the description of joint motion, it is suggested that the guidelines of the International Federation of Societies for Surgery of the Hand (1972) be adopted. *Flexion* and *extension* should be confined to motion at the interphalangeal or metacarpo-

phalangeal joints (**7.119**A–C). The carpometacarpal joint has the motions of *palmar abduction* (**7.119**D, E), in which the first metacarpal moves away from the second at right angles to the plane of the palm, and *radial abduction* (**7.119**D, F), in which the first metacarpal moves away from the second with the thumb in the plane of the palm. The opposite of radial abduction is *ulnar adduction*, or *transpalmar adduction*, in which the thumb crosses the palm towards its ulnar border. In clinical practice the term *adduction* is generally used without qualification. *Circumduction* describes the angular motion of the first metacarpal, solely at the carpometacarpal joint, from a position of maximal radial abduction in the plane of the palm towards the ulnar border of the hand, maintaining the widest possible angle between the first and second metacarpals (**7.119**G, H). *Lateral inclinations* of the first phalanx maximize the extent of excursion of the circumduction arc. *Opposition* is a composite position of the thumb achieved by circumduction of the first metacarpal, internal rotation of the thumb ray and maximal extension of the metacarpophalangeal and interphalangeal joints (**7.119**I). *Retroposition* is the opposite to opposition (**7.119**J). *Flexion adduction* is the position of maximal transpalmar adduction of the first metacarpal; the metacarpophalangeal and interphalangeal joints are flexed and the thumb is in contact with the palm (**7.119**K).

Rotary movements occur during circumduction. The simple angular movements described above combine with rotation about the long axis of the metacarpal shaft: in opposition, the shaft must rotate medially into pronation; in retroposition, the thumb must rotate laterally into supination. Axial rotation of the thumb metacarpal is due to:

- Muscle activity, which moves the thumb through its arc of circumduction
- The geometry of the articular surfaces of the trapezio-metacarpal joint
- Tensile forces in the ligaments, which combine with forces exerted by the muscles of opposition and retroposition to produce axial rotation (see below).

The stability of the first metacarpal is greatest after complete pronation in the position of full opposition, when ligamentary tension, muscular contraction and joint congruence combine to maximal effect.

Position of rest. The hand has a well-recognised position of rest, with the wrist in extension and the digits in some degree of flexion. The precise position of the thumb in the position of rest appears to be rather variable but has been defined by Duchenne (1867) as the midpoint between maximal palmar abduction and maximal retroposition. In this position the carpometacarpal joint lies within 20° of radial

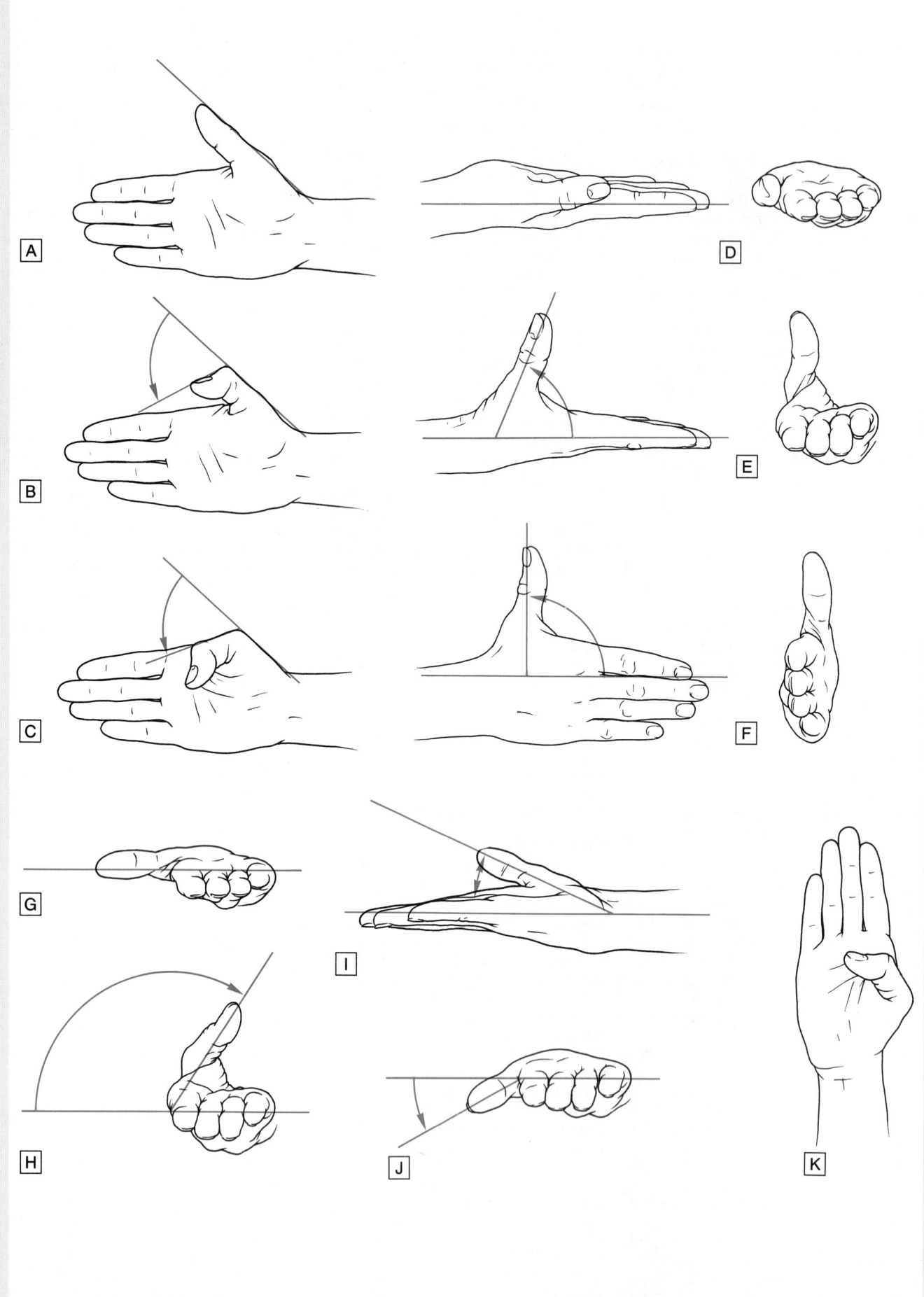

7.119 Movements of the thumb. A–C: Flexion and extension. A. Extension at the metacarpophalangeal and interphalangeal joints. B. Flexion at the interphalangeal joint. C. Added flexion at the metacarpophalangeal joint. D–F: Abduction at the carpometacarpal joint. D. Starting position. E. Palmar abduction. F. Radial abduction. G–H: Circumduction. I. Opposition. J. Retroposition. K. Flexion adduction. (For further detail see text.)

abduction and 30° of palmar abduction, and from clinical observations it seems that the metacarpophalangeal joint lies within about 40° of flexion and the interphalangeal joint between extension and 10° of flexion. Obviously many forces contribute to this position of balance, which would be upset by division or palsy of the corresponding structures.

Grips

From the position of rest, the tip of the thumb can approach the radial aspect of the fingers without incurring axial rotation because the palmar and dorsal trapezio-metacarpal ligaments remain relaxed (see below).

From different positions of the arc of circumduction, numerous different types of pinch grip are possible (**7.**120). In clinical practice these have been classified into two main types: *tip pinch* and *lateral (or key) pinch*. Again, many forces contribute to these configurations.

Srinivasan & Landsmeer (1982) have tackled the very difficult question of the dynamic role of the intrinsic muscles in maintaining stability and movement by the use of a mathematical model combined with clinical observations in leprosy patients. They have emphasised that the thumb is not a biarticular system, like the finger, as the distal two joints are not linked mechanically. It is, rather, a tri-articular system activated by mono-articular muscles (abductor pollicis longus and opponens pollicis), biarticular muscles (extensor pollicis brevis, adductor pollicis, abductor pollicis brevis and flexor pollicis brevis), and triarticular muscles (extensor pollicis longus and flexor pollicis longus). It appears, however, that even a mono-articular muscle can change posture in all three joints by altering the overall balance of forces, and it is therefore very difficult to attribute function to the individual

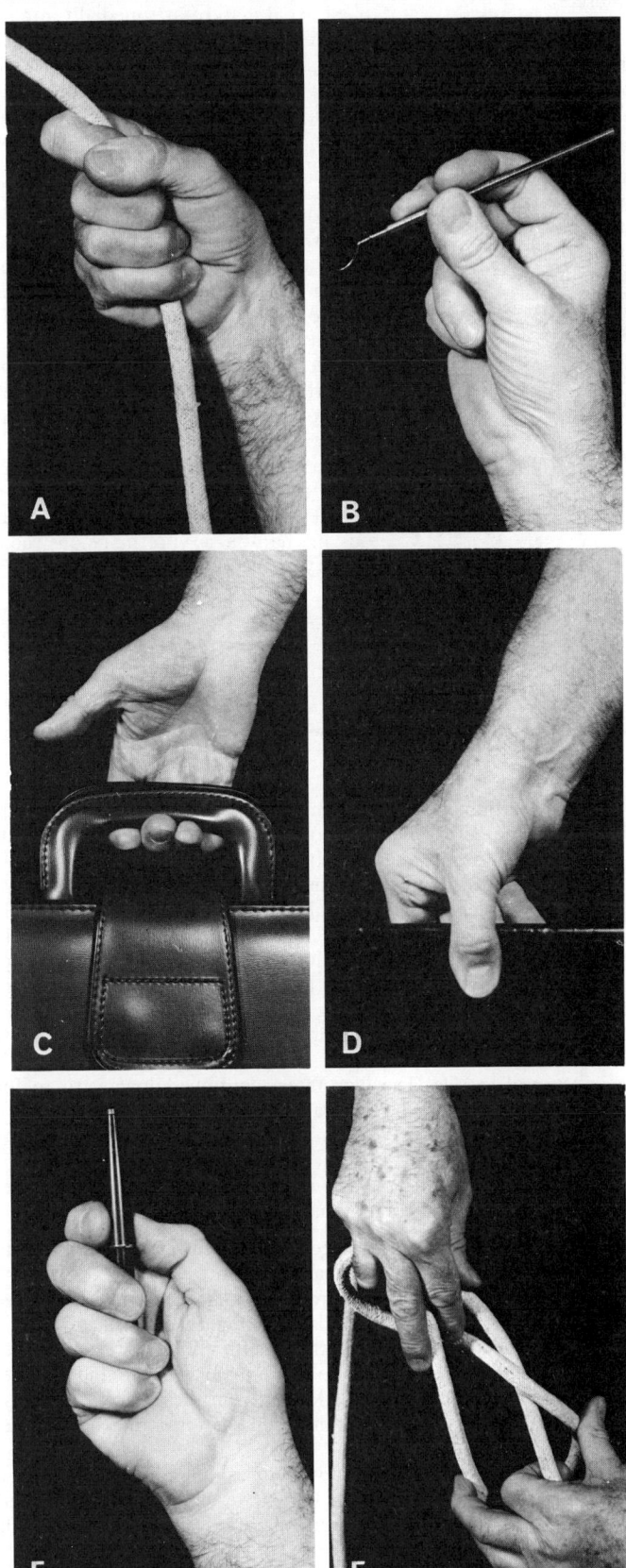

7.120 Some of the many varieties of functional posture that may be adopted by the human hand. A. In the **power grip**, the fingers are flexed around an object, with counter pressure from the thumb. Any skill in wielding the object derives from the limb, including the wrist; relative movements of the thumb and fingers are not involved. B. The **precision grip**, which varies considerably with the task, stabilizes the object between the tips of one or more fingers and the thumb. The gross position of the object may be adjusted by movements at the wrist, elbow or even shoulder, but the most skilled manipulations are carried out by the digits themselves—for example in advancing a thread to the eye of a needle. C. The **hook grip** is used to suspend or to pull open objects. The fingers are flexed around the object; the thumb may or may not be involved. It is a grip for the transmission of forces, not for skilful manipulation. D. Powerful opposition of the thumb to the radial side of the index finger produces a **lateral pinch grip**—used, for example, to hold a door key; here the object is larger, and all the fingers are involved. E. Many activities involve a **combination** of grips. Here a fountain pen is stabilized in a power grip by flexion of digits 4–5 against the palm, while the index finger and thumb, used in a precision grip, unscrew the cap. F. Complex manipulation. For further discussion, see Grips (above).

intrinsic muscles. The thumb muscles do, however, seem to provide two broad functions:

- Control of metacarpal positioning (the guy-rope function). This is automatically accompanied by rotation
- Control of the axial stability of the skeleton of the thumb.

The present account follows the analysis of thumb function by Zancolli (1979), in which the muscles are classified into those used for retroposition, opposition and pinch grip.

Retroposition muscles. The muscles that bring about retroposition are:

- extensor pollicis longus
- extensor pollicis brevis
- abductor pollicis longus.

As the thumb moves into retroposition there is automatic axial rotation to produce supination of the first metacarpal. This is brought about by the off-axis action of two parallel, but oppositely directed, forces: one exerted by extensors pollicis longus and brevis and the other by abductor pollicis longus and the anterior

oblique carpometacarpal ligament.

Opposition muscles. There is a succession of activity in thenar muscles during the movement of opposition. Zancolli has described three subgroups of radial, central and ulnar muscles:

- radial: abductor pollicis longus and extensor pollicis brevis
- central: abductor pollicis brevis and opponens pollicis
- ulnar: flexor pollicis brevis.

These forces act simultaneously but with different intensities, depending on the situation of the thumb. As the thumb moves into opposition there is automatic axial rotation of the first metacarpal shaft to produce pronation. This is again brought about by the paired action of oppositely directed forces: in this case the opposition muscles provide one force, and the posterior oblique carpometacarpal ligament provides the other.

Pinch grip muscles. Zancolli has subdivided the muscles of pinch grip into lateral, medial and intermediate subgroups:

- lateral: opposition muscles

- medial: abductor pollicis and first dorsal interosseous
- intermediate: flexor pollicis longus.

The lateral subgroup moves the first metacarpal into palmar abduction. The metacarpal shaft rotates medially into pronation. Radial angulation at the metacarpophalangeal joint increases the span of the hand. The metacarpophalangeal joint is stabilized, principally by extensor pollicis brevis and flexor pollicis brevis. Flexion of the proximal and distal phalanges is controlled. Muscles of the medial subgroup produce an approach of the first metacarpal towards the palm. Since they act with the lateral group they have a strong controlling effect on the position and rotation of the first metacarpal. The intermediate subgroup consists simply of the flexor pollicis longus, which flexes powerfully the interphalangeal or metacarpophalangeal joint, as described earlier. Palpating the thenar eminence during tip and lateral pinch provides some appreciation of the action of the pinch grip muscles. An understanding of this ingenious mechanism is vital in reconstructive surgery of the hand.

MUSCLES AND FASCIAE OF THE LOWER LIMB

Muscles of the lower limb may be grouped as follows:

- Muscles of the iliac region
- Muscles of the thigh and gluteal region
- Muscles of the leg
- Muscles of the foot.

(Note that, according to anatomical convention, 'leg' refers to the part of the lower limb between knee and ankle.)

See Table **7.2**A, B, pages 896, 897 for notes and further information on the segmental innervation of muscles of the lower limb.

MUSCLES OF THE ILIAC REGION

Although there is no 'iliac region' as such, this heading conveniently describes a group of three muscles that originate from the lumbar vertebral column (psoas major and minor) and the iliac bone (iliacus). Two (psoas major and iliacus) are attached together on the femur as flexors; psoas minor falls short of this and acts on the spine and sacro-iliac joint.

Iliac fascia

The iliac fascia covers psoas and iliacus. It is thin above, but thickens progressively towards the inguinal ligament. The *part covering psoas* is thickened above as the *medial arcuate ligament* (p. 816). Medially, the fascia over psoas is attached by a series of fibrous arches to the intervertebral discs, margins of vertebral bodies, and the upper part of the sacrum. Laterally, it blends with the fascia anterior to quadratus lumborum (p. 829) above the iliac crest, and with the fascia covering iliacus below the crest.

The *iliac part* is connected laterally to the whole of the inner lip of the iliac crest and medially to the pelvic brim, where it blends with the periosteum. It is attached to the iliopectineal eminence, where it receives a slip from the tendon of psoas minor, when that muscle is present. The external iliac vessels are anterior to the fascia

but the branches of the lumbar plexus are posterior; it is separated from the peritoneum by loose extraperitoneal tissue. Lateral to the femoral vessels, the iliac fascia is continuous with the posterior margin of the inguinal ligament and the transversalis fascia. Medially it passes behind the femoral vessels to become the pectineal fascia, attached to the pecten pubis. At the junction of its lateral and medial parts it is attached to the iliopectineal eminence and the capsule of the hip joint. It thus forms a septum between the inguinal ligament and the hip bone, dividing the space here into a lateral part, the *lacuna musculorum*, containing psoas major, iliacus and the femoral nerve, and a medial part, the *lacuna vasorum*, transmitting the femoral vessels. The iliac fascia continues downward to form the posterior wall of the femoral sheath (p. 871).

Psoas major

Psoas major (**7.121**) is a long muscle that lies on either side of the lumbar vertebral column and the pelvic brim. It arises:

- from the anterior surfaces and lower borders of the transverse processes of all the lumbar vertebrae
- by five digitations, each from the bodies of two adjoining vertebrae and their intervertebral disc. The highest slip arises from the lower margin of the body of the twelfth thoracic vertebra, the upper margin of the body of the first lumbar vertebra and the interposed thoracolumbar disc; the lowest from the adjacent margins of the bodies of the fourth and fifth lumbar vertebrae and the interposed disc
- from a series of tendinous arches extending across the narrow parts of the bodies of the lumbar vertebrae between the digitations already described. The lumbar arteries and veins, and filaments from the sympathetic trunk, pass medial to these arches.

The upper four lumbar intervertebral foramina bear important relations to these attachments of the muscle. The foramina lie anterior to the transverse processes and posterior to the attachments to vertebral bodies, discs and tendinous arches. Thus, the roots of

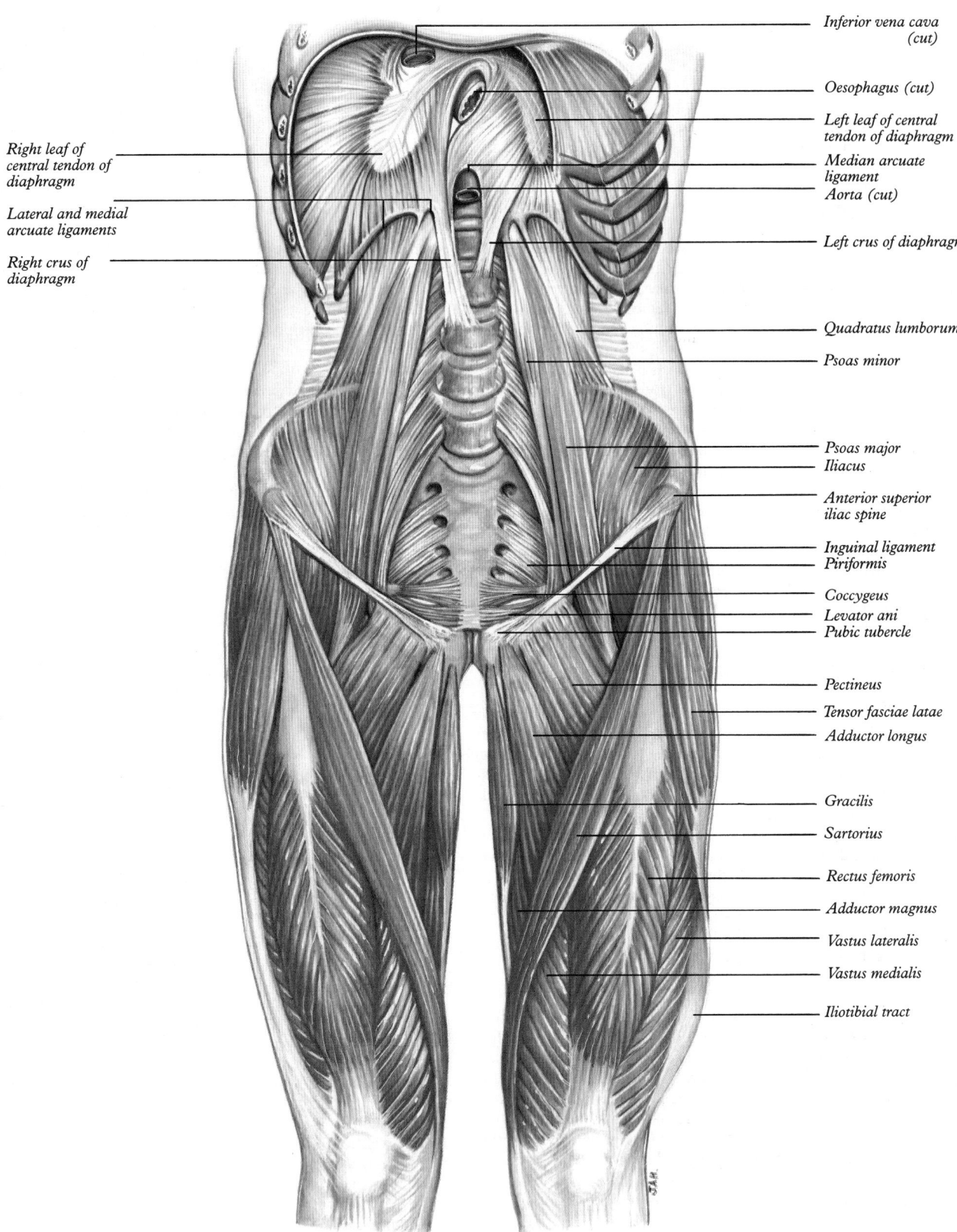

7.121 View of the abdomen, pelvis and thigh, showing abdominal aspect of the diaphragm, flexors of the hip and superficial muscles of the thigh.

the lumbar plexus enter the muscle directly; the plexus is lodged within it, and its branches emerge from its borders and surfaces.

The muscle descends along the pelvic brim, continues posterior to the inguinal ligament and anterior to the capsule of the hip joint, and converges to a tendon which, having received on its lateral side nearly all the fibres of iliacus, becomes attached to the lesser trochanter of the femur. The large subtendinous iliac bursa, which occasionally communicates with the cavity of the hip joint, separates the tendon from the pubis and the capsule of the joint.

Variations. The complex vertebral attachments of psoas major sometimes display minor numerical variations.

Relations. The upper limit of psoas major is posterior to the diaphragm in the lowest part of the posterior mediastinum. It may be in contact with the posterior extremity of the pleural sac. In the abdomen its **anterolateral surface** is related to the medial arcuate ligament—an arched thickening in the general psoas fascia, extra-peritoneal tissue and peritoneum, the kidney, psoas minor, renal vessels, ureter, testicular or ovarian vessels and genitofemoral nerve.

869

In front the right psoas is overlapped by the inferior vena cava and traversed by the end of the ileum; the left is crossed by the colon. Its **posterior surface** is in relation with the transverse processes of the lumbar vertebrae and the medial edge of quadratus lumborum. As already noted, the lumbar plexus is embedded posteriorly in the substance of the muscle (p. 1277). **Medially** the muscle is related to the bodies of the lumbar vertebrae and lumbar vessels. Along its anteromedial margin it is in contact with the sympathetic trunk, aortic lymph nodes and, along the pelvic brim, with the external iliac artery. This margin is covered by the inferior vena cava on the right side, and lies posterior and lateral to the abdominal aorta on the left side. In the thigh it is related: **in front**, to the fascia lata and the femoral artery; **behind**, to the capsule of the hip joint, from which it is separated by a bursa; at its **medial border**, to pectineus and the medial circumflex femoral artery, and the femoral vein, which may overlap it slightly; at its **lateral border**, to the femoral nerve and iliacus. The femoral nerve descends at first through the fibres of psoas major, and then in the furrow between it and iliacus.

Branches of the lumbar plexus diverge from the abdominal part of psoas. Emerging from the **lateral border**, from above downwards, are: the iliohypogastric, ilio-inguinal and lateral femoral cutaneous and femoral nerves; from the **anterolateral surface**, the genitofemoral nerve; from the **medial border**, the obturator and accessory obturator nerves and the upper root of the lumbosacral trunk.

Blood supply. Lumbar arteries 1–4 (p. 1558); variably arteria lumbalis ima (p. 1558); twigs from the renal artery (p. 1557); common iliac artery (p. 1558); external iliac artery (p. 1563); lumbar branch of iliolumbar artery (p. 1562); variably, obturator artery (p. 1560) and medial circumflex femoral artery (p. 1567).

Nerve supply. Ventral rami of the lumbar spinal nerves, L1, **2** and 3.

Actions. Psoas major acts together with iliacus, the combination being referred to *as iliopsoas* (see below).

Psoas minor

Psoas minor (**7.**121) lies anterior to psoas major, entirely within the abdomen. It arises from the sides of the bodies of the twelfth thoracic and first lumbar vertebrae and from the disc between them. It ends in a long, flat tendon which is attached to the pecten pubis and iliopectineal eminence and, laterally, to the iliac fascia.

Variations. The muscle is absent in about 40% of subjects.

Blood supply. Lumbar arteries (p. 1558); arteria lumbalis ima (p. 1558); the lumbar branch of the iliolumbar artery (p. 1562); common iliac artery (p. 1558); sometimes the obturator artery (p. 1560) and deep circumflex artery (p. 1563).

Nerve supply. A branch from the first lumbar nerve.

Action. Psoas minor is probably a weak flexor of the trunk.

Iliacus

Iliacus (**7.**121) is a triangular sheet of muscle which arises from the superior two-thirds of the concavity of the iliac fossa, the inner lip of the iliac crest, the ventral sacro-iliac and iliolumbar ligaments, and the upper surface of the lateral part of the sacrum (**6.**111A). In front, it reaches as far as the anterior superior and anterior inferior iliac spines, and receives a few fibres from the upper part of the capsule of the hip joint. Most of its fibres converge into the lateral side of the strong tendon of psoas major, and the muscles then insert together into the lesser trochanter, but some fibres are attached directly to the femur for about 2.5 cm below and in front of the lesser trochanter.

Relations. In the abdomen, the **anterior surface** of iliacus is related to: its fascia, which separates the muscle from extraperitoneal tissue and peritoneum; the lateral femoral cutaneous nerve; on the right, the caecum; on the left, the iliac part of the descending colon. On its **posterior surface** is the iliac fossa; at its **medial** border, psoas major and the femoral nerve. In the thigh, its **anterior surface** is in contact with the fascia lata, rectus femoris, sartorius and arteria profunda femoris, its **posterior surface** with the capsule of the hip joint, from which it is separated by a bursa common to it and psoas major.

Blood supply. Iliac branch of iliolumbar artery (p. 1562); iliac branches of obturator artery (p. 1560); lateral circumflex femoral artery (p. 1567); arteria profunda femoris (p. 1566).

Nerve supply. Branches of the femoral nerve, **L2** and 3.

Actions. Psoas major, acting from above together with iliacus, flexes the thigh upon the pelvis. Electromyographic studies do not support the common view that psoas major acts as a medial rotator of the hip joint, but activity has been described in **lateral** rotation, particularly in the young. When psoas major and iliacus of both sides act from below, they contract powerfully to bend the trunk and pelvis forwards against resistance, as in raising the trunk from the recumbent to the sitting posture.

Geometrical reasoning suggests that, with the body erect and the lower limb fixed, contraction of one psoas major might flex the trunk forwards and laterally; however, electromyography does not support such a prediction, but indicates maximum activity when the lumbar curvature is increased. Direct electromyographic recording from the muscle during sympathectomy in the lumbar region suggests that in addition to its role as a hip flexor, psoas major is active in balancing the trunk while sitting (Keagy et al 1966).

In symmetrical standing, iliopsoas might be expected to act from below to maintain the vertebral column upright. This would be in accordance with the principle that a muscle which is so close to a joint centre is likely to have an important postural or stabilizing function (Basmajian & De Luca 1985). Basmajian and Greenlaw (1968) confirmed this by reporting continuous slight to moderate electrical activity during relaxed standing. The fact that there is so little activity in most subjects can be understood by drawing a vertical line through the centre of gravity of the body. Such a line falls behind the transverse axis of the hip joints, which are near their close-packed positions, with spiralization and tautening of the ligaments (especially the iliofemoral) and marked compression and congruence of the articular surfaces. Thus the extending torque exerted by the weight of the trunk is balanced mainly by passive mechanisms.

Clinical anatomy. When the neck of the femur is fractured psoas major acts as a lateral rotator of the femur, producing a characteristic posture of the lower limb.

MUSCLES OF THE THIGH AND GLUTEAL REGION

Although muscles of the thigh and hip can be classified on functional and morphological grounds as flexors and extensors, the division into flexor and extensor columns that was clearly evident in the upper limb has been lost. The underlying reason is the evolutionary change that took place in land vertebrates, during which the lower limb rotated through 180° into a new working position (p. 613). This change has not affected the muscles of the pelvic girdle: iliopsoas, a flexor already described, is still ventral in position, and the gluteal muscles, which represent primitive extensors, remain dorsal, so the hip flexes to the front. However, the thigh has rotated so that the original dorsal or extensor surface has become anterior, and the ventral aspect, containing the flexor muscles, posterior; the knee therefore flexes to the rear. Muscles that cross both joints can extend at the hip and flex at the knee. The further development of multiaxial function at the hip has been coupled with the appearance of adductors and abductors, so that the joint is surrounded on all sides, not merely ventrally and dorsally, by muscles capable of moving the femur in any direction or maintaining it in static postures, in particular the erect position. Superimposed on these activities is the influence of gravity, which aids some movements and opposes others, so the muscle groups are not equal in power.

MUSCLES OF THE THIGH—ANTERIOR GROUP

Included in this group (**7.**121) are tensor fasciae latae, sartorius and rectus femoris, which can act at both hip and knee joints, and vastus medialis, lateralis, and intermedius, which act only at the knee. Articularis genus, a derivative of vastus intermedius, completes the group; it retracts the synovial capsule of the knee joint. Rectus femoris and the vasti extend the knee joint through a common tendon and are hence considered as one muscle: quadriceps femoris.

Superficial fascia

The superficial fascia of the thigh consists, as elsewhere in the limbs, of loose areolar tissue containing a variable amount of fat. In some regions, particularly near the inguinal ligament, it splits into recognizable layers, between which may be found the branches of superficial vessels and nerves. It is thick in the inguinal region and between the two layers are the superficial inguinal lymph nodes, great saphenous vein and other smaller vessels. Here the **superficial layer** is continuous with the abdominal superficial layer. The **deep layer**, a thin fibro-elastic stratum, is most marked medial to the great saphenous vein and inferior to the inguinal ligament, and extends between the subcutaneous vessels and nerves and the deep fascia, with which it fuses a little below the ligament. (The line of fusion lies in the floor of the ventral flexure line or groove associated with the hip joint.) This membranous fascia completes the saphenous opening (see below), blending with its circumference and with the femoral sheath (p. 1564). Over the opening it is multiply perforated by the great saphenous vein and other vessels—hence the term *cribriform fascia* (Latin: *cribrum* = a sieve).

Fascia lata

The fascia lata, the deep fascia of the region, so called because of its width, is thicker in the proximal and lateral parts of the thigh where tensor fasciae latae and an expansion from gluteus maximus are attached to it. It is thin posteriorly, and over the adductor muscles, but thicker around the knee, where it is strengthened by expansions from the tendon of biceps femoris laterally, sartorius medially, and quadriceps femoris in front. The fascia lata is attached: above and behind, to the back of the sacrum and coccyx; laterally, to the iliac crest; in front, to the inguinal ligament and superior ramus of the pubis; medially, to the inferior ramus of the pubis, the ramus and tuberosity of the ischium, and the lower border of the sacrotuberous ligament. From the iliac crest it descends as a dense layer over gluteus medius to the upper border of gluteus maximus, where it splits into two layers, one passing superficial and the other deep to this muscle; at its lower border the layers reunite. Over the flattened lateral surface of the thigh, the fascia lata thickens to form a strong band, the *iliotibial tract*. The upper end of the tract splits into two layers, where it encloses and anchors tensor fasciae latae and receives, posteriorly, most of the tendon of gluteus maximus. The superficial layer ascends lateral to tensor fasciae latae to the iliac crest; the deeper layer passes up and medially, deep to the muscle, and blends with the lateral part of the capsule of the hip joint. Distally, the iliotibial tract is attached to a smooth, triangular, anterolateral facet on the lateral condyle of the tibia, where it is superficial to and blends with an aponeurotic expansion from vastus lateralis. When the leg is extended it stands out as a strong, visible ridge on the anterolateral aspect of the knee (Kaplan 1958). Below, the fascia lata is attached to all exposed bony points around the knee joint, such as the condyles of the femur and tibia, and the head of the fibula; this applies particularly to the iliotibial tract. On each side of the patella the deep fascia is reinforced by transverse fibres which attach the vasti to it; the stronger lateral fibres are continuous with the iliotibial tract. The fascia lata is continuous with two intermuscular septa, which are attached to the whole of the linea aspera and its prolongations above and below: the lateral, stronger septum, which extends from the attachment of gluteus maximus to the lateral condyle, lies between vastus lateralis in front and the short head of biceps femoris behind and provides partial attachment for them; the medial, thinner septum lies between vastus medialis and the adductors and pectineus. Numerous smaller septa pass between the individual muscles, ensheathing them and sometimes providing partial attachment for their fibres.

Saphenous opening (7.122). The saphenous opening is an aperture in the deep fascia, lateral and a little distal to the medial part of the inguinal ligament, which allows passage to the great saphenous vein and other smaller vessels. The cribriform fascia, which is pierced by these structures, fills in the aperture and must be removed to reveal it. Adjacent subsidiary openings may exist, to transmit venous tributaries, but these openings are more usually in the floor of the fossa. In the adult the approximate centre of the opening is some 3 cm inferior and 3 cm lateral to the pubic tubercle. It varies considerably in size, with a height of 1.5–9 cm and a width of 1–4 cm. The fascia lata in this part of the thigh displays *superficial* and *deep strata* (not to be confused with the superficial and deep layers of the superficial fascia described above). They lie respectively anterior and posterior to the femoral sheath; the somewhat spiral circum-

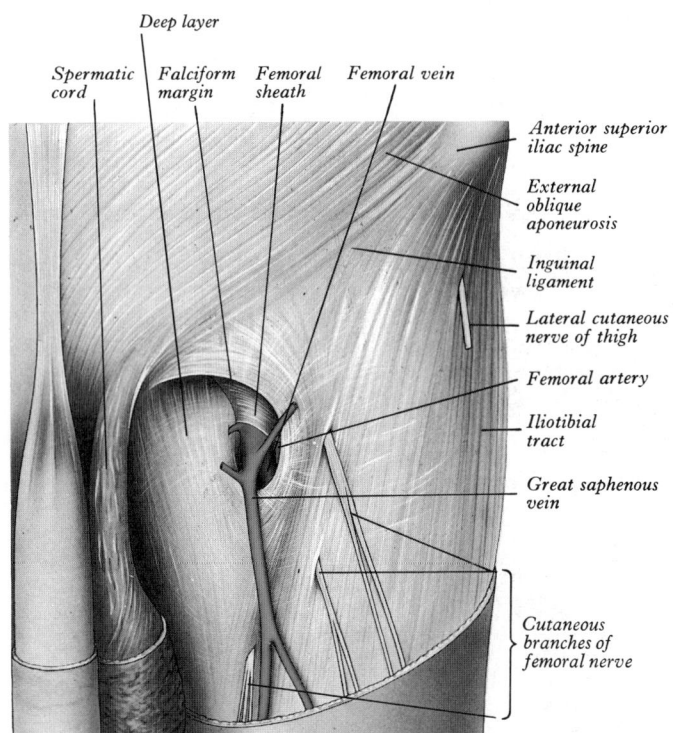

7.122 The left saphenous opening, after the removal of the cribriform fascia. Note the superficial and deep layers of the deep fascia (see text).

ference of the saphenous opening is formed where the two are in continuity.

The *superficial stratum*, lateral to the saphenous opening, is attached to the crest and anterior superior spine of the ilium, to the whole length of the inguinal ligament, and to the pecten pubis together with the lacunar ligament (p. 822). From the pubic tubercle it is reflected inferolaterally as the arched *falciform margin*, which forms the superior, lateral and inferior boundaries of the saphenous opening (7.122); this margin adheres to the anterior layer of the femoral sheath, and the cribriform fascia is attached to it. The falciform margin is considered to have *superior* and *inferior cornua*. The latter *cornu* is well defined, and is continuous behind the great saphenous vein with the deep stratum of the fascia lata.

The *deep stratum* is medial to the saphenous opening and is continuous with the superficial stratum at its lower margin. Traced upwards, it covers pectineus, adductor longus and gracilis, passes behind the femoral sheath, to which it is closely united, and continues to the pecten pubis.

Tensor fasciae latae

Tensor fasciae latae (7.121) arises from the anterior 5 cm of the outer lip of the iliac crest, from the lateral surface of the anterior superior iliac spine and part of the border of the notch below it between gluteus medius and sartorius, and from the deep surface of the fascia lata; proximal attachments may extend to the aponeurotic fascia superficial to gluteus medius. It descends between, and is attached to, the two layers of the iliotibial tract of the fascia lata and usually ends about one-third of the way down the thigh, although it may reach as far as the lateral femoral condyle.

Blood supply. Superior and inferior gluteal arteries and some of their gluteal anastomoses (p. 1562).

Nerve supply. Superior gluteal nerve, L**4**, **5** and S1.

Actions. Tensor fasciae latae, acting through the iliotibial tract, extends the knee with lateral rotation of the leg; it may also assist in abduction and medial rotation of the thigh, but its role as an abductor has been contested (Kaplan 1958). The muscle helps to maintain upright posture: when the subject is standing it acts from below to steady the pelvis on the head of the femur and, through the iliotibial tract, to steady the condyles of the femur on the tibial condyles. When the thigh is flexed against gravity and the knee is

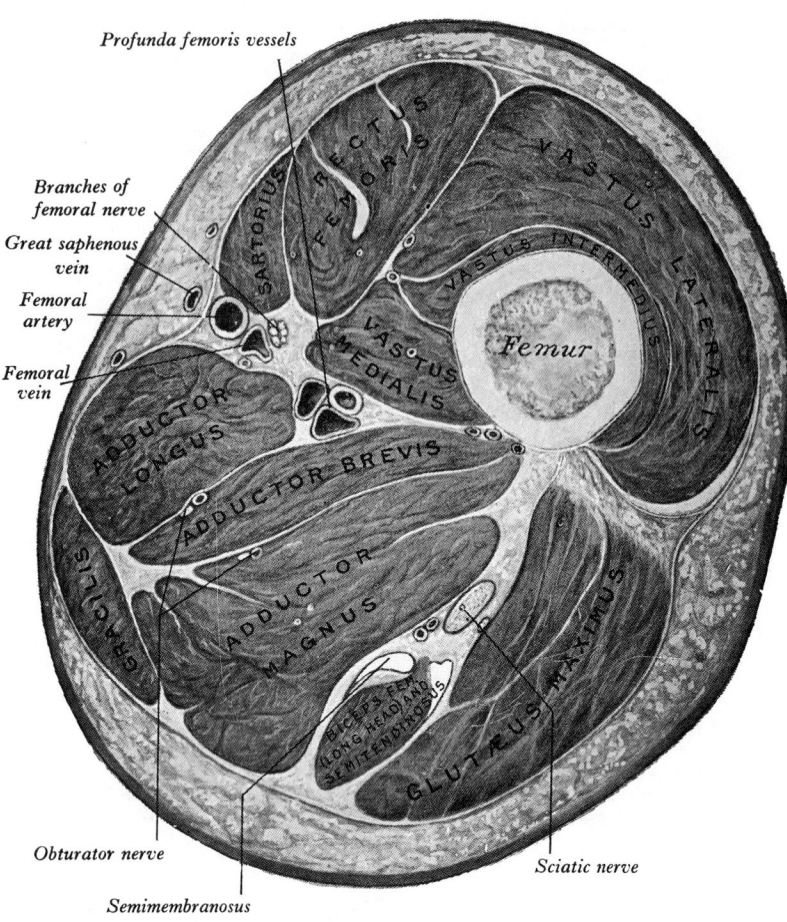

Profunda femoris vessels

Branches of
femoral nerve

Great saphenous
vein

Femoral
artery

Femoral
vein

Obturator nerve

Semimembranosus

7.123 Transverse section through the right thigh at the level of the apex of the femoral triangle: proximal (superior) aspect.

extended, an angular depression appears immediately below the anterior superior iliac spine; its lateral boundary is tensor fasciae latae. The muscle aids gluteus medius in postural abduction at the hip (see p. 875). Some authors consider the iliotibial tract to be more important in steadying the pelvis than tensor fasciae latae.

Sartorius

Sartorius (**7.121, 123, 124**) is a narrow strap muscle—the longest in the body. It arises by tendinous fibres from the anterior superior iliac spine and the upper half of the notch below it. It crosses the thigh obliquely over to the medial side, then descends more vertically to the medial side of the knee. The muscle fibres terminate at this point and a thin, flattened tendon curves obliquely forwards and expands into a broad aponeurosis. The aponeurosis attaches to the proximal medial surface of the tibia in front of gracilis and semitendinosus (**7.135**). A slip from its upper margin blends with the capsule of the knee joint, and another from its lower margin merges with the fascia on the medial side of the leg. Its upper part curves backwards over the upper edge of the gracilis tendon and attaches behind it.

Variations. In some cases the muscle is absent while in others it is doubled, the extra head being attached to the pectineal line or to the femoral sheath (Bergman et al 1988; Tillmann 1987). Variations in the insertion of the sartorius in relation to the knee axis are known to occur and may account for the observation that in some subjects electromyographic activity increases during extension of the knee rather than during flexion, as is usually the case (Johnson et al 1972; Basmajian & De Luca 1985).

Relations. The *femoral triangle*, in the upper third of the thigh, is formed by the medial border of sartorius (lateral side), the medial border of adductor longus (medial side), and the inguinal ligament (base). The femoral artery descends through this triangle from the middle of the base to the apex. In the middle third of the thigh, the femoral artery is contained in the adductor (subsartorial) canal, covered anteriorly by a strong stratum of deep fascia and by sartorius (**7.124**). The fascia bridges the interval between the adductors and quadriceps; it must be incised to expose the vessels.

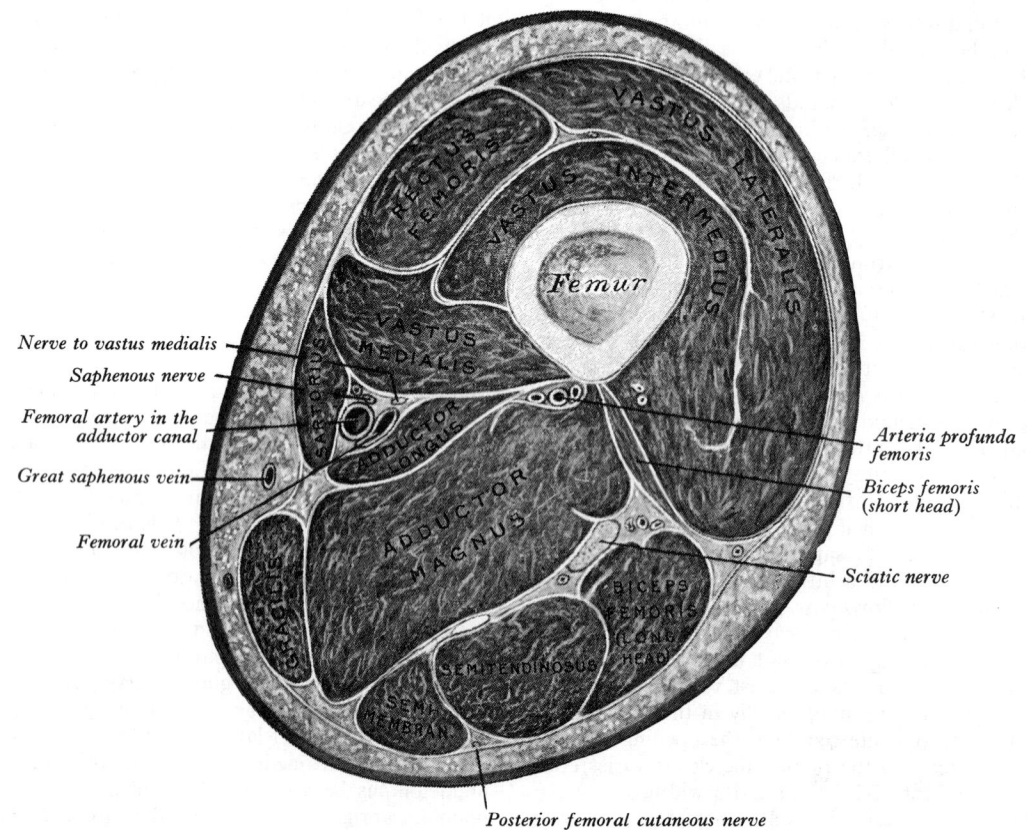

Nerve to vastus medialis

Saphenous nerve

Femoral artery in the
adductor canal

Great saphenous vein

Femoral vein

Arteria profunda
femoris

Biceps femoris
(short head)

Sciatic nerve

Posterior femoral cutaneous nerve

7.124 Transverse section through the middle of the right thigh: proximal (superior) aspect.

Blood supply. Femoral artery (p. 1564); saphenous and direct branches of the descending genicular artery (p. 1568); superficial and deep circumflex iliac arteries (pp. 1563, 1564); superior and inferior medial genicular arteries (pp. 1569, 1570).

Nerve supply. Femoral nerve, L2 and 3.

Actions. Sartorius assists in flexing the leg at the knee, and the thigh on the pelvis, particularly when these two movements are combined. It also helps to abduct the thigh and to rotate it laterally. (Together with inversion of the foot these movements bring the sole of the foot into direct view.) When it contracts against gravity, as it usually does, the muscle can be both seen and felt in the living subject. The fact that sartorius represents only 1% of the physiological cross-sectional area of all muscles crossing the hip or knee joint (Winter 1990) suggests that its role in walking is a minor one. In a subject ascending steps, electromyographic activity of sartorius increases during lateral rotation of the thigh at the end of the swing phase immediately preceding heel strike (Carvalho et al 1972); thus the muscle may well have a substantial involvement in climbing.

Quadriceps femoris

Quadriceps femoris (7.121, 123, 124), the great extensor muscle of the leg, covers almost all of the front and sides of the femur. It can be divided into four parts, each named individually. One arises from the ilium and travels straight down the middle of the thigh; hence the name *rectus femoris*. The other three arise from the shaft of the femur and surround it (apart from the linea aspera) from the trochanters to the condyles: lateral to the femur is *vastus lateralis*, medial to it *vastus medialis*, and in front *vastus intermedius.* Rectus femoris crosses both hip and knee joints; the three vasti cross the knee joint only.

The tendons of the four components of quadriceps unite in the lower part of the thigh to form a single strong tendon attached to the base of the patella, some fibres continuing over it to blend with the ligamentum patellae. The patella is a sesamoid bone in the quadriceps tendon, and the 'ligamentum' patellae, which extends from the patellar apex to the tubercle of the tibia, is in fact the continuation of the tendon, the medial and lateral patellar retinacula (p. 691) being expansions from its borders. The suprapatellar bursa (a synovial extension of the knee joint) lies between the femur and the suprapatellar part of the quadriceps tendon; the deep infrapatellar bursa lies between the ligamentum patellae and the proximal end of the tibia (6.309).

Quadriceps is not subject to appreciable variation.

Rectus femoris. Rectus femoris (7.121, 123, 124) is fusiform. Its superficial fibres are bipennate, the deep fibres parallel. It has a double origin on the ilium: a *straight tendon* arises from the anterior inferior iliac spine, and a thinner, flatter *reflected tendon* from a groove above the acetabulum and from the fibrous capsule of the hip joint. The two unite at an acute angle and spread into an aponeurosis which is prolonged downwards on the **anterior surface** of the muscle; from this the muscular fibres arise. The fibres end in a broad, thick aponeurosis that forms over the lower two-thirds of its **posterior surface**, and gradually narrows into the thick, flat tendon by which it is attached to the base of the patella. This constitutes the superficial central part of the quadriceps tendon.

Variations. Rectus femoris may arise from the anterior superior iliac spine and its reflected head may be absent.

Blood supply. Arteria profunda femoris directly, and rami from the descending branch of the lateral circumflex femoral artery (p. 1567). Distally, by rami from vessels contributing to the genicular anastomoses (p. 1570).

Vastus lateralis. Vastus lateralis (7.121, 123) is the largest component of quadriceps femoris. It arises by a broad aponeurosis from the upper part of the intertrochanteric line, the anterior and inferior borders of the greater trochanter, the lateral lip of the gluteal tuberosity, and the proximal half of the lateral lip of the linea aspera (7.124). This aponeurosis covers the proximal three-quarters of the muscle, and from its deep surface many additional fibres arise. A few fibres also arise from the tendon of gluteus maximus and the lateral intermuscular septum between vastus lateralis and the short head of biceps femoris. The muscular mass thus formed is attached to a strong aponeurosis on the deep surface of the lower part of the muscle; this narrows to a flat tendon which is attached to the base and lateral border of the patella, and blends into the compound

quadriceps femoris tendon (see above). It contributes to the capsule of the knee joint an expansion that descends to the lateral condyle of the tibia and blends with the iliotibial tract.

Blood supply. Intimate supply (dual, superficial and deep) from the descending branches of the lateral circumflex femoral artery (p. 1567) and also from its transverse and ascending branches; lateral superior genicular branch of the popliteal artery (pp. 1569, 1570); terminations of the perforating arteries (p. 1567).

Vastus medialis. Vastus medialis (7.121, 123, 124) arises from the lower part of the intertrochanteric line, spiral line, medial lip of the linea aspera, proximal part of the medial supracondylar line, the tendons of adductor longus and magnus, and the medial intermuscular septum (p. 871). Its fibres pass downwards and forwards at an angle of about 15° to the long axis of the femur, most of them into an aponeurosis on the deep surface of the muscle which is attached to the medial border of the patella and quadriceps tendon. An expansion from this aponeurosis reinforces the capsule of the knee joint and is attached below to the medial condyle of the tibia. The lowest fibres are much more horizontal and form a bulge in the living subject, medial to the upper half of the patella. Some authors distinguish this part of the muscle as the *vastus medialis oblique*, with fibres that originate largely from the tendon of adductor magnus and insert into the medial border of the patella.

Blood supply. The femoral artery (p. 1564); the descending genicular artery (p. 1568); the medial superior (and inferior) genicular branches of the popliteal artery (p. 1570).

Vastus intermedius. Vastus intermedius (7.123, 124) arises from the anterior and lateral surfaces of the upper two-thirds of the femoral shaft, and from the lower part of the lateral intermuscular septum. Its fibres end in an aponeurosis on the anterior surface of the muscle; this aponeurosis forms the deep part of the quadriceps tendon and is attached to the lateral border of the patella and the lateral condyle of the tibia.

Vastus intermedius appears to be inseparable from vastus medialis, but when rectus femoris is reflected a narrow cleft can be seen extending upwards from the medial border of the patella between the two muscles, sometimes as far as the lower part of the intertrochanteric line, beyond which the two muscles are frequently fused.

Blood supply. The femoral artery (p. 1564); arteria profunda femoris and descending and transverse branches of the lateral circumflex femoral artery (p. 1567); vessels contributing to the genicular anastomoses (p. 1570).

Articularis genus. Articularis genus, a small muscle that is usually distinct from vastus intermedius but occasionally blends with it, consists of several muscular bundles which arise from the anterior surface of the lower part of the femoral shaft and are attached to a proximal reflexion of the synovial membrane of the knee joint (DiDio et al 1967).

Nerve supply. Quadriceps femoris and articularis genus are supplied by the femoral nerve, L2, **3** and **4**.

Actions. Quadriceps femoris extends the knee. Rectus femoris helps to flex the thigh on the pelvis; if the thigh is fixed, it helps to flex the pelvis on the thigh. Rectus can flex the hip and extend the knee simultaneously. During knee extension the patella tends to be displaced laterally because of the change of angle between the shaft of the femur and the bones of the lower leg (Lieb & Perry 1968). The horizontally opposed forces of vastus lateralis and the lower fibres of vastus medialis counteract this tendency, retaining the patella in its groove on the surface of the femur (Speakman & Weisberg 1977). Weakness of one or the other of these muscles (due, for example, to arthritis or trauma of the knee joint) can result in abnormal patellar movement and a loss of joint stability. Electromyographic studies indicate that the three vasti are not equally active in different phases of extension or rotation. There is little or no activity in quadriceps during standing (see Standing, walking and running, p. 895). Articularis genus retracts the synovial suprapatellar bursa proximally during extension of the leg, presumably to prevent interposition of redundant synovial folds between patella and femur (cf. articularis cubiti at the elbow, p. 844).

MUSCLES OF THE THIGH—MEDIAL GROUP

This group has evolved, as its nerve supply suggests, from both flexor and extensor columns. All five muscles—gracilis, pectineus, adductor longus, adductor brevis, and adductor magnus—cross the hip joint, but only gracilis reaches beyond the knee. They are known collectively as the adductors of the thigh, although their actions are more complex than this.

Gracilis

Gracilis (**7**.121, 123, 124) is the most superficial of the adductor group. It is thin and flat, broad above, narrow and tapering below. It arises by a thin aponeurosis from the medial margins of the lower half of the body of the pubis, the whole of the inferior pubic ramus, and the adjoining part of the ischial ramus (**6**.295). The fibres descend vertically into a rounded tendon which passes across the medial condyle of the femur posterior to the tendon of sartorius. It then curves around the medial condyle of the tibia, where it fans out and attaches to the upper part of the medial surface of the tibia, just below the condyle. A few fibres from the lower part of the tendon continue into the deep fascia of the lower leg. The attachment is immediately proximal to that of semitendinosus, and its upper edge is overlapped by the tendon of sartorius, with which it is partly

blended. It is separated from the tibial collateral ligament of the knee joint by the tibial intertendinous bursa (p. 700).

Blood supply. Obturator artery (p. 1560); medial circumflex femoral artery (p. 1567); descending genicular artery (p. 1568); superior and inferior medial genicular arteries (pp. 1569, 1570); femoral artery (p. 1564).

Nerve supply. Obturator nerve, L2 and 3.

Actions. Gracilis flexes the leg and rotates it medially; it may also act as an adductor of the thigh.

Pectineus

Pectineus (**7**.121) is a flat, quadrangular muscle in the femoral triangle. It arises from the pecten pubis, from the bone in front of it between the iliopectineal eminence and the pubic tubercle, and from the fascia on its own anterior surface. The fibres descend posterolaterally to attach along a line from the lesser trochanter to the linea aspera.

Variations. The muscle may be bilaminar, as it is in some other mammals, the two layers receiving separate nerve supplies (see below). Proximally it may be partially or wholly attached to the capsule of the hip joint.

Relations. It is related **anteriorly** to the fascia lata, which separates it from the femoral vessels and great saphenous vein; **posteriorly** to the capsule of the hip joint, adductor brevis, obturator externus and the anterior branch of the obturator nerve; **laterally** to psoas major and the medial circumflex femoral vessels; **medially** to the lateral margin of adductor longus.

Blood supply. Obturator artery (p. 1560); medial circumflex femoral artery (p. 1567); first perforating branch of arteria profunda (p. 1567); deep external pudendal artery (p. 1566); femoral artery (p. 1564).

Nerve supply. Femoral nerve, L2 and 3; and accessory obturator, L3, when present. Occasionally it receives a branch from the obturator nerve. The muscle may be incompletely divided into dorsal and ventral strata, supplied respectively by obturator and femoral (or accessory obturator) nerves. Woodburne (1960) found only 69 out of 800 cases with a partial supply from an accessory obturator nerve.

Actions. Pectineus adducts the thigh and flexes it on the pelvis.

Adductor longus

Adductor longus (**7**.124, 125), the most anterior of the three adductors, is a large, fan-shaped muscle in the same plane as pectineus. It arises by a narrow tendon with a flattened (sometimes C-shaped) cross-section, which is attached to the front of the pubis in the angle between the crest and the symphysis. It expands into a broad fleshy belly which descends posterolaterally and inserts by an aponeurosis into the linea aspera in the middle third of the femur, between vastus medialis and the other two adductors (magnus and brevis), usually blending with all of them.

Variations. The muscle is occasionally double.

Relations. **Anterior** to adductor longus are the spermatic cord, fascia lata (which separates it from the great saphenous vein) and, near its attachment, the femoral artery and vein and sartorius. **Posterior** to it are adductor brevis and adductor magnus, the anterior branch of the obturator nerve and, near its attachment, the profunda femoris vessels. **Lateral** is pectineus; **medial** is gracilis.

Blood supply. Femoral artery (p. 1564); arteria profunda femoris, direct branches and, variably, first to third perforating arteries (p. 1567); medial circumflex femoral artery (p. 1567); obturator artery (p. 1560).

Nerve supply. Anterior division of the obturator nerve, L2, **3** and 4.

Adductor brevis

Adductor brevis (**7**.123, 125) lies posterior to pectineus and adductor longus. It arises by a narrow attachment from the external aspect of the body and inferior ramus of the pubis, between gracilis and obturator externus. Like adductor longus it is somewhat triangular, and expands as it descends posterolaterally to insert via an aponeurosis into the femur, along a line from the lesser trochanter to the linea aspera, and on the upper part of the linea immediately behind pectineus and the upper part of adductor longus.

Variations. Adductor brevis often has two or three separate parts, or it may be integrated into adductor magnus.

Pectineus

Iliofemoral ligament

Groove for tendon of psoas major

Posterior branch of obturator nerve

Anterior branch of obturator nerve

Obturator externus

Adductor brevis

Adductor magnus

Adductor longus

Opening in adductor magnus

7.125 The adductor muscles of the left thigh: anterior aspect. Most of adductor longus has been excised; its borders are indicated by dashed lines.

Relations. **Anterior** are pectineus, adductor longus, arteria profunda femoris, and the anterior branch of the obturator nerve; **posterior** are adductor magnus and the posterior branch of the obturator nerve. The **upper border** of adductor brevis is related to the medial circumflex femoral artery, obturator externus, and the conjoined tendon of psoas major and iliacus; its **lower border**, to gracilis and adductor magnus. The second, or first and second, perforating arteries pierce it near its femoral attachment.

Blood supply. Femoral artery (p. 1564); arteria profunda femoris, direct branches and, variably, first to third perforating arteries (p. 1567); medial circumflex femoral artery (p. 1567); obturator artery (p. 1560).

Nerve supply. Obturator nerve, L2, 3.

Adductor magnus

Adductor magnus (**7.**123, 124, 125), a massive triangular muscle, arises from a small part of the inferior ramus of the pubis, from the conjoined ischial ramus, and from the inferolateral aspect of the ischial tuberosity. The short, horizontal fibres from the pubic ramus insert into the medial margin of the gluteal tuberosity of the femur, medial to gluteus maximus; this part of the muscle, in a plane anterior to the rest, is sometimes called *adductor minimus.* The fibres from the ischial ramus fan out downwards and laterally, to insert via a broad aponeurosis into the linea aspera and the proximal part of the medial supracondylar line. The medial part of the muscle, composed mainly of fibres from the ischial tuberosity, is a thick mass which descends almost vertically, and ends in the lower third of the thigh in a rounded tendon, which can be palpated proximal to its attachment to the adductor tubercle (p. 681) on the medial condyle of the femur. The tendon is connected by a fibrous expansion to the medial supracondylar line.

The long, linear attachment of the muscle is interrupted by a series of osseo-aponeurotic openings, bridged by tendinous arches attached to the bone. The upper four are small, and transmit the perforating branches and the termination of arteria profunda femoris. The lowest is large, and allows the femoral vessels to cross to the popliteal fossa.

Variations. The vertical, ischiocondylar part of the muscle varies in its degree of separation from the rest. The upper border of adductor magnus may fuse with quadratus femoris.

Relations. **Anterior** are pectineus, adductor brevis and adductor longus, the femoral and profunda vessels, and the posterior branch of the obturator nerve; a bursa separates the proximal part of the muscle from the lesser trochanter of the femur. **Posterior** are the sciatic nerve, gluteus maximus, biceps femoris, semitendinosus and semimembranosus. The **superior border** is parallel with quadratus femoris, the transverse branch of the medial circumflex femoral artery passing between the muscles. The **medial border** is related to gracilis, sartorius and the fascia lata.

Blood supply. Femoral artery (p. 1564); arteria profunda femoris, direct branches and *all* perforating arteries (p. 1567); medial circumflex femoral artery (p. 1567); obturator artery (p. 1560).

Nerve supply. Adductor magnus is composite and is doubly innervated by the obturator nerve and the tibial division of the sciatic nerve (**L2, 3** and 4); the latter nerve supplies the ischiocondylar part. Both nerves are derived from **anterior** divisions in the lumbosacral plexus, indicating a primitive flexor origin for both parts of the muscle.

Actions. Extensive or forcible adduction of the femur is not often called for, and although the adductors can act in this way when required, they are more commonly synergists in the complex patterns of gait activity, and to some degree controllers of posture. They are, for example, active during flexion and extension of the knee (Janda & Stara 1965). Magnus and longus are probably medial rotators of the thigh, according to de Sousa and Vitti (1966), who also observed that whereas the adductors are inactive during adduction of the abducted thigh in the erect posture (when gravity assists), they are active in other postures, such as the supine position, or during adduction of the flexed thigh when standing. The adductors are also active during flexion (longus) and extension (magnus) of the thigh at the hip joint. In symmetrical easy standing their activity is minimal.

GLUTEAL MUSCLES

The glutei—maximus, medius and minimus (**7.**126, 127)—are the larger muscles of this group; they serve as extensors and abductors at the hip joint. The smaller muscles, which are lateral rotators of the joint, are situated more deeply; they include piriformis, obturators internus and externus, the superior and inferior gemelli, and quadratus femoris. (These actions are, however, modified by the initial position of the thigh.)

Gluteus maximus

Gluteus maximus (**7.**126) is the largest and most superficial muscle in the region. It is a broad, thick quadrilateral mass which, with its overlying adipose fascia, forms the familiar prominence of the buttock. Gluteus maximus is thicker and more extensive in man than in any non-human primate, developments that are associated with the evolutionary transition to bipedality and a permanently upright posture. The muscle has a coarse fascicular architecture, with large bundles of fibres separated by fibrous septa. It arises from the posterior gluteal line of the ilium, and the rough area of bone, including the crest, immediately above and behind it, from the aponeurosis of erector spinae, from the dorsal surface of the lower part of the sacrum and the side of the coccyx, from the sacrotuberous ligament and from the fascia (gluteal aponeurosis) that covers gluteus medius. The fibres descend laterally, the upper and larger part of the muscle, together with the superficial fibres of the lower part, ending in a thick tendinous lamina which passes lateral to the greater trochanter and attaches to the iliotibial tract of the fascia lata. The deeper fibres of the lower part of the muscle are attached to the gluteal tuberosity between vastus lateralis and adductor magnus.

A large, usually multilocular, bursa separates the muscle from the greater trochanter (*trochanteric bursa of gluteus maximus*); a second bursa lies between the tendon of the muscle and that of vastus lateralis (*gluteofemoral bursa*); a third bursa, when present, lies between the muscle and the ischial tuberosity (*ischial bursa of gluteus maximus*).

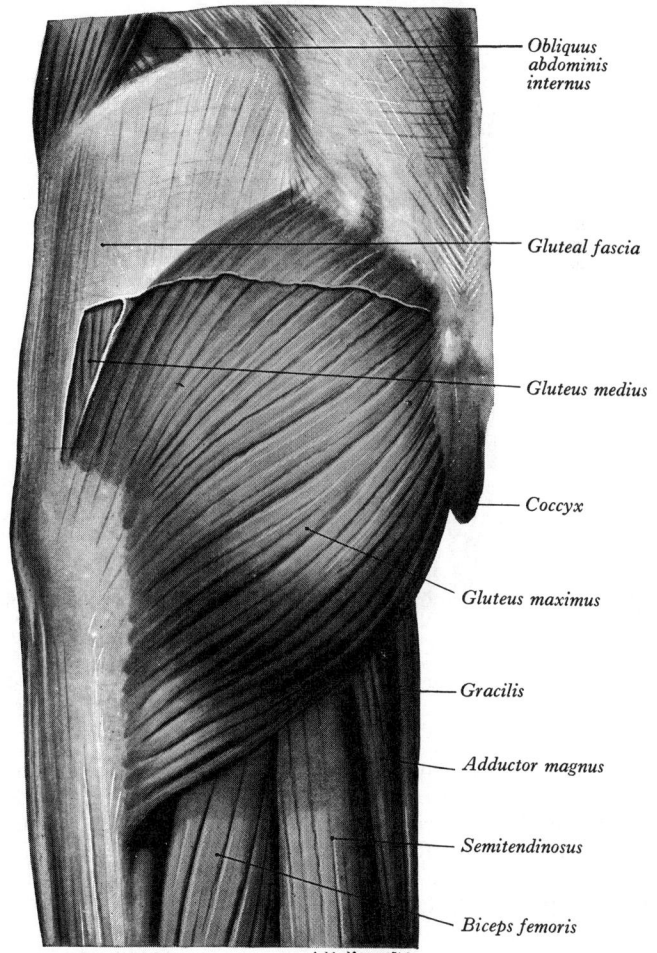

Obliquus abdominis internus

Gluteal fascia

Gluteus medius

Coccyx

Gluteus maximus

Gracilis

Adductor magnus

Semitendinosus

Biceps femoris

A·K· MAXWELL

7.126 The left gluteus maximus. A triangular piece of gluteal fascia has been removed to expose part of gluteus medius.

875

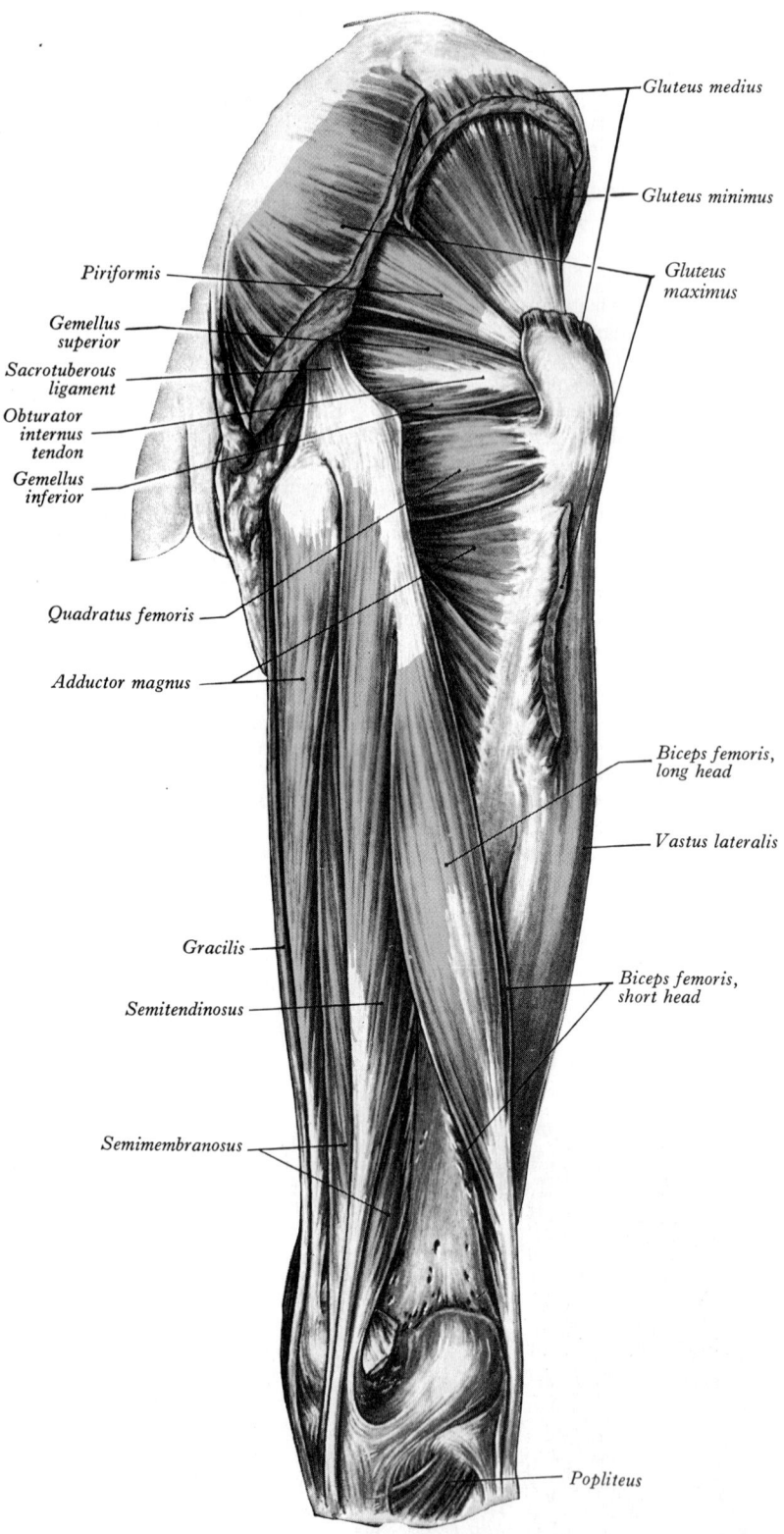

Gluteus medius

Gluteus minimus

Gluteus maximus

Piriformis

Gemellus superior

Sacrotuberous ligament

Obturator internus tendon

Gemellus inferior

Quadratus femoris

Adductor magnus

Biceps femoris, long head

Vastus lateralis

Gracilis

Semitendinosus

Biceps femoris, short head

Semimembranosus

Popliteus

7.127   Muscles of the gluteal region and posterior aspect of the right thigh.

Variations. There may be additional slips from the lumbar aponeurosis or ischial tuberosity. The muscle may also be bilaminar.

Relations. A thin fascia separates the superficial surface of gluteus maximus from the overlying thick adipose subcutaneous tissue. Its **deep** surface is related to the ilium, sacrum, coccyx, and sacrotuberous ligament, part of gluteus medius, piriformis, gemelli, obturator internus, quadratus femoris, the ischial tuberosity, greater trochanter, and the attachments of biceps femoris, semitendinosus, semimembranosus and adductor magnus. The superficial division of the superior gluteal artery reaches the deep surface of the muscle between piriformis and gluteus medius; the inferior gluteal and internal

pudendal vessels, the sciatic, pudendal and posterior femoral cutaneous nerves, muscular branches from the sacral femoral cutaneous nerves, and muscular branches from the sacral plexus leave the pelvis below piriformis. The first perforating artery and the terminal branches of the medial circumflex femoral artery are also deep to the lower part of gluteus maximus. Its **upper border** is thin, and overlies gluteus medius. Its prominent **lower border** is free and slopes downwards and laterally; it is crossed by the *horizontal gluteal fold* (the *posterior flexure line* of the hip joint) which marks the upper limit of the back of the thigh on the surface (**7**.71). (The *anterior flexure line* corresponds to the fusion of fascial layers below the inguinal ligament, see p. 822.)

Blood supply. Inferior gluteal artery (p. 1562); superior gluteal artery (p. 1562); dorsal branches of the lateral sacral arteries (p. 1562); rami from vessels forming the cruciate anastomosis, in particular the lateral circumflex femoral artery (p. 1567); rami from the internal pudendal artery (gluteal part; p. 1526).

Nerve supply. Inferior gluteal nerve, **L5** and **S1** and 2. For details of the intramuscular distribution of the gluteal nerves see Menning et al (1974).

Actions. Acting from the pelvis, gluteus maximus can extend the flexed thigh and bring it into line with the trunk. Acting from its distal attachment, it may prevent the forward momentum of the trunk from producing flexion at the supporting hip during bipedal gait. The muscle is inactive during standing, swaying forwards at the ankle joints, or bending forwards at the hip joints to touch the toes. However, it acts with the hamstrings in raising the trunk after stooping, by rotating the pelvis backwards on the head of the femur (Joseph & Williams 1957). It is intermittently active in the walking cycle and in climbing stairs, and continuously active in strong lateral rotation of the thigh. Its upper fibres are active in powerful abduction of the thigh. It is a tensor of the fascia lata, and through the iliotibial tract it stabilizes the femur on the tibia when the knee extensor muscles are relaxed. The morphological specializations that distinguish the human gluteus maximus from that of other primates are confined to the upper part of the muscle, and the overall functional significance of these changes seems to be that the human muscle can exert greater control over lateral stability of the trunk (Stern 1972).

Gluteus medius

Gluteus medius (**7**.126, 127) is a broad, thick muscle. Its posterior third is covered by gluteus maximus, but it is superficial in its anterior two-thirds, being covered there only by a strong layer of deep fascia (**7**.126). It arises from the outer surface of the ilium between the iliac crest and posterior gluteal line above and the anterior gluteal line below, and also from the strong fascia superficial to its upper part. The fibres converge to a flat tendon, which attaches to a ridge that slants downwards and forwards on the lateral surface of the greater trochanter. Where the tendon glides on the anterosuperior part of the lateral surface of the trochanter, a bursa (*trochanteric bursa of gluteus medius*) separates it from the bone.

Variations. A deep slip of the muscle may be attached to the upper border of the trochanter. The posterior edge of gluteus medius sometimes blends with piriformis.

Blood supply. Superior gluteal artery (p. 1562); rami from the inferior gluteal artery (p. 1562); internal pudendal artery (p. 1562); upper rami from vessels forming the cruciate anastomosis, in particular the lateral circumflex femoral artery (p. 1567).

Nerve supply. Superior gluteal nerve, L4, **5** and S1.

Actions. Considered below with gluteus minimus.

Gluteus minimus

Gluteus minimus (**7**.127) lies deep to gluteus medius, which it resembles. The fan-shaped muscle arises from the outer surface of the ilium between the anterior and inferior gluteal lines and, behind, from the margin of the greater sciatic notch. The fibres converge below to the deep surface of an aponeurosis; this ends in a tendon which attaches to an anterolateral ridge on the greater trochanter, and contributes an expansion to the capsule of the hip joint. A bursa (*trochanteric bursa of gluteus minimus*) separates the tendon from the medial part of the anterior surface of the greater trochanter.

Variations. The muscle may divide into anterior and posterior parts. Separate slips may pass to piriformis, gemellus superior, or vastus lateralis.

Relations. Between gluteus medius and gluteus minimus are the deep branches of the superior gluteal vessels, and the superior gluteal nerve. The reflected tendon of rectus femoris and the capsule of the hip joint are deep to gluteus minimus.

Blood and nerve supplies. As for gluteus medius.

Actions. Both glutei medius and minimus, acting from the pelvis, abduct the thigh, and their anterior fibres rotate it medially. They play an essential part in maintaining the trunk upright when the foot of the opposite side is raised from the ground in walking and running. In this phase the body weight tends to make the pelvis sag downwards on the unsupported side; this is counteracted by the gluteus medius and minimus of the supporting side, which, acting from below, exert such powerful traction on the hip bone that the pelvis is actually raised a little on the unsupported side. In symmetrical standing 'at ease' with the feet somewhat separated, the abductor muscles are usually electrically 'silent', but with the feet placed parallel and close together (the position adopted for Romberg's Test) they are active (Jonsson & Steen 1962).

Clinical relevance. The supportive effect of the glutei (medius and minimus) on the pelvis when the contralateral foot is raised, depends on the following:

(1) the two muscles, and their innervation, must be functioning normally

(2) the components of the hip joint, which forms the fulcrum, must be in their usual relation

(3) the neck of the femur must be intact, with its normal angulation to the shaft.

When any one of these conditions is not fulfilled—e.g. (1) paralysis of the glutei (2) congenital dislocation of the hip (3) non-united fracture of the neck of the femur or coxa vara—the supporting mechanism is upset and the pelvis sinks on the unsupported side when the patient tries to stand on the affected limb. This is known clinically as *Trendelenberg's sign.* Paralysis of gluteus medius and minimus is the most serious muscular disability affecting the hip: sufferers have a characteristic lurching gait. Provided that these muscles are intact, paralysis of other muscles acting on the hip joint produces remarkably little deficit in walking, and even running.

Piriformis

Piriformis (**7.127**) occupies a central position in the buttock, where it lies in the same plane as gluteus medius. It arises from the anterior surface of the sacrum by three digitations, which are attached to the portions of bone between the pelvic sacral foramina, and to the grooves leading from the foramina (**6.111A**): it also arises from the gluteal surface of the ilium near the posterior inferior iliac spine, from the capsule of the adjacent sacro-iliac joint and sometimes from the upper part of the pelvic surface of the sacrotuberous ligament. The muscle passes out of the pelvis through the greater sciatic foramen, which it substantially fills; here it constitutes an important point of reference for structures that emerge above and below it. It inserts into the medial side of the upper border of the greater trochanter of the femur via a rounded tendon, which lies behind and above, but is often partially blended with, the common tendon of obturator internus and the gemelli. The muscle itself may be fused with gluteus medius.

Relations. **Within the pelvis**: the **anterior surface** of piriformis is related to the rectum (especially on the left), the sacral plexus of nerves and branches of the internal iliac vessels; the **posterior surface** is against the sacrum. **Outside the pelvis**: its **anterior surface** is in contact with the posterior surface of the ischium and capsule of the hip joint; its **posterior surface**, with gluteus maximus. Its **upper border** is in contact with gluteus medius, and the superior gluteal vessels and nerve; its **lower border**, with coccygeus and gemellus superior. The inferior gluteal and internal pudendal vessels, the sciatic, posterior femoral cutaneous and pudendal nerves, and muscular branches from the sacral plexus appear in the buttock in the interval between piriformis and gemellus superior. The muscle is frequently pierced by the common peroneal nerve, which may divide it into two parts.

Variations. The variable relationship between the sciatic nerve and piriformis has been documented by Anson (1963) and by Lee and Tsai (1974). They observed variations in which the undivided nerve emerged above the muscle, through the muscle, with its divisions above and below, or with one division between the heads of a divided muscle and one division either above or below; the last was the most common configuration.

Blood supply. **In the pelvis**: inferior gluteal artery (p. 1562); superior gluteal artery (p. 1562); internal pudendal artery (p. 1562); lateral sacral artery (p. 1562). **In the buttock**: inferior gluteal artery (p. 1562); superior gluteal artery (p. 1562); internal pudendal artery (p. 1562); vessels forming the cruciate anastomosis (see lateral and medial circumflex femoral arteries, p. 1567).

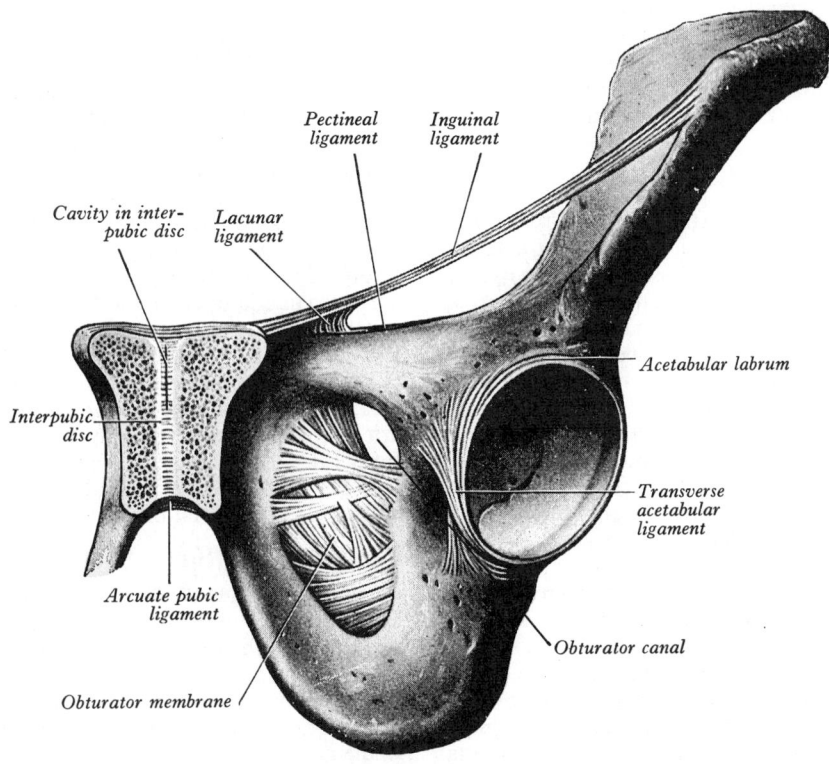

7.128 The left obturator membrane: ventral aspect.

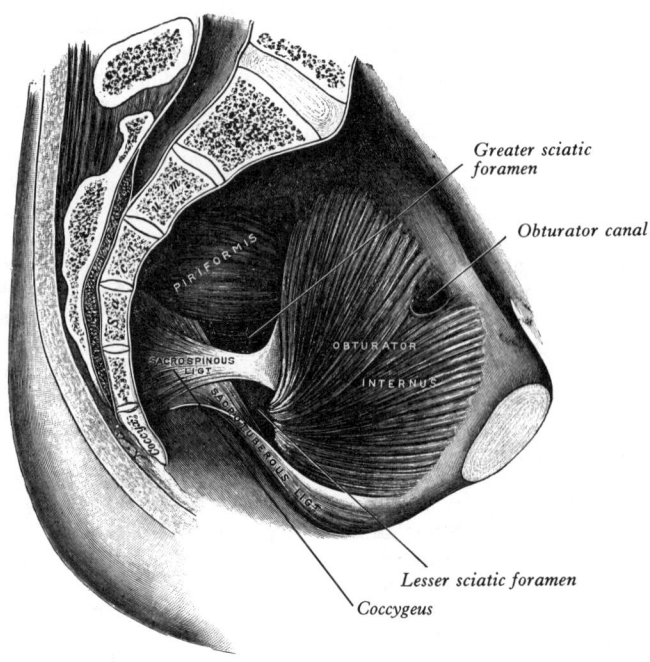

Greater sciatic foramen

Obturator canal

Lesser sciatic foramen

Coccygeus

7.129 The left obturator internus: pelvic aspect. Note that the muscle fibres of coccygeus are blended and coextensive with the sacrospinous ligament on their gluteal aspect.

Nerve supply. Branches from L5, S1 and 2.

Actions. Piriformis rotates the extended thigh laterally, but abducts the flexed thigh.

Obturator membrane

The obturator membrane (7.128) is a thin aponeurosis which closes (*obturates*) most of the obturator foramen, leaving an anterosuperior aperture, the obturator canal, through which the obturator vessels and nerve leave the pelvis and enter the thigh. The membrane is attached to the sharp margin of the obturator foramen except at its inferolateral angle, where it is fixed to the pelvic surface of the ischial ramus, i.e. internal to the foramen. Its fibres are arranged mainly transversely in interlacing bundles; the uppermost bundle, which is attached to the obturator tubercles, completes the obturator canal. The two surfaces of the obturator membrane provide attachment for the two obturator muscles, internus and externus, and some fibres of the pubofemoral ligament of the hip joint are attached to the external surface.

Obturator internus

Obturator internus (7.129) is situated partly within the true pelvis and partly posterior to the hip joint. It arises from the internal surface of the anterolateral wall of the lesser pelvic cavity; its attachments, which almost surround the obturator foramen, are to the inferior ramus of the pubis, the ischial ramus, and the pelvic surface of the hip bone below and behind the pelvic brim, to the upper part of the greater sciatic foramen above and behind, to the obturator foramen below and in front (**6.295**). It also arises from the medial part of the pelvic surface of the obturator membrane, from the tendinous arch which completes the obturator canal, and, to a small extent, from the obturator fascia that covers the muscle. The fibres converge rapidly towards the lesser sciatic foramen and end in four or five tendinous bands on the deep surface of the muscle; these bands make a lateral right-angled turn around the grooved surface of the ischium between its spine and tuberosity. The grooved surface is covered with a smooth layer of hyaline cartilage and is separated from the tendon by a bursa; ridges on the surface correspond to furrows between the tendinous bands. These bands leave the pelvis through the lesser sciatic foramen and unite to form a single flattened tendon, which passes horizontally across the capsule of the hip joint. The gemelli fuse with this tendon before it inserts into an anterior impression on the medial surface of the greater trochanter anterosuperior to the trochanteric fossa. A long, narrow trochanter anterosuperior to the trochanteric fossa. A long, narrow

bursa is usually interposed between the tendon and the capsule of the hip joint; it occasionally communicates with the bursa between the tendon and the ischium.

Relations. **Within the pelvis**, the **anterolateral surface** of the muscle is in contact with the obturator membrane and inner surface of the lateral wall of the pelvis; its **posteromedial surface** contacts the obturator fascia, the origin of levator ani, and the sheath that surrounds the internal pudendal vessels and pudendal nerve (p. 1287), and forms the lateral wall of the ischiorectal fossa. **Outside the pelvis**, the muscle is covered by gluteus maximus, is crossed posteriorly by the sciatic nerve and passes behind the hip joint. As the tendon of obturator internus emerges from the lesser sciatic foramen it is overlapped both above and below by the two gemelli, which form a muscular canal for it; near its termination the gemelli pass anterior to the tendon and form a groove in which it lies.

Blood supply. **In the pelvis**: inferior gluteal artery (p. 1562); superior gluteal artery (p. 1562); internal pudendal artery (p. 1562). **In the buttock**: inferior gluteal artery (p. 1562); vessels forming the cruciate anastomosis (p. 1567).

Nerve supply. Nerve to obturator internus, L5 and S1.

Actions. Considered below with obturator externus.

Gemellus superior

Gemellus superior (7.127), the smaller of the two gemelli, arises from the dorsal surface of the ischial spine, blends with the upper border of the tendon of obturator internus, and inserts with it into the medial surface of the greater trochanter. It is sometimes absent.

Gemellus inferior

Gemellus inferior (7.127) arises from the upper part of the ischial tuberosity, immediately below the groove for the obturator internus tendon. It blends with the lower border of this tendon, and inserts with it into the medial surface of the greater trochanter.

The two gemelli can be regarded as accessory to obturator internus, to which they add attachments external to the pelvis.

Blood supply. Both gemelli are supplied by the inferior gluteal artery (p. 1562), superior gluteal artery (p. 1562), internal pudendal artery (p. 1562) and vessels forming the cruciate anastomosis (p. 1567).

Nerve supply. Gemellus superior is supplied by the nerve to obturator internus, L5 and S1; gemellus inferior is supplied by the nerve to quadratus femoris, L5 and S1.

Actions. The gemelli rotate the extended thigh laterally; they abduct the flexed thigh.

Quadratus femoris

Quadratus femoris (7.127) is a flat, quadrilateral muscle lying between gemellus inferior and the upper margin of adductor magnus, from which it is separated by the transverse branch of the medial circumflex femoral artery. It arises from the upper part of the external aspect of the ischial tuberosity and passes behind the hip joint and the neck of the femur, separated from them by the tendon of obturator externus and the ascending branch of the medial circumflex femoral artery. It inserts into a small tubercle a little above the middle of the trochanteric crest of the femur and into the bone for a short distance below. A bursa is often present between the muscle and the lesser trochanter. The muscle may be absent.

Blood supply. Internal pudendal artery (p. 1562); inferior gluteal (p. 1562), lateral and medial circumflex femoral, and first perforating arteries, i.e. vessels forming the cruciate anastomosis (p. 1567). For further detail see Leborgne et al (1973).

Nerve supply. Nerve to quadratus femoris, L5 and S1.

Action. Lateral rotation of the thigh.

Obturator externus

Obturator externus (7.130) is a flat, triangular muscle covering the external surface of the anterior pelvic wall. It arises from the medial two-thirds of the external surface of the obturator membrane, and from the adjacent bone of the pubic and ischial rami, extending for a short distance onto their pelvic surfaces between the margin of the obturator foramen and the obturator membrane (see above). The whole muscle, and the tendon into which its fibres converge, spirals backwards, laterally and upwards, and crosses the back of the neck of the femur and lower part of the capsule of the hip joint to end in

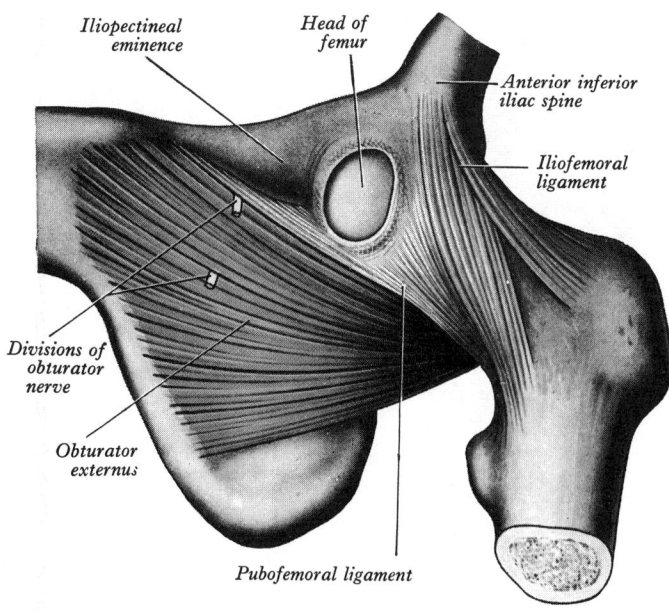

7.130   The left obturator externus: antero-inferior aspect. The bursa of the psoas major tendon, which in this specimen communicated with the synovial cavity of the hip joint, has been opened to expose the head of the femur.

the trochanteric fossa of the femur. A bursa, which communicates with the hip joint, may be interposed between this tendon and the hip joint capsule and femoral neck. The obturator vessels lie between the muscle and the obturator membrane; the anterior branch of the obturator nerve reaches the thigh by passing in front of the muscle, and the posterior branch by piercing it (**7.130**).

Blood supply. Obturator artery (p. 1560); medial circumflex femoral artery, particularly its ascending branch (p. 1567); at the **insertion** of the muscle, anastomosis of the latter with branches of the gluteal and lateral circumflex femoral arteries (p. 1567).

Nerve supply. Posterior branch of the obturator nerve, L3 and **4**.

Actions. It has been suggested that the short muscles around the hip joint—pectineus, piriformis, obturators, gemelli and quadratus femoris—are more important as postural muscles than as prime movers, acting as adjustable ligaments to maintain the stability and integrity of the hip. However, these muscles are largely inaccessible to direct observation, and because of the hazards presented by their close relationship to important neurovascular structures there is a total lack of electromyographic data in man. A comparative electromyographic study of the obturator muscles, conducted mainly in apes, has indicated that earlier speculations about the function of these muscles may be inaccurate (Stern & Larson 1993). In both bipedal walking and vertical climbing obturator externus was recruited during the early part of swing phase: in climbing it effected lateral rotation of the thigh, and in walking it probably counteracted the tendency to medial rotation produced by the anterior adductor muscles at this stage of the cycle. Obturator internus differed from externus in its pattern of use but its role in bipedal walking remains unclear. Its attachments suggest that it—like the gemelli—is a lateral rotator of the extended thigh and an abductor of the flexed thigh; these actions may be used to antagonize unwanted components of movement produced by the primary locomotor muscles.

MUSCLES OF THE THIGH—POSTERIOR GROUP

The posterior femoral muscles (**7.127**)—biceps femoris, semi-tendinosus, and semimembranosus, familiarly referred to as the 'hamstrings'—cross both hip and knee joints, integrating extension at the hip with flexion at the knee. As the muscles span the back of the knee, they form the proximal lateral and medial margins of the popliteal fossa (p. 1568). The actions of these muscles will be considered as a group after they have been described individually.

Biceps femoris

Biceps femoris (**7.123, 124, 127, 131A, B**) occupies a posterolateral

position in the thigh. It has two proximal attachments: one, the *long head*, arises from an inferomedial impression on the upper area of the ischial tuberosity (**6.267A**), via a tendon which it shares with semi-tendinosus, and from the lower part of the sacrotuberous ligament; the other, the *short head*, arises from the lateral lip of the linea aspera, between adductor magnus and vastus lateralis, the attachment extending proximally almost to gluteus maximus and distally along the lateral supracondylar line to within 5 cm of the lateral femoral condyle, and from the lateral intermuscular septum. The long head forms a fusiform belly that descends laterally across the sciatic nerve, the fibres ending in an aponeurosis that covers the posterior surface of the muscle; this aponeurosis receives on its deep surface the fibres of the short head, and gradually narrows to a tendon (the lateral hamstring). The main part of the tendon splits round the fibular collateral ligament and is attached to the head of the fibula. The remainder splits into three laminae: the intermediate lamina fuses with the fibular collateral ligament; the others pass superficial and deep to the ligament to attach to the lateral condyle of the tibia (Sneath 1955). The common peroneal nerve descends along the medial border of the tendon and separates it distally from the lateral head of gastrocnemius.

Variations. The short head may be absent. Additional slips may arise from the ischial tuberosity, linea aspera, or medial supra-condylar line.

Blood supply. **Ischial attachment and proximal part**: obturator artery, posterior branch (p. 1560); inferior gluteal artery and cruciate anastomosis (p. 1567). **Both heads, central part**: first to fourth perforating arteries and longitudinal anastomotic chain (p. 1567); superior muscular branches of popliteal artery (p. 1569). **Insertion**: superior and inferior lateral genicular arteries (p. 1570); circumflex fibular artery (p. 1573).

Nerve supply. Sciatic nerve, L5, S1 and 2, the long head through the tibial division and the short head through the common peroneal division, reflecting the composite derivation from flexor and extensor musculature. (See also nerve supply of semimembranosus.)

Semitendinosus

Semitendinosus (**7.124, 127**), notable for the length of its tendon, is posteromedial in the thigh. It arises from an inferomedial impression on the upper area of the ischial tuberosity (**6.267B**), by a tendon shared with the long head of biceps femoris, and from an aponeurosis connecting the adjacent surfaces of the two muscles for about 7.5 cm from their origin. The belly is fusiform and ends a little below midthigh in a long, rounded tendon, which runs on the surface of semimembranosus; the tendon curves around the medial condyle of the tibia, passes over the tibial collateral ligament of the knee joint (from which it is separated by a bursa) and inserts into the upper part of the medial surface of the tibia behind the attachment of sartorius and distal to that of gracilis (**7.135**). At its termination it is united with the tendon of gracilis and gives off a prolongation to the deep fascia of the leg. A tendinous interruption is usually present near the midpoint of the muscle, which may also receive a muscular slip from the long head of biceps femoris.

Blood supply. **Ischial attachment and proximal part**: obturator artery, posterior branch (p. 1560); inferior gluteal artery and cruciate anastomosis (p. 1567). **Central part**: first to fourth perforating arteries and longitudinal anastomotic chain (p. 1567); superior muscular branches of popliteal artery (p. 1568). **Insertion**: inferior medial genicular artery, and the arteries that anastomose with it (p. 1570).

Nerve supply. Sciatic nerve, L5, S1 and 2, through its tibial division. (See also nerve supply of semimembranosus.)

Semimembranosus

Semimembranosus (**7.124, 127, 131A, B**), named after the flattened form of its upper attachment, is also posteromedial in the thigh. It arises by a long, flat tendon from a superolateral impression on the ischial tuberosity (**6.267A**). Inferomedially the tendinous fibres intermingle to some extent with those of biceps femoris and semi-tendinosus. The tendon receives, from the ischial tuberosity and ramus, two fibrous expansions which flank the adductor magnus. It then broadens and descends deep to semitendinosus and the long head of biceps femoris. Muscle fibres arise from the tendon at about midthigh and converge to a second aponeurosis on the posterior aspect of the lower part of the muscle; this tapers to the heavy,

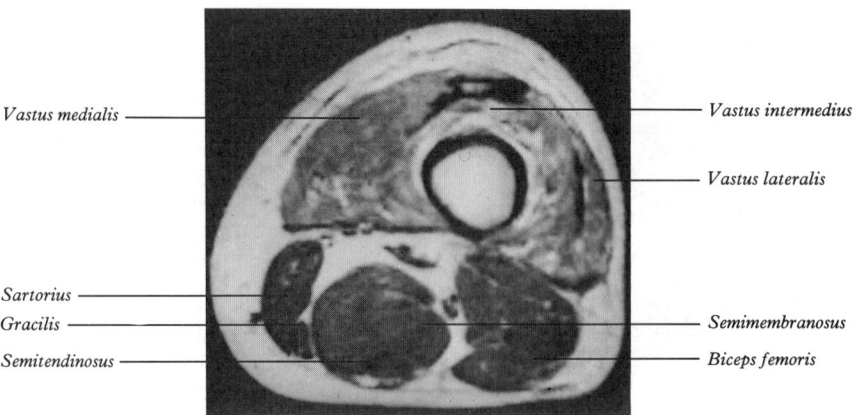

Vastus medialis

Vastus intermedius

Vastus lateralis

Sartorius

Gracilis

Semitendinosus

Semimembranosus

Biceps femoris

7.131A Transverse magnetic resonance image of the right thigh, proximal to the section illustrated in **7.131B**: proximal (superior) aspect. (Supplied by Shaun Gallagher, Guy's Hospital; photography by Sarah Smith.)

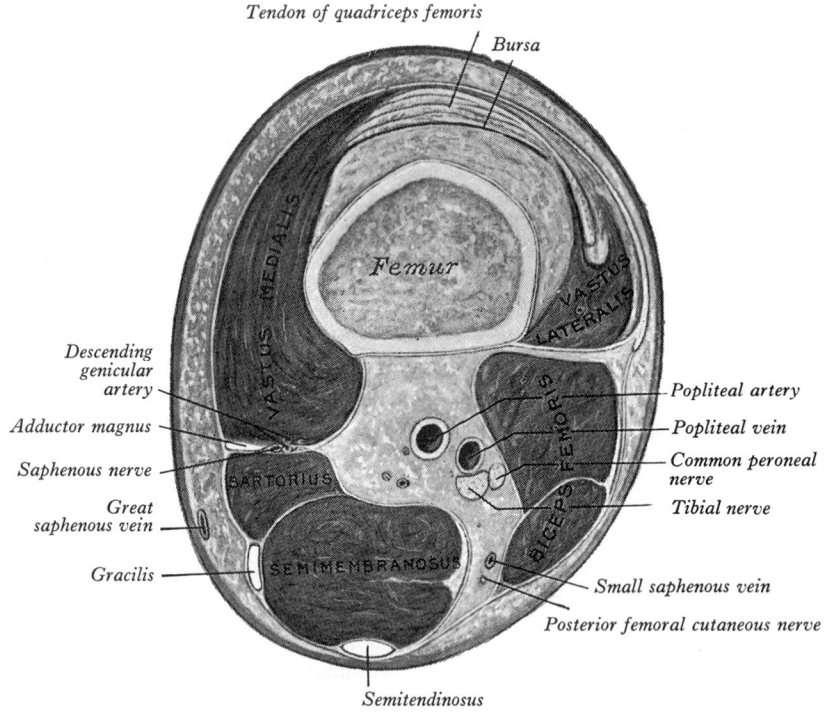

Tendon of quadriceps femoris

Bursa

Femur

VASTUS MEDIALIS

VASTUS LATERALIS

Descending genicular artery

Adductor magnus

Saphenous nerve

Great saphenous vein

Gracilis

SARTORIUS

SEMIMEMBRANOSUS

BICEPS FEMORIS

Popliteal artery

Popliteal vein

Common peroneal nerve

Tibial nerve

Small saphenous vein

Posterior femoral cutaneous nerve

Semitendinosus

7.131B Transverse section through the right thigh, about 4 cm superior to the adductor tubercle of the femur: proximal (superior) aspect.

rounded tendon of the distal attachment. The tendon divides at the level of the knee into five components, the main one being attached to a tubercle (sometimes called the *tuberculum tendinis*) on the posterior aspect of the medial tibial condyle (Cave & Porteous 1958). The other components are: a series of slips to the medial margin of the tibia, immediately behind the tibial collateral ligament; a thin fibrous expansion to the fascia over popliteus; a cord-like tendon to the inferior lip and adjacent part of the groove on the back of the medial tibial condyle, deep to the tibial collateral ligament; and a strong expansion which passes obliquely upward to the femoral intercondylar line and lateral femoral condyle, and forms much of the *oblique popliteal ligament* of the knee joint. The muscle overlaps the popliteal vessels and is itself partly overlapped by semitendinosus throughout its extent (**7.127**). (The distal tendons of semitendinosus and semimembranosus form the medial 'hamstring'.)

Variations. Semimembranosus varies considerably in size, and may be absent. It may be double, arising mainly from the sacrotuberous ligament. Slips to the femur or adductor magnus may occur.

Blood supply. **Ischial attachment and proximal part**: obturator artery, posterior branch (p. 1560); inferior gluteal artery and cruciate

anastomosis (p. 1567). **Central part**: first to fourth perforating arteries and longitudinal anastomotic chain (p. 1567); superior muscular branches of popliteal artery (p. 1569). **Insertion**: medial superior and medial inferior genicular arteries, and anastomoses of the latter with the anterior tibial recurrent artery and saphenous branch of the descending genicular artery (p. 1568).

Nerve supply. Sciatic nerve, L5, **S1** and 2, through its tibial division. The detailed intramuscular distributions of the nerves supplying the posterior femoral muscles have been described by Himstedt et al (1974).

Actions. Acting from above, the posterior femoral muscles flex the knee. Acting from below, they extend the hip joint, pulling the trunk upright from a stooping posture against the influence of gravity; the biceps is the most active in this. When the knee is semiflexed, biceps femoris can act as a lateral rotator, and the semimembranosus and semitendinosus as medial rotators, of the lower leg on the thigh at the knee. When the hip is extended, biceps is a lateral rotator, and semimembranosus and semitendinosus are medial rotators, of the thigh. As is the case with quadriceps femoris, the adductors and gluteus maximus, the hamstrings are quiescent in easy symmetrical standing. However, any action which takes the centre of gravity in front of a transverse axis through the hip joints—for example, forward reaching, forward sway at the angle joints, or forward bending at the hips—is immediately accompanied by strong contraction of the hamstrings. (This is in marked contrast to gluteus maximus, which contracts only when there is a call for powerful extension at the hip joint.)

When the knee is flexed against resistance, the tendon of biceps can be felt lateral to the popliteal fossa. Medial to the fossa, the tendons of gracilis (which is the more medial) and semitendinosus stand out sharply, and in the interval between them (and also by deep pressure from a 'pincer' grip beyond their margins) the semimembranosus tendon is just palpable.

There is some evidence that semimembranosus, semitendinosus and biceps femoris, although they cross both hip and knee joints, may produce movement at one of these joints without resisting antagonists at the other (Markee et al 1955). Usually, however, each of these muscles contracts as a whole, and whether or not movement takes place at hip or knee is determined by other muscles that act as fixators of these joints.

Clinical relevance. In disease of the knee joint, contracture of the flexor tendons is a frequent complication; this causes flexion of the leg, and a partial dislocation of the tibia backwards, with slight lateral rotation, probably due to biceps femoris. When the flexor tendons require surgical manipulation it is important to remember the close relationship of the common peroneal nerve to the medial border of the biceps femoris tendon. The flexors, when relaxed, show considerable variation in length and in some individuals the muscles are so short that they impose a serious limitation on flexion of the trunk at the hip joints when the knees are kept extended. Movements such as stooping must then be accomplished by flexing the vertebral column or squatting.

MUSCLES OF THE LEG

This group consists basically of an anterior set of extensor muscles, which produce dorsiflexion of the foot, a posterior set of flexor muscles, which produce plantar flexion, and a lateral set of muscles derived from the extensors, the peronei. The greater bulk of the muscles in the calf is consistent with the powerful propulsive role of the plantar flexors in walking and running.

Fascia cruris

The fascia cruris (Latin: *crus* = leg or shin), the deep fascia of the leg, is continuous with the fascia lata, and is attached around the knee to the patella, the ligamentum patellae, the tubercle and condyles of the tibia, and the head of the fibula. Posteriorly, it forms the popliteal fascia that covers the popliteal fossa; here it is strengthened by transverse fibres and perforated by the small saphenous vein. It receives lateral expansions from the tendon of biceps femoris, and multiple medial expansions from the tendons of sartorius, gracilis, semitendinosus and semimembranosus. It blends with the periosteum on the subcutaneous surface of the tibia and the head and malleolus of the fibula. It is continuous below with the extensor and flexor retinacula (pp. 888–889). It is thick and dense in the proximal and anterior part of the leg, and some fibres of tibialis anterior and extensor digitorum longus are attached to its deep surface; it is thinner posteriorly, where it covers gastrocnemius and soleus. On the lateral side it is continuous with the intermuscular septa of the lower leg, the *anterior* and *posterior crural intermuscular septa*, which are attached respectively to the anterior and posterior borders of the fibula; the fascia also has several slender extensions which enclose individual muscles. A broad, transverse, intermuscular septum, the *deep transverse fascia of the leg*, passes between the superficial and deep muscles in the calf. These named sheets, united to one another and to bone, form a kind of auxiliary, connective tissue 'skeleton'.

MUSCLES OF THE LEG—ANTERIOR GROUP

The anterior group (**7.132**) consists of: a common digital extensor, an extensor of the hallux, and two muscles—tibialis anterior and peroneus tertius—whose actions include dorsiflexion of the foot.

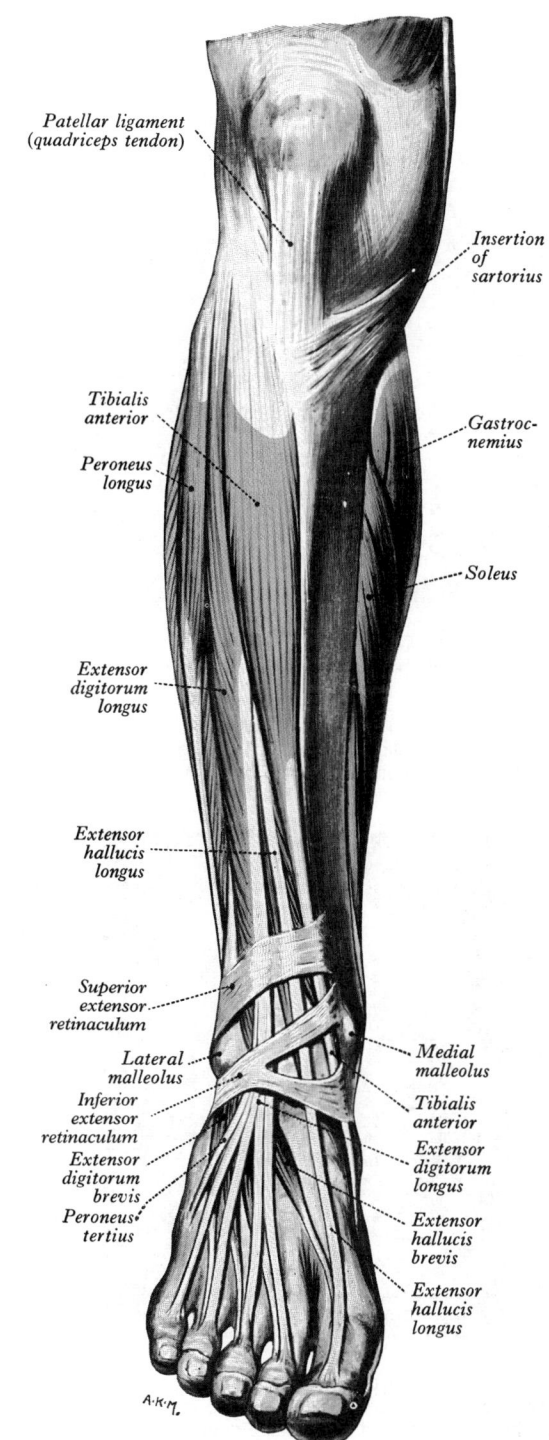

7.132 Muscles of the right leg: anterior aspect (from Quain's *Anatomy*, 11th edn).

Tibialis anterior

Tibialis anterior (**7.132, 133A, B**) is a superficial muscle and is therefore readily palpable lateral to the tibia. It arises from the lateral condyle and proximal half to two-thirds of the lateral surface of the tibial shaft, from the adjoining anterior surface of the interosseous membrane, from the deep surface of the fascia cruris and from the intermuscular septum between it and extensor digitorum longus. The muscle descends vertically to end in a tendon on its anterior surface in the lower third of the leg; this passes through the medial compartments of the superior and inferior retinacula, inclines medially, and inserts into the medial and inferior surfaces of the medial cuneiform and the adjoining part of the base of the first metatarsal bone (**7.135**). The muscle overlaps the anterior tibial vessels and deep peroneal nerve in the upper part of the leg.

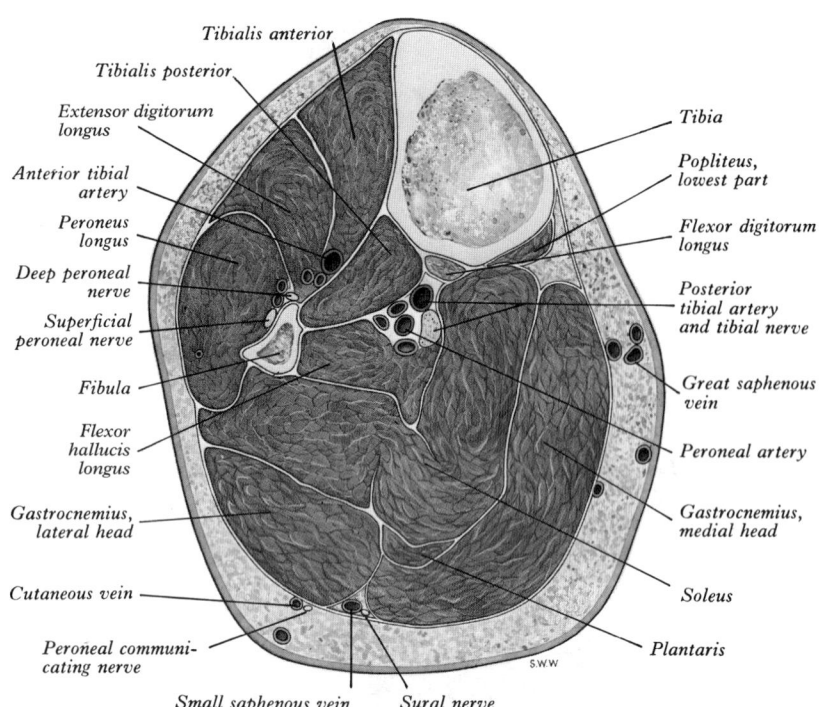

7.133A Transverse section through the right leg, about 10 cm distal to the knee joint: proximal (superior) aspect.

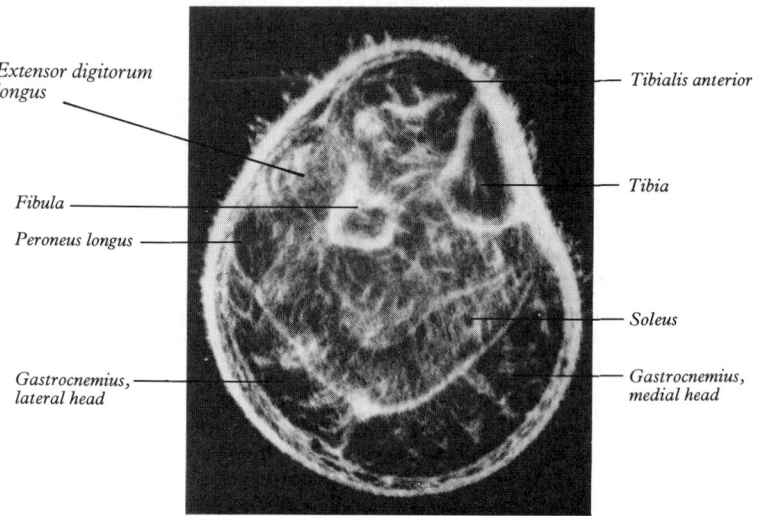

7.133B Transverse ultrasonic scan of the right leg of an adult man, at a level similar to that of the section illustrated in 7.133A: proximal aspect. (Supplied by H-D Rott and Siemens, Erlangen; photography by Sarah Smith.)

Variations. Attachments to the talus, first metatarsal head, or base of the proximal phalanx of the hallux have been recorded.

Blood supply. Numerous direct branches of the anterior tibial artery (p. 1570); anterior tibial recurrent artery (p. 1571). **Tendon**: anterior medial malleolar artery and network (p. 1571); arteria dorsalis pedis (p. 1572); medial tarsal arteries (p. 1572); posterior tibial artery, medial malleolar and calcaneal branches (pp. 1572–1573).

Nerve supply. Deep peroneal nerve, L4 and 5.

Actions. Tibialis anterior is a dorsiflexor of the ankle (tibiotalar) joint and invertor of the foot. It is most active when both movements are combined, as in walking. Its tendon can be seen through the skin lateral to the anterior border of the tibia and can be traced downwards and medially across the front of the ankle to the medial side of the foot. It elevates the first metatarsal base and medial cuneiform and rotates their dorsal aspects laterally.

The muscle is usually quiescent in a standing subject, since the weight of the body acts through a vertical line that passes anterior to the ankle joints. Acting from below, it helps to counteract any tendency to overbalance backwards by flexing the leg forwards at the ankle. It has a role in supporting the medial longitudinal arch of the foot, and although electromyographic activity is minimal during standing, it is manifest during any movement which increases the arch, such as toe-off in walking and running.

Extensor hallucis longus

Extensor hallucis longus (7.132, 134) lies between, and partly deep to, tibialis anterior and extensor digitorum longus. It arises from the middle half of the medial surface of the fibula, medial to extensor digitorum longus, and to a similar extent from the adjacent anterior surface of the interosseous membrane. The anterior tibial vessels and deep peroneal nerve lie between it and tibialis anterior. Its fibres run distally and end in a tendon which forms on the anterior border of the muscle. The tendon passes deep to the superior extensor retinaculum and through the inferior extensor retinaculum, crosses to the medial side of the anterior tibial vessels near the ankle, and inserts into the dorsal aspect of the base of the distal phalanx of the hallux. At the metatarsophalangeal joint a thin prolongation from each side of the tendon covers the dorsal surface of the joint. An expansion from the medial side of the tendon to the base of the proximal phalanx is usually present.

Variations. The muscle is sometimes united with extensor digitorum longus; it may send a slip into the second toe.

Blood supply. Numerous direct branches of the anterior tibial artery (p. 1570); anterior medial malleolar artery and network (p. 1571); arteria dorsalis pedis (p. 1572); first dorsal metatarsal artery (p. 1572), sometimes supplemented by proximal and distal perforating arteries from the sole; medial and lateral hallucial dorsal digital arteries (p. 1572); in some cases, perforating branch of peroneal artery (p. 1573).

Nerve supply. Deep peroneal nerve, L5.

Actions. Extensor hallucis longus extends the phalanges of the hallux and dorsiflexes the foot. When the hallux is actively extended, relatively little external force is required to overcome the extension of the distal phalanx, whereas considerable force is needed to overcome the extension of the proximal phalanx. When these movements are resisted, the tendon can be seen and felt on the lateral side of the tendon of tibialis anterior.

Extensor digitorum longus

Extensor digitorum longus (7.132, 133A, B, 134) is a pennate muscle that arises from the lateral condyle of the tibia, the proximal three-quarters of the medial surface of the fibula, the adjacent anterior surface of the interosseous membrane, the deep surface of the fascia cruris, the anterior crural intermuscular septum, and the septum between it and tibialis anterior; these origins form the walls of an osteo-aponeurotic tunnel. In the upper part of the leg the anterior tibial vessels and deep peroneal nerve lie between the muscle and tibialis anterior; at a lower level, extensor hallucis longus also comes between them. Extensor digitorum longus becomes tendinous at about the same level as tibialis anterior, and the tendon passes behind the superior extensor retinaculum and within a loop of the inferior extensor retinaculum (p. 889) with peroneus tertius (7.139, 140). It divides into four slips, which run forward on the dorsum of the foot and are attached in the same way as the tendons of extensor digitorum in the hand (pp. 849–850). At the metatarsophalangeal joints the tendons to the second, third and fourth toes are each joined on the lateral side by a tendon of extensor digitorum brevis. The *dorsal digital expansion* thus formed on the dorsal aspect of the proximal phalanx, like that on the fingers, receives contributions from the lumbrical and interosseous muscles (p. 860). The expansion narrows as it approaches a proximal interphalangeal joint, and divides into three slips: an intermediate slip, attached to the base of the middle phalanx, and two collateral slips, which reunite on the dorsum of the middle phalanx and are attached to the base of the distal phalanx.

Variations. The tendons to the second and fifth toes are sometimes doubled. There may be accessory slips attached to metatarsals or to the hallux.

Blood supply. Direct branches of the anterior tibial artery (p. 1570); anterior lateral malleolar artery and network (pp. 1571–1572), the latter joined by lateral tarsal branches of arteria dorsalis pedis (p. 1572); second to fourth dorsal metatarsal arteries (p. 1572), supplemented by proximal and distal perforating arteries from the sole (p. 1572); dorsal digital arteries of the second and fourth toes (p. 1572); perforating branch of peroneal artery, joining lateral anterior malleolar and lateral tarsal artery (p. 1572).

Nerve supply. Deep peroneal nerve, **L5**, S1.

Actions. Extensor digitorum longus extends the toes, and dorsiflexes the foot synergistically with tibialis anterior and extensor hallucis longus. Acting with the latter it tautens the plantar aponeurosis (p. 893).

Peroneus tertius

Peroneus tertius (**7.**132, 134, 140) is part of extensor digitorum longus, and might be described as its fifth tendon. The muscle fibres that operate on this tendon arise from the distal third or more of the medial surface of the fibula, the adjoining anterior surface of the interosseous membrane and the anterior crural intermuscular septum. The tendon passes behind the superior extensor retinaculum and within the loop of the inferior extensor retinaculum that it shares with extensor digitorum longus (**7.**139, 140). It inserts into the medial part of the dorsal surface of the base of the fifth metatarsal bone, but a thin expansion usually extends forwards along the medial border of the shaft of the leg.

Variations. The muscle is highly variable, but is completely absent only in about 4.4% of cases (Werneck 1957).

Blood supply. Direct branches of the anterior tibial artery (p. 1570); anterior lateral malleolar artery and network (pp. 1571–1572); lateral tarsal artery (p. 1572), joining the anterior lateral malleolar artery; perforating branch of the peroneal artery (p. 1573); termination of the arcuate artery (p. 1572); fourth dorsal metacarpal artery (p. 1572), supplemented by proximal and distal perforating arteries from the sole (p. 1575).

Nerve supply. Deep peroneal nerve, L5, S1.

Actions. During the swing phase of gait (**7.**149), electromyographic studies show that peroneus tertius acts with extensor digitorum longus and tibialis anterior to produce dorsiflexion and eversion of the foot (Jungers et al 1993). This levels the foot and helps the toes to clear the ground, an action that improves the economy of bipedal walking. Peroneus tertius is not active during stance phase, a finding that contradicts suggestions that it acts primarily to support the lateral longitudinal arch or to transfer the foot's centre of pressure medially.

Clinical relevance. The common peroneal nerve is easily traumatized at the fibular neck. The resultant loss of function, particularly of the major dorsiflexors of the foot, produces 'foot-drop'. Affected patients will circumduct at the hip when walking, in order to avoid tripping over their toes.

MUSCLES OF THE LEG—LATERAL GROUP

The lateral group of leg muscles consists of peroneus longus and peroneus brevis, both evertors of the foot.

Peroneus longus

Peroneus longus (**7.**132, 133A, B, 134, 136, 137), the more superficial of the two muscles, arises from the head and proximal two-thirds of the lateral surface of the fibula, from the deep surface of the fascia cruris, from the anterior and posterior crural intermuscular septa, and occasionally by a few fibres from the lateral condyle of the tibia. Between its attachments to the head and shaft of the fibula there is a gap through which the common peroneal nerve passes. The muscle belly ends in a long tendon, which runs distally behind the lateral malleolus in a groove shared with the tendon of peroneus brevis. The groove is converted into a canal by the superior peroneal retinaculum, so that the tendon of peroneus longus, and that of peroneus brevis which lies behind it, are contained in a common synovial sheath (**7.**140). The peroneus longus tendon runs obliquely forwards across the lateral side of the calcaneus, below the peroneal trochlea and the tendon of peroneus brevis, and beneath the inferior peroneal retinaculum (p. 889). It crosses the lateral side of the cuboid, and then runs under it in a groove converted into a canal by the long plantar ligament (**6.**347). It crosses the sole of the foot obliquely, and is attached by two slips to the lateral side of the base of the first

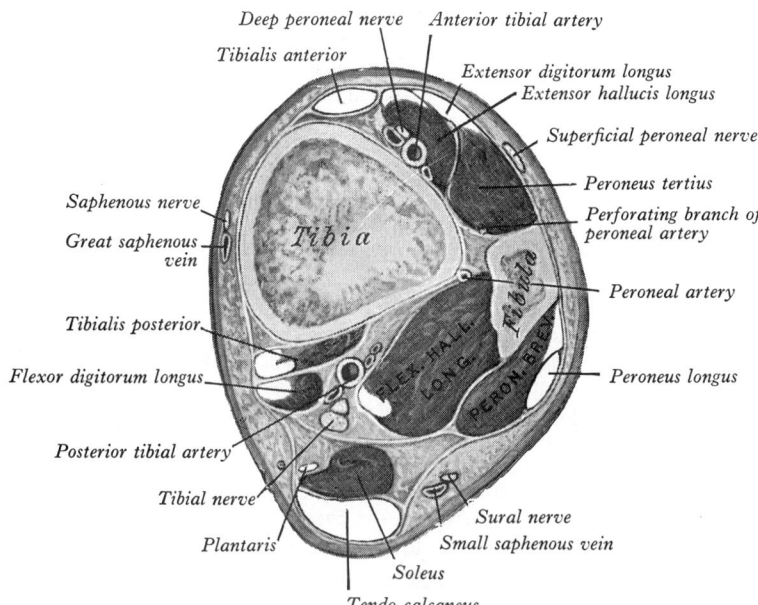

7.134 Transverse section through the right leg, about 6 cm superior to the tip of the medial malleolus: proximal (superior) aspect.

metatarsal bone and the medial cuneiform; occasionally a third slip is extended to the base of the second metatarsal bone. The tendon changes direction at two points:

- below the lateral malleolus
- on the cuboid bone.

At both sites it is thickened and at the second a sesamoid fibrocartilage (sometimes a bone) usually develops within it. A second synovial sheath invests the tendon as it crosses the sole of the foot.

Variations. Tendinous slips may extend to the base of the third, fourth or fifth metatarsal bone, or to adductor hallucis. Fusion of peroneus longus and brevis can occur, but is rare.

Blood supply. **Proximal end**: variably supplied by: inferior lateral genicular artery (p. 1570); stem of anterior and posterior tibial arteries (pp. 1570, 1572); anterior and posterior tibial recurrent artery (p. 1571); circumflex fibular artery (p. 1573). **Main belly**: peroneal artery directly, its perforating branch joining the anterior lateral malleolar artery (pp. 1571, 1572). **Tendon**: peroneal perforating artery with anterior lateral malleolar artery (pp. 1571, 1572); lateral calcaneal artery (p. 1573); lateral tarsal artery (p. 1572); lateral plantar artery and its branches (p. 1574); medial plantar artery (p. 1574).

Nerve supply. Superficial peroneal nerve, L5, S1.

Actions. There is little doubt that peroneus longus can evert and plantar-flex the foot, and possibly act on the leg from its distal attachments. The oblique direction of its tendon across the sole would also enable it to support the longitudinal and transverse arches of the foot. How are these potentialities actually deployed in movement? With the foot off the ground, eversion is visually and palpably associated with increased prominence of both tendon and muscle. It is not clear to what extent this helps to maintain plantigrade contact of the foot in standing, but electromyographic records show little or no peroneal activity under these conditions. On the other hand, peroneus longus and brevis come strongly into action to maintain the concavity of the foot during toe-off and tip-toeing. If the subject deliberately sways to one side, the peronei contract on that side, but their involvement in postural activity between the foot and leg remains uncertain.

Peroneus brevis

Peroneus brevis (**7.**134, 136, 137) arises from the distal two-thirds of the lateral surface of the fibula, anterior to peroneus longus, and from the anterior and posterior crural intermuscular septa. It passes vertically downwards and ends in a tendon which passes behind the lateral malleolus together with, but anterior to, that of peroneus longus, the two tendons running deep to the superior peroneal

883

retinaculum in a common synovial sheath (p. 891). It then runs forwards on the lateral side of the calcaneus above the peroneal trochlea and the tendon of peroneus longus, to insert into a tubercle on the base of the fifth metatarsal bone, on its lateral side.

On the lateral surface of the calcaneus the tendons of peronei longus and brevis occupy separate osseo-aponeurotic canals formed by the calcaneus and the inferior peroneal retinaculum; each tendon is enveloped in a separate forward prolongation of the common synovial sheath (7.140).

Blood supply. Peroneal artery directly, its perforating branch joining the anterior lateral malleolar artery (p. 1571). **Tendon**: peroneal perforating artery with anterior lateral malleolar artery (p. 1571); lateral calcaneal artery (p. 1573, **10**.150); lateral tarsal artery (p. 1572); lateral plantar artery and its branches (p. 1574); tip of arcuate artery (**10**.150).

Nerve supply. Superficial peroneal nerve, L5, S1.

Action. Peroneus brevis may limit inversion of the foot and so relieve strain on the ligaments that are tightened by this movement (lateral part of interosseous talocalcanean, lateral talocalcanean and calcaneofibular). It participates in eversion of the foot and may help to steady the leg on the foot (but see above, peroneus longus—Actions).

MUSCLES OF THE CALF—SUPERFICIAL GROUP

The muscles in the posterior compartment of the lower leg form superficial and deep groups, separated by the deep transverse fascia (p. 886).

Muscles of the superficial group (7.136)—gastrocnemius, plantaris and soleus—form the bulk of the calf. They constitute a powerful muscular mass, whose main function is plantar flexion of the foot. Their large size is one of the most characteristic features of the musculature of man, being related directly to his upright stance and mode of progression. Gastrocnemius and plantaris act on both knee and ankle joints, soleus on the latter alone.

Gastrocnemius

Gastrocnemius (7.133A, B, 135, 136) is the most superficial muscle of the group, and forms the 'belly' of the calf. It arises by two heads, which are connected to the condyles of the femur by strong, flat tendons. The medial and larger head is attached to a depression at the upper and posterior part of the medial condyle behind the adductor tubercle, and to a slightly raised area on the popliteal surface of the femur just above the medial condyle. The lateral head is attached to a recognizable area on the lateral surface of the lateral condyle and to the lower part of the corresponding supracondylar line. Both heads also arise from subjacent areas of the capsule of the knee joint. The tendinous attachments expand to cover the posterior surface of each head with an aponeurosis, from the anterior surface of which the muscle fibres arise. The fleshy part of the muscle extends to about midcalf, the muscle fibres of the larger medial head extending lower than those of the lateral head. As the muscle descends, the muscle fibres begin to insert into a broad aponeurosis that develops on its anterior surface; up to this point the muscular masses of the two heads remain separate. The aponeurosis gradually contracts and receives the tendon of soleus on its deep surface to form the *tendo calcaneus* or *tendon of Achilles* (see below).

Variations. On occasion the lateral head, or the whole muscle, is absent. A more frequent variation is a third head, arising from the popliteal surface of the femur.

Relations. Proximally, the heads of gastrocnemius form the lower boundaries of the popliteal fossa. The lateral head is partially overlaid by the tendon of biceps femoris, the medial head by semimembranosus. Over the rest of its length the muscle is superficial, and the two heads can easily be seen in the living subject. The *superficial surface* of the muscle is separated by the fascia cruris from the small saphenous vein and the peroneal communicating and sural nerves; the common peroneal nerve crosses the lateral head of the muscle, partly under cover of biceps femoris. The *deep surface* lies posterior to the oblique popliteal ligament, popliteus, soleus, plantaris, popliteal vessels and the tibial nerve. A bursa, which sometimes communicates with the knee joint, is located anterior to the tendon of the medial head. The tendon of the lateral head sometimes contains a fibrocartilaginous or bony sesamoid where it

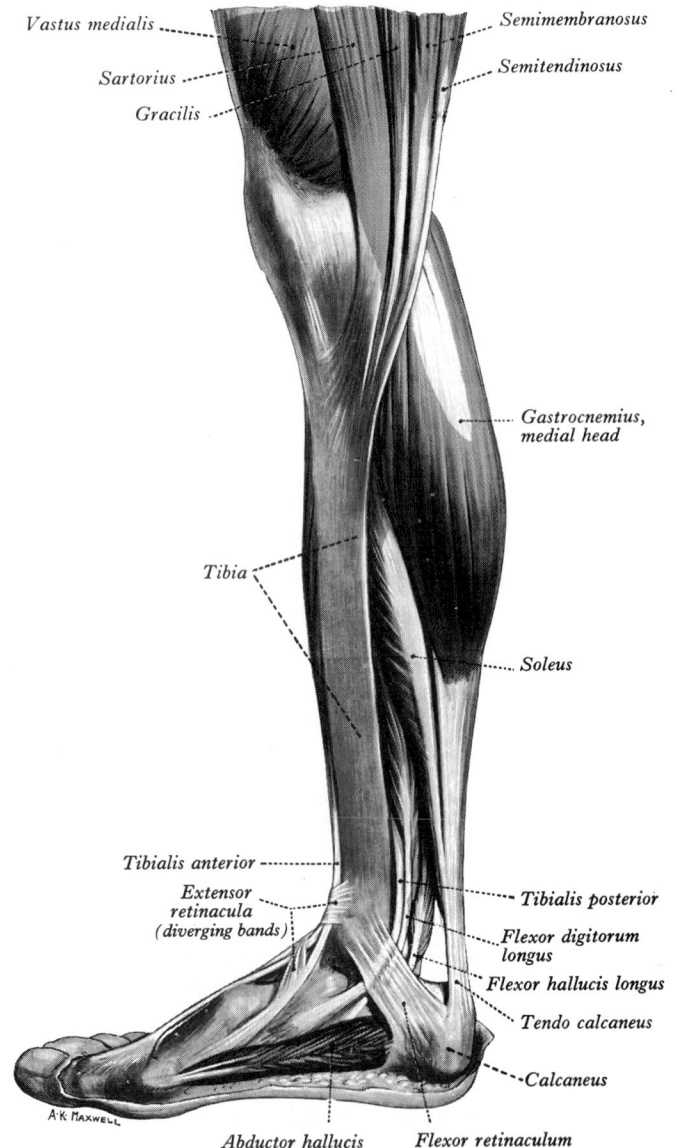

7.135   Muscles of the right leg: medial aspect.

plays over the lateral femoral condyle; occasionally one is also present in the tendon of the medial head.

Blood supply. Sural arteries, from the popliteal artery (p. 1569); medial and lateral inferior genicular arteries (pp. 1569, 1570); posterior tibial artery (p. 1572); peroneal artery (p. 1573) and its upper and lower communicating branches. **Tendon**: anterior and posterior, medial and lateral malleolar arteries (**10**.150); calcanean branches of posterior tibial, peroneal and lateral plantar arteries (**10**.150).

Nerve supply. Tibial nerve, S1 and **2**.

Actions. Considered with soleus, below.

Soleus

Soleus (7.133A, B, 135, 136, 137) is a broad flat muscle situated immediately deep or anterior to gastrocnemius. It arises from the posterior surface of the head and proximal quarter of the shaft of the fibula, from the soleal line and the middle third of the medial border of the tibia, and from a fibrous band between the tibia and fibula which arches over the popliteal vessels and tibial nerve. This origin is aponeurotic, and most of the muscular fibres arise from its posterior surface and pass obliquely to the tendon of insertion, which is on the posterior surface of the muscle. Other muscle fibres arise from the anterior surface of the aponeurosis; they are short, oblique and bipennate in arrangement, and converge on a narrow, central intramuscular tendon which merges distally with the principal tendon. The latter gradually becomes thicker and narrower, and joins with the tendon of gastrocnemius to form the tendo calcaneus

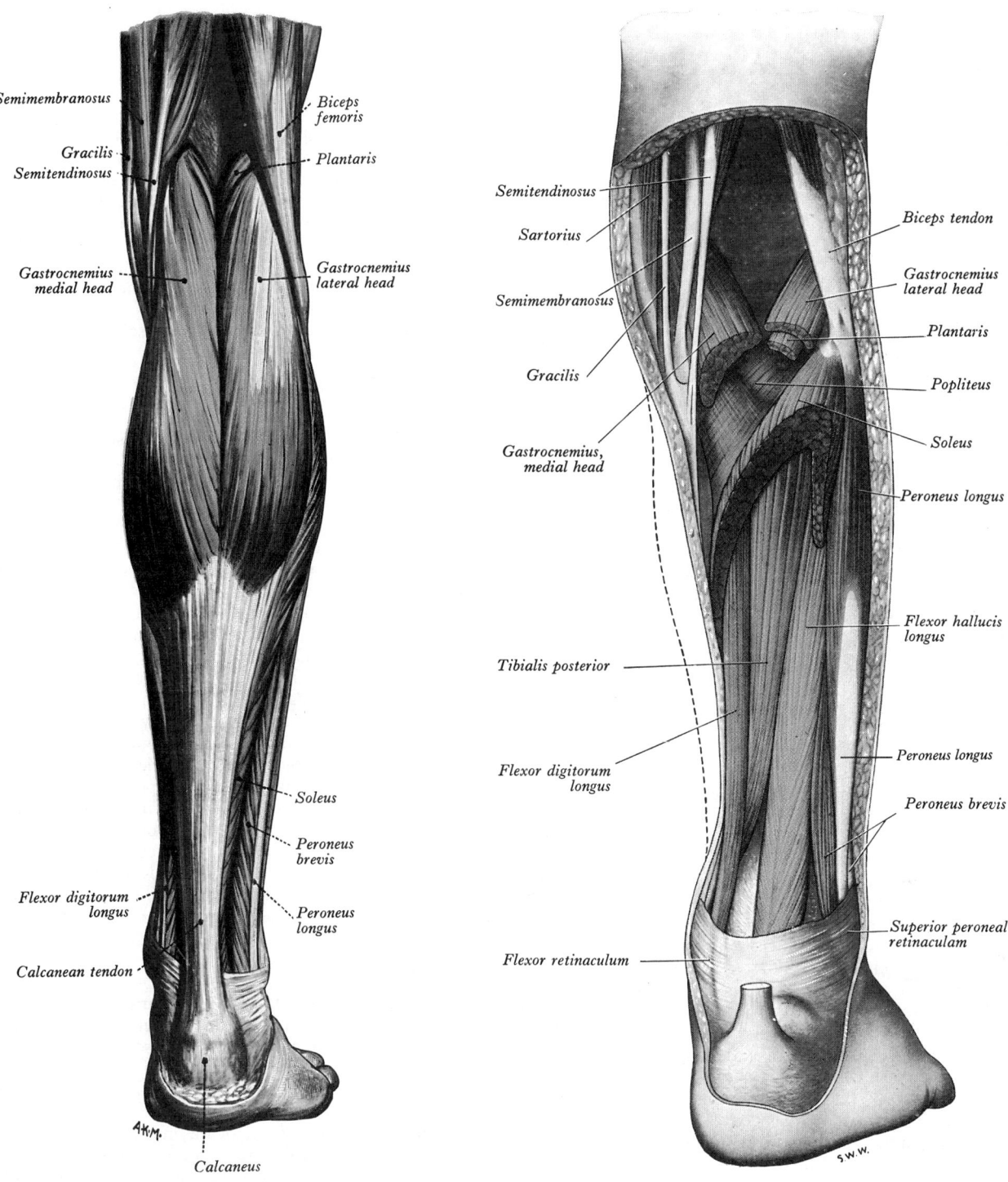

7.136 Muscles of the right calf: superficial group (from Quain's *Anatomy*, 11th edn).

7.137 Muscles of the right calf, deep group, in a child aged eight years.

(see below). The muscle is covered proximally by gastrocnemius, but below midcalf it is broader than the tendon of gastrocnemius and is accessible on both sides—a convenient feature for studies by biopsy, electromyography or nuclear magnetic resonance spectroscopy, for example.

Relations. The **superficial surface** of soleus is in contact with gastrocnemius and plantaris; its **deep surface** is related to flexor digitorum longus, flexor hallucis longus, tibialis posterior and the posterior tibial vessels and tibial nerve, from all of which it is separated by the deep transverse fascia of the leg.

Blood supply. Sural arteries, from the popliteal artery (p. 1569); posterior tibial artery (p. 1572) and peroneal artery (p. 1573) and upper and lower communicating arteries between them. **Tendon:** anterior and posterior, medial and lateral malleolar arteries (**10.**150);

calcanean branches of posterior tibial, peroneal and lateral plantar arteries (**10.**150).

Nerve supply. Two branches from the tibial nerve, S1 and 2.

Actions. The two heads of gastrocnemius, together with soleus, form a tripartite muscular mass sharing the tendo calcaneus, and hence sometimes termed the *triceps surae*. These muscles are the chief plantar flexors of the foot, and the gastrocnemius is also a flexor of the knee. They are usually large and correspondingly powerful.

Gastrocnemius provides force for propulsion in walking, running and leaping. Soleus is said to be more concerned with steadying the leg on the foot in standing. This postural role is also suggested by its high content of slow, fatigue-resistant (Type 1) muscle fibres (see The fibre types of adult skeletal muscle, pp. 753–756); in the soleus

885

muscle of many adult mammals the proportion of this type of fibre approaches 100%. In man, at least, such a rigid separation of functional roles seems unlikely; soleus probably participates in locomotion, and gastrocnemius in posture. Nevertheless, the talotibial joint is loose-packed in the erect posture, and since the weight of the body acts through a vertical line that passes anterior to the ankle joint, a strong brace is required behind the joint to maintain stability. Electromyography shows that these forces are supplied mainly by soleus: during symmetrical standing, soleus is continuously active, whereas gastrocnemius is recruited only intermittently (Joseph et al 1955; Joseph 1960). The relative contributions of soleus and gastrocnemius to phasic activity of the triceps surae in walking has yet to be analysed satisfactorily.

Tendo calcaneus

The *tendo calcaneus* or *Achilles tendon* (**7.135, 136**) is the thickest and strongest tendon in the human body. It is about 15 cm long, and begins near the middle of the calf, but its anterior surface receives muscle fibres from soleus almost to its lower end. It gradually becomes more rounded to about 4 cm above the calcaneus; below this it expands and becomes attached to the posterior surface of the calcaneus at its midlevel. A bursa usually separates the tendon from the upper part of the bony surface. The tendon fibres spiral laterally through 90° as they descend, so that the fibres associated with gastrocnemius come to insert on the bone more laterally, and those associated with soleus more medially. The tendon plays an important part in reducing the energy cost of locomotion by storing energy elastically and releasing it at a subsequent point in the gait cycle (see Standing and walking and Running, pp. 898).

Plantaris

Plantaris (**7.136, 137**) arises from the lower part of the lateral supracondylar line and the oblique popliteal ligament. Its small fusiform belly is 7 to 10 cm long and ends in a long slender tendon; this crosses obliquely between gastrocnemius and soleus, runs distally along the medial border of the tendo calcaneus, and fuses or inserts with it.

Variations. The muscle is sometimes double. It is absent in about 10% of cases (Daseler & Anson 1943). Occasionally, its tendon merges with the flexor retinaculum (p. 891) or with the fascia of the leg.

Blood supply. Sural arteries, from the popliteal artery (p. 1569); posterior tibial artery (p. 1572) and peroneal artery (p. 1573) and upper and lower communicating arteries between them. **Tendon:** anterior and posterior, medial and lateral malleolar arteries (**10.150**); calcanean branches of posterior tibial, peroneal and lateral plantar arteries (**10.150**).

Nerve supply. Tibial nerve, often from the ramus that supplies the lateral head of gastrocnemius, S1 and 2.

Actions. Plantaris is the lower limb's equivalent of palmaris longus: in many mammals it is well developed and inserts directly or indirectly into the plantar aponeurosis. In man the muscle is almost vestigial and normally inserts well short of the plantar aponeurosis, usually into the calcaneus. It is therefore presumed to act with gastrocnemius.

MUSCLES OF THE CALF—DEEP GROUP

The deep flexors of the calf (**7.135, 137**) include one, popliteus, which acts on the knee joint; the others—flexor hallucis longus, flexor digitorum longus and tibialis posterior—act on the ankle joint and other joints of the foot.

Deep transverse fascia

The deep transverse fascia of the leg is a fibrous stratum between the superficial and deep muscles of the calf that extends transversely from the medial margin of the tibia to the posterior border of the fibula. Proximally, where it is thick and dense, it is attached to the soleal ridge of the tibia and to the fibula, inferomedial to the attachment of soleus. Between these bony attachments it is continuous with fascia covering popliteus and receives an expansion from the tendon of semimembranosus. At intermediate levels it is thin, but distally, where it covers the tendons behind the malleoli, it

is again thick and continuous with the flexor and superior peroneal retinacula (p. 889).

Popliteus

Popliteus (**6.307, 7.137**) is a flat muscle that forms the floor of the lower part of the popliteal fossa. It arises within the capsule of the knee joint by a strong tendon, about 2.5 cm long, which is attached to a depression at the anterior end of the groove on the lateral aspect of the lateral condyle of the femur (**6.307**); medially this tendon is joined by collagenous fibres from the arcuate popliteal ligament (p. 702) and from the fibrous capsule adjacent to the lateral meniscus; there is also some attachment to the outer margin of the meniscus itself. Fleshy fibres expand from this point to form a somewhat triangular muscle which descends medially to insert into the medial two-thirds of the triangular area above the soleal line on the posterior surface of the tibia, and into the tendinous expansion that covers its surface.

Variations. An additional head may arise from the sesamoid in the lateral head of gastrocnemius.

Relations. The popliteal tendon is intracapsular and is overlapped by the fibular collateral ligament of the knee and the tendon of biceps femoris (**6.314**). Invested on its deep surface by synovial membrane, it grooves the posterior border of the lateral meniscus and the adjoining part of the tibia, and emerges inferior to the posterior band of the arcuate ligament (**6.307**). On the floor of the popliteal fossa it is covered by a strong layer of fascia derived mostly from the tendon of semimembranosus.

Blood supply. Popliteal artery, directly and via the sural arteries (p. 1569); medial and lateral inferior genicular arteries (p. 1570); posterior tibial recurrent artery (p. 1572).

Nerve supply. Tibial nerve, L4 and 5 and S1.

Actions. Popliteus rotates the tibia medially on the femur or, when the tibia is fixed, rotates the femur laterally on the tibia. It is usually regarded as the muscle that 'unlocks' the joint at the beginning of flexion of the fully extended knee, and electromyography supports this view. Its connection with the arcuate popliteal ligaments, fibrous capsule and lateral meniscus suggests that it may retract the posterior cornu of the meniscus during lateral rotation of the femur and flexion of the knee joint, protecting the meniscus from being crushed between the femur and the tibia during these movements (Last 1950). The muscle is markedly active in crouching, indicating that it may share the load on the posterior cruciate ligament in preventing forward dislocation of the femur.

Flexor hallucis longus

Flexor hallucis longus (**7.133A, 134, 137**) arises from the distal two-thirds of the posterior surface of the fibula (except for the lowest 2.5 cm or so), from the adjacent interosseous membrane and the posterior crural intermuscular septum, and from the fascia covering tibialis posterior, which it overlaps to a considerable extent. Its fibres pass obliquely down to a tendon that occupies nearly the whole length of the posterior aspect of the muscle. This tendon grooves the posterior surface of the lower end of the tibia, then successively the posterior surface of the talus and the **inferior** surface of the sustentaculum tali of the calcaneus (**7.138, 139**). The grooves on the talus and calcaneus are converted by fibrous bands into a canal, lined by a synovial sheath. Distal to this, in the sole of the foot, it crosses the flexor digitorum longus from the lateral to the medial side, curving obliquely **superior** to it; at the crossing point the long digital flexor receives a fibrous slip from the flexor hallucis longus tendon. The tendon then crosses the lateral part of flexor hallucis brevis to reach the interval between the sesamoid bones under the head of the first metatarsal. It continues on the plantar aspect of the hallux, running in an osseo-aponeurotic tunnel to be attached to the plantar aspect of the base of the distal phalanx. The tendon is retained in position over the lateral part of flexor hallucis brevis by the diverging stems of the distal band of the medial intermuscular septum.

Variations. The connecting slip to flexor digitorum longus varies in size; it usually continues into the tendons for the second and third toes, but is sometimes restricted to the second, and occasionally extends to the fourth.

Relations. **Superficial** are soleus and the tendo calcaneus, from which it is separated by the deep transverse fascia; **deep** are the fibula, tibialis posterior, the peroneal vessels, the distal part of the interosseous membrane and the tibiotalar joint; **lateral** are the peronei; **medial** are tibialis posterior, the posterior tibial vessels and the tibial nerve.

Blood supply. Posterior tibial (p. 1572) and peroneal (p. 1573) arteries, and upper and lower communicating arteries between them; anterior and posterior medial malleolar arteries and network (**10.**109, pp. 1571, 1572); medial tarsal arteries (p. 1572); medial plantar artery (p. 1573); first plantar metatarsal artery (p. 1574) and its hallucial plantar digital arteries.

Nerve supply. The tibial nerve, L5, **S1** and **2**.

Actions. Considered with flexor digitorum longus, below.

Flexor digitorum longus

Flexor digitorum longus (**7.**133A, 134, 135, 137) lies medial to flexor hallucis longus. It is thin and pointed proximally, but gradually widens as it descends. It arises from the posterior surface of the tibia medial to tibialis posterior from just below the soleal line to within 7 or 8 cm of the distal end of the bone; it also arises from the fascia covering tibialis posterior. The muscle ends in a tendon that extends along almost the whole of its posterior surface; this gradually crosses tibialis posterior and passes behind the medial malleolus, where it shares a groove with tibialis posterior but is separated from it by a fibrous septum, each tendon in its own compartment lined by a synovial sheath. It then curves obliquely forwards and laterally, in contact with the medial side of the sustentaculum tali (**7.**138), passes deep to the flexor retinaculum, and enters the sole of the foot (**7.**145). Here it crosses superficial to the tendon of flexor hallucis longus and receives a strong slip from it. It continues across the sole to form the whole of the long flexor tendon of the fifth toe and to contribute to those of the second, third and fourth toes. It may also send a slip to the tendon of flexor hallucis longus. The tendons of flexor accessorius insert into long flexor tendons of the second, third and fourth digits, and flexor hallucis longus makes a variable contribution through the connecting slip already mentioned. The long flexor tendons of the lateral four digits are attached to the plantar surfaces of the bases of their distal phalanges, each passing through a divarication in the corresponding tendon of flexor digitorum brevis at the base of the proximal phalanx (cf. the arrangement in the hand).

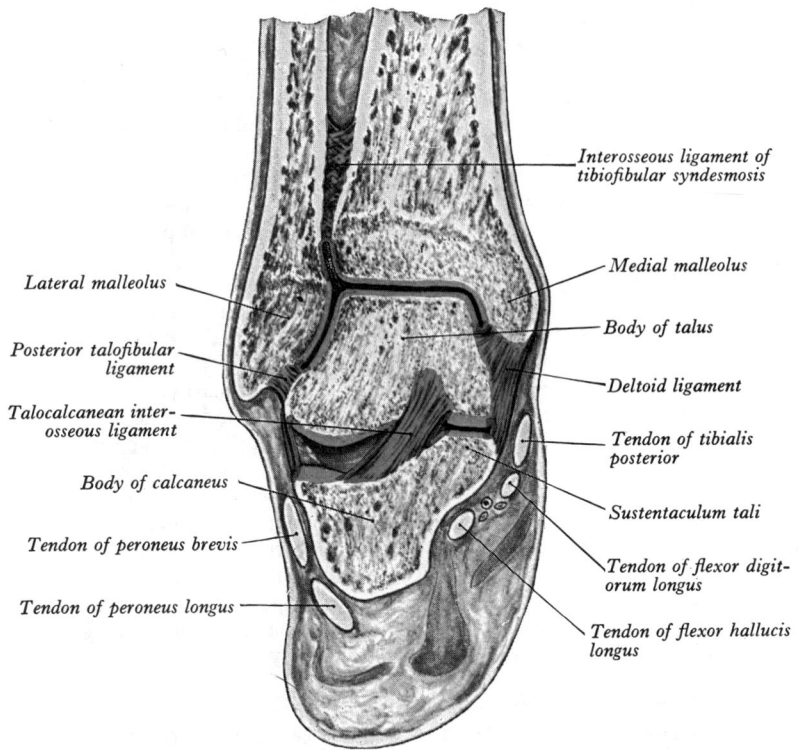

7.138 Coronal section through the left talocrural, talocalcanean and subtalar joints: posterior aspect. Ligaments are shown in green, articular cartilage in blue and synovial membrane in red.

Variations. The lateral head of flexor accessorius may be inserted into the lateral border of the flexor digitorum longus tendon.

Relations. In the leg the **superficial surface** of the muscle is in contact with the deep transverse fascia, which separates it from soleus and distally from the posterior tibial vessels and tibial nerve; its **deep surface** is related to the tibia and to tibialis posterior. In the

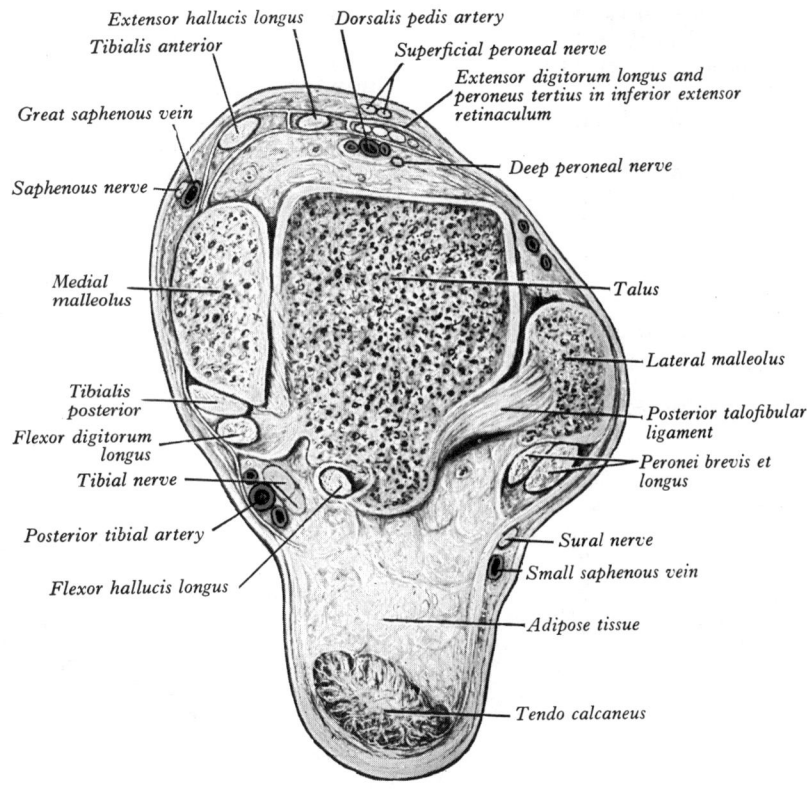

7.139 Horizontal section through the inferior part of the left talocrural joint: inferior (distal) aspect.

foot it is covered by abductor hallucis and flexor digitorum brevis and, as noted, crosses superficial to flexor hallucis longus.

Blood supply. Many direct branches from the posterior tibial artery (p. 1572, **10.**144); peroneal artery (p. 1573); upper and lower communicating arteries between posterior tibial and peroneal arteries; medial malleolar network and its tributaries (**10.**109, p. 1571); stem of medial plantar artery (p. 1573); lateral plantar artery and plantar arch (p. 1574); four plantar metatarsal arteries, (proximally three, distally four, perforating arteries, p. 1574); eight plantar digital arteries (to lateral four toes, p. 1574).

Nerve supply. The tibial nerve, L5, S1 and S2.

Actions. Both flexor hallucis longus and flexor digitorum longus can act as plantar flexors, but this action is weak compared with gastrocnemius and soleus. **When the foot is off the ground**, both muscles flex the phalanges of the toes, acting primarily on the distal phalanges. **When the foot is on the ground** and under load, they act synergistically with the small muscles of the foot and—especially in the case of flexor digitorum longus—with the lumbricals and interossei (p. 860) to maintain the pads of the toes in firm contact with the ground, enlarging the weight-bearing area and helping to stabilize the heads of the metatarsal bones, which form the fulcrum on which the body is propelled forwards. Activity in the long digital flexors is minimal during quiet standing, so they apparently contribute little to the static maintenance of the longitudinal arch, but during toe-off and tip-toe movements they become very active.

Tibialis posterior

Tibialis posterior (**7.**133A, 137) is the most deeply placed muscle of the flexor group. At its origin it lies between flexor hallucis longus and flexor digitorum longus, and is overlapped by both, but especially by the former. Its proximal attachment consists of two pointed processes, separated by an angular interval which is traversed by the anterior tibial vessels. The medial process arises from the posterior surface of the interosseous membrane, except at its most distal part, and from a lateral area on the posterior surface of the tibia between the soleal line above and the junction of the middle and lower thirds of the shaft below. The lateral part arises from a medial strip of the posterior fibular surface in its upper two-thirds. The muscle also arises from the deep transverse fascia, and from the intermuscular septa that separate it from adjacent muscles. In the distal quarter of the leg its tendon passes deep to that of flexor digitorum longus, with which it shares a groove behind the medial malleolus, each enclosed in a separate synovial sheath. It then passes deep to the flexor retinaculum (p. 889) and superficial to the deltoid ligament (**7.**138) to enter the foot. In the foot it is at first inferior to the plantar calcaneonavicular ligament, where it contains a sesamoid fibrocartilage. The tendon then divides into two. The more superficial, larger division, a direct continuation of the tendon, is attached to the tuberosity of the navicular, from which fibres continue to the inferior surface of the medial cuneiform. A tendinous band also

passes laterally and a little proximally to the tip and distal margin of the sustentaculum tali. The deeper, lateral division gives rise to the tendon of origin of the medial limb of flexor hallucis brevis, and then continues between this muscle and the navicular and medial cuneiform bones to end on the intermediate cuneiform and the bases of the second, third and fourth metatarsals, the slip to the fourth metatarsal being the strongest.

Variations. The slips to the metatarsals vary in number. Slips to the cuboid and lateral cuneiform have also been described (Lewis 1964b; see also **6.**349).

Relations. The **superficial surface** of the muscle is in relation to soleus, from which it is separated by the deep transverse fascia, and to flexor digitorum longus, flexor hallucis longus, the posterior tibial vessels, tibial nerve and the peroneal vessels. The **deep surface** is in contact with the interosseous membrane, tibia, fibula and tibiotalar joint.

Blood supply. Anterior tibial stem, at the most proximal part of the muscle (p. 1570); posterior tibial (p. 1572) and peroneal arteries (p. 1573), and upper and lower communicating branches between the two; medial malleolar network and its tributaries (p. 1571, **10.**109); medial plantar artery (p. 1573).

Nerve supply. Tibial nerve, L4 and 5.

Actions. Tibialis posterior is the principal invertor of the foot, although it may assist in vigorous plantar flexion. By reason of its insertions into the cuneiform bones and the bases of the metatarsals it has long been considered to assist in elevating the longitudinal arch of the foot, although electromyography shows that it is actually quiescent in standing. It is phasically active in walking, during which it probably acts with the intrinsic foot musculature and the lateral calf muscles to control the degree of pronation of the foot and the distribution of weight through the metatarsal heads. It is said that when the body is supported on one leg, the invertor action of tibialis posterior, exerted from below, helps to maintain balance by resisting any tendency to sway laterally. However, any act of balancing demands the co-operation of many muscles, including groups acting on the hip joints and vertebral column.

FASCIAE AND RETINACULA OF THE ANKLE JOINT

In the vicinity of the tibiotalar joint, the tendons of the muscles of the leg are bound down by localized thickenings of the deep fascia which constitute retinacular bands, comparable, in both form and function, with the retinacula of the wrist (p. 854). They consist of superior and inferior extensor, flexor, and peroneal retinacula.

Superior extensor retinaculum

The superior extensor retinaculum (**7.**132, 140) binds down the tendons of tibialis anterior, extensor hallucis longus, extensor digitorum longus and peroneus tertius immediately above the anterior aspect of the tibiotalar joint. The anterior tibial vessels and deep peroneal nerve also pass deep to the retinaculum. **Laterally**, it is attached to the distal end of the anterior border of the fibula;

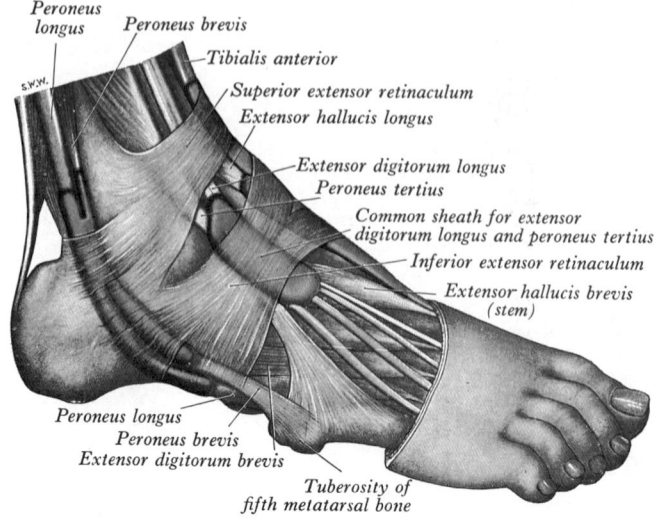

7.140 The synovial sheaths of the tendons of the right ankle: lateral aspect. The superior and inferior peroneal retinacula are not labelled.

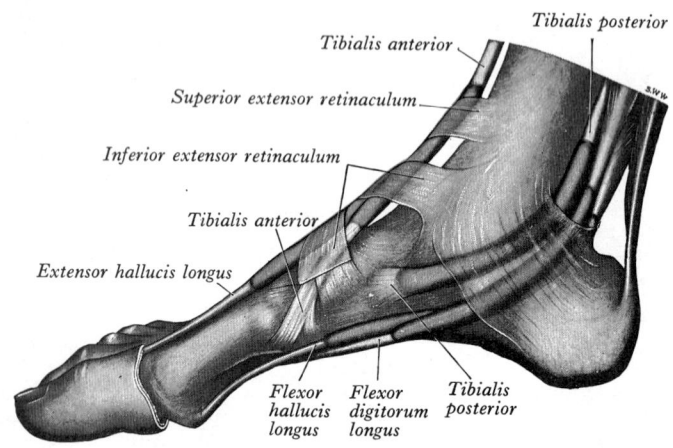

7.141 The synovial sheaths of the tendons of the right ankle: medial aspect.

medially, to the anterior border of the tibia. Its **proximal border** is continuous with the fascia cruris, and dense connective tissue of a similar type connects its **distal border** to the inferior extensor retinaculum. Only the tendon of tibialis anterior has a synovial sheath here (7.140).

Inferior extensor retinaculum

The inferior extensor retinaculum (7.132, 140) is a Y-shaped band lying anterior to the tibiotalar joint. The stem of the Y is at the lateral end, where it is attached to the upper surface of the calcaneus, in front of the sulcus calcanei. The band passes medially, forming a strong loop around the tendons of peroneus tertius and extensor digitorum longus (7.139). From the deep surface of the loop a band passes laterally behind the interosseous talocalcanean ligament and the cervical ligament and is attached to the sulcus calcanei (Stamm 1931). At the medial end of the loop the Y is completed by two diverging bands, which continue further medially. The more **proximal band** has two layers. The **deep** layer passes deep to the tendons of extensor hallucis longus and tibialis anterior, but superficial to the anterior tibial vessels and deep peroneal nerve, to reach the tibial malleolus. The **superficial** layer crosses superficial to the tendon of extensor hallucis longus and then adheres firmly to the deep one; in some cases it continues superficial to the tendon of tibialis anterior to reach the tibia. The more **distal band** extends downwards and medially and is attached to the plantar aponeurosis. It is superficial to the tendons of extensor hallucis longus and tibialis anterior, the arteria dorsalis pedis and the terminal branches of the deep peroneal nerve.

Flexor retinaculum

The flexor retinaculum (7.135, 141) is attached anteriorly to the tip of the medial malleolus, distal to which it is continuous with the deep fascia on the dorsum of the foot; it continues posteriorly to the medial process of the calcaneus and the plantar aponeurosis. **Proximally**, there is no clear demarcation between its border and the deep fascia of the lower leg, especially the latter's deep transverse layer. **Distally**, its border is continuous with the plantar aponeurosis, and many fibres of abductor hallucis are attached to it. The flexor retinaculum converts grooves on the tibia and calcaneus into canals for the tendons, and bridges over the posterior tibial vessels and tibial nerve. As these structures enter the sole they are, from medial to lateral: the tendon of tibialis posterior, the tendon of flexor digitorum longus, the posterior tibial vessels, tibial nerve and the tendon of flexor hallucis longus (7.139).

Peroneal retinacula

The peroneal retinacula (7.137, 140) are fibrous bands that retain the tendons of peroneus longus and brevis in position as they curve round the lateral side of the ankle.

Superior peroneal retinaculum. The superior peroneal retinaculum extends from the back of the lateral malleolus to the deep transverse fascia of the lower leg and the lateral surface of the calcaneus.

Inferior peroneal retinaculum. The inferior peroneal retinaculum is continuous in front with the inferior extensor retinaculum, and is attached posteriorly to the lateral surface of the calcaneus; some of its fibres are fused with the periosteum on the peroneal trochlea of the calcaneus, forming a septum between the tendons of peroneus longus and brevis.

Synovial sheaths in the ankle region

The tendons that cross the ankle joint are all deflected to some degree from a straight course, and must therefore be held down by retinacula and enclosed in synovial sheaths.

Anterior to the ankle, the sheath for tibialis anterior extends from the proximal margin of the superior extensor retinaculum to the interval between the diverging limbs of the inferior retinaculum (7.141). A common sheath encloses the tendons of extensor digitorum longus and peroneus tertius, starting just above the level of the malleoli, and reaching to the level of the base of the fifth metatarsal bone (7.140). The sheath for extensor hallucis longus starts just below that for extensor digitorum longus and reaches to the base of the first metatarsal bone (7.140, 141).

Medial to the ankle (7.141), the sheath for tibialis posterior starts about 4 cm above the malleolus and ends just proximal to the

attachment of the tendon to the tuberosity of the navicular. The sheath for flexor hallucis longus reaches the level of the malleolus proximally, and the base of the first metatarsal bone distally. The sheath for flexor digitorum longus starts slightly above the malleolus and ends at the navicular.

Lateral to the ankle (7.140), the tendons of peroneus longus and brevis are enclosed in a sheath which is single proximally but double distally. From the tip of the malleolus it extends for about 4 cm both proximally and distally.

MUSCLES OF THE FOOT

The *intrinsic* muscles, i.e. those contained entirely within the foot, follow the primitive limb pattern of dorsal extensors and plantar flexors. The tendons of the *extrinsic* muscles, which have already been considered, are associated with them topographically and functionally. The intrinsic extensor musculature is limited, but, as in the hand, some intrinsic flexor muscles are involved in extensor activities.

As in the hand, the muscles in the plantar region of the foot can be divided into medial, lateral and intermediate groups, the medial and lateral groups comprising the intrinsic muscles of hallux and minimus, and the central or intermediate group including the lumbricals, interossei and short digital flexors. However, it is customary to group them in four layers, as they are encountered during dissection. These 'layers' can be overemphasized, and in functional terms the former grouping will often be found more useful. Their actions are considered together (see Actions of the intrinsic muscles of the foot, p. 897).

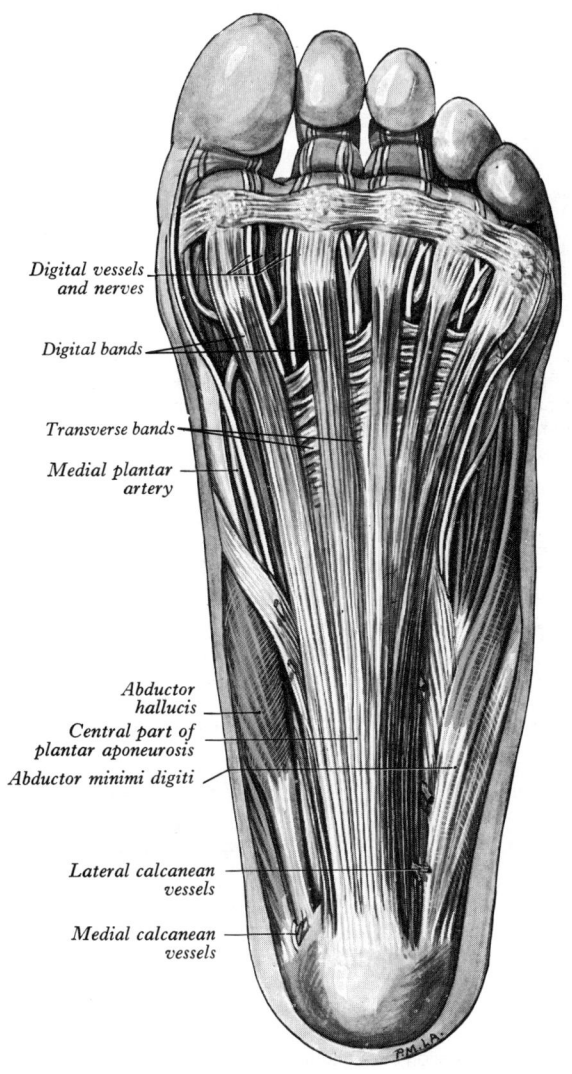

Digital vessels and nerves

Digital bands

Transverse bands

Medial plantar artery

Abductor hallucis

Central part of plantar aponeurosis

Abductor minimi digiti

Lateral calcanean vessels

Medial calcanean vessels

7.142   The plantar aponeurosis of the left foot.

DORSAL MUSCLE AND FASCIA OF THE FOOT

Deep dorsal fascia

The deep fascia on the dorsum of the foot (*fascia dorsalis pedis*) is a thin layer, continuous above with the inferior extensor retinaculum; it covers the dorsal extensor tendons.

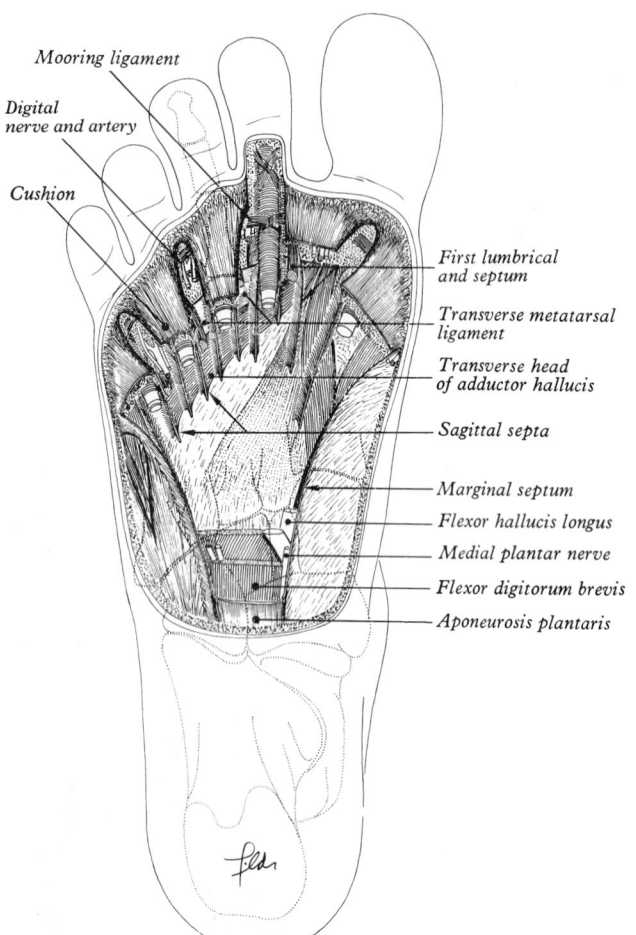

Extensor digitorum brevis

Extensor digitorum brevis (7.132, 140) is a thin muscle, arising from the anterior superolateral surface of the calcaneus, in front of the shallow lateral groove for peroneus brevis, from the interosseous talocalcaneal ligament, and from the stem of the inferior extensor retinaculum. It slants distally and medially across the dorsum of the foot, and ends in four tendons. The medial part of the muscle is usually a more or less distinct slip ending in a tendon which crosses the dorsalis pedis artery superficially to insert into the dorsal aspect of the base of the proximal phalanx of the hallux; this slip is sometimes termed *extensor hallucis brevis*. The other three tendons attach to the lateral sides of the tendons of extensor digitorum longus for the second, third and fourth toes.

Variations. The muscle is subject to much variation. There may be accessory slips from the talus and navicular, an extra tendon to the fifth digit, or a lack of one or more tendons. The muscle may be connected to the adjacent dorsal interosseous muscles.

Blood supply. Perforating branch of peroneal artery (p. 1573); anterior lateral malleolar artery (pp. 1571–1572); lateral tarsal arteries (p. 1572); arteria dorsalis pedis (p. 1572); arcuate artery (p. 1572); first, second and third dorsal metatarsal arteries (p. 1572); proximal and distal perforating arteries (p. 1572); dorsal digital arteries to **medial four** toes (including hallux; p. 1574).

Nerve supply. The lateral terminal branch of the deep peroneal nerve, L5, S1.

Actions. The muscle assists in extending the phalanges of the middle three toes via the tendons of extensor digitorum longus; in the hallux, it acts only on the proximal phalanx.

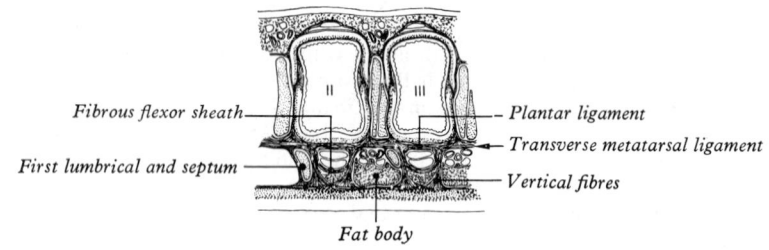

7.143A, B, C Details of the tendinous and fibrous architecture of various regions on the plantar aspect of the right foot. A. Plantar aspect of the central compartment and the structures forming the ball of the foot. Of the plantar interdigital ligament, only the mooring ligament is shown.

7.143B Transverse section through the heads of the second and third metatarsal bones showing the course of the collagen fibre bundles in the submetatarsal cushions and around the joints. Fat covers the fibrous flexor sheath inside the cushion; the digital nerves and vessels are lodged between the cushions.

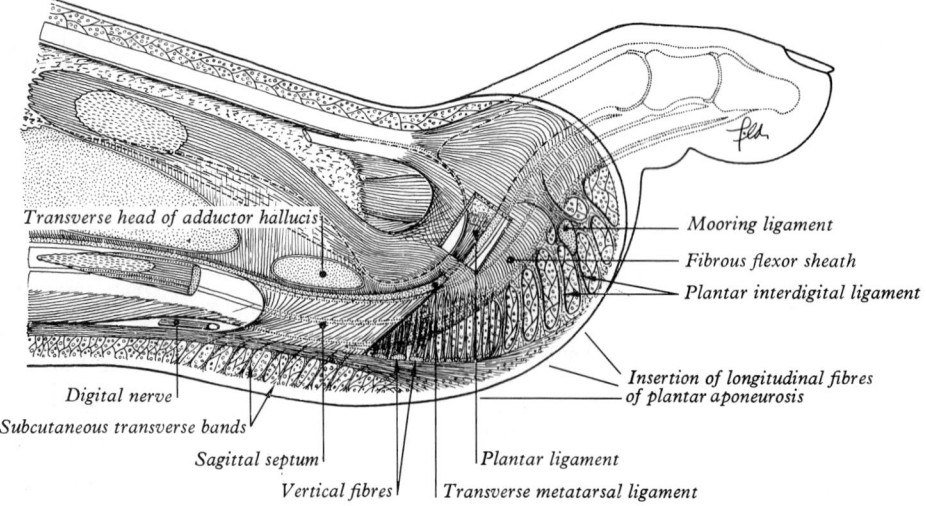

7.143C Sagittal section through the second interosseous cleft showing the internal architecture of the three major areas of the ball of the foot. The sagittal septum is attached to the proximal phalanx through the transverse metatarsal ligament and the plantar ligament of the joint. The vertical fibres

and the lamellae of the plantar interdigital ligament are attached to the proximal phalanx through the fibrous flexor sheath (from Bojsen-Møller & Flagstad 1976, by courtesy of the authors and the Cambridge University Press).

PLANTAR FASCIAE OF THE FOOT

Deep and superficial plantar fasciae

The deep and superficial plantar fasciae are arranged similarly to those in the hand (7.142, 143A–C), with some small differences due to the absence of opposition and grasping functions in the foot. Fasciae are arranged: to limit the tangential mobility of the skin; to provide 'skin joints'—linear flexure lines (p. 662) at which soft tissue angulation is permitted; to hold down muscles, and especially tendons, in the concave surfaces of the sole and digits; to facilitate the excursion of these tendons; to avoid excessive compression of plantar and digital vessels and nerves; and possibly to aid venous return. The plantar skin is repeatedly subjected to shearing and impact stresses in locomotion, particularly over the posterior calcaneal tubercles, the metatarsal heads, and the pulps of the terminal segments of the toes. As in the hand, these regions contain pads of adipose tissue. This is specialized, containing 19–25% more unsaturated fatty acids than other human tissues, the unsaturation being mainly in the triglyceride fraction. From a determination of kinematic viscosities of synthetic triolein and trilinolein, it could be inferred that adipose tissue of the foot has a lower viscosity than that elsewhere (Bojsen-Møller & Jorgensen 1991). The fat pads are diffusely pervaded by fine but collectively strong connective tissue strands, which tether the skin and limit displacement of fat, augmenting its resilient cushioning effect. These strands extend from the deep fascia through the subcutaneous tissues to the dermis of the skin, and their orientation reflects the prevailing stresses, as has been clearly demonstrated in the submetatarsal region (the 'ball of the foot') by Bojsen-Møller and Flagstad (1976) (7.143C).

The parts of the deep fascia inferior to the plantar structures are usually referred to collectively as the *plantar aponeuroris* (see below); but only the central part is extensively aponeurotic, and some anatomists reserve the name for this part alone. The medial and lateral parts are aponeurotic only proximally, where they provide for attachment of muscles (see below).

Plantar aponeurosis

The plantar aponeurosis (7.142) is composed of densely compacted collagen fibres orientated mainly longitudinally, but also transversely. Its medial and lateral parts overlie the intrinsic muscles of the hallux and minimus; its dense central part overlies the long and short digital flexors.

The **central part** is the strongest and thickest. It is narrow posteriorly, where it is attached to the medial process of the calcaneal tuberosity proximal to flexor digitorum brevis; it becomes broader and somewhat thinner as it diverges towards the metatarsal heads. Just proximal to these it divides into five bands, one for each toe. These five bands are united by transverse fibres where they begin to diverge below the metatarsal shafts (7.142). Proximal, ventral and a little distal to the metatarsal heads and their joints the *superficial stratum* of each band is connected to the dermis by *skin ligaments* (*retinacula cutis*), which reach the skin of the ball of the foot proximal to, and in the floors of, the furrows that separate the toes from the sole (7.143D). These cutaneous retinacula condense proximally to form a sagittal septum but diverge distally into numerous bundles and lamellae which pass at right-angles through bundles of the plantar interdigital ligament (see below). The *deep stratum* of each digital band of the aponeurosis divides into two septa which flank the digital flexor tendons, separating them from the lumbrical muscles and the digital vessels and nerves. These septa pass deeply to fuse with the interosseous fascia, the deep transverse metatarsal ligaments, the plantar ligaments of the metatarsophalangeal joints, and the periosteum and fibrous flexor sheaths at the base of each proximal phalanx. Pads of fat develop in the webs between the metatarsal heads and the bases of the proximal phalanges; these cushion the digital nerves and vessels from adjoining tendinous structures and extraneous plantar pressures. Vertical strands of collagen from the digital fibrous flexor sheaths tie these four fat pads to the superficial stratum of the plantar aponeurosis and, through this, to the skin. Just distal to the metatarsal heads a *plantar interdigital ligament* (*superficial transverse metatarsal ligament*) blends progressively with the deep aspect of the superficial stratum of the plantar aponeurosis, where it enters the toes (7.143B, C). The central part of the plantar

aponeurosis thus provides an intermediary structure between the skin and the osteoligamentous framework of the foot, via numerous cutaneous retinacula and deep septa extending to the metatarsals and phalanges. It is also continuous with the medial and lateral parts, and at the junctions two *intermuscular septa*, medial and lateral, extend in oblique vertical planes between the medial, intermediate and lateral groups of plantar muscles to reach bone (see below). Thinner horizontal intermuscular septa, passing between muscle layers, are derived from the vertical intermuscular septa.

The **lateral part** of the plantar aponeurosis, which covers abductor digiti minimi, is thin distally and thick proximally, where it forms a strong band, sometimes containing muscle fibres, between the lateral process of the calcanean tuberosity and the base of the fifth metatarsal bone. It is continuous medially with the central part of the aponeurosis, and with the fascia on the dorsum of the foot around its lateral border.

The **medial part** of the plantar aponeurosis, which covers abductor hallucis, is thin; it is continuous proximally with the flexor retinaculum, medially with the fascia dorsalis pedis and laterally with the central part of the plantar aponeurosis.

Lateral intermuscular septum. This septum is incomplete, especially at its proximal end; distally its deep attachments are to the fibrous sheath of peroneus longus and to the fifth metatarsal bone.

Medial intermuscular septum. This septum is also incomplete and divides into three bands, proximal, intermediate and distal, each of which displays lateral and medial divisions as it approaches its deep attachment. The *proximal band* is attached laterally to the cuboid and blends medially with the tendon of tibialis posterior. The *middle band* is attached laterally to the cuboid and the long plantar ligament

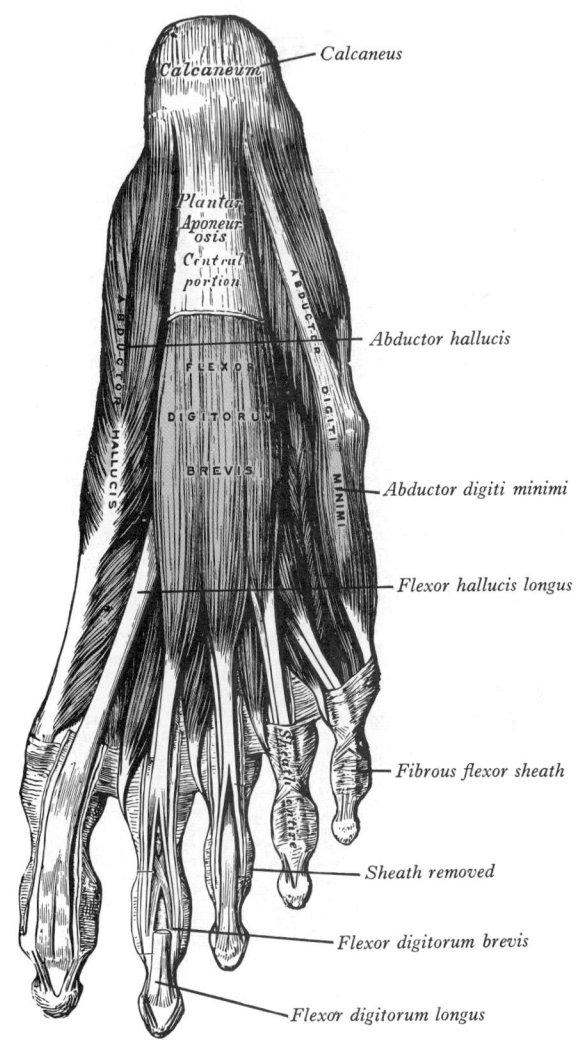

7.144 The superficial plantar muscles of the right foot.

and medially to the medial cuneiform bone. The *distal band* divides to enclose the tendon of flexor hallucis longus and is attached to the fascia over flexor hallucis brevis.

PLANTAR MUSCLES OF THE FOOT—FIRST LAYER

This superficial layer (7.144) includes abductor hallucis, abductor digiti minimi and flexor digitorum brevis. All three extend from the calcanean tuberosity to the toes, and therefore, in this case, comprise a functional group that assists in maintaining the concavity of the foot.

Abductor hallucis

Abductor hallucis (7.144) lies along the medial border of the foot and covers the origins of the plantar vessels and nerves. It arises principally from the flexor retinaculum, but also from the medial process of the calcanean tuberosity, the plantar aponeurosis, and the intermuscular septum between this muscle and flexor digitorum brevis. The muscle fibres end in a tendon which is attached, together with the medial tendon of flexor hallucis brevis, to the medial side of the base of the proximal phalanx of the hallux. Some fibres are attached more proximally to the medial sesamoid bone of this toe. The muscle may also derive some fibres from the dermis along the medial border of the foot.

Blood supply. Medial malleolar network and its tributaries (p. 1571); medial calcaneal branches of the lateral plantar artery (pp. 1573, 1574, **10**.150); *medial plantar artery*, directly and via *superficial* and *deep* branches (p. 1574); first plantar metatarsal artery and perforators; end of plantar arch (p. 1574, **10**.151A).

Nerve supply. Medial plantar nerve, S1 and 2.

Flexor digitorum brevis

Flexor digitorum brevis (7.144) lies immediately superior (deep) to the central part of the plantar aponeurosis. Its deep surface is separated from the lateral plantar vessels and nerves by a thin layer of fascia. It arises by a narrow tendon from the medial process of the calcanean tuberosity, from the central part of the plantar aponeurosis, and from the intramuscular septa between it and adjacent muscles. It divides into four tendons, which pass to the lateral four toes; these enter digital tendon sheaths (see below) accompanied by the tendons of flexor digitorum longus, which lie deep to them. At the bases of the proximal phalanges, each tendon divides around the corresponding tendon of flexor digitorum longus; the two slips then reunite and partially decussate, forming a tunnel through which the tendon of flexor digitorum longus passes to the distal phalanx. The short flexor tendon divides again and attaches to both sides of the shaft of the middle phalanx. The way in which the tendons of flexor digitorum brevis divide and attach to the phalanges is identical to that of the tendons of flexor digitorum superficialis in the hand.

Variations. The slip to a given toe may be joined by a second, supernumerary slip, be absent, or be replaced by a small muscular slip from the long flexor tendon or from flexor accessorius. Nathan and Gloobe (1974) found the slip to the fifth toe to be the most susceptible to such variation (63%); those to the third and fourth less so (10%), and that to the second almost invariable.

Blood supply. Lateral plantar artery (p. 1573); medial plantar artery (p. 1573); plantar metatarsal arteries (p. 1572); plantar digital arteries to lateral four toes.

Nerve supply. Medial plantar nerve, S1 and 2.

Abductor digiti minimi

Abductor digiti minimi (7.144) lies along the lateral border of the foot, and its medial margin is related to the lateral plantar vessels and nerve. It arises from both processes of the calcanean tuberosity, from the plantar surface of the bone between them, from the plantar aponeurosis, and from the intermuscular septum between the muscle and flexor digitorum brevis. Its tendon glides in a smooth groove on the plantar surface of the base of the fifth metatarsal and is attached, with flexor digiti minimi brevis, to the lateral side of the base of the proximal phalanx of the fifth toe; hence it is more a flexor than an abductor. Some of the fibres arising from the lateral calcaneal process usually reach the tip of the tuberosity of the fifth metatarsal (6.353) and may form a separate muscle, *abductor ossis metatarsi digiti quinti*. An accessory slip from the base of the fifth metatarsal is not infrequent.

Blood supply. Medial plantar artery (to medial 'head'; p. 1573); lateral plantar artery (**10**.151A; p. 1573); plantar digital artery to lateral side of minimus from beginning of plantar arch (p. 1574); fourth plantar metatarsal artery; end twigs of arcuate and lateral tarsal arteries (p. 1572, **10**.150).

Nerve supply. Lateral plantar nerve, S1, 2 and 3.

Flexor tendon sheaths

The terminations of the tendons of the long and short flexor muscles are contained in osseo-aponeurotic canals similar to those in the fingers. These canals are bounded above by the phalanges, and below by fibrous bands—the *digital fibrous sheaths*—which arch across the tendons and attach on each side to the margins of the phalanges (7.144). Along the proximal and intermediate phalanges the fibrous bands are strong, and the fibres are transverse (*annular part*); opposite the joints they are much thinner and the fibres decussate (*cruciform part*). Each osseo-aponeurotic canal has a synovial lining, which is reflected around its tendon; within this sheath vincula tendinum are arranged as in the fingers.

PLANTAR MUSCLES OF THE FOOT—SECOND LAYER

Beneath the first layer is a second group of intrinsic muscles that consists of flexor digitorum accessorius and four lumbrical muscles. Intimately associated with them are the preterminal tendons of flexor hallucis longus and flexor digitorum longus.

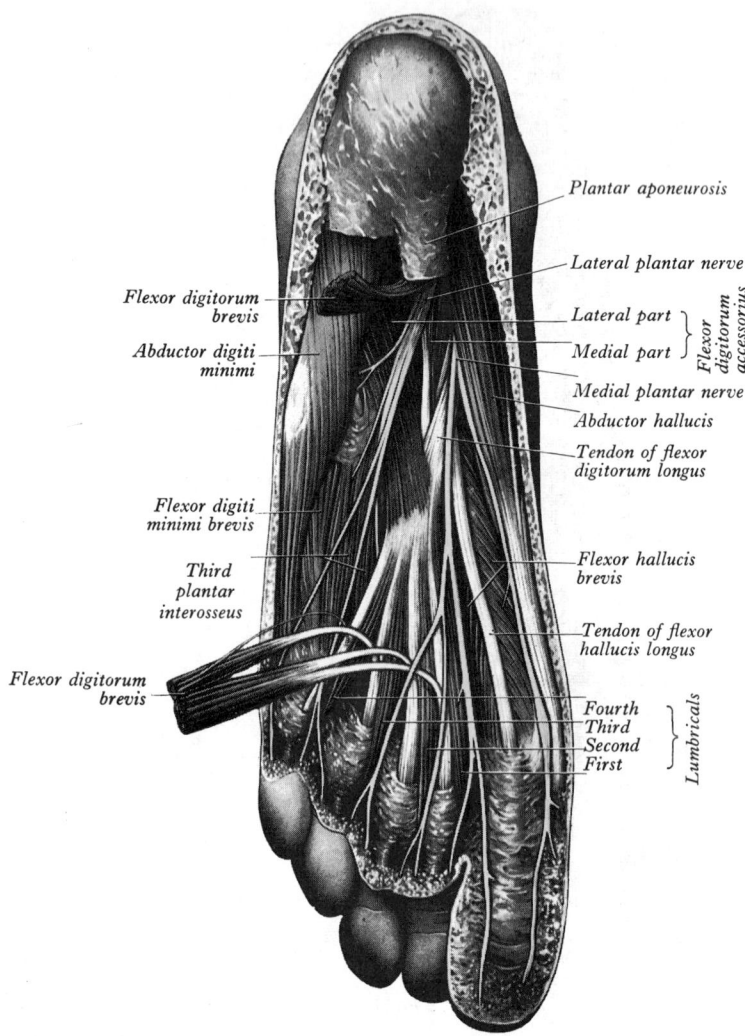

Flexor digitorum brevis
Abductor digiti minimi
Flexor digiti minimi brevis
Third plantar interosseus
Flexor digitorum brevis

Plantar aponeurosis
Lateral plantar nerve
Lateral part
Medial part } Flexor digitorum accessorius
Medial plantar nerve
Abductor hallucis
Tendon of flexor digitorum longus
Flexor hallucis brevis
Tendon of flexor hallucis longus
Fourth
Third
Second
First } Lumbricals

7.145 The plantar muscles of the left foot: first and second layers.

Flexor digitorum accessorius

Flexor digitorum accessorius (**7**.145) arises by two heads separated by the long plantar ligament. The medial head is larger and more fleshy: it is attached to the medial concave surface of the calcaneus below the groove for the tendon of flexor hallucis longus. The lateral head is flat and tendinous: it is attached to the lateral process of the tuberosity, and to the long plantar ligament. In some cases the medial head ends in a fibrous lamina which passes deep to the tendon of flexor digitorum longus and divides into tendinous slips which join the long flexor tendons to the second and third, and sometimes fourth, digits. Almost as frequently the medial head joins the lateral border of the tendon of flexor digitorum longus. The lateral head either joins this fibrous lamina, on its superficial surface or its lateral border, or fuses with the lateral border of the long flexor tendon (Lewis 1962), perhaps 'correcting' the diagonal vector of this muscle.

Variations. In addition to the variations already noted, the muscle is sometimes absent altogether. It also varies in the number of digits that it supplies: the slip to the fourth is often absent; a slip to the fifth is sometimes present.

Blood supply. Stem of medial plantar artery (to medial 'head'; p. 1573); lateral plantar artery (p. 1573); plantar arch (p. 1574).

Nerve supply. Lateral plantar nerve, S1, 2 and 3.

Lumbrical muscles

The lumbrical muscles (**7**.145) are four small muscles (numbered from the medial side of the foot) which are accessory to the tendons of flexor digitorum longus. They arise from these tendons as far back as their angles of separation, each springing from the sides of two adjacent tendons except for the first, which arises only from the medial border of the first tendon. The muscles end in tendons which pass distally on the medial sides of the four lesser toes, to be attached to the dorsal digital expansions on their proximal phalanges.

Blood supply. Lateral plantar artery and plantar arch (p. 1573); four plantar metatarsal arteries (four distal perforating joined by three proximal perforating arteries). **Tendons**: dorsal digital arteries (and their dorsal metacarpal origins) to the lateral four toes (p. 1574).

Nerve supply. The first lumbrical is supplied by the medial plantar nerve and the rest by the deep branch of the lateral plantar nerve, S2 and 3.

PLANTAR MUSCLES OF THE FOOT—THIRD LAYER

The third layer comprises the shorter intrinsic muscles of the hallux and minimus: flexor hallucis brevis, adductor hallucis and flexor digiti minimi brevis (**7**.146, 147). These are the most deeply situated

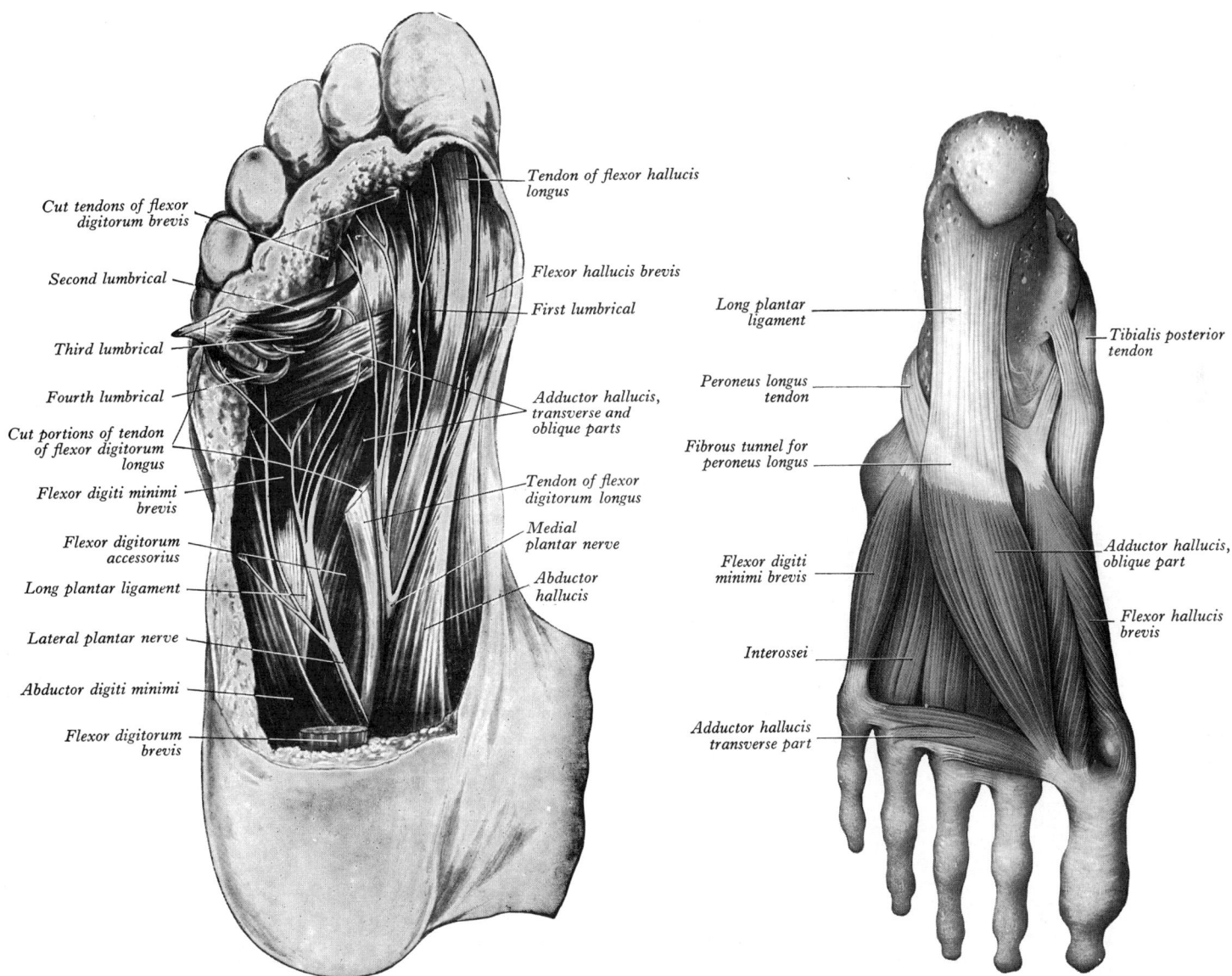

7.146   The plantar muscles of the right foot and their nerve supply. Most of flexor digitorum brevis has been removed. The tendon of flexor digitorum longus has been divided and its distal end has been turned forwards together with the second, third and fourth lumbricals.

7.147   The plantar muscles of the left foot: third layer.

muscles in the sole, except for the interossei, which are superior to them.

Flexor hallucis brevis

Flexor hallucis brevis (**7.**145, 147) has a bifurcate tendon of origin. The lateral limb arises from the medial part of the plantar surface of the cuboid, posterior to the groove for the peroneus longus tendon, and from the adjacent part of the lateral cuneiform. The medial limb has a deep attachment directly continuous with the lateral division of the tendon of tibialis posterior, and a more superficial attachment to the middle band of the medial intermuscular septum (Lewis 1964b). The belly of the muscle divides into medial and lateral parts whose twin tendons are attached to the sides of the base of the proximal phalanx of the hallux, with a sesamoid bone usually occurring in each tendon near its attachment. The medial part blends with abductor hallucis, the lateral with adductor hallucis, as they reach their terminations.

Variations. Accessory slips may arise proximally from the calcaneus or long plantar ligament. A tendinous slip may extend to the proximal phalanx of the second toe.

Blood supply. Medial plantar artery (p. 1573); first plantar metatarsal artery (p. 1574). (**Origins**): lateral plantar artery and plantar arch (p. 1574).

Nerve supply. Medial plantar nerve, S1 and 2.

Adductor hallucis

Adductor hallucis (**7.**146, 147) arises by oblique and transverse heads. The *oblique head* springs from the bases of the second, third and fourth metatarsal bones, and from the fibrous sheath of the tendon of peroneus longus. The *transverse head*, a narrow, flat fasciculus, arises from the plantar metatarsophalangeal ligaments of the third, fourth and fifth toes (sometimes only from the third and fourth), and from the deep transverse metatarsal ligaments between them. The oblique head has medial and lateral parts: the medial part blends with the lateral part of flexor hallucis brevis and is attached to the lateral sesamoid bone of the hallux; the lateral part joins the transverse head and is also attached to the lateral sesamoid bone and directly to the base of the first phalanx of the hallux. Cralley et al (1975) were unable to identify a phalangeal attachment for the transverse part of the muscle; fibres that failed to reach the lateral sesamoid bone were attached with the oblique part.

Variations. In the study by Cralley et al (1975), the transverse part of this muscle was absent in 6% of feet. Part of the muscle may be attached to the first metatarsal, constituting an *opponens hallucis.* A slip may also extend to the proximal phalanx of the second toe.

Blood supply. Medial plantar artery (p. 1573); lateral plantar artery (p. 1573); plantar arch (p. 1574); first to fourth plantar metatarsal arteries (p. 1574).

Nerve supply. The deep branch of the lateral plantar nerve, S2 and 3.

Flexor digiti minimi brevis

Flexor digiti minimi brevis (**7.**145, 147) arises from the medial part of the plantar surface of the base of the fifth metatarsal bone, and from the sheath of peroneus longus. It has a distal tendon which inserts into the lateral side of the base of the proximal phalanx of the minimus; this tendon usually blends laterally with that of abductor digiti minimi. Occasionally some of its deeper fibres extend to the lateral part of the distal half of the fifth metatarsal bone, constituting what may be described as a distinct muscle, *opponens digiti minimi.*

Blood supply. End twigs of arcuate and lateral tarsal arteries (p. 1572; **10.**150); lateral plantar artery (p. 1573) and its digital (plantar) branch to the lateral side of minimus (p. 1574; **10.**151A).

Nerve supply. The superficial branch of the lateral plantar nerve, S2 and 3.

PLANTAR MUSCLES OF THE FOOT—FOURTH LAYER

The fourth layer comprises the plantar and dorsal interossei. They resemble their counterparts in the hand, but they are arranged relative to an axis through the second digit and not the third, as in the hand, the second being the least mobile of the metatarsal bones.

Dorsal interossei

The dorsal interossei (**7.**148A) are situated between the metatarsal bones. They comprise four bipennate muscles, each arising by two heads from the sides of the adjacent metatarsal bones. Their tendons are attached to the bases of the proximal phalanges and to the dorsal digital expansions. The first inserts into the medial side of the second toe; the other three pass to the lateral sides of the second, third and fourth toes. Between the heads of each of the three lateral muscles, there is an angular space through which a perforating artery passes to the dorsum of the foot; between the heads of the first muscle the same space transmits the terminal part of the dorsalis pedis artery to the sole.

Plantar interossei

The plantar interossei (**7.**148B), of which there are three, lie below rather than between the metatarsal bones, and each is connected to one metatarsal bone only. They arise from the bases and medial sides of the third, fourth and fifth metatarsal bones, and insert into the medial sides of the bases of the proximal phalanges of the same toes, and into their dorsal digital expansions.

Blood supply. Dorsal interossei are supplied by the arcuate artery (p. 1572); lateral tarsal arteries (p. 1572); medial tarsal arteries (p. 1572); first to fourth plantar **and** first to fourth dorsal metacarpal arteries (receiving proximal and distal perforating arteries, see p. 1574); dorsal digital arteries of lateral **four** toes. Plantar interossei are supplied by the lateral plantar artery (p. 1573); plantar arch (p. 1574); second to fourth plantar metacarpal arteries; dorsal digital arteries of lateral **three** toes.

Nerve supply. Dorsal and plantar interossei are supplied by the deep branch of the lateral plantar nerve (S2 and 3), except those in the fourth interosseous space, which are supplied by the superficial branch of the same nerve. The first dorsal interosseus frequently receives an extra filament from the medial branch of the deep peroneal nerve on the dorsum of the foot, and the second a twig from the lateral branch of the same nerve.

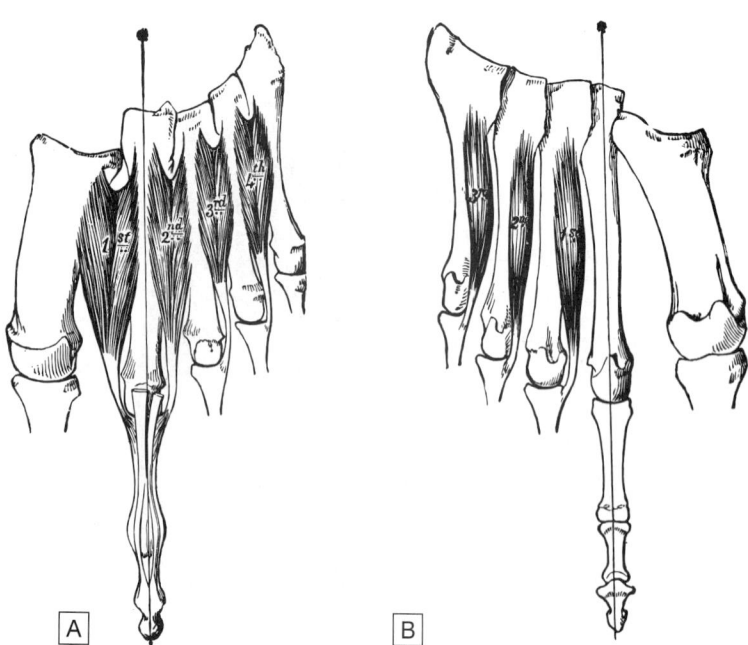

7.148 The interossei of the left foot. A. Dorsal interossei viewed from the dorsal aspect. B. Plantar interossei viewed from the plantar aspect. The axis to which the movements of abduction and adduction are referred is indicated.

Actions of the intrinsic muscles of the foot

The main intrinsic muscle mass of the foot consists of abductor hallucis, adductor hallucis, flexor digitorum brevis, flexor hallucis brevis and abductor digiti minimi. These muscles are particularly difficult to study by the normal methods of investigation (see The study of muscle action). The geometry of a muscle and its attachments may suggest its potential actions—and this is the basis for the names applied to some of them—but such deductions must take account not only of the influence of other muscles but also of the modifying effects of contact with the ground.

When a subject is standing quietly, with the feet flat on the ground, the feet serve as platforms for the distribution of weight, the centre of gravity of the body being maintained above them by suitable adjustment of tension and length in muscles of the leg and trunk. Under these conditions, the skeleton of the foot—with interosseous and deep plantar ligaments only—is capable of supporting several times body weight without failure (Walker 1991). The intrinsic muscles show no electrical activity other than sporadic bursts at intervals of 5 to 10 seconds associated with postural adjustment.

When the heel lifts clear of the ground in beginning to take a step, whether in walking or running, the whole of the weight and muscular thrust is transferred to the forefoot region of the metatarsal heads and the pads of the toes. This shifts the role of the foot from platform to lever, and intensifies the forces acting on the fore part of the foot, especially in running and jumping. There has been so much argument about the nature and behaviour of the 'arches' of the foot and the muscles and ligaments that act as 'tie-beams' or trusses across them, that the essential role of the foot as a lever is often overlooked. At first sight it appears ill-suited to act as a lever, being composed of a series of links, although there are good mechanical precedents for its curved or arched form. As the heel lifts, the concavity of the sole is accentuated, at which point available electromyographic evidence indicates that the intrinsic muscles become strongly active. This would slacken the plantar aponeurosis, but dorsiflexion of the toes tightens it up. The foot is also supinated, and the position of close-packing of the intertarsal joints is reached as the foot takes the full effects of leverage. The toes are held extended at the meta-tarsophalangeal and interphalangeal joints. In this position the foot loses all its pliancy and so becomes effective as a lever.

The intrinsic muscles are the main contributors to the muscular support of the arch. Their line of pull lies essentially in the long arch of the foot and perpendicular to the transverse tarsal joints; thus they can exert considerable flexion force on the fore part of the foot, and are also the principal stabilizers of the transverse tarsal joint. (This includes the abductors of the hallux and minimus, since both act as flexors and probably have little abductor effect.) The pronated or flat foot requires greater activity in the intrinsic muscles to stabilize the midtarsal and subtalar joint than does the normal foot (Suzuki 1972). This can be shown in walking. In a subject with a normal foot, activity in the intrinsic muscles begins at approximately 30% of the gait cycle and increases at the time of toe-off (7.149). In an individual with flat feet, these muscles begin to function much earlier, at approximately 15% of the cycle, and their action ceases when the arch again drops at toe-off (Mann & Inman 1964).

Table 7.2A, B (pp. 896–897) has two main purposes:

a. to complement the mainly topographical description of muscles in the text with a listing that groups the major muscles according to their functions;
b. to bring together for easy reference, information about the innervation of muscles by their peripheral nerves and nerve roots.

To achieve this, some simplification has been necessary.

Movements. At the central nervous level of control, muscles are not recognised as individual actuators but as components of movement. Muscles may contribute to several types of movement, acting variously as prime movers, antagonists, fixators or synergists. For example, in the movement of the scapula around the thorax, serratus anterior acts as an antagonist of trapezius, but in the forward rotation of the scapula the two muscles combine as prime movers. Moreover, a muscle that crosses two joints can produce more than one movement: the hamstring muscles, for example, can both extend the hip and flex the knee. One or other of these functions may be emphasized when the origin or insertion is fixed by the action of gravity or other muscles. Even a muscle that acts across one joint can produce a combination of movements, such as flexion with medial rotation, or extension with adduction. Some muscles have therefore been included in more than one place in the tables, but even these listings are not exhaustive.

Nerve roots. The reader should not be dismayed to find variation between texts in the spinal roots listed as contributing to the innervation of the muscles; this is a reflection of the often unreliable nature of the information available. The most positive identifications have been obtained by stimulating spinal roots electrically, and recording the evoked electro-myographic activity in the muscles (Thage 1965). This is, however, a laborious process and data of this quality is in limited supply. Much of the information in the tables is based on neurological experience gained in examining the effects of lesions, and some of it is far from new (Foerster 1913).

Major and minor contributions. Spinal roots have been given the same shading when they innervate a muscle to a similar extent or when differences in their contribution have not been described. Heavy shading has been used to indicate roots from which there is known to be a dominant contribution. From a clinical viewpoint, some of these roots may be regarded as innervating the muscle almost exclusively: for example, deltoid by C5, brachioradialis by C6, and triceps by C7. Minor contributions have nevertheless been retained in the table in order to increase its utility in other contexts, such as electromyography and comparative anatomy.

Clinical testing. For diagnostic purposes, it is neither necessary nor possible to test every muscle, and the experienced neurologist can cover every clinical possibility with a much shorter list. Red has been used to highlight those muscles or movements that have diagnostic value. The emphasis in these tables is on the differentiation of lesions at different root levels. Other lists may be developed to differentiate lesions at the level of the root, plexus or peripheral nerve, at different sites along the length of a nerve, or between different peripheral nerves. The preferred criteria for including a given muscle on such a list are that it is visible and palpable; that its action is isolated or can be isolated by the examiner; that it is innervated by one peripheral nerve or (predominantly) one root; that it has a clinically elicitable reflex; and that it is useful in differentiating between different nerves, roots or levels of lesion. In practice, such tests would of course be combined with tests of sensory function (Aids to the Examination of the Peripheral Nervous System, 1986).

Table 7.2A

JOINT	MOVEMENT	MUSCLE	INNERVATION	C3	C4	C5	C6	C7	C8	T1
SCAPULA	ELEVATION	Upper trapezius	Spinal accessory n.	▓	▓					
		Levator scapulae	Dorsal scapular n.	▓	▓	▓				
	DEPRESSION	Lower trapezius	Spinal accessory n.	▓	▓					
	RETRACTION	Middle trapezius	Spinal accessory n.	▓	▓					
		Rhomboids	Dorsal scapular n.		▓	▓				
SHOULDER	PROTRACTION	Serratus anterior	Long thoracic n.			▓	▓	▓		
	FLEXION	Anterior deltoid	Axillary n.			▓	▓			
		Pectoralis major (clavicular head)	Medial & lateral pectoral nn.			▓	▓			
		Pectoralis major (sternocostal head)	Medial & lateral pectoral nn.				▓	▓	▓	▓
		Coracobrachialis	Musculocutaneous n.			▓	▓	▓		
	EXTENSION	Posterior deltoid	Axillary n.			▓	▓			
		Infraspinatus	Suprascapular n.			▓	▓			
		Teres minor	Axillary n.			▓	▓			
		Teres major	Lower subscapular n.			▓	▓	▓		
		Latissimus dorsi	Thoracodorsal n.				▓	▓	▓	
	VERTICAL ABDUCTION	Middle deltoid	Axillary n.			▓	▓			
		Supraspinatus	Suprascapular n.			▓	▓			
	VERTICAL ADDUCTION	Pectoralis major (sternocostal head)	Medial & lateral pectoral nn.				▓	▓	▓	▓
		Latissimus dorsi	Thoracodorsal n.				▓	▓	▓	
		Coracobrachialis	Musculocutaneous n.			▓	▓	▓		
	HORIZONTAL ABDUCTION	Posterior deltoid	Axillary n.			▓	▓			
	HORIZONTAL ADDUCTION	Pectoralis major (clavicular head)	Medial & lateral pectoral nn.			▓	▓			
		Pectoralis minor	Medial & lateral pectoral nn.					▓	▓	▓
		Anterior deltoid	Axillary n.			▓	▓			
	MEDIAL ROTATION	Subscapularis				▓	▓			
		Teres major	Brachial plexus			▓	▓	▓		
		Latissimus dorsi	Thoracodorsal n.				▓	▓	▓	
		Anterior deltoid	Axillary n.			▓	▓			
	LATERAL ROTATION	Infraspinatus	Suprascapular n.			▓	▓			
		Teres minor	Axillary n.			▓	▓			
		Posterior deltoid	Axillary n.			▓	▓			
ELBOW	FLEXION	Biceps brachii	Musculocutaneous n.			▓	▓			
		Brachialis	Musculocutaneous & radial nn.			▓	▓			
		Brachioradialis	Radial n.			▓	▓	▓		
	EXTENSION	Triceps	Radial n.				▓	▓	▓	
	SUPINATION	Biceps brachii	Musculocutaneous n.			▓	▓			
		Supinator	Posterior interosseus n.				▓	▓		
	PRONATION	Pronator quadratus	Anterior interosseus n.					▓	▓	▓
		Pronator teres	Median n.				▓	▓		
WRIST	FLEXION	Flexor carpi radialis	Median n.				▓	▓		
		Palmaris longus	Median n.					▓	▓	
		Flexor carpi ulnaris	Ulnar n.					▓	▓	▓
	EXTENSION	Extensor carpi radialis longus	Radial n.				▓	▓		
		Extensor carpi radialis brevis	Posterior interosseus n.				▓	▓		
		Extensor carpi ulnaris	Posterior interosseus n.					▓	▓	
	ABDUCTION	Extensor carpi radialis longus	Radial n.				▓	▓		
		Extensor carpi radialis brevis	Posterior interosseus n.				▓	▓		
		Flexor carpi radialis	Median n.				▓	▓		
	ADDUCTION	Extensor carpi ulnaris	Posterior interosseus n.					▓	▓	
		Flexor carpi ulnaris	Ulnar n.					▓	▓	▓
FINGERS	FLEXION (MP/PIP Joints)	Flexor digitorum superficialis	Median n.					▓	▓	▓
	FLEXION (DIP Joints)	Flexor digitorum profundus (lateral)	Anterior interosseus n.					▓	▓	▓
		Flexor digitorum profundus (medial)	Ulnar n.					▓	▓	▓
		Dorsal interossei	Ulnar n.						▓	▓
		Palmar interossei	Ulnar n.						▓	▓
	FLEXION (MP Joint)	Flexor digiti minimi brevis	Ulnar n.						▓	▓
	EXTENSION (MP/PIP/DIP Joints)	Extensor digitorum	Posterior interosseus n.					▓	▓	
		Extensor indicis	Posterior interosseus n.					▓	▓	
	EXTENSION (MP/PIP/DIP Joints)	Flexor digiti minimi	Posterior interosseus n.					▓	▓	
	EXTENSION (PIP/DIP Joints)	Lumbricals I & II	usu. Median n.					▓	▓	
		Lumbricals III & IV	usu. Ulnar n.						▓	▓
	ABDUCTION	Dorsal interossei	Ulnar n.						▓	▓
	ABDUCTION (thumb fixed)	Abductor pollicis brevis	Median n.						▓	▓
	ABDUCTION	Abductor digiti minimi	Ulnar n.						▓	▓
	ADDUCTION	Palmar interossei	Ulnar n.						▓	▓
	OPPOSITION	Opponens digiti minimi	Ulnar n.						▓	▓
THUMB	FLEXION (IP Joint)	Flexor pollicis longus	Anterior interosseus n.					▓	▓	▓
	FLEXION/ROTATION (MP Joint)	Flexor pollicis brevis	Median n. and/or ulnar n.						▓	▓
	EXTENSION (MP Joint)	Extensor pollicis brevis	Posterior interosseus n.					▓	▓	
	EXTENSION (IP Joint)	Extensor pollicis longus	Posterior interosseus n.					▓	▓	
	ABDUCTION	Abductor pollicis longus	Posterior interosseus n.					▓	▓	
	ABDUCTION/ROTATION	Abductor pollicis brevis	Median n.						▓	▓
	ADDUCTION/ROTATION	Adductor pollicis	Ulnar n.						▓	▓
	ADDUCTION/FLEXION (MP Joint)	Palmar interosseus I	Ulnar n.						▓	▓
	OPPOSITION	Opponens pollicis	Median n. and ulnar n.						▓	▓

Table 7.2B

JOINT	MOVEMENT	MUSCLE	INNERVATION	L1	L2	L3	L4	L5	S1	S2	S3
HIP	FLEXION	Psoas major	Spinal nn. L1, 2, 3	■	■	■					
		Iliacus	Femoral n.		■	■					
		Pectineus	Femoral n.		■	■					
		Rectus femoris	Femoral n.		■	■	■				
		Adductor longus	Obturator n.		■	■	■				
		Sartorius	Femoral n.		■	■					
	EXTENSION	Gluteus maximus	Inferior gluteal n.					■	■	■	
		Adductor magnus	Obturator & tibial nn.		■	■	■				
		Hamstrings	Mainly tibial nn.					■	■	■	
	MEDIAL ROTATION	Iliacus	Femoral n.		■	■					
		Gluteus medius & minimus	Superior gluteal n.				■	■	■		
		Tensor fasciae latae	Superior gluteal n.				■	■	■		
	LATERAL ROTATION	Superior & inferior gemelli	Lumbosacral plexus					■	■	■	
		Quadratus femoris	Lumbosacral plexus					■	■		
		Piriformis	Lumbosacral plexus						■	■	
		Obturator internus	Lumbosacral plexus					■	■		
		Obturator externus	Obturator n.			■	■				
		Sartorius	Femoral n.		■	■					
	ADDUCTION	Gracilis	Obturator n.		■	■					
		Adductor longus	Obturator n.		■	■	■				
		Adductor magnus	Obturator & tibial nn.		■	■	■				
		Adductor brevis	Obturator n.		■	■	■				
		Pectineus	Femoral n.		■	■					
	ABDUCTION	Tensor fasciae latae	Superior gluteal n.				■	■	■		
		Gluteus medius & minimus	Superior gluteal n.				■	■	■		
		Piriformis	Lumbosacral plexus						■	■	
KNEE	FLEXION	Hamstrings:									
		Semimembranosus	Tibial n.					■	■	■	
		Semitendinosus	Tibial n.					■	■	■	
		Biceps femoris	Tibial & common peroneal nn.					■	■	■	
		Gastrocnemius	Tibial n.						■	■	
	EXTENSION	Quadriceps femoris:									
		Rectus femoris	Femoral n.			■	■				
		Vastus lateralis	Femoral n.			■	■				
		Vastus intermedius	Femoral n.			■	■				
		Vastus medialis	Femoral n.			■	■				
ANKLE	DORSIFLEXION	Tibialis anterior	Deep peroneal n.				■	■			
		Extensor digitorum longus	Deep peroneal n.				■	■	■		
		Extensor hallucis longus	Deep peroneal n.				■	■	■		
		Peroneus tertius	Deep peroneal n.					■	■		
	PLANTAR FLEXION	Gastrocnemius	Tibial n.						■	■	
		Soleus	Tibial n.						■	■	
		Flexor digitorum longus	Tibial n.						■	■	■
		Flexor hallucis longus	Tibial n.						■	■	■
		Peroneus longus	Superficial peroneal n.					■	■		
		Tibialis posterior	Tibial n.				■	■			
	INVERSION	Tibialis anterior	Deep peroneal n.				■	■			
		Tibialis posterior	Tibial n.				■	■			
	EVERSION	Peroneus longus	Superficial peroneal n.					■	■		
		Peroneus tertius	Deep peroneal n.					■	■		
		Peroneus brevis	Superficial peroneal n.					■	■		
TOES	FLEXION	Flexor digitorum longus	Tibial n.						■	■	■
		Flexor hallucis longus	Tibial n.						■	■	
		Flexor hallucis brevis	Medial plantar n.						■	■	
		Flexor digitorum brevis	Medial plantar n.						■	■	■
		Flexor digitorum accessorius	Lateral plantar n.						■	■	■
		Flexor digiti minimi brevis	Lateral plantar n.							■	■
		Abductor hallucis	Medial plantar n.						■	■	
		Abductor digiti minimi	Lateral plantar n.							■	■
		Lumbricals	Medial & Lateral plantar nn.							■	■
	EXTENSION	Extensor digitorum longus	Deep peroneal n.					■	■		
		Extensor hallucis longus	Deep peroneal n.					■	■		
		Extensor digitorum brevis	Deep peroneal n.					■	■		
	ABDUCTION	Abductor hallucis	Medial plantar n.						■	■	
		Abductor digiti minimi	Lateral plantar n.							■	■
		Dorsal interossei	Lateral plantar n.							■	■
	ADDUCTION	Plantar interossei	Lateral plantar n.							■	■
		Adductor hallucis	Lateral plantar n.							■	■

STANDING AND WALKING

The human species is not unique in being bipedal. Many lizards run on their hind legs when travelling fast. Birds run or hop bipedally, and kangaroos and some rodents also hop. Chimpanzees occasionally rise to walk on their hind legs, especially when carrying things in their hands, and gibbons sometimes walk bipedally on horizontal branches (Alexander 1991).

Human bipedalism is unique in that we stand and walk with the trunk erect and the knees almost straight. In contrast, birds, kangaroos, apes and other non-human bipeds stand and move with their knees bent and the trunk sloping or even horizontal (Jenkins 1972). Another unusual feature is that we are plantigrade, setting down the whole length of the foot on the ground. Most medium to large mammals (e.g. dogs) are digitigrade, standing and walking on their toes, and ungulates such as horses and cattle stand on hooves on the tips of their toes. Many small mammals are plantigrade, but the only large plantigrade mammals are primates and bears.

When we stand motionless, the ground exerts on the feet a force equal and opposite to body weight. The weight acts at the centre of gravity, a little above the hip joints, and the force on the ground is centred vertically below it, at the centre of pressure. When people stand comfortably, the centre of pressure is usually midway between the insteps of the two feet. We do not remain absolutely still, but sway slightly, so the centre of pressure moves, but it normally remains within a circle of 25 mm diameter (Debrunner 1985). Because we stand so steadily, we could easily balance on smaller feet.

Body weight acts along a line that passes a few centimetres anterior to the tibiotalar joint, exerting a moment that must be balanced by the plantar flexor muscles. Some electromyographic investigations of standing have found activity mainly in soleus, but others have found moderate activity in gastrocnemius as well (Soames & Atha 1981; Basmajian & De Luca 1985). In either case it seems likely that the activity is mainly in type I (slow oxidative) fibres, which can maintain tension more economically than faster fibres could do under the same conditions (Heglund & Cavagna 1987; Barclay et al 1993). The soleus contains about 80% of type I fibres, and gastrocnemius about 50% (Yamaguchi et al 1990).

In normal standing, the weight of those parts of the body that are above the knee joint acts slightly anterior to the axes of the knees, exerting a moment which is balanced passively by tension in the liga-

ments that prevent hyperextension (Smith 1956). If the knees are kept straight, there is little or no electrical activity in the hamstrings and only moderate levels in the quadriceps (Soames & Atha 1981; Basmajian & De Luca 1985). The combined weight of the trunk, arms and head seems generally to act slightly behind the hip joints, exerting a small moment that is balanced largely by iliopsoas (Basmajian & De Luca 1985). Thus a relaxed stance, with trunk erect and knees straight, requires very little activity in thigh muscles. This should help to make our standing economical of energy, but it seems to be less economical than that of some domestic animals. The difference in metabolic rate between standing and lying is about 0.21 watts/kg body mass for humans but only 0.10 watts/kg for cattle and 0.14 watts/kg for sheep (Blaxter 1962).

When we stand on one leg, or when we walk, the weight of the upper parts of the body exerts a moment about the supporting hip which must be balanced by abductor muscles, especially tensor fasciae latae and gluteus medius and minimus (McLeish & Charnley 1970).

In walking, each foot is on the ground (stance phase) for about 60% of the stride, and off (swing phase) for about 40% (Alexander & Jayes 1980; **7.149**). Thus single-support phases (one foot on the ground) alternate with double-support phases (two feet). Each knee remains nearly straight (150–170°) for most of the stance phase of that leg, bending more only immediately before toe-off (Debrunner 1985). In this respect we contrast markedly with chimpanzees, whose knees are bent to 120° or beyond for most of the stance phase of bipedal walking (Jenkins 1972). We are also peculiar in our habit of setting the heel down before the toes: apes set down the whole length of the sole almost simultaneously. However, apes and other plantigrade mammals, like ourselves, lift the heel before the toes.

Force plate records of walking (Cavagna et al 1977; Alexander & Jayes 1980) show that the forces exerted on the ground are always more or less in line with the leg (**7.150**). Early in the stance phase, while the foot is in front of the trunk, it pushes downwards and forwards on the ground, decelerating the body as well as supporting it. Later, when it is behind the trunk, it pushes downwards and backwards, re-accelerating the body (**7.149**). The speed, and so the kinetic energy, of the body passes through a maximum in each double-support phase and a minimum in each single-support phase.

The height of the centre of gravity, and so the potential energy of the body, also fluctuates. This is inevitable if the knee is kept nearly straight, making the hip move in a near-circular arc about the ankle of

the supporting foot. The vertical component of the total force on the ground (exerted by both feet) in the double-support phase is greater than body weight, giving the body an upward acceleration, but the vertical component of the ground force during the single-support phase is less than body weight, giving the body a downward acceleration (Cavagna et al 1977). The force fluctuations have to be larger at higher speeds, to give the same vertical movement in less time (Alexander & Jayes 1980).

The potential energy of the body is high when its kinetic energy is low, and vice versa. Thus energy can be swapped back and forth between the two forms, as in a swinging pendulum (Cavagna et al 1977). A frictionless pendulum (if such a thing existed) would continue swinging forever with no fresh input of energy. In walking, the exchange of potential and kinetic energy is less perfect, and the leg muscles have to do work to replace energy lost at each impact of a foot with the ground (McGeer 1992). Even so, much less work is needed because of the pendulum principle. A second pendulum effect can be seen in the forward swing of the legs (Mochon & McMahon 1980). If the leg were a rigid rod swinging from a fixed pivot it would swing forward too slowly for normal walking, but because it is free to bend at the knee and because the hip from which it swings rises and falls, it swings forward faster with very little need for muscular work.

These pendulum effects ensure that rather little work is needed to drive the fluctuations of kinetic and potential energy that occur in walking. The additional work needed to overcome air resistance and joint friction is tiny, because we travel slowly and have well-lubricated joints. Consequently, human walking is economical of energy. Measurements of oxygen consumption show that 70-kg men use only about 230 joules of metabolic energy for every metre they walk at their most economical speed, about 1.3 metres per second (Margaria 1976). This is about 140 J/m more than they would use if they stood still. Running uses about 260 J/m more than standing. Measurements on non-human mammals ranging from shrews to cattle show that a typical 70-kg mammal could be expected to use about 200 J/m more when walking or running than when standing (Taylor et al 1982). In energy terms, therefore, human walking is rather economical, and running rather expensive, compared to animals.

Walking is economical only near the optimum speed. The energy cost of fast walking overtakes that of running at about 2 m/s (Margaria 1976). Accordingly, adults break into a run at about this speed (Thorstensson & Roberthson 1987). Children, with their shorter legs, start running at lower speeds: the theoretical expectation is that the critical speed should be proportional to the square root of leg

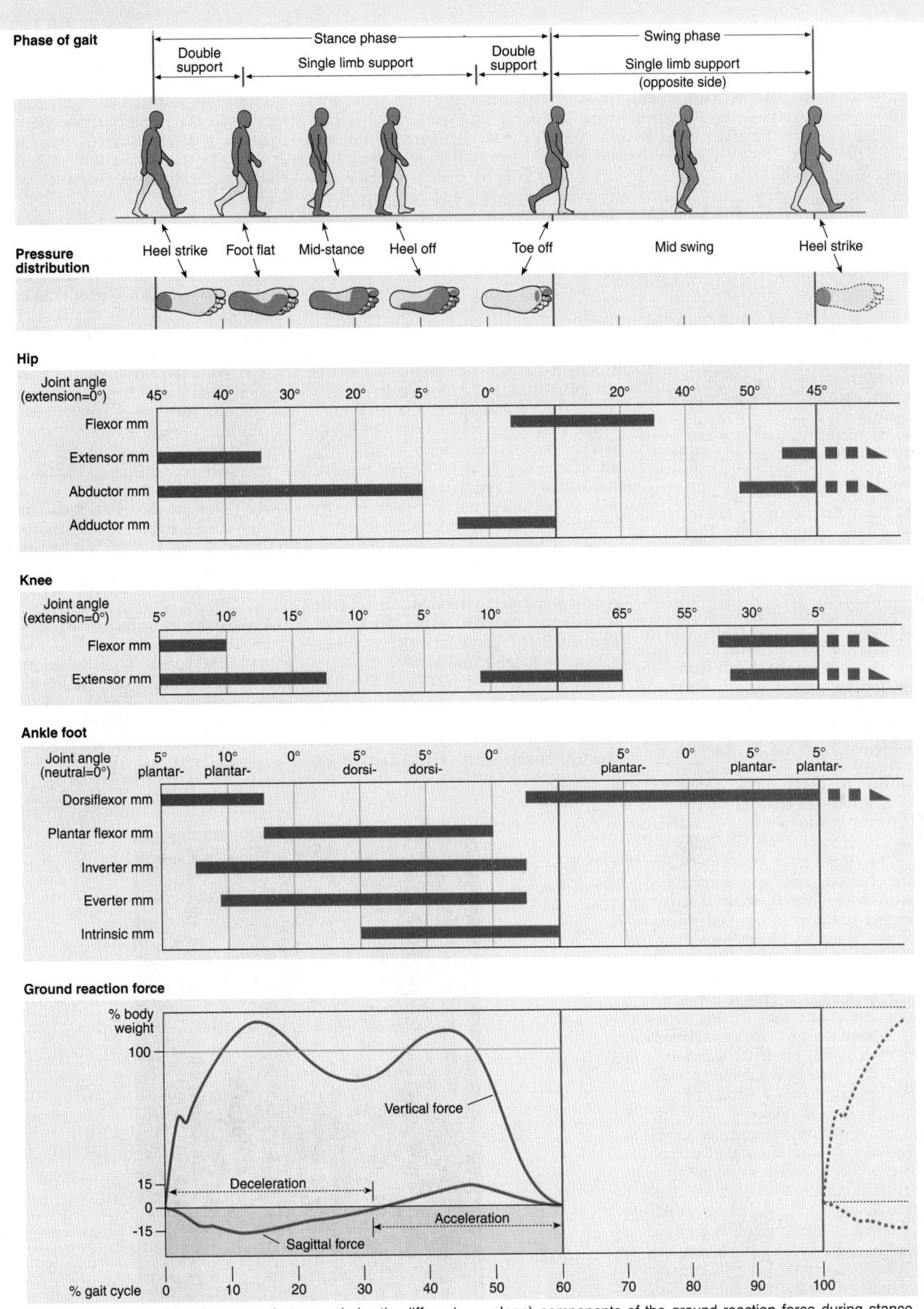

7.149 Diagram to show the events that occur during the different phases of a normal gait cycle. Depicted are: distribution of pressure on the plantar surface of the foot; changes in the angles of hip, knee and ankle joints, together with activity in the corresponding muscle groups; and vertical and horizontal (sagittal plane) components of the ground reaction force during stance phase. (For a more detailed listing of muscles in each of the groups shown, see Table 7.2.) (Chart collated from various sources by Michael Gunther, Department of Human Anatomy and Cell Biology, University of Liverpool.)

length (Alexander & Jayes 1983). Adults in small villages usually walk at speeds well below the most economical, averaging 0.8 m/s, but in large cities they walk faster, at 1.5–1.8 m/s (Bornstein & Bornstein 1976). This was originally interpreted as reflecting the stress of city life, but it has since been shown that it is explained largely by the higher proportion of elderly people in villages (Wirtz & Ries 1993). The function of arm swinging in walking is not fully understood (Jackson 1983).

For further discussion of standing and walking see Alexander (1992).

RUNNING

Walking involves dual-support phases, but in running each foot is on the ground for 40% (jogging) to 27% (sprinting) of the stride, so there are aerial phases when neither foot is on the ground (Högberg 1952). During each aerial phase the body rises and then falls under gravity, so its height and potential energy are maximal in the middle of this phase. They have their minimum values at midstance when (in contrast to walking) the knee of the supporting leg bends to 130–140° (Brandell 1973; Debrunner 1985).

The mean vertical force on the ground during a complete stride cycle of any gait must equal body weight. If the foot is on the ground for only a small fraction of the stride, the forces must then be high. Peak vertical forces on one foot are about 1.0 times body weight in walking, 2.5 times in jogging, and 3.5 times in sprinting (Alexander & Jayes 1980; Debrunner 1985). Leg muscles have to exert much larger forces in running than in walking because the ground forces are higher and also because (for a given ground force) the bending of the knee increases the moments about it. There is strong electrical activity in the gastrocnemius and soleus, and also in the quadriceps and hamstring groups, during the stance phase of running (Brandell 1973).

As in walking, the ground force acts more or less in line with the leg, so the body is decelerated and reaccelerated during each stance phase (Cavagna et al 1977). Kinetic energy is minimal at midstance when (as already explained) potential energy is also minimal. Thus the pendulum principle cannot be used. Instead, energy is saved by the principle of the pogo stick: elastic strain energy is stored up in stretched tendons and ligaments as kinetic and potential energy fall, and returned by elastic recoil as they rise again (Alexander 1988). Muscle elasticity may contribute a little but is very much less important than tendon elasticity (Alexander & Bennet-Clark 1977).

Tendon is fairly strong, capable of withstanding stresses (force per unit cross-sectional area) of at least 100 N/mm^2 (10 kg force/mm^2). It stretches elastically by about 8% before breaking, and its recoil returns 93% of the energy used to stretch it (Ker 1981; Alexander 1988). This high energy return is important, not only because it reduces the work required from the muscles, but also because the lost mechanical energy becomes heat: leg tendons with poor energy return would overheat in running, and be damaged.

The Achilles tendon is the most important spring in the leg. Most runners strike the ground first with the heel, but the centre of pressure moves rapidly forward to the distal heads of the metatarsals, where it remains for most of the stance phase (Cavanagh & Lafortune 1980). A large force is then required in the Achilles tendon to balance the moments about the tibiotalar joint. For a 70-kg man running at middle-distance speed, the peak force in the tendon is about 5000 N (0.5 tonne force), which is enough to stretch it by about 6% (Ker et al 1987). The parts of the tendon that run alongside the gastrocnemius and soleus muscle bellies must be stretched, as well as the free distal part.

The ground force acts upward on the metatarsal heads and the Achilles tendon pulls upwards on the calcaneus. The necessary balancing reaction occurs at the ankle, where the tibia presses downwards on the talus. Together these three forces flatten the longitudinal arch of the foot, forcing the ankle 10 mm nearer the ground than it could go if the foot were rigid (Alexander 1992). Mechanical tests on amputated feet have shown that the foot is a reasonably good spring, giving an energy return of about 78% (Ker et al 1987). Further tests in which ligaments were cut showed that the plantar aponeurosis, the long and short plantar ligaments and the plantar calcaneonavicular ligament were all involved in the spring action. They consist largely of collagen and presumably have elastic properties similar to those of tendon.

It was estimated from the tests that, of the kinetic and potential energy lost and regained in each stance phase, 35% is stored temporarily as elastic strain energy in the Achilles tendon and 17% in the ligaments of the arch of the foot. Thus, together these springs approximately halve the work required from the muscles. Similar percentage savings are made by tendon elasticity in hopping kangaroos. Larger savings are probably made in camels and horses, in which the muscle fibres of some distal leg muscles are only a few millimetres long, although their tendons are 700 mm or more (Alexander 1988). The length changes of these muscle–tendon complexes during the stance phase must be almost entirely due to passive elastic stretching of the tendons, with very little active contribution from the muscle fibres.

A runner's foot is still moving, typically at about 1.5 m/s, when the heel hits the ground. The impact is cushioned by the subcalcaneal foot pad, supplemented (when shoes are worn) by the compliance of the heel of the shoe (Ker et al 1989).

For further discussion of running see Cavanagh (1990) and Alexander (1992).

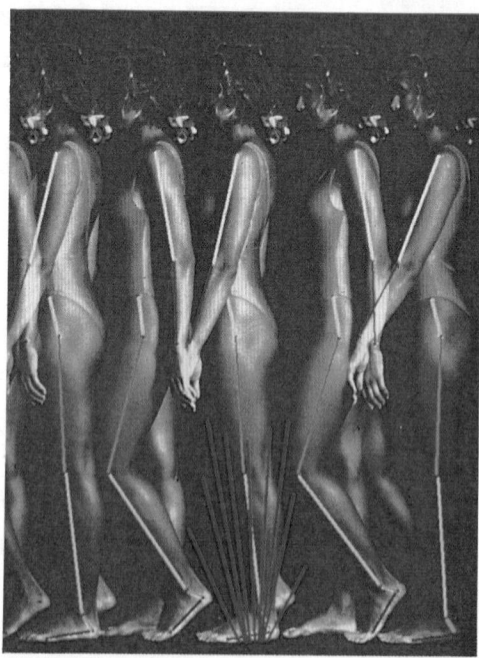

7.150 A stroboscopic sequence of body positions during normal gait. Data from sensors were processed automatically and superimposed upon the image in real time to show the movement of body segments and the resultant ground reaction forces. (Photograph by Antonio Pedotti, Bioengineering Centre of Milan, Italy.)

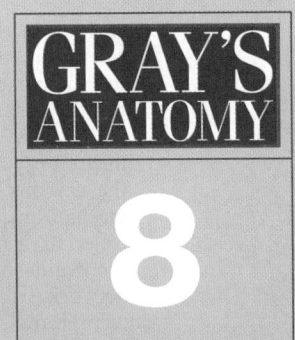

GRAY'S ANATOMY

8

NERVOUS SYSTEM

Section Editors: Martin Berry, Lawrence H Bannister, Susan M Standring

G Burnstock (Autonomic nervous system), Stuart Butler (Electrical activity of the brain), Arthur Butt (Neuroglia), Malcolm B Carpenter (Spinal tracts), Alan Colchester (Imaging), Barry Everitt (Limbic lobe), Heidi Felix (Membranous labyrinth), D Gaffan (Learning and memory), Michael Gleeson (Membranous labyrinth), M H Glickstein (Cerebellum), N A Gregson (CNS myelin), Carole Hackney (Cochlear nerve), Wolfgang Hamann (Cutaneous sensory endings), P Harrison (Cerebral asymmetry), R Haskell (Trigeminal nerve), M Hastings (Circadian clocks), Joe Herbert (Stress), Robin Howard (Glossopharyngeal nerve), N Jones (Facial nerve), C Kennard (Oculomotor, trochlear, abducens nerves), Roger Lemon (Neural control of complex movement), Olle Lindvall (Transplantation and Parkinson's disease), S McMahon (Neural basis of pain), T Matthews (Oculomotor, trochlear, abducens nerves), P Milner (Autonomic nervous system), J Morris (Hypothalamus), M O'Brien (Peripheral nerves and plexuses), C Pearson (Cerebral cortex, thalamus), G D Perkin (Accessory nerve), G Raisman (Neural transplantation), E L Rees (Spinal medulla), G Ruskell (Accessory visual apparatus), K Smith (Neurons, physiology), J Voogd (Cerebellum), K E Webster (Basal nuclei), R O Weller (Fluid compartments).

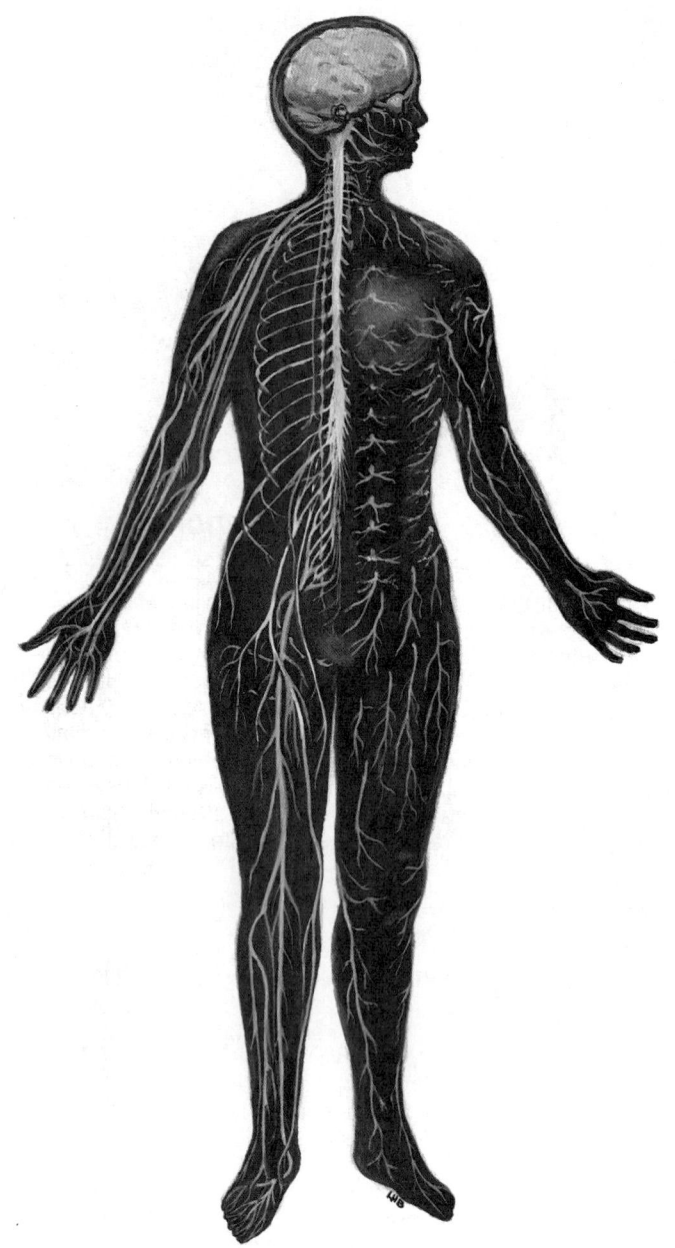

8.1　Schema illustrating the anatomical arrangement of the human nervous system, including its main central and peripheral components. The deep structures are shown on the left, and the superficial, mainly cutaneous nerves on the right. The innervation of the viscera and many minor branches of other parts of the peripheral nervous system have been omitted for clarity.

INTRODUCTION

Overview of the section

The human nervous system (8.1) is the most complex physical system known to mankind; it consists of many billions of interactive units whose constantly changing patterns of activity are reflected in every aspect of human behaviour and experience. Investigators from many disciplines, and with many different methods, motives and persuasions have converged in its study, yet our understanding of neural organization must at present be considered still quite rudimentary, and our ability to deal with its pathologies extremely limited. What is known about the nervous system has been gleaned from many centuries of anatomical study, experiment and clinical observation, beginning in classical antiquity, faltering for many centuries but accelerating from the second half of the nineteenth century, until at present tens of thousands of scientists around the world are occupied with various aspects of this most complex entity.

The present account of the nervous system is, of course, directed primarily towards its structure, but at every level of organization

various methodological approaches have to be taken into consideration because the mechanisms within it can only be understood in dynamic terms. At the very minimum a combination of anatomical, physiological and molecular techniques is required for its appraisal, and we may also have to draw on clinical observations and experimental psychology. At the same time, while it is essential to reduce the nervous system to its parts in order to understand its detailed mechanisms, such analyses provide only a partial and, if taken in isolation, a misleading picture of the nervous system; ultimately we are dealing with an immensely structured, integrated and coherent network which is itself a functional unity rather than merely a complicated assembly of individual components. Even at a less comprehensive level, we have to consider the interactive behaviour of subordinate systems within it, each composed of large cell populations which together can produce effects not readily predicted from its individual cellular units. Such holistic concepts are only gradually coming into focus within current neuroscience, and there is much to do before we begin to appreciate neural behaviour on such a scale. However, there is also much value in a traditional approach, and indeed, it is essential to understand the basic parts of the nervous system and their major pathways of conduction and transmission to have any grasp of neural function at all.

This section of Gray's begins with a general overview of the nervous system's chief features, including its cellular basis, functional roles, phylogenetic and embryonic origins, and some of the ways in which cells interact to form functional units within it. After this, the historical roots and methods of modern neuroscience are briefly considered, followed by a description of the general structure and behaviour of the cells of the nervous system. We then proceed to the main subject of the section, the detailed structural organization of the central and peripheral nervous components of the human nervous system. Using the customary (and in some instances rather arbitrary) subdivisions, the parts of the central nervous system are described in caudal to rostral sequence—spinal cord, hind-, mid- and forebrain. In each of these regions topography is considered first, then the enclosed populations of cells, their connections and, briefly, their functions. This consideration of the central nervous system is concluded with a description of its vascular system and meninges. After the central nervous system the peripheral nervous system is described including its subdivisions—cranial and spinal nerves, autonomic nervous system, and special senses (gustatory, olfactory, visual and vestibulocochlear organs and their accessory structures). Within this descriptive framework a number of essays on topics of special interest are placed where relevant to particular regions of the nervous system.

CELLULAR NATURE OF THE NERVOUS SYSTEM

To appreciate the organization of the nervous system it is essential to understand something of its cellular composition, as the immense complexity of its organization is due to its vast population of intercommunicating cells (8.2A–C). These are the nerve cells or *neurons*, which can encode information, conduct it over considerable distances and then transmit it to other neurons or to various non-neural cells. The movement of such information within the nervous system depends on the rapid conduction of minute transient electrochemical fluctuations along neuronal surface membranes. Its transmission to other cells is effected by the secretion of neurotransmitters at special junctions with other neurons (*synapses*) or with cells outside the nervous system, for example muscle cells (*neuromuscular junctions*), gland cells, adipose tissue, etc. to cause various changes in their behaviour. Besides the large population of neurons, there is also a great army of supporting cells (*neuroglia*, etc.) which, whilst not electrically active in the same way, are responsible for creating and maintaining an appropriate environment in which the neurons can operate efficiently (see p. 937).

As alluded to above, the unique features of the nervous system include the high interconnectivity of its neurons, each of them receiving information from and transmitting it to great numbers of others. In the cerebral cortex, for example, a single cortical pyramidal neuron may receive afferent contacts from many hundreds of other neurons and may itself make efferent contacts with a similar number. This degree of interaction is only possible because of the shapes of neurons, whose surface areas are very extensive due to the numerous

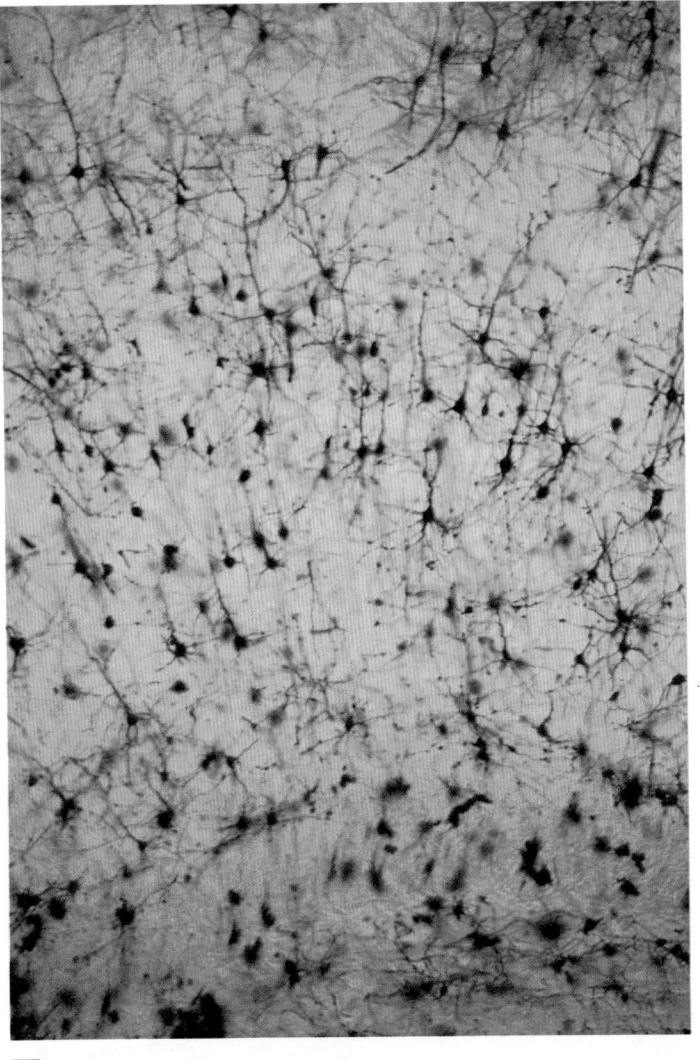

A

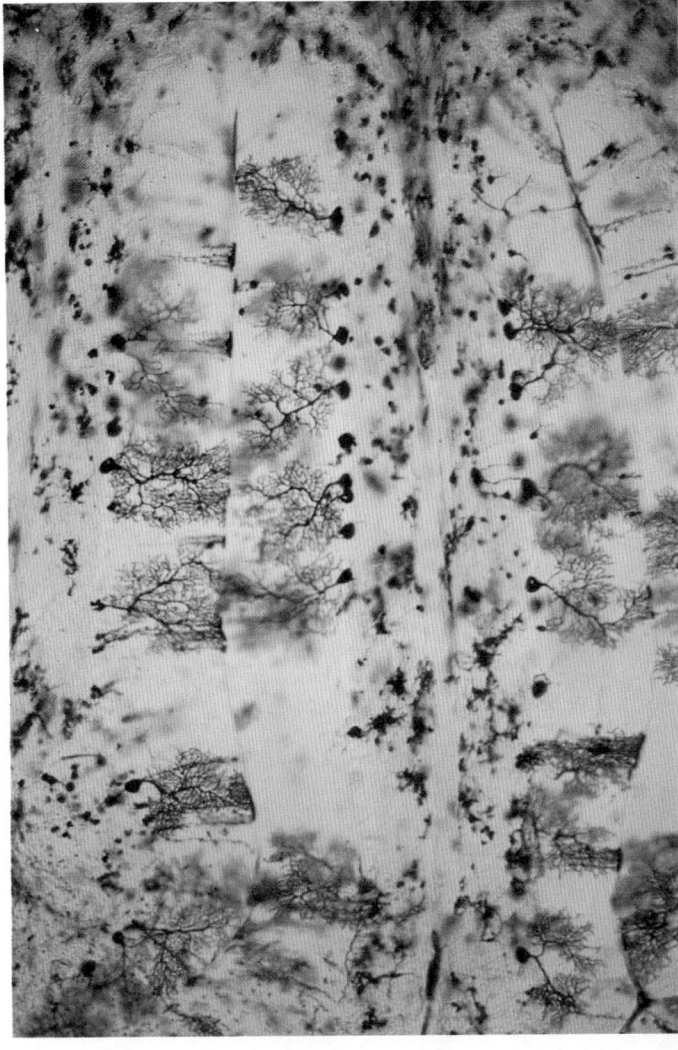

B

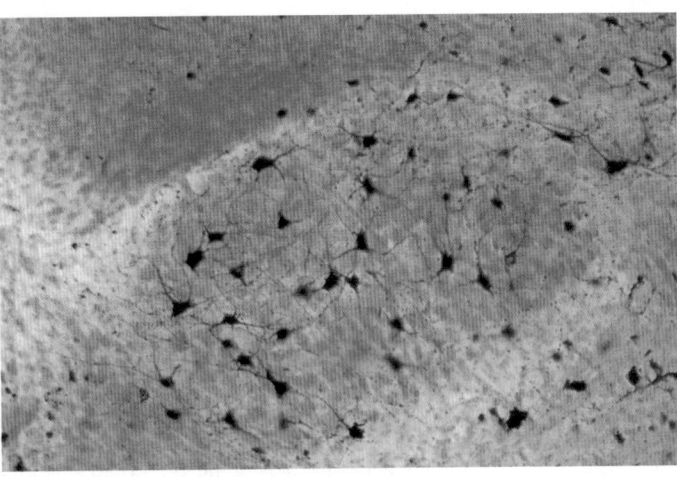

C

8.2A–C Cellular basis of the nervous system in the central nervous system: neuronal variety and complexity.

A is a micrograph of a section through the cerebral cortex (mouse) stained by the Golgi method which demonstrates only a small proportion of the total neuronal population.

B is a similar section from the cerebellum, showing rows of large tree-like Purkinje cells and small granular cells (see also p. 1040).

c. A Golgi preparation of a deep cerebellar nucleus containing a group of multipolar neurons counter-stained with a Nissl stain which colours all cell bodies blue. Magnifications: A and B: ×150; c: ×450. (All specimens prepared by M Sadler, Division of Anatomy and Cell Biology, UMDS London.)

narrow branched cell processes projecting from their perimeters. Most neurons, therefore, have a rounded central mass of cytoplasm enclosing the cell's nucleus (the *cell body* or *soma*), giving off long, branched extensions, collectively termed *neurites*, with which most of the intercellular contacts are made. In most instances one of these processes, the *axon*, is much longer than the others, which are termed *dendrites* (**8.3**). Dendrites typically conduct electrical changes towards the soma, and axons conduct away from it, under normal physiological conditions. The precise arrangement of the different elements in the neuron vary considerably, as indicated in **8.4**.

Neurons exist in huge populations, estimated at more than 10^{12} within the brain; the sum total of synapses within the nervous system is, therefore, truly astronomical. However, within this community of cells there is also much variation in detailed shape, electrical behaviour, chemistry and connectivity. The pathways formed by the axons and dendrites of these different categories of neurons are arranged in orderly and largely predictable patterns, defining discrete pathways, microcircuits, and special areas of synaptic interaction within the great mass of cells.

Functional arrangements of neurons

Nervous systems in all animals have three basic functional elements

903

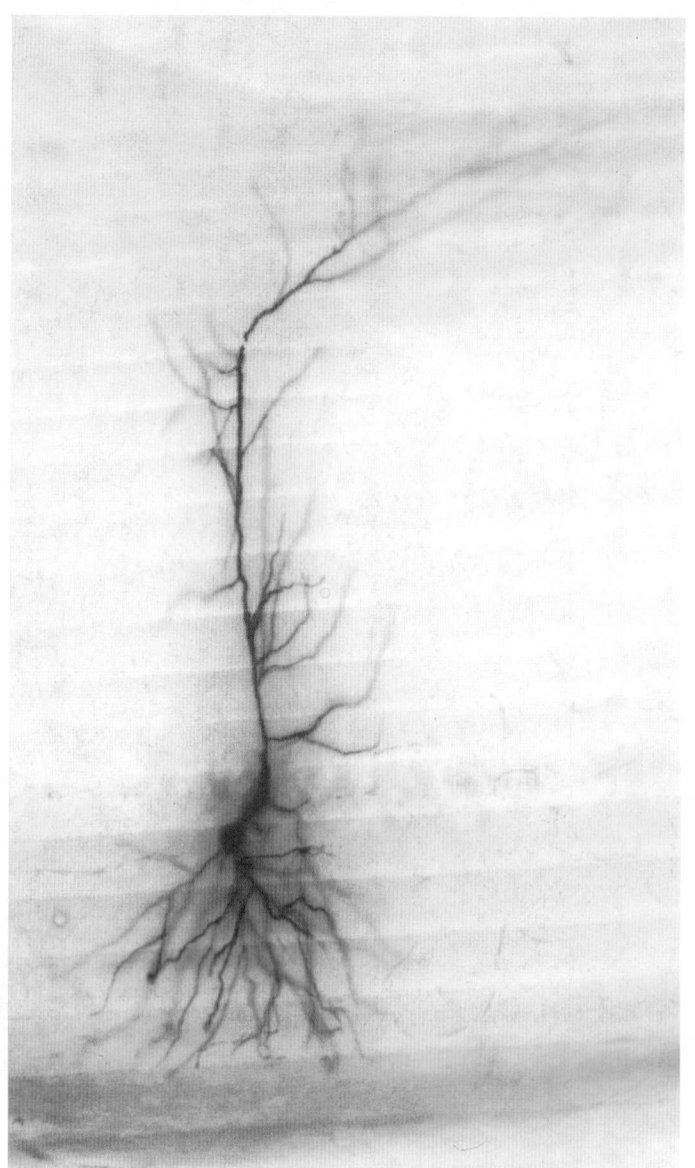

8.3 A large pyramidal neuron from the hippocampal cortex (rat), showing the central soma and radiating branched dendrites. The neuron was present in a living brain slice maintained in vitro, and had been injected with lysine conjugated to biotin, then visualized with streptavidin-peroxidase. The large transverse striations are artefacts caused when the slice was cut from the hippocampus prior to culture. (Provided by Neil Bannister, Department of Physiology, University of Oxford.)

which can be defined as sensory, motor and processing or integrative (8.5). At the simplest level of operation, these components allow the nervous system to detect changes in the environment and make appropriate effector responses to them. The sensory elements are able to detect a wide range of energy forms which are customarily classed as mechanical, chemical, thermal and electromagnetic (including photic). Some sensory channels detect these stimuli using specialized receptor cells which transmit through synapses to sensory neurons (e.g. visual, taste, auditory and vestibular systems) whereas in other situations, for example spinal nerves, the peripheral end of a sensory neuronal process is itself the sensory detector. The conversion of external energy into an electrical change in the receptor is termed *transduction*; it involves various molecular mechanisms, often complex, whose details vary considerably in different receptor cells. *Motor neurons* (*motoneurons*) send axons from the central nervous system to the effector organs (chiefly muscles and glands); they may also have more subtle influences on the functions of many other tissues in the body, for example the immune and endocrine systems, by mechanisms at present poorly understood. Neurons

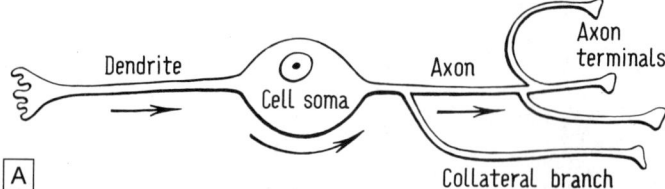

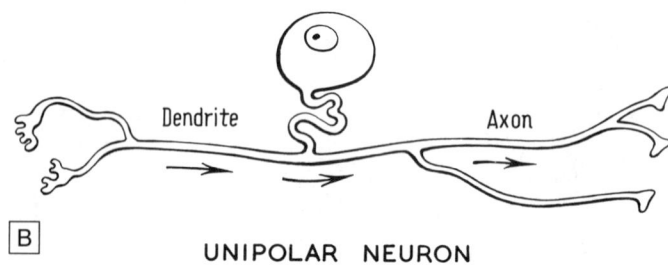

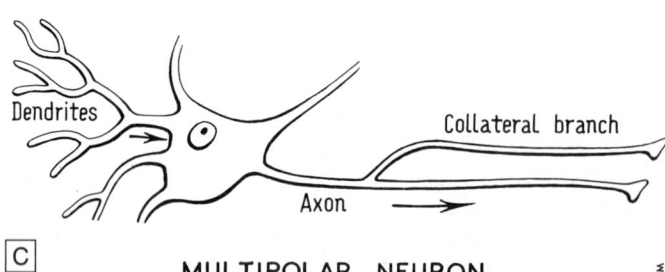

8.4 Three general morphological groups of neurons classified according to the number of neurites which arise from the surface of the cell soma; A. bipolar neuron; B. unipolar neuron; C. multipolar neuron. For a more detailed analysis of the branching patterns of neurites, see 8. 33.

which are confined to the central nervous system, possessing neither direct sensory nor motor terminals, are called *interneurons*; they engage in various intermediary operations, integrating and analysing the inputs of information, distributing them to other parts of the nervous system, storing sensory information and processing it in various ways. Such neurons are responsible for selecting appropriate motor responses to stimulation and issuing them to motor neurons, although in some instances sensory neurons may activate motor neurons directly without the need for a third, processing set (a monosynaptic pathway, e.g. for muscle strength reflexes, see p. 907). The great majority of the neurons within the human nervous system are interneurons. Because most of the nervous system's activities are determined by this population, their degree of organization corresponds closely to behavioural complexity in any animal species.

The 'processing' part of the nervous system is not merely an interface between sensory and motor elements, but can initiate and entrain many complex activities depending on stored memory resulting from experience, or by genetically programmed outputs depending on intrinsically self-directed mechanisms, for example respiratory centres controlling the ventilation cycle, circadian time-keeping 'clocks' and neurally controlled cyclic release of reproduction-related hormones.

Adaptive structuring of the nervous system

The formation of the principal interconnections and functional behaviour of the sensory, motor and central processing pathways are essentially under genetic control, and are determined during ontogenesis by a series of interlocked, interactive processes, as described on page 217 et seq. Of course, during the many millions of years in which the phylogenetic development of any species has

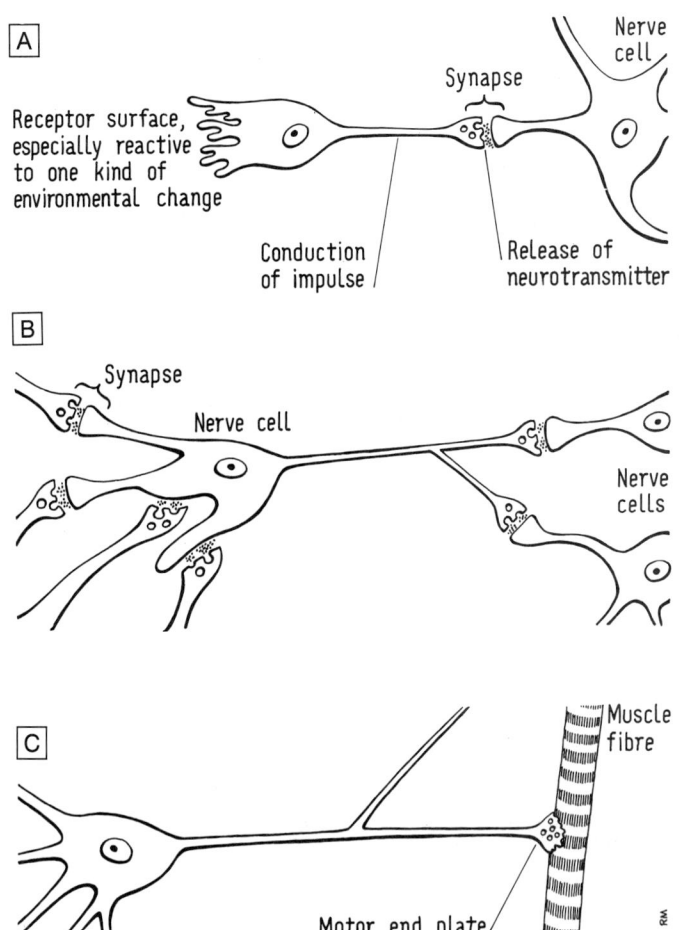

8.5 The three main avenues of differentiation which may be followed by a primitive neuroblast: A. a receptor neuron; B. an interneuron; C. an effector neuron.

occurred, it appears that the genetic information specifying this neural organization has been finely sculpted by the process of natural selection, an interaction between the gene complement and its environment which has generated a genetic 'memory' built into the essential fabric of the nervous system, related to survival and successful reproduction within the constraints of a particular environment.

However, in any individual, the details of neural organization and behaviour are clearly not all determined by the genetic code; there is considerable adaptation by neurons to external or internal influences during individual development and, in some parts of the nervous system, extending throughout life. This adaptability or *plasticity*, is seen at its most extreme in the mechanisms of cognitive and motor memories mediated by nerve cells whose electrical behaviour and perhaps structure can be modified for long periods of time by appropriate inputs of information; but recent evidence suggests that some degree of plasticity is present in many parts of the mature system to a more modest extent. The balance between genetic determinance and environmentally influenced plasticity in determining behaviour is a matter for ongoing, often heated debate; the nervous system is complex, and its different components show varying amounts of plasticity, so this broad issue is not likely to be brought to a satisfactory conclusion in the immediate future.

PHYSIOLOGICAL PROPERTIES OF NEURONS (8.6)

All cells generate a steady electrochemical potential across their plasma membranes (a membrane potential) because of the different ionic concentrations inside and outside the cell. Neurons use minute fluctuations in this potential to receive, conduct, and transmit information across their surfaces.

Resting potential

The membrane potential (8.6) of a neuron, known as the resting potential, is similar to that of non-excitable cells. In most neurons it is about 80 mV, inside negative. Such bioelectrical potentials result from the selectively permeable nature of the plasma membrane, which prevents large molecules, predominantly with negative charges (non-diffusible anions) from leaving the cell. For electrostatic neutrality within the cytoplasm an equal number of positive charges is needed to establish electrical neutrality. The cell uses potassium ions for this purpose (it actively excludes sodium, the other major cation of the body), so that there is a high concentration of potassium within cells. However, outside the cell there is little potassium, and these ions tend to leak out through the plasma membrane along their diffusion gradient, carrying positive charges and creating a net negative charge within the cell. Outward potassium ion leakage continues until an equilibrium (the Gibbs-Donnan equilibrium) is reached when the electrical energy within the cell is sufficient to prevent any further diffusion of this ion. Various other ions also play a part in establishing the level of the resting potential, although their roles are minor. The size of the resting potential matches that calculated according to the concentrations of the different ions inside and outside the cell.

Modulation of the membrane potential

Any activity which causes a change in the distribution of ion across the plasma membrane inevitably affects the resting potential. The entry into neurons of sodium or, in some sites, calcium ions causes depolarization of the cell, while an increased chloride influx or an increased potassium efflux results in hyperpolarization. Alterations in plasma membrane permeability to these ions are brought about by the opening or closing of ion-specific transmembrane channels, triggered by a number of agents which may be chemical or electrical. Chemically triggered ionic fluxes occur at synapses (p. 926), and may either be direct, the chemical agent (neurotransmitter) binding to the channel itself to cause it to open, or else the neurotransmitter is bound by a transmembrane receptor molecule which is not itself a channel; this then activates a complex second messenger system within the cell to open separate transmembrane channels. Electrically induced changes in membrane potential depend on the presence of voltage sensitive ion channels which, when the transmembrane potential reaches a critical level, open to allow the influx or efflux of specific ions. In all cases, the channels remain open only for a brief instant, the numbers opening and closing determining the total flux of ions across the membrane.

The types and concentrations of transmembrane channels and related proteins, and therefore the electrical activity of the membranes, vary in different parts of the cell. Dendrites and neuronal cell bodies depend mainly on neurotransmitter action and show graded potentials, whereas axons have voltage-gated channels which give rise to action potentials.

Graded potentials. Graded potentials are changes in membrane potential which can vary in size, duration and charge polarity. Depolarizing potentials result from excitatory neurotransmitters eliciting an increased inflow of sodium or calcium ions from high extracellular concentrations, reducing the membrane towards zero (but not beyond). Alternatively, hyperpolarizing (inhibitory) neurotransmitters cause the influx of negatively charged chloride ions or the efflux of positively charged potassium ions, to increase the total number of internal negative charges. The amplitude and duration of a graded potential at a particular site depends on a number of factors: the chemical nature and dynamics of neurotransmitter release from the presynaptic membrane, and the numbers and classes of receptor molecule and ion channels on the post-synaptic side. Because of the electrical properties of the neuronal cytoplasm and its plasma membrane, there is a flow of current from or into adjacent areas of the cell when a synapse is activated, and this contributes to the total degree of polarization of the membrane covering the cell body. However, the influence of an individual synapse on neighbouring regions decreases with distance so that, for instance, synapses on the distal tips of dendrites may, on their own, have relatively little effect on the total outcome. As can be imagined, the electrical state of a neuron therefore depends on a mathematically complex equation in which the many variables include the numbers and positions of the

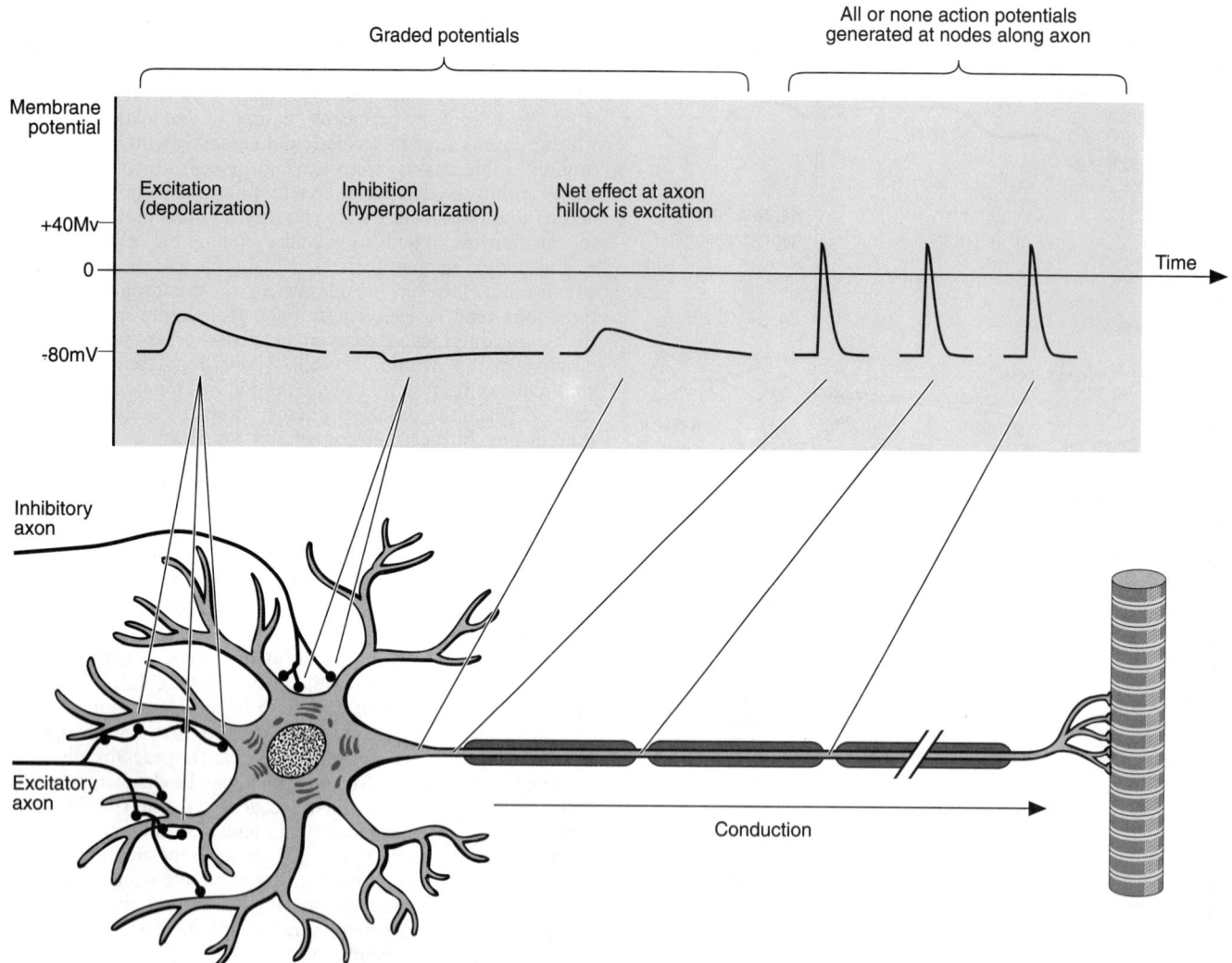

8.6 The types of change in electrical potential which can be recorded across the cell membrane of a motor neuron at the points indicated by the arrows. Excitatory and inhibitory synapses on the surfaces of the dendrites and soma cause local graded changes of potential which summate at the axon hillock and may initiate a series of all-or-none action potentials, which in their turn are conducted along the axon to the effector terminals.

many thousands of excitatory and inhibitory synapses, their degree of activation and effects, the branching pattern of the dendritic tree and the geometry of the cell body. The target of all these processes is a small but crucial part of the neuron surface, that of the axon hillock where, unlike the dendrites or cell body, a high concentration of voltage sensitive channels is found. This is the site where action potentials are generated prior to their conduction down the axon.

Action potential. The action potential, nerve impulse or spike potential, as studied most extensively in peripheral nerves, is a brief, complete reversal of polarity which propagates itself along membranes. Its mechanism, first described in the squid giant axon by Hodgkin and Huxley (1952) depends on an initial influx of sodium ions which causes the reversal of polarity to about 40 mV (positive inside), followed by a rapid return to the resting potential as potassium ions flow out to restore the number of internal negative charges. The whole process is completed in about 5 msec. (It should be noted however, that variations may occur in the detail of ionic conductance changes; thus in central axons, the recovery phase of the action potential appears not to depend on potassium efflux but on general current leakage.)

For a particular neuron, the size and duration of action potentials are always the same ('all or none') no matter how much a stimulus exceeds the threshold value. Once initiated, an action potential spreads rapidly and at constant velocity because the electrotonic spread of current triggers the opening of neighbouring voltage-sensitive channels of the same sort. It is therefore said to be a *propagating potential*. The velocity of conduction, ranging from about 4–120 m/sec, depends on a number of factors related to the

way in which the electrotonic current spreads, e.g. axonal cross sectional area, membrane capacitance (influenced by the presence of myelin in some fibres), and to the numbers and positioning of ion channels (see p. 919). At the end of an action potential, there is an irreducible delay, the *refractory period*, during which another action potential cannot be elicited. This determines the maximum frequency at which action potentials can be conducted along a nerve fibre; its value differs in different neurons so that their upper and lower limits of their action potential frequency range (dynamic range) may differ. This affects the amount of information which can be carried by an individual fibre.

It will be seen from this account that once the cell body has been depolarized below a certain threshold voltage it can initiate action potentials at its axon hillock, and in general, as long as the depolarization is maintained it will continue to do so, rather like an automatic gun being fired by pressure on its trigger. The frequency of firing is thus a measure of the state of excitation of the neuron cell body, and this is the fundamental principle of information conduction within the nervous system. When an action potential reaches the axonal terminals, it causes a graded depolarization of the presynaptic membrane and as a result, quanta of neurotransmitter are released to change the degree of excitation of the next neuron, muscle fibre or glandular cell. At synapses, closely grouped action potentials (trains or volleys) are usually more effective because they maintain higher levels of neurotransmitter release, countering its rapid removal by extracellular enzymes, uptake or diffusion.

Axonal conduction is naturally unidirectional, from dendrites and soma to axon terminals (orthodromic conduction); when artificially

906

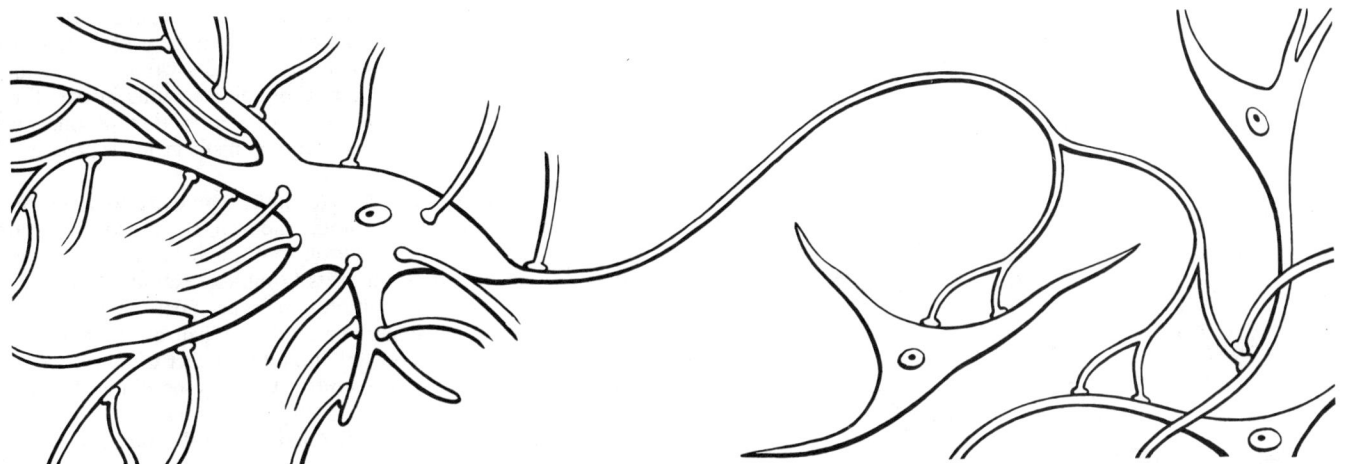

8.7 A generalized multipolar neuron and the parts of its surface upon which synaptic terminals from other neurons may converge. These include the surfaces of the dendrites, the cell soma, the initial segment of the axon and the proximal surface of its own axonal synaptic terminals.

stimulated in their periphery, axons can also conduct centripetally (antidromic conduction). In *amacrine neurons* and other small neurons lacking true axons, all excitation may be conducted in any direction from the locus of stimulation. The dendrites of some large neurons have regions where action potentials are conducted over limited distances to assist the electrotonic spread of excitation.

Sensory transduction. The distal ends of sensory neurons also have regions where extracellular changes are converted into graded electrochemical responses (sensory transduction) and thence into frequency-coded action potentials. The depolarizing or hyperpolarizing graded potential (*receptor potential*, p. 980) is elicited by the action of various agents on transmembrane proteins, causing the opening of ion channels. More proximally, the axonal membrane has numerous voltage-sensitive channels which initiate the action potential when the receptor potential reaches a threshold value. Sensory transduction also occurs at the surfaces of specialized receptor cells which are linked synaptically with the distal ends of sensory neurons. This condition is found in the receptors of taste buds, the inner ear and the retina.

Synaptic interactions between neurons

The types of synaptic interaction between neurons clearly determine the behaviour of the complex networks which compose the nervous system. In a given neural pathway there may be many or only a few synaptically linked neurons. At one extreme, as in the synapses between Ia muscle spindle afferents and a motor neurons, only two cells are concerned (therefore this is a *monosynaptic pathway*). In most instances, three or more neurons form synaptically interactive sequences (*polysynaptic pathways*) which may be linear, leading from

one part of the nervous system to another (as in the somatosensory pathways from the spinal cord to the somatosensory cortex) or may form localized multineuronal functional units (*microcircuits*) with complex recurrent interactions between a number of different cell types, for example as in cortical columns (p. 1151) and the cerebellar cortex (p. 1038).

Divergence and convergence. A neuron may possess axon terminals or collaterals which spread to synapse with many cells—*divergence*—or may concentrate their terminals on only one; in other instances, the axons of many neurons may synapse with a single postsynaptic neuron—*convergence* (**8.7**). The 'many to one' convergent channels can integrate information from many sources, for example complex pyramidal neurons of the visual cortex able to detect shapes (p. 1142). The 'one to many' divergent channels can

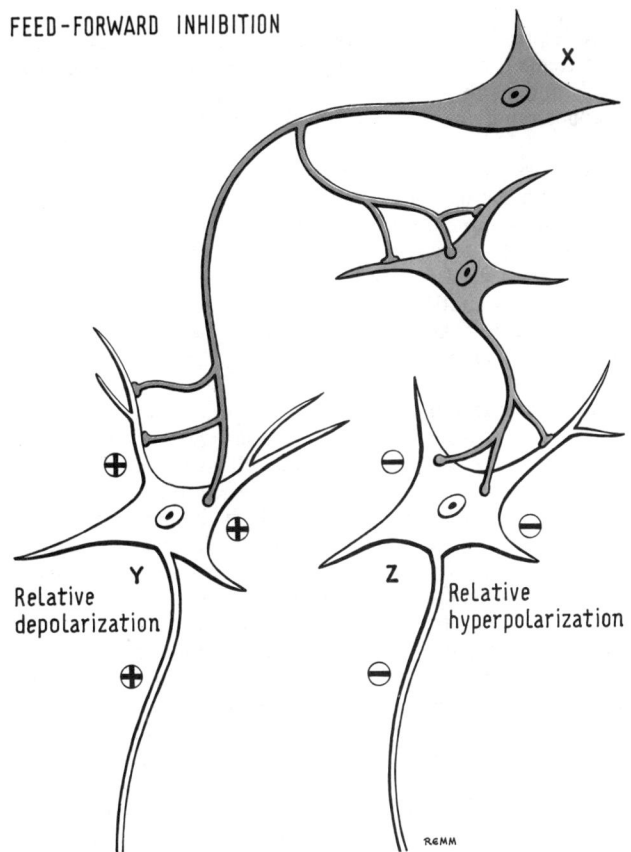

8.9 In this example of an elementary circuit a direct excitatory circuit (left) is compared with a simple feed-forward inhibitory circuit (right). Pink = excitatory neuron; blue = inhibitory neuron.

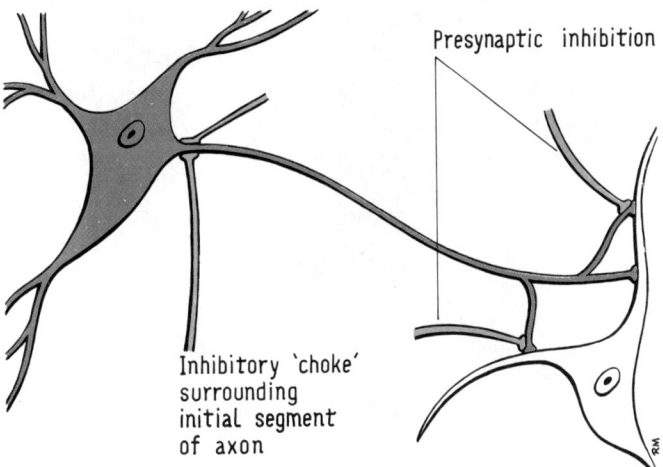

8.8 The multipolar neuron (shown in red), has inhibitory synaptic terminals (blue) applied to the initial segment of its axon and others to the surfaces of its axonal synaptic terminals.

907

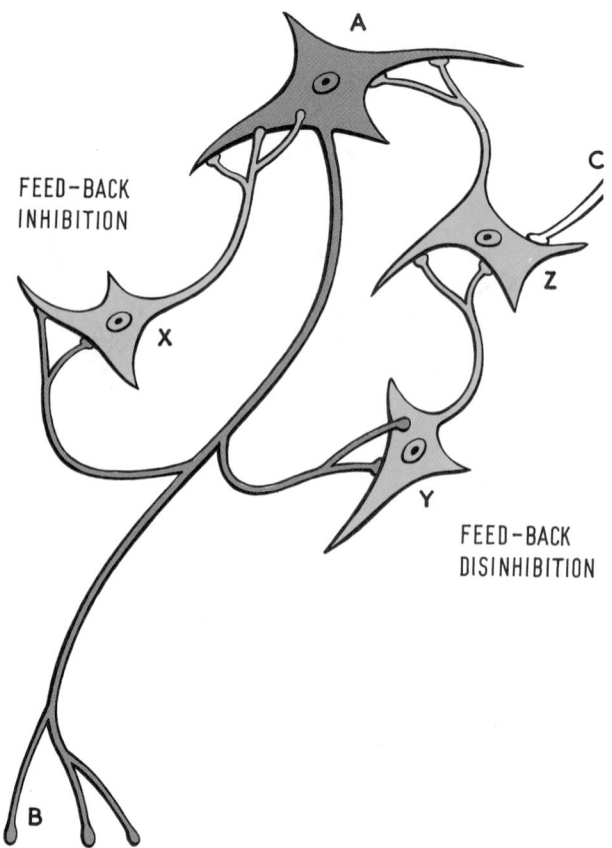

FEED—BACK
INHIBITION

FEED—BACK
DISINHIBITION

8.10 Feedback circuits of two orders of complexity with, on the left, one, and on the right, two inhibitory interneurons interposed on the recurrent pathway. Excitatory, neuron = pink; inhibitory neuron = blue.

exert widespread effects in many parts of the nervous system, seen in an extreme form in, for example, neurons in the locus coeruleus (p. 1077) and of the ascending reticular pathways (p. 1078) which have axons ramifying widely through many different regions of the brain.

In all types of interaction a single axon typically forms many synapses with the neurons it innervates, even when there is a one-to-one relationship between pre- and postsynaptic neurons; the excitatory or inhibitory power of individual synapses is rather limited and many are needed for the adequate transmission of information from one cell to another (although there are a few places where a single, particularly large synapse occurs between neurons, for example at the endings of some auditory fibres in the cochlear nuclear complex).

Synaptic excitation and inhibition. In the simplest case, involving just two neurons, one may cause *postsynaptic excitation* (depolarization) of the second neuron at synapses on either its dendrites or its cell body; this excitation leads to an increase in the probability of initiating action potentials at the base of the second neuron's axon, to be conducted in turn to its synaptic terminals. Secondly, a neuron may cause *postsynaptic inhibition* (hyperpolarization) of another neuron, again either on its dendrites or its cell body, or often also on the initial part of its axon where inhibition can completely stop action potential formation, whatever the electrical state of the rest of the neuron (**8.8**). In a more complex set of interactions, a number of neurons may be involved. To the simple two neuron arrangement, a third may be added, synapsing on the *presynaptic* terminal of the first to silence its action, therefore either causing *presynaptic inhibition*, if the first neuron was excitatory, or *presynaptic disinhibition* if the first neuron was inhibitory.

Interactions between three or more neurons are used by the nervous system to produce a number of different effects by different arrangements of excitatory and inhibitory synapses. For example, in *feedforward inhibition* as illustrated in **8.9** an excitatory neuron (X) is linked with two others, Y and Z, the latter being inhibitory to a

third cell, Z. When the excitatory neuron is active, the inhibitory neuron on the second path reduces the excitatory level of Z, while that of Y rises. In reality other local circuits would also be active but the principle illustrated here probably accounts in part for, for example, the increase in the force of contraction of one muscle group, while the contraction in an antagonistic group is progressively reduced.

In *feedback inhibition* as depicted in **8.10** an excitatory neuron (A) has direct axon terminals on another neuron (B), and also a collateral which excites an inhibitory neuron (X); this in turn inhibits the first neuron to limit the duration of its firing. An example of this is seen in the Renshaw loop of *a* motor neurons. Such feedback circuits vary in complexity; in some, two inhibitory neurons (Y and Z, **8.10**) may form a recurrent loop; the inhibitory effect of neuron Z on A, perhaps from an alternative source (C), may be diminished by the inhibitory neuron Y. Such a release from an inhibitory effect by a second neuron, in series with the first, is called *disinhibition*.

Lateral inhibition. **8.11** shows a special form of feedforward inhibition, *lateral inhibition* or an *inhibitory surround*, prominent in many sites in the nervous system, and well researched in sensory pathways such as the visual system including the retina (p. 1333),

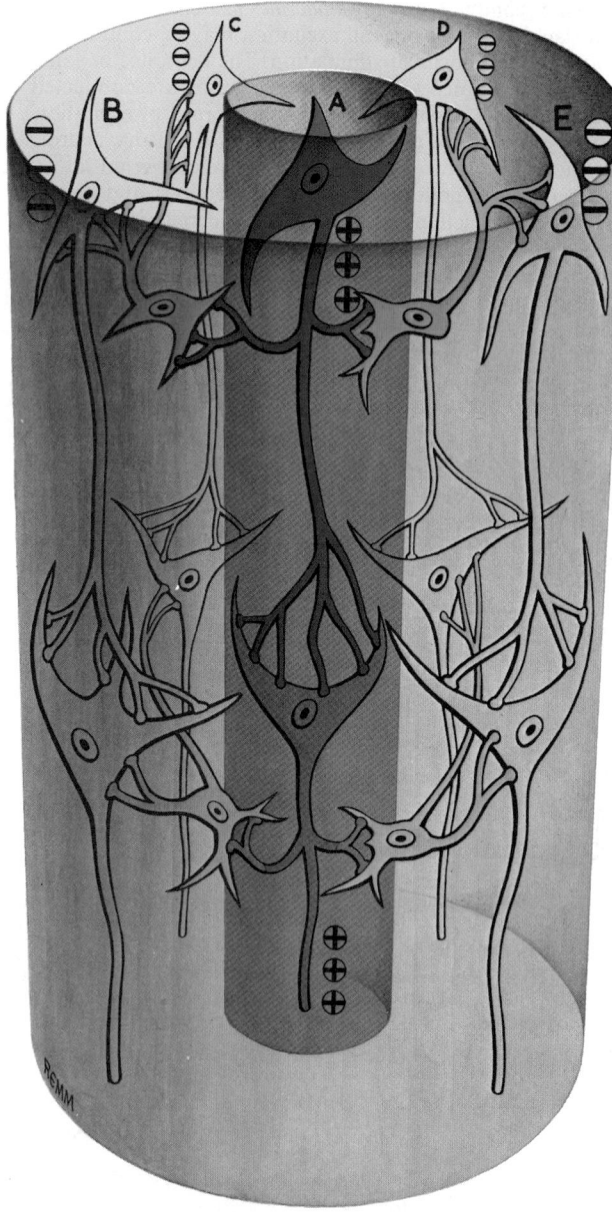

8.11 Examples of lateral inhibition. A central excitatory train of neurons (pink) is surrounded by a hollow cylindrical zone of inhibition, mediated by shells of inhibitory interneurons (blue) which are activated by the central column.

and in the olfactory bulb (p. 1317). Parallel paths A–E carrying functionally similar information may be imagined to transmit sporadically with a low information content; if the excitatory state of one (e.g. A) significantly exceeds that in the others, activity in B–E is reduced by adjacent 'surrounds' of interposed inhibitory neurons. The central activated path is thus surrounded by a quiescent zone, reducing confusion caused by random activity in the others. The discriminative value of the central channel is thus greatly increased, a phenomenon termed *neural sharpening*.

Repetitive microcircuits. Another common feature of the central nervous system is the clustering of repetitive assemblies of interactive cells (microcircuits) each with similar sets of excitatory and inhibitory neurons and connections within it, and with similar but topically varied inputs and outputs. Examples of these are the *neuronal columns* of the visual and somatosensory cortices, and the repetitive sequences of Purkinje and related cells of the cerebellar cortex. Many other instances occur in the body, although they may not always be as clearly recognizable as they are in the sensory cortex and cerebellum.

SUBDIVISIONS OF THE NERVOUS SYSTEM AND TERMINOLOGY

The nervous system is customarily divided into two major parts the central nervous system (CNS), containing the great majority of neuronal cell bodies, and the peripheral nervous system (PNS), composed mainly of the axons of sensory and motor neurons passing from the central nervous system into all parts of the body.

The *central nervous system* is further divisible, though rather artificially, into the spinal cord and the brain, the latter being defined by its enclosure within the cranium. Both are derived embryonically from the neural tube (p. 217). The cell bodies of neurons are often grouped together in areas termed *nuclei*, or they may form more extensive layers or masses of cells collectively called *grey matter*. Neuronal dendrites and synaptic activity are mostly confined to

nuclei and areas of grey matter, while their axons pass into bundles of nerve fibres which tend to be grouped separately to form *tracts*. In the spinal cord, cerebellum, cerebral cortices and some other areas, concentrations of tracts constitute the *white matter*, so called because the axons are often ensheathed in myelin (p. 951) which glistens white in the fresh state. When tracts are flattened structures they are termed *lemnisci* (Latin: ribbon), and when rounded or thicker, sometimes, *funiculi* (Latin: rope). Tracts within the nervous system often cross the midline (a *decussation*). Connections between corresponding areas of the brain across the midline are *commissures*.

The *peripheral nervous system* comprises the cranial and spinal nerves and the peripheral part of the *autonomic nervous system* (see p. 1292) including the *enteric nervous system* (composed of plexuses of nerve fibres and cell bodies in the wall of the alimentary tract). The peripheral nervous system is composed of the axons of motor neurons situated inside the central nervous system, and the cell bodies and processes of neurons grouped together as *ganglia* (swellings). Sensory ganglion cells in posterior (dorsal) roots give off both centrally and peripherally directed processes, and do not have synapses on their cell bodies, whilst ganglionic neurons of the autonomic nervous system receive synaptic contacts from various sources. The cell bodies situated in peripheral ganglia are all derived embryonically by migration from the neural crest (p. 147).

OUTLINE OF CENTRAL NERVOUS SYSTEM ORGANIZATION (8.12)

As noted above, the general plan of central nervous system organization can be discerned most clearly in its embryonic development, and also by comparison with its mature condition in the various groups of living vertebrates with simpler nervous systems. The brain and spinal cord are formed as a bilaterally symmetrical dorsal hollow tube with neurons primarily clustered along its internal wall. Within this framework neuronal populations are functionally divided into longitudinal columns which stretch from the most caudal part of the

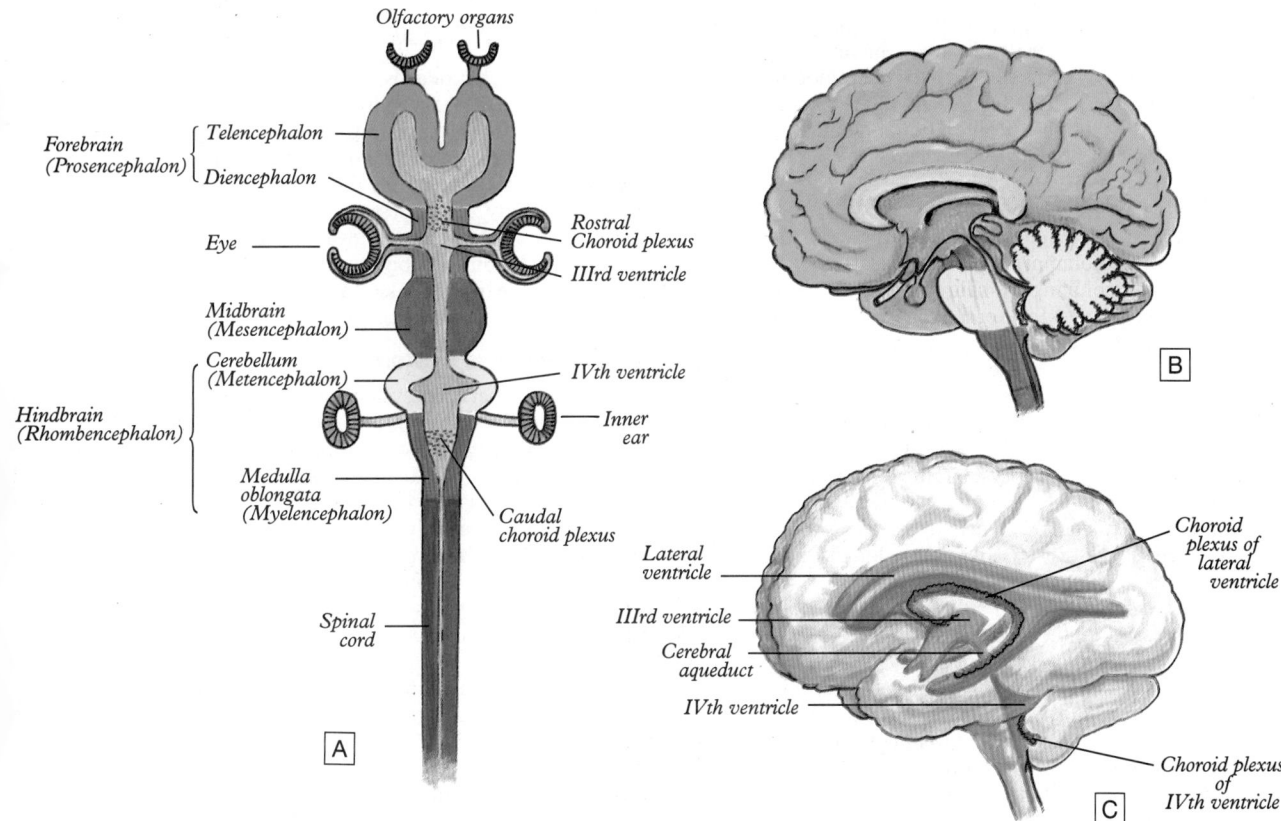

8.12 Diagrams showing the nomenclature and arrangement of the different areas of the brain.

A depicts the major features of the theoretical basic vertebrate brain plan, including the relationships of its parts to the major special sensory organs of the head.

B shows how the same regions are arranged in the human brain, seen in sagittal section.

C illustrates the organization of the ventricular system in the human brain, which is depicted as a semi-transparent structure.

spinal cord into the brain, terminating some distance from the end of the neural tube at the boundary between mid- and forebrain (see below). In the forebrain the columnar system appears to be absent or much modified, and other more complex types of subdivision exist. As well as this longitudinal alignment the neurons also have a segmental level of organization where the same neuronal pattern is repeated at regular intervals along the length of the central nervous system, corresponding to the series of somites flanking it (p. 225). From these neuronal concentrations emerge the segmental spinal and cranial nerves, one motor nerve to each myotome and a corresponding sensory nerve to the dermatome arising from each somite. Within the nervous system each segment contains the interneuronal microcircuits needed to handle the sensory and motor activities of that region, and these are repeated throughout the spinal cord and the brain as far as the rostral limit of the midbrain. The homeobox genes controlling the development of this segmental pattern are discussed on page 225. These segments are also linked together by longitudinally directed neurons, and to more distant regions by ascending and descending axons.

As described in greater detail later, the brain is traditionally divided into three major regions: forebrain, midbrain and hindbrain, each associated with expansions of the anterior part of the neural tube related to the sensory inputs of the olfactory organ, eyes and ears respectively. The mid- and hindbrain have the same segmental organization as the spinal cord, with which they are continuous; however, the roofs of these two regions are specialized areas (the colliculi and cerebellum) on which sensory inputs from different parts of the body form two-dimensional maps of those regions. The floor areas of the mid- and hindbrain contain the major sensory and motor neurons, as well as many longitudinal fibre tracts passing through or terminating there; this region is called the *brainstem*. In humans, during prenatal development the primitive tubular form of the brain becomes highly distorted by the unequal growth of different areas within its wall; from the rostral end of the tube the two cerebral hemispheres bulge out on either side as the neuronal populations in their walls increase greatly in number, and grow back to overshadow the more caudal parts of the brain. The cerebellum also expands considerably and grows forwards to meet the cerebrum, hiding the midbrain roof from surface view. The expansion of cerebral and cerebellar surface areas achieved in this way are further increased by their pleating to form complex folds (gyri and folia), to accommodate the large number of fibres growing into them from other regions of the central nervous system, and the proliferation of neuronal microcircuits and output neurons associated with them.

Longitudinal organization of neuronal populations

As already mentioned, there are functional similarities between the neurons in any one longitudinal column; this is seen clearly in the spinal cord, where the dorsal columns of neurons are primarily concerned with sensory functions and the ventral ones with motor activities. Both dorsal and ventral components can be subdivided into those which are connected directly or indirectly to the 'external' parts of the body such as the skin, muscles, joints and associated connective tissue (somatosensory and somatomotor neurons) and those concerned with the body's interior, mainly the alimentary tract and its derivatives such as the respiratory system and many glands (viscerosensory and visceromotor). The neurons in these columns may be concentrated into discrete nuclei in some areas, for example the brainstem, or may form more diffuse continuous longitudinal bands of grey matter, as in much of the spinal cord (8.13). The existence of longitudinal columns in the brainstem, proposed by Herrick and Johnson at the end of the nineteenth century, is well established, although some problems still remain about their precise form and homologies as these depend on interpretations of cranial development, at present a lively area of experiment and debate (see e.g. the extensive review of this subject by Nieuwenhuys 1994). In the traditional scheme of columnar organization (for details see p. 979), the *somatomotor* column contains motor neurons whose axons serve muscles derived from head somites (although some argue for a special origin of some extrinsic eye muscles), while the visceral motor column becomes divided into two longitudinal columns related to specialized features of head morphology: a *branchiomotor* column innervating muscle derived from the wall of the embryonic pharynx (branchial muscle) and another *general visceromotor* column sup-

plying parasympathetic fibres to glands and visceral smooth muscle. The *visceral sensory* column deals largely with chemoreceptor information from taste buds (general visceral sensory) and other visceral sensory endings (special visceral sensory), and the *somatosensory* column deals with general sensory information from the surface of the head, the interior of the oral cavity and pharynx, and the musculoskeletal apparatus of most of the anterior head region. Another most dorsally placed column is found in the brainstem; in its primitive condition in fishes, it deals with sensory inputs from mechanoreceptors in the lateral line and inner ear (the acousticolateralis system), and proprioceptive data from much of the body; part of this column fuses with its contralateral partner across the midline to form the cerebellum, and much of the rest is composed of nuclei receiving the vestibulocochlear nerve. In terrestrial vertebrates the cerebellum becomes very elaborate and assumes a major role in the co-ordination of motor function, while the lateral line, an aquatic adaptation, disappears. The rest of this acousticolateralis-derived column is retained as the vestibular and cochlear nuclear complexes.

The ventricular system

When the neural tube is formed during prenatal development, its walls thicken greatly but do not completely obliterate the cavity within it. It remains in the spinal cord as the narrow central canal, but in the brain it becomes greatly expanded to form a series of interconnected cavities, the ventricular system (p. 910). In two regions, the fore- and hindbrains, parts of the neural tube roof do not generate nerve cells but become thin, folded sheets of highly vascular secretory tissue, the choroid plexuses. These secrete cerebrospinal fluid which fills the ventricles and permeates the intercellular spaces of the brain and spinal cord to create its extracellular fluid determining the neuronal environment. The central nervous system also has a rich blood supply, as might be expected of an organ with such a high metabolic rate, although there are severe restrictions on the substances which can diffuse from the bloodstream into the nervous tissue (the blood–brain barrier, see p. 1221).

PHYLOGENETIC ORIGINS AND EVOLUTION OF THE NERVOUS SYSTEM

A central endeavour of neuroscience is to uncover the general principles underlying the exceedingly complicated arrangement of the nervous system. In the past, important clues have come from a study of how it is assembled during development (neuroembryology) and what its simpler origins were during evolutionary history, as surmised from a study of the less complicated nervous systems of other species (comparative neuroanatomy). More recently molecular genetics has added considerably to the available tools for such investigations, and clearly possesses much potential when combined with the more traditional approaches.

Invertebrate nervous systems

The emergence of a nervous system appears to have been a very early event in animal evolution, and probably occurred soon after the arrival of the multicellular state of organization. Most cells show electrical responses when suitably stimulated, and this is true of even simple unicellular organisms such as the ciliate *Paramecium*, which possesses ion channels sensitive to mechanical and other types of stimulation, controlling the direction of ciliary beating (and therefore swimming). In some of the simplest multicellular animals, such as the coelenterates (e.g. polyps such as sea anemones, jellyfish and the freshwater *Hydra*), differentiation of cell types is found so that in addition to cells involved in nutrition, protection, movement, secretion, reproduction, etc. there are diffuse networks of neurons which co-ordinate these activities. In the least differentiated state, the nerve systems found in coelenterates are composed of neurons with several radiating processes which individually make reciprocal synaptic connections with neighbouring neurons to create a diffuse two-dimensional system (*a nerve net* 8.14, 17) spreading over the body between the two cell layers (ectoderm and endoderm) of which these animals are constructed. Some ectodermal cells are specialized sensory receptors which can detect various types of stimuli, and others are contractile; both are linked synaptically by neurons. Some species also have specialized sensory organs such as gravity receptors (statocysts) linked in to the nerve net. Even at this unsophisticated level, such animals have a surprisingly wide repertoire of activities, enabling them to perform co-ordinated motor responses to the presence of food and threats, gravity and other biologically important stimuli. In some coelenterates the neurons are locally concentrated into linearly conducting systems to produce rapid escape responses or to co-ordinate complex sets of swimming muscles (**8**.15).

Next in the degree of complexity, it can be seen that in simple triploblastic (p. 5) animals the simple nerve net is exchanged for the grouping of neuronal cell bodies into a central nervous system often composed of ganglia which issues axons to various parts of the body (**8**.16, 17). Typically, such ganglia are situated in the head where specialized sense organs including chemoreceptors and photoreceptors are also concentrated. In bilaterally symmetric animals there are typically two longitudinal, interconnected nerve trunks which distribute axons to all parts of the body. This pattern of organization has been extensively studied in a species of nematode worm, *Caenorhabditis elegans*, a creature sufficiently small (1 mm long and consisting of a total of about 3000 cells), to allow a comprehensive analysis of the numbers, types and connections of its entire nervous system. The use of molecular genetics to examine the effects of gene mutations on the development of the nematode nervous system indicates that many of its ground rules are also observed in the construction of the mammalian nervous system, indicating a phylogenetic continuity between the two.

A further development in neural complexity emerges when segmented animals are examined, where there is a repetition of structures, for example muscles, nerve trunks, appendages, etc., along the body (see p. 119). This is of particular interest because all vertebrates also show the same segmental pattern of organization. In the segmented invertebrates (annelid worms, arthropods, molluscs, echinoderms, etc.) the convention of paired neuronal ganglia and nerve trunks is retained, but their arrangement is now segmentally repeated so that each segment has its own neural control centre receiving sensory stimuli, integrating them and giving local motor commands. These are co-ordinated by neural connections to large paired ganglia in the head, also linked closely to eyes, chemoreceptors and specialized mechanoreceptors of the head region. The segmental ganglia have a complex internal organization which allows a fair degree of autonomy, so that many activities can be performed even if the head is removed. In some bivalve molluscs this independence is pushed to extremes, with relatively little cephalic interference on local ganglionic function. On the other hand, centralized neural control and extreme elaboration of the nervous system is seen in the cephalopod molluscs such as the species of octopus, which parallel the vertebrates in the complexity of their behaviour.

Within the segmentally organized invertebrates, insects, particularly the fruit fly *Drosophila melanogaster*, have been a major source of information regarding the construction of segmental order in the nervous system (see also p. 115). Many of the genes responsible for it, for example the homeobox genes, have considerable homology to those of vertebrates, and it appears that such developmental phenomena as routing of axonal growth, decussation, grouping of neuronal cell bodies and patterns of synaptic connectivity have origins which are deeply buried in the invertebrate past. However, there are also differences; one of these is that the precise pattern of nerve cells and their connections is quite predictable, and relatively little influenced by environmental changes. Correspondingly, behavioural patterns tend to be rather stereotyped; genetically determined routines dominate the behavioural repertoire, learning having only a very restricted role, and problem solving is extremely limited or non-existent. (It must be admitted, however, that the cephalopods are again an exception to this and represent a unique development amongst the invertebrates). Besides these purely phylogenetic considerations, the relatively simple and predictable circuitry of many segmented invertebrate nervous systems has provided neuroscience with some powerful experimental models, for example synaptic facilitation in the mollusc *Aplysia*, and electrical behaviour of neuroglial cells in the leeches.

Nervous systems in chordates (8.17, 18)

The search for the phylogenetic origins of the vertebrate nervous system has focused on the phylum widely believed to contain the closest living relatives among the invertebrates; for various reasons

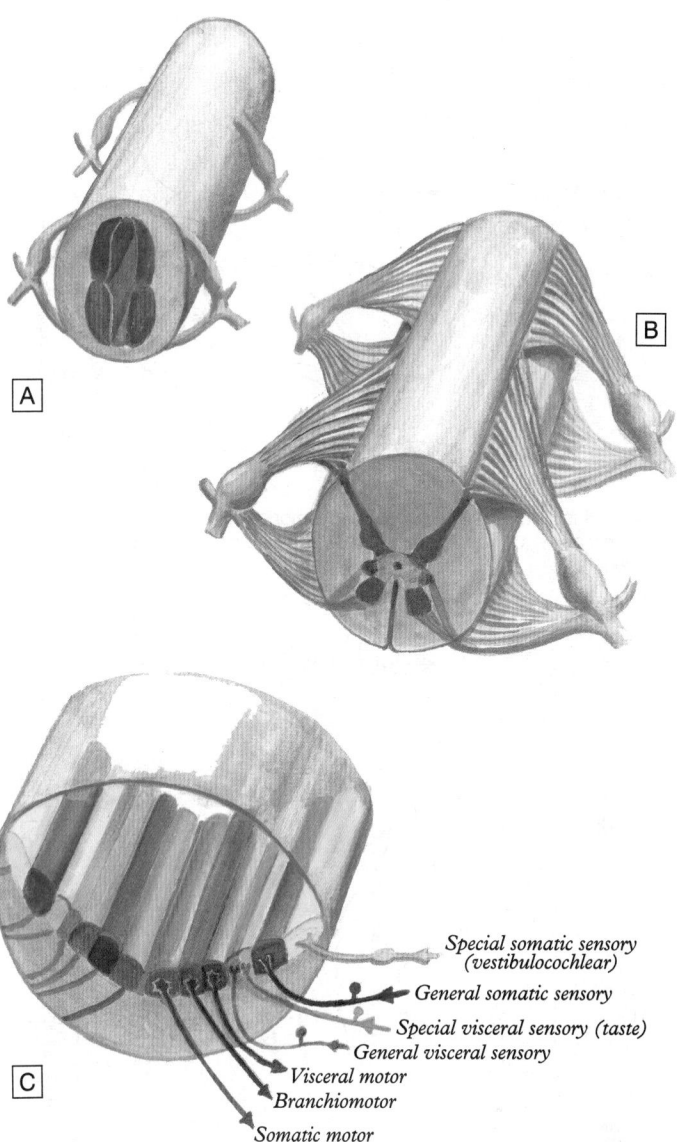

8.13   Schema showing the arrangement of sensory and motor columns in the spinal cord and brain stem.

A shows the organization of the primitive spinal cord with a dorsal sensory column (blue), a ventral column (red), and segmentally arranged dorsal and ventral nerve roots.

B depicts the arrangement of adult spinal cord serving the thorax and lumbar region, with sensory and somatic motor columns colour coded in the same way, and an additional intermediate (lateral) visceral motor column (brown).

C indicates the arrangement of multiple longitudinal columns in the brainstem, where the motor column is now subdivided into three, and the sensory column into four. For further information about the embryological aspects of the early nervous system see p. 217 and **3**.3.

to do with comparative anatomy and embryology, this is thought to be the Echinodermata (starfish, sea-urchins and related species), and it is interesting that in this group the nervous system is in essence a flat epidermally-derived superficial plate of neurons and glial cells, connected to a ring of ganglia around the mouth. In some species (the crinoids: sea lilies) this plate is rolled into a tube, an arrangement strongly suggesting how the hollow central nervous system of the chordates might have arisen. The simplest chordates also show some intriguing features; the larval ascidians (sea-squirts) each have a simple hollow nerve cord connected to a photoreceptor and a statocyst at the head end, issuing synaptic connections to blocks of muscle cells along each side of a stiff notochord, and so allowing the larva to swim vigorously like a fish for a brief period while it selects a site on which to cement its head and undergo a metamorphosis to a sedentary filter-feeding form. A prolongation of this larval period and suppression of the adult might have given rise to

Labels on figure C:
Special somatic sensory (vestibulocochlear)
General somatic sensory
Special visceral sensory (taste)
General visceral sensory
Visceral motor
Branchiomotor
Somatic motor

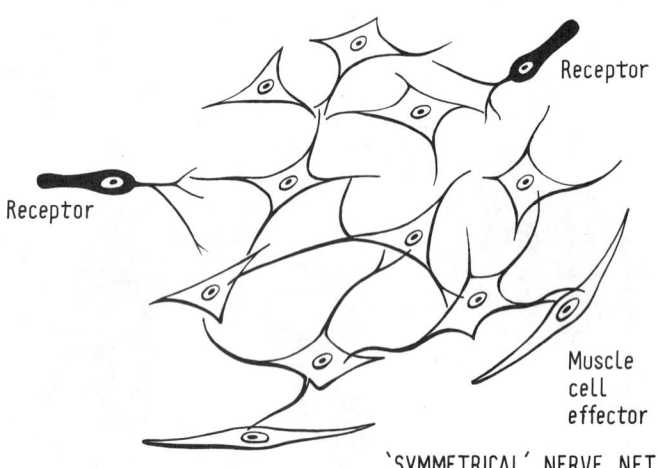

'SYMMETRICAL' NERVE NET

8.14 In this simple nervous system receptor cell terminals feed into a fairly symmetrical network of interneurons which in turn makes contact with the effectors.

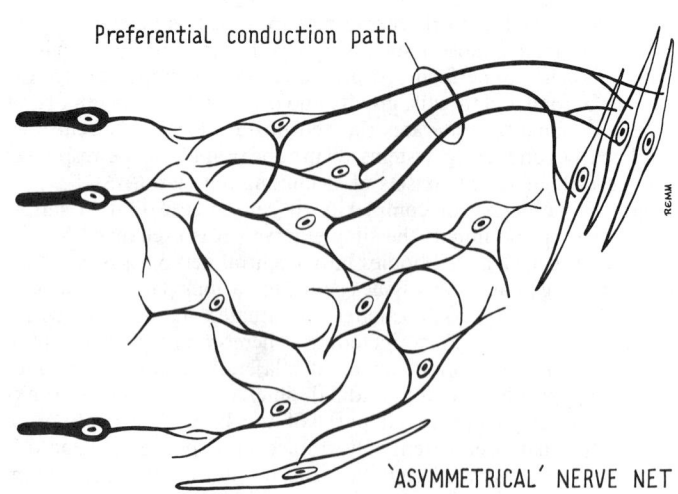

'ASYMMETRICAL' NERVE NET

8.15 In this simple nervous system interneurons between receptors and effectors are organized so that diffuse multisynaptic conduction pathways predominate but more direct routes are also present.

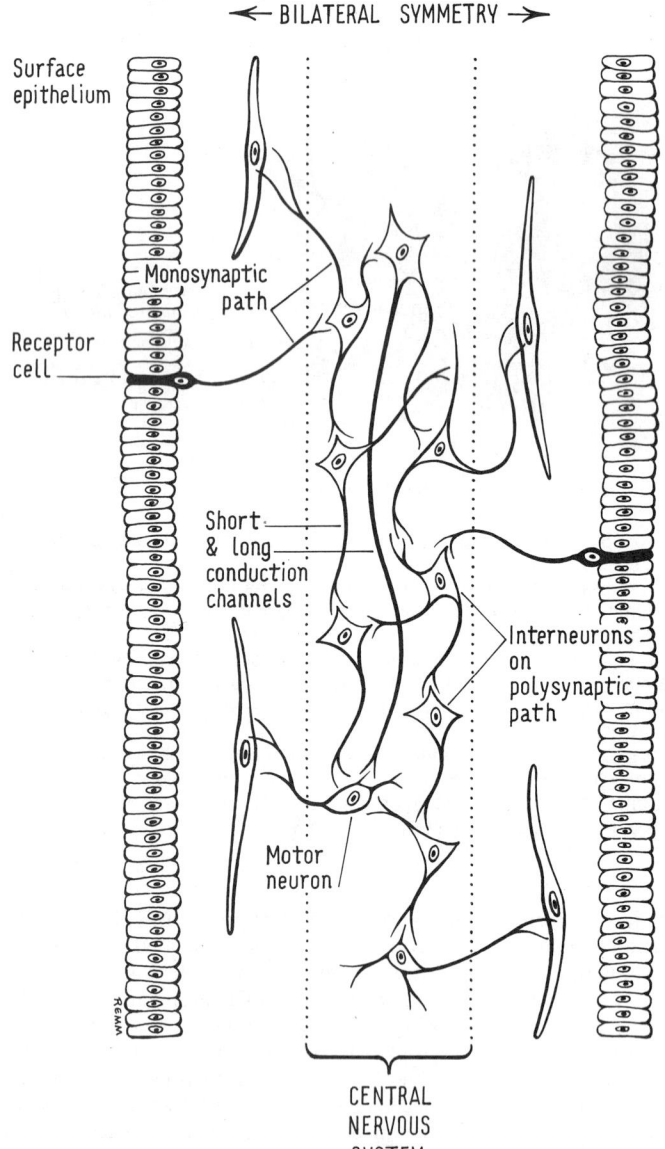

8.16 Some features of the nervous system in a primitive organism with bilateral symmetry. Note the intra-epithelial positions of the receptor cells and the aggregation of interneurons and motor neurons near the plane of symmetry as a central nervous system. Note also the different orders of complexity of the conduction pathways and the possibility of co-operative actions involving both sides of the body.

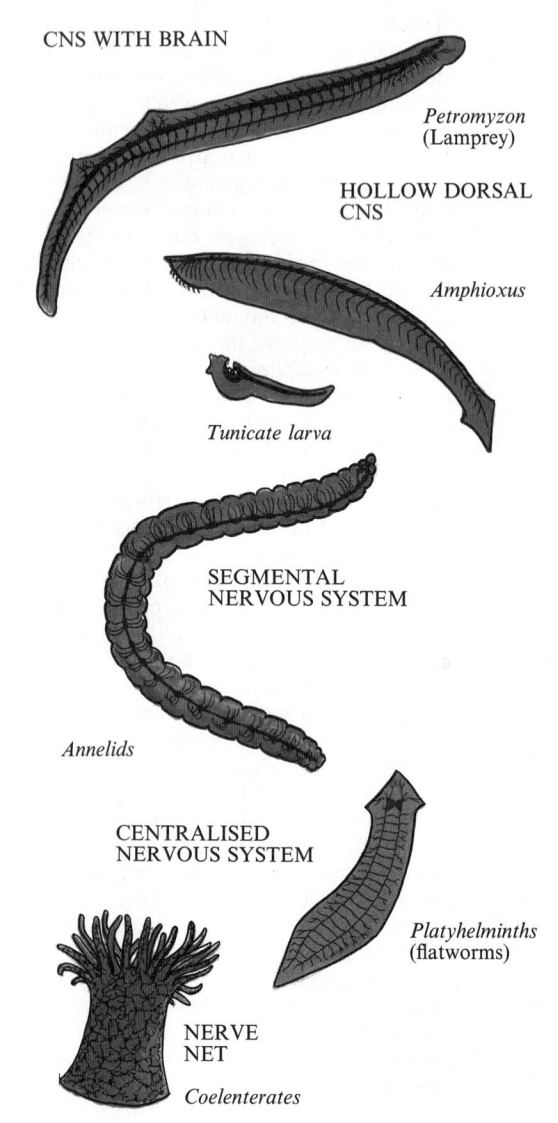

8.17 Schema of the different grades of neural organization found in the invertebrates and primitive vertebrates such as the Lamprey. Red = neural structures.

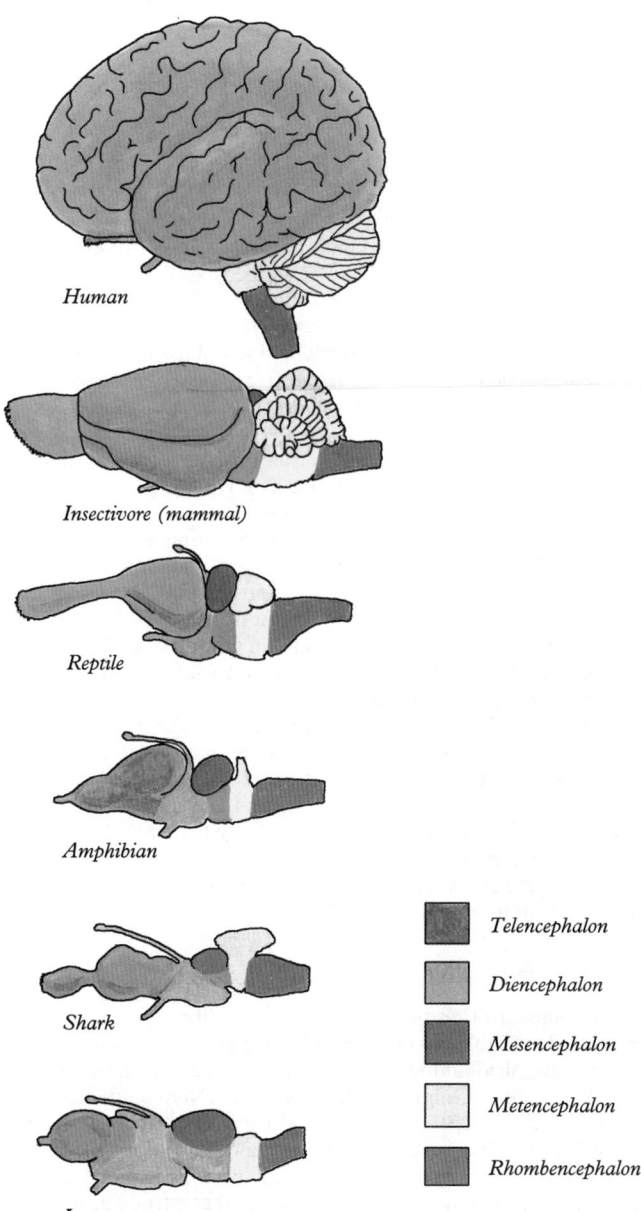

Human

Insectivore (mammal)

Reptile

Amphibian

Shark

Lamprey

■ *Telencephalon*

■ *Diencephalon*

■ *Mesencephalon*

□ *Metencephalon*

■ *Rhombencephalon*

8.18 Schema comparing the external appearances of the major regions in the brains of different groups of vertebrates related to the human lineage. Note that while the term metencephalon is applied to the cerebellum and pons in mammals, it is, strictly speaking, only applicable to the cerebellum in submammalian forms, which lack a pons. However, the area of the hindbrain which is homologous with the pontine region of mammals is coloured yellow in this diagram, for purposes of comparison.

the earliest vertebrates, and indeed there are groups of tunicates, such as the salps (Larvacea, e.g. *Oikopleura*) which never metamorphose but spend their lives as free swimming oceanic forms. Closer to the vertebrates, the protochordate *Branchiostoma* (Amphioxus) is a simple fish-like form whose organization suggests how the ancestral chordate nervous system might have looked. It has a hollow dorsal spinal cord, segmentally arranged and with a slightly expanded anterior region suggesting the beginnings of a brain. However, there are some odd features, for example the absence of peripheral motor nerves (the central nervous system is linked to muscles by thin extensions of the muscle cells reaching into the spinal cord: and the presence of photoreceptive cells within the spinal cord; these and various other aspects of body structure indicate that Amphioxus is a specialized offshoot of the main evolutionary line, albeit a fascinating one.

In whatever way the ancestral vertebrates arose, we find that all living vertebrates including humans have a similar plan of neural

organization which has varied little in its essential features over the evolution of this group. The neuronal cell bodies are concentrated into a dorsal hollow neural tube which is derived embryonically from an epithelium-like plate of neurectoderm, forming the central nervous system; ganglionated nerve cells of the peripheral nervous system and their ensheathing peripheral glial elements are all derived from the neural crest (a chordate development which has had considerable consequences for vertebrate organization in the nervous system and elsewhere). Within the central nervous system the cell populations are segmentally arranged (see p. 911), except most rostrally, a pattern clearly visible in probably all vertebrates in the rhombomeres of the hindbrain (p. 240), and in fishes in the development of the spinal cord. In adults the segmentation is shown in the symmetrically paired repetitive dorsal and ventral roots and corresponding sensory and motor neuron populations of the brainstem and spinal cord. The rostral end of the neural tube is expanded into three paired regions associated with three major special sensory systems, the olfactory organ, eyes and ears (or their homologues; the fore-, mid- and hindbrain respectively); the segmental pattern is present in all except the forebrain, whose origins are a matter of some speculation.

The peripheral nervous system has dorsal roots which are sensory and bear ganglia, and ventral roots that contain motor neurons. The head has a predictable pattern of cranial nerves, although in the fishes there are only ten pairs because the skull is not so extensive (the cranial accessory and hypoglossal nerves thus constitute the first and second spinal nerves), and there is a complete autonomic system with sympathetic, parasympathetic and enteric components. While the general pattern seen throughout the vertebrates was achieved at an early stage, there have also been some fundamental changes within this group of animals. For example, in the earliest vertebrates, the fossil record shows that only two semicircular canals were present in the inner ear, as occurs also in the modern Agnatha such as *Petromyzon* (lampreys) and *Myxine* (hagfish); the fusion of dorsal and ventral nerve roots to form common trunks seems also to have occurred secondarily, these being separate in the primitive hagfish. The conversion of the branchial arch and cleft system of the pharynx into a musculoskeletal feeding mechanism by the development of jaws also had a considerable impact on the organization of the central and peripheral connections of this part of the body, although the basic pattern common to all vertebrates is still detectable.

Within the brain it is possible to follow a progression from a simple plan of neural organization, seen in primitive fishes, to its rather more elaborate condition in humans. Such changes can be related to environmental needs and the increasing elaboration of behaviour, although caution has to be exercised in making generalizations, since all living lower vertebrates have been subject to further evolutionary changes since their lineage branched from the line leading to mammals. In the most primitive forms (e.g. lampreys such as *Petromyzon*) the wall of the brain is relatively thin except where major tracts are concentrated, neuronal cell bodies being generally clustered against the ventricular surface close to their mitotic origins from neural stem cells, and their axons being more superficially placed, away from the ventricular surface, so forming, respectively, mantle and marginal zones resembling that of the human embryonic brain and cord (see p. 217). In these cell populations the sensory and motor organization is represented rather like a map of the body, in an essentially two-dimensional *somatotopic* pattern; in more complex vertebrates, an increase in the numbers of neuronal circuits handling these activities has been gained by an enlargement in the brain's surface area, often with an elaborate folding, giving rise to expansions such as the cerebellum, the cerebral hemispheres and midbrain roof. Indeed, the retina is mostly such an expanded part of the brain. Elaboration of neural organization and complexity of connections has led to a thickening of the brain wall as neuronal cell bodies migrate away from their point of ventricular origin to established discrete nuclei, layers or more diffuse systems (e.g. the reticular nuclei of the brainstem).

Alongside this proliferation of neuronal numbers and increase in the complexity of microcircuits, there is a trend for novel connections to be made within the brain, linking hitherto unconnected regions and exploiting old neuronal populations in new ways. One of the most spectacular of these innovations is the mammalian neocortex, part of the telencephalon, which in fishes and amphibians and, to a lesser extent, reptiles is dominated by the olfactory sense, with the non-olfactory parts of the cerebrum being relatively small. The elaboration of neocortical circuitry, especially the development of cortical columns (p. 1151) and the enlargement of sensory and motor inputs from the thalamus, converted this region of the brain into an area with a dominant role in sensory analysis and motor control which, in lower forms, is mainly the prerogative of the thalamus and midbrain roof (tectum). We see further trends within the mammalian cerebral cortex as additional areas of cortex devoted to activities other than primary sensory analysis or motor control are elaborated. In the simplest mammals (e.g. insectivores) the cerebrum is chiefly a region of sensory and motor centres, with relatively small regions of associative cortex where integration between the different inputs and outputs can be accomplished. In some other groups of mammals, especially the primates, the association area has become greatly expanded, increasing the size of the cerebrum relative to the rest of the brain and to body size. In addition, some cortical functions have been allocated to different sides of the brain (e.g. speech recognition and motor control in the left hemisphere), presumably increasing the efficiency of integration. The elaboration of the cortex is also associated with the increase in commissural fibres within the corpus callosum, co-ordinating the activities of the two cerebral hemispheres. The formation of such new connections has allowed the generation of novel types of activity within these areas, associated with various forms of complex behaviour, for example problem solving, and in humans, the gamut of intellectual activity.

Many other transformations can also be traced through the vertebrate neural lineage, for example the increased size and changes of connectivity of the motor co-ordination centres: (1) in the hindbrain, the cerebellum of mammals gains incoming and outgoing connections with the motor centres of the cerebral cortex via the pons and thalamus, modulating and correcting cortical motor control in accordance with incoming sensory information; (2) in the forebrain, the basal nuclei (p. 1186) of tetrapods, particularly mammals, have become elaborate mechanisms for initiating and patterning cortical motor commands.

More generally, we can also discern evolutionary trends towards increased absolute numbers of neurons, and the duplication, or rather multiplication, of parallel pathways. This contrasts with the condition in insects where the circuits are generally very parsimonious (but their behaviour limited and mostly stereotyped). Non-mammalian vertebrates grow continually throughout life, and the nervous system also increases in size and neuronal number to cope with the increased sensory and motor demands. Mammals, perhaps because of the complexity of the brain's circuitry, restrict neurogenesis to prenatal or very early postnatal life, after which individual neurons may grow in size and connectivity but not in number. The price to pay for this extreme elaboration is that regeneration does not take place in the mature mammalian central nervous system (see p. 944), but perhaps this is a small fee for the versatility of the mammalian brain, and in our species, for conscious awareness and the ability to think and create.

DEVELOPMENT OF NEUROHISTOLOGICAL TECHNIQUE AND LIGHT MICROSCOPY

Initially, nerve fibres were examined using a simple lens (Leeuwenhoek 1674; Swammerdam 1675). Fontana (1781) described nerve fibres but did not distinguish between axons and their myelin sheaths. Further advances during the nineteenth century were dependent upon the development and refinement of microscope design and of techniques for preparing and staining neural tissues.

Preparation of material for microscopy

Early microscopists used teased or squashed samples of fresh or, at most, partially preserved, material to examine the structure of nervous tissue. The introduction of alcohol (Reil 1809) and chromic acid (Hannover 1840) as tissue hardeners were important steps in improving the morphological integrity of sectioned tissues. Stilling (1846) cut transverse and longitudinal sections of the spinal cord, and advocated the use of serial sections, as did Virchow (1846) in

studies of neuroglia. Stilling and Wallach (1842) devised a simple microtome for cutting sections of tissue: improvements in design meant that Von Gudden and Catsch (1875) were able to cut sections of whole cerebral hemispheres. The subsequent semi-automation of microtomes and the introduction of novel embedding media (paraffin wax, collodion, celloidin) were significant methodological advances which followed before the end of the century.

Tissue staining methods in neuroanatomy

The earliest investigations of neural tissue were carried out on unstained specimens. Remak (1836) described axons and their sheaths in unstained embryonic material; Purkinje (1837) reported the eponymous cerebellar neurons using acetic alcohol for clearing and Canada balsam for permanent mounts. Waller's study of axonal degeneration (1850) was carried out on teased unfixed, unstained nerves, and Kuhne (1862) discovered motor endings in tissues treated simply with weak hydrochloric acid.

The first neurohistological stain was probably the carmine and gold method of Gerlach (1858). Deiters (1865) used carmine to distinguish between axons and dendrites. Ranvier's classic work on nodes (1871) depended upon silver impregnation of chromic acid fixed tissue, and Golgi developed silver staining methods which enabled him to visualize neurons in their entirety. Ramón y Cajal (1908) adopted and refined Golgi's methods and used Nissl's methylene blue protocol for staining 'chromatin granules'. Earlier, Ehrlich (1886) had used methylene blue, as the first *vital stain*, to delineate peripheral nerve fibres to their terminals.

Weigert's (1892) technique for staining *normal* myelin sheaths (consisting of pretreatment with potassium bichromate followed by acid fuchsin), Marchi's osmic acid method for staining *degenerating* myelin (Marchi & Algeri, 1885–1886), and the methods developed by Glees (1946) and by Nauta and Gygax (1951) for staining degenerating axon terminals and synaptic boutons, have all proved invaluable in the study of experimentally lesioned animal tissues and post mortem human material **8.19, 20**.

NEURON TRACING TECHNIQUES (8.19–24)

Waller's demonstration that damage to nerve fibres produced microscopically identifiable changes heralded the start of a brilliant period of neuroanatomical and neuropathological research. The subsequent work of Gudden, Golgi, Weigert, Marchi, Nissl and others, all published in the last 30 years of the nineteenth century, established the broad basis of neuronal morphology and the major experimental techniques which were to be employed in investigations into the organization of the nervous system until the introduction of the modern alternatives of retrograde or anterograde tracing using axonally transported reporter molecules (see Mesulam 1982). Of particular significance in the development of tracing techniques was Nissl's discovery (1892) of the acute response of the nerve cell soma to axonal damage, typified by the breakdown of Nissl or chromatin granules (*chromatolysis*): recognition of these changes remains an important tool when tracing axons back to their somata.

It is difficult to place small experimental lesions in a mass of nervous tissue: there is no means of ablating somata alone, and in all experiments, dendritic trees, synaptic terminals from other neurons and blood vessels are inevitably affected. Clearer results follow when axons are cut along their course. Certain terms are used for the various regions of the degeneration that is produced, and these will be briefly summarized. Effects distal to a lesion are said to be *anterograde*, whereas those proximal to a lesion are *retrograde* changes. After a suitable interval, these changes may be examined by the methods of Marchi, Glees, Nauta, Fink-Heimer and by various histochemical and ultrastructural research techniques **8.22**. Changes in undamaged neurons connected synaptically with the damaged one are *transneuronal* changes and may be *primary, secondary,* etc. depending upon the number of cells interposed; they may also be anterograde or retrograde. Anterograde transneuronal degeneration occurs in the visual pathway: retinal lesions affect not only the fibres of the injured ganglion cells as far as the lateral geniculate body, but also the geniculate neurons with which they synapse; the process may even involve neurons in the striate cortex in a chain of primary and secondary transneuronal degenerations.

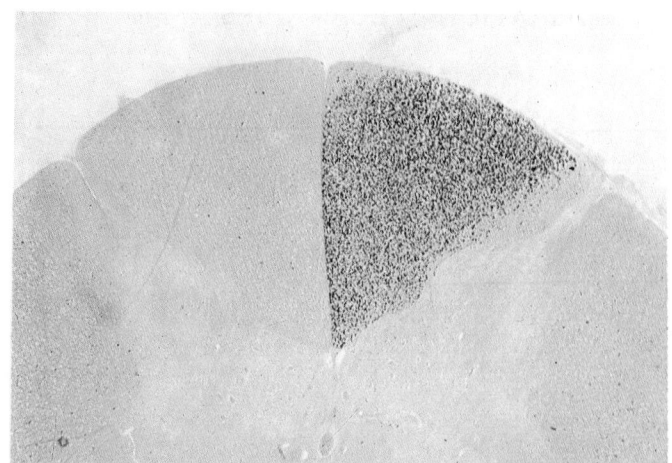

8.19 Transverse section through dorsal funiculi of feline cervical spinal cord, after unilateral dorsal column section at a more caudal level. Note anterograde Wallerian degeneration of ascending nerve fibres: degenerating myelin sheaths are stained black by Marchi technique. (Provided by E W Baxter, Department of Biology, Guy's Hospital Medical School, London.)

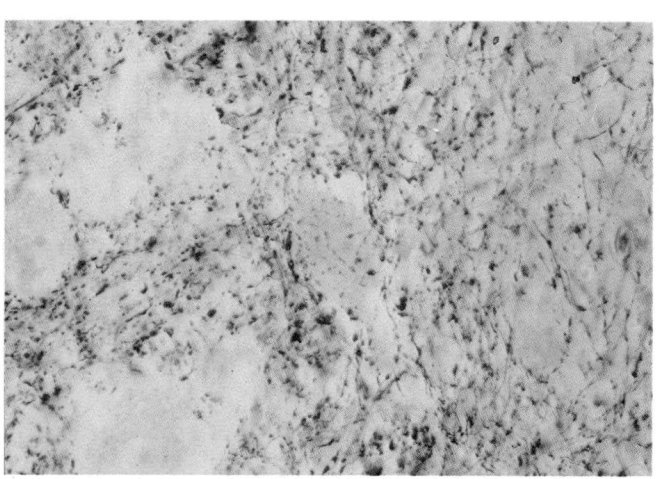

8.20 A high-power light micrograph showing preterminal degeneration of afferent axons ending in relation to neurons of the red nucleus of a rat, after the previous placing of a cerebellar lesion. The preparation was stained by the Nauta-Gygax method. (Supplied by K E Webster, King's College, University of London.)

Selective lesions and stereotaxis

Tracing techniques require a consistently accurate method of gaining access to and subsequently lesioning the target neurons. Whereas nerve section or ablation under direct vision may suffice in peripheral nerves or superficial central tracts, it is inappropriate for most regions of the central nervous system, where targets are at some depth, and where unplanned damage to surrounding tissue during the surgical approach may invalidate experimental findings.

Most methods of making focal lesions entail the use of *stereotaxis*: the head of an experimental animal is fixed in a rigid frame in which an electrode or micropipette can be adjusted in three planes to previously established co-ordinates and thus aligned with a target within the brain (e.g. Carpenter & Whittier 1952). Since Horsley and Clarke (1908) constructed the prototype stereotactic apparatus the technique has been widely exploited both in research and in neurosurgery. Experimentally, stereotactically placed focal lesions have been produced using: fine electrodes, for stimulation and electrocoagulation; probes which produce intense cold at their tips;

implants of destructive substances such as alcohol, hydrocyanide, carbon dioxide snow, radioactive yttrium; focused ultrasound or proton beams.

However, traditional lesioning techniques are limited in their selectivity. Recently, two related approaches, suicide transport and immunolesioning, both based on the use of ribosome-inactivating proteins, have been reported which address the problem of achieving greater selectivity. Both techniques are designed to target cytotoxins to neurons. Suicide transport has obviously developed out of the widespread use of lectins in neuroanatomical tract tracing. The technique depends on axonal uptake and transport to neuronal perikarya of cytotoxic lectins such as ricin, abrin, viscumin or volkensin, and can produce the selective death of neurons which project into the site of application of the lectin. Although reasonably effective as a technique (see Wiley 1992 for references), it is not without danger to laboratory personnel. In immunolesioning, monoclonal antineuronal antibodies conjugated to various toxin moieties (immunotoxins) have been used to knock out specific groups of neurons.

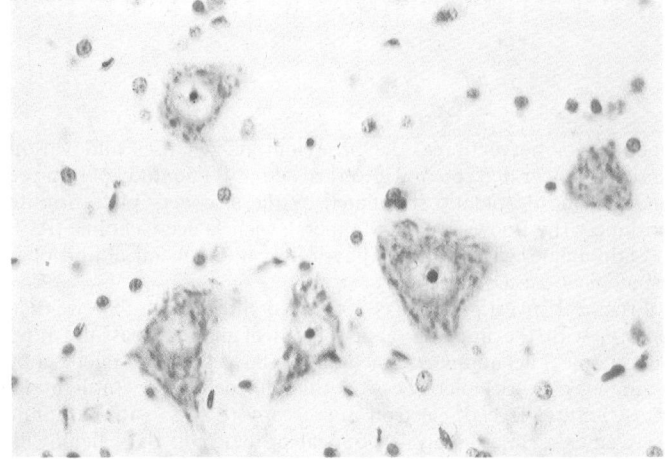

8.21A Large multipolar neuronal perikarya in the magnocellular part of the feline red nucleus, showing prominent Nissl's granules, bases of dendrites and axon hillocks. The nuclei are euchromatic and vesicular, with prominent nucleoli. The small nuclei scattered in the surrounding neuropil are characteristic of the various categories of neuroglial cells.

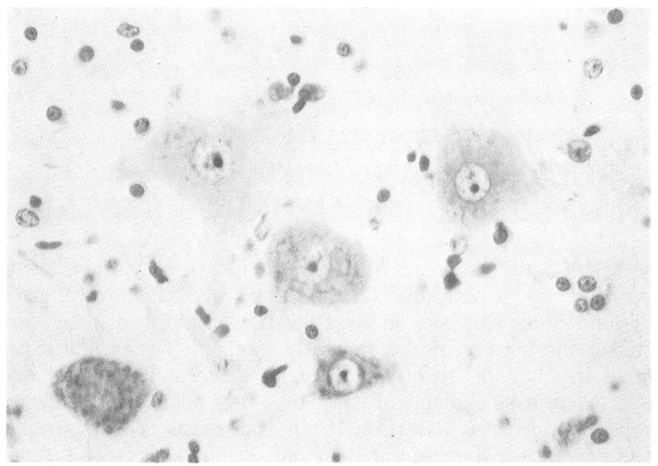

8.21B A field similar to that depicted in A but after previous contralateral hemisection of the spinal cord at the level of the fifth cervical segment, thereby severing the rubrospinal tract. The section shows characteristic chromatolytic retrograde changes in the cytoplasm of three large neurons. Two smaller neurons are unaffected. (Photography by Kevin Fitzpatrick, Division of Anatomy and Cell Biology, UMDS, Guy's Campus, London.)

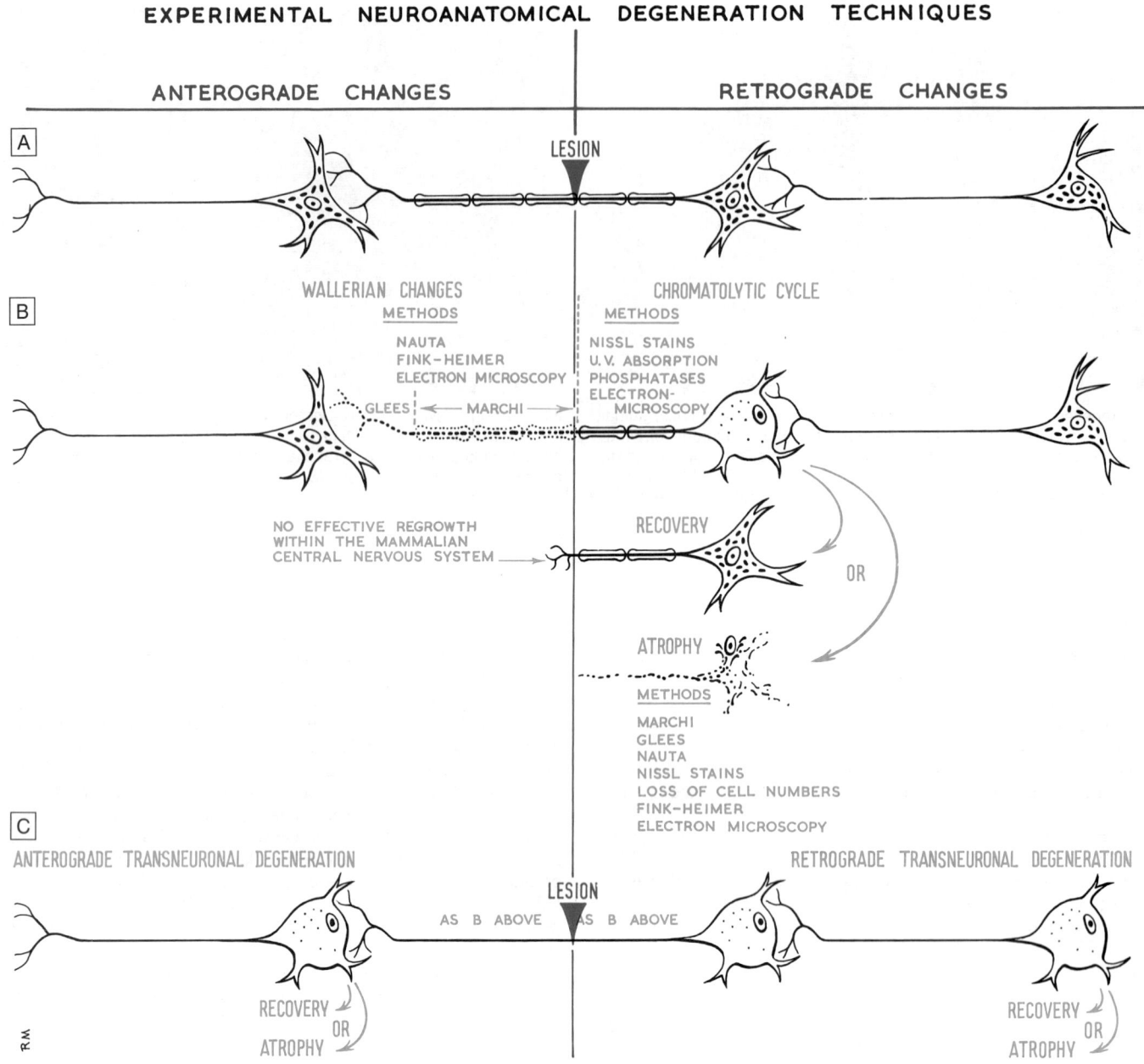

8.22 The sequelae of interruption of the fibres of central nervous system neurons. As shown, regeneration or atrophy may follow the response to injury, both in the neurons primarily damaged and in those affected trans-neuronally. Transneuronal effects may occasionally supervene in neurons more remotely associated with the damaged neuron.

MODERN DEVELOPMENTS IN STRUCTURAL AND FUNCTIONAL ANALYSES OF THE NERVOUS SYSTEM

By the 1900s the disciplines of structural analysis of neural tissue by microscopy were well advanced and the general features of nerve cells and fibres had been in large measure established, their types detailed and the neuron theory widely accepted. The earliest experiments in what was to become recognized as 'tissue culture' were undertaken using explants of embryonic frog neural tube grown in drops of frog lymph (Harrison 1907). The overall cellular arrangement of the central nervous system and peripheral nervous systems, including their autonomic components, had been defined in terms sufficient to be highly useful in clinical diagnosis, though the underlying mechanisms remained largely obscure. Moreover, neurophysiological studies were proving very successful in localizing function and reflex activity. The spectacular evolution of electronics was beginning to provide accurate instrumentation for examining the functions of nerve fibres, the behaviour of synapses and various aspects of integrated cerebral electrical activity. The study of synapses was even more potently stimulated by the discovery of transmitter substances (by Loewi, Dale and others), such as acetylcholine (ACh) and adrenaline, with immense physiological, biochemical and pharmacological consequences.

Structural investigation has continued throughout the twentieth century, with the impetus of new types of microscopes and novel microscopic techniques, including fluorescence microscopy; (scanning) confocal microscopy; immunohistochemistry (at light and ultrastructural levels); electron microscopy (transmission, scanning and elemental microanalysis); optical probes (e.g. the calcium fluorophore fura-2) in conjunction with digitized fluorescence imaging for quantitative analyses of the dynamic intracellular biochemistry of vital cells (see Mason, 1993). What follows is a brief and by no means exhaustive account of recent developments in experimental approaches to examining structure and function in the vertebrate nervous system.

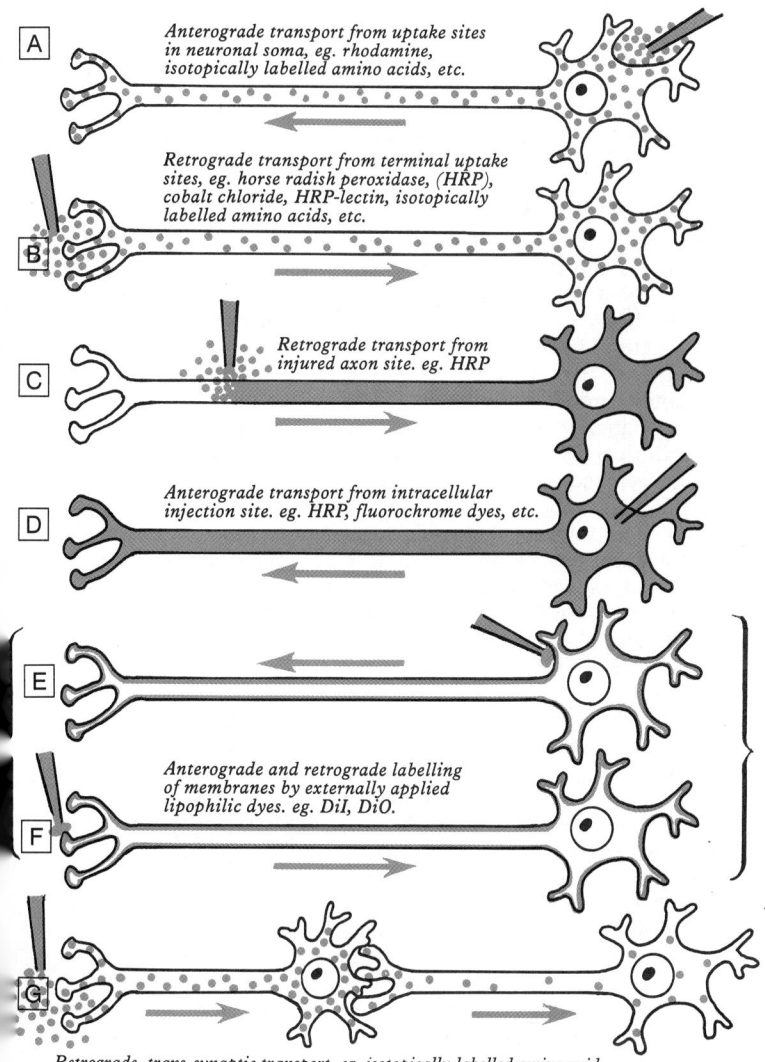

8.23   Some widely used methods of tracing the connections of neurons by intracellular labelling.

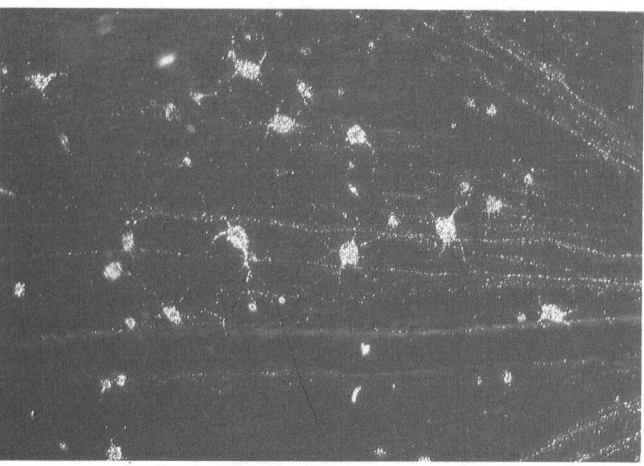

8.24   Part of a whole-mount preparation of a retina (rat) after prior horse-radish peroxidase injection into the optic nerve. The tracer has passed in retrograde fashion to fill many ganglion cells and their processes. Polarizing illumination. (Provided by E L Rees, Division of Anatomy and Cell Biology, UMDS, Guy's Campus, London.)

MODERN MICROSCOPY AND RELATED TECHNIQUES

The light microscope has now become a highly flexible instrument, with refined optics, dark-field illumination, polarization, phase contrast, contrast interference (Nomarski), ultraviolet fluorescence, and other auxiliary techniques including: warmed stages for tissue culture, recording cameras for still, cine and time-lapse photography, computer-linked devices for micromeasurement, microdensitometry and equipment for microdissection and microinjection. The phase-contrast microscope and its congeners, the interference and contrast interference (Normarski) microscopes, initiated a new era in cytology. Phase microscopy has been extensively applied to nerve cells and glia (Geiger 1963a,b; Murray 1965). Interference and contrast interference microscopy have been used to assess the refractive index, even in parts of one cell, and concentration, water content and dry mass in living cells (Ross 1967). Incident illumination of living tissue in situ is also a powerful method for analysis, and has been used to examine myelinated nerves in the adult mouse (e.g. Williams & Hall 1970, 1971a,b).

Ultraviolet microscopy can offer increased resolving power and, far more importantly, selective absorption of frequencies by various substances, especially nucleoproteins. Caspersson (1936) evolved a technique applicable to single cells, which was widely applied in quantitative assessments of DNA and RNA in nerve cells by Hydén (1960), although it is now little used.

Preparing tissue samples for conventional light microscopy normally involves cutting thin sections of appropriately fixed material and then staining the sections so obtained. Because the sections must of necessity be thin, any attempts at reconstructing 3-D relationships of structures within the original tissue from photomicrographs of serial sections are tedious and rarely undertaken. However, recently a new breed of microscope has appeared, the confocal microscope, which 'optically sections' thick samples. Basically, these microscopes produce 3-D reconstructions of material which can be viewed in stereo, from any orientation, within a few minutes of collecting the images (which may have been obtained using fluorescence, reflectance or transmitted light). For example, intracellular dye injection in vivo is a technique for displaying whole cell morphology (of neurons and/or glia) which may now be analysed using the confocal microscope. Not surprisingly, given the enormous potential of this instrument, there is wide interest in the ways in which confocal microscopy is being applied in experimental neuroanatomy and in neuropathology (Murray 1992).

Fluorescent dyes such as diI and diO have been used in tracing connections (**8.23**). They are also of value in cell lineage studies, when a 'mother' cell in an early embryo is injected with a dye that is retained within all of the cellular progeny of that cell, wheresoever they may be located when tissue sections of the neonate are examined microscopically.

HISTOCHEMISTRY AND IMMUNOHISTOCHEMISTRY

Phase, interference and ultraviolet microscopy are adjuncts to histochemistry, especially cytochemistry. Histochemistry perhaps began with Raspail, a botanist, as long ago as 1830 but accelerated greatly with the discovery of methods for the identification of biological compounds (Pearse 1968). Many such tests are available for nervous tissues, both normal and pathological (Adams 1965). Specially valuable are the methods for identification of neurotransmitters and their enzymes; pituitary hormones and their releasing factors; and other specific proteins, with resolution often superior to conventional staining or biochemical assays (Jones & Hartman 1978). Using these techniques, the mammalian brain has been 'mapped' extensively in terms of the distribution of many classes of transmitter-specific neurons and tracts (pp. 987, 1005).

Immunohistochemical methods involve the production and identification of sites of antibody–antigen interaction in tissue sections. Several factors influence the distribution of such sites, thereby complicating interpretation. These factors include the following:

- Antibody specificity. The use of monoclonal antibodies has largely circumvented this problem, although there are other problems in their use, e.g. cross-reaction with other proteins which may share some amino acid sequences. Recently, molecular genetics has provided a relatively simple means of preparing highly purified antigens which can be used to refine antibody specificity greatly.

917

- Tissue preparation, especially during fixation. Fixation is mostly designed to achieve an optimum compromise between preservation of structure and retention of antigenicity. The commonest fixative in use is formaldehyde; other aldehydes, with stronger cross-linking abilities, have proved less effective, although such combinations as periodate-lysine-paraformaldehyde have been used with advantage (Nakane & Kawaoi 1974). Freeze-drying, freeze-substitution and cryosectioning can minimize exposure to chemicals before labelling.
- Selection of an appropriate visual marker, e.g. fluorescein isothiocyanate (FITC), rhodamine, horseradish peroxidase (HRP) or colloidal gold. FITC emits a high yield of green fluorescence (517 nm) when excited with blue light (peak excitation 490–500 nm), which in combination with modern fluorescence microscopes permits examination of, e.g., fine adrenergic fibres (Hartman 1973). However, preparations are not permanent (fluorescence may sometimes quench, i.e. diminish in intensity, in mountant or undergo photodecomposition with time) and fluorescent markers cannot be used in electron microscopy. Immunolabelling with HRP (a 40 kDa glycoprotein) or with colloidal gold provides a permanent preparation. HRP was initially conjugated directly with antibodies via bifunctional cross-linking reagents, a step which results in partial inactivation of peroxidase activity. The later introduction of the peroxidase-antiperoxidase method (PAP) in which antibodies to HRP are bound to peroxidase without inactivating it, marked a methodological breakthrough in immunohistochemistry, especially at the ultrastructural level. The PAP technique became probably the most widely used pre-embedding technique for tracing neuronal connections (Priestley 1984). The large size of the PAP molecule (~420 kDa) may, however, produce problems of penetration (e.g. in fine nerve terminals). Further methodological refinements have included the introduction of colloidal gold particles prepared in a wide range of sizes (5–50 nm) and subsequently amplified using silver intensification techniques, and the highly sensitive avidin-biotin systems.

Pre-embedding labelling for electron microscopy, i.e. immunolabelling the tissue prior to embedding, is methodologically complex. Moreover, the process involves fixing and then permeabilizing tissue slices to ensure maximum antibody penetration, two steps which are clearly diametrically opposed in their aims. After these rigorous fixation and permeabilization protocols many antigens may be lost or denatured at sites of low concentration, while some cell surface antigens are so fragile that no on-grid method of immunolabelling preserves them. In recent years, the scope of electron microscope immunocytochemistry has been extended by the introduction of post-embedding techniques (e.g. Newman & Hobot 1989) for the examination of the subcellular localization of antigens: as the name implies, in these techniques, tissue is fixed, embedded and sectioned before sections are immunolabelled. Many research publications bear witness to the fact that while pre-embedding techniques are not ideal for either the preservation of myelin sheaths or for the localization of myelin-associated antigens, epoxy resins are suboptimal for post-embedding labelling. Recent developments which may provide better preservation of myelin sheaths for post-embedding include the use of the progressive lowering of temperature (PLT) technique combined with UV-polymerization of a methacrylate-based resin.

Immunolabelling techniques are not restricted to conventional tissue sections, and they have been applied to neurons and satellite cells, either in suspension after isolation from whole tissue or growing and differentiating in vitro prior to fixation. In this way, oligodendrocytes have been labelled in vitro with anti-galactocerebroside, anti-carbonic anhydrase II, and RIP, while astrocytes can be stained using monoclonal or polyclonal antibodies against glial fibrillary acidic protein (GFAP). It has proved more difficult to find a reliable marker for Schwann cells: they can be labelled in vitro using anti-RAN I and antibodies against the low affinity nerve growth factor receptor (NGF-R), but in tissue sections they are best labelled with antibodies against S-100 (which will also label other cells in different tissues). Some neurons may be labelled with antitetanus toxin (Raff et al 1978). Antisera, to certain components of the myelin sheath and to neurotrophins have been used in studies of the control of myelinogenesis and of ontogenetic and pathological mechanisms in nervous tissues.

Other relevant techniques include: autoradiography (Rogers 1967, 1973), cine and time-lapse photography (Rose 1963), microreconstruction (Gaunt & Gaunt 1978), microphotometry, micromanipulation, neuronal counting techniques (Konigsmark 1970; Corsellis et al 1975), morphometric analysis (Weibel & Elias 1969), the construction of models as functional analogues (Weiner & Schade 1963) and various methods of computerized image analysis.

In situ hybridization

Since the first reports of its potential in 1969, this powerful technique has been used extensively for the cellular localization of both DNA and mRNA within tissue sections. Probes may be single-stranded cDNA/cRNA or shorter oligonucleotide sequences of 30–50 bases (the length of the probe sequence is governed by cost, specificity and strength of the DNA–RNA hybrid formed). The use of oligonucleotide probes has brought the technique out of the molecular biology laboratory and into routine pathology and neuroscience laboratories. Oligonucleotides can be produced readily on a DNA synthesizer and can be made specific for individual members of a gene family. Probes can be labelled with isotopic (using [^{35}S] or [^{32}P]) or non-isotopic (using biotin, digoxigenin or enzymes such as alkaline phosphatase) reporter molecules. It is possible to use the technique semi-quantitatively to evaluate the amount of target in a cell or tissue. Thus it has been possible to analyse changes in gene expression during normal development, and also during postinjury repair and in response to drug administration (Emson 1993).

Tissue culture

The technique of tissue culture, which was derived very largely from the pioneering work of Harrison (1907a,b, 1910) and of Carrel (1912), proved vital in settling the controversial question of axonal origin: Harrison's description of nerve fibres growing out directly from explanted neural tubes made it abundantly clear that axons were derived from neurons and were not composed of independent axonal segments. In the period before World War II, most studies of neural tissue in vitro examined aspects of neuronal growth in relatively simple systems. The technique provided a useful adjunct to conventional microscopical examinations, but was not considered to be at the cutting edge of neurobiological research. However, the numerous methodological advances that have taken place since the 1950s, in particular the development of methods for growing cells in chemically defined media, often in sophisticated organotypic cultures (which permit recombinations of cells of different lineages), has significantly altered the status of tissue culture as a research tool (refer to Freshney 1994). The reductionist approach of studying cells in vitro has frequently attracted the criticism that tissue culture probably reveals what neurons and glia can do, rather than what they actually do in vivo in an intact and complex nervous system. Nonetheless, it is generally acknowledged that the experimental manipulation of selected populations of cells in tissue culture has provided valuable insights into many aspects of neural function, including the regulatory factors affecting glial and neuronal development; the mechanisms of myelination and of demyelination; the nature of neuron/glia interactions with each other and with substrates derived from extracellular matrix components; the mechanisms that regulate cortical connectivity.

Advances in neurophysiology

With improving neurophysiological instrumentation the study of electrical activity has been revolutionized, while the refinement of electrodes has meant that smaller groups of fibres and single cells can be examined in great detail. For example, information derived from longitudinal current analyses of undissected mammalian nerve fibres can be converted into membrane current contour maps, from which internodal lengths and conduction times can be calculated. The techniques of evoked potential measurement by controlled stimulation at one point with recording elsewhere have been used extensively and the impact of computer-based analysis has been particularly effective in this area.

The insertion of microelectrodes or micropipettes into single neurons allows the recording of their activity and such cells can be marked with tracers for subsequent structural work (at light or electron microscope level) by injecting them iontophoretically with dyes or other substances from the recording electrode (**8.3**). By recording simultaneously from several cells linked together in small 'integrative units' or 'microcircuits' and combining the results with those from detailed studies of neuronal connections, a new era of analysis began (e.g. Lissäk 1967a, b; Shepherd 1974; Rakic 1975; Schmitt et al 1976).

The first description of the voltage clamp technique by Huxley and Hodgkin in 1952 marked an important milestone in neurophysiology. In the last two decades, developments in voltage clamp techniques have further clarified our still imperfect understanding of the ionic events that occur during the propagation of the action potential. In particular, numerous studies have examined the density of nodal Na^+ channels in normal mammalian and amphibian nerves; and the axonal distribution of Na^+ and K^+ channels (using tetrodotoxin, (TTX) and tetraethyl ammonium (TEA) to selectively block Na^+ and K^+ channels respectively). Results have been correlated with elegant analyses of freeze fractured myelinated nerve fibres in normal and dysmyelinating mutant models and with cytochemical studies to demonstrate putative Na^+ channels using ferric ion/ferricyanide staining or saxitoxin-binding to intact and homogenized nerves (see, for example, Waxman 1981).

Non-invasive imaging of the brain

In the last two decades, it has become possible to examine the activity of neuronal populations by relatively non-invasive methods which, for many purposes, have superseded the more conventional X-ray analyses of the skull and its contents. The tremendous impact of techniques such as magnetic resonance imaging (MRI) has meant that the visualization of the behaviour of even small areas of the brain in conscious normal human subjects is now routine in many research centres and neurology departments. The development and refinement of techniques has acquired its own momentum, in particular in the drive to use these methods to relate psychological models ('processes') to cerebral anatomy in normal and brain-injured subjects (see, for example, Frackowiak 1994) and to produce atlases of normal brain using computer-assisted segmentation. In 1980 nuclear magnetic resonance (NMR) spectroscopy was used to study brain biochemistry in vivo in the rat brain. Since then the technique has developed rapidly into a versatile non-invasive tool for investigating brain biochemistry and physiology in health and disease in a range of samples, from perfused tissue slices to the human brain. In clinical ^{31}P and ^1H NMR spectroscopy of the brain, metabolites in defined regions can be observed, and in parallel with the development of the technique in animal studies, diffusion weighted imaging has also been used to investigate human stroke (Kauppinen et al 1993). Single motor units in muscle can be caused to fire by magnetic stimulation of the cortex, a technique which may provide information about the nature of the corticospinal projection in man (Mills 1991). Modifications in MRI have made it possible to study not only cerebral vessels as small as 1 mm in diameter, but also to examine blood flow within the larger cerebral vessels. There have been significant advances in functional mapping of the human brain. Although currently much of these data have been acquired from positron emission tomography (PET), spatially detailed maps from

which functional connectivity may be deduced have also been derived from functional MRI (fMRI), single photon emission computed tomography (SPECT), electroencephalography (EEG), event related potential mapping (ERP) and magnetoencephalography (MEG) (p. 2072). All of these approaches have limitations in terms of temporal and spatial resolution and/or sensitivity.

Neural transplantation techniques

Intracerebral transplantation into mammalian brain was attempted before the end of the last century, but did not enter mainstream neuroscience research until the 1970s, when it emerged from relative obscurity. It is now widely used as a research tool for analysing the factors that may be involved in neuronal development and in the restitution of function after injury in the brain and spinal cord. It is in this latter role that the use of neural transplantation has excited worldwide attention as a potentially powerful clinical tool for the treatment of neurodegenerative diseases.

Numerous studies have now shown that transplants of fetal central nervous system tissue (in the form either of solid pieces or cell suspensions) into preformed cavities within a host brain can become functionally integrated with the host tissue to the extent that the behaviour of the grafted cells is influenced by the host. Sometimes the integration is so successful that transplanted cells take part in the reconstruction of simple functional circuitry; for example, in the Purkinje cell-deficient (*pcd*) mutant mouse, grafted E12 isogeneic Purkinje cells selectively invade the deprived cerebellar cortex, induce axonal sprouting of target populations of neurons and can occasionally become synaptically integrated within the *pcd* cerebellar cortex (Sotelo & Alvarado-Mallart 1991).

Transplanted cells can act as 'biological minipumps', to deliver molecules (e.g. neurotrophic factors or neurotransmitters) that can compensate for specific deficits induced experimentally in the host animal, for example in the use of intrastriatal transplants of fetal dopamine-rich nigral tissue in a Parkinsonian rat, or to encourage axonal regeneration after injury (p. 944).

The power of the technique may be enhanced by the use of genetically modified cells, in effect using 'customized' cells capable of delivering a required neuroactive molecule into sites where it is deficient. Currently studies have shown that such cells can survive in the cerebral microenvironment, express the selected transgene, synthesize and release the expected gene product and exert a measurable functional effect.

Glial cells (either mixed or defined populations of central nervous or peripheral nervous system glia) have also been transplanted into host brains in order to examine their interactions with other glia and/or with neurons. Two basic experimental approaches have been adopted. Cells have either been introduced to repopulate areas which have been rendered totally aglial (in the irradiation-gliotoxin model) or they have been transplanted into the brain or spinal cord and their interaction with endogenous glia has been observed (in these models, transplanted glia carry a phenotypic marker, or inherent repair mechanisms that would ordinarily obtain in the lesion have been modified).

Neural Transplantation

The central nervous system (CNS) is the most complex structure in the body. In response to injury, the tissues of the brain and spinal cord were for a long time considered as inert, capable only of degeneration, or at best passivity. However, it is now known that in fact injury causes vigorous formation of new synapses by surviving axons (Raisman 1969).

One of the first convincing demonstrations that new connections form in the adult brain after injury came from electron microscopic studies counting normal and degenerating synapses in the rat hippocamposeptal system. Normally, the hippocampal axons are distributed on both sides of the septal nuclei. When the fimbria of one side is cut, the degenerating axon terminals are removed by astroglial phagocytosis and completely replaced by new synapses, which arise as sprouts from

the terminal regions of the local axonal arborizations formed by the crossed fibres of the remaining, contralateral fimbria. The formation of new synapses was confirmed in a second experiment. Normally the axosomatic synapses in the septal nuclei are formed by axons from the medial forebrain bundle, but not by axons from the hippocampus. After lesions of the medial forebrain bundle, however, the hippocampal afferents to the septal nuclei are induced to reinnervate denervated axosomatic postsynaptic sites (**8.25**).

Although these newly formed synapses result in abnormal patterns of con-

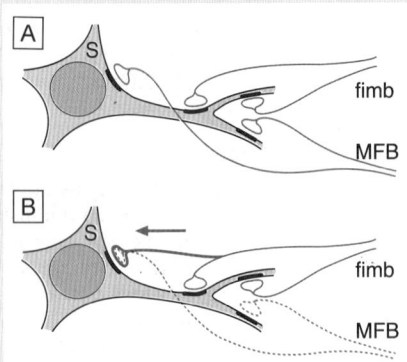

8.25 A. The normal pattern of distribution of synapses of the fimbrial axons (fimb) and the medial forebrain bundle (MFB). B. The formation (heavy line) of axosomatic synapses by fimbrial axons after deafferentation of axosomatic postsynaptic sites (broken lines) by a lesion of the adult MFB.

nectivity, which may be functionally valueless or even deleterious, the demonstration that the damaged adult brain is capable of forming new synapses after injury has encouraged experimental interventions designed to restore lost connections. These

have largely focused on intracerebral transplantation. Experimentally, the response to the transplantation of embryonic central or peripheral nervous tissue provides a way of investigating the latent capacity for regenerative reorganization in the adult brain and spinal cord.

Embryonic neurons survive transplantation into adult hosts, and both give and receive normal patterns of specific functional synaptic connections which integrate them into the host brain circuitry. This is illustrated by experiments in which embryonic mouse tissue from a Thy-1.1 strain was transplanted into the hippocampal neuropil of adult mice of a congenic Thy-1.2 strain (Zhou et al 1985). The specific Thy-1.1 epitope recognized by the OX7 monoclonal antibody marks the axons of the donor tissue, and shows that appropriate types of embryonic tissue can correctly reinnervate host tissue which has been deprived of those specific types of axons (8.26).

Where degenerative conditions result in the loss of a fairly specific category of neurons (as in Parkinson's disease) attempts have been made to replace the lost cells by injections of embryonic neurons of a similar type, or by cells genetically engineered to secrete sub-

stances required for amelioration of the symptoms (see p.1200). But where there is damage to central fibre tracts — as in strokes affecting the internal capsule, or damage to long spinal tracts — different strategies will be needed to induce the cut axons to regrow and re-establish the severed connections. It is known that cut axons can regenerate if severed in the peripheral nervous system. A comparable regenerative response does not occur after damage to central fibre tracts, but can be elicited by implantation of segments of peripheral nerve. In the most successful experiments, transplanted sciatic nerve segments provided bridges which led cut optic nerve fibres to regenerate functional connections with their central targets (Vidal-Sanz 1987), but even in the best situations only a minor proportion of the cut axons were able to regenerate to their original targets.

While such peripheral tissue transplants might be developed into a useful approach for restoring connections in systems where a discrete group of nerve cells projects to a similarly discrete target, they would not be sufficient for situations such as lesions of the long ascending and descending spinal tracts which recruit axons from multiple sites at all levels of the brain and

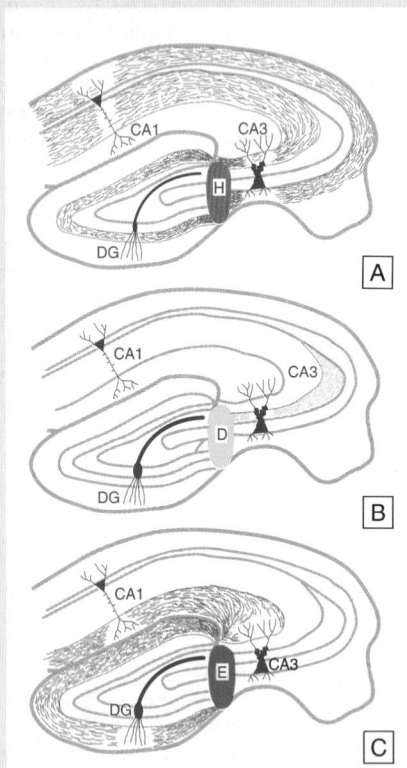

8.26 The complementary, contiguous but mutually exclusive territories of projections arising from transplants of late embryonic hippocampal (H), dentate (D) or entorhinal (E) tissue into the denervated adult hippocampus.

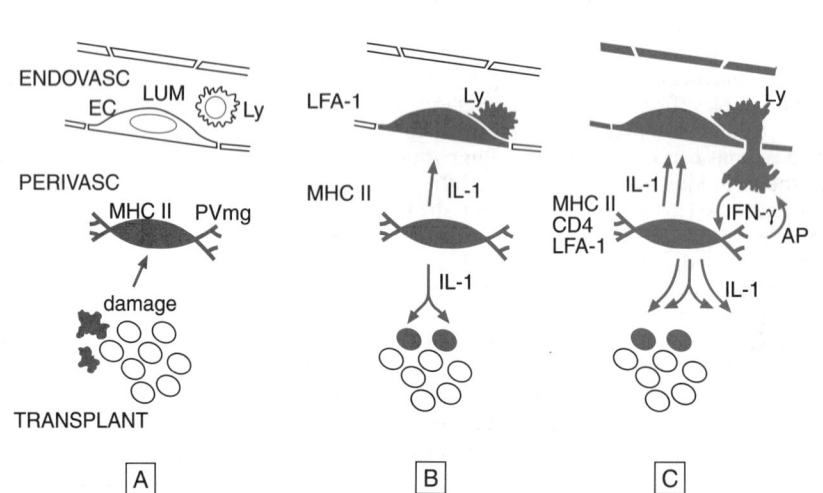

8.27 Role of perivascular microglia (PVmg) in the immune response. A. Tissue damage induces the PVmg to express MHC I and II antigens, and to secrete a number of cytokines (such as IL-I).

B. Cytokines secreted by the activated PVmg now activate (upper arrow) the adjacent endothelial cells (EC) to induce luminal adhesion (via factors such as LFA-I) of activated lymphocytes (Ly), and also (lower arrows) induce the immediately adjacent, underlying graft cells to begin to express MHC I antigens.

C. This leads to diapedesis of the activated lymphocytes, whose arrival in the perivascular space now exposes the PVmg to further stimulation by secreted lymphocytic factors such as gamma interferon (IFNγ). This twist in the spiral of activation enables the PVmg to extend the activation to the entire vascular system of the graft region, and to spread MHC I induction throughout the entire population of grafted cells. In turn, the diapedetic population of activated lymphocytes of mixed specificities is now subjected to selective activation of allospecific lymphocytes by transplant-specific alloantigen presentation (AP) by the perivascular microglia in the context of microglial molecules such as MHC 11, LFA-I, and CD4. Ultimately, this initial microglial antigen-presenting function will be reinforced and perpetuated by the arrival of the constitutively MHC 11 expressing dendritic cells in the perivascular space.

spinal cord and deliver them to similarly dispersed targets. Here, repair would only be possible if (in addition to bridging the lesion) the regenerating axons were able to regrow correctly through their normal spinal tracts.

Until recently, it seemed that the cause of the failure of central axon regeneration lay in the properties of the adult fibre tracts along which the cut axons had to regenerate. The tracts along which axons grow during their normal development have a completely different structure from adult tracts, whose constituent glial cells are largely formed after birth. The rat fimbria illustrates the remarkable regularity of structure of both embryonic and adult central tracts. The fimbria develops from an embryonic structure consisting of radial glial cells traversed at right angles by axons. This is superseded in the adult fimbria by a glial skeleton made up of interfascicular rows of glial cells, in which solitary astrocytes are spaced between roughly eight contiguous oligodendrocytes (Suzuki & Raisman 1992; (**8.47**). The individual interfascicular glial rows are spaced regularly; each row is associated with about 1200 axons (one-third unmyelinated). Astrocytes and oligodendrocytes each have both longitudinal and radial processes, which form an interlocking meshwork.

Transplanted astrocytes and Schwann cells are highly migratory in adult host brain, and readily enter central fibre tracts and migrate along them, Schwann cells becoming transformed into elongated, threadlike cells (Brook et al 1993). Further, it has now been shown that transplanted embryonic neurons not only innervate adult host neuropil, but also produce axons which can grow for long distances along adult fibre tracts. The donor axons are confined to the longitudinal tissue axis defined by the host tract structure (Davies et al 1994). Whether cut adult central axons (with or without initial stimulation by peripheral nerve grafts or Schwann cells) can do so is still not known.

The recent rapid developments in the use of neuronal, glial and Schwann cell transplantation raise the question of immune compatibility. The mechanism of the immune response in the adult central nervous system is less well understood than in other tissues, such as skin. The same rules of genetic histocompatibility seem to apply, but the mechanism of immune presentation is different, and although it is sometimes less effective, it cannot be ignored: serious clinical conditions, such as multiple sclerosis, are caused by immune attack directed at specific cell types in the central nervous system. Transplantation of allogeneic embryonic central nervous tissue (Lawrence et al 1990) induces the expression of major histocompatibility antigens on central neurons. Perivascular microglia are induced to express the phenotype of facultative immune presenting cells. Perivascular cuffs of immune cells accumulate in the region of the transplants, and their rapid invasion of the allografts leads to complete destruction of the donor cells (**8.27**).

CYTOLOGY OF THE NERVOUS SYSTEM

The cells of the nervous system comprise neurons, glia, and those associated with blood vessels and related connective tissues. Conventionally, descriptions of the cytology of the nervous system cover the central and peripheral parts separately. This division is justified for glia in the two systems, because they have different embryological origins and phenotypes, for intrinsic peripheral and central neurons many of which are specialised, and for many neural structures in the two systems which may also have unique features. However, many central neurons project to the periphery and, likewise, many peripheral neurons ramify centrally. Naturally, the axons of such neurons relate to central and peripheral glia over the respective parts of their trajectory paths. Nonetheless, the general pathology, including reactions to injury, of all central and peripheral neural elements are distinct and this dichotomy is not only attributable to the diverse properties of their associated glia, but also to functional specialisation of neural elements in the two systems.

CYTOLOGY OF THE CENTRAL NERVOUS SYSTEM

CENTRAL NEURONS

Most of the neurons in the central nervous system are either clustered (into nuclei, or laminae), or dispersed within grey matter. Their dendritic processes are usually confined within grey matter, but their axons often project in tracts over varying distances within white matter. Axons may be intrinsic to the central nervous system or come from or go into the periphery. Neurons interrelate at specialized junctions between their processes and cell bodies called synapses. The entire neuropil (white and grey matter) is pervaded by glia and their processes, glia outnumber neurons by some 10–50 times and comprise microglia and macroglia. The latter are further subdivided into the main forms of oligodendrocytes, astrocytes and ependymal cells.

Perikaryon or soma

The plasma membrane of the soma or perikaryon is generally smooth but may possess minute spinous postsynaptic elevations called *gemmules*. Somata are unmyelinated in man but in other species may be myelinated, for example the spiral ganglion cells of the guinea pig cochlea (p. 1393). The soma is engaged by inhibitory and excitatory axosomatic synapses (see **8.36**) and in some sites, somasomatic and dendrosomatic contacts. The non-synaptic surface is overlain by either astrocytic or satellite oligodendrocyte processes (**8.23**).

The cytoplasm of a typical soma is rich in granular and agranular endoplasmic reticulum (**8.28, 29c, 30a**) and free polyribosomes. The latter often congregate in large groups associated with the granular endoplasmic reticulum; these aggregates of RNA-rich structures are visible by light microscopy as basophilic *Nissl* (*chromatin*) *bodies* or *granules*; these are more obvious in large, highly active cells, such as spinal motor neurons, where stacks of granular endoplasmic reticulum occur. These features of neurons indicate high levels of protein synthesis. The significance of this is probably manifold. Maintenance and repair of cytoplasm are necessary in all cells and the huge total

921

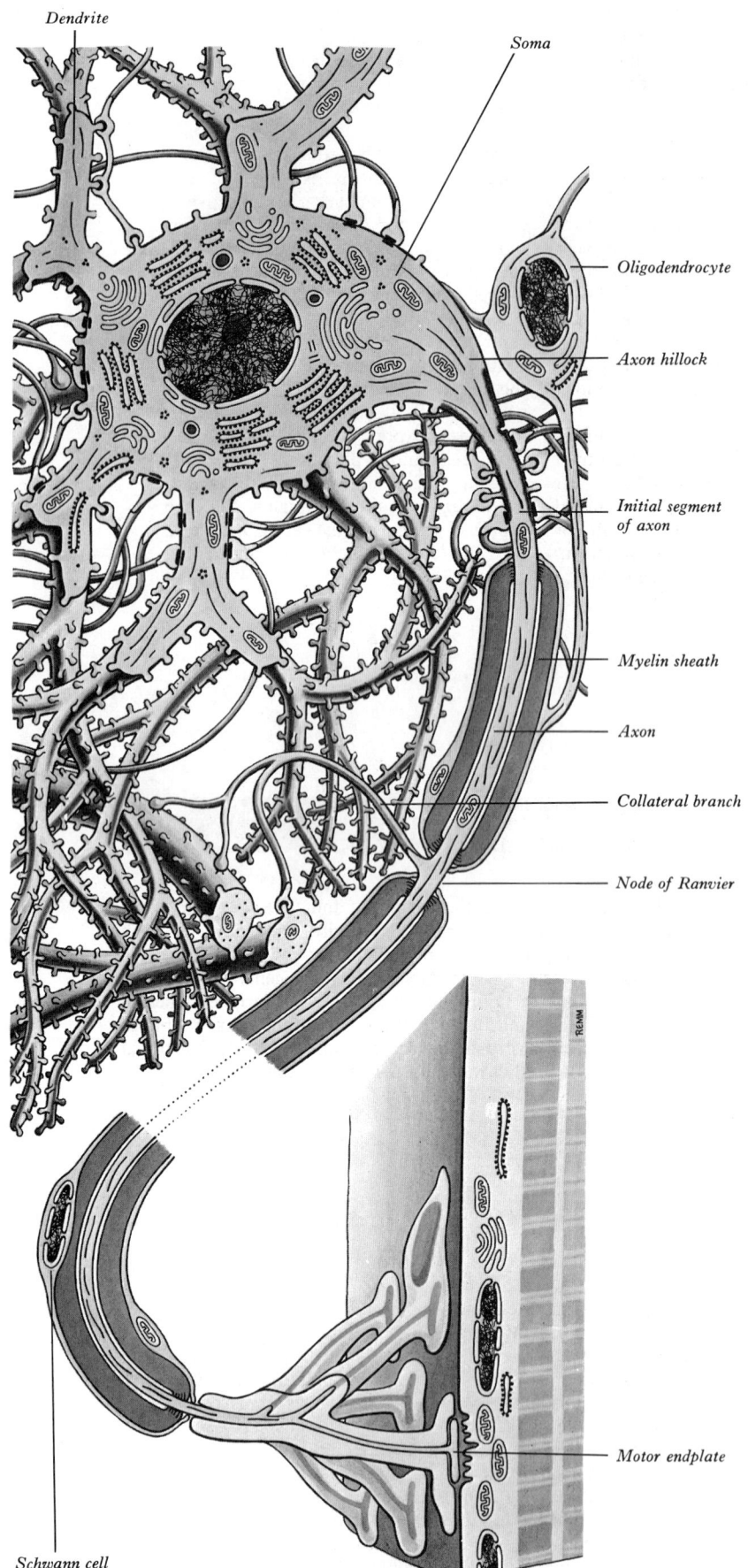

Dendrite

Soma

Oligodendrocyte

Axon hillock

Initial segment
of axon

Myelin sheath

Axon

Collateral branch

Node of Ranvier

Motor endplate

Schwann cell

8.28 Schematic drawing of the ultrastructure of a motor neuron, showing part of its dendritic field (above left); the dendrites are studded with spines which are contacted by different types of synaptic terminal. The cytoplasm of the neuronal soma contains stacks of rough endoplasmic reticulum and other organelles. See text for full description.

volume of cytoplasm within the soma and processes of many neurons must demand a high level of protein synthesis simply for these routine activities. Other proteins (enzyme systems, etc.) are involved in the elaboration of neurotransmitters and in the reception of stimuli. Various enzymes occur at the surfaces of neurons where they are associated both with ionic transport, for example sodium and potassium activated adenosine triphosphate (ATP)-ase, and with the 'second messenger' systems mediated by the adenylatecyclase and phosphoinositol pathways. Although the apparatus for protein synthesis (including RNA and ribosomes) occurs throughout the soma and dendrites, it is usually absent from axons, leading to the question of how transmitter substances and other materials are differentially transported within neuronal processes. (See Axoplasmic flow, p. 925, and Dendritic transport, p. 923).

The *nucleus* is characteristically large, round and euchromatic, with one or more prominent *nucleoli*, as in all cells engaged in a marked degree of protein synthesis (**8.28**, 29D, 30A, B). The nuclear envelope is double-layered with numerous prominent pores. In the cytoplasm, there are many mitochondria which act as sources of energy for cellular activities. Lysosomes occur in moderate numbers and Golgi complexes form distinct groups, particularly close to the nucleus, near the bases of main dendrites and opposite the axon hillock, and are the sites of both glycosylation of proteins and glycoprotein incorporation into membrane-bound vesicles for transport into the processes (see also p. 925).

Neurofilaments (7–10 nm in diameter) and *microtubules* (25 nm in diameter) are abundant, bundles of the former being the 'neurofibrils' of light microscopy. Both occur in the soma and extend along *dendrites* and *axons*, in proportions varying with the type of neuron and cell process. Neurofilaments are polymers of triplet proteins assembled from three polypeptide subunits, NF-L (68 kDa), NF-M (95 kDa) and NF-H (115 kDa). Antineurofilament subunit antibodies are used to specifically identify neurons using immunohistochemical methods (**8.31**). Dendrites are usually richer in microtubules than axons, which may be almost filled by neurofilaments. Though their bundles diverge at neuritic branch points, tubules and filaments do not themselves branch. Actin microfilaments (4 nm in diameter) are also found in neurons, as in most cells.

Centrioles, formerly believed absent from mature neurons, have been seen in every type examined, perhaps concerned in the generation or maintenance of the microtubular apparatus during development and subsequent life, rather than in cell division. (Neurons cannot undergo mitosis, once they are formed in the prenatal period, see p. 229.) In some neurons, centrioles associated with ciliary projections have been reported; though such structures are common on the surfaces of developing neuroblasts, cilia also occur in mature cells; their significance, except at some sensory terminals (p. 1317), is obscure.

Other inclusions are also common in the neuronal cytoplasm; *pigment granules* appear in certain regions; for example, neurons of the substantia nigra (p. 1067) contain a *neuromelanin*, probably a waste product of catecholamine synthesis. In the locus coeruleus a similar pigment, rich in copper, gives a bluish colour to the neurons. Some neurons are unusually rich in certain metals, for example zinc in the hippocampus, iron in the oculomotor nucleus. These metals may form a component of special enzyme systems. Ageing neurons accumulate granules of *lipofuscin* (senility pigment), especially in spinal ganglia. They represent residual bodies, the lysosomes packed with partially degraded lipoproteinaceous cellular material (corpora amylaceae).

DENDRITES

Dendrites are highly branched short processes stemming from the soma (**8.32**). The branching patterns of many dendritic arrays are probably established by random adhesive interactions between dendritic growth cones and afferent axons during development. There is an overproduction of dendritic segments in early development, and as the animal matures and information is processed through the tree, the arbors become pruned and segments redistributed, perhaps in response to functional demand. There is also some evidence that dendritic trees may be plastic structures throughout adult life, expanding and contracting as the traffic of synaptic activity varies through afferent axodendritic contacts (for review see Berry 1991).

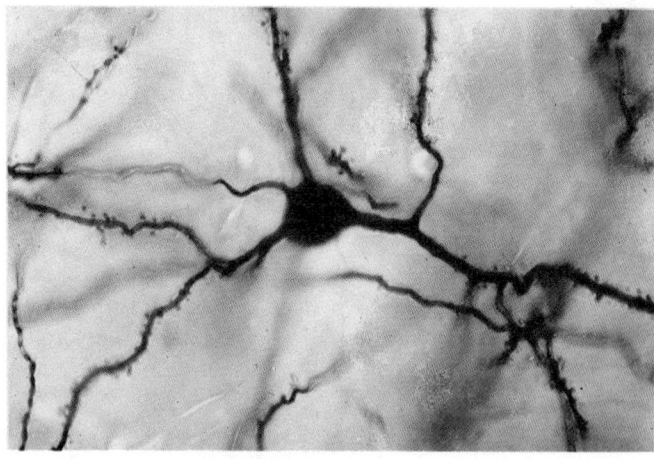

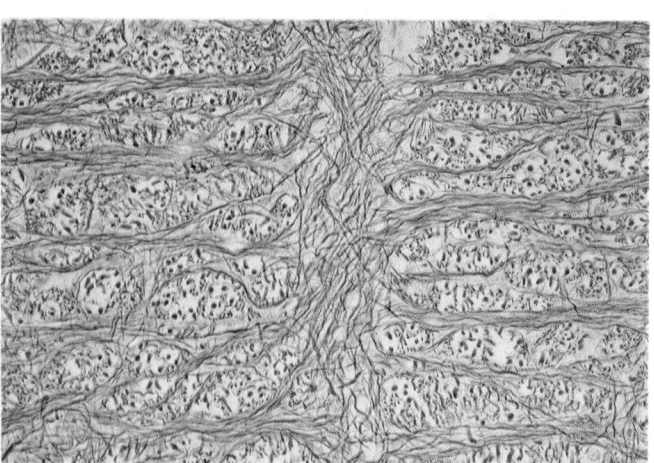

8.29 Different neurohistological methods.

A. A high-power light micrograph showing part of a pyramidal neuron from the cerebral cortex of a rat, prepared by the rapid method of Golgi. The bases of several dendrites covered with dendritic spines and a thin axon (left) are visible. (Preparation supplied by A R Lieberman of University College, London.)

B. A low-power light micrograph of groups of interweaving axons from the medulla oblongata of a cat, stained by the Holmes' silver method. (Preparations B–D supplied by E L Rees, Division of Anatomy and Cell Biology, UMDS, Guy's Campus, London.)

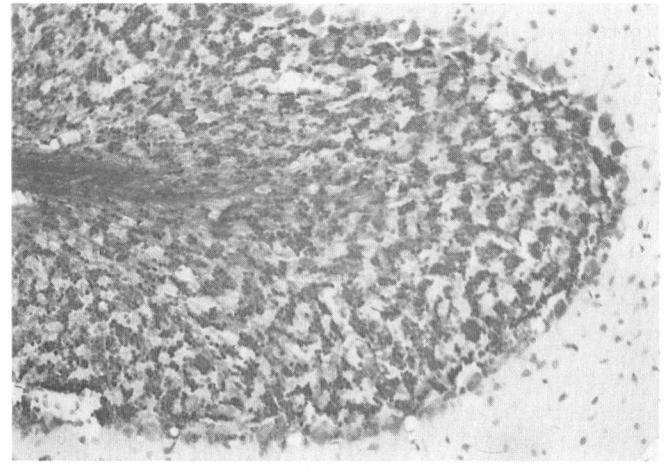

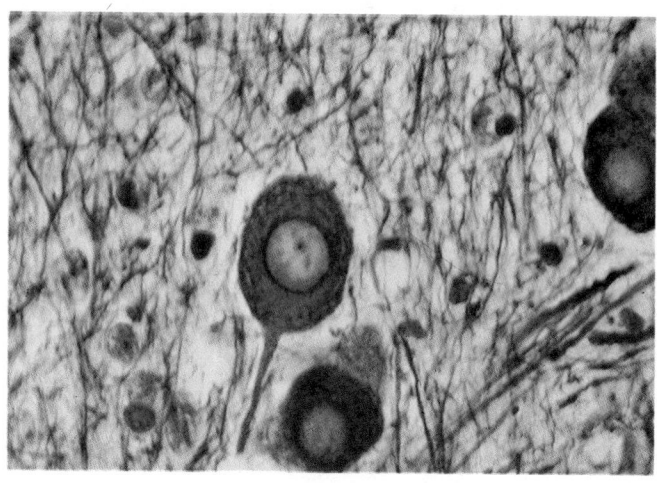

C. A group of neuronal perikarya (purple) amongst bundles of myelinated fibres (blue), from the cerebellum of rat. Stained by the cresyl fast violet-Luxol fast blue method.

D. A section through the mesencephalic nucleus of the trigeminal nerve (rat), stained with the Holmes' silver nitrate method to show large unipolar neurons from one of which a dendro-axonal process is emerging.

Nonetheless, the overall pattern of branching established has a precise topology which has been defined mathematically (Berry 1992). Groups of neurons with similar functions have a similar stereotypic tree structure (**8.33**), suggesting that the branching patterns of dendrites, together with the lengths and frequencies of segments, are all important determinants of the integration of afferent inputs converging on the tree.

Dendrites differ from axons in many respects. In representing the afferent rather than the efferent system of the neuron, they are engaged by both excitatory and inhibitory axodendritic contacts and may also make dendrodendritic and dendrosomatic engagements, some of which are reciprocal. Synapses occur either on small projections called dendritic spines (axospinous synapses) or on the smooth dendritic surface (**8.28**). Dendrites contain ribosomes, smooth endoplasmic reticulum (SER), microtubules, neurofilaments, actin filaments and Golgi membranes. The neurofilament proteins are of high and medium molecular weights and are poorly phosphorylated. Dendrites do not contain growth-associated proteins (GAP-43) but do possess the microtubule associated protein (MAP-2) almost exclusively. Accordingly, MAP-2 antibodies are used immunocytochemically to identify dendrites. Spine shapes range from sessile protrusions to structures with a slender stalk or neck and

expanded distal ends; most spines are not more than 2 μm long, with one or more terminal expansions; but they can also be short and stubby, branched and bulbous. Some, for example cortical spines, contain aggregates of SER which can form a specialized structure called the *spine apparatus*. Free ribosomes and polyribosomes are concentrated at the base of the spine. Dense arrays of actin filaments radiate from both the SER endoplasmic reticulum and spine apparatus into the subsynaptic region in typical globular spines. In sessile spines, actin filaments are orientated in parallel arrays, along the long axis, proximally associated with microtubules in the dendritic shaft and with the SER and coated vesicles in the spine base, passing distally into the region of synaptic apposition. The presence of contractile actin filaments probably explains the changes in width of the spine neck seen after experimental modification of afferent axospinous stimulation.

Various experimental and theoretical studies have so far failed to demonstrate an unequivocal role for spines in dendritic function. It has been proposed that they may limit the impact of individual synapses on the electrical state of the postsynaptic cell so that no single synapse dominates the total input. However, it has been calculated that a change in the width of a spine's stalk could change the effective synaptic current transmitted to the dendritic shaft

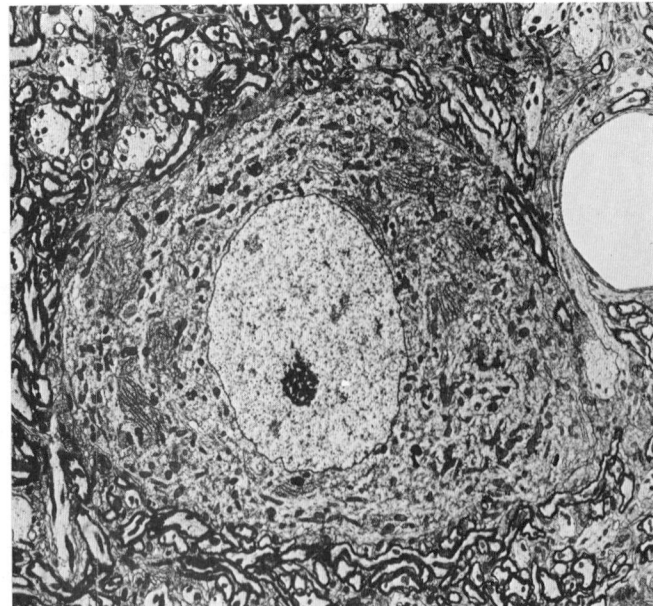

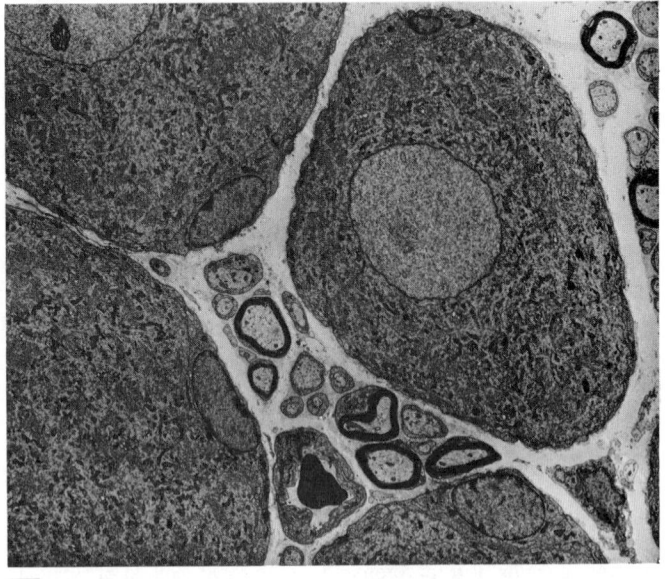

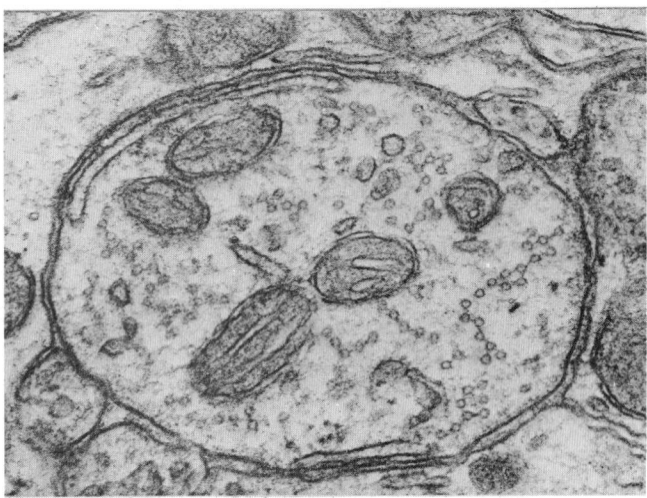

8.30 Electron micrographs of neuronal perikarya of the rat.

A. Typical ventral grey column multipolar neuron placed amongst numerous profiles of dendrites and axons, including myelinated nerve fibres. Note the prominent nucleolus and in the cytoplasm the clusters of rough endoplasmic reticulum.

B. A section through the somata of a number of unipolar spinal ganglionic neurons, associated with which are small flattened capsular (satellite) cells. Myelinated and non-myelinated nerve fibres and a capillary are also present.

C. An electron micrograph of a transverse section through the initial segment of an axon, showing the rows of linked microtubules which characterize this region. (Specimens provided by A R Lieberman of University College, London.)

(Crick 1982), providing a possible means of modulating neuronal excitability, for example in memory formation (see Koch & Poggio 1983).

The microtubules in dendrites are not uniformly orientated in a single direction; instead they have equal numbers with (+) and (−) ends within the soma (p. 925). It has been proposed that ribosomes and elements of the Golgi apparatus may be preferentially transported towards the (−) end accounting for the presence of these organelles in dendrites but not axons. The intracellular distribution of mRNA suggests a highly selective transport. For example, only mRNA actively encoding MAP-2 and the subunit of Ca^{2+}/calmodulin-dependent protein kinase and a polymerase III non-translated RNA transcript (called BC 1 in rats, BC 200 in man) of unknown function are found in dendrites. There are three possible mechanisms for the control of the differential distribution of mRNA: a sorting system in the soma; a mechanism for selective transport into dendrites over microtubules; and a docking mechanism for siting mRNA in specific regions, for example subsynaptically. Ribosomal accumulations near synaptic sites provide a mechanism for activity-dependent synaptic plasticity through the local regulation of protein synthesis.

AXONS

The axon stems either from the soma or from the proximal segment of a dendrite. At the point of origin on the neuron, there is a specialized region called the *axon hillock* which is free of Nissl bodies (**8.28**). This first part of the axon is called the *initial segment* (**8.30**c). Here, the axolemma is undercoated and is spike-generating (p. 906). Undercoating is thought to be attributable to a concentration of cytoskeletal molecules, including spectrin and F-actin, possibly important in anchoring numerous voltage sensitive channels to the plasmalemma (Hildebrand et al 1992). The initial segment is unmyelinated and often engaged by inhibitory axo–axonal synapses. This region of the axon is unique in that it is the only part

8.31 Neurofilaments in basket cell axons in the Purkinje cell layer of the adult human cerebellar cortex shown with the immunofluorescent technique using a primary antibody, RT97 which recognizes the high molecular weight (200 kDa) component of the neurofilament triplet. Magnification ×50×print size. (Prepared by Jonathan Carlile, Division of Anatomy and Cell Biology, UMDS, Guy's Campus, London.)

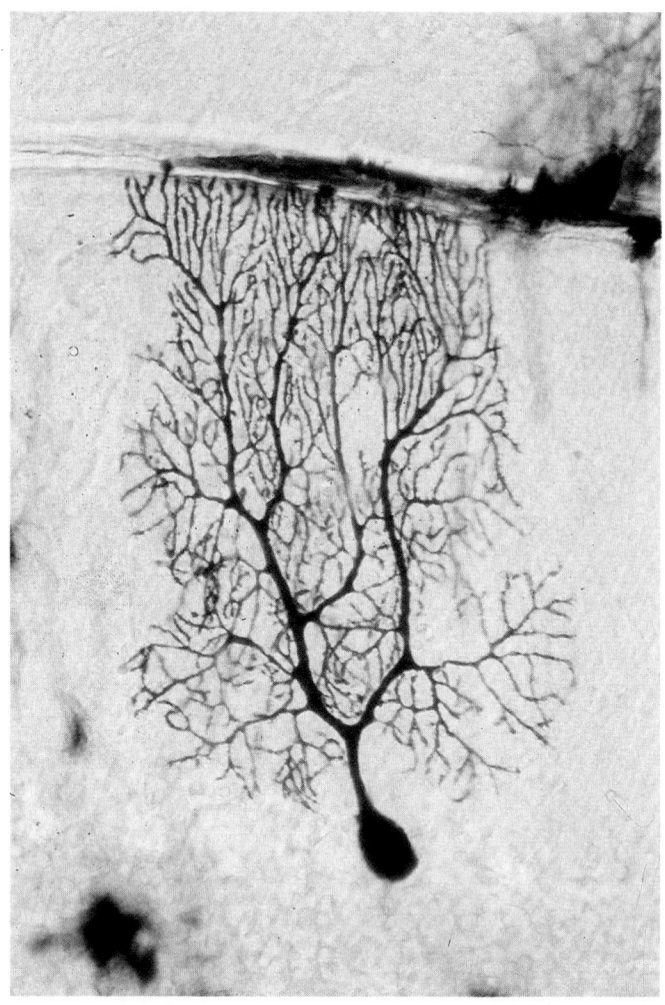

8.32 Purkinje neuron from the cerebellum of the rat stained by the Golgi-Cox method, showing the extensive two-dimensional array of dendrites. Magnification ×40. (Provided by Martin Sadler and M Berry, Division of Anatomy and Cell Biology, UMDS, Guy's Campus, London.)

which contains ribosomal aggregates sited below the postsynaptic membranes. When present, myelin (p. 951) begins at the distal extremity of the initial segment; each oligodendrocyte myelin segment is separated along the length of axon by a node of Ranvier. Myelin thickness and internodal segment lengths are positively correlated with axon diameter. Unmyelinated central nervous system axons may be as large as 0.8 μm in diameter, myelinated fibres as small as 0.2 μm in diameter. Unlike unmyelinated axons in the periphery which are embedded in Schwann cell cytoplasm, those in the central nervous system lie free in the neuropil. Nodes are specialized constricted regions of myelin-free axolemma (p. 942) exhibiting undercoating where unit potentials are regenerated and where an axon may branch. There is probably a high concentration of sodium channel density in the axolemma at nodes of Ranvier associated with a high density of E-face intramembranous particles (possible morphological correlates of sodium channels) both in the nodal and paranodal attachment regions. Fast potassium channels are also present in the paranodal regions. Fine astrocyte processes surround the nodal axolemma (p. 939). The terminals of an axon are also unmyelinated and expand into presynaptic specializations which may engage axons, dendrites, perikarya and, in the periphery, muscle fibres and glands and lymphoid tissue. They may themselves be engaged by axo–axonal contacts subserving presynaptic inhibition.

Axons contain microtubules, neurofilaments, mitochondria, membrane vesicles and cisterns, and lysosomes, but no ribosomes or Golgi elements, except in the initial segment (see above). Ribosomes are also found in the neurosecretory fibres of hypothalamo–hypophyseal neurons which contain the mRNA of neuropeptides. These organelles are differentially distributed along the axon. In the initial segment, at nodes and in presynaptic endings, there is a greater density of mitochondria and membrane vesicular aggregates. Axonal microtubules are interconnected by cross-linking microtubule associated proteins (MAP) of which *tau* is the most abundant, and this is particularly obvious in the initial segment (**8**.30c) where MAP elements are often visible, in electronmicrographs, interconnecting microtubules. Microtubules have an intrinsic polarity derived from the asymmetry of the tubulin molecule. Tubulin addition occurs preferentially at the (+) end of the microtubule and in axons all microtubules are uniformly orientated with their rapidly growing (+) ends directed away from the soma towards the axon terminal. Neurofilament proteins ranging from high to low molecular weights are phosphorylated in mature axons and antibodies raised to these molecules are important specific markers for defining axons and neuronal phenotype. Growing and regenerating axons also contain a calmodulin-binding membrane-associated phosphoprotein, growth-associated protein-43 (GAP-43), which was also thought to be an exclusive neuron marker until it was found to be expressed in some glia. Nonetheless, antibodies raised against the GAP-43 molecule are useful for identifying growing and regenerating axons.

Axoplasmic flow

Neuronal cytoplasm, as in other cells, is in continual motion; in tissue culture bidirectional streaming of vesicles along axons is clearly visible and there is indisputable evidence that similar movements occur in vivo, resulting in a net transport of materials from the soma to the terminals, with a lesser movement in the opposite direction (Weiss 1970). Experiments with radioactive substances (e.g. from the retina along the visual pathway) and investigations involving the ligature of peripheral nerves (Kapeller & Mayor 1967) showed that two major types of transport occur: one slow, the other relatively fast. The first, the *slow transport*, is a *bulk flow of axoplasm* which occurs only in the anterograde direction, transporting cytoskeletal proteins and soluble, non-membrane bound proteins at a rate of about 0.1–3 mm a day. In contrast, *rapid transport*, which has several components, carries vesicular material at about 100–400 mm a day and in the hypothalamo–hypophyseal tract (p. 1099) at a maximum of 2800 mm a day; it is bidirectional along the axon. This rapid flow is abolished by local treatment with colchicine, indicating that microtubules are involved. Ultrastructurally (and most clearly demonstrated in lampreys), vesicles with side projections can be seen to line up along the outside of microtubules and may be transported by the shearing forces generated between their side-arms and microtubules. Since ligature experiments show a build-up of vesicles on both sides, the mechanism must allow *bidirectional movement* of organelles.

Two microtubular based motor proteins with adenosine triphosphate (ATP)-ase sites have been identified, *kinesin* and cytoplasmic *dynein*. It has been suggested that kinesin-coated organelles are moved specifically towards the (+) end of microtubules, dynein-coated organelles towards the (−) end of microtubules, accounting for both the fast retrograde and orthograde flow of material in axons. The molecule which mediates slow transport has not been identified but is probably one of the microtubule associated motor proteins of the kinesin superfamily (KIF) (Hirokawa 1993). Kinesin and dynein bind to different membrane receptors and exist in active and inactive forms on the same vesicle. The direction of fast movement of an organelle could thus be determined by activation of one or other of the motor molecules, whereas speed of transport might be governed by differential activation of both dynein and kinesin simultaneously.

Axoplasmic flow is the means by which molecules and organelles (e.g. synaptic vesicle precursors, mitochondria, plasma membrane and receptor proteins) formed in the soma are transported into the axon. Since Golgi membranes and ribosomes are largely absent from axons, a sorting mechanism must be available in the soma to account for the differential distribution of these elements within the neuron (p. 1023). Retrograde axonal transport accounts for flow of mitochondria, endosomes and autophagic vacuoles from the axonal terminals into the soma and, pathologically, is a mechanism for the movement and concentration of neurotrophic viruses (e.g. herpes zoster and polio) intraneuronally. Axoplasmic flow is utilized experimentally in both orthograde and retrograde tracer studies for the demonstration of axonal and dendritic arbors, for the identification

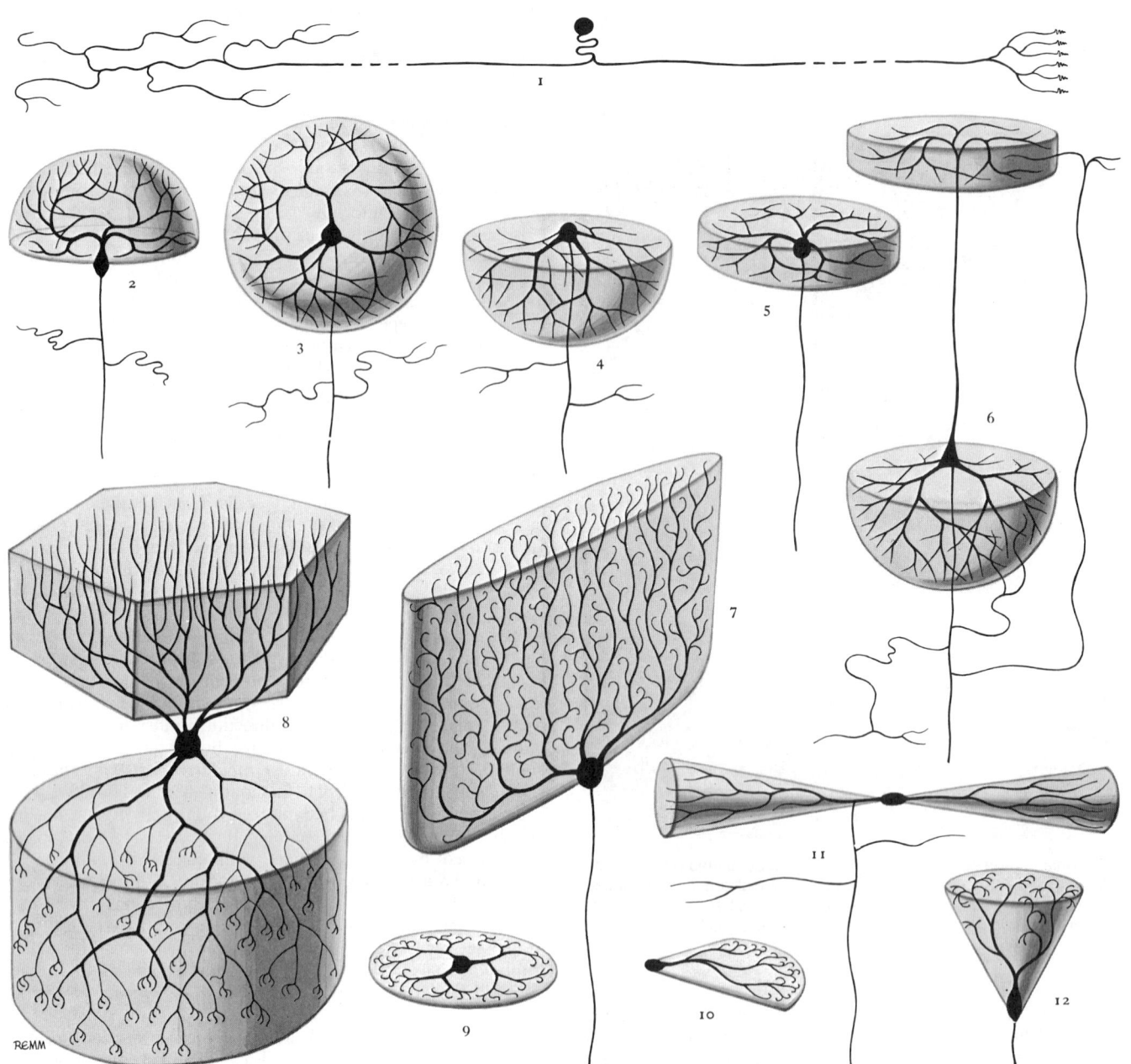

8.33 Scheme showing pattern variations of neuronal geometry: (1) uni-polar, sensory ganglionic neuron; (2) bipolar neuron; (3) stellate (isodendritic) neuron, with (4), (5), and (11) which are modifications of this pattern; (6) pyramidal neuron with an apical and a series of basal dendrites and recurrent axon collaterals from the cerebral cortex; (7) Purkinje neuron from the cerebellar cortex (see **8.32**); (8) Golgi neuron from the cerebellar cortex; (9) and (10) amacrine cells lacking axons; (12) glomerular neuron (mitral cell) from the olfactory bulb, showing recurved dendritic tips.

of the parent neurons of afferents terminating in a given centre (**8.23**) and for defining the connectivity of axonal projection systems.

The nature of synapses

The concept of an interruption in conduction at specific junctions, synapses, arose from the observations that there is an irreducible delay in reflex responses to sensory stimuli and that along a multi-neuronal pathway conduction generally occurs in only one direction (Sherrington 1947; Eccles 1964a, b). With the general acceptance of this neuron doctrine, attention focused on the cellular structures responsible for synaptic transmission. Studies by the Golgi technique (**8.2**, 32) demonstrated structural specializations at axonal terminals, while other methods showed similar endings in muscles. Later, the use of electron microscopy, correlated with physiological, pharmacological and biochemical studies, established the major features of synaptic structure (**8.34–38**) and molecular organization, although there are still many unsolved questions. By the mid-1940s it was known that neurotransmission is very largely chemical, depending on the release of neurotransmitters from the presynaptic side to cause a change in the electrical state of the postsynaptic neuron, either its depolarization or hyperpolarization.

Synapses can be formed between almost any surface regions of the two participating neurons. The most common type (**8.34**, 35, 37) occurs between an axon and either a dendrite or a soma, the axon being expanded as a small bulb or bouton. This may be a terminal of an axonal branch (*bouton terminal*) or one of a row of bead-like endings, the axon making contact at several points, often with more than one neuron (*bouton de passage*). Boutons may synapse with:

- dendrites, including dendritic spines or the flat surface of a den-dritic shaft
- a soma, usually its flat surface, and infrequently on spines
- the axon at its initial segment
- the terminal boutons of other axons.

The patterns of axonal termination vary considerably; a single axon may synapse with one neuron, for example climbing fibres ending on cerebellar Purkinje neurons (p. 1062), or more often with many, for example cerebellar parallel fibres, an extreme instance of

926

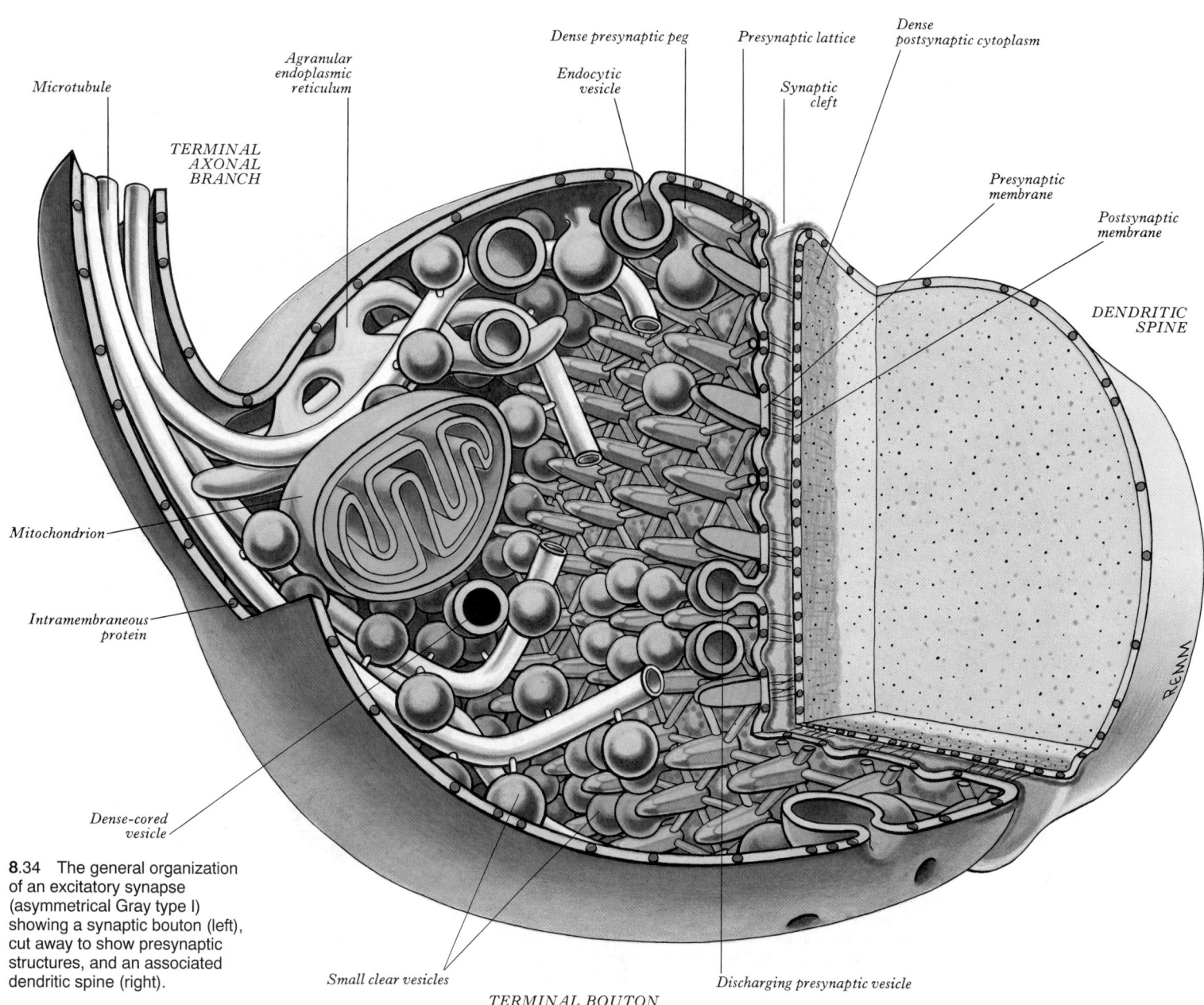

8.34 The general organization of an excitatory synapse (asymmetrical Gray type I) showing a synaptic bouton (left), cut away to show presynaptic structures, and an associated dendritic spine (right).

this phenomenon (p. 1038). An axon may synapse primarily with a dendritic tree or with a soma. Afferent axons of different origins may synapse with specific parts of a neuron, for example pyramidal neurons of the visual cortex, where optic afferents synapse chiefly with the basal segments of apical dendrites. (See also afferent terminals in the cornu ammonis, p. 1128). In *synaptic glomeruli* and *synaptic cartridges* groups of synapses between two or many neurons form interactive units, encapsulated by neuroglia (8.39, 40; see also below).

SYNAPTIC STRUCTURE

As seen by electron microscopy, synapses are defined structurally as specialized appositions between two or more neurons, with evidence of some form of neurotransmission. The overwhelming majority of them are of the chemical type, although electrical synapses also occur throughout the central nervous system (see p. 932) in much smaller numbers.

Chemical synapses

Chemical synapses have an asymmetric structural organization (8.35–38) in keeping with the unidirectional nature of their transmission. Typical chemical synapses have important common features as well as differences. In all of them an area of presynaptic membrane is

apposed to a corresponding postsynaptic membrane, the two being separated by a narrow gap, the *synaptic cleft*. *Synaptic vesicles* containing neurotransmitter are present on the presynaptic side, clustered near zones or patches of dense material coating the cytoplasmic aspect of the presynaptic membrane; a corresponding region of submembrane density is present on the postsynaptic side and these together define the *active zone*, the area of the synapse at which neurotransmission takes place.

Chemical synapses can be classified according to a number of different considerations, including:

- which neuronal regions participate in forming the synapse
- ultrastructural details
- the chemical nature of their neurotransmitter(s)
- their effects on the electrical state of the postsynaptic neuron.

The present account will be limited to associations between neurons, although neuromuscular junctions have many (though not all) features in common, and are often referred to as peripheral synapses. They are described separately on pages 957–960.

Neuron region. These can be axodendritic (most commonly), axosomatic (also frequent), or, less often, all other possible combinations: axoaxonic, dendroaxonic, dendrodendritic, somatodendritic or somatosomatic (Shepherd 1974; Gray 1974). Axodendritic and axosomatic synapses occur in all regions of the

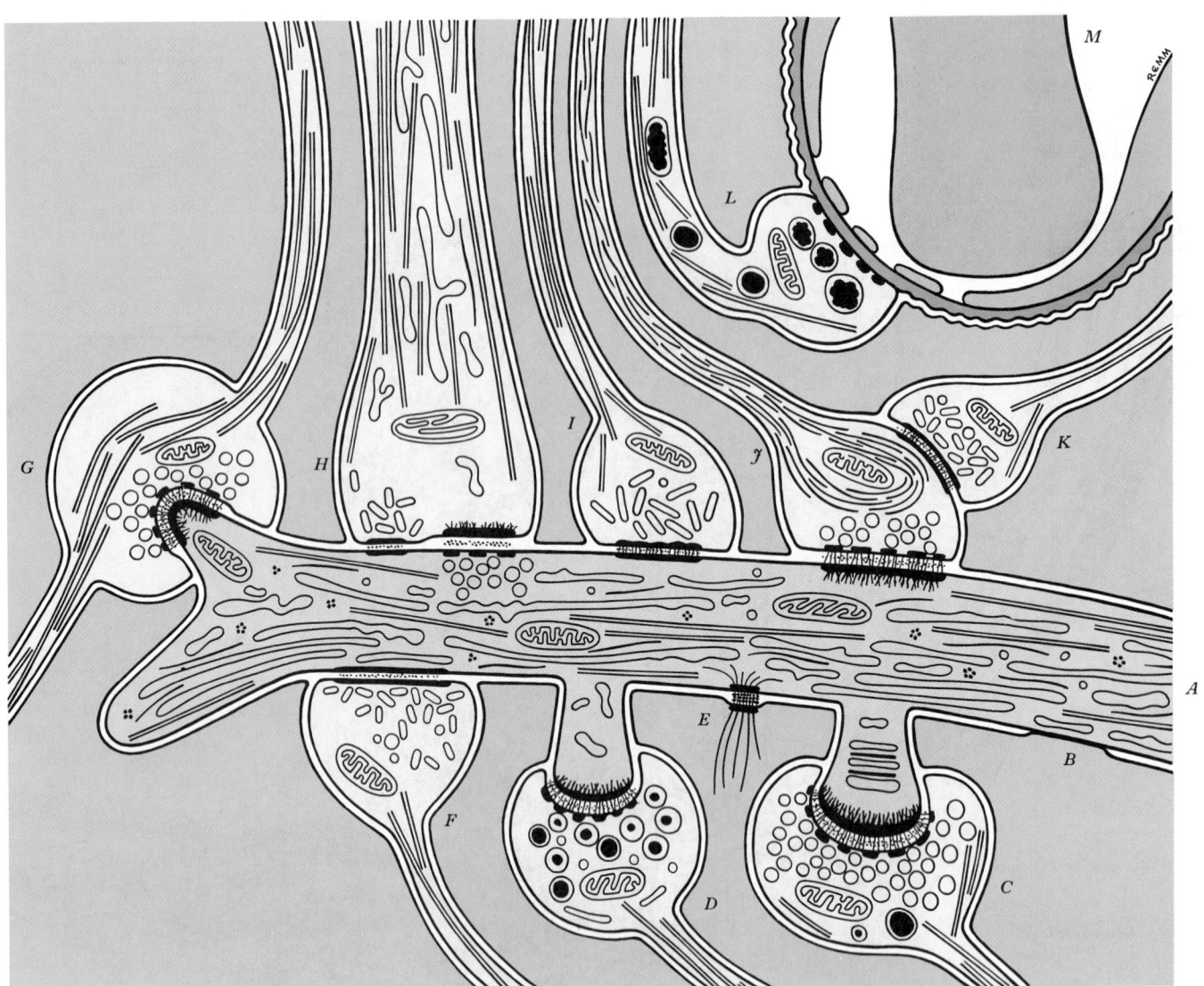

8.35 A scheme of the ultrastructure of chemical synapses, showing various junctional structures, grouped around a dendrite (A). The gap junction (B) and the desmosome (E) are without synaptic significance. Excitatory synaptic boutons are shown (C, G) containing small spherical translucent vesicles. D: a bouton with dense-cored, catecholamine-containing vesicles; F: an inhibitory synapse containing small flattened vesicles; H: a reciprocal synaptic structure between two dendritic profiles, inhibitory towards dendrite A and excitatory in the opposite direction; I: an inhibitory synapse containing large flattened vesicles. J and K: two serial synapses; J is excitatory to the dendrite; K is inhibitory to J; L: a neurosecretory ending adjacent to a vascular channel (M), surrounded by a fenestrated endothelium. All the boutons in this diagram are of the terminal type, except G which is a *bouton de passage*.

central nervous system and in autonomic ganglia including those of the enteric nervous system. Axoaxonic synapses can occur between boutons of two axonal terminals or between axon terminals and the initial segments of other axons (**8.8**, 36). The other types appear restricted to regions of complex interaction between larger sensory neurons and microneurons, for example in the thalamus.

In detailed structure. Ultrastructurally, synaptic vesicles may be internally clear or dense, and of different sizes (loosely categorized as small or large) and shapes (round, flat or pleomorphic i.e., irregularly shaped). The submembrane densities may be thicker on the postsynaptic than on the presynaptic side (*asymmetric synapses*), or equivalent in thickness (*symmetrical synapses*). The pre- and postsynaptic densities may also be interrupted by a dendritic extension (*perforated synapses*). Most synapses fall into one of two categories, those with round vesicles and asymmetric submembrane densities (RA or Gray Type I synapses), and those with flat vesicles and symmetric densities (SF or Gray Type II synapses). Other combinations also exist; for example, pleomorphic vesicles can occur in symmetric synapses, and dense-cored vesicles may be present in small numbers in either type. In a few instances Types I and II synapses are found in close proximity, orientated in opposite directions across the synaptic cleft (a *reciprocal synapse*: see p. 834).

Other subtypes have also been distinguished in various parts of the brain, depending upon bouton size, multiple areas of pre- and postsynaptic densities, vesicle contents and size, and various detailed features in the postsynaptic cytoplasm (see e.g. Starr & Wolpaw 1994).

Synaptic ribbons (**8.36**) are found at the neurotransmitting sites in the retina and inner ear. They are synapses with a distinctive internal morphology, the synaptic vesicles being grouped around a ribbon- or rod-like density orientated perpendicular to the cell membrane (Borg et al 1974; Boycott & Kolb 1973; see also p. 1381) which has a presynaptic dense undercoating, the arciform density. How this synapse operates is not yet clear, but the ribbon may act as some form of docking or guidance apparatus directing vesicles to the presynaptic surface. In the retina each ribbon synapse engages more than one postsynaptic process (p. 1344), although vestibular and cochlear hair cells make only one-to-one synaptic contacts.

In addition to the boutons which are in close contact with postsynaptic structures, as described above, there are many terminals lacking specialized contact zones; these are areas of transmitter release from the varicosities of non-myelinated axons, such effects sometimes being diffuse (paracrine, see p. 1294) as in the aminergic pathways of basal nuclei (p. 1192). In some instances, such axons

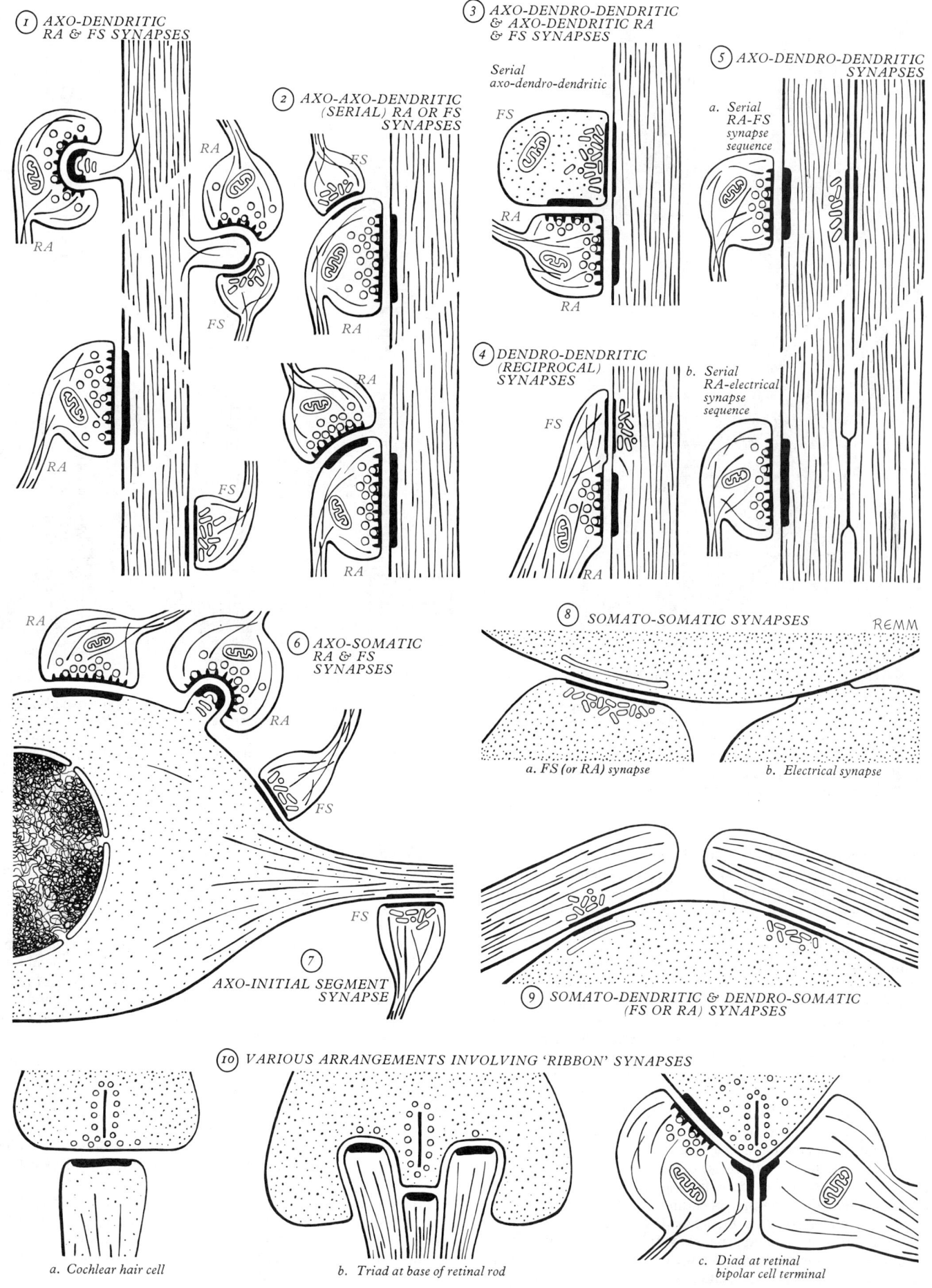

1 AXO-DENDRITIC RA & FS SYNAPSES

2 AXO-AXO-DENDRITIC (SERIAL) RA OR FS SYNAPSES

3 AXO-DENDRO-DENDRITIC & AXO-DENDRITIC RA & FS SYNAPSES

Serial axo-dendro-dendritic

5 AXO-DENDRO-DENDRITIC SYNAPSES

a. Serial RA-FS synapse sequence

4 DENDRO-DENDRITIC (RECIPROCAL) SYNAPSES

b. Serial RA-electrical synapse sequence

6 AXO-SOMATIC RA & FS SYNAPSES

7 AXO-INITIAL SEGMENT SYNAPSE

8 SOMATO-SOMATIC SYNAPSES

a. FS (or RA) synapse
b. Electrical synapse

9 SOMATO-DENDRITIC & DENDRO-SOMATIC (FS OR RA) SYNAPSES

10 VARIOUS ARRANGEMENTS INVOLVING 'RIBBON' SYNAPSES

a. Cochlear hair cell

b. Triad at base of retinal rod

c. Diad at retinal bipolar cell terminal

REMM

8.36 Various types of simple and multiple arrangements of synapse involving 'asymmetrical' synapses with rounded vesicles (RA), 'symmetrical' synapses with flattened vesicles (FS) and electrical synapses. For further details, see text.

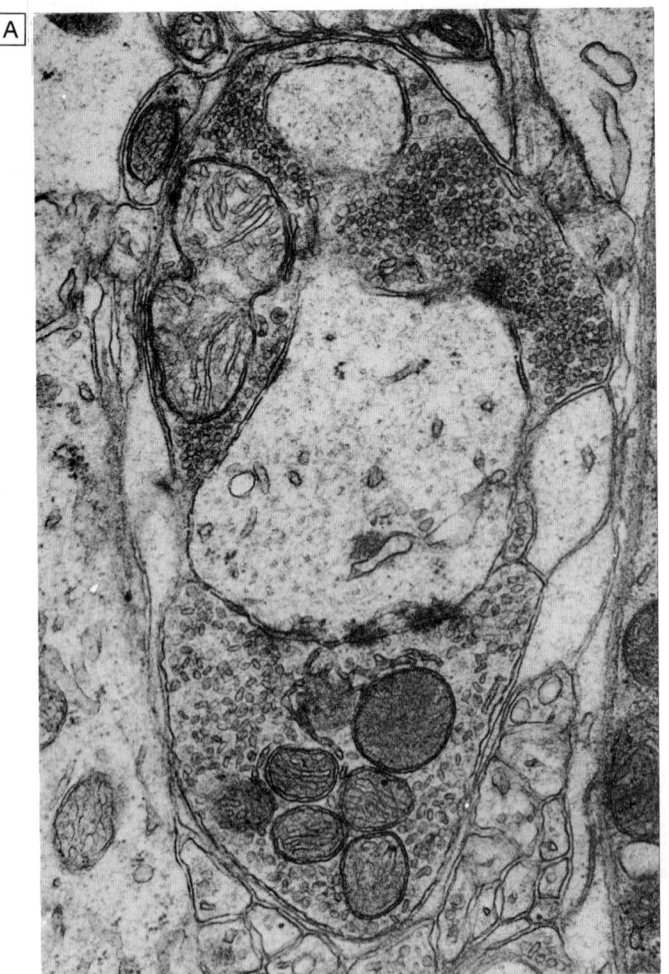

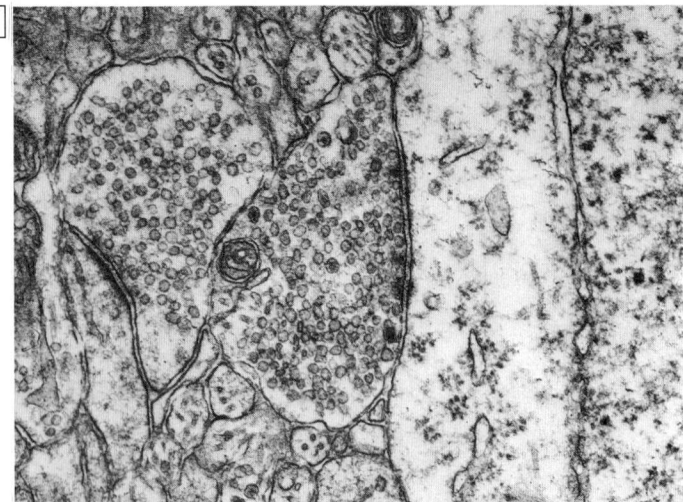

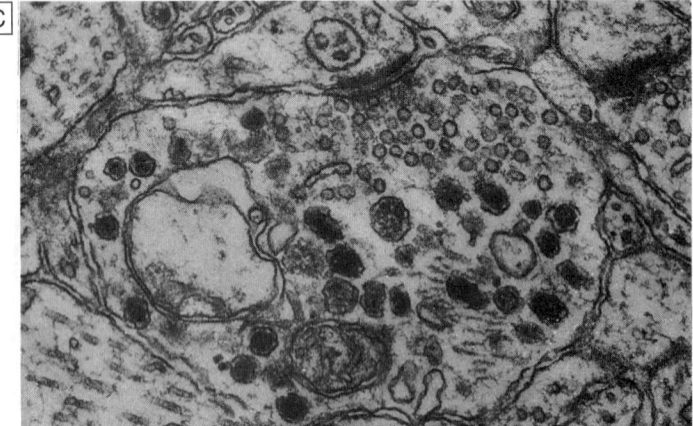

8.37 Electron micrographs demonstrating various types of synapse.

A. This shows a pale cross-section of a dendrite upon which end two synaptic boutons. One of them (above) contains round vesicles, and the other (below) contains flattened vesicles of the small type. A number of pre- and postsynaptic thickenings mark the specialized zones of contact.

B. Two types of synaptic structures; one of them (left) is a type I synapse between an axon terminal containing round vesicles and a dendritic spine; the other (right) is a type II synapse between an axon terminal containing pleomorphic vesicles, and the surface of a neuronal soma.

C. A type I synapse containing both small, round, clear vesicles and also large dense-cored vesicles of the neurosecretory type. (A and B provided by A R Lieberman, Department of Anatomy, University College, London.)

may ramify widely throughout extensive areas of the brain and, therefore, affect the behaviour of very large populations of neurons, an example being the diffuse cholinergic innervation of the cerebral cortices (p.1141). A negative aspect of this is that pathological degeneration of such pathways can cause widespread disturbances in neural function.

Chemical nature. A wide variety of transmitters or putative transmitters occur within neurons, either as one class of neurotransmitter per cell or more often as multiples. Good correlations exist between some of these chemicals and specialized structural features of synapses, as shown by immuno-electron microscopic localization of related enzyme systems, or autoradiographic detection of the neurotransmitters themselves. This information is very incomplete at present, and in some cases is contradictory, or variable in different regions of the brain. In general, asymmetric synapses with relatively small spherical vesicles are associated with several neurotransmitters, including acetylcholine (ACh), glutamate, 5-HT, and some amines; those with dense-cored vesicles included many peptidergic synapses and other amines (e.g. noradrenaline, adrenaline, dopamine), although the appearances of dense-cored vesicles are dependent on preparation methods. Frequently, a few dense-cored vesicles are also found in synapses with a predominance of the spherical type. Symmetrical synapses with flattened or pleomorphic vesicles have been shown to contain either γ-aminobutyric acid (GABA) or glycine.

Neurosecretory endings found in various parts of the brain and in neuroendocrine glands also have many features like those of pre-

synaptic boutons. They all contain peptides or glycoproteins within dense-cored vesicles of characteristic sizes and appearances, which are often ellipsoidal or irregular in shape, and may be relatively huge: oxytocin and vasopressin vesicles in the neurohypophysis, for example, range up to 200 nm across (see p.915).

Electrophysiological categories. Synapses may cause depolarization or hyperpolarization of the postsynaptic membrane, depending on the neurotransmitter released and the classes of receptor molecule in the postsynaptic membrane. Subtle variations in these responses may also occur at synapses where mixtures of neuromediators are present (p.935).

Axodendritic synapses

For clarity the structure of a typical axodendritic synapse of the asymmetric type will first be detailed (8.34–36), this category being the most intensively investigated (see, e.g., Gray 1959, 1961, 1969, 1974; Uchizono 1965; Akert et al 1972; Shepherd 1974; Rakic 1975; Jones 1978; Landis et al 1988).

In these synapses, the axonal ending forms a rounded presynaptic expansion or bouton (synaptic bag) attached strongly to the membrane of a dendritic spine or shaft. Glial processes commonly surround the synaptic structures but do not normally enter the synaptic clefts. The presynaptic surface is flat where it adjoins the smooth surface of a dendrite or soma but at endings on postsynaptic spines it may be highly curved around one or more of these projections (8.35–37). In some sites the dendritic surface forms a

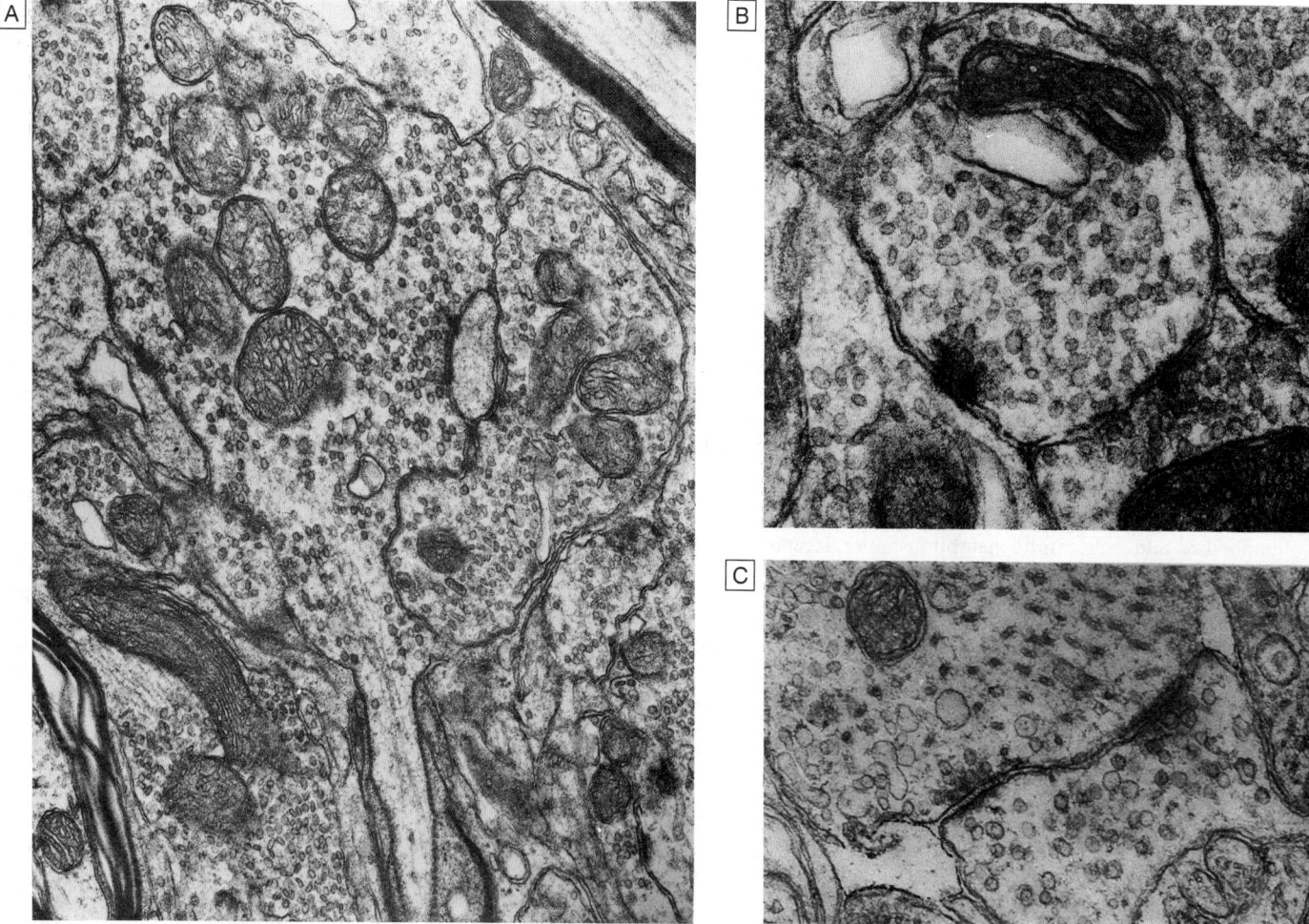

8.38 Electron micrographs of complex arrangements of synapses.

A. This shows a large terminal bouton of an optic nerve afferent fibre, which is making contact with a number of postsynaptic processes, in the dorsal lateral geniculate nucleus of the rat. One of the postsynaptic processes (right) also receives a synaptic contact from a bouton containing flattened vesicles.

B. Three neuronal processes in serial contact. On the lower right, a large spinule, interdigitating with the presynaptic surface. Conversely, process containing round vesicles synapses with a second process (centre) containing flattened vesicles; in turn the latter makes contact with a third process (lower left): specimen from the dorsal lateral geniculate nucleus of the rat.

C. This demonstrates reciprocal synapses between two neuronal processes in the olfactory bulb. (A and B provided by A R Lieberman of University College, London.)

dendritic expansions may be deeply invaginated by axonal terminals.

In sections across the synaptic junction, the submembrane density of the presynaptic side appears divided into a number of smaller patches, although when sectioned parallel to its plane it is seen to be a perforated plate termed the *presynaptic grid*, with discontinuities allowing direct access of synaptic vesicles to the membrane surface.

On the postsynaptic (dendritic) side, the submembrane density has an irregular cytoplasmic surface which is continuous with a system of interwoven filaments, the *subsynaptic web*. Associated with this are actin filaments, microtubules and microtubule-associated proteins, cisternae of smooth endoplasmic reticulum and, often, granular endoplasmic reticulum. In some subtypes of synapse a dense rodlet or plate lies parallel and immediately deep to the subsurface cisterna(e), known as a Taxi body (see, e.g., Starr & Wolpaw 1994), of unknown function. Where synapses are made with dendritic spines, a series of flattened membranous cisternae and associated dense material often (e.g. in cortical neurons) lies beneath this, constituting the *spine apparatus*.

The synaptic cleft is 20–30 nm wide, and occupied by granular or filamentous material, in which fine fibrils running between the presynaptic and postsynaptic surfaces have been described (see also below).

Synaptic vesicles are clustered against the presynaptic membrane, sometimes filling almost the whole bouton; mitochondria, irregular, agranular (smooth) endoplasmic reticulum cisternae, coated vesicles, endosomes and, occasionally, small lysosomes also occur.

Axonal microtubules continue into the bouton and may participate in the shuttling of transport vesicles into it, and also possibly in taking the synaptic vesicle to the presynaptic surface (Gray 1975); neurofilaments may also pass into the bouton, sometimes forming loops visible by light microscopy after silver impregnation.

Cytochemical methods (see, e.g., Pfenninger & Rees 1976) have also revealed other details of presynaptic organization: the presynaptic and postsynaptic submembrane densities are proteinaceous, and the presynaptic density consists of a hexagonally interconnected array of small pillars which may guide synaptic vesicles to dock with the presynaptic membrane (**8.34**; see also below).

Freeze-fracture techniques (see, e.g., Akert et al 1972; Landis & Reese 1974) show small rings of intramembranous particles (IMPs) in presynaptic membranes corresponding to sites of vesicular fusion. On the postsynaptic side, high densities of IMPs represent concentrations of receptor molecules and functionally linked ion channels.

Various proteins have been isolated from presynaptic boutons, and many others are anticipated. Important to synaptic activity are the filamentous cytoskeletal proteins F-actin and spectrin which form a network immobilizing synaptic vesicles except when needed for neurotransmission, and numerous other proteins associated with vesicle docking and fusion with the presynaptic membrane, such as synapsins I and II, synaptotagmin, syntaxin, neurexin(s), synaptophysin, synaptobrevin and SNAP-25 (Walch-Solimena et al 1993; see also p. 933). The membrane of the bouton also contains voltage-sensitive calcium channels and numerous other components associated with the complex activities of synaptic terminals.

Within the postsynaptic side, especially in spinous synapses, is a cytoskeleton of actin and actin-binding proteins, calmodulin, fodrin, MAP2 and some tubulin. Various enzymes are also characteristic of this region, for example calmodulin-dependent kinase II, and protein kinase C, and these are thought to be active in the plastic responses of synapses to changes in transmission rates. In addition, various molecules engaged in neurotransmitter actions are present, i.e. receptors, ion channels and second messenger systems, and may be bound to the underlying cytoskeleton by other proteins, including eutrophin, a molecule similar to dystrophin (found at neuromuscular junctions, p. 748).

The *synaptic cleft* also contains a range of characteristic macromolecules, consisting of the extracellular ends of transmembrane proteins from either side, and extracellular matrix molecules; these various components have not yet been fully characterized, but include neural cell adhesion molecules (N-CAMs: Persohn et al 1989) and integrins (Bahr & Lynch 1992) responsible for the strong attachment between pre- and postsynaptic membranes (p. 27). At skeletal muscle motor end plates an extracellular protein called *agrin* causes clustering of ACh receptors in the postsynaptic membrane, and an isoform may also be present in synaptic clefts, with similar functions, binding to transmembrane proteins which in some as yet unknown way immobilize and concentrate neurotransmitter receptors. For further information on synaptic proteins see the reviews by Walch-Solimena et al (1993) and Harris and Kater (1994).

Type I and II synapses. In his classical studies of mammalian central nervous system ultrastructure, Gray (1959, 1961) recognized the existence of the two broad categories of synapse already mentioned: Type I in which the subsynaptic zone of dense cytoplasm is thicker than on the presynaptic side; and Type II in which the two zones are more symmetrical but thinner (**8.35**). Other differences include the widths of their synaptic clefts, about 30 nm in Type I and 20 nm in Type II, and their vesicle content. After fixation by aldehyde perfusion, Type I boutons have a predominance of small spherical vesicles about 50 nm in diameter and Type II a variety of flat forms. Limited electrophysiological data initially linked Type I synapses with excitation and Type II with inhibition (Uchizono 1965); although this was later found to be a considerable oversimplification, the general principle has been found to apply in broad outline throughout the whole central nervous system. Type I synapses are now known to contain a wide variety of neurotransmitters, and a range of vesicle shapes. Different vesicle sizes and forms have also been reported for Type II synapses, including large (25–60 nm) and small (15–40 nm) flat vesicles (Pinching & Powell 1971), and also discoidal, fusiform and irregular types (Dennison 1971). Preparative procedures may also affect vesicle appearance (Bodian 1970a, b). GABA and glycine have been persistently reported to occur in Type II synaptic endings.

Of these two classes of synapse, the Type IIs are still the most intriguingly problematical; freeze-fracture studies show a lack of pre- and postsynaptic intramembrane particles typical of Type I, suggesting basic differences in the mechanisms of release and actions of their transmitters at the postsynaptic membrane (Landis et al 1974).

Electrical synapses

In mammals chemical transmission at synapses is by far the most common, but in lower vertebrates and some invertebrates electrical synapses are abundant where speed or synchrony of neural response is a requisite, for example in the medulla at the 'club' endings of Mauthner cells in fish, and between electromotor neurons of electric fish. They are also found in many areas of the mammalian brain, including the inferior olive, vestibular nuclei, cerebellar and cerebral cortex, mesencephalon and olfactory bulb, and they occur in the retina. Such synapses are like 'gap' or electrical junctions in cardiac (pp. 769, 1496) and smooth muscle (p. 779); because they are regions of direct ionic coupling at cell surfaces they transmit much more rapidly than chemical synapses. Ultrastructurally they are seen as patches of close membrane apposition between cell bodies, dendrites or axons. At such areas the lipid bilayers of the apposed surfaces are separated by a narrow gap of about 4 nm, communication being achieved by tubular assemblies of proteins called *connexins* embedded in each membrane so that each is in register with another in the opposite cell, thus creating a small open channel between the two.

Such assemblies usually comprise hexagonally packed clusters of many thousand units, but may also contain just a few, when they are difficult to detect by electron microscopy. Their presence can be shown functionally by their enhancement of neuronal membrane conductances or by the injection into one of the coupled cells of a fluorescent dye which then rapidly diffuses into adjacent coupled cells.

Connexins form a family of gap junction-forming proteins, several of which are present in the different cells of the central nervous system, as demonstrated by immunohistology with specific antibodies. Neurons synthesize a 32 kDa protein, Connexin 32, which is also found in oligodendrocytes, other classes being found in different non-neuronal central nervous system cells. Functionally, the significance of such interneuronal contact is not altogether clear. The larger of them undoubtedly serve as true synapses, mediating large interactions between the membrane potentials of coupled cells, so that, for example, the action potentials of a group can be synchronized, as in inferior olivary neurons projecting to the cerebellum which possibly provide a timing device for that structure. Smaller areas of contact may give more subtle interactions of a less dramatic kind either by the transfer of ions or of second messengers from one neuron to another. Thus populations of coupled neurons may affect each other's excitation thresholds or their responses to trophic factors and other more general metabolic influences. This is of considerable interest, because in a number of instances gap junctions have been found to be sensitive to extracellular chemicals; for example, dopamine uncouples retinal horizontal cells in lower vertebrates, so that diffuse 'paracrine' systems of the brain may affect the co-ordination of neuronal populations as well as influencing individual neurons.

For a recent review of electrical junctions in the central nervous system, see Dermietziel and Spray 1993.

FUNCTIONAL CLASSIFICATION OF SYNAPSES

The search for a correlation between synaptic structure and neurotransmitter content was initially dominated by the notion that each neuron secreted just one type of neurotransmitter (at all its endings), but more recently it has been found that multiple neuromediators may coexist at a single synapse, although usually one predominates. Moreover, the effects of a synapse depend ultimately on the types of postsynaptic receptor molecules present, and these are only distinguishable by immuno-electron microscopy. In spite of these caveats, a partial correlation can be made between the structures of synapses and the neurotransmitters which they release (see, e.g., the review by Jones & Cowan 1983).

Asymmetric synapses with spherical vesicles are associated with several neurotransmitters, including ACh, glutamate, 5-HT, and some amines; those with dense-cored vesicles include many peptidergic synapses and also some amines (e.g. noradrenaline, adrenaline, dopamine (when fixed appropriately)). Neurosecretory endings of the posterior pituitary contain relatively huge (50–200 nm), irregular dense-cored vesicles (see p. 1887).

Mixed populations of small, clear vesicles and large, dense-cored ones commonly occur, sometimes correlated with peptide transmitter substance P, serotonin, or enkephalins (Beaudet & Descarries 1979; Pickel et al 1979; see below).

MECHANISMS OF SYNAPTIC ACTIVITY

The molecular dynamics of neurotransmission are at present understood only in outline and many pieces of the functional jigsaw have yet to be placed. The mechanisms also are thought to vary with different types of synapse, with a range of response times and postsynaptic consequences. In fast-acting synapses, for example those releasing glutamate or ACh, the mechanisms are probably quite similar (see the reviews by Walch-Solimena et al 1993; Jahn & Südhof 1994). Activation begins with arrival of one or more action potentials at the presynaptic bouton, causing the opening of voltage-sensitive calcium channels in the presynaptic membrane. The response time is then very rapid, neurotransmitter being released in less than a millisecond, too fast to be accounted for by any activation of a classical second messenger system on the presynaptic side. It is currently thought that the influx of calcium activates Ca-dependent protein kinases (e.g. Ca^{2+} calmodulin-dependent kinase II) which uncouple synaptic vesicles from the spectrin-actin meshwork within the presynaptic ending. Prior to this, vesicles are bound to this meshwork via synapsins I and II which span the vesicle membrane; kinase activity causes synapsin phosphorylation which inhibits this binding, setting the vesicles free to move to the presynaptic membrane. How vesicles get to that target is not known; their movements may be randomly Brownian in nature or they may be directed by some preformed structure (e.g. microtubules, see above). Having arrived at a suitable site, the vesicles now dock with the presynaptic membrane, then the vesicle membrane fuses with it to open a pore ('synaptopore') allowing neurotransmitter to diffuse into the synaptic cleft. Other synaptic vesicle membrane proteins are involved in these processes, including synaptotagmin, synaptophysin, synaptobrevin and SNAP-25 which together bind to proteins within the presynaptic membrane (e.g. syntaxin) and possibly induce membrane fusion, in the presence of intracellular Ca^{2+}.

Once the vesicle has discharged its contents, its membrane joins with the presynaptic vesicle membrane and is then more slowly recycled back into the bouton by endocytosis around the edges of the active site (Heuser & Reese 1975). This membrane is then used to form new synaptic vesicles filled with neurotransmitter. Using fluorescence labelling of membranes, Betz and Bewick (1992) have shown in vitro that the time taken between endocytosis and re-release may be about 30 seconds, and that there is no queuing system for vesicle usage, newly recycled ones competing randomly with previously stored vesicles for the next cycle of neurotransmitter release. The recycling phenomenon can also be used experimentally to investigate the rate of synaptic activity by introducing an electron-dense (or for light microscopy, fluorescent) tracer into the extracellular space; its rate of endocytosis into the bouton is then a measure of the rate of vesicle fusion and hence of synaptic activity (see also, e.g., Dodson et al 1991).

The existence of synaptic vesicles of predictable size has provided a satisfactory basis for the observed quantal release of neurotransmitter at nerve endings, although it proved surprisingly difficult to demonstrate unequivocally the presence of neurotransmitter within the vesicles. It is now generally accepted that they do indeed contain neurotransmitters, and that at least in the major types of synapses, their fusion with the presynaptic membrane is responsible for the observed quantal behaviour both during neural activation and, spontaneously, in the slightly leaky resting condition.

Having described these activities, it must be noted that other scenarios may exist for more slowly acting synapses, for example in the release of neuropeptides, where vesicles are generally larger and their contents highly concentrated, and in nitric oxide release (p. 936).

Postsynaptically, the events vary greatly, depending on the receptor molecules and their related molecular complexes. Receptors are generally classed as either ionotropic or metabotropic; ionotropic receptors double as ion channels, so that conformational changes induced in the receptor protein by binding the neurotransmitter cause the opening of an ion channel within the same protein assembly, thus causing a voltage change within the postsynaptic cell. Examples are the nicotinic ACh receptor and the N-methyl-D-aspartate (NMDA) glutamate receptor. Alternatively, the receptor and ion channel may be separate molecules, coupled by a complex cascade of chemical interactions (a second messenger system), for example the adenylate cyclase pathway. This topic is considered again elsewhere (p. 24).

Neurochemical Transmission

Neurotransmission at all the synapses so far described in this account is chemical, involving the release of neurotransmitters from synaptic vesicles into a synaptic cleft to cause a change in the permeability and therefore the electrical polarization of the postsynaptic membrane. Such alterations may be excitatory (depolarizing) or inhibitory (hyperpolarizing), and are generally rapid and short-lived, as the transmitter is quickly inactivated either by an extracellular enzyme (e.g. acetylcholinesterase; AChE) or by uptake into the presynaptic process or into neuroglial cells. The presynaptic ending may also have more complex actions on the target cell, causing much more prolonged or even permanent changes in cell behaviour and structure. Indeed it is becoming increasingly clear that classic, rapid neurotransmission, measured in milliseconds, represents one extreme of

a broad spectrum of neural effects which also include slower electrical changes lasting for seconds or minutes, or much longer. They may even cause permanent cellular changes due to alterations in gene expression, resulting, for example, in the synthesis of more receptor molecules for the postsynaptic surface, or altering the numbers of synapses, the extent of the dendritic tree, the growth of axons and the overall metabolism of the cell. Permanent or semi-permanent changes of these types provide a physical basis for memory processes in the nervous system; they are also reflected in the trophic interactions between neurons which not only occur during development (where they are most obvious, e.g. see growth factors, p. 233) but form the constantly fluctuating background to the day-to-day activities of the mature nervous system, seen most dramatically when neurons alter their behaviour and morphology after damage has deprived them of their normal synaptic input. Neurohormones must also be included in this range; these are synthesized in neurons and released into the blood circulation by exocytosis at synaptic terminal-like structures and, of course, may act at great distances from their site of secretion. Similarly, neurons may also secrete into the cerebrospinal fluid or into the intercellular spaces of the nervous system (see below) to affect many other neurons, diffusely and at a distance. To encompass this wide range of phenomena the general term *neuromediation* has been used, the chemicals involved being *neuromediators*.

All such changes affect the electrical behaviour of individual cells and, if multiplied by similar responses in large neuronal populations, enable neural networks to modulate their behaviour according to the types and magnitudes of the influences reaching them.

Neuromodulators

A further twist in the story is that some neuromediators do not themselves have noticeable effects on the postsynaptic membrane but affect its responses to other neuromediators, either enhancing their activity (increasing the immediate response in size, or causing a prolongation) or perhaps limiting or inhibiting their action. Such substances have been called neuromodulators: a single synaptic terminal may contain one or more neuromodulators in company with a neurotransmitter, usually (though not always) in separate vesicles; the mode of action of neuromodulators is still not entirely clear but may involve either a direct binding to, and alteration in the response of, the receptor for the neurotransmitter or it may cause a second messenger-mediated change in the postsynaptic membrane which would then alter its response to the neurotransmitter. In some cases there may be a difference in the number of nerve impulses needed for the release, the neuromodulator only being secreted after more sustained stimulation of the ending.

Neuropeptides, which are extremely numerous (see pp. 936–937), are apparently nearly all modulators, at least in some of their actions. They are stored within dense granular synaptic vesicles of various sizes and appearances. Although they are distributed widely through the nervous system, certain areas have high concentrations and large numbers of different types. This finding has been analysed in detail by Nieuwenhuys (1986) in an extensive review and theoretical discussion of neuromediators in relation to classic neuroanatomy (see also p. 935). It is well known that in many parts of the nervous system, both central and peripheral, axon terminals have zones of transmitter release which are not closely apposed to a postsynaptic membrane but separated from it by a variable intercellular gap, perhaps as much as 200 nm ('synapses à distance', see, e.g., Chan-Palay 1983). Chemicals released from such axons may diffuse quite widely through the intercellular spaces to arrive at receptor sites on the surfaces of several neighbouring cells. Such effects are analogous to those of neuroendocrine endings, although the chemicals released are of course restricted to a limited volume and are said to be paracrine.

In a given area of grey matter (or of smooth muscle), several different neurotransmitters and neuromodulators from different sources may impinge on the mixed population of receptor molecules on a particular target cell, giving a great variety of possible responses, so that the level of excitation and, therefore, of action potential generation in a neuronal population fluctuates constantly as information from different sources converges on its dendrites and somata. Such areas of multiple interaction are frequently associated with neural activities directed towards homeostasis (e.g. ionic regulation, cardiovascular control), the survival of the individual in more extreme circumstances and the continuance of the genes, i.e. reproduction.

Synaptosomes

The term synaptosomes (synaptic 'bags') is the name given to an experimental preparation consisting of axon terminals, separable by fractionation techniques from brain homogenates. Where ACh is the transmitter, enzymes (e.g. choline acetyltransferase, CAT) able to synthesize it from choline exist in synaptosomes, the transmitter being stored in or near the synaptic vesicles. Catecholamines and other possible transmitters have also been demonstrated thus in synaptosomes (see below).

Organization of Synaptic Groups

The effects of synaptic endings on other neurons partly depend on their arrangement and relation to other synapses. In *serial synapses* (8.35, 36, 38) some terminal bulbs end on others to modify their response to afferent volleys, a possible basis of presynaptic inhibition (e.g. in the spinal cord) and of presynaptic facilitation, depending on the type of synapse. Reciprocal synapses (8.35, 36, 38c, 39), first found in the olfactory bulb and lateral geniculate body and later in many other sites, transmit both ways by staggered synaptic zones on opposite sides of the synaptic cleft; they are usually excitatory in one direction and inhibitory in the other. They are often the basis of lateral inhibition (Rall et al 1966; Shepherd 1974, 1978). Other varieties of serial synapses between different axonal, dendritic and somal structures have been described, some of them depicted in 8.36 (Gray 1974; Colonnier 1974; Shepherd 1974, 1978). In synaptic glomeruli (8.39) several boutons synapse with dendrites and some-

times with each other in localized regions of neuropil, usually within layers of gliocytes (Szentágothai 1970). Where microneurons are involved, synaptic patterns may become exceedingly complex, including various excitatory and inhibitory relations between neurites; these may occupy extensive zones as synaptic clusters. In synaptic or neuropil cartridges (8.40) part of a dendrite is enclosed by a glial sheath to isolate a cylindrical zone of synaptic endings on the spines and dendritic surface between them. Astrocytes (p. 939) may also isolate or juxtapose groups of interacting neurons. Though such arrangements of synapses in circumscribed areas is well established, the disposition of different types of synapse on neuronal surfaces is less certain. Inhibitory synapses can reduce the excitability of a neuron by their actions on dendrites and the soma, or may exert a total inhibitory blockade at some strategically-placed sites such as the initial segment of the axon (8.36), or the terminals of basket neuron axons synapsing with the 'pre-axons' of Purkinje neurons (p. 1040).

Synaptic spines (gemmules)

Synaptic spines are short projections (8.35, 36, 39) from the surfaces of dendrites, and to a lesser extent, neuronal cell bodies and axon hillocks, which form receptive synaptic contacts with afferent boutons. Spines usually have slender stalks and expanded distal ends; most spines are not more than 2 μm long, with one or more terminal expansions, but they can also be short and stubby, branched and bulbous. They contain the postsynaptic structures described above, although with much variation in detailed structure, even on a single neuron: there may be more than one postsynaptic density, or it may have a central non-dense zone (in perforated synapses),

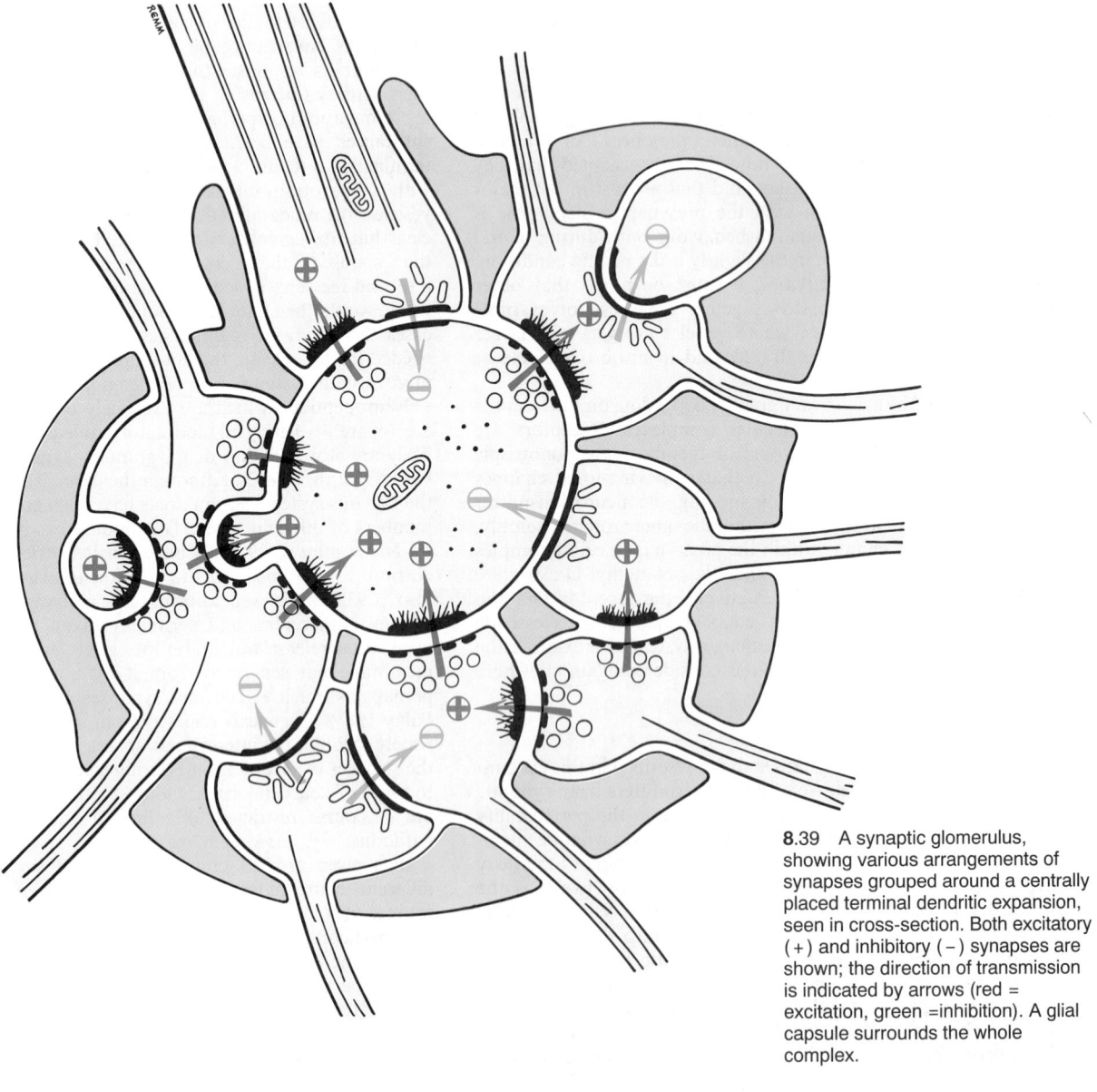

8.39 A synaptic glomerulus, showing various arrangements of synapses grouped around a centrally placed terminal dendritic expansion, seen in cross-section. Both excitatory (+) and inhibitory (−) synapses are shown; the direction of transmission is indicated by arrows (red = excitation, green =inhibition). A glial capsule surrounds the whole complex.

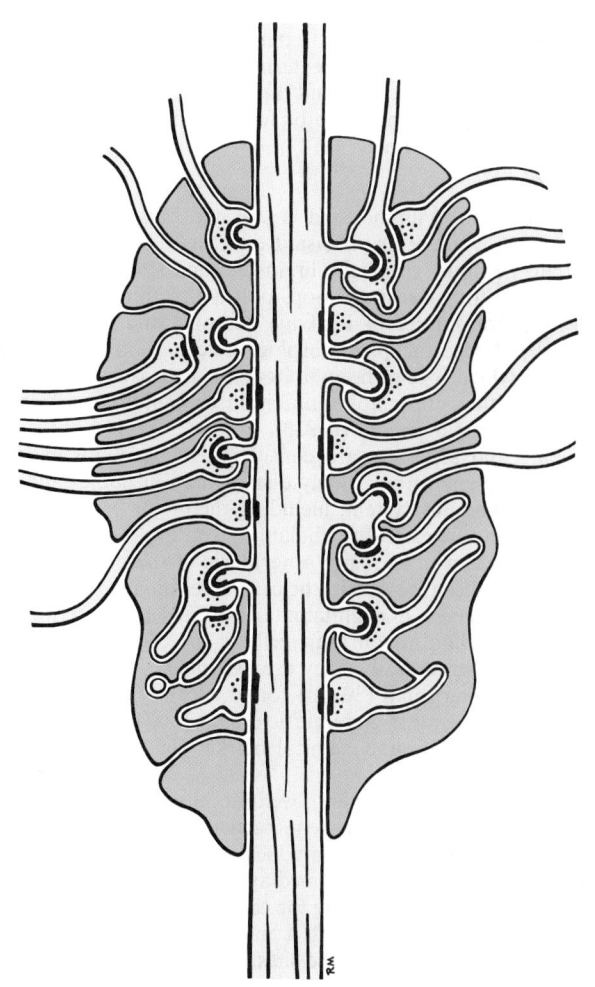

8.40 A synaptic cartridge, with synapses grouped around a segment of a dendrite and enclosed within a glial capsule (green).

establish preferential conduction pathways. Recording from hippocampal neurons suggests that in some locations even a brief synaptic activity (e.g. 1 second) can increase the strength of the synapse for some hours or longer (long-term potentiation). The mechanism of this appears to involve cytoskeletal changes modulated by calcium activation of protein kinases within the postsynaptic process (see e.g. Smith 1987). However, such dramatic changes may be limited to regions of the nervous system involved in memory storage; in other areas smaller adjustments may occur with the use or disuse of synapses, for example in the number of postsynaptic receptor sites. During early postnatal life it is well-established that a normal increase in numbers and sizes of synapses and dendritic spines depends on the degree of neural activity, as shown in the visual cortex of young animals temporarily blinded in one eye, where dendritic spines of cortical neurons show a greatly impaired development (Rothblat & Schwarz 1979).

NEUROMEDIATORS OF THE CENTRAL AND PERIPHERAL NERVOUS SYSTEM

Until recently the classes of chemicals known to be involved in chemical synapses were limited to a fairly small group of 'classic' neurotransmitters: ACh, noradrenaline, adrenaline, dopamine and histamine, all with quite well-defined 'fast' effects on other neurons, muscle cells or glands and satisfying the criteria laid down by the classic pharmacologists such as Henry Dale. With increasing research into the chemistry of the brain and more detailed electrophysiological and pharmacological studies, it became increasingly obvious that within the nervous system there are many synaptic interactions that cannot be explained in terms of these neurotransmitters and that other substances, particularly some amino acids such as glutamate, glycine, aspartate, GABA and the monoamine, serotonin, were good transmitter candidates. With the development of monoclonal antibody technology it was found that many substances which hitherto had been observed only in relation to the hormonal secretions of the hypophysis, or of the enteroendocrine system of the alimentary tract, can be detected widely and often systematically throughout the central and peripheral parts of the nervous system (see, e.g., Nieuwenhuys 1986; see also p. 958). Many of these are peptides, some of them closely related to each other chemically or even derived from a single large 'parent' molecule by its fragmentation. When isolated and tested by neuropharmacological methods, these substances have been shown to have a great range of effects on neurons, smooth muscle and glands, frequently as neuromodulators (see above). There are in excess of 60 known neuropeptides at the time of writing and their numbers are likely to increase as the techniques of molecular genetics are applied to the nervous system. However, it is highly problematical as to which of these substances actually represent functional neuromediators; some of them may be intermediate metabolites, or even the breakdown products of other neuromediators. Because more than one may be present at a single synapse, it has proved difficult to apply the rigorous criteria of classic neuropharmacology and many of these chemicals are therefore often referred to as only *putative* neuromediators. Nevertheless, various of these chemicals have been localized within synaptic vesicles of specific terminals and it has been possible to relate their presence to the physiological properties of known cells. Some of the postsynaptic receptor molecules which bind these substances have also been characterized, giving the corresponding neuromediator a measure of pharmacological respectability.

A comprehensive view of this field, were it indeed possible, is clearly outside the scope of the present account. It must be noted, though, that these substances, their neurobiology and distributions within the nervous system are of major importance in the functional organization of the brain, spinal cord and peripheral nerves and of neural interactions with the rest of the body. Before discussing these topics in the context of neuroanatomical pathways and centres, we will consider some of the better known neuromediators (see below).

Acetylcholine (ACh)

ACh is perhaps the most extensively studied neurotransmitter of the classic type; its precursor, choline, is synthesized in the neuronal cell body and transported to the axon terminals where it is acetylated

and the size may vary by an order of magnitude, as determined from serially sectioned nervous tissue: (see Harris et al 1992). The function of spines has excited much speculation, and it has been suggested that because of their narrow necks (possibly restricting current flow) they may limit the electrochemical impact of individual synapses on the electrical state of the postsynaptic cell so that no single synapse dominates the total input. It has been calculated that a change in the width of a spine's stalk could change its effect markedly and it has been suggested that spines (which contain actin) might be contractile (Crick 1982), providing a possible means of modulating neuronal excitability, for example in memory formation (see Koch & Poggio 1983). However, there is little experimental evidence for these suggestions, and calculations indicate that the narrow neck would not usually hinder electrotonic spread from the synapse into the main dendrite. The constriction might serve to limit the diffusion of chemicals involved in synaptic reception, or in synaptic modification, and changes in spine size might also affect the excitability of the neuron as a whole. Indeed, studies on hippocampal neurons involved in memory and showing long-term potentiation (LTP) when repetitively stimulated (e.g. area CAI pyramidal cells) have supported the view that spines can change size and other structural characteristics as a result of such stimulation, and that this may be an important factor in the memory process (see the review by Lisman & Harris 1993).

Development and plasticity of synapses

Embryonic synapses first appear as inconspicuous dense zones flanking synaptic clefts (Bodian 1970a, b; Pfenninger & Rees 1976). Immature synapses often appear after birth, suggesting that they may be labile, recruitable for transmission and dispensable when redundant. This is implicit in some theories of memory, which postulate that synapses are modifiable by frequency of use, to

and stored in 'clear' spherical vesicles about 50 nm in diameter. This neurotransmitter is synthesized by motor neurons and released at all their motor terminals on skeletal muscle and at synapses in parasympathetic and sympathetic ganglia. Many parasympathetic and some sympathetic ganglionic neurons are also cholinergic, as are some of the terminals of the efferent olivocochlear tract ending on cochlear hair cells. ACh has been demonstrated in many major non-motor systems of the brain and spinal cord, using immuno-histochemical methods, by labelling neurons with antibodies directed against the enzyme choline acetyl transferase (CAT) which is involved in its synthesis; in some sites ACh is also associated with the degradative extracellular enzyme acetyl cholinesterase (AChE), for example at neuromuscular junctions (p. 957), an association that has been used extensively to indicate the presence of the transmitter. There has been much recent clinical interest in the central cholinergic pathways, since there is evidence that damage to this neurochemical system, particularly in the basal forebrain, may be a causative agent in some degenerative conditions such as Alzheimer's disease.

The effects of ACh on nicotinic receptors (i.e. those in which nicotine is an agonist) are rapid and excitatory; in the peripheral autonomic system, the slower, more sustained excitatory effects of cholinergic autonomic endings are mediated by different (muscarinic, m_1) receptors via a second messenger system (see above) which results in the closure of a potassium channel.

Monoamines

Monoamines, often termed *biogenic amines* because of their import-ance to nervous function, consist of: the *catecholamines* nor-adrenaline, adrenaline and dopamine; the *indoleamine* serotonin (5-hydroxytryptamine); and histamine. Before suitable monoclonal antibody labels were available, catecholamines were localized by the formaldehyde-induced fluorescence (Falck et al 1962) or the glyoxylic acid methods (e.g. Axelsson et al 1973; Lindvall & Björklund 1974) but now it is possible to detect specifically the synthetic enzymes associated with each substance, using immunohistochemistry. Neurons which synthesize the monoamines include sympathetic ganglia and their homologues, the chromaffin cells of the adrenal medulla and paraganglia; within the central nervous system, their cell bodies lie chiefly in the brainstem, although their axons spread and ramify exceedingly widely into all parts of the central nervous system. Monoamine cells are also present in the retina (p. 442).

Noradrenaline is the chief transmitter present in sympathetic gangli-onic neurons and is released at their endings in various tissues, notably smooth muscle and glands but also in other sites including adipose and haemolymphopoietic tissues and the corneal epithelium. This neuromediator is also present at synaptic endings widely dis-tributed within the central nervous system; many of them are ter-minals of neuronal somata situated in the locus coeruleus in the medullary floor. The actions of noradrenaline depend on its site of action, varying with the type of postsynaptic receptor. In some cases, for example the neurons of the submucosal plexus of the intestine and of the locus coeruleus, it is strongly inhibitory due to its actions in closing a potassium channel via the α2 adrenergic receptor, whereas the β receptors, for example of vascular smooth muscle, mediate depolarization and therefore vasoconstriction.

Adrenaline is also present in central and peripheral nervous path-ways and occurs alongside noradrenaline in the adrenal medulla. Both of these monoamines are found in dense-cored synaptic vesicles about 50 nm across.

Dopamine is a neuromediator of considerable neurobiological and clinical importance, present mainly in the central nervous system, where it occurs in neurons with cell bodies in the telencephalon, diencephalon and mesencephalon. A major dopaminergic neuronal population in the midbrain constitutes the *substantia nigra*, so called because its cells contain neuromelanin, a black granular by-product of dopamine synthesis (p. 1067). Dopaminergic endings are par-ticularly numerous in the corpus striatum, limbic system and cerebral cortex, and pathological reductions of dopaminergic activity have widespread effects on motor control, affective behaviour and other neural activities, as seen in Parkinson's syndrome. Structurally, dopaminergic synapses contain numerous dense-cored vesicles resem-bling those of noradrenaline.

Serotonin and *histamine* occur in neurons mainly in the central nervous system; serotonin is synthesized chiefly in small median

neuronal clusters of the brainstem (mainly in the raphe nuclei), but their axons spread and branch extensively throughout the entire brain and spinal cord. Synaptic terminals contain rounded, clear vesicles about 50 nm across and are of the asymmetrical type. Histaminergic neurons appear to be relatively few and are restricted largely to the hypothalamus.

Amino acids

The best understood amino acid is γ-amino butyric acid (GABA) which is a major inhibitory transmitter released at the terminals of local circuit neurons within the brainstem and spinal cord (e.g. the recurrent inhibitory Renshaw loop, p. 1004), within the cerebellum (as the main transmitter of Purkinje neurons) and elsewhere. It is located in flattened or pleiomorphic vesicles within symmetrical synapses, at which it may be inhibitory to the postsynaptic neuron or may give either presynaptic inhibition or facilitation, depending on the synaptic arrangement (p. 933).

Glutamate and *aspartate* are considered to be major excitatory transmitters present within widely distributed cell bodies and fibres of the central nervous system, including the major projection path-ways from the cortex to the thalamus, tectum, substantia nigra, pontine nuclei, as well as many other parts of the brain and spinal cord. They have been located in the central terminals of the auditory and trigeminal nerves, and glutamate is present in the terminals of parallel fibres ending on Purkinje cells in the cerebellum, amongst other locations. Structurally, they are associated with asymmetrical synapses containing small (30 nm) round, clear synaptic vesicles. A major synthetic enzyme is glutamic acid decarboxylase (GAD) which can be used as an immunochemical marker for the localization of glutamate.

Glycine is another important, well-established inhibitory trans-mitter of the central nervous system, particularly the lower brainstem and spinal cord, where it is mainly located in local circuit neurons.

Taurine, an inhibitory neuromediator, is present widely in the central nervous system, including the cerebral cortex and cerebellum; there is evidence, however, that it may act as a neuromodulator rather than a transmitter at these sites.

Nitric oxide (NO)

An unexpected addition to the list of neuromediators, NO has been implicated in a wide variety of situations within the nervous system (see Bredt & Snyder 1992), although the full extent of its activities have yet to be clarified. It is of considerable importance at autonomic and enteric synapses, mediating smooth muscle relaxation in a number of well-authenticated instances. The enzyme responsible for its generation from arginine, nitric oxide (NO) synthase is identical to the NAD diaphorase; antibodies against this enzyme have located it in numerous sites within the central nervous system, and it is likely that it is of major importance in neuronal interactions, including long-term potentiation (p. 935). However, there are problems of a technical and conceptual nature; technical, because it is possible that NAD diaphorase/NO synthase may have other metabolic functions, and conceptual because the gas is able to diffuse freely through cell membranes, and is presumably not under such tight quantal control as vesicle-mediated neurotransmission. However, this is a rapidly moving area of research and a more stable view of the role of nitric oxide is to be expected in the next few years.

Neuropeptides

As already mentioned, the number of peptide neuromediators, either established or putative, is large (see Table 8.1). Many of them coexist with other neuromediators in the same synaptic terminals, from one to three types often sharing a particular ending with a well-established neurotransmitter; in some cases they have been shown to be present within the same synaptic vesicles. Some of them occur both centrally and peripherally in the nervous system and are particularly rep-resented in the ganglion cells and peripheral terminals of the auto-nomic system (see Burnstock 1986), where their physiological actions are more accessible to study; others are entirely restricted to the central nervous system. In view of the vast scope of this subject, only a few examples will be considered; for further details the reader is referred to some recent reviews of this subject (e.g. Emson 1983; Martin & Barches 1986; Nieuwenhuys 1985).

For convenience of description, most of the neuropeptides are classified according to the site where they were first discovered. Thus

Table 8.1 A summary of the main classes of neuromediators or putative neuromediators found in the nervous system

Non-peptidergic neuromediators

Acetylcholine

Nitric oxide

Monoamines

Noradrenaline
Adrenaline
Dopamine
Serotonin
Histamine

Amino acids

Glutamate
Aspartate
Glycine
Gamma aminobutyric acid (GABA)
Taurine

Purines

Adenosine triphosphate (ATP)

Peptides

Peptides first found in the gastrointestinal tract

Bombesin
Cholecystokinins (CCK)
Gastrin
Glucagon
Insulin
Motilin
Neurotensin (NT)
Pancreatic polypeptide (PP)
Substance P (SP)
Vasoactive intestinal polypeptide (VIP)

Peptides first associated with the hypothamalo-hypophyseal complex

Hypothalamic releasing hormones:
Corticotropin-releasing factor (CRF)
Growth hormone releasing hormone (GHRH)
Luteinizing hormone releasing hormone (LHRH)
Somatostatin (SST)
Thyrotropin-releasing hormone (TRH)
Neurohypophyseal peptides:
Vasopressin (arginine vasopressin; AVP)
Oxytocin (OXT)
Pro-opiomelanocortin (POMC) derivatives:
Corticotropin (ACTH)
Corticotropin-like intermediate lobe peptide (CLIP)
β-endorphins (β-END)
β-lipotropin (β-LPH)
γ-lipotropin (γ-LPH)
Met-enkephalin (M-ENK)
Leu-enkephalin (L-ENK)
α-melanocyte stimulating hormone (α-MSH)
γ-melanocyte stimulating hormone (γ-MSH)
Prodynorphin derivatives:
Neodynorphins α and β (α, β-NE)
Dynorphins (DYN) A and B

Other peptides

Angiotensin II (ANG-II)
Bradykinin
Calcitonin-related gene peptide (CGRP)
Carnosine
Gallinine
Natriuretic peptide
Neuropeptides Y and YY
Sleep peptide(s)

Growth factors

Nerve growth factor (NGF)
Platelet derived growth factor (PDGF)

there are the 'gastrointestinal' peptides found initially in the gut wall (p. 1787), then a group first associated with the hypophysis cerebri (including releasing hormones, adenohypophyseal and neuro-hypophyseal hormones) and finally peptides discovered first in the nervous system. Some of these peptides are closely related to each other in their chemistry because they are derived from the same gene products (e.g. the pro-opiomelanocortin group) which are cleaved in various ways to provide smaller peptides. The significance of the presence of these substances in both neural and non-neural tissue can at present only be guessed at: perhaps it represents a genetic economy in that the same molecule can be used for quite different purposes in different biological situations; alternatively it has been suggested that at least in certain instances the same peptide is present in regions with related biological functions.

Substance P (SP) was the first of the peptides to be characterized as a 'gastrointestinal' neuromediator. It consists of 11 amino-acid residues and is a major neuromediator in the brain and spinal cord. It occurs in about 20% of spinal and trigeminal ganglion cells, in particular those small neurons giving off narrow unmyelinated (class C) or myelinated (Aδ) axons, nociceptive in function. It is also present in some fibres of the facial, glossopharyngeal and vagal nerves. Within the central nervous system, SP is present in several apparently unrelated major central nervous pathways. It is contained within large granular synaptic vesicles in multineuromediator synapses; its known action on neurons is prolonged postsynaptic excitation.

Vasoactive intestinal polypeptide (VIP), another gastrointestinal peptide, is also widely present in the central nervous system, where it is probably an excitatory neurotransmitter or neuromodulator. Its distribution includes, among many other areas, distinctive bipolar neurons of the cerebral cortex, small spinal ganglion cells, particularly of the sacral region, and the median eminence of the hypothalamus where it may be involved in endocrine regulation. It is also present in intramural ganglion cells of the gut wall and sympathetic ganglia.

Somatostatin (ST, somatotropin release inhibiting factor) has a broad distribution within the nervous system and may be a central neurotransmitter or neuromodulator. It has also been detected in small spinal ganglion cells.

β-endorphin, leu-enkephalin and *met-enkephalin* and the *dynorphins* belong to a group of peptides ('naturally-occurring opiates') which have aroused much interest because of their pharmacological properties in relation to analgesia. They bind to opiate receptors in the brain and can induce analgesia if infused into appropriate areas of the brainstem. Although their distribution in the brain is complex, they coincide frequently with the opiate receptor sites, as determined by biochemical and radioactive labelling methods. In general their action seems to be inhibitory. The enkephalins have been localized in many areas of the brain, particularly the septal nuclei, amygdaloid complex, basal ganglia and hypothalamus; they therefore appear to be important mediators in the limbic system and in the control of endocrine function. They are also strongly implicated in the central control of pain pathways, including the periaqueductal grey matter of the midbrain, a number of reticular raphe nuclei (e.g. nucleus raphe magnus, the medial reticular formation of the rhombencephalon) and the spinal nucleus of the trigeminal with its spinal continuation into the substantia gelatinosa. Among other means of modulating the nociceptive channels, the enkephalinergic pathways appear to exert an important presynaptic inhibitory action on the nociceptive afferents in the spinal cord and brainstem (see p. 1004). Like many other neuromediators, the enkephalins also occur widely in other parts of the brain, though in lower concentrations, being present throughout the neocortex, the olivocochlear bundle and many other sites in the nervous system.

Cholecystokinin (CCK) is present throughout the brain but is particularly concentrated in the cerebral cortex, amygdaloid complex, hippocampus, periaqueductal grey and the dorsal grey columns of the spinal cord. Its precise functions in these sites are as yet uncertain.

CENTRAL NEUROGLIA

Neuroglial cells vary considerably in abundance and types in different regions of the central nervous system. In earlier times, their small

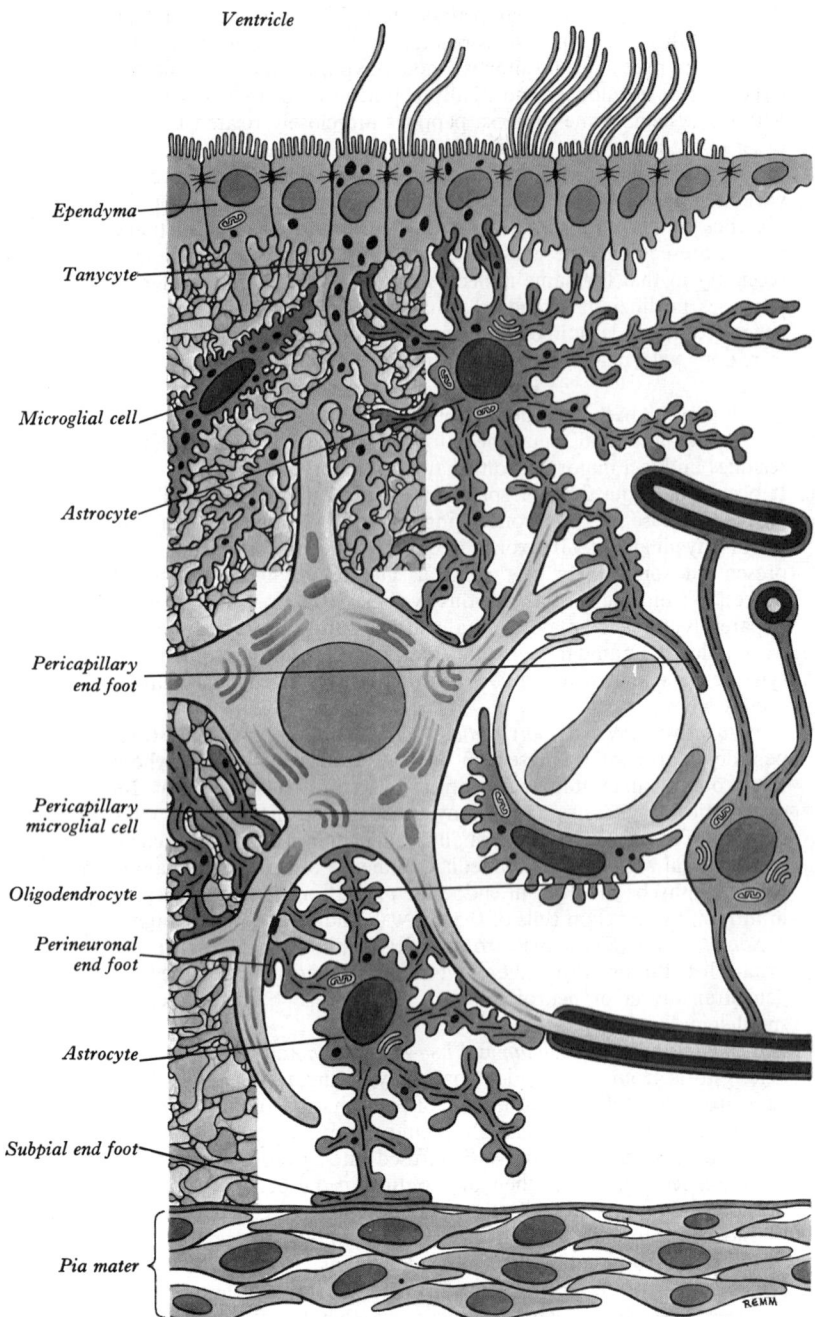

Ventricle

Ependyma

Tanycyte

Microglial cell

Astrocyte

Pericapillary
end foot

Pericapillary
microglial cell

Oligodendrocyte

Perineuronal
end foot

Astrocyte

Subpial end foot

Pia mater

8.41 Schema showing the types of non-neuronal cells in the central nervous system. The ependymal and glial cells are shown in green. The ependyma includes examples of ciliated and non-ciliated cells and one tanycyte, with a centrally directed basal process. Two astrocytes are shown apposed to a neuronal soma and dendrites; one (above) also contacts a capillary, the other (below) expands on the pial surface. An oligodendrocyte (middle right) provides myelin sheaths for two axons. Two flattened microglial cells, one adjacent to a capillary (middle right), and the other within the neuropil at the top left, are also illustrated.

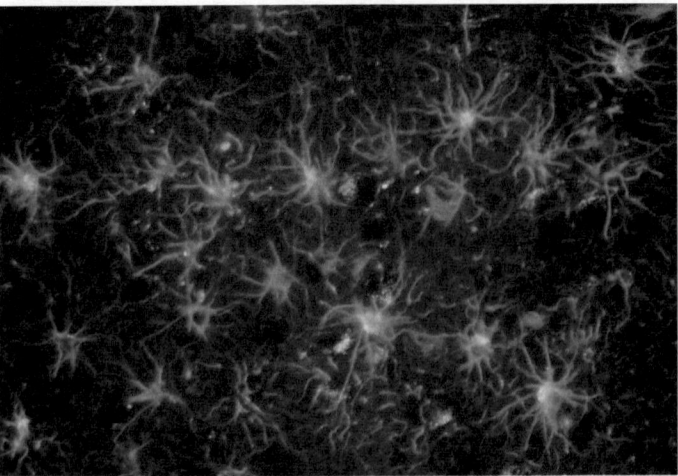

8.42 Section of the human cerebral cortex stained by immunofluorescence to show astrocytes containing glial fibrillary acidic protein (GFAP). Magnification ×400. (Preparation by Jonathan Carlile, Division of Anatomy and Cell Biology, UMDS, Guy's Campus, London.)

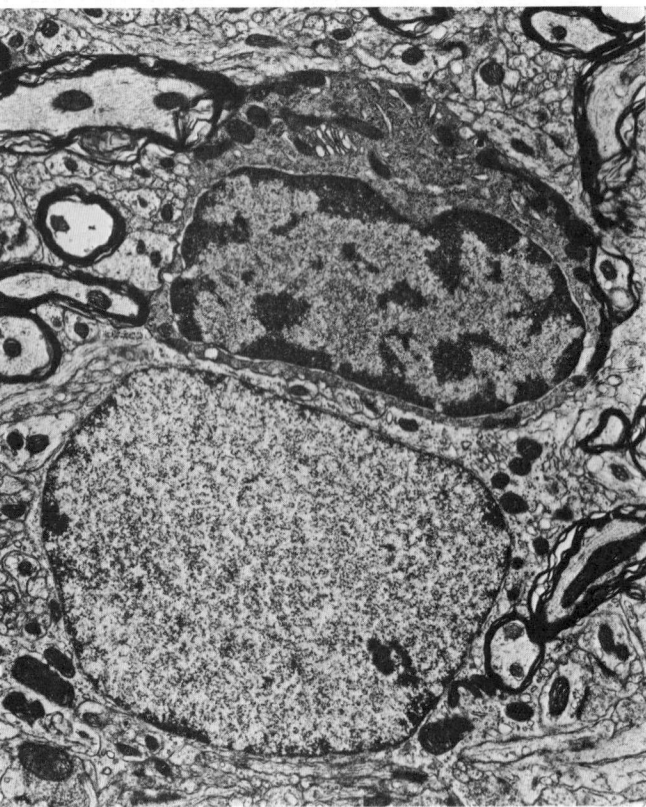

8.43 An electron micrograph of two neuroglial cells situated amongst myelinated and non-myelinated nerve fibres in the rat thalamus. A darkly staining oligodendrocyte containing numerous mitochondria, a well-developed endoplasmic reticulum and an indented nucleus is shown below; a larger, paler astrocyte with a vesicular nucleus and scanty cytoplasm is demonstrated above. (Provided by A R Lieberman of University College, London.)

size, and variable reactions to the special staining methods needed to demonstrate them, made them less accessible than neurons to histologists. With the application of electron microscopy, biochemistry and, more recently, immunohistochemistry, cell culture and intracellular dye injection methods, great advances on the classic descriptions (e.g. by del Rio Hortega 1924) have been made. Even now there are many uncertainties about the number of classes of neuroglia, their origins and their functions. There are two major groups classified according to origin: *macroglia* arise within the neural plate, in parallel with neurons, and constitute the great majority; *microglia* are smaller cells and generally considered to be a type of mononuclear phagocyte (p. 1414) (8.41).

MACROGLIA

The cells of this division are *astrocytes* and *oligodendrocytes*; the former also include specialized types such as *Müller cells* of the retina, *Bergmann glia* of the cerebellum, *pituicytes* of the neurohypophysis and *ependymal cells* and *choroidal cells* of the ventricles. In addition to these there are the stem cells from which macroglial cells originate during development and throughout postnatal life.

Astrocytes

Astrocytes are star-shaped glia whose radicular and vellate processes ramify throughout the entire central neuropil (8.41, 42). Their processes are functionally coupled at gap junctions and form an interconnected network intimately ensheathing all neuronal plasmalemmae except at synapses and along the myelinated segments of axons. Astrocyte processes terminate as end-feet at the basal laminae of the glia limitans of blood vessels and the pial surface where they are bound together by desmosomal junctions. Specialized fine processes also ramify around nodes of Ranvier. Ultrastructurally astrocytes are typified by a pale nucleus with a narrow rim of heterochromatin (8.43), pale cytoplasm rich in glycogen, lysosomes (granules or gliosomes of light microscopy), Golgi complexes and (in fibrous astrocytes) bundles of intermediate (10-nm) filaments throughout their processes (Mori & Leblond 1970; Ling et al 1973).

Although two distinct morphological and functional astrocytic phenotypes have been described in tissue culture (Raff et al 1989), only one cell type is seen in vivo which appears capable of subserving all astrocytic functions. Intracellular microinjection of dyes into astrocytes (8.49) in vivo demonstrates a wide range of process geometries and orientations (Butt et al 1994a,b). In the optic nerve, for example, when this technique is combined with electron microscopy, the processes of astrocytes, in addition to terminating as classical end-feet on blood vessels and pial surface, also possess protoplasmic extensions which surround nodes of Ranvier. Perinodal astrocytic contacts include fine filopodial processes, 50–60 nm thick, end-feet terminations and en passant associations with large processes. A single node has a cluster of such filopodia originating from several astrocytes embedded in a proteoglycan matrix. Some of these processes contact the oligodendrocyte paranodal loops by gap junctions indicating functional coupling. Astrocyte perinodal processes have high densities of potassium and sodium channels and intramembranous particles. Astrocytic Na^+ currents can be generated by ephaptic transmission at perinodal sites and their activation could be important for neuronal/glial signalling (Chao et al 1994). The injection technique has also shown that the processes of astrocytes are dye-coupled, dye passing from one cell to the next across low resistance intercellular gap junctional complexes. Astrocytes may thus form a functional network in the brain. Accordingly, although astrocytes are morphologically diverse, existing in at least two forms, protoplasmic and fibrous, they probably serve the common functions of maintenance of the glia limitans externa and blood–brain barrier (p. 1221), and also serve an unidentified function at nodes probably related to nodal activity.

Astrocytes appear to signal to each other through gap junctions using intracellular Ca^{2+} wave propagation at a rate of 7–27 μm/sec (Cornell-Bell & Finkbeiner 1991), triggered by synaptically released glutamate (Dani et al 1992). The source of intracellular Ca^{2+} is by release of stores from the endoplasmic reticulum, probably mediated through G protein linked receptors. Astrocyte Ca^{2+} signals could mediate a host of normal astrocyte functions like, for example, the regulation of synaptic activity and plasticity (Mennerick & Zorumski 1994), neurotransmitter uptake and metabolism, membrane transport, secretion of peptides, amino acids, eicosanoids, trophic factors, nitric oxide, regulation of astrocytic energy metabolism, vascular interactions etc. (Dani et al 1992).

In addition to Na^+ channels, astrocytes express all other types of voltage and ligand (e.g. glutamate and γ-aminobutyric acid (GABA)) gated ion channels (Barres 1991), providing a means of neuronal/astrocyte interaction. For example, Chao et al (1994) have suggested that astrocytic ion channels are important in sensing glial membrane depolarizations resulting from either damage or neuronal activation. Ion channels may amplify and transduce these signals to control glial function by increasing the amplitude of depolarization, activation of Ca^{2+} influx, increasing intracellular Na^+ concentration and activation of G-protein coupled receptors and thereby releasing Ca^{2+} intracellularly.

Astrocyte end-feet secrete heparan sulphate proteoglycan, laminin and fibronectin and thus assist in the formation of the basal lamina e.g., of blood vessels, against which the end-feet abut (Sievers et al 1994). Astrocytes also express S100 protein, vimentin and glial fibrillary acid protein (GFAP), a glial-specific intermediate filament cytoskeletal protein (8.44). There are regional differences in the levels

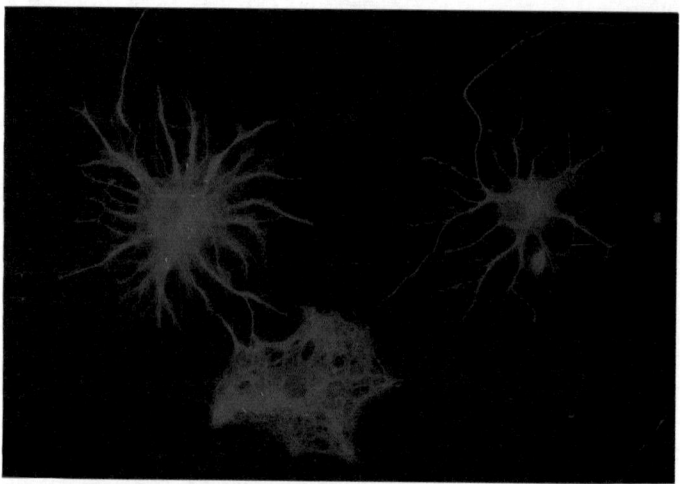

8.44 Astrocytes cultured from neonatal rat cerebral cortex, demonstrating glial fibrillary acidic protein (GFAP) intermediate filaments visualized with antibodies coupled to rhodamine. Magnification ×165 ×print mag. (Provided by Caroline Wigley, Division of Anatomy and Cell Biology, UMDS, Guy's Campus, London.)

of GFAP and GFAP-mRNA found in astrocyte processes; those of hippocampal astrocytes possess higher titres than elsewhere. GFAP may be required for the formation of stable processes and expression is upregulated after injury even in areas far from the site of direct damage. Injury induced astrocytosis is attributable to a local increase in the number of cells expressing GFAP at the lesion site, rather than to either an influx of new cells or increased mitotic activity in local astrocytes, and is accompanied by an upregulation of a battery of other proteins, implying that astrocytes may have a protective role in the central nervous system injury response (Eddleston & Mucke 1993). For example, astrocytes secrete:

- proteases and protease inhibitors which could remodel the extracellular matrix of the developing scar, regulate the protein content of the parenchyma and clear debris
- many key cytokines which mediate immunity and inflammation and which could also regulate the blood–brain barrier
- neurotrophic factors to enhance neuron survival
- transporter molecules and enzymes to metabolize excitotoxic amino acids

and activate the antioxidant pathway, to protect against neuronal cell death. Astrocytes also respond to injury by re-establishing the glia limitans externa along the open faces of a penetrant wound thereby preserving the integrity of the brain/cerebrospinal fluid barrier.

The first astrocytes to come from the neurectoderm are called *radial glia* because their apical and basal processes interconnect with the ventricular and pial surface respectively. These first formed astrocytes are important for guidance of migrating neuroblasts to the definitive positions within the walls of the primitive neural tube (p. 225). A secondary radial glial scaffold is formed in the late developing cerebellum and dentate gyrus which serves to translocate neuroblasts, formed in secondary germinal centres, to their definitive adult locations (Sievers et al 1992, 1994). When migration ceases, most radial glia (except those persisting in the retina as *Müller cells*, in the cerebellum as *Bergmann glia* (8.45), and in the hypothalamus as *tanycytes*) first retract their apical and later their basal processes, and differentiate into mature astrocytes. All the morphologically diverse types of astrocytes probably develop from a single lineage of germ cells in the ventricular, subventricular, and later, subependymal layers (Luskin et al 1993, 1994). When neurogenesis is complete, the ventricular zone differentiates into the ependymal cell layer although the exact lineage origin of ependymal cells is unknown, and the subventricular zone forms the subependymal plate (layer).

Ependymal cells (*ependymocytes*) line the ventricles and central canal. They form a unicellular epithelium varying from squamous to columnar in form according to locality. At the ventricular surface cells are in contact by means of gap junctions and occasional

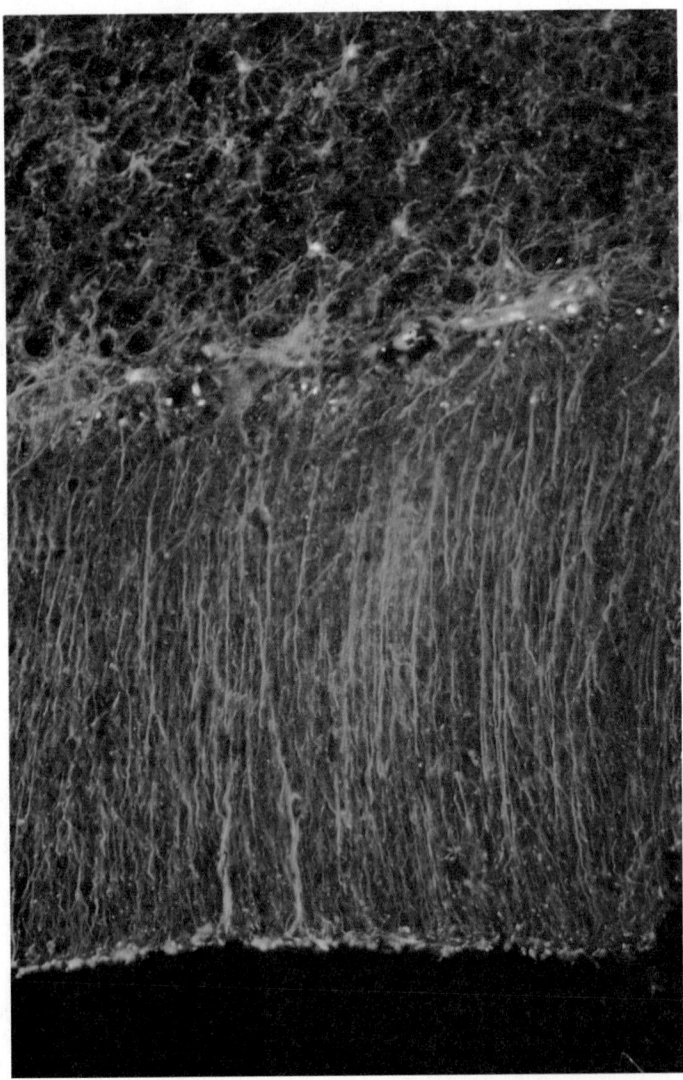

8.45 Radial Bergman glia fibres in the molecular layer of the adult human cerebellar cortex demonstrated by an immunofluorescent technique using an anti-glial fibrillary acidic protein (GFAP) antibody. Magnification × 200. (Prepared by Jonathan Carlile, Division of Anatomy and Cell Biology, UMDS, Guy's Campus, London.)

desmosomes; their apical surfaces have numerous microvilli and cilia, the latter often motile and contributing to the flow of cerebrospinal fluid. Ultrastructurally (Brightman & Palay 1963; Bleier 1977) the nucleus is heterochromatic and indented; the cytoplasm abounds in mitochondria, lysosomes, microtubules and microfilaments. There is much regional variation in the ependymal lining of the ventricles but four major varieties have been distinguished in mammals (see Scott et al 1974a; Page et al 1979). These consist of:

• general ependyma overlying areas of grey matter
• general ependyma lining white matter
• specialized areas of ependyma in the third and fourth ventricles
• choroidal epithelium.

Firstly, the ependymal cells overlying areas of grey matter are cuboidal, each cell bearing about 20 cilia in its apical centre, surrounded by short microvilli. The cell margins are not extensively folded, and cells are joined by gap junctions and desmosomes; their contents are as stated above. They do not have a basal lamina, but beneath them a *subependymal zone* may be present, from two to three cells deep, consisting of cells resembling ependymal cells in their organelles and nuclei; the blood vessels beneath them have no fenestrations and few transcytotic vesicles, i.e. they are typical of the central nervous system (p. 932). Where the ependyma lines myelinated tracts, cells are much flattened and even squamous and fewer of them are ciliated; again there are gap junctions and desmosomes but

the lateral margins of cells are highly folded and interdigitating. No subependymal zone is present but blood vessels are as described for the previous type. It has been suggested that these differences may be related to a greater role in the exchange of metabolites between grey matter and cerebrospinal fluid than occurs for white matter, the former being metabolically more demanding than the latter.

Specialized areas of ependymal cells are found in four areas around the margins of the third ventricle (the circumventricular organs) including the lining of the median eminence of the hypothalamus and forming the subcommissural organ, the subfornical organ and the organum vasculosum of the lamina terminalis and other related areas (see p. 1101). At the inferoposterior limit of the fourth ventricle is the area postrema, which has a similar structure. In these sites the ependymal cells are only rarely ciliated and their ventricular surfaces have many microvilli and apical blebs. They have many mitochondria and well-formed Golgi complexes lying apical to a rather flattened basal nucleus. The cells are joined laterally by tight junctions forming a barrier to the passage of materials across the ependyma, and desmosomes. Many of these cells are *tanycytes (ependymoglial cells, ependymal astrocytes)* with basal processes projecting into the perivascular space surrounding underlying capillaries, which are fenestrated and therefore do not form a blood–brain barrier. It is thought probable that these areas constitute special zones by which substances can pass from the nervous tissue and vascular supply into the cerebrospinal fluid within the ventricle by active transport through the ependymal cells; many of the neurons in the vicinity of such areas liberate neuropeptides and other biogenic substances, which may therefore pass into the ventricles to gain access to a much wider population of neurons via the permeable ependymal lining of the rest of the ventricle; a reverse process is also likely by this route (see also p. 1204). High concentrations of receptor sites for certain neuropeptides are present at the surfaces.

Finally, the ependyma is highly modified where it lies adjacent to the vascular layer of the *choroid plexuses* (p. 1203). Here the cells resemble those of the circumventricular organs, except that they do not have basal processes but constitute a cuboidal epithelium resting on a basal lamina adjacent to the externally applied pia and capillary layer (with fenestrated endothelium). Cells have numerous long microvilli with a few cilia interspersed; they have many mitochondria and large Golgi complexes and their nuclei are basally placed. Tight junctions forming a transepithelial barrier and desmosomes occur between cells and the lateral margins of cells are highly folded. All of these structural features accord with the secretory activity of these cells, which are responsible for the formation of most of the cerebrospinal fluid.

A small population of cells is found within the ventricles lying on the apical surfaces of ependymal cells called *supra-ependymal cells*. They are probably a mixed population of glia, neurons and macrophages. The latter cells which overlie the choroid plexus are called *Kolmer (epiplexus) cells*. The subventricular zone transforms into the *subependymal plate*, a layer of primitive, mitotically active cells containing light or dark nuclei. The layer contains the stem cells of the oligodendrocyte and astrocyte lineages (Luskin et al 1994) and replication therein continues production of both types of macroglia into the mature animal. The layer is important because it is probably the source of most periventricular glial tumours in man.

Pituicytes are found in the pituitary, infundibulum and neurohypophysis. They resemble astrocytes but their processes end mostly on vascular endothelial cells of the neurohypophysis and tuber cinereum. These cells together with the glia of the olfactory nerve are presently attracting much interest because they both permit axon regeneration. Transplantation studies are presently underway to discover if transplantation of pituicytes and/or olfactory nerve glia into central lesions will promote regeneration of otherwise nonregenerating systems of axons. If the permissive nature of these glia is induced only by the axons with which they are normally associated (Kiss et al 1993) then the findings of these experiments may be disappointing.

Oligodendrocytes

As *intrafascicular* cells in myelinated tracts, the major role of oligodendrocytes is to lay down myelin around central nervous axons and thus they are the central counterpart of peripheral myelinating Schwann cells (**8.46**). However, both the composition and detailed

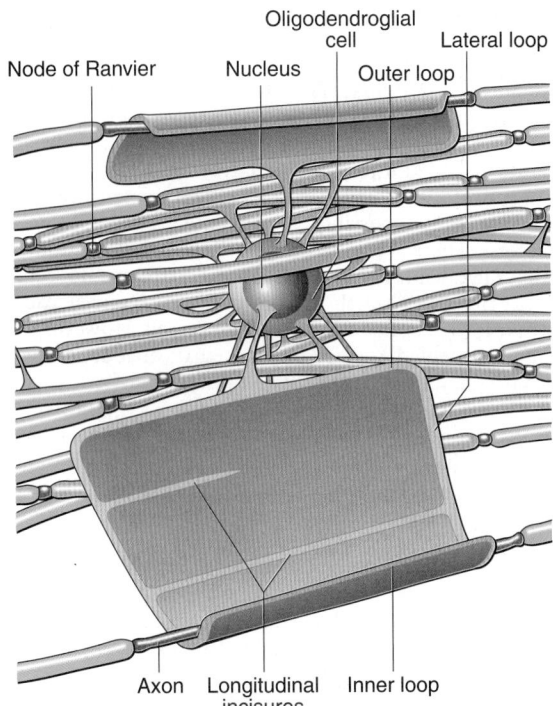

Node of Ranvier   Nucleus   Oligodendroglial cell   Lateral loop   Outer loop

Axon   Longitudinal incisures   Inner loop

8.46 Oligodendrocyte soma (top centre) attached to numerous myelin sheaths that have been unfolded to various degrees to demonstrate the enormous surface area they occupy. Note also the displacement of oligodendrocyte cytoplasm to narrow ridges in the flattened sheet of myelin. This analysis is a composite of those given by Bunge et al (1961) and Hirano and Dembitzer (1967). (Modified from Morell & Norton 1980 by Ramie 1984 with permission.)

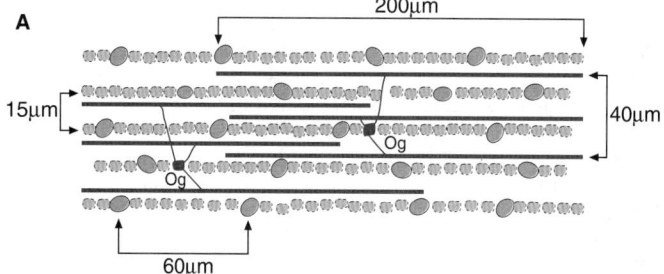

A   200μm   15μm   40μm   Og   Og   60μm

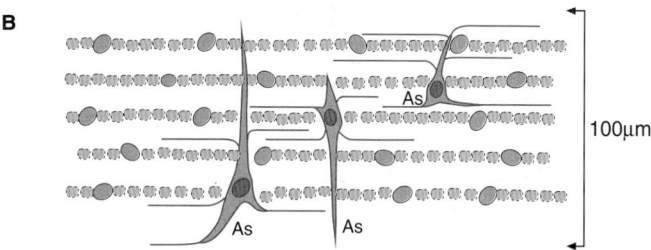

B   100μm   As   As   As

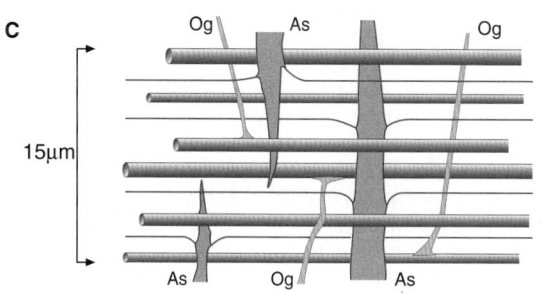

C   Og   As   Og   15μm   As   Og   As

8.47 Arrangement of radial and longitudinal processes of oligodendrocytes (A) and astrocytes (B) to form a 'woven' meshwork of processes (C)

A. Shown against a background of the interfascicular glial nuclear rows, the types of radial (stem) and longitudinal (myelinating) processes of two oligodendrocytes (Og, black squares) are illustrated.

B. Three astrocytes (As) illustrating typical radial and longitudinal processes.

c. Higher magnification view of 'woven' meshwork of oligodendrocytic (Og) and astrocytic (As) processes. *Typical dimensions*: Core-to-core distance between interfascicular glial rows, 15 μm; interastrocytic distance within a row, 60 μm; oligodendrocytic radial span, 40 μm; length of internode, 200 μm; astrocytic radial span, 100 μm. (From Suzuki & Raisman 1992 with permission.)

form of central and peripheral myelin differ (p. 952) and the relation between the axon and the myelinating cell is also dissimilar: an oligodendrocyte may enclose several axons in separate myelin sheaths, whereas Schwann cells ensheath only one axon. Some oligodendrocytes are not associated with axons, and some of these are either an adult form of the oligodendrocyte precursor cell or a perineuronal (satellite) oligodendrocyte with processes ramifying about neuronal somata, with unknown functions.

The densities of oligodendrocytes vary widely from region to region throughout the nervous system; in the heavily myelinated human pontocerebellar tract, for example, the estimate is $64\,000/\text{mm}^3$ (Friede 1961). Within tracts, interfascicular oligodendrocytes are disposed in long rows (Suzuki & Raisman 1992). Single astrocytes are inserted at regular intervals; in the rat, for example, between approximately eight consecutive oligodendrocytes (**8.47**). Oligodendrocyte units in the rows myelinate the surrounding axons with processes radially aligned to the axis of the row. Thus, myelinated tracts are comprised of groups of cables of axons all predominantly myelinated by a row of oligodendrocytes running down the axis of the cable. The domains of the units of oligodendrocyte in the axes of adjacent cables overlap and interaxial distances are around 15 μm.

Ultrastructurally oligodendrocytes have a round nucleus and a cytoplasm rich in mitochondria, microtubules and glycogen (**8.43**). Like astrocytes, they vary from cells with large euchromatic nuclei and pale cytoplasm to those with heterochromatic nuclei and dense cytoplasm. Tritium labelling shows that they can proliferate in mature animals and at this late stage both maturing and degenerating cells are seen.

Oligodendrocytes express galactocerebroside (gal C), carbonic anhydrase II (CAII), myelin basic protein (MBP), 2'3'-cyclic nucleotide 3'-phosphodiesterase (CNPase) and transferrin. Antibodies to these molecules, in addition to RIP, a monoclonal antibody to an unidentified intracellular epitope (**8.48**), are used for identification. The myelin sheaths formed by oligodendrocytes differ from those of Schwann cells in many important ways (p. 952). Antibodies against many of the constituents of central myelin (e.g. MBP, myelin associated glycoprotein (MAG) and Wolfgram protein) are also found in

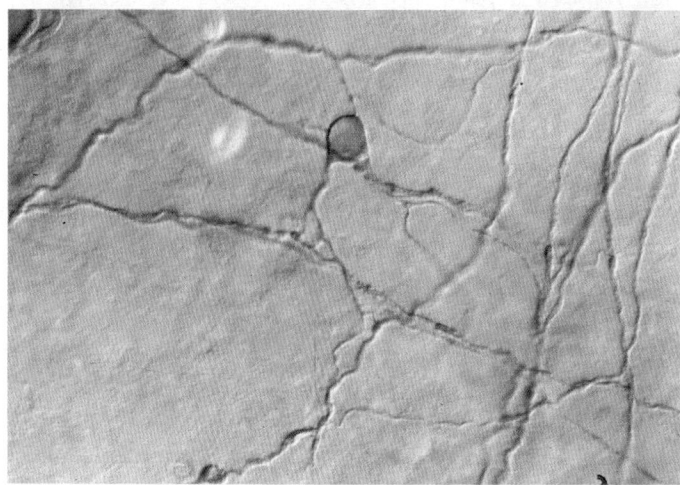

8.48 Type II oligodendrocyte unit in the anterior medullary velum of the rat demonstrated by the peroxidase-anti-peroxidase technique using the Rip antibody and DIC microscopy. This oligodendrocyte has 7 processes which engage and unsheath axons to form their Rip-positive myelin sheaths. Magnification × 660. (Prepared by Fiona Ruge, Division of Anatomy and Cell Biology, UMDS, Guy's Campus, London.)

the periphery. For the unequivocal identification of central myelin, antibodies to specific constituents such as proteolipid protein (PLP), MAG, CNPase, myelin-oligodendrocyte-associated glycoprotein (MOG) and myelin-oligodendrocyte-specific protein (MOSP) are used. The myelin of small-diameter fibres differs in chemical composition, lamellar compaction and detailed structure of Schmidt-Lanterman clefts from that of large calibre axons perhaps reflecting differential production by oligodendrocytes associated with the different types (I–IV, see below) of oligodendrocyte units. No basal lamina surrounds central myelin, and minor dense lines are found at points of contact between adjacent myelin sheaths.

As with Schwann cells, the terminal loops, identified in longitudinal sections of central nervous system nodes, are the cytoplasmic rim of the oligodendrocyte plasma membrane, which is spiralled around some 4 μm of the perinodal axolemma. The zone of contact of the oligodendrocyte cytoplasm with the axolemma thus forms a linear spiral junctional complex seen in freeze fracture preparations. The zone gives attachment to some 40 paranodal loops; more paranodal loops than this become piled up on each other without attachment to the axolemma. The nodal gap is 0.8–1.1 μm in length. The astrocytic and axonal specializations in this region are described on pages 934, and 924 respectively.

Oligodendrocyte units have been classified according to the number of axons engaged. Type I units are formed by a multibranched cell myelinating many axons; type IV units are Schwann cell-like myelinating one axon; types II (**8.48**) and III are intermediate forms (del Rio Hortega 1928; Penfield 1932). Since type IV units are associated with large-diameter and types I–III units with smaller diameter axons, the concept has arisen that all oligodendrocyte units (I–IV) produce the same quantity of myelin—since large-diameter fibres induce thicker myelin sheaths (with more lamellae) and longer internodal lengths than do small-diameter fibres. Serial reconstruction studies in the spinal cord of the cat (Remahl & Hildebrand 1990a,b) indicate that the myelinated axons of a unit share a similar diameter, and dye injection of oligodendrocytes in rat and mouse optic nerve (**8.49**) show that all internodal myelin segments of a given unit have similar lengths (Butt & Ransom 1993; Butt et al, 1994a, c). These observations appear to suggest that type I–IV oligodendrocytes recruit similar numbers of similar-sized axons into each type of unit. The frequency of myelin lamellae is positively correlated with axon diameter according to a curvilinear function (Hildebrand & Hahn 1978) and internodal lengths show a positive linear correlation with axon diameter (Murray & Blakemore 1980).

Oligodendrocytes originate from the ventricular neurectoderm and the subependymal layer (p. 939) in the fetus and continue to be generated from the subependymal plate postnatally. Some stem cells may migrate and seed into white and grey matter to form a pool of adult progenitor cells which may later differentiate to replenish lost oligodendrocytes and possibly remyelinate pathologically demyelinated regions. There is a huge literature from culture studies maintaining that oligodendrocytes, and a special astrocyte, found in white matter with processes which engage nodes of Ranvier exclusively, are both formed from a common progenitor cell. However, this view is no longer accepted and it appears that oligodendrocytes and astrocytes originate from different cell lineages in vivo (Luskin et al 1993, 1994) and that only one astrocytic phenotype probably exists able to subserve nodal as well as many other functions (Butt et al 1994a,b). Nonetheless, in vitro studies have provided data which could indicate how oligodendrocyte production and differentiation is controlled in vivo (see Goldman 1992 for review).

Oligodendrocyte stem cells are defined in culture as motile primitive cells reacting with a monoclonal antibody A2B5, recognizing a tetrasialoganglioside, but not expressing the sulphatide presumed to react with the O₄ antibody. They do express platelet derived growth factor (PDGF) α receptor, and respond to PDGF, basic fibroblast growth factor (FGF) and insulin-like growth factor (IGF) I and II as mitogens. Progenitor cells differentiate into A2B5-negative, O₄-positive, galactocerebroside gal C-positive oligodendrocytes through an intermediate pro-oligodendrocyte stage which has an A2B5-positive/negative, O₄-positive, gal C-negative phenotype. Astrocytes and neurons secrete PDGF and thus may help control proliferation. In the presence of PDGF, stem cells can differentiate into oligodendrocytes, but basic FGF blocks differentiation and promotes proliferation by maintaining PDGF α receptors. IGF-I and II induce the differentiation of pro-oligodendrocytes into oligodendrocytes. Both PDGF and IGF-I also promote the survival of stem cells and are therefore implicated in a mechanism matching numbers of oligodendrocytes with numbers of axons to be myelinated.

The processes of oligodendrocytes initially engage axons with uncompacted cytoplasmic ensheathments with at least one complete turn, called E-sheaths. Later, these become compacted M-sheaths exhibiting major and minor dense lines (Remahl & Hildebrand 1990a,b). The first axons to become ensheathed ultimately reach larger diameters than those engaged later. The critical minimal axon diameter for myelination is smaller and more variable in the central than in the peripheral nervous system and is about 0.2 μm (compared with 1–2 μm in the periphery).

An oligodendrocyte unit is defined as all the axons myelinated by one oligodendrocyte unit; axon diameters and myelin segment lengths are fairly uniform but can also show wide variation. When the change from E to M-ensheathment occurs, there is a reduction in unit axon number indicating that the E-state is a plastic phase during which sheaths may be eliminated to equate available axonal surface area with number of oligodendrocyte units (Bjartmar et al 1994). Although it is generally believed that axons control oligodendrocyte behaviour during myelination, determining parameters like internodal length and number of lamellae, it is not understood what factors control the spacing of internodal myelin segments along axons. One plausible thesis proposes that nodal regions are formed before myelination commences and that the axolemma of each internode will accept only one oligodendrocyte process. As axons elongate, the thesis subsumes that some internodal myelin segments may be added to small diameter fibres and lost from large-diameter fibres.

MICROGLIA

Microglia are small dendritic cells found throughout the central nervous system (**8.50**) including the retina (p. 1346). A large body of evidence supports the view that microglia are derived from fetal monocytes, and/or their precursors, which invade the developing nervous system (Boya et al 1991; Theele & Streit 1993; Ling & Wong 1993). Haematogenous cells pass through the walls of parenchymal, and probably also meningeal, blood vessels and invade neural tissue initially as amoeboid cells, prenatally. Later they lose their motility

8.49 Confocal micrographs of mature myelin forming oligodendrocyte (A) and astrocyte (B) iontophoretically filled in the adult rat optic nerve with an immunofluorescent dye by intracellular microinjection. 1 cm = 30 μm. (Prepared by Dr A Butt and Kate Colquhoun, Division of Physiology, UMDS, London and photographed by Sarah Smith using the pseudocolour technique, Division of Anatomy and Cell Biology, UMDS, Guy's Campus, London.)

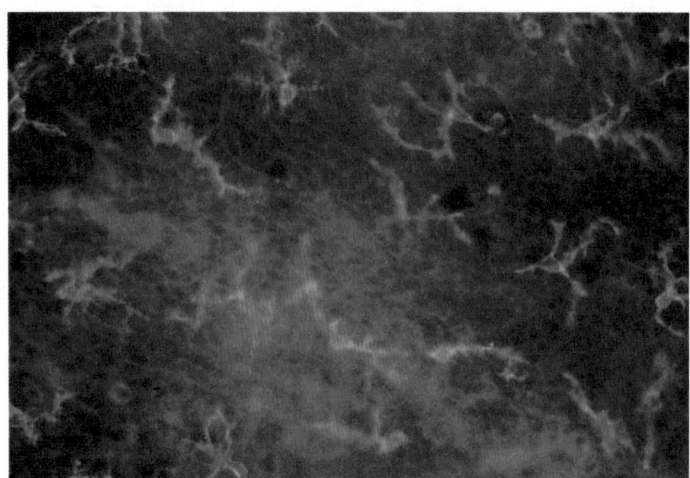

8.50 Microglia in the rat anterior medullary velum demonstrated using the lectin *Griffonia simplicifolia* and a peroxidase avidin-biotin amplification second step. Magnification ×125 ×print size. (Prepared by Fiona Ruge, Division of Anatomy and Cell Biology, UMDS, Guy's Campus, London.)

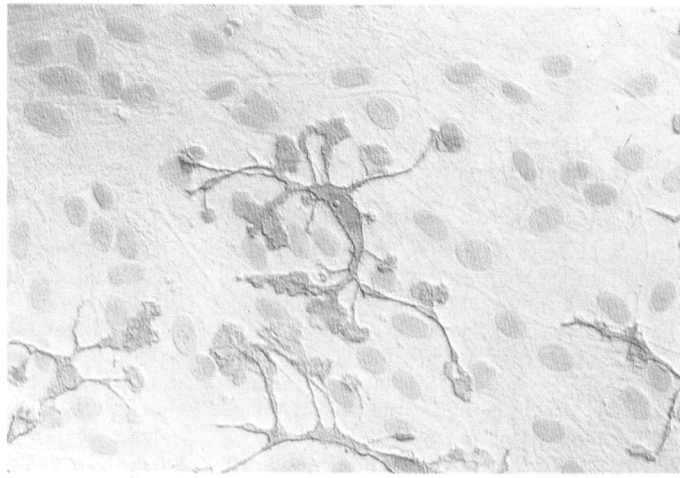

8.51 Rat microglia on a monolayer of astrocytes (nuclei stained with cresyl violet) in tissue culture. Microglia have been stained with the OX42 antibody against the Fc-receptor and developed with the peroxidase-anti-peroxidase technique. All microglia have differentiated from haematogenous monocytes after seeding on to the astrocytes. Magnification ×100. (Prepared by J Sievers, Anatomy Department, University of Kiel, Kiel, Germany.)

and transform into typical microglia bearing branched processes which ramify in non-overlapping territories within the brain. All microglia domains, defined by their dendritic fields, are equivalent in size and form a regular mosaic throughout the brain (**8.50**). It is possible that no new microglia are added from exogenous bone marrow sources in the mature animal, even after injury and inflammation (Lassman et al 1993; Matsumoto & Fugiwara 1987)—new microglia are thus probably recruited in the adult from the endogenous population by proliferation. The consensus is that mature monocytes invading the postnatal brain become macrophages not microglia. The expression of microglia-specific antigens changes with age, many becoming down regulated as microglia attain the mature dendritic form. Evidence that the transformation of haematogenous cells into microglia within the brain may be astrocyte-induced is provided by the work of Richardson et al (1993) and Sievers et al (1994). For example, the latter group have shown that monocytes seeded on to an astrocyte monolayer in culture transform into dendritic cells with a similar morphology, antigenic phenotype and unique inwardly rectifying K^+ membrane channels characteristic of microglia (**8.51**).

In the rodent, and probably also the human brain, 10–20% of all glia are microglia, distributed more frequently in grey than white matter. They form a stable population, in the normal brain, in which turnover is barely detectable. In electron micrographs, microglia have elongated nuclei with peripheral hetero-chromatin. The cytoplasm is diminutive and pale staining, containing granules and scattered tubules of rough endoplasmic reticulum (RER), with the Golgi apparatus collected at both poles. Two or three primary processes stem predominantly from opposite poles of the soma which serially bifurcate to form short claw-like terminal branches. Microglia may be identified morphologically using classical silver stains particularly the silver carbonate technique (del Rio Hortega 1932). More recently, several immunocytological and lectin markers have been used to identify microglia, including antibodies to the leucocyte common antigen (Ox-1), CR-3 complement receptor (Ox-42), a macrophage cytosolic protein (ED1) and IgG Fc receptors (e.g. G2 and Mac-1), and also the plant lectins *Bandeiraea* (*Griffonia*) *simplicifolia* agglutinin (BS-1, see **8**.49, 52) and *Ricinus communis* agglutinin-120 (RCS-1).

The function of microglia in the normal brain remains a mystery (see Nakajima & Kohsaka 1993 for review) but, like astrocytes, they are activated by traumatic and ischaemic injury and in many diseases including Parkinson's disease, Alzheimer's disease, multiple sclerosis, acquired immuno deficiency syndrome (AIDS), amiotrophic lateral sclerosis and paraneoplastic encephalitis (**8.52**) they become phagocytotic and some transform into the amoeboid, motile type. They then become actively involved in synaptic stripping and neuronophagia. Activation is also characterized both by the upregulation of expression of the ED1, Ox-42, leucocyte common and major histocompatibility complex I and II (MHCI and II) antigens

(Lassman et al 1993); and by the secretion of proteases, cytokines and reactive oxygen and nitrogen intermediates (Banati et al 1993). Activated microglia and brain macrophages also express increased numbers of peripheral benzodiazepine binding sites (see Dubois et al 1988). A ligand for the latter ($[^{11}C]$ PK 11195) allows activated microglia/macrophages to be PET-scanned in human brains with infarcts (Ramsay et al 1992).

There is little turnover of resident microglia in response to damage to the neuropil. Thus, microglia form a relatively stable network of potential antigen-presenting cells throughout the brain and spinal cord. Antigen expression is both functionally and phenotypically heterogeneous amongst reactive microglia in different brain locations and according to the nature of the insult. Microglia are very sensitive to depolarizing events since in the absence of outward currents, large inward currents are generated by relatively small membrane currents. Microglia probably possess ion-channel linked P_2 purinoceptors and, during injury, could become activated by adenosine 5'-triphosphate released from damaged cells. The ensuing pronounced depolarization of microglia could trigger activation, in response to tissue damage (Kettenmann et al 1993).

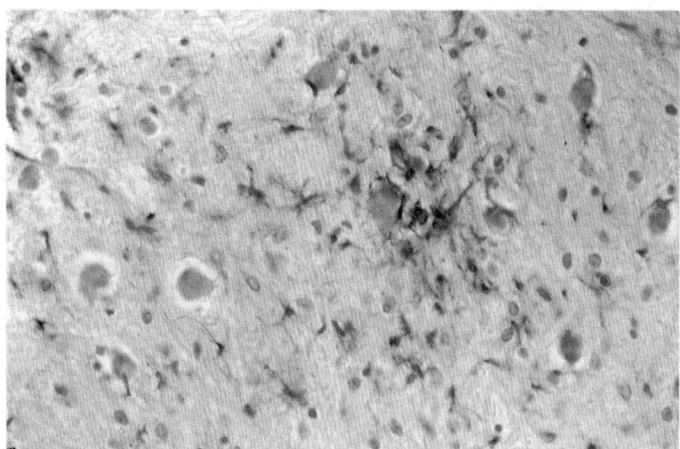

8.52 Activated microglia expressing MHC class II antigen in the human brain. The specimen is from a patient with paraneoplastic encephalitis and autoimmune neuronal degeneration. Activated microglia cells are demonstrated in association with neurons of the inferior olive using indirect immunoperoxidase with a monoclonal antibody against a non polymorphic HLA-DR determinant. Magnification ×100. (Prepared by Dr N Gregson, Division of Anatomy and Cell Biology, UMDS, Guy's Campus, London.)

Regeneration of axons in the central nervous system

Neurons will not replicate in the mature human central nervous system nor will central axons regrow if severed by injury. Accordingly, recovery from brain and spinal cord trauma is limited to a rectification of transitory ischaemia and a reorganization of surviving circuitry by plasticity. The reasons why central axons will not regenerate after damage are unknown, but some interesting findings have been reported from research laboratories which do offer hope for reconnecting the lesioned brain and cord in the future. The classical view of the injury response of the brain was dominated by the concept that axons were inherently incapable of regrowth after damage except for a transient period of abortive regeneration in the immediate postinjury period (Ramón y Cajal 1928). It was also generally held that the deposition of scar tissue in the lesion established an impenetrable tissue mass impeding the growth of axons (Clemente 1964). Both tenets were refuted by Aguayo and colleagues (Richardson et al 1980) who have demonstrated unequivocally that most, if not all, central axons will regenerate into peripheral nerve grafts implanted into either the brain or spinal cord. This work suggested that the failure of regeneration might be attributable either to a lack of neurotropic/neurotrophic factors in the mature system essential for axon growth, and/or the presence of inhibitory substances which actively arrest axon regrowth after the abortive phase. All current research is directed to defining which of the above issues are the most important determinants of axon growth failure in the damaged central nervous system.

The propensity for central axons to regenerate into peripheral nerve grafts is directly correlated with the presence of viable Schwann cells which secrete both soluble growth promoting factors and a basal lamina substrate rich in neurotropic molecules (Berry et al 1988). If there is an absence in the mature brain of cells with properties similar to those of Schwann cells, a growth promoting environment may never be recreated in the adult central nervous system. If

Schwann cells are transplanted (Brook et al 1993) or become naturally seeded into the central nervous system (Berry et al 1992) axon sprouting and elongation is readily promoted.

Substrate maps exist in the developing central nervous system which guide growing axons into targets (Cohen et al 1987), but we do not know if such maps either persist, or are re-established in the adult after injury, nor is there any evidence that mature axons can recapitulate a growth status equivalent to that of the pioneering phase of early development. Some neurotrophins (molecules which maintain neuronal survival and promote axonal growth) are found in the mature brain which have the potential for supporting a regenerative response.

Contact inhibition is another explanation for regenerative failure in which collapse of axonal growth cones occurs, probably by interaction of surface axonal transmembrane receptors with glial ligands (Berry et al 1994; Johnson 1993). Secondary messenger transduction within the growth cone may be mediated by G protein receptor links with ion channels on cisternal membranes, leading to the release of intracellular Ca^{++} stores (Igarashi et al 1993) causing F-actin depolymerization leading to an arrest of microtubule assembly and membrane incorporation.

The inhibitory ligand probably resides on macroglial membrane surfaces and the development of either receptor and/or inhibitory ligand must be delayed until late in ontogeny to allow connections between brain centres to become established. It has been proposed that oligodendrocytes and central myelin have a major axon growth inhibitory role (Berry 1982; Schwab 1990). Both elements develop late, long after the major central tracts have been laid down. Two axon growth-inhibitory proteins have been isolated from central myelin, and monoclonal antibodies to one of these appears to promote regeneration in the spinal cord when administered intrathecally over the immediate postinjury period (Schnell & Schwab 1990, 1993). Presumably, the neutralizing antibody

engages the inhibitory ligand and thereby blocks the receptor, allowing axon regrowth to proceed unimpeded. Since, however, axon growth failure is as complete in grey matter as it is in white matter, it seems unlikely that inhibition of axon growth by contact with central myelin/oligodendrocytes provides a complete explanation for the failure of regeneration. Indeed, adult optic fibres will not regenerate in a mutant rat in which both central myelin and oligodendrocytes are absent (Berry et al 1992). Moreover, the axons of adult central neurons are also incapable of growing over cryosections of optic nerve taken from both pre- and postmyelination phases (Shewan et al 1993, 1994). These findings implicate astrocytes in the failure of axon regeneration in the brain, but the nature of the 'stop signal' for growth (Luizzi & Lasek 1987) is unknown.

Immediately, postmitotic neuroblasts, transplanted into adult brain, produce processes which exhibit florid growth over this putative inhibitory substrate (Wictorin et al 1992; Davies et al 1993). A possible explanation for this paradoxical growth might be that axons growing de novo normally do not express the receptor for the inhibitory ligand. Pioneering axons may connect with their targets even if the ligand is already incorporated into the membranes of immature astrocytes. Shewan et al (1994) have proposed that inhibitory receptor expression occurs on axons after target encounter, raising the intriguing possibility that the target may provide the signal for receptor production. The signalling molecule may be taken up by target-docked terminals and retrogradely transported to the soma.

There is now good evidence from neural transplantation studies (p. 919) in which axons are made to invade adult host denervated targets, that precise reinnervation of postsynaptic sites occurs to re-establish old connectivity (Zhou et al 1985, 1989) and restore lost function (Lund et al 1991). Thus, if regeneration could be promoted in the brain and spinal cord and if regrowing axons were successful in homing into old denervated targets, functional recovery might ensue.

CYTOLOGY OF THE PERIPHERAL NERVOUS SYSTEM

Cellular organization

The peripheral nervous system (PNS) includes the craniospinal and autonomic nerves and their associated ganglia, together with their connective tissue sheaths. All lie peripheral to the pial covering of the central nervous system, through which the central and peripheral nerve fibres are continuous (**8.53, 61**).

Afferent nerve fibres connect receptors to the central nervous system: their neuronal somata are located either in special sense organs (e.g., the retina) or in the sensory ganglia of craniospinal nerves. *Efferent nerve fibres* connect the central nervous system to the effector apparatus: they are the peripheral axons of neurons with somata in the central grey matter. In man, there are 12 pairs of cranial nerves issuing from the brain and 31 pairs of spinal nerves. The sympathetic trunks, ganglia and splanchnic nerves are part of this system but will be described separately (pp. 1298).

In the most primitive vertebrates the spinal cord gives off a series of *ventral motor nerve roots*, arising from a ventral (anterior) grey column, and a series of *dorsal sensory nerve roots* which are connected to a dorsal (posterior) column. The ventral and dorsal roots are not co-incident: a ventral root is segmental and is distributed to the myotome corresponding to its original neuromere, whereas dorsal roots are intersegmental. In most fishes and all higher vertebrates the corresponding ventral and dorsal roots unite to form individual *spinal nerves*, whose arrangement has been relatively little modified during evolution. In contrast, the arrangement of the cranial nerves has undergone profound modification during the development of the head region.

In the brain, the corresponding ventral and dorsal nerves never fuse, although adjoining ventral or dorsal nerves sometimes do. Because some myotomes disappear, the corresponding ventral nerves are suppressed: dorsal nerves, originally sensory to the skin of the head and the mucous membrane of the mouth and pharynx, acquire motor fibres which they distribute to branchial arch musculature. The incorporation of some precervical segments into the head has resulted in the fusion of corresponding ventral nerves, giving rise to the hypoglossal nerve.

Craniospinal nerve fibres run in small bundles called *fasciculi* which pursue uninterrupted courses from the centre to the periphery: single fibres or groups may leave one fasciculus to join another, often at acute angles. Nerves divide into branches, frequently communicating with branches of nearby nerves, forming *plexuses*. Such a plexus is formed by the ventral rami of spinal nerves, e.g., cervical, brachial, lumbar and sacral plexuses; terminal fasciculi may form peripheral plexuses. In forming a plexus, the component nerves divide, join and again subdivide, often in such a complex manner that individual fasciculi are intricately interwoven. Each branch leaving a plexus may hence contain filaments from more than one or even all the 'roots' of the plexus. In smaller plexuses in the periphery there is free interchange of fibres. Through this interchange every nerve leaving a plexus gains more extensive connections with the spinal cord.

The origin of a nerve is a phrase usually implying its site of exit from or entry into the central nervous system.

Ganglia are aggregations of neuronal somata associated with some peripheral nerves, occurring in the dorsal roots of spinal nerves and the sensory roots of the trigeminal, facial, glossopharyngeal, vagal and vestibulocochlear cranial nerves. They also occur in autonomic nerves (p. 1292). They vary in form and size, each ganglion being invested by a smooth, firm capsule of fibrous connective tissue. Each ganglion contains neuronal somata and neuronal processes: some ganglia, particularly those found in the autonomic system, contain fibres from cells located elsewhere which pass through or terminate within them.

Sensory ganglia. The sensory ganglia of dorsal spinal roots (**8.54**) and the ganglia of the trigeminal, facial, glossopharyngeal and vagal cranial nerves are enclosed in periganglionic connective tissue, resembling perineurium (p. 947). Their neurons are unipolar, with spherical or ovoid somata of varying size, aggregated in groups interspersed with fasciculi of myelinated and non-myelinated nerve

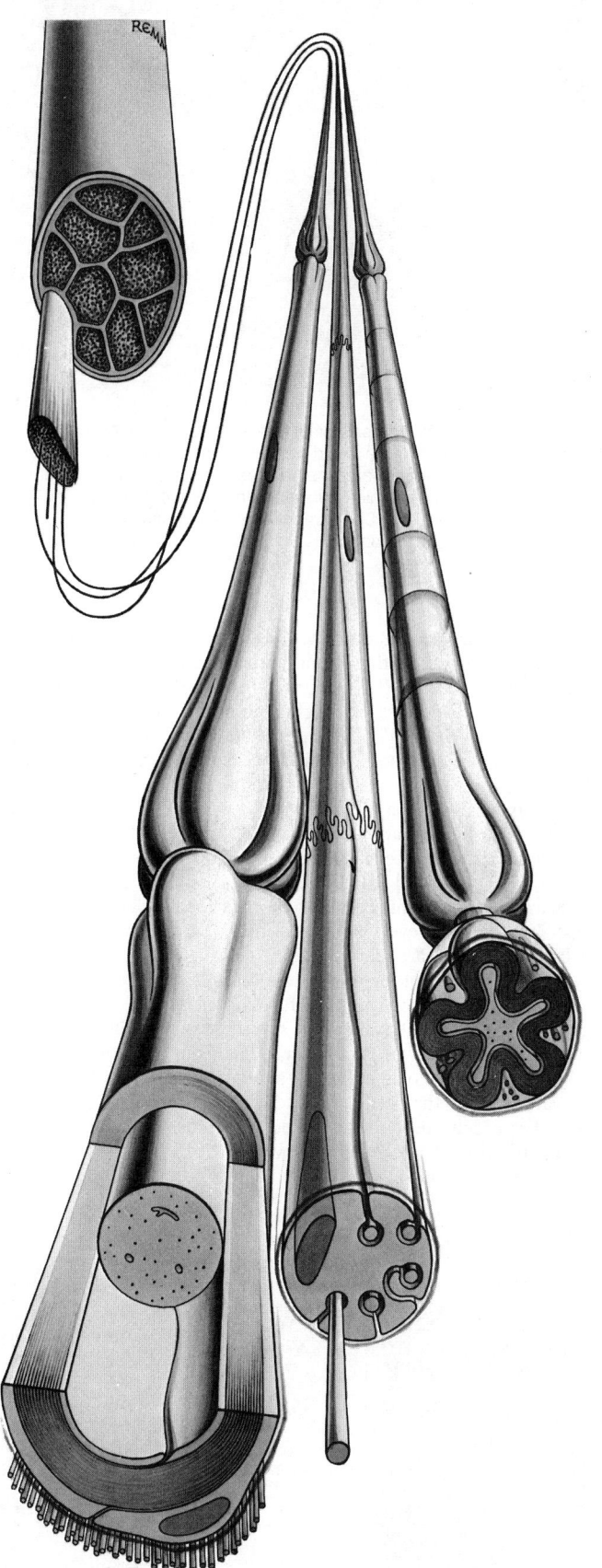

8.53 Some structural features of peripheral nerve fibres. A nerve trunk (top left) is cut away to expose a single fasciculus, from which three fibres are indicated in detail. These include two myelinated axons, one on each side of a group of non-myelinated axons enclosed within a Schwann cell sheath. The myelinated fibre on the left has been cut away at various points to demonstrate the relationship between the axon, the Schwann cell and its sheath of myelin.

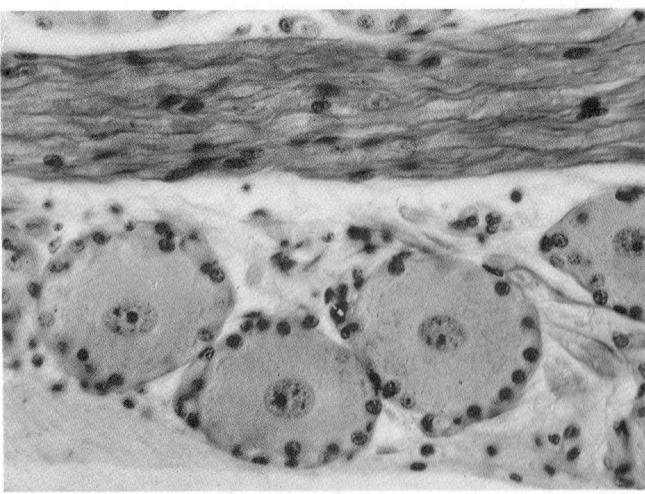

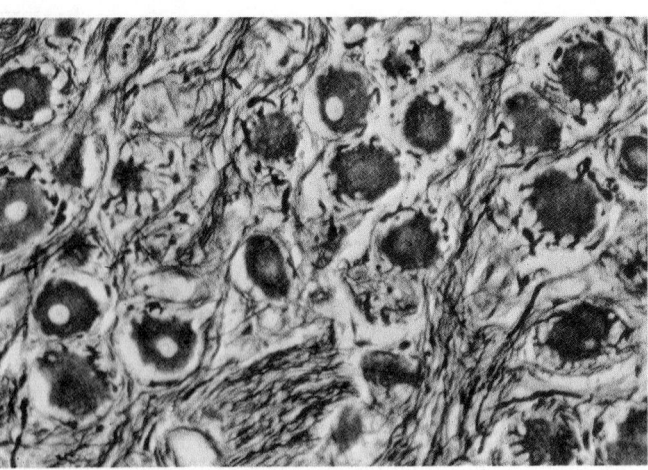

8.54 A typical field in a dorsal spinal nerve root ganglion. Note the characteristic juxtaposition of large ovoid nerve cell somata and the fascicles of myelinated and non-myelinated nerve fibres. Note also the nuclei of the capsular (satellite) cells which surround each nerve cell. Grübler's stain. (Provided by Lyn Gregson, Department of Anatomy and Cell Biology, Guy's Hospital Medical School, London.)

8.55 Typical field in an autonomic ganglion (human ciliary ganglion), showing nerve cells evenly scattered among fascicles of nerve fibres. Stained by Bielschowsky's silver and erythrosin technique. (Material supplied by N A Locket, Institute of Ophthalmology, London.)

fibres. Their structure is described elsewhere (p. 960); a single non-myelinated axon (a 'dendro-axonal' process) leaves each soma, highly convoluted at its origin before bifurcating at a T-junction into central and peripheral processes. In myelinated fibres the junction occurs at a node of Ranvier (p. 951). The peripheral process reaches a sensory ending; since it conducts towards the soma it is functionally an elongated dendrite but has the structural and functional properties of a peripheral axon and, following common usage, it will be so termed here. Each unipolar soma has a nucleated capsule of flat, epithelioid capsular cells (ganglionic gliocytes or satellite cells). (Many cells are called satellite cells. The list includes small round extracapsular ganglionic cells; ganglionic capsular cells and Schwann cells; some authors even include all non-neuronal cells, central and peripheral, which are perineuronal; cells associated with striated myocytes.) The cytoplasm of capsular cells resembles that of Schwann cells (see below); their deep surfaces interdigitate with reciprocal irregularities in the exteriors of the subjacent nerve cells. The capsular layer is continuous with similar cells enclosing the convoluted part (initial glomerulus) of the dendro-axonal process and then with the Schwann cells of the peripheral and central processes. Outside these layers lies a delicate vascular connective tissue continuous with the endoneurium of the peripheral nerve and nerve root.

Sensory ganglionic neurons are not entirely confined to the discrete craniospinal ganglia; singly or in small groups they often occupy 'heterotopic' positions distal or proximal to their ganglia.

Autonomic ganglia. These have a different structure; their neurons are multipolar, with dendritic trees on which preganglionic autonomic motor fibres synapse. They are surrounded by a mixed neuropil of afferent and efferent fibres, dendrites, synapses and non-neural cells (**8.55, 56**).

Nerve fibres (i.e. axons with their ensheathing Schwann cells). These are grouped into fasciculi of widely variable numbers. The size, number and pattern of fasciculi vary in different nerves and at different levels along their paths; their number increases and their size decreases some distance proximal to a point of branching (see Sunderland 1978). Similarly, where nerves are subjected to pressure, e.g. deep to a retinaculum, fasciculi are increased in number but reduced in size and the associated connective tissue and vascularity also increase; such a nerve shows a pink, fusiform dilatation, sometimes termed a pseudoganglion or gangliform enlargement.

STRUCTURE OF PERIPHERAL NERVES

CONNECTIVE TISSUE SHEATHS OF PERIPHERAL NERVES

Nerve trunks, whether uni- or multi-fascicular, are surrounded by an *epineurium*; individual fasciculi are enclosed by a multilayered *perineurium*, which in turn surrounds the *endoneurium* or intra-fascicular connective tissue (**8.57**) (for a detailed review, refer to Thomas & Lansky 1993).

Epineurium

This is a condensation of areolar connective tissue, and is derived from mesoderm. In humans, the epineurium normally constitutes 30–70% of the total cross-sectional area of the nerve bundle. As a general rule, the more fasciculi present in a peripheral nerve, the thicker the epineurium. The epineurium contains fibroblasts, collagen (types I and III), and variable amounts of fat. It has been suggested that the epineurial fat functions to 'cushion' the nerve it surrounds, and that loss of this protective layer may be associated with pressure palsies seen in wasted bedridden patients. The epineurium also contains lymphatics, which probably pass to regional lymph nodes, and blood vessels, the *vasa nervorum*, which pass across the perineurium to communicate with the network of arterioles and venules within the endoneurium.

Perineurium

This extends from the CNS–PNS transitional zone to the periphery,

8.56 Cells in the superior cervical sympathetic ganglion of rabbit. Semi-thin section of araldite-embedded material stained by toluidine blue. (Material supplied by J S Dixon, Department of Anatomy, University of Manchester.)

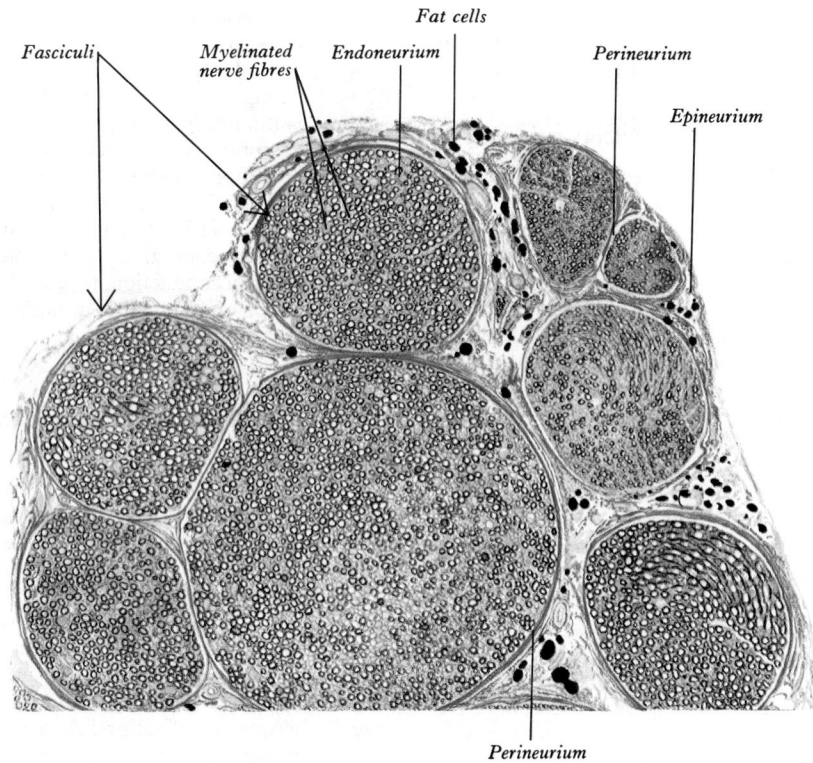

8.57 Transverse section of a peripheral nerve (cat). Stained with osmic acid and van Gieson's technique. Note the nerve fasciculi, the epi-, peri- and endoneurial connective tissue sheaths and the variations in the calibre of the myelinated nerve fibres. Magnification *c.* ×55.

where it is continuous with the capsules of muscle spindles and encapsulated sensory endings. At unencapsulated endings and neuromuscular junctions the perineurium ends openly. The perineurium consists of alternating layers of flattened polygonal cells (which are thought to be derived from fibroblasts) and collagen: in humans, the perineurium can often contain 15–20 layers of cells. Each layer of cells is enclosed by a basal lamina; in human nerves this can be up to 0.5 μm thick. Freeze-fracture studies have revealed that contiguous cells in each layer interdigitate along extensive tight junctions (zonulae occludentes). The cells characteristically contain numerous pinocytotic vesicles and often contain bundles of microfilaments. The ubiquitous presence of pinocytotic vesicles and the finding that perineurial cells are rich in phosphorylating enzymes underlie the assumption that the perineurium functions as a metabolically active diffusion barrier. It is probable that the perineurium, together with the blood–nerve barrier, plays an essential role in maintaining the osmotic milieu and the fluid pressure within the endoneurium.

Endoneurium

Strictly speaking, the term 'endoneurium' should be restricted to interfascicular connective tissue excluding the perineurial partitions within fascicles (Thomas & Lansky 1993). Endoneurium consists of a fibrous matrix composed predominantly of Type I collagen fibres, mainly organized in bundles lying parallel to the long axis of the nerve, and condensed around individual Schwann cell-axon units and endoneurial vessels. Bundles of unbranched fibrils, 10–12.5 nm in diameter, identified as oxytalan fibres, have been found in the endoneurial spaces of all species examined. The fibrous and cellular components of the endoneurium are bathed in endoneurial fluid (Low 1984). Endoneurial fluid pressure is slightly higher than that of the surrounding epineurium: it is believed that the resulting pressure gradient functions to minimize endoneurial contamination by toxic substances external to the nerve bundle (Powell et al 1979). The major cellular constituents of the endoneurium are Schwann cells, associated with axons, and endothelial cells. Schwann cell-axon units and endothelial cells are enclosed within basal laminae. Other cells which are always present within the endoneurium are fibroblasts (constituting approximately 4% of the total endoneurial cell population); resident macrophages, some of which are considered to

have a dendritic cell lineage (4%) (Monaco et al 1992); and mast cells (relatively common in the rat, but uncommon in human nerves). The proportion of intrafascicular cells in the human sural nerve has been assessed by Ochoa and Mair (1969).

BLOOD VESSELS OF PERIPHERAL NERVES

The blood vessels supplying a nerve end in a capillary plexus whose members pierce the perineurium and run largely parallel with the fibres, connected by short transverse vessels, to form narrow, oblong meshes similar to those found in muscle. The blood supply of peripheral nerves is highly unusual in several ways. First, endoneurial capillaries have atypically large diameters and intercapillary distances greater than those in many other tissues (Bell & Weddel 1984a, b). Second, peripheral nerves have two separate, functionally independent vascular systems: an extrinsic system (regional nutritive vessels and epineurial vessels) and an intrinsic system (longitudinally running microvessels in the endoneurium) (Lundborg & Branemark 1968; McManis et al 1993). There are rich anastomoses between the two systems, resulting in considerable overlap between the territories of the segmental arteries. This unique pattern of vessels, together with the high basal nerve blood flow relative to the metabolic requirements of the nerve, confer a high degree of resistance to ischaemia on peripheral nerves. It is still not known which of the systems is more important in maintaining nerve perfusion.

Endoneurial arterioles have a poorly developed smooth muscle layer, which supports the observation that they do not autoregulate well. In sharp contrast, epineurial and perineurial vessels have a dense perivascular plexus of peptidergic, serotoninergic and adrenergic nerves (McManis et al 1993).

Blood–nerve barrier

Just as the neuropil within the central nervous system is protected by a blood–brain barrier, so the endoneurial contents of peripheral nerve fibres are protected by a blood–nerve barrier and by the cellular elements of the perineurium (see above). The blood–nerve barrier operates at the level of the endoneurial capillary walls: these vessels are non-fenestrated, the endothelial cells are joined by tight junctions, and surrounded by continuous basal laminae. The barrier

947

is much less efficient in dorsal root and autonomic ganglia (Jacobs et al 1976), and in the distal parts of peripheral nerves (Hughes 1990). For a recent review of the barrier consult Poduslo (1993).

CLASSIFICATION OF PERIPHERAL NERVE FIBRES

Several schemes of classification of peripheral nerve fibres have been used, based on various parameters such as conduction velocity, function, fibre diameter and other attributes. Of two classifications in common use, the first, devised by Erlanger and Gasser (1937) from conduction speeds in amphibian axons, divides fibres into three major classes, designated A, B and C, corresponding to peaks in the distribution of their conduction velocities. Group A fibres are subdivided into α, β and γ subgroups; B group fibres are preganglionic autonomic efferents, and C fibres are non-myelinated. Since diameter and conduction velocity are in most fibres proportional (in myelinated fibres conduction in metres per second is approximately equal to six times the fibre diameter expressed in micrometres), the group Aα fibres are widest and most rapid and C fibres the narrowest and slowest. In mammals, Aβ fibres were found to be negligible but a subclass of non-autonomic fibres similar in conduction speed to B fibres, termed Aδ fibres, was discovered.

In Erlanger and Gasser's scheme afferent fibres are confined to Aα, Aδ and C groups, the largest (Aα fibres) including the axons of the encapsulated cutaneous, joint and muscle receptors and some large alimentary enteroceptors. Aδ fibres belong to thermoreceptors and nociceptors, including those in dental pulp, skin and connective tissue; C fibres have thermoreceptive, nociceptive and interoceptive functions. Somatic efferent fibres include Aα, Aβ and Aγ axons. Aα fibres innervate only extrafusal muscle fibres, being maximally 22 μm in diameter and conducting at a maximum of 120 m/s. Fibres to 'fast' twitch muscles are larger than those to 'slow' muscle. Aβ fibres are restricted to collaterals of Aα fibres, forming plaque endings on some intrafusal muscle fibres; Aγ fibres are exclusively fusimotor to plate and trail endings on intrafusal muscle fibres (see below). Autonomic efferents comprise preganglionic B fibres and postganglionic sympathetic and parasympathetic axons of the C (non-myelinated) group. This scheme can be applied to all fibres of spinal and cranial nerves except perhaps those of the olfactory nerve, whose fibres form a uniquely small and slow group.

Another classification, used for afferent fibres of somatic muscles, was introduced by Lloyd in 1943: myelinated fibres are divided into groups I, II and III, non-myelinated fibres forming group IV. Group I fibres are large (12–22 μm) and include primary sensory fibres of muscle spindles (Group Ia) and smaller fibres of Golgi tendon organs (Ib). Group II comprises fibres of secondary sensory terminals of muscle spindles, with diameters of about 6–12 μm. Group III fibres, 1–6 μm in diameter, have free sensory endings in the connective tissue sheaths around and within muscles and appear to be nociceptive, related to 'pressure-pain' in externally stimulated muscles. Paciniform (encapsulated) endings of muscle sheaths may also contribute fibres to this class. Group IV includes non-myelinated fibres below 1.5 μm with 'free' endings in muscles, being chiefly nociceptive.

While these general schemes of classification are valuable in neurophysiology, a single structural parameter such as diameter, measured at one point, cannot adequately categorize nerve fibres throughout the whole course of a nerve. Many values quoted are related only to velocity peaks or sampled diameters. The figures quoted are relative, and there is some overlap between the functional classes; however, these schemes reveal that a general pattern of organization exists in peripheral nerves.

CONDUCTION IN PERIPHERAL NERVES

When a nerve is stimulated, the sum of the action potentials of the constituent fibres, the compound action potential, can be recorded using electrodes placed near the surface of the nerve or on the overlying skin. Since action potentials travel at different speeds in fibres of different diameters, and since large fibres create greater electrical signals than small fibres, the compound action potential can be of complex waveform, with at least four sequential waves of different amplitude and velocity, known as α, β, γ and δ waves. In general, fibre types are classified primarily by their conduction

velocities, although fibres of different function may have similar velocities (see above).

A number of different factors govern the conduction of velocities of nerve fibres. Thus in non-myelinated fibres the action potential sweeps continuously over the axolemma as depolarization of one area of membrane triggers depolarization of adjacent areas: the rate of spread is proportional to the axonal cross-sectional area (Hodgkin 1964). However, in myelinated fibres the myelin sheath limits excitation to the nodes of Ranvier, and conduction proceeds from node to node in sequence along the axon. This mode of conduction, termed saltatory conduction, is much faster and more energy efficient than the mode of conduction in unmyelinated axons (Stämpfli 1954; Schmidt & Thews 1989; Kandel 1991).

PERIPHERAL NEUROGLIA

SCHWANN CELLS

Schwann cells are satellite cells of the peripheral nervous system; peripheral axons are ensheathed by them and are separated from the endoneurium by the Schwann cell plasma membrane. In a mature peripheral nerve fibre, Schwann cells are distributed along the axons in longitudinal chains: the geometry of this association depends on whether the axon is myelinated or non-myelinated. Myelinated axons have a 1:1 relationship with their ensheathing Schwann cells, and the territory of an individual Schwann cell defines an *internode*. The interval between myelinating Schwann cells is a *node of Ranvier*. The internodal Schwann cell cytoplasm surrounds the myelin sheath in a delicate network of interlacing strips which radiate from an approximately mid-internodal perinuclear region towards the paranodal collar, from whence finger-like processes of cytoplasm extend across the nodal gap to interdigitate with processes from the neighbouring Schwann cell. Helical strands of cytoplasm wind from the abaxonal layer of cytoplasm through the myelin sheath to the adaxonal layer of cytoplasm at the *Schmidt-Lanterman incisures*. There is evidence to suggest that the maintenance of the periaxonal space and of the adaxonal layer of Schwann cytoplasm in myelinated fibres is dependent upon the presence of myelin associated glycoprotein (MAG) in Schwann cell adaxonal membranes (Griffin et al 1993).

In non-myelinated fibres the structural relationship between axons and Schwann cells is quite different. Individual Schwann cells are usually associated with groups of small calibre axons; however, it is not uncommon to find single, non-myelinated axons up to 1.5 μm in diameter in human peripheral nerves.

Immunohistochemical staining has revealed that the molecular phenotype of mature myelin-forming Schwann cells is different from that of the mature non-myelin forming Schwann cell. Not surprisingly, adult myelin-forming Schwann cells are characterized by the presence of several myelin proteins including the major myelin protein Po; myelin basic protein (MBP); myelin-associated glycoprotein (MAG); peripheral myelin protein (PMP-22). They do not express the low affinity nerve growth factor receptor (NGF-R); neural cell adhesion molecule (N-CAM); a glial fibrillary acidic protein-like (GFAP) intermediate filament protein; the transmembrane glycoprotein L1; growth-associated protein (GAP-43), all of which are characteristic of adult non-myelin forming Schwann cells. The L2/HNK-1 carbohydrate epitope is apparently expressed preferentially on Schwann cells in ventral spinal roots and motor axon-related Schwann cells of muscle nerves, but only rarely in dorsal roots and in predominantly sensory, cutaneous nerves (Martini et al 1988). All Schwann cells express a Ca^{2+}-binding protein S-100; galactocerebroside (GC); and the sulphatide recognized by the O4 monoclonal antibody. The molecules characteristic of the non-myelin forming cell are expressed by all Schwann cells prior to myelination but are downregulated at the onset of myelination (Jessen & Mirsky 1992). Recent in vitro studies have shown that expression of P_o protein can be regulated at both transcriptional and translational/post-translational stages.

Schwann cell lineage

Clonal analysis of avian neural crest cells in vitro (Anderson 1989) and in vivo studies using either microinjection with a vital dye of

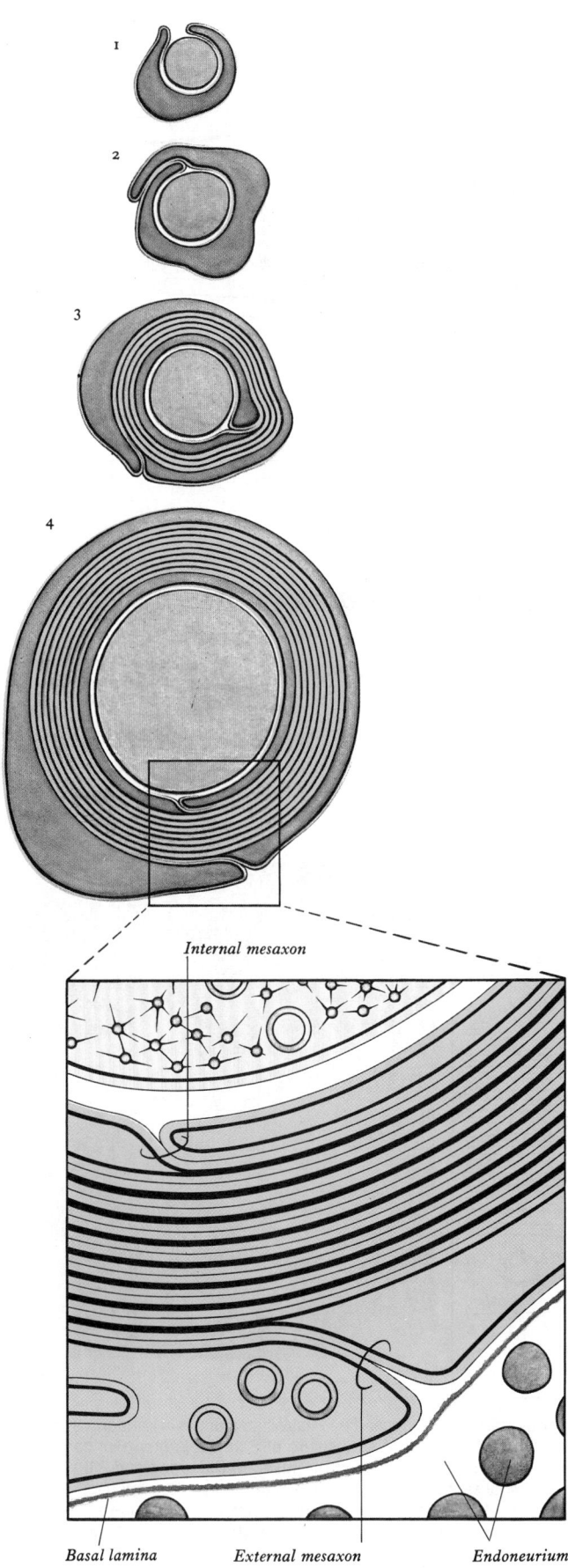

Internal mesaxon

Basal lamina *External mesaxon* *Endoneurium*

8.58 The development and organization of the myelin sheath of a peripheral nerve fibre. In stages 1–4 myelin formed by a Schwann cell (blue) progressively envelops the growing axon (yellow), to form the final pattern of spirally disposed myelin lamellae: see enlarged detail at the base of the diagram.

single migrating cells (Fraser & Bronner-Fraser 1991) or labelling crest cells by retrovirus-mediated gene transfer (Frank & Sanes 1991) all support the concept that many of the cells in the very early migrating neural crest are multipotent, and possess the ability to give rise to neurons and Schwann cells. The regulatory events involved as precursor cells become committed to the Schwann cell lineage have yet to be established. It is known that axon-associated signals are critical in controlling the proliferation of Schwann cells (Ratner et al 1988) and in influencing gene expression in Schwann cells during their differentiation. Myelinating Schwann cells that are deprived of axonal contact either in vivo after nerve transection, or in vitro in dissociated cell culture, lose their myelinating phenotype and display a phenotype more typical of a non-myelinating Schwann cell (i.e. they express the NGF-R, N-CAM and GFAP genes). Conversely, myelin protein genes are upregulated in Schwann cells that have been contacted either by regenerating axons in vivo (Mitchell et al 1990), or by exploratory neurites in vitro (Morrison et al 1991; Suter et al 1992).

Other interactions between axons and Schwann cells are equally precisely regulated. Recent work suggests that neurons may regulate developmentally programmed death of Schwann cell precursors (Jessen & Mirsky 1992) possibly as a mechanism for matching numbers of axons and glia within each peripheral nerve bundle. Neuronal signals appear to control the production of basal laminae by Schwann cells, the induction and maintenance of myelination, and Schwann cell survival (few Schwann cells persist in chronically denervated nerves). Schwann cell signals may influence axonal calibre, and are of crucial importance in repair of damaged peripheral nerves.

Schwann cell development can be divided into perinatal migratory and proliferative phases, succeeded by a final axon-associated state, in which myelin formation and maintenance may occur. Immature Schwann cells are large and rounded, with an oval nucleus and dense cytoplasm. As they migrate from the neural crest they are first fusiform in appearance and then irregular, as they insinuate their processes between the outgrowing axons. This process of axonal segregation continues, producing *pro-myelinated axons* (i.e. axons which have established a 1:1 relationship with their ensheathing Schwann cells, and which are probably committed to myelination) and *non-myelinated axons* with a mature configuration. For a recent review of the development of peripheral nerves, consult Webster (1993).

All larger mammalian axons are myelinated: myelin is responsible for the glistening whiteness of peripheral nerves and central white

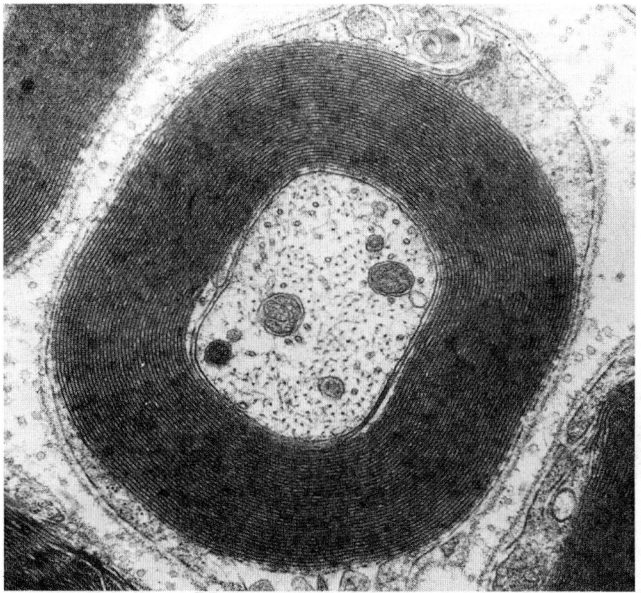

8.59 An electron micrograph of a myelinated peripheral nerve fibre, showing an axon containing neurofilaments, microtubules and mitochondria, surrounded by a myelin sheath, enclosed in turn by Schwann cell cytoplasm and endoneurial space. Magnification ×25 000. (Provided by S Standring, Division of Anatomy and Cell Biology, UMDS, Guy's Campus, London.)

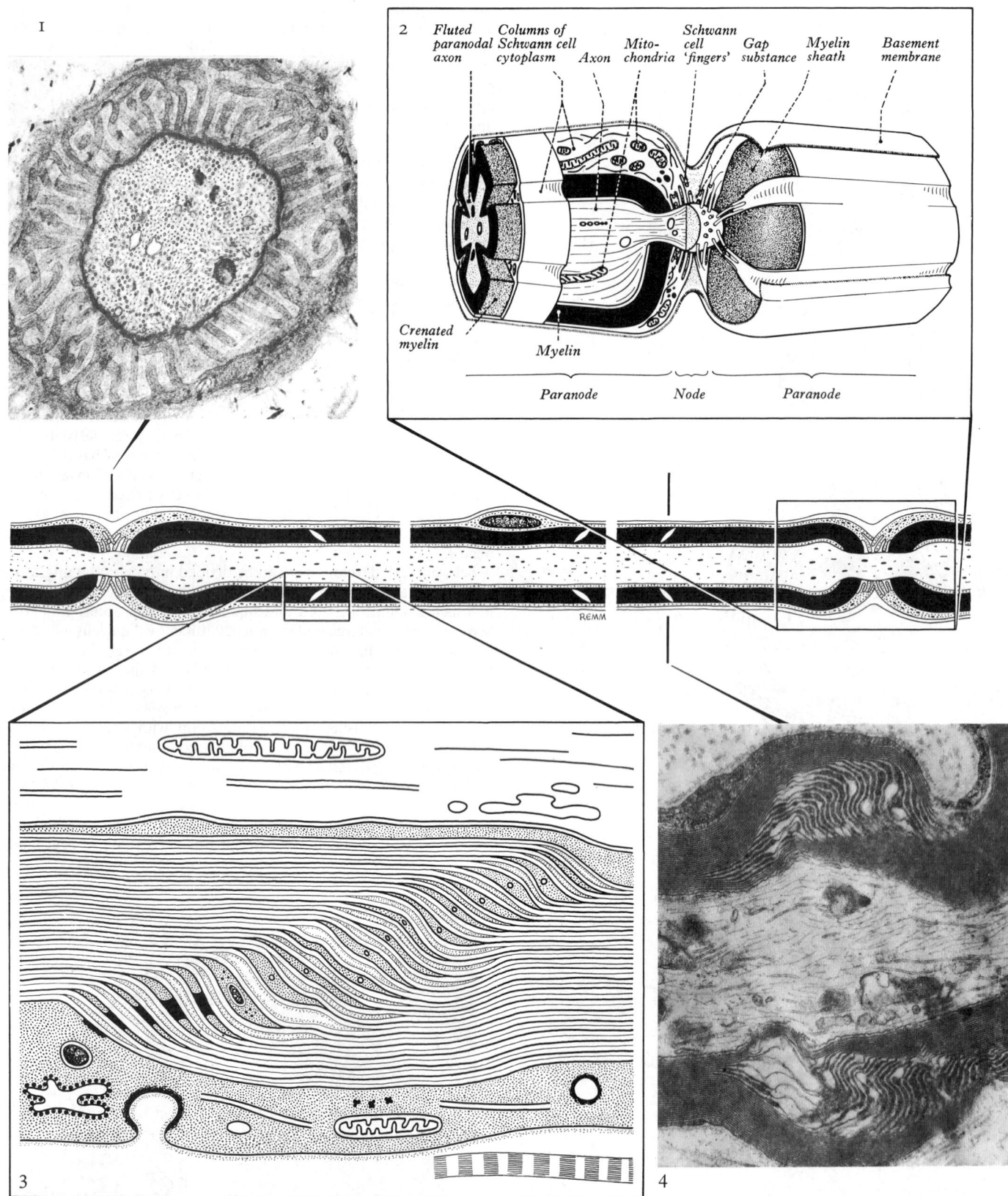

8.60 General plan of a myelinated nerve fibre in longitudinal section including one complete internodal segment and two adjacent paranodal bulbs, used as a key for the more detailed microarchitecture of specific subregions. 1: a transverse section through the centre of a node of Ranvier, with numerous finger-like processes of adjacent Schwann cells converging towards the nodal axolemma. Many microtubules and microfilaments are visible within the axoplasm. 2: a diagram showing the arrangement of the axon, myelin sheath and Schwann cell cytoplasm at the node of Ranvier in the paranodal bulbs. (Supplied by P L Williams and D N Landon.) 3: detailed substructure of one-half of an incisure of Schmidt-Lanterman; consult text for further information. (Supplied by Susan M Standring and P L Williams.) 4: longitudinal section of part of a myelinated nerve fibre (mouse), including an incisure of Schmidt-Lanterman; this appears as oblique zones in the myelin sheath on both sides of the fibre. Consult text for structural details. (Nos. 1 and 4 supplied by Susan M Standring.)

matter. Axons smaller than 1 μm in diameter are usually non-myelinated.

Non-myelinated fibres

In cutaneous nerves and dorsal spinal roots, about 75% of mammalian axons are non-myelinated; they form about 50% of the fibres of nerves to muscles and 30% in ventral spinal roots. Autonomic postganglionic axons are almost exclusively non-myelinated and preganglionic nerves contain significant numbers of these fibres. A non-myelinated 'fibre' is really a group of small axons (0.15–2.0 μm in diameter) within a sequential series of Schwann cells. In mature nerves the mode of enclosure of each group of axons shows inter- and intraspecific variation. Axons are usually separated from each other by tongues of Schwann cell cytoplasm, but are sometimes further isolated by separate processes of cytoplasm which converge in the perinuclear region (Gamble & Eames 1964).

The line of invagination during development is marked by a *mesaxon*, a double layer of Schwann cell plasma membrane, its apposed intucked surfaces lying parallel to each other and separated by about 15–20 nm. These layers separate to enclose the axon, separated from it by a periaxonal space of similar dimensions. At the exterior of the Schwann cell the layers separate and are continuous with the plasma membrane. Because of this arrangement, endoneurial tissue fluid reaches the periaxonal space between the mesaxonal membranes. These intercellular spaces allow the movement of ions when action potentials are conducted along the enclosed axon. In the absence of a myelin sheath and nodes, saltatory conduction does not occur, and the uninterrupted passage of impulses is relatively slow, with velocities of about 0.5–4.0 m/s.

A three-dimensional reconstruction from sections of somatic autonomic nerves revealed that the spatial relationships between axons and Schwann cells alter continuously within each cell (Aguayo et al 1973). The transfer of axons between Schwann cells usually occurs at the extremities of adjacent glial cells, where their cytoplasmic processes interdigitate (Gamble et al 1978).

Myelinated fibres

Myelination increases the conduction velocity of the action potential along an axon. Myelinated nerve fibres are a feature of the nervous systems of all chordates above the Acraniata. Although some invertebrates do have large axons (particularly those involved in activating fast muscle responses), which may be ensheathed by glial processes, these bear only a superficial resemblance to the vertebrate myelinated nerve fibre.

Within the peripheral nervous system, myelin is produced by the Schwann cells. The myelin sheath can be thought of as a flat glial process which becomes spirally wrapped around the axon: the intracellular and extracellular spaces of the glial process are lost as the external and internal faces of the membrane become tightly apposed. In the electron microscopic image of myelin the compacted external surfaces produce the *minor dense lines* alternating with the compacted inner cytoplasmic surfaces which correspond to the *major dense lines* (**8.58**, **8.59**). These in turn correspond to the intraperiod

and period lines defined in earlier X-ray studies of the myelinated fibre. The inner and outer zones of occlusion of the spiral process are continuous with the minor dense line and are called the *inner* and *outer mesaxons*. The major dense line is continuous with the cytoplasmic face of the membrane at all regions where compaction is lost and appears to be quite stable. In contrast, the minor dense line appears to be labile (Napolitano & Scallen 1969; Williams & Hall 1971a,b; Blaurock et al 1986).

Nodes of Ranvier. In myelinated fibres, the territory of the Schwann cell defines an *internode*, the interval between internodes being the *node of Ranvier* (**8.60**). The internodal length varies directly with the diameter of the fibres, from 150 to 1500 μm (Kashef 1966). When axons branch, they do so at nodes of Ranvier. In the peripheral nervous system, the myelin sheaths on both sides of a node terminate in *paranodal bulbs*, which often show an asymmetry related to growth. The surfaces of the bulbs and of the underlying axon are fluted as they approach the nodes. The grooves in the external surface of the myelin sheath that are produced by fluting are filled by Schwann cell cytoplasm which is rich in mitochondria (Landon & Williams 1963; Berthold 1968). Expanded *terminal loops* of paranodal cytoplasm containing microtubules, membranous vesicles and microfilaments abut the paranodal axolemma. There is a structural complex of cytoskeletal elements and membrane-bridging structures at the paranode which are concerned with the adhesion and maintenance of the sheath and which may also reflect Schwann cell involvement with nodal functioning (Ichima & Ellisman 1991). The paranodal regions contain high levels of Na^+ and Ca^{2+}. Fine villous processes arise from the paranodal collar of Schwann cell cytoplasm and curve into the *nodal gap* to contact the nodal axolemma; these finger-like processes are numerous in large fibres, where they form regular hexagonal arrays. The nodal gap contains a *gap substance* rich in acidic proteoglycans (Landon & Langley 1971). Each myelinated segment is separated from the enclosed axon by a narrow *periaxonal space* (15–20 nm) which although nominally part of the extracellular space, is isolated functionally from the extracellular space at the paranodes.

Schmidt-Lanterman incisures. Schmidt-Lanterman incisures are oblique interruptions of interparanodal myelin, in which the membrane compaction is lost (**8.60**). The major dense line of the sheath separates to enclose a continuous spiral band of granular cytoplasm which passes between the abaxonal and adaxonal layers of Schwann cytoplasm. There is often an oblique row of desmosomoid attachments near the abaxonal surface of the incisure, and the cytoplasm frequently contains a microtubule. The minor dense line is usually split throughout an incisure, thereby creating a helical conduit connecting the periaxonal and endoneurial spaces.

The dimensions and relationships of all of these features of the myelinated segment are altered to varying degrees in pathological conditions. Thus following nerve crush or the induction of primary demyelination the paranodal myelin loses contact with the axon and the Schmidt-Lanterman incisures dilate as the adjacent minor dense line opens and there is an irreversible collapse of the myelin periodicity (Williams & Hall 1971; Hall & Gregson 1971).

Myelin

Myelin is effectively an intracellular structure, produced by Schwann cells in the peripheral nervous system (PNS) and oligodendrocytes in the central nervous system (CNS). There are significant differences between central and peripheral myelin, reflecting the fact that oligodendrocytes and Schwann cells use different proteins during myelinogenesis.

The basic dimensions of the myelin membrane are different: mammalian PNS myelin has a period to period line thickness of 18.5 nm whereas CNS myelin has a period repeat thickness of 15.7 nm. The major structural protein of PNS myelin, P_0, is glycosylated whereas the major structural protein of CNS myelin, proteolipid protein (PLP), is not. The larger periodicity of PNS myelin can be accounted for by the glycosylated extracellular portion of P_0, producing a minor dense line space in a number of species of 4.0 nm compared

to 2.4 nm in CNS myelin (Blaurock 1981). The major dense line space has average values of 2.5 and 1.7 nm in PNS and CNS myelin respectively. The greater thickness of the major dense line in PNS myelin is variable and is likely to result from the presence of both P_1 and P_2 basic proteins and the cytoplasmic globular region of the protein P_0 at the surface. CNS myelin is distinguished by the presence of a tight junction complex extending through the radius of the compact internodal myelin segment—the radial component (Peters

1961) which maintains the apposition across intraperiod and period densities after the distension of the sheath following hexachlorophene poisoning (Tabira et al 1978). The periodicity across this zonula adherens as determined by X-ray diffraction is 3.04 nm compared to the bulk periodicity of 15.7 nm (Inouye & Kirschner 1984).

THE COMPOSITION OF MYELIN

Myelin membrane contains protein, lipid and water (which forms at least 20% of the wet weight).

Myelin lipids

Myelin is a relatively lipid-rich membrane and contains 70–80% lipid in the PNS and CNS respectively. All classes of lipid have been found. The major lipid species are cholesterol (40 moles%), the commonest single molecule; phospholipids (40–48 moles%) and glycosphingolipids (12–19 moles%). Minor lipid species include galactosylglycerides, phosphoinositides and gangliosides. The lipid composition of PNS and CNS myelin is different. The proportion of cholesterol and glycospingolipid is particularly high in myelin. The major glycolipids are galactocerebroside and its sulphate ester, sulphatide: although these lipids are not unique to myelin they are present in characteristically high concentrations. The fatty acid components of the phosphoglycerides, sphingomyelin and ceramides are variable but there is a preponderance of C18 fatty acids in the phosphoglycerides and C24 acids in the ceramides. Galactocerebroside and sulphatide also contain long chain hydroxy fatty acids. Both CNS and PNS myelin contain acidic glycolipids; although these are only present in low concentrations, they are important as antigens in myelin. The gangliosides, glycosphingolipids characterized by the presence of sialic acid (N-acetylneuraminic acid), account for less than 1% of the lipid. The concentrations and the specific gangliosides vary between species. In the human, LM1 (sialosyl paragloboside), is characteristic of PNS myelin whereas GM4 (sialosylgalactocerebroside) is the major ganglioside of CNS myelin. PNS myelin of most vertebrates contains sulphated glucuronylparagloboside lipids, bearing a carbohydrate hapten which is also found in a number of myelin glycoproteins (MAG, P_0 and PMP-22).

Inherited disorders of lipid metabolism, particularly those involving lipid catabolism leading to abnormal accumulations of lipid, such as metachromatic leucodystrophy, Krabbe's disease and Niemann-Pick's disease, are frequently characterized by severe demyelination.

Alterations in fatty acid composition that occur in Refsum's disease and impairment of long chain fatty acid oxidation, seen in adrenoleucodystrophy, may also be associated with diffuse demyelination.

Myelin proteins

A relatively small number of protein species account for the majority of the myelin protein. Some of those proteins are common to both PNS and CNS myelin, but the major structural proteins are different in these regions of the nervous system (Table **8**.2). However, this simplicity in composition is deceptive since most myelin proteins exist in multiple forms: variability arises from alternative splicing and from variable post-translational modification. Many other proteins are present in low overall concentration and are probably localized in specific regions of the myelin segment. The major proteins represent structural proteins and are found throughout the sheath.

On the basis of their structure and distribution, membrane proteins fall roughly into three types: proteins bound mainly to the surface (extrinsic membrane proteins); proteins with a hydrophobic portion penetrating and possibly spanning the hydrophobic region of the membrane with the larger part of the polypeptide superficial to the membrane; and proteins with multiple stretches of hydrophobic regions so that the protein threads backwards and forwards across the membrane. All three types of protein occur as structural proteins in myelin. The basic proteins P_1 and P_2 are charged proteins localized at the 'cytoplasmic' face of the membrane. Myelin basic protein P_1 is found in both PNS and CNS myelin (accounting for 5–15% of PNS myelin protein and 30% of CNS myelin protein) and occurs in multiple forms as a result of alternative splicing with at least six forms of m-RNA. It is also modified post-translationally by phosphorylation and methylation to generate charged isoforms. P_1 is considered to be responsible for the compaction at the major dense line in CNS myelin where it is thought to interact with the major CNS myelin protein—proteolipid protein (PLP). P_1 is the major antigen producing experimental allergic encephalitis (EAE) which has been studied as a model of multiple sclerosis. P_2 is found mainly in the PNS; the amount varies with species, ranging from <2% in the guinea pig to 15% in bovine PNS myelin. The protein is found at a much lower level in the CNS, particularly in the spinal cord. It is related to the fatty-acid binding protein of the liver and is a major myelin antigen responsible for producing experimental allergic neuritis, a model for acute idiopathic demyelinating polyneuropathy (Guillain-Barré syndrome). The proteins P_0 and MAG are members of the immuno-

globulin supergene family and are membrane proteins of the second type (see above). They are both glycosylated, and the large glycosylated globular region of the protein extends into the space of the minor dense line. P_0 is the major structural protein of PNS myelin where it accounts for 50% of the total protein. It is not found in the CNS, except in fish. It may be modified post-translationally by variable glycosylation, phosphorylation, sulphation or acylation. The protein has a single membrane-spanning region and a highly basic portion lying in the major dense line which may play a role in the compaction of the major dense line in PNS myelin analogous to that of P_1 in CNS myelin. This would suggest that P_0 acts in the PNS as the structural equivalent of PLP/DM20 and P_1 in the CNS. In terms of abundance, PLP and the splice variant DM20 are the CNS myelin equivalent of P_0, and account for 50% of CNS myelin protein. Unlike P_0, PLP/DM20 is not glycosylated (except in the lung fish where a glycosylated version of DM20 occurs in CNS myelin) but it is acylated. PLP/DM20 is considered to have four membrane spanning stretches and large portions of polypeptide at both 'extracellular' and 'cytoplasmic' interfaces. The amino-acid sequence of PLP/DM20 is highly conserved between species indicating a high level of adaptation to its function, suggesting that it may be more than a structural protein in myelin. The gene is expressed in neural tissues and extraneural tissues during early development before myelination starts. It is expressed in Schwann cells but not incorporated into the myelin. Peripheral myelin contains a structurally similar but unrelated protein, PMP22, which accounts for 5% of the PNS myelin proteins. Unlike the PLP/DM20 proteins it is glycosylated on the 'extracellular' interface. It is identical to the growth arrest protein found in fibroblasts, heart, lung and gut, and may have a similar role in the Schwann cell.

A number of other significant proteins occur in myelin which are more restricted in their localization. In both CNS and PNS sheaths, MAG, another member of the immunoglobulin supergene family, is localized at those regions of the myelin segment where compaction starts, namely, the mesaxons and inner periaxonal membranes, paranodal loops and incisures, in both CNS and PNS sheaths. The glycosylated globular part of the molecule extends into the extracellular space. Cytoskeletal elements, F-actin and spectrin, co-localize with MAG at the cytoplasmic face of the membranes, consistent with the proposed functional role of MAG in membrane adhesion (Trapp et al 1989). CNP (2',3'-cyclic nucleotide 3'-phosphodiesterase) is also localized mainly at the incisures and paranodes. It is more concentrated in CNS (5%) than PNS (1%) myelin. Like

P_1 it is phosphorylated and may be a guanosine triphosphate (GTP)-binding protein. It has been suggested that it functions in the organization of cytoskeletal networks and may assist in the incorporation of P_1 into myelin (Braun et al 1990). There are many other enzymes and glycoproteins associated with the myelin segment, but their localization and functional significance are not clearly understood.

Mutations of the major myelin structural proteins have now been recognized in a number of inherited human neurological diseases (Table 8.2). As would be expected, these mutations, and others found in rodents, produce defects in myelination consistent with the suggested functional roles of the relevant proteins in the myelin sheath.

Table 8.2 The proteins of the myelin sheath

Protein	Mol.wt (kD)	Features of protein	Localization, concentration	Pathological significance
P_0	ca 29[1]	Variably glycosylated Ig-like transmembrane protein	PNS High, major protein	Mutated in Charcot-Marie-Tooth type 1b neuropathy. Possible autoantigen in GBS[2]
P_1	14–22[1]	Phosphorylated, methylated, deiminated	PNS & CNS Cytoplasmic face. High, major protein	Possible autoantigen in multiple sclerosis (MS)
P_2	14.5[1]	Member of fatty acid binding proteins	PNS, Cytoplasmic face. High. CNS, regional low	Possible autoantigen in GBS
Proteolipid protein & DM20	28 & 21[1]	Acylated Transmembrane hydrophobic protein	CNS High, major protein	Defects in expression in Pelizaeous-Merzbacher syndrome. Possible autoantigen in MS
Myelin associated glycoprotein (MAG)	67 & 72[3]	Glycosylated Ig-like transmembrane protein	PNS & CNS Located at uncompacted regions. Low	Possible autoantigen in demyelinating neuropathy associated with IgM paraprotein
CNPase (2', 3' cyclic AMP phosphodiesterase)	46 & 48[1]	Phosphorylated, amidated	CNS high levels, PNS low. Cytoplasmic face	
Myelin-oligodendrocyte glycoprotein (MOG)	26, 28[3]	Glycosylated Ig-like protein	CNS Transmembrane. Low	Possible autoantigen in MS
Oligodendrocyte-myelin glycoprotein (OMGP)	120[1]	Glycosylated GPI-linked protein	CNS, extracellular face. Low	
PMP22	22[1]	Glycosylated transmembrane protein	PNS. High (ca 5%)	Mutated in Charcot-Marie-Tooth type 1a neuropathy. Possibly involved in some other inherited neuropathies

[1] Native protein molecular weight.
[2] Guillain-Barré syndrome.
[3] Polypeptide molecular weight.

MYELINATION

In general myelination is seen only in axons above a certain diameter, about 1.5 μm in the PNS and 1 μm in the central nervous system (e.g. Matthews 1968) (**8**.61). It was considered that axonal diameter was critical in determining myelination; however, since there is considerable overlap between the size of the smallest myelinated and the largest unmyelinated axons, axonal calibre is unlikely to be the only factor. In man and other mammals there is a reasonable linear relationship between axon diameter and internodal length and myelin sheath thickness (Williams & Wendell-Smith 1971; Murray & Blakemore 1980). In the peripheral nervous system, the division and association of Schwann cells with axons stops before myelination starts, each glial cell elongating in adaptation to further linear and radial growth of the axon (Vizoso & Young 1948; Williams & Kashef 1966). The final dimensions of any particular axon are determined by the neuron; presumably therefore the nodal regions must also be determined by the neuron before myelination (Ellisman 1979; Wiley-Livingston & Ellisman 1980). Since the myelin segment dimensions are related to the axonal dimensions it is reasonable to assume that

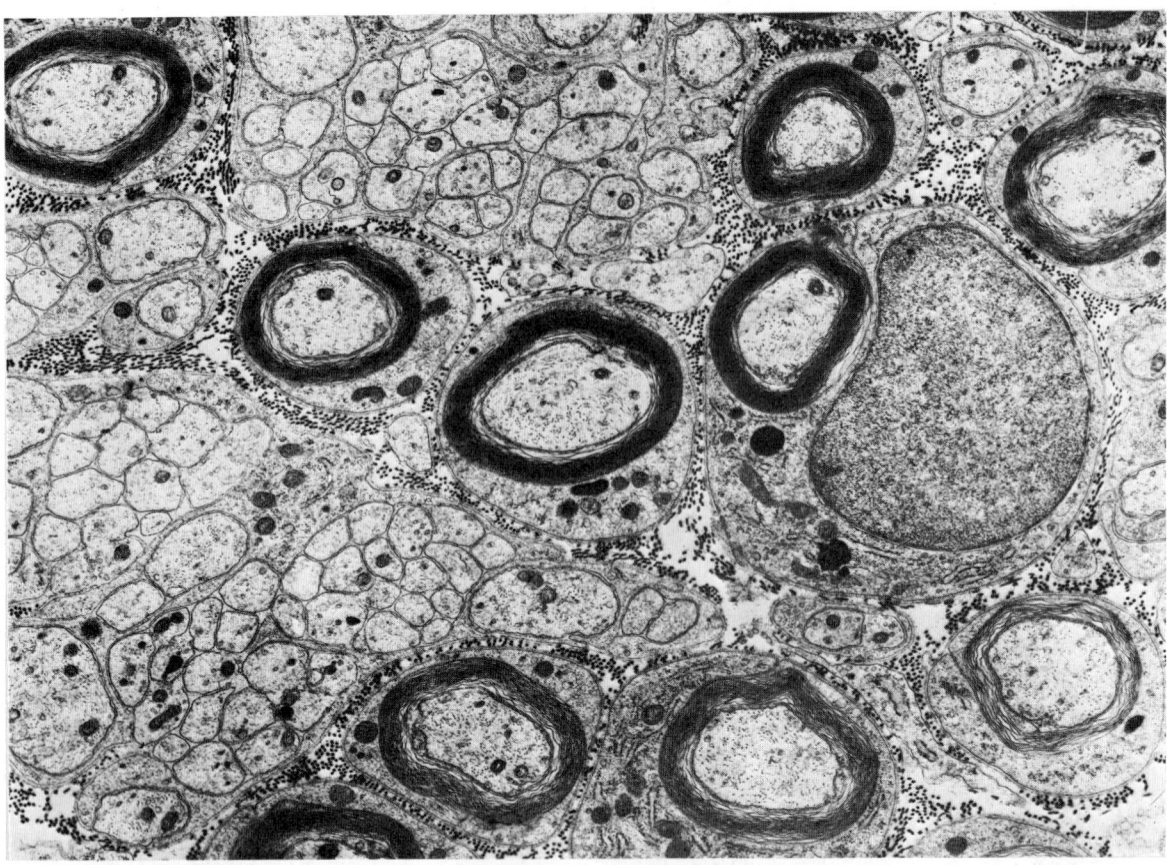

8.61 Transverse section of an immature peripheral nerve of a rat, taken one week after birth, showing the profiles of numerous axons. Some of the latter are non-myelinated and, either singly or in groups, are invaginated into the surfaces of cytoplasmic processes of adjacent Schwann cells. Other axons are in the process of myelination. Note the Schwann cell nucleus (right) to one side of a myelin sheath and the ultrastructure of the Schwann cell cytoplasm at this stage of development.

the numbers and spacing of the Schwann cells associated with the axon before myelination starts are also neuronally determined. The precise dimensional relationships between axon and myelin segment vary with the function of the fibre (Williams & Wendell-Smith 1971).

The most obvious difference between the peripheral and central nervous systems with regard to myelination is the fact that Schwann cells are associated with axons during their outgrowth to their targets, whereas in the central nervous system axon outgrowth to target precedes the migration of oligodendrocyte precursors; consequently the oligodendrocyte associates with and myelinates axons after their phase of elongation. In the Schwann cell the transcription of myelin protein genes is upregulated by axon association, and may reflect the action of elevated cAMP levels in downregulating suppressor regulatory genes as well as upregulating transcription-promoting factors. The level of expression of the regulatory genes reverts when axonal contact is lost. In the oligodendrocyte, myelin genes are not invoked by axon-association. Axons, and in particular axonal activity, may be more important for promoting the proliferation and survival of oligodendrocytes and their precursors either directly, or indirectly, via astrocytes (Barres & Raff 1993). Adhesion/recognition molecules such as MAG, L1 and P_0 appear to play distinct roles in the inductive events leading to the initial ensheathment of axons by myelinating glia, and in the subsequent formation of compact myelin (Colman 1991). In the central nervous system a 72 kD form of MAG is initially produced in the oligodendrocyte, before the expression of the 67 kD polypeptide version which predominates in the adult. In the peripheral nervous system the 67 kD form is always the major form. It is possible that the larger form of MAG is important in the first association of the oligodendrocyte process with axons, and that the 67 kD version is concerned with maintaining axon association.

The mechanism by which myelin is formed is unknown. Early models of myelinogenesis, derived from tissue culture data, proposed that Schwann cells first formed a loop of cytoplasm around their target axons, then migrated around them many times to wrap the axons in a tight spiral of membrane (Geren 1954). It is assumed that cytoplasm is subsequently extruded from the sheath at all points other than incisures and paranodes. In the central nervous system this is unlikely to be the only mechanism because a single oligodendrocyte ensheathes several separate axons (Bunge 1968). It has also been proposed that myelin grows by interstitial deposition of individual molecular components within lamellae. The amphiphilic proteins, e.g. P_0, PLP, MAG, which are synthesized on rough endoplasmic reticulum after processing in the Golgi, are transported as separate vesicles to the myelin membrane at the region of the external mesaxon. Soluble proteins such as MBP are produced on free polysomes at the paranodal regions to become incorporated at the major dense line interface, possibly with the help of CNP.

While the sheath thickens from a few lamellae to perhaps 300 in the peripheral nervous system, the axon may also grow from 1 to 15 μm in diameter and internodal segments increase from 150 μm to 1500 μm in length (Williams & Wendell-Smith 1971). Actin and tubulin are found in myelin, particularly in association with the paranodal regions and the Schmidt-Lanterman incisures and it is possible that spiralling involves a contractile process. However, since overall growth must be in length and internal and external radii as well as in thickness, it may be that constituents are added to the growing membrane with slippage at the minor dense line as the radius increases.

In late fetal and early postnatal development, myelination does not occur simultaneously in all parts of the body. Nerves and tracts have their own specific temporal patterns, which can be related to their degree of functional maturity (Ochoa & Mair 1969a,b).

THE CENTRAL–PERIPHERAL TRANSITION REGION

The transition between central and peripheral nervous systems is gradual, and usually occurs some distance from the point at which

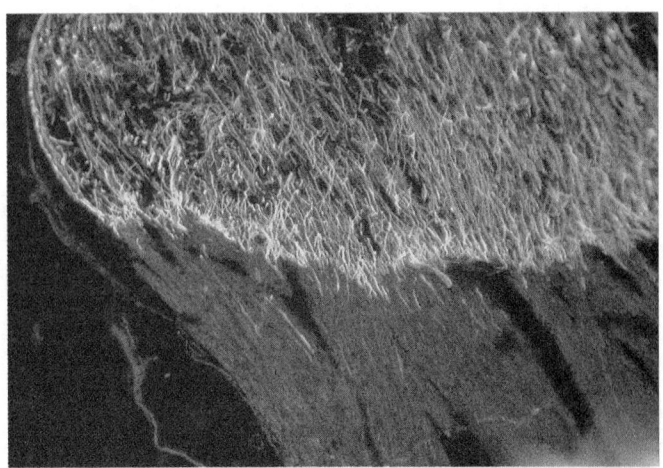

8.62 Section through the junction between the central and peripheral nervous system in the sensory root of the trigeminal nerve (rat) demonstrated by immunofluorescence of glial fibrillary acidic protein (GFAP). This is present in the astrocytes of the central nervous system but not in Schwann cells of the peripheral nerve. (Provided by Martin Sadler, Division of Anatomy and Cell Biology, UMDS, Guy's Campus, London.)

the roots emerge from the brain or the spinal cord (**8.62**). The segment of nerve root which contains components of both central nervous system (CNS) and peripheral nervous system (PNS) tissue is called the CNS–PNS transitional region (TR). All axons in the PNS, other than postganglionic autonomic neurons, traverse a TR. Macroscopically, as a nerve root is traced towards the spinal cord

or the brain, it can be seen to split into several thinner *rootlets* which may, in turn, subdivide into *minirootlets*. The TR is located within either rootlet or minirootlet (**8.63**). The arrangement of roots and rootlets varies according to whether the root trunk is ventral, dorsal or cranial. Thus, in dorsal roots, the main root trunk separates into a fan of rootlets and minirootlets which enter the spinal cord in sequence along the dorsolateral sulcus, whereas in certain cranial nerves the minirootlets come together central to the TR and enter the brain as a stump of white matter (Berthold et al 1993).

Microscopically, the TR is characterized by an axial CNS compartment surrounded by a PNS compartment. In humans, the TR lies more peripherally in sensory than in motor nerves: in both situations, the apex of the TR is described as a *glial dome*, whose convex surface is directed distally. Ultrastructurally the centre of the dome consists of fibres with a typical CNS organization, surrounded by an outer mantle of astrocytes (corresponding to the external glial limiting membrane). From this mantle numerous processes, the *glial fringe*, project into the endoneurial compartment of the peripheral nerve where they interdigitate with the Schwann cells. The astrocytes form a loose reticulum through which axons pass. Peripheral myelinated fibres usually cross the TR at a node of Ranvier, termed a *PNS–CNS compound node* (Carlstedt 1977). At such a node distally there is a corona of Schwann cell microvilli and mitochondria-laden paranodal cytoplasm; centrally are a few astrocyte processes, typically making contacts with the axolemma. In the first sacral spinal nerve roots (of cats) an average of four or five nodes are associated with the processes of a single astrocyte and these node–astrocyte relations may be specific to such borderline nodes. In some myelinated fibres, however, the central–peripheral transition occurs at an internode, the central myelin being telescoped within an external peripheral myelin sheath. Considerable rearrangement of axons occurs in the rootlets; moreover, many of the largest non-myelinated axons are invested with a thin myelin sheath as they traverse the TR.

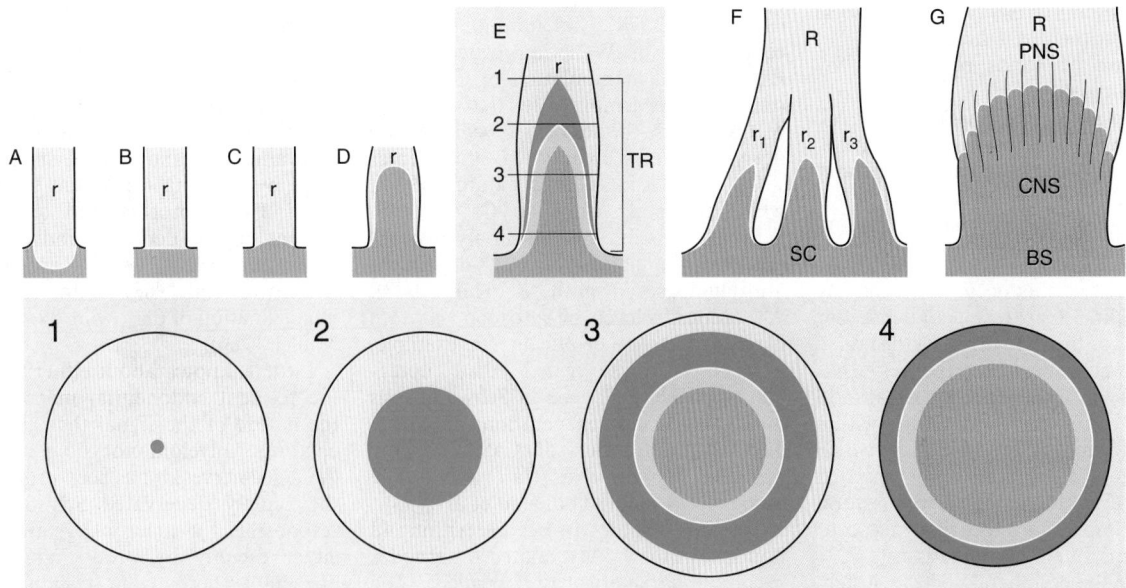

8.63 Schematic representation of the nerve root–spinal cord junction. A to E, Different CNS-PNS borderline arrangements, A, Concave borderline (*white line*) and inverted TR. B, Flat borderline situated at the level of the rootlet (r)–spinal cord junction. C and D, Convex, dome-shaped borderline; the CNS expansion into the rootlet is moderate in C and extensive in D. Brown denotes CNS tissue. The glial fringe is not shown, E, Pointed borderline. The extent of the transitional zone (TR) is indicated. The cross-sectional appearance at four different TR levels (*A, B, C,* and *D*) and the distribution of the different TR zones are shown in the lower part of the illustration. Yellow = endoneurial zone; dark green =glial fringe; light green = mantle zone; brown = core zone. F, Root–spinal cord junction. The root (R) splits into rootlets (r), each with its own TR and attaching separately to the spinal cord (SC). G, Arrangement noted in several cranial nerve roots (e.g., accoustic nerve). The PNS component of the root separates into a bundle of closely packed minirootlets, each equipped with a TR. The minirootlets reunite centrally. BS = brain stem.

Regeneration of axons in the peripheral nervous system

When a mammalian peripheral nerve is crushed or transected, all of the fibres distal to the injury, both myelinated and non-myelinated, undergo Wallerian degeneration. Since Waller's description of the phenomenon in 1850, the spatio-temporal sequence of cellular changes that occur within a nerve during the injury response has been extensively documented; more recently, the techniques of molecular biology and molecular genetics have begun to reveal the molecular basis of these changes.

Responses that occur within the neuronal cell body after axotomy and factors determining the specificity of re-innervation are both outside the scope of this essay: the reader is directed to Lieberman (1971); Sunderland (1978); Fawcett and Keynes (1990).

The major events that may occur within a nerve fascicle after injury may be summarized as follows:

- axonal fragmentation and myelinolysis
- recruitment of haematogenously derived myelomonocytic cells into the endoneurium
- invasion of Schwann cell basal lamina tubes by macrophages which remove the cellular debris
- Schwann cell gliosis at the tip of the proximal stump and throughout the distal stump
- axonal sprouting and outgrowth of axons and Schwann cells from the proximal stump
- formation of bands of Büngner (columns of quiescent Schwann cells disposed within basal lamina tubes) throughout the distal stumps
- penetration of bands of Büngner by regenerating axons
- establishment of axon–Schwann cell relationships and onset of myelination, in a proximo distal sequence throughout the distal stump
- re-innervation of target structures and restitution of function.

The first six events occur constitutively during the first 2 or 3 weeks after injury irrespective of the type of injury sustained by the nerve (i.e. whether the nerve has been crushed, when the proximal and distal stumps remain in continuity within the perineurium, or transected, in which case the stumps are inevitably separated by a gap). Clearly, axonal recolonization of distal stumps is far more likely to occur after crush than after transection.

Repair in the peripheral nervous system involves two sequential but overlapping processes; an acute 'wound healing' phase, and a chronic phase when axons seek out their targets. The cascade of molecular and cellular events which take place at the lesion site is very similar to those which occur in other tissues after damage. At the same time, axonal outgrowth from the proximal stump begins: this will continue long after the initial wound has healed, and may ultimately prove unsuccessful. For example, in clinical practice injuries may involve soft tissue damage, often in association with severe contusion of the nerve stumps; loss of tissue, resulting in long gaps between nerve ends; foreign body contamination and infection, particularly when the injury has been produced by shot gun or high velocity rounds. Moreover, distances to be regrown (whether across an interstump gap or within a distal stump) may be many centimetres long; chronically denervated Schwann cells may be unable to respond to ingrowing axons when they finally arrive. In humans, therefore, functional recovery may be disappointing (Sunderland 1978). What follows is a brief account of what is currently known about repair of damaged peripheral nerve fibres in laboratory animals: there is no reason to believe that the basic response to injury is significantly different in humans.

Early changes

One of the earliest morphological changes that occurs after transection or crush is a disintegration of the axonal cytoskeleton throughout the distal stump and at the extreme distal tip of the proximal stump. This is probably mediated by an influx of Ca^{2+} into the severed axons, activating Ca^{2+}-dependent proteases which are responsible for the disruption of axoplasmic microtubules and neurofilaments (Schlaepfer 1974). Calcium ions play a central role in Wallerian degeneration. Experimental manipulation of Ca^{2+} concentration has demonstrated that exclusion of Ca^{2+} from the lesion site significantly delays axonal breakdown (Schlaepfer 1979; de Medinacelli & Church 1984), while increasing cytosolic Ca^{2+} within Schwann cells initiates myelinolysis probably via the action of Ca^{2+}-dependent phospholipases (Smith & Hall 1988). Alterations in levels of cytosolic Ca^{2+} are likely to have other effects: for example, it has been suggested that upregulation of NGF-R gene in Schwann cells during Wallerian degeneration is a consequence of an influx of Ca^{2+}, possibly mediated by the Na^+/Ca^{2+} membrane exchanger protein (Thomson et al 1993).

Myelin breakdown begins within 48 hours of injury. Myelinated internodes become characteristically beaded. The beads (myelin 'ovoids') are subsequently degraded into fragments of lamellar debris and droplets of neutral lipid which are sequestered by phagocytosis within intratubal cells. In vivo, myelin breakdown begins within the Schwann cell, before the appearance of exogenous macrophages (Stoll et al 1989), perhaps as a result of the activation of Schwann cell-derived Ca^{2+}-dependent phospholipase A_2 (PLA2) (Paul & Gregson 1992). However, recruited macrophages appear to be responsible for the bulk of myelin degradation and removal and for the substantial increase in the levels of PLA2 detected in distal stumps during the first week of Wallerian degeneration (Trotter & Smith 1986).

Role of macrophages

Many of the intratubal debris-laden cells seen within the Schwann cell basal lamina tubes during the first 2 weeks after injury are recruited macrophages. These cells subsequently leave the basal lamina tubes and slowly disappear from the endoneurium, although some lipid-laden foamy macrophages persist within the endoneurium for several months after injury. Experimental manipulation of macrophage numbers during Wallerian degeneration has demonstrated that these cells are essential components of the injury response (Beuche & Friede 1984; 1988; Lunn et al 1989). It is well known that during wound repair in other tissues, macrophages release a wide variety of biologically active substances which facilitate the recruitment of additional inflammatory cells; augment macrophage-mediated tissue debridement; increase the expression of genes implicated in extracellular matrix formation; and stimulate angiogenesis (ten Dijke & Iwata 1989). In addition to these general functions, activated macrophages which enter the growing end of the proximal stump and ramify throughout the distal stump may also have 'tissue-specific' functions. There is evidence that they may stimulate Schwann cells and fibroblasts to secrete NGF by releasing interleukin-1 (Heumann et al 1987); process and subsequently present myelin-derived products to the Schwann cells, either as mitogens (Baichwal et al 1988), or for reutilization in myelination of regrowing axons (Stoll & Muller 1986).

Little is known about either the role of the resident endoneurial macrophage or the nature of the signal that attracts circulating myelomonocytic cells into damaged nerves. It has been proposed that the acutely denervated Schwann cell is responsible for macrophage recruitment, either directly by producing a chemoattractant (perhaps in response to loss of axonal contact), and/or indirectly, by initiating myelin breakdown (Hall 1993).

Schwann cell proliferation

The number of cells within the endoneurium rises dramatically during the first 2 postoperative weeks. This increase is due in part to proliferation of endogenous Schwann cells, fibroblasts and endothelial cells, and in part to the rapid recruitment of exogenous myelomonocytic cells. Schwann cells begin to divide 3–4 days after injury. The factors that regulate Schwann cell proliferation during nerve regeneration have not been established. Schwann cells may respond initially to mitogens derived from myelin or axonal debris (Baichwal et al 1988); or to cytokines such as TGFβ_1 present at the wound site (Ridley et al 1989). Later, as the Schwann cells migrate out of the nerve stumps, they may continue to divide in response to elevated levels of fibronectin in the wound site (Lefcort et al 1992) or to a neuronally derived mitogen (Ratner et al 1989) as they interact with regrowing axons. Recently several glial growth factors (GGF), members of the neuregulin family, have been identified and shown to be Schwann cell mitogens at least in vitro (Marchionni et al 1993). It has been suggested that GGF stimulate Schwann cell division by activating a tyrosine kinase receptor encoded by the proto-oncogene *neu/erbB2*. [The neu oncogene encodes a 185kD tyrosine kinase receptor, p185^{erbB2}, which is expressed in the peripheral nervous system on the Schwann cell surface.] Neuregulin transcripts are expressed in both motor and sensory systems during development, but are downregulated in the adult nerve (Mudge 1993). It may be significant that neu is expressed at high levels after injury in the nervous system; a finding which is consistent with a role for neu and GGF in peripheral nervous system regeneration (Cohen et al 1992).

Regenerating axons do not immediately enter the microenvironment of a distal stump unless the two ends of the nerve remain in continuity. Instead, they grow out from the proximal stump accompanied by newly generated Schwann cells and perineurial-like cells in small bundles (minifascicles). This exodus of Schwann cells and axons may be facilitated by the upregulation of the fibronectin receptor $\alpha_5\beta_1$ on both Schwann cells and regenerating axons after transection, and the concomitant increase in expression of fibronectin that occurs within the wound region (Komiyama et al 1991; Lefcort et al 1992). Schwann cells appear to be essential: if Schwann cells are prevented from migrating with the axons then significant axonal outgrowth does not occur (Hall 1986).

The distal stump

Regenerating axons exhibit directed growth towards the distal stump (providing the interstump gap is no more than 1–1·5 cm long), presumably responding to diffusable tropic factors released from cells within the stump and from cells which grow out from the stump. The powerful neurotropic and neurotrophic influence that the distal stump exercises over regrowing axons (Politis et al 1982; Scaravilli 1984) is thought to be primarily a function of the Schwann cell. Schwann cells are a major source of neurotrophic factors such as the neurotrophins NGF and BDNF, and CNTF (Korsching 1993). Although levels of BDNFmRNA and NGFmRNA are barely detectable in normal nerve, there is a significant upregulation of expression of both factors after axotomy and final levels of BDNF are up to ten times higher than those of NGF (Meyer et al 1992). Levels of CNTF, which are high in normal myelinating Schwann cells, fall dramatically in the distal stump of a transected nerve (Friedman et al 1992): since CNTF lacks a signal sequence and is not normally secreted, it has been suggested that CNTF acts as a 'lesion factor' released by injured Schwann cells and presented to axons (Thoenen 1991; Curtis et al 1993).

The Schwann cells generated during post-traumatic gliosis display a molecular phenotype which resembles that of the normal adult non-myelinating cell: NGF-R, GAP-43, GFAP, L1 and N-CAM genes are upregulated in Schwann cells throughout the distal stump, while the myelin protein genes are profoundly downregulated until the onset of myelination (Tacke & Martini 1990; Thomson et al 1993). The reappearance and upregulation of molecules which are thought to mediate functionally important axon–glial interactions during development is consistent with the pivotal role that Schwann cells play during axonal regeneration (e.g. Johnson et al 1988). Schwann cells not only produce neurotrophic factors (see above) but also provide molecular cues which are known to facilitate axonal elongation, either directly by surface expression (e.g. L1, N-CAM, NGF-R), or indirectly by insertion into their basal laminae (e.g. laminin, tenascin).

If axons fail to reach the distal stump, or are delayed for several months, then the Schwann cells lying within chronically denervated bands of Büngner do not continue to divide but soon become quiescent, and may ultimately disappear. The implications for the repair of human nerve, particularly for secondary repair, are obvious.

Clearly, regenerating axons in the peripheral nervous system, whether growing out from the proximal stumps in association with their comigrating Schwann cells, or entering bands of Büngner in the distal stumps, encounter an appropriate substrate upon which to grow. In the central nervous system, the microenvironment of a traumatized axon does not usually permit its regeneration. However, many central nervous system axons will regrow into grafts of vital peripheral nerves, presumably responding to the favourable environment provided by the Schwann cells contained therein (Benfey & Aguayo 1982).

PERIPHERAL ENDINGS OF EFFECTOR NEURONS

Of the various types of effector endings the most intensively studied are those which innervate muscle, particularly the skeletal variety. All such *neuromuscular* or *myoneural junctions* are regions of neuronal cytoplasm specialized for the release of neurotransmitter on to surfaces of adjacent muscle fibres, causing a change in their electrical state leading to contraction. Because of their similarity to central nervous synapses and the relative ease with which functional studies can be carried out on them, much of our general knowledge of neurotransmission comes from the ultrastructural, physiological, biochemical and pharmacological analysis of neuromuscular junctions rather than central synapses.

In addition to their innervation of muscle, effector neurons also have terminals in or near other cells capable of various types of activity, for example glands (secretomotor endings), myoepithelial cells and adipose tissue. It has been proposed on the basis of experimental evidence that nerve fibres may also contribute to the regulation of immune responses (p. 1430), by their effects on T-lymphocyte maturation in the thymus, and to many other poorly understood activities of tissues not classically considered to be under nervous control. The hormonal contribution of neuro-endocrine cells has, of course, long been known, but more subtle neural effects elsewhere may play a major role in the maintenance of homeostasis in many other sites in the body.

NEUROMUSCULAR JUNCTIONS OF SKELETAL MUSCLE

The general structure of these has already been outlined on page 752. The terminals are end branches of somatic motor fibres, each innervating from a few to many hundreds of muscle fibres, a numerical relationship determining the precision of motor control. The precise structure of a motor terminal varies with the type of muscle innervated. Two major endings are recognized: 'en plaque' terminals typical of extrafusal muscle fibres and *plate endings* of intrafusal fibres, the latter including 'en grappe' terminals of extra-ocular muscle fibres and 'trail' endings on intrafusal fibres (Harker 1972; Barker 1974). In the first type each axonal terminal (*telodendron*) usually ends midway along a muscle fibre in a discoidal *motor end plate* (**8.64–66**). In the second type, the axon has numerous subsidiary branches forming a cluster of small expansions extending along the muscle fibre (**8.64**). *En plaque* endings usually initiate action potentials which are rapidly conducted to all parts of muscle fibres, whereas *en grappe* endings, in the absence of propagated muscle excitation, excite the fibre at several points. Both types have a specialized region, the *sole plate*, in which a number of muscle cell nuclei are grouped within the granular sarcoplasm. Ultrastructurally the sole plate contains numerous mitochondria, endoplasmic reticulum and Golgi complexes (**8.65, 66**). The neuronal terminal branches are received into shallow grooves in the surface of the sole plate (primary clefts), from which numerous pleats extend for a short distance into the underlying sarcoplasm (secondary clefts); the axon terminal contains mitochondria and many clear 60 nm spherical vesicles like those in presynaptic boutons, clustered against the membrane over the zone of apposition. Ensheathing the motor terminal are Schwann cells (*teloglia*), with cytoplasmic projections extending into the synaptic cleft. The membranes of the nerve terminal and the muscle cell are separated by a 30–50 nm gap, with a basal lamina interposed; the basal lamina follows the surface folding of the sole plate membrane into the secondary clefts; various adhesion molecules synthesized by both participating cells are present here.

En plaque endings of 'fast' and 'slow' twitch muscle fibres differ in details, the sarcolemmal grooves being deeper and the presynaptic vesicles more numerous in the former (Padykula & Gauthier 1970). Freeze-fracture studies show numerous intramembranous particles, which represent the ACh receptors, in the crests of the sarcolemmal folds nearest to presynaptic membrane (Heuser et al 1974). Opposite these the axon membrane is slightly invaginated and vesicles cluster along borders of the groove so formed, probably the main site of their release (cf. the 'active zone' of synapses). Microtubular arrays bearing synaptic vesicles, as in central synapses, have also been described (Gray 1978).

Physiological and pharmacological studies (Katz & Miledi 1965) show that junctions with skeletal muscle are *cholinergic*, the release of ACh changing the ionic permeability of the muscle fibre. The earliest change occurring after neurotransmitter release is a *graded potential*; when the depolarization of the sarcolemma reaches a particular threshold, it initiates an all-or-none action potential in the sarcolemma, which is then propagated rapidly over the whole cell surface and also within its substance via the invaginations (transverse tubules) of the sarcolemma (see p. 749), causing contraction. The amount of ACh released by the arrival of a single nerve impulse is sufficient to trigger an action potential; however, because ACh is very rapidly hydrolysed by the enzyme *acetylcholinesterase* (AChE) present at the sarcolemmal surface of the sole plate, a single nerve impulse only gives rise to one muscle action potential, so that there is a one-to-one relationship between neural and muscle action potentials. Thus the contraction of a muscle fibre is controlled by the firing frequency of its motor neuron. However, even in quiescent muscle fibres, sporadic depolarizations continually occur (*miniature end plate potentials*), although too small to cause contraction. Their measured amplitudes occur at a series of preferential levels, indicating that multiples of *quanta* of transmitter are released even in resting stages, presumably a process of slow leakage. The amount of ACh necessary to cause these unitary changes is calculated to be equivalent to the volume of a single synaptic vesicle (Katz & Miledi 1965).

AChE can be shown cytochemically to be present in myoneural clefts. Experiments with specialized motor endings in electric organs of the Electric Ray *Torpedo* locate the enzyme to the sarcolemma near the sites of action. The neurotransmitter can be blocked by *curare*, by a sea-snake venom α-bungarotoxin, by black widow spider venom and various other toxins, all combining irreversibly with the nicotinic ACh receptor molecules to paralyse the neuromuscular junctions (Miledi et al 1971). If acetylcholinesterase is inhibited, e.g. by *eserine* (*physostigmine*), transmitter action is cumulative and tetanus may ensue. Neuromuscular junctions are partially blocked by high concentrations of lactic acid, as in some types of muscle

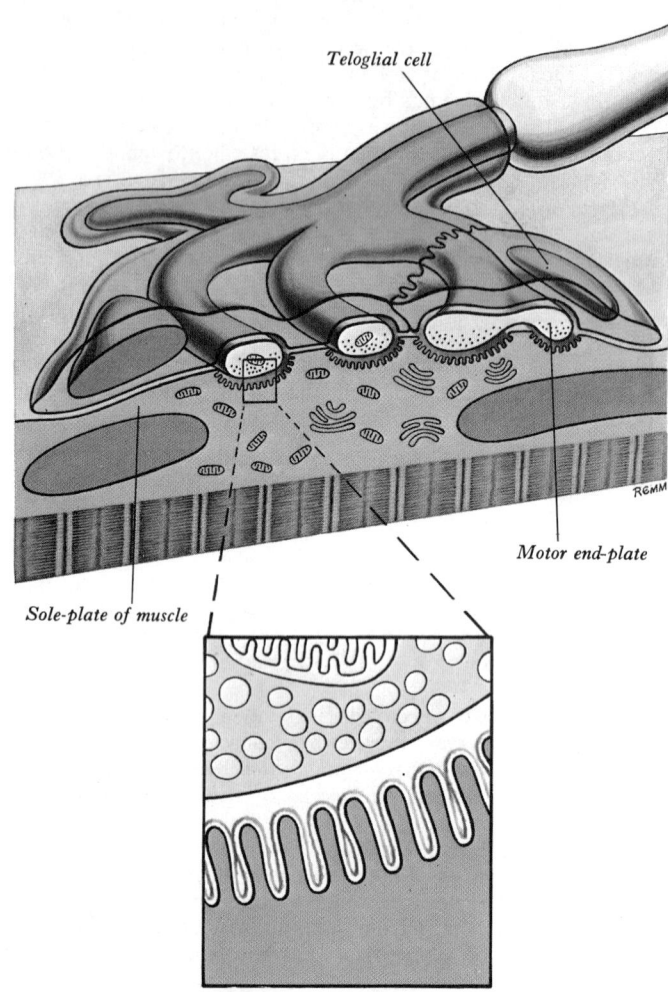

Teloglial cell

Motor end-plate

Sole-plate of muscle

8.64 Diagram showing some types of innervation of striated muscle, including the 'en plaque' terminals of α efferents (below), and the more widely spread 'trail' and 'en grappe' endings of γ efferents (above).

8.65 Diagram of the detailed structure of an 'en plaque' neuromuscular junction. An enlarged portion of the terminal is shown below; note the folding of the sarcolemma to form subsynaptic gutters, the disposition of the basal lamina and synaptic vesicles within the axon terminal.

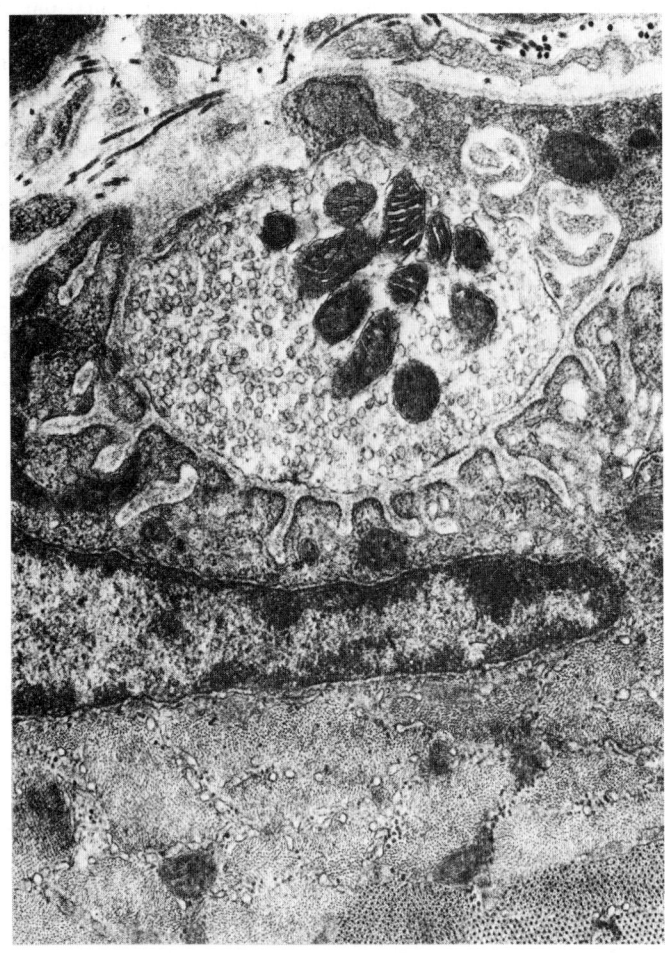

8.66 Electron micrograph of a neuromuscular junction in striated muscle, showing part of a motor end-plate containing synaptic vesicles (above). The latter is situated in a groove in the sarcolemma; this is further convoluted to form the subsynaptic gutters of the sole-plate (below). (Provided by D N Landon, Neurobiological Unit, National Hospital for Nervous Diseases, London.)

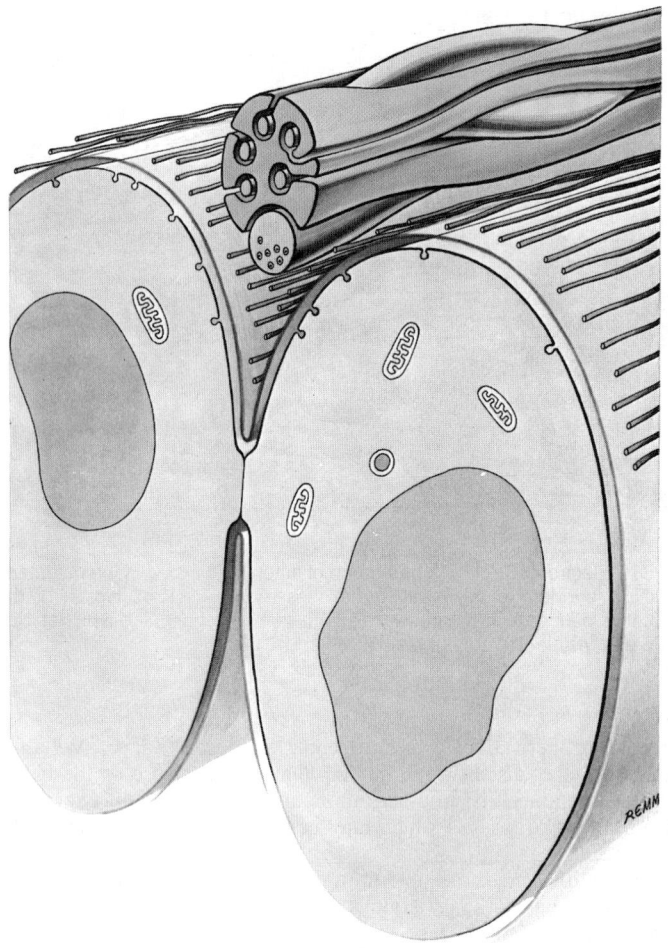

8.67 Diagram of an autonomic neuromuscular junction between a group of non-myelinated axons (above) and smooth muscle cells (below). The Schwann cell (blue) is reflected at intervals to expose enlargements of the axons (yellow) which contain synaptic vesicles.

fatigue (Miledi et al 1971). Clustering of ACh receptors at the neuromuscular junction depends on (amongst other factors) the presence of an extracellular protein, agrin, synthesized by the motor neuron, which induces changes in the cytoskeletal attachments to the ACh receptor molecules within the muscle cell, preventing their lateral diffusion out of the junction (see Nastuk & Fallon 1993). For further review of structure see Duchen & Gale 1985.

AUTONOMIC MOTOR TERMINATIONS

Unlike those in skeletal muscle, autonomic terminals are not usually closely applied to smooth myocytes but end at variable distances from their surfaces (Richardson 1962). Non-myelinated autonomic axons branch into tapering, varicose collaterals (**8.67**). At the zone of transmission, clusters of synaptic vesicles exist in expanded regions of axoplasm and the Schwann cell is retracted to leave the axon in a shallow groove, providing a path of diffusion between axon and myocytes. In *sympathetic fibres* the vesicles are usually *dense-cored* (p. 930), and correspond in position to the characteristic fluorescence of catecholamines seen when preparations fixed in formalin vapour are viewed with ultraviolet light (Falck & Owman 1965), or to the positive reaction to the glyoxylic acid method. Besides noradrenaline, they contain enzymes involved in catecholamine synthesis and degradation. Other vesicles, 100 µm across, often also occur.

Noradrenaline is the usual transmitter at sympathetic postganglionic endings while *adrenaline* occurs in some of the *chromaffin cells* of the adrenal glands. Synaptic vesicles containing each catecholamine can be distinguished by electron microscopy. Catecholamines can be released experimentally be treatment with the drug *reserpine*, which is a valuable research tool and also clinically useful. After release some of the transmitter is reabsorbed into the axon by endocytosis and may be re-used, or broken down. Sympathetic endings contain *monoamine oxidases* degrading catecholamines, the control of these enzymes being important in the clinical regulation of sympathetic function both in the peripheral and central nervous systems.

At *parasympathetic* endings are clear spherical vesicles, like those in motor end plates of striated muscle. Much evidence indicates that they are *cholinergic*; similar terminals also occur in sympathetic endings. In addition to their action on non-nervous tissues, some cholinergic endings may perhaps cause the release of catecholamines from neighbouring sympathetic endings.

A third category of autonomic neurons differing from noradrenergic or cholinergic cells has been described by Burnstock and colleagues (Burnstock 1975). These can be described as 'non-adrenergic, non-cholinergic endings', and are now recognized to contain a wide variety of chemicals with transmitter properties (see Burnstock 1986), contained within vesicles of different forms. The conjugated purine adenosine triphosphate (ATP; a nucleoside), probably the neurotransmitter at these terminals, is classed as *purinergic*. Typically, their axons contain large, dense vesicles 80–200 nm across ('*large opaque vesicles*'), congregated in varicosities at intervals along nerve fibres (**8.68**). Such fibres occur in many sites in mammals, including the alimentary external muscle layers and sphincters, lungs, vascular walls, urogenital tract and central nervous system. In the intestinal wall their neuronal cell bodies lie in the myenteric plexus, their axons spreading caudally for a few millimetres, chiefly to innervate circular muscle. Purinergic neurons are under cholinergic control from preganglionic sympathetic neurons. Purinergic endings mainly hyperpolarize myocytes, causing their relaxation, for example

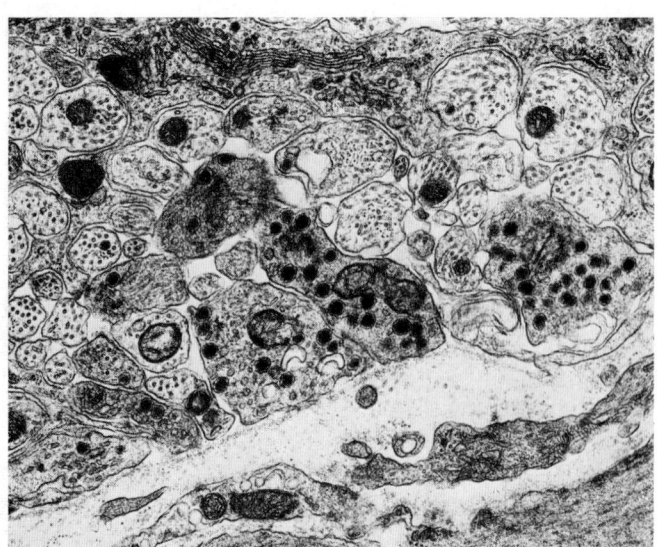

8.68 Electron micrograph of a group of autonomic axons in the myenteric plexus, showing profiles with large dense-cored vesicles typical of the putative purinergic system (see text); smaller, catecholamine-type vesicles are also visible (lower left). Magnification ×40 000.

preceding peristaltic waves, opening sphincters and, probably, causing reflex distension in gastric filling. The release of the transmitter resembles that in other autonomic endings, i.e. by exocytosis from axon varicosities which may be up to 100 nm away from the target cell.

In addition to these ubiquitous neurotransmitters, many others are released in different regions of the body; serotonin, substance P(SP), somatostatin, vasoactive intestinal polypeptide (VIP), calcitonin-related gene product (CRGP) and nitric oxide. These chemicals or related enzyme systems can be demonstrated by immunohistochemistry and by pharmacology.

The pattern of terminal branching of autonomic efferents is related to their effects (Burnstock 1970). In smooth muscles with a slow widespread action, a single neuron may innervate a large number of myocytes, the distance between synaptic varicosities and myocytes being large (50 nm or more). In rapid smooth muscle, with greater precision of control, for example the iris or ductus deferens, innervation is more localized, with less branching and close apposition to myocyte surfaces (15–20 nm), the ending sometimes being invaginated into the sarcolemma (Burnstock 1975). Other tissues innervated by autonomic efferents include glands, myoepitheliocytes, adipose and lymphoid tissue.

PERIPHERAL ENDINGS OF SENSORY NEURONS

GENERAL FEATURES OF SENSORY RECEPTORS

As frequently stated, an organism's reaction to changes in its environment requires the presence of suitable receptors to scan the parameters important to survival. Though single-celled organisms such as protozoa have no such specialization, they can detect changes in temperature, osmotic pressure, concentrations, light and other environmental properties by means of the specialized components of their membranes. In more elaborate animals these fluctuations are recorded by cells which have differentiated to respond selectively and with great precision. Such cells are sensory receptors; they take many forms but in mammals, with minor exceptions, they have a common pattern which will be outlined below.

Sense organs have three major forms, according to the relation of the nervous system to the receptor cells. In *neuroepithelial receptors* the receptors are neurons with somata situated peripherally near a sensory surface and axons extending into the central nervous system to connect with second order neurons. The only example of this type

in mammals is the sensory cell of the olfactory epithelium but in many invertebrates it is the main type and can thus be regarded as phylogenetically primitive. Secondly, the sensory cell may be an *epithelial receptor*, modified from the cells of a non-nervous sensory epithelium and innervated by a primary sensory neuron, the soma of which lies near the central nervous system. Activity in this type of receptor causes the passage of excitation from the receptor by neurotransmission across a synaptic gap; examples are gustatory and auditory receptors. In gustatory receptors individual cells are constantly being renewed from the surrounding epithelium, as may also occur in other similar sensory systems (p. 1314). Visual receptors are in many ways similar in their form and relations, formed from the ventricular lining in the fetal brain, although no replacement occurs. Thirdly, a *neuronal receptor* is a primary sensory neuron, with a soma in a craniospinal ganglion and a peripheral axon whose end is the sensory terminal. All cutaneous sensors and proprioceptors are probably of this type, but the sensory terminals may be encapsulated or linked to special mesodermal or ectodermal elements forming a part of the sensory apparatus. These extraneural cells are not necessarily excitable, but rather create the right environment for the excitation of the neuronal dendrite or modify its excitation in some way.

Receptor responses

The events which occur between the incidence of a stimulus and the conduction of an electrical signal to the CNS have been extensively studied (e.g. Granit 1962), although much remains to be understood. It is convenient to divide these processes into a number of stages: first the preservation of an effective stimulus, then the transduction of the stimulus at the receptor surface into a graded change of electrical potential (*receptor potential*) and next the initiation of an all-or-none action potential passing to the CNS. All of these processes may occur in the receptor, where this is a neuron, or some may occur partly in the receptor and partly in the neuron innervating it, in the case of epithelial receptors.

Transduction varies with the modality of stimulus, but in all receptors there is a stimulus-induced change in permeability of the receptor membrane to certain ions, usually causing its depolarization (or, in the retina, hyperpolarization). How a stimulus effects this is uncertain. In mechanoreceptors it may involve the deformation of membrane structure perhaps with strain- or voltage-sensitive transducing protein molecules opening ion channels as a result; in chemoreceptors, receptor action may resemble that postulated for ACh at neuromuscular junctions (p. 958), involving receptor proteins altered by binding stimulant molecules, again with the opening of ionic channels. Visual receptors appear to resemble chemoreceptors in many respects; light causes changes in receptor proteins (p. 1343) which may cause the release of *second messengers* to affect membrane permeability.

Osmoreceptors may resemble mechanoreceptors but react instead to mechanical deformation from osmotic inflow or outflow of water. In some fishes a remarkable type of transduction occurs in electroreceptors, capable of sensing changes in electric fields set up by the animal's own bioelectric processes or those of other individuals or prey (Lissmann & Machin 1958). So far, no sensory mechanism of this type has been reported in humans.

The quantitative responses of sensory endings to stimuli vary greatly and give added flexibility to the functional design of sensory systems. Although increase of excitation with the increase of a stimulus level is a common pattern ('on' response) some receptors respond to decrease in stimulus (the '*off*' response). Even unstimulated receptors show varying spontaneous activity, against the background of which an increase or decrease in activity occurs with changing levels of stimulus. When stimulation is maintained at a steady level, there is, in all receptors studied, an initial burst (the *dynamic phase*) followed by a gradual *adaptation* to steady level (the *static phase*). Though all receptors show these two phases, one or other may predominate, giving a distinction between *rapidly-adapting* endings accurately recording the *rate* of stimulus onset and *slowly-adapting* endings which signal the constant amplitude of a stimulus, for example the position sense. Dynamic and static phases are reflected in the *amplitude* and *duration* of the generator or sensory potential and also in the *frequency* of action potentials in the sensory fibres. The stimulus strength necessary to elicit a response in a receptor (i.e. its *threshold level*) varies greatly between receptors, providing an extra level of information about stimulus strength.

Functional classification of receptors

Receptors are classified in several ways; for example, by the specific energy forms or '*modalities*' to which they are especially sensitive, such as *mechanoreceptors* responsive to deformation (touch, pressure, sound waves, etc.), *chemoreceptors*, *photoreceptors*, *thermoreceptors* and *osmoreceptors* (reacting to osmotic pressure changes). Some receptors respond selectively to more than one modality (*polymodal receptors*), usually having high thresholds and responding to damaging stimuli, associated with irritation or pain (i.e. *nociceptors*).

Another widely used, though somewhat arbitrary classification divides receptors on the basis of their distribution in the body and their role in its sensory activities into *exteroceptors*, *proprioceptors* and *interoceptors*. Exteroceptors and proprioceptors are receptors of somatic afferent components of the nervous system; interoceptors are receptors of the visceral afferent pathways.

Exteroceptors. These respond to external stimuli and are at or close to surfaces (Sinclair 1967). They can be subdivided into the *general* or *cutaneous sense organs* and *special sensory organs*. The general sensory receptors include the 'free' and the encapsulated terminals in skin and near hairs; special sensory organs are the olfactory, visual, acoustic, vestibular and gustatory receptors.

Proprioceptors. They respond to stimuli *proper* to deeper tissues, especially of the locomotor system, and are concerned with detecting movement, mechanical stresses and position; they include the neuro-tendinous organs of Golgi, neuromuscular spindles, Pacinian corpuscles, other endings in joints and vestibular receptors. Proprioceptors are stimulated by the contraction of muscles, movements of joints and changes in the position of the body or of its parts; they are essential to the co-ordination of muscles, the grading of muscular contraction and maintenance of equilibrium.

Interoceptors. Included in these are receptors in the walls of the viscera, glands and vessels, where their terminations include 'free' nerve endings, encapsulated terminals and endings associated with specialized epithelial cells. Nerve terminals occur in all the layers of visceral walls and are numerous in the adventitia of blood vessels; the functional nature of many of these endings, and indeed their detailed structure in many cases, is not well established. Encapsulated (lamellated) endings occur in the heart, adventitia, pancreas and mesenteries; 'free' terminal arborizations also occur in the endocardium, loose connective tissue, the endomysium of all muscles and connective tissue generally.

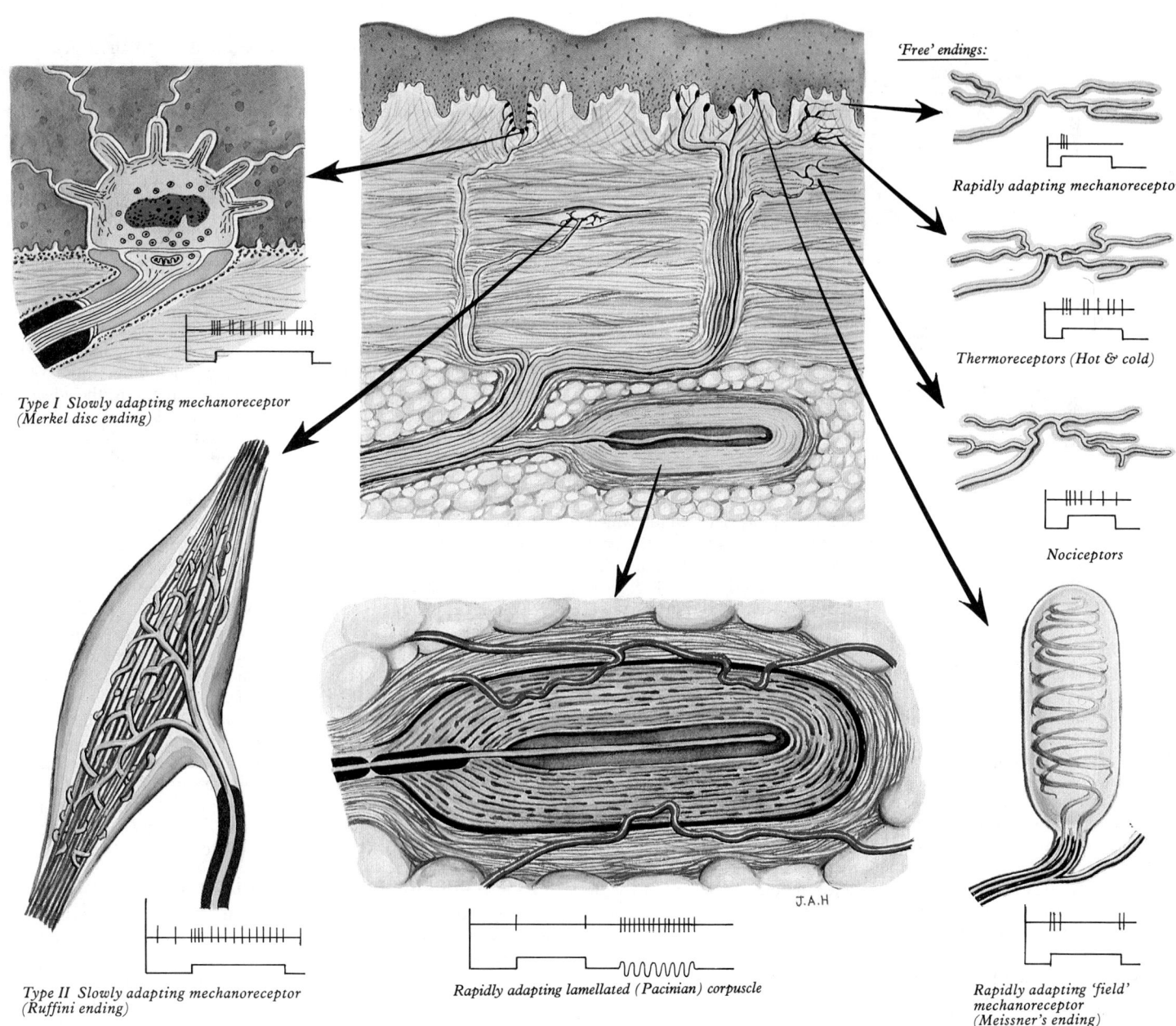

Free' endings:

Rapidly adapting mechanoreceptor

Thermoreceptors (Hot & cold)

Nociceptors

Type I Slowly adapting mechanoreceptor (Merkel disc ending)

Type II Slowly adapting mechanoreceptor (Ruffini ending)

Rapidly adapting lamellated (Pacinian) corpuscle

Rapidly adapting 'field' mechanoreceptor (Meissner's ending)

J.A.H

8.69   Some major types of sensory endings of general afferent fibres (omitting neuromuscular, neurotendinous and hair-related types).

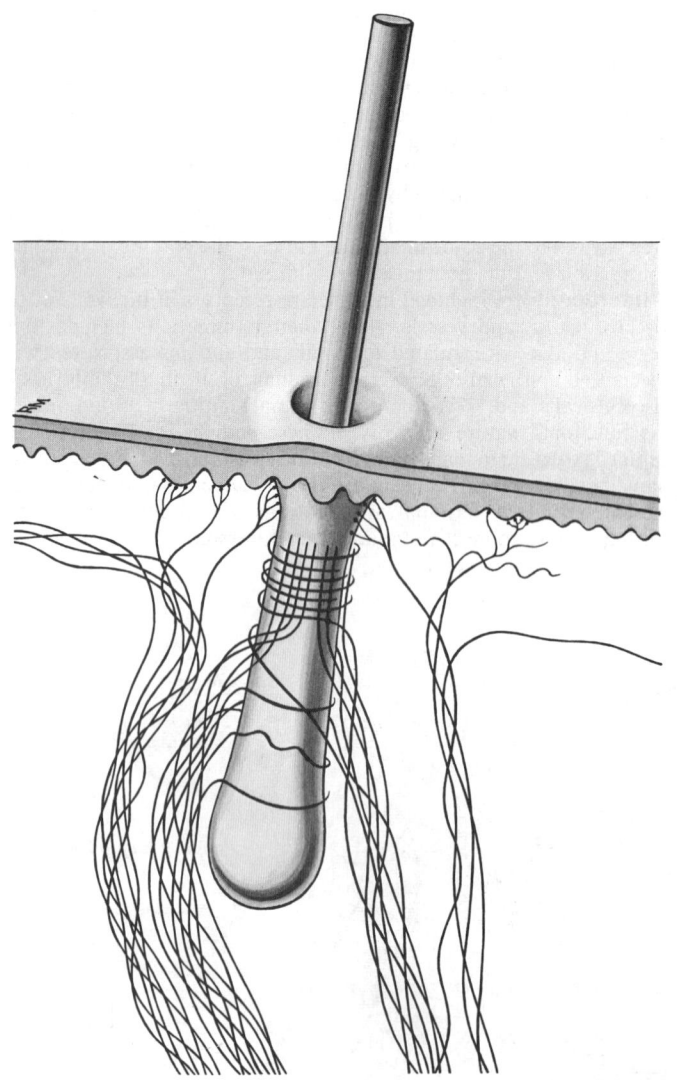

8.70 The innervation of a large hair follicle; fine and coarse axons terminate around the intermediate and superficial regions, some branching in a circular direction and others pursuing a longitudinal course. Nerve terminals associated with Merkel's cells are also shown surrounding the neck of the follicle.

Visceral nerve terminals are not usually responsive to stimuli which act on exteroceptors and do not respond to localized mechanical and thermal stimuli. But tension produced by excessive muscular contraction often causes visceral pain, particularly in pathological states, which is frequently poorly localized and of the deep-seated variety.

Interoceptors include vascular chemoreceptors and baroceptors concerned in the regulation of blood flow and pressure and in the control of respiration.

Irritant receptors responding polymodally to noxious chemicals or damaging mechanical stimuli are widely distributed in the epithelia of the alimentary and respiratory tracts and they may initiate protective reflexes.

Summary. This scheme of classification may seem arbitrary, since many *structural* types of end-organ occur in all three classes and their activities may be closely linked in the central nervous system. For convenience, therefore, the structural classification is followed here. But this in turn is arbitrary since in some cases endings with similar structure may be physiologically distinct and a functional classification may be regarded as of deeper significance.

STRUCTURAL CLASSIFICATION OF GENERAL SENSORY ENDINGS

In addition to the division of receptors into functional categories, the receptors (apart from those of the special senses) can be grouped by structural features on morphological grounds (**8.**69–77). How

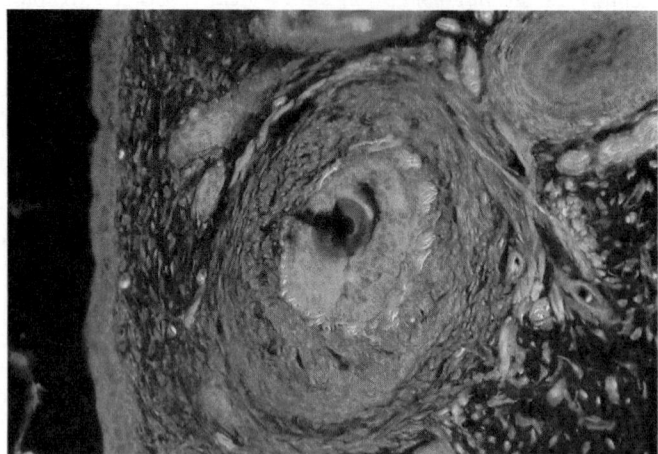

8.71 Sensory endings around a hair follicle, in transverse section. The axon terminals have been demonstrated by immunofluorescence using an antibody directed against neurofilaments (yellow). Magnification ×250. (Material provided by Samantha Negus, UMDS, Guy's Campus, London.)

much functional significance can be attached to these features is debatable. Factors which complicate this issue include variations in receptor structure linked with ageing, regeneration, local topography and with species differences. The terminology is further confused by a lack of agreement on the structural definition of many sensory endings. Some receptors are limited to one tissue or combination of tissues; others occur in many sites. Generally, one may distinguish between *free nerve endings* which form plexuses or spread without any particular association with other types of cell, *encapsulated endings* where groups of specialized non-nervous cells invest neural process, and *epidermal endings*, where sensory fibres are attached to specific non-nervous cells or tissues (Bannister 1976).

Free nerve endings

Sensory endings, branching to form plexuses, occur in many sites. They are found in all connective tissues including: those of the dermis, fasciae, capsules of organs, ligaments, tendons, the adventitia of blood vessels, meninges, articular capsules, periosteum, perichondrium, Haversian systems, parietal peritoneum, the visceral wall and endomysial spaces of all types of muscle. They also innervate the epithelium of the skin, cornea, buccal cavity, and alimentary and respiratory tracts and their glands, though within epithelia they are devoid of Schwann cells and are enveloped instead by epitheliocytes (and so are perhaps not 'free' endings, see Cauna 1966).

Afferent fibres from free terminals are either myelinated or non-myelinated but are always of small diameter and low conduction velocity, belonging to group III (Aδ) or IV (C) (p. 948). Where afferent axons are myelinated, their terminal arborizations are not and are probably devoid of Schwann cells at their ends. Electrophysiological recordings show that such terminals serve several sensory modalities. In the dermis, some are responsive to moderate cold or heat (*thermoreceptors*), to light mechanical touch (*mechanoreceptors*), to damaging heat, cold or deformation (*unimodal nociceptors*), or to damaging stimuli of several kinds (*polymodal nociceptors*). Similar fibres in deeper tissues may also signal extreme conditions, experienced, as with all nociceptors, as pain. Free endings in the cornea, dentine and periosteum may be exclusively nociceptor in function (see also Kruger 1987 and below, Dermal receptors).

Special endings associated with epidermal structures

Terminals associated with hair follicles are those of myelinated fibres in the deep dermal cutaneous plexus; the number, size and form of the endings are related to the size and type of hair follicle innervated (Cauna 1966). In *lanceolate* or *palisade endings* (see below) fibres approach the follicle from different directions just below the sebaceous duct, where they divide to run parallel to the hair in the outer follicular layer (**8.**70, 71). In many mammals there are fine *down hairs*, coarser *guard hairs* and *whiskers* or *vibrissae* which have erectile vascular tissue around their follicles and are the most

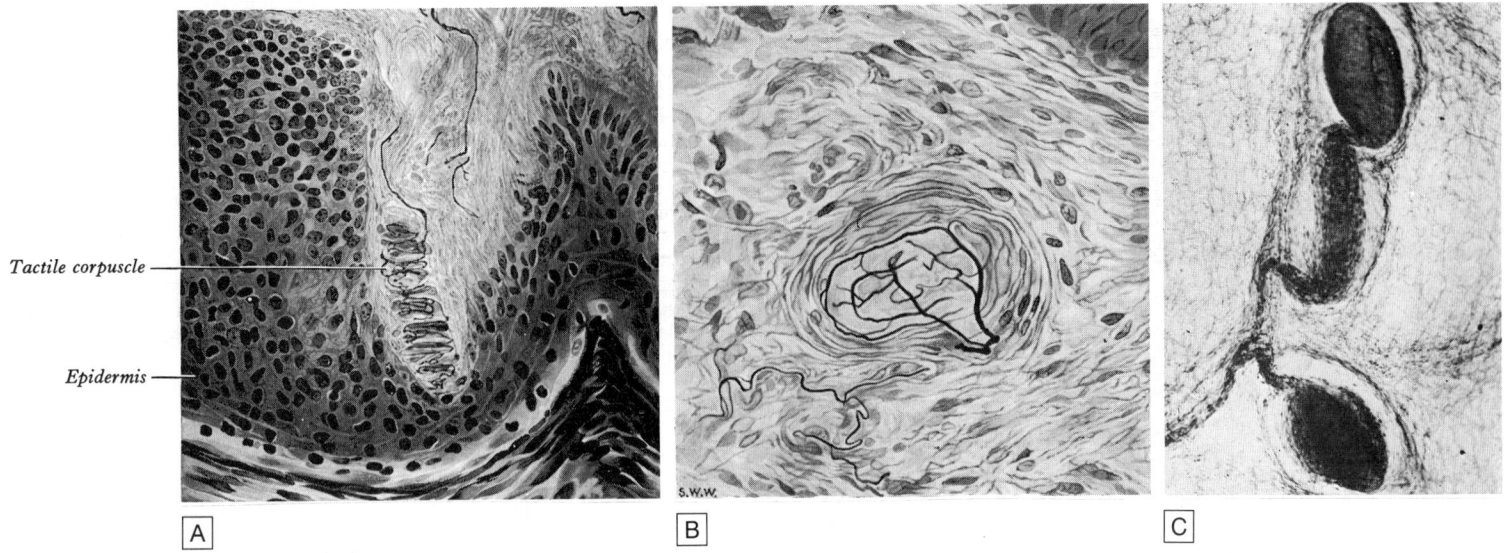

8.72 Specialized sensory end-organs. A. Tactile corpuscle of Meissner in human skin. Gros-Bielschowsky technique. Magnification *c.* ×250. B. Bulbous corpuscle from human anal canal. Gros-Bielschowsky and haematoxylin. Magnification *c.* ×480. (Material supplied by M J T FitzGerald, University College, Galway.) c. Whole mount of developing Pacinian corpuscles in feline mesentery. Gros-Bielschowsky technique. Magnification *c.* ×120. (Specimens A and c provided by N Cauna, University of Pittsburgh.)

complex, with at least three types of ending (see **8.70, 76**). Human hair is probably of the first two types. Lanceolate endings respond mainly to rapid movements when hair is deformed and belong to the rapidly adapting mechanoreceptor group (see also **8.75**).

Tactile menisci (*Merkel cell* (*disc*) *endings*) lie just below the epidermis or around the apical ends of some hair follicles (**8.73**c). Their nerve fibre expands into a disc applied closely to the base of a specialized cell (Merkel cell) inserted into the base of the epidermis, bearing spike-like protrusions which interdigitate with the surrounding keratinocytes. The Merkel cells contain many large (50–100 nm) dense-cored vesicles, particularly congregated near the junction with the nerve fibre. In many mammals, groups of such units are assembled at the base of dome-like epidermal discs (*touch domes*) supplied by single, highly branched nerve fibres, also often associated with specialized hairs (*tylotrichs*). These endings are slow-adapting (Type I) mechanoreceptors responsive to vertical pressure and served by large myelinated (Aβ) afferents. The ending's structure suggests some form of synaptic transmission but attempts to demonstrate this unequivocally have failed (see Iggo & Muir 1969; English 1978; Diamond et al 1988; see, however, Baumann et al 1988). For further details, see below.

Encapsulated nerve endings

These are a major group of special end organs exhibiting considerable variety in their size, shape and distribution but they all have a common feature: the axon terminal is encapsulated by non-excitable cells. Included in this category of ending are lamellated corpuscles of various kinds (e.g. Pacinian, see below), neurotendinous endings, neuromuscular spindles and Ruffini endings.

Tactile corpuscles (of Meissner). These are found in the dermal papillae of all parts of the hand and foot, the front of the forearm, the lips, palpebral conjunctiva and mucous membrane of the apical part of the tongue, although they occur mainly in thick hairless skin. Mature corpuscles are cylindrical in shape, with their long axes perpendicular to the skin surface, and are about 80 μm long and 30 μm broad. The corpuscle has a connective tissue capsule and central core (**8.72, 74**), the capsule being loosely attached to the core and absent at the extremities. Light microscopy indicates an external capsule of fine elastic fibres orientated mainly in the long axis of the corpuscle, interspersed with fibrocytes. The elastic fibres may anchor the corpuscle to the epidermis (Quilliam 1966). Further details are described below with other dermal receptors.

Large lamellated corpuscles of Vater-Pacini (Pacinian corpuscles) (**8.72**c, **73**A, B). These are sited subcutaneously in the ventral aspects of the hand and foot and their digits, the genital organs of both sexes, arm, neck, nipple, periostea, interosseous membranes, near the joints and in the mesentery and pancreas (cat). They are oval, spherical or irregularly coiled and are relatively huge, up to 2 mm in length and 100–500 μm or more across, the larger ones being visible to the naked eye. Each has a capsule, an intermediate growth zone and a central core containing an axon terminal. The capsule is formed by about 30 concentrically arranged lamellae of flat cells about 0.2 μm thick. Adjacent cells overlap at their edges and successive lamellae are separated by an amorphous proteoglycan matrix containing collagen fibres, the latter disposed circularly and closely applied to the surfaces of lamellar cells, especially their external surfaces. The amounts of collagen increase with age. The intermediate zone is cellular; occasional mitoses appear in it and the cells are incorporated into a capsule or core; the intermediate zone is not conspicuous in mature corpuscles. The core consists of about 60 bilateral, compacted lamellae, lying on both sides of the central nerve terminal and separated by two longitudinal clefts. Nucleated cell bodies exist in the outermost core, at the junction with the intermediate zone; from these arise cylindrical cytoplasmic arms passing into the clefts, where they extend as flat processes passing to one or both sides to form core lamellae, interdigitating with the processes from other arms. Adjacent lamellae do not arise from the same arm.

Each corpuscle is supplied by one or, rarely, two thick myelinated fibres (Aβ), the unbranched terminals of peripheral nerves. This fibre loses its myelin sheath, and at the junction with the core the Schwann cell also ends. The naked axon then runs along the central axis of the core, usually without any branching, to end in a slightly expanded bulb. The axon is in contact with the innermost core lamellae and is transversely oval, with the long axis in the plane of the clefts between lamellae; into these clefts the axon sends short spinous projections, of unknown function. It contains numerous large mitochondria, of which the most superficial are usually arranged radially beneath the axolemma. Minute vesicles of about 5 nm in diameter also occur, aggregated opposite the clefts. Cells of the capsule and core lamellae are actually modified fibroblasts, as distinct from Schwann cells (Pease & Quilliam 1957). Lamellated corpuscles may lie close to glomeral arteriovenous anastomoses (p. 1467) and are supplied by capillaries accompanying the nerve fibre as it enters the capsule. A condensation of richly elastic fibrous tissue forms an external capsule.

Lamellated corpuscles develop in the third fetal month; the terminal fibre is first surrounded by capsular lamellae which continue

963

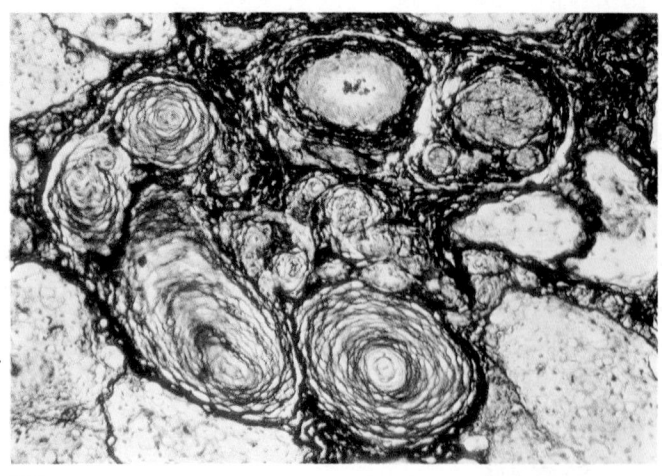

A

8.73 Structure of some peripheral sensory terminals.

A. A cluster of Pacinian corpuscles stained with the Glees and Marsland silver technique to show the capsules and the central axons, sectioned in various planes. (Rhesus monkey finger.) Magnification ×150. (Provided by R Bilous, Guy's Hospital Medical School, London.)

B. Electron micrograph of a Pacinian corpuscle in transverse section, showing the central core region with lamellar cells surrounding the axon. Note the presence of large intercellular spaces between the lamellar cells and the numerous mitochondria in the axon. (Rhesus monkey finger.) Magnification ×5000.

C. Electron micrograph showing a Merkel cell (M) associated with a Type I slowly-adapting cutaneous mechanoreceptor nerve terminal (N) from a rabbit touch-dome. Note the numerous dense vesicles clustered near the sensory nerve ending (arrowheads) and epidermal keratinocytes (K). Magnification ×5000. (Material provided by W Hamann, Department of Anaesthetics, Guy's Hospital Medical School, London.)

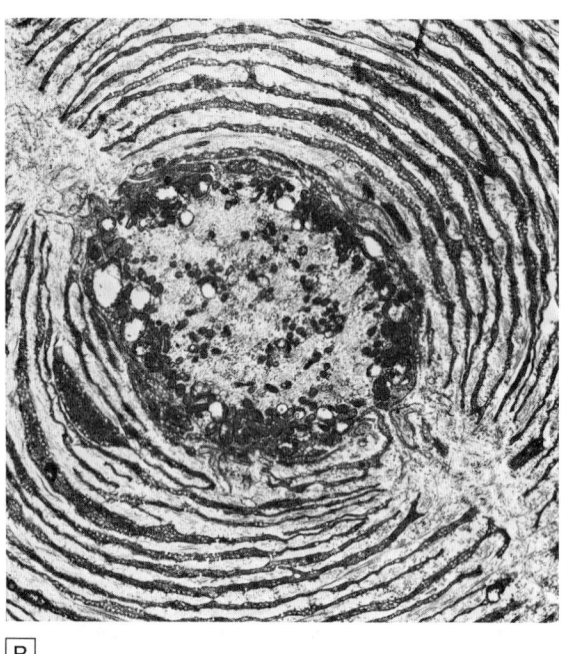

B

C

to accumulate into adult life, increasing the size of the corpuscle (Cauna & Mannan 1959). The corpuscles are said to exhibit turgidity due to fluid pressure between lamellae. Extensive studies show these endings to behave as very rapidly adapting mechanoreceptors, responding only to sudden disturbances and especially sensitive to vibration (Loewenstein 1971; Gray & Sato 1973). The rapidity may be partly due to the lamellated capsule acting like a 'high pass' frequency filter, damping slow distortions by fluid movements between lamellar cells. If the capsule is removed, the rate of adaptation, though still rapid, is considerably lessened.

Various other smaller *lamellated endings* have been described in various species of mammal and different sites but there is little physiological evidence about their functional nature. Some, which have been described in detail, have a circumferential, concentric, lamellar pattern like the large lamellated (Pacinian) endings but are perhaps less regular and certainly smaller. Examples are found in the endings in the connective tissue sheaths of the vibrissae in cats and in other mammals (Gottschaldt et al 1973) in joint capsules and other such sites (see Poláček & Halata 1970), where they have often been called *paciniform endings*. Endings with similar organization are the *end-bulbs of Krause*, *bulbous corpuscles*, *genital corpuscles* and probably the '*innominate corpuscles*' and *Golgi-Mazzoni endings* (see Bannister 1976).

Type II slowly adapting cutaneous mechanoreceptors (Ruffini endings). These occur in the dermis of hairy skin, consisting of highly branched, non-myelinated endings of Aβ (or II) myelinated afferents, which invade and ramify among bundles of collagen fibres

within a spindle-shaped structure enclosed partly by a fibrocellular sheath derived from the perineurium of the nerve (Chambers et al 1972). Their detailed structure is described below. Though less organized, these structures resemble the neurotendinous ending of Golgi (see below) and appear electrophysiologically similar, being responsive to maintained stresses in dermal collagen. Similar structures appear in joint capsules.

Neurotendinous endings (Golgi tendon organs). These are found chiefly near musculotendinous junctions (8.77). More than 50 may occur at any one such site. Each terminal is related closely to a group of muscle fibres (up to 20) which insert into the tendon fasciculus enclosing the ending. Neurotendinous endings are about 500 μm long and 100 μm in diameter, consisting of small bundles of tendon fibres enclosed in a delicate capsule. The collagen bundles (*intrafusal fasciculi*) are less compact than elsewhere in the tendon, the collagen fibres being smaller and the fibroblast larger and more numerous. The capsule consists of concentric cytoplasmic sheets, about 100–300 nm thick, belonging to capsular cells which are closely opposed, the successive layers being separated by intervals of variable width containing basal laminae. Numerous endocytic vesicles occur, suggesting that capsular cells may assist in maintaining the ending's internal environment. Outside is a thin layer of collagen fibres. One or more thickly myelinated group Iβ nerve fibres pierce the capsule and divide. Their ramifications, which may lose their Schwann cell sheaths, terminate in clasp- or leaf-like enlargements, rich in vesicles and mitochondria and wrapped round the tendon fasciculi with a basal lamina or Schwann cell cytoplasm intervening (Schoultze &

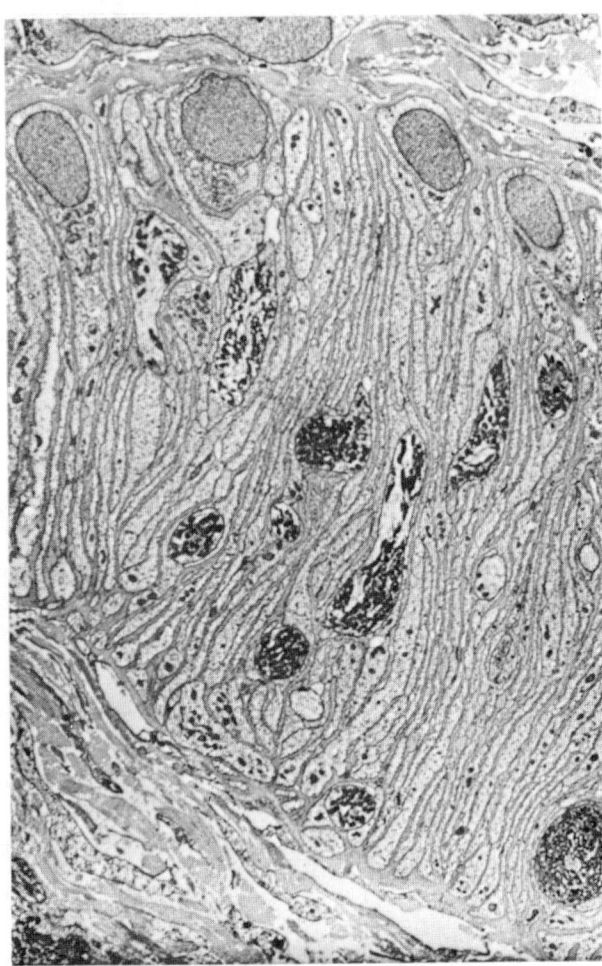

8.74 Ultrastructure, near the apex, of a tactile corpuscle of Meissner in vertical section, showing flattened lemmal cells arranged horizontally, with their nuclei to the right of the field. The sectional profiles of the terminal nerve fibres, appearing between the lemmal cells, contain numerous dense mitochondria. Magnification *c.* ×5000. (From Cauna 1966 with permission.)

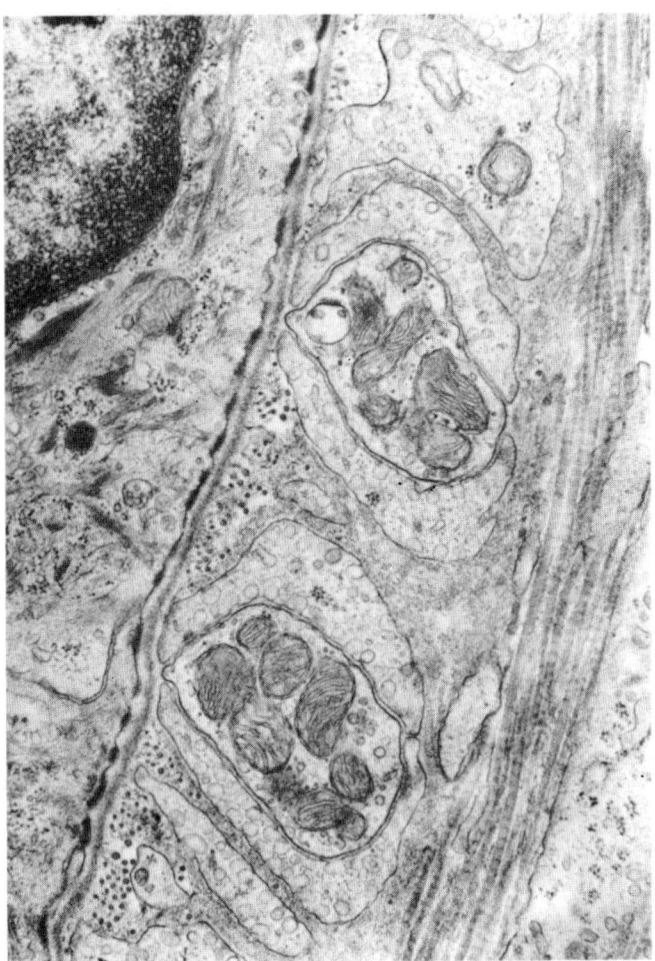

8.75 Ultrastructure of lanceolate terminal nerve fibres in close association with a hair follicle in the auricle of a rat. Note (above) part of the nucleus and cytoplasm of a keratinocyte; the plasma membrane adjoins a well-defined basal lamina and presents a series of hemidesmosomes. The two nerve fibres contain numerous mitochondria and are enveloped by Schwann cell processes. Surrounding the latter are basal laminae, reticulin fibres (above) and collagen fibres (below). Magnification ×35 000. (From Cauna 1966, with permission.)

Swett 1972, 1974). The endings are activated by passive stretch of the tendon but are much more sensitive to active contraction of the muscle. Classically, they were considered to initiate myotactic reflexes inhibiting the development of excessive tension during muscle contraction, but it has now been shown that they are important in providing proprioceptive information complementing that from neuromuscular endings (p. 969), in all condition of muscle activity (see, e.g., Prochazka & Wand 1980). Their responses are slowly-adapting, signalling maintained tension well (see Matthews 1973). The structural and physiological evidence indicates that the endings may be deformed by surrounding collagen fibres as they straighten under tension.

SPECIAL ARRAYS OF SENSORY ENDINGS

Now that varieties of individual sensory endings have been considered separately, *arrays* of several types of ending, being functionally significant, must be briefly described. Although our knowledge of such multiple patterns is as yet only partial, there are at least three well-studied receptive arrays providing sensory data on the forces acting on a particular locality and analysed, finally, together in the central nervous system. These are the receptors of skin, joints and muscles.

CUTANEOUS SENSORY RECEPTORS

The skin is a major organ of communication with the outside world. Functionally and structurally a number of sensory receptors have been identified to subserve this task. Cutaneous receptors should, however, not be regarded as a self-contained group, because the same or similar receptor structures can be found among the proprio- and interoreceptors (For recent reviews, see Munger & Ide 1988; Hamann 1992; Halata 1992.)

Specificity of nerve endings

Our understanding of the sensory mechanisms in the skin has developed against the background of scientific arguments between specificity and non-specificity in various sensory pathways. In these engagements, dogma often gained the upper hand against the evidence of nature's diversity in employing a solution most appropriate for a given need. It is now generally accepted that cutaneous sensory receptors are specific in the sense that there is always one type of stimulus for which they are most receptive by orders of magnitude compared with other forms of stimulation. In the skin, somatosensory receptors generally have stable and predictable responses to stimuli. However, in certain cases, inflammation or sympathetic nervous activity may enhance the responsiveness of the sensory receptor, an example at the extreme of this principle being the 'silent' nociceptor, a not uncommon type of sensory fibre, which although normally

965

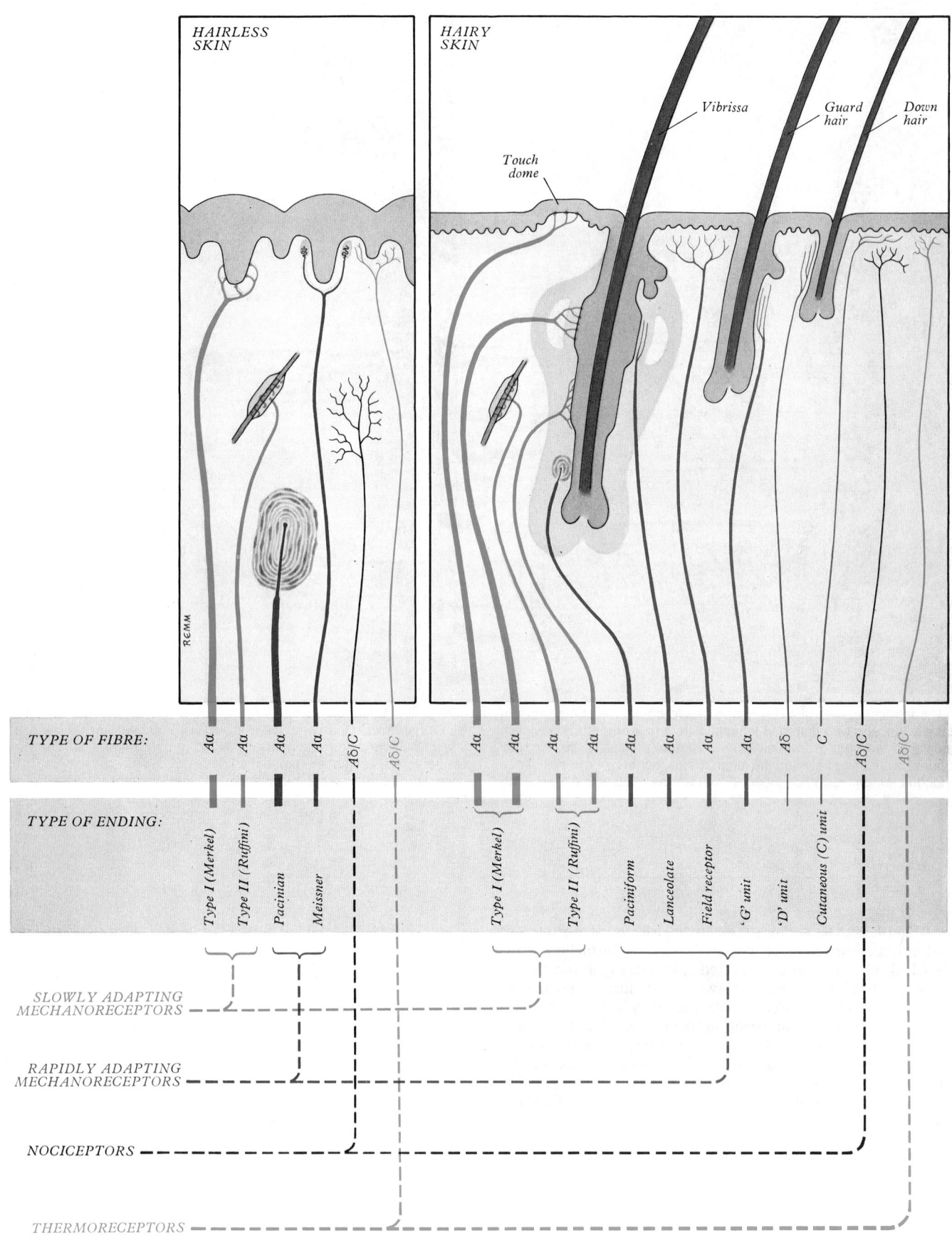

8.76 Schematic survey of the major types of mammalian cutaneous sensory endings and their afferent fibres. The endings are depicted symbolically according to their structural features and their mode of response to specific types of stimulus is indicated by colour coding, i.e. slowly-adapting mechanoreceptors, green; rapidly-adapting mechanoreceptors, red; nociceptors, black; thermoreceptors, blue. The classes of afferent fibre are according to the classification of Erlanger and Gasser see text. Note that the fibres designated *Aa* extend into the *Ab* range and that the field receptors may also be considered as hair receptors. Hairless skin is on the left and hirsute skin on the right.

966

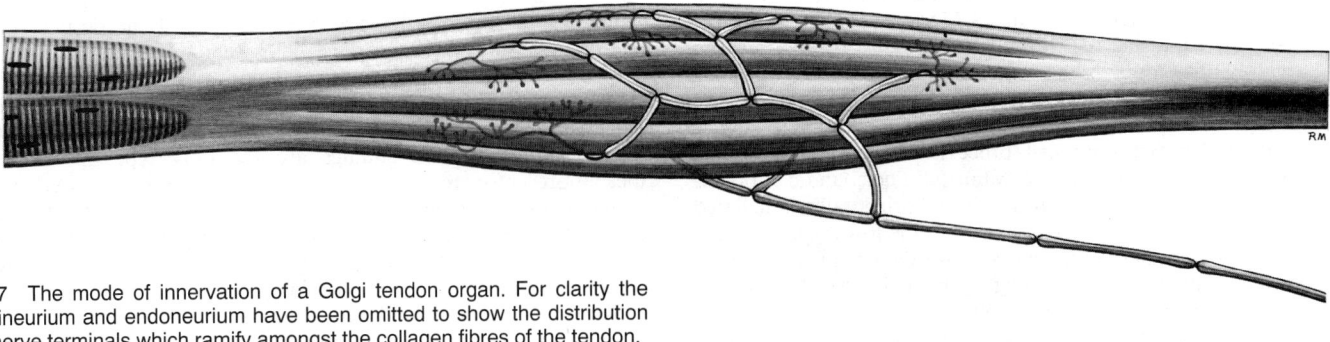

8.77 The mode of innervation of a Golgi tendon organ. For clarity the perineurium and endoneurium have been omitted to show the distribution of nerve terminals which ramify amongst the collagen fibres of the tendon.

inactive, becomes responsive in the presence of inflammatory mediators.

All cutaneous sensory receptors with structurally elaborate secondary structures are sensitive mechanoreceptors with afferent nerve fibres in the Group II and III range (**8.76**, see below). Pacinian corpuscles respond to vibration with frequencies of 40–1000 Hz. Meissner corpuscles cover the lower frequency range, while Merkel cell receptors and Ruffini type endings are slowly adapting mechanoreceptors although they also respond to vibration. Movement of hair is detected by the collar of lanceolate endings around the hair bulb just below the sebaceous gland (p. 962).

Free nerve endings are present in the epidermis as well as the dermis. Even in this structurally less developed group there is specificity of function. These receptors are either nociceptors (polymodal nociceptor, heat receptor or high-threshold mechanoreceptor), thermoreceptors or low-threshold mechanoreceptors. The function of sensory receptors is to transform specific stimuli into nervous impulses. In the skin, this process takes place with the possible exception of Merkel cell receptors in specialized terminals of primary afferent fibres (primary sensory receptors). There is considerable variation in the numbers of sensory receptors per cm^2 between different areas of the body surface, and with advancing age the density of receptors decreases. There is also considerable diversity in the specific histological arrangement between glabrous and hairy skin as well as between species. This account has been written with strong emphasis on human cutaneous sensory receptors.

TYPES OF CUTANEOUS RECEPTORS

Epidermal receptors

Free nerve endings (FNE). These are the terminal receptor structures of sensory C-fibres (Group IV) or Aδ fibres (Group III). They can be found within the basal and spiny cell layers of the epidermis as well as in the dermis, and are present in both glabrous and hairy skin (**8.69**). FNE cannot always be discriminated from passing autonomic nerve fibres with certainty, but a number of morphological criteria indicating sensory endings are now generally accepted for nervings in this and other situations (Halata 1992). These are

- presence of an incomplete Schwann cell sheath
- increased electron density on the internal aspect of the plasma membrane
- an increase in diameter of the parent axon as it becomes a sensory terminal
- increased numbers of mitochondria
- an irregular arrangement of microtubules and neurofilaments.

FNE of afferent fibres in the non-myelinated range are mainly nociceptive, but also include thermoreceptors and mechanoreceptors, so that electrical stimulation of primary afferent C-fibres will not excite pain-fibres exclusively.

Merkel-cell receptors. These consist of Merkel cells in close apposition to terminal enlargements of primary afferent Aβ (Group II) fibres (**8.69**, 73c, **5.35**). Merkel cells are located between the basement membrane and keratinocytes of the epidermis or bulbar epithelium of hair follicles. They are disc-shaped cells with a diameter of 10–15 μm in the long axis. They possess a large lobulated nucleus. At the dermal side they are resting in a bowl-shaped terminal enlargement of the primary afferent neuron. The interface between a Merkel cell and its primary afferent terminal shows some structural features of chemical synapses, and this notion is further supported by the presence of dense-cored vesicles, predominantly at the dermal side of Merkel cells (Iggo & Muir 1969). The contents of these vesicles is not known with certainty. There appear to be differences between species. The electron-dense contents of the vesicles can be depleted by hypoxia (see also p. 394).

The nerve terminals making contact with Merkel cells are richly endowed with mitochondria. They also contain clear vesicles of unknown function. At the interface between Merkel cells and keratinocytes there are evenly spaced cytoplasmic spikes protruding in between or into neighbouring cells. Functionally, Merkel cell receptors are slowly adapting. They are very sensitive to perpendicular indentation of the skin or to bending of sinus hairs or vibrissae.

Against the anatomical evidence largely in favour of a chemical synaptic relationship there is no clear physiological evidence either against or in favour of this concept (Baumann et al 1990). If there were a functioning chemical synapse at its interface with the nerve terminal, the transducer-mechanism of a Merkel cell receptor would be in the Merkel cell itself. In a non-synaptic arrangement Merkel cells would subserve a trophic or support function. If the latter notion proves to be correct it follows that Merkel cell receptors could be classified as free nerve endings. In hairy skin Merkel cell receptors are organized in clusters of Merkel cell–nerve terminal complexes, supplied by one or two primary afferent nerve fibres. These complexes are known under a variety of names (slowly-adapting Type I cutaneous mechanoreceptor, haarscheibe, touch corpuscle, Iggo corpuscle). In glabrous skin slowly adapting Type I mechanoreceptor neurons commonly contact only one Merkel cell.

Dermal receptors

Dermal and dermis-associated receptors include free nerve endings, Meissner corpuscles, lanceolate endings, Ruffini endings, and Pacinian and paciniform corpuscles. Before the development of the electron microscope several other types of lamellar receptors were also described (e.g. Golgi-Mazzoni and Dogiel corpuscles). However, they all follow the lamellar design pattern of the paciniform receptor and are considered part of this group (see also p. 963).

Free nerve endings (FNE). All layers of the skin contain FNE. These appear to be identical with the FNE of the epidermis (see above), and will not be described further.

Meissner corpuscles. This type of rapidly adapting mechanoreceptor can be found typically in the superficial dermis in glabrous skin (**8.69**, 72A). Meissner corpuscles have been described in the glabrous skin of plantar and volar surfaces, the preputium penis and also in the oral mucosa (Halata 1992). The most highly developed are found in the finger pads, where there may be up to 24 corpuscles per cm^2 in young adults. Meissner corpuscles are egg-shaped lamellar structures positioned closely below the epidermis, with the long diameter (100–150 μm) oriented perpendicularly to the surface of the skin. The short diameter measures 40–70 μm. Up to 7 nerve fibres (Aβ or Group II) enter a Meissner corpuscle through its dermal pole. On losing their myelin sheaths they branch and run in a helical manner towards the epidermal pole. On their way they develop disc-shaped enlargements which contain mitochondria and clear vesicles. The spirals of non-myelinated sensory terminals are ensheathed by flat Schwann cell processes originating from the corpuscle's periphery where the Schwann cell nuclei and cell bodies are clustered to resemble a capsule. The horizontally lamellated appearance of this type of receptor is due to the low angle at which the nerve fibres take their spiral course towards the epidermal pole.

The perineurium of the approaching myelinated nerve fibres widens to form a chalice of perineureum covering the dermal fifth of a Meissner corpuscle. The remaining 4/5ths of a corpuscle are devoid of perineural covering layer. Meissner corpuscles are rapidly adapting receptors providing information about rapidly fluctuating mechanical forces acting on the ventral surfaces of the hands and feet (Vallbo et al 1979). They are particularly sensitive to vibrations at frequencies ranging from 10–400 Hz with maximum sensitivity between 100 and 200 Hz.

Lanceolate endings of hair follicles. Structurally and functionally there is much similarity between Meissner corpuscles and lanceolate endings (Andres 1966; Halata 1992; (8.70, 75). Approaching the area just below the sebaceous gland, their Aβ (Group II) myelinated sensory nerve fibres lose their myelin sheaths, each branching to form up to 4 flat lanceolate sensory terminals. Their flattened profiles are orientated so that a narrow edge makes direct contact with the basement membrane of the epithelium of the hair bulb. Between individual lanceolate endings there are flat processes from Schwann cell bodies which tend to be positioned close to the circular connective tissue surrounding the hair follicle. The whole structure gives the appearance of a lamellar ring around the hair bulb. Physiologically lanceolate endings are rapidly adapting receptors responding to the bending of hairs.

Corpuscles of Vater-Pacini (Pacinian corpuscles). These are the largest type of receptors in the diverse group of lamellar endings with complete perineural capsules. The afferent nerve fibres are myelinated with diameters between 3 and 6 μm (Group II). The Pacinian corpuscle was one of the first somatosensory receptors to be investigated physiologically at the transducer level (Loewenstein 1971). They are rapidly adapting mechanoreceptors with an optimal response in the higher range of frequencies. Their detailed structure has already been described (see p. 963).

Ruffini endings. These can be found in the glabrous as well as hairy skin. They are also present in the gingiva, glans penis, joint capsule and tendinous insertions, where their appearance is similar to Golgi tendon organs. The structure of cutaneous Ruffini endings is best understood by considering their function as dermal stretch receptors (**8.69, 78**). Each consists typically of a perineural cylinder positioned around dermal collagen strands into which one or two myelinated sensory nerve fibres enter (Chambers et al 1972). The perineural cylinder tapers at either end, and more than one cylinder may contribute to a single receptor, following the course of collagen fibres with different orientations. Afferent nerve fibres are 5–6 μm in diameter (Group II or Aβ). Within a cylinder nerve fibres branch and lose their myelin sheath. Terminal non-myelinated branches are arranged in a shrub-like manner. They show the above characteristics of somatosensory receptor endings. Nerve fibres enter the perineural capsule either at the ends or laterally. Because of their shrub-like termination, Ruffini receptors are sometimes referred to as spraylike endings. Ruffini endings are slowly-adapting mechanoreceptors. In the skin they respond best to stretching of the skin. However, they may also be excited by perpendicular indentation.

RECEPTIVE FIELDS

The configuration of its receptive field is an important factor determining the performance of a sensory receptor. In the older literature there are many descriptions of receptive fields in animals. More recently, since the advent of recording techniques from human peripheral nerves, knowledge has become available about receptive

fields in man (Johannsen & Vallbo 1979). Of the four major types of mechanoreceptor responding to perpendicular cutaneous stimulation, i.e. Merkel cell receptors, Meissner and Pacinian corpuscles, and Ruffini endings, the latter two are receptors of the deeper dermis and hypodermis; their receptive fields tend to be larger than the preceding two types, and are represented in the cortex as having low contrast edges. Pacinian corpuscles are thus much more suitable to detect mechanical vibrations rather than the precise spatial extent of a stimulus. Ruffini endings are the only type of cutaneous mechanoreceptor readily excited by dermal stretch. Merkel cell receptors and Meissner corpuscles are receptors well suited to tactile exploration. Particularly in the fingertips they have small receptive fields with high contrast at the edges. Both properties are likely to enhance the power of tactile discrimination.

Tactile receptors with afferent C-fibres are known to be present in glabrous as well as hairy skin. This type of unit has ill-defined borders and may be discontinuous. It is therefore, unlikely to serve consciously perceptual or cognitive functions. It has been speculated that the C-fibre tactile system subserves subcortical, and possibly limbic and hypothalamic centres of the brain.

EFFERENT FUNCTIONS OF SENSORY NERVE FIBRES AND PEPTIDE CONTENTS

The concept of sensory nerve fibres having an efferent function was first established with the discovery of axon reflexes. A new dimension was added to this mechanism with the growing awareness that primary afferent fibres contain a range of neuropeptides and that, apart from their central action, some of these are released from peripheral nerve endings. Peptides are likely to be involved in inflammation, repair, autonomic and trophic functions, although our knowledge about these mechanisms is still incomplete (see also p. 936), or the evidence somewhat contradictory. The role of substance P (SP) in this response has been much studied; many non-myelinated (C) afferent nerve fibres contain this neuropeptide, and when in experimental animals this fibre population is eliminated by systemic treatment with capsaicin, plasma extravasation in response to cutaneous noxious stimulation is also abolished. However, the assignment of neuropeptides to particular classes of nerve fibres is a complex matter; it is necessary in the first instance to identify the type of primary afferent neuron by recording their electrophysiological responses to natural stimulation, then to label them intracellularly and determine their peptide content using immunohistological procedures. In an initial study of this nature in the cat, Leah et al (1985) were not able to find a correlation between SP-content and type of primary afferent unit. More recently, Lawson et al (1994) were able to correlate afferent fibre type with SP contents in guinea pigs; SP was found in high-threshold mechanoreceptors and C-fibre mechano-heat receptors in the glabrous skin. Surprisingly, no SP was present in polymodal nociceptor units in hairy skin. Other peptides that have been shown in primary afferent nerve fibres or Merkel cells are calcitonin gene related peptide (CGRP) and vasoactive intestinal peptide (VIP).

Cutaneous receptors in other species

It is remarkable how much uniformity there is in the types of cutaneous sensory receptors between species. However, there are some exceptions. Eimer's organ is a special form of epidermal free nerve ending found in a number of nocturnal animals or burrowing animals with rudimentary eyes like the mole (*Talpa*). In this structure, free nerve endings extend through straight channels in cones of thickened epidermis beyond the stratum basale. These are probably mechanoreceptors (Halata 1992).

Vibrissae (whiskers), found in many mammals in groups on the head and also scattered individually over the body, are a specialized sensory form of hair provided with a battery of receptors around their follicles, which are also provided with a vascular sac (hence the term sinus hair). Sensory endings in contact with follicles include lanceolate endings, Merkel cell receptors and so called pilo-Ruffini endings. Paciniform corpuscles are also present in the follicle sheath. In response to bending, two types of slowly adapting and two types of rapidly adapting response can be elicited from the vibrissal

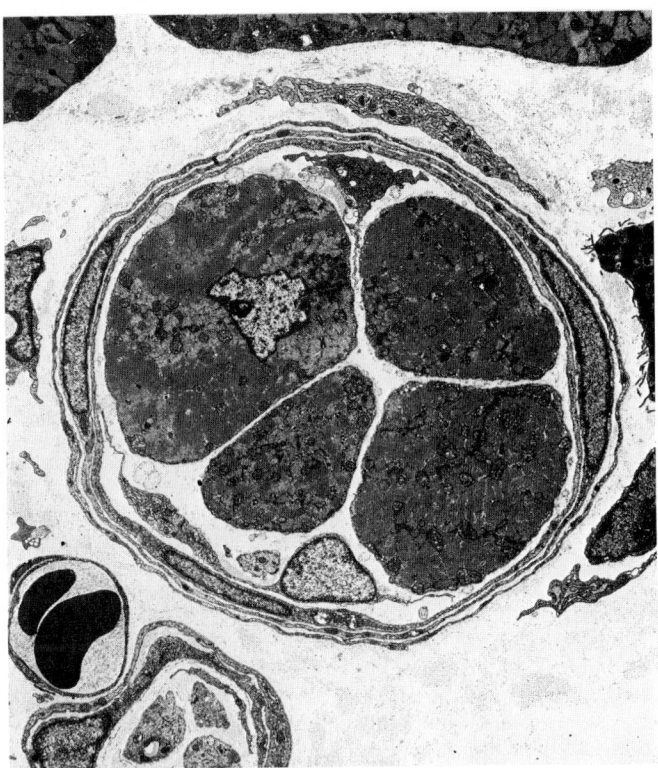

8.78   An electron micrograph of a neuromuscular spindle of a rat, in transverse section, showing the capsule, capsular space and four intrafusal muscle fibres, one with a centrally positioned nucleus. (Provided by D N Landon, National Hospital for Nervous Diseases, London.)

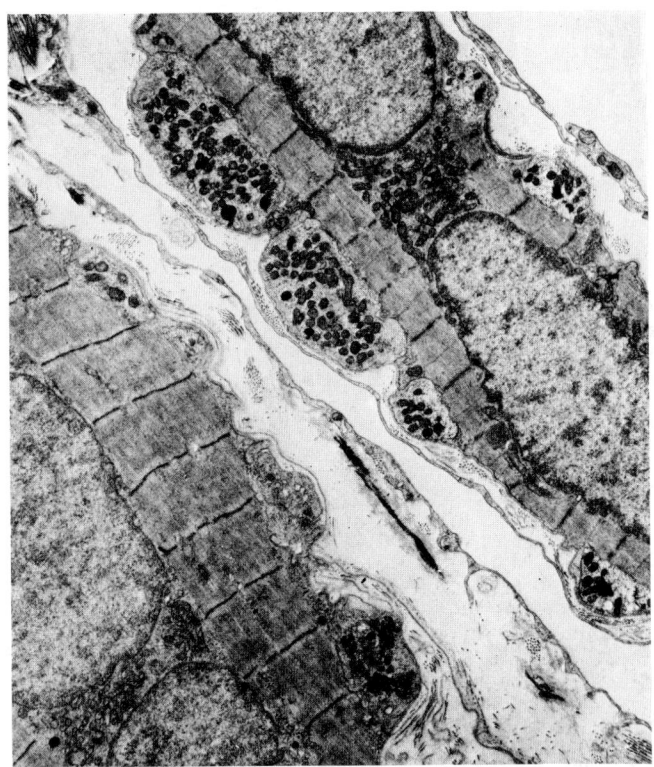

8.79   An electron micrograph of a longitudinal section through two intrafusal muscle fibres from a neuromuscular spindle of a rat. Note the primary (annulospiral) afferent nerve fibre endings cut in cross-section as they spiral around the equatorial region of a nuclear chain fibre (top right) and of a nuclear bag fibre (lower left). Note also the large numbers of mitochondria present in the sensory fibres. (Provided by D N Landon, National Hospital for Nervous Diseases, London.)

receptor complex (Gottschaldt et al 1973), the slowly adapting corresponding to Merkel and Ruffini endings and the rapidly adapting, to lanceolate and paciniform endings.

Grandry and Herbst corpuscles are mechanoreceptors present in the beaks of birds. Structurally, Grandry corpuscles resemble an agglomeration of Merkel endings, in that they have clusters of specialized epidermal cells associated with axon terminals. However they have two unexpected features, firstly that not all of the Merkel-like cells are in contact with an afferent fibre, and secondly, that these receptors are rapidly adapting. Herbst corpuscles are the equivalent of Pacinian corpuscles in birds. Numerous other variations of the pattern described above have been described in different mammals. It is interesting that in the primitive mammal *Ornitho-rhynchus*, the duck-billed platypus, electroreceptors capable of detecting action potentials generated by the muscles of its prey (e.g. worms) are present; such sensory structures are common amongst fish, but have not yet been found in more advanced mammals.

JOINT RECEPTORS

The arrays of receptors placed in and near articular capsules provide information on the position, movements and stresses acting in their vicinity (Wyke 1967). Structural and functional studies have demonstrated at least four types of such receptors, their proportions and distribution varying with site. Three are encapsulated endings, the fourth a free terminal arborization.

Type I endings. These are capsulated corpuscles of the Type II slowly adapting mechanoreceptor (Ruffini) type (see p. 964), situated in the superficial layers of fibrous capsules in small clusters and supplied by myelinated afferent fibres of the group II class. Being slowly adapting, they provide awareness of joint position and movement, responding, it is thought, to patterns of stress in articular capsules (Skoglund 1973) and particularly common in articulations

where static positional sense is necessary for the control of posture (e.g. hip, knee, etc.).

Type II endings. They are lamellated (Paciniform) receptors, like but smaller than the large (Pacinian) terminals elsewhere in connective tissue (p. 963). They occur in small groups throughout the joint capsules, particularly in the deeper layers and other articular structures (e.g. the fat pad of the temporomandibular joint). They are rapidly adapting, low-threshold mechanoreceptors, sensitive to movement and pressure changes and responding to joint movement and transient stresses in the joint capsule. They are supplied by Group II or III myelinated afferent fibres, but are probably not concerned in the conscious awareness of joint sensation.

Type III endings. Identical with neurotendinous organs (Golgi) in structure and function (p. 964), they occur in articular ligaments, but not their capsules. They are high-threshold, slowly adapting receptors and apparently serve, at least in part, to prevent excessive stresses at joints by reflex inhibition of the adjacent muscles. They receive large myelinated Group Ib afferent nerve fibres.

Type IV endings. Free terminals of Group III myelinated fibres and Type IV non-myelinated fibres, they ramify in articular capsules, the adjacent fat pads and around the blood vessels of the synovial layer. These are high-threshold, slowly adapting receptors and are considered to respond to excessive movements, providing a basis for articular pain.

NEUROMUSCULAR SPINDLES

Neuromuscular spindles are essential to the control of muscle contraction, a complex activity reflected in the structure and function of the spindle, which are not entirely understood. Their structure varies much in submammalian species and this account applies only to mammals (Bowden 1966; Landon 1966; Matthews 1971; Barker 1974; Banks et al 1975; Boyd 1985; Hunt 1990; Kanamuru 1993).

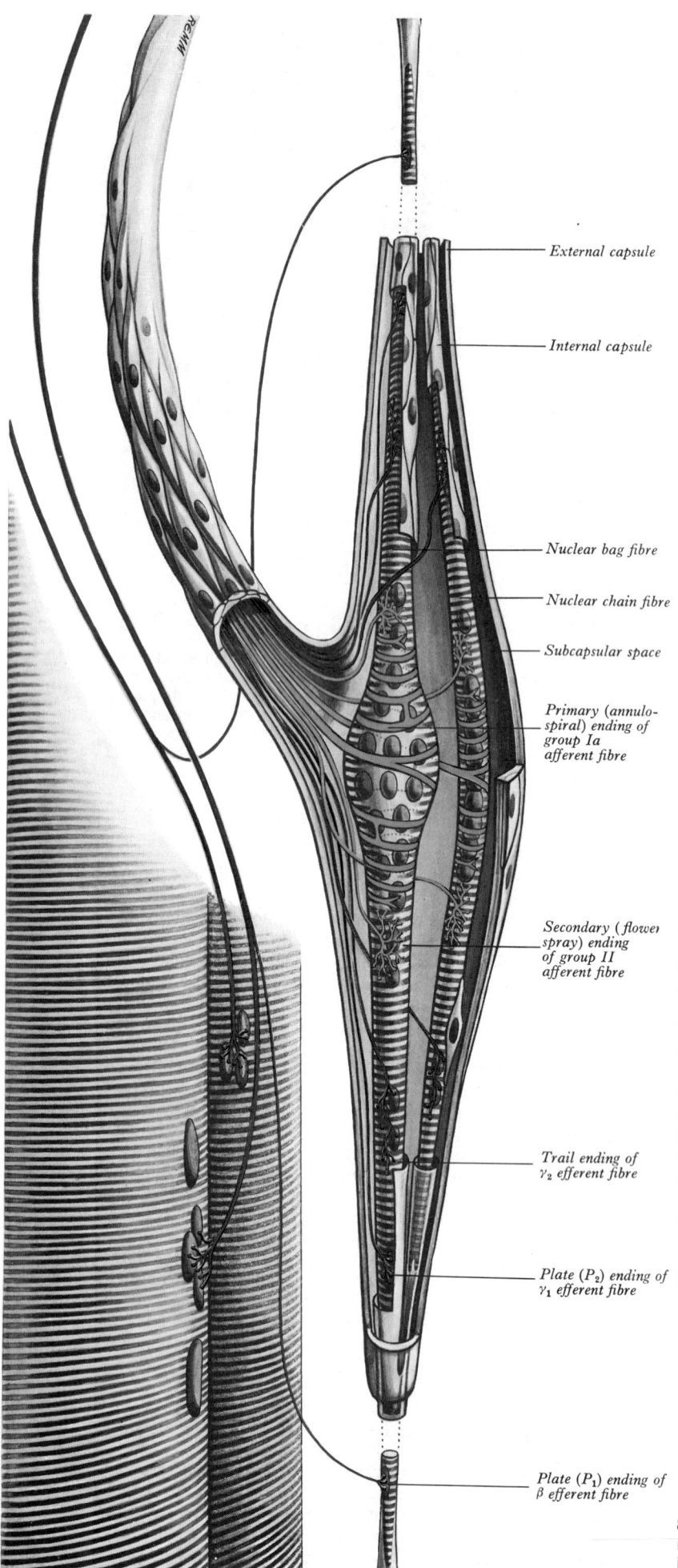

External capsule

Internal capsule

Nuclear bag fibre

Nuclear chain fibre

Subcapsular space

Primary (annulo-
spiral) ending of
group Ia
afferent fibre

Secondary (flower
spray) ending
of group II
afferent fibre

Trail ending of
γ_2 efferent fibre

Plate (P_2) ending of
γ_1 efferent fibre

Plate (P_1) ending of
β efferent fibre

Each spindle contains a few, small, specialized *intrafusal muscle fibres*, innervated by both sensory and motor nerve fibres (**8.78–81**). This complex is surrounded equatorially by a fusiform *spindle capsule* of connective tissue, arranged as an *external capsule* of flat fibroblasts and collagen, as in the perineurium (p. 946), and an *internal capsule* (axial sheath of Sherrington) forming delicate tubes around individual intrafusal fibres. Between the two sheaths is a fluid rich in glycosaminoglycans of gelatinous consistency.

There are usually 6–14 intrafusal fibres, varying in muscles and species, and two major types of muscle fibre, *nuclear bag* and *nuclear chain fibres*, distinguished by the arrangement of nuclei in their equatorial sarcoplasm. In the former the equatorial cluster of nuclei makes the fibres bulge slightly, whereas in the latter the nuclei form a single axial row. Nuclear bag fibres are greater in diameter than chain fibres and extend beyond the surrounding capsule to the endomysium of nearby extrafusal muscle fibres; nuclear chain fibres are attached at their poles to the capsule or to the sheaths of nuclear bag fibres. Two subtypes of nuclear bag fibres have more recently been demonstrated, the bag_1 (or *dynamic* bag_1 fibres) and bag_2 (*static* bag_2 fibres), distinguishable by their ultrastructure, histochemistry and physiological properties. Human spindles may contain three or four bag_1 and bag_2 fibres and as many as 10 chain fibres.

In their contractile apparatus the intrafusal fibres resemble the extrafusal, except that the zone of myofibrils is thin where they surround the nuclei. Ultrastructurally, intrafusal dynamic nuclear bag_1 fibres generally lack M lines, possessing little sarcoplasmic reticulum but having an abundance of mitochondria and oxidative enzymes; they have a low alkaline adenosine triphosphate (ATP)-ase activity and little glycogen. 'Static' bag_2 fibres have distinct M lines and a moderate to high level of alkaline ATP-ase and glycogen. Nuclear chain fibres have marked M lines, sarcoplasmic reticulum and T-tube elements, more glycogen and higher alkaline ATP-ase activity; they also have fewer mitochondria and lower oxidative enzyme levels. There are also differences in the extracellular environments of the fibre types, static bag_2 fibres being surrounded in their polar regions by prominent elastic fibres, whereas dynamic bag_2 fibres are not. These variations in the structural and other properties of intrafusal fibres are reflected in their contractile properties (see below).

Sensory innervation of muscle spindles.

This is of two types, both of which are the non-myelinated terminations of large myelinated axons. *Primary annulospiral* endings are equatorially placed and form spirals around the nucleated parts of intrafusal fibres; they are the endings of large sensory fibres (Group Ia), each of which gives branches to a number of intrafusal muscle fibres. Each terminal lies in a deep sarcolemmal groove beneath the basal lamina and contains mitochondria, vesicles, neurofilaments, microtubules and a pervading flocculent material. *Secondary* (*flower spray* and *annulospiral*) endings, largely confined to nuclear chain fibres, are the branched terminals of somewhat thinner myelinated (Group II) afferents; they are beaded and spread in a narrow band on both sides of the primary endings. Ultrastructurally, the varicosities are like the primary endings and lie close to the sarcolemma, though not in grooves. Primary endings are rapidly adapting, while secondary endings have a regular, slowly adapting response to static stretch (Matthews 1972; Hunt 1974). However, this statement is an oversimplification of the complex properties of the primary and secondary endings of different types of intrafusal fibres, since these depend on:

8.80 Schematic three-dimensional reconstruction of a mammalian neuromuscular spindle, showing nuclear bag and nuclear chain fibres; these are innervated by the sensory annulospiral and 'flower-spray' terminals (blue) and by the γ and β fusimotor terminals (red). See also **8.81**.

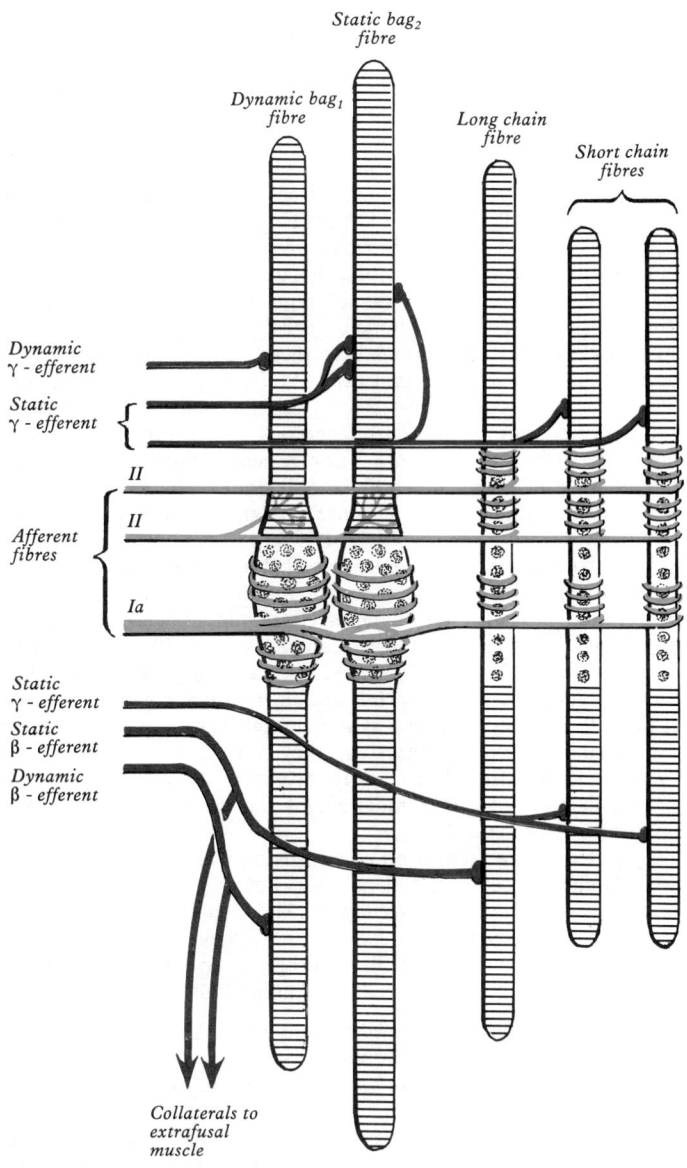

Static bag₂
fibre

Dynamic bag₁
fibre

Long chain
fibre

Short chain
fibres

Dynamic
γ - efferent

Static
γ - efferent

II

II

Afferent
fibres

Ia

Static
γ - efferent

Static
β - efferent

Dynamic
β - efferent

Collaterals to
extrafusal
muscle

8.81 Schematic diagram of the organization of intrafusal fibres and their innervation within a neuromuscular spindle.

- the mechanical properties of different regions of the bag₁, bag₂ and chain fibres on which they end
- the contractile characteristics of these muscle fibres when stimulated by their efferent terminals
- variations in the numbers and patterns of afferent primary and secondary endings and of the efferent terminals.

To give an example of this complexity, the primary spiral endings of the dynamic bag₁ fibres are highly sensitive to small stretches but rapidly adapt, probably because of mechanical 'creep' in the bag fibre on either side of it which decreases the tension of the central part of the fibre. In static bag₂ fibres, this tendency is much less marked, presumably due to the presence of elastic fibres surrounding the bag fibre and also because of differences in bag fibre cytology.

Motor endings in muscle spindles

These include three types, two from fine, but myelinated, fusimotor (γ-) efferents and one from β-efferent (also myelinated) collaterals of extrafusal slow twitch muscle. The first two are situated nearest to the equatorial region, ramifying to form cholinergic motor terminals with no obvious end plate or sole; the P_2 endings placed further away from the equator, have a typical 'en plaque' end plate and sole. At the extreme ends of nuclear bag fibres are P_1 endings of the β-efferents, forming 'en grappe' end plates (p. 958). Stimulation of

efferent endings causes the contraction of intrafusal fibres, with the activation of their sensory endings. Bag₁, bag₂ and chain fibres contract differently and their motor endings reflect this. The terminals of γ-efferents on dynamic bag₁ and static bag₂ fibres differ in their detailed structure, the bag₁ fibres receiving distinct synaptic end plates (P_2, or m_b terminals) and bag₂ fibres (usually) long 'trail' (m_a) endings; chain fibres have a third (m_c) type of more complex form or in many cases share branches of m_a terminals. For further details of structure and ultrastructure, see Arbuthnott et al (1982).

Muscle spindles signal the length of extrafusal muscle both at rest and throughout activity and relaxation, the velocity of their contraction and changes in velocity. These modalities may be related to the different behaviours of the three major types of intrafusal fibres and their sensory terminals. Dynamic nuclear bag₁ fibres are particularly concerned with signalling rapid changes in length occurring during movement; static bag₂ fibres, in contrast, are less responsive to movement; chain fibres have relatively slowly adapting responses at all times. These elements therefore can detect complex changes in the state of the extrafusal muscle surrounding spindles and can signal fluctuations in length, tension, velocity of length change and acceleration. Moreover, they are under complex central control; recently, sympathetic endings have been described in muscle spindles, adding further possibilities of changes in sensitivity mediated by the central nervous system. *Nuclear bag fibres* are probably concerned with *position, velocity* and *acceleration*, giving responses of a rapidly adapting, *dynamic* type, while *nuclear* efferent nerve fibres can adjust the length of the intrafusal fibres and therefore the activity of sensory fibres by causing contraction of the polar regions, thus compensating for the shortening caused by the contraction of extrafusal fibres during normal muscle activity. Such changes in tension can also magnify or reduce the responses of the afferent endings (see Boyd 1984). In summary the organization of spindles is such that they are capable of **actively** monitoring muscle conditions to allow **comparisons** between intended and actual movements and to provide a detailed input to the spinal, cerebellar, extrapyramidal and cortical centres of the nervous system concerning the state of the locomotor apparatus.

Development of neuromuscular spindles

This has been studied in detail by various investigators (Zelená & Szentágothai 1957; Landon 1972; Milburn 1973). Initially, intrafusal fibres form by the fusion of myoblasts, as in extrafusal muscle; the primary sensory endings are established (in rodents) before birth, followed by motor terminals, secondary sensory endings and the opening of the capsular space. Early development is absolutely dependent on the formation of primary sensory endings (Zelená & Szentágothai 1957) but later spindles may survive denervation, although they may undergo marked changes even if regenerating crushed nerves reinnervate them (Schiaffino & Pierobon Bormiolo 1976).

CAROTID BODIES (GLOMERA CAROTICA)

The two carotid bodies are reddish-brown, ellipsoid and lie near the carotid sinuses in the neck (p. 1514). Each is 5–7 mm in height and 2.5–4 mm in width and either posterior to the carotid bifurcation or between the start of its branches, being attached to or sometimes partly embedded in their adventitia. Occasionally it is a group of separate nodules. Aberrant 'miniglomera', microstructurally similar but with diameters of 600 μm or less, may appear in the adventitia and adipose tissue near the carotid sinus in human cadavers (Garfia 1980). Each glomus is innervated by glossopharyngeal carotid branches, including the *carotid sinus nerve*, and by a *plexus* of glossopharyngeal, vagal and sympathetic components (pp. 1297, 1301). Its abundant blood supply is derived from the adjacent external carotid rami.

Structure and function

The carotid glomus is an *arterial chemoreceptor*. When stimulated by hypoxia, hypercapnia or increased hydrogen ion concentration, it elicits reflex increase in the rate and volume of ventilation via connections with brainstem respiratory centres. Although this main role is certain, which of its components are chemoreceptors is obscure

(Chen et al 1976). It may also be *endocrine*; its *glomus cells* (see below) are in the amine precurser uptake and decarboxylation (APUD) series (p. 1898), which has been extended to include virtually all cells specialized for peptide hormone production (Pearse 1976); but no specific peptide hormone has yet been assigned to them. A suggested controlling role in erythropoiesis (Tramezzani et al 1971) has been disproved (Paulo et al 1973).

The glomus has a fibrous capsule whose septa lobulate it, each lobule being a collection of epithelioid '*glomus*' (Type I) cells enveloped by *sustentacular* (Type II) cells (8.82) and separating the former from extensive anastomoses of fenestrated sinusoids. Between sustentacular cells and the sinusoidal endothelium are non-myelinated nerve fibres, neurolemmocytes, attenuated processes of fibrocytes and collagen fibres (Chen et al 1976). Many of the nerve fibres are afferent, passing between the sustentacular to synapse with the 'glomus' (glomeral) cells. Preganglionic efferent fibres reach a sparse population of parasympathetic and sympathetic *ganglion cells*; these fibres are derived from the carotid sinus and sympathetic nerves (McDonald & Mitchell 1975), while the ganglion cells are either separate or in small groups near the body's surface. Axons proceed from the ganglion cells to local blood vessels, the parasympathetic efferent fibres probably being vasodilatory (Biscoe et al 1969) and the sympathetic ones vasoconstrictor (Purves 1970).

Glomeral cells (8.83), more numerous than sustentacular cells, are moderately large, with much cytoplasm and a few dendritic processes extending into intercellular spaces. Membrane-bound, electron-dense granules adjoin the Golgi apparatus and plasma membrane. Fusions of the limiting membranes of the granules and plasma membranes have been seen (Hansen 1977). Glomeral cells store dopamine (Kobayashi 1969), some other neurotransmitters (Fidone et al 1988) and the protein 'glomin' (Pearse 1969), presumably in their granules. They are accepted as chromaffin (Böck & Gorgas 1976) but a positive chromaffin response can be detected only ultrastructurally. They have also been regarded as paraneurons (Fujita 1976). Granular endoplasmic reticulum is not abundant but arrangements resembling neuronal Nissl substance have been described in human glomeral cells (Böck et al 1970). In rats, two types of glomeral cell are recognized (McDonald & Mitchell 1975): Type A have larger, more numerous electron-dense granules than Type B and usually a smooth, globular contour with a few short dendrites; Type B cells are more irregular with several long thin processes. Nerve endings seldom synapse with Type B cells but at least two kinds of fibre synapse with Type A, over 95% being *chemoafferent axons* leaving in the carotid sinus nerve, their cell bodies being in the sensory glossopharyngeal ganglia. Less than 5% are *preganglionic efferent axons* from the cervical sympathetic trunk, entering the glomus with postganglionic axons from the superior cervical sympathetic ganglion. No efferent glossopharyngeal axons appear to synapse with glomeral cells but some are preganglionic to parasympathetic ganglion cells. In rabbits ultrastructurally efferent fibres of uncertain origin, presumed inhibitory, synapse with the chemoafferent axons (Verna 1975). Among 'afferent' nerve endings some are presynaptic to Type A glomeral cells, others postsynaptic and some form *reciprocal synapses* with them. Such synapses have also been found between glomeral cells (McDonald & Mitchell 1975); they are dendrodendritic (Reese & Shepherd 1972). Similar connections occur in the central nervous system (pp. 928, 934) but not hitherto in the *peripheral*. Various neural circuits described in the glomus of rats and rabbits (McDonald & Mitchell 1975; Verna 1975, Fidone et al 1988) are shown in 8.83. Human details are awaited with interest (see also Kumnor & Habeck 1993).

Ultrastructural and neurophysiological evidence ascribes at least three functions to glomeral cells. Firstly, they release neurotransmitters in response to hypoxia (Eyzaguire et al 1972) and may be *sensory*. Secondly, in ultrastructure they are like APUD cells (Pearse 1969) and may be *effector cells*, modifying the sensitivity of chemoreceptive nerve endings by variable release of dopamine (Biscoe et al 1970). Thirdly, having a synaptic input and output, a gliaform sheath and dendritic processes, they may act as *interneurons* (McDonald & Mitchell 1975). Involvement in several functions, as postulated above, is reminiscent of the presumed phylogenetic progenitor neuronal cell.

As stated above there is no consensus on which carotid glomeral cell is a chemoreceptor; *glomeral cells* (Lever et al 1959; Eyzaguire et al 1972), *afferent nerve terminals* (McDonald & Mitchell 1975) and *sustentacular cells* (Mills & Jöbsis 1972) have all been favoured. McDonald & Mitchell (1975) hypothecate co-operation between afferent axons and glomeral cells, proposing that:

- afferent nerve endings, connected with glomeral cells by reciprocal synapses, are the true chemoreceptors
- glomeral cells are dopaminergic interneurons which modify the sensitivity of the chemoreceptive endings
- the reciprocal synapses between the glomeral cells and the afferent axons may form an inhibitory feedback, the glomerular cells inhibiting the activities of the axons with dopamine, the axons releasing an excitatory transmitter when stimulated, e.g. by hypoxia
- preganglionic sympathetic neurons may decrease chemoreception by evoking dopamine release from glomeral cells
- synaptic interconnections between adjacent glomeral cells could mediate reciprocation.

Another hypothesis (Mills & Jöbsis 1972), implicating sustentacular cells, suggests that hypoxia may affect these cells, initiating 'firing' of adjacent 'free' afferent nerve endings; glomeral cells, with their efferent sympathetic innervation, could be part of a feedback modifying the activity of the afferent axons. Half the cytochrome (a_3) of the glomus has a low affinity for oxygen and appears to be located in sustentacular cell mitochondria, which would make such cells sensitive to hypoxia, cytochrome remaining reduced in oxygen shortage and depressing oxidative metabolism. This might make them release, for example, potassium, activating adjacent afferent axons whose many mitochondria, containing a cytochrome a_3 with a high affinity for oxygen, might sustain normal function even in hypoxia. It is interesting to speculate on the role of local haemodynamic control in such a monitoring system.

The carotid glomus develops from mesenchyme in the third pharyngeal arch (Boyd 1937), as a condensation around its artery; its nerve supply is mainly glossopharyngeal, the nerve being of that arch.

Other small bodies, resembling carotid glomera, occur near the arteries of the fourth and sixth pharyngeal arches and hence near the aortic arch, ductus arteriosus and right subclavian artery and are supplied by the vagus nerve. They are also considered to be chemoreceptors.

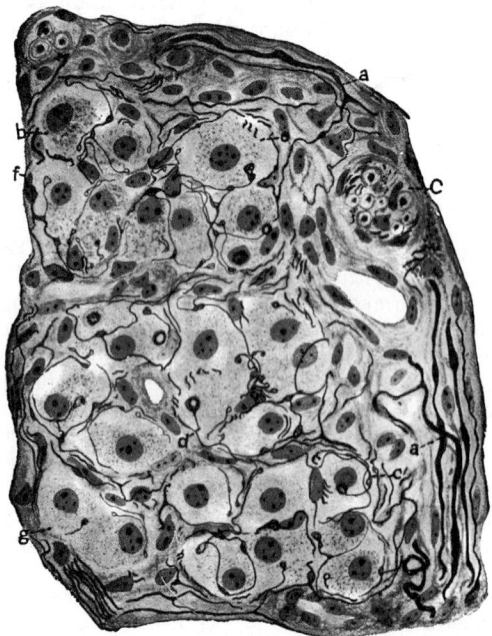

8.82 A section of the carotid body, showing nerve fibres distributed to the cells (de Castro): a, myelinated fibre dividing into two fine branches; b, cell closely surrounded by nerve fibrils; c, section of a small nerve, composed of several myelinated fibres; f, a nerve fibre apparently ending within the cytoplasm of a cell; g, a nerve fibre ending between the cells.

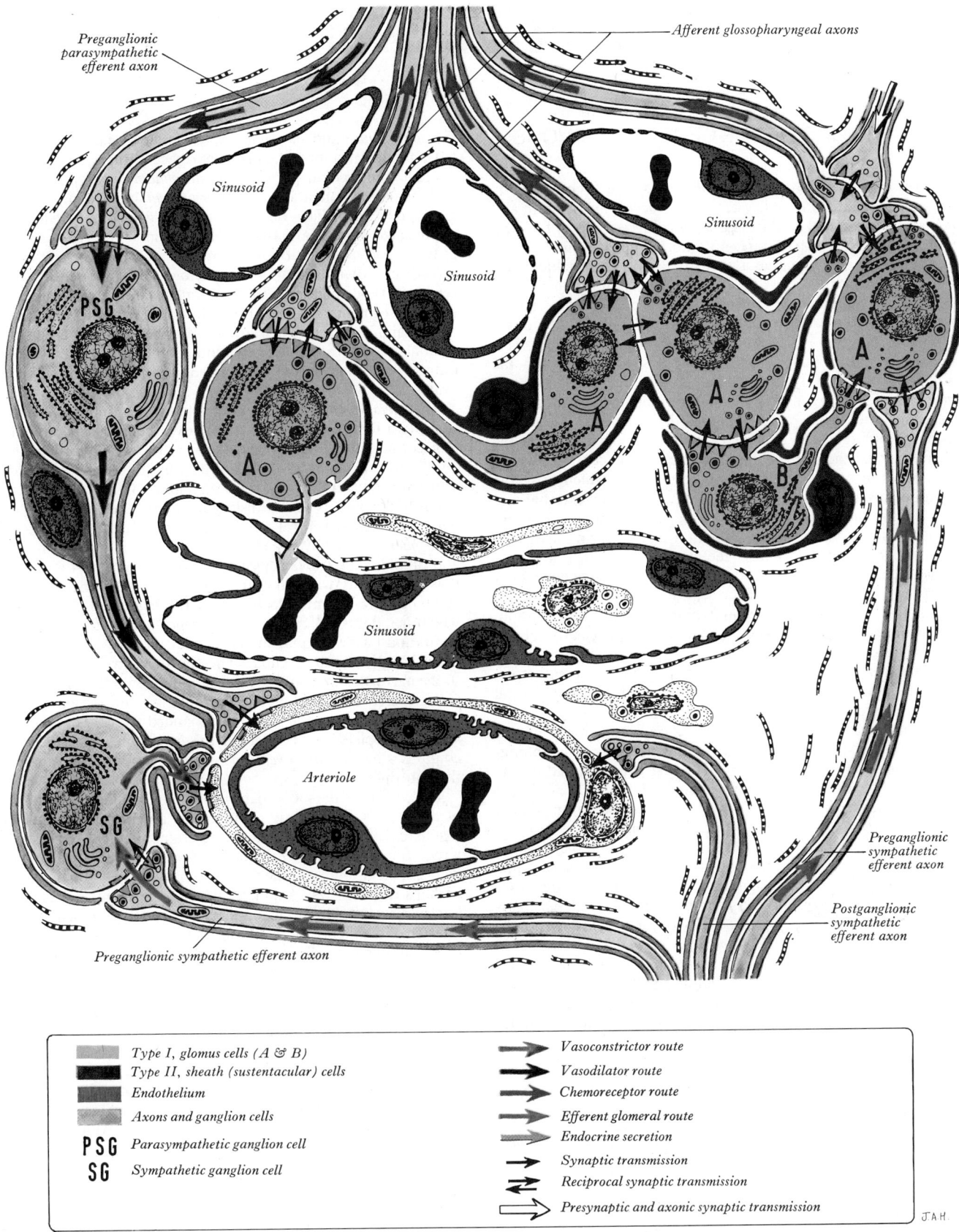

Preganglionic
parasympathetic
efferent axon

Afferent glossopharyngeal axons

Sinusoid

Sinusoid

Sinusoid

PSG

A

A

A

A

A

B

Sinusoid

Arteriole

SG

Preganglionic
sympathetic
efferent axon

Postganglionic
sympathetic
efferent axon

Preganglionic sympathetic efferent axon

Type I, glomus cells (A & B)	Vasoconstrictor route
Type II, sheath (sustentacular) cells	Vasodilator route
Endothelium	Chemoreceptor route
Axons and ganglion cells	Efferent glomeral route
PSG Parasympathetic ganglion cell	Endocrine secretion
SG Sympathetic ganglion cell	Synaptic transmission
	Reciprocal synaptic transmission
	Presynaptic and axonic synaptic transmission

J.A.H.

8.83 The cellular, neural and vascular architecture of the carotid body.
Functional pathways are indicated.

REGIONAL ORGANIZATION OF THE CENTRAL NERVOUS SYSTEM

MAJOR DIVISIONS OF THE CENTRAL NERVOUS SYSTEM

Although essentially a continuum, the nervous system is conveniently divided into parts, regions and systems. The *encephalon* or brain and *medulla spinalis* or spinal cord form the *central nervous system* (CNS). Extending from this in pairs are: 12 cranial and 31 spinal nerves constituting a peripheral nervous system (PNS). This includes not only all the ramifications of these nerves, which mediate *somatic sensory* and *motor* functions, but also *visceral* or *splanchnic* nerves connected to the central nervous system through the somatic channels, thus forming a *peripheral autonomic nervous system*. This division into central and peripheral parts is justifiable, for the latter consists of relatively simple conductors connecting peripheral receptor and effector organs to each other through the intermediation of the brain and spinal cord. Though the spinal cord contains extensions of afferent and efferent pathways deployed through the peripheral nerves, the particular significance of the central nervous system resides in complex networks of neurons in which arise the appropriate patterns of response to stimuli of both the external and internal environment. This same intricate area of intermediation, between incoming patterns of information and emerging arrays of 'commands' to effectors, is also the domain in which learning, memory and consciousness are intrinsic, each to a degree dependent upon the level of development of the central apparatus. Elaboration of these activities, which has increased along the lines of evolution, especially along that leading to the human animal, is clearly related to a population of vastly increased central interneurons, rather than to changes in the peripheral afferent and efferent conductors. Nevertheless, the essential continuity and interdependence of all parts of the nervous system is never to be overlooked.

The spinal cord occupies about the cranial two-thirds of the vertebral canal and is arbitrarily continuous with the medulla oblongata just below the foramen magnum. The first pair of spinal nerves emerge from the cord immediately caudal to this. The walls of the cord are thick, the central cavity being reduced to an almost microscopic *central canal*, extending nearly throughout the cord.

The encephalon or brain (**8.84, 85**) lying wholly within the cranium is divided, for convenience, into regions which are of considerable morphological and functional significance. Ascending in order from the spinal cord these are: the *rhombencephalon* or *hindbrain*, *mesencephalon* or *midbrain* and *prosencephalon* or *forebrain*. The rhombencephalon includes the *myelencephalon* or *medulla oblongata*, *metencephalon* or *pons* and the *cerebellum*. The prosencephalon comprises the *diencephalon* ('between brain') and the *telencephalon*. The former is the central connecting part corresponding approximately to the *dorsal thalamus* and *hypothalamus*, but also includes

the *epithalamus* and *subthalamus*; the latter is mainly composed of a left and right cerebral 'hemisphere' or cerebrum, and also contains a small transmedian part, the *telencephalon impar*. Midbrain, pons and medulla oblongata form the *brainstem*, connecting the forebrain and spinal cord. The relation of these divisions to each other is appreciated more clearly from their development (p. 218). The pattern of fore-, mid- and hindbrain is not only an expression of ontogenetic growth in individuals; it is also phylogenetic, representing the basic central nervous hierarchy in vertebrates. These levels are sometimes termed 'segments' of the brain; the telencephalon, particularly its cortex and connections, is often described as 'suprasegmental', a term also applied to the cerebellum. Both are phylogenetically later outgrowths of the basically elongated form of the primitive vertebrate brain.

The *medulla oblongata* is the most caudal (inferior) part of the brainstem, situated immediately above the basilar occipital bone, and continuous with the pons above and spinal cord below. The *pons* is also related to the basi-occiput, and to the sphenoidal dorsum sellae; it is greater in transverse and anteroposterior dimensions than the medulla and is easily distinguished by the mass of transverse nerve fibres on its ventral aspect. The *cerebellum*, consisting of paired *hemispheres* united by a median *vermis*, is dorsal to the pons, medulla and caudal midbrain, occupying the posterior cranial fossa. Ventrally it is continuous with all three: midbrain, pons and medulla. The cavity of the rhombencephalon is the expanded *fourth ventricle*, which lies dorsal to the pons and upper half of the medulla, being continuous with a canal in the caudal medulla and, through this, with the spinal central canal. The fourth ventricle contracts above to the narrow channel of the midbrain, the somewhat inappropriately termed *cerebral aqueduct*. The *midbrain* is a short segment of brainstem, narrower than the pons but expanded above. The *diencephalon*, almost completely embedded in the cerebrum and largely hidden, contains a median *third ventricle* which communicates caudally with the aqueduct.

The *cerebrum*, the most rostral part, is in mankind a major fraction of the brain's volume and occupies the anterior and middle cranial fossae and is directly related to the cranial vault. It consists of two large convoluted *cerebral hemispheres*. (Strictly its halves are not hemispherical but together form approximately one hemisphere; perhaps the term was originally used in the singular, but the plural however unsuitable is customary.) Each half is equal to about a quarter of a sphere, and contains a crescentic *lateral ventricle* which is continuous medially with the third ventricle in the diencephalon. Each hemisphere has an external grey layer, the *cerebral cortex*, and a central white core of *medullary substance*, in which are several large *basal nuclei* of grey matter (earlier, incorrectly, called 'ganglia').

As noted, the PNS contains a somatic *cerebrospinal* and a visceral *autonomic* system. In the former, efferent nerve fibres pass from extrinsic neurons of the CNS to effector organs, mostly muscles. Efferent autonomic fibres terminate in the peripheral ganglia, forming synapses with neurons whose axons innervate cardiac and non-striated muscle as well as glandular tissue. Autonomic efferent pathways thus have *pre-* and *postganglionic* neurons, though autonomic ganglia also sometimes include a variety of interneurons (p. 1299). The arrangement of afferent fibres is similar in both cerebrospinal and autonomic systems.

The autonomic nervous system has *sympathetic* and *parasympathetic* divisions, often functionally opposed. Preganglionic sympathetic efferent fibres issue from a spinal region extending from the first thoracic to the second or sometimes third lumbar segments. Preganglionic parasympathetic efferent fibres emerge only in certain cranial nerves (oculomotor, facial, glossopharyngeal, vagus with accessory) and the second to fourth sacral spinal nerves. These groups of autonomic efferents are usually designated *thoracolumbar* (sympathetic) and *craniosacral* (parasympathetic) *outflows*. A detailed description of the autonomic system appears on page 1292 et seq. The autonomic nervous system is integrated with the enteric nervous system, a plexus of neurons within the alimentary tract (p. 1310).

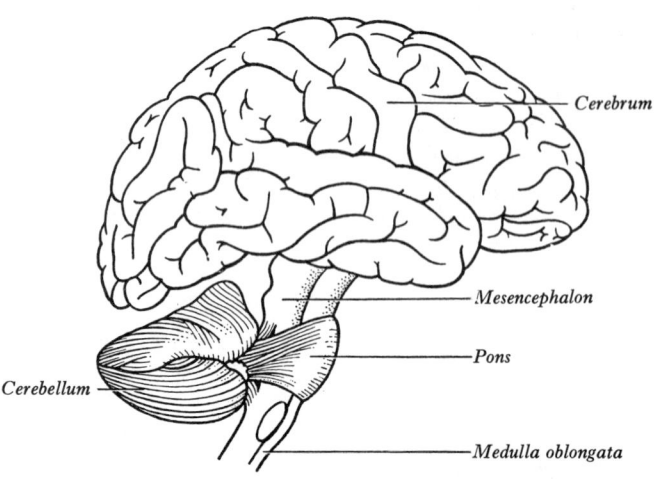

8.84   Semi-diagrammatic scheme of the main divisions of the brain.

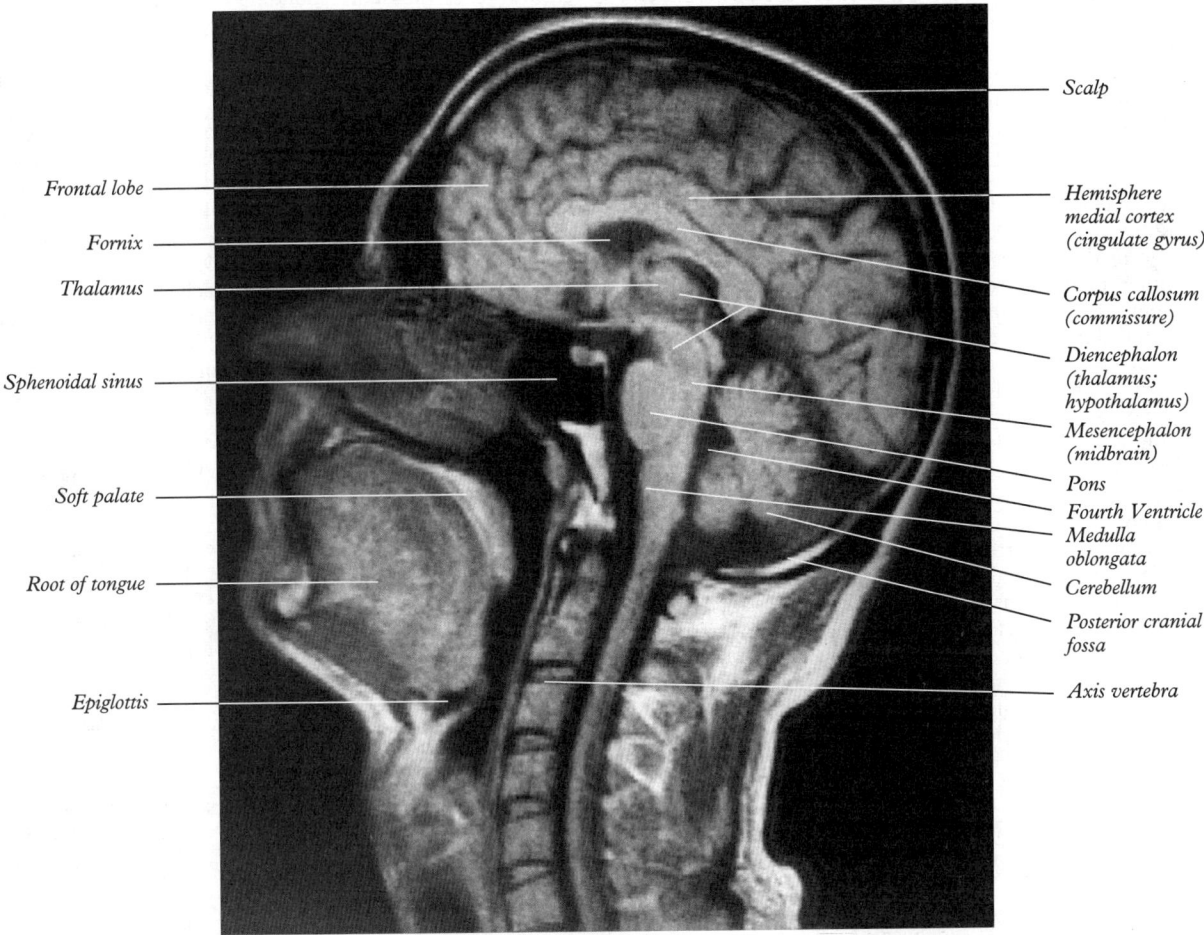

Scalp

Frontal lobe

Hemisphere medial cortex (cingulate gyrus)

Fornix

Thalamus

Corpus callosum (commissure)

Diencephalon (thalamus; hypothalamus)

Sphenoidal sinus

Mesencephalon (midbrain)

Pons

Fourth Ventricle

Medulla oblongata

Soft palate

Cerebellum

Root of tongue

Posterior cranial fossa

Axis vertebra

Epiglottis

8.85 Midline sagittal magnetic resonance imaging (MRI) scan of the head and neck. (Supplied by Siemens, Erlangen, West Germany; photography by Sarah Smith.)

SPINAL MEDULLA OR CORD

EXTERNAL FEATURES AND RELATIONS

The spinal cord is an elongated, approximately cylindrical part of the CNS, occupying the superior two-thirds of the vertebral canal (**8.86**–**8.91**). Its average length in European males is 45 cm, its weight about 30 g. (For dimensional data consult Barson & Sands 1977.) It extends from the upper border of the atlas to the junction between the first and second lumbar vertebrae, the lower level varying, with some correlation with length of trunk, especially in females (Jit & Charnalia 1959). The termination may be as high as the caudal third of the twelfth thoracic vertebra or as low as the disc between the second and third lumbar vertebra; its position rises slightly in vertebral flexion. The spinal cord is enclosed in the *dura, arachnoid* and *pia maters,* separated from each other by the *subdural* and *subarachnoid spaces,* the former being merely potential, the latter containing cerebrospinal fluid (CSF; p. 1204). Continuous cranially with the medulla oblongata, the cord narrows caudally to the *conus medullaris,* from whose apex a connective tissue filament, the filum terminale, descends to the dorsum of the first coccygeal vertebral segment (**8.86**). In *transverse width* the spinal cord varies, gradually tapering craniocaudally, except at the levels of the enlargements. It is not cylindrical, being widest transversely at all levels and especially in the cervical segments.

The *cervical enlargement* is the source of large spinal nerves supplying the upper limbs and extends from the third cervical to the second thoracic segments, its maximum circumference (about 38 mm) is in the sixth cervical segment. (A spinal cord segment provides the attachment of the rootlets of a pair of spinal nerves.)

The *lumbar enlargement* similarly corresponds to the innervation of the lower limbs, extending from the first lumbar to the third sacral segments, the equivalent *vertebral* levels being the ninth to twelfth thoracic. The greatest circumference (about 35 mm) is near the lower part of the body of the twelfth thoracic vertebra, below which it rapidly dwindles into the conus medullaris.

Fissures and *sulci* extend along most of the external surface; an anterior median fissure and a posterior median sulcus and septum almost completely separate the cord into right and left halves but these are joined by a *commissural band* of nervous tissue containing a *central canal* (**8.90**).

The *anterior median fissure* extends along the whole ventral surface with an average depth of 3 mm, although deeper at caudal levels. It contains a reticulum of pia mater. Dorsal to it is the *anterior white commissure.* Perforating branches of the spinal vessels pass from the fissure to the commissure to supply the central spinal region. The *posterior median sulcus* is shallower; from it a *posterior median septum* of neuroglia penetrates more than halfway into the cord, almost to the central canal. The septum varies in anteroposterior extent from 4 to 6 mm, diminishing caudally as the canal becomes more dorsally placed and the cord contracts.

A *posterolateral sulcus* exists from 1.5 to 2.5 mm lateral to each side of the posterior median sulcus; along it dorsal roots (strictly rootlets) of spinal nerves enter the cord. The white substance between the posterior median and posterolateral sulcus on each side is the *posterior funiculus.* In cervical and upper thoracic segments a longitudinal *posterointermediate sulcus* marks a septum dividing each posterior funiculus into two large tracts: the *fasciculus gracilis* (medial) and *fasciculus cuneatus* (lateral). Between the posterolateral sulcus and anterior median fissure is the *anterolateral funiculus*, subdivided into *anterior* and *lateral funiculi* by issuing ventral spinal roots. The anterior funiculus is medial to (and includes) the emerging ventral roots, whilst the lateral funiculus lies between the roots and the posterolateral sulcus (8.90, 91). In upper cervical segments, nerve radicles emerge through each lateral funiculus to form the spinal accessory nerve which ascends in the vertebral canal lateral to the spinal cord to enter the posterior cranial fossa via the foramen magnum (8.122).

The *filum terminale* (8.86, 87, 89), a filament of connective tissue about 20 cm long, descends from the apex of the conus medullaris. Its upper 15 cm, the *filum terminale internum*, is surrounded by extensions of the dural and arachnoid meninges and reaches the caudal border of the second sacral vertebra. Its final 5 cm, the *filum terminale externum*, fuses with the investing dura mater, and then descends to the dorsum of the first coccygeal vertebral segment. The filum is continuous above with the spinal pia mater; adherent to its upper part are a few strands of nerve fibres probably representing roots of rudimentary second and third coccygeal spinal nerves. The central canal is continued into the filum for 5–6 mm. A capacious part of the subarachnoid space surrounds the filum terminale internum; it is the site of election for spinal (lumbar) puncture.

Continuous with the cord is a series of paired dorsal and ventral *roots* of the spinal nerves (8.91). These cross the subarachnoid space and traverse the dura mater separately, uniting in or close to their intervertebral foramina to form the (mixed) spinal nerves. Since the spinal cord is shorter than the vertebral column, the more caudal spinal roots descend for varying distances around and beyond the cord to reach their corresponding foramina; thus, they form, largely distal to the apex of the cord, a divergent sheaf of spinal nerve roots, the *cauda equina*, which is gathered round the filum terminale in the *spinal theca*. (For developmental changes consult p. 238 and Pearson & Sauter 1971b.)

Ventral spinal roots contain efferent somatic and, at some levels, efferent sympathetic nerve fibres which emerge from their spinal sources. The presence of afferent nerve fibres in these roots has been reported (see Willis & Coggeshall 1991). The rootlets comprising each ventral root emerge from the anterolateral sulcus over an elongated vertical elliptical area. *Dorsal spinal roots* have ovoid swellings, the *spinal ganglia*, one on each root proximal to its junction with a corresponding ventral root in an intervertebral foramen; each fans out into six to eight rootlets before entering the cord in a *vertical row* in the posterolateral sulcus. Dorsal roots are usually

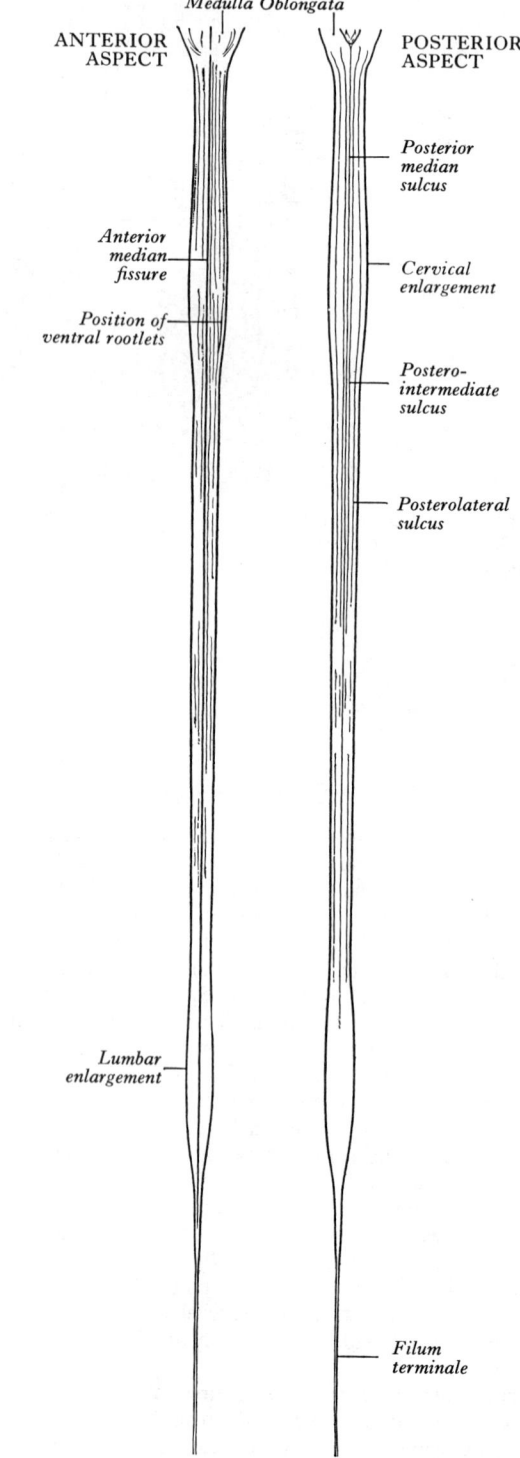

8.86 Median sagittal section of the lumbosacral part of the vertebral column to show the conus medullaris and filum terminale. The section has opened up the subarachnoid space as far as the first sacral vertebra. Note the difference in levels between the inferior limits of the spinal cord and its meninges. This illustration retained from an earlier edition has two major inaccuracies. The periosteum lines the vertebral canal and is separated from the dura by internal vertebral venous plexuses etc: at lumbar levels the fibres of interspinous ligaments slope dorsocranially.

8.87 The main features of the spinal cord.

said to contain only afferent axons (both somatic and visceral) from unipolar neurons in spinal root ganglia; but a small number (3%) may be efferent (Young & Zuckermann 1936) and autonomic vaso-dilator fibres may issue in them. These views with regard to efferent fibres have received little support. Each ganglionic neuron has a single short stem (axon) which at once divides into a medial branch entering the spinal cord via a dorsal root and a lateral one passing peripherally to a sensory end organ. The central branch is an axon; the peripheral one is an elongated dendrite (but when traversing a peripheral nerve is, in general structural terms, indistinguishable from an axon). The region of spinal cord associated with the emergence of a pair of nerves is a *spinal segment*, but there is no actual surface indication of segmentation. (Further, the deep neural sources or destinations of radicular fibres may lie far beyond the confines of the 'segment' so defined.) Recent researches show that ventral spinal nerve roots contain only one neuromediator (acetylcholine; ACh), whereas dorsal roots contain many, which include calcitonin gene-related peptide (CGRP), bombesin, substance P, vasoactive intestinal polypeptide (VIP), cholecystokinin (CCK), somatostatin, dynorphin and angiotensin II (see p. 937).

The arterial blood supply and venous drainage of the spinal cord are reviewed on p. 918 and p. 920, respectively.

INTERNAL STRUCTURE OF THE SPINAL CORD

Internally the spinal cord may be considered from several complementary points of view. Ignoring blood vessels and neuroglia, the arrangement of neurons and their processes can be studied by dissection and macroscopic inspection of sections, by light and electron microscopy, neurohistochemical approaches of great variety, by experimental techniques and combinations of these. Dissection reveals little more than the general layout of fibres and cells; microscopy details cellular types, fibre calibres and their intimate disposition. While light and electron microscopy have greatly clarified connections between neurons, their potential can only be fully exploited with experimental manoeuvres, such as degeneration, microelectrode and chemical tracing methods. Spinal organization is hence considered in steps:

- the general arrangement of grey and white matter
- the distribution of neurons in grey matter
- the deployment of tracts of fibres in white matter
- the detailed organization of the spinal neurons.

General arrangement of grey and white matter

Spinal grey matter is central (i.e. deep to the white matter) and shaped like a fluted column, except where modified at its continuation into the medulla oblongata and conus medullaris. In transverse sections (**8.92**) this column has symmetrical right and left comma-shaped masses connected by a narrow transverse *grey commissure*, the whole resembling a letter H. The commissure is traversed by the central canal, which may be just visible to the unaided eye. Each lateral crescentic mass has a lateral concavity and *anterior* and *posterior columns*. At some levels a small, intermediate *lateral column* projects from the concavity. In transverse sections the columns appear as projections and are often called 'horns' (*cornua*). The

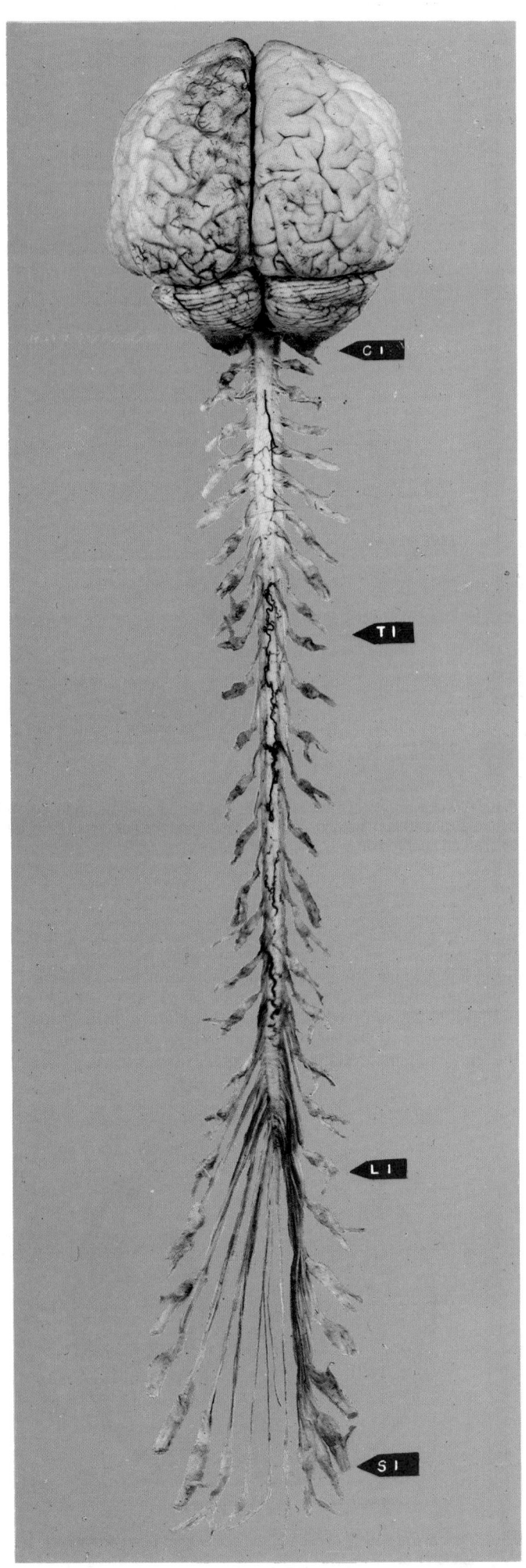

8.88 (*right*) The brain and spinal cord with attached spinal nerve roots and dorsal root ganglia, photographed from the dorsal aspect. Note the relative sizes of the cerebral and cerebellar hemispheres and the fusiform cervical and lumbar enlargements of the spinal cords. The median longitudinal fissure between the hemispheres which receives the falx cerebri and falx cerebelli is visible, together with the horizontal cleft between cerebrum and cerebellum which receives the tentorium cerebelli. Contrast the irregular pattern and dimensions of the cerebral gyri and sulci with the more regular, largely transverse pattern of the smaller cerebellar folia and their intervening fissures. Note also the changing obliquity of the spinal nerve roots in their rostrocaudal progression, the stouter roots attached to the limb enlargements and the formation of the cauda equina and filum terminale. The cauda is undisturbed on the right and has been fanned out on the left to facilitate identification of its individual components. (Dissection by M C E Hutchinson, photograph by Kevin Fitzpatrick, both of Division of Anatomy and Cell Biology, Guy's Hospital Medical School, London.)

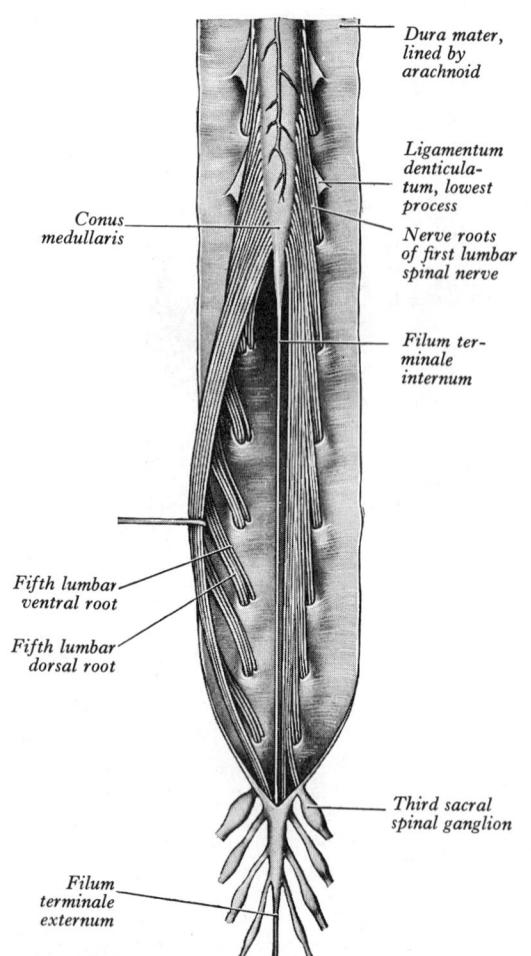

Dura mater, lined by arachnoid

Ligamentum denticula- tum, lowest process

Conus medullaris

Nerve roots of first lumbar spinal nerve

Filum ter- minale internum

Fifth lumbar ventral root

Fifth lumbar dorsal root

Third sacral spinal ganglion

Filum terminale externum

8.89 The lower end of the spinal cord, the filum terminale and the cauda equina exposed from behind. The dura mater and the arachnoid have been opened and spread out.

central grey matter is surrounded by white matter, the latter consisting largely of nerve fibres, many of which (but by no means all) being longitudinal and grouped into *funiculi* or *white columns*. The general arrangement of these as dorsal, lateral and ventral funiculi has been noted and further details appear later (p. 987 et seq).

The *anterior* or *ventral grey column* projects ventrolaterally from the grey commissure. It is short, broad and separated from the

surface by part of the anterior funiculus (**8.92**). Its anterior and posterior regions are sometimes named its head and base.

The *posterior* or *dorsal grey column*, projecting dorsolaterally, is transversely narrow and extends almost to the surface near the posterolateral sulcus, separated from it by a thin *dorsolateral tract* (of Lissauer) (**8.103,104**). It also is considered to have a *base* where it is continuous with the *intermediate* grey region, a constricted neck which expands into an oval or fusiform *head*, and an apex which is capped by a crescent of semitranslucent nervous tissue, the *substantia gelatinosa* (*Rolandi*). The latter is intimately connected with incoming afferent nerve fibres (p. 980).

The *lateral grey column* is a small, angular projection extending between the second thoracic and first lumbar *spinal cord segments*, and does not appear at other levels.

The boundary between white and grey matter is usually clear but, at cervical levels, strands of grey matter invade the lateral funiculus from the base of the dorsal grey column, separated by interlacing nerve fibres like a net, whence its name, the *reticular formation*. Similar regions appear at lower spinal levels; brainstem reticular formations also exist, where physiological investigations have led to a concept of an extensive *reticular 'system'* widely deployed throughout the neuraxis (p. 1073).

This main pattern of white and grey matter is what might be expected in simple terms of peripherally placed conductors, i.e. longitudinally arranged spinal tracts of fibres, but with their sources and interconnections centrally placed; however, it is also an expression of spinal development (p. 238). Dimensions and relative volumes of peripheral (white) fibres and centrally aggregated neurons at different levels (**8.92**) can be explained partly by the amounts of muscle, skin and other tissues innervated by different segments and by the sequential expansion of longitudinal tracts (both ascending and descending) as progression is made in a cranial direction. At thoracic levels, the volume of the grey matter is absolutely and relatively small, while the white substance shows an ascending increase. In the cervical and lumbar enlargements, the amount of grey matter, especially of the ventral columns, is augmented by large accumulations of neurons innervating the limbs; but while white matter at cervical levels is also pronounced, in the lumbar enlargement and particularly the conus medullaris, the white funiculi contain many fewer fibres passing through these segments. **8.92** shows the details in representative segments; it is obvious that various levels can easily be distinguished. It is, however, more useful to recognize the explanation of these differences in terms of the criteria noted above.

The *central canal* traverses the whole spinal cord and caudal half of the medulla oblongata, opening above into the fourth ventricle (p. 1208). In the conus medullaris it expands as a fusiform *terminal ventricle*, triangular in section with a ventral base, and is 8–10 mm in length, obliterating at about 40 years. At cervical and thoracic levels, the canal is slightly ventral to the midpoint of the cord, and

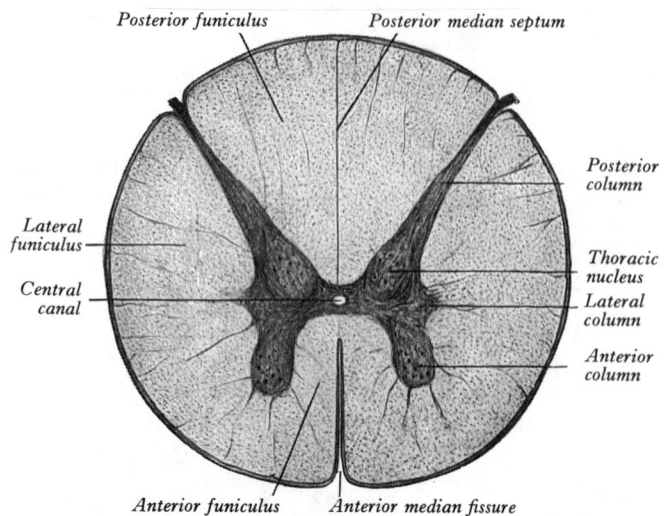

Posterior funiculus

Posterior median septum

Posterior column

Lateral funiculus

Thoracic nucleus

Central canal

Lateral column

Anterior column

Anterior funiculus

Anterior median fissure

8.90 Typical transverse section of the spinal cord at a mid-thoracic level. Magnification × 8.

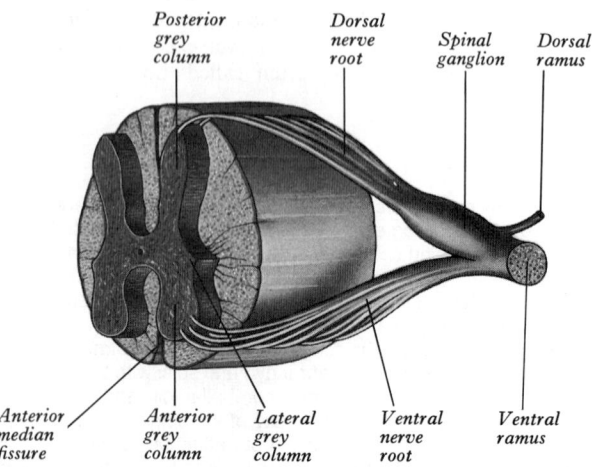

Posterior grey column

Dorsal nerve root

Spinal ganglion

Dorsal ramus

Anterior median fissure

Anterior grey column

Lateral grey column

Ventral nerve root

Ventral ramus

8.91 Diagram of a spinal cord segment showing mode of formation of a typical spinal nerve and the gross relationships of the grey and white matter. Note dorsal nerve rootlets in a single linear row; ventral rootlets in three or more rows.

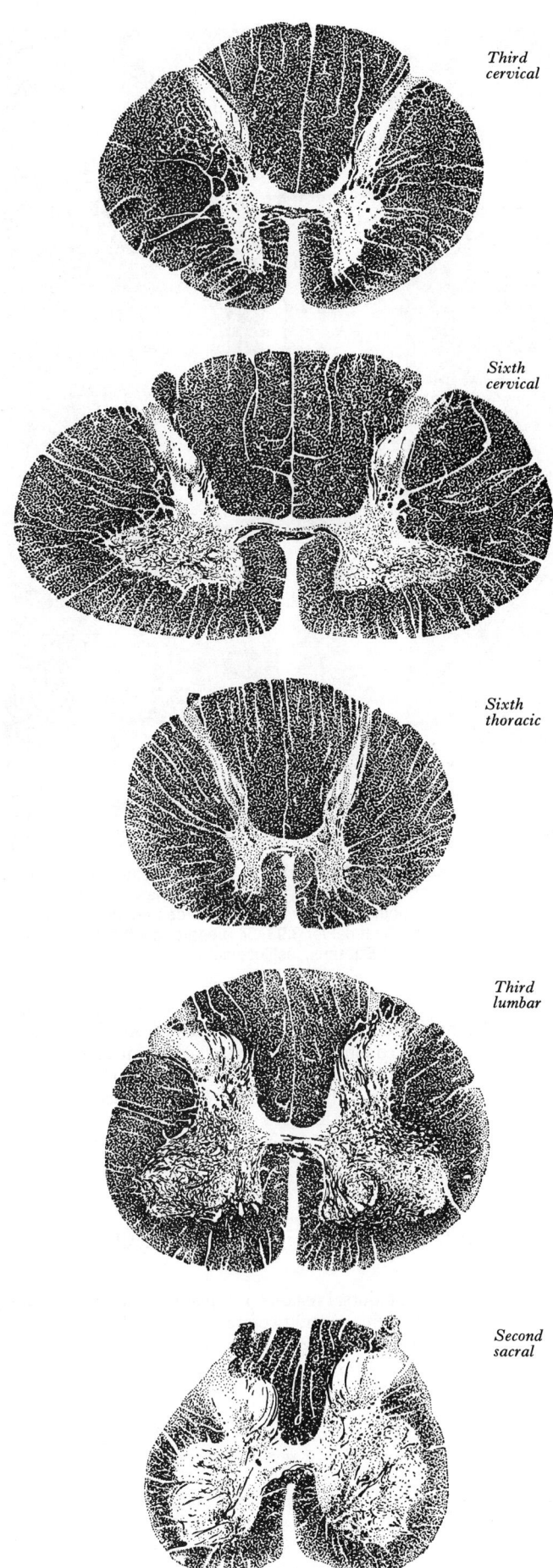

*Third
cervical*

*Sixth
cervical*

*Sixth
thoracic*

*Third
lumbar*

*Second
sacral*

8.92 Transverse sections through the spinal cord at representative levels. Note changes in overall profile and the relative changes in grey and white regions, their shape, size and proportions. Magnification × 5.

central in the lumbar enlargement, but more dorsal in the conus medullaris; it extends for 5–6 mm into the filum terminale. It contains CSF, and is lined by columnar, ciliated epithelium, the *ependyma*, which is encircled by a zone of neuroglia containing a few neurons and a network of fine nerve fibres, the *substantia gelatinosa centralis.* This is traversed by processes spreading from the basal aspects of ependymal cells. The grey matter around the canal, external to the *substantia*, is the *grey commissure* which is thin ventrally. Anterior to the grey commissure is the *ventral white commissure*. The grey commissure is traversed by two longitudinal veins and, dorsal to the canal, it is contiguous with the posterior median septum; it is thinnest at the thoracic level, thickest in the conus medullaris. The grey commissure is permeated by transverse myelinated nerve fibres, which collectively are sometimes termed the *dorsal white commissure.*

GREY MATTER OF THE CORD

Spinal grey matter (**8.93, 94**) is a complex mixture of neurons and neurites, neuroglia and blood vessels. The predominance of neuronal somata is responsible for the so-called grey appearance. Neuroglia (p. 937) form an intricate lattice among the somata and their neurites, being particularly condensed in the gelatinous substance around the central canal. Neurites will be described in detail later, with the tracts (p. 987) and with the organization of interneurons (p. 985); they include axons arriving from or departing to the fibre tracts of the white funiculi, the initial part of efferent peripheral fibres and the termination of afferent peripheral fibres together with their collaterals, and a most complex neuropil. The latter is composed of many neurites of neurons which are mainly confined to the grey matter. Many neurites cross the midline in the commissures, and the right and left halves of the cord, including its grey matter, are a functional continuum. Neurons in the grey substance are multipolar, varying in size and in other features, particularly length and the arrangement of axons and dendrites. Many are Golgi types I and II neurons, axons of the former passing out of the grey matter into ventral spinal roots or spinal tracts. Axons and dendrites of Golgi type II neurons are largely confined to the nearby grey matter. Some neurons are *intrasegmental*, deployed within a single segment; others spread through several segments, thus being *intersegmental* in distribution (p. 1008).

In much of the central nervous system, nerve cell somata are grouped, often in large numbers, usually indicating a common function. A large group may be divided with a constancy justifying specific names. Such constant patterns of distribution inevitably suggest functional implications, though the influence of developmental constraints may sometimes be of greater significance. Neurons of the spinal grey matter are not distributed uniformly: they occur in major and minor aggregations, some of which have obvious functional significance, whilst others are subject to controversy. The following cytoarchitecture of the spinal grey substance is first described in purely topographical terms and, for convenience, separately in ventral, dorsal and lateral grey columns. Functional interpretations of some groups in these columns will be considered later.

NEURONAL GROUPS OF THE ANTERIOR GREY COLUMNS

Neurons in the ventral columns vary in size. The average dimensions of the largest somata of multipolar cells exceed 25 μm; their axons emerge in ventral roots to innervate the striated skeletal muscles as *α*-efferents. Large numbers of smaller neurons of 15–25 μm also occur and some of their axons are *γ*-efferents innervating the intrafusal fibres of neuromuscular spindles. By the evidence of retrograde degeneration, many smaller neurons in this column do not have such efferents and most are interneurons.

The ventral column neurons are arranged in elongated groups, forming a number of separate longitudinal columns extending through several segments. These are seen most easily in transverse sections (**8.93**); although longitudinal sections are rarely depicted, these clearly show that the neuronal columns are not uniformly continuous (**8.94**), each is a series of small aggregations, too dim-

979

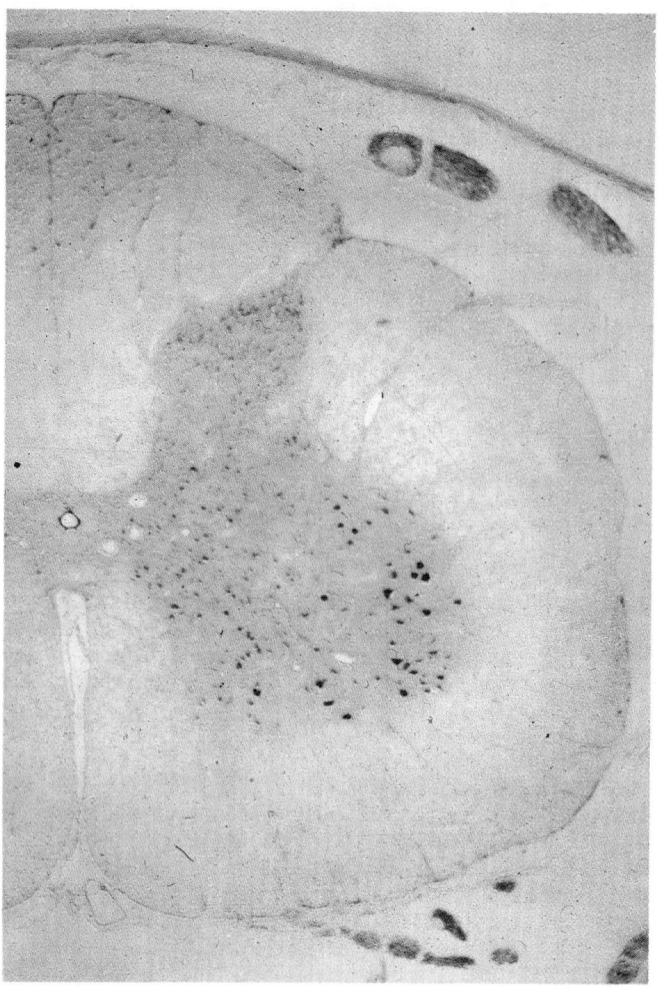

8.93 Transverse section of left half of human spinal cord at a mid-lumbar level. Note dorsal and ventral grey columns and commissural grey mass. The larger motor neurons in the ventral grey column are visibly grouped. For details see text. Stained with cresyl fast violet.

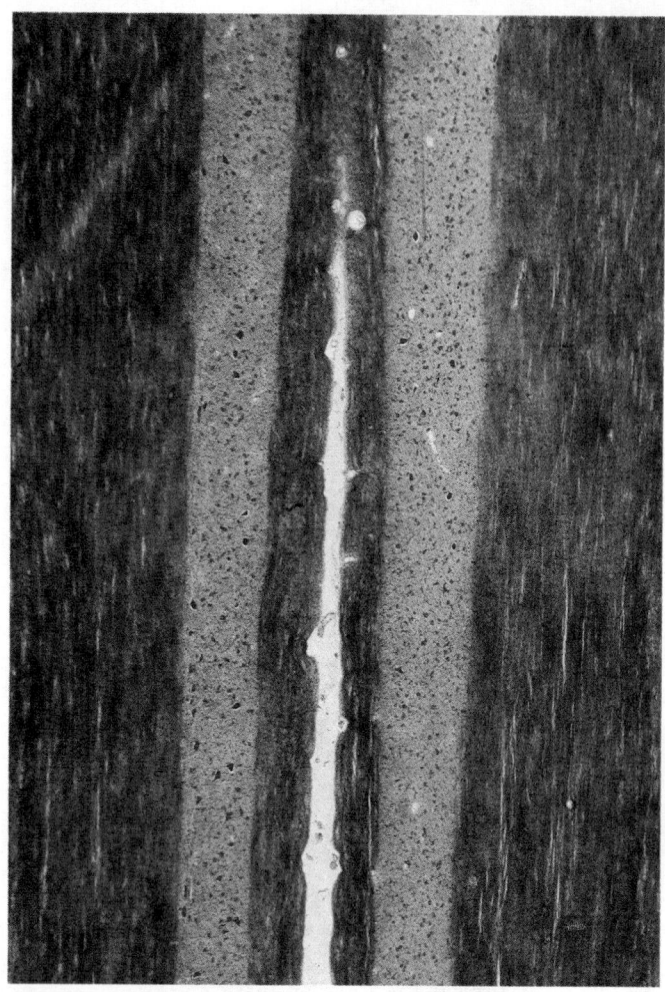

8.94 Longitudinal section of feline spinal cord showing the anterior median fissure and anterior white columns and lateral to these the ventral grey columns, in which motor neurons show some degree of grouping into longitudinal columns. (Material for **8**.93, 94 prepared by the late L Laruelle and supplied by J André-Balisaux, Institut Neurologique Belge, Brussels.)

inutive for segmental significance (Laruelle & Reumont 1933). The basic division of the ventral grey region is into *medial, central* and *lateral* columns and all exhibit subdivision at certain levels, usually into dorsal and ventral parts. As can be seen in **8**.95, the *medial group* extends throughout the cord, being perhaps absent in the fifth lumbar and first sacral segments. In the thoracic and the upper four lumbar segments, it is subdivided into *ventromedial* and *dorsomedial groups*; in segments cranial and caudal to this, the medial group has only a ventromedial moiety, except in the first cervical where only the dorsomedial group exists. The *central group*, the least extensive, is found only in some cervical and lumbosacral segments. In the cervical cord, through the third to seventh segments, is a centrally situated columnar *phrenic nucleus*; abundant experimental and clinical evidence shows that its neurons innervate the diaphragm, being probably the least controversial motor pool in the entire cord. For experimental data in mammals, including primates, see Kohnstamm (1898), Sharrard (1955), Keswani and Hollinshead (1956), Warwick and Mitchell (1956), Ullah (1978), and Kuypers (1985). The *lumbosacral nucleus*, in the second lumbar to first sacral segments, is also central; the distribution of its axons is unknown. Neurons whose axons are said to enter the spinal accessory nerve form an irregular *accessory group*, in the upper five or six cervical segments, at the ventral border of the anterior grey column and intermediate in position but lateral to the dorsomedial group in the first cervical segment; the ventral siting of this nucleus may be due to the absence of lateral groups from the first three cervical segments (**8**.95).

The *lateral group* in the ventral column is subdivided into *ventral, dorsal* and *retrodorsal groups*, all largely confined to the spinal segments innervating the limbs. Their extents are indicated in **8**.95

and their significance will be discussed later (p. 982). Onufrowicz (1899), who later called himself Onuf, described a ventrolateral group in the first and second sacral segments, considered to innervate the perineal striated muscles. This '*nucleus of Onuf*' has been confirmed in mankind by Mannen et al (1977) and Schrøder (1981), and by Konishi et al (1978) and Holstege and Tan (1987) in cats (see p. 1078).

NEURONAL GROUPS OF THE POSTERIOR GREY COLUMNS

Two groups are in the dorsal regions of spinal grey matter extending the whole length of the cord and two are limited to the thoracic and upper lumbar segments. No less than 15 neuromediators have been identified in the spinal dorsal grey column.

Substantia gelatinosa (of Rolando), present at all levels, consists of small Golgi type II neurons with some larger ones. Connections with afferents of the dorsal roots and the spinothalamic tract complex have long been accepted, but a revision of the details has followed experimental work (pp. 986–990). A second long group of large neurons, ventral to the *substantia*, is the *dorsal funicular group* or *nucleus proprius* (**8**.95). A thin lamina of neurons, distinguishable from those of the substantia by their larger size, is the *marginal zone* of some observers, sited dorsal to the substantia.

Nucleus dorsalis or *thoracicus* ('Clarke's column') is basal in the posterior grey column, immediately dorsal to the intermediate zone in laminae VI–VII (p. 984). At most levels, it is near the dorsal white funiculus and may project into it. In the human spinal cord, it can

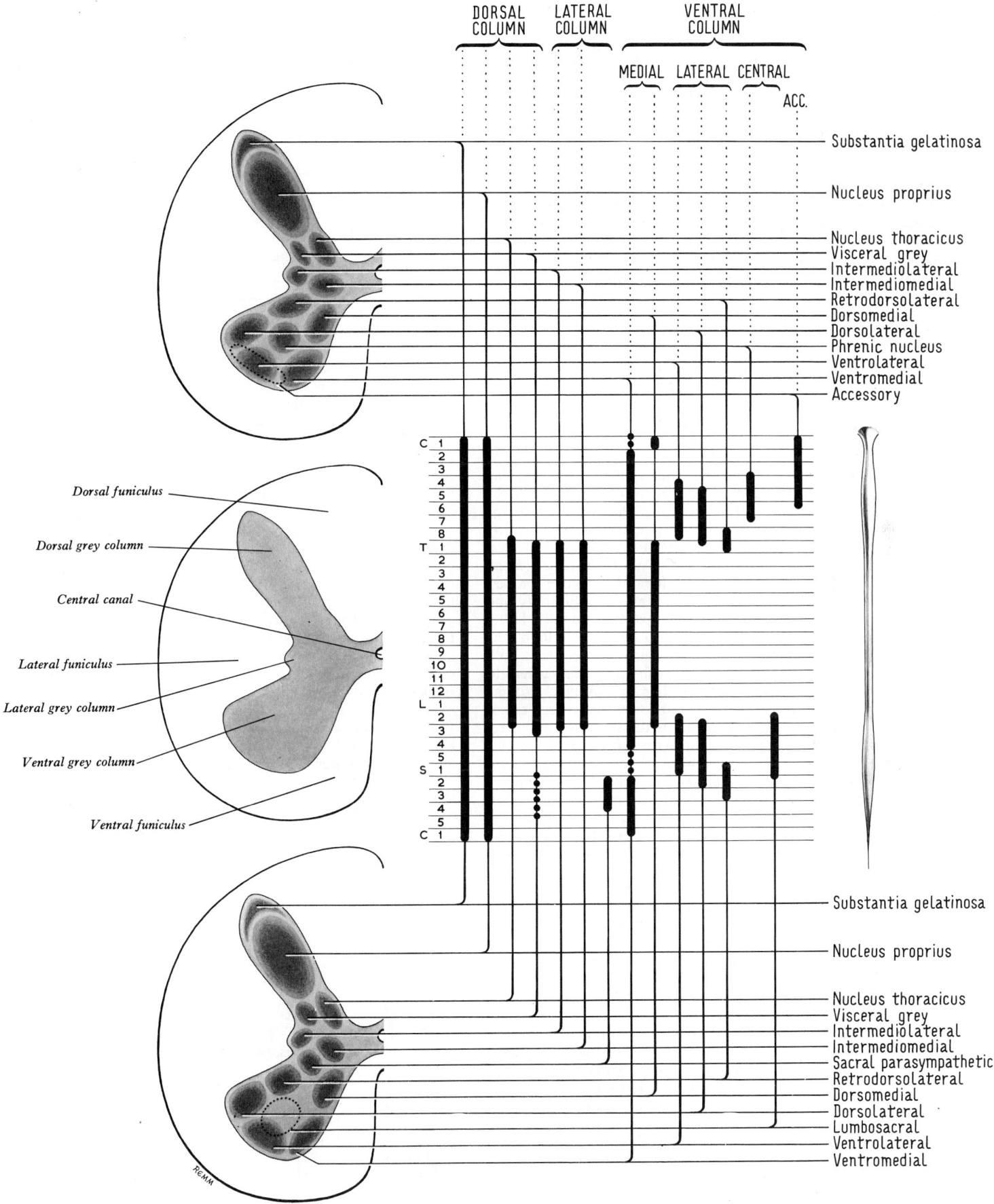

8.95 The groups or nuclei of nerve cells in the grey columns of the human spinal cord as generally accepted. Relative positions of these columnar groups, as well as their extension through varying series of spinal segments, are as indicated. (Adapted from data in Crosby et al 1962, with permission of the authors and publishers.)

usually be identified from the eighth cervical to the third or fourth lumbar segments. Similar groups have been described at cervical levels superior to the nucleus dorsalis; also prolongations at caudal levels appear to exist in some long-tailed monkeys (Chang 1951). But these 'cervical' and 'sacral' nuclei consist of different neurons and have been described only in some mammals; hence it is premature to extrapolate such groups to the human spinal cord. Neurons of the dorsal nucleus itself vary, most being large, especially in the lower thoracic and lumbar segments; some send axons into the dorsal spinocerebellar tracts (p. 990) while some are interneurons. Petras and Cummings (1977) have described the neurons and connections of this nucleus in neonatal dogs, confirming a role as a 'relay' in the dorsal spinocerebellar paths; they ascribed a similar role to the *nucleus centrobasalis*, which is in the dorsal grey column like the nucleus thoracicus, but situated in the lower cervical and lumbosacral segments. These groups have not been established in human spinal cord.

Lateral to the nucleus dorsalis and dorsal to the intermediolateral column (**8**.95), a small region of neurons of medium size extends through the same segments (first thoracic to third lumbar) as the intermediate columns (Takahashi 1913); this group is identifiable in the human cord, but is functionally obscure.

NEURONAL GROUPS OF THE INTERMEDIATE GREY MATTER

The intermediate region of spinal grey matter (**8**.93, 95), including the lateral grey columns, contains small neurons, many with the features of autonomic preganglionic cells. These develop in the embryonic cord at first dorsolateral to the central canal. Many migrate lateral to it, forming an *intermediolateral column*. An *intermediomedial column* is formed from neurons nearer the central canal. The intermediolateral is the projecting lateral grey column proper; many of its neurons send axons into ventral spinal roots and via white rami communicantes to the sympathetic trunk (p. 1298). Preganglionic fibres are similarly derived from some cells of the intermediomedial column (the remainder being interneurons). Both groups extend from the eighth cervical or first thoracic segment to the second or third lumbar, corresponding approximately to the thoracolumbar outflow. In the second to fourth sacral segments a similar group, intermediate in position, is the source of the sacral outflow of parasympathetic preganglionic nerve fibres (p. 1297). This *sacral parasympathetic grey column* also lies lateral to the central canal and substantia gelatinosa centralis in the zone between the bases of the anterior and posterior grey columns and shows no mediolateral division, nor does it project like the thoracolumbar lateral grey column. The emergence of parasympathetic preganglionic nerve fibres from other segments has been described by Kuré et al (1930) and Sheehan (1933), their origins being ascribed to the basal region of the dorsal grey column and perhaps the intermediate grey zone; the fibres were stated to issue in the *dorsal* roots, to be vasodilator and to synapse in the corresponding dorsal spinal root ganglia (Kiss 1932; Kuré et al 1934). These interesting views have received neither general acceptance nor confirmation.

This description of spinal cytoarchitecture largely depends on material stained to show the *somata* of neurons rather than their processes; it has been amplified by a *laminar concept* of spinal organization (p. 983). More widely based on interconnections, its structural data are correlated with the results of degeneration experiments and microelectrode studies. The laminar pattern yields a more precise definition of spinal cord activities; but the two modes of description are not exclusive, the older scheme of columnar groups being in most features adaptable into the newer description. The main modifications concern the structural relations between the dorsal grey column neurons and the fibres of dorsal roots and spinal tracts.

FUNCTIONAL IMPLICATIONS OF ANTERIOR GREY COLUMN CELL GROUPS

Even in the earliest accounts of spinal columnar arrays of neurons, mostly based on Nissl-stained transverse sections (from a miscellany of animals, including tadpoles, an ostrich, a gorilla and even man), a somatotopic interpretation was advanced with confidence (Elliot

1942). Thus, an early tenet was that medial groups innervate the axial musculature, the limbs being innervated from lateral groups. This speculation, based initially on structural data, has been confirmed experimentally in mammalian studies, mainly in the cat, using retrograde degeneration (Romanes 1951) and the retrograde tracing methods (for reviews see Kuypers 1981; Holstege 1991). The basic building block of the somatic motor neuronal populations is represented by a longitudinally disposed group of neurons that innervate a given muscle, and in which the α and γ motor neurons are intermixed. The various groups innervating the different muscles are aggregated into two major longitudinal columns, medial and lateral, which in transverse section form the medial and lateral cell groups in the ventral grey column (**8**.96).

The *medial longitudinal motor column* extends throughout the length of the spinal cord, its neurons innervating epaxial and hypaxial muscle groups. The epaxial muscles are innervated by branches of the dorsal primary rami of spinal nerves; the hypaxial muscles by branches of the ventral primary rami. In the medial column, motor neurons supplying epaxial muscles are sited ventral to those supplying hypaxial muscles (Sprague 1948; Smith & Hollyday 1983). Basically, epaxial muscles include, amongst others, the erector spinae which extend the head and vertebral column, while hypaxial muscles flex the neck and the trunk; the latter include prevertebral muscles of the neck, intercostal and anterior abdominal wall muscles.

The *lateral longitudinal motor column* is found only in the enlargements of the spinal cord; the motor neurons of this column in the cervical and lumbar enlargements innervate muscles of the fore- and hindlimbs respectively. In the cervical enlargement, motor neurons supplying muscles intrinsic to the forelimb are situated dorsally in the ventral grey column, those innervating the most distal (hand) muscles are sited further dorsally, whereas motor neurons of the girdle muscles are found in the ventrolateral part of the ventral grey matter (**8**.96). There is also a further somatotopic organization in that the proximal muscles of the limb are supplied from motor cell groups located more rostrally in the enlargement than those supplying the distal muscles; for example, motor neurons innervating intrinsic muscles of the hand are sited in segments C8 and T1, while motor neurons of shoulder muscles are in segments C5 and 6. A similar overall arrangement of motor cell locations of hindlimb muscles obtains in the lumbosacral cord.

In mankind, data on the location of spinal motor neurons are few and less precise than those obtained from animal experiments. Such information has been gleaned mainly from clinicopathological studies

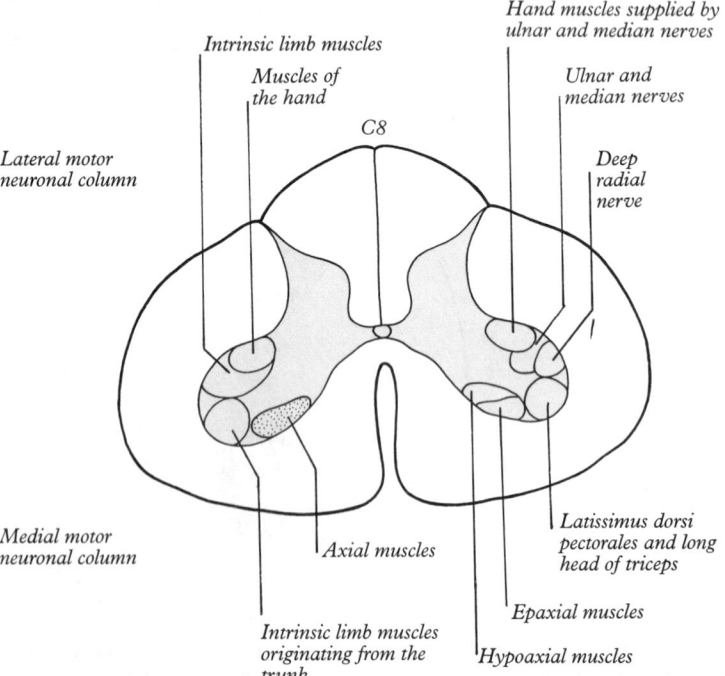

8.96 Schematic overview of the location of motor cells groups at C8 of segmental level of the spinal cord of the cat. The left side of the figure shows the subdivision of the lateral and medial longitudinal motor columns; the right side depicts these in more detail. (Redrawn and modified from Holstege 1991 with permission of Elsevier Science Publishers B.V.)

on patients dying from poliomyelitis which induces chromatolytic changes in motor neurons, ultimately leading to the death and loss of these virus-infected cells. The most detailed studies were undertaken by Sharrard (1955, 1956, 1964); his findings are illustrated in **8.97**, **98**, and in general confirm the pattern of motor neuronal localization obtained in the cat.

FURTHER ASPECTS OF SPINAL ORGANIZATION

The preceding introduction to the organization of the spinal cord must now be expanded and partly modified in the light of recent studies using both neuroanatomical and neurophysiological techniques, often in parallel (for reviews with extensive references see Brown 1981; Willis & Coggeshall 1991). Such studies include comparisons in many vertebrates, alternative schemes for the classification of spinal grey matter based on cytoarchitectonics and more precise analyses of dendritic and axonal arborizations using modified Golgi techniques or intraneuronal injection of a variety of markers. Newer tracing techniques have also augmented our knowledge of the terminations of dorsal root afferents and collaterals, and of ascending and descending supraspinal projections. Minute focal lesions have been placed to unravel the intricacies of spinal cord circuitry; and light microscopical techniques together with detailed ultrastructural studies of synapses have been improved by quantification. The distribution of putative transmitters has also shown much progress; see Ruda et al (1986) and Tohyama and Shiotani (1986).

LAMINAR ARCHITECTURE

The general outline of spinal grey regions, as seen in transverse section, has long provided a useful but arbitrary terminological basis for morphology and experiment. Dorsal, lateral and ventral columns with their arbitrary subdivisions have been recognized (p. 979) and named. Such entities as the substantia gelatinosa, thoracic nucleus and subgroups of anterior grey column neurons have been named, with a terminology which, if arbitrary, is still used. Much basic work has been carried out within this topographical scheme but increasing analysis, both structural and functional, reveals a lack of precision, prompting attempts to re-describe the grey matter of the cord (Rexed 1952, 1954, 1964). The currently adopted scheme stems initially from studies in thick and thin sections, stained by the Nissl method for neuronal somata in spinal cords of neonatal, young and adult cats. Based on neuronal size, shape, cytological features and density in

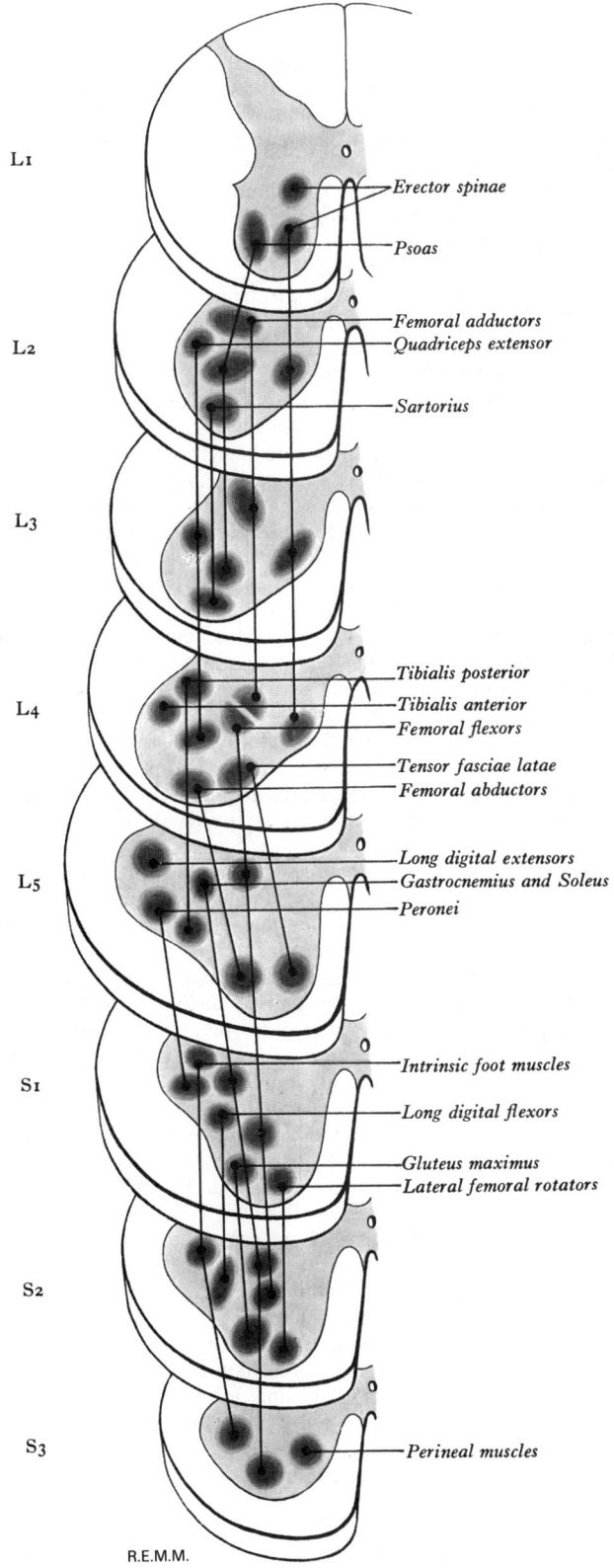

8.97 The approximate location in the transverse plane, and in longitudinal extent, of the nerve cell groups innervating muscles, chiefly in the leg, in the lumbosacral segments of the human spinal cord. Based on clinico-pathological studies of poliomyelitis (Sharrard 1955).

THE INNERVATION OF THE LOWER LIMB MUSCLES

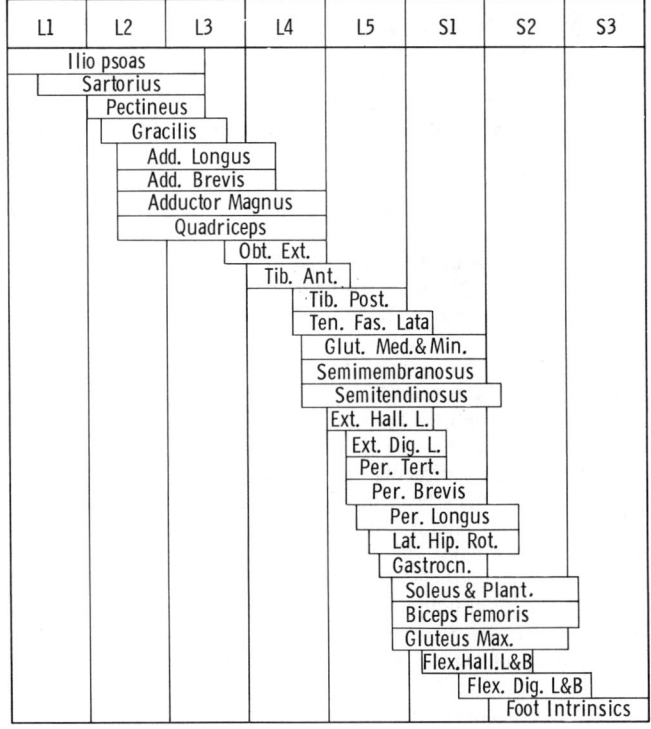

8.98 The segmental arrangement of the innervation of the lower limb muscles (Sharrard 1964).

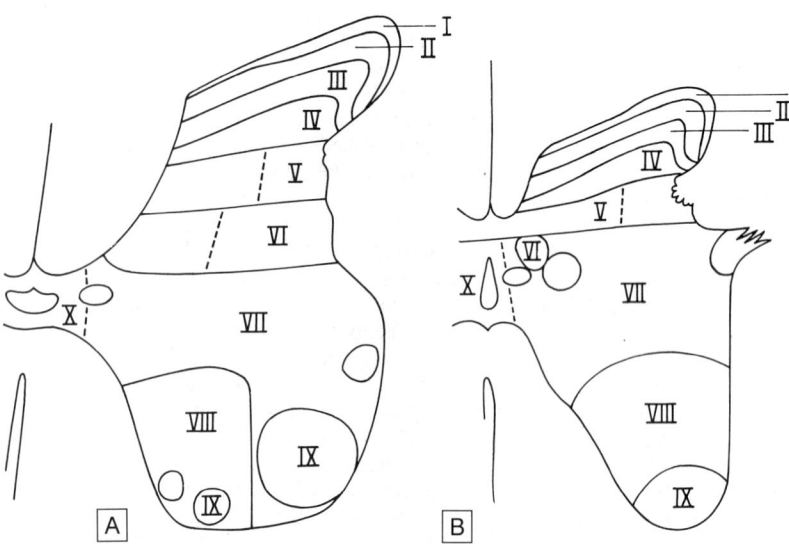

8.99 The pattern of lamination proposed by B Rexed (1964) for the spinal cord grey matter of the cat, viewed in transverse section: A. the fifth lumbar segment; B. the third thoracic segment. (Reproduced with the permission of B Rexed and Elsevier.)

different regions, nine laminae have been distinguished, which are arrayed more or less parallel with the dorsal and ventral limits of the grey matter and extend throughout most of the length of the cord, together with a region (lamina X) surrounding the central canal. These laminae, as they appear in the transverse section of a fifth lumbar segment, are shown in **8.99A**. General confirmation of the laminar pattern in human material has been provided by Schoenen (1973) and Schoenen and Faull (1990). Briefly the structure of laminae is as follows:

Lamina I is a very thin layer with an ill-defined boundary. It adjoins the white matter (which outlying neurons invade) and has a reticular appearance due to bundles of coarse and fine nerve fibres intermingling in many directions. It contains small, intermediate and large neuronal somata, many being fusiform in shape. Alternative names are *lamina marginalis* or *layer of Waldeyer* (who recognized a similar zone in 1888).

Lamina II occupies most of the head of the dorsal column and consists of densely packed, small neurons which give rise to its dark appearance in Nissl-stained sections. With myelin stains it is characteristically distinguished from adjacent laminae by the almost total lack of myelinated fibres which accounts for its gelatinous appearance.

Lamina III consists of somata mostly larger, more variable and less closely arrayed than those in lamina II. It also contains many myelinated fibres.

Lamina IV is a thick, loosely packed, heterogeneous zone permeated by fibres. Neuronal somata vary much in size and shape, from small and round, through intermediate triangular, to very large stellar types.

Laminae I–IV correspond to the head of the dorsal column. Lamina II (and some workers consider in addition part or all of lamina III) corresponds to the *substantia gelatinosa*; whilst the ill-defined *nucleus proprius* of the dorsal grey column corresponds to some of the cell constituents of laminae III and IV.

Lamina V is a thick layer including the neck of the dorsal column, is divisible into a lateral third and medial two-thirds. Both have a mixed population but the former contains many prominent well-stained somata interlaced by numerous bundles of transverse, dorsoventral and longitudinal fibres: hence the term 'formatio reticularis' for this region, particularly prominent at cervical levels and recognized first by Deiters in 1865; this term is now used more widely, p. 1073.

Lamina VI is most prominent in the limb enlargements, particularly in young animals; it has a medial third of small densely packed neurons and a lateral two-thirds containing larger, more loosely packed, triangular or stellate somata. The medial part hence stains more heavily, in contrast to lamina V, where the converse applies.

Lamina VI corresponds approximately to the *base* of the dorsal column.

Laminae VII–IX show a variety of complex forms in the limb enlargements (**8.99A**); to assist explanation, the simpler arrangement at thoracic levels is included for comparison (**8.99B**).

Lamina VII includes much of the intermediate grey column. It contains prominent neurons of the *thoracic nucleus* and *intermediomedial* and *intermediolateral columns* at their spinal levels (**8.95**). The remaining areas (between these columns and, in limb enlargements, between lamina VIII and groups of IX) contain a uniform array of medium-sized triangular or stellate somata.

Lamina VIII spans the base of the thoracic ventral column but is restricted in limb enlargements to the medial aspect of this column. It contains a heterogeneous mixture of cell sizes and shapes from small to moderately large.

Lamina IX is a complex array of columns (**8.97**) which comprise the very large somata of α motor neurons and numerous smaller cells. The smaller ones include motor neurons with small-diameter efferent fibres (γ efferents) for muscle spindles, and numerous interneurons, some of which were thought to be inhibitory in nature (see below). The location of γ motor neurons was long in doubt but studies of the retrograde changes following peripheral trauma (Nyberg-Hansen 1965a) and intracellular recording (Eccles et al 1960) show them to be dispersed among α neurons in the motor columns.

Lamina X surrounds the central canal, including the *dorsal and ventral grey commissures* and the *substantia gelatinosa centralis*.

The preceding description outlines the scheme, originally described in the spinal cord of the cat (Rexed 1952, 1954), but which has been applied *de facto* to spinal cords of other mammals, for example the monkey (Kuypers & Brinkman 1970; Miller & Strominger 1973) and the rat (Brichta & Grant 1985); and has been formally confirmed in the mouse (Sidman et al 1971) and man (Schoenen 1973; Schoenen & Faull 1990). Rexed proposed the following tentative functional analysis (though some conclusions have been revised, see below).

Laminae I–IV are the main receiving areas for cutaneous primary afferent terminals and collateral branches (see below). From this region start many complex polysynaptic reflex paths, ipsilateral and contralateral, intrasegmental and intersegmental: and from it many long ascending tracts to higher levels are considered to arise (but see below).

Laminae V and VI receive most of the terminals of proprioceptive primary afferents and profuse corticospinal projections from the motor and sensory cortex and subcortical levels, suggesting intimate involvement in the regulation of movement.

Lamina VII in its lateral part has extensive ascending and descending connections with the midbrain and cerebellum (via the spinocerebellar, spinotectal, spinoreticular, tectospinal, reticulospinal and rubrospinal tracts) and is thus involved in the regulation of posture and movement. Its medial part has numerous propriospinal reflex connections with the adjacent grey matter and segments concerned both with movement and autonomic functions (p. 1292). Intracellular recordings indicate inhibitory interneurons in the ventral extension of lamina VII, insinuated between VIII and IX (Willis & Willis 1966). Golgi staining in this region (Scheibel & Scheibel 1966c) has not revealed typical Golgi type II neurons, long assumed to be the basis of 'Renshaw loop' inhibition. Nevertheless, Szentágothai (1967a) considers that neurons with longer axons are not incompatible with inhibitory function and that the extension of lamina VII receives most initial collateral branches from axons of α motor neurons (assumed to synapse with Renshaw cells). More recently, Renshaw cells have been identified and located precisely in this ventral extension, just medial to the motor column (Jankowska & Lindström 1971); furthermore, the so-called 1a inhibitory neurons are found in the ventral part of lamina VII, just dorsal and medial to the motor column (Hultborn et al 1971; Jankowska & Lindström 1972).

Lamina VIII, a mass of propriospinal interneurons, receives terminals from the adjacent laminae, many commissural terminals from the contralateral lamina VIII and descending connections from the interstitiospinal, reticulospinal and vestibulospinal tracts and the medial longitudinal fasciculus. Their axons influence motor neurons of both sides, perhaps directly but more probably by excitation of small neurons supplying γ efferent fibres to muscle spindles.

Lamina IX contains a and γ motor neurons and many interneurons. Large *a motor neurons* supply motor end plates of extrafusal muscle fibres in the motor units of striated muscle (p. 969); they vary in size. Recording techniques have demonstrated *tonic* and *phasic* a neurons (Granit et al 1956). The former, with a lower rate of firing and lower conduction velocity, are assumed to be smaller in size. Attempts to correlate these varieties of a motor neurons with structural and functional types of striated muscle fibre show that the small motor neurons with a low conduction velocity tend to innervate type S muscle units and large motor neurons with a high conduction velocity tend to supply fast twitch (type FR, FF) muscle units. Some large motor neurons (β *motor neurons*) have been held to supply extrafusal and intrafusal fibres.

There are also several functionally distinct types of γ *motor neuron*, the fusimotor fibres of which innervate the intrafusal fibres in muscle spindles. The 'static' and 'dynamic' responses of muscle spindles (p. 971) have separate controls mediated by *static* and *dynamic fusimotor fibres* distributed variously to *nuclear chain* and *bag* fibres; but it is impossible histologically to differentiate types of γ motor neuron somata, though *plate* and *trail* endings have been recognized as have two varieties of γ-efferent myelinated nerve fibre (γ 1 and γ 2) in nerves to muscle (Boyd 1962). For reviews on the innervation of muscle spindles see Barker (1974b) and Boyd and Gladden (1985).

GEOMETRY OF SPINAL NEURONS

Since Cajal's classic investigations (1908), foreshadowing so much and still a primary source of information, more precise data on spinal neurons have accumulated. As has been shown, much has been learned about the sizes, shapes, distribution, packing density and the cytological features of the neuronal *somata* from studies using the Nissl method or its modifications. Such methods provide only limited information and need to be supplemented by other methods which show analyses (preferably morphometric) of the dendroarchitecture, and of the arborizations and sites of the termination of axons and their collaterals. Furthermore, degenerative and other techniques (p. 915) are necessary for the precise determination of their connections with other neurons.

Examples of such quantitative approaches were made by Aitken and Bridger (1961) and Schadé (1964) in which the lumbosacral spinal cord of the cat was studied. The former authors found that in the ventral zone of the ventral grey column of one complete spinal segment (lumbar 6) the total neuronal population was about 7000; of these 700 were considered to be fusimotor cells giving rise to γ efferent fibres to muscle spindles; of the larger cells 3276 were propriospinal (interneurons), 126 were classed as 'spinal border' cells, whilst 2898 were a motor neurons. Thus, in this region about half of the cells were interneurons and half motor neurons; in the whole ventral column, the ratio was about seven interneurons to one motor neuron and, with the intermediate zone and base of the dorsal column included, the ratio rises to 13 to 1. The neuronal density was highest in the intermediate zone (7 cells per $100\,\mu m$ cube of tissue), and lowest in the ventral column (1–2 cells per $100\,\mu m$ cube). The *total* surface area of individual cell somata and their dendrites ranged from 11 000 to 97 000 μm^2, whereas the surface area of *cell somata* alone ranged up to 25 000 μm^2; stem dendrites varied in number to a maximum of 13, whilst *dendritic* surface area ranged up to about 76 000 μm^2. Dendritic surfaces formed about 80% of the total *receptive* neuronal surface (i.e. excepting axonal surface), the dendrites sometimes extending as far as 1000 μm from the parent soma, in which cases the terminal dendrites entered the adjacent white matter; as much as 50% of the estimated receptor surface was more than 300 μm from the parent soma. The latter figure is especially interesting, since many types of neurons have very wide ranging dendritic fields; and neurophysiological evidence (Rall 1967) shows that the excitation of these distal branches exerts a critical influence on impulse generation at the axon hillock. Schadé (1964) estimated the percentage of grey matter occupied by cell somata and their surface areas, and the percentage occupied by their dendrites and their surface areas. A mean value of 7500 μm^3 was estimated for the volume of the soma of an interneuron and 29 000 μm^3 for a soma of a motor neuron. The surface area of the 'average' soma ranged from 4.4 to $5.9 \times 10^3\,\mu m^2$ and that of the 'average' dendritic tree from 59 to $73 \times 10^3\,\mu m^2$.

Other investigations (Romanes 1964; Sprague & Ha 1964; Scheibel & Scheibel 1969) have also shown the complex dendritic patterns of ventral column motor neurons and interneurons in adjacent cell laminae, emphasizing the wide dendritic fields of motor neurons, seen to best advantage when both transverse and, particularly, longitudinal sections are examined. Recent Golgi studies (Schoenen 1982; Schoenen & Faull 1990) on motor neurons of the lumbar enlargement of the human spinal cord illustrate the complex

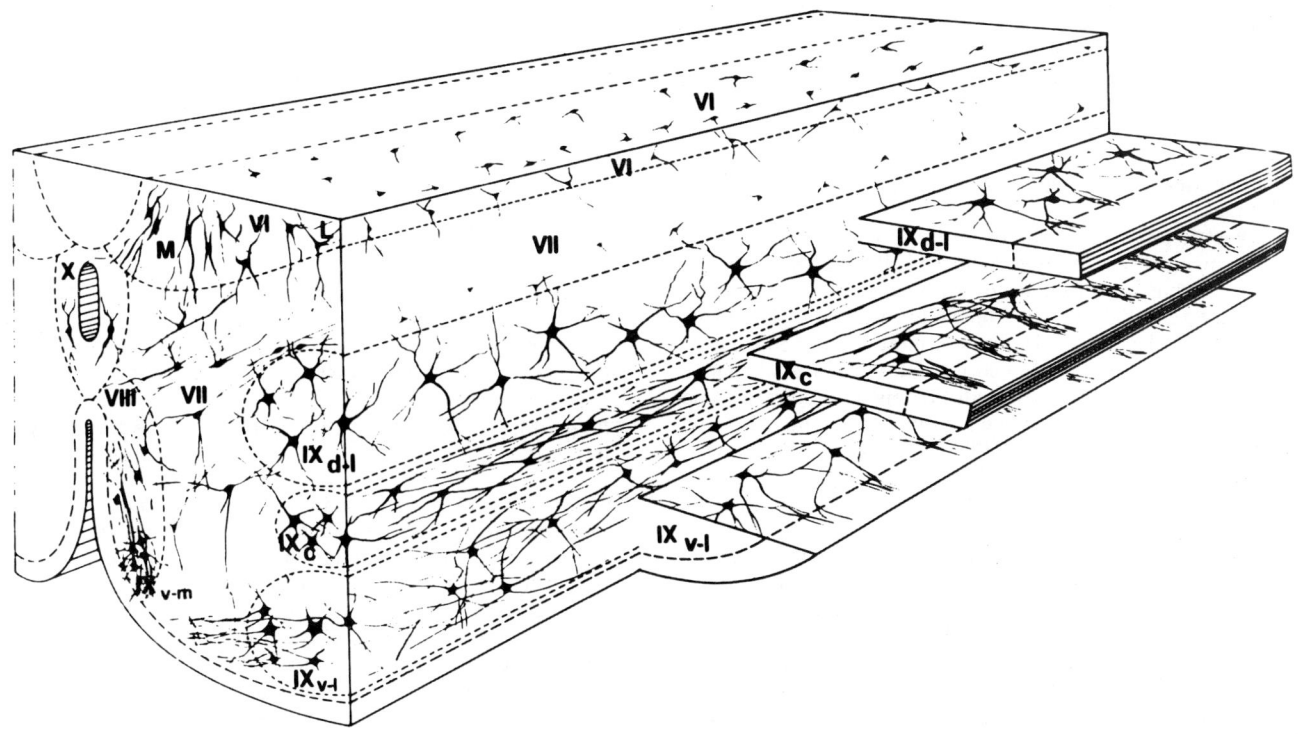

8.100 Three dimensional representation of the spinal dendroarchitecture in the intermediate and anterior grey columns. IXv-m = ventromedial; IXv-l = ventrolateral; IXc = central; and IXd-l = dorsolateral columns of motor neurons; m = medial; L = lateral. (From Schoenen 1982 with permission of Wiley-Liss Inc, a subsidiary of John Wiley & Sons Ltd.)

nature of their dendritic fields, and also show that each motor neuronal column has a distinct dendroarchitecture (8.100). Thus:

(1) Motor neurons in the *ventromedial column* have long, dorsally projecting branches emerging from one or two primary apical dendrites, and numerous, short basal dendrites which branch in a fan-like manner. Dendrites of these motor neurons aggregate into vertical and longitudinal bundles. The vertical bundles, composed of 10–30 dendrites, arise from adjacent motor cells within the column and project dorsally, for some 2–3 mm, penetrating lamina VIII to reach as far as the ventral grey commissure. The longitudinal dendrites, arising from neighbouring or distant ventromedial motor neurons, interweave to form a rostrocaudal dendritic plexus which extends throughout the length of the motor column. The plexus contains dendritic 'microbundles', only a few tens of micrometres in length, which are formed by some 5 dendrites.

(2) Motor neurons of the *central column* show a radial, multipolar dendritic configuration in the transverse plane, but characteristically have numerous, rostrocaudally directed dendrites, and also project dendrites laterally through the ventral grey column into the surrounding ventrolateral white funiculus. The rostrocaudally orientated dendrites form a longitudinal plexus similar to that of the ventromedial column.

(3) Dendrites of motor neurons of the *ventrolateral column* are disposed radially in the transverse plane; most dendrites in the medial part of the column spread medially, those in the lateral part spread laterally. In the sagittal plane there are numerous, long dendrites running rostrocaudally. Motor neurons of this column like those of the central column give rise to both transverse and longitudinal dendritic bundles.

(4) Motor neurons of the *dorsolateral column* greatly differ from those of other columns. In transverse and horizontal planes, their dendrites are numerous and spread radially showing little polarization; in the sagittal plane, most dendrites display a ventrodorsal orientation. Bundles of dendrites are not conspicuous in this column.

In motor columns within which the preferential dendritic array is longitudinal, the dendrites overlap over a long distance. Functionally, this dendritic network would favour spatial summation along the length of the column. The findings in the human lumbosacral cord show that the longitudinal network is common to motor neurons within each of the ventromedial, central and ventrolateral columns. These neurons supply axial, proximal and crural muscles whose main functions, among others, are the maintenance of posture where synchronization and synergy, provided by spatial summation, are necessary requirements. In contrast, the radial dendritic organization of the dorsolateral column permits only minimal interaction between motor neurons because only dendrites of adjacent neurons are close to each other. Motor neurons of this column supply distal muscles of the limb, concerned with delicate and fractionated movements; thus their dendritic arrangement allows precise and selective contacts with afferents.

Morphometric analyses of the dendritic spread of adult human motor neurons (for details, see Schoenen 1982b) show that in the central column, lateral dendrites are about 1400 μm in length penetrating the ventrolateral white funiculus, whilst the global span of the longitudinal dendrites is 1800 μm or more. In the ventrolateral motor column, the longitudinal dendrites can reach a total span of 3 mm forming the most extensive dendritic domain in human spinal grey matter. In an earlier morphometric study on the human spinal cord Abdel-Maguid and Bowsher (1979) have shown, on the basis of dendritic field size and dendritic branch pattern, two types of α and two types of γ motor neurons (consult the original paper for details).

Scheibel and Scheibel (1968) have analysed the dendritic fields in spinal grey matter, Szentágothai and Albert (1955) and Böhme (1962) have similarly examined Clarke's column, and Szentágothai (1964) and Ralston (1965) have analysed the substantia gelatinosa. Ralston (1974) has reviewed the field.

The general neuronal arrangement in the *substantia gelatinosa* is as follows. The neurons of lamina I usually have large dendritic networks which spread tangentially across the dorsal aspect of the posterior grey column, where they mix with the deepest fibres of the dorsolateral tract and some of the dorsal root afferents; their axons mainly ramify in the subjacent laminae, but some decussate and

ascend to the brainstem and diencephalic levels in the ventrolateral white columns (8.103). Dendrites of small neurons in lamina II and larger ones in lamina III are predominantly radially disposed, forming longitudinal 'sheets' perpendicular to the dorsal column; some of their axons may pass ventrally to the deeper laminae but most remain in the substantia gelatinosa (see below). These fine axons ascend or descend a short distance within lamina II or pass into the dorsolateral tract and then return to either lamina II or III before ramifying. Between the radial dendrites of the small neurons are two other components also radially disposed: the terminal parts of long dendrites of the larger, more deeply sited neurons in lamina IV and terminal branches of many primary cutaneous dorsal root fibres. The fine non-myelinated afferents approach the substantia gelatinosa from its dorsal aspect, their terminal branches travelling ventrally; afferents of larger diameter curve around the substantia to its ventral aspect.

A detailed study of the substantia gelatinosa (Réthelyi & Szentágothai 1969) was based on the Golgi technique and ultrastructural methods combined with dorsal root transection or isolation of the dorsal grey columns. Neurons in laminae II and III were examined with special reference to the larger pyramidal neurons sited at the junction between laminae III and IV. The latter have recurrent axons entering lamina II, where they expand to form cores of large *glomerular synaptic complexes* which contain various kinds of synapses. Features of these synapses, the inputs from dorsal root afferents, the connections of gelatinosal neurons, the main output channels via lamina IV neurons and terminals of fibres from supraspinal sources, are summarized in **8.101**.

Szentágothai (1964) claimed that the gelatinosa was a 'closed' system in which all the axons stemming from gelatinosal cells either remained in the system or left it only to re-enter at other levels of the cord. An important corollary was that the small gelatinosal cells influenced the dorsal dendrites of antenna-type neurons in laminae IV and V, the main output of the system. The concept of the 'closed' system, although germinal to the development of ideas about gelatinosal organization, has been modified, since it is now known that axons of some lamina II cells project to the thalamus, brainstem and also to lamina I and deeper laminae. Furthermore, the views on the structure of glomerular synaptic complexes (glomeruli), prominent features of the lamina II neuropil, have also been modified. Basically, glomeruli consist of a central ending or core which is an *en passant* primary afferent terminal having the morphological characteristics of an excitatory terminal. The central ending is in synaptic contact with a group (usually four to eight) of surrounding dendrites and other (peripheral) axonal terminals. The source of these dendrites is controversial, but all appear to arise from spinal cells which include gelatinosal cells and probably antenna-type cells in laminae IV and V. The origin of the peripheral axonal terminals is unknown, but it is presumed that they arise from lamina II cells; these terminals have the morphological features of inhibitory synapses. Glomerular circuitry is further complicated by the presence of 'triads' where the central terminal makes contact with two abutting dendrites, one of which is presynaptic to the other. Glomeruli, the key elements in dorsal grey column synaptology, allow for both pre- and postsynaptic modification of primary afferent input. Note that the detailed roles of the substantia gelatinosa remain obscure, but see below. (For a recent review consult Willis & Coggeshall 1991.)

TERMINATIONS OF DORSAL ROOT AFFERENT FIBRES

The formation, topography and division of dorsal spinal roots have been described (p. 976) and confirmed in man (Sindou et al 1974). Terminations of these in spinal grey matter must now be detailed. Approaches to this problem have been anatomical and neurophysiological. In the former, terminations at different levels have been followed by such techniques as those of Glees, Nauta and Fink-Heimer after the severance of individual dorsal roots. In the latter, the focal electrical potentials generated in spinal grey matter have been explored by microelectrodes to record the results of stimulation of the muscle, cutaneous nerves and dorsal roots. Most of the informative studies of dorsal root terminals (Sprague 1958; Sprague & Ha 1964) were on spinal cords of cats; similar arrays probably exist in other mammals but details cannot be transferred without reserve to the human spinal cord. The findings were related to laminar architecture (p. 983), with the proviso that the degenerating terminals seen are only those near cell somata and dendrite trunks, although the branches of many dendrites radiate widely (8.101). Dendrites are covered by synaptic contacts along all their course (Armstrong et al 1956; Wyckoff & Young 1956; Rasmussen 1957; Young 1958; Illis 1964; Gelfan & Rapisarda 1964), numbering thousands in large neurons, but these are not revealed by the degeneration techniques mentioned above. Such studies must be combined with Golgi and other techniques.

The fields of termination, after section of cats' sixth right lumbar dorsal roots, are shown at three levels (lumbar 5, 6 and 7) in 8.102. All large dorsal funicular fibres (except some placed medially) have collaterals which traverse the medial two-thirds of laminae I, II and III, many curving around the medial aspects of these laminae to form a dense plexus of degenerating fibres of passage and terminals round most neurons in lamina IV. Many fibres of passage recurve into the substantia gelatinosa from its ventral aspect and are seen as degenerating terminals between the radial dendrites of small neurons in laminae II and III and terminal segments of long dorsally directed dendrites from lamina IV. Degeneration also occurs in some fine fibres of the dorsolateral tract over three segments both cranial and caudal to the level of the severed root; from these, collaterals pass into laminae I, II and III, appearing in all these laminae as degenerating terminals.

From lamina IV many larger fibres pass to the medial zones of V and VI (containing commissural interneurons), whilst many others form a mass of degenerating terminals in the central zones of these laminae. From this concentration 'fingers' of degenerating terminals radiate into laminae VII and VIII; and running with them are fibres of passage which then converge on motor neuron pools and their interneurons in lamina IX. Sprague (1958) demonstrated degenerating synaptic terminals from dorsal root afferents terminating on the somata and dendrites of large multipolar motor neurons, where they are interspersed between numerous terminals from interneurons of other laminae and other cord levels. In the cat, such monosynaptic terminals of dorsal root afferents were found to extend on motor neurons two segments above and below a severed root; whereas terminals on interneurons in other laminae were also identified one or two segments beyond this. Similar studies in rhesus monkeys (Shriver et al 1968; Carpenter et al 1968) show comparable findings but differ in detail.

NERVE FIBRE TRACTS OF THE SPINAL CORD

The spinal 'white matter', containing nerve fibres, neuroglia and blood vessels, surrounds the fluted column of grey matter and owes its hue to large numbers of myelinated nerve fibres. Its arrangement into anterior, lateral and posterior funiculi has been noted (8.90). Fibres vary in calibre, many being small and lightly- or non-myelinated. Some tracts are typically of small fibres, for example the dorsolateral tract, fasciculus gracilis and central part of the lateral funiculus. Nerve fibres in the fasciculus cuneatus, anterior funiculus and peripheral zone of the lateral funiculus all contain many large diameter fibres. Most 'white' regions show a wide *spectrum of fibre diameters*, from 1 μm or less to about 10 μm. Fibres of 3 μm or less predominate; the larger (few exceeding 10 μm) form a small fraction. Detailed studies of the distribution of fibre diameters in human spinal cord are few (Häggqvist 1936; Giok 1956) but many tracts are claimed to be identifiable on this basis. The proportions of fibres of particular diameters have been established (Szentágothai-Schimert 1941) but data of this kind are few. In the past much information regarding the spinal tracts in animals has been derived from selective damage to the spinal cord, or to dorsal roots, or to regions of brain which may make fibre connections with the cord. In such experiments retrograde degeneration indicates the neurons from which particular axons proceed, anterograde terminal degeneration indicating the sites of termination. More recently, the source, course and terminations of spinal tracts in experimental animals can be shown by a plethora of anterograde or retrograde tracing techniques involving the use of horseradish peroxidase (HRP) or wheatgerm agglutinin-(WGA)-

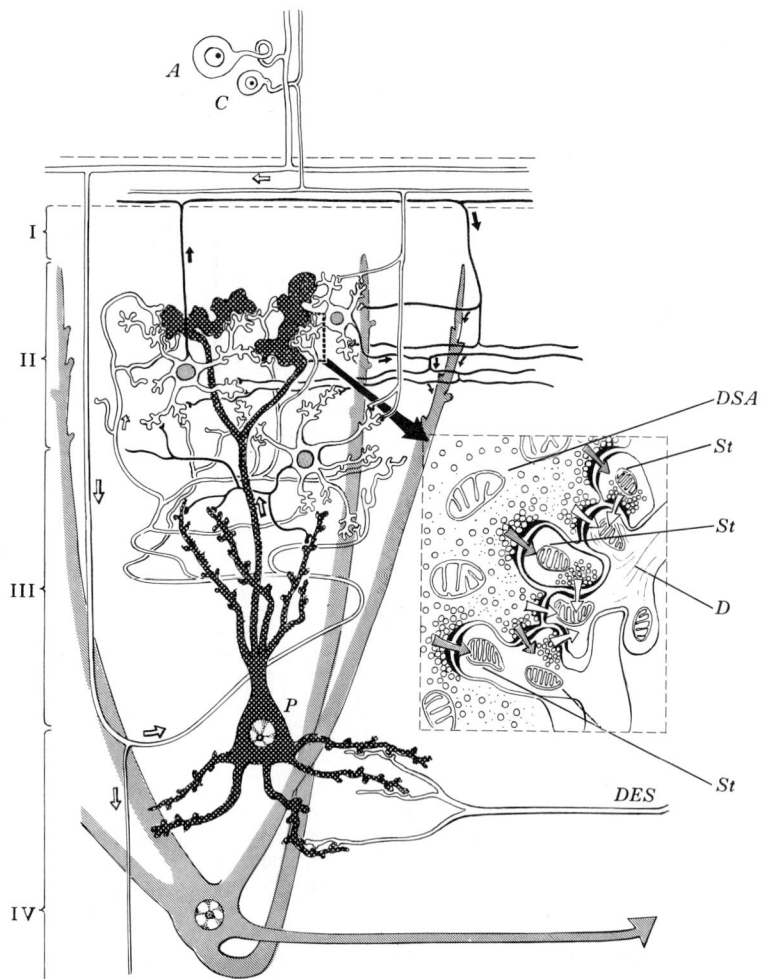

8.101 The arrangement of neurons and their interconnections in a longitudinal section through the dorsal grey column of the spinal cord, which includes the substantia gelatinosa and adjacent neuronal laminae (Roman numerals I–IV). Inset (right) shows synaptic detail of the area indicated. Two primary sensory afferent fibres are shown: a cutaneous afferent of large calibre (A) and a small calibre non-myelinated afferent (C). Small substantia gelatinosa interneurons are in white with black outline; their axons are single black lines. A pyramidal cell with dendrites and spines and a recurrent axon expanding into synaptic complexes is shown in black with white dots. A large multipolar neuron of lamina IV with long radial dendrites and initial axon is in cross-hatch. DES = axon descending from a supraspinal source. Arrows on main diagram show presumed direction of impulse conduction. Note (1) the different sites of synaptic termination of primary afferents A and C, (2) the axonal pattern and terminals of substantia gelatinosa interneurons, (3) the synaptic complexes formed between the recurrent axon expansibns of the pyramidal cell, the small gelatinosa interneuron dendrites and the primary sensory axon terminals. See inset for details. DSA = pyramidal cell axon terminal; D = dendrite of gelatinosa interneuron; St = primary afferent fibre axon terminal; white arrows = axo-dendritic synapses; cross-hatched arrows = axoaxonic synapses. Consult text for a discussion of the 'gate' theory and structural details. (From Szentágothai 1975.)

conjugated HRP, fluorescent dyes or fluorescent labelled compounds, certain lectins and other compounds which are transported in nerve processes (for details, see p. 914). While certain tracts are largely discrete and the central regions of most are regularly located in funiculi, reciprocal overlap usually occurs at their fringes (see below). This partly accounts for variation in their extent as seen in diagrams of transverse spinal sections according to different authors; in all such diagrams arbitrary boundaries delineate the supposed limits of tracts, especially in the human cord, where deliberate experimentation is impossible; the data available result only from disease and injury, or selective cordotomy for pain relief. Such investigations, particularly experiments (see p. 915) on other primates, are likely to provide results similar to human arrangements; but it is unwise to assume that they are identical. Evidence from the examination of

NEUROPHYSIOLOGICAL CORRELATIONS

NEUROPHYSIOLOGICAL CORRELATIONS

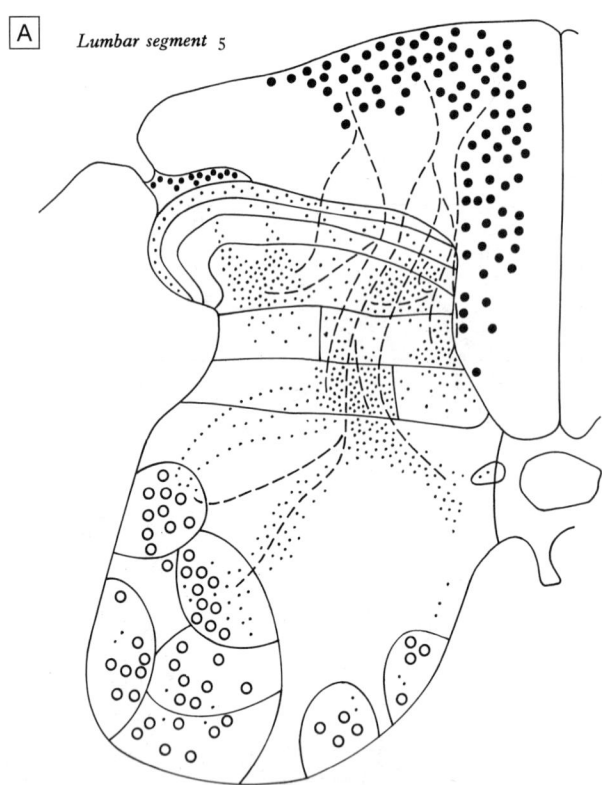

A Lumbar segment 5

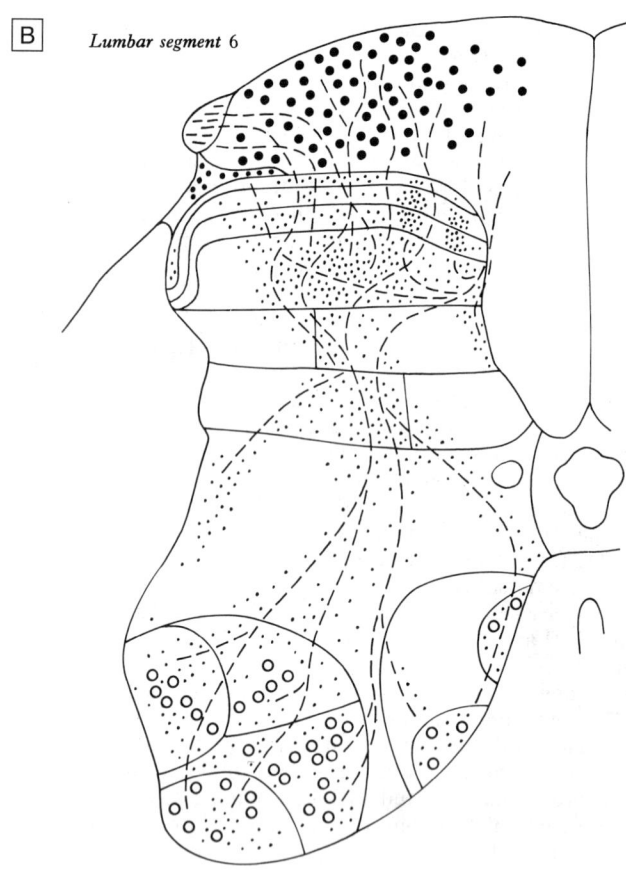

B Lumbar segment 6

8.102 The pattern of degeneration of nerve fibres and their terminals, demonstrated with the Nauta-Laidlaw technique in the ipsilateral half of the spinal cord at various segmental levels, five days after surgical division of the *sixth* lumbar dorsal spinal nerve root of the cat. A. The fifth lumbar segment; B. the sixth lumbar segment; C. the seventh lumbar segment. The large dots indicate degeneration of fibres in the dorsal funiculus; smaller dots = degenerating fibres in the dorsolateral tract of Lissauer; smallest dots = degenerating nerve terminals; dashed lines = degenerating fibres of passage; circles = neuronal somata of motor neurons. (From Sprague & Ha 1964, with the permission of the authors and Elsevier.)

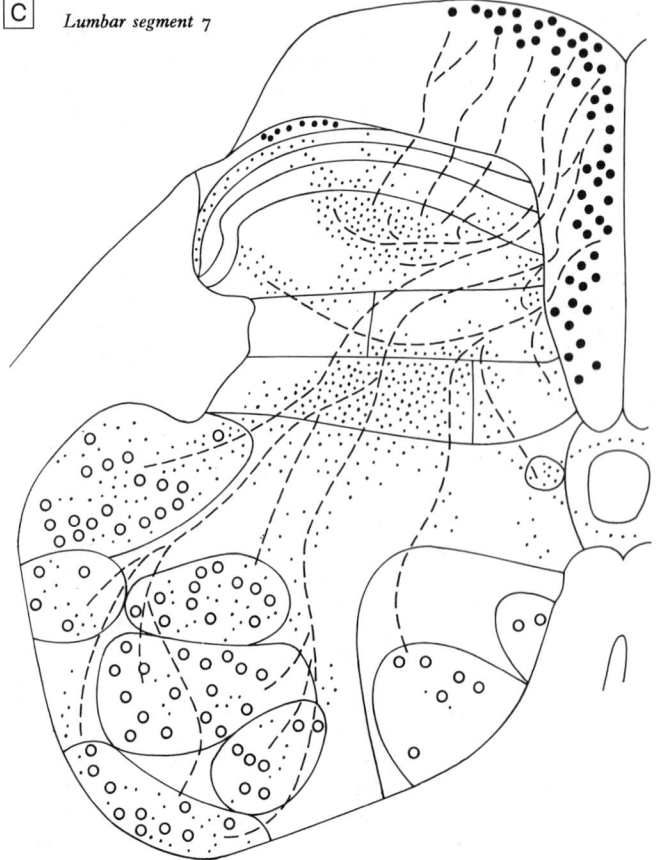

C Lumbar segment 7

human spinal cords affected by disease or injury does support the presumption that the general layout of tracts in the human primate is much the same as in others. Information from this source is surprisingly abundant, though usually less precise; it was the principal source of early data and large numbers of reports are scattered through the neurological literature (Nathan & Smith 1955b, 1959).

The following account of spinal tracts is concerned with the human cord; but reference to findings in animal experimentation must often be made where adequate clinicopathological data are unavailable. In a later section (p. 1007), dealing with the finer details of neuronal organization in the spinal cord, evidence from animals other than man must predominate, but it is probable that deductions from this source are in many instances applicable to the human spinal cord (but with some notable exceptions). As a convenient simplification, nerve fibres in spinal white matter are assigned to five groups:

- afferent fibres from neurons in dorsal root ganglia entering by dorsal roots and extending variable spinal distances
- long ascending fibres, derived from spinal neurons conducting afferent impulses to supraspinal levels
- long fibres descending from supraspinal sources to synapse with spinal neurons
- fibres effecting intrasegmental and intersegmental connections
- fibres from motor neurons in ventral and lateral grey columns issuing in ventral nerve roots.

Fibres in all except the last category form *longitudinal tracts*. Arrangements are not, however, so simple. Examination in different planes reveals that many fibres proceed in oblique and even horizontal directions, particularly across the midline in grey and white commissures, many being *decussating* fibres. Many others are *commissural* intrasegmental connections linking the neurons in grey columns to contralateral neurons. Some longitudinal tracts are polysynaptic, i.e. composed of trains of neurons. Most, if not all, fibres entering by the dorsal root divide into ascending and descending branches, all with collaterals extending into the grey matter, in which the number of neurons sending axons into ventral nerve roots or long projection tracts is a mere fraction of the total, most being propriospinal in nature.

In the following account, the tracts are considered under the three main headings for descriptive and functional convenience: ascending, descending and propriospinal tracts. However, both the topography and the interrelations of the tracts are important to consider in the context of neurological diagnosis, experimental and phylogenetic studies.

For comprehensive reviews on spinal pathways in mammals see: Fyffe (1984), Clark (1984), Tracey (1986), and Willis and Coggeshall (1991) on ascending tracts and pathways; and Kuypers (1964, 1973, 1981) and Holstege (1991) on descending and propriospinal pathways. An extensive review as well as a compilation of experimental data on the corticospinal tract has been published by Phillips and Porter (1977). The classic reviews on the descending tracts and fasciculi proprii by Nathan and Smith (1955b, 1959) are still current sources of information on the human spinal cord.

The general disposition of the major tracts is shown in **8**.103 and in greater detail at two transverse levels in **8**.104. Some features are further summarized in **8**.105–107.

ASCENDING TRACTS

Dorsal funiculus

The dorsal funiculus (or column) contains the large fasciculi gracilis and cuneatus on each side, separated by the posterointermediate septum (**8**.108). It comprises several systems of ascending fibres, namely:

- long primary afferent fibres of spinal ganglion cells, projecting to the dorsal column nuclei in the medulla oblongata
- shorter primary afferent fibres, projecting to neurons of the thoracic nucleus of Clarke and other spinal neurons
- axons from secondary neurons of the spinal cord ascending to the dorsal column nuclei.

In addition the funiculus contains axons of propriospinal neurons (see p. 1003).

The *fasciculus gracilis* (**8**.108) begins at the caudal end of the spinal cord. It contains long ascending branches of medially placed bundles of dorsal spinal roots, and also ascending axons of *secondary* neurons in laminae IV–VI of the ipsilateral dorsal grey column (Rustioni & Dekker 1974). All ascend the dorsal funiculus, augmented by axons of each dorsal root. Fibres entering in coccygeal and lower sacral regions are shifted medially by successive additions of fibres which enter at higher levels (**8**.109). The fasciculus gracilis is derived from fibres of the coccygeal, sacral, lumbar and lower thoracic segments. It lies medial to the fasciculus cuneatus in the upper spinal cord (**8**.104A).

The *fasciculus cuneatus* (**8**.108) begins at the midthoracic cord level

and lies lateral to the fasciculus gracilis. It is derived from fibres of the upper thoracic and cervical dorsal roots. Some of its axons arise from secondary neurons in laminae IV–VI of the ipsilateral dorsal grey column (Rustioni et al 1979).

The fasciculus gracilis at upper cervical levels contains a larger proportion of afferents from cutaneous receptors than from deep (proprioceptive) ones (Whitsel et al 1969, 1970). The dearth of proprioceptive fibres at this level is due to axons leaving the fasciculus at lower segments to synapse on the nucleus dorsalis of Clarke. Note that proprioception from the lower limb mostly reaches the thalamus by relaying in Clarke's nucleus and then in the nucleus Z (p. 1017). Long ascending gracile axons from both primary and secondary neurons terminate in the nucleus gracilis. In contrast, the fasciculus cuneatus at upper cervical levels contains a large population of afferents from both deep and cutaneous receptors of the upper limb. Long ascending cuneate axons (primary and secondary) end in the nucleus cuneatus; some also end in the lateral (external or accessory) cuneate nucleus; the neurons of the latter project to the cerebellum via the cuneocerebellar pathway. Both fasciculi contain myelinated fibres; in the cuneate fasciculus, many are of large diameter due to the high content of proprioceptive fibres.

As noted previously, many ascending fibres of the gracile and cuneate fasciculi end by synapsing on cells of their respectively named nuclei which are situated in the medulla oblongata (p. 1015). Axons from neurons of these dorsal column nuclei arch ventro-medially round the central grey matter of the medulla as *internal arcuate fibres* (**8**.131) to decussate in the *sensory* or *lemniscal decussation*. They then ascend, as the *medial lemniscus*, to the ventro-posteriolateral nucleus of the thalamus, and there are relayed to the postcentral gyrus (areas 3, 1 and 2). Some neurons of the dorsal column nuclei form *posterior external arcuate fibres* which enter the cerebellum (**8**.131).

The dorsal column–medial lemniscal pathway mediates pro-prioception (position sense and kinaesthesia) and exteroceptive (touch-pressure) information, as well as vibratory sensation. Nathan et al (1986) reviewed cases of patients with lesions involving the dorsal half of the spinal cord. Their findings were loss of pro-prioception; tactile stimuli were still felt but there were disturbances in two-point touch discrimination and gross deficits in both ster-eognosis and graphaesthesia; vibratory sense was lost. The segmental organization of the gracile and cuneate fasciculi, according to animal studies, is more complex than described above. Caudally in both bundles, the afferent fibres are organized in a dermatomal manner and, by means of resorting, acquire a somatotopic pattern at high rostral levels (Whitsel et al 1970). Smith and Deacon (1984), in a study on the dorsal columns in the human cord, found a certain degree of segmental lamination with extensive overlapping of fibres from different segments within each fasciculus; but found no, or

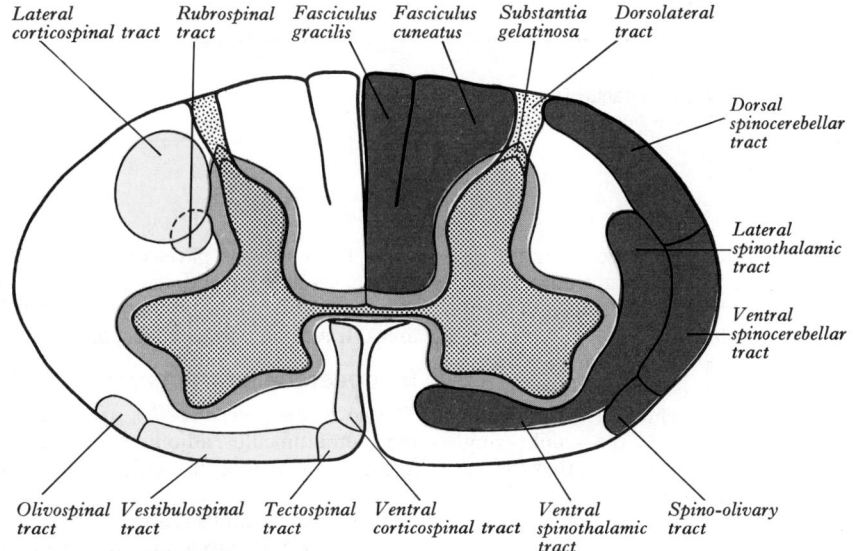

8.103   Simplified diagram of the main tracts of the spinal cord. The ascending tracts are shown in red on the right side of the figure; the descending tracts are shown in yellow on the left side; the 'intersegmental' tracts are in orange on both sides. Many tracts are omitted (see **8**.104 A, B).

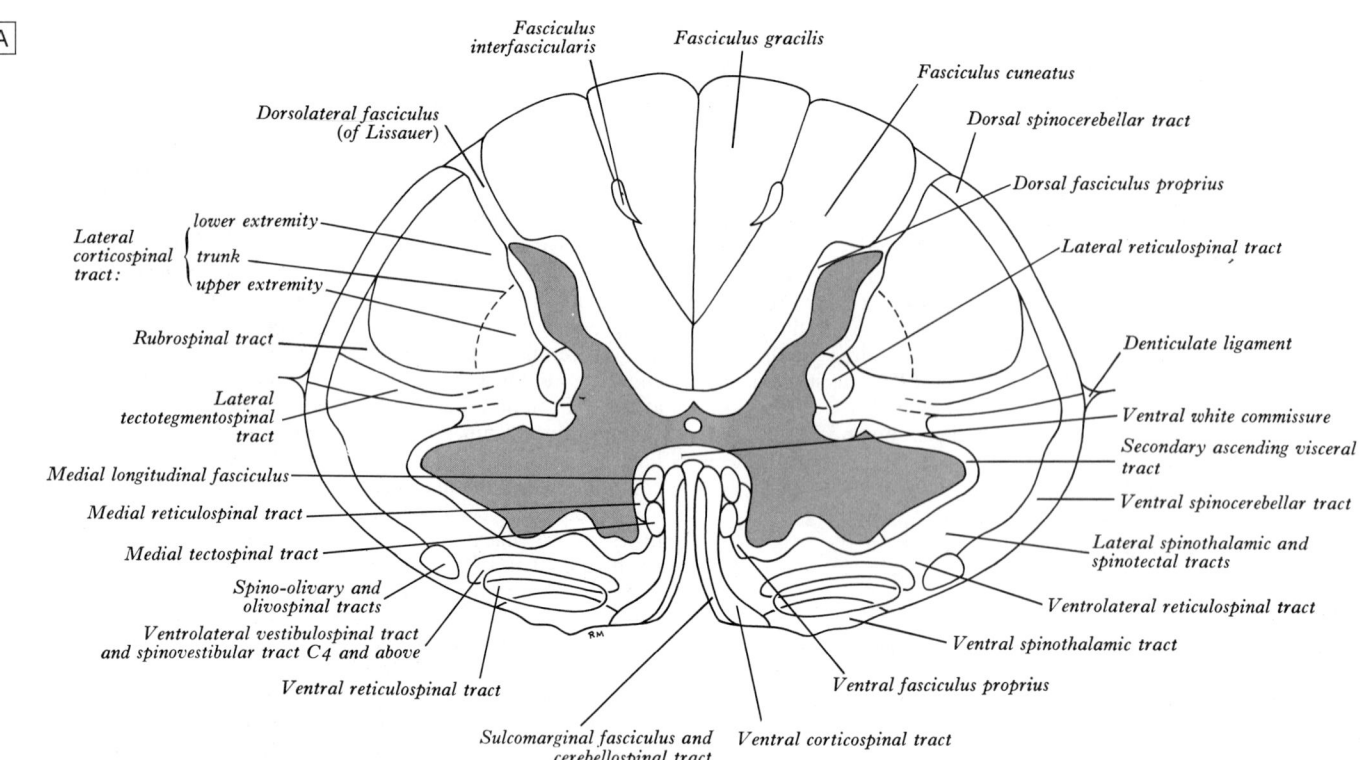

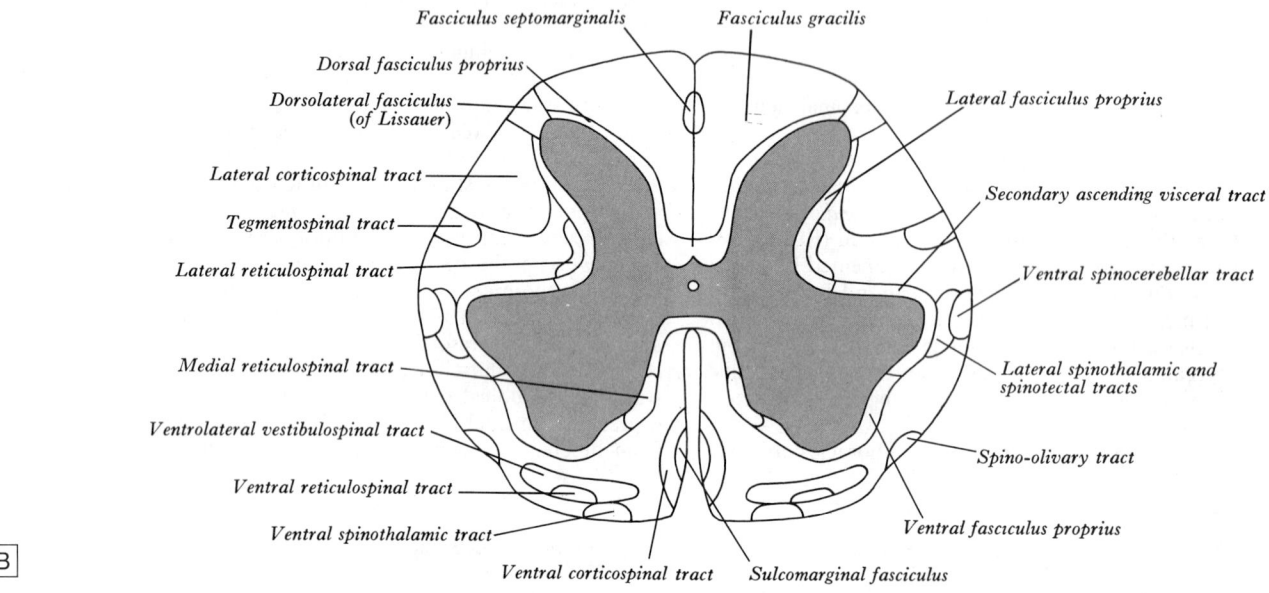

8.104   The approximate relative positions of nerve fibre tracts of the human spinal cord at mid-cervical (A) and lumbar (B) levels. (Adapted from Crosby et al 1962.)

minimal, overlapping of fibres of the cuneate with those of the gracile funiculus, and regarded each fasciculus as a separate anatomical entity. They tentatively suggest that resorting of fibres as described above by Whitsel et al (1970) may take place.

Somatotopy is preserved through the pathway from the dorsal column nuclei to, and including, the primary sensory cortex. In the dorsal column nuclei, the lower limb is represented medially in the gracile nucleus, the upper limb in the cuneate, the trunk lying between. Segregation of fibres by modality is also reported in the dorsal column, those from hair receptors being most superficial, those from tactile and vibratory receptors lying in deeper layers (Uddenberg 1968).

Sensory information transmitted via neurons of the dorsal column nuclei may be modulated (inhibited or facilitated) by descending fibres from various parts of the brain which include the cerebral cortex, cerebellum and the reticular formation. The cortical projections arise from the primary and supplementary motor and sensory areas, travelling with corticospinal fibres.

Spinocerebellar tracts (8.110)

The *posterior spinocerebellar tract* ascends in the peripheral part of the lateral funiculus, adjoining the lateral corticospinal tract medially and the dorsolateral fasciculus dorsally (8.103). It begins about the level of the second or third lumbar segment, and enlarges as it ascends to the medulla oblongata. Here it passes through the inferior cerebellar peduncle to terminate ipsilaterally in the rostral and caudal parts of the cerebellar vermis (p. 1128). Axons of the tract stem from the larger neurons of the nucleus thoracis ('Clarke' column), in

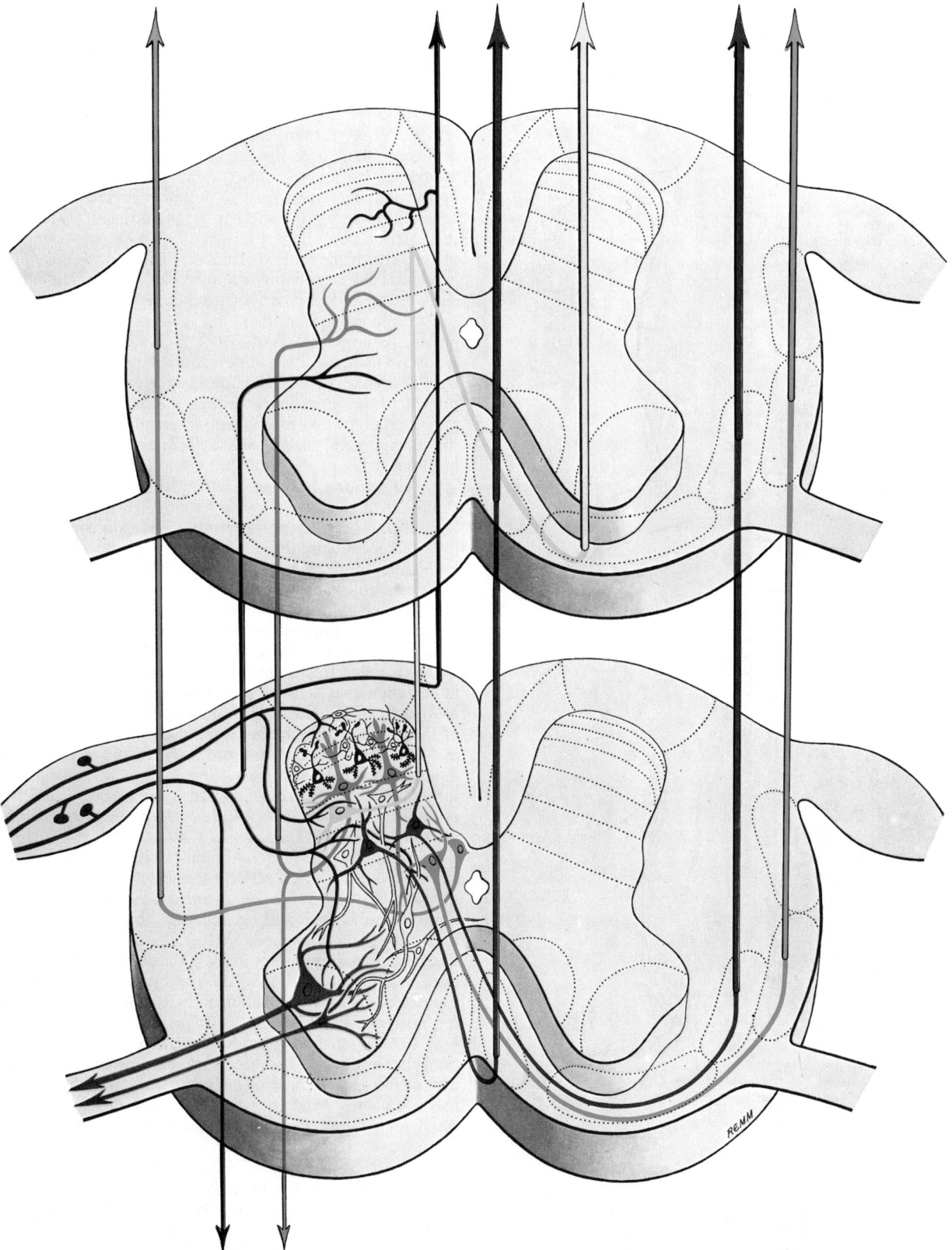

8.105 Simplified scheme of some of the major ascending tract systems of the spinal cord and some features of grey matter organization. Within the grey matter the dotted lines show the laminar pattern; within the white matter they are an approximate guide to the topography of the tracts. Attempts have been made to indicate in a simplified manner the overlapping of dendritic fields described in the text. An alpha and a gamma motor neuron (grey) are included, together with some of the structural features of the substantia gelatinosa which are described and illustrated more fully in **8**.101.

Some of the small substantia gelatinosa neurons are uncoloured, as are some interneurons in the deeper laminae. The larger substantia gelatinosa neurons are solid black. Large lamina IV cells and associated ascending and descending intersegmental fibres are green. Primary sensory afferent fibres, including a fibre in the fasciculus gracilis, are purple. Spinotectal fibre—orange; anterior spinothalamic fibre—yellow; lateral spinothalamic fibre—magenta; and dorsal and ventral spinocerebellar fibres—blue. Compare with **8**.107.

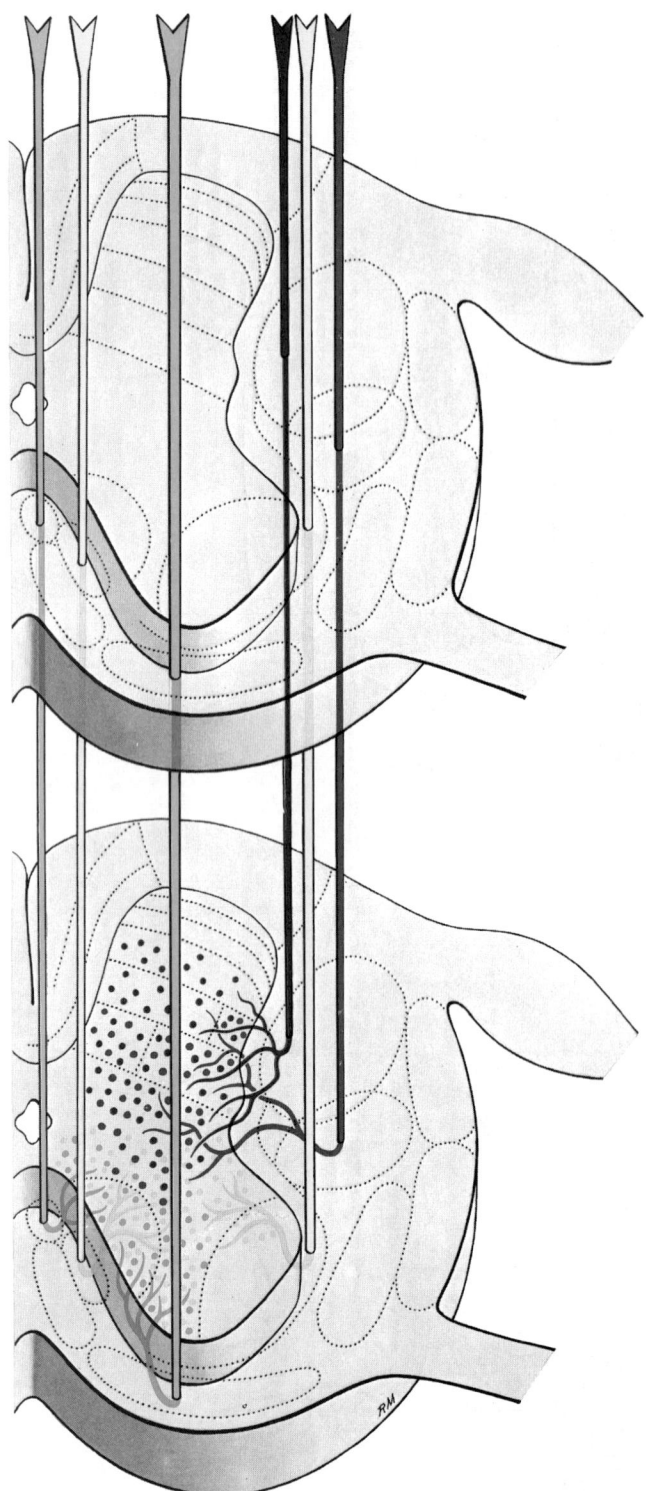

The *anterior spinocerebellar tract* (**8**.110) occupies a crescentic area in the periphery of the lateral funiculus, anterior to the posterior spinocerebellar tract (**8**.103). Animal studies (Ha & Liu 1968 in the cat; Matsushita & Hosaya 1979 in the rat) show that cells of origin of the tract are in the lumbosacral region of the cord in laminae V–VII; some are the 'spinal border cells' of Cooper and Sherrington (1940). Axons forming the tract mostly decussate: a few remain ipsilateral (Jansen & Brodal 1954). The tract begins in the upper lumbar region and ascends through the medulla oblongata to the upper pontine level where it descends in the dorsal part of the superior cerebellar peduncle to terminate mainly contralaterally in the anterior cerebellar vermis (p. 1028). The primary afferent fibres to the cells of the anterior spinocerebellar tract enter the fasciculus gracilis and are probably arranged like those of the posterior tract (see above), and carry information concerning the lower limb.

The spinocerebellar tracts are laminated; fibres from lower segments are superficial (Yoss 1952, 1953; Smith 1957). Smith (1957) reports in man, a dorsal shift of anterior tract fibres into the posterior tract at high cervical levels: fibres of the tracts intermingle and most project to the cerebellum through the inferior cerebellar peduncle; only a small, medial component of the anterior tract passes through the superior cerebellar peduncle. Both tracts contain large diameter, myelinated fibres; those of the posterior tract are more numerous, finer calibre fibres being associated with the anterior tract (Häggqvist 1936).

Both tracts convey proprioceptive and exteroceptive information, but are functionally different. Neurons of the thoracic nucleus are excited monosynaptically by Ia and Ib primary afferent fibres (from muscle spindles and tendon organs respectively) and also group II muscle afferents, and cutaneous touch and pressure afferents. The proprioceptive impulses often arise from a single muscle or from synergistic muscles acting at a common joint. Thus, the posterior spinocerebellar tract transmits modality-specific and space-specific information that is used in the fine co-ordination of posture and movement of individual limb muscles. On the other hand the cells of the anterior tract are activated monosynaptically by Ib afferents and transmit information from large receptive fields that include different segments of a limb. The anterior tract lacks subdivisions for different modalities and forwards impulses used for the co-ordinated movement and posture of the entire lower limb (for details see Lundberg 1971; Oscarsson 1973).

Since the thoracic nucleus diminishes rostrally (**8**.95) and does not extend above the lowest cervical segment, it follows that the posterior spinocerebellar tract carries information from the trunk and lower limb. Proprioceptive and exteroceptive information from the upper limb travels in primary afferent fibres of the fasciculus cuneatus. These fibres end somatotopically in the accessory (external or lateral) cuneatus nucleus and the adjoining part of the cuneate nucleus situated in the medulla oblongata. Cells of these nuclei give rise to the posterior external arcuate fibres forming the *cuneo-cerebellar tract* (**8**.110) which enters the cerebellum via the ipsilateral inferior cerebellar peduncle. The accessory cuneate nucleus and the lateral part of the cuneate nucleus are considered to be homologous to the thoracic nucleus; and thus the cuneocerebellar tract is functionally allied to the posterior spinocerebellar tract, being its upper limb equivalent.

A *rostral spinocerebellar tract* functionally associated with the anterior spinocerebellar tract, but conveying information from the forelimb, is found in animals (Oscarsson & Uddenberg 1964; Hirai et al 1976). Its fibres enter the cerebellum through the inferior and superior peduncles. The tract cells are in the nucleus cervicalis centrobasalis, situated in lamina VII of the lower four cervical segments (Petras & Cummings 1977; Matsushita & Hosaya 1979). Cells of the nucleus receive forelimb, dorsal root terminals.

A further *cervicospinocerebellar pathway* is reported in animals (Wiksten 1975; Cummings & Petras 1977). It arises from neurons of the nucleus cervicalis centralis, situated in lamina VII of the upper four cervical segments and receives primary afferents from neck muscles. The tract cells project contralaterally to the cerebellum via the superior cerebellar peduncle.

Axons of all the spinocerebellar tracts and the cuneocerebellar tract form part of the 'mossy fibre system'. They end in the cerebellar cortex in a highly organized, somatotopical and functional pattern (p. 1042).

8.106 A simplified scheme of some of the major descending tract systems of the spinal cord including their overlapping zones of termination in the grey matter. The significance of the dotted lines is the same as for **8**.105. Corticospinal tract—mauve; rubrospinal tract—magenta; reticulospinal tracts—yellow; vestibulospinal tracts—blue.

lamina VII throughout spinal segments T1–L2. The nucleus thoracis receives input from:

- collaterals of long ascending primary afferents of the posterior column
- terminals of shorter ascending primary afferents of the posterior column.

Many of these afferent fibres ascend from segments caudal to the termination of the nucleus thoracis at L2.

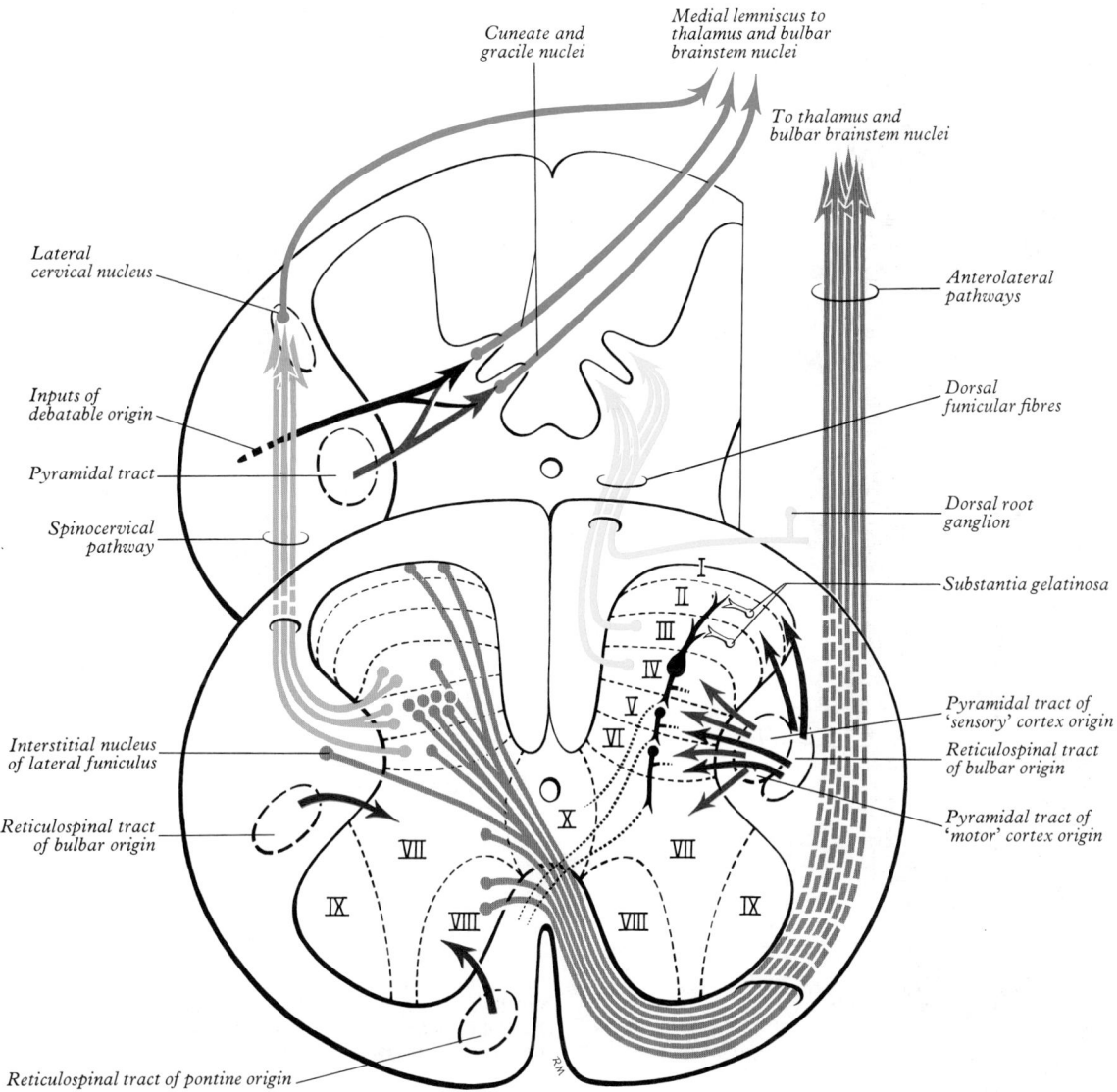

8.107 A more detailed analysis of the principal somaesthetic pathways. Descending corticospinal and reticulospinal tracts involved in sensory modulation are also indicated. (Modified from data provided by K E Webster, King's College, University of London.)

Descending pathways from the cerebral cortex and brainstem can modify the activity of spinocerebellar tract neurons. For example, on the exteroceptive division of the thoracic nucleus, corticospinal fibres may excite or inhibit; lateral vestibulospinal and rubrospinal fibres facilitate excitation.

Spinothalamic tracts (8.111, 112)

The *anterior spinothalamic tract* (**8**.111), located in the anterior funiculus of the spinal cord, lies medial to fibres of the ventral nerve roots and dorsal to the vestibulospinal tract (**8**.103) which it overlaps with all neighbouring tracts. Intermingled with the spinothalamic tract are descending reticulospinal and ascending spinoreticular fibres. Laterally, the tract is continuous with the *lateral spinothalamic tract* (**8**.112) which is sited in the lateral funiculus lying medial to the anterior spinocerebellar tract (**8**.103). On the basis of clinical evidence, the anterior spinothalamic tract conveys impulses subserving crude tactile and pressure modalities and the lateral tract subserves pain and temperature sensibilities. However, this is not entirely in agreement with physiological investigations. According to Applebaum et al (1975) modality segregation within the anterior/lateral spinothalamic complex is not supported by experimental data and these tracts are to be considered as a structural and functional continuum. This view is supported by other investigators.

Basically axons forming the spinothalamic pathway arise from a heterogeneous collection of neurons, distributed in diverse laminae in all segments of the cord (see below). Although there is a small ipsilateral projection, the majority of spinothalamic axons cross the midline in the anterior white commissure and then project to the thalamus in the ventral quadrant of the spinal cord. Evidence from human cordotomies shows that the decussation is completed in the segment above the entrance of the dorsal root fibres (Foerster 1936). On reaching the lower brainstem, spinothalamic tract axons separate: those of the anterior tract join the medial lemniscus, while the axons of the lateral tract continue as the spinal lemniscus (p. 1019); both lemnisci ascend to end in the thalamus (**8**.111, 112). There is a clear somatotopic organization of the fibres in the spinothalamic tract (Walker 1940; Morin et al 1951; Nathan 1963). Fibres crossing at any level join the deep aspect of those already crossed and both tracts are thus segmentally laminated (**8**.113); the fibres from the lower segments of greater total length are superficially placed. A slight spiral twist is also described, the superficial fibres becoming progressively more dorsal as they ascend. Somatotopy is maintained throughout the medulla oblongata and pons. In the midbrain, fibres in the spinal lemniscus conveying pain and temperature sensation from the lower limb extend dorsally, while those from the trunk and upper limb are more ventrally placed (Walker 1943).

Distribution of spinothalamic neurons. Following a large injection of wheatgerm agglutinin-conjugated horseradish peroxidase (WRA-HR) into the somatosensory thalamus on one side, Apkarian and Hodge (1989a) studied the distribution of the cells of origin of the spinothalamic tract in the monkey. The distribution pattern is shown in **8**.114. A similar pattern has also been reported in the

993

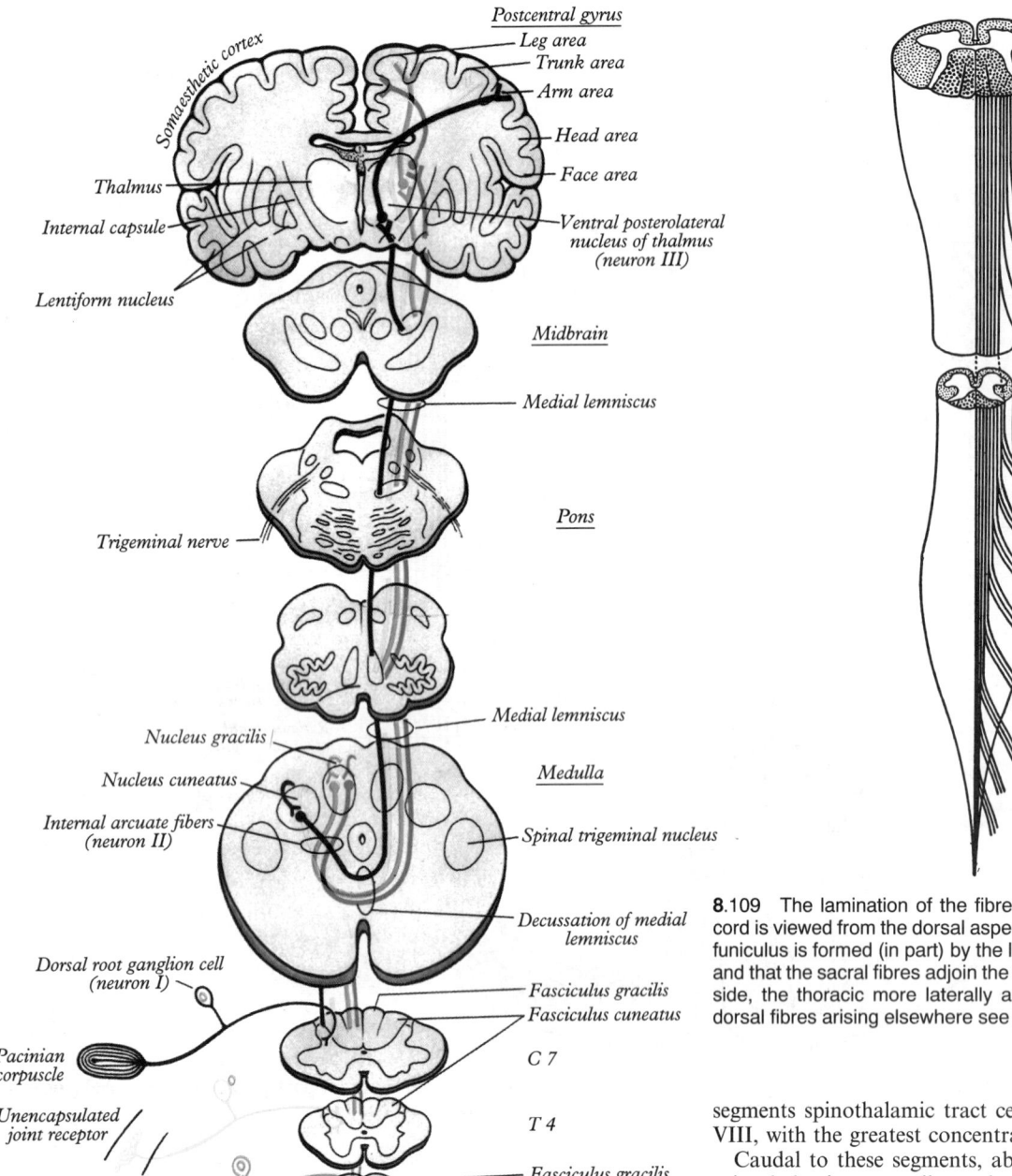

8.108 Schematic diagram of the dorsal column—medial lemniscus pathway. The dorsal white column contains ascending and descending fibres of dorsal root ganglion cells. Ascending fibres in the fasciculi gracilis and cuneatus synapse on neurons of the nuclei gracilis and cuneatus respectively. Axons from neurons of these nuclei cross in the lower medulla oblongata to form the medial lemniscus which ascends to end in the ventroposterolateral nucleus of the thalamus. Neurons of this nucleus then project axons via the internal capsule to the somaesthetic cortex. Impulses mediated by this pathway are concerned with discriminative touch and pressure sense, and also with proprioceptive sense. Dorsal root ganglia and their fibres entering the spinal cord at various levels are colour-coded (red = sacral; blue = lumbar; yellow = thoracic; black = cervical). Letters and numbers show the segmental levels of the spinal cord. (From Carpenter M B 1991. Core text of neuroanatomy, Williams & Wilkins, with permission of author and publisher.)

8.109 The lamination of the fibres in the posterior funiculus. The spinal cord is viewed from the dorsal aspect. The drawing shows that the posterior funiculus is formed (in part) by the long ascending fibres of the dorsal roots and that the sacral fibres adjoin the median plane, the lumbar to their lateral side, the thoracic more laterally and the cervical most lateral of all. For dorsal fibres arising elsewhere see p. 989.

monkey (Trevino & Carstens 1975; Willis et al 1974; and others). Just over 30% of the entire population of spinothalamic tract cells are found in the upper three cervical segments. Many of these cells are located ipsilateral to the thalamic injection, largely in lamina VIII, and represent about 50% of the total population of ipsilateral labelled cells. Contralateral to the injection site in these cervical segments spinothalamic tract cells are found in laminae I and IV–VIII, with the greatest concentration in laminae VI and VII.

Caudal to these segments, about 20% of the total population of spinothalamic tract cells are located in the lower cervical segments (C4–8), about 20% in the thoracic region (mostly in segments T1–3); while some 20% and 10% are found in the lumbar and sacrococcygeal regions respectively (Apkarian & Hodge 1989a). In the lower cervical and lower lumbar regions, contralateral spinothalamic tract cells are concentrated in laminae I and V, and also in the ventral column laminae VII–VIII; while in the thoracic region the contralateral moiety is found mainly in laminae V and VII. Cell bodies giving rise to spinothalamic tract axons are predominantly contralateral; only 10% of the total population of labelled cells are ipsilateral, the highest ipsilateral concentrations being in the upper three cervical segments (Hodge & Apkarian 1990). Physiological studies using antidromic activation of spinothalamic tract axons have largely confirmed the distribution maps produced by retrograde tracers. In the monkey spinothalamic tract cells are activated antidromically from parts of the ventroposterolateral and ventrolateral nuclei, the centrolateral and parafascicular nuclei of the thalamus (p. 1086; for references see Willis & Coggeshall 1991).

In man, the distribution of spinothalamic tract cells is less well known. Data from clinicopathological studies following anterolateral cordotomy (Foerster & Gagel 1932; Kuru 1949) depict degenerated cell bodies in the apical region (lamina I), the neck and base (probably laminae IV–VI) of the dorsal grey column, and also in the ventral grey column; while Smith (1976) showed degenerated neurons, distributed mostly in laminae I, IV, V and VII. However, much of this evidence is flawed because anterolateral cordotomy severs ascending fibres other than spinothalamic, for example spi-

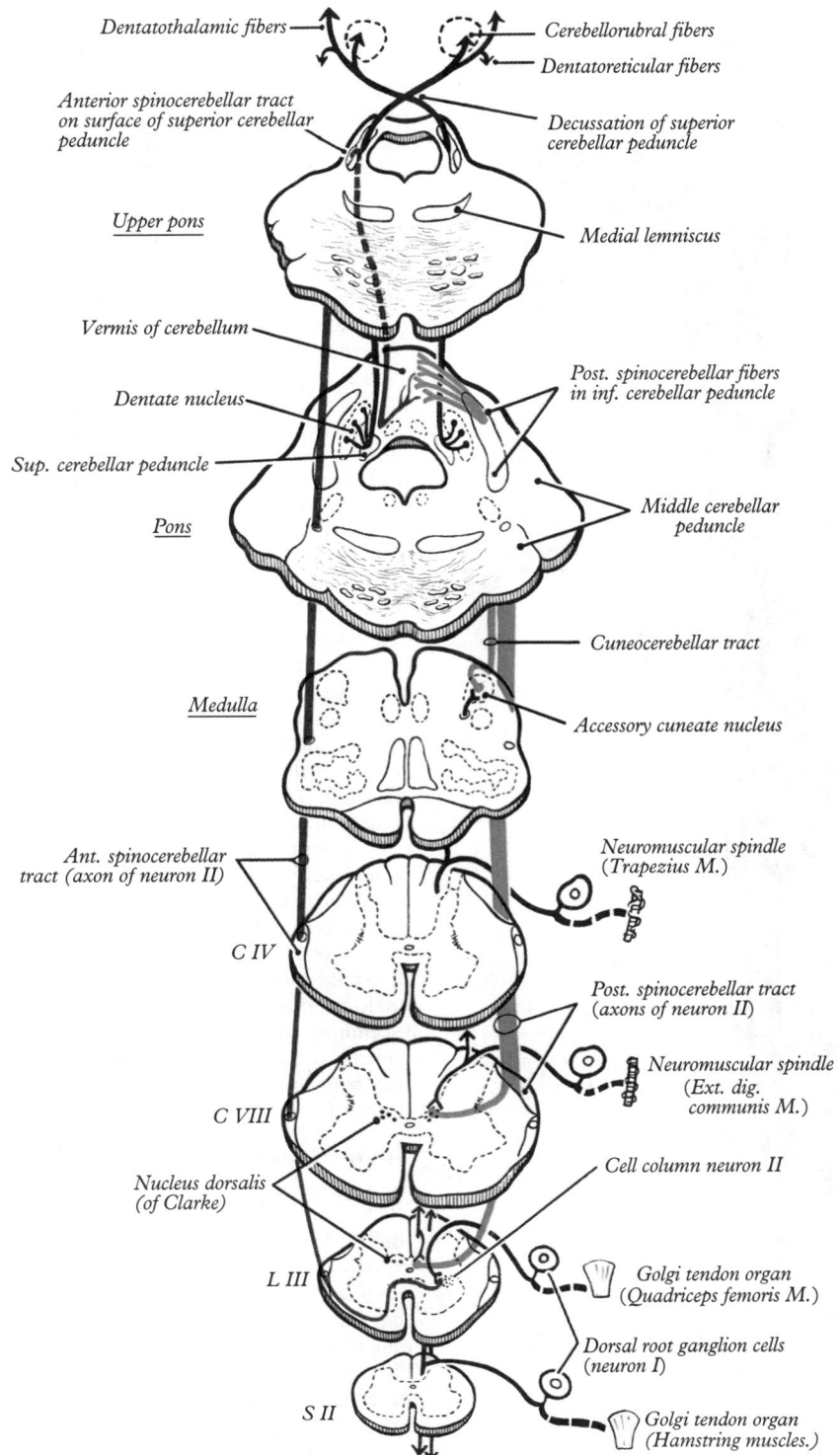

8.110 Schematic diagram of the anterior (red) and posterior (blue) spino-cerebellar tracts, and also the cuneocerebellar tract (blue). Fibres forming the posterior spinocerebellar tract arise from neurons of the thoracic nucleus, and are mainly uncrossed; this tract carries information from muscle spindles and Golgi tendon organs. The anterior spinocerebellar tract, composed of crossed fibres, arises mainly from cells in laminae V to VII of the lumbosacral cord; it conveys impulses from Golgi tendon organs. The cuneocerebellar tract, composed of uncrossed fibres, originates from cells of the accessory cuneate nucleus, and is regarded as the upper limb equivalent of the posterior spinocerebellar tract. Letters and numbers denote the segmental levels of the spinal cord. (For details of these tracts see p. 990.) (From Carpenter M B, 1991. Core text of neuroanatomy, Williams & Wilkins, with permission of author and publisher.)

noreticular, spinocerebellar and propriospinal fibres. Thus, the precise laminar and segmental location of human spinothalamic tract neurons remains uncertain. The major spinothalamic projections in man are to the ventroposterolateral nucleus, and also to the centrolateral intralaminar nucleus of the thalamus (p. 1087; Walker 1940; Bowsher 1957; Mehler 1962, 1974).

Of particular interest is the discovery of a *dorsolateral spinothalamic tract* in the rat, cat and monkey from studies using both retrograde and anterograde tracing, and antidromic activation techniques (see reviews of Hodge & Apkarian 1990; Willis & Coggeshall 1991). In the monkey, axons forming the tract arise mainly from lamina I neurons and then cross to ascend in the dorsolateral funiculus to end in the thalamus, largely in the ventroposterolateral complex (p. 1086; Apkarian & Hodge 1989b,c). These neurons respond maximally to noxious, mechanical and thermal cutaneous stimuli (Willis et al 1974). The finding of a dorsolateral spinothalamic

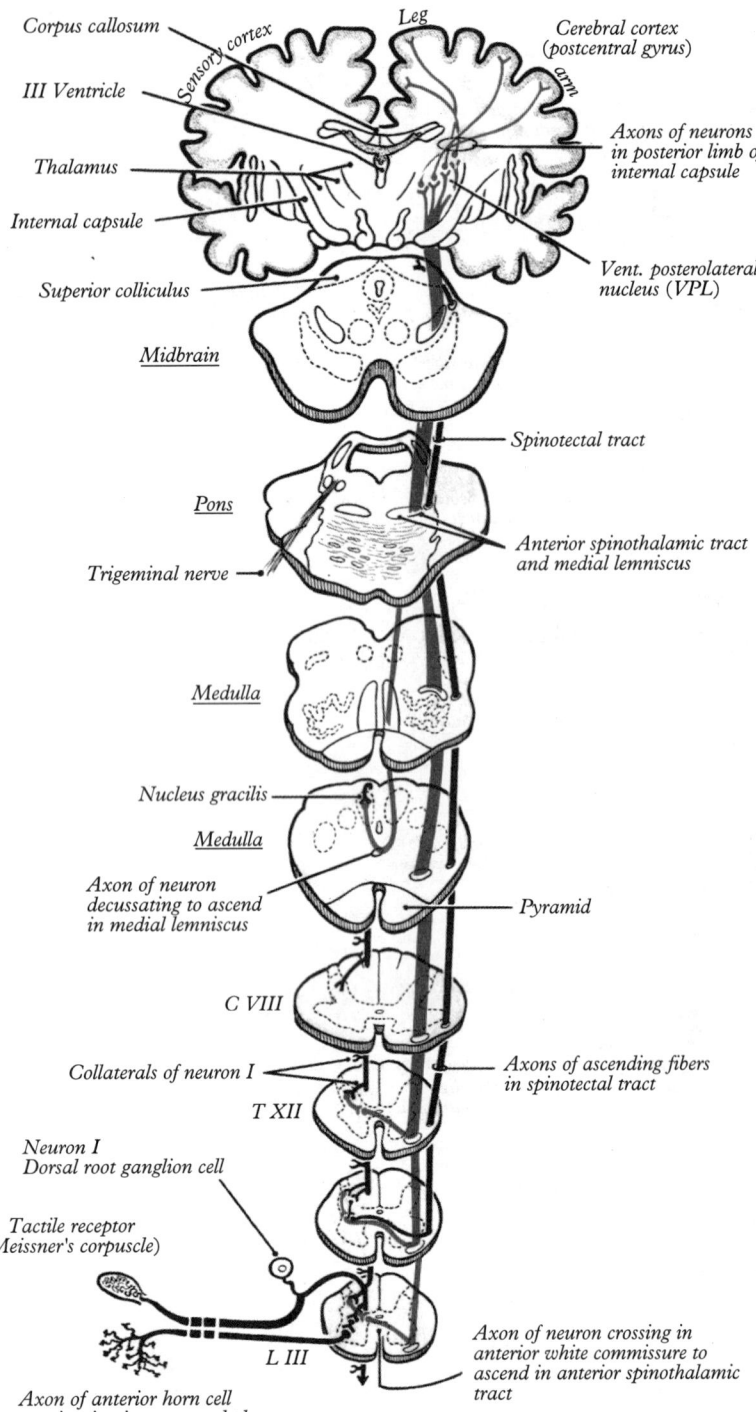

Corpus callosum

Sensory cortex

Leg

Cerebral cortex
(postcentral gyrus)

III Ventricle

arm

Thalamus

Axons of neurons
in posterior limb of
internal capsule

Internal capsule

Superior colliculus

Vent. posterolateral
nucleus (VPL)

Midbrain

Spinotectal tract

Pons

Trigeminal nerve

Anterior spinothalamic tract
and medial lemniscus

Medulla

Nucleus gracilis

Medulla

Axon of neuron
decussating to ascend
in medial lemniscus

Pyramid

C VIII

Collaterals of neuron I

Axons of ascending fibers
in spinotectal tract

T XII

Neuron I
Dorsal root ganglion cell

Tactile receptor
(Meissner's corpuscle)

L III

Axon of neuron crossing in
anterior white commissure to
ascend in anterior spinothalamic
tract

Axon of anterior horn cell
terminating in motor end plates

8.111   Schematic diagram of the anterior spinothalamic tract (red), and the
spinotectal tract (black). The anterior spinothalamic tract, composed of
mainly crossed fibres arises from cells in laminae I, IV to VIII (for details of
segmental location and functional significance of these cells see p. 983,
8.99). The spinotectal tract arises from neurons of laminae I, IV to VIII and
is composed of crossed fibres which intermingle and ascend with those of
the spinothalamic system. Spinotectal fibres project to the superior colliculus, and functionally convey nociceptive information. Letters and
numbers represent the segmental levels of the spinal cord. (From Carpenter
M B 1991. Core text of neuroanatomy, Williams & Wilkins, with permission
of author and publisher.)

tract in all mammals so far investigated may imply that a similar
tract exists in man. Kuru (1949) described such a tract in man arising
from lamina I cells and suggested that it was concerned with pain
and temperature perception; furthermore, several examples of clinical
pain relief following dorsolateral cordotomy are recorded (Sweet
1973, 1975; Moffie 1975).

Modulation of spinothalamic tract cells by descending path-

ways. The activity of spinothalamic tract neurons may be selectively
modulated by pathways descending from the brain to the spinal
cord. Many studies show that the response of spinothalamic tract
cells to noxious stimuli is inhibited by stimulation of certain regions
of the brain (for reviews see Besson & Chaouch 1987; Willis 1988).
This is obviously of considerable clinical interest in the treatment of
chronic, intractable pain. In the brainstem, these regions include
the nucleus raphe magnus, the periaqueductal grey, parts of the
mesencephalic and medullary reticular formation including the parabrachial region (see p. 1077); these neuronal groups together with
their connections constitute the endogenous analgesic system
(p. 1005). In the forebrain, sites that on stimulation inhibit spinothalamic tract cells include the periventricular grey, ventroposterolateral nucleus of the thalamus and the primary sensory
(SI) and posterior parietal cortex. Note that inhibition of spinothalamic tract neurons is also produced by electrical stimulation
of peripheral nerves, the most effective being volleys from A-delta
fibres (see gate control theory, p. 1004). In contrast some spinothalamic tract cells are excited by stimulation of the medullary
reticular formation, and also the primary motor cortex; in the latter,
data suggest the involvement of the corticospinal tract. Functional
aspects of spinothalamic neurons are further considered on p. 1004.

Spinocervicothalamic pathway

The *lateral cervical nucleus*, small in man, lies in the lateral funiculus
ventrolateral to the dorsal grey column in the upper two cervical
segments (Kircher & Ha 1968; Truex et al 1970). In some human
cord specimens the nucleus is not distinctly defined, possibly being
incorporated into the dorsal grey column. It receives axons from the
spinocervical tract which ascends in the dorsolateral funiculus. The
tract cells are found in laminae III–V at all levels of the spinal cord,
ipsilateral to the nucleus. Most neurons of the nucleus project to the
contralateral thalamus via the medial lemniscus, and some to the
contralateral midbrain. Specific thalamic targets include the ventroposterolateral nucleus (p. 1086) and part of the posterior complex.
Spinocervical tract neurons respond to hair movement, pressure,
pinch and thermal stimuli (Brown & Franz 1969, 1970), and to high
threshold muscle input (Kniffki et al 1977); many also respond to
noxious stimuli (Brown & Gordon 1977). Like tract cells of other
ascending pathways, they are under tonic descending inhibitory
control. In carnivores this system is an important tactile and nociceptive pathway; in man the distribution of the tract cells and their
function are less well known.

Spinoreticular fibres

Spinoreticular fibres are intermingled with those of the spinothalamic
tracts, and ascend in the ventrolateral quadrant of the spinal cord
(**8.**115). In a study on the monkey using the retrograde horseradish
peroxidase tracing method, Kevetter et al (1982) found labelled cells
at all levels of the spinal cord, but particularly in the upper cervical
segments. Most labelled neurons are in lamina VII, some in VIII,
and also in the dorsal grey column, especially lamina V. In the
lumbar and cervical enlargements most axons cross the midline, but
in cervical regions there is a large uncrossed component. Most
axons are myelinated. Anterograde degeneration studies in man
and animals following anterolateral cordotomy show spinoreticular
projections to many nuclei of the medial pontomedullary reticular
formation. There is also a projection to the lateral reticular nucleus,
a precerebellar relay nucleus (p. 1078). No somatotopic arrangement
is reported. Spinoreticular neurons respond to inputs from the skin
or deep tissues; innocuous cutaneous stimuli may inhibit or excite a
particular cell, whereas noxious stimuli are often excitatory (Fields
et al 1977). A spino–reticulo–thalamo–cortical pathway has been
proposed as an important route serving pain perception. Like other
ascending pathways, the tract cells are influenced by descending
control. For example, electrical stimulation of the periaqueductal
grey inhibits responses of certain spinoreticular cells to input from
cardiopulmonary afferents; stimulation of the reticular formation
also alters the activity of spinoreticular neurons.

Spinomesencephalic tract

The spinomesencephalic tract comprises a number of pathways
ascending from the spinal cord to various regions of the midbrain.
It includes the *spinotectal tract* (**8.**111) projecting to the superior

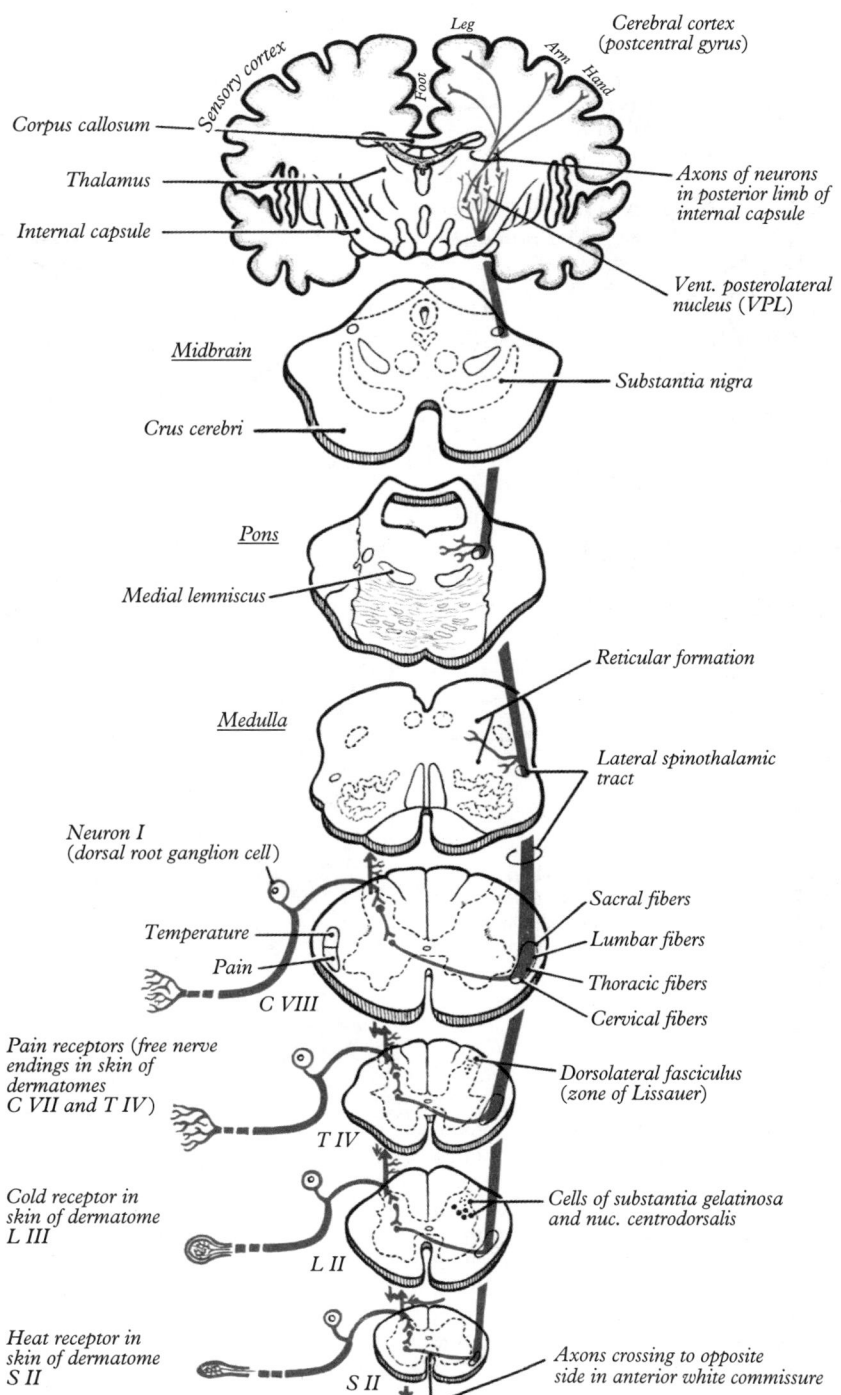

8.112 Schematic diagram of the lateral spinothalamic tract. This tract, arising from cells in laminae I, IV to VIII is composed mainly of crossed fibres. Letters and numbers indicate the segmental levels of the spinal cord. For details of segmental location of the cells and their functional significance see p. 983, 8.99. (From Carpenter M B 1991. Core text of neuroanatomy, Williams & Wilkins, with permission of author and publisher.)

colliculus, the *spinoannular tract* synapsing on neurons of the periaqueductal grey, and also other spinal cord projections that end in the parabrachial nucleus, the pretectal nuclei and the nucleus of Darkschewitsch. Studies in the monkey following horseradish peroxidase injections into the intercollicular region and superior colliculus show retrogradely labelled cells throughout the length of the spinal cord. Many of the cells are concentrated in the cervical segments and the lumbosacral enlargement, the majority in lamina I, but also in laminae IV–VIII, with a large number in lamina V. Most of the labelled cells are contralateral to the injection site but a prominent ipsilateral group is also found at upper cervical levels. Fibres of the spinomesencephalic tract, mostly myelinated, ascend in the white matter of the anterolateral quadrant of the spinal cord, associated with the spinothalamic and spinoreticular tracts.

Spinomesencephalic tract neurons are low-threshold, wide-dynamic range, or high-threshold classes (see p. 1014). Their receptive fields may be small, or very complex encompassing large surface areas of the body. Many spinomesencephalic tract cells are nociceptive and are likely to be involved in the motivational-affective component of pain. Electrical stimulation of spino-annular terminals in the periaqueductal grey results in severe pain in man (Nashold et al 1969). Furthermore, the cells of the deeper layers of the superior colliculus, where spinotectal fibres synapse, are activated by noxious stimuli (Stein & Dixon 1978). For details of the distribution and projection targets of spinomesencephalic tract neurons in the monkey see Wiberg et al (1987).

Spino-olivary tract

The spino-olivary tract is described in animals as arising from neurons in the deeper laminae of grey matter. Axons forming the

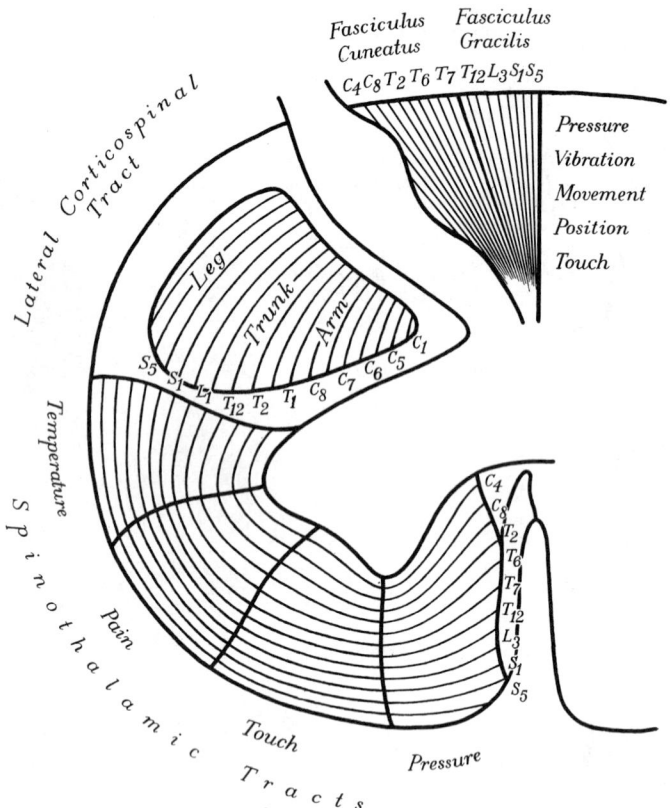

8.113 The general plan of segmental organization of the fibres in the posterior funiculus, the lateral corticospinal tract and the lateral and anterior spinothalamic tracts. The probable cross-sectional areas of these tracts are enlarged to provide adequate space. This general plan applies to *all* segmentally organized tracts whether ascending, descending, ipsilateral or contralateral. (After Foerster 1936, with permission.)

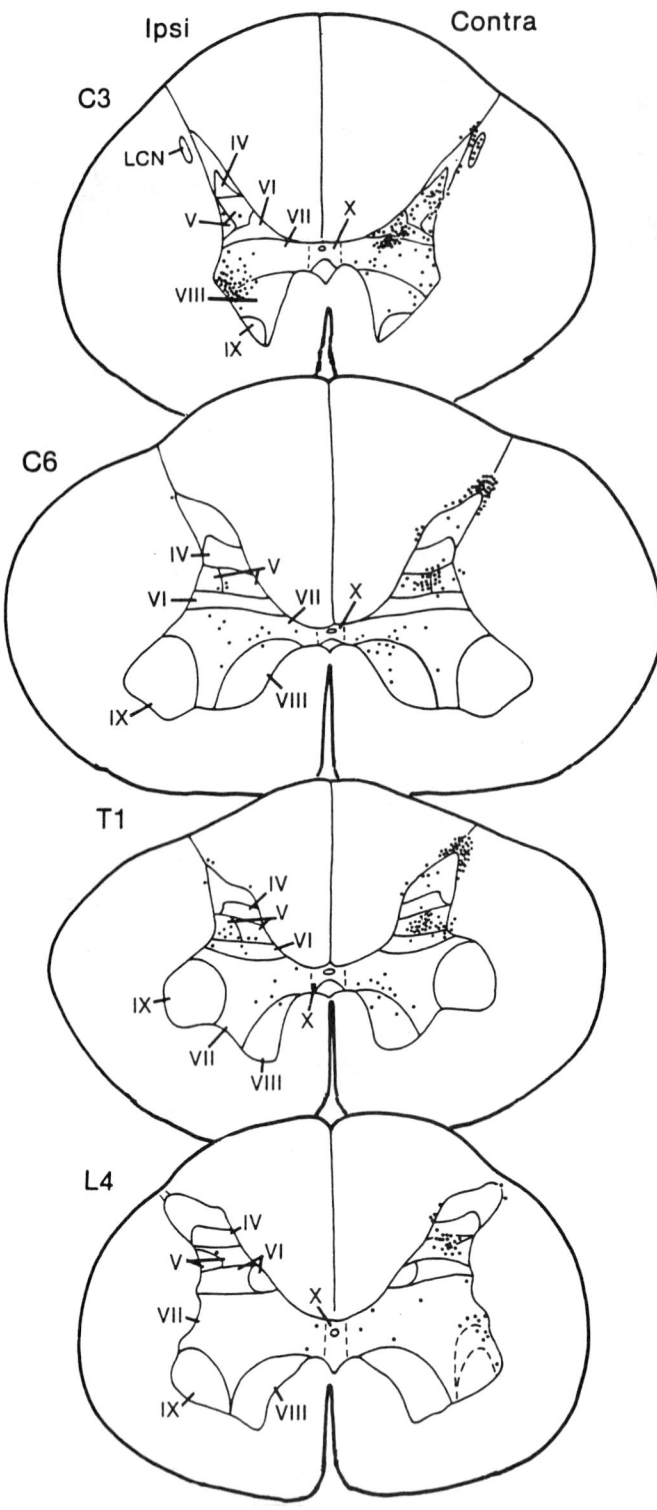

8.114 The distribution of spinothalamic neurons in four selected sections of the spinal cord of the monkey. Letters and numbers indicate the segmental levels; LCN, the lateral cervical nucleus. (Extracted from Apkarian and Hodge, 1989, with permission of Wiley-Liss, Inc. a subsidiary of John Wiley & Sons Ltd.)

tract cross and then ascend superficially at the junction of the anterior and lateral white funiculi, to end in the 'spinal' regions of the dorsal and medial accessory olivary nuclei (Boesten & Voogd 1975). The tract carries information from muscle and tendon proprioceptors, and also from cutaneous receptors (Grant & Oscarsson 1966b). A functionally similar route, the *dorsal spino-olivary tract*, ascends in the dorsal white funiculi, and relays in the dorsal column nuclei to the contralateral inferior olive (Berkeley & Hand 1978). Information on these tracts in primates is scant, but evidence from cordotomies in man show degenerating axonal terminals in the inferior olive (p. 1020).

DESCENDING TRACTS (8.115, 116, 117)

Corticospinal tracts

Corticospinal fibres arise from cells of the cerebral cortex and project to neurons in the spinal cord (8.116). En route they descend at first through the posterior crus of the internal capsule, traverse the cerebral peduncle of the midbrain, the pons and then, at the rostral level of the medulla oblongata, form a discrete bundle, the *pyramid* (8.124). Just rostral to the level of the spinomedullary junction, about 75%–90% of the corticospinal fibres in the pyramid cross the median plane in the *pyramidal decussation* to continue as the *lateral corticospinal tract*; the rest of the fibres continue uncrossed as the *anterior corticospinal tract*. The lateral tract also contains some uncrossed corticospinal fibres. Corticospinal tracts, thus defined, are commonly termed the *pyramidal tracts*, because their fibres traverse the medullary pyramids. However, the term also embraces not only the corticospinal tracts, but also *corticobulbar* fibres which diverge above this level to end in association with cranial motor nuclei.

The *lateral corticospinal tract* (8.117) descends in the lateral funiculus throughout most of the length of the spinal cord, progressively

diminishing to end at about the fourth sacral spinal segment. It occupies an oval area, anterolateral to the posterior grey column and medial to the posterior spinocerebellar tract (8.104); in the lumbar and sacral regions, where the latter tract is absent, it reaches the dorsolateral surface of the cord.

The *anterior corticospinal tract* (8.116), usually small and inverse in size to the lateral tract, descends in the anterior funiculus. It adjoins the anterior median fissure, but is separated from it by the sulcomarginal fasciculus (8.104). Present in the upper spinal cord, it

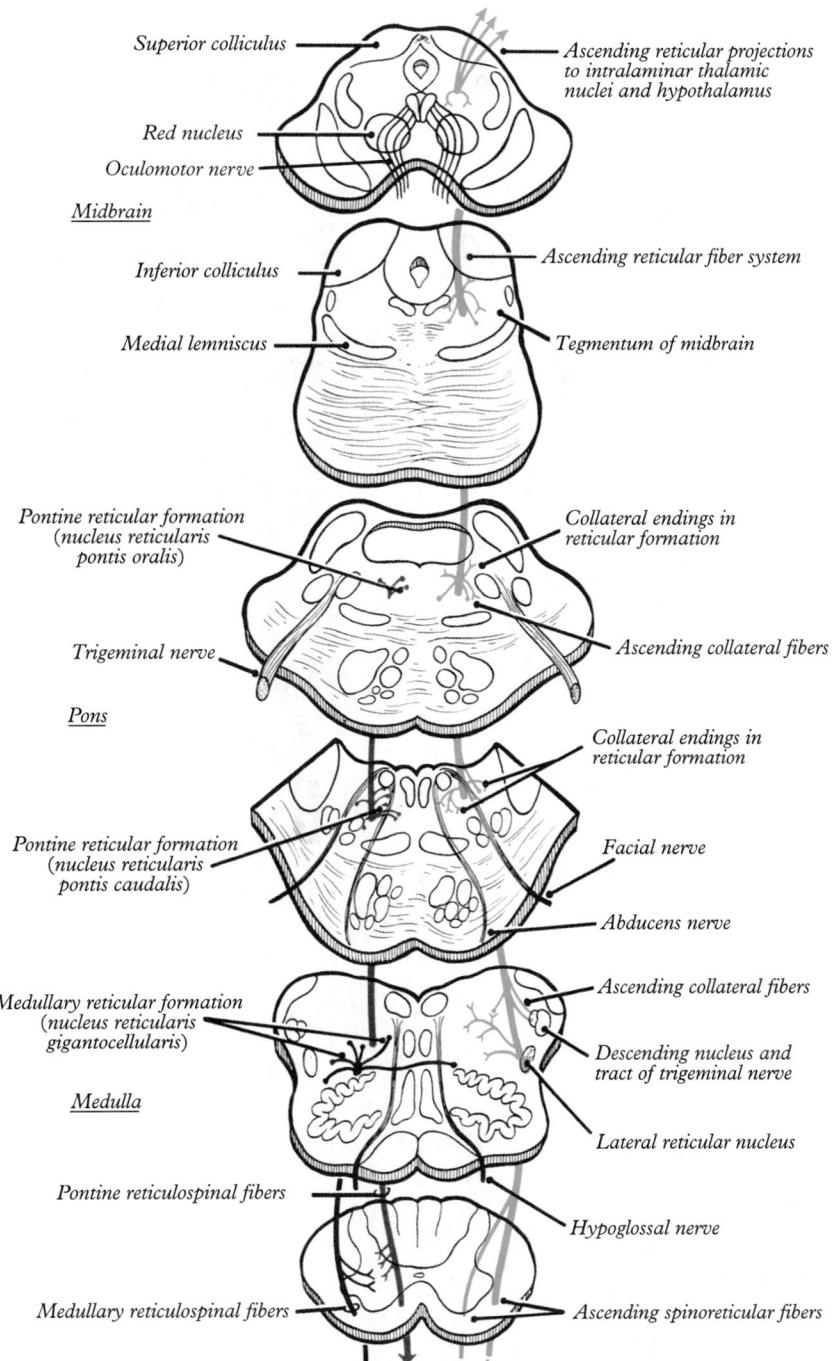

8.115 Schematic diagrams of ascending (blue) and descending (red) and medullary (black) reticular tracts. Reticular axons give off abundant collaterals at various levels of the brainstem and spinal cord. Medullary reticulospinal fibres originate from the gigantocellular reticular nucleus and descend bilaterally in the anterolateral quadrant of the spinal cord. Pontine reticulospinal fibres descend ipsilaterally in the anterior funiculus of the spinal cord and arise from the oral and caudal pontine nuclei. The pontine and medullary descending fibres collectively form the medial reticulospinal tract. For details of the ascending and descending reticular fibres (see **8**.192–195). (From Carpenter M B 1991. Core text of neuroanatomy, Williams & Wilkins, with permission of author and publisher.)

diminishes as it descends and peters out at midthoracic cord levels; it may be absent or, very rarely, contains almost all the corticospinal fibres (Nyberg-Hansen & Rinvik 1963).

At spinal levels, most fibres of the anterior corticospinal tract cross the median plane to synapse with spinal neurons, doing so in the anterior white commissure, whereas fibres of the lateral tracts mostly end on ipsilateral cord neurons. Somatotopy is found throughout the cerebrum and brainstem, except perhaps in the pons. Details are to be found in the appropriate sections of the text. Whether the arrangement is identical in the medullary pyramids and spinal cord is uncertain (Foerster 1936; Barnard & Woolsey 1956). However, there appears to be a laminar organization in the spinal cord; longer fibres are superficial, shorter ones lying internally (**8**.113).

Each pyramid contains about a million fibres of varying diameter, 70% being myelinated; about 90% have a diameter 1–4 μm, about 9% 5–10 μm and less than 2% 11–22 μm. The largest diameter fibres arise from the giant pyramidal neurons of Betz (see below).

Cells of origin. The majority of corticospinal fibres arise from cells situated in the upper two-thirds of the precentral motor cortex (area 4), and from the premotor cortex (area 6); a small contribution of fibres stems from cells of the postcentral gyrus (somatosensory cortex, areas 3, 1, and 2) and the adjacent parietal cortex (area 5) p. 1154. In the monkey 30% of descending fibres in the pyramid arise from area 4, 30% from area 6, and 40% from the parietal regions (Russell & DeMeyer 1961). Cells of origin of corticospinal fibres vary in size in the different cortical areas and cluster into groups or

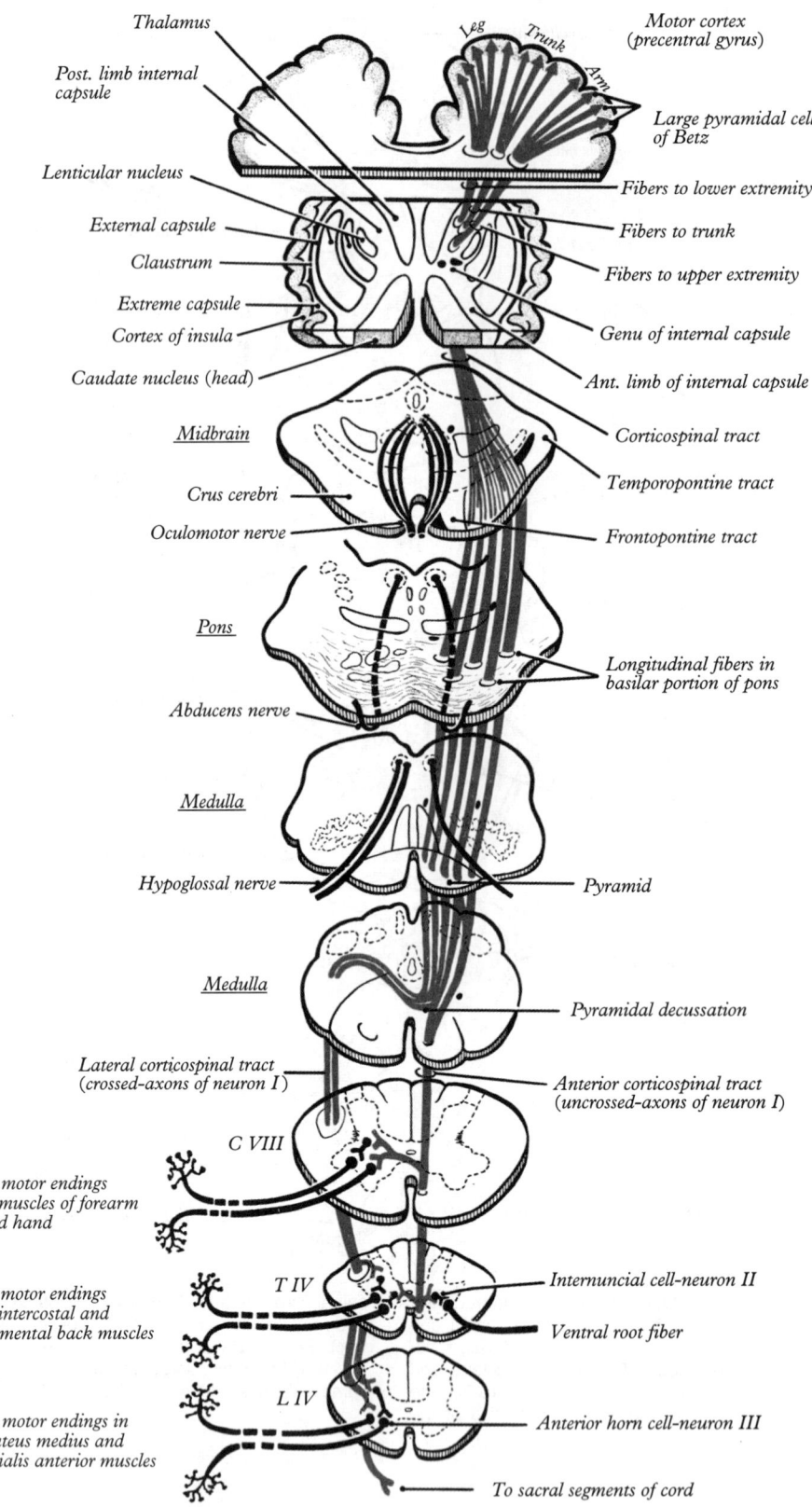

8.116 Schematic diagram of lateral and anterior corticospinal tracts (red) ventral and motor neurons and axons (black). Letters and numbers indicate the various levels of the spinal cord. For details of these tracts see p. 998.

(From Carpenter M B 1991. Core text of neuroanatomy, Williams & Wilkins, with permission of author and publisher.)

strips (Jones & Wise 1977); the largest cells (giant pyramidal neurons of Betz) are in the precentral cortex.

Terminal distribution. Corticospinal fibres synapse with interneurons and also, in some mammalian species including man, directly with spinal motor neurons. The distribution in the human spinal cord has been shown in clinicopathological studies using anterograde degeneration methods (Schoen 1964, 1969; Schoenen 1981). Corticospinal fibres are found to end mainly contralaterally in the lateral

parts of laminae IV–VI, lamina VII and, with regard to motor neurons, in the dorsolateral group, and the lateral parts of both central and ventrolateral groups of lamina IX (8.106). Some terminals are distributed to the medial parts of lamina VII contralaterally, and to lamina VIII bilaterally (Schoen 1969). The small contribution of fibres from parietal sources ends mainly in the lateral parts of laminae IV–VI and lamina VII.

In the monkey, fibres from cells of the parietal cortex end mainly in the contralateral dorsal grey column in laminae IV–VI (Kuypers 1960; Coulter & Jones 1977). They represent phylogenetically the oldest part of the corticospinal system (Martin & Fisher 1968), and modulate the transmission of afferent impulses to higher centres, including the motor cortex (Lundberg 1975). Corticospinal fibres from the frontal cortex (areas 4 and 6) end more ventrally mainly in the contralateral laminae VII and VIII throughout the cord, and also on motor neurons particularly those in the spinal enlargements (Schoen 1964; Kuypers & Brinkman 1970). These fibres subserve motor control—i.e. the modulation of spinal reflex activity and the direction of movements.

Evidence from animal studies shows that direct projections from the precentral cortical areas to spinal motor neurons are concerned with highly-fractionated movements of the limbs. In the *rhesus* monkey precentral corticospinal fibres are mainly distributed to motor neurons supplying the distal extremity muscles. Transection of corticospinal fibres at the pyramids (bilateral pyramidotomy) in the *rhesus* monkey results in a flaccid paresis of the distal extremities and, after a recovery period, in the permanent loss of independent hand and finger movements (Lawrence & Kuypers 1968). In the chimpanzee and man, direct projections of precentral corticospinal fibres to motor neurons are distributed not only to ventral horn neurons innervating distal muscles but also to those supplying proximal muscles of the limbs. In the chimpanzee (Tower 1949) pyramidotomy produces a flaccid paralysis of the whole limb. However, after pyramidotomy in the cat, which has few direct cortical connections with motor neurons, results in minimal paresis (Liddell & Phillips 1944; Lundberg & Voorhoeve 1962; Flindt-Egebak 1977).

Precentral corticospinal projections influence the activities of both α and γ motor neurons, facilitating flexor muscles and inhibiting extensors—the reverse effects are mediated by the lateral vestibulospinal fibres (see below). Immunocytological studies suggest that glutamate or aspartate, often colocalized, may be the excitatory neurotransmitters in some corticospinal neurons.

Postnatal development. Myelination of corticospinal axons in the human neonate starts at 10 to 14 days in the internal capsule and cerebral peduncles, and then proceeds simultaneously in both tracts; longer axons appear to myelinate first. Myelination is completed in the second year. In the *rhesus* monkey direct cortical connections with motor neurons are gradually made during the first 6 postnatal months (Kuypers 1962), and occur in parallel with the capacity to execute relatively independent hand and finger movements (Lawrence & Hopkins 1976). In the human neonate, this motor capacity develops only gradually during the first 2 years of postnatal life (Touwen 1976), and is often attributed to a learning process. However, in view of these experimental findings in the monkey it may represent the external manifestation of the postnatal establishment of direct cortico–motor–neuronal connections.

Clinical signs of damage to the corticospinal system. Destruction of corticospinal fibres at the level of the internal capsule, commonly caused by a cerebral vascular accident or 'stroke', results in a contralateral hemiplegia. The paralysis is initially flaccid, later becoming spastic, and is most marked in the distal muscles of the extremities, especially those concerned with individual movements of the fingers and hand. Associated signs on the paralysed side are:

- hyperactive deep tendon reflexes
- the loss of superficial abdominal and cremasteric reflexes
- the appearance of dorsiflexion of the toes (Babinski's sign) in response to stroking the sole of the foot.

The Babinski sign is usually interpreted as pathognomonic of corticospinal damage, but it is not always present in patients with confirmed corticospinal lesions (Nathan & Smith 1955a). This sign is normally present in human infants up to about 2 years of age, its disappearance possibly being due to the completion of myelination of the corticospinal fibres or to the establishment of direct cortico–motor–neuronal connections.

Vestibulospinal tracts

The large complex of vestibular nuclei (p. 1024), which lies in the floor of the fourth ventricle and abounds on the pontomedullary junction of the brainstem, gives rise to two spinal tracts, each functionally and topographically distinct (**8.117**). The *lateral vesti-*

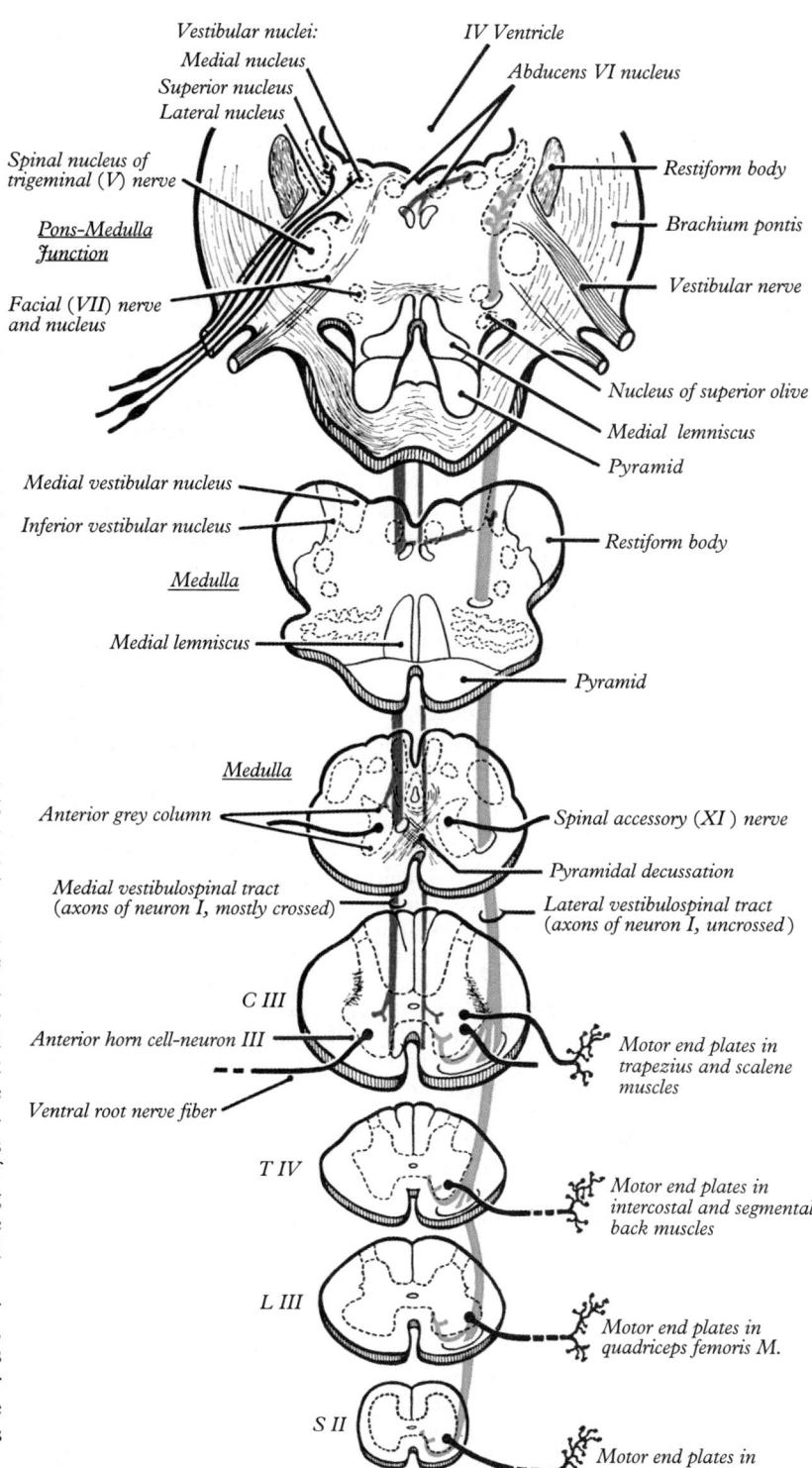

8.117 Schematic diagram of the vestibulospinal tracts. The lateral vestibulospinal tract (blue) projects ipsilaterally in the spinal cord. The medial vestibulospinal tract (red) descends in the medial longitudinal fasciculus at brainstem levels and then projects bilaterally in the spinal cord. Letters and numbers indicate the segmental levels of the spinal cord. (From Carpenter M B 1991. Core text of neuroanatomy, Williams & Wilkins, with permission of author and publisher.)

bulospinal tract (**8.117**) descends ipsilaterally in the periphery of the anterolateral funiculus and then shifts into the medial part of the anterior funiculus at lower spinal levels. Fibres of this tract stem from small and large neurons of the lateral vestibular nucleus (Nyberg-Hansen 1964b; Nyberg-Hansen & Mascitti 1964), and are somatotopically organized (Pompeiano & Brodal 1957b; Akaike 1983). In the cat, fibres projecting to the cervical, thoracic, and lumbosacral segments of the cord arise respectively from neurons in the rostroventral, central, and dorsocaudal parts of the lateral vestibular nucleus. Similar somatotopy with minor differences also obtains in humans (Foerster & Gagel 1932; Løken & Brodal 1970). Lateral vestibulospinal fibres end ipsilaterally in the medial part of the anterior grey column, i.e. lamina VIII and the medial part of lamina VII. The *medial vestibulospinal tract* (**8**.117) descends via the medial longitudinal fasciculus (p. 1041) into the anterior funiculus of the spinal cord where it lies close to the midline in the so-called sulcomarginal fasciculus (**8**.104A). Unlike the lateral tract it contains both crossed and uncrossed fibres, and does not extend beyond the midthoracic cord level. Neurons giving rise to medial vestibulospinal fibres are found mainly in the medial vestibular nucleus (Pompeiano & Brodal 1957b; Nyberg-Hansen 1964b), but some are also located in the inferior (spinal or descending) and lateral vestibular nuclei (Rasmussen 1932; Peterson & Coulter 1977; Gerrits 1990). Fibres of the medial tract project mainly to the cervical cord segments, ending in lamina VIII and the adjacent posterior part of lamina VII.

Data from stimulation of vestibular nuclei (Wilson & Yoshida 1969a,b, 1970; Hultborn 1976) show that axons of the medial tract inhibit monosynaptically motor neurons innervating axial muscles of the neck and upper part of the back. On the other hand, axons of the lateral vestibulospinal tract excite, through mono- and polysynaptic connections, motor neurons of extensor muscles of the neck, back and limbs, but inhibit disynaptically motor neurons of flexor limb muscles, via 1a inhibitory interneurons.

Other descending tracts

Medial reticulospinal tract. (**8**.115) This tract originates from the medial tegmental field of oblongata and the pons, the main sources being the gigantocellularis reticular nucleus in the medulla, and the oral and caudal pontine reticular nuclei (see p. 1075). Medullary reticulospinal fibres, both ipsilateral and contralateral, descend in the anterior and anterolateral funiculi, whereas pontine ones (mainly ipsilateral) descend in the anterior funiculus. These fibres furnish many collaterals, so that two-thirds of the reticulospinal neurons that distribute to the cervical anterior grey matter also project to the lumbosacral cord. The terminals of the reticulospinal fibres are bilaterally distributed to lamina VIII, and the central and medial parts of lamina VII. The medullary reticulospinal terminals are more widely distributed, ending additionally in the lateral parts of laminae VI and VII and also directly on motor neurons. Both *a* and *γ* motor neurons are influenced by reticulospinal fibres, through polysynaptic and monosynaptic connections. Physiological evidence shows that reticulospinal fibres from pontine sources excite motor neurons of axial and limb muscles; on the other hand, medullary fibres excite or inhibit motor neurons of cervical muscles, and excite those of axial muscles (Wilson & Peterson 1981). Functionally, the medial reticulospinal tract is concerned with posture, the steering of head and trunk movements in response to external stimuli and crude, stereotyped movements of the limbs.

Tectospinal tract. This tract arises from the intermediate and deep layers of the superior colliculus of the midbrain (p. 1070). It crosses ventral to the periaqueductal grey in the dorsal tegmental decussation to descend in the medial part of the anterior funiculus of the spinal cord (**8**.103). Fibres of the tract project only to the upper cervical cord segments, ending in laminae VI–VIII. They make polysynaptic connections with motor neurons that facilitate contralateral neck muscles and inhibit ipsilateral ones. Turning of the head to the contralateral side results from unilateral, electrical stimulation of the superior colliculus in the cat, and is mainly effected through the tectospinal tract. For reviews of this tract consult Kuypers (1981) and Holstege (1991), and for a quantitative study on the evolutionary status of the mammalian tectospinal tract see Nudo and Masterton (1989).

Interstitiospinal tract. This tract arises from cells of the interstitial nucleus of Cajal (p. 1070) and the immediate surrounding area, and descends via the medial longitudinal fasciculus into the anterior funiculus of the spinal cord. Its fibres, mainly ipsilateral, project as far as lumbosacral levels, and are mainly distributed to the dorsal part of lamina VIII and the dorsally adjoining part of lamina VII. They establish some monosynaptic connections with motor neurons of neck muscles, but mainly disynaptic connections with motor neurons of limb muscles. Although this tract has long been identified in

the human cord (Muskens 1914) no details are available; the above information is derived from animal studies (see Holstege 1991).

Rubrospinal tract. This arises from the *red nucleus*, an ovoid mass of cells situated in the midbrain tegmentum. The nucleus (p. 1068) consists of a rostral parvocellular part and a caudal magnocellular part, the latter being poorly developed in man. Rubrospinal fibres cross in the *ventral tegmental decussation* and descend into the lateral funiculus of the cord, where they lie anterior to, and intermingled with, fibres of the lateral corticospinal tract (**8**.104). Rubrospinal fibres are distributed to the lateral parts of laminae V–VI and the dorsal part of lamina VII (Nyberg-Hansen & Brodal 1964). In the monkey, the rubrospinal fibres also connect directly with motor neurons supplying the distal muscles of the limbs (Holstege et al 1988).

Somatotopy is well established in the cat (Pompeiano & Brodal 1957a; Nyberg-Hansen & Brodal 1964). Thus, rubrospinal neurons projecting to the cervical and lumbosacral segments of the cord are located respectively in the dorsomedial and ventrolateral parts of the red nucleus; somewhat similar findings obtain in the *rhesus* monkey (Castiglioni et al 1978). Physiological evidence in the cat shows that rubrospinal fibres facilitate flexor muscles and inhibit extensor ones (Thulin 1963).

In man (Stern 1938), the rubrospinal fibres originate from the 'so-called' caudal magnocellular part of the red nucleus which consists of some 150–200 large neurons (Grofová & Maršala 1960), interspersed with small neurons. From the large neurons arise axons of the rubrospinal tract; whether the small neurons also contribute is uncertain, but the tract in man appears to project only to the upper three cervical cord segments (Nathan & Smith 1982). As the evolutionary scale is climbed the 'rubrospinal part' of the red nucleus regresses, due possibly to the development of the corticospinal system which in man is substantial (see Massion 1988).

Lateral reticulospinal tract. This is situated in the lateral funiculus of the spinal cord, closely associated with the rubrospinal and lateral corticospinal tracts (**8**.104). Its fibres arise from neurons of the ventrolateral tegmental field of the pons. Crossing in the rostral medulla oblongata the fibres project, with a high degree of collateralization, throughout the length of the spinal cord. Axons of this tract terminate in laminae I, V and VI, and also bilaterally in the lateral cervical nucleus (Holstege & Kuypers 1982; Tan & Holstege 1986). Evidence suggests that this pathway is involved in the control of pain perception and also in motor functions.

The *solitariospinal tract*, a small group of mostly crossed fibres, arises from the ventrolateral part of the solitary nucleus (p. 1018). Descending in the anterior and anterolateral funiculi of the cord these fibres innervate phrenic motor neurons supplying the diaphragm, and also thoracic motor neurons of intercostal muscles (for details see Holstege 1991). A pathway, with somewhat similar course and terminations to that of the solitariospinal one, originates from the nucleus retroambiguus. Both pathways subserve respiratory activities by driving inspiratory muscles; some descending retroambiguus fibres facilitate expiratory ones. Clinical evidence shows that bilateral anterolateral cordotomy at high cervical levels abolishes rhythmic respiration (Nathan 1963).

Hypothalamospinal fibres have been shown by tracing and immunohistochemical methods in the rat, cat and monkey (for reviews see Kuypers 1981; Saper 1990). Arising from the paraventricular nucleus and other areas of the hypothalamus the fibres descend ipsilaterally, mainly in the posterolateral funiculus of the cord, to be distributed to sympathetic and parasympathetic preganglionic neurons of the intermediolateral column. Fibres from the paraventricular nucleus show oxytocin and vasopressin immunoreactivity and are also distributed to laminae I and X. Descending fibres from the dopaminergic cell group (A11), situated in the caudal hypothalamus, innervate sympathetic preganglionic cells and also cells of the posterior grey column. That similar pathways exist in man may be inferred from ipsilateral sympathetic deficits (e.g. Horner's syndrome) resulting from lesions of the hypothalamus, the lateral tegmental brainstem and the lateral spinal funiculus (Nathan & Smith 1986).

Catecholaminergic spinal pathways. These arise from several sources (**8**.191):

- The coeruleospinal projections originate from noradrenergic cell groups A4 and A6 of the locus coeruleus complex of the pons, and descend via the anterolateral funiculus to innervate all cord segments bilaterally. They end in the posterior grey (laminae IV–VI), and the intermediate and anterior grey columns; while an extensive input is received by preganglionic parasympathetic cells of the sacral cord. Other descending noradrenergic fibres from the lateral tegmental cell groups A5 and A7 of the pons travel in the posterolateral funiculus to be distributed to laminae I–III, and massively to the intermediate grey column.

- Descending fibres from adrenergic cell groups C1 and C3 of the medulla oblongata have been traced into the anterior funiculus of the cord where they are extensively distributed to the inter-mediolateral column.
- Dopaminergic fibres projecting to the spinal cord have already been described (see above under hypothalamospinal fibres).

The precise functional role of these catecholaminergic spinal pathways needs clarification, but they appear to be concerned with the modulation of sensory transmission, and the control of autonomic and somatic motor neuronal activities (for reviews see Kuypers 1981; Lindvall & Björklund 1983; Pearson et al 1990).

Raphespinal tracts. These form part of the serotonergic system. The raphe nuclei pallidus (B1), obscura (B2) and magnus (B3) cell groups situated in the brainstem (p. 1074) give rise to two descending bundles (**8.192**):

- The lateral raphespinal bundle from B3 cells, concerned with the control of nociception, descends close to the lateral corticospinal tract; its fibres end in the posterior grey column (laminae I, II and V).
- The ventral bundle, composed mainly of axons from B1 cells, travels in the medial part of the anterior white column and ends in the anterior grey column (laminae VIII and IX). This bundle subserves the facilitation of extensor and flexor motor neurons.

Some descending serotonergic fibres project to sympathetic pre-ganglionic cells and are concerned with the central control of cardiovascular function. For data, mostly from animal studies, consult Holstege and Kuypers (1982), Törk and Hornung (1990) and Holstege (1991).

Olivospinal tract of Helweg. This tract, as described in transverse sections of the human cervical cord, occupies a triangular zone lying lateral to emerging ventral root fibres in the superficial part of the lateral funiculus. There is no evidence, in man or animals to show the presence of olivospinal fibres in this tract. It was once considered to comprise spino-olivary fibres, possibly on account of their close proximity to the tract. However, Smith and Deacon (1981) in the human spinal cord find that Helweg's tract consists mostly of small, finely myelinated, descending axons; the source and terminations of these are undetermined. No homologous tract appears to exist in animals.

Summary of the major descending pathways

In an analysis of the descending pathways in mammals Kuypers (1981) subdivided the descending brainstem pathways into groups, A and B, on the basis of their terminal distribution and functional attributes.

Group A or the ventromedial brainstem pathways. These comprise both vestibulospinal tracts, the medial reticulospinal tract, the tectospinal and interstitiospinal tracts, all of which pass through the medial and ventral parts of the lower brainstem tegmentum to descend in the ventral and ventrolateral funiculi of the spinal cord. Fibres of these tracts end, often with a bilateral distribution, in the ventromedial part of the intermediate zone (laminae V–VII) of the spinal grey matter. This region contains both long and intermediate propriospinal neurons (see below), the axons of which are to some degree distributed bilaterally. The fibres of most of these tracts are highly collateralized, and some make monosynaptic connections with motor neurons innervating muscles of the limbs. The cells of origin of group A axons receive cortical projections mainly from areas rostral to the precentral gyrus. Functionally, this system is concerned with the maintenance of posture, the integration of movements of the body and limbs, and synergistic whole-limb movements; it also subserves the orientation movements of the body and head, and the direction of the course of progression.

Group B or the lateral brainstem pathways. Descending through the ventrolateral part of the lower brainstem tegmentum these pathways continue in the dorsolateral funiculus of the spinal cord. They consist of the rubrospinal tract, and the lateral reticulospinal tract, i.e. the crossed pontospinal tract arising from the ventrolateral pontine tegmentum. Fibres of these tracts end, mainly ipsilaterally, in the dorsal and lateral parts of the intermediate zone of spinal grey matter (laminae V–VII), a region containing short propriospinal neurons (see below). Rubrospinal fibres in the monkey also establish monosynaptic connections with motor neurons of distal muscles of the limbs. Rubrospinal neurons receive cortical afferent fibres mainly from the precentral gyrus. Data obtained in the freely moving monkey (Lawrence & Kuypers 1968) show that group B pathways are functionally instrumental in providing the capacity for independent, flexion-biased movements of the limbs and of the shoulder but, especially, of the elbow and hand. Thus, pathways of group B supplement the motor control carried out by those of group A. Furthermore, the corticospinal pathway arising from motor areas of the frontal lobe terminate in the region which largely overlaps those of the two groups of brainstem pathways. Functionally, this part of the corticospinal system enhances the brainstem controls but, additionally, provides the capacity for fractionation of movements, as exemplified by individual finger movements, which are probably executed through direct corticospinal motor neural connections (p. 1000).

PROPRIOSPINAL TRACTS

Propriospinal neurons are confined to the spinal cord. Thus, their ascending or descending fibres, both crossed and uncrossed, begin and end within the spinal grey matter; they constitute the propriospinal or intersegmental tracts, sometimes referred to as fasciculi proprii. The fibres interconnect with local cells within the same segment and/or with other cells in more distant segments of the spinal cord. The majority of spinal neurons are propriospinal neurons which are mostly located in laminae V–VIII. Propriospinal or intersegmental fibres are mainly concentrated around the margins of the grey matter (**8.103**) but are also dispersed diffusely in the white funiculi. The propriospinal system plays an important role in spinal functions as exemplified by the distribution of descending pathways to specific subgroups of propriospinal neurons which in turn relay to motor neurons and other spinal cells (see below). Furthermore, the system mediates all those automatic functions that continue after transection of the spinal cord, such as sudomotor and vasomotor activities, bowel and bladder functioning.

Many of the data on the source and distribution of propriospinal fibres come from experimental studies in the cat and monkey (for reviews see Kuypers 1981; Holstege 1991). Propriospinal neurons are categorized according to the length of their axons into long, intermediate, and short propriospinal neurons:

- The long propriospinal neurons distribute their axons throughout the length of the cord, mainly via the ventral and ventrolateral funiculi; their cell bodies are in lamina VIII and the dorsally adjoining part of lamina VII. Axons from the long propriospinal neurons of the cervical cord descend bilaterally, whereas those from the corresponding lumbosacral neurons ascend mainly contralaterally.
- The intermediate propriospinal neurons occupy the central and medial parts of lamina VII; they project, mainly ipsilaterally, over shorter distances.
- The short propriospinal neurons that project their axons over a distance of eight segments are found in the lateral parts of laminae V–VIII; these axons run ipsilaterally in the lateral funiculus.

Propriospinal fibres in the different parts of the white funiculi are distributed preferentially to specific regions of the spinal grey matter. In the spinal enlargements, the propriospinal fibres in the dorsolateral funiculus project to the dorsal and lateral parts of the intermediate zone, and also to spinal motor neurons supplying distal muscles of limbs, especially those of the hand and the foot. In contradistinction, the propriospinal fibres in the ventral part of the ventrolateral funiculus are distributed to the central and medial parts of lamina VII and to motor neurons of proximal limb and girdle muscles. A further component of propriospinal fibres runs in the medial part of the ventral funiculus. These fibres are delivered mainly to the ventromedial part of the intermediate zone which characteristically contains long propriospinal neurons, and also to motor neurons innervating axial and girdle muscles.

Less is known about the precise source and distribution of the propriospinal fibre system in the human spinal cord. Most of the available data are extensively reviewed by Nathan and Smith (1959) and considered below.

Ground bundles

The *anterior ground bundle* is present throughout the length of the spinal cord and comprises all fasciculi proprii fibres that descend or ascend in the anterior white funiculus. The length of the fibres ranges from short ones, spanning only one segment, through to those that run the length of the cord. The shortest fibres lie immediately adjacent to the grey matter, the longer ones being situated more peripherally. The sites of the cells of origin are poorly known, but are probably in the more medial and posterior parts of the anterior grey column, the lateral part of the intermediate grey zone and, possibly, in the posterior grey column. The fibres of this bundle terminate in the anterior grey columns throughout the spinal cord. The anterior ground bundle is the first spinal tract to myelinate; most of its fibres are fine, less than 3 μm in diameter.

The *lateral ground bundle*, situated in the lateral white funiculus, is present throughout the length of the cord. It consists of both ascending and descending fibres of varying length, and is well developed at the enlargements of the cord. The cells of origin are in the intermediate grey zone, the posterior grey column and, to a lesser extent, in the anterior grey column; their axons, both ipsilateral and contralateral, have many collaterals distributed throughout the grey matter. Myelinated fibres are present in the lateral ground bundle in the 5-month-old fetus.

The *posterior ground bundle*, as defined by Nathan and Smith (1959), comprises only the fine fibres of the fasciculi proprii scattered throughout much of the area of the posterior white column. These fibres, both ascending and descending, are short, unmyelinated and of fine diameter (0.5–2.0 μm). They probably stem from cells in the posterior grey column, and are distributed to the grey matter of the medial part of the posterior grey column. However, the existence of these propriospinal fibres is disputed by some authors.

Dorsolateral tract

This bundle, sometimes called Lissauer's tract, consists of fine myelinated and non-myelinated fibres; it lies between the apex of the posterior grey column and the surface of the spinal cord, surrounding the entering dorsal root fibres (8.99). Present throughout the spinal cord, it is most developed in the upper cervical regions. The tract is formed in part by fibres of the lateral bundles of dorsal roots which bifurcate into ascending and descending branches. The branches travel one or two segments projecting collaterals to and around the cells of the posterior grey column (p. 980, 8.100, 101). The tract also contains many propriospinal fibres as first suggested by Flechsig (1876) who considerably predated Lissauer's original description of 1885. The presence of propriospinal fibres has been confirmed in animal studies (Earle 1952; Poirier & Bertrand 1955; Szentágothai 1965). Findings in the cat show that about 75% of fibres in the tract are of intrinsic origin (Earle 1952); many of these are short axons of small neurons of the substantia gelatinosa which then re-enter the posterior grey column (see 8.101).

Other propriospinal tracts

A somewhat confusing number of small tracts consisting of an admixture of propriospinal and other fibres have been described in the dorsal funiculus by a variety of authors who worked chiefly in the late nineteenth century and based their accounts on pathological appearances in human spinal cord. Thus, extending through cervical and thoracic levels, in the medial part of the cuneate fasciculus, is the *comma tract* (of Schultze), also known as the *semilunar tract* or, more recently, the *interfascicular fasciculus* (8.104). Whether it consists of branches of dorsal roots and/or intrinsic fibres has been a matter of debate. Most evidence suggests that the comma tract contains descending branches of the cervical and upper thoracic dorsal roots.

At lower thoracic levels in the dorsal funiculus, a thin superficial strand of fibres has been described which is the rostral end of the *septomarginal tract* (8.104). At lumbar levels it abuts the posterior median septum. The so-called 'oval field of Flechsig' and the 'triangular field of Gombault and Philippe' are also merely different levels of the septomarginal tract which appears to alter its shape and position as the cord is descended. The tract consists of a mixture of propriospinal fibres and descending branches of dorsal roots.

The *cornu-commissural tract*, present throughout the cord, is most developed in the lower lumbar segments. It lies along the medial side of the posterior grey column abutting the posterior commissure; and consists mainly of ipsilateral, ascending and descending propriospinal fibres, mostly of short length; some dorsal root branches are also present in the tract.

NEUROPHYSIOLOGICAL CORRELATIONS

In addition to being a prime site for retrograde degeneration studies, large multipolar neurons of motor columns in lamina IX were also the targets for classic studies of reflex responses (Sherrington 1906), from which emerged the first clear evidence of *integration* of contacts between neurons, and the concepts of *excitation* and *inhibition*. Their large size made them most suitable for microelectrode recording; so they could be excited *orthodromically* by stimulation of the peripheral nerves or dorsal spinal roots or invaded *antidromically* by stimulation of the ventral roots. Thus detailed analyses have been made of the electrical and ionic events occurring at synapses during the generation of *excitatory* and *inhibitory postsynaptic potentials* (EPSPs and IPSPs). Similarly, recognition of adjacent inhibitory interneurons (Renshaw 1941, 1946) has led to the enquiry into *lateral* and *feedback* inhibitory phenomena.

Since 1940, evidence of *presynaptic inhibition* has grown, for which spinal neurons have provided a major experimental source (for reviews see Eccles 1964b). In presynaptic inhibition, the synaptic terminals (A) which contact a neuron (B) are themselves subjected to the action of synaptic terminals (C) of other neurons, through axoaxonic synapses. When the inhibitory terminals (C) are active they cause a relative depolarization of terminals (A), thus reducing the effectiveness of terminals (A) in producing a postsynaptic response in neuron (B). In common with postsynaptic excitation and inhibition, presynaptic inhibition is also effected by descending fibres from supraspinal sources.

Presynaptic inhibition influences many, possibly all, primary afferent terminals. Thus, sensory information entering the CNS does not simply reflect environmental changes but is continually modified at the first synapse depending on local conditions in the grey matter. A much investigated site of presynaptic effects is in the substantia gelatinosa (Wall 1964; Mendell & Wall 1964; Melzack & Wall 1965; Mendell 1966; Heimer & Wall 1968; Ralston 1974; Nathan 1976; Wall 1978, 1985). As noted elsewhere (p. 1007), it has been proposed that impulses from cutaneous (and other) afferents are here subjected to tonic control involving the relative depolarization and hyperpolarization of primary afferent terminals, mediated by small neurons of the substantia gelatinosa; but precise synaptic events are still under investigation. A *gate control theory*, first proposed by Melzack and Wall (1965) as a possible gelatinosal mechanism in providing a 'gate' to the inflow of impulses along nociceptive and other afferent pathways, has promoted much discussion. The mechanisms initially envisaged are summarized in 8.118.

It was proposed that large-diameter afferents (e.g. from hairs and touch corpuscles) are excitatory to gelatinosal interneurons (SG) and to the larger neurons (T cells) of lamina IV (from which spinothalamic fibres arise). In contrast fine non-myelinated afferents are excitatory to T cells but inhibitory to the SG cells; the axons of the latter were presumed to inhibit presynaptically terminals of all afferents which synapse with T cells. In such a system, a low activity in the fine afferents inhibits SG cells so that they are prevented from inhibiting T cells; hence the 'gate' to T cells in lamina IV is open to transmit intermittent small volleys of impulses from the large fibres. A prolonged high-frequency volley of impulses in the large-diameter afferents, however, is transmitted to lamina IV T cells initially, but this soon ceases as activity in the SG cells closes the gate. Conversely, a persistent high activity in the fine afferents opens the gate resulting

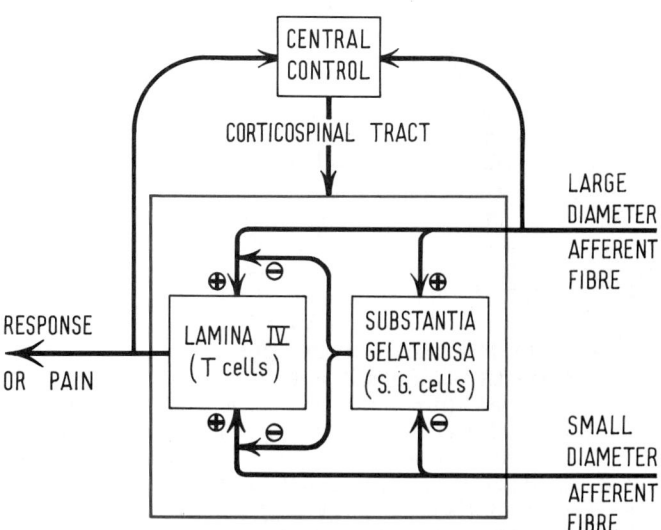

8.118 The sensory 'gate' mechanism as *originally* proposed by R Melzack and P D Wall for the modus operandi of the dorsal laminae of grey matter of the spinal cord. See text for a discussion of the effects of an imbalance in the sensory inflow along the large and small diameter afferent fibres. (From an illustration in Melzack & Wall 1965, with permission of the authors and publishers.) Consult references for a critical review of the gate theory by Nathan (1976) and a comprehensive reappraisal of the evidence and subsequent re-statement of the theory by Wall (1978).

in massive bombardment of neurons of lamina IV. The latter include some neurons of high threshold which are only activated by such bombardment; it is presumed that the onward transmission in the lateral spinothalamic tract will evoke pain at supraspinal centres. Pain would thus result from an *imbalance* between the varieties of afferent impulses when there is a disproportionally large traffic along the fine afferents. These fibres should perhaps not be regarded as 'specific pain afferents' but as information mediators of the *state of the tissues* innervated. Thus, in addition to *interaction* and *comparison* of information flowing along different fibre types, other features of gate control theory involve the *presynaptic inhibition* of primary afferent terminals. Overall 'sensitivity' of the gate may be varied by *descending supraspinal control systems* (see below and p. 1007).

Since its origin the theory has been modified and refined (Melzack 1973; Wall 1973, 1974, 1976). Nevertheless, Nathan (1976) was prompted to write a lengthy criticism. Subsequently Wall (1978) presented a *re-statement* of the gate control theory of pain mechanisms: 'In 1965, we proposed that transmission of information about injury from the periphery to the first central neurons was under control. The setting of this control or gate was influenced by peripheral afferents, other than those which signalled injury. The gate was also influenced by impulses descending from the brain.

Subsequent work has fully supported and enlarged this view. All the cells so far discovered which transmit information from nociceptors are inhibited by low-threshold afferents and by descending controls. The mechanism by which this control is achieved remains completely unknown. Presynaptic inhibition as a phenomenon isolated from postsynaptic inhibition is in doubt. Whether the inhibitions and facilitations are presynaptic or postsynaptic or both is unknown. The role of the substantia gelatinosa in any function is unknown. That a gate control exists is no longer open to doubt but its functional role and its detailed mechanism remain open for speculation and for experiment.'

The endogenous analgesia system

Much information has accumulated concerning a descending pain control system (for extensive reviews see Basbaum & Fields 1979, 1984; Wall & Melzack 1988). Three principal, interconnected regions are involved and each receives a variety of afferents and contains an array of neuromediators.

In the midbrain the *periaqueductal grey matter* together with the dorsal raphe nucleus, and part of the cuneiform nucleus comprise neuron populations containing serotonin (5HT), γ-aminobutyric acid (GABA), substance P, CCK, neurotensin, enkephalin and dynorphin. The periaqueductal grey matter receives afferents from the frontal somatosensory and cingulate neocortex, the amygdala, numerous local reticular nuclei and the hypothalamus (afferents from the latter are separate bundles carrying histamine, luteinizing hormone-releasing hormone (LHRH), vasopressin, oxytocin, adrenocortico-trophic hormone (ACTH), melanocyte-stimulating hormone (γ-MSH), endorphin, and angiotensin II). From the periaqueductal grey matter some fibres descend to rhombencephalic centres, others pass directly to the spinal cord.

In the rhombencephalon, the raphe magnus nucleus and the medial reticular column is an important multineuromediator centre, containing serotonin, substance P, CCK, thyrotrophin-releasing hormone (TRH), enkephalin and dynorphin. Some neurons contain two or even three neuromediators. Descending bulbospinal fibres pass to the nucleus of the spinal tract of the trigeminal nerve and its continuation, the substantia gelatinosa, throughout the length of the cord. Here, there are again populations of neurons containing many different neuromediators, such as GABA, substance P, neurotensin, enkephalin and dynorphin (see Fields et al 1991, and for a review Akil & Lewis 1987). There is now abundant physiological and pharmacological evidence that these regions are intimately concerned with the control of nociceptive (and probably other modality) inputs.

Other general electrophysiological investigations have involved the exploration of spinal grey matter by microelectrodes during stimulation of muscle and cutaneous nerves (Eccles et al 1954; Coombs et al 1956) and during 'natural' stimulation of peripheral receptors (Kolmodin 1957; Kolmodin & Skoglund 1960). The focal extracellular potentials thus evoked correlate well with the specific laminar regions and terminations of dorsal spinal afferents determined by degeneration techniques.

Pain and nociception

It is nearly a century since the publication of Sherrington's influential work 'The integrative action of the nervous system'. What is surprising is how little the conceptual ideas about pain mechanisms changed over most of that period, and how much they have changed in the last few years.

For most of this century, textbooks have expounded a view with its roots in the writings of Descartes and couched in neurophysiological terms by Sherrington, who wrote that 'Pain appears the psychical adjunct to protective reflexes'. He (as Descartes before him) envisaged pain as an alarm system, triggered by stimuli which threaten or damage the body, and drive avoidance behaviour. Sherrington postulated the existence of *nociceptors*, sensory neurons that would not respond to normal physiological events or innocuous stimuli, but would be recruited specifically by immediate threats. With this guidance researchers sought and found evidence for just such a population of afferent neurons, initially in skin and then in deep somatic

tissues. There was a lag of several decades, however, because of the technical difficulties in making recordings from these thin fibres (conducting in the Aδ and C range of velocities). These findings were seen as vindicating the so-called specificity theory, over its rival, the pattern theory (which proposed that sensory information was encoded in a combinatorial way in groups of broadly tuned afferent neurons). Parenthetically, recent work on the properties of sensory neurons innervating visceral tissues suggests that specific nociceptors are very rare in many organs, and rather that noxious events are mostly signalled by 'intensity-encoding' neurons that respond to innocuous physiological stimuli and, with a higher frequency of action potential discharge, to noxious ones.

The idea of a specific pathway for pain was by most writers implicitly applied also to the central nervous system. The Gate Control theory of Melzack and Wall was the first serious challenge to the specific pathway theory. This theory emphasized that pain was a subjective experience, dependent on the context in which it occurred and, therefore, modifiable by other events. The particular 'wiring diagram' (8.118) which illustrated the theory focused on interactions between different afferent fibre types, and proposed that the activity of large diameter innocuous afferents would modify (inhibit) the central transmission of information carried by small diameter fibres.

In the last decade a major shift in thinking has occurred, driven by a recognition that mechanisms of acute pain (also called physiological pain) might differ substantively from those of chronic (also called pathophysiological) pain. It is not so much that earlier facts have been refuted, but rather that their applicability to clinically relevant pain states has been challenged. What has become very clear is that the signalling system is itself strongly modified by the very injury that it reports upon.

This plasticity in the injury-signalling system is being intensively studied at two loci: firstly, at the peripheral terminals of nociceptors; secondly, at the first central site of processing, in the posterior horn of the spinal cord. The changes at these sites are generally referred to as peripheral and central sensitization, respectively.

Peripheral sensitization, as its name implies, relates to an increase in the sensitivity of the peripheral endings of nociceptors. One new development, however, has been the description of a novel class of nociceptors that is not activated by traditional noxious stimuli (i.e. excessive mechanical or thermal stimuli), but which is recruited when tissue becomes inflamed. These sensory neurons have been dubbed 'silent afferents', 'sleeping nociceptors' and, rather more prosaically, 'mechanically insensitive afferents'. They are ubiquitous. In the presence of tissue injury, some of these fibres become mechanosensitive and this is likely to constitute an important new source of afferent barrage. For instance, in an arthritic joint, normally innocuous movements may activate sensitized afferents. These afferent neurons are obviously primarily chemosensitive. The chemical changes in damaged tissue usually persist long after the precipitating cause. These afferents cannot, therefore, function as classical Sherringtonian nociceptors, triggering 'protective reflexes'. A still uncertain issue is exactly what chemical mediators are responsible for recruiting these silent afferents. The list of potential candidates has merely lengthened, actually more a mark of research failure than success. Alongside traditional mediators such as bradykinin, prostaglandins, and serotonin, evidence is growing for the involvement of new molecules—cytokines and growth factors, such as tumour necrosis factor (TNF) and nerve growth factor (NGF).

The second major area of current interest is that of central sensitization. The basis of this phenomenon is that repetitive activity in unmyelinated primary sensory neurons is capable of producing a long-lasting facilitation in the responsiveness of the neurons in the spinal cord that process nociceptive information, which includes a lowering of the threshold of peripheral stimuli necessary to excite the cells. The process provides a ready explanation for some features of the increased sensitivity that is commonly seen after tissue damage in man (so-called *hyperalgesia*, some aspects of which, such as spread around a focal peripheral lesion, are not easily explained by peripheral mechanisms). The significance of the time course of central sensitization (prolonged action after only a brief initiating stimulus) is, of course, that the principal site of pathophysiology in persistent pain states may effectively move from a peripheral to a central locus, and attempts to 'correct' a peripheral pathology may be futile. It is also notable that the role of large tactile afferents changes from inhibitory to excitatory as one moves from the normal to the injured state.

Central sensitization appears to be a very general phenomenon, and has been seen in a large number of models of persistent pain and under a wide variety of conditions. Rather remarkably, all forms of central sensitization seen to date share a common pharmacology. It is now known that most primary sensory neurons release excitatory amino acids (glutamate and aspartate) as neutrotransmitters. There are different classes of receptors for these transmitters. Most second-to-second signalling in spinal cord neurons appears to depend critically on one receptor subtype (the so-called a-amino-3-hydroxy-5-methyl-4-isoxalone proprionic acid (AMPA) receptor). In contrast, the various manifestations of central sensitization depend on a different subtype— the N-methyl-D-aspartate (NMDA) receptor. Hence, blockade of NMDA receptors has little effect on sensory processing under resting conditions, but completely prevents central sensitization. The reason for this dichotomy appears to be that the NMDA receptor is only recruited during repetitive firing in unmyelinated afferents. Once recruited, however, it allows Ca^{2+} to enter the postsynaptic cell, and this in turn triggers a cascade of change that maintains the central hyperexcitable state. One of the second messengers activated by the increased intracellular Ca^{2+} levels under these conditions is nitric oxide (NO), a diffusible transmitter the production of which also appears to be critical for the development of central sensitization. It is interesting just how many parallels there are between these changes in spinal cord function in persistent pain states, and other forms of neuronal plasticity in the adult nervous system, such as long-term potentiation in the hippocampus.

This new knowledge is changing the emphasis of those interested in developing therapies to help treat patients in pain. There is a growing realization that rather than seek analgesic drugs (which aim to block injury-related neuronal signals at some point), there is a great opportunity to develop a new class of agents that are actually antihyperalgesic. Such drugs will, it is hoped, restore the signalling system to its normal level of excitability, and, therefore, retain the protective features of the pain signalling system.

Unit recording with intracellular microelectrodes

Recordings from microelectrodes inserted into individual neurons have provided much information about their properties and activities. Neurons contributing axons to long tracts, such as the spinothalamic, have a complex functional organization and are generally classified according to the types of cutaneous or deep afferent stimuli that activate them. Low-threshold (LT) units are neurons which respond only to either hair movement or gentle cutaneous pressure, and do not increase their firing rate when more intensely noxious stimuli are applied. Wide dynamic range (WDR) units are activated by hair movement or gentle mechanical stimulation, but, in addition, increase their activities when noxious stimuli are applied to the skin, so that they respond maximally to noxious stimuli. High-threshold (HT) units refer to neurons that respond only to intense mechanical or thermal stimulation of the skin. Neurons receiving stimulation from deeper tissues (muscles, tendons or joints) are designated deep (D) units. Other functional subclasses within these classes are also defined. Some neurons that receive exclusively or additionally visceral input are termed visceral specific or somatovisceral units respectively; others that record innocuous warming or cooling of their receptive fields are thermoreceptive units.

COMPARISON OF THE DORSAL COLUMN–MEDIAL LEMNISCUS COMPLEX WITH THE SPINOTHALAMIC PATH

It is instructive to compare, in these two 'systems', the size of the receptive fields, somatotopy, specificity of channels, and forms of control of transmission.

Neurons of dorsal column nuclei

Neurons of dorsal column nuclei (Mountcastle 1968; Norton 1968) receive terminals of long, uncrossed, primary afferent fibres of the fasciculi gracilis and cuneatus (p. 989), which carry information concerning deformation of skin, movement of hairs, joint movement and vibration. In the cat, fibres from hair receptors are superficial, those for touch and vibration more deeply placed. The somatotopy of fibres in the dorsal white columns has been noted (8.109, 113); the connections of dorsal column nuclei are further detailed with the medulla oblongata (p. 1015).

Unit recording in the neurons of dorsal column nuclei shows that their tactile *receptive fields* (i.e. the skin area in which a response can be elicited) vary in size, being mostly small and smallest in the digits. Some fields have *excitatory centres* and *inhibitory surrounds*; thus stimulation just outside its field inhibits the neuron. Neurons in the nuclei are spatially organized into a somatotopic map of the periphery (in accord with the similar localization in the dorsal columns). In general specificity is high. Many cells receive input from one or a few specific receptor types, for example hair, type I and II slowly adapting receptors and Pacinian corpuscles; some cells respond to Ia muscle spindle input. However, some neurons do receive convergent input from tactile pressure and hair follicle receptors.

The transmission of impulses through the dorsal column–medial lemniscus pathway is subjected to a variety of control mechanisms (Jabbur & Towe 1961; Andersen et al 1964c; for review see Willis & Coggeshall 1991). Concomitant activity in adjacent dorsal column fibres may result in presynaptic inhibition by depolarization of the presynaptic terminals of one of them. Stimulation of the sensory–motor cortex also modulates the transmission of impulses by both pre- and postsynaptic inhibitory mechanisms, and sometimes by facilitation. These descending influences are mediated by the corticospinal tract. Modulation of transmission by inhibition also results from stimulation of the reticular formation, raphe nuclei and other sites.

The dorsal column nuclei are not merely 'relay nuclei', as was long supposed. They have been pictured as a highly reliable telephone system in which afferent information is separated in channels which are discrete both for spatial origin and stimulus specificity. In this the dorsal columns strongly contrast with the spinothalamic tracts (see below).

Neurons of the spinothalamic tract

Neurons of the spinothalamic tract have very different receptive fields (see below). Specificity of separate channels, as it exists in the dorsal column nuclei, is absent in the laminae of the cord. Convergence of different functional types of afferent fibres onto an individual tract cell is a common feature in the cord. On the basis of laminar site, functional properties and specific thalamic termination of their axons, spinothalamic tract neurons may be divided into three separate groups, namely:

- apical cells of the dorsal grey column (lamina I)
- deep dorsal column cells (laminae IV–VI)
- cells in the ventral grey column (laminae VII, VIII).

Although there are species differences the data given below pertain to the monkey. For a critical review on the spinothalamic tract and its neurons see Hodge and Apkarian (1990).

Lamina I cells projecting to the thalamus show the following characteristics. In essence they respond maximally to noxious or thermal cutaneous stimulation, and consist mainly of high threshold, but also some wide dynamic range units. Their receptive fields are usually small, comprising a part of a digit or a small area of skin involving several digits. Lamina I spinothalamic tract neurons receive input from A-δ and C fibres, and some respond to convergent input from deep somatic and visceral receptors. Marked viscerosomatic convergence is shown in spinothalamic tract cells in the thoracic cord. Lamina I spinothalamic tract neurons project preferentially to the ventroposterolateral nucleus of the thalamus with limited projections to the centrolateral and mediodorsal thalamic nuclei.

Deep dorsal column (laminae IV–VI) spinothalamic neurons studied in the lumbar cord comprise 60% wide dynamic range, 30% high threshold, and 10% low threshold type units. They can code accurately both innocuous and noxious cutaneous stimuli. Some cells respond also to input from deep somatic and visceral receptors. In the lumbar cord their receptive fields are small or medium sized, being larger than the area of the foot but smaller than the entire leg; in the thoracic cord the fields of these laminar cells are larger, often including the entire upper limb plus part of the chest. Many of the deep dorsal column spinothalamic tract neurons in the thoracic segments receive convergent input from sympathetic afferent fibres. Laminae IV–VI spinothlamic tract units project to either the ventroposterolateral (VPL) nucleus or to the centrolateral nucleus of the thalamus, and sometimes to both nuclei. Units projecting to the ventroposterolateral nucleus receive input from all classes (A-β, A-δ and C) of cutaneous fibres.

Ventral grey column (laminae VII and VIII) spinothalamic tract cells respond mainly to deep somatic (muscle and joint) stimuli, but also to innocuous and/or noxious cutaneous stimuli. In the thoracic regions of the spinal cord they also receive convergent input from visceral sources. The majority of laminae VII and VIII spinothalamic tract neurons have large, complex receptive fields (often bilateral) which encompass widespread areas of the body. Cells of this group that project exclusively to the medial thalamus receive input from A–β, A-δ, and C classes of afferent fibres, and many respond to convergent input from receptors of deep structures. These neurons were found to comprise 25% wide diframic range, 63% high threshold, and 12% low threshold or deep type. Most of the spinothalamic tract cells in the ventral grey column project to the intralaminar nuclei of the thalamus.

Note that the wide dynamic range type neurons are particularly effective for the discrimination of different intensities of painful stimulation. Furthermore, it is suggested that the spinothalamic projection to the ventroposterolateral nucleus is concerned with the discriminative aspects of pain perception, whereas the projection to other thalamic regions, particularly the intralaminar nuclei, may be involved in arousal and/or aversive behaviour.

The control of impulse transmission is modulated in a variety of ways. First, the cutaneous afferents are influenced by a tonic regulating mechanism in the substantia gelatinosa described previously; additionally, transmission is influenced by a variety of descending fibres from the sensory–motor cortex and brainstem centres.

The roles of dorsal columns and spinothalamic tracts have aroused much controversy. The classic view (Mountcastle 1968) regards the dorsal columns as the *essential discriminatory pathway*, without which a mechanical stimulus is recognized but assigned no specific location, intensity or pattern. This view is strongly challenged (Wall 1970; Wall & Noordenbos 1977) because complete section of the dorsal column does not abolish discrimination of weight, texture, two-point stimulation, vibration or position (but see Nathan et al 1986). Environmental stimuli may be classified into those 'passively impressed' and those which 'must be actively explored by motor movement or sequential analysis' for successful discrimination. The former is considered the spinothalamic role, that of the dorsal columns is to initiate and plan exploration of the stimulus for the subsequent transmission of information.

SPINAL TERMINATIONS OF TRACTS DESCENDING FROM SUPRASPINAL SOURCES

Degeneration techniques such as Nauta's have much illuminated the spinal terminations of descending tracts (Nyberg-Hansen 1964a,b, 1965b, 1966a,b, 1969; Nyberg-Hansen & Brodal 1963, 1964; Nyberg-Hansen & Mascitti 1964; Brodal 1969). Most investigations have been in cats, rarely primates. Results, while probably generally applicable, cannot be transferred in toto to human structures. The

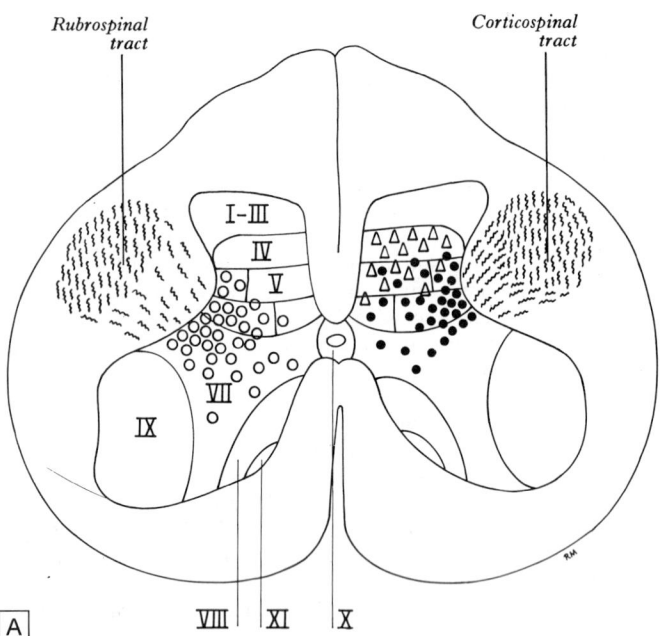

8.119 The spinal terminations of various descending tracts of the spinal cord determined experimentally in the cat and referred to the laminar pattern of the grey matter which is described elsewhere in the present section. (Redrawn from Brodal 1969, by courtesy of the author and publishers. The original papers and illustrations stemmed from the numerous publications by R Nyberg-Hansen and his collaborators to whom we are grateful. Consult bibliography under 'Spinal Terminations of Descending Tracts from Supra-

spinal Sources'.) A. Termination of corticospinal fibres from 'motor' areas of the cerebral cortex—black dots; corticospinal fibres from 'sensory' areas of the cerebral cortex—white triangles; rubrospinal fibres—white dots. B. Terminations of vestibulospinal fibres; those from the lateral vestibulospinal tract—black dots; those from the medial vestibulospinal tract are shown on the opposite side of the cord as white dots.

principal findings are summarized in **8.119**, in which the distributions of terminals are related to laminar architecture. The following points, some already mentioned, are noteworthy.

Corticospinal fibres. Almost all these terminate, in cats, on interneurons in laminae IV–VII; but because of the widespread dendrites of multipolar neurons in lamina IX, which penetrate lamina VII, the existence of a few axodendritic contacts with motor neurons cannot be ignored. Corticospinal fibres from the 'sensory' cortex terminate chiefly in laminae IV and V, those from the 'motor' cortex in V–VII, with the densest concentration laterally in lamina VI. Thus, despite some overlap, corticospinal fibres from these two regions end differently—findings of interest in view of increasing evidence involving corticospinal tracts in the supraspinal *modulation of sensory inflow*; this may be mediated by presynaptic inhibition of primary afferent terminals or the postsynaptic inhibition or facilitation of subsequent neurons. In contrast, there is anatomical (Hoff & Hoff 1934; Kuypers 1960; Liu & Chambers 1964) and physiological (Bernhard et al 1953; Preston & Whitlock 1961; Landgren et al 1962) evidence, that in monkeys some corticospinal fibres end monosynaptically on large a motor neurons (see p. 1000). Less is known quantitatively about human synaptic terminals; most end on interneurons but many end directly on motor neurons (see p. 1000 for details). Physiological studies (Corazza et al 1963) indicate that feline corticospinal tracts influence a and γ motor neurons, mainly via interneurons. The increased flux of impulses in corticospinal axons is excitatory to motor neurons of flexors and inhibitory to those supplying extensors. Converse effects of decreased flux are equally essential in normal function.

Rubrospinal fibres. These arise from large and small neurons in the contralateral red nucleus, with some degree of somatotopic order. Degeneration after nuclear lesions in cats shows the tract descending to lumbosacral levels, with terminals on interneurons in laminae V–VII. Its terminal zones correspond to those of corticospinal fibres from the 'motor' cortex, with similar effects on a and γ motor neurons. In some animals a somatotopic *corticorubral projection* has been demonstrated from the sensory–motor cortex, suggesting dual routes from cortex to cord, *direct corticospinal* and *indirect corticorubrospinal*, with similar spinal terminations and common functions. But the origin, localization, termination and functions of human rubrospinal connections are poorly defined, and the tract appears to be rudimentary (see p. 1069).

Vestibulospinal tracts. Medial and lateral are much investigated in other animals, but are less clarified in man. The lateral, from the ipsilateral *lateral vestibular nucleus*, descends the whole cord, ending at successive levels largely in laminae VII and VIII and less so in lamina IX. The medial tract, mainly from both medial vestibular nuclei, descends perhaps only to midthoracic levels, terminating less widely in parts of laminae VII and VIII (**8.119**). Activation of the lateral tract excites extensor and inhibits flexor motor neurons.

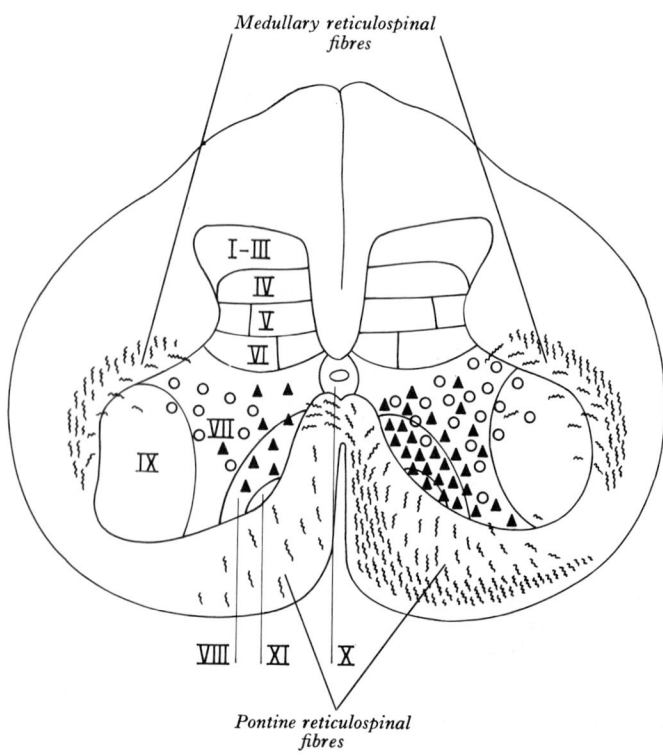

8.120 Terminations of reticulospinal fibres; those originating in the medulla oblongata (white dots) are in general more dorsally placed than those originating in the pons (black triangles).

Excitation is monosynaptic, indicating that vestibulospinal terminals synapse with the extensive dendrites of some motor neurons penetrating laminae VII and VIII. Gamma motor neurons are also probably facilitated; the inhibitory effect on flexors is presumably by inhibitory interneurons in their laminae of termination.

Reticulospinal tracts. Notably difficult to evaluate in human spinal cords, these have been mainly examined in cats, by retrograde degeneration in spinal neurons after spinal trauma and by anterograde effects following brainstem lesions. Pontine and medullary reticulospinal fibres from one side apparently pass to both sides of the spinal cord; the pontine fibres are the more concentrated on the ipsilateral side; the medullary fibres have also a substantial contralateral component. The zones of termination are summarized in **8.120**. (For non-aminergic, noradrenergic, serotonergic, enkephalinoid and other neuromediator substances associated with reticulospinal fibres, see pp. 1002, 1073.) Similar experiments indicate that tectospinal and interstitiospinal tracts both terminate in laminae VI–VIII (see p. 1072).

SUMMARY OF SPINAL ORGANIZATION

Szentágothai (1967) has considered spinal grey matter as a *central core* with paired *dorsal* and *ventral appendages*, each with distinctive features (**8.121**), terms which of course cut across the usual description but are held to be less arbitrary. The core has a diffuse, non-discriminative, reticular organization, with great divergence and convergence of paths; most interneurons connect with hundreds, perhaps thousands, of others distributed in a substantial length of cord. In contrast, dorsal and ventral appendages are more discriminatively organized in terms of somatotopy and functional localization. The precise limits to core and appendages are indefinable. The concept will undoubtedly need revision and perhaps lose relevance as knowledge increases. The central core includes interneurons of laminae VII and VIII (i.e. the intermediate zone and the areas between the motor neuron columns). But interneurons of dorsal columns and in motor neuron columns should also be included in this postulated reticular core. The ventral appendage corresponds to the neuronal columns of lamina IX; the dorsal appendage includes laminae I–VI.

Dorsal appendage (p. 986). This is a main receptive zone of exteroceptive, proprioceptive and interoceptive dorsal spinal root fibres. Laminae I–IV are the main cutaneous receptive areas; lamina V receives fine afferents from the skin, muscle and viscera; lamina VI receives proprioceptive and some cutaneous afferents. But few appropriate investigations have yet been made; hence the functional boundaries are uncertain and interneuronal complexities are

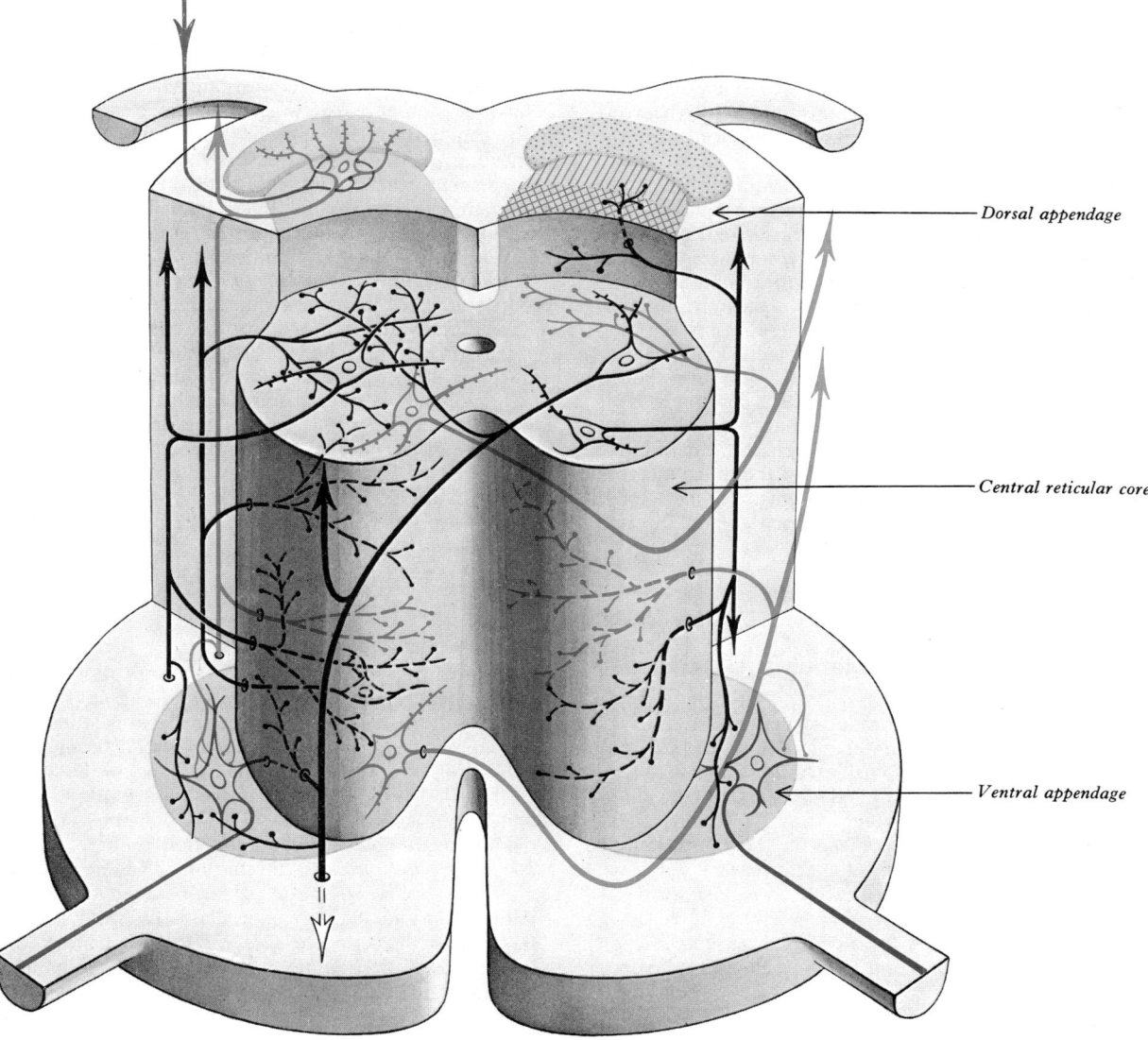

8.121 A highly simplified stereodiagram illustrating the concept of the spinal cord as consisting of a central 'reticular' core of grey matter, with related dorsal and ventral 'appendages' of grey matter. Many structural features are omitted and only a few examples, relevant to the concept, are included. A dorsal column neuron and others, more ventrally placed, which give rise to descending, long ascending and local collateral branches, are shown in blue. Varieties of interneuron are in black. Two motor neurons are shown in red; also in red is a single example of a fibre descending from a supraspinal source. See text for a more detailed description; see also **8.107** for the origin and termination of some tracts and **8.101** for one view of the fine structure of the substantia gelatinosa. (Redrawn from Szentágothai 1967 by courtesy of the author and publishers.)

postulated but as yet undemonstrated. Intracellular recording has its difficulties; some neurons may long remain out of technical reach.

Nevertheless, the available recordings suggest that neurons in the dorsal appendages abstract data from internal and external environments. Neuronal groups show varying somatotopic array, size and response of receptive fields, specificity, convergence and interaction. Clearly, simple views of spinal neurons as merely relays in invariant, discrete, 'unimodality' channels, transmitting a punctate replica of the environment to the spinal cord or brain, are inadequate. Complex transformations of input occur in the dorsal appendage, whose output spreads to many destinations: directly to the ventral motor neuron columns, or indirectly, via laminae including complex interneurons of the reticular core, to both sides of the cord, cranial and caudal to the input. Neurons in the dorsal appendage and reticular core contribute to the ascending tracts, reaching many brainstem centres.

Transmission to and through the dorsal appendage may be modified by mutual interaction and control. Facilitatory and inhibitory effects, due to simultaneous activity in various afferent fibres converging on a single neuron, have been noted, as has tonic modulation by the substantia gelatinosa. Much evidence suggests that transmission in all laminae is influenced by supraspinal sources, with excitation or inhibition provided by a wide array of neuromediators. The functional significance of these mechanisms is obscure; they may eliminate redundancy, reduce confusion or be linked to central 'states of readiness' or temporary 'preoccupation' with immediately significant transformations. It is increasingly clear that most descending tracts, which influence motor behaviour, do so indirectly by modifying transmission in the primary afferents, and in interneurons in the spinal laminae, less often than by direct influence on motor neurons.

Interneurons of the reticular core. These form an intricate net in which each neuron receives inputs from and transmits to large numbers of others (pp. 1073–1079) and is characterized by one or more neuromediators. The core receives input from some axons of the dorsal appendage, the proprioceptive dorsal root fibres and some descending fibres. This plethora of connections makes investigation difficult but an earlier view of *random nerve networks* is receding with newer methods, which include minute stereotactic lesions, intracellular recording, the inspection of thousands of Golgi-stained sections and the mapping of somata or terminals according to their content of established or putative neuromediators (p. 1073). An aspect of organization has emerged that concerns the quantitative analysis of connectivity ('transmitting power') of the different types of interneurons and some of the descending tracts. Some axonal terminals have very long courses in the grey matter and through

successive branches give two or three synaptic end-bulbs to each of many hundreds of interneurons encountered; others concentrate many end-bulbs on one or a small group of neurons; while others have widespread paracrine effects. Diffuse, 'non-discriminative' connections hence contrast with 'discriminative' ones. Many proprioceptive terminals in the core are 'segmentally' localized in *transverse* 'sheets' of grey matter, in contrast to dorsal appendage cutaneous afferents which terminate in *longitudinal* sheets. In such complex interneuronal congeries, sensory input probably interacts with supraspinal influences to set in train the multivarious locomotor responses. This analysis is largely speculative but the modern technical armamentarium will doubtless effect some progress.

Ventral appendage (pp. 979, 982, 984). This is a columnar array of α and γ motor neurons and interneurons. Evidence points to 'tonic' and 'phasic' types of neurons innervating striated muscle and to different types of neurons for 'static' and 'dynamic' responses in muscle spindles and their independent controls; but their detailed synaptic patterns remain uncertain.

The main connections of the *motor neurons* are:

- direct monosynaptic terminals of proprioceptive dorsal root afferents in the same or nearby segments
- terminals from axonal collaterals from dorsal appendage interneurons
- terminals of interneurons of the reticular core: 'discriminative' from the same segment, 'non-discriminative' from adjacent segments
- direct monosynaptic terminals from the vestibulospinal and (in primates including man) corticospinal tracts.

The interaction of such converging channels for integrated motor behaviour is obscure. A few generalizations can be made; descending paths can be grouped into those wherein impulses are excitatory to flexors, inhibitory to extensors (cortico-, rubro- and medullary reticulospinal tracts) and those with the opposite effect (vestibulo- and pontine reticulospinal tracts). But this simple dualistic view ignores much investigation reported on the complex modification of reflex activities by descending tracts.

Muscle is made to contract or relax by two routes: the pathway produces a direct, immediate change in the excitatory level of α motor neurons innervating motor units, but probably acts infrequently, in sudden forceful responses; usually a γ pathway also operates by sequential activity in local interneurons and activity (or inhibition) of the efferents to muscle spindles which, via local muscle 'servo-loop' mechanism (p. 971), causes the appropriate change in tonic and phasic motor neurons by maintaining or breaking the α–γ linkage (Granit 1970). Available reports indicate that during voluntary actions initiation of activity in the α system may be more frequent than previously recognized (p. 971).

Level of spinal injury is a determinant of clinical severity

The segmental level of spinal cord injury may be determined from clinical data and accurate anatomical knowledge. Complete division above the fourth cervical segment causes respiratory failure by the loss of activity in the phrenic and intercostal nerves. Lesions between C5 and T1 paralyse all four limbs (quadriplegia), the effects in the upper limbs varying with the site of injury: at the fifth cervical segment paralysis is complete; at the sixth each arm is positioned in abduction and lateral rotation, with the elbow flexed and the forearm supinated, due to unopposed activity in the deltoid, spinatus, rhomboid and brachial muscles (all supplied by the fifth cervical spinal nerves). In lower cervical lesions upper limb paralysis is less. Lesions of the first thoracic segment paralyse small muscles in the hand and damage the sympathetic outflow, resulting in contraction of the pupil, recession of the eyeball, narrowing of the palpebral fissure and loss of sweating in the face and neck (Horner's syndrome); sensation is retained in areas

innervated by segments above the lesion; thus cutaneous sensation is retained in the neck and chest down to the second intercostal space, because this area is innervated by the supraclavicular nerves (C3 and C4). At thoracic levels, division of the cord paralyses the trunk, below the segmental level of the lesion, and both lower limbs (paraplegia). The first sacral neural segment is approximately level with the thoracolumbar vertebral junction; injury, commonly occurring here, paralyses the urinary bladder, rectum and muscles supplied by the sacral segments; cutaneous sensibility is lost in the perineum, buttocks, the back of the thighs and the legs and soles of the feet. The roots of lumbar nerves descending to join the cauda equina may be damaged at this level, causing complete paralysis of both lower limbs. Lesions below the first lumbar vertebra may divide or damage the cauda equina, but severe nerve damage is uncommon and is usually confined to the spinal roots at the level of the trauma. Neurological symptoms may also be due to interference with the spinal blood supply, particularly in the lower thoracic and upper lumbar segments.

Vertebral levels of spinal cord segments

The level of spinal segments relative to the vertebrae is clinically important. A useful approximation is: in the cervical region the tip of the vertebral spine corresponds to the succeeding cord segment (i.e. the *sixth* cervical spine is opposite the *seventh* spinal segment); at upper thoracic levels a tip of a vertebral spine corresponds to the cord two segments lower (i.e. the *fourth* spine is level with the *sixth* segment); in the lower thoracic region there is a difference of three segments (i.e. the *tenth* thoracic spine is level with the *first* lumbar segment). The *eleventh* thoracic spine overlies the *third* lumbar segment, the *twelfth* is opposite the first *sacral* segment. The neonatal spinal cord extends to the upper border of the third lumbar vertebra. Barson and Sands (1970), in a series of 258 pre- and postnatal subjects, found the perinatal level at the third lumbar vertebra, rising during the first 2 postnatal months. Individual variation was marked: first to fourth lumbar at birth, first to third in children (3 months–15 years of age).

RHOMBENCEPHALON OR HINDBRAIN

The rhombencephalon, which includes the medulla oblongata, pons and cerebellum, occupies the posterior cranial fossa, its ventral surface lying on the clivus; its cavity is the fourth ventricle. The medulla and pons contain tracts connecting all parts of the central nervous system and also nuclei of several cranial nerves and many other groups of neurons. Emerging superficially from the pons and medulla are: the trigeminal, abducent, facial, vestibulocochlear, glossopharyngeal, vagus, cranial accessory and hypoglossal nerves. Lying among the nuclei and tracts is the *reticular formation* (p. 1073), a mass of neurons and axons continuous caudally with its spinal counterpart; some of its nuclei are concerned in cardiac, respiratory and alimentary control, others in aspects of many neural activities. Both the spinothalamic (spinal lemniscal) and medial lemniscal systems for somaesthesia together with the trigeminal systems ascend to the thalamus (**8.108, 132**). The special sensory systems for the auditory and vestibular pathways are also present (**8.140**). Massive afferent and efferent cerebellar projections are found in all parts of the hindbrain (**8.110**) and the extrapyramidal, corticospinal and corticonuclear motor pathways are a prominent feature of this part of the nervous system (**8.116**). Clinically, lesions of the brainstem are devastating and life threatening since they can destroy vital cardio/respiratory centres, disconnect rostral servo-motor centres from the more caudal executive areas for movement and sever incoming sensory fibres from higher centres of consciousness, perception and cognition. Irreversible cardiac and respiratory arrest ensue after complete destruction of the neural respiratory and cardiac centres in the hindbrain. Clinically this is called *brainstem death*, a condition which requires accurate diagnosis since it may occur in patients on life support machines whose respiratory and cardiac functions can paradoxically be maintained indefinitely.

Criteria for the diagnosis of brainstem death

The traditional criteria of cardiac and respiratory arrest for the certification of death are appropriately used in the huge majority of cases, but the development and widespread use of cardiac resuscitation and artificial ventilation in the late 1960s created a need to redefine the criteria of death in the very small numbers of patients in apnoeac coma, who could be maintained on a ventilator for days or weeks; a need made more pressing by the demand for organs for transplantation.

Twenty years ago many such patients were ventilated until asystole supervened, by which time the brain had often liquefied. Over several years the concept that patients in deep apnoeac coma, due to irreversible destruction of the brainstem, was incompatible with life, led to the establishment of criteria to diagnose brainstem death at the bedside with absolute reliability and without the use of special techniques such as electroencephalogram, evoked responses or blood flow measurements, provided that the appropriate protocol is rigorously followed. If these criteria are met, life support systems may be withdrawn with the confidence that recovery cannot occur. Organs may then be removed for transplantation and better use can be made of intensive care facilities. Relatives should be kept fully informed of each stage in this process.

The preconditions are of critical import-ance and must be fulfilled before proceeding further. This demands negative answers to the following questions:

- Could primary hypothermia, drugs, or metabolic/endocrine abnormalities be contributing significantly to the apnoeic coma? (Where appropriate, check plasma and urine for drugs, plasma pH, glucose, sodium, and calcium.)
- Have any neuromuscular blocking drugs been administered during the preceding 12 hours?
- Is the rectal temperature below 35°C? (If so, warm the patient and reassess.)

The tests of reflex brainstem function should only be carried out when the cause of brain damage is established and if consciousness is irrecoverable. Although the occulocephalic reflex (doll's head eye movement) was not part of the United Kingdom code (Conference of Medical Royal Colleges and their Faculties in the UK, 1976), it is a simple and easy test to elicit and if positive there is no need to proceed further. The response to light and corneal stimulation, the gag reflex, cough reflex and motor responses both in the cranial nerve distribution, to stimulation in 5th nerve territory, and in the limbs, should all be to adequate stimuli. Ice-cold water irrigation of the tympanic mem-brane should not elicit any eye movement; tonic deviation of either eye indicates some residual brainstem function. The test for spontaneous ventilation is usually carried out by an anaesthetist and preferably with blood gas analysis, which should be available in all intensive care units where these problems are likely to arise.

Accordingly, the criteria for brainstem death are met when two clinicians independently obtain negative answers to the following questions:

- When the head is gently, but fully, rotated to either side is there contraversive conjugate deviation of the eyes (doll's head eye movement)?
- Do the pupils react to light?
- Is there any response to corneal stimulation on either side?
- Do the eyes deviate when either ear is irrigated with 50 ml of ice cold water for 30 seconds (first confirm tympanic membranes visible and intact)?
- Is there a gag reflex?
- Is there a cough reflex following bronchial stimulation by a suction catheter?
- Are there any motor responses within the cranial nerve distribution following adequate stimulation of any somatic area (supraorbital and nail bed pressure)?
- Are there any spontaneous respiratory movements?

The patient is then pre-oxygenated for 10 minutes with either 100% oxygen (O_2) or 95% O_2 and 5% carbon dioxide (CO_2)

and blood gases (Pa_{CO_2} and Pa_{O_2}) are recorded. Pa_{CO_2} before disconnection must exceed 5.3 kPa—if not, ventilation rate should be slowed until Pa_{CO_2} rises to this level. The patient is then disconnected from the ventilator and given oxygen,

at 6 l/min through a suction catheter in the trachea. After 10 min blood gases are again measured. If the Pa_{CO_2} exceeds 6.65 kPa at the end of the disconnection period and no spontaneous respiratory movements are observed,

brainstem death has occurred.

The background to the concept of brainstem death, the historical aspects and its validation, has been fully discussed by Pallis (1983, 1990); see also *British Medical Journal* (1976).

MEDULLA OBLONGATA

EXTERNAL FEATURES AND RELATIONS

The medulla oblongata extends from the lower pontine margin to a transverse plane, above the first pair of cervical spinal nerves, which

intersects the upper border of the atlas dorsally and the centre of the dens ventrally (**8.122**). At this point, the internal structure is similar to that of the spinal cord below but changes rostrally. The anterior surface of the medulla is separated from the basilar part of the occipital bone and apex of the dens by the meninges and occipito-axial ligaments. Caudally, the dorsal surface occupies the midline

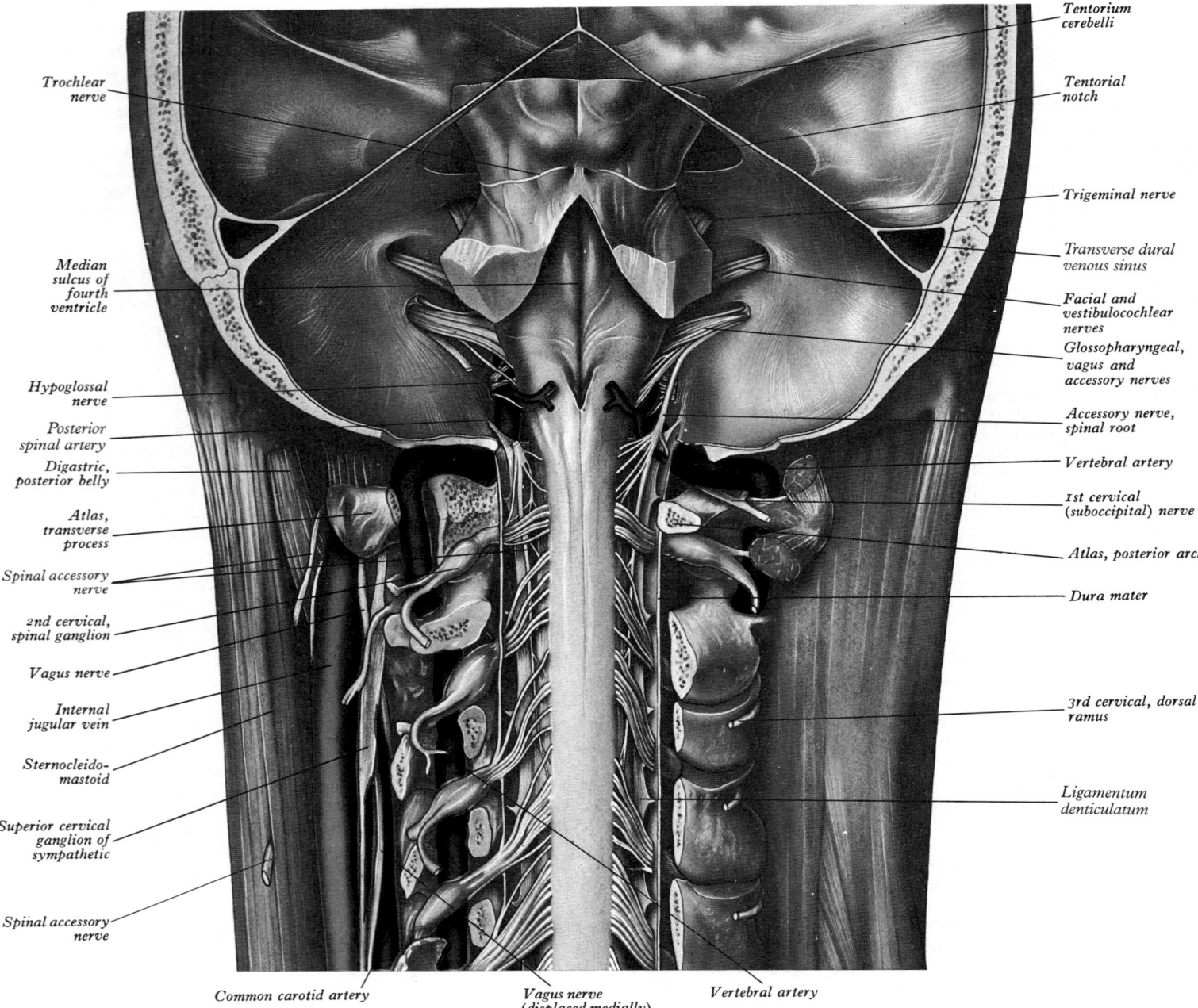

8.122 Dissection exposing the brain stem and upper five cervical spinal segments after removal of large portions of the occipital and parietal bones and the cerebellum together with the roof of the fourth ventricle. On the left, the foramina transversaria of the atlas and the third, fourth and fifth cervical

vertebrae have been opened to expose the vertebral artery. On the right, the posterior arch of the atlas and the laminae of the succeeding cervical vertebrae have been removed.

notch between the cerebellar hemispheres; the rostral upper part forms the lower half of the floor of the fourth ventricle (rhomboid fossa) (8.122, 123). It is about 3 cm in length, 2 cm at its widest and sagittally some 13 cm thick. The spinal central canal is prolonged into its lower half, expanding above as the fourth ventricle; this divides the medulla into a closed part containing the central canal and an open part containing the lower half of the fourth ventricle. After piercing the posterior atlanto-occipital membrane, spinal dura and arachnoid, the vertebral arteries lie against the lateral medullary surfaces (8.122), giving off the small posterior spinal arteries. They then run rostro-anteriorly anterior to the ligamentum denticulatum between the roots of the hypoglossal and first spinal nerves and on the ventrolateral surface give off the anterior spinal arteries and the tortuous posterior inferior cerebellar arteries, damage to which gives rise to the medial and lateral medullary syndromes respectively (p. 1021). They meet in the midline at the pontomedullary junction to form the basilar artery.

The anterior and posterior surface has a median fissure and sulcus respectively.

Anterior median fissure. This contains a shallow fold of pia mater, and extends throughout, continuous below with the spinal anterior median fissure; it ends above at the lower pontine border in a small triangular *foramen caecum* (8.124). Inferiorly, it is interrupted by the obliquely crossing fascicles of the *pyramidal decussation*. *Anterior external arcuate fibres* emerge from the fissure above this and curve laterally over the medullary surface as the stria medullaris (8.123).

Posterior median sulcus. Present only in the closed part, this is continuous below with the spinal posterior median sulcus (8.123); it rapidly shallows above, ending at the midlevel of the medulla, where the central canal expands into the fourth ventricle.

Anterior region (8.124). Between the anterior median fissure and the anterolateral sulcus, the anterior region shows an elongated ridge inappropriately named the *pyramid*. At its slightly narrowed rostral end, at the junction with the pons, the abducent nerve emerges; caudally it tapers into the spinal anterior funiculus. Each pyramid contains ipsilateral corticospinal fibres, approximately 70–90% of which leave the pyramids in successive bundles, crossing in and deep to the anterior median fissure as the *pyramidal decussation*. They then descend dorsally in the contralateral spinal lateral funiculus as the crossed lateral corticospinal tract. The remaining lateral fibres do not cross; some descend as the anterior corticospinal tract (8.125) into the ipsilateral anterior funiculi, others incline posterolaterally to join the lateral corticospinal tracts as a lesser uncrossed component (p. 1014). The corticospinal tracts display somatotopy at almost all levels; in the pyramids the arrangement is like that at higher levels, the most lateral fibres subserving the most medial arm and neck movements. How far this pattern is carried into either the anterior corticospinal tracts or the decussating fibres is unknown; but similar somatotopy is ascribed to the lateral corticospinal tracts within the spinal cord.

The last four cranial nerves emerge from the medulla. Hypoglossal rootlets are in line with the ventral spinal roots, emerging from an *anterolateral sulcus* of the spinal cord. The accessory, vagus and glossopharyngeal nerves are in line with the dorsal spinal roots (p. 976), entering through a *posterolateral sulcus* (8.126). These features are used to divide each half medulla into anterior, middle and posterior regions. Though these appear to be continuous with the corresponding spinal funiculi, they do not contain precisely the same fibres; some spinal tracts either end, begin or alter course in the medulla.

Lateral region (8.126). This is between the anterolateral sulcus (with the emerging hypoglossal roots) and the posterolateral sulcus (with roots of the accessory, vagus and glossopharyngeal nerves). Its upper part contains an oval prominence, the olive; its lower part is only partly continuous with the spinal lateral funiculus; the lateral corticospinal tract is mainly from the contralateral pyramid and the posterior spinocerebellar tract mostly leaves it to enter the inferior cerebellar peduncle. The lateral intersegmental anterior spinocerebellar and other tracts continue into the lateral region.

Olive. A smooth, oval elevation between the anterolateral and posterolateral sulci, this is formed by the underlying *inferior olivary complex of nuclei* (p. 1020). It lies lateral to the pyramid, separated by the anterolateral sulcus and hypoglossal fibres, and is about 125 cm

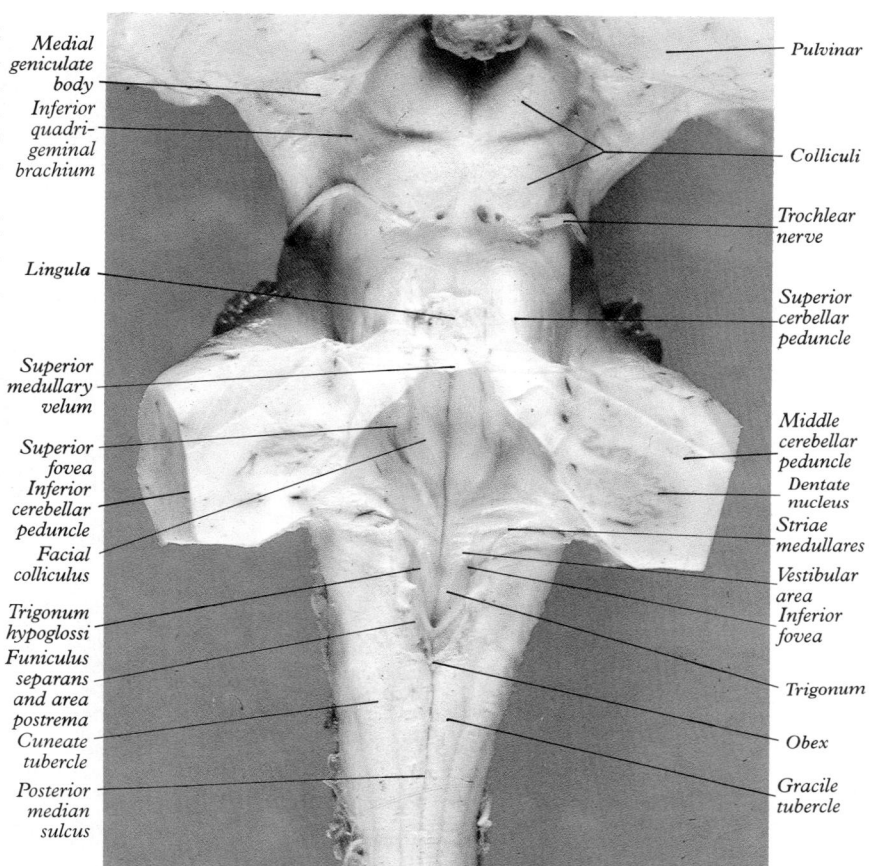

Labels around image (left side, top to bottom): *Medial geniculate body*, *Inferior quadrigeminal brachium*, *Lingula*, *Superior medullary velum*, *Superior fovea*, *Inferior cerebellar peduncle*, *Facial colliculus*, *Trigonum hypoglossi*, *Funiculus separans and area postrema*, *Cuneate tubercle*, *Posterior median sulcus*

Labels around image (right side, top to bottom): *Pulvinar*, *Colliculi*, *Trochlear nerve*, *Superior cerebellar peduncle*, *Middle cerebellar peduncle*, *Dentate nucleus*, *Striae medullares*, *Vestibular area Inferior fovea*, *Trigonum*, *Obex*, *Gracile tubercle*

8.123   A dorsal view of the brain stem including the floor of the rhomboid fossa. Note: (1) the crenated outlines of the right and left dentate nuclei in the sectioned surface of the cerebellar white matter opposite the widest part of the rhomboid fossa; (2) the midline pineal gland cranial to the superior colliculi; (3) the rounded pulvinar of the dorsal thalami which encroach on the uppermost part of the photograph; (4) the right and left habenular trigones immediately lateral to the base of the pineal; (5) the medial geniculate bodies, lateral to the superior colliculi. (Dissection by E L Rees, photography by Kevin Fitzpatrick, both of the Division of Anatomy and Cell Biology, UMDS, Guy's Campus, London.)

long. The roots of the facial nerve emerge between its rostral end and the lower pontine border, in the pontocerebellar angle. Anterior external arcuate fibres course from the anterior median fissure across the pyramid and olive to the inferior cerebellar peduncle (8.126).

Posterior region (8.122, 123). Dorsal to the posterolateral sulcus this region, like the lateral, is divisible into rostral and caudal parts. The *caudal part* is an upward continuation of the *fasciculi gracilis* and *cuneatus*. The former flank the posterior median fissure, separated from the cuneate fasciculus on each side by the cranial continuation of the postero-intermediate sulcus and septum of the cervical spinal cord (p. 975). Both fasciculi are first vertical and parallel; but at the caudal end of the fourth ventricle they diverge, each developing an elongated swelling, the *gracile* and *cuneate tubercles*, produced by the subjacent *nuclei gracilis* and *cuneatus* (8.127, 128). Most fibres in both fasciculi synapse with neurons in their respective nuclei and are relayed on to the contralateral primary somaesthetic cortex through the thalamus (8.108). The *tuberculum cinereum* (8.126) is an inconspicuous raised area, between the fasciculus cuneatus and the rootlets of the accessory nerve; narrow below, it widens upwards and overlies a nucleus and tract continuous with the substantia gelatinosa and tract of Lissauer in the spinal cord; the nucleus and overlying fibres of the spinal trigeminal tract (8.129); and, most superficially, the posterior spinocerebellar tract (p. 990; 8.110). The rostral posterior medullary structure is the *inferior cerebellar peduncle*, a rounded ridge between the fourth ventricle and the glossopharyngeal and vagal rootlets. The two peduncles diverge and incline to enter the cerebellar hemispheres, where they are

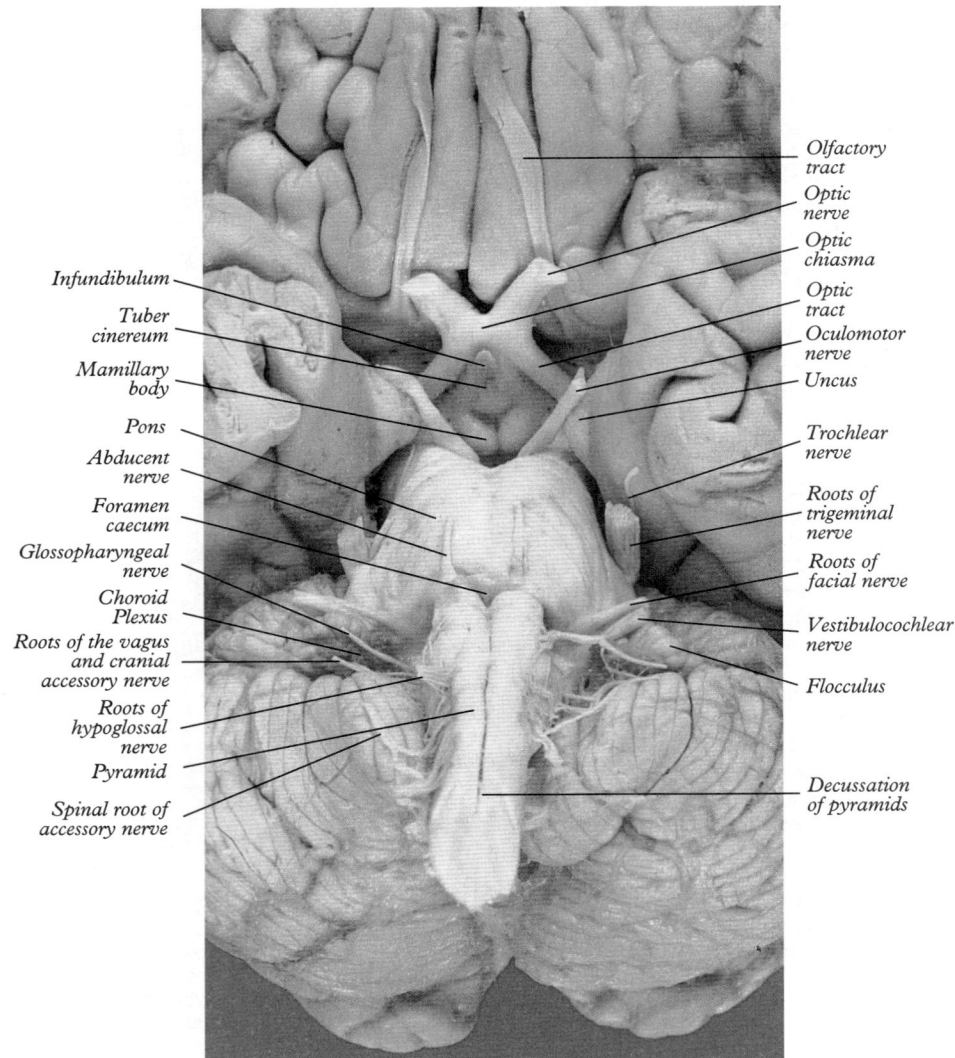

Infundibulum

Tuber cinereum

Mamillary body

Pons

Abducent nerve

Foramen caecum

Glossopharyngeal nerve

Choroid Plexus

Roots of the vagus and cranial accessory nerve

Roots of hypoglossal nerve

Pyramid

Spinal root of accessory nerve

Olfactory tract

Optic nerve

Optic chiasma

Optic tract

Oculomotor nerve

Uncus

Trochlear nerve

Roots of trigeminal nerve

Roots of facial nerve

Vestibulocochlear nerve

Flocculus

Decussation of pyramids

8.124 The ventral aspect of the brain stem, interpeduncular fossa and adjacent parts of the cerebellar and cerebral hemispheres. (Dissection by E L Rees, photograph by Kevin Fitzpatrick, both of the Division of Anatomy and Cell Biology, UMDS, Guy's Campus, London.)

crossed by the *striae medullares*, running to the median ventricular sulcus (**8.**123). Here also the peduncles form the anterior and rostral boundaries of the lateral recess of the fourth ventricle which becomes continuous with the subarachnoid space through the lateral apertures of the fourth ventricle, the foramina of Luschka. Protruding from the foramina, and lying between the roots is a tuft of choroid plexus which is continuous with that of the fourth ventricle. The composition of the inferior peduncle is described on page 1035.

INTERNAL STRUCTURE

It is customary and convenient to describe the medulla in sample transverse sections taken at four successive levels. The general disposition of some principal brainstem nuclei is shown in **8.**129.

A transverse section in the lower medulla oblongata

A transverse section in the lower medulla oblongata intersects the dorsal, lateral and ventral funiculi contiguous with those of the spinal cord (**8.**127). The ventral is separated from the central grey matter by corticospinal fibres crossing in the *pyramidal decussation* to opposite lateral funiculi (**8.**125). Usually, at least 75% of all corticospinal fibres cross in the *pyramidal decussation* and descend in the lateral funiculus as the crossed lateral corticospinal tract. In the rostral medulla, fibres cross by inclining ventromedially, more caudally they pass dorsally, decussating ventral to the central grey matter. The decussation is orderly: the fibres ending in the cervical

segments decussate first. Uncrossed fibres descend either ventromedially in the ipsilateral anterior funiculus as the anterior corticospinal tract or join the crossed fibres in their ipsilateral lateral funiculus. The decussation displaces the anterior intersegmental tract, the central grey matter and central canal dorsally. Continuity between the ventral grey column and central grey matter, maintained throughout the spinal cord, is lost; the column subdivides into the *supraspinal nucleus* (continuous above with that of the hypoglossal nerve) the efferent source of the first cervical nerve, and the *spinal nucleus of the accessory nerve*, which provides some spinal accessory fibres and merges rostrally with the nucleus ambiguus (p. 1021).

The dorsal grey column (**8.**108) is also modified as the *gracile nucleus* and appears at this level as a grey lamina in the fasciculus gracilis. The nucleus extends upwards to the caudolateral limit of the fourth ventricle, forming the gracile tubercle (p. 1026) which is more laterally placed, beginning and ending at a higher level than the gracile complex. The *nucleus cuneatus* invades the fasciculus cuneatus from its ventral aspect and forms the cuneate tubercle.

The substantia gelatinosa and tract of Lissauer are continuous with the caudal end of the *spinal nucleus* and *spinal tract* respectively of the trigeminal nerve (p. 1027) (**8.**129, 132).

A transverse section just above the pyramidal decussation

A transverse section just above the pyramidal decussation shows an increase in changes already noted and some new features (**8.**128).

The *nucleus gracilis* is broader and the fibres of its fasciculus are located on the dorsal, medial and lateral surfaces; the *nucleus cuneatus* is also larger. Here, both retain continuity with the central grey matter but lose it at higher levels. Gracile and cuneate uncrossed fascicular fibres synapse in their respective nuclei at different levels. Axons emerge from the nuclei as internal arcuate fibres, at first curving ventrolaterally around the central grey matter and then ventromedially between the trigeminal spinal tract and the central grey matter and decussate, constituting an ascending contralateral tract, the medial lemniscus. The *lemniscal decussation* is located dorsal to the pyramids and ventral to the central grey matter and thus the latter becomes more dorsally displaced than in the previous section. The gracile and cuneate nuclei are not simple sensory relay stations on a path widely considered the major route for the discriminative aspects of tactile and locomotor sensation. Taber (1961) and Kuypers & Tuerk (1964) have described several types of neurons in the nuclei and Biedenbach (1972) defined upper and lower zones of contrasting cytoarchitecture. In all the species examined, including monkeys, the upper regions of both nuclei are *reticular*, containing small and large multipolar neurons with long dendrites, and clusters of large round neurons with short and profusely branching dendrites in the lower regions, the last predominating. Upper and lower zones differ in their connections; both receive terminals from the dorsal spinal roots at all levels but inferiorly they have a denser input. Dorsal funicular fibres from neurons in the spinal grey matter (p. 980) terminate only in the superior, reticular zone. In both zones there is variable ordering of terminals on the basis of spinal root levels with variable overlap (Millar & Basbaum 1975). In monkeys, the hindleg and tail are represented medially, the trunk ventrally and digits dorsally. There is also modal specificity; lower levels respond to low-threshold cutaneous stimuli, upper reticular levels to inputs from fibres serving receptors in the skin, joints and muscles. The cuneate nucleus of primates is divided into:

- a middle zone, containing a large pars rotunda, in which rostrocaudally elongated medium-sized neurons are clustered between bundles of densely myelinated fibres

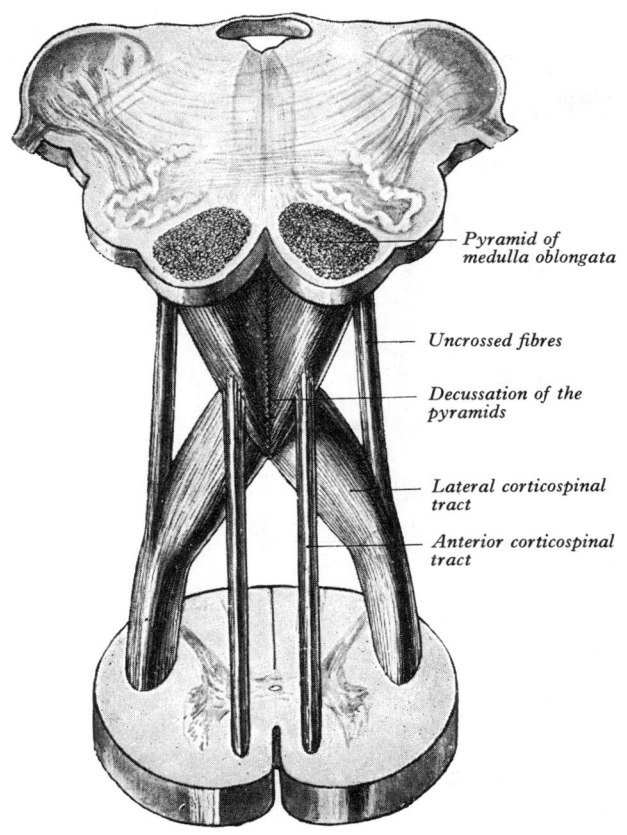

Pyramid of medulla oblongata

Uncrossed fibres

Decussation of the pyramids

Lateral corticospinal tract

Anterior corticospinal tract

8.125 Schematic dissection to show the decussation of the pyramids.

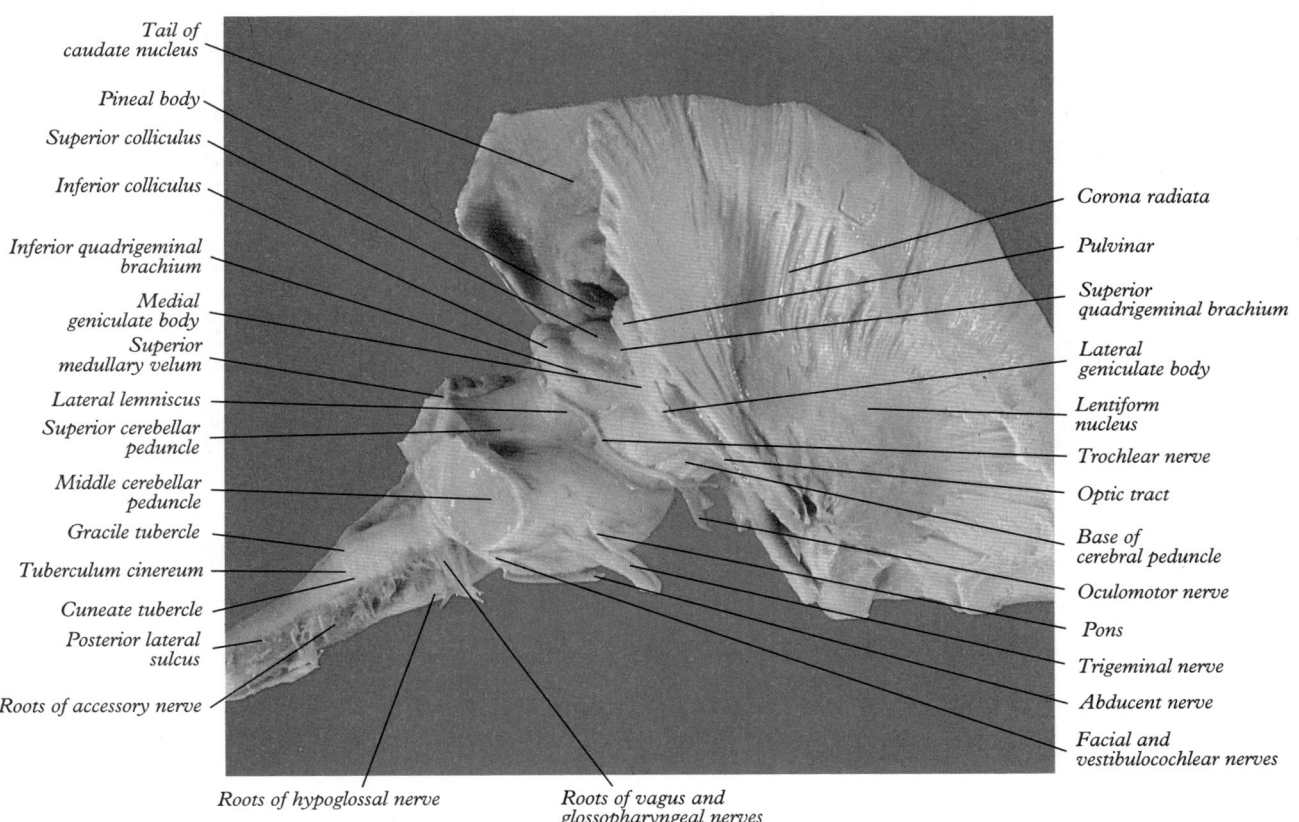

Tail of caudate nucleus

Pineal body

Superior colliculus

Inferior colliculus

Inferior quadrigeminal brachium

Medial geniculate body

Superior medullary velum

Lateral lemniscus

Superior cerebellar peduncle

Middle cerebellar peduncle

Gracile tubercle

Tuberculum cinereum

Cuneate tubercle

Posterior lateral sulcus

Roots of accessory nerve

Corona radiata

Pulvinar

Superior quadrigeminal brachium

Lateral geniculate body

Lentiform nucleus

Trochlear nerve

Optic tract

Base of cerebral peduncle

Oculomotor nerve

Pons

Trigeminal nerve

Abducent nerve

Facial and vestibulocochlear nerves

Roots of hypoglossal nerve

Roots of vagus and glossopharyngeal nerves

8.126 The brain stem, posterolateral aspect.

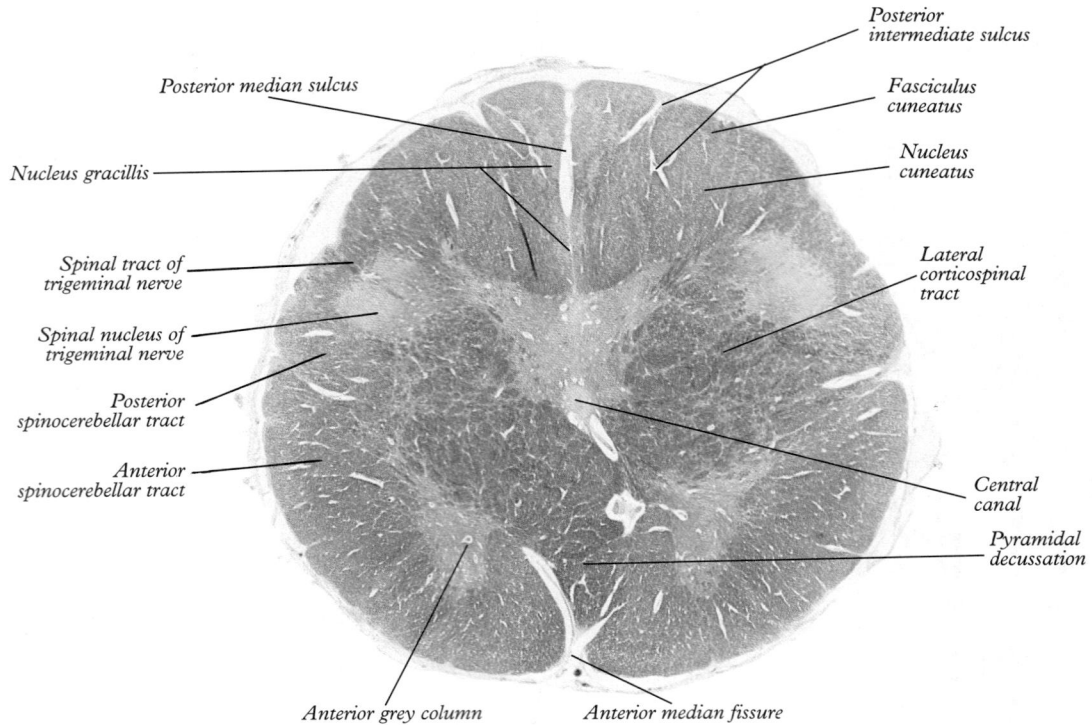

8.127 Transverse section through medulla oblongata at the level of the pyramidal decussation. Magnification × 8. (Solochrome cyanin preparation by J Carlile, and photographed by Kevin Fitzpatrick, Division of Anatomy and Cell Biology, UMDS, Guy's Campus, London.)

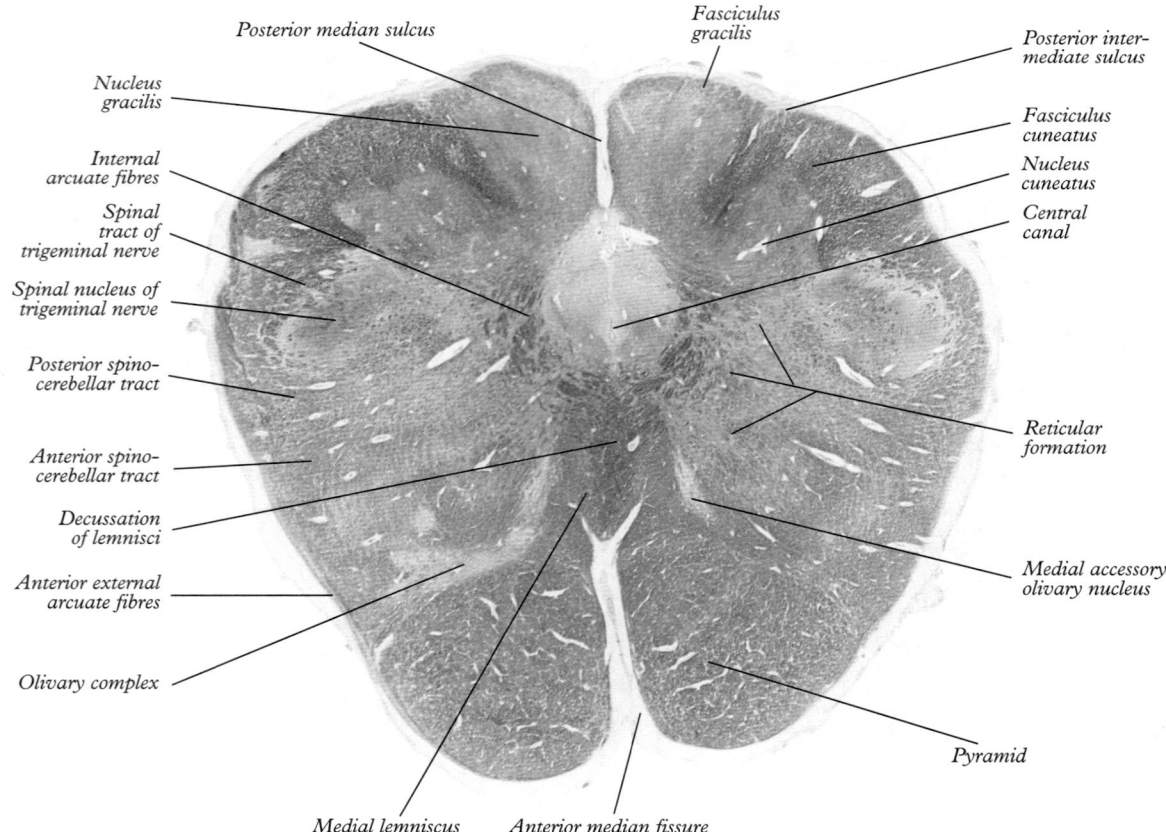

8.128 Transverse section through the medulla oblongata at the level of the decussation of the lemnisci. Magnification × 8. (Solochrome cyanin preparation by J Carlile and photographed by Kevin Fitzpatrick, both of the Division of Anatomy and Cell Biology, UMDS, Guy's Campus, London.)

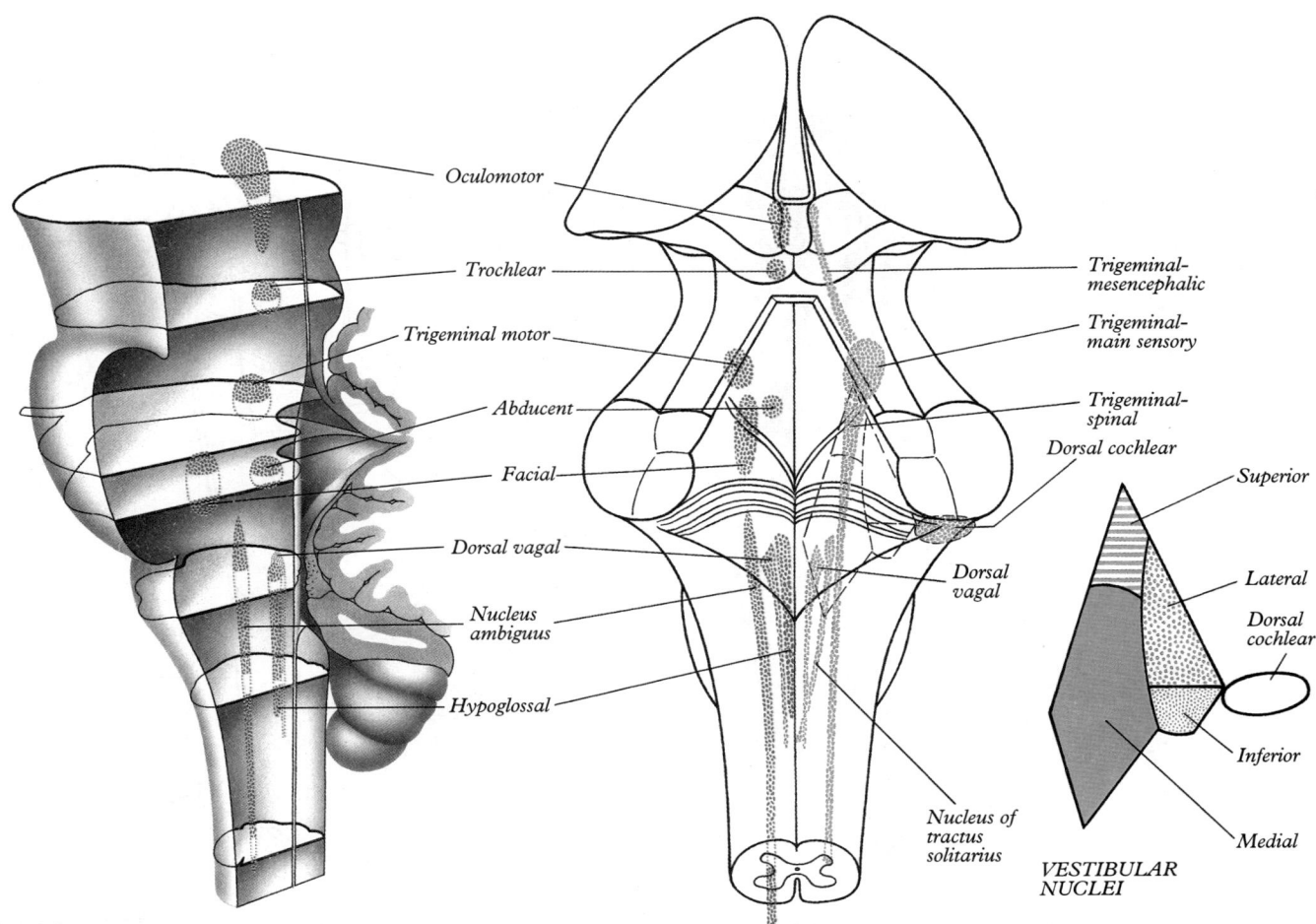

8.129 Surface projection of some cranial nerve nuclei on the dorsal aspect of the brain stem. Motor nuclei are in red, sensory in blue. The vestibular nuclei are indicated in the main diagram by interrupted lines and are shown in detail in the small diagram. The olfactory and optic centres are not shown.

- a smaller laterally placed pars triangularis, with little or no cell clustering
- reticular poles of the rostral and caudal zones, containing scattered, evenly distributed neurons of various sizes.

The pars triangularis in man is more differentiated into cell clusters than that of monkeys. There is a somatotopic pattern of termination of cutaneous inputs from the forelimb into the cell clusters of the pars rotunda (**8**.130) (Florence et al 1989). Terminations are diffuse in the reticular poles. Both the gracile and cuneate nuclei contain interneurons (Andersen et al 1964; Rustioni & Sotelo 1974); many are inhibitory, but primary spinal afferents synapse with multipolar neurons forming the major nuclear efferent projection, as a relay between the spinal cord and higher levels. Descending afferents from the somatosensory cortex (p. 1155), reaching the nuclei through the corticospinal tracts, appear restricted to the upper, reticular zones. Since these afferents both inhibit and enhance activity, the nuclear region is clearly one of sensory modulation. The reticular zones also receive connections from the reticular formation proper (Spacek & Lieberman 1974). It is probable that 'feed back' from the gracile and cuneate nuclei to the spinal cord also exists. By antidromic stimulation (Dart 1971), retrograde horseradish peroxidase (Kuypers & Maisky 1975) and anterograde isotopic transport (Burton & Loewy 1977), it has been shown in cats and monkeys that neurons of these nuclei project to the ipsilateral spinal dorsal appendage (p. 1009), by fibres presumably involved in the observed depression of dorsal column activity (Hillman & Wall 1969).

The *accessory cuneate nucleus*, dorsolateral to the cuneate, is part of the spinocerebellar system of precerebellar nuclei (pp. 1059, 1078, **8**.131) and contains large neurons like those in the spinal thoracic nucleus; these form the posterior external arcuate fibres (p. 1031), which enter the cerebellum by its ipsilateral inferior peduncle. The nucleus receives lateral fibres of the fasciculus cuneatus, derived from cervical segments. It provides the *cuneocerebellar tract* for fibres carrying proprioceptive impulses from the upper limb which enter the spinal cord above its thoracic nucleus. A group of neurons, 'nucleus Z', was identified in cats by Brodal & Pompeiano (1957) between the upper pole of the nucleus gracilis and the inferior vestibular nucleus and said to be present in the human medulla (Webster 1977). Its input is probably from the dorsal spinocerebellar tract (Rustioni 1973); it may be a separated part of the gracile reticular zone, which it resembles; it receives proprioceptive fibres from the ipsilateral hind limb (Landgren & Silfvenius 1971) and projects through the internal arcuate fibres to the contralateral medial lemniscus.

The *nucleus of the spinal tract of the trigeminal nerve* (**8**.129, 132) is separated from the central grey matter by internal arcuate fibres and from the lateral medullary surface only by the trigeminal spinal tract, which ends in it, and by some dorsal spinocerebellar tract fibres; the latter progressively incline dorsally and at a higher level enter the inferior cerebellar peduncle (p. 990).

Two other nuclei occur at this level. One is dorsolateral to the pyramid, the other medial to it and near the median plane; these are parts of the precerebellar *medial accessory olivary nucleus*, described with the inferior olivary nuclear complex (p. 1020). Precerebellar nuclei of the vestibular, pontine and reticular system are described on pages 1024, 1022, 1059, 1078 respectively.

The central grey substance, at this level near the dorsal medullary surface, contains three bilateral nuclei. The prominent *hypoglossal nucleus*, of large motor neurons interspersed with myelinated fibres, is ventromedial in the central grey matter. It extends into the open part of the medulla, subjacent to the *trigonum hypoglossi* in the floor of the fourth ventricle (**8**.122, 123). Near it are several smaller groups, perhaps misnamed '*perihypoglossal complex*' or '*perihypoglossal grey*', for none is known to be connected with the hypoglossal nerve

A Macaque

B Human

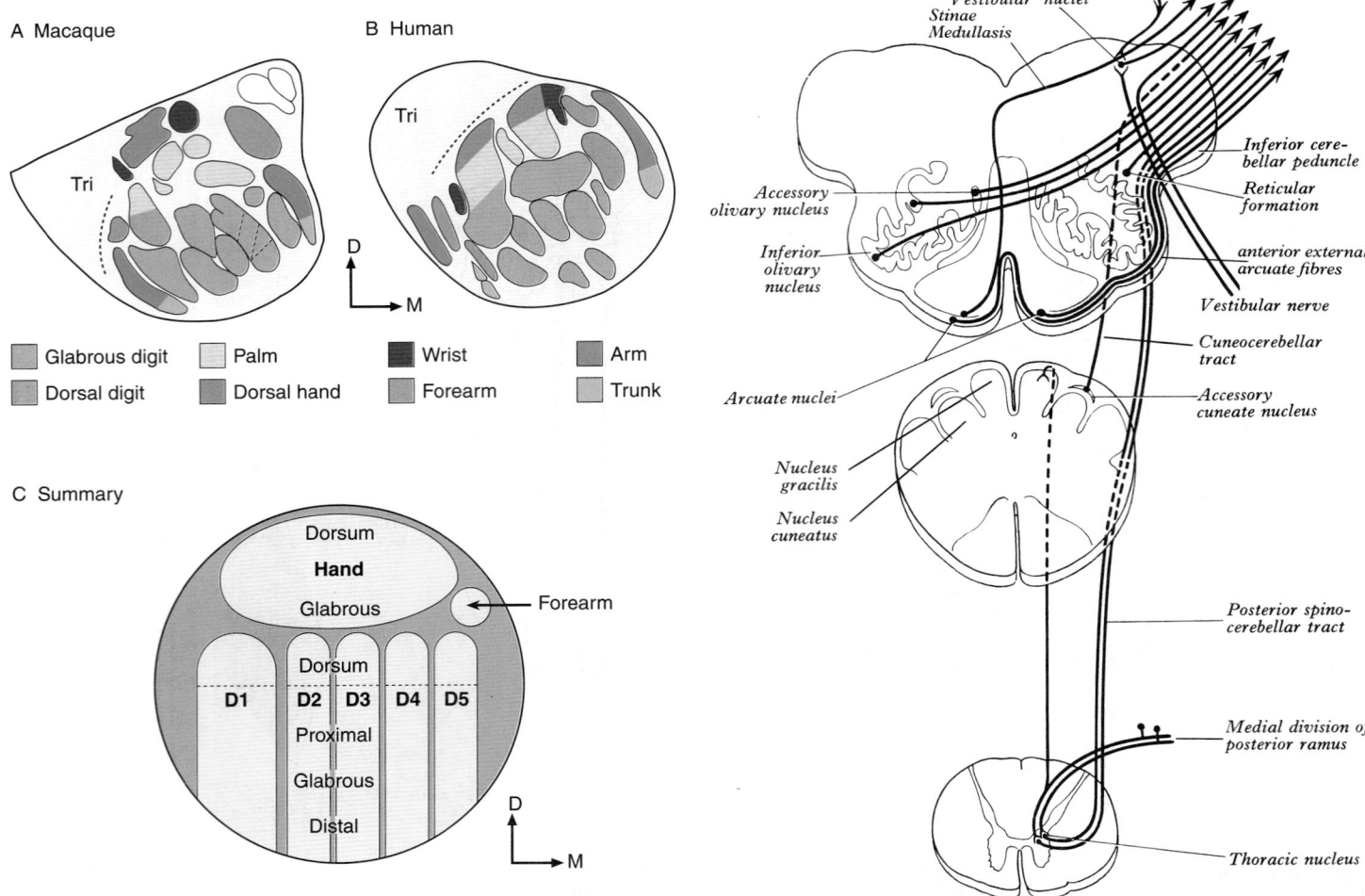

Glabrous digit
Palm
Wrist
Arm

Dorsal digit
Dorsal hand
Forearm
Trunk

C Summary

Dorsum
Hand
Glabrous
— Forearm

Dorsum
D1 | D2 | D3 | D4 | D5
Proximal
Glabrous
Distal

Vestibular nuclei
Stinae
Medullasis

Accessory olivary nucleus

Inferior olivary nucleus

Arcuate nuclei

Nucleus gracilis

Nucleus cuneatus

Inferior cerebellar peduncle
Reticular formation

anterior external arcuate fibres

Vestibular nerve

Cuneocerebellar tract

Accessory cuneate nucleus

Posterior spinocerebellar tract

Medial division of posterior ramus

Thoracic nucleus

8.130 A. Schematic summary of the relation of cutaneous inputs from different regions of the forelimb to cell clusters in the pars rotunda of the cuneate nucleus of a Macaque monkey. B. The proposed relation of cutaneous inputs to cell clusters in the pars rotunda of human. Although information is available for the representations of the arm and trunk in monkeys, limited data are available for the forearm and representations of the latter are tentatively depicted as split around the hand. C Summary of the somatotrophic pattern of representation in elongated cell columns of the pars rotunda of Macaque monkeys assessed with subcutenous injections of the forelimb coronal view; D = dorsal, M = medial, Tri = nucleus triangularis. (From Florence et al (1989) with permission of author and publisher.)

8.131 Some of the afferent components of the inferior cerebellar peduncles; the efferent components have been omitted.

or nucleus. These small groups include the *nucleus intercalatus, sublingual nucleus, nucleus prepositus hypoglossi* and *nucleus paramedianus dorsalis (reticularis),* all containing neurons suggestive of reticular connections, definitely ascribed to the paramedian nucleus (Brodal 1957). Gustatory and visceral connections are attributed to the nucleus intercalatus; there is more convincing evidence that the perihypoglossal nuclei project to the cerebellum, at least in cats (Torvik & Brodal 1954) and monkeys (Mehler et al 1960). Representation of lingual musculature has been described in the hypoglossal nucleus (p. 1225).

Dorsolateral to the hypoglossal is the *dorsal vagal nucleus* containing neurons of at least two types, the larger with fine preganglionic parasympathetic fibres innervating non-striated muscle and smaller fusiform neurons possibly concerned with visceral afferents. But many believe that all vagal visceral afferent fibres end in the nucleus solitarius (see below). Superiorly, the dorsal vagal nucleus is lateral to the hypoglossal, in the floor of the fourth ventricle subjacent to the *trigonum vagi* (8.122, 123). Dorsolateral to it at this level is the *nucleus of the tractus solitarius,* intimately related to the descending *tractus solitarius.* At the lower end of the medulla these nuclei fuse dorsal to the central canal. As the nucleus solitarius

ascends it lies deeper in the medulla, ventrolateral to the dorsal vagal nucleus and almost coextensive with it. The tractus solitarius receives afferent fibres from the facial, glossopharyngeal and vagus nerves, entering it in descending order and conveying gustatory information from the lingual and palatal mucosa and, according to many, visceral impulses from the pharynx (glossopharyngeal and vagus) and from the oesophagus and abdominal alimentary canal (vagus). In this vertical representation there is some overlap (Schwartz et al 1951; Kerr 1962). Neurons in the solitary nucleus are smaller than those in the dorsal vagal nucleus; their axons may project to the thalamus and thence to the cerebral cortex, but attempts to establish this in cats have failed (Morest 1967). The dorsal vagal nucleus and nucleus ambiguus are connected. The solitary nucleus may project to the upper levels of the spinal cord through a *solitariospinal tract* (p. 1002) in man (Collier & Buzzard 1903) and cat (Torvik 1957). This nucleus is considered to receive fibres from the spinal cord, cerebral cortex and cerebellum (Angaut & Brodal 1967). A neuronal group ventrolateral to the solitary nucleus has been termed the *nucleus parasolitarius* (Crosby et al 1962). Numerous islets of grey matter are scattered centrally in the ventrolateral medulla, an area intersected by nerve fibres in all directions and hence termed the *reticular formation.* It exists at all medullary levels, extending to the pontine tegmentum and midbrain. The connections of the nucleus of the tractus solitarius and dorsal motor nucleus of the vagus with the reticular formation are considered later (p. 1077).

The medullary white matter is rearranged above the corticospinal decussation. The *pyramids* contain ipsilateral corticospinal and corticonuclear fibres (8.125), the latter distributed to nuclei of cranial nerves and other medullary nuclei; they form two large ventral bundles flanking the anterior median fissure; dorsal are the accessory olivary nuclei and lemniscal decussation.

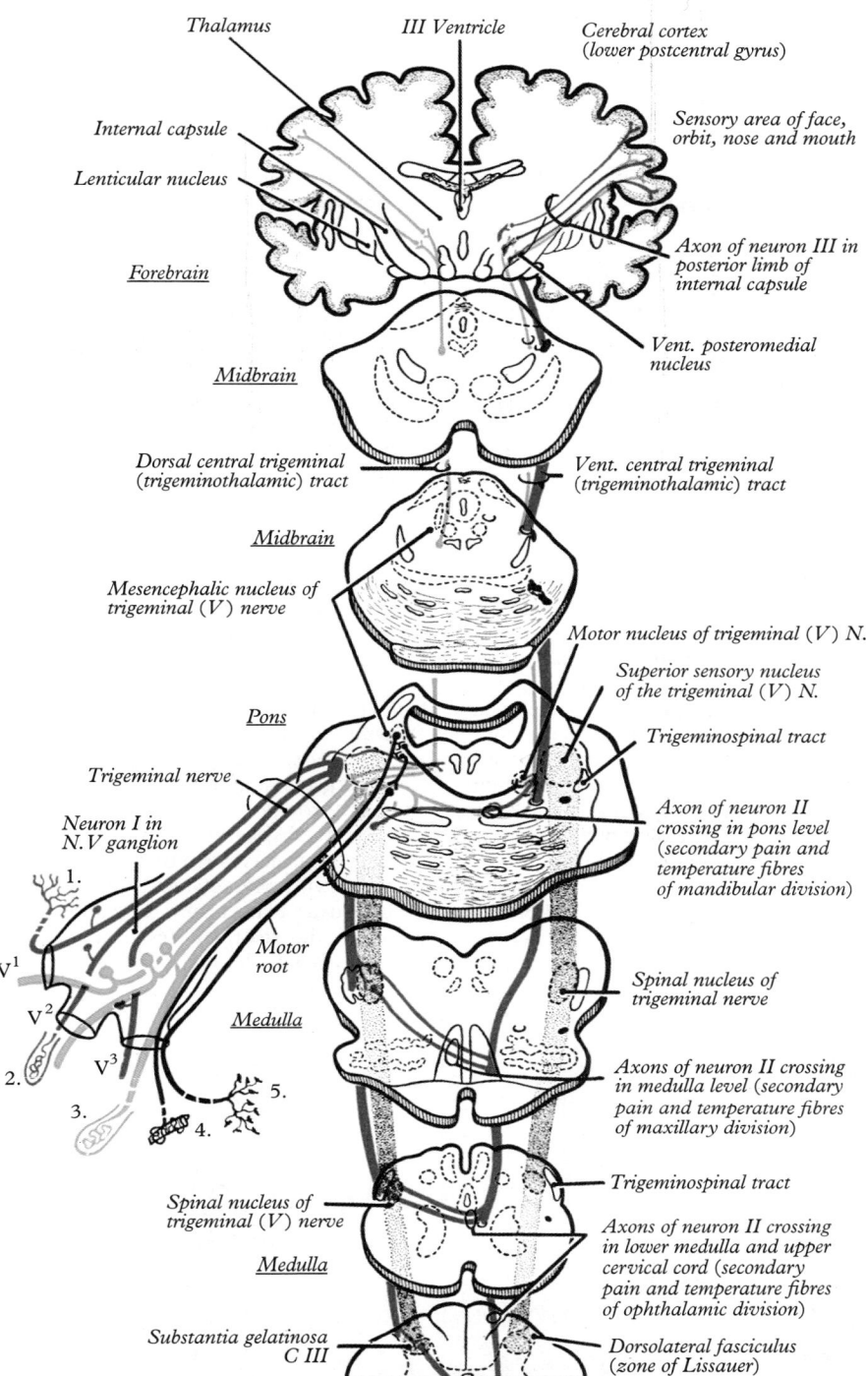

8.132 Diagram of the secondary trigeminal tracts. The ventral trigeminal tract (red) conveys pain, thermal and tactile sense. These fibres originate from the spinal trigeminal nucleus, cross in the lower brain stem at various locations and ascend in association with the contralateral medial lemniscus. Secondary trigeminothalamic fibres from the principal sensory nucleus, conveying touch and pressure (blue) ascend by two separate pathways. Fibres from the ventral part of the principal sensory nucleus of N. V cross and ascend in association with the contralateral medial lemniscus. Fibres from the dorsomedial part of the same nucleus ascend uncrossed as the dorsal trigeminal tract. Both the ventral and dorsal trigeminal tracts project to the ventral posteromedial nucleus of the thalamus. The brain stem location of the ascending lateral spinothalamic tract is indicated in black on the right side. The ophthalmic (V^1), maxillary (V^2), and mandibular (V^3) divisions of the trigeminal nerve are identified. 1, Free nerve ending; 2, thermal receptor; 3, Meissner's corpuscle; 4, neuromuscular spindle; 5, motor end plate in muscle of mastication (from Truex and Carpenter 1964, Strong and Elwyn's human neuroanatomy, Williams & Wilkins, with permission of authors and publisher.)

The *medial lemniscus* (p. 1015) (**8.108**) ascends from the lemniscal decussation on each side as a flattened tract, near the median raphe. The tracts ascend to the pons, increasing as fibres join from upper levels of the decussation. Ventral are the corticospinal fibres and dorsal the medial longitudinal fasciculus and tectospinal tract. In the decussation, fibres are rearranged; those from the gracile are ventral to those from the cuneate nucleus; above this the medial lemniscus is also rearranged (p. 1021): ventral (gracile) fibres become lateral, dorsal (cuneate) fibres medial. At this level, medial lemniscal fibres in monkeys (Ferraro & Barrera 1936) and chimpanzees (Walker 1937) show a laminar somatotopy on a segmental basis, as fibres from C1 to S4 spinal segments are segregated sequentially from medial to lateral respectively. This arrangement is almost certainly present in man.

The *medial longitudinal fasciculus*, a small compact tract near the midline and ventral to the hypoglossal nucleus, is continuous with the ventral spinal intersegmented tract; at this medullary level it is displaced dorsally by the pyramidal and lemniscal decussations. It ascends in the pons and midbrain in the same relation to the central grey matter and midline and is therefore near the somatic efferent nuclear column. Fibres course for short distances in the tract, being from a variety of sources, and are detailed on page 1027 and in **8.141**.

The *spinocerebellar*, *spinotectal*, *vestibulospinal*, *rubrospinal* and *lateral spinothalamic (spinal lemniscal)* tracts are all in the ventrolateral area, limited dorsally by the spinal trigeminal nucleus, ventrally by the pyramid.

A transverse section level with the lower end of the fourth ventricle

A transverse section level with the lower end of the fourth ventricle (8.133) shows some new features with most of those already described. The total area of grey matter is increased by the large olivary nuclear complex, arcuate nucleus and nuclei of the vestibulocochlear, glossopharyngeal, vagus and accessory nerves.

The *inferior olivary nuclear complex*, comprising the inferior, medial accessory and dorsal accessory olivary nuclei, is one of several brainstem precerebellar nuclear complexes which include the pontine (p. 1060), arcuate, vestibular (p. 1058), reticularcerebellar (p. 1059) and spinocerebellar p. 1058) nuclei, all of which receive afferents from specific sources and project to the cerebellum. The *inferior olivary nucleus* is a hollow, irregularly crenated grey mass, with a longitudinal medial hilum, surrounded by myelinated fibres which form the *olivary amiculum*. Dorsolateral to the pyramid, it underlies the olive but ascends within the pons. It contains small neurons, most of which form the *olivocerebellar tract*, emerging from the hilum or through the adjacent wall to run medially, intersecting the medial lemniscus (8.131). Its fibres cross the midline, and either sweep dorsal to or traverse the opposite olivary nucleus, intersecting the lateral spinothalamic and rubrospinal tracts and spinal trigeminal nucleus to enter and constitute the major component of the contralateral inferior cerebellar peduncle. Fibres of the contralateral inferior olivary complex terminate on Purkinje cells in the cerebellum as climbing fibres forming a one-to-one relationship between Purkinje cells and neurons in the complex. The afferent olivary connections are ascending and descending; ascending fibres, mainly crossed, arrive from all spinal levels in the *spino-olivary tracts*; ascending connections also arrive via the dorsal white columns (Hand & Liu 1966). Descending ipsilateral fibres come from the cerebral cortex, thalamus, basal nuclei, red nucleus and central grey of the midbrain

(Walberg 1960); the latter two projections in part comprise the *central tegmental fasciculus* (p. 1070) (Jansen & Brodal 1954), which forms the olivary amiculum.

The *medial accessory olivary nucleus* is a curved grey lamina, concave laterally, between the medial lemniscus and pyramid and the ventromedial aspect of the inferior olivary nucleus. The *dorsal accessory olivary nucleus* is a similar lamina dorsomedial to the inferior olivary nucleus. Both nuclei are connected with the cerebellum. The accessory nuclei are phylogenetically older than the inferior, connecting with the paleocerebellum (p. 1067); the inferior nucleus occurs only in mammals, enlarging caudally during its evolution. In all connections, cerebral, spinal and cerebellar, the olivary nuclei sometimes display very specific somatotopy, particularly in their cerebellar connections, detailed later (pp. 1056, 1058, 1062). The *arcuate nuclei* are curved, interrupted bands, anteromedial to the pyramids; they are said to be displaced pontine nuclei (Rasmussen & Peyton 1946). Anterior external arcuate fibres and those of the striae medullaris are derived from them and project mainly to the contralateral cerebellum through the inferior cerebellar peduncle (8.131).

The central grey matter, at this level spreads over the ventricular floor, contains sequentially from medial to lateral the *hypoglossal nucleus*, *dorsal vagal nucleus* and the *nucleus solitarius* ventrolateral to the vagal; these and the inferior cerebellar peduncle are near the caudal ends of the *inferior and medial vestibular nuclei* (p. 1024). Between the hypoglossal nucleus and dorsal vagal nucleus is the *nucleus intercalatus* (p. 1018).

The tractus solitarius and its associated circumferential nucleus extends throughout the length of the medulla. The tract (8.134) is composed of general visceral afferents from the vagus and glossopharyngeal nerves (p. 1018), and the nucleus and its central connections with the reticular formation subserve the reflex control of cardiovascular, respiratory and cardiac functions (p. 1077). In addition, the rostral fibres of the tract comprise gustatory fibres from the facial, glossopharyngeal and vagal nerves projecting to the

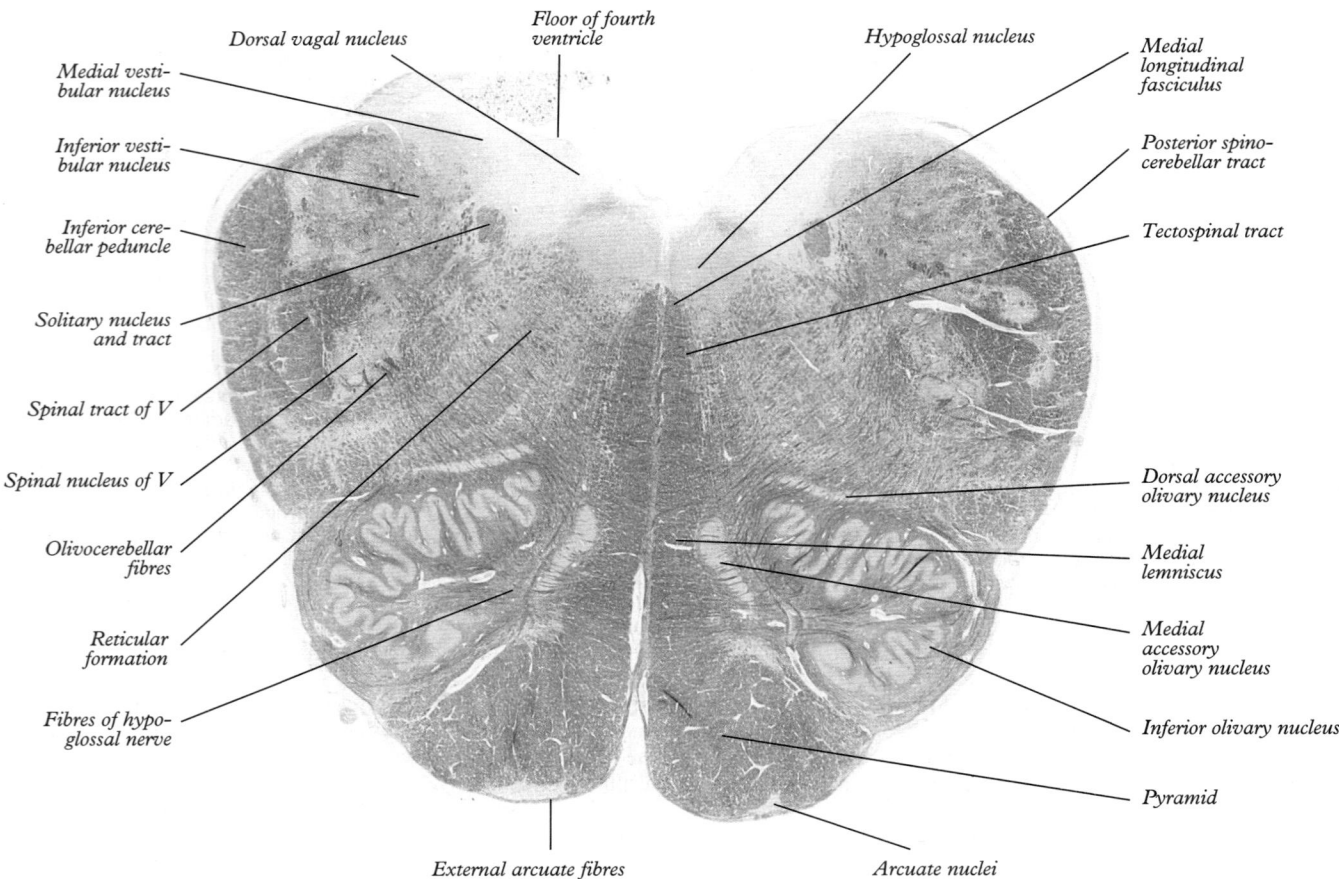

Dorsal vagal nucleus

Floor of fourth ventricle

Hypoglossal nucleus

Medial vestibular nucleus

Medial longitudinal fasciculus

Inferior vestibular nucleus

Posterior spinocerebellar tract

Inferior cerebellar peduncle

Tectospinal tract

Solitary nucleus and tract

Spinal tract of V

Spinal nucleus of V

Dorsal accessory olivary nucleus

Olivocerebellar fibres

Medial lemniscus

Reticular formation

Medial accessory olivary nucleus

Fibres of hypoglossal nerve

Inferior olivary nucleus

Pyramid

External arcuate fibres

Arcuate nuclei

8.133 Transverse section through the medulla oblongata at the mid-olivary level. Weigert Pal preparation. Magnification × 4.5.

rostral pole of the solitary nucleus, *the gustatory nucleus*.

A group of large motor neurons, *the nucleus ambiguus*, is isolated deep in the reticular formation and descends as far as the upper end of the dorsal vagal nucleus. Caudally, it is continuous with the spinal accessory nucleus (p. 980). Fibres emerging from it pass dorsomedially, then curve laterally, rostral fibres join the glossopharyngeal nerve, those at a caudal level join the vagus and cranial accessory nerves and innervate striated muscle of branchial arch origin (p. 238). The nucleus displays several groups of neurons in man and other mammals; some representation of the muscles innervated has been established (p. 1250). At its upper end, between this and the facial nucleus, is a small *retrofacial nucleus*; though in line with the special visceral efferent nuclei, it is a reputed source of general visceral efferent vagal fibres.

The gracile and cuneate nuclei, diminishing and irregular, fill the dorsolateral region; ventral is the *spinal trigeminal* tract and nucleus. The cochlear nuclei are superficial to the inferior cerebellar peduncle (p. 1024). The white matter shows little change except for the development of the inferior cerebellar peduncles lateral to the fourth ventricle. The pyramid, medial lemniscus, tectospinal tract and medial longitudinal fasciculus are unchanged in position. Olivocerebellar tracts sweep across the midline, turning dorsally to join the inferior peduncles (8.131). *Anterior external arcuate fibres* arising from both ipsilateral and contralateral arcuate nuclei emerge from the anterior median fissure to pass dorsolaterally over the surface of the pyramid, olive and spinal trigeminal tract to reach the posterior spinocerebellar tract, then together ascend into the inferior cerebellar peduncle (8.131).

Hypoglossal fibres emerge ventrally from their nucleus, traverse the reticular formation lateral to the medial lemniscus and medial to (sometimes through) the inferior olivary nucleus and curve laterally to emerge superficially as rootlets in the ventrolateral sulcus.

Medullary syndromes

The *medial medullary syndrome* results from infarction of the ventral medulla at this level and involves the corticospinal tract and hypoglossal nerve, causing characteristic crossed paralyses in ipsilateral lingual muscles (lower motor neuron) and contralateral limbs (upper motor neuron type). The medial lemniscus is also involved resulting in contralateral loss of discriminatory touch, and both movement and position senses. The medullary branches of the anterior spinal arteries are usually occluded.

Occlusion of the medullary branches of the posterior inferior cerebellar artery causes the *lateral medullary (Wallenberger) syndrome*. The infarcted area includes the spinal nucleus and tract of the trigeminal nerve, nucleus ambiguus and lateral spinothalamic tract and descending pathway to the preganglionic sympathetic intermediolateral cell column in the thoracic cord; this results respectively in an ipsilateral loss of pain and temperature over the trigeminal area, dysphagia and dysarthria, contralateral loss of pain and temperature below the neck and Horner's syndrome. The reticular formation is traversed dorsally by vagal fibres from the dorsal nucleus, the nucleus ambiguus and nucleus solitarius, all emerging as rootlets in the dorsolateral sulcus. The lateral spinothalamic tract (*spinal lemniscus*) (p. 1019), dorsal to the inferior olivary nucleus, is separated from the surface by the anterior spinocerebellar and spinotectal tracts. Clinical and experimental evidence indicates somatotopy among its fibres: those for the lower limb are superficial, for the upper limb deep and for the trunk intermediate.

A transverse section of the medulla at its upper limit

A transverse section of the medulla at its upper limit (8.135) shows

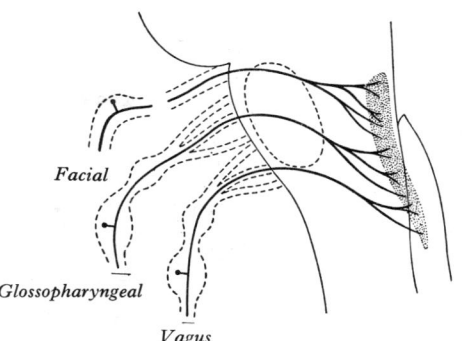

8.134 Afferent fibres of the facial, glossopharyngeal and vagus nerves, conveying gustatory impulses of the tractus solitarius. The cell bodies of these fibres lie in the geniculate ganglia of the facial nerves and the inferior ganglia of the glossopharyngeal and vagus nerves.

little change; the dorsal surface is relatively flat but undulant and may show a few fibres of the stria medullaris (p. 1026). The inferior olivary nucleus is unchanged, but accessory olivary nuclei are diminishing. The medial vestibular nucleus is wider and dorsolateral to the dorsal vagal nucleus, separating the latter from the floor of the rhomboid fossa. The inferior vestibular nucleus lies between the medial vestibular nucleus and the inferior cerebellar peduncle. At the pontomedullary junction, the *lateral vestibular nucleus* (p. 1024) replaces the inferior vestibular nucleus and the *cochlear nuclei* are usually present. The nucleus solitarius, spinal trigeminal tract and nucleus and the nucleus ambiguus are almost unchanged in position.

The white substance at this level is also little changed: the lateral spinothalamic tract (spinal lemniscus) ascends dorsal to the olivary nucleus, its fibres retaining their somatotopic arrangement (p. 1019). The *inferior cerebellar peduncle* (p. 1027) is a large dorsolateral bulge. The *medial lemniscus* (8.108) widens ventrally and moves between the pyramid and the narrowing olivary nucleus, its dorsal part receding from the tectospinal tract and medial longitudinal bundle. Entering the pons, it spreads coronally in the ventral tegmentum (8.136). It contains fibres for proprioceptive and tactile sensibility. As it ascends in the medulla it is probably joined by the anterior spinothalamic tract. In the pons, therefore, it contains fibres serving proprioception, tactile and pressure sense from the contralateral lower limb, trunk and upper limb; fibres from the lower limb are lateral, from the upper limb intermediate and from the neck medial in position.

The *medullary reticular formation* is described on pages 173–179.

PONS

EXTERNAL FEATURES AND RELATIONS

The pons lies ventral to the cerebellum, below the midbrain and above the medulla, with which it is continuous. The site of transition is demarcated superficially by a transverse ventrolateral sulcus in which the abducent, facial and vestibulocochlear nerves emerge. Its ventral surface (8.124), separated from the clivus (basisphenoid and dorsum sellae) by the cisterna pontis, is markedly convex transversely, less so vertically and grooves the petrous temporal bone laterally up to the internal acoustic meatus. Bundles of transverse fibres bridging the midline originate from neurons in the nuclei pontis and are projected contralaterally into the cerebellum, converging on each side into a large compact *middle cerebellar peduncle*. The surface has a shallow vertical median *sulcus basilaris*, usually containing the basilar artery and bounded bilaterally by prominences due partly to the corticospinal fibres descending in the pons. The superior cerebellar and labyrinthine arteries run over the ventral surface of the pons. The former courses below the tentorium cerebelli, the latter takes a tortuous course to the internal acoustic meatus and often lies in the cerebellopontine angle in which the facial, vestibulocochlear and glossopharyngeal roots are located together with the nervus intermedius, all lying on the choroid plexus of the fourth

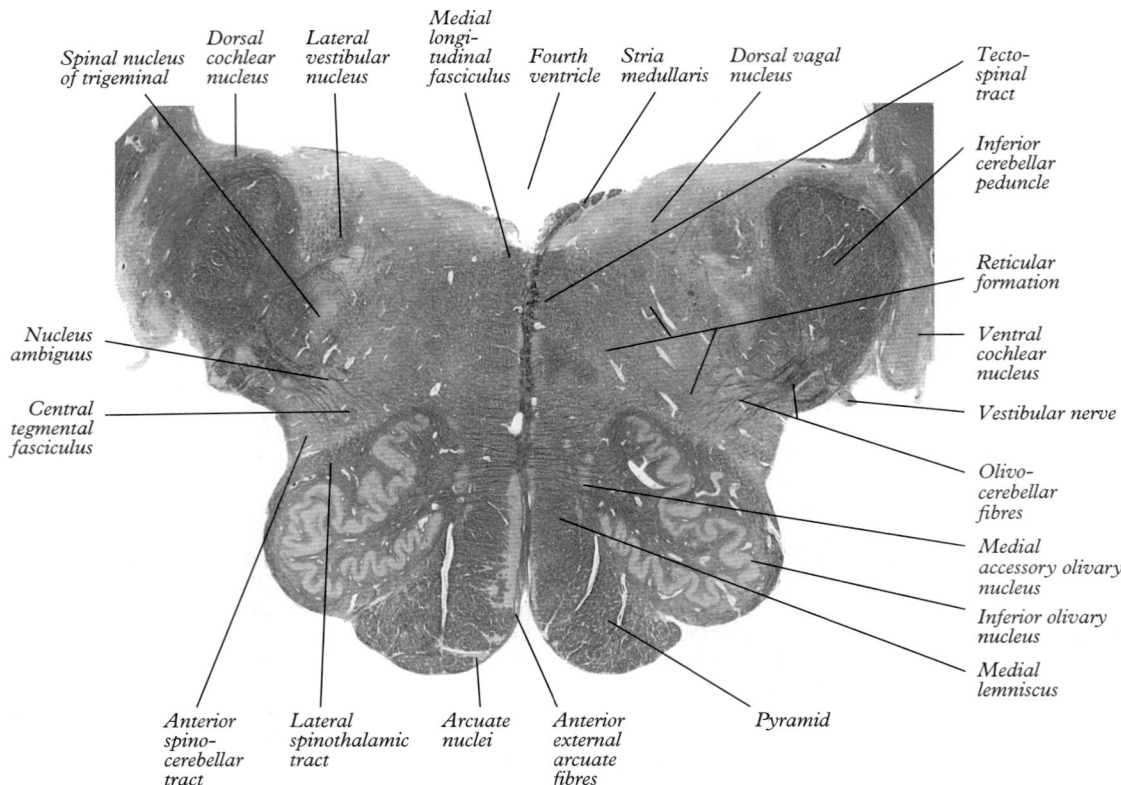

Spinal nucleus of trigeminal
Dorsal cochlear nucleus
Lateral vestibular nucleus
Medial longitudinal fasciculus
Fourth ventricle
Stria medullaris
Dorsal vagal nucleus
Tecto-spinal tract
Inferior cerebellar peduncle
Reticular formation
Ventral cochlear nucleus
Vestibular nerve
Olivo-cerebellar fibres
Medial accessory olivary nucleus
Inferior olivary nucleus
Medial lemniscus
Pyramid
Anterior external arcuate fibres
Arcuate nuclei
Lateral spinothalamic tract
Anterior spinocerebellar tract
Central tegmental fasciculus
Nucleus ambiguus

8.135   Transverse section through the superior half of the medulla oblong-ata. Magnification × 4.5. (Solochrome cyanin preparation by J Carlile and photographed by Kevin Fitzpatrick, Division of Anatomy and Cell Biology, UMDS, Guy's Campus, London.)

ventricle (8.122, 123) which protrudes from the foramen of Luschka into the subarachnoid space. The auditory nerve lies anterior to the vestibular and facial nerves when it emerges from the internal acoustic meatus. In the pontocerebellar angle it moves posteriorly to align with the vestibular nerve; both nerves then lie posterior to the facial nerve as they enter the brainstem (Silverstein 1984). Near the midpontine level, the trigeminal nerves emerge, each with a small superomedial motor root and a large inferolateral sensory root. The abducent nerves emerge at the pontomedullary junction near the midline and ascend on the ventral surface of the pons before piercing the dura over the basisphenoid. The dorsal surface, hidden by the cerebellum, roofs the rostral half of the rhomboid fossa into which the aqueduct of the midbrain empties. The roof is formed by a thin sheet of tissue, the *anterior (superior) medullary velum*, in which the IVth nerves decussate, and is overlain by the lingula of the vermis of the cerebellum. The velum is attached on each side to the superior cerebellar peduncles and enclosed by pia mater above and ependyma below (8.123). Transverse sections show a dorsal *tegmentum* and a *ventral (basilar) part*, the former a continuation of the medulla, excluding the pyramids. The ventral pons contains bundles of *longitudinal fibres*, some continued into the pyramids, some ending in many pontine or medullary nuclei; also present are many *transverse* fibres and the scattered *nuclei pontis*.

INTERNAL STRUCTURE

Ventral (basilar) pons

The ventral (basilar) pons is similar in structure at all levels. Descending from the crus cerebri of the midbrain (p. 1067), the longitudinal fibres (8.116, 136) of the corticopontine, corticonuclear and corticospinal tracts enter the pons compactly but rapidly disperse into fascicles, separated by the *pontine nuclei* and transverse pontine fibres. *Corticospinal fibres* traverse the pons to the medullary pyramids, converging again here into compact tracts (p. 1013); *corticonuclear fibres* accompany them, some diverging to both contralateral (and some ipsilateral) nuclei of cranial nerves and other nuclei in the pontine tegmentum, the rest reaching the pyramids. Clinical evidence

supports the contention that the facial and other nuclei (p. 1026) receive ipsilateral corticonuclear fibres. *Corticopontine fibres*, from the frontal, temporal, parietal and occipital cortex, end in the nuclei pontis (8.137); axons from the latter are the *transverse pontine fibres* (pontocerebellar) which after decussation continue to form the contralateral middle cerebellar peduncle. Frontopontine axons end in the nuclei pontis above the level of the emerging trigeminal roots and are relayed to the contralateral cerebellum forming the upper transverse pontine fibres. All pontocerebellar fibres end as mossy fibres in the cerebellar cortex (p. 1060). A degree of somatotopy is maintained in these connections (see below).

The precerebellar *pontine nuclei* include all the neurons scattered in the ventral pons. Varying in size and shape, they are, as indicated, relays of paths from the cerebral cortex to the contralateral cerebellum. The nucleus develops by migration ventrally and upwards of neuroblasts from the rhombic lip (p. 238) but they do not all reach the ventral pons; some remain in an ectopic oblique dorsolateral disposition across the inferior cerebellar peduncle, forming the *nucleus of the circumolivary bundle* (pontobulbar body), whose axons are said to ascend vertically on the surface between the emerging facial nerve and eighth cranial nerve on its lateral side. Afferents to the nucleus have been claimed to traverse the pons descending longitudinally with the corticospinal fibres, leaving in the medulla to ascend, recurving dorsally over the olive to the nucleus, as part of the *pyramidal circumolivary fasciculus* (8.154).

Brodal and Bjaalie (1992) have reviewed the organization of the pontine nuclei in mammals including primates and man. Corticopontine fibres arise mainly from neurons in layer V of the premotor, somatosensory, posterior parietal, extrastriate visual and cingulate neocortex. Projections from prefrontal, temporal and striate cortex are sparse. The terminal fields although divergent form topographically segmented patterns resembling overlapping columns, slabs or lamellae within the pons. About half the pontine neurons are activated from more than one cortical site but this convergence of input is limited. There is no integration at the level of the pons of cortical inputs from the motor, posterior parietal cortex, visual, somatosensory, or auditory areas. In primary sensory cortex, there is an inverse relation between the density of projection and cortical

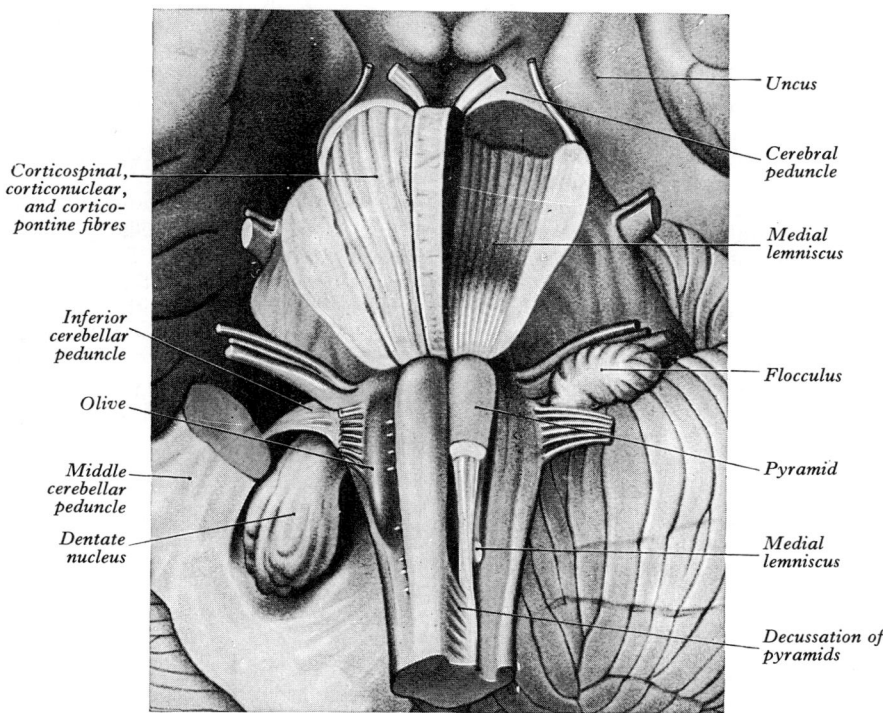

8.136 Ventral aspect of a dissection of the pons, the medulla oblongata and the right cerebellar hemisphere. In the pons and medulla, the dissection is deeper on the left (right side of figure). Note the spiralling of the medial lemniscus from sagittal (below) to oblique coronal (in pons).

magnification factor. Discrete subcortical projections to the pontine nuclei include superior colliculus to dorsolateral pons, medial mamillary nucleus to rostromedial pons and pretectal nuclei; ventrallateral geniculate nucleus, dorsal column nuclei; trigeminal nuclei; hypothalamus and intracerebellar nuclei also project to restricted neurons of the pons. Functionally related subcortical and cerebrocortical afferents converge, e.g. those from somatosensory cortex and dorsal column nuclei, medial mamillary nucleus and angulate gyrus. There is also non-specific input from the reticular formation, raphe nuclei, locus coeruleus and paraqueductal grey (pp. 1074–1079). The density of the subcortical input declines with ascent of the phylogenetic scale. There are some 5% γ-aminobutyric acid (GABA-ergic) inhibitory interneurons in the pontine nuclei forming

type II axodendritic and dendrodendritic synapses with pontocerebellar projection neurons. The latter are engaged monosynaptically by type I axodendritic synapses. In man, there are some 20 million pontine neurons; all are probably glutaminergic mostly projecting to the cerebellar cortex with some input to the deep cerebellar nuclei. The high degree of divergence and convergence of pontine connections, the presence of inhibitory interneurons and complex synaptology suggest an information processing function of the pons, probably of task related inputs from various sources which are then delivered to cerebellar cortical regions for further processing.

Tegmental pons

The tegmental pons varies at different levels, especially in cytoar-

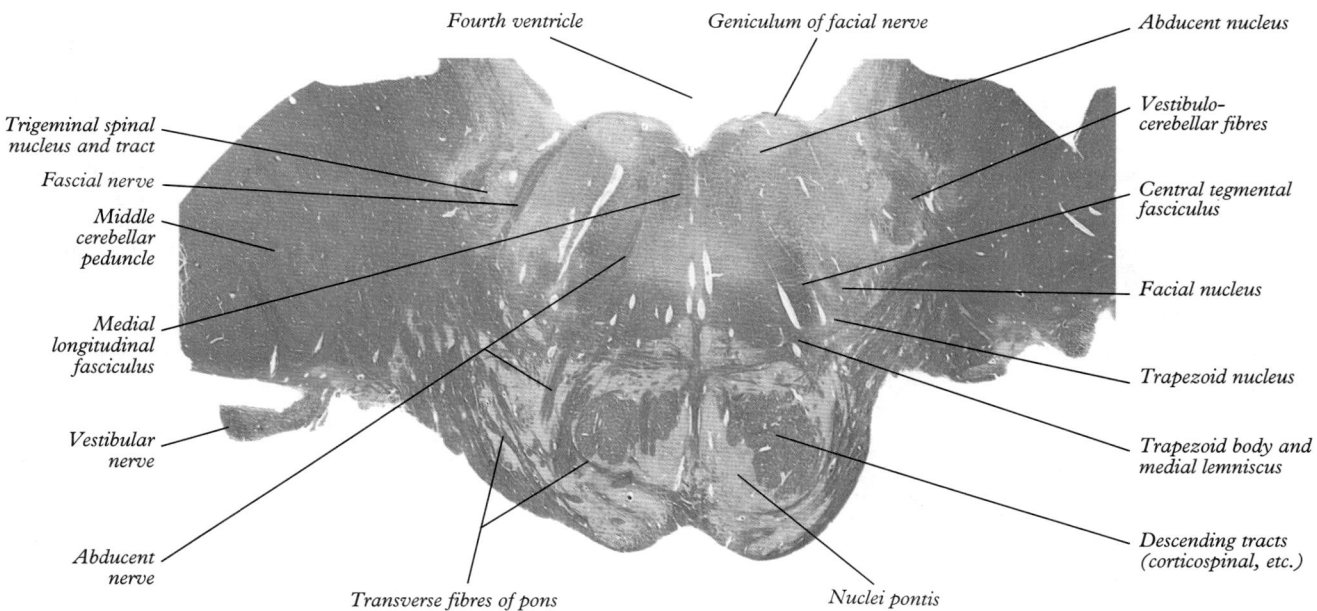

8.137 Transverse section through the pons at the level of the facial colliculus. Magnification ×3.5. (Solochrome cyanin stained preparation by J Carlile and photographed by Kevin Fitzpatrick, Division of Anatomy and Cell Biology, UMDS, Guy's Campus, London.)

chitecture, but is adequately described for general purposes by examples of the lower and upper sections.

Transverse section through the pontine lower segment

A transverse section through the pontine lower tegmentum transects the facial colliculi (**8.**137, 138), each containing the motor nucleus of the abducent and the geniculum of the facial nerves. More deeply placed are the facial nuclei, the nearby vestibular and cochlear nuclei and other isolated neuronal groups. The *medial vestibular nucleus* thus continues a little from the medulla into the pontine tegmentum, with the *lateral vestibular nucleus* between it and the inferior cerebellar peduncle.

The precerebellar vestibular nuclei are laterally placed in the rhomboid fossa of the fourth ventricle, subjacent to the roughly rhomboid vestibular area which spans the rostral medulla and caudal pons (**8.**129). They comprise medial, lateral (Deiter's nucleus), superior and inferior vestibular groups all receiving fibres from the vestibular nerve and sending axons to the cerebellum, medial longitudinal fasciculus, spinal cord and lateral lemniscus. Evidence favours spatial representation of the vestibular apparatus in the nuclei (p. 1380). The *medial vestibular nucleus* broadens, then narrows as it ascends from the upper olivary level into the lower pons, separating the dorsal vagal nucleus from the fourth ventricular floor. It is crossed by the striae medullares nearer the floor. Below, it is continuous with the nucleus intercalatus. The *inferior vestibular nucleus* (the smallest) lies between the medial vestibular nucleus and inferior cerebellar peduncle, from the level of the upper end of the nucleus gracilis to the pontomedullary junction. It is traversed by descending fibres of the vestibular nerve and the vestibulospinal tract. The *lateral vestibular nucleus* is just above the inferior, ascending almost to the level of the abducent nucleus, and is composed of large multipolar neurons, which are the main source of the vestibulospinal tract. The *superior vestibular nucleus* is small and lies above the medial and lateral nuclei.

Vestibular fibres of the vestibulocochlear nerve enter the medulla between the inferior cerebellar peduncle and the trigeminal spinal tract and approach the vestibular area, bifurcating into descending and ascending fascicles. The former descend medial to the inferior cerebellar peduncle and end in medial, lateral and inferior vestibular nuclei; the latter enter the superior and medial nuclei. A few vestibular fibres enter the cerebellum directly through the inferior peduncle, (superficially in the *juxtarestiform body*) to end in the nucleus fastigii, flocculonodular lobe and uvula (p. 1033). Vestibular nuclei project extensively to the cerebellum (p. 1058) and also receive axons from its cortex and fastigial nuclei (p. 1050). Their uncrossed spinal projections in the vestibulospinal tracts have been described (p. 1001); vestibular axons also reach the spinal cord in the medial longitudinal fasciculus (**8.**117) and some also reach cerebral levels, possibly for bilateral cortical representation. The vestibular nuclear complex also

projects to the pontine reticular nuclei (pp. 1075, 1059) and to motor nuclei of the ocular muscles and cervical cord in the medial longitudinal fasciculus.

Discrete small neuronal groups near the vestibular nuclei have been observed; only the *interstitial nucleus* is known to receive primary vestibular axons. The *nucleus parasolitarius* (p. 1018) may be linked to the vestibular complex by afferent fastigial connections (p. 1050).

Fibres of the cochlear division of the vestibulocochlear nerve partially encircle the inferior cerebellar peduncle laterally and end in *dorsal* and *ventral cochlear nuclei*. The *dorsal cochlear nucleus* forms a bulge, the auditory tubercle, on the posterior surface of the peduncle and is continuous medially with the vestibular area in the rhomboid fossa. The *ventral cochlear nucleus* is ventrolateral to the dorsal cochlear nucleus, between the cochlear and vestibular fibres of the eighth cranial nerve, both parts of which, with the cochlear nuclei, are usually at the level of the pontomedullary junction (Moore & Osen 1979; Terr & Edgerton 1985a,b).

Ventral cochlear nucleus

The ventral cochlear nucleus is complex in cytoarchitecture (Moore & Osen 1979), containing many neuronal types (e.g. giant, large and small spherical, multipolar, granular) with distinct dendritic field characteristics (Adams 1986), the variants being segregated in separate nuclear regions. Marked topographical order has been demonstrated in cochlear nerve terminals within the nucleus, different parts of the spiral organ and differing stimulation frequencies being related to neurons serially arrayed antero-inferiorly in the ventral nucleus (Schuknecht 1960, Whitfield 1967). All cochlear nerve fibres enter the nucleus both by bifurcating and twisting into ascending branches which end in the ventral nucleus, and by descending traversing it to reach the dorsal nucleus. Fibres from the base of the cochlear bifurcate ventrally, those from the apex divide rostrally (Moore & Osen 1979). There are some 25 000 axons in the human cochlear nerve projecting into a much larger number of neurons in the cochlear nucleus. Thus, the number of cochlear fibres in the lateral lemniscus greatly exceeds that in the cochlear nerve (Ferraro & Minckler, 1977a,b). A minor fraction of the cochlear neurons receive terminals from the nerve, though each fibre may connect with several (Lewy & Kobrak 1936). Terminals are limited to the antero-inferior region of the ventral nucleus, whose elements are probably in large part local interneurons.

Dorsal cochlear nucleus

The dorsal cochlear nucleus is almost continuous with the ventral, separated only by a thin stratum of nerve fibres. Unlike that of other mammals, the human dorsal cochlear nucleus has no laminar pattern. Giant cells predominate whose dendritic fields are aligned with the incoming auditory fibres (Adams 1986).

Though the cellular origins are not precisely known, axons of most neuronal types in the cochlear nuclei leave to end at pontine levels in the superior olivary, trapezoid and lateral lemniscal nuclei (**8.**139, 140). They leave the cochlear nuclei by three routes:

(1) A ventral contingent is the larger, the fibres of which decussate as the *trapezoid body*, level with the pontomedullary junction (**8.**137, 139). These axons ascend slightly while decussating; a few, however, do not cross, synapsing in the ipsilateral superior olivary nuclei. Those decussating, relay in the contralateral nuclei; and in both the next order of axons ascend in the corresponding *lateral lemniscus*. A few decussating fibres traverse the contralateral superior olive into the lateral lemniscus to relay in lemniscal nuclei.

(2) Some axons from ventral cochlear neurons pass dorsally, superficial to the descending trigeminal spinal fibres, the cerebellar fibres in its inferior peduncle and to axons of the *dorsal* cochlear nucleus (see below). The bundle of ventral cochlear fibres is smaller than that of the trapezoid decussation, and swerves ventromedially across the midline, ventral to the medial longitudinal fasciculus as *intermediate acoustic striae* (Held 1863); its further path is uncertain but is probably ascends in the opposite lateral lemniscus.

(3) The most dorsal fibres, from the dorsal nucleus, curve dorsomedially round the inferior cerebellar peduncle towards the midline as *dorsal acoustic striae* (Monakow 1905), not to be confused with the striae medullares (p. 1026), to which they are ventral. They incline ventromedially and cross the midline to ascend in the opposite lateral

8.138 Diagram of the central course of the fibres of the facial nerve, superior aspect, in a transverse section of the pons.

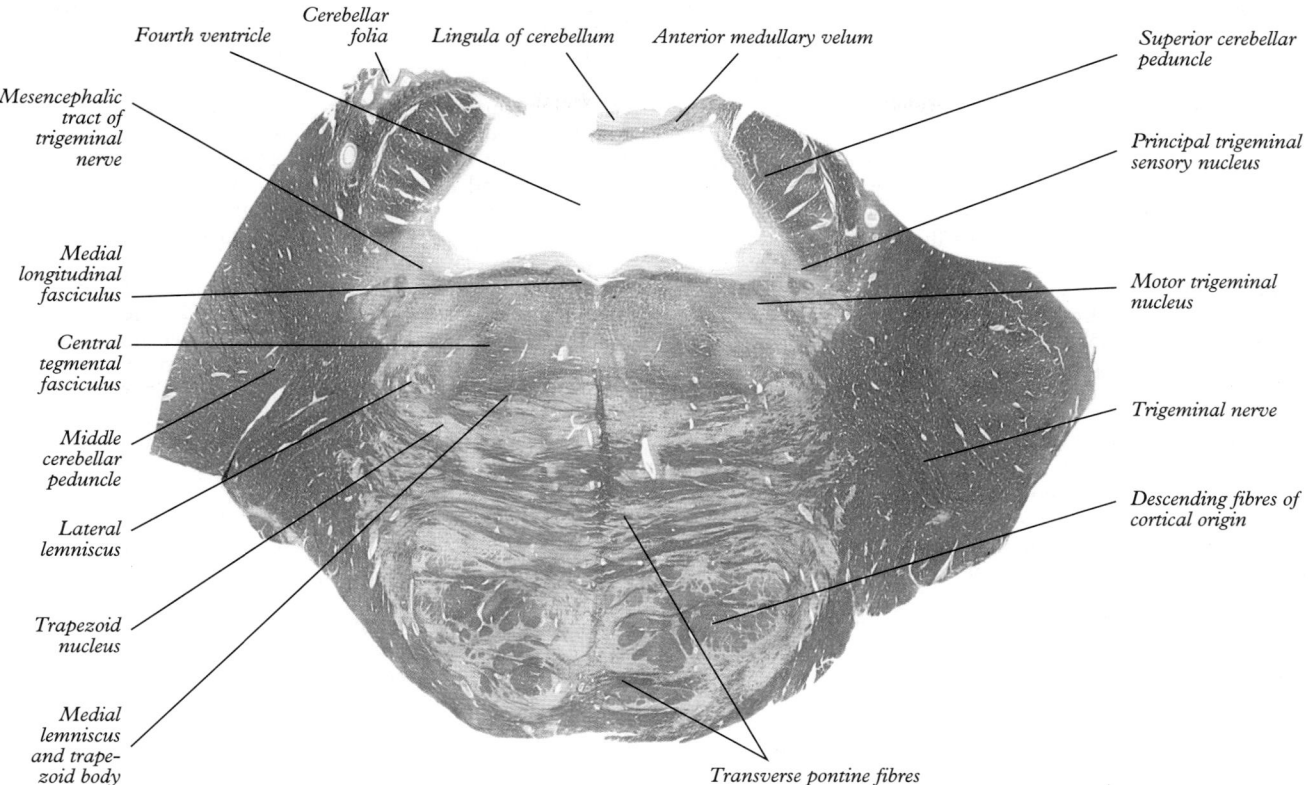

Cerebellar
Fourth ventricle *folia* *Lingula of cerebellum* *Anterior medullary velum* *Superior cerebellar peduncle*

Mesencephalic tract of trigeminal nerve

Principal trigeminal sensory nucleus

Medial longitudinal fasciculus

Motor trigeminal nucleus

Central tegmental fasciculus

Middle cerebellar peduncle

Trigeminal nerve

Lateral lemniscus

Descending fibres of cortical origin

Trapezoid nucleus

Medial lemniscus and trapezoid body

Transverse pontine fibres

8.139   Transverse section of the pons at the level of the trigeminal nerve. Magnification × 3. (Solochrome cyanin stained preparation by J Carlile and photographed by Kevin Fitzpatrick, Division of Anatomy and Cell Biology, UMDS, Guy's Campus, London.)

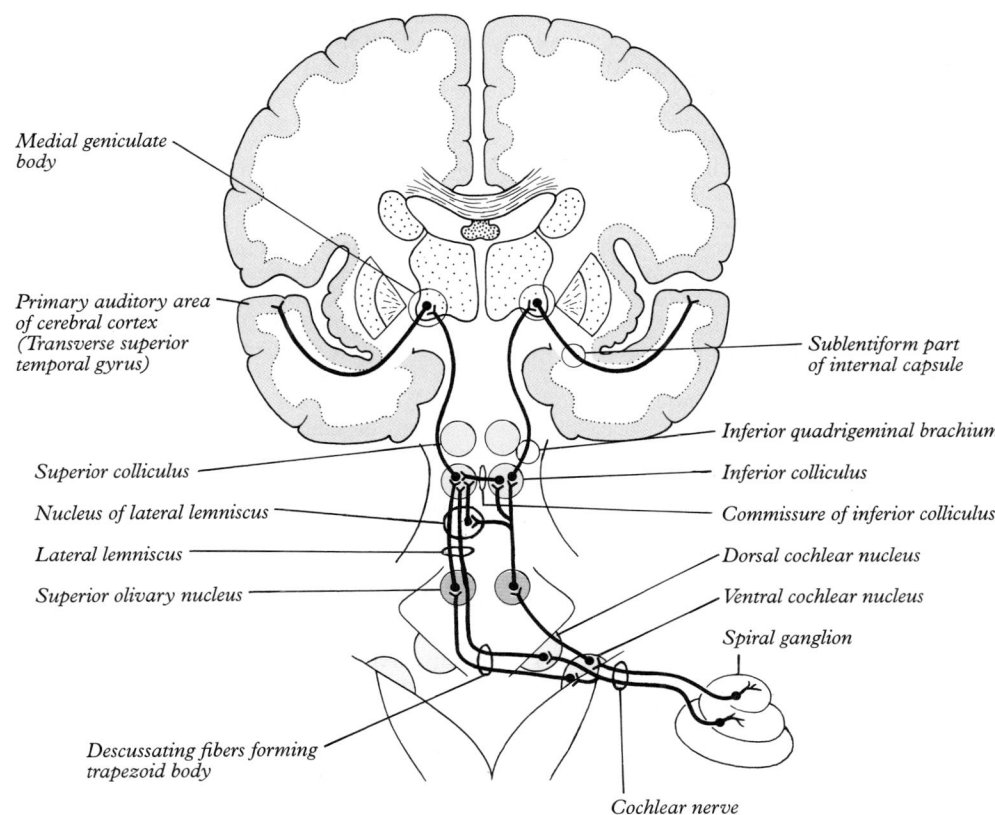

Medial geniculate body

Primary auditory area of cerebral cortex (Transverse superior temporal gyrus)

Sublentiform part of internal capsule

Inferior quadrigeminal brachium

Superior colliculus

Inferior colliculus

Nucleus of lateral lemniscus

Commissure of inferior colliculus

Lateral lemniscus

Dorsal cochlear nucleus

Superior olivary nucleus

Ventral cochlear nucleus

Spiral ganglion

Descussating fibers forming trapezoid body

Cochlear nerve

8.140   Ascending auditory pathway. (With permission from Kiernan J A: Introduction to Human Neuroscience, p. 119. Philadelphia, J B Lippincott Co 1987.)

lemniscus, probably relaying in its nuclei. The auditory projection to the primary auditory cortex is summarized in **8**.140 (p. 1025).

The *superior olivary complex* is sited in the tegmentum of the caudal pons, lateral in the reticular formation at the level of the pontomedullary junction. The superior complex includes several named nuclei and nameless smaller groups (Irving & Harrison 1967; Stromberg & Hurwitz 1976). The *lateral superior olivary nucleus* is made up of some six small cellular clusters in humans. The *medial (accessory) superior olivary nucleus* (para-olivary nucleus of Minckler) is large and compact in man. Medial to the latter is the trapezoid nucleus (see below). Dorsal in the complex is a *retro-olivary group*, the reputed origin of some efferent cochlear fibres described below. Some internuclear connections have been described. Unit recording from the feline lateral nucleus (Warr 1966) demonstrated a tonotopical organization, adjoining neurons being connected to the ipsilateral cochlear fibres concerned with different but related frequencies. The medial superior olivary nucleus receives impulses from both spiral organs; evidence suggests its involvement in auditory sound source localization. With the trapezoid nuclei, superior olivary complexes are the main relay stations of the ventral and the largest cochlear projection. These intricate connections are not yet well established in man. Neuronal counts of certain human nuclei have been recorded by Ferraro and Minckler (1977 a,b).

The *medial nucleus* of the trapezoid body is small in man (Richter et al 1983; Paxinos et al 1990) and has large neurons in a ventral component scattered among the trapezoid fascicles and a more compact dorsal nucleus, medial to the superior olivary complex. The nucleus lies at the level of the exiting abducent nerve roots, anterior to the central tegmental tract. It is uncertain if the human trapezoid nuclei function in the auditory relay. Some trapezoid axons may enter the medial longitudinal fasciculus, ascending to end in trigeminal, facial, oculomotor, trochlear and abducent nuclei, mediating reflexes involving the stapedius, tensor tympani and extraocular muscles.

The *nucleus of the lateral lemniscus* consists of small groups of neurons among the lateral lemniscal fibres. Dorsal, ventral and intermediate groups probably receive afferent axons from both cochlear nuclei; their efferents enter the midbrain along the lateral lemniscus and terminate in the inferior colliculi (Geniec & Morest 1971) (**8**.125, p. 1071). Total neuronal counts of 18 000–24 000 have been recorded in human lemniscal nuclei (Ferraro & Minckler 1977a,b).

Efferent cochlear axons travel in the cochlear nerves to the spiral organ (Held 1863; Rasmussen 1967). Though few (about 500 in cats), they may be involved in hearing, perhaps by inhibitory and excitatory reflexes via cochlear nuclei (Allanson & Whitfield 1955). Lateral inhibition has been demonstrated by unit recording at trapezoid levels. In the squirrel monkey (Carpenter et al 1987), all cochlear efferent neurons contain choline acetyltransferase (AChE) and some also colocalize leucine encephalin. They are located at the hilus and along the lateral border of the lateral superior olivary nucleus and lateral edge of the ventral trapezoid nucleus, probably corresponding to the AChE-positive medial periolivary nucleus in man (Paxinos et al 1990). Fibres from both sides proceed to both cochleae. Borg (1973) has confirmed projection to the cochlea, in rabbits, from neurons both dorsal and ventral to the superior olivary nucleus, describing also a descending connection from the inferior colliculus to the olivary complex (confirming Munzer & Wiener 1902). Since a descending projection from the medial geniculate body to the inferior colliculus has been demonstrated, a complete efferent corticocochlear pathway appears established (p. 1090).

Striae medullares of the fourth ventricle are an *aberrant cerebropontocerebellar* connection, in which arcuate nuclei (p. 1020), the pontobulbar body (p. 1022) and external arcuate fibres (p. 1021) are involved. Embryological evidence (p. 241) suggests that some neurons, migrating ventrally to the pons from the rhombic lip to form the pontine nuclei, remain near the fourth ventricle as the pontobulbar nucleus. Others migrate farther, scattered ventrally over much of the surface of the pyramids as precerebellar arcuate nuclei, just below the pons. Both groups may receive corticobulbar projections, descending to the arcuate nuclei in the pyramids with the corticospinal fibres. Axons from both arcuate groups spread round the medulla, above and below the inferior olive, their fascicles being superficially visible. All these fibres, collectively the external arcuate

fibres, enter the inferior cerebellar peduncle (**8**.131). Some so-called '*external*' arcuate fibres pass dorsally from arcuate nuclei through the medulla near its midline; near the floor of the fourth ventricle they decussate, turn laterally under the ependyma and enter the cerebellum through the inferior peduncle They constitute the striae medullares, also known as the *arcuatocerebellar tract* (**8**.123, 133, 135). This may end in the flocculus (Szentágothai 1965); some fibres are said to end in the pontobulbar nucleus but may be confused with its projection fibres: some may travel ventrally, usually visible on the surface in the *circumolivary fasciculus*, which skirts below the inferior olive. The fasciculus and pontobulbar nucleus have been found absent in pontine aplasia, a confirmation of their pontocerebellar association (Baumgarten 1959). Efferent circumolivary fibres, passing ventrally, join the arcuatocerebellar tract, also reaching the striae medullares to enter the contralateral inferior cerebellar peduncle. However, as noted (above), pontobulbar afferents have also been ascribed to the circumolivary fasciculus; the precise relations of efferent and afferent fibres to the fasciculus remains uncertain.

Abducent nucleus

The abducent nucleus is paramedian in the central grey matter, in line with the trochlear, oculomotor and hypoglossal nuclei with which it forms a *somatic motor column* (**8**.129). It lies ventromedial to the medial longitudinal fasciculus by which vestibular, cochlear and other cranial nerve nuclei, especially the oculomotor, connect with the abducent. Efferent abducent axons pass ventrally, descend through the reticular formation, trapezoid body and medial lemniscus and traverse the ventral pons to emerge at its inferior border (p. 1240) (**8**.138).

Facial nucleus

The facial nucleus is deeper, lying ventrolateral in the pontine reticular formation, posterior to the dorsal trapezoid nucleus; the trigeminal spinal tract and nucleus are dorsolateral. The facial nucleus receives both crossed corticonuclear fibres and a smaller ipsilateral number (p. 1243) and ipsilateral rubroreticular tract fibres. Axons of its large motor neurons form the facial nerve. At first they incline dorsomedially towards the fourth ventricle, below the abducent nucleus (**8**.138) and ascend medial to it near the medial longitudinal fasciculus, through which the facial may communicate with other cranial nerves. Its fibres now curve anterolaterally round the upper pole of the abducent nucleus, as the *geniculum of the facial nerve*, and descend anterolaterally through the reticular formation. Finally, they pass between their own nucleus medially and the spinal trigeminal nucleus. This unusual course provided apparent evidence for neurobiotaxis (p. 237). In 10-mm human embryos the nucleus lies in the floor of the fourth ventricle, in the branchial (special visceral) efferent column, and is above the abducent nucleus in the somatic efferent column. As growth proceeds, the facial nucleus migrates at first downwards, dorsal to the abducent, then ventrally to its final position. As it migrates its axons elongate, their subsequent course marking the path of migration.

The facial nucleus receives corticonuclear fibres for volitional control and (among other sources) afferents from its own sensory root (via the nucleus solitarius) and the spinal trigeminal nucleus. These infracortical afferents complete local reflex loops, as in the spinal segments.

Facial neurons are grouped; those innervating muscles in the scalp and upper face are dorsal and believed to receive bilateral corticonuclear fibres; the ventral group has a contralateral corticonuclear innervation and supplies lower facial musculature (Papez 1927; Buskirk 1945). The groups may represent discrete motor pools (p. 1243). Clinically, upper and lower motor-neuron lesions of the facial nerve are differentiated since the former results in paralysis confined to the contralateral lower face, the latter in a complete ipsilateral paralysis (Bell's palsy).

Salivary nucleus

The salivary nucleus is near the upper pole of the dorsal vagal nucleus, just above the pontomedullary junction (Lewis & Shute 1959) and near the inferior pole of the facial nucleus. It is customarily divided into *superior and inferior salivary nuclei*, sending secretomotor fibres to the salivary and lacrimal glands via the facial and glossopharyngeal nerves (pp. 1243, 1249).

Trigeminal spinal nucleus

The trigeminal spinal nucleus ascends in the lower pons, has the trigeminal tract immediately lateral, the lateral vestibular nucleus ventral, and is traversed by vestibular nerve fibres. The inferior cerebellar peduncle is lateral, but inclines dorsally as it ascends into the cerebellum. The nucleus continues rostrally to expand into the superior sensory trigeminal nucleus. The spinal 'tract' consists not of endogenous fibres but of descending axons from the trigeminal ganglion and is continuous below with the tract of Lissauer in the cord. Collaterals and terminals enter the spinal nucleus, which is continuous below with the spinal substantia gelatinosa. It is mainly concerned with the mediation of pain and thermal sensibility in the trigeminal area and shows well-established topographical organization (p. 1230); the projection pathway to cortex is summarized in **8.132**.

Other structures

In addition to the tracts already noted at lower levels, the lower pontine tegmentum contains the trapezoid body, lateral lemniscus and emerging fibres of the abducent and facial nerves. The *medial lemniscus* is ventral; its now transverse outline, a flat oval, extends laterally from the median raphe (**8.136, 137, 139**); its vertical fibres are traversed by horizontal trapezoid axons; it is laterally related to the *lateral spinothalamic tract* and *trigeminal lemniscus*. The latter originate from neurons of the contralateral spinal nucleus, serving pain and thermal sensibility in facial skin and mucosae of the conjunctiva, tongue, mouth, nose, etc. The lemnisci together here form a transverse band composed, in lateral order from the midline, of medial and trigeminal lemnisci, the lateral spinothalamic tract and lateral lemniscus (**8.108, 112, 140**).

The *trapezoid body* contains cochlear fibres (**8.140**), mainly from the ventral cochlear and trapezoid nuclei. These ascend transversely in the ventral tegmentum; traversing or passing ventral to the vertical medial lemniscal fibres, they decussate with the contralateral fibres in the median raphe. Below the emerging facial axons, the trapezoid fibres turn up into the *lateral lemniscus*, in the *ascending* auditory pathway (**8.140**).

The *medial longitudinal fasciculus* is paramedian, ventral to the fourth venticle, near the abducent nucleus and facial fibres ascending medial to this. It is the main 'intersegmental' tract in the brainstem, particularly for interactions between nuclei of extraocular muscles and the vestibular system (**8.141**). In the lower pons it receives fibres from vestibular and perhaps dorsal trapezoid nuclei through its peduncle. Vestibulocochlear contributions form its greater part (p. 1024).

A transverse section at an upper pontine tegmental level contains trigeminal elements (**8.139**) but otherwise shows no notable alteration.

Trigeminal motor nucleus

The trigeminal motor nucleus is in the reticular formation, under the lateral part of the floor of the fourth ventricle in line with trigeminal fibres traversing the ventral pons (**8.139**).

Principal (superior) trigeminal sensory nucleus

The principal (superior) trigeminal sensory nucleus is lateral to its motor nucleus, between it and the middle cerebellar peduncle, continuous below with the spinal nucleus of the trigeminal nerve. Secondary axons from it decussate to ascend in the trigeminal projection system to the thalamus (**8.132**).

The small *lateral lemniscal nucleus* is medial to its tract in the upper pons, receiving some lemniscal terminals; some of its efferent fibres enter the medial longitudinal fasciculus, others return to the lemniscus. It is a relay station in the auditory pathway (**8.140**) associated with the trapezoid nucleus.

Tegmental white matter in the upper pons contains the lateral lemnisci, replacing the trapezoid body; its dorsolateral parts are invaded by the superior cerebellar peduncles.

The *medial lemniscus* (**8.108, 139**), ventral in the pontine tegmentum, lies a little lateral to the median raphe and is joined medially by fibres from the principal trigeminal sensory nucleus serving proprioceptive, tactile and pressure receptors in its area. Dorsolateral are the trigeminal lemniscus and lateral spinothalamic tract, serving

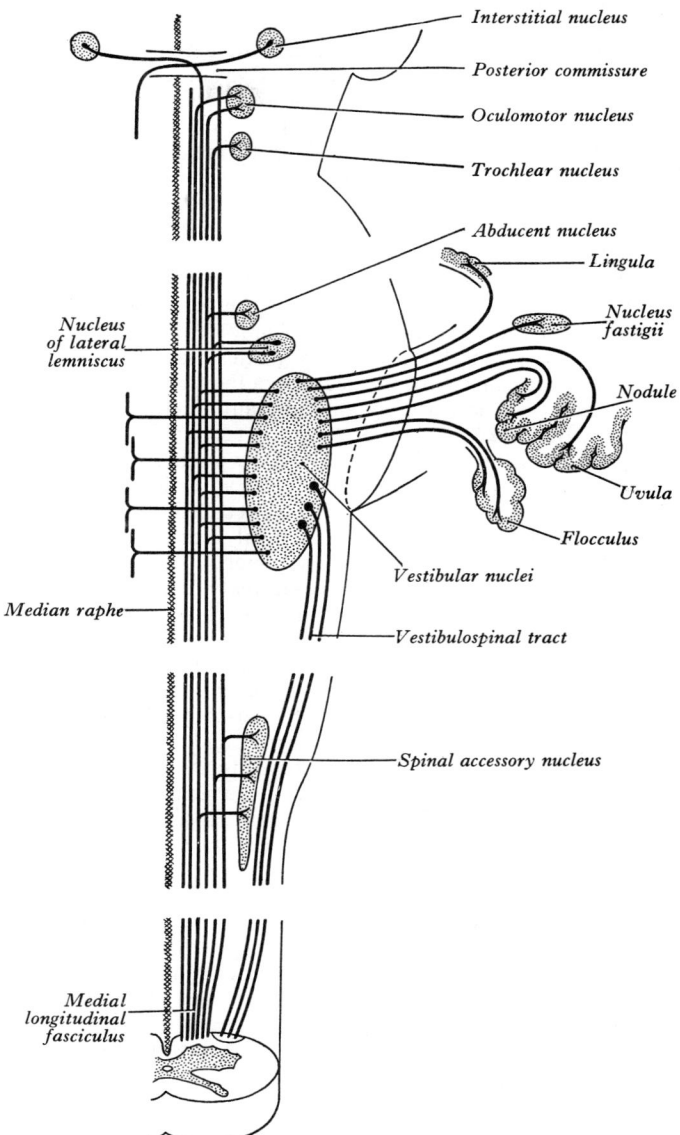

8.141 Simplified diagram of some of the components of the medial longitudinal fasciculus and of the distribution of its fibres to cranial nerve nuclei.

pain and thermal senses, and the lateral lemniscus and its nucleus. As the *lateral lemniscus* ascends it is near the dorsolateral surface of the brainstem. Above, its fibres enter the inferior colliculus and medial geniculate body (**8.132**). The *medial longitudinal fasciculus* (**8.141**) retains its paramedian position.

The *superior cerebellar peduncle*, a mass of fibres, many from the intracerebellar dentate nucleus (p. 1052) (**8.123, 139**), ascends into the lateral part of the roof of the fourth ventricle. It also inclines ventromedially into the dorsolateral tegmentum; the *ventral spinocerebellar tract* is closely associated with it. In the medulla it is dorsal to the olivary nucleus, separated from the surface only by anterior external arcuate fibres. In the lower pons it inclines dorsally between the trigeminal sensory nucleus medially and middle cerebellar peduncle laterally. Its fibres then recurve to descend dorsally into the cerebellum. It gives attachment to the anterior (superior) medullary velum laterally.

The *reticular formation* is continuous throughout the pons and is considered on pages 1073–1079.

CEREBELLUM

The cerebellum, the largest part of the hindbrain, is dorsal to the pons and medulla, its median region being separated from them by   **1027** the fourth ventricle. It occupies the posterior cranial fossa, covered by the tentorium cerebelli (p. 1210) and is roughly spherical, but somewhat constricted in its median region and flattened, the greatest diameter being transverse. The average weight of the cerebellum in males is about 150 g. In adults the ratio of cerebellum to cerebrum is about 1 to 10, in infants about 1 to 20.

The cerebellum is part of a side loop to major circuits linking sensory to motor areas of the brain. It receives sensory information through spinal, trigeminal, and vestibulocerebellar pathways and via the pontine nuclei, from the cerebral cortex and the tectum. The output of the cerebellum is almost exclusively to those structures of the brain which control movement. Although the human cerebellum comprises only about one-tenth of the entire brain by weight, the surface area of the cerebellar cortex, if unfolded, would be about half that of the cerebral cortex; much greater than the 10% might imply. The great majority of the neurons in the cerebellar cortex are the small and extremely densely packed granule cells. Granule cells are so densely packed that the cerebellar cortex contains many more neurons than the cerebral cortex. Unlike the cerebral cortex, which has a large number of diverse cell-types which are arranged differently in different regions, there are only a few types of cells in the cerebellar cortex and these are interconnected in a highly stereotyped way. One region of the cerebellar cortex looks very much like another.

The cerebellum is required for the co-ordination of fine movement. In health, it provides corrections during motion which are the basis for precision and accuracy, and it is critically involved in motor learning and reflex modification. Disease of the cerebellum or its connections leads to inco-ordination. Movements of the eyes, speech apparatus, individual limbs and balance are usually affected resulting in nystagmus, dysarthria, inco-ordination, and ataxia. All these movements become defective in widespread disease of the cerebellum or its connections but topographical arrangements within the cerebellum lead to a variety of clinically recognizable disease patterns. In cerebellar hemisphere disease, the ipsilateral limbs show rhythmical tremor during movement, but not at rest. The tremor increases as the target is approached; reaching and accurate movements of the arm are especially difficult. Diseases which affect the ascending spinocerebellar pathways or the midline vermis have a disproportionate effect on axial structures leading to severe loss of balance. Lesions of outflow tracts in the superior cerebellar peduncles result in wide amplitude, severely disabling proximal tremor which interferes with all movements and may even disturb posture leading to rhythmic oscillations of the head or trunk so that the patient is unable to stand or sit without support. But although cerebellar lesions may initially cause profound motor impairment, a great deal of recovery is possible. There are clinical reports of large cerebellar

lesions caused by trauma or surgical excision, in which the initial symptoms improve progressively over time.

Although the basic structure of the cerebellum and its importance for normal movement have been recognized for many years, many of the details of how it functions remain obscure. The goal of this chapter is to describe the known structure and connections of the cerebellum. Further understanding of the functions of the cerebellum in health and disease will ultimately be based on knowledge of the cells it contains, their neurochemical properties and their connections.

GENERAL FORM OF THE CEREBELLUM

Like the cerebral hemispheres, the cerebellum is covered by a cortex, which is a laminated sheet of neurons and supporting cells. The interior of the cerebellum consists of white matter, containing the cerebellar nuclei (8.146). If the cerebellar cortex is thought of as unrolled and flattened it is easier to visualize its major subdivisions (8.142–145). The cerebellum can be subdivided into medial–lateral, or anterior–posterior divisions. Midline cerebellum is called the *vermis* (Latin: a worm). The remainder of the cerebellar cortex constitutes the *cerebellar hemispheres*. Vermis and hemispheres are separated by the *paramedian sulci*. Orthogonal to this scheme of subdivisions, the cerebellum is divided by the deep transverse primary fissure into the *anterior* and *posterior lobes*, each of which can be further subdivided into lobules and folia.

The cortical surface of the cerebellum is very extensive. Ventrally the cerebellum borders on the fourth ventricle, which penetrates as a transverse cleft (*fastigium*: a sloping roof) into the cerebellar white matter. The ventricular surface of the cerebellum is relatively small and covered with ependyma (8.151). Caudally, where the cerebellar cortex and the ventricular surface meet, the ependymal roof of the fourth ventricle is attached to the cerebellum (the taenia of the fourth ventricle).

The white matter in the rostral wall of the fastigium is known as the *anterior medullary velum* (8.147). The anterior (or superior) medullary velum extends as a thin sheet beyond the cerebellum in the roof of the rostral part of the fourth ventricle. Laterally the anterior medullary velum is bordered by the massive, superior cerebellar peduncles. Rostrally, at the border with the tectum, the anterior medullary velum contains the decussation of the trochlear nerve. The caudal part of the velum is covered by cerebellar cortex of the lingula (8.149).

The superior surface of the cerebellum, which would constitute the anterior part of the unrolled cerebellar cortex, is relatively flat. The paramedian sulci are shallow and the borders between vermis and hemispheres are indicated by kinks in the transverse fissures.

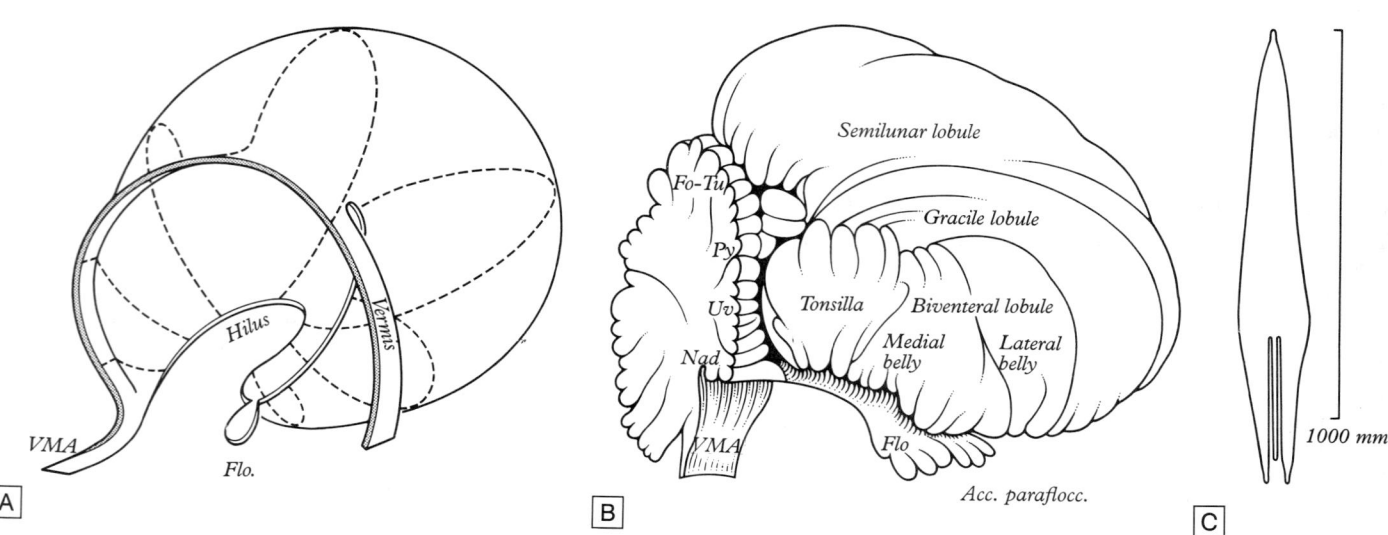

8.142 A. Diagram of the cortical sheet of the right half of the human cerebellum, as viewed from the medial side. For graphic purposes, the discontinuous portion of the cortex of the vermis is bent posteriorly. Dotted lines show the direction of the folia. The midline margin of the cerebellar cortical sheet is cut. (From Braitenberg and Atwood, 1958).
B. Right half of the human cerebellum. From Voogd (1967).

C. Plane representation of the human cerebellar cortical sheet, in which the maximum length and width of the unfolded cortical sheet are represented in their true proportions (about 7:1). From Braitenberg and Atwood (1958). Acc p flocc = accessory paraflocculus; Fo = folium vermis; Nod = nodule; Py = pyramis; Tu = tuber vermis: Uv = uvula; Vma = anterior medullary velum.

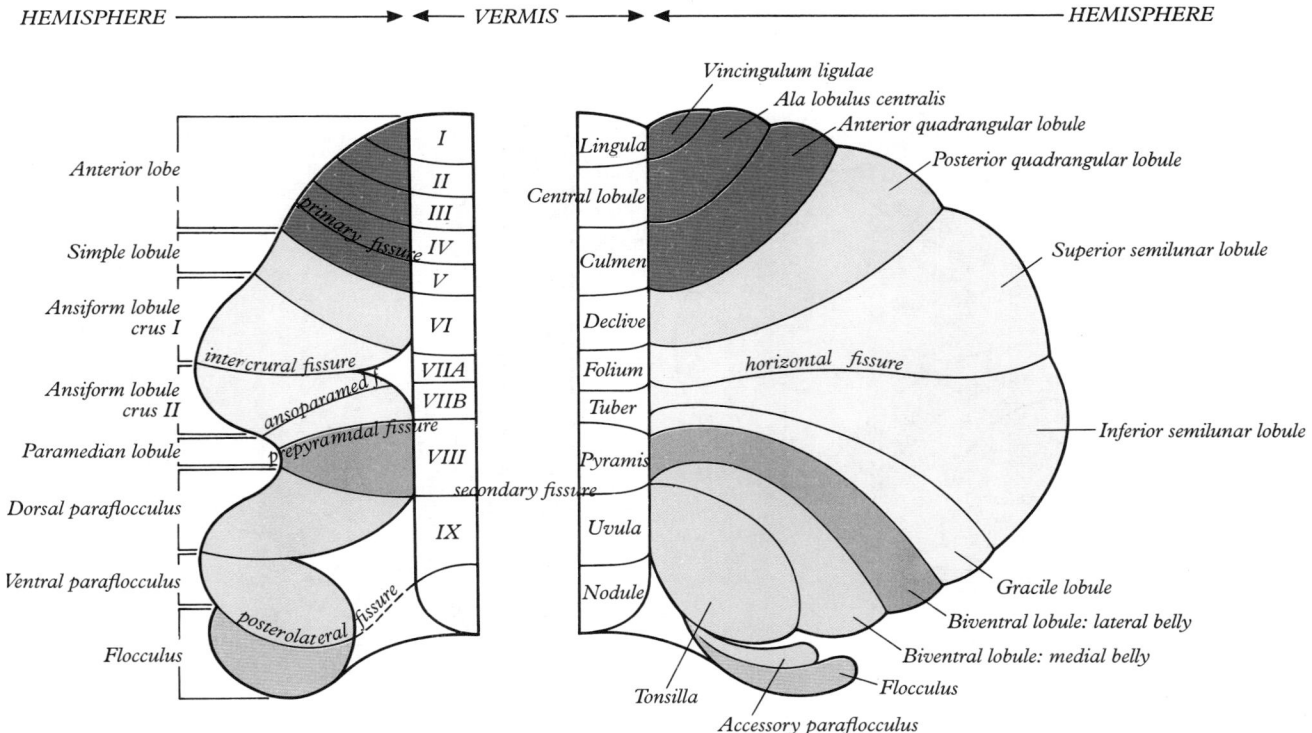

8.143 Diagram of the flattened cerebellar surface showing Bolk's comparative anatomical nomenclature for the lobules of the cerebellar hemisphere and Larsell's roman numerals (I–X) for the lobules of the vermis (left panel) and the human gross anatomical nomenclature for the lobules of the cerebellum (right panel). Corresponding lobules are indicated with the same colours.

The superior surface adjoins the tentorium cerebelli and projects beyond its free edge. The transverse sinus borders the cerebellum at the point where the superior and inferior surfaces meet. The inferior surface is characterized by a massive enlargement of the cerebellar hemispheres, which extend medially to overlie some of the vermis. Deep paramedian sulci demarcate the vermis from the hemispheres. Dorsally the hemispheres are separated by the *posterior cerebellar notch*, deep, narrow, and containing the dural *falx cerebelli*. The inferior cerebellar surface adjoins the occipital squama. The shape of the ventral surface is irregular. It includes the narrow ventricular surface of the cerebellum which extends laterally as the roof of the lateral recess. Rostrally the area of the cerebellar peduncles borders

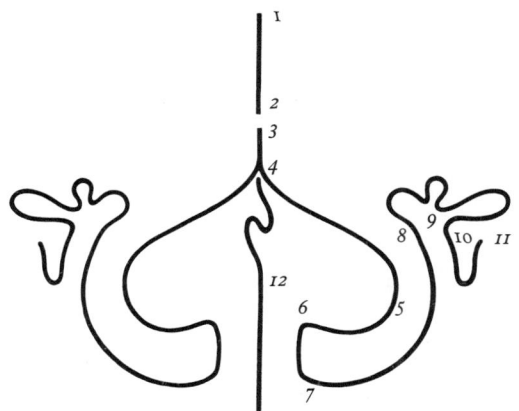

8.144 Bolk's schematic diagram of the relationship between the folial chains of the vermis and the hemispheres. Vermis and hemispheres cannot be separated in the anterior lobe (1–2) and the lobulus simplex (3–4). The posterior lobe vermis (12) and hemisphere (4–11) behave like two independent folial chains. The lobules of the posterior lobe correspond to the following line segments: 4–5: crus I of the ansiform lobule; 5–6: crus II of the ansiform lobule; 6–7: paramedian lobule; 7–10 paraflocculus (Bolk's crus circumcludens); 10–11: flocculus (Bolk's uncus terminalis). (From Bolk 1906.)

on the ventricular surface of the cerebellum. Ventrally the cerebellum adjoins the posterior surface of the *petrosal temporal bone.*

SURFACE CEREBELLAR TOPOGRAPHY

The cerebellar surface is divided by numerous curved, transverse fissures, giving it a laminated appearance and separating its folia. Deeper fissures divide it into lobules. One conspicuous fissure, the *horizontal fissure*, extends around the dorsolateral border of each hemisphere from the middle cerebellar peduncle to the posterior cerebellar notch separating the superior and inferior surfaces. Although the horizontal fissure is prominent, it appears relatively late in embryological development, and it does not mark the boundary between major functional subdivisions of the cerebellar cortex.

Superior surface (8.148, 149)

The deepest fissure in the vermis is the *fissura prima*, or *primary fissure*. The fissure curves ventrolaterally around the superior surface of the cerebellum to meet the horizontal fissures. The fissura prima is identifiable in virtually all mammals, appears early in embryological development and marks the boundary between the anterior and posterior lobes.

Because the cerebellar cortex has a roughly spherical shape, the true relations between its parts can sometimes be obscured. Thus, the most anterior lobule of the cerebellar vermis, the *lingula*, lies very close to the most posterior lobule, the *nodulus*. As a convention the term anterior will be used to refer to an 'unrolled' cerebellum when discussing its fissures and subdivisions.

Deep fissures divide the superior vermis into lobules. The lobules of the superior vermis in sequential order from anterior are called *lingula, central lobule, culmen, declive* and *folium vermis*. Each, except the lingula, is continuous bilaterally with an adjoining lobule in each hemisphere (8.149, 150). The fissura prima marks the boundary between the culmen which is the caudalmost lobule of the anterior lobe and declive which is the most rostral lobule of the posterior lobe. The lingula is a single lamina of four or five shallow folia, its white core continuous with the anterior medullary velum. The next

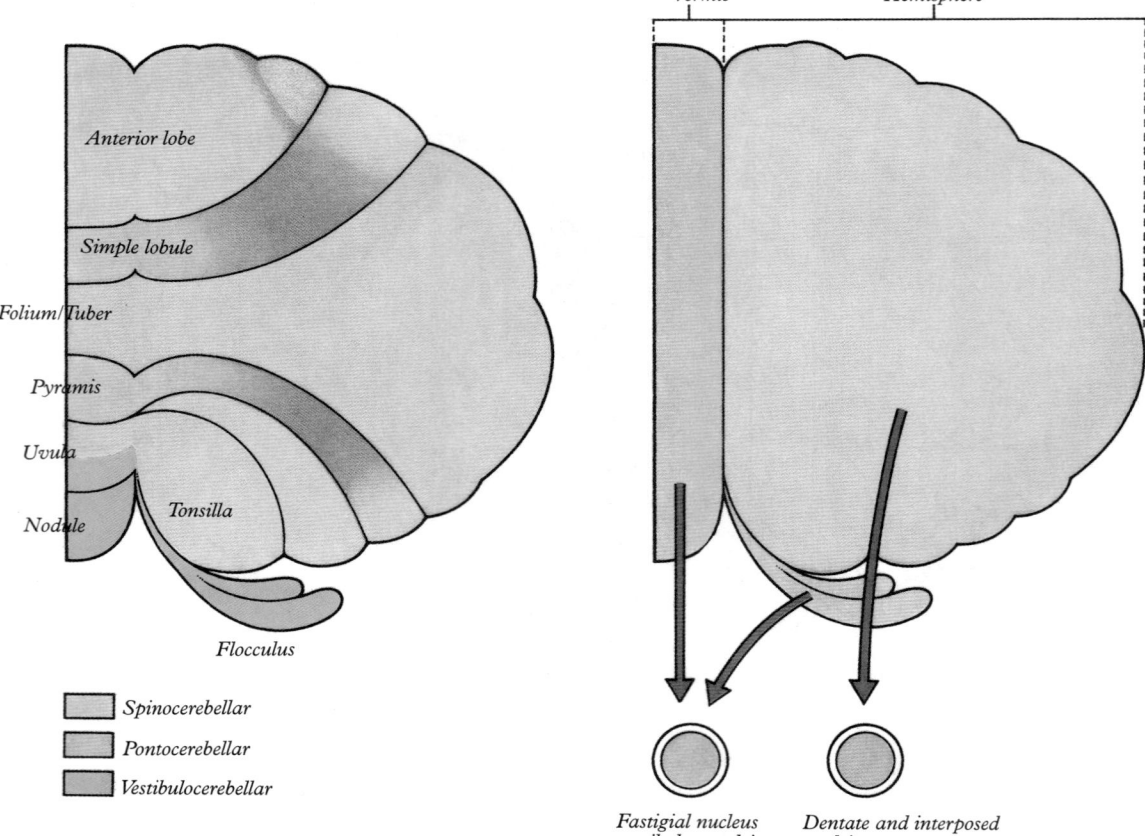

Vermis *Hemisphere*

Anterior lobe

Simple lobule

Folium/Tuber

Pyramis

Uvula

Tonsilla

Nodule

Flocculus

Spinocerebellar

Pontocerebellar

Vestibulocerebellar

Fastigial nucleus
vestibular nuclei

Dentate and interposed
nuclei

8.145 Diagrams of the flattened cerebellar surface showing two modes of functional subdivision of the cerebellum. The left panel illustrates the transverse, lobular organization of the afferent spino-, ponto- and vestibulo- cerebellar connections of the cortex. In the right panel the longitudinal zonal organization of the efferent connections of the cortex of vermis and hemispheres with the cerebellar and vestibular nuclei is indicated.

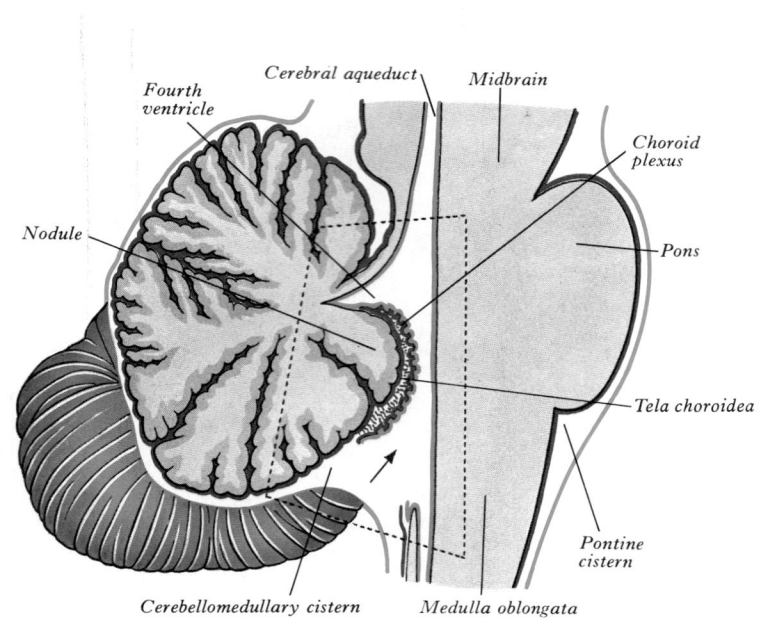

Cerebral aqueduct

Fourth ventricle

Midbrain

Choroid plexus

Nodule

Pons

Tela choroidea

Pontine cistern

Cerebellomedullary cistern

Medulla oblongata

8.146 Sagittal section through the brain stem and the cerebellum close to the median plane. The black arrow is placed in the median aperture of the fourth ventricle. Blue = arachnoid mater; Red = pia mater; Green = ependyma.

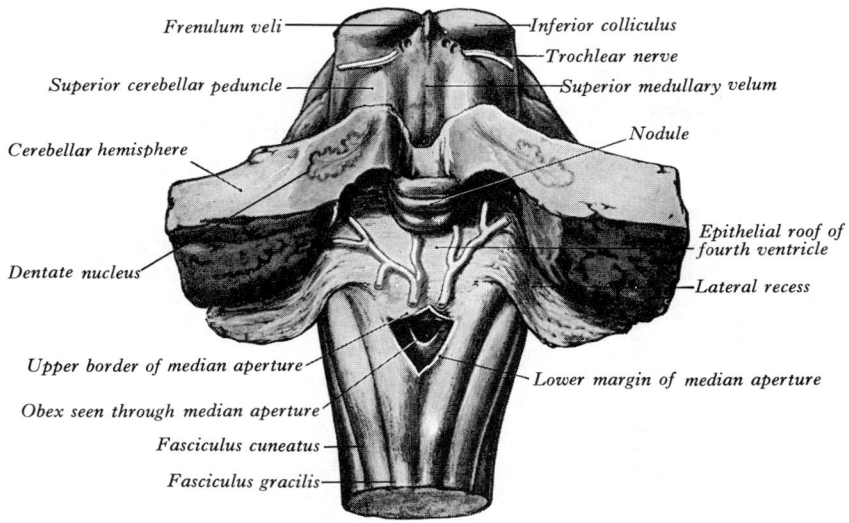

8.147 Dorsal aspect of the roof and the lateral recesses of the fourth ventricle, exposed by removal of part of the cerebellum.

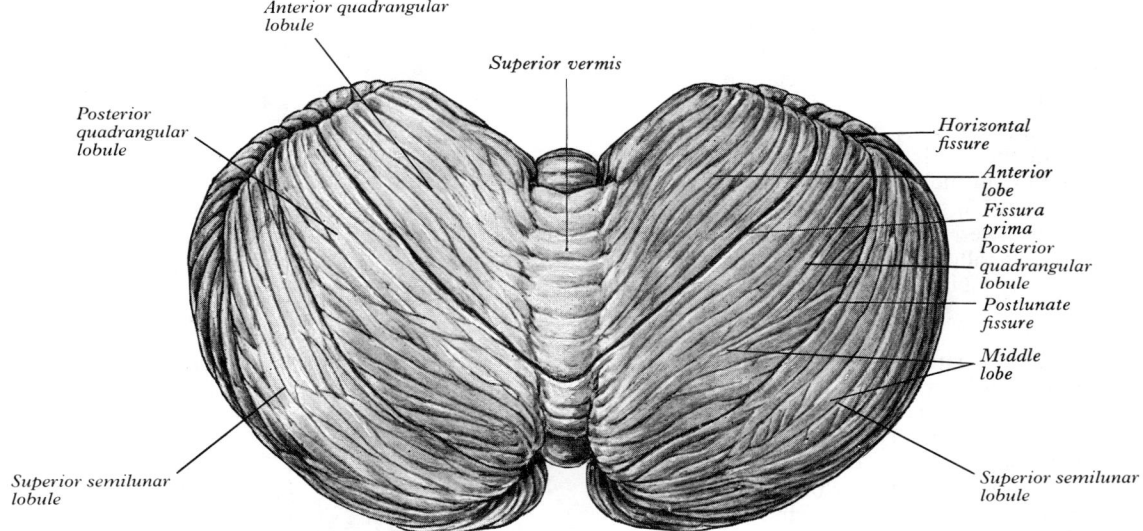

8.148 Superior aspect of the cerebellum to show major fissures and lobes.

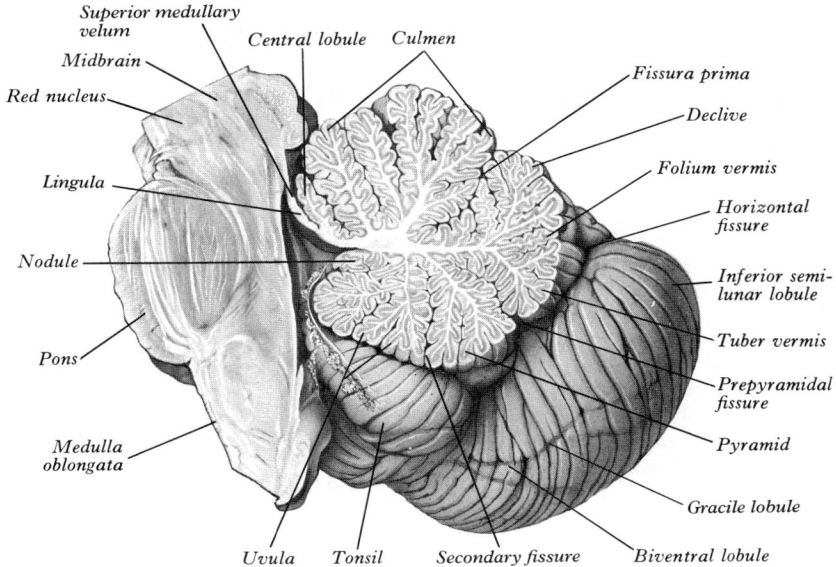

8.149 Median sagittal section of the cerebellum and brain stem.

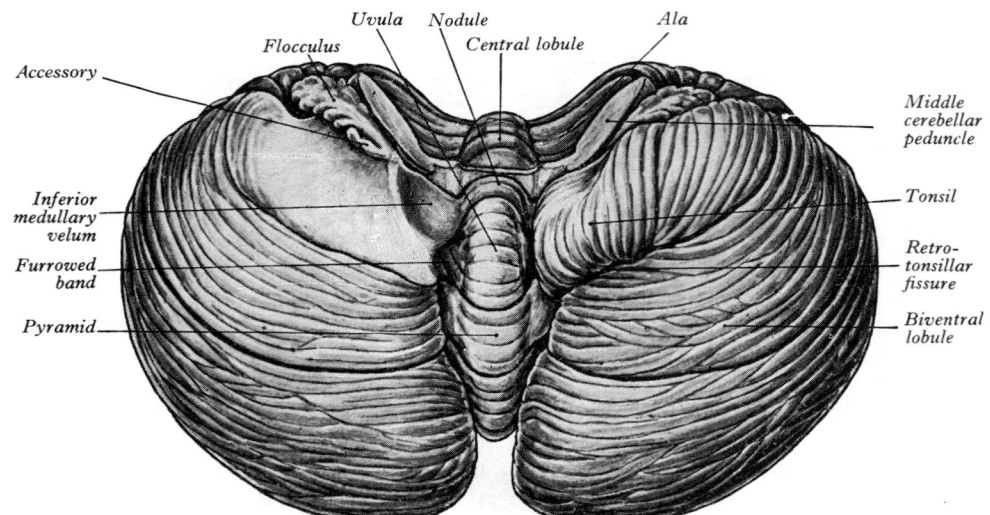

8.150   Inferior aspect of the cerebellum. The tonsil and the adjoining part of the biventral lobule of the right side have been removed.

lobule is the central lobule which is separated from the lingula by a *postlingual fissure*. The central lobule is continuous on each side with its alae and bounded caudally by the *postcentral fissure*. Between the postcentral fissure and the fissura prima is the culmen and laterally the anterior quadrangular lobules.

The region just behind the primary fissure consists of the declive and the posterior quadrangular lobule. Bolk (1906) called them jointly the *lobules simplex*, to indicate the lack of a clear division into vermis and hemispheres in this region, which makes it appear similar in structure to the anterior lobe. Caudal to the declive is the narrow folium vermis. Laterally the folium vermis is connected to the wide superior semilunar lobule.

Inferior surface (8.150)

The inferior vermis is divided into the *tuber vermis, pyramis, uvula* and *nodule*, in that order. The vermian tuber is continuous laterally with the inferior semilunar and gracile lobules which are bounded rostrally by the horizontal fissure. The tuber vermis is bounded caudally by the *prepyramidal fissure*. The pyramid is separated from the uvula by the *postpyramidal fissure (fissura secunda)* and is continuous laterally with a biventral lobule, visible on each inferior hemispheric surface. Behind the uvula, separated by the median part of the *posterolateral fissure*, is the nodule.

The *tonsil* is a roughly spherical lobule located on the inferior aspect of the hemisphere of the posterior lobe. It is separated from the biventral lobule by the deep retrotonsillar fissure. The cortex of the tonsil is continuous with that of the biventral lobule in the depth of this fissure. Medially the tonsil is connected with the uvula by a strip of cortex in the floor of the paramedian sulcus, the *furrowed band* (8.150). Adjacent to the furrowed band, the cortex between the pyramis and the tonsil is interrupted by white matter coming to the surface.

The *flocculus* is a small cerebellar lobule, located caudal to the tonsil, applied to the caudal surface of the *brachium pontis* (middle cerebellar peduncle). It is located in the roof of the lateral recess of the fourth ventricle, and dorsal to the cochlear nuclei and the stato-acoustic nerve, which are situated ventral to the recess. A small folial rosette between the flocculus and the tonsil is known as the *accessory paraflocculus of Henle* (8.150).

The *nodule*, the last of the vermian divisions, is separated from the uvula by the posterolateral fissure. Where its cortex ends it forms the attachment (taenia) of the ependymal roof of the fourth ventricle. Lateral to the nodule the floor of the paramedian sulcus is formed by a sheet of white matter, known as the *posterior medullary velum*, which extends beneath the tonsil, between the nodule and the flocculus (8.147). The internal surface of the velum is the *ventricular ependyma*; its outer surface is covered by *pia mater* (8.151). The taenia of the fourth ventricle continues from the nodule, along the caudal margin of the posterior medullary velum, onto the flocculus.

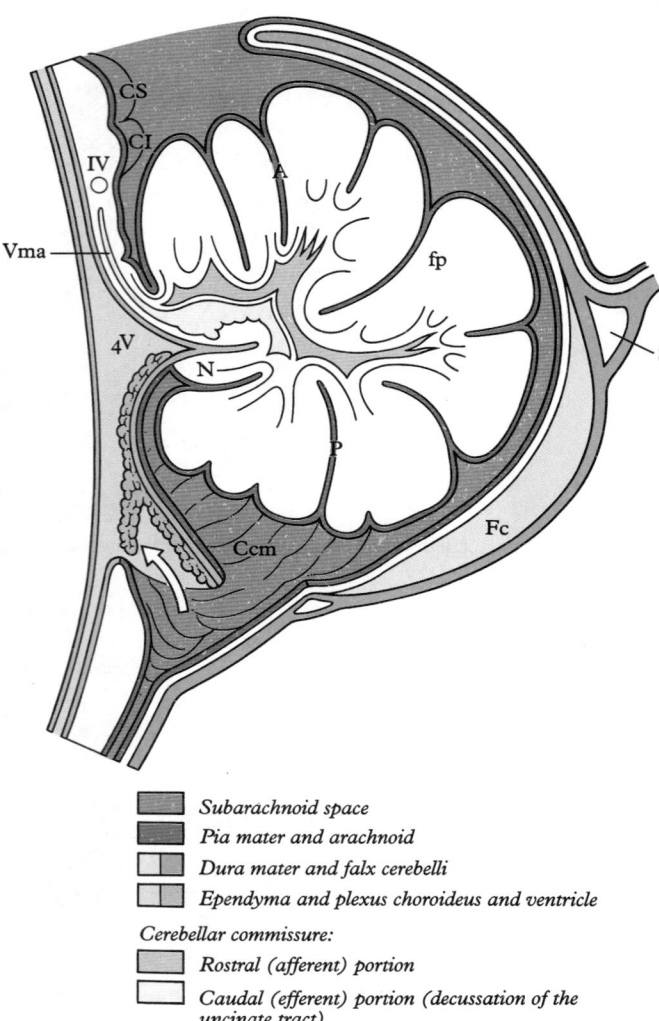

Subarachnoid space
Pia mater and arachnoid
Dura mater and falx cerebelli
Ependyma and plexus choroideus and ventricle

Cerebellar commissure:

Rostral (afferent) portion
Caudal (efferent) portion (decussation of the uncinate tract)

8.151   Anatomical relationships between the cerebellum, the fourth ventricle, the meninges and the cisterna cerebello-medullaris. 4V = fourth ventricle; A = anterior lobe; Ccm = cisterna cerebello-medullaris; CI = inferior colliculus; CS = superior colliculus; cx = cerebellar commissure; Fc = falx cerebelli; fp = primary fissure; IV = decussation of trochlear nerve; N = nodulus; P = posterior lobe; St = transverse sinus; Tc = tentorium cerebelli; Vma = anterior medullary velum. The arrow points to the median aperture of the fourth ventricle of Magendie. Compare with 8.147.

Lobulation of the cerebellum according to the schemes of Bolk and Larsell

The Dutch anatomist Lodewijk Bolk (1906) established the fact that despite its lumps and folds there is a simple underlying plan of cerebellar cortical organization which can be applied to all mammals. He showed that the cerebellar cortex is a continuous but highly convoluted sheet. The vermian cortex is continuous from its anterior to its posterior end. In the anterior lobe, the vermis is continuous laterally with that of the hemispheres often without any obvious transition. Immediately behind the anterior lobe, in the first division of the posterior lobe, there is also continuity between vermis and hemispheres. In the remainder of the posterior lobe the continuity between vermis and hemispheres is broken in places. Although the medio-lateral continuity between the vermis and hemispheres may be broken, the cortex of the hemispheres, like that of the vermis, is continuous in the rostrocaudal direction, although its complex folding makes it hard to follow the continuity. It was Bolk's major contribution to establish that even in the most convoluted hemispheres of mammals the cerebellar cortex is basically a continuous sheet. The continuity between vermis and hemispheres in the anterior lobe is obvious. In the region of the posterior lobe, which lies just behind the primary fissure, there is a similar continuity between vermis and hemispheric cortex which led Bolk to call this region the lobulus simplex, or simple lobule.

Bolk's nomenclature (8.143, 144)

In the human cerebellum and that of many other mammals the hemispheric cortex just behind the simple lobule forms a loop; bending first laterally and then curving back towards the midline. Bolk called this region of the cerebellum the *ansiform* or *loop-shaped lobule*. He named the laterally directed loop *crus I*, the returning, medially directed, loop *crus II*. The next division of the cerebellar hemisphere lies parallel to the vermis hence it is called the paramedian lobe. Behind the paramedian lobe the hemispheres again bend outward and then back again towards the vermis. Bolk called this whole region the *formatio vermicularis*, a name which is no longer commonly used. The outwardly directed part of the loop and part of the returning loop is now called the *paraflocculus*. The very last folia of the cerebellar hemispheres constitute the flocculus.

The pattern of lobules and fissures which is seen in a midsagittal section formed the basis for Bolk's scheme of cerebellar subdivisions. In almost all mammals the fissura prima is the deepest fissure (8.149) and it divides the anterior from the posterior lobe. A smaller fissure, the posterolateral, separates the nodulus from posterior lobe.

Larsell's nomenclature

The vermis typically has a straightforward organization in which the transversely oriented fissures and folia follow one another in a regular way. The cerebellar hemispheres vary greatly among different species of mammals. In the anterior lobe the vermis is directly continuous with the hemispheres, often without an obvious boundary. The adjacent region of the posterior lobe, the simple lobule, resembles the anterior lobe in that the vermian cortex is directly continuous with the hemispheres. The remainder of the posterior lobes varies greatly among different species of mammals, and although the continuity between vermis and hemispheres is often broken. Larsell (1934, 1947, 1952) assumed that each hemispheric lobule can be related to one of the vermian lobules and he devised a numbering scheme which he applied to the vermis and hemispheres. Larsell prefixed the hemispheric component of each lobule with the letter H. Lobules I through V of Larsell constitute the anterior lobe. Lobule VI is lobulus simplex. The ansiform lobule is associated with vermian lobule VII (H VII) of Larsell. Similarly, the paramedian lobule, which lies parallel to the vermis and behind the ansiform lobule, is the hemispheric extension of lobule VIII (H VIII). The paraflocculus is partly the hemispheric extension of lobule VIII, partly lobule IX. The flocculus is the hemispheric extension of lobule X.

The comparative anatomical nomenclatures of Bolk and Larsell and the classical nomenclature of the human cerebellum are compared in 8.143.

FUNCTIONAL DIVISIONS OF THE CEREBELLUM

The division of the cerebellum into anterior and posterior lobes (8.145) is useful for descriptive reasons, but it does not have any immediate functional significance. A functional division of the cerebellum into a *corpus cerebelli*, with inputs from the spinal cord, the trigeminal and pontine nuclei, and a *flocculonodular lobe*, which has strong afferent and efferent connections with the vestibular nuclei, was introduced by Herrick (1924) and Larsell (1937). The concept of the flocculonodular lobe as the vestibulocerebellum is a useful approximation, but it should not obscure the fact that the vestibular nuclei are also connected with other parts of the cerebellum, and that there are important functional differences between vermis and hemisphere.

The corpus cerebelli can be subdivided into a rostrocaudal series of regions dominated by their spinal or pontine inputs (8.145). These regions correspond roughly to certain of the lobules which were described in the section on the gross anatomy of the cerebellum. The anterior lobe, the simple lobule, and the pyramis with the gracile lobule are the main recipients of spinal and trigeminal cerebellar connections. Pontocerebellar input dominates in folium and tuber vermis, in the uvula and in the entire hemisphere, including those regions of the hemisphere which receive a projection from the spinal cord.

The mediolateral subdivision of the cerebellum into vermis and hemispheres represents another functionally important mode of subdivision which is closely related to the output of the cerebellum (8.144, 145). In parallel with the development of the cerebral cortex in mammals there is a great increase in size of the cerebellar hemispheres, reflecting the importance of the corticopontocerebellar input and the efferent connections of the hemisphere, through the dentate and interposed cerebellar nuclei and the thalamus, to the cerebral cortex.

INTERNAL STRUCTURE OF THE CEREBELLUM: THE WHITE CORE, THE CEREBELLAR COMMISSURE AND THE CEREBELLAR NUCLEI

The white core of the cerebellum branches in diverging medullary laminae, which occupy the central part of the lobules and are covered by the cerebellar cortex. In a sagittal section through the cerebellum the highly branched pattern of medullary laminae is known as the *arbor vitae* (8.149). The white core consists of the efferents (Purkinje cell axons) and afferents of the cerebellar cortex. Fibres crossing the midline in the white core of the cerebellum and the anterior medullary velum constitute the *cerebellar commissure* (8.151). The commissure consists of an efferent portion, containing decussating fibres of the fastigial nucleus, and an afferent portion, containing fibres of the restiform body and the middle cerebellar peduncle. In neuroanatomy the word commissure may have two meanings. In one sense a commissure like the corpus callosum is thought of as connecting homotopic points on the two sides of the brain. In the cerebellum, commissural afferent and efferent fibres are simply crossing the midline. The cerebellum has no callosum-like commissure connecting haemotopic points on the two sides.

Laterally, the medullary laminae merge into a large, central white mass which contains the four *cerebellar nuclei* (**8.152, 153**). The most lateral and largest of these cerebellar nuclei is the *nucleus dentatus*, or *lateral nucleus*, medial to which are the smaller *nuclei emboliformis*, *globose* and *fastigii*. The emboliform, or anterior interposed nucleus, is continuous laterally with the dentate. The globose, or posterior interposed nucleus is located caudal and medial to the emboliform nucleus. It is continuous with the fastigial (medial or roof) nucleus, which is located next to the midline, bordering on the fastigium (roof) of the fourth ventricle. The globose and emboliform nuclei collectively are known as the *interposed nucleus.*

The nucleus dentatus (**8.153**), within the white core of its hemi-sphere, is an irregularly folded sheet of neurons which encloses a mass of white fibres largely derived from dentate neurons. The dentate resembles a leather purse, whose opening is directed medially. Through this so-called 'hilum' fibres stream out to form much of the superior cerebellar peduncle (**8.153–155**). The nucleus emboliformis partially covers the dentate hilum; the nucleus globosus is located on its dorsomedial side. Efferent fibres of the emboliform and globose nuclei also join the superior cerebellar peduncle.

A large proportion of the efferent fibres of the fastigial nucleus cross within the cerebellar white matter and the anterior medullary velum in the cerebellar commissure. After their decussation they constitute the *uncinate tract* (hook bundle) which passes dorsal to the superior cerebellar peduncle to enter the vestibular nuclei of the opposite side (**8.154, 155**). Uncrossed fastigiobulbar fibres enter the vestibular nuclei by passing along the lateral angle of the fourth ventricle. Some fibres of the fastigial nucleus ascend in the superior cerebellar peduncle.

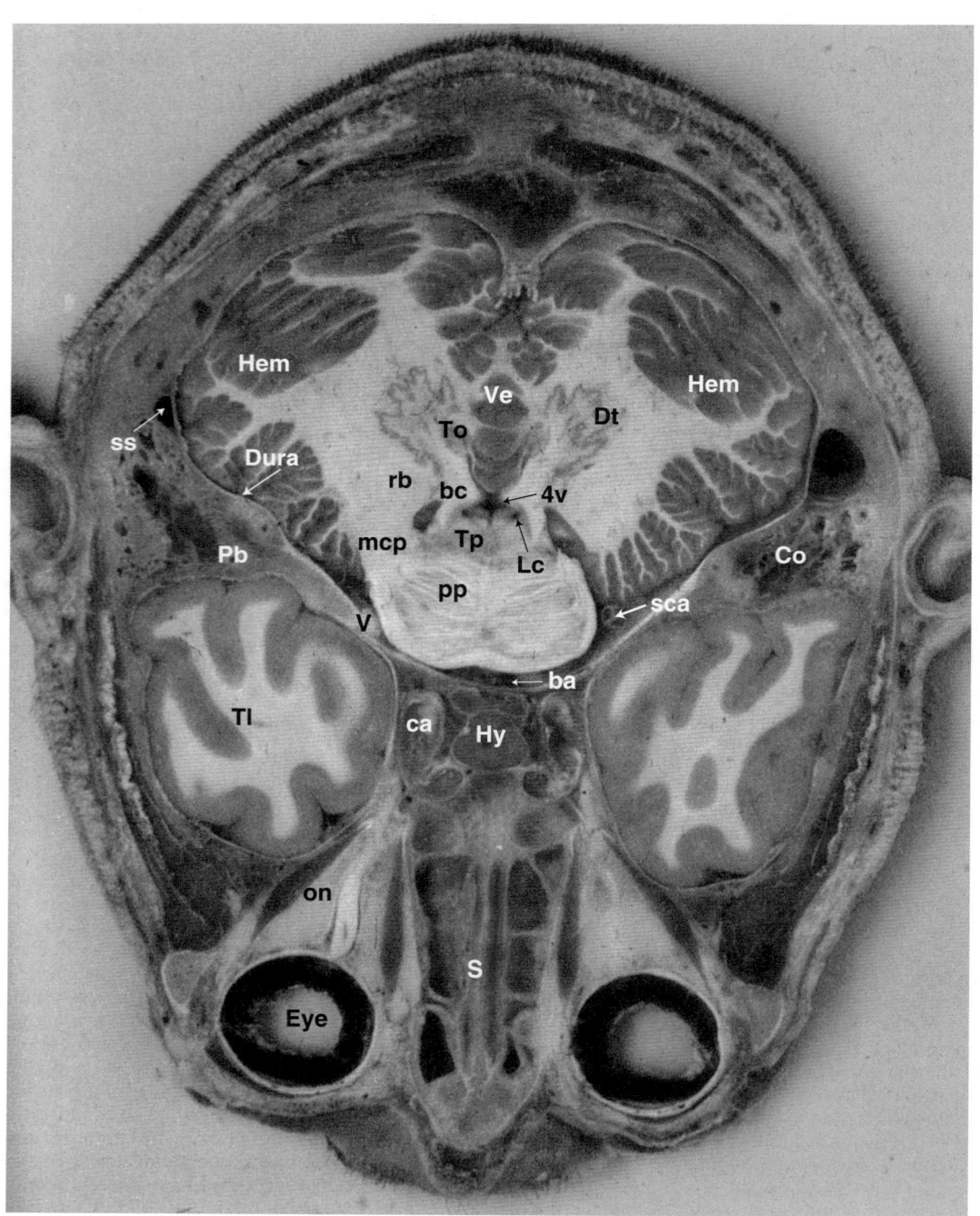

8.152 Horizontal section through the cerebellum and brain stem. Courtesy of Dr. G. J. R. Maat. Abbreviations:
4v = 4th ventricle;
ba = basilar artery;
bc = brachium conjunctivum;
ca = carotid artery;
Co = cochlea;
Dt = dentate nucleus;
Dura = dura mater;
Eye = eyeball;
Hem = cerebellar hemisphere;
Hy = hypophysis;
Lc = locus coeruleus;
mcp = middle cerebellar peduncle;
Pb = petrosal bone;
pp = pes pontis with pontine nuclei;
rb = restiform body;
S = nasal septum;
sca = superior cerebellar artery;
ss = sigmoid sinus;
Tl = temporal lobe;
Tp = tegmentum pontis;
V = trigeminal nerve;
Ve = vermis.

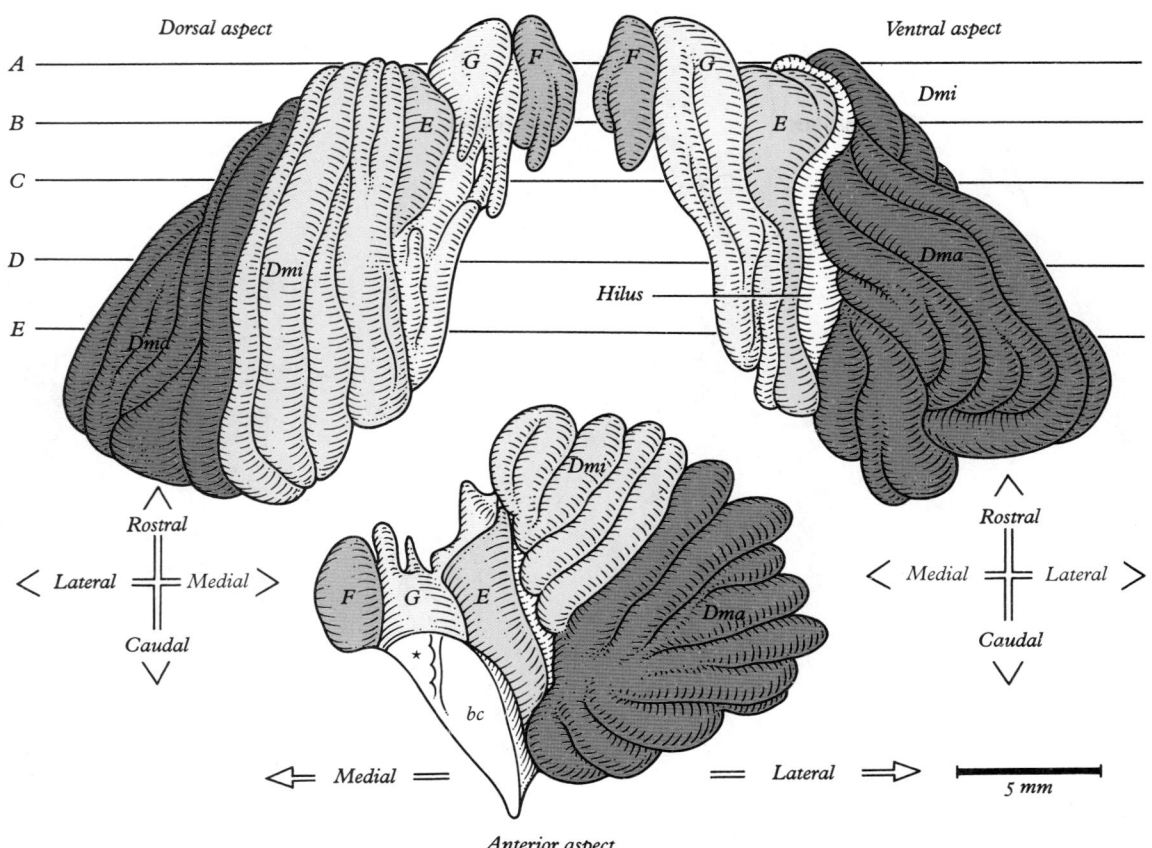

Dorsal aspect

Ventral aspect

Anterior aspect

8.153 Reconstruction (dorsal, ventral, and anterior views) of the central nuclei of the human cerebellum. The medial component of the brachium conjunctivum (bc) is indicated by an asterisk. (Redrawn from Voogd et al 1990.) F = fastigial nucleus; G = globose nucleus; E = emboliform nucleus; Dma = Ventrolateral, macrogyric part of dentate nucleus; Dmi = dorsomedial, microgyric part of the dentate nucleus.

CEREBELLAR PEDUNCLES

The attachment of the cerebellum to the brainstem is located rostral to the fourth ventricle and its lateral recess. Three peduncles connect the cerebellum with the rest of the brain (8.154, 155). In addition, the vestibular nuclei located in the floor of the fourth ventricle and the fastigial nucleus located in its roof, merge in this region around the lateral angle of the fourth ventricle. The *middle peduncle* passes obliquely from the basal pons to the cerebellum. It is the most lateral and by far the largest of the three peduncles. The middle peduncle is composed almost entirely of fibres of the basal pontine nuclei, with a smaller addition from nuclei in the pontine tegmentum. The *inferior cerebellar peduncle* is located medial to the middle peduncle. It consists of an outer, compact fibre tract, located on the dorsolateral aspect of the upper medulla (the *restiform body*; Latin: rope-like) and a medial portion, consisting of scattered fibre bundles which enter the cerebellum by passing through the vestibular nuclei (*juxtarestiform body*). The restiform body is a purely afferent system containing fibres from the spinal cord and the medulla. It consists of the *spinocerebellar, trigeminocerebellar, cuneocerebellar, reticulocerebellar* and *olivocerebellar tracts*. The juxtarestiform body is a mainly efferent system. Apart from the primary afferent vestibulocerebellar fibres of the vestibular nerve and secondary vestibulocerebellar fibres from the vestibular nuclei, it is made up almost entirely of efferent Purkinje cell axons from the vermis and the vestibulocerebellum on their way to the vestibular nuclei and the uncrossed fibres of the fastigial nucleus. The crossed fibres of the fastigial nucleus enter the brainstem as the uncinate tract at the border of the juxtarestiform and restiform body, after their passage dorsal to the superior cerebellar peduncle.

The *superior cerebellar peduncle* (8.146) contains all of the efferent fibres from the dentate, emboliform and globose nuclei and a small fascicle of the fastigial nucleus. The superior cerebellar peduncle decussates in the caudal mesencephalon. Although the superior peduncle consists mainly of efferent fibres from the cerebellar nuclei, some spinocerebellar fibres pass ventral and rostral to the entrance of the trigeminal nerve and enter the cerebellum in this peduncle. Within the cerebellum these afferent fibres join the spinocerebellar fibres entering the cerebellum through the restiform body.

GENERAL CEREBELLAR DEVELOPMENT

The cerebellum develops from a dorsal ridge (rhombic lip) of the alar plate of the metencephalon, which constitutes the rostral margin of the diamond-shaped fourth ventricle (8.156). Initially the ven-

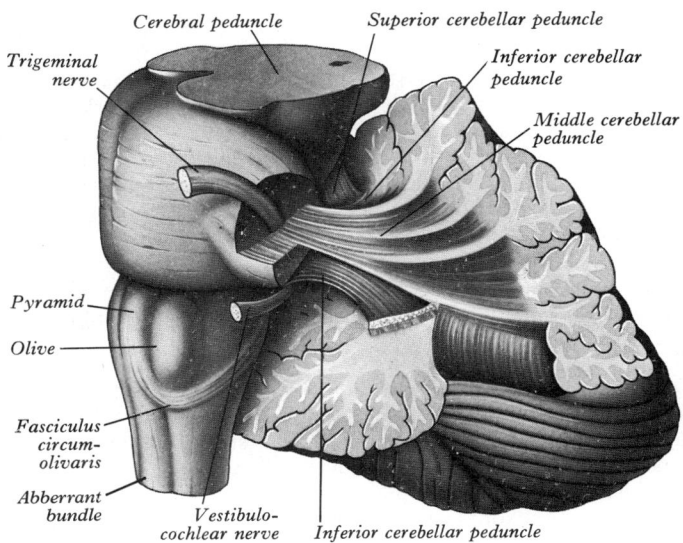

Cerebral peduncle
Superior cerebellar peduncle
Trigeminal nerve
Inferior cerebellar peduncle
Middle cerebellar peduncle
Pyramid
Olive
Fasciculus circum-olivaris
Abberrant bundle
Vestibulo-cochlear nerve
Inferior cerebellar peduncle

8.154 Dissection of the left cerebellar hemisphere and its peduncles (by Dr E B Jamieson, University of Edinburgh).

1035

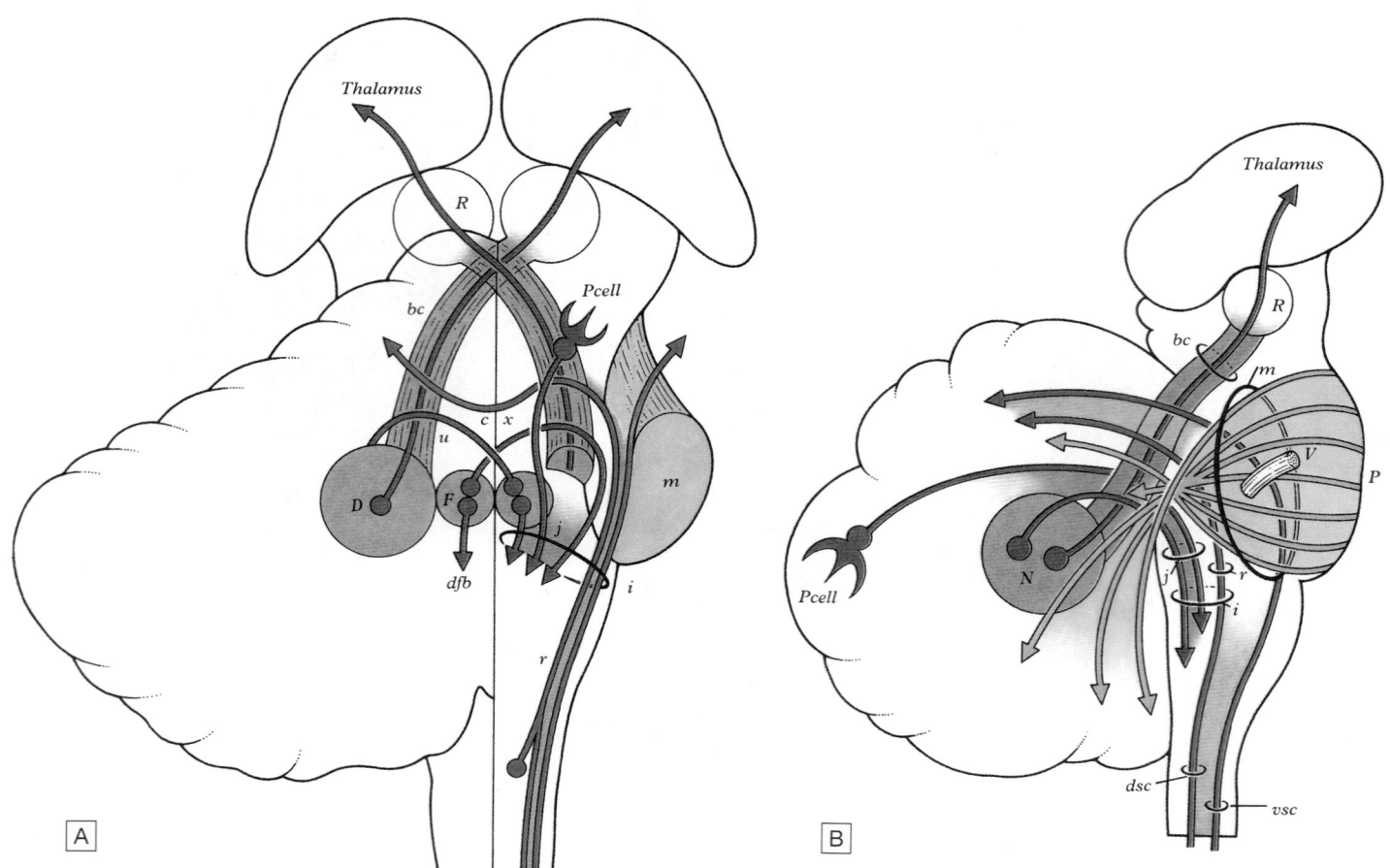

8.155 Diagrams showing the cerebellar peduncles in dorsal, A, and lateral, B, views. The inferior cerebellar peduncle (i) consists of the juxtarestiform body (j) and the restiform body (r). The juxtarestiform body is an efferent pathway, containing uncrossed fibres from the fastigial nucleus (dfb), the crossed uncinate tract (u) from the same nucleus, and axons from Purkinje cells of the cerebellar vermis (P cell). The restiform body (r) is an afferent pathway, containing fibres originating from the medulla oblongata and the spinal cord. The dorsal spinocerebellar tract (dsc) enters the cerebellum in the restiform body; the ventral spinocerebellar tract (vsc) passes rostral to the entrance of the trigeminal nerve (v) and enters the cerebellum more rostrally along the brachium conjunctivum. The brachium conjunctivum is the efferent pathway from the dentate and interposed nuclei (D in A). In B the dentate and the fastigial nucleus are represented by (n). bc = brachium conjunctivum; cx = cerebellar commissure; D = dentate and interposed nuclei; dcs = dorsal spino-cerebellar tract; dfb = direct (uncrossed) fastigiobulbar tract; F = fastigial nucleus; i = inferior cerebellar peduncle; j = juxtarestiform body; N = cerebellar nuclei; P = pontine nuclei; Pcell = Purkinje cell of the cerebellar vermis; r = restiform body; R = red nucleus; u = uncinate tract; V = trigeminal nerve; vsc = ventral spinocerebellar tract.

tricular surface of these ridges expands on both sides and the midline region retains its structure of a thin, epithelial roof plate. The bilateral expansion of the ventricular surface reflects the production by the ventricular epithelium of the *neurons of the cerebellar nuclei*, the *efferent neurons of the cerebellar cortex* (the Purkinje cells) and the *radial glia*. The radial glia play a role in guiding the Purkinje cells to the meningeal surface of the cerebellar anlage. Another group of cells is produced at the attachment of the roof of the fourth ventricle to the cerebellar anlage. These cells migrate over the meningeal surface, where they constitute the external germinative layer (**8.156**A). This layer does not start to produce cells till much later in development. At this stage the primitive cerebellar cortex consists of a multicellular layer of migrated *Purkinje cells* and the *superficial external germinative layer* (**8.156**B) The bilateral anlage is changed into a unitary structure by fusion of the bilateral intra-ventricular bulges and the disappearance of the ependyma at this site, the merging of the left and right primitive cerebellar cortex over the midline and the development of the cerebellar commissure by ingrowth of afferent fibres and the outgrowth of efferent axons of the medial cerebellar nucleus.

During this early stage of the cerebellar development, which is dominated by the production and migration of efferent cerebellar neurons, the surface of the cerebellar anlage remains smooth. At a later stage, which coincides with the period of cell production by the external germinative layer, the transverse folial pattern begins to emerge. The main cell type produced by the external layer is the *granule cell.* Millions of granule cells migrate inwards, from the cerebellar surface along the radial glia, through the layer of the Purkinje cells, to settle beneath the Purkinje cells in the granular layer (**8.156**c). Production of the granule cells leads to a great rostrocaudal expansion of the meningeal surface of the cerebellum, to the formation of transverse fissures and the transformation of the multicellular layer of Purkinje cells into a monolayer. Purkinje cells and nuclear cells are formed prior to the granule cells, and granule cells serve as the recipient of the main afferent (mossy fibre) system of the cerebellum. Thus the development of the efferent neurons of the cerebellar cortex and nuclei precedes the development of its afferent organization.

DEVELOPMENT OF LONGITUDINAL PURKINJE CELL ZONES

During the early stage of cerebellar development, when the Purkinje cells settle beneath the external germinative layer, the multicellular layer of Purkinje cells is not uniform, but subdivided into clusters, which form rostrocaudally extending columns (**8.157**). The medial Purkinje cell clusters develop into the future vermis. These Purkinje cells will grow axons which connect to neurons in the vestibular nuclei and the fastigial nucleus. The lateral clusters belong to the future hemisphere and will grow axons terminating in the interposed and dentate nuclei. The sharp border in the efferent projections from

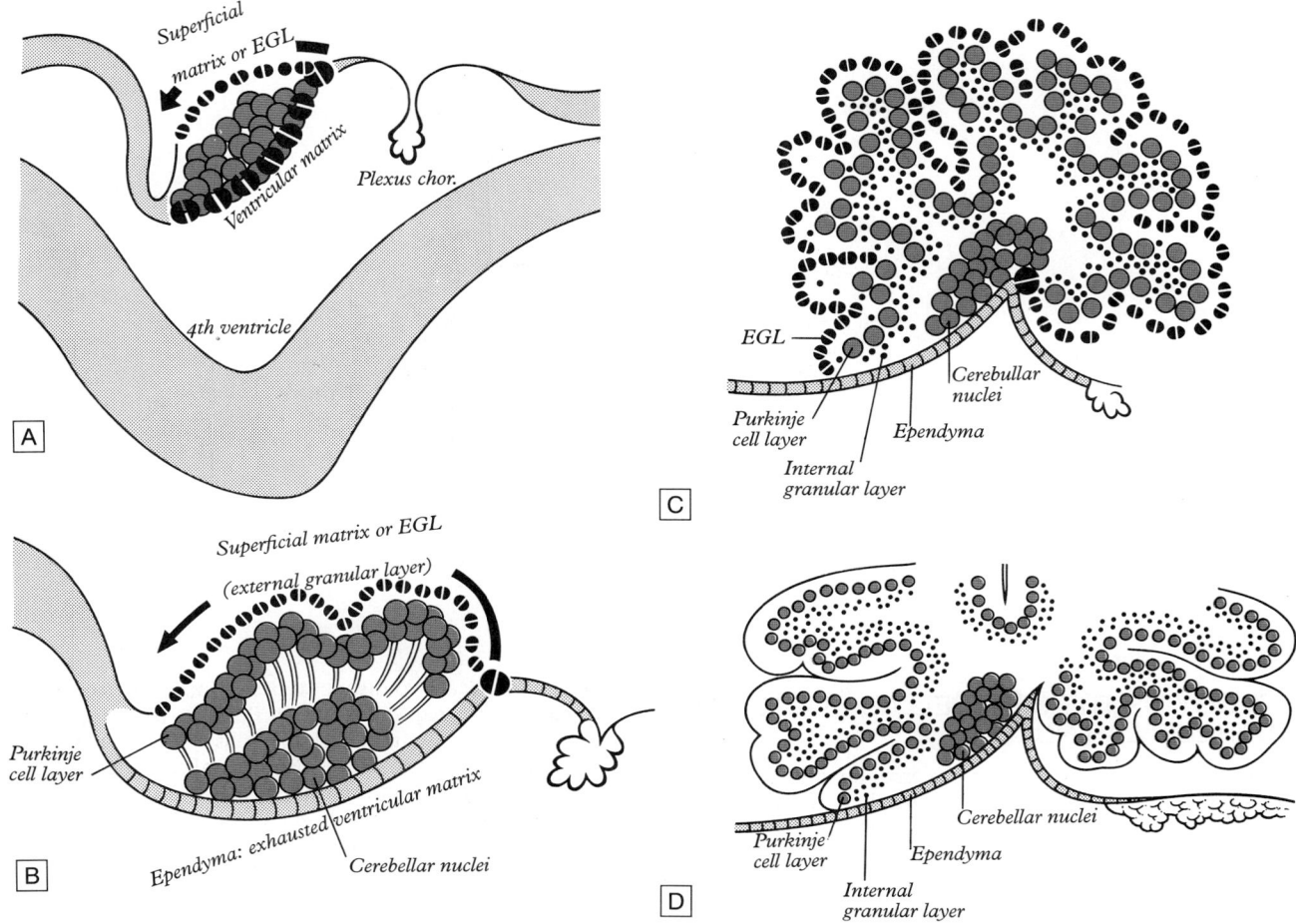

8.156 Four stages in the histogenesis of the cerebellar cortex and the cerebellar nuclei.
A. Purkinje cells and cells of the cerebellar nuclei are produced by the ventricular epithelium and are in the process of migration to their future positions. The cells of the superficial matrix (the external granular layer) take their origin from the ventricular epithelium at the caudal pole of the cerebellar anlage and migrate rostrally over its surface.

B. After migration the Purkinje cells constitute a multicellular layer, beneath the external granular layer. Cell production in the ventricular epithelium has stopped. The remaining cells transform into ependymal cells.
c. Granule cells are produced by the external granular layer and migrate inwards, through the Purkinje cell layer to their position in the granular layer. Purkinje cells spread into a monolayer.
D. Adult position of cortical and nuclear neurons.

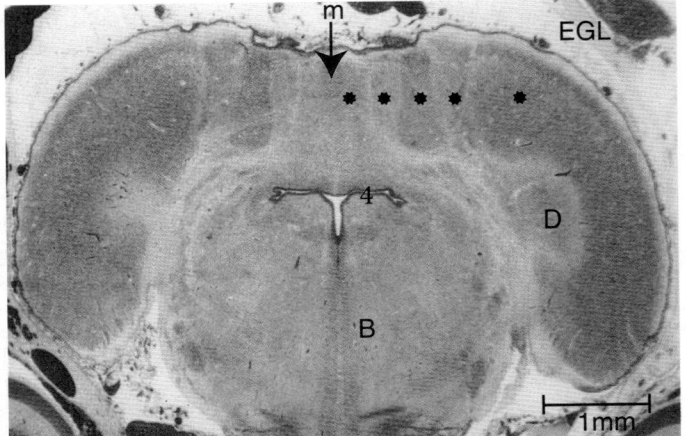

8.157 Photograph of a coronal section through the cerebellum and the brain stem of 65 mm human fetus. The Purkinje cells are located in 5 multicellular clusters (stars) on both sides of the midline. The anlage of the dentate nucleus occupies the centre of the most lateral Purkinje cell cluster. B = brain-stem; D = dentate nucleus; EGL = external granular layer; m = midline; 4 = fourth ventricle. (Schenk collection, Department of Pathology, Erasmus University, Rotterdam.)

the vermis and hemispheres is thus established at an early age. These clusters will give rise to Purkinje cell zones in the adult cerebellum which project to a single vestibular or cerebellar nucleus.

Development of fissures and lobes

The first fissure to appear on the cerebellar surface (8.158) is the lateral part of the posterolateral fissure which forms the border of a caudal region corresponding to the flocculi of the adult. The right and left parts of this fissure subsequently meet in the midline, where they form the boundary between the most caudal vermian lobule, the nodulus, and the rest of the vermis. The *flocculonodular lobe* can now be recognized as the most caudal cerebellar subdivision at this stage, which serves as the attachment of the epithelial roof of the fourth ventricle. Because of the expansion of the other divisions of the cerebellum the flocculonodular lobe comes to occupy an antero-inferior position in adults. As the third month ends, a transverse sulcus deepens to form the fissura prima, invading the vermis and both hemispheres and forming the border between the anterior and posterior lobes. About the same time, two transverse grooves appear in the caudal vermis. The fissura secunda forms the rostral border of the uvula; the prepyramidal fissure forms that of the pyramid (8.158). The cerebellum continues to expand dorsally, rostrally, caudally and laterally, the hemispheres enlarging much more than their adjacent vermian surface. Numerous other transverse grooves develop, most having little taxonomic significance; the most extensive is the horizontal fissure.

1037

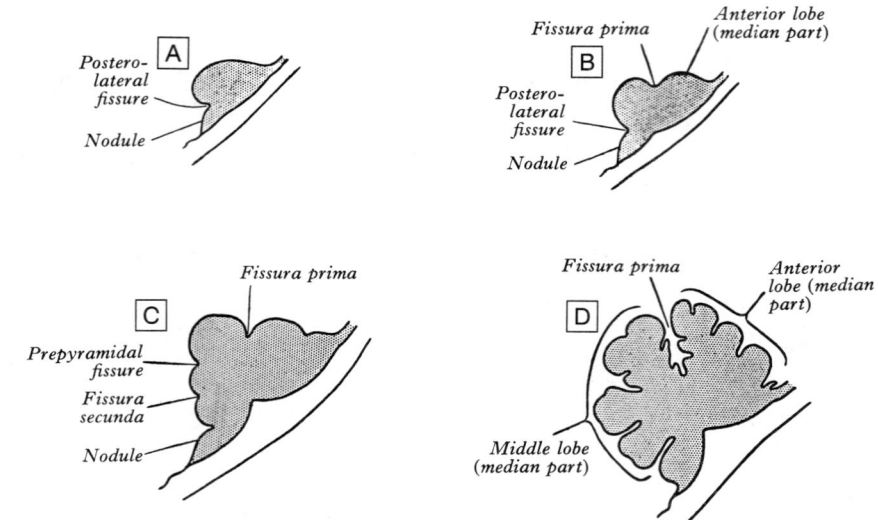

8.158   Median sagittal sections through the developing cerebellum at four successive stages.

HISTOLOGY OF THE CEREBELLAR CORTEX AND THE CEREBELLAR NUCLEI

The cerebellar cortex is folded by many predominantly transversely curved fissures, closely arranged, approximately parallel and varying in depth. The smallest laminae and their curved overlying cortex are the cerebellar folia. So complexly pleated is the cortex that its 'unfolded' dorsoventral (caudorostral) extent would exceed over a metre, and transversely measure about a sixth of this (**8.142c**) (Braitenberg & Atwood 1958). On first appearance the whole cortex appears almost uniform in microscopic structure. Local differences, obvious in the cerebral cortex, do not occur, and sections from different areas are indistinguishable. The same homogeneity obtains throughout all mammals and, with only minor differences, throughout the vertebrates.

The elements of the cerebellar cortex have a precise geometric order which is arrayed relative to the tangential, longitudinal and transverse planes in individual folia (**8.159**). It contains:

- the terminations of afferent 'climbing' and 'mossy' fibres
- five varieties of neuron: granular, outer stellate, basket, Golgi, and Purkinje (only the Purkinje cell axons leave the cortex, the other neurons are completely intrinsic)
- neuroglia and blood vessels.

The cerebellar cortex has three main strata, the *molecular layer*, the *Purkinje layer*, and the *granular layer*. Anatomical and physiological research on the cerebellar cortex has accumulated a wealth of data which can only be abbreviated here. For details and extensive bibliographies consult Jansen and Brodal (1954); Dow and Moruzzi (1958); Eccles et al (1967); Fox and Snider (1967); Llinas (1967); Larsell and Jansen (1972); Braitenberg and Atwood (1958); Palay and Chan-Palay (1982); Ito (1984); Glickstein et al (1987); Strata (1989).

The main circuit of the cerebellum involves the granule cells, the Purkinje cells and the cells of the cerebellar nuclei (**8.160, 8.161A**). Granular neurons receive one of the two main cerebellar cortical inputs, the terminals of the mossy fibre afferents (i.e. all afferent systems except the olivocerebellar fibres). The axons of the granule cells ascend to the molecular layer where they bifurcate into *parallel fibres*. Parallel fibres are so called because they are oriented parallel to the transverse fissures and perpendicular to the dendritic trees of the Purkinje cells on which they terminate. Purkinje neurons are large and are the sole output cells of the cerebellar cortex; their axons terminate on the cerebellar nuclei, and certain vestibular nuclei. In addition to the dense array of parallel fibres, the dendritic trees of Purkinje cells receive terminals from *climbing fibres* whose cells of origin are in the inferior olivary nucleus. The cerebellar

cortex thus has two distinct types of input: olivocerebellar climbing fibres which synapse directly on Purkinje neurons, and *mossy fibres* which connect to the Purkinje cells via granular neurons whose axons are the parallel fibres. Both parallel and climbing fibres excite the Purkinje cells, but they differ greatly in their firing characteristics and their effect on the Purkinje cells. Purkinje cell axons inhibit the neurons of the intracerebellar nuclei and constitute the sole output from the cerebellar cortex. Cerebellar nuclei, in turn, project to all the major motor control centres in the brainstem and cerebrum. The remaining neurons of the cerebellar cortex (external stellate, basket and Golgi cell (**8.161B**)) are inhibitory interneurons, connecting the cortical elements in complex geometrical patterns with the exception of the brush cell.

LAYERS OF THE CEREBELLAR CORTEX

Molecular layer. The molecular layer, about 300–400 μm thick, has a sparse population of neurons, dendritic arborizations, non-myelinated axons and radial fibres of the epithelial (Bergmann) glial cells. By ordinary histological technique, it is almost featureless, contrasting with the granular layer's immense cellular population. It contains the following elements (**8.161, 162**):

- Purkinje cell dendritic trees: these extend towards the surface and spread out in a plane, perpendicular to the long axis of the cerebellar folia. Purkinje cell dendrites are flattened. The lateral extent of the Purkinje cell dendrites is about 30 times greater in the transverse plane than it is in a plane parallel to the cerebellar folia.
- Parallel fibres: these are the axons of granule cells, the stems of which ascend into the molecular layer where they bifurcate at T-shaped branches. The two branches extend in opposite directions as parallel fibres along the axis of a folium. Parallel fibres terminate on the dendrites of the Purkinje cells and Golgi cells which they pass on their way, and on the basket and stellate cells of the molecular layer.
- Dendritic trees of Golgi neurons: these reach towards the surface. Unlike the flattened dendritic tree of the Purkinje cell, Golgi cell dendrites span the territory of many Purkinje neurons longitudinally as well as transversely. These dendrites receive synapses from parallel fibres. Some Golgi cell dendrites enter the granular layer where they are contacted by mossy fibre terminals. The cell bodies of Golgi neurons are below, in the superficial part of the granular layer.
- Somata, dendrites and axons of external stellate neurons: these are located superficially within the molecular layer.
- Somata, dendrites and axons from the basket cells: the somata of these lie deeper within the molecular layer.

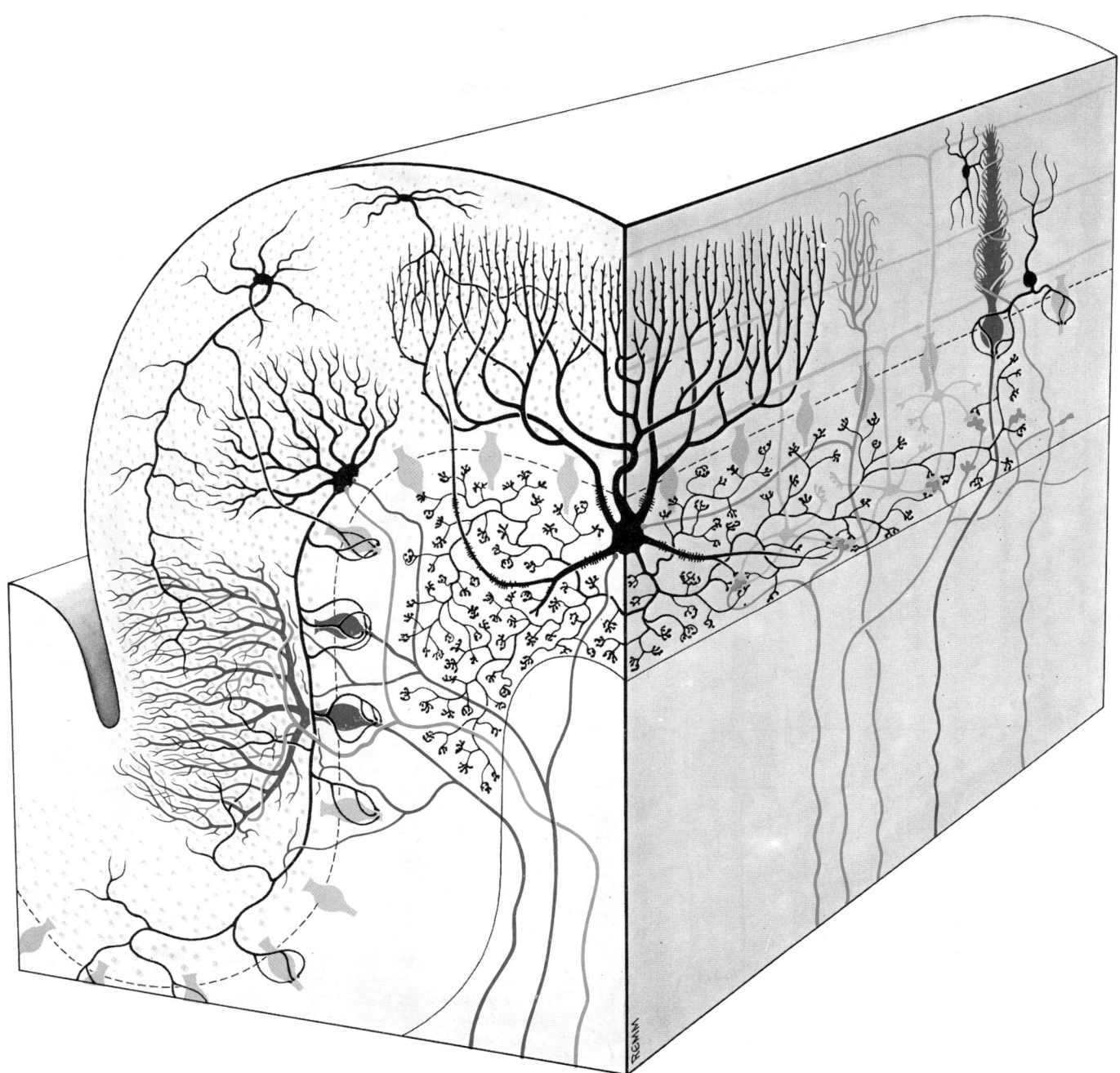

8.159   The general organization of the cerebellar cortex; a single cerebellar folium has been sectioned vertically, both in its longitudinal axis (right part of the diagram) and transversely (on the left). Red = Purkinje cells; black = inhibitory interneurons, including outer stellate, basket and Golgi cells; yellow = granule cells and their ascending axons which bifurcate into longi- tudinally disposed horizontal fibres; blue = climbing fibres and mossy affer- ents. Note also the synaptic glomeruli formed between the terminals of the mossy afferent fibres, the complex dendrite tips of the granule cells and the ramifications of the Golgi cell axon. (Redrawn from Eccles et al 1967 with the permission of the authors and publishers.)

- Climbing fibres: these are the terminals of olivocerebellar fibres which ascend through the granular layer to contact Purkinje dendrites in the molecular layer.
- Radiating branches from large epithelial (Bergmann) glial cells: these give off processes which surround all neuronal elements except at the synapses; at the surface their conical expansions join to form an external limiting membrane.

The general disposition of the above elements is summarized in 8.159, 161, 162.

Purkinje cell layer. The Purkinje cell layer contains the large, pear-shaped perikarya of the Purkinje cells. Smaller somata of epithelial (Bergmann) glial cells are located at this level. Clumps of granule cells and occasional Golgi cells penetrate between the Pur- kinje cell somata.

Granular layer. The granular layer (8.159) is about 100 μm thick in fissures and 400–500 μm on folial summits; it contains an enormous number of granular neurons: about 2.4 million per cubic millimetre in the simian cerebellar cortex, 2 to 7 million in the human cortex (Fox & Barnard 1957; Braitenberg & Atwood 1958). In the human cerebellum it has been estimated that there are a total of about 4.6×10^{10} granule cells (Zagon et al 1977) and about 3000 granule cells for each Purkinje cell (Lange 1975). In summary the granular layer consists of:

- the somata of granular neurons and their axons as they ascend to the molecular layer where they branch to form parallel fibres (8.160)
- the dendrites of granular neurons, with their terminal expansions
- the branching terminal axons of afferent mossy fibres

1039

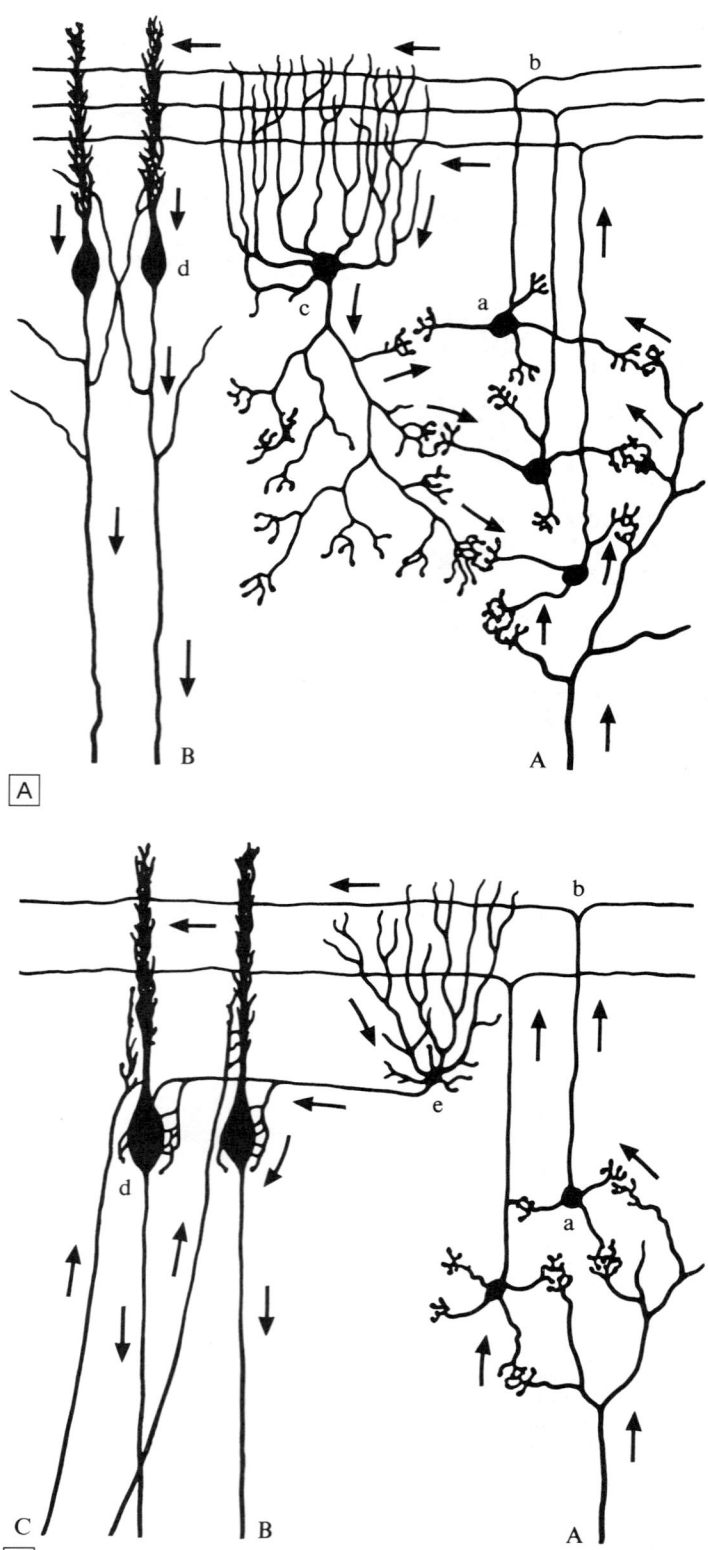

8.160 A. Diagrams of Golgi-stained neurons, showing the main circuits of the cerebellar cortex. The direction of impulse conduction is shown by arrows. Purkinje cells are drawn as seen en face with their compressed dendritic trees. In A a mossy fibre contacts several granule cells (a). The axon of a granule cell bifurcates in two parallel fibres (b) that terminate on dendrites of a Golgi cell (c) and two Purkinje cells (d). Axonal arborizations of the Golgi cell terminate on granule cell dendrites. The axons of the Purkinje cells (b) leave the cortex. In B a basket cell and its axon (e), that forms baskets around the somata of two Purkinje cells (d), and two climbing fibres, terminating on the Purkinje cell dendrites, are illustrated. Basket cell axons are oriented in a plane perpendicular to the long axis of the folia (see **8.156, 162**). This diagram is only schematic because parallel fibres, that run in the long axis of the folia, and basket cell axons cannot be seen in a single section. (Redrawn from Cajal 1955.)

- climbing fibres passing through the granular layer en route to the molecular layer
- somata, basal dendrites and complex axonal ramifications of Golgi neurons
- monodendritic or brush cells
- cerebellar glomeruli: these are synaptic complexes with four types of neurite: at the centre is a mossy fibre terminal which synapses with the granular and Golgi cell dendrites, while granular dendrites also receive synaptic contacts from Golgi terminals (p. 1042)
- collateral ramifications of Purkinje cell axons.

CELL TYPES OF THE CEREBELLAR CORTEX

Purkinje neuron

Purkinje cells have a specific geometry and occur in their typical form in all vertebrate classes (**8.160–163**). Arranged in a single layer between the molecular and granular layer, (**8.165A**) individual Purkinje cells are separated by about 50 μm transversely and longitudinally 50–100 μm. Their somata measure vertically about 50–70 μm, transversely 30–35 μm.

One or sometimes two large primary dendrites arise from the 'neck', the superficial pole of the Purkinje cell. From these a most abundant arborization, with several orders of subdivision, extends towards the surface. Branches of each neuron are confined to a narrow sheet in a plane transverse to the long axis of the folium. Proximal first and second order dendrites have smooth surfaces with short, stubby spines which are contacted by the climbing fibres; distal branches show a dense array of short-necked dendritic spines which receive synapses from the terminals of parallel fibres (see below). These *spiny branchlets* carry about 45 spines on each 10 μm of length; thus, on average (Fox & Barnard 1957), each Purkinje neuron has about 180 000 spines on its dendritic tree.

The subcellular structure of the Purkinje cell is similar to that of other neurons. One distinguishing feature is the *subsurface cisterns*, which are present below the plasma lemma of soma and dendrites and which may penetrate into the spines and are often associated with a mitochondrion. These cisterns represent intracellular calcium stores which are important links in the second messenger systems of the cell. Excitatory (asymmetric) synapses of the climbing fibres contact the proximal spines of the spiny branchlets; parallel fibres contact the distal spines of the spiny branchlets. In addition there are inhibitory (symmetric) synapses of basket and stellate cells and recurrent collaterals of the Purkinje cell axon which contact the shafts of the proximal dendrites. Excitatory synapses are rare on the soma of the Purkinje cell, but there are inhibitory synapses from basket cell axons and recurrent collaterals. The non-synaptic area of the surface of the soma and dendrites of the Purkinje cell is covered by lamellar protrusions of the Bergmann glial fibres.

From a Purkinje neuron's base, the axon traverses the granular layer into the subjacent white matter. Its initial portion is narrow, unmyelinated and has the typical features of an initial axon segment. It is surrounded by the distal branches of the basket cell axons as the so-called 'pinceau' (brush). Beyond the initial segment, the axon suddenly enlarges, acquires a myelin sheath and gives off collateral branches. The main axon proceeds into the white matter and finally forms a plexus in one of the cerebellar or vestibular nuclei. Collateral branches of Purkinje axons form plexuses above and below their somata (**8.163**). These collaterals are oriented in the same plane as the Purkinje cell dendritic tree and the inhibitory synapses from basket and stellate cells. Purkinje cell axon recurrent collaterals end on Purkinje neurons and on basket and Golgi neurons.

Granule cell

Each granule cell has a spherical nucleus, 5–8 μm in diameter, with a mere shell of cytoplasm containing a few small mitochondria, ribosomes and a diminutive Golgi complex. Granule cells usually give rise to 3–5 dendrites, each about 10–30 μm in length, which end in claw-like terminal expansions; these synapse with the terminals of mossy fibres and Golgi cell axons to form complex synapses, known as *cerebellar glomeruli*, which are visible by light microscopy in the intervals between groups of granular neurons. The fine axons of granule cells pass from their superficial aspect into the molecular layer and branch at a T-junction to form a parallel fibre (**8.156, 157**),

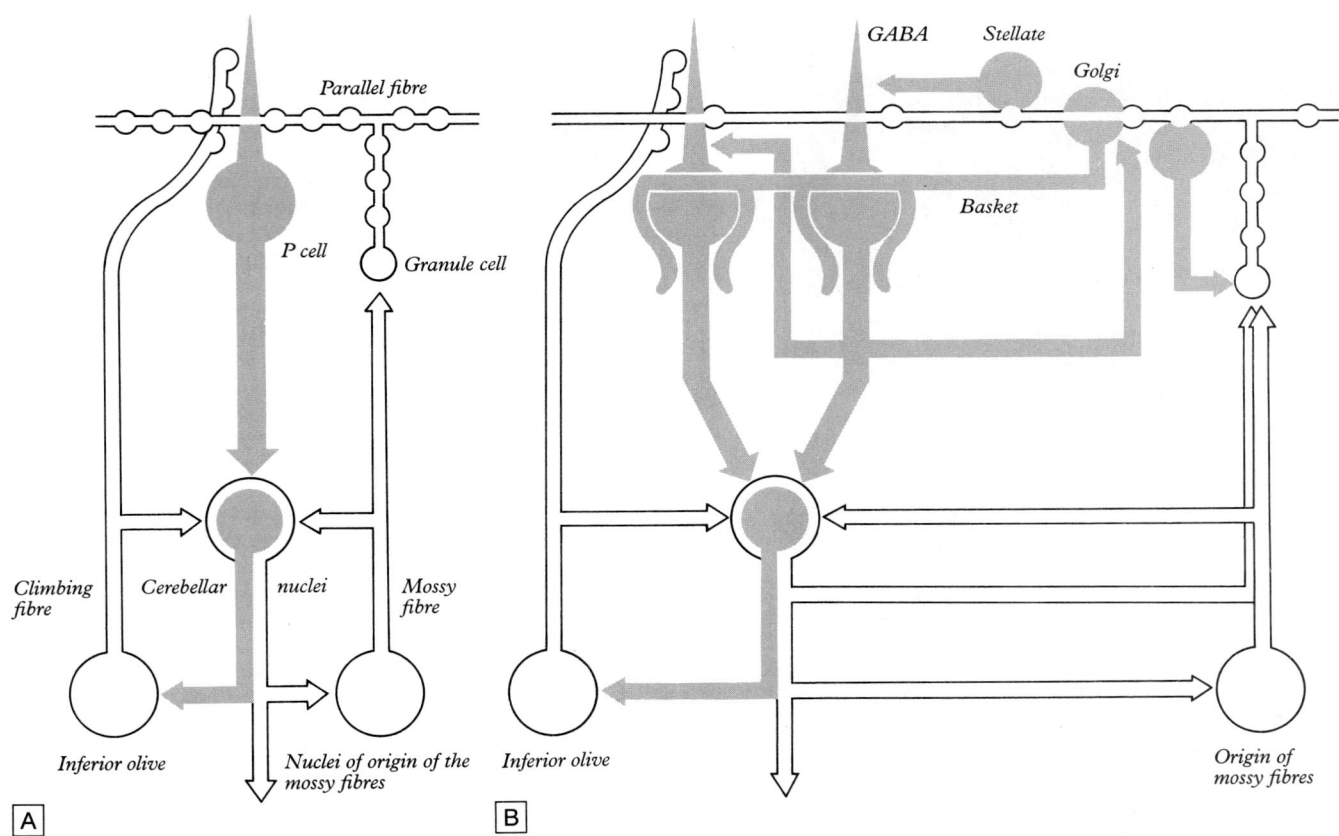

8.161 A. Diagram of the main circuits of the cerebellar cortex.
B. Connections of the inhibitory interneurons (stellate, basket and Golgi cells) of the cerebellar cortex and the recurrent collaterals of Purkinje cell axons. Inhibitory neurons are indicated in black.

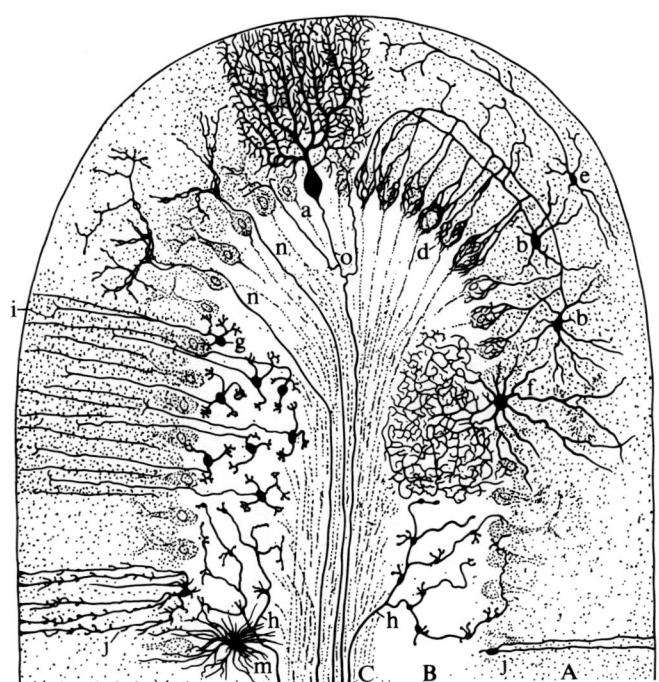

8.162 Diagram of cell types in the cerebellar cortex oriented perpendicular to the long axis of a folium. a = Purkinje cell; A = molecular layer; b = basket cell; B = granular layer; C = cerebellar white matter; d = baskets formed by a basket cell axon; e = superficial stellate cell; f = Golgi cell; g = granule cell; h = mossy fibre; i = axon of granule cell bifurcating in parallel fibres; j = Bergmann glial cell; m = astroglial cell; n = climbing fibre; o = collateral branching of a Purkinje cell axon. (Redrawn from Cajal 1955.)

passing in opposite directions over a distance of several millimetres. Terminals located along the parallel fibre give it a beaded appearance. These terminals are sites of synapses between the parallel fibres and the dendrites and somata of Purkinje, stellate, basket and Golgi cells in the molecular layer. Most numerous are the synapses with Purkinje dendritic spines. It had been estimated that about 250 000 parallel fibres cross a single Purkinje dendritic tree, although every parallel fibre may not synapse with the dendritic tree which it crosses.

Basket and stellate cells

Basket and stellate cells (8.159, 162) are the neurons of the molecular layer. Their sparsely branched dendritic trees and the ramifications of their axons are located in a plane approximately perpendicular to the long axis of the folium, i.e. in the same plane as the Purkinje cell dendritic tree and the ramifications of the Purkinje cell recurrent collaterals. Both basket and stellate cells are inhibitory, γ-amino-butyric acid (GABA)-ergic neurons which also share certain other neurochemical features. Stellate cells are located in the superficial molecular layer and their axons synapse with the shafts of Purkinje cell dendrites. Both stellate and basket cells receive excitatory (asymmetrical) synapses from parallel fibres as they pass through their dendritic tree. Basket cells are located in the lower third of the molecular layer. Their somata receive synapses from Purkinje cell recurrent collaterals, climbing and mossy fibres in addition to the parallel fibres. Basket cell axons increase in size away from their somata. The thick axons run deep in the molecular layer just above the Purkinje cells. Continuing for about 1 mm each covers the territories of 10–12 Purkinje neurons. Collaterals of the basket cell axon ascend along the Purkinje cell dendrites, and descend towards the Purkinje cell soma forming pericellular networks, or 'baskets', around them. The terminal branches of the basket cell axons surround the Purkinje cell axon as the 'pinceau' (8.162). Branches from each basket cell axon also extend in the direction of the long axis of the folium to a further 3–6 rows of Purkinje neurons flanking the

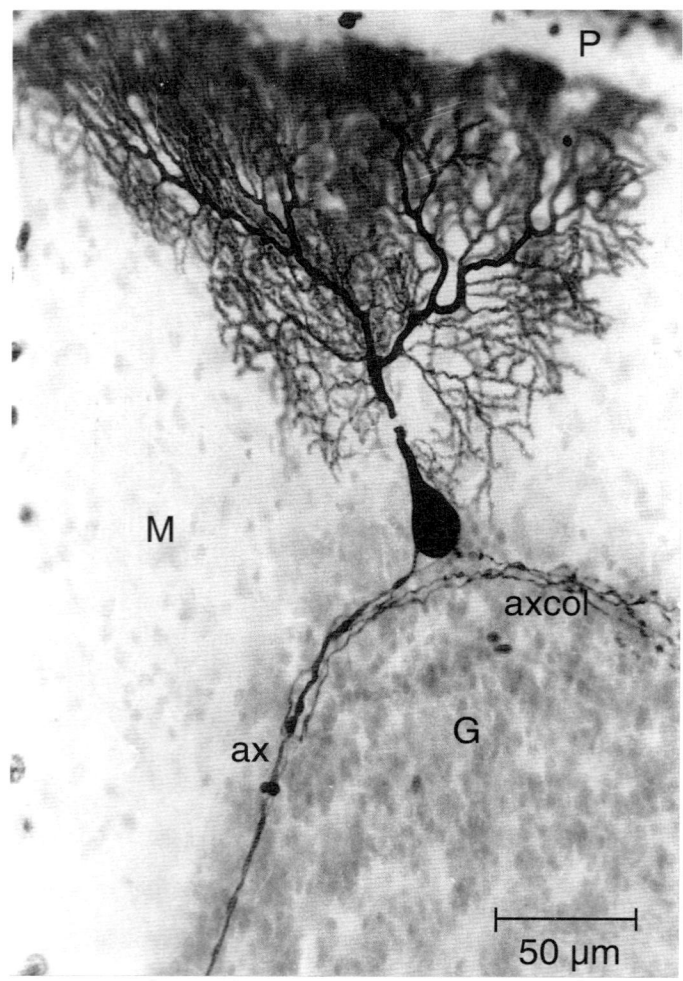

8.163 Photograph of an intracellularly labelled Purkinje cell of rat cerebellum. The plexus of Purkinje cell axon collaterals (axcol) is located in the superficial granular layer. ax = axon, axcol = axon collaterals, G = granular layer, M = molecular layer, p = pia mater. (Courtesy of Dr T J H Ruigrok.)

axon. Hence an estimated 72 Purkinje cell neurons may receive synapses from a single basket neuron.

Golgi cell

Golgi cells (8.159, 162) are inhibitory, GABAergic interneurons, whose somata are located in the granular layer. Most Golgi cells are found in the superficial zone of the granular layer, adjoining the Purkinje cell somata. Their dendrites radiate into the molecular layer to arborize, their courses predominantly at right angles to the surface. Unlike the Purkinje cell, Golgi cell dendritic trees are not flattened, appearing much the same in transverse and longitudinal foliar section; in both planes they overlap the territories of several Purkinje cells and neighbouring Golgi cells. Some Golgi dendrites, however, do not enter the molecular layer, dividing in the granular layer to join the cerebellar glomeruli (see below).

A Golgi neuron's axon arises from the base of the cell body or a central dendrite, immediately dividing into a profuse arborization which extends through the entire thickness of the granular layer. The territory occupied by the axonal ramifications is of a volume which corresponds approximately to its dendritic tree in the molecular layer, and which overlaps with the axonal arborizations of adjacent Golgi cells. The main synaptic input to Golgi cell dendrites is from parallel fibres in the molecular layer. Purkinje cell recurrent collaterals and mossy and climbing fibres also terminate on their proximal dendrites and, more sparsely, on their somata.

Monodendritic or brush cells

Monodendritic or brush cells (8.164) have been described only

recently (Altman & Bayer 1977; Braak & Braak 1993; Mugnaini & Floris 1994). These cells are located in the granular layer. The soma of the neuron contains a faintly stained nucleus and issues a single short dendrite terminating in a tuft or brush. Mossy fibres make large synaptic contacts with the brush-like process. The cells are strongly immunoreactive with antibodies against calretinin. Brush cells are especially numerous in the nodulus and the flocculus. They give rise to a thin axon, whose termination is presently unknown.

INPUTS TO THE CEREBELLAR CORTEX

Two very different excitatory inputs serve the cerebellar cortex, mossy fibres and climbing fibres (8.165A,B).

Climbing fibres

These arise only from the inferior olivary nucleus. Olivocerebellar fibres traverse the white matter and granular layer where they branch to form climbing fibres. Each climbing fibre innervates a single Purkinje cell. There are about ten times as many Purkinje cells as there are cells in the inferior olive and each olivocerebellar fibre branches into about 10 climbing fibres, each innervating a Purkinje cell. The climbing fibre passes along the soma of the Purkinje cell without terminating. Its terminal branches divide and are applied to the smooth, proximal Purkinje cell dendrites over most of their length, where they make numerous synapses with the short stubby spines which are present on these areas.

Mossy fibres

These take their origin from the spinal cord, the trigeminal, dorsal column, and reticular nuclei of the medulla and the pontine tegmentum and basal pons. Like climbing fibres they are excitatory, but otherwise they contrast sharply in their anatomical distribution and physiological properties. As each mossy fibre traverses the white matter its branches diverge to enter several adjacent folia. Within each folium mossy fibre branches supply ramifications to the granular layer and expand into grape-like synaptic terminals (mossy fibre rosettes) which occupy the centre of a cerebellar glomerulus.

Cerebellar glomeruli are complex synaptic sites containing a central mossy fibre 'rosette', dendrites of several granular neurons, terminals of Golgi axons and sometimes a Golgi dendrite. Each glomerulus, roughly spherical or ovoid, is about 10 μm in its greatest diameter; they occur in a ratio to granular neurons of about 1 to 5. All synapses are axodendritic. The central mossy fibre 'rosette' establishes synaptic contact with a surrounding spray of up to 20 granule cell dendrites and, when present, the spine-studded surface of a Golgi cell dendrite.

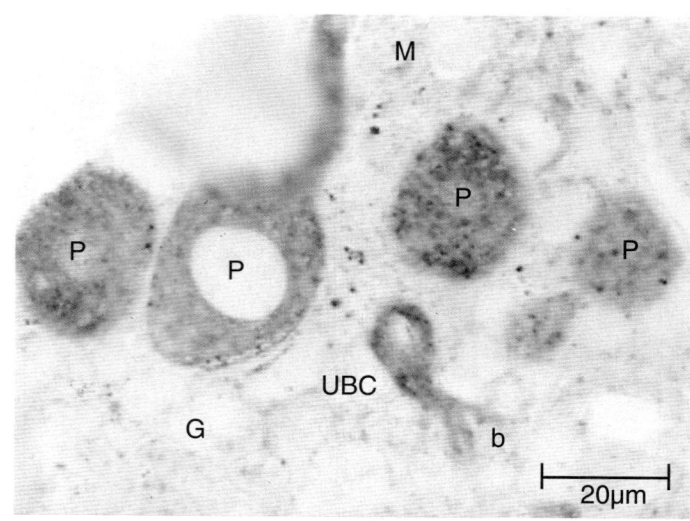

8.164 Unipolar brush cell (UBC) from the superficial granular layer. Semithin section of rat cerebellum immunostained with antibody against calretinin. Note the medium-sized cell body and the brush-like tip (b) of the single dendrite of the UBC. b = brush-like tip of the single dendritic process; G = granular layer; M = molecular layer; P = Purkinje cell; UBC = unipolar brush cell. (Courtesy of Dr E Mugnaini.)

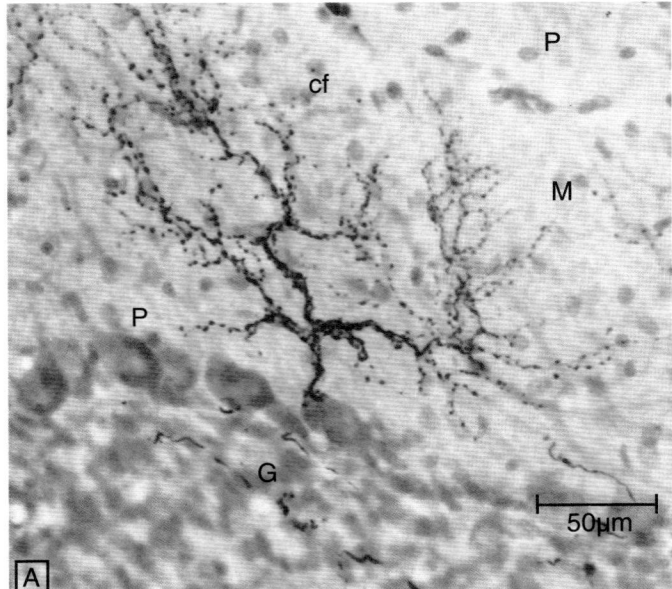

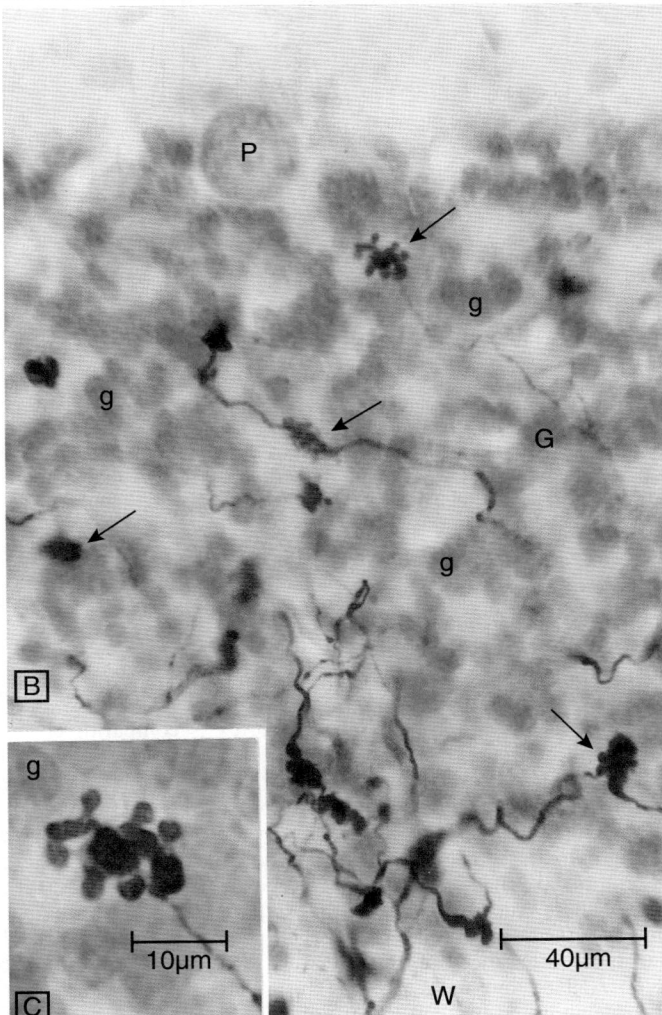

8.165 Photographs of (A) phaseolus vulgaris lectin-labelled climbing fibres, and (B, C) mossy fibres of the cerebellum of the rat. The varicosities along the climbing fibre (A) are the sites of synaptic contact with the proximal dendrites of the Purkinje cell. Purkinje cell somata and proximal dendrites are lightly immunostained with an antibody against Zebrin. Mossy fibres enter the granular layer from the white matter (W) and terminate with multiple complex terminals, that are known as mossy fibre rosettes (arrows in B). Each rosette occupies an empty space between the granule cells, the so-called islands of Geld. One of these islands with its mossy fibre rosette is enlarged in c. cf = climbing fibre; G = granular layer; g = granule cell nucleus; M = molecular layer; P = Purkinje cell soma; p = pia mater; W = white matter. (Courtesy of Dr T J H Ruigrok.)

These synapses are excitatory (asymmetric). The Golgi cell's axonal terminals establish inhibitory (symmetric) synapses with several dendrites of granular neurons, as shown in diagram **8.166**.

NEURONS OF THE CEREBELLAR NUCLEI

The main neuronal population of the cerebellar nuclei consists of multipolar neurons of different sizes, with long ramifying dendrites and an axon that leaves the cerebellum through the superior cerebellar peduncle, the uncinate tract or the juxtarestiform body. Some collaterals of these efferent axons enter the cortex, where they terminate rather sparsely as mossy fibres. Another population of small, GABAergic neurons gives rise to the pathway terminating in the contralateral inferior olive (**8.161**). Most of these so-called nucleoolivary fibres travel with the superior cerebellar peduncle. The question of the presence of local interneurons (Golgi type II cells) in the cerebellar nuclei has not been definitely settled. Neurochemical evidence on the presence of glycinergic interneurons in the cerebellar nuclei is presented in the section on the chemoarchitecture of the cerebellum. Purkinje cell axons are the main input to the neurons of the cerebellar nuclei; they terminate with inhibitory synapses both on dendrites and somata. Collaterals of climbing and mossy fibres terminate on proximal and distal dendrites and provide the cerebellar nuclei with an excitatory input.

QUANTITATIVE ASPECTS OF THE CEREBELLAR CORTEX

In its regular, repetitive cytoarchitecture, the cerebellar cortex lends

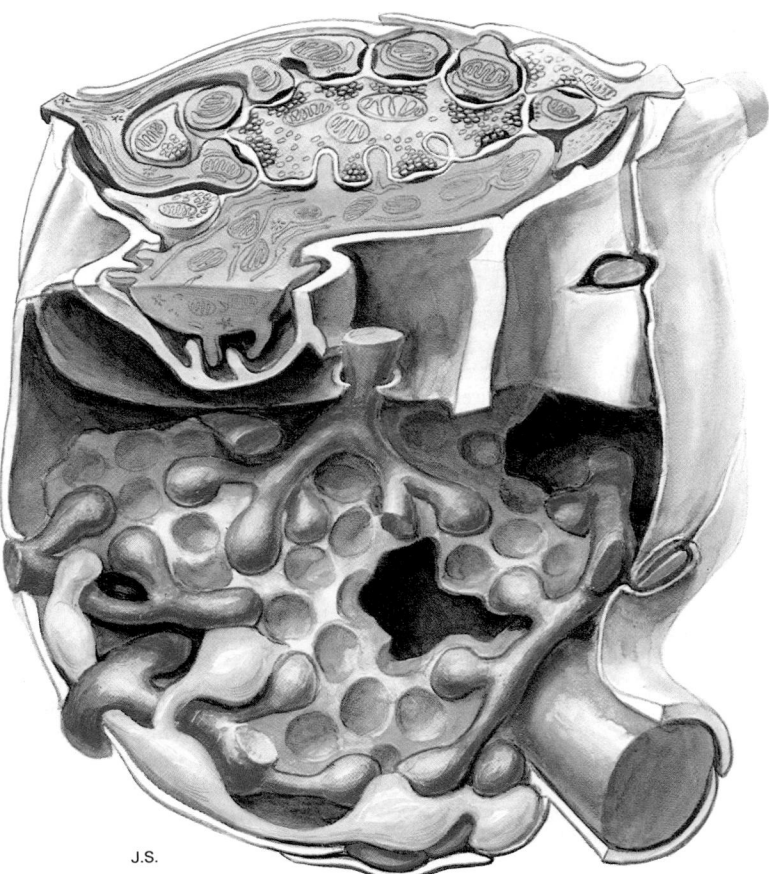

J.S.

8.166 A stereodiagram illustrating the structure of a cerebellar synaptic glomerulus. Blue = mossy afferent fibre rosette; red = granule cell dendrites; yellow = terminals of Golgi cell axon; green = Golgi cell dendrite; grey = neurological capsule. Note that the essential synaptic contacts are axodendritic between: mossy afferent fibres and granule cell dendrites; mossy afferents and Golgi cell dendrites; Golgi cell axons and granule cell dendrites. (From Eccles et al 1967, by courtesy of the authors and publishers.)

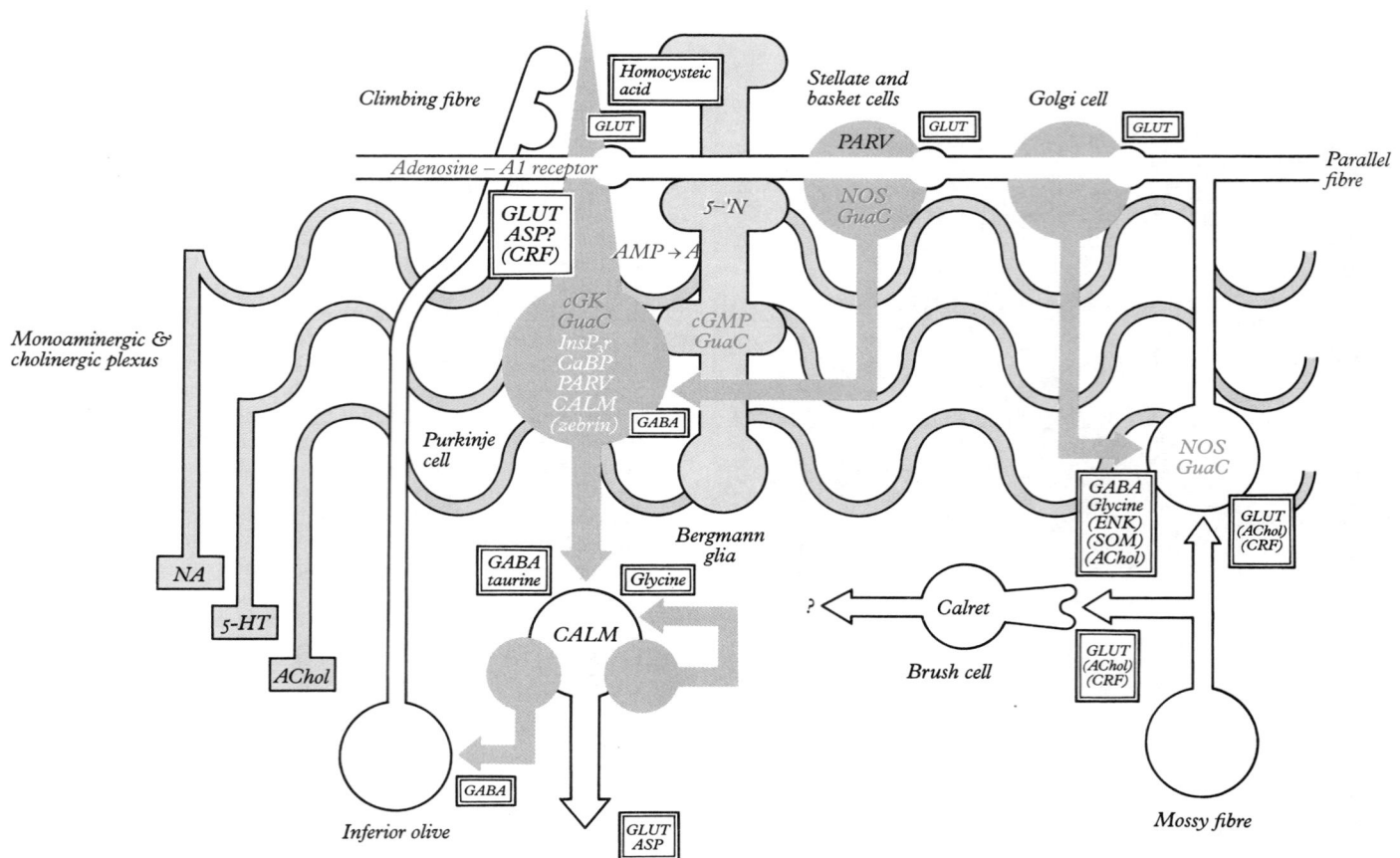

8.167 Diagram of the chemoarchitecture of the cerebellum. Substances involved in the nitric oxide system are indicated in blue. Substances involved in adenosine-transmission are indicated in red: Adenosine (A) is formed extracellularly by 5'-nucleotidase-catalyzed breakdown of adenosine monophosphate (AMP). The source of AMP is not indicated. Neurotransmitters and peptides active at the various synapses are indicated in boxes. Neurotransmitters and peptides that are present in subpopulations of neurons are indicated between brackets. Calcium binding proteins and certain other substances are indicated in the neurons that contain them. The nor-

adrenergic, serotoninergic and cholinergic plexus are drawn as green, wavy lines. 5'N = 5'-nucleotidase; 5-HT = serotinin; A = adenosine; AChol = acetylcholine; AMP = adenosine monophosphate; ASP = aspartate; CaBP = 28K vitamin D-dependent calcium binding protein; CALM = calmodulin; Calret = calretinin; cGK = cyclic GMP-dependent protein kinase; cGMP = cyclic guanosine monophosphate; CRF = corticotrophin releasing factor; ENK = enkephalin; GABA = gamma-amino-butyric acid; GLUT = glutamate; GuaC = guanylyl cyclase; InsP₃rNA = noradrenalin; NOS = nitric oxide synthase; PARV = parvalbumin; SOM = somatostatin.

itself to quantitative analysis (Fox & Bernard 1957; Eccles et al 1967; Fox et al 1967; Braitenberg 1967, 1977).

A vertical column of human cerebellar cortex, 1 mm square in area at a folia summit, contains about 500 Purkinje, 600 basket, 50 Golgi and perhaps 3 000 000 granular neurons, with about 600 000 glomeruli. It is difficult to estimate the total cerebellar cortical area, but since its sagittal dimension (8.142c) is said to be over a metre, and its transverse, unrolled extent about one-sixth of a metre the total surface area would be about 200 000 square millimetres. By these calculations there would be over 10^{11} granule cells and their associated circuitry in the cerebellar cortex.

On the *input side* a single olivary afferent gives rise to ten climbing fibres; each climbing fibre synapses with only one Purkinje neuron, and by collaterals with an undetermined number of interneurons. In contrast, a single mossy fibre diverges greatly, synapsing with 400 or more granular neurons in one folium; if branches to adjacent folia are included, the number is probably several thousand. Conversely, each granule cell receives synapses from four or five different mossy fibre terminals.

Ascending axons of granule cells bifurcate into parallel fibres, synapsing with Purkinje, Golgi, basket (internal) and external stellate neurons. In cats, parallel fibres have been reported to extend about 7 mm and synapses with 300–450 Purkinje neurons. Thus, there is divergence from a mossy fibre through the granular neurons to perhaps hundreds of thousands of Purkinje neurons; there is uncertainty about the amount of overlap between parallel fibre territories, but enormous convergence of paths to individual Purkinje neurons exists, a dendritic tree of one Purkinje cell receiving an estimated

total of 175 010 synapses from different parallel fibres in the rat (Napper & Harvey 1988).

CEREBELLAR CHEMOARCHITECTURE

The neurochemistry of the cerebellar cortex is comparatively well understood but gaps remain. The main cerebellar circuit consists of the climbing fibre and mossy fibre–parallel fibre afferents of the Purkinje cells and the Purkinje cell output to the cerebellar nuclei. Mossy, climbing and parallel fibres are excitatory and, probably, all use L-glutamate as a neurotransmitter. Purkinje cells are GABAergic and inhibit the neurons of their cerebellar and vestibular target nuclei. These nuclei contain both excitatory (glutamatergic) and inhibitory (GABAergic and glycinergic) neurons. GABA is also the neurotransmitter mediating feedforward or feedback inhibition by Golgi, stellate and basket cells. This relatively simple scheme is further elaborated by the distribution of different functional classes of glutamate and GABA receptors, by the presence of certain peptides or proteins in particular (sub)populations of neurons and by the monoaminergic and cholinergic innervation of the cerebellar cortex and the nuclei (8.167).

L-glutamate appears to be the neurotransmitter in most mossy fibre systems, including the spinocerebellar tracts, the pontocerebellar system and the primary vestibulocerebellar projection, the latter consisting of root fibres of the vestibular nerve. Acetylcholine (ACh) has been identified as the neurotransmitter of secondary vestibulocerebellar mossy fibres arising from the vestibular nuclei (Barmack et al 1992a,b). Receptors in the granular layer mediating

Table 8.3   The localization of subunits of glutamate receptors and GABA-A receptors in neurons of the cortex and the cerebellar nuclei and in Bergmann glia

Type	Subunit	P cells	Gran cells	Golgi cells	Basket & stellate cells	Bergmann glia	Cerebellar nuclei
AMPA	GluRA	+	–	–	–	+	–
	GluRB	+	+	+	+	–	+
	GluRC	+	–	+	+	–	+
	GluRD	–	+	–	–	+	+
KAINATE	Ka1	±	–	–	–	–	–
	Ka2	–	+	–	–	–	+
	GluR5	+	–	–	–	–	–
	GluR6	–	+	–	–	–	–
	GluR7	–	–	–	+	–	+
NMDA	NR1	+	+	+	+	–	+
	NR2A	–	+	–	–	–	+
	NR2B	–	+[1]	–	–	–	–
	NR2C	–	+	–	–	–	–
	NR2D	–	–	–	+	–	±
METABOTROPIC	mGluR1	+	±	±	±	–	±
	mGluR2	–	–	+	–	–	–
	mGluR3	–	–	+	–	–	–
	mGluR4	–	+	–	–	–	–
	mGluR5	–	–	+[2]	–	–	–
	mGluR7	+	–	–	–	–	–
GABA$_A$	alpha1	+	+	–	+	–	+
	alpha2	–	–	–	–	+	–
	alpha3	±	–	–	±	–	+
	alpha4	–	±	–	–	–	–
	alpha5	–	–	–	–	–	–
	alpha6	–	+	–	–	–	–
	beta1	–	±	–	–	+	+
	beta2	+	+	–	+	–	+
	beta3	±	+	–	–	–	–
	gamma1	–	–	+	–	+	–
	gamma2	+	+	–	+	–	+
	gamma3	–	±	–	–	–	–
	delta	–	+	–	–	–	–

+ indicates distinct labelling
± indicates weak labelling
– indicates absent or unknown labelling
1 = only present during development
2 = present in subpopulation of Golgi cells

glutamatergic and cholinergic transmission include ionotropic (coupled to ion channels in the cell membrane) glutamate receptors of the NMDA (N-methyl-D-aspartate) and non-NMDA type, metabotropic (coupled to second messenger systems) glutamate receptors and ionotropic (nicotinic) and metabotropic (muscarinic) ACh receptors (glutamate receptors reviewed by Sommer & Seeburg 1992; Nakanishi 1992), see also Table 8.3; ACh receptors reviewed by Neustadt et al (1988), Levey et al (1991) and Cimino et al (1992)). Metabotropic receptors in granule cells (mGluR4 type of metabotropic glutamate receptor, Kristensen et al 1993; and the M_2 muscarinic receptor, Cortès et al 1987) inhibit cyclic adenosine monophosphate (cAMP) formation. Their precise function in mossy fibre-granule cell transmission is not known. NMDA receptors are the dominant type of ionotropic glutamate receptor in developing granule cells (Garthwaite & Brodbelt 1989). NMDA receptors are voltage dependent and cause slow depolarizations and the opening of Ca^{2+} channels in the postsynaptic neuron. Non-NMDA glutamate receptors mediate fast excitatory amino-acid neurotransmission. They include α-amino-3-hydroxy-5-methyl-4-isoxalone proprionic acid (AMPA) and the high affinity kainate types. Both types occur in granule cells, but kainate receptors prevail in the granular layer.

Certain subpopulations of mossy and climbing fibres contain peptides, apart from their amino acid transmitter. Corticotrophin releasing factor (CRF) has been located in mossy and climbing fibres of many species. It has a facilitatory effect on responses of neurons to excitatory amino acids (Bishop 1990; King et al 1992).

Parallel fibres synapse with dendrites of inhibitory interneurons and the distal spiny branchlets of the Purkinje cell dendritic tree in the molecular layer. Parallel fibre to Purkinje cell transmission is mediated by ionotropic glutamate receptors of the AMPA type and by metabotropic receptors (types mGluR2 and 7) which are coupled to the phosphoinositide hydrolysis second messenger system. NMDA receptors on basket and stellate cells mediate the parallel fibre-induced inhibition of Purkinje cells by these neurons (Quinlan & Davis 1985). Parallel fibre–Purkinje cell transmission is blocked by adenosine which binds to A_1-adenosine receptors present on the parallel fibres (Weber et al 1990). Release of adenosine in the molecular layer is conditional on climbing fibre activity (Cuénod et al 1989).

The weight of the evidence at present favours L-glutamate as the neurotransmitter of the climbing fibres (Zhang & Ottersen 1993), but L-aspartate remains a possible candidate. Glutamate receptors at the climbing fibre to Purkinje cell synapse are of a non-NMDA type, but so far have not been sufficiently characterized. Stimulation of climbing fibre synapses leads to an influx of calcium ions into the Purkinje cell dendrites.

The components of the phosphoinositide second messenger system, which forms inositol 1,4,5-triphosphate (InsP3) and diacylglycerol by hydrolysis of phosphatidyl inositol 4,5 biphosphate, are enriched in Purkinje cells (Blackstone et al 1989; Ito 1991). These include the receptor for InsP3, which mobilizes calcium from the subsurface cisterns, and protein kinase C, which is activated by diacylglycerol. The reason for the concentration of these elements, presumably, is the presence of metabotropic glutamate receptors mediating parallel fibre–Purkinje cell transmission, which are coupled to the phosphoinositide cycle. Ca^{2+} concentration in Purkinje cells, therefore, may increase from metabotropic receptor, parallel fibre induced release from subsurface cisterns, and by climbing fibre mediated influx from calcium channels. Several calcium-binding proteins are prominent in Purkinje cells (Lawson 1981; Celio & Heizmann 1981; Seto-Oshima et al 1983). Calbindin-D_{28k} occurs exclusively in Purkinje cells, and is often used as a marker substance for this cell type. Parvalbumin is present in Purkinje, stellate and basket cells; calmodulin is found in Purkinje cells and in neurons of the cerebellar nuclei.

Cell-specific substances in Purkinje cells

Several Purkinje cell-specific substances are present in a subset of the Purkinje cells. This is the case with the Zebrins, a group of proteins which were recognized with immunocytochemistry in rat Purkinje cells by Hawkes and Leclerc (1987). Zebrin-containing Purkinje cells are distributed in a symmetrical pattern of longitudinal bands, separated by Zebrin-negative Purkinje cells (**8.168**). These bands are identical to the Purkinje cell zones which can be distinguished on the basis of their efferent corticonuclear or afferent, climbing fibre connections. A similar banding pattern was observed much earlier for the distribution of the enzyme 5'-nucleotidase in the cerebellum of the mouse (Scott 1967). This enzyme, however, appears to be localized in Bergmann glial fibres, and not in the Purkinje cells. 5'-Nucleotidase in Bergmann glia increases if climbing fibres are destroyed and disappears in mutant mice in which the Purkinje cells die.

Conjunctive activation of parallel fibres and climbing fibres leads to a reduction of the transmission in parallel fibre–Purkinje cell synapses as a result of the desensitization of Purkinje cell AMPA receptors (Ito 1991). This process is known as long-term depression

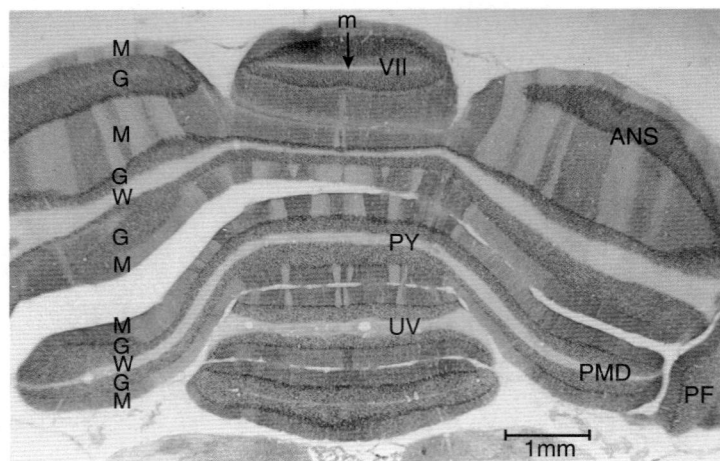

8.168 Photograph of a coronal section through the posterior lobe of the cerebellum of the rat, immunostained with an antibody against the Purkinje cell specific marker Zebrin I (Hawkes and Leclerc, 1987). Note alternation of stripes of Zebrin-positive and Zebrin-negative Purkinje cells in vermis and hemisphere. In the paraflocculus (PF) all Purkinje cells are Zebrin-positive. ANS = ansiform lobule; G = granular layer; M = molecular layer; m = midline; PF = paraflocculus; PMD = paramedian lobule; PY = pyramis; UV = uvula; VII, lobule VII = folium and tuber.

and is thought to be responsible for the plastic changes in cerebellar circuitry, involved in adaptation and learning. Long-term depression is dependent on an increase of intracellular Ca^{2+} and on the presence of cyclic guanosine 3',5'-monophosphate (cGMP)-dependent protein kinase in Purkinje cells. Long-term depression is abolished by the inhibition of the production of cGMP by nitric oxide (NO) in the cerebellar cortex (see Dawson et al 1992 for a review of NO in neural transmission). Purkinje cells are enriched in cGMP-dependent protein kinase, which has been used as another marker for this cell type (de Camilli et al 1984), but stable levels of cGMP have not been demonstrated in these cells. The formation of cyclic GMP is catalysed by soluble guanylate cyclase, and this enzyme in its turn is stimulated by NO. Synthesis of this diffusable messenger by NO-synthase has been located in basket cells and in certain populations of granule cells, but not in Purkinje cells (Bredt et al 1990). Guanylate cyclase is present in all cerebellar cell types, but cGMP in the cerebellum is mainly located in Bergmann glia and astrocytes (De Vente et al 1989). Two mechanisms which suppress parallel fibre–Purkinje cell transmission are thus available: the presynaptic blockage of parallel fibres by climbing fibre dependent release of adenosine and long-term depression.

The feedback inhibition of granule cells is accomplished by the Golgi cells and the postsynaptic inhibition of the Purkinje cells by the basket and stellate cells. Golgi cells differ from basket and stellate cells in various respects. Colocalization of GABA and glycine has been demonstrated in a large proportion of the Golgi cells but not in basket or stellate cells (Ottersen et al 1987). Subpopulations of Golgi cells contain choline acetyl transferase (ChAT), the synthetizing enzyme of ACh (De Lacalle et al 1993) or display a colocalization of GABA with enkephalin or somatostatin. Golgi cells lack calcium binding proteins, whereas parvalbumin is present in basket and stellate cells. AMPA glutamate receptors have been demonstrated in all cell types; the involvement of NMDA receptors in basket and stellate cell mediated inhibition of Purkinje cells has been shown in physiological experiments. A large proportion of the Golgi cells uniquely contains the mGluR2 class of the metabotropic glutamate receptor and, therefore, may react with inhibition of cyclic adenosine monophosphate formation on stimulation of glutamatergic parallel fibre or mossy fibre afferents (Ohishi et al 1993).

$GABA_A$ and $GABA_B$ receptors have been localized in the cerebellum by specific ligand binding. A precise localization of the different subunits of the $GABA_A$ receptor was obtained with in situ hybridization and immunocytochemistry in small rodents. $GABA_A$ receptors are coupled to chloride channels and possess a benzodiazepine binding site. GABA_B receptors are negatively linked to the phosphoinositide and cyclic AMP second messenger systems. Specific binding of [³H]muscimol to GABA_A receptors prevails over the granular layer, but specific binding to the benzodiazepine site of the GABA_A receptor is stronger over the molecular layer. This indicates a diversity in the GABA_A receptor, which can be further analysed by studying the localization of its subunits. GABA_B receptor binding studies in the rat revealed its localization on zonally distributed Purkinje cells in the caudal vermis (Turgeon & Albin 1993).

Different combinations of subunits of the GABA_A receptor have been found in cerebellar neurons (reviewed by Laurie et al 1992; Fritschy et al 1992; Persohn et al 1992; see also Table 8.3). The α1 and 3, β2 and μ2 subunits. α1 Subunits occur in Purkinje cells. α1 subunits are localized in the soma, i.e. opposite the basket cell terminals and α3 subunits in the proximal dendrites, i.e. opposite stellate cell terminals. The α1-β2-μ2 combination produces GABA_A receptors displaying high affinity binding for benzodiazepine ligands (Pritchett et al 1989). The α1, β2 and γ2 subunits also are expressed by granule cells, but, in addition, these cells express the α6, β3 and δ subunits. The α1, β2 and 3 subunits are distributed over the synaptic and non-synaptic surface of the cell, but the α6 subunit is limited to the synapses of the Golgi cell axons. The combination of α6, β2 and γ2 forms a receptor complex which is insensitive to benzodiazepine agonists. The prevalence of the α6 subunit in Golgi cell to granule cell synapses, therefore, may explain the lack of benzodiazepine-sensitive GABA_A receptors in the granular layer (Baude et al 1992).

Bergmann glial cells are involved in several signalling pathways in the cerebellar cortex. Their membrane contains the enzyme 5'-nucleotidase, which catalyses the production of adenosine by hydrolytic cleavage of 5'-nucleotide monophosphates (Schoen et al 1988). Bergmann glia are the main source of cGMP in the cerebellar cortex (De Vente et al 1989). Homocysteic acid, a putative aminoacid neurotransmitter, is released in a climbing fibre dependent manner from these cells (Cuénod et al 1990). Bergmann glial cells are

equipped with specific uptake systems for glutamate and convert it into glutamine, which again is used for the synthesis of glutamate by glutamatergic terminals (Ottersen et al 1992). Bergmann glia possess kainate receptors, with a unique subunit composition and specific ionic conductances and contain the α2 subunit of the GABA_A receptor as the only cell type in the cerebellar cortex (Table 8.3).

Neurons of the cerebellar nuclei can be divided into excitatory relay cells projecting to the brainstem, the thalamus and the spinal cord and small GABAergic neurons, which give rise to the nucleo-olivary projection (Nelson & Mugnaini 1989). Recently a third cell type was identified as an interneuron, which contains glycine, often colocalized with GABA. It projects to large, aspartate containing, relay cells, which are equipped with glycine receptors (Chen & Hillman 1993). GABA_A receptors composed of α1-β2 or 3-μ2 subunits (Persohn et al 1992) and ionotropic glutamate receptors of the NMDA and non-NMDA types (Audinat et al 1992) are present on neurons of the cerebellar nuclei.

Noradrenergic and serotonergic fibres form a rich plexus in all layers of the cerebellar cortex (Takeuchi et al 1982; Bishop & Ho 1985; Grzanna & Fritschy 1991). The aminergic fibres are fine, varicose and form extensive cortical plexuses; their release of noradrenalin and serotonin is assumed to be non-synaptic and their effects are paracrine involving volumes of tissue. The serotoninergic afferents of the cerebellum take their origin from neurons in the medullary reticular formation, but not from the raphe nuclei. The noradrenergic, coeruleocerebellar projection, when active, inhibits Purkinje cell firing not by direct action but via β-adrenergic receptor mediated inhibition of adenylatecyclase in the Purkinje cells. The presence of dopamine in elements of the cerebellar cortex is still disputed. Cerebellar afferents have been traced from dopaminergic cells in the ventral tegmental area (Ikai et al 1992) and dopamine D2 and D3 receptors are present in the molecular layer (Bouthenet et al 1991). A similar plexus of thin, ChAT-containing fibres is centred on the Purkinje cell layer (De Lacalle et al 1993). The origin of this cholinergic plexus is not known.

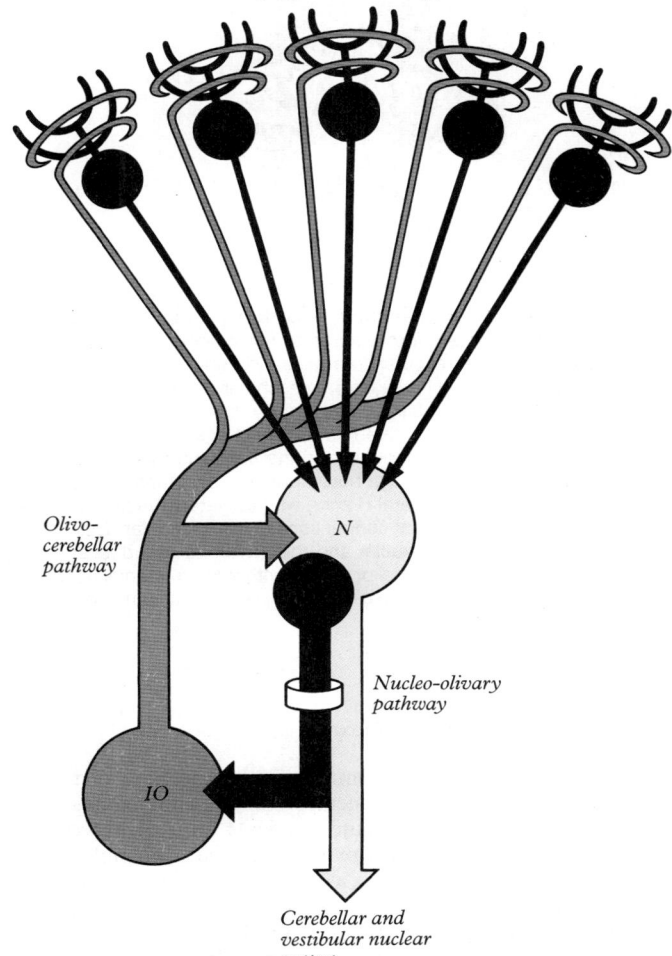

Purkinje cells and climbing fibres

Olivo-cerebellar pathway

N

Nucleo-olivary pathway

IO

Cerebellar and vestibular nuclear output

8.169 Diagram of a cerebellar module. Purkinje cells are shown in a single longitudinal oriented strip projecting onto a single cerebellar or vestibular target nucleus (N). A set of olivocerebellar fibres terminates on these Purkinje cells and sends a collateral projection to their target nucleus. A recurrent nucleo-olivary GABA-ergic pathway connects the target nucleus with the inferior olive. Inhibitory connections are indicated in black.

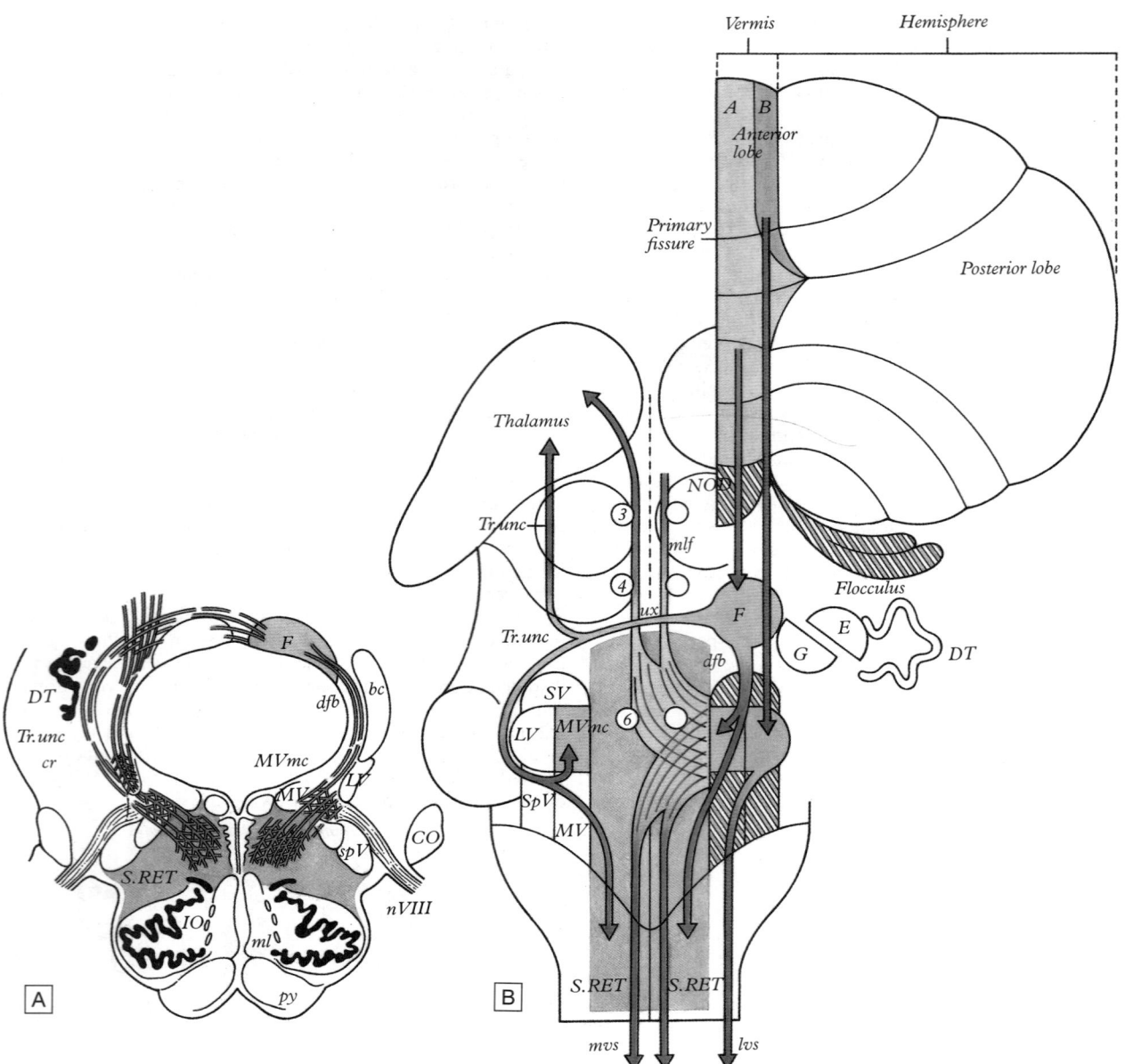

8.170 A. Transverse section through the fastigial nucleus, showing the bilateral distribution of its efferent fibres to the magnocellular medial vestibular nucleus and the reticular formation. Purkinje cell axons from the ventral B zone, terminating in the lateral vestibular nucleus, are indicated in red. The reticular formation is indicated in grey.

B. Efferent connections of the vermis. Connections of the medial A zone of the vermis (blue) and the nodulus and the flocculus (blue hatched) with the fastigial nucleus, the vestibular nuclei and the reticular formation (grey), and the connections of the lateral B zone with the lateral vestibular nucleus (red) are indicated. The efferent connections of the vestibular nuclei ascend bilaterally to the oculomotor nuclei and the thalamus and descend to the spinal cord. 3, 4, 6 = motor nuclei of the 3rd, 4th and 6th cranial nerves; A = Purkinje cell zone A; B = Purkinje cell zone B; bc = brachium conjunctivum;

CO = cochlear nuclei; cr = restiform body; dfb = (direct uncrossed) fastigiobulbar tract; DT = dentate nucleus; E = emboliform (anterior interposed) nucleus; F = fastigial nucleus; G = globose (posterior interposed) nucleus; IO = inferior olive; LV = lateral vestibular nucleus; lvs = lateral vestibulospinal tract; ml = medial lemniscus; mlf = medial longitudinal fascicle; MV = medial vestibular nucleus; MVmc = magnocellular part of the medial vestibular nucleus; mvs = medial vestibulospinal tract, NOD = nodulus; nVIII = statoacoustic nerve; SpV = spinal vestibular nucleus; py = pyramid; sp V = spinal tract of the trigeminal nerve; S.RET = reticular formation; SV = superior vestibular nucleus; Tr.unc.(al) = (ascending limb of the) uncinate tract: ux = decussation of the uncinate tract.

CEREBELLAR CIRCUITRY

Most of our knowledge of the anatomical connections of the cerebellum is derived from experimental studies with axonal tracing techniques in non-human primates, rodents and carnivores. Verification in human pathological material has been possible in some cases (see Voogd et al 1990 for a review). The connections of the cerebellum are organized in two perpendicular planes, corresponding to the planar organization of the cerebellar cortex. Efferent connections of the cortex are disposed in parasagittal sheets or bundles.

They connect longitudinal strips of Purkinje cells with certain cerebellar or vestibular nuclei. The climbing fibre afferents of these Purkinje cell zones from the inferior olive display a similar zonal disposition. This arrangement also can be designated as the *modular organization of the cerebellar output* (8.169). A module consists of one or more Purkinje cell zones, their cerebellar or vestibular target nucleus and their olivocerebellar climbing fibre input. The function of such a module is determined by the projections to the brainstem of the cerebellar or vestibular target nucleus. A general feature of the modular organization of the cerebellum is that GABAergic

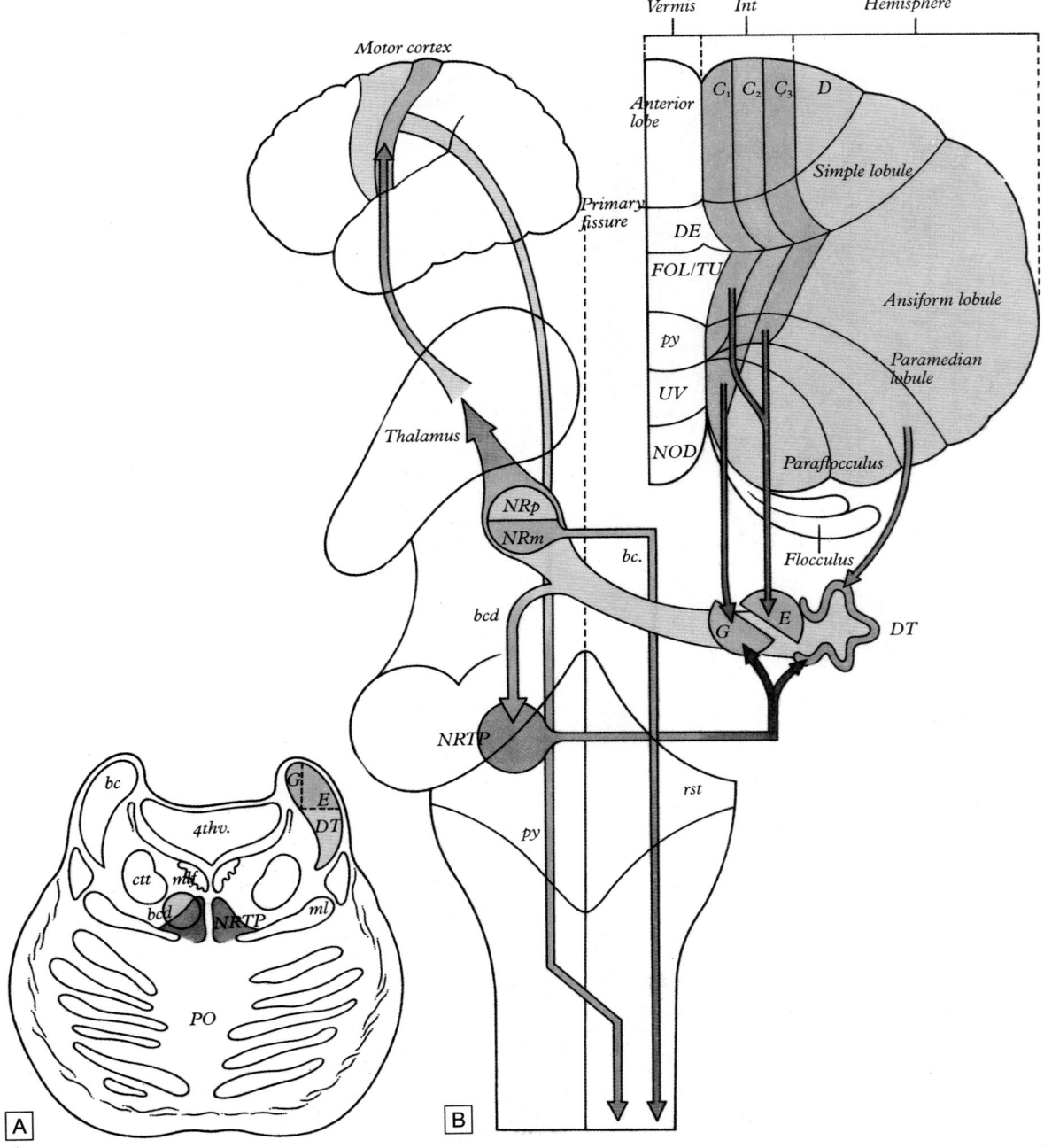

8.171A. Transverse section through the rostral pons, showing the components of the brachium conjunctivum from the globose (G), emboliform (E) and dentate nuclei (DT), the brachium conjunctivum descendens and its termination in the nucleus reticularis tegmenti pontis.

B. Efferent connections of the cerebellar hemisphere. Purkinje cell zones of the hemisphere and their target nuclei are indicated with the same colours. The brachium conjunctivum takes its origin from these nuclei, decussates and divides in ascending and descending branches. The ascending branch terminates in the red nucleus and the thalamus. The descending branch terminates in the nucleus reticularis tegmenti pontis. Motor pathways from the red nucleus and the motor cortex recross and descend to the spinal cord. Purkinje cell zones C₁ and C₃ (red) project to the emboliform nucleus. The emboliform nucleus is preferentially connected with the magnocellular

red nucleus and the caudal bank of the motor cortex. The connections of the globose nucleus resemble the emboliform nucleus with respect to the projection to the red nucleus, and the dentate, with respect to the motor cortex. bc = brachium conjunctivum; bcd = descending branch of the brachium conjunctivum; C_{1-3} = Purkinje cell zones C_{1-3}; ctt = central tegmental tract; D = Purkinje cell zone D; DE = declive; DT = dentate nucleus; E = emboliform (anterior interposed) nucleus; FOL/TU = folium/tuber; G = globose (posterior interposed) nucleus; Int = pars intermedia; ml = medial lemniscus; mlf = medial longitudinal fascicle; NOD = nodulus; NRm = magnocellular red nucleus; NRp = parvicellular red nucleus; NRTP = nucleus reticularis tegmenti pontis; PO = pontine nuclei; py = pyramidal tract; PY = pyramis; UV = uvula; 4th v = fourth ventricle.

neurons contained in the cerebellar nuclei project to the subnuclei of the contralateral inferior olive, which give rise to their respective climbing fibre afferents. These recurrent connections are known as nucleo-olivary pathways.

Mossy fibre afferent systems from precerebellar nuclei in the spinal cord and the brainstem terminate in the granular layer of certain lobules in transversely oriented terminal fields. The transverse lobular arrangement of the mossy fibre afferents is enforced by the transverse orientation of the parallel fibres, which are axons of the granule cells

and constitute the second link in the mossy fibre–parallel fibre input of the Purkinje cells. Parallel fibres cross and terminate on Purkinje cells belonging to several successive modules on their course through the molecular layer.

EFFERENT CONNECTIONS OF THE CEREBELLUM

The efferent connections of the cerebellum comprise the inhibitory projections of the Purkinje cells to the cerebellar and the vestibular

1049

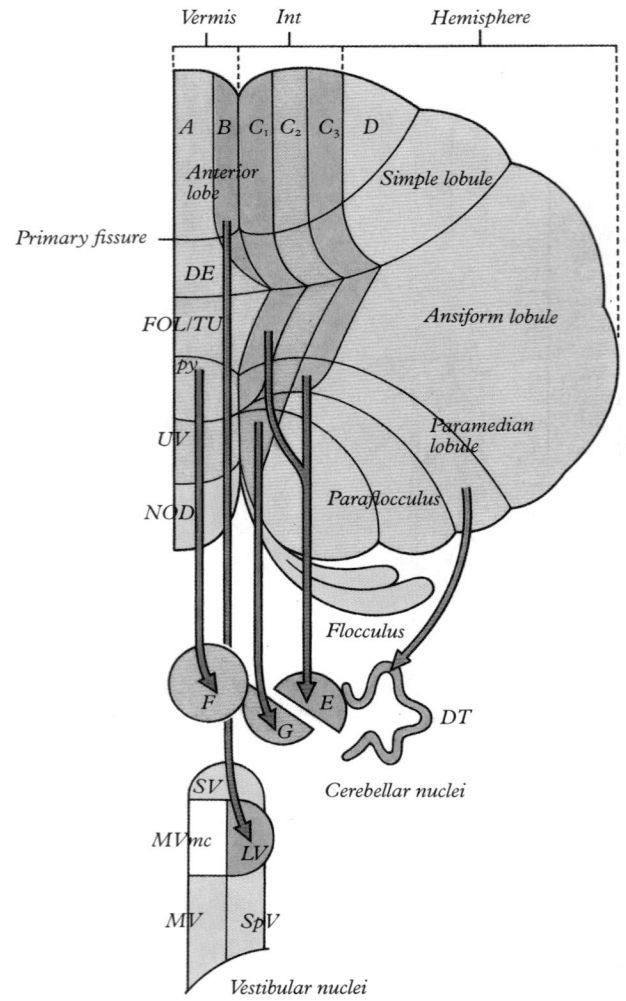

8.172 Diagram of the corticonuclear and corticovestibular projection. The subdivision of the cerebellar cortex in vermis, pars intermedia (Int) and hemisphere is indicated at the top of the diagram. Purkinje cell zones A–D and their target nuclei are indicated with the same colours. The projection of the nodulus and the flocculus to the vestibular nuclei is indicated in green. (Based on data from the cat from Voogd 1964 and Voogd and Bigaré 1980). A = Purkinje cell zone A; B = Purkinje cell zone B; C_{1-3} = Purkinje cell zones C_{1-3}; D = Purkinje cell zone D; DE = declive; DT = dentate nucleus; E = emboliform (anterior interposed) nucleus; F = fastigial nucleus; Fol/Tu = folium/tuber; G = globose (posterior interposed) nucleus; Int = pars intermedia; LV = lateral vestibular nucleus; MV = medial vestibular nucleus; MVmc = magnocellular part of the medial vestibular nucleus; NOD = nodulus; PY = pyramis; SpV = spinal vestibular nucleus; SV = superior vestibular nucleus; UV = uvula.

nuclei, and the efferent connections of the cerebellar nuclei. The cerebellar nuclei are connected with motor centres in the brainstem and, through the thalamus, with the motor cortex. Their effects on movement are always indirect, there are no direct projections from the cerebellar nuclei to motor neurons. Disynaptic connections of Purkinje cells of the anterior vermis and the vestibulocerebellum with motor neurons of the eye muscle nuclei and axial and proximal limb muscles are mediated by the vestibular nuclei. In addition, the vermis exerts an influence on motor neurons of these muscles bilaterally through multisynaptic pathways involving the fastigial nucleus, the vestibular nuclei and the reticular formation (**8.**170B). The vermis cannot be considered as a single module. Each half of the vermis is composed of several modules (each comprising a longitudinal Purkinje cell zone and a target nucleus) and their supporting climbing fibre afferent projections.

The hemisphere influences movements of the ipsilateral extremities by way of projections to the dentate and interposed (emboliform and globose) nuclei, and from these cerebellar nuclei to the contralateral red nucleus, thalamus and motor cortex. The red nucleus

and motor cortex in turn give rise to the crossed rubrospinal and corticospinal pathways (**8.**171B).

The paravermal region projecting to the interposed nucleus was distinguished from the rest of the hemisphere as the *pars intermedia* (Jansen & Brodal 1940, 1942). The pars intermedia and the hemisphere were further subdivided into modules, with the globose, the emboliform and subdivisions of the dentate as their target nuclei (Voogd & Bigaré 1980; see also **8.**172). The pars intermedia is mainly responsible for the control of movements of the ipsilateral extremities, through the rubrospinal and corticospinal tracts. The function of the rest of the hemisphere and the dentate nucleus is more difficult to define. Lesions of the dentate nucleus in primates do not lead to gross motor disturbances. The dentate nucleus may be involved in the preprogramming of movements or in the motor aspects of cognitive functions, such as speech.

Corticonuclear and corticovestibular projections

Purkinje cells of each hemivermis project to the ipsilateral fastigial nucleus and the vestibular nuclei, Purkinje cells of the hemisphere to the interposed and dentate nuclei. Although the cerebellar cortex is organized in strips of Purkinje cell zones projecting to the different cerebellar and vestibular nuclei, the borders between these strips are not apparent in the structure of the cortex with conventional staining methods. The vermis of the anterior lobe and the simple lobule consists of two parallel strips *A* and *B* of Purkinje cells (**8.**170, 172). The medial strip (A zone) projects to the rostral pole of the fastigial nucleus, the lateral strip (B zone) to the lateral vestibular (Deiters') nucleus. The B zone does not continue beyond the simple lobule. The cortex of the entire caudal vermis, which projects to the fastigial nucleus, is included in the A zone. Folium and tuber vermis, which represent a region of the cerebellum which receive a visual input, and which are involved in the accurate calibration of saccades, project to the caudal pole of the fastigial nucleus. Pyramis, uvula and nodule can be subdivided into several Purkinje cell zones (see Cerebello-vestibular connections p. 1051), but the significance of their connections with the cerebellar and vestibular nuclei is not completely understood. Projections from the pyramis to the fastigial and lateral vestibular nuclei strongly overlap with the projections of the anterior vermis; projections from the uvula extend beyond the fastigial nucleus to the interposed and dentate nuclei. Corticovestibular projections to the superior, spinal and medial vestibular nuclei, but not to the lateral vestibular nucleus, take their origin from the nodule and the adjacent region of the uvula (**8.**170, 172).

The pars intermedia consists of two strips of Purkinje cells (C1 and C3 zones) which project to the emboliform (anterior interposed) nucleus, flanking a single C2 zone which projects to the globose (posterior interposed) nucleus (**8.**171, 172). C1 and C3 zones with their projection to the emboliform nucleus are well developed in the anterior lobe, the simple lobule and the gracile lobule (corresponding to the paramedian lobule of Bolk), scarce in the semilunar lobules (Bolk's ansiform lobule), but absent from the biventral lobule and the tonsil (corresponding to the paraflocculus). The rest of the hemisphere projects to the dentate nucleus. There are indications for a subdivision of the hemisphere into two zones (D1 and D2) projecting to the caudolateral (D1) zone and rostromedial parts of the dentate nucleus. The caudolateral and rostromedial parts of the dentate nucleus differ in average cell size (the neurons of the caudolateral dentate are generally smaller), the shape of the convolutions of the nucleus (broader in the caudolateral dentate) and in their projections to the thalamus. The efferent connections of the flocculus are mainly with the superior, spinal and medial vestibular nuclei and resemble those from the nodule and the adjacent uvula.

Efferent connections of the fastigial nucleus

The *fastigial nucleus* is connected bilaterally with the vestibular nuclei and the medullary and pontine reticular formation (**8.**171B, 172). Smaller, crossed connections ascend to the mesencephalon and diencephalon and descend into the spinal cord. Small GABAergic neurons give rise to nucleo-olivary fibres, which terminate in the medial accessory olive (**8.**174). The nucleo-olivary projection of the fastigial nucleus is less developed than for the other cerebellar nuclei.

The uncinate tract is the major efferent pathway of the fastigial nucleus. Its fibres cross in the rostral part of the cerebellar com-

Table 8.4 Summary of the projections of the cerebellar nuclei to the brain stem, the thalamus and the spinal cord. The afferent connections of the cerebellar nuclei are indicated in the left two columns. Projections are arranged into functional systems: projections to motor nuclei in the brain stem, projections to the spinal cord, direct and indirect projections to precerebellar nuclei and projections to the thalamus. Abbreviations DAO = dorsal accessory olive; MAO = medial accessory olive; NRTP = nucleus reticularis tegmenti pontis; nuu = nucleus; tr = tract; VL = ventrolateral thalamic nucleus.

Corticonuclear projection from:	Cerebellar nucleus	Motor nuclei in the brain stem			Spinal cord	Direct and indirect connections with precerebellar connections			Thalamus
		Subcortical motor systems	Visuomotor systems	Visceromotor systems		Precerebellar (mossy fibre nuclei)	Inferior olive	Mesencephalo-olivary pathways	
Vermis — A zone	fastigial nu.	medial medullary reticular formation: reticulospinal tr. medial and spinal vestibular nuclei: medial vestibulospinal tr.	horizontal gaze centre (PPRF) vertical gaze centre (riMLF) superior colliculus	central grey parasolitary nu. raphe nuclei nucleus of the locus coeruleus	cervical cord	NRTP lateral reticular nu.	caudal MAO	Darkschewitsch nu.: medial tegmental tr.	bilateral VL and intralaminar nuclei
B zone		lateral vestibular nu.: lateral vestibulospinal tr.					caudal DAO		
Pars intermedia — C₁ & C₃ zone	emboliform nu. (anterior interposed nu.)	magnocellular red nu.: rubrospinal tr.				pontine nuclei NRTP	rostral DAO		contralateral VL and intralaminar nuclei
C₂ zone	globose nu. (posterior interposed nu.)		superior colliculus	central grey raphe nuclei	cervical cord		rostral MAO	Darkschewitsch nu.: medial tegmental tr.	contralateral VL and intralaminar nuclei
Hemisphere — D zone	dentate nu.		contralateral nu. III (from group y)			pontine nuclei NRTP	principle olive	parvicellular red nu.: central tegmental tr.	contralateral VL and intralaminar nuclei
Vestibulo cerebellum: nodulus and flocculus			superior and medial vestibular nuclei: ascending pathways to oculomotor nuclei						

missure (**8**.151) and pass dorsal to the superior cerebellar peduncle, to enter the vestibular nuclei from laterally. Direct (uncrossed) fastigiobulbar fibres enter the cerebellar nuclei through the juxtarestiform body (**8**.155). The distribution of the fibres of the uncinate tract and the direct fastigiobulbar fibres is bilateral with a contralateral preponderance (**8**.170B): both terminate in the medial and spinal vestibular nuclei and traverse these nuclei to distribute to the medial reticular formation where they terminate. Some crossed fibres can be traced caudally into the spinal cord. A small fascicle of crossed fibres of the fastigial nucleus ascends along the superior cerebellar peduncle. It separates from the peduncle at its decussation and is distributed to the dorsal tegmentum, the central grey and bilaterally in the intercollicular region and the deep layers of the superior colliculus and the nuclei of the posterior commissure. In the thalamus, fibres terminate bilaterally in the ventrolateral nucleus and the intralaminar nuclei; the ipsilateral components recross in the commissure of the superior colliculus, the posterior commissure and the massa intermedia.

Cerebello-vestibular connections

The relations of the cerebellum to the vestibular nuclei are complex (**8**.170). In addition to the vestibulocerebellum (nodule, adjacent folia of the uvula and the flocculus), the vermis and the fastigial nucleus also project to the vestibular nuclei. The vestibulocerebellum projects to the rostral pole of vestibular nuclei, represented by the superior vestibular nucleus, and to the caudal tail of this complex, containing the medial and spinal vestibular nuclei (**8**.170). Neurons of these nuclei, which receive an input from the vestibular nerve and which project to the eye muscle nuclei (vestibulo-ocular relay cells) are among the main targets of the Purkinje cells of the flocculus. Purkinje cell axons from the nodule and the flocculus terminate in the same vestibular nuclei, but in different regions. Through its connections with vestibulo-ocular relay cells, the flocculus is involved in long-term adaptation of compensatory eye movements, in the generation of smooth eye movements used to pursue an object and in the suppression of the vestibulo-ocular reflex during smooth pursuit. The function of the nodulus in eye movement control is less well understood.

Both flocculus and nodulus receive mossy fibre projections from the same vestibular nuclei which receive their Purkinje cell axons. The vestibular nuclei are the main source of mossy fibre afferents for the nodulus; the vestibular mossy fibre projection to the flocculus is a relatively minor one. Most mossy fibres terminating in the flocculus take their origin from the reticular formation and relay optokinetic and visual information. The flocculus is included in the vestibulocerebellum because it uses the vestibular nuclei as its efferent pathway. The nodule has strong afferent as well as efferent connections with the vestibular nuclei.

Although the central, magnocellular region of the vestibular nuclei is often considered to be a single nucleus, this terminology is misleading, because it is made up of two completely different nuclei. A dorsal portion corresponds to *Deiters' lateral vestibular nucleus* and a ventral portion corresponds to the magnocellular part of the *medial vestibular nucleus*. Deiters' nucleus which lacks an input from the labyrinth and receives the Purkinje cell axons of the B zone of the anterior vermis can be considered as a

displaced, cerebellar nucleus. Deiters' nucleus gives rise to an ipsilaterally descending excitatory pathway (lateral vestibulospinal tract) to all levels of the spinal cord. Deiters' nucleus is avoided by the bilateral efferent pathways of the fastigial nucleus, which terminate more ventrally on large neurons which belong to the magnocellular part of the medial vestibular nucleus and in the medial reticular formation (8.170). The medial cerebellar nucleus (including its magnocellular part) and the spinal vestibular nucleus receive a strong input from the vestibular nerve and give rise to bilaterally ascending and descending tracts, which course in the medial longitudinal fascicle. Some of these pathways are inhibitory. The ascending

fibres include the axons of the vestibulo-ocular relay cells from the medial and spinal vestibular nuclei. The descending fibre systems from these nuclei are known as the medial vestibulospinal tract. Through Deiters' nucleus and the magnocellular medial nucleus, the vermis exerts an influence on postural and labyrinth reflexes. In lower mammals the lateral vestibulospinal tract is the dominant efferent pathway, and lesions of the cerebellum including the B zone, which disinhibit Deiters' nucleus, lead to ipsilateral extensor hypertonia. In primates and in man this is no longer the case, and lesions of the anterior lobe usually induce hypotonia.

Via the fastigial nucleus each hemivermis influences different functional systems (Table 8.4). The fastigial nucleus projects bilaterally to several subcortical motor centres, which give rise to descending brainstem pathways. They include the medial and spinal vestibular nucleus (see Cerebello-vestibular connections p. 1051) and the medial bulbar reticular formation, which gives rise to the bilaterally descending medial reticulospinal tracts. Through these pathways the A zone of the vermis exerts a bilateral influence on ventromedially located spinal interneurons and motor neurons, which innervate axial, truncal and proximal limb muscles (Kuypers' medial motor system). Some fibres of the uncinate tract descend as far as the cervical cord, where they terminate on the same neurons. Through its projection to the lateral vestibular nucleus and the lateral vestibulospinal tract, the B zone exerts an influence on ipsilateral interneurons and motor neurons of the same system (8.167).

The projections of the fastigial nucleus to the thalamus are relatively minor. They are bilateral, due to the recrossing of the crossed ascending fibres of the uncinate tract. They include parts of the ventrolateral nucleus and the intralaminar nuclei (centrolateral and parafascicular nuclei), where they overlap with the terminations of other cerebellar nuclei. The termination in the ventrolateral nucleus is medial with respect to the projections of the dentate and interposed nuclei. This region of the ventrolateral nucleus projects to the rostral motor cortex, which gives rise to a component of the pyramidal tract which terminates bilaterally in the bulbar medial reticular formation and the ventromedial interneurons and motor neurons of the spinal cord. Motor centres in the brainstem and regions of the motor cortex which exert a bilateral control over the medial motor system of the spinal cord, therefore, are influenced by the fastigial nucleus.

The caudal region of the fastigial nucleus which receives Purkinje cell axons from the folium and tuber, an area of the vermis which receives visual inputs, (8.175) projects to regions of the contralateral pontine and rostral mesencephalic reticular formation that contain the horizontal gaze centre (paramedian pontine reticular formation; PPRF) and the vertical gaze centre (rostral interstitial nucleus of the medial longitudinal fascicle; riMLF) and, bilaterally, to deep layers of the superior colliculus. These projections probably mediate the adaptation of saccades by the vermal visual area.

Cerebellar influences on visceromotor systems are mediated by the projections of the fastigial nucleus to the parasolitary nucleus, a region bordering on the viscerosensory nuclei of the solitary tract, and to the dorsal visceromotor nucleus of the vagus nerve, the central grey, the serotoninergic raphe nuclei and the noradrenergic nucleus of the locus coeruleus (Table 8.4).

Other pathways from the cerebellar nuclei terminate on precerebellar relay nuclei which give rise to mossy or climbing fibres. Recurrent circuits involving the fastigial nucleus include the nucleus reticularis tegmenti pontis (8.173B) and the so-called 'nucleo-olivary'

projection from the fastigial nucleus to the medial accessory olive (8.174). The nucleo-olivary projections, which take their origin from all cerebellar nuclei, are crossed and contain GABA as a neurotransmitter. The connections of the fastigial nucleus with the reticular nuclei are excitatory.

A third system which takes its origin from the cerebellar nuclei terminates on cells which are located at the border of the mesencephalon and the diencephalon and which give rise to uncrossed descending pathways to the inferior olive (8.173). These pathways are known as the tegmental tracts. The medial tegmental tract originates from cell groups located in or around the central grey. The *nucleus of Darkschewitsch* is the main representative of this group. The medial tegmental tract terminates in the medial accessory olive. The central tegmental tract arises from the rostral, parvicellular part of the red nucleus; it is one of the major descending pathways in the human brainstem and terminates on the principal nucleus of the inferior olive. The tegmental tracts are excitatory pathways that complement the inhibitory nucleo-olivary projection. Through its nucleo-olivary projection and its connections with the contralateral nucleus of Darkschewitsch, the fastigial nucleus controls the climbing fibre output of the medial accessory olive.

Efferent connections of the dentate and interposed nuclei

The axons of neurons in the dentate and interposed nucleus are contained in the superior cerebellar peduncle. Fibres from the globose nucleus occupy a medial position; those from the emboliform and dentate nucleus are successively more lateral (8.171A). Axons of excitatory vestibulo-ocular relay cells of the superior vestibular nucleus occupy the extreme lateral pole of the peduncle. Nucleo-olivary fibres of the interposed and dentate nuclei are located in a separate bundle, ventral to the peduncle. The superior cerebellar peduncle including its nucleo-olivary component decussates in the caudal mesencephalon (8.171B). The decussation consists of dorsal and ventral portions. The dorsal portion consists of fibres of the medial two-thirds of the peduncle, which start to cross the midline at the level of the inferior colliculus, ventral to the medial longitudinal fasciculus. The ventral portion consists of fibres of the lateral third of the peduncle, which decussate in the ventral tegmentum, immediately dorsal to the interpeduncular nucleus. Rostrally, at the level of the caudal red nucleus, the ventral and dorsal portions of the decussation merge and the entire decussation is displaced ventrally by the dorsal tegmental (tectospinal) decussation.

After its decussation the peduncle divides into ascending and descending branches. The descending branch terminates in the medial reticular formation of the pons and the medulla and in the reticular tegmental nucleus of the pons (8.171). The nucleo-olivary fibres join the descending branch to terminate in the inferior olive in a strictly orderly manner (see below). The much larger, ascending branch

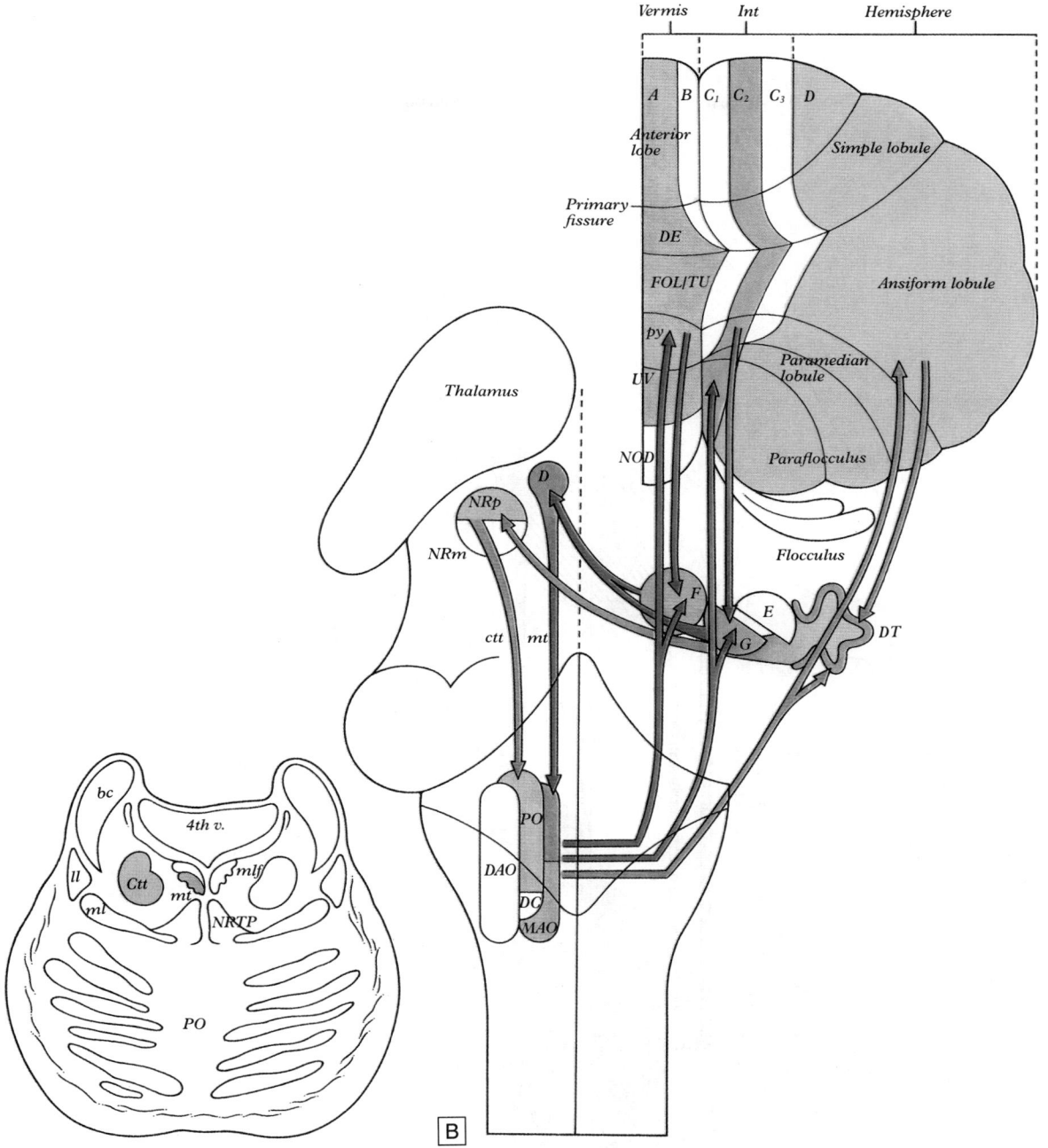

Vermis · Int · Hemisphere

A B C₁ C₂ C₃ D

Anterior lobe

Simple lobule

Primary fissure

DE

FOL/TU

Ansiform lobule

py

Paramedian lobule

UV

NOD

Paraflocculus

Flocculus

Thalamus

NRp

NRm

D

F

E

G

DT

ctt mt

PO

DAO

DC

MAO

bc

4th v.

mlf

ll

Ctt

mt

ml

NRTP

PO

A

B

8.173   The tegmental tracts.

A.   Transverse section through the pons, showing the localization of the central and medial tegmental tracts.

B.   The medial and the central tegmental tract project to different divisions of the inferior olive. The central tegmental tract is a link in a circuit involving the dentate nucleus, the parvicellular red nucleus, the principal olive and the D zone of the hemisphere. The medial tegmental tract is a link in a circuit including the globose nucleus, Darkschewitsch nucleus, the rostral medial accessory olive and the C2 zone. The fastigial nucleus, the caudal medial accessory olive and the A zone participate to some degree in the latter circuit. For connections of the cerebellar nuclei with the magnocellular red

nucleus and the thalamus see **8**.170. 4th v = fourth ventricle; A = Purkinje cell zone A; B = Purkinje cell zone B; C₁₋₃ = Purkinje cell zones C₁₋₃; ctt = central tegmental tract; D = Purkinje cell zone D; DA = Darkschewitsch nucleus; DAO = dorsal accessory olive; DC = dorsal cap; DE = declive; DT = dentate nucleus; E = emboliform (anterior interposed) nucleus; FOL/Tu = folium/tuber; G = globose (posterior interposed) nucleus; Int = pars intermedia; ll = lateral lemniscus; MAO = medial accessory olive; ml = medial lemniscus; mlf = medial longitudinal fascicle; mt = medial tegmental tract; NOD = nodulus; NRm = magnocellular red nucleus; NRp = parvicellular red nucleus; NRTP = nucleus reticularis tegmenti pontis; PO = pontine nuclei; PO = principal nucleus of the inferior olive; UV = uvula.

distributes to the mesencephalon and the diencephalon, with the red nucleus and the thalamus as its main targets. The dentate and interposed nuclei influence different functional systems, although they share some of their target nuclei (Table **8**.4). The emboliform nucleus (anterior interposed nucleus), which receives Purkinje cell axons from the pars intermedia (C1 and C3 zones) of the anterior lobe and the simple lobule (lobulus quadrangularis posterior), projects to the contralateral magnocellular red nucleus. The caudal, magnocellular part of the red nucleus is a subcortical motor centre,

which gives rise to the rubrospinal tract. This tract crosses in the mesencephalon, and terminates on laterally located spinal interneurons and motor neurons which innervate distal limb muscles.

The emboliform nucleus projects to lateral parts of the ventrolateral nucleus, which are connected with the caudal motor cortex: pyramidal tract fibres which take their origin from the caudal motor cortex terminate contralaterally on laterally located interneurons and motor neurons. Control of the ipsilateral limbs by the pars intermedia is effectuated by the emboliform nucleus through two different

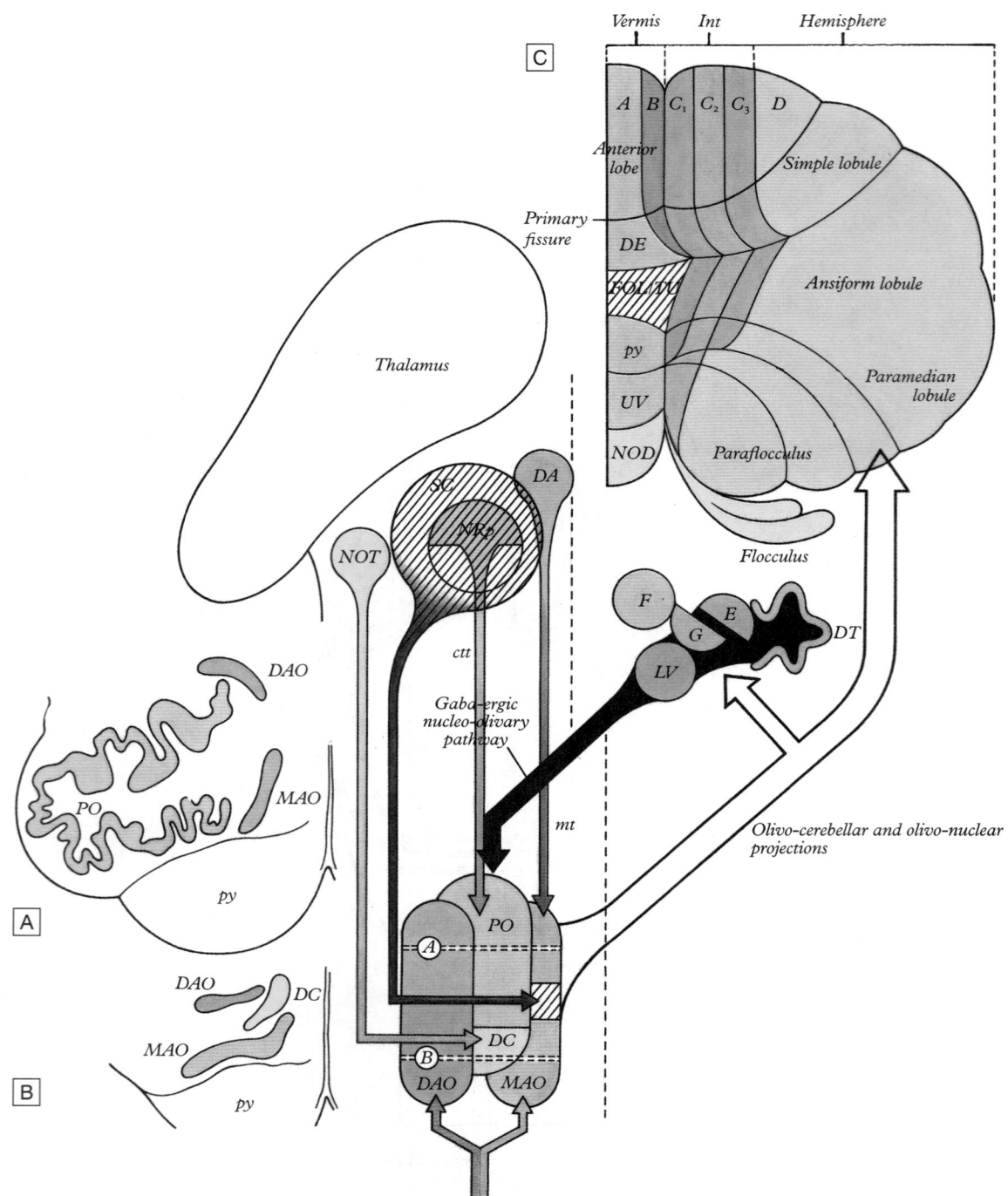

8.174 Diagram of the olivocerebellar projection.

A and B. Transverse sections through the left inferior olive, showing its subdivisions. Levels indicated in C.

C. The principal olive and the accessory olive, drawn as three cylinders. The olivocerebellar projection is indicated with an open arrow, the reciprocal GABAergic nucleo-olivary pathway as a filled arrow. Interconnected subdivisions of the inferior olive, their main afferent connections, their terminations as climbing fibres on Purkinje cell zones of vermis and hemispheres, and their collateral projections to the cerebellar nuclei are indicated with the same colours. A = Purkinje cell zone A; B = Purkinje cell zone B; C_{1-3} = Purkinje cell zones C_{1-3}; ctt = central tegmental tract; D = Purkinje cell zone D; DA = Darkschewitsch nucleus; DAO = dorsal accessory olive; DC = dorsal cap; DE = declive; DT = dentate nucleus; E = emboliform (anterior interposed) nucleus; FOL/TU = folium/tuber; G = globose (posterior interposed) nucleus; Int = pars intermedia; MAO = medial accessory olive; mt = medial tegmental tract; NOD = nodulus; NRp = parvicellular red nucleus; NOT = nuclei of the optic tract; on = olivonuclear collateral connection; PO = principal nucleus of the inferior olive; py = pyramidal tract; SC = superior colliculus; UV = uvula.

pathways: the rubrospinal and the corticospinal tracts, which converge upon the same interneurons and motor neurons (**8.171B**).

The emboliform nucleus projects to the nucleus reticularis tegmenti pontis and the basal pontine nuclei; precerebellar nuclei which give rise to mossy fibres. Its nucleo-olivary efferents terminate in the rostral half of the dorsal accessory olive (**8.171, 179**). The emboliform nucleus does not participate in the recurrent cerebello–mesencephalon–olivary circuits.

The efferent connections of the globose nucleus (posterior interposed) are very similar to those of the fastigial nucleus. The two nuclei share projections to the cord, the superior colliculus, the central grey and the raphe nuclei. Nucleo-olivary projections from the globose nucleus and the recurrent globose nucleus–Darkschewitsch nucleus–inferior olivary pathway converge upon the rostral half of the medial accessory olive (**8**.173, 174). Thalamic projections overlap with those from the fastigial and anterior interposed nuclei.

The main projections from the dentate nucleus include the *contralateral, parvicellular red nucleus*, the *thalamus* and the *oculomotor nucleus*. The central tegmental tract takes its origin from the parvicellular red nucleus and terminates on the principal nucleus of the olive (**8**.173, 174). The thalamic projection to the ventrolateral nucleus overlaps with other cerebellar nuclei, but also extends in the most medial region of this nucleus, which projects to the premotor area of the frontal lobe. Projections of the dentate to the most medial part of the ventrolateral nucleus are derived from caudal and lateral parts of the dentate nucleus. Direct projections from the dentate nucleus to the contralateral oculomotor nucleus take their origin from group Y: a cell group located ventral to the dentate nucleus located within the floccular peduncle.

In addition to the cerebellar projections, the thalamus receives a massive input from other major motor systems. In particular, the output of the basal ganglia is relayed to the thalamus by a projection from the globus pallidus. The evidence suggests that these two great subcortical motor systems terminate on different regions of the ventral thalamus and project to different targets in the motor and premotor cortex (p. 1164).

AFFERENT CONNECTIONS TO THE CEREBELLUM

Afferent connections of the cerebellum include the mossy fibres and the climbing fibres. The monoaminergic afferents were considered in the section on the chemoarchitecture of the cerebellum. The organization of the mossy fibre systems differs substantially from that of the climbing fibres. Mossy fibre systems terminate bilaterally in transversely oriented 'lobular' areas. The terminations of different mossy fibre systems overlap considerably (**8**.145A). Climbing fibres from different subnuclei of the inferior olive terminate contralaterally, on discrete, longitudinal strips of Purkinje cells (**8**.174). This longitudinal pattern closely corresponds with the zonal arrangement in the corticonuclear projection (**8**.172).

Cerebellar localization

During the early years of this century it was generally thought that the cerebellum was concerned primarily with proprioceptive and

vestibular functions. The presence of tactile, visual and acoustic inputs and their localization in specific parts of the cerebellum was demonstrated with evoked potential methods in anaesthetized laboratory animals in the 1940s and 1950s (**8**.175). Somaesthetic, tactile and proprioceptive input was found in two areas. One area comprised the anterior lobe and the adjoining simple lobule; the other, located in the posterior lobe, included the paramedian lobule and the pyramis. Each area displays a crude somatotopic localization. The hindlimb is located in the most anterior parts of the anterior lobe and the posterior part of the posterior lobes. There is an orderly somatotopic organization with the head in the simple lobule, caudal to the primary fissure, and in the dorsal part of the paramedian lobule. This mirrored somatotopy in anterior and posterior lobes of the cerebellum is more distinct in the medial hemisphere (the pars intermedia, the paramedian lobule) than it is in the vermis. Tactile and proprioceptive input from the periphery was studied by stimulation of peripheral nerves or by natural stimulation. Evoked potentials on stimulation of the contralateral sensory and motor cortex were found in the same two areas with a similar somatotopy. Visual evoked potentials on flash stimulation of the eye were located in a vermal visual area corresponding to folium and tuber (lobule VII of Larsell). This visual area may extend into the hemisphere (the semilunar or ansiform lobule). A second visual area, corresponding to the paraflocculus (the biventral lobule and the tonsil) was added much later on the basis of input relayed to it from the visual association cortex of the cerebral hemisphere. Acoustic areas, containing evoked potentials to sound and/or afferent connections from the acoustic cortex, seem to overlap with the visual areas. Vestibular input was mainly localized in the nodulus and the flocculus, i.e. the lobules of the vestibulocerebellum.

At the time, the mossy and climbing fibre inputs of the cerebellum

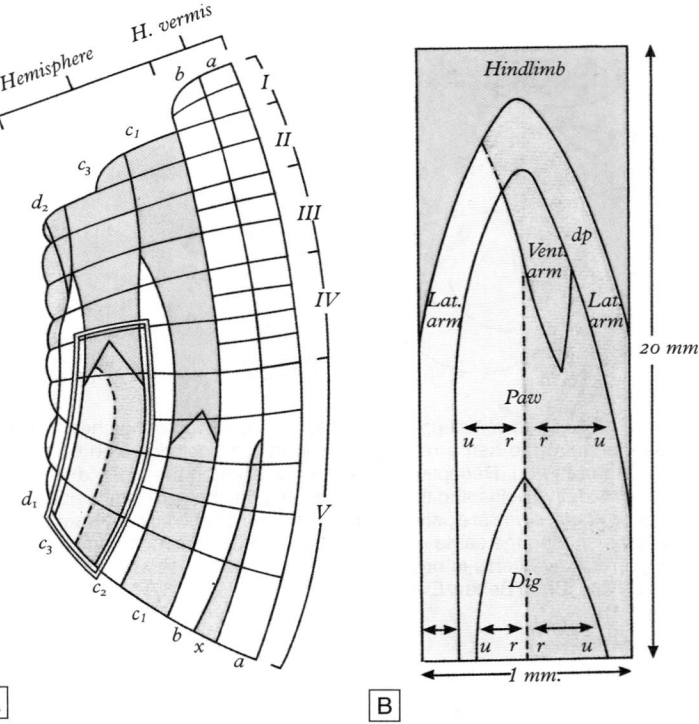

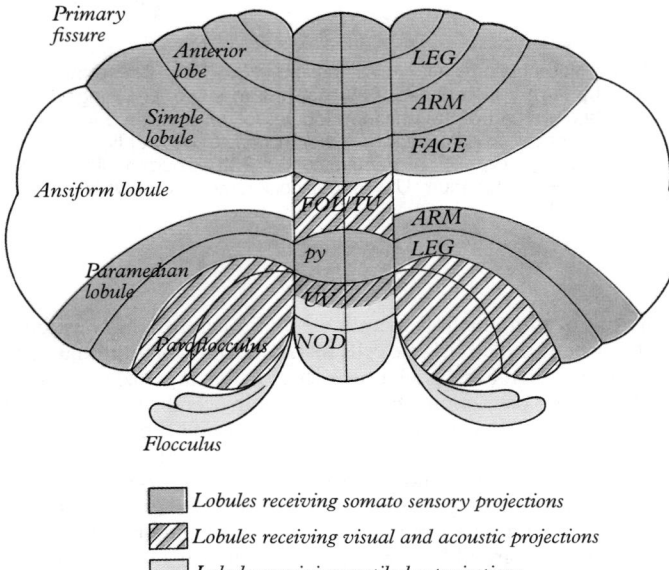

8.175 Diagram of the localization of somatosensory (red), acoustic and visual (blue) and vestibular (yellow) evoked potentials and the crude somatotopic localization in the somatosensory areas of the cerebellum. FOL/TU, folium tuber; NOD, nodulus; PY, pyramis; UV, uvula.

8.176 A. Diagram of the zonal organization of the cutaneous climbing fibre input to lobules I–V of the anterior lobe of the cerebellum of the cat. Input from the forelimb is indicated in yellow, of the hindlimb in blue. Empty zones do not receive a somatotopically organized climbing fibre cutaneous input. Redrawn from Ekerot and Larson (1982).
B. Diagram of the somatotopic organization of nociceptive climbing fibre input from the forelimb to part of the c_3 zone. The forelimb is represented twice, once in the medial and once in the lateral half of the c_3 zone. The regions indicated in the diagram can be further subdivided into microzones representing climbing fibres with identical receptive fields. From Garwicz et al (1991). a = climbing fibre zone a; b = climbing fibre zone b; $c_{1–3}$ = climbing fibre zones, $c_{1–3}$; d = distal; $d_{1,2}$ = climbing fibre zones d_1 and d_2; dig, digits; I–Va, lobules I–Va of Larsell; lat = lateral; p = proximal; r = radial; u = ulnar; vent, ventral; x = climbing fibre zone x.

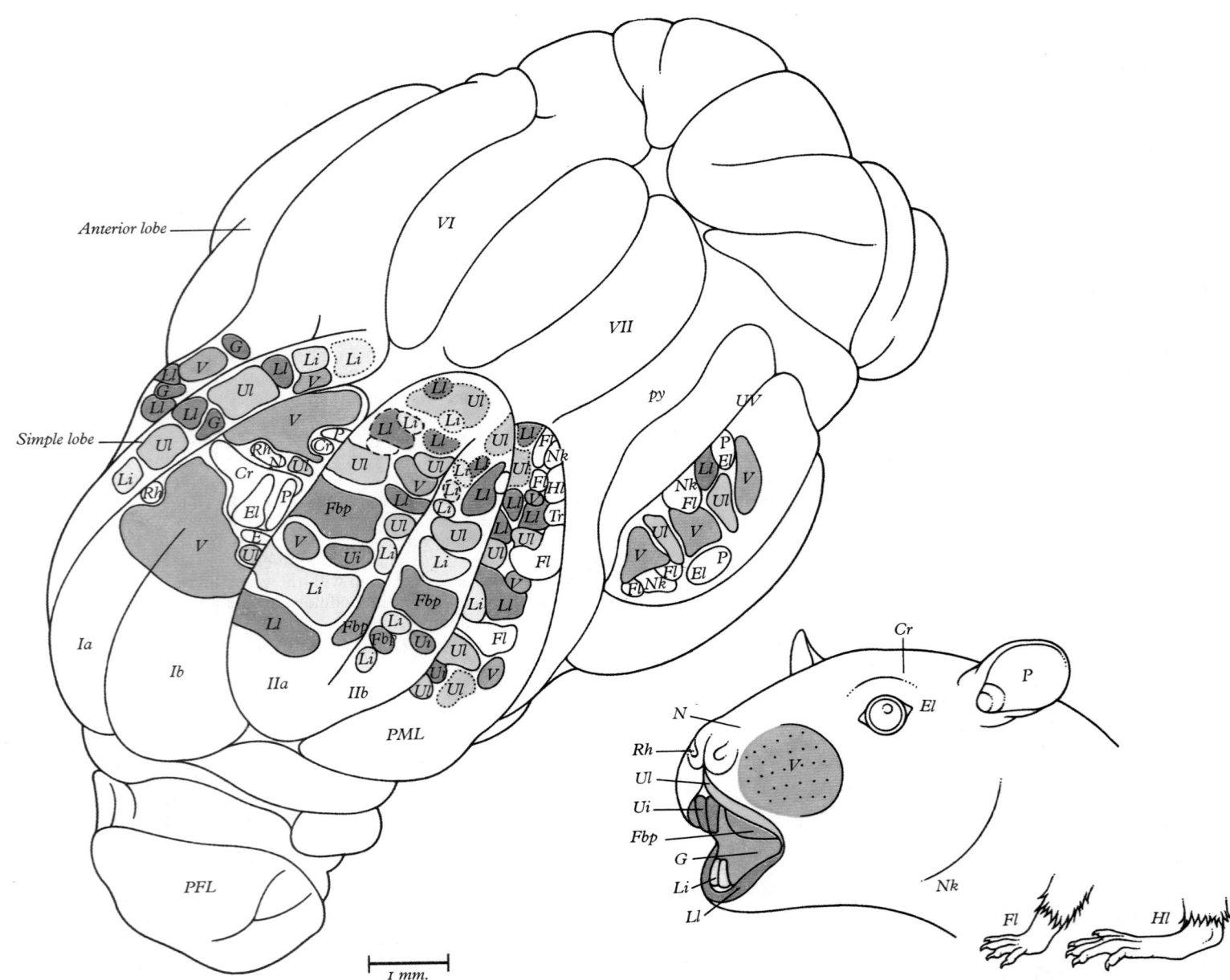

8.177 Fractured somatropy: Somatotopic distribution of patches of mossy fibres sharing the same receptive fields in the posterior lobe of the cerebellum of the rat. Receptive fields are indicated on the figurine of the rat. Major receptive fields and the corresponding patches are indicated with the same colours, some are only indicated with their abbreviations. Note multiple patches sharing the same receptive field, and the loss of common borders of the receptive fields in ordering of the patches. Redrawn from Shambes et al (1978, Brain Behav. Evol., 15: 94) and Welker (1987, New Concepts in Cerebellar Neurobiology, Alan Liss Inc. pp. 239–280). Cr = crown; El = eyelids; Fbp = furry buccal pad; Fl = foot and forelimb; G = gingiva; Hl = hindlimb; Ia,c = crus I of the ansiform lobule, folium a, b; IIa,b = crus II of the ansiform lobule, folium a, b; Li = lower incisor; Ll = lower lip; N = nose; Nk = neck; P = pinna; PFL = paraflocculus; PML = paramedian lobule; py = pyramis; Rh = rhinarium; Ui = upper incisor; uv = uvula; VI, VII =lobule VI, VII of Larsell.

could not be distinguished with physiological or anatomical methods. The distinction between the typical short burst of spikes (the complex spike) which characterizes the climbing fibre evoked potential in Purkinje cells, and the single (simple) spikes evoked by the parallel fibres, and the characterization of the mossy fibre responses in the granular layer followed from the work of Granit and Philips, and Eccles in the 1960s. Anatomical tracing methods allowing for the distinction of mossy and climbing fibres became available at the same time.

Localization in the olivocerebellar system: zones and microzones

Physiological and anatomical studies showed that climbing fibres originate exclusively from the contralateral inferior olive. The fibres from the different subnuclei of the inferior olive terminate as climbing fibres on longitudinal strips of Purkinje cells in the cerebellar cortex.

Collaterals of climbing fibres terminate on the cerebellar or vestibular target nuclei of these Purkinje cells (8.174, 176). A longitudinal zonal arrangement, therefore, is characteristic of the organization of the olivocerebellar projection (8.172). The olivocerebellar projection zones, moreover, correspond precisely to the corticonuclear projection zones described in the previous section of this chapter. The cerebellar output was found to be organized in a modular fashion, each module comprising one or more Purkinje cell zones, with their target nucleus and its efferent systems (8.169). Climbing fibres from the inferior olive are able to modify the cerebellar output in such a way that each subnucleus of the inferior olive monitors the output of a single cerebellar module.

The inferior olive and its climbing fibres can be activated by tactile and proprioceptive, visual and vestibular stimulation and from the sensory, motor and visual cortex and brainstem relays. Detailed maps have been constructed for several of the climbing fibre zones in the anterior lobe of the cat, showing the somatotopic organization of their tactile or nociceptive input (8.176). Climbing fibres activated from the same receptive field constitute long and narrow strips (microzones) within the climbing fibre zone. The size of these microzones in the cat, where they are continuous from the base, over the apex of single lobules, can be estimated at 80–200 × 20.000 μm, corresponding to 1–4 × 350 Purkinje cells. The receptive fields are mapped in an orderly manner in microzones from the medial to the lateral border of the climbing fibre zone. The representation of the body in a single climbing fibre strip, therefore, is stretched out over a great length. The representation of the body in the climbing fibre zones of the anterior lobe is multiple. Each tactile zone contains one or sometimes two symmetrical representations of the body (8.176B). The border between the representation of the hindlimb in the anterior part of the anterior lobe and of the forelimb in its posterior part can be recognized. Identical somatotopical patterns are present in these climbing fibre zones on stimulation of the contralateral somatosensory and motor cortex. The climbing fibre zones with somatosensory input alternate with zones innervated from other subnuclei of the inferior olive. These zones do not receive a short-latency somatotopically organized climbing fibre input, but their internal organization in mediolaterally arranged microzones, probably, is very similar.

In the adult each climbing fibre innervates a single Purkinje cell. Olivocerebellar parent fibres branch sparingly, each parent fibre innervating 10 Purkinje cells. Purkinje cells innervated by the same climbing fibre are located in somatotopically equivalent sections (microzones) of single or multiple climbing fibre zones.

Localization in mossy fibre systems

Mossy fibres are by far the main input to the cerebellum. Mossy fibres take their origin from different precerebellar nuclei in the brainstem and the spinal cord. Most mossy fibres enter the cerebellum in the middle and inferior cerebellar peduncles. In the cerebellum they are positioned lateral, rostral and dorsal to the cerebellar nuclei. Medially some of the mossy fibres cross in the rostral, afferent portion of the cerebellar commissure to terminate in the contralateral half of the cerebellum. The caudal, efferent portion of the cerebellar commissure contains the fibres of the uncinate tract (8.151). The afferent portion of the cerebellar commissure extends from the anterior medullary velum and the white matter of the anterior lobe, into the white matter of folium and tuber. Mossy fibres branch repeatedly. Branches entering the white matter of the lobules and folia are oriented in a parasagittal plane and may give rise to longitudinally oriented terminal fields in the granular layer, which resemble the longitudinal climbing fibre zones. Mossy fibre terminal zones are always multiple, and are more variable and less well defined than the climbing fibre zones (8.180).

The main characteristic of the mossy fibre terminal fields is their transverse or 'lobular' arrangement. This transverse arrangement is enhanced by the transverse orientation of the parallel fibres, which constitute the second link in this afferent pathway. Mossy fibre systems are distributed in different, dorsoventrally arranged tiers in parasagittal sections of the cerebellum (8.178). As a consequence mossy fibre projections differ with respect to the localization of their terminal fields along the baso–apical axis of the individual lobules. Vestibulocerebellar fibres terminate in a ventral tier, including the nodulus and the ventral portion of the uvula, the ventralmost lobules of the anterior lobe and the granular layer in the bottom of the deep interlobular fissures. Spinocerebellar fibres terminate more dorsally and apically in the lobules of the anterior lobe, the declive and in the pyramis of the caudal vermis. Pontocerebellar fibres terminate superficially in the lobules of the anterior lobe, and more strongly in folium and tuber and in the dorsal half of the uvula. There is extensive overlap of the different fields in a single lobule, but the general baso–apical disposition of the terminals of the different mossy fibre systems remains obvious (8.180).

Mossy fibres terminate both in the granular layer and in the cerebellar nuclei. Unlike climbing fibres, which always give rise to collateral projections to the cerebellar target nuclei of the Purkinje cells they innervate, the mossy fibre collateral projections to the nuclei are not provided by all mossy fibre systems. Reticulocerebellar mossy fibres from the lateral reticular nucleus and the nucleus reticularis tegmenti pontis are the main sources of mossy fibre

collaterals (8.179); pontocerebellar and cuneocerebellar mossy fibres project sparsely if at all to the nuclei.

Somatotopical localization in mossy fibre systems: fractured somatotopy

Somatotopic localization in tactile mossy fibre terminal fields has been studied in great detail. Evoked potentials on stimulation of a cutaneous source were found in multiple, discrete patches in the granular layer. Contiguity of adjacent body areas is not maintained in the localization of the corresponding patches: representations of the hindlimb may border on representations of the lower lip and the facial whiskers. This type of localization was called 'fractured somatotopy' by Shambes et al (1978); (8.180). The mosaic of somatotopically defined patches is fairly constant in different individuals. Mossy fibre projections from the somatosensory cortex and the superior colliculus to the cerebellar cortex conform to the same patchy mosaic.

The precise relationship between the fractured somatotopy in tactile mossy fibre projections and the multiple, mediolaterally arranged somatotopic representations in tactile and nociceptive climbing fibre zones has not been studied. There is a tendency for a crude somatotopical pattern in the anterior and posterior lobes for both afferent systems, but at a more detailed level mossy and climbing fibre somatotopical patterns do not coincide precisely.

Relation of mossy fibre–parallel fibre input to the output systems of the cerebellum

With respect to the relation of the mossy fibre–parallel fibre systems to the output systems of the cerebellar cortex it should be remembered that the Purkinje cell layer of each cerebellar lobule is subdivided into longitudinal zones, which belong to different cerebellar modules, project to different cerebellar nuclei and receive their climbing fibre input from different subnuclei of the inferior olive (8.181A). There is a strong convergence in the projection of the Purkinje cells along a zone (or microzone) on their target nucleus. Axons of Purkinje cells, belonging to the same zone but located in the apex or at the base of a lobule, probably terminate on the same nuclear cells (8.181B).

A patch of mossy fibre terminals activates a transversely oriented beam of parallel fibres, which terminate on Purkinje cells belonging

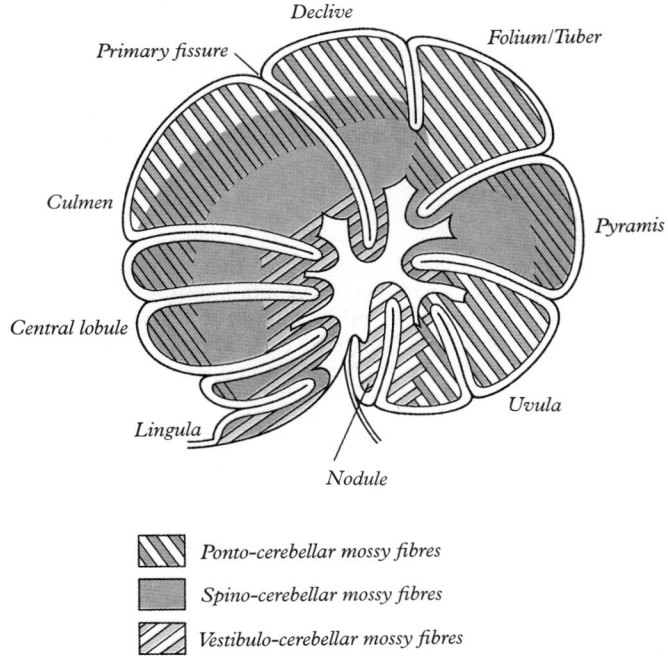

Declive

Folium/Tuber

Primary fissure

Culmen

Pyramis

Central lobule

Uvula

Lingula

Nodule

||||| Ponto-cerebellar mossy fibres

▨ Spino-cerebellar mossy fibres

▨ Vestibulo-cerebellar mossy fibres

8.178 Concentric, or tiered distribution of different mossy fibre systems in a diagram of a sagittal section of the cerebellum. Pontocerebellar mossy fibres (see also 8.184) terminate superficially, vestibulocerebellar mossy fibres (see also 8.182) terminate in the cortex in the bottom of the fissures, spinocerebellar mossy fibres (see also 8.183) terminate in an intermediate position.

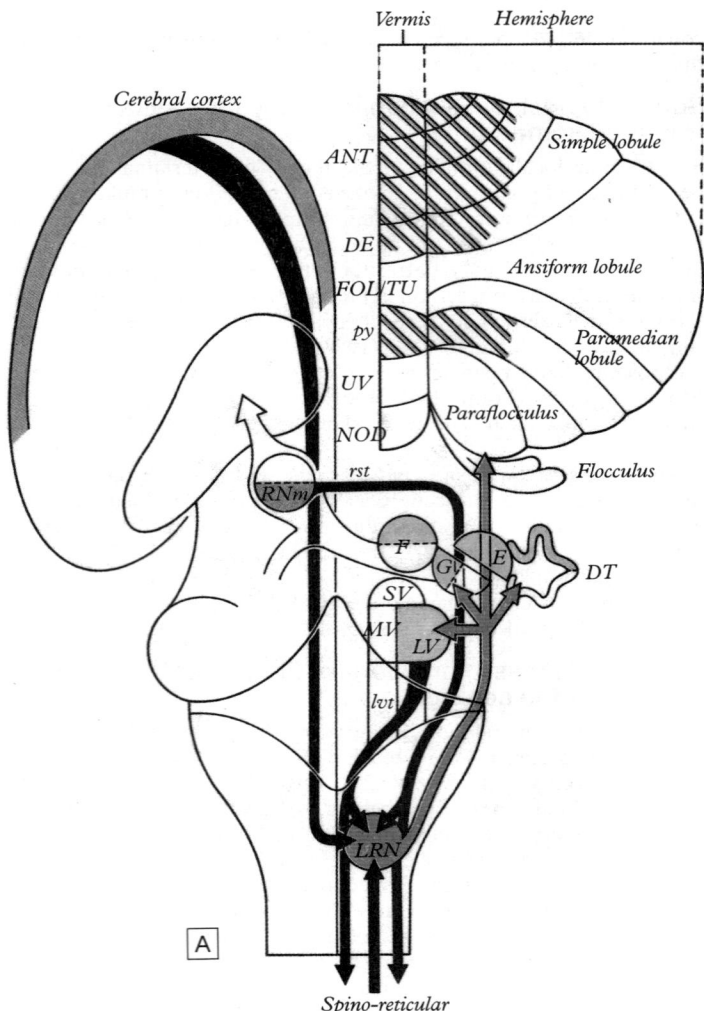

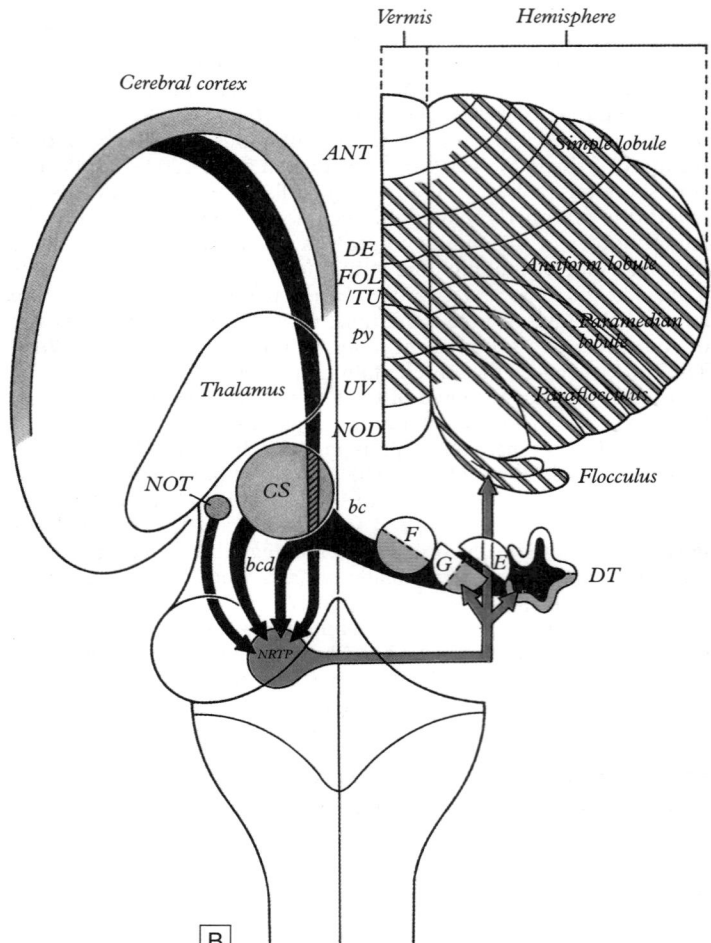

8.179 Reticulocerebellar projections: reticulocerebellar mossy fibres terminate in the cerebellar cortex; their collaterals terminate in the cerebellar nuclei.

A. The lateral reticular nucleus receives collateral projections from the rubrospinal and lateral vestibulospinal tracts, a strong spinoreticular projection and a projection from the cerebral cortex. It projects to the anterior lobe and the paramedian lobules and has collaterals to the rostral part of the fastigial nucleus, part of the globose, the dentate and to the emboliform nucleus.

B. The nucleus reticularis tegmenti pontis receives afferents from the nucleus of the optic tract, the tectum, the cerebral cortex and the descending limb of the brachium conjunctivum. It projects to all lobules of the cerebellum, with the exception of some parts of the anterior lobe and the nodulus, and with a collateral projection to parts of the fastigial, globose and dentate nuclei. Note complementarity in the collateral projections of the nucleus reticularis tegmenti pontis and the lateral reticular nucleus to the cerebellar nuclei. Whether such a complementarity also exists for their mossy fibre projections in the cerebellar cortex, is not known. The diagrams are based on studies in the cat, reviewed in Brodal (Neurological Anatomy, third edition, Oxford University Press, 1981), and Gerrits and Voogd (J. Comp. Neurol. 258: 52, 1986). ANT = anterior lobe; bc = brachium conjunctivum; bcd = descending branch of the brachium conjunctivum; CS = superior colliculus; DE = declive; DT = dentate nucleus; E = emboliform (anterior interposed) nucleus; F = fastigial nucleus; FOL/TU = folium/tuber; G = globose (posterior interposed) nucleus; LRN = lateral reticular nucleus; LV = lateral vestibular nucleus; lvt = lateral vestibulospinal tract; MV = medial vestibular nucleus; NOD = nodulus; NOT = nucleus of the tractus opticus; NRTP = nucleus reticularis tegmenti pontis; PY = pyramis; RNm = red nucleus, magnocellular division; rst = rubrospinal tract; SV = superior vestibular nucleus; UV = uvula.

to several different modules. Parallel fibre beams, activated by mossy fibre systems which differ in their termination deeply or superficially within a lobule, will activate different baso–apical segments of the Purkinje cell zones, or the microzones, present in that lobule (**8.181B**). The Purkinje cells of each of these zones converge upon a common group of nuclear cells. The Purkinje cell zones of a lobule, therefore, sample mossy fibre–parallel fibre input from widely different sources, but the results of this operation, in terms of the output of their cerebellar target nuclei to particular motor systems, are largely independent of the source of the mossy fibre input (**8.181A**).

Primary and secondary vestibulocerebellar mossy fibres

Primary vestibulocerebellar mossy fibres are fibres of the vestibular nerve, which enter the cerebellum with the ascending branch of this nerve, passing through the superior vestibular nucleus and the juxtarestiform body. They terminate, mainly ipsilaterally, in the granular layer of the nodule, the caudal part of the uvula, in the ventral part of the anterior lobe and in the bottom of the deep fissures of the vermis (**8.182A**). Secondary vestibulocerebellar mossy fibres take their origin from the superior vestibular nucleus and the caudal portions of the medial and spinal vestibular nuclei. They terminate bilaterally in the same regions which receive primary

vestibulocerebellar fibres, but also in the flocculus and the adjoining paraflocculus, which lack a primary vestibulocerebellar projection (**8.182B**). Some of the mossy fibres from the medial and spinal vestibular nuclei are cholinergic. In this respect they differ from the projections of the superior vestibular nucleus. Collateral projections of vestibulocerebellar mossy fibres to the cerebellar nuclei are still disputed.

Spinal and trigeminocerebellar mossy fibre systems

The spinal cord is connected with the cerebellum through spinocerebellar tracts and through indirect mossy fibre pathways, which are relayed by the lateral reticular nucleus. The spinocerebellar tracts are classified on the basis of their origin, their decussation within the spinal cord, their position in the lateral funiculus, their entrance route into the cerebellum and their lobular and zonal distribution

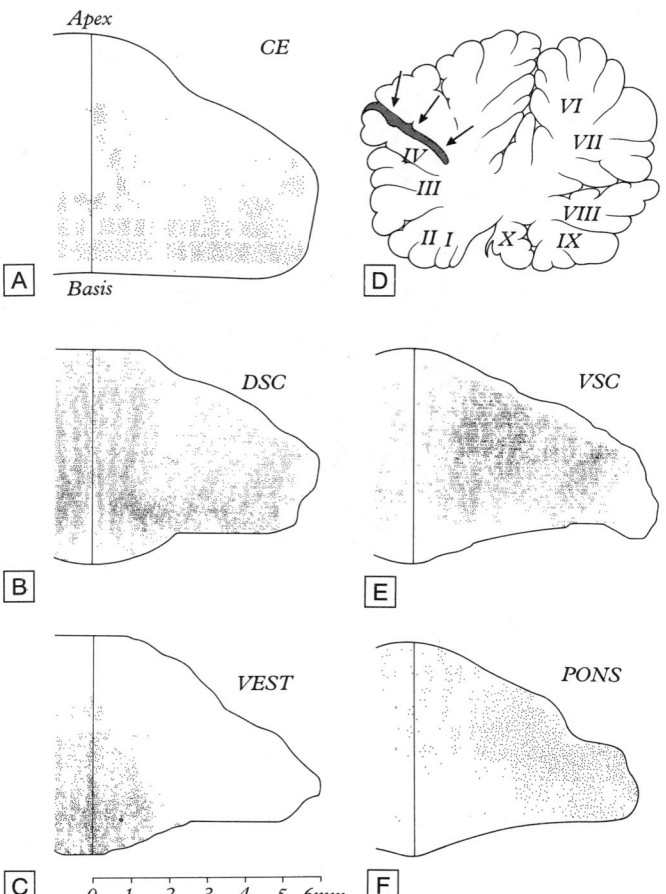

8.180 Distribution of different mossy fibre systems on the dorsal surface of lobule IV of the anterior lobe of the cat. The dorsal surface of lobule IV is indicated in the sagittal section of the cerebellum of the cat in panel D. Plots were reconstructed from serial sections with labelling of mossy fibre terminals of a specific pathway. A: cuneocerebellar mossy fibres (CE: from N M Gerrits, Brainstem control of the cerebellar flocculus. Thesis, Leiden University 1985), B: dorsal spinocerebellar tract (DSC, from Yaginuma and Matsushita, J. Comp. Neurol. 258: 1, 1987), C: secondary vestibulo-cerebellar mossy fibres (VEST, from Matsushita and Wang, Neurosci. Lett 74: 25, 1987), E: ventral spinocerebellar tract (VSC, component from spinal border cells, from Yaginuma and Matsushita, Brain Res. 384: 175, 1986) and F: pontocerebellar mossy fibres (from Gerrits, 1985).

(8.183). In addition to the classical dorsal and ventral spinocerebellar tracts, two more spinocerebellar tracts can be distinguished: the cuneocerebellar tract, which transmits forelimb information, and a rostral spinocerebellar tract from the cervical enlargement (8.183). The cuneocerebellar tract has similar properties to the dorsal spinocerebellar tract; the rostral spinocerebellar tract is similar in function to the ventral spinocerebellar tract. These tracts differ principally in the region of the body which they serve. The rostral spinocerebellar and cuneocerebellar tracts serve the forelimbs; the ventral and dorsal spinocerebellar tracts serve the hindlimbs. The dorsal spinocerebellar and cuneocerebellar tracts transmit pro-prioceptive and exteroceptive information from the limbs. The ventral and rostral spinocerebellar tracts both arise from the inter-mediate zone of the spinal cord and may provide the cerebellum with information from the interneurons located in this region. A fifth spinocerebellar tract arises from the central cervical nucleus in the upper cervical cord.

The dorsal spinocerebellar tract takes its origin from Clarke's column and from neurons in the dorsal horn (8.183). It terminates, mainly ipsilaterally, in the vermis, the pars intermedia and the extreme lateral part of the anterior lobe, bilaterally in the pyramis and the adjoining lobules of the posterior lobe hemisphere. The dorsal spinocerebellar tract transmits proprioceptive and extero-ceptive information about the lower extremity. The forelimb-equi-valent of the dorsal spinocerebellar tract is the cuneocerebellar tract.

The ventral spinocerebellar tract is a composite pathway which contains crossed components from lower sacrococcygeal segments, from lumbar spinal border cells and from different cell groups in the lumbar intermediate zone (8.183). The lower lumbar and sac-rococcygeal component terminates preferentially in the apical part of the lingula and the central lobule of the anterior lobe. The terminations of the spinal border cells are mainly ipsilateral to their origin, i.e. the fibres recross in the cerebellar commissure. They terminate extensively throughout the entire anterior lobe. The ventral spinocerebellar tract transmits information about the status of inter-neuronal pools in the lumbar and sacral cord.

The rostral spinocerebellar tract takes its origin from cell groups of the intermediate zone and the dorsal horn at the cervical enlargement. Although in some ways it can be thought of as the forelimb-equivalent of the ventral spinocerebellar tract, unlike the ventral tract, most of its fibres ascend ipsilaterally. It terminates dorsal to the dorsal and ventral spinocerebellar tracts, in the culmen and the simple lobule and the dorsal part of the pyramis and the paramedian lobule. Its distribution is mainly ipsilateral.

The fifth spinocerebellar tract takes its origin from the central cervical nucleus. This nucleus is located in the upper cervical segments and receives an input from neck muscle proprioceptors (8.183). The tract decussates within the cord and distributes bilaterally to the granular layer in the bottom of the fissures of the anterior lobe where it overlaps with primary and secondary vestibulocerebellar mossy fibres.

The cuneocerebellar tract, like the dorsal spinocerebellar tract, consists of exteroceptive and proprioceptive components, which take their origin from the internal and external cuneate nucleus respectively. The component which arises from the dorsal column nuclei is predominantly uncrossed and directed at the culmen, the simple lobule and the dorsal parts of the pyramis and the paramedian lobule, where it overlaps with the rostral spinocerebellar tract (8.180, 183) and with trigeminocerebellar mossy fibres. Exteroceptive and proprioceptive mossy fibre components of the cuneocerebellar tract terminate differentially in the apical and basal part of the folia. The exteroceptive component overlaps with the pontocerebellar mossy fibre projection in the apices of the folia of the anterior lobe.

All of the tracts discussed so far have their origin from the body by way of the spinal cord. There is a parallel system of cerebellar projections from the trigeminal system. Anatomical tracing studies in several mammalian species have demonstrated direct trigeminal nucleus inputs to the cerebellar cortex terminating as mossy fibres. There are also inputs from the trigeminal nuclei to the inferior olive relayed as somatosensory information from the face to the cerebellar cortex. Thus the trigeminal nuclei pass both mossy and climbing fibre information to the cerebellum.

The termination of spino- and trigeminocerebellar fibres in the granular layer is not uniform but organized in parasagittal strips of mossy fibre rosettes which alternate with regions containing few or no labelled mossy fibre terminals (8.180). Collaterals of ventral and rostral spinocerebellar mossy fibres terminate in the fastigial, emboliform and medial globose nuclei.

Reticulocerebellar mossy fibres

Three nuclei in the reticular formation, the lateral reticular nucleus, the paramedian reticular nucleus and the reticular nucleus of the tegmentum pontis, give rise to mossy fibres. The lateral reticular nucleus and the reticular nucleus of the tegmentum pontis give rise to major collateral projections to the cerebellar nuclei (8.179).

The lateral reticular nucleus and the paramedian reticular nucleus are located in the caudal medulla, the lateral reticular nucleus in the lateral funiculus, the paramedian reticular nucleus in the medial longitudinal fasciculus. The lateral reticular nucleus is surrounded by the ascending fibre systems of the lateral funiculus and by the rubrospinal and lateral vestibulospinal tracts. Spinoreticular fibres terminate in a somatotopical pattern within the entire lateral reticular nucleus, where they overlap with collaterals from the rubrospinal and the lateral vestibulospinal tracts and a projection from the cerebral cortex.

The lateral reticular nucleus projects bilaterally to the vermis and hemispheres of the cerebellum. The projection of the dorsal part of the nucleus, which receives collaterals from the rubrospinal tract in addition to spinal afferents, is centred on the ipsilateral hemisphere.

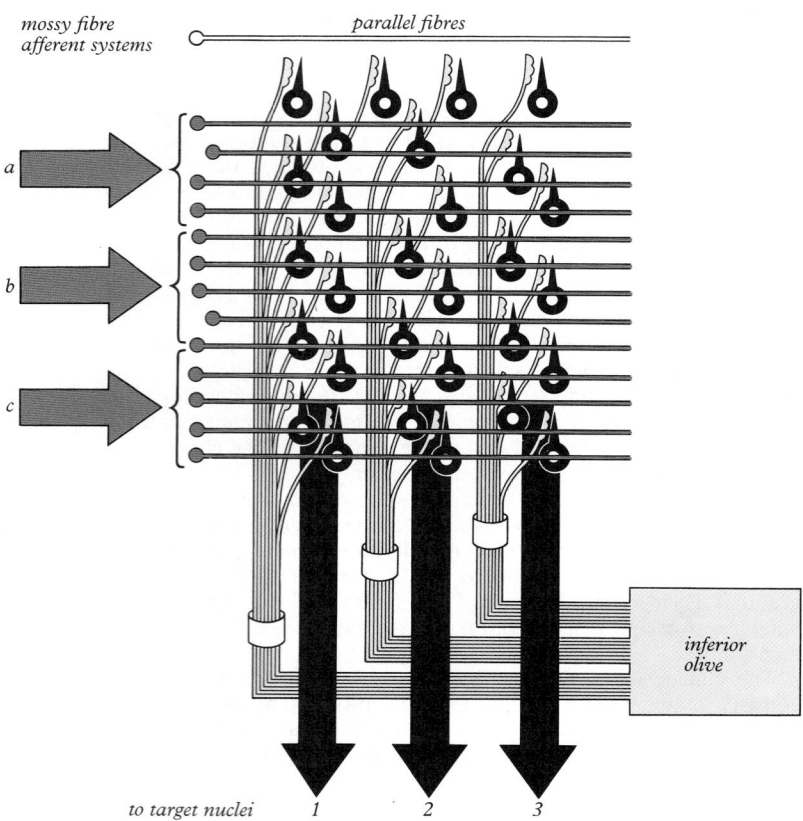

mossy fibre afferent systems

parallel fibres

a

b

c

inferior olive

to target nuclei   1   2   3

8.181   Diagram of the organization of mossy fibre-parallel fibre and climbing fibre inputs to Purkinje cell longitudinal zones. Three cerebellar modules (1–3), consisting of a Purkinje cell zone, each with an output to a cerebellar target nucleus and its climbing fibre input from the inferior olive, are indicated. The transverse arrangement of three mossy fibre (large red arrows)-parallel fibre systems (a–c) guarantees that each of these systems has access to Purkinje cells and may interact with climbing fibres of each module.

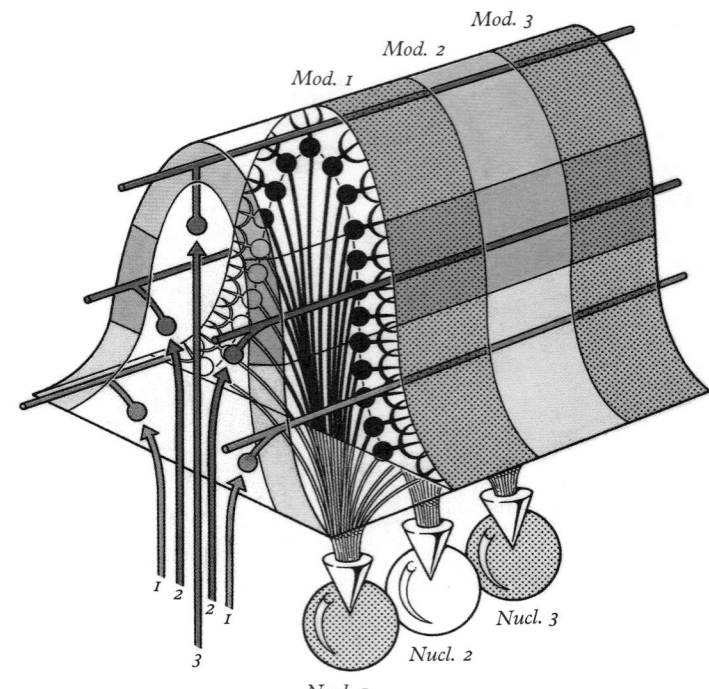

Mod. 1 *Mod. 2* *Mod. 3*

1 2 *2 1* *Nucl. 3*

3 *Nucl. 2*

Nucl. 1

B.   Diagram of the organization of mossy fibre-parallel fibre inputs to Purkinje cell longitudinal zones in a single lobule. Beams of parallel fibres, activated by mossy fibres terminating in the base (green), the intermediate part (red) and the apex of a lobule (blue), traverse Purkinje cells belonging to three different modules (Mod. 1–3). Purkinje cells of each module project to their target nuclei (Nucl 1–3). At the level of the cortex the different mossy fibre-parallel fibre inputs of a module are clearly separated along the long axis of the Purkinje cell zone of each module. At the level of the target nuclei there is strong convergence of these different inputs upon the neurons of the target nucleus.

The ventral part of the nucleus, which receives a strong projection from the spinal cord and a collateral projection from the lateral vestibulospinal tract, projects bilaterally, mainly to the vermis. The lateral reticular nucleus gives rise to a strong projection to the rostral fastigial nucleus, the emboliform nucleus and the medial pole of the globose nucleus (**8**.179A).

The paramedian reticular nucleus consists of cell groups at the lateral border of the medial longitudinal fasciculus. It receives fibres from the vestibular nuclei and the interstitiospinal and tectospinal tracts, which descend in the medial longitudinal fasciculus, and from the spinal cord and the cerebral cortex. It projects to the entire cerebellum, with the possible exception of the paraflocculus.

The reticular nucleus of the pontine tegmentum pontis is located next to the midline, dorsal to the pes pontis, in the caudal half of the tegmentum (**8**.167A). It receives afferent connections from the cerebral cortex, the tectum and nucleus of the optic tract and from the cerebellar nuclei through the crossed descending branch of the superior cerebellar peduncle. Efferents from this nucleus reach the cerebellum through the middle cerebellar peduncle. They terminate superficially in the cortex of the anterior lobe, and more strongly in the simple lobule, the folium and tuber vermis, with the adjoining semilunar lobules in the flocculus and in the adjoining region of the paraflocculus, which probably corresponds to the human accessory paraflocculus. In addition, efferent fibres from the reticular nucleus of the tegmentum pontis terminate in the caudal fastigial nucleus, dentate nucleus and the lateral parts of the globose nucleus (**8**.175B). Their termination in these nuclei is complementary to the projection of the lateral reticular nucleus.

Mossy fibre projections of the basal pontine nuclei

By far the largest single source of fibres projecting to the pontine nuclei (**8**.184A–C) is from the cerebral cortex. Many corticopontine

fibres are collaterals of axons which project to other targets in the brain or spinal cord. For example, it is likely that all corticospinal fibres give off collaterals to the pontine nuclei. All corticopontine axons arise from lamina V pyramidal cells, but the projection from different areas of the cerebral cortex is highly uneven. Some cortical areas project heavily to the pons, some very lightly or not all. The areas of cerebral cortex that project to the pontine nuclei are those that are particularly involved in the control of movement. In the case of visual areas for example, the input arises from those extra-striate visual areas in the parietal lobe whose cells are responsive to movement, and which function as important links in the visual guidance of movement. Although the projection from the cerebral cortex to the pontine nuclei and from the pons to the cerebellar cortex is not precise, there is an overall rough pattern which is summarized in **8**.184.

The pontine nuclei give rise to the middle cerebellar peduncle or brachium pontis which is by far the largest afferent system of the human cerebellum. The projection of rostral and caudal parts of the pontine nuclei to the cerebellum is reversed (Bechterew 1995; Spitzer & Karplus 1907; Voogd 1964). Fibres originating in the ventral and superficial layers of the pontine nuclei travel in superficial layers of the middle cerebellar peduncle and terminate preferentially in caudal and ventrolateral parts of the cerebellum. Bechterew (1885) was able to distinguish this pathway (his 'cerebral', i.e. rostral, system) because it acquires its myelin after birth. One of its main constituents is the corticopontocerebellar projection from visual areas of the cerebral cortex to the paraflocculus and caudal vermis.

Corticopontine projections from extra-striate visual areas terminate in the dorsolateral parts of the pontine grey of the monkey (Glickstein et al 1985; Stein & Glickstein 1992). In all mammals that have been studied, the paraflocculus and lobules IX and VII of the vermis are the main recipients of the visual corticopontocerebellar

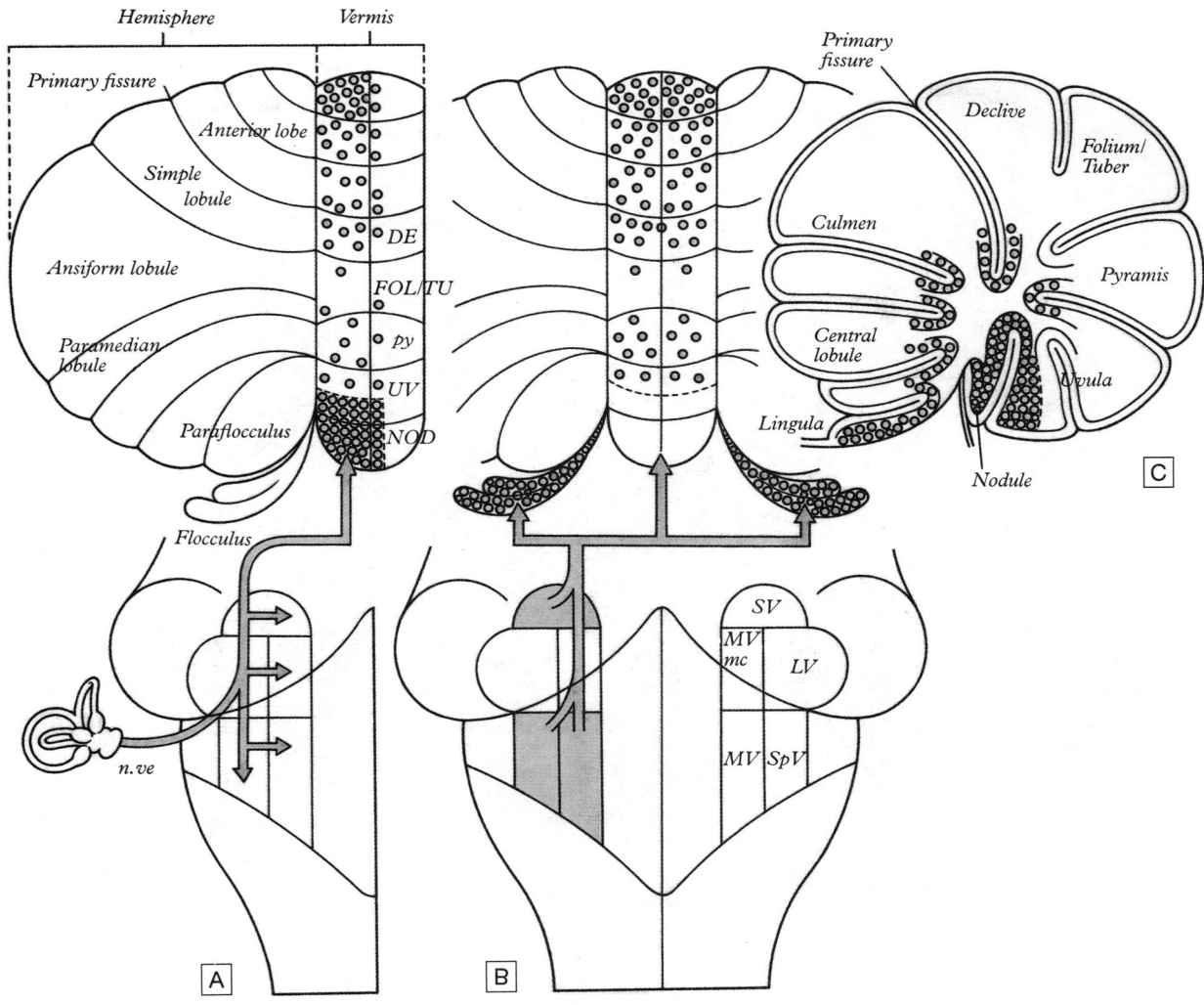

8.182   Vestibulo-cerebellar mossy fibre projections.

A.   Primary vestibulocerebellar mossy fibre projection from root fibres of the vestibular nerve.

B.   Secondary vestibulo-cerebellar mossy fibre projection from neurons of the vestibular nuclei.

C.   Sagittal section showing the distribution of primary and secondary vestibular mossy fibre projections.   De = declive;   FOL/TU = folium/tuber; LV = lateral vestibular nucleus; MV = medial vestibular nucleus; MVmc = magnocellular part of the medial vestibular nucleus; NOD = nodulus; n.ve = vestibular nerve; PY = pyramis; SpV = spinal vestibular nucleus; SV = superior vestibular nucleus; UV = uvula.

projection (Hoddevik 1977; Burne et al 1978; Robinson et al 1984). The basal pontine nuclei do not project to the flocculus.

In addition to its input from extrastriate visual areas, the pons also has collateral branches from corticotectal fibres. Fibres from the parietal, temporal and frontal areas of the cerebral cortex which project to the superior and inferior colliculus also give rise to branching axons to the pons (Baker et al 1983; Keizer et al 1987). Auditory corticopontocerebellar connections are far less prominent than the visual pathways. The paraflocculus is the main target of the auditory pontocerebellar projection in the rat (Azizi et al 1985). Direct tectopontine connections from the inferior colliculus terminate in the dorsal lateral pons which projects to the vermal lobules VI and VII (Kawamura 1975; Burne et al 1981; Azizi et al 1985). The tectopontine pathways from the superior colliculus (Münzer & Wiener 1902; Kawamura & Brodal 1973; Mower et al 1979) terminate in the dorsolateral pons, which also projects to lobules VI and VII.

Fibres from caudal and central portions of the pontine nuclei occupy deeper layers of the peduncle and distribute to more rostral parts of the cerebellum. This pathway corresponds to the early myelinating 'spinal' (i.e. caudal) component of the middle cerebellar peduncle of Bechterew (1885). An interesting confirmation of Bechterew's subdivision of the brachium pontis can be found in the dissection of Jamieson (1910) of the middle cerebellar peduncle. The spinal system conveys the corticopontocerebellar projection to the anterior lobe. It also includes projections from the nucleus reticularis

tegmenti pontis (the papilliform nucleus of Olszewski & Baxter 1954) and the paramedian pontine reticular formation. These nuclei send their fibres through the midline raphe into the pes pontis where they deflect laterally to occupy the deep stratum of the middle cerebellar peduncle (8.179B). Both these nuclei receive connections from subcortical visual centres. Fibres from the superior colliculus and from different parts of the cerebral cortex terminate in the nucleus reticularis tegmenti pontis. It also receives a strong projection from the cerebellar nuclei by way of the descending limb of the brachium conjunctivum (8.171B). The paramedian pontine reticular formation of the cat projects bilaterally to lobule VII and the caudal part of lobule VI and to the ansiform lobule, i.e. to the areas of the caudal vermis which are involved in control of saccades (Gerrits et al 1984). Fibres of the reticular nucleus of the pons distribute bilaterally, with ipsilateral predominance, to all lobules of the cerebellum, with the exception of the lobules I and X (Kawamura & Hashikawa 1981; Gerrits et al 1984). This projection includes the flocculus and the adjacent part of the ventral paraflocculus (Gerrits et al 1985a) and parts of the central nuclei (Gerrits & Voogd 1987; Dietrichs & Walberg 1987). Only in the apex of the lobules of the anterior vermis are the terminals distributed in longitudinal zones.

The sensory and motor cortex and their adjoining areas, which give origin to the pyramidal tract in the cat (Van Crevel & Verhaart 1963; Catsman-Berrevoets & Kuypers 1981), also give rise to a corticopontine projection which is relayed principally to the anterior

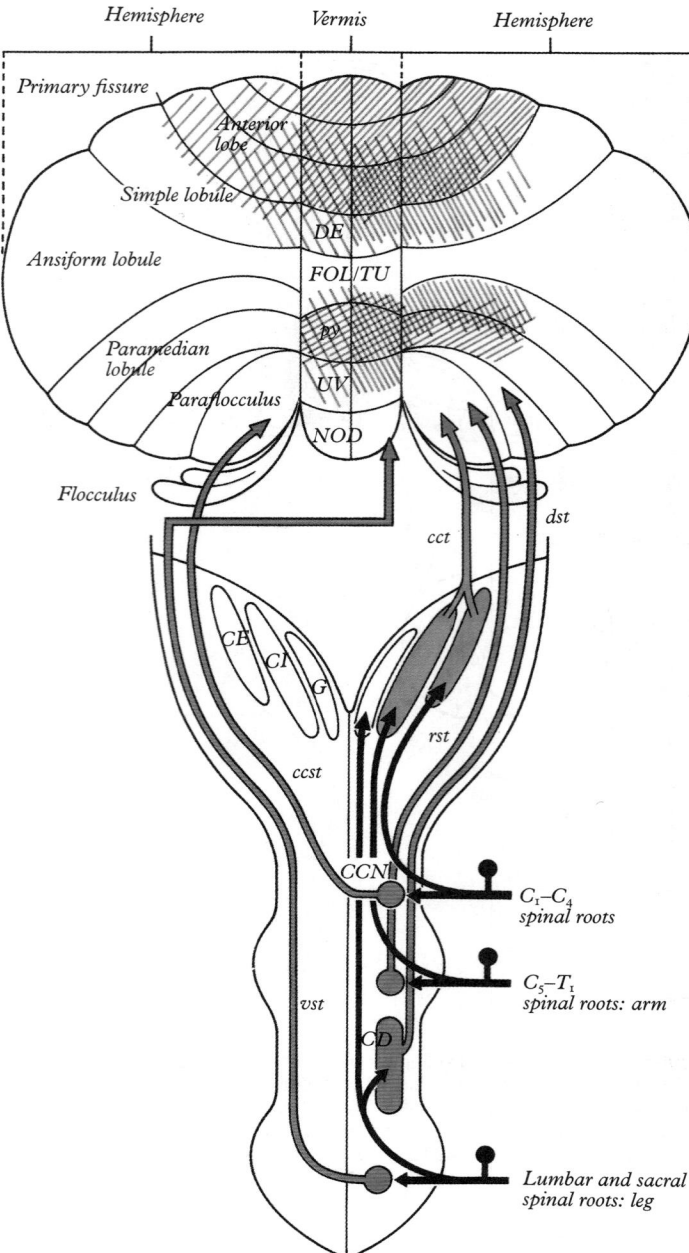

8.183 Spino- and cuneocerebellar mossy fibre projections. The four spino-cerebellar systems (red) and the cuneocerebellar projection (blue) project to largely overlapping regions in the anterior lobe, the lobulus simplex and the paramedian lobule. CCN = central cervical nucleus; ccst = central cervical spinocerebellar tract; cct = cuneocerebellar tract; CD = dorsal column of Clarke; CE = external cuneate nucleus; CI = internal cuneate nucleus; DE = declive; dst = dorsal spinocerebellar tract; FOL/TU = folium/tuber; G = gracile nucleus; NOD = nodulus; PY = pyramis; rst = rostral spinocerebellar tract; UV = uvula; vst = ventral spinocerebellar tract.

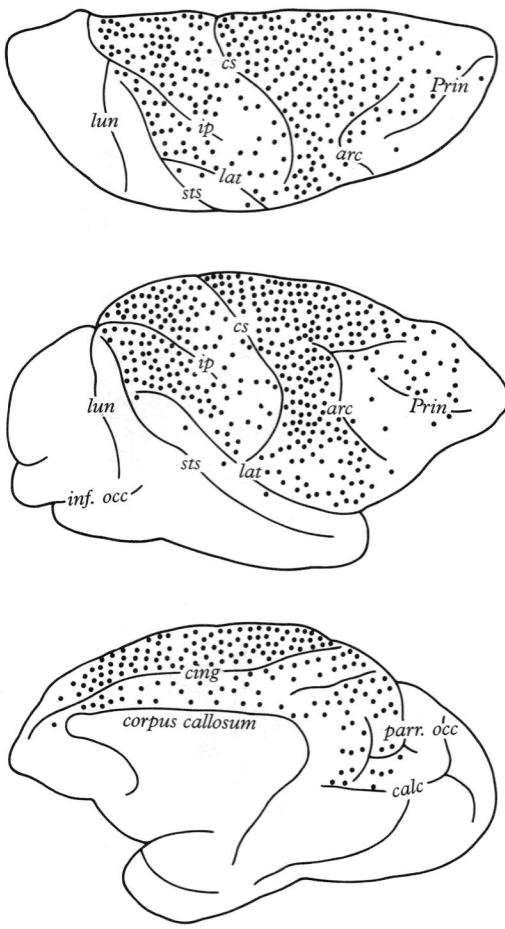

8.184 A. The distribution of cortico-pontine cells on the cerebral cortex of the Macaque monkey. The pontine projections arise principally from a centrally located region of the cerebral cortex. There are relatively few cortico-pontine fibres arising from the bulk of the occipital lobe or the infero-temporal cortex. The projections from the areas of frontal cortex which are rostral to the arcuate sulcus are sparse. Abbreviations of sulci: arc = arcuate; calc = calcarine; cing = cingulate; cs = central; inf. occ = inferior occipital; ip = intraparietal; lat = lateral; lun = lunate; parr, occ = parieto-occipital; Prin = principal; sts = superior temporal.

lobe. These corticopontine fibres terminate in the peripeduncular region of the pes pontis (Brodal 1968a,b, 1971; 1982, 1987). Spino-pontine fibres and collaterals from the medial lemniscus terminate in this same area. The collateral origin of the corticopontine fibres from the pyramidal tract was demonstrated by Ugolini and Kuypers (1986) with a retrograde fluorescent fibre labelling technique. The corticopontocerebellar projections from the sensory–motor cortex include the paramedian lobule and extend into the ansiform lobule and the paraflocculus.

In man the corticopontine fibres are contained in the cerebral peduncle. Fibres from the pericentral cortex occupy the central region of the peduncle, frontopontine fibres are located more medially and the parietotemperopontine tract forms the lateral part of the

peduncle (Dejerine & Dejerine-Klumpke 1901; Lankamp 1967). The extensive termination of the corticopontine fibres in the pontine nuclei and the nucleus papillioformis can be observed in cases with large hemispheric lesions (Schoen 1969, case H.5671). Tem-poropontine fibres were degenerated in a case with a temporal abscess. Terminations are found in the lateral part of the pontine grey but are absent from the papillioform nucleus (reticular pontine nucleus). Frontopontine connections are more extensive in man than in experimental animals. Their terminations are found in the medial portion of the pes pontis and in the papillioform nucleus. The terminal localization of these degenerated tracts is in accordance with reports on the corticopontine projection in non-human primates (Spitzer & Karplus 1907; Sunderland 1940; Nyby & Jansen 1951; Künzle & Akert 1977; Künzle 1978; Wiesendanger et al 1979; Glickstein et al 1985).

Olivocerebellar climbing fibre connections

The inferior olive can be subdivided into the principal olive, a convoluted structure, and medial and dorsal accessory olives (8.174A,B). The olivocerebellar projection terminates as climbing fibres and is completely crossed. In addition, olivary fibres give off collaterals to the lateral vestibular nucleus of Deiters and to the cerebellar nuclei. The topography in the olivocerebellar projection was studied in human cases with gun-shot wounds of the cerebellum and in many subsequent experimental investigations. Climbing fibres

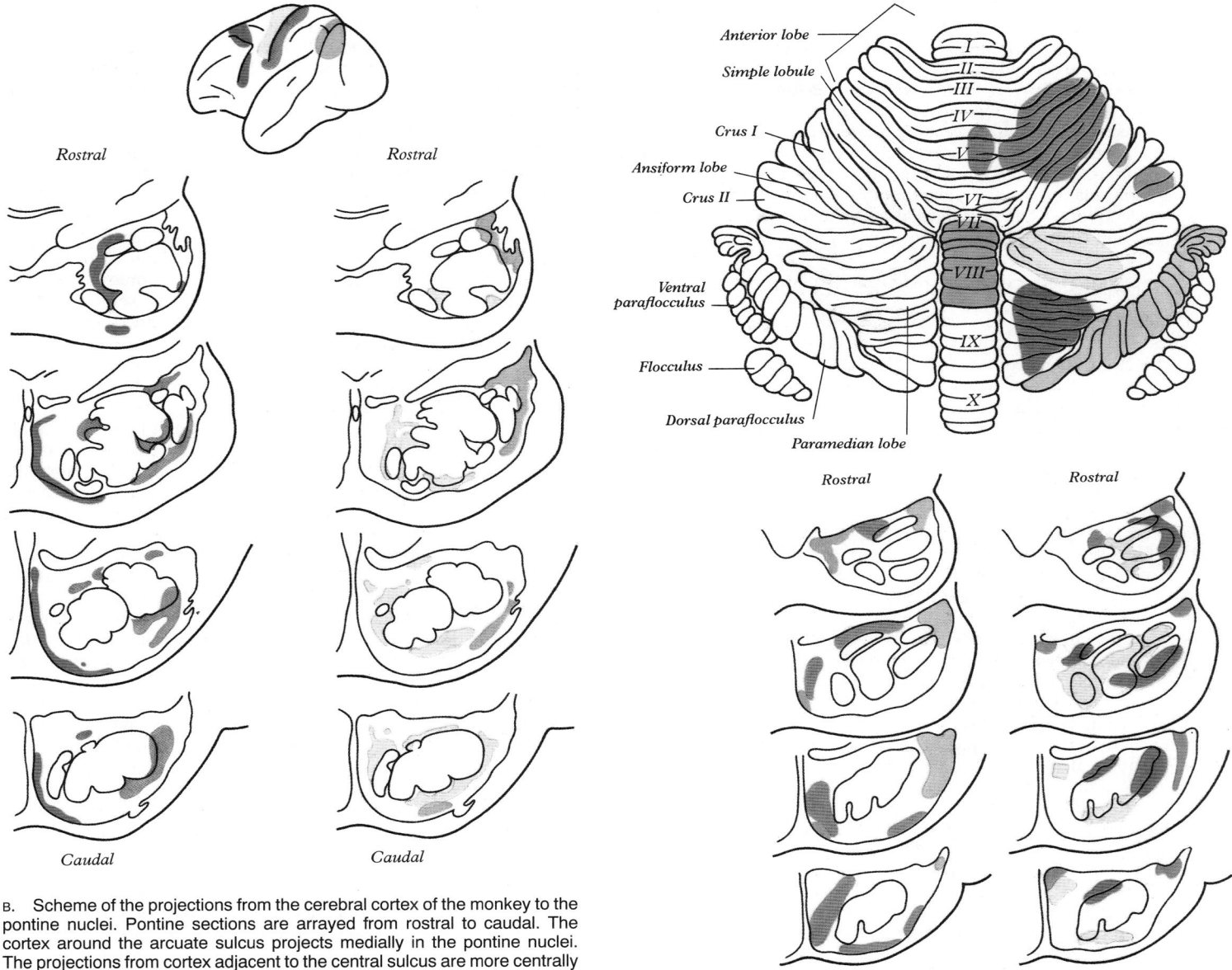

Rostral   *Rostral*

Caudal   *Caudal*

B.   Scheme of the projections from the cerebral cortex of the monkey to the pontine nuclei. Pontine sections are arrayed from rostral to caudal. The cortex around the arcuate sulcus projects medially in the pontine nuclei. The projections from cortex adjacent to the central sulcus are more centrally located. The major projections from the parietal lobe terminate dorsolaterally.

Rostral   *Rostral*

Caudal   *Caudal*

c.   Projections from the pontine nuclei to the cerebellar cortex based in part on Brodal (1992) and Glickstein (1985). arc = arcuate sulcus; cing = cingulate sulcus; CS = central sulcus; Inf. occ. = Inferior occipital sulcus; Lat = lateral fissure; lun = lunate sulcus; Par = parieto-occipital sulcus; Prin = principal sulcus; sts = superior temporal sulcus.

from subnuclei of the inferior olive terminate on longitudinal strips of Purkinje cells. The zonal patterns in the corticonuclear and olivocerebellar projections correspond precisely. The accessory olives project to the vermis and the pars intermedia. The caudal halves of the medial and dorsal accessory olive innervate the vermis (**8**.174c). The caudal part of the dorsal accessory olive projects to Deiters' nucleus and to the B zone of the anterior vermis; the caudal half of the medial accessory olive gives rise to a projection to the fastigial nucleus and provides climbing fibres to the A zone. The rostral halves of the accessory olives project to the pars intermedia; climbing fibres from the rostral dorsal accessory olive, with collateral projections to the emboliform nucleus, terminate in zones (C1 and C3) which flank a climbing fibre zone innervated by the rostral medial accessory olive (C2 zone), which provides a collateral projection to the globose nucleus. The principal olive projects to the contralateral hemisphere (D zone) with collaterals to the dentate nucleus (**8**.174c).

The inferior olive receives afferent connections from the spinal cord, from sensory relay nuclei in the brainstem, such as the dorsal column, and sensory trigeminal nuclei and descending connections from the superior colliculus, the parvicellular red nucleus and related nuclei in the mesencephalon (**8**.173, 174c). In addition, the cerebellar nuclei and certain vestibular nuclei give rise to a mainly crossed, GABAergic projection to the inferior olive (**8**.174c). This nucleo-

olivary pathway is topically organized. The dentate nucleus projects to the principal olive, the emboliform nucleus to the rostral dorsal accessory olive and the globose nucleus to the rostral medial accessory olive. Connections of the fastigial nucleus with the caudal medial accessory olive are less numerous. The caudal dorsal accessory olive receives a nucleo-olivary projection from the lateral vestibular nucleus of Deiters.

The dorsal accessory olive and the caudal half of the medial accessory olive are provided with spinal and sensory input. A middle region of the medial accessory olive receives a projection from the superior colliculus and projects to folium and vermis. The parvicellular red nucleus and related nuclei project to the olive through the ipsilateral descending central and medial tegmental tracts projects to follow form and nerves (**8**.173, 174c). They terminate in the rostral half of the medial accessory olive and the principal olive. The parvicellular red nucleus receives converging projections from the cerebellar nuclei and from the motor and premotor cortex. Direct pathways from the cerebral cortex to the inferior olive are very sparse. Indirect pathways from cerebral cortex to olive, which synapse in the region of the parvicellular red nucleus, are much stronger.

Climbing fibres terminating in the vestibulocerebellum (flocculus and nodule) are derived from small subnuclei, belonging to the medial accessory olive. Two of these nuclei (dorsal cap and ventrolateral outgrowth collectively indicated as the dorsal cap, DC in **8.**174B,C), which receive a strong descending afferent connection from optokinetic centres in the mesencephalon, project to the flocculus and the nodulus. Optokinetic information is used by the flocculus in long-term adaptation of compensatory eye movements. Two other subnuclei (group β and dorsomedial cell column) are under vestibular control and project to the nodulus and the adjoining uvula only.

MECHANISMS OF THE CEREBELLAR CORTEX

The cerebellar cortex has two distinct inputs, climbing and mossy fibres, and only one output, the axons of Purkinje neurons (p. 1049).

The electrical responses of Purkinje cells make it apparent that one of the traditional tenets of neurophysiology—the all-or-none law—must be modified. In its original formulation the all-or-none law held that if a neuron reaches threshold it will fire an action potential. All action potentials were thought to be like all others. Purkinje cells violate this rule since there are two totally different ways in which they can be activated. One of these, the simple spike, resembles the response of other cells in the brain. When Purkinje cells are activated by way of their mossy fibre–parallel fibre input they fire a simple spike. Activation of the Purkinje cell by a climbing fibre is different. The spike produced by a climbing fibre, called the complex spike, is a prolonged depolarization of the cell upon which are superimposed several spike-like waves. In addition to these differences in the character of their electrical activity, the rate of firing of single and complex spikes differs markedly. While the Purkinje cell may fire simple spikes at a rate of hundreds per second, Purkinje cells are activated by complex spikes at very low frequencies, seldom more than three or four spikes per second. The low frequency of complex spike activities suggests that they cannot provide detailed sensory information; they must play a very different role in the function of the cerebellum from that of the simple spike (Gibson et al 1987).

Purkinje cell activity is regulated by local inhibitory neurons: Golgi cells, basket cells and stellate cells. Like Purkinje cells, Golgi cells have a rich dendritic tree which extends through the molecular layer. Unlike the Purkinje cells, the dendrites of the Golgi cell are not restricted to a plane transverse to the folia and their axons do not leave the cerebellar cortex. Golgi cells regulate firing by presynaptic inhibition of the mossy fibre afferents. By inhibiting the mossy fibre input Golgi cells can thus act as a governor or rate limiter on the activity of Purkinje cells. Stellate and basket cells are also inhibitory in function. Unlike the Golgi cells, they synapse directly on Purkinje cells exerting a powerful inhibition on them. **8.**160A is a drawing from Cajal showing the axons of basket cells surrounding the cell body of the Purkinje cell. Some 80 years after Cajal made these drawings physiological experiments began to reveal the nature of basket cell control in suppressing the firing of Purkinje cells.

Structural and functional cerebellar localization

Since the cerebellar cortex is largely uniform in microstructure and microcircuitry, it seems likely that its basic mode of operation is also uniform. However, the nature of this operation is still unknown. It is clear that the main input for this operation is provided by the numerous mossy fibre afferents which carry information from all levels of the spinal cord including the activity of interneuronal pools, as well as specialized sensory and motor information relayed from the cerebral cortex and subcortical motor centres. It is equally clear that the output of the cerebellum is directed at motor systems. Mossy fibres are distributed according to transversely oriented, lobular patterns. Their transverse distribution is enhanced by the transverse spread of the parallel axons of the granule cells, on which they terminate (**8.**181A). The mossy–parallel fibre terminal fields in the molecular layer cover many Purkinje cells. These Purkinje cells are organized in modules: discrete, parallel zones, which converge upon different output nuclei of the cerebellum which, in turn, are coupled to different motor systems in the brainstem, the spinal cord and the cerebral cortex. Cerebellar function, therefore, is determined by the temporal and spatial factors which regulate the access of a particular

combination of mossy fibre–parallel fibre inputs to an appropriate output. Some of these factors may be found in the inhibitory interneurons of the cerebellar cortex, which restrict the mossy–parallel fibre input in space and time. Plastic changes in the response properties of Purkinje cells, in the form of long-term depression of the parallel fibre–Purkinje cell synapses, may equally contribute. Short-term and long-term changes in the response properties of Purkinje cells are under the influence of the climbing fibres. The physiological properties of the climbing fibres make them less suitable for fast transmission of detailed information, but they may serve as a level-setting device, adjusting the excitability of the Purkinje cells. The precise register between the spatial organization of the olivocerebellar climbing fibre system and the Purkinje cell output are in accordance with this view (**8.**172, 174, 181A). Moreover Purkinje cells deprived of their climbing fire input fire at very high rates (Colin et al 1980; Montarolo et al 1982), thus effectively shutting off the output from the cerebellar nuclei.

Some functional aspects of the subdivision of the cerebellum were discussed at the beginning of this chapter (**8.**175). One feature is the presence of a double, mirrored localization in the anterior and posterior cerebellum (**8.**175). The anterior lobe and the simple lobule and the pyramis with the adjoining lobules of the hemisphere of the posterior lobe (the paramedian lobule) receive branches from the same mossy and climbing fibres and project to the same cerebellar nuclei. The mossy fibres are derived from sensory and motor nuclei in the cord and the brainstem and the motor and sensory corticopontine system. The efferent pathways of these regions monitor the activity in the corticospinal and rubrospinal tracts and the subcortical motor systems from the vestibular nuclei and the reticular formation. The inputs to the cerebellum and the outputs from it are organized according to the same somatotopical patterns, but the orientation of these patterns is reversed: the representation of the head is found principally in the simple lobule, and caudally in a corresponding region of the posterior lobe. The double representation of the body follows in rough somatotopic order. Vestibular connections of the cerebellum display a similar, double representation: in the most rostral lobules of the anterior lobe and far caudally in the vestibulocerebellum (**8.**182).

Two regions in the vermis, the folium/tuber and the uvula, intervene between the somatotopically organized and vestibular areas of the cerebellum. These lobules receive an almost pure pontine mossy fibre input. Climbing fibres from the inferior olive and mossy fibres from the basal and reticular tegmental pontine nuclei relay visual cortical and tectal information to the folium and tuber vermis, which, therefore, have been considered as a vermal visual area (**8.**174, 175). Its efferent connections are directed, through the fastigial nucleus, to the gaze centres in the reticular formation (Table **8.**4). The uvula has an important cortical visual pontocerebellar input which it shares with the paraflocculus: the homologue of the biventral lobule and the tonsil of the human cerebellum. The output of the uvula and the paraflocculus is directed at all cerebellar nuclei, but its terminations are complementary to the projections of the somatotopically organized regions in the anterior and posterior lobes.

Although there is a rough somatotopic organization of spinocerebellar afferent pathways, there is incomplete understanding of the functional differences and principles of localization in the cerebellum. Cerebellar localization has been much studied; foundations were laid by comparative, developmental and connectivity studies (Smith 1903; Riley 1930; Larsell 1937, 1953; Jansen & Brodal 1954; Nieuwenhuys 1967) and detailed analysis of patterns of connection (Brodal 1969).

Most of our understanding of cerebellar connections is based on research on experimental animals but in general is applicable to the human cerebellum; interesting physiological parallels have already been shown. Cerebellar stimulation often modifies movements generated by simultaneous reflex or cerebral cortical stimulation; cerebellar stimulation in decerebrate animals can elicit discrete movements. Again, rostral and caudal areas corresponding to the spinocerebellum display a somatotopic order (Hampson et al 1950). The rostral area mediates ipsilateral responses, the caudal bilateral responses.

Such investigations, combined with effects of ablation (Chambers & Sprague 1955a,b), suggest that the vermis controls posture, tone, locomotion and equilibrium in the whole body, the intermediate zone controlling posture and movements in ipsilateral limbs. The lateral zone's function remains obscure.

Cerebellar dysfunction

Innumerable reports on the behavioural effects of human cerebellar disease and of selective experimental ablations are available and have been reviewed by Holmes (1939), Wyke (1947), Brown (1949), Dow and Moruzzi (1958), Dow (1969), etc. The cerebellum has inputs from motor and sensory areas of the cerebral cortex from cutaneous receptors, proprioceptors, and brainstem reticular formation. This input is integrated and discharged to motor centres in the cerebrum and brainstem. Its normal action is necessary for smooth, co-ordinated, effective movement. The more obvious effects of cerebellar dysfunction include:

- disturbance in equilibrium
- disturbance of muscle 'tone', or resistance to stretch, tendon reflexes and ability to stabilize joints
- motor inco-ordination (*ataxia*) due to irregularities in timing, rate and force of the contraction in synergistic muscles.

Disequilibrium shows as a tendency to fall when standing and perhaps unsteady gait, with sensations of spinning, nausea, etc. The affected muscles are soft, tendon reflexes diminished and muscles tire easily (*asthenia*). Lowering of joint control may progress to pendular swinging of a limb segment after displacement or to 'flail' joints. *Muscular inco-ordination* is basic in most cerebellar dysfunction, affecting the regions variably. Hence symptoms vary. *Asynergia* is a diminished capacity for smooth, orderly action between muscle groups. A complex act may become an irregular sequence, *decomposition of movements*. A defect in rapid alternating movements, e.g. supination and pronation, may develop, called *dysdiadochokinesis* by Babinski. Control of range of movement may be lost, *dysmetria*. Locomotor disturbances, a tendency to fall and (with closed eyes) deviations from the intended course are common. So is an inability to point accurately, *past-pointing*. Tremor is usually absent at rest but *intention tremor* may appear, intensified by movement; tremor may also affect the head or trunk. Muscular inco-ordination produces *defects of speech. Cerebellar nystagmus* may occur, conjugate drift of the gaze followed by a rapid return. But attempts to correlate clinical phenomena with different cerebellar regions, or with experimental results, have had limited success.

In the *flocculonodular syndrome*, with damage to the nodule, uvula and flocculus in man and other animals, the main feature is imbalance: swaying, staggering and a tendency to fall backwards. Positional nystagmus is often present. These effects are attributable to upset of the integration between vestibular nuclei and the 'vestibulocerebellum'.

In experimental animals, *ablation* of the vermis in the anterior lobe exaggerates tendon reflexes and rigidity, already present in decerebrate preparations; vermian stimulation reduces rigidity. The converse results from ablation or stimulation of paravermian parts of the anterior lobe. These effects show somatotopy but have not been clearly demonstrated in man.

Most human cerebellar disorder is *neocerebellar*, involving one or both hemispheres or their outflows. In unilateral disease, if severe, the hypotonia and inco-ordination noted above appear on the side of the lesion, but gross intention tremor and staggering only appear if the dentate nucleus or superior cerebellar peduncle are involved. Small cortical lesions have little effect; even quite extensive disease, though causing transient dysfunction, is followed by rapid improvement in locomotor control. Such *cerebellar compensation* is not yet explained.

Lesions of the cerebellum impair movement. The motor system must deal with two rather different sorts of controls. One is positional. If you lift a feather, a glass, or a heavy book from a table, the trajectory of your arm would still be similar for all three tasks, but in this case the brain and spinal cord would have to adapt to these different loads. If one recorded from a neuron it would be difficult to tell whether an active cell is involved with position or load control; hence it is useful to study neuronal activity associated with simpler movements. Eyes do not change their weight; hence the analysis of eye movements is simpler than that of movements of the limbs.

There are two distinct kinds of voluntary conjugate eye movements. An object appears in the corner of the eye and the eyes make a fast jump, a *saccade*, to inspect it. Pursuit movements are slower. A bird flies across the field of view and the eyes follow it as it flies.

The cerebellum plays an important role in both. In monkeys and in people, destruction of the cerebellum virtually abolishes smooth pursuit (Westheimer & Blair, 1973, 1974). A target can still be followed but only using saccadic movement. Cerebellar lesions do not abolish saccadic movement, but they make it impossible to correct inappropriate saccades. If one of the extraocular muscles becomes weakened, saccades are at first inaccurate. If a target appears 20° to the left, the eye might move only 10° towards it. Saccade amplitude can correct itself over time. There is evidence from cerebellar lesions that the ability to recalibrate saccades requires the cerebellum (Optican & Robinson 1980).

One of the fundamental questions which remain to be solved is why the cerebellum has two totally different types of afferent fibre. There is no agreement, but there is no lack of speculation as to why there are two such different afferents to the cerebellar cortex. One suggestion was put forward by David Marr (1969) and modified shortly thereafter by James Albus (1971). They suggested that the cerebellar cortex is the major site in the brain for motor learning and reflex modification. The role of the cerebellum in plasticity has been studied in modifiability of the vestibulo-ocular reflex. When the head is turned to the left there is a reflex tendency for the eyes to move to the right. A three-neuron arc connects the horizontal semicircular canals to the extraocular motor neuron, so that rotation of the head tends to produce an equal and opposite movement of the eyes thus stabilizing the gaze. If the vestibulo-ocular reflex fails to compensate completely for head movement the image on the retina would slip when the head is turned. Ito (1982) suggested that a mismatch of this sort between the vestibular input and the eye movement would be detected and relayed by climbing fibres to the flocculus. Flocculus Purkinje cells would then serve to adjust the gain of the vestibulor-ocular reflex.

The cerebellum also plays an important role in Pavlovian conditioning. One such conditioning task involves the external eyelids and the nictitating membrane of rabbits (McCormick et al 1981; McCormick & Thompson, 1987; Yeo et al 1985a,b). In the conditioning a tone is presented, and followed shortly thereafter by a puff of air to the cornea. With repeated pairing of the tone followed by the air puff the animal learns to blink when the tone alone is presented. One interpretation is that the mossy fibres relay the tone signal, the climbing fibre the air puff, to the cerebellar cortex. The climbing fibre input changes the synaptic efficiency of the parallel fibre synapses so that the tone comes to elicit the blink.

Thus the cerebellum and its associated circuitry is necessary for normal movement. Lesions of the cerebellum impair movement and motor learning. The challenge for future experimental and clinical studies is to relate the known anatomical, physiological properties of the cerebellum to those functions.

MESENCEPHALON OR MIDBRAIN

EXTERNAL FEATURES AND RELATIONS

The midbrain traverses the hiatus in the tentorium cerebelli, connecting the pons and cerebellum with the forebrain. It is the shortest brainstem segment, not more than 2 cm in length, and most of it lies in the posterior cranial fossa. Lateral to it are the parahippocampal gyri, hiding its sides when the inferior surface of the brain is examined. Its long axis inclines ventrally as it ascends. For description, it is divided into the right and left *cerebral peduncles*, each demarcated into a ventral *crus cerebri* and a dorsal *tegmental part* by a bilateral pigmented lamina, the *substantia nigra*. The two crura are separate, the tegmental parts united and traversed by the *cerebral aqueduct* connecting the third with the fourth ventricles. The region dorsal to an oblique coronal plane, including the aqueduct, is the *tectum*, consisting of the pretectal area and the *corpora quadrigemina* comprising four *rounded colliculi* in superior and inferior pairs.

Crura cerebri are superficially corrugated and emerge from the cerebral hemispheres, converging as they descend to meet where they enter the pons, forming here the caudolateral boundaries of the *interpeduncular fossa* (8.185, 186). At the level of the tentorial incisure, the basilar artery divides in the interpeduncular fossa into the posterior cerebral arteries. The superior cerebellar arteries branch from the basilar artery immediately behind. Both arteries run laterally around the ventral (basilar) crural surfaces, the former passing above the tentorium cerebelli, the latter below. The oculomotor and trochlear nerves lie between the two arteries. The posterior communicating artery joins the posterior cerebral artery on the medial surface of the peduncle in the interpeduncular fossa. The median caudal part of the interpeduncular fossa is a greyish area, the *posterior perforated substance*, through which pass central branches of the posterior cerebral arteries. Near the crural entry into the hemispheres, the optic tract winds dorsolaterally around the crus.

Near the pons, a thin white *taenia pontis* often appears, extending from the crus into the cerebellum between its middle and superior peduncles. Each crus bears a *medial sulcus*, from which roots of the oculomotor nerve emerge (8.124, 185, 186). Its lateral surface adjoins the parahippocampal gyrus and is crossed by the trochlear nerve (8.123, 126); it bears a longitudinal *lateral sulcus*, in which fibres of the lateral lemniscus reach and form a surface elevation which inclines rostrodorsally and in part joins the inferior colliculus; the rest continues into the inferior quadrigeminal brachium (8.123, 126).

The *colliculi* (*corpora quadrigemina*) (8.123, 126) are two paired eminences, rostral to the superior medullary velum, inferior to the pineal gland and caudal to the posterior commissure, the whole sloping ventrally as it ascends. Below the splenium, they are partly overlapped on each side by the pulvinar of the dorsal thalamus. Superior and inferior pairs are separated by a cruciform sulcus, whose upper limit expands into a depression for the *pineal gland*; from its caudal end a median *frenulum veli* is prolonged down over the superior medullary velum; lateral to the frenulum the trochlear nerves emerge; they pass ventrally over the lateral aspects of the cerebral peduncles and traverse the interpeduncular cistern to the petrosal end of the cavernous sinus. The *superior colliculi*, larger and darker, are stations for visual responses (p. 1072). The *inferior colliculi*, smaller but more prominent, are associated with auditory paths (p. 1071). The difference in colour is due to the superficial layers of neurons in the superior colliculi.

From the lateral aspect of each colliculus a *brachium ascends ventrolaterally* (8.123, 126). *The brachium of the superior colliculus* (*superior quadrigeminal brachium*) passes below the pulvinar, partly overlapping the medial geniculate body, continuing partly into the lateral geniculate body (p. 1090) and partly into the optic tract. It conducts fibres from the retina and optic radiation to the superior colliculus. *The brachium of the inferior colliculus* (*inferior quadrigeminal brachium*) ascends ventrally, conveying fibres from the lateral lemniscus and inferior colliculus to the medial geniculate body.

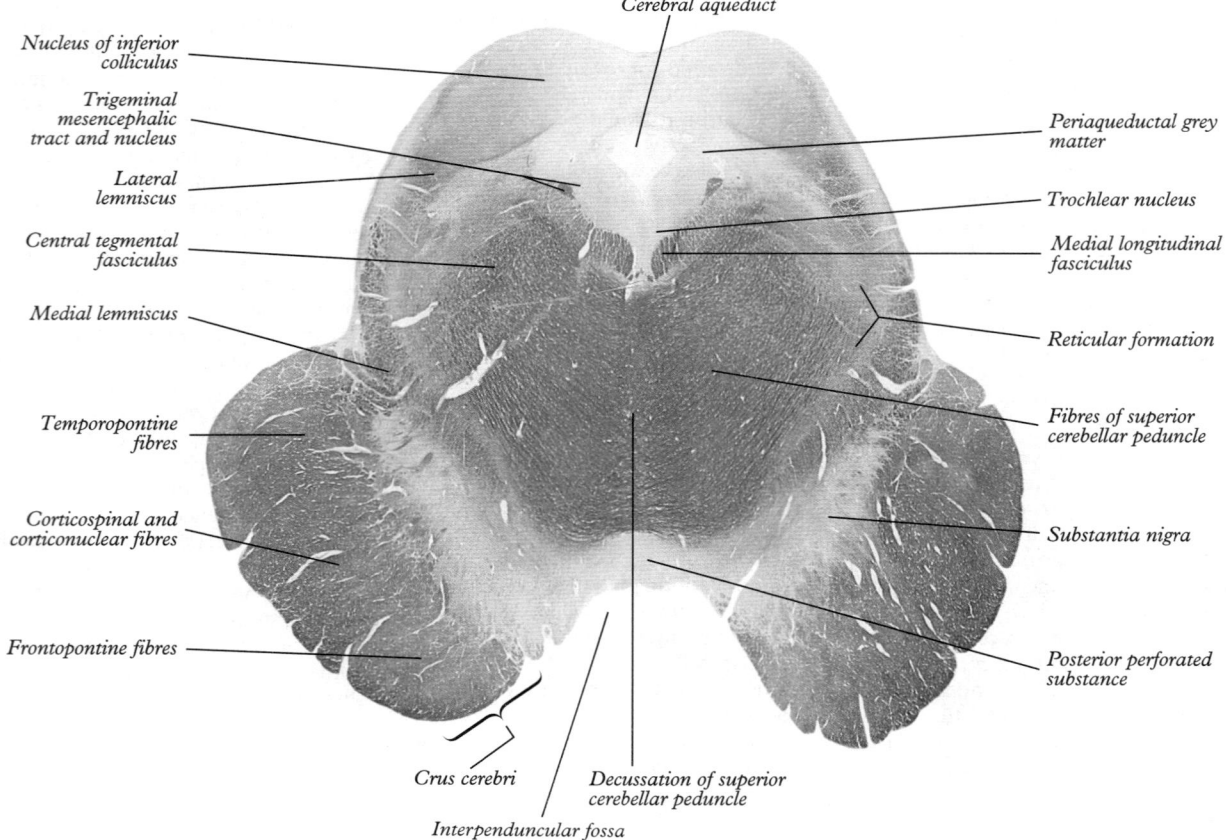

Nucleus of inferior colliculus

Trigeminal mesencephalic tract and nucleus

Lateral lemniscus

Central tegmental fasciculus

Medial lemniscus

Temporopontine fibres

Corticospinal and corticonuclear fibres

Frontopontine fibres

Cerebral aqueduct

Periaqueductal grey matter

Trochlear nucleus

Medial longitudinal fasciculus

Reticular formation

Fibres of superior cerebellar peduncle

Substantia nigra

Posterior perforated substance

Crus cerebri

Decussation of superior cerebellar peduncle

Interpeduncular fossa

8.185 Transverse section of the midbrain through the inferior colliculi. Magnification × 3. (Solochrome cyanin stained preparation by J Carlile, and photographed by Kevin Fitzpatrick, Division of Anatomy and Cell Biology, UMDS, Guy's Campus, London.)

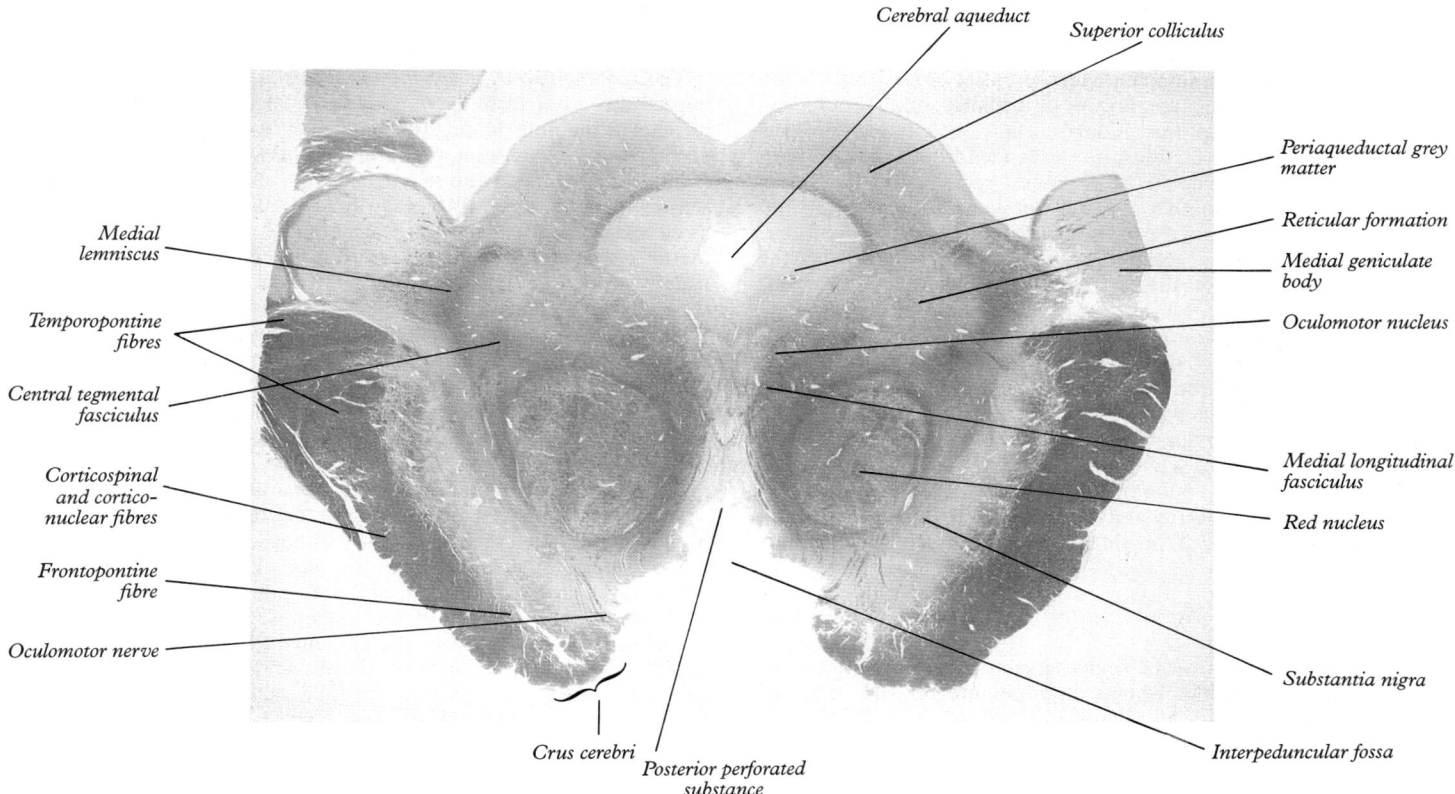

8.186 Transverse section of the midbrain through the superior colliculi. Magnification × 3.4. (Solochrome cyanin stained preparation by J Carlile, and photographed by Kevin Fitzpatrick, Division of Anatomy and Cell Biology, UMDS, Guy's Campus, London.)

INTERNAL STRUCTURE

In transverse section (**8**.185, 186), the cerebral peduncles have, as noted above, dorsal and ventral regions separated by the *substantia nigra*, the dorsal being the *tegmenti* and the ventral the *crura cerebri*. The crura are separated while the tegmenti are continuous across the midline.

Crus cerebri

Each crus cerebri, semilunar in section, contains corticospinal, corticonuclear and corticopontine fibres. The first two occupy the middle crural two-thirds, descending via the pons and medulla: corticonuclear fibres end in nuclei of the cranial nerves and other brainstem nuclei; corticospinal fibres continue into the medullary pyramid (**8**.116). Corticopontine fibres arise in the cerebral cortex and end in the nuclei pontis (p. 1022). They form two groups: the *frontopontine* from the frontal lobe, principally areas 6 and 4, traversing the internal capsule and then occupying the medial sixth of the ipsilateral crus cerebri, and *temporopontine* fibres from the temporal lobe, also traversing the internal capsule but coming to occupy the lateral sixth of the crus; both end in the pontine nuclei. *Parieto-* and *occipitopontine* fibres are also described in the crus, medial to the temporopontine, which are largely from the posterior region of the temporal lobe; corticopontine projections include few fibres from the primary sensory cortex (Verhaart & Mechelse 1954; Brodal & Bjaalie 1992).

Tractus peduncularis transversus. This band of fibres, the tractus peduncularis transversus, may be visible emerging from the optic tract on the lateral peduncular aspect to pass round its ventral surface midway between the pons and the optic tract and disappearing into the interpeduncular fossa dorsolateral to the mamillary body, where it terminates in a small *nucleus of the transverse peduncular tract*, medial to the substantia nigra. The tract, constant in many lower mammals, is identifiable in only 30% of human brains. Since it degenerates after ocular enucleation, it may be part of the visual pathway; it projects to oculomotor nuclei in some mammals (Gillilan 1941, p. 1227).

Substantia nigra

The substantia nigra, a bilateral lamina of numerous pigmented (neuromelanin-containing) multipolar neurons, extends through the whole midbrain. Its pigmentation is easily visible in transverse or coronal sections (**8**.185, 186). The pigment is related to the aminergic status of many mesencephalic reticular neurons, increases with age, is more abundant in primates, maximal in man and present even in albinos (Marsden 1961). The nucleus is semilunar in transverse section, concave dorsally; from its convex ventral surface extensions pass between fibres of the crus cerebri. Thicker medially, it reaches from the medial to the lateral crural sulcus and from the pons to the subthalamic region; its medial part is traversed by radicular oculomotor fibres streaming ventrally to their oculomotor sulcus in the interpeduncular fossa. The substantia nigra is divisible into a dorsal *pars compacta* of medium-sized dopaminergic and cholinergic neurons, which contain melanin pigment granules, and a ventral *pars reticularis*, intermingled with fibres of the crus cerebri, containing fewer neurons grouped in clusters, some of which are dopaminergic and contain small amounts of pigment but the majority are γ-aminobutyric acid (GABA-ergic). The ventral part reaches the subthalamic region and is considered continuous with the globus pallidus, which it structurally resembles. The neurons in both nuclei contain unusually high levels of iron and have smooth dendrites with few branches which overlap in the pars reticularis. In submammalian vertebrates, a well-developed *pars lateralis* is recognizable but is insignificant in man (Huber Crosby 1933), though it has been shown to project to the tectum in primates (Woodburne et al 1946).

The substantia nigra is connected with the cerebral cortex, spinal cord and hypothalamus and has a massive reciprocal projection with the basal ganglion (Parent et al 1983a,b; 1984). Corticonigral fibres arise from precentral and probably postcentral gyri, a few terminating on neurons in the *pars reticularis* and many being fibres of passage to the red nucleus and reticular formation. Collaterals from fibres in sensory tracts from the spinal cord are also said to end in the substantia nigra; fibres from the mamillary peduncle have also been traced to its neurons.

Afferent connections with the basal ganglia (p. 1191) pass to the caudate nucleus, putamen, lateral segment of the globus pallidus and subthalamus. The largest group form the striatonigral pathway from the caudate nucleus and putamen which projects into the substantia nigra topographically, the rostral third of the substantia nigra receiving fibres from the head of the caudate nucleus, the putamen projects to all parts. Striatonigral fibres form axodendritic contacts with neurons in the pars reticularis. The lateral segment of the globus pallidus sends a small number of GABA-ergic pallidonigral fibres to both the pars compacta and pars reticularis; most end in the latter. Subthalamonigral fibres terminate in scattered regions of the pars reticularis; most of these fibres also project to the globus pallidus.

Dopaminergic nigrostriatal fibres from the pars compacta constitute a topographically segregated projection onto the striatum providing an exclusive innervation to either the globus pallidus or caudate nucleus. In Parkinson's disease the levels of dopamine in the substantia nigra and striatum are virtually absent. Striatal dopamine levels may be raised by the administration of L-dihydroxyphenylalanine (Levodopa), a precursor of dopamine which passes the blood–brain barrier and is concentrated in the nigrostriatal closed loop system. GABA-ergic neurons in the pars reticularis project through:

- a nigrothalamic tract to the ventral anterior and dorsomedial thalamic nuclei
- a nigrotegmental path to the *pedunculopontine nucleus* (see below) and reticular formation, whence impulses are relayed to spinal ventral column neurons
- a nigrotectal projection to the ipsilateral superior colliculus which may control saccadic eye movements.

The pars compacta of the substantia nigra contains the dopaminergic cell group A9 of Dahlström and Fuxe (1964) (**8.296**, p. 293). Two other dopaminergic cell groups are found in the ventral tegmentum: cell group A10 in the rostromedial region constituting the ventral tegmental area of Tsai and cell group A8 in the dorsolateral reticular area forming the nucleus parabrachialis pigmentosus (Oades & Halliday 1987). The A10 dopaminergic cell group lies over the pedunculopontine tegmental nucleus (Ch5 cell group) caudally and the lateral dorsal tegmental nucleus (Ch6 cell group) laterally. The whole ventral tegmental system appears to act as an integrative neural centre for adaptive behaviour reciprocally projecting both caudally through a mesorhombencephalic pathway to the cerebellum and to most brainstem monoaminergic cell clusters (p. 1073), and also through mainly ipsilateral fibres in the medial forebrain bundle as:

- a mesodiencephalic system terminating in thalamic and hypothalamic nuclei
- a mesostriatal projection
- a mesorhombic pathway to the nucleus accumbens, olfactory tubercle, lateral septum, interstitial nucleus of the stria terminalis, amygdala and entorhinal cortex
- mesocortical fibres to most cortical areas particularly prefrontal, orbitofrontal and cingulate cortex.

Mesencephalic tegmentum

The mesencephalic tegmentum is directly continuous below with the pontine tegmentum and contains the same tracts. At inferior collicular levels, grey matter is restricted to the environs of the cerebral aqueduct, as scattered collections in the reticular formation (p. 1073) and the tectum (p. 1071). The *trochlear nucleus* is in the ventral grey matter near the midline, in a position corresponding to the abducent and hypoglossal nuclei. With the medial longitudinal fasciculus running immediately ventral, it extends through the lower half of the midbrain, just caudal to the oculomotor nucleus. In some primates, these nuclei are merged and distinguished only by the arrangement of their neurons, the trochlear cells being also smaller. Trochlear *efferent fibres* pass *laterodorsally* round the central grey matter, then descend medial to the trigeminal mesencephalic nucleus to reach the upper end of the superior medullary velum, where they decussate and emerge lateral to the frenulum (p. 1098, 1100). A few fibres remain ipsilateral in all vertebrates. The trochlear nerve may

originally have supplied muscles of a pineal eye, accounting for its dorsal course. Embryological evidence and phylogenetic data support a more dorsal origin of its nucleus.

The *trigeminal mesencephalic nucleus* is lateral in the central grey matter, ascending from the upper pole of the main trigeminal sensory nucleus in the pons to superior collicular level in the midbrain. It is accompanied by a tract of both peripheral and central branches from its axons. Its large ovoid neurons are unipolar, as in peripheral sensory ganglia, and arranged in many small groups which extend as curved laminae on each lateral margin of the periaqueductal grey matter. Neurons are most numerous in its lower level, and are usually so close that somato-somatic contacts have been suggested (Hinrichsen & Larramendi 1969). For connections see p. 1230, **8.132**. Apart from these nuclei the mesencephalic tegmentum contains many scattered neurons; most are included in the reticular formation (p. 1073).

The *white matter* contains all the tracts mentioned in the pontine tegmentum; prominent is the large decussation of the superior cerebellar peduncles (p. 135) (**8.154**), which enter the tegmentum and pass ventromedially round central grey matter to the median raphe, where most fibres cross in the *decussation of the superior cerebellar peduncles* and then separate into ascending and descending fascicles. Some ascending fibres end in or give collaterals to the red nucleus, which they encapsulate and penetrate; many others ascend to the nucleus ventralis lateralis of the thalamus. Some, uncrossed, have branches believed to end in the circumaqueductal grey matter and reticular formation, interstitial nucleus and posterior commissural nucleus (sometimes, perhaps mistakenly, called the nucleus of Darkschewitsch); the latter nucleus may send efferent fibres to the medial longitudinal fasciculus and posterior commissure. Descending fascicles end in the pontine and medullary reticular formation, the olivary complex and possibly cranial motor nuclei (p. 1070, **8.141**).

The *medial longitudinal fasciculus* (**8.141**) adjoins the somatic efferent column, dorsal to the decussating superior cerebellar peduncles. The *medial, trigeminal* and *lateral lemnisci* and *lateral spinothalamic tract* (spinal lemniscus) form a curved band dorsolateral to the substantia nigra. Fibres in the medial and trigeminal lemnisci continue a rostral course to synapse with neurons in the lateral and medial ventral posterior nuclei respectively (**8.110, 132**). Some fibres of the lateral lemniscus end in the inferior collicular nucleus, encapsulating it and synapsing with its neurons. The remaining direct lemniscal and inferior collicular-derived fibres enter the inferior quadrigeminal brachium, which commences at this level and conducts them to the medial geniculate body. Some fibres to the inferior colliculus are collaterals of direct lemniscal fibres.

Superiorly, level with the superior colliculus, the tegmentum contains the *red nucleus*, extending into the subthalamic region. *Central grey matter* round the aqueduct contains ventromedially the *oculomotor nucleus*, elongated and related ventrolaterally to the medial longitudinal fasciculus; below, it reaches the trochlear nucleus. The oculomotor is divisible into neuronal groups partially correlated with the nerve's motor distribution; they include a parasympathetic preganglionic visceral efferent *accessory oculomotor* (*Edinger-Westphal*) *nucleus*, dorsal to the main nucleus (p. 1227).

Red nucleus

The red nucleus is an ovoid mass with a pink tinge, about 5 mm in diameter, dorsomedial to the substantia nigra (**8.186**). The tint appears only in fresh material and is due to a ferric iron pigment in the multipolar neurons of varying size, mostly large or small. Their proportions and arrangements vary in mammalian groups; in primates the magnocellular element is decreased, with a reciprocal increase of the parvocellular complement. Small multipolar neurons occur in all parts, but in human nuclei the larger neurons are restricted to the lower level and have been estimated to be as few as 200 (Grofová & Marsala 1960). Condé and Condé (1973) classified feline rubral cells as multipolar, pyramidal, fusiform and spherical, emphasizing also a heterogeneous nuclear cytoarchitecture; multipolar neurons predominated below, pyramidal and spherical at higher levels, but all occurred at all levels. Superiorly the red nucleus is poorly demarcated, blending into the reticular formation and caudal pole of the interstitial nucleus (Davenport & Ranson 1930). Inferior compact and superior *diffuse* architectonic regions have been

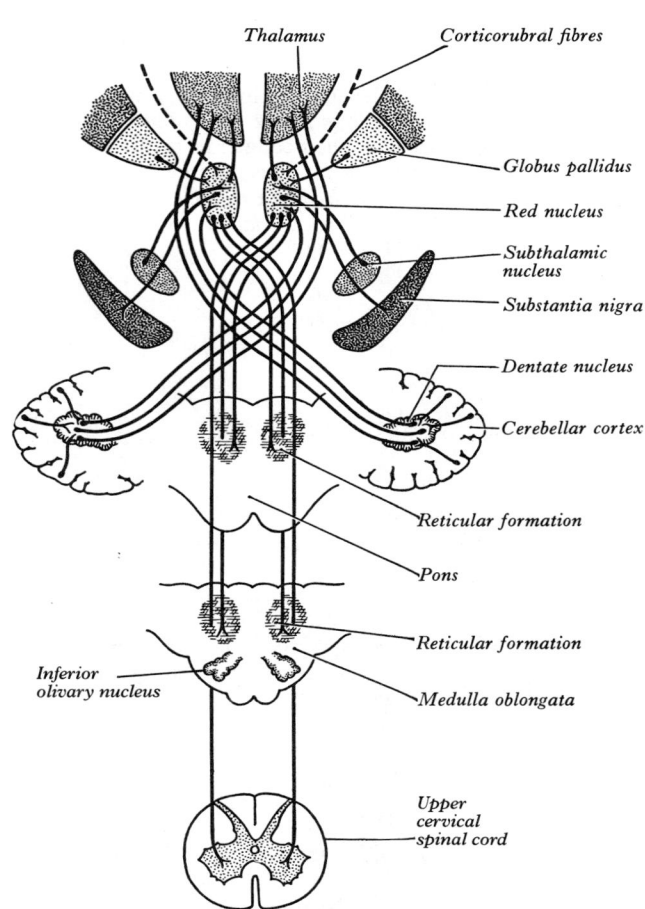

8.187 Simplified diagram of the principal connections of the red nucleus in man.

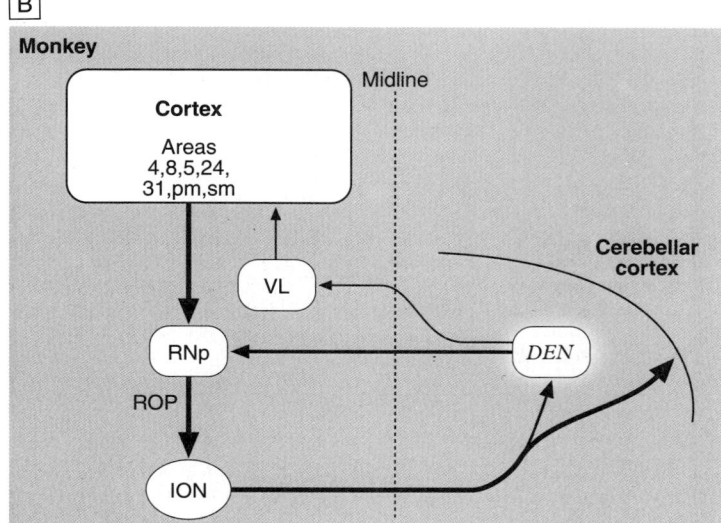

A

8.188A. Crossed corticospinal tract (CST) of the monkey sends collaterals to neurons of origin of the rubrospinal tract (RST) in the magnocellular division of the red nucleus (RNm). This division also receives some direct input from areas 4 and 6 of the motor cortex, and a more dominant input from the interposed nucleus (IP) of the cerebellum which in man is represented by the globose and emboliform nuclei.
B. Distinct system in the monkey originates from widespread areas of the cortex which send a massive input to neurons of origin of the rubro-olivary projection (ROP) located in the parvocellular division of the red nucleus (RNp). There is not a relay in the spinal cord, but instead to the inferior olivary nucleus (ION) which projects to the cerebellum. The cerebellum, including its dentate nucleus (DEN), projects back onto neurons of RNp, and also to the ventrolateral nucleus of the thalamus (VL) for relay back to the cortex. pm = premotor area; sm = supplementary motor area. (From Kennedy (1990) with permission of author and publisher.)

described; the whole mass is traversed and surrounded by fascicles of nerve fibres, including many from the oculomotor nucleus. This makes the red nucleus appear reticular. Its magnocellular element is considered phylogenetically old, which accords with the parvocellular predominance in primates. *Afferent connections* are complex and many (**8**.187). Uncrossed corticorubral fibres from the sensorimotor cortex appear in cats (and other mammals); an area frontal to the precentral gyrus (p. 1166), termed supplementary motor area in the feline cerebrum, projects bilaterally to the red nuclei; somatotopy has been shown in these fibres and nuclear terminations, conforming with localization in the rubrospinal tract (see below). The cortical projection is from primary somatomotor and somatosensory areas. Brown (1974) has described their terminations as axodendritic and largely in peripheral parts of the red nucleus. There are also bilateral, probably reciprocal connections with the superior colliculi. Feline red nuclei also receive nerve fibres from the contralateral nucleus interpositus, corresponding to human globose and emboliform nuclei, and from the contralateral dentate nucleus. All these cerebellar connections and perhaps others (p. 1135, 1178) traverse the superior cerebellar peduncle and display some somatotopy. Other reputed sources of afferents are the globus pallidus, subthalamic and hypothalamic nuclei, substantia nigra and spinal cord. (Rubral connections are outlined in **8**.187, 188.)

Rubrospinal tract

The crossed rubrospinal tract is small in man (Nathan & Smith 1982) and originates from the caudal magnocellular part of red nucleus; few fibres gain the cervical cord. After decussation, the fibres run obliquely laterally in the ventral tegmental decussation ventral to the tectospinal decussation, where they lie dorsal to the medial lemniscus. On reaching the grey matter ventral to the inferior cerebellar peduncle, the tracts turn caudally to enter the lateral part

of the lateral lemniscus. They continue descending ventral to the tract and nucleus of the trigeminal nerve through the medulla and enter the upper part of the cervical cord intermingled with fibres of the lateral corticospinal tract. In experimental animals, tract and nuclear origins show somatotopy, by the recording of antidromic impulses evoked in the nucleus after stimulation of the tract. Some efferent axons form a *rubrobulbar tract* to motor nuclei of the trigeminal, facial, oculomotor, trochlear and abducent nerves; many 'rubrobulbar' fibres may end throughout the brain-stem reticular formation. Associated with rubrospinal tracts are the *tegmentospinal fibres* from tegmental reticular elements lateral to the red nuclei, probably to be grouped with other medullary and pontine reticulospinal tracts (p. 1070).

Central tegmental fasciculus

The largest group of efferents from the red nucleus in man is found in the massive uncrossed central tegmental fasciculus lying ventral in the midbrain, at first lateral to the medial longitudinal fasciculus and dorsolateral to both the red nucleus and the decussation of the superior cerebellar peduncles (8.135, 137, 139, 185). Most descending fibres arise from the parvocellular part of the red nucleus (Nathan & Smith 1982) as the fasciculus traverses this nucleus on its path to the ipsilateral inferior olivary nucleus in the medulla from the motor cortex and lenticular nucleus, via the ansa lenticularis and field of Forel. Some fibres also terminate in the brainstem reticular nuclei. Traversing the red nucleus, the ansa lenticularis (p. 1191) and lenticular nucleus, the fasciculus forms a path from the motor cortex to the brainstem reticular nuclei and inferior olivary nuclear complex. Some ascending and descending axons from brainstem reticular formation run in the fasciculus, their collaterals and terminals innervating other 'reticular' or adjacent 'specific' nuclei. They include: *dorsal* and *ventral ascending noradrenergic bundles*, a *ventral ascending serotonergic bundle* and some fibres of *dorsal* and *ventral ascending cholinergic bundles* (pp. 1074–1076).

Function of the rubro-olivary projection

Kennedy (1990) has proposed a unifying hypothesis for the projections of the corticospinal, rubrospinal and rubro-olivary systems (8.188). Lesions of the corticospinal system in man result in permanent paresis but in monkeys, although initially complete, the paralysis disappears and good recovery ensues. The explanation for this interprimate variability in recovery of corticospinal lesions could lie in the differential capacity of the rubrospinal system to compensate. Monkeys never fully recover from combined lesions of both the corticospinal and rubrospinal tracts suggesting that the two systems are functionally interrelated in the control of movement. Both encode force, velocity and direction parameters, but the rubrospinal system primarily directs activity both during the terminal phase of a move-ment and preceding a movement. There is thus overlap of activity in the two systems for all parameters during movements of limbs and even of individual digits. The corticospinal system is most active during the learning of new movements, the rubrospinal during the execution of learnt automated movements.

The rubro-olivary projection, contained in the central tegmental fasciculus, connects the red nucleus to the contralateral cerebellar cortex (8.187, 188) and also indirectly to the ipsilateral motor cortex from whence both the corticospinal and central tegmental tracts originate. The cerebellum is thought to play a role in motor learning; thus the rubro-olivary system could switch the control of movements from the corticospinal to the rubrospinal system for programmed automation. The rubro-olivary switch is two-way to allow the corticospinal system to break-in, in response to environmental changes during on-going automated learnt movements executed by the rubrospinal system.

After a specific corticospinal tract lesion in monkeys, error signals ascending to the cortex would be routed to the rubro-olivary projection (8.188) and on to the cerebellum and back to the rubrospinal system. Following cerebellar relearning, recovery of motor control would ensue as proper contextual motor commands are fed into the spinal cord by the rubrospinal system which in monkeys is substantial, projecting to ventral horn cells in all segments. The relative absence of a rubrospinal system in man could thus explain the poor recovery of motor function after stroke.

Tectospinal and tectobulbar tracts

The tectospinal and tectobulbar tracts also start at this level, from neurons in the superior colliculi, sweeping ventrally round the central grey matter to decussate ventral to the oculomotor nuclei and medial longitudinal fasciculi as part of the *dorsal tegmental decussations*. The tectospinal tract descends ventral to the medial longitudinal fasciculus as far as the medial lemniscal decussation in the medulla, where it diverges ventrolaterally to reach the spinal ventral white column near the ventral lip of the anterior median fissure. The tectobulbar tract, mainly crossed, descends near the tectospinal tract, ending in the pontine nuclei and motor nuclei of the cranial nerves, particularly those innervating the orbital muscles, and serves reflex ocular movements (see references to lateral tectotegmentospinal tract, p. 1002).

Medial longitudinal fasciculus

The medial longitudinal fasciculus (8.141). A heavily myelinated composite tract, is ventrolateral to the oculomotor nucleus at this level, where its fibres are more dispersed than at lower levels, though its relation to efferent nuclei is retained. The fasciculus ascends to the *interstitial nucleus* (of Cajal) in the lateral wall of the third ventricle, just above the cerebral aqueduct. (Closely related to its upper ends and the decussation of the fasciculi are also the *interstitial* and *dorsal* parts of the nuclear groups *of the posterior commissure* which probably exchange fibres with these complex fasciculi and additionally the *nuclei of Darkschewitsch*, whose status remains uncertain.) The fasciculus retains its position relative to the central grey matter through the midbrain, pons and upper medulla, but is displaced ventrally by successive decussations of the medial lemnisci and lateral corticospinal tracts, to enter the ventral spinal intersegmental fasciculus.

The medial longitudinal fasciculus interconnects the oculomotor, accessory oculomotor, trochlear, abducent, spinal accessory, vestibular and reticular nuclei, co-ordinating conjugate eye movements. Continuity with the ventral spinal intersegmental tract provides for connections between these nuclei and cervical motor neurons, especially those innervating the nuchal musculature. For example, co-ordination between facial and hypoglossal nerves in movements of the lips and tongue in speech is often attributed to connections via the medial longitudinal fasciculus; but this is doubtful. Long established are substantial contributions to it by all *vestibular nuclei* and, to a lesser extent, the lateral lemniscal nucleus, its chief function being to co-ordinate movements of the eyes and head in response to vestibulocochlear stimulation (Maciewicz et al 1975; Yamamoto et al 1978; and p. 1024). Fascicular lesions may cause internuclear ophthalmoplegia. Bilateral vestibular connections ascend or descend in the fasciculus or divide into ascending and descending branches, which send collaterals to nuclei of the third to sixth cranial nerves and the spinal nucleus of the eleventh. All four vestibular nuclei contribute ascending fibres, those from the superior remaining uncrossed (McMasters et al 1966), the others partly crossed. Some fibres reach the interstitial and posterior commissural nuclei, some decussating to the contralateral nuclei (see also p. 1248). Descending axons, from medial vestibular nuclei and perhaps the lateral and inferior, partially decussate and descend in the fasciculus as a *medial vestibulospinal tract* (Brodal et al 1962, and pp. 101, 108, 8.117). Fibres join from the dorsal trapezoid, lateral lemniscal and posterior commissural nuclei. Therefore the cochlear as well as the vestibular nerve may influence movements of the eyes and head via the fasciculus. Some vestibular fibres may ascend in it up to the thalamus.

Unmyelinated longitudinal fasciculus

The unmyelinated longitudinal fasciculus (of Schütz) runs in the central grey matter of the midbrain, pons and medulla, ventrolateral to the aqueduct and fourth ventricle, as a path for descending and ascending connections, largely uncrossed, between hypothalmic and dorsal thalamic and brainstem nuclei, including the accessory oculomotor, superior collicular, ambigual, salivatory, facial, solitary, hypoglossal brainstem reticular nuclei and autonomic nuclei in the spinal cord (Crosby & Woodburne 1951). Some *cholinergic* fibres are described as *descending* from hypothalamic nuclei to enter the cerebellum via its superior peduncle. A *dorsal ascending serotonergic* bundle accompanies the dorsal fasciculus to the diencephalon (p. 996).

Inferior quadrigeminal brachium

The inferior quadrigeminal brachium is a rounded superficial lateral strand in the upper midbrain (8.123, 126); this ascends from the inferior colliculus and lateral lemniscus to the medial geniculate body. It separates dorsolateral fibres of the medial lemniscus from the surface. Quantitative examination by Ferraro and Minckler (1977) in 28 autopsy specimens (from newborn to 97 years) revealed a fibre count of 3.5–5.6 million and a fibre density of about 68000/mm, with little variation between left and right and no significant diminution until the ninth decade. Ramon-Moliner and Dansereau (1974) have examined the 'peribrachial' region at the pontomesencephalic junction and proposed an arbitrary topological division of this part of the tegmental brainstem.

TECTUM OF THE MIDBRAIN

Though the tectum exhibits dorsal swellings from the earliest vertebrate stages, differentiation into superior and inferior colliculi (corpora quadrigemina) appears only in mammals. In prototherian monotremes, only a single pair of swellings exists, the *optic lobes* (corpora bigemina). Optic lobes are highly developed in fishes and are larger than the olfactory lobes in Osteichthyes. At this and later levels of vertebrate evolution the olfactory lobes are, in volume, the major forebrain developments; with the emergence of cerebral hemispheres, i.e. further forebrain development with more than olfactory connections, the optic lobes are relatively small but still remain substantial in amphibians, reptiles and birds. Their connections and functions show a progressive forward neural migration, passing from reptiles to mammals, a process called *telencephalization*. This initial dominance of the optic lobes (in earlier vertebrates probably concerned with all sensory modalities other than olfactory) gradually diminishes, perhaps coupled with a decrease in complexity of their cytoarchitecture. These processes are considered most advanced in primates, in whom the highly developed cerebrum has taken over much primal tectal activity. Differentiation of the optic lobes into superior and inferior colliculi appears in eutherian mammals.

Inferior colliculus

The structure, connections and function of the inferior colliculus have been reviewed by Irvine (1986) and Webster and Garey (1990) and are partly illustrated in 8.189. There is a central ovoid main nucleus, continuous with the periaqueductal grey matter, surrounded by a laminar zone of nerve fibres, many from the lateral lemniscus (8.140), which terminate in it. Nuclear and neuronal organization have been detailed in cats (Morest 1965 and Oliver 1984; Oliver & Morest 1984) and to a lesser extent in man (Geniec & Morest 1971). The central nucleus has *dorsomedial* and *ventrolateral* zones covered by *dorsal cortex*. In humans, the dorsal cortex has four cytoarchitectonic layers: layer I contains small neurons with flattened radial dendritic fields; layer II, medium-sized neurons with ovoid dendritic fields aligned parallel to the collicular surface; layer III, medium-sized neurons with spherical dendritic fields; and layer IV, large neurons with variably-shaped dendritic fields. The central nucleus is laminated; bands of cells with disc-shaped or stellate dendritic fields orthogonally span the fibre layers in which the terminals of lateral lemniscal fibres ramify. The neurons are sharply tuned to frequency

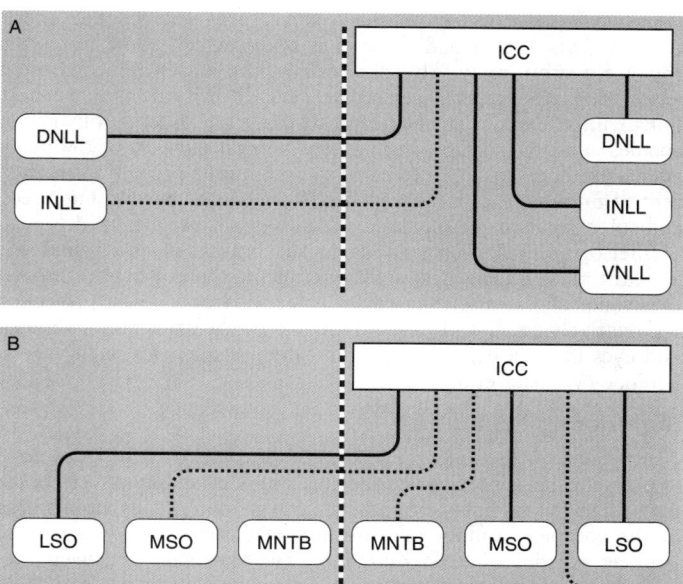

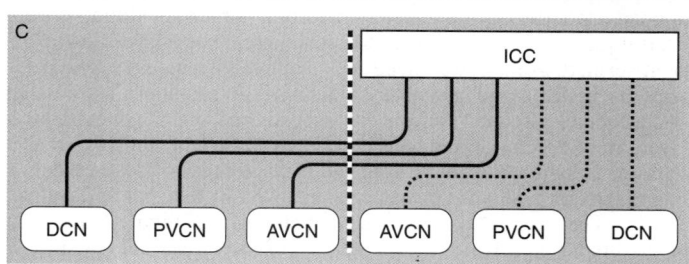

8.189 Summaries of major (solid lines) and minor (broken lines) ascending projections to the central nucleus of the inferior colliculus (ICC) from ipsilateral and contralateral (shown to left of bold vertical broken line) nuclei of (A) lateral lemniscus, (B) superior olivary complex and (C) cochlear nucleus. (AVCN = anteroventral cochlear nucleus; DCN = dorsal cochlear nucleus; DNLL = dorsal nucleus of lateral lemniscus; ICC = central nucleus of inferior colliculus; INLL = intermediate nucleus of lateral lemniscus; LNTB = lateral nucleus of trapezoid body; LSO = lateral superior olivary nucleus; MNTB = medial nucleus of trapezoid body; MSO = medial superior olivary nucleus; PVCN = posterior ventral nucleus of cochlear nucleus; VNLL = ventral nucleus of lateral lemniscus). (From Irvine (1986) with permission from author and publishers.)

and the laminae may represent the structural basis of tonal discrimination since cells driven by low frequencies are found in the dorsal laminae and those driven by high frequencies in the ventral laminae (Webster et al 1984a, b). Neurons are broadly frequency tuned in the dorsal cortex and lateral nucleus. In cats, most cells are binaurally stimulated: 41% are delay sensitive and/or bilaterally excited, 31% are contralaterally excited and ipsilaterally inhibited. Binaural excitatory/inhibitory inputs are probably organized in parallel with the tonotopic cell bands. In cats also, there has been some success in the spatial mapping of auditory receptive fields within the inferior colliculus but this has not been examined in primates. Lesions of either the inferior colliculus or its brachium produce tonal, sound localization, auditory motor reflex and learning defects in experimental animals but in man the effects of such lesions are poorly documented.

Efferent fibres largely traverse the inferior brachium to the *ipsilateral medial geniculate body* (8.189); a crossed connection, via the intercollicular commissure, may exist (Ades 1944). Lemniscal fibres relay only in the central nucleus (Goldberg & Moore 1967); some pass without relay to the medial geniculate body; similarly some colliculogeniculate fibres do not relay in the geniculate body but continue with those which do via the auditory radiation to the auditory cortex, area 42 (8.140). As in other sensory systems a *descending* projection from this cortical area reaches the inferior colliculus via the medial geniculate body, which some fibres may traverse without relay. This descending path may produce effects at levels from the medial geniculate body downwards; it probably links with efferent cochlear fibres, through the superior olivary and cochlear nuclei (p. 1026). In man, the ventral division of the medial geniculate body (p. 1090) receives a topographic projection from the central nucleus, the dorsal division from dorsal cortex, but precise collicular input to the medial division has not been defined.

Inferior collicular projections to the brainstem and spinal cord appear to first traverse the superior colliculi, thereby connecting with the origins of tectospinal and tectotegmental tracts. These projections are relatively small and probably mediate reflex turning of the head and eyes in response to sounds and high frequencies in the ventral laminae (Webster et al 1984).

Superior colliculus

The superior colliculus, unlike the inferior which is fully developed in mammals, is generally regarded as simplified in higher vertebrates, particularly in primates; but nevertheless in man it still exhibits much of the complex laminar organization of earlier forms. At least six laminae are described in human superior colliculi and even more intricate arrangements in other mammals (Ramon y Cajal 1909–1911; Angaut & Repérant 1976). Human collicular laminae are termed at successive depths from the exterior as the strata zonale, cinereum, opticum and lemnisci. The stratum lemnisci itself is often divided into the strata griseum medium, album medium, griseum profundum and album profundum. These seven layers have also been termed: zonal, superficial grey, optic, intermediate grey, deep grey, deep white and periventricular strata (Crosby et al 1962). The two schemes do not completely accord but, as a generalization, layers may be considered alternately composed of neurons or their fibres and dendrites, though some admixture occurs. The connections of the superior colliculi have been reviewed by Huerta and Harting (1984). The *zonal layer* consists chiefly of myelinated and non-myelinated fibres from the occipital cortex (areas 17, 18 and 19, p. 1158), arriving as the *external corticotectal tract*, but among these fibres are a few small neurons, horizontally arrayed. The *superficial grey layer* (stratum cinereum) has many small multipolar interneurons, with which cortical fibres partly synapse, the whole being a crescentic lamina (centrally thicker) over the deeper layers. The *optic layer* consists partly of fibres from the optic tract. As they terminate, they invade the entire anterior–posterior extent of the superficial layers with numerous collateral branches providing a retinotopic map of the contralateral visual field in which the foveal is represented anterolaterally. Retinal axons terminate in clusters from specific retinotectal neurons and as collaterals of retino-geniculate fibres (Garey 1990). Most axons are from slow W cells, a minority are from fast Y cells. The layer also contains some large multipolar neurons; efferent fibres to the retina are said to start in this layer (Wolter & Liss 1956) in man and other mammals. The internal four layers are sometimes considered together as a stratum lemnisci but will be briefly outlined. The *intermediate grey* and *white layers* are collectively the main reception zone, consisting of neurons of various sizes mixed with axons and dendrites. Its main afferent source is the *medial corticotectal path* from the layer V neurons of the ipsilateral occipital cortex (area 18) and other neocortical areas concerned with ocular following movements. These layers also receive mainly contralateral spinal afferents through spinotectal and spinothalamic routes (Yezierski 1988) and probably from the inferior colliculus together with noradrenergic and serotonergic neurons in the locus coeruleus and raphe nuclei (pp. 1075, 1077). The *deep grey* and *deep white layers*, adjacent to the periaqueductal grey substance, are collectively called the parabigeminal nucleus. They contain a mixture of neurons with dendrites extending into the optic layer, but their axons form many of the collicular efferents. (For details of the neonatal superior colliculus consult Labriola & Laemle 1977.)

The superior colliculus thus receives *afferents* from a wide area (Wolter & Liss 1956; Garey 1990), including the retina, spinal cord, inferior colliculus and occipital and temporal cortex; the first three of these pathways convey visual, tactile and probably thermal, pain and auditory impulses, the cortical projection acting as a 'command' and possibly modulating path. Collicular *efferents* pass to the retina

and a wide array of brainstem and spinal neurons, inferior, medial and lateral pulvinar, lateral geniculate nucleus, pretectum and parabigeminal nucleus. Fibres passing from the pulvinar are relayed to primary and secondary visual cortex forming an extrageniculate retinocortical pathway for visual orientation and attention. *Tecto-oculomotor* fibres project to the motor nuclei of ocular muscles. In cats (Edwards & Henkel 1978) neurons in the upper third project to the periaqueductal grey substance dorsal to the upper end of the oculomotor complex, some also synapsing directly with dendrites of oculomotor neurons. Neurons in this central grey region also project to both abducent nuclei. *Tectospinal* fibres (p. 1070) descend to cervical segments while *tectotegmental* fibres reach various tegmental reticular nuclei and also the substantia nigra, red nucleus and probably the spinal cord. *Tectopontine* fibres, probably descending with the tectospinal tract, terminate in dorsolateral pontine nuclei, with a relay to the cerebellum (p. 1022). All descending fibres cross, mostly in the *dorsal tegmental decussation*, but to a lesser extent through an intercollicular commissure. Kawamura et al (1974), reviewing these connections, have studied tectoreticular projections in cats by collicular lesions, producing degeneration in ipsilateral mesencephalic and contralateral pontomedullary reticular nuclei (gigantocellular reticular, caudal pontine reticular, oral pontine reticular and other nuclei). Distribution of these projections corresponded to those from cortical, fastigial and vestibular neurons and thus to the main sources of reticulospinal fibres. A tecto-olivary projection, from deeper collicular laminae to the upper third of the medial accessory olivary nucleus, exists in primates (Frankfurter et al 1976); it is crossed and links with the posterior vermis in ocular movements.

Central collicular stimulation produces 'normal' contralateral head movement in cats (Hess et al 1946). Many similar responses like those of intact animals have been observed in several species, involving the eyes, ears, head, trunk and limbs, thus implicating the superior colliculus in complex integrations between vision and widespread bodily activity (Schaefer & Schneider 1968). In view of the bilateral representation of retinae in the colliculi, results of brain-splitting experiments are of special interest; e.g. tegmental division leads in cats to profound changes in visual behaviour, not so much in reflex responses as in the ability to interpret the environment and adapt to it (Voneida 1965). Response to threatening stimuli and an ability to locate edges and follow them are lost. Similar results appear in monkeys and resemble those of the split-brain syndrome in human patients (p. 1183).

A descending projection from the auditory cortex has been described in some mammals, including cats (Diamond et al 1969) and monkeys (Whitlock & Nauta 1956). Paula-Barbosa and Sousa-Pinto (1973) have confirmed this and explored the projection in greater detail in cats, in which a bilateral projection from secondary auditory areas (AII) reaches the superficial laminae in both superior colliculi; no such projection from the primary auditory area (AI) was observed. Though these are from parts of the auditory cortex which, as far as is known, have no visual connections, this corticocollicular pathway may be involved, via known connections between superior and inferior colliculi, in integrations between visual and auditory behaviour.

Pretectal nucleus

The pretectal nucleus is a poorly defined mass of neurons at the junction of the mesencephalon and diencephalon, extending from a position dorsolateral to the posterior commissure caudally towards the superior colliculus, with which it is partly continuous. It receives fibres through the superior quadrigeminal brachium from the visual cortex, the lateral root of the optic tract from the retina (Kuhlenbeck & Miller 1949) and the superior colliculus. Its efferent fibres reach both accessory oculomotor nuclei (Ranson & Magoun 1933); those which decussate pass ventral to the aqueduct or through the posterior commissure. By this autonomic outflow through the oculomotor nerve, with a relay in ciliary ganglia (p. 1227), sphincters of the iris in both eyes are made to contract in response to impulses from either eye (**8**.119). This bilateral light reflex may not be the sole activity of the pretectal nucleus; some of its efferents project to the pulvinar and deep laminae of the superior colliculus providing another extrageniculate cortical path through the retinotecto-parabigeminopulvinocortical projection (Garey 1990).

Extrageniculate visual pathways

As a corrective codicil to the above it is apposite to refer briefly to data accumulated in regard to visual paths in mammals and particularly birds (Webster 1974). It is almost certain that the vertebrate visual system was primarily mesencephalic in its connections. The concept of 'telencephalization' is part of a greater process of 'encephalization', the evolutionary cranial migration of 'centres' mediating sensorimotor activities, from spinal to *encephalic* levels. Intrusion of visual projections into the *telencephalon* via the thalamus in mammals, with a reciprocal reduction in *mesencephalic* visual connection, remains the major example of *telencephalization*. The change is often regarded as more advanced in mammals, especially primates, than in birds. Compared with mammalian conditions, avian colliculi or optic lobes are relatively larger and more complex in laminar pattern, and the avian corpus striatum is more developed than the superincumbent cortex, proportions apparently reversed in mammalian cerebral hemispheres. The generalizations thus engendered have tended to assign avian and mammalian visual systems to opposite balances in a supposed *duality of pathways*: one integrated at mesencephalic level, vaguely termed 'reflex', the other telencephalic and loosely labelled 'perceptual'. This is an oversimplification. Avian visual structure and function show that both types of path, whether through the midbrain tectum or direct to the dorsolateral thalamus, involve thalamic and cortical projection and striatal connections. In mammals both retinocortical paths exist, the indirect taking a pretectal route, in addition to the superior collicular path, via the pulvinar of the thalamus to the occipital cortex. Functional studies also show that it is erroneous to consider the two visual paths, either in birds or mammals, as being in the one case perceptual and in the other reflexive. In both vertebrate classes the mesencephalic level appears involved in perception and not merely as a level for ocular reflexes, e.g. in avian brains neurons of a tecto-striate projection exhibit responses to movement and to colour, though not to shape or orientation. In contrast, a more direct route via the thalamus to a cortical region known as the 'wulst' in birds (equivalent to the mammalian geniculostriate pathway) has not been shown to evince any special sensitivities, except perhaps to movement. After destruction of primary striate cortex patients may point at objects and also discern different levels of luminosity without consciously seeing. This phenomenon is called blind sight and might be explained if visual stimuli excite extrastriate occipital cortex via the indirect retinotectopulvinocortical routes. In mammals, including mankind perhaps more than in birds, the complex paths of visual information and multiplicity of collateral and descending interconnections provide a 'system' of intricate projection and 'feed-back' which remains speculative. Despite a mass of data particularly concerning the peculiarities of response in individual neurons at every level, it is difficult to ascribe aspects of visual information to identifiable neuronal groups; perhaps it is misleading to seek to do so. Even in man, clinical evidence from injury to the visual cortex suggests that the customary assignment of 'conscious' vision to cortical levels may impede recognition of the intimate interactions between the occipital cortex, tectum and pretectum. Though no functional synthesis can be discerned in the structural and physiological findings so far amassed, visual function must involve most widespread networks of neurons at all levels.

RETICULAR FORMATION OF THE BRAIN STEM

GENERAL ORGANIZATION

Among the more conspicuous tracts and nuclei throughout the brainstem are extensive fields of intermingled neurons and nerve fibres collectively termed the reticular formation. The reticular regions are often regarded as phylogenetically ancient, representing a supposed primitive random nerve network, upon which background more organized, selective routes have appeared during evolution. But, as noted elsewhere (p. 100), the most primitive nervous systems show both diffuse and highly organized regions, which co-operate in response to different demands. Clearly both evolved together, each providing indispensable and interdependent contributions to the total response of the organism.

The general characteristics of reticular regions are:

- Deeply placed, ill-defined collections of neurons and fibres with diffuse connections.
- Conduction paths which are difficult to define, complex and often polysynaptic having ascending and descending widely dispersed components which are partly crossed and uncrossed; unilateral stimulation often resulting in bilateral responses.
- Distinct chemoarchitectonic nuclear groups including clusters of serotoninergic cell bodies (group B cells) which synthesize and secrete the indolamine 5-hydroxytryptamine (serotonin), cholinergic neurons (group Ch cells) which contain acetyltransferase, the enzyme which catalyses the synthesis of acetylocholine, and three catecholaminergic groups, containing noradrenergic (group A) adrenergic (group C) and dopaminergic (group A) cell types which synthesize respectively noradrenaline, adrenaline and dopamine as neurotransmitters.
- Components subserving *somatic* and *visceral* functions.

Modern reviews of the components of the reticular formation, their organization and connections are provided by Niewenhuys (1985); Nieuwenhuys et al (1988); Martin et al (1990), Holstege and Griffiths (1990); Törk and Hornung (1990); Pearson et al (1990); Saper (1990) and what follows is largely a synopsis of these works.

Studies with the Golgi technique show that few brainstem reticular neurons are classic Golgi type II, with short axons branching locally; their dendrites are long and usually spread across the long axis of the brainstem in transverse sheets. Usually dendrites have a simple pattern classified as the *isodendritic configuration* by Ramón-Moliner and Nauta (1966) and described as forming an *isodendritic core*, its territory encompassing many ill-defined, 'diffusely' connected reticular nuclei. These radiating dendrites may spread into 50% of the cross-sectional area of their half of the brainstem and are intersected by, and may synapse with, a complex of ascending and descending fibres. Many axons of the reticular neurons ascend or descend or bifurcate to do both, travelling far, perhaps through the whole brainstem and often beyond. As an example, a bifurcating axon from a cell in the magnocellular medullary nucleus (see below) may project rostrally into the upper medulla, pons, midbrain tegmentum, subthalamus, hypothalamus, dorsal thalamus, septum, limbic system and neocortex, while the descending branch innervates the reticular core of the lower medulla and may reach the cervical spinal intermediate grey matter (laminae V and VI). Many reticular neurons have unidirectional, shorter axons, synapsing with the radiating dendrites of innumerable other neurons en route, and also collaterals which synapse with cells in 'specific' brainstem nuclei or cortical formations, such as the cerebellum. Multitudes of afferent fibres converging on individual neurons and their myriad synapses and destinations provide the structural basis for the polymodal responses elicited by experiment, and also for such terms as 'diffuse', 'non-specific' polysynaptic systems.

A contrasting dendritic form is an *idiodendritic configuration*, in which dendrites are short, sinuous or curved, branch profusely and pursue re-entrant courses at the perimeter of a nuclear group, defining a boundary between it and its environs. Neurons with an intermediate dendritic complexity occur in and near such nuclei and vary in density in much of the remaining reticular formation, being termed allodendritic. In different zones, the proportion of different sizes of neuronal somata varies, some regions containing only small to intermediate multipolar cells ('parvocellular' regions) while, in a few areas, these mingle with large multipolar neurons in 'gigantocellular' or 'magnocellular' nuclei.

In general terms the reticular formation is a continuous isodendritic core traversing the whole brainstem, continuous below with the reticular intermediate spinal grey laminae and divisible into three bilateral longitudinal columns: one *median*, a second *medial* (containing mostly large reticular neurons) and a third *lateral* (containing mostly small to intermediate neurons) columns on the basis of cytoarchitectonic, chemoarchitectonic and functional criteria (**8**.190, 191).

MEDIAN COLUMN OF RETICULAR NUCLEI

This extends throughout the medulla, pons and midbrain and contains neurons largely aggregated in bilateral, vertical sheets, blended

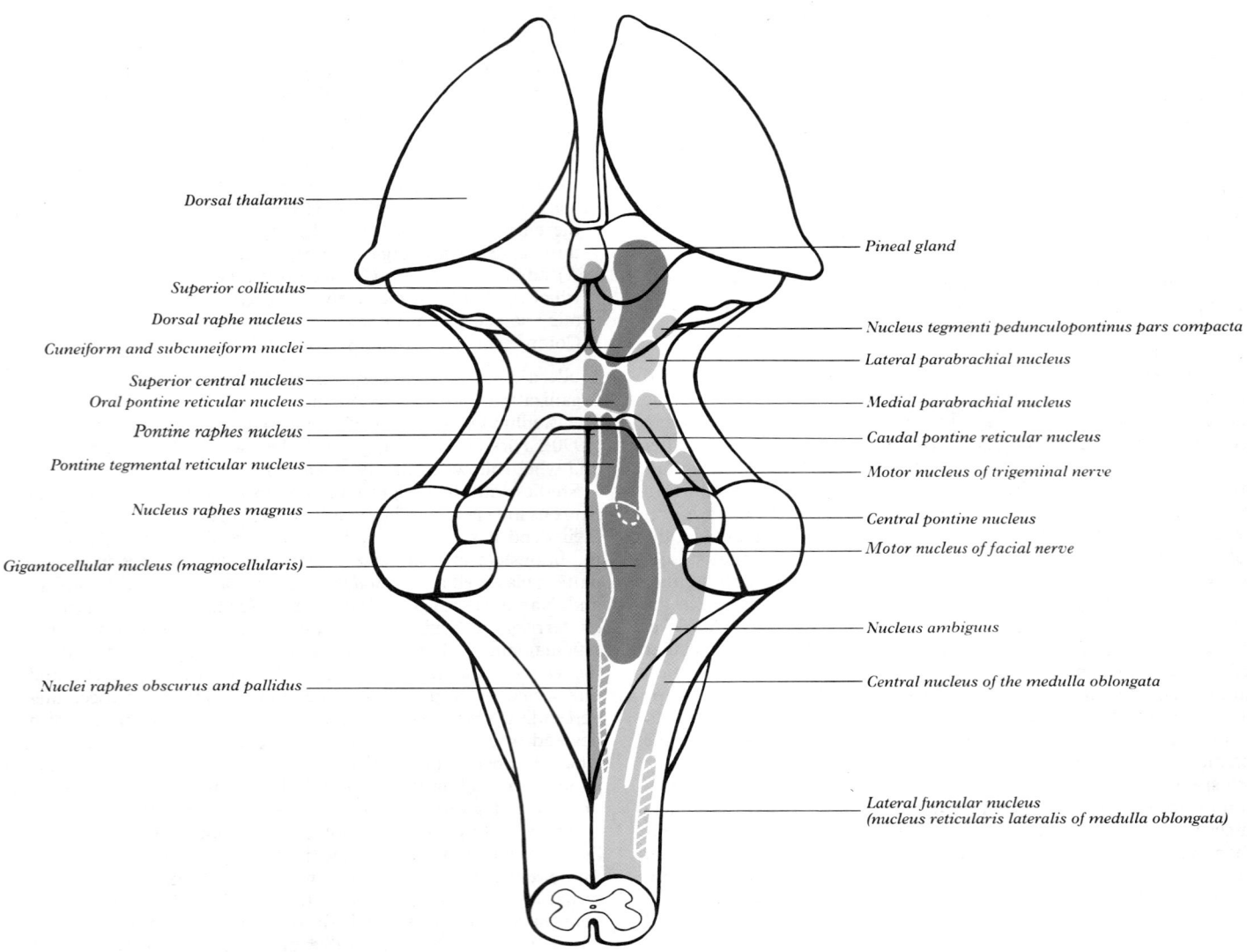

Dorsal thalamus

Superior colliculus

Dorsal raphe nucleus

Cuneiform and subcuneiform nuclei

Superior central nucleus
Oral pontine reticular nucleus

Pontine raphes nucleus

Pontine tegmental reticular nucleus

Nucleus raphes magnus

Gigantocellular nucleus (magnocellularis)

Nuclei raphes obscurus and pallidus

Pineal gland

Nucleus tegmenti pedunculopontinus pars compacta

Lateral parabrachial nucleus

Medial parabrachial nucleus

Caudal pontine reticular nucleus

Motor nucleus of trigeminal nerve

Central pontine nucleus

Motor nucleus of facial nerve

Nucleus ambiguus

Central nucleus of the medulla oblongata

Lateral funicular nucleus
(nucleus reticularis lateralis of medulla oblongata)

8.190   An outline of the human brain stem (black) extending from the caudal end of the medulla to the dorsal thalami; note the margins of the rhomboid fossa, the lateral angles of which indicate the pontomedullary junction; note also the profiles of the transected surfaces of the cerebellar penducles, the colliculi and pineal gland. The principal nuclear derivatives of the brain stem reticular formation are indicated in approximate outline, those from the median and paramedian nuclear column are in magenta; medial column derivatives are purple, lateral column derivatives blue. In reality, of course, considerable overlap of the nuclear profiles would be present when the third dimension is considered. A number of 'non-reticular' nuclei are also included.

in the midline and occupying the paramedian zones; collectively they are *nuclei of the raphe*. (8.190, 192). Many neurons in raphe nuclei are serotonergic and grouped into 9 clusters B1–9 (Dahlström & Fuxe 1964, 1965). In the upper two-thirds of the medulla and crossing the pontomedullary junction is the *raphe pallidus nucleus* and associated *raphe obscurus nucleus*; partly overlapping this and ascending into the pons is the *raphe magnus nucleus*, containing many B3 neurons, and above it the *pontine raphe nucleus* formed by the cell group B5. Also located in the pons is the *central superior raphe nucleus* containing parts of cell groups B6 and B8; finally the *dorsal (rostral) raphe nucleus* approximating to cell group B7 ascends, expanding then narrowing through much of the midbrain.

The serotoninergic raphe system ramifies extensively throughout the entire central nervous system. Although many of these fibres may be diffusely distributed recent work has shown substantial preferential innervation by discrete parts of the system. For example, whereas the central superior raphe nucleus projects divergently to all areas of the cortex, different neurons in the dorsal raphe nucleus not only project specifically to circumscribed regions of the frontal, parietal and occipital cortex but also to functionally related regions of the cerebellar cortex. Similarly, the caudate nucleus and putamen receive a preferential input from the dorsal raphe nucleus; the hippocampus, septum and hypothalamus, on the other hand, are innervated mainly by cells in the central superior mesencephalic raphe nucleus.

All raphe nuclei provide mainly serotoninergic descending projections which terminate in the brainstem and spinal cord. Brainstem connections are multiple and complex. For example, the dorsal raphe nucleus, in addition to sending a large number of fibres to the locus coeruleus (p. 1077), projects together with the central superior, pontine raphe and raphe magnus nuclei to the dorsal tegmental nucleus and most of the rhombencephalic reticular formation.

Raphespinal serotoninergic axons originate mainly from neurons in the raphe magnus, pallidus and obscurus nuclei, projecting as ventral, dorsal and intermediate spinal tracts in the ventral and

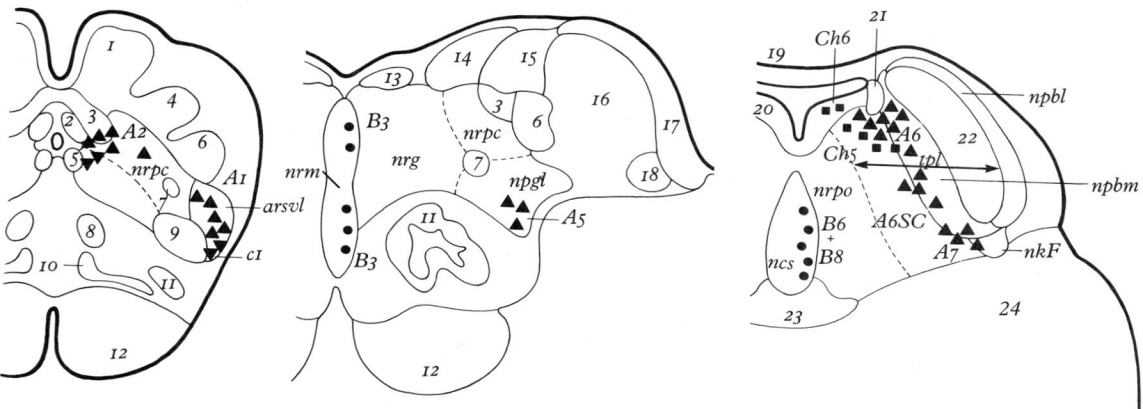

8.191 The reticular formation. Diagrammatic transverse sections through the caudal (A), intermediate (B) and rostral (C) rhombencephalon, to show the position of the reticular formation and the various monoaminergic (noradrenergic: ▲, adrenergic: ▼, serotoninergic: ●) and cholinergic: ■ cell groups located within the confines of that structure. 1. Gracile nucleus. 2. Dorsal nucleus of vagus nerve. 3. Solitary nucleus. 4. Medial cuneate nucleus. 5. Hypoglossal nucleus. 6. Spinal nucleus of trigeminal nerve. 7. Nucleus ambiguus. 8. Anterior funicular nucleus. 9. Lateral funicular nucleus. 10. Medial accessory olivary nucleus. 11. Inferior olivary nucleus. 12. Pyramidal tract. 13. Hypoglossal prepositus nucleus. 14. Medial vestibular nucleus. 15. Inferior vestibular nucleus. 16. Inferior cerebellar peduncle. 17. Dorsal cochlear nucleus. 18. Pontobulbar body. 19. Anterior medullary velum. 20. Central pontine grey. 21. Mesencephalic trigeminal nucleus. 22. Superior cerebellar peduncle. 23. Pontine trigeminal reticular nucleus. 24. Pontine nuclei. A1, A2, A5, A7 = Noradrenergic cell groups, showing no relation to cytoarchitectonic entities; A6 = Noradrenergic cells, constituting the locus coeruleus; A6 sc = Noradrenergic cells confined to the subcoeruleus area; B3, B6, B8 = Serotoninergic cell groups; arsvl = Ventrolateral superior reticular area; ncs = Superior central nucleus; nKF = Kölliker-Fuse nucleus; npbl = Lateral parabrachial nucleus; npbm = Medial parabrachal nucleus; npgl = Lateral paragigantocellular reticular nucleus; nrm = Raphe magnus nucleus; nrpc = Parvocellular reticular nucleus; nrpo = Oral pontine reticular nucleus; tpl = Lateral pontine tegmentum. From Nieuwenhuys et al 1988, The Human Nervous System, Springer Verlag, with permission of publisher and author.

lateral funiculi, terminating respectively in the ventral horns and laminae I, II and V of the dorsal horns of all segments, and in the thoracolumbar intermediolateral sympathetic and sacral parasympathetic preganglionic cell columns. The dorsal raphe spinal projections function as a pain control pathway descending from the mesencephalic pain control centre, located in the periaqueductal grey, dorsal raphe and cuneiform nuclei. The intermediate raphe spinal projection is inhibitory and, in part, modulates central sympathetic control of cardiovascular function. The ventral raphespinal system excites ventral horn cells and could function to enhance motor responses to nociceptive stimuli and to promote the flight and fight response.

The mesencephalic serotoninergic raphe system is principally reciprocally interconnected rostrally with the limbic system, septum, prefrontal cortex and hypothalamus (**8**.192). Efferents ascend forming a large ventral and diminutive dorsal pathway. Both originate from neurons in the dorsal and central superior raphe nuclei, with the raphe magnus nucleus also contributing to the dorsal ascending serotoninergic pathway which is at first incorporated into the dorsal longitudinal fasciculus of Schütz (p. 1071). A few fibres terminate in the central mesencephalic grey matter and posterior hypothalamus, but most continue into the medial forebrain bundle merging with the axons of the ventral pathway which are distributed to the same targets (**8**.192). The fibres of the ventral ascending serotoninergic pathway exit the ventral aspect of the mesencephalic raphe nuclei and then course rostrally through the ventral tegmentum from whence fibres pass to the ventral tegmental area, substantia nigra and interpeduncular nucleus. A large number of fibres then enter the habenulo-interpeduncular tract running rostrally to innervate the habenular nucleus, intralaminar, midline, anterior, ventral and lateral dorsal thalamic nuclei and lateral geniculate body. The ventral ascending serotoninergic pathway then enters the median forebrain bundle in the lateral hypothalamic area and splits to pass medially and laterally. The fibres in the medial tract terminate in the mamillary body, dorsomedial, ventromedial, infundibular, anterior and lateral hypothalamic, medial and lateral preoptic and suprachiasmatic nuclei. Those in the lateral tract take the ansa peduncularis–ventral amygdalofugal path to the amygdala, striatum and caudal neocortex. The medial forebrain bundle carries the remaining ventral ascending serotoninergic axons into the medullary stria (p. 1026), stria terminali (p. 1098), fornix (p. 1129) diagonal band (p. 1129), external capsule (p. 1197), cingulate fasciculus (p. 1175) and medial olfactory stria to terminate in all the structures these systems interconnect.

Major afferents into the mesencephalic raphe nuclei include those from: the interpeduncular nucleus linking the limbic and serotoninergic systems; the lateral habenular nucleus linking the septum, preoptic hypothalamus and prefrontal cortex through the habenulo-interpeduncular tract and the medial forebrain bundle; and the pontine central grey.

The ascending raphe system probably functions to moderate forebrain, particularly limbic, septal and hypothalamic activities. Recent demonstrations of specificity of connectivity suggests that precise as well as tonal control is exerted.

MEDIAL COLUMN OF RETICULAR NUCLEI

This column (**8**.190, 193) is composed of neurons of medium size but in some regions very large neurons are found; most are isodendritic with processes orientated in the transverse plane. In the lower medulla the column is indistinct, perhaps represented by the thin lamina lateral to the raphe nuclei; in the upper medulla, however, it expands into the *medullary gigantocellular (magnocellular) nucleus*, lateral to the raphe nuclei, ventrolateral to the hypoglossal, ventral to the dorsal vagal nuclei and dorsal to the inferior olivary complex. Ascending farther, the column continues as the *pontine gigantocellular (magnocellular) nucleus* lying medially in the tegmentum; its neurons suddenly diminish in size forming, in rostral order, the almost coextensive *caudal and oral pontine tegmental reticular nuclei* from which the medial column expands into the *cuneiform nucleus* and *subcuneiform nucleus*, fading away in the midbrain tegmentum. A narrow medial strip of the central nucleus of the medulla oblongata is also included.

Axons of the medial reticular column neurons form a multisynaptic ascending and descending system within the column, ultimately entering the spinal cord and diencephalon (**8**.193). All cranial motor neurons are heavily innervated and descending fibres of the medial reticular zone comprise two major systems, the pontospinal, or lateral reticulospinal, and bulbospinal, or medial reticulospinal tracts. The former is constituted by axons from neurons in the caudal and oral parts of the pontine reticular nucleus which descend uncrossed in the anterior spinal funiculus and terminate in spinal cord laminae VII, VIII and IX. The latter originate from the medullary reticular formation and descend bilaterally to terminate in laminae VII, VIII, IX, and X and ipsilaterally to end in laminae IV, V and VI. The system modulates spinal motor function and segmental nociceptive input.

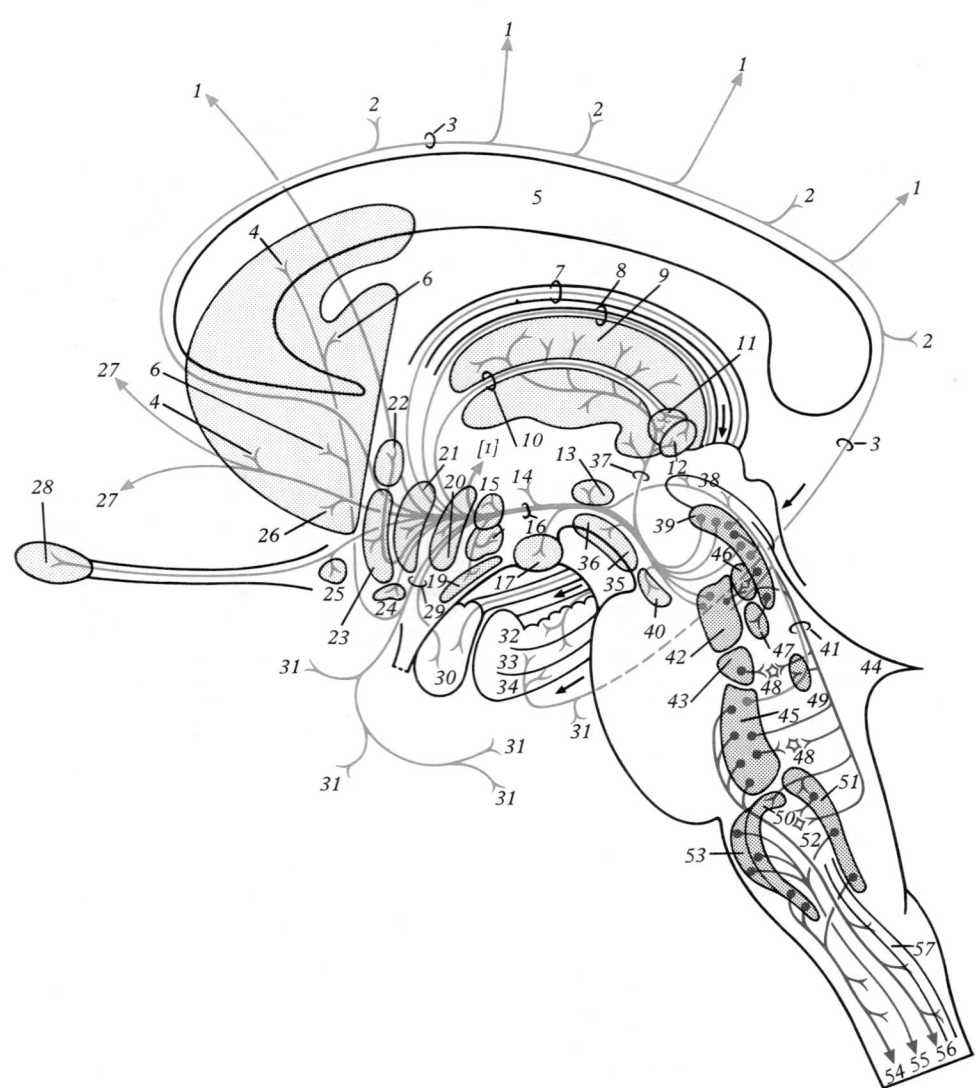

8.192   Ascending (blue) and descending (red) fibres of the raphe reticular system. 1. Neocortex. 2. Cingulate gyrus. 3. Longitudinal striae and cingulum. 4. Caudate nucleus. 5. Corpus callosum. 6. Putamen. 7. Fornix. 8. Stria terminalis. 9. Thalamus. 10. Stria medullaris. 11. Lateral habenular nucleus. 12. Medial habenular nucleus. 13. Ventral tegmental area. 14. Lateral hypothalamic area. 15. Dorsomedial nucleus. 16. Medial telencephalic fasciculus. 17. Mamillary body. 18. Ventromedial nucleus. 19. Infundibular nucleus. 20. Anterior hypothalamic nucleus. 21. Lateral and medial preoptic nuclei. 22. Lateral and medial septal nuclei. 23. Nucleus of the diagonal band. 24. Suprachiasmatic nucleus. 25. Anterior olfactory nucleus. 26. Nucleus accumbens. 27. Prefrontal cortex. 28. Olfactory bulb. 29. Ansa peduncularis and ventral amygdalofugal fibres. 30. Amygdala. 31. Parahippocampal gyrus. 32. Dentate gyrus. 33. Ammon's horn. 34. Subiculum. 35. Substantia nigra. 36. Pars compacta of substantia nigra. 37. Habenulo-interpeduncular tract. 38. Mesencephalic central grey. 39. Dorsal raphe nucleus. 40. Interpenducular nucleus. 41. Dorsal longitudinal fasciculus. 42. Superior central nucleus B6–B8. 43. Pontine raphe nucleus B5. 44. Fourth ventricle. 45. Raphe magnus nucleus B3. 46. Dorsal tegmental nucleus. 47. Locus coeruleus. 48. Mesencephalic reticular formation. 49. Central pontine grey. 50. Raphe pallidus nucleus. 51. Raphe obscurus nucleus. 52. Medullary reticular formation. 53. Arcuate nucleus. 54. Ventral raphe spinal projection. 55. Intermediate raphe spinal projection. 56. Dorsal raphe spinal projection. 57. Substantia gelatinosa. From Nieuwenhuys et al 1988, The Human Nervous System, Springer Verlag, with permission of publisher and author.

Specific afferent components to the medial reticular nucleus include the spinoreticular projection and those from all central nuclei of the sensory components of the cranial nerves. The former are non-specific and stem from neurons in the intermediate grey matter of the spinal cord, decussate in the anterior white commissure, ascend in the anterolateral funiculus, usually via several neurons, and terminate not only at all levels of the medial column of reticular nuclei but also in the intralaminar nuclei of the thalamus. Three areas of the medial reticular zone receive particularly high densities of terminations; these are the combined caudal and rostral ends of the gigantocellular and central nuclei respectively, the caudal pontine reticular nucleus, and the pontine tegmentum. Collaterals of centrally projecting spinal trigeminal, vestibular and cochlear fibres end in the medial reticular formation. Retinotectal and tectoreticular fibres relay visual information and the medial forebrain bundle transmits olfactory impulses.

Efferents from the medial column of reticular nuclei project through a multisynaptic pathway within the column to the thalamus (8.188). Areas of maximal termination of spinoreticular fibres also project directly to the intralaminar thalamic nuclei. The multisynaptic pathway is integrated into the lateral column of reticular nuclei with cholinergic neurons in the lateral pontine tegmentum. The intralaminar thalamic nuclei project directly to the striatum and neocortex.

LATERAL COLUMN OF RETICULAR NUCLEI

This column (8.185, 194, 195) contains six nuclear groups: the parvocellular reticular area, superficial ventrolateral reticular area, lateral pontine tegmental noradrenergic cell groups A1, A2, A4–A7 (A3 is absent in primates), adrenergic cell groups C1–C2 and cholinergic cell groups Ch5–Ch6. The small neurons of the parvocellular reticular area are allodendritic or idiodendritic. Descending through the lower two-thirds of the lateral pontine tegmentum and upper medulla, the column lies between the gigantocellular nucleus medially, and sensory trigeminal nuclei laterally; continuing caudally, it expands to form most of the reticular formation lateral to the raphe nuclei, abuts the superficial ventrolateral reticular area, nucleus solitarius, nucleus ambiguus and dorsal motor nucleus of the vagus. Here it contains the adrenergic cell group C2 and noradrenergic group A2.

At the rostral pole of the diffuse *superficial ventrolateral reticular area* (lying at the level of the facial nucleus), is the *lateral paragigantocellular nucleus*. The zone extends caudally as the *nucleus retroambiguus* and on into the spinal cord. The ventrolateral reticular area is involved in cardiovascular, respiratory, vasoreceptor and chemoreceptor reflexes and in the modulation of nociception. Noradrenergic cell groups A1, A2, A4 and A5 and the adrenergic cell group C1 are located in this reticular zone. The *A2* or *noradrenergic dorsal medullary cell group* lies in the nucleus of the tractus solitarius, dorsal motor nucleus of the vagus and adjoining parvocellular reticular area. Adrenergic group C1 lies rostral to the A2 cell group. *Noradrenergic cell group A4* extends into the lateral pontine tegmentum, along the subependymal surface of the superior cerebellar peduncle. *Noradrenergic group 5* forms part of the *paragigantocellular nucleus* in the caudolateral pontine tegmentum. *Noradrenergic cell group A5* and *adrenergic cell group C1* probably function as centres of vasomotor control. The entire region is subdivided into functional areas on the basis of stimulation experiments, in which vasoconstrictor, cardioaccelerator, depressor, inspiratory, expiratory and sudomotor pools of neurons are located (McAllen 1986a,b).

The *lateral pontine tegmental reticular grey matter* is related to the superior cerebellar peduncle forming the *medial and lateral parabrachial nuclei* and the ventral *Kölliker-Fuse nucleus*, a pneumotaxic centre. The *locus coeruleus (noradrenergic cell group A6)*, *area subcoeruleus, noradrenergic cell group A7* and *cholinergic group Ch5* in the *pedunculopontine tegmental nucleus* (p. 1026) are all located in the lateral pontine and mesencephalic tegmental reticular zones — the mesencephalic group Ch5 is continuous caudally with *cell group Ch6* in the pontine central grey matter.

Cell group A6 contains all the noradrenergic cells in the central region of the *locus coeruleus*. Group A6 has ventral (*nucleus subcoeruleus, A6 Sc*), rostral and a caudolateral extension merging with the A4 group. The locus coeruleus probably functions as an attention centre focusing neural functions to the prevailing needs of the alert animal (see later). The *noradrenergic A7 group* occupies the rostroventral part of the pontine tegmentum continuous with A5 and A1 through the lateral rhombencephalic tegmentum. The A7, A5, A1 complex is also connected by noradrenergic cell clusters with group A2, caudally, and group A6, rostrally. The A5 and A7 groups largely lie within the medial parabrachial and Kölliker-Fuse nuclei. Reticular neurons in the lateral pontine tegmental reticular area, like those of the ventrolateral zone, function to regulate respiratory, cardiovascular and gastrointestinal activity. In addition, there are two micturition centres, the M- and L-regions located in the dorsomedial and ventrolateral parts respectively of the lateral pontine tegmentum.

The connections of the lateral column reticular nuclei are complex. The short ascending and descending axons of the parvocellular reticular area constitute bulbar reflex pathways through a propriobulbar system interconnecting all branchiomotor nuclei and the hypoglossal nucleus with central afferent cranial nerve complexes. The area also receives descending afferents from contralateral motor cortex in the corticotegmental tract and from the contralateral red nucleus in the rubrospinal tract. The longitudinal catacholamine bundle also passes through the parvocellular reticular formation.

The *superficial ventrolateral reticular area* receives some input from the spinal cord, insular cortex and amygdala but the principal projection is from the nucleus of the tractus solitarius subserving cardiovascular, baroreceptor, chemoreceptor and respiratory reflexes (**8.194**). Reticulospinal afferents from the region terminate bilaterally on sympathetic preganglionic neurons in the thoracic spinal cord. Afferents from the pneumotaxic centre (the Kölliker-Fuse nucleus) project to an inspiratory centre in the ventrolateral part of nucleus solitarius and a mixed expiratory–inspiratory centre in the superficial ventrolateral reticular area. Inspiratory neurons in both centres monosynaptically project to the phrenic and intercostal motor neurons; the axons of expiratory neurons terminate on lower motor neurons innervating intercostal and abdominal musculature. The superficial ventrolateral area is also the seat of the visceral alerting response. Fibres from the hypothalamus, periaqueductal grey matter

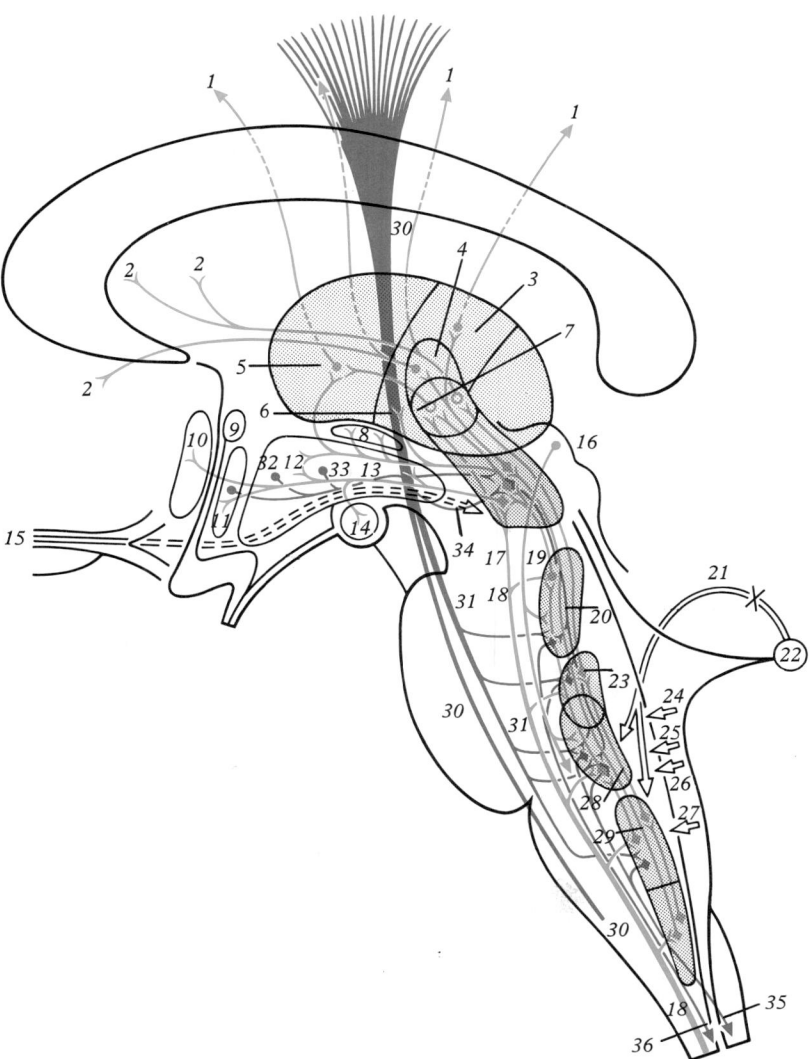

8.193 Ascending (blue) and descending (red) fibre systems of the medial reticular formation. 1. Neocortex. 2. Corpus striatum. 3. Posterior lateral nucleus of thalamus. 4. Intralaminar nuclei of thalamus. 5. Lateral ventral and anterior ventral nuclei of thalamus. 6. Posterior ventral nucleus of thalamus. 7. Centromedian nucleus of thalamus. 8. Zona incerta. 9. Anterior commissure. 10. Septal nuclei. 11. Preoptic nucleus. 12. Lateral hypothalamic area. 13. Ventral tegmental area. 14. Lateral nucleus of mamillary body. 15. Olfactory tract. 16. Superior colliculus. 17. Mesencephalic reticular formation. 18. Spino-reticular tract. 19. Tectobulbar and tectospinal tracts. 20. Pontine oral reticular nucleus. 21. Uncinate fasciculus of cerebellum. 22. Fastigeal nucleus. 23. Pontine caudal reticular nucleus. 24. Trigeminal input. 25. Acoustic input. 26. Vestibular input. 27. Input from nucleus solitarius. 28. Gigantocellular nucleus. 29. Central nucleus of medulla oblongata. 30. Pyramidal tract. 31. Corticotegmental fibres. 32. Anterior hypothalamic nucleus. 33. Hypothalamus. 34. Medial telencephalic fasciculus. 35. Pontospinal tract. 36. Bulbospinal tract. From Nieuwenhuys et al 1988, The Human Nervous System, Springer Verlag, with permission of publisher and author.

and midbrain tegmentum mediate increased respiratory activity, raised blood pressure, tachycardia, vasodilation in skeletal muscle and renal and gastrointestinal vasoconstriction. Ascending efferents of the superficial ventrolateral area synapse on neurons of the supraoptic and paraventricular hypothalamic nuclei. Excitation of these cells causes release of vasopressin from the neurohypophysis. Medullary noradrenergic cell groups A1 and A2 also innervate directly and indirectly the median eminence and control the release of growth hormone, luteinizing hormone and adrenocorticotrophic hormone (ACTH).

The lateral pontine tegmentum, particularly the parabrachial region, is reciprocally connected with the insular cortex (**8.189**). There are also reciprocal projections from the amygdala through the ventral amygdalofugal pathway, medial forebrain bundle and central tegmental fasciculus; and from the hypothalamic, median preoptic and paraventricular nuclei which preferentially project to the lateral parabrachial nucleus and the micturition M-region.

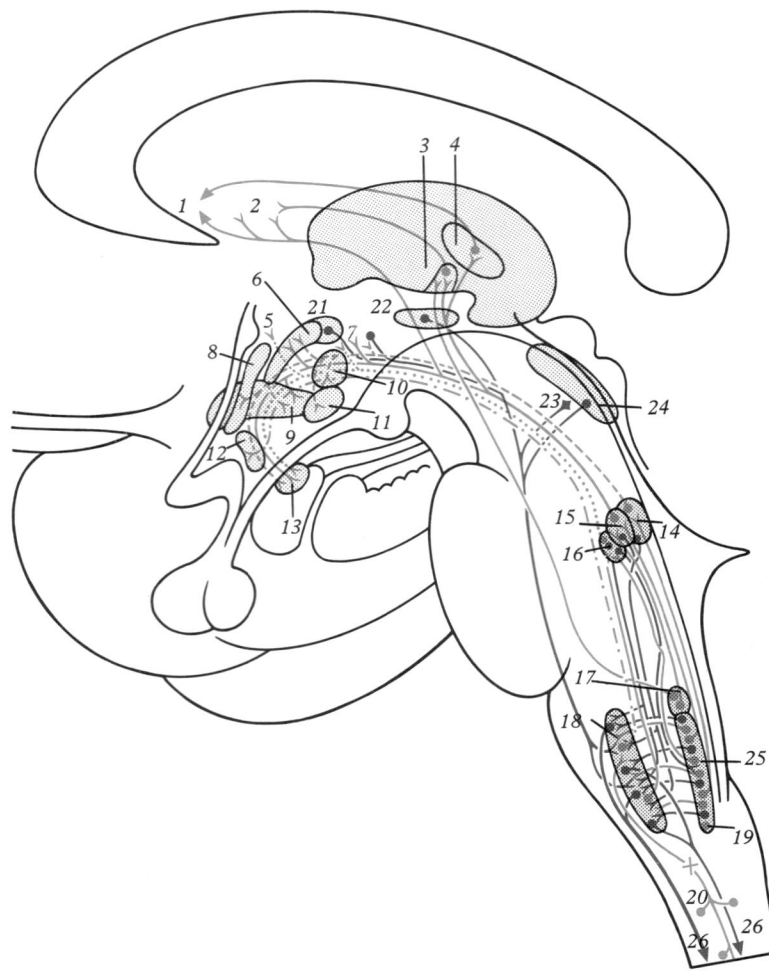

8.194 Ascending (blue) and descending (red) projections from the super-ficial ventrolateral and parabrachial areas of the reticular formation. 1. Lateral part of prefrontal cortex. 2. Visceral cortex of frontoparietal operculum. 3. Posterior medial nucleus of thalamus (pars parvocellularis). 4. Intralaminar nuclei of thalamus. 5. Lateral preoptic nucleus. 6. Paraventricular nucleus (pars magnocellularis). 7. Lateral area of hypothalamus. 8. Median preoptic nucleus. 9. Substantia innominata. 10. Dorsomedial nucleus. 11. Ventromedial nucleus. 12. Supraoptic nucleus. 13. Central nucleus of the amygdala. 14. Lateral parabrachial nucleus. 15. Medial parabrachial nucleus. 16. Kölliker-Fuse nucleus. 17. Gustatory part of nucleus solitarius. 18. Ventrolateral superficial area of reticular formation. 19. Cardiorespiratory part of nucleus solitarius). 20. Spinoreticular fibres. 21. Paraventricular nucleus (pars parvocellularis). 22. Zona incerta. 23. Mesencephalic reticular formation (cuneiform nucleus). 24. Central grey of midbrain. 25. Cardiorespiratory part of the nucleus solitarius. 26. Bulbospinal fibres. From Nieuwenhuys et al 1988, The Human Nervous System, Springer Verlag, with permission of publisher and author.

Reciprocal bulbar projections, many from the Kölliker-Fuse nucleus, are to the nucleus solitarius and superficial ventrolateral reticular area.

Reticulospinal fibres descend from the lateral pontine tegmentum. A mainly ipsilateral subcoeruleospinal pathway is distributed to all spinal segments of the cord through the lateral spinal funiculus. Crossed pontospinal fibres descend from the ventrolateral pontine tegmentum, decussating in the rostral pons and occupying the contralateral dorsolateral spinal funiculus to terminate in laminae I, II, V and VI of all spinal segments of the cord. As mentioned above, spinal fibres of the Kölliker-Fuse nucleus innervate the phrenic nucleus and also T1–T3 sympathetic preganglionic neurons bilaterally through this fibre projection system. There are also bilateral projections in the lateral spinal funiculus from the micturition M- and L-regions. The former terminate in the preganglionic parasympathetic neurons in the sacral cord innervating the detrusor muscle, the latter in the nucleus of Onuf which sends fibres to the musculature of the pelvic floor and the anal and urethral sphincters. Descending fibres of the A6 noradrenergic neurons of the locus coeruleus project both into the longitudinal dorsal fasciculus, as the caudal limb of the dorsal periventricular pathway, and also into

the caudal limb of the dorsal noradrenergic bundle, as part of the longitudinal catecholamine bundle, to innervate, mainly ipsilaterally, all other rhombencephalic reticular areas, principal and spinal trigeminal nuclei, pontine nuclei, cochlear nuclei, nuclei of the lateral lemniscus, and bilaterally all spinal preganglionic autonomic neurons and the ventral region of the dorsal horn of all segments. Other axons contributing to the longitudinal catecholamine bundle originate from cell groups C7, A1, A2, A5 and A7. The main projection is, however, a descending one from cell groups C1 and A5, which are sudomotor neural control centres, innervating preganglionic sympathetic neurons.

Most ascending fibres from the locus coeruleus pass in the dorsal noradrenergic (or tegmental) bundle, others run in either the rostral limb of the dorsal periventricular pathway or in the superior cerebellar peduncle (**8.195**). The latter fibres terminate on the deep cerebellar nuclei. The dorsal noradrenergic bundle is large and runs through the ventrolateral periaqueductal grey matter, to join the medial forebrain bundle in the hypothalamus, where fibres continue forward to innervate all rostral areas of the brain. For example, the pathway contains efferent and afferent axons reciprocally connecting the locus coeruleus with adjacent structures along its course, e.g. central mesencephalic grey matter, dorsal raphe nucleus, superior and inferior colliculi, interpeduncular nucleus, epithalamus, dorsal thalamus, habenular nuclei, amygdala, septum, olfactory bulb and anterior olfactory nucleus, entire hippocampal formation and neocortex. Fibres from the locus coeruleus in the rostral limb of the dorsal periventricular pathway ascend in the ventromedial periaqueductal grey matter adjacent to the longitudinal dorsal fasciculus to terminate in the parvocellular part of the paraventricular nucleus in the hypothalamus.

The functions of the locus coeruleus and related tegmental noradrenergic cell groups are poorly understood. The diversity of their rostral and caudal projections suggests an holistic role in central processing which might be understood if the location of the afferent neurons providing the major drive to the neurons of the locus coeruleus could be detected (Saper 1987). Firing rates of the neurons peak when the animal is awake and decrease when falling asleep to almost completely disappear during rapid eye movement (REM) sleep. During wakefulness firing rates are augmented when novel stimuli are presented. The locus coeruleus may then function to control the level of attentiveness, enhancing the signal processing capacity of target neurons by increasing their signal-to-noise ratio. Other functions have also been ascribed to the locus coeruleus which include control of the wake–sleep cycle, regulation of blood flow and maintenance of synaptic plasticity.

The A1, A2, A5 and A7 noradrenergic cell groups project rostrally mainly through the central tegmental fasciculus as a major longitudinal catecholamine pathway which continues through the medial forebrain bundle to terminate in the amygdala, lateral septal nucleus, bed nucleus of the stria terminalis, nucleus of the diagonal band and the hypothalamus.

The ascending dorsal periventricular pathway also contains a few non-coerulean noradrenergic fibres which terminate in the periventricular region of the thalamus. Dopaminergic cell groups A9 in the substantia nigra, dopaminergic cell groups A8 and A10, and the cholinergic Ch5 cell group, in the ventral mesencephalic tegmental area are described on pages 168, 293.

Propriobulbar projections (p. 996) also receive a contribution from the diffusely organized dorsal medullary and lateral tegmental noradrenergic cell groups interconnecting cranial nerve nuclei and other reticular cell groups, particularly those of the vagus, facial and trigeminal and the rhombencephalic raphe and parabrachial nuclei.

Within the reticular formation are three precerebellar nuclei involved in the relay of spinal information into the vermis and paravermal regions of the ipsilateral cerebellar hemispheres: the lateral and paramedian reticular nuclei and the nucleus of the pontine tegmentum. These reticular nuclei receive fibres from the contralateral primary motor and sensory neocortex, ipsilateral cerebellar and vestibular nuclei and also ipsilateral spinal cord through the ascending spinoreticular pathway. This system thus augments that of the dorsal and ventral spinocerebellar projection systems, the cuneocerebellar and accessory cuneocerebellar projections and trigeminocerebellar tracts.

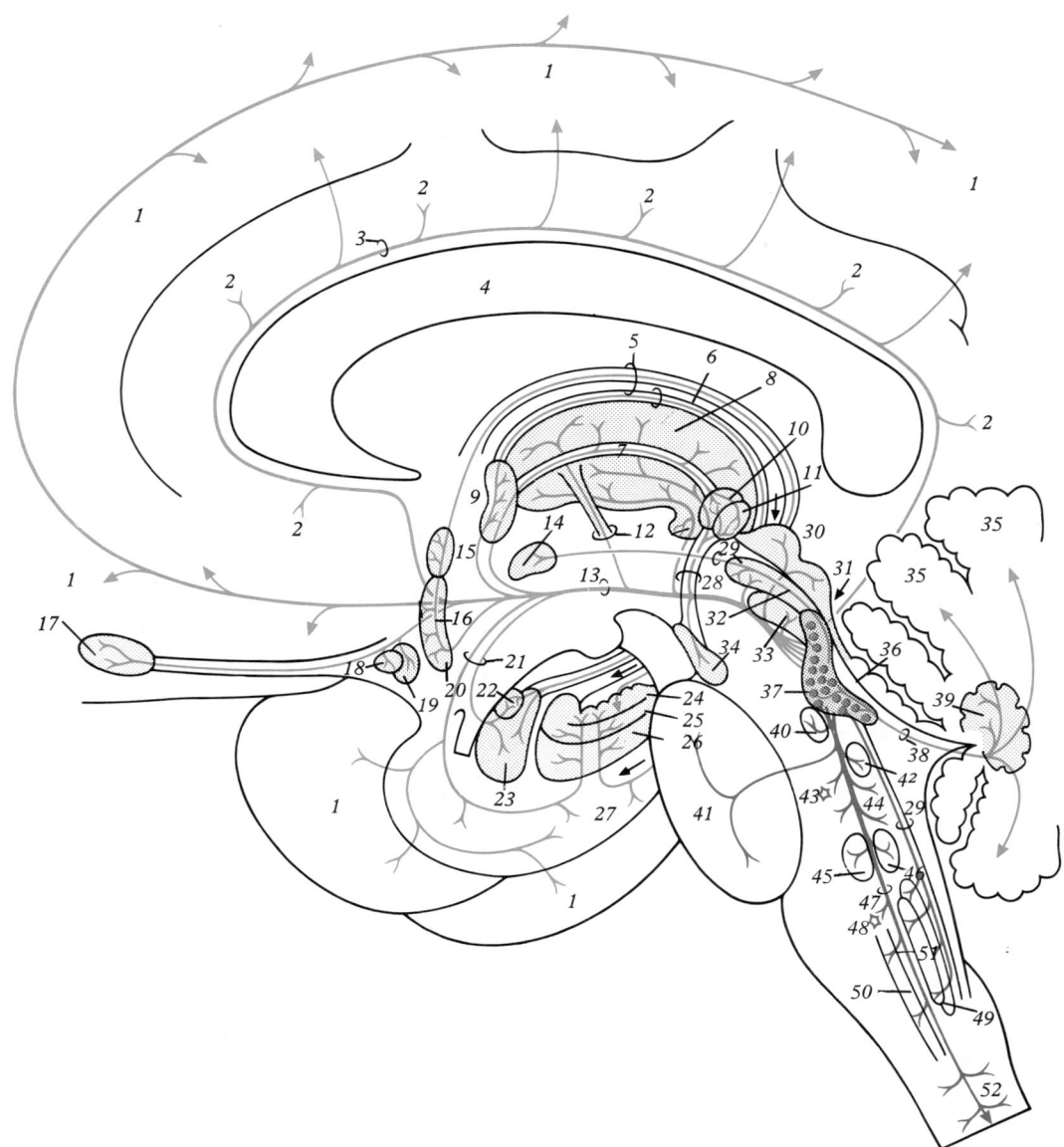

8.195 Ascending (blue) and descending (red) noradrenergic projections from the locus coeruleus of the reticular formation. 1. Neocortex. 2. Cingulate gyrus. 3. Longitudinal striae. 4. Corpus callosum. 5. Fornix. 6. Stria terminalis. 7. Medullary stria. 8. Thalamus. 9. Interstitial nucleus of the striae terminalis. 10. Lateral habenular nucleus. 11. Medial habenular nucleus. 12. Mamillothalmic tract. 13. Medial telencephalic fasciculus. 14. Parvocellular paraventricular nucleus. 15. Medial septal nucleus. 16. Diagonal band. 17. Olfactory bulb. 18. Anterior olfactory nucleus. 19. Anterior perforated substance. 20. Nucleus of the diagonal gyri. 21. Ventral amygdalo-fugal fibres of the ansa peduncularis. 22. Central nucleus of the amygdala. 23. Basal nucleus of the amygdala. 24. Dentate gyrus. 25. Ammons horn. 26. Subiculum. 27. Parahippocampal gyrus. 28. Habenulointerpenduncular tract. 29. Dorsal longitudinal fasciculus. 30. Superior colliculus. 31. Inferior colliculus. 32. Mesencephalic central grey. 33. Dorsal raphe nucleus. 34. Interpeduncular nucleus. 35. Cerebellar cortex. 36. Locus coeruleus. 37. Subcoerulear area. 38. Superior cerebellar peduncle. 39. Central cerebellar nuclei. 40. Nucleus of lateral lemniscus. 41. Pontine nuclei. 42. IVth ventricle. 43. Upper medullary reticular formation. 44. Parvocellular reticular nucleus. 45. Ventral cochlear nucleus. 46. Dorsal cochlear nucleus. 47. Longitudinal catecholamine bundle. 48. Medullary reticular formation. 49. Nucleus solitarius. 50. Spinal nucleus of the trigeminal nerve. 51. Dorsal nucleus of vagus. 52. Reticulospinal fibres. From Nieuwenhuys et al 1988, The Human Nervous System, Springer Verlag, with permission of publisher and author.

DIENCEPHALON

The diencephalon is part of the prosencephalon which develops from the foremost primary cerebral vesicle (p. 1072). This *forebrain vesicle* and its cavity, the future *third ventricle*, soon differentiate into a caudal *diencephalon* and rostral *telencephalon*. From the latter's sides, right and left diverticula develop into cerebral hemispheres, each with a contained ventricle. The sites of evagination become the interventricular foramina, by which all three ventricles are continuous. The diencephalon corresponds largely to most of the third ventricle and its adjacent structures; the *telencephalon* comprises a median *telencephalon medium* (*impar*), containing a limited forward extension of the third ventricle and massive *bilateral telencephalic hemispheres*, each containing a lateral ventricle. (For development see p. 245.)

TERMINOLOGY

The development, structure and connections of the thalamus have been extensively and elegantly reviewed by Jones (1985), and the terminology relating specifically to the human thalamus brought into line with that relating to the subhuman primate thalamus on the basis of histochemical staining (Hirai & Jones 1989). His terminology will be largely followed in this description, and the reader is referred to his book for a more extensive bibliography than that provided here (Jones 1985).

The prosencephalon of the developing brain gives rise to the telencephalon anteriorly, and the diencephalon behind the origin of the cerebral vesicles. The lateral walls of the developing diencephalon exhibit four somewhat distinct regions of growth, which separably form the epithalamus most superiorly, the dorsal and ventral thalamus centrally and hypothalamus most inferiorly. These subdivisions in the adult have connectional and functional validity. The epithalamus in the mature brain comprises the anterior and posterior paraventricular nuclei, the medial and lateral habenular nuclei, the stria medullaris thalami and the pineal body. The developing dorsal thalamus undergoes a second phase of cellular proliferation during which it subdivides into pronuclear masses, which in turn develop into the major principal nuclei of the thalamus. The ventral thalamic rudiment gives rise in the adult to the reticular and ventral geniculate (pregeniculate) nuclei of the thalamus, the zona incerta and the cell bodies within the fields of Forel. The term subthalamus is sometimes used synonymously with ventral thalamus, and taken to include the subthalamic nucleus. However, this latter nucleus, despite its close anatomical relationship to the ventral thalamus, has a distinct developmental origin, and functionally is closely related to the basal nuclei and substantia nigra, with which it should be considered (p. 1186). The hypothalamic rudiment gives rise to most of the subdivisions of the adult hypothalamus. It should be noted, however, that the preoptic region develops from the telencephalon impar (p. 247), although it is usually considered, for functional reasons, as part of the hypothalamus.

DORSAL THALAMUS

The thalamus of each side (8.196–199), an obliquely lying ovoid

nuclear mass about 4 cm long, borders the third ventricle. The narrow *anterior pole* lies close to the midline, forming the posterior boundary of the interventricular foramen. Posteriorly, there is an expansion, directed dorsolaterally, which extends beyond the third ventricle to overhang the superior colliculus (8.200). This expanded *posterior pole* is the *pulvinar*. The brachium of the superior colliculus (superior quadrigeminal brachium) separates the pulvinar above from the medial geniculate body inferiorly. Lateral to this latter structure is a small oval elevation, the lateral geniculate body.

The *superior (dorsal) surface* (8.198), covered by a thin layer of white matter, the *stratum zonale*, extends laterally from the line of reflection of the ependyma (*taenia thalami*), forming the roof of the third ventricle. This curved surface is separated from the overlying body of the fornix by the choroid fissure with the tela choroidea within it; more laterally it forms part of the floor of the lateral ventricle. The lateral border of the superior surface is marked by the *stria terminalis* and overlying thalamostriate vein, separating the thalamus from the body of the caudate nucleus. Laterally, a slender white matter sheet, the *external medullary lamina*, separates the main

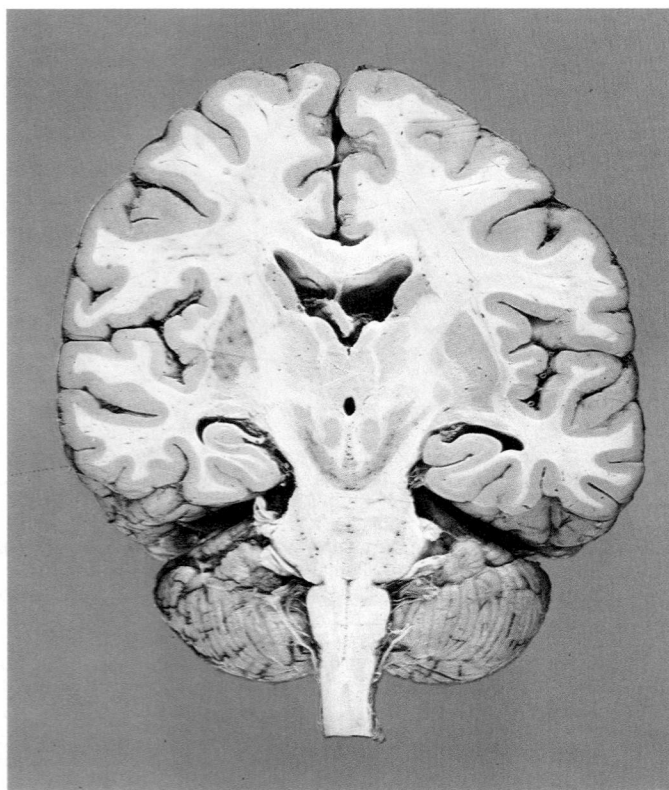

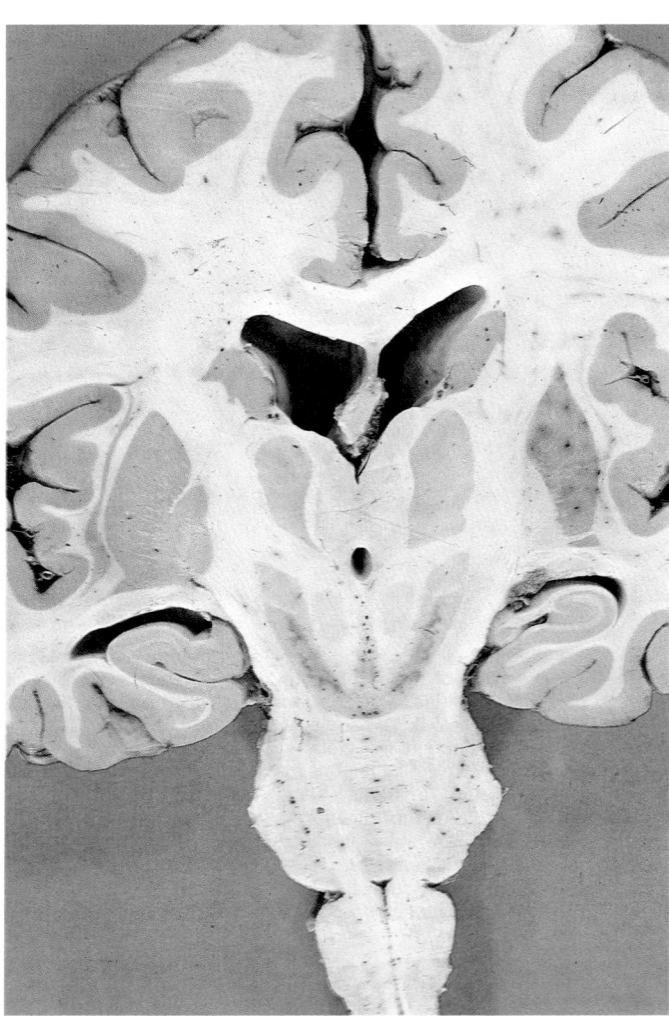

8.196 The dorsal half of a brain sectioned in an oblique coronal plane which passes through the cerebral hemispheres, diencephalon, midbrain, pons and medulla oblongata, to show the general disposition of main structures, some of which are labelled on 8.199. Note: (1) the complex folding of the cerebral cortical gyri and sulci of the frontoparietal, insular and temporal regions; (2) the sectioned surfaces of the corpus callosum, septum pellucidum, body of the fornix, the corona radiata, internal capsule, ventral pons and medulla oblongata; in the latter, part of the decussation of the corticospinal tracts is visible. Note also: (3) the body and inferior horn of the lateral ventricle; (4) the lentiform and caudate nuclei and the dorsal thalami which are fused across the midline. This illustration includes features referred to at many points in the text which are too numerous to include in a caption; these should be studied as appropriate. (Dissection by E L Rees, photography by Kevin Fitzpatrick, both of the Department of Anatomy, Guy's Hospital Medical School, London.)

8.197 The central area of the ventral part of the oblique coronal section of the brain shown in 8.196, photographed at higher magnification to show some structural features in greater detail; compare with 8.199 for appropriate labelling. Note in particular: (1) the anterior, medial and lateral parts of the dorsal thalamus, separated by the internal medullary laminae; (2) the relation of the caudate nucleus to the anterior and inferior horns of the lateral ventricle; (3) the lentiform nucleus, divided into an external putamen and an internal globus pallidus, the latter again divided into internal and external parts; (4) the internal capsule, external capsule, claustrum, extreme capsule and insular cortex; (5) the profiles of the sectioned subthalamic and red nuclei and substantia nigra; (6) the hippocampus projecting into the floor of the inferior horn of the lateral ventricle. Other structural features of this section are referred to at many points throughout the text. (Dissection by E L Rees, photography by Kevin Fitzpatrick, both of the Department of Anatomy, Guy's Hospital Medical School, London.)

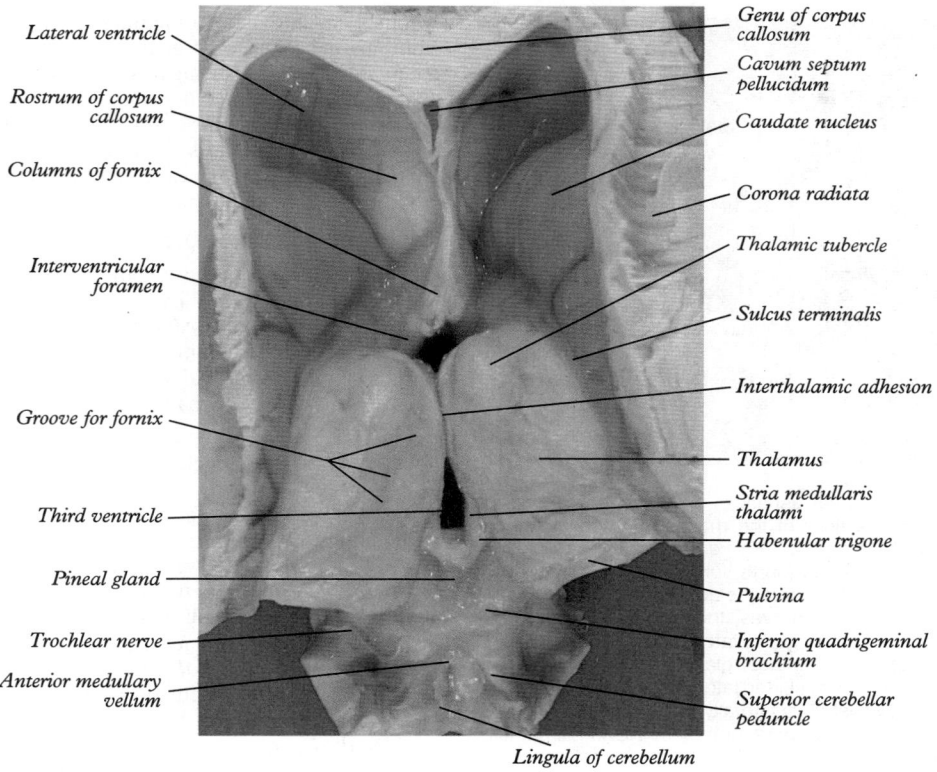

Lateral ventricle

Rostrum of corpus callosum

Columns of fornix

Interventricular foramen

Groove for fornix

Third ventricle

Pineal gland

Trochlear nerve

Anterior medullary vellum

Genu of corpus callosum

Cavum septum pellucidum

Caudate nucleus

Corona radiata

Thalamic tubercle

Sulcus terminalis

Interthalamic adhesion

Thalamus

Stria medullaris thalami

Habenular trigone

Pulvina

Inferior quadrigeminal brachium

Superior cerebellar peduncle

Lingula of cerebellum

8.198 Dorsal aspect of the caudate nuclei, thalami, pineal gland and tectum, revealed by removal of most of the corpus callosum, the body of the fornix and of the tela choroidea.

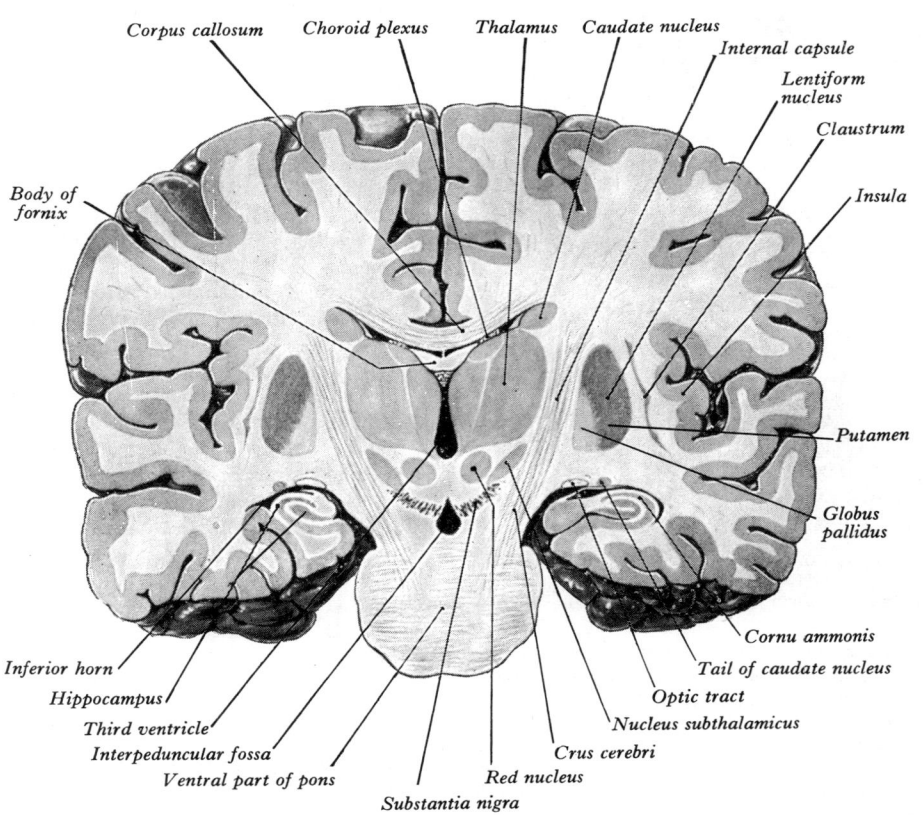

Corpus callosum   Choroid plexus   Thalamus   Caudate nucleus

Internal capsule

Lentiform nucleus

Claustrum

Insula

Body of fornix

Putamen

Globus pallidus

Cornu ammonis

Tail of caudate nucleus

Optic tract

Nucleus subthalamicus

Inferior horn

Hippocampus

Third ventricle

Interpeduncular fossa

Ventral part of pons

Substantia nigra

Red nucleus

Crus cerebri

8.199   Coronal section of the brain through the ventral part of the pons.

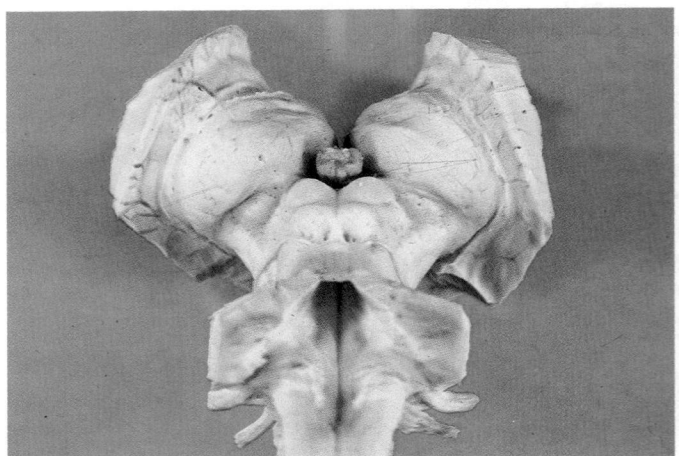

8.200 An oblique view of the dorsal aspect of the brain stem looking cranially. In the foreground is the floor of the rhomboid fossa, bounded laterally by the sectioned white matter of the cerebellum containing the dentate nuclei; the cranial recess of the fourth ventricle passes inferior to the superior medullary velum to continue into the aqueduct of the midbrain. More cranially, the emerging trochlear nerves, the colliculi, superior and inferior brachia, the medial and lateral geniculate bodies and the pineal gland may be identified. Lateral to the pineal gland on each side is the rounded pulvinar of the dorsal thalamus, skirted laterally by the curving body and tail of the caudate nucleus, whilst most laterally is the cut surface of the corona radiata. (Dissection by E L Rees, photography by Kevin Fitzpatrick, both of the Department of Anatomy, Guy's Hospital Medical School, London.)

body of the thalamus from the reticular nucleus. Lateral to this, the thick posterior limb of the internal capsule (**8.126, 201**) lies between the thalamus and the lentiform nucleus more laterally.

The *medial surface* (**8.202**A, B) is the superior (dorsal) region of the lateral wall of the third ventricle, usually connected to the opposite thalamus by a flat, grey *interthalamic adhesion* behind the interventricular foramen; its anteroposterior dimension is on average

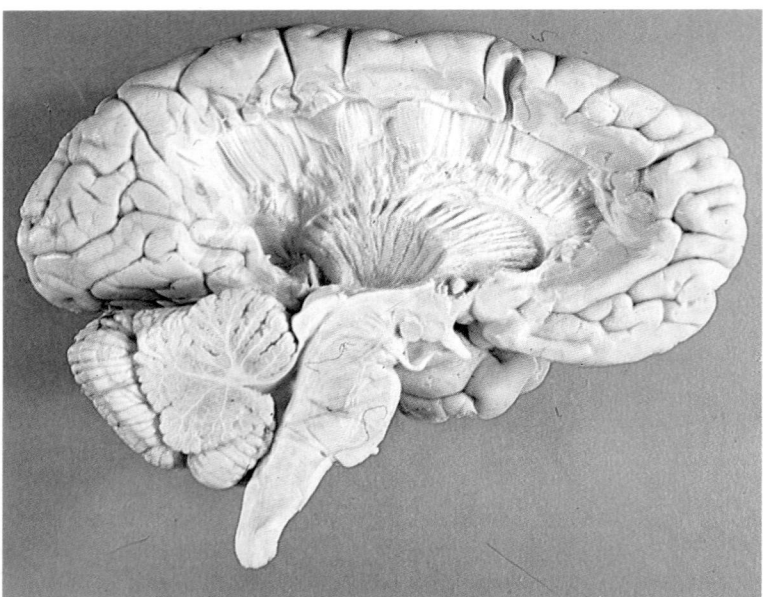

8.201 After median hemisection of the cerebrum, the left cerebral hemisphere has been dissected from its *medial* aspect to display the fibre bundles of the corona radiata and internal capsule. This entailed the removal of the cingulate gyrus and subjacent white matter, much of the paramedian corpus callosum and fornix, the dorsal thalamus and the head and body of the caudate nucleus. The oval depression previously occupied by the dorsal thalamus can clearly be seen within the curved depression left after removal of the caudate nucleus. (Dissection by Andrew Seal, photography by Kevin Fitzpatrick, both of the Department of Anatomy, Guy's Hospital Medical School, London.)

about 1 cm and it is sometimes multiple, occasionally absent and contains neurons, some of their axons crossing the midline, though many recurve back from this. The medial surface is limited below by an often indistinct *hypothalamic sulcus*, which curves from the upper end of the cerebral aqueduct to the interventricular foramen. Inferiorly, the thalamus is continuous with the rostral continuation of the midbrain tegmentum most posteriorly, the ventral thalamus and, more anteriorly, the superior part of the hypothalamus.

Major structure of the thalamus

The thalamus is composed, in the main, of grey matter, covered superiorly and laterally by thin sheets of white matter, the *stratum zonale* and *external medullary lamina* respectively. Internally, the substance of the thalamus is incompletely divided into its major subdivisions by a vertical Y-shaped sheet of white matter, the *internal medullary lamina*. The thalamus comprises the following main nuclear groups (**8.203**):

- *Anterior* (rostral) nuclei;
- *Medial* nuclei;
- *Lateral nuclei* in the dorsal half of the lateral nuclear mass extending posteriorly to include the pulvinar;
- *Ventral nuclei* in the ventral half of the lateral nuclear mass;
- *Medial geniculate body*, separated from the lateral nuclear mass by the superior quadrigeminal brachium and lateral and ventral to this, the *lateral geniculate body*. Together, the geniculate bodies comprise the *metathalamus*, but use of this historic anatomical term serves little useful purpose, and both the medial geniculate nuclear complex and the lateral geniculate nucleus are best considered as components of the thalamus proper;
- *Intralaminar nuclei*, nerve cell groups embedded within and surrounded by the internal medullary lamina;
- *Midline nuclei* which either abut the ependyma of the lateral walls of the third ventricle medially, or lie adjacent to (and to some extent within) the interthalamic adhesion;
- *Reticular nuclei*, separated from the main nuclear mass of the thalamus by the external medullary lamina which, together with the ventral geniculate (pregeniculate) nucleus and the zona incerta, form the ventral thalamus.

Thalamic nuclei and their connections

The dorsal thalamic nuclei both project to and receive fibres from the cerebral cortex (**8.204**). The whole cerebral cortex, not only neocortex but also the phylogenetically older paleocortex of the piriform lobe and archicortex of the hippocampal formation, are reciprocally connected with the dorsal thalamus (Jones 1985).

The projection to the thalamus from the cortex is precisely reciprocal; each cortical area projects in a topographically organized manner to all sites in the dorsal thalamus from which it receives an input. Corticothalamic fibres reciprocating 'specific' thalamocortical pathways (see below) arise from modified pyramidal cells of layer VI; those reciprocating 'non-specific' inputs arise from typical pyramidal cells of layer V, and may in part be axon collaterals of other cortico–subcortical pathways (Swadlow & Weyand 1981).

In addition to their cortical targets, the intralaminar nuclei (and possibly some others; Jones 1985) also send fibres to the striatum. In contrast, the components of the ventral thalamus do not project to, though they receive fibres from, the cerebral cortex.

It has for many years been customary to classify thalamic nuclei as specific or non-specific, and further to subdivide specific nuclei into relay nuclei and association nuclei. It is perhaps time for both of these rigid parcellations to be abandoned in favour of a description more securely based upon functional considerations. It is clear that there are different types of thalamic projection upon the cerebral cortex; (Macchi 1983; see also Jones 1985) has recognized four major patterns of thalamocortical projection: dense projections to single cortical areas from identified thalamic nuclei; projections from single thalamic nuclei which terminate densely in one cortical area and diffusely in another; nuclei which project diffusely to several cortical areas, but with a predominant projection to one or more targets; and, finally, nuclei which project diffusely over widespread regions of the cerebral cortex. It is clear that both specific, dense, focused projections as well as non-specific light, diffuse thalamocortical projections exist; indeed all cortical areas probably receive more than one such type of thalamic input. However, it is also apparent

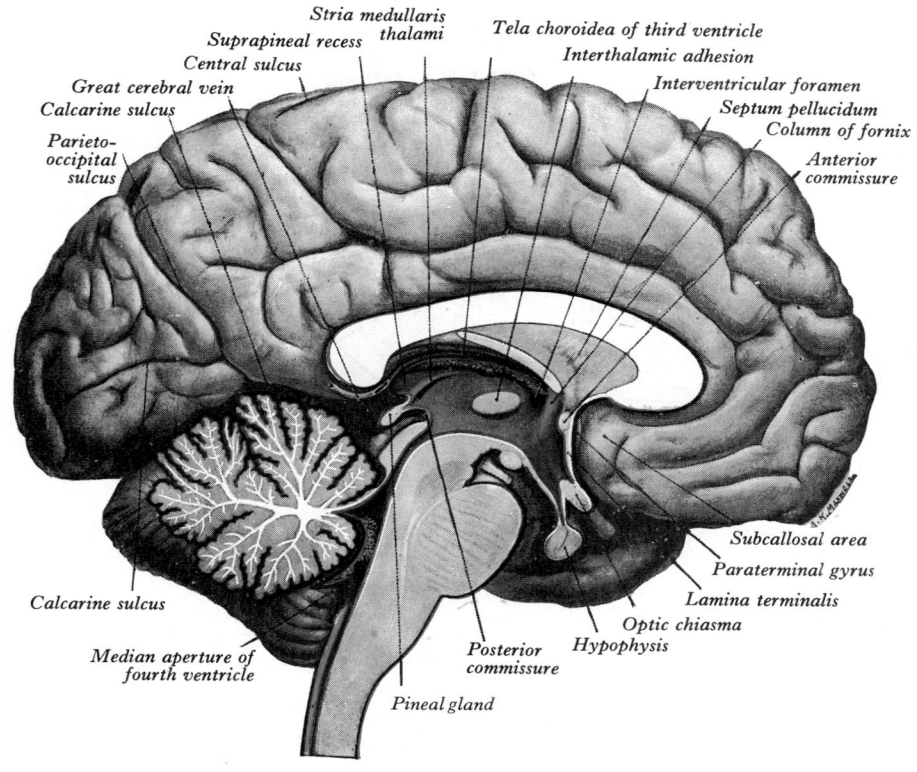

Stria medullaris
thalami
Suprapineal recess
Central sulcus
Great cerebral vein
Calcarine sulcus
Parieto-
occipital
sulcus

Tela choroidea of third ventricle
Interthalamic adhesion
Interventricular foramen
Septum pellucidum
Column of fornix
Anterior
commissure

Subcallosal area
Paraterminal gyrus
Lamina terminalis
Optic chiasma
Hypophysis

Calcarine sulcus

Median aperture of
fourth ventricle

Posterior
commissure

Pineal gland

A

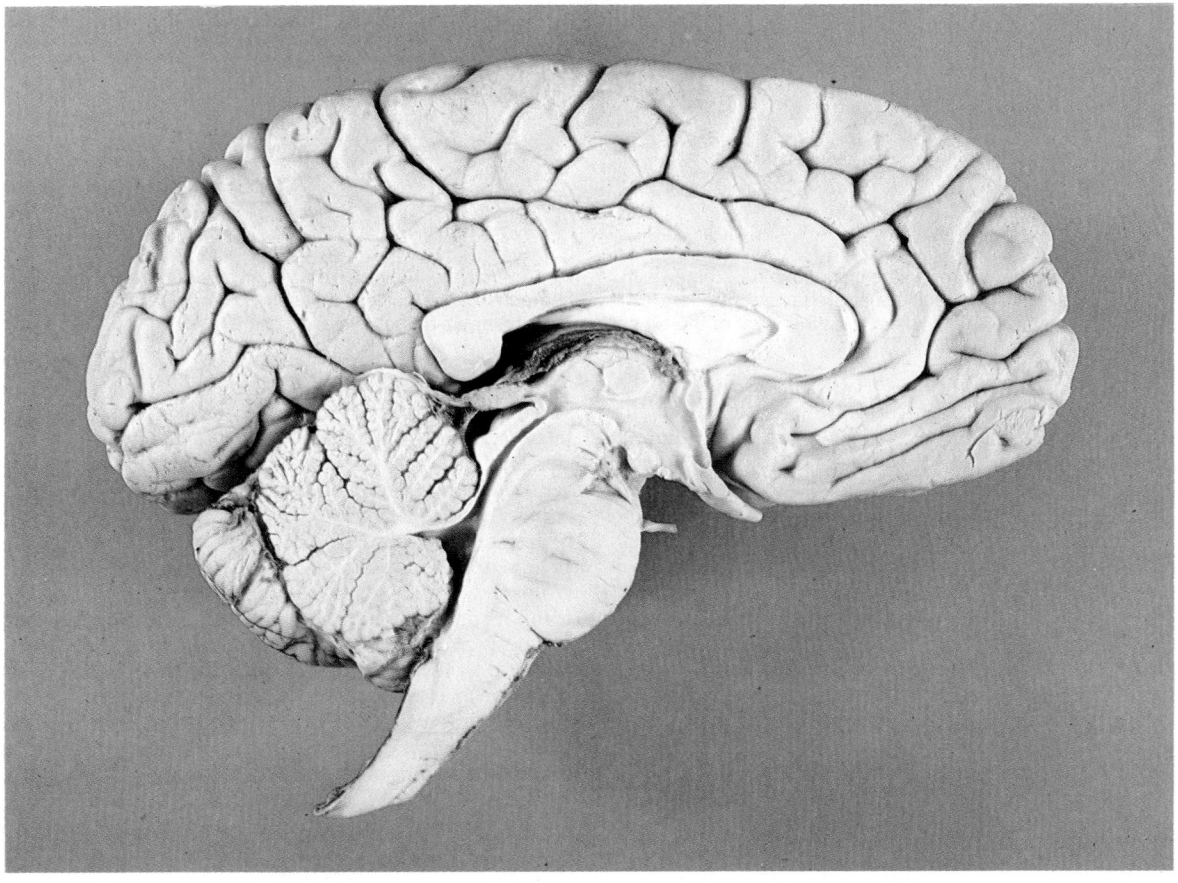

B

8.202A.   Median hemi-section of the brain to show the third and fourth ventricles. The pia mater is indicated in red, the ependyma in blue.
B. A sagittal hemi-section through the brain. For detailed labelling of the structures visible on this specimen compare with 8.202A. (Dissection by E L Rees, photography by Kevin Fitzpatrick, both of the Department of Anatomy, Guy's Hospital Medical School, London.)

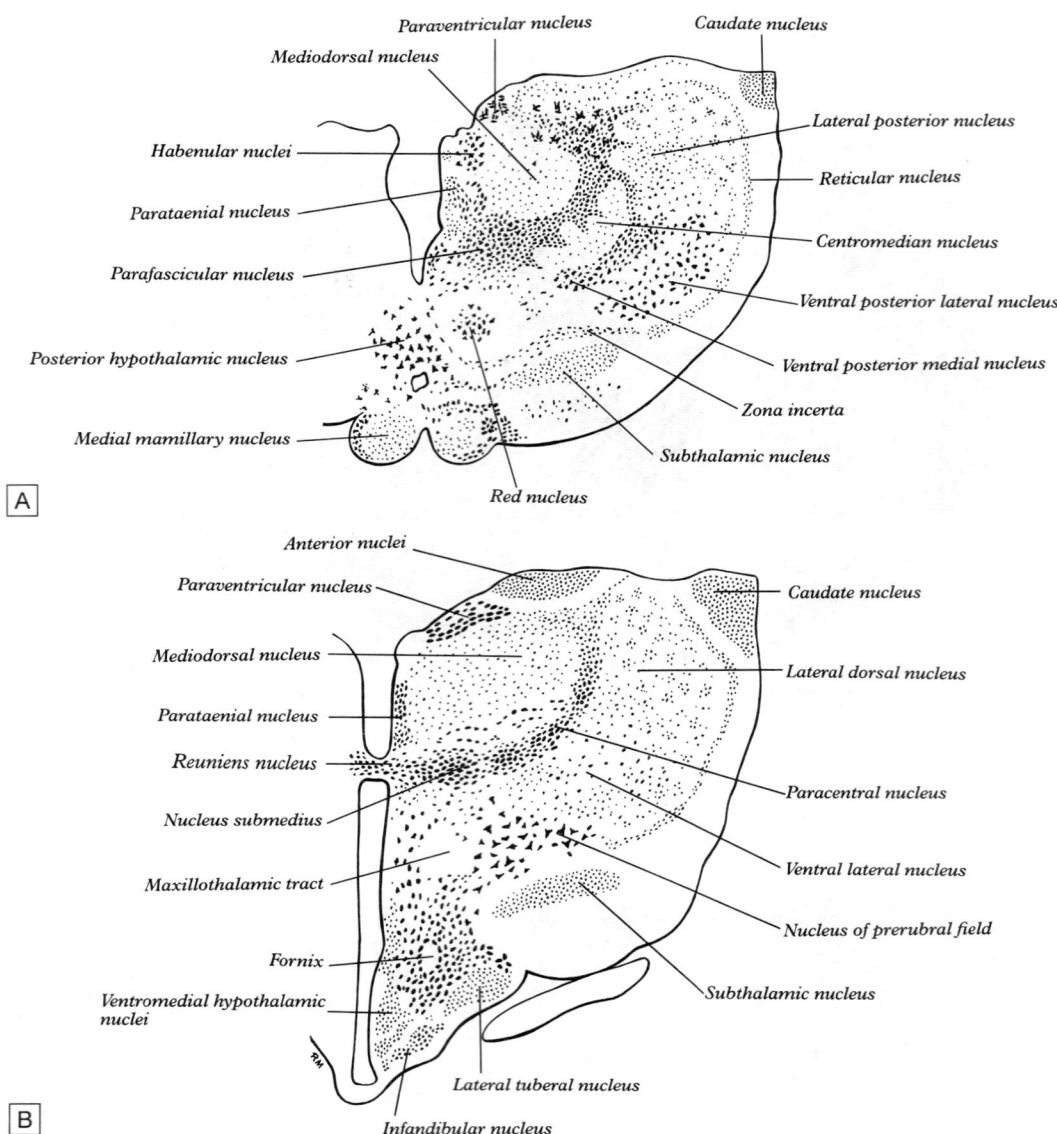

8.203 Drawings of coronal sections through the diencephalon, stained with the method of Nissl to show the main nuclear aggregations of nerve cell somata: A. at the level of the mamillary bodies; B. at the level of the tuber cinereum. Note the variations in cell size, shape and packing density, which characterize the nuclear masses of the dorsal thalamus, subthalamus and hypothalamus at these levels.

that the diffuse, non-specific projections do not arise from a single, readily definable group of thalamic nuclei, and that many nuclei previously classified as 'specific' may also send 'non-specific' projections to widespread cortical areas (see below). Any such classification is, therefore, best reserved for the description of thalamocortical terminations, rather than of their nuclei of origin (Macchi 1983; Jones 1985; Bentivoglio et al 1991). Similarly, the historic subdivision of the principal thalamic nuclei into relay and association groups is no longer useful. This classification rested upon the assumption that relay nuclei received a major subcortical pathway, whereas association nuclei received their principal non-cortical input from other thalamic nuclei. There is little evidence on the one hand for significant intrathalamic connectivity between different nuclei, and on the other increasingly significant non-cortical afferent pathways to so-called association nuclei are being identified (Jones 1985).

Synaptic organization of thalamic nuclei

All thalamic nuclei exhibit aggregations of synapses usually encapsulated and separated from the surrounding less organized neuropil by extensive astrocytic processes. These *synaptic glomeruli* are most prominent in subprimate species but are recognizable in primates. Jones (1985) has recently described a fundamental pattern of organization which will be followed here. Central to the glomerulus

structure is a primary dendrite (or dendritic spine) of a thalamic relay cell, surrounded by a cluster of two types of presynaptic element. The first of these, usually the least numerous, is a conventional axon terminal derived from the principal subcortical afferent system to the nucleus. These large terminals are usually packed with spherical vesicles and have dense cytoplasm. They make multiple asymmetric synapses with both the dendritic element of the glomerulus and with the second type of presynaptic profile. This second component comprises the dendrites of thalamic interneurons which are both presynaptic to the dendrites of the relay cells and postsynaptic to the incoming afferent terminals. They contain flattened, pleiomorphic vesicles, free ribosomes, rough endoplasmic reticulum and microtubules. They make symmetric synapses with the dendrites of the thalamic relay cells and sometimes with each other and are probably γ-aminobutyric acid (GABA)-ergic (O'Hara et al 1989). Frequently, a further type of synaptic profile is seen at the periphery of the glomerulus. These are axon terminals containing flattened vesicles, thought to arise from thalamic interneurons, and making symmetric synapses with one or more presynaptic dendritic elements in the glomerulus. In addition to the conventional synaptic contacts seen, numerous specialized, non-synaptic contacts occur between the various neuritic elements within the glomerulus.

Corticothalamic axons form round-vesicle containing terminals which make asymmetric synapses on the dendrites of both relay cells

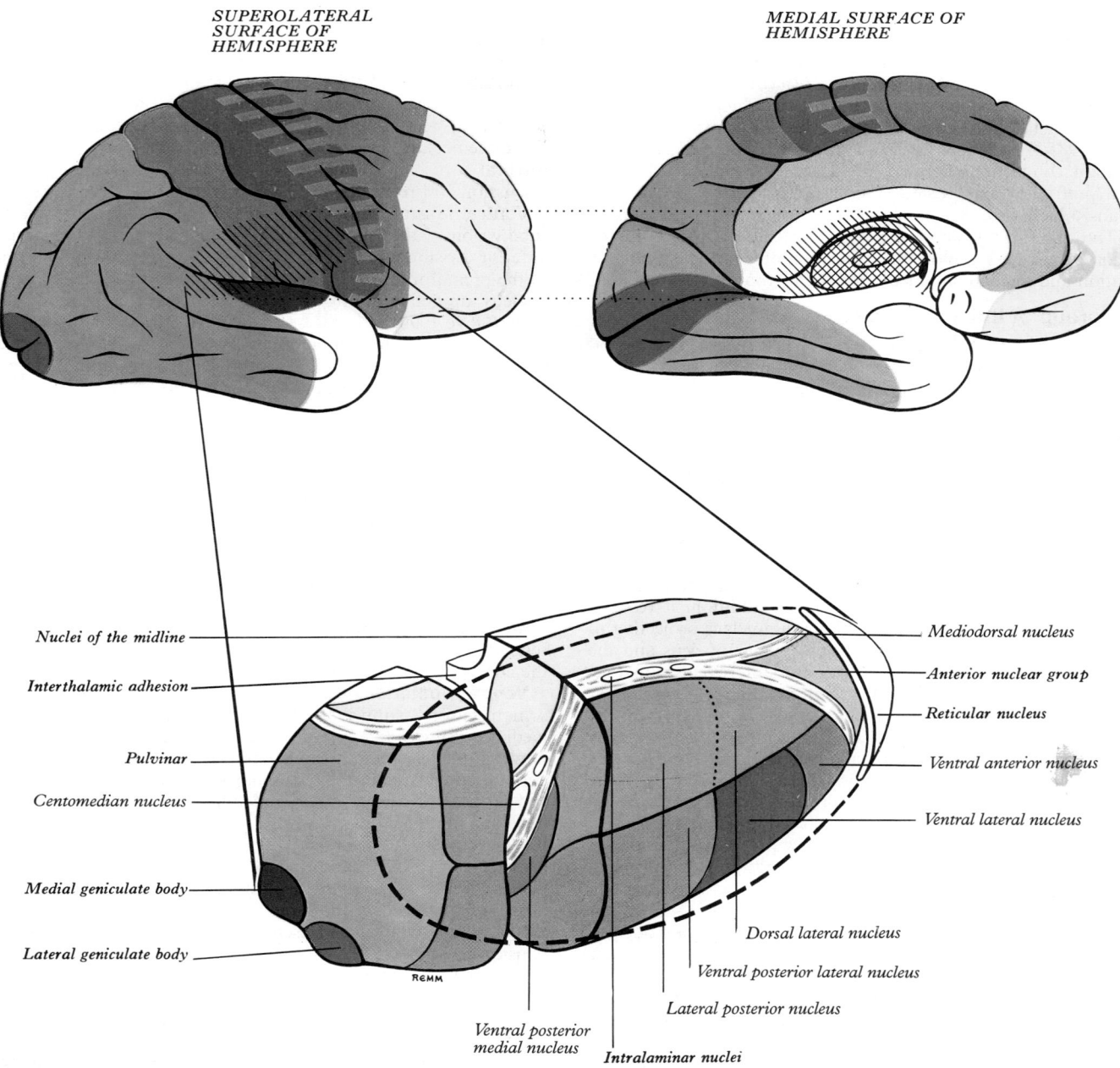

SUPEROLATERAL
SURFACE OF
HEMISPHERE

MEDIAL SURFACE OF
HEMISPHERE

Nuclei of the midline

Interthalamic adhesion

Pulvinar

Centomedian nucleus

Medial geniculate body

Lateral geniculate body

REMM

Mediodorsal nucleus

Anterior nuclear group

Reticular nucleus

Ventral anterior nucleus

Ventral lateral nucleus

Dorsal lateral nucleus

Ventral posterior lateral nucleus

Lateral posterior nucleus

Ventral posterior
medial nucleus

Intralaminar nuclei

8.204 The main nuclear masses of the dorsal thalamus (below) have been labelled and colour coded and the same colours have been used to indicate the areas of cerebral neocortex interconnected with these nuclei. The lack of colour in the centromedian, intralaminar and reticular nuclei and in restricted areas of the frontal and temporal lobes are *not* related to the colour code. The boundaries of the coloured cortical zones may well need revision in the future as experimental and pathological data accumulate.

and thalamic interneurons within the neuropil outside the glomerular structure. Similarly, the axons within the dorsal thalamic nuclei arising from the reticular nucleus are probably also confined to the extra-glomerular neuropil, where they form flattened vesicle containing terminals making symmetric GABA-ergic synapses with the dendrites of thalamic neurons (O'Hara et al 1989).

Anterior group of thalamic nuclei

The anterior group of nuclei are enclosed between the arms of the Y-shaped internal medullary lamina as it divides anteriorly and underlie the anterior thalamic tubicle (**8**.198). Three subdivisions are recognized in the human thalamus (Hirai & Jones 1989). The largest is the anteroventral nucleus; also prominent is the anteromedial nucleus. These two nuclei are sometimes grouped together as the principal anterior nucleus (Armstrong 1990). The anterodorsal nucleus is small, but is also clearly seen as a crescentic cluster of cells immediately deep to the ependyma of the third ventricle (Hirai & Jones 1989). The laterodorsal nucleus is also considered by some to be functionally a part of the anterior nuclear group (Jones 1985;

Hirai & Jones 1989). However, the laterodorsal nucleus will not be included with the anterior nuclei in this account, but will be described later, with the lateral group of nuclei (p. 1087).

Connections of the anterior nuclei. The anterior nuclei are the principal recipients of the mamillothalamic tract (Jones 1985). The mamillary nuclei receive fibres from the hippocampal formation via the fornix. The medial mamillary nucleus projects to anteroventral and anteromedial nuclei on the same side, and the lateral mamillary nucleus projects to anterodorsal nuclei bilaterally. Fornical fibres which bypass the mamillary nuclei to terminate directly in the thalamus, are essentially corticothalamic in nature. In addition, the component nuclei of the anterior group are prominently stained using acetylcholinesterase histochemistry (Hirai & Jones 1989). They do not appear to contain cholinergic cell somata, but receive a prominent cholinergic input from the basal forebrain (Parent et al 1988) and the brainstem (Woolf et al 1990). The anteromedial and anteroventral nuclei may also receive a few fibres from the ventral pallidum (Alheid et al 1990).

The cortical targets of efferent fibres from the anterior nuclei lie

1085

largely on the medial surface of the hemisphere, and include the anterior limbic area, in front of and inferior to the corpus callosum, the cingulate gyrus, and the parahippocampal gyrus, including medial entorhinal cortex and the pre- and para-subiculum (Thompson & Robertson 1987; Yanagihara et al 1987; Schmahmann & Pandya 1990; Armstrong 1990). These thalamocortical pathways are reciprocal (Jones 1985; Yeterian & Pandya 1988). In addition, there appear to be minor connections between the anterior nuclei and the dorsolateral prefrontal and posterior areas of neocortex (Selemon & Goldman-Rakic 1988; Schmahmann & Pandya 1990; Armstrong 1990). The anterior thalamic nuclei appear to be involved in the regulation of alertness, and in the acquisition of information, that is in attention and in encoding memories (Armstrong 1990).

Medial group of thalamic nuclei

The single component of this thalamic region is the large mediodorsal nucleus. Jones (1985) has considered the midline nuclei as part of this group but these will be considered separately in this account. The mediodorsal nucleus is particularly large in man; laterally it is limited by the internal medullary lamina and component nuclei of the intralaminar group (p. 1087). Medially, it abuts the midline parataenial and reuniens (medioventral) nuclei. It is divisible into small anteromedial magnocellular and large posterolateral parvocellular portions.

Connections of the anteromedial magnocellular mediodorsal nucleus. The magnocellular division receives an olfactory input from the piriform and adjacent cortex (Price 1990) and responds to olfactory stimuli (Jones 1985; Price 1990). In addition, it receives fibres from the amygdala, with the mediobasal nucleus projecting to the dorsal part of the anteromedial magnocellular nucleus and the lateral nuclei passing to the more central and anteroventral regions (Armstrong 1990; de Olmos 1990). Furthermore, there is a prominent projection to the anteromedial magnocellular nucleus from the ventral pallidum (Alheid et al 1990). The anteromedial magnocellular nucleus projects to the anterior and medial prefrontal cortex (Giguere & Goldman-Rakic 1988; Ray & Price 1993), notably to the lateral posterior and central posterior olfactory areas on the orbital surface of the frontal lobe (Jones 1985). In addition, fibres pass to the ventromedial cingulate cortex; only a few project to the inferior parietal cortex, the superior temporal sulcus and the anterior insula (Giguere & Goldman-Rakic 1988). These cortical connections are reciprocal.

Connections of the posterolateral parvocellular mediodorsal nucleus. The non-cortical afferents to the posterolateral parvocellular nucleus are not clear. However, there is little evidence of the intrathalamic connections once postulated (Jones 1985; Armstrong 1990). This nucleus does appear to receive fibres from the internal segment of the globus pallidus (Alheid et al 1990) and connects reciprocally with the dorsolateral and dorsomedial prefrontal cortex, the anterior cingulate gyrus and the supplementary motor area (Giguere & Goldman-Rakic 1988; Wiesendanger & Wiesendanger 1985). In addition, fibres pass to the posterior parietal cortex (Schmahmann & Pandya 1990).

The mediodorsal nucleus appears to be involved in a wide variety of higher functions. Damage may lead to a decrease in anxiety, tension, aggression or obsessive thinking. There may also be transient amnesia, particularly with confusion developing over the passage of time (Armstrong 1990). It is, perhaps, not surprising that much of the neuropsychology of medial nuclei damage reflects defects in functions similar to those performed by the prefrontal cortex, with which it is so closely linked, with ablation of the medial nuclei paralleling, in part, the results of prefrontal lobotomy.

Ventral nuclear group

The ventral group of thalamic nuclei is functionally and anatomically heterogeneous comprising three major subdivisions: the ventral anterior nucleus, the ventral lateral nuclear complex and the ventral posterior complex. These are best considered separately.

Ventral anterior nucleus. This is a region of large cells at the anterior pole of the ventral group, limited anteriorly by the reticular nucleus, posteriorly by the ventral lateral nucleus and lying between the external and internal medullary laminae, respectively lateral and medial. The connections of this nucleus remain largely unknown, although afferents from the deep cerebellar nuclei and the internal

segment of the globus pallidus have at various times been suggested. The destination of its efferent fibres is also uncertain; it may be related to the striatum and to the anterior parietal cortex (Jones 1985; Ohye 1990). As with the connections, the functions are also unclear. However, it may play a central role in the transmission of the cortical 'recruiting response' whereby long-lasting, high voltage, repetitive negative electrical waves can be initiated over much of the cerebral cortex by stimulation of the thalamus (see Jones 1985 for discussion and references).

Ventral lateral nuclear complex. This comprises three major subdivisions with distinctly different connections and functions. The anterior division receives fibres from the globus pallidus and projects to the premotor and supplementary motor cortices. Cells within this nucleus are active during voluntary movement of the contralateral body (Ohye 1990).

The posterior division receives fibres from the deep cerebellar nuclei in a precisely ordered topographic way. Additional projections come from the spinothalamic tract and the vestibular nuclei. The primary motor cortex (Brodmann's area 4) projects to and receives from the nucleus wherein responses can be recorded during both passive and active movement of the contralateral body. The topography of its connections, and recordings made within the nucleus, suggest that the posterior ventral lateral nucleus contains a body representation comparable to that in the ventral posterior nucleus (see below). Stereotaxic surgery of the posterior ventral lateral nucleus is sometimes used in the treatment of Parkinson's disease, particularly for the relief of tremor.

The medial division of this complex is analogous to the ventral medial nucleus of lower animals, and receives fibres from the pars reticulata of the substantia nigra. It projects somewhat diffusely to the cortex particularly of the dorso-lateral and medial frontal lobe.

Ventral posterior nucleus. The principal relay nucleus for the somatosensory pathway is the lateral division, which receives the medial lemniscal and spinothalamic pathways and the medial part, in which the trigeminothalamic pathway terminates. Most anteriorly and ventromedially taste fibres synapse, and this region of the medial ventral posterior nucleus has sometimes been designated a separate nucleus, the mediobasal ventral posterior nucleus (Jones 1985; Norgren 1990). A further subdivision, the ventral posterior inferior nucleus along the ventral surface of ventral posterior nucleus, receives connections from the vestibular nuclei, as well as lemniscal fibres. It has been suggested in the monkey that this latter nucleus contains an additional complete representation of the body including the face (Cusick & Gould 1990).

The nucleus contains a well-ordered topographic representation of the body, with sacral segments most laterally and cervical segments most medially, abutting the face area of representation (trigeminal territory) in the medial ventral posterior nucleus. At a more detailed level, single body regions are represented as curved lamellae of neurons, parallel to the lateral border of the ventral posterior nucleus, such that there is a continuous overlapping progression from dorsolateral to ventromedial of adjacent receptive fields. Considerably less change in location of receptive field on the body is seen when passing anteroposteriorly through the nucleus. Whilst not precisely dermatomal in nature, these curvilinear lamellae of cells probably derive from afferents related to a few adjacent spinal segments. Because of the differences in peripheral innervation density of different body regions, there is therefore considerable distortion of the body map within the nucleus, with many more neurons responding to stimulation of the hand, for example, than of the trunk. Within a single lamella, neurons in the anterodorsal part of the nucleus respond to deep stimuli, including movement of joints, tendon stretch, and manipulation of muscles. Most ventrally, probably including cells in the ventral posterior inferior nucleus, neurons once again respond to deep stimuli, particularly tapping. Between these two, cells within a single lamella respond only to cutaneous stimuli. This organization has been confirmed by recordings made in the human ventral posterior nucleus (Lenz et al 1988). Single lemniscal axons have an extended anteroposterior terminal zone within the nucleus. Rods of cells running the length of the anteroposteriorly dorsoventrally oriented lamellae respond with closely similar receptive field properties and locations, derived from a small bundle of lemniscal afferents. It appears, therefore, that each lamella contains the complete representation of a single body part, for example a finger; lamellae are further comprised of multiple narrow rods of neurons, oriented anteroposteriorly, each of which receives input from the same small part of that body region represented within the lamella, and from the same type of receptors. These thalamic 'rods' form the basis for both the place and modality specific input to columns of cells in the somatic sensory cortex (see below). Spinothalamic tract afferents to the lateral ventral posterior nucleus terminate throughout the nucleus. The neurons from which these axons originate appear to be mainly of the 'wide dynamic range' class with responses to both low threshold mechanoreceptors and high threshold nociceptors. A smaller proportion are solely high threshold nociceptors. Some neurons respond to temperature changes. In the human, around 5–6% of neurons respond to noxious heat stimuli in regions where microstimulation elicits painful sensations (Lenz et al 1993).

The ventroposterior nucleus projects to the primary somatic sensory cortex (SI) of the postcentral gyrus and to the second somatic sensory area (SII) in the parietal operculum. Within the primary sensory cortex, the central cutaneous core of the ventral posterior nucleus projects solely to area 3b; dorsal and ventral to this, a narrow band of cells projects to both 3b and area 1. The deep stimulus receptive cells most dorsally and ventrally project to areas 3a and 2. The whole nucleus projects additionally to the second somatic sensory area.

Medial geniculate complex

The medial geniculate body (Jones 1985; Webster & Garey 1990) is a rounded elevation posteriorly on the ventrolateral surface of the thalamus, separated from the pulvinar by the superior quadrigeminal brachium. It receives the inferior quadrigeminal brachium. Histologically, three major nuclei are recognizable within it: the medial, ventral and dorsal nuclei. The inferior brachium separates the medial (magnocellular) nucleus, comprising sparse, deeply staining neurons, from the lateral nucleus, which is made up of medium sized, densely packed and darkly staining cells. The dorsal nucleus overlies the ventral nucleus and expands posteriorly; hence it is sometimes known as the posterior nucleus of the medial geniculate. It contains small to medium sized, pale staining cells, less densely packed than those of the lateral nucleus. The ventral nucleus receives fibres from the central nucleus of the ipsilateral inferior colliculus via the inferior quadrigeminal brachium, with an additional contribution from the contralateral inferior colliculus. The nucleus contains a complete tonotopic representation with low-pitched sounds represented laterally and progressively higher pitched sounds encountered as the nucleus is traversed from lateral to medial. The dorsal nucleus receives afferents from the pericentral nucleus of the inferior colliculus and from other brainstem nuclei of the auditory pathway. A tonotopic representation has not been described in this subdivision and cells within the dorsal nucleus respond to a broad range of frequencies. The magnocellular medial nucleus receives fibres from the inferior colliculus and from the deep layers of the superior colliculus. Neurons within the magnocellular subdivision may respond to modalities other than sound. Many cells, however, respond to auditory stimuli, usually to a wider range of frequencies than neurons in the ventral nucleus. Many units show evidence of binaural interaction with the leading effect arising from stimuli in the contralateral cochlea. The ventral nucleus projects primarily and perhaps solely to the primary auditory cortex. The dorsal nucleus projects to auditory areas surrounding the primary auditory cortex. The magnocellular division projects diffusely to auditory areas of cortex and to adjacent insular and opercular fields.

Lateral geniculate nucleus and the visual pathway

The optic nerves pass posteromedially into the cranial cavity to meet in the midline, forming the *optic chiasma*. This flat mass of decussating fibres lies at the junction of the anterior wall and floor of the third ventricle. Behind, the optic tracts pass posterolaterally from the chiasma. The lamina terminalis, continuous with its upper surface, is crossed, dorsal to the chiasma, by the anterior communicating artery. Ventral, is the diaphragma sella, a little behind the optic groove of the sphenoid bone in about one subject in ten; the chiasma is either in the groove or altogether posterior, always near the hypophysis. Posterior to the chiasma are the tuber cinereum and infundibulum, with the third ventricle dorsal to them. Lateral is the end of the

internal carotid artery and anterior perforated substance. The optic recess of the third ventricle passes over its superior surface to reach the lamina terminalis.

Optic nerve fibres arising from the nasal half of each retina, including half the macula, cross in the chiasma to enter the contralateral optic tract. Fibres from the temporal retinae continue into the ipsilateral optic tract. Decussating fibres loop a little backwards into their ipsilateral optic tract before crossing and then pass forwards into the contralateral optic nerve after crossing. Macular fibres, and those from an adjacent central area, form a flat band occupying almost two-thirds of the central chiasma, dorsal to all peripheral decussating fibres, ventral to which are fibres from the extramacular parts of both nasal half retinae; most ventral are the nasal fibres concerned with monocular fringes of the binocular field.

The optic chiasma is supplied with blood from a pial plexus receiving branches from the superior hypophyseal, internal carotid, posterior communicating, anterior cerebral and anterior communicating arteries; its veins drain into the basal and anterior cerebral venous system.

The *optic tracts* continue dorsolaterally from the chiasma, each passing between the anterior perforated substance and tuber cinereum as the ventrolateral boundary of the interpenduncular fossa. Each flattens and curves round its cerebral peduncle, to which it adheres, hidden from view on the ventral cerebral surface by both the uncus and the parahippocampal gyrus.

Optic tract fibres terminate in the lateral geniculate nucleus of the thalamus, the superior colliculus, pretectal area and nuclei of the accessory optic tract in the midbrain, and in the suprachiasmatic nucleus of the hypothalamus. A direct retinal input to the inferior pulvinar has also been reported (p. 1087).

A relay of fibres from neurons in the lateral geniculate nucleus traverses the posterior limb of the internal capsule, emerging as a broad *optic radiation* of axons of secondary visual neurons, curving dorsomedially to the occipital cortex. They are separated from the posterior cornu of the lateral ventricle only by the tapetum of the corpus callosum.

Some fibres in the optic radiation, from neurons in the occipital cortex, descend to the superior colliculus, which therefore receives *cortical* and *retinal paths*. From this a relay travels by tectobulbar tracts to motor nuclei of the third, fourth, sixth and eleventh cranial nerves and the spinal anterior grey column. Details of the organization of the visual pathway are shown in **8.205** and further references to the lateral geniculate nucleus and visual pathway are Jones (1985) and Garey (1990).

Lateral geniculate body

The lateral geniculate body is visible as a small ovoid ventral projection from the posterior thalamus (**8.206**), separated from the lateral aspect of the crus cerebri by the fibres of the optic tract passing to the midbrain. The *superior quadrigeminal brachium* enters the posteromedial part of the lateral geniculate body dorsally, lying between the medial geniculate body and the pulvinar.

The lateral geniculate body comprises the dorsal lateral geniculate nucleus. There is no ventral lateral geniculate nucleus in man; its equivalent, the pregeniculate nucleus, is part of the ventral thalamus and will be considered later. The lateral geniculate nucleus is an inverted U-shaped nucleus, somewhat flattened in man, and is characteristically laminated. In Old World monkeys, six layers are recognized in coronal sections, though the arrangement is somewhat more complex in man where seven or even eight laminae may be seen (Garey 1990). The laminae are numbered 1 to 6 from the innermost ventral to the outermost dorsal. This appearance is shown in **8.**207, 208. Laminae 1 and 2 comprise larger cells, the magnocellular layers, whereas 4 to 6 have smaller neurons, the parvocellular laminae. The apparent gaps between laminae are not free of neuronal processes, and are called the *interlaminar zones*. Most ventrally an additional *superficial* or *S lamina* can be recognized.

The lateral geniculate nucleus receives a major afferent input from the retina. The contralateral nasal retina projects to laminae 1, 4 and 6, whereas the ipsilateral temporal retina projects to laminae 2, 3 and 5. The parvocellular laminae receive predominantly axons of X-type retinal ganglion cells, that is more slowly conducting cells with sustained responses to visual stimuli. The faster conducting, rapidly adapting Y-type retinal ganglion cells project mainly to the

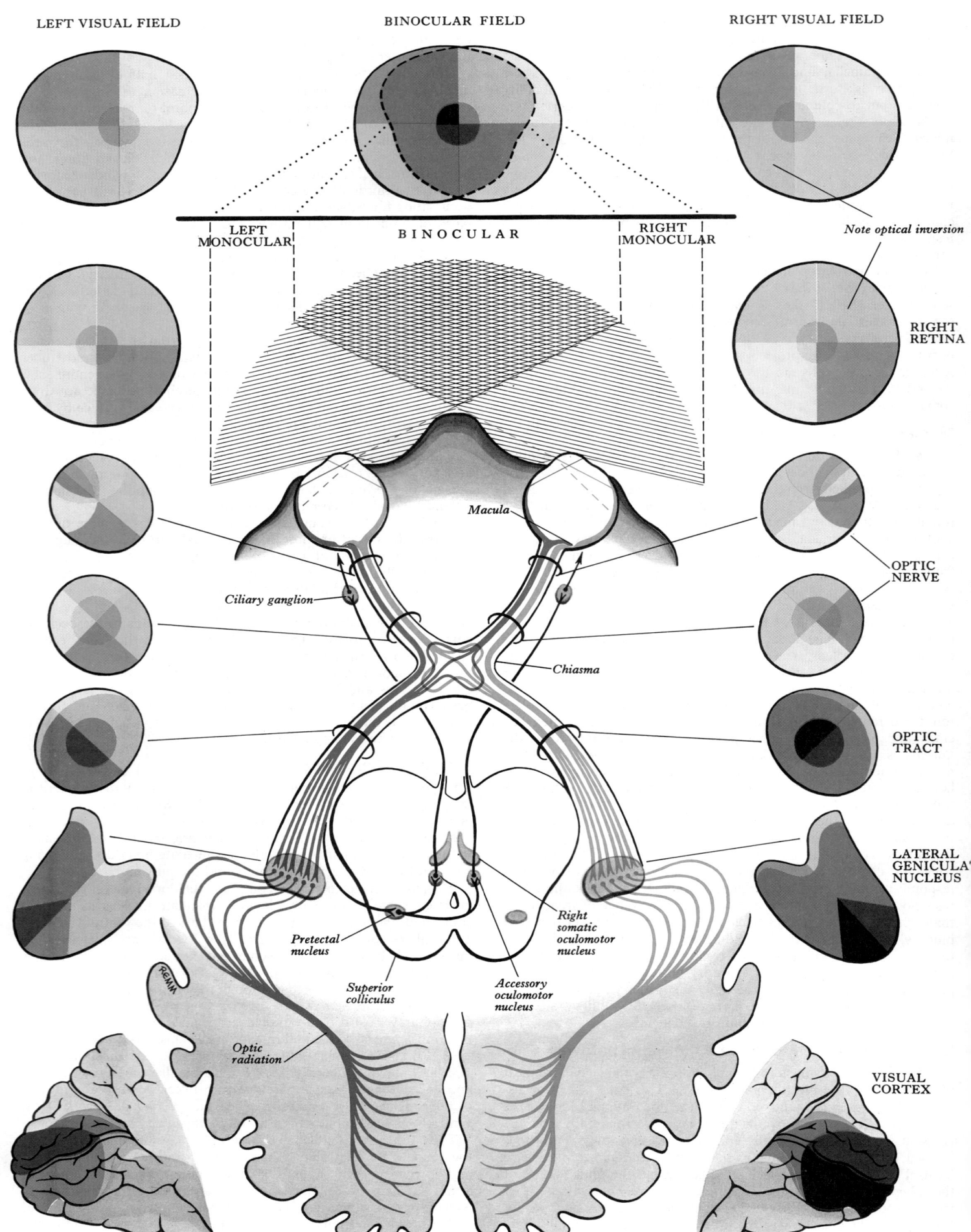

LEFT VISUAL FIELD

BINOCULAR FIELD

RIGHT VISUAL FIELD

LEFT
MONOCULAR

BINOCULAR

RIGHT
MONOCULAR

Note optical inversion

RIGHT
RETINA

Macula

Ciliary ganglion

OPTIC
NERVE

Chiasma

OPTIC
TRACT

LATERAL
GENICULATE
NUCLEUS

*Right
somatic
oculomotor
nucleus*

*Pretectal
nucleus*

*Superior
colliculus*

*Accessory
oculomotor
nucleus*

*Optic
radiation*

VISUAL
CORTEX

magnocellular laminae 1 and 2, with axon branches passing also to the superior colliculus. A third type of retinal ganglion cell, the W cells, which show large receptive fields and slow responses, project to both the superior colliculus and the lateral geniculate nucleus, where they terminate particularly in the interlaminar zones and in the S lamina.

The lateral geniculate nucleus is organized in a visuotopic manner, that is, it contains a map of the contralateral visual field. The vertical meridian lies posteriorly, the peripheral anteriorly with the upper field laterally, and the lower field medially (see 8.206). Similarly, precise point-to-point representation is also found in the projection of the lateral geniculate nucleus to the visual cortex, with radially arranged inverted pyramids of neurons in all laminae, responding to a single small area of the contralateral visual field, projecting to a circumscribed area of cortex. The termination of geniculocortical axons in the visual cortex will be considered in detail later.

Aside from retinal afferents, the lateral geniculate nucleus receives a major corticothalamic projection, the axons of which ramify densely in the interlaminar zones. The major part of this projection arises from the primary visual cortex, Brodmann's area 17, but smaller projections from extrastriate visual areas pass to the magnocellular and S laminae (Jones 1985). Other afferents include fibres from the superficial layer of the superior colliculus, which terminate in the interlaminar zone between laminae 1 and 2, and 2 and 3, and around lamina S, noradrenergic fibres from the locus (coeruleus,

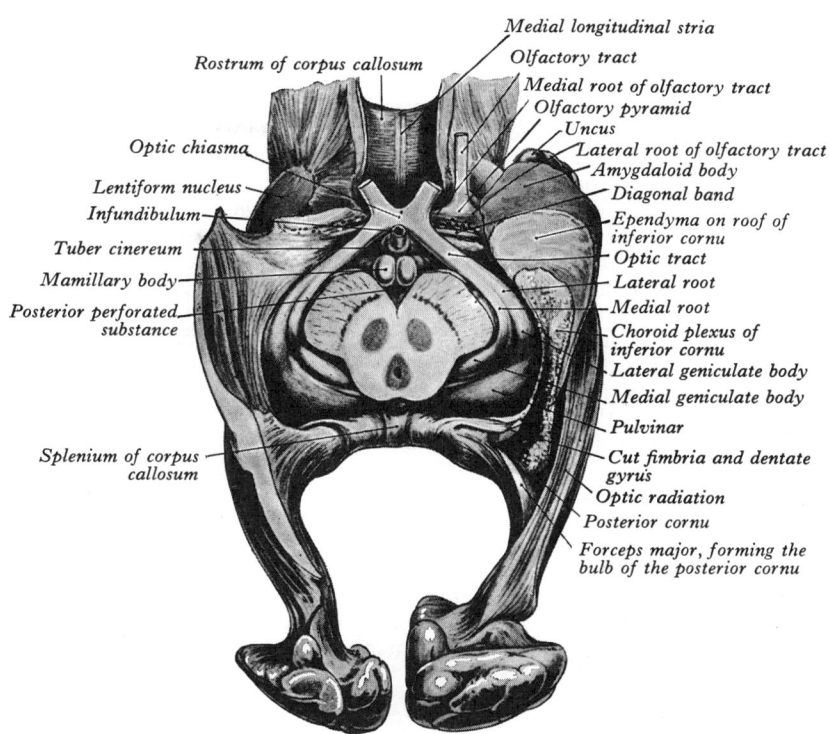

8.205 A diagram (left) of the visual pathway to show the spatial arrangement of nerve cells and their fibres in relation to the quadrants of the retinae and visual fields. The proportions at various levels are not exactly to scale and in particular the macula is exaggerated in size in the visual fields and retinae. In each quadrant of the visual field, and the parts of the visual pathway subserving it, two shades of the respective colour are used, the paler for the peripheral fields and a darker shade for the macular part of the quadrant. From the optic tract onwards these two shades are both made more saturated to denote intermixture of neurons from both retinae, the palest shade being reserved for parts of the visual pathway concerned with uniocular vision. The path of the light reflex has also been indicated.

8.206 A ventral dissection of the brain showing the metathalamus and the optic tracts. On the right side of the figure the inferior horn of the ventricle is exposed. The floor has been removed but the choroid plexus is in situ and obscures most of the roof.

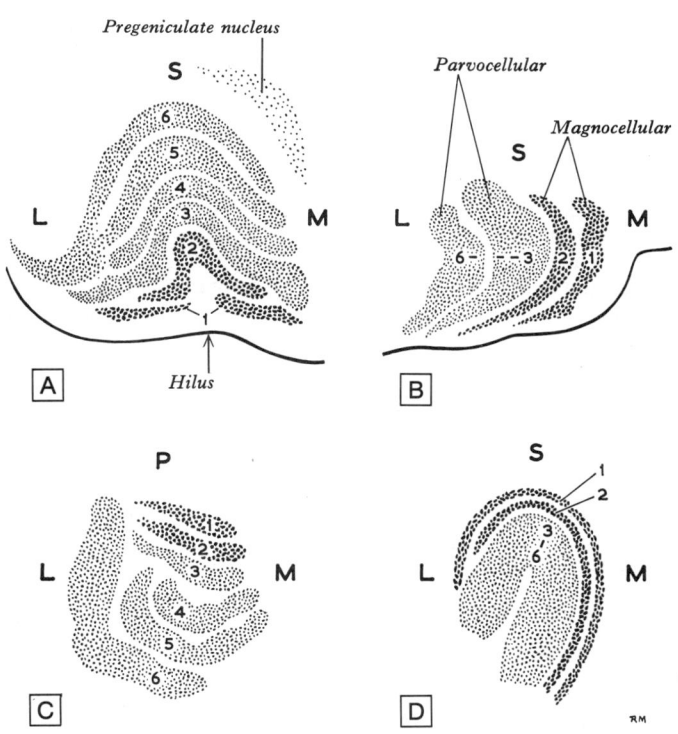

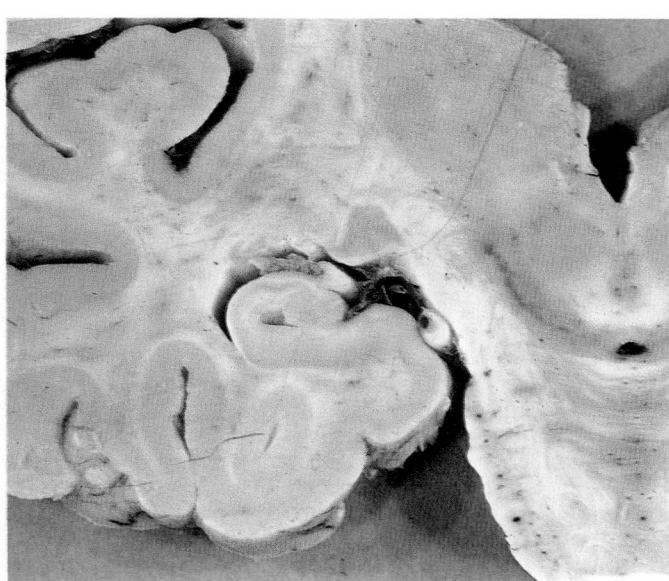

8.207 The lateral geniculate body, shown in coronal section in the human brain to display its general position and orientation: it is the cap-shaped mass of grey and white matter near the centre of the field. Note its relationship to the inferior horn of the lateral ventricle, the structures visible on the sectioned surface of the midbrain tegmentum and the dorsal thalamus. Even at this low magnification the lamination of the lateral geniculate body is visible. 8.209 shows the lateral geniculate nucleus in section.

8.208A. A mature human nucleus in coronal section near its central region and B. near its posterior pole. Note the reduction in the number of discernible laminae in the latter. The lamination is also visible in C, in an approximately horizontal section at the time of birth. In some primates, e.g. *Tarsius* (D), the magnocellular layers (1 and 2) are curved externally around the parvocellular layers (3–6); the higher primate arrangement is almost the reverse of this when examined in the coronal plane. (See text and Le Gros Clark (1932), Cooper (1945), Chacko (1955). Dissection by E L Rees, photography by Kevin Fitzpatrick, Department of Anatomy, Guy's Hospital Medical School, London.

serotoninergic afferents from the midbrain raphe nuclei (Garey 1990) and cholinergic fibres from the pontine and mesencephalic reticular formation (Woolf et al 1990).

The efferent fibres of the lateral geniculate nucleus pass principally to the primary visual cortex (area 17) in the banks of the calcarine sulcus (see below). It is possible that additional small projections pass to extrastriate visual areas in the occipital lobe, possibly arising primarily in the interlaminar zones (Jones 1985).

Interactions in the lateral geniculate nucleus (Jones 1985). It is clear from the above description that there is a well-demarcated segregation of retinal afferents to the lateral geniculate nucleus arising from each eye. Terminations of optic tract axons arising in the contralateral nasal retina are confined to laminae 1, 4 and 6, whereas those from the ipsilateral temporal retina are restricted to laminae 2, 3 and 5. The lack of anatomical overlap between the input to the lateral geniculate nucleus from the two eyes does not, however, preclude functional binocular interaction. Indeed, such interaction has been observed in cats, with both excitatory convergence and inhibition from the non-projecting (non-dominant) eye having been reported. In primates, perhaps including man, such interactions may be confined to inhibition of magnocellular Y-type cells by activation of the non-dominant eye. The anatomical substrate for such interaction is uncertain; it may be via dendrites of neurons crossing the interlaminar zones to encroach upon the adjacent lamina, or via long-axoned interneurons within the lamina passing to adjacent laminae.

Lateral group of thalamic nuclei

This group comprises the lateral dorsal nucleus, the lateral posterior nucleus and the pulvinar, which is further subdivided into medial, lateral and inferior nuclei. A further subdivision, the anterior or oral pulvinar, is considered part of the posterior group (see below).

Lateral dorsal nucleus. The most anterior of the lateral group of nuclei, the anterior pole of this nucleus lies within a splitting of the internal medullary lamina. Posteriorly, it merges with the anterior lateral posterior nucleus. Subcortical afferents to the lateral dorsal nucleus are from the pretectum and superior colliculus (Jones 1985; Thompson & Robertson 1987). It is connected with the cingulate, retrosplenial and posterior parahippocampal cortex, the presubiculum of the hippocampal formation (Yeterian & Pandya 1988; Jones 1985) and the parietal cortex (Schmahmann & Pandya 1990; Selemon & Goldman-Rakic 1988).

Lateral posterior nucleus. Lying dorsal to the ventral posterior inferior nucleus, the lateral posterior nucleus receives its subcortical afferents from the superior colliculus. It is reciprocally connected with the superior parietal lobe (Brodmann area 5; Pearson et al 1978; Schmahmann & Pandya 1990). Additional connections have been reported with the inferior parietal (Jones 1985), cingulate and medial parahippocampal (Yeterian & Pandya 1988) cortex.

Pulvinar. The posteriorly expanded mass of the thalamus is the *pulvinar* which, in man, overhangs the superior colliculus. Three major subdivisions are recognized histologically: dorsomedially lies the *medial pulvinar* nucleus comprising compact evenly spaced neurons; laterally and to some extent inferiorly, the *lateral pulvinar* nucleus is traversed by bundles of axons in the mediolateral plane, giving a characteristically fragmented appearance, with horizontal cords or sheets of cells separated by these white matter bundles; most inferiorly and laterally, the *inferior pulvinar* nucleus is a more homogeneous collection of cells.

Connections of the pulvinar. The subcortical afferents to the pulvinar are uncertain. However, medial and lateral pulvinar nuclei may receive from the superior colliculus. It has been suggested that the inferior pulvinar nucleus receives both from the superior colliculus and directly from the retina in monkeys, and it certainly contains a complete retinotopic representation (Jones 1985; Cusick et al 1993).

The cortical targets of efferent fibres from the pulvinar are widespread. In essence, the medial pulvinar nucleus projects to association areas of the parietotemporal cortex, whereas lateral and inferior pulvinar nuclei project to visual areas in the occipital and posterior temporal lobes. Thus, the inferior pulvinar nucleus connects with the striate and extrastriate cortex in the occipital lobe (Trojanowski & Jacobson 1976; Jones 1985) and with visual association areas in the posterior part of the temporal lobe (Ungerlieder et al 1984; Cusik et

al 1993; Baizer et al 1993). The lateral pulvinar nucleus connects with extrastriate areas of the occipital cortex (Trojanowski & Jacobson 1976; Jones 1985), with posterior parts of the temporal association cortex (Cusick et al 1993; Ungerlieder et al 1984; Baizer et al 1993) and also with the parietal cortex (Schmahmann & Pandya 1990). The medial pulvinar nucleus connects with the inferior parietal cortex (Pearson et al 1978; Schmahmann & Pandya 1990; Selemon & Goldman-Rakic 1988; Trojanowski & Jacobson 1976; Jones 1985; Baizer et al 1993), with the posterior cingulate gyrus (Yeterian & Pandya 1988) and with the widespread areas of the temporal lobe (Trojanowski & Jacobson 1976; Jones 1985; Cusick et al 1993; Baizer et al 1993), including the posterior parahippocampal gyrus, perirhinal (Yeterian & Pandya 1988) and entorhinal cortex (Insausti et al 1987b). It is also now clear that the medial pulvinar nucleus has extensive connections with prefrontal and orbitofrontal cortex (Trojanowski & Jacobson 1976; Yeterian & Pandya 1988). Similarly, the lateral pulvinar nucleus may also connect with the rostromedial prefrontal cortex (Yeterian & Pandya 1988).

The functions of the main subdivisions of the pulvinar are poorly understood. The inferior pulvinar nucleus contains a complete retinotopic representation, and lateral and medial pulvinar nuclei also contain visually responsive cells. The latter nucleus at least is not however, purely visual; other modality responses can be recorded, and some cells may be polysensory (Mathers & Rapisardi 1973). Given the complexity of functions of the association areas to which they project, particularly in the temporal lobe, including perception, cognition and memory, it is likely that the role of the pulvinar in modulating these functions is equally complex.

Anteriorly, the major subdivisions of the pulvinar blend into a poorly differentiated region, within which several nuclear components have been variously recognized by different authorities (see Jones 1985 for review). These include the anterior or oral pulvinar, the suprageniculate/limitans and the posterior nuclei. Together these ill-defined elements form the *posterior group*. The connectivity of this complex is also poorly understood, but different components receive subcortical afferents from the spinothalamic tract and the superior and inferior colliculi. Cortical connections centre primarily on the insula and adjacent parts of the parietal operculum posteriorly. The significance of this poorly understood region of the thalamus centres on physiological studies in cats which suggest the presence of nociceptive neurons (Poggio & Mountcastle 1960). Recent studies do not support a major role for these nuclei in a central pain pathway, although stimulation in man has been reported to elicit pain, and large lesions in this region may alleviate painful conditions (Hassler 1960). Similarly, excision of its cortical target in the parietal operculum (Talairach et al 1949; Lende et al 1971) or small infarcts in this cortical region (Biemond 1956) may result in hypoalgesia suggesting that exclusion of such a functional role for this thalamic area might be premature.

Intralaminar nuclei

The term intralaminar nuclei refers to collections of neurons forming nuclei within the internal medullary lamina of the thalamus. Two groups of nuclei are recognized in primates, including man, the anterior (rostral) and posterior (caudal) intralaminar nuclei. The former comprises the central medial, paracentral and central lateral nuclei, the latter the centromedian and parafascicular nuclei. The designations central medial and centromedian are open to confusion, but are an accepted part of the terminology of thalamic nuclei in common usage; it is important to emphasize that the centromedian nucleus is much larger, is considerably expanded in man in comparison with other species and is importantly related to the globus pallidus, deep cerebellar nuclei and motor cortex. Anteriorly, the internal medullary lamina separates the mediodorsal nucleus from the ventral lateral complex and is occupied by the paracentral nucleus laterally, and the central medial nucleus ventromedially, as the two laminae converge towards the midline. A little more posteriorly, the central lateral nucleus appears dorsally in the lamina as the latter splits to enclose the lateral dorsal nucleus. More posteriorly, at the level of the ventroposterior nuclei, the lamina splits to enclose the ovoid centromedian nucleus, with the smaller parafascicular nucleus lying more medially.

The anterior intralaminar nuclei, central medial, paracentral and central lateral, have reciprocal connections with widespread cortical areas, with some evidence of areal preference (Macchi & Bentivoglio 1986). Thus, the central lateral nucleus projects mainly to parietal and temporal association areas, the paracentral nucleus to occipitotemporal and prefrontal, and the central medial nucleus to orbitofrontal and prefrontal cortex and to the cortex on the medial surface. In contrast, the posterior nuclei, centromedian and parafascicular, have more restricted connections, principally with the motor, premotor and supplementary motor areas. Both anterior and posterior intralaminar nuclei project to the striatum in addition to the cortex. Many cells throughout the anterior nuclei have branched axons to the cortex on the one hand, and to the striatum on the other (Macchi et al 1984), though such dual projections are less frequent in the posterior (centromedian and parafascicular) nuclei. The thalamostriate projection is topographically organized. The posterior intralaminar nuclei (centromedian and parafascicular) receive a major input from the internal segment of the globus pallidus. Additional afferents come from the pars reticulata of the substantia nigra, the deep cerebellar nuclei, the pedunculopontine nucleus of the midbrain and possibly the spinothalamic tract. The anterior nuclei have widespread subcortical afferents, with the central lateral nucleus receiving afferents from the spinothalamic tract, and all component nuclei receiving fibres from the brainstem reticular formation, the superior colliculus and several pretectal nuclei. Afferents to all intralaminar nuclei from the brainstem reticular formation include a prominent cholinergic pathway (Woolf et al 1990).

The functional role of the intralaminar nuclei is complex and unclear. This pathway appears to mediate cortical activation from the brainstem reticular formation, and to play a part in sensorimotor integration. In man, damage of the intralaminar nuclei may contribute to thalamic neglect—a true unilateral neglect of stimuli originating from the contralateral body or extrapersonal space. This may arise particularly from unilateral damage of the centromedian–parafascicular complex. Bilateral injury to the posterior intralaminar nuclei leads to a kinetic mutism with apathy and loss of motivation. A second syndrome associated with damage involving the intralaminar nuclei is that of unilateral motor neglect, with contralateral paucity of spontaneous movement and motor areactivity. Detailed consideration of the functional mechanisms in which the intralaminar nuclei may participate is beyond the scope of the present account and readers are referred to reviews by Jones (1985) and Macchi and Bentivoglio (1986) for further information.

Midline nuclei

There is considerable divergence between different authors as to which elements of the medial diencephalon constitute the component nuclei of the midline thalamic group. Candidates for inclusion are the paraventricular nuclei, the central medial nucleus and a group of nuclei ventral to the latter, the reuniens, rhomboid and parataenial nuclei. On developmental grounds, following the terminology of Jones (1985), the paraventricular nuclei are here considered part of the epithalamus. The central medial nucleus, although located at the midline, is embedded in the fibres of the internal medullary lamina. This and its efferent connections with the cortex justify its inclusion as part of the anterior intralaminar group of thalamic nuclei (see above; Bentivoglio et al 1991). For the purposes of the present account, therefore, the midline group of nuclei comprises those medial thalamic structures ventral to the central medial nucleus, viz. the rhomboid and reuniens nuclei together with the parataenial nuclei more dorsolaterally.

The midline nuclei receive subcortical afferent fibres from the hypothalamus, the periaqueductal grey matter of the midbrain, the spinothalamic tract and the medullary and pontine reticular formation. The midline nuclei are the major thalamic target of ascending noradrenergic and serotoninergic axons from the locus coeruleus and raphe nuclei respectively, and they also receive a cholinergic input from the midbrain. Efferents from the midline nuclei pass to the hippocampal formation, the amygdala and the nucleus accumbens. Additional thalamocortical axons reach the cingulate, and possibly orbitofrontal cortex. The dual cortical and basal nuclear relationship of these nuclei has often led to their being considered a part of the intralaminar system. The cortical projections are reciprocal. The relationships of these nuclei clearly demarcate them as part of the limbic system. There is some evidence that the midline nuclei may play a role in memory and arousal, and,

pathologically, may be important in the regulation of seizure activity (Miller et al 1989).

GENERAL CONCLUSIONS

The dorsal thalamus is the major, though far from the sole, route by which subcortical neuronal activity influences the cerebral cortex. It has been traditional to separate thalamocortical relationships into specific, mediating particularly finely organized and securely transmitted sensory information, and non-specific, mediating a general arousal system. As discussed above, this classification is no longer of value. In the major sensory relay nuclei which clearly relate to a single modality of sensation (viz. the lateral and the medial geniculate and the ventroposterior nuclei), their cortical target areas are restricted to clear single modality functional regions. None of these nuclei is, however, restricted to a single cortical target. Perhaps somewhat similarly, the ventrolateral nucleus, particularly the posterior division, has a relatively restricted projection to motor areas of the frontal cortex. Just as with the cortical areas which are the primary targets of these nuclei (p. 1149), the above examples are perhaps the least typical of the mode of projection of the majority of the main thalamic nuclei. The largest expansion of thalamic nuclei in man, reflecting the growth of the cortical lobes to which they project, is seen in the mediodorsal and pulvinar nuclei. These two large nuclear masses exemplify the complexity of organization of thalamocortical connections which is now apparent. Undoubtedly the major target of the mediodorsal nucleus is the prefrontal cortex, but it also sends fibres to association cortex of the parietotemporal lobes. More markedly, the pulvinar provides the major thalamic input to the majority of the so-called association areas in occipital, parietal and temporal cortex, yet it also projects (particularly the medial pulvinar) to prefrontal cortex. These projections appear to be a linking of the thalamus to functionally related but topographically separate cortical areas, similar to that seen in other subcortical connections, with the striatum, the claustrum and other nuclei (see below, p. 1186). Thus, the thalamus appears to be a key component of the distributed neural networks subserving specific cognitive and behavioural functions (Selemon & Goldman-Rakic 1988; Goldman-Rakic 1988).

Perhaps the greatest impediment to our understanding the role of the thalamus, at least in terms of its connectivity, is the knowledge that numerically the greatest input to most if not all nuclei derives from the cortex. Added to this is the dual nature of this projection, a direct excitatory pathway and an indirect inhibitory one via the reticular nucleus. It is presumably via corticothalamic fibres that the cerebral cortex in some way regulates its own thalamic afferents. Perhaps, when the cortex is quiescent, the subcortical pathways alone are insufficient to activate the thalamus, whereas with an already activated cortex, thalamic input is enhanced. Within such a framework, a mechanism of selective attention could be hypothesized. The simple corticothalamic thalamocortical loop is excitatory at both ends, and may require the equal and equivalent, but delayed, inhibition provided indirectly via the reticular nucleus, to prevent a crescendo effect of mutual recurrent activation of thalamus and cortex.

Whatever the value or otherwise of such speculation, it is clear that the thalamus is more than a simple stepping stone for sensory input en route to the cortex. Much more remains to be established of the synaptic organization, physiological properties and functional roles of the thalamus in perception and behaviour. Perhaps the techniques of electrophysiological recording in awake, behaving animals will be applied to this problem as they have to unravelling the mysteries of cerebral cortical functioning. With ever improving spatial and temporal resolution of modern neuroimaging techniques such as PET and MRI (p. 919), their role in man may become more clearly elucidated.

VENTRAL THALAMUS

The main nuclear groups of the ventral thalamus comprise the reticular nucleus, the zona incerta, the fields of Forel and the pregeniculate nucleus and also include the upper pole of the red nucleus and substantia nigra and the entopeduncular nucleus. The subthalamic nucleus is excluded on both developmental grounds and because of its close functional and connectional relationship to the basal nuclei with which it is considered (Jones 1985, see below).

The main subthalamic tracts are:

- the upper parts of the medial, spinal and trigeminal lemnisci and the solitariothalamic tract, approaching their terminations in the thalamic nuclei
- the dentatothalamic tract from the contralateral superior cerebellar peduncle accompanied by ipsilateral rubrothalamic fibres
- the fasciculus retroflexus
- the fasciculus lenticularis;
- the fasciculus subthalamicus
- the ansa lenticularis
- fascicles from the prerubral field (H field of Forel)
- the continuation of the fasciculus lenticularis (in the H_2 field of Forel)
- the fasciculus thalamicus (the H_1 field of Forel).

All, of course, are bilateral.

Subthalamic topography is complex and best appreciated in solid models or in coronal and sagittal serial sections. A parallel study of the corpus striatum, from which prominent subthalamic tracts are derived, is also helpful. Figure **8.209** may clarify the region's complicated terminology but three-dimensional topography is difficult to appreciate from flat (two-dimensional) diagrams.

As the upper ends of the red nucleus and substantia nigra pass into the subthalamus they diminish in area, ending a little below the mamillary bodies. The changing relation of the lemnisci to the red nucleus and substantia nigra as they ascend in the midbrain has been described (p. 1068). Lemniscal fibres enter the subthalamus largely lateral to the red nucleus; as they ascend they approach the dorsal aspect of the nucleus to reach the ventral surface of the thalamic nucleus ventralis posterior, in which most fibres end. Dentatothalamic and rubrothalamic run with pallidothalamic fibres in the *thalamic fasciculus*, which ascends beyond the lemnisci to distribute largely to the ventral lateral and ventral anterior thalamic nuclei (p. 1066, and see below).

Reticular nucleus

The reticular nucleus is a curved lamella of large, deeply-staining fusiform cells which wraps around the lateral margin of the dorsal thalamus, separated from it by the external medullary lamina. Anteriorly, it curves around the rostral pole of the dorsal thalamus to lie between it and the prethalamic nuclei, notably the bed nucleus of the stria terminalis. Posterio-inferiorly, it becomes displaced from its close approximation to the dorsal thalamus by the intervening geniculate bodies. The nucleus is criss-crossed by bundles of fibres passing between thalamus and cortex; this confers a reticular appearance upon the nucleus and hence its name.

The nucleus receives collateral branches of all corticothalamic, thalamocortical and probably thalamostriatal and pallidothalamic fibres that traverse it. An additional afferent pathway arises from the nucleus cuneiformis of the midbrain, and this pathway may be cholinergic. The efferent fibres from the reticular nucleus pass into the dorsal thalamus and are GABA-ergic (p. 1084). The afferents from the cortex and thalamus are broadly speaking topographically arranged, and the reticular nucleus shows visual, somatic and auditory regions, each of which contains a crude topographic representation of the sensorium concerned. Cells within these parts of the nucleus respond to visual, somatic or auditory stimuli with a latency suggesting that these properties arise from activation by thalamocortical axon collaterals. Only in areas where representations abut do cells show modality convergence. The projections into the main thalamic nuclei broadly, but not entirely, reciprocate the thalamoreticular connections. There may also be projections to the contralateral dorsal thalamus (Paré & Steriade 1993). The nucleus is believed to function in gating information relayed through the thalamus. For a more detailed account and for references, readers should consult Jones (1985).

Pregeniculate (ventral geniculate) nucleus

The pregeniculate nucleus of primates is homologous with the ventral lateral geniculate nucleus of subprimate species and is particularly large in highly visual animals such as the tree-shrew in which it is distinctly laminated (Jones 1985; Conley & Friederich-Ecsy 1993a,

b). It receives a prominent input from the retina, and contains a retinotopic representation. Additional afferents come from visual cortical areas, and from the pretectum, the superior colliculus, the cerebellum, the vestibular nuclei and possibly from the subthalamic nucleus and the locus coeruleus. Efferent projections pass to the superior colliculus, the pretectal nuclei, the pontine nuclei and parts of the hypothalamus, notably the suprachiasmatic nucleus. Within the dorsal thalamus there is evidence of projections to the pulvinar, the dorsal lateral geniculate nucleus and the lateral dorsal nucleus and the anterior intralaminar group. On the basis of its connectivity, the pregeniculate nucleus may play a role in visuosensory and oculomotor processes. (For further discussion and references see Jones 1985; Conley & Friederich-Ecsy 1993a, b).

Zona incerta and the fields of Forel

Between the ventral part of the external medullary lamina of the thalamus and the cerebral peduncle lies an aggregation of small cells, the nucleus of the zona incerta. It is tenuously linked to the reticular nucleus dorsolaterally, and this continuity is more easily seen following staining for acetylcholinesterase, glutamic acid decarboxylase, somatostatin and other histochemical markers. More medially lie a scattered group of cells in a matrix of fibres known as the H field of Forel. Dorsally, on either side of the zona incerta lie the field H_1 of Forel, comprising the thalamic fasciculus, and ventrally the field H_2 of Forel, between the zona incerta and the subthalamic nucleus, containing the fasciculus lenticularis (see below and **8.209**).

The nucleus of the zona incerta receives from the sensorimotor cortex, the pregeniculate nucleus, the deep cerebellar nuclei, the trigeminal nuclear complex and the spinal cord. It projects to the spinal cord and the pretectal region. Its functions are unknown (for references see Jones 1985).

The neurons of the H field of Forel receive afferents from the internal segment of the globus pallidum, the spinal cord and the reticular formation of the brainstem. They may project to the spinal cord. Like the zona incerta, their functions are unknown (Jones 1985).

The zona incerta is functionally associated with neurons grouped along its inferomedial border, collectively called the *nucleus of the prerubral* or *tegmental field*, and other groups between fascicles of the ansa lenticularis (see below), sometimes regarded as 'detached' parts of the globus pallidus but collectively termed the *entopeduncular nucleus*. These nuclei are mainly relays on discharge pathways from the globus pallidus to the mesencephalic reticular formation; some of their fibres descend in the central tegmental fasciculus to the inferior olivary complex (p. 1020), numerous branches leaving to innervate the 'reticular' and 'non-reticular' brainstem nuclei.

In addition to terminal parts of the lemniscal, dentatothalamic and rubrothalamic tracts, the subthalamus is typified by white fascicles, often containing small groups of neurons of complex topography. Conflicting terminologies have been proposed. The approach adopted here is to consider the fascicles in relation to the main striatal outflows (p. 1193). These are derived partly from the putamen but mostly from the globus pallidus and appear at the latter's surface, fanning out medially; the radiation's dorsal and intermediate fibres intersect those of the internal capsule, while the ventral ones curve round the capsule's posteroventral border. Earlier investigators (von Monakow 1882) termed the whole radiation the *ansa lenticularis* with dorsal, intermediate and ventral divisions, a term now restricted to the ventral radiation, the intermediate radiation being the fasciculus subthalamicus, the dorsal radiation the fasciculus lenticularis (**8.209**).

The fasciculus lenticularis is the dorsal division of pallidofugal fibres traversing the internal capsule; it turns medially near the capsule's medial aspect, partly intermingled with the dorsal zone of the subthalamic nucleus and ventral part of the zona incerta, where the fasciculus traverses the H_2 *field of Forel*. Reaching the medial border of the zona incerta, the fasciculus intermingles with fibres of the ansa lenticularis, scattered elements of the prerubral nucleus and with dentatothalamic and rubrothalamic fibres. This merging of diverse pathways and associated cell groups is variously called the *prerubral, tegmental* or *H field of Forel*.

The *ansa lenticularis* has a complex origin from both parts of the globus pallidus, from the putamen and possibly other adjacent structures; its fibres partly relay in neurons along its course, the

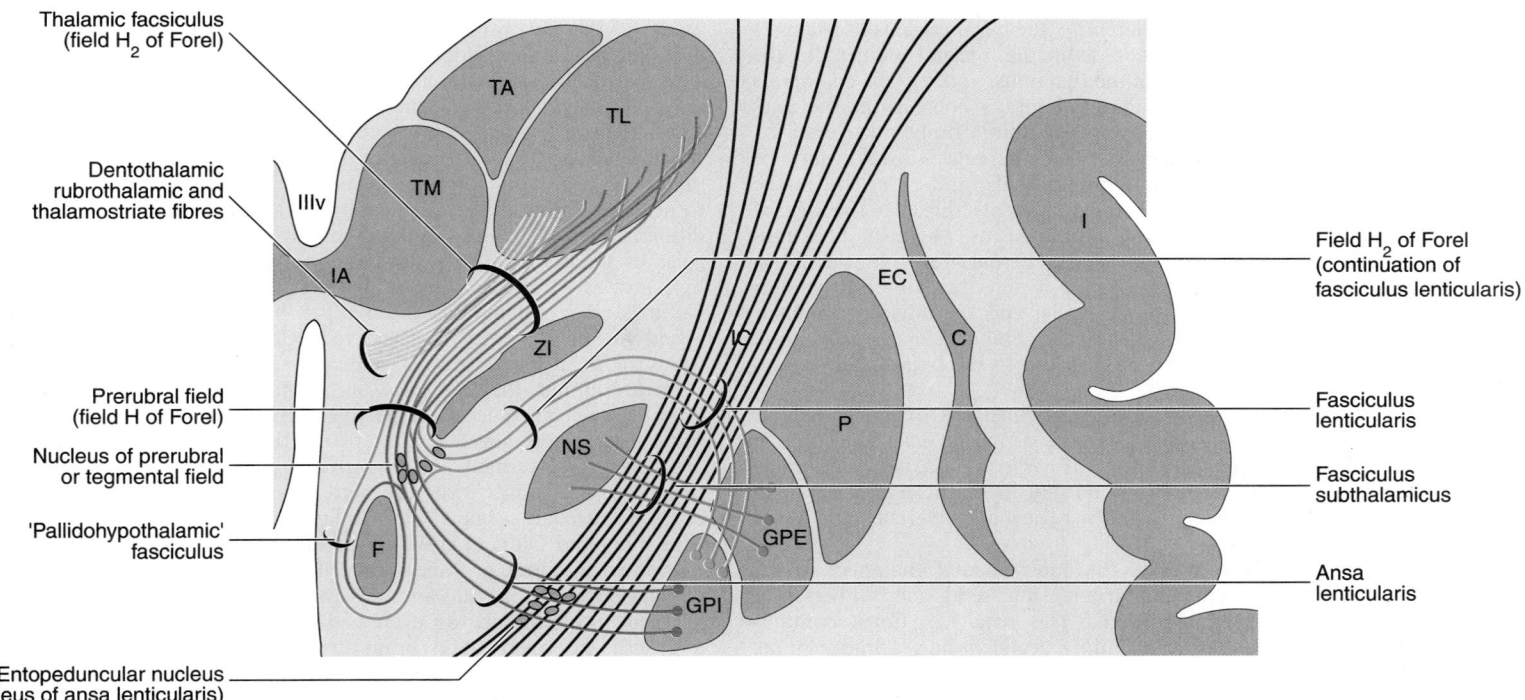

Thalamic facsiculus
(field H$_2$ of Forel)

Dentothalamic
rubrothalamic and
thalamostriate fibres

Prerubral field
(field H of Forel)

Nucleus of prerubral
or tegmental field

'Pallidohypothalamic'
fasciculus

Entopeduncular nucleus
nucleus of ansa lenticularis)

Field H$_2$ of Forel
(continuation of
fasciculus lenticularis)

Fasciculus
lenticularis

Fasciculus
subthalamicus

Ansa
lenticularis

8.209   The nuclear masses of grey matter and fibre tract systems associated with, or closely related topographically to, parts of the dorsal thalamus, subthalamus and globus pallidus. The information presented is compounded from a series of closely spaced coronal sections through this region, attempts being made to include what are essentially three-dimensional structures in a two-dimensional diagram; it must be emphasized that all the structures shown would not appear on the same single coronal section. The significance of the letters is as follows: IIIv = third ventricle; M = medial nuclear group of thalamus; TA = anterior nuclear group of thalamus; TL = lateral nuclear group of thalamus; IA = interthalamic adhesion; ZI = zona incerta; F = column of fornix; NS = nucleus subthalamicus; IC = internal capsule; GPI and GPE = internal and external parts of globus pallidus; P = putamen; EC = external capsule; C = claustrum; I = cortex of insula.

entopeduncular nucleus. It curves medially round the ventral border of the internal capsule, continuing dorsomedially to mingle with other fibres noted above in the prerubral field. Some fibres in both fasciculus lenticularis and ansa lenticularis synapse in the nucleus subthalamicus, prerubral field and zona incerta; the remainder continue laterally with other fascicles into the thalamic nuclei, particularly the intermediate anterior ventral and central medial nuclei.

The *thalamic fasciculus* is a complex extending from the prerubral field, dorsal to and also partly traversing the zona incerta and related dorsally to the ventral thalamic nuclei. It contains continuations of the fasciculus lenticularis and ansa lenticularis, dentatothalamic and rubrothalamic fibres and thalamostriate fibres. Its territory is sometimes termed the *H$_1$ field of Forel*.

The *'pallidohypothalamic' fasciculus* leaves the main pallidofugal system in the prerubral field and pursues a curious course, curving ventromedially round the column of the fornix towards the hypothalamus (Bard & Rioch 1937; Vidal 1940; Ingram 1940), where it was long assumed to end in the mediodorsal nucleus. But evidence is inconclusive and experiments in monkeys (Nauta & Mehler 1966) show that it recurves laterally below the column, turning dorsally to rejoin the H$_1$ field of Forel.

The fasciculus subthalamicus is an abundant two-way array of fibres traversing the internal capsule, interweaving with it at right angles, to connect the subthalamic nucleus with the globus pallidus and, to a lesser extent, the putamen (p. 1193).

EPITHALAMUS

The epithalamus, following the terminology reviewed by Jones (1985), comprises the anterior and posterior paraventricular nuclei, the medial and lateral habenular nuclei, the stria medullaris thalami and the pineal body. The posterior commissure is also included. The axons of the latter cross in anterior and posterior laminae of the pineal peduncle. Pineal development is briefly mentioned on page 245, its structure, neuroendocrine roles and innervation on page 1889 with accompanying illustrations.

The *trigonum habenulae* is a small, bilateral triangular depression, anterior to the superior colliculus, medial to the pulvinar but separated by a *sulcus habenulae*; anteromedial is the posterior end of a ridge occupied by the stria medullaris thalami and by the pineal peduncle.

Paraventricular nuclei

The paraventricular nuclei are small, darkly stained neurons which form a densely cellular region immediately underlying the ependyma of the third ventricle dorsally. They are often considered as part of the midline thalamic nuclei (Bentivoglio et al 1991). Afferents to the paraventricular nuclei come from the hypothalamus, particularly the anterior and lateral hypothalamic areas, the septal nuclei, the bed nucleus of the stria terminalis and the hippocampal formation (p. 1123). Additional inputs are from the brainstem and may include noradrenergic fibres from the locus coeruleus. They project to the nucleus accumbens, the amygdala and the hippocampal formation. Their functions are unknown but are best considered with the midline thalamic nuclei (see above; for reviews see Jones 1985; Bentivoglio et al 1991).

Habenular nuclei and stria medullaris

The habenular nuclei lie posteriorly at the dorsomedial corner of the thalamus, immediately deep to the ependyma of the third ventricle, with the stria medullaris thalami above and laterally. From the ventral margin of the nuclei, a white matter bundle emerges, the habenulopenduncular tract, passing caudally and inferiorly towards the interpeduncular region of the midbrain. The medial habenular nucleus is a densely-packed, deeply staining mass of neurons, whereas the lateral nucleus is more dispersed and paler staining. The nuclear complex is limited laterally by a fibrous lamina which enters the habenulopenduncular tract. Typically, the tela choroidea of the third ventricle arises from the ependyma at the superolateral corner of the medial habenular nucleus. Posteriorly, the nuclei of the two sides and the internal medullary laminae are linked across the midline by the habenular commissure.

Afferent fibres to the habenular nuclei travel in the stria medullaris from the prepiriform cortex bilaterally, the basal nucleus of Maynert and the hypothalamus. Afferents from the internal segment of the globus pallidus ascend through the thalamus, and may be collaterals of pallidothalamic axons. Additional inputs come from the pars compacta of the substantia nigra, the midbrain raphe nuclei and the lateral dorsal tegmental nucleus. The afferent pathways may be somewhat segregated in their terminal fields, and most end in the lateral nucleus. The only identified afferent fibres to the medial habenular come from the septofimbrial nucleus. The medial habenular nucleus is cholinergic and sends efferent fibres to the interpeduncular nucleus of the midbrain. From the lateral habenular nucleus, fibres pass to the raphe nuclei and the adjacent reticular formation of the midbrain, to the pars compacta of the substantia nigra and the ventral tegmental area and to the hypothalamus and basal forebrain.

Little is known of the physiological functions of the habenular nuclei. Lesions which include this area of the medial diencephalon indicate a role in the regulation of visceral and neuroendocrine functions. It has also been suggested that these nuclei play a part in the control of sleep mechanisms (for review and references see Jones 1985).

The *stria medullaris* crosses the superomedial thalamic aspect, skirts medial to the habenular trigone and sends many fibres into the ipsilateral habenular nucleus. The stria has fibres containing several neuromediators including acetylcholine, noradrenaline, serotonin, γ-aminobutyric acid (GABA), luteinizing hormone releasing hormone (LHRH), somatostatin, vasopressin and oxytocin. Other strial fibres cross in the anterior pineal lamina, decussating as the *habenular commissure* to reach the contralateral habenular nucleus. Some fibres are really commissural and interconnect the amygdaloid complexes and hippocampal cortices; crossed tectohabenular fibres accompany them in the commissure. Serotonin(5-hydroxytryptomine)ergic fibres from the *ventral ascending tegmental serotonergic bundle*, which join the habenulopeduncular tract (see below) to reach the nuclei, may exert some control over neurons of the *habenulopineal tract*, thus influencing innervation of the pinealocytes (p. 1889), as may also the habenular nuclear afferents from the *dorsal ascending tegmental noradrenergic bundle* (p. 996). The gland is also innervated by sympathetic fibres from the superior cervical ganglia (see p. 1077). Though the human habenulas is relatively small, it is a focus of integration of diverse olfactory, visceral and somatic afferent paths.

The main habenular outflow reaches the interpeduncular nucleus, mediodorsal thalamic nucleus, mesencephalic tectum and reticular formation, the largest being the *habenulopeduncular tract* or *fasciculus retroflexus* (8.213). This courses ventrally and upwards, skirts the inferior zone of the thalamic nucleus mediodorsal and traverses the superomedial region of the red nucleus to the interpeduncular nucleus; this provides relays to the midbrain reticular formation, from which tectotegmentospinal tracts and dorsal longitudinal fasciculi connect with autonomic preganglionic neurons controlling salivation, gastric and intestinal secretory activity and motility; others pass to motor nuclei for mastication and deglutition. Ablation of habenular complexes causes extensive changes in metabolism, endocrine and thermal regulation (Szentágothai et al 1962).

Posterior commissure

The posterior (dorsal) commissure is a complex fasciculus decussating in the posterior pineal lamina, relatively reduced in primates and of unknown constitution in man. It myelinates early; estimates of fibres in several species have been made (Tomasch & Malpass 1958). Various nuclei are associated with it: small groups scattered along it as the *interstitial nuclei of the posterior commissure*, accumulations in the periventricular grey matter forming *dorsal nuclei of the posterior commissure nucleus of Darkschewitsch* in the periaqueductal grey, and the *interstitial nucleus* (of Cajal) near the upper end of the oculomotor complex, closely linked with the medial longitudinal fasciculus (p. 1070). Fibres from all these nuclei and the fasciculus cross in the posterior commissure. Other contributors to it include dorsal thalamic nuclei, pretectal nuclei, superior colliculi and connections between the tectal and habenular nuclei. The destinations and functions of many of these fibres are obscure.

Ventral to and below the posterior commissure (i.e. near the inferior wall of the pineal recess), ependymal cells on the dorsal aspect of the cerebral aqueduct are tall, columnar and ciliated with granular basophilic cytoplasm and specific histochemical reactions. This patch, possibly secreting into the cerebrospinal fluid, is the *subcommissural organ* (Keene & Hewer 1935; Wislocki & Leduc 1953; Mollgard et al 1973). Its cells may be involved in the transport of materials to the cerebrospinal fluid from adjoining axonal terminals or capillaries; or substances may be transported from fluid to neurons, blood vessels or pinealocytes (p. 1888, and cf. the infundibular recess of the third ventricle, p. 1207). Possible neuroendocrine roles of these specialized ependymal *tanycytes* have been reviewed by Knowles (1974), Reichlin et al (1978), Joseph and Knigge (1978), Collins and Woollam (1981 and see p. 940). Other patches of similar ependyma project into the third ventricle from its secondary roof (body of fornix) and from its anterior wall between the diverging fornical columns: the *subfornical organ* and the organum vasculosum or *intercolumnar tubercle* respectively. These and, in some vertebrates, other specialized regions of the third ventricular ependyma are collectively termed *circumventricular organs*. For a review of the disposition, ultrastructure and possible functional roles of circumventricular organs see Collins and Woollam (1981) and McKinley and Oldfield (1990); they indicate that circumventricular organs are a mosaic of three main cell varieties: 'basic' ciliated ependymal cells, secretory cells and tanycytes, the latter, however, varying in their ultrastructure as each is location specific. In summary, a generalized mammalian brain displays, in median section, the following specialized ependymal circumventricular organs; the median eminence, and variable infundibular recess; the collicular recess organ; the aqueductal recess organ; the subcommissural organ; the habenular ependyma; the habenular commissural organ; the subfornical organ; the organum vasculosum of the lamina terminalis or intercolumnar tubercle. Recall, also, the area postrema and funiculus separans in the fourth ventricle (p. 1208).

HYPOTHALAMUS

The human hypothalamus comprises only 4 cm³ of neural tissue, or 0.3% of the total brain. Nevertheless, it contains the integrative systems controlling fluid and electrolyte balance, food ingestion and energy balance, reproduction, thermoregulation, and immune and many emotional responses, via the autonomic and endocrine effector systems. Many of its nuclei and functions appear to have changed little from their form in lower animals.

The hypothalamus extends posteriorly from the lamina terminalis to a vertical plane posterior to the mamillary bodies and from the hypothalamic sulcus to the base of the brain beneath the third ventricle. This region's anterior part, the preoptic area, strictly belongs to the telencephalon impar but is included here for functional reasons. The hypothalamus is bordered laterally by the anterior part of the subthalamus, internal capsule and optic tract; posteriorly by the tegmental part of the subthalamus and the mesencephalic tegmentum; dorsally by the dorsal thalamic nuclei (8.210, 211). Anteriorly the optic chiasm, lamina terminalis and anterior commissure separate the preoptic area from the precommissural septum, the continuation of the diagonal band into the paraterminal and paraolfactory gyrus (p. 1129). However, many functional systems are continuous across these arbitrary boundaries.

Structures in the floor of the third ventricle reach the pial surface in the interpeduncular fossa (8.212); from front to back they are: the optic chiasm; the tuber cinereum, tuberal eminences and the infundibular stalk; the mamillary bodies; and the posterior perforated substance. The latter, included here for convenience, lies in the interval between the diverging crura cerebri, pierced by small central branches of posterior cerebral arteries. Within it is the interpeduncular nucleus, small in man and homologous with a more extensive complex in submammalian forms, which receives terminals of the fasciculus retroflexus (see above) of both sides and has other connections with the mesencephalic reticular formation and mamillary bodies. The *mamillary bodies* are smooth, hemispherical, pea-sized eminences, lying side by side, anterior to the posterior perforated substance, each with nuclei enclosed in white fascicles derived largely from the fornix. The *tuber cinereum*, between the mamillary bodies and the optic chiasm, is a convex mass of grey matter; its ventral aspect presents a series of eminences with inter-

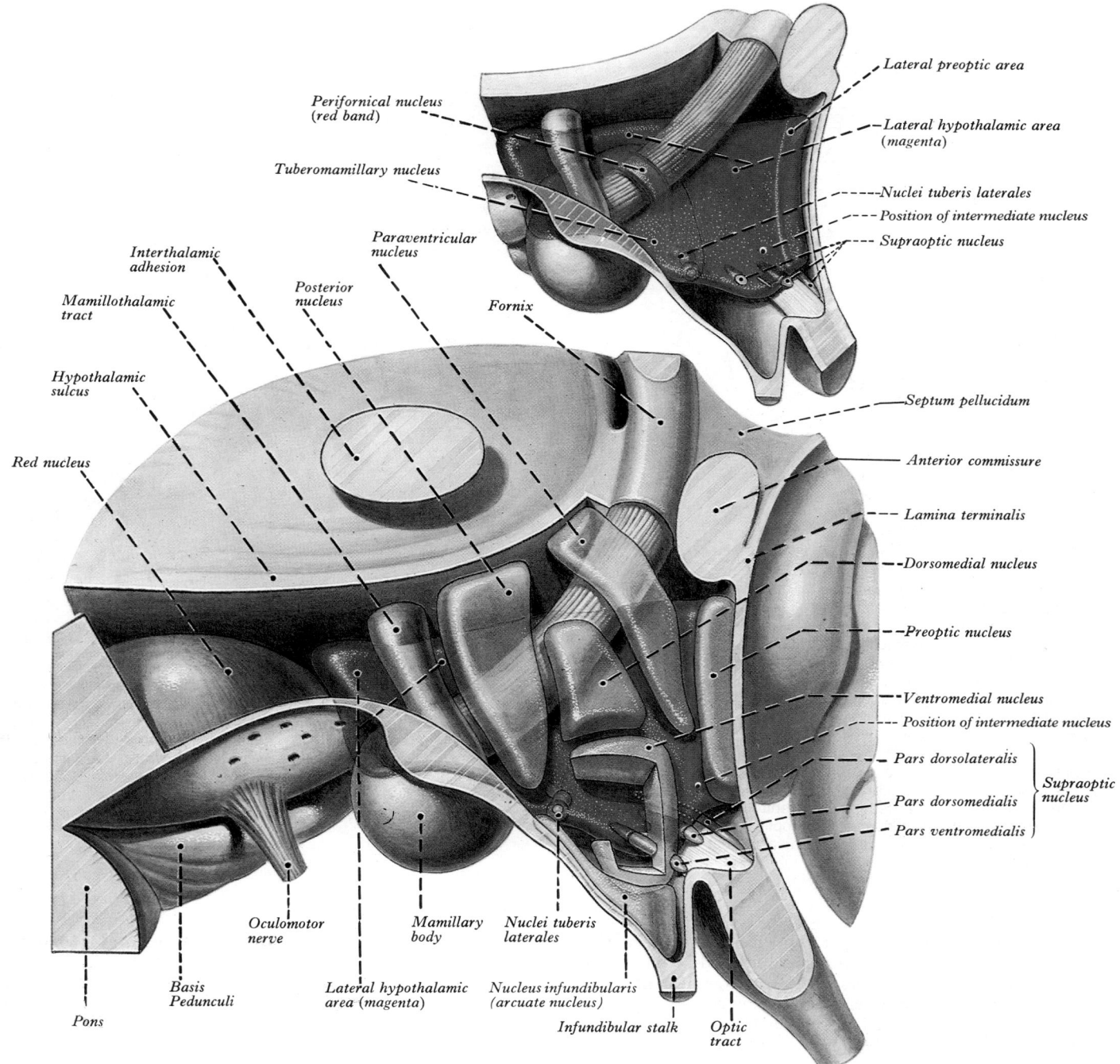

Perifornical nucleus
(red band)

Tuberomamillary nucleus

Paraventricular
nucleus

Interthalamic
adhesion

Mamillothalamic
tract

Posterior
nucleus

Fornix

Hypothalamic
sulcus

Red nucleus

Lateral preoptic area

Lateral hypothalamic area
(magenta)

Nuclei tuberis laterales

Position of intermediate nucleus

Supraoptic nucleus

Septum pellucidum

Anterior commissure

Lamina terminalis

Dorsomedial nucleus

Preoptic nucleus

Ventromedial nucleus

Position of intermediate nucleus

Pars dorsolateralis

Pars dorsomedialis

Pars ventromedialis

Supraoptic
nucleus

Oculomotor
nerve

Mamillary
body

Nuclei tuberis
laterales

Basis
Pedunculi

Lateral hypothalamic
area (magenta)

Nucleus infundibularis
(arcuate nucleus)

Infundibular stalk

Optic
tract

Pons

8.210 Schemata of the hypothalamic region of the left cerebral hemisphere from the medial aspect dissected to display the major hypothalamic nuclei. In the upper diagram the medially placed nuclear groups have been removed; in the lower diagram both lateral and medial are included. Lateral to the fornix and the mamillothalamic tract is the lateral hypothalamic region (magenta), in which the tuberomamillary nucleus is situated posteriorly, and the lateral preoptic nucleus rostrally. Surrounding the fornix is the perifornical nucleus (red band), which joins the lateral hypothalamic area with the posterior hypothalamic nucleus. The medially placed nuclei (yellow) fill in much of the region between the mamillothalamic tract and the lamina terminalis, but also project caudally to the tract. The lateral tuberal nuclei (blue) are situated ventrally, largely in the lateral hypothalamic area. The supraoptic nucleus (green) may form three rather separate parts. The intermediate nuclei (p. 1096) form three groups between the supraoptic and paraventricular nuclei. (Modified from Nauta & Haymaker 1969, by courtesy of the authors and publishers.)

vening grooves of varying depth. From it, the median, conical, hollow *infundibulum* becomes continuous ventrally with the solid posterior lobe of the pituitary (p. 1883). Because of the foreshortening of the human skull and face, the pituitary gland lies immediately beneath the hypothalamus rather than posterior to it, and the infundibulum may be angled forward, downward or backward. Around the base of the infundibulum is the *median eminence*, demarcated by a shallow tubero-infundibular sulcus. The tuber cinereum also has a pair of *lateral eminences* which mark the lateral tuberal nuclei, and a small median postinfundibular eminence.

Hypothalamic divisions and nuclei

The hypothalamus contains a number of neuronal groups classified on phylogenetic, developmental, cytoarchitectonic, synaptic and histochemical grounds into named nuclei, many of which are not very clearly delimited, especially in the adult. A few large, myelinated tracts are present, but many of the connections are diffuse and unmyelinated, and the precise path of many afferent, efferent, and intrinsic connections is uncertain. The region has been difficult to study, hence its varied terminology (Le Gros Clark et al 1938; 1095

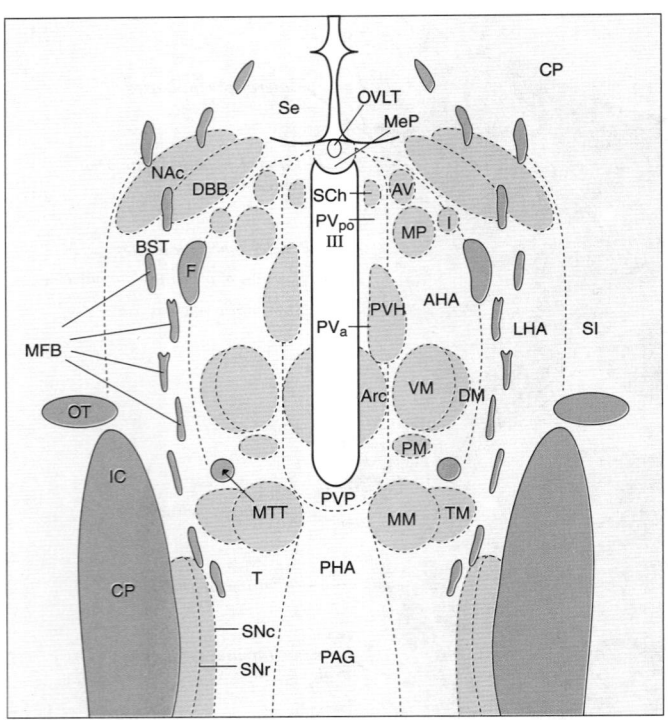

8.211 Schematic horizontal section to show the major cell groups and tracts in and around the hypothalamus. NAc = nucleus accumbens; AH = anterior hypothalamic area; Arc = arcuate nucleus; AV = anteroventral preoptic nucleus; BST = bed nucleus of stria terminalis; CP = caudate nucleus and putamen; DBB = nucleus of diagonal band; DM = dorsomedial nucleus; LHA = lateral hypothalamic area; MB = mamillary body (mainly medial mamillary nucleus); MeP = median preoptic nucleus; MP = medial preoptic nucleus; OVLT = vascular organ of the lamina terminals; PAG = periaqueductal grey; PHA = posterior hypothalamic area; PV = periventricular nucleus (PVpo = preoptic part; PVa = anterior part, PVp = posterior part); PVH = paraventricular (hypothalamic) nucleus; Se = septal cortex; SCh = suprachiasmatic nucleus; T = midbrain tegmentum; TM = tuberomamillary nucleus; VM = ventromedial nucleus; VTA = ventral tegmental area. Fibre tracts (shaded) CP = cerebral peduncle; OT = optic tract; F = fornix; MFB = medial forebrain bundle; MTT = mamillo-thalamic tract. (Modified from Swanson 1991)

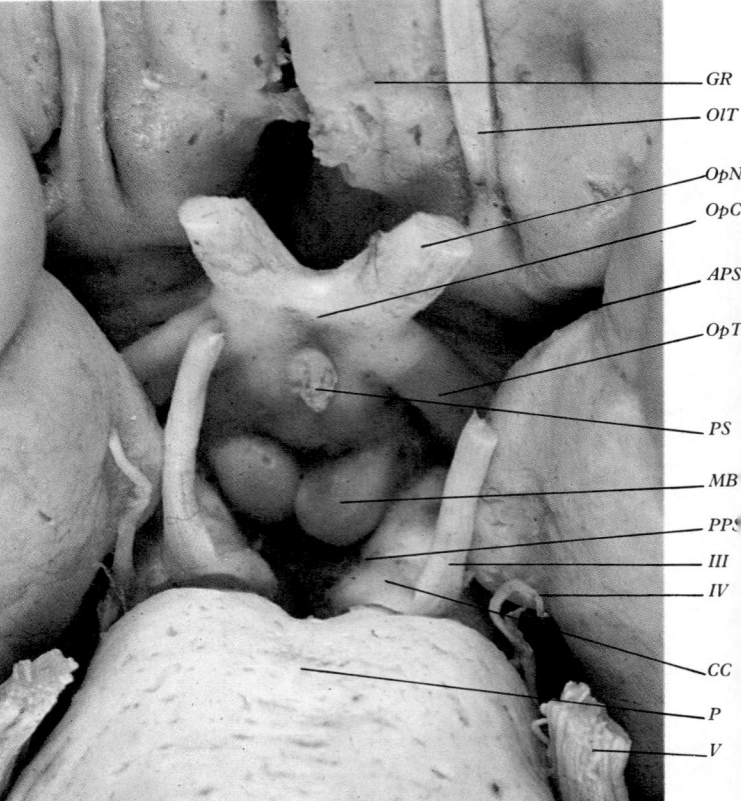

8.212 The interpeduncular fossa and surrounding structures. From above downward note the gyri recti of the frontal lobes (GR), olfactory tracts (OIT); optic nerve (OpN), chiasm (OpC) and tract (OpT); anterior perforated substance (APS); tuber cinereum with attached infundibular stem (pituitary stalk, PS); mamillary bodies (MB); posterior perforated substance (PPS) between the mamillary bodies and diverging crura cerebri (CC); oculomotor (III) and trochlear (IV) cranial nerves; pons (P) and trigeminal nerves (V). (Dissection by E L Rees, photography by Kevin Fitzpatrick, both of the Department of Anatomy, Guy's Hospital Medical School, London.)

Brockhaus 1942). However, the use of histochemical, immunochemical, and hybridization-histochemical methods, with anterograde and retrograde tracer studies (p. 918), is now defining many cell groups and tracts more precisely, showing many similarities with and some differences from those in other animals. Only major nuclei and connections can be described here. More detailed anatomical studies include those of Nauta and Haymaker (1969), Braak and Braak (1987, 1992), Saper (1990) Loewy (1991), Swaab et al (1992).

The hypothalamus can be divided anteroposteriorly into *chiasmatic* (supraoptic), *tuberal* (infundibulo-tuberal) and *posterior* (mamillary) regions, and mediolaterally into *periventricular, intermediate (medial),* and *lateral* zones (Saper 1990). Between the intermediate and lateral zones is a paramedian plane which contains the prominent myelinated fibres of the column of the fornix, the mamillothalamic tract and the fasciculus retroflexus. For this reason, some authors group the periventricular and intermediate zones as a single medial zone. These divisions are, of course, artificial and functional systems cross them. The main nuclear groups and myelinated tracts are illustrated in **8**.210, 211, 213, 214.

Periventricular zone. This borders the third ventricle. In the anterior wall of the ventricle are the *vascular organ* (OVLT, *organum vasculosum) of the lamina terminalis* which is continuous dorsally with the *median preoptic nucleus* and *subfornical organ.* On each side in the chiasmatic region are part of the *preoptic nucleus,* the small *suprachiasmatic nucleus,* and periventricular neurons medial to and blending with the paraventricular nucleus. In the tuberal region the periventricular cell group expands around the base of the third ventricle to form the *arcuate nucleus* overlying the median eminence.

In the posterior region, the narrow periventricular zone is continuous laterally with the posterior hypothalamic area and behind that with midbrain periaqueductal grey matter. The periventricular zone also contains a prominent periventricular fibre system (p. 1098). In man, the suprachiasmatic nucleus is difficult to define in Nissl preparations but obvious with vasopressin, vasoactive interstitial polypeptide somatostatin or neurotensin immunocytochemistry, and is sexually dimorphic (Essay p. 1106).

Intermediate zone. This contains the best differentiated nuclei: the *paraventricular* and *supraoptic nuclei,* 'intermediate' nuclear groups which show sex dimorphism (see **8**.215), the *ventromedial* and *dorsomedial* nuclei, and the *mamillary body* and *tuberomamillary nuclei.* In the chiasmatic region the large paraventricular nucleus forms a thick sheet of cells that extends upward and posteriorly from near the base of the ventricle to the hypothalamic sulcus. The discrete subnuclei seen in rodents cannot be distinguished, but its parvicellular neurons tend to lie medially, and its magnocellular neurons ventrolaterally (**8**.208). Similar magnocellular neurons form the supraoptic nuclei which lie dorsolateral to the optic tract. The rostral poles of the paraventricular and supraoptic nuclei lie nearly adjacent, but the main part of the supraoptic nucleus diverges laterally with the optic tract while its retrochiasmatic portion lies more medially in the floor of the tuberal region. The paraventricular and supraoptic nuclei are both more heavily vascularized than the surrounding neural tissue. At the tuberal level, the ventromedial nucleus is well defined by a surrounding neuron-poor zone, but the dorsomedial nucleus above it is much less distinct. The *medial mamillary nuclei* which form the bulk of the mamillary bodies are

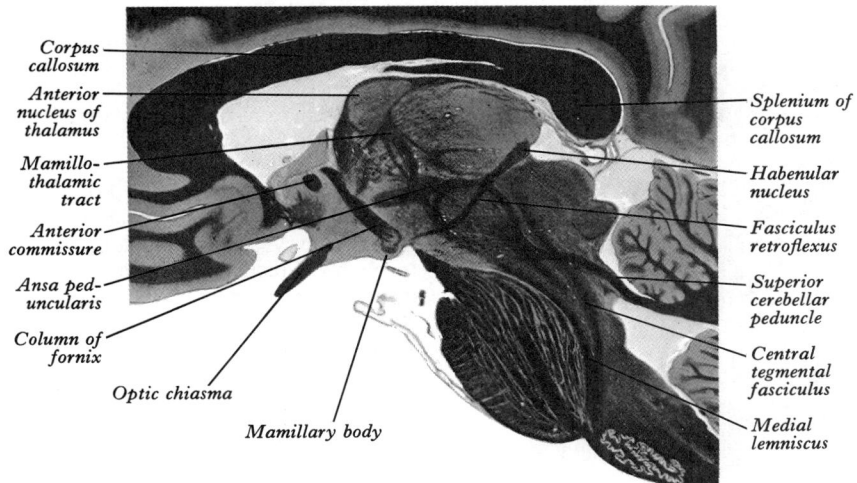

8.213 Sagittal paramedian section of the right cerebral hemisphere through the mamillary body, viewed from the left. Myelin stain. The fasciculus retroflexus is seen crossing medial to the red nucleus, which is surrounded by a capsule of white fibres derived chiefly from the superior cerebellar peduncle. The column of the fornix is seen descending to the mamillary body, and part of the mamillothalamic tract passing to the anterior thalamus is seen above. (After Foix & Nicolescu 1925.)

very prominent in man. There is controversy as to the composition of a lateral mamillary nucleus, though a group of larger cells can be distinguished along the lateral border of the medial mamillary nucleus. Lateral to this, neurons of the *tuberomamillary nucleus* are

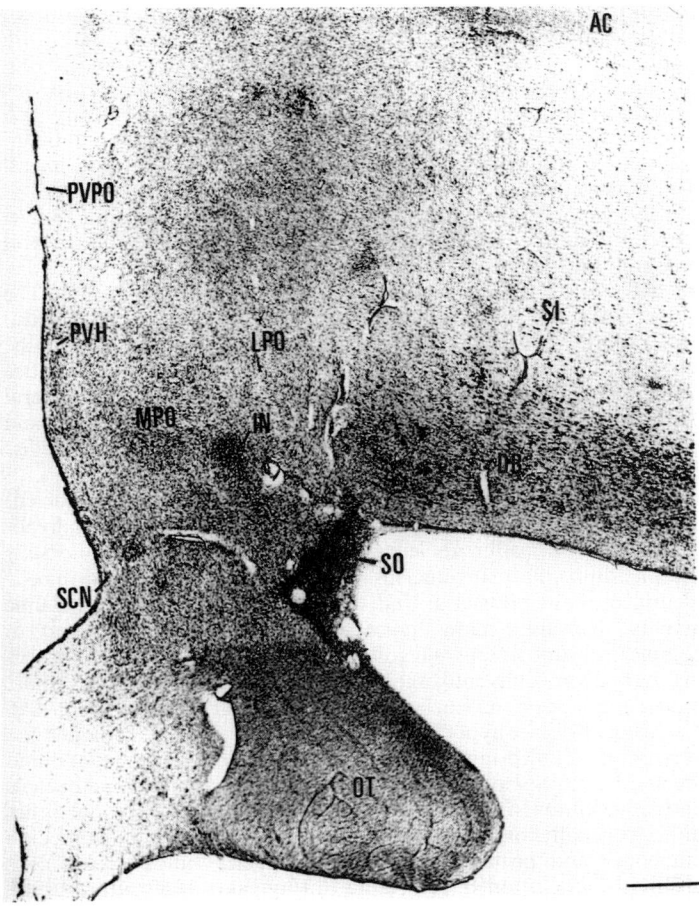

8.214 Nissl-stained coronal section through the tuberal region of the hypothalamus. Anterior commissure AC; nucleus of diagonal band DB; intermediate nucleus IN; lateral preoptic area LPO; medial preoptic area MPO; optic tract OT; periventricular preoptic nucleus PVPO; paraventricular hypothalamic nucleus PVH; suprachiasmatic nucleus SCN; substantia innominata SI; supraoptic nucleus SO. (From Saper 1990 in Paxinos G, The Human Nervous System, Academic Press with permission)

characterized immunocytochemically by their content of histamine, γ-aminobutyric acid (GABA) and galanin. Like the monoamine neurons of the locus coeruleus and raphe, they give rise to widespread axons that diffusely innervate the entire cerebral cortex, hypothalamus and brainstem. (The supraoptic and tuberomamillary nuclei were previously included in the lateral zone (Gray's 37th edn.) but are now included in the intermediate zone for functional reasons.)

Lateral zone. This forms a continuum that runs from the preoptic nucleus through the *lateral hypothalamic area* to the posterior hypothalamus. In the tuberal region, the *lateral tuberal nuclei* are large and well defined in man. They are surrounded by fine fibres and bulge the base of the brain; in Huntingdon's chorea they atrophy markedly.

The preoptic, anterior, dorsomedial and ventromedial nuclei all comprise mainly small or medium neurons, whereas the posterior and lateral hypothalamus consists of sparse large neurons scattered amongst smaller ones.

None of these nuclei will be described further here except where they form part of functional systems; for details see the references quoted.

The neuronal somata, axons and the fibre terminals in the preopticohypothalamic region contain in toto (and in many subregions) many different neuromediators, each (within technical limits) having been localized ('mapped') and each with a large and increasing literature. These include: angiotensin II, delta sleep-inducing peptide, dynorphin, enkephalin, endorphin and α melanocyte-stimulating hormone (αMSH), galanin, adrenocorticotrophic hormone (ACTH), vasopressin, oxytocin, gonadotrophin-releasing hormone (GnRH; = luteinizing hormone-releasing hormone LHRH), thyrotrophin-releasing hormone (TRH), somatostatin, corticotrophin-releasing factor (CRF), neurotensin, cholecystokinin (CCK), vasoactive intestinal peptide (VIP), substance P (SP), glycine, glutamate and aspartate, GABA, histamine, serotonin, adrenalin, noradrenaline, dopamine and acetylcholine (ACh). Clearly, it is not possible to describe their locations individually in this volume (for review see Nieuwenhuys 1985). More recently the various receptors for many of these ligands have also been mapped. In addition, functional hypothalamic neuroanatomy has been considerably advanced by the detection of the c-fos mRNA and protein, which is rapidly switched on when some neural systems are activated.

CONNECTIONS OF THE HYPOTHALAMUS

The hypothalamus has afferent and efferent connections with the rest of the body via two quite distinct routes: neural connections, and the bloodstream (and probably also the cerebrospinal fluid; CSF).

Some hypothalamic neurons have specific receptors which sense

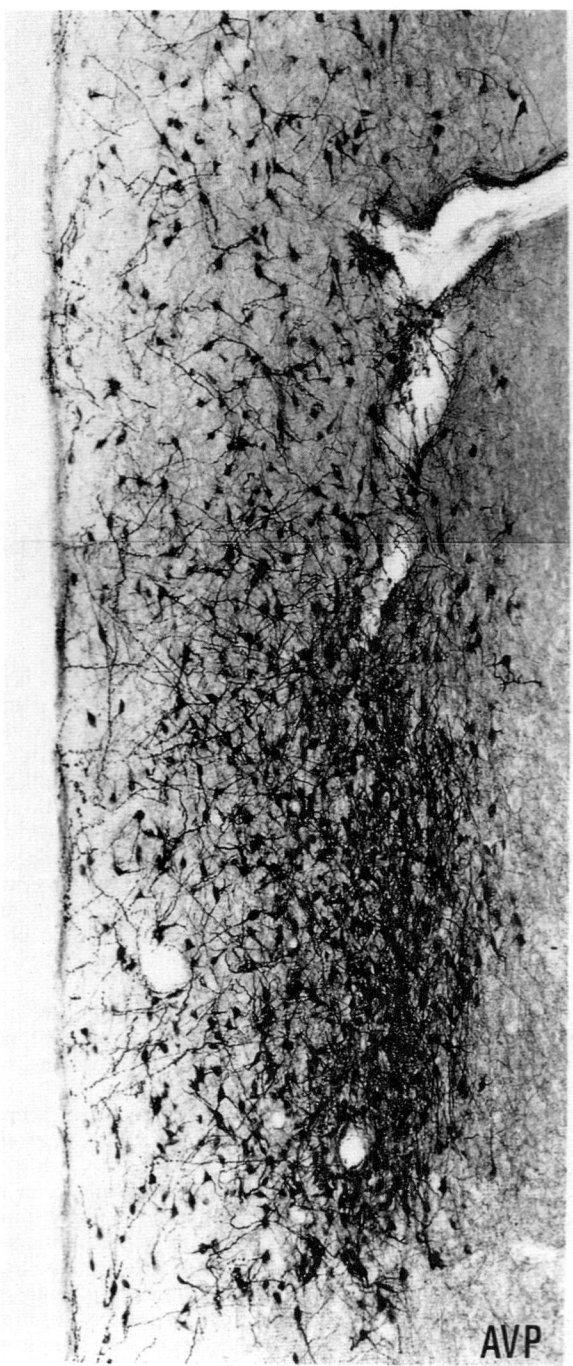

8.215 Human paraventricular nucleus; the vasopressin immunostained neurons form a cluster in the ventrolateral part of the nucleus. (From Saper 1990 in Paxinos G, The Human Nervous System, Academic Press with permission.)

the temperature, osmolarity, glucose and free fatty acid, and hormone content of the blood; and neurosecretory neurons secrete into the blood neurohormones which control the anterior pituitary and act on organs such as the kidney, breast, uterus and blood vessels. Some of its neural connections, especially those to the mamillary bodies, form discrete myelinated fascicles but most are diffuse, unmyelinated and uncertain in origin and termination except where they can be defined chemically in humans and/or by (anterograde and retrograde) tracer methods in animals. Most pathways are multisynaptic so that the majority of synapses on any neuron type are derived from hypothalamic interneurons.

Broadly, neural inputs to the hypothalamus are derived from the ascending visceral and somatic sensory systems, the visual and olfactory systems, and numerous tracts from the brainstem, thala-

mus, 'limbic' structures and neocortex. Efferent neural projections are reciprocal to most of these sources; in particular they impinge on and control the central origins of peripheral autonomic nerve fibres. The hypothalamus therefore exerts control via the autonomic and endocrine systems and through its connections to the telencephalon.

Afferent connections

From the spinal cord and brainstem the hypothalamus receives visceral, gustatory and somatic sensory information. It receives largely polysynaptic projections from the nucleus tractus solitarius (probably directly and indirectly via the parabrachial nucleus and medullary noradrenergic cell groups (ventral noradrenergic bundle)), collaterals of lemniscal somatic afferents (to the lateral hypothalamus), and projections from the dorsal longitudinal reticular formation. Many enter via the *medial forebrain bundle* (**8.**211) and *periventricular fibre system*; others converge in the midbrain tegmentum, forming the *mamillary peduncle* to the mamillary body.

Direct projections reach the hypothalamus from ipsilateral and contralateral subthalamic nuclei and zonae incertae, and perhaps from the thalamic dorsomedial nuclei via periventricular fibres.

The major forebrain inputs to the hypothalamus are derived from structures often grouped as the *limbic system* (p. 1115), including the hippocampal formation, amygdala and septum, and also from the piriform lobe and adjacent neocortex (Rolls 1985). These connections, which are reciprocal, form prominent fibre systems: the *fornix*, *stria terminalis*, and *ventral amygdalofugal tracts*.

The *hippocampal formation*, in particular the subiculum and CA1 (p. 1114) is reciprocally connected to the the hypothalamus by the fornix (p. 1129), a complex tract which also contains commissural connections. As the fornix curves ventrally towards the anterior commissure it is joined by fascicles from the cingulate gyrus, indusium griseum and the septal areas, then divides around the anterior commissure into pre- and postcommissural parts. The precommissural fornix distributes to the septum and preoptic hypothalamus. The septum in turn sends numerous fibres to the hypothalamus. The postcommissural fornix passes ventrally and posteriorly through the hypothalamus to the medial mamillary nucleus, giving in its course many fibres to the medial and lateral hypothalamic nuclei.

The *amygdala* (p. 1131) innervates most hypothalamic nuclei anterior to the mamillary bodies. Its corticomedial nucleus innervates preoptic and anterior hypothalamic areas and the ventromedial nucleus; the central nuclei project to the lateral hypothalamus. The fibres reach the hypothalamus by two routes. The short ventral amygdalofugal path passes medially over the optic tract, beneath the lentiform nucleus, to reach the hypothalamus. The long curved stria terminalis runs parallel to the fornix, separated from it by the lateral ventricle, passes through the bed nucleus of the stria terminalis, and is then distributed to the anterior hypothalamus via the medial forebrain bundle.

Olfactory afferents reach the hypothalamus largely via the nucleus accumbens and septal nuclei; most terminate in the lateral hypothalamus. Visual afferents leave the optic chiasm and pass dorsally into the suprachiasmatic nucleus. No auditory connections have been identified, though it is clear that such stimuli influence hypothalamic activity. However, many hypothalamic neurons respond best to complex sensory stimuli, suggesting that sensory information reaching the neocortex has converged and been processed by the amygdala, hippocampus and neocortex (Jones & Powell 1970; Rolls 1985). Neocortical corticohypothalamic afferents to the hypothalamus are very poorly defined in primates, but probably arise from frontal and insular cortex. Some may relay in the mediodorsal thalamic nucleus and project into the hypothalamus via the periventricular route, other direct corticohypothalamic fibres may end in lateral, dorsomedial, mamillary and posterior hypothalamic nuclei, but all these connections are questioned (see Nauta & Haymaker 1969; Saper 1990).

Like the rest of the forebrain, the hypothalamus also receives diffuse aminergic inputs from the locus coeruleus (noradrenaline), and raphé nuclei (5-HT). In addition, it receives: a cholinergic input from the ventral tegmental ascending cholinergic pathway; a noradrenergic input to dorsomedial, periventricular, paraventricular, supraoptic and lateral hypothalamic nuclei from the ventral tegmental noradrenergic bundle; dopamine fibres from the mesolimbic dopaminergic system (p. 1193); group A11 innervates the medial hypothalamic nuclei, and groups A13 and A14 supply the dorsal and rostral hypothalamic nuclei. Many of these fibres also run in the medial forebrain bundle.

The medial forebrain bundle (**8**.211) is actually neither medial nor a bundle. Rather, it is a loose grouping of fibre pathways which run mostly longitudinally through the lateral hypothalamus, connecting forebrain autonomic and limbic structures with the hypothalamus and brainstem, receiving and giving small fascicles throughout its course. It contains many different classes of fibre: descending afferents from the septal area and orbitofrontal cortex, ascending afferents from the brainstem, efferents from the hypothalamus (see below) and numerous chemically defined pathways. Indeed, the medial forebrain bundle contains many neuromediators including: acetylcholine, dopamine, noradrenaline, adrenaline, serotonin, histamine, SP, VIP, CCK, neurotensin, CRF, GnRH, somatostatin, ACTH and enkephalin (Nieuwenhuys 1985).

Efferent connections

Hypothalamic efferents in primates have been studied rather more than its afferents. They include reciprocal paths to the limbic system, descending polysynaptic paths to autonomic and somatic motor neurons, and neural and neurovascular links with the pituitary.

Septal areas and the amygdaloid complex have reciprocal hypothalamic connections along the paths described above. The medial preoptic and anterior hypothalamic areas give short projections to nearby hypothalamic groups. The ventromedial nucleus has more extensive projections which pass via the medial forebrain bundle to the bed nucleus of the stria terminalis, basal nucleus of Meynert, central nucleus of the amygdala, and midbrain reticular formation. The posterior hypothalamus projects largely to midbrain central grey matter. Some tuberal and posterior lateral hypothalamic neurons project directly to the entire neocortex and appear to be essential for maintaining cortical arousal, but the topography of these projections is unclear. Most of the hypothalamocortical projection cells appear to contain cholinesterase but not choline acetyltransferase (CAT). In addition, many of the tuberal lateral hypothalamic cells also contain an αMSH-like peptide, and the tuberomamillary neurons contain histamine, GABA, galanin and brain natriuretic peptide. The transmitter in the posterior lateral hypothalamic group is not known. These cholinesterase-positive hypothalamocortical neurons selectively undergo neurofibrillary degeneration in Alzheimer's disease.

Hypothalamic neurons projecting to autonomic motor neurons are found in the paraventricular nucleus (oxytocin and vasopressin neurons), perifornical and dorsomedial nuclei (atrial natriuretic peptide neurons), lateral hypothalamic area (αMSH neurons), and zona incerta (dopamine neurons). These fibres run through the medial forebrain bundle into the tegmentum, ventrolateral medulla and dorsal lateral funiculus of the spinal cord. In the brainstem, fibres innervate the parabrachial nucleus, nucleus ambiguus, nucleus of the solitary tract and dorsal motor nucleus of the vagus. In the spinal cord, they end on sympathetic and parasympathetic preganglionic neurons in the intermediolateral column. Both oxytocin and vasopressin fibres can be traced to the most caudal spinal autonomic neurons.

The medial mamillary nucleus gives rise to a large ascending fibre bundle which diverges into: a *mamillothalamic tract* (**8**.211, 213, and see p. 185) which ascends through the lateral hypothalamus to reach the anterior thalamic nuclei, whence massive projections radiate to the cingulate gyrus (p. 1114); and a *mamillotegmental tract*, which curves inferiorly into the midbrain ventral to the medial longitudinal fasciculus and is distributed to tegmental reticular nuclei. Small mamillosubthalamic fascicles reach the subthalamic prerubral field; their destinations are uncertain.

Neuroendocrine connections of the hypothalamus with the pituitary gland

The concept of neurosecretion, in which neurons secrete their bioactive products into the perivascular space around capillaries rather than into synaptic clefts, is now entirely accepted although when first proposed it was roundly opposed (see Scharrer & Scharrer 1940). Neurosecretory neurons were first discovered through their structural characteristics and the affinity of magnocellular neurosecretory neurons for Gomori's chromalum-haematoxylin stain (Bargmann 1949). This revealed the cell bodies and axons with a beaded appearance. The largest irregular distended masses of neurosecretory material in the axons in the neurohypophysis are termed Herring bodies. Subsequent experiments involving transection of the axons in the infundibulum, hypophysial transplantation, culture of neurohypophysial explants, autoradiography with labelled cysteine, fractionation and extraction with biological, chemical, and immunoassays, the effects of dehydration, drugs and stress, chemical and electrical stimulation and ablation of focal points, electron microscopic, immunocytochemical and hybridization histochemical analyses, and electrophysiological recording have all demonstrated the essential elements of neurosecretion. Neurosecretory peptides are synthesized as precursors on the rough endoplasmic reticulum in the neuronal somata, packaged with proteolytic enzymes into neurosecretory granules by the Golgi complexes, transported in the granules along the axons by fast axonal transport, then released by exocytosis as a result of the electrical activity of the neurons generating calcium influx at terminals, and absorbed into adjacent capillaries. The perivascular nerve terminals also contain 50 nm microvesicles of uncertain function; they do not appear to contain a neurotransmitter, but may act in the control of intraterminal calcium. Neurosecretory peptides are very similar throughout mammals, so that antisera raised against them can be used to identify homologous cell groups in different species, including man.

Nerve fibres from hypothalamic neurosecretory neurons end on blood vessels throughout the median eminence, infundibulum and posterior lobe. Those ending in the posterior lobe secrete vasopressin and oxytocin into the inferior hypophysial capillary plexus which drains directly into the systemic circulation. Those ending in the median eminence and infundibulum secrete peptides and amines which regulate the anterior pituitary into the superior hypophysial capillary plexus which drains via the long and short portal veins into the vascular sinusoids among the endocrine cells forming the anterior lobe of the pituitary (p. 1883 and **8**.230). The anterior lobe receives no major nerve supply (though some fibres of hypothalamic origin and uncertain function have recently been described in mammals (Ju & Liu 1989). Almost all its blood comes from the hypothalamohypophysial portal vessels in which the predominant flow is from median eminence and infundibulum to anterior lobe. However, flow reversal may occur, allowing anterior pituitary and other blood-borne hormones access to the hypothalamus through the median eminence, which lacks a blood–brain barrier (see below).

The neurons which secrete vasopressin and oxytocin into the systemic vessels of the posterior lobe are large magnocellular neurosecretory neurons with extensive rough endoplasmic reticulum. Golgi zones and very large numbers of 160 nm secretory granules, particularly in the extensive dilated terminal arborizations of the neurosecretory axons in the posterior lobe. Magnocellular neurons are found in the supraoptic and paraventricular nuclei, and in groups of neurons which lie between them. This reflects the phylogenetic origin of these two nuclei from a single nucleus in amphibia.

The neurons which secrete the peptides and amines which control the anterior lobe have an essentially similar morphology but are smaller—parvocellular neurosecretory neurons—because much less peptide needs to be produced to achieve an equivalent concentration in the small volume portal venous circulation. Compared with magnocellular neurons they are rather more widely distributed within the hypothalamus but are situated mainly in the medial zone, in the arcuate nucleus, medial parvocellular part of the paraventricular nucleus, and periventricular nucleus.

The activity of neurosecretory systems is now known to be much more complex than the secretion of a single active product at their axonal terminal:

- Neurosecretory neurons have simple dendritic trees, and the peptides that they secrete can be found not only in their axons and somata, but also in their dendrites. There is now evidence that the release of vasopressin and oxytocin is not restricted to their perivascular axonal terminals, but also occurs from many parts of the dilated axons, and from the dendrites and somata, exerting local effects in the hypothalamus (Morris & Pow 1990; see Plasticity in the adult hypothalamus p. 1107).
- Neurosecretory neurons may also give axon collaterals which form classical synaptic boutons and synapses in the hypothalamus.

- Nearly all neurosecretory neurons have been shown to cosecrete more than one active compound. In general, these copackaged peptides are produced in much smaller quantities than the main peptide and probably exert paracrine or autocrine effects at the site of their release.
- Neurosecretion is controlled not only by the synaptic input to the cells, but also by the glia that surround their somata, dendrites and terminals.

It should also be remembered that the peptides released by neurosecretory neurons are not restricted to such neurons, but are also produced by other neurons to be released as neurotransmitters or neuromodulators at classical synapses.

Magnocellular neurosecretion

Magnocellular neurosecretory neurons are located in the *supraoptic nucleus, paraventricular nucleus*, and as isolated clusters of cells between (8.214). The supraoptic nucleus, curved over the lateral part of the optic chiasm, has a uniform population of large neurons which may form three subgroups. Behind the chiasm, a thin plate of cells in the floor of the brain forms its retrochiasmatic part. Supraoptic neurons all appear to project to the neurohypophysis. The paraventricular nucleus extends from the hypothalamic sulcus downward across the medial aspect of the column of the fornix, its ventrolateral angle reaching towards the supraoptic nucleus. Its neurons are more diverse: magnocellular neurons projecting to the neurohypophysis tend to lie laterally, parvocellular neurons projecting to the median eminence and infundibulum lie more medially and intermediate-sized neurons, which may project caudally, lie posteriorly. The axons of the paraventricular magnocellular neurons pass toward the supraoptic nucleus (paraventriculohypophysial tract) where they join axons of supraoptic neurons to form a supraopticohypophysial tract which runs down the infundibulum superficially, and into the neural lobe where the axons are distended and branch repeatedly around the capillaries. Vasopressin and oxytocin are produced by separate neurons. Vasopressin neurons tend to cluster in the ventrolateral part of the paraventricular nucleus (8.215), with the oxytocin cells around them, but the cells are much less tightly grouped than in rats.

If data from other mammals can be extended to man, the vasopressin neurons are themselves osmosensitive, receive osmosensory afferents from the median preoptic nucleus and subfornical organ, and receive cardiovascular afferents from brainstem noradrenergic neurons. They are excited by glutamate, acetylcholine, angiotensin II and α2-adrenergic inputs, and inhibited by GABA. The vasopressin is synthesized as part of a precursor which also contains a neurophysin (which binds the hormone in the granule) and a glycopeptide of unknown function. In addition to vasopressin, the neurons cosecrete smaller amounts of other peptides (dynorphin, galanin, CCK, peptide histidine isoleucine (PHI), and TRH in amounts that vary with the physiological state. Oxytocin is produced with its neurophysin from a precursor that is very similar but lacks a glycopeptide moiety. It is co-secreted with smaller amounts of enkephalins, CCK, CRH, galanin, dynorphin and TRH, and its neurons receive excitatory polysynaptic afferents from the nipple, uterine cervix and vagina for the milk-ejection and Ferguson reflexes (see below). The neurons are excited by glutamate and oxytocin, and inhibited by GABA and opioid peptides. Stress causes the release of vasopressin but inhibits the release of oxytocin.

Parvocellular neurosecretion and control of the anterior pituitary

Parvocellular neurosecretory neurons lie within the periventricular zone, in particular the medial *parvocellular part* of the *paraventricular nucleus* (see above), and the *arcuate (infundibular)* nucleus. Their peptide-containing neurosecretory granules are smaller (80–100 nm) than those of the magnocellular neurons; their perivascular nerve terminals also contain 50 nm microvesicles, and are also partly surrounded by astrocytic processes. The arcuate nucleus is median in the postinfundibular part of the tuber cinereum, extending forward into the median eminence and almost encircling the infundibular base, but not meeting anteriorly, where the infundibulum adjoins the median part of the optic chiasm. Its numerous neurons are all small and round in coronal section, oval or fusiform in sagittal

section. No glial layer intervenes between the nucleus and the ependymal tanycytes lining the infundibular recess of the third ventricle. (For the neuroendocrine role of tanycytes see Joseph & Knigge 1978; Everitt & Hökfelt 1986.) Afferents controlling the parvocellular neurons have to be inferred largely from studies in rodents, and secretion of releasing factors cannot be measured in man. However, circadian variation in the secretion of all anterior pituitary hormones suggests that suprachiasmatic nucleus projections must reach parvocellular neurosecretory neurons, afferents from the limbic system probably mediate the widespread effects of stress, and serotonin and noradrenalin from the brainstem influence the output of most anterior pituitary hormones. The afferent control may be exerted either by influencing electrical activity synaptically via the soma/dendrites or by influencing release from the axonal terminals. The axons of parvocellular neurons converge on the infundibulum, forming a *tubero-infundibular* tract ending on the capillary loops which form the hypophysial portal vessels.

Neurons producing *growth hormone-releasing hormone* (GHRH) are largely restricted to the arcuate nucleus, some extending dorsally into the periventricular nucleus and laterally into the retrochiasmatic area. Their fibres run through the periventricular region to the neurovascular zone of the median eminence. The neurons receive afferent information from glucose receptors in the ventromedial nucleus, and inputs from the hippocampal/amygdala/ septal complex could explain release of growth hormone (GH) during stress. In man, midline defects such as septo-optic dysplasia are associated with defective growth hormone secretion. Central dopamine probably has a stimulatory effect, and Levodopa (L-dopa) and bromocriptine cause release of growth hormone.

Neurons producing *somatostatin* (-14 and -28; growth hormone release-inhibiting hormone) are located in the periventricular nucleus. GHRH and somatostatin are secreted in intermittent (3–5 hour) reciprocal pulses, but the origin of the pulses is unclear. A large pulse of GH is secreted at the onset of slow wave sleep. Somatostatin also inhibits release of pituitary thyroid-stimulating hormone (TSH).

Neurons producing GnRH and projecting to the median eminence are also located in the periventricular and arcuate nuclei. Other GnRH neurons are found in the periventricular preoptic area but these appear to project to the vascular organ of the lamina terminalis. Luteinizing hormone (LH) and follicle-stimulating hormone (FSH) are secreted in circhoral pulses which are stimulated by GnRH and are influenced by central monoamines, GABA, by oestrogen and progesterone acting indirectly through other neurons, and by corticotrophin-releasing factor, and endogenous opioids.

Corticotrophin-releasing hormone (CRH) neurons are located primarily in parvocellular paraventricular neurons. They are profoundly stimulated by neurogenic (limbic input) and hypoglycaemic (ventromedial nucleus) stress, and are also controlled by negative feedback by cortisol. Vasopressin facilitates ACTH release, and in rodents is cosecreted with CRH from parvocellular neurons, particularly when plasma cortisol is depleted. ACh appears to stimulate and noradrenalin, 5-HT, GABA, somatostatin-28 and opioids to inhibit centrally the release of ACTH.

Thyrotrophin-releasing hormone (TRH) neurons are rather more widely distributed in the periventricular, ventromedial and dorsomedial nuclei. TRH release is influenced by core temperature, sensed in the anterior hypothalamus, and by negative feedback of thyroid hormones; there is little consensus concerning neurotransmitter control of TRH release. It stimulates release of pituitary TSH and also acts to excite cold- and inhibit warm-sensitive neurons in the preoptic area (see p. 1105).

Other tubero-infundibular arcuate neurons contain neuropeptide Y (NPY) and neurotensin; arcuate neurons containing proopiomelanocortin peptides project to the periventricular nucleus rather than the median eminence.

Some of these peptides have other central motor effects which are related to their neuroendocrine effects. Thus oxytocin is involved in parturition and milk ejection and, when injected centrally, promotes nest building and maternal behaviour. Similarly GnRH facilitates reproductive sexual behaviour.

In addition to these peptide-containing cells, dopamine neurons in the arcuate nucleus (A12 group) have terminals in the median eminence and infundibulum. Dopamine acts as the principal prolactin-inhibiting hormone, and also inhibits secretion of TSH (likewise, TSH acts as a prolactin-releasing hormone). Noradrenergic terminals are also found in the median eminence, where they may act largely in a paracrine manner.

CIRCUMVENTRICULAR ORGANS

The posterior pituitary and median eminence/infundibulum are only two of a series of periventricular neurohaemal organs which lack a blood–brain barrier (McKinley & Oldfield 1980). The vascular organ of the lamina terminalis (OVLT) lies in the lamina terminalis between the optic chiasm and anterior commissure. Its external zone contains a rich fenestrated vascular plexus; deep to this are glia and a network of nerve fibres. The ependymal cells of the vascular organ (organum vasculosum) of the lamina terminalis, like those of other circumventricular organs, are flattened and have few cilia. The major inputs appear to come from the subfornical organ, locus coeruleus and a number of hypothalamic nuclei; some contain GnRH, angiotensin II, somatostatin and atrial natriuretic peptide. It projects to the median preoptic and supraoptic nuclei, binds angiotensin II strongly and is involved in the regulation of fluid balance. The tiny *subfornical organ* lies in the midline at the level of the interventricular foramen. It contains many neurons, glial cells, a dense fenestrated capillary plexus, and is covered by flattened ependyma. In the rat it has widespread hypothalamic connections. Like the vascular organ of the lamina terminalis it binds angiotensin II, has an AII-containing innervation from the lateral hypothalamus, and induces water drinking and vasopressin secretion.

The other circumventricular organs, the pineal gland (p. 1888), subcommissural organ (p. 996) and area postrema (p. 1209) lie outside the hypothalamus.

FUNCTIONS OF THE HYPOTHALAMUS

The nervous system acts to preserve the individual in a changing environment so that the species is maintained. This implies long-term homeostasis of bodily functions, appropriate feeding, drinking and reproductive behaviour, and an ability to respond to and overcome various forms of stress. It also implies control of the growth of the individual to physical and reproductive maturity. Any skeletal motor behaviour is complemented by appropriate changes in autonomic and endocrine functions. Hypothalamic lesions have long been linked with widespread and bizarre endocrine syndromes and with metabolic, visceral, motor and emotional disturbances. It has been assumed that these effects result from interruption of paths or 'centres' which, though independent, are structurally associated in the hypothalamus. The neuroendocrine role of the hypothalamus has gradually emerged during this century (Cushing 1912; Harris 1955; Scharrer & Scharrer 1963; Lightman & Everitt 1986), also the role of the hypothalamus in controlling ('the head ganglion of') the autonomic nervous system (Sherrington 1947; Loewy 1991). However, although many of these systems function reasonably well in the absence of the cerebral cortex, finer aspects of control are missing, and it is now clear that the hypothalamus acts to integrate responses to both internal and external afferent stimuli with the complex analysis of our world provided by the cerebral cortex.

Thus the hypothalamus is only one of a hierarchically arranged set of 'centres' which together provide visceral and somatic control, and reference is often made to lower, intermediate and higher 'centres' of control. The concept of a 'centre' is a functional one, based on the effects of stimulation, lesions and on recording of neural activity. We have seen that, except in a few instances such as the neuroendocrine output neurons, the hypothalamus lacks clearly defined nuclei, and there is an even greater ignorance of the connections of most hypothalamic neurons. Progress in linking what is known of the structural and chemical anatomy of the hypothalamus with the functional data has therefore been difficult. The literature is large and often contradictory, putative 'centres' often overlap and bear little relationship to described cell groups, and many uncertainties remain.

Experimental transections of the nervous system show that, as progressively higher levels are included with the spinal cord below the section, more effective homeostasis is retained. After transection between the cord and medulla there is spinal shock, the blood pressure falls and the bladder and rectum become atonic. As the spinal shock diminishes the blood pressure returns toward normal, the bladder and rectum empty automatically, but there is no co-ordination and minor stimuli may produce a 'mass reflex' with limb withdrawal, sweating, defaecation and micturition. Transections between the midbrain and hypothalamus cause little fall in blood pressure, and basic cardiovascular, respiratory and alimentary reflexes survive. However, normal temperature is not maintained, the reflexes are not integrated with somatic behaviour or emotional affect and there is no anticipation. Provided that the hypothalamus is intact, some circadian variation of endocrine function occurs. Transections above the hypothalamus, separating it from the limbic system but leaving the connections with the pituitary, brainstem, and spinal cord, permit homeostatic responses within a moderate range; these include thermoregulation, resistance to stress, organized visceromotor and endocrine responses, and 'rage' reactions. Some 'motivated behaviour' such as feeding, drinking and even copulation is preserved, but may become abnormally directed. If the connections of the hypothalamus and limbic structures are preserved, homeostasis is preserved in a wide range of adverse conditions. Although these studies do throw light on the functions of the various areas, lesions in humans are almost never so localized.

The hypothalamus controls the *endocrine system* in a variety of ways: through magnocellular neurosecretory projections to the

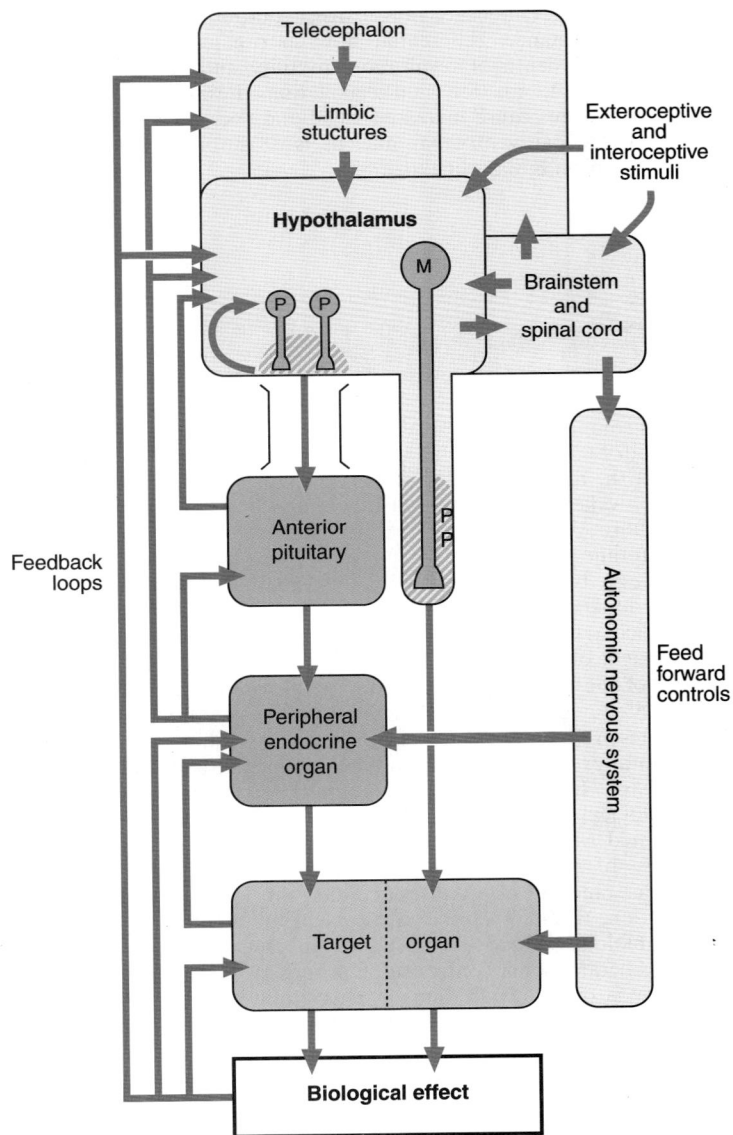

8.216 Scheme to show the ways in which the hypothalamus controls the autonomic and endocrine systems and is itself controlled by exteroceptive and interoceptive endocrine and neural stimuli. Note the numerous feedback loops which control the systems.

posterior pituitary; through parvocellular neurosecretory projections to the median eminence which control the endocrine output of the anterior pituitary and thereby the peripheral endocrine organs; and via the autonomic nervous system. Control through the pituitary has been recognized for many years, but it is now becoming increasingly clear that most peripheral endocrine glands also receive autonomic nerve fibres which modulate their activity. The posterior pituitary neurohormones, vasopressin and oxytocin, are primarily involved, respectively, in the control of osmotic homeostasis and various aspects of reproductive function (see below). Through its effects on the anterior pituitary (see above) the hypothalamus influences the thyroid gland (TSH), adrenal cortex (ACTH), gonads (LH, FSH, prolactin), mammary gland (prolactin), and influences the processes of growth and metabolic homeostasis (GH). Every hierarchical level of feed-forward control is also subject to feedback control (8.216) either by the hormones involved (e.g. cortisol has effects in the hippocampus, hypothalamus, and pituitary gland) or by the controlled variable (e.g. plasma glucose influences the secretion of CRH and GH). For further details see Lightman and Everitt (1986).

The hypothalamus influences both *parasympathetic* and *sympathetic autonomic systems*. In general, parasympathetic effects predominate when the anterior hypothalamus is stimulated; sympathetic effects depend more on the posterior hypothalamus. However, this does not imply discrete parasympathetic and sympathetic 'centres'. Stimuli in many different parts of the hypothalamus can cause profound changes in heart rate, cardiac output, vasomotor tone, peripheral resistance, differential flow in organs and limbs, the frequency and depth of respiration, motility and secretion in the alimentary tract, erection and ejaculation. Lesions of the ventromedial nucleus cause increased vagal and decreased sympathetic tone; and the paraventricular nucleus is an important integrative centre (Swanson & Sawchenko 1983).

Biological rhythms

The suprachiasmatic nucleus appears to be the neural substrate for the day–night cycles in motor activity, body temperature, plasma concentration of many hormones, renal secretion, sleeping and waking and many other variables. The nuclei receive glutamatergic afferents from retinal ganglion cells which entrain the rhythm to the light–dark cycle, but they are not essential for the production of the rhythm, which persists in the blind. In animals, some retinal axons also project farther back to the anterior, lateral and arcuate nuclei. The suprachiasmatic nuclei contain many different neurotransmitters including vasopressin, VIP, NPY and neurotensin, and very complex synaptic connections including dendrodendritic synapses. As yet, the mechanism by which the nuclei produce these rhythms is not known. Axons from the suprachiasmatic nuclei pass to many other hypothalamic nuclei including the paraventricular, ventromedial, dorsomedial and arcuate nuclei. For futher details see Moore (1989) and van den Pol and Dudek (1993).

The suprachiasmatic nuclei also influence the activity of preganglionic sympathetic neurons at C8,T1 level. These project to the superior cervical ganglion neurons which, in turn, project to the pineal gland. In the pineal, which contains modified photoreceptors, circadian variation in the postganglionic sympathetic input causes parallel variation in pineal N-acetyltransferase activity and thus pineal melatonin production. The role of the pineal in man is uncertain (see p. 1888), but pineal tumours can influence reproductive development, and administration of melatonin has been advocated to alleviate jet-lag.

In ageing and especially in Alzheimer's dementia there is a marked loss of vasopressin neurons in the suprachiasmatic nucleus (Swaab et al 1993) which may be associated with diminished circadian rhythms and sleep disturbances.

Circadian clocks

It is common experience that the functions of our body show regular, recurrent cycles over the day and night. For example, you are awake and able to read this sentence because your internal clock has defined this time as your active phase. Nevertheless, biological rhythmicity is often overlooked: to the experimentalist and clinician the variation it entails is often thought of as 'noise', complicating analysis of the underlying steady-state. Unfortunately, this view of daily rhythms represents a failure to understand a fundamental property of life in both health and disease. In recognizing the ubiquity of biological rhythms the clinician is confronted with the question of how knowledge of rhythmicity might advance the understanding of disease and its prevention, whilst the principal problem for the biologist is to identify how rhythmicity is generated and controlled. One possibility is that daily rhythms in physiology and behaviour occur in direct response to regular alterations in the immediate social and physical environment. However, under conditions in which the environment is held constant, overt rhythms, from the daily rhythm in body temperature to sleep–wake cycle, continue with a period very close to 24 hours, demonstrating that

the ability to keep time is an endogenous property. This in turn implies the existence of biological clocks, which under conditions of temporal isolation free-run with a periodicity of approximately (Latin *circa-*) one day (Latin *dies*), hence, *circadian*. The accuracy of the circadian clock can be quite remarkable, varying by only 1–2% after several months of isolation. Nevertheless, to be effective in life it has to be synchronized or *entrained* to external time, such that its period is exactly 24 hours and the various rhythms which it drives are held in their most appropriate temporal (phase) relationships. The internal clock thereby enables the body to anticipate, and so prepare for predictable changes in the environment. A major advance of the last 20 years has been to recognize the importance of rhythmicity and to identify the tissues which function as our biological clocks.

Light and rhythms

The definitive characteristic of an endogenous clock is the ability to express a free-running circadian rhythm when isolated from other tissues. In vertebrates, the principal entraining stimulus or *Zeitgeber* (from the German, time-giver) is the light–dark cycle and so it is not surprising that circadian clocks are intimately associated with photoreceptive structures. In lower vertebrates, photoreceptors are expressed

in both the retina and the pineal, and depending upon species, one or other of these tissues when held in culture will express robust, free-running rhythms, e.g. the synthesis of the hormone melatonin. The rhythms can also be synchronized by illumination of the tissues, demonstrating that both the clock and its entrainment pathways are present. The significance of the pineal clock has been demonstrated in sparrows where removal of the gland destroys the circadian pattern of activity and rest, and transplantation of a pineal from a donor restores circadian rhythmicity to the recipient, possibly via the rhythmic release of melatonin. The mammalian pineal also secretes melatonin in a circadian pattern, but it is not a self-sustaining clock, nor is it necessary for the expression of other circadian rhythms. Lesion studies had suggested that the light-entrained clock was contained not in the pineal but within the hypothalamus and with the advent of modern tract-tracing methods it became possible to demonstrate the *retinohypothalamic tract*, a large proportion of which terminates in small, bilaterally paired nuclei immediately dorsal to the optic chiasm; the *suprachiasmatic nuclei* (8.217). Following their identification as a retinal target, lesion studies quickly demonstrated that the integrity of the suprachiasmatic nuclei was critical to circadian function. Their destruction in experimental animals disrupted endocrine and behavioural rhythms, whilst lesions of the suprachiasmatic region in humans lead to a similar syndrome, often presenting as a disordered sleep–wake cycle.

Suprachiasmatic nuclei

Although they each contain only a few thousand neurons, the suprachiasmatic nuclei are remarkable structures. Held in isolation, they express pronounced circadian rhythms of electrical activity, metabolism and the synthesis and secretion of neuropeptides. Even more dramatic was the demonstration that tissue grafts of fetal hypothalamus containing the suprachiasmatic nuclei are able to restore free-running circadian rhythms of activity and rest in arrhythmic, lesioned rodents. Given the precise quality of the restored rhythms, it could be argued that suprachiasmatic grafts are one of the best examples of restoration of function by transplantation into the central nervous system. The definitive test that the grafts of suprachiasmatic nuclei do contain the circadian clock came with the isolation of a mutant strain of hamster, *tau*, with a circadian period of approximately 20 hours in a constant environment. Reciprocal grafting of suprachiasmatic nuclei between wild type and *tau* showed that the restored circadian period always mirrored the genotype of the graft and not of the host, thereby confirming that the clock was in the grafted tissue. This raises the question of how the clock works, and how it communicates its signal to the rest of the body.

In mammals, including humans, the suprachiasmatic nuclei are composed of two principal subdivisions. Retinal fibres terminate in a ventrolateral subdivision, characterized by neurons immunoreactive for vasoactive intestinal polypeptide (VIP). This appears to be a general input zone also receiving afferents from the midbrain raphe and parts of the lateral geniculate nucleus of the thalamus. The dorsomedial subdivision has relatively sparse afferent innervation, and characteristically contains parvocellular neurons immunoreactive for arginine vasopressin (AVP) (8.217A, B). Both VIP- and AVP-immunoreactive fibres course out of the nucleus, but for a structure which regulates such an array of processes, the suprachiasmatic nuclei have surprisingly few efferent connections. Circadian control of the autonomic nervous system (including secretion of melatonin by the pineal) is probably relayed through connections to the paraventricular nuclei of the hypothalamus, but the pathways conveying the signal elsewhere remain unclear. Neurons within the suprachiasmatic nuclei in receipt of direct retinal input do not respond to pattern, movement or colour. Instead, they operate as luminance detectors, responding to the onset and offset of light, and their firing rates vary in proportion to light intensity, thereby synchronizing to the light–dark cycle. In common with other retinal terminal fields, excitatory amino acids are important transmitters in the afferent fibres, and recent studies have revealed a role for both N-methyl D aspartate (NMDA)- and non-NMDA-types of glutamate receptor in photic entrainment of the clock, neurons within the suprachiasmatic nuclei expressing a specific complement of subunits for the NMDA receptor which distinguishes them from the surrounding hypothalamus. Considerable effort is now being applied to understanding the cellular consequences of photic activation within the suprachiasmatic nuclei. An important advance was the finding that presentation of light pulses during the night that would reset the clock also induced the expression of a category of immediate-early genes, e.g. *c-fos*, within the suprachiasmatic nuclei. The induction of these transcription-regulatory factors is spatially specific, occurring only

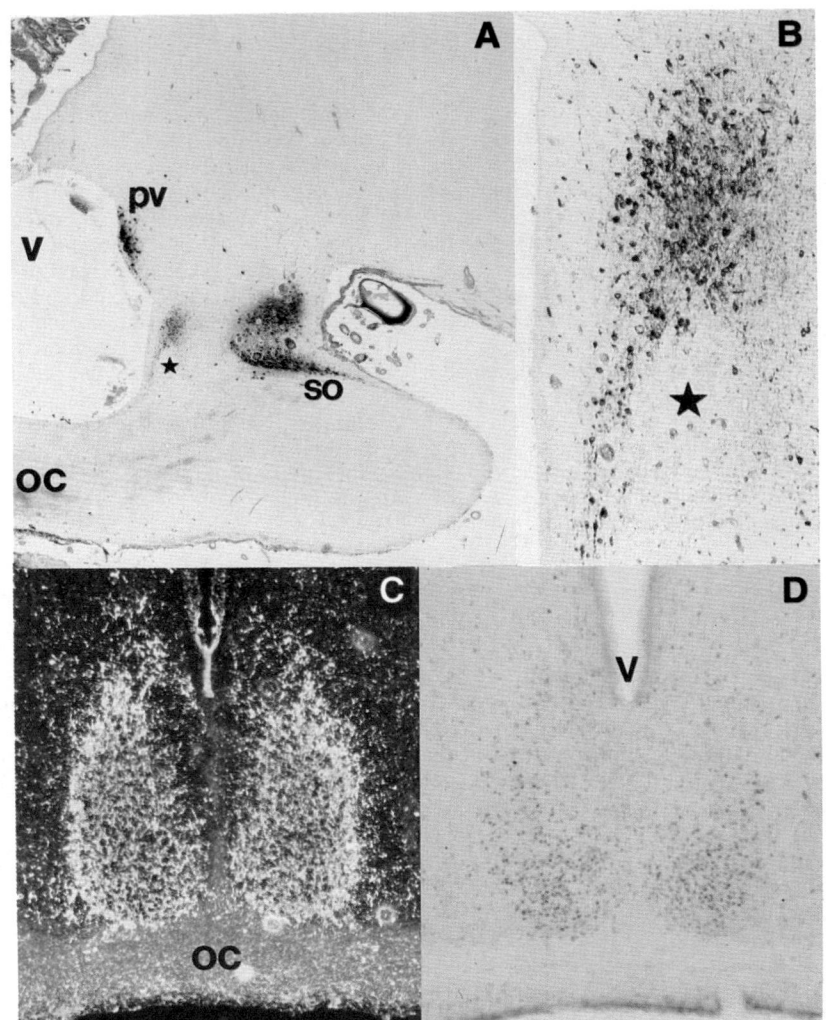

8.217A. Coronal section of human hypothalamus immunostained for arginine vasopressin-neurophysin. oc = optic chiasm; pv = paraventricular nucleus; so = supraoptic nucleus; v = third ventricle. The suprachiasmatic nucleus (SCN) is identified by the asterisk. Material kindly provided by Dr M V Sofroniew, Department of Anatomy, University of Cambridge.
B. Higher power view of the SCN in (A) to illustrate neurophysin-immunoreactive perikarya in the dorso-medial division of the nucleus. The asterisk identifies the ventrolateral subdivision where retinal and other afferent fibres terminate.
c. Dark field view of coronal section of hamster hypothalamus following intraocular injection of cholera toxin tracer, immunostained to reveal the termination of the retinohypothalamic tract within the ventro-lateral suprachiasmatic nuclei.
D. Adjacent section immunostained for Fos protein to identify light-responsive cells of the suprachiasmatic nuclei. Note overlap between Fos-immunoreactive nuclei and the retinal input zone.

in the retinoreceptive zone of the nucleus (**8.217c, d**), and also temporally specific, insofar as light presented at phases of the circadian cycle when it would not reset the clock was ineffective. Identification of the neurochemical inputs, peptidergic phenotype and connectivity of these light-responsive neurons will provide new insights into the neural basis to entrainment.

Non-photic entrainment

In contrast to our knowledge of photic entrainment, understanding of the mechanisms underlying non-photic entrainment is rudimentary. For some time, social interaction and arousal of the individual have been identified as important in synchronizing the human clock, but only recently has the full impact on the clock of non-photic cues been recognized. They may be particularly important during fetal life. The clock starts to oscillate long before retinal fibres grow into the suprachiasmatic nuclei and synaptogenesis is complete. At this stage, synchrony between mother and fetus is established by transplacental signals, including the maternal rhythm of melatonin: an interesting reflection of the role of melatonin in lower vertebrates. The expression of circadian rhythmicity in human neonates has been a topic of debate but recent work has been a shown that under appropriate conditions, circadian rhythms are expressed soon after birth even in preterm infants, a finding which has important implications for the design of facilities for neonatal care. In adults, the loss of synchrony between internal circadian time and the external environment following shift work or transmeridional flights contributes to temporary disorders of cognition and mood. A disruption of circadian timing may also underlie a more intractable pathology, depression. Depressives typically have disordered sleep–wake and endocrine cycles, often with abnormal phase relationships or blunted amplitude. Whether precipitated by life events or spontaneous changes in behaviour (e.g. social withdrawal), changes in non-photic social cues and subsequent circadian dysfunction may be a causal link in the aetiology of some depressive illness.

An important question still to be resolved is whether the clock is a property of individual neurons, or of their networked activities. Evidence from the pineal of lower vertebrates and from unicellular organisms suggests that individual cells may act as circadian oscillators. In mammals, studies in vivo and in vitro using tetrodotoxin to block sodium channels have produced very surprising results: the clock continues to function in the absence of action potentials within the suprachiasmatic nuclei, suggesting that the timing mechanism is divorced from electrical and synaptic activity within the nucleus. Another striking feature observable in the suprachiasmatic nuclei in vitro is the spontaneous generation of rhythmic, high-frequency waves of intracellular concentrations of calcium which are propagated between cells (neurons and glia), probably via gap junctions. Theoretically, a long-period circadian oscillation could be produced by coupled interactions within such a population of high-frequency oscillators. Another suggestion is that the time-keeping process is a self-sustaining transcriptional cycle, a hypothesis consistent with the observation that transcriptional inhibitors can reset the clock, and that phase-shifting by light induces transcriptional-regulators (e.g. the protein c-Fos). To test these, models will require an exhaustive genetic analysis of the clock, but to date only the *tau* hamster and the *clock* strain of mouse provide a good example of a circadian mutation in mammals. In lower organisms a variety of spontaneous and induced mutations of the circadian system have been isolated. In *Drosophila*, mutations of the *per* gene lead to lengthening, shortening or obliteration of circadian periodicity, and although the function and sites of expression of the gene have yet to be characterized in full, it is known that the protein product is able to regulate transcription, including that of its own gene. Whether transcriptional cycles linked to the *per* gene are part of the clockwork remains to be determined. Nevertheless, it is certain that dissection of the clock will rely upon a combination of anatomical and molecular approaches.

Sleep–wake cycle

The alternation of sleeping and waking is a fundamental circadian rhythm. During the waking state electroencephalograms (EEG) show a *desynchronized* low amplitude undulatory activity at about 10 Hz, upon which bursts of irregular activity are superimposed. Four stages and two main types of sleep are recognized. First, the EEG pattern becomes *synchronized*, larger in amplitude and slower. From this 'slow-wave sleep' the subject can be aroused easily, and does not dream. Slow-wave sleep is interrupted by periods of '*paradoxical sleep*' in which muscle tone (especially in the neck) is reduced, but rapid eye movements occur (REM sleep) in conjunction with fast, low amplitude EEG waves; the subject dreams and is difficult to rouse. Three or four episodes of REM sleep occur each night. Much effort has gone into investigating sleep, and sleep patterns are disturbed in many people. It is thought that the level and type of sleep depend on a balance between the activity of the brainstem reticular activating system (p. 1173), which projects to the cerebral cortex and causes wakefulness, arousal, and desynchronization of the EEG, and various hypnogenic (sleep) 'centres' distributed throughout the brainstem. An anterior hypothalamic 'sleep centre' may act by inhibiting the reticular activating system, causing EEG synchronization and behavioural phenomena characteristic of sleep. Certainly, lesions of the anterior hypothalamus are associated with insomnia and lesions of the posterior hypothalamus with hypersomnia. A variety of different transmitters are involved. An intact locus coeruleus, rich in noradrenalin, appears to be important in generation of REM sleep. Serotonin secretion from the midbrain raphe nuclei varies with sleep, and serotonin axons form a prominent projection to the suprachiasmatic nucleus. A hypothalamic peptide (delta sleep-inducing peptide) is very potent in inducing sleep when introduced into the cerebrospinal fluid; CRH appears to suppress slow-wave sleep, consistent with insomnia in stress situations; prostaglandins D2 and E2 appear to have actions, respectively, in the sleep centres of the anterior hypothalamus and the wake centres in the posterior hypothalamus, and benzodiazepines administered to the preoptic area induce sleep, but when administered in the dorsal raphe induce wakefulness. However, despite many studies, we are still far from having either a neuroanatomical or neurochemical understanding of the control of sleep.

Regulation of plasma osmotic pressure, blood volume and water intake

Regulation of the osmotic environment of central neurons is crucial and plasma osmotic pressure is normally regulated very tightly. Hypothalamic osmoreceptors (Verney 1947) in the anterior hypothalamus and including the magnocellular vasopressin neurons themselves (Leng et al 1982) detect as little as 1% increase in the osmotic pressure of the blood and stimulate release of vasopressin from the posterior pituitary. The integrity of the anterior hypothalamus, including the vascular organ of the lamina terminalis and median preoptic nucleus (Renaud et al 1993) is crucial. Peripheral osmoreceptors, probably in the portal vein, contribute to control via the vagus nerve and brainstem. Raised plasma osmotic pressure also stimulates *drinking behaviour*. The vascular organ of the lamina terminalis and subfornical organ are again involved, together with the medial preoptic area. The lack of a blood–brain barrier in these organs allows angiotensin II access to the anterior hypothalamus, and a brain renin–angiotensin system uses angiotensin II as a neurotransmitter in the system. A fall in blood volume or blood pressure of greater than 5–10% also stimulates the release of vasopressin and drinking, via volume receptors in the walls of the great veins and atria and baroreceptors in the carotid sinus. These project via the vagus and glossopharyngeal nerves to the nucleus tractus solitarius and thence, via brainstem monoaminergic pathways, to the magnocellular nuclei. Osmotic and volume signals interact, more vasopressin being released for a given change in osmotic pressure if the blood volume is also diminished. Nausea, pain and emotional stress also cause the release of vasopressin. The osmoreceptor set-point may be abnormal, and a biochemical defect in vasopressin production or interruption of the supraopticohypophysial pathway (e.g. by a head injury) can cause cranial diabetes insipidus. However, after injury this condition may recover as the magnocellular neurons have the ability to regrow axonal terminals toward the blood vessels of the median eminence, creating a new miniature neural lobe. Excessive drinking caused by psychological disturbance has to be differentiated from cranial diabetes insipidus.

Regulation of the cardiovascular system

In addition to controls on blood volume, the hypothalamus exerts marked effects on the cardiovascular centres of the medulla. Stimulation of almost any part of the hypothalamus causes cardiovascular changes, making analysis of the control mechanisms difficult. Stimulation of the anterior hypothalamus and paraventricular nucleus can cause decreased blood pressure and in some experiments decreased heart rate. Stimulation of the lateral hypothalamic area has similar effects, but influences primarily the coronary circulation. The posterior hypothalamus used to be thought of as a pressor region; more recent experiments have shown small depressor responses (Loewy 1991) but stimulation of the tuberomamillary nuclei raises blood pressure and heart rate (Atkins & Bealer 1993).

Temperature regulation

In all homeothermic animals production and loss of heat are balanced, the hypothalamus providing a central thermoreceptor and controlling the autonomic, endocrine and metabolic responses to a change in core temperature. Raised temperature induces heat loss by cutaneous vasodilatation, sweating, panting and depressed heat production; lowered temperatures provoke the opposite changes with shivering and, if prolonged, increased thyroid activity. Central thermoreceptors are located in the preoptic area; these respond to the temperature of the blood perfusing the hypothalamus. Peripheral thermoreceptor afferents and limbic afferents also reach thermosensitive areas, but the central receptors override peripheral information if the two are contradictory. Hypothalamic neurons in the same region react to various bacterial and toxic pyrogens; cytokines appear to act on the vascular organ of the lamina terminalis. Central prostaglandins are important in this reaction (Rothwell 1992), hence the use of aspirin to lower body temperature. Stimulation in the anterior hypothalamus induces panting, sweating and vasodilatation and thus heat loss, via projections which pass through the medial forebrain bundle to autonomic centres in the brainstem and cord; projections to the ventromedial hypothalamus conjointly regulate food intake. Damage to the anterior hypothalamus, as in surgery for suprasellar extensions of pituitary tumours, can result in an uncontrollable rise in body temperature (Clar 1985). Stimulation in the posterior part of the hypothalamus induces sympathetic arousal with vasoconstriction, piloerection, shivering and increased metabolic heat production. The motor 'centre' for shivering is in the dorsomedial posterior hypothalamus (Stuart et al 1961). Experiments suggest that there are no thermoreceptors in the posterior region, so that both heat loss and heat conservation appear to be controlled from the more anterior thermoreceptors. Central catecholamines appear to stimulate heat loss, and central serotonin to stimulate heat production and conservation.

Regulation of food intake and metabolism

Most animals regulate their food intake to maintain a stable body weight despite considerable changes in energy expenditure. In humans, obesity and eating disorders are common and may be linked with stress and emotional disturbance; much feeding behaviour is socially conditioned and food intake increases if more varied food is available. The complex balance between energy intake and expenditure involves many factors: eating behaviour, autonomic control of the alimentary tract and pancreas, and endocrine control via growth hormone, the thyroid, and glucocorticoids, all of which are influenced by the hypothalamus. The ventromedial nucleus contains neurons receptive to plasma levels of glucose and other nutrients and receives visceral somatic afferents via the nucleus tractus solitarius; the lateral hypothalamus receives olfactory afferents which act as important food signals; and both receive extensive inputs, from limbic structures. Stimulation and lesion experiments, together with human case studies, suggest that the ventromedial nuclei act together as a 'satiety centre'. Bilateral ventromedial nucleus damage promotes over-eating (hyperphagia) and restricting food intake may provoke rage-like outbursts. The resultant obesity is usually coupled with hyposexuality (Fröhlich's syndrome). Interestingly, in infants, ventromedial damage can lead to emaciation despite apparent normal feeding (Carmel 1985). Experimental lesions in the lateral hypothalamus promote hypophagia or aphagia and stimulation there can prolong feeding. Thus the concept of a lateral hypothalamic 'feeding centre' arose. Although re-evaluation of the effects of electrolytic lesions has been necessary, more recent studies support the involvement of the lateral and ventromedial areas and also the paraventricular nucleus in the control of feeding but many refinements of the initial concepts have been required (Robbins 1986). Neurochemically, serotonin, CCK and CRF appear to decrease, and noradrenaline-$\alpha 2$ and NPY to promote food/carbohydrate intake. This may be related to an apparent decrease in serotonin activity in anorexia and a blunting of 5HT responses in bulimia.

The ventromedial nucleus, lateral hypothalamic area and paraventricular nucleus also influence intermediate metabolism through the autonomic and endocrine systems. These appear to complement the effects on feeding behaviour. Thus, ventromedial stimulation facilitates glucagon release and increases glycogenolysis, gluconeogenesis and lipolysis, whereas lateral hypothalamic stimulation causes insulin release and opposite metabolic effects (see Shimazu 1986). A high-calorie diet also promotes increased basal metabolism through release of TRH and thus increased thyroid hormone action.

Sexual behaviour and reproduction

The hypothalamus is essential for the control of pituitary oxytocin, gonadotrophin and prolactin secretion. The release of oxytocin from neurosecretory nerve terminals in the neurohypophysis induces contraction of the uterus at term, and of myoepithelial cells surrounding the mammary gland alveoli. Two neuroendocrine reflexes are involved: stretching of the cervix of the uterus during childbirth stimulates a multisynaptic afferent pathway that passes via the pelvic plexus, anterolateral column and brainstem to the magnocellular oxytocin neurons (the Ferguson reflex); the milk ejection reflex involves stimulation of the intercostal nerves of the nipples by suckling, and a similar central pathway. The Ferguson reflex is a positive feedback mechanism terminated by the birth of the child; the milk ejection reflex can be conditioned to a baby's cry, and can be inhibited by stress. In animals central oxytocin also facilitates maternal behaviour.

Gonadotrophin and prolactin secretion are controlled by their respective hypothalamic factors (see above). GnRH is released around birth but is then inhibited by unknown mechanisms until puberty when it is released in a pulsatile manner, first at night and then circhorally. The onset of GnRH secretion at puberty is influenced by body mass, and starvation, like many other types of stress, can disrupt normal GnRH secretion and thus reproductive functions. Many hypothalamic neurons are responsive to sex steroids but their effect on GnRH neurons is apparently indirect. Central GnRH provokes sexual behaviour in animals. Hypothalamic disease can either inhibit reproductive development and function or lead to precocious puberty depending on the nature of the lesion. Prolactin is also released in response to the sucking stimulus, which inhibits the release of dopamine from arcuate neurons. A vast reproductive neuroendocrine literature exists (see Lightman & Everitt 1986; Knobil & Neill 1988, 1994).

Hunger, thirst, and the urge to reproduce are all strong elementary drives which require an intact hypothalamus. However, their full integration into behaviours such as searching out food, drink, and mates, home-building and the rearing of young also requires the neocortex, in particular the limbic system. In man the massive development of the neocortex and limbic structures means that these have a proportionally much greater influence on hypothalamic function than in lower animals.

1105

Hypothalamic dimorphism in relation to gender and sexual orientation

Sex differences in the human brain have been assumed since ancient times but only recently has evidence for them started to emerge. Such differences could result either from differentiation or activation and therefore be, respectively, either irreversible or reversible. Research in animals has, to a certain extent, distinguished between these possibilities and has revealed that the postnatal brain remains plastic in its structure (see also Plasticity in the adult hypothalamus). Most studies on the human hypothalamus necessarily involve correlation of structure post-mortem with gender, sexual orientation and factors such as exposure to sex hormones during life (Swaab et al 1992).

Total adult brain weight is sexually dimorphic (Swaab and Hofman 1984) and numerous sex dimorphisms have been described. One of the first sex hormone-dependent differences to be demonstrated was a difference in the synaptic connectivity in the bed nucleus of the stria terminalis (Raisman & Field 1973). Dimorphic nuclei have been investigated largely in animals, mainly rodents. A classic example is the sexually dimorphic nucleus (SDN) of the rat preoptic area,

which differentiates in early postnatal life under the influence of circulating androgens (converted to oestrogens in the hypothalamus) to become eight times larger in the male than in the female (Gorski et al 1978; Gorski 1985). The putative human homologue of the rat sexually dimorphic nucleus (SDN-POA; intermediate nucleus (Braak & Braak 1987); INAH-1 (Allen et al 1989)) is located between the supraoptic and para-ventricular nuclei at the level of the suprachiasmatic nucleus and contains twice as many cells in men as in women. From birth to 4 years, the number of cells in the SDN-POA increases rapidly in both sexes, but at about 4 years in girls the number of cells starts a decline to 50% of that found in males in whom it remains constant until the age of 50 years. In both sexes, the number of cells declines still further in later life. A similar sex difference has been described for part of the bed nucleus of the stria terminalis (Allen et al 1989) and another interstitial nucleus of the hypothalamus, INAH-3 (LeVay 1991). The suprachiasmatic nucleus differs in shape in men (spherical) and women (elongated) but, interestingly, there is no

difference in the total volume or number of cells (Swaab et al 1992). At present, the functional implications of these sex differences are far from clear, but lesion experiments suggest that the rat sexually dimorphic nucleus has a role in male sexual behaviour.

It has been proposed that an interaction between the developing brain and sex hormones influences sexual orientation and that male homosexuals have a 'female' hypothalamus (Dörner 1988). Anatomical evidence for this is controversial: Swaab and Hofman (1990) did not find the SDN-POA to differ in homosexual and control heterosexual men, but their morphometric analysis did show the suprachiasmatic nucleus in male homosexuals to be almost twice as large as in male heterosexuals. LeVay (1991), however, reports that interstitial nucleus INAH-3 is smaller in homosexual than heterosexual men.

Such is the complexity of human sexual behaviour and the difficulty of obtaining evidence for humans, that understanding the functional relationships between anatomical differences and behaviour presents an enormous challenge for the future.

Response to stress

Stress can be defined as anything which threatens homeostasis (Stress, p. 1139). Given the above, the hypothalamus is clearly essential for orchestrating the body's responses to stresses via the sympathetic nervous system and the endocrine system, in particular the control of the adrenal cortex and medulla (Swanson 1991).

Emotions: fear, rage, aversion, pleasure, reward

An emotional state can be considered to have two main components: a subjective feeling and its objective physical accompaniments, which together form emotional expression. For these, an intact hypothalamus, limbic structures and frontal neocortex appear to be essential. It is clear that much of the autonomic output associated with different emotional states is profoundly influenced by the hypothalamus, driven by the limbic structures, and some information has been gained by focal stimulation and lesion experiments in animals and by observations of human pathology. Early studies showed that 'sham' rage (hissing, growling, baring of claws and fangs, piloerection, pupil dilatation and other signs of sympathetic arousal) could be elicited in decorticate dogs and cats by mild peripheral stimulation, and could be abolished by obliteration of the posterior hypothalamus. The term 'sham' was used because it was assumed that the emotional feelings could not occur in decorticate animals, and because the reaction subsided almost immediately when the stimulation ceased.

Behaviour can also be thought of as being driven by subjectively perceived 'rewards' and the existence of positive and negative 'reward' centres has been postulated. Thus, when hungry, ingestion of food produces through taste, gastric filling, and a rise in blood glucose pleasurable sensations of positive reward, but ingestion of something

that tasted unpleasant would be aversive (negative reward). Through such mechanisms we learn what stimuli lead to positive reward and which to avoid. Indeed, emotions have been defined as 'states elicited by reinforcing stimuli' (Rolls 1990). A stimulus may produce a positive reward in one situation and a negative reward in another—ingestion of food would produce a negative reward if the stomach is already overdistended. Experiments to detect such 'reward centres' have involved the placement of stimulating electrodes in different regions of the brain, with the animal able to activate the stimulation by pressing a bar in its cage. When electrodes are placed in certain locations ('pleasure centres', 'positive reward centres') an animal will self-stimulate until exhausted, ignoring food and drink even after prolonged deprivation. The main regions which support such self-stimulation include parts of the catecholaminergic complex of the brainstem, the medial forebrain bundle of the hypothalamus, and septal, orbitofrontal and entorhinal neocortex (Rolls 1975; Olds 1976). The most effective of these is the median forebrain bundle (see above) with its multiple ascending and descending systems and neurotransmitters. The ventral (limbic) striatum, substantia innominatum and nucleus accumbens (Nucleus accumbens dopamine reward and addiction, p. 1137) have also been implicated (Murray 1991). Stimulation of these areas in man can cause sensations of well-being, with sometimes strong erotic content. Stimulation of the posterior hypothalamus can cause sympathetic arousal and may be associated with negative 'reward'; experimental animals actively avoid repeatedly stimulating such areas. The neurochemical basis for these effects is not known, but dopaminergic paths ascending from the substantia nigra pars compacta may be important (Routtenberg & Santos Anderson 1977) and pharmacological manipulation of brain monoamines is widely used clinically to manipulate mood.

Plasticity in the adult hypothalamus

Cajal's view that 'in adult centres, the nerve paths are something fixed, ended, immutable' has profoundly influenced neuroanatomical thinking for many decades. Now, however, there is a considerable body of evidence that, at least in some systems, the arrangement of neurons and glia, neuronal dendritic trees, synaptic connections, and receptors expressed by the neurons are all subject to quite marked function-related changes (Theodosis & Poulain 1993). The evidence has been derived largely from studies in rodents, but there is no reason to believe that the general principles do not also apply to humans.

In the hypothalamic magnocellular nuclei, during parturition and lactation when the release of oxytocin is increased, the hypertrophied magnocellular oxytocin neurons and their dendrites form extensive neuron–neuron contacts without the intervening astrocyte lamellae which separate the neurons in the resting system. In addition, an increased number of γ-aminobutyric acid (GABA-ergic) synaptic boutons contact two adjacent oxytocin soma, or dendrites ('shared synapses') and the number of GABA-ergic synapses upon oxytocin neurons increases (Hatton & Tweedle, 1982; Theodosis et al 1986a). The number of terminals making axosomatic contacts also increases in aged animals in which many magnocellular neurons are hyperactive (Silverman & Sladek 1991). Adjacent vasopressin neurons do not, however, show these changes. The plasticity is not restricted to the somata and dendrites but, when hormone release is increased, the neurosecretory nerve terminals in the neural lobe also become less surrounded by processes of the astrocyte-like pituicytes and thereby make more contact with the perivascular basal lamina. The changes are rapid: synaptic plasticity in the hypothalamus occurs within 48 hours of the stimulus, and release of terminals from pituicyte envelopment within 1 hour. The soma/dendrite changes appear to be caused by intrahypothalamic release of oxytocin (Theodosis et al 1986b) from dendrites of the oxytocin neurons (Pow & Morris 1989) or oxytocin synapses, whereas the neurohypophysial plasticity involves β-adrenergic stimulation. Similar plastic changes occur in the system of gonadotrophin-releasing hormone (GnRH) neurons and their terminals in the median eminence and probably other releasing factor neurons. The rapidity of synapic plasticity is well illustrated in the arcuate nucleus, where oestrogen-receptive neurons become more ensheathed in astrocytic glial lamellae and the number of axosomatic GABA synapses on them decreases markedly on the day when oestrogen increases during the 4-day reproductive cycle (Olmos et al 1989).

Oestrogen also modifies the structure, size and synaptic organization of ventromedial hypothalamic neurons, causing an increase in axodendritic synapses and in the density of dendritic spines (Frankfurt & McEwen 1991), and causes a redistribution of oxytocin receptors on the neurons (McEwen et al 1990).

These few examples suggest that rapid and substantial changes in the synaptic, receptor, and neuron/glia organization may be widespread within the adult hypothalamus and probably play an important role in modulating its control mechanisms.

TELENCEPHALON

Expansion of the telencephalon and development of the cerebral hemispheres are described in page 1147. In earlier vertebrates each hemisphere is predominantly concerned with olfactory signals, entering it rostrally at the *olfactory lobe*. This lobe is elongated as an *olfactory bulb* connected to the hemisphere by an *olfactory tract*. Basally in each hemisphere masses of grey matter, *basal nuclei*, form early motor centres. The wall of the hemisphere is the *pallium*, where olfactory and other information are presumably integrated. During evolution visual, auditory and other paths have extended through the thalamus to the cerebral pallium, an instance of encephalization. Each hemisphere is thus enlarged by an additional *neopallium*, the largely olfactory pallium being confined to a *piriform lobe*, sited inferolaterally. The hemisphere's medial wall becomes specialized as the *hippocampal formation*, long regarded as primarily olfactory, a view now untenable (see p. 1115). In higher mammals the neopallium is greatly enlarged and the piriform lobe relatively reduced; neopallial motor paths develop from it but the basal nuclei remain essential parts of motor control. This mammalian neopallial expansion is largely due to the growth of *association areas* concerned with interaction between afferent and efferent connections. The hippocampal formation is often termed *archipallium* or *primal* cortex and the piriform lobe *palaeopallium* or *ancient* cortex; some, however, group both as *archipallium*.

The telencephalon includes:

- the cerebral hemispheres, their commissures and their cavities
- the anterior part of the third ventricle, including the preoptic regions in the telencephalon impar (p. 1080).

Each cerebral hemisphere has an external stratum of neurons, the *cortex*, an internal mass of neuronal processes (*centrum semiovale*), deeply situated *basal nuclei* and a *lateral ventricle*. The cerebral hemispheres are the largest part of the brain and, viewed from above, have an ovoid shape, broader behind, the greatest transverse diameter being between the parietal tuberosities. They are incompletely separated by a deep median cleft, the *longitudinal cerebral fissure*, each hemisphere containing a *lateral ventricle*.

The longitudinal cerebral fissure. It contains a crescentic fold of the dura mater, the *falx cerebri*, and anterior cerebral vessels; in front and behind, the fissure completely separates the hemispheres; centrally it descends to a large commissure, the *corpus callosum*, connecting the hemispheres.

SURFACES OF THE CEREBRUM

Each cerebral hemisphere presents superolateral, medial and inferior surfaces or aspects.

The *superolateral surface* is adapted to the concavity of its half of the cranial vault. The *medial surface*, flat and vertical, is separated from its fellow by the longitudinal fissure and falx cerebri. The *inferior (basal) surface* is irregular and divided into orbital and tentorial regions; the orbital part of the frontal lobe is concave and lies above the orbital and nasal roofs. The tentorial region is the concavoconvex inferior surface of the temporal and occipital lobes, anteriorly adapted to its half of the middle cranial fossa; posteriorly it is above the tentorium cerebelli which is interposed between it and the superior cerebellar surface.

The surfaces are separated by the following borders:

- *superomedial*, between the superolateral and medial surfaces
- *inferolateral*, between the superolateral and basal surfaces (its anterior part separates the superolateral from the orbital surface in the frontal lobe, as the *superciliary* border)
- *medial occipital*, between the tentorial region of the inferior surface and the medial
- *medial orbital*, separating the orbital region of the inferior surface from the medial.

1107

The anterior and posterior hemispheric extremities are the *frontal* and *occipital poles* respectively; the temporal pole is the anterior extremity of the temporal lobe. About 5 cm anterior to the occipital pole on the inferolateral border is the *preoccipital incisure*.

A paramedian line, from a point a little superolateral to the inion to one just superolateral to the nasion, marks the superomedial margin. The superciliary border is at the level of the eyebrows as far as the zygomatic process of the frontal bone, ascending thence to the pterion. The temporal pole corresponds to a line, convex forwards, on the surface of the head, from the pterion to the midpoint of the upper border of the zygomatic arch; it then continues back above the arch to cross the ear a little above the external acoustic meatus; it corresponds to the inferolateral margin, which then curves down to the posterior end of the superomedial margin (**10.159**).

Hemispheric surfaces are moulded into a number of *gyri* or *convolutions*, separated by *sulci* or *fissures*. This familiar appearance is gradually achieved. Until the end of the third fetal month, the surfaces are smooth, as in the brains of reptiles and birds. Thereafter, localized depressions appear, deepen and extend over the surfaces as sulci (see p. 247). Each sulcus is an infolding of the cortex, increasing the cortical grey matter about three times. Some sulci develop along the zones separating areas differing in details of structure and functions (Le Gros Clark 1945) and may be termed *limiting sulci*. The central is a limiting sulcus, being between two areas differing in thickness enough to be visible to the eye (**8.218**). Some sulci develop in the long axis of a rapidly growing area and are *axial sulci*; the posterior part of the calcarine sulcus is merely a fold in the centre of the striate area. In other sites a sulcus may be between two structurally different areas; but its lip, not its floor, may divide two areas and then a third area may be in the walls of the sulcus without appearing on the surface; such a sulcus is *operculated*, exemplified in the human brain by the lunate sulcus, separating striate from peristriate areas on the surface and containing the submerged parastriate area, which intervenes between them. These varieties include all sulci on the surface, except the lateral sulcus and parieto-occipital sulci; the former results from the slower expansion of the insular cortex with consequent submersion by adjoining areas, which eventually come into contact to delimit the lateral sulcus. The parieto-occipital sulcus is associated with the development of the corpus callosum. The posterior end of this commissure conveys not only fibres from the occipital lobes but also a large number from the temporal lobes. Hence, several smaller axial and limiting sulci are crowded together and some are buried in the walls of the parieto-occipital sulcus. These are really *secondary sulci*, depending on factors other than exuberant growth in the adjoining areas.

Some sulci are deep enough to produce elevations in the ventricular walls; the anterior part of the calcarine sulcus, which thus produces the calcar avis of the posterior cornu, and the collateral fissure, producing the collateral eminence in the inferior cornu, are therefore termed *complete fissures*; but no special morphological or functional significance is attached to the fact that some sulci are complete and others incomplete.

Gyri and their intervening sulci are approximately constant in their general overall arrangement but vary in their dimensions and minor details (or even their occurrence in the smaller cases), not only in different individuals but in the hemispheres of one brain. The gyral pattern is an inevitable result of the greater increase in volume of the pallium or mantle of neurons in the cortex compared with the much smaller increase in the subjacent white matter. The area of the human cortex is about 2200 cm², a third of this being

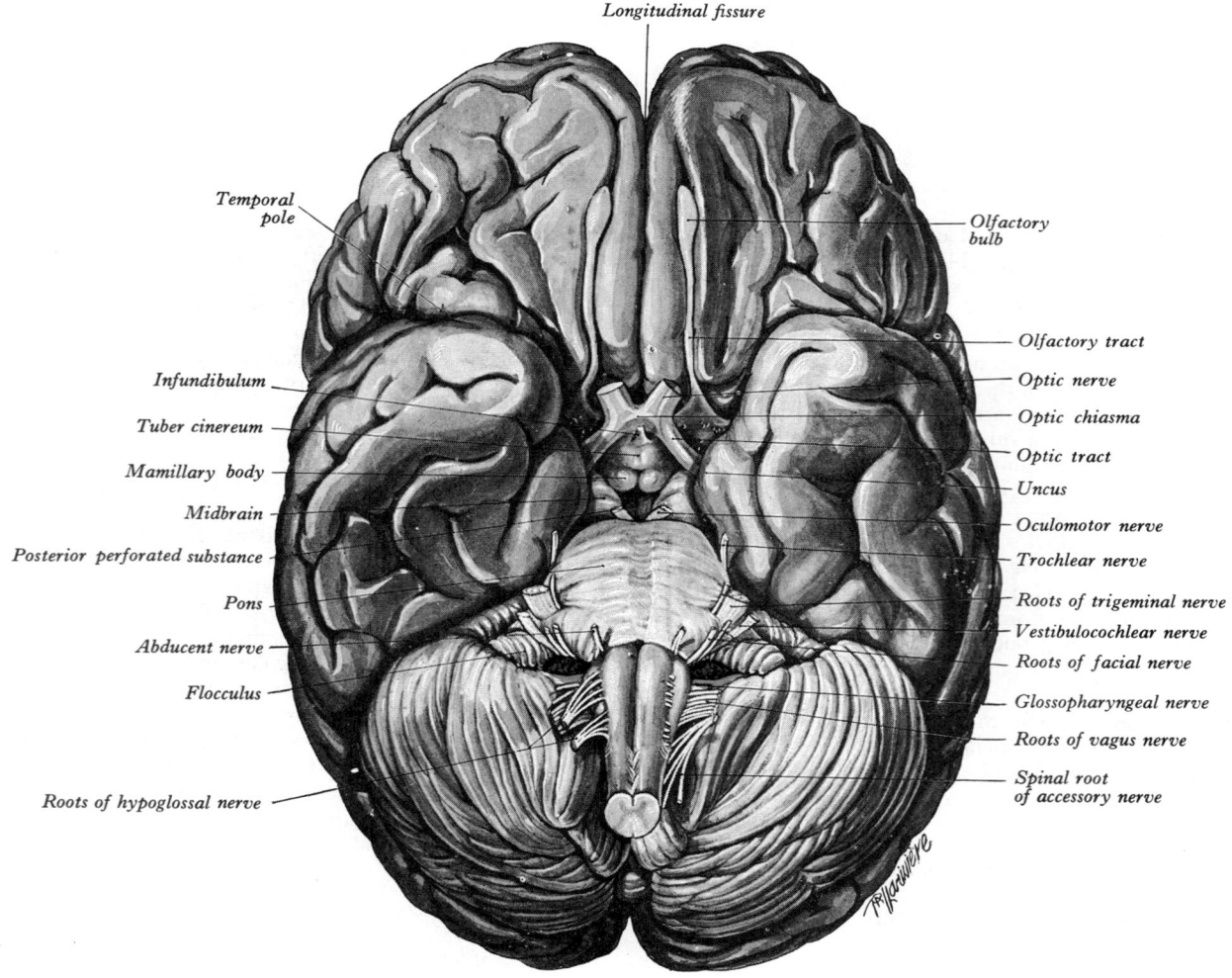

Longitudinal fissure

Temporal pole

Olfactory bulb

Olfactory tract

Infundibulum

Optic nerve

Tuber cinereum

Optic chiasma

Mamillary body

Optic tract

Uncus

Midbrain

Oculomotor nerve

Posterior perforated substance

Trochlear nerve

Pons

Roots of trigeminal nerve

Vestibulocochlear nerve

Abducent nerve

Roots of facial nerve

Flocculus

Glossopharyngeal nerve

Roots of vagus nerve

Spinal root of accessory nerve

Roots of hypoglossal nerve

8.218 Basal aspect of the brain. The anterior perforated substance (unlabelled) is between the diverging lateral and medial roots of the olfactory tract and anterolateral to the optic tract.

visible on the surface while the rest is obscured in the sulci and fissures. By this mode of evolution a large increase in the cortical area entails a lesser change in cranial capacity; but it is misleading to explain the arrangement in this teleological manner. Similarly, a presumed association of high intelligence with great complexity of convolutional pattern is fallacious; the most intricate arrays of sulci and gyri occur in the cerebra of the elephant and whale (Hammelbo 1972), both of which also have larger brains than man, though not so in relation to total size. No close relation between gyral complexity and brain size with cerebral abilities has been established in mankind; abundant examples of highly able individuals with relatively small brains and the reverse of this are attested. Attempts to draw deductions from endocranial casts of fossil forms, as an indication of development of certain gyri and hence abilities (e.g. capacity for speech), have likewise proved misleading and are largely abandoned except by anthropologists.

It is convenient to separate the cerebral hemisphere into a number of lobes but this division is purely descriptive; nor do lobes precisely correspond in surface extent to the cranial bones from which they take their names.

SUPEROLATERAL CEREBRAL SURFACE

Two sulci—the *lateral* and *central*—are the outstanding features of this surface and the main factors used in limiting its surface divisions (**8**.219, 220).

Lateral sulcus

The lateral sulcus is a deep cleft on the inferior and lateral surfaces, and has a short stem dividing into three rami (**8**.219, 220). The *stem* commences inferiorly at the anterior perforated substance, extending laterally between the frontal lobe's orbital surface and the anterior pole of the temporal lobe. It is adapted to the posterior border of the lesser wing of the sphenoid and contains the sphenoparietal venous sinus. Reaching the lateral surface it divides into anterior horizontal, anterior ascending and posterior rami. The *anterior ramus* runs forwards for 2.5 cm or less into the inferior frontal gyrus while the *ascending ramus* ascends for an equal distance into the same gyrus; the *posterior ramus*, the longest, runs posteriorly and slightly up across the lateral surface for about 7 cm, turning up to end in the parietal lobe. Its floor is the limen insulae and insula; it conducts the middle cerebral vessels from the inferior to the superolateral surface. It is represented by a line sloping back and slightly up for about 7 cm from the pterion, then curving up to the parietal eminence.

Central sulcus

The central sulcus (**8**.219, 220) starts in or near the superomedial border a little behind the midpoint between the frontal and occipital poles (i.e. midway between the nasion and inion). It runs sinuously downwards and forwards for about 8–10 cm to end a little above the posterior ramus of the lateral sulcus, from which it is always separated by an arched gyrus. Its general direction makes an angle of about 70° with the median plane (**8**.219, 220). It demarcates the primary motor and somatosensory areas of the cortex (pp. 1154, 1164). When the sulcus is opened up, its opposed walls are seen to be marked by small gyri which alternate like gears in mesh, hence termed *interlocking gyri*. This provides an additional cortex without the corresponding increase in the surface area. About the middle of the sulcus its walls are usually connected by a transverse gyrus; this is due to the mode of development of the central sulcus. When it appears in the sixth month, it is in the superior and inferior parts, at first separated by a transverse gyrus connecting the precentral to the postcentral gyrus. The two occasionally remain separate but usually coalesce, the transverse gyrus being buried as a *deep transitional gyrus*.

Frontal lobe

The frontal lobe, the rostral region of the hemisphere, is limited behind by the central sulcus, above by the superomedial border and below by the superciliary border and stem of the lateral sulcus. Its superolateral surface is traversed by three sulci and four gyri. The *precentral sulcus* is parallel to the central, separated from it by a precentral gyrus and usually divided into upper and lower parts, which may be confluent. The *superior frontal sulcus* curves forwards from about midway in the upper precentral sulcus; the *inferior frontal sulcus* is parallel but at a lower level. The area of the frontal lobe anterior to the precentral sulcus is thus divided into the superior, middle and inferior frontal gyri; an incomplete sulcus often divides the middle gyrus (**8**.219, 220).

The *precentral gyrus*, with the central sulcus posterior and precentral sulcus anterior to it, extends from the superomedial border, where it is continuous with the paracentral lobule on the medial surface, down to the posterior ramus of the lateral sulcus. Its cortex is the origin of many of the fibres of large corticonuclear and corticospinal tracts, in addition to a multitude of other connections.

The *superior frontal gyrus*, above the superior frontal sulcus, is continuous over the superomedial margin with the medial frontal gyrus. It may be incompletely divided (**8**.219, 220). The *middle frontal gyrus* is between the superior and inferior frontal sulci. The *inferior frontal gyrus* is below the inferior frontal sulcus and is invaded by the anterior and ascending rami of the lateral sulcus. The areas around these rami on the left are the *speech area of Broca* (areas 44 and 45), associated with the motor aspects of speech (p. 1183). The region below the anterior ramus is the *pars orbitalis*, curving round the superciliary margin to the orbital surface. The area between the ascending and anterior rami is the *pars triangularis* and that posterior

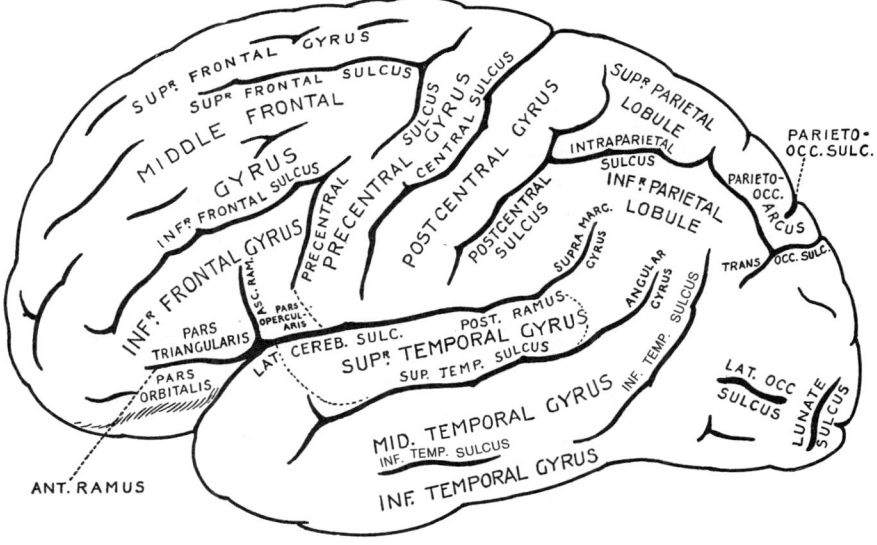

8.219   Lateral aspect of the superolateral surface of the left cerebral hemisphere.

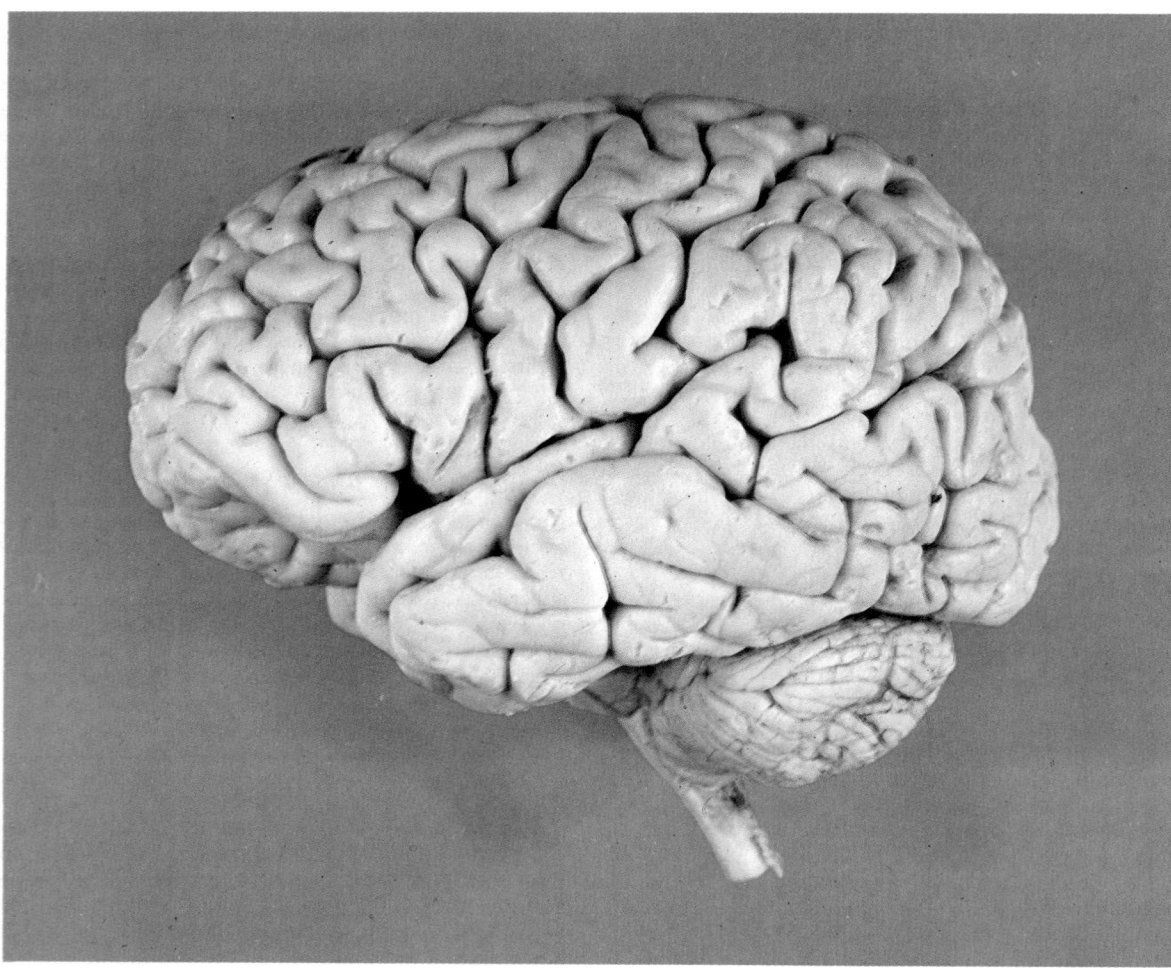

8.220   A left lateral view of the brain to show the pattern of gyri and sulci on the superolateral aspect of the cerebral hemisphere. Compare with **8.219**, which was drawn from a different specimen, for labelling of the many structures visible. Note also the contrasting cortical patterns of the cerebrum and cerebellum. (Dissection by E L Rees, photography by Kevin Fitzpatrick, both of the Department of Anatomy, Guy's Hospital Medical School, London.)

to the ascending ramus is the *pars opercularis* (*posterior*), continuous posteriorly with the inferior end of the precentral gyrus.

Temporal lobe

The temporal lobe is inferior to the lateral sulcus and limited behind by an arbitrary line from the preoccipital incisure to the parieto-occipital sulcus, meeting the superomedial margin about 5 cm from the occipital pole. Its lateral surface is divided into three parallel gyri by two sulci.

The *superior temporal sulcus* begins near the temporal pole and slopes slightly up and backwards parallel to the posterior ramus of the lateral sulcus. Its end curves up into the parietal lobe. The *inferior temporal sulcus* is subjacent and parallel to the superior and often broken into two or three short sulci; its posterior end also ascends into the parietal lobe, posterior and parallel to the upturned end of the superior sulcus.

The lateral surface is thus divided into three parallel *superior*, *middle* and *inferior temporal gyri*. Along its superior margin the superior temporal gyrus is continuous with gyri in the floor of the posterior ramus of the lateral sulcus; these vary in number, extending obliquely anterolaterally from the *circular sulcus* around the insula as *transverse temporal gyri* (**8.221**), usually two (anterior and posterior), but sometimes single on one or both sides (Campian & Minckler 1976). The anterior transverse temporal gyrus and adjoining part of the superior temporal gyrus are auditory in function (p. 1161) and considered to be Brodmann's area 42; the anterior gyrus is approximately area 41.

Parietal lobe

The parietal lobe extends from the central sulcus in front to a lobe

joining the preoccipital incisure to the superomedial margin where it is crossed by the parieto-occipital sulcus. Inferior is the posterior ramus of the lateral sulcus and an imaginary posterior prolongation from its straight part. Parts of its boundaries are thus arbitrary. Its lateral aspect is subdivided into three areas by *postcentral* and *intraparietal sulci*.

The *postcentral sulcus* (**8.212, 213**), often divided into upper and lower parts, is posterior and parallel to the central sulcus. Inferiorly it ends above the posterior ramus of the lateral sulcus some distance in front of its upturned end, dividing the parietal lobe into the postcentral gyrus and a large posterior area, subdivided by the *intraparietal sulcus*, which usually starts in the postcentral sulcus near its midpoint or at the upper end of its lower part. It extends postero-inferiorly across the parietal lobe, dividing it into superior and inferior parietal lobules. Posteriorly, as its *occipital ramus*, it extends into the occipital lobe, joining the *transverse occipital sulcus* at right angles. The *postcentral gyrus* is between the central and postcentral sulci. Its cortex receives somatosensory impulses (p. 1155) and has numerous other connections.

The *superior parietal lobule*, between the superomedial margin and the intraparietal sulcus, is continuous anteriorly with the postcentral gyrus round the upper end of the postcentral sulcus; posteriorly it often joins the *arcus parieto-occipitalis*, surrounding the lateral part of the parieto-occipital sulcus (**8.219, 220**).

The *inferior parietal lobule*, below the intraparietal sulcus and behind the lower part of the postcentral sulcus, is divided into three: the *anterior part* is the *supramarginal gyrus* arching over the upturned end of the lateral sulcus and is continuous anteriorly with the lower part of the postcentral gyrus and postero-inferiorly with the superior temporal gyrus; it may be limited behind by a small *sulcus intermedius*

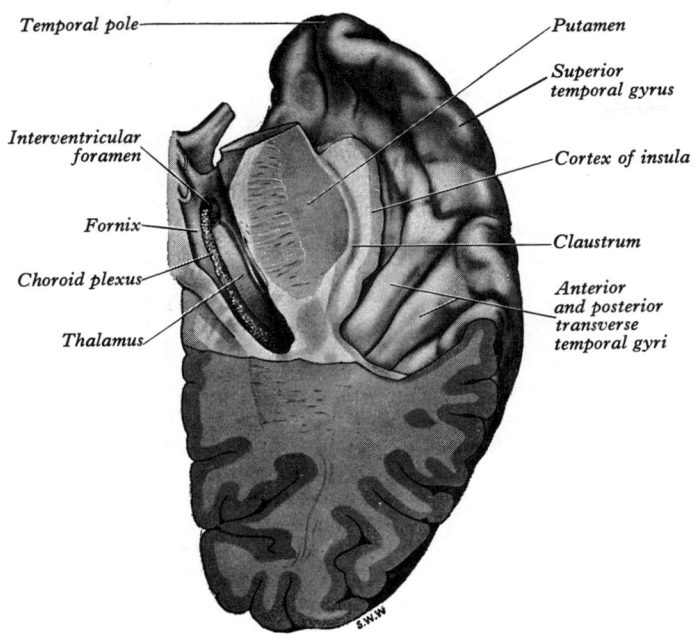

Temporal pole
Putamen
Superior temporal gyrus
Interventricular foramen
Cortex of insula
Fornix
Claustrum
Choroid plexus
Anterior and posterior transverse temporal gyri
Thalamus

8.221   Horizontal section showing the superior surface of the right temporal lobe.

primus descending from the intraparietal sulcus. The *middle* part, the *angular gyrus* (believed to be concerned with the visual element in stereognosis, p. 1158) arches over the end of the superior temporal sulcus and is continuous postero-inferiorly with the middle temporal gyrus; sometimes a small *sulcus intermedius secondus* appears at its posterior end. (Anterior and middle parts of the inferior parietal lobule are subjacent to the parietal tuberosity, p. 593.) The *posterior part* arches over the upturned end of the inferior temporal sulcus on to the occipital lobe, forming an *arcus temporo-occipitalis*.

Occipital lobe

The occipital lobe is behind the arbitrary line joining the preoccipital incisure to the parieto-occipital sulcus. The *transverse occipital sulcus* descends from the superomedial margin behind the parieto-occipital sulcus and is joined about its midpoint by the intraparietal sulcus. Its superior part is behind the arcus parieto-occipitalis, an arched gyrus surrounding the end of the parieto-occipital sulcus. The lateral occipital sulcus, short and horizontal on the lateral aspect of the occipital lobe, divides it into *superior* and *inferior occipital* gyri (**8.**219, 220). The *lunate sulcus*, when present, is just in front of the occipital pole, placed vertically and sometimes joined to the calcarine

sulcus, but the two are more often separate; its lips, which are opercular, separate *striate* from *peristriate areas* but the *parastriate area* is buried in the sulcus between the other two striate areas. The lunate sulcus is posterior to the *gyrus descendens*, which is behind the superior and inferior occipital gyri. Curved superior and inferior polar sulci often appear near the ends of the lunate sulcus. The *superior polar sulcus* arches up on to the medial occipital surface near the upper limit of the lunate sulcus; the *inferior polar sulcus* arches down and forwards on to the inferior cerebral surface from the lunate's lower limit. These polar sulci enclose semilunar extensions of the striate area (p. 1158), indicating the expansion of the visual cortex associated with the large cortical macular area (Smith 1930).

Insula

The insula (**8.**221, 223B), deep in the floor of the lateral sulcus, is almost surrounded by a *circular sulcus* and is overlapped by growth of the adjacent cortical areas and is thus only visible when the lateral sulcus is artificially widely opened; these overlapping areas are therefore termed the *opercula of the insula*, separated by ascending and posterior rami of the lateral sulcus. The *frontal* operculum or *lid* is between the anterior and ascending rami, forming the pars triangularis of the inferior frontal gyrus; it is small when the rami arise by a common stem. The *frontoparietal operculum*, between ascending and posterior rami of the lateral sulcus, is the pars posterior of the inferior frontal gyrus and lower ends of the precentral and postcentral gyri, also the lower end of the anterior part of the inferior parietal lobule. The *temporal operculum*, below the posterior ramus of the lateral sulcus, is formed by superior temporal and transverse temporal gyri. Anteriorly the inferior region of the insula adjoins the pars orbitalis of the inferior frontal gyrus.

When the opercula are removed, the insula appears as a pyramidal area, its apex inferior and near the anterior perforated substance (**8.**222, 223B), where the circular sulcus is deficient and the medial part of the apex is termed the *limen insulae* (*gyrus ambiens*). The *insular surface* is divided into a larger *anterior* and a smaller *posterior* part by the *sulcus centralis insulae*, slanting posterosuperiorly from the apex. The anterior part is divided by shallow sulci into three or four *short gyri*, the posterior being one *long gyrus*, often divided at its upper end. The cortex of the insula is continuous with that of its opercula in the circular sulcus. The insula is approximately coextensive with the subjacent claustrum and putamen (**8.**223, p. 1121, 1123).

The angioarchitecture of the primate insula has been studied by Vlahovitch et al (1973). Despite the development of the opercula in man and their exiguous size in, for example, the baboon or chimpanzee, these observations indicated great similarity of vascular pattern in all primates examined.

MEDIAL CEREBRAL SURFACE

The medial surface (**8.**224, 225) is clearly visible only when the cerebral hemispheres are separated by division of all the commissures

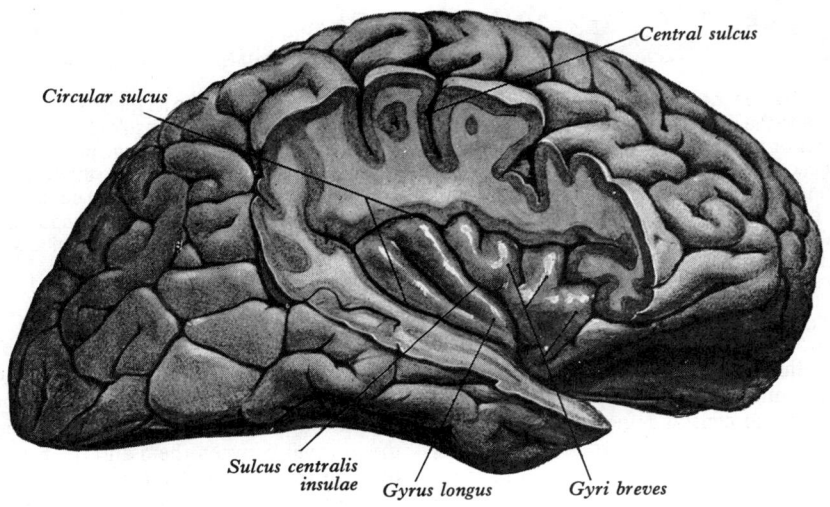

Circular sulcus
Central sulcus
Sulcus centralis insulae   *Gyrus longus*   *Gyri breves*

8.222   The right insula, exposed by the removal of its opercula.

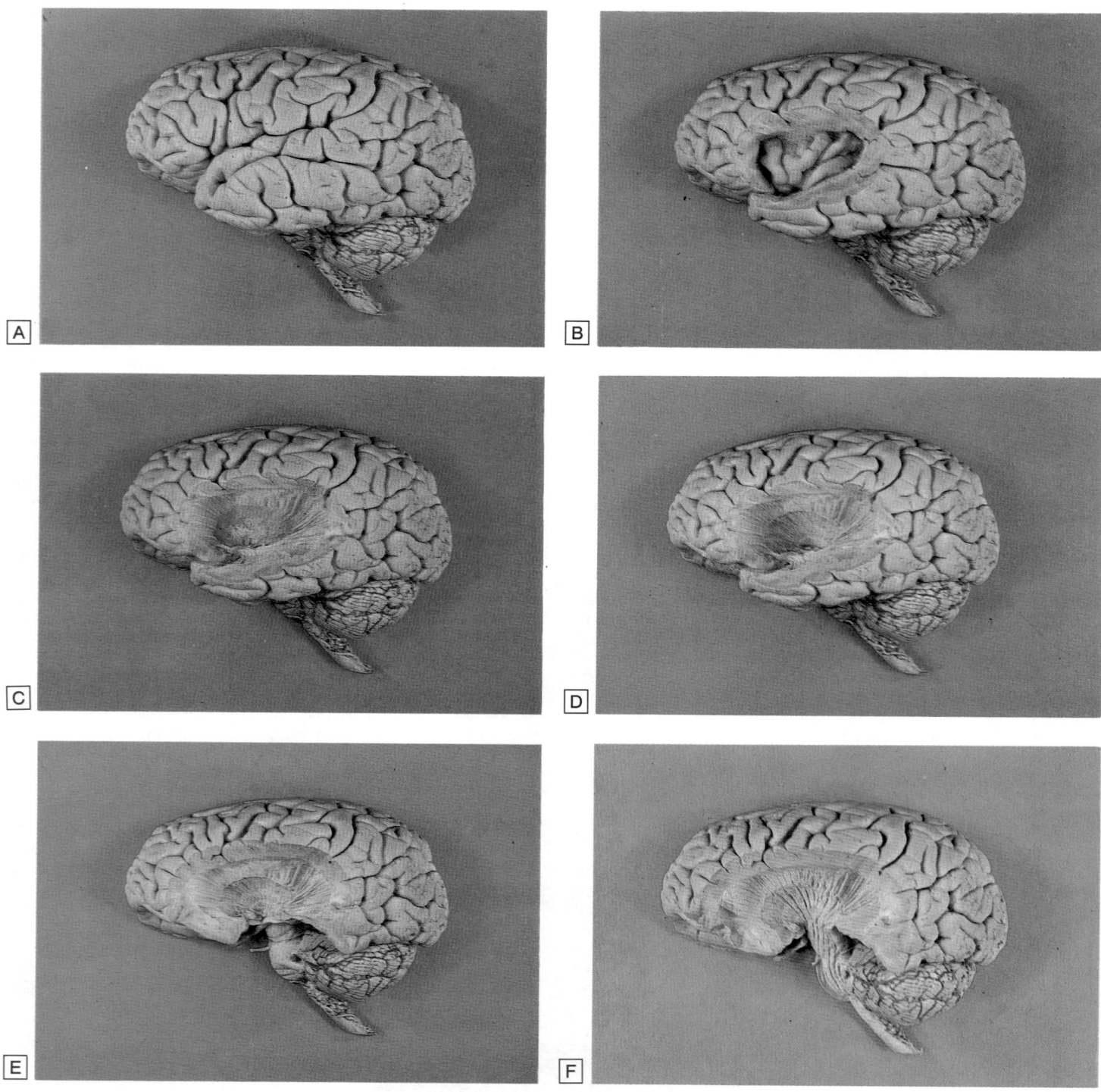

8.223 A series of dissections of the left cerebral hemisphere at progressively deeper levels to demonstrate the insula and subjacent structures: A. the intact brain; note the position of the posterior ramus of the lateral cerebral sulcus on which the dissections are centred; B. the cortical gyri of the insula exposed by removal of the frontal, temporal and parietal opercula; C. the removal of the insular cortex, extreme capsule, claustrum and external capsule has exposed the lateral aspect of the lentiform nucleus (the putamen); D. removal of the lentiform nucleus displays fibres of the internal capsule coursing across its medial aspect; E. removal of part of the temporal lobe shows the internal capsular fibres converging on the crus cerebri of the midbrain; F. removal of the optic tract, and superficial dissection of the pons and upper medulla, emphasizing the continuity of the corona radiata, internal capsule, crus cerebri, longitudinal pontine fibres and the medullary pyramid. (Dissection by E L Rees, photography by Kevin Fitzpatrick, both of the Department of Anatomy, Guy's Hospital Medical School, London.)

and the structures around the third ventricle (**8.289**). The most conspicuous feature is the great commissure, the *corpus callosum*, a broad arched band in the floor of the central region of the longitudinal fissure (**8.202A, B**). Its curved anterior part is the *genu*, continuous below with the *rostrum* and narrowing rapidly as it passes back to the upper end of the lamina terminalis. The genu continues above into the *trunk*, the main part of the commissure, which arches up and back to a thick, rounded posterior extremity, the *splenium*. To the concave surfaces of the trunk, genu and rostrum the bilateral vertical laminae of the septum pellucidum are attached, occupying the interval between them and the fornix, a curved, flat band inferior to it. In front of the lamina terminalis, almost coextensive with it, is a narrow triangle of grey matter, the *paraterminal gyrus* (p. 1129), separated from the rest of the cortex by a shallow *posterior par-*

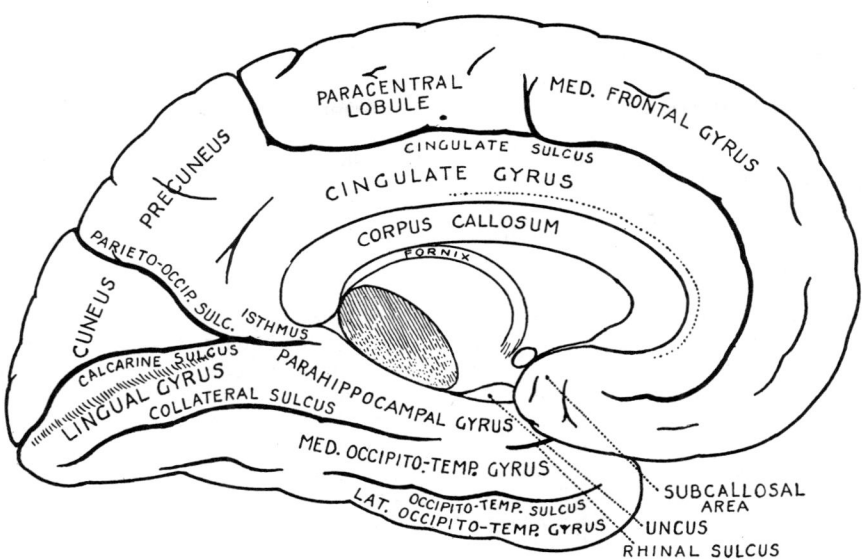

8.224 The medial surface of the left cerebral hemisphere, after sagittal section of the brain and removal of the brain stem.

olfactory sulcus. A little anterior to this a short, vertical sulcus may occur, the *anterior parolfactory sulcus;* the cortex between these two sulci is the *subcallosal area (parolfactory gyrus)* (**8.**202, 222, 230). The anterior sloping edge of the paraterminal gyrus is sometimes called the *prehippocampal rudiment* (p. 1115).

The anterior region of the medial surface is divided into outer and inner zones by the curved *cingulate sulcus,* starting below the rostrum and passing first forwards, then up and finally backwards, con-

forming to the callosal curvature. Its posterior end turns up to the superomedial margin about 4 cm behind its midpoint and is posterior to the upper end of the central sulcus (**8.**140, 145). The outer zone, except for its posterior extremity, is part of the frontal lobe, subdivided into anterior and posterior areas by a short sulcus ascending from the cingulate sulcus above the midpoint of the corpus callosum. The larger, anterior area is the *medial frontal gyrus,* the posterior being the *paracentral lobule.* The superior end of the central

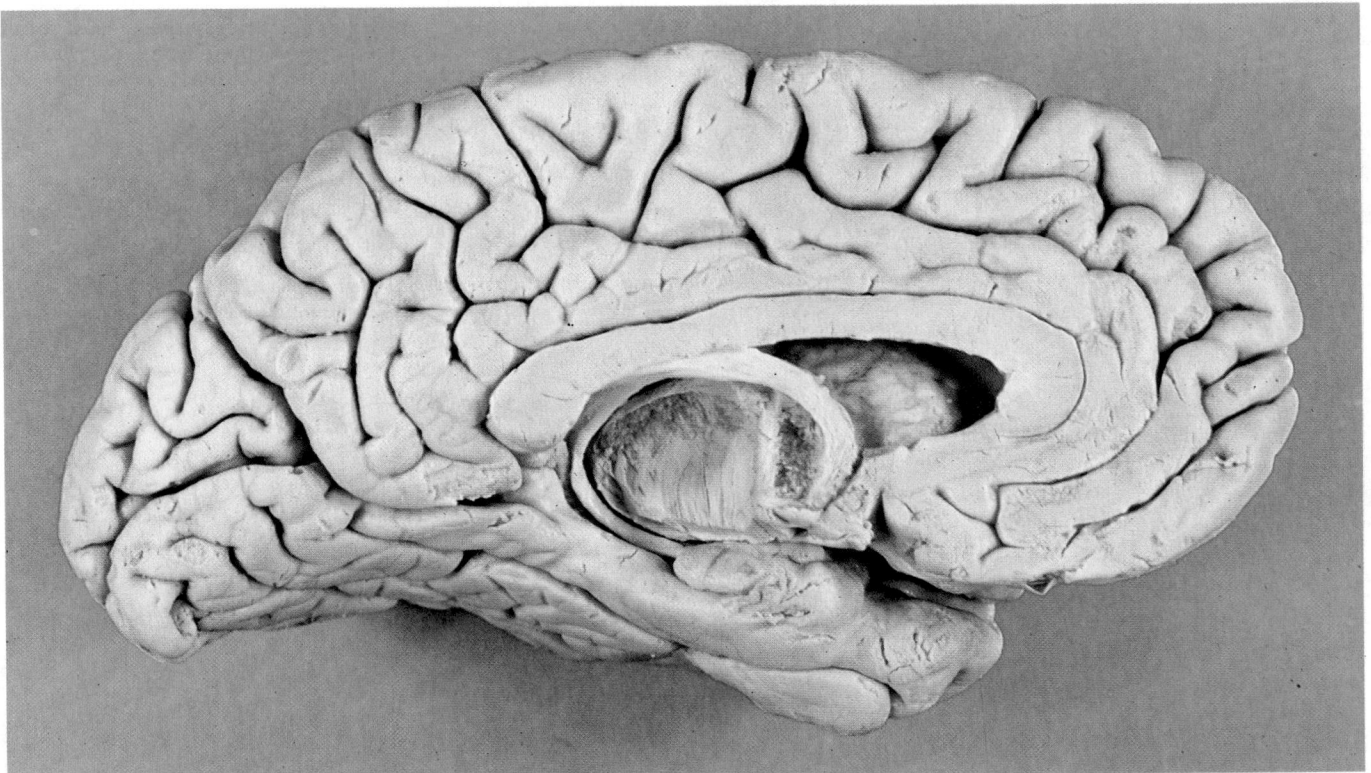

8.225 The medial surface of the left cerebral hemisphere after sagittal section of the brain, followed by removal of the brain stem and septum pellucidum. (For identification of the principal gyri and sulci of the cerebral cortex, compare with **8.**224.) The dissection has been deepened in the region of the dorsal thalamus and hypothalamus to demonstrate the column, body, crus and fimbria of the fornix and the mamillothalamic fasciculus (compare with **8.**228, 229). The head of the caudate nucleus is visible bulging into the floor of the anterior horn of the lateral ventricle. (Dissection by E L Rees, photography by Kevin Fitzpatrick, both of the Department of Anatomy, Guy's Hospital Medical School, London.)

sulcus usually invades the paracentral lobule posteriorly and the precentral gyrus is continuous with the lobule. This area is concerned with movements of the contralateral lower limb and perineal region; clinical evidence suggests that it exercises voluntary control over defaecation and micturition (pp. 1375, 1420).

The zone under the cingulate sulcus is the *cingulate gyrus*. Starting below the rostrum this follows the callosal curve, separated by the *callosal sulcus*, and continues round the splenium to the inferior surface, continuing into the parahippocampal gyrus through the narrow *isthmus* (8.122). The cingulate sulcus is interrupted posterior to the paracentral lobule but partially continued by a variable *subparietal (suprasplenial) sulcus*.

The posterior region of the medial surface is traversed by two deep sulci converging anteriorly to meet a little posterior to the splenium. These are the parieto-occipital and the calcarine sulci. The *parieto-occipital sulcus* starts on the superomedial margin about 5 cm anterior to the occipital pole, sloping down and slightly forwards to the calcarine sulcus. When opened it is clear that the parieto-occipital and calcarine sulci, though on the surface apparently continuous, are separated by the deeply sited *cuneate gyrus*. The walls of the sulcus also show two or more vertical sulci, originally exposed on the medial surface but included in the parieto-occipital sulcus by growth of the splenium. The walls of the parieto-occipital sulcus thus resemble those of the lateral sulcus, though its contained sulci and gyri are fewer and smaller.

The *calcarine sulcus* starts near the occipital pole. Though usually restricted to the medial surface, its posterior end may reach the lateral. Directed anteriorly a little above the inferomedial margin in a slightly curved course with an upward convexity, it joins the

parieto-occipital sulcus at an acute angle behind the splenium. Continuing forwards it crosses the inferomedial margin to the interior aspect of the hemisphere, forming the inferolateral boundary of the *isthmus* (which, as noted, connects the cingulate with the parahippocampal gyrus). At its junction with the parieto-occipital sulcus the calcarine sulcus is crossed by a buried *anterior cuneolingual gyrus*. Its posterior part, behind the junction with the parieto-occipital, is an axial sulcus in the long axis of the visual cortex (p. 1158); but the anterior part is a limiting sulcus separating the striate (visual) cortex from that of the isthmus. The anterior part of the calcarine is a complete sulcus, producing the *calcar avis*, an elevation in the posterior cornu of the lateral ventricle.

The quadrilateral area, posterior to the upturned end of the sulcus cinguli, anterior to the parieto-occipital sulcus, inferior to the superomedial margin and superior to the suprasplenial sulcus, is the *precuneus*; with the part of the paracentral lobule behind the central sulcus it forms the medial surface of the parietal lobe. The wedge of cortex bounded in front by the parieto-occipital sulcus, below by the calcarine sulcus and above by the superomedial margin, is the *cuneus* (its surface usually indented by one or two irregular sulci); it is the medial surface of the occipital lobe.

INFERIOR CEREBRAL SURFACE

The inferior cerebral surface is divided by the stem of the lateral fissure into smaller and larger parts, respectively anterior and posterior to it (8.218, 226, 227). The anterior is the orbital region of the inferior surface, transversely concave and above the cribriform plate of the ethmoid, the orbital plate of the frontal and lesser wing of the sphenoid. A rostrocaudal *olfactory sulcus* traverses it near its medial margin, overlapped by the olfactory bulb and tract. The medial strip thus marked off is the *gyrus rectus*. The rest of this surface bears irregular *orbital sulci*, generally H-shaped, dividing it into *orbital gyri*, usually four: the anterior, medial, posterior and lateral orbital gyri (8.227).

The larger, posterior region of the inferior cerebral surface is partly superior to the tentorium but also to the middle cranial fossa and traversed by the anteroposterior collateral and occipitotemporal sulci (8.224, 225). The *collateral sulcus* starts near the occipital pole, extending anteriorly and parallel to the calcarine sulcus, separated by the *lingual gyrus*. Anteriorly it may continue into the *rhinal sulcus* (fissure) but they are usually separate. The rhinal sulcus runs forwards in the line of the collateral, separating the temporal pole from a somewhat hook-shaped *uncus* posteromedial to it. This sulcus is the lateral limit of the *piriform lobe* (8.230).

The *occipitotemporal sulcus* is parallel to the collateral sulcus and lateral to it. It usually does not reach the occipital pole and is frequently divided.

The *lingual gyrus*, between the calcarine and collateral sulci, passes into the *parahippocampal gyrus*, which commences at the *isthmus* where it is continuous with the cingulate gyrus and passes forwards

8.226   The base of the brain. For labelling compare with 8.211. (Dissection by E L Rees, photography by Kevin Fitzpatrick, both of the Department of Anatomy, Guy's Hospital Medical School, London.)

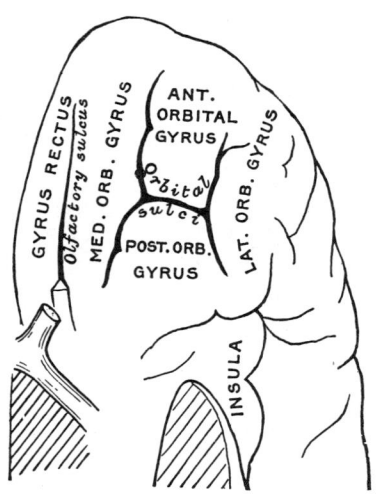

8.227   The orbital surface of the left frontal lobe.

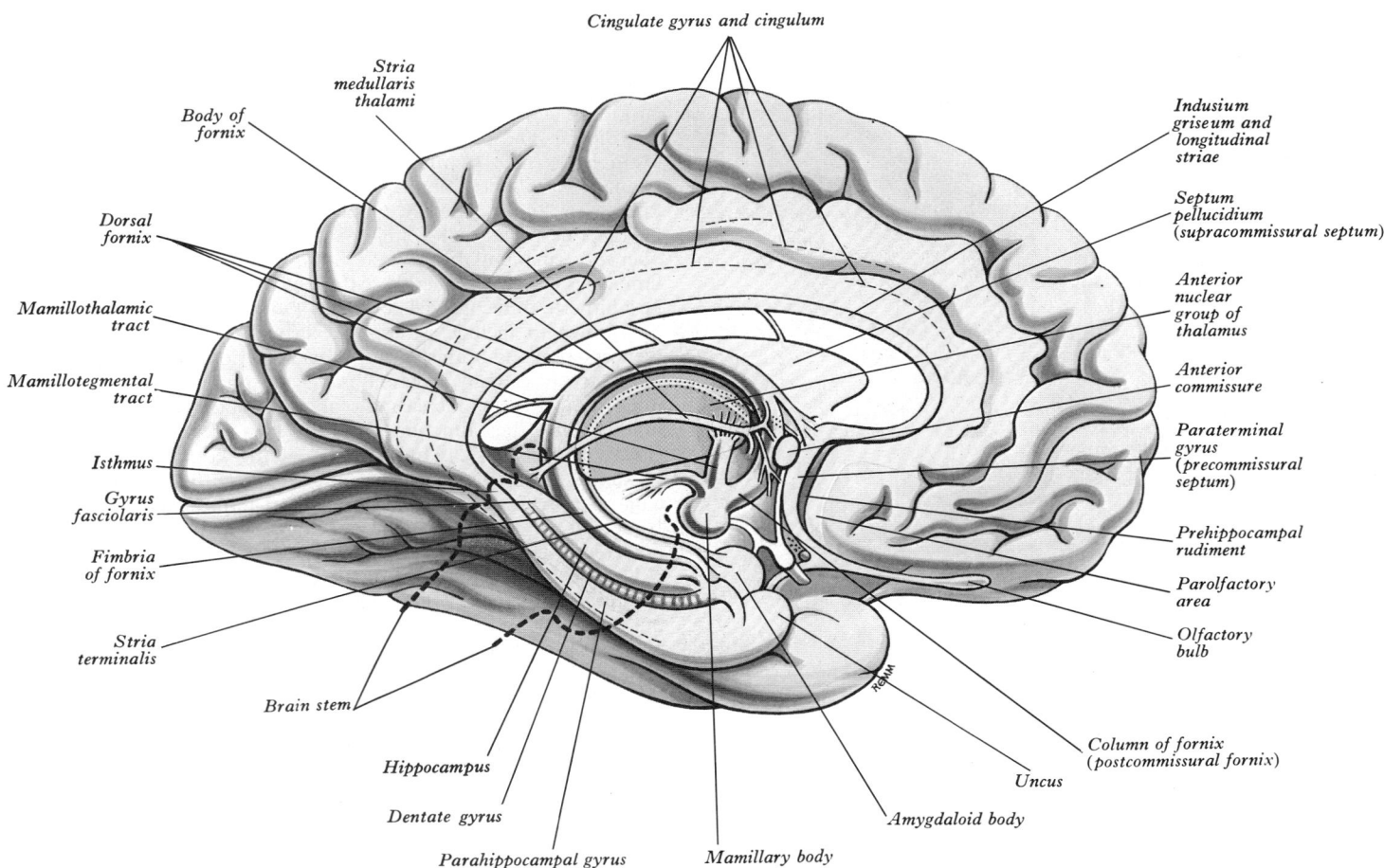

8.228 Diagram of a dissection of the medial aspect of a cerebral hemisphere to demonstrate some limbic lobe structures; these are coloured yellow. The anterior nuclear group of the dorsal thalamus is coloured orange and is closely related to the limbic cortex; the remainder of the dorsal thalamus is magenta. The approximate position of the brainstem is outlined in a heavy interrupted line.

medial to the collateral and rhinal sulci. Anteriorly the parahippocampal gyrus continues into the uncus, its medial edge lying lateral to the midbrain. The uncus, the anterior end of the parahippocampal gyrus, is the posterolateral boundary of the anterior perforated substance. The medial part of the uncus extends laterally above its lateral part and will be described later (**8.230**); its inferior surface is exposed only when its lateral, more superficial part has been removed (**8.239**). The uncus is part of the *piriform lobe* of the olfactory system (see below), phylogenetically one of the oldest parts of the pallium. (For details of the uncal region and complex terminology, consult illustrations **8.228** and **8.230**.)

The *medial occipitotemporal gyrus* extends from the occipital to the temporal poles, limited medially by the collateral and rhinal sulci and laterally by the occipitotemporal. Lateral in this area is the *lateral occipitotemporal gyrus*, which is continuous round the inferolateral margin with the inferior temporal gyrus.

LIMBIC LOBE AND OLFACTORY PATHWAYS

During development, the superolateral aspects of the diencephalon gradually merge with central areas of the inferomedial surfaces of the hemispheres. Bordering the whole area of fusion on each side, a series of structures develops in the hemisphere's wall which Broca (1878) described as 'le grand lobe limbique' and which included the subcallosal, cingulate and parahippocampal gyri together with the underlying hippocampus and dentate gyrus (**8.228**). Broca described the remarkable constancy of these structures across the brains of a wide variety of mammalian species and, because of the close spatial relationships between these phylogenetically old cortical structures

and the termination of the olfactory tract in the medial temporal lobe, the term 'rhinencephalon' (smell brain) was introduced by Bargmann and Schadé (1963) to imply their collective function as an olfactory system. This is now known to be incorrect, but it does explain why the olfactory pathways continue to be treated in the context of the limbic lobe in many neuroanatomical texts.

However, the two most significant events in the evolution of the limbic lobe concept were hypotheses of the function of these cortical structures put forward by Papez (1937) and later MacLean (1952). On the basis of observations of emotional disturbance in patients with apparent damage to the hippocampus and cingulate gyrus, Papez described a closed circuit (still called the circuit of Papez) linking the hippocampus, via the hypothalamic mamillary bodies and anterior thalamus, with the cingulate cortex. He proposed the hippocampus to be the site where programmes of emotional expression were organized; the mamillary bodies to be the site responsible for the expression of emotions; and the cingulate cortex to be the cortical receptive area for experiencing emotion, just as the striate cortex is the visual receptive area. In this way, the first step was taken in transforming Broca's anatomical definition of a limbic lobe into a functional system that depended upon the interconnectedness of its component parts. Although the limbic system theory of emotion is not formally stated, it was Paul MacLean who took Papez' circuit, added associated subcortical regions and proposed the concept of a 'visceral brain' to explain how 'the affective qualities of experience could act on autonomic centres'. The focal point of the visceral brain was the hippocampus (with which MacLean also included the amygdala) where, he suggested, 'the possibility exists for correlating not only olfactory, gustatory and visceral sensations, but auditory, visual somesthetic, and perhaps sexual sensations as well'. As for many earlier and subsequent

1115

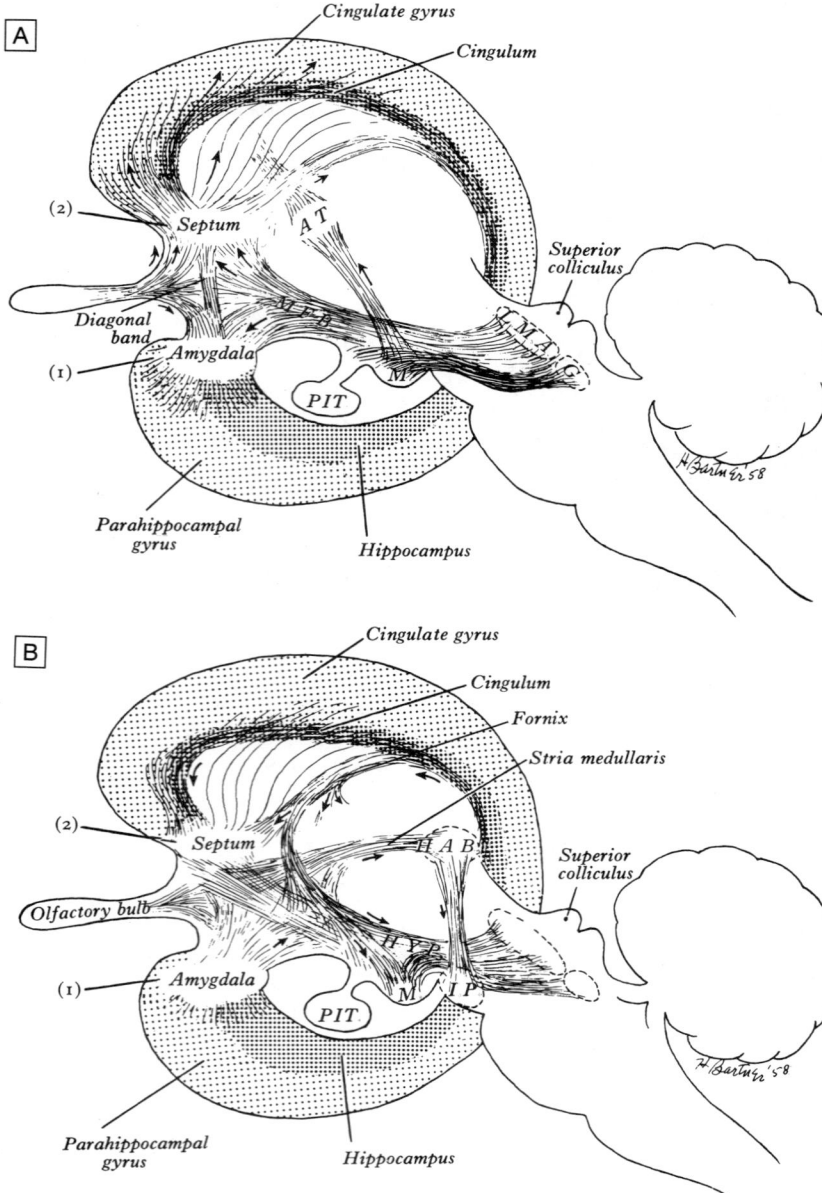

8.229 Schematic drawings of MacLean's 'limbic system' concept. Emphasis is placed on the medial forebrain bundle (MFB) as a major line of communication between the limbic cortex, hypothalamus and midbrain. Note the relationship between the fornix and the cingulum. The limbic cortex, which is considered as a hierarchical system of concentric strips, is indicated by heavy and light stipple. The neocortex is not shown.

A. The ascending pathways to the limbic structures, with emphasis on the divergence of fibres from the MFB to the amygdala (1) and to the septal area (2). Note also the input from the olfactory bulb and tract.

B. Descending pathways from the limbic system. AT = anterior group of thalamic nuclei; G = tegmental reticular nuclei; HAB = habenular nucleus; HYP = hypothalamus; IP = interpeduncular nucleus; LMA = limbic midbrain area (of Nauta); M = mamillary body; PIT = pituitary gland. (From MacLean, 1958.)

researchers on emotion, the hypothalamus was assumed to be the site where hippocampal processes gained access to co-ordinators of autonomic outflow that control the peripheral manifestations of emotional states. Finally, in 1952, MacLean proposed that the term 'limbic system' be used instead of 'visceral brain' to describe Broca's limbic lobe, together with associated subcortical nuclei including the amygdala, septum, hypothalamus, habenula, anterior thalamic nuclei and parts of the basal ganglia (8.229). It is quite clear from MacLean's many papers on the subject that he regarded this group of structures truly as an anatomical system that had a special involvement in emotion through its role in visceral regulation.

Whether or not the primary function of the limbic system is to mediate emotional experience and expression is the subject of ongoing debate and controversy (see below). However, the very existence of the limbic system concept has had, and continues to have, an enormous impact on the way that neuroanatomists, psychologists, neurologists and psychiatrists view the neural basis of emotion. For example, as neuroanatomists have discovered new and important connections of these core limbic structures, they too have become known as 'limbic' and are immediately suspected or speculated to have a role in emotion. Similarly, an emotional or affective consequence of manipulating a neural structure not within the original limbic system has frequently led to the suggestion that it, too, must be a hitherto unrecognized component of it. And so the limbic system has grown to include widespread structures in the telencephalon, diencephalon and brainstem. Yet there is serious doubt as to whether these structures truly function as a system and, perhaps even more important, it seems increasingly obvious that, even if they do, it is unlikely that they function primarily as a mechanism of emotion (LeDoux 1986, 1991). Indeed, one of the key elements, the hippocampus, contributes much more importantly and obviously to cognitive processes, such as spatial short-term memory (O'Keefe & Nadel 1978), there being little contemporary evidence that it is involved in emotional processes per se (see LeDoux 1991).

Despite this background of a changing view of the nature and emotional functions of the limbic system, there is a widespread implicit acceptance of its existence and this provides a pragmatic basis for describing its component parts and their connections under the heading 'limbic lobe'. It seems likely that structures will be described as 'limbic' for many years to come, but readers should bear in mind that a 'limbic' grouping should not be taken to indicate that the primary function of such a structure is in emotional processing.

OLFACTORY PATHWAYS

Olfactory bulb

The olfactory bulb (8.230) is situated inferior to the anterior end of the olfactory sulcus on the orbital surface of the frontal lobe. It receives all the input from the olfactory sensory neurons, the nerve fibres of which collect into about 20 bundles, pass through the foramina in the cribriform plate and enter its inferior surface. The olfactory bulb and tract, through which the output of the bulb passes directly to the olfactory cortex, develop as a hollow diverticulum from the floor of the primitive cerebral hemisphere. The basal part elongates to form the olfactory tract and, in human embryos, the cavity of the olfactory bulb ('olfactory ventricle') and of the elongating tract are gradually obliterated by fusion of their walls. The site of the original cavity is sometimes marked by vestigial groups of modified ependymal cells. Therefore the olfactory bulb has a radial organization with a number of superimposed layers. This laminar pattern is well defined in many mammals including the human fetus, but becomes less distinct as the brain matures. Detailed histology of the olfactory bulb has been known since the turn of the century (Blanes 1898; Ramón y Cajal 1890, 1911, 1955), but its organization has recently become exceptionally well understood through the use of immunocytochemical, in situ hybridization, tract-tracing and electron microscopical and electrophysiological techniques (Takagi 1989; Halász 1990; Shepherd & Greer 1990).

There is a clear laminar structure in the olfactory bulb (8.231). From the surface inwards the laminae are as follows:

- *The olfactory nerve layer* which consists of the unmyelinated axons of the olfactory neurons. Because of the ongoing turnover of receptor cells (p. 1317), the axons in this layer are at different stages of growth, maturity or degeneration.
- *The glomerular layer*, comprised of a thin sheet of glomeruli is penetrated by the incoming olfactory nerve fibres which divide only within glomeruli and synapse on terminal dendritic tufts of secondary olfactory neurons, namely mitral, tufted and periglomerular cells.
- *The external plexiform layer*, comprised of the principal and secondary dendrites of mitral and tufted cells. It is divided into two layers: the superficial layer principally contains the somata of

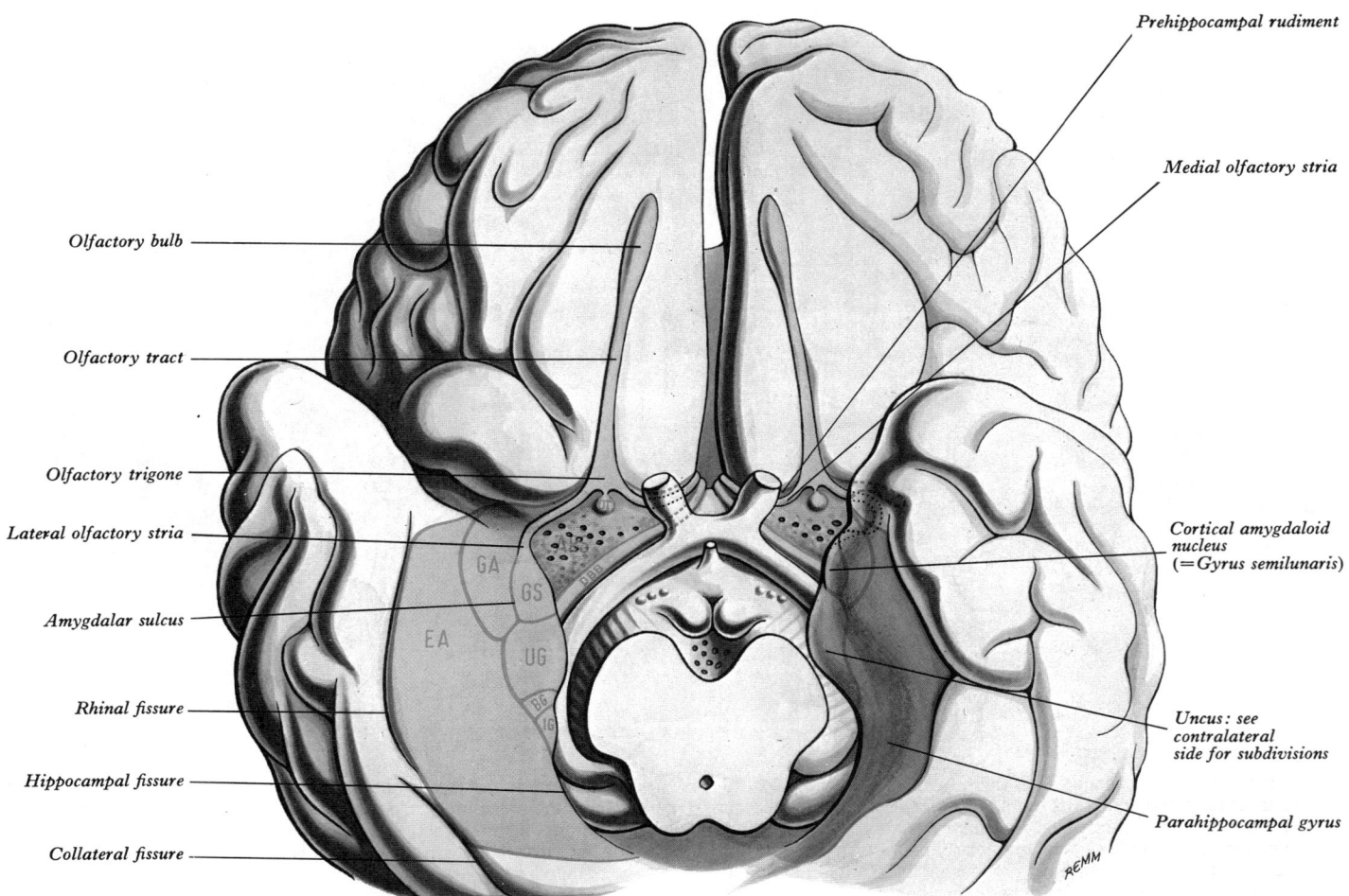

8.230 A diagram of structures on the inferior aspect of the human brain in the area immediately surrounding the optic nerves, chiasma, optic tracts and interpeduncular fossa. Many of these structures are intimately related to the olfactory and limbic systems; they are coloured blue. The right temporal pole has been displaced laterally to expose underlying structures. In addition to the features which have been labelled fully, the abbreviations used have the following significance: OT = olfactory tubercle; APS =anterior perforated substance; DBB = diagonal band of Broca. The uncus hippocampi is divided into three areas: IG = the intralimbic gyrus; BG = the band of Giacomini; UG = the uncinate gyrus. The lateral olfactory stria continues into the gyrus semilunaris (GS); this is bordered laterally by the gyrus ambiens (GA); whilst further laterally is the entorhinal area (EA) which is the rostral extension of the parahippocampal gyrus. Note the curved extensions of the prehippocampal rudiments, medial olfactory striae and diagonal bands of Broca on the medial aspect of the hemisphere. The triangular midline zone between the converging diagonal bands and superior to the optic chiasma is the lamina terminalis. The occasional intermediate olfactory stria which merges with the olfactory tubercle is illustrated but unlabelled. (After Kuhlenbeck; redrawn and modified from Nauta and Haymaker, 1969, with permission of the authors and publishers.)

tufted cells, while the deep layer contains many secondary dendrites, and also some misplaced cell bodies, of mitral cells.

- *The mitral cell layer*, made up of a thin sheet of the somata of large mitral cells, each of which sends a single principal dendrite to a glomerulus, many secondary dendrites to the external plexiform layer and single axons to deep layers of the bulb. Some granule cell bodies are also found in this layer.
- *The internal plexiform layer*, composed of axons, recurrent and deep collaterals of mitral and tufted cells and some granule cell bodies.
- *The granule cell layer* contains the majority of granule cells, together with their superficial and deep processes. They are present in large number, for example 3×10^6 in the rat, arranged in small tightly packed clusters. Deep short axon cells are also present in this layer and numerous centripetal and centrifugal nerve fibres pass through it.
- For the sake of completeness, a *periventricular* or *subependymal layer* is the deepest layer of the bulb and it surrounds the intrabulbar (obliterated) part of the ventricle.

The *neuronal elements* in the bulb, as in other regions of the brain, fall into three categories: input, output and intrinsic. The early descriptions of these neuronal elements were based upon examination of Golgi-impregnated material, but they have been confirmed by more recent investigations that have also used Golgi material and horseradish peroxidase injections and extended by immunocytochemical techniques that have allowed the definition of the chemical phenotype of many neurons.

As noted above, the inputs to the olfactory bulb arise primarily from the olfactory sensory neurons, but there are also central inputs arising from a variety of sites. The sensory axons are all unmyelinated and grouped in bundles that separate and interweave when they enter the bulb surface, and terminate in the glomeruli. These olfactory glomeruli are a clear example of the principle of grouping of neural elements and synapses and are analogous to 'barrels' and 'columns' in the cerebral cortex (p. 1153). They represent a higher level of organization than the synaptic glomeruli of the thalamus and cerebellum (Shepherd & Greer, 1990). The olfactory axons only branch within the glomeruli. An important and exceptional feature of olfactory sensory neurons is that they are continuously replaced from stem cells in the olfactory epithelium throughout life, indicating that the specificity of synaptic connections within the glomeruli must be achieved in the face of this constant remodelling. This degree of plasticity is not to be found in other areas of the mammalian central nervous system (CNS) and its molecular basis is as yet uncertain. The sensory olfactory neurons contain a special peptide, the *olfactory*

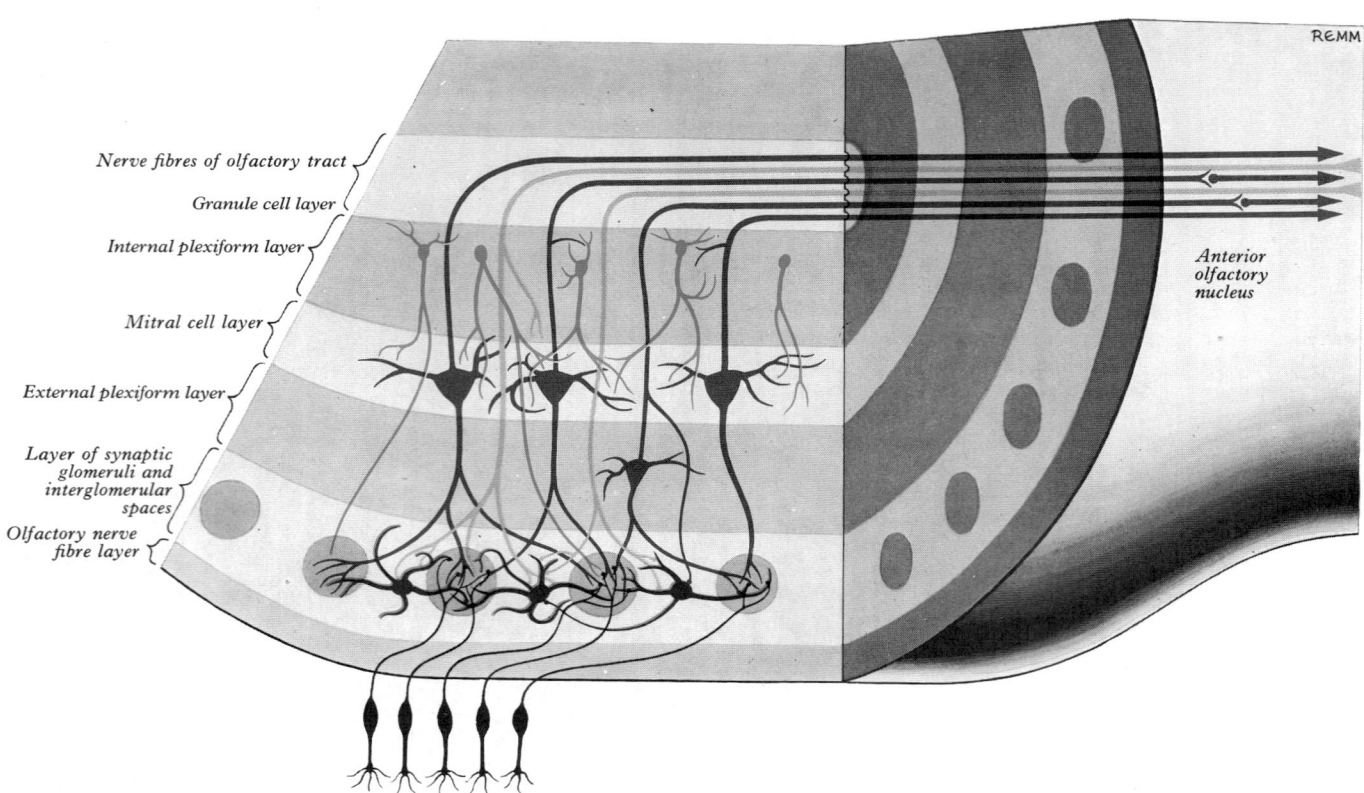

8.231 A scheme of the olfactory bulb based upon neurocytological and experimental studies in a number of mammalian species. The radial organization of the bulb into 'layers', with their principal neuron types, and an approximate indication of their main connectivity patterns is shown. Red = mitral and tufted neurons and their processes; blue = internal granule neurons; purple = dopaminergic periglomerular neurons; black = olfactory receptor neurons and their processes. Note that the olfactory tract consists of (1) centripetal axons of mitral and tufted cells, some of which synapse with neurons in the anterior olfactory nucleus and (2) centrifugal axons (yellow) which terminate in the different zones indicated. Refer to text for a more detailed description of both the organization of the bulb and the destinations of olfactory tract fibres.

marker protein, and also high concentrations of the dipeptide carnosine, although neither substance appears to be a neurotransmitter within the glomeruli. The olfactory nerve glia also contains the glial fibrillary acidic protein, similar to astrocytes in the central nervous system. Laminin is also expressed in adulthood in the olfactory nerve layer and it has been suggested that this may be correlated with the continuous turnover of olfactory nerve axons entering the bulb from the olfactory epithelium.

The centrifugal (i.e. arising from the brain and projecting outwards to the bulb) inputs arise from a variety of sites at several levels of the neuraxis, and each has a quite distinctive laminar termination pattern (Macrides & Davis 1983; Mori 1987; Shepherd & Greer 1990). The *anterior olfactory nucleus* projects extensively to the olfactory bulb and there is evidence that terminations in its different laminae are related to different populations of granule cells. Collaterals of pyramidal neuron axons in the *olfactory cortex* (see below) also arrive in the olfactory bulb and terminate largely in the granule cell layer. Cholinergic neurons in the *horizontal limb nucleus of the diagonal band of Broca*, part of the basal forebrain cholinergic system, project to the granule cell layer and also to the glomerular layer, especially its periglomerular parts. Other important, chemically defined afferents arise from the pontine *locus coeruleus* and the mesencephalic *raphe nucleus*. The noradrenergic and serotoninergic fibres, respectively, are distributed diffusely to the granule cell layer and also to the interiors of the glomeruli (see Shepherd & Greer 1990). These centrifugal afferents to the olfactory bulb mediate the considerable degree of control by the brain, the functional importance of which has been established, for example, in a variety of reproductive contexts in rodents and sheep (Brennan et al 1990; Kendrick et al 1992).

The principal neurons in the olfactory bulb are the *mitral* and *tufted* cells, and their axons form its output which passes centripetally via the olfactory tract. In general, each mitral cell gives rise to a single *primary dendrite* which passes through the external plexiform layer to terminate as a tuft of branches within a glomerulus. The tuft extends across most of the glomerulus and is a more or less unique characteristic among principal neurons in the brain. Each mitral cell also gives rise to laterally directed *secondary dendrites* which branch to a much more limited extent than the primary dendrite, and terminate within the external plexiform layer. There appear to be subtypes of mitral cells identified on the basis of secondary dendritic branching pattern (Mori et al 1983; Shepherd & Greer 1990). Mitral cells have *aspiny* primary and secondary dendrites, and their axons pass to the depths of the olfactory bulb, giving off recurrent collaterals as they go, ultimately gathering together to emerge as the olfactory tract. Experiments in which mitral cells have been filled with HRP indicate, in contrast to the earlier Golgi studies (Ramón y Cajal 1911), that the axon collaterals tend to remain within the granule cell and internal plexiform layers and are distributed quite diffusely. The transmitter used by mitral cells at both its somatodendritic output within the bulb (see below) and its axon terminals within the olfactory cortex is widely assumed to be an amino acid, probably glutamate or aspartate.

The tufted cells and mitral cells are morphologically similar, but are situated more superficially in the external plexiform layer. Three main groups of tufted cell have been identified (Shepherd & Greer 1990):

- *Middle tufted cells* form the main population, having several thin basal dendrites and a primary dendrite that ends in a confined tuft of branches within a glomerulus. Their axons join the olfactory tract, but also give off collaterals that are mainly confined within the internal plexiform layer. It is important to note that they project to sites in the olfactory cortex different from those of mitral cells.
- *External tufted cells* have dendrites with distinctive branching patterns and give off collaterals within the internal plexiform layer and adjacent granule cell layer. They are essentially an intrabulbar

association system (Schoenfeld et al 1985) and, according to Shepherd and Greer (1990), should be classified as intrinsic neurons.

• *Internal tufted cells* overlap in appearance and position with some outwardly placed mitral cells. Like mitral cells, tufted cells also appear to use glutamate/aspartate as a transmitter at their dendritic and axon terminal output sites, but some tufted cells appear to be dopaminergic (Halász et al 1977)

The main types of intrinsic neuron in the olfactory bulb are *periglomerular cells* and *granule cells*. The periglomerular cell axons are among the shortest in the brain and they have short bushy dendrites that arborize within a glomerulus (Pinching & Powell 1971 a,b) interweaving among both the dendritic branches of mitral and tufted cells, and also the terminals of olfactory nerve axons. The axons of periglomerular cells are distributed laterally to terminate within extraglomerular regions. Immunocytochemical studies have revealed the majority of periglomerular cells to be dopaminergic (Halász et al 1977; cell group A15 according to the nomenclature of Dahlström & Fuxe 1965), but some also contain glutamic acid decarboxylase- (GAD-) immunoreactivity and are γ-aminobutyric acid-(GABA)ergic. Indeed, some periglomerular cells appear to contain both dopamine and GABA (tyrosine hydroxylase and GAD immunoreactivities), as do some neurons elsewhere, for example in the hypothalamic arcuate nucleus (Everitt et al 1984).

Granule cells are similar in size to periglomerular cells and tend to be grouped in clusters. Their most characteristic feature is the lack of an axon and they resemble, therefore, amacrine cells in the retina (p. 1345). Granule cells have two principal spine-bearing dendrites that pass radially in the bulb, to ramify and terminate in the external plexiform layer, and also a deep process that branches but little in the granule cell layer. Detailed analysis in rodents, using intra- and extracellular HRP injections, has revealed *superficial*, *intermediate* and *deep* granule cells. The former appear primarily to contact the dendrites of tufted cells within the superficial external plexiform layer, whereas the latter interact mainly with the dendrites

of mitral cells in the deep external plexiform layer. Intermediate granule cells appear not to reach specific regions of the external plexiform layer and their dendrites ramify throughout its depth. Thus, mitral and tufted cells have both segregated and overlapping circuits through granule cells (Macrides et al 1983; Shepherd & Greer 1990). Granule cells have been demonstrated to contain GAD-immunoreactivity and presumably release GABA as a neurotransmitter.

There is also a relatively small population of *short-axon cells* that are distributed within the glomerular and granule cell layers. They appear to be of several subtypes and their short axons are distributed within the external plexiform or granule cell layers.

In addition to classical transmitters, many neuropeptides have been localized to the olfactory bulb and the majority appear to be in intrinsic neurons, often coexisting with the classical transmitters GABA, dopamine or glutamate/aspartate (**8.232**). Enkephalin has been demonstrated in some granule and periglomerular cells and substance P (SP) in tufted cells. In addition, luteinizing hormone releasing hormone (LHRH) and SP are also present in centrifugal afferents to the bulb (Halász 1990).

The synaptic organization and an overview of the basic circuitry of the olfactory bulb are illustrated in **8.233**. As emphasized by Shepherd and Greer (1990) in their excellent review (which the reader should consult for a more detailed consideration of olfactory processing in the bulb), the basic plan depends upon the fact that the mitral cell spans the layers of the bulb, receiving the sensory input superficially at its glomerular tuft, while giving rise to the output of the bulb from its cell body. Thus, the two important functions of input processing and output control are spatially separated at two distinct levels, superficial and deep, in the olfactory bulb.

The processing of inputs occurs within the glomeruli through the apposition of the olfactory nerve axon, mitral and tufted cell dendrite and periglomerular cell dendrite. This *synaptic triad* involves synapses from separate olfactory nerve axons onto a principal neuron (mitral or tufted cell) or an intrinsic neuron (periglomerular cell). The

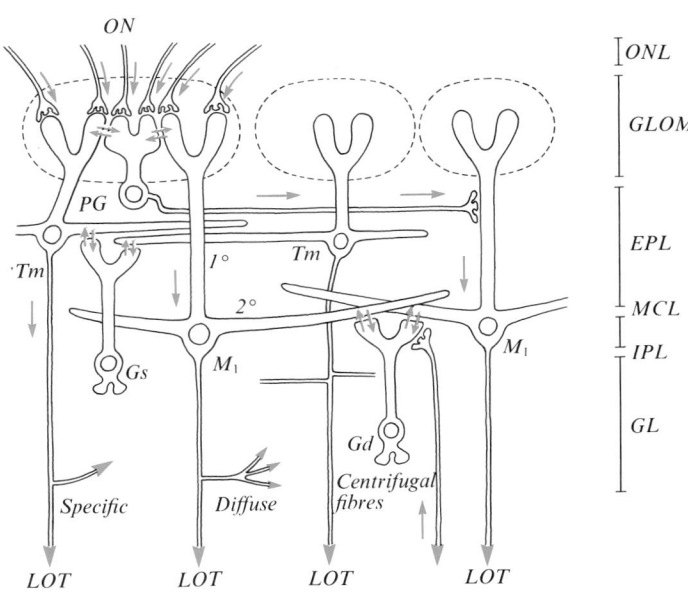

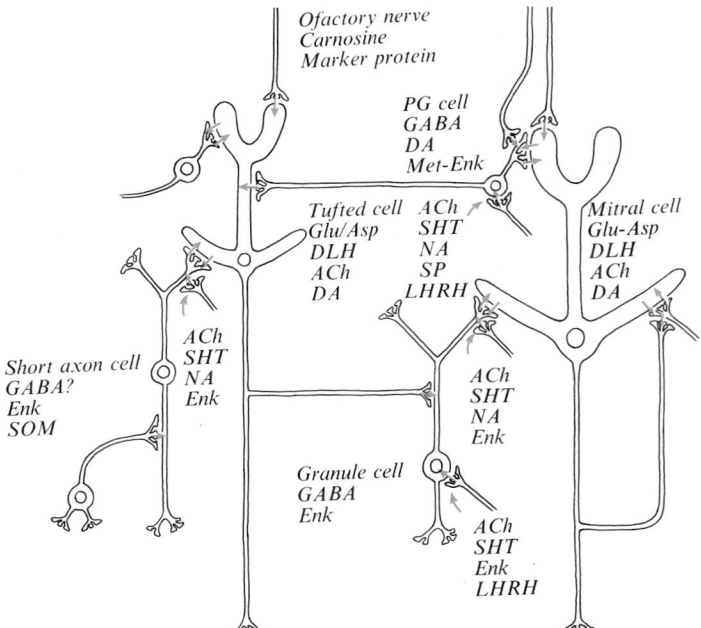

8.232 Schematic diagram of the olfactory bulb, showing cell types, some connections and the putative neurotransmitter substances each contain, as evidenced by immunocytochemical investigations. The terminals of afferent projections from the brainstem and basal forebrain are also shown, but the listed transmitter substances found in these terminals should *not* be taken to indicate coexistence, but instead the different transmitters found in each category of distinctive afferent. ACh = acetylcholine; DA = dopamine; DLH = DL-homocysteate; Enk = met-enkephalin; Glu-Asp = glutamate-aspartate; 5HT = 5-hydroxytryptamine; LHRH = luteinizing hormone releasing hormone; NA = noradrenaline; SOM = somatostatin; SP = substance P. (Redrawn from Shepherd & Greer, 1990, after Halasz & Shepherd, 1983).

8.233 Schematic diagram of the basic synaptic circuits of the olfactory bulb. Olfactory nerve afferents enter the bulb at the top of the diagram, while corticofugal efferents from the bulb leave from its depths, at the bottom of the diagram. (a) Layers of the bulb—ONL = olfactory nerve layer; GLOM = glomerular layer; EPL = external plexiform layer; MCL = mitral cell layer; IPL = inner plexiform layer; GL = granule cell layer. (b) Cell types—ON = olfactory nerve; PG = periglomerular cell; T_M = middle tufted cell; M_1 = mitral cell; G_s, superficial granule cell; G_d, deep granule cell; LOT = lateral olfactory tract; 1° & 2° = primary and secondary dendrites of mitral cell; centrifugal fibres are those arising in the brainstem and basal forebrain (e.g. noradrenergic afferents from the locus coeruleus). (Redrawn from Shepherd & Greer 1990).

1119

glomerulus is also characterized by reciprocal dendrodendritic synapses between periglomerular cells and mitral/tufted cells. Interglomerular connections are formed by the axons of periglomerular cells and onto the primary dendrites of other mitral and tufted cells as they leave the glomeruli. In this way, processing in one glomerulus can affect the output of neighbouring glomeruli. Centrifugal fibres, like those arising from the noradrenergic locus coeruleus, also make synaptic contact with periglomerular cells.

At the level of output control, the key synaptic interaction involves reciprocal synaptic contacts between the secondary dendrites of mitral/tufted cells with the spines of granule cell dendrites in the external plexiform layer. There is considerable evidence that the mitral/tufted cell-to-granule cell synapse is excitatory, while the reciprocal granule cell-to-mitral/tufted cell synapse is inhibitory. Since the latter represents the sole output of the granule cell, it is likely that its inhibitory influence on the output neurons is a powerful primary method of controlling output from the olfactory bulb (Shepherd & Greer 1990). Other synaptic interactions in the external plexiform layer involve intrinsic short axon cells and again centrifugal afferents to the bulb from monoaminergic and cholinergic neurons in the brainstem and basal forebrain. In the granule cell layer, the spines and shafts of granule cell dendrites receive synaptic contacts from the axon collaterals of mitral/tufted cells and from the axons of deep short-axon cells. Noradrenergic, serotoninergic, cholinergic and other centrifugal afferents also terminate richly on granule cells in this layer (Shepherd & Greer 1990). In the granule cell layer, the dendritic spine of the granule cell is a most important site for the modulation by the brain of olfactory information processing, through the synaptic triad formed between the spine, mitral/tufted cell dendrites and the centrifugal afferent terminal. Such centrifugal control is also exerted at the level of the glomeruli themselves, especially in the case of serotoninergic afferents arriving directly within the glomeruli from the mesencephalic raphé nuclei.

The axons of mitral and tufted cells appear to serve parallel output pathways from the olfactory bulb. While it remains uncertain as to whether these two types of cell receive inputs from different populations of olfactory receptor-bearing sensory neurons, it is now established that different populations of granule cell affect output processing of these two types of principal neuron in the external plexiform layer. Furthermore, superficial and deep populations of mitral and tufted cells have differential projections to the anterior olfactory nucleus, piriform cortex, amygdala and entorhinal cortex (see below), strongly suggesting the parallel processing of chemosensory information that is analogous to that seen in visual, auditory and somatosensory systems (Shepherd & Greer 1990).

Olfactory tract

The olfactory tract (8.230) leaves the posterior pole of the olfactory bulb to run on the inferior (orbital) surface of the frontal lobe, along the olfactory sulcus. As we have seen, it consists of centripetal axons of mitral and tufted cells and centrifugal axons from a variety of sources, such as the opposite bulb and anterior olfactory nucleus, which have all crossed in the anterior commissure, and also of neurons in the basal forebrain, including the cholinergic horizontal limb nucleus of the diagonal band of Broca and brainstem nuclei, especially the noradrenergic locus coeruleus in the pons and the serotoninergic dorsal raphe nucleus in the midbrain. Posteriorly, characteristic cell layers of the olfactory bulb disappear, but the granule cell layer is represented in the olfactory tract by scattered medium-sized multipolar neurons, the *anterior olfactory nucleus*; these continue into the olfactory striae and trigone (see below) to the grey matter of the prepiriform cortex, the anterior perforated substance and precommissural septal areas. Many centripetal axons from mitral and tufted cells relay in, or give collaterals to, the anterior olfactory nucleus, the axons of which continue with the remaining direct fibres from the bulb into the olfactory striae.

Anterior perforated substance. This is an important landmark on the cerebral base; it is caudal to the olfactory trigone and diverging olfactory stria, in the angle between the optic chiasma and tract medially and the uncus caudally (8.257). It is continuous medially, above the optic tract, with the grey matter of the tuber cinereum and, more anteriorly, with the paraterminal gyrus. Laterally, it reaches the limen insulae to continue into the prepiriform cortex; more caudally it merges with the periamygdaloid area (gyrus

semilunaris). Superiorly, it is continuous with the grey matter of the corpus striatum and claustrum through aggregations of grey and white matter forming the substantia innominata. Part of the latter, with fascicles of the ansa lenticularis and anterior commissure, separate the anterior perforated substance from the globus pallidus. The aggregates of grey matter in the substantia innominata are grouped as the magnocellular corticopetal system (primarily the cholinergic nucleus basalis of Meynert, cell group Ch4 according to the nomenclature of Mesulam 1989a,b), the ventral globus pallidus and, according to Alheid and Heimer (1988) and de Olmos (1990), an extension of the medial and lateral divisions of the central nucleus of the amygdala in a sublenticular position that merges rostrally with the bed nucleus of the stria terminalis (p. 1135); they have termed this the 'extended amygdala'. The anterior perforated substance is related to the bifurcation of the internal carotid artery into the anterior and middle cerebral arteries, from which central arteries pierce the surface to supply deeper structures (p. 1219). Caudal to the olfactory trigone, the anterior perforated substance displays a small olfactory tubercle, variable in prominence, into the base of which the occasional intermediate olfactory stria sinks. The tubercle is large in macrosomatic animals but greatly reduced and sometimes difficult to locate in the human brain. The intermediate stria, though sometimes absent, is occasionally comprised of two or three fine striae radiating into the perforated substance. The caudal zone of the substance, adjoining the optic tract, is the smooth surface of the diagonal band of Broca. Caudolaterally the band is continuous with the periamygdaloid area; rostromedially it continues above the optic chiasma into the paraterminal gyrus (precommissural septum).

As the olfactory tract approaches the anterior perforated substance it flattens and splays out into the olfactory trigone (olfactory pyramid), from the caudal angles of which fibres of the tract continue as diverging medial and lateral olfactory striae bordering the anterior perforated substance (8.230). In some brains, a small *intermediate stria* passes from the centre of the trigone to sink into the anterior perforated substance. The lateral olfactory stria follows the anterolateral margin of the anterior perforated substance as a visible bundle continuing into the limen insulae (p. 1111), where it bends posteromedially to merge with an elevated region, the gyrus semilunaris, at the rostral margin of the uncus hippocampi (8.230). A tenuous grey layer covering the lateral olfactory stria is the lateral olfactory gyrus, merging laterally with the gyrus ambiens, part of the limen insulae. The lateral olfactory gyrus and gyrus ambiens form the prepiriform region of the cortex, passing caudally into the entorhinal area of the parahippocampal gyrus. The prepiriform and periamygdaloid regions and the entorhinal area (area 28) together comprise the so-called piriform lobe. The lobe is bounded laterally by the rhinal sulcus and is relatively prominent both in macrosmatic mammals and during fetal development. The relative positions of these structures will be clarified by reference to 8.230. The medial olfactory stria, covered thinly by the grey matter of the medial olfactory gyrus, passes medially along the rostral boundary of the anterior perforated substance towards the medial continuation of the diagonal band of Broca. Together, they curve up on the medial aspect of the hemisphere, anterior to the attachment of the lamina terminalis (see p. 1112). The diagonal band enters the paraterminal gyrus, the medial stria becoming indistinct as it approaches the boundary zone, which includes the paraterminal gyrus, parolfactory gyrus and, between them, the prehippocampal rudiment (8.230).

Olfactory cortex

The olfactory cortex (8.230) is generally defined as an area that receives direct input from the olfactory bulb arriving via the olfactory tract and, in contrast to other sensory systems, without relay in the thalamus. However, this apparent uniqueness of the olfactory cortex is not so absolute as it once seemed, since it is clear that the primary olfactory cortex projects both directly and via the medial dorsal nucleus of the thalamus to areas of the orbitofrontal neocortex that have been demonstrated to be involved in olfactory information processing. The largest olfactory area is the *piriform cortex* (it is also called the prepiriform cortex in some accounts), but the *anterior olfactory nucleus*, *olfactory tubercle*, regions of the *entorhinal* and *insular cortex*, as well as specific nuclei of the *amygdala*, are also in receipt of direct projections from the olfactory bulb (Haberly 1990).

The *anterior olfactory nucleus* is the most rostral of the structures innervated by the olfactory bulb. It is a poorly laminated cortical structure, having a superficial plexiform layer (layer I), a compact pyramidal cell layer (layer II) and a polymorphic cell layer (layer III). Efferents from the olfactory bulb terminate exclusively in the superficial half of the superficial plexiform layer (layer Ia), while centrifugal efferents to the bulb arise from layers II and III. Central projections of the anterior olfactory nucleus include the piriform cortex, but not, apparently, the entorhinal cortex or amygdala which, in non-primate species, are sites that receive a projection from the accessory olfactory bulb.

The *piriform cortex* is generally described as trilaminar (palaeocortex), comprising a superficial plexiform layer (layer I), a superficial compact cell layer (layer II) and a deeper, more sparsely packed cell layer (layer III). In some species, an endopiriform nucleus has been defined that contains densely packed multipolar cells resembling those in layer III. It is sometimes referred to as layer IV (Haberly 1990). The superficial parts of layer I (Ia) receive fibres from the olfactory tract, principally the axons of mitral cells, which terminate on the distal dendrites of pyramidal cells in deep layer II and layer III. Deeper parts of the superficial plexiform layer (layer Ib) receive association fibres from olfactory cortical areas and these terminate on the more proximal segments of the apical dendrites of pyramidal cells. Projections from this primary olfactory cortex are widespread, including those to the neocortex and thalamus (especially the orbitofrontal cortex and medial dorsal thalamic nucleus, see below), the hypothalamus and amygdala (see below). The projection from pyramidal cells in the piriform cortex to the insular neocortex overlaps somewhat afferents to the same area from gustatory pathways. The synaptic arrangements and patterns of information processing occurring in the piriform cortex have been studied in great detail and the interested reader is referred to the excellent review by Haberly (1990). In speculating on the functions of the piriform cortex, Haberly (1990) emphasizes the non-topographical nature of the input from the olfactory bulb and the presence of intrinsic associational fibre systems that mediate spatially distributed positive feedback onto pyramidal cells. He suggests that this kind of circuitry, together with an 'ensemble code' for odour quality (one consequence of the non-topographical arrangement of olfactory bulb inputs), indicates that the olfactory cortex is a locus for the association of odour stimuli with memory traces of previous odour stimuli (Haberly 1985, 1990).

The *olfactory tubercle* is a relatively mysterious structure in the human brain and its functions are not particularly well understood in other species. It is generally included as part of the piriform lobe and regarded as one of the constituents of the olfactory cortex. In macrosmatic animals, such as rats, the olfactory tubercle is a conspicuous eminence on the base of the brain, immediately caudal to the olfactory peduncle. As with the rest of the primary olfactory cortex, it has a trilaminar structure. However, in the rat this structure is best known for its rich dopaminergic innervation from the ventral tegmental area (cell group A10) and its close relationship to the overlying ventral striatum (Alheid et al 1990). In microsmatic primates, only a small anterolaterally situated area of the olfactory tubercle receives a direct projection from the olfactory bulb and its laminar structure is not obvious. In man, the olfactory tubercle is even harder to define, lying just posterior to the point of attachment of the olfactory tracts on the base of the frontal lobes (see Alheid et al 1990) in the region usually termed the anterior perforated substance. It has been suggested that the olfactory tubercle uniquely receives inputs from, but does not project to, other olfactory areas. In addition to the olfactory bulb, afferents arise from the amygdala (see below) and medial dorsal thalamus, while its efferents reach the septal area and extend into the stria medullaris thalami and medial forebrain bundle (MFB), the entorhinal area, amygdaloid complex and hippocampal formation. Although electrophysiological studies in rodents show that olfactory tubercle neurons respond to odours, their role in olfaction is far from clear.

The *amygdala* in primates and man is not dominated by olfaction as it is in many other mammals, but it retains substantial connections with the olfactory system (see below). The accessory olfactory bulb, with its exclusive connections with the vomeronasal system, projects richly to the corticomedial amygdaloid field in non-primates and has important functions in reproductive neuroendocrine integration in

many species (Brennan et al 1990; Kendrick et al 1992). However, this system is lacking in man and in the old world monkeys and apes in which there are direct projections from the main olfactory bulb to the anterior cortical nucleus, nucleus of the lateral olfactory tract and to much of the periamygdaloid cortex (see below). The latter two areas also project back to the olfactory bulb. There are also important association projections between all parts of the primary olfactory cortex, including the piriform cortex, and the nucleus of the lateral olfactory tract, anterior cortical nucleus and the periamygdaloid cortex (Haberly 1990).

The *entorhinal cortex* (Brodmann's area 28) is the most posterior part of the piriform cortex. It comprises two regions, medial and lateral (Brodmann's areas 28a and 28b, respectively; Brodmann 1909; Kretteck & Price 1977; Brodal 1981). It is generally considered to consist of six layers, but the marked cytoarchitectonic changes that occur over the rostrocaudal extent of the entorhinal cortex have resulted in the description of up to 23 fields (see Amaral & Insausti 1990). Lateral parts of the entorhinal cortex mainly receive fibres from the olfactory bulb, as well as from the piriform and peri-amygdaloid cortex. There are also rich projections to the entorhinal cortex from widespread neocortical areas and it is itself a major source of afferents to the dentate gyrus and cornu ammonis of the hippocampal formation (see below) and also to the frontal lobe via the uncinate fasciculus.

The above areas represent the major sites of processing of olfactory information relayed directly from the olfactory bulb. However, of particular interest is the demonstration that discrete areas of the frontal lobe are also in receipt of olfactory information, relayed via the piriform cortex. Two such areas have been particularly well characterized in monkeys: the *lateroposterior* and the *centroposterior orbitofrontal cortex*. Although the precise details of the projections have still to be confirmed, it appears that the lateroposterior orbitofrontal cortex receives projections from the piriform cortex that do not pass through the thalamus, perhaps arriving directly or through the dorsal posterior hypothalamus (Tanabe et al, 1975; Takagi 1989). Better established, perhaps, is the major projection from the piriform cortex to the magnocellular division of the medial dorsal nucleus of the thalamus. The projections of the medial dorsal thalamus onto the frontal lobes define the prefrontal cortex in general (see p. 1164). However, that part of the prefrontal cortex which has a medial dorsal thalamus-dependent olfactory representation has been shown to be the centroposterior orbitofrontal cortex (Tanabe et al 1975). Furthermore, damage to this area of cortex in man is associated with major disturbances in odour identification and discrimination (Zatorre et al 1993). An in vivo imaging study of the cortical representation of olfactory processing in man using positron emission tomography (PET) to measure regional cerebral blood flow has also pointed to the importance of the orbitofrontal cortex. Thus, olfactory stimulation strongly activates the piriform cortex bilaterally in the temporal lobes, as would be expected of a primary olfactory area. However, there is also a region of markedly increased blood flow within the orbitofrontal cortex but only on the right side of the brain (**8.234**; Zatorre et al 1992). This lateralized response of the orbitofrontal cortex to bilaterally presented olfactory stimuli indicates hemispheric specialization and a functional asymmetry in olfactory processes that arises at the level of the secondary, but not the primary, olfactory cortex.

LIMBIC CORTEX

Broca's limbic lobe is usually included with other structures, notably the hippocampus, amygdala and their subcortical connections, and referred to as the 'limbic system', with its putative unitary function related to emotion. It was discussed earlier that for pragmatic reasons, this tendency to group these structures will not be resisted here. Therefore, in this section the general organization of the limbic cortex will be considered, followed by a more detailed consideration of the structure, organization and connections of the hippocampal formation and the amygdaloid nuclear complex.

There are several definitions of 'limbic cortex', each of which is based upon variations in cortical nomenclature, different criteria of what a limbic system is or should be and, therefore, different inclusion criteria for various cortical and related subcortical areas (see MacLean 1952; Nauta 1958; Stephan 1975; Nauta & Domesick

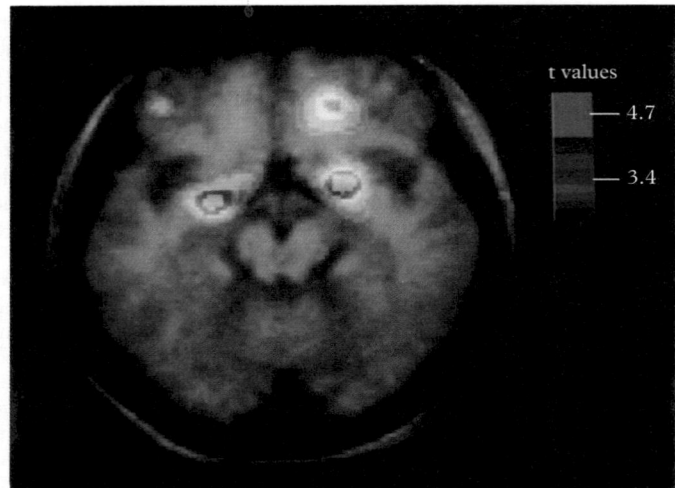

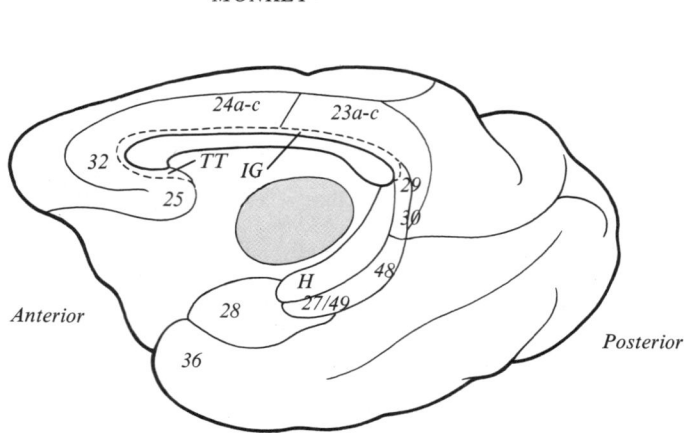

MONKEY

Anterior

Posterior

8.234 Cortical regions activated by olfactory stimulation. The composite figure shows the averaged PET subtraction image superimposed on the average horizontal MRI scan, taken at a vertical level 17 mm below the commissural plane. The three areas of activation are found within the piriform cortex bilaterally, and unilaterally in the right orbitofrontal cortex. (PET image provided by Robert Zattore; from Nature 360: 339–340, 1992.)

8.235 Schematic representation of the ventromedial aspect of the brain of an old world monkey to illustrate subdivisions of the limbic cortex. H = hippocampal formation; IG = indusium griseum; TT = taenia tecta; numbers refer to Brodmann's areas. (Redrawn from Lopes da Silva et al 1990.)

1981; Isaacson 1982; Swanson 1983; Nauta & Fiertag 1986; LeDoux 1986; Lopes da Silva et al 1990). However, some features of the limbic cortex have consistently surfaced in these accounts. The first is that one of its most central components, the hippocampus, is three-layered allocortex (archicortex in more classical terminology) and that, emerging from this medial position in the temporal lobe, the cortex of Broca's limbic lobe is juxtallocortical, that is transitional between primitive trilaminar cortex and the six-layered structure of the neocortex (isocortex). Thus, for the most part, when considering limbic cortex, the focus is on allocortical and juxtallocortical structures on the medial wall of the hemisphere (**8.235**). The amygdala, as a central component of the limbic system, presents a difficulty in this definition of the limbic cortex or the limbic lobe, as it has generally been regarded as a collection of subcortical nuclei. But it has been suggested that the anatomical and chemical structure, together with the afferent and efferent connections, of basolateral parts of the amygdala indicate that it, too, may be viewed as a cortical structure—'quasicortical' in the terms of Carlsen and Heimer (1986; see also Alheid & Heimer 1988). A second feature of the limbic system reflects the dependency of its definition on the notion of connectedness (Swanson 1983; Lopes da Silva et al 1990). One of the major characteristics of all juxtallocortical areas is that they are strongly connected with each other, with the hippocampal formation and with the anterior thalamic nuclei (particularly the anterodorsal, anteroventral and reuniens nuclei) which are often referred to as the truly limbic domain of the thalamus (Nauta & Domesick 1981; Lopes da Silva et al 1990). It has been pointed out that these juxtallocortical areas also share the characteristic of receiving inputs from polymodal association cortex (areas of sensory convergence; see Mesulam et al 1977), which are primarily represented by adjacent areas of proisocortex and isocortex, and they may thus function as supramodal association areas.

In this account, the limbic cortex (**8.235**) is taken to include:

- The hippocampal formation, which includes the dentate gyrus, the hippocampus proper (Ammon's horn), the subicular complex (subiculum, presubiculum, parasubiculum) and entorhinal cortex (area 28). These areas are often referred to as archicortical (dentate gyrus, Ammon's horn and, in some classifications, the subiculum) and periarchicortical (pre- and parasubiculum, entorhinal cortex), the former being incorporated within the term 'allocortical' and the latter 'juxtallocortical'.
- Large parts of the cortex on the medial wall of the hemisphere (Broca's limbic lobe), including medial parts of the perirhinal cortex (area 35a), the granular part of the posterior cingulate or

retrosplenial cortex (area 29), ventral parts of the anterior cingulate cortex (areas 24a, b, c) and the infralimbic cortex (area 25).

Pandya and Seltzer (1982) have suggested the term 'paralimbic cortex' to include the proisocortical areas that occupy an intermediate position between second-and-third-order association areas of the neocortex and the archicortical/periarchicortical areas that comprise the limbic cortex. Included among these areas on the medial surface of the hemisphere are the prelimbic cortex, parts of the cingulate cortex (23, 29d) and the caudal part of the parahippocampal gyrus (e.g. 35b, 36).

The organization and connections of the hippocampal formation will be considered in detail below. The structure, interconnections and thalamic relationships of the periarchicortical components of the limbic cortex will first be summarized briefly. In primates, including man, only parts of the cingulate and parahippocampal gyri usually are afforded the limbic notation. In the classical description of Brodmann (1878, 1909), the cingulate gyrus was divided rostrocaudally into several cytoarchitectonically discrete areas: the prelimbic (area 32) and infralimbic (area 25) cortex, the anterior cingulate cortex (areas 23 and 24) and part of the posterior cingulate or retrosplenial cortex (area 29). Areas 23 (posterior cingulate cortex) and 32 are generally taken to be isocortical. Only areas 25 and parts of 24 (a, b, c) and 29 (mainly c) that directly border the *induseum griseum* are periallocortical (see Vogt 1985 for a detailed account of the primate cingulate cortex). The *indusium griseum* (supracallosal gyrus) is a poorly differentiated layer of grey matter covering the superior aspect of the corpus callosum. Laterally, on each side, it enters the callosal sulcus to continue into the cortex of the cingulate gyrus. Anteriorly, it passes around the genu and rostrum of the corpus callosum to merge with the superior ends of each paraterminal gyrus, which are continuous below with the diagonal band of Broca and, through this, with the anterior perforated substance (see **8.238**) and periamygdaloid area. Posteriorly, the indusium griseum diverges on the splenium to merge with the gyrus fasciolaris (splenial gyrus), a delicate strip of grey matter curving down, forwards and laterally to the posterior extremity of the dentate gyrus. Embedded in the indusium, ridging its free surface, are two narrow bundles of fibres on each side, the medial and lateral longitudinal striae (**8.228**). The medial striae are near the midline, the lateral in the callosal sulci. The striae are regarded as the reduced white matter of a vestigial indusium. Anteriorly, they pass towards the paraterminal 'gyri'; posteriorly they continue through the gyrus fasciolaris to the fimbriae of the fornix. The indusium griseum is considered to be the vestige of the dorsal hippocampus, partially obliterated by the marked growth of the corpus callosum in primates and man. The complex parahippocampal gyrus includes areas 27, 28 (entorhinal cortex), 35, 36, 48, 49 and temporal cortical fields TF and TH (von Bonin & Bailey 1947). Of these, areas 35b, 36 and the TF and TH fields are proisocortical, the remainder are periarchicortical according to most accounts.

Schematically represented in **8.236** are the rich interconnections within the cingulate and parahippocampal cortices, as well as with the hippocampal formation (see below) and Lopes da Silva et al (1990) have suggested that this interconnectedness sets limbic cortical areas apart from the paralimbic areas. The infralimbic cortex (area 25) has been shown in monkeys to project to areas 24a and 24b and to the retrosplenial or posterior cingulate cortex (areas 29a, b, c) in non-primate species (Vogt and Miller 1983; Vogt et al 1986, 1987). Area 25 also has reciprocal connections with the entorhinal cortex. Projections between the paralimbic area 32 and the limbic cortex (anterior, retrosplenial and entorhinal cortex) are somewhat less prominent. Whereas in non-primate species there are significant interconnections between areas 24 and 29, this does not appear to be the case in monkeys, but both are connected with the paralimbic posterior cingulate area 23 (Vogt 1985). A similar marked species difference in interconnections involves the retrosplenial cortex, especially areas 29b, c and d. These areas are clearly interconnected with the subicular complex in rats and rabbits, but not apparently in monkeys (Vogt 1985). The strong connections between subicular and entorhinal areas will be discussed in the context of the hippocampal formation itself. Reference to **8.236** emphasizes the way that the proisocortical cingulate and related areas (32, 24c, 23, 29d, 35b, 36) interface between the limbic archi- and periarchicortex and widespread areas of the neocortex. This pattern of cortical connection outwards from the hippocampus, via the entorhinal cortex to the perirhinal cortex, caudal parahippocampal gyrus and posterior cingulate gyrus has taken on enormous functional importance so far as the hippocampus is concerned, as will be discussed below. The parahippocampal gyrus in particular projects to virtually all association areas of the cortex in primates (van Hoesen 1982) as well as providing the major funnel through which polymodal sensory inputs converge on the hippocampus.

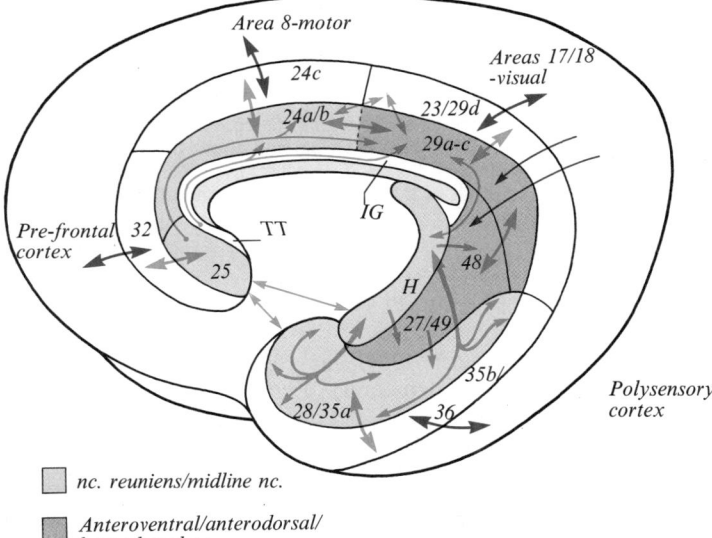

nc. reuniens/midline nc.

Anteroventral/anterodorsal/laterodorsal nc.

8.236 Schematic representation of the limbic cortex illustrating major connections within its constituent parts, as well as with major thalamic and extra-limbic cortical areas. The connections represent an overview of the *major features* of the limbic cortex and do not take account of species differences. There is a clear dichotomy in the limbic cortex with respect to its connections with the so-called 'limbic thalamus', indicated by different densities of stippling. Major connections with extra-limbic cortices are such that, within the limbic cortex, at least four functionally different domains can be recognized. Abbreviations as for **8.225**. (Redrawn from Lopes da Silva, et al, 1990.)

HIPPOCAMPAL FORMATION

The last decade has seen major advances in understanding the organization and functions of not only the rodent, but also the primate and even the human hippocampal formation. In addition to the classical literature on hippocampal structure (Cajal 1890, 1911; Lorente de Nó 1934; Rose 1927; Braak 1974), there are now exquisitely detailed and increasingly complete accounts of the primate and human hippocampal formation (Amaral 1987; Amaral & Insausti 1990; Duvernoy 1988; Rosene & van Hoesen 1987; Swanson & Köhler 1987). For more information than is possible to summarize here, readers are especially referred to Amaral and Insausti (1990), which provides special detail of experimental investigations of the structure and connections of the monkey hippocampal formation in the context of this structure in man. There are several definitions of the hippocampal formation, but the one used here again reflects the interconnectedness of the component structures by a series of associational projections, namely with the dentate gyrus, cornu ammonis, subicular complex and entorhinal cortex. But, as emphasized by Amaral (1987), this grouping remains somewhat arbitrary; for example the perirhinal cortex is rarely included as part of the hippocampal formation, even though it provides a major projection to the hippocampus and receives efferents from the subicular complex and entorhinal cortex.

The name hippocampus stems from the supposed resemblance of the complex, in coronal section, to the profile of a seahorse (Arantius 1587; cited in Amaral & Insausti 1990). The cornu ammonis lies above the subiculum and medial parahippocampal gyrus, forming a curved elevation about 5 cm long along the floor of the inferior cornu of the lateral ventricle (**8.237**). Its anterior end is expanded and here its margin may have two or three shallow grooves giving a paw-like appearance, the pes hippocampi. The ventricular aspect is coronally convex and covered by ependyma, beneath which fibres of the alveus converge medially on a longitudinal bundle of fibres, the fimbria of the fornix. The general order of these cell layers and fasciculi in coronal section are illustrated in **8.238**. Passing medially from the collateral sulcus, the neocortex of the parahippocampal gyrus merges with the transitional juxtallocortex of the subiculum, which curves superomedially to the inferior surface of the dentate gyrus, continuing laterally to the laminae of the cornu ammonis; this continues the curvature, first superiorly then medially above the dentate gyrus, and ends pointing towards the centre of the superior surface of the dentate gyrus. The degree of curvature varies somewhat along the length of the hippocampus and in different specimens. The dentate gyrus (**8.238, 239**) is a crenated strip of cortex related inferiorly to the subiculum, laterally to the cornu ammonis, superiorly to the recurved cornu ammonis, the alveus and, more medially, the fimbria of the fornix (**8.239**). The form of the fimbria is quite variable, but medially it is separated from the crenated medial margin of the dentate gyrus by the fimbriodentate sulcus (**8.240**). The hippocampal sulcus, of variable depth, lies between the dentate gyrus and the subicular extension of the parahippocampal gyrus. Posteriorly, the dentate gyrus is continuous with the gyrus fasciolaris and thus with the indusium griseum. Anteriorly, it is continued into the notch of the uncus, turning medially across its inferior surface, as the tail of the dentate gyrus (band of Giacomini), vanishing on the medial aspect of the uncus (**8.239**). The tail separates the inferior surface of the uncus into an anterior uncinate gyrus and posterior intralimbic gyrus (**8.239**).

In terms of the structure of the hippocampal formation, there are at least three nomenclatures still in use for the various hippocampal fields (Ramón y Cajal 1893, 1955; Rose 1926; Rose 1939 and Lorente de Nó 1934). Part of the reason for the confusion is that descriptions that are accurate for one species are not easily transferable to another, indicating that the hippocampal formation has undergone considerable species-specific specialization (Stephan 1983; Amaral 1987). Amaral (1987) presents a lucid description of the relationships of these schema to each other as well as providing the nomenclature adopted here.

The trilaminar cortex of the dentate gyrus is the least complex of the hippocampal fields, and its major cell type is the granule cell, found in the dense granule cell layer. Granule cells (approximately 9×10^6 in the human dentate gyrus; Seress 1988) have unipolar dendrites that extend into the overlying molecular layer which

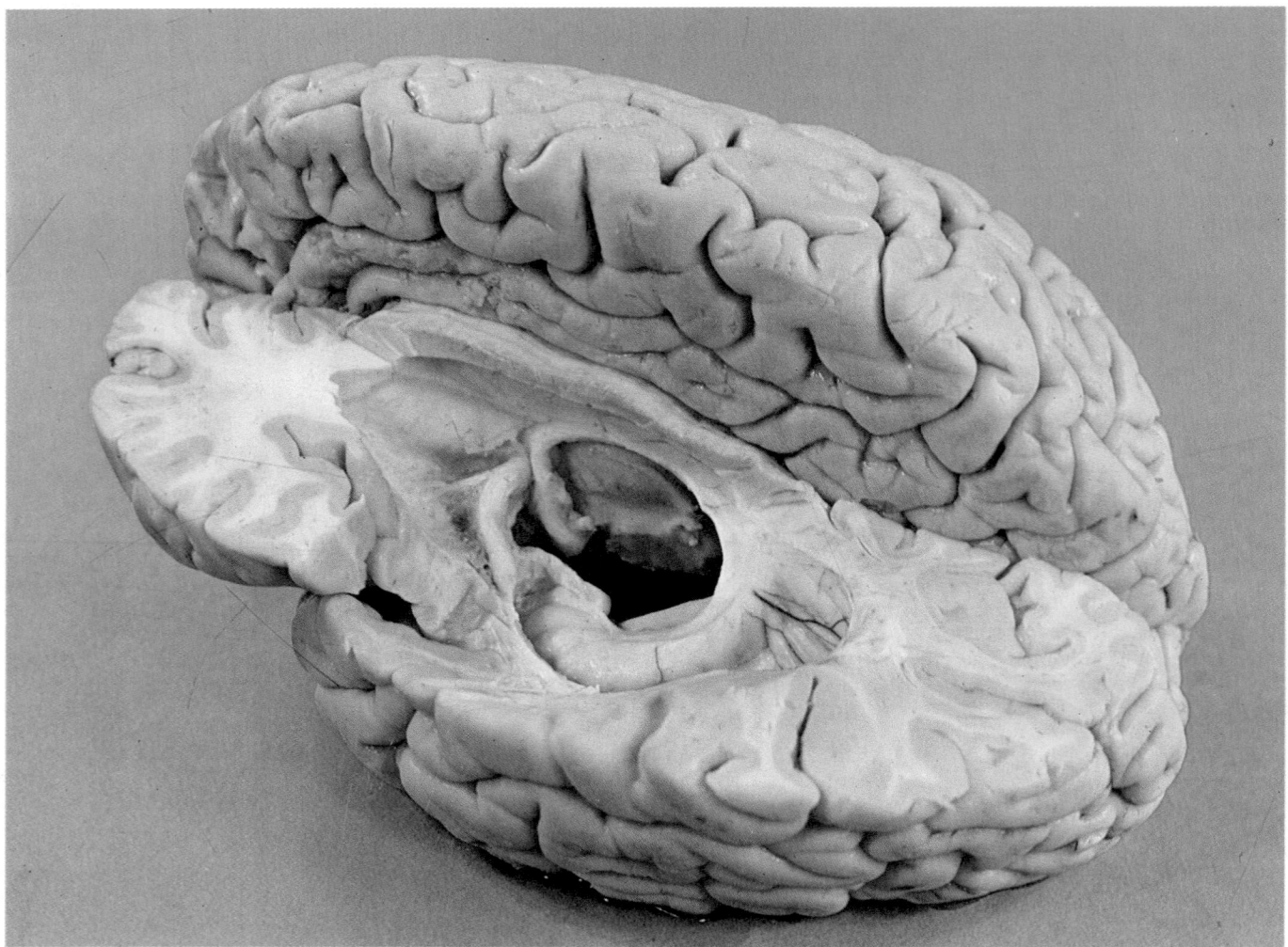

8.237 A dissection of the left cerebral hemisphere from the superolateral aspect to demonstrate various structural features of the limbic forebrain. The corpus callosum is divided sagitally in the region of its body only; the frontal, temporal and occipital lobes have been sectioned horizontally and their superior parts removed. The left lentiform nucleus, much of the caudate nucleus and dorsal thalamus have been removed and the floor of the inferior horn of the lateral ventricle laid open. Note: (1) the horizontally sectioned head of the caudate nucleus; (2) the spiral disposition of the fornix as it curves from the mamillary body through its left column, body, crus and fimbria; (3) the curved elevation of the hippocampus projecting into the floor of the inferior horn of the ventricle and ending anteriorly as the grooved pes hippocampi; (4) the anterior commissure entering the left hemisphere immediately anterior to the column of the fornix and passing laterally, to diverge into small anterior and large posterior components; between the latter the deep aspect of the anterior perforated substance is visible; (5) within the curve of the fornix the medial aspect of the right thalamus crossed superiorly by the stria medullaris thalami; (6) coursing above the corpus callosum a longitudinal white stria is visible and above this arches the right gyrus cinguli. Compare with **8**.228. (Dissection by A M Seal, photography by Kevin Fitzpatrick, both of the Department of Anatomy, Guy's Hospital Medical School, London.)

receives most of the afferent projections to the dentate gyrus (primarily from the entorhinal cortex, see below). The granule cell and molecular layers are sometimes referred to as the fascia dentata. The polymorphic layer, or hilus of the dentate gyrus, contains cells that give rise primarily to ipsilateral association fibres that remain within the dentate gyrus and do not extend into other hippocampal fields. The granule cell layer encloses a portion of the pyramidal cell layer of the cornu ammonis, which Lorente de Nó (1934) called the CA4 field.

The human hippocampus proper (cornu ammonis) is trilaminar archicortex and has essentially a single cellular layer, the pyramidal cell layer, with plexiform layers above and below it. It may best be divided into three distinct fields, following the nomenclature of Lorente de Nó (1934), namely CA1, CA2 and CA3 (**8**.240, 241). Field CA3 borders the hilus of the dentate gyrus at one end, and field CA2 at the other. In early accounts a field CA4 was also identified. However, there appear to be no cytoarchitectonic or connectional reasons to distinguish field CA3 from CA4 (Blackstad 1956, Amaral & Insausti 1990) and so the term CA4 has been dropped from most contemporary accounts of the hippocampal formation. Field CA3 pyramidal cells are the largest in the hippocampus and the whole pyramidal cell layer in this field is about 10 cells thick. The most important feature of pyramidal cells in CA3 is that they receive the mossy fibre input from dentate granule cells on their proximal dendrites. The border between CA3 and CA2 is not well marked as the pyramidal cells of the former appear to extend under the border of the latter for some distance. The CA2 field has the most compact layer of pyramidal cells. It completely lacks a mossy fibre input from dentate granule cells and receives a major input from the supramamillary region of the hypothalamus. Field CA1 is usually described as the most complex of the hippocampal subdivisions and its appearance varies along its transverse and rostrocaudal axes. The CA1/CA2 border is not sharp and at its other end CA1 overlaps the subiculum for some distance. The thickness of the pyramidal cell layer varies from about 10 to more than 30 cells and about 10% of neurons in this field are interneurons.

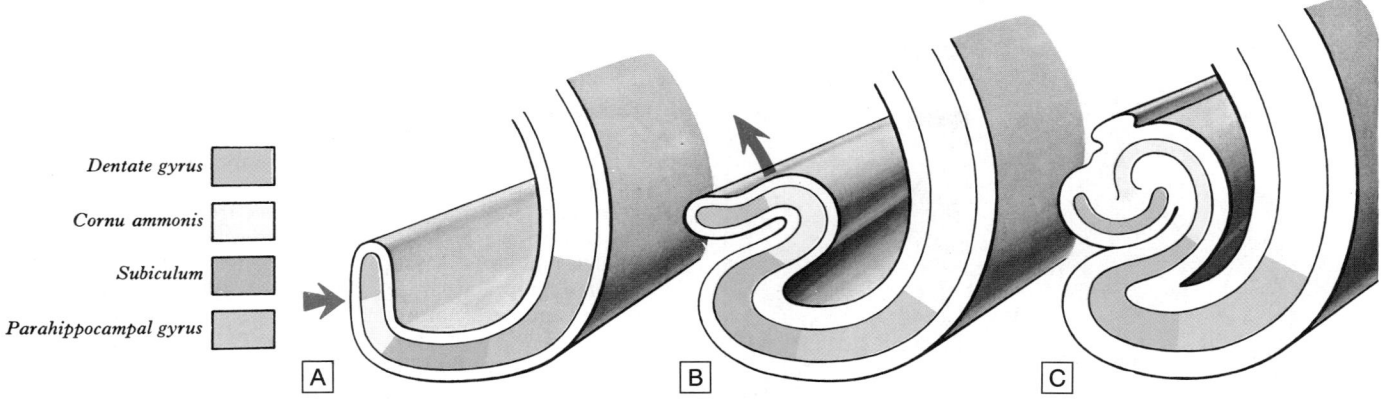

8.238A–C The hippocampus and related structures seen in coronal sections: A, B and C are a series of diagrams to assist understanding of the assumption of the definitive positions of the dentate gyrus, cornu ammonis, subiculum and parahippocampal gyrus in the floor of the inferior horn of the lateral ventricle in the human brain. Note that these are *not* tracings from a series of embryonic sections and that they have been somewhat simplified in the interests of clarity. Note also that the amount of curvature and infolding which occurs varies along the length of the hippocampus and in different specimens. It is important to appreciate that, following folding, the original *external* surfaces of the dentate gyrus and part of the subiculum are in contact and that the degree of tissue fusion which occurs along the line of the hippocampal sulcus is variable.

It is common to describe several stratal divisions of the layers of the cornu ammonis beginning from its ventricular aspect, as follows (**8**.240, 241):

- The *ependyma*
- The *alveus*, comprised of subicular and hippocampal pyramidal cell axons converging on the fimbria of the fornix
- The *stratum oriens*, comprised mainly of the basal dendrites of pyramidal cells and some interneurons.
- The *stratum pyramidalis*
- The *stratum lucidum*, in which mossy fibres pass to make contact with the proximal dendrites of pyramidal cells in field CA3 (it is not as prominent in man as in other primates and is not present in fields CA1 and CA2)
- The *stratum radiatum* and *stratum lacunosum-moleculare*.

In the stratum radiatum and stratum oriens, CA3 and CA2 cells receive associational connections from other rostrocaudal levels of the hippocampus, as well as afferents from subcortical structures, such as the septal nuclei and supramamillary region. The projections from pyramidal cells of fields CA3 and CA2 to CA1, often called Schaffer collaterals, also terminate in the stratum radiatum and stratum oriens. The projections from the entorhinal cortex to the dentate gyrus (the perforant pathway) travel in the stratum lacunosum-moleculare, where its fibres make synaptic contact en passant with the distal apical dendrites of hippocampal pyramidal cells.

The subicular complex is generally viewed as comprising three main subdivisions, namely the subiculum, presubiculum and parasubiculum (**8**.240, 241). The pyramidal neurons of the subicular complex are the origin of major subcortical projections of the hippocampal formation (to the septal nuclei, mamillary nuclei, nucleus accumbens and anterior thalamus), as well as to the entorhinal cortex. The subiculum can be divided into three layers: a superficial molecular layer containing apical dendrites of subicular pyramidal cells, a pyramidal cell layer that is about 30 cells thick and a deep polymorphic layer. The presubiculum is medial to the subiculum and has the distinctive feature of a densely packed superficial layer of pyramidal cells. There is a plexiform layer that is superficial to this dense cell layer, but cells deep to it are best regarded as either a medial extension of the subiculum or a lateral extension of the deep layers of the entorhinal cortex (Amaral & Insausti 1990). The parasubiculum also has a superficial plexiform layer and a primary cell layer and it forms the boundary between the subicular complex as a whole and the entorhinal cortex. The cell layers deep to the parasubiculum are indistinguishable from the deep layers of the entorhinal cortex (Amaral & Insausti 1990).

The entorhinal cortex (Brodmann's area 28; **8**.230, 240, 241) has undergone considerable laminar, as well as regional, differentiation in the primate brain when compared with non-primate species (Stephan 1983). As mentioned above, the human entorhinal cortex has recently been partitioned into many more than Brodmann's original medial and lateral fields and there is clearly a rostrocaudal gradient of cytoarchitectonic differentiation. It extends rostrally to the anterior limit of the amygdala and caudally overlaps only a portion of the hippocampal fields. The more primitive levels of the entorhinal cortex (below the amygdala) receive projections from the olfactory bulb (see above), but more caudal regions do not generally receive primary olfactory inputs. In man, there is no easily identifiable lateral border to the entorhinal cortex, in contrast to the monkey and rat, where this is marked by the rhinal sulcus. Indeed, as pointed out by Amaral and Insausti (1990), in man the rhinal sulcus is actually situated rostral to the entorhinal cortex and is therefore spatially dissociated from it. The collateral sulcus lies lateral to all of the entorhinal cortex, but does not form its natural border either. It is laterally adjacent to the perirhinal cortex (Brodmann's areas 35 and 36) over much of its length. The entorhinal cortex is a multilaminated structure, but one that is quite distinct from those of other neocortical regions. According to Amaral and Insausti (1990), the entorhinal cortex can be divided into six layers:

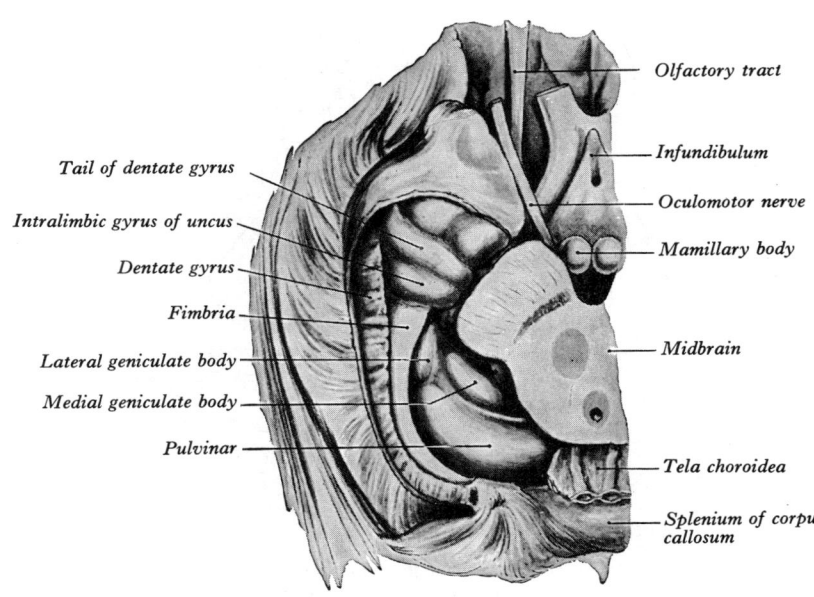

8.239 Basal aspect of part of the brain dissected to display the uncus, dentate gyrus, fimbria etc.

Olfactory tract

Infundibulum

Oculomotor nerve

Mamillary body

Tail of dentate gyrus

Intralimbic gyrus of uncus

Dentate gyrus

Fimbria

Lateral geniculate body

Medial geniculate body

Midbrain

Pulvinar

Tela choroidea

Splenium of corpus callosum

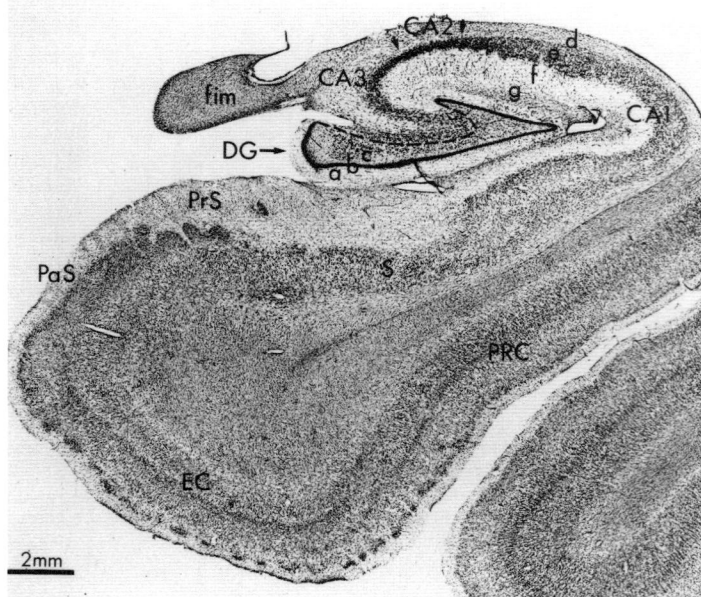

8.240 Photomicrograph of a coronal, thionin-stained section of the human hippocampal formation. DG = dentate gyrus; a, b, c layers of the dentate gyrus—a = molecular layer; b = granule cell layer; c = plexiform layer; CA1–3 = fields of the hippocampus; d, e, f, g, layers of the hippocampus—d = stratum oriens; e = pyramidal cell layer; f = stratum radiatum; g = stratum lacunosum-moleculae; S = subiculum; PrS = presubiculum; PaS = parasubiculum; EC = entorhinal cortex; PRC = perirhinal cortex; fim = fimbria. (Photomicrograph provided by David Amaral; see Amaral & Insausti, 1990.)

- An acellular plexiform layer (I).
- A narrow cellular layer comprised of islands of large pyramidal and stellate cells that is a distinguishing feature of the entorhinal cortex (II). These cell islands form small bumps on the surface of the brain that can be seen by the naked eye (verrucae hippocampae) and provide an indication of the boundaries of the entorhinal cortex.

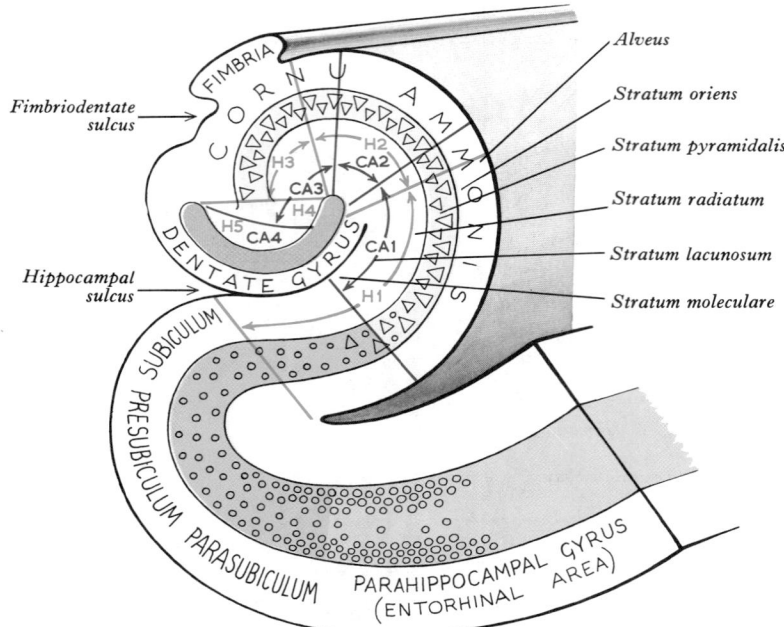

8.241 Schematic diagram of the hippocampal formation showing the disposition of the various cell fields. Colour coding: pink = dentate gyrus; yellow = hippocampus proper (cornu ammonis); green = areas of the subicular complex; blue = entorhinal cortex. CA1–3 = hippocampal cell fields.

- A layer of medium-sized pyramidal cells (III).
- There is no internal granular layer, another classical feature of the entorhinal cortex, and in its place is an acellular region of dense fibres called the lamina dissecans (Rose 1927) which some authors label as layer IV.
- In regions where the lamina dissecans is not present, layers III and V are apposed, layer V being comprised of large pyramidal cells five or six deep.
- Layer VI is only readily distinguishable from layer V close to the border with the perirhinal cortex. Its cells continue around the angular bundle (subcortical white matter deep to the subicular complex comprised largely of perforant path axons) to lie beneath the pre- and parasubiculum.

Chemical anatomy. This is a rapidly changing scene and only a few, selected features of the chemical phenotype of neurons of the hippocampal formation will be presented here (see Swanson & Köhler 1987; Amaral & Insausti 1990). In addition to the monoaminergic, cholinergic and GABAergic extrinsic afferents described below, other classical neurotransmitter substances are also found in the hippocampal formation, most studies having been conducted using rats. Glutamate and/or aspartate appears to be the major excitatory transmitter in three pathways in the hippocampal formation: the perforant pathway arising in the entorhinal cortex and terminating primarily in the dentate gyrus; the mossy fibres running from the dentate granule cells to the pyramidal cells of the CA3 field and in the Schaffer collaterals of CA3 pyramidal cells that terminate on CA1 pyramidal cells. GABAergic (GAD-immunoreactive) neurons are found in the deep portions of the granule cell layer in the dentate gyrus (basket cells) and the highest concentration of GABA receptors is found in the molecular layer of the dentate gyrus. In the hippocampus proper, GAD-immunoreactive cells are found mostly in the stratum oriens, but also in the pyramidal cell layer and stratum radiatum. There are many peptide-containing neurons in the hippocampal formation, including that in man. Granule cells in the dentate gyrus appear to contain the opioid peptide dynorphin, which is also present in mossy fibres running to the CA3 field, while enkephalin or a related peptide may be present in fibres arising in the entorhinal cortex. There is a dense plexus of somatostatin-immunoreactive fibres in the molecular layer of the dentate gyrus and also in the stratum lacunosum-moleculare of the hippocampus. There are quite numerous somatostatin-immunoreactive neurons in the polymorphic layer of the dentate gyrus, stratum oriens of the cornu ammonis and the deep layers of the entorhinal cortex. This somatostatin-immunoreactivity is also found in many neurons that also contain GAD-immunoreactivity, while the distribution of these neurons is very similar to that of neurons containing neuropeptide-Y (NY). In many species, NY and somatostatin coexist in many cortical and striatal neurons (Everitt et al 1984; Everitt & Hökfelt 1989), and this may also be the case for these peptides in the hippocampal formation. Neurons containing the vasoactive intestinal polypeptide (VIP) are also plentiful in many hippocampal fields, being especially common in the superficial layers of the entorhinal cortex. Cells containing CCK-immunoreactivity are found in the hilar region of the dentate gyrus, in all layers of the cornu ammonis, especially in the pyramidal cell layer, and also throughout the subicular complex and entorhinal cortex. There are also substantial plexuses of CCK-immunoreactive fibres in the stratum lacunosum-moleculare, subicular complex and entorhinal cortex. Hippocampal CCK-immunoreactive cells may give rise to extrinsic projections, for example, to the lateral septum and medial mamillary nucleus, since CCK-immunoreactive fibres are found in the fimbria/fornix in rats, monkeys and man, while transection of the fornix results in decreases in CCK in these structures.

Intrinsic circuitry. As shown in **8.236**, one important feature of hippocampal circuitry is the apparently unidirectional progression of synaptic activation (Amaral & Insausti 1990). The point of entry into the hippocampal circuitry is the dentate gyrus, which receives via the perforant path projections from layers II and III of the entorhinal cortex. The axons terminate in an orderly way in the outer two-thirds of the molecular layer of the dentate gyrus on the dendritic spines of granule cells (there are also terminations on the distal dendrites of CA1 and CA3 pyramidal cells, but these are fewer in number). The dentate granule cells project heavily via their mossy fibres on to the proximal dendrites of CA3 pyramidal cells. These pyramidal cells of field CA3 give rise, via the so-called Schaffer collaterals, to an equally impressive projection that terminates mainly in the stratum radiatum of the CA1 hippocampal field. In its turn, the CA1 field projects heavily to the subicular complex which, to complete the circuitry, projects to the entorhinal cortex. The unidirectionality of intrinsic hippocampal connections is further emphasized by the absence of feedback projections from, for example, CA3 to the dentate gyrus, or CA1 back to CA3. This intrinsic circuitry, then, appears to form a closed loop of connections, but it is essential to bear in mind that each of the hippocampal fields, except the dentate gyrus, also gives rise to extrinsic projections. Thus, pyramidal cells in the cornu ammonis project to the lateral septal nucleus, while the subicular complex gives rise to major projections inter alia to the mamillary bodies, ventral striatum, anterior thalamus and amygdaloid complex.

Extrinsic connections. The perception of extrinsic hippocampal connections has changed markedly over the past decade. Dominated by the circuit of Papez and MacLean's notion of the limbic system, the hippocampal formation was generally perceived as receiving sensory information from neocortical association cortices, while sending its output through the fimbria and fornix to the mamillary

bodies. As will be described below, this early view is not only too simple, but also inaccurate. For example, the subiculum, rather than hippocampus proper, projects to the mamillary complex, whereas the hippocampus proper gives rise principally to efferents destined for the septal complex. Parts of the striatal complex have also been identified recently as a major target of subicular outflow. Furthermore, the fimbria and fornix do not represent the sole vehicle of hippocampal outflow, there being major projections from the subicular complex and entorhinal cortex to neighbouring cortices such as the perirhinal cortex, parahippocampal gyrus and, further afield, to the orbitofrontal cortex. Amaral (1987) makes the general point that the dentate gyrus and cornu ammonis receive little or no direct neocortical afferents. Instead, the subicular complex and entorhinal cortex receive such projections from temporal, frontal and parietal cortices and from the insula. By contrast, all hippocampal fields receive subcortical afferents. Summaries of hippocampal circuitry, formation of the fornix and connections are shown schematically in **8**.242–244.

Hippocampal subcortical connections

Afferents. There are two prominent sources of subcortical afferents to the hippocampal formation: the medial septal complex and the

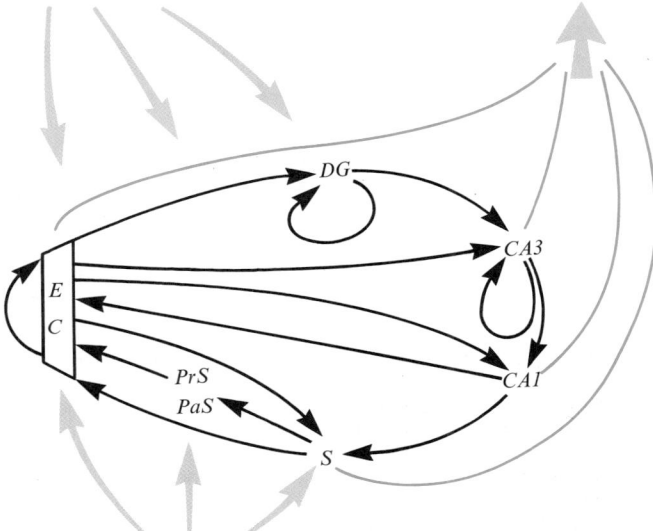

Subcortical input	Subcortical output
Amygdala	*Olfactory regions*
Claustrum	*Claustrum*
Septal nuclei	*Amygdala*
Basal nucleus (Meynert)	*Septal nuclei*
Supramammillary nucleus	*Nucleus accumbens*
Anterior thalamus	*Caudate/Putamen*
Midline thalamus	*Hypothalamus*
Ventral tegmental area	*Anterior thalamus*
Raphe nucleus	*Mammillary nuclei*
Locus coeruleus	

Cortical input
Perirhinal cortex (areas 35 and 36)
Parahippocampal gyrus (areas TF and TH)
Cingulate cortex
Piriform cortex
Insular cortex
Orbitofrontal cortex
Superior temporal gyrus

8.242 Schematic illustration of the major intrinsic connections of the hippocampal formation and a listing of prominent afferent and efferent connections. Curved arrows in the dentate gyrus (DG) and in the CA3 field of the hippocampus indicate the presence of associational projections that link different levels of the fields. The curved arrow in the entorhinal cortex (EC) indicates the presence of associational projections between different levels of the field and projections from deep layers to superficial layers. Dashed lines at the right represent efferent projections carried by the fornix. Several of the subcortical afferents listed at the left enter the hippocampal formation through the fornix. A separate list of cortical outputs has not been listed, but Amaral and Insausti (1990) suggest that most, if not all, areas listed as afferents to the hippocampal formation receive return projections from the subiculum and entorhinal cortex. Other abbreviations: S, PrS, PaS = subiculum, presubiculum and parasubiculum, respectively. (Reproduced with permission from Amaral and Insausti, 1990.)

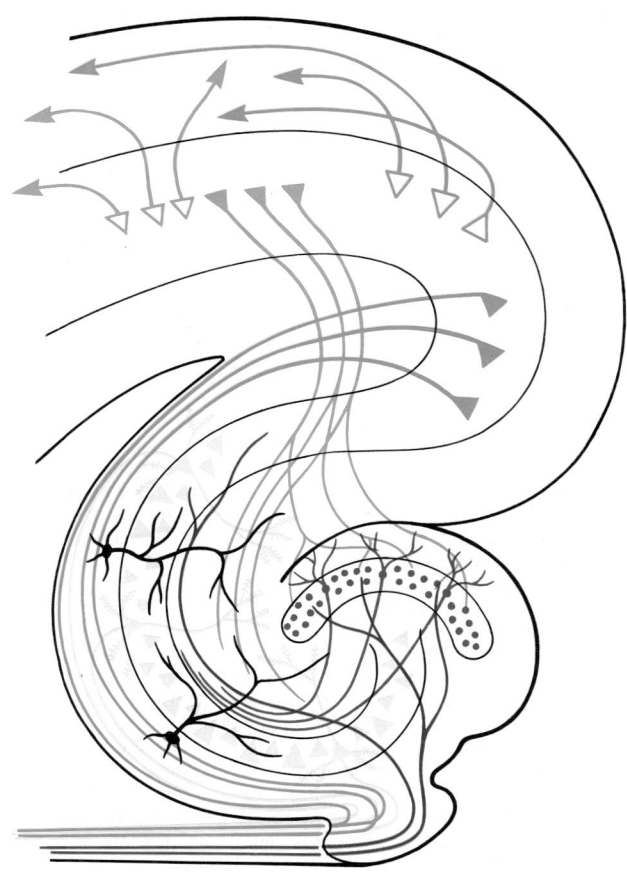

8.243 Some of the main features of the neuronal organization and connectivity patterns of the dentate gyrus, cornu ammonis, subiculum and parahippocampal gyrus. The cell somata, dendrites and axons of the pyramidal neurons of the cornu ammonis are yellow; their axons form the efferent hippocampal fibres of the alveus and fimbria. Afferent fibres to the cornu ammonis from the fimbria are purple; afferents from the entorhinal cortex via the perforant path are blue. Basket neurons are in black. The neurons of the dentate gyrus and their axons which form the mossy fibres of the hippocampus are in magenta. Subicular efferents to the fornix via the alveus are in green.

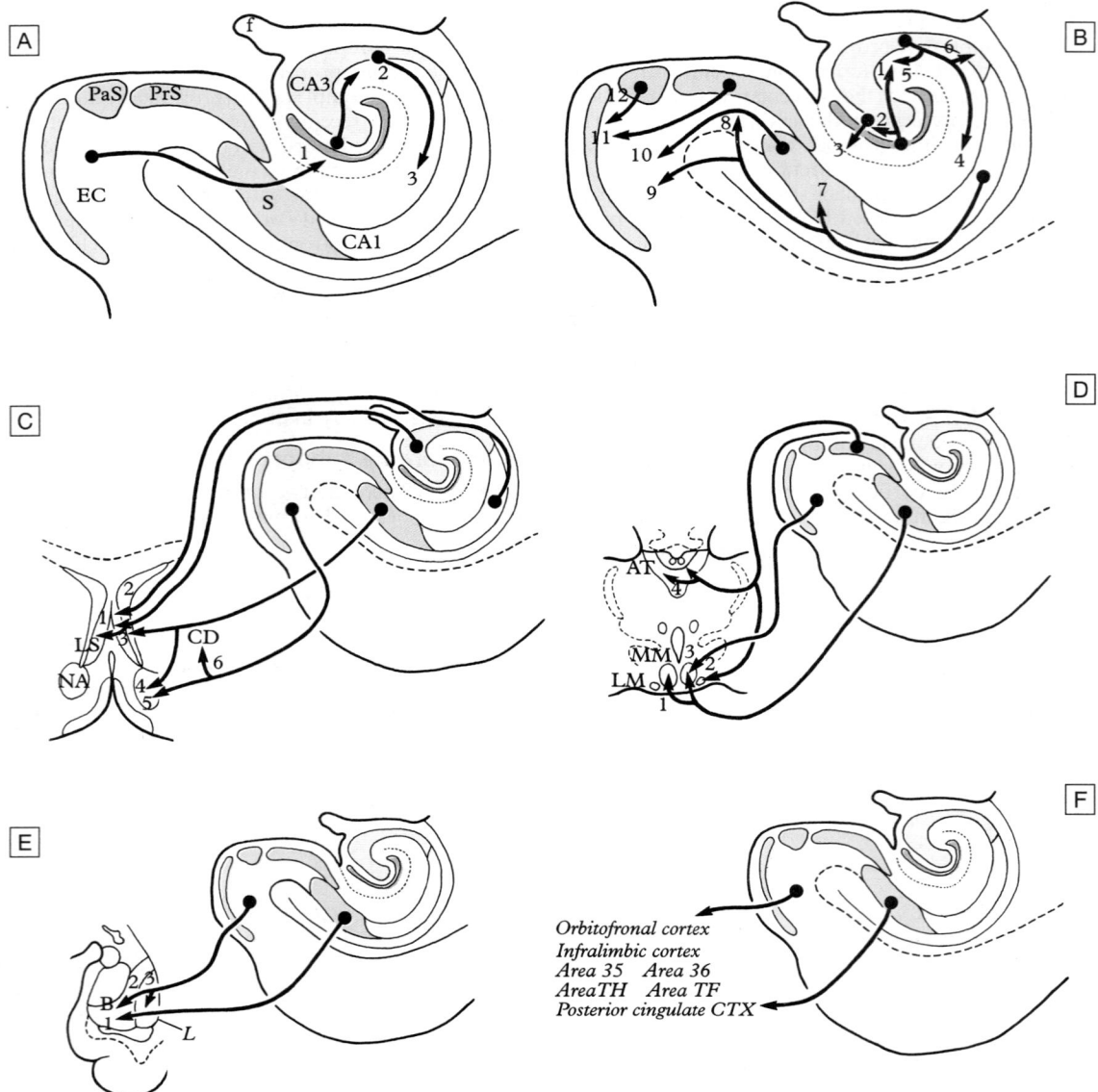

8.244 Line drawing of a coronal section through the monkey hippocampal formation on which major intrinsic and extrinsic efferents are illustrated. A. various fields that comprise the hippocampal formation are labelled and the fundamental trisynaptic circuit is drawn (entorhinal cortex to dentate gyrus (1), dentate gyrus to hippocampal field CA3 (2), field CA3 to CA1 (3)). B. in addition to projecting to field CA3 (1), mossy fibres arising from dentate granule cells terminate on polymorphic cells of the hilar region (2); these cells give rise to ipsilateral associational and commissural projections that terminate in the molecular layer (3). CA3 pyramidal cells give rise to associational projections to other levels of field CA3 (5, 6) in addition to their projection to field CA1 (4). CA1 pyramidal cells project to subiculum (7), presubiculum (8) and entorhinal cortex (9). Cells in subiculum, presubiculum and parasubiculum send a major projection to entorhinal cortex (10, 11 and 12, respectively). c. Projections to septal nuclei are diagrammed. Field CA3 of the hippocampus projects bilaterally to the lateral septum (1) and field CA1 projects ipsilaterally (2). The subiculum also projects to the lateral septum (3) and to the nucleus accumbens (4). The entorhinal cortex projects to the nucleus accumbens (5), the caudate nucleus and putamen (6).

D. projections to the diencephalon. The subiculum projects bilaterally to the medial mamillary nucleus (1), whereas the presubiculum projects primarily to the lateral mamillary nucleus (2). The presubiculum also projects lightly to the medial mamillary nucleus, as does the entorhinal cortex (3). The projection to the anterior thalamus originates primarily in the presubiculum and it terminates bilaterally (4). E. projections to the amygdaloid complex. Both the subiculum (1) and the entorhinal cortex (2) project to the parvicellular portion of the basal nucleus; the entorhinal cortex also projects to the lateral nucleus (3). F. projections to the neocortex. Although corticopetal projections of the hippocampal formation are relatively unstudied, there is evidence for projections from both the subicular complex and the entorhinal cortex to the cortical fields listed. AT = anterior thalamic nuclei; B = basal nucleus of the amygdala; CA1, CA3 = fields of the hippocampus; DG = dentate gyrus; f = fornix; LM = lateral mamillary nucleus; LS = lateral septal nucleus; MM = medial mamillary nucleus; NA = nucleus accumbens; PaS = parasubiculum; PrS = presubiculum; S = subiculum. (Reproduced with permission from Amaral and Insausti, 1900.)

supramamillary area of the posterior hypothalamus (see Amaral & Insausti 1990). There are also projections from the amygdaloid complex (see below) and claustrum to the subicular complex and entorhinal cortex, as well as monoaminergic projections from the ventral tegmental area (possibly dopaminergic), the mesencephalic raphe nuclei (serotoninergic) and the locus corruleus (noradrenergic). The noradrenergic and serotoninergic projections reach all hippocampal fields, but are especially dense in the dentate gyrus.

The projections from the septal complex arise in the medial septal and vertical limb nuclei of the diagonal band of Broca and travel via four routes, namely the dorsal fornix, fimbria, supracallosal striae and a ventral route through the amygdaloid complex. While these projections reach all hippocampal fields, the most prominent terminations are in the dentate gyrus, field CA3, the presubiculum, parasubiculum and entorhinal cortex. Many of these medial septal/diagonal band neurons contain choline acetyltransferase (ChAT) immunoreactivity and are cholinergic, forming a part of the topographically organized basal forebrain cholinergic system (cell groups Ch1 and Ch2, according to the nomenclature of Mesulam et al 1983a, b). They also contain nerve growth factor receptor (NGF-R) immunoreactivity, indicating the dependence of these neurons on NGF derived from the hippocampus, at least for part of their life. However, it is also clear that many neurons in the medial septal/diagonal band complex innervating the hippocampal formation are not cholinergic, but contain GAD-immunoreactivity and are therefore GABAergic (Köhler et al 1984). Neurons in the supramamillary area also provide a significant innervation of the hippocampal formation, arriving partly through the fornix and partly through a ventral route, terminating most heavily in the dentate gyrus, and fields CA2 and CA3 of the cornu ammonis.

Retrograde tracing studies in monkeys have revealed that all divisions of the anterior thalamic nuclear complex and associated lateral dorsal nucleus project to the hippocampal formation, directed predominantly to the subicular complex. Some midline thalamic nuclei, particularly the parataenial, central medial and reuniens nuclei, also project to the hippocampal formation, especially to the entorhinal cortex (Amaral 1987; Amaral & Insausti 1990).

Efferents. The fornix contains about 1.2 million fibres in man (Powell et al 1957). Cells in the CA3 field project bilaterally to the lateral nucleus of the septal complex, via the precommissural fornix. These CA3 cells are the same as those giving rise to the Schaffer collaterals to CA1 cells and to the commissural projections to the contralateral hippocampus (Swanson et al 1981). Neurons in the subicular complex and entorhinal cortex give rise to projections to the nucleus accumbens and to parts of the caudate nucleus and putamen (Groenewegen et al 1982; Kelley & Domesick 1982). The subicular complex gives rise to the major, postcommissural fibre system of the fornix (Swanson & Cowan 1975). The presubiculum in particular projects to the anterior thalamic nuclear complex (anteromedial, anteroventral and laterodorsal nuclei), while both the subiculum and presubiculum provide the major extrinsic input to the mamillary complex (Simpson 1952; Swanson & Cowan 1975; Poletti & Cresswell 1977; Rosene & van Hoesen 1977). Both the lateral and the medial mamillary nuclei receive afferents from the subicular complex.

Commissural connections are not as evident in the primate as in the non-primate hippocampal formation. Only the rostral part of the hippocampus proper and associated dentate gyrus appear to be connected by commissural fibres in monkeys and, presumably, in humans. This contrasts with the rich commissural projections in rats, arising from CA3 neurons to reach CA3 and CA1 neurons in the opposite hippocampus, and from the polymorphic layer of the dentate gyrus to the inner molecular layer of the opposite dentate gyrus. The subicular complex also gives rise to a commissural projection that terminates in layer III of the opposite entorhinal cortex in monkeys.

Cortical connections. In primate species, there is increasing evidence of phylogenetically new projections constituting substantial direct connections between the neocortex, subicular complex and entorhinal cortex (van Hoesen et al 1975a,b,c; Amaral & Insausti 1990). Several fields in the temporal lobe neocortex, especially TF and TH of the parahippocampal gyrus, the dorsal bank of the superior temporal gyrus, the perirhinal cortex (Brodmann's area 35) and the temporal polar cortex, together with the agranular insular cortex and posterior orbitofrontal cortex (Walker's areas 12, 13, 14) all project to the entorhinal cortex. There are also projections to the entorhinal cortex arising from the dorsolateral prefrontal cortex (Brodmann's areas 9, 10, 46), the medial frontal cortex (Brodmann's areas 25, 32), the cingulate cortex (Brodmann's areas 23, 24) and retrosplenial cortex. The subicular complex also receives direct cortical inputs, for example, from the temporal polar cortex, perirhinal cortex, parahippocampal gyrus, superior temporal gyrus and dorsolateral prefrontal cortex. Efferent projections from the primate entorhinal cortex have not been extensively studied, but it seems that most areas projecting to the entorhinal cortex receive reciprocal projections from it (Amaral & Insausti 1990). There are projections from the entorhinal cortex to the perirhinal cortex (Learning and memory, p.1130), as well as to temporal polar cortex, caudal parahippocampal and cingulate gyri. In monkeys, the subicular complex also projects to a number of cortical areas, including perirhinal cortex, parahippocampal gyrus, caudal cingulate gyrus, medial frontal and medial orbitofrontal cortex. It should also be borne strongly in mind that the parahippocampal gyrus is an important and nodal point for these projections from the hippocampal formation, since it gives rise to projections to virtually all association cortices in the primate brain (van Hoesen 1982).

SEPTAL AREA

In subprimate mammals, the septal area is the thick medial wall of the cerebral hemispheres, anterior and superior to the lamina terminalis and anterior commissure, consisting of nuclear masses and fibre bundles, divisible into pre- and supracommissural parts. In higher primates, particularly in the human brain, septal areas are modified by the expansion of the neocortex and corpus callosum. The human supracommissural septum corresponds largely to the bilateral laminae of fibres, sparse grey matter and neuroglia, forming the septum pellucidum. The precommissural septum corresponds partly to the paraterminal gyrus, a narrow vertical strip between the anterior surface of the lamina terminalis and the posterior parolfactory sulcus. Its anterior slope passing into the sulcus is sometimes called the prehippocampal rudiment and inferiorly, the gyrus and rudiment are continuous with the diagonal band of Broca and the medial olfactory stria (8.230); superiorly they narrow, spreading round the rostrum and genu of the corpus callosum to the indusium griseum.

The septal region is comprised of four main nuclear groups: dorsal, ventral, medial and caudal. Each is subdivided into a number of more or less discrete nuclei, the full details of which may be found in Andy and Stephan (1968, 1974) and Stephan and Andy (1962). The dorsal group is essentially the dorsal septal nucleus (which has four parts); the ventral group is comprised of the lateral septal nucleus (which has internal and external parts); the medial group contains the medial septal nucleus and the nucleus of the diagonal band of Broca (dorsal and ventral parts); the caudal group contains the fimbrial and triangular septal nuclei. Andy and Stephan include the bed nucleus of the stria terminalis in this caudal group, but it is considered separately here in the context of the amygdala, since it shows structural and connectional features in common with the centromedial nuclei (see below).

The connections of the septal region have been defined largely in experiments on the rat and they are poorly understood in primates, especially in man. The major afferents to the region terminate primarily in the lateral septal nucleus. As we have seen, these include fibres carried in the precommissural fornix that arise from hippocampal fields CA3 (a bilateral projection) and CA1, and the subiculum. There are also afferents arising from the preoptic area, anterior, paraventricular and ventromedial hypothalamic nuclei, and also the lateral hypothalamic area. The projection from the paraventricular nuclei contains the neuropeptide, arginine vasopressin (AVP), and is both sexually dimorphic and responsive to changes in circulating levels of sex steroids, this region also being rich in receptors for androgenic and oestrogenic hormones. The lateral septum is also in receipt of a rich monaminergic innervation, including noradrenergic afferents arising from the locus coeruleus, as well as medullary cell groups (A1, A2), serotoninergic afferents arising from the midbrain raphe nuclei and dopaminergic afferents arising from the ventral tegmental area (A10). The laterodorsal tegmental, parabrachial, Kölliker-Fuse and dorsal vagal nuclei have all been demonstrated to project to the lateral septal nucleus.

There are generally considered to be three major efferent systems originating from the lateral septal nucleus. Hitherto, one of them has been assumed to be a relatively massive projection to the medial septal and diagonal band nuclei. However, this has recently been questioned following detailed investigations in the rat involving a combination of immunocytochemistry and anterograde tract tracing with *Phaseolus vulgaris* leucoagglutinin (Leranth et al 1992). The results of this study suggest that the lateral to medial septal projection is relatively sparse, and this observation has quite major implications for theories of septohippocampal function that are yet to have their full impact. Projections to the medial and lateral preoptic areas, anterior hypothalamus, supramamillary and midbrain ventral tegmental area from the lateral septum run via the medial forebrain bundle. There is also a projection via the stria medullaris thalami, which runs on the dorsomedial wall of the third ventricle, to the medial habenular nucleus and some midline thalamic nuclei. The projections from the habenula via the fasciculus retroflexus to the interpeduncular nucleus and adjacent ventral tegmental area in the midbrain provide a very distinctive route through which forebrain limbic structures can influence midbrain nuclear groups. However, the functions of this system are particularly obscure.

One of the most distinctive features of the medial septal/diagonal band complex is that a large proportion of its neurons are cholinergic and they project richly onto the hippocampal formation (see above) and also the cingulate cortex (Mesulam et al 1983; Wainer et al 1985). Many of them also contain the neuropeptide galanin and the enzyme nitric oxide synthase, revealed immunocytochemically, as well as by the NADPH-diaphorase histochemical procedure (Vincent & Kimura 1992). However, many medial septal neurons contain not acetylcholine, but the amino acid GABA, and these neurons also provide an important source of afferents to these cortical structures, as well as to the lateral septal nuclei (Leranth & Frotscher 1989; Leranth et al 1992). A similar organization of cholinergic and GABAergic neurons is found in the magnocellular corticopetal system (that includes the cholinergic nucleus basalis of Meynert), emphasizing the continuum of related neurons that provide a topographically organized cholinergic, and probably GABAergic,

innervation of the cortical mantle. In addition to receiving the projection from the lateral septal nucleus, which is in part also GABAergic, the medial septum/diagonal band complex appears to be in receipt of afferents from the dorsal tegmental nucleus, medial mamillary nucleus, lateral preoptic and anterior hypothalamic areas, which largely run in the medial forebrain bundle together with limited monoaminergic projections arising from pontine and medullary noradrenergic cell groups. The majority of the latter pass through the medial septum and run dorsally over the genu of the corpus callosum.

The substantial reciprocal interactions with the hippocampal formation through the medial septal cholinergic/GABAergic efferents from, and precommissural fornix afferents to, the lateral septum indicate that the functions of the septal complex must be considered at least in part in the context of the septohippocampal system (as suggested by Gray 1982). However, the close relationship between the septal complex and hypothalamus, together with its steroid hormone sensitivity, suggest that its functions must also be viewed in a broader neuroendocrine and behavioural context, although these functions are poorly understood at present.

Systems for learning and memory

At the cellular level, the capacity for long-lasting functional changes is widespread in the central nervous system. Analysis of the cognitive effects of brain damage shows, however, that in some ways memory is not simply a diffuse property of nervous tissue, but is a specialized function of discrete anatomical systems in the brain. The evidence in favour of the concept of memory systems in the brain came in the first place from patients with acquired memory disorder ('organic amnesia'). Memory disorder is often produced as one component of a general loss of mental ability ('dementia'), but in some patients amnesia is a discrete disorder, leaving intact many other cognitive abilities such as reasoning, perception and intelligence. Relatively pure amnesia of this kind is caused by correspondingly circumscribed brain damage, as opposed to the diffuse damage which is seen in dementia. Neuropathological analysis of the brain damage responsible for producing discrete amnesia suggests that the critical lesion for producing this disorder is any bilateral interruption of a system of interconnected structures which was first clearly identified by Delay and Brion in 1969. The Delay–Brion system consists of the hippocampal formation in the medial temporal lobe, including the subiculum as well as the hippocampus proper; the fimbria and fornix; the mamillary bodies; the mamillothalamic tract; the anterior group of thalamic nuclei; and the cingulate bundle and cingulate cortex. In different patients, amnesia can be caused by different lesions which are quite distinct from each other in gross topography in the brain: for example, by temporal lobe infarctions due to posterior cerebral artery occlusion in one patient,

and in another patient by lesions to the mamillary bodies, adjacent to the midline. Delay and Brion proposed that this apparent heterogeneity of the causative lesions in amnesia could be explained by the neural connections of the structures involved. For example, the subiculum of the hippocampus sends a heavy projection to the mamillary bodies through the fornix, and interruption of the fornix also causes amnesia (Gaffan & Gaffan 1991).

Modern evidence on the neuropathology of amnesia has largely supported the interpretation put forward by Delay and Brion (Mair et al 1979; Gaffan & Gaffan 1991). However, since their time our understanding of memory systems in the brain has significantly advanced in two important ways, which are further discussed below. Experimental work with non-human primates has given a much clearer picture than clinical evidence can as to the effects of particular localized brain lesions upon memory. At the same time, psychological analysis of these effects has shown that the type of memory deficit which is seen in the organic amnesic syndrome is only one kind of memory impairment, and that impairment in other kinds of memory can follow lesions outside the Delay–Brion system.

Amnesia in non-human primates

The functional relationship between brain systems and memory is revealed only imperfectly in clinical material. The interpretation of such material has necessarily remained to some extent controversial, since the causative lesions are produced by the vagaries of disease and trauma, while the consequent memory impairments must be assessed against the background of wide individual variation

in memory ability, in patients whose pre-morbid memory ability is usually unknown. For these reasons, a considerable effort has been devoted to the investigation of experimentally produced amnesia in non-human primates.

The results of early studies were puzzling in that macaque monkeys (*Macaca mulatta* and *M. fascicularis*) appeared to show little impairment in some simple tests of object memory after experimentally produced ablations in the Delay–Brion system. However, more recent experiments, investigating a wider range of memory tasks, have shown that these ablations produced a severe impairment in monkeys' memory for complex spatially organized scenes. These impairments are revealed in a wide variety of tasks, including spatial memory tasks in mazes (Murray et al 1989), memory for the location of hidden food rewards (Gaffan & Harrison 1989), memory for complex naturalistic scenes such as frames from a cinema film (Gaffan 1992), and memory for artificial scenes generated by a formal algorithm on a computer-driven display (Gaffan 1994); this last kind of experiment is particularly valuable in allowing the effects of brain lesions on memory for objects, backgrounds and spatial organization to be separately analysed. After interruption of the Delay–Brion system monkeys are not impaired in remembering objects independently of the scenes in which the objects were presented, but they are impaired in scene-specific object memory. In terms of cognitive psychology, the 'episodic memory' in which amnesic patients are severely impaired—that is, memory for discrete personally experienced events—is analogous to the monkeys' memory for complex events involving some specific objects set in a specific background or scene. This type of memory is contrasted with 'semantic memory'—that is, acquired general knowledge about objects, independent of any specific background or any specific discrete event. The experimental and clinical evidence indicates that the Delay-Brion system is specially involved in memory for events, as opposed to general knowledge which is not specific to some discrete event in a particular scene. The discovery leads naturally on to the idea that some other memory system or systems, independent of the Delay-Brion system, might be responsible for the kind of memory which is manifested in general knowledge about objects, independent of any one specific scene.

Impairments of semantic memory

Patients with lesions in the neocortex of the anterior temporal lobe, sparing the Delay-Brion system, can show a syndrome which is in some respects complementary to the classical amnesic syndrome. Unlike amnesic patients, these patients do not show striking impairments in remembering discrete events such as the visit of a family member or some particular meal; but, again unlike amnesic patients, they are deficient in general knowledge ('semantic memory') as tested, for example, by the ability to identify and describe a family member or a well-known food item (Hodges et al 1992). The anatomical basis of this type of impairment has been elucidated by experiments with macaque monkeys.

Monkeys with discrete ablation of the perirhinal cortex (a strip of cortex in the anterior temporal lobe, lateral to the rhinal sulcus) show disorders of knowledge about objects. These disorders are revealed in discrimination learning tasks, in which the animal learns for food reward to choose the objects which the experimenter has arbitrarily designated as correct, in preference to other objects which the experimenter has designated as incorrect (Gaffan 1994); a similar disorder is also revealed in the matching-to-sample task with objects, in which the monkey learns to choose the object which is identical to a given sample object (Gaffan & Murray 1992). Both of these impairments occur when the animal has to deal with a large population of objects, requiring an accurate specification of individual objects in order to perform the task correctly; the impairments in the same tasks disappear if only one pair of objects is repeatedly used throughout the experiment (Eacott et al 1994). This kind of impairment was first discovered in experiments with delayed matching (or non-matching) to sample, and with large ablations of the medial temporal lobe, involving not only the perirhinal cortex but also the hippocampus and amygdala (Mishkin 1978). It is now known, however, that damage to the perirhinal cortex alone, sparing the hippocampus and amygdala, produces in these tasks an impairment of almost equal severity to that produced by large medial temporal ablations (Meunier et al 1993). It is also now known that the delay component of delayed matching-to-sample, as tested in early experiments, is not crucial since an impairment is also seen in matching-to-sample with no delay (Eacott et al 1994).

The memory impairment produced by discrete perirhinal cortex ablation in the monkey is qualitatively dissimilar from that which follows discrete interruption of the Delay-Brion system, by fornix transection, for example. Monkeys with fornix transection are severely impaired in memory for the spatial organization of scenes, and only mildly impaired in matching-to-sample with objects, whereas monkeys with perirhinal cortex ablations show the opposite pattern (Gaffan 1994). Thus, there is clear evidence for at least two distinct specialized memory systems in the primate temporal lobe, and the functions of these discrete anatomical structures correspond, at least in part, to the discrete cognitive functions of episodic memory and object knowledge.

Multiple memory systems

The Delay-Brion system and the perirhinal cortex are two of the most important and best understood memory systems of the primate brain, but there are also other identifiable systems with specialized functions, including the amygdala and the prefrontal cortex (Gaffan 1994). In general, therefore, the primate brain should be thought of as containing multiple (that is, more than two) specialized memory systems. Memory has frequently been classified in a binary way, for example into 'memory' and 'habit' but any such binary classification appears to be too simple as a summary of the multiple diversity of the memory systems in the primate brain.

AMYGDALOID COMPLEX

The amygdaloid nuclear complex (amygdaloid body) comprises a group of distinct nuclei found in the dorsomedial temporal pole, anterior to the hippocampus and in close proximity with the tail of the caudate nucleus (8.228). It forms the ventral, superior and medial walls of the tip of the inferior cornu of the lateral ventricle. The relations of the amygdala are complicated. It is partly continuous above with the inferomedial margin of the claustrum; fibres of the external capsule and substriatal grey matter, including the cholinergic magnocellular nucleus basalis (of Meynert), incompletely separate it from the putamen and globus pallidus; laterally, it is close to the optic tract. It is partly deep to the gyrus semilunaris, gyrus ambiens and uncinate gyrus (8.230).

In terms of the original limbic system concept discussed above, the amygdala remains very much at its heart as a structure of major importance in the neural mechanisms underlying emotional behaviour. As with the hippocampus, however, the traditional view of its organization and connections has changed quite markedly following detailed tract-tracing experiments, some of them conducted in primates. As with the hippocampal formation, there have been several detailed and elegant studies of the organization and connections of the primate, including the human, amygdaloid complex (Amaral 1987; Price et al 1987; de Olmos 1990; Sims & Williams 1990; Amaral et al 1992) and the reader is directed to these sources for more detailed information.

Nuclear organization

The amygdaloid complex is comprised of a number of irregularly shaped nuclei, leading Amaral (1987) to comment that it has a thalamic appearance. There is no consistent nomenclature for the amygdaloid nuclei, there having been two major approaches to the anatomy of this part of the temporal lobe. The first has tended to divide the amygdala into a number of small subdivisions (Volsch 1906, 1910; Uchida 1950a,b; Brockhaus 1938), whereas the second, following Johnston (1923), has tended to divide the complex into fewer, inclusive regions (Crowby & Humphrey 1941, 1944; Lauer 1945). Moreover, amygdaloid nuclei have different spatial interrelationships in non-primate and primate species that appear to have been brought about by a ventromedial rotation of the complex as a result of the differentiation of the neocortex. The most notable consequence of this rotation is that the lateral nucleus has moved ventrolateral to the basal nucleus in man, whereas it is dorsal to the basal nucleus in rats and in an intermediate position in cats (Amaral 1987). The nomenclature adopted here is that of Amaral (1987; Amaral et al 1992), which in turn is adapted from the early descriptions of Crosby and Humphrey (1941) and Lauer (1945). Figure 8.245 shows a schematic view of the monkey amygdaloid complex with a summary of some of the many names used to describe the various nuclei, while 8.246 shows a photomicrograph of the Macaque monkey's amygdala alongside that of the human amygdala and these should be referred to in the description that follows.

The lateral nucleus is clearly the largest nucleus in the amygdaloid

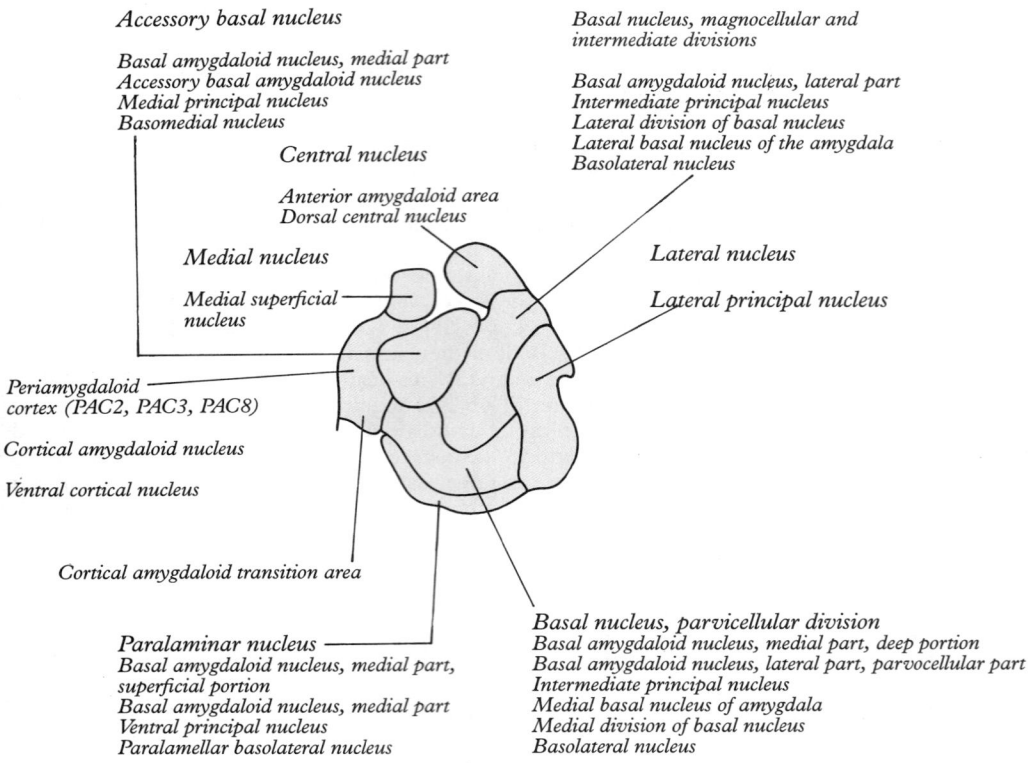

Accessory basal nucleus

Basal amygdaloid nucleus, medial part
Accessory basal amygdaloid nucleus
Medial principal nucleus
Basomedial nucleus

Basal nucleus, magnocellular and
intermediate divisions

Basal amygdaloid nucleus, lateral part
Intermediate principal nucleus
Lateral division of basal nucleus
Lateral basal nucleus of the amygdala
Basolateral nucleus

Central nucleus

Anterior amygdaloid area
Dorsal central nucleus

Medial nucleus

Medial superficial
nucleus

Lateral nucleus

Lateral principal nucleus

Periamygdaloid
cortex (PAC2, PAC3, PAC8)

Cortical amygdaloid nucleus

Ventral cortical nucleus

Cortical amygdaloid transition area

Basal nucleus, parvicellular division
Basal amygdaloid nucleus, medial part, deep portion
Basal amygdaloid nucleus, lateral part, parvocellular part
Intermediate principal nucleus
Medial basal nucleus of amygdala
Medial division of basal nucleus
Basolateral nucleus

Paralaminar nucleus
Basal amygdaloid nucleus, medial part,
superficial portion
Basal amygdaloid nucleus, medial part
Ventral principal nucleus
Paralamellar basolateral nucleus

8.245 A prototypical coronal section through the monkey amygdala with outlines around the major nuclei and cortical regions. For each area, a window indicates the term used in this chapter (in bold lettering) and then several additional terms used by others to label similar regions. The list of alternative terms is not intended to be comprehensive but rather indicates those terms that are significant for historical reasons or because they are commonly used in current literature.

complex and, as indicated above, it lies ventrolateral to the basal nucleus. The latter is commonly divided into three subnuclei: a dorsal magnocellular basal nucleus; an intermediate parvicellular basal nucleus and a ventral band of darkly staining cells usually referred to as the paralaminar basal nucleus, since it borders the white matter ventral to the amygdaloid complex. The accessory basal nucleus lies medial to the basal nuclear divisions and it, too, is usually divided into a dorsal, magnocellular and ventral, parvicellular part. These lateral and basal nuclei are often referred to collectively as the basolateral area (nuclear group) of the amygdaloid complex.

It has been suggested by several anatomists that the basolateral complex of nuclei (lateral, basal, accessory basal) shares several characteristics with the cortex and may best be considered as a quasi-cortical structure (see Alheid & Heimer 1988 for discussion). Although this region does not have a laminar structure, some of its cortical features include direct, often reciprocal, connections with adjacent temporal and other areas of cortex and it projects to the motor or premotor cortex. It receives a direct cholinergic and non-cholinergic input from the magnocellular corticopetal system in the basal forebrain and has reciprocal connections with the mediodorsal thalamus that are also similar to cortical structures. The distribution of small peptidergic neurons in the basolateral nuclear complex, for example, those containing neuropeptide-Y (NY), somatostatin (SOM) and CCK, are also similar in form and density to those found in the adjacent temporal lobe cortex. Projection neurons from this part of the amygdala also appear to utilize, at least in part, the excitatory amino acid glutamate/aspartate as a transmitter and they are directed, in addition to cortical sites, to the ventral striatum rather than to hypothalamic and brainstem sites (see below). Thus, it may be appropriate to consider this part of the amygdaloid complex as a polymodal cortical-like area that is separated from the cerebral cortex by fibres of the external capsule.

The central nucleus is present through the caudal half of the amygdaloid complex and it lies dorsomedial to the basal nucleus. It is divided into medial and lateral divisions, with the former, which contains larger cells than the latter, resembling the adjacent putamen. The central nucleus, together with the medial nucleus, also appears to have an extension across the basal forebrain, as well as within the stria terminalis, that merges with the bed nucleus of the stria terminalis, which can also be divided into medial and lateral divisions, that resemble very closely the same divisions of the central nucleus. This extensive nuclear complex, called the 'extended amygdala', is illustrated in **8.247**. It can be considered as a macrostructure formed by the centromedial amygdaloid complex (medial nucleus, medial and lateral parts of the central nucleus), the medial bed nucleus of the stria terminalis and the cell columns traversing the sublenticular substantia innominata between them (Alheid & Heimer 1988; Alheid, Heimer & Switzer 1990; de Olmos, 1990). Alheid, Heimer and Switzer have also suggested that portions of the medial nucleus accumbens may be included in the extended amygdala, but this suggestion has yet to gain uniform acceptance. The central nucleus is also continuous rostrally within the complex with a so-called anterior amygdaloid area. The cortical region of the amygdaloid complex is usually divided into a medial nucleus, cortical nuclei and the periamygdaloid cortex. The nucleus of the lateral olfactory tract is a relatively minor structure in the rostral part of the primate amygdaloid complex, being much more substantial in the brain of macrosmatic mammals. In the caudal half of the amygdala, the basal nucleus appears to merge with deeper parts of the periamygdaloid cortex and is called, therefore, a transitional zone. A similar transitional zone appears between the amygdala and hippocampus caudally—the so-called amygdalohippocampal area. There are also several nuclei comprised of darkly staining neurons, called the intercalated cell masses, the largest of which is found in the anterior amygdaloid area.

Chemical anatomy

As in other areas of the CNS, most studies of transmitter distribution in the amygdaloid complex have involved rats. However, there is now a considerable body of information on the chemical anatomy of the primate amygdala which will be summarized here (further

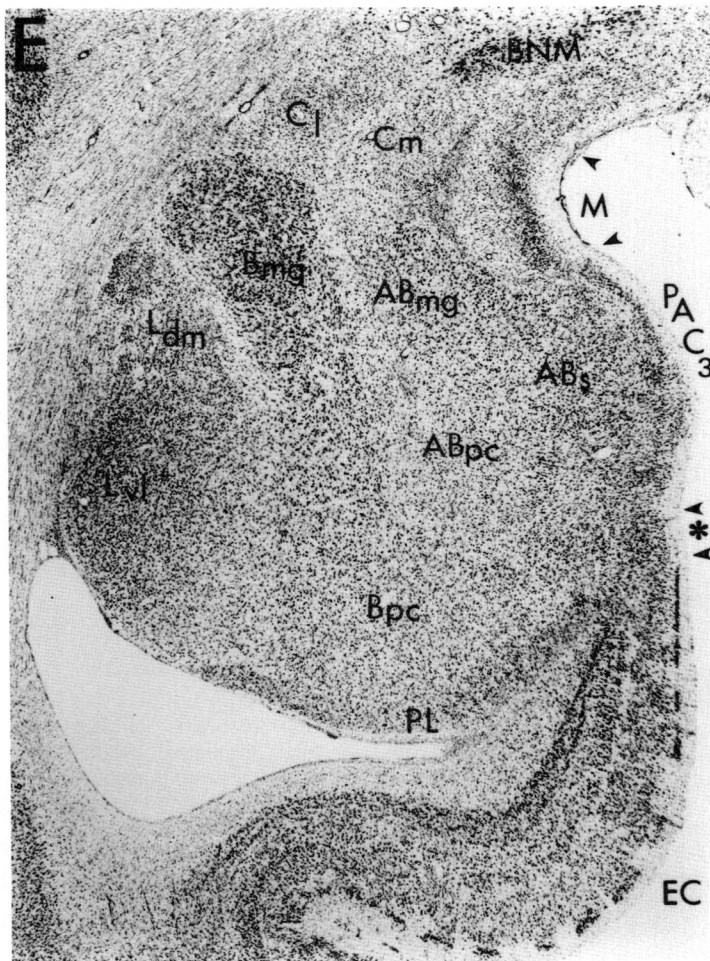

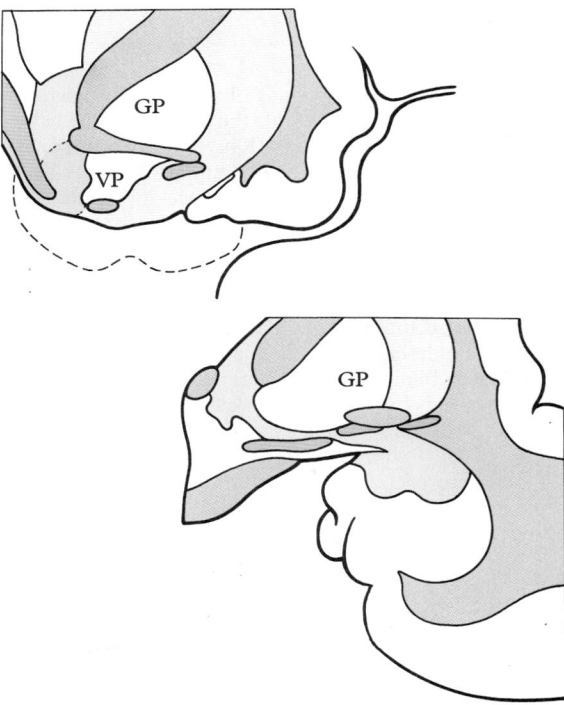

8.247 Schematic diagram of the relationship between the striatum (yellow), pallidum (GP = dorsal globus pallidus; VP = ventral pallidum), extended amygdala (blue) and the magnocellular corticopetal basal forebrain system (magenta). Note that the medial part of the nucleus accumbens-olfactory tubercle area (green) may possibly be a mixed zone of the ventral striatopallidal system and the extended amygdala. (From Alheid & Heimer 1988.)

8.246 Coronal section through the Nissl-stained amygdaloid complex of the Macaque monkey. The major subdivisions indicated are: lateral nucleus, which has dorsomedial (Ldm) and ventrolateral (Lvl) subdivisions; basal nucleus, which has magnocellular (Bmg), parvicellular (Bpc), superficial (ABs) and paralaminar (PL) subdivisions; accessory basal nucleus, which has magnocellular (ABmg) and parvicellular (ABpc) subdivisions; central nucleus, which has medial (Cm) and lateral (Cl) subdivisions; medial nucleus (M); cortical nucleus or periamygdaloid cortex (PAC, 3rd subdivision shown). Other abbreviations: EC = entorhinal cortex; BNM = basal nucleus of Meynert. (Photograph provided by David Amaral; see Price et al 1987.)

details may be found in Price et al 1987; Amaral et al 1992). The amygdala is in receipt of a rich monoaminergic innervation. The noradrenergic projection arises primarily from the locus coeruleus (with some contribution from the lateral tegmental cell groups) that runs mainly through the medial forebrain bundle before sweeping laterally into the temporal lobe. The central nucleus, intercalated nuclei and periamygdaloid cortex show the greatest levels of dopamine-β-hydroxylase immunoreactivity, while deeper nuclei contain rather few noradrenergic fibres (Sadikot & Parent 1990). There is apparently also a sparse adrenergic innervation of the central nucleus.

The dorsal and, to some extent the median, raphe nuclei are the origin of the serotoninergic innervation of the amygdala which runs in the medial forebrain bundle along with noradrenergic projections (Mehler 1980). The densest serotonin-immunoreactive plexuses are found in the lateral, parvicellular basal, magnocellular accessory basal and central nuclei, as well as in the amygdalohippocampal area. It has been suggested that the serotoninergic innervation of the amygdala is quantitatively greater than either the noradrenergic or dopaminergic innervations.

The dopaminergic innervation of the amygdala arises primarily in the midbrain ventral tegmental area (A10), and the highest levels of TH-immunoreactivity (which provides a good indication of the dopaminergic innervation even though found in all catecholaminergic neurons) are found in the lateral, central and intercalated nuclei, with smaller numbers of fibres in the parvicellular basal nucleus (Sadikot & Parent 1990).

The basal and parvicellular accessory basal nuclei, the amygdalohippocampal area and nucleus of the lateral olfactory tract receive a very dense cholinergic innervation arising from the magnocellular nucleus basalis of Meynert, particularly its anterolateral part (Mesulam et al 1983). Other amygdaloid nuclei are relatively devoid of (Ch AT)-immunoreactivity and have only low levels of acetylcholinesterase.

The monkey amygdala contains high concentrations of GABA, glutamate and aspartate, but the precise anatomical distribution of neurons and fibres have not been clearly established in this species (Amaral et al 1992). In rats, most GAD-immunoreactivity is found in terminal plexi in the central and medial nuclei and in the anterior amygdaloid area, with lower levels in the accessory basal, basal and lateral nuclei. In addition, GAD- or GABA-immunoreactive cell bodies are found in all amygdaloid nuclei, especially in basal, lateral and cortical nuclei, and these probably give rise to a substantial proportion of the GABAergic terminal plexi in the amygdaloid complex generally (Otterson et al 1987). Much interest has focused on the GABAergic system of the amygdala because of the high concentration of benzodiazepine binding sites, especially $GABA_A$-binding sites in the lateral and accessory basal nuclei. Many of the anxiolytic actions of the benzodiazepines can be demonstrated in experimental animals following their infusion directly into the amygdala and these data represent an interesting point of contact between contemporary analysis of the neural basis of fear and anxiety and early observations of the changes in fear in temporal lobectomized monkeys, part of the Klüver-Bucy syndrome.

The Klüver-Bucy syndrome

The Klüver-Bucy syndrome was observed following bilateral removal of the temporal lobes in rhesus monkeys (Klüver & Bucy 1937, 1939). The lesioned animals apparently no longer showed fearful reactions and approached humans, other animals and inanimate objects readily; the commonly held notion that these animals showed decreased aggressive behaviour is, however, not accurate, nor consistent with the original description. The animals, although not blind, apparently failed to recognize objects by sight and picked them up indiscriminately and repeatedly, usually without realization that they had been seen before. Such objects were often placed in the mouth. They also showed marked changes in ingestive behaviour, eating faeces, meat, fish and other foods not usually eaten by rhesus monkeys. Patterns of sexual behaviour were also altered markedly: lesioned monkeys attempted to copulate with members of the same sex, or with animals of other species. Klüver and Bucy described their syndrome as one of 'psychic blindness' (visual agnosia), 'hypermetamorphosis' (compulsive attentiveness to visual stimuli), 'hyperorality', 'hypersexuality' (a rather misleading description of the disturbed sexual behaviour these animals showed) and of marked alterations in ingestive behaviour. Because of the dominant presence of the hippocampal formation in the temporal lobe, Klüver and Bucy not unreasonably attributed these changes in behaviour to damage to this structure. While this reinforced subsequent theorists in their attempts to rationalize the role of the limbic system in emotional behaviour, it is now known that the majority of the symptoms characterizing the syndrome depend upon damage to the amygdala. Weiskrantz (1956) was the first to propose a general function of the amygdala in evaluating the significance of environmental events, most particularly the association between environmental stimuli and reinforcement. More recently, it has been demonstrated that such stimulus–reward associations are markedly impaired following lesions of the amygdala (Jones & Mishkin 1972; Gaffan & Harrison 1987; Everitt & Robbins 1992) and Gaffan (1992) has presented a compelling argument that this fundamental deficit underlies many of the cardinal signs of the Klüver-Bucy syndrome.

The nuclear distribution of glutamate/aspartate is unknown in the monkey and not very certain in the rat brain. It may be assumed that the corticoamygdaloid projection (see below) is glutamatergic and this is related to the high affinity uptake system for the amino acids, especially in the lateral and basal nuclei, anterior cortical nucleus and periamygdaloid cortex. Presumably, the many neurons in the basal and accessory basal nucleus that project to the striatum also use glutamate/aspartate as a transmitter and there is a considerable body of evidence supporting glutamate-dependent changes in ventral striatal activity following excitation of the amygdala.

There are many neuropeptide-containing neurons in the amygdaloid complex (see Amaral 1987; Amaral et al 1992 for reviews). Somatostatin-immunoreactive fibres are found in greatest density in the lateral nucleus with moderate levels in the basal nucleus. The lateral central nucleus contains more somatostatin-immunoreactive neurons than the medial division, there also being large numbers of cell bodies in the dorsomedial lateral nucleus. NY has a very similar distribution to that for somatostatin and this reflects the strong degree of coexistence of these peptides in many central neurons. Vasopressin-immunoreactive neurons are found in the medial nucleus of the amygdala, which also receives a vasopressin-containing projection from the suprachiasmatic nucleus. The central nucleus also contains vasopressin- as well as oxytocin-immunoreactive terminals that appear to originate in the hypothalamic paraventricular nucleus. As in the lateral septum, the vasopressin innervation is sexually dimorphic. There are neurons and fibres containing corticotrophin releasing hormone, vasoactive intestinal polypeptide and cholecystokinin in the amygdala, again especially in the medial and central nuclei. The corticotrophin releasing hormone-containing afferents also appear to arise largely from the hypothalamic paraventricular nucleus. Similar distributions of peptide containing neurons to those found in the central nucleus are also found in the bed nucleus of the stria terminalis, as might be expected. Among the opioid peptides, there is a rich enkephalin-immunoreactive plexus, as well as numbers of cell bodies, in the central nucleus, whereas there is little enkephalin-immunoreactivity in the lateral and basal nuclei. There are appreciable amounts of β-endorphin immunoreactivity in the medial and central nuclei of the amygdala and this appears to originate from the pro-opiomelanocortin-immunoreactive neurons in the mediobasal hypothalamus.

A particularly characteristic feature of parts of the amygdaloid complex is the presence of quite high numbers of steroid hormone concentrating neurons and binding sites (Pfaff et al 1976). Thus, the medial, accessory basal and posterior cortical nuclei contain many oestrogen-concentrating neurons, while neurons concentrating dihydrotestosterone are found especially in the medial nucleus, but also in the accessory basal, parvicellular basal and lateral nuclei. There is also a high level of activity of the enzymes 5a-reductase, which converts testosterone into the non-aromatisable 5a-dihydrotestosterone, and aromatase, which converts testosterone and androstenedione to oestradiol (Michael & Rees 1982). This steroid chemical address system of neurons in parts of the amygdala suggests that some of its functions, like those of the hypothalamus, are considerably affected by changes in endocrine state, such as those accompanying the menstrual cycle.

Intrinsic connections

An important and consistent feature of the intrinsic connections among amygdaloid nuclei is that they arise primarily in lateral and basal nuclei and terminate in the central and medial nuclei (Amaral 1987). There are a few, weak projections in the reverse direction suggesting, as with the hippocampal formation, a largely unidirectional flow of information. These intrinsic connections are summarized in 8.248. In brief, the lateral nucleus projects to all divisions of the basal nucleus, accessory basal nucleus, paralaminar and anterior cortical nuclei, and less heavily to the central nucleus. The lateral nucleus receives few afferents from other nuclei and there appear to be quite complex intralateral nucleus connections. The magnocellular, parvicellular and intermediate parts of the basal nucleus project to the accessory basal, central (especially the medial part) and medial nuclei as well as to the periamygdaloid cortex and the amygdalohippocampal area. The basal nucleus also has substantial intranuclear connections. The accessory basal nucleus projects densely to the central nucleus, especially its medial division, as well as to the medial and cortical nuclei. Its major intra-amygdaloid afferents arise from the lateral nucleus. The medial nucleus projects to the accessory basal, anterior cortical and central nuclei as well as to the periamygdaloid cortex and amygdalohippocampal area, while afferents arise especially from the lateral nucleus. The intrinsic connections of the cortical nucleus are not very well understood. The posterior part of the cortical nucleus projects to the medial nucleus, but it has been difficult to differentiate this projection from that arising in the amygdalohippocampal area. The central nucleus projects to the anterior cortical nucleus and the various

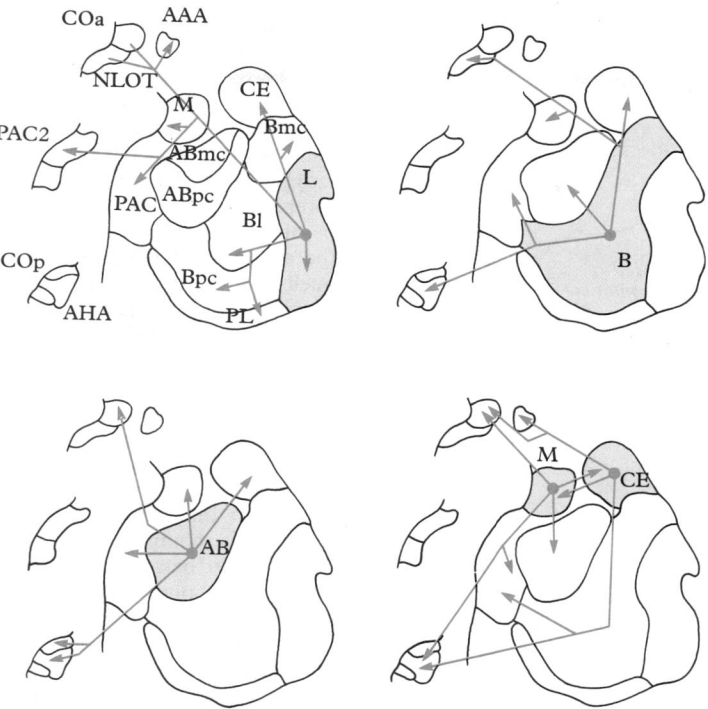

8.248 Line drawings of a prototypical section through the amygdala to illustrate the organization of the *major* efferent intrinsic connections of the monkey amygdala. Windows around the left side of the amygdala indicate additional regions that are not usually observed at the midrostrocaudal level illustrated in the prototypical section. A: Intrinsic efferent connections of the lateral nucleus. Note the arrow which ends within the nucleus indicates that there are significant intranuclear connections. B: Intrinsic efferent connections of the basal nucleus. C: Intrinsic efferent connections of the accessory basal nucleus. D: Intrinsic efferent connections of the central and medial nuclei. (Reproduced with permission from Amaral et al 1992.)

cortical transition zones, while it forms, as we have seen, an important focus for afferents from many of the amygdaloid nuclei, especially the basal and accessory basal nuclei; it has major extrinsic connections (see below).

Extrinsic connections

Hitherto, the amygdaloid complex has been viewed largely as a structure that receives afferents from temporal lobe cortical fields and the olfactory system, and projects via two major outflow systems, the stria terminalis and ventral amygdalofugal pathway (**8.228, 229**), primarily to the hypothalamus and brainstem. As we will see, although these are indeed its major output pathways, the amygdala also has rich interconnections with a much wider variety of structures than hitherto appreciated, particularly in the forebrain, and this has changed hypotheses concerning its functions markedly. Amaral (1987) has pointed out that although most of the extrinsic connections of the amygdala are reciprocal, there are three apparently important exceptions: the striatum and thalamus receive marked projections from the amygdala, but do not return these projections, while the amygdala projects to several cortical fields that also are not reciprocated. The following description relies heavily on Amaral's accounts (Amaral 1987; Amarel et al 1992).

Amygdaloid subcortical connections

Brainstem. The central nucleus provides the major relay for projections from the amygdala to the brainstem and also receives many of the return projections. No other amygdaloid nucleus contributes significantly to these projections but, as might be expected, the bed nucleus of the stria terminalis has a very similar pattern of efferents and is, therefore, a similar relay for amygdaloid connections with brainstem autonomic and other nuclei. In the midbrain, the periaqueductal grey, ventral tegmental area and substantia nigra pars compacta, peripeduncular nucleus and tegmental reticular formation all receive afferents from the central nucleus. In the pons, the parabrachial nuclei receive a particularly prominent projection while in the medulla, the nucleus of the solitary tract and dorsal motor nucleus of the vagus receive afferents from the central nucleus.

The heaviest brainstem projection to the amygdala arises in the peripeduncular nucleus, terminating in the central and medial nuclei in rats, but apparently in the lateral and medial nuclei in monkeys, as well as to the bed nucleus of the stria terminalis. The parabrachial nuclei also project richly to the central nucleus. In the monkey, the nucleus of the solitary tract does not project to the central nucleus (whereas this is a substantial projection in the rat), but it does send many fibres to the parabrachial nuclei and is, therefore, indirectly connected with the amygdala. These connections are consistent with a role in the regulation of cardiovascular, respiratory and gustatory processes with which the amygdala has always been associated. As described above, the amygdala is in receipt of serotoninergic afferents from the midbrain raphe, dopaminergic afferents from the ventral tegmental area and substantia nigra (which mostly terminate in the medial central nucleus) and noradrenergic afferents from the locus coeruleus and subcoeruleus.

Hypothalamus and bed nucleus of the stria terminalis. The central nucleus is again the major relay for amygdaloid projections to the hypothalamus. The bed nucleus of the stria terminalis, which also has medial and lateral divisions that are virtually identical in cytoarchitectural and chemical organization to the central nucleus, is also best viewed in this way. That is, it is an extension of the central nucleus with which it retains cellular continuity via the stria terminalis and the sublenticular basal forebrain (the 'extended amygdala'; **8.247**). Amygdaloid fibres reach the bed nucleus primarily via the stria terminalis, but also via the ventral amygdalofugal pathway. In general, central and basal nuclei project to the lateral part of the bed nucleus, while medial and posterior cortical nuclei project to the medial bed nucleus.

Anterior cortical and medial nuclei project largely to the medial preoptic area and anterior medial hypothalamus, including the paraventricular and supraoptic nuclei. There is a particularly prominent projection to the ventromedial and premamillary nuclei. The medial

1135

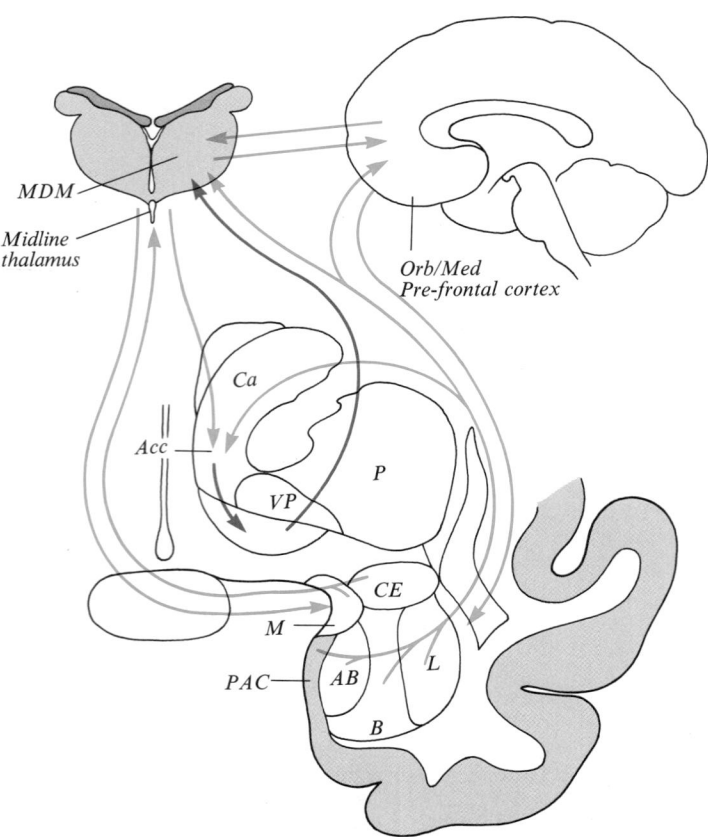

8.249 Various routes through which the amygdaloid complex can influence the function of the frontal lobe. (i) The amygdala has direct reciprocal connections with various regions of the orbital and medial frontal lobe. (ii) The amygdala projects to the mediodorsal nucleus (MD) of the thalamus which, in turn, projects to the same regions of the frontal lobe that receive a direct amygdaloid input. (iii) Many amygdaloid nuclei project to the nucleus accumbens either directly, or via the midline thalamus. The nucleus accumbens projects heavily to the ventral pallidum which, in turn, projects to the medial dorsal nucleus of the thalamus. (Reproduced with permission from Amaral et al, 1992.)

and accessory basal nuclei primarily project to the cell dense 'core' of the ventromedial nuclei, while the amygdalohippocampal area projects to its cell sparse 'shell'. The amygdala projects to the rostrocaudal extent of the lateral hypothalamus, with the majority of the fibres originating in the central nucleus and running principally in the ventral amygdalofugal pathway and medial forebrain bundle. Return projections from the hypothalamus to the amygdala are sparse in comparison to amygdalohypothalamic projections. They arise largely in the ventromedial nucleus and lateral hypothalamic area and terminate in central, medial, basal and accessory basal nuclei.

Thalamus. There is a particularly rich projection to the mediodorsal nucleus of the thalamus that both gives access to the prefrontal cortex and complements direct projections from the amygdala to the same cortical domain (see below). The projection to the mediodorsal nucleus arises from most amygdaloid nuclei, but particularly from the lateral, basal and accessory basal nuclei and the periamygdaloid cortex. The major termination of amygdaloid afferents is in the medial, magnocellular part of mediodorsal nucleus, especially rostrally. This part of mediodorsal nucleus projects to the identical medial and orbital prefrontal cortical areas that receive amygdaloid afferents directly (8.249). This projection to mediodorsal nucleus is not reciprocated. The central and medial nuclei project not to the mediodorsal nucleus, but to the midline nuclei, especially nucleus centralis and also nucleus reuniens. These midline thalamic nuclei do project to the amygdala, primarily to central and basal nuclei. The parvicellular ventral posterior medial nucleus of the thalamus also projects to the lateral nucleus (in the

cat) and provides a second route through which gustatory information reaches the amygdala. The medial geniculate nucleus has also been shown to project to lateral, accessory basal and central nuclei in rats and cats.

Basal forebrain. Among the more recent neuroanatomical observations that have had an impact on functional perspectives of the amygdala are the substantial, reciprocal connections with the basal forebrain. The anterolateral part of the magnocellular nucleus basalis of Meynert (Ch4) sends a dense, cholinergic projection to the amygdala that terminates primarily in the magnocellular basal nucleus and less densely in the accessory basal nucleus. It has been suggested that the magnocellular basal nucleus receives the heaviest cholinergic innervation of any forebrain structure. The parvicellular division of the basal nucleus, magnocellular accessory basal nucleus (but not the magnocellular basal nucleus) and also the central nucleus in turn project to basal forebrain cholinergic cell groups, notably the nucleus basalis of Meynert and the horizontal limb nucleus of the diagonal band. These fibres do not terminate in the cholinergic cell groups, but make en passant synapses while continuing to thalamic, hypothalamic and brainstem nuclei. Amaral (1987) has commented that the amygdala seemingly provides the nucleus basalis of Meynert with its major cortical input, although the prefrontal cortex afferents to this cell group are also substantial.

Striatum. Although not embodied in neuroanatomical concepts of the limbic system until recently (Mogenson et al 1984; Everitt & Robbins 1992; Groenewegen et al 1982, 1990), it has long been established that the striatum receives prominent projections from the amygdaloid complex (Nauta 1962; Heimer & Wilson 1975; Nauta & Domesick 1981, 1984; Kelley et al 1982). The nucleus accumbens in particular, but also the ventromedial caudate and putamen, as well as more caudal parts of the dorsal striatum including the entire body and tail of the caudate nucleus (p. 1186), receive afferents from the amygdala. Indeed, these striatal projections represent one of the most substantial components of amygdaloid outflow. The basal and accessory basal nuclei are the most important contributors to this projection and studies in the rat suggest there is enormous complexity in the pattern of termination within the nucleus accumbens, there being precise interdigitation with afferents from the midline thalamic nuclei, prefrontal cortex and subiculum, as well as with dopaminergic afferents from the ventral tegmental area (Groenewegen et al 1990). The ventral striatum sends many fibres to the ventral pallidum which in its turn projects to the mediodorsal nucleus of the thalamus. Thus, the ventral striatopallidal system provides a second route through which the amygdala can influence mediodorsal thalamic-prefrontal cortical processes (8.234).

The anterior commissure. This is a compact bundle of myelinated nerve fibres crossing anterior to the columns of the fornix and embedded in the lamina terminalis, where it is part of the anterior third ventricular wall, 1·5–2·0 cm above the optic chiasma (8.228). In sagittal section it is oval, its long diameter (about 1·5 mm) vertical. Its fibres twist and entwine like the strands of a rope and laterally it separates into two bundles: the smaller *anterior bundle* curves forwards on each side to the anterior perforated substance and olfactory tract; the *posterior bundle* curves posterolaterally on each side for some distance in a deep groove on the antero-inferior aspect of the lentiform nucleus, beyond which it fans out into the anterior part of the temporal lobe, including the parahippocampal gyrus. Commissural fibres have been described in mammals, including primates, as interconnecting the following structures with their fellows: (1) the olfactory bulb and anterior olfactory nucleus, (2) the anterior perforated substance, olfactory tubercle and diagonal band of Broca, (3) the prepiriform cortex, (4) the entorhinal area and adjacent parts of the parahippocampal gyrus, (5) part of the amygdaloid complex, especially the nucleus of the lateral olfactory stria, (6) the bed nucleus of the stria terminalis and nucleus accumbens septi, (7) the middle and inferior temporal gyri in their anterior regions, (8) possibly other neocortical areas, including the frontal lobe.

The inter-temporal neocortical connections are the largest component of the anterior commissure in primates, including mankind. However, many detailed connections in the human commissure remain unknown. Some fibres may not be commissural but decussating pathways between dissimilar structures.

Nucleus accumbens, dopamine, reward and addiction

The nucleus accumbens, which is part of the ventral striatum, together with its dopaminergic innervation which originates in the midbrain ventral tegmental area (cell group A10), has become intimately associated with theories of reward (sometimes called incentive motivation). Indeed, the dopaminergic innervation of the nucleus accumbens, often called the 'mesolimbic dopamine system', is believed by many researchers to represent a critical neural substrate for the rewarding effects of several classes of drugs of abuse and, therefore, to be a major determinant of their addictive potential.

An initial impetus to the systematic study of neural mechanisms of reward was the discovery by Olds and Milner (1954) of the phenomenon of intracranial electrical self-stimulation (ICSS) of the brain, whereby rats would work to the point of exhaustion to deliver small electrical currents to specific neural loci. Especially high rates of responding were obtained from the lateral hypothalamus and also the ventral tegmental area. Subsequent studies revealed that lesions of the dopaminergic projections to the nucleus accumbens, which originate in the ventral tegmental area and run through the medial forebrain bundle in the lateral hypothalamus, or treatment with dopamine receptor blockers systemically or within the nucleus accumbens, greatly attenuated ICSS. More recently, using the techniques of in vivo dialysis and electrochemistry to measure transmitter release directly in the brains of freely moving animals, it has become clear that dopamine levels in the nucleus accumbens are markedly elevated in subjects engaged in ICSS. Such data strongly link the rewarding effects of ICSS to increased activity in the dopaminergic innervation of the nucleus accumbens.

The observation that the locomotor activating effects of psychomotor stimulant drugs, such as amphetamine and cocaine, are dependent on dopamine transmission in the nucleus accumbens also led directly to the hypothesis that the reinforcing or rewarding properties of these drugs are similarly mediated by the mesolimbic dopamine system. There are insurmountable problems in equating the behavioural properties of rewarding stimuli with subjective feelings of pleasure or hedonism in experimental animals, although it is possible to make inferences about such covert states through an experimental analysis of behaviour that provides operational measures of reward evaluation; for example, measurement of ICSS thresholds has been used in this way. Another set of such operational measures includes the propensity to approach, to work or to show a preference for particular environmental stimuli, which can,

thus, be termed incentives. These stimuli may be intrinsically associated with primary goals, such as the sight or smell of food, or arbitrary stimuli that have gained incentive value because they predict the occurrence, in time and place, of such primary goals. There is now considerable evidence to support the view that mesolimbic dopamine subserves this specific behavioural function by promoting appetitive behaviour in the presence of both conditioned and unconditioned incentive stimuli. This function is to be contrasted with the co-ordination of the more stereotyped responses which occur following direct contact with the goal itself, such as chewing or sexual mounting, that appear to depend more on dopamine transmission in the dorsal striatum. The description of these latter responses as consummatory denotes their position at the end of the motivational sequence, in contrast to the more flexible forms of appetitive behaviour which serve to bring the animal into contact with the goal.

Early examples of this dichotomy include the reductions both in locomotor excitement in the presence of food and also in food hoarding, in the absence of any decremental effect on eating, following experimentally-induced depletion of dopamine in the ventral striatum. It has also been demonstrated that the appetitive (or preparatory) responses to a stimulus conditioned to food presentation (a conditional stimulus or CS) are selectively disrupted by systemic treatment with dopamine receptor antagonists at doses without effect on ingestion. A more direct assessment of the relationship between ventral striatal dopamine activity and incentive motivational processes has become possible through the use of single-unit recording of identified dopamine neurons and in vivo electrochemistry. The former approach has revealed in monkeys marked changes in the activity of dopamine neurons in response to food reward, or a CS paired with food. In vivo neurochemical studies in rats have shown an increased dopamine signal in the nucleus accumbens, but not in the dorsal striatum, in the presence of a CS signalling a meal or in the presence of food itself, or a sexual partner.

In the face of the above data, which strongly implicate the dopaminergic innervation of the nucleus accumbens in the neural mechanisms of reward, it is perhaps not surprising to discover that drugs interacting with the dopaminergic system are powerful reinforcers, are self-administered by man and by animals and have significant abuse potential. Such drugs include, of course, the psychomotor stimulants amphetamine and cocaine, which act presynaptically on dopaminergic neurons

to enhance dopamine release (amphetamine) or block reuptake (cocaine). But narcotic opiates, such as heroin, also interact with midbrain dopamine neurons, as well as with receptors in the nucleus accumbens. In addition, nicotine and also alcohol are able to increase dopamine levels in the nucleus accumbens. This has led some theorists to the conclusion that increasing dopamine transmission may be a common, even necessary, property of all drugs of abuse. But full discussion of this complex issue is beyond the scope of this brief review.

The discovery that experimental animals such as rats and monkeys will self-administer intravenously drugs such as cocaine and heroin has provided an extremely important opportunity to study the neural basis of their rewarding effects. The results of such experiments bring the mesolimbic dopamine system and the nucleus accumbens powerfully into view, but the precise mechanisms that mediate the reinforcing effects of each class of drug remain the subject of intense study. Thus, the intravenous self-administration of cocaine is dose-dependently increased by treatment with a dopamine receptor antagonist given either systemically, or infused directly into the nucleus accumbens, but not into the overlying dorsal striatum. This result, perhaps, needs a little explanation: in the presence of the dopamine receptor antagonist, the self-administered cocaine becomes less effective (competitive antagonism in pharmacological terms), so the animal self-administers more cocaine to obtain the same reinforcing effect. As the dose of the dopamine receptor antagonist increases, the rate of intravenous cocaine self-administration increases—up to the point when receptor blockade is total and the self-administration behaviour extinguishes. The opiate receptor antagonist naloxone is completely without effect on cocaine self-administration—i.e. there is neurochemical selectivity in these effects. It has also been demonstrated that amphetamine is self-administered directly into the nucleus accumbens and together such data strongly support the view that dopaminergic mechanisms in the nucleus accumbens are critical for the reinforcing effects of psychomotor stimulants.

The picture for heroin is more complex and this may reflect the possibility that the reinforcing effects of opiates depend upon actions at more than one site in the brain. Intravenously self-administered heroin increases dopamine release in the nucleus accumbens and also the firing of midbrain dopamine neurons, most likely through interactions with μ opiate receptors on neurons in the ventral tegmental area. In addition, morphine is self-administered directly into the ventral tegmental area. Thus, these data have been taken as evidence that the reinforcing effects of heroin depend upon the integrity of the dopaminergic innervation of the nucleus accumbens. However, infusion of methyl-naloxonium (a lipophobic form of naloxone) directly into the nucleus accumbens results in a dose-dependent increase in heroin self-administration, indicating that a large part of the reinforcing effect of the opiate is mediated directly within this site. Moreover, dopamine receptor antagonists given systemically failed to modify intravenous heroin self-administration in some studies. At present, it seems reasonable to conclude that the reinforcing effects of narcotic opiates may involve both opiate receptor mechanisms within the nucleus accumbens that are independent of interactions with dopamine neurons and also a second, opiate receptor-dependent mechanism in the midbrain that results in the activation of mesolimbic dopamine transmission.

Conditioning

Another important aspect of addiction is the impact of conditioning on drug-seeking behaviour. Thus, stimuli that have reliably been paired with the pharmacological effects of self-administered cocaine may invoke intense craving for the drug. This is particularly the case in the later stages of abstinence, when such drug-associated cues are especially important in relapse and the re-establishment of the drug-taking habit. In the case of opiates, previously neutral stimuli may not only become associated with the positive reinforcing effects of the drug, but also with the negative consequences of its absence, i.e. withdrawal. Such stimuli, which may include the general context in which withdrawal has been experienced, are subsequently able to precipitate withdrawal (so-called 'conditioned withdrawal') and thereby powerfully motivate drug-seeking behaviour or relapse in previously abstinent individuals. Clearly,

understanding the neural basis of such conditioned influences on drug self-administration is of considerable importance.

One of the functions of a CS paired with the positive, or rewarding, effects of a drug such as cocaine is to act as a *conditioned reward* or *conditioned reinforcer* that serves to maintain responding in the absence of the primary goal. Such stimuli acquire conditioned reinforcing properties by virtue of their predictive temporal association with primary reward, a process that presumably depends on higher-order associative processes known to occur in limbic forebrain sites, especially the amygdala (see p. 1131).

A number of experiments have now determined the role of the mesolimbic dopamine system in mediating the control over behaviour by conditioned reinforcers, using a procedure in which the acquired reinforcing efficacy of the conditioned reinforcer is measured in the absence of the primary goal, by its capacity to support the learning of a new response. Thus, systemic psychomotor stimulants, or infusions of d-amphetamine directly into the nucleus accumbens, powerfully enhance responses that provide the conditioned reinforcer, an effect that is behaviourally, neurochemically and neuroanatomically specific. For example, ventral, but not dorsal, striatal dopamine depletion significantly attenuates this potentiation of responding with conditioned reinforcement produced by intra-accumbens amphetamine. Moreover, the effects are mimicked by intra-accumbens infusions of dopamine (but not noradrenaline) and also by selective D_1 and D_2 receptor agonists. These observations indicate why psychomotor stimulants in particular may exert such powerful motivational effects: not only do they exert their pharmacological action of increasing dopaminergic activity in the nucleus accumbens, but they also enhance the salience, and hence control over drug-seeking behaviour, of cues paired with the unconditioned (rewarding) effects of the drug.

These findings clearly indicate that the effects of conditioned, as well as primary, aspects of rewards are modulated by dopamine-dependent functions of the ventral striatum, and raise the issue of whether this effect of learning impinges directly on the mesolimbic dopamine neurons, or whether it is mediated by other neural systems converging on the ventral striatum. It has been demonstrated that the potentiative effects of ventral striatal dopamine release on behaviour controlled by reward-related stimuli or conditioned reinforcers is greatly diminished by lesions to limbic structures, particularly the basolateral amygdala, which provide the major source of cortical afferents to the ventral striatum. This suggests the operation of a 'limbic–ventral striatal loop' that is concerned with mediating the impact of affective processes on behaviour. Thus, the associative processes that underlie the ability of drug-paired stimuli to gain reinforcing efficacy and thereby control drug-seeking behaviour (often called craving when applied to man) appear to depend upon interactions between limbic and ventral striatal structures that are in turn strongly modulated by alterations in transmission in the mesolimbic dopamine pathways.

For general reference see the following: Di Chiara and North (1992); Edwards and Lader (1990); Eikelboom and Stewart (1982); Everitt and Robbins (1992); Goldberg and Stolerman (1986); Goudie and Emmett-Ogelsby (1989); Hurd et al (1989); Koob and Bloom (1988); Koob et al (1989); Koob (1992a,b,c,d); Koob et al (1992); Lader (1988); Markou and Koob (1991); Markou et al (1993); O'Brien et al (1986); Phillips et al (1989); Phillips and Fibiger (1990); Robbins et al (1989); Robbins and Everitt (1992); Robins et al (1975); Robinson and Berridge (1993); Samson and Harris (1992); Schuster (1986), Siegel (1988); Stolerman (1992); Stewart and Eikelboom (1987); Stewart (1987); Wikler (1965); Wise (1981); Wise (1982).

Cortical connections

The amygdala has rich interconnections with allocortical, juxtallocortical and, especially, neocortical areas (Amaral 1987; Amaral et al 1992). In addition to direct projections from the olfactory bulb to the nucleus of the lateral olfactory tract, anterior cortical nucleus and the periamygdaloid cortex (piriform cortex), there are also associational connections between all parts of the primary olfactory cortex and these same superficial amygdaloid structures.

The hippocampal formation has only recently been shown to have direct connections with the amygdala (see Amaral et al 1992). The lateral, magnocellular accessory basal and parvicellular basal nuclei contribute the largest proportion of efferents to the hippocampal formation. The main projection is from the lateral nucleus to the rostral entorhinal cortex, but many fibres also terminate in the hippocampus proper and the subiculum. The return projection from the hippocampus to the amygdala is less

extensive, the border zone of the CA1 field and adjacent subiculum, and perhaps also the entorhinal cortex, projecting mainly to the parvicellular basal nucleus. Amaral et al (1992) point out the rather marked polarity in amygdalohippocampal connections, with the amygdala having a greater influence on hippocampal processes than vice versa.

The amygdaloid complex has particularly extensive and rich connections with many areas of the neocortex. In contrast to the commonly held view that the subcortical connections of the amygdala are the most dominant, it is now clear that a large proportion of the inputs to the amygdala arise in unimodal and polymodal regions of the frontal, cingulate, insular and temporal neocortex while its outputs are directed to even more widely dispersed neocortical fields (Amaral et al 1992). The amygdalocortical projections take origin principally in the basal nucleus and to a smaller extent in the lateral and cortical nuclei as well. The extent of these connections with the neocortex is, as might be expected, much greater in the monkey than in the rat and other non-primate species.

Temporal and occipital cortical connections. The amygdala projects to virtually all levels of the visual cortex in both temporal and occipital lobes (**8**.249). The magnocellular basal nucleus gives rise to the largest component of these projections. According to Amaral, they are distributed in a gradient manner, with the heaviest projections being directed from the accessory basal nucleus to rostral levels of the visual cortex in the anterior temporal lobe, and progressively lighter projections arising from the magnocellular basal nucleus directed at more caudal levels of the visual cortex (Amaral et al 1992). The amygdala projects to more of these visual cortical areas than from which it receives afferents; moreover, the lateral nucleus receives from, but does not project to, these visual cortical areas. While studied in less detail, the amygdala also reciprocates projections to the auditory cortex in the rostral half of the superior temporal gyrus. Projections to the polymodal sensory areas of the temporal lobe generally reciprocate the amygdalopetal projections. Thus, efferents from the lateral and accessory basal nuclei are directed at the temporal pole, particularly the medial perirhinal area, and the density of this projection diminishes more caudally in the perirhinal cortex. Amygdala afferents generally terminate in layers I and II of the temporal and occipital cortex.

The anterior temporal lobe provides the largest proportion of the cortical input to the amygdala, predominantly to the lateral nucleus. Area TE projects richly to the lateral nucleus and provides the channel through which visual information is relayed to the amygdala (**8**.250). Rostral parts of the superior temporal gyrus, which may represent unimodal auditory association cortex, project to parts of the lateral nucleus that are distinct from those receiving from field TE. There are also projections from polymodal sensory association cortices of the temporal lobe, including perirhinal cortex (areas 35 and 36), areas TF and TH that lie in the caudal half of the parahippocampal gyrus, the dorsal bank of the superior temporal sulcus and both the medial and lateral areas of the cortex of the temporal pole. The latter two projections terminate in the accessory basal nucleus as well as in the lateral nucleus.

Frontal, insular and cingulate cortical connections. There are four fields that receive especially rich projections from the amygdala. The agranular insular cortex is in particular very heavily innervated

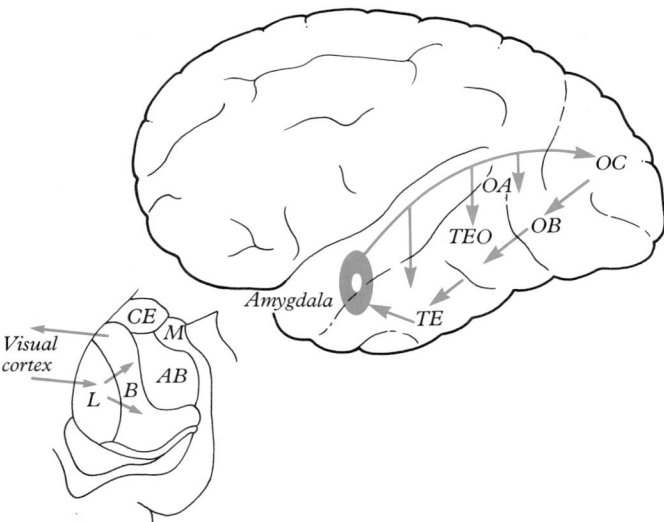

8.250 Schematic illustration showing the relationship of the amygdala with the visually related cortices of the temporal and occipital lobes. Visual information is processed in a hierarchical fashion in cortical regions at progressively greater distances (OB, OA, TEO, TE) from the primary visual cortex (OC). The amygdaloid cortex receives a substantial input from the highest level of the hierarchy (area TE). This information enters the amygdala via the lateral nucleus (drawing at lower left). A projection back to the visual cortex originates in the basal nucleus and this projection extends to all levels of the visually related cortex in the temporal and occipital lobes. Within the amygdala prominent projections between the lateral and basal nuclei potentially 'close the loop' on amygaloid interconnections with the visual cortex.

by the amygdaloid medial and anterior cortical nuclei. The lateral orbital cortex (Walker's area 12) and the medial orbital cortex (Walker's areas 14 and part of 13) as well as the medial frontal cortical areas 24, 25 and 32, including parts of the anterior cingulate gyrus, also receive a heavy projection. Areas 8, 9, 45 and 46 of the dorsolateral prefrontal cortex, as well as the premotor cortex (area 6), receive a patchy innervation arising in the amygdala. The basal nucleus is an important source of these projections that generally terminate in layers I and II of the frontal cortex. However, the accessory basal (magnocellular and parvicellular divisions) and lateral nuclei also contribute to frontal and prefrontal cortical projections, the latter being targeted largely on the medial orbital cortex.

The frontal, cingulate and insular cortices generally reciprocate their amygdala afferents. It is not yet clear, however, whether the amygdaloid nuclei that originate corticopetal projections also receive cortical afferents. The rostral insula projects heavily to the lateral, parvicellular basal and medial nuclei. The caudal insula, which is reciprocally connected with the second somatosensory cortex, also projects to the lateral nucleus, thus providing a route by which somatosensory information reaches the amygdala. The caudal orbital cortex projects to the basal, magnocellular accessory basal and lateral nuclei. The medial prefrontal cortex projects to both the magnocellular divisions of the accessory and basal nuclei. The complex interactions between the amygdala and prefrontal cortex, both direct and via the mediodorsal thalamus and ventral striatopallidal system, are summarized in **8**.249.

SUMMARY

Amygdala. The organization and connections of the amygdala are extremely consonant with a role in emotional behaviour, much as enshrined in the original limbic system concept. It receives highly processed sensory information in all modalities from the thalamus, unimodal and polymodal sensory and association cortices, as well as olfactory information from the bulb and piriform cortex, visceral and gustatory information relayed via brainstem structures and the thalamus. Its projections reach widespread areas of the brain, including the endocrine and autonomic domains of the hypothalamus and brainstem that have formed the linchpin of theories of emotional expression for many years. However, more recently it has been demonstrated that the amygdala has even richer projections to the striatum and to many areas of the neocortex. Thus, its influences on motor outflow and cortical processes are likely to be much more diverse and pervasive than previously thought.

Limbic system. The description here, under the heading 'limbic lobe', of a series of structures having more or less close connections reflects the force of the widely held view that the brain contains a limbic system, rather as it contains motor and sensory systems, and that its integrated function is to mediate emotional expression and, perhaps, experience. There have been several attempts to deal with this limbic system theory of emotion over the decades since it first made an appearance. Brodal (1981) is clear in his view that the concept should be expunged from neural texts and that the functions of the component parts should be explored in their own right. MacLean, on the other hand, continues to evolve the concept and apparently sees no real problem in progressively extending the definition of its constituent parts (e.g. MacLean 1992; **8**.229). By contrast, Swanson (1983) has suggested a reorganization of the concept and proposes a 'limbic telencephalon' comprising first, the hippocampal formation, second, a rim of association cortex adjacent to the hippocampal formation (essentially Broca's limbic lobe) and third, subcortical limbic nuclei including the amygdala. One positive feature of the latter scheme is that it designates as extrinsic those connections with the diencephalic and brainstem areas (hypothalamus, thalamus, midbrain) commonly incorporated within the original limbic system concept and so helps to limit its exponential growth.

What is undeniable is that the hypotheses of Papez and MacLean have served the essential function of stimulating enormous amounts of research on the neural basis of emotion, so much so that the belief in a limbic system is entrenched in the literature and attempts to reappraise it may seem eccentric. This is not really a problem if it is made clear at the outset what is being studied. If the major goal of research is to explore the neural basis of emotion, then studies can be designed to identify the structures involved and thence the systems of which they are a part. Undoubtedly, some of the structures identified in this way will be part of the currently defined limbic system. The amygdala is one such structure and it is seen by many to be both at the heart of the limbic system concept and of the brain's emotional system. But it is now equally clear that the areas included within the limbic system do not function as a system specialized for emotional processing, as opposed to other forms of information processing. Indeed, the hippocampus, while clearly the centrepiece of the limbic system concept, is not at all the centrepiece of the brain's emotional system. This structure and some of those connected with it, including those of the Papez circuit, are now widely accepted to be involved more with cognitive processes including mnemonic functions, perhaps especially spatial short-term memory. In this context, it would appear to be of doubtful utility to continue to explore the function, or functions, of the limbic system since the

anatomical criteria for defining it are at best imprecise and its purported unitary function in emotion is untenable.

It has been emphasized most elegantly by LeDoux (1986, 1991) that the limbic system concept of emotion has survived for so long primarily because of the inclusion of the amygdala, but that great caution must be exercised before it is replaced with an amygdala concept of emotion. What is required is an open-minded and thorough analysis of the neural structures involved in a much wider variety of emotional processes than have been studied hitherto, including those underlying emotional experience. Systematic study of the frontal, especially orbitofrontal, cortex as well as the medial limbic cortex, the functions of which remain obscure so long after Broca, Papez and MacLean drew attention to them, may well prove to be exceptionally important in this regard. Furthermore, studies of emotional and motivational processes must be integrated with those of cognitive processes if a broader understanding of the brain's emotional system is to emerge.

Stress

Animals, including man, live in an environment in which features such as temperature, humidity and energy supply can vary widely and unpredictably. Claude Bernard recognized that defending the internal environment, which is relatively intolerant to such changes, was a prerequisite for existence in a hostile world — one, for example, that can be dry, cold and in which food may be scarce. Whilst the concept of homeostasis has undergone some modifications (particularly that some features of the internal milieu can vary within wider limits than others, and that these limits may themselves not be fixed) nevertheless it remains accepted that defence against disturbances in the external environment is critical. Added to these are other, more recently recognized sources of potential disruption. An important one is the social environment in which animals and man live. A social structure of some sort is an almost universal attribute of mammals (and most other animals). Whilst it provides well-recognized advantages (defence against predators, ease of reproduction, help in foraging, etc.), the presence of potential competitors can regulate or limit an individual's actions or access to available resources. Finally, animals also need defences against parasites and infection, and many have to avoid predation.

All these disturbances, as well as the processes by which individuals encounter, recognize and respond to such events that threaten their well-being, have been encompassed by the general term 'stress'. The term itself has been through a series of definitions, to the point where it is used with reluctance by some. Cannon recognized that, to survive such vicissitudes, animals must call on a set of emergency responses, and that these included both physiological and behavioural ('flight or fight') adaptations. Selye focused on

the secretions of the adrenal cortex (in particular, glucocorticoids such as cortisol). He echoed Cannon in supposing that all stress responses were essentially undifferentiated (that is, the same response occurred in the presence of any type of stress). More recently, however, the concept of stress has evolved in important ways.

Variations in responses to stress

First, it has become clear that, even though many stresses may induce the same reaction in some systems (e.g. the adrenal cortex), stress responses occur across a much wider spectrum than originally imagined. Furthermore, some of these responses are highly differentiated — that is, they reflect the specific features of the stressor. For example, the physiological and behavioural adaptations to water deprivation have features distinct from, say, the response to extreme heat or cold, or to the presence of a threatening conspecific. Secondly, stress itself is not an absolute or invarying process. Much of the earlier confusion derived from arguments over whether 'stress' should be defined by external conditions (e.g. a drop in temperature, the receipt of aggression, etc.), or the nature of the response (e.g. whether the adrenal cortex or the cardiovascular system was activated). It now seems that whether or not a particular set of conditions are stressful may depend on a whole range of ancillary circumstances. For example, in man the response to adverse events may depend not only on the event itself, but upon the way that the event is perceived, upon the degree of social support available and upon the previous experience or history of the individual concerned. Observations on animals show that stress is modulated in them by similar factors. The response to a persistent or recurring stress may change with time as a consequence of alterations ('transactions') in the relation between the individual and the stress or its source. Finally, the distinction between a 'stressed'

and an 'unstressed' individual is not absolute; indeed, it could be said that any living animal is always under some degree of stress, in that it has to maintain its internal environment in the face of an external one with a very different composition, to compete with others for resources and to undergo periodic energetic demands such as those associated with reproduction.

Adaptations to stress

Despite all these reservations and qualifications, it is important to understand how the body handles stress. There is now overwhelming evidence that persistent stress, particularly in those having difficulty in coping with it, is a major risk factor for a range of both somatic and psychological illnesses. Experimental evidence that stress can alter gastric secretion and induce erosions is consistent with clinical findings that gastric ulcers are associated with persistent stress. Exaggerated cardiovascular reactions to stress occur in some strains of rats. A parallel finding in man is that certain types of personality (those that react markedly to demand) may also have a higher incidence of heart disease. Experiencing a major adversity (particularly on top of chronic social or other difficulties) is a well-established risk factor for major depressive disorders. Current work is attempting to provide a detailed account of the physiological and pathological events that are responsible both for effective adaptation to stress, and for the ill health that may follow inadequate responses. Even seemingly adequate adaptations to stress may carry a 'cost' measured as increased vulnerability to later ill health or tissue damage.

It is obvious that the brain plays a central role in the response to stress. Whilst the pervasive nature of stress ensures that most, if not all, of the brain will be involved in some way in the processes of recognizing, evaluating and responding to stress or stressful events, certain areas seem to be particularly important. The limbic system has both the receptor and the effector mechanisms to detect and respond to threats to the internal environment, such as those on body temperature, blood glucose, acid–base balance and state of hydration. For more complex stressors, such as those derived from the social environment, analysis by cortical mechanisms seems likely. But there are well-recognized major neural pathways from the cortex (e.g. through the amygdala) that allow such information access to other limbic structures, such as the hypothalamus. Damage to the limbic system results in disturbances in the internal environment, or to inadequate responses to demands from the external world.

The organization of responses to stress has three main components: changes in behaviour which allow the individual to engage in appropriate behavioural responses to demand or imbalance, such as eating, drinking, seeking shelter, avoiding attack, etc.; alterations in endocrine function, including generalized responses such as increased adrenal cortical hormone secretion and more specialized ones, such as those to hypoglycaemia, or cooling, or dehydration, etc., each of which evoke distinct patterns of endocrine response; and changes in cardiovascular activity, via the autonomic nervous system, which tend to be fairly undifferentiated with respect to the type of stress. The hypothalamus, through its output to the pituitary, brainstem autonomic centres and behavioural mechanisms, occupies a critical position

in the organization of the triadic response to stress.

Some progress is being made in understanding how different patterns of response are formulated to meet specific demands. These seem to depend on the intrinsic neurochemical signalling systems in the limbic system. The limbic system has an unusually rich content of peptides, and it is becoming apparent that these may form the chemical architecture of stress responses. The structure and variety of peptides makes them ideal as carriers of specific information, allowing a single molecule to activate selectively the particular pattern of dispersed neural mechanisms responsible for the appropriate behavioural, endocrine and autonomic responses. For example, angiotensin II (an octapeptide) is activated in the brain by dehydration, and stimulates drinking, vasopressin release and increased blood pressure—all part of the co-ordinated response to this particular stress. Other peptides seem able to formulate patterns of responses appropriate to hypoglycaemia (neuropeptide Y), low environmental temperatures (thyrotrophin-releasing factor), or to anxiety-inducing situations (corticotrophin-releasing factor) and so on. Yet other peptides, such as oxytocin or β-endorphin, may be particularly concerned with regulating the demands imposed by reproduction.

Peptides do not act alone. The limbic system also expresses high concentrations of steroid hormone receptors. Some of these, such as those responsive to gonadal

hormones, may be concerned with integrating reproduction, though associated stress-related behaviour (such as aggression) may also be involved, and levels of gonadal hormones are easily reduced by stress. Corticoids, which usually increase during stress, also bind to receptors in the limbic system, and it is likely that these play a role in the neural regulation of stress (such as modifying the actions of peptides). It is strange that, although the involvement of corticoids in stress responses has been recognized for decades, their precise role is still not well understood (though some think that they limit the stress response in target tissues). Finally, the ascending monoaminergic systems, such as those containing noradrenaline, serotonin or dopamine, are also known to be activated by unpredictable or exceptional demands such as stress. Whilst these systems provide a rich nerve supply to the limbic system, they also innervate large areas in other parts of the brain. Their role in stress is thus likely to be distinct from that of the chemically more complex, and anatomically more localized, peptides; experiments on monoamines have shown that they are involved in a wide range of neural activity. Taken together, it seems that the great neurochemical diversity of the limbic system is the basis for the equally diverse variety in adaptive responses to stress. Understanding how these different neurochemical signals interact, and how their effects differ in the various structures that make up the limbic system, is a major goal of current work.

CEREBRAL CORTEX

INTRODUCTION

The cerebral cortex or pallium is often divided into a phylogenetically old, original part, the allocortex, consisting of the archicortex and palaeocortex (archipallium and palaeopallium), and a newer development, the neocortex (isocortex or neopallium). The latter may be equated with systems of sensory and motor activity which originally had little or no connection with the forebrain, but have acquired these by an evolutionary process of prosencephalization. The remarks which follow apply only to the neocortex.

The cerebral cortex has been studied over several centuries. It was examined by the pioneering microscopists; the first recorded structural detail was the stria in the occipital cortex named by Gennari in 1776. Improved microscopes in the 1830s made investigation of cortical organization more effective. In recent years, increasing emphasis has come to be placed on findings which combine physiological/functional studies with the examination of structure and connectivity. Improved methods for tracing axonal connections, the use of awake behaving primates for physiological studies, the advent of newer electrophysiological and histochemical, immuno-cytochemical and other microscopic techniques have combined with ever advancing methods for studying the functioning human brain in vivo, notably the electroencephalogram (EEG) positron emission topography (PET) and magnetic resonance imaging (MRI) (p. 1171). The most meaningful subdivisions of the cerebral neocortex are those where significant changes in microscopic appearance are shown to reflect connectivity, where these

changes coincide with functional specialization and where similar areas are identifiable in vivo in the human neocortex. There is little doubt that both improving spatial resolution in techniques for imaging the functioning human brain, and increasingly detailed structural, connectional and functional understanding of subhuman primate neocortex will radically alter our view of the cerebral cortex in coming decades. Much of the way in which ideas are evolving and changing has been recently discussed in a stimulating account concentrating on visual sensation and perception (Zeki 1993). In the interim, however, while we await a resolution of controversies and a crystallization of knowledge based on advancing technology, it is necessary to give a somewhat traditional account of the structure and organization of the cerebral cortex, at least in part to clarify the terminology and knowledge base on which such improved understanding will be built.

NEURONS OF THE CEREBRAL CORTEX

To the unaided eye, the cerebral cortex forms a complete mantle or pallium covering the hemispheres, obviously variable in thickness (15–45 mm) when seen in section, being thicker on the summits of gyri than in the depths of sulci (in which most of the cortex is hidden). Such thickness variations might well correspond to microstructural variations in the pallium; and it has been suggested that the positioning of gyri and sulci is conditioned by structural differences (Le Gros Clark 1945), but this cannot be claimed with respect to functionally differentiated areas, which often depart in outline from the sulcal pattern. In the freshly cut cerebral cortex, some laminar details can be appreciated even without a lens (e.g.

the visual stria of Gennari); elsewhere finer horizontal layers of nerve fibres, the inner and outer bands of Baillarger (p. 1146), can usually be discerned. It has even been claimed that more than a score of structurally distinct areas can be identified by simple visual inspection (Smith 1907).

The microscopic structure of the cerebral cortex, like 'grey matter' elsewhere, is an intricate blend of nerve cells and fibres, neuroglia and blood vessels. Neuroglia and vascular arrangements have been dealt with elsewhere (pp. 937, 1219). The neuronal features, connections and distributions must now be considered. However, it is to be noted that variation in vascular distribution has also been utilized as a criterion in differentiating cortical areas (Pfeifer 1940) and many other finer features of its microarchitecture show corresponding variations in angioarchitecture (Duvernoy et al 1981).

The cortex comprises essentially three cell groups. The most abundant (c. 66%; Rockel et al 1980; Powell 1981) are pyramidal cells. Non-pyramidal cells, called stellate or granule cells, are subdivided into spiny and non-spiny groups. All subtypes have been grouped into variable subdivisions on the basis of size, shape and neuritic array (8.251A, B).

Pyramidal cells (Feldman 1984) (8.252) have a flask-shaped or triangular cell soma giving rise to a single apical and multiple basal dendrites. The cell bodies vary in size from around 10 μm to as much as 80 μm in diameter. A single, thick apical dendrite ascends from the superficial pole of the soma, tapering and branching, to end in a spray of terminal dendritic twigs in the most superficial lamina, the molecular layer. From the basal, deeper surface of the cell, basal dendrites spread almost horizontally, or at a shallow angle, directed towards the white matter for variable distances, but up to almost 1 mm for the largest pyramidal cells. Like the apical dendrite, and perhaps more so, the basal dendrites branch profusely along their length. All pyramidal cell dendrites are studded with a myriad of dendritic spines, which become more numerous as distance from the parent cell soma increases. A single, slender, non-tapering axon arises from the axon hillock, usually situated centrally on the basal surface of the pyramidal neuron. Ultimately, in the vast majority if not all cases, the axon leaves the cortical grey matter to enter the white matter. Pyramidal cells are thus, perhaps universally, *projection* neurons. As their axons traverse the grey matter, however,

they branch profusely, with many collaterals passing horizontally or diagonally for considerable distances within the grey matter. Other neurons which diverge somewhat from this rigid description but share such common features as spiny dendrites, one dendrite ascending towards the pia, and an axon entering the white matter, can reasonably be considered as modified pyramidal cells. This group includes many of the pleiomorphic cells of lamina VI.

The spiny stellate cells (Lund 1984) are the second most numerous cell type in the neocortex and for the most part occupy lamina IV. They have relatively small cell bodies, commonly 6 to 10 μm in diameter which are essentially multipolar, with several primary dendrites radiating for variable distances. As implied by their name, the dendrites are profusely spinous. Their axons ramify within the grey matter predominantly in the vertical plane.

Numerically, the smallest group comprises the heterogenous, non-spiny or sparsely-spinous stellate cells. All are interneurons, with axons confined to grey matter. In morphological terms, this is not a single class of cell, but a multitude of different forms, including basket, chandelier, double bouquet, neurogliaform, bipolar/fusiform and horizontal cells (8.251A). Various types may have horizontally, vertically or radially ramifying axons. It is on this basis, perhaps, that it is reasonable to attempt some form of initial subclassification:

- A group with mainly *horizontally dispersed axons* includes the basket and horizontal cells. The *basket cells* (Jones & Hendry 1984) have a short, vertical axon which rapidly divides into a horizontal family of collaterals, which end in large terminal sprays synapsing with the somata and proximal dendrites of pyramidal cells. The cell bodies of *horizontal cells* (Marin-Padilla 1984) lie mainly at the superficial border of lamina II, occasionally deep in lamina I, (the molecular or plexiform layer). They are small and fusiform; their dendrites spread short distances in two opposite directions in lamina I. Their axons often stem from a dendrite, then divide into two branches which travel away from each other for great distances in the same layer.
- Neurons with an *axonal arborization predominantly perpendicular* to the pial surface include chandelier, double bouquet and bipolar/fusiform cells. *Chandelier cells* (Peters 1984) have a variable morphology, although most are ovoid or fusiform with dendrites

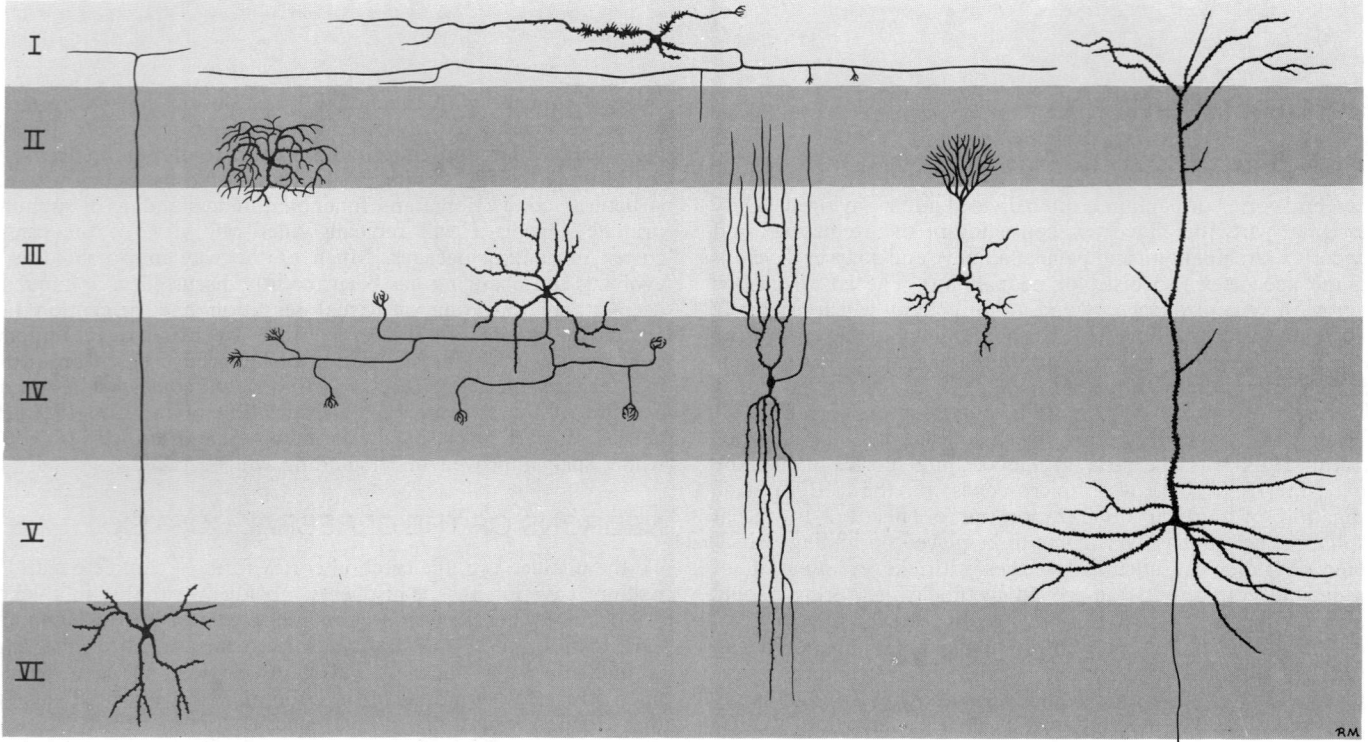

8.251A Typical outlines of characteristic neocortical neurons as seen in sections prepared by the metallic impregnation techniques introduced by Golgi and Cajal. From left to right are shown Martinotti, neurogliaform, basket, horizontal, fusiform, stellate and pyramidal types of neuron. Many other forms and variants have been described. See text for literature.

arising from the upper and lower poles of the cell body. A characteristic axonal arborization which emerges from the cell body or a proximal dendrite identifies these neurons. A few cells in the more superficial lamina (II and IIIa) have descending axons, whereas deeper cells (laminae IIIc and IV) have ascending axons, with intermediate neurons (IIIb) often having both. The axons ramify within the vicinity of the parent cell body and terminate in numerous vertically oriented strings of axonal swellings, the 'candles of the chandelier'. These vertical strings of terminals run alongside the axon hillocks of pyramidal cells with which they synapse. *Double bouquet* (or bitufted) cells (Somogyi & Cowey 1984) are found in laminae II and III and have axons traversing laminae II and V. Generally, but not exclusively, these neurons have two or three main dendrites giving rise to a superficial and deep dendritic tuft (hence bitufted). A single axon arises usually from the oval or spindle-shaped cell soma and rapidly divides into an ascending and descending branch. These branches collateralize extensively, but the axonal arbour is confined to a perpendicularly extended, but horizontally confined cylinder, about 50 to 80 μm across. *Bipolar cells* (Peter 1984b) are ovoid cells with a single ascending and a single descending dendrite arising from the upper and lower poles respectively. These primary dendrites branch sparsely with the branches also running vertically, giving a narrow dendritic tree, rarely more than 100 μm across, which may extend through most of the cortical thickness. Commonly, the axon originates from one of the primary dendrites, and rapidly branches to give a vertically elongated, horizontally confined axonal arbor which closely parallels the dendritic tree in extent.

- The principal recognizable neuronal type with a *radially ramifying axon* is the *neurogliaform* or spiderweb cell (Jones 1984a). These small sperical cells, 10–12 μm in diameter, are found mainly in

laminae II to IV, depending on cortical area. Seven to ten thin dendrites typically radiate out from the cell soma, some branching once or twice, but many not, to form a spherical dendritic field of about 100–150 μm diameter. The slender axon arises from the cell body or a proximal dendrite and almost immediately branches profusely within the vicinity of the dendritic field and usually somewhat beyond to give a spherical axonal arbor up to 350 μm in diameter. Other varieties of non-spiny or sparsely spinous non-pyramidal cells with local axonal plexi occur which are not easily included in any of the preceding categories (Peters & Saint Marie 1984), but do not fit into a single additional subtype. This perplexing heterogeneity will not be considered further here, except to note that the preceding description is of necessity a simplification and is also incomplete.

Considerable recent data have accumulated concerning the characterization of different neuronal types within the cortex according to content of specific identifiable intracellular molecules. For the most part, such studies have centred on neurotransmitters, or neurotransmitter-related molecules, such as transmitter receptors, synthesizing and degrading enzymes. In addition, important new findings relate to the presence of calcium related proteins such as calbindin in specific neuronal types (DeFelipe 1993; Andressen et al 1993; Condé et al 1994). Pyramidal neurons appear exclusively to use excitatory amino acids as their neurotransmitters, either glutamate or aspartate (Streit 1984). It may be possible to subclassify pyramidal cells on the basis of the presence of either glutaminase or aspartate aminotransferase (Donoghue et al 1985; Conti et al 1987; Najlerahim et al 1990), though this is uncertain at present. In addition, specific receptor populations may be concentrated on subsets of pyramidal neurons (Francis et al 1992; Chessell et al 1994).

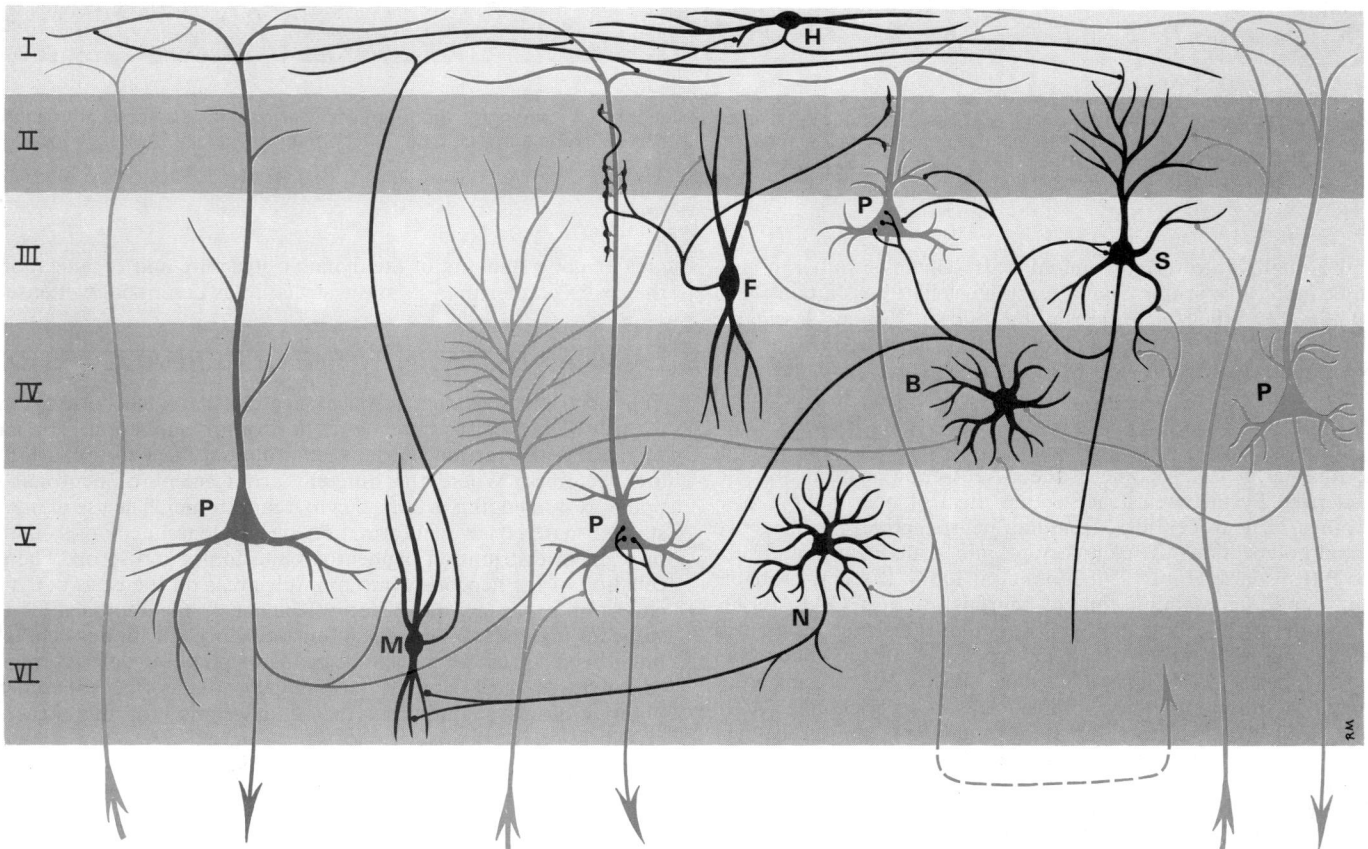

8.251B A diagrammatic representation of the most frequent types of neocortical neuron, showing typical connections with each other and with afferent fibres (blue). Neurons limited to the cortex in their distribution are indicated in black. Efferent neurons are in magenta. The right and left afferent fibres are association or cortico-cortical connections, the central afferent is a specific sensory fibre. Neurons are shown in their characteristic lamina, but many have somata in more than one layer. They are indicated thus: P = pyramidal, M = Martinotti, F = fusiform, H = horizontal, N = neurogliaform, B = basket, S = stellate. See text for details and compare with illustration **8.257** et seq.

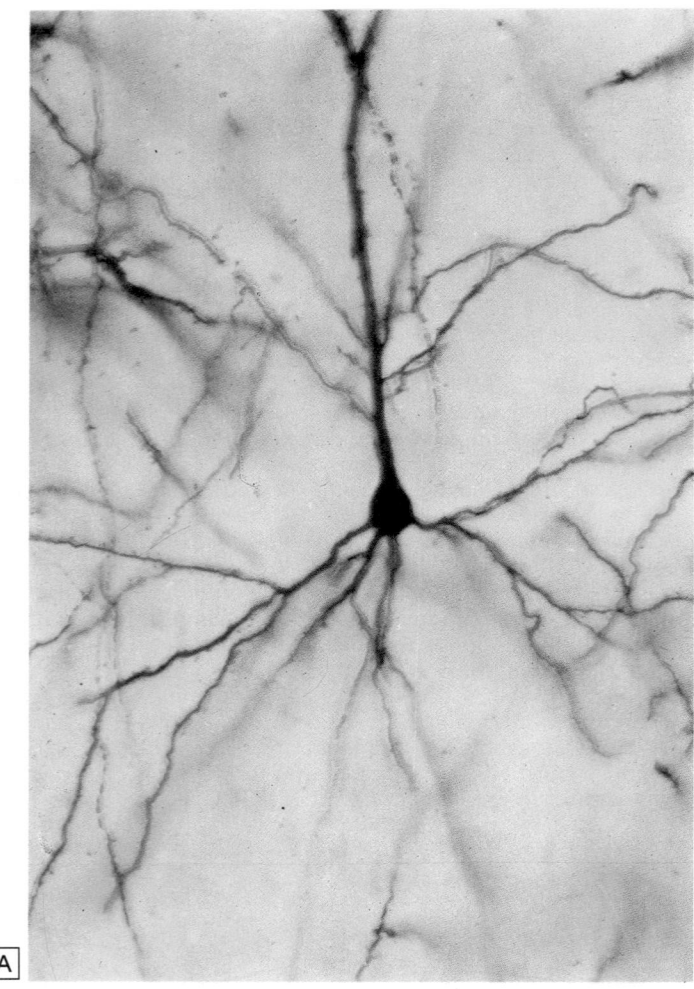

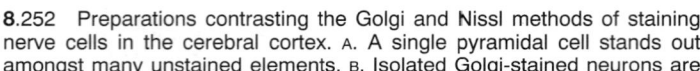

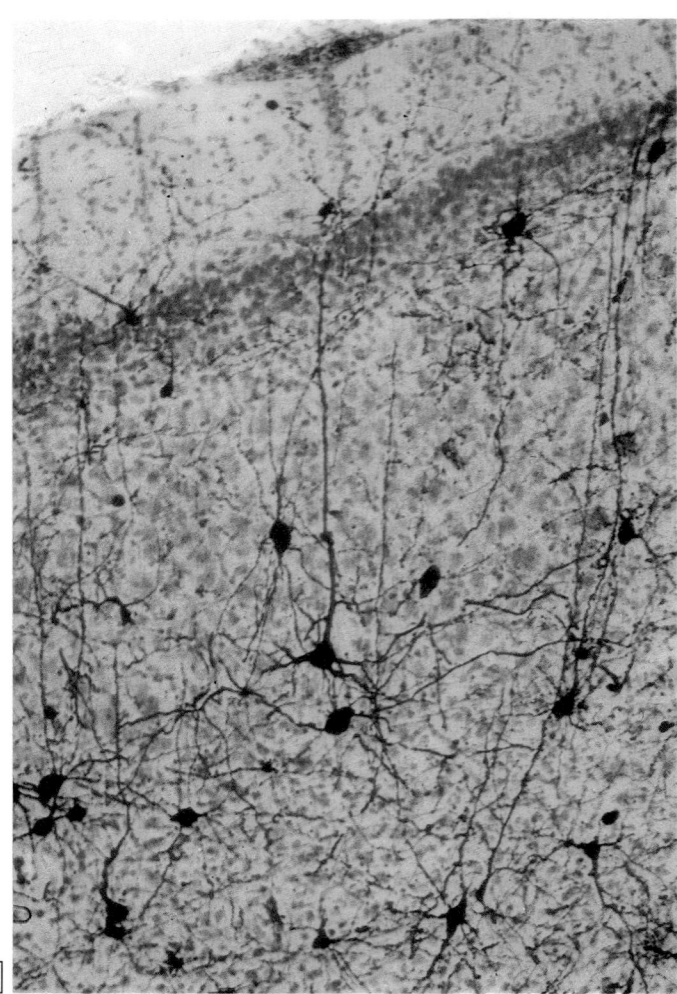

8.252 Preparations contrasting the Golgi and Nissl methods of staining nerve cells in the cerebral cortex. A. A single pyramidal cell stands out amongst many unstained elements. B. Isolated Golgi-stained neurons are prominent amongst the remaining Nissl-stained cortical elements. (Preparations provided by A R Lieberman, University College, London.)

In the main, however, pyramidal cells remain a rather homogeneous, indivisible group. Similarly, spiny stellate cells are likely to use glutamate as their neurotransmitter, and are not subclassifiable on the basis of other known neurochemical markers. Of the nonspiny or sparsely spinous non-pyramidal cells, probably the great majority, if not all, use γ-aminobutyric acid (GABA) as a principal neurotransmitter. This is almost certainly the case for basket, chandelier, double bouquet, neurogliaform and bipolar cells (Houser et al 1984; Jones et al 1987). Some of the GABA-ergic neurons are also characterized by the coexistence within them of one or more of a wide range of neuropeptides, including neuropeptide Y, vasoactive intestinal polypeptide (VIP), cholecystokinin, somatostatin and substance P (Emson & Hunt 1984; Jones et al 1987). It seems probable that all peptide containing cortical neurons are also GABA-ergic. Furthermore, it appears that most if not all of these can be classified as bipolar cells; other GABA-ergic cell types probably do not contain peptides (Jones et al 1987). An additional 'classical' neurotransmitter present in a subpopulation of bipolar cells is acetylcholine (ACh; Houser et al 1985; Eckenstein & Baughman 1984); these cells may additionally be GABA-ergic (Kosaka et al 1988; Kubota & Jones 1992) and may also contain VIP (Eckenstein & Baughman 1984). The occurrence of different calcium binding proteins within cortical neurons may well be a method for further subdivision of GABA-ergic neurons (DeFelipe 1993; Andressen et al 1993).

The advent of neurochemical markers for specific neuronal types, together with increasing knowledge of their connectivity and physiology, will undoubtedly allow a more systematic and rational classification into families of similarly functional cells. The role of each such type in modulating cortical function will become clearer and a greater understanding of the dynamic structure and organization of the cortex, rather than its static structure as described, will ensue.

LAMINAR PATTERN IN THE CEREBRAL CORTEX

The most apparent microscopical feature of the neocortex stained for cell bodies or for fibres is its horizontal lamination. The study of the different arrangements seen within the neocortex is termed architectonics. Where the different arrangement of neuronal cell bodies is studied, this is termed cytoarchitectonics. The use of myelin-stained material gives information on myeloarchitectonics, the use of pigment distribution pigmentoarchitectonics and so on. The parcellation of the neocortex into multiple areas on the basis of cytoarchitectonics has a long history (Kemper & Galaburda 1984). Its value for understanding cortical functional organization is debatable, but the use of cytoarchitectonic maps to pinpoint different regions of cortex, and of laminar terminology to describe experimental observations is so universal that a description of this structural classification is essential.

Typical neocortex is described as having six layers or laminae lying parallel to the surface (**8.253–255, 567, 158**). These are as follows:

I The molecular or plexiform layer is cell sparse, containing only scattered horizontal cells and their processes (see above) enmeshed in a compacted mass of tangential, principally horizontal axons and dendrites (Marin-Padilla 1984). These comprise afferent fibres arising from outside the cortical area, as well as intrinsic fibres from cortical interneurons (see above), and the apical

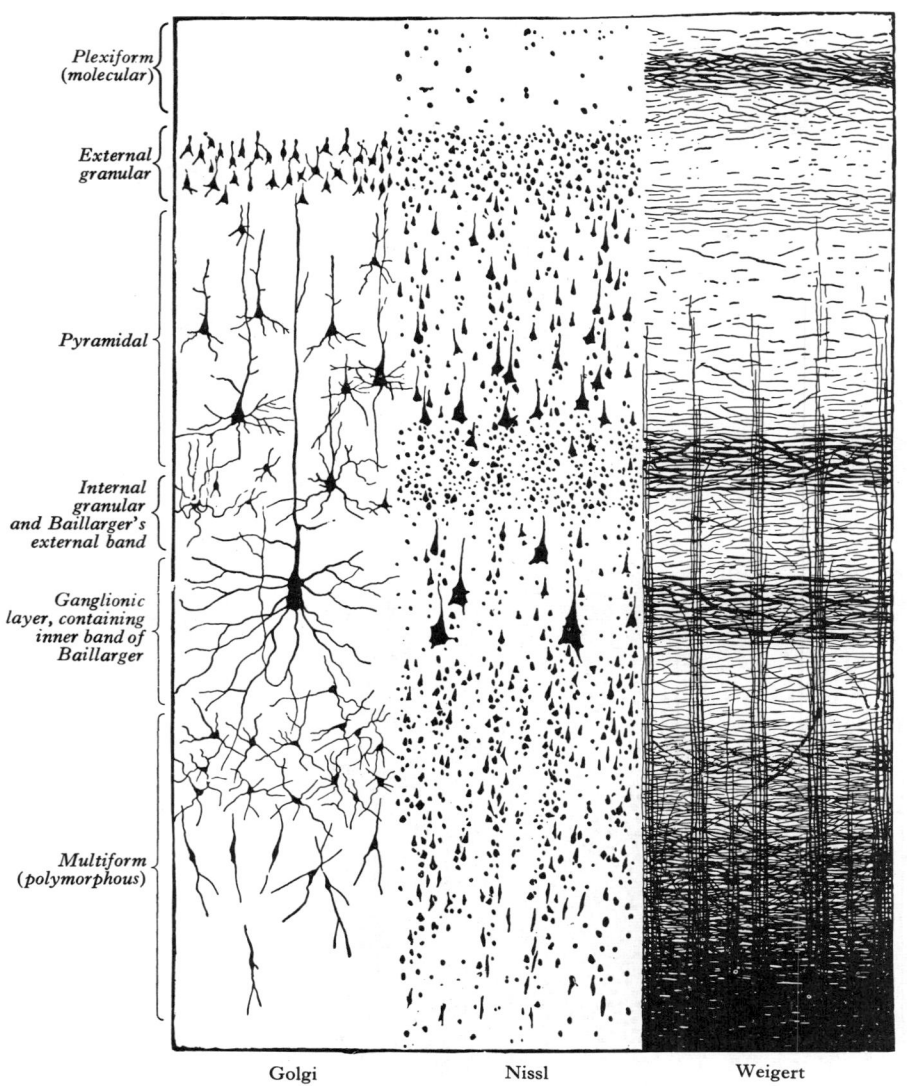

Plexiform (molecular)

External granular

Pyramidal

Internal granular and Baillarger's external band

Ganglionic layer, containing inner band of Baillarger

Multiform (polymorphous)

Golgi   Nissl   Weigert

8.253 Representations of the layers of the human cerebral cortex, as stained by the techniques of Golgi, Nissl and Weigert.

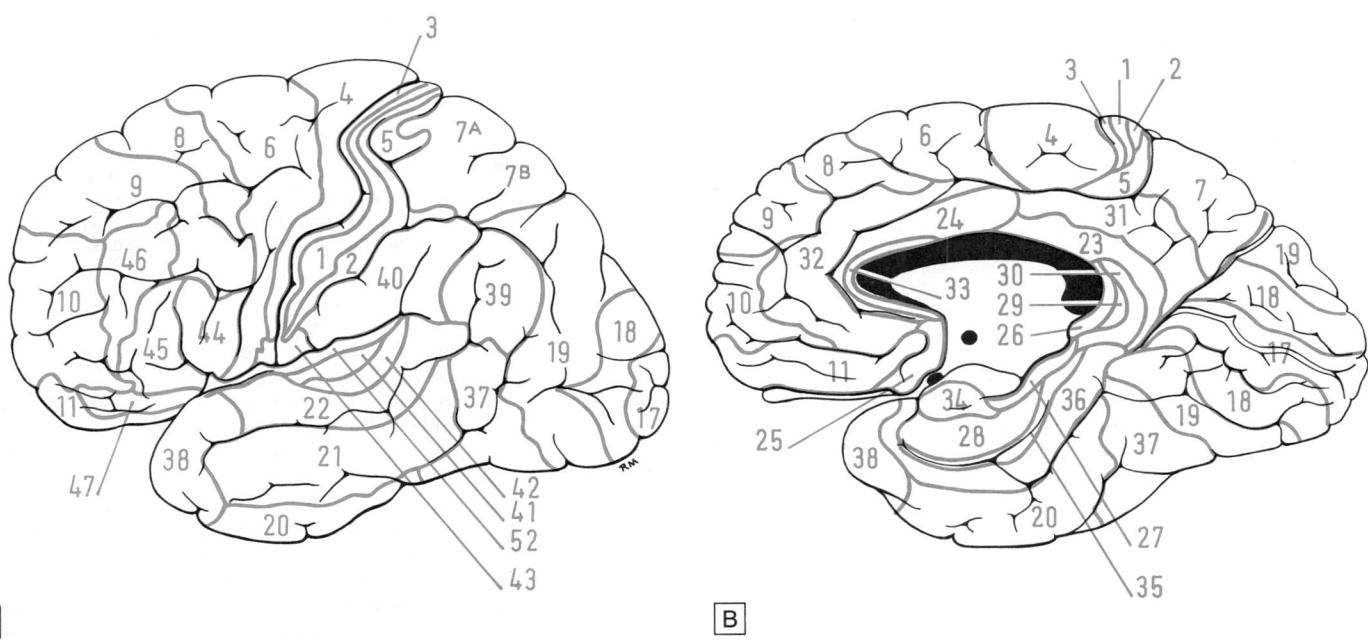

A

B

8.254 The superolateral (A) and medial (B) surfaces of the human cerebral hemisphere demonstrating the cytoarchitectonic areas identified and designated numerically by K Brodmann (1909). Compare with **8**.249A.

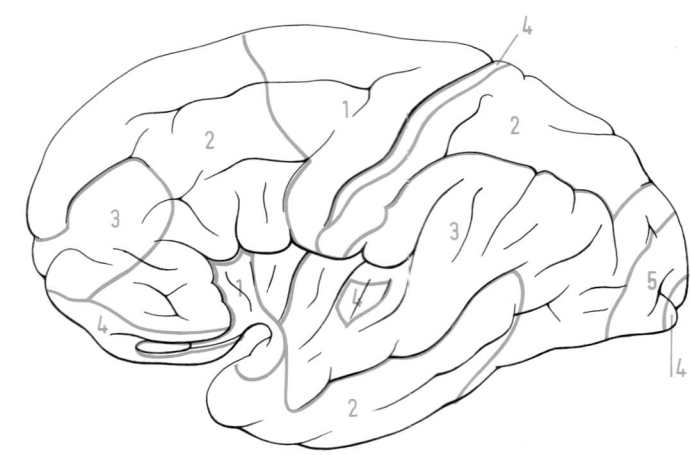

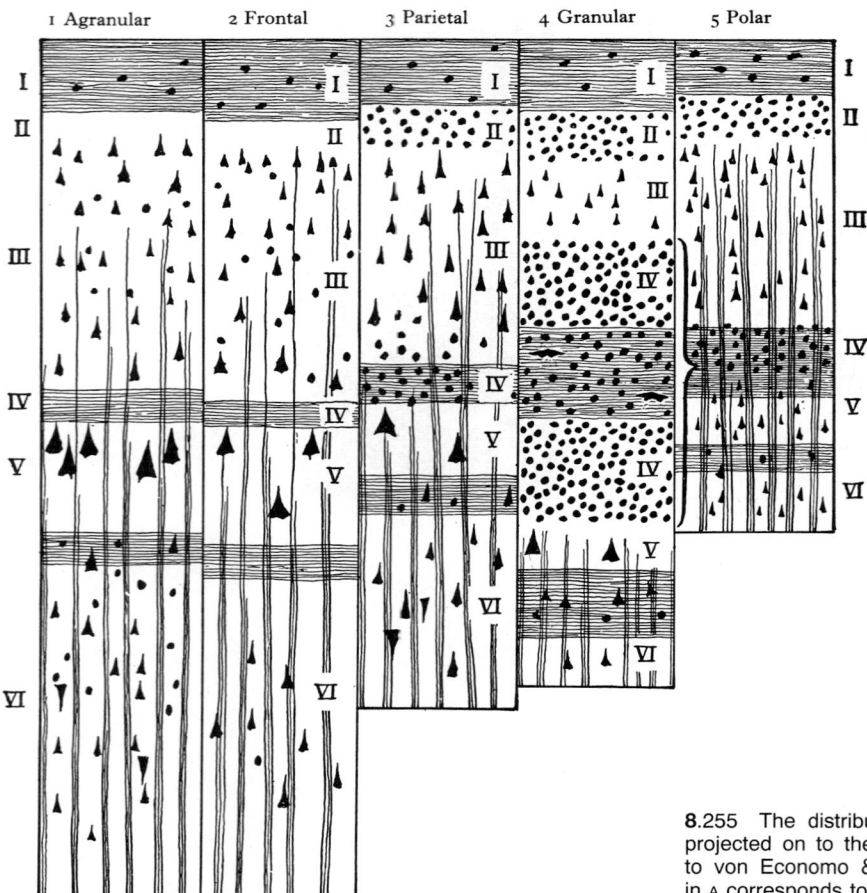

1 Agranular	2 Frontal	3 Parietal	4 Granular	5 Polar

8.255 The distribution of the five major types of cerebral cortex, as projected on to the superolateral surface of the hemisphere, according to von Economo & Koskinas (1925). The numbering of cortical areas in A corresponds to the cytoarchitectonic types shown in B. Compare with **8.254**A, B

dendritic arbors of virtually all pyramidal neurons of the cerebral cortex. In myelin stained sections, layer I appears as a narrow horizontal band of fibres.

II   The external granular lamina contains a varying density of small neuronal cell bodies. These include both small pyramidal as well as non-pyramidal cells, although the latter may predominate. Fibre stains show mainly vertically arranged processes traversing the layer.

III The external pyramidal lamina contains pyramidal cells of varying sizes, together with scattered non-pyramidal neurons. The size of the pyramidal cells is smallest in the most superficial part of the layer and greatest in the deepest part. This lamina is frequently further subdivided into IIIa, IIIb and IIIc, with IIIa most superficial and IIIc deepest. As in layer II, myelin stains reveal a mostly vertical organization of fibres.

IV   The internal granular lamina is usually the narrowest of the cellular laminae and contains densely packed small, round cell bodies of non-pyramidal cells, notably spiny-stellate cells and some small pyramidal cells. Within the lamina, in myelin stained sections, a prominent band of horizontal fibres is seen, the outer band of Baillarger.

V   The internal pyramidal lamina (or ganglionic lamina) typically contains the largest pyramidal cells in any cortical area, though actual sizes vary considerably from area to area. Scattered non-pyramidal cells are also seen. In myelin stains, ascending and descending vertical fibres traverse the layer, but a prominent central band of horizontal fibres is seen, the inner band of Baillarger.

VI   The multiform (or fusiform/pleiomorphic) layer is comprised of neurons with a variety of shapes, including recognizable pyramidal, spindle, ovoid and many other shaped somata. Typically, most cells are small to medium in size. This lamina blends gradually with the underlying white matter, and a clear demarcation of its deeper boundary is not always possible.

REPRESENTATIVE VARIANTS OF CORTICAL STRUCTURE

While it is impossible, and probably unprofitable, to detail and discuss here the almost endless nuances of cortical structure based on full-blown architectonics, a smaller number of variant types must be indicated. These were recognized in the classic studies of Campbell (1905) and corroborated by Economo and Koskinas (1929). Five fundamental types are described in the neocortex (**8.255A, B**). While all these are said to develop from the same sexalaminar pattern, two are regarded as virtually lacking certain laminae when differentiated and are hence heterotypical; these are the granular and agranular types. Homotypical variants, in which all six laminae persist, are called frontal (premotor), parietal (postcentral) and polar (visuopsychic), names linking them with specific regions in a misleading manner, as illustration **8.255A** shows (e.g. the frontal type occurs in parietal and temporal lobes).

The *agranular* type is considered to have diminished or to lack altogether granular laminae (II and IV) but always contains scattered stellate somata. The large pyramidal neurons are found in the greatest densities in agranular cortex. Originally identified in the precentral gyrus (area 4), it also occupies areas 6, 8 and 44 (**8.254A, B**) and occurs elsewhere, including parts of the limbic system (p. 1121). It is typified by the efferent projection of particularly large numbers of axons from its pyramidal cells; but like all neocortical areas, many varieties of both efferent and afferent projections are present. Agranular cortex is thus often equated with cortical motor areas.

In *granular* type of cortex (koniocortex) the granular layers are maximally developed and contain densely packed stellate cells, amongst which are dispersed small pyramidal neurons. Laminae III and IV are poorly developed or unidentifiable. This type of cortex is particularly associated with afferent projections but does have efferent fibres, although less numerous than elsewhere, derived from the scattered pyramidal cells.

Despite the relative lack of different laminae, granular and agranular cortices represent opposite extremes of a gradation, in which the pyramidal and stellate neurons are reciprocally prominent. A typical granular cortex appears in the postcentral gyrus (somatosensory area), striate area (visual area) and superior temporal gyrus (acoustic area) and in small parts of the parahippocampal gyrus (p. 1114). Despite its very high density of stellate cells, especially in the striate area, it is almost the thinnest of the five main types. In the striate cortex the external band of Baillarger (lamina IV) is well defined as the stria of Gennari (or Vicq d'Azyr).

The remaining three types of cortex are intermediate forms. In the frontal type large numbers of small and medium-sized pyramidal neurons appear in laminae III and V, granular layers (II and IV) being less prominent. The relative prominence of these major forms of neuron vary reciprocally wherever this form of cortex exists. It is not confined to the frontal region (**8.255A, B**). The parietal type of cortex contains pyramidal cells which are mostly smaller in size than in the frontal type; granular laminae are, on the contrary, wider and contain more of the stellate cells. This kind of cortex occupies large areas in the parietal and temporal lobes (**8.255A, B**). The polar type is classically identified with small areas near the frontal and occipital poles, hence its name. It is the thinnest form of cortex (**8.255B**). All six laminae are represented but the pyramidal layer (III) is reduced in width and not so extensively invaded by stellate cells as in the granular type of cortex. As in the latter, the multiform layer (VI) is more highly organized than in other types.

While subdivision of these five basic types of cortical 'organization' may sometimes be useful, it must be re-emphasized again that in microscopic sections where they are customarily distinguished, whether stained to show somata or processes, the finer and more significant details of true organization are not so apparent in studies of the whole thickness of the cortex. Functional organization is naturally linked to the spatial distribution of cells but it is in their actual patterns of connection that any real enlightenment about cortical mechanisms must be sought. Golgi stained preparations have yielded an immense amount of information indicating the probable circuit design for neuronal interaction. Functional hypotheses deduced from such structural data, however intricate, require confirmation in terms of the precise nature of the synapses, their distribution and mode of action. Such details depend on electron microscopy and unit recording, techniques which deal only with much smaller volumes of cortical tissue, and also on the rapidly expanding techniques of neurohistochemistry. Nevertheless, exciting results have accrued in this field in recent years and doubtless more is to come. The cytoarchitectural approach to cortical activity was a necessary prelude and the resulting definitions of forms of organization in structural terms remain the bases of orientation to which ultrastructural and other details must be referred.

BASIC UNIFORMITY OF THE CEREBRAL CORTEX

Despite considerable variations in cytoarchitectonic appearance between different neocortical areas, it is becoming apparent that a fundamental architectural plan underlies the structure and organization of all neocortical areas.

The most extensive, which include comparative, quantitative studies of cortical and laminar thickness, absolute neuronal numbers in standard full-thickness cortical strips and pyramidal/non-pyramidal ratios are by Rockel et al (1980) and Powell (1981). Their data (and reviewed literature) must provoke much radical reappraisal. The cortical areas (frontal, motor, somatosensory, parietal, visual (area 17) and temporal) were studied in the mouse, rat, cat, monkey and man; additionally area 17 received further study in tupaia, galago, marmoset, squirrel monkey, baboon and chimpanzee. Total and differential counts were made in strips $30 \mu m$ wide and $25 \mu m$ thick cut perpendicular to the pial surface and passing to the subcortical white matter. The outstanding findings were that the total neuronal populations of standard strips (and therefore perpendicularly beneath a unit area of pial surface), with the exception of primate area 17, are so close as to be regarded as virtually identical, whether from different regions in the same brain, the same species or from those as remote as mouse and man. Additionally, in all cases, about two-thirds of the neurons are pyramidal, the remainder non-pyramidal (varieties of stellate neurons, Winfield et al 1980). Interestingly, the parts of area 17 concerned with primate binocular vision have a neuronal population that is about 2.5 times greater than other areas. Later studies (Powell & Hendrickson 1981) showed that both monocular and binocular parts of area 17 in the macaque monkey have the same high density of neurons, whereas area 18 and other visual areas are like all remaining regions of the neocortex. The numerical neuronal homogeneity (both absolute and the ratio of two principal varieties) of almost all the neocortex in a wide range of mammals, in standardized full-thickness strips or columns, despite marked variations in cortical thickness and subjectively described laminar patterns, must profoundly affect the interpretation of the classically described variations in structure ascribed to different regions (see below). It also stimulates speculation concerning the phylogeny, ontogeny, structural definition and integrative operation of fundamental cortical units; the establishment of absolute criteria for their universal definition presents many difficulties.

A more recent study in the rat (Beaulieu 1993) has questioned the uniformity of neuronal numbers in a given cortical area, suggesting that the increased numbers seen in primate primary visual cortex is paralleled by an increase in numbers in parietal (somatosensory barrel field) cortex in the rat. The suggestion was made that this increase might reflect specialization in the sensory area preferentially used by each species. Despite this modification, the observation of a general uniformity of neuronal numbers remains of fundamental importance for understanding neocortical architecture. The constancy of proportions of pyramidal versus non-pyramidal cells (Sloper et al 1979; Winfield et al 1980) has been confirmed (Braak & Braak 1986; Schuz & Palm 1989) and extended to include a constancy in number of inhibitory GABA-ergic interneurons in different areas (Beaulieu 1993; Jones et al 1987, Hendry et al 1987).

Given this uniformity in overall cell number and in the proportions of different cell classes which make up that number, it is important to consider the changes which give rise to what can be striking differences in the histological appearance of different cortical areas. It is axiomatic that the size of a neuronal cell soma is dependent on the total volume of that cell's processes, axon and dendrites. In cortical neurons projecting to distant targets, the vast majority of the extrasomatic volume is contributed by the axon. A large calibre axon originating in the neocortex and terminating in the sacral spinal cord would, for example, arise from a very large pyramidal cell. The corresponding axonal volumes and soma sizes of neurons whose axons ramify entirely within a single cortical area, i.e. the vast majority of non-pyramidal cells in the cortex, are relatively small. It is, therefore, the population of neocortical pyramidal cells which would show the greatest variation in somatic volume according to the calibre and destination of their axons. Medium and larger sized pyramidal cells are much more readily identifiable in Nissl-stained material, whereas very small pyramidal cells are largely indistinguishable from non-pyramidal cells. The packing density of non-pyramidal cells is markedly affected by changes in the soma size of the surrounding pyramidal cell population, being densely packed where the pyramidal cells are small (granular cortex), and most dispersed where the pyramidal cells are largest (agranular cortex).

It follows from the above that changes in the cytoarchitectonic appearance of cortical areas reflect, largely, variations in the soma size of pyramidal cells within those areas, which in turn is determined by the calibre and destination of pyramidal cell axons. Thus, cytoarchitectonics reflects (principally efferent) connectivity of a cortical area. Where the histological differences are great, the differences in connectivity are also likely to be great, and so cytoarchitectonic parcellation has functional validity. Where the differences are subtle, the changes in connectivity, at least in terms of the distance travelled by efferent axons, are also likely to be subtle.

The preceding argument is undoubtedly an oversimplification. It is unlikely that neurite volume is the sole determinant of neuronal soma volume, although it may be the major one. Similarly, factors which govern the calibre or profusion of collateral branching of an axon are unknown, although these factors would be an important influence on soma size. In addition, patterns of afferent and intrinsic connectivity might reasonably be expected to influence cortical architecture quite dramatically. However, in relation to this last question, there is also some evidence of a measure of cortical uniformity. In the mouse, the synaptic density in three widely different cytoarchitectonic areas has been shown to be almost constant and the number of synapses per neuron surprisingly similar (Schuz & Palm 1989). In studies on the pattern of local axonal degeneration following microelectrode lesions in the monkey neocortex, Powell and colleagues described a qualitatively very similar appearance in the primary visual, somatic sensory and motor cortices (Fisken et al 1975; Gatter & Powell 1978; Shanks et al 1985). In an important recent study using more sophisticated anatomical methods, Lund and colleagues (Lund et al 1993) have further demonstrated a qualitatively similar pattern of intraareal, laterally spreading projections in the same and additional neocortical areas in the monkey. Intriguingly, these authors conclude that the quantitative features of the spread of these connections are determined by the lateral spread of the dendritic field of single pyramidal neurons within an area.

OVERVIEW OF CORTICAL CONNECTIVITY

It follows from the above discussion that neocortical connectivity defines cortical cytoarchitectonics, although many extrinsic cortical connections are shared by all areas. It is worth, therefore, examining the common pattern of connections of all cortical areas before either discussing the relationship of these connections to cortical cytoarchitecture, or considering the differences in connectivity between individual areas. All neocortical areas have axonal connections with other cortical areas on the same side (ipsilateral corticocortical or association connections), the opposite side (contralateral corticocortical or commissural connections), and with subcortical structures. It is convenient to consider each of these in turn.

Ipsilateral corticocortical connections

The fundamental organization of ipsilateral corticocortical (or association) connections of the neocortex of the subhuman primate was elucidated by Jones and Powell (1970). In this scheme, the primary sensory areas of the cerebral cortex, somatic sensory, visual and auditory, represent the starting point for a series of stepwise, area-to-area connections, progressing through the association areas of the parietal, occipital and temporal lobes, towards the medial temporal limbic areas, notably the parahippocampal gyrus, entorhinal cortex, and hippocampus. Thus, the first somatic sensory area (SI, see below) projects to the superior parietal cortex (Brodmann's area 5). This in turn projects to the inferior parietal cortex (BA7). From here connections pass to cortex in the walls of the superior temporal sulcus, and so on to the posterior parahippocampal gyrus, and on into limbic cortex. Similarly, for the visual system, the striate cortex (primary visual; BA17; see below) projects to the parastriate (BA18), then to peristriate (BA19), to inferotemporal (BA20), to cortex in the walls of the superior temporal sulcus, then to medial temporal cortex in the posterior parahippocampal gyrus, and so to limbic areas. The auditory system showed a similar progression from primary auditory cortex, through surrounding areas to temporal association cortex and so to the medial temporal lobe. In addition to this stepwise outward progression from sensory areas through posterior association cortex, Jones and Powell (1970) also proposed that each stage in this cascade of ongoing association connections is linked to a part of the frontal cortex. Thus, taking the somatic sensory cortical route as an example, primary somatic sensory cortex (SI) in the postcentral gyrus is reciprocally connected with the primary motor cortex (BA4) in the precentral gyrus. The next step in the outward progression, the superior parietal lobule (BA5), is interconnected with the premotor cortex (BA6). The next step, area 7 in the inferior parietal lobule, has reciprocal connections with prefrontal association cortex on the lateral surface of the hemisphere (BA 9/46), and temporal association areas connect with more anterior prefrontal association areas and, ultimately in the sequence, with orbitofrontal cortex. Similar stepwise links between areas on the visual and auditory association pathways in the occipitotemporal lobe and areas of the frontal association cortex were defined. It is also apparent that a similar cascade of projections within the frontal lobe may exist, with prefrontal association areas projecting progressively more posteriorly ultimately to premotor cortex, and so feeding into the precentral gyrus.

With the advent of more sophisticated neuroanatomical tracing techniques and further more detailed studies, this general scheme has been extended and modified, particularly in two general ways. Firstly, the connections between sensory and association areas are reciprocal, and the precise nature of termination and origin within a cortical area is different according to whether it is in the line of flow from sensory to limbic cortex (feedforward) or in the reverse direction (feedback; see below). Secondly, the singularity of outward progression of connectivity is complex. Single sensory and perisensory areas do not project to other single areas of cortex in the same or adjacent lobes; there are multiple cortical sensory pathways in parallel, perhaps subserving different criteria of perception. This has been particularly defined in the visual areas of the occipital, parietal and temporal cortex (Zeki 1993). However, the general principle of a stepwise outflow of sensory information through progressive association areas of posterior cortex, each linked with a related area of frontal cortex, remains a fundamentally important scheme of considerable anatomical and functional significance for understanding the organization of cerebral neocortex.

Contralateral corticocortical (commissural) connections

The corpus callosum is the largest fibre pathway of the brain in man and links the cerebral cortex of each hemisphere. Cortical regions not linked via the corpus callosum send and receive fibres to/from the contralateral cortex through other commissures. Contralateral connections, however, are not a simple linking of a point on one hemisphere to the same point on the other. In areas containing a clear representation of a contralateral sensorium (e.g. body surface, visual field), only those areas functionally related to midline representation are linked to the contralateral hemisphere. This is most clearly seen for the visual areas (Zeki 1993) where the cortex containing the representation of each midline retinal zone is linked to its counterpart on the contralateral side. A similar arrangement is seen in somatic areas, where the trunk representation is callosally linked, but the peripheral limb areas (hand and foot) are not (Shanks et al 1985a). The auditory and olfactory pathways show no such laterality, since in both cases, the sensory receptor of either side can detect stimuli from the full 360° of the surrounding world in relation to the body. As specific spatial representation within the somatosensory and visual cortices breaks down in relation to specific function, so does this particular connectional relationship. Where it persists, the callosal connections can be viewed as the anatomical 'glue' that joins the separate cerebral representation of the left and right halves of the sensory world.

In addition to such connections, linking the same or similar areas on each side (homotopic connections), the corpus callosum also interconnects heterogeneous cortical areas on the two sides (heterotopic connections). These may serve to connect functionally similar but anatomically different loci in the two hemispheres (Schwartz & Goldman-Rakic 1982, 1984), or to connect functional areas in one hemisphere with regions which are specialized for a unilaterally confined function in the other. Such connections could be predicted to be more extensive in man than in other animals (see below).

Subcortical connections

Certain connections with subcortical nuclei are common to all cortical areas, although the quantity of such connections may vary markedly. First among these are connections with the thalamus. All areas of the neocortex receive afferents from more than one thalamic nucleus, and all such connections are reciprocal; that is, each cortical area projects back to the thalamic nuclei from which it receives an input. Historically, such thalamocortical connections were regarded as originating from specific and non-specific nuclei. In relation to the classification of thalamic nuclei, this terminology has been discussed previously (see p. 1882). It is now probably more acceptable to suggest that thalamocortical afferents be classified according to their mode of termination in the cortex and that many, if not all thalamic nuclei give rise to more than one such thalamocortical pathway. All cortical areas receive more than one such set of connections. The types of thalamocortical termination are illustrated in **8.238**. The relative contribution of each pattern of termination of thalamocortical fibres to the input into any area is highly variable.

In addition to the thalamus, all cortical areas are reciprocally connected with the claustrum (Pearson et al 1982; Sherk 1986). Broadly speaking, there is a topographic relationship between the cortex and the claustrum, with anterior parts of the nucleus connecting with the frontal cortex, posterior parts with the occipital lobe and so on. The more detailed point-to-point relationship in this pathway, however, is more complex (Pearson et al 1982; see below). The density of claustrocortical connections is variable between different cortical areas, but it is probably not the case that any area, such as the primary auditory cortex, lacks such connections entirely (Neal et al 1986a).

As well as reciprocal connections between the cortex, thalamus and claustrum, all cortical areas project to the striatum (caudate/putamen) and to the pons (and so on to the cerebellum). Once again, the relative contributions of different cortical areas to these corticostriate and corticopontine pathways varies greatly, but the vast majority, if not all, cortical areas contribute fibres. As with the claustrum, these projections are topographically organized, but at a complex level (Selemon & Goldman-Rakic 1985; Brodal 1978). Similarly, perhaps most or even all neocortical areas send fibres to the tectum. Certainly, virtually all cortical areas project to the reticular formation of the brainstem (p. 1073).

Of particular pharmacological interest are a group of afferents to the neocortex from subcortical nuclei which contain specific neurotransmitters within their axons. These include a topographically organized cholinergic projection from the basal forebrain to all cortical areas (Pearson et al 1983a,b,c; Mesulam et al 1983), which represents a major source of acetylcholine within the cortex (Struble et al 1986), and which is profoundly affected by the neurodegenerative processes of Alzheimer's disease (see Pearson & Powell 1989 for review). Similarly, noradrenergic fibres pass to all cortical areas from the locus coeruleus of the hindbrain (Gatter and Powell 1977; Morrison et al 1984), as do serotoninergic fibres from the midbrain raphe nuclei (Morrison et al 1984), and histaminergic fibres from the posterior hypothalamus (Onodera et al 1994). Although concentrated in the frontal and limbic cortical areas, dopaminergic

fibres to the cortex from the ventral midbrain probably reach more widespread areas of cortex than previously thought (Richfield et al 1989). The particular interest of these generalized and rather diffusely organized projections to the cortex lies in their relationship to the pharmacology, or at least the pharmacotherapy, of a broad spectrum of neuropsychiatric diseases, ranging from Alzheimer's disease, through depression to schizophrenia.

Of course, different cortical areas have widely different afferent and efferent connections, and some areas have connections, however small, which are unique. Perhaps most obvious is the corticospinal motor projection (the corticospinal tract) from pyramidal cells in a restricted area around the central sulcus (see below). More generally, the quantitative contribution to cortical connections of different pathways and the topographical restriction of their origins and terminations in individual cortical areas or in subcortical nuclei profoundly alter the functional connectivity of different areas. Nonetheless, there is considerable underlying similarity in the global pattern of extrinsic connections of many cortical areas. It is perhaps salutary that the most studied areas, the sensory and the motor cortex, are also the most untypical in architecture, representing extremes of both cortical cytoarchitectonic types, (granular (sensory) and agranular (motor)) and overall patterns of connectivity.

Cortical lamination and cortical connections

It is clear from the above discussion that changes in cortical cytoarchitectonics (that is, variations in laminar appearance) reflect quantitative and qualitative differences in connectivity. The cortical laminae therefore represent, to some extent, horizontal aggregations of neurons with common connections. This is most clearly seen in the lamination of cortical efferent (pyramidal) cells (Jones 1984). The internal pyramidal lamina, layer V, gives rise to corticosubcortical fibres, notably corticostriate, corticobulbar, corticopontine, and corticospinal axons. In addition, a significant proportion of feedback corticocortical axons arise from cells in this layer, as do some corticothalamic fibres. Layer VI, the multiform lamina, is the major source of corticothalamic fibres. Supragranular pyramidal cells, predominantly layer III, but also lamina II, give rise primarily to both ipsilateral (association) and contralateral (commissural) corticocortical pathways. Short corticocortical fibres arise more superficially, and long corticocortical (both association and commissural) axons come from cells in the deeper parts of layer III. Major afferents to a cortical area tend to terminate in layers I, IV and VI, with quantitatively lesser projections ending in the intervening laminae II/III and V, or sparsely throughout the depth of the cortex (Pandya & Yeterian 1985). Within this overall framework, specific points merit mention. Numerically, the major single input to a cortical area tends to have its main termination field in layer IV, with interrupted tufts or flares of heavy termination extending into the overlying deep parts of layer III. Such a pattern of termination is seen in the major thalamic input to visual and somatic sensory cortex (see below). In so-called 'association' areas such as those of the parietal lobe, this pattern is seen in feedforward association connections (Pearson & Powell 1985). Feedback corticocortical fibres terminate almost exclusively in lamina I (Pandya & Yeterian 1985; Rockland 1994), and this has important functional implications which require further elucidation (Cauller & Connors 1994). In general, non-thalamic subcortical afferents to the neocortex, which are shared by widespread areas, tend to terminate throughout all cortical layers, but the laminar pattern of their endings still varies considerably from area to area (Mesulam et al 1984; Morrison et al 1984). The preceding statements on laminar segregation of cortical connections are not absolute, but represent the predominant laminae of origin or termination of connections. For example, 'feedforward' corticocortical association fibres come from some pyramidal cells in layer V (Hiorns et al 1991) and layer III pyramidal neurons give rise to a few corticostriate fibres (Yeterian & Pandya 1994), even though a much greater proportion of such fibres arise from cells in layers III (association) and V (corticostriate) respectively.

There is some evidence that widely separated but functionally interconnected areas share common patterns of connections with subcortical nuclei, and within the neocortex. In particular, this relates to areas of prefrontal association cortex and the areas in the (postRolandic) parietal, occipital and temporal lobes with which they are interconnected. Thus, contiguous zones of the striatum

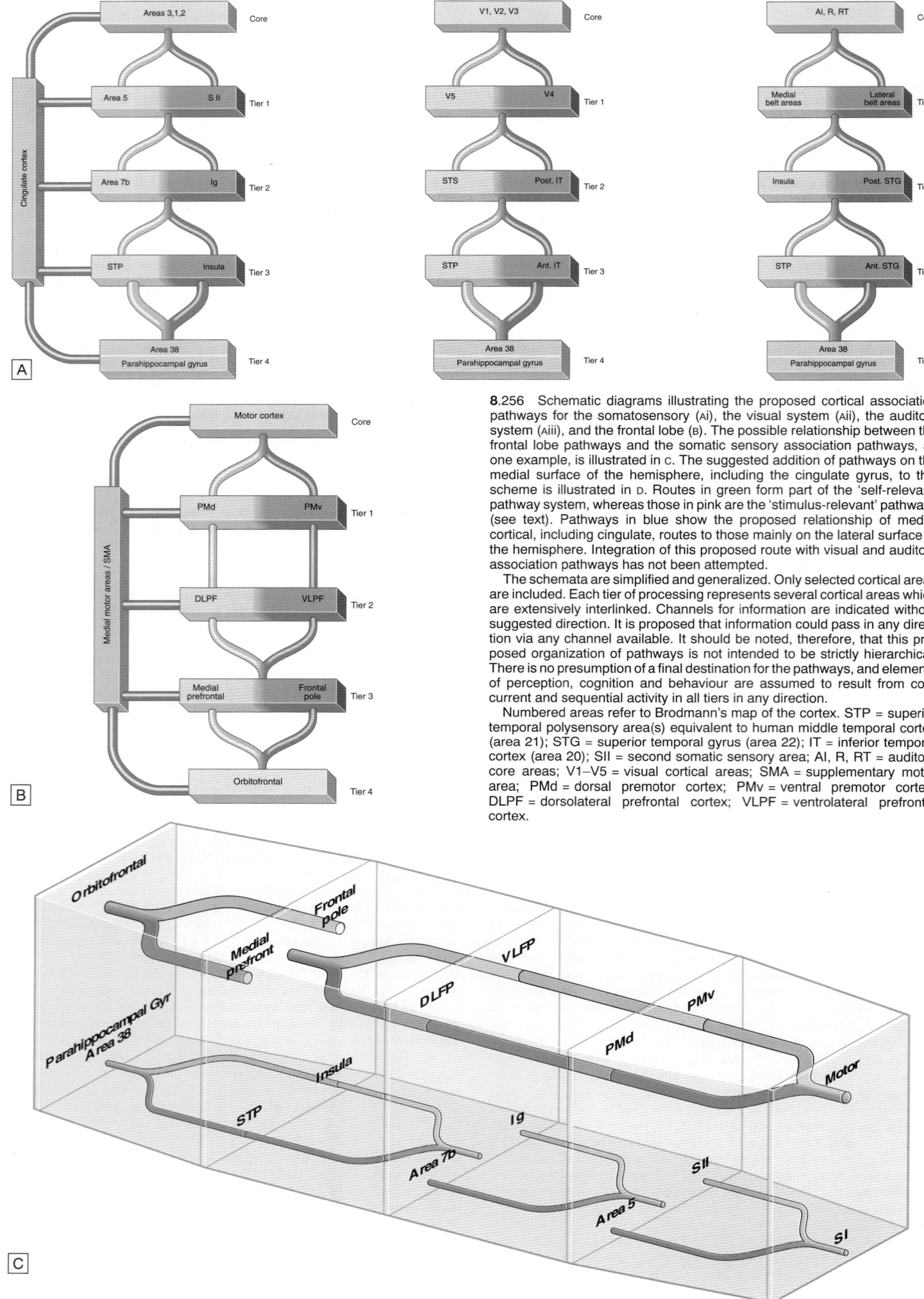

8.256 Schematic diagrams illustrating the proposed cortical association pathways for the somatosensory (Ai), the visual system (Aii), the auditory system (Aiii), and the frontal lobe (B). The possible relationship between the frontal lobe pathways and the somatic sensory association pathways, as one example, is illustrated in C. The suggested addition of pathways on the medial surface of the hemisphere, including the cingulate gyrus, to this scheme is illustrated in D. Routes in green form part of the 'self-relevant' pathway system, whereas those in pink are the 'stimulus-relevant' pathways (see text). Pathways in blue show the proposed relationship of medial cortical, including cingulate, routes to those mainly on the lateral surface of the hemisphere. Integration of this proposed route with visual and auditory association pathways has not been attempted.

The schemata are simplified and generalized. Only selected cortical areas are included. Each tier of processing represents several cortical areas which are extensively interlinked. Channels for information are indicated without suggested direction. It is proposed that information could pass in any direction via any channel available. It should be noted, therefore, that this proposed organization of pathways is not intended to be strictly hierarchical. There is no presumption of a final destination for the pathways, and elements of perception, cognition and behaviour are assumed to result from concurrent and sequential activity in all tiers in any direction.

Numbered areas refer to Brodmann's map of the cortex. STP = superior temporal polysensory area(s) equivalent to human middle temporal cortex (area 21); STG = superior temporal gyrus (area 22); IT = inferior temporal cortex (area 20); SII = second somatic sensory area; AI, R, RT = auditory core areas; V1–V5 = visual cortical areas; SMA = supplementary motor area; PMd = dorsal premotor cortex; PMv = ventral premotor cortex; DLPF = dorsolateral prefrontal cortex; VLPF = ventrolateral prefrontal cortex.

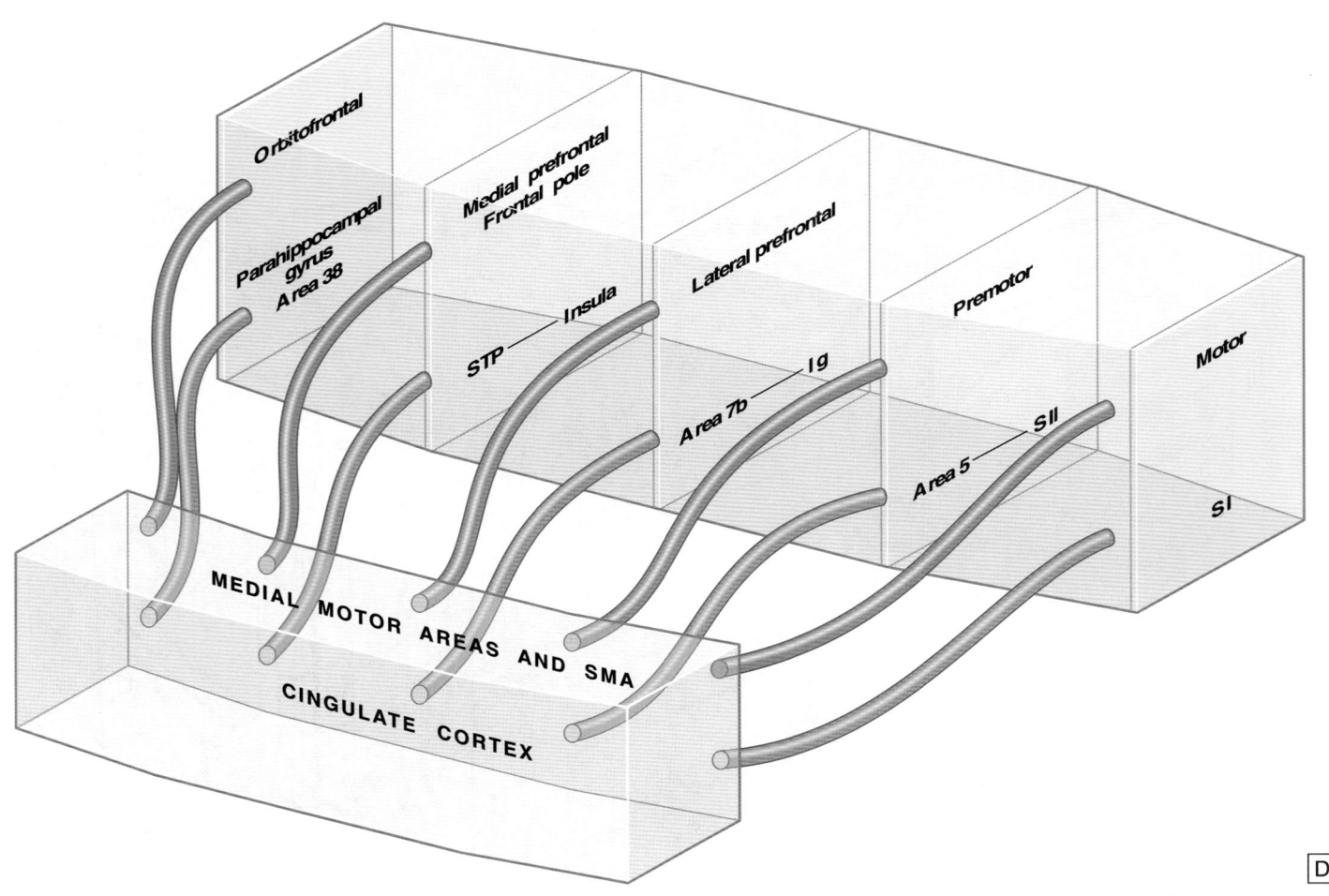

D

(Selemon & Goldman-Rakic 1985; Goldman-Rakic & Selemon 1986), thalamus (Selemon & Goldman-Rakic 1988), claustrum (Pearson et al 1982; Sherk 1986), cholinergic basal forebrain (Pearson et al 1983), superior colliculus and pontine nuclei (Selemon & Goldman-Rakic 1988) connect with geographically widely separated areas in the prefrontal and parietal cortex which are themselves interconnected (Selemon & Goldman-Rakic 1988). In contrast, other cortical regions which are functionally distinct, for example areas in the temporal and parietal cortex, do not share such marked contiguity in their subcortical connections, but appear well segregated (Baizer et al 1993). It should be emphasized that the concern here is not with convergent projections from heterogeneous cortical areas onto single neurons, or divergent projections from single neurons to multiple, widely separated target areas, but with the regional organization of connections to contiguous or closely adjacent parts of individual nuclei. Whether this represents overlapping connectivity, or complex separated interdigitation (Goldman-Rakic & Selemon 1986), though important, is a secondary issue. More importantly, this general pattern of shared connectivity of physically separated but functionally related cortical areas in the prefrontal and post-Rolandic cortex gives rise to the concept of distributed neural networks which serve specific cognitive and behavioural functions (Selemon & Goldman-Rakic 1988; Goldman-Rakic 1988).

CONCEPTS OF CORTICAL ARCHITECTURE — COLUMNS AND MODULES

Histologically, the overwhelming dimension of cortical organization has been conceived as mainly an array of elements parallel to the pial surface (horizontal) constrained within laminae as discussed above. However, physiological and connectional studies in recent decades have emphasized an organization at right angles to the pial surface (vertical) into columns or modules running through the depth of the cortex. Functional columns were first described in the somatosensory cortex (Mountcastle 1957; Mountcastle & Powell 1959; Powell & Mountcastle 1959). The term column refers to the observation that all cells encountered by a microelectrode penetrating and passing perpendicularly through the cortex respond to a single peripheral stimulus. The concept of columnar physiological organization was extended in the visual cortex by Hubel and Wiesel (1977), who described narrow (50 μm) vertical strips of neurons responding to a bar stimulus of the same orientation (orientation columns), and wider strips (500 μm) responding preferentially to stimuli detected by one eye (ocular dominance columns). Adjacent orientation columns were further conceived as aggregating within an ocular dominance column to form a hypercolumn, responding to all orientations of stimulus for both eyes for one point in the visual field (Hubel & Wiesel 1977). Despite modifications to incorporate later data (Livingstone & Hubel 1984; Zeki 1993), the concept of functional columns in the sensory cortex is widely accepted, and a similar functional columnar organization has been described in widespread areas of neocortex, including motor cortex and so-called association areas.

The neurophysiological description of the columnar organization of the cerebral cortex led to a search for an anatomical basis for this functional arrangement. Once again studies of the visual cortex led the way, with the demonstration of discrete patches of geniculocortical axons related to one eye alternating in layer IV in a regular way with patches related to the other eye (Hubel & Wiesel 1977) underlying the functional organization manifested as ocular dominance columns. Considerable further work on connectivity and chemoarchitecture (notably the occurrence of cytochrome oxidase

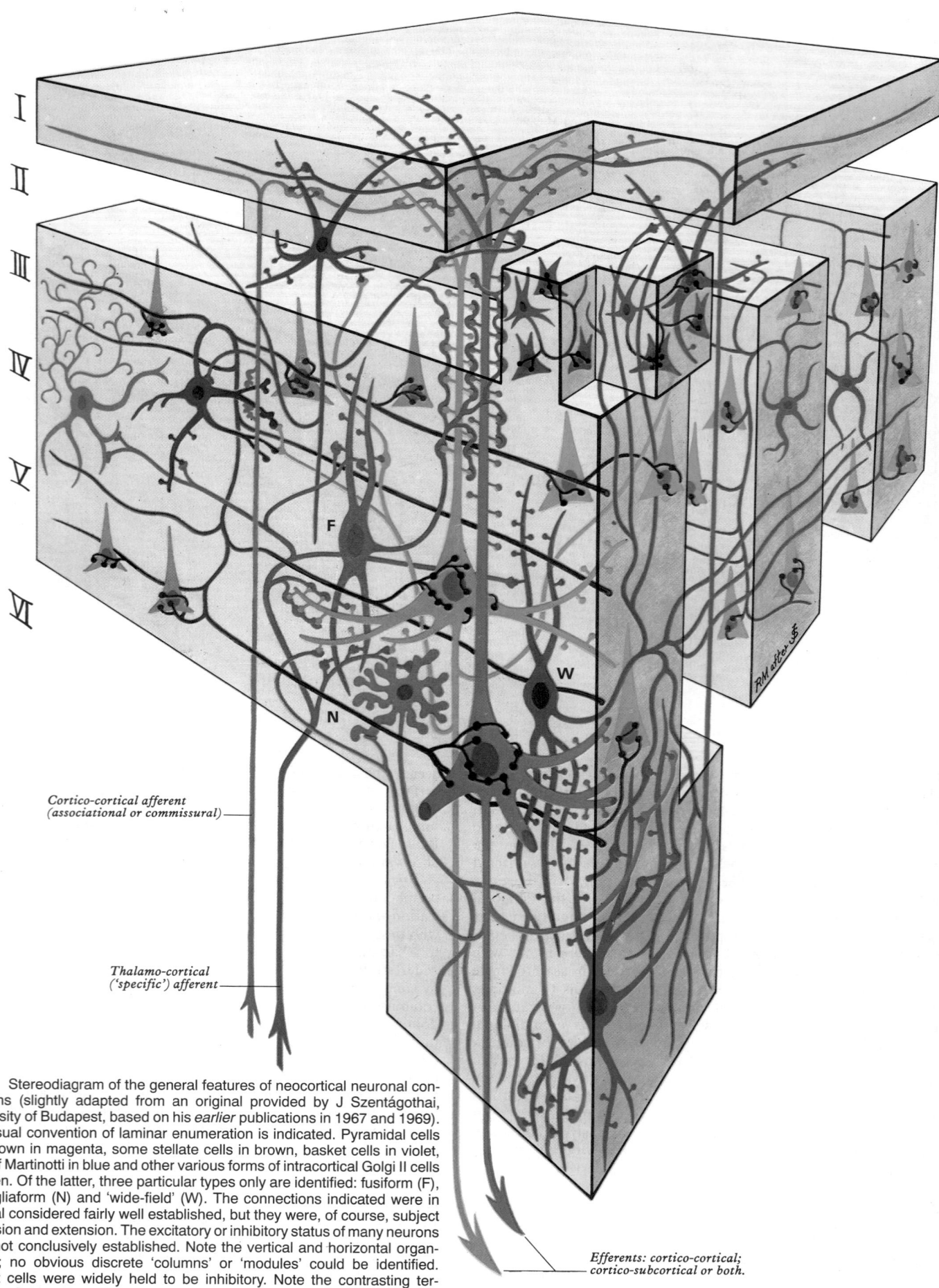

8.257 Stereodiagram of the general features of neocortical neuronal connections (slightly adapted from an original provided by J Szentágothai, University of Budapest, based on his *earlier* publications in 1967 and 1969). The usual convention of laminar enumeration is indicated. Pyramidal cells are shown in magenta, some stellate cells in brown, basket cells in violet, cells of Martinotti in blue and other various forms of intracortical Golgi II cells in green. Of the latter, three particular types only are identified: fusiform (F), neurogliaform (N) and 'wide-field' (W). The connections indicated were in general considered fairly well established, but they were, of course, subject to revision and extension. The excitatory or inhibitory status of many neurons were not conclusively established. Note the vertical and horizontal organization; no obvious discrete 'columns' or 'modules' could be identified. Basket cells were widely held to be inhibitory. Note the contrasting termination fields of 'specific' and cortico-corticol afferents; also of intracortical recurrent collaterals of pyramidal neuron axons.

Cortico-cortical afferent (associational or commissural)

Thalamo-cortical ('specific') afferent

Efferents: cortico-cortical; cortico-subcortical or both.

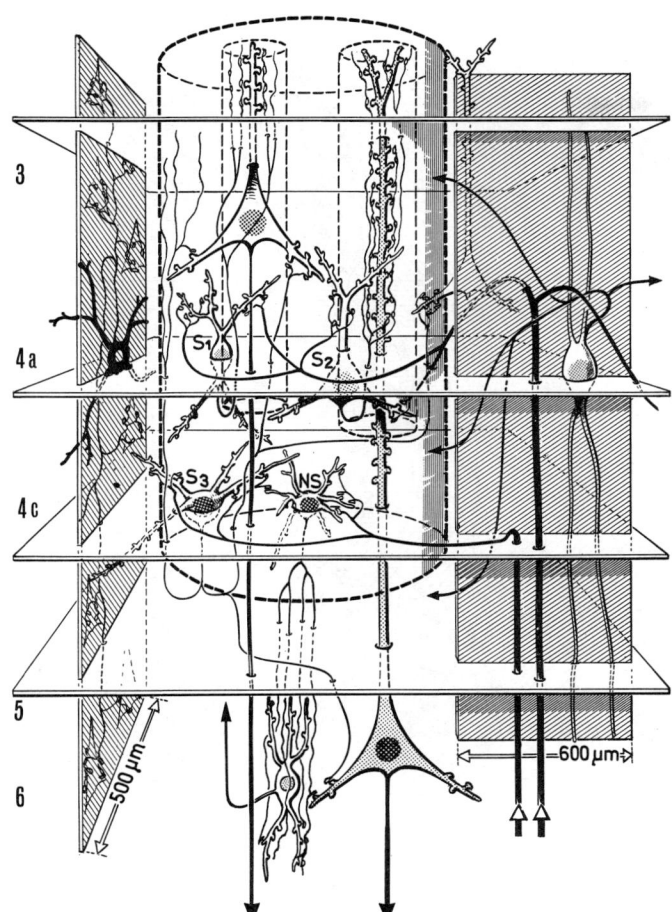

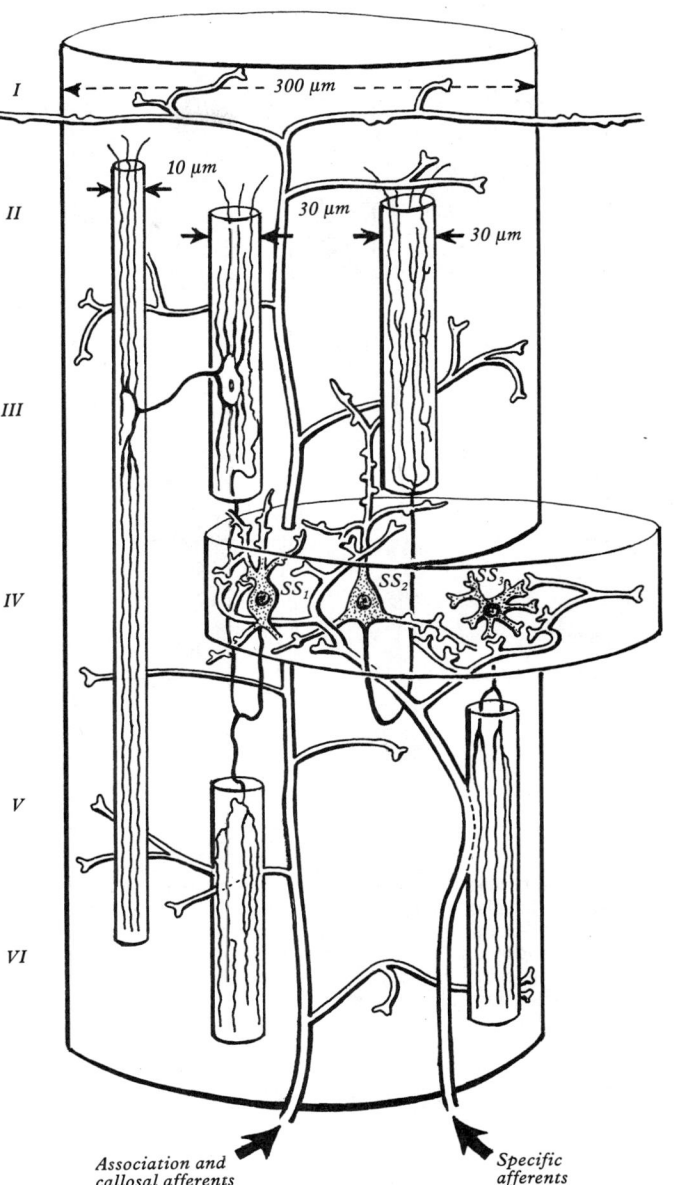

8.258A A steroscopic view of the elementary neuron circuit in sensory cortical areas. The horizontal planes are entirely arbitrary and are included to aid stereoscopic visualization; they are unrelated to the cortical lamination (arabic numerals on the left, indicating the 'non-absolute' character of the lamination in such a diagram). Specific sensory afferents (heavy black vertical lines on the right) terminate (separately) on the spiny stellate neurons (S1) and the so-called star pyramids (S2) of upper lamina IV and in lower lamina IV on another type of spiny stellate neuron (S3) as well as on neurogliaform non-spiny stellate neurons (NS). Ascending relay of sensory afferent impulses is twofold: (1) within *narrow* cylindrical spaces (indicated with dashed outlines) by horsetail-shaped axon arborizations of S1 and S2 type neurons and primarily to selected individual (or small groups of) pyramid cell and (2) within *wider* cylindrical spaces (heavier dashed outline) from ascending S2 type neurons, probably mainly to basal dendrites of a much larger group of pyramidal cells. Descending relay is more widely and more indiscriminately distributed by descending branches of the spiny stellate neurons and star pyramidal neurons and occurs in narrow columns by the vertically orientated axonal lacework of neurogliaform non-spiny stellate neurons (NS). The vertical plane on the left shows the strictly orientated axonal arborization of a large basket cell: the vertical plane on the right, orientated at right angles to the basket cell plane, shows a large stellate neuron with vertically orientated dendrites and part of its extended axonal arborization which is strictly confined to this plane. (From Szentágothai 1975 with permission.)

8.258B Some features of a cortico-cortico module redrawn from a stereodiagram (provided by Szentágothai 1978). All neurons and contacts shown are presumed to be excitatory. Pyramidal neurons, their axonal efferents and inhibitory interneurons are not included for clarity. The module consists of a tall cylinder 300 μm in diameter extending through the full thickness of the cortex; ascending centrally, with lateral and terminal branches is one representative of a cortico-cortical afferent (either association or callosal). The 'flat cylinder' also about 300 μm in diameter is the 'termination space' of a specific thalamocortical afferent; overlap of the latter and the module varies greatly from minimal, through the condition illustrated, to virtual coincidence. Synaptic contacts through one or more excitatory interneurons transforms the flat (almost tangential) termination space of the specific afferent into narrow (10–30 μm), *radial* cylindrical spaces or submodules. Stellate interneurons SS2 has a recurrent axon, its arborization ascending to lamina II; the microglioform neuron (right) has a descending arborization; SS1 has both a descending and an ascending arborization, the latter synapsing with a *cellule fusiforme à double bouquet dendritique*, the axon of which again bifurcates forming a long vertical slender (10 μm) arborization and which possibly encloses, and is excitatory to, a single pyramidal neuron. It should be noted, however, that a significant proportion of neurons with all these cytomorphologies have been demonstrated as having inhibitory counterparts (see **8.259**).

patches) in visual cortex has elucidated much of the anatomical framework underlying the functional organization seen physiologically (see Zeki 1993 for review, and see below). Similar studies in many cortical areas permit the generalization that most cortical afferents end in discrete patches or bands, alternating with patches of afferents from other sources, and that the majority of cortical efferents arise from clusters of cells, alternating with clusters projecting to other destinations. In most cases, the dimensions of these afferent or efferent bands or patches in the monkey neocortex are of the order of 400 to 600 μm in width. These and other observations, notably on the distribution and organization of intrinsic cortical axons, led several investigators to construct detailed models of the

anatomical and functional organization or the neocortex into modules (Szentágothai 1969, 1975, 1978; Jones 1981; Eccles 1984; **8.**257, 258, 259). In general terms, the central ideal of such models is that a discrete block of cortex encompassing all layers, and probably

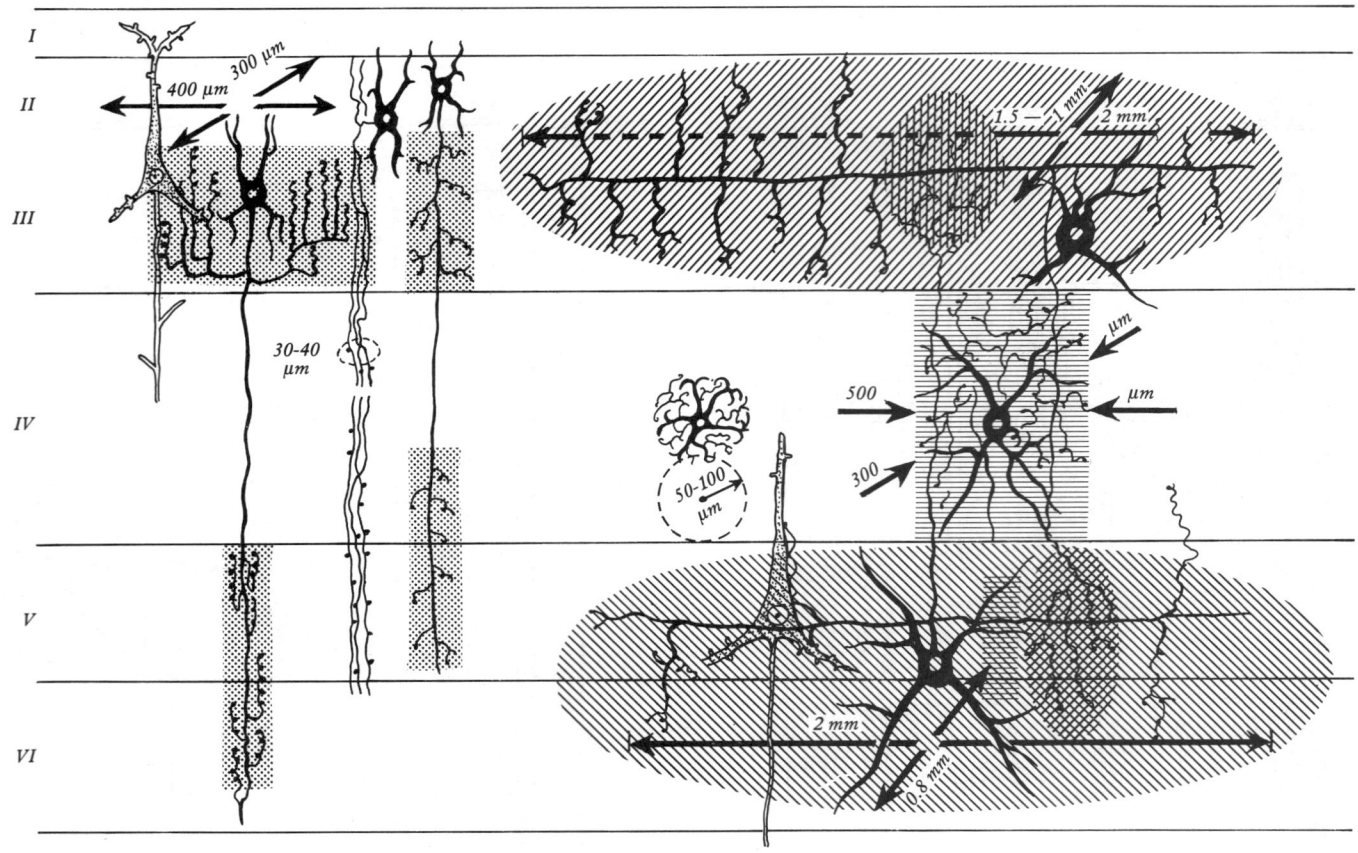

8.259 Diagrammatic illustration of the seven types of well characterized (GABA-ergic) inhibitory interneurons. In order to facilitate recognition of dendrites and axons, the dendritic trees are simplified and drawn with exaggerated thickness. Fields of axonal arborization (where necessary) are indicated by hatching and stippling. Horizontal arrows indicate maximal (observed) extension of the axonal arborizations in the sagittal and oblique arrows in the coronal directions; the extension of the axons in depth can be derived from the cortical layering indicated at left margin. (1) Large basket cell of the upper (supragranular) group (Somogyi et al 1983) (2) large basket cell of the infragranular group (3) 'clutch cell' terminating mainly in lamina IV (Kisvárday et al 1985) (4) columnar basket cell (Szentágothai 1938) (5) microglioform cell (both dendritic and axonal arborization most generally spherical) (6) 'cellule a double bouquet' of Ramón y Cajal (7) axo-axonic interneuron (Szentágothai 1978). There are more local interneuron types known that are probably also GABA-ergic, but they were not included, because their axonal arborizations have not yet been sufficiently well characterized. The spatial relations between cell types 1–3 have been adapted from a diagram of Somogyi & Soltész (1986). (After Szentágothai 1987 with permission.)

under something of the order of 0.5×0.5 mm of pial surface area receives a discrete set of afferents, performs its physiological operations in relation to that afferent information in a standard way, and distributes efferents to all appropriate destinations via association, commissural and corticosubcortical pathways. In such a scheme, the function of any cortical module is dependent on the source of its afferent input; its operation is uniform. The operational capacity of the neocortex is then increased by adding more such modules, so that a large cortical surface area, such as that of man, does more than the small cortical surface area of lower animals. The actual operation of a module is hypothesized to be constant in all mammalian species.

Such theories accord well with much of the physiological data on cortical organization and with the concept of cortical uniformity (see above). They have also stimulated much important and detailed work on cortical structure and connectivity. However, it must be emphasized that there is no clearly defined anatomical basis for such cortical modularity. Structurally, the cortex in any given area is a continuum. It is not possible to define sharp boundaries where one module ends and another begins; neurons do not abruptly change the orientation of their dendrites, for example, to confine themselves to a single modular unit. For example, pyramidal cells in layers III and V of the monkey parietal cortex projecting to a common target, although clustered in both laminae, are not in strict vertical register with one another (Hiorns et al 1993), as predicted by input–output modular theory. Moreover, columnar physiological organization is subserved by a mosaic of cortical connections more complex than permitted by a circumscribed modular arrangement.

THE MAIN CORTICAL AREAS

In considering the parcellation of the neocortex into major functional areas, a lobar sequence will be followed, beginning with parietal, then occipital, temporal and finally frontal lobes. This will allow, as near as is possible, the description of connectivity to follow the pattern proposed by Jones and Powell (1970), beginning with the primary sensory areas (somatosensory with the parietal lobe; visual with the occipital lobe; auditory with the temporal lobe) and following their outflow into post-Rolandic association cortex, with more distant parts of these pathways passing to areas of the temporal lobe, and ultimately to limbic structures in the medial temporal lobe. After this, the linked areas in the frontal lobe will be considered. Throughout the description, the area parcellation of Brodmann will be used, as far as is possible, as a reference grid (**8.254**). Discussion will centre on ipsilateral corticocortical (association) connections passing in the feedforward direction, that is out from the primary sensory areas towards the temporal pole; reciprocal feedback connections are taken as read. Commissural connections will only be discussed where specific differences from a pattern of connection to the homotopic area of the other side are known. Similarly, connections with subcortical nuclei which are considered elsewhere, will only be discussed in detail where they are known to be important for understanding the specific organization and function of an area or pathway.

Parietal lobe

The cortex of the posterior wall of the central sulcus and of the surface of the postcentral gyrus forms the primary somatosensory cortex (SI). Cytoarchitectonically within this lie Brodmann's areas 3a, 3b, 1 and 2. Area 3a lies most anteriorly, adjoining area 4 (the motor cortex); area 3b is buried in the posterior wall of the central sulcus, and is of the granular type of cortex (see above). Areas 1 and 2 are more homotypic in cytoarchitectonic appearance, with quite prominent pyramidal cells in layers III and V; area 1 lies essentially along the posterior lip of the central sulcus, and area 2 occupies the crown of the postcentral gyrus. The term primary somatosensory cortex is derived historically, being the first cortical area from which evoked potentials were recorded after physiological stimulation of the periphery. The term primary does not, or should not, impute peculiar or pre-eminent functional significance to the postcentral gyrus in terms of its role in somatic sensation.

The primary somatosensory cortex contains within it a topographical map of the contralateral body, with the most sacral segments medially, in the paracentral lobule, the trunk and upper limb represented on the lateral surface with the face, tongue and lips most laterally. This localization, first observed by recording evoked potentials with surface electrodes, gave rise to the traditional 'homunculus' map of sensory representation in SI (**8.260, 261**). The microelectrode single-unit recording studies of Mountcastle (1957); Mountcastle and Powell (1959) and Powell and Mountcastle (1959) identified a submodality segregation of cortical columns, with single vertical columns of neurons through the depth of the cortex responding to either cutaneous or deep stimuli (but not both) of the same place on the body. Superficial (cutaneous) units were found more anteriorly, and deep columns more posteriorly. The mosaic of cortical columns, each receiving input from one class of receptors in a particular body region, implied the existence in SI of rostrocaudal dermatomal strips, forming a lateral to medial sequence representing all spinal segments. Such an arrangement was clearly incompatible in detail with an 'homunculus' type of representation. Further electrophysiological studies led to an elaboration of a complex topographical hypothesis of sensory representation in SI (Werner & Whitsel 1968) related to a shifting but overlapping rostrocaudal dermatomal map. This was later proposed to be continuous and to follow the dermatomal sequence (Dreyer et al 1975). More recent work has modified this considerably, and the precise mode of body representation in SI will be discussed below in relation to more detailed anatomical studies of the connectivity of SI.

The somatosensory response properties of SI depend firstly on its

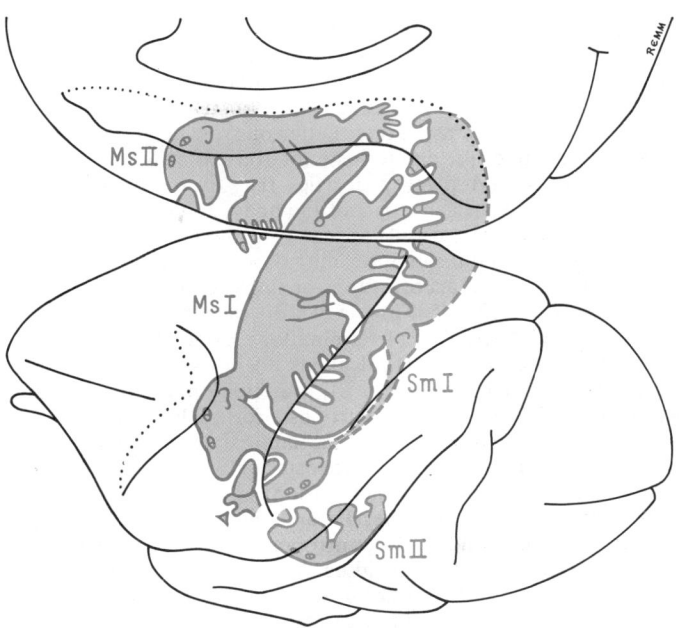

8.260 The main sensorimotor areas projected diagrammatically upon the superolateral surface of the simian cerebral hemisphere. Note the somatotopic arrangement in all four areas. (Adapted from Woolsey 1964.)

thalamic input from the ventroposterior nucleus of the thalamus, which in turn receives the medial lemniscal, spinothalamic and trigeminothalamic pathways. Within the ventroposterior nucleus, neurons in the central core respond to cutaneous stimuli and those in the most dorsal anterior and posterior parts, arching as a 'shell' over this central core, respond to deep stimuli. This is reflected in the differential projections to SI with the cutaneous central core projecting to 3b, the deep tissue-responsive neurons sending fibres to areas 3a and 2, and an interviewing zone projecting to area 1 (Jones 1986). This corresponds well with the response properties of SI neurons described by Mountcastle and Powell (1959); Powell and

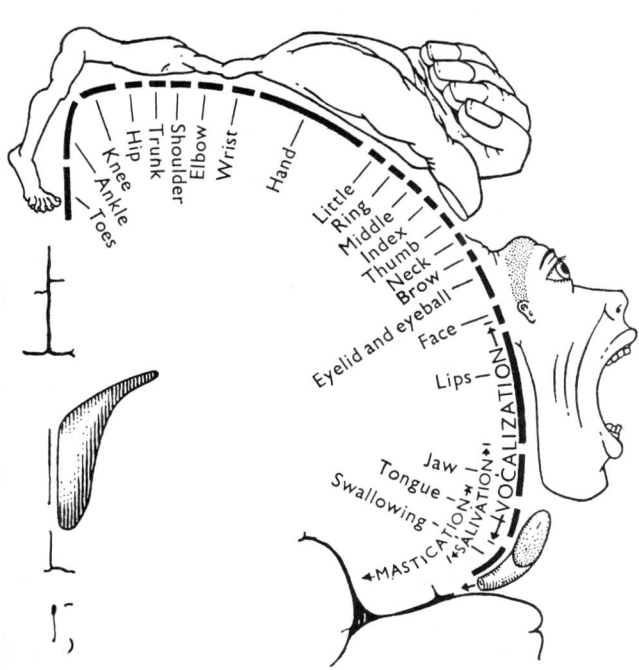

8.261A The *motor homunculus* showing proportional somatotopical representation in the main motor area. (After Penfield & Rasmussen 1950.)

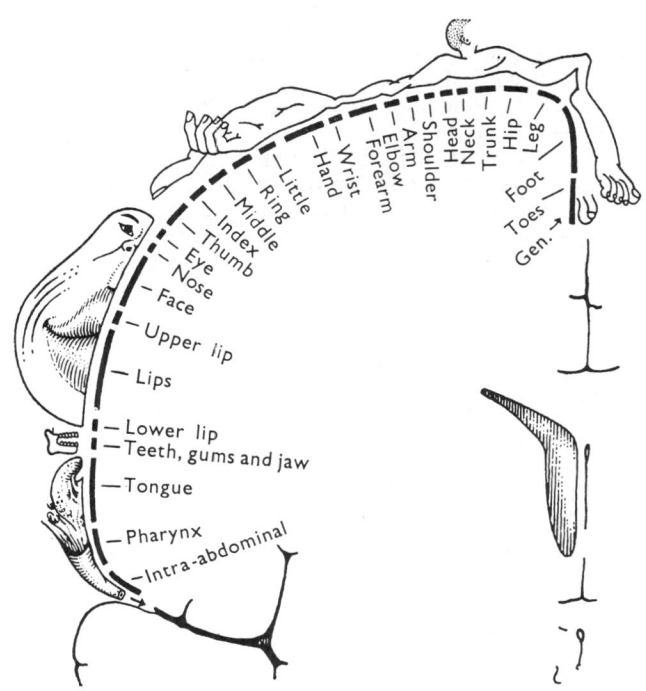

8.261B The *sensory homunculus* showing proportional somatotopical representation in the somaesthetic cortex. (After Penfield & Rasmussen 1950.)

Mountcastle (1959), with vertical columns of neurons in area 3b responding to cutaneous stimuli arising from a common location, and those in area 2 responding predominantly to deep stimuli; columns in area 1 were found to be either superficial or deep responsive (not both), giving a mixed population of submodality specific cortical columns, either cutaneous or deep. Within the ventroposterior nucleus, anteroposterior rods of cells respond with similar modality and place properties (i.e. to the same type of stimulus applied to the same part of the body; Jones 1985, 1986 and see above). These rods of cells appear to project to restricted focal patches in SI of about 0.5 mm, forming narrow strips mediolaterally along SI. Indeed, focal arborizations of single axons appear to form three or more foci 350–500 μm in width, each separated by 250–350 μm gaps relatively free of terminations (Jones 1986). It is also clear that single thalamocortical axons do not branch to different cytoarchitectonic subdivisions of SI, preserving place and modality specific channels through the ventroposterior nucleus to the cortex. It is also important to note that the laminar termination of thalamocortical axons from the ventroposterior nucleus is different in the separate cytoarchitectonic subdivisions of SI. In 3a and 3b these axons terminate mainly in layer IV and the adjacent deep part of layer III; in areas 1 and 2, the ventroposterior afferents end in the deeper half of layer III, avoiding lamina IV. Additional thalamocortical fibres to SI arise from the intralaminar system, notably the centrolateral nucleus, and possibly from the oral pulvinar nucleus, at least to area 2.

Interareal corticocortical fibres within SI of one side are specific, highly organized and reinforce the validity of the subdivision of SI into different cytoarchitectonic areas (Shanks et al 1985b; Jones 1986). Throughout these connections, topographical representation is maintained, with the part of one area containing representation of a body region connecting only with parts of other subdivisions of SI containing the same representation. Area 3b projects to areas 3a, 1 and 2, and these projections are of the feedforward type, terminating densely in layer IV and the adjacent deep part of layer III. Area 1 projects to areas 3a and 2, again with a feedforward distribution of termination, and also to 3b; in the latter case, the mode of termination is of the feedback type, ending mainly in lamina I. Area 2 sends feedforward connections only to area 3a within SI, and feedback connections to areas 1 and 3b. It is worth noting in this context that area 3b receives no ipsilateral corticocortical fibres terminating in the pattern of feedforward connections, and the thalamocortical fibres in this subdivision terminate densely in layer IV. Areas 1 and 2 receive feedforward connections from 3b, and 3b and 1 respectively, which terminate in lamina IV, and the thalamic afferents to these latter areas are less dense and specifically avoid layer IV, ending in the middle of lamina III. This is an example of the reciprocity in connections of cortical areas discussed earlier, with the quantitatively greatest input centring on layer IV (see above: 'Cortical lamination and cortical connections').

This complexity in the organization of interareal connections within SI, with an apparently stepwise, hierarchical progression from area 3b through area 1 to area 2, overlying a parallel, non-hierarchical distribution of thalamocortical afferents between areas, is in line with more recent physiological findings in SI. These relate to five sets of observations:

(1) The recognition of two categories of sensory neuron, slowly adapting and rapidly adapting, segregated within different columns or modules in primate SI (Sur et al 1984).

(2) The proposal from multiunit recording studies that SI contains several maps of the contralateral body, perhaps even one in each cytoarchitectonic area (Paul et al 1972; Merzenich et al 1978; Kaas et al 1979; Nelson et al 1980).

(3) Studies on injury-induced changes in somatotopic maps in SI, showing a dramatic amount of resulting reorganization of representation (Dykes & Ruest 1986; Garraghty & Kaas 1992; Wall et al 1992a,b; Garraghty et al 1994).

(4) The observation of use-dependent changes in response properties of cells with, for example, training, movement, or selective attention (Garraghty & Kaas 1992; Lin et al 1994a,b; Cohen et al 1994; Prud'homme et al 1994).

(5) The findings, particularly of Iwamura and colleagues (1993), of increasing complexity of response properties, including convergence of cutaneous and deep responses (see Jones 1986 for review) along a rostrocaudal (anteroposterior) gradient in SI.

The difficulties in reconciling the variety of physiological and anatomical findings into a single cohesive account of the functional organization of SI has been discussed in a stimulating article by Dykes and Ruest (1986). It is clear that there is a point-to-point topographical organization within the somatosensory pathway up to and including SI. There is, therefore, within the cortex some measure of topographical representation resulting from the anatomical organization of both thalamocortical and interareal connections. The precise relationship of these connections to functional representation, and the exact nature of any physiological map or maps may be variable, and is certainly dependent on the experimental circumstances and techniques used in any investigation. Suffice it to say that the anatomical connections provide the scaffolding upon which state-dependent physiological representations are built, via both thalamocortical and interareal corticocortical pathways in parallel. The sensory 'homunculus' remains broadly correct and is at present sufficient for the understanding of major dysfunction of the somatosensory cortex of man, at least until the spatial resolution of in vivo imaging approaches that of experimental physiology.

Outside the postcentral gyrus, SI has ipsilateral corticocortical association connections with the second somatosensory area (SII), with area 5 in the superior parietal lobe, with area 4, the motor cortex in the precentral gyrus, and with the supplementary motor cortex in the medial part of area 6 of the frontal lobe. All cytoarchitectonic areas project to and receive from SII, in a point-to-point topographical manner, reflecting the presence of a topographical representation of the body in the latter area. From SI to SII, the corticocortical fibres terminate in a feedforward manner, concentrating in layer IV and the adjacent deep part of layer III. Projections from SII to SI have a feedback distribution being concentrated in lamina I (see Burton 1986 for review). The projection from SI to area 5 in the superior parietal lobe comes from all cytoarchitectonic subdivisions of SI and ends in a feedforward distribution centred on layer IV. The topography of SI appears to be largely maintained in this projection and is a mirror-image, with area 3a projecting most posteriorly in area 5, and area 2 most anteriorly. The reciprocal connections from area 5 to SI are of the feedback type (Pearson & Powell 1985). Some of the fibres passing to area 5 may be collaterals of axons branching to other cytoarchitectonic subdivisions of SI (DeFelipe et al 1986). The projection from SI to the motor cortex also preserves topographical organization and is of the feedforward type. It arises mostly from areas 1 and 2 (Jones 1986).

All cytoarchitectonic subdivisions of SI both send and receive callosal commissural fibres from all the cytoarchitectonic subdivisions of the other side. Not all parts of any one cytoarchitectonic area, however, are callosally connected. Cortex containing the representation(s) of the distal limbs in all areas are relatively devoid of such connections, neither sending fibres to, nor receiving from the contralateral hemisphere. Extensions of connections into the hand and foot areas of representation as seen on the homuncular map, particularly along the borders of cytoarchitectonic areas, may reflect the interconnection of regions containing representations of the proximal limbs and trunk when a dermatomal-type map is considered (Shanks et al 1985a; Jones 1986). SI is also connected with the contralateral area 5, though again, avoiding the representations of the hand and foot. SI as well sends fibres to, but does not receive axons from the contralateral SII (Jones 1986).

Callosal fibres in SI arise mainly from the deep part of layer III and terminate in layers I to IV. This termination, which is densest in layers IV and III, forms characteristic patchy, discontinuous bands (Shanks et al 1985a; Jones 1986). It has been shown that callosally projecting pyramidal cells receive monosynaptic thalamic and commissural connections (Jones 1986).

In addition to having reciprocal subcortical connections with the thalamus and claustrum and receiving afferents from the basal nucleus of Meynert, the locus coeruleus and the midbrain raphe, SI has prominent subcortical projections (Jones 1986). Corticostriatal fibres, arising in layer V, pass mainly to the putamen of the same side. Corticopontine and corticotectal fibres from SI are also prominent and arise in layer V. As well as the main pontine nuclei (Brodal

1978), SI also projects to the pontine tegmental reticular nucleus (Brodal 1980). In addition, axons arising in SI pass to the brainstem, notably the dorsal column nuclei, and to the spinal cord. Cortico-spinal pyramidal cells are found in layer V in all cytoarchitectonic subdivisions of SI in distinct clusters (Murray & Coulter 1981), and the topographical representation in the cortex is preserved in terms of the spinal segments to which different parts of the postcentral gyrus project; thus the arm representation projects to the cervical enlargement, the leg representation to the lumbosacral enlargement, and so on. Within the grey matter of the spinal cord, fibres from SI terminate in the dorsal horn, Rexed's laminae 3 to 5, with fibres from 3b and 1 ending more dorsally, and those from area 2 more ventrally (Jones 1986).

The second somatosensory area (SII; see Burton 1986, for references), numbered according to the historic sequence of its discovery, lies along the upper bank of the lateral sulcus (Sylvian fissure) posterior to the central sulcus, hence in the parietal operculum. Its location to this region has recently been confirmed in man (Burton et al 1993). SII contains a somatotopic representation of the body, with the head and face most anteriorly, adjacent to SI, and the sacral regions most posteriorly (8.260). More recent data suggest that actually there may be two mirror-image body maps within SII (see Burton et al 1993 for references). SII is reciprocally connected with the ventroposterior nucleus of the thalamus in a topographically organized fashion. Probably a percentage of thalamic neurons project to both SI and SII via axon collaterals. Other thalamic connections are with the posterior group of nuclei and with the intralaminar central lateral nucleus. SII sends fibres to subcortical areas which also receive inputs from all other cortical areas (p. 1149). SII also projects to the cervical and thoracic spinal cord (where axons terminate in Rexed's lamina IV–VII of the dorsal horn), the dorsal column nuclei, the principal trigeminal nucleus and the periaqueductal grey matter of the midbrain.

Within the cortex, SII is reciprocally connected with SI in a topographically organized manner (see above), and projects to the motor cortex (area 4). SII also projects in a topographically organized way and with a feedforward connection to the lateral part of area 7 (area 7b) in the inferior parietal lobe (Neal et al 1987, 1990b). There are also connections with the posterior cingulate gyrus. Across the corpus callosum, both right and left SII areas are interconnected; distal limb representations are probably excluded. There are additional callosal projections to SI and area 7b.

Before considering the possible functions of SII, two adjacent but separate areas require description. In the upper bank of the lateral sulcus of subhuman primates the retro-insular area (Ri) lies immediately posterior to SII. Anterior and lateral to SII, in the most posterior part of the insular cortex proper, lies the granular insular cortex (Ig). SII projects to and receives from both the retro-insular cortex and the granular insular cortex (Burton 1986). Both are reciprocally connected with area 7b (see below) in the inferior parietal lobe (Neal et al 1987, 1990b). The thalamic projections to both areas are uncertain, but probably include axons from the posterior group of nuclei, including the oral part of the pulvinar.

Neurons in SII respond particularly to transient, moderate-to-high velocity cutaneous stimuli, such as brush strokes or tapping, with little response to maintained stimuli. Perhaps the most effective stimulus for many SII neurons is vibration or flutter, characteristic of Pacinian corpuscle responses in the periphery (Burton 1986). Responses in the retro-insular cortex are best to hair stimulation or low-threshold skin stimulation, with little convergence between hairy and glabrous skin receptive fields (Burton 1986). The insular granular cortex of monkeys also shows responses to tactile stimuli, and an area has been identified in humans by positron emission tomography (PET) responding similarly (Burton et al 1993).

Area 5 in the superior parietal lobe receives a dense feedforward projection from all cytoarchitectonic areas of SI, in a topographically organized manner (Pearson & Powell 1985). The thalamic afferents to this area come from the lateral posterior nucleus and from the central lateral nucleus of the intralaminar group (Pearson et al 1978). Ipsilateral corticocortical fibres from area 5 go to the lateral part of area 7, area 7b in the inferior parietal cortex (Neal et al 1986b, 1990b), the premotor and supplementary motor cortex, area 6, in the frontal lobe, the posterior cingulate gyrus, and the insular granular cortex (Mesulam & Mufson 1985). Commissural con-

nections between area 5 on both sides tend to avoid the areas of representation of the distal limbs (Shanks et al 1985a), and additional heterotopic contralateral connections are with the premotor cortex. The response properties of cells in area 5 are more complex than in SI (Hyvarinen 1982) with larger receptive fields and evidence of submodality convergence. The responses to passive stimulation are considerably enhanced when a voluntary movement causes the cell to discharge, and thus this region is probably important in the control of skilled movements (Mountcastle et al 1975; Georgopoulos et al 1984, 1985; Singh & Knight 1993). Aside from subcortical projections general to the majority of cortical areas (p. 1149), area 5 contributes to the corticospinal tract (Murray & Coulter 1981).

In monkeys, the inferior parietal lobe comprises area 7. In man, this area is more superior, with areas 39 and 40 intervening in the inferior parietal lobe. The counterparts for these areas in monkeys are unclear, if they exist at all. Little experimental evidence is available on the connections and functions of these latter areas. Their role in human cerebral processing will be discussed below. The lateral part of area 7, area 7b in the monkey, receives somatosensory inputs from area 5, SII, and the retro-insular cortex. The projections are of the feedforward type, and appear to conform to a topographical body map in each area (Neal et al 1986b, 1987, 1990b). Additional feedforward connections pass to the posterior cingulate gyrus (area 23). The relationship with the granular insular cortex is of a feedforward type from area 7b to the insula, reciprocated by a feedback pathway. Onward connections of area 7b to the temporal cortex pass to cortex in the depths of the superior temporal sulcus and appear to be feedforward types in both directions (Neal et al 1987, 1990b); these will be discussed later, when temporal cortex is considered. Area 7b is reciprocally connected with the frontal lobe, area 46 in the prefrontal cortex and the lateral part of the premotor cortex, area 6. Parietofrontal projections are feedforward, and are reciprocated by feedback connections (Neal et al 1990a). Commissural connections of area 7b are with the contralateral homologous area and with SII, the insular granular cortex and area 5. It has been suggested that these connections avoid representations of the distal limbs (Neal 1990). Thalamic connections are with the medial pulvinar nucleus and the intralaminar paracentral nucleus (Pearson et al 1978). Other subcortical connections conform to those general to the majority of neocortical areas.

The medial part of the inferior parietal lobe in monkeys, area 7a, is not related to the cortical pathways for somatosensory processing, but instead forms part of a dorsal cortical pathway for spatial vision. The major feedforward ipsilateral corticocortical connections to area 7a derive from visual areas in the occipital and temporal lobes and these will be considered in more detail below. It has been suggested on the basis of connections in the monkey that area 7a contains an approximate retinotopic map (Neal et al 1988a, 1990c). In essence, this part of the cortex is not at all interconnected with the somaesthetic cortical pathway passing through the more laterally placed area 7b (Neal et al 1990b). In the ipsilateral hemisphere, aside from connections with the occipital and temporal areas, to be considered in detail below, area 7a has connections with the posterior cingulate cortex (area 24; Neal et al 1988a) and with the frontal lobe. In the latter pathway, area 7a sends a feedforward projection to area 8 and area 46 dorsomedially and a second locus in area 46 more laterally. These connections are reciprocated in a feedback manner (Neal et al 1990a). The commissural connections of 7a are with its homotopic contralateral cortex and with other areas in the opposite hemisphere with which it shares ipsilateral corticocortical connections. Aside from general projections to subcortical nuclei, area 7a is connected with the medial pulvinar and intralaminar paracentral nuclei of the thalamus (Pearson et al 1978). In line with the cortical connectivity of 7a, the majority of neurons within this area are visually responsive, and largely relate to peripheral vision and respond to stimulus movement. They are also modulated significantly by eye movement (see Stein 1992 for refs). The significance of these responses is discussed below.

Before considering the cortical route for somatosensory processing and the role of the parietal lobe in man, it is important to address the sometimes controversial issue of cortical representation of two important somaesthetic pathways: the vestibular and the spinothalamic pain and temperature pathways. There is no doubt that a cortical vestibular area exists in subhuman primates around the tip of the intraparietal sulcus (Fredrickson & Rubin 1986). It is likely that this functional area is within area 2 of the primary somatosensory cortex, and shows that area's connectivity although this region has been included as part of area 5 (Pearson & Powell 1985). The thalamic pathways for transmission of vestibular information have been considered previously (see thalamus; but see Fredrickson & Rubin 1986 for discussion). It is interesting that, regardless of cytoarchitectonic localization, the postulated vestibular region lies in close proximity to the area of representation of the scalp over the occiput. A better definition of this proprioceptive pathway for the optimal perception and regulation of eye and body position is required for both man and experimental animals. More controversial but similarly ill-defined is the area of termination and cortical representation of the pain pathway. The spinothalamic tract(s), which convey information relating to pain and temperature, terminate in the ventroposterior and other thalamic nuclei, including the posterior group and certain of the intralaminar nuclei (see above). Theoretically, therefore, any cortical area receiving afferents from these diverse origins could participate in the perception of pain. Of the possible cortical regions, perhaps SII and its surroundings are the best candidates as areas of pain and temperature representation (see Stevens et al 1993 and Burton et al 1993 for discussion). Ethical issues properly restrict investigation of cortical mechanisms of pain perception in experimental animals, and the best hope for future understanding rests with the in vivo study of human subjects (see for example Jones et al 1991). The concept that pain perception is a property of subcortical structures like the thalamus seems inherently unlikely. It is not improbable, however, that the perception of pain might involve multiple cortical areas and subcortical nuclei (Coghill et al 1994), whereas its localization is more likely to be represented focally in the neocortex.

The cortical outflow of somatosensory information from SI through parietal areas to temporal cortex (Jones & Powell 1970) requires modification. There are at least two routes for the processing of somatosensory information through the parietal lobe: a dorsal path from SI through area 5 to area 7b, and a ventral route from SI through SII to the insular cortex and area 7b (area 7a in the medial part of the inferior parietal lobe of monkeys is essentially visual in function). The dorsal route through area 5 seems to function in the active exploration of extrapersonal space (Georgopoulos et al 1984, 1985; Singh & Knight 1993). The ventral route through SII appears to be concerned with tactile discrimination. Both routes converge on lateral area 7 and area 7b in subhuman primates, and the outflow continues on into the temporal lobe (see below).

No convincing homologues for larger regions of the human inferior parietal association cortex, areas 39 and 40, exist in commonly investigated subhuman primates. Injury of the superior parietal cortex in man can lead to the inability to recognize the shape of objects by touch (astereognosis), difficulty with assimilation of spatial perception of the body (amorphosynthesis) and sensory neglect of the contralateral body (asomatognosia), leading to a variety of syndromes, including dressing apraxias. More complex perceptional disturbances follow damage of the inferior parietal cortex, including areas 39 and 40. These include difficulties in language, since Wernicke's speech area includes parts of the inferior parietal lobe (8.262, see below) of the dominant hemisphere, and dyscalculia if the non-dominant hemisphere is involved. Contralateral sensory neglect extends to include the visual appreciation of the world, such as the omission of one side of a drawing when the patient is asked to copy a sketch, for example, of a clock face. Difficulties with complex orientation in space, such as map-reading, are also seen. The visual components of perception and awareness presumably involve pathways passing via posteromedial area 7 and area 7a. The more somatosensory disturbances following superior parietal lobe damage accord well with the dorsal pathway via area 5 observed in subhuman primates, mediating active touch. The role of the parietal cortex in the orientation and awareness of the body and the surrounding world has been recently reviewed (Stein 1992).

Occipital lobe

The occipital lobe of the human brain comprises almost entirely Brodmann's areas 17, 18 and 19. However, perhaps in these areas more than in any other part of the neocortex, the usefulness of cytoarchitectonics has been superseded by recent anatomical, physio-

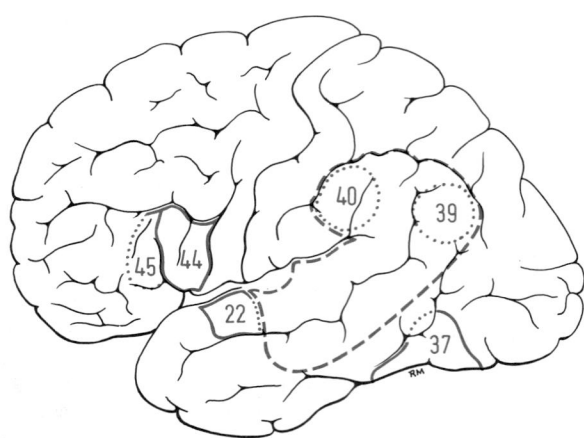

8.262 The superolateral surface of the left hemisphere showing the motor speech areas of Broca (44, 45) and Wernicke. The latter is variously depicted by different authorities and is tentatively indicated by the large parieto-temporal area enclosed in an interrupted outline, which itself includes areas 39 and 40. Areas 22 and 37 are considered by some to be respectively auditory and visuo-auditory areas associated with speech and language.

logical and functional investigations. A host of distinct visual areas reside in occipital and temporal cortex, at least 20 in the monkey (Baizer et al 1991; Rosa et al 1993). Only area 17, the striate cortex, retains good correspondence between its cytoarchitectonic boundaries and the boundaries of the functional primary visual cortex, VI. Functional subdivisions V2, V3 (dorsal and ventral) and V3A (Zeki 1993) lie within Brodmann's area 18. Other functional areas at the junction of occipital cortex within the parietal or temporal lobes lie wholly or partly in area 19. This progressive difficulty in aligning cytoarchitectonic with functional subdivisions is a clear illustration of the view stated earlier, that clear cytoarchitectonic changes, such as between area 17 and area 18, reflect clear connectional and hence functional differences, whereas subtle changes in cytoarchitectonics, which can be impossible to define consistently or accurately, parallel subtle connectional gradients and appropriately complex functional diversity. For the purposes of the following account, the terminology of the multiple visual areas presented by Baizer et al (1991) will be followed, with references to both Brodmann's cytoarchitectonic map and to other nomenclatures as appropriate.

The primary visual cortex (area 17; VI) is coextensive with the visual stria of Gennari, hence its alternative name, the striate cortex. It occupies the upper and lower lips and depths of the posterior part of the calcarine sulcus (8.263A, B), extending into the cuneus and lingual gyrus. Posteriorly it is limited by the lunate sulcus (and polar sulci above and below this), extending only to the occipital pole in the human, though reaching the lateral surface of the occipital lobe in other primates. As a cytoarchitectonic area it can easily be defined by the visual stria and by the thinness of the cortex (from pia to white matter). The stria becomes less obvious towards the occipital pole, a change correlated with retinotopic organization (see below), its prominence being inversely related to distance from the area of central retinal representation.

The status of area 17 as the primary visual area is long established, both by electrical stimulation in man and by its connections with the lateral geniculate body, and through this with the retinae (p. 1087). Each cortical area receives impulses from two half retinae, representing the contralateral half of the binocular visual field. The patterns of retinal impulses do not undergo simple relay in the geniculate bodies, where some processing occurs, but exclude interaction of a biretinal nature. Such processing has been studied most intensively in the striate cortex, especially by the single unit recording technique. The geniculate radiation spreads as it swerves through the white core of the occipital lobe, its fibres terminating in strict point-to-point deployment in the striate area: the peripheral parts of the retinae activate the most anterior parts in the calcaneal cortex, the macular regions activating a relatively large part adjoining its posterior end. Moreover, superior and inferior retinal quadrants are

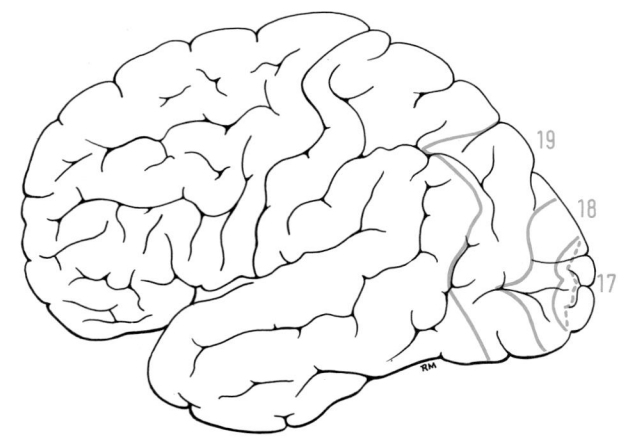

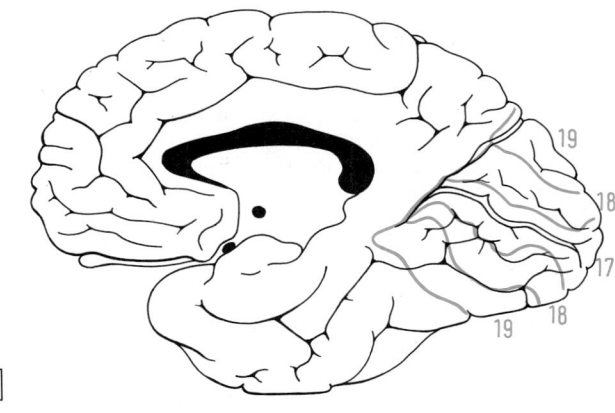

8.263 Superolateral (A) and medial (B) surfaces of the cerebral hemispheres showing the visual areas in the occipital lobe. The striate (17), parastriate (18) and peristriate (19) areas correspond approximately to the Brodmann areas as indicated and also to visual areas I, II and III.

connected with corresponding areas of the striate cortex. In the classic studies of the effects of injuries of the occipital lobe in warfare, similar retinotopic results were obtained (Holmes & Lister 1916; Teuber et al 1960). More recent studies in human patients, using modern imaging techniques, confirm the retinotopic organization, but suggest that a much greater extent (60%) of the striate cortex is occupied by the central 15° of the visual field, with a corresponding reduction in the representation of the periphery (McFadzean et al 1994).

Experimental findings in a wide range of mammals, especially primates, were corroborated by stimulation of the human cortex (Penfield & Jasper 1954); the visual impressions thus elicited were simple, such as flashes of light, but were referred to a specific locus in the visual field according to the location of the cortical stimulus. Eye movements are also produced by such stimulation. When areas 18 and 19 are stimulated more complex visual images are reported, indicating that they are concerned with the integration of the information reaching area 17.

The striate cortex (area 17) is granular or koniocortex, with difficulty in distinguishing layer III from layer II. Layer IV, bearing the prominent bundle of white matter parallel to the pial surface, the stria of Gennari, is commonly divided into three sublayers passing from superficial (pial) to deep: IVA, IVB containing the stria, and IVC. The densely cellular IVC is further subdivided into a superficial IVCα and a deep IVCβ. Layer IVB contains only sparse, mainly non-pyramidal neurons (Garey 1990). Perhaps the most significant recent advance in understanding the architecture of the striate cortex came with the application of cytochrome oxidase histochemistry (Wong-Riley 1979). Using this technique, layer IVC stains darkly, IVB is lightly stained and IVA is characterized by darkly staining patches, which extend in a columnar fashion through layers II and III. These cytochrome oxidase rich patches or columns in the superficial laminae are commonly referred to as 'blobs'. This chemoarchitecture, first described in the monkey, is also seen in human striate cortex (Horton & Headley-White 1984; Burkhalter & Bernardo 1989; Wong-Riley et al 1993). The same pattern of blobs is demonstrated by a number of other staining methods (see Martin 1988 for references).

The major input to area 17 comes from the lateral geniculate nucleus, organized in a retinotopic manner. The geniculocortical axons terminate predominantly in layers IVA and IVC. Axons arising in the parvocellular laminae of the lateral geniculate nucleus terminate in IVA and IVCβ, whereas those from the magnocellular laminae end in IVCα. Additional geniculocortical axons from the intralaminar zones and S laminae terminate in layers I, III and IVA. Other thalamic afferents pass to layers I and VI from the inferior pulvinar nucleus and the intralaminar group (see Garey 1990 for references).

Geniculocortical afferents terminate in alternating bands with the axons from geniculate laminae from the ipsilateral eye (2, 3 and 5) segregated from those of laminae from the contralateral eye (1, 4

and 6). Within layer IVC neurons are monocular, that is, they respond to stimulation of only the ipsilateral or contralateral eye, not both. This horizontal segregation forms the anatomical basis of the ocular dominance column (Hubel & Wiesel 1977) whereby neurons encountered in a vertical strip from pia to white matter, although binocular outside layer IV, exhibit a preference for stimulation of one or other eye. These ocular dominance columns in monkey are of the order of 400 μm across. The other major functional basis for visual cortical columnar organization first described by Hubel and Wiesel is the orientation column (see Hubel & Wiesel 1977 for review). This describes the observation that neurons encountered by an electrode passing through the depth of the cortex at right angles to the plane, from pia to white matter, all respond preferentially to a stationary or moving straight line segment of a given orientation within the visual field. They further described the occurrence of circularly symmetric, simple, complex and hypercomplex receptive fields in area 17. Circularly symmetric receptive fields are analogous to those encountered in the lateral geniculate nucleus of the thalamus. Simple cells respond to lines or bars of optimal orientation in a narrowly defined position. Complex cells respond to a line of specific orientation anywhere within a (usually) rectangular receptive field. Hypercomplex cells are similar to complex cells except that the length of the line or bar stimulus is also critical for an optimal response. They observed a relationship between complexity of response properties and the position of cells in relation to the cortical laminae, with circularly symmetric cells in layer IVC, simple cells mainly in other subdivisions of layer IV and complex and hypercomplex cells predominating in supragranular (II/III) and infragranular (V/VI) laminae. In their Ferrier Lecture to the Royal Society, Hubel and Wiesel (1977) concluded that the striate cortex is made up of multiple hypercolumns of more or less identical structure, made up of a block of cortex containing either sufficient numbers of 50 μm orientation columns, shifting 10° from column to column in an orderly sequence, to cover the full 180°, or two ocular dominance columns, one for each eye, representing one locus in the visual field. In both cases, the dimension of an orientation or an ocular dominance hypercolumn approached 1 mm in width. Although both types of hypercolumn were illustrated on a single (oft reproduced) diagram, the authors emphasized that there was at that time no evidence as to how the two proposed sets of hypercolumns were related.

This model of functional organization of the visual cortex has changed considerably since the 1977 Ferrier lecture. Many of the alterations in concepts of striate cortex architecture and physiology relate to the further elucidation of cortical structure by cytochrome oxidase histochemistry. It is beyond the scope of the present account to give a detailed review of all the different studies which have contributed to the development of present concepts. A brief summary will therefore be given of the major salient features. Readers are referred to recent reviews for further detail and for references (Martin 1988; DeYoe & Van Essen 1988; Goodale 1993; Merigan & Maunsell

1993; Zeki 1993). Essentially three somewhat separate zones are recognized, the cytochrome oxidase rich blobs, the interblob zones with less cytochrome oxidase staining and layer IVB. Within the blobs, neurons are not orientation selective, and many are wavelength-sensitive, i.e. colour responsive. Neurons in the interblob zones are orientation but not wavelength selective. Neurons in layer IVB, which is more clearly seen in cytochrome oxidase sections, are sensitive to movement, and many are direction selective. The blobs lie at the centre of the ocular dominance columns. Blobs of a certain wavelength selectivity connect with other blobs of the same wavelength selectivity via often comparatively long intracortical connections. Neurons in the interblob zones and in layer IVB may show binocular disparity, and evidence exists that area 17 participates in binocular disparity (depth) discrimination in man (Gulyas & Roland 1994).

It has been suggested that the separate geniculocortical pathways from the magnocellular laminae to layer ICVα on the one hand, and from the parvocellular laminae to IVCβ on the other, remain segregated within area 17 and contribute to separate streams passing through the parietal and dorsal temporal cortex and the inferior temporal cortex respectively. These two distinct pathways are proposed to mediate the analysis of different types of visual information (Merigan & Maunsell 1993; Goodale 1993; Zeki 1993; see below). Such a segregation would be mediated by separate intrinsic connectivities between the sublaminae of layer IV and neurons in deeper and more superficial layers, segregated in blob and interblob zones. It is clear, however, that whilst such parallel pathways exist to some degree, the segregation is incomplete, both physiologically (Nealey & Maunsell 1994) and anatomically (Gilbert 1993a,b), with both magnocellular and parvocellular geniculocortical routes contributing to more complex processing in the supragranular and infragranular layers (Nealey & Maunsell 1994; see also Ohzawa et al 1990; DeAngelis et al 1991; Lamme et al 1993a,b, 1994; Celebrini et al 1993). Although information gained on the functioning and organization of the striate cortex in the last decade or so has led to considerable modification of the description proposed by Hubel and Wiesel (1977), much of their original proposal remains valid. Orientation selectivity of neurons has been repeatedly confirmed with cells of common orientation grouped in narrow vertical columns in the supragranular and infragranular interblob zones. Similarly, the existence of ocular dominance stripes is not questioned. Recent studies using optical recordings in monkey cortex (Blasdel 1992a,b) have presented a new scheme of functional organization in the striate cortex interrelating ocular dominance and orientation selectivity in a way which permits segmentation by distinguishing surfaces from contours (see also Lamme et al 1993a,b, 1994).

Ipsilateral corticocortical (association) fibres pass from area 17 to a variety of functional areas within areas 18 and 19 and in the parietal and temporal cortices. Consideration of visual pathways through the association cortex is a daunting task, with 32 visual or partly visual areas identified in subhuman primates, interconnected by 305 pathways (Van Essen et al 1992). The precise partitioning of these areas and the terminology by which they are known is variable between groups of investigators, and relatively few of these have clearly identified homologues in the human brain. Only a few of the more clearly demarcated areas will therefore be considered in detail here. Readers are referred to several recent accounts for further information (Van Essen et al 1992; Zeki 1993; Merigan & Maunsell 1993; Goodale 1993; Van Essen 1985; DeYoe & Van Essen 1988; Baizer et al 1993). Fibres from area 17 pass to area 18, containing visual areas V2, V3 and V3a, and area 19 containing V4, the posterior intraparietal and the parieto-occipital areas, and to parts of the posterior temporal lobe, the middle temporal (MT) area and the medial superior temporal (MST) area. Where it is known, these projections are predominantly of the feedforward type. Recent detailed studies of feedback projections to area 17 have shown such pathways to be extensive, reciprocal and non-reciprocal (Rockland 1994; Rockland & Van Hoesen 1994; Rockland et al 1994). Contralateral connections of V1 pass to and from the representation of the vertical meridian at the anterior border of area 17. This restriction of commissural connections to representation of the vertical meridian is common to many visual responsive areas containing a retinotopic map, and has been used, in part, to identify distinct areas containing separate representations of the visual hemifield (see Zeki 1993 for

review). Subcortical efferents of the striate cortex pass to the superior colliculus, pretectum and parts of the brainstem reticular formation. Projections to the striatum (notably the tail of the caudate nucleus) and to the pontine nuclei are respectively sparse, but do exist. Geniculo- and claustrocortical afferents are reciprocated by prominent descending projections arising in layer VI.

The second visual area (V2) occupies much of area 18 but is not coextensive with it. It contains a complete retinotopic representation of the visual hemifield which is a mirror image of that in area 17, with the vertical meridian represented most posteriorly along the border between areas 17 and 18. The architecture of V2 visualized by cytochrome oxidase histochemistry is distinctive, with a coarse array of stripes most obvious in layers III–V, running away from the border with VI. Thick stripes are distinguished from thin cytochrome oxidase rich stripes, and these are separated by stripes of low staining, referred to as interstripes or pale stripes (De Yoe & Van Essen 1988; Martin 1988; Zeki 1993). The major ipsilateral corticocortical feedforward projection to V2 comes from V1, and there is segregation of these inputs relating to the pattern of cytochrome oxidase staining in both areas (Merigan & Maunsell 1993; Goodale 1993; Zeki 1993). The blob regions of V1 project to the thin stripes, the interblob regions to the pale stripes (interstripes) and layer IVB of V1 passes to the thick stripes. Feedforward projections from V2 pass to several other visual areas (and are reciprocated by feedback connections) including the third visual area (V3) and its various subdivisions (V3/V3d; V3v/VP; V3a; see below), the fourth visual area (V4), areas in the temporal (MT; MST; FST) and parietal (PO; PIP; VIP) association cortices and to the frontal eye fields (area 8; Van Essen et al 1992). Of these, the projection to the middle temporal area (V5; see below) arises from the thick stripes, whereas that to V4 comes from the thin stripes and pale stripes (interstripes; Goodale 1993; Merigan & Maunsell 1993; Zeki 1993). Thalamic afferents to V2 come from the lateral geniculate nucleus, the inferior and lateral pulvinar nuclei and parts of the intralaminar group of nuclei. Additional subcortical afferents are as for cortical areas in general (see above). Subcortical efferents arise predominantly in layers V and VI and pass to the thalamus, the claustrum, the superior colliculus, the pretectum, the brainstem reticular formation, the striatum and the pons. As in area 17, the callosal connections of V2 are restricted predominantly to the cortex containing the representation of the vertical meridian.

The third visual area (V3) is a narrow strip adjoining the anterior margin of V2, probably still within area 18 of Brodmann. On the basis of projections from V1, myeloarchitecture, callosal and association connections and receptive field properties, V3 is further subdivided into a dorsal (V3/V3d) and a ventral (VP/V3v) subdivision (Van Essen 1985; Zeki 1993). Notably, the dorsal subdivision receives from V1 whereas the ventral does not, the dorsal subdivision is delimited by the presence of a distinctive pattern of heavy myelination and V3/V3d shows a more irregular pattern of callosal connectivity than does VP/V3v. Functionally, the dorsal part shows less wavelength selectivity, greater direction selectivity and smaller receptive fields than does the ventral subdivision. Both areas receive a moderate to strong feedforward projection from V2, and they are interconnected by association fibres. A further visual area, area V3a, lies anterior to the dorsal subdivision of V3 (V3/V3d). This area receives afferent association connections from V1, V2, V3/V3d and VP/V3v, and has a complex and irregular topographic organization. All subdivisions project to diverse visual areas in the parietal, occipital and temporal cortices, including V4 (see below) and to the frontal eye fields. This V3 complex of multiple visual areas remains poorly understood in subhuman primates, and the existence of homologous multiple areas in the human is unproven. All receive thalamic afferents from the inferior and lateral pulvinar nuclei and from intralaminar nuclei, and share the other subcortical afferent and efferent connections common to the majority of cortical areas. Differences between subdivisions of V3 in these connections are not known. In considering the routes that visual processing takes through the association cortical areas, V3 is often omitted from the account (Goodale 1993; Merigan & Maunsell 1993).

The fourth visual area, V4, lies within area 19 anterior to the V3 complex. It has no defining architectural features. It receives a major ipsilateral feedforward projection from the thin stripes and pale stripes (interstripes) of V2 but not from the thick stripes. This route from the blob and interblob zones of V1 through the thin and pale stripes of V2 to V4 suggests that wavelength (colour) selectivity as well as orientation selectivity might be transmitted to V4, as is found (Van Essen 1985; Zeki 1993). This area has been equated with a colour discrimination area in man, bilateral damage of which causes achromatopsia, located in the fusiform gyrus of the inferior occipital lobe (Zeki et al 1991; Zeki 1993; Allison et al 1993). V4 is more complex than a simple colour discrimination area since it is also involved in the discrimination of orientation and form and even movement (Heywood et al 1992; Cheng et al 1994). It is likely that several subareas in this region group together to form a V4 complex, perhaps with different functional specializations localized to different regions. V4 sends a conspicuous feedforward projection to the inferior temporal cortex and receives a feedback projection (Steele et al 1991; Distler et al 1993). It also connects with other visual areas in the temporal lobe more dorsally and in the parietal lobe (Steele et al 1991). Thalamocortical connections are with the lateral and inferior pulvinar and the intralaminar nuclei. Other subcortical connections conform to the general pattern for all cortical areas. Callosal connections are with the contralateral V4 and other occipital visual areas.

A fifth visual area, V5 or the middle temporal area (MT), is found towards the posterior end of the superior temporal sulcus on its posterior bank in subhuman primates, and has a characteristic myeloarchitecture, with heavy myelination in the deep layers (Van Essen 1985). It receives ipsilateral association connections from area 17, V2, V3 and V4, in a topographically organized way. Other lesser projections are received without a clear topographical organization from widespread visual areas in the temporal and parieto-occipital lobes and from the frontal eye fields (Rosa et al 1993). Of these, the projections from V1 and V2 are of the feedforward type, and come from layer IVB of the striate cortex and from the cytochrome oxidase thick stripes of V2. V5 is primarily a movement detection or discrimination area, with a high proportion of movement-sensitive, direction-selective cells within it (Lagae et al 1993; Cheng et al 1994), equated with a visual motion discrimination area in man, situated at the occipitotemporal junction, near the ascending limb of the inferior occipital sulcus (Zeki et al 1991; Shipp et al 1993; Watson et al 1993; Probst et al 1993). In subhuman primates, V5 is known to contain a representation of the visual field, with overemphasis on those parts that would be 'maximally stimulated during visually guided hand movements' (Maunsell & Van Essen 1987). Feedforward projections go to surrounding temporal and parietal areas, and to the frontal eye field (area 8, Kaas & Morel 1993). Thalamic connections are with the lateral and inferior pulvinar and intralaminar group of nuclei. Other connections follow the general pattern of all neocortical areas.

Detailed consideration of further cortical visual association areas is beyond the scope of the present account, and crosses into lobes other than that under consideration in the present section. Before moving on to a description of the temporal lobe, beginning with the auditory cortex, it is appropriate to give a somewhat cursory summary of current concepts of visual processing in inferior temporal and temporoparietal cortical areas. From the occipital lobe two broadly parallel but interwoven pathways emanate, a dorsal pathway through multiple parieto-occipital, parietal and neighbouring temporal areas, which is concerned primarily with visuospatial discrimination, and a ventral route via inferior temporal cortical areas dealing with perception and object recognition (Merigan & Maunsell 1993; Goodale 1993). Although extensive and complex interconnections between areas in each stream of connections occur at all hierarchical levels (Van Essen et al 1992), towards the latter parts of the two pathways, in inferior temporal and inferior parietal cortices, there is a remarkable segregation of neurons projecting to the two systems (Baizer et al 1993).

Turning first to the dorsal tier of connections, these essentially emanate from V1 and V2 to the superior temporal and surrounding parietotemporal areas and ultimately to area 7a of the parietal cortex. Surrounding the middle temporal area (MT, V5) within the superior temporal cortex are a so-called fundal superior temporal area (FST) antero-inferiorly, and a medial superior temporal area (MST) antero-superiorly. The medial area (MT) receives a feedforward projection from the middle temporal area (MT) and projects to parietal visual association areas, including area 7a (Van Essen

1985) and to more anterior superior temporal association areas (Seltzer & Pandya 1994). Its cells have large receptive fields and there is no obvious retinotopic organization (Van Essen 1985). The fundal area (FST) is subdivided into dorsal and ventral parts. The dorsal region receives from the middle temporal area (V5) and the medial area (MST) and projects to the parietal cortex. The ventral subdivision connects with the inferior temporal cortex, as well as a fringe region around V5 (Kaas & Morel 1993). These connectional differences correlate with an interesting functional segregation, with cells in the dorsal subdivision responding in relation to movement of the animal through visual space, and those in the ventral part are activated by objects moving in visual space (Tanaka et al 1993). Several of the areas in this dorsal pathway show prominent connections with the frontal eye fields (Van Essen et al 1992). Damage to these dorsal visuospatial pathways and areas disrupts motion perception (Cowey & Marcar 1992; Marcar & Cowey 1992) and causes optic ataxia (Goodale 1993). (For a discussion of the role of the parietal cortex in orientation and action in extrapersonal space see above and also see Stein 1992.) Lesions may also disrupt learning of visuospatial tasks (Gattan & Harrison 1993; but see also Pu et al 1993).

The fourth visual area, V4, is a key relay station for the ventral (perceptual) pathway, with connections passing forwards into inferior temporal cortex (Steele et al 1991; Distler et al 1993). In general, these connections pass predominantly sequentially along the inferior temporal gyrus in a feedforward manner, from V4 to posterior, intermediate and then anterior inferior temporal cortex, finally feeding into the temporal polar and medial temporal areas (Webster et al 1991; Saleem et al 1993) and so interfacing with the limbic system (see p. 1121). Visual functions in this ventral pathway relate to complex visual discrimination and perception (Young 1993a; Kobatake & Tanaka 1994), including colour as a contributor to visual discrimination (Komatsu et al 1992). These functions include tasks as complex as face discrimination (Mikami et al 1994; Allison et al 1994; Seeck et al 1993), visual search (Haglund et al 1994) and recognition memory (Sobotka & Ringo 1993; Fahy et al 1993). There is a broad gradient of responses, with more complex properties most anteriorly (Nakamura et al 1994; Kobatake & Tanaka 1994). More detailed consideration of the anatomical connections and functions of inferior, superior and medial temporal areas will be given below.

Temporal lobe

The temporal lobe extends from the lateral sulcus superolaterally to the hippocampal formation ventromedially. It includes the cortex of the lower bank of the lateral sulcus in the temporal operculum, and is limited posteriorly by the inferior occipital sulcus. Two major sulci groove the lateral surface of the temporal lobe, a superior and an inferior temporal sulcus. In general, five topographic areas can therefore be described: the temporal operculum, superior temporal (area 22), middle temporal (area 21) and inferior temporal (area 20) regions are on the lateral and inferior surfaces; the temporal pole (area 35) lies in front of the termination of these sulci. Cortex of the medial temporal lobe includes major subdivisions of the limbic system, including the hippocampus and entorhinal cortex, which has been described (see p. 1123). Areas of neocortex adjacent to these limbic regions can be grouped together as medial (or mesial) temporal association cortex. The temporal lobe is expanded enormously in man, along with the frontal lobe (Zilles et al 1988), which poses the problem of relating physiological and anatomical studies of subhuman primates to human brain topography. In general, the commonly studied old world monkeys lack a middle temporal gyrus. For the purposes of the present description, the term middle temporal cortex will be taken to include experimental evidence of function and connections of area 21 in the banks of the superior temporal sulcus. Area 20 equates with the inferior temporal cortex from the surface, adjacent to area 21, round to the rhinal fissure. The superior temporal region (area 22) extends from the fundus of the superior temporal sulcus superiorly to the lip of the lateral sulcus. The terms temporal pole and operculum are as in man.

The temporal operculum houses the primary auditory cortex, AI. This is coextensive with the granular (koniocortex) area 41 in the transverse temporal gyri of Heschl (Webster & Garey 1990). Layer IV is thick and prominent in cell stains. The inner and outer bands of Baillarger, particularly the former, are clearly seen on sections stained for myelin. Layer IV is also prominently stained by acetylcholinesterase and cytochrome oxidase histochemistry (Morel et al 1993). The primary auditory cortex is reciprocally connected with all subdivisions of the medial geniculate nucleus (Morel & Kaas 1992; Morel et al 1993; Pandya et al 1994) and may receive additional thalamocortical projections from the medial pulvinar and the posterior group of nuclei. The geniculocortical afferents terminate densely in layer IV, with high-density patches alternating with less dense zones of terminals with a periodicity in the monkey of approximately 200 μm (Pandya & Rosene 1993). AI contains a tonotopic representation with high frequencies encountered posteriorly and low frequencies anteriorly. Single cell responses are to single tones of a narrow frequency band (Morel et al 1993) and cells in single vertical electrode penetrations share an optimum frequency response. There is evidence of equally sharp frequency tuning in the human auditory cortex (Sams & Salmelin 1994). There is a suggestion, at least in the cat, that cells in strips at right angles to the isofrequency axis respond to different tone intensity (Heil et al 1994). A third functional response property, besides frequency and tone intensity responses, is binaural interaction for the localization of sound in space. At least in the cat, neurons in AI show two types of binaural interaction; the first is a summation response with single cells excited by stimuli to both ears, the second is a suppression of response, with cells excited by stimulating the contralateral ear but inhibited by sounds detected in the ipsilateral ear. In both cases, there may be a time lag between ipsilateral and contralateral responses (interaural time and level). Bands of cells showing excitation–excitation responses (E–E; summation) alternate with bands showing excitation–inhibition responses (E–I; suppression). These bands run approximately orthogonal to the isofrequency lines, and their alternating distribution may relate to the patchy or banded organization of callosal terminations in AI (Seldon 1985; Webster & Garey 1990; Brugge 1992; Pandya & Rosene 1993). Theoretically at least, the temporal firing pattern of neurons may also be important in encoding sound location in the cortex (Middlebrooks et al 1994). More complex response properties are likely to occur, particularly perhaps outside layer IV, including the encoding of phonetic features (Steinschneider et al 1993).

The anatomical and functional subdivision of the cortex surrounding AI in the temporal operculum has received the attentions of several groups of investigators, with the result that several different schemes for the parcellation of auditory association areas in the monkey exist (Pandya & Yeterian 1985; Cippoloni & Pandya 1989; Morel & Kaas 1992; Morel et al 1993; Pandya & Rosene 1993; Pandya et al 1994). It would be inappropriate in the present account to introduce yet another such classification, and yet there is no evidence to indicate which scheme might be more applicable to man. For no other reason than that their studies combine physiological and anatomical data from the same animals, the following discussion will follow the terminology of Kaas and colleagues (Morel & Kaas 1992; Morel et al 1993), though certain essential features of the organization are similar (though not identical) in other recent accounts (Pandya & Yeterian 1985; Pandya & Rosene 1993; Pandya et al 1994). Passing anteriorly along the temporal operculum from the primary auditory area (AI), a second tonotopically organized auditory responsive area, the rostral (R) area, is encountered. This shares many architectonic features with AI and may lie within the koniocortex but the tonotopic representation is reversed, with low frequency responses encountered posteriorly and higher frequencies more anteriorly. This mirror-image pattern of peripheral representation is strongly reminiscent of those seen in adjacent cortical somatosensory and visual areas (see above) and may well represent a fundamental principle of cortical organization of contiguous representations in neighbouring fields. Anterior to this lies a third rostrotemporal (RT) area, which is cytoarchitectonically distinct, and which contains a further mirror-image reversal of tonotopic representation. Posterior to AI is a further caudal (C) area, which is architectonically distinct, with less dense myelination. This may also contain a crude tonotopic representation; certainly neurons close to and on either side of the border of AI and the caudal area have similar frequency responses, possibly suggesting yet another mirror-image representation. Cortex surrounding these auditory areas, both medially, on the temporal operculum, and laterally, on the superior temporal gyrus, appear to be auditory in function. A caudomedial

(CM) area lies parallel with AI on the operculum, and a posterolateral (PL) area on the superior temporal gyrus; similarly the rostral area has a rostromedial subdivision (RM) medially and an anterolateral area (AL) laterally; the rostrotemporal area is flanked by an opercular medial rostrotemporal zone (MRT) and a superior temporal lateral rostrotemporal zone (LRT). The central opercular areas (AI, R and RT) are designated the 'core' and the surrounding areas (C, CM, RM, MRT, PL, AL and LRT) are termed 'belt' regions. Another recent classification by Pandya and colleagues (Pandya & Yeterian 1985; Cippoloni & Pandya 1989; Pandya & Rosen 1993; Pandya et al 1994) is largely cytoarchitectonic and connectional, but also identifies core regions. In this classification, the 'belt' regions are redefined as a medially situated 'root' zone, comprising four subdivisions, and a laterally placed 'belt' zone, also comprising four subdivisions. The two schemes, though similar, are not identical, and individual areas cannot necessarily be equated with each other. There may also be species differences. The following account of connectivity ignores these difficulties of detail, and hence may contain inaccuracies. All core and belt areas are reciprocally connected with the subdivisions of the medial geniculate nucleus of the thalamus. The projection of the ventral division of the medial geniculate nucleus is mostly to the core areas, and much less to belt areas; the dorsal and magnocellular divisions project both to belt and core; connections of the medial pulvinar, and suprageniculate-limitans nuclei are mostly with belt areas. In addition to subcortical connections common to the majority of cortical areas, both core and belt auditory areas project to the inferior colliculus, with the core projecting to the central nucleus and the belt projecting to other subdivisions.

Ipsilateral corticocortical connections between auditory areas are numerous. Essentially, the primary auditory area, AI, only receives feedback types of projections. It sends prominent feedforward connections to all adjacent areas in both the core and belt regions. The rostral area, R, projects forwards to the rostrotemporal area (RT) and to adjacent core areas. The medially placed core areas project onwards to parts of the insula; laterally placed core areas project into auditory association areas of the superior temporal gyrus. Where clear tonotopic representations have been identified, the association projections are point-to-point, from one best frequency representation to the same best frequency representation in the adjacent area. Overall, the auditory areas interconnect with prefrontal cortex, though the projections from core regions, particularly AI, are small. In general, posterior parts of the operculum project to area 8 and to adjacent area 9 more anteriorly, central areas project to area 8, area 9 and area 46, and more anterior areas project to area 9, area 46, area 12 on the orbital surface and to the anterior cingulate gyrus on the medial surface (Petrides & Pandya 1988). Contralateral corticocortical connections are with the same area in the other hemisphere, and to adjacent areas with which each area has feedforward association connections.

Injury of the auditory cortex in man has a variety of manifestations, including cortical deafness, verbal auditory agnosia and non-verbal auditory agnosia. The markedly bilateral nature of the auditory pathway means that noticeable deficits occur with bilateral damage only (Webster & Garey 1990).

It is tempting to draw parallels between the different sensory systems within the cortex. Thus, it is possible that the medial belt areas and their onward projections to the insula represent a dorsal pathway, analogous to the visual route to parietal cortex, and the somatic sensory pathway through the superior parietal lobe. Certainly, damage of the temporoparietal junction has effects on auditory selective attention (Woods et al 1993), which might be analogous to mechanisms of redirection of visual attention in parietal cortex (Steinmetz et al 1994) or 'active touch' mechanisms in the somatic sensory pathway. The ventral pathway, via laterally placed belt areas, would be presumed to be important in auditory perception. Onward connections of the auditory association pathway converge with those of the other sensory association pathways in areas in the superior temporal sulcus (Seltzer & Pandya 1994). Undoubtedly, any such scheme would prove to be as much of a simplification in the auditory association pathway as it is in the visual cortical areas. Perhaps the most difficult question is the contribution of auditory association areas to the perception of speech and language, a topic for which no clear animal experimental paradigm is available. Cortical areas contributing to language perception and speech are discussed below. Whatever the validity of proposing a dorsal and ventral auditory association pathway, analogous to those in the visual and somaosensory areas, it is of little doubt that auditory cortical areas, like those in the other two systems mentioned, show a complex hierarchical series, interlinked at all levels in parallel, but conforming to the underlying principle of an outflow of connections from the primary sensory areas towards the medial temporal lobe.

Evidence suggests that area 21, the middle temporal cortex of man, is polysensory, connecting with auditory, somatosensory and visual cortical association pathways. It is analogous to the cortex buried in the walls of the superior temporal sulcus in monkeys. A number of distinct architectonic subdivisions of this cortex have been described and their connections analysed (Seltzer & Pandya 1989, 1991, 1994; Baines & Pandya 1992). Detailed consideration of these studies is beyond the scope of the present account, but a simplified general overview is appropriate. Broadly speaking, the middle temporal cortex (of the superior temporal sulcus in monkeys) can be divided into three or four areas from posterior to anterior, and three parallel zones at right angles to these from superomedial to inferolateral. These long parallel zones may be overlapping in connectivity but, in general, the auditory association areas project to the most superomedial of these zones, the inferotemporal cortex to the most inferolateral and the parietal cortex to the intermediate zone. Within three or four areas running consecutively posterior to anterior, there is an approximate stepwise progression of feedforward projections from the most posterior to the most anterior via the intervening area or areas. This may in fact represent a gradient of connectivity rather than an absolute area-to-area sequence. The inferotemporal projection to the inferolateral zone mirrors this progression, with the posterior inferotemporal projecting most posteriorly and the anterior inferotemporal projecting most anteriorly. Similarly, the auditory association areas of the superior temporal gyrus project in the same fashion to the superomedial zone. Projections to the intermediate zone from parietal cortex are much the same, with area 7b projecting most anteriorly (Neal et al 1988a, b, 1990b, c). Such a gradient of connectivity is also seen in the connections with the frontal lobe, with the most posterior areas projecting to posterior prefrontal cortex, areas 8 and 9, and intermediate areas connecting more anteriorly with areas 19 and 46; further forwards, the middle temporal region again has connections with anterior prefrontal areas 10 and 46 and with anterior orbitofrontal areas 11 and 14. The most anterior middle temporal area is connected with the posterior orbitofrontal cortex, area 12 and with the medial surface of the frontal pole (Seltzer & Pandya 1989). Further onward projections of this middle temporal region are to the temporal pole (Moran et al 1987) and the entorhinal cortex (Van Hoesen & Pandya 1975a; Insausti et al 1987a). Thalamic connections are with the medial (and possibly lateral) pulvinar nuclei and with elements in the intralaminar group. Other subcortical connections follow the general pattern for all cortical areas, although some projections (e.g. to the pons), particularly from anteriorly in the temporal lobe, are minimal. Physiological responses of cells in this middle temporal region are complex (Baylis et al 1987) and include convergence of different sensory modalities. Many neurons respond to faces (Baylis et al 1987; Mikami et al 1994) and may be 'viewer-centred', more often tuned for full-face or profile views (Perrett et al 1991). In line with this complexity, lesions of the temporal lobe in man can lead to considerable disturbance of intellectual function, particularly when the dominant hemisphere (p. 1183) is involved. These disturbances can include visuospatial difficulties, prosopagnosia, hemisomatognosia and severe sensory dysphasia.

The inferior temporal cortex, area 20, is a higher visual association area. It is divided in monkeys into posterior and anterior areas, with some investigators including an intermediate area between these. The posterior inferior temporal area receives major ipsilateral corticocortical fibres from occipitotemporal visual areas, notably V4. It contains a coarse retinotopic representation of the contralateral visual field (Boussaoud et al 1991). It sends a major feedforward pathway to the anterior part of the inferior temporal cortex (Webster et al 1991; Distler et al 1993) and this projection has a patchy, columnar pattern of axonal termination (Saleem et al 1993). There

is physiological evidence of functional clustering of neurons in 500 μm patches in the inferior temporal cortex (Gochin et al 1991). The anterior inferior temporal cortex projects on to the temporal pole and to paralimbic areas on the medial surface of the temporal lobe (Insausti et al 1987a; Webster et al 1991; Distler et al 1993). Additional ipsilateral association connections of the inferior temporal cortex are with the anterior middle temporal cortex, in the walls of the superior temporal gyrus and with visual areas of the dorsal pathway in the parietotemporal cortex (Distler et al 1993). Frontal lobe connections are with area 46 in the dorsolateral prefrontal cortex (posterior inferior temporal) and with the orbitofrontal cortex (anterior inferior temporal; Pandya & Yeterian 1985). Additional connections of the posterior area are with the frontal eye fields (Distler et al 1993). Reciprocal thalamic connections are with the pulvinar nuclei, with the posterior part related mainly to the inferior and lateral nuclei, and the anterior part to the medial and adjacent lateral pulvinar. Intralaminar connections are with the paracentral and central medial nuclei. Other subcortical connections conform to the general pattern of all cortical areas (Steele & Weller 1993; Baizer et al 1993). Callosal connections are between the same areas and adjacent visual association areas of each hemisphere.

As discussed earlier (see above, Occipital lobe), the inferior temporal cortex is part of the ventral visual pathway which functions in visual perception. Neurons respond to form, with more complex forms recognized anteriorly than posteriorly (Nakamura et al 1994; Kobatake & Tanaka 1994). The precise function of these areas in relation to memory tasks has attracted considerable experimental attention. It seems that the inferior temporal cortex is not associative, in the sense of responding in a specific way to paired stimuli (Sobotka & Ringo 1993; Gochin et al 1994). Cells do, however, show a significant recognition memory with a decreased response to repeated images (Miller et al 1991; Sobotka & Ringo 1993). It has been proposed that the inferior temporal cortex has two populations of neuron, one set which are suppressed when a presented stimulus matches a familiar image, and the other smaller set showing the opposite effect. Such a dual population could provide on the one hand a sensory 'filter', selecting stimuli which have appropriate features, but which are unfamiliar or unexpected, and on the other a 'sensory referent'. Interaction between the two populations permits a temporal 'figure-ground' mechanism to occur, that is a separation or selection of stimuli on the basis of their contrast with previous stimuli (Miller et al 1993).

The cortex of the temporal pole receives feedforward projections from widespread areas of temporal association cortex immediately posterior to it. The dorsal part receives predominantly auditory input from the anterior part of the superior temporal gyrus; the inferior part receives visual input from the anterior area of the inferior temporal cortex. The middle temporal cortex, in the depths of the superior temporal sulcus, projects largely between these two. Other ipsilateral connections are with the anterior insular, the posterior and medial orbitofrontal, and the medial prefrontal cortex (Moran et al 1987). The temporal pole projects onwards into limbic and paralimbic areas (Insausti et al 1987a). Thalamic connections are mainly with the medial pulvinar nucleus, and elements of the intralaminar/midline nuclei. Other subcortical connections are as for cortex in general, although some projections, such as that to the pontine nuclei, are very small. Physiological responses of cells in this and more medial temporal cortex are complex. In particular, responses correspond to behavioural performance (Nakamura et al 1994), and to the recognition of high level aspects of social stimuli (Brothers & Ring 1993).

The further relationship of the temporal neocortex to limbic and paralimbic structures has been described earlier (see p. 1121). One connectional relationship, not previously mentioned here, deserves description. That is the neocortical connections of the amygdala (Turner et al 1980; Aggleton et al 1980; Moran et al 1987; Baizer et al 1993; Steele & Weller 1993). Nuclei of the amygdala project to and receive from neocortical areas, predominantly of the temporal lobe, but also perhaps including inferior parietal cortex. The intensity of these pathways increases towards the anterior temporal pole, so that the heaviest connections are with higher order association areas of each pathway, and with multimodal areas. The role of these connections and the functions of the amygdala have been discussed earlier (see Limbic system p. 1121).

Frontal lobe

The frontal lobe is limited posteriorly by the central sulcus and laterally by the lateral sulcus (Sylvian fissure). Anterior to the central sulcus, the precentral sulcus can usually be identified running parallel, from medial to lateral. Further forwards, two major sulci are commonly seen, the superior and inferior frontal sulci, running antero-posteriorly. In front of the sulci lies the frontal pole. The ventral surface of the lobe overlies the bony orbit, and the medial surface extends from the frontal pole anteriorly to the paracentral lobule behind. The frontal cortex can thus be divided into precentral motor cortex (area 4), and premotor (area 6) cortex in the gyrus in front of the precentral sulcus, superior, middle and inferior frontal gyri, the frontal pole, orbitofrontal cortex and medial frontal cortex, including the anterior cingulate cortex. The cortex in front of the premotor area (area 6) is termed the prefrontal cortex. Even more than in the temporal lobe, the expansion of the frontal lobe in man (Zilles et al 1988) makes the topographic relevance to the human of experimental data obtained in subhuman primates problematic. For the purposes of the present description, the divisions of motor and premotor cortex, frontal eye fields (area 8), medial motor areas including the supplementary motor cortex, medial, dorsolateral and ventrolateral prefrontal and orbitofrontal cortex will be used. Wherever possible cytoarchitectonic subdivisions of Brodmann will be cited.

Before describing separate motor areas in the frontal lobe, it is worth considering the cortical origin of direct fibres to the spinal cord, the corticospinal (pyramidal) tract. As mentioned previously, several areas in the parietal lobe project to the spinal cord, including SI, area 5 of the superior parietal lobe and SII in the parietal operculum. There is a similarly widespread origin from the frontal lobe, including that from the motor cortex (area 4), the premotor cortex, and the supplementary motor area and adjacent regions (see below; Murray & Coulter 1981; Dum & Strick 1991). The actual percentage of corticospinal fibres arising from the motor cortex may actually be quite small. Between 40 and 60% arise from parietal areas, particularly area 3a (Murray & Coulter 1981). Within the cervical enlargement, at least of New World monkeys, more than 60% of frontal lobe fibres have cells of origin outside area 4 (Dum & Strick 1991). On this basis, only between 20 and 30% of the axons in the pyramidal tract arise from cells in area 4, the primary motor cortex. In all areas, the cells of origin are virtually confined to lamina V. There is a marked difference between cortical areas in the size of pyramidal cells contributing axons, with the largest corticospinal neurons residing in area 4 and the smallest in area 3b (Murray & Coulter 1981). This is reflected in the origin of the largest diameter pyramidal tract fibres originating from motor cortex.

It appears that the majority of parietal fibres to the spinal cord terminate in the deeper layers of the dorsal horn, at least in subhuman primates (see above). At least a percentage of those from the frontal cortex, notably the motor cortex, terminate in spinal cord laminae of the ventral horn, in close relationship to motor neuronal groups. This is especially true in cord segments mediating dexterous hand and finger movements. Terminations of motor cortical pyramidal tract fibres in the segments innervating the hand and finger muscles concentrate in the lateral part of the ventral horn. This relationship appears to evolve phylogenetically in relation to increasing manual dexterity (Bortoff & Strick 1993), and so would be expected to be most marked in man.

In considering the role of different cortical areas in the innervation of spinal cord motor neurons, caution should be exercised in adducing functional correlates of anatomical observations. Although the primary motor cortex may contribute a relatively small percentage of corticospinal tract axons, the vast majority of post-central axons to the spinal cord terminate in the dorsal horn of the cord, distant from the motor neuronal cell, whereas the motor cortex contributes the largest diameter fibres, and these terminate predominantly in the grey matter of the ventral horn, close to and around the motor neurons. The relative functional significance of these contributions to the corticospinal tract in controlling the activity of motor neurons may therefore be much greater than consideration of their numbers might imply.

The primary motor cortex (MI) was first described as the area of cortex with the lowest threshold for stimulation of the surface to produce peripheral muscle contraction. It is coextensive with area 4 of the precentral gyrus. The cortex of area 4 is agranular, with layers II and IV difficult to recognize. The most characteristic feature is the presence in lamina V of some extremely large pyramidal cell bodies, the Betz cells. In monkeys, these approach 60 μm in diameter (Murray & Coulter 1981) and are even larger in man.

The major thalamic connections of area 4 are with the posterior ventrolateral nucleus, which in turn receives afferents from the deep cerebellar nuclei, and possibly from the cord through the spinothalamic tracts (Jones 1986). This nucleus contains a topographic representation of the contralateral body, which is preserved in its point-to-point projection to area 4. Stimulation studies of motor cortex showed the existence of a topographic body map in area 4, with the head most laterally, and the legs and feet on the medial surface, analogous to the homunculus of body representation in SI (see above; see 8.260, 261). Neurons in area 4 are responsive to peripheral stimulation, and have receptive fields similar to those in SI. Cells posteriorly in motor cortex have cutaneous receptive fields, whereas more anteriorly situated neurons respond to stimulation of deep tissues. It has been suggested that there is in fact a dual representation of the contralateral body half throughout area 4 (for review, see Jones 1986). Lamina IV is difficult to identify in the agranular motor cortex, but there is a major thalamic afferent pathway from the posterior ventrolateral nucleus which terminates heavily in the central laminae, probably centred on lamina IV. Other thalamic connections of area 4 are with the centromedian and parafascicular nuclei of the posterior intralaminar nuclei (see above). The latter provide the only route through which pallidal output, routed via the thalamus, might impinge directly on the motor cortex. Evidence strongly suggests that the projection of the internal segment of the globus pallidus to the ventrolateral nucleus of the thalamus is confined to the anterior division of the nucleus, with no overlap with cerebellothalamic terminations. Furthermore, this anterior ventrolateral nucleus projects to the premotor and supplementary motor areas of cortex with no projection to area 4. This absolute segregation of cerebellothalamocortical and pallidothalamocortical pathways has, however, been questioned recently (Rouiller et al 1994).

The ipsilateral somatosensory cortex, SI, projects in a topographically organized way to area 4; the pathway is reciprocal. The projection to the motor cortex arises in areas 1 and, predominantly, area 2, with little or no contribution from area 3b (Jones 1986). Fibres from SI terminate in layers II and III of area 4, where they contact mainly pyramidal neurons. Evidence suggests that neurons activated monosynaptically by fibres from SI, as well as those activated polysynaptically, make contact with layer V pyramidal cells giving rise to corticospinal fibres, including Betz cells (Kaneko et al 1994a,b). There appears to be little convergence of SI input on to cells activated from the supplementary motor cortex. Movement related neurons in the motor cortex, showing activation from SI, tend to have a late onset of activity, perhaps mainly during the execution of a movement, and it has been suggested that this pathway plays a role primarily in making motor adjustments during a movement (Aizawa & Tanj 1994). Additional ipsilateral corticocortical fibres to area 4 from behind the central sulcus come from the second somatic sensory area, SII, and possibly from area 5 in the superior parietal lobe (Jones 1986).

The motor cortex receives major frontal lobe association fibres from the premotor cortex and the supplementary motor area (see below; Morecraft & Van Hoesen 1993; Lu et al 1994) and from the insula (Pandya & Yeterian 1985). The role of these areas, and of their input to area 4 in motor control, will be considered in more detail later; in summary, it is probable that these pathways modulate motor cortical activity in relation to the preparation, guidance and temporal organization of movements (Kurata 1994; Tanji 1994).

Area 4 sends fibres to and receives from its counterpart on the opposite side, and also projects to the contralateral supplementary motor cortex. There is some absence by callosal connections of parts of the motor cortex containing the representations of the distal limbs, particularly posteriorly in area 4, where neurons with cutaneous receptive fields are found. However, this lack of commissural connectivity is much less marked than equivalent regions in the somatosensory areas, with much smaller acallosal areas (Jones 1986). This is perhaps not surprising in view of the fact that the motor cortex in man is active during movements of the ipsilateral hand (Kim et al 1993), appears to contain a motor representation of the ipsilateral upper limb (Wassermann et al 1994), and shows evidence of interhemispheric facilitation within the hand area (Ugawra et al 1993).

As stated previously, stimulation studies of the motor cortex in both man and experimental animals revealed the presence of a topographic map within the motor cortex of the contralateral body half (see Zeffiro 1990 for review), with the leg representation in the paracentral lobule on the medial surface, and the face most inferolaterally in the precentral gyrus. Controversy in the interpretation of microstimulation studies has centred on the nature of the somatotopic organization with reference to the representation of either movements or of specific muscles. Current ideas of motor cortical function have derived most from experiments recording the activity of neurons in area 4 in awake, behaving monkeys, pioneered by Evarts and his colleagues (see Zeffiro 1990 for references). A detailed discussion of the activity of motor cortical neurons in relation to movement is beyond the scope of the present account. However, some consideration of these data is essential. Broadly speaking, the results of unit recording experiments in monkey motor cortex can be considered under two categories: firstly, observations on the activity of neurons with direct monosynaptic connections with spinal cord motor neurons, so-called corticomotor neuronal cells, as a subset of neurons projecting to the spinal cord, but not necessarily making such monosynaptic contacts, known as pyramidal tract neurons; secondly, observations on motor cortical neuronal activity in relation to active movement without reference to the connectivity or otherwise with the spinal cord. Considering first the corticomotor neuronal system, approximately 18% of motor cortex cells give monosynaptic contact on motor neurons, especially in the innervation of hand and arm motor neuronal pools (Georgopoulos 1991). Corticomotor neuronal cells are active in relation to agonist muscle force of contraction, whereas the relationship is less clear in other pyramidal tract neurons; the activity in cortical output neurons precedes the onset of related electromyographic activity by 50–100 mseconds, suggesting a role for cortical activation in generating rather than monitoring movement; finally, the relationship of cortical activity to movement holds true for complex as well as simpler single-joint movements (Zeffiro 1991). A recent study specifically of hand area corticomotor neuronal cells in area 4 of the monkey (Maier et al 1994) has elucidated their modes of activity further. Neurons facilitating electromyographic activity of finger and forearm muscles during a low-force precision grip task, and having evidence of monosynaptic inputs to spinal motor neurons, were studied. Activity in all cells correlated with muscle contraction. One-third of the cells examined showed a significant positive correlation with the static force exerted, whereas a further 20% showed a significant negative correlation. Each cell facilitated activity in one to five target muscles, with those neurons showing a high correlation with grip force having a restricted muscle field. These data show that even amongst the corticomotor neuronal population in area 4, a direct

relationship of cells to single muscles is rare, and quantitative encoding of muscle contraction in the sense here of force, is also far from universal amongst these cells. It is not surprising, therefore, that the control of finger movement, when examined by unit recording in the motor cortex without reference to the cells' efferent connections to the cord or elsewhere, 'appears to utilize a population of neurons distributed throughout (the motor cortex) hand area rather than a somatotopically segregated population' (Schieber & Hibbard 1993). Thus, single pyramidal tract neurons influence several motor neuron pools and, conversely, single motor neurons are influenced by a relatively large cortical area (Georgopoulos 1991). When the response proportion of motor cortical neurons in general, as distinct from pyramidal tract cells, are considered, changes in activity in preparation for a movement are selective for direction of movement, independent of the pattern of muscle contraction needed to effect that movement (Georgopoulos 1991). Indeed, in one recent study, nearly 80% of neurons 'were modulated significantly by movement direction' (Fu et al 1993). The relation between activity of motor cortical cells and the amplitude of movement is less clear, and it has been suggested that the basal nuclei provide signals for the proper amplitude of movement (Georgopoulos 1991). However, the majority of cortical neuronal activity may be significantly modulated by the range of movement (amplitude), though not necessarily in the cell's preferred movement direction. Correlation with distance may also occur later in the neuron's activity, notably during the execution of the movement, indicating separate processing of direction and amplitude (Fu et al 1993). Perhaps the most intriguing aspects of motor cortical neuronal activity relates to memorized delay tasks. In a recent study, Georgopoulos and colleagues (Smyrnis et al 1992) compared the responses in motor cortex associated with a non-delay task, a memorized delay task and a non-memorized delay task. The neuronal population signal showed direction selectivity in all tasks. In the delay tasks, the population activity increased during the delay prior to movement, and was maintained at a higher level where the cue to movement signal had to be memorized for a short period (450–750 msec). These data 'indicate that the motor cortex is involved in encoding and holding memory directional information concerning visually cued arm movement' (Smyrnis et al 1992).

Aside from its contribution to the corticospinal tract, the motor cortex has diverse subcortical projections. The connections to the striatum and pontine nuclei are predictably heavy. It also projects to the subthalamic nucleus. It is important to emphasize that the motor cortex sends significant projections to all nuclei in the brainstem which make a major contribution to the extrapyramidal descending pathways to the spinal cord, namely the reticular formation, the red nucleus, the superior colliculus, the vestibular nuclei and the inferior olive. Other connections of area 4 conform to the general pattern for all cortical areas.

Immediately in front of the primary motor cortex lies area 6 of Brodmann (8.264); this area is also agranular but was originally distinguished on the grounds of the presence in lamina V of Betz

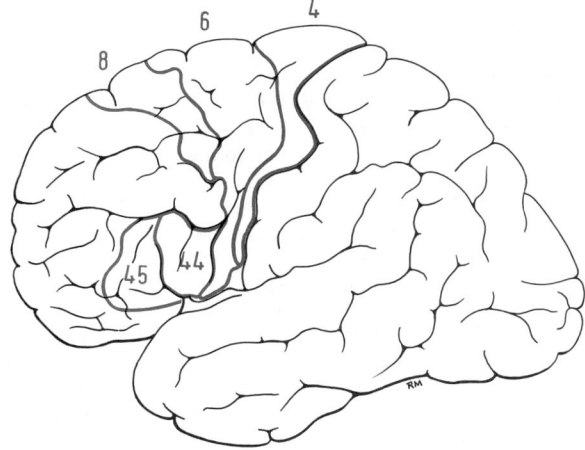

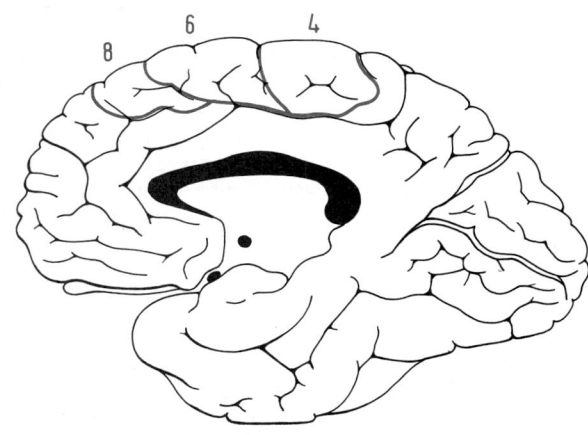

8.264 Superolateral (A) and medial (B) surfaces of the cerebral hemispheres, showing approximate correspondence of the Brodmann areas to the main motor area (4) or MsI, the premotor area (6, 8) and motor speech area of Broca (44, 45). Compare with **8.254**.

cells, and their absence in area 6. The validity of this distinction, and the confidence with which Betz cells can be identified, is questionable (Zilles 1990). Area 6 extends on to the medial surface, where it becomes contiguous with area 24 in the cingulate gyrus, anterior and inferior to the paracentral lobule. A number of functional motor areas are contained within this cortical region. Lateral area 6, the area over most of the lateral surface of the hemisphere, corresponds to the premotor cortex, which is often further subdivided in experimental monkeys into dorsal (superior) and ventral (inferior) premotor areas. Medial to area 6, from the most superolateral part of area 6 adjoining the medial margin and on to the medial surface of the hemisphere, is the supplementary motor area (SMA; MII **8.260**). Area 24 in the cingulate gyrus adjacent to area 6 contains several motor areas, termed cingulate motor areas, and anterior to the supplementary motor area on the medial surface, an addition functional subdivision, the preSMA, is recognized (Tanji 1994). For the purposes of the present discussion, the additional medial motor areas will be included with the supplementary motor cortex. It is recognized that this enlarged SMA includes areas with prefrontal connections and oculomotor functions which are not strictly within the functional supplementary area (see Tanji 1994 for discussion). However, since the major ipsilateral corticocortical efferents of the surrounding motor areas are with the supplementary motor cortex, it is felt a justified simplification to consider this expanded medial motor area as a single anatomical entity.

The supplementary motor area receives its major thalamic input from the anterior part of the ventrolateral nucleus, which in turn is the major recipient of fibres from the internal segment of the globus pallidus (Jones 1985). Additional thalamic afferents are from the ventral anterior nucleus, the intralaminar nuclei, notably the centrolateral and centromedial nuclei, and possibly lateralis posterior and the oral pole of the pulvinar (Wiesendanger & Wiesendanger 1985). The mediodorsal nucleus also projects to medial motor areas, both the supplementary motor cortex and surrounding region (Wiesendanger & Wiesendanger 1985; Giguere & Goldman-Rakic 1988). The connections with the thalamus are reciprocal. The medial motor areas, including the supplementary motor cortex, receive widespread connections from the ipsilateral frontal lobe, including from the primary motor cortex, the dorsal premotor area, the dorsolateral and ventrolateral prefrontal, medial prefrontal and orbitofrontal cortex and the frontal eye field (area 8) (Morecraft & Van Hoesen 1993; Bates & Goldman-Rakic 1993; Lu et al 1994). These connections are reciprocal, but the major ipsilateral efferent pathway is to the motor cortex. Parietal lobe connections of the medial motor areas are with the superior parietal area 5 and possibly inferior parietal area 7b (Tanji 1994). Contralateral connections are with the medial motor areas of the other hemisphere and with the motor and premotor cortex. Subcortical connections, other than with the thalamus, pass to the striatum, subthalamic nucleus and pontine nuclei, the brainstem reticular formation and the inferior olive (Tanji 1994). The supplementary motor area also makes a substantial contribution to the corticospinal (pyramidal) tract, as discussed earlier, contributing as much as 40% of the fibres from the frontal lobe (Dum & Strick 1991).

The human supplementary motor area contains a representation of the body with the leg posterior, the face anterior and the upper limb between these two (Fried et al 1991). The role of the supplementary motor cortex in the control of movement is primarily important in complex tasks, requiring temporal organization of sequential movements and retrieval of motor memory (Halsband et al 1993; Shibasaki et al 1993; Tanji 1994). Damage to the supplementary motor area in human patients bears some striking similarities to the effects of basal ganglia dysfunction, with akinesia being common. Also seen are problems with the performance of sequential, complex movements. Stimulation of the supplementary motor area in conscious patients has been reported as eliciting the sensation of an 'urge' to move, or of 'anticipation that a movement was about to occur' (Fried et al 1991). A region anterior to the supplementary motor area for face representation is important in vocalization and speech production (Fried et al 1991; Ojemann 1991; Grasby et al 1993; Demonet et al 1993).

The premotor cortex, within area 6, is subdivided into a dorsal and a ventral area (PMd and PMv respectively) on functional grounds, and on the basis of ipsilateral corticocortical association connections. The connections of the premotor cortex as a whole will, therefore, be considered, and the reported differences in connectivity highlighted where appropriate. The major thalamic connections of the premotor cortex are with the anterior division of the ventrolateral nucleus and with the centromedian, parafascicular and centrolateral components of the intralaminar nuclei. Subcortical projections to the striatum and pontine nuclei are prominent, and this area also projects to the superior colliculus and the reticular formation. Both dorsal and ventral areas contribute to the corticospinal (pyramidal) tract (see above). Other subcortical connections are as for all neocortical areas. Commissural connections are with the contralateral premotor, motor and superior parietal (area 5) cortex. Ipsilateral corticocortical (association) connections with area 5 in the superior parietal cortex, and inferior parietal area 7b are common to both dorsal and ventral subdivisions of the premotor cortex (Neal et al 1990a), and both send a major projection to the primary motor cortex, area 4 (Morecraft & Van Hoesen 1993; Lu et al 1994). The dorsal premotor area also receives from the posterior superior temporal cortex (Petrides & Pandya 1988) and projects to the supplementary motor cortex (Morecraft & Van Hoesen 1993). The frontal eye field (area 8) projects to the dorsal subdivision (Barbas & Pandya 1989; Arikuni et al 1988). Perhaps the greatest functionally significant difference in connectivity between the two premotor area subdivisions is that the dorsal premotor area receives from the dorsolateral prefrontal cortex, whereas the ventral subdivision receives from the ventrolateral prefrontal cortex (Barbas & Pandya 1989; Lu et al 1994). All of these association connections are likely to be, or are known to be, reciprocal.

Neuronal activity in the premotor cortex in relation to preparation for movement and to movement itself have been extensively studied in recent years (for reviews see Georgopoulos 1991; Kurata 1994). Direction selectivity for movement appears to be a common feature for many neurons. In behavioural tasks, neuronal populations in the dorsal premotor cortex show anticipatory activity and task-related discharge as well as direction selectivity, but little or no stimulus-related changes, related to the retention of visual information (di Pellegrino & Wise 1991). The response properties are modulated by visuospatial attention (di Pellegrino & Wise 1993). A consensus is emerging that the dorsal premotor cortex is important in establishing a motor set or intention, contributing to motor preparation in relation to internally guided movement (Boussaoud & Wise 1993a,b; Kurata 1993). This includes encoding the attributes of intended movement, such as direction and amplitude (Crammond & Kalaska 1994; Kurata 1994), and may extend to a role in the ongoing control of movement (Flament et al 1993). In contrast, ventral premotor cortex is more related to the execution of externally (especially visually) guided movements in relation to a specific external stimulus (Boussaoud & Wise 1993b; Kurata 1993, 1994).

The frontal eye field lies predominantly within Brodmann's area 8, anterior to the superior premotor cortex (**8.244**). It receives its major thalamic projection from the parvocellular mediodorsal nucleus, with additional afferents from the medial pulvinar, the ventro-anterior nucleus and the suprageniculate–limitans complex. It connects with the paracentral nucleus of the intralaminar group (Barbas et al 1991). The thalamocortical pathways to the frontal eye field form part of a pathway from the superior colliculus, the substantia nigra and the dentate nucleus of the cerebellum (Lynch et al 1994). It has extensive ipsilateral corticocortical connections, receiving from several visual areas in the occipital, parietal and temporal lobes including the medial temporal area (V5) and the adjacent areas (Rosa et al 1993), area 7a (Neal et al 1990a) and several occipital visual areas (Van Essen et al 1992). There is also a projection from the superior temporal gyrus, which is auditory rather than visual in function (Deacon 1992). Within the frontal lobe it receives from the ventrolateral (Barbas & Pandya 1989; Deacon 1992) and dorsolateral prefrontal cortex (Barbas & Pandya 1989; Arikuni et al 1988). It projects to the dorsal (Arikuni et al 1988; Barbas & Pandya 1989) and ventral premotor cortex (Arikuni et al 1988), and to the medial motor area, probably to the supplementary eye field adjacent to the supplementary motor area proper (Bates & Goldman-Rakic 1993). It projects prominently to the superior colliculus, to the pontine gaze centre within the pontine reticular formation, and to other oculomotor related nuclei in the brainstem. Other subcortical connections follow the pattern common to the neocortex in general. As its name implies, it is important in the control of eye movements.

The prefrontal cortex on the lateral surface of the hemisphere comprises essentially Brodmann's areas 9, 46 and 45 from superior to inferior (**8.264, 265**). In subhuman primates, two subdivisions of the lateral prefrontal cortex are recognized, a dorsal area equivalent to area 9 and perhaps including the superior part of area 46, and a ventral area, comprising the inferior part of area 46 and area 45. Both the dorsolateral and ventrolateral prefrontal areas receive their major thalamic afferents from the mediodorsal nucleus, with additional contributions from the medial pulvinar and the ventro-anterior nuclei, and from the paracentral nucleus of the anterior intralaminar group (Barbas et al 1991). The dorsolateral area receives long association fibres from the posterior and middle superior temporal gyrus, including auditory association areas (Petrides & Pandya 1988), from parietal area 7a (Neal et al 1990a) and from much of the anteroposterior extent of the cortex in the superior temporal sulcus (Seltzer & Pandya 1989) which, in the present account, has been taken to be the equivalent of the middle temporal cortex. Within the frontal lobe, it receives projections from the frontal pole (area 10) and from the medial prefrontal cortex (area 32) on the medial surface of the hemisphere (Barbas & Pandya 1989). It projects to the supplementary motor area, the dorsal premotor cortex and the frontal eye field (Barbas & Pandya 1989; Lu et al 1994; Bates & Goldman-Rakic 1993; Morecraft & Van Hoesen 1993). All these thalamic and corticocortical connections are reciprocal. Commissural connections are with the homologous area and with the inferior parietal cortex of the opposite side. The ventrolateral prefrontal area receives long association fibres from both area 7a and area 7b of the parietal lobe (Neal et al 1990a), from auditory association areas of the temporal operculum (Petrides & Pandya 1988), from the insula (Pandya & Yeterian 1985) and from the anterior part of the lower bank of the superior temporal sulcus (Seltzer & Pandya 1989). Within the frontal lobe it receives from the anterior orbitofrontal cortex (Barbas & Pandya 1989) and projects to the frontal eye field, and the ventral premotor cortex (Barbas & Pandya 1989; Deacon 1992; Lu et al 1994). It connects

with the contralateral homologous area via the corpus callosum. Once again these connections are probably all reciprocal. Non-thalamic subcortical connections for both the dorsal and ventral areas conform to the general pattern for neocortical connectivity.

The physiological response properties of lateral prefrontal neurons reflect the distribution of long association afferents, with somatic responses concentrated ventrally, response to moving visual stimuli dorsally, oculomotor responses more caudally in both, and other responses more scattered (Tanila et al 1993). The major difference appears to be a segregation of functional contributions to the ordering of motor tasks. The dorsolateral prefrontal cortex is important for spatial processing of afferent information (Wilson et al 1993) and for the organization of self-ordered working memory tasks, including verbal working memory (Petrides et al 1993a,b), whereas the ventrolateral prefrontal cortex is concerned with mnemonic processing of objects (Wilson et al 1993). This is consistent with the projections of the dorsolateral area to the supplementary and dorsal premotor areas, and of the ventrolateral to the ventral premotor area (see above).

The cortex of the frontal pole (area 10) receives its thalamic input from the mediodorsal nucleus, the medial pulvinar and the paracentral nucleus. It is reciprocally connected with the cortex of the temporal pole (Moran et al 1987), the anterior orbitofrontal cortex, and the dorsolateral prefrontal cortex (Barbas & Pandya 1989). Other connections follow the general pattern for the neocortex as a whole. The orbitofrontal cortex connects with the mediodorsal, anteromedial, ventro-anterior, medial pulvinar, paracentral and midline nuclei of the thalamus. Cortical association pathways come from the inferotemporal cortex (Weller & Steele 1992), the anterior superior temporal gyrus (Petrides & Pandya 1988), the temporal pole and the anterior superior temporal sulcus (Seltzer & Pandya 1989). Within the frontal lobe it has connections with the frontal pole, the medial prefrontal cortex, the ventrolateral prefrontal cortex and medial motor areas (Barbas & Pandya 1989; Bates & Goldman-Rakic 1993; Morecraft & Van Hoesen 1993). Commissural and other connections follow the general pattern for all neocortical areas. The medial prefrontal cortex is connected with the mediodorsal, ventro-anterior, anterior medial pulvinar, paracentral, midline and supra-geniculate–limitans nuclei of the thalamus. It receives from cortex in the walls of the superior temporal sulcus anteriorly (Seltzer & Pandya 1989) and from the anterior cortex in the superior temporal gyrus (Petrides & Pandya 1988). Within the frontal lobe, it has connections with the orbitofrontal cortex (Barbas & Pandya 1989), with the medial motor areas (Morecraft & Van Hoesen 1993) and with the dorsolateral prefrontal cortex (Barbas & Pandya 1989). Once again, other connections conform to a general pattern.

Information on the detailed functions of the subregions of the prefrontal cortex are sparse. Evidence from surgical isolation (prefrontal lobotomy) or pathological damage suggests a role in the appreciation or understanding of time, the normal expression of emotions (affect), and the ability to predict the consequences of actions. Both hemispheres interact in these functions, so deficits following unilateral damage may be relatively slight. Medial prefrontal cortex as a whole is important in auditory and visual associations (Gaffan & Harrison 1991), and widespread changes in prefrontal activation are associated with calculating and thinking (Sasaki et al 1994b). Changes in potential, probably primarily in relation to lateral prefrontal cortex are associated with Go/No-Go decision making (Sasaki et al 1993, 1994a). For a detailed and thorough consideration of the organization and functions of the frontal lobe, readers should consult Passingham (1993).

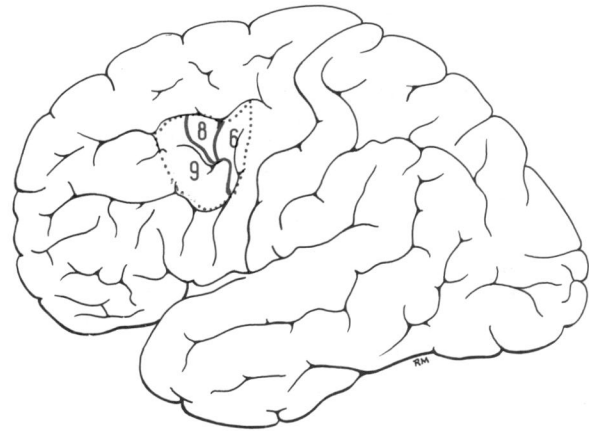

8.265 Superolateral surface of the left cerebral hemisphere showing the frontal motor eye field, corresponding to parts of Brodmann areas 6, 8 and 9. The perimeter of this area is delineated by an interrupted line to indicate uncertainty as to its precise extent.

Neural control of complex movements

Consider the act of reaching and grasping a glass of water, raising it to your lips and drinking. For normal individuals this is a simple exercise, but it can be extremely difficult for brain damaged patients. As individuals, we have very little insight as to how our own motor system generates this sequence of movements, and our understanding of the brain operations involved is still rudimentary. Some progress has been made by trying to construct models of the brain's motor control system.

Some models of motor control envisage the system as carrying out three different processes: the *idea* or *plan* of action, the *programme* required to bring this plan about, and finally, the *execution* of the movement. In our example, the *idea* describes the objective of the movement: acquiring the glass of water. This could be achieved in a variety of ways: with either arm, or even by gripping the glass between the teeth. Thus the idea of the movement is quite general and is not mapped out in terms of specific muscles or joints. It is known that some parts of the brain involved in motor control, such as the posterior parietal lobe of the cerebral cortex, are more concerned with the idea or plan than with issues such as which limb or which set of muscles to use. The concept of a plan for movement predicts that when an action is carried out, then some feature of the plan will be present irrespective of the particular limb or body segments used to perform it. This common plan is assumed to underlie the phenomenon of *equivalence of movement*, by which a movement pattern, e.g. your own signature, is preserved whatever particular effector system you use to write with (Rosenbaum 1991; Rothwell 1994).

The *programme* of the movement must control the entire motor act: once the plan has been adopted then the whole sequence of movements is expressed. The reaching movement might employ the right hand, passing along a straight-line path towards the glass. To programme this movement, it has been proposed that the brain has to solve the *inverse kinematics problem*, calculating the timing and scale of changes in angle of appropriate joints (shoulder, elbow and wrist) that will be needed to make the hand follow the selected path of movement. Once the desired angular changes are specified, how are the muscles to produce them? This is not a trivial problem since the torque that contraction of a muscle exerts at a joint will, in general, also have mechanical influences on remote joints (look at what happens to your wrist during rapid elbow flexion, for example). Thus the solution of this *inverse dynamics problem* is exceedingly complex. The forces and movements resulting from a neural command to contract a given muscle will vary greatly depending, for instance, on the length of the muscle, the speed at which it is shortening, and the contractile state of other muscles acting with it (its synergists) or against it (its antagonists). For this reason, some models of motor control assume that movement proceeds by programming a series of successive approximations to a desired trajectory of movement. One possibility is that the brain defines a series of *equilibrium points* or postures, each of which is fixed by the length–tension curves of the muscles acting at a given joint. The final component of the elements making up the

motor control sequence is the *execution*: activating selected sets of muscles in a manner that will achieve the objective of the programme (Rosenbaum 1991).

There are so many different muscles in the body that the control system could adopt a very large number of possible solutions to achieve the reaching movement required. The adoption of *functional muscle synergies* helps to reduce this 'degrees of freedom' problem. These synergies are a well-recognized and important part of our motor control system; they are used for the co-ordination of activity within a limb (e.g. the contraction of triceps during forearm supination), between limbs (e.g. weight-bearing by one leg during walking) and for the co-ordination of eye, head and body movements. Interestingly, many central motor structures, including the primary motor cortex and cerebellum, appear to have a motor representation that involves control of muscle groups rather than single muscles. All purposeful motor acts involve the contraction of multiple muscles.

The *execution* of all movements, from the simplest reflex to the most highly skilled, must finally employ the 'final common path', the motor neurone and the muscle fibres which it innervates. We can recognize a hierarchical organization in the different parts of the motor system. Mechanisms within the spinal cord and brainstem are concerned with reflex activity; these mechanisms can subserve complex patterns of movement such as locomotion and swallowing. These movements are encoded by activity within specific groups of interneurons and this activity can be modulated by descending motor pathways from the brainstem, midbrain and cerebral cortex (such as the corticospinal tract). Descending pathways exert specific influences over groups of interneurons and motor neurones concerned with trunk, girdle and distal limb (hand or foot) movements. The hierarchy is completed by higher order motor centres, including the cerebellum, basal ganglia and non-primary regions of the cerebral cortex: the latter include the premotor cortex, supplementary motor area and posterior parietal cortex, which are all involved in the preparation and guidance of movement. Measurement of regional cerebral blood flow (by positron emission tomography; PET) suggest that most of the areas mentioned are active in human volunteers performing complex movements (Porter & Lemon 1993; Rothwell 1994).

Damage at different levels of the motor hierarchy causes characteristic changes in movement performance: for instance, patients with damage to the basal ganglia exhibit very slow movements, while those with cerebellar damage show deficits of timing and co-ordination. Damage to the primary motor cortex and its descending

motor pathways often results in the complete loss of skilled hand movements, while characteristic disturbances of head and body posture result from lesions of other descending pathways, such as the vestibulospinal tract. These results can best be interpreted in terms of the site of termination of the different motor pathways described above (Porter & Lemon 1993).

Neurophysiological recordings in experimental animals show that neurons in different parts of the motor system are active before and during movement and that their rate of discharge encodes different parameters of movement, such as force or direction. However, this coding is not sufficiently specific to allow precise control of a given movement parameter by single cells, and it is probable that whole assemblies or populations of neurons co-operate for this purpose. Although particular motor structures are concerned with specific aspects of movement generation and control, a given parameter of movement is represented in many different structures.

The organization of the motor system is characterized by *re-entrant loops*. This means that the output of a particular structure is sent to a number of other regions which process this information and then feed it back, directly and indirectly, to the structure from which it originated. The two most important loops are those involving the cerebral cortex (primary motor and premotor regions) with the cerebellum and basal ganglia (Rothwell 1994). Since there is detectable activity in the brain up to a second before the onset of a voluntary movement, there is time for information to traverse these loops several times over before the final command for output is generated. All this evidence suggests that movement control is a parallel distributed process, with many parts of the motor system processing information simultaneously to produce the final outcome. The distributed nature of this system may explain why damage to the central nervous system rarely causes a permanent loss of a particular motor function; the motor system also has a considerable capacity to reorganize following damage.

An important aspect of motor control is the incorporation of sensory input into the different parts of the idea–programme–execute sequence. Visual and auditory information, and sensory inputs from the eyes, ears and from skin, muscle and joint receptors can characterize the location, size, weight and texture of the object forming the goal of the movement (in our example, the glass of water). While some movements may rely on sensory feedback for their control, others may be driven by a 'feedforward' mechanism — a neural process based entirely on the brain's model of the required movement.

Feedforward mechanisms are evidently more important for rapid movements (in which there is no time for feedback to play any part) or for highly predictable movements, such as saccadic eye movements, where no external loads or disturbances are likely to impede the production of the programmed movement. However, it is important to realize that sensory feedback must be used to create the brain's model of the movement in the first place and this process contributes to the acquisition of new motor skills (Rosenbaum, 1991). Feedback is important for updating the model and for controlling unpredictable or novel movements (e.g. moving underwater). Deafferented patients who have completely normal motor innervation can perform complex movements under visual control, but have great difficulty in doing so.

OTHER AREAS OF CORTEX

The *cingulate cortex* has been considered earlier with the limbic system (see p. 1122). However, a few points about its relationship to the neocortex are worth mentioning here. The cingulate gyrus in relation to the medial surfaces of the frontal lobe contains within it specific motor areas, and has extensive connections with neocortical areas of the frontal lobe. The cingulate gyrus on the medial surface of the parietal lobe has equally extensive connections with somatosensory and visual association areas of the parietal, occipital and temporal lobes. These are predominantly afferents to the cingulate gyrus from neocortical areas on the lateral surface of the hemisphere. Within the cingulate cortex, projections pass predominantly caudally, and ultimately into the posterior parahippocampal gyrus. This system, therefore, presents a second route whereby afferents from widespread areas of association cortex converge, ultimately leading to the medial temporal lobe and hippocampal formation, other than via parallel stepwise routes through cortical areas on the lateral surface.

The *insula* is buried in the floor of the lateral sulcus by the relative expansion of the frontal, parietal and temporal lobes (8.215, 216B, 266). It is separated from the frontoparietal operculum by the superior limiting sulcus and from the temporal operculum by the inferior limiting sulcus. Posteriorly, where these two sulci meet, is the caudal limit of the insula. Together these two sulci are known as the circular sulcus (of Reill). The anterior margin, the limen insulae, blends into the orbitofrontal cortex, with no clear boundary. The structure, connections and functions have been recently reviewed (Mesulam & Mufson 1985), and many of the connections with other cortical areas have been mentioned earlier. Only a brief summary will be given here (see Mesulam & Mufson 1985 for references). Cytoarchitectonically, three zones are recognized: anteriorly and extending caudally into the central insula, the cortex is agranular;

surrounding this is a belt of cortex called dysgranular, in which laminae II and III can be recognized; finally, a surrounding zone, extending to the caudal limit of the insula, is homotypical cortex, referred to as granular. Thalamic afferents to the insula come from subdivisions of the ventroposterior nucleus and of the medial geniculate body, from the oral and medial parts of the pulvinar, the suprageniculate nucleus limitans complex, the mediodorsal nucleus and nuclei of the intralaminar and midline groups. The topographic distribution of these connections is not clear, but it seems that the anterior (agranular) cortex is connected predominantly with the mediodorsal and ventroposterior nuclei, and the posterior (granular) cortex predominantly with the pulvinar and the ventroposterior nuclei. The other nuclear groups mentioned appear to connect with all areas. Ipsilateral cortical connections of the insula are diverse. Somatosensory connections are with SI, SII and surrounding areas, area 5 of the superior parietal lobe and area 7b of the inferior parietal lobe. The somatosensory nature of the granular insular cortex has been discussed earlier (see parietal lobe above), but later stages of this pathway, notably area 7b, are connected with the caudal dysgranular area of the insula. These areas of the insula cortex, the granular and dysgranular cortex posteriorly also have connections with the orbitofrontal cortex. Several auditory regions in the temporal lobe interconnect with the insula, both the posterior granular insula and the dysgranular cortex more anteriorly. Connections with visual areas are virtually absent, except for a small input to the agranular and adjacent dysgranular cortex from the medial inferior temporal cortex. The sensory association functions of the insula in the somatic sensory and auditory pathways clearly require considerable further elucidation. At least for the somatosensory pathway, areas in the insula appear to be key waystations in the discriminative-touch pathway passing via SII (see above). It is possible, though far from certain, that a similar second auditory association pathway, other than that passing into the superior temporal lobe, might also crucially involve parts of the insula (see above, Temporal lobe). The anterior agranular cortex of the insula appears to have connections primarily with olfactory, limbic and paralimbic structures, including most prominently, the amygdala. Information on the functions of the insula in man are sparse. The somatosensory functions of the posterior part are clearly present in man (Burton et al 1993), and anterior insular cortex appears to have a role in olfaction and taste (see Mesulam & Mufson 1985 for references). The posterior regions of the insula have also been implicated in language functions, which might accord well with the possibility that higher order auditory association pathways may pass via areas in the insula (see above, Temporal lobe).

GENERAL CONCLUSIONS

Drawing general conclusions about the organization of the cerebral cortex from diverse observations is at best hazardous. It is particularly dangerous to extract simple concepts from what must, by its very nature, be the most complex and least comprehensible of organs. However, it is possible, having reviewed recent years' progress in understanding, to draw some broad conclusions and abstract some general proposals which might at least stimulate the urgent desire in some students to challenge overbold and simplistic statements. It is a dichotomy that only by summary and simplification at the expense of detail do concepts become accessible, yet only by examination of the detail are inconsistencies recognized and new and better concepts developed.

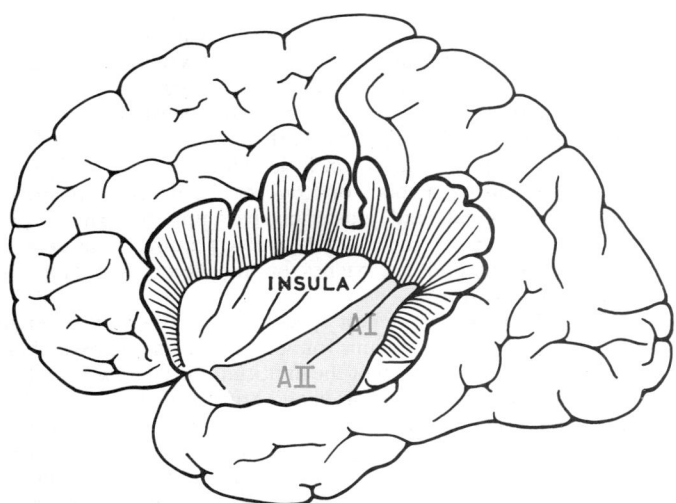

8.266 Superolateral surface of the left cerebral hemisphere from which the opercula have been cut away to expose the insula and the adjoining anterior and posterior transverse temporal gyri and their continuity with the superior temporal gyrus. The area shown in blue contains the classic acoustic area, AI (equal to Brodmann area 41 and parts of areas 42 and 52) and the secondary acoustic area, AII (extending into area 22).

The original suggestion (Jones & Powell 1970) of a stepwise, hierarchical progression of cortical sensory processing, from primary areas via association areas towards the medial temporal lobe, has proved to be an oversimplification. Multiple pathways in parallel issue from the sensory areas to surrounding regions, where subsets of functional processing occur. This being said, the principle of a feedforward, progressive outflow, now via multiple routes, to the temporal lobe and then to parahippocampal gyrus remains. Indeed, the very definition of feedforward or feedback connections rests on the existence of such a hierarchical progression of pathways through association areas. In what way should this important conceptual description of convergent sensory pathways be modified in the light of newer information? The sensory pathways with initial recipient zones within neocortex, i.e. somatosensory, visual and auditory modalities, share certain features in common. In each there is a koniocortical, heavily thalamo-recipient zone which has few or no feedforward corticocortical afferents, which has minimal or no connections with frontal cortex and which contains a well characterized point-to-point representation of the sensorium. These are area 3b for the somatosensory pathway, area 17 for the visual pathway and AI (area 41) for the auditory pathway. Each of these is surrounded by areas which share a representative organization and an, albeit lesser, thalamic input from the same nucleus or nuclei, and to which the first area projects in a point-to-point feedforward manner. Using terminology common in the discussion of auditory areas, these might be called the core areas; for the auditory pathway, they are AI, R and RT, for the somatic sensory, areas 3, 1 and 2 and for the visual V1, V2 and the V3 complex (see above). From these 'core' areas the pathways diverge, largely speaking, into two streams of onward projections. In the visual system these have been termed the dorsal and ventral pathways, but the separation may not be geographically the same (i.e. dorsal and ventral) when one considers the other two sensory modalities. For the purpose of the present discussion, let us coin the terms 'self-relevant' and 'stimulus-relevant' to distinguish the two. In the former, stimulus information relevant to the body is transmitted. In the visual system, this becomes movement of the stimulus in relation to self (or of self in relation to the stimulus) and is the major component of the so-called dorsal stream. In the somatosensory system, this would relate to stimuli arising from self, for example, joint position sense or the detection of body movement passing via a superior parietal pathway. In the auditory system, the distinction is less clear (and may not exist), but one could postulate localization of sound as one such egocentric parameter. This is probably too simplistic, and perhaps one could speculate that egocentrically relevant sound patterns, such as speech, would be relevant to such an 'associative stream'. The auditory equivalent of the dorsal visual pathway, the self-relevant route, would be postulated to pass into the insula. The stimulus-relevant pathways would, in such a scheme, concentrate on the analysis of the specific features of a stimulus (feature extraction) without reference to self. In the somatosensory system, this would be form and texture of cutaneous stimuli, and would be proposed to pass through SII and on to the insular somatosensory area(s). In the visual pathway, contour, colour, texture and shape perception are mediated by the ventral pathway through V4 and the inferior temporal cortex. Once again, analogies in the auditory system are less clear, but 'chasing the hare', this route would be predicted to be related to frequency analysis and combination, and to pass through the auditory 'belt' areas to auditory related superior temporal cortex. One might speculate that music would, for example, present a non-self-relevant stimulus of this type, requiring stimulus-relevant processing.

The self-relevant pathways converge on middle temporal cortex, in the depths of the superior temporal sulcus of monkeys, where separate but overlapping modality related zones exist, as they must, since self-orientated analysis of the surrounding world requires, a priori, fairly rapid distillation of signals from the separate sensory systems. Within the stimulus-relevant pathways, discriminative and recognition processes occur. Intermodality convergence is less important than stimulus identification and so is delayed. The two pathways reconverge in two centres, the temporal pole and the medial temporal parahippocampal cortex. Even the most loosely worded of functional descriptions of this stage of cortical processing are likely to prove damagingly irrelevant, but clearly memory is one such probable function, as is, perhaps, significance interpretation,

i.e. the relating of stimulus features to self in a meaningful way. Schematic diagrams of the proposed generalized pathways are shown in **8.256**.

It hardly needs stating that the dual pathways described, even if they truly exist, cannot be independent. Stimulus-relevant features are not unimportant to self, any more than self-relevant features are insignificant in the comprehension of a stimulus. Therefore, predictably, there is considerable cross-talk (anatomical interconnection) between the proposed pathways. At the same time, like navigating a route using a detailed map, it is necessary, perhaps, to identify the best itinerary to achieve a given goal or destination, though several possible routes might exist, and circumstance could easily alter one's choice. To stretch the analogy, the reader should compare the detailed and unquestionably correct route map for visual processing offered by Van Essen et al (1992) with the simpler, and undoubtedly oversimplified, itineraries offered by others (Menigan & Maunsell 1993).

Having summarily discussed three cortical lobes (parietal, occipital and temporal) is it possible to introduce the frontal lobe into the proposed scheme? The second strand of the Jones and Powell (1970) sensory convergence hypothesis was that each successive step in the hierarchical post-Rolandic stream of connections was linked to an equivalent area in the frontal lobe.

Once again, this has proved to be an oversimplification, and a more complex hierarchical and parallel set of processing streams can be postulated, with at one extreme the orbitofrontal cortex, linked to medial temporal paralimbic cortex and, at the other, the motor cortex linked to the primary somatosensory cortex, SI. The principal direction of flow of processing is assumed to be towards the motor cortex. The orbitofrontal cortex projects to the frontal pole and to the medial prefrontal cortex. These in turn project to the ventrolateral and dorsolateral prefrontal cortex respectively, which in turn feed into the two subdivisions of the premotor cortex, and so reconverge on to the motor cortex. There is therefore a dorsomedial stream via medial prefrontal, dorsolateral prefrontal and dorsal premotor cortex, and a ventral stream via the frontal pole, the ventrolateral prefrontal and the ventral premotor cortex reconverging on the motor cortex as the final step. These may be analogous to the proposed self-relevant and stimulus-relevant pathways in the posterior (post-Rolandic) association areas, with the first interconnecting stepwise with the dorsomedial frontal stream and the second relating stepwise to the anteroventral pathway. In general, the long association pathways conform to this relationship, at least to some extent, with successive self-relevant areas connected with more anterior dorsomedial frontal regions, and successive stimulus-relevant areas connected with more anterior anteroventral frontal regions. The dorsomedial frontal pathway is thus an internally-generated (self-relevant) route, and the anteroventral an externally-generated (stimulus-relevant) pathway for action.

A third frontal stream of connections exists, via the medial motor area, including the supplementary motor cortex and surrounding motor zones. This is more closely related to the dorsolateral pathway than to the anteroventral. Is there an analogous third parallel tier in the sensory processing streams of the parietal, occipital and temporal lobes? It is tempting to suggest, on little evidence, that it might be in the form of sensory association connections with the posterior cingulate, retrosplenial and posterior parahippocampal cortex. Proper consideration of such a suggestion requires considerable further investigation and encroaches on the description and discussion of limbic pathways.

The above discussion is at best speculative, and a very different view of parallel processing streams for action is given by Passingham (1993). However, consideration of the multitudinous pathways within the neocortex and between the cortex and other structures is fruitless without equal consideration of the functional role of such pathways. This requires extra weight to be given to some connections, and less specific functional significance attributed to others. In anatomical terms, this can be relatively simple where clear differences in origin and termination are defined, as in feedforward and feedback connections in sensory association pathways. However, many association connections are of intermediate type, with mixed origins from infragranular and supragranular pyramidal cells and terminations through supragranular laminae, but avoiding layer IV. These 'intermediate' pathways may predominate in connections between the frontal lobe and the postRolandic sensory association areas, although all types of connection have been described. In the absence of such a clear categorization, the selection of predominant direction of processing, or choice of predominant pathway, becomes almost impossible. Three approaches may offer hope of future understanding. The study of simpler systems, where understanding is not so confounded by complexity, may elicit rules for functional processing in neuronal networks that elucidate fundamental principles still at work in the mammalian brain (Heiligenberg 1991). Similarly, theoretical approaches to unravelling the basis of functional neuronal networks and the processes which govern connectivity may shed welcome light on the neuroanatomical maze which is sometimes encountered (Young 1993a; Griffin 1994). Finally, functional neuroimaging holds out the hope of deciphering the distributed systems operational both temporally and spatially in the brain during specific events, either of perception or action, in the human brain.

Imaging and computerized visualization of the brain

Imaging modalities

For many years conventional X-rays provided the only widely available technique for imaging the interior of the body. The X-rays emanate from a small focal spot in a conical beam which passes through the patient and casts a 2-dimensional (2-D) shadow of the 3-dimensional (3-D) structures. Interpretation of the 3-D anatomy is difficult, and information in images obtained from more than one viewpoint must be combined if the 3-D location of structures is to be deduced. For sparse structures such as blood vessels filled with contrast medium during an angiogram this can be achieved with two images if the viewpoints are favourable.

Conventional X-ray imaging of the head has been supplemented and indeed largely superseded in the past 20 years by tomographic techniques which have revolutionized the imaging of the skull and brain (Raichle 1994). With X-ray computerized tomography (CT), a thin collimated X-ray beam is shone through the patient and the intensity of the beam emerging at the far side is measured by a detector positioned in line with the beam. The emitter/detector pair is rotated around the long axis of the patient and a large number of readings of X-ray intensity are obtained. From these an image in the plane of the rotation is reconstructed by computer processing. Brain tissue, cerebrospinal fluid (CSF), air and bone can be discriminated in these well known tomographic images. Multiple adjacent slices are obtained and this allows a 3-D data set to be built up. The excellent contrast between bone and the other tissues allows good 3-D reconstructions of the skull to be obtained with minimal user interaction (8.267).

During the same period, other imaging modalities have developed, each with advantages and disadvantages. Ultrasound is attenuated by the dense bone of the skull, although Doppler signals from the basal cerebral arteries can be obtained through the thinner temporal bone. Certain gamma- and positron-emitting isotopes which can be injected into the living body accumulate in the brain in sufficient concentration to be localized by external radiation detectors. With traditional isotope brain scanning, a 2-D emission image is obtained by a gamma

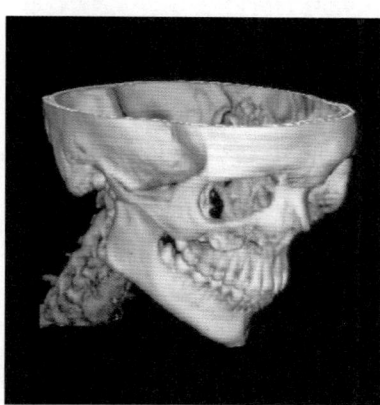

8.267 Computer-generated surface view of the skull of a patient studied with X-ray CT head scanning. A patient with abnormal skull development underwent a high resolution, clinically standard CT head scan. A simple threshold was used to extract the bone tissue, which has high intensity values in CT, and was then 'rendered' to show the surface from a chosen viewpoint. This figure illustrates what can currently be achieved with routinely acquired data and minimal user interaction (rendering routine: UMDS Guy's Campus Dept of Neurology).

camera, but tomographic techniques are now increasingly used for gamma imaging and are usually referred to as single photon emission computed tomography (SPECT). Positron emission tomography (PET) is much more technically demanding and expensive and this has restricted its use, but available positron-emitting isotopes include ^{15}O, ^{11}C and ^{18}F, which can be incorporated into a wide variety of molecules. Physiological indices including regional cerebral blood flow, blood volume, metabolic rate, and the distribution of different receptors can all be measured. The readings can be localized to within a 5–10 mm cube of brain and the results displayed as a 'functional' image. Activation of specific brain areas can be shown by comparing images obtained during a task (such as viewing an alternating checker-board pattern on a screen) with those obtained in a control state. PET is thus a modality for functional rather than structural imaging. An import-

ant body of information about localization of brain activation in humans has been obtained using PET; figure **8.268** is an example which shows maps of changes in local brain blood flow in the normal human brain during the processing of words (Peterson et al 1988). The four lateral views of the human brain shown in **8.268** are averages of the brain activities of nine normal subjects. The receptive components of language—seeing a written word or hearing it—activate the regions of the brain shown in the upper two images. The expressive components of language and the mental activity associated with this activate the regions shown in the lower two images in **8.268**. The availability of PET is increasing as its cost is reducing, but recent developments in magnetic resonance imaging (MRI) (see below) may provide an alternative method of functional imaging which could have higher spatial and temporal resolution and avoid ionizing radiation altogether.

Of all the imaging modalities, it is MRI that has made the greatest impact on imaging the brain. The subject lies in a very strong magnetic field and radio wave pulses are transmitted through the subject; this stimulates hydrogen atoms within the patient to emit a radio signal of their own and from this signal it is possible to reconstruct an image. The data may be acquired as a sequence of 2-D slices (as with X-ray CT) or directly as a 3-D volume. There are several parameters which can be adjusted, and can have an important effect on the resulting image. The techniques are evolving rapidly, leading to improved spatial, temporal and contrast resolution. Good contrast between brain tissue and CSF, and between grey and white matter within the brain, can be obtained. With appropriate selection of parameters, the pial surface of the brain can be seen within sulci as well as on the superficial aspect of the brain. The anatomy of the basal ganglia is shown well. Nuclei within the brainstem or within the thalamus cannot be resolved with current techniques. The radiation and field strengths currently used are believed to be harmless to humans and multiple repeated MRI studies can be carried out on healthy volunteers as well as patients and cadavers.

A number of special modifications of

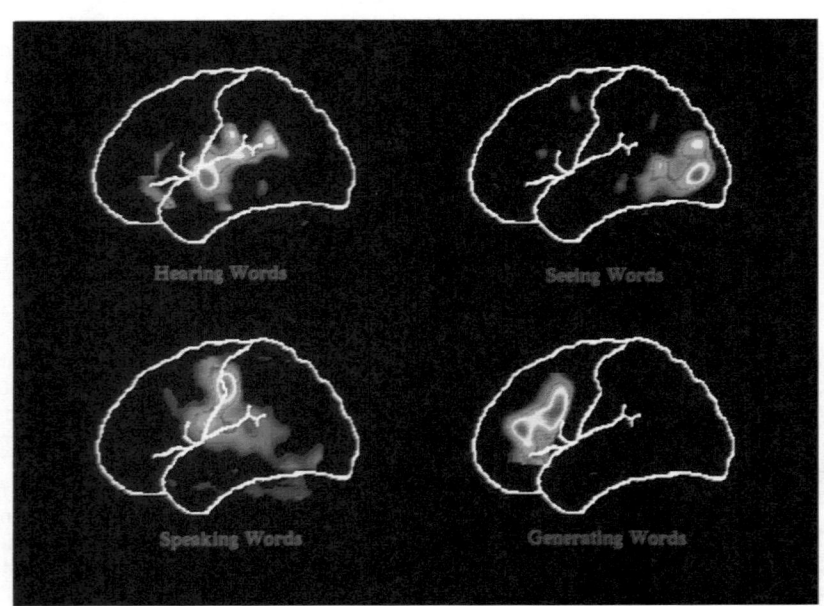

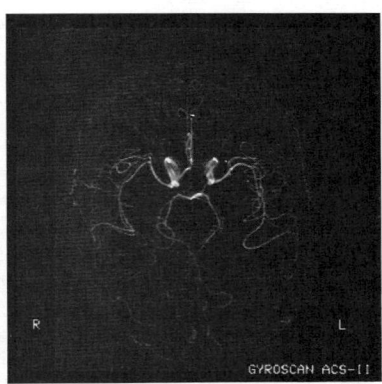

8.268 Functional imaging using PET in a normal volunteer while seeing words, hearing words, speaking words and generating words. Top left: temporal and temporo-patietal cortex active while hearing a list of nouns being spoken. Top right: primary visual cortex and association cortex active while reading nouns presented on a screen. The control scans, obtained while the subject merely looked at the blank screen, have been subtracted. Bottom left: in addition to hearing or seeing nouns, as in the upper images, the subject had to say them out loud. The image shown is the result of subtracting the visual or auditory activation scans, revealing some of the additional brain areas activated during speaking. Bottom right: the antero-inferior frontal cortex becomes active during mental operations such as consciously analysing the meaning of a word. The subjects were asked to respond to seen or heard words (common English nouns) with the first appropriate verb or action word that came to mind (for example, the word *hammer* might elicit the response *hit*). The visual and auditory activity that occurred when the subjects read or heard the words as well as the motor system activity resulting from responding have been subtracted away. (Reproduced by permission of Professor Raichle, Washington University, St Louis.)

8.269 Magnetic resonance (MR) angiography in a patient. This was obtained in a patient from a 10-minute MR scan without the injection of any contrast medium. A simple threshold was used to extract the vessels, which are the main structures to produce a high signal with this type of scan. This view is termed a 'maximum intensity projection', as if the user is looking through a fixed slab of tissue and only seeing the brightest feature along each line of sight. Despite the apparent high quality of this picture, rendered views showing the surface of the threadlike vessels draw attention to noise and discontinuities in the vessel image, and are not at present used routinely for MR angiography. This figure illustrates the state-of-the-art in routine MR angiography.

the basic MRI imaging technique are under development for different applications. The MRI signal can be made sensitive to moving fluid and can be tuned to arterial or venous blood velocities making it possible to obtain MRI angiograms of cerebral vessels down to about 2 mm or even 1 mm in diameter (8.269). Methods for quantitative vascular measurements, as opposed to simple imaging, have limitations but are improving steadily. In individual large vessels, satisfactory blood flow velocity measurements can be made, but geometric measurements (vessel calibre) are unreliable and, where detailed demonstration of vessel structure is required, X-ray angiography remains the technique of choice. With different selection of parameters, total CSF volume can be measured or low-velocity CSF motion can be imaged. Another class of motion-sensitizing MRI techniques which may become important for the imaging of brain anatomy is referred to as diffusion weighted imaging. The signal obtained within white matter is influenced by the predominant direction of nerve fibres, so that major tracts may be distinguished where they are adjacent

to fibres running in different directions. Image quality is currently poor, but these techniques are in their infancy. Degenerating fibre tracts may also be detected by alteration in their signal both anterograde and retrograde to a lesion.

A further exciting development in MRI has emerged recently. The MRI signal can be made sensitive to changes which take place in blood flow during activation, and, as with PET, functional images can be obtained which show neurologically active areas.

Visualization of 3-D images

The fundamental difficulties of depicting 3-D anatomical structure are essentially the same for morbid anatomy and for medical imaging. Serial slices, whether obtained from physically cut tissue (microscopic or macroscopic) or from imaging (CT or MRI), have traditionally been viewed as a sequence and then mentally reconstructed into a stack, allowing the observer to imagine the 3-D surface and internal structure of organs. Explicit reconstruction of the surface appearance of 3-D structures can also be carried out by an artist or using computers. The com-

puter techniques have advanced rapidly and principles are outlined below.

In order to generate a realistic view of the surface of an object from a specific viewpoint, a method for identifying the location of the surface of the structures of interest in each slice has to be established. The process of identifying objects and their boundaries in images is referred to as segmentation. In the case of identifying bone on CT scan images, as in 8.267, this is straightforward: all picture elements (pixels) where the CT intensity is above a certain threshold can be labelled as bone, and all those below as non-bone. MR angiograms can be segmented by thresholding in the same way (8.270). However, for most other tissues some more elaborate segmentation is required. This may be an entirely manual process, or an initial approximation computer segmentation may be edited. Until recently, an experienced observer had to outline selected boundaries slice by slice for accurate results. For a large data set, this was a very time-consuming process. Advances in computer segmentation techniques can dramatically reduce the amount of human interaction required. An example, using a technique developed at UMDS (Guy's Hospital) in London, is shown in **8.270**. The computer initially analysed the image and stored a large list of objects of different sizes together with their boundaries. The same algorithm is used for all types of images: for this initial processing no special adjustments (e.g. setting of thresholds) were used. The user then interacted with the computer and was able to select and identify the boundaries of the chosen object (the lateral ventricle) with just three 'mouse' clicks, within a few seconds.

Computer-assisted segmentation was also used by a group at the University of Hamburg to segment MRI of a complete cadaver brain. A large number of structures were outlined and stored to form a digital brain atlas. The atlas can be used by a non-expert, for example, a medical student, in several ways. Displays like those in **8.271A, B** can be pre-stored or created by a user who can construct a display by selecting from various options, including the objects to be displayed, magnification, colours, text labels, cut planes

etc. Only after these choices have been made can the process of constructing the final screen image take place.

Medical image acquisition systems, data transfer and storage methods, and computer processing techniques including segmentation and synthesis of displays, are all evolving rapidly. The methods are increasingly used in clinical decision making and also have an important role in teaching and research for revealing the neuroanatomy of healthy volunteers, patients and cadavers.

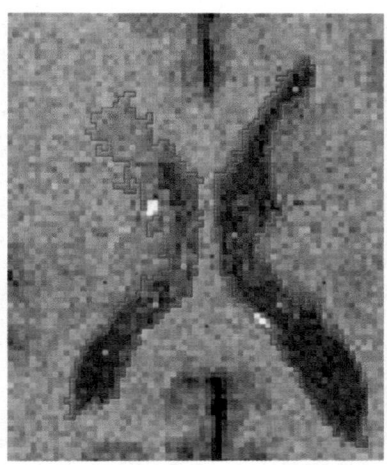

8.270 Computer-assisted segmentation of a transaxial MR slice through the brain of a patient. Initial fully automatic processing by computer was followed by very simple user interaction (just three mouse-button clicks) to select from the initial computer segmentation the object (lateral ventrical) of current interest. The computer boundary is overlaid in red on the MR image.

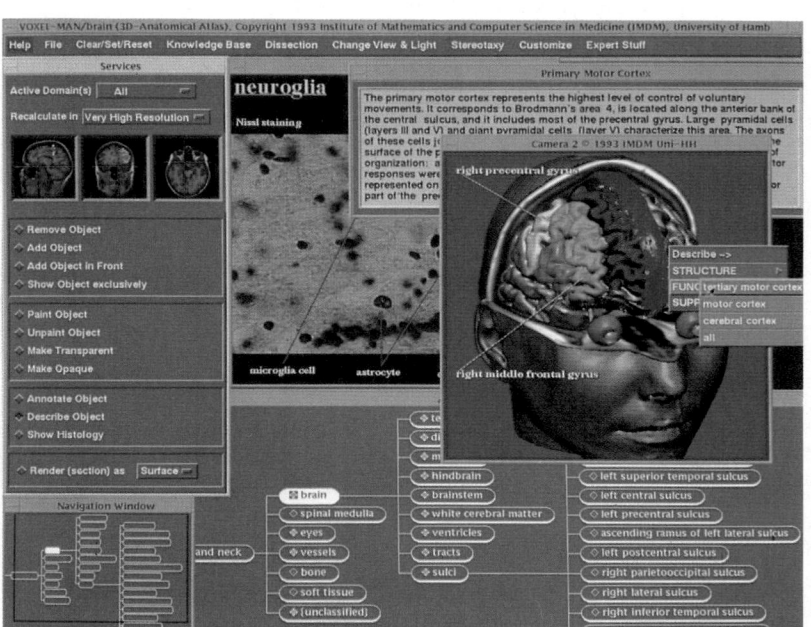

8.271 Composite view synthesized by the user from the 3-D digital atlas 'Voxel Man' derived from MR images of a cadaver. This represents the state-of-the-art that is achievable with high resolution MR of a cadaver and lengthy manual segmentation. With the pre-segmented atlas already stored in a computer workstation, user interaction and subsequent computer processing needed to generate a view of this complexity is still time consuming. Top: combination of surface and cut away views help to reveal complex 3-D relationships. Bottom: other types of information about selected structures, e.g. microscopic images or physiological data, can be summoned using 'hypermedia' techniques and viewed at the same time as anatomical images. (Reproduced by permission of Professor K-H Höhne, University of Hamburg.)

Electrical activity of the brain

The electroencephalogram (EEG) provides a recording of the electrical activity of the brain from electrodes attached to the scalp. The signals which appear on the scalp arise from the extraneuronal currents associated with neuronal activity which are strong enough to generate magnetic fields detectable by gradiometers situated outside the skull. This provides an alternative method of recording the brain's

electrical activity, the magnetoencephalogram (MEG).

The waveforms of the EEG and MEG vary in both amplitude and frequency as a function of cerebral activity and changing levels of arousal. Many different 'rhythms' have been described (Buser 1987), which appear during various behavioural states and have different distributions over the brain. Four major

frequency bands (**8.272**) are recognized:

(1) *Beta activity* is a waveform with a frequency >13 Hz normally present during alert wakefulness, intense cognitive activity, and rapid eye movement (REM) sleep when the individual is presumed to be dreaming. It is sometimes referred to as beta rhythm though the oscillations are seldom regular. Its amplitude is usually less than $10 \mu V$ and is maximal over frontal areas of the cerebral cortex.

(2) *Alpha rhythm* is the predominant

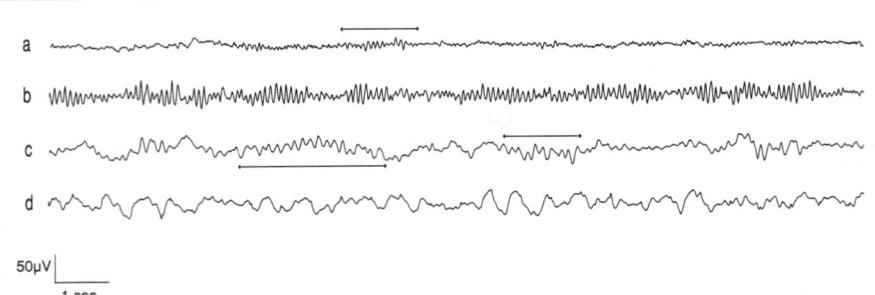

8.272   Rhythmic activity in the EEG (a) beta activity, and a burst of low amplitude alpha rhythm (arrowed); (b) spindles (bursts) of alpha rhythm at 10.5 Hz; (c) periods of· theta rhythm at 6.3 Hz (arrowed) amid delta waves in a patient with subarachnoid haemorrhage; (d) delta waves at about 1.5 Hz in coma due to traumatic brain injury.

waveform of relaxed wakefulness and reaches its greatest amplitude when the eyes are closed. It is defined as a rhythmic oscillation of 8–12 Hz but is usually close to 10 Hz in healthy adults. Its amplitude (up to 50 μV) is maximal over occipital areas. Opening the eyes results in 'alpha blocking', and beta activity takes its place. A homologous *mu rhythm* appears over the somatosensory and motor cortex and blocks during voluntary movement. A similar effect can be obtained over the auditory cortex in response to auditory stimulation.

(3) *Theta rhythm* is defined as activity between 4 and 7 Hz. Normally, it does not occur as a continuous oscillation in the EEG though individual waves appear in the early stages of falling asleep.

(4) In deep sleep the EEG is dominated by irregular slow waves (1–3 Hz) of high amplitude referred to as *delta rhythm*.

The amplitude of the EEG increases and its frequency decreases as the level of arousal falls, but this is not a true continuum. The alpha rhythm, for example, may persist during mental activity and even increase in amplitude during selective attention and cognitive processes (Ray & Cole 1985). It has a remarkably stable frequency which does not vary with the intensity of mental activity.

In epilepsy, encephalitis, encephalopathies and other neurological disorders the EEG may show abnormal waveforms including spikes, slow waves and complexes which have diagnostic and localizing significance.

Anatomical generators of the EEG

The membrane phenomena, which form the basis of neuronal activity, give rise to ion currents whose circuits are completed through the extracellular volume conductor. The density of these currents diminishes rapidly with distance from their origin. The principal generator of the electrical signals which reach the scalp is therefore the cerebral cortex; the contribution of deeper structures is at least an order of magnitude smaller.

The voltage detected by an electrode on the scalp represents the average of signals originating in neurons distributed over a considerable area of the underlying cortex, weighted in favour of the closest. Alpha and delta rhythms are therefore believed to reflect the operation of synchronous rhythmic discharges of large numbers of neurons in the cortex. The low amplitude and high frequency of beta activity is the result of neurons firing more independently during mental activity.

Postsynaptic potentials on the soma of pyramidal cells are thought to be the principal source of the scalp EEG (Creutzfeld et al 1966). Both the magnitude of dendritic currents is believed to be too small to contribute significantly to voltages at the scalp, and the ionic events associated with propagation of action potentials are too brief (Thatcher & John 1977). Periods of sustained neuronal activity result in the accumulation of extracellular potassium, an effect which may be amplified by glia (Speckmann & Elger 1987), and contribute to the slow potentials of the EEG which accompany sustained mental activity (McCallum 1988).

The cells with axes and extraneuronal currents oriented at right angles to the surface of the brain contribute most to the EEG. Those oriented parallel to the surface of the brain, at right angles to the axis of the gradiometer contribute most to the MEG. The EEG is therefore influenced chiefly by cells in the gyri, while the MEG detects mainly the activity of cells in sulci. For this reason the MEG and EEG may detect rather different signals from the same area of brain.

Arousal and thalamocortical mechanisms of cortical synchrony

Bursts of activity at 6–10 Hz, termed spindles, appear in the early stages of normal sleep and during low levels of barbiturate anaesthesia. These synchronous discharges of cortical neurons are under the control of thalamic oscillators which act as pacemakers. Thalamocortical relay cells appear to function in two modes. During

the waking state, they relay action potentials from specific afferents in a manner which codes sensory input or feedback from subcortical systems. In a second mode of operation, the same cells deliver bursts of action potentials which synchronize the discharge of the cortical neurons to produce a rhythmic waveform in the EEG and the cortex is deprived of inputs from specific afferents. The oscillatory behaviour of the thalamocortical relay cells is produced by a circuit which involves interneurons local to the thalamocortical relay neurons as well as cells in the reticular nucleus of the thalamus (Lopes da Silva 1991). Feedback to the thalamus from the cerebral cortex and modulation of the excitability of elements of this circuit by projections from the brainstem determine whether the discharges in the cortex occur as spindles, alpha rhythm or delta rhythm (Steriade et al 1993).

The projections from the brainstem are also responsible for switching the system between the waking mode, in which afferents reach the cerebral cortex through the thalamic relay, and the drowsy or sleeping mode, in which the cortex receives rhythmic discharges instead (Monizz & Magoun 1949). The pathways from the brainstem correspond to the physiologically identified reticular activating system (Lindsley et al 1950; Rogawski & Aghajanian 1980), and include cholinergic fibres from the ventral tegmentum and basal forebrain as well as noradrenergic axons from the locus coeruleus and serotonergic axons from the raphe nuclei. The noradrenergic fibres appear to enhance transmission of information via specific afferents in the waking state (Rogawski & Aghajanian 1980), while the cholinergic and serotonergic pathways modulate discharges in the oscillatory mode (Steriade et al 1993). The cholinergic inputs from the tegmentum have a particular role in preventing the oscillatory discharges to enable dreaming to take place in REM sleep (Webster & Jones 1988) although the thalamocortical relays remain closed to specific afferents.

The binding problem

Different stimulus features of a sensory input are processed in parallel in anatomically separate areas of the brain. In the visual system, for example, cells which respond to wavelength, orientation and movement are clustered in separate groups within areas V1 and V2. They project to different supplementary areas in occipital, posterior parietal and inferotemporal cortex where colour, form, orientation and movement are further analysed separately. This raises the question of how the perception of a stimulus retains its unity. How do we know that the movement, redness and round shape of the approaching ball are related if they are detected by anatomically separate systems? This is known as the binding problem.

It has been observed in animals that neurons which process the same sensory input in different regions of cerebral cortex discharge in a highly correlated fashion at frequencies between 30 and 70 Hz (Engel et al 1992). Oscillation in this frequency band can be seen in the MEG in humans (Tesche & Hari 1993). The rhythms alter little with the level of arousal or the physical characteristics of the stimulus. The correlated discharges have been interpreted as evidence for temporal coding of the association between stimulus features processed at different cortical locations (Engel et al 1992) (**8.274**).

Evoked Potentials

Large populations of nerve cells contribute to the signals recorded at the individual EEG electrodes and the MEG gradiometers. Since all areas of the brain are electrically active all the time, the activity of particular anatomical systems cannot normally be distinguished in the realtime EEG or MEG. For example, in recordings from occipital regions, the responses of the visual cortex to flashes of light or patterned stimuli are obscured by ongoing alpha and beta rhythms. However, the electrical waveforms evoked by specific sensory stimuli or which accompany cognitive and motor activity can be discriminated from this 'noise' by using computational techniques such as a signal averaging. The waveforms, known as evoked potentials (EPs) or event related potentials, have made it possible to study the neuronal activity of individual sensory systems, the motor cortex and associated areas non-invasively in man.

The earliest inflections in the waveform of EPs can be detected milliseconds after a stimulus and arise from the first relays in the sensory pathway. Thus the brainstem auditory evoked potential to click stimuli consists of a series of waves generated in the cochlear, cochlea nucleus, the lateral lemniscus and midbrain. Homologous potentials are generated in the visual and somaesthetic pathways. The arrival of afferent volleys at the primary sensory and supplementary areas of the cerebral cortex gives rise to medium latency (20–150 msec) inflections, sometimes known as the 'exogenous' components of the EP. The amplitude and waveform of these components are stimulus dependent and reflect the early stages of automatic processing in the cortex. They are followed by long latency 'endogenous' components such as the contingent negative variation, P300 (a positive wave with a latency of about 300 msec), N400 and mis-match negativity whose occurance is a function of cognitive processes such as attention, expectancy, and semantic analysis. A slow wave known as the bereitschaftspotential is generated in the region of supplementary motor cortex in the moments preceding voluntary movement.

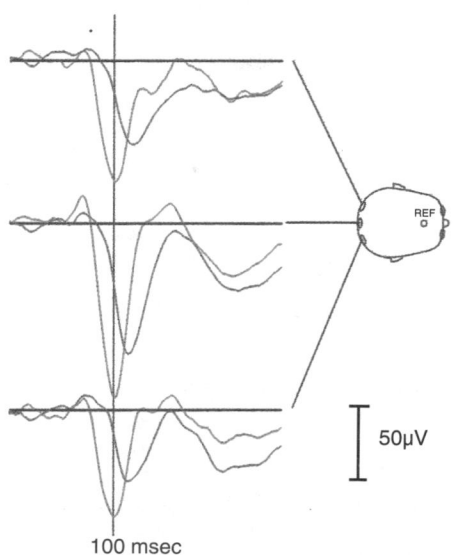

8.273 Visual evoked potentials to stimulation of the right eye (green trace) and left eye (red trace) reveal damage in the visual pathway. The stimulus, a black and white checkerboard pattern, is presented at the beginning of the trace. The response of the cerebral cortex to stimulation of the normal right eye peaks at a latency of 100 msec. Demylination in the left optic tract has delayed the response to stimulation of the left eye.

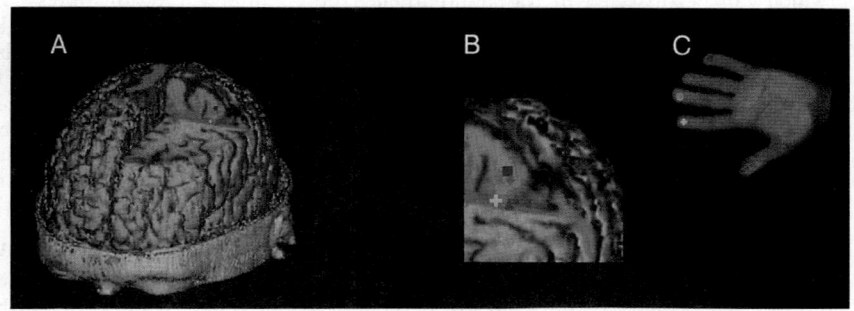

8.274 The location of the digits of the hand in the somatosensory cortex. Stimulation of each digit gives rise to an electrical response in the cortex which is detected by magnetoencephalography. Its location is calculated and superimposed on a three-dimensional magnetic resonance image (MRI) of the subject's brain (A and B) using colour key in C. The procedure reveals the somatotopic organization of this cortex. (From Mogilner et al, with permission.)

The high temporal resolution of EPs finds important clinical applications in the measurement of neuronal conduction times. For example, **8.273** shows the visual evoked potential at the occipital scalp (computed from the EEG) in a patient with demyelination in one optic nerve. The impairment in conduction is clearly revealed by the delayed cortical response evoked by stimulation of this eye. For reviews of the EP phenomena and their clinical applications the reader is referred to Chiappa (1989) and Halliday (1993).

The anatomical source of evoked potentials can be computed from measurements of their topography at the scalp (Henderson et al 1975; Scherg et al 1990). However, the path of extraneuronal currents is distorted and attenuated by the high resistance of the skull. The magnetic field of magnetic currents within the brain is not affected in this way. MEG therefore promises to yield more precise information than the EEG about the location of electrical activity within the brain (Wiskwo et al 1993). Figure **8.274** illustrates the high spatial resolution with which the somatosensory cortex can be non-invasively mapped with MEG (Moligner et al 1993). This type of functional imaging is potentially an important tool in areas such as neurosurgery where it may be used to map abnormalities such as epeleptic foci which are to be removed and normal tissue which must be spared. In practice, its place among alternative and perhaps complementary imaging techniques such as positron emission tomography, echoplanar magnetic resonance imaging and magnetic resonance spectroscopy has still to be established.

NERVE FASCICLES OF THE CEREBRUM

In a hemisphere sliced horizontally about 1.25 cm above the corpus callosum, the central white substance appears as an oval area surrounded by a narrow, much folded lamina of grey matter and studded by red *puncta vasculosa* due to the escape of blood from divided vessels. Transected at the level of the corpus callosum, there is continuity of white matter of the two sides, containing nerve fibres of varying size described according to their course and connections, as:

- *association* (arcuate) *fibres* connecting different cortical areas in the same hemisphere; some are collaterals of the projection and commissural fibres but most are main axons
- *projection fibres*, connecting the cerebral cortex with the corpus striatum, diencephalon, brainstem and the spinal cord in both directions.
- *commissural fibres*, linking corresponding or *homotopic* loci and *heterotopic* loci in both hemispheres

Association (arcuate) fibres

Association (arcuate) fibres (**8.186**A, B), confined to one hemisphere and all ipsilateral, are grouped as *short*, connecting adjacent gyri, or *long*, connecting more widely separated gyri. The details of many association pathways appear with their cortical areas.

Short arcuate fibres may be entirely intracortical but many pass subcortically between adjacent gyri, some merely from one wall of a sulcus to the other. They are very numerous and easily, but crudely, displayed by blunt dissection in fixed brain tissue.

Long arcuate fibres are grouped, somewhat indistinctly, into bundles which can be dissected in formalin-hardened brains after removal of the cortex and subjacent short arcuate fibres. Fibres in each fasciculus vary in length, the longest usually being deepest. Concerning the connections of these bundles little information is available; they are difficult to follow by histological technique and any form of dissection reveals only the crudest details. The following large fasciculi can usually be distinguished: the uncinate fasciculus, the cingulum, the superior longitudinal fasciculus, the inferior longitudinal fasciculus, the fronto-occipital fasciculus.

- The *uncinate fasciculus* connects the motor speech area and orbital gyri of the frontal lobe with the cortex in the temporal pole; the fibres follow a sharply curved course across the stem of the lateral sulcus. They are near the antero-inferior part of the insula (**8.275**, **276**).
- The *cingulum*, a long, curved fasciculus starting in the medial cortex below the rostrum, then lies in the gyrus cinguli and follows its curve. Inferiorly it enters the parahippocampal gyrus and spreads into the adjoining temporal lobe. From its convexity fibres enter and leave in groups, giving it a spiked irregular appearance when dissected.
- The *superior longitudinal fasciculus*, largest of the arcuate bundles, commences in the anterior frontal region and arches back above the insular area and lateral to the massive cortical projection fibres of the internal capsule (corona radiata, see below). Contributing fibres to the occipital cortex (areas 18 and 19), it curves down and forwards behind the insular area to spread out in the temporal lobe. Like other long fasciculi, fibres leave and join it throughout its extent but it is impossible to determine the precise connections by gross methods (**8.276**); even with the modern techniques of fibre tracing little progress has yet been made in this field.
- The *inferior longitudinal fasciculus* commences near the occipital pole, its fibres derived perhaps mostly from areas 18 and 19. They sweep forwards, separated from the lateral ventricle's posterior cornu by the optic radiation and commissural tapetal fibres and, after being crossed by the superior longitudinal fasciculus, are then distributed throughout the temporal lobe.
- The *fronto-occipital fasciculus* starts from the frontal pole, passing back deep to the superior longitudinal fasciculus but separated from it by the projection fibres in the corona radiata (see below). It is lateral to the caudate nucleus and therefore near the central part of the lateral ventricle. Posteriorly it fans out into the occipital and temporal lobes, lateral to the posterior and inferior ventricular cornua and the criss-crossing fibres of the tapetum.

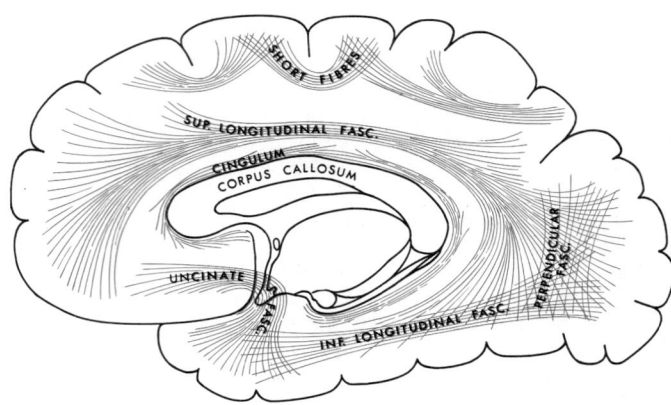

8.275 The principal arcuate (association) fibres in the cerebrum.

Accurate knowledge of association fibres can only be established by experimental methods not yet applied to most cortical regions. Studies of visual areas (Le Gros Clark 1941, Zeki 1970, 1974) and the main somatosensory areas (SmI) (see Jones & Powell 1968) suggest a high degree of specificity in such connections.

Projection fibres

Projection fibres connect the cerebral cortex with lower levels in the brain and spinal cord; they are *corticofugal* and *corticopetal*. Projection fibres converge from all directions to the corpus striatum (**8.277**), mostly (but not exclusively) medial to association fibres, and intersect commissural fibres of the corpus callosum and anterior commissure. At the periphery of the corpus striatum, they form the *corona radiata*; its medial aspect is, however, separated from the lateral ventricle by the fronto-occipital fasciculus and its lateral aspect covered by the superior longitudinal fasciculus. It is continuous with the internal capsule, a curved zone including almost all the projection fibres (see below).

Internal capsule

In horizontal cerebral section the internal capsule is seen as a broad white band, with a lateral concavity adapted to the convex medial aspect of the lentiform nucleus (**8.278–283**). It has an anterior limb, genu, posterior limb, retrolentiform and sublentiform parts. Both limbs are, of course, medial to the lentiform nucleus; medial to the anterior limb is the head of the caudate nucleus and medial to the posterior limb the thalamus. Fibres of the capsule continue to converge as they descend, the frontal fibres tending to pass posteromedially, temporal and occipital fibres anterolaterally. At a lower lentiform level, they are crossed by the optic tract and enter the midbrain, many (but not all) of the corticofugal fibres lying in the crus cerebri, where the frontal fibres are medially placed while temporal, parietal and occipital fibres are laterally situated.

The *anterior limb* contains *frontopontine fibres*, from the cortex in the frontal lobe, which synapse with cells in the nuclei pontis and the axons of which enter the opposite cerebellar hemisphere. Anterior thalamic radiations interconnect the medial and anterior thalamic nuclei and various hypothalamic nuclei and limbic structures with the frontal cortex.

The *genu* is usually regarded as containing *corticonuclear* fibres mainly from area 4 and terminating in the largely contralateral motor nuclei of cranial nerves. Anterior fibres of the superior thalamic radiation, between the thalamus and cortex, also extend into the genu.

The *posterior limb* includes the *corticospinal tract* in scattered bundles, the fibres concerned with the upper limb being anterior and followed by those for the trunk and lower limbs. This location of corticospinal fibres anterior in the posterior limb has been accepted since the observations of Charcot (1883) and Déjerine and Déjerine-Klumpke (1901); but more evidence from stereotactic lesions in man suggests that these fibres are posterior in the posterior limb. The evidence has been reviewed by Smith (1967) and Hanaway and Young (1977). Other descending fibres include the frontopontine,

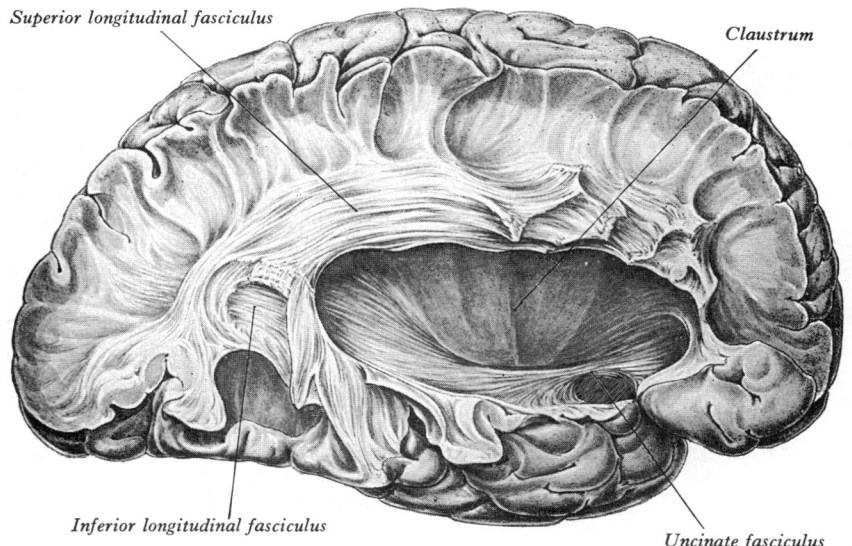

Superior longitudinal fasciculus

Claustrum

Inferior longitudinal fasciculus

Uncinate fasciculus

8.276 A dissection showing some of the long arcuate fasciculi of the right cerebral hemisphere.

particularly from areas 4 and 6, *corticorubral* fibres from the frontal lobe to the red nucleus and fibres from the globus pallidus in the subthalamic fasciculus. Most of the posterior limb also contains fibres of the superior thalamic radiation (the somaesthetic radiation) ascending to the postcentral gyrus.

In the *retrolentiform part* are the *parietopontine, occipitopontine, occipitocollicular* and *occipitotectal* and also the *posterior thalamic radiation*, including the optic radiation, and interconnections between the occipital and parietal lobes and caudal parts of the thalamus, especially the pulvinar.

The *optic radiation* arises in the lateral geniculate body and sweeps back in the concavity between central and inferior cornual parts of the lateral ventricle, intimately related to the superolateral aspect of the ventricle's inferior cornu and the lateral aspect of the posterior cornu, separated from it by the tapetum.

The *sublentiform part* contains *temporopontine* and some parieto-pontine fibres, the *acoustic radiation* from the medial geniculate body to the superior temporal and transverse temporal gyri (areas 41 and 42) and a few fibres connecting the thalamus with the temporal lobe and insula. Fibres of the acoustic radiation sweep anterolaterally below and behind the lentiform nucleus to reach the cortex.

Connections between cortex and thalamus are detailed on page 1082 et seq, corticohypothalamic connections on page 1094 and corticostriate connections on page 1086. Corticoreticular connections, corticonuclear fibres to all varieties of sensory integrating and relay nuclei in the brainstem and spinal laminae are mentioned throughout the text at numerous points. All the foregoing have reciprocal projections but their internal capsular location, in man, is as yet conjectural.

Corpus callosum

The corpus callosum is the major transverse commissure connecting

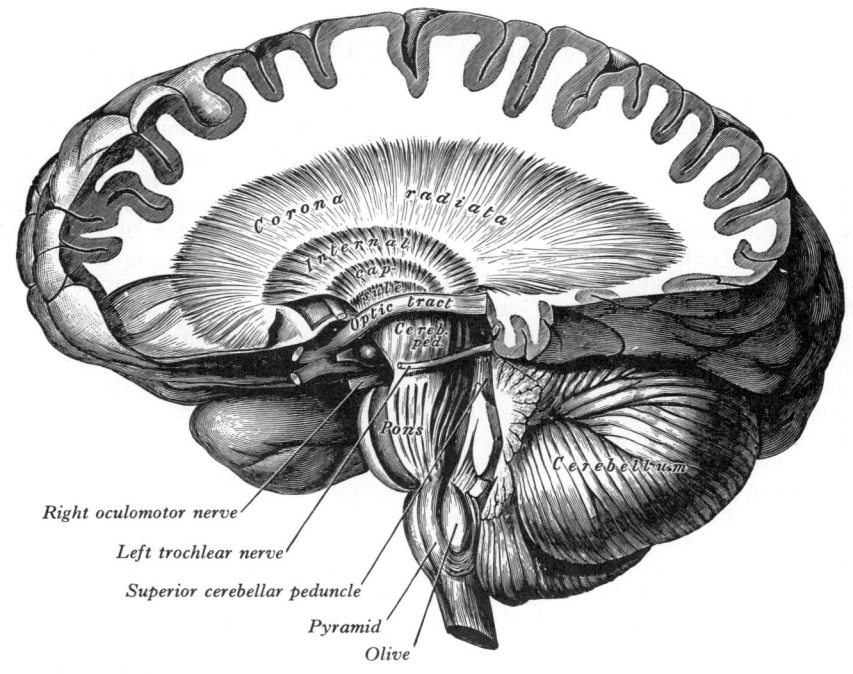

Corona radiata

Internal cap.

Optic tract

Cereb. ped.

Pons

Cerebellum

Right oculomotor nerve

Left trochlear nerve

Superior cerebellar peduncle

Pyramid

Olive

8.277 A dissection showing the convergence of cortical projection fibres through the corona radiata into the cerebral peduncle and pons.

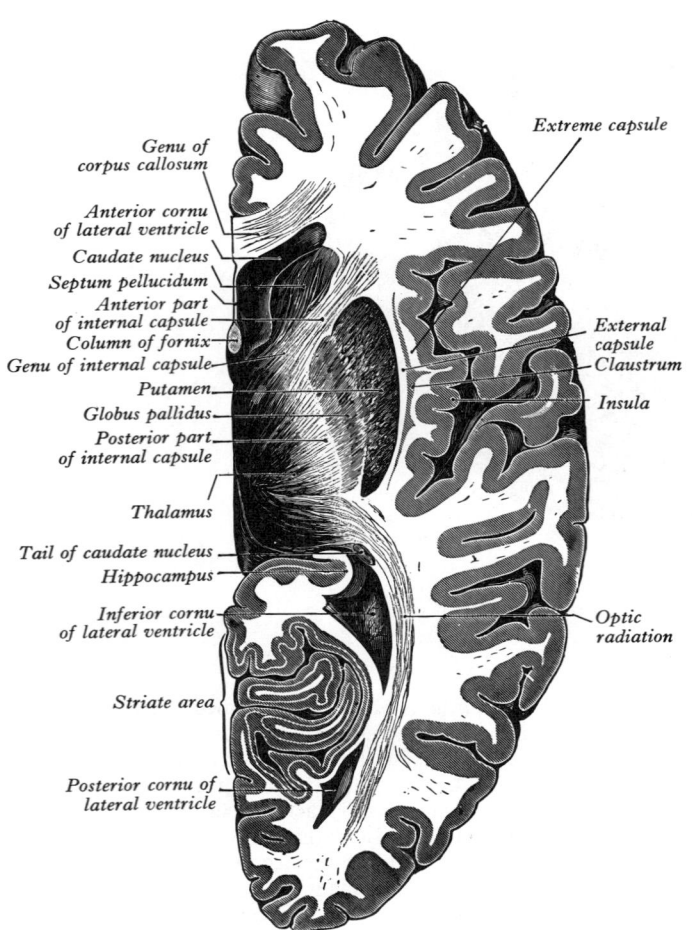

Genu of
corpus callosum

Anterior cornu
of lateral ventricle

Caudate nucleus

Septum pellucidum

Anterior part
of internal capsule

Column of fornix

Genu of internal capsule

Putamen

Globus pallidus

Posterior part
of internal capsule

Thalamus

Tail of caudate nucleus

Hippocampus

Inferior cornu
of lateral ventricle

Striate area

Posterior cornu of
lateral ventricle

Extreme capsule

External
capsule

Claustrum

Insula

Optic
radiation

8.278 Superior aspect of a horizontal section through the right cerebral hemisphere.

the cerebral hemispheres; it incidentally roofs in the lateral ventricles. Its mammalian development is proportional to the surface area and volume of the neocortex; it is maximal in human brains (Rakic & Yakovlev 1968). Its position and size is well appreciated in median sections (**8**.85, 202A, B, 224, 225). It forms an arch about 10 cm in length, its anterior end being about 4 cm from the frontal poles and its posterior end about 6 cm from the occipital poles. The *genu*, its anterior end, recurves posteroinferiorly in front of the septum pellucidum, then diminishes rapidly in thickness and is prolonged posteriorly to the upper end of the lamina terminalis as the *rostrum*. The *trunk* arches back and is convex above, ending posteriorly in the expanded *splenium*, its thickest part.

The superior surface of the callosal trunk (**8**.284) is covered by the *indusium griseum*, extending anteriorly around the genu, then on the inferior aspect of the rostrum, to continue into the paraterminal gyrus; in it are narrow longitudinal bundles of fibres, two on each side, the medial and lateral longitudinal striae (p. 1120); posteriorly the indusium griseum is continuous with the dentate gyrus and hippocampus through the gyrus fasciolaris (**8**.285).

In the median region the trunk is the floor of the great longitudinal fissure, where it is related to anterior cerebral vessels and lower border of the falx cerebri, which may contact it behind. On each side the trunk is overlapped by the gyrus cinguli, separated by the callosal sulcus. Its inferior surface is concave in its long axis but convex transversely. The septum pellucidum is attached to it anteriorly to an extent depending on septal length and disposition of the fornix (**8**.202). Posteriorly it is fused with the fornix and its commissure. On each side its inferior surface roofs the lateral ventricle (**8**.281, and **7**.198), covered by ependyma.

The genu connects the trunk to the rostrum. Its anterior surface, related to the anterior cerebral vessels, is covered by the indusium griseum and longitudinal striae. To its posterior surface the median

septum pellucidum is attached; on each side it is the *anterior* wall of the lateral ventricle's anterior cornu.

The rostrum connects the genu and lamina terminalis; its superior surface is attached to the septum pellucidum and, on each side, forms part of the narrow floor of the lateral ventricle's anterior cornu (**8**.224, 225). On its inferior surface the indusium griseum and longitudinal striae pass back to the paraterminal gyrus.

The splenium overhangs the posterior ends of the thalami, the pineal gland and tectum but is separated from them by several structures. On each side the crus of the fornix and gyrus fasciolaris (**8**.285) curve up to the splenium; the crus continues forwards on the *inferior* surface of the callosal trunk but the gyrus fasciolaris skirts above the splenium, then rapidly diminishing into the indusium griseum. The tela choroidea of the third ventricle advances below the splenium through the transverse fissure, the internal cerebral veins emerging between its two layers to form the great cerebral vein. Above, the splenium is covered by the commencing indusium griseum and is related to the falx cerebri with the inferior sagittal sinus and to the cingulate gyrus on each side of it. Posteriorly the splenium is near the tentorium cerebelli, great cerebral vein and the beginning of the straight sinus.

Nerve fibres of the corpus callosum radiate into the white core of each hemisphere, dispersing to the cerebral cortex. Commissural fibres forming the rostrum extend laterally **below** the ventricular anterior cornua, connecting the orbital surfaces of the frontal lobes; fibres in the genu curve **forwards** to connect the lateral and medial surfaces of the frontal lobes, as the *forceps minor*; fibres of the trunk pass laterally across (intersecting with) the projection fibres of the corona radiata (**8**.201, 277), connecting wide neocortical areas of the hemispheres. Fibres of the trunk and splenium which form the roof and lateral wall of the posterior cornu and the lateral wall of the inferior cornu constitute the *tapetum* (p. 1205). The remaining fibres of the splenium curve back medially into the occipital lobes as the *forceps major*, which bulges into the *medial* wall of the posterior cornu as a curved *bulb of the posterior horn*.

Despite its size and the enormous number of its commissural fibres, limited information is available concerning the precise functional roles of the corpus callosum, apart from the obvious inference that it links the hemispheres, perhaps to ensure that they act as an entity (however, see below). The total of its fibres is unknown in man, but in cats there are 700 000 in each square millimetre (Myers 1959). A detailed analysis of callosal connections is lacking for many regions; but initial investigations have been made in the visual area (Zeki 1970, 1974) and postcentral gyrus (Jones & Powell 1969). In somatic sensory areas (SmI and SmII) connections are limited to the same contralateral area, but right and left loci concerned with the hand and foot appear to lack commissural connection. These views have been strongly confirmed and amplified (Dr T P S Powell, Oxford, personal communication 1983): 'there is considerable experimental evidence, and from use of modern techniques, that there are no callosal connections between the cortex containing the representations of the distal limbs. These conclusions are based not only from a correlation of the experimental anatomical work with the maps of the representations from the evoked potential states but also from a correlation of anatomical tracing and microelectrode recording in the same animal. Not only is this so for the somatosensory cortex in the postcentral gyrus but it is also true for the motor cortex and area 4 in the precentral gyrus.

'It is totally definite that the callosal connections between the visual cortex of the two hemispheres connect only representations of the vertical meridian of the retina (or visual field). The callosal connections are restricted to narrow bands of cortex, each only 1–2 mm wide, precisely at the boundaries between the different visual areas of the occipital lobe. There is such a band at the boundary between area 17, the primary visual cortex and the adjoining area 18, and also bands between the other three or four visual areas that have been identified in the prestriate cortex. It is probably true to say that the regions of cortex connected are related to the very narrow middle region of the retina within which the ganglion cells are now known to send axons which branch and send a branch into the optic tract of both sides.' Commissural linkages are considered highly specific, both associating the 'corresponding' columnar cortical units in bilateral functions, in addition to heterotopic loci.

A congenital absence of corpus callosum is rare, usually found at

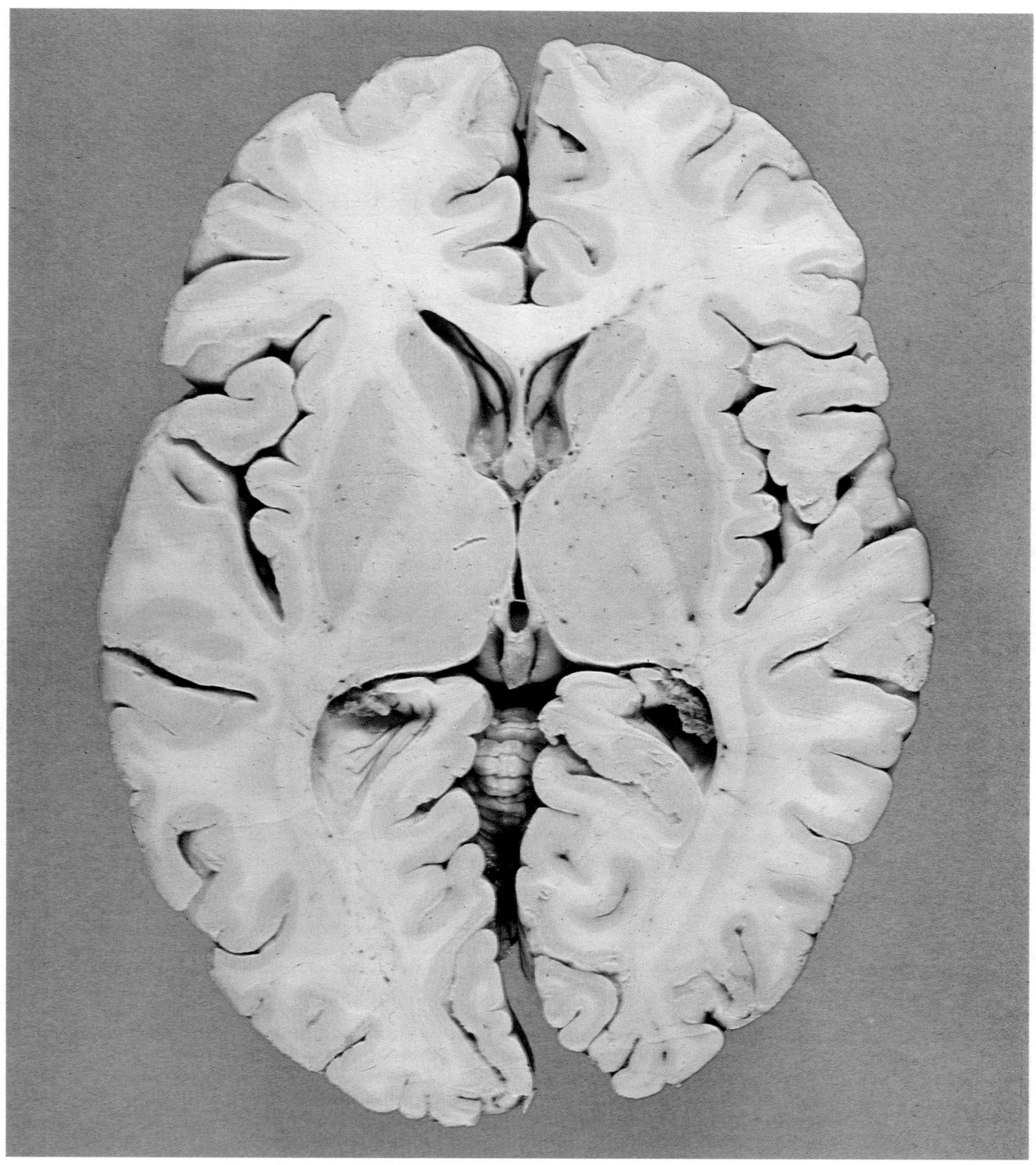

8.279 A horizontal section through the brain including the frontal and occipital poles of the cerebral hemispheres. Features appearing in this section are discussed at many points throughout the text. For appropriate labelling compare with **8.278**. (Dissection by E L Rees, photography by Kevin Fitzpatrick, both of the Department of Anatomy, Guy's Hospital Medical School, London.)

autopsy, and the clinical history lacks diagnostic features (Unterharnscheidt et al 1968). In recent decades large parts, and in some cases all of the corpus callosum, have been divided with apparently little disturbance of function. Nevertheless, the accumulated experience of the results of brain damage (Milner 1974), especially to the temporal lobe and corpus callosum, experimental studies of commissurotomized cats (Butler 1966) and chimpanzees (cerebral asymmetry) and particularly the studies of Sperry (see

below for references) on the effects of the division of the human corpus callosum—all this evidence has not only illumined the function of this great commissure in the transfer of information (including memorized data) across the midline of the cerebrum but has also confirmed a long-suspected asymmetry of function, leading to a concept of 'dominance' usually by the left hemisphere. This has become a major arena of cerebral research. Though it is impossible even to survey here the profuse and even prolix literature recorded

1179

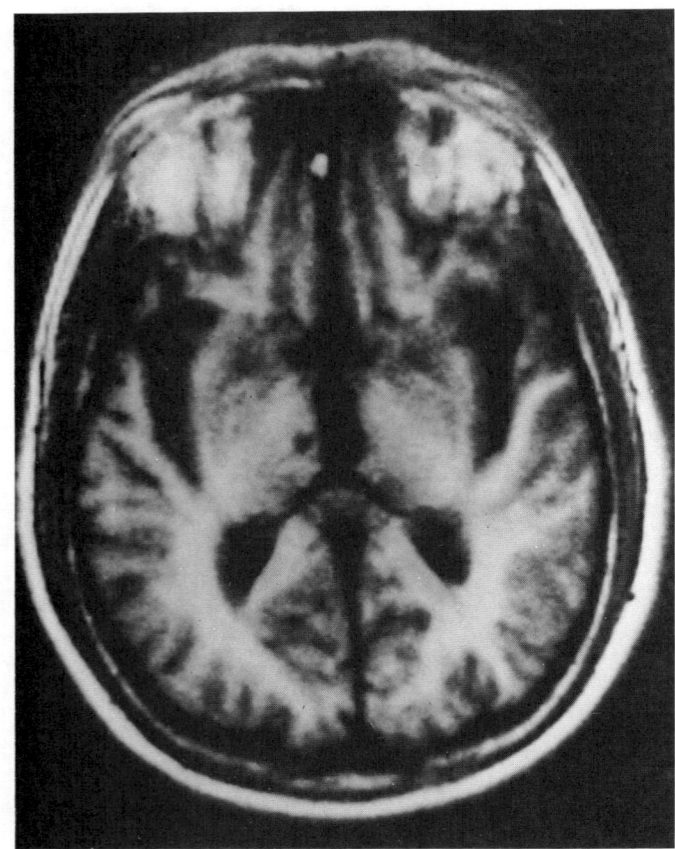

8.280A Horizontal magnetic resonance scan of the head at the level of the third ventricle. Supplied by Philips Medical Systems; photography by Sarah Smith.

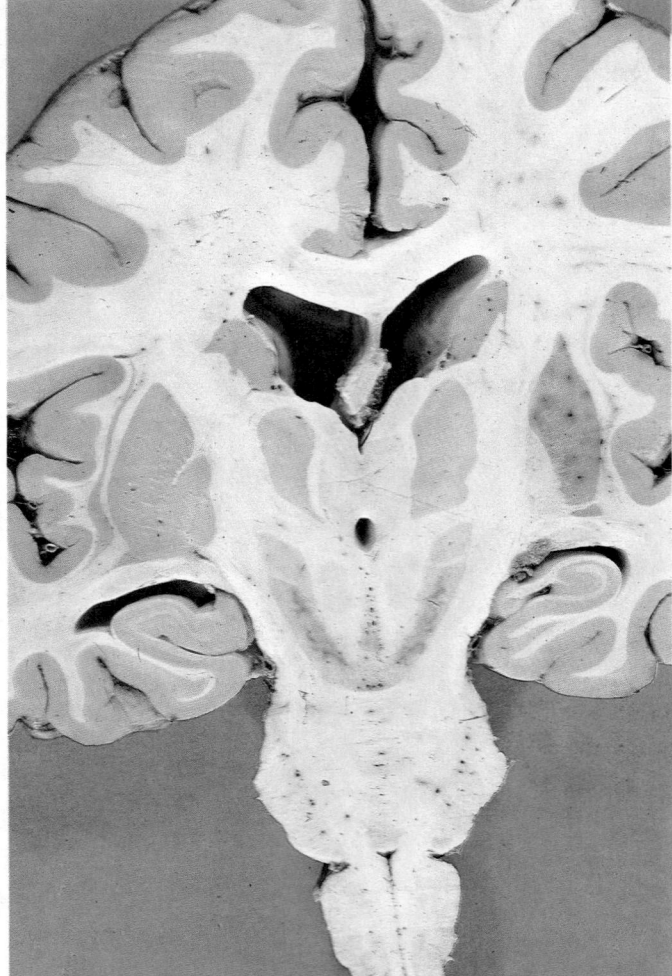

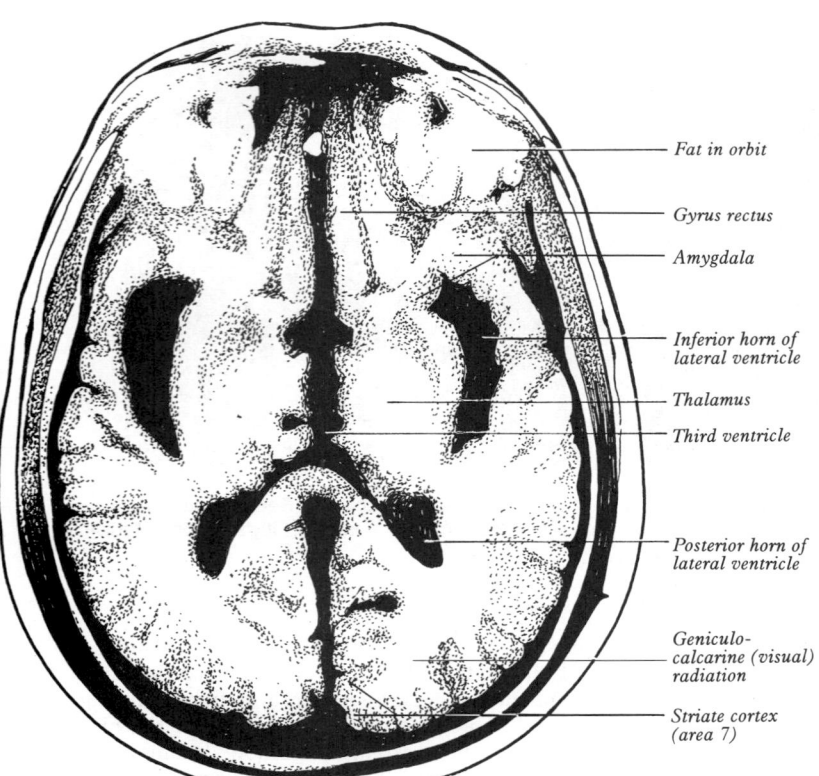

Fat in orbit

Gyrus rectus

Amygdala

Inferior horn of lateral ventricle

Thalamus

Third ventricle

Posterior horn of lateral ventricle

Geniculo-calcarine (visual) radiation

Striate cortex (area 7)

8.281 The central area of the ventral part of the oblique coronal section of the brain shown in **8.**190, photographed at higher magnification to show some structural features in greater detail; compare with **8.**199 for appropriate labelling. Note in particular: (1) the anterior, medial and lateral parts of the dorsal thalamus, separated by the internal medullary laminae; (2) the relation of the caudate nucleus to the anterior and inferior cornua of the lateral ventricle; (3) the lentiform nucleus, divided into an external putamen and an internal globus pallidus; the latter again divided into internal and external parts; (4) the internal capsule, external capsule, claustrum, extreme capsule and insular cortex; (5) the sectioned profiles of the subthalamic and red nuclei and the substantia nigra; (6) the hippocampus projecting into the floor of the inferior cornu of the lateral ventricle. Other structural features on this section are discussed at many points throughout the text. Compare also with **8.**279. (Dissection by E L Rees, photography by Kevin Fitzpatrick, both of the Department of Anatomy, Guy's Hospital Medical School, London.)

8.282 (Facing page; top.) Horizontal computed tomogram through the head at the level of the orbits and middle ears. (Kindly supplied by Dr Shaun Gallagher, Guy's Hospital; photography by Miss Sarah Smith.)

8.283 (Facing page; bottom.) Diagram of the main components of the internal capsule. Descending motor fibres are shown in yellow, corticofugal fibres to the thalamus and pons, etc. in red and ascending fibres in blue. From Strong & Elwyn's *Human Neuroanatomy* and Kretschmann (1988). However, see also in text references concerning alternative views about the position of the corticospinal and other fibres.

by clinicians, experimenters (anatomical and physiological), psychologists, behaviourists and others, references to major contributions will enable the interested reader to enlarge his knowledge elsewhere. Other commissural fibres include those of the posterior (dorsal) commissure (p. 1094); the anterior commissure (p. 1136); and the commissure of the fornix (p. 1129), and the optic chiasma (p. 1087).

8.280B Diagram of **8.**280A. Illustration: J Halstead.

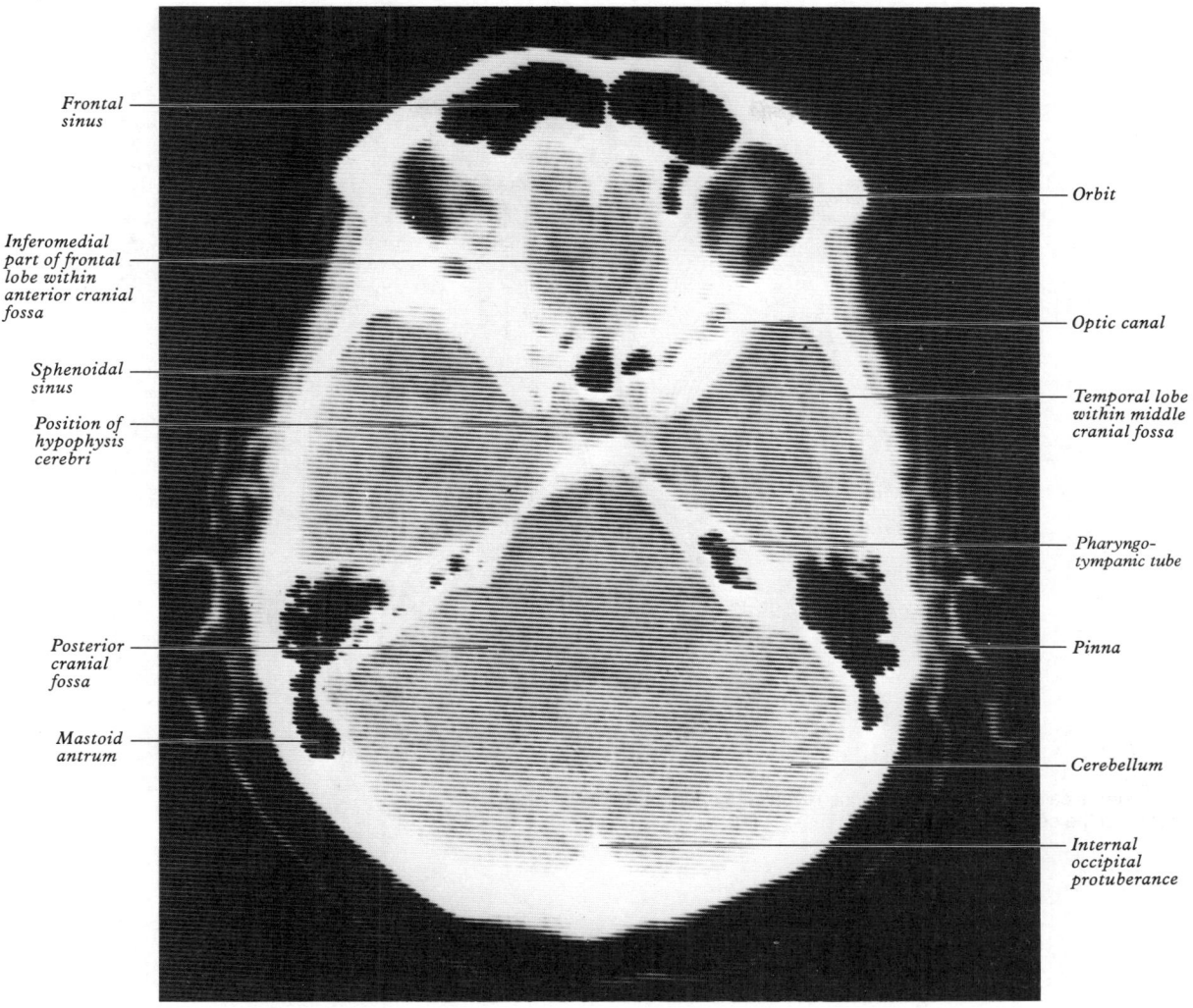

Frontal sinus

Inferomedial part of frontal lobe within anterior cranial fossa

Sphenoidal sinus

Position of hypophysis cerebri

Posterior cranial fossa

Mastoid antrum

Orbit

Optic canal

Temporal lobe within middle cranial fossa

Pharyngo-tympanic tube

Pinna

Cerebellum

Internal occipital protuberance

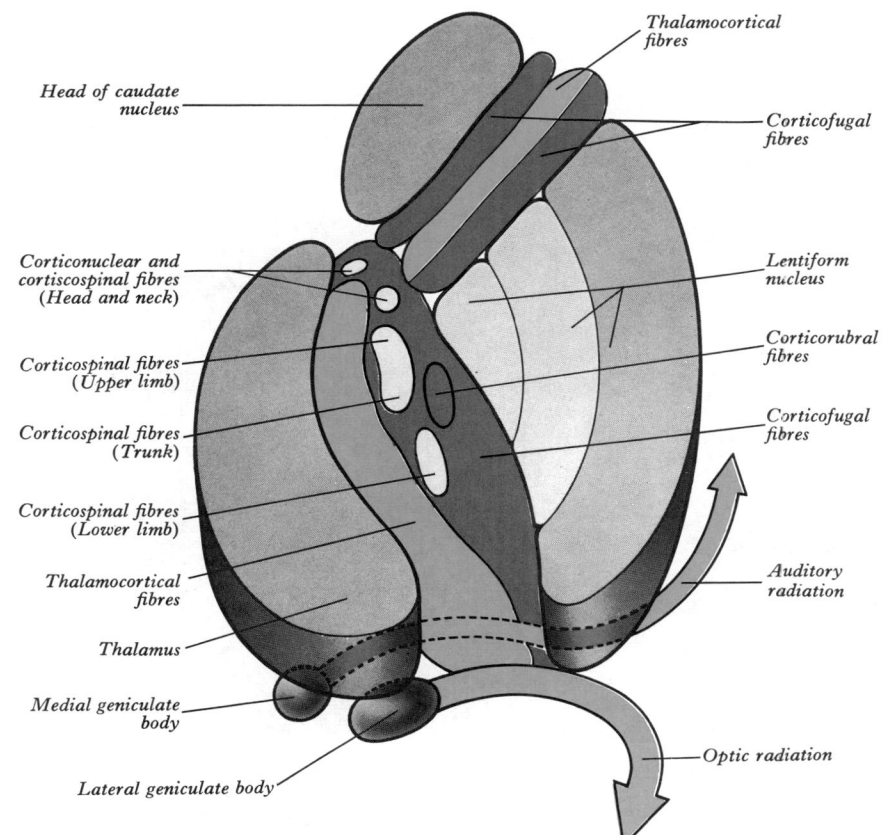

Thalamocortical fibres

Head of caudate nucleus

Corticofugal fibres

Corticonuclear and cortiscospinal fibres (Head and neck)

Lentiform nucleus

Corticospinal fibres (Upper limb)

Corticorubral fibres

Corticospinal fibres (Trunk)

Corticofugal fibres

Corticospinal fibres (Lower limb)

Thalamocortical fibres

Auditory radiation

Thalamus

Medial geniculate body

Lateral geniculate body

Optic radiation

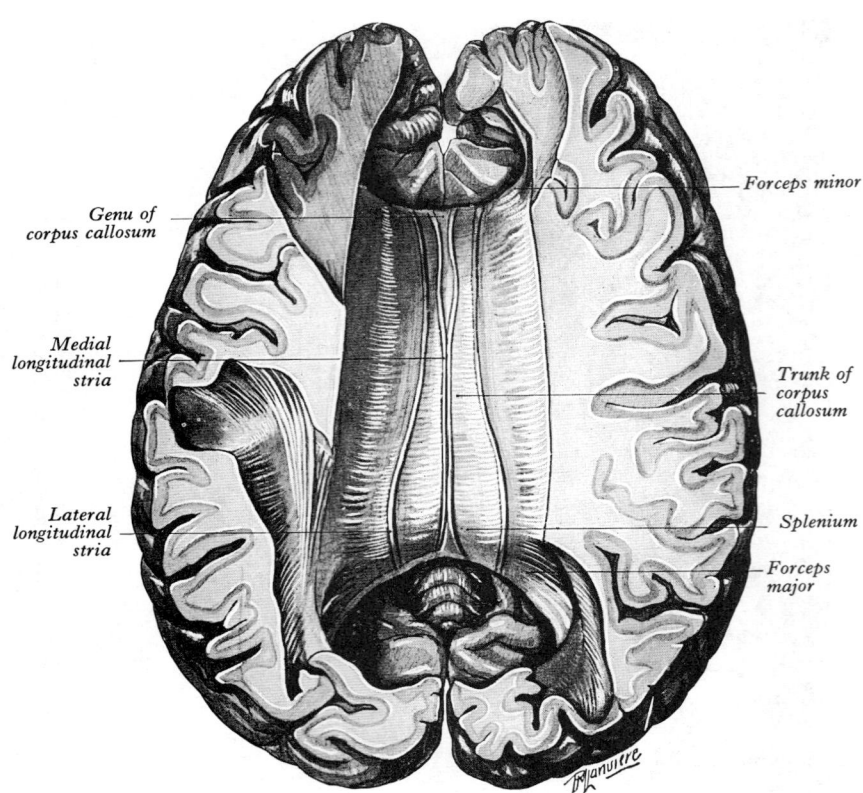

Genu of
corpus callosum

Forceps minor

Medial
longitudinal
stria

Trunk of
corpus
callosum

Lateral
longitudinal
stria

Splenium

Forceps
major

8.284   The corpus callosum, superior aspect, revealed by partial removal
and dissection of the cerebral hemispheres.

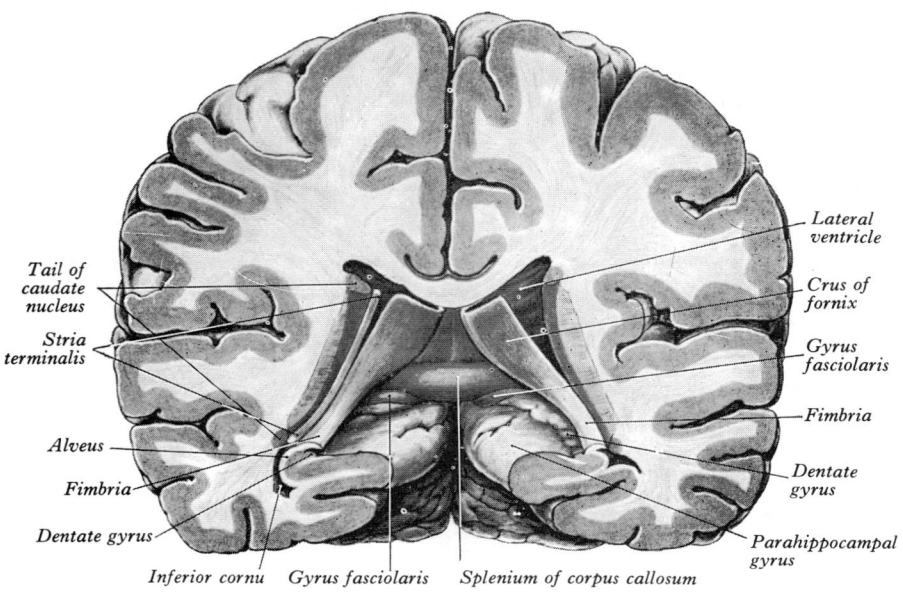

Tail of
caudate
nucleus

Stria
terminalis

Alveus

Fimbria

Dentate gyrus

Inferior cornu   Gyrus fasciolaris   Splenium of corpus callosum

Lateral
ventricle

Crus of
fornix

Gyrus
fasciolaris

Fimbria

Dentate
gyrus

Parahippocampal
gyrus

8.285   Anterior aspect of a coronal section of the cerebrum from which the
posterior parts of the thalami have been removed to reveal the splenium
and parts of the limbic system. (Note that the denate gyrus is not equally
exposed on the two sides.)

Cerebral asymmetry

The two human cerebral hemispheres are not mirror images of each other. This simple yet profound fact adds an intriguing dimension to the study of the central nervous system. Although the principle of functional lateralization in the brain is now universally accepted, the magnitude and number of asymmetries, as well as the interpretation of their significance, continue to generate controversy. Another central issue of particular relevance here concerns the anatomical asymmetries which may accompany these hemispheric specializations.

Historical background

The concept of cerebral asymmetry has a rich and complex history. The first phase comprised the initial suggestions by Dax and others in the 1830s that some functions might indeed be lateralized in the brain, a fact which became established by the seminal study of Broca in 1861. He described a case of expressive aphasia resulting from an infarct within the left posterior inferior frontal lobe, which thereby became known as Broca's area. The later discovery of Wernicke's area in the left posterior temporal and inferior parietal lobe provided another unequivocally lateralized function and demonstrated an asymmetry for language comprehension as well as for speech production.

The association of language impairment with left hemisphere lesions helped lead to the more general concept of a dominant left and a minor right hemisphere. This was intuitively appealing with regard to the prevalence of right handedness and its relationship, if not virtual equivalence, to left hemisphere dominance. Cerebral dominance thereby became at times synonymous with cerebral asymmetry. Even in the nineteenth century this generalization was counselled against by Hughlings Jackson on the grounds that other functions might be subserved mainly by the right hemisphere. His caution proved perspicacious, as discussed below. Simplistic models of left hemisphere dominance could also not readily address the issue of left handedness and speech representation in left handers. For further discussion of cerebral asymmetry from the perspective of handedness, see Annett (1991).

Functional asymmetries

Apart from these initial findings, little progress in our comprehension of functional asymmetries was made until the 1950s. Since then advances have continued apace, though understanding remains far from complete. One important conclusion of the contemporary research is that cerebral lateralization is neither simple nor restricted to a particular functional domain and hence it is more appropriate to speak of asymmetry in the plural.

Research has relied largely on the traditional technique of inferring the functions of an area from studying the consequences of damage to it, whether the lesion be natural, pathological or therapeutic in origin. Firstly, naturalistic clinicopathological data have been collected about how the functional impairment occurring after a lesion in a given brain area differs according to the hemisphere affected. Focal injuries arising from strokes, tumours, epilepsy, gunshot wounds as well as congenital abnormalities have all been studied. The work has been enhanced by the advent of brain imaging, allowing accurate in vivo localization of the lesion contemporaneously with neuropsychological testing. The second technique, pioneered by Wada in the 1940s, is unilateral injection of a barbiturate into the carotid artery. This allows the ipsilateral hemisphere briefly to be 'put to sleep' in a reasonably, though not entirely, selective way. Its contributions to functions, especially speech, can thereby be deduced. Thirdly, and crucially, division of the corpus callosum and other neocortical commissures has been used. Commissurotomy, as it is called, was developed in animals in the 1950s and subsequently used in patients as a treatment for intractable bilateral epilepsy. Persons with congenital absence of part or all of the corpus callosum have also been studied. The commissurotomy procedure severs all contralateral corticocortical connections and produces the 'split-brain' syndrome (8.286; Sperry 1974). Such subjects have been extensively and repeatedly investigated by various experimental manoeuvres, since they allow for the functions of the two hemispheres to be studied virtually independently. All these methods are, of course, not without their limitations, especially regarding extrapolation of the data to people with entirely normal brains. However, collectively they have provided a convergent body of evidence supporting the existence of abilities or functions predominantly associated with one or other hemisphere. The recent arrival of functional brain imaging provides a further and corroborative form of investigation, since these techniques can identify and localize changes in metabolic activity occurring during particular (lateralized) mental tasks.

The functional asymmetries of the brain still remain to be fully characterized, but the following general principles are well established. The left hemisphere prevails for verbal and linguistic functions, for mathematical skills and for analytical thinking. The right hemisphere is mostly non-verbal, and is more involved in spatial and holistic or 'Gestalt' thinking, in many aspects of music, and in some emotions. Memory also shows lateralization; as might have been predicted, verbal memory is primarily a left hemisphere function, whilst non-verbal memory is represented in the right hemisphere (Milner 1974). These asymmetries are relative, not absolute, and vary in degree according to the function and individual concerned. Moreover, these conclusions apply primarily to right-handed men. Those with left-hand preference, or mixed handedness, comprise a heterogeneous group. As an approximation, they show reduced or anomalous lateralization, rather than a simple reversal of the situation in right handers. For example, speech representation can occur in either or both hemispheres. Similarly, women show on average less functional asymmetry than men, especially on right hemisphere tasks (Kimura 1992). To complicate the issue there are also interactions of sex with handedness on several measures.

The significance of hemispheric asymmetry may spread well beyond the functions mentioned, although the evidence becomes increasingly less convincing. For example, the two hemispheres may play different roles in regulation of the immune system, and reduced cerebral asymmetry has been reported in association with homosexual orientation in both sexes. Many scientists and philosophers have also been tempted to speculate upon the relationship between cerebral asymmetry and more expansive concepts such as consciousness, creativity, and the unity of the self (see David 1989). Certainly the data, especially from the split-brain patients, provide fertile ground for such debate (Sperry 1984).

Anatomical asymmetries

Starting with Broca himself, many early investigators attempted to find anatomical substrates to accompany the emerging discoveries of functional asymmetries. Lengths, weights and other parameters were compared between the two hemispheres or parts thereof. However, a series of negative or unreplicated positive studies eventually gave rise to scepticism and even to a belief that anatomical asymmetries were undetectable—and probably nonexistent. It remains true that no qualitative differences in structure, connectivity or neuronal physiology between the hemispheres have been found. Nor, parenthetically, have robust neurochemical asymmetries in the cerebral cortex been demonstrated, despite reports of various minor differences. Where progress has been made is with the discovery of convincing quantitative anatomical asymmetries. These are apparent at both the macroscopic and histological levels, and their recognition has been facilitated by methodological improvements in imaging and morphometry.

The revival of interest in anatomical asymmetry can be traced to the work of Sperry and of Geschwind. In a key paper, Geschwind and Levitsky (1968) measured the size of the planum temporale in 100 brains and found it to be larger on the left than the right in 65, with no asymmetry in 24 and with a reversed pattern in 11 (**8.287**A). Probably as a result of the larger planum temporale, the sylvian fissure is longer and more horizontal in the left

hemisphere (**8.287**B) and provides a surface marker of temporal lobe asymmetry, as does the orientation of the overlying vasculature. The limits of asymmetry in the superior temporal lobe remain uncertain, but appear to include Heschl's gyrus and some other structures adjacent to (or sometimes considered to be an extension of) the planum temporale. Attempts to interpret and summarize the data are complicated by the range of overlapping terminologies and precise areas measured: for example, Brodmann areas 42, 41 and

posterior 22, areas TA–TD of von Economo, Wernicke's area, and auditory cortex, have all been used in studies of superior temporal lobe asymmetry, sometimes without clear definition. Some clarification can be found in chapters 22 and 27 of Paxinos (1990).

Galaburda and colleagues have provided more detailed descriptions of planum temporale asymmetry (Galaburda et al 1978). They showed that it originates almost entirely from right–left differences in size of a cytoarchitectonic subfield

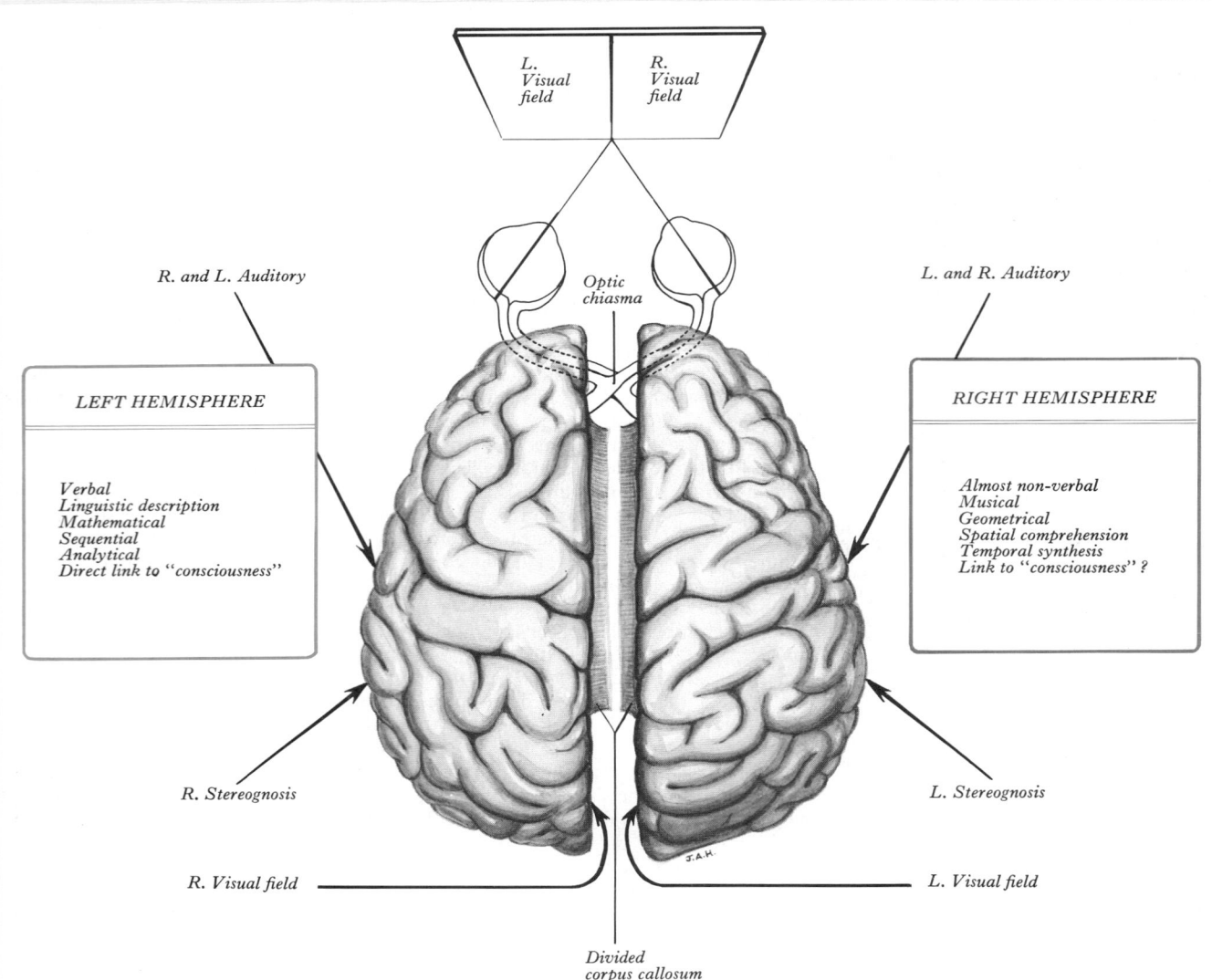

8.286 A summary of the split-brain schema by Sperry, showing the functions which are lateralized to one or other hemisphere (adapted with the permission of the author). Split-brain patients have been studied by presenting stimuli selectively to one or other hemisphere and comparing the subject's responses to them. For instance, a stimulus presented briefly to one visual field, or placed in one hand, is only accessible to the opposite hemisphere (since the projections are contralateral and all commissural connections have been severed). Objects in the right visual field or right hand are recognized and named easily by the 'verbal' left hemisphere. In contrast, patients cannot name, and appear to lack knowledge of,

objects placed in the left visual field or left hand, as these are available only to the 'non-verbal' right hemisphere. However the object has undoubtedly been identified correctly since the person can later point to it from a selection of objects.

These functional specializations are relative and apply to people with left hemisphere language representation. Subsequent studies since this original formulation have added more detail and complexity. Overall, the split-brain work has been central in establishing the extent and nature of functional asymmetries. Its importance was highlighted by the award of a Nobel prize to Sperry in 1981. For more extensive discussion see Sperry (1974, 1984).

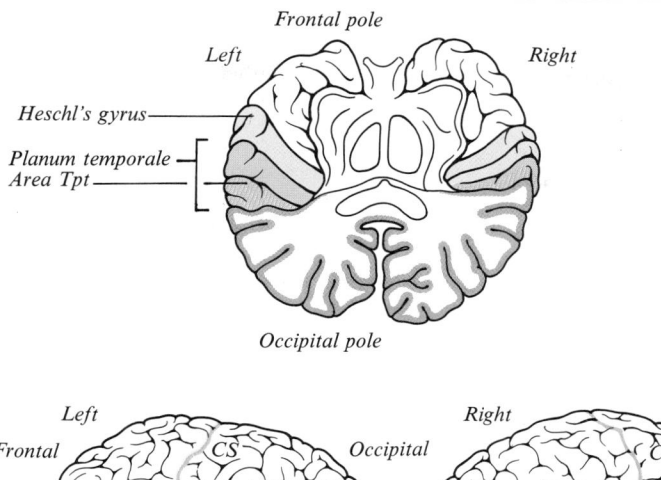

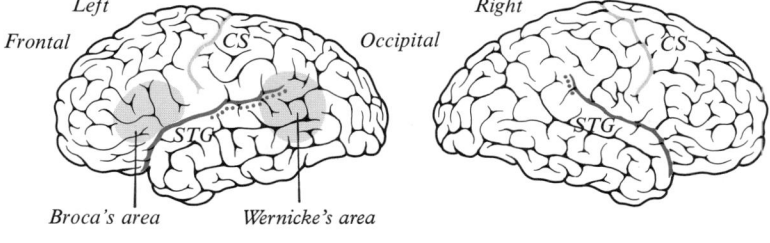

8.287 Examples of anatomical asymmetries in the cerebral cortex. A. Horizontal section showing the exposed upper surface of the temporal lobes. The planum temporale (shown stippled in red) forms the upper posterior part of the temporal lobe, bordered anteriorly by Heschl's gyrus (stippled in blue), laterally by the sylvian fissure, and posteriorly by the end of the sylvian fissure. The brain shown here demonstrates a marked asymmetry in size of the planum temporale, which is larger on the left in a majority of brains. This brain also shows asymmetry of Heschl's gyrus. The asymmetrical length of the lateral border of the planum temporale underlies the asymmetries in the sylvian fissure itself (see also B). Asymmetry of the planum temporale arises mostly from differences in the size of the cytoarchitectonic field Tpt (shown shaded in green). Tpt forms much of the posterior part of the planum temporale, though it also extends onto the lateral surface of the posterior superior temporal gyrus. (Redrawn and adapted from Geschwind and Levitsky 1968.)
B. Lateral views of the left and right hemisphere emphasizing differences between the two sylvian fissures, in red. Compared to the left hemisphere, the right sylvian fissure is shorter and turns upwards. This results from the planum temporale asymmetries (represented by the adjacent red stippling). STG = superior temporal gyrus. CS = central sulcus. The approximate locations of Broca's and Wernicke's areas in the left hemisphere are indicated; however, much of Wernicke's area is buried within the sulcal folds and is not visible on a lateral view.

called Tpt (**8.287**A). Subtle asymmetries in dendritic organization and the neuropil have also been reported (Seldon 1982). Thus, asymmetries in the superior temporal lobe—whichever terminology is adopted—have been demonstrated in terms of overall size and shape, sulcal pattern, cytoarchitecture and at the neuronal level. It seems reasonable to assume that these differences underlie some of the functional asymmetry for language representation.

Asymmetries in areal size, cytoarchitecture or neurocytology also occur elsewhere in the cerebral cortex as well as subcortically (for summary see Witelson & Kigar 1988). A few recent examples are given here. Many brains show a counterclockwise rotation, sometimes called Yakovlevian torque, with a wider right frontal pole and a wider left occipital pole. Brodmann area 45 in the inferior frontal lobe, corresponding to Broca's area, contains a population of large pyramidal neurons found only on the left side (Hayes & Lewis 1993). The complexity of dendritic trees is also asymmetrical (Scheibel et al 1985). The cortical surface surrounding the central sulcus is larger in the left hemisphere, especially in the areas containing the primary somatosensory and motor maps of the arm (White et al 1994); these data suggest that one cerebral manifestation of hand preference is a larger amount of neural circuitry in the relevant parts of the cortex. Histological asymmetries are also found in areas not usually considered to be closely related either to language or handedness. The entorhinal cortex has significantly more neurons in it in the left than the right hemisphere, especially affecting the pre-a cells of lamina II (Heinsen et al 1994). The magnitude of the difference reached 51% in one individual, with an average in the 22 cases of 13%. This study is noteworthy in that the entorhinal cortex is sometimes (erroneously) thought of as a primitive cortical structure and, therefore, perhaps less likely to be asymmetrical. No hemispheric differences in the total number of neurons in the neocortex were found in an initial stereological study (Pakkenberg 1993).

The work summarized here makes it clear that localized anatomical asymmetries of several kinds do exist in the cerebral cortex. They are of a robustness and magnitude suggesting that they represent at least part of the structural substrate of functional asymmetries. It is, however, important to emphasize that whilst these anatomical asymmetries are demonstrable in the majority of cases, they are not invariable and their magnitude varies markedly from one brain to another. This parallels the situation for functional lateralization, as does the fact that anatomical asymmetries are less clearcut in left handers and in women.

Mechanisms of asymmetry

Phylogenetically, asymmetry is not restricted to the human brain—a fact which bears upon the nature of its relationship with language—but asymmetries are much greater in, and have a particular significance for, humans (Corballis 1989). The genetics of cerebral asymmetry are unclear, although a single gene model with autosomal dominant inheritance is favoured, at least with regard to handedness (Annett 1991). Some clues as to the gene(s) involved may come from sex chromosome aneuploidies such as Turner's syndrome (45X0), in which alterations in functional and structural asymmetry are found.

Environmental factors may modify the development of asymmetry and handedness too. Geschwind proposed an elaborate and attractive unifying hypothesis, whereby testosterone in early life slows development of the left hemisphere, affects cerebral lateralization and has a number of other effects (Geschwind & Galaburda 1987). His hypothesis continues to be influential (McManus & Bryden 1991), though in truth little has been established regarding the importance of the hormonal milieu or other environmental factors upon cerebral asymmetry. Similarly, the mechanisms by which a gene or genes could produce asymmetry is unknown, as is the nature of any interaction between putative environmental influences and the predominant genetic determinants. In terms of mediating structures, the corpus callosum plays a role in ontogenesis of cerebral asymmetry (Lent & Schmidt 1993). This is thought to be related to the loss of callosal connections which is a characteristic of asymmetrical cortical areas (Witelson & Nowakowski 1991). Whatever processes underlie cerebral asymmetry, they must operate largely prenatally, in that human brains show anatomical asymmetries as early as the second trimester in utero, and babies exhibit functional lateralization. It is not known if, when, or how asymmetry of form or function becomes immutable.

Regardless of the ultimate explanation for their occurrence, there are several features which appear common to asymmetrical brain structures (Galaburda 1994). Firstly, size asymmetry is accounted for primarily by differences in neuronal number rather than by neuronal density or other possible explanations, such as neuronal size. Secondly, when a brain area is more symmetrical than usual it is associated with the area being bilaterally large, not bilaterally small; it is therefore suggested that asymmetry is related primarily to production of the smaller side. Thirdly, a given brain tends to show a similar direction and magnitude of asymmetry for all parameters which can be asymmetrical.

Clinical and pathological implications of asymmetry

Once it is accepted that the cerebral hemispheres are not structurally or functionally identical, the possibility is raised that disorders of the brain may affect and be affected by its asymmetries. This could occur in a number of ways. The first category comprises the classic neurological disorders where the clinical consequences of a lesion differ depending on the side affected, as discussed above. Another example of a disease interaction with asymmetry is provided by Rasmussen's syndrome, an idiopathic degenerative disorder of childhood which affects one or other hemisphere. Other conditions, such as Alzheimer's disease, can also show marked clinical and/or pathological asymmetries in a small percentage of cases. The mechanisms underlying these seemingly random forms of asymmetrical disease involvement are unknown.

Notwithstanding these examples, the most interesting clinical implications of cerebral asymmetry occur where disturbed lateralization appears to be inherent in the nature and even aetiology of a disorder. It is schizophrenia where this relationship is most striking. A number of studies suggest that the disease is associated with a failure to develop normal structural and functional cerebral asymmetry, and its pathology is characterized by a greater affliction of the left than the right hemisphere. Schizophrenia has thereby been proposed to be caused by an abnormality in the cerebral asymmetry gene and to be related to the rapid evolutionary emergence of asymmetry itself (Crow 1993); this hypothesis, however, remains to be established and separate explanations for altered cerebral asymmetry in schizophrenia exist. Other putative neurodevelopmental disorders, including dyslexia and autism, may also be associated with asymmetrical cerebral abnormalities and similar causative mechanisms, though the evidence is less convincing (Geschwind & Galaburda 1987).

Summary

Cerebral structural and functional asymmetry is a remarkable phenomenon, yet paradoxically its existence and its diverse implications are sometimes overlooked. It is stressed that the nature of cerebral lateralization, its anatomical basis, and the underlying mechanisms, remain far from clear. Nevertheless, some important conclusions can be drawn and are listed below:

- There are structural asymmetries between the cerebral hemispheres. These are localized and often subtle, affecting areal size, cytoarchitecture, neuronal number, and possibly size and dendritic arborization of constituent neurons.
- There are many functions for which one hemisphere plays the major role. These particularly relate to aspects of language comprehension and production, but also involve memory, spatial thinking and other domains. Presumably the known anatomical asymmetries underlie, at least partially, the functional ones, though their concordance remains uncertain.
- Both the anatomical and the functional asymmetries vary in magnitude from one person and one parameter to another, resist simplistic dichotomous classification, and are too complex to support an unqualified concept of cerebral dominance. This is especially so given the need to account for left handedness and its frequent association with reduced rather than reversed cerebral asymmetry, as well as the finding that asymmetries are generally larger in men than women.
- Developmentally, asymmetries are present at or before birth, further constraining hypotheses as to the mechanisms underlying them.
- Schizophrenia is associated with a disturbance of cerebral asymmetry, seemingly in a causally important way. Understanding schizophrenia may therefore tell us much about the origins, nature and consequences of human cerebral asymmetry as a whole.

BASAL NUCLEI

These are the subcortical grey masses lateral to the thalamus in the inferior parts of each cerebral hemisphere (8.288A). In this sense they include the *corpus striatum*, the *claustrum*, and the *amygdaloid complex*. (This last is an integral part of the limbic system and is dealt with on p. 1131.) The corpus striatum is functionally intimately related to the subthalamus of the diencephalon, and to the midbrain substantia nigra, both of which will be dealt with here.

The *corpus striatum* comprises the *lentiform* and *caudate nuclei*, separated from one another by the internal capsule (8.288B). The lentiform nucleus is subdivided into the medially placed *globus pallidus*, or *pallidum* (so named because of its pale colour due to a relative lack of perikarya and a preponderance of myelinated axons) and a lateral part, the *putamen* (named probably because it appears 'pruned' from the caudate nucleus, which it resembles in general

8.288 The topographical anatomy of the corpus striatum.

A. The general position of the corpus striatum in the cerebral hemisphere in lateral view. Notice that the greater part of the corpus striatum is above the lateral fissure and in front of the postcentral sulcus. The general topography of the cortico-striate projection is determined by this (arrows).

B. The corpus striatum seen from the lateral side. Notice (a) the relationship of the head of the caudate nucleus and fundus striati to the anterior perforated substance; (b) the prominent cell bridges joining the caudate nucleus and putamen anteriorly and disrupting the anterior limb of the internal capsule; and (c) the position of the anterior commissure. (i)–(v) indicate planes of section for E–H (below) and for 8.292.

C. A schematic representation of the lentiform nucleus seen from the lateral side and behind.

D. As in (c) but the globus pallidus has been detached from the putamen.

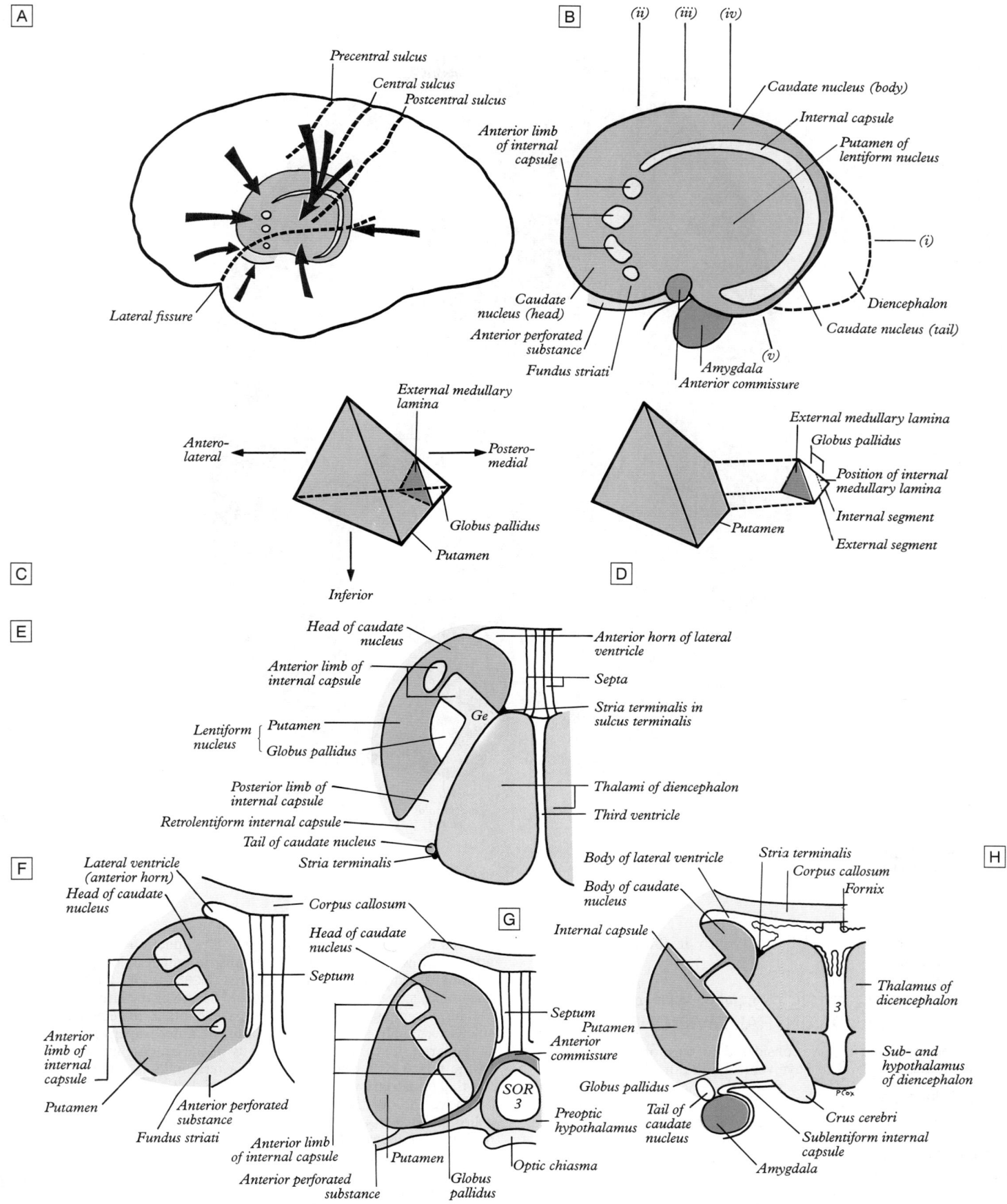

A

Precentral sulcus
Central sulcus
Postcentral sulcus

Lateral fissure

B

(ii) (iii) (iv)

Anterior limb of internal capsule

Caudate nucleus (body)
Internal capsule
Putamen of lentiform nucleus

(i)

Diencephalon
Caudate nucleus (tail)

Caudate nucleus (head)
Anterior perforated substance
Fundus striati

(v)
Amygdala
Anterior commissure

C

External medullary lamina
Antero-lateral
Postero-medial
Globus pallidus
Putamen
Inferior

D

External medullary lamina
Globus pallidus
Position of internal medullary lamina
Internal segment
Putamen
External segment

E

Head of caudate nucleus
Anterior limb of internal capsule
Anterior horn of lateral ventricle
Septa
Stria terminalis in sulcus terminalis
Lentiform nucleus { Putamen / Globus pallidus
Ge
Posterior limb of internal capsule
Thalami of diencephalon
Third ventricle
Retrolentiform internal capsule
Tail of caudate nucleus
Stria terminalis

F

Lateral ventricle (anterior horn)
Head of caudate nucleus
Corpus callosum
Head of caudate nucleus
Septum
Anterior limb of internal capsule
Putamen
Anterior perforated substance
Fundus striati
Anterior limb of internal capsule

G

Septum
Putamen
Anterior commissure
Globus pallidus
Preoptic hypothalamus
Putamen
Globus pallidus
Anterior perforated substance
SOR 3
Optic chiasma

H

Body of lateral ventricle
Body of caudate nucleus
Internal capsule
Stria terminalis
Corpus callosum
Fornix
Thalamus of dicencephalon
Sub- and hypothalamus of diencephalon
Globus pallidus
Tail of caudate nucleus
Amygdala
Crus cerebri
Sublentiform internal capsule
3

The globus pallidus could be similarly dismembered into its internal (medial) and external (lateral) segments, separated by the internal medullary lamina (dotted line).

E. Semi-schematic horizontal section in plane (i)—see B, above. Ge = genu of internal capsule. Compare with **8**.257, 258.

F, G, H. Three semi-schematic frontal sections in planes (ii), (iii), (iv) respect-

ively—see B, above, and compare **8**.293, 294. Notice that the anterior limb of the internal capsule is disrupted by the continuities between putamen and caudate nucleus (F, G); that the basal nuclei lie immediately above the anterior perforated substance (F, G); and that the pallidum appears in only the more posterior sections (G, H). SOR3 = supraoptic recess of third ventricle; 3 = third ventricle.

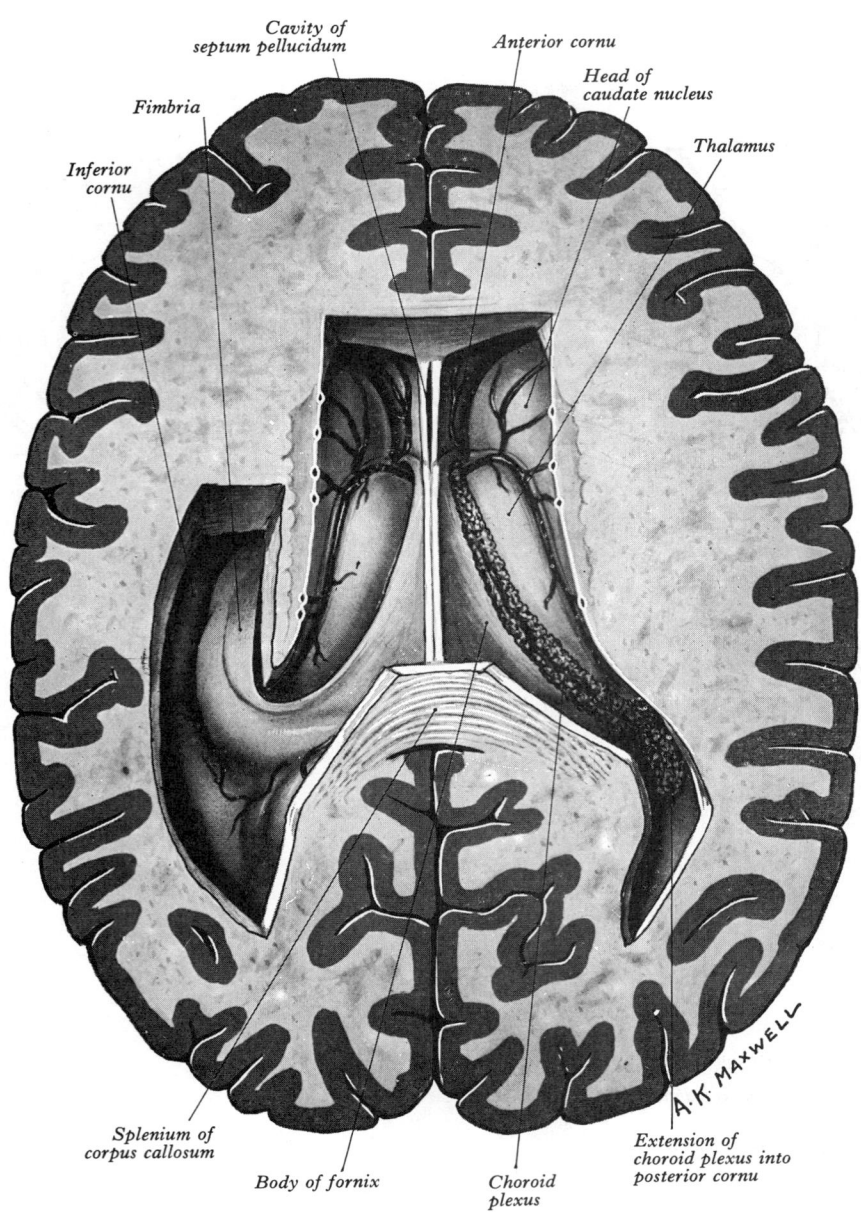

Cavity of
septum pellucidum

Anterior cornu

Fimbria

Head of
caudate nucleus

Inferior
cornu

Thalamus

Splenium of
corpus callosum

Body of fornix

Choroid
plexus

Extension of
choroid plexus into
posterior cornu

8.289 Horizontal section of the cerebrum dissected to remove the roofs of
the lateral ventricles.

texture and appearance, and with which it forms a structural/
functional unit).

TOPOGRAPHY OF THE CORPUS STRIATUM:
THE DORSAL AND VENTRAL DIVISIONS

The corpus striatum is now considered to be more extensive than
previously believed, and to have ventral and dorsal moieties.

Dorsal division

A division of the corpus striatum, it is identical with the classical
corpus striatum, i.e. the caudate and lentiform nuclei.

Caudate nucleus. This is an arcuate mass with a large anterior
head which tapers to a body and a downcurving tail (**8.288**B). The
head lies, covered with ependyma, in the floor and lateral wall of the
anterior horn of the lateral ventricle in front of the interventricular
foramen. The tapering body of the nucleus is in the floor of the
body of the ventricle; the tail follows the curve of the inferior horn
and so is in the ventricular roof in the temporal lobe. The tail is
slender, except in the anterior part of the temporal lobe, where it
expands considerably. Medially, the greater part of the caudate

nucleus abuts the thalamus (**8.288**B). This junction is marked by a
groove known as the sulcus terminalis, in which is lodged the stria
terminalis, lying deep to the ependyma (**8.288**E, H, 289–291). The stria
terminalis is one margin of the choroid fissure of the lateral ventricle,
the hippocampal fimbria and fornix the other (**8.288**H, 290). The
sulcus terminalis is especially prominent anterosuperiorly (because
of the large size of the head and body of the caudate nucleus relative
to the tail; **8.290**), and here the stria terminalis is accompanied by
the thalamostriate vein (**8.289–291** and p. 1581).

Above the head and body of the caudate nucleus is the corpus
callosum (**8.288**F–H): the two are separated laterally by the fronto-
occipital bundle (p. 1176), and medially by the bundle of thin axons
capping the caudate nucleus and known as the subcallosal fasciculus
(**8.290**, 292). The caudate nucleus is for the most part separated from
the lentiform nucleus by the anterior limb of the internal capsule
(p. 1176 and **8.288–292**). The inferior part of the head of the nucleus
does, however, become substantially continuous with the most
inferior putamen immediately above the anterior perforated substance. This junctional region is the fundus striati of Brockhaus
(**8.288**, 292A). The continuity is echoed by the bridges of cells which
connect the putamen to the caudate nucleus for most of its length;

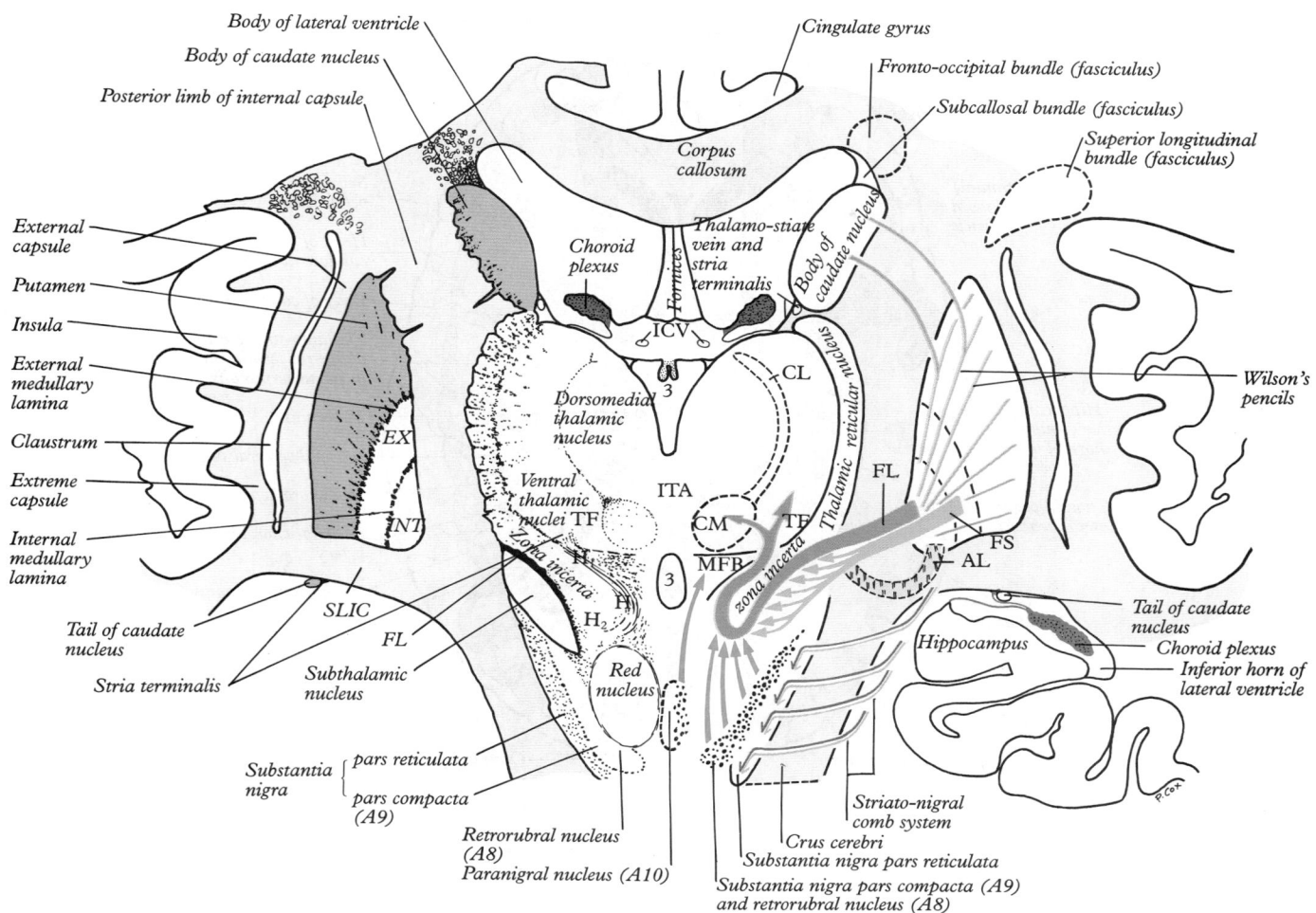

8.290 An oblique section of the brain (plane v of **8.288B**), which is an enlargement of the central area of **8.281, 294**. On the left, the figure is presented as of a myelin-stained preparation (white matter is black). On the right, the important fibre systems of the basal nuclei and substantia nigra are represented schematically. Wilson's pencils, shown schematically on the right, are prominent in the putamen on the left; compare with **8.292**. A8, 9, 10 = dopaminergic cell groups; AL = ansa lenticularis; CL = centrolateral nucleus of thalamus; CM = centromedian nucleus of thalamus; EX = external pallidal segment; FL = fasciculus lanticularis; FS = fasciculus subthalamicus; H, H_1, H_2 = subthalamic fields of Forel; ICV = internal cerebral veins in the transverse fissure; INT = internal pallidal segment; ITA = interthalamic adhesion; MFB = median forebrain bundle; SLIC = sublentiform internal capsule; TF = thalamic fasciculus; 3 = 3rd ventricle.

bridges which are, moreover, most prominent anteriorly, in the region of the fundus striati and the head and body of the caudate nucleus, where they break up the anterior limb of the internal capsule (**8.288B, E–G, 292**). In the temporal lobe, the anterior, enlarged part of the tail of the caudate nucleus becomes continuous with the postero-inferior putamen. Together, the caudate nucleus and putamen are referred to as the *dorsal striatum*. The tail of the nucleus contacts but remains distinct from the amygdaloid complex.

Lentiform nucleus. It lies immediately deep to the insular cortex, from which it is separated by white matter and by the grey matter of the claustrum. The *claustrum* is roughly coextensive with the insular cortex and outer surface of the lentiform nucleus (**8.290, 292**). The claustrum splits the insular subcortical white matter to create the extreme and external capsules, the latter of which separates the claustrum from the lentiform nucleus (**8.278, 279, 281, 290, 292–294**). The name of the lentiform ('lens-shaped') nucleus belies its true shape, which is nearer that of a distorted tetrahedral prism, lying on one side, its apex directed medially and slightly backwards, and its somewhat convex base laterally and forwards (**8.288C, D**). This is why the nucleus appears roughly triangular in most sections in conventional horizontal and coronal planes (**8.205, 278, 279, 281, 288E–H, 290, 292–294**), and its medial part (the globus pallidus) is not visible in more anterior transverse sections (compare **8.288F** with **G** and **H**). The nucleus is separated from the medially placed caudate nucleus by the internal capsule, the latter surrounding it almost completely (**8.288**). The laterally-placed putamen is separated from

the globus pallidus by a sheet of myelinated axons known as the external medullary lamina (**8.288C, D, 290, 292B**). A similar but less substantial sheet, the internal medullary lamina, divides the globus pallidus (or *dorsal pallidum*) into lateral (or external) and medial (or internal) segments (**8.288D, 290, 292B**). Inferiorly, a little behind the fundus striati, the lentiform nucleus is grooved by the anterior commissure interconnecting inferior parts of the temporal lobes and the anterior olfactory cortex of the two sides (**8.288, 292B**).

Ventral division

This division of the corpus striatum is the smaller. It has been categorized in many animals, including humans (Heimer & Van Hoesen 1979; Heimer et al 1982; Alheid et al 1990). In front of the anterior commissure, much of the grey of the anterior perforated substance (and especially the olfactory tubercle) previously included with olfactory cortex is, in terms of cellular composition, histochemistry and interconnections (see below), indistinguishable from and continuous with the fundus striati (**8.288B**). The caudate nucleus is also continuous medially with the nucleus accumbens (**8.292**), which literally, as its name implies, leans against the nuclei of the septum (p. 1129), close by the paraolfactory area and diagonal band of Broca (**8.292A**) and the fornix (p. 1129). The nucleus accumbens and the olfactory tubercle comprise the *ventral striatum*. In the more posterior of the anterior perforated substance, superolateral to the nucleus basalis of Meynert (**8.292B** and p. 1120), is the *ventral pallidum*, partially separated from its dorsal equivalent by the anterior commissure (**8.292B**). Unlike the spatial relationship in the dorsal

1189

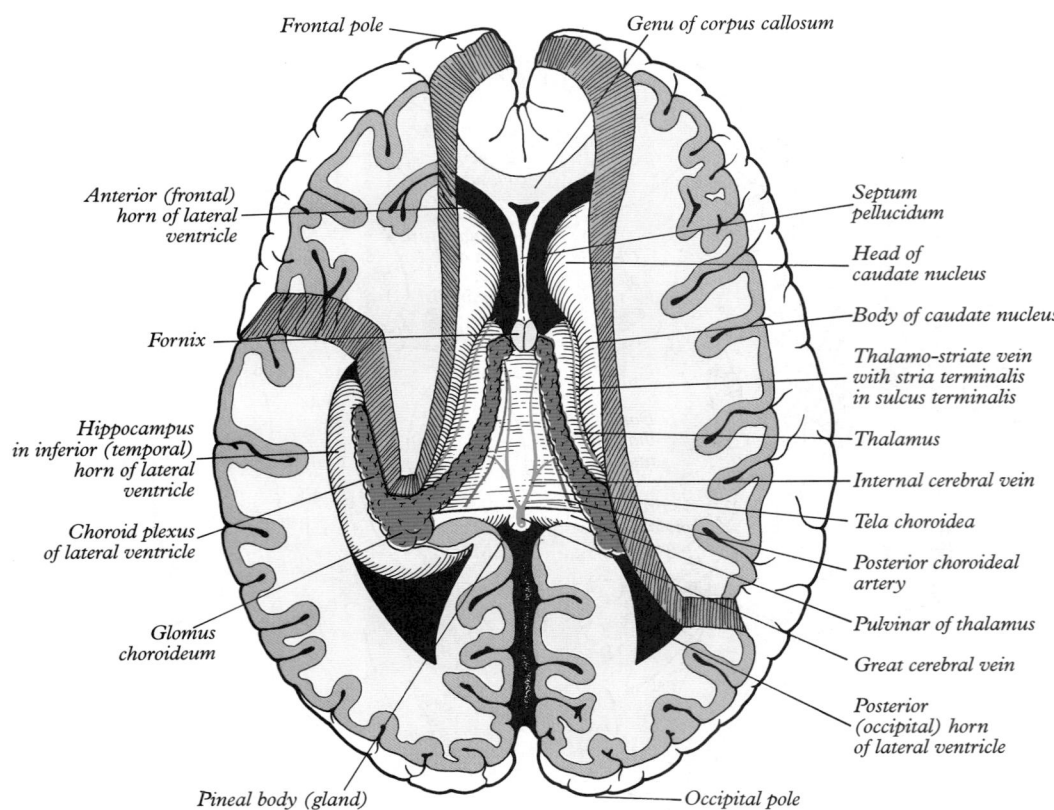

8.291 The tela choroidea of the third ventricle and the choroid plexus of the lateral ventricle.

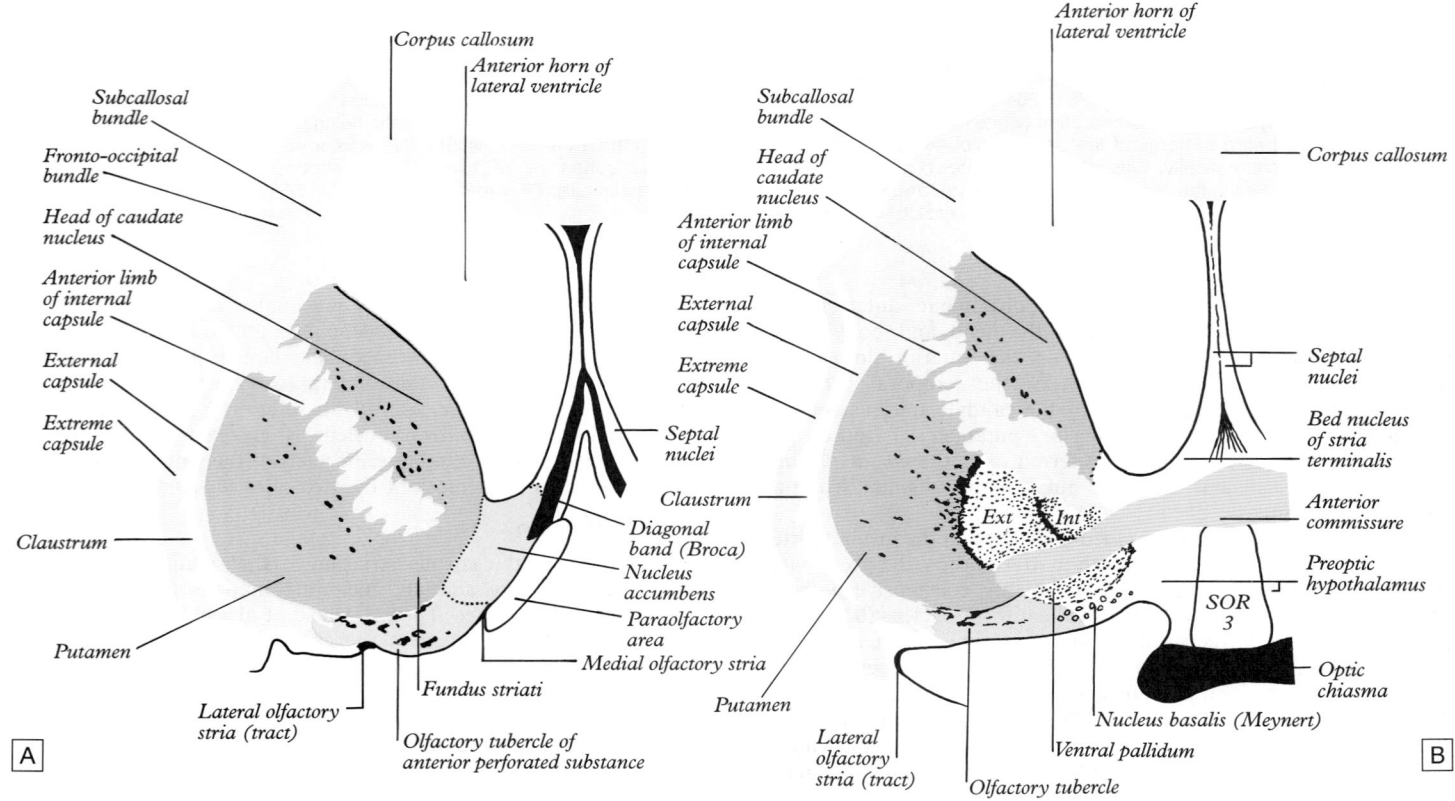

8.292 Myelin preparations (white matter is black) of coronal sections through the corpus striatum and anterior perforated substance. A is anterior to B, corresponding to: A. plane (ii); B. plane (iii) in **8**.288B. Compare with **8**.289F, G and **8**.293 respectively. In A, notice the inferior continuities of the caudate nucleus and putamen (the fundus striati) and their extension into the anterior perforated substance (as the olfactory tubercle). Together with the nucleus accumbens, the tubercle forms the ventral striatum. The pal-lidum is shown in B, where EX = the external and INT = the internal segment of the dorsal pallidum (globus pallidus): note the internal medullary lamina separating them, and the external medullary lamina between the putamen and external pallidal segment. The ventral pallidum is in the anterior per-forated substance, inferior to the anterior commissure. The fibre bundles in the caudate-putamen are Wilson's pencils. SOR3 = supraoptic recess of the third ventricle.

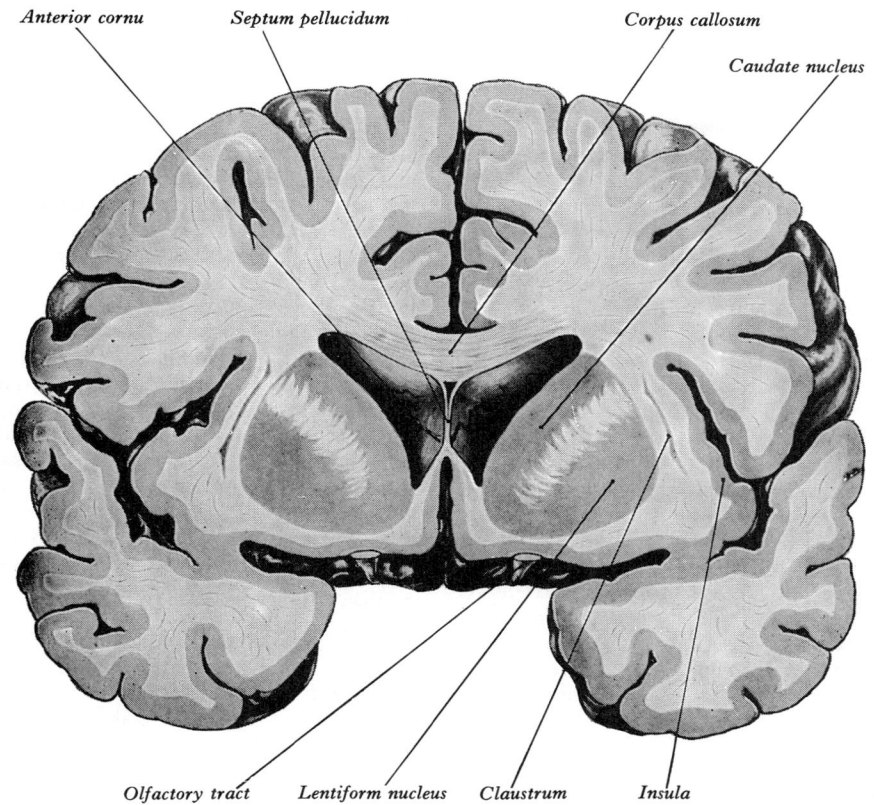

8.293   Posterior aspect of a coronal section through the anterior cornua of the lateral ventricles.

corpus striatum, the ventral pallidum is therefore predominantly posterior to the ventral striatum.

Arterial blood supply

The most important arterial supply comprises the lenticulostriate vessels, which are commonly involved in cerebral haemorrhage. They are derived from the roots of middle and anterior cerebral arteries and enter through the anterior perforated substance. They also supply the anterior limb and much of the posterior limb of the internal capsule. The caudate nucleus also receives blood from the anterior and posterior choroidal arteries. The postero-inferior part of the lentiform nucleus is supplied by the thalamostriate branches of the posterior cerebral artery. (See also p. 1534.)

Fibre systems of the basal nuclei

All efferent and some afferent connections of the corpus striatum are made with the diencephalon and midbrain, from both of which the basal nuclei are separated by the internal capsule and crus cerebri (8.205, 290). The fibre connections negotiate these either by running around their anterior border (as the ansa lenticularis: marked AL in 8.290), or by penetrating the capsule directly (the fasciculus lenticularis: FL; and fasciculus subthalamicus: FS, which is related exclusively to the subthalamic nucleus), or by slipping obliquely through the crus (the striatonigral comb system). The ansa and fasciculus lenticularis unite in the subthalamus, where they follow a horizontal hairpin trajectory before turning upwards to enter the thalamus (as the thalamic fasciculus: marked TF in 8.290). The trajectory delineates the subthalamic zona incerta (which is continuous above with the thalamic reticular nucleus) and creates the so-called 'H' fields ('Haubenregionen': 'hat plume regions') of Forel (marked H, H₁, H₂ in 8.290). These fields are descriptive only, and do not define particular nuclear targets of the system. From field H, the so-called pallido-hypothalamic bundle enters the hypothalamus only to leave and rejoin the H fields without synapsing (8.205). Finally, the median forebrain bundle lies medial to the subthalamus and carries important ascending fibres to the striatum (median forebrain bundle in 8.290).

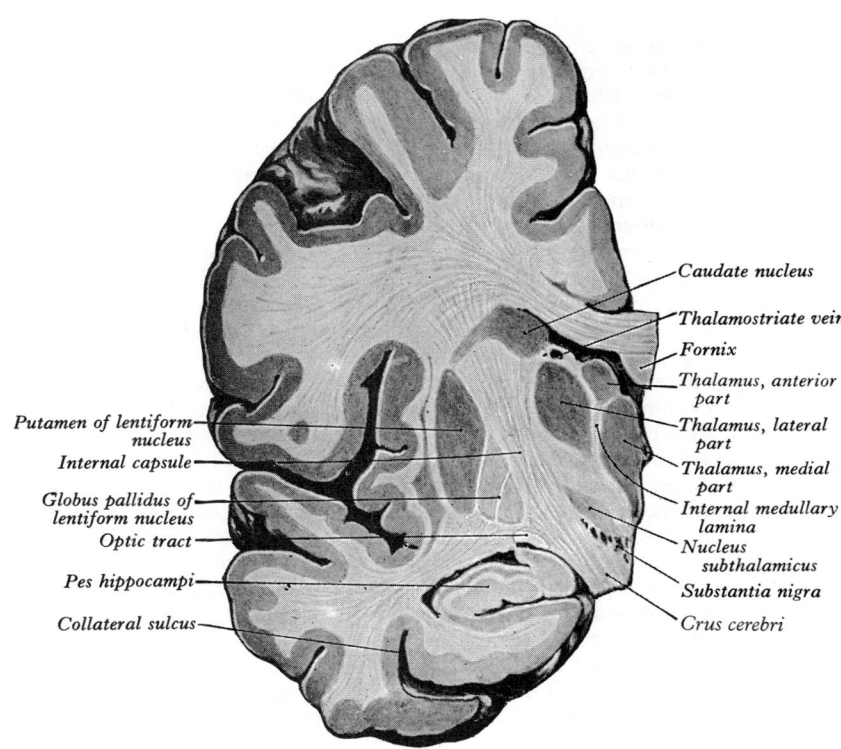

8.294   Anterior aspect of a coronal section through the right cerebral hemisphere.

1191

STRUCTURE OF THE CORPUS STRIATUM

Striatum

The caudate nucleus, putamen and ventral striatum are the striatum. They are highly cellular and well-vascularized. The caudate-putamen is permeated by small bundles of finely myelinated or non-myelinated, small-diameter fibres which are striatal afferents and efferents, and which radiate through its substance as though converging on or radiating from the globus pallidus. These bundles are 'Wilson's pencils' (**8.290, 292**) and, together with the cellular bridges linking the two nuclei, account for much of the striated appearance of the human corpus striatum.

Although the overall connections of the striatum with other regions are now well-known (see below), little is known in detail of its intrinsic organization. However, it is possible to make some general points. (For references, see Pasik et al 1979; Graybiel & Ragsdale 1983; Alheid et al 1990; Di Figlia & Aronin 1990; Saper 1990; Webster 1990; Gerfen 1992.)

Neurons of both dorsal and ventral striatum are mainly small multipolar cells with round, triangular or fusiform somata, mixed with a smaller number of large multipolar cells; the ratio of small:large cells is at least 20:1. The large neurons have extensive spherical or ovoid dendritic trees up to 600 μm across. The small neurons also have spherical dendritic trees, about 200 μm across, which receive the synaptic terminals of many striatal afferents. The dendrites of both small and large striatal cells may be either spiny or non-spiny, which allows the identification of four subtypes of striatal neuron, although most authors describe more. The most common neuron (comprising about 75% of the whole) is a small cell with spiny dendrites. These cells contain γ-aminobutyric acid (GABA), and either enkephalin or substance P (SP). Enkephalinergic neurons appear to express D_2 dopamine receptors, SP neurons have D_1 receptors. These neurons are the chief and perhaps exclusive source of striatal efferents (to the pallidum and substantia nigra; see below). The remaining small neurons are aspiny and are intrinsic cells containing acetylcholinesterase (AChE), choline acetyl-transferase (CAT), somatostatin and avian pancreatic polypeptide. Large neurons with spiny dendrites contain AChE and CAT. Most, perhaps all, are intrinsic neurons, as are aspiny large neurons, about which little is known.

Intrinsic synapses are probably largely asymmetric (Type II), and those derived from external sources symmetric (Type I). The aminergic afferents from the substantia nigra, raphe and locus coeruleus end as profusely branching axons with varicosities containing dense-core vesicles—the presumed store of amine transmitters. Many of these varicosities have no conventional synaptic membrane specializations and may release transmitter in a way analogous to that found in peripheral postsynaptic sympathetic axons (pp. 924–925).

Striosomes and the striatal mosaic. (See Graybiel & Ragsdale 1983; Graybiel 1984; Alexander et al 1986; Pearson et al 1990; Pioro et al 1990; Saper 1990; Törk & Hornung 1990; Webster 1990; Gerfen 1992 for references.) Neuroactive chemicals, whether intrinsic or derived from afferents, are not distributed uniformly in the striatum. For example, serotonin and glutamic acid decarboxylase (GAD) concentrations are highest caudally and SP, acetylcholine (ACh) and dopamine rostrally. There is, however, a finer grain organization in that the striatum may be considered as a mosaic of 'islands' or *striosomes* (sometimes referred to as 'patches'), each 0.5–1.5 mm across, packed in a 'matrix' in such a way that the latter appears as patches of about the same size. Striosomes contain SP and enkephalins. During development, the first dopamine terminals from the substantia nigra are found in striosomes, and although this exclusivity does not persist after birth, striosomes in the caudate nucleus still contain a higher concentration of dopamine than does the matrix. Non-striosomal islands (i.e. the matrix) contain ACh and somatostatin and are the targets of thalamostriate axons (see below). Receptor sites for at least some neurotransmitters are also differentially distributed: for example, opiate receptors are found almost exclusively within striosomes, muscarinic receptors predominantly so. Moreover, the distributions of neuroactive substances within the striosomes of primates are not uniform. The striosome/matrix patchwork is less evident in the primate (including human) putamen

than caudate nucleus: the putamen in these species seems to comprise predominantly matrix.

All afferents to the striatum terminate in a 'mosaic' manner, although the size of a cluster of terminals is usually only ~100–200 μm across. These afferent terminal clusters are not, however, always arranged with the clear striosome/matrix distributions seen in nigrostriate and thalamostriate axons. For example, in general it can be said that afferents from neocortex end in striatal matrix and those from allocortex in striosomes. The distinction is not, however, absolute: afferents from the neocortex arise in layers V and VI; but whereas those from superficial layer V end predominantly in striatal matrix, those from deeper neocortex project to striosomes (Gerfen 1992). Striatal cell bodies which are the sources of efferents also form clusters, but again are not uniformly related to striosomes. For example, the cell bodies of some striatopallidal and striatonigral axons lie clustered within striosomes, some outside them, but still in clusters. The neurons and neuropil of the ventral striatum are essentially similar to those of the dorsal striatum. The striosomal/matrix organization is, however, less well defined and seems to be comprised predominantly of striosomes. Gerfen (1992) has suggested that the matrix compartment so well developed in the dorsal striatum is, in fact, a relatively 'new' addition in evolutionary terms.

Pallidum

(See Webster 1990 for references.) The cell density of the human dorsal pallidum (i.e. globus pallidus) is less than one-twentieth of that of the striatum. Further, although it is about twice the volume of the internal segment (see above, and **8.288**D, **290, 292**B), the density of neurons in the external segment is 50% higher. The morphology of the majority of cells, however, seems identical in the two segments: they are large multipolar neurons closely resembling those of the substantia nigra pars reticulata (see below and **8.296**). The dendritic fields are discoid, with their planes at right angles to Wilson's pencils (**8.290, 292**), which contain afferents from the striatum. Each of these striatally derived afferents therefore potentially contacts many

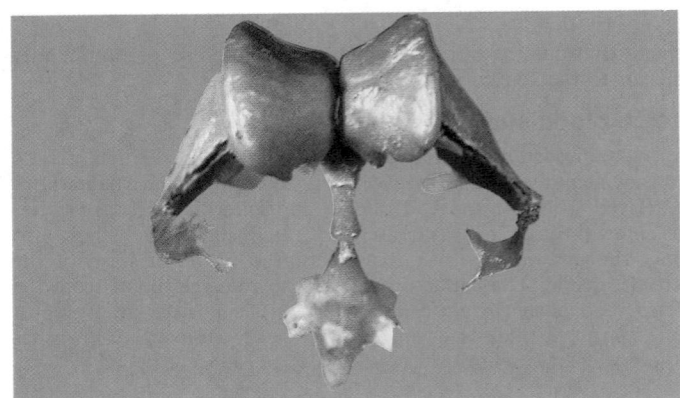

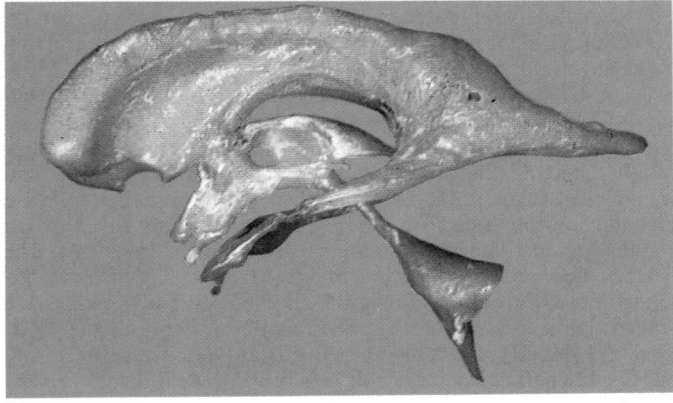

8.295 Resin casts of the ventricular system of the human brain (prepared by D H Tompsett of the Royal College of Surgeons of England): A. ventral view; B. left lateral view.

pallidal dendrites en passant, and this and the diameters of the dendritic fields (> 500 μm) would seem to predicate against a precise topical organization within the nucleus. Scarce small interneurons are also present.

Knowledge of the distributions of neurotransmitters in the dorsal pallidum is best documented in relation to those associated with afferents from the striatum: SP in the internal segment, enkephalin in the external segment, and GABA throughout. Pallidal neurons appear to utilize either GABA or (less frequently) ACh as transmitters. Axons from the ventral striatum containing either enkephalin or SP are found intermingled throughout the ventral pallidum. Of the pallidal neurons themselves, both GABA and SP are associated with their efferents to the substantia nigra pars reticulata. Ventral pallidal neurons, like those of the dorsal pallidum, utilize either GABA or ACh, but in this case the cholinergic population predominates.

Substantia nigra

(See Dray 1979; Graybiel 1984; Hökfelt et al 1984; Björklund & Lindvall 1984; Törk & Hornung 1990; Pearson et al 1990; Saper 1990; Pioro et al 1990; Di Figlia & Aronin 1990; and Webster 1990 for references.)

The substantia nigra is a nuclear complex deep to the crus cerebri in each cerebral peduncle. It comprises a deep, cell-rich pars compacta and a superficial, larger but less cellular pars reticulata (8.296). The pars compacta, together with the smaller pars lateralis, is the cell group A9 of Dählstrom and Fuxe (1964, 1965); together with the retrorubral nucleus (A8) (8.290) it comprises most of the dopaminergic neuron population of the midbrain, and is the source of the *mesostriatal* dopamine system (8.297). All these neurons are thought to contain ACh in addition to dopamine, and there is evidence that up to 25% of them are in fact cholinergic. The pars compacta of each side is continuous with its opposite fellow through the ventral tegmental dopamine group A10, sometimes known as the paranigral nucleus (8.290, 296, 297), which represents the remaining midbrain dopamine population and is the source of the *mesolimbic* dopamine system (8.297). This system in fact also supplies the ventral striatum and neighbouring parts of the dorsal striatum, as well as the prefrontal and anterior cingulate cortex. The dopaminergic neurons of the pars compacta (A9) and paranigral nucleus (ventral tegmental group A10) also contain cholecystokinin (medial cells) or somatostatin (lateral cells).

Within the pars reticulata are large multipolar neurons very similar to those of the pallidum: their disc-like dendritic trees are also orientated at right angles to afferents from the striatum. These afferents comprise the comb system, and run through the length of the nucleus (8.290), probably making en passant contacts. Like the striatopallidal axons, of which they may be collaterals, striatonigral comb axons utilize GABA and SP or enkephalin, and also distribute differentially in the pars reticulata: the enkephalinergic axons to the medial part, SP axons throughout. The projection neurons of the pars reticulata appear to be GABAergic. The dendrites of many of the dopaminergic pars compacta neurons extend down into the pars reticulata (8.297), making dendrodendritic in addition to the conventional axodendritic contacts. The large reticulata neurons are the source of efferents from this part of the nigral complex. As in the pallidum, small interneurons are present but rare.

Subthalamic nucleus

(See Webster 1990 for references.)

This is a biconvex lens-shaped nucleus in the subthalamus of the diencephalon medial to the crus cerebri (8.290). It is encapsulated by axons, many of which derive from the subthalamic fasciculus. Small interneurons are intermingled with large multipolar cells with dendrites which, in humans, extend for about one-tenth the diameter of the nucleus. Little is known of its neurochemistry.

CONNECTIONS OF THE CORPUS STRIATUM

The connections are summarized in 8.298, and presented in simplified form in 8.299. Three important general points need to be made. First, although the connections of the dorsal and ventral divisions overlap, those of the ventral division are predominantly with the limbic system and orbitofrontal and temporal cortex. Secondly, for both dorsal and ventral systems, it is important to realize that both the pallidum and substantia nigra pars reticulata are key nodal areas on the efferent side. Thirdly, the fundamental arrangement is the same for both divisions: cerebral cortex projects to the striatum, which in turn projects to the pallidum and substantia nigra pars reticulata, whence efferents leave to control the ultimate 'effector' targets of the system, primarily cerebral cortex (either the supplementary motor area or prefrontal and cingulate cortex) and superior colliculus. Extensive bibliographies will be found in Divac and Öberg 1979; Alexander et al 1986; Carpenter 1981, 1984; Nauta

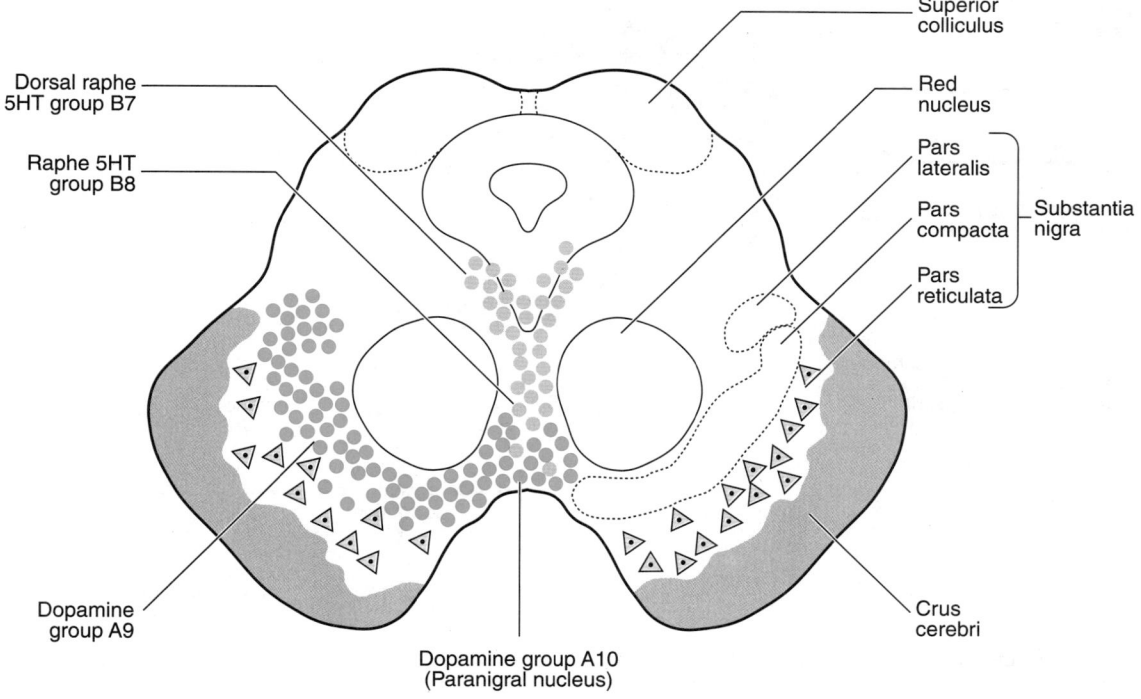

8.296   Transverse section through the midbrain to show the arrangement of the substantia nigra (right) and the position of dopaminergic cell groups (A9, 10) and the serotonergic cell groups B7, 8 in the raphe (left and centre). (Modified from Webster, 1990, with permission of the author and publisher.)

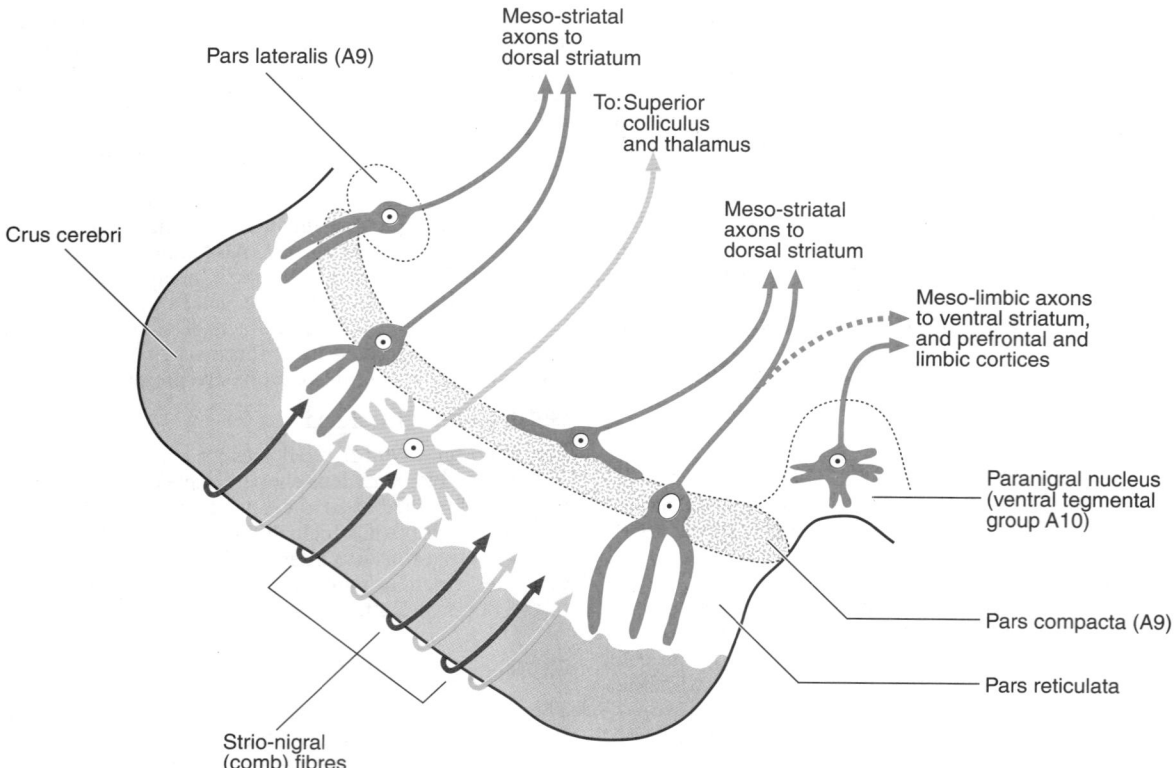

8.297 A scheme of the organization of the substantia nigra in transverse section. Compare with **8.296**. Notice that, medially, there is no sharp distinction between dopaminergic cells projecting to the dorsal striatum (pars compacta, A9) and those projecting to the ventral striatum and limbic system (paranigral nucleus, A10). Note, too, the intrusion of the dendrites of dopaminergic neurons into the pars reticulata and the distinctive projection systems from the latter. (Modified from Webster, 1990, with permission of the author and publishers.)

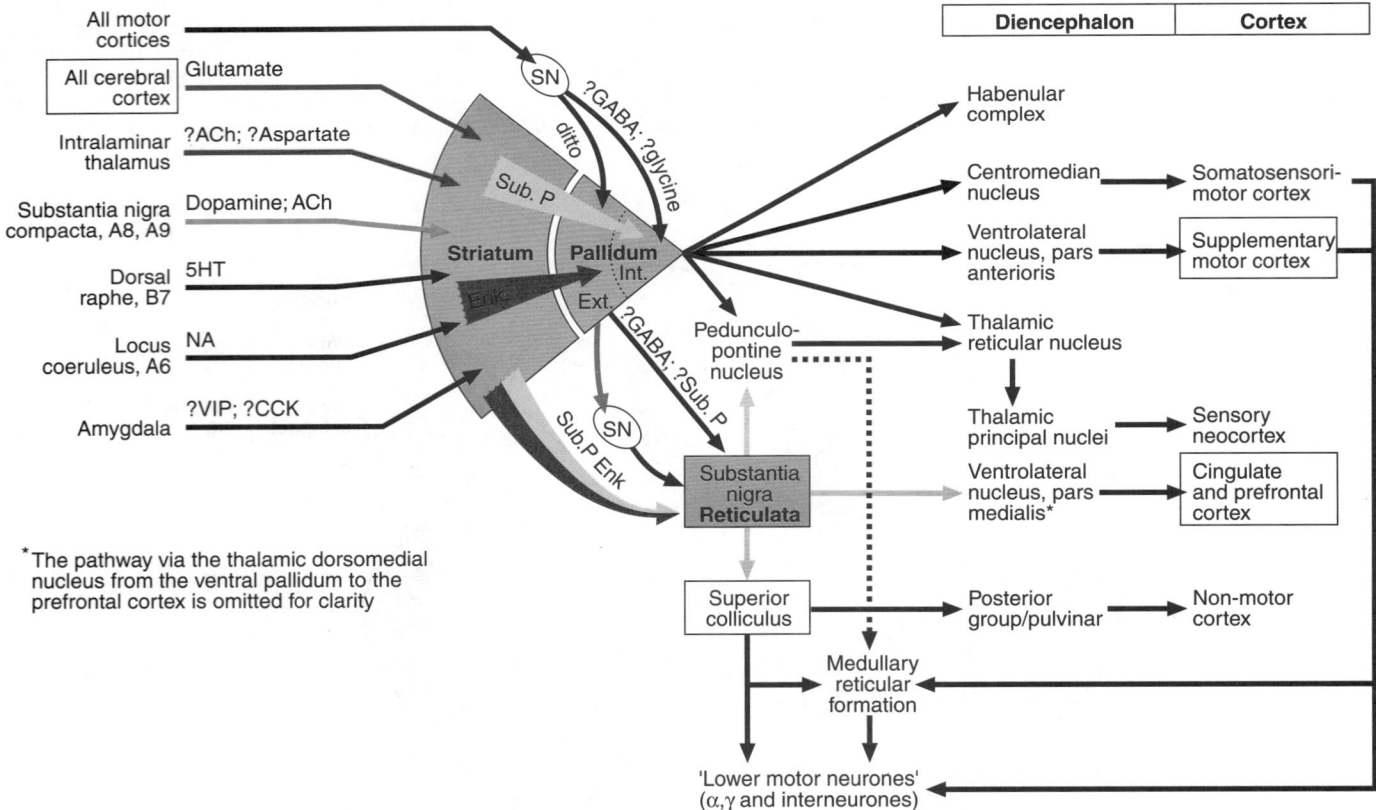

8.298 A scheme of the connections of the basal ganglia. Notice the efferent nodal point represented by the substantia nigra pars reticulata as well as the pallidum. The transmitters known or suspected to be associated with various pathways are indicated. ACh = acetylcholine; Enk = enkephalins; Ex = external pallidal segment; GABA = γ-aminobutyric acid; CCK = cho-lecystokinin; NA = noradrenaline; SN = subthalamic nucleus; Sub P = substance P; VIP = vasoactive intestinal polypeptide; 5HT = 5-hydroxytryptamine. (Modified from Webster, 1990, with permission of the author and publishers.)

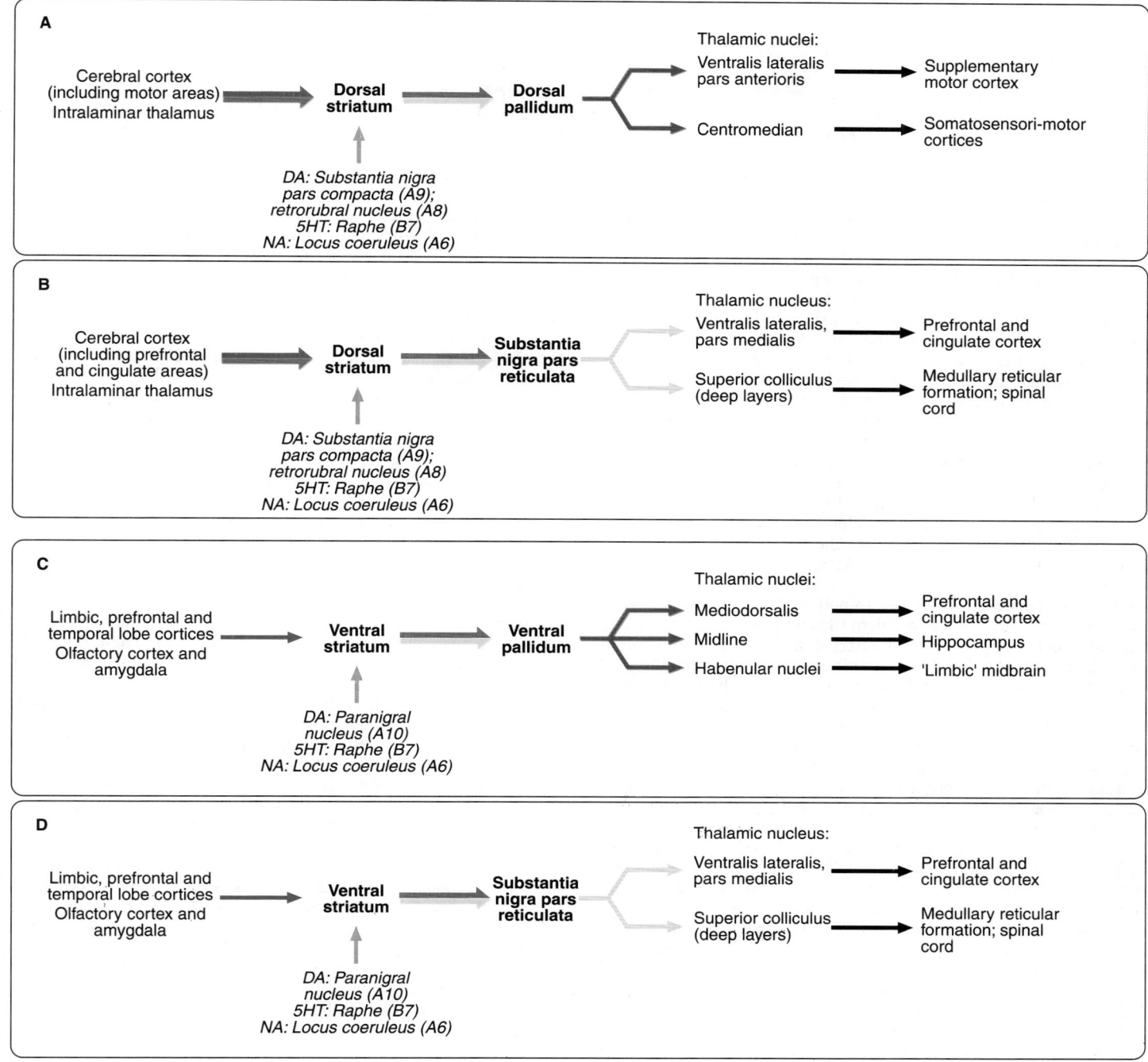

8.299 Schemes of the principal connections of the dorsal (A, B) and ventral (C, D) divisions of the basal ganglia. In each case pathways established through the pallidum are distinguished from those passing through the substantia nigra pars reticulata. The colour coding corresponds to that in **8.290**, 296–300. DA = dopamine; NA = noradrenaline; 5HT = hydroxy-tryptamine.

and Domesick 1984; Alheid et al 1990; Webster 1990; and Parent and Hazrati 1993.

Dorsal system

The entire neocortex sends glutaminergic axons to the striatum of its own hemisphere. For a long time, these axons were thought to be collaterals of other cortical efferents, but it is now known that they arise exclusively from small pyramidal cells in layers V and VI—although it has been suggested that some of the cells of origin are in the supragranular 'cortical association' layers II and III. The entire projection is organized topographically. In non-human primates, the spatial ordering of the corticostriate projection and the topography of the caudate–putamen and cerebral hemisphere mean that the greater part of the input from the cerebral cortex to the dorsal striatum is derived from the frontal and parietal lobes, and that the volume of striatum occupied by occipitotemporal inputs is relatively small (**8.288**A). Thus, the orbitofrontal association cortex projects to the inferior part of the head of the caudate nucleus neighbouring the ventral striatum; the dorsolateral frontal associ-ation cortex and frontal eye fields to the rest of the head of the caudate nucleus; much of the parietal lobe to the body of the nucleus, and so on. The somatosensory and motor cortices of primates project predominantly to the putamen, in which these afferents establish a somatotopic pattern, with 'lower body axons' ending laterally and 'upper body' medially. The motor cortex is also unique in sending axons through the corpus callosum to the opposite putamen, where they end with the same spatial ordering. The occipital and temporal cortices project to the tail of the caudate nucleus and to the inferior putamen. Also, regions of cortex which establish reciprocal association connections with each other have a dual input to the striatum. Thus, each zone of the striatum receives a heavier, primary input determined by corticostriate topography; and a secondary, much lighter projection from that cortex with which the primary source establishes reciprocal corticocortical connections. In all cases, the mosaic or cluster patterns of ending (see above) ensure that overlapping projections in effect interdigitate rather than overlap in the true sense.

The striatum also receives afferents from the polysensory intralaminar thalamus. These afferents are again, if more crudely, spatially organized: the cerebello-receptive nucleus centralis lateralis projects to the anterior striatum (especially caudate nucleus) and the cerebello- and pallido-receptive centromedian nucleus to the putamen.

It is important to note that through these two inputs, the dorsal striatum gains access to all sensory (except olfactory) as well as cognitive information. One of the functions of the system is to process and to pass this information to the supplementary motor cortex, which is otherwise almost entirely deprived of such inputs.

The aminergic inputs to the caudate–putamen are derived from the retrorubral nucleus (dopaminergic group A8; 8.290) and substantia nigra pars compacta (dopaminergic group A9; 8.290, 296, 297), the dorsal raphe nucleus (serotonergic group B7; 8.296), and the locus coeruleus (noradrenergic group A6. The nigral input is often referred to as the 'mesostriatal' dopamine pathway. It reaches the striatum by traversing the H fields of the subthalamus. These aminergic inputs appear to modulate the responses of the striatum to cortical and thalamic afferent barrages, without which the striatal neurons are almost silent.

Efferents from the striatum pass to both segments of the pallidum, where they end in a topically ordered fashion but neurochemically segregated between internal and external segments (see above and 8.298). The internal pallidal segment sends efferents through the ansa lenticularis, fasciculus lenticularis, the H fields of the subthalamus and so through the thalamic fasciculus to both the intralaminar centromedian nucleus and the principal nucleus ventralis lateralis pars anterioris (8.290, 299A). The latter projects to the supplementary motor area on the dorsomedial side of the frontal lobe, the former diffusely to the somatosensorimotor cortices. A second outflow is established from striatum to the pars reticulata of the substantia nigra both directly (8.298, 299B), and indirectly via the pallidum (8.300). The axons of the direct striatonigral projection constitute the laterally placed comb system which is thus spatially quite separate from the ascending dopaminergic nigrostriate pathway (8.290). Direct striatonigral fibres end in a spatially ordered way in the pars reticulata. The indirect pathway centres on the pallidum, which sends axons from its external segment through the subthalamic fasciculus to the subthalamic nucleus and from its internal segment to the midbrain pedunculopontine nucleus. Both of these nuclei in turn project to the nigra pars reticulata (8.300), which in turn projects both to the deep (polysensory) layers of the superior colliculus, and so to the brainstem and spinal cord; and to the thalamic nucleus ventralis lateralis pars medialis, which projects to the anterior cingulate cortex and the prefrontal association cortex. This last represents an overlap with the organization of the ventral striatal system.

(Additional outflows from the basal nuclei are indicated in 8.298. See Webster 1990, for discussion and references.)

Ventral system

(Heimer & Van Hoesen 1979; Heimer et al 1982; Alheid et al, 1990; see also Alexander et al 1986; Rolls 1990.) As in the dorsal system, the ventral striatum is the primary target of cortical afferents (8.299C,D). In this case, these afferents are from limbic cortices, including allocortex or, for the most part, from limbic associated regions: the hippocampus (through the fornix) and orbitofrontal cortex (through the internal capsule) project to the nucleus accumbens, and the olfactory, entorhinal, anterior cingulate and temporal visual cortices to both nucleus accumbens and olfactory tubercle in varying degrees. The tubercle also receives afferents from the amygdala. The contiguities of the cortical areas projecting to the ventral striatum and neighbouring dorsal striatum emphasize the imprecise nature of the boundaries between the two divisions (8.292); all the cortical regions overlap and abut one another and project to neighbouring parts of the dorsal striatum as well as to the ventral striatum. Thus, the fundus striati and ventromedial caudate nucleus abut the olfactory tubercle and nucleus accumbens (8.292) and receive connections from the orbito-frontal cortex and, to a lesser extent, the lateral prefrontal and anterior cingulate cortex, which also project to the contiguous head of the caudate nucleus, which is dorsal striatum.

This continuity of ventral with dorsal striatum, as evidenced by the arrangements of corticostriate projections, is reinforced by consideration of the aminergic inputs to the ventral striatum, which derive from the dorsal raphe (serotonergic group B7), the locus coeruleus (noradrenergic group A6), and from the paranigral nucleus (dopamine group A10), as well as the most medial part of the substantia nigra pars compacta (A9) (8.296, 297). These dopamine projections constitute the 'mesolimbic' dopamine pathway, which also projects to the septal nuclei, hippocampus and amygdala and prefrontal and cingulate cortex through the medial forebrain bundle (8.290). The lateromedial continuity of cell groups A9 and 10 (8.296) is thus reflected in the relative positions of their ascending fibres in the sub- and hypothalamus (the H fields and median forebrain bundle respectively; 8.290), as well as in the lateromedial topography of the dorsal and ventral striata (8.292), which in turn have contiguous and overlapping sources of cortical afferents.

As in the dorsal system, efferents leave the striatum to find both the pallidum (in this case the ventral pallidum) and the substantia nigra pars reticulata (8.292C, D). In the latter case, the connection is again both direct, and indirect via the subthalamic nucleus. The projections from the pars reticulata are as described for the dorsal system, but axons from the ventral pallidum reach the thalamic mediodorsal nucleus (which projects to cingulate and to prefrontal association cortex) and midline nuclei (which project to the hippocampus). Ventral pallidal axons also reach the habenular complex of the limbic system.

The brain areas beyond the basal nuclei, substantia nigra and subthalamic nucleus to which both ventral and dorsal systems would seem to project are therefore the prefrontal association and cingulate cortex and the deep superior colliculus.

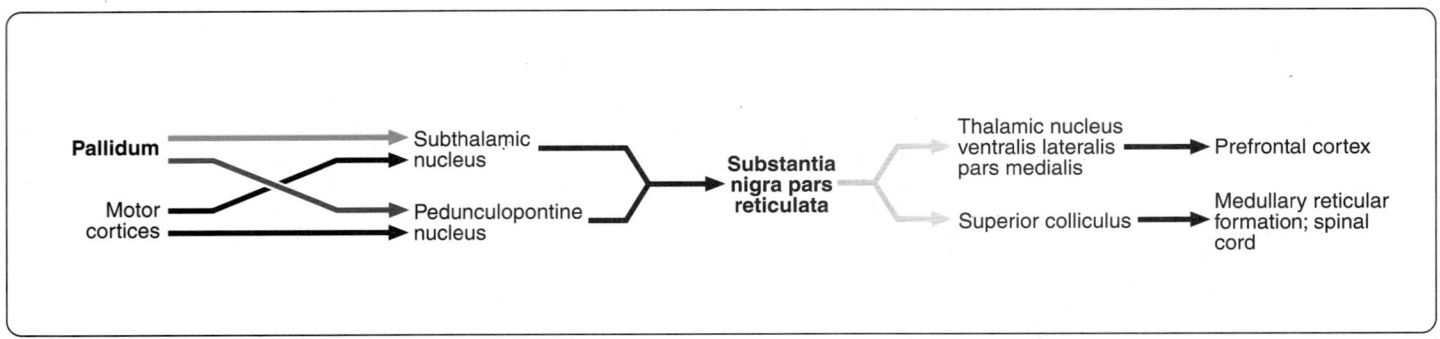

8.300 A scheme of the additional pathways which pass to the substantia nigra pars reticulata via the subthalamic and pedunculo-pontine nuclei. Note the direct projections to these nuclei from the motor cortex. Compare with 8.301.

Claustrum

The claustrum is a thin sheet of grey matter coextensive with the insula and putamen, from which it is separated by the external capsule. Thickest below and in front, it becomes continuous here with the anterior perforated substance, amygdala and prepiriform cortex. It is regarded by some as belonging to the corpus striatum, by others as a detached part of the insular cortex, but detailed studies suggest that it may have at least two structurally and functionally distinct zones, the 'insular' claustrum and the 'temporal' or 'prepiriform' claustrum. In experimental animals, the insular part has been shown to have reciprocal, topically organized cortico-claustral and claustrocortical connections with many regions of the neocortex. Its connections and functional significance are unknown in the human brain.

Some functional and pathophysiological correlates

(For references see Divac & Öberg 1979; DeLong & Georgopoulos 1981; Marsden 1990; Alexander at al 1986; Rolls 1990.)

Striatal dopamine and glucose metabolism

Positron emission tomography (PET) studies of Parkinsonian patients reveal an expected deficit of dopamine storage and reuptake, due to loss of nigrostriate terminals, but normal dopamine receptor levels (Brooms & Frackowiack 1989). In progressive supranuclear gaze palsy, however, in which the mesostriatal projection can be normal, it is the striatal dopamine receptor sites which are deficient. At first sight, it seems paradoxical that the general metabolic state of the striatum (as determined by PET scan studies of glucose uptake) in Parkinson's disease is often normal, whereas in other disorders, including progressive supranuclear gaze palsy, Huntington's chorea and Wilson's disease, it is always depressed. Increased glucose uptake is associated with increased synaptic activity, and dopamine terminals (depleted or absent in Parkinson's disease) account for only about 10% of the total in the striatum: the resolution of the technique is too poor to detect such small changes. However, the other disorders mentioned are associated with loss of striatal cells and their intrinsic synapses, which accounts for the greater (and therefore detectable) change in glucose metabolism. The loss of striatal neurons presumably also accounts for the loss of dopamine receptor sites (which are associated with their membranes) in, for example, progressive supranuclear gaze palsy and Huntington's chorea.

Bradykinesia, abnormal movements and disturbances of gaze

The remarkably limited nature of cortical inputs to the motor cortices from any but the somatosensory areas has been remarked above. Since the basal nuclei receive afferents from the entire cerebral cortex (including limbic system), they provide a channel for sensory and for cognitive, affective and mnemonic information to reach the (dorsomedial) supplementary motor area. The importance of this channel is underlined by the observation from imaging studies of humans that mental planning of a movement induces increased activity in the supplementary motor area before any of the other motor cortices, none of which become active until overt movement begins. This becomes more significant in the context of akinesia—one of the difficulties faced by patients with severe Parkinson's disease (or severe MPTP (N-methyl 4-phenyl 1,2,3,6-tetrahydropyridine) poisoning, which destroys the mesostriatal and mesolimbic systems). All parkinsonian patients suffer from bradykinesia: they find it difficult to start (or to stop) a movement. In extreme cases, the result is an akinetic or 'frozen' patient, unable to move or to speak, limbs and body rigidly held in often bizarre postures. What is more, when such patients are 'released' by Levodopa treatment, they report that they were always fully conscious and aware, and constantly thinking of and planning movements but quite incapable of carrying them out. It has been pointed out that the (lateral) premotor cortex (receiving ascending information, like the primary motor area, from the cerebellum) does receive a direct input from the visual cortices and that this may be why parkinsonian patients, deprived of effectively functioning (dorsomedial) supplementary motor areas, come to rely overmuch on visual clues for the control of movement: for example, such patients are better able to walk between two tramlines painted on the floor than when given a free choice of path (see Iversen 1979). This interpretation does, of course, focus on the relationship of the pallidal outflow with the supplementary motor area. It ignores the parallel pallidal outflow to the thalamic intralaminar centromedian nucleus, which in turn projects onto the entire somatosensorimotor cortex. The significance of this second projection is unknown: it is diffuse and ends in different cortical layers from the projections arising in the principal thalamic nuclei (ventralis lateralis pars anterioris et posterioris, and the ventroposterior nucleus).

The pathway from the striatum to the superior colliculus via the substantia nigra pars reticulata presumably bears a similar functional relationship to cortical control of gaze as does that pathway influencing the supplementary motor cortex and therefore the initiation of general body movement. The uncontrolled or fixed gaze disturbances of supranuclear gaze palsy, Huntington's chorea and advanced Parkinson's disease readily attest to this. The appearance of uncontrolled movements such as athetosis and chorea is mimicked by over-dosing with Levodopa or its agonists, which suggests that the system may in such cases begin the 'free-run' downstream and independent of the non-motor cortical control.

Muscle tone and tremor

All these disturbances are, of course, accompanied by changes in muscle tone, and specific disturbances of gait and eye movements. Eye movements are spectacularly impaired in progressive supranuclear palsy and Huntington's chorea, in both of which striatal dysfunction is implicated: the connections though the substantia nigra pars reticulata to the superior colliculus is presumably of crucial significance in this regard. The changes in muscle tone presumably reflect a disturbance of the relationship between the activities of the somatosensorimotor cortex and the brainstem reticular formation—the latter influenced by the basal nuclei in a direct way only tenuously (through the pedunculo-pontine nucleus— see 8.298) and indirectly through the motor cortex and superior colliculus. The tremor of Parkinson's disease, superimposed on the rigidity, produces the characteristic 'cog-wheel' resistance to passive movement. The tremor is itself interesting because no experimental destruction of the nigrostriatal system or interference with the basal nuclei in any species produces it. Additional damage to the cerebellorubral and cerebellothalamic pathway is required. The evidence in humans is indirect, but points in the same direction. First, tremor is not a striking symptom of MPTP poisoning (see above). Secondly, recording from the ventrolateral thalamic nucleus of parkinsonian patients reveals neurons firing periodically in bursts, the frequency of the bursts corresponding to the frequency of the tremor (~5 Hz). Thirdly, the cerebello-receptive ventrolateral nucleus pars posterioris projects to the primary motor cortex, and destruction of this cortex (as in a stroke superimposed on the parkinsonian syndrome) abolishes the tremor. Finally, therapeutic thalamotomy abolishes parkinsonian tremor if the lesion is in the posterior (cerebello-receptive) ventrolateral nucleus; whereas rigidity is alleviated only when the lesion extends into the more anterior (pallido-receptive) ventrolateral nucleus. This, of course, leaves unanswered the question of why, if it is due to nigrostriatal degeneration, Parkinson's disease usually has tremor as one of its features.

Gait

Locomotion in non-primates is certainly based upon the existence in the spinal cord of 'central pattern generators'—pools of interneurons which are able to drive the somatic efferent neurons to produce the required patterns of limb movements (Grillner & Wallén 1985). The existence of such generators in primates (including humans) is less well established. The mechanisms of supraspinal control of the generators confer on the patterns of movement the requisite power as well as 'goal directedness'. It is not clear, however, that given the existence of this basic arrangement in humans, exactly how the basal ganglia would control such pattern generator mechanisms, and specifically, why one of the features of Parkinson's disease should be the characteristic impairment of gait (including the loss of associated arm-swinging movements). Experimental evidence, however, indicates dopamine systems descending from the brainstem are crucial in activating the cord pattern generators (and will, in fact, trigger the onset of quadripedal walking patterns, of which the arm-swinging associated with human gait is a reflection). It has to be remem-

bered that in Parkinson's disease, the degeneration is not confined to the nigrostriatal system, but involves aminergic neurons throughout the brainstem, including, presumably, the source of these descending 'trigger' axons.

Behavioural disorders

Other, and of late largely ignored, experimental observations are also beginning to appear clinically significant. There are scattered in the literature numerous reports of experiments in various species (including primates) in which ablation or stimulation of especially the caudate nucleus induced uncontrollable hyperactivity (e.g. obstinate progression, head turning, incessant pacing and even more elaborate and constantly repeated behaviour, and—in cats—'ecstatic kneading', a rhythmical pumping with alternate forepaws of cushions, owner's clothes or, in suckling kittens, the mother's abdomen around the nipple). These and other results have led some workers to the generalization that in terms of motor activity, the corpus striatum enables the animal to make motor choices and to avoid 'stimulus-bound' behaviour (see Webster 1975; Divac & Öberg 1979; Iversen 1979, for references). Recent PET scanning studies have shown defects in the uptake of dopamine by the striatum in patients suffering from at least some (repetitive movement) dystonias (Brooks & Frackowiack 1989). (It is also noteworthy that focal dystonias—such as writer's cramp—represent the disordered execution of a planned movement, and respond well to dopamine-related therapies.) PET scanning studies in humans have also produced evidence that sufferers from obsessional-compulsive disorders (accompanied by meaningless

but repeated ritualistic motor behaviour and intrusive thoughts) show signs of hyperactivity in the prefrontal cortex and caudate nuclei (Bench et al 1990). There are similar suggestive observations in the hyperactive child syndrome. It is worthwhile remembering that the basal nuclei, besides receiving connections from the frontal lobe and limbic cortices, also have an ascending influence on the prefrontal and cingulate cortex through the substantia nigra pars reticulata and dorsomedial and ventromedial thalamus (8.298, 299B, C, D). These pathways may also be of significance for the finding that in the large number of parkinsonian patients who become clinically depressed the prefrontal cortex is hypofunctional (Bench et al 1990)—although again it must be remembered that the disease process destroys mono-amine neurons of all types and in widespread sites in the brainstem, many of which (including the raphe, paranigral nucleus and locus coeruleus) project directly to the cortex.

Sensory disturbances

Finally, examination of 8.298 reveals other connections which do not fit easily into the category of 'motor', even when this is interpreted broadly in the sense of the motor realization of cognitive events: for example, the relationships with the pulvinar and sensory relay nuclei of the thalamus. In this context, the minority school of thought which ascribes sensory functions to the corpus striatum is interesting (Krauthamer 1979), as is the observation that parkinsonian patients are unable accurately to judge the perpendicular by visual inspection alone (Teuber & Proctor—see Webster 1975).

Heterogeneity, loops and channels in basal ganglia circuits

Open and closed feedback loops

(8.298–300), illustrating the principal connections of the basal ganglia, are laid out in linear fashion on the assumption that such schemes are more easily followed. Close examination will reveal that these are in fact only 'opened out' versions of more usual illustrations which emphasize the existence of reciprocal feedback connections and apparently closed loops. One might also usefully ask if such 'loop' or 'feedback' arrangements are really what they seem. For example, detailed examination of the 'to and fro' interconnections between the pallidum, on the one hand and the subthalamic and pendunculo-

pontine nuclei, on the other, reveals them to be substantially linear or 'feedforward' pathways to the pars reticulata and superior colliculus (compare 8.300, 301). It is possible that 'feedback' connections of this sort are examples of spatial separation between interneurons (the subthalamus and pedunculopontine nuclei) and the projection neurons (the pallidum) they control. (The arrangements in the substantia gelatinosa of the spinal cord or the thalamic reticular nucleus serve as paradigms for such organizations.) In this light, notice that the system as illustrated in 8.301 is not quite straightforward: it confers on the motor cortices the 'privilege' of influencing the general pallidal

and pars reticulata outflows over and above the influences these same cortices exercise through the putamen. This subtlety is obscured by drawing the connections in simple linear fashion (8.300).

Probably the most significant of such 'feedback loops' in the system are those which are essentially cerebral cortex ⇒ basal nuclei ⇒ thalamus ⇒ cerebral cortex. Their significance depends, in part, on the possibility that basal nuclei connections are established by means of more or less discrete channels or pathways through the system. In this case, the loops might be 'open' or 'closed'. In the 'closed' arrangement (8.302A), the connections through the system would be organized

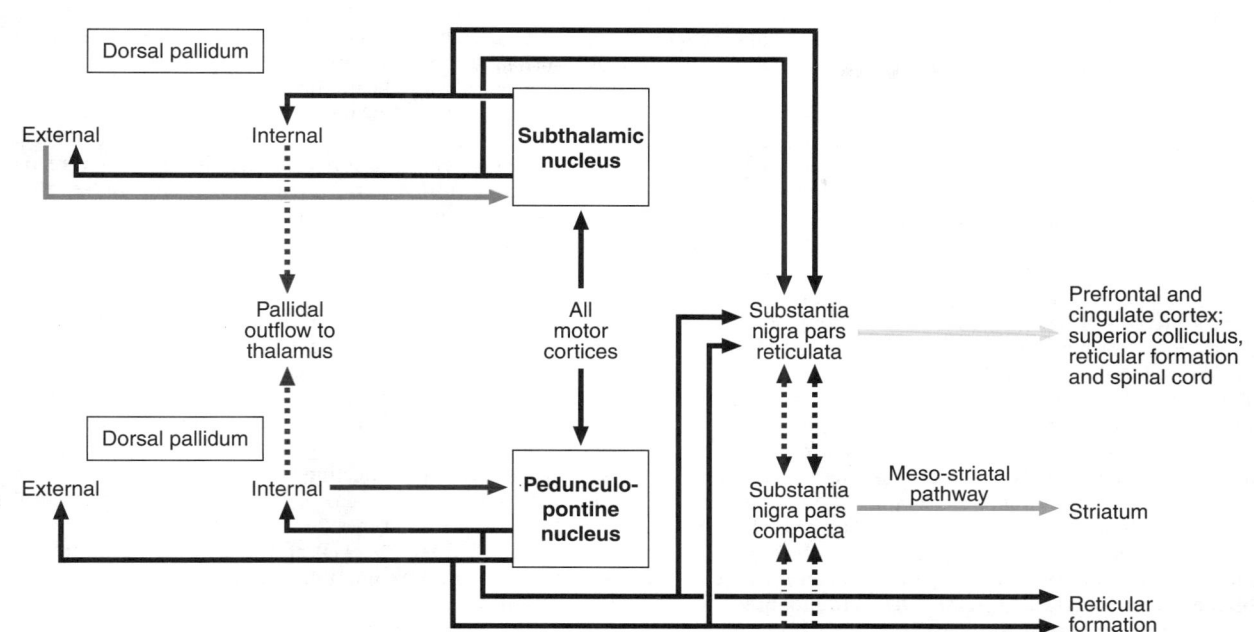

8.301 Scheme to show how an apparently closed feedback loop between the pallidum and the subthalamic and pedunculo-pontine nuclei is an elaborate feedforward projection: the feed forward and feedback axons are in fact collaterals. Notice, however, that the connections as shown here confer on the motor cortices the ability to control, independent of the cortico-striatopallidal pathway, (a) the outflow from the internal pallidal segment to the thalamus; and (b) the meso-striatal dopamine system (through the interactions between the pars compacta and pars reticulata of the substantia nigra). These subtleties are obscured by presenting the connections in simple linear fashion, as in **8**.300.

into channels arranged to ensure that an area of cerebral cortex which receives from the system (i.e. the supplementary motor area, via the thalamic nucleus ventralis lateralis pars anterioris; the general somatosensorimotor cortex via the centromedian nucleus; and prefrontal and anterior cingulate cortex via the dorsomedial and ventromedial thalamic nuclei) would project into that channel which ultimately leads back to itself. In the 'open' arrangement (**8.302**B), the opposite would apply, and the channels would ensure that, for example, cortical areas which ultimately feed back onto supplementary motor cortex are those outside the supplementary motor area, but not the supplementary motor area itself. There might exist, of course, a mixture of the two arrangements (**8.302**C). What is the evidence for the existence of such channels and loops?

Heterogeneity and channels

That the basal nuclei are not homogeneous is crucially evidenced by the parcellation of the corticostriatal projection, which confers a functional heterogeneity on the striatum, such that, in non-human primates, quite distinct behavioural and performance deficits result from dysfunction of different parts. This goes beyond what might be called the simple motor control associated with the putamen. It seems that different regions of the striatum enable the cognitive 'decisions' of related cerebral

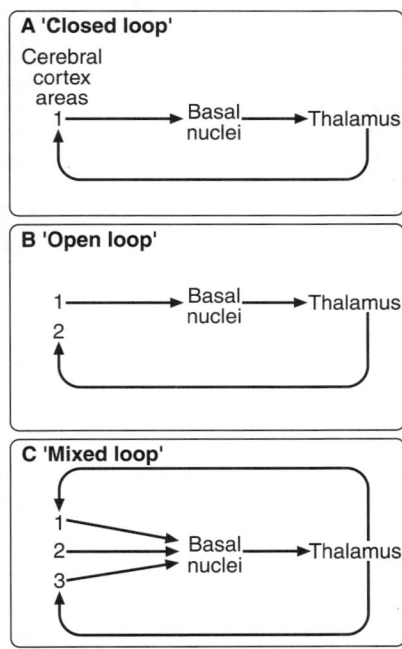

8.302 Simplified schemes to illustrate possible permutations of corticocortical loop–feedback configurations through the basal ganglia. In each case the cortical areas 1, 2, 3 are hypothetical and do not relate to any cytoarchitectural or physiological scheme. A. Closed loop— area 1 could represent, for example, either the medial supplementary motor

cortex to be translated into appropriate overt (motor) behaviour and for midaction adjustments to be made as necessary. Thus, the head of the caudate nucleus (related to prefrontal cortex) is essential for overt performance of a response which involves planning, strategy and 'working memory'; the inferior putamen for the responses dependent on detailed visual analysis; and so on. The striatal topical heterogeneity also appears to be carried through into the pallidum, despite the marked convergence implied by the ratio of striatal to pallidal neurons and the dendritic/afferent relationships within the latter. Spatial arrangements of afferents in the substantia nigra pars reticulata are less certainly known (compare accounts in Nauta & Domesick 1984; Alexander et al 1986; Webster 1990; and Gerfen 1992),

cortex or the orbito-frontal cortex. B. Completely open configuration: area 1 could represent the entire cerebral cortex less that represented by area 2. c. Mixed loop: if area 3 denotes, for example, the medial supplementary motor cortex, and area 1 the orbito-frontal and anterior cingulate cortices, these represent the sources and terminations of closed loops. Area 2 would denote all other cortices: for loop 3 ⇒ 3, area 2 could subsume area 1; for loop 1 ⇒ 1, area 2 could subsume area 3.

and those of the pallidothalamic projection equally contentious (compare accounts in Carpenter 1981, 1984; Jones 1985; and see Webster 1990).

In spite of these reservations, Alexander et al (1986) have proposed that the projection systems of the basal nuclei involve at least five distinct channels. Moreover, these are based on complex loops, each with a 'closed' component (supplementary motor area ⇒ supplementary motor area; frontal eye fields ⇒ frontal eye fields; dorsolateral prefrontal cortex ⇒ dorsolateral prefrontal cortex; anterior cingulate cortex ⇒ anterior cingulate cortex), each loop passing through the basal nuclei, but with an 'open loop' component peculiar to itself, in as far as the relevant part of the striatum in each channel is assumed to have a separate set of afferents from additional and distinctive areas of cortex (8.302c). For example, the 'closed' supplementary motor loop runs through that part of the putamen which also receives from the (lateral) premotor and primary motor areas as well as from the somatosensory cortices. The 'closed' frontal eye field loop begins by entering that part of the caudate nucleus which also receives from dorsolateral prefrontal cortex and posterior parietal areas, whereas the dorsolateral prefrontal cortex 'closed' loop involves another part of the caudate nucleus, which additionally receives from the (lateral) premotor area and posterior parietal cortex, and so on. Alexander et al also point out that the differential regional developments of the striosome/matrix mosaic and of the relationships of afferents and efferents to it may provide an additional basis for the channelling in the striatum. This had been proposed by Graybiel (1984) who also suggested that the differential distributions of neuroactive

substances in the pallidum and substantia nigra pars reticulata may be possible extensions of this principle downstream of the striatum. This theme has been elaborated by Gerfen (1992). First, he distinguishes, on the basis of their dopamine receptor types, pathways of striatal origin which control either the pallidum or substantia nigra pars reticulata. Secondly, he proposes that, in the latter case, it is possible further to differentiate two efferent streams: those striatal efferents arising from within striosomes, themselves controlled through allocortex, which modulate, through the pars reticulata, the ascending mesostriatal system at its origin in the pars compacta; and those efferents from striatal matrix which control pars reticulata cells which are the source of efferents to the superior colliculi and ventromedial thalamus.

Moreover, although differential distributions are not exclusive, striosomes are found predominantly in the ventral and neighbouring dorsal striatum, and receive most of their cortical input from allocortex and from deeper in layer V of the neocortex, whereas the matrix predominates in the dorsal striatum, especially the putamen, and receives cortical axons largely from cells of the superficial layer V of the neocortex. Gerfen suggests that there may therefore exist three channels which, although not isolated from one another, are nevertheless distinct: the first, articulated through striosomes is limbic, and deeper neocortex-related, and controls the overall activity of the striatum (and therefore of the whole system) through the mesostriatal dopamine pathway (and perhaps even the mesolimbic projection, too); the second, funnelled through the striatal matrix, allows superficial layer V of the neocortex to

influence, through the substantia nigra pars reticulata, the deeper layers of the superior colliculus (and therefore eye and head movements); the third, again synapsing in the matrix, permits neurons of the superficial layer V of the neocortex to influence activity in the entire pallidal outflow (including control of the supplementary motor cortex). One speculative, but potentially important aspect of such arrangements, is that, since such parcellations imply chemospecificities along each path, it becomes possible to anticipate that 'basal nuclei disease' will present as a variety of pathophysiological syndromes, depending on the combinations of functional channels disordered by more or less subtle pathologies affecting, for example, neurons with particular neurochemical and receptor phenotypes.

Even if the idea of such precise parcellation proves ultimately untenable, it represents an important and challenging conceptual framework against which experimental results and clinical findings can be interpreted. That the basal nuclei are heterogeneous is beyond question and this has an important practical consequence for the future of treatments involving the grafting of dopaminergic cells. The effective radius of activity of such implants is a few millimetres: all other things equal, attempts to restore complete function to a striatum deprived of its ascending dopaminergic input must involve the introduction of several implants scattered as widely as possible through the caudate–putamen, so as to reactivate as many subchannels as possible. Without this, the successful survival of a single graft will promote functional recoveries of only limited sorts.

Cell transplantation in Parkinson's disease

Intrastriatal implants of embryonic ventral mesencephalic tissue, rich in dopamine neurons, reinnervate the dopamine denervated striatum of rodents and monkeys with experimental Parkinson's disease, form synaptic contacts with host striatal neurons, release dopamine and improve motor and sensorimotor function (Dunnett 1991; Dunnett & Annett 1991). In the animal models, the neural grafts reverse both behavioural deficits of unclear clinical relevance (mainly apomorphine- and amphetamine-induced rotational asymmetry in animals with a unilateral lesion of the mesostriatal dopamine system), and those deficits probably

or definitely relevant for Parkinson's disease in humans (sensory neglect, spontaneous rotation, tremor, rigidity and hypokinesia). Also, human embryonic dopamine neurons implanted into rats reinnervate the striatum, release dopamine and improve motor deficits (Brundin et al 1988). However, not all motor symptoms in animals can be reversed by neural grafts.

The improvement after transplantation in animal models of Parkinson's disease is dependent both on the number of surviving grafted dopamine neurons and the density and extent of the graft-derived reinnervation. Poor graft survival and

limited reinnervation of the striatum by the graft lead to much less symptomatic relief than if many grafted dopamine cells have survived and given rise to a reinnervation of high density throughout most parts of the striatum. Furthermore, the improvement disappears after destruction of the graft. Thus, the symptomatic relief is dependent on the continuous presence of the graft.

From the clinical point of view, the most attractive feature of neural grafting in Parkinson's disease is the possibility of restoration of the physiological release of dopamine at synaptic sites in the striatum deprived of intrinsic dopaminergic innervation. Such a specific local effect, just in the area with deficient dopamine transmission and not in brain regions outside the striatum, cannot be obtained with any other approach.

Cell grafts in humans

The major scientific objective in the first human grafting studies has been to explore if survival and function of human embryonic mesencephalic grafts are at all possible in patients with Parkinson's disease, i.e. whether the basic principles of cell replacement, established in animal experiments, are valid also in the diseased human brain. More than 150 patients have so far been grafted, either uni- or, in a few cases, bilaterally in the caudate nucleus and/or putamen (for references, see Lindvall 1994). Most patients have been immunosuppressed. Minor to moderate alleviation of motor symptoms has been reported in almost all patients after transplantation, but the mechanisms of improvement are unknown in most cases. Using positron emission tomography (PET), significant increase of [18F] fluorodopa uptake in the grafted striatum has been demonstrated in about 20 cases (8.303). This is most likely due to survival and growth of the grafted dopamine neurons, as previously demonstrated in animal experiments. In support of this hypothesis, a patient with sustained improvement of motor function and a progressive increase of [18F] fluorodopa uptake showed surviving grafts and extensive dopaminergic reinervation of the striatum at neurological examination 18 months post-grafting (Kardower et al 1995).

Since idiopathic Parkinson's disease is an ongoing degenerative disorder it has been unclear whether the disease process will destroy also the grafted dopamine neurons. In two patients with unilateral implants into the putamen (8.303A), repeated PET scans demonstrated a marked increase of [18F] fluorodopa uptake in the grafted putamen up to 3 years after surgery despite a progressive fall of tracer uptake in non-grafted striatal regions (Lindvall et al 1994). Clinical assessment showed improved motor performance on the side contralateral to the graft but, after an initial improvement during the first postoperative year, a worsening of Parkinson's disease symptoms on the ipsilateral side (8.303B). These data indicate that grafts can survive and have long-term functional effects but that the graft-induced improvement is counteracted by degeneration of the patient's own dopamine neurons.

The clinical observations made so far support the idea that cell transplantation can be developed into an effective treatment for Parkinson's disease, but further improvements are necessary before this procedure should be performed in a large number of patients. At present, the symptomatic relief produced by neural grafts is incomplete both in animal models and in patients. Increased survival and reinnervation volume of grafted dopamine neurons, and testing of alternative sources of cells suitable for implantation are some current research strategies for the further development of a transplantation therapy in Parkinson's disease. The survival of embryonic dopamine neurons is low (only 5–20%) after transplantation with available procedures. Why up to 95% of the dopamine neurons die is unknown. Due to this low survival rate, it seems that mesencephalic tissue from 3–4 embryos needs to be implanted on each side in a patient with Parkinson's disease in order to obtain a major improvement, which restricts the clinical usefulness of neural grafting. Survival of dopamine neurons might be increased by the addition of neurotrophic factors, such as brain-

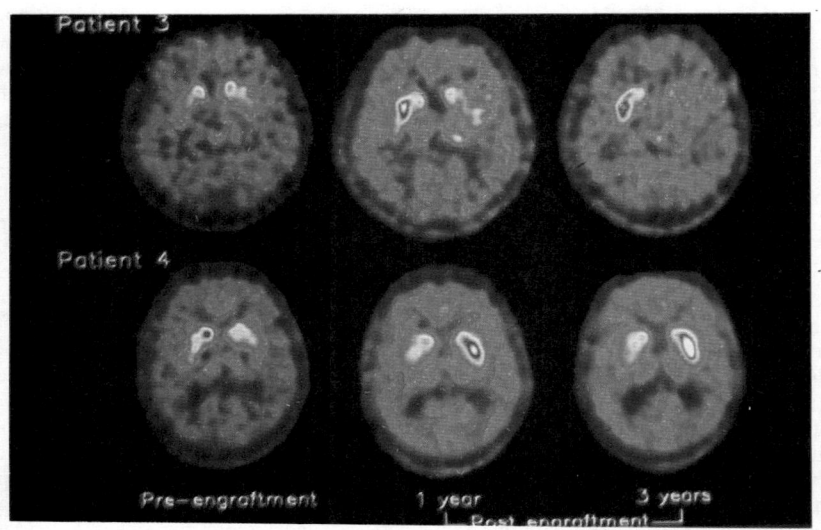

8.303A PET scans showing [18F] fluorodopa uptake in two patients implanted with human embryonic mesencephalic tissue in the left (Patient 3) or right (Patient 4) putamen. At 1 year after surgery there is increased fluorodopa uptake in the grafted putamen indicating survival of implanted dopaminergic neurons. This increase is stable at 3 years in Patient 3 but has become more pronounced in Patient 4. However, there is also a progressive fall of tracer uptake in non-grafted striatal regions, especially in Patient 3, suggesting degeneration of the patient's own DA neurons (from Lindvall et al 1994).

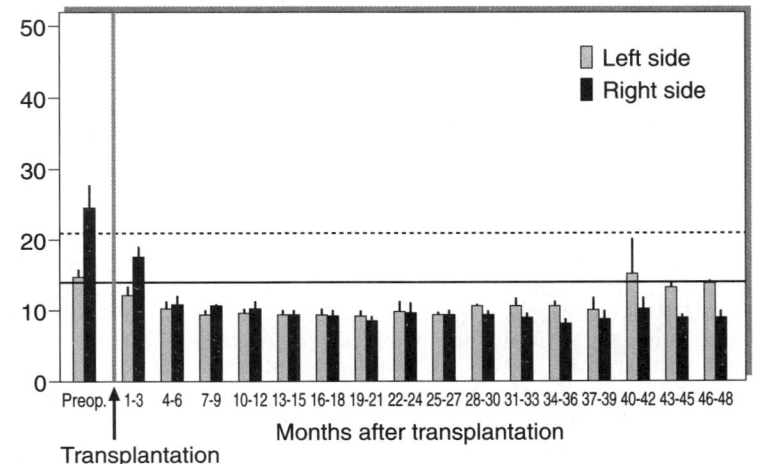

8.303B Time needed to perform 20 pronation-supination movements in the 'off' state in Patient 3. This task started to improve during the second postoperative month, mainly on the right side, contralateral to the graft. In good agreement with the PET data there was a worsening on the left (ipsilateral) side from 28 months after surgery.

derived neurotrophic factor (Hyman et al 1991) and glial cell line-derived neurotrophic factor (Lin et al 1993). This effect can already be achieved in vitro and in the future it may be possible to supply the graft with these factors to increase dopamine neuron survival in vivo.

When human embryonic dopamine neurons are implanted along three tracts in the putamen (as in the patients illustrated in **8.303**), probably only about 25% of the total volume of this structure is reached by graft-derived axons, achieving a reinnervation density of 25% or more of normal (Lindvall 1994). This density could be a critical level for obtaining a clear, long-lasting functional effect. One strategy for more complete reinnervation of the striatum is to distribute the graft material more efficiently over larger areas and bilaterally. Another possibility could be to stimulate growth and branching of axons from the grafted dopamine neurons by the addition of neurotrophic factors.

Alternative sources of cells

If cell transplantation is going to become a clinically useful treatment for a large number of parkinsonian patients and be applied also in other neurological disorders, alternative sources of cells suitable for transplantation must be found. The main interest is presently focused on adrenal medulla cells and genetically engineered cells.

Several hundred patients with Parkinson's disease have received intrastriatal implants of autologous adrenal chromaffin cells, intended to provide a new source of catecholamines (for references see Lindvall 1994). In agreement with the animal experimental data, only modest symptomatic relief has been detected in grafted patients

and survival of the implants has been poor. Further improvement of the adrenal medulla autotransplantation procedure, e.g. by increasing cell survival and function through the addition of nerve growth factor to the graft tissue, has to be demonstrated in animal models before more patients with Parkinson's disease should be operated on.

One possible future strategy could be to implant cells that have been genetically engineered to synthesize and release Levodopa (L-dopa) or dopamine. Such cells are made through insertion of the gene encoding for tyrosine hydroxylase (TH); they can be produced in large numbers and, if derived from the patient's own tissues, are not at risk for immunological rejection. The first attempts at testing the functional capacity of genetically engineered cells revealed that various cell lines (producing either L-dopa or dopamine; Wolff et al 1989; Horellou et al 1990) and primary fibroblasts (secreting L-dopa; Fisher et al 1991) or myoblasts (producing dopamine; Jiao et al 1993) have been shown to ameliorate apomorphine-induced rotational asymmetry after implantation into the dopamine denervated striatum of rats. Although these data support the potential usefulness of gene transfer in combination with the intracerebral transplantation approach, from the perspective of a clinical application two major issues must be considered apart from the risks for adverse effects. Firstly, the duration of the symptomatic relief produced by the implants has been too short. The major limiting factor is the decline of the expression of the inserted TH gene as well as of the functional improvement over a few months. Recent evidence indicates,

however, that a stable and high level of TH-gene expression can be obtained in muscle cells for at least 6 months after grafting (Jiao et al 1993). Secondly, the capacity of genetically engineered cells to reverse the functional deficits relevant for the human disorder is unknown. Critical criteria for the ability of such cells to improve a particular symptom in a parkinsonian patient include ability of the graft to restore well-regulated or partly regulated synaptic release and to integrate anatomically and functionally into the host brain.

Summary

In conclusion, available data indicate that grafts of embryonic mesencephalic neurons can partly restore dopamine transmission in the striatum and reverse, though still incompletely, symptoms in experimental parkinsonism as well as in patients with Parkinson's disease. The major objectives in this field of research are:

- to optimize the neural grafting procedures in order to normalize dopamine transmission in the basal ganglia and achieve maximum symptomatic recovery
- to explore the possibility that similar functional effects can be induced after implantation of other cell types, e.g. genetically engineered cells.

Cell transplantation will become a useful treatment for patients with Parkinson's disease if the degree, pattern and duration of functional improvement observed using this strategy is comparable to or better than the symptomatic relief induced by other therapeutic approaches. An essay on the biology of neural transplantation is to be found on p. 919.

FLUID COMPARTMENTS AND FLUID BALANCE IN THE CENTRAL NERVOUS SYSTEM

There are two major extracellular fluid compartments in the central nervous system (CNS); they contain the *cerebrospinal fluid* (CSF) and *interstitial fluid*. Although the compartments are connected and the fluid in both is originally derived from the blood, the functions and the drainage pathways of the two fluids differ. Substantially greater in volume, CSF is derived from the blood and secreted by the choroid plexus. CSF fills the ventricles and passes through the craniospinal subarachnoid spaces and drains back into the blood largely through the arachnoid granulations and villi. The CSF plays a major buoyancy role in the mechanical support of the central nervous system. Interstitial fluid is also derived from the blood and may alter substantially, both in composition and in amount, when there is breakdown of the blood–brain barrier. Animal experiments suggest that major pathways for the drainage of interstitial fluid, particularly from grey matter regions of the brain, are along perivascular spaces and through paravascular compartments of the

subarachnoid space to regional lymph nodes, i.e. cervical lymph nodes for the brain and lumbar lymph nodes for the spinal cord. Although the evidence from tracer studies is scarce in man, there are anatomical pathways in the human central nervous system which correspond to the *lymphatic drainage pathways of the brain* identified in experimental animals.

The functional anatomy of the meninges, fluid compartments and fluid balance in the central nervous system is reviewed here by:

- tracing the production, circulation and drainage of CSF from the choroid plexus, through the ventricles and subarachnoid spaces to the arachnoid granulations
- examining the structural aspects of the blood supply of the brain, the blood–brain barrier, the extracellular spaces and evidence for lymphatic drainage of the interstitial fluid from the central nervous system.

CHOROID PLEXUS AND THE PRODUCTION OF CEREBROSPINAL FLUID

CHOROID PLEXUS

The choroid plexus (8.291, 304–307) is located in the lateral ventricles, the third ventricle and the fourth ventricle. In the embryo, it develops initially from an invagination of mesenchyme in the thin roof area of the myelencephalon during the sixth week of intrauterine life. In the 7–9 week human embryo, the telencephalic choroid plexus starts to develop with a loose mesenchymal stroma covered by a layer of cells derived from ependyma (Shuangshoti & Netsky 1966; Dohrmann 1970). During the second half of gestation the choroid plexus develops a stroma consisting of leptomeningeal cells, connective tissue and blood vessels (Shuangshoti & Netsky 1966).

In the lateral and third ventricles, the choroid plexus is part of the *tela choroidea* (8.291, 304, 305), which has a core of meninges invaginated during development along a linear region of the medial hemispheric wall where no nervous tissue develops. Hence, leptomeninges (pia mater) are directly in contact with the ventricular *ependyma* as the two tissues fuse to form the choroid plexus, which otherwise consists chiefly of small blood vessels, capillaries and nerve fibres. In the *lateral ventricle*, the choroid plexus extends anteriorly to the interventricular foramen where it is continuous across the third ventricle with the plexus of the opposite ventricle. From the foramen, it passes posteriorly in contact with the thalamus, curving round its posterior end into the ventricle's inferior horn and reaching the pes hippocampi. When the plexus is removed from the hemisphere, the line of invagination becomes the *choroid fissure*. Through the central part of the ventricle, the fissure is between the fornix superiorly and the thalamus inferiorly (8.304). The choroid fissure is the first groove to appear on the surface of the cerebrum; in coronal sections of the brain at 8 weeks of gestation, it is already in contact with the lateral margin of the ependymal roof of the third ventricle, its overlying pia mater and accompanying blood vessels. At this stage, before the development of the commissures and expansion of the lamina terminalis, single layers of pia and ependyma form the roof of the *third ventricle*. The corpus callosum and the body of the fornix expand posteriorly above the choroid fissure, carrying a layer of pia mater on their inferior surfaces which overlie the third ventricle pial layer and fusing with it to form the central part of the tela choroidea; the lateral extensions of this, also double layered, invaginate the choroidal fissures and form a choroid plexus in the lateral ventricles (8.304). Posteriorly, the two pial layers separate the inferior (original) layer following the ventricular roof to the pineal gland and tectum; the superior layer cleaves to enclose the corpus callosum and passes round the splenium to the superior callosal surface.

As described above, two layers of pia mater fuse to form the *tela choroidea of the third ventricle* (as usually termed, although the choroid plexus of the *lateral* ventricles are extensions of it). From above, it is triangular with a rounded apex between the interventricular foramina, often indented by the anterior columns of the fornices (8.291). Its lateral edges are irregular, containing choroid vascular fringes. At the posterior basal angles of the tela, these fringes continue and curve on into the inferior cornu of the ventricle (8.291, 305), while centrally the pial layers depart from each other as described above. When the tela choroidea is removed, a transverse slit is left between the splenium and the junction of the ventricular roof with the tectum, the *transverse fissure* (not a cerebral fissure in the ordinary sense, for cortex is not involved). It marks the posterior limit of the *extracerebral* space enclosed by the posterior extensions of the corpus callosum above the third ventricle; in this, enclosed between the two layers of pia mater, are the roots of the choroid plexus of the third ventricle and of the lateral ventricles (8.304). The choroid plexus of the third ventricle is attached to the tela choroidea which is, in effect, the thin roof of the third ventricle as it develops during fetal life. In coronal sections of the cerebral hemispheres, the choroid plexus of the third ventricle can be seen in continuity with the choroid plexus of the lateral ventricles (8.304).

As in the roof of the third ventricle and the medial walls of the lateral ventricles, the roof of the *fourth ventricle* develops as a thin sheet in which the pia mater is in contact with the ependymal lining of the ventricle and there is no intervening neural tissue. This thin sheet forms the *tela choroidea of the fourth ventricle* and is between the cerebellum and the inferior part of the roof of the ventricle. A dorsal layer covers the inferior vermis and, reaching the nodule, is reflected ventro-inferiorly in direct contact with the ependyma. The choroid plexus thus has vertical and horizontal limbs in the fourth ventricle. Two longitudinal, vertical parts of the choroid plexus flank the midline, fusing at the cranial margin of the median aperture (foramen of Magendie) and are often prolonged on to the ventral aspect of the vermis to which they adhere. The horizontal parts of the plexus are continuous and project into the ventricle, passing into the lateral recesses and emerging through the lateral apertures (foramina of Luschka) still covered by ependyma. The entire structure is like a T, with a double vertical limb, but this form varies widely (Lang & Schäfer 1977).

Blood supply

The blood supply of the choroid plexus in the *tela choroidea of the third and lateral ventricles* is from the anterior choroidal branch of

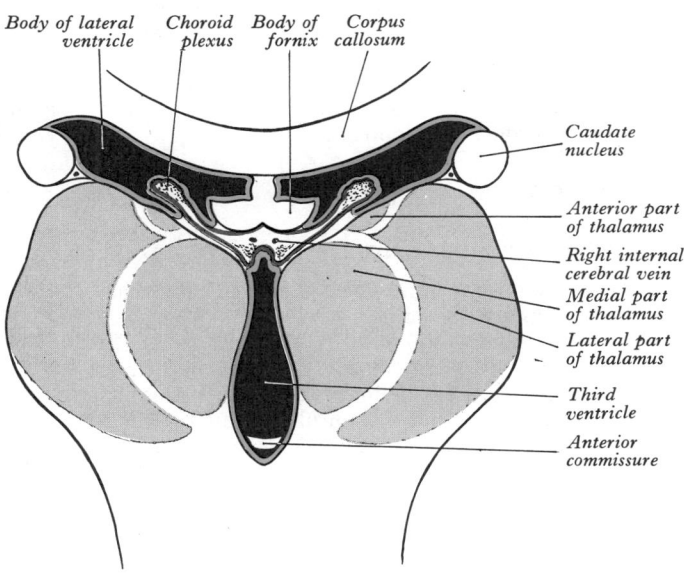

8.304   Diagram of a coronal section through the lateral and third ventricles. The pia mater of the tela choroidea is shown in red and the ependyma in blue.

Body of lateral ventricle — Choroid plexus — Body of fornix — Corpus callosum — Caudate nucleus — Anterior part of thalamus — Right internal cerebral vein — Medial part of thalamus — Lateral part of thalamus — Third ventricle — Anterior commissure

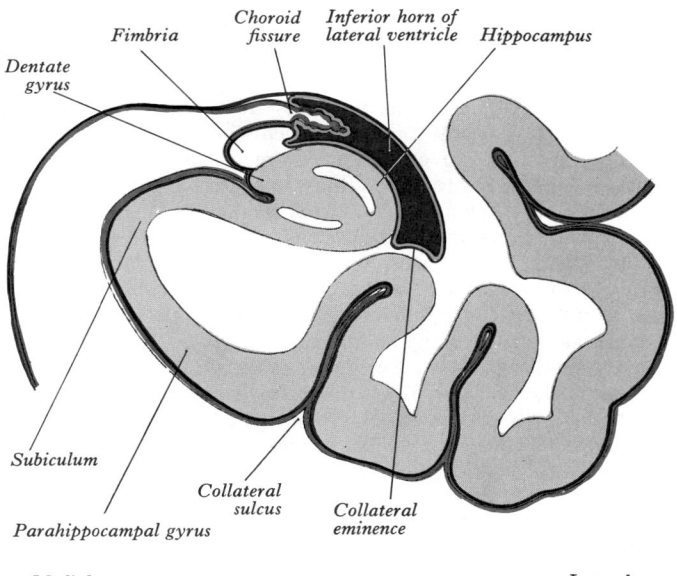

8.305   Diagram of a coronal section through the inferior cornu of the lateral ventricle. The pia mater is shown in red and the ependyma in blue.

Fimbria — Choroid fissure — Inferior horn of lateral ventricle — Hippocampus — Dentate gyrus — Subiculum — Collateral sulcus — Collateral eminence — Parahippocampal gyrus

←Medial   Lateral→

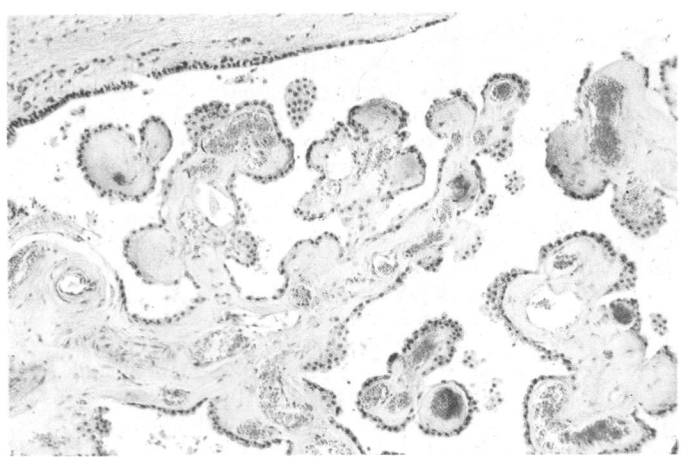

8.306 A section of part of the choroid plexus of the lateral ventricle, stained with haematoxylin and eosin. Note the ependyma lining the ventricular wall above and covering the loose connective tissue cores of the processes of the plexus, which contain numerous small blood vessels, including many capillaries. A calcareous deposit (dark blue) is present in one process. Owing to the complexity of the ramification of the processes, several appear as disconnected islands of tissue.

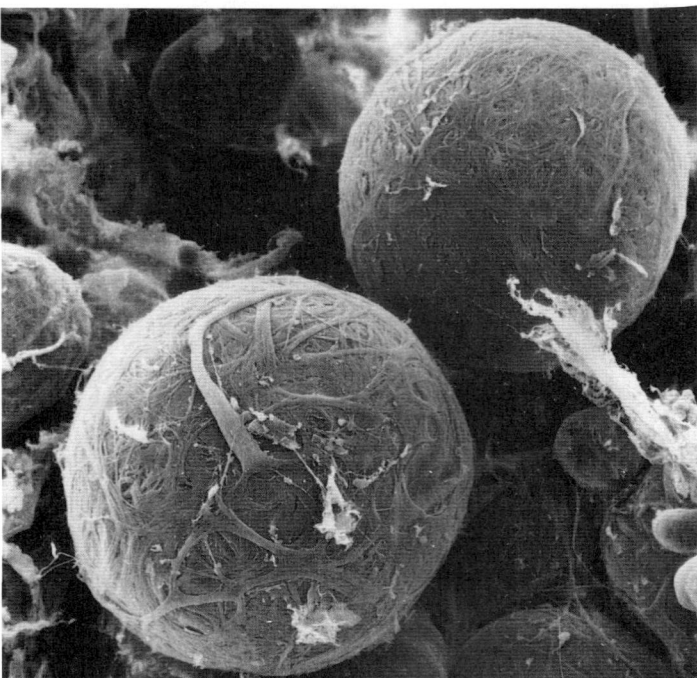

8.307 Psammoma bodies in the choroid plexus stroma of a 74-year-old female showing their spherical form and matted collagenous structure. SEM × 290 (reprinted from Alcolado et al 1986).

the internal carotid and choroidal branches of the posterior cerebral artery. The former usually forms a single vessel and the latter 3–5 in number (Millen & Woollam 1953). The two sets of vessels anastomose to some extent. Capillaries drain into a rich venous plexus served by a single choroidal vein leaving the tela choroidea, commencing near each basal (posterior lateral) angle of the tela. This region corresponds to the margin between territories of anterior and posterior choroidal arteries and here also (on each side) a solitary so-called 'glomus' tissue is situated near the free edge of the choroid plexus; many tributaries of the choroidal vein converge towards it.

The blood supply of the fourth ventricular choroid plexus is from the inferior cerebellar arteries (Maillot et al 1976).

Microscopic structure

The choroid plexus has a villous structure with a *stroma* composed of meningeal cells derived from pia mater (Alcolado et al 1986), bundles of collagen and blood vessels (8.306). During fetal life, there is erythropoiesis in the stroma of the choroid plexus with bone marrow-like cells occupying the stroma. Transmission electron microscopy has shown that the *leptomeningeal cells* within the stroma have a clear cytoplasm and round nuclei, and are joined by intervening desmosomes and gap junctions. Small packets and whorls of collagen form within the stroma and many are completely surrounded by arachnoid cell processes. Such collagen whorls vary in size from 2–3 μm in diameter to 60 μm or more (Alcolado et al 1986). Capillaries within the stroma are thin-walled and mostly fenestrated (Dermitziel & Schinke 1975; Van Deurs 1979) although the endothelial cells are joined by tight junctions.

An *epithelium*, derived from ependyma, coats the surface of the choroid plexus. It is a low cuboidal epithelium with numerous microvilli but few cilia on the surface (Clementi & Marini 1972). The epithelial cells are tightly packed, joined by tight junctions (zonulae occludentes) and covered on the basal aspect by basement membrane (Peters et al 1976). Immunocytochemistry has shown that the epithelial cells contain S100 protein and the enzyme carbonic anhydrase C (Weller et al 1986). In this way, the choroid plexus epithelium can be distinguished from ependyma which does not express carbonic anhydrase C. Epithelial cells in tumours of the choroid plexus may also express glial fibrillary acidic protein and low molecular weight cytokeratins as intermediate filaments (Weller 1990).

Phagocytic cells are present in the stroma of the choroid plexus, and as epiplexus (Kolmer) cells on its surface in man and in other species (Allen 1975; Sturrock 1978). Both choroid plexus epithelium

and epiplexus cells pinocytose particles and proteins from the ventricular lumen (Lu et al 1993).

Ageing changes occur in the human choroid plexus which have considerable relevance for imaging of the brain. Calcification of the human choroid plexus can be detected by skull X-ray (Dyke 1930) and more readily by computerized axial tomography (CT) in 0.5% of individuals in the first decade of life and in 86% in the eighth decade (Modic et al 1980). There is a sharp rise in the incidence of calcification from 35% of CT scans in the fifth decade to 75% in the sixth decade. The visible calcification is usually restricted to the glomus region of the choroid plexus, i.e. the vascular bulge in the choroid plexus as it curves to follow the anterior wall of the lateral ventricle into the temporal horn. Scanning and transmission electron microscopy have shown that the calcification is in the form of calcospherites or psammoma bodies 30–50 μm in diameter within the choroid plexus stroma (8.307) (Alcolado et al 1986). Such psammoma bodies are formed by the deposition of calcium hydroxyapatite in collagen whorls originally formed by the meningeal cells within the stroma (Alcolado et al 1986).

CEREBROSPINAL FLUID

Composition and secretion

CSF is a clear, colourless liquid which in normal individuals contains a very small amount of protein and differs from blood in its electrolyte content (Davson et al 1987). The intracranial CSF volume has been estimated at 123 ml, some 25 ml in the ventricles and 98 ml in the subarachnoid space (Condon et al 1986). Its ionic composition suggests that the CSF is not just an ultrafiltrate of blood but that there is active secretion by the choroid plexus epithelium (Davson et al 1987; Bradbury 1993). Choroid plexus epithelial cells have the characteristics of transport and secretory cells with microvilli on the apical surfaces and interdigitations and folding of the basal aspects of the cells (Peters et al 1976). There are tight junctions at the apical ends of the epithelial cells which are permeable to small molecular weight substances. Fenestrated capillaries in the stroma of the choroid plexus are just beneath the epithelial cells. CSF is secreted from the apical surface of the epithelial cells at a rate of 0.35–0.4 ml per minute; this means that 50% of the CSF is replaced in 5–6 hours (Bradbury 1993). The mechanism of secretion involves carbonic anhydrase C within the epithelial cells; the Na-K-pump is the main motive force of CSF secretion (Saito & Wright 1983). The enzyme, Na-K-ATPase, has been localized in the microvillous ventricular surface of the choroid plexus epithelium (Bradbury 1993).

A blood–CSF barrier, therefore, exists and is sited at the choroid plexus epithelium. A dramatic demonstration of the blood–CSF barrier is seen at postmortem in jaundiced adult patients in whom the stroma of the choroid plexus is stained yellow by bile whereas CSF and brain remain unstained. As extracellular fluid from the brain parenchyma also drains into CSF, some 11% of CSF (in the rat) is derived from this *extrachoroidal source* (Szentistvanyi et al 1984). Other estimates vary from 30–60% (Davson et al 1987; Bradbury 1993).

Circulation and drainage

CSF secreted by the choroid plexuses in the lateral, third and fourth ventricles passes through the ventricular system and into the cisterna magna and subarachnoid cisterns over the front of the pons by passing through the exit foramina of Luschka and Magendie from the fourth ventricle. Mixing of CSF within the ventricles appears to be effected by cilia on the ependymal cells lining the ventricles and by arterial pulsations. Thus layers of fluid adjacent to the ependyma are agitated and mixed with the bulk of CSF. Radio-isotope scanning after cisternal injection indicates that it takes 1–2 hours for fluid to reach the basal cisterns, 3–5 hours to reach the subarachnoid space of the lateral fissure and 10–12 hours to spread over the cerebral surface. By 24 hours, labelled albumin becomes concentrated along the superior sagittal sinus and is being cleared from the basal cisterns (Milhorat 1972).

There is a free communication between the cerebral and spinal subarachnoid compartments but the mode of circulation of CSF in the spinal canal is uncertain. Some arachnoid villi exist in the spinal canal and absorption of some 16% may occur through the spinal meninges in the cat (Marmarou et al 1975).

The use of magnetic resonance imaging (MRI) to study CSF flow patterns in healthy volunteers has led to reconsideration of the classical concepts outlined above (Greitz et al 1993). Such studies suggest that extraventricular CSF flow is mainly caused by pulsatile movements of arteries and not by convective movements (bulk flow); pulsatile flow in the ventricles is smaller and bulk flow can only be identified in the aqueduct.

VENTRICULAR SYSTEM

The ventricular system in the cerebral hemispheres and hindbrain consists of two lateral ventricles and the midline third and fourth ventricles connected by the aqueduct of Sylvius (**8.308**). The third and fourth ventricles, together with the aqueduct, are derived from the central lumen of the neural tube but the lateral ventricles originate from the central lumen of the cerebral vesicles and are connected to the third ventricle by the foramina of Monro.

LATERAL VENTRICLES

Viewed from its lateral aspect, each lateral ventricle has a C-shaped morphology with an occipital tail (**8.308**). The shape is due to the expansion of the primate and human brain with enlargement of the frontal, parietal and occipital regions of the hemispheres displacing the temporal lobe inferiorly and anteriorly. Both the caudate nucleus and fornix have adopted a similar C-shaped morphology. The tail of the caudate nucleus encircles the thalamus in a C-shape and the outflow from the hippocampus, the fornix, traces the outline of the ventricles forwards to the pillars anterior to the *interventricular foramina of Monro* en route to the mamillary bodies of the hypothalamus.

When a cast of the ventricles is viewed from above, the lateral ventricles are seen to splay laterally as they curve into the temporal horns (**8.309**). Anatomically, the ventricles are divided into several regions, the *anterior horns, body, posterior or occipital horns* and the *temporal horns* (**8.289, 309**). The bodies of the lateral ventricles are separated by the septum pellucidum, which extends from the splen-

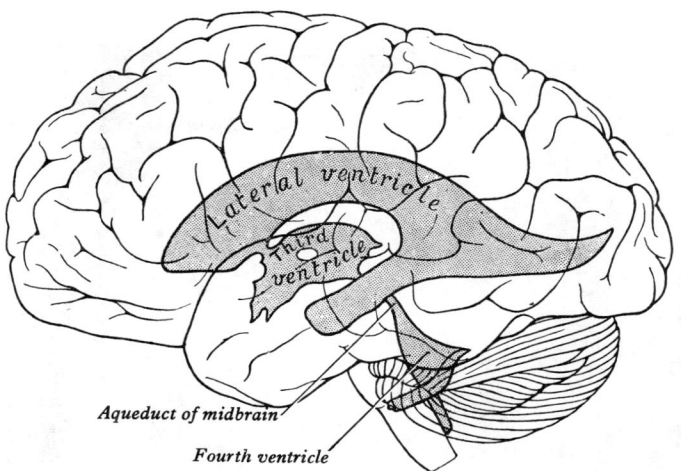

8.308 Projection of the ventricles on to the left surface of the brain.

ium of the corpus callosum forwards to the foramina of Monro; the fornices are suspended from the septum.

Structures forming the walls of the lateral ventricles can be seen in **8.310–312**.

Anterior horns (cornua) of the lateral ventricles. These extend from their most anterior limits back to the foramina of Monro; they are bounded anteriorly by the posterior aspect of the genu of the corpus callosum and the rostrum. The roof of each ventricle is formed by the anterior part of the callosal trunk and most of the lateral wall and floor is formed by the rounded head of the caudate nucleus. But, medially, part of the floor is formed by the upper aspect of the rostrum. The medial boundary of each lateral ventricle is the septum pellucidum, which contains the columns of the fornices in its posterior edge. The body of the lateral ventricle extends from the interventricular foramina (of Monro) to the splenium of the corpus callosum. Like the anterior part of the lateral ventricle, the coronal profile of the body of the ventricle is a flattened triangle (**8.310**) with an inward bulging lateral wall, formed by the thalamus inferiorly and the tail of the caudate nucleus superiorly. There are two grooves in the lateral wall of the lateral ventricle; the upper

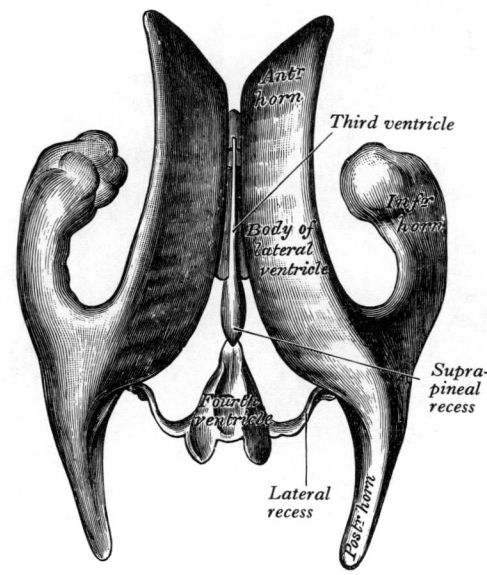

8.309 A drawing of a cast of the ventricular cavities: superior aspect (Retzius). Note that, where the lateral recess joins the fourth ventricle, the lateral dorsal recesses of the roof of the ventricle project dorsally on each side beyond the posterior margin of the median dorsal recess. The superior angle of the fourth ventricle and the aqueduct of the midbrain are hidden by the suprapineal recess.

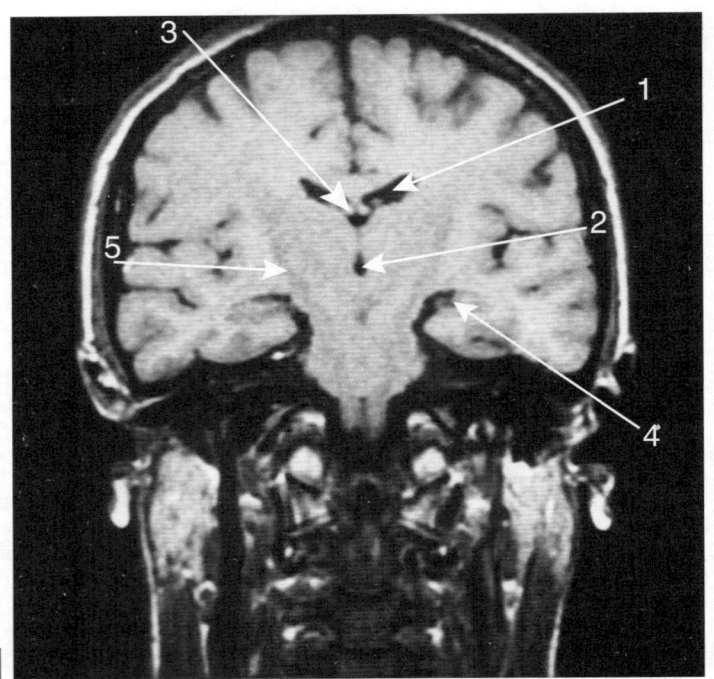

A

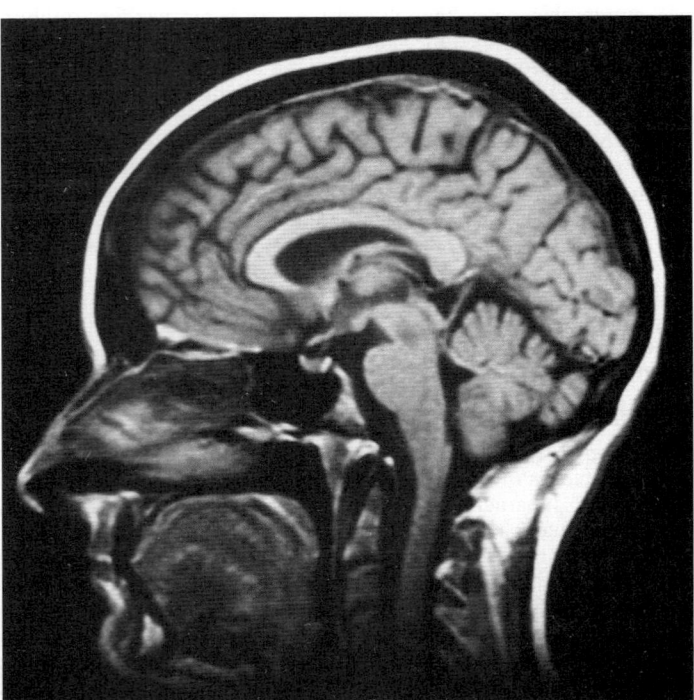

B

8.310 Magnetic resonance images of the brain. A. A coronal section through the level of the thalamus. Cerebrospinal fluid in the ventricles and cerebral sulci appears black. Key: 1 lateral ventricles; 2 third ventricle; 3 fornices suspended from the corpus callosum; 4 hippocampus in the tem-

poral horn of the lateral ventricle; 5 internal capsule. B. Sagittal section through the brain showing the ventricular system and the subarachnoid cisterns. The structures visible in this MRI are labelled in 8.313.

groove is occupied by the stria terminalis, a bundle of white fibres, and the thalamostriate vein (8.291); this groove separates the caudate nucleus from the thalamus. The inferior limit of the lateral ventricle and its medial wall is formed by the body of the fornix, which is separated from the thalamus by the choroidal fissure—a structure occluded by the choroid plexus. In an intact brain (8.289—right

side), the choroid plexus covers part of the thalamus and part of the fornix. Just posterior to the interventricular foramen, a small bulge on the surface of the thalamus may be seen representing the anterior nucleus of the thalamus.

Posterior or occipital horn of the lateral ventricle. This curves posteromedially into the occipital lobe (8.289). There is often asymmetry between the two posterior horns but, when present, they are usually diamond shaped or square in outline (8.311). The *roof* and *lateral wall* of the posterior horn is formed by fibres of the tapetum separating them from the optic radiation.

Splenial fibres forming the forceps major pass medially as they sweep back into the occipital lobe, producing a rounded *bulb* of the

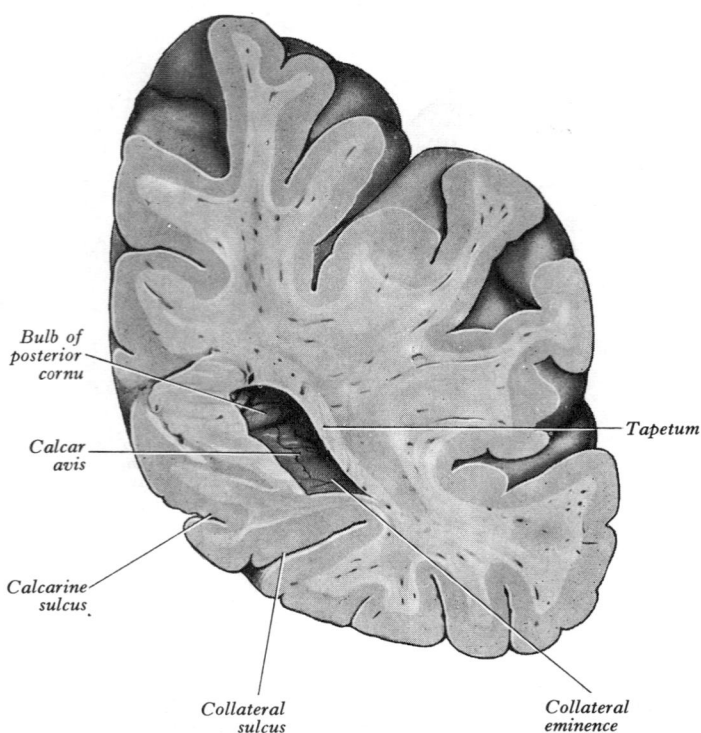

Bulb of posterior cornu

Calcar avis

Calcarine sulcus

Collateral sulcus

Collateral eminence

Tapetum

8.311 Anterior aspect of a coronal section through the posterior cornu of the left lateral ventricle.

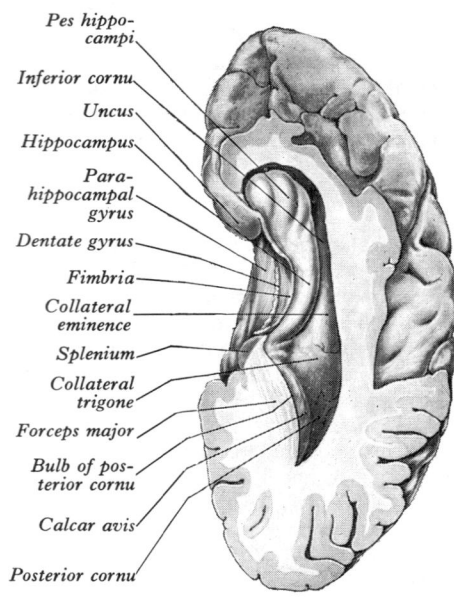

Pes hippo-campi

Inferior cornu

Uncus

Hippocampus

Para-hippocampal gyrus

Dentate gyrus

Fimbria

Collateral eminence

Splenium

Collateral trigone

Forceps major

Bulb of pos-terior cornu

Calcar avis

Posterior cornu

8.312 The posterior and inferior cornua of the right lateral ventricle, exposed from above.

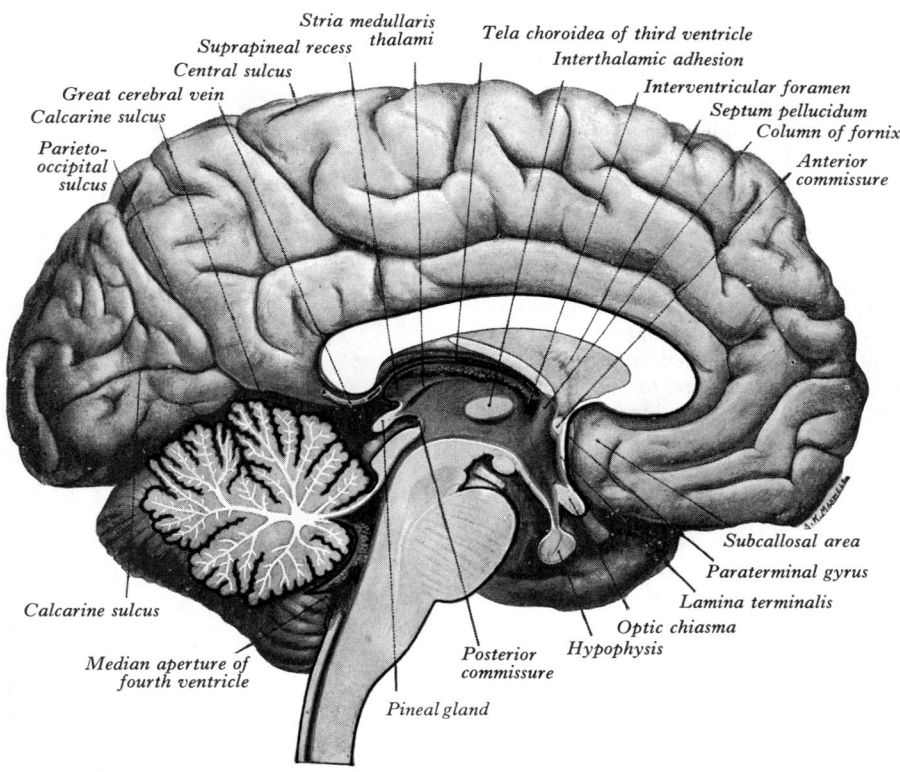

Stria medullaris
thalami
Suprapineal recess
Central sulcus
Great cerebral vein
Calcarine sulcus
Parieto-
occipital
sulcus

Tela choroidea of third ventricle
Interthalamic adhesion
Interventricular foramen
Septum pellucidum
Column of fornix
Anterior
commissure

Subcallosal area
Paraterminal gyrus
Lamina terminalis
Optic chiasma
Hypophysis

Calcarine sulcus

Median aperture of
fourth ventricle

Posterior
commissure

Pineal gland

8.313 Median hemi-section of the brain to show the relationship of the third and fourth ventricles. The pia mater is indicated in red and the ependyma in blue. [cf **8.310B**].

posterior horn in its upper medial wall (**8.289**) below which is a second elevation, the *calcar avis*, corresponding to the infolded cortex of the anterior calcarine sulcus (**8.311**).

Temporal or inferior horn of the lateral ventricle. The largest compartment, this extends forward into the temporal lobe. It curves round the posterior aspect of the thalamus (pulvinar) and at first passes downwards and posterolaterally before curving anteriorly to end within 2.5 cm of the temporal pole near the uncus. Its position on the surface of the hemisphere usually corresponds to the superior temporal sulcus.

The *roof* of the temporal horn is formed mainly by the tapetum of the corpus callosum but the tail of the caudate nucleus and stria terminalis also extend forwards in the roof to terminate in the amygdala at the anterior end of the ventricle. The floor of the ventricle consists of the collateral eminence laterally and the hippocampus medially (**8.312**). The fimbria of the hippocampus extend back on the superior medial surface of the hippocampus to become the alveus and then the crus of the fornix. Between the stria terminalis in the roof of the temporal horn and the fimbria, is the inferior part of the choroid fissure and the temporal extension of the choroid plexus filling the fissure and covering the outer surface of the hippocampus (**8.305**). In coronal section, the temporal horn of the lateral ventricle is flattened and, when opened superiorly, it can be seen that the *collateral eminence* (**8.312**) forms a long swelling lateral and parallel to the hippocampus and overlies the collateral sulcus. The eminence continues posteriorly into the flattened triangular *collateral trigone* forming the floor of the ventricle between its temporal and posterior horns.

THIRD VENTRICLE

The third ventricle (**8.289, 304, 308, 309, 313**) is a midline, slit-like cavity which is derived from the primitive forebrain vesicle. It lies between the two thalami and it is bordered inferiorly by the hypothalamus. Structures in the walls of the third ventricle are illustrated in **8.308** and **8.313** and the outline shape of the third ventricle is depicted in **8.308** and **8.309**. Anteriorly, the third ventricle extends to the lamina terminalis and interventricular foramina;

posteriorly the third ventricle is connected to the fourth ventricle by the cerebral aqueduct (of Sylvius). The *pineal gland* is at the apex of the thin walled *epiphyseal recess* of the third ventricle.

In the *roof* of the third ventricle is a thin ependymal layer extending from the lateral wall of the third ventricle to the *choroid plexus* which spans the *choroidal fissure*. Above this is the body of the fornix. The choroid plexus projects vertically down into the roof of the third ventricle (**8.304**).

Anteriorly, the *floor* of the third ventricle is lower than in its caudal portion and is formed mainly by hypothalamic structures which, passing rostrocaudally, are: the optic chiasm, infundibulum and tuber cinereum, and the mamillary bodies at the posterior limit of the hypothalamus. Posterior to the mamillary bodies is the *posterior perforated substance* and the tegmentum of the cerebral peduncles. The ventricle is prolonged into the infundibulum as the *infundibular recess*.

Rostrally (**8.310, 313**) the third ventricle is bounded ventrally by the *lamina terminalis* which is the rostral end of the neural tube. It is a thin structure stretching from the dorsum of the optic chiasm to the rostrum of the corpus callosum. Above this, the anterior wall is formed by the diverging columns of the fornices and the transversely orientated *anterior commissure* (**8.304, 313**) which crosses the midline rostral to the columns of the fornices. A small angular optic recess is seen in the third ventricle, just dorsal to the optic chiasm. At the junction of the roof and the anterior wall of the third ventricle are the *interventricular foramina* of Monro, connecting the lateral ventricles with the third ventricle. This is the site of the original outgrowth of the telencephalon to form the cerebral hemispheres. The interventricular foramina are relatively large and circular in the human embryo, but in the adult, they are slit-like and bounded anteriorly by the columns of the fornices and posteriorly by the anterior nucleus of the thalamus.

The pineal gland, posterior commissure and the cerebral aqueduct form the *posterior boundary* of the third ventricle (**8.310, 313**). The *pineal recess* projects into the pineal stalk and there is a *suprapineal recess* above it. Laterally, the third ventricle is bordered by the medial surface of the anterior two-thirds of the thalamus and the lower part of the lateral wall is formed by the hypothalamus anteriorly and the subthalamus posteriorly. A *hypothalamic sulcus* extends from the interventricular foramen to the cerebral aqueduct; it separates the *pars dorsalis diencephali* (dorsal thalamus and epithalamus) from the *pars ventralis diencephali* (hypothalamus and subthalamus). Dorsally, the lateral wall is limited by a ridge covering the *stria medullaris thalami* (p. 1093). In many cases, the lateral walls of the third ventricle are joined by an *interthalamic adhesion*, a band of grey matter extending from one thalamus to the other. An account of the phylogeny and development of the third ventricle has been compiled by Kier (1977).

Below the hypothalamus and the third ventricle is the *interpeduncular fossa* of the subarachnoid space. This is a trapezoid-shaped area, limited posteriorly by the anterior/superior surface of the pons and by the diverging cerebral peduncles. Anteriorly, is the optic chiasm. The mamillary bodies, posterior perforated substance, and tuber cinereum are in the roof of the interpeduncular fossa and the infundibulum and pituitary stalk pass through it.

FOURTH VENTRICLE

The fourth ventricle (**8.308, 313–316**) has a complex shape with a rhomboid floor and a tented roof. Viewed in sagittal section (**8.310, 313**), the narrow circular aqueduct passing through the midbrain is seen to expand ventrally into the fourth ventricle. Triangular in sagittal section, the ventricle has its apex protruding into the inferior aspect of the cerebellum. When the cerebellum is removed from the brainstem and the floor of the ventricle exposed, it is seen as a diamond-shaped or rhomboidal structure, continuous with the central canal of the spinal cord at the obex at its lower end and the lateral foramina of Luschka at the lateral extremities, just above the striae medullaris (**8.316**). The superior apex of the ventricle narrows to become the aqueduct, joining it with the third ventricle.

Developmentally, the fourth ventricle has three parts: *superior*, part of the isthmus rhombencephali; *intermediate*, the metencephalic (pontine) portion; and the *inferior* myelencephalic (medullary) section. The wall of the ventricle is lined by ependyma, continuous below with the central canal of the medulla and above with the cerebral aqueduct and extending into the lateral foramina.

The ventricle has lateral boundaries, a roof and a rhomboidal ventral floor — the *rhomboid fossa*.

Lateral boundaries of the ventricle. These are formed inferiorly by the gracile and cuneate tubercles and then by the diverging inferior cerebellar peduncles and, lastly, the lateral apertures of the foramina of Luschka. Superiorly, the lateral walls are formed by the superior cerebellar peduncles as they converge towards the aqueduct.

Roof (**8.314, 315**) A thin sheet of tissue which stretches across the roof of the ventricle between the superior cerebellar peduncles, this is formed superiorly by the superior cerebellar peduncles which, as they diverge inferiorly, are joined by the superior medullary velum.

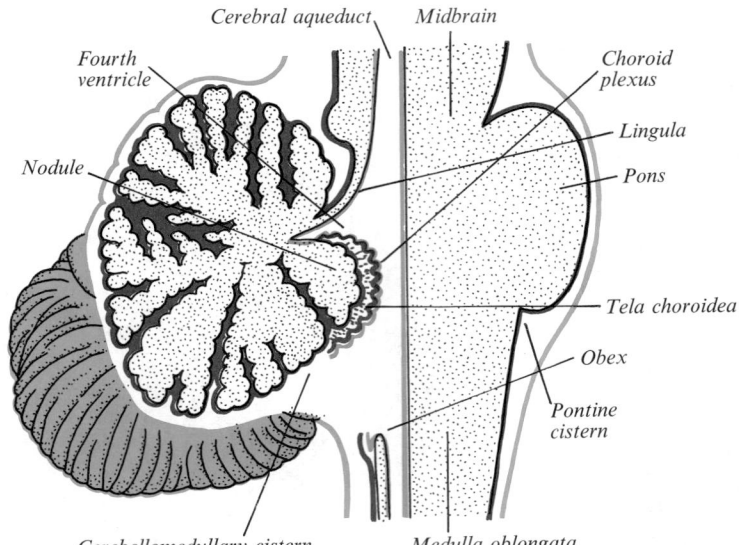

8.314 Sagittal section of the brainstem and the cerebellum close to the median plane. A median aperture below the tela choroidea allows drainage from the fourth ventricle into the cerebellomedullary cistern.

The *superior medullary velum* is continuous with the cerebellar white matter and is covered dorsally by the lingula of the superior vermis (**8.314, 316**). Inferiorly, the roof is more complex and is mostly composed of a thin sheet devoid of neural tissue and formed by ventricular ependyma and the pia mater of the tela choroidea which covers it dorsally (**8.314**). A *median aperture* (foramen of Magendie) (**8.314, 315**) in the roof of the ventricle allows CSF to flow from the ventricle into the *cerebellomedullary cistern* (*cisterna magna*) and thus into the subarachnoid space. Although difficult to demonstrate in dissected brains, this foramen is well seen during surgical approaches to the fourth ventricle. The *tela choroidea of the fourth ventricle* is formed by the apposition of leptomeninges (pia mater) and the ependyma of the roof of the fourth ventricle due to the disappearance of neural tissue from the roof; it is the root of the choroid plexus of the fourth ventricle. Mainly in the midline, the choroid plexus also extends laterally out through the lateral foramina of Luschka to present on the anterior surface of the brain at the pontomedullary junction. This protrusion of choroid plexus marks the anterior aperture of each foramen of Luschka. On each side, the tela choroidea is in contact with the ependyma until it reaches the inferolateral border of the ventricular floor where it is marked by a narrow ridge, the *taenia*. The paired taeniae are continuous below with a curved margin, the *obex*, which overlaps the inferior angle and is covered by ependyma on both its aspects (**8.314, 316**). Superiorly, this ridge (the taenia) where the tela choroidea of the roof joins the floor of the fourth ventricle extends along the inferior aspect of the lateral recess.

Fourth ventricular foramina

There are three openings in the caudal part of the fourth ventricle through which CSF flows from the ventricular system into the subarachnoid space. The *median aperture* (foramen of Magendie) is large and is a perforation in the posterior medullary velum just inferior to the nodule (**8.314, 315**). It varies in size with an irregular upper border drawn dorsally towards the inferior medullary velum; it connects the fourth ventricle with the cerebellomedullary cistern (cisterna magna) (**8.314**). The *lateral apertures* of the ventricle (foramina of Luschka) are at the apices of the lateral recesses of the ventricle and are partly occupied by choroid plexus which protrudes through them into the subarachnoid space. The ependyma and pia are continuous at their margins. Occasionally, a lateral recess may fail to open but the median aperture is constant. Following haemorrhage into the fourth ventricle, the cisterna magna fills with blood via the median aperture and the lateral apertures can be identified on the front of the brainstem as blood escapes from them into the subarachnoid space at the pontomedullary junction. The median and lateral apertures are normally the only connections between the ventricular system and the subarachnoid space.

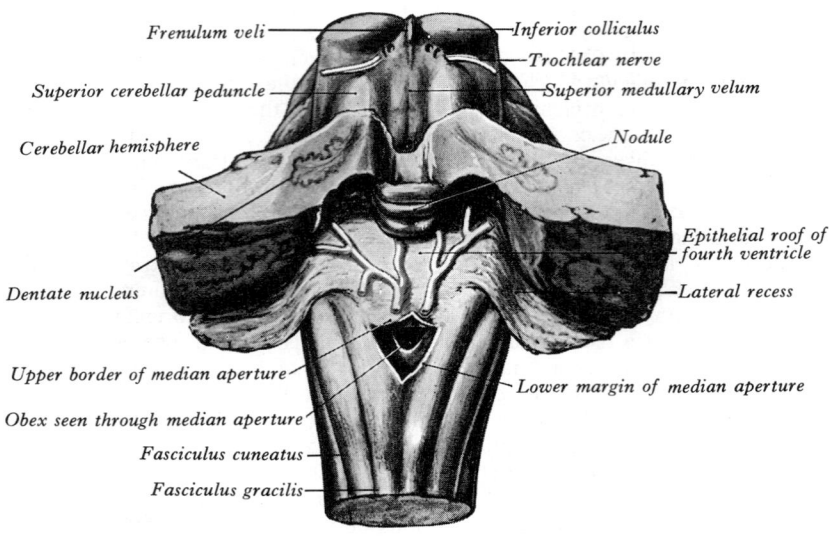

8.315 Dorsal aspect of the roof and the lateral recesses of the fourth ventricle, exposed by removal of parts of the cerebellum.

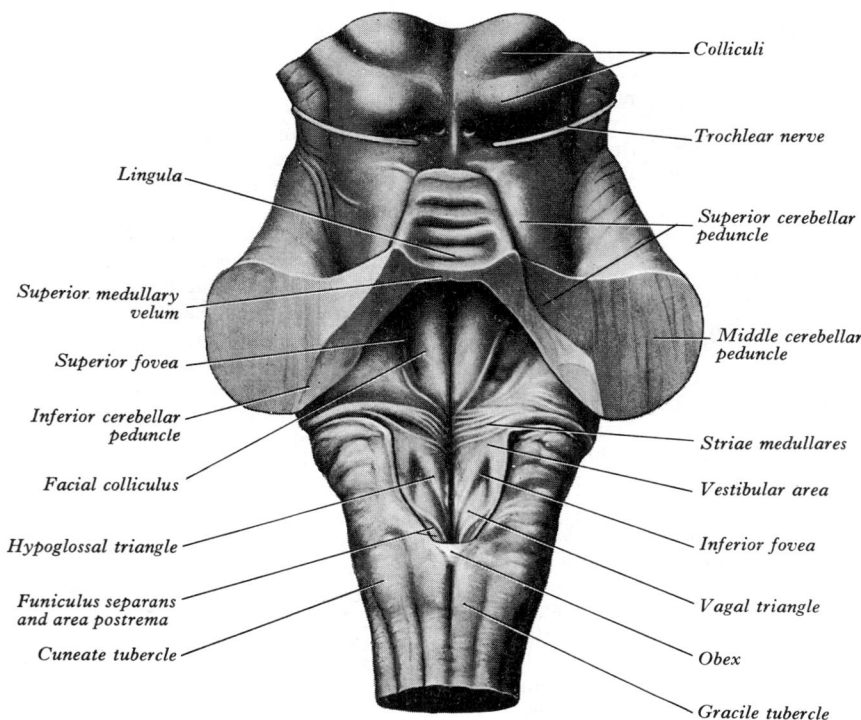

Colliculi

Trochlear nerve

Lingula

Superior cerebellar
peduncle

Superior medullary
velum

Superior fovea

Middle cerebellar
peduncle

Inferior cerebellar
peduncle

Striae medullares

Facial colliculus

Vestibular area

Hypoglossal triangle

Inferior fovea

Funiculus separans
and area postrema

Vagal triangle

Cuneate tubercle

Obex

Gracile tubercle

8.316   The rhomboid fossa or 'floor' of the fourth ventricle.

Choroid plexus of the fourth ventricle

The choroid plexus in the fourth ventricle (8.314) is similar in structure to the choroid plexus in the lateral and third ventricles. It is a T-shaped structure with longitudinal limbs flanking the midline and adherent to the roof of the fourth ventricle. Here it fuses at the superior margin of the median aperture in the roof of the fourth ventricle and is often prolonged on to the ventral aspect of the vermis (Hewitt 1960). In its cranial extension, the choroid plexus reaches the tent-like apex in the roof of the ventricle. Horizontal parts of the T-shaped choroid plexus project laterally into the lateral recesses and into the subarachnoid space. There is a wide variation in the form of the fourth ventricular choroid plexus (Lang & Schäfer 1977). The inferior cerebellar arteries supply the fourth ventricular choroid plexus (Maillot et al 1976).

The *floor of the fourth ventricle* (rhomboid fossa) (8.313, 316) is formed by the dorsal surfaces of the pons and the cranial half of the medulla. It consists of grey matter which is homologous with the anterior and posterior horns of grey matter in the spinal cord. The most superficial layers of the floor of the fourth ventricle are an ependymal lining and a subependymal layer of glia. The floor can be divided into superior, intermediate and inferior areas. The *superior* (rostral) area is triangular, and is limited laterally by the superior cerebellar peduncles; its apex is continuous with the walls of the cerebral aqueduct and its base is an arbitrary line drawn through the upper ends of two small *superior foveae*. An *intermediate* area descends from this level to the taeniae where they extend horizontally into the lateral recesses. The *inferior* (caudal) area is also triangular and is continuous below with the walls of the central canal at the lower medulla and spinal cord. A *median sulcus* divides the floor of the fourth ventricle vertically and is flanked by paired *medial eminences* each bounded laterally by a *sulcus limitans*. In the superior area, each eminence occupies its half of the floor; but medial to the superior fovea, it is expanded into a long *facial colliculus*, superficial to the abducent nucleus but partly produced by radicular facial nerve fibres. In the inferior area of the floor, each medial eminence is a *hypoglossal triangle* (*trigonum hypoglossi*) with medial and lateral parts separated by faint oblique furrows. The medial area corresponds to the upper pole of the hypoglossal nucleus and lateral to the *nucleus intercalatus*.

Each sulcus limitans lies lateral to the medial eminence and in its

upper part is itself the lateral limit of the floor of the fourth ventricle. Here it presents a bluish-grey *locus coeruleus* overlying a group of pigmented nerve cells of the reticular formation.

At the level of the facial colliculus, the sulcus limitans widens into the *superior fovea* and inferiorly presents an *inferior fovea*. Lateral to the fovea is a rounded *vestibular area*, extending into the lateral recess where it becomes the *auditory tubercle*, produced by the subjacent dorsal cochlear nucleus and cochlear part of the eighth cranial nerve, winding round the inferior cerebellar peduncle and across the vestibular area and medial eminence to enter the median sulcus at the *striae medullaris*. Caudal to the inferior fovea, between the hypoglossal triangle and the vestibular area, is the *vagal triangle* (*trigonum vagi*), overlying the dorsal vagal nucleus. The triangle is crossed below by a narrow translucent ridge, the *funiculus separans*; between this and the gracile tubercle is a small *area postrema*. The funiculus is covered by thickened ependyma-containing tanycytes; the area postrema has a similar tanycyte covering and contains neurons; the blood–brain barrier is modified in these regions (p. 1222). The specialized ependyma is similar to that in the third ventricle and cerebral aqueduct (p. 1094). Ependyma and tanycytes may be involved in:

* secretion into the CSF
* transport of neurochemicals from subjacent neurons, glia or vessels to the CSF
* transport of neurochemicals from CSF to the same subjacent structures
* chemoreception.

The caudal ventricular floor, towards its inferior apex at the obex, resembles a pen nib and hence the term *calamus scriptorius* for this region. For further phylogenetic and ontogenetic development see Kier (1977).

MENINGES

The brain and spinal cord are enveloped by three membranes — the meninges. From without inwards, the meninges comprise the dura mater (pachymenix) and the leptomeninges — the arachnoid mater and pia mater.

PACHYMENINX — DURA MATER

The dura mater is a thick dense inelastic membrane and is the most external of the meninges. The cranial dura mater encloses the brain and differs from the spinal dura mater mainly in its relationship to the surrounding bones. The cranial and spinal dura mater are continuous with each other at the foramen magnum.

Cranial dura mater

The cranial dura mater lines the cranial cavity. It is composed of two layers, an *inner* or *meningeal* layer and an *outer* or *endosteal layer*. These two layers are united except where they separate to enclose the venous sinuses draining blood from the brain (p. 1111). Dura mater adheres to the internal surfaces of the cranial bones and blood vessels and fibrous bands pass from it into the bones. Adhesion of the dura to bone is firmest at the sutures, the cranial base and around the foramen magnum. In children, it is difficult to remove the dura from the suture lines but in adults, the dura becomes separated from the suture lines as they fuse. With increasing age, the dura becomes thicker, less pliable and more firmly adherent to the inner surface of the skull, particularly of the calvarium. Vessels and fibrous bands connecting the dura mater to the skull are torn across when the dura is detached from the bone so the outer surface of the dura is rough and fibrillated, whereas the inner surface of the dura is smooth. The endosteal layer of the dura is continuous through the cranial sutures and foramina with the pericranium and through the superior orbital fissure with the orbital periosteum. The meningeal layer provides tubular sheaths for the cranial nerves as they pass out through the cranial foramina; these sheaths fuse with the epineurium as nerves emerge from the skull. The dural sheath of the optic nerve is continuous with the ocular sclera (p. 1322).

The meningeal layer of the dura is folded inwards as four septa that partially divide the cranial cavity into freely communicating spaces in which subdivisions of brain are lodged.

(1) The *falx cerebri* is a strong, crescentic sheet of dura mater descending vertically in the longitudinal (sagittal) fissure between the cerebral hemispheres (**8.317**). It is narrow in front, where it is fixed to the *crista galli*, and broad behind, where it blends in the midline with the tentorium cerebelli; the anterior part is thin and may have a number of irregular perforations. Its convex upper margin is attached to the internal cranial surface on each side of the midline, as far back as the internal occipital protuberance; the superior sagittal sinus (p. 1582) runs along this margin in a cranial groove and the falx is attached to the lips of this groove. At its lower edge, the falx is free and concave and contains the inferior sagittal sinus; the straight sinus runs along its attachment to the tentorium cerebelli (**8.317**).

(2) The *tentorium cerebelli* (**8.317, 318**) is a crescentic, 'tented' sheet of dura mater covering the cerebellum and passing under the occipital lobes of the cerebral hemispheres. Its concave, anterior edge is free and between it and the dorsum sellae of the sphenoid bone is a large hiatus of the tentorium cerebelli (or *tentorial incisure*), occupied by the midbrain and the anterior part of the superior aspect of the cerebellar vermis. The convex outer limit of the tentorium cerebelli is attached posteriorly, to the lips of the transverse sulci of the occipital bone and the posterior-inferior angles of the parietal bones, where it encloses the transverse sinuses; laterally, to the superior borders of the petrous temporal bones, where it contains the superior petrosal sinuses (**8.318**). Near the apex of the petrous temporal bone, the lower layer of the tentorium is evaginated anteriolaterally under the superior petrosal sinus to form a recess between the endosteal and meningeal layers in the middle cranial fossa. This recess is the *trigeminal cave* (p. 591) containing the roots and ganglion of the trigeminal nerve. The evaginated meningeal layer fuses in front with the anterior part of the ganglion. At the apex of the petrous temporal bone, the free border and attached periphery of the tentorium cross each other (**8.318**); the anterior ends of the free border are fixed to the anterior clinoid processes and the attached periphery to the posterior clinoid processes. In the groove between them, lies the oculomotor nerve. Details of the comparative anatomy, phylogeny and development of the tentorium cerebelli are described by Klintworth (1967, 1968).

(3) The *falx cerebelli* is a small crescentic fold of dura mater below the tentorium cerebelli, which projects forward into the posterior cerebellar notch. Its base is directed upwards and attached to the posterior part of the inferior surface of the tentorium cerebelli in the midline; its posterior margin is attached to the internal occipital crest and contains the occipital sinus; its apex frequently divides into two

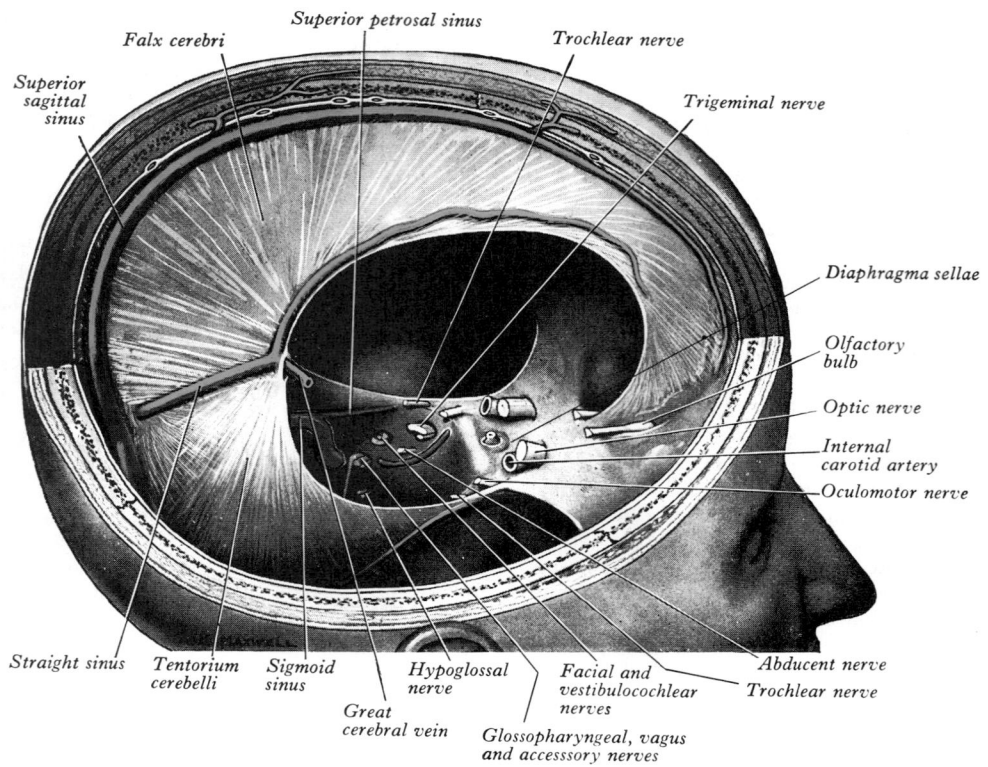

Falx cerebri
Superior petrosal sinus
Trochlear nerve
Superior sagittal sinus
Trigeminal nerve
Diaphragma sellae
Olfactory bulb
Optic nerve
Internal carotid artery
Oculomotor nerve
Straight sinus
Tentorium cerebelli
Sigmoid sinus
Hypoglossal nerve
Great cerebral vein
Facial and vestibulocochlear nerves
Glossopharyngeal, vagus and accesssory nerves
Abducent nerve
Trochlear nerve

8.317 The cerebral dura mater and its reflexions, exposed by the removal of a part of the right half of the skull and brain.

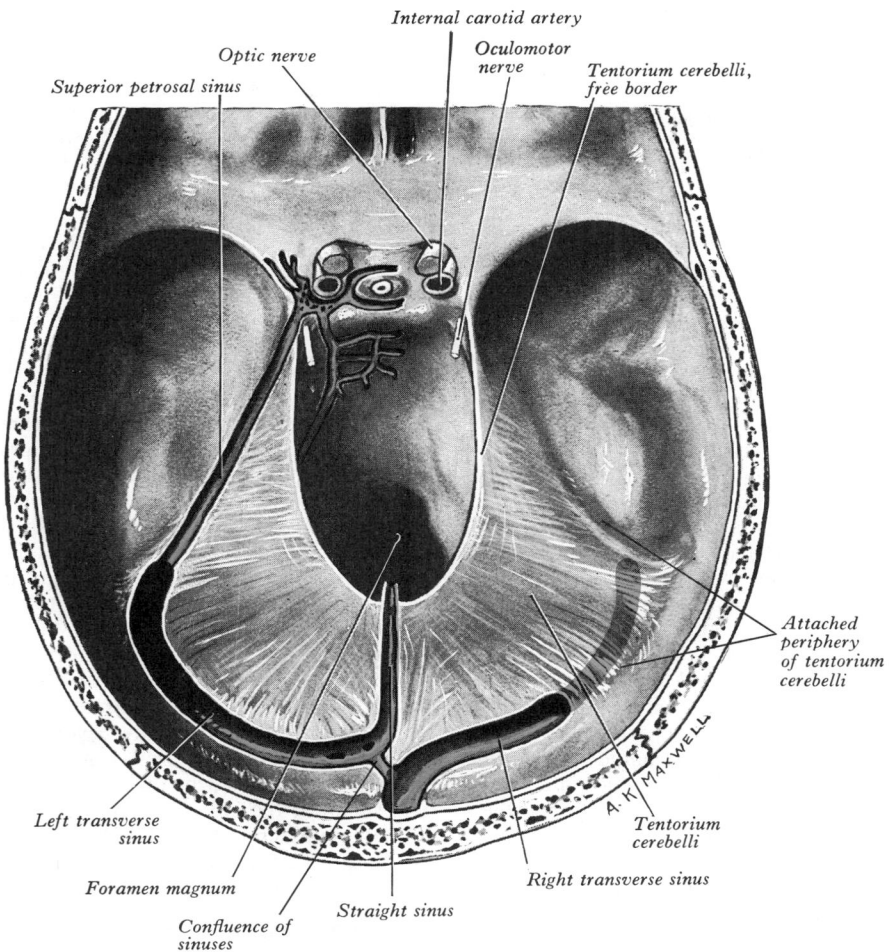

Internal carotid artery

Optic nerve

Oculomotor nerve

Superior petrosal sinus

Tentorium cerebelli, free border

Attached periphery of tentorium cerebelli

Left transverse sinus

Tentorium cerebelli

Foramen magnum

Right transverse sinus

Confluence of sinuses

Straight sinus

A.K.MAXWELL

8.318   The superior aspect of the tentorium cerebelli.

small folds which disappear at the sides of the foramen magnum. Hassan and Das (1969) found that the falx cerebelli was double in 76 of 100 cadavers.

(4) The *diaphragma sellae* (**8.317**) is a small, circular, horizontal sheet of dura mater which forms a roof to the sella turcica and, in many cases, almost completely covers the hypophysis (pituitary). The central opening in the diaphragma allows the infundibulum and pituitary stalk to pass into the pituitary fossa. There is wide individual variation in the size of the central opening. The diaphragma has become an important surgical structure with the increase in trans-phenoidal hypophysectomies.

The arrangement of the dura mater in the central part of the *middle cranial fossa* is complex (**8.318**). The tentorium cerebelli forms a large part of the floor of the middle cranial fossa, filling much of the gap between the ridges of the petrous temporal bones. The rim of the tentorial incisure is attached on both sides to the apex of the petrous temporal bones and continues forward as a ridge of dura mater to attach to the anterior clinoid processes. This ridge marks the junction of the roof and the lateral part of the cavernous sinus (**8.317, 318**). The periphery of the tentorium cerebelli is attached to the superior border of the petrous temporal bone and, crossing under the free border of the tentorial incisure, the peripheral attachment continues forward to the posterior clinoid processes as a rounded, indefinite ridge of the dura mater. Thus, an angular depression exists between the anterior parts of the peripheral attachment of the tentorium and the free border of the tentorial incisure (**8.317, 318**); this depression in the dura mater is part of the roof of the cavernous sinus and is pierced in front by the oculomotor and behind by the trochlear nerves, which remain in contact with the deep surface of the dura mater and proceed antero-inferiorly into the lateral wall of

the cavernous sinus (**10.164–166**). In the *anteromedial* part of the middle cranial fossa, the dura mater ascends as the lateral wall of the cavernous sinus. Reaching the ridge produced by the anterior continuation of the free border of the tentorium, it runs medially as the roof of the cavernous sinus and here is pierced by the internal carotid artery (**8.317, 318**). *Medially*, the roof of the sinus is continuous with the upper layer of the diaphragma sellae. At, or just below, the opening in the diaphragma for the infundibulum and pituitary stalk, the dura, arachnoid and pia mater blend with each other and with the capsule of the pituitary gland (p. 1883); within the sella turcica it is not possible to distinguish the layers of the meninges, and the subdural and subarachnoid spaces are obliterated.

In addition to its role as periosteum for the skull, the dura also encloses the major *venous sinuses*. Through its projections as the falx cerebri and tentorium cerebelli, the dura may also stabilize the brain within the cranial cavity. Although the brain itself is effectively suspended within a bath of CSF, the falx and tentorium may form an outer stabilizing jacket for the brain. Such an arrangement, however, does cause problems when there is focal brain swelling or a focal space-occupying lesion within one cerebral hemisphere. Herniation of brain may occur under the falx cerebri, or more significantly, through the tentorial incisure with consequent compression of the oculomotor nerve, midbrain and arteries on the inferior medial surface of the temporal lobe. Despite their origin as tumours from arachnoid cells, most meningiomas are firmly adherent to the inner surface of the dura or attached to the falx cerebri or tentorium cerebelli.

Structure of the dura mater. It is that of a dense, fibrous sheet, composed of collagen but containing some elastic fibres. The collagen fibres are densely packed in fascicles, which are arranged in laminae. The fascicles run in different directions in adjacent laminae which

1211

results in a lattice-like appearance. This is well seen in the tentorium cerebelli and around the perforations in the anterior portion of the falx cerebri. Although *endosteal* and *meningeal* layers are described, they are mainly distinguishable as separate layers of the dura at the venous sinuses, the foramen magnum and optic canals. There is little histological difference between the two layers; the smaller branches of the meningeal vessels are largely in the endosteal layer since they are primarily periosteal vessels. Although largely acellular, fibroblasts are distributed throughout the dura mater but osteoblasts are confined to the endosteal layer. Nevertheless, focal ossification may occur in the falx cerebri. Although the endosteal element of the dura mater is continuous with the external periosteum and with the periosteum through the sutures, for the most part there is no clear plane of separation between the meningeal part of the dura and the endosteal portion. The meningeal element is continuous with the dural sheaths of the spinal cord and the optic nerves; at other foramina, the meningeal dura fuses with the epineurium of the peripheral nerves. At sites where major vessels, such as the carotid and vertebral arteries, pierce the dura to enter the cranial cavity, the collagenous dura is firmly fused with the adventitia of the vessel (Alcolado et al 1988).

Although the inner aspect of the dura is closely applied to the arachnoid over the surface of the brain, the two layers are easily separated and are joined only at sites where veins pass from the brain into venous sinuses, especially the superior sagittal sinus, or connect brain to dura as at the anterior pole of the temporal lobe. Similar separation of dura and arachnoid occurs during the formation of subdural haematomas. Despite the ease of separation of the two layers and the potential subdural space, the outer layer of subdural mesothelium on the surface of the arachnoid appears to be part of the dura (Schachenmayr & Friede 1978; Alcolado et al 1988). It probably marks the plane of separation between the dura and leptomeningeal mesenchyme that occurs during embryonic development (O'Rahilly & Müller 1986).

Arterial supply and venous drainage of the cranial dura mater. It is derived from numerous vessels. In the anterior cranial fossa, the dura is supplied by the anterior meningeal branches of the anterior and posterior ethmoidal and internal carotid arteries and a branch of the middle meningeal artery. In the middle cranial fossa, the middle and accessory meningeal branches of the maxillary artery, a branch of the ascending pharyngeal artery (entering via the foramen lacerum), branches of the internal carotid and a recurrent branch of the lacrimal artery all supply the dura. Dura mater in the posterior fossa is supplied by the meningeal branches of the occipital artery (one entering the skull by the jugular foramen and another by the mastoid foramen), the posterior menin branches of the vertebral artery and occasional small branches of the ascending pharyngeal artery which enter by the jugular foramen and hypoglossal canal. The meningeal arteries are chiefly distributed to bone, in contrast to those in spinal dura mater; they are therefore unsuitably named. Only very fine arterial branches are distributed to the cranial dura mater itself.

Veins return blood from the cranial dura mater. (See pp. 1225, 1580–1589.)

Nerves of the cranial dura mater. These are derived mostly from the three divisions of the *trigeminal nerve*, the first three *cervical spinal nerves* and the *cervical sympathetic* trunk. Less well-established meningeal branches have been described arising from the vagus and hypoglossal nerves and possibly from the facial and glossopharyngeal nerves.

In the *anterior cranial fossa*, there are meningeal branches of the anterior and posterior ethmoidal nerves and anterior filaments of the meningeal rami of the maxillary (*nervus meningeus medius*) and mandibular (*nervus spinosus*) trigeminal divisions. *Nervi meningeus medius et spinosus* are, however, largely distributed to the dura of the *middle cranial fossa*, which also receives filaments from the trigeminal ganglion. A recurrent *tentorial nerve* (a branch of the ophthalmic division) supplies the *tentorium cerebelli*. The dura in the *posterior cranial fossa* is innervated by ascending meningeal branches of the upper cervical nerves which enter it through the anterior part of the foramen magnum (second and third cervical nerves) and through the hypoglossal canal and jugular foramen (first and second cervical nerves).

All meningeal nerves contain a postganglionic sympathetic com-

ponent, either from the superior cervical sympathetic ganglion or by communication with its perivascular intracranial extensions.

Various dural receptor terminals, including simple end-bulbs and Meissner's and Pacinian corpuscles, have been described in various mammals, but there is little information available concerning man. The roles of the sensory and autonomic nerve supply of the cranial dura mater remain uncertain.

Spinal dura mater

The single layer of dura that lines the cranial cavity divides into two layers as it passes downwards through the foramen magnum, although it is still a single layer as it forms the anterior and posterior atlanto-occipital membranes. Within the spinal column, the outer endosteal layer becomes the periosteum of the vertebral canal, which is separated from the spinal dura mater by an *extradural* (*epidural*) *space*. The spinal dura mater thus forms a tube, the upper end of which is attached to the edge of the foramen magnum and to the posterior surfaces of the second and third cervical vertebral bodies and also by fibrous bands to the posterior longitudinal ligament, especially towards the caudal end of the vertebral canal (Parkin & Harrison 1985). At the lower border of the second sacral vertebra, the dural tube narrows to invest the thin spinal filum terminale to descend to the back of the coccyx and blend with the periosteum. The spinal dura mater has tubular prolongations around the spinal roots and nerves as they pass out of the intervertebral foramina. These prolongations of dura are short in the upper vertebral column but gradually become longer with the increasing obliquity of the spinal roots. The dural sheaths of the spinal nerves fuse with the epineurium, within or slightly beyond the intervertebral foramina. At the cervical level, where the nerves are short and the vertebral movement is greatest, the dural sheaths are strongly adherent to the periosteum of the adjacent transverse processes (Sunderland 1974). In the lumbosacral region, however, there is no strong adherence of the dura to the periosteum and there is free connection between the epidural space and the extraspinal connective tissue.

Extradural (epidural) space

This lies between the spinal dura mater and the periosteum and ligaments within the vertebral canal. It contains loose connective tissue, fat and a venous plexus. In the lumbar region, the dura mater is apposed to the walls of the vertebral canal and attached by connective tissue in a manner that permits displacement of the dural sac during movement and venous engorgement. Adipose tissue is present posteriorly, in recesses between the ligamentum flavum and the dura (Parkin & Harrison 1985). The connective tissue extends for a short distance through the intervertebral foramina along the spinal nerves. Dyes and other fluids injected into the epidural space at the sacral level can spread up to the cranial base; local anaesthetics injected near the spinal nerves, just outside the intervertebral foramina, may spread up or down to affect the adjacent spinal nerves or pass to the opposite side. In each case, spread is through the epidural space.

Subdural space

Between the spinal dura and arachnoid mater, this is only a potential space (Haines et al 1993) in the normal spine as the arachnoid and dura are closely apposed. It does not connect with the subarachnoid space but continues for a short distance along the cranial and spinal nerves. Accidental subdural catheterization may occur during extradural injections (McMenemin et al 1992). Injection of fluid into the subdural space may either damage the cord from direct toxic effects or by compression of the vasculature.

LEPTOMENINGES—ARACHNOID AND PIA MATER

Whereas the dura is a thick, collagenous sheet covering the surface of the brain and spinal cord, the leptomeninges are thin and, for the most part, almost transparent. There are two major layers of leptomeninges, the *arachnoid mater* and the *pia mater*. They are separated by the *subarachnoid space* and joined by *trabeculae*. The anatomical relationships of the arachnoid and pia mater differ, to some extent, in the cerebral and spinal regions. However, the basic cell type and fine structure of the arachnoid and pia mater have many similarities, as do the associated structures.

Cranial arachnoid mater

The cerebral part of the arachnoid mater invests the brain but does not enter the sulci or fissures, except for the longitudinal fissure. On the upper surface of the brain in younger individuals, the arachnoid is transparent but in older people it may become white and opaque, particularly near the midline. The arachnoid is thicker on the basal aspect of the brain and is also slightly opaque where it extends between the temporal lobes and the front of the pons; here there is a large space between arachnoid and pia mater. The arachnoid is easily separated from the dura over the surface of the brain. However, at the sites where the carotid and the vertebral arteries enter the subarachnoid space, the arachnoid mater is adherent to the adventitia of the vessel. From this point, it is reflected on to the surface of blood vessels in the subarachnoid space and is eventually continuous with the pia mater (Hutchings & Weller 1986; Alcolado et al 1988). The arachnoid also coats the superior surface of the pituitary fossa.

Subarachnoid space. This is the space between the arachnoid and the pia mater, which contains CSF and the larger arteries and veins which traverse the surface of the brain. Arteries and veins are coated by a thin layer of leptomeninges, often only one cell thick (Zhang et al 1990). The pia mater, the blood vessels and the arachnoid mater are connected by collagenous trabeculae and sheets (Arutinov et al 1974; Alcolado et al 1988), also coated by leptomeningeal cells (8.319, 320). Arachnoid and pia mater are at closest association over the summits of the gyri but the arachnoid bridges the sulci so that only blood vessels and pia extend into the sulci. Wherever the brain and the cranium are not closely applied to each other, the arachnoid is separated from the pia by a wide interval to form *subarachnoid cisterns*. Such cisterns are continuous with each other through the general subarachnoid space of which they are dilatations. Subarachnoid trabeculae are either absent or long and filamentous (8.320) as they cross the subarachnoid cisterns. There is evidence from experimental studies that the trabeculae which cross the subarachnoid space may form well-defined compartments, particularly in the perivascular regions, to enable directional flow of CSF through the subarachnoid space by, in effect, the formation of channels (Zhang et al 1992).

Subarachnoid cisterns. The *cerebellomedullary cistern* (*cisterna cerebellomedullaris*, or *cisterna magna*) (8.314) is formed as the arachnoid bridges the interval between the medulla oblongata and the inferior cerebellar surface. It is triangular in its sagittal section and is continuous below with the subarachnoid space of the spinal cord and with the fourth ventricle through the foramen of Magendie. The *pontine cistern* (8.314, 321) is an extensive space ventral to the pons, continuous below with the spinal subarachnoid space, behind with the cerebellomedullary cistern and, rostral to the pons, with the interpeduncular cistern. The basilar artery runs through the pontine cistern into the interpeduncular cistern. As the arachnoid passes between the two temporal lobes it is separated from the cerebral peduncles and structures of the interpeduncular fossa by the *interpeduncular cistern*, which contains the circulus arteriosus (circle of Willis). Anteriorly, the interpeduncular cistern continues rostrally to the optic chiasm and is continuous with the subarachnoid space and the supracallosal cistern over the superior surface of the corpus callosum (8.321). The anterior cerebral arteries are contained within this cistern. The *cistern of the lateral fossa* contains the middle cerebral artery and is formed by the arachnoid bridging the lateral sulcus. Posterior to the brain stem and third ventricle is the *cistern of the great cerebral vein* (*cisterna ambiens* or *superior cistern*), which occupies the interval between the splenium of the corpus callosum and the superior cerebellar surface (8.321); the great cerebral vein traverses this cistern and the pineal gland protrudes into it.

Smaller cisternae have been described, including the *prechiasmatic* and *postchiasmatic cisterns* related to the optic chiasm, and the *cisterna of the lamina terminalis* and the *supracallosal cistern*; all are extensions of the interpeduncular cistern and contain the anterior cerebral arteries.

The cerebral subarachnoid space connects with the ventricles of the brain by three openings: the median aperture (foramen of Magendie) (8.314. 315) in the median plane in the inferior part of the roof of the fourth ventricle, and the two lateral apertures (foramina of Luschka) at the ends of the lateral recesses, behind the upper roots of the glossopharyngeal nerves. There is normally no

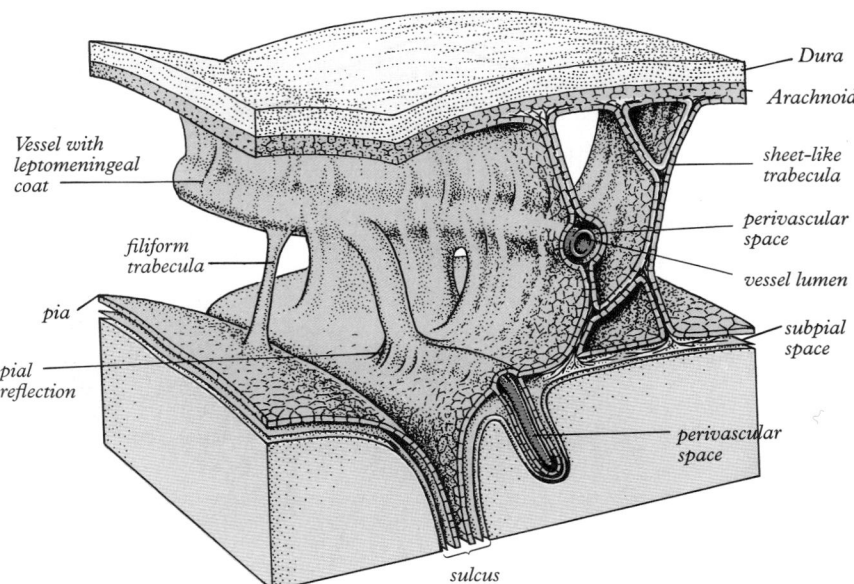

8.319   Relationships of pia and arachnoid mater to the dura, brain and vessels. (Modified from Alcolado et al 1988 according to Zhang, Inman & Weller 1990.)

communication between the subdural and subarachnoid spaces as the tight junctions (zonulae occludentes) between the cells of the outer layer of the arachnoid (Alcolado et al 1988) prevent the escape of CSF from the subarachnoid space.

The subarachnoid space also extends along the optic nerves to the back of the globe at which point the dura fuses with the sclera of the eye. There is a connection between the subarachnoid space and the ear through the cochlear duct and, in experimental animals, both bacteria and tracers in the subarachnoid CSF may enter the cochlea through this pathway (Kida et al 1993b).

The well-characterized connection between the subarachnoid space and nasal lymphatics have been described in experimental animals

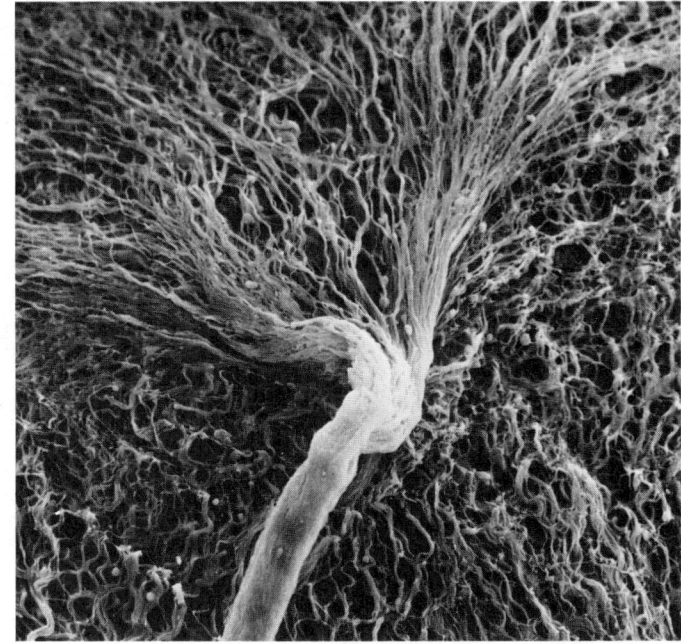

8.320   Scanning electron micrograph (× 240) of an arachnoid trabecula. Collagen fibres fan out into the internal aspect of the arachnoid. (Alcolado et al 1988.)

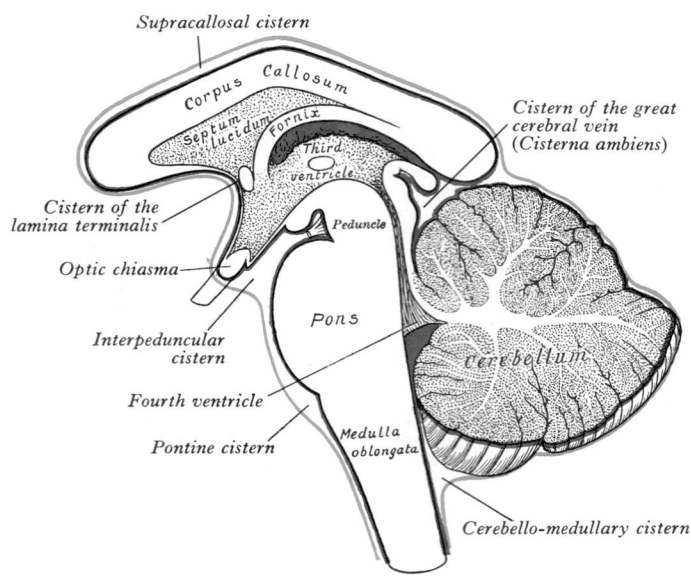

8.321 The positions of the principal subarachnoid cisterns. Red = pia mater, Blue = arachnoid mater.

sinus endothelium. *Microscopic villi* are present in the superior sagittal sinus of the fetus and newborn infant (Le Gros Clark 1920; Turner 1961) and granulations are visible by the age of 18 months in the parieto-occipital region of the superior sagittal sinus and by the age of 3 years in the lateral sinuses of the posterior fossa (Le Gros Clark 1920). The arachnoid granulations become more lobulated and complex with increasing age (Turner 1961). Similar drainage pathways exist in other mammals but do not exhibit the complexity of human arachnoid granulations (Tripathi & Tripathi 1974; Davson et al 1987; Kida et al 1993b).

At the base of each arachnoid granulation, a thin neck of arachnoid mater projects through an aperture in the dural lining of the venous sinus and expands to form a core of collagenous trabeculae and interwoven channels (8.323) (Le Gros Clark 1920; Upton & Weller 1985; Kida & Weller 1994a). An *apical cap* of arachnoid cells, some 150 μm thick, surmounts the collagenous core and channels extend through the cap to reach the subendothelial regions of the granulation (Upton & Weller 1985) (8.323). Channels within the granulation are lined by compacted collagen and are coated by arachnoid cells (Kida et al 1988). The cap region of each granulation is attached to the endothelium of the sinus over an area some 300 μm in diameter, whereas the rest of the granulation core is separated from the endothelium by fibrous dural cupola and potential subdural space. Physiological and tracer studies (Tripathi & Tripathi 1974; Davson et al 1987) suggest that there is bulk flow of CSF through the channels of the collagenous core of the granulations and by either

(Cserr et al 1992; Weller et al 1992; Kida et al 1993b) and possibly exists in man also but direct evidence is, as yet, sparse.

Cranial and spinal nerves traversing the subarachnoid space to pass out of cranial or intervertebral foramina are coated by a thin layer of leptomeninges which fuses with the arachnoid at the exit foramina.

Arachnoid granulations and villi. Classical studies have defined the arachnoid granulations and villi as the major pathways for the bulk flow of CSF back into the blood in man (Davson et al 1987). These structures are most prominent along the margins of the longitudinal fissure from which they project into the superior sagittal sinus. However, arachnoid villi have been located in other cerebral venous sinuses and in the spinal region (Kiddo et al 1976). If the superior sagittal sinus is opened longitudinally and the lateral recesses of the sinus are examined, the arachnoid granulations in adult individuals can be observed protruding into the sinus lumen (8.322) (Upton & Weller 1985). Arachnoid villi and granulations are, in effect, extensions of the subarachnoid space and arachnoid through the dural wall of the sinus to present an exchange surface with the

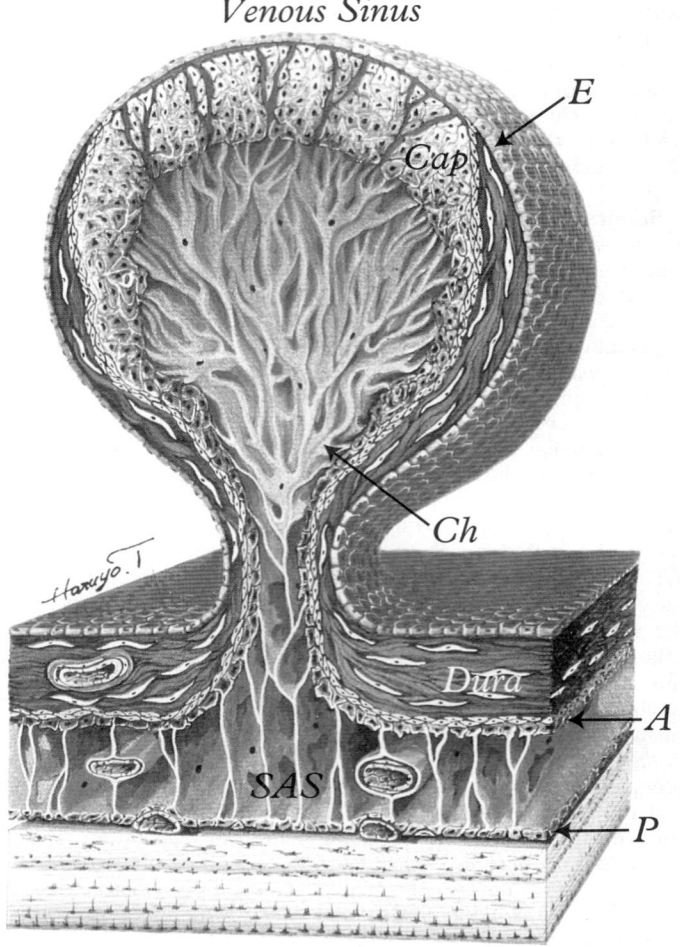

8.323 Diagram of an arachnoid granulation. The subarachnoid space (SAS) between the arachnoid (A) and pia mater (P) is highly trabeculated and is continuous with the channel (Ch) in the centre of the granulation. Narrow channels traverse the cap region of the granulation to come into contact with the endothelium (E) of the venous sinus. It is through the endothelium that the fluid finally drains. (Reproduced with permission from Kida & Weller 1994a.)

8.322 A coronal section through the vertex of the skull to show the arrangement of the veins and the meninges of the brain and arachnoid granulations.

macrovesicular or microvesicular transport across the sinus endothelium into the blood. The passage of particulate matter through
this pathway has also been suggested. Following subarachnoid haemorrhage, erythrocytes may be found in drainage channels within the
arachnoid granulations (Upton & Weller 1985). However, there is
no firm evidence that arachnoid granulations become permanently
blocked following subarachnoid haemorrhage (Torvik et al 1978).

If the dura and the superior sagittal sinus is torn away from the
surface of the brain at postmortem, arachnoid granulations become
evulsed; they thus lose the arachnoid cap attachment and the granulations remaining attached to the arachnoid are only partially preserved.

Cranial pia mater

The pia mater is a delicate membrane which closely invests the
surface of the brain and the spinal cord. It follows the contours of
the brain into the sulci (**8.319**) and also, during development, becomes
apposed to the ependyma in the roof of the telencephalon and fourth
ventricle to form the stroma of the choroid plexus (p. 1203).

Pia mater over the surface of the brain is formed from a layer of
leptomeningeal cells often only 1–2 cells thick (Alcolado et al 1988).
Individual cells are joined by *desmosomes* and *gap junctions* but few,
if any, tight junctions. Over the apices of the cerebral gyri, the pia
mater is in continuity with the deep layers of the arachnoid via the
trabeculae which traverse the subarachnoid space (**8.319**). Pia mater
is separated from the brain by the *subpial space*; thus, between the
basement membrane of the glia limitans on the surface of the brain
and the pia mater are fine bundles of collagen and small arteries and
veins which are entering and leaving the surface of the brain
(Alcolado et al 1988; Zhang et al 1990). When stripped from the
surface of the cerebral cortex, the pia mater, the subpial space
containing blood vessels and the collagen and the *basement membrane
of the glia limitans* all separate as one unit from the surface of the
brain (Hutchings & Weller 1986). This gives the impression that the
pia mater is 'a vascular membrane'.

Trabeculae in the form of sheets or fine filiform structures traverse
the arachnoid space from the deep layers of the arachnoid mater to
the pia mater and are also attached to large blood vessels within the
subarachnoid space (Arutinov et al 1974). Each trabecula has a core
of collagen and is coated by leptomeningeal cells. The collagen core
fans out into the deep layer of the arachnoid (**8.320**) and also fans
out to become intermingled with the fine collagen bundles of the
subpial space (Alcolado et al 1986).

Relationships of the pia mater to cerebral blood vessels.
Following the tracer experiments of Weed (1923) and others, it was
long thought that the subarachnoid space connected directly with
the *perivascular spaces* (*Virchow-Robin spaces*) in the brain. Scanning
and transmission electron microscopy (Krahn 1982; Hutchings &
Weller 1986), however, have shown that the pia mater is reflected
from the surface of the brain on to the surface of blood vessels in
the subarachnoid space (**8.324**). Thus the subarachnoid space is
separated by a layer of pia from the subpial and perivascular spaces
of the brain (**8.319, 325**). Physiological evidence suggests that the pia
forms an effective barrier to pharmacological agents (Aird 1984),
and particulate matter in the subarachnoid space is for the most
part prevented by the pia mater from entering the perivascular spaces
of the brain (Hutchings & Weller 1986).

As arteries enter the brain from the subpial space, they are coated
by a layer of pia mater cells subtended from the deep aspect of the
pia mater proper (Zhang et al 1990). This layer follows the vessels
into the brain forming a perivascular sheath which becomes discontinuous and eventually disappears as the vessels become capillaries (**8.325**). Thus, a layer of leptomeningeal cells separates arteries
from the surrounding brain and may form a regulatory interface
between blood vessels and brain (Feuer & Weller 1991). In particular,
such a layer may play a role in limiting the spread of neurotransmitters from nerves supplying the vessels, such that the surrounding brain remains unaffected (Kaplan et al 1981; Feuer &
Weller 1991). No similar layer of leptomeninges surrounds veins
(Zhang et al 1990).

Lymphatic drainage of the brain

Some 50% of the CSF in a number of mammalian species drains to
the *cervical lymph nodes* (Cserr et al 1992). Simple arachnoid villi

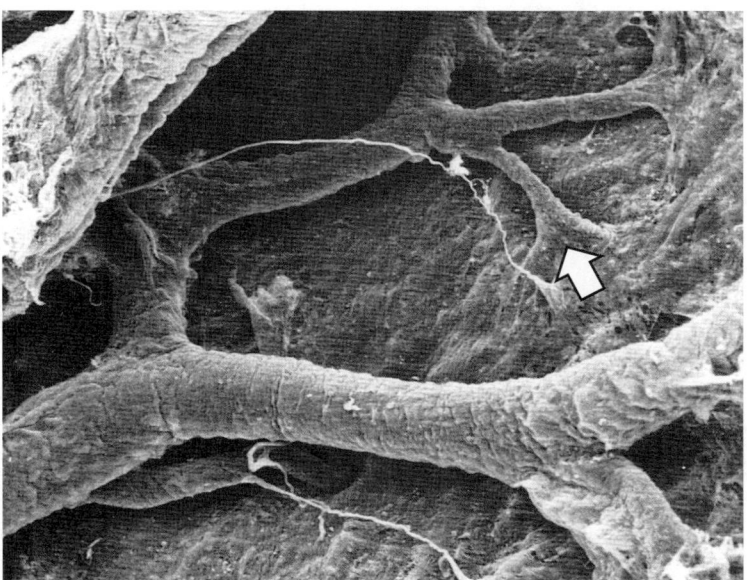

8.324 Scanning electron micrograph of the pial surface within a human
cerebral sulcus. An artery branches within the subarachnoid space over the
surface of the pia and, as branches descend into the brain, the pia mater
(arrow) is reflected on to the surface of the vessel, thus separating the
subarachnoid space from the perivascular and subpial spaces (× 96).
(Reproduced with permission from Hutchings & Weller 1986.)

and distinct arachnoid lymphatic channels are present in the rat
(Kida et al 1993b). In these animals, the volume of CSF is relatively
small whereas in man there is a high volume of ventricular and
subarachnoid CSF, which drains largely into blood through the
arachnoid granulations and villi. The development of the high volume
and flow of CSF through arachnoid granulations appears to have
largely overshadowed the lymphatic drainage of interstitial fluid
from the brain in man.

Experiments in the rat have shown that proteins injected into the
caudate putamen of one cerebral hemisphere drain to the cervical
lymph nodes on the same side of the body (Yamada et al 1991;
Cserr et al 1992). The anatomical pathways for such drainage appear
to lie centrifugally along perivascular spaces within the brain and
thence in paravascular compartments following branches of the
major cerebral arteries to the circle of Willis. Highly directionalized
flow of CSF alongside arteries to the cribriform plate under the
olfactory bulbs (Zhang et al 1992) allows CSF and tracers to enter
arachnoid channels continuous with the *lymphatic vessels* of the *nasal
mucosa*, which drain into the *deep cervical lymph nodes* (Kida et al
1993b).

Although similar tracer experiments cannot be performed in man,
the anatomical pathways for comparable lymphatic drainage are
present in man (Zhang et al 1990). Not only are there well-defined
perivascular spaces, but also the subarachnoid space is highly compartmentalized (Alcolado et al 1988) and possibly allows directional
flow of CSF for lymphatic drainage.

Spinal leptomeninges

The arachnoid mater surrounding the spinal cord (**8.326, 327**) is
continuous with the cranial arachnoid mater. It is closely applied to
the deep aspect of the dura mater. At sites where vessels and nerves
enter or leave the subarachnoid space, the arachnoid mater is
reflected on to the surface of these structures to form a thin coating
of leptomeningeal cells over the surface of both vessels and nerves
(**8.327**). Thus a *subarachnoid angle* is formed as nerves pass through
the dura into intervertebral foramina (McCabe & Low 1969). At
this point, the layers of leptomeninges fuse and become continuous
with the perineurium. The epineurium is in continuity with the dura.
Such an arrangement seals the subarachnoid space and particulate
matter does not pass directly from the subarachnoid space into
nerves (Brierley & Field 1948; Brierley 1950). There is an, as yet,
unspecified route of lymphatic drainage for CSF from the spine to

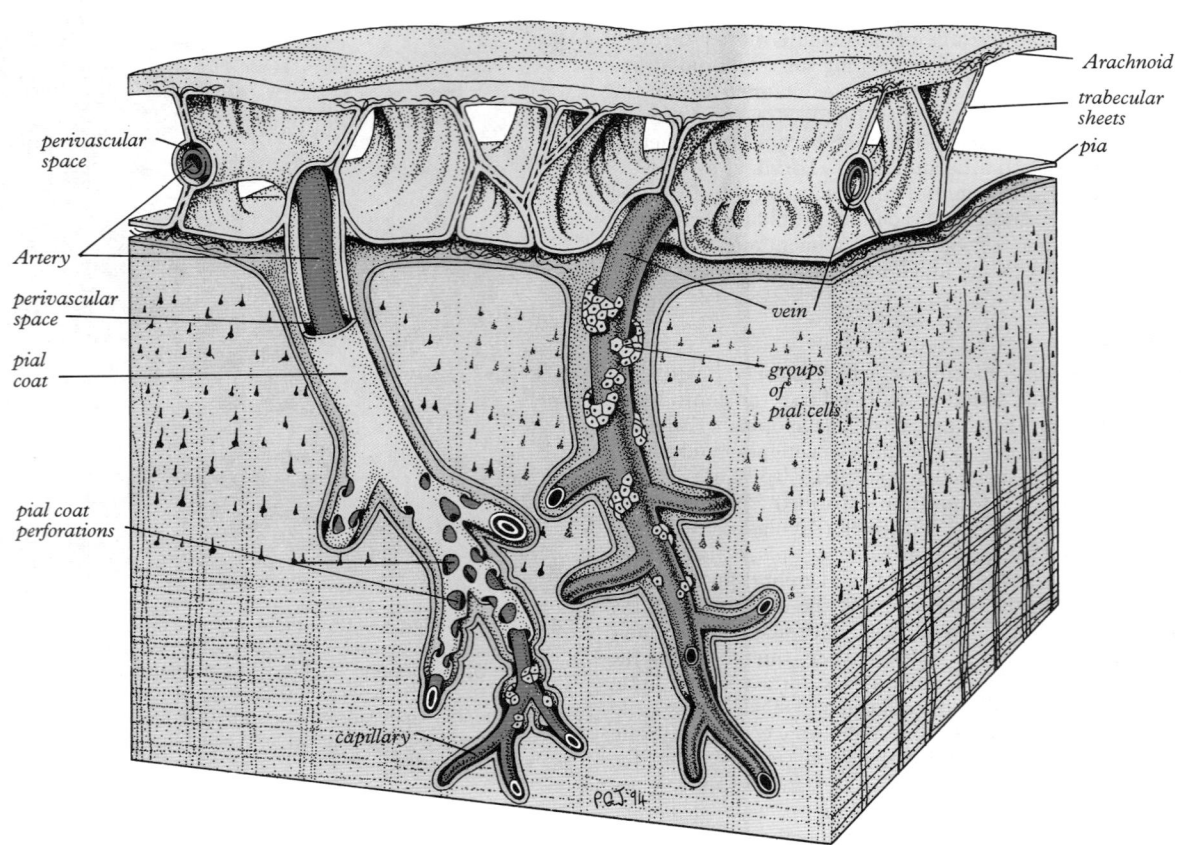

8.325 A diagram to show the interrelationships between leptomeninges and blood vessels entering and leaving the cerebral cortex. The sub-arachnoid space is divided by trabeculae and, as the artery enters the cortex, a layer of pia mater accompanies the vessel into the brain. With decreasing size of the vessel, the pial coating becomes perforated and finally disappears at capillary level. The perivascular space between the artery and the pia mater inside the brain is continuous with the perivascular space around the meningeal vessel. Veins do not have a similar coating of pia mater. (Reproduced and modified, with permission from Zhang, Inman & Weller 1990.)

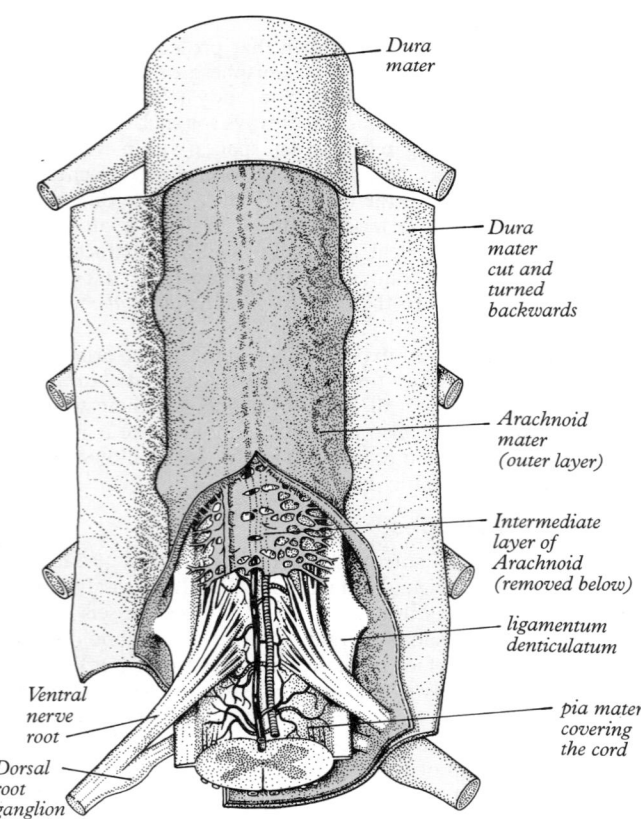

8.326 Part of the spinal cord exposed from the ventral aspect showing its meningeal coverings.

lumbar lymph nodes in the rat (Brierley & Field 1948; Kida et al 1993b).

The *spinal pia mater* closely invests the surface of the spinal cord and passes into the anterior median fissure. As in the cranial region, there is a *subpial space* but over the surface of the spinal cord the subpial collagenous layer is thicker than in the cerebral region and is continuous with the collagenous core of the ligamentum denticulatum (Nicholas & Weller 1988).

The *ligamentum denticulatum* is a flat, fibrous sheet situated on each side of the spinal cord between the ventral and dorsal spinal roots (Epstein 1966; Nicholas & Weller 1988) (**8.326, 327**). Its medial border is continuous with the subpial connective tissue of the cord and its lateral border forms a series of triangular processes, the apices of which are fixed at intervals to the dura mater. There are usually *21 processes on each side*; the first crosses behind the vertebral artery where it is attached to the dura mater and is separated by the artery from the first cervical ventral root. Its site of attachment to the dura mater is above the rim of the foramen magnum, just behind the hypoglossal nerve (**8.327**); the spinal accessory nerve ascends on its posterior aspect (**8.122**). The last of the dentate ligaments is between the exits of the twelfth thoracic and the first lumbar spinal nerve and is a narrow, oblique band descending laterally from the conus medullaris (p. 976). Changes in the form and position of the dentate ligaments during spinal movements has been demonstrated by cine-radiography (Epstein 1966).

Beyond the conus medullaris, the pia mater continues as a coating of the *filum terminale* (p. 976) with no dentate ligaments.

In addition to the well-defined arachnoid and pia mater coating the cord, there is an extensive *intermediate* layer of leptomeninges around the cord (**8.326, 327**). It is concentrated in the dorsal and ventral regions and forms a highly perforated, almost lace-like structure which is focally compacted to form the *dorsal, dorsolateral and ventral ligaments* of the spinal cord. Dorsally, the intermediate

Intermediate layers
of arachnoid
Dorsal ligament
Dura
Outer layer
of arachnoid
Pia mater
Dorsal
root
Ligamentum
denticulatum
Ventral
root
Intermediate layers
of arachnoid

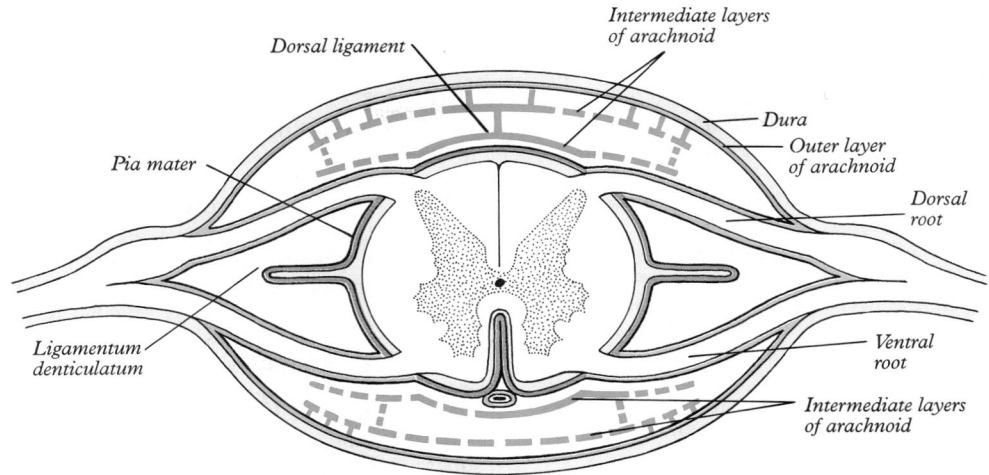

8.327 Transverse section through the spinal cord and meninges to show the relationships between the leptomeninges and ligaments with the spinal cord and nerves; dura mater (yellow); arachnoid mater, outer layer (pale blue) arachnoid mater – intermediate layer (bright blue); pia mater (red); subpial connective tissue (yellow).

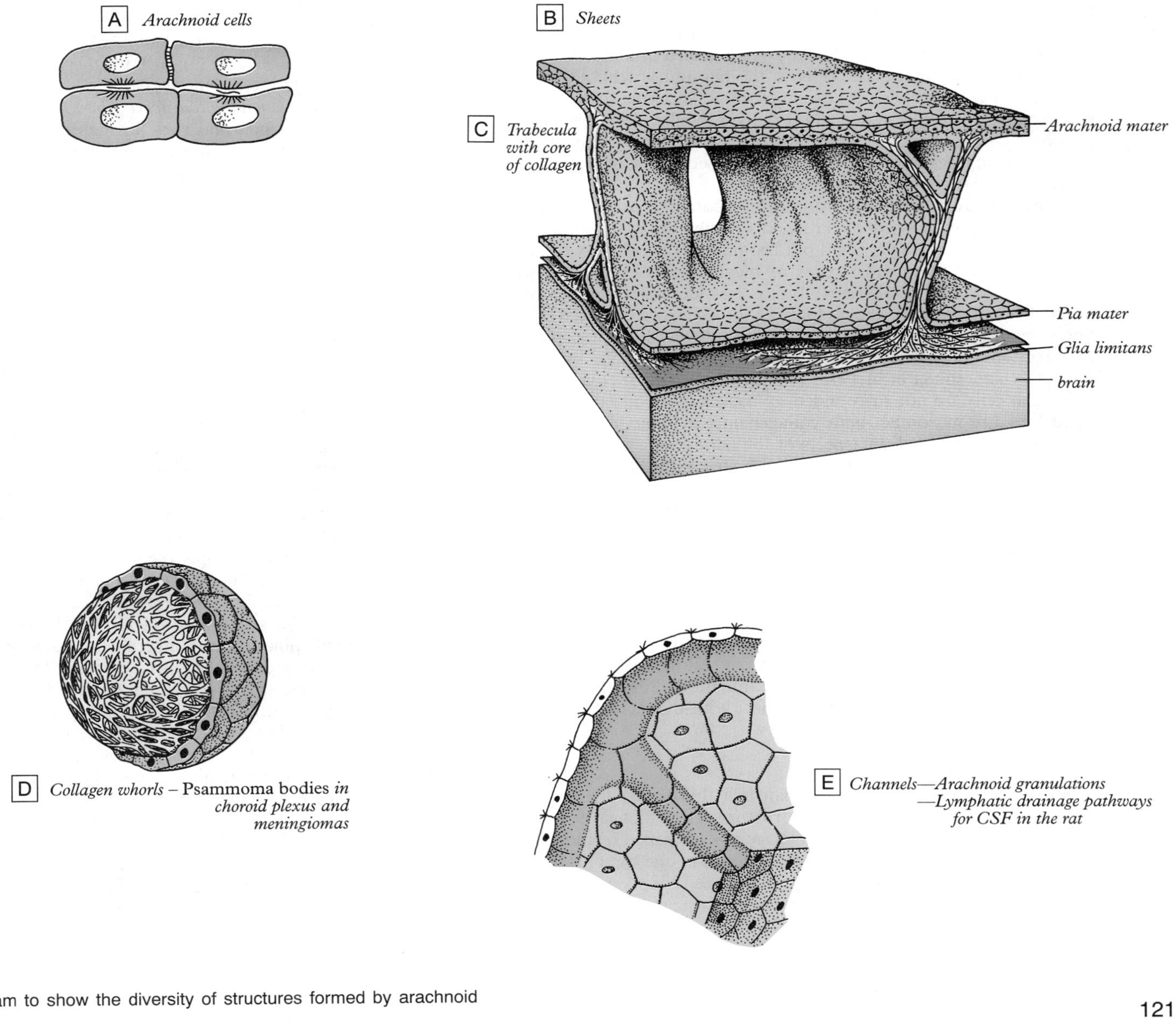

A Arachnoid cells
B Sheets
C Trabecula
with core
of collagen
Arachnoid mater
Pia mater
Glia limitans
brain
D Collagen whorls – Psammoma bodies in
choroid plexus and
meningiomas
E Channels—Arachnoid granulations
—Lymphatic drainage pathways
for CSF in the rat

8.328 Diagram to show the diversity of structures formed by arachnoid cells.

layer is adherent to the deep aspect of the arachnoid mater and forms a discontinuous series of dorsal ligaments which attach the spinal cord to the arachnoid. The dorsolateral ligaments are more delicate and fenestrated; they extend from dorsal roots to the parietal arachnoid. As the intermediate layer spreads laterally over the dorsal surface of the dorsal roots, it becomes increasingly perforated and eventually disappears.

Ventrally, the intermediate layer is less substantial (Nicholas & Weller 1988).

The *intermediate layer* is, in effect, in two parts. A lacy outer layer (adherent to the inner aspect of the arachnoid mater) and an inner layer, which lies over the arteries and nerve roots. The two intermediate layers are joined by discontinuous dorsal and dorsolateral ligaments and laterally both layers become highly perforated and eventually disappear. A similar arrangement is seen over the ventral aspect of the spinal cord. Fine trabeculae forming intermediate layers of spinal meninges are seen in other mammals (Andres 1967; Cloyd & Low 1974).

The structure of the intermediate layer resembles that of the trabeculae which traverse the cranial subarachnoid space; a collagenous core is coated by leptomeningeal cells. The intermediate layers of leptomeninges around the spinal cord may act as a baffle within the subarachnoid space to dampen waves of CSF in the spinal column. Inflammation within the spinal subarachnoid space may result in extensive fibrosis within the intermediate layer and the complications of chronic arachnoiditis.

Microscopic structure of the leptomeninges

The leptomeninges, comprising the pia and arachnoid mater, are composed of the same basic cell type—here called *arachnoid cells*—and bundles of collagen. The cells of the pia and arachnoid mater hava a common embryological origin from mesenchyme surrounding the developing nervous system (O'Rahilly & Müller 1986). Formed initially as a network of mesenchymal cells, the leptomeninges separate during development into two distinct layers of arachnoid and pia mater with connecting trabeculae.

General structure of leptomeninges. Both the pia and arachnoid mater are composed of flattened or cuboidal cells with oval nuclei and usually a single, small but prominent nucleolus. A similar morphology is seen in most types of meningiomas (Weller 1990). *Vimentin* intermediate filaments can be identified by immunocytochemistry within the cytoplasm of these cells which also express *epithelial membrane antigen*. Joined together by desmosomes, gap junctions and, in the outer layer of the arachnoid, by tight junctions (Nabeshima et al 1975; Parrish et al 1986; Alcolado et al 1988) such cells are not surrounded by basement membrane, except where they are in contact with collagen in the inner layers of the arachnoid and on the deep aspects of the pia mater.

Arachnoid cells form a diversity of structures (**8.328**), which include *sheets of cells*, as in the arachnoid mater and the pia mater, and trabeculae with cores of collagen and coated by arachnoid as seen in the trabeculae extending across the subarachnoid space. Within the stroma of the choroid plexus, and occasionally within the arachnoid itself, *spherical collagen whorls* are formed by arachnoid cells which subsequently become calcified to form the *calcospherites* or *psammoma bodies* of the choroid plexus and in meningiomas. Channels for the drainage of CSF form within the arachnoid caps of arachnoid granulations and allow CSF to percolate to the subendothelial layers of the granulation. Similar channels form in the arachnoid in rats and connect with the nasal lymphatic vessels.

Arachnoid mater

Although the arachnoid mater in man is a thin transparent membrane, it has a defined microscopic structure. The outer layer of the arachnoid — the dura–arachnoid interface — is formed from five or six layers of cells joined by numerous desmosomes and tight junctions (Rascol & Izard 1976; Schachenmayr & Friede 1978; Alcolado et al 1988). This layer forms the barrier layer of the arachnoid which prevents permeation of CSF through the arachnoid. Closely apposed to the outer layer is the central portion of the arachnoid, formed from polygonal cells closely packed and joined by desmosomes and gap junctions. On the inner layer of the arachnoid, the cells are more loosely packed and intermingled with bundles of collagen which are continuous with the trabeculae that cross the subarachnoid space (Alcolado et al 1988).

Pia mater

Mostly composed of a membrane one-cell thick, the pia mater cells are flattened and joined by *desmosomes* and *gap junctions* (Alcolado et al 1988). They are continuous with the coating of the subarachnoid trabeculae and separated from the basal lamina of the glia limitans by the collagen bundles, fibroblast-like cells, arteries and veins of the subpial space (**8.325**) (Alcolado et al 1988; Zhang et al 1990). The collagen fibres of the subpial space and the basal lamina of the glia limitans can be stained by reticulin techniques and separate as distinct layers especially when there is inflammation of the leptomeninges (*leptomeningitis*) (Hutchings & Weller 1986). Macrophages and other inflammatory cells passing out of the subpial and subarachnoid blood vessels accumulate initially beneath the pia mater and the leptomeningeal coatings of the vessels in the subarachnoid space and then penetrate between the cells of the pia mater into the subarachnoid space (Krahn 1981). Despite its delicate and thin nature, the pia mater appears to form a *regulatory interface* between the subarachnoid space and the brain. Not only does it separate the subarachnoid space from the subpial and perivascular spaces but cells of the pia mater exhibit pinocytotic activity and ingest particles up to 1 μm in diameter and also contain enzymes such as catechol-O-methyl-transferase and glutamine synthetase which will degrade neurotransmitters (Kaplan et al 1981; McCormick et al 1990; Feuer & Weller 1991). Further evidence of the intact nature of the pia mater and its effectiveness as a barrier is seen in subarachnoid haemorrhages (Hutchings & Weller 1986) and in subpial haemorrhages in infants (Friede 1989); in both these instances red blood cells do not penetrate the pia mater.

Small bundles of *unmyelinated nerve fibres*, surrounded by their Schwann cells and perineurium pass through the cranial and spinal leptomeninges and are thought to be mainly supplying the blood vessels within the subarachnoid and subpial spaces.

BLOOD VESSELS

The arterial supply and venous drainage of the brain and spinal cord are described in this section.

ARTERIAL BLOOD SUPPLY OF THE SPINAL CORD

Blood reaches the spinal cord along spinal branches of the vertebral, deep cervical, intercostal and lumbar arteries; these, with the anterior and posterior spinal arteries, form longitudinal anastomotic channels along the cord (pp. 1532, 1546; Gillilan 1972). Spinal arteries send anterior and posterior radicular branches to the spinal cord along ventral and dorsal roots. Most anterior radicular arteries are small, ending in the ventral nerve roots or the cord's pial plexus. The posterior radicular arteries supply the dorsal root ganglia; according to Somogyi et al (1973) these ganglionic ramules enter at both ganglionic poles and are distributed around ganglion cells and nerve fibres; the same authors and Undi et al (1973) have described the arterial supplies of spinal roots. Some radicular arteries (usually four to nine), mainly situated in the lower cervical, lower thoracic and upper lumbar regions, are large enough to reach the anterior median sulcus where they divide into slender ascending and large descending branches. These branches anastomose with the anterior spinal arteries to form a single or partly double, longitudinal vessel of uneven calibre along the anterior median sulcus. The largest anterior radicular artery, *arteria radicularis magna*, varies in level; but it arises from an intersegmental branch of the aorta at the lower thoracic or upper lumbar level. In about 65% of cases it arises on the left. Reaching the spinal cord, it sends a branch to the anterior spinal artery below and another to anastomose with the ramus of the posterior spinal artery lying anterior to the dorsal roots. It is sometimes the main supply to the lower two-thirds of the cord. Central branches of the anterior spinal artery enter the anterior median fissure, turning right or left to supply the ventral grey column, the base of the dorsal grey column, including the dorsal nucleus, and the adjacent white matter (**8.329**).

Each posterior spinal artery contributes to a pair of longitudinal anastomotic channels, anterior and posterior to the dorsal spinal roots. These are reinforced by posterior radicular arteries, variable in number and size but more numerous than the anterior radicular arteries. The anterior channel is also joined by a ramus from the descending branch of the arteria radicularis magna. Lazorthes et al (1971) have largely confirmed this description but emphasize the uneven calibre and interruptions in longitudinal spinal arteries. At the conus medullaris they communicate by anastomotic loops. The authors also emphasized the importance of anastomoses other than those between the pial or peripheral spinal arterial branches, such as a posterior spinal series of anastomoses between rami of the dorsal divisions of segmental arteries near the spinous processes.

The central branches of the anterior spinal artery supply about two-thirds of the cross-sectional area of the cord. The rest of the dorsal grey and white columns and peripheral parts of lateral and ventral white columns are supplied by numerous small radial vessels from posterior spinal arteries and the pial plexus (Torr 1957; Gillilan 1958). In a microangiographic study of the human spinal cord at cervical levels (Turnbull et al 1966) there were 1–6 anterior and 0–8 posterior radicular spinal arteries. From each centimetre of anterior spinal artery arose 5–8 central branches. No internal anastomoses were seen but overlapping of territories of central arteries was confirmed, and similar longitudinal overlap was also emphasized.

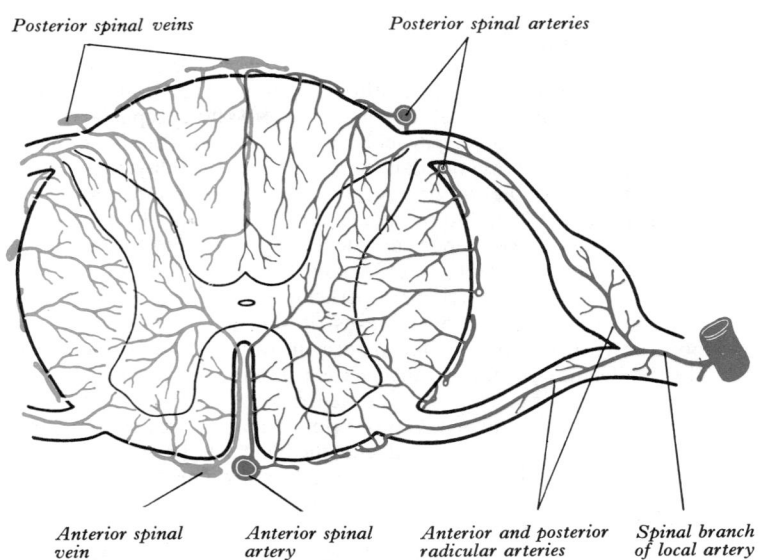

8.329 The intrinsic blood vessels of the spinal cord. The position of the veins is quite variable.

ARTERIAL BLOOD SUPPLY OF THE BRAIN

The arterial supply of the brain (pp. 1523, 1530) is derived from the *internal carotid* and *vertebral arteries* which lie in the subarachnoid space (p. 1213). The vertebral and basilar arteries supply branches to the spinal cord, brainstem and cerebellum; the basilar artery ends at the upper border of the pons by dividing into two posterior cerebral arteries. The internal carotid artery divides at its end into *anterior* and *middle cerebral arteries*; the anterior are interconnected by the *anterior communicating artery*. Just before its end, the internal carotid artery connects via the *posterior communicating artery* with the *posterior cerebral artery*, completing a vascular circle, the *circulus arteriosus* (*circle of Willis*), around the interpeduncular fossa (see **10.88**). The dimensions of vessels forming the circulus arteriosus were studied in 100 fixed brains from cadavers by Kamath (1981). The greatest variation in length was found in the anterior communicating artery and in diameter in the posterior communicating artery. Abnormal narrowing of vessels was commoner on the right than on the left, the posterior cerebral artery being particularly affected. In keeping with the dominance of the left hemisphere, this side appeared to have the more abundant blood supply, all arteries except the posterior communicating being of larger mean diameter on the left. Although the circulus arteriosus offers a potential shunt in abnormal conditions, such as during an occlusion or spasm, in normal circumstances it is not an equalizer and distributor of blood from different sources. For details of collateral circulation following blockage of the main feeders of this circle, see Fields et al (1965) and Gillilan (1974). From the circulus arteriosus, or vessels near it, *central branches* arise to supply the interior of the cerebral hemisphere and the thalamus. These vessels form six principal groups:

- the *anteromedial group*, from the anterior cerebral and anterior communicating arteries (see p. 1528)
- the *posteromedial group*, from the posterior cerebral and posterior communicating arteries
- the right and left *anterolateral groups*, from the middle cerebral arteries
- the right and left *posterolateral groups*, from the posterior cerebral arteries.

(For details consult Kaplan & Ford 1966.) Lang & Brunner (1978) have described a recurrent central ramus, often double, arising from the anterior cerebral artery beyond the origin of its anteromedial group of central rami and returning to join these; they name this vessel *arteria recurrens anterior*.

Cerebral cortex

The entire blood supply of the cerebral cortex, described in detail by Duvernoy et al (1981), comes from *cortical branches* of the anterior, middle and posterior cerebral arteries. Subarachnoid vessels

pass into the subpial space without piercing the pia mater (**8.319, 324**). They enter the cortex and divide in its substance; branches penetrating the cortex perpendicularly are divisible into long and short rami (von Bonin 1950). The *long* and *medullary arteries* traverse the cortex and penetrate the subjacent white matter for 3 or 4 cm (Lewis 1957) without communicating and thus form many small independent systems. *Deep medullary vessels* extending from central branches to the cortex have been described but these are recurrent branches of the long or medullary vessels (Lewis 1957). The *short arteries* are confined to the cortex, forming with the long vessels a compact network in the middle zone of the grey matter, the outer and inner zones being sparingly supplied. Lazorthes (1949) and de Reuck (1972) have described the differences in angioarchitecture in iso- and allocortical areas, the former being more elaborate with arterioles ending in different strata. Vessels of the cortex are not so strictly 'terminal' as those in the white matter or central system (Sunderland 1938) but, although adjacent vessels anastomose on the surface of the brain, they become end arteries as soon as they enter it. Even superficial anastomoses occur in general only between microscopic branches of the cerebral arteries; there is little evidence that they can provide an effective alternative circulation after the occlusion of larger vessels. The blood supply of the grey matter is more copious than that of the white.

The lateral surface of the hemisphere is mainly supplied by the *middle cerebral artery*; a strip next to the superomedial border as far back as the parieto-occipital sulcus is supplied by the *anterior cerebral artery*; the occipital lobe and most of the inferior temporal gyrus (excluding the temporal pole) is supplied by the *posterior cerebral artery* (**10.87**). Medial and inferior surfaces are supplied by the *anterior*, *middle* and *posterior cerebral arteries*, the area supplied by the anterior extending almost to the parieto-occipital sulcus and including the medial part of the orbital surface. (For detailed distribution of the anterior cerebral artery in 53 hemispheres and 300 angiograms consult Farnarier et al 1977.) The rest of this surface and the temporal pole are supplied by the middle cerebral artery. The remaining medial and inferior surfaces are supplied by the posterior cerebral artery (**10.87A**). The junctional zone near the occipital pole between the territories of the middle and posterior cerebral arteries corresponds to the striate visual cortex concerned with the macula. The phenomenon known clinically as 'sparing of the macula' may be due to the collateral circulation of blood from branches of the middle cerebral artery into those of the posterior, when the latter vessel is blocked. The middle cerebral artery may itself supply the macular area (Smith & Richardson 1966).

Most of the *corpus striatum* and *internal capsule* is supplied by the medial and lateral striate rami of the middle cerebral artery's central branches, the rest being supplied by central branches of the anterior cerebral artery. A ramus of the middle cerebral is Charcot's 'artery of cerebral haemorrhage' (p. 1528).

The *choroid plexuses* of the *third* and *lateral ventricles* are supplied by branches of the internal carotid and posterior cerebral arteries.

Finer details of the vessels of some parts of the diencephalic region have been well explored, particularly in relation to the hypophysis cerebri and related hypothalamic nuclei (p. 1095) (Haymaker et al 1969). Detailed studies of the vascularization of the lamina terminalis (Duvernoy et al 1969) and of the posterior wall of the third ventricle (Plets 1969) have been reported. The arterial supply to the lamina is from the anterior cerebral arteries and their communicating vessel and is described as supplying a superficial pial capillary plexus which drains into a second, deeper plexus of sinusoidal capillaries, with loops or vortices which drain in turn into the hypothalamic veins. The significance of these arrangements is unknown. The main artery to the posterior parts of the third ventricle is the medial branch of the posterior choroidal artery; this supplies the posterior commissure, habenular region, pineal gland and medial parts of the thalamus, including the pulvinar. The *thalamus* is supplied chiefly by branches of the posterior communicating, posterior cerebral and basilar arteries; their pattern of branches, and varying details of angioarchitecture in the different thalamic nuclei, have been described in extenso in human brains, with a critique of literature by Plets et al (1970) and Percheron (1977). The latter has denied the often noted thalamic supply by the anterior choroidal artery, deriving almost the entire thalamic supply from branches of the posterior cerebral and basilar arteries (p. 1528).

Brainstem

The vessels supplying the brainstem have been described in detail by Duvernoy (1978).

Midbrain

The midbrain is supplied by the posterior cerebral, superior cerebellar and basilar arteries. The crura cerebri are supplied by vessels entering on their medial and lateral sides; the medial vessels enter the medial side of the crus and also supply the superomedial part of the tegmentum, including the oculomotor nucleus, lateral vessels supplying the lateral part of the crus and the tegmentum. The colliculi are supplied by three vessels on each side from the posterior cerebral and superior cerebellar arteries. An additional supply to the crura, the colliculi and their penduncles comes from the posterolateral group of central branches of the posterior cerebral artery.

Pons

The pons is supplied by the basilar artery and the anterior inferior and superior cerebellar arteries. Direct branches of the basilar enter along the basilar sulcus; branches also enter along the trigeminal, abducent, facial and vestibulocochlear nerves and nervus intermedius. There is also a supply from the subpial plexus.

Medulla oblongata

The medulla oblongata is supplied by the vertebral, anterior and posterior spinal, posterior inferior cerebellar and basilar arteries. Some branches enter along the anterior median fissure and the posterior median sulcus. Other vessels enter along radicles of the last four cranial nerves to supply the central substance. There is also a supply via a pial plexus from the same main arteries.

Cerebellum

The cerebellum is supplied by three pairs of cerebellar arteries which, like the cerebral, form superficial anastomoses. Anastomoses between deeper, medullary branches, as distinct from cortical, have been postulated. The anatomy and development of the cerebellar arteries have been reviewed by Gillilan (1974). According to Kielbasinski (1976) the vermis is supplied by one or both inferior cerebellar arteries. The vascularization of the human cerebellar cortex has been investigated in detail by Duvernoy et al (1983).

Choroid plexus of the fourth ventricle. The choroid plexus of the fourth ventricle is supplied by the posterior inferior cerebellar arteries.

Optic chiasma tract and radiation

The blood supplies of the optic chiasma, tract and radiation are of

marked clinical interest. The chiasma is supplied in part by the anterior cerebral arteries but its median zone depends upon rami from the internal carotids reaching it via the stalk of the hypophysis cerebri. Anterior choroidal and posterior communicating arteries supply the optic tract, while the optic radiation receives blood through deep branches of the middle and posterior cerebral arteries. For further details consult Abbie (1938), and Bergland and Ray (1969).

VENOUS DRAINAGE

Venous drainage of the spinal cord

Spinal veins drain into six tortuous, often plexiform longitudinal channels, one each in the anterior and posterior median fissures and four others, often incomplete, one pair being posterior, the other anterior to the ventral and dorsal nerve roots. These vessels connect together freely and above with the cerebellar veins and cranial sinuses. The veins accompanying the anterior spinal artery receive large venules from the central grey matter; much of the blood from the cord's periphery enters the pial veins (p. 1595).

The venous drainage of the brain (pp. 1580–89) can be divided into veins receiving blood from the cerebrum and from the cerebellar–brainstem arena. The veins are thin-walled, devoid of valves and most of them cross the subarachnoid space to join the dural venous sinuses.

External cerebral veins

The veins of the cerebrum are either external or internal. External cerebral veins are grouped as three sets:

- the *superior*, draining forwards into the superior sagittal sinus
- the *inferior*, draining principally into the transverse and cavernous sinuses
- the *middle*, which are subdivided into superficial and deep.

The *superficial middle cerebral vein* drains most of the lateral surface of the hemisphere, following the lateral sulcus to end in the cavernous sinus. The *deep middle cerebral vein* drains the insular region and joins the *anterior cerebral* and *striate veins* to form a *basal vein*. Regions drained by the anterior cerebral and striate veins correspond approximately to those supplied by the anterior cerebral artery and the central branches entering the anterior perforated substance. These striate veins have been described in detail by Rosa and Borzone (1973). The basal veins pass back alongside the interpeduncular fossa and midbrain, receive tributaries from this vicinity and join the *great cerebral vein*.

Internal cerebral veins

The two internal cerebral veins are formed near the interventricular foramina by union of the *thalamostriate* and *choroidal veins* draining the choroid plexuses of the third and lateral ventricles. They travel back parallel to one another between the layers of the tela choroidea and unite to form the great cerebral vein, which enters the straight sinus.

The veins of the *midbrain* join the basal or great cerebral veins. *Pontine* veins drain into the basal vein, cerebellar veins, the petrosal sinuses, transverse sinus or the venous plexus of the foramen ovale. Veins of the *medulla oblongata* drain into the veins of the spinal cord, the adjacent dural venous sinuses or along the last four cranial nerves via radicular veins to the inferior petrosal sinus or superior bulb of the jugular vein. For systematic accounts of the superficial veins of the brainstem consult Tournade et al (1972) and Duvernoy (1975).

The *veins of the cerebellum* drain mainly into sinuses adjacent to them or, from the superior surface, to the great cerebral vein.

NERVE SUPPLY

Though the *innervation* of the intracranial arteries (including those supplying the brain) remains obscure, a considerable supply of postganglionic sympathetic fibres accompanies the carotid and vertebral arterial trees and some myelinated fibres accompany them. A parasympathetic supply is doubtful (Nelson & Rennels 1970; Purves 1972).

MICROSCOPIC STRUCTURE

Major branches of cerebral arteries in the subarachnoid space over the surface of the brain have a thin outer coating of leptomeningeal cells, usually one layer thick; adjacent leptomeningeal cells are joined by desmosomes and gap junctions (Zhang et al 1990). Such arteries have a smooth muscle media and a distinct elastic lamina. Veins on the surface of the brain have very thin walls; often the smooth muscle layers in the wall are discontinuous. These vessels are also coated externally by a monolayer of leptomeningeal cells.

As arteries enter the subpial space and penetrate the brain, they lose their elastic laminae so that only *arterioles* and *capillaries* are seen within the cerebral cortex and white matter (Dahl et al 1965; Dahl 1986). The exceptions are the large penetrating vessels in the basal ganglia; many of these arteries retain their elastic laminae and thick smooth muscle media. It is around these large arteries that enlarged perivascular spaces (*état lacunaire*) form in ageing individuals. Arterioles and venules in the cortex and white matter can be distinguished from each other by the presence of a smooth muscle coat surrounding arterioles and the larger lumen and thinner wall of veins and venules (Roggendorf & Cervos-Navarro 1977; Roggendorf et al 1978).

Capillaries in the brain are the site of the blood–brain barrier (Risau 1991). They are lined by endothelium joined by tight junctions (zonulae occludentes); the endothelial cytoplasm contains a few pinocytotic vesicles. Zonulae occludentes in cerebral capillaries have a denser array of intramembranous particles than do capillaries elsewhere (Goldstein & Betz 1986; Risau & Wolburg 1990). A basal lamina surrounds the endothelial cells (**8.330**), and where the endothelial cells are in contact with the perivascular astrocytes, the basal lamina separating them is formed by fusion of the endothelial and glial basal lamina. *Pericytes*, completely surrounded by basal lamina, are present around capillaries; such cells contain few, if any, lysosomes (Kida et al 1993a) and their function is not fully known. *Perivascular cells* are also attached to the outer walls of capillaries and to other vessels; they are an immunophenotypically distinct group of cells, originally derived from monocytes, and forming part of the population of resident histiocytes in the brain (Graeber et al 1992; Kida et al 1993a, 1994b). A thin layer of leptomeningeal cells derived from the pia mater surrounds arterioles but is no longer present around capillaries (Zhang et al 1990) (**8.325, 230**).

Endothelial cells can be identified by immunocytochemistry due to the presence of *factor VIII related antigen* in the cytoplasm and they can be stained using the lectin derived from *Ulex europaeus*. There are no markers for pericytes but perivascular cells in man express the antigen recognized by *PGM-1 antibody* (Kida et al 1994b) and, from experimental studies, appear to be the scavengers of the perivascular fluid drainage pathways and remain distinct from haematogenous macrophages and from microglia (Kida et al 1993a).

Venules are thin-walled vessels which resemble capillaries but have larger lumina.

CEREBRAL BLOOD FLOW

Cerebral blood flow in the human brain is approximately 50 ml/100 g/min. Due to a complex system of autoregulation, blood flow remains constant despite the variation in blood pressure over a relatively broad range. For example, in normal individuals cerebral blood flow may remain constant even though mean arterial blood pressure may vary from 8.7–18.7 kPa, (65–140 mmHg) (Graham 1992). If blood pressure falls below this range, cerebral blood flow decreases; alternatively if the pressure rises above this range, cerebral blood flow may increase.

Cerebral blood flow may be measured in a variety of ways in experimental animals but in man positron emission tomography (PET) is a major technique which not only measures regional cerebral blood flow but also oxygen and glucose metabolism. By the use of isotopes such as fluorine-18-labelled deoxyglucose, glucose metabolism can be estimated in both healthy individuals and in patients with a variety of brain disorders such as epilepsy (Henry et al 1990). An illustration of this technique is seen in **8.331**. Control of cerebral blood flow is through innervation of blood vessels in the subarachnoid space by sympathetic nerves and by the supply of adrenergic intrinsic fibres to blood vessels within the brain. Oxygen and carbon dioxide are also important for determining blood flow. The relationships between intracranial pressure and cerebral blood flow are complex but autoregulation maintains, within limits, a constant cerebral blood flow despite rising intracranial pressure (Graham 1990).

BLOOD–BRAIN BARRIER

It was recognized over a century ago that protein-bound dyes circulating in the blood entered most tissues of the body but not the brain, spinal cord or peripheral nerves (p. 947). This concept of a blood–brain barrier has been extended to many substances, some of which are actively transported across the blood–brain barrier whereas others are actively blocked.

The blood–brain barrier is located at the capillary endothelium within the brain and depends upon the presence of tight junctions

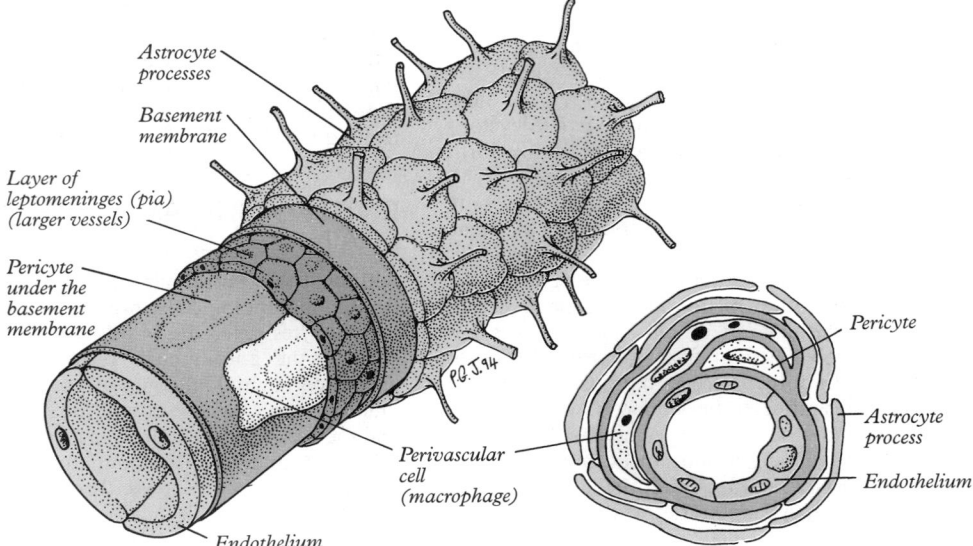

8.330 Diagrams to show the relationship between the glia limitans, perivascular cells and blood vessels within the brain. A. longitudinal view, B, transverse view. A sheath of astrocyte foot processes (blue) is firmly applied to the basement membrane (red). In larger vessels, a sheath of leptomeninges (purple) coats the vessel but this is lost from around capillaries.

Perivascular cells (yellow) lie free of basement membrane within the perivascular space but the pericytes lie enclosed in basement membrane (red). Endothelial cells (green) are joined by tight junctions and surrounded by basement membrane.

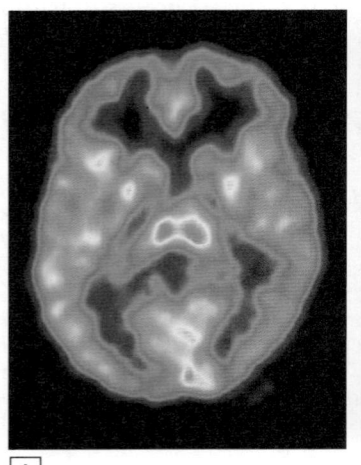 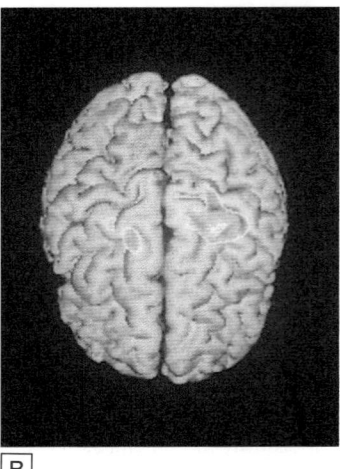

A B

8.331 Cerebral blood flow demonstrated by Positron Emission Tomography (PET).
A. A PET scan showing regional blood flow—red is high flow and purple is low flow. (Courtesy of Dr Ralph Myers, MRC Cyclotron Unit, Hammersmith Hospital, London.)
B. 'State-of-the-art' superimposition of a PET scan on to an MRI of the same subject. Water labelled with oxygen 15 was used as a tracer showing increased blood flow, particularly in the right motor cortex, during movement of the left arm. Scale: red—high; yellow—intermediate; white—lower. (Courtesy of Drs John Kew and Ralph Myers, MRC Cyclotron Unit, Hammersmith Hospital, London.)

between endothelial cells and a relative lack of vesicular transport. There are three major functions of the blood–brain barrier:

• Protection of the brain from circulating substances in the blood— this is effected by the complex tight junctions between endothelial cells which prevent non-specific passage of molecules
• Selective transport of substances by specialized transport systems (Goldstein & Betz 1986; Betz & Goldstein 1986; Risau & Wolburg 1990)
• Metabolism or modification of blood or brain-borne substances (Hardebo & Owman 1980).

There are certain areas of the brain in which the endothelial cells do not have tight junctions and there is a free exchange of molecules between blood and adjacent brain. Most of these areas are situated close to the ventricles and are, therefore, *circumventricular organs*. They include the median eminence of the hypothalamus, the pituitary, choroid plexus, pineal gland, subfornical organ, organum vasculosum lamina terminalis and the area postrema (Bouchard & Bosler 1986).

The presence of the blood–brain barrier depends upon the close apposition of astrocytes to blood capillaries. Such a barrier develops during embryonic life but may not be fully completed by birth (Janzer & Raff 1987; Risau 1991).

Unrestricted diffusion through the blood–brain barrier is only possible for substances that can cross biological membranes by virtue of their lipophilic character, although mechanisms may exist to actively export lipophilic molecules as soon as they enter the brain endothelium. *P-glycoprotein* is a transmembrane glycoprotein that actively exports lipophilic molecules out of cells and may prevent drugs (e.g. cancer chemotherapy agents) from entering the brain (Cordon-Cardo et al 1989)). Endothelial cells may also metabolize substances such as neurotransmitters (Hardebo & Owman 1980), thus preventing their entry into the brain. Specific carrier systems that allow control over the exchange of substances between blood and the nervous system are present in brain endothelial cells (Risau 1991). Such transporters may depend upon the presence of *clathrin-coated vesicles* and involve substances such as amino acids, glucose, insulin, and low-density lipoproteins (Risau 1991). During development there appears to be a co-ordinated induction of complex tight junctions and transporter mechanisms (Stewart & Hayakawa 1987).

In areas in which the blood–brain barrier is not present, specialized ependymal and glial cells, in some organs called 'tanycytes', build up a barrier (Risau 1991). The influence of astrocytes on the blood–

brain barrier has been tested in vitro and in vivo (Janzer & Raff 1987; Risau 1991) and is associated with orthogonal arrays of particles on astrocyte end-feet. The regulation of protein phosphorylation in brain endothelial cells may be associated with the phosphorylation of proteins associated with the cytoplasmic portion of tight junctions between the endothelial cells (Stevenson et al 1986).

Breakdown of the blood–brain barrier occurs following brain damage due to ischaemia or infection with the consequent influx of fluid, ions, protein and other substances into the brain. This is also a feature associated with primary and metastatic cerebral tumours. *Experimentally*, the blood–brain barrier breakdown can be demonstrated by the injection of protein-binding dyes such as trypan blue or the protein horseradish peroxidase (HRP). Such *vasogenic brain oedema* is mediated largely by *bradykinin* (Wahl et al 1993) and results in the influx of protein into the brain with swelling of astrocytes in the cortex and expansion of the extracellular space in the white matter. CT and MRI are used in man to demonstrate breakdown of the blood–brain barrier. Contrast media are injected into the blood and then visualized by the appropriate imaging technique. In this way, anatomical and functional attributes of pathological lesions within the central nervous system can be characterized.

A similar example of breakdown of the blood–brain barrier may be seen at postmortem in patients who are jaundiced and have a high serum bilirubin. Normal brain, spinal cord and peripheral nerves remain unstained by the bile, except for the choroid plexus which is often stained a deep yellow. However, if there are areas of recent infarction (1–3 days) these areas will be stained by bile pigment due to breakdown of the blood–brain barrier.

A discussion of the blood–nerve barrier is given on p. 947.

EXTRACELLULAR SPACE OF THE BRAIN

Electron microscope studies have shown that stainable portions of cell membranes of neurons, glia and their processes in grey matter areas are 15–20 nm apart (Peters et al 1976). This may not represent the true extracellular space in the brain, as components of the cell membrane that remain unstained or are removed during preparation may influence the apparent size of the space. Within the white matter, myelinated fibres and astrocyte processes are less closely applied to each other and in pathological circumstances in which there is cerebral oedema, white matter fibres are more readily separated from each other to accommodate oedema fluid. In the grey matter, astrocytes initially take up the fluid and protein so that the extracellular space does not alter significantly in the initial phases.

Physiological studies emphasize that the extracellular space of the brain is in continuity with the CSF (Davson et al 1987) such that substances entering the extracellular spaces of the brain may drain either into ventricular CSF or along the perivascular and, ultimately, lymphatic drainage pathways (Szentistvanyi et al 1984). The size of the extracellular space in the brain, as measured by physiological techniques, depends upon the substance used (Davson et al 1987).

ENTRY OF INFLAMMATORY CELLS INTO THE BRAIN

Although the central nervous system has always been considered to be an immunologically privileged site, it is well established that lymphocytes enter the brain in response to virus infections and as part of the autoimmune response in multiple sclerosis in man and experimental allergic encephalomyelitis in animals. Such an inflammatory response entails the entry of lymphocytes into the brain and the presentation of antigens. Small numbers of lymphocytes enter the brain, and in an inflammatory response activated, though not resting, lymphocytes pass through the endothelium and migrate into brain tissue. Within the central nervous system, microglia and astrocytes can be induced by T-cell cytokines to act as efficient antigen-presenting cells (Wekerle 1993). Following surveillance of the brain, lymphocytes probably drain along lymphatic pathways to regional cervical lymph nodes (Cserr et al 1992; Weller et al 1992).

Lymphocytes enter the central nervous system through venules. Such entry requires the expression of recognition and adhesion molecules (p. 27) which may be induced following cytokine activation

(Hughes et al 1988). Adhesion molecules include intercellular adhesion molecule 1 (ICAM-1), vascular cell adhesion molecules (VCAM) and, in chronic immunological diseases, addressins (Male 1992; Shimizu et al 1992). There is species variation in the expression of adhesion molecules by endothelia but ICAM expression has been reported in human endothelium in multiple sclerosis (Sobel et al 1990). The adhesion of lymphocytes and their passage through the endothelium may also entail changes in charge on the endothelial cells (Male 1992). Following adhesion, lymphocytes pass through endothelial cells in regions adjacent to tight junctions but do not appear to pass through the tight junctions themselves. Once through the endothelium, lymphocytes penetrate the basement membrane of the perivascular space and activated lymphocytes pass into the central nervous system parenchyma.

Polymorphonuclear leukocyte entry into the central nervous system is less common than lymphocyte entry (Perry & Andersson 1992) but is seen in the early stages of infarction and autoimmune disease and, in particular, in pyogenic infections. Such cells probably enter the nervous system following expression of adhesion molecules on endothelium and passage through the endothelium. In the later stages of inflammation, monocytes may follow similar pathways.

Within the subarachnoid space, polymorphonuclear leucocytes and lymphocytes pass through the endothelium of large veins into the CSF during the inflammatory phase of meningitis.

Sequelae of major cerebral lesions: trauma, neoplasia, vascular disease and infection

Tissue destruction, oedema, and *brain displacement* are the three major secondary effects of trauma, neoplasia, vascular disease and infection which may result in further brain damage or death of the patient. An understanding of intracranial anatomy is essential for interpretation of the causes and clinical signs arising from such pathological changes within the brain (see also Graham 1990; Miller 1992).

Destruction of neurons and axons occurs after cerebral infarction, haemorrhage, abscess and from viral encephalitis (Table **8**.5); the resulting clinical signs and symptoms depend upon the site of the brain damage. *Cerebral oedema* causes brain swelling and is mainly due either to breakdown of the blood–brain barrier associated with tissue damage, or to an increase in vascular permeability in malig-

nant tumours (Table **8**.5). Cerebral oedema produces a space-occupying lesion (SOL) either alone, or together with a tumour, abscess or focal haemorrhage; this results in raised intracranial pressure and herniation of brain tissue between intracranial compartments.

The three major intracranial compartments are separated by sheets of dura (**8.332**). The *tentorium cerebelli* separates the posterior fossa (infratentorial compartment), containing the pons, medulla and cerebellum, from the supratentorial compartment which is itself divided into two halves by the falx cerebri, separating the two cerebral hemispheres. Herniation of brain tissue from one compartment to the other is a major consequence of focal SOL (**8.332**).

Raised intracranial pressure due to a

SOL initially results in the expulsion of cerebrospinal fluid (CSF) from the ventricular system and subarachnoid space. Gyri on the surface of the brain become flattened and, as the subarachnoid space itself becomes occluded around the tentorial incisure and the foramen magnum, intracranial pressure starts to rise. If the increase in mass of the SOL is rapid, intracranial pressure quickly reaches that of arterial blood pressure, cerebral blood flow then ceases and the brain dies before significant internal herniation occurs.

Internal herniae

The site of herniation and its effect upon brain function depend largely upon the site of the SOL, and the rapidity with which it increases in size. An SOL in the superior part of one cerebral hemisphere (**8.332**) initially causes distortion of the brain with shift in the midline structures to the other side, narrowing of the ipsilateral ventricle and occlusion of the foramina of Monro resulting in dilatation of the contralateral ventricle. Further increase in the size of the SOL and its area of surrounding oedema results in herniation of the cingulate gyrus under the falx cerebri with depression of the corpus callosum and downward distortion of the roof of the lateral ventricle. As a consequence of *subfalcine herniation*, a wedge-shaped infarct may develop on the cingulate gyrus (**8.332**). Furthermore, the pericallosal arteries may be occluded with consequent infarction of the medial aspects of one or both cerebral hemispheres resulting in weakness or paralysis of one or both legs.

Herniation of brain tissue through the *tentorial incisure* frequently results in severe brain damage which may either kill the patient or induce severe neurological deficit due to compression of structures within and around the incisure. The uncus and the medial parahippocampal gyrus herniate through the tentorial incisure with unilateral intracerebral SOL, or lesions such as subdural haematoma or

Table 8.5 Consequences of major cerebral and cerebellar lesions

Type of primary cerebral or cerebellar lesion	Degree or type of tissue damage	Resulting space-occupying lesion (SOL)
Trauma		
a) Diffuse axonal injury & contusion	+ + +	Oedema
b) Haematomas		
i) subdural	–	Haematoma
ii) extradural	–	Haematoma
iii) intracerebral	+	Haematoma
Intracranial tumours		
a) Intracerebral	+/+ + +	Tumour & oedema
b) Extracerebral	–/+	Tumour +/– oedema
Vascular disease (stroke)		
a) Infarction 85%	+/+ + +	Oedema
b) Intracerebral haemorrhage 15%	+	Haematoma +/– oedema
Infections		
a) Encephalitis	+/+ + +	Oedema
b) Meningitis	Infarction +/+ + +	Oedema
c) Abscess	+/+ +	Abscess and oedema

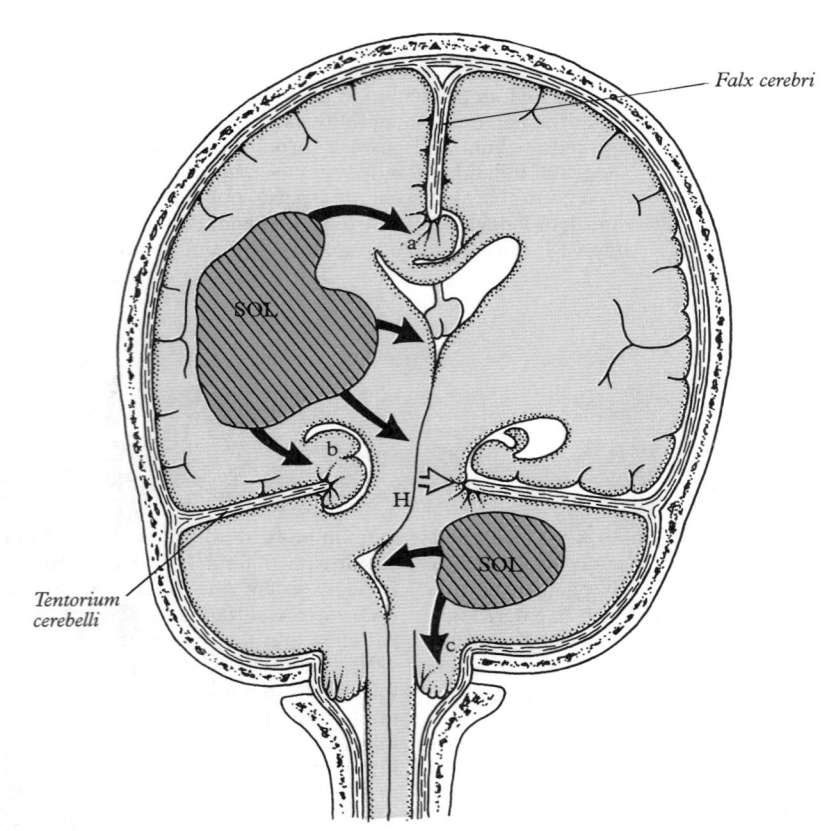

Falx cerebri

SOL

Tentorium cerebelli

SOL

8.332 Consequences of a space occupying lesion (SOL).
a) Herniation of the cingulate gyrus under the falx
b) Tentorial herniation of the parahippocampal gyrus
c) Herniation of cerebellar tonsils through the foramen magnum.
H: haemorrhage into the midbrain.
Open arrow: compression of cerebral peduncle against the free edge of the tentorium cerebelli.

leads to infarction of the superior aspect of the cerebellum.

Severe, and often fatal, damage to the midbrain may complicate tentorial herniation. Most dramatic is a flame-shaped haemorrhage in the centre of the midbrain extending into the thalamus and into the tegmentum of the pons. Ischaemic areas of infarction are also seen in the midbrain; both haemorrhage and infarction are probably due to stretching of branches of the basilar artery and the draining veins by the displaced brain.

Posterior fossa SOL in the cerebellum, fourth ventricle, cerebellopontine angle, medulla or pons cause dilatation of the supratentorial ventricles due to compression or distortion of the fourth ventricle (**8.333**). The other major effect of a posterior fossa SOL is *herniation of the cerebellar tonsils* as they are forced down through the foramen magnum, compressing and kinking the medulla and resulting in infarction of the tips of the cerebellar tonsils themselves. Apnoea due to compression of the medulla may be fatal. Longstanding protrusion of the cerebellar tonsils through the foramen magnum, often due to a congenital defect, may result in impedance of flow of the CSF through the foramen magnum, with consequent syringomyelia or hydrocephalus.

meningioma pressing on the cerebral hemisphere. Temporal lobe lesions cause the maximum effect. The degree of herniation depends upon the size of the individual's tentorial incisure and the size of the SOL and its surrounding oedema. Initially the midbrain, which passes through the incisure, will be compressed from one side by herniation of the parahippocampal gyrus; compression of the aqueduct may impede CSF flow and result in dilatation of the ventricular system. Compression of the contralateral cerebral peduncle against the free edge of the tentorium can cause infarction of the corticospinal tract with hemiparesis on the same side as the SOL. More commonly, it is the ipsilateral oculomotor nerve which is compressed against the free edge of the tentorium, resulting in ptosis, dilatation of the pupil, loss of the pupillary response to light (parasympathetic paralysis) and deviation of the eye laterally and downwards due to paralysis of extraocular muscles supplied by the third nerve on the same side as the SOL. Such effects are

important clinical signs and an indication of tentorial herniation.

As pressure in the supratentorial compartment increases, infarction of the parahippocampal gyrus occurs in the groove formed on its undersurface by compression against the free edge of the tentorium cerebelli also (**8.333**). At this point, arteries on the undersurface of the temporal lobe and around the brainstem become compressed. Damage to the anterior choroidal artery in this way results in infarction of the medial aspect of the globus pallidus, part of the internal capsule, and the optic tract. Compression of branches of the posterior cerebral artery as they traverse the inferior aspect of the temporal lobe results initially in infarction of the visual cortex on the same side as the SOL; there is a residual homonymous hemianopia if the patient survives. More severe compression of the arteries results in infarction of the whole inferior aspect of the temporal lobe and the thalamus. The superior cerebellar artery is also vulnerable, and compression of this vessel

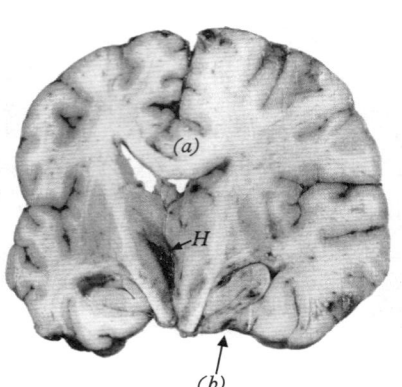

8.333 Coronal section of a brain showing severe cerebral oedema in the right hemisphere.
The oedematous post-mortem brain of a patient, 7 days after head injury and extradural haematoma. There is a shift of the midline towards the left and the cingulate gyrus (a) has herniated under the falx cerebri. The parahippocampal gyrus on the right has herniated through the tentorial opening and a groove with a patch of haemorrhage (b) is seen at the site of the herniation. Haemorrhage into the midbrain, extending into the thalamus (H), is seen near the midline.

PERIPHERAL NERVOUS SYSTEM

The peripheral nervous system comprises the afferent or centripetal nerve fibres connecting receptors to the central nervous system and efferent, centrifugal nerve fibres connecting the central nervous system to the effector apparatus. In man these are grouped into 12 pairs of cranial nerves issuing from the brain and 31 pairs of spinal nerves. The sympathetic trunks, ganglia and splanchnic nerves are part of this system but will be described in a separate section (pp. 1292–1311).

In the most primitive vertebrates the spinal cord has a series of ventral motor nerve roots, arising from a ventral (anterior) grey column, and a series of dorsal sensory nerve roots, connected to the dorsal (posterior) grey column. The ventral and dorsal roots do not unite or coincide exactly in position; a ventral root is segmental and distributed to the myotome corresponding to its neuromere of origin while dorsal roots are intersegmental, running in the intersegmental connective tissue to their cutaneous distribution.

The arrangement of the cranial nerves is more complex and reflects the profound modifications that have occurred during the development of the branchial system. In the brain, the corresponding ventral and dorsal nerves never fuse, though adjoining ventral or dorsal nerves sometimes do. Owing to the disappearance of some myotomes, the corresponding ventral nerves are suppressed; and dorsal nerves, originally sensory to the skin of the head and the mucous membrane of the mouth and pharynx, acquire motor fibres which they distribute to the musculature arising in the branchial region (p. 277). With growth and modification of the brain and elaboration of the head, the cutaneous areas are transferred from one nerve to a neighbour, altering the functions of the individual dorsal nerves.

The incorporation of some precervical segments into the head leads to the fusion of corresponding ventral nerves; the hypoglossal nerve, so formed, is thus added to the cranial series.

CRANIAL NERVES

There are twelve pairs of cranial nerves, all of which pass through foramina in the skull base. The names of the cranial nerves are:

I	Olfactory	II	Optic	III	Oculomotor
IV	Trochlear	V	Trigeminal	VI	Abducens
VII	Facial	VIII	Vestibulocochlear	IX	Glossopharyngeal
X	Vagus	XI	Accessory	XII	Hypoglossal

The **motor** or efferent fibres of the cranial nerves arise from groups of neurons in the brainstem which are termed their *nuclei of origin*. Corticonuclear fibres arising from neurons of cortical motor areas influence neurons in the motor nuclei of the trigeminal, facial and hypoglossal nerves and in the nucleus ambiguus and the spinal accessory nucleus. In general, these nuclei receive a bilateral corticonuclear innervation (however, the motor neurons of the facial nucleus which innervate the lower facial muscles are influenced mainly by the contralateral motor cortex). The motor nuclei of the trigeminal and hypoglossal nerves and the trapezius motor neurons of the accessory nucleus receive a preponderance of crossed (contralateral) fibres, while the sternocleidomastoid motor neurons of the accessory nucleus often receive a preponderance of doubly crossed fibres (Nolte 1993). The oculomotor, trochlear and abducens nuclei receive no direct corticonuclear fibres.

The **sensory** or afferent cranial nerves typically arise from neurons located outside the brain, either in ganglia or in peripheral sensory organs such as the eye, nose and ear. The central processes of these neurons enter the brain and end with their *nuclei of termination*.

Fibres of most cranial nerves begin to myelinate about the fourteenth week in utero, but not until the twenty-second week in utero in the sensory part of the trigeminal nerve and cochlear division of the vestibulocochlear, and even later in the optic nerve.

OLFACTORY NERVES

The olfactory nerves serving the sense of smell (**8.334**) have their cells of origin in the olfactory mucosa in the nasal cavity; this olfactory region comprises the mucosa of the superior nasal concha and the opposite part of the nasal septum. The nerve fibres originate as the central or deep processes of the olfactory cells (**8.231**) and collect into bundles which cross in various directions, forming a plexiform network in the mucosa, finally forming about 20 branches, which traverse the cribriform plate in lateral and medial groups and end in the glomeruli of the olfactory bulb (**8.231**). Each branch has a sheath consisting of dura mater and pia-arachnoid, the former continuing into the nasal periosteum, the latter into the perineural sheaths of the nerve bundles. Tissue spaces in these sheaths connect with those in the nasal mucous membrane and with the subarachnoid space.

The olfactory nerves are non-myelinated and are bundles of fine axons enfolded within Schwann cells. They are unique in the peripheral origin of their neurons in ectoderm, where they remain throughout life in all vertebrates.

Clinical anatomy. In severe injuries involving the anterior cranial fossa the olfactory bulb may be separated from the olfactory nerves or the nerves may be torn, producing *anosmia*, loss of olfaction. Fractures may involve the meninges, admitting cerebrospinal fluid (CSF) into the nose resulting in cerebrospinal rhinorrhoea. Such injuries also open up avenues for infection from the nasal cavity. The extensions of the subarachnoid space around bundles of olfactory nerve fibres, sometimes regarded as a lymphatic drainage, may favour the spread of infection into the cranial cavity. Evidence for this route of infection is equivocal.

Associated with the olfactory nerves are two small *nervi terminales* (Pearson 1941). These were discovered in lower vertebrates but they exist in the human embryo and adult, consisting mainly of non-myelinated nerve fibres with small groups of bipolar and multipolar neurons. Each nerve lies medial to an olfactory tract and its branches traverse the cribriform plate to be distributed to the nasal mucosa. The nerve is connected to the brain near the anterior perforated substance and septal areas; in some animals its fibres reach the lamina terminalis, in others the hypothalamic region. Peripherally it passes to the mucosa of the nasal cavity (see p. 1317). Ganglion cells have been associated with the nerve by Pearson (1941) and others and ganglia have been observed in mice by Gruneberg (1973), who did not, however, equate them with the ganglion cells which are scattered along the human terminal nerve. The connections and significance of the latter 'ganglion terminale' are unknown. Bojsen–Møller (1975) considered the nerve to be entirely sensory and recent evidence suggests a role in pheromonal detection in some mammals. The *vomeronasal nerve*, with which the nervus terminalis is frequently confused, is probably absent in adults.

The detailed structure and central connections of the olfactory bulb are described on pages 1116–1121 and the structure of the olfactory mucosa on page 1634.

OPTIC NERVE

The optic nerve, mediating vision, is distributed to the eyeball. Most of its fibres are afferent, originating in retinal ganglionic neurons, but some may be efferent, their origin uncertain. Developmentally, the optic nerves and retinae are outgrowths of the brain (p. 259),

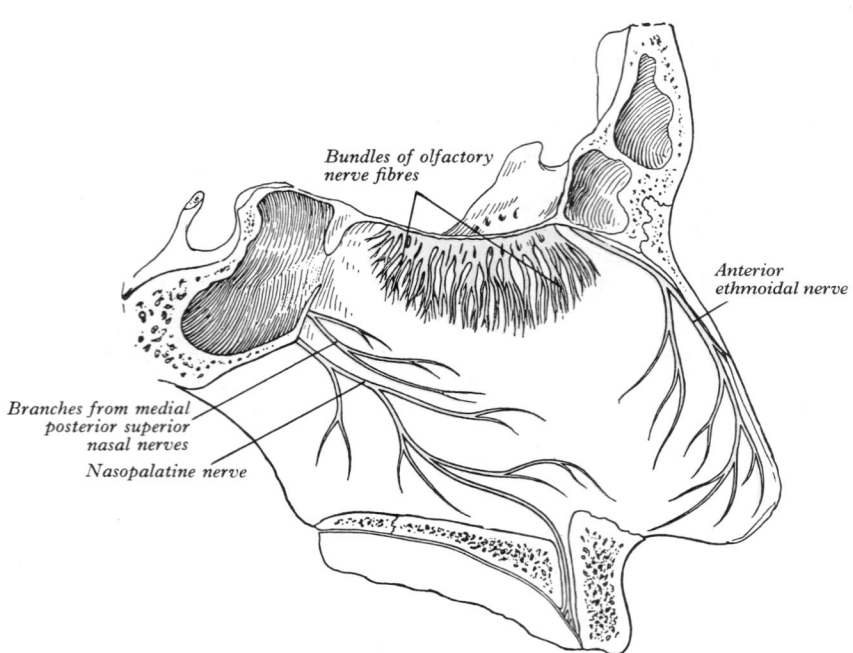

8.334 Bundles of olfactory nerve fibres and nerves of the septum of the nose (right side).

Bundles of olfactory nerve fibres

Anterior ethmoidal nerve

Branches from medial posterior superior nasal nerves

Nasopalatine nerve

their fibres are covered by oligodendrocytes (p. 940). Optic nerve fibres form the internal layer (*stratum opticum*) of the retina, being the axons of cells in its ganglionic layer; they converge on the optic disc, pierce the outer layers of the retina, the choroid coat, and lamina cribrosa near the posterior pole of the eyeball, about 3 or 4 mm nasal to its centre. As they traverse the lamina cribrosa they develop myelin sheaths and run in fascicles which collectively form the optic nerve. This nerve is about 4 cm long (Parraveno et al 1993) and is directed posteromedially through the back of the orbital cavity, where it runs through the optic canal into the cranial cavity to join the optic chiasma. Its intraorbital part, about 25 mm long, has a slightly sinuous course, the nerve being about 6 mm longer than the distance between the optic canal and the eyeball. Posteriorly it is surrounded by the four recti and separated from them anteriorly by fat, in which the ciliary vessels and nerves are embedded. The ciliary ganglion lies between the optic nerve and the lateral rectus. The nerve is pierced inferomedially about 12 mm behind the eyeball by the central retinal artery and vein, which pass along the centre of the nerve to the optic disc. In the optic canal, which is about 5 mm long, the nerve lies superomedial to the ophthalmic artery and is separated medially from the sphenoidal and posterior ethmoidal sinuses by a thin osseous lamina; anterior to the canal the nasociliary nerve and ophthalmic artery run forward and medially, usually crossing above the optic nerve, whilst a branch from the inferior division of the oculomotor nerve passes below it to the medial rectus. In a study of 71 dissected Caucasian orbits, it was found that the incidence of the ophthalmic artery passing in the orbit medially under the optic nerve was 18.6% (Lang & Kageyama 1990).

The intracranial part of the optic nerve, which is about 10 mm long, runs posteromedially from the optic canal to the optic chiasma. The posterior parts of the olfactory tract and gyrus rectus and, near the chiasma, the anterior cerebral artery, are above the nerve, the internal carotid artery being lateral to it.

The optic nerve is enclosed in three sheaths continuous with the meninges and prolonged to the eyeball. The outer *sheath*, from the dura mater, is thick and fibrous, blending with the sclera. The *intermediate sheath* from the arachnoid mater is thin, separated from the outer by the subdural space and from the inner by the subarachnoid space. The inner *sheath* from the pia mater is vascular and closely invests the nerve. From its deep surface septa enter the nerve, dividing and reuniting to enclose, as seen in transverse sections, polygonal areas which are occupied by fascicles of fibres, about 1000 fascicles in all. The inner sheath also invests the central vessels of the retina as far as the optic disc.

The ultrastructure of the optic meninges resembles that of meninges elsewhere (Anderson & Hoyt 1969) but the amount of collagen fibres in the pia and arachnoid is greater than in the intracranial leptomeninges. As elsewhere the subarachnoid space is lined completely by epitheliocytes of the pia-arachnoid, resembling fibroblasts and forming multilaminar membranes of 'mesothelium' or 'meningothelium'.

Near the eye the macular fibres (*papillomacular bundle*) are lateral in the nerve, but they gradually become medial and just anterior to the chiasma lie close to the medial margin. Fibres from the upper and lower retinal areas are, respectively, above and below; the fibres from the temporal quadrants are lateral, and those from the nasal quadrants medial.

Counts of optic nerve fibres in man (Oppel 1963; Kupfer et al 1967; Jonas et al 1990) show that there are about 1 200 000 myelinated axons, about 92% being about 1 μm in diameter, the rest varying from 2 to 10 μm. The mean minimal fibre diameter is smaller in the temporal and inner region of the optic nerve than in the nasal and outer area, and the nerve fibre count/unit area is correspondingly higher in the temporal and inner parts of the optic nerve than in the nasal and outer parts (Jonas et al 1990). About 53% cross in the chiasma. Most end in the lateral geniculate body but some pass to the pretectal nucleus, superior colliculus and hypothalamic nuclei. A small number are efferent but of unknown origin. Such centrifugal fibres reaching the retina have attracted much interest in birds, where they arise from the *isthmo-optic nucleus*, which lies dorsolaterally at the junction of the mid- and hindbrain (Cowan & Clarke 1976).

The optic nerve is supplied with arterial blood by the plexus in its pial sheath and by direct intraneural branches. The pial plexus is supplied by a superior hypophysial and the ophthalmic artery intracranially, by recurrent ophthalmic branches in the optic canal and by posterior ciliary arteries and the extraneural part of the central retinal artery in the orbit. Intraneural branches are from the central artery but their actual contribution to the nerve is probably small (Belmonte 1968; Francois & Neetens 1969). The rich supply of the optic papilla and lamina cribrosa has been emphasized (Henkind & Levitsky 1969). Venous drainage is by the central retinal vein (Steele & Blunt 1956; Taylor et al 1993). Image analysis coupled with three-dimensional reconstructions of human eyes has shown that whereas the retinal artery has a uniform perimetric length and cross-sectional area at the lamina cribrosa, the retinal vein is constricted at this site, and adopts a crescentic shape. It has been suggested that the constriction of the vein at the lamina cribrosa acts as a 'throttle' mechanism on venous flow, serving to maintain a relatively high intraocular venous pressure, and so ensuring the patency of the retinal venules and capillaries (Taylor et al 1993).

The optic chiasma and the optic tract have been described elsewhere.

Papilloedema. This is often a consequence of an intracranial neoplasm, and is probably caused by increased pressure due to excess fluid in the general subarachnoid space, which extends as far as the lamina cribrosa. The latter has also been termed the primary site of glaucomatous damage to the optic nerve (see Jonas et al 1991, for an account of the morphometry of the human lamina cribrosa).

OCULOMOTOR NERVE

The oculomotor nerve supplies all the extraocular muscles except the obliquus superior and rectus lateralis; it also supplies, through the ciliary ganglion, the sphincter pupillae and ciliaris. It contains about 15 000 axons. Its fibres arise from a *complex of nuclei* in the grey matter of the midbrain, ventral to the cranial part of the cerebral aqueduct and extending rostrally for a short distance into the floor of the third ventricle. From this region fibres pass forwards through the tegmentum, red nucleus and the medial part of the substantia nigra, curving with a lateral convexity to emerge from the sulcus on the medial side of the cerebral peduncle. Peripherally the nerve contains afferent fibres from neurons in the trigeminal ganglion, which are considered to be proprioceptive (Bortolami et al 1977; Manni et al 1978). Sensory ganglion cells have recently been demonstrated in the rootlets of the oculomotor nerve (Lanzino et al 1993). Their fibres probably arise from the ophthalmic division of the trigeminal nerve, join the oculomotor nerve in the lateral wall of the cavernous sinus and terminate in the spinal trigeminal nucleus.

The nuclear complex from which efferent fibres arise consists of several paired groups of large multipolar neurons (12–20 dendrites in man; Abdel-Maguid & Bowsher 1979, 1984), with paired masses of smaller multipolar neurons, not so easily identified but well developed in primates (Burde 1983) and other mammals which are the source of the parasympathetic outflow in the oculomotor nerves. On each side the large-celled mass contains motor neurons and innervates, in dorsoventral order, the ipsilateral rectus inferior, obliquus inferior and rectus medialis. There is also a medially placed column almost in the long axis of the midbrain which innervates the contralateral rectus superior (Crosby & Henderson 1948; Warwick 1950b). The medial rectus subnucleus consists of three distinct anatomical subpopulations: the ventral portion, which contains the largest number of motor neurons, occupies the rostral two-thirds. A subpopulation of smaller diameter motor neurons lies dorsally throughout the rostral two-thirds of the nucleus. These motor neurons innervate the small orbital fibres of the medial rectus and are thought to be involved in vergence movements (Büttner-Ennever & Akert 1981). A further population lies dorsolaterally in the caudal two-thirds of the nucleus. The neurons innervating the contralateral superior rectus muscle lie medially, next to each other, and their axons decussate in the caudal part of the nucleus (Bienfang 1975). These subnuclei are identifiable in early fetal life in man (Pearson 1944).

At the dorsal-caudal pole of the oculomotor nucleus lies a median nucleus of large neurons, the *caudal central nucleus* adjacent to the superior rectus and dorsal medial rectus subnuclei (Warwick 1950, 1953). Within this subnucleus motor neurons innervating the levator palpebrae superioris on both sides are completely intermixed; some 30% send axons to both muscles (Sekiya et al 1992), which is a unique condition among all paired skeletal muscles (Schmidtke & Büttner-Ennever 1992).

Dorsal to the main oculomotor nuclei is the accessory or autonomic nucleus (of Edinger and Westphal) composed of smaller multipolar neurons, whose axons travel in the oculomotor nerve to relay in the ciliary ganglion (Warwick 1954a); these are largest rostrally, fusing together to arch ventrally over the main oculomotor nuclei (8.335). In their caudal paired parts these autonomic columns have a tendency to further splitting in man and other primates. Sugimoto et al (1977), using the retrograde horseradish peroxidase technique, suggest that many oculomotor parasympathetic neurons may be sited near but outside these nuclei. Burde (1983) has defined the origin of these fibres in monkeys as the anteromedian nucleus,

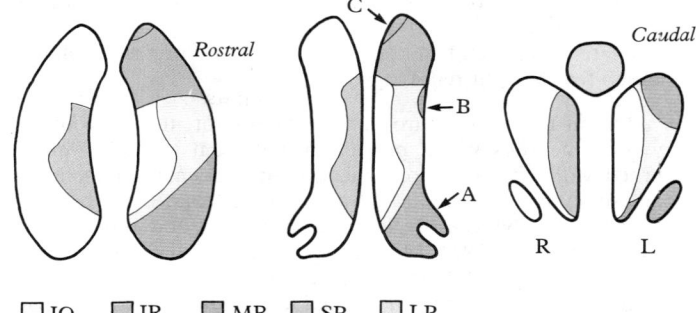

□ IO   ▨ IR   ▨ MR   ▨ SR   □ LP

8.335 Coronal sections of the oculomotor nucleus of the monkey (*Macaca mulatta*) illustrating the position of motorneurons innervating the extraocular muscles of the left eye. Note that the extraocular muscles are all innervated by ipsilateral motorneurons with the exception of the SR and LP. These are innervated by contralateral motorneurons and centrally placed motorneurons respectively. The motorneurons innervating the medial rectus are divided into three subpopulations A, B & C. The largest number of neurons are in group A located in the ventral portion of the rostral two thirds of the nucleus, also in the rostral two thirds but located dorsally is group C, which innervate the small orbital fibres of the medial rectus and are thought to subserve vergence movements. The third subpopulation, group B, lies dorsolaterally through the caudal two thirds of the nucleus. IO = inferior oblique; IR = inferior rectus; MR = medial rectus; SR = superior rectus; LP = levator palpebrae. (From Büttner Ennever J A (ed) 1988 Neuroanatomy of the Oculomotor System Ch 5 Eringer C. Elsevier, with permission.)

the nucleus of Perlia and the lateral visceral columns of the Edinger-Westphal nucleus; equivalent areas in the human are yet to be fully characterized.

Though reference to a median group of larger motor neurons has been a standard feature of oculomotor topography for decades, this 'central nucleus of Perlia' is most variable in mammals, even in the same species. The function of convergence ascribed to it was based on inadequate and fallacious evidence, and it is more likely that this role is subserved by the dorsal medial rectus subnucleus (Büttner-Ennever & Akert 1981). Its development in primates is not commensurate with its supposed function, nor is it possible to equate its size with binocular vision (Le Gros Clark 1926). Moreover, it is often unidentifiable in the human midbrain (Tsuchida 1906; Crosby & Woodburne 1943). There are always a few scattered large motor neurons between the right and left oculomotor masses but these never constitute a clear nucleus, like the caudal central nucleus; in any case, they appear to innervate the superior, not the medial, rectus (Warwick 1955).

From the subnuclei separate fascicles course forward in the midbrain to emerge on the surface of the brainstem in the interpeduncular fossa. The fascicles are most probably arranged from medial to lateral as fibres subserving the following structures: the pupil, the inferior rectus, the medial rectus, the levator palpebrae superioris and superior rectus, and the inferior oblique. Vascular lesions of individual fascicles or groups of fascicles in the midbrain have recently been reported (Keane 1988; Shuaib et al 1989; Castro et al 1990), corroborating this arrangement.

Connections

The afferent inputs to the oculomotor nuclei include fibres from:

- the rostral interstitial nucleus of the medial longitudinal fasciculus (riMLF) and the interstitial nucleus of Cajal (INC), both of which are involved in the control of vertical and torsional gaze
- the nuclei of the posterior commissure, both directly and via the INC, and, via these nuclei, from the frontal eye fields, the superior colliculus, the dentate nucleus and other cortical areas
- the medial longitudinal fasciculus, including fibres from the trochlear, abducent and vestibular nuclei
- the ascending tract of Deiters directly linking the medial and lateral vestibular nuclei to the medial rectus subnucleus
- directly from the superior colliculus in the descending predorsal bundle

- the nucleus prepositus hypoglossi, again primarily to the medial rectus subnucleus
- the bilateral pretectal nuclei (primarily the pretectal olivary nucleus) for the light reflex.

In addition to motor neurons, the oculomotor nucleus contains many other neurons which project to and from the other nuclei concerned with ocular motor function. In particular, horseradish peroxidase studies have indicated a reciprocal connection between oculomotor and abducent nuclei, both ipsilateral and contralateral (Graybiel & Hartwig 1974; Maciewicz et al 1975). Such internuclear connections are expected from the results of experimental stimulation of or damage to the medial longitudinal fasciculus, and from clinico-pathological data derived from cases of internuclear ophthalmo-plegia.

Course

As it emerges from the brain, often by several rootlets which fuse to form a single trunk (Tschabitscher & Hocker 1991), the oculomotor nerve lies in the interpeduncular fossa covered by the pia mater. It passes in the subarachnoid space between the posterior cerebral and superior cerebellar arteries (10.86), runs forwards, downwards and laterally through the basal cistern lateral to the medial inferior surface of the posterior communicating artery, and below the temporal lobe uncus. During its subarachnoid course the parasympathetic pupillary fibres lie peripherally in the dorsomedial part of the nerve (Sunderland & Hughes 1946; Kerr & Hollowell 1964).

The nerve then perforates the arachnoid in the triangular interval between the free and attached borders of the tentorium cerebelli. It then pierces the inner dural layer lateral to the posterior clinoid process to traverse the roof of the cavernous sinus. Anteriorly, it descends into the lateral wall of the cavernous sinus, where it lies above the trochlear nerve (10.165). Here it receives one or two filaments from the internal carotid sympathetic plexus and connects with the ophthalmic division of the trigeminal. It divides into superior and inferior rami, which enter the orbit by the superior orbital fissure within the annulus tendineus communis (of Zinn), with the nasociliary and abducent nerves between them (8.336).

The smaller *superior ramus* ascends on the lateral side of the optic nerve, dividing into multiple branches which run for several millimetres before entering the rectus superior and levator palpebrae superioris. The *inferior ramus* divides into three branches: one passes under the optic nerve to the rectus medialis, another to the rectus inferior, the third and longest passes forwards between the rectus inferior and lateralis to the obliquus inferior. The branches enter the muscles on their ocular surfaces, except that to the obliquus inferior, which enters its posterior border. From the nerve to obliquus inferior a short (sometimes double or treble) branch passes to the lower part of the ciliary ganglion as its *motor, parasympathetic root*. It contains finely myelinated fibres from the autonomic portion of the oculomotor nucleus, which synapse with the ganglionic neurons, whose postganglionic fibres pass in the short ciliary nerves to the sphincter pupillae and ciliaris (pp. 1328, 1332).

The vascular supply of the oculomotor nuclei and fascicles is via a median group of arteries that arise from the terminal bifurcation of the basilar artery. After entering the brainstem they ascend dorsally supplying the midline structures up to and along the sylvian aqueduct. In the subarachnoid space the nerve receives vascular twigs from the posterior cerebral artery, the superior cerebellar artery and the tentorial and dorsal meningeal branches of the meningohypophyseal trunk of the internal carotid artery. In the cavernous sinus the latter two branches together with branches from the ophthalmic artery supply the nerve (Asbury et al 1970; Nadeau & Trobe 1983).

CILIARY GANGLION

This is a small, flat reddish-grey irregular-shaped ganglion (8.336, 337) measuring between 1 and 2 mm in diameter, situated near the orbital apex in loose fat about 1 cm in front of the medial end of the superior orbital fissure. It lies between the optic nerve and the rectus lateralis, usually lateral to the ophthalmic artery (Sinnreich & Nathan 1981). It is a peripheral parasympathetic ganglion. Its neurons, which are multipolar, are larger than in typical autonomic ganglia; a very small number of more typical neurons are also present (Warwick 1954b). Its *connections* or *roots* (8.337) enter or leave it posteriorly. Sympathetic and sensory fibres merely pass through (and may be absent in some mammals). The *parasympathetic root*, derived from the branch of the oculomotor nerve to the inferior oblique, consists of preganglionic fibres from the Edinger-Westphal nucleus, which relay in the ganglion, the postganglionic fibres travelling in the short ciliary nerves to the sphincter pupillae and ciliaris. More than 95% of these fibres supply the ciliaris, which is much the larger muscle in volume (Warwick 1954b), hence this motor pathway is

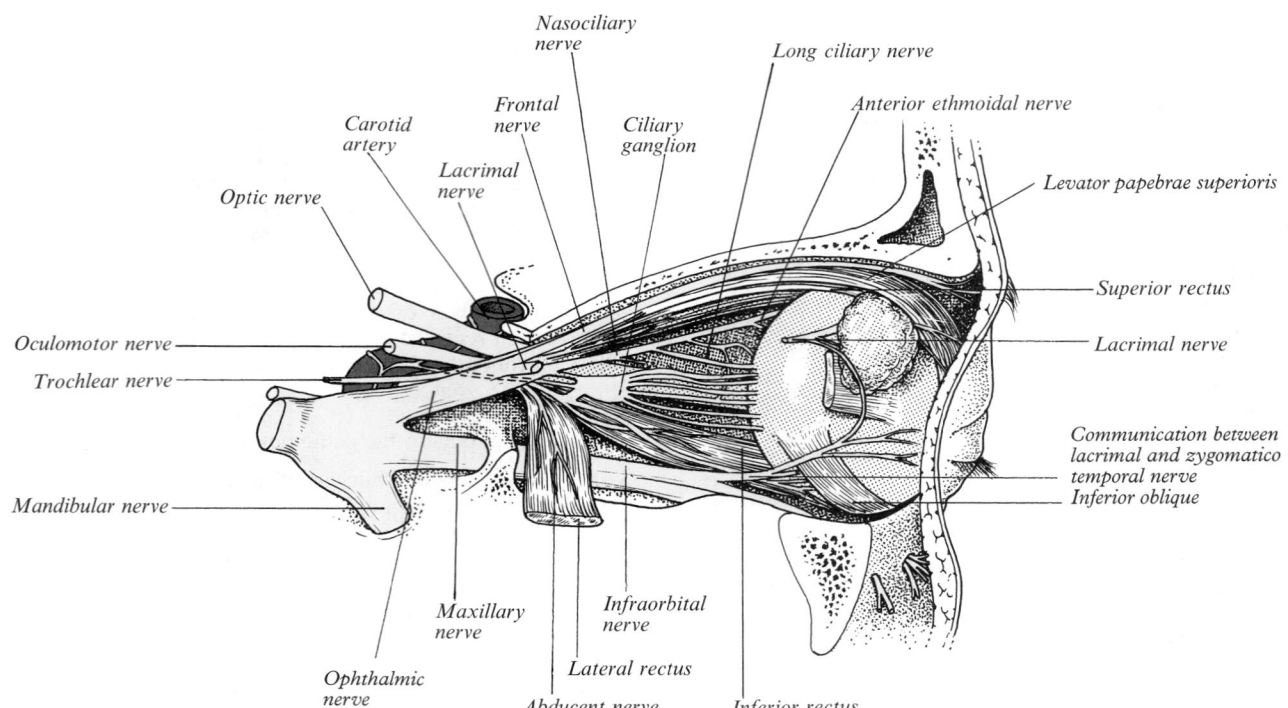

8.336   The nerves of the right orbit and the ciliary ganglion: lateral aspect.

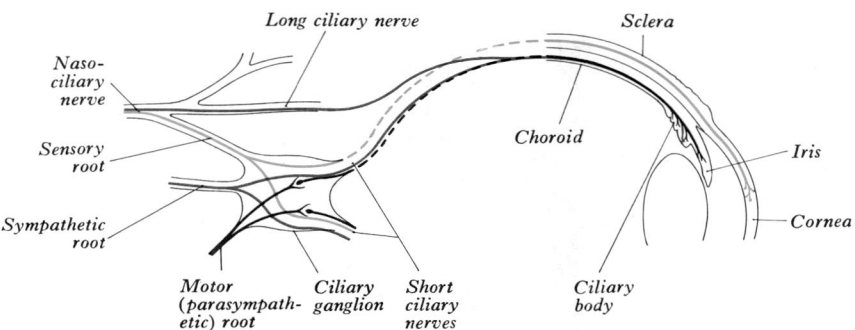

8.337 The ciliary ganglion, with its roots and branches of distribution. Red = sympathetic fibres, heavy black = parasympathetic fibres, blue = sensory (cerebrospinal) fibres. Alternative pathways are given for the sym-pathetic fibres to the dilator pupillae. A schematic sagittal section is shown in the upper lateral quadrant of the eyeball but the retina has not been included.

more concerned with accommodation than with the light reflex. The *sympathetic root* is a branch from the internal carotid plexus, which either passes direct to the ganglion or joins the sensory root to reach it indirectly; it consists of postganglionic fibres from the superior cervical ganglion, which traverse the ganglion without synapsing, to emerge into the short ciliary nerve. They are distributed to blood vessels of the eyeball but may include axons supplying the dilator pupillae when these do not follow their usual course in the ophthalmic, nasociliary and long ciliary nerve. The *sensory root* is a *ramus communicans* of the nasociliary nerve, containing sensory fibres from the eyeball which reach the ganglion in short ciliary nerves and traverse it without synapsing. The ramus leaves the ganglion posteriorly and runs back to join the nasociliary nerve near its orbital entry.

The *branches* of the ganglion are eight to ten delicate filaments which emerge anteriorly in two or three bundles, the lower being larger, termed *short ciliary nerves*. The postganglionic parasympathetic fibres are myelinated. With the ciliary arteries they run forwards sinuously, above and below the optic nerve, dividing into 15–20 branches which pierce the sclera around the optic nerve and run in small grooves on the internal scleral surface. They contain motor (parasympathetic and sympathetic) and afferent sensory fibres, the former distributed to sphincter pupillae and ciliaris and to choroidal and iridial blood vessels. The existence of proprioceptive fibres in the oculomotor nerve can no longer be doubted, since stretch endings occur in the extraocular muscles (p. 1353). How far such fibres travel in the nerve, and their central terminations, remain unsettled. The blood supply of the ciliary ganglion, investigated in man by Elišková (1973), is from small rami of muscular, posterior ciliary and central retinal arteries.

Lesions of the oculomotor nerve and nuclei

Palsies of the oculomotor nerve can be largely subdivided into:

- incomplete palsies where there is usually no involvement of the pupillomotor fibres and only partial paralysis of the supplied extraocular muscles
- complete palsies involving the pupillomotor fibres with complete paralysis of the supplied extraocular musculature.

Incomplete palsies, by far the most common, are usually due to infarction of the nerve either in its intramedullary, intracranial or intraorbital course, the site of the lesion being determined by any additional signs. Complete palsies are generally due to compression of the nerve by either a tumour (directly or indirectly due to raised intracranial pressure causing herniation of the uncus) or an aneurysm, most commonly of the posterior communicating artery. Because of the position of the parasympathetic fibres in the nerve in relation to the artery, the pupil is paralysed in 95–97% of complete oculomotor nerve palsies due to aneurysmal compression (Trobe 1988).

Oculomotor nuclear lesions are rare but cause a characteristic constellation of physical signs. There is paralysis of the ipsilateral inferior oblique, medial and inferior recti and the contralateral superior rectus with bilateral ptosis. Brainstem infarction may cause

a fascicular lesion of the oculomotor nerve. This may be restricted to an isolated muscle, i.e. the inferior oblique (Castro et al 1990), or it may involve both elevators (the inferior oblique and the superior rectus), the medial rectus and the levator palpebrae superioris (Shuaib & Murphy 1987). Finally all of the extraocular muscles supplied by the oculomotor nerve may be involved but the pupil spared (Breen et al 1991).

The clinical features of an oculomotor palsy are ptosis and a divergent strabismus with vertical diplopia, the false image being the higher. There is also difficulty with reading due to loss of accommodation and an ipsilateral loss of the pupil response to light shone in either eye.

TROCHLEAR NERVE

The trochlear nerve (**8.336, 338**), the thinnest cranial nerve, supplies the ocular superior oblique muscle. According to Mustafa and Gamble (1979), the adult human nerve contains about 2400 fibres, fetal counts being 4000 (at CR length 9.2 cm), 6000 (at CR length 10 cm) and 3200 (at CR length 24 cm). Many fibres therefore degenerate after an initial increase. The orbital part of the nerve contains more fibres than its stem, a disparity also observed in fetal trochlear nerves.

The trochlear nucleus lies in the grey matter in the floor of the cerebral aqueduct, level with the upper part of the inferior colliculus (**8.129, 180**), and is in line with the ventromedial part of the oculomotor nucleus, in the position of the somatic efferent column. The medial longitudinal fasciculus is ventral and lateral to it. The oculomotor and trochlear nuclei often overlap slightly but can be distinguished by the smaller size of the trochlear neurons.

Connections

The afferent inputs to the trochlear nucleus include fibres from:

- the rostral interstitial nucleus of the medial longitudinal fasciculus (riMLF) and the interstitial nucleus of Cajal (INC), both of which are involved in the control of vertical and torsional gaze
- the nuclei of the posterior commissure, both directly and via the INC, and, via these nuclei, from the frontal eye fields, the superior colliculus, the dentate nucleus and other cortical areas
- the medial longitudinal fasciculus including fibres from the oculomotor, abducent and vestibular nuclei (p. 1070)
- directly from the superior colliculus in the descending predorsal bundle
- the nucleus prepositus hypoglossi.

Course

After leaving its nucleus the trochlear nerve pursues an unusual course, at first passing laterally through the tegmentum and then curving dorsocaudally round the aqueduct into the anterior medullary velum. Here it decussates with its fellow, crossing the midline to emerge as one or more rootlets from the velum at the side of the frenulum veli, below the inferior colliculus (**8.123**). It is the only

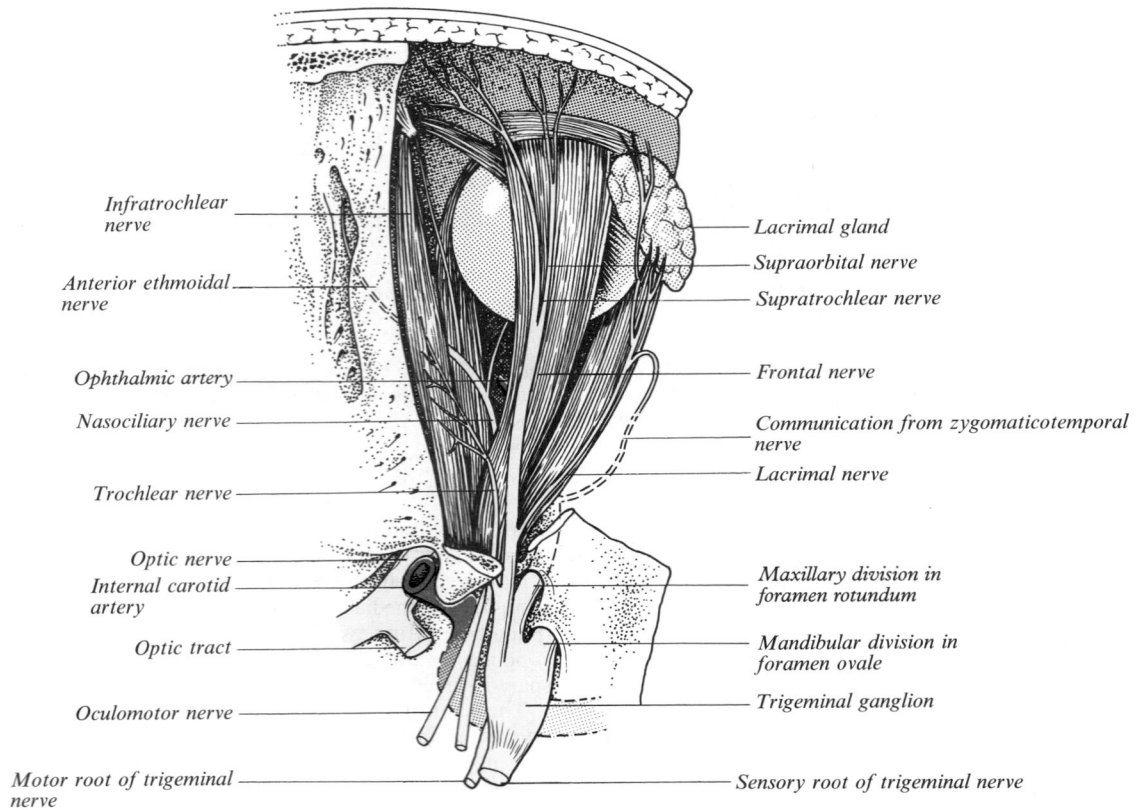

8.338 The nerves of the right orbit: superior aspect.

Labels on figure:
Infratrochlear nerve
Anterior ethmoidal nerve
Ophthalmic artery
Nasociliary nerve
Trochlear nerve
Optic nerve
Internal carotid artery
Optic tract
Oculomotor nerve
Motor root of trigeminal nerve
Lacrimal gland
Supraorbital nerve
Supratrochlear nerve
Frontal nerve
Communication from zygomaticotemporal nerve
Lacrimal nerve
Maxillary division in foramen rotundum
Mandibular division in foramen ovale
Trigeminal ganglion
Sensory root of trigeminal nerve

cranial nerve to emerge dorsally from the brainstem, and it supplies the *contralateral* superior oblique muscle. Recent studies in non-primate mammals have shown a small (2–4%) projection to the ipsilateral superior oblique muscle (Miyazaki 1985). The nerve crosses to the lateral side of the superior cerebellar peduncle and winds round the cerebral peduncle just above the pons, between the posterior cerebral and superior cerebellar arteries, appearing between the upper pontine border and the temporal lobe. It pierces the inner dural stratum below the free edge of the tentorium cerebelli, just behind the posterior clinoid process, and then passes forwards in the lateral wall of the cavernous sinus, inferior to the oculomotor nerve and above the ophthalmic division of the trigeminal (**10**.164). Here it is adherent to the tentorial branch of the ophthalmic nerve, which lies below it. Near the anterior end of the sinus it crosses the oculomotor nerve, entering the orbit by the superior orbital fissure above the annulus of Zinn and medial to the frontal nerve (**8**.338). In the orbit it inclines medially, above the origin of the levator palpebrae superioris, to enter the orbital surface of the obliquus superior (**8**.336).

In the lateral wall of the cavernous sinus the nerve communicates with the ophthalmic division of the trigeminal and with the internal carotid sympathetic plexus. In the superior orbital fissure it occasionally sends a branch to the lacrimal nerve. Though an exchange of fibres in the cavernous sinus has been denied (Sunderland & Hughes 1946), fibre analysis in human material (Zaki 1960) has demonstrated that a substantial component of large nerve fibres, possibly proprioceptive, exists in the trochlear nerve *distal* to the sinus; this part contains 3500 fibres but only 2400 proximal to the sinus. It is sometimes assumed that proprioceptive fibres (from the superior oblique) enter the brainstem in the trochlear nerve. However, Manni et al (1970) have suggested that these leave the nerve peripherally to join the ophthalmic division of the trigeminal.

Eye movements after trochlear lesions. Interruption of the trochlear nerve paralyses the superior oblique, limiting inferomedial ocular movement; the affected eye takes up a position of excyclotorsion (the superior pole of the eye rotating laterally), producing *diplopia*. Single vision prevails as long as the eyes move above the horizontal; diplopia occurs on looking downwards. To counteract this the sufferer holds his head forwards and inclined to the other side.

TRIGEMINAL NERVE

The trigeminal, the largest cranial nerve, is the sensory supply to the face, the greater part of the scalp, the teeth, the oral and nasal cavities, the dura mater and the cerebral blood vessels, certainly in the rat (Arbab et al 1986) and the monkey (Ruskell & Simons 1987). It gives the motor supply to the masticatory muscles, and the anterior belly of digastric and mylohyoid, and contains proprioceptive nerve fibres from the masticatory and probably the extraocular and facial muscles. It has three divisions: ophthalmic, maxillary and mandibular. The ophthalmic division contains 26 000 myelinated fibres, the maxillary 50 000 and the mandibular 78 000. The trigeminal sensory root contains 170 000 fibres and the motor root 7700 (Pennisi et al 1991).

Baumel (1974) has reviewed the functions of the widespread peripheral connections between the trigeminal and facial nerves. Despite the voluminous literature on this topic, uncertainties still exist; however, the preponderant view is that fibres joining the trigeminal from the facial are afferent and arise largely from the facial musculature, a minority being proprioceptive, the majority pain fibres. Sensory input from mechanoreceptors in the facial skin, oral mucosa and periodontal membranes to a large extent replaces the intramuscular proprioception usual in skeletal muscles.

The trigeminal nerve emerges from the ventral surface of the pons, near its upper border, as a large sensory and a small motor root, the latter lying anteromedial to the former. There may be contact or apparent compression of the sensory root by either the superior cerebellar or anterior inferior cerebellar arteries or by pontine branches of the basilar artery which may be important in trigeminal neuralgia (Dandy 1934; Jannetta 1967; Klun & Prestor 1986).

Fibres in the *sensory root* are mainly axons of cells in the trigeminal (semilunar) ganglion, which (**8**.336, 338–340) occupies a recess in the trigeminal cave (of Meckel), in the dura mater covering the trigeminal impression near the apex of the petrous temporal bone.

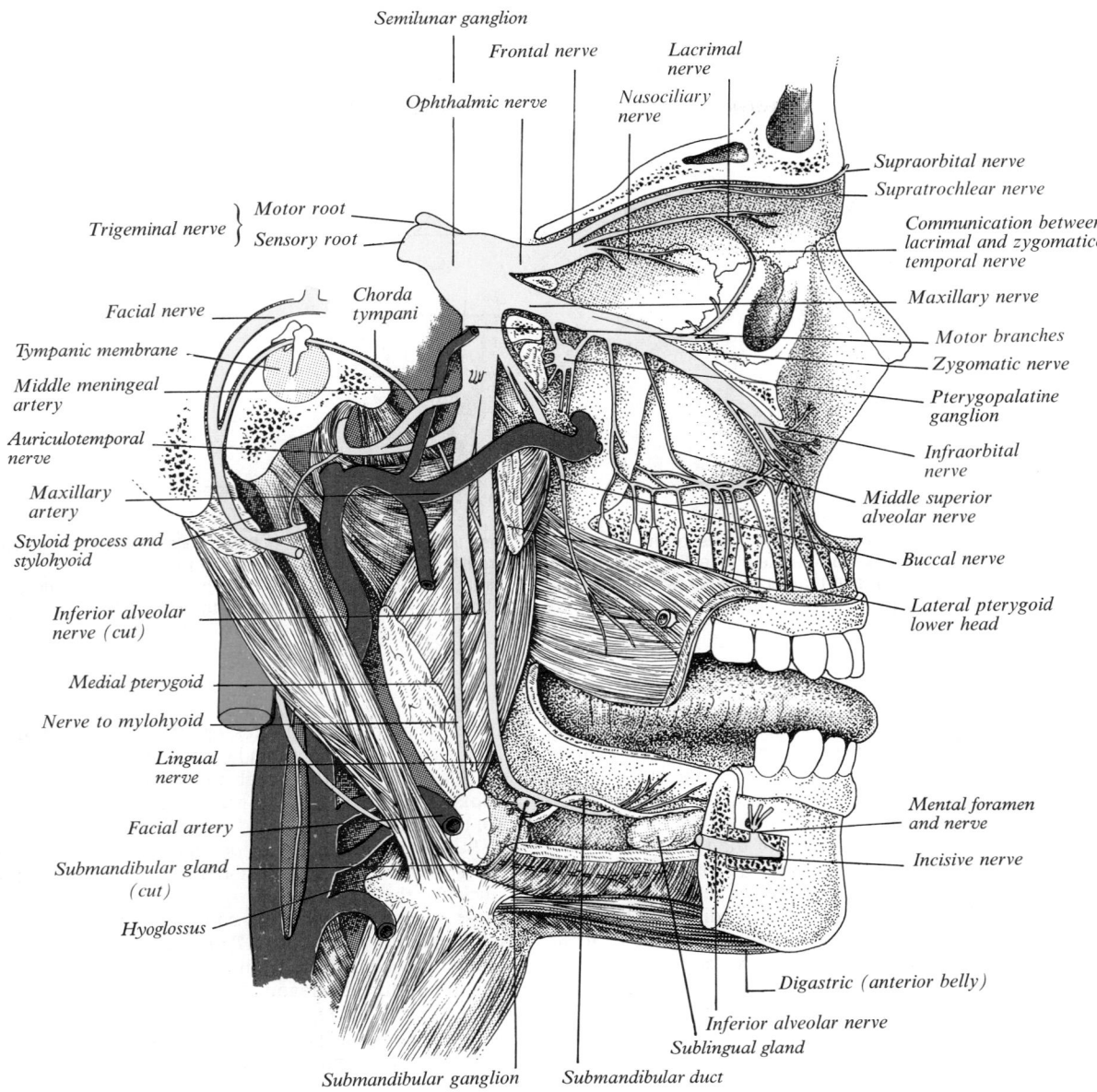

8.339 The right ophthalmic, maxillary and mandibular nerves and the submandibular and pterygopalatine ganglia (semi-diagrammatic). Note that the zygomatic and superior alveolar nerves are not labelled in this diagram.

The ganglion lies at a depth of 4.5–5 cm from the lateral surface of the head deep to the posterior end of the zygomatic arch; it is crescentic, with its convexity directed anterolaterally and on its surface interlacing nerve fascicles are visible.

Medial to it are the internal carotid artery within the posterior part of the cavernous sinus; inferior are the motor root of the nerve, the greater (superficial) petrosal nerve, the apex of the petrous temporal bone and the foramen lacerum, and the carotid artery in its bony canal. It receives filaments from the internal carotid sympathetic plexus and supplies twigs to the tentorium cerebelli.

Axons of unipolar cells in the trigeminal ganglion divide into peripheral and central branches, the former being grouped to form the *ophthalmic* and *maxillary* nerves and the sensory part of the *mandibular nerve*. The central branches constitute the fibres of the sensory root. They leave the concave margin of the ganglion to run posteromedially under the superior petrosal sinus and tentorium cerebelli to enter the pons. Some proprioceptive fibres from the masticatory muscles traverse the ganglion without interruption to pass to the trigeminal mesencephalic nucleus (p. 1068). Sensory fibres from the extraocular muscles may do likewise: electrophysiological observations (Manni et al 1970) indicate that most if not all of such proprioceptive axons have somata in the trigeminal ganglion.

The sensory nuclei

On entering the pons, the fibres of the sensory root run dorsomedially towards the *principal sensory nucleus* situated at this level (8.139); before reaching the nucleus about 50% of the fibres divide into ascending and descending branches, the others ascending or descending without division. The descending fibres, of which 90% are less than 4 μm in diameter (Sjoquist 1938), form the spinal tract of the trigeminal nerve which reaches the upper cervical spinal cord. The tract embraces the *spinal trigeminal nucleus* (8.127–129, 133, 135, 137, 340), in the lower medulla oblongata where it is superficial and lies under the tuberculum cinereum. In the tract there is a precise somatotopic organization. Fibres from the ophthalmic root lie ventrolaterally, those from the mandibular lie dorsomedially, and the maxillary fibres lie between them. The tract is completed on its dorsal rim by fibres from the sensory roots of the facial, glossopharyngeal and vagus nerves: these fibres synapse in the nucleus caudalis.

The detailed anatomy of the trigeminospinal tract excited early clinical interest since it was known that dissociated sensory loss could occur in the trigeminal area. For example, in Wallenberg's syndrome, occlusion of the posterior inferior cerebellar branch of

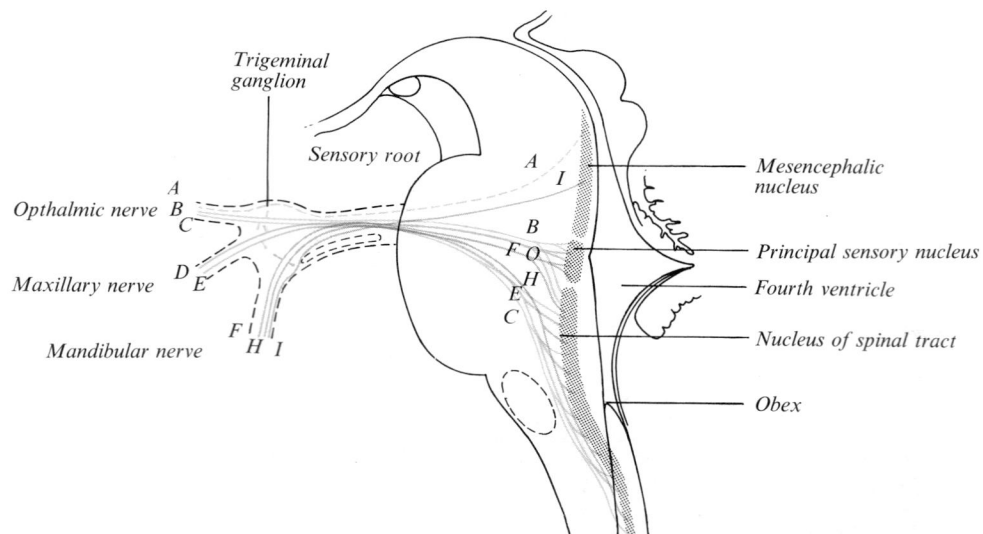

8.340 The nuclei receiving the primary afferent fibres of the trigeminal nerve: A. proprioceptive fibres from ocular muscles; B. tactile and pressure fibres from ophthalmic areas; C. pain and temperature fibres from the oph-thalmic area; D. tactile and pressure fibres from the maxillary area; E. pain and temperature fibres from the maxillary area; F. tactile and pressure fibres from the mandibular area; H. pain and temperature fibres from the mandibular area; I. proprioceptive fibres from the muscles of mastication. Proprioceptive fibres are believed to occur in all three divisions of the trigeminal nerve.

the vertebral artery leads to loss of pain and temperature sensation in the ipsilateral half of the face with retention of common sensation. Neurosurgery in the 1890s originated largely in attempts to alleviate paroxysmal trigeminal neuralgia; the introduction of medullary tract-otomy (Sjoquist 1938) confirmed that dissociated thermoanalgesia of the face was associated with destruction of the tract.

There are conflicting opinions on the pattern of termination of the fibres in the spinal nucleus. It has long been held that fibres are organized rostrocaudally within the tract: according to this view, ophthalmic fibres are ventral and descend to the lower limit of the first cervical spinal segment; maxillary fibres are central and do not extend below the medulla oblongata; mandibular fibres are dorsal and do not extend much below the midmedullary level (8.340). The results of section of the spinal tract in cases of severe trigeminal neuralgia (Smyth 1939; Brodal 1947; Falconer 1949) support this distribution. It was found that a section 4 mm below the obex rendered the ophthalmic and maxillary areas analgesic but tactile sensibility, apart from the abolition of 'tickle', was much less affected; to include the mandibular area, it was necessary to section at the level of the obex.

More recently, it has been proposed that fibres are arranged dorsoventrally within the spinal tract. There appear to be sound anatomico-physiological (Kerr 1963, 1970; Yokota & Nishikawa 1977) and clinical (Kunc 1970) reasons for believing that all divisions terminate throughout the whole nucleus, although the ophthalmic division may not project fibres as far caudally as the maxillary and mandibular divisions. Fibres from the posterior face (adjacent to C2) terminate in the lower (caudal) part, whilst those from the upper lip, mouth and nasal tip terminate at a higher level. This can give rise to a segmental (cross-divisional) sensory loss in syringobulbia and was apparently common in tertiary syphilis (Dejerine 1914). Tractotomy of the spinal tract, if carried out at a lower level, can spare the perioral region (Torvik 1956; Kerr 1963; Kunc op. loc. cit.; Brodal 1981), a finding which would accord with the 'onion-skin' pattern of sensory loss of pain sensation. However, in clinical practice, the progression of anaesthesia on the face is most commonly 'divisional' rather than onion-skin in distribution.

Fibres of the glossopharyngeal, vagus and facial nerves subserving common sensation (general visceral afferent) form a column dorsally within the spinal tract of the trigeminal and synapse with cells in the lowest part of the spinal trigeminal nucleus (Bossy 1968; Brodal 1981). Consequently, operative section of the dorsal part of the spinal tract results in analgesia which extends to the mucosa of the tonsillar sinus, the posterior third of the tongue and adjoining parts of the pharyngeal wall (glossopharyngeal nerve) and the cutaneous area supplied by the auricular branch of the vagus.

Other afferents that reach the spinal nucleus are from the dorsal roots of the upper cervical nerves; and from the sensorimotor cortex (p. 1148).

It is appropriate to divide the spinal nucleus into three parts: the *subnucleus oralis*, (most rostral adjoining the principal sensory nucleus), the *subnucleus interpolaris* and the *subnucleus caudalis* (the most caudal part which is continuous below with the dorsal gray column of the spinal cord (Olszewski 1950)). The subnucleus caudalis is different in structure from the other trigeminal sensory nuclei, and has a structure analogous to the posterior horn of the spinal cord with a similar arrangement of cell laminae, and is certainly involved in trigeminal pain perception. Neuroanatomical tracing shows that cutaneous nociceptive afferents, and small-diameter muscle afferents terminate in layers I, II, V and VI of the subnucleus caudalis. Low-threshold mechanosensitive afferents of Aβ neurons terminate in layers III/IV of subnucleus caudalis and rostral (interpolaris, oralis and main sensory) nuclei.

Many of the neurons in the subnucleus caudalis that respond to cutaneous or tooth-pulp stimulation are also excited by noxious electrical, mechanical or chemical stimuli derived from the jaw or tongue muscles, demonstrating that there is convergence of superficial and deep afferent inputs via wide-dynamic range or nociceptive-specific neurons. Similar convergence of superficial and deep inputs occurs in the rostral nuclei and may account for the poor localization of trigeminal pain, and for the spread of pain which often makes diagnosis difficult.

There are distinct subtypes of cells in lamina II. Afferents from 'higher-centres' arborize within it as do axons from nociceptive and low-threshold afferents. 'Descending' influences from these higher centres include particularly fibres from the periaqueductal gray matter and from the nucleus raphe magnus and associated reticular formation.

The nucleus raphe magnus projects directly to the subnucleus caudalis, probably via enkephalin, noradrenaline and 5-HT con-taining terminals; these fibres directly or indirectly (through local interneurons) influence pain perception. Stimulation of peri-aqueductal gray matter or nucleus raphe magnus inhibits the jaw opening reflex to nociception, and may induce primary afferent depolarization in tooth-pulp afferents and other nociceptive facial afferents. Enkephalins are involved—some of these effects are naloxone-reversible—but not primary afferent depolarization of tooth-pulp neurons. Neurons in the subnucleus caudalis can be suppressed by stimuli applied outside their receptive field, particularly by noxious stimuli. The subnucleus caudalis is an important site for relay of nociceptive input, which functions by defined intranuclear (rostral) projection as part of the pain 'gate-control'. But rostral nuclei also have a nociceptive role. Tooth-pulp afferents, wide-dynamic range and nociceptive-specific neurons may terminate in rostral nuclei. All the rostral trigeminal nuclei project to the subnucleus caudalis.

Some ascending trigeminal fibres, many of them heavily myelinated, synapse around the small neurons in the principal sensory nucleus, which lies lateral to the motor nucleus and medial to the middle cerebellar peduncle, and it is continuous inferiorly with the spinal nucleus (**7.86, 217**). This nucleus is considered to be mainly concerned with tactile stimuli.

Other ascending fibres enter the *mesencephalic nucleus*, a column of unipolar cells, whose peripheral branches may convey proprioceptive impulses from the masticatory muscles; it is also stated (Corbin & Harrison 1940; Pearson 1949) that similar impulses reach it from the teeth and from the facial and ocular muscles (**8.129, 180**). Its neurons are unique in being the only primary sensory neurons with somata in the CNS (Johnston 1909). It is the relay for the only supraspinal monosynaptic reflex, namely the 'jaw-jerk' (Szentágothai 1948). If, however, the primary proprioceptive neurons of extraocular muscles are in fact situated in their motor nerves or in the trigeminal ganglion (pp. 1230, 1311), some mesencephalic trigeminal neurons may be 'secondary' in status. Small multipolar cells, possibly interneurons, occur near the unipolar neurons.

Connections

Most fibres arising in the trigeminal sensory nuclei cross the midline to ascend in the trigeminal lemniscus (p. 1068) to the contralateral thalamic nucleus ventralis posterior medialis (p. 1086), relaying to the cortical postcentral gyrus (areas 3, 1 and 2, p. 1155). Some, however, ascend to the nucleus ventralis posterior medialis of the ipsilateral thalamus.

Fibres from the subnucleus caudalis, especially from laminae I, V and VI, project to the cerebellum; periaqueductal gray of the midbrain; parabranchial area of pons; brainstem reticular formation; spinal cord; and the rostral trigeminal nuclei. Fibres from lamina I of the subnucleus caudalis project to the subnucleus medius of the medial thalamus.

Collateral branches of primary and secondary afferent trigeminal neurons probably reach many other central regions, such as the other cranial nerve nuclei, the reticular formation, cerebellum, tectum, subthalamus, hypothalamus, etc., but details have not been established in the human brain (Humphrey 1969; Webster 1977; Nieuwenhuys et al 1988; p. 1311.)

Nerve fibres ascending to the mesencephalic nucleus may give collaterals to the motor trigeminal nucleus and cerebellum. Electrophysiological evidence suggests that the mesencephalic nucleus is modulated during masticatory reflexes by connections with the vagus nerve but anatomical confirmation of this is lacking (Manni et al 1977).

The motor nucleus

This is ovoid, and contains characteristic large multipolar cells interspersed with smaller multipolar cells. It lies in the upper pons medial to the principal sensory nucleus, separated from it by fibres of the trigeminal nerve. It occupies the position of the branchial (special visceral) efferent column (**8.129, 139**) and consists of a number of relatively discrete subnuclei whose axons innervate individual muscles (Szentágothai 1949).

Connections. The motor nucleus receives fibres from *both* corticonuclear tracts; these fibres leave the tracts at the nuclear level or higher in the pons (aberrant corticospinal fibres), descending in the medial lemniscus. They may end on motor neurons or interneurons. The motor nucleus receives afferents from the sensory nuclei, including some possibly from the mesencephalic nucleus, the latter forming monosynaptic reflex arcs for proprioceptive control of the masticatory muscles. It also receives afferents from the reticular formation, red nucleus and tectum, the medial longitudinal fasciculus and possibly from the locus coeruleus: collectively these represent pathways by which salivary secretion and mastication may be coordinated.

OPHTHALMIC NERVE

The ophthalmic nerve (**8.338, 339, 341**), the superior and smallest trigeminal division, is wholly sensory. It supplies the eyeball, lacrimal gland and conjunctiva, part of the nasal mucosa and the skin of the nose, eyelids, forehead and part of the scalp. It arises from the anteromedial end of the trigeminal ganglion as a flat band, about 2.5 cm long, passing forwards in the lateral wall of the cavernous sinus, below the oculomotor and trochlear nerves (**10.164**); just before entering the orbit by the superior orbital fissure it divides into *lacrimal, frontal* and *nasociliary* branches.

The ophthalmic nerve is joined by filaments from the internal carotid sympathetic plexus and communicates with the oculomotor, trochlear and abducent nerves; the latter communication may be the route by which proprioceptive fibres from extraocular muscles enter the trigeminal nuclear complex. The recurrent meningeal branch (*tentorial nerve*), crosses below and adheres to the trochlear nerve and is distributed to the tentorium cerebelli (p. 1212).

Lacrimal nerve

The smallest of the main ophthalmic branches, the lacrimal nerve (**8.336, 338, 346**) sometimes receives a filament from the trochlear nerve. The lacrimal nerve enters the orbit through the lateral part of the superior orbital fissure (**8.338**) and runs along the upper border of the rectus lateralis with the lacrimal artery, receiving a twig from the zygomaticotemporal branch of the maxillary nerve, which is often said to contain lacrimal secretomotor fibres. It enters and supplies the lacrimal gland and the adjoining conjunctiva. It pierces the orbital septum and ends in the upper eyelid, where it joins filaments of the facial nerve. It is occasionally absent, being replaced by the zygomaticotemporal nerve; conversely, when the latter is absent it is replaced by a branch of the lacrimal nerve.

Frontal nerve

This is the largest branch of the ophthalmic division, (**8.336, 338**) and enters the orbit by the superior orbital fissure (**8.338, 346**) above the annular tendon (of Zinn). It proceeds between the levator palpebrae superioris and the periosteum, dividing about midway between the apex and base of the orbit into a small supratrochlear and a large supraorbital branch.

The *supratrochlear nerve* runs anteromedially, passing above the trochlea, and supplies a descending filament to the infratrochlear branch of the nasociliary nerve. It then emerges between the trochlea and the supraorbital foramen, curving up on the forehead close to the bone with the supratrochlear artery and supplying the conjunctiva and the skin of the upper eyelid; it ascends beneath the corrugator and the frontal belly of occipitofrontalis, dividing into branches which pierce these muscles to supply the skin of the lower forehead near the midline.

The *supraorbital nerve* proceeds between the levator palpebrae superioris and the orbital roof and traverses the supraorbital notch or foramen, supplying palpebral filaments to the upper eyelid and conjunctiva. It ascends on the forehead with the supraorbital artery, dividing into (smaller) medial and lateral branches, which supply the skin of the scalp nearly as far back as the lambdoid suture. These branches are at first deep to the frontal belly of the occipitofrontalis; the medial branch perforates it, while the lateral pierces the epicranial aponeurosis. The main nerve and both branches supply small rami to the mucosa of the frontal sinus and to the pericranium; some enter the sinus by foramina in the floor of the supraorbital notch.

Nasociliary nerve

Intermediate in size between frontal and lacrimal, the nasociliary nerve (**8.336–338**) is more deeply placed in the orbit, which it enters through the annular tendon, lying between the two rami of the oculomotor nerve (**8.336, 346**). It crosses the optic nerve with the ophthalmic artery and runs obliquely below the rectus superior and obliquus superior to the medial orbital wall. Here, as the *anterior ethmoidal nerve*, it traverses the anterior ethmoidal foramen and canal, enters the cranial cavity and runs forwards in a groove on the upper surface of the cribriform plate beneath the dura mater; it descends through a slit lateral to the crista galli into the nasal cavity, where it occupies a groove on the internal surface of the nasal bone. It supplies two *internal nasal branches*: a medial to the anterior septal mucosa and a lateral to the anterior part of the lateral nasal wall. It emerges, as the *external nasal nerve*, at the lower border of the nasal bone, descending under the transverse part of the nasalis to supply the skin of the nasal ala, apex and vestibule.

The nasociliary nerve connects with the ciliary ganglion and has long ciliary, infratrochlear and posterior ethmoidal branches.

The *ramus communicans* to the ganglion (**8.**337) usually joins the nerve as it enters the orbit lateral to the optic nerve. As it emerges from the posterosuperior angle of the ganglion (**8.**337) it is sometimes joined by a filament from the internal carotid sympathetic plexus or from the superior oculomotor ramus.

Two or three long ciliary nerves branch from the nasociliary as it crosses the optic nerve. They accompany the short ciliary nerves to pierce the sclera near the attachment of the optic nerve. Running forwards between sclera and choroid, they supply the ciliary body, iris and cornea and usually contain postganglionic sympathetic fibres for the dilator pupillae (p. 1332) from neurons in the superior cervical ganglion. In view of the susceptibility of the corneal epithelium to damage, the corneal distribution of the long ciliary nerves is of great importance.

The *infratrochlear nerve* branches from the nasociliary near the anterior ethmoidal foramen and runs forwards along the medial orbital wall above the rectus medialis. It is joined, near the trochlea, by a small branch from the supratrochlear nerve. Leaving the orbit below the trochlea, it supplies the skin of the eyelids and the side of the nose above the medial canthus, the conjunctiva, lacrimal sac and lacrimal caruncle.

The *posterior ethmoidal nerve* leaves the orbit by the posterior ethmoidal foramen and supplies the ethmoidal and sphenoidal sinuses.

Fractures causing craniofacial disjunction may damage all or some of the branches of the ophthalmic division in the superior orbital fissure. Usually the trochlear and abducent nerves are also damaged, and there is a partial oculomotor palsy. This is the superior orbital fissure 'syndrome' which is readily diagnosed by the galaxy of neurological signs, although it may be overlooked initially because of associated head injury.

Stimulation of the branches of the ophthalmic division during operations on the orbit may elicit the *oculocardiac reflex*. The efferent limb of this reflex is the vagus nerve: profound bradycardia may occur, sometimes with prolonged asystole. To a lesser extent this reflex may occur with stimulation of other trigeminal branches and has been referred to as the *trigeminocardiac reflex* (Lang et al 1991).

MAXILLARY NERVE

The maxillary nerve (**8.**336, 339), the intermediate division of the trigeminal, is wholly sensory; it leaves the trigeminal ganglion between the ophthalmic and mandibular divisions as a flat plexiform band which passes horizontally forwards, and slightly medially, low in the lateral wall of the cavernous sinus (**10.**164), to traverse the foramen rotundum, where it becomes more cylindrical and compact. The foramen rotundum leads directly into the posterior wall of the pterygopalatine fossa. Crossing the upper part of the pterygopalatine fossa, it gives off two large ganglionic branches containing fibres destined for the nose, palate and pharynx, which pass through the pterygopalatine ganglion without synapsing; it then inclines sharply laterally on the posterior surface of the orbital process of the palatine bone and on the upper part of the posterior surface of the maxilla in the inferior orbital fissure (which is continuous posteriorly with the pterygopalatine fossa), outside the orbital periosteum giving off its *zygomatic*, and then *posterior superior alveolar* branches. About halfway between the orbital apex and the orbital rim the nerve turns medially to enter the infraorbital canal as the *infraorbital nerve* through which it is conveyed progressively further below the orbital floor, in the roof of the maxillary antrum, until it emerges onto the face through the infraorbital foramen about 1 cm below the inferior orbital rim (in line with the pupil). It emerges below the origin of levator labii superioris, and divides into branches which are distributed to the nasal ala and lower eyelid and to the skin and mucous membrane of the cheek and upper lip; these rami communicate with the facial nerve.

Since the mouth is regarded as having evolved from a pair of fused visceral clefts, the maxillary nerve can be described as the

pretrematic and the mandibular nerve as the post-trematic branch of the trigeminal nerve. In the early fetus the maxillary nerve primarily supplies structures of the maxillary process but later extends into the adjoining frontonasal process (p. 237 and **3.**100).

Branches of the maxillary nerve

These can be divided into four groups corresponding to their origins, as follows:

In the cranial cavity	Meningeal
In the pterygopalatine fossa	Ganglionic
	Zygomatic
	Posterior superior alveolar
In the infraorbital canal	Middle superior alveolar
	Anterior superior alveolar
On the face	Palpebral
	Nasal
	Superior labial

Meningeal nerve

Also known as *nervus meningeus medius* (Kimmel 1961a,b), the meningeal nerve leaves the maxillary nerve near the foramen rotundum. It receives a ramus from the internal carotid sympathetic plexus and accompanies the frontal branch of the middle meningeal artery to supply the dura mater in the middle cranial fossa. Its anterior twigs just reach the anterior fossa.

Two ganglionic branches connect the maxillary nerve to the pterygopalatine (sphenopalatine) ganglion situated just below it in the pterygopalatine fossa (**8.**339). They contain lacrimal secretomotor fibres (see below) and sensory fibres from the orbital periosteum and the mucosae of the nose, palate and pharynx (p. 1732).

Zygomatic nerve (**8.**339)

The zygomatic nerve starts in the pterygopalatine fossa, enters the orbit through the inferior orbital fissure, runs along its lateral wall and divides into two branches, zygomaticotemporal and zygomaticofacial.

The *zygomaticotemporal* nerve passes along the inferolateral angle

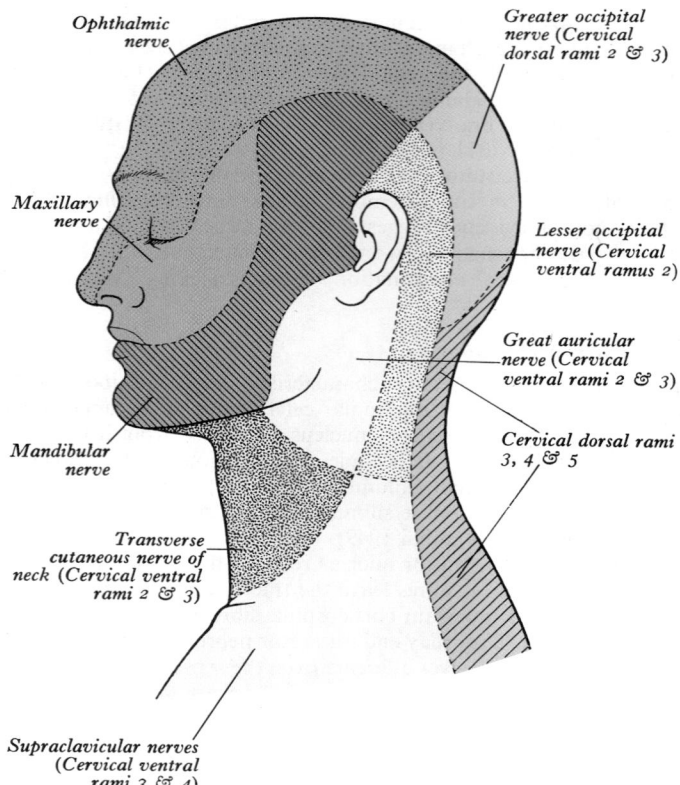

8.341 The cutaneous nerve supply of the face, scalp and neck. Magenta = trigeminal nerve, blue = cervical dorsal rami, yellow = cervical ventral rami.

of the orbit, supplies a ramus to the lacrimal nerve, traverses a canal in the zygomatic bone into the temporal fossa, ascends between the bone and temporalis and pierces the temporal fascia about 2 cm above the zygomatic arch, to supply the skin of the temple. It communicates with the facial and auriculotemporal nerves. As it pierces the deep layer of the temporal fascia it sends a slender twig between the two layers of the fascia towards the lateral angle of the eye. The lacrimal ramus conveys parasympathetic postganglionic fibres from the pterygopalatine ganglion to the lacrimal gland.

The *zygomaticofacial nerve* also traverses the inferolateral angle of the orbit, emerging on the face through a foramen in the zygomatic bone; perforating the orbicularis oculi, it supplies the skin on the prominence of the cheek. It forms a plexus with zygomatic branches of the facial nerve and palpebral branches of the maxillary nerve. Occasionally it is absent.

Superior alveolar (dental) nerves (8.339)

These arise from the maxillary nerve in the pterygopalatine fossa or in the infraorbital groove (canal). *The posterior superior alveolar (dental) nerve* leaves the maxillary nerve in the pterygopalatine fossa and runs antero-inferiorly to pierce the infratemporal surface of the maxilla (p. 1706), descending under the mucosa of the maxillary sinus. After supplying the sinus the nerve divides into small branches which link up as the molar part of the superior dental plexus supplying twigs to the molar teeth. It also supplies a branch to the upper gum and the adjoining part of the cheek.

The *middle superior alveolar (dental) nerve* arises from the infra-orbital nerve as it runs in the infraorbital groove, and runs down and forwards in the lateral wall of the maxillary sinus. Like the posterior, it ends in small branches which link up with the superior dental plexus, supplying small rami to the upper premolar teeth. This nerve is variable: it may be duplicated or triplicated or absent (Wood-Jones 1939a,b; Fitzgerald 1956; Pacini & Gremigni 1975).

The *anterior superior alveolar (dental) nerve* (8.339) leaves the lateral side of the infraorbital nerve near the midpoint of its canal and traverses the canalis sinuosus in the anterior wall of the maxillary sinus. Curving first under the infraorbital foramen, it passes medially towards the nose, turns downwards and divides into branches supplying the incisor and canine teeth. It assists in the formation of the superior dental plexus and gives off a nasal branch, which passes through a minute canal in the lateral wall of the inferior meatus to supply the mucous membrane of the anterior area of the lateral wall (as high as the opening of the maxillary sinus) and the floor of the nasal cavity, communicating with the nasal branches of the pterygopalatine ganglion. Finally it emerges near the root of the anterior nasal spine to supply the adjoining part of the nasal septum.

The *palpebral branches* ascend deep to the orbicularis oculi, piercing the muscle to supply the skin in the lower eyelid and join with the facial and zygomaticofacial nerves near the lateral canthus.

Nasal branches supply the skin of the side of the nose and of the movable part of the nasal septum, joining the external nasal branch of the anterior ethmoidal nerve.

Superior labial branches, large and numerous, descend behind the levator labii superioris, to supply the skin of the anterior part of the cheek, upper lip, oral mucosa and labial glands, and are joined by branches from the facial nerve to form the infraorbital plexus.

Local analgesia and lesions of the infraorbital nerve. The infraorbital nerve may be readily blocked by injection of local anaesthetic solution. The needle is introduced in the upper labial vestibule over the premolar teeth in line with the pupil and directed upwards and backwards to enter the foramen. One finger should be kept on the infraorbital rim to ensure that the needle does not pass the mark. The nerve is invariably damaged in depressed fractures of the zygomatic bone. It may also be compromised in blow-out fractures of the orbital floor, and is at considerable risk during their surgical repair. Damage leads to numbness of the cheek, lower eyelid and the ipsilateral incisor teeth and associated gingivae. Malignant tumours of the maxillary sinus may present with pain and numbness over the distribution of the infraorbital nerve.

PTERYGOPALATINE GANGLION (8.339, 342)

The largest of the peripheral parasympathetic ganglia, it is placed deeply in the pterygopalatine fossa, near the sphenopalatine foramen

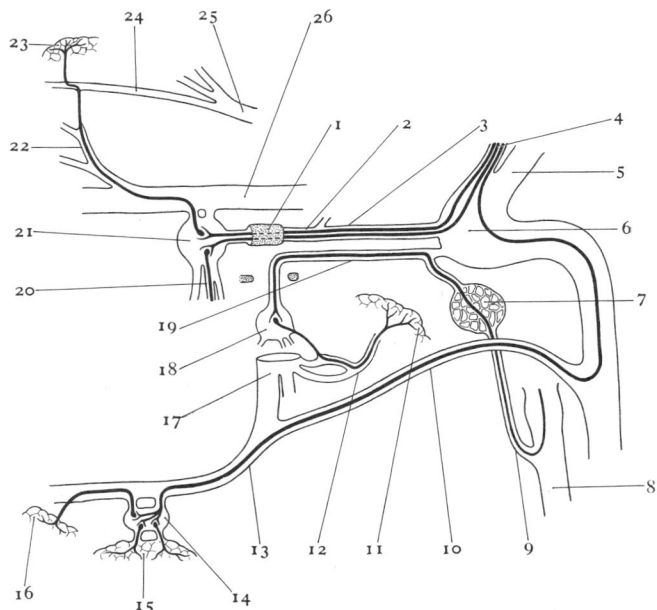

8.342 The parasympathetic connections of the pterygopalatine, otic and submandibular ganglia. The parasympathetic fibres, both pre- and post-ganglionic, are shown as heavy black lines. The parasympathetic fibres in the palatine nerves (20) are secretomotor to the nasal, palatine and pharyngeal glands. Consult text for recent views on the supply to the lacrimal gland.

1. Pterygoid canal.
2. Nerve of pterygoid canal.
3. Greater petrosal nerve.
4. Sensory root of facial nerve.
5. Motor root of facial nerve.
6. Ganglion of facial nerve.
7. Tympanic plexus.
8. Glossopharyngeal nerve.
9. Tympanic nerve.
10. Chorda tympani nerve.
11. Parotid gland.
12. Auriculotemporal nerve.
13. Lingual nerve.
14. Submandibular ganglion.
15. Submandibular salivary gland.
16. Sublingual salivary gland.
17. Mandibular nerve.
18. Otic ganglion.
19. Lesser petrosal nerve.
20. Palatine nerves.
21. Pterygopalatine ganglion.
22. Zygomaticotemporal nerve.
23. Lacrimal gland.
24. Lacrimal nerve.
25. Ophthalmic nerve.
26. Maxillary nerve.

and anterior to the pterygoid canal and foramen rotundum. It is flattened, reddish-grey and lies just below the maxillary nerve as it crosses the fossa. Though connected functionally with the facial nerve, it is so closely related to the maxillary nerve in position that it may conveniently be described here. Indeed, the majority of the 'branches' of the ganglion are maxillary division sensory fibres from the palate, nasal mucosa, pharynx and orbit which pass through the ganglion without synapsing and enter the maxillary nerve through its ganglionic branches (8.343).

The motor or parasympathetic root is the *nerve of the pterygoid canal* (p. 1245), which enters the ganglion posteriorly. Preganglionic fibres probably arise from a special lacrimatory nucleus in the lower pons, emerging in the sensory root of the facial nerve (*nervus intermedius*) to run in its greater petrosal branch (p. 1245), which unites with the deep petrosal nerve (8.342) to form the nerve of the pterygoid canal. These fibres synapse in the pterygopalatine ganglion, the postganglionic fibres following a complicated course to their destination. They leave the ganglion in one of its branches, join the maxillary nerve and pass into its zygomatic branch and thence probably into the zygomaticotemporal nerve in its communicating ramus to reach the lacrimal nerve. Thus they supply secretomotor fibres to the gland (see below). Secretomotor fibres (of uncertain origin) for the palatine, pharyngeal and nasal glands are also believed to follow a similar route to the ganglion, where they synapse. The postganglionic fibres are distributed in the palatine and nasal branches (8.342).

The *sympathetic root* is also incorporated in the nerve of the pterygoid canal. Its postganglionic fibres arise in the superior cervical

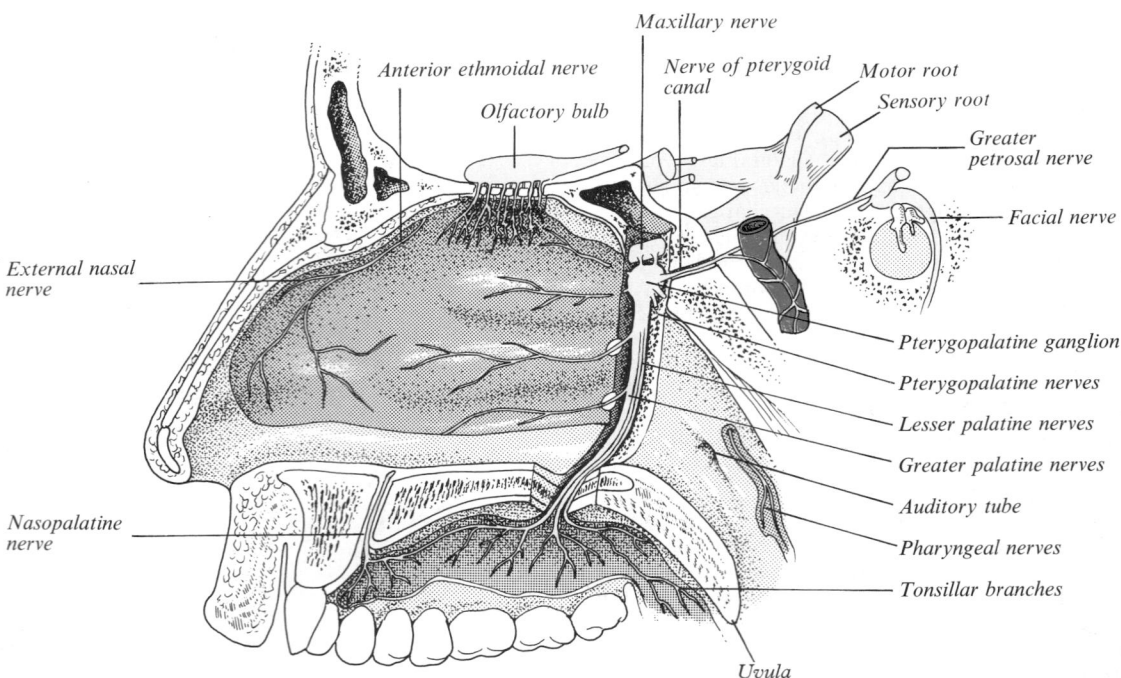

8.343 The right pterygopalatine ganglion and its branches.

ganglion and travel via the internal carotid plexus and deep petrosal nerve.

The branches of the ganglion include the orbital, palatine, nasal and pharyngeal.

The *orbital branches* are two or three fine rami which enter the orbit by the inferior orbital fissure and are distributed to the periosteum and orbitalis muscle; some fibres traverse the posterior ethmoidal foramen to supply the sphenoidal and ethmoidal sinuses. The fibres supplying the orbitalis are from the sympathetic root. Experiments in monkeys and post-mortem dissections of human material suggest that the orbital rami form, with branches of the internal carotid sympathetic nerve, a 'retro-orbital' plexus (Ruskell 1970, 1971a) which supplies parasympathetic and sympathetic branches to orbital structures, including the lacrimal gland.

Palatine nerves (8.220)

These are distributed to the roof of the mouth, the soft palate, tonsil and the nasal mucosa. The *greater palatine nerve* descends through the greater palatine canal, emerges on the hard palate from the greater palatine foramen, runs forwards in a groove on the inferior surface of the bony palate almost to the incisor teeth and supplies the gums and the mucosa and glands of the hard palate; it also communicates with the terminal filaments of the nasopalatine nerve. In the greater palatine canal it supplies posterior inferior nasal branches, which emerge through the perpendicular plate of the palatine bone and ramify over the inferior nasal concha and the walls of middle and inferior meatuses; as it leaves the canal, palatine branches are distributed to both surfaces of the soft palate. The much smaller *lesser (middle and posterior) palatine nerves* descend through the greater palatine canal, from which they diverge low down to emerge through the inconspicuous lesser palatine foramina (in the tubercle of the palatine bone) and give branches to the uvula, tonsil and soft palate. Fibres conveying taste impulses from the palate probably pass via the palatine nerves to the pterygopalatine ganglion and through it to the nerve of the pterygoid canal and greater petrosal nerve to the facial ganglion, where their somata are situated. The central processes of these neurons traverse the sensory root of the facial nerve (nervus intermedius) to pass to the gustatory nucleus in the nucleus of the tractus solitarius (p. 1018).

The **surface marking** of the greater palatine nerve as it enters the palate is midway from the midline to the gingival margin level with the posterior surface of the second molar tooth. Nerve block at this point almost inevitably involves the middle and lesser palatine nerves.

Nasal branches enter the nasal cavity through the sphenopalatine foramen, forming lateral and medial groups.

Approximately six *lateral posterior superior nasal nerves* innervate the mucosa of the posterior parts of the superior and middle nasal conchae and the lining of the posterior ethmoidal sinuses. Two or three *medial posterior superior nasal nerves* cross the nasal roof below the opening of the sphenoidal sinus to supply the mucosa of the posterior part of the roof and of the nasal septum. The largest of these nerves is the *nasopalatine (long sphenopalatine) nerve*, which runs antero-inferiorly on the nasal septum in a groove in the vomer. It descends to the roof of the mouth through the incisive fossa in the anterior hard palate. When an anterior and a posterior incisive foramen (p. 562) exist in this fossa, the left nasopalatine nerve traverses the anterior and the right nerve the posterior foramen. The nasopalatine nerves supply a few filaments to the nasal septum and end by supplying the mucosa of the anterior part of the hard palate, there communicating with the greater palatine nerves.

Pharyngeal nerve

This arises from the posterior part of the ganglion, traverses the palatinovaginal canal with a pharyngeal branch of the maxillary artery and supplies the mucosa of the nasopharynx behind the auditory tube. The maxillary nerve, and to a lesser extent the ophthalmic, appear to transmit the principal sensory supply from the Eustachian tube and middle ear cavity, presumably through the pharyngeal branch (Eden 1981; Saunders & Weider 1985).

It is convenient to discuss here the innervation of the tympanic membrane, middle ear, and Eustachian (auditory) tube. The Eustachian tube is largely innervated by the trigeminal but also receives fibres from the glossopharyngeal. The middle ear is also largely innervated by the trigeminal, but some sensory fibres are transmitted via the facial nerve (nervus intermedius, chorda tympani and direct to the facial nerve trunk in the temporal bone). The glossopharyngeal and vagus via Jacobsen's nerve, and the nerve of Arnold respectively also make a contribution. All these somatic sensory afferents however converge in the brainstem to synapse in the descending trigeminal sensory nucleus, and in the nucleus of the tractus solitarius. The tympanic glomus body (which is analogous in structure to the carotid and aortic bodies) is connected to the glossopharyngeal nerve, and has afferent connections to the 'respiratory centre' in the tractus solitarius.

The tympanic membrane is almost exclusively innervated by the auriculotemporal nerve, and appears to perceive only pain. There is a minor, inconstant, overlapping sensory supply from the seventh, ninth and tenth cranial nerves.

MANDIBULAR NERVE

The mandibular nerve, the largest trigeminal division, (8.339, 341, 344), supplies the teeth and gums of the mandible, the skin in the temporal region, part of the auricle, including the external meatus and tympanum; the lower lip, the lower part of the face and the muscles of mastication; the mucosa of the anterior two-thirds, (presulcal part) of the tongue and the mucosa of the floor of the oral cavity. It has a large sensory root which proceeds from the lateral part of the trigeminal ganglion to emerge almost at once from the foramen ovale, and a small motor root which passes under the ganglion to unite with the sensory root just outside the skull. The nerve immediately passes between the tensor veli palatini (medial) and the lateral pterygoid. Just beyond this junction a meningeal branch and the nerve to the medial pterygoid leaves the medial side of the nerve, which then divides into a small **anterior** and large **posterior trunk**. As it descends from the foramen ovale, the nerve is about 4 cm from the surface and a little anterior to the neck of the mandible.

Meningeal branch (*nervus spinosus*). This re-enters the cranium through the foramen spinosum with the middle meningeal artery, dividing into anterior and posterior branches which accompany the main divisions of the artery and supply the dura mater in the middle cranial fossa and to a lesser extent in the anterior fossa and calvarium. The posterior branch also supplies the mucous lining of the mastoid air cells, while the anterior communicates with the meningeal branch of the maxillary nerve. The nervus spinosus contains sympathetic postganglionic fibres from the middle meningeal plexus.

Nerve to the medial pterygoid. This is a slender ramus entering

the deep aspect of its muscle. It supplies one or two filaments which pass through the otic ganglion (p. 1250) without interruption to supply the tensor tympani and tensor veli palatini (**8.344**).

Anterior trunk

The anterior trunk of the mandibular nerve gives rise to the buccal nerve, which is sensory, and the masseteric, deep temporal and lateral pterygoid nerves, which are all motor.

Buccal nerve (8.345). This proceeds between the two parts of the lateral pterygoid, descending deep then anterior to the tendon of the temporalis muscle; it then passes laterally in front of the masseter muscle to unite with the buccal branches of the facial nerve. It supplies the lateral pterygoid while passing through it and may give off the anterior deep temporal nerve. It supplies the skin over the anterior part of the buccinator and the buccal mucous membrane, together with the posterior part of the buccal gingivae adjacent to the second and third molar teeth.

Masseteric nerve (8.345). This passes laterally, above the lateral pterygoid, on the skull-base, anterior to the temporomandibular joint and posterior to the tendon of the temporalis; it crosses the posterior part of the mandibular coronoid notch with the masseteric artery, ramifies on and enters the deep surface of masseter. It also supplies the temporomandibular joint.

Deep temporal nerves. Usually an anterior and a posterior branch pass above the lateral pterygoid to enter the deep surface of the temporalis. The small posterior nerve sometimes arises in common with the masseteric nerve. The anterior nerve is frequently a branch of the buccal nerve; it ascends over the upper head of the lateral pterygoid. A middle branch often occurs.

Nerve to the lateral pterygoid. This enters the deep surface of the muscle. It may arise separately from the anterior division or with the buccal nerve.

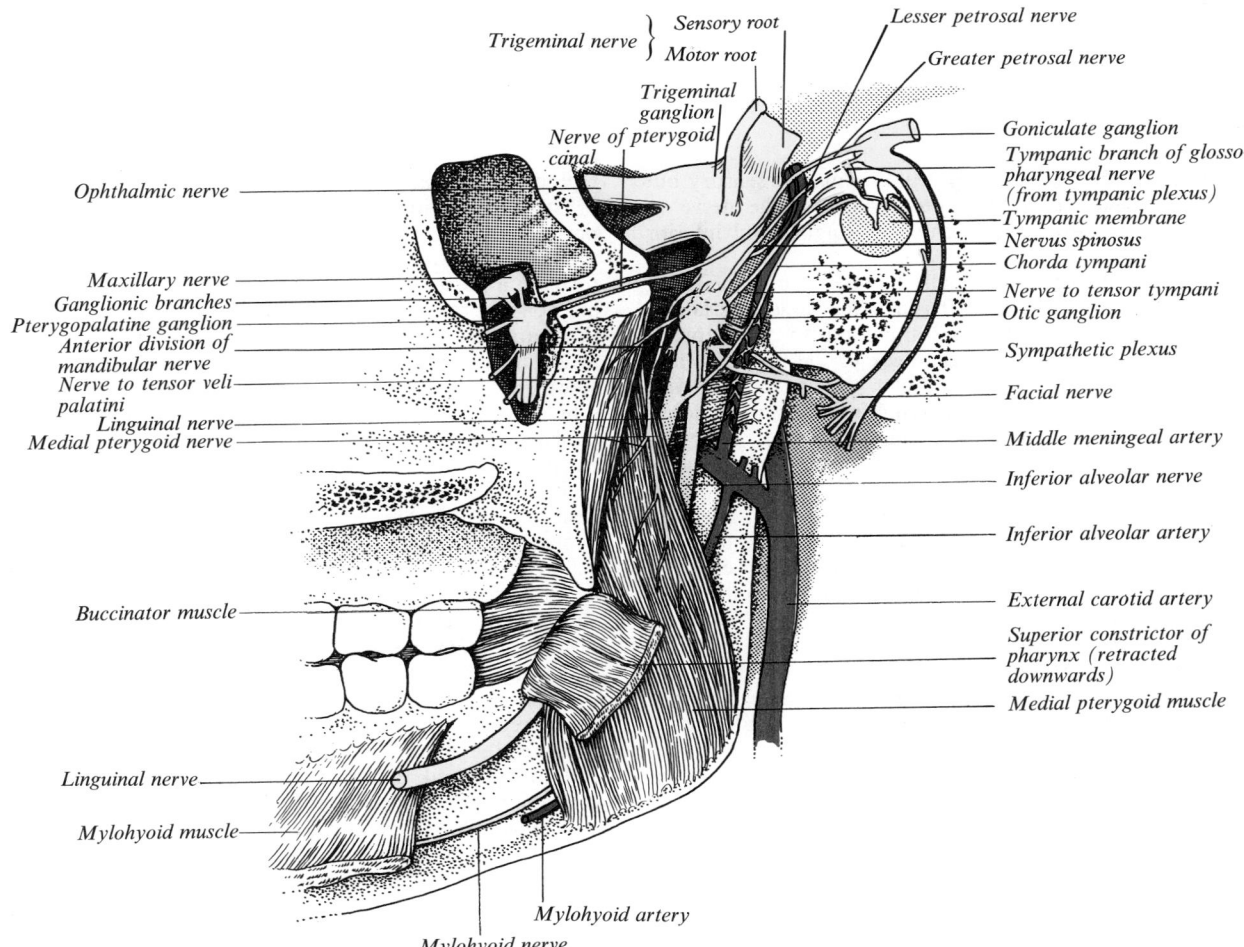

8.344 The right otic and pterygopalatine ganglia and their branches displayed from the medial side (semi-diagrammatic).

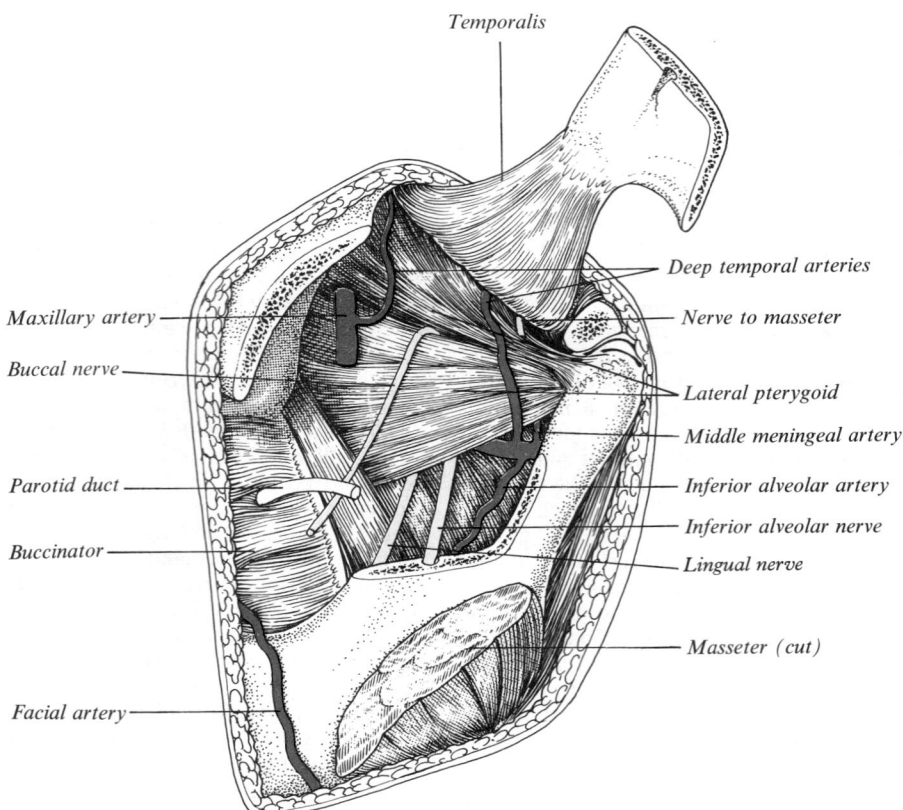

Temporalis

Maxillary artery

Buccal nerve

Parotid duct

Buccinator

Facial artery

Deep temporal arteries

Nerve to masseter

Lateral pterygoid

Middle meningeal artery

Inferior alveolar artery

Inferior alveolar nerve

Lingual nerve

Masseter (cut)

8.345 A dissection of the left pterygoid region, showing some of the branches of the mandibular nerve and maxillary artery.

Posterior trunk

The posterior, and larger, mandibular trunk is mainly sensory but receives a few filaments from the motor root (for the nerve to mylohyoid). It divides into auriculotemporal, lingual and inferior alveolar (dental) nerves.

Auriculotemporal nerve. This usually has two roots, encircling the middle meningeal artery (**8.339**). It runs back under the lateral pterygoid on the surface of the tensor veli palatini to pass between the sphenomandibular ligament and the neck of the mandible and then laterally behind the temporomandibular joint in relation with the upper part of the parotid gland. Emerging from behind the joint, it ascends posterior to the superficial temporal vessels, over the posterior root of the zygoma, and divides into superficial temporal branches.

It communicates with the facial nerve and otic ganglion. The rami to the facial nerve, usually two, pass anterolaterally behind the neck of the mandible to join the facial nerve at the posterior border of the masseter. Filaments from the otic ganglion join the roots of the auriculotemporal nerve close to their origin (**7.226**).

The branches of the auriculotemporal nerve are: the anterior auricular, branches to the external acoustic meatus, articular, parotid and superficial temporal. Usually two *anterior auricular branches* supply the skin of the tragus (**8.341**) and sometimes a small part of the adjoining helix. Two *branches to the external acoustic meatus* pass between the osseous and cartilaginous parts of the meatus to supply the skin of the meatus; the upper sends a twig to the tympanic membrane. The *articular branches* are one or two filaments which enter the posterior part of the temporomandibular joint. The parotid branches convey secretomotor fibres to the gland; preganglionic fibres come from the glossopharyngeal nerve by its tympanic branch, travelling via the lesser petrosal nerve to the otic ganglion, whence postganglionic fibres pass to the auriculotemporal nerve to reach the gland (**8.342**). Vasomotor fibres to the blood vessels of the parotid gland are from the sympathetic root of the otic ganglion (p. 1250).

The *superficial temporal branches* accompany the superficial temporal artery and its terminal branches, supply the skin in the temporal region and connect with the facial and zygomaticotemporal nerves.

The innervation of the temporomandibular joint. The temporomandibular joint capsule, lateral ligament and retro-articular tissue contain mechanoreceptors of three types, and pain fibres forming a plexus with free nerve endings. Axons of the pain fibres are non-, or thinly myelinated (4–5 μm). As in all mammalian joints there are no sensory receptors in the synovial membrane or intra-articular disc. The input from mechanoreceptors provides the major source of proprioceptive sensation underlying the control of mandibular posture and movement. There are three groups of mechanoreceptors (Clark & Wyke 1973). Type I are small globular receptors distributed throughout the joint capsule. Clusters of 3–6 such endings are served by branches from one axon 5–8 μm in diameter. These are very low-threshold, slowly adapting mechanoreceptors. Type II are thickly encapsulated conical receptors occurring singly or in small groups associated with axons 8–12 μm in diameter. These are low-threshold, rapidly adapting mechanoreceptors. Type III are large, thinly encapsulated, high-threshold, slowly adapting mechanoreceptors, found only in the ends of the lateral ligament and responsive to excessive tension therein.

Type I receptors provide the principal source of input that mediates the perception of mandibular position and movement. They strongly influence the actions of the muscles of mastication, both ipsilateral and contralateral, either directly through connections with the trigeminal motor nucleus, or by influencing tone in the intrafusal muscle spindles. Type II receptors fire briefly at the onset of mandibular movement and cause recruitment of motor neurons to reinforce the movement pattern. Type III receptors are only activated when the lateral ligament is overstretched and then result in reflex inhibition of jaw closing muscles, and increased activity of mylohyoid and lateral pterygoid.

Sensory inputs from the oral mucosa and mechanoreceptors in the periodontal ligament also influence the actions of the muscles of mastication, as does limited proprioceptive sensation from the muscles themselves. These are necessary for the extremely delicate control of mandibular posture required for articulation and mastication. The rest-position of the mandible is largely determined by the tone in the musculature controlled by the discharges from the Type I mechanoreceptors. Most joints in the body can move in isolation, the temporomandibular joint cannot, since both joints are inevitably involved in *all* mandibular movements.

Lingual nerve (8.339). This is sensory to the mucosa of the presulcal part of the tongue, the floor of the mouth and the mandibular lingual gingivae. It arises from the posterior trunk of the mandibular nerve and at first runs between the tensor veli palatini and the lateral pterygoid, where it is joined by the chorda tympani branch of the facial nerve and often by a branch of the inferior alveolar nerve. Emerging from the cover of the lateral pterygoid it proceeds down and forwards lying on the surface of medial pterygoid and is progressively carried closer to the medial surface of the mandibular ramus until it is intimately related to the bone a few millimetres below and behind the junction of the vertical and horizontal rami of the mandible. Here it lies anterior to, and slightly deeper than, the inferior alveolar (dental) nerve. It then passes below the mandibular attachment of the superior pharyngeal constrictor and pterygomandibular raphe, closely applied to the periosteum of the medial surface of the mandible, until it lies opposite the posterior root of the third molar tooth, where it is covered only by the gingival mucoperiosteum. At this point it lies usually 2–3 mm below the alveolar crest and 0.6 mm from the bone but in 4.6% of cases it lies **above** the alveolar crest (Kiesselbach & Chamberlain 1984). It then passes medial to the mandibular origin of the mylohyoid muscle which carries it progressively away from the mandible, and separates it from the alveolar bone covering the mesial root of the third molar tooth. It passes downward and forward on the deep surface of the mylohyoid to cross the lingual sulcus, submucosally, where it lies on the deep portion of the submandibular gland and then passes below the submandibular duct which crosses it from medial to lateral. The nerve next curves upward, forward and medially to enter the tongue. It lies first on styloglossus and then the lateral surface of the hyoglossus and genioglossus, before dividing into terminal branches which supply the overlying lingual mucosa (8.339). In addition to receiving the chorda tympani and a branch from the inferior alveolar nerve, the lingual nerve is connected to the submandibular ganglion (p. 1247) by two or three branches (8.339) and, at the anterior margin of the hyoglossus, it forms connecting loops with twigs of the hypoglossal nerve.

Branches of the lingual nerve supply the mucosa of the floor of the mouth, lingual gingivae and the mucosa of the anterior two-thirds (presulcal part) of the tongue, being overlapped slightly posteriorly by lingual fibres of the glossopharyngeal nerve (p. 1250). It also carries postganglionic fibres from the submandibular ganglion (p. 1247) to the sublingual and anterior lingual glands.

The lingual nerve is at great risk during surgical removal of (impacted) lower third molars. After such operations up to 10% of patients may have symptoms, which are usually temporary, of nerve damage. The nerve is also at risk during operations to remove the submandibular salivary gland, during which the duct must be dissected from the lingual nerve.

Inferior alveolar (dental) nerve. This descends medial to the lateral pterygoid and then, at its lower border, passes between the sphenomandibular ligament and the mandibular ramus to enter the mandibular canal via the mandibular foramen. Below the lateral pterygoid it is accompanied by the inferior alveolar artery, a branch of the maxillary, which, with associated veins, also enters the canal. In the canal, the nerve runs downward and forward, generally below the apices of the teeth until below the first and second premolars it divides into terminal *incisive* and *mental* branches. The former continues forward in a bony canal or in a plexiform arrangement, giving off branches to the first premolar, canine and incisor teeth, and the associated labial gingivae.

Variation in the inferior alveolar nerve in man has been described by Nortje et al (1977) and by Khaledpour (1984). In many cases there is a single nerve which lies a few millimetres below the roots of the teeth; in an almost equal number the nerve takes a course much lower in the mandible to lie near the lower border of the bone; only rarely is it plexiform. Branches leave the nerve and interconnect

in a plexus to innervate the teeth and associated gingivae. The nerve may lie on the lingual or buccal side of the mandible, slightly more commonly on the buccal (Miller 1990). Even when the third molar tooth is in a normal position the nerve may be so intimately related to it that it grooves its root. Exceptionally the nerve may be so related to the second molar.

The *mental nerve* passes upward, backward and outward to emerge from the mandible via the mental foramen between and just below the apices of the premolar teeth. Here it may be visible, and is invariably palpable, through stretched oral mucosa. It immediately divides into three branches, two of which pass upward and forward close to the mucosal surface of the lower lip, branching freely and communicating widely with terminal filaments of the mandibular branch of the facial nerve. The third branch passes through the intermingled fibres of depressor anguli oris and platysma muscles to supply the skin of the lower lip and chin.

Just before entering the mandibular canal the inferior alveolar nerve gives off a small *mylohyoid* branch which pierces the sphenomandibular ligament and enters a shallow groove on the medial surface of the mandible following a course roughly parallel to its parent. It passes below the origin of mylohyoid to lie on the superficial surface of the muscle, between it and the anterior belly of digastric, both of which it supplies. It gives a few filaments to supply the skin over the point of the chin (Roberts & Harris 1973).

The **surface marking** of the inferior alveolar nerve from the inside of the oral cavity is important in giving nerve blocks. The mandibular foramen lies midway between the anterior and posterior borders of the ascending ramus of the mandible about 1 cm above the occlusal surfaces of the lower teeth. The ascending ramus diverges from the sagittal plane from front to back; consequently once the needle engages the medial surface at this level it must be diverted laterally. However at a higher level, near the base of the coronoid process, the nerve is sufficiently medial to be accessible to a needle in the sagittal plane. With either technique the buccal and lingual nerves can be blocked en passant.

The inferior dental nerve may be damaged during the extraction of an impacted lower third molar tooth. The roots of such teeth are commonly grooved and, very rarely, perforated by the nerve. It is also frequently damaged in fractures of the posterior tooth-bearing part of the mandible.

Tooth sensation. The teeth appear to be subserved exclusively by pain sensation. The nerves of the dental pulps form plexuses with free nerve endings. The principal controversy surrounding dental sensibility concerns the dentine. Two hypotheses have existed, either that there are free nerve endings in the dentinal tubules or that there are no nerves in the dentine, but that the odontoblasts themselves, through their protoplasmic processes in the tubules, transmit sensation to nerves connected to the odontoblast cell bodies in the pulp. This latter hypothesis can be further subdivided into consideration as to whether the odontoblasts merely transmit hydrodynamically the effects of mechanical, hot or cold damage, or osmotic effects which are detected by the nerves; or whether the odontoblast process has a 'nervous' or 'receptor' function.

The treatment of trigeminal neuralgia

The trigeminal nerve is subject to the common but nevertheless enigmatic condition of paroxysmal trigeminal neuralgia, in which agonizingly severe paroxysmal pains radiate over one, or occasionally two divisions; the ophthalmic division is rarely affected. It is a condition of the fifth decade onward and females are affected more commonly than males. Drug treatment is usually successful but if it fails surgical measures are called for: the multiplicity of surgical treatments suggests that none is satisfactory (for references concerning facial pain, consult Sessle 1987; Aghabei 1992).

Peripheral procedures involving cryoprobe application to the infraorbital or inferior alveolar (dental) nerves may be helpful, as may chemical neurolysis of those branches, using alcohol or phenol. Closed percutaneous procedures under radiological control on the trigeminal ganglion, via the foramen ovale, include the injection of chemicals, the application of a radiofrequency probe, and recently the application of pressure alone, applied by an inflatable balloon.

In 1967 Jannetta resurrected an observation of Dandy (1934) that a direct approach to the sensory root via the posterior fossa may indicate compression of the root by a blood vessel (usually arterial) which can be moved and held aside; this obviously has the advantage of preserving all sensation. In the absence of such apparent compression fractional root section may be performed: section of the outer fibres (portio major) may produce analgesia without anaesthesia, since the fibres responsible for tactile sensation in the medial part (portio minor) are preserved.

ABDUCENT NERVE

The abducent nerve (8.336, 346) supplies the lateral rectus, its fibres arising from a small nucleus in the superior part of the floor of the fourth ventricle, near the midline and beneath the facialis colliculus (8.129, 137, 138, p. 1209). They descend ventrally through the pons, emerging in the sulcus between the caudal border of the pons and the superior end of the pyramid of the medulla oblongata.

The *abducens nucleus* contains large and small multipolar neurons which are intermixed, although the latter are most heavily concentrated in the lateral and ventral aspects of the nucleus. The former are motor neurons of the abducent nerve and the latter are interneurons, the axons of which cross the midline at the level of the nucleus and ascend in the medial longitudinal fasciculus to all three medial rectus subnuclei of the oculomotor nucleus. The total number of neurons in the nucleus is about 6500 (Vijayashankar & Brody 1977). Claims that all abducent neurons react to division (Warwick 1964 and others) are based on differing considerations of which cells should be included as 'abducent'. In a patient with a congenital absence of an abducent nerve, 2110 cells were found in the nucleus. Since the nerve normally contains approximately 4000 axons, there

appears to be a 2:1 split between motor neurons and interneurons (Miller et al 1982).

Connections

The abducent nucleus receives afferent connections from:

- the corticonuclear tract, principally contralateral (some of these fibres are aberrant corticospinal fibres which descend from the midbrain to this level in the medial lemniscus (p. 1015) and interneurons may link them to the nucleus)
- the medial longitudinal fasciculus, connecting it to oculomotor and trochlear nuclei and to the vestibular nuclei
- the tectobulbar tract, from the deep layers of the superior colliculus (see also p. 1072)
- the paramedian pontine reticular formation lying rostral and caudal to the nucleus (see below Neural control of conjugate gaze)
- the nucleus prepositus hypoglossi (see section on conjugate gaze)
- the contralateral medullary reticular formation.

Course

Axons projecting to the ipsilateral lateral rectus muscle leave the medial aspect of the nucleus and course ventrally, laterally and caudally, passing through the pontine tegmentum, lateral to the corticospinal tract, to emerge at the caudal border of the pons. After leaving the brainstem, the abducent nerve ascends anterolaterally through the cisterna pontis along the clivus, usually dorsal to the anterior inferior cerebellar artery. It pierces the dura mater lateral to the dorsum sellae and bends sharply forwards over the superior border of the petrous temporal bone, near its apex medial to the trigeminal nerve. Here it enters a fibro-osseous canal (Dorello's canal) formed by the apex of the petrous temporal bone and the petrosphenoidal ligament. The latter is a fibrous band connecting the lateral margin of the dorsum sellae to the upper border of the petrous temporal bone near its medial end. The nerve next traverses the cavernous sinus, lying lateral to and running parallel with the internal carotid artery to which it is loosely attached (10.164, 165). The nerve lies in the body of the sinus in contradistinction to the oculomotor and trochlear nerves which lie in the lateral wall of the sinus. It enters the orbital cavity via the medial end of the superior orbital fissure within the annulus of Zinn, between the superior and inferior divisions of the oculomotor nerve and inferolateral to the nasociliary nerve, finally sinking into the ocular surface of the lateral rectus (8.346). The nerve may be divided into two or more trunks in any part of its intracranial course in up to 58% of patients.

In the cavernous sinus the nerve is joined by one or two branches

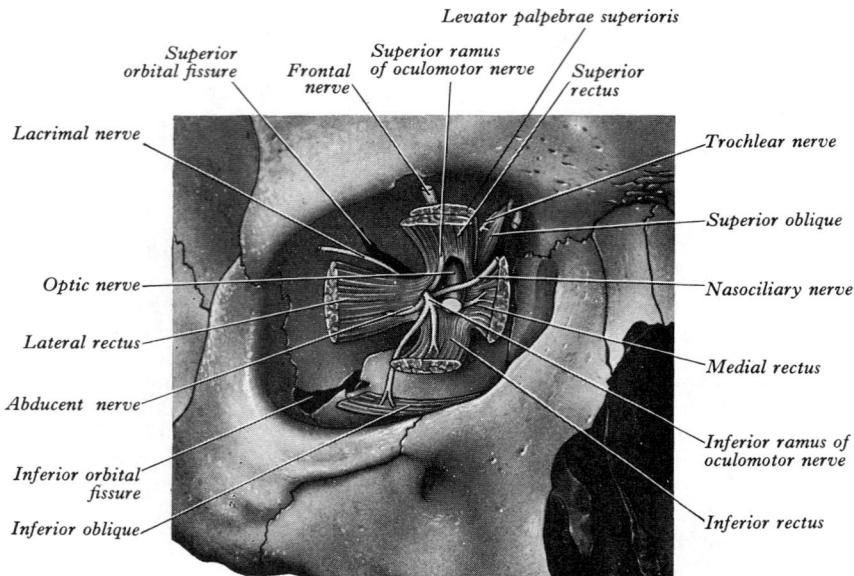

Levator palpebrae superioris
Superior ramus
of oculomotor nerve
Superior
orbital fissure
Frontal
nerve
Superior
rectus
Lacrimal nerve
Trochlear nerve
Superior oblique
Optic nerve
Nasociliary nerve
Lateral rectus
Medial rectus
Abducent nerve
Inferior ramus of
oculomotor nerve
Inferior orbital
fissure
Inferior rectus
Inferior oblique

8.346 A dissection of the right orbit, viewed from in front, to show the origins of the orbital muscles and the relative positions of the nerves of the orbit.

from the internal carotid sympathetic plexus. A branch leaves the abducent nerve a few millimetres distal to this sympathetic communication to join the ophthalmic division of the trigeminal nerve. This would accord with the passage of sympathetic nerve fibres to the eye via the long ciliary branches of the nasociliary nerve.

Lesions of the abducent nerve

The long intracranial course of the abducent nerve and its sharp bend over the petrous temporal bone make the nerve peculiarly liable to injury through a variety of aetiologies including: microvascular

infarction, vascular and tumoral compression, direct trauma and infection. Raised intracranial pressure may indirectly cause a sixth nerve palsy through traction on the nerve as the brainstem is pushed caudally. A unilateral abducent nerve palsy produced in this manner can be caused by a lesion on either side of the midline and has therefore been called a 'false localizing' sign.

The clinical features of an abducent nerve palsy are diplopia with horizontal separation of the images and a convergent squint due to failure of abduction of the eye.

Neural control of conjugate gaze

The development of a high acuity region in the retina, the fovea, and the presence of forward looking eyes, has demanded highly accurate neural control systems to keep the two eyes yoked together so that the image of the object of interest is simultaneously held on both foveae despite movement of the object or the observer. A number of separate neural systems are involved: first, to shift gaze to the object of interest using rapid movements, called *saccades*; and second, those that stabilize the image on the fovea either during movement of the object of interest, the *smooth pursuit system*, and/or during movement

of the head or body, the *vestibulo-ocular and optokinetic systems*. Although the anatomical substrates for these systems differ, they have a final common pathway which lies mainly in the pons and midbrain for horizontal and vertical gaze movements respectively (**8.347**).

Neuroanatomical substrates for gaze movements

The final common pathway for all types of horizontal gaze movements is the abducent nucleus. This contains both motor neurons innervating the ipsilateral lateral rectus muscle, and internuclear

neurons which project to the contralateral medial rectus subnucleus of the oculomotor nucleus via the medial longitudinal fasciculus (MLF). A lesion of the abducent nucleus leads to a total ipsilateral loss of horizontal conjugate gaze. A lesion of an MLF would produce slowed or absent adduction of the ipsilateral eye, usually associated with jerky movements, nystagmus, of the abducting eye, a syndrome called an internuclear ophthalmoplegia.

The gaze motor command is prepared in specialized areas of the reticular formation of the brainstem, which receive a variety of supranuclear inputs from different areas. The main premotor region for horizontal gaze is the *paramedian pontine reticular formation (PPRF)*, which

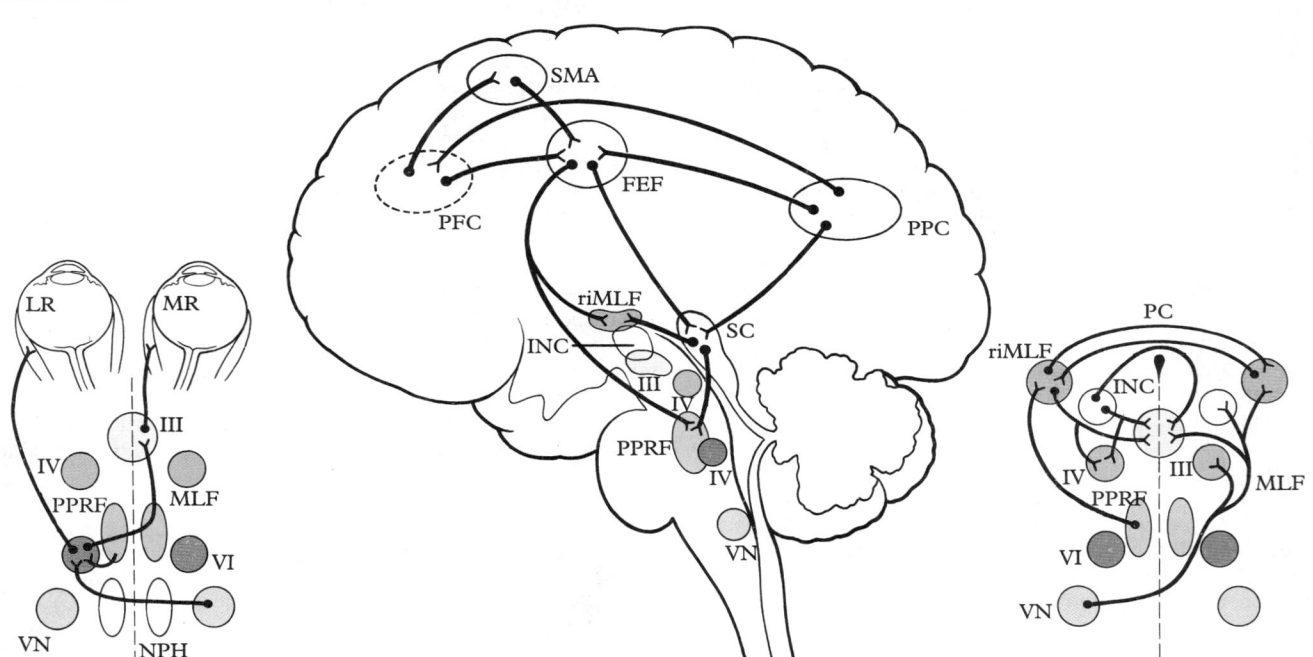

8.347 Summary of eye movement control. The centre figure shows the supranuclear connections from the frontal eye fields (FEF) and the parieto-occipital-temporal junction region (POT) to the superior colliculus (SC) rostral interstitial nucleus of the medial longitudinal fasciculus (riMLF) and the paramedian pontine reticular formation (PPRF). The FEF and SC are involved in the production of saccades, while the POT is thought to be important in the production of pursuit. The schematic drawing on the left shows the brainstem pathways for horizontal gaze. Axons from the cell bodies located in the PPRF travel to the ipsilateral lateral rectus muscle (LR) and with abducens

internuclear neurons whose axons cross the midline and travel in the medial longitudinal fasciculus (MLF) to the portion(s) of the oculomotor nucleus (III) concerned with the medial rectus (MR) function (in the contralateral eye). The schematic drawing on the right shows the brainstem pathways for vertical gaze. Important structures include the riMLF, PPRF, the interstitial nucleus of Cajal (INC), and the posterior commissure (PC). Note that axons from cell bodies located in the vestibular nuclei (VN) travel directly to the abducens nuclei and, mostly via the MLF, to the oculomotor nuclei. IV = trochlear nucleus.

is located on each side of the midline in the central paramedian part of the tegmentum, extending from the pontomedullary junction to the pontopeduncular junction. The equivalent region for vertical gaze is the *rostral interstitial nucleus* of the medial longitudinal fasciculus (riMLF), located at the level of the upper pole 'of the red nucleus. Each PPRF contains excitatory burst neurons which discharge at high frequencies just prior to and during ipsilateral saccades, and provide the eye velocity commands, known as the pulse. Pause neurons, which are located in a midline caudal pontine nucleus called the *nucleus raphe interpositus*, discharge tonically except just before and during saccades. They appear to exert an inhibitory influence on the burst neurons preventing extraneous saccades occurring during fixation.

The vestibular nuclei and the perihypoglossal complex (especially the nucleus prepositus hypoglossi) project directly to the abducent nuclei. These projections probably carry both smooth pursuit signals, via the cerebellum, and vestibular signals. In addition these nuclei, via reciprocal innervation with the PPRF, contain integrator neurons which control the step change in innervation required to maintain the eccentric position of the eye against the viscoelastic forces in the orbit, tending to move the eyeball back to the looking straight ahead position (the primary position), after a saccade. Abducent motor neurons would, therefore, show a pulsestep pattern of neural discharge during, for example, an ipsilateral horizontal saccade to move the eye rapidly to its desired position (pulse) and then maintain it in its new position (step).

The final common pathway of vertical gaze movements is formed by the oculomotor and trochlear nuclei. The premotor riMLF contains neurons that discharge in relation to up-and-down vertical saccadic movements. The riMLF projects through the posterior commissure to its equivalent on the other side of the mesencephalon, as well as directly to the oculomotor nucleus. Lesions within the posterior commissure will, therefore, give rise to a disturbance in vertical gaze, especially up-gaze. Lesions placed more ventrally in the region of the riMLF again give rise to vertical gaze disorders which may be mixed up-and-down or mainly down-gaze. Slightly caudal to the riMLF, and directly connected to it, lies the *interstitial nucleus of Cajal*. This nucleus contains neurons which appear to be involved in vertical gaze holding and vertical pursuit.

Generation of saccades

The cerebral hemispheres are extremely important for the programming and coordination of both saccadic and pursuit conjugate eye movements. Since different areas are involved in these two types of eye movements they will be dealt with separately, always realizing that for fully effective ocular motor control, coordination between these subtypes of eye movement is essential.

There appear to be four main cortical areas in the cerebral hemispheres involved in the generation of saccades. In the frontal lobe in man there is the frontal eye field (FEF) which lies laterally at the caudal end of the second frontal gyrus, in the premotor cortex (Brodmann area 8), and the supplementary eye field (SEF) which lies mesially at the anterior region of the supplementary motor area in the first frontal gyrus (Brodmann area 6). The third area is in the dorsolateral prefrontal cortex (DLPFC), which lies anterior to the FEF in the second frontal gyrus (Brodmann area 46). Finally, a posterior eye field (PEF) lies in the parietal lobe, possibly in the superior part of the angular gyrus (Brodmann area 39), and the adjacent lateral intraparietal sulcus. Studies in monkeys reveal that these areas are all interconnected with each other, and they all appear to send projections to the superior colliculus (SC) and the premotor areas in the brainstem controlling saccades.

It appears that there are two parallel pathways involved in the cortical generation of saccades. An anterior system originating in the FEF projecting both directly, and via the SC, to the brainstem saccadic generators. This pathway also passes indirectly via the basal ganglia to the SC. The second or posterior pathway originates in the PEF passing to the brainstem saccadic generators via the SC. Only after bilateral lesions to both the FEF and SC in monkeys is there a failure to trigger saccades.

Although the precise functions of these various cortical areas in saccade generation have not been determined, a number of general statements can be made. The FEF is involved in triggering volitional saccades which, for example, may be predictive (in anticipation of the appearance of a target), memory-guided (to a previously seen target), or scanning (searching for a particular target of interest). The PEF could be involved in triggering reflexive saccades to the sudden appearance of novel visual or auditory stimuli, and appears to be involved in visuo-spatial integration. The DLPFC may be responsible for maintaining a spatial map of the environment in short-term memory providing spatial information for memory-guided saccades and other volitional saccades. There is also evidence that it contains circuits responsible for inhibiting unwanted misdirected reflexive saccades. The SEF appears to be involved in the generation of sequences of saccades.

A subsidiary neural circuit related to saccade generation is from the frontal lobe to the superior colliculus via the basal ganglia. Projections from the frontal cortex pass to the substantia nigra, pars reticularis (SNpr), via a relay in the caudate nucleus. An inhibitory pathway from the SNpr projects directly to the SC. This appears to be a gating circuit related to volitional saccades, especially of the memory-guided type.

Smooth pursuit system

To maintain foveation of a moving target the smooth pursuit system has developed relatively independently of the saccadic oculomotor system, although there have to be interconnections between the two. It is first necessary to identify and code the velocity and direction of a moving target. This is carried out in the extrastriate visual area known as the middle temporal visual area (MT) (also called visual area V5), which contains neurons sensitive to visual target motion. In man, this lies immediately posterior to the ascending limb of the inferior temporal sulcus at the occipitotemporal border (Brodmann area 19/37 junction). Area MT sends this motion signal to the medial superior temporal visual area (MST), which in monkeys is located on the anterior bank of the superior temporal sulcus, but in man is considered to lie superior and a little anterior to area MT within the inferior parietal lobe. Damage to this area results in an impairment of smooth pursuit of targets moving towards the damaged hemisphere. Evidence for a possible contribution of the FEF to the generation of smooth pursuit has recently been obtained in the monkey.

Both area MST and the FEF send direct projections to a group of nuclei which lie in the basis pontis of the pons. In the monkey, the dorsolateral and lateral groups of pontine nuclei receive direct cortical inputs related to smooth pursuit. Lesions of similarly located nuclei in man result in abnormal pursuit. These nuclei transfer the pursuit signal bilaterally to the posterior vermis, contralateral flocculus and fastigial nuclei of the cerebellum. Finally, the pursuit signal passes from the cerebellum to the brainstem, specifically the medial vestibular nucleus and nucleus prepositus hypoglossi, and thence to the PPRF and possibly directly to the ocular motor nuclei. This circuitry therefore involves a double decussation, firstly at the level of the midpons (pontocerebellar neuron) and secondly in the lower pons (vestibulo-abducent neuron).

Vestibular-ocular reflex

The final conjugate gaze type to consider is that of the vestibular-ocular reflex, the function of which is to maintain clear vision during movement of the head. It results in a compensatory conjugate eye movement which is equal but opposite to the movement of the head. This is essentially a three-neuron arc consisting of the primary vestibular neuron which projects to the vestibular nuclei; the secondary neuron which projects from these nuclei directly to the abducent nucleus; and the tertiary neuron which is the abducent motor neuron itself. Although this is the primary excitatory reflex arc there are other connections with polysynaptic circuits as well as inhibitory connections.

FACIAL NERVE

The facial nerve (8.348–351) has a motor and a sensory root. The sensory root, the *nervus intermedius* (8.349), gains its name from its position between the facial and vestibulocochlear nerves at the cerebellopontine angle. The two roots arise from the pons, lateral to the recess between the inferior olive and inferior cerebellar peduncle, and lie superior and slightly anterior to the vestibulocochlear nerves. The nervus intermedius usually cleaves at first to the vestibulocochlear rather than the facial nerve, passing to the latter as it approaches the internal acoustic meatus, often as more than one filament. In approximately one-fifth of 73 dissections it was not a separate nerve until the meatus was reached, a point of surgical importance (Rhoton et al 1968). These nerves have no epineurium and are covered by pia mater and surrounded by cerebrospinal fluid (CSF).

The *motor root* supplies: the muscles of the face, scalp and auricle, the buccinator, platysma, stapedius, stylohyoid, and the posterior belly of the digastric.

The *sensory root* conveys gustatory fibres from the presulcal area (anterior two-thirds) of the tongue via the chorda tympani and, via the palatine and greater petrosal nerves, taste fibres from the soft palate; it also carries the preganglionic parasympathetic (secretomotor) innervation of the submandibular and sublingual salivary glands, lacrimal gland and glands of the nasal and palatine mucosa.

Motor nucleus

The nucleus from which most facial motor fibres are derived lies deep in the reticular formation of the caudal part of the pons (p. 1027), posterior to the dorsal trapezoid nucleus (8.129, 137) and ventromedial to the spinal tract nucleus of the trigeminal nerve. It represents the branchial efferent column but lies deeper in the pons than might be expected and its efferent fibres have a most unusual course (8.138). Both these features have been explained by invoking neurobiotaxis (p. 242). The nucleus receives fibres from both corticonuclear tracts in the lower pons and is reputedly supplied by aberrant pyramidal fibres which descend in the medial lemniscus. Contralateral corticonuclear fibres end in the part of the nucleus innervating the muscles of the lower part of the face (p. 1026) while the corticonuclear projection to neurons for muscles around the eyes and forehead is bilateral. Some facial efferent fibres proceed from the *superior salivatory nucleus* (see p. 1026), said to be in the reticular formation, dorsolateral to the caudal end of the motor nucleus. Neurons of the facial nucleus have been described as clustered along the intrapontine part of the nerve distal to its loop round the abducent nucleus (Crosby & Dejonge 1963); it belongs to the general visceral efferent column, sending its fibres to the sensory root, by which they ultimately, via the chorda tympani, reach the submandibular and sublingual salivary glands and perhaps also the parotid (p. 1297). Other preganglionic fibres in the sensory root reach the pterygopalatine ganglion in the greater petrosal nerve and the nerve of the pterygoid canal (see below). From this double origin, the *motor root* passes dorsomedially to the caudal end of the abducent nucleus and ascends superficial to it and deep to the facial colliculus. At the upper limit of the abducent nucleus the nerve swerves into a caudoventral course to its emergence between the olive and the inferior cerebellar peduncle (8.124, 138) at the cerebellopontine angle.

The facial motor nucleus is a complex consisting of lateral, intermediate and medial subnuclei (Marinesco 1899; Papex 1927). A further division of the medial nucleus into ventral, dorsal and intermediate groups has been described. (For details consult Vraa-Jensen 1942.) These subsidiary groups of neurons are arranged in columns, like those in the spinal cord or oculomotor nucleus. There is general agreement that they innervate individual muscles or correspond to branches of the nerve, but observers disagree about

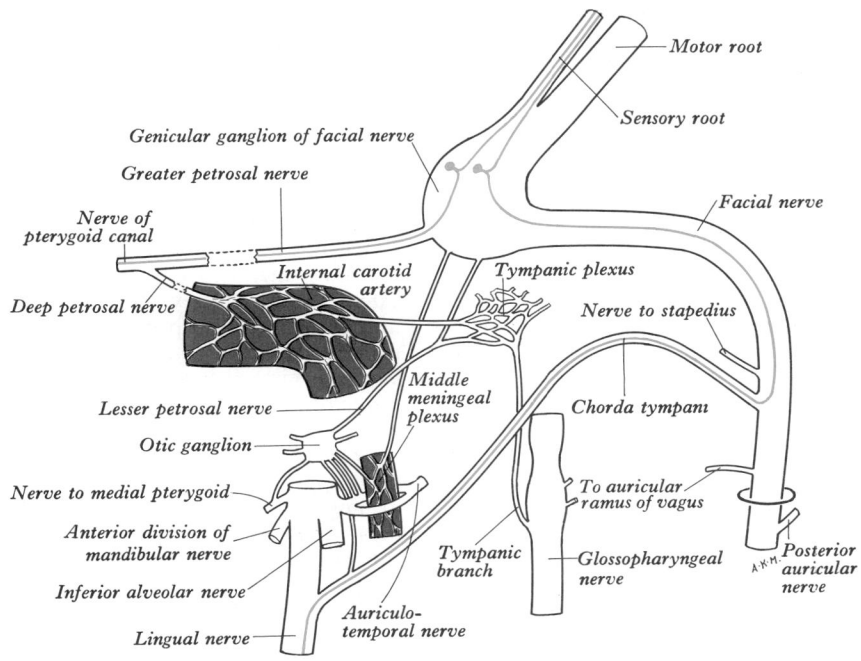

8.348   A plan of the intrapetrous section of the facial nerve, its branches and communications. The course of the taste fibres from the mucous membrane of the palate and from the anterior, oral or presulcal part of the tongue is represented by the blue lines.

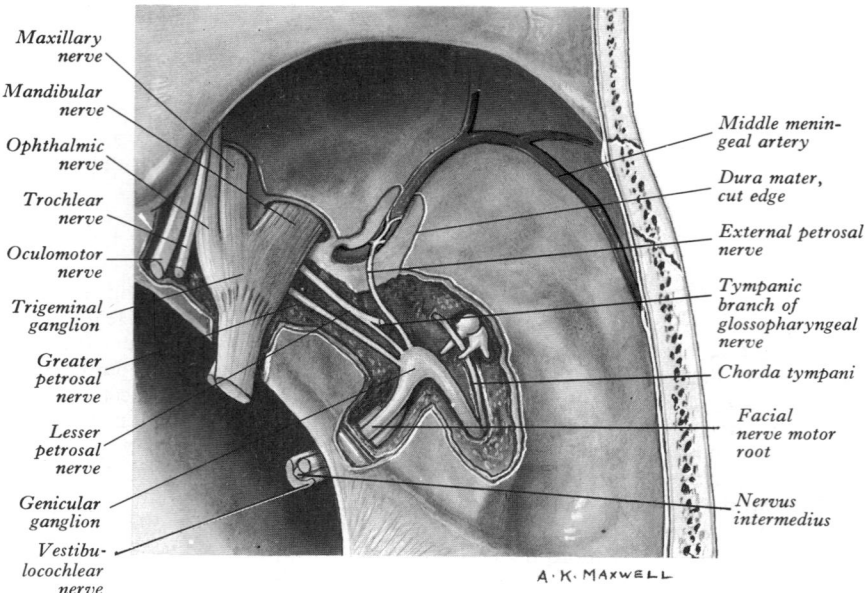

Labels on figure:
Maxillary nerve
Mandibular nerve
Ophthalmic nerve
Trochlear nerve
Oculomotor nerve
Trigeminal ganglion
Greater petrosal nerve
Lesser petrosal nerve
Genicular ganglion
Vestibulocochlear nerve

Middle meningeal artery
Dura mater, cut edge
External petrosal nerve
Tympanic branch of glossopharyngeal nerve
Chorda tympani
Facial nerve motor root
Nervus intermedius

A·K·MAXWELL

8.349 A dissection of the right middle cranial fossa, showing the course and some of the connections of the facial nerve within the temporal bone.

details. Retrograde changes following division of different branches of the nerve in dogs (Yagita 1910; Vraa-Jensen 1942) and cats (Papex 1927; Courville 1966) have provided most of the evidence; the effects on the motor terminals of selective nuclear lesions have also been studied in cats. The lateral subnucleus is said to innervate the buccal musculature, the intermediate sends axons into the temporal, orbital and zygomatic facial branches and the medial group into the posterior auricular and cervical rami and probably the stapedial nerve. Nuclear lesions have produced a roughly similar but more detailed schema (Szentágothai 1948).

Sensory nucleus

This is the rostral end of the *nucleus solitarius* in the medulla oblongata (p. 1018). It receives gustatory and possibly other afferents from the sensory root and sends fibres to the contralateral ventral lateral thalamic nuclei. As they ascend in the midbrain and subthalamic regions, these fibres pass near the midline (Harris 1952). From the thalamus they are relayed to the inferior part of the postcentral gyrus. For other connections, see p. 1311.

The *sensory root* (*nervus intermedius*) contains the centripetal processes of unipolar neurons in the genicular ganglion, which leave the trunk of the facial nerve in the internal acoustic meatus in one or more slender bundles either between the motor root and the vestibulocochlear nerve or adherent to the latter, and enter the brainstem at the caudal border of the pons. The peripheral branches of the ganglion cells are mainly taste fibres travelling in the chorda tympani and greater petrosal nerve and a few somatic afferent fibres from the auricular concha (p. 1368). The sensory root also contains **efferent** preganglionic parasympathetic fibres for the submandibular and sublingual salivary glands, lacrimal gland, and pharyngeal, nasal and palatine glands.

Course. From their emergence from the brain, the two roots pass anterolaterally with the vestibulocochlear nerve to the internal acoustic meatus; here the motor root is in an anterosuperior groove on the vestibulocochlear nerve, with the sensory root between them. The facial nerve is in close and variable contact with the anterior inferior cerebellar artery (Brunsteins & Ferreri 1990) which usually lies in a ventral position between the nerves and the pontine surface. In 12.3% of 1327 temporal bones the anterior inferior cerebellar artery looped within the internal auditory canal (Reisser & Schuknecht 1991). Within the internal auditory canal the facial nerve appears whiter than the cochlear nerve. The facial nerve is connected to the superior vestibular nerve by the fibres of Rasmussen whose function is unknown. While the cochlear and vestibular nerves rotate

90° from the brainstem (Silverstein et al 1986) to the inner ear, the facial nerve remains anterior in its course. At the lateral fundus of the meatus it pierces the arachnoid and dura mater to enter the facial canal superior to the transverse crest and separated from the superior vestibular nerve by a vertical bar of bone. In its intratemporal course its bony canal is narrowest at the meatal foramen. It is accompanied by the labyrinthine branch of the anterior inferior cerebellar artery although this can occasionally originate from the basilar artery. The labyrinthine segment of the nerve runs across the axis of the petrous pyramid to the geniculum, here the nerve presents a reddish asymmetrical swelling, the *genicular ganglion* (**8.348**), which lies just medial to the tip of the cochleariform process. It then turns 130° and forms the tympanic or horizontal segment which is 10–12 mm long and passes lateral to the vestibule, above the oval window, and below the lateral semicircular canal. It rarely lies lateral to the horizontal semicircular canal. In the medial wall of the middle ear it slopes down from anterior to posterior forming an angle of approximately 10° with the lateral semicircular canal. It lies medial to the malleus head anteriorly, the incudo-malleolar joint, incus and attic posteriorly. The pyramidal part connects the horizontal and mastoid segments at an angle between 95–125° and here it gives off the nerve to the stapedius muscle. It then descends to the stylomastoid foramen and gives off the chorda tympani nerve approximately 5 mm proximal to it although the exact position varies and in 2% lies distal to the foramen (Nager & Proctor 1982). Emerging from the stylomastoid foramen, the nerve runs forwards in the parotid gland (p. 1691), lateral to the styloid process, retromandibular vein and external carotid artery and divides behind the neck of the mandible into branches which pierce the anteromedial surface of the parotid gland and diverge under cover of it. They form a network (*parotid plexus*) which distributes to the facial musculature. At the stylomastoid foramen the nerve is about 2 cm deep to the middle of the anterior border of the mastoid processes.

Arterial supply and venous drainage. The facial nerve is supplied in its canal by the superficial petrosal branch of the middle meningeal artery which enters the hiatus for the greater petrosal nerve and passes to the facial canal at the geniculum. It is also supplied by the stylomastoid branch of the posterior auricular or occipital arteries, extracranially by branches from the stylomastoid, posterior auricular, occipital, superficial temporal, transverse facial, and tympanic branch of the ascending pharyngeal arteries, which are linked longitudinally by free anastomoses within the epineurium of the nerve. Venous drainage is into the venae comitantes of the superficial petrosal and stylomastoid arteries (Blunt 1954).

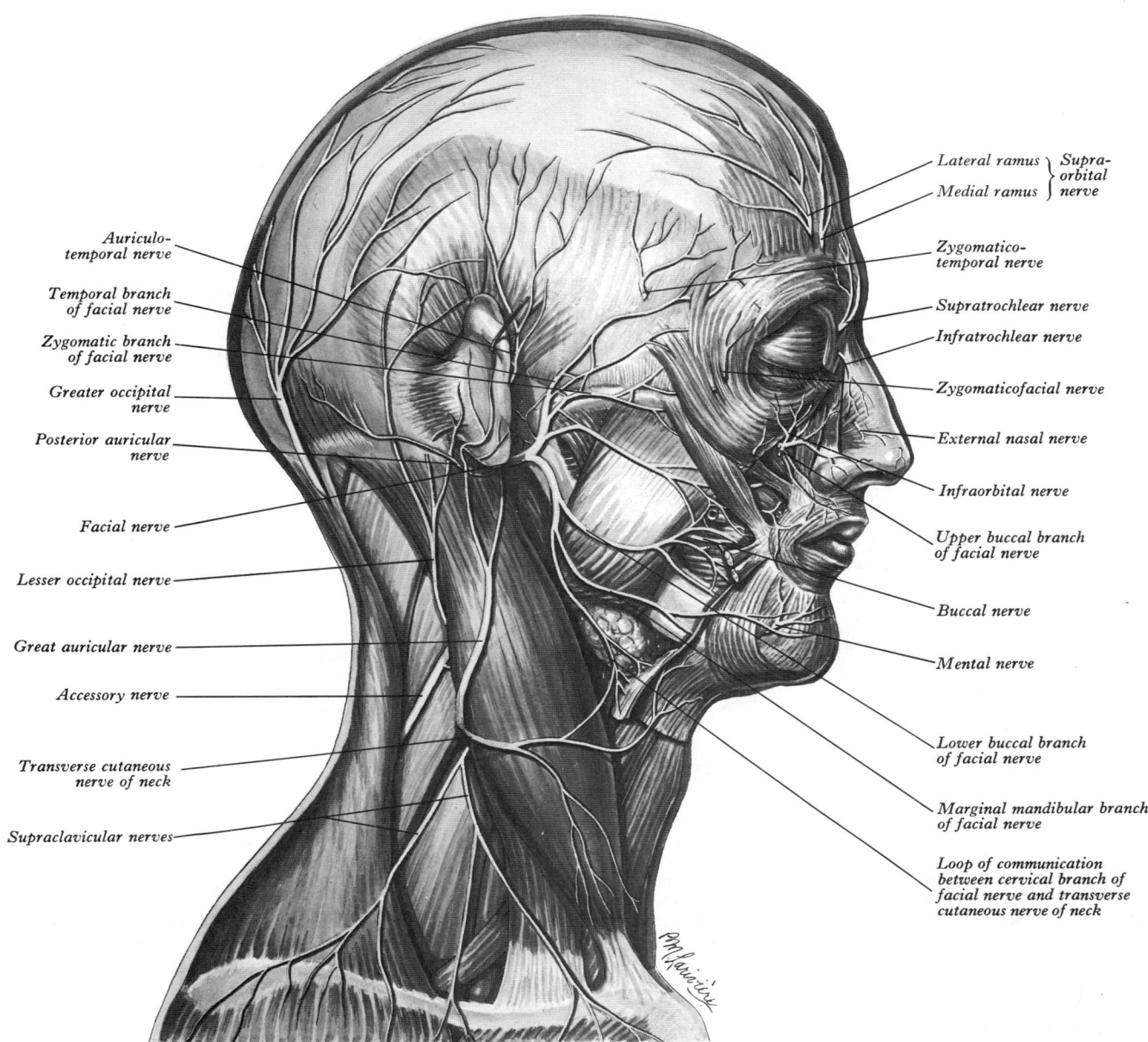

8.350 The nerves of the right side of the scalp, face and neck. Compare with **8.351**.

Communicating branches

Intracranial	Vestibulocochlear
Genicular ganglion	Pterygopalatine ganglion via the greater petrosal nerve
	Otic ganglion via the lesser petrosal nerve
	Middle meningeal sympathetic plexus
Facial canal	Auricular branch of vagus
At exit from stylomastoid foramen	To glossopharyngeal, vagus, great auricular and auriculotemporal nerves
Postauricular	To the lesser occipital nerve
Facial	With the trigeminal nerve
Cervical	With the transverse cervical nerve

In the internal acoustic meatus minute filaments connect the facial nerve with the vestibulocochlear nerve.

Greater petrosal nerve. This starts from the genicular ganglion and contains mainly taste fibres from the palatal mucosa and also preganglionic parasympathetic fibres travelling to the pterygopalatine ganglion and said to be relayed through the zygomatic and lacrimal nerves to the lacrimal gland (p. 1237) and through the nasal and palatine nerves to the nasal and palatine mucosal glands (**8.342**). It receives a ramus from the tympanic plexus, traverses the hiatus on the anterior surface of the petrous temporal bone and enters a groove on it, passing under the trigeminal ganglion to the foramen lacerum; here it is joined by the *deep petrosal nerve* (**8.348**) from the internal carotid sympathetic plexus to become the Vidian nerve or *nerve of the pterygoid canal* which traverses the pterygoid canal to end in the pterygopalatine ganglion. Gustatory fibres pass without interruption through or over the pterygopalatine ganglion into its palatine branches.

From the facial nerve near the genicular ganglion, the ganglion itself or the root of the greater petrosal nerve (Vidić & Young 1967),

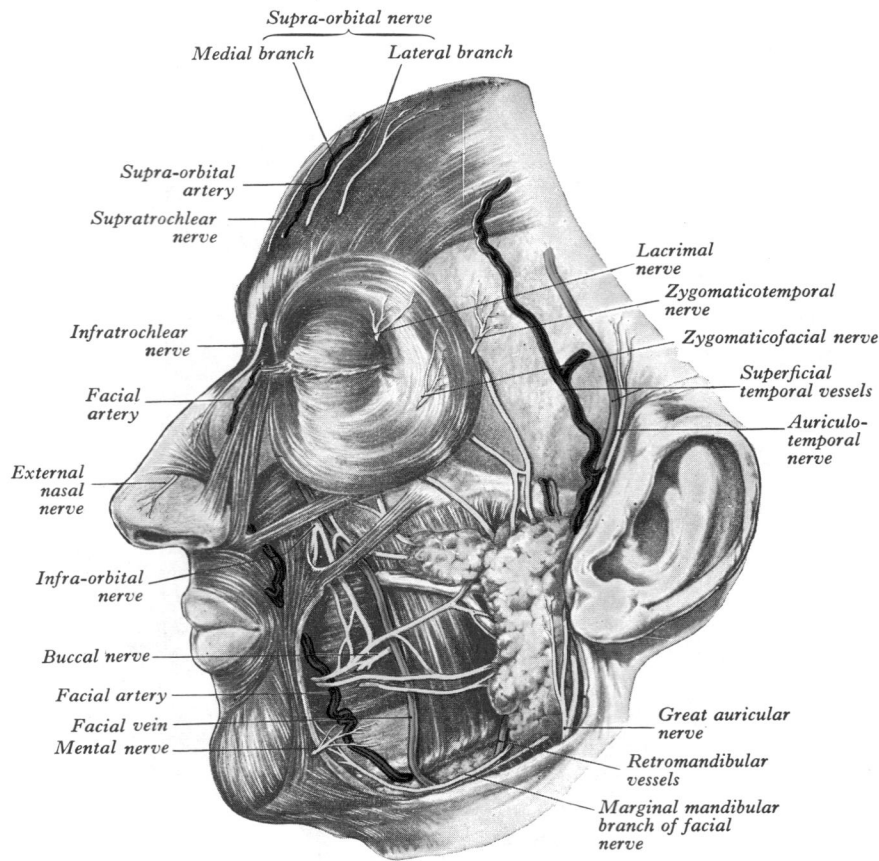

8.351   The terminal branches of the left trigeminal and facial nerves in the face.

a branch runs to the lesser petrosal nerve (**8.**348) by which it reaches the otic ganglion. However, fibres in this small communication are not facial but come from the vagal auricular branch. In 24 out of 25 human dissections the fibres approached the facial nerve through the stapedius, travelling in its fascial sheath almost to the genicular ganglion, before departing to join the lesser superficial petrosal nerve (Vidić 1968).

The middle meningeal sympathetic plexus is joined to the genicular ganglion by an inconstant *external petrosal nerve*.

Before leaving the stylomastoid foramen the facial nerve receives another branch from the vagal auricular nerve. After leaving the foramen, it receives a twig from the glossopharyngeal, communicating with the great auricular and auriculotemporal nerves in the parotid gland, with the lesser occipital nerve behind the ear, with terminal trigeminal branches on the face and with the transverse cutaneous cervical nerve in the neck.

Branches of distribution (8.348, 350)

In the facial canal	Nerve to stapedius
	Chorda tympani
At exit from stylomastoid foramen	Posterior auricular
	Digastric, posterior belly
	Stylohyoid
On the face	Temporal
	Zygomatic
	Buccal
	Marginal mandibular
	Cervical

Nerve to the stapedius. This arises behind the pyramidal eminence of the posterior wall of the tympanic cavity, passing forwards through a small canal to reach the muscle (p. 1375).

Chorda tympani (**8.**342). This leaves the facial nerve about 5 mm above the stylomastoid foramen, ascending forwards in a canal to perforate the posterior wall of the tympanic cavity via its posterior canaliculus near the posterior border of the medial aspect of the tympanic membrane, where it crosses over the incus and deep to the upper end of the handle of the malleus. Passing forwards it re-enters the bone via its anterior canaliculus at the medial end of the petrotympanic fissure. It now descends ventrally on the medial surface of the sphenoid spine (which it sometimes grooves) and passes deep to the lateral pterygoid. Here the nerve is posterolateral to the tensor veli palatini and is crossed medially by the middle meningeal artery, the roots of the auriculotemporal nerve and by the inferior alveolar nerve. It joins the posterior aspect of the lingual nerve at an acute angle. It contains efferent preganglionic parasympathetic (secretomotor) fibres which enter the submandibular ganglion, from which postganglionic fibres are relayed to the submandibular and sublingual glands. However, most of its fibres are afferent from the mucosa of the anterior two-thirds of the tongue, except the vallate papillae, and it constitutes the nerve of taste for this lingual region. Before uniting with the lingual nerve the chorda tympani is joined by a small branch from the otic ganglion.

Posterior auricular nerve. This arises near the stylomastoid foramen, ascends in front of the mastoid process to be joined by a filament from the auricular branch of the vagus, and communicates with posterior branches of the great auricular and lesser occipital nerves. As it ascends between the external acoustic meatus and mastoid process it divides into auricular and occipital branches. The *auricular branch* supplies the auricularis posterior and the intrinsic muscles on the cranial aspect of the auricle which are rudimentary in 10% of the population; the larger *occipital branch* passes back along the superior nuchal line to supply the occipital belly of occipitofrontalis.

The *digastric branch* also starts near the stylomastoid foramen, dividing into several filaments which supply the posterior belly of the digastric, one joining the glossopharyngeal nerve.

The *stylohyoid branch*, long and slender, frequently arises with the digastric branch; it enters the middle part of the stylohyoid muscle.

The *frontal branch* leaves the parotid 1.5 cm in front of the tragus then traverses an area 1 cm in width at the midpoint between the radix helicis and the lateral canthus.

The *temporal branches* cross the zygomatic arch to the temple, supplying intrinsic muscles on the lateral surface of the auricle, the anterior and superior auricular muscles, and join with the zygomaticotemporal branch of the maxillary nerve and the auriculotemporal branch of the mandibular nerve. The more anterior branches supply the frontal belly of the occipitofrontalis, orbicularis oculi and corrugator and join the supraorbital and lacrimal branches of the ophthalmic nerve.

Zygomatic branches cross the zygomatic bone to the lateral canthus, supplying the orbicularis oculi and joining filaments of the lacrimal nerve and zygomaticofacial branch of the maxillary nerve.

Buccal branches pass horizontally to a distribution below the orbit and around the mouth. *Superficial branches* run deep to subcutaneous fat and the superficial muscular and aponeurotic system over the superficial muscles which they supply; some pass to the procerus, joining with the infratrochlear and external nasal nerves. *Upper deep branches* pass under the zygomaticus major and levator labii superioris, supplying them and forming an *infraorbital plexus* with the superior labial branches of the infraorbital nerve; they also supply the levator anguli oris, zygomaticus minor, levator labii superioris alaeque nasi and the small nasal muscles. These branches are sometimes described as lower zygomatic branches. *Lower deep branches* supply the buccinator and orbicularis oris, joining filaments of the buccal branch of the mandibular nerve.

The *marginal mandibular branch* runs forwards below the angle of the mandible under the platysma, at first superficial to the upper part of the digastric triangle, then turning up and forwards across the body of the mandible to pass under the depressor anguli oris (**8.351**). It supplies the risorius and the muscles of the lower lip and chin, joining the mental nerve (p. 1239).

The *cervical branch* issues from the lower part of the parotid gland and runs antero-inferiorly under the platysma to the front of the neck, supplying the platysma and communicating with the transverse cutaneous cervical nerve.

The *cutaneous fibres* of the facial nerve accompany the auricular branch of the vagus and probably innervate the skin on both auricular aspects, in the conchal depression and over its eminence; however, details of this are uncertain, as is a supply to the external acoustic meatus and tympanic membrane.

Submandibular ganglion

This is a small, fusiform body which lies on the upper part of the hyoglossus; there are further ganglion cells in the hilum of the submandibular gland. Like the ciliary, pterygopalatine and otic ganglia, the submandibular is a peripheral parasympathetic ganglion. It is superior to the deep part of the submandibular gland and inferior to the lingual nerve, suspended from the latter by anterior and posterior filaments (**8.339**). Though related to the lingual nerve, the ganglion is connected functionally with the facial nerve and chorda tympani. Its motor, parasympathetic root is the posterior filament connecting it to the lingual nerve; it conveys preganglionic fibres from the superior salivatory nucleus travelling in the facial, chorda tympani and lingual nerves to the ganglion, which they synapse. The postganglionic fibres are secretomotor to the submandibular and sublingual salivary glands. (Some fibres may also reach the parotid gland, see p. 1297.) The sympathetic root is derived from the plexus on the facial artery; it consists of postganglionic fibres from the superior cervical ganglion, which traverse the submandibular ganglion without synapsing. They are vasomotor to the blood vessels of the submandibular and sublingual glands. Five or six branches from the ganglion supply the submandibular gland and its duct; other fibres pass through the anterior filament connecting the gland to the lingual nerve and are carried to the sublingual and anterior lingual glands.

Surgical anatomy of the facial nerve

In parotid surgery the facial nerve is reliably found between the mastoid process and the bony part of the external auditory meatus where it lies approximately 4 mm deep to the junction of the bony and cartilaginous segments of the external auditory meatus, above the upper border of the posterior belly of the digastric muscle. It can then be traced forwards following all its branches. Using this method the likelihood of inadvertent damage to the nerve is minimized (Shaheen 1984). The following anatomical points are helpful when undertaking facial plastic procedures. In front of the parotid the facial nerve lies deep to subcutaneous fat and the superficial muscular and aponeurotic system. There is a fascial plane which extends from the frontalis muscle down to the platysma and forwards to the orbicularis oculi. It also covers the parotid but is separate from the parotid fascia (Bernstein 1986). The marginal mandibular branch can descend up to 2 cm below the inferior border of the mandible, particularly when the head is rotated to the other side as in submandibular gland excision; this is the most common site of iatrogenic damage to the nerve. The frontal branch lies under the superficial temporal fascia, an extension of the superficial muscular and aponeurotic system, and it lies superficial as it crosses the zygomatic arch. Dissection in this area is best undertaken on the deep temporal fascia (Stuzin et al 1989) and within the temporal fat pad until the zygomatic arch is reached. Surface landmarks have been described for this branch of the facial nerve more than the others but its course is too varied for these to be of any practical use (May 1986).

Facial paralysis, often unilateral, may be due to:

- *supranuclear lesions* in the corticonuclear fibres from the frontal lobe, variably combined with numerous other descending fibres converging on the facial nucleus
- *nuclear* or *infranuclear lesions* involving lower motor neurons.

Supranuclear facial paralysis involving 'upper motor neuron' pathways is usually part of a hemiplegia. Movements in the lower part of the face are usually more severely affected, voluntary movements being weak or absent though emotional expression is little affected. Occasionally supranuclear lesions may abolish or weaken emotional movements but not voluntary movements. This dissociation shows that the supranuclear control of expressive movements is separate from the corticonuclear path for voluntary movements. At this level cerebrovascular accidents and tumours are the most likely cause.

Nuclear or infranuclear lesions vary in their effects according to the site of the lesion. If the nucleus or facial pontine fibres are involved, neighbouring structures are inevitably also involved. Facial muscles are represented in cell groups within the nucleus, and their degree of involvement governs the extent of paralysis, which is ipsilateral; otherwise the effects are identical with those of more peripheral lesions. Lesions due to adjacent damage include paralysis of the lateral rectus because of the involvement of the abducent nucleus (around which the facial nerve loops); paralysis of the masticatory muscles by involvement of the motor trigeminal nucleus; sensory loss on the face from involvement of the principal sensory and spinal trigeminal nuclei or spinothalamic tract; and paralysis of the upper or lower limbs due to corticospinal lesions. Due to the proximity of the facial sensory root to the vestibulocochlear nerve, lesions in the posterior cranial fossa or in the internal acoustic meatus may cause ipsilateral deafness, tinnitus and imbalance. Loss of the corneal reflex is an early sign whereas facial paralysis is often a late sign. Petrous temporal bone fractures are described as being either longitudinal, running parallel to, or transverse to the axis of the bone. Longitudinal fractures are more common and involve the middle ear and ossicles, while transverse fractures often damage the inner ear and are more likely to disrupt the facial nerve. A facial palsy can only be called a 'Bell's palsy' when other pathology has been excluded; it is synonymous with the term idiopathic palsy. Lower motor neuron lesions are more equally distributed between the upper and lower divisions of the facial nerve. The angle of the mouth sags and may drool, food accumulates in the cheek from paralysis of the buccinator, while paralysis of the upper eyelid may fail to protect and lubricate the cornea which

will ulcerate quickly unless it is both protected and lubricated—this must be given a high priority. The site of a lesion can be determined by testing whether the branches of the facial nerve are functioning. Objective tests of lacrimation (Schirmer's test), stapedius (stapedial reflex), and taste (electrogustometry) exist.

The arrangement of the nerve fibres throughout the course of the facial nerve remains in dispute (Gacek & Radpour 1982; May 1986). While cadaver and intraoperative stimulation studies have supported a topographic arrangement, the retrograde transport of horseradish peroxidase from individual nerves has failed to confirm this (Thomander et al 1982).

Variations in the intratemporal course of the facial nerve should be anticipated if there is an associated malformation of the external or middle ear. A number of variations exist (Fowler 1961; Proctor & Nager 1982), but mention should be made of the dehiscent facial nerve which is

present in up to 55% of normal temporal bones (Baxter 1971) and is usually sited above the oval window. Other not infrequent variations include the posterior displacement of the junction of the tympanic and mastoid segments, and a large chorda tympani which may contain motor fibres and should therefore be preserved. Extratympanic variations have been subdivided into five main groups: 24% have straight branching patterns off the two main branches of the temporofacial and cervicofacial divisions (Katz & Catalano 1987); 14% had loops involving the zygomatic division; 44% involving the buccal division; 14% had complex patterns with multiple interconnections; and 3% had two main trunks. An awareness of these variations is essential for the operating surgeon. At birth the mastoid process is absent, leaving the facial nerve superficial and vulnerable. Before the age of four, particular care is needed when operating in this area.

VESTIBULOCOCHLEAR NERVE

The vestibulocochlear nerve (**8.**129, 133, 135, 137) contains two major sets of afferent fibres differing in their principal central connections but both transmitting impulses from the inner ear to the brain. Both sets innervate specialized sensory end organs containing ciliated mechanoreceptors (called *hair cells*) but the end organs have specific adaptations so that the two divisions of the nerve carry different types of information. The vestibular division indicates positions and movements of the head in space whereas the cochlear division carries auditory information. The vestibular nerve arises from the neurons in the vestibular (or *Scarpa's*) ganglion in the outer part of the internal auditory meatus whilst the auditory or cochlear nerve arises from neurons in the spiral ganglion of the cochlea. Both ganglia contain bipolar neurons, each with central and peripheral processes: the former pass to the brainstem, the latter to the inner ear. The nerve also contains efferent fibres passing from neuronal cell bodies in the brainstem to each part of the labyrinth. The peripheral arrangement of the vestibulocochlear nerve is described on pp. 1337, 1392.

Centrally, the vestibulocochlear nerve (**8.**129, 133, 135, 137) can be identified emerging in the groove between the pons and the medulla oblongata, slightly lateral and posterior to the facial nerve (**8.**124). Leaving the medulla oblongata, it crosses the posterior border of the middle cerebellar peduncle with the facial nerve, partially separated from the latter by the labyrinthine artery. The nerves enter the internal acoustic meatus together. At the outer end of the meatus, the vestibulocochlear nerve splits into its *cochlear* and *vestibular* parts, the distribution of which will be described with the internal ear (pp. 1392–1394). The glial-Schwann cell border of the vestibulocochlear nerve is situated at the inner end of the internal acoustic meatus.

VESTIBULAR NERVE

Vestibular fibres enter the brain adjacent to those of the cochlear nerve and pass through the pons between the inferior cerebellar peduncle and spinal trigeminal tract to divide into ascending and descending branches ending mainly in the vestibular nuclei, although some go direct to the cerebellum through its inferior peduncle (p. 1035).

The vestibular nuclear complex comprises the following:

- The *medial vestibular nucleus* (p. 1024) lies under the vestibular area of the floor of the fourth ventricle, crossed dorsally by the striae medullares. The largest subdivision of the complex, it extends

up from the medulla oblongata into the pons.
- The *inferior vestibular nucleus* (p. 1024), lateral to the medial, reaches to a lower medullary level and lies between the medial nucleus and inferior cerebellar peduncle; descending branches of afferent vestibular fibres end among its cells
- The *lateral nucleus* (p. 1024) is ventrolateral to the upper part of the medial and it is characterized by its large neurons; its rostral end is continuous with the caudal end of the *superior nucleus*, which extends higher into the pons than other subdivisions, occupying the upper part of the vestibular area.

Several minor subdivisions have been described in feline vestibular nuclei (Brodal & Pompeiano 1957) and a tentative somatotopic pattern has been suggested in the lateral nucleus (Løken & Brodal 1970).

Connections

All vestibular nuclei receive *radicular fibres* from the nerve; they also receive *afferent cerebellovestibular fibres* through the inferior cerebellar peduncle, mainly derived from the flocculus and nodule (posterior lobe), together with others from the anterior lobe and fastigial nucleus. The vestibular nuclei also receive afferent fibres from the spinal cord and the reticular formation. From the nuclei, cerebellar fibres enter the inferior cerebellar peduncle, most destined for the flocculus and nodule. As noted, some vestibular fibres bypass the nuclei and reach the flocculus and nodule directly via the inferior cerebellar peduncle.

As a whole, the vestibular nuclear complex is a relay station on an afferent cerebellar path and a distributing station for efferent cerebellar fibres. Fibres from vestibular nuclei also enter the medial longitudinal fasciculus (**8.**141), ascending and descending to motor nuclei of the ocular and nuchal muscles. The 'octavo-oculomotor system' has attracted much attention and dissension exists regarding the vestibular nuclei involved, routes of projections, decussation and destinations. Tarlov (1972, 1975) has described a projection from the medial and superior vestibular nuclei to specific motor pools in the feline oculomotor nucleus and has also reviewed the literature; it is suggested that excitatory and inhibitory projections exist, mediating complex and subtle integration between vestibular signals and eye movements. From the vestibular nuclei, and the lateral nucleus in particular, fibres descend in the ventral funiculus of the spinal cord to form vestibulospinal tracts (p. 1001). Fibres from the vestibular nuclei also reach the cerebral cortex by way of the thalamus (for connections in man, see Hawrylshyn et al 1978; squirrel monkey,

Akbarian et al 1992). The thalamic relay of the vestibular system in primates seems to involve posterior parts of the ventroposterior complex and the medial pulvinar. The primary vestibular cortical area is located in the parietal lobe at the junction between the intraparietal and the postcentral sulci; this is adjacent to the portion of the postcentral gyrus where the head is represented. This makes sense functionally as this region of the somatosensory cortex is concerned with conscious appreciation of body position. There may be an additional representation of the vestibular system in the superior temporal gyrus near the auditory cortex. Through its connections, the vestibular system influences movements of the eyes and head, and the muscles of the trunk and limbs, to maintain equilibrium.

COCHLEAR NERVE

The cochlear nerve consists of afferent axons of spiral ganglion cells Types I and II. Type I cells (95%) supply the *inner hair cells* and have myelinated central axons. Type II cells (5%) supply the *outer hair cells* and have unmyelinated central axons. The cochlear nerve also contains efferent fibres to the sensory epithelium. These fibres leave the brainstem in the vestibular nerve and enter the cochlear nerve via the vestibulocochlear (*Oort's*) anastomosis which bridges the vestibular and cochlear portions of the nerve in the internal auditory meatus (see Arnesen 1984 for details in man). The olivocochlear bundle consists of medial olivocochlear fibres which are myelinated and supply the outer hair cells by means of large terminals, and lateral olivocochlear fibres which are unmyelinated and supply the afferent fibres of the inner hair cells.

Each Type I fibre bifurcates and supplies a number of different cell types in the cochlear nuclei, each type giving rise to a specific ascending pathway to auditory centres in the pons and mesencephalon. The dorsal cochlear nucleus projects via the dorsal acoustic stria to the contralateral inferior colliculus. The ventral cochlear nucleus projects via the trapezoid body or the intermediate acoustic stria to relay centres in the superior olivary complex, the nuclei of the lateral lemniscus, or the inferior colliculus (**8**.352) (see Moore & Osen 1979 for a description of the cytoarchitecture of the human cochlear nuclear complex and Morest 1993 for a review of

the structure and function of the brainstem auditory nuclei). In man, the superior olivary complex is dominated by the medial superior olive (Moore 1987) which receives direct input from the ventral cochlear nucleus on both sides and is involved in localization of sound by measuring the time difference between the two ears. The inferior colliculus consists of a central nucleus and two cortical areas, the dorsal cortex which is situated dorsomedially and the external cortex which is situated ventromedially (Faye-Lund & Osen 1985). Secondary and tertiary fibres ascend in the lateral lemniscus and converge in the central nucleus which projects to the ventral division of the medial geniculate body. The fibres which run between the dorsal nuclei of the lateral lemniscus and also project to the contralateral inferior colliculus form the commissure of Probst. The external cortex of the inferior colliculus receives both auditory and somatosensory input and projects to the medial division of the medial geniculate body. The external cortex and the central nucleus also are the origin of descending pathways to the olivocochlear cells in the superior olivary complex or to cells in the cochlear nuclei. The dorsal cortex of the inferior colliculus receives input from the auditory cortex and projects to the dorsal division of the medial geniculate body (Faye-Lund & Osen 1985). Connections also run from the dorsal nucleus of the lateral lemniscus to the deep part of the superior colliculus (Bajo et al 1993) to co-ordinate auditory and visual responses.

The ascending auditory pathway crosses the midline at several points below and at the level of the inferior colliculus. However, the input to the central nucleus of the inferior colliculus and higher centres has a clear contralateral dominance. The medial geniculate body is connected reciprocally to the primary auditory cortex, which is located in the superior temporal gyrus buried in the lateral fissure.

GLOSSOPHARYNGEAL NERVE

The glossopharyngeal nerve (**8**.124, 135, 137, 353, 354) is both motor and sensory, supplying motor fibres to the stylopharyngeus, parasympathetic secretomotor fibres to the parotid gland and sensory fibres to the tympanic cavity, Eustachian tube, fauces, tonsils, naso-

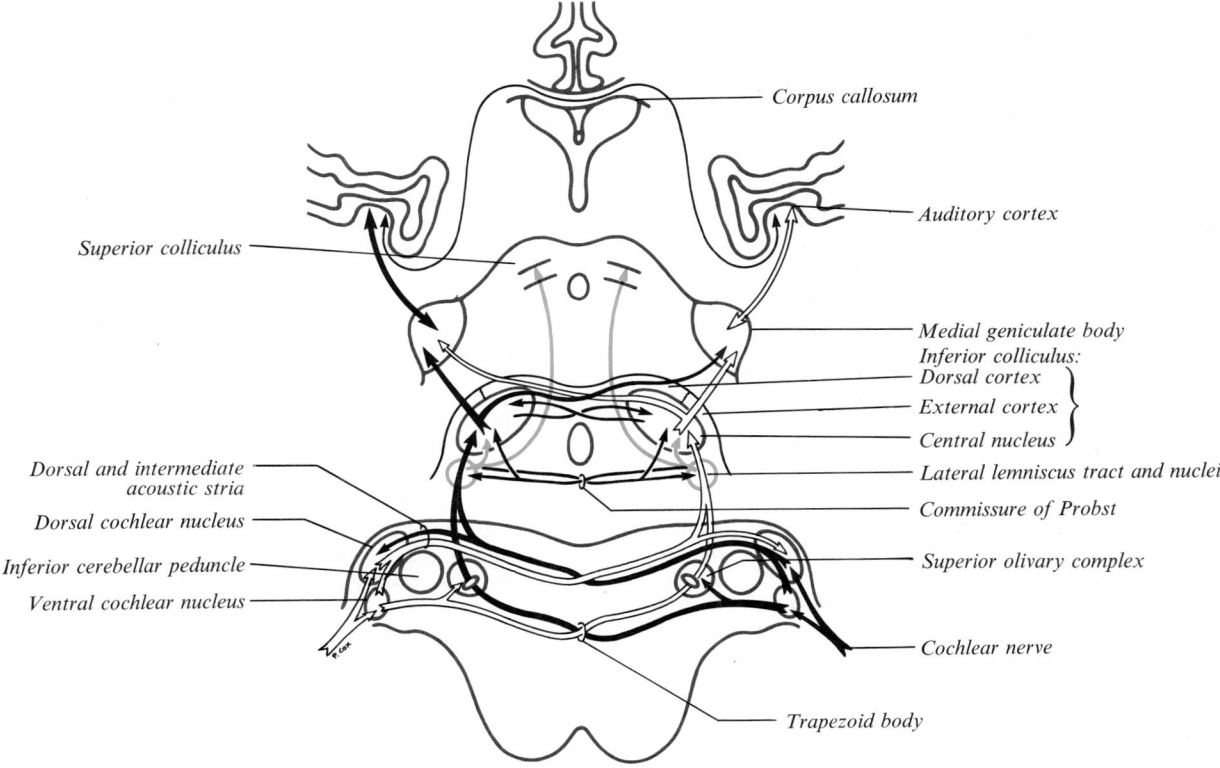

Corpus callosum

Auditory cortex

Superior colliculus

Medial geniculate body
Inferior colliculus:
Dorsal cortex
External cortex
Central nucleus
Lateral lemniscus tract and nuclei
Commissure of Probst

Dorsal and intermediate acoustic stria
Dorsal cochlear nucleus
Inferior cerebellar peduncle
Ventral cochlear nucleus

Superior olivary complex

Cochlear nerve

Trapezoid body

8.352 A simplified diagram to show the main features of the ascending auditory pathway in man. Ipsilateral and commissural connections appear to occur at most levels in this system as well as the pronounced contralateral projections which occur in the brainstem.

pharynx, uvula, inferior surface of the soft palate and posterior (postsulcal) third of the tongue; it is also the gustatory nerve for this part of the tongue. It emerges as three or four rootlets from the rostral part of the medulla oblongata in a groove between the olive and the inferior cerebellar peduncle above the rootlets of the vagus nerve.

Sensory nuclei. These receive the central processes of unipolar neurons in the superior and inferior glossopharyngeal ganglia; fibres concerned with taste end in the rostral part of the nucleus tractus solitarius (Nageotte 1906; Norgren 1978; Hamilton & Norgren 1984) whilst those concerned with general visceral afferents probably terminate both in the caudal part, possibly with a connection to the contralateral commissural nucleus (Rhoton et al 1966), and in the spinal trigeminal nucleus (Brodal 1947). Afferents from the carotid body and sinus project to the middle third of the nucleus tractus solitarius (Cottle 1964; Panneton & Loewy 1980) although some terminate on large neurons of the paramedian reticular formation of the medulla (Miura & Reis 1969).

Motor nucleus. The rostral part of the nucleus ambiguus, it is situated deep in the reticular formation medial to the spinal tract and nucleus of the trigeminal nerve. It receives both crossed and uncrossed corticonuclear fibres which leave their tracts at the level of the nucleus ambiguus or in the pons to descend in the medial lemniscus. The glossopharyngeal portion of the nucleus ambiguus lies level with, but ventrolateral to, the rostral tip of the main column (Getz & Sirnes 1949; Lawn 1966). It supplies the stylopharyngeus.

Parasympathetic fibres join the motor fibres from the inferior salivatory nucleus, a component of the visceral efferent column, located in the reticular formation below the superior salivatory nucleus; fibres from the nucleus travel via the glossopharyngeal tympanic branch and the tympanic plexus to the lesser petrosal nerve and otic ganglion, where they relay; postganglionic fibres join the auriculotemporal nerve to supply the parotid gland.

From the medulla oblongata the glossopharyngeal nerve passes anterolaterally to the triangular depression for the cochlear aqueduct on the inferior surface of the petrous temporal bone. At first it lies under the flocculus, resting on the jugular tubercle of the occipital bone, sometimes grooving it. It then turns abruptly down, leaving the skull through the anteromedial part of the jugular foramen, anterior to the basus and accessory nerves, in a separate dural sheath (**8.355**); in the foramen it is lodged in a deep groove leading from the cochlear aqueductual depression, separated by the inferior petrosal sinus from the vague and accessory nerves; the groove is bridged by fibrous tissue, ossified in about 25% of skulls. After exit the nerve passes forwards between the internal jugular vein and internal carotid artery and then descends anterior to the latter, deep to the styloid process and its attached muscles, to reach the posterior border of the stylopharyngeus. It curves forwards on the stylopharyngeus and either pierces the lower fibres of the superior pharyngeal constrictor or passes between it and the middle constrictor (**7.58**) to be distributed to the tonsil, the mucosae of the pharynx and postsulcal part of the tongue, the vallate papillae, and oral mucous glands.

Two ganglia are situated on the nerve as it traverses the jugular foramen (**8.355**): superior and inferior.

Superior ganglion. This is in the upper part of the groove occupied by the nerve in the jugular foramen. It is small, has no branches and is usually regarded as a detached part of the inferior ganglion.

Inferior ganglion. This is larger and lies in a notch in the lower border of the petrous temporal bone (**6.141**). Its cells are typical unipolar neurons, whose peripheral branches convey gustatory and tactile signals from the mucosa of the tongue (posterior third including the sulcus terminalis and vallate papillae) and general sensation only from the oropharynx, soft palate and fauces.

The glossopharyngeal nerve communicates with the sympathetic trunk, vagus and facial nerves. The inferior ganglion is connected with the superior cervical sympathetic ganglion. Two filaments from the inferior ganglion pass to the vagus, one to its auricular branch and the other to its superior ganglion. A branch to the facial arises from the glossopharyngeal nerve below the inferior ganglion, perforating the posterior belly of the digastric to join the facial nerve near the stylomastoid foramen.

Branches of distribution

These are: tympanic, carotid, pharyngeal, muscular, tonsillar and lingual.

Tympanic nerve. This leaves the inferior ganglion, ascends to the tympanic cavity through the inferior tympanic canaliculus and divides in the cavity into branches forming the *tympanic plexus*, contained in grooves on the surface of the promontory. This plexus supplies a branch to the greater superficial petrosal branch of the facial nerve; branches to the mucosa of the tympanic cavity, auditory tube and mastoid air cells and a branch to the lesser petrosal nerve.

Carotid branch. Often double, this arises just below the jugular foramen and descends on the internal carotid artery to the wall of the carotid sinus and to the carotid body. It contains primary afferent fibres from chemoreceptors in the carotid body and from the baroreceptors lying in the carotid sinus wall. It may communicate with the vagus (inferior ganglion or one of its branches) and with a sympathetic branch from the superior cervical ganglion. Another branch joins a plexus which also supplies the carotid body; other branches to this plexus come from the sympathetic (superior cervical sympathetic ganglion) and vagus. For distribution of the carotid nerve consult Willis & Tange (1959).

Lesser petrosal nerve. This contains parotid secretomotor fibres (see below). It enters a canal inferior to that for the tensor tympani, receives a connecting branch from the facial ganglion and reaches the anterior surface of the petrous bone through a small opening lateral to the hiatus for the greater petrosal nerve, passing thence via the foramen ovale or the canaliculus innominatus (p. 586) to join the otic ganglion.

Pharyngeal branches. These are three or four filaments uniting, near the middle pharyngeal constrictor, with the pharyngeal branch of the vagus and the laryngopharyngeal branches of the sympathetic trunk to form a pharyngeal plexus, through which the glossopharyngeal nerve supplies sensory fibres to the pharyngeal mucosa.

Muscular branch. This supplies the stylopharyngeus.

Tonsillar branches. These form a plexus with branches of the middle and posterior palatine nerves around the tonsil; from this, filaments supply the tonsil, soft palate and fauces.

Lingual branches. One branch supplies the vallate papillae and mucosa near the sulcus terminalis (p 1314), the other supplies the mucosa of the postsulcal (posterior) part of the tongue, communicating with the lingual nerve. It is the nerve of special sense (gustation) and general sensibility to the posterior lingual region.

Otic ganglion

This is a small, oval, flat reddish-grey ganglion (**8.344, 348**) situated just below the foramen ovale. It is a peripheral parasympathetic ganglion intimately related topographically to the mandibular nerve, but functionally connected with the glossopharyngeal. Lateral to it is the mandibular nerve near its junction with the trigeminal motor root, the ganglion usually surrounding the origin of the nerve to the medial pterygoid; medial is the tensor veli palatini, separating the ganglion from the cartilaginous auditory tube; posterior is the middle meningeal artery.

The motor, parasympathetic root of the otic ganglion is the lesser petrosal nerve, conveying preganglionic fibres from the glossopharyngeal nerve. These fibres originate from neurons in the inferior salivatory nucleus. They relay in the otic ganglion, post-ganglionic fibres passing by a communicating branch to the auriculotemporal nerve and so to the parotid gland (**8.342**). The sympathetic root is from the plexus on the middle meningeal artery; it contains postganglionic fibres, from the superior cervical sympathetic ganglion, which traverse the otic ganglion without relay; emerging with parasympathetic fibres in the connection to the auriculotemporal nerve, they supply blood vessels in the parotid gland.

Branches. A twig connects the ganglion to the chorda tympani, another ascends to join the nerve of the pterygoid canal; these may form an additional pathway by which gustatory fibres from the presulcal area of the tongue may reach the facial ganglion without traversing the middle ear; they are not relayed in the otic ganglion. Motor branches to the tensor veli palatini and tensor tympani, derived from the nerve to the medial pterygoid (mandibular division of the trigeminal nerve) also pass through the ganglion.

Lesions of the glossopharyngeal nerve

Damages to the glossopharyngeal nerve rarely occurs without involvement of other lower cranial nerves. Transient or sustained hypertension may follow surgical section of the nerve, reflecting involvement of the carotid branch (Ripley et al 1977). Isolated lesions of the glossopharyngeal nerve lead to loss of sensation over the ipsilateral soft palate, fauces, pharynx and posterior third of the tongue. Taste is also lost over the ipsilateral postsulcal portion although this is difficult to assess clinically and requires galvanic stimulation. The palatal and pharyngeal (gag) reflexes are reduced or absent and salivary secretion from the parotid gland may also be reduced. Weakness of stylopharyngeus cannot be tested individually. Glossopharyngeal neuralgia consists of episodic brief but severe pain, often precipitated by swallowing, and experienced in the throat, behind the angle of the jaw and within the ear.

VAGUS NERVE

The vagus nerve (**8**.124, 129, 133–135, 354, 355) contains motor and sensory fibres and has a more extensive course and distribution than any other cranial nerve, traversing the neck, thorax and abdomen. It emerges as eight or ten rootlets from the medulla oblongata, below the glossopharyngeal nerve in the groove between the olive and the inferior cerebellar peduncle. It has four nuclei in the medulla oblongata, namely the dorsal nucleus, the nucleus ambiguus, the nucleus tractus solitarius, the spinal trigeminal nucleus.

Dorsal nucleus. This is a general visceral efferent nucleus with 80% of its neurons giving rise to the parasympathetic preganglionic fibres of the vagus nerve and the remainder being interneurons or projecting centrally (Hopkins 1987). It is the largest parasympathetic nucleus of the brainstem and is sited in the central grey matter of the lower dorsomedial portion of the medulla oblongata close to the floor of the IVth ventricle. It extends caudally to the first cervical spinal segment and rostrally to the open part of the medulla under the vagal triangle and separated from the hypoglossal nucleus by the nucleus intercalatus. Its motor fibres are distributed to the non-striated muscle of the viscera of the thorax (heart, bronchi, lungs and oesophagus) and abdomen (stomach, liver, pancreas, spleen, small intestine and proximal part of the colon). In man, neurons within the nucleus are heterogeneous and can be classified into nine subnuclei that are regionally grouped into rostral, intermediate and caudal divisions (Huang et al 1993). Topographic maps of visceral representation in other species suggest the heart and lungs are represented in the more caudal and lateral part of the nucleus whereas gastric and pancreatic representation occupies intermediate regions and the remaining abdominal organs are represented in the rostral and medial part of the nucleus (Getz & Sirnes 1949; Mitchell & Warwick 1955; Katz & Karten 1985; Laughton & Pewley 1987; Hopkins 1987; Okumura & Namiki 1990). There may be a sparse sensory afferent supply which arises in the nodose ganglion and projects directly to the dorsal and lateral edges of the nucleus (Shapiro & Miselis 1985) and possibly beyond into the nucleus tractus solitarius.

Nucleus ambiguus. Below the origin of the fibres joining the glossopharyngeal nerve, neurons of the nucleus ambiguus contribute fibres to the vagus for distribution to striated muscle: the pharyngeal constrictors, intrinsic laryngeal muscles and striated muscles of the palate and upper oesophagus. The nucleus is connected to corticonuclear tracts bilaterally and to many brainstem centres. There is topographical organization in the dorsal nucleus ambiguus, with the individual laryngeal muscles being innervated by relatively discrete groups in more caudal zones (Szentágothai 1943; Getz & Sirnes 1949; Lawn 1966), those to the pharynx lying in the intermediate group and those to the oesophagus and soft palate being rostral (Holstege et al 1983). Most caudally there is also a group of preganglionic parasympathetic fibres ventrolateral to the main cell column which is the main site of origin of cardioinhibitory neurons (Hopkins 1987).

Nucleus tractus solitarius (**8**.155, 157). This receives special visceral gustatory afferents from facial glossopharyngeal and vagus nerves which terminate in a viscerotopic pattern predominantly in the rostral region (Norgren 1978; Hamilton & Norgren 1984). Experimental evidence suggests that fibres from the anterior two-thirds of the tongue and the roof of the oral cavity (via chorda tympani and greater superficial petrosal branches of the facial nerve) terminate in the extreme rostral part of the solitary complex. Those from the circumvallate and foliate papillae of the posterior third of the tongue, tonsils, palate and pharynx (via the lingual branch of the glossopharyngeal nerve) are distributed throughout the rostrocaudal extent of the nucleus tractus solitarius predominantly rostral to the obex whilst gustatory afferents from the larynx and epiglottis in the superior laryngeal branch of the vagus have a more caudal and lateral distribution (Rhoton et al 1966; Hamilton & Norgren 1984; Whitehead 1986). Vagal afferents terminate throughout the nucleus, although the most rostral fibres appear to be somewhat denser laterally (Beckstead & Norgren 1979). The cytoarchitectural characteristics of the subnuclei of the human nucleus tractus solitarius correspond well with the nuclei described in experimental studies (Loewy & Burton 1978; Kalia & Mesulam 1980a,b; Tork et al 1990; Hyde & Miselis 1992). The medial and commissural nuclei in the caudal nucleus tractus solitarius appear to be the primary site of termination for gastrointestinal afferents (Gwyn et al 1979, 1985). Ventral and interstitial subnuclei probably receive tracheal, laryngeal and pulmonary afferents (Kalia & Richter 1985) and have an important role in both respiratory control and possibly rhythm generation (Euler et al 1973; Merrill 1974; Feldman et al 1985; Feldman 1986; McCrimmon et al 1987). The carotid sinus and aortic body nerves terminate in the dorsal and dorsolateral region of the solitary complex which may have an important role in cardiovascular regulation (Ciriello et al 1981; Ciriello 1983).

Spinal trigeminal nucleus. The vagus contains somatic afferent nerve fibres from the skin of the concha of the external ear and from the meninges of the posterior fossa and foramen magnum. These are believed to terminate in the pars caudalis of the spinal trigeminal nucleus together with visceral afferent pain fibres from the larynx (Brodal 1947).

Vagal rootlets unite to form a flat cord which passes below the flocculus to the jugular foramen, by which it leaves the cranium. As it emerges it accompanies the accessory nerve, sharing an arachnoid and dural sheath; both lie anterior to a fibrous septum which separates them from the glossopharyngeal nerve. After emerging from the foramen the vagus has two marked enlargements, the small round superior ganglion and the larger inferior ganglion.

Superior (jugular) ganglion. This is greyish, spherical and about 4mm in diameter in man. It is connected to the cranial root of the accessory nerve, the inferior glossopharyngeal ganglion, and to the sympathetic trunk by a filament from the superior cervical ganglion. The significance of these connections is not entirely clear but the first probably contains aberrant motor fibres from the nucleus ambiguus which issue in the accessory nerve, to be distributed to the palatal, pharyngeal, laryngeal and upper oesophageal musculature via the vagus; the sympathetic connection may be like the one between this sympathetic ganglion and the inferior vagal ganglion. As it leaves the superior ganglion the auricular branch gives off an ascending filament to the facial nerve. In cats the jugular ganglion contains about 8 700 unipolar neurons, 73% of which appear to form the auricular nerve, which is composed of heavily myelinated somatic afferents, and 15% contribute to the vagus itself (Foley & DuBois 1937). Counts are apparently not available for the human ganglion; but since the human vagus nerve contains, at midcervical level, about 16 500 (Rt) and 20 000 (Lt) myelinated fibres, counted in 17 paired nerves, it follows that human ganglionic neurons must be more numerous (Schnitzlein et al 1958).

Inferior (nodose) ganglion. This is larger than the superior ganglion, being elongated and cylindrical in shape with a length of about 25 mm and a maximum breadth of 5 mm. It is connected with the hypoglossal nerve, the loop between the first and second cervical spinal nerves, and with the superior cervical sympathetic ganglion. The cranial root of the accessory nerve passes over the inferior ganglion, attached only by fibrous tissue. Beyond the ganglion the cranial accessory blends with the vagus nerve, its fibres distributed mainly in pharyngeal and recurrent laryngeal vagal branches. Most visceral afferent fibres are located in the nodose ganglion; in cats it is estimated to contain about 30 000 neurons (Jones 1937; DuBois & Foley 1937), most are unipolar but a few are fusiform or bipolar; most are in the range of 35–45μm (Mohiuddin 1953).

Both vagal ganglia are exclusively sensory, containing somatic, special visceral and general visceral afferent neurons which are unipolar (Ramon y Cajal 1909; Gabella 1976). The superior ganglion is chiefly somatic, most of its neurons entering the auricular nerve, whilst neurons in the inferior ganglion are concerned with visceral sensation from the heart, larynx, lungs and alimentary tract from the pharynx to the transverse colon; some fibres transmit impulses from taste endings in the vallecula and epiglottis. In addition there are large afferent fibres derived from muscle spindles in the laryngeal muscles (Lucas Keene 1961; Grim 1967; Mei 1970). Vagal sensory neurons in the nodose ganglion may have a topographical layout (Collman et al 1992). Both ganglia are traversed by parasympathetic and perhaps some sympathetic fibres but there is no evidence that vagal parasympathetic components relay in the inferior ganglion. Preganglionic motor fibres from the dorsal vagal nucleus and the special visceral efferents from the nucleus ambiguus, which descend to the inferior vagal ganglion, commonly form a visible band, skirting the ganglion in some mammals (Hoffman & Kuntz 1957; Mei & Dussardier 1966). These larger fibres appear to provide motor innervation to the larynx in the recurrent laryngeal nerve with some contribution to the superior laryngeal nerve supplying cricothyroid.

In man the superior laryngeal nerve contains 15 000 fibres with 30% being myelinated afferents (Ogura & Lam 1953). In contrast only 3% of fibres in the recurrent laryngeal nerve appear to be afferent (Brocklehurst & Edgeworth 1940. The abdominal vagus is composed almost entirely of unmyelinated fibres (Sharma & Thomas 1975).

Course

The vagus nerve descends vertically in the neck in the carotid sheath, between the internal jugular vein and the **internal** carotid artery to the upper border of the thyroid cartilage and then passes between the vein and the **common** carotid artery to the root of the neck. Its further course differs on the two sides.

The *right* vagus nerve descends posterior to the internal jugular vein to cross the first part of the subclavian artery, entering the thorax and descending through the superior mediastinum, at first behind the right brachiocephalic vein, then right of the trachea and posteromedial to the right brachiocephalic vein and superior vena cava. The right pleura and lung are lateral to it above but are separated from it below by the azygos vein, which arches forwards above the right pulmonary hilum (**10**.173). The nerve then passes behind the right principal bronchus to the posterior aspect of the right hilum and divides into the posterior pulmonary (bronchial) branches, which unite with rami from the second to fifth or sixth thoracic sympathetic ganglia to form the *right posterior pulmonary plexus*. From the caudal part of this plexus two or three branches descend on the dorsal surface of the oesophagus, where, with a left vagal ramus, they form the *posterior oesophageal plexus*, from which a trunk is re-formed and continued posterior to the oesophagus to traverse the diaphragmatic oesophageal opening. This posterior vagal trunk contains fibres from both vagus nerves (p. 1253).

(Details of the cardiac plexuses are on pp. 1302, 1306.)

In the abdomen the posterior vagal trunk divides into a small gastric and a larger coeliac branch. The former supplies the posteroinferior gastric surface except the pyloric canal. The coeliac branch ends chiefly in the coeliac plexus but sends twigs to the splenic, hepatic, renal, suprarenal and superior mesenteric plexuses (p. 1367).

The *left* vagus enters the thorax between the left common carotid and subclavian arteries and behind the left brachiocephalic vein. It descends through the superior mediastinum and crosses the left side of the aortic arch to pass behind the left pulmonary hilum. Above the aortic arch it is crossed anterolaterally by the left phrenic nerve and on the arch by the left superior intercostal vein (**10**.26). Behind the hilum it divides into the posterior

pulmonary (or bronchial) branches, which unite with rami of the second to fourth thoracic sympathetic ganglia; this forms the *left posterior pulmonary plexus*, two branches of which descend anteriorly on the oesophagus forming, with a ramus from the right posterior pulmonary plexus, the *anterior oesophageal plexus*. From this a trunk containing fibres from both vagus nerves continues anterior to the oesophagus, entering the abdomen through the oesophageal diaphragmatic opening (p. 816).

In the abdomen the *anterior vagal trunk* supplies the cardiac antrum of the stomach and then divides into right and left branches. The left group follows the lesser gastric curvature to supply the anterosuperior surface of the stomach. The right group has three main branches. The first, sometimes duplicated, proceeds between the layers of lesser omentum towards the porta hepatis, dividing into: (*a*) upper branches entering the porta, and (*b*) lower branches supplying chiefly the pyloric canal, pylorus, superior and descending parts of the duodenum and the head of the pancreas. The second is distributed to the anterosuperior surface of the body of the stomach; the third branch follows the lesser curvature to the angular notch (see also p. 1763).

Branches of distribution

In the jugular fossa	Meningeal
	Auricular
In the neck	Pharyngeal
	Branches to carotid body
	Superior laryngeal
	Recurrent laryngeal (right)
	Cardiac
In the thorax	Cardiac
	Recurrent laryngeal (left)
	Pulmonary
	Oesophageal
In the abdomen	Gastric
	Coeliac
	Hepatic
	Renal

Meningeal branch or branches. These appear to start from the superior vagal ganglion and are distributed to the dura mater in the posterior cranial fossa. However, evidence suggests (Kimmel 1961a) that they are in fact recurrent sensory and sympathetic nerves from the upper cervical spinal nerves and superior cervical sympathetic ganglion, which run for a short distance in the sheath of the vagus nerve (pp. 1212, 1261).

Auricular branch. This also arises from the superior vagal ganglion and is joined soon after by a ramus from the inferior ganglion of the glossopharyngeal nerve. It passes behind the internal jugular vein and enters the mastoid canaliculus on the lateral wall of the jugular fossa. Traversing the temporal bone thus, it crosses the facial canal about 4 mm above the stylomastoid foramen and here supplies an ascending branch to the facial nerve. (Here fibres of the nervus intermedius may pass to the auricular branch, perhaps explaining the cutaneous vesiculation which sometimes accompanies geniculate herpes.) The auricular branch then traverses the tympanomastoid fissure, dividing into two rami: one joining the posterior auricular nerve and the other distributed to the skin of part of the cranial auricular surface and to the posterior wall and floor of the external acoustic meatus and adjoining part of the outer surface of the tympanic membrane. The vagal auricular branch thus contains somatic afferent nerve fibres, which probably terminate in the spinal trigeminal nucleus.

Pharyngeal branch. The main motor nerve of the pharynx, it emerges from the upper part of the inferior vagal ganglion and consists chiefly of filaments from the cranial accessory nerve. It passes between the external and internal carotid arteries to the upper border of the middle pharyngeal constrictor, dividing into numerous filaments which join rami of the sympathetic trunk and glossopharyngeal and external laryngeal nerves to form a *pharyngeal plexus* by which vagal fibres are distributed to the pharyngeal and palatal muscles, except the tensor veli palatini. A minute filament, the ramus lingualis vagi, joins the hypoglossal nerve as it curves round the occipital artery.

Branches to the carotid body (p. 971). Variable in number, these may arise from the inferior ganglion or travel in either the pharyngeal branch or the superior laryngeal nerve, though rarely in the latter. They form a plexus with the glossopharyngeal rami and branches of the cervical sympathetic trunk (Sheehan et al 1941; also pp. 1250, 1300).

Superior laryngeal nerve. Larger than the pharyngeal branch, this issues from the middle of the inferior vagal ganglion and receives a branch from the superior cervical sympathetic ganglion. It descends alongside the pharynx, first posterior, then medial to the internal carotid artery, and divides into the internal and external laryngeal nerves.

The *internal laryngeal nerve* is sensory to the laryngeal mucosa down to the level of the vocal folds. It also carries afferent fibres from the laryngeal neuromuscular spindles and other stretch receptors (Lucas Keene 1961; Scheuer 1964). It descends to the thyrohyoid membrane, pierces it above the superior laryngeal artery and divides into an upper and lower branch; the upper is horizontal and supplies the mucosa of the pharynx, the epiglottis, vallecula and laryngeal vestibule; the lower descends in the medial wall of the piriform recess, supplying the aryepiglottic fold, the mucosa on the back of the arytenoid cartilage and one or two branches to the arytenoideus, which unite with twigs from the recurrent laryngeal to supply the same muscle (p. 1647). The internal laryngeal nerve ends by piercing the inferior constrictor muscle to unite with an ascending branch from the recurrent laryngeal nerve. As it ascends in the neck it supplies branches, more numerous on the left, to the mucosa and tunica muscularis of the oesophagus and trachea and to the inferior constrictor. There is little constant topography within the recurrent laryngeal nerve and separate nerve bundles to individual laryngeal muscles not having been traced in man (Sunderland 1952; Bowden 1955). However, in the equine nerve there is clear separation of fibres proximally with mixing occurring approximately 15 cm from the larynx (Dyer & Duncan 1987).

The *external laryngeal nerve*, smaller than the internal, descends posterior to the sternothyroid with the superior thyroid artery but on a deeper plane; it lies at first on the inferior pharyngeal constrictor and then, piercing it, curves round the inferior thyroid tubercle to reach and supply the cricothyroid. It also supplies the pharyngeal plexus and inferior constrictor; behind the common carotid artery it connects with the superior cardiac nerve and superior cervical sympathetic ganglion.

Recurrent laryngeal nerve

This differs, in origin and course, on the two sides. On the **right** it arises from the vagus anterior to the first part of the subclavian artery, curving backwards below and then behind it to ascend obliquely to the side of the trachea behind the common carotid artery. Near the lower pole of the thyroid lateral lobe it is near the inferior thyroid artery, crossing **either** in front of or behind it, or between its branches. On the **left**, the nerve arises from the vagus on the left of the aortic arch, curves below it immediately behind the attachment of the ligamentum arteriosum to the concavity of the arch and ascends to the side of the trachea. On both sides the recurrent laryngeal nerve ascends in or near a groove between the trachea and oesophagus and is closely related to the medial surface of the thyroid gland before passing under the lower border of the inferior constrictor to enter the larynx behind the articulation of the inferior thyroid cornu with the cricoid cartilage. It supplies all laryngeal muscles, except the cricothyroid; it communicates with the internal laryngeal nerve, supplying sensory filaments to the laryngeal mucosa below the vocal folds. It also carries afferent fibres from laryngeal stretch receptors.

As the recurrent laryngeal nerve curves round the subclavian artery, or the aortic arch, it gives cardiac filaments to the deep cardiac plexus.

The varying relations of the recurrent laryngeal nerves near the larynx are important in thyroid surgery. The nerve does not always lie in a protected position in the tracheo-oesophageal groove but may be slightly anterior to it (more often on the right) and it may be markedly lateral to the trachea at the level of the lower part of the thyroid gland. On the right the nerve is as often anterior to, or posterior to, or intermingled with terminal branches of the inferior thyroid artery, while on the left the nerve is usually posterior to the artery, though occasionally anterior to it. The nerve may supply extra-laryngeal branches to the larynx, arising before the nerve passes behind the inferior thyroid cornu. Outside its capsule the thyroid gland has a distinct covering of pretracheal fascia (p. 804), which splits into two layers at the posterior border of the gland. One layer covers the entire medial surface of its lobe and, at or just above the isthmus, has a conspicuous thickening, the *lateral ligament of the thyroid gland* (p. 1892) which attaches the gland to the trachea and the lower part of the cricoid cartilage. The other layer is posterior, passing behind the oesophagus and pharynx and attached to the prevertebral fascia. By this splitting of the fascia, a compartment is formed on each side, lateral to the trachea and oesophagus, and it is in the fat that this contains that the recurrent laryngeal nerve and terminal parts of the inferior thyroid artery lie. The nerve may be lateral or medial to the lateral ligament of the thyroid gland, or sometimes may be embedded in it.

Cardiac branches. Two or three in number, these arise from the vagus at superior and inferior cervical levels. The small *superior branches* join sympathetic cardiac branches and reach the deep cardiac plexus. The *inferior branches* arise in the root of the neck, the right passing in front or by the side of the brachiocephalic artery to the deep cardiac plexus, the left descending across the left side of the aortic arch to join the superficial cardiac plexus. Additional cardiac branches arise from the right vagus nerve near the trachea and from both recurrent laryngeal nerves, ending in the deep cardiac plexus. The cardiac plexuses are described on p. 1306.

Anterior pulmonary branches. Two or three in number, and small, these reach the anterior surface of the hilum of the lung, forming with sympathetic rami the anterior pulmonary plexus.

Posterior pulmonary branches. More numerous and larger, these pass behind the hilum, forming with sympathetic rami from the second to fifth or sixth thoracic sympathetic ganglia the posterior pulmonary plexus, branches from which accompany the bronchial ramifications and supply the constrictor muscles and other tissues of the pulmonary tree (pp. 1307, 1664, 1675).

Oesophageal branches. These arise above and below the pulmonary, the lower being numerous and larger. They form the oesophageal plexus, from which filaments supply the oesophagus and the back of the pericardium (p. 1252).

Gastric branches. These supply the anterosuperior surface of the stomach (mainly from the left vagus) and postero-inferior surface (mainly from the right) (p. 1307). Brizzi et al (1973) described separate 'cardiac' branches to the cardia; they found that both gastric branches supplied the fundus and body, while the pylorus received a complex innervation mainly from the anterior gastric nerve and vagal hepatic branches, less frequently from the posterior gastric nerve. Both anterior and posterior gastric nerves lie within the hepatogastric ligament, respectively anterior and posterior to the peri-arterial nerves that surround the left gastric artery.

Coeliac branches. These branches of the posterior vagal trunks join the coeliac plexus.

Hepatic branches. Coming from both vagi (p. 1307) they join the hepatic plexus and supply the liver.

Renal branches. Also from both nerves, these join the renal plexus (p. 1307).

For details of the abdominal distribution of the vagus nerves, see pages 1298, 1307, 1308. For lesions of the vagal nerve see p. 1647.

ACCESSORY NERVE

The accessory nerve (8.353–357) is conventionally described as a single entity though its two components (which join for a relatively short part of its course) are of quite separate origin. The **cranial root** (the internal ramus), which joins the vagus, has been considered to be a branchial or special visceral efferent nerve, though in animals

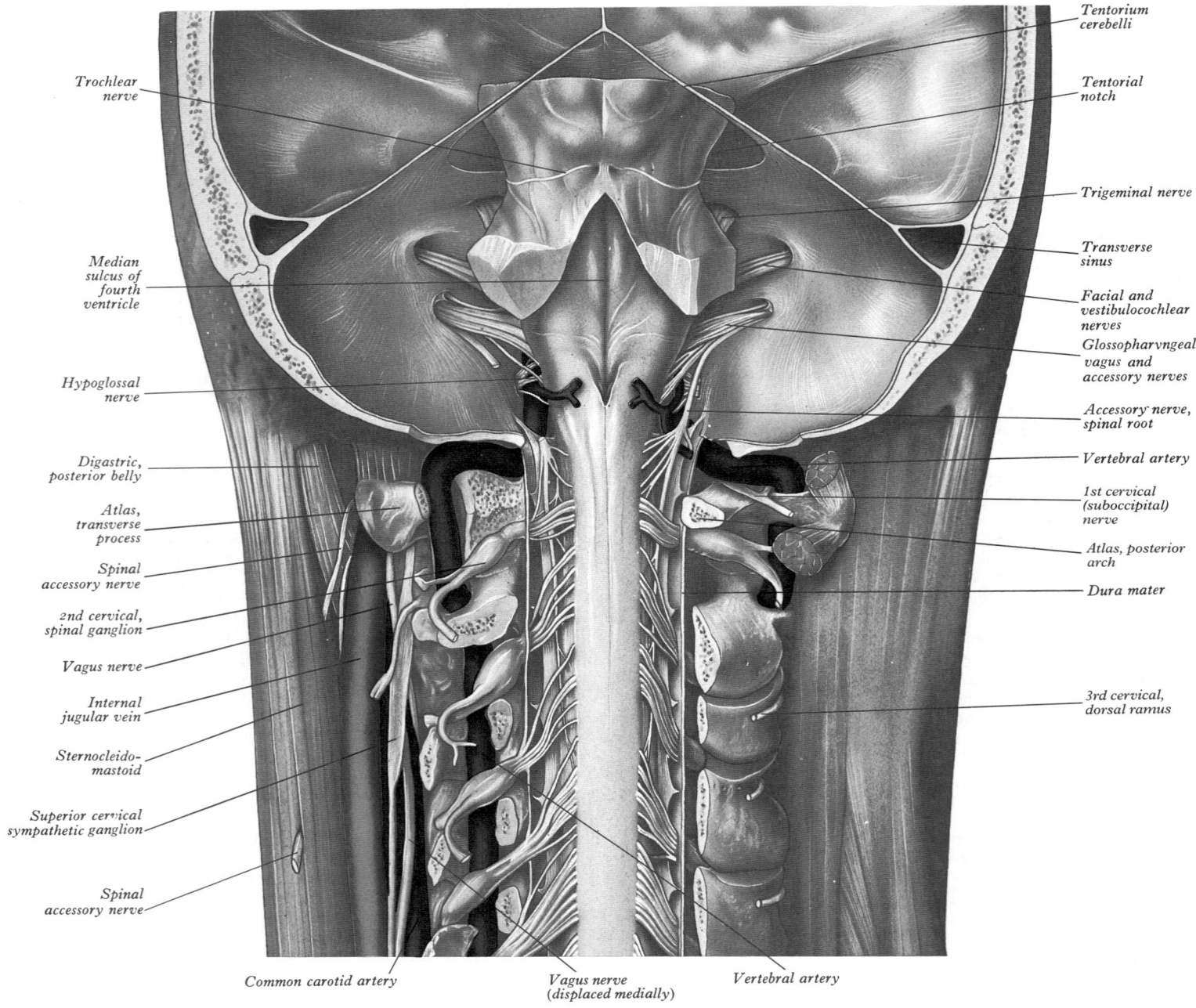

Trochlear
nerve

Median
sulcus of
fourth
ventricle

Hypoglossal
nerve

Digastric,
posterior belly

Atlas,
transverse
process

Spinal
accessory nerve

2nd cervical,
spinal ganglion

Vagus nerve

Internal
jugular vein

Sternocleido-
mastoid

Superior cervical
sympathetic ganglion

Spinal
accessory nerve

Tentorium
cerebelli

Tentorial
notch

Trigeminal nerve

Transverse
sinus

Facial and
vestibulocochlear
nerves

Glossopharyngeal,
vagus and
accessory nerves

Accessory nerve,
spinal root

Vertebral artery

1st cervical
(suboccipital)
nerve

Atlas, posterior
arch

Dura mater

3rd cervical,
dorsal ramus

Common carotid artery

Vagus nerve
(displaced medially)

Vertebral artery

8.353   A dissection exposing the brain stem and the upper part of the spinal cord after removal of large portions of the occipital and parietal bones and the cerebellum, together with the roof of the fourth ventricle. On the left side the foramina transversaria of the atlas and the third, fourth and fifth cervical vertebrae have been opened to expose the vertebral artery. On the right side the posterior arch of the atlas and the laminae of the succeeding cervical vertebrae have been divided and have been removed together with the vertebral spines and the laminae of the opposite side. The tentorium cerebelli and the transverse sinuses have been divided and their posterior portions removed.

it contains, in addition, a general visceral efferent component. The **spinal root** (the external ramus) can be considered as a somatic, special visceral efferent, or mixed nerve, depending on the view taken of the embryological origin of the muscles it supplies, sterno-cleidomastoid and trapezius. The assumption that the spinal component is purely motor is almost certainly incorrect. In human embryonic material, sensory ganglia have been located along the course of the spinal root (Pearson 1938).

Cranial root (8.355)

The smaller root, this arises from the caudal two-thirds of the nucleus ambiguus (Kitamura et al 1987), the caudal four-fifths of the dorsal nucleus of the vagus (at least in animals) and its caudal extension, the nucleus retroambigualis (Kitamura et al 1989). The nucleus ambiguus is connected with the corticonuclear tracts of both sides,

some fibres from this source descending from the midbrain in the medial lemniscus (aberrant pyramidal fibres, p. 1019). The cranial root emerges as four or five fine rootlets from the dorsolateral surface of the caudal medulla oblongata below the vagal roots. They are possibly joined by a small number of roots which emerge from the upper cervical cord and run along the trunk of the spinal root before joining the internal ramus. These roots derive from the caudal dorsal vagal nucleus and the nucleus retroambigualis (Kitamura et al 1989). The cranial root runs laterally to the jugular foramen uniting for a short distance with the spinal root. It also connects with the superior vagal ganglion. It traverses the foramen, separates from the spinal part and immediately joins the vagus nerve superior to the inferior vagal ganglion. Those fibres distributed in the pharyngeal branches of the vagus, and derived from the nucleus ambiguus, probably innervate the palatal muscles, except tensor veli palatini. Other

1254

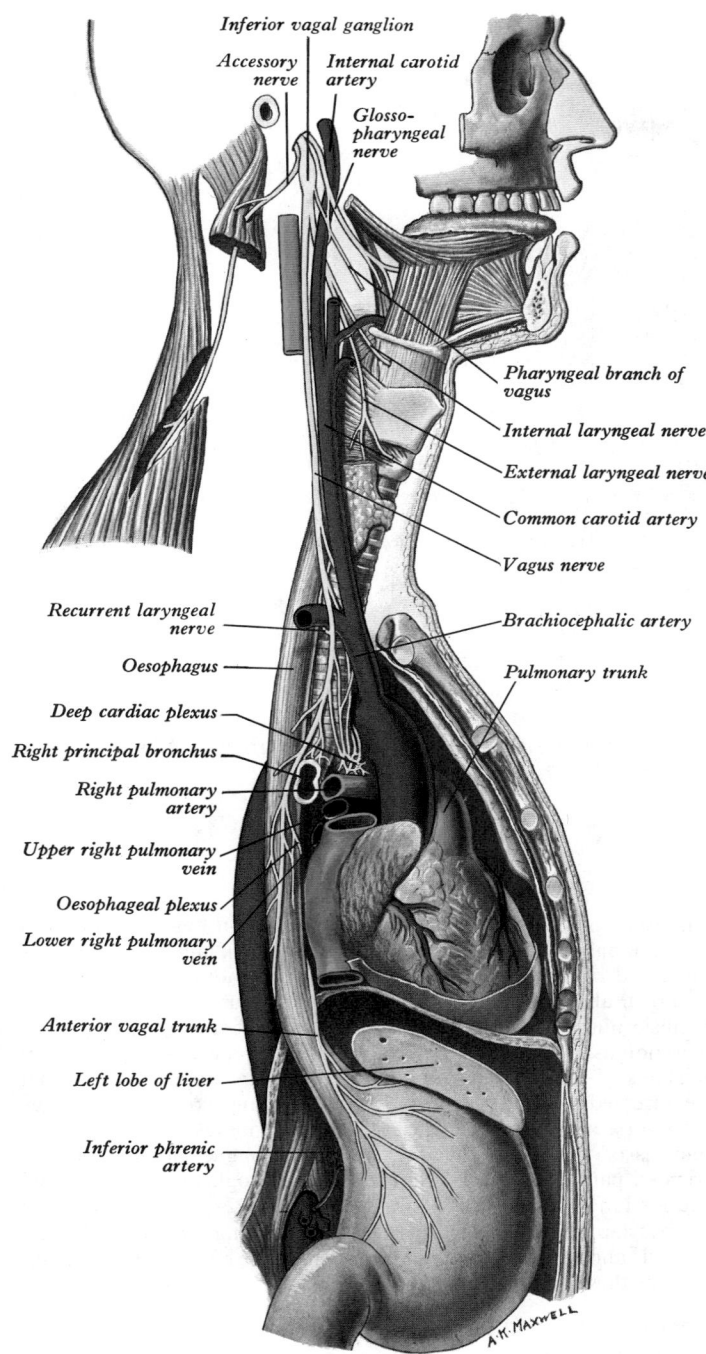

Inferior vagal ganglion
Accessory nerve | *Internal carotid artery*
Glosso-pharyngeal nerve

Pharyngeal branch of vagus
Internal laryngeal nerve
External laryngeal nerve
Common carotid artery
Vagus nerve
Brachiocephalic artery
Pulmonary trunk

Recurrent laryngeal nerve
Oesophagus
Deep cardiac plexus
Right principal bronchus
Right pulmonary artery
Upper right pulmonary vein
Oesophageal plexus
Lower right pulmonary vein
Anterior vagal trunk
Left lobe of liver
Inferior phrenic artery

A.K. MAXWELL

8.354 The course and distribution of the glossopharyngeal, vagus and accessory nerves.

accessory fibres enter the recurrent laryngeal nerve to supply the adductor muscles of the vocal cords, thyroarytenoid and the lateral crico-arytenoid. The destination of the general visceral efferent fibres within the internal ramus that originate from the dorsal vagal nucleus is less certain. Animal studies suggest a considerable contribution to the innervation of the abdominal viscera, heart, trachea and thoracic oesophagus (Kitamura et al 1989).

Spinal root (8.353)

This arises from a cell column in the lateral aspect of the ventral horn, extending from the junction of the spinal cord and medulla to the sixth cervical segment (Pearson 1938; Ullah & Salman 1986). The supranuclear pathway of fibres destined for sternocleidomastoid appears to undergo a double decussation in the brainstem (Willoughby & Anderson 1984), though cortical stimulation exper-

iments in humans have suggested a bilateral projection from each hemisphere.

Some rootlets emerge directly, others turn cranially before exiting. The line of exit is irregular rather than linear. The roots form a trunk which lies close to the dorsal roots. There is a variable relationship to the first cervical dorsal root and ganglion—usually the accessory trunk passes through the ganglion. In both animals and man, sensory ganglia are found along the course of the spinal root which enters the skull via the foramen magnum, behind the vertebral artery. It then turns up and laterally to the jugular foramen, traversing this in a single dural sheath with the vagus but separated from it by a fold of arachnoid. Some fibres from the upper cervical cord that run along with the trunk of the spinal accessory finally join the internal ramus. As the spinal root exits from the jugular foramen it runs posterolaterally passing either medial or lateral to the internal jugular vein, or rarely through it. The nerve then crosses the transverse process of the atlas and is itself crossed by the occipital artery. It descends obliquely, medial to the styloid process, stylohyoid and the posterior belly of the digastric. With the superior sterno-cleidomastoid branch of the occipital artery, it reaches the upper part of the sternocleidomastoid and enters its deep surface, there forming an anastomosis with fibres from C2 alone, C3 alone or both—the ansa of Maubrac (Soo et al 1986; Caliot et al 1989). Rarely the nerve terminates in the muscle but more commonly it emerges a little above the midpoint of the posterior border of the muscle, generally above the emergence of the great auricular nerve and usually within 2 cm of it, and between 4–6 cm from the tip of the mastoid. The point of emergence is, however, very variable. It crosses the posterior triangle on levator scapulae separated from it by the prevertebral layer of deep cervical fascia and adipose tissue. Here the nerve is relatively superficial and related to the superficial cervical lymph nodes. About 3–5 cm above the clavicle it passes behind the anterior border of the trapezius, often dividing to form a plexus on its deep surface which has contributions from C3 and C4, or C4 alone, before entering the deep surface of the muscle. In about a quarter of subjects the nerve receives no fibres from the cervical plexus (Krause et al 1991). The cervical course of the nerve follows a line from the lower anterior part of the tragus to the tip of the atlantal transverse process and then across the sternocleidomastoid and the posterior triangle to a point on the anterior border of the trapezius 3–5 cm above the clavicle.

The spinal root has been considered to provide the sole motor supply to the sternocleidomastoid, the second and third cervical nerves conveying proprioceptive fibres from it (Fitzgerald et al 1982). The innervation of the trapezius is more complex. The motor supply to the upper and middle portions of the muscle is primarily from the accessory nerve. The lower two-thirds of the muscle, however, in up to three-quarters of subjects, receives an innervation from the cervical plexus (Soo et al 1990; Krause et al 1991). On the basis of the incomplete denervation of the muscle in some individuals following sacrifice of both the accessory nerve and the cervical plexus, it has been suggested that the trapezius receives a partial motor supply from other sources, possibly via thoracic roots. In addition to their motor contribution, cervical roots 3 and 4 supply proprioceptive fibres to the trapezius.

Lesions affecting the accessory nerve and its nucleus

As a consequence of the double decussation of the supranuclear fibres reaching that part of the spinal accessory nucleus concerned with innervation of the sternocleidomastoid, a lesion of the pyramidal system above the pons results in a hemiplegia with weakness of the ipsilateral sternocleidomastoid. The trapezius weakness is contralateral to the hemiplegia, however. In spasmodic torticollis, one of the focal dystonias, episodic contraction of the sterno-cleidomastoid and trapezius occurs, often accompanied by contraction of other muscle groups, for example splenius capitis.

In the jugular foramen syndrome, lesions of the eleventh, tenth and ninth cranial nerves coexist. Causative pathologies include nasopharyngeal carcinoma and a glomus tumour. Distally the eleventh nerve can be injured by trauma or surgical exploration. An isolated palsy of the eleventh nerve has been described, with pain followed by weakness of the relevant muscles. Recovery occurs in the majority of patients.

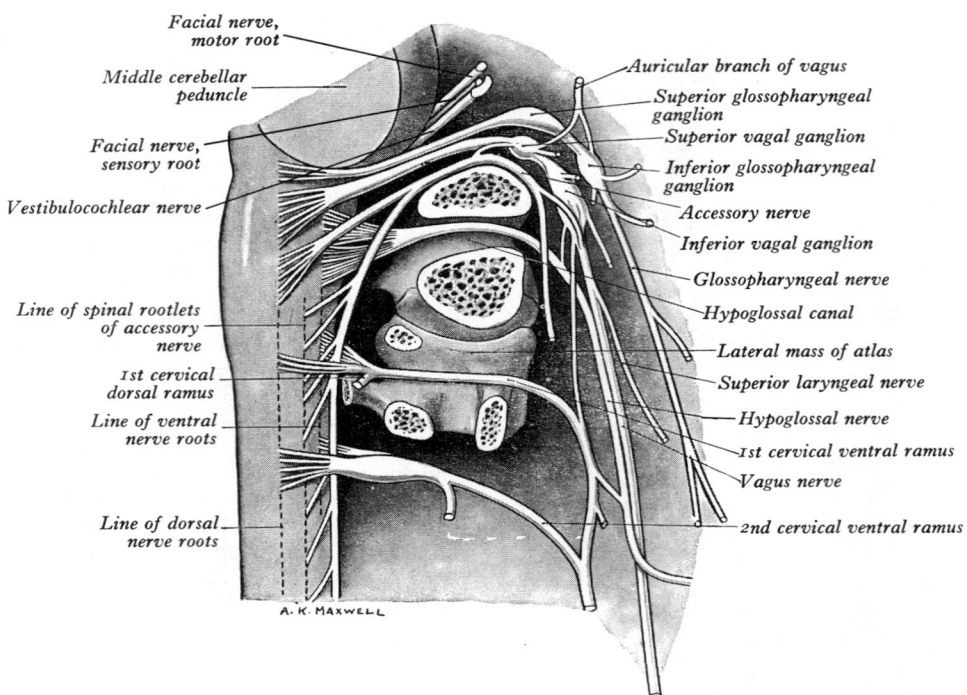

Facial nerve,
motor root

Middle cerebellar
peduncle

Facial nerve,
sensory root

Vestibulocochlear nerve

Line of spinal rootlets
of accessory
nerve

1st cervical
dorsal ramus

Line of ventral
nerve roots

Line of dorsal
nerve roots

A. K. MAXWELL

Auricular branch of vagus

Superior glossopharyngeal
ganglion

Superior vagal ganglion

Inferior glossopharyngeal
ganglion

Accessory nerve

Inferior vagal ganglion

Glossopharyngeal nerve

Hypoglossal canal

Lateral mass of atlas

Superior laryngeal nerve

Hypoglossal nerve

1st cervical ventral ramus

Vagus nerve

2nd cervical ventral ramus

8.355   The communications between the last four cranial nerves of the right side viewed from the dorsolateral aspect. The hypoglossal canal has been split in its long axis and the transverse process of the atlas has been divided close to the lateral mass. The descending branch of the hypoglossal nerve is not shown.

HYPOGLOSSAL NERVE

The hypoglossal nerve (**8**.129, 357, 358) is motor to all the muscles of the tongue, except the palatoglossus. (It has been suggested that the palatoglossus is innervated from two sources, namely from the nucleus ambiguus and also from the lateral hypoglossal nucleus (Sokoloff & Deacon 1992).) The hypoglossal lies in series with the oculomotor, trochlear and abducent nerves and the ventral nerve roots of the spinal nerves and represents the fused ventral roots of probably four precervical or spino-occipital nerves whose dorsal roots have disappeared.

The hypoglossal nucleus

This is in line with the spinal anterior grey column. It is about 2 cm long, its rostral part corresponding with the hypoglossal triangle in the floor of the fourth ventricle (p. 1209), its caudal part extending into the closed part of the medulla oblongata, where it is ventral and paramedial in the central grey matter (**8**.128). Its fibres pass ventrally through the medulla to emerge as a linear series of 10–15 rootlets in the anteriolateral sulcus between the pyramid and olive (**8**.124).

The hypoglossal nucleus is organized into two main nuclear tiers, either ventral and dorsal or ventromedial and dorsolateral (according to species studied), each divisible into a medial–lateral sequence of subnuclei (Kosaka & Yagita 1903; Sturman 1916; Barnard 1940; O'Reilley & Fitzgerald 1990). In the hypoglossal nucleus of the cynomolgus monkey, the medial nucleus consists of a pars medialis and a pars intermedialis and the lateral nucleus contains a pars ventralis and a pars dorsalis with, in addition, cell columns constituting small ventral and ventrocaudal nuclei (Sokoloff & Deacon 1992).

There is a musculotopic organization of motor neurons within the hypoglossal nuclei which corresponds to structural and functional divisions of tongue musculature. Thus, motor neurons innervating tongue retrusor muscles are located in dorsal or dorsolateral nuclei, whereas motor neurons innervating the main tongue protrusor muscle are located in ventral, ventromedial or intermediate regions of the nucleus (Krammer et al 1979; Uemura et al 1979; Lowe 1981).

This basic pattern of musculotopic organization has been found in all mammals studied (cat, dog, monkey, rat), and is apparently conserved in non-mammalian vertebrates. Although relatively little is known about the organization of motor neurons innervating the intrinsic muscles of the tongue, a recent tract-tracing study in the cynomolgus monkey has revealed that motor neurons of the medial divisions of the hypoglossal nucleus innervate tongue muscles that are oriented in planes transverse to the long axis of the tongue (transverse and vertical intrinsics and genioglossus), whereas motor neurons of the lateral divisions innervate tongue muscles that are oriented parallel to this axis (styloglossus, hyoglossus, superior and inferior longitudinal) (Sokoloff & Deacon 1992). It is possible that the overlap of motor neuron pools innervating similarly oriented extrinsic and intrinsic muscles may facilitate the simultaneous recruitment of these muscles.

Connections and course

The hypoglossal nucleus receives corticonuclear fibres from the precentral gyrus and adjacent areas of mainly the contralateral hemisphere, some fibres leave the tract in the pons to travel in the medial lemniscus; they connect with the nucleus directly or via internuncial neurons. Evidence indicates that the most medial subnuclei receive projections from both hemispheres. The nucleus may connect with the cerebellum via adjacent perihypoglossal nuclei (Torvik & Brodal 1954) and perhaps also with the medullary reticular formation, the trigeminal sensory nuclei and the solitary nucleus.

The hypoglossal rootlets run laterally behind the vertebral artery, collected into two bundles which perforate the dura mater separately opposite the hypoglossal (anterior condylar) canal in the occipital bone, uniting after traversing it; the canal is sometimes divided by a bony spicule. The separate dural sheaths confirm the composite character of the nerve. It emerges from its canal in a plane medial to the internal jugular vein, internal carotid artery, ninth, tenth and eleventh cranial nerves and passes inferolaterally behind the internal carotid artery and glossopharyngeal and vagus nerves to the interval between the artery and the internal jugular vein. Here it makes a half-spiral turn round the inferior vagal ganglion, being united with it by connective tissue. It then descends almost vertically between the vessels and anterior to the vagus to a point level with the mandibular angle, becoming superficial below the posterior belly of the digastric and emerging between the internal jugular vein and internal carotid artery. It loops round the inferior sterno-cleidomastoid branch of the occipital artery (p. 1515), crosses lateral to both internal and external carotid arteries and the loop of the lingual artery a little above the tip of the greater cornu of the hyoid (8.357) and is itself crossed by the facial vein. It inclines up and forwards on the hyoglossus by passing deep to the digastric tendon, stylohyoid and the posterior border of the mylohyoid. Between the hyoglossus and mylohyoid the nerve is inferior to the deep part of the submandibular gland, submandibular duct and lingual nerve. It then passes on to the lateral aspect of the genioglossus, continuing forwards in its substance as far as the tip of the tongue and distributing fibres in the muscle.

The hypoglossal nerve communicates with the sympathetic trunk, vagus, first and second cervical nerves and lingual nerve. Near the atlas it is joined by branches from the superior cervical sympathetic ganglion and by a filament from the loop between the first and second cervical nerves which leaves the hypoglossal as the upper root of the ansa cervicalis (8.337). The vagal connections occur close to the skull, numerous filaments passing between the hypoglossal nerve and the inferior vagal ganglion in the connective tissue uniting them. As the hypoglossal nerve curves round the occipital artery it receives from the pharyngeal plexus the ramus lingualis vagi (p. 1252). Near the anterior border of hyoglossus it is connected with the lingual nerve by many filaments ascending on the muscle (p. 1239).

Branches

The branches of distribution of the hypoglossal nerve are: meningeal, descending, thyrohyoid and muscular.

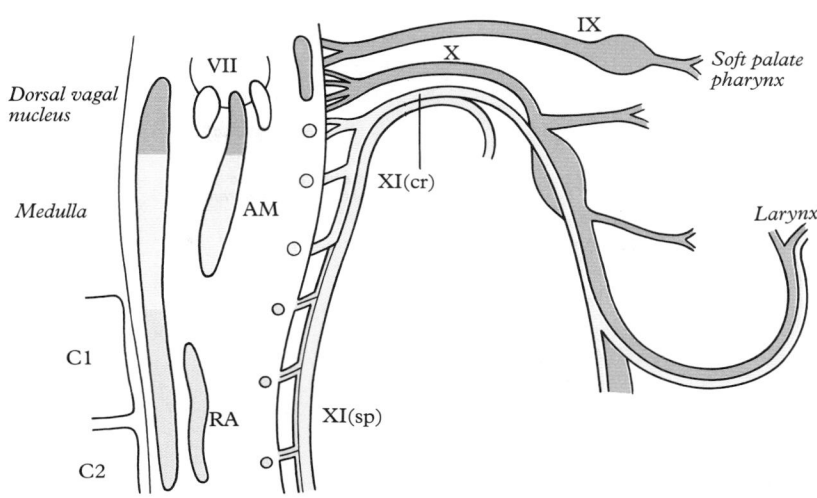

8.356 Schematic drawing showing the distribution of neurons of origin of the vago-glossopharyngeal rootlets and those of the internal ramus of the accessory nerve. AM = nucleus ambiguus; RA = nucleus retroambigualis; blue = spinal accessory root; mauve = origin and distribution of neurons of the vago-glossopharyngeal rootlets; yellow = neurons of the internal ramus traversing the rootlets of the cranial root of the accessory nerve; green = neurons traversing the spinal extension of the cranial accessory root. (After Kitamura et al 1983.)

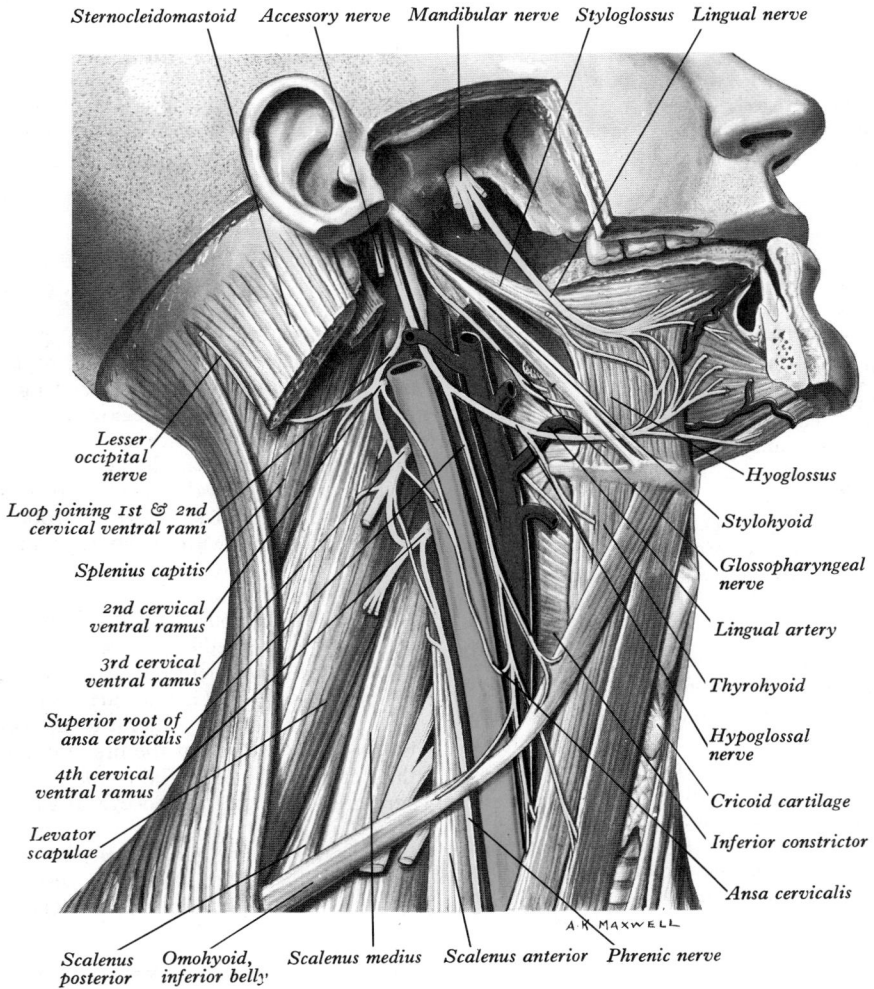

8.357 A dissection to show the general distribution of the right hypoglossal and lingual nerves and the position and constitution of some parts of the cervical plexus of the right side.

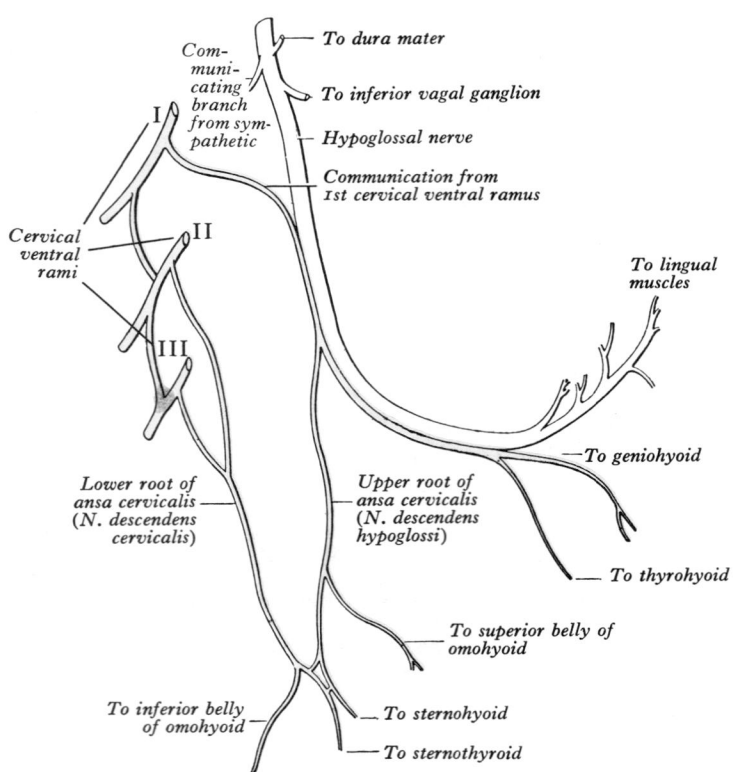

8.358 A plan of the right hypoglossal nerve and ansa cervicalis.

The meningeal branch or branches. These leave the hypoglossal nerve in its canal, returning through it to supply the diploë of the occipital bone, the dural walls of the occipital and inferior petrosal sinuses and much of the floor and anterior wall of the posterior cranial fossa. These meningeal rami (pp. 1212, 1300) may not contain hypoglossal fibres but ascending, mixed sensory and sympathetic fibres from the upper cervical nerves and superior cervical sympathetic ganglion (Kimmel 1961a,b).

The descending branch (descendens hypoglossi or upper root of the ansa cervicalis (**8.358**)). This leaves the hypoglossal nerve where it curves round the occipital artery and then descends anterior to or in the carotid sheath. It contains only fibres from the first cervical spinal nerve. After giving a branch to the superior belly of the omohyoid, it is joined by the lower root of the ansa from the second and third cervical spinal nerves. The two roots form the ansa cervicalis (ansa hypoglossi), from which branches supply the sternohyoid, sternothyroid and the inferior belly of the omohyoid; another branch is said to descend anterior to the vessels into the thorax to join the cardiac and phrenic nerves.

The nerves to the thyrohyoid and geniohyoid. These arise near the posterior border of the hyoglossus and cross obliquely the greater cornu of the hyoid to supply the thyrohyoid and geniohyoid; they contain fibres of the first cervical spinal nerve. Motor neurons innervating the geniohyoid have been demonstrated (using HRP) in subnuclei of the ventral tier of the hypoglossal nuclear complex in the macaque and in the rat (Uemura at al 1979; Uemura-Sumi et al 1981; Kitamura et al 1983; O'Reilly & Fitzgerald 1990; Sokoloff & Deacon 1992).

Muscular branches. These are distributed to the styloglossus, hyoglossus and genioglossus. Numerous slender rami ascend into the tongue to supply its intrinsic muscles; all contain true hypoglossal fibres.

Lesions of the hypoglossal nerve. Complete hypoglossal division causes unilateral lingual paralysis and hemiatrophy; the protruded tongue deviates to the paralysed side; on retraction, the wasted and paralysed side also rises higher than the unaffected side. The larynx may deviate towards the active side in swallowing, due to unilateral paralysis of the hyoid depressors. If paralysis is bilateral, the tongue is motionless. Taste and tactile sensibility are unaffected but articulation is slow and swallowing very difficult.

THE SPINAL NERVES

General organisation

Spinal nerves are united ventral and dorsal spinal roots, attached in series to the sides of the spinal cord. There are 31 pairs: 8 cervical, 12 thoracic, 5 lumbar, 5 sacral, 1 coccygeal (**16.8**). The abbreviations C, T, L, S and Co, with appropriate numerals, are commonly applied to individual nerves. These emerge through intervertebral foramina; C1 leaves the vertebral canal between the occipital bone and atlas and is hence often termed the *suboccipital nerve*; C8 passes between the seventh cervical and first thoracic vertebrae (p. 1275). Each nerve is continuous with the spinal cord by the ventral and dorsal roots, the latter each bearing a *spinal ganglion*.

Ventral (anterior) roots

These contain axons of neurons in the anterior and lateral spinal grey columns. Each emerges as a series of *rootlets* in two or three irregular rows in an area about 3 mm in horizontal width. In rats the rootlets of lumbar ventral roots are each ensheathed by a single fenestrated layer of cells. At the spinal cord surface the rootlets are separated by a labyrinth of interradicular spaces lined by this sheath. Between adjacent rootlets the interradicular spaces, which contain small blood vessels, taper distally. The interradicular spaces communicate with the endoneurial spaces of the rootlets and with the subpial space but are isolated from the subarachnoid space by the multilayered, unfenestrated sheath which surrounds the aggregations of rootlets which comprise each ventral root (Kaar & Fraher 1986).

Dorsal (posterior) roots

These contain centripetal processes of neurons sited in the spinal ganglia. Each consists of medial and lateral fascicles both diverging into rootlets entering along the posterolateral sulcus. In many mammals, including humans, the rootlets of adjacent dorsal roots are often connected by oblique filaments, especially in the lower cervical and lumbosacral regions (Pallie & Manuel 1968).

Each root is covered by the pia mater and is loosely invested by the arachnoid mater prolonged to where the roots pierce the dura mater. The dorsal and ventral roots do so separately, each receiving a dural sheath (**8.361**); where the roots unite to form spinal nerves these sheaths fuse with the epineurium.

Spinal ganglia

These are large groups of neurons on the dorsal spinal roots (**8.359**). Each is oval and reddish, its size being related to that of its root; it is bifid medially where the two fascicles of the dorsal root emerge to enter the cord. Ganglia are usually sited in the intervertebral foramina, immediately lateral to the perforation of the dura mater by the roots (**8.89**), but the first and second cervical ganglia are on the vertebral arches of the atlas and axis, the sacral inside the vertebral canal and the coccygeal ganglion usually within the dura mater.

The first cervical ganglia may be absent. Small aberrant ganglia sometimes occur on the upper cervical dorsal roots between the spinal ganglia and cord. (Heterotopic ganglionic neurons also occur in other sites, see p. 782.)

Internal structure of sensory ganglia

The cytological organization within cranial and spinal ganglia is similar (p. 846 and consult Van Gehuchten 1892; Marinesco 1909; Cajal 1911; De Castro 1932; Scharf 1958; Lieberman 1976). Each sensory ganglion has a laminar connective tissue capsule continuous

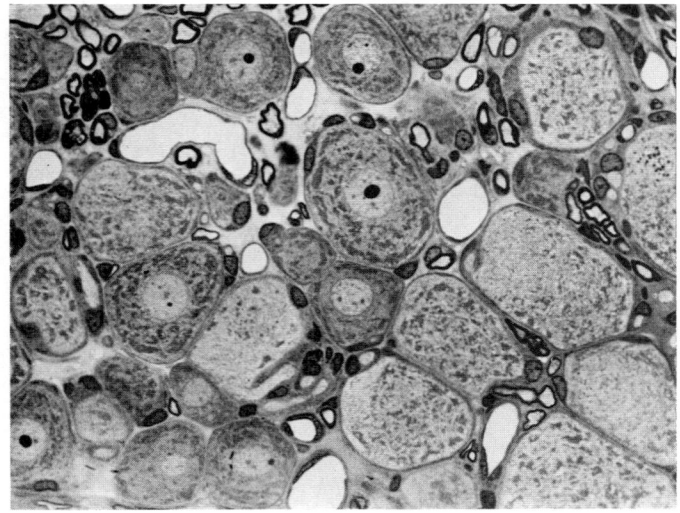

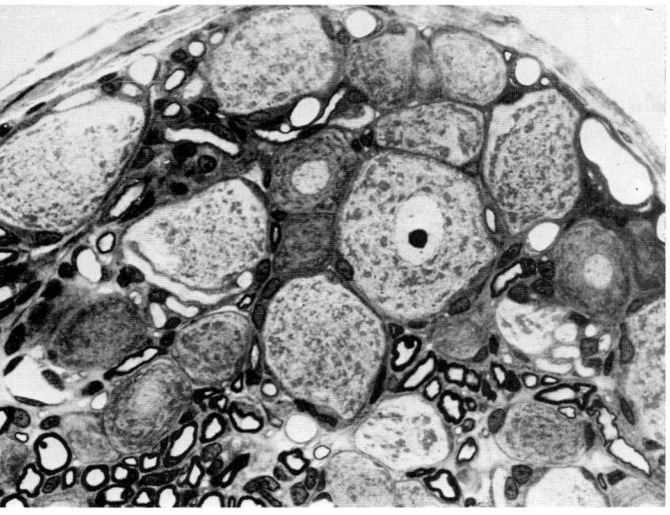

8.359 Two photographs of fields in normal rat cervical dorsal root ganglion to show contrasting features of light and dark neuronal somata. Note the capsules of satellite cells; the darkly stained multiple profiles between many of the nerve cells represent glomeruli in repeated transverse section. Interneuronal capillary profiles are also visible. Cresyl fast violet staining of semithin sections of material embedded in araldite. (Photographs supplied by J M Jacobs, National Hospital for Nervous Diseases, London.)

with the epineurium of the spinal root. Endoneurial stroma permeates the ganglion, supporting its neuronal and axonal population; perineurial capsular trabeculae extend between groups of these elements. The stroma is intimately related to the satellite cells (amphicytes); it contains a few mast cells and a dense vascular network, denser around ganglion cells, into which capillary loops may be invaginated (Scharf 1958). These capillaries are non-fenestrated in rodents (Lieberman 1968) but commonly fenestrated in primates (Olsson 1971). Ganglionic vascular permeability varies among species, amounting to a 'blood–nerve' barrier in some, largely dependent on the junctional complexes between endothelial cells; details are not available for mankind. Ganglionic neurons vary in size (15–110 μm in man, Ohta et al 1974); most are spheroidal but smaller cells appear ellipsoidal or angular in section.

Ganglionic neurons resemble other neurons but vary greatly in the distribution of cytoplasmic chromatin, from fine dispersal to concentration in large masses (Nissl granules); this has been the chief basis of many classifications, which remain conflicting. Melanin and lipofuchsin pigments occur in some but less than in some cranial sensory ganglia. Dense-cored vesicles are common (Lieberman 1968), despite the apparent absence of catecholamines. However, the occurrence of two extreme types is agreed: large 'light' neurons (A cells) and small 'dark' ones (B cells). In 'light' cells the granular

endoplasmic reticulum is more dispersed but highly concentrated in 'dark' cells. The latter are sometimes mimicked by artefact, perhaps due to poor fixation. Both types appear in prenatal material. Functional differences remain unclarified but the axons of A cells are said to be myelinated and those of B cells non-myelinated. It has been suggested that B cells are visceral. 'Atypical' neurons have been described in dorsal root and other sensory ganglia, the most interesting being reputed to be multipolar neurons; but since synapses have not been identified in dorsal root ganglia, this is improbable and is unconfirmed. Almost all ganglionic neurons are unipolar (p. 904), many with a coiled 'stem' process close to the parent soma, forming an axonal 'glomerulus' before branching into peripheral and central parts (p. 945). Spinal ganglionic cells have been submitted to ultrastructural studies (Duce & Keen 1977), assessment of specific intracellular substances (Hokfelt et al 1976), preferential glutamine absorption (Duce & Keen 1978) and specific reactions to neurotoxins (Jancsco et al 1977). Such data, while confirming 'light' and 'dark' cells, collectively suggest a subdivision into further types, particularly of 'dark' cells. Small dark cells may occur in at least two variants, differentiated by production of either SP or somatostatin. Different cells respond also to different neurotoxins or differ in glutamine metabolism.

Counts of cells in the dorsal root ganglia show specific variation, as expected; few estimates exist for human ganglia. Maximal counts are reached about 3 years after birth; but the subsequent supposed loss has not been confirmed. The distribution of somata and axons is variable, the former often being peripherally concentrated; but grouping of the somata between large fascicles of axons is described as more usual in human ganglia. Such grouping may indicate somatopic organization, sometimes described in terms of somata and axons. Burton and McFarlane (1973), by injection of labelled amino acids into ganglia, associated local groups of neurons in lumbar ganglia of the cat with branches of spinal nerves and also with particular spinal roots. Horseradish peroxidase injections near peripheral receptor endings have produced more exact results in rodent sensory ganglia; no results are available for primates.

Appearance and orientation of spinal roots

The size and direction of spinal nerve roots vary. The upper four *cervical* roots are small, the lower four large. Cervical dorsal roots have a thickness ratio to the ventral roots of three to one, greater than in other regions. The first dorsal root is an exception, being smaller than the ventral; in about 8% it is absent. The first and second cervical roots are short, running almost horizontally to their exits from the vertebral canal. From the third to the eighth cervical they slope obliquely down, obliquity and length increasing successively; the distance between spinal attachment and vertebral exit never exceeds the height of one vertebra.

Thoracic roots, except the first, are small, the dorsal only slightly exceeding the ventral in thickness. They increase successively in length and in the lower thoracic region descend in contact with the spinal cord for at least two vertebrae before emerging from the vertebral canal (but see below).

Kubik and Müntener (1969) consider that the cervicothoracic part of the spinal cord grows more in length than other parts and thus explain their observations which differ from the above remarks. They state that upper cervical roots **descend**, the fifth being horizontal, and that the sixth to eighth actually **ascend**, that the first two thoracic roots are horizontal, the next three ascend, the sixth is horizontal and the rest descend.

Lower *lumbar* and upper *sacral roots* are the largest and their radicles the most numerous, while the *coccygeal roots* are the smallest. Kubik and Müntener (1969) confirm that lumbar, sacral and coccygeal roots descend with increasing obliquity to their exits; since the spinal cord ends near the lower border of the first lumbar vertebra, the lengths of successive roots rapidly increase. The consequent collection of roots is the *cauda equina* (**8.88**).

The largest roots and the hence largest spinal nerves are continuous with the spinal cervical and lumbar swellings and innervate the upper and lower limbs.

Immediately distal to the spinal ganglia, ventral and dorsal roots unite to form *spinal nerves* which emerge through intervertebral foramina and give off recurrent meningeal branches (see below), dividing immediately into *dorsal* and *ventral rami* (**8.361**). (From

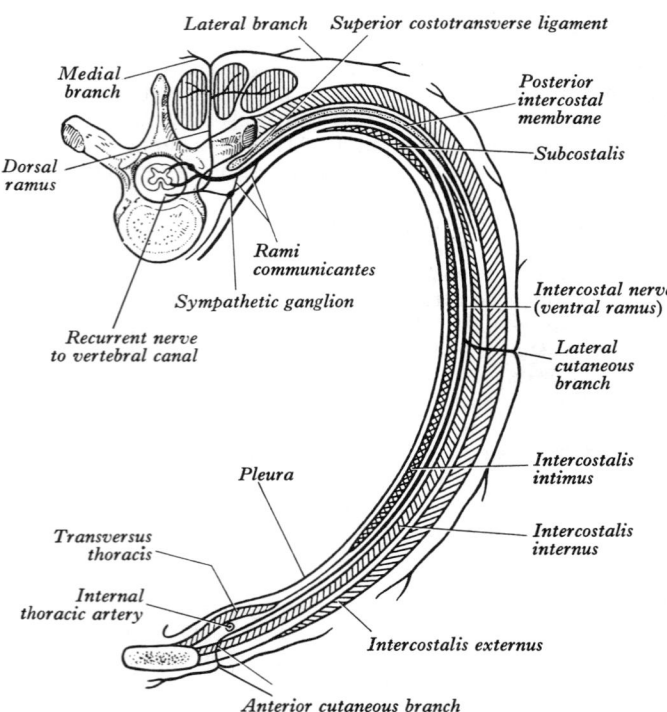

8.360 The course of a typical intercostal nerve. The muscular and the collateral branches are not shown.

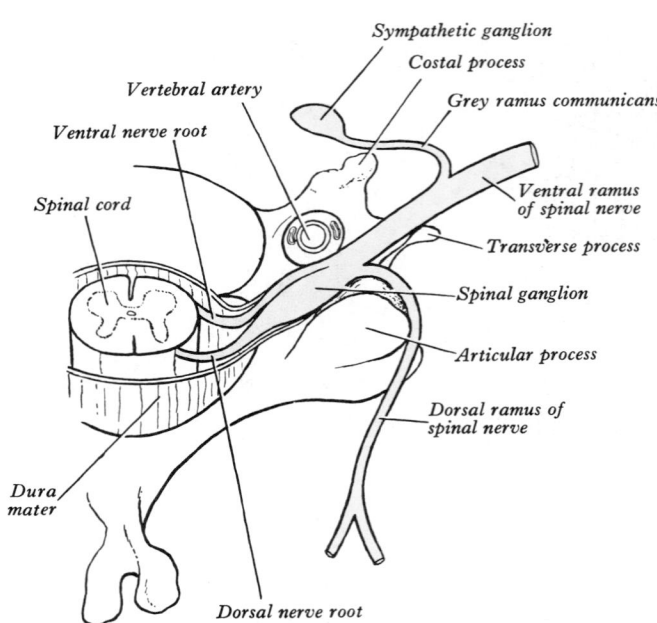

8.361 Scheme showing the relations of a cervical nerve and its ganglion to a cervical vertebra.

limited dissections Sato (1974) has described the *trifurcation* of spinal nerves at some cervical and thoracic levels, the third branch being a *ramus intermedius*.) At or distal to its origin each ventral ramus receives a *grey ramus communicans* from the corresponding sympathetic ganglion, while the thoracic and first and second lumbar ventral rami each contribute a *white ramus communicans* to the corresponding ganglia (**8**.361, 362). The second, third and fourth sacral nerves also supply visceral branches, unconnected with sympathetic ganglia, which carry a parasympathetic outflow direct to the pelvic plexuses (pp. 1298, 1309).

Cervical spinal nerves enlarge from the first to the sixth, the seventh and eighth cervical and first thoracic being like the sixth cervical in size. The remaining thoracic nerves are relatively small. Lumbar nerves are large, increasing in size from the first to the fifth. The first sacral is the largest spinal nerve, thereafter they decrease to the coccygeal, the smallest.

Intervertebral foramina. Here spinal nerves have clinically important relations. Anterior are the intervertebral discs and adjacent vertebral bodies. Posterior are the synovial zygapophysial joints. Superior and inferior are vertebral notches of the pedicles of adjoining vertebrae. Each nerve, accompanied by a spinal artery, a small venous plexus and its own meningeal branch or branches together traverse a foramen.

Lesions of the conus and cauda equina

These lesions cause bilateral deficit, often with pain in the back extending into the sacral segments and to the legs. Loss of bladder function and impotence are early features. There are lower motor neuron signs in the legs with fasciculation and muscle atrophy. Sensory loss usually involves the peroneal or 'saddle area' as well as involving other lumbar and sacral dermatomes. Tumours which may affect the conus and cauda equina include neurofibroma, meningioma, ependymoma, astrocytoma and metastatic carcinoma. There may be congenital abnormalities such as spina bifida, lipomata or dystematomyelia with the conus extending below the lower border of L1, often with a tethered filum terminalae. Extramedullary lesions include prolapsed intervertebral discs. A midline disc protrusion in the lumbar region may present with involvement of the sacral segments only.

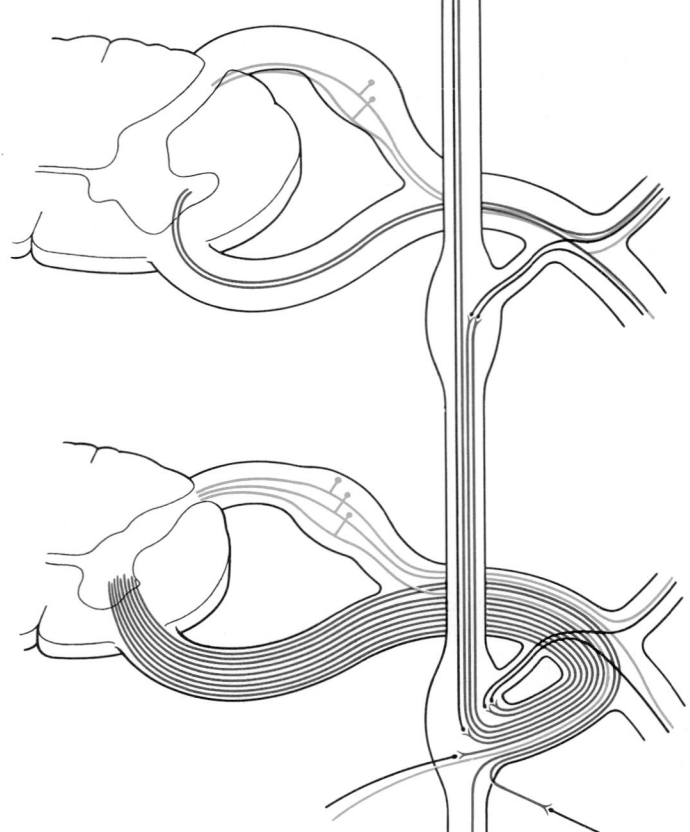

8.362 Scheme showing the constitution of a typical spinal nerve. In the upper part of the diagram the spinal nerve roots show the somatic components; in the lower part of the diagram the spinal roots show the visceral components. Red = somatic efferent and preganglionic sympathetic fibres, blue = somatic afferent and visceral afferent fibres, black = post-ganglionic sympathetic fibres.

Lesions of the spinal roots

The spinal roots may be damaged as they leave the vertebral column through the foraminae. In the cervical region the nerve root exits above the correspondingly numbered vertebra, so that the C5 root would be affected by prolapse of the C4/5 disc. However, since there are eight cervical nerve roots and only seven cervical vertebrae, this relationship changes at the cervicothoracic junction, so that below this level the nerve root emerges below the correspondingly numbered vertebra. In the lumbar spine the nerve root leaves the vertebral column laterally above the disc and is affected by a prolapsed disc at one level above its exit. For example the L5 root, which emerges between L5 and S1, is usually affected by disc prolapse between L4 and 5. The nerve roots lie alongside the disc, so that rupture of the annulus with disc herniation causes root compression, usually where the nerve still lies within the dura in a root sleeve (the lateral recess syndrome): compression of the nerve root can be demonstrated with intrathecal contrast material. The dorsal root ganglion is situated in the foramen just outside the dura. Neurofibromas may occur on the nerve roots in the exit foraminae, and as they enlarge become dumbbell in shape with both an intra- and extraspinal component. Plain X-rays show enlargement of the foramina.

Root compression usually presents acutely with pain which may be severe and this pain is felt in the myotome, not in the dermatome, whereas paraesthesiae and numbness occurs in the dermatome. It may be difficult to demonstrate sensory loss due to extensive overlap of the dermatomes. The spinal reflex is lost early. Traction injury may cause avulsion of spinal roots from the spinal cord in the cervical region and this is not recoverable.

FUNCTIONAL COMPONENTS OF SPINAL NERVES

Each typical spinal nerve contains somatic and visceral fibres.

Somatic components. These are efferent and afferent. Somatic efferent fibres for the innervation of skeletal muscles are axons of a, β and γ neurons in the spinal anterior grey column. Somatic afferent fibres convey impulses into the CNS from receptors in the skin, subcutaneous tissue, muscles, fasciae, joints, etc. (pp. 962–965); they are peripheral processes of unipolar neurons in the spinal ganglia.

Visceral components. These are also afferent and efferent, and belong to the autonomic nervous system (p. 1292). They include sympathetic or parasympathetic fibres at different spinal levels. Preganglionic *visceral efferent* sympathetic fibres are axons of neurons in the spinal lateral grey column in the thoracic and upper two or three lumbar segments; they join the sympathetic trunk along corresponding white rami communicantes to synapse with postganglionic neurons distributed to non-striated muscle or glands. The preganglionic *visceral efferent* parasympathetic fibres are axons of cells in the spinal lateral grey column of the second to fourth sacral segments; they leave the ventral rami of corresponding sacral nerves to synapse in pelvic ganglia, the postganglionic axons being distributed mainly to muscle or glands in the walls of the pelvic viscera. *Visceral afferent* fibres are from neurons in the spinal ganglia. Their peripheral processes pass through white rami communicantes and, without synapsing, through one or more sympathetic ganglia to end in viscera. Some visceral afferent fibres may enter the spinal cord in ventral roots; Coggeshall et al (1973) claim that almost 30% of fibres in the feline seventh lumbar and first sacral ventral roots are nonmyelinated afferents, which may project into the cord from neurons in the corresponding dorsal root ganglia.

Central processes of ganglionic unipolar neurons enter the spinal cord by posterior roots and connect with somatic or sympathetic efferent neurons, usually through interneurons, completing reflex paths, or they synapse with other neurons in the spinal or brainstem grey matter which provide a variety of ascending tracts.

Little detail of the dendrites of spinal autonomic neurons is available. Schramm et al (1976) showed that sympathetic efferent neurons have largely horizontal dendritic arrays in newborn rats, reorientated into longitudinal arrays in the next 5 or 6 postnatal weeks. No such data are available for the human spinal cord.

After emerging from its intervertebral foramen each spinal nerve supplies small *meningeal branches* and splits almost at once into *dorsal* and *ventral rami*, both receiving fibres from both roots.

Meningeal branches. The *recurrent meningeal* or *sinuvertebral nerves*, numbering two to four filaments on each side, occur at all vertebral levels (Kimmel 1961a,b). Each receives one or more rami from a nearby grey ramus communicans or from a thoracic sympathetic ganglion directly; most then pursue a recurrent (often perivascular) course into the spinal canal through the intervertebral foramen ventral to the dorsal root ganglion. Here these mixed sensory and sympathetic nerves divide into transverse, ascending and descending branches distributed to the dura mater, the walls of blood vessels, the periosteum, ligaments and intervertebral discs in the ventrolateral region of the spinal canal. Fine meningeal branches occasionally pass dorsal to the spinal ganglia to the dorsal dura, periosteum and ligaments, others passing ventrally to the posterior longitudinal ligament. Ascending branches of the upper three cervical meningeal nerves are large and distributed to the dura mater in the posterior cranial fossa (p. 1212). Meningeal nerves are important in relation to the referred pain characteristic of many spinal disorders and in occipital headache.

DORSAL RAMI OF THE SPINAL NERVES

Dorsal (posterior primary) rami of spinal nerves, usually smaller than the ventral and directed posteriorly, divide (except for the first cervical, fourth and fifth sacral and the coccygeal) into medial and lateral branches to supply the muscles and skin (**8.363**) of the posterior regions of the neck and trunk.

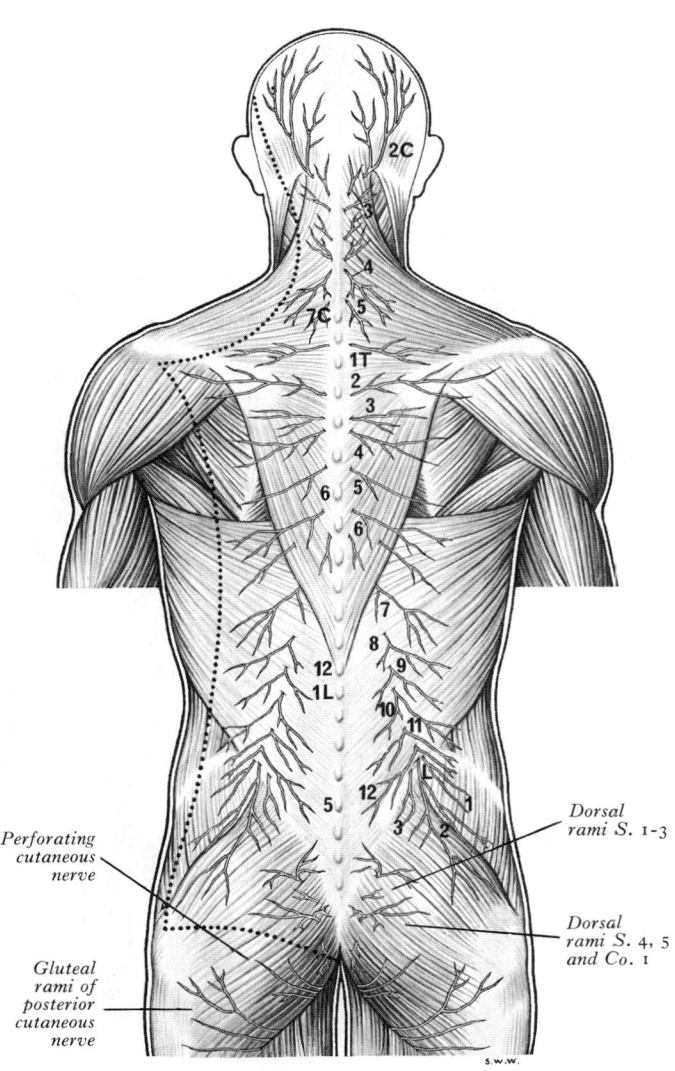

8.363 The cutaneous distribution of the dorsal rami of the spinal nerves. The nerves are shown lying on the superficial muscles; on the left side the limit of the skin area supplied by these nerves is indicated by the dotted line. The nerves are numbered on the right side and the spines of the seventh cervical, sixth and twelfth thoracic and first and fifth lumbar vertebrae are labelled on the left side.

CERVICAL DORSAL RAMI

Each cervical spinal dorsal ramus, except the first, divides into medial and lateral branches, all innervating muscles; but in general only medial branches of the second to fourth and usually the fifth supply the skin. Except for the first and second, each dorsal ramus passes back medial to a posterior intertransverse muscle, curving round the articular process into the interval between the semispinalis capitis and semispinalis cervicis.

First cervical dorsal ramus (suboccipital nerve). Larger than the ventral, this emerges superior to the posterior atlantal arch and inferior to the vertebral artery. It enters the suboccipital triangle to supply local muscles: the rectus capitis posterior major and minor, superior and inferior oblique and the semispinalis capitis. A filament from the branch to the inferior oblique joins the second dorsal ramus. The suboccipital nerve occasionally has a cutaneous branch which accompanies the occipital artery to the scalp, connecting with the greater and lesser occipital nerves.

Second cervical dorsal ramus. Slightly larger than the ventral and all other cervical dorsal rami, this emerges between the posterior atlantal arch and the lamina of the axis, below the inferior oblique which it supplies, receiving a connection from the first cervical dorsal ramus, and divides into a large medial and smaller lateral branch. Its ganglion is extradural. The medial branch, termed the greater occipital nerve (**8.363, 364**), ascends between the inferior oblique and semispinalis capitis, pierces the latter and the trapezius near their occipital attachments and is joined by a filament from the medial branch of the third dorsal ramus; ascending with the occipital artery, it divides into branches which connect with the lesser occipital nerve and supply the skin of the scalp as far forward as the vertex. It supplies the semispinalis capitis and occasionally the back of the auricle. The lateral branch supplies the splenius, longissimus capitis and semispinalis capitis and is often joined by the corresponding third cervical branch.

Greater occipital neuralgia. This syndrome of pain and paraesthesiae felt in the distribution of the greater occipital nerve is usually due to an entrapment neuropathy of the nerve as it pierces the attachment of the neck extensors to the occiput. A similar syndrome may be due to upper apophyseal arthritis involving the second cervical root.

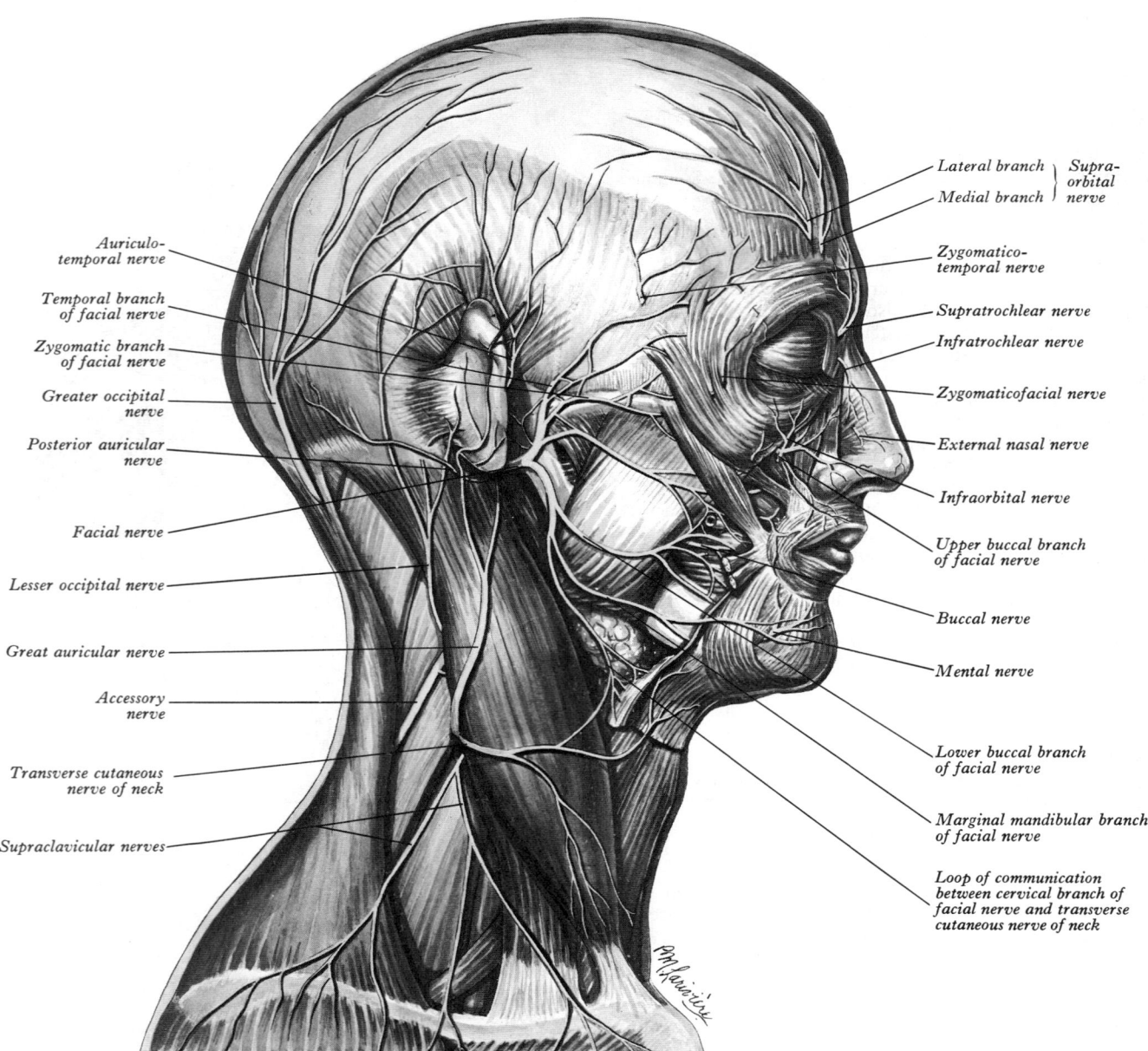

8.364 The nerves of the right side of the scalp, face and side of the neck.

Third cervical dorsal ramus. This is between the second and fourth in size, and courses back round the third cervical articular pillar, medial to the posterior intertransverse muscle, dividing into medial and lateral branches. Its medial branch runs between the spinalis capitis and semispinalis cervicis, piercing the splenius and trapezius to end in the skin. Deep to the trapezius it gives rise to a branch, the third occipital nerve, which pierces the trapezius to end in the skin of the lower occipital region (**8.363**), medial to the greater occipital nerve and connected to it. The lateral branch often joins that of the second cervical dorsal ramus. The dorsal ramus of the suboccipital and medial branches of the dorsal rami of the second and third cervical nerves are sometimes joined by loops to form the posterior cervical plexus.

Dorsal rami of the lower five cervical nerves. These curve back round the vertebral articular pillars and divide into medial and lateral branches. Medial branches of the fourth and fifth run between the semispinalis cervicis and semispinalis capitis, reach the vertebral spines and pierce the splenius and trapezius to end in the skin (**8.363**). The fifth medial branch may not reach the skin. The medial branches of the lowest three cervical nerves are small and end in the semispinalis cervicis, semispinalis capitis, multifidus and interspinales. The lateral branches supply the iliocostalis cervicis, longissimus cervicis and longissimus capitis.

THORACIC DORSAL SPINAL RAMI

Thoracic dorsal rami pass backwards close to the vertebral zygapophyseal joints to divide into medial and lateral branches. Each medial branch emerges between a joint and medial edges of the superior costotransverse ligament and intertransverse muscle, but each lateral branch runs in the interval between ligament and muscle before inclining posterior on the medial side of the levator costae.

Medial branches of the upper six thoracic dorsal rami pass between and supply the semispinalis thoracis and multifidus; they pierce the rhomboids and trapezius, reaching the skin near the vertebral spines (**8.363**).

Medial branches of the lower six thoracic dorsal rami chiefly supply the multifidus and longissimus thoracis and occasionally skin in the median region. Lateral branches increase inferiorly in size, running through or deep to the longissimus thoracis to the interval between it and the iliocostalis cervicis, supplying these muscles and the levatores costarum; the lower five or six also have cutaneous branches, piercing the serratus posterior inferior and latissimus dorsi in line with the costal angles (**8.363**). Some upper thoracic lateral branches also supply the skin. The twelfth thoracic lateral branch sends a filament medially along the iliac crest, then passes down to the anterior gluteal skin. Medial cutaneous branches of the thoracic dorsal rami descend close to the vertebral spines before reaching the skin; lateral branches descend as far as the level of four ribs before becoming superficial, the branch of the twelfth thoracic reaching the skin a little above the iliac crest.

LUMBAR DORSAL SPINAL RAMI

Lumbar dorsal rami pass back medial to the medial intertransverse muscles, dividing into medial and lateral branches.

Medial branches run near the vertebral articular processes to end in the multifidus; they are related to the bone between the accessory and mamillary processes and may groove it, traversing a distinct notch or even a foramen. **Lateral** branches supply the erector spinae (sacrospinalis). In addition, the upper three give rise to cutaneous nerves which pierce the aponeurosis of the latissimus dorsi at the lateral border of the erector spinae and cross the iliac posteriorly to reach the gluteal skin (**8.363**), some reaching as far as the level of the greater trochanter.

SACRAL DORSAL SPINAL RAMI

Sacral dorsal rami are small, diminishing downwards; excepting the fifth, they emerge though the dorsal sacral foramina. The upper three are covered at the exit by the multifidus, dividing into medial and lateral branches. Medial branches are small and end in the multifidus. Lateral branches join together and with lateral branches of the last lumbar and fourth sacral dorsal rami form loops dorsal to the sacrum; from these loops branches run dorsal to the sacrotuberous ligament to form a second series of loops under the gluteus maximus; from these two or three gluteal branches pierce the gluteus maximus (along a line from the posterior superior iliac spine to the coccygeal apex) to supply the posterior gluteal skin (**8.363**).

The dorsal rami of the fourth and fifth sacral nerves are small and lie below the multifidus. They unite with each other and the coccygeal dorsal ramus to form loops dorsal to the sacrum; filaments from these supply the skin over the coccyx. Berthold and Carlstedt (1977) have recorded a detailed study of the feline first sacral nerve at its junction with the spinal cord.

COCCYGEAL DORSAL SPINAL RAMUS

This does not divide into medial and lateral branches. Its connections and distribution are noted above.

VENTRAL RAMI OF THE SPINAL NERVES

The ventral rami of spinal nerves supply the limbs and the anterolateral aspects of the trunk; they are mostly larger than the dorsal rami. The thoracic are independent and retain, like all dorsal rami, a largely segmental distribution. The cervical, lumbar and sacral connect near their origins to form plexuses. Dorsal rami do not join these plexuses.

CERVICAL VENTRAL RAMI

Cervical ventral rami, except the first, appear between the anterior and posterior intertransverse muscles. The upper four form a *cervical plexus*; the lower four, with most of the first thoracic ventral ramus, form a *brachial plexus*. Each receives at least one grey ramus communicans, the upper four from the superior cervical sympathetic ganglion, the fifth and sixth from the middle ganglion and the seventh and eighth from the cervicothoracic ganglion (p. 1302).

The *first cervical ventral ramus* (suboccipital nerve) emerges above the posterior arch of the atlas, passes forwards lateral to its lateral mass and medial to the vertebral artery. It supplies the rectus lateralis, emerges medial to it, descends anterior to the atlantal transverse process and posterior to the internal jugular vein and joins the ascending branch of the second cervical ventral ramus.

The *second cervical ventral ramus* issues between the vertebral arches of the atlas and axis, ascends between their transverse processes, passes anterior to the first posterior intertransverse muscle and emerges lateral to the vertebral artery generally between the longus capitis and levator scapulae, but when scalenus medius is attached to the atlas it intervenes between the nerve and the levator scapulae. The ramus divides into an ascending branch which joins the first cervical nerve and a descending one which joins the ascending branch of the third cervical ventral ramus.

The *third cervical ventral ramus* appears between the longus capitis and scalenus medius. The remaining ventral rami emerge between the scalenus anterior and the scalenus medius.

CERVICAL PLEXUS

The cervical plexus (**8.365**), formed by the upper four cervical ventral rami, supplies some nuchal muscles, the diaphragm and areas of skin in the head, neck and chest (**8.341**). Level with the first four vertebrae, it is deep to the internal jugular vein and sternocleidomastoid and anterior to the scalenus medius and levator scapulae. Each ramus, except the first, divides into ascending and descending parts, which unite in communicating loops. From the first loop (C2 and 3) superficial branches supply the head and neck; from the second (C3 and 4) arise cutaneous nerves of the shoulder and chest. Muscular and communicating branches arise from the same nerves. The branches are superficial or deep; the superficial perforate the cervical fascia to supply the skin while the deep branches mostly supply muscles. The superficial form ascending and descending groups and form the deep medial and lateral series.

ASCENDING SUPERFICIAL BRANCHES

These branches of the cervical plexus (8.364–366) are:

Lesser occipital	C2
Greater auricular	C2, 3
Transverse (anterior) cutaneous	C2, 3

Lesser occipital nerve (8.364, 365). Coming from the second cervical ventral ramus and sometimes also from the third, this curves around the accessory nerve and ascends along the posterior border of the sternocleidomastoid. Near the cranium it perforates the deep fascia and ascends the scalp behind the auricle, supplying the skin and connecting with the great auricular and greater occipital nerves and the posterior auricular branch of the facial. It varies in size and is sometimes double. Its *auricular branch* supplies the skin on the upper third of the medial auricular aspect and connects with the posterior branch of the great auricular nerve. The auricular branch is occasionally derived from the greater occipital nerve.

Great auricular nerve (8.364, 365). This is the largest ascending branch. It arises from the second and third cervical rami, encircles the posterior border of the sternocleidomastoid, perforates the deep fascia and ascends on the muscle beneath the platysma with the external jugular vein. It passes to the parotid gland, dividing into anterior and posterior branches. The *anterior branch* is distributed to the facial skin over the parotid gland, connecting in the gland with the facial nerve. The *posterior branch* supplies the skin over the mastoid process and on the back of the auricle (except its upper

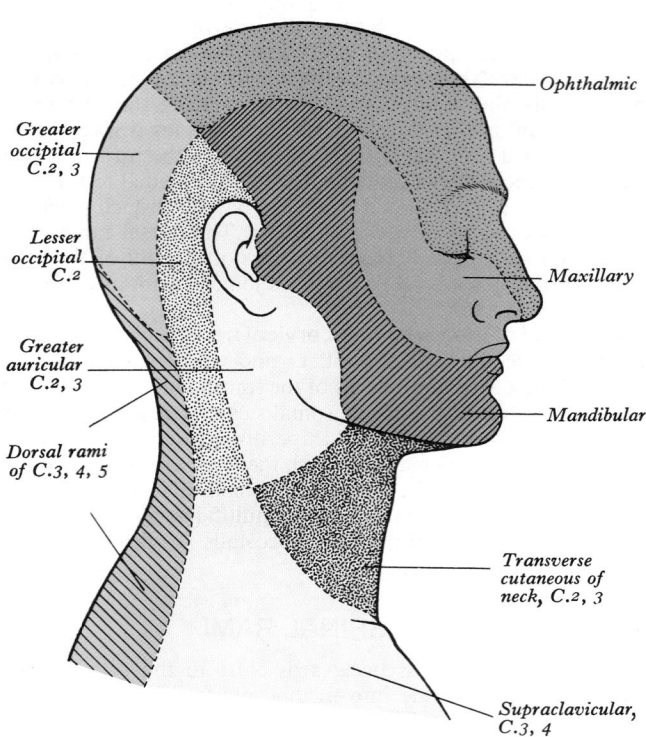

8.366 A diagram showing the cutaneous nerve supply of the face, scalp and neck. Magenta = trigeminal nerve, yellow = cervical ventral rami, blue = cervical dorsal rami.

part); a filament pierces the auricle to reach its lateral surface where it is distributed to the lobule and concha. The posterior branch communicates with the lesser occipital, the auricular branch of the vagus and the posterior auricular branch of the facial nerve.

Transverse cutaneous nerve of the neck (8.364, 365). This arises from the second and third cervical rami, curves round the posterior border of the sternocleidomastoid near its midpoint and runs obliquely forwards, deep to the external jugular vein, to the anterior border of the muscle. It perforates the deep cervical fascia, dividing under the platysma into ascending and descending branches distributed to the anterolateral areas of the neck. The *ascending branches* ascend to the submandibular region, forming a plexus with the cervical branch of the facial nerve beneath the platysma; others pierce the platysma and are distributed to the skin of the upper anterior areas of the neck. The *descending branches* pierce the platysma and are distributed anterolaterally to the skin of the neck, as low as the sternum.

DESCENDING SUPERFICIAL BRANCHES

These are supraclavicular (C3, 4): medial, intermediate and lateral.

Supraclavicular nerves (8.364, 365). These arise by a common trunk from the third and fourth cervical ventral rami and emerge from the posterior border of the sternocleidomastoid, to descend under the platysma and the deep cervical fascia; they divide into medial, intermediate and lateral (posterior) branches, which diverge to pierce the deep fascia a little above the clavicle.

The *medial supraclavicular nerves* run inferomedially across the external jugular vein and the clavicular and sternal heads of the sternocleidomastoid to supply the skin as far as the midline and as low as the second rib. They supply the sternoclavicular joint. The *intermediate supraclavicular nerves* cross the clavicle to supply the skin over the pectoralis major and deltoid down to the level of the second rib, next to the area of supply of the second thoracic nerve (8.367). Overlap between these nerves is minimal. The *lateral supraclavicular nerves* descend superficially across the trapezius and acromion, supplying the skin of the upper and posterior parts of the shoulder.

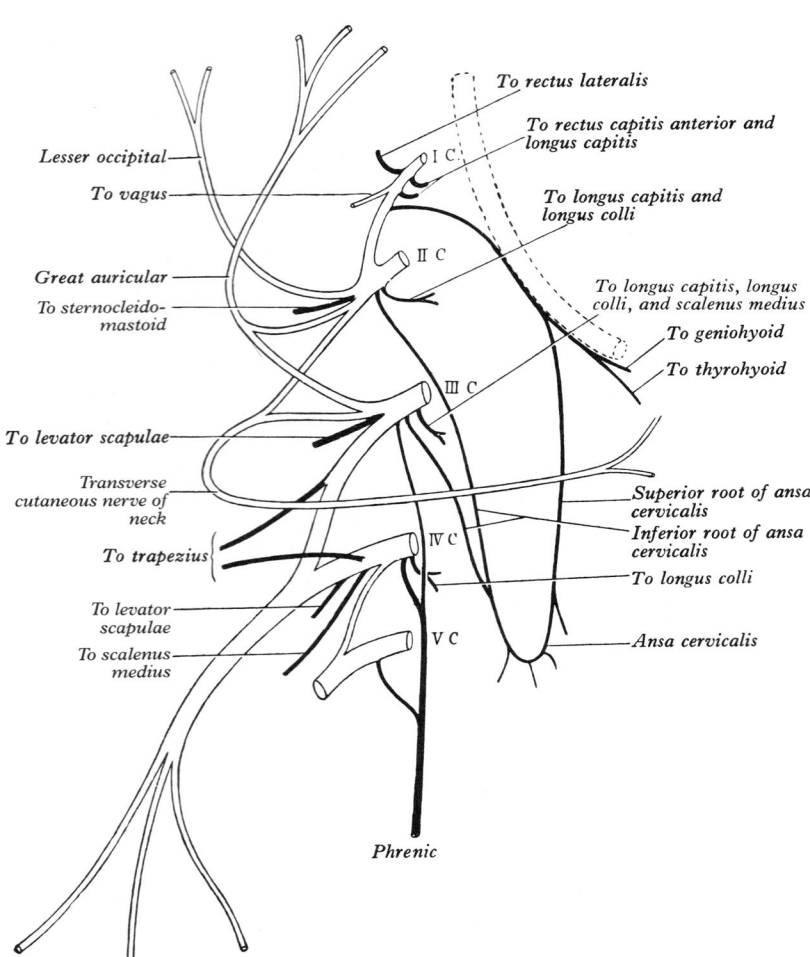

8.365 A plan of the cervical plexus. The hypoglossal nerve is shown by interrupted lines and the muscular branches by solid black lines. The roman numerals and letters I C to V C indicate the ventral rami of these cervical spinal nerves.

DEEP BRANCHES—MEDIAL SERIES

Communicating and muscular branches

Communicating branches with	Hypoglossal	C1, 2
	Vagus	C1, 2
	Sympathetic	C1–4
Muscular branches to	Rectus capitis lateralis	C1
	Rectus capitis anterior	C1, 2
	Longus capitis	C1–3
	Longus colli	C2–4
	Inferior root of ansa cervicalis	C2, 3
	Phrenic nerve	C3–5

Communicating branches. These pass from the loop between the first and second cervical rami to the vagus and hypoglossal nerves and to the sympathetic trunk. The hypoglossal branch later leaves it as a series of branches, viz. the meningeal, *superior root of ansa cervicalis*, nerves to the thyrohyoid and probably to the geniohyoid (p. 807). A branch also connects the fourth and fifth cervical rami; the first four cervical ventral rami each receive a grey ramus communicans from the superior cervical sympathetic ganglion.

Muscular branches

These supply the rectus capitis lateralis, rectus capitis anterior, longus capitis and longus colli.

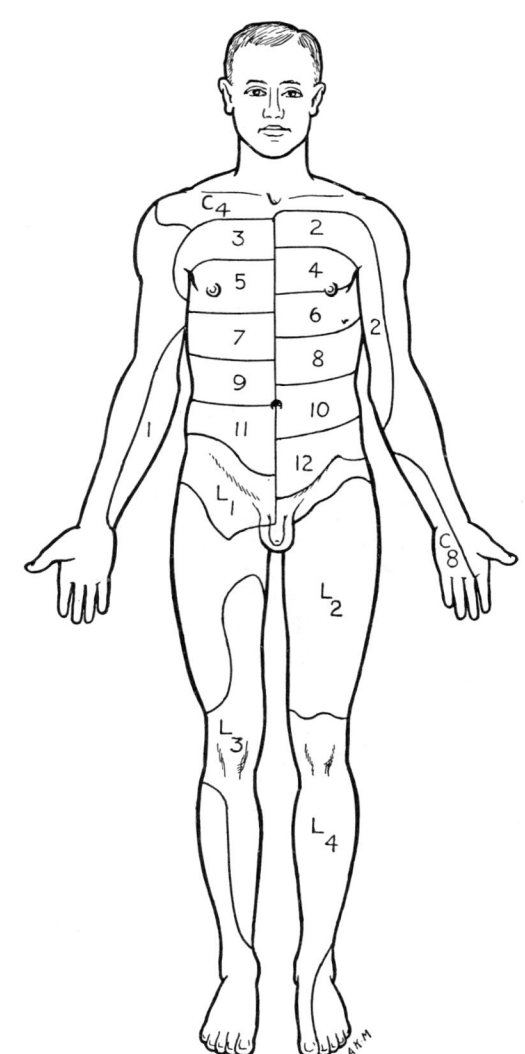

8.367 The cutaneous areas supplied by the ventral rami of the thoracic and upper four lumbar nerves (after Foerster 1933). By comparing both sides the degree of overlapping and the area of exclusive supply of any individual nerve may be estimated. See text for the areas supplied by T1 on the trunk.

Inferior root of the ansa cervicalis (nervus descendens cervicalis) (**8.365**). This is formed by the union of a branch from the second with another from the third cervical ramus. It descends on the lateral side of the internal jugular vein, crosses it a little below the middle of the neck, and continues forwards to join the superior root anterior to the common carotid artery, forming the *ansa cervicalis* (*ansa hypoglossi*) (**10.74**), from which all infrahyoid muscles are supplied, except the thyrohyoid. In 160 dissections, the inferior root was from the second and third cervical ventral rami in 74%, from the second to fourth in 14%, from the third alone in 5%, from the second yalone in 4% and from the first to third in 2% (Poriraer & Chernikov 1965).

The phrenic nerve. This is the sole motor supply to the diaphragm, and also contains widespread sensory fibres. It arises chiefly from the fourth cervical ramus but also has contributions from the third and fifth (**8.365**). Formed at the upper part of the lateral border of the scalenus anterior, it descends almost vertically across it **behind** the prevertebral fascia on its anterior surface. It descends posterior to the sternocleidomastoid, the inferior belly of omohyoid (near its intermediate tendon), the internal jugular vein, transverse cervical and suprascapular arteries (**10.73**) and, on the left, the thoracic duct. It then runs anterior to the subclavian artery, posterior to the subclavian vein and enters the thorax by crossing medially in front of the internal thoracic artery (**10.95**), after which it descends anterior to the pulmonary hilum, between the fibrous pericardium and mediastinal pleura, to the diaphragm, accompanied by the pericardiacophrenic vessels. The right and left phrenic nerves differ in their intrathoracic relations.

The *right phrenic nerve*, shorter and more vertical, is separated at the root of the neck from the second part of the right subclavian artery by the scalenus anterior. It is then lateral to the right brachiocephalic vein, the superior vena cava and the fibrous pericardium covering the right surface of the right atrium and inferior vena cava.

The *left phrenic nerve*, at the root of the neck, is commonly stated to leave the medial edge of the scalenus anterior to pass anterior to the first part of the left subclavian artery and behind the thoracic duct. However, Quist (1977) claims that both right and left nerves are **symmetrical** in their cervical course and that at the thoracic inlet the left crosses anterior to the second part of the left subclavian artery, separated by the scalenus anterior. Thereafter the left phrenic crosses anterior to the left internal thoracic artery, descending across the medial aspect of the apex of the left lung and its pleura to the first part of the subclavian artery, which it crosses obliquely to reach a groove between the left common carotid and subclavian arteries. It passes anteromedially superficial to the left vagus nerve just above the aortic arch and behind the left brachiocephalic vein. It then passes superficial to the aortic arch and the left superior intercostal vein, anterior to the left pulmonary hilum, to lie between the fibrous pericardium covering the left surface of the left ventricle and the mediastinal pleura (p. 1531).

In the neck each nerve receives variable filaments from the cervical sympathetic ganglia or their branches and may also connect with internal thoracic sympathetic plexuses (Pearson & Sauter 1971); these connections may represent a devious course of sympathetic fibres to these plexuses (p. 1303). In its thoracic course each nerve supplies sensory branches to the mediastinal pleura, fibrous pericardium and parietal serous pericardium.

Diaphragmatic relations (Merendino et al 1956; Perera & Edwards 1957). The right phrenic nerve traverses the central tendon of the diaphragm, either by the caval orifice or just lateral to it. The left phrenic nerve traverses the muscular part of the diaphragm anterior to the central tendon, just lateral to the left cardiac surface and more anterior than the right phrenic. At the diaphragm or slightly above it, each phrenic nerve supplies fine branches to the parietal pleura above, and the parietal peritoneum below, the central diaphragm. The trunk of each nerve then divides as it traverses the diaphragm into commonly three branches arranged as follows, with some variation:

(1) An *anterior* (sternal) branch runs anteromedially towards the sternum, connecting with its fellow.

(2) An *anterolateral* branch runs laterally anterior to the lateral leaf of the central tendon.

(3) A short *posterior* branch divides into a posterolateral ramus coursing behind the lateral leaf and a posterior (crural) ramus supplying the crural fibres; posterolateral and crural branches may arise separately from the phrenic nerve.

These main branches are often submerged in diaphragmatic muscle or below it; they supply motor fibres to the diaphragmatic muscle and sensory fibres to the peritoneum and pleura related to the central part of the diaphragm. They also contain proprioceptive fibres from the musculature. Location of the main branches is of importance in avoiding surgical damage. The right crus splits to enclose the oesophagus (p. 816); the right phrenic nerve supplies the part of it to the right of the oesophagus, the left supplying the left crus and the part of the right crus on the left of the oesophagus (Collis et al 1954; Thornton & Schweisthal 1969).

On the diaphragm's inferior surface phrenic rami connect with branches of the coeliac plexuses (p. 1307); on the right, at the junction of the plexuses, is a small *phrenic ganglion*. Rami from the plexuses supply the suprarenal glands and, on the right, the hepatic falciform and coronary ligaments and the inferior vena cava and possibly (via connections with coeliac and hepatic plexuses) the gallbladder (pp. 1307, 1811).

Accessory phrenic nerve. Fibres for the phrenic nerve from the fifth cervical ventral ramus often pass in a branch of the nerve to the subclavius, the accessory phrenic nerve. This lies lateral to the main nerve and descends posterior, or sometimes anterior, to the subclavian vein; it usually joins the phrenic near the first rib but may not do so until near the pulmonary hilum or beyond. An accessory phrenic nerve may be derived from the fourth or sixth cervical rami or from the ansa cervicalis (p. 1265).

Lesions of the phrenic nerve. Division of the phrenic nerve in the neck completely paralyses the corresponding half of the diaphragm, which atrophies. If an accessory phrenic nerve exists, section or crushing of the main nerve as it lies on the scalenus anterior will *not* produce complete paralysis. The phrenic nerve may be involved

with traumatic lesions of the upper brachial plexus and this can be demonstrated by X-ray screening of the diaphragm.

DEEP BRANCHES—LATERAL SERIES

Communicating—Accessory		C2, 3, 4
Muscular branches	Sternocleidomastoid	C2, 3, 4
	Trapezius	C2, (3)
	Levator scapulae	C3, 4
	Scalenus medius	C3, 4

Communicating branches. Lateral deep branches of the cervical plexus connect with the spinal accessory nerve in the sternocleidomastoid, posterior triangle and under the trapezius.

Muscular branches. These are distributed to sternocleidomastoid and to the trapezius, levator scapulae and scalenus medius. Trapezial branches cross the posterior triangle obliquely below the spinal accessory nerve.

BRACHIAL PLEXUS

The brachial plexus (**8.368, 369**) is a union of the lower four cervical ventral rami and the greater part of the first thoracic ventral ramus (p. 1263); the fourth ramus usually gives a branch to the fifth and the first thoracic frequently receives one from the second. Contributions to the plexus by C4 and T2 vary; when the branch from C4 is large, that from T2 is frequently absent and the branch from T1 is reduced, forming a *prefixed* type of plexus. If the branch from C4 is small or absent, the contribution of C5 is reduced but that of T1 is larger and one from T2 is always present; this arrangement constitutes a *postfixed* type of plexus. These ventral rami are the roots of the plexus, almost equal in size but variable in their mode of junction. The commonest arrangement is as follows:

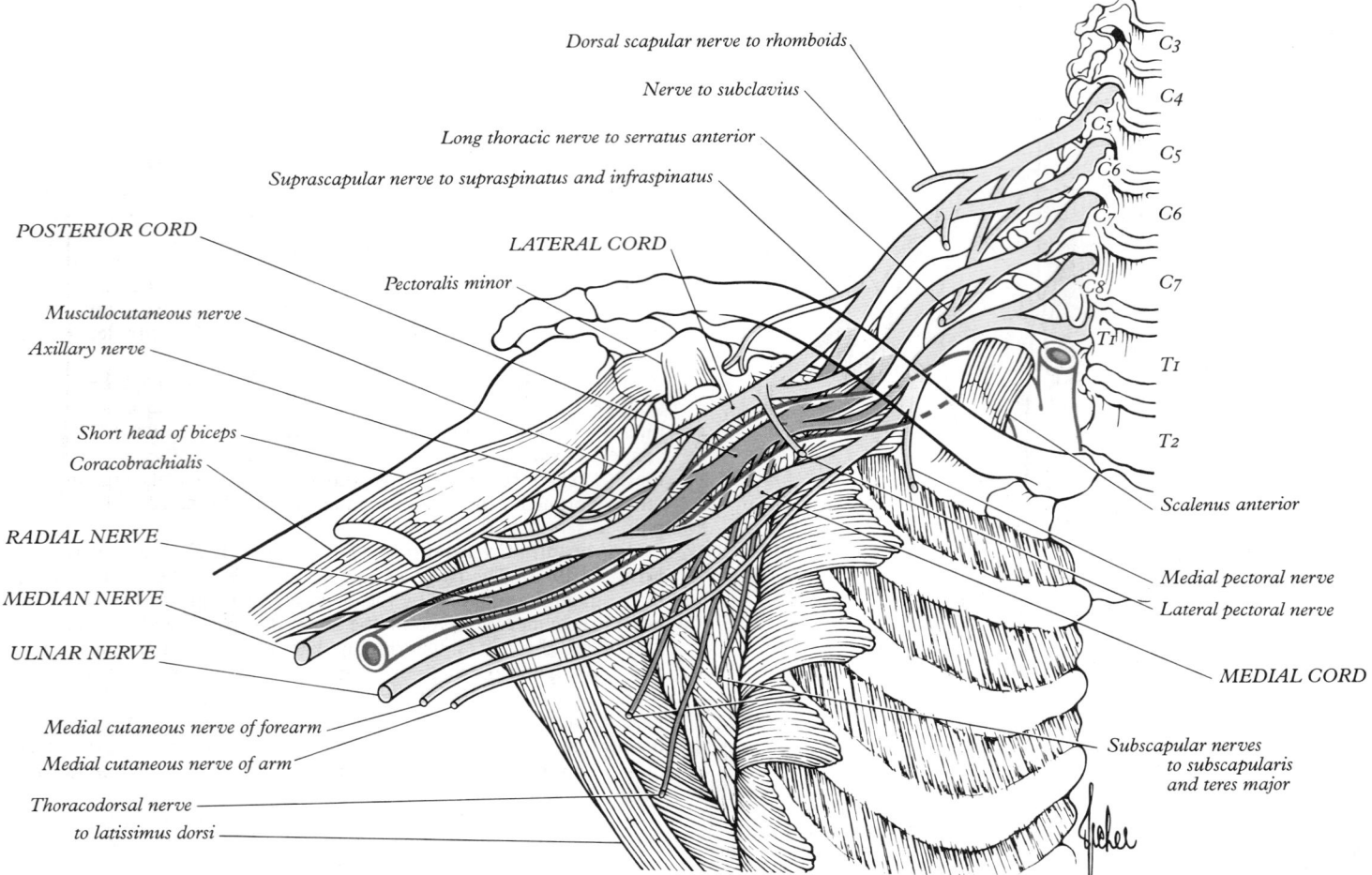

Dorsal scapular nerve to rhomboids
Nerve to subclavius
Long thoracic nerve to serratus anterior
Suprascapular nerve to supraspinatus and infraspinatus
POSTERIOR CORD
LATERAL CORD
Pectoralis minor
Musculocutaneous nerve
Axillary nerve
Short head of biceps
Coracobrachialis
RADIAL NERVE
MEDIAN NERVE
ULNAR NERVE
Medial cutaneous nerve of forearm
Medial cutaneous nerve of arm
Thoracodorsal nerve to latissimus dorsi
C3
C4
C5
C5
C6
C6
C7
C7
C8
T1
T1
T2
Scalenus anterior
Medial pectoral nerve
Lateral pectoral nerve
MEDIAL CORD
Subscapular nerves to subscapularis and teres major

8.368 Diagram of the brachial plexus, its branches and the muscles which they supply. (From O'Brien 1988. With permission of Baillière Tindall.)

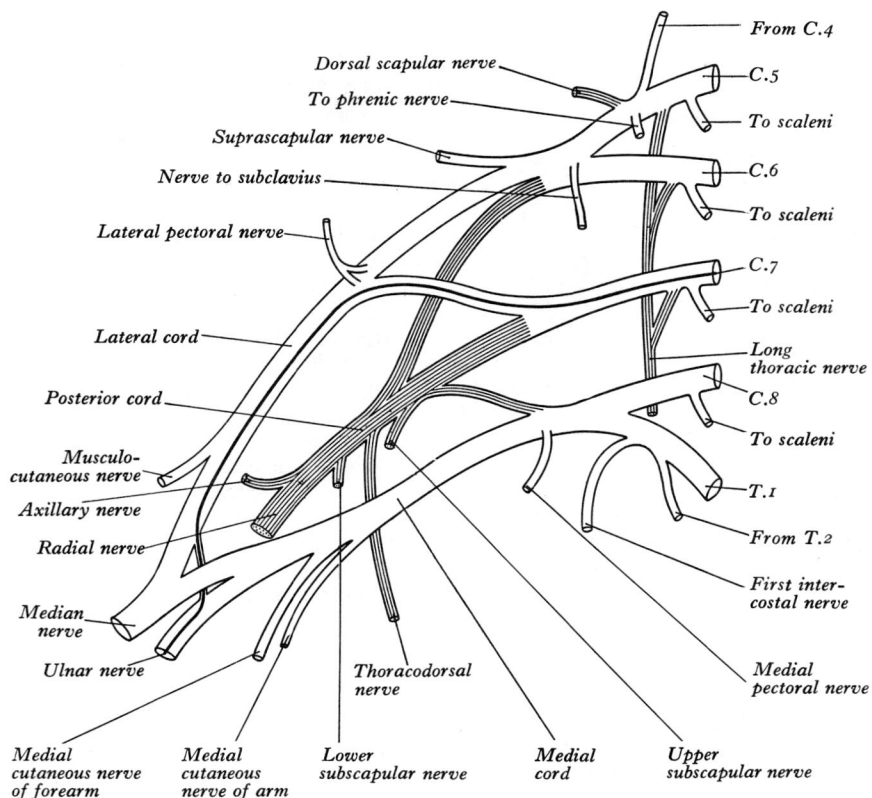

Dorsal scapular nerve
To phrenic nerve
Suprascapular nerve
Nerve to subclavius
Lateral pectoral nerve
Lateral cord
Posterior cord
Musculo-cutaneous nerve
Axillary nerve
Radial nerve
Median nerve
Ulnar nerve
Thoracodorsal nerve

From C.4
C.5
To scaleni
C.6
To scaleni
C.7
To scaleni
Long thoracic nerve
C.8
To scaleni
T.I
From T.2
First intercostal nerve
Medial pectoral nerve

Medial cutaneous nerve of forearm   Medial cutaneous nerve of arm   Lower subscapular nerve   Medial cord   Upper subscapular nerve

8.369 A plan of the brachial plexus. The posterior division of the trunks and their derivatives are shaded and the fibres from C.7 which enter the ulnar nerve are shown as a heavy black line. Letters and numbers C.4–C.8 and T.1–T.2 indicate the ventral rami of these cervical and thoracic spinal nerves.

the fifth and sixth rami unite at the lateral border of the scalenus medius as the *upper trunk*; the eighth cervical and first thoracic rami join behind the scalenus anterior as the *lower trunk*; the seventh cervical becomes the middle trunk. These three trunks incline laterally; just above or behind the clavicle each bifurcates into anterior and posterior divisions; the anterior divisions of the upper and middle trunks form a *lateral cord*, lateral to the axillary artery. The anterior division of the lower trunk descends at first behind, then medial to the axillary artery, forming the *medial cord* which often receives a branch from the seventh cervical ramus. Posterior divisions of all three form the *posterior cord*, at first above and then behind the axillary artery. The posterior division of the lower trunk is much smaller than the others, containing few, if any, fibres from the first thoracic ramus. It is frequently derived from the eighth cervical before the trunk is formed.

Despite the adaptation to evolutionary changes in upper-limb musculature, the human brachial plexus reflects the original flexor–extensor organization of a primitive fin. The posterior cord is the extensor supply, the medial and lateral cords the flexor supply. Migration of muscle masses has modified this pattern; e.g. brachialis and the anterior part of the deltoid are supplied (the former in part) from 'extensor' nerves. For comparative morphology of the plexus consult Harris (1939).

Relations of the brachial plexus

In the neck, the plexus is in the posterior triangle, in the angle between the clavicle and lower posterior border of the sternocleidomastoid, covered by platysma, deep fascia and skin, through which it is palpable. It is crossed by the supraclavicular nerves, the nerve to the subclavius, the inferior belly of the omohyoid, the external jugular vein and the superficial ramus of the transverse cervical artery (**10.92**). It emerges between the scaleni anterior and medius; its proximal part is superior to the third part of the subclavian artery, the lower trunk posterior to it; the plexus passes posterior to the medial two-thirds of the clavicle, the subclavius and the suprascapular vessels and lies on the first digitation of the serratus anterior and the subscapularis.

In the axilla the lateral and posterior cords are lateral to the first part of the axillary artery, the medial cord being behind it. The cords surround the second part of the artery, related according to their names. In the lower axilla the cords divide into nerves for the upper limb. Except for the median nerve's medial root, these nerves are related to the artery's third part as their cords are to the second; i.e. branches of the lateral cord are lateral, of the medial cord medial and of the posterior cord posterior, to the artery.

Close to their exit from the intervertebral foramina, the fifth and sixth cervical ventral rami receive grey rami communicantes from the middle cervical sympathetic ganglion, the seventh and eighth from the cervicothoracic ganglion (p. 1303). The first thoracic ventral ramus also receives a grey ramus from and contributes a white ramus to the cervicothoracic ganglion.

Branches of the brachial plexus may be described as supraclavicular and infraclavicular.

SUPRACLAVICULAR BRANCHES

These arise from roots or from trunks:

From roots	1. Nerves to scaleni and longus colli	C5, 6, 7, 8
	2. Branch to phrenic nerve	C5
	3. Dorsal scapular nerve	C5
	4. Long thoracic nerve	C5, 6 (7)
From trunks	1. Nerve to subclavius	C5, 6
	2. Suprascapular nerve	C5, 6

Branches to the scaleni and longus colli arise from the lower cervical ventral rami near their exit from the intervertebral foramina. Anterior to the scalenus anterior the phrenic nerve is joined by a branch from the fifth cervical ramus.

Dorsal scapular nerve. This comes from the fifth cervical ventral ramus, pierces the scalenus medius, passes behind the levator scapulae, which it occasionally supplies, and runs with the deep branch of the dorsal scapular artery to the rhomboids, which it supplies.

Long thoracic nerve (8.370). This is usually formed by roots

Lesions of the brachial plexus

Lesions of the brachial plexus commonly affect either the upper part of the plexus, that is the C5 and C6 roots and the upper trunk, and these are usually traumatic; or the lower part of the brachial plexus, that is the C8 and T1 roots and the lower trunk, when lesions may be caused by trauma but may also be produced by malignant infiltration or a thoracic outlet syndrome. Severe trauma may affect the whole plexus.

Upper plexus palsies. Rucksack palsy is due to a traction on the upper trunk of the brachial plexus from heavy and maladjusted rucksacks. Since axonal continuity is preserved recovery is usually complete. Severe traction injuries may occur in motorcycle accidents with lateral flexion of the head away from downward displacement of the shoulder, causing a traction injury of the upper part of the brachial plexus. The whole plexus may be involved in these injuries and sometimes the nerve roots are avulsed from the cervical spinal cord. There is gross wasting and weakness of the shoulder girdle muscles (C5) with inability to abduct the arm, and with marked weakness of elbow flexion and wrist extension (C5 and 6).

Lesions of the lower part of the brachial plexus. Malignant infiltration of the brachial plexus may result from extension of an apical lung carcinoma (Pancoast tumour) or from metastatic spread, often from carcinoma of the breast. There is

slowly progressive weakness usually starting in the small hand muscles (T1) and spreading to involve the finger flexors (C8). This is usually a painful condition and the pain may be severe. There is sensory loss on the medial aspect of the forearm (T1) extending into the medial side of the hand and to the little finger (C8). A Horner's syndrome may occur if there is involvement of the cervical sympathetic ganglia. A similar syndrome may occur following radiotherapy for breast carcinoma, but this is usually painless. Thoracic surgery involving a sternal split may cause traction on the brachial plexus and usually affects the lower part of the plexus.

The lower trunk of the brachial plexus (C8, T1) may be angulated over a cervical rib, together with the subclavian artery (the thoracic outlet syndrome). Patients may present with vascular symptoms due to kinking of the subclavian artery (this is more likely to occur with large bony ribs), or they may present with neurological deficit (this is more likely in patients with small rudimentary ribs which extend into a fibrous band which joins the first rib anteriorly). Cervical ribs are quite common and are rarely associated with symptoms. There is a slow insidious onset of wasting of the small hand muscles, often starting on the lateral side with involvement of the thenar eminence and first dorsal interosseous, with pain and

paraesthesiae in the medial aspect of the forearm extending to the little finger, which is often aggravated by carrying shopping or suitcases. A bruit may be heard over the subclavian artery and the radial pulse may be easily obliterated by movements of the arm, particularly with the arm extended and abducted at the shoulder.

Neuralgic amyotrophy. This is a demyelinating neuropathy which principally affects branches of the brachial plexus, so that a characteristic feature is the dense involvement of some muscles within a myotome while others in the same myotome are not affected. For example, involvement of the suprascapular nerve causes marked weakness of supraspinatus and infraspinatus, but deltoid may be normal. More rarely the median, radial or ulnar nerves may be affected and the condition may present with an anterior or occasionally a posterior interosseous nerve palsy. There is severe pain in the shoulder girdle initially and the weakness may not become evident until the pain starts to subside after a week or so. Wasting of the affected muscles then becomes evident. The weakness may take up to 18 months to recover and is sometimes permanent. Some wasting usually persists. There may be more than one branch of the brachial plexus involved, either clinically or electrophysiologically, and electromyography can confirm the dense involvement of some muscles with sparing of others in the same myotome.

---

from the fifth to the seventh cervical rami; the last may be absent. (70 dissections demonstrated all three roots in only 42%, Alexandre et al 1968.) The upper two roots pierce the scalenus medius obliquely, uniting in or lateral to it; the nerve descends dorsal to the brachial plexus and the first part of the axillary artery. Crossing the superior border of serratus anterior to reach its lateral surface, it may be joined by the root from C7, which emerges between the scaleni anterior and medius and descends on the latter's lateral surface. The nerve continues downwards to the lower border of the serratus anterior, supplying branches to each of its digitations.

Neuralgic amyotrophy. The long thoracic nerve is the most common nerve to be affected by neuralgic amyotrophy. Winging of the scapula may be the only clinical manifestation: it is best demonstrated by asking the patient to push against resistance with the arm extended at the elbow and flexed to 90° at the shoulder.

Nerve to the subclavius. Small and arising near the junction of the fifth and sixth cervical ventral rami, this descends anterior to the plexus and the third part of the subclavian artery and is usually connected to the phrenic nerve. It passes above the subclavian vein to supply the subclavius.

Suprascapular nerve (10.92, 8.371). A large branch of the superior trunk, this runs laterally deep to the trapezius and omohyoid, enters the supraspinous fossa through the suprascapular notch inferior to the superior transverse scapular ligament, runs deep to the supraspinatus and curves round the lateral border of the scapular spine with the suprascapular artery to reach the infraspinous fossa, where it gives two branches to the supraspinatus and articular rami to the shoulder and acromioclavicular joints. The suprascapular nerve was found to have a cutaneous branch in six upper limbs out of 61 Japanese cadavers (Horiguchi 1980). When present, it pierced

the deltoid muscle close to the tip of the acromion; in the one case where its peripheral distribution was examined, it was found to supply the skin of the proximal third of the arm within the territory of the axillary nerve.

Lesions of the suprascapular nerve. The commonest cause involving the suprascapular nerve is neuralgic amyotrophy, but an entrapment neuropathy may occur in the scapular notch or the nerve may be damaged by trauma to the scapula and shoulder. There is pain in the shoulder and wasting and weakness of supraspinatus and infraspinatus.

INFRACLAVICULAR BRANCHES

These branch from the cords but their fibres may be traced back to the spinal nerves:

Lateral cord	Lateral pectoral	C5, 6, 7
	Musculocutaneous	C5, 6 7
	Lateral root of median	C(5), 6, 7
Medial cord	Medial pectoral	C8, T1
	Medial cutaneous of forearm	C8, T1
	Medial cutaneous of arm	C8, T1
	Ulnar	C(7), 8, T1
	Medial root of median	C8, T1
Posterior cord	Upper subscapular	C6, 6
	Thoracodorsal	C6, 7,8
	Lower subscapular	C5, 6
	Axillary	C5, 6
	Radial	C5, 6, 7, 8, (T1)

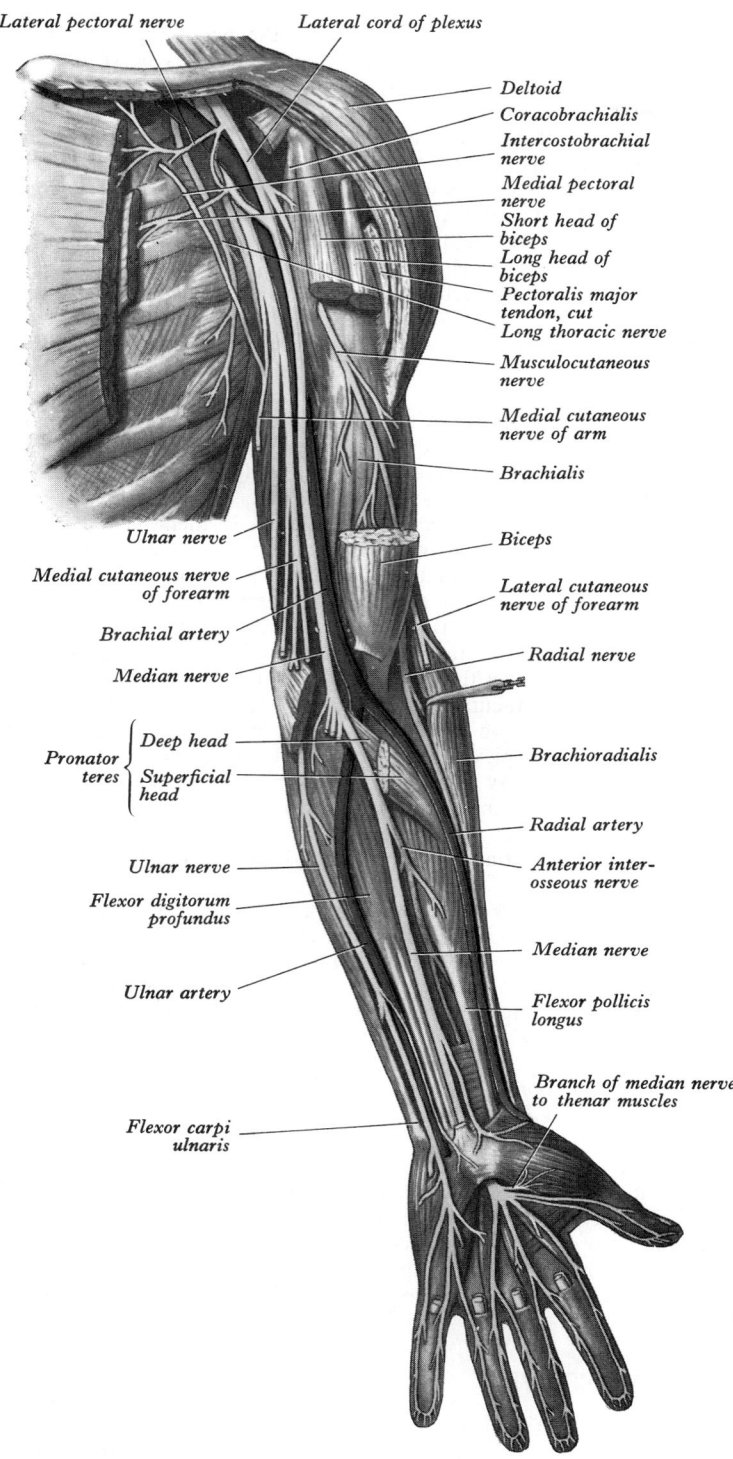

Lateral pectoral nerve
Lateral cord of plexus
Deltoid
Coracobrachialis
Intercostobrachial nerve
Medial pectoral nerve
Short head of biceps
Long head of biceps
Pectoralis major tendon, cut
Long thoracic nerve
Musculocutaneous nerve
Medial cutaneous nerve of arm
Brachialis
Ulnar nerve
Biceps
Medial cutaneous nerve of forearm
Lateral cutaneous nerve of forearm
Brachial artery
Median nerve
Radial nerve
Pronator teres { Deep head / Superficial head
Brachioradialis
Radial artery
Ulnar nerve
Anterior interosseous nerve
Flexor digitorum profundus
Median nerve
Ulnar artery
Flexor pollicis longus
Branch of median nerve to thenar muscles
Flexor carpi ulnaris

8.370 The nerves of the left upper limb, dissected from the anterior aspect.

Lateral pectoral nerve (8.370). This is larger than the medial, and may arise from the anterior divisions of the upper and middle trunks or by a single root from the lateral cord; its fibres are from the fifth to seventh cervical rami. It crosses anterior to the axillary artery and vein, pierces the clavipectoral fascia and supplies the deep surface of the pectoralis major. It sends a ramus to the medial pectoral nerve forming a loop in front of the first part of the axillary artery (8.370), to supply some fibres to the pectoralis minor.

Medial pectoral nerve. Derived from the eighth cervical and first thoracic ventral rami, this branches from the medial cord while the latter is posterior to the axillary artery. It curves forwards between the axillary artery and vein; anterior to the artery it joins a ramus of the lateral pectoral nerve, entering the deep surface of the pectoralis minor to supply it. Two or three branches pierce the pectoralis minor and others may pass round its inferior border to end in the pectoralis major.

Superior subscapular nerve. Smaller than the inferior, this arises from the posterior cord (C5 and 6), enters the subscapularis at a high level and is frequently double.

Inferior subscapular nerve. This is also from the posterior cord (C5 and 6), and supplies the lower part of the subscapularis, ending in the teres major, which is sometimes supplied by a separate branch.

Thoracodorsal nerve. Coming from the posterior cord, this derives its fibres from the sixth to eighth cervical ventral rami, arises between the subscapular nerves and accompanies the subscapular artery along the posterior axillary wall to supply the latissimus dorsi, reaching its distal border.

Axillary (circumflex humeral) nerve (8.371). This arises from the posterior cord, its fibres being derived from the fifth and sixth cervical ventral rami. It is at first lateral to the radial nerve, posterior to the axillary artery and anterior to the subscapularis, at whose lower border it curves back inferior to the humeroscapular articular capsule and, with the posterior circumflex humeral vessels, traverses a quadrangular space bounded **above** by the subscapularis (anterior) and teres minor (posterior), **below** by the teres major, medially by the long head of triceps and **laterally** by the humeral surgical neck. The nerve finally divides into anterior and posterior branches. The *anterior branch*, with the posterior circumflex humeral vessels, curves round the humeral neck, deep to the deltoid, to its anterior border, supplying it and giving a few small cutaneous branches which pierce the muscle to ramify in the skin over its lower part. The *posterior branch* supplies the teres minor and the posterior part of the deltoid; on the branch to the teres minor an enlargement or pseudoganglion usually exists. The posterior branch pierces the deep fascia low on the posterior border of the deltoid, continuing as the *upper lateral cutaneous nerve of the arm* and supplying the skin over the lower part of the deltoid and the upper part of the long head of triceps (8.372, 373). The axillary trunk supplies a branch to the shoulder joint below the subscapularis.

Lesions of the axillary nerve. The commonest causes of axillary nerve lesions are trauma and neuralgic amyotrophy. There is wasting and weakness of deltoid, which is usually clinically evident, and a patch of sensory loss on the outer aspect of the arm. This can be differentiated from a C5 root lesion by finding normal function in the distribution of the suprascapular nerve.

Musculocutaneous nerve (8.370). This comes from the lateral cord opposite the lower border of the pectoralis minor and is derived from the fifth to the seventh cervical ventral rami. It pierces the coracobrachialis and descends laterally between the biceps and brachialis to the lateral side of the arm; just below the elbow it pierces the deep fascia lateral to the tendon of biceps, continuing as the *lateral cutaneous nerve of the forearm*. A line drawn from the lateral side of the third part of the axillary artery across the coracobrachialis and biceps to the lateral side of the biceps tendon is a surface projection for the nerve, but this is varied by its point of entry into the coracobrachialis (Latarjet et al 1967). It supplies the coracobrachialis, both heads of biceps and most of the brachialis. The branch to the coracobrachialis leaves the musculocutaneous before it enters the muscle; its fibres are from the seventh cervical ramus and may branch directly from the lateral cord. Branches to the biceps and brachialis leave after the musculocutaneous pierces the coracobrachialis; the branch to the brachialis supplies the elbow joint. The nerve also supplies a small branch to the humerus, entering with the nutrient artery.

Lesions of the musculocutaneous nerve. An isolated lesion of the musculocutaneous nerve is rare, but may occur in injuries to the upper arm and shoulder including fracture of the humerus, and it may also be found in patients with neuralgic amyotrophy. There is marked weakness of elbow flexion because of paralysis of the biceps brachii and much of brachialis. There is sensory impairment on the extensor aspect of the forearm in the distribution of the lateral cutaneous nerve of the forearm. The pain and paraesthesiae may be aggravated by elbow extension.

Lateral cutaneous nerve of the forearm (8.372, 373). This passes deep to the cephalic vein, descending along the radial border of the

1269

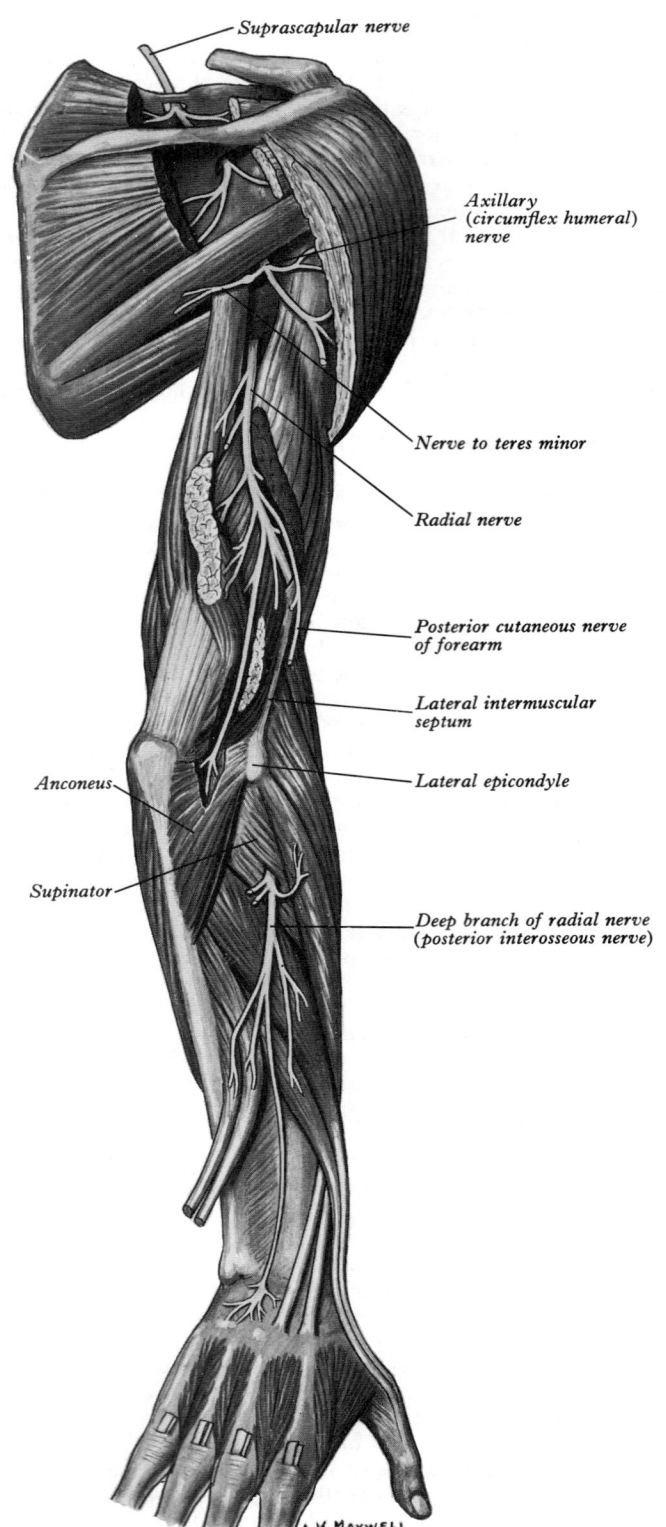

Suprascapular nerve

Axillary
(circumflex humeral)
nerve

Nerve to teres minor

Radial nerve

Posterior cutaneous nerve
of forearm

Lateral intermuscular
septum

Lateral epicondyle

Anconeus

Supinator

Deep branch of radial nerve
(posterior interosseous nerve)

A·K·MAXWELL

8.371 The suprascapular, axillary and radial nerves of the right upper limb, dissected from the posterior aspect.

forearm to the wrist, supplying the skin of the forearm's anterolateral surface and connecting by branches around its radial border with the posterior cutaneous nerve of the forearm and the terminal branch of the radial nerve. Its trunk gives rise to a slender recurrent branch which extends along the cephalic vein as far as the middle third of the upper arm, distributing filaments to the skin over the distal third of the anterolateral surface of the upper arm close to the vein (Horiguchi 1981). Although observed in the nineteenth century

(Arnold 1851; Bolk 1898), this recurrent branch has more recently been omitted from most descriptions of the nerve supply of the upper limb. At the wrist joint the lateral cutaneous nerve of the forearm is anterior to the radial artery and some filaments, piercing the deep fascia and accompanying this to the dorsum of the carpus. The nerve then passes to the base of the thenar eminence, ending in cutaneous rami. It connects with the terminal branch of the radial nerve and the palmar cutaneous branch of the median nerve.

The musculocutaneous nerve has frequent variations. It may run behind the coracobrachialis or adhere for some distance to the median nerve and pass behind the biceps. Some fibres of the median nerve may run in the musculocutaneous nerve, leaving it to join their proper trunk; less frequently the reverse occurs, the median nerve sending a branch to the musculocutaneous. Occasionally it supplies the pronator teres and may replace radial branches to the dorsal surface of the thumb.

Medial cutaneous nerve of the arm. Supplying the skin in that area (**8.**372) and the smallest branch of the plexus, this arises from the medial cord and contains fibres from the eighth cervical and first thoracic ventral rami. It traverses the axilla, crossing anterior or posterior to the axillary vein, to which it is then medial, and communicating with the intercostobrachial nerve; it descends medial to the brachial artery and basilic vein (**8.**370) to a point midway in the upper arm, where it pierces the deep fascia to supply a medial area in the arm's distal third, extending on to its anterior and posterior aspects. Some rami reach the skin anterior to the medial epicondyle, others over the olecranon. It connects with the posterior branch of the medial cutaneous nerve of the forearm. Sometimes the medial cutaneous nerve of the arm and the intercostobrachial nerve are connected in a plexiform manner in the axilla. Sometimes the intercostobrachial nerve is large and reinforced by part of the lateral cutaneous branch of the third intercostal nerve, replacing the arm's medial cutaneous nerve and receiving from the brachial plexus a connection representing the latter; occasionally this connection is absent.

Medial cutaneous nerve of the forearm (**8.**370). Coming from the medial cord, this is derived from the eighth cervical and first thoracic ventral rami. At first it is between the axillary artery and vein and supplies a ramus piercing the deep fascia to supply the skin over the biceps, almost to the elbow. The nerve descends medial to the brachial artery, pierces the deep fascia with the basilic vein midway in the arm and divides into anterior and posterior branches. The larger, *anterior branch* usually passes in front of, occasionally behind, the median cubital vein, descending anteromedial in the forearm to supply the skin as far as the wrist and connecting with the palmar cutaneous branch of the ulnar nerve (**8.**372). The *posterior branch* descends obliquely medial to the basilic vein, anterior to the medial epicondyle, and curves round to the back of the forearm, descending on its medial border to the wrist, supplying the skin. It connects with the medial cutaneous nerve of the arm, the posterior cutaneous nerve of the forearm and the dorsal branch of the ulnar (**8.**373).

MEDIAN NERVE

The median nerve (**8.**370) has two roots from the lateral (C(5), 6, 7) and medial (C8, T1) cords, which embrace the third part of the axillary artery, uniting anterior or lateral to it. Some fibres from C7 often leave the lateral root in the lower part of the axilla passing distomedially posterior to the medial root, usually anterior to axillary artery, to join the ulnar nerve; they may branch from the seventh cervical ventral ramus. Clinically they are believed to be mainly motor to the flexor carpi ulnaris. If the lateral root is small, the musculocutaneous nerve (C5, 6, 7) connects with the median nerve in the arm.

The median nerve enters the arm at first lateral to the brachial artery; near the insertion of the coracobrachialis it crosses in front of (rarely behind) the artery, descending medial to it to the cubital fossa where it is posterior to the bicipital aponeurosis and anterior to the brachialis, separated by the latter from the elbow joint. It usually enters the forearm between the heads of the pronator teres, crossing to the lateral side of the ulnar artery and separated from it by the deep head of pronator teres. It proceeds behind a tendinous bridge between the humero-ulnar and radial heads of the flexor

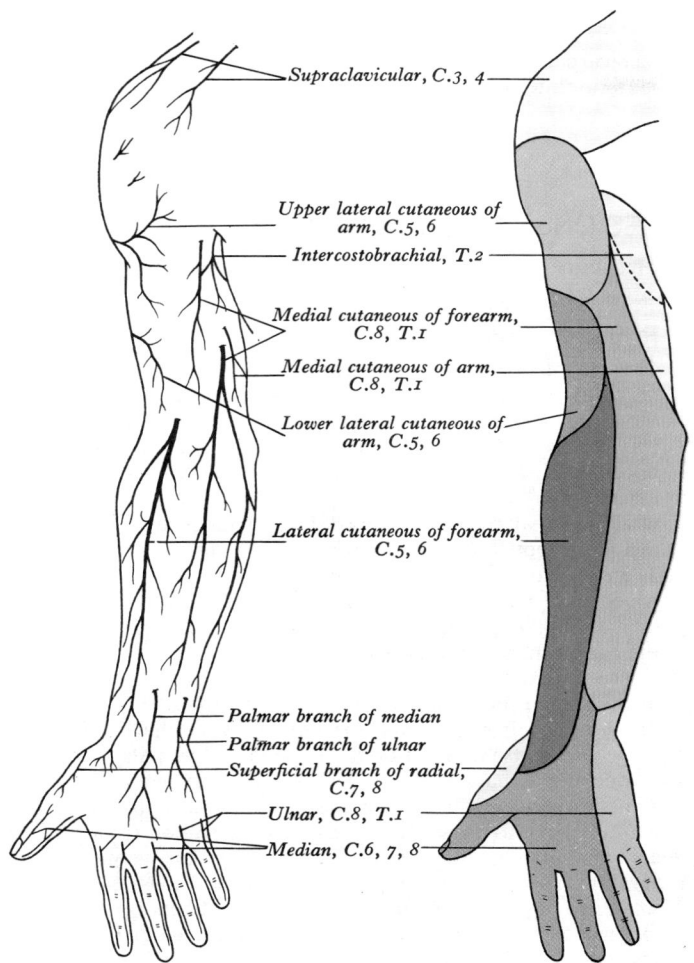

8.372 The cutaneous nerves of the right upper limb, their areas of distribution and segmental origins, viewed from the anterior aspect.

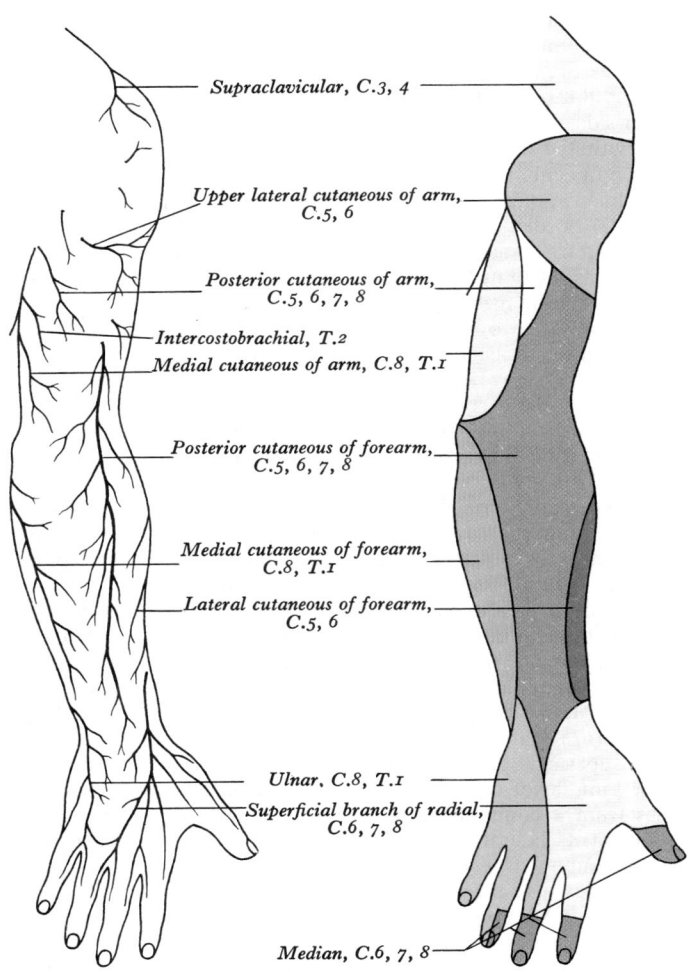

8.373 The cutaneous nerves of the upper right limb, their areas of distribution and segmental origins, viewed from the posterior aspect.

digitorum superficialis, descending posterior and adherent to the flexor digitorum superficialis and anterior to the flexor digitorum profundus. About 5 cm proximal to the flexor retinaculum it emerges from behind the lateral edge of the flexor digitorum superficialis, becoming superficial just proximal to the wrist between the tendons of the flexores digitorum superficialis and carpi radialis, projecting laterally from behind the tendon of the palmaris longus. It then passes deep to the flexor retinaculum into the palm. In the forearm it is accompanied by the median branch of the anterior interosseous artery. Its course can be marked on the surface by a line from the medial side of the brachial artery in the cubital fossa along the forearm's midline (16.10).

Relations as the median nerve enters the forearm are variable. According to Anson (1963) the route described above occurred in 82.8% of 1000 dissections; in 10.8% the nerve was posterior to the humeral head of the pronator teres, the ulnar slip being absent. In 4.6% the nerve was posterior to both heads, and in 1.8% traversed **through** the humeral head.

Branches in the arm

These are vascular branches to the brachial artery and usually a branch to the pronator teres, a variable distance proximal to the elbow joint.

Branches in the forearm

These are muscular, articular, anterior interosseous, palmar cutaneous and communicating. *Muscular branches*, except one, are given off proximally (near the elbow) to the superficial flexor muscles (except the flexor carpi ulnaris), i.e. to the pronator teres, flexor carpi radialis, palmaris longus and the flexor digitorum superficialis. The branch to the part of the flexor digitorum superficialis for the

index finger arises near midforearm but may be from the anterior interosseous nerve. *Articular branches*, arising at or just distal to the elbow joint, supply it and the proximal radio-ulnar joint.

Anterior interosseous nerve. This branches posteriorly from the median nerve between the two heads of pronator teres, just distal to the origin of branches to the superficial forearm flexors. With the anterior interosseous artery it descends anterior to the interosseous membrane, between and deep to the flexores pollicis longus and digitorum profundus and supplying both; branches to the latter are limited to its lateral part, which sends tendons to the index and middle fingers. Terminally it is posterior to the pronator quadratus, supplying its deep surface, and supplies the distal radio-ulnar, radio-carpal and carpal joints.

Palmar cutaneous branch. This starts just proximal to the flexor retinaculum, pierces it or the deep fascia and divides into *lateral branches* supplying the thenar skin and connecting with the lateral cutaneous nerve of the forearm; and *medial branches* supplying the central palmar skin and connecting with the palmar cutaneous branch of the ulnar nerve.

Communicating branches, which may be multiple, often arise (sometimes from the anterior interosseous branch) in the proximal forearm and pass medially between flexores digitorum superficialis and profundus and behind the ulnar artery to join the ulnar nerve. This communication is a factor in explaining anomalous muscular innervation in the hand (see below).

Branches in the hand

Proximal to the flexor retinaculum the nerve is lateral to the tendons of flexor digitorum superficialis but further distally it lies between the retinaculum and tendons in the 'carpal tunnel' (see p. 852), i.e. the space between the flexor retinaculum and the anterior carpal

1271

surface. The nerve may become compressed here (see below). Distal to the retinaculum the nerve enlarges and flattens, usually dividing into five or six branches, but the mode and level of division are variable.

Muscular branch. This is short and thick, and is from the nerve's lateral side; it may be the first palmar or a terminal branch arising level with the digital branches. It runs laterally, just distal to the flexor retinaculum, with a slight recurrent curve beneath the part of the palmar aponeurosis covering the thenar muscles. It turns round the distal border of the retinaculum to lie superficial to the flexor pollicis brevis, usually supplying it and either continuing superficial to it or traversing it. It gives a branch to the abductor pollicis brevis, which enters the medial edge of the muscle and then passes deep to it to supply the opponens pollicis, entering its medial edge. Its terminal part occasionally gives a branch to the first dorsal interosseous, which may be its sole or partial supply. The muscular branch may arise in the carpal tunnel and pierce the flexor retinaculum, a point of surgical importance (Papathanassion 1968).

Palmar digital branches. (In this account of cutaneous innervation of the digits, the distinction between proximal, penultimate, undivided rami, termed *common palmar digital nerves*, and their ultimate branches to individual digits, the *proper palmar digital nerves*, must be noted. The corresponding terms for the foot are *common plantar digital nerves* and *proper plantar digital nerves*.) The median nerve divides into four or five digital branches, though it often divides first into two: a lateral ramus providing digital branches to the pollex and the radial side of the index finger; and a medial, supplying digital branches to adjacent sides of the index, medius and annularis. Other modes of termination occur (Poisel 1974). Digital branches are commonly arranged as follows. They pass distally, deep to the superficial palmar arch and its digital vessels, at first anterior to the long flexor tendons. Two *proper* palmar digital nerves, sometimes from a common stem, pass to the sides of the pollex, that supplying its lateral side crossing in front of the tendon of flexor pollicis longus. The proper palmar digital nerve to the lateral side of the index also supplies the first lumbrical muscle. Two *common* palmar digital nerves pass distally between the long flexor tendons: the lateral divides in the distal palm into two proper palmar digital nerves traversing adjacent sides of the index and medius; the medial one divides into two proper palmar digital nerves supplying adjacent sides of the medius and annularis. The lateral common digital nerve supplies the second lumbrical muscle; the medial receives a communicating twig from the common palmar digital branch of the *ulnar* nerve and may supply the third lumbrical muscle. In the distal part of the palm the digital arteries pass deeply between the divisions of the digital nerves; on the sides of the digits the nerves are anterior to the arteries. The median nerve usually supplies palmar cutaneous digital branches to the lateral three and one-half digits (pollex, index, medius and the lateral side of the annularis); sometimes the lateral side of the ring finger is supplied by the ulnar nerve. The proper palmar digital nerves that pass along the medial side of the index, both sides of the medius and the lateral side of the annularis, enter these digits in fat between slips of the central palmar aponeurosis (p. 854). They pass, with the lumbricals and palmar digital arteries, dorsal to the superficial transverse metacarpal ligament (p. 855) and ventral to the deep transverse metacarpal ligament (p. 658). In the digits, the nerves run distally beside the long flexor tendons, outside their fibrous sheaths, level with the anterior phalangeal surfaces and anterior to the digital arteries. Each nerve gives off several branches to the skin on the front and sides of the digit, many ending in lamellated corpuscles (p. 963), and branches to the metacarpophalangeal and interphalangeal joints. They also supply the fibrous sheaths of the long flexor tendons, digital arteries (vasomotor) and sweat glands (secretomotor). Distal to the base of the distal phalanx the digital nerve gives off a branch passing dorsally to the nail bed, the main nerve dividing to supply the pulp and skin of the terminal part of the digit. Distal to the base of the proximal phalanx, each proper digital nerve also gives off a dorsal branch to supply the skin over the back of the middle and distal phalanges (**8**.373). The proper palmar digital nerves to the pollex and the lateral side of the index emerge with the long flexor tendons from under the lateral edge of the central palmar aponeurosis and are arranged in the digits as described above; but in the pollex small distal branches supply the skin on the back of the distal phalanx only.

In addition to the branches of the median nerve described above,

variable vasomotor branches supply the radial and ulnar arteries and their branches. Some of the intercarpal, carpo-metacarpal and intermetacarpal joints are said to be supplied by the median nerve or its anterior interosseous branch, the precise details being uncertain.

LESIONS OF THE MEDIAN NERVE

Median nerve lesions occur at two sites, in the forearm and at the wrist.

Pronator syndrome

This is an uncommon entrapment neuropathy of the median nerve as it passes alongside the fibrous band connecting the biceps tendon to the forearm fascia, then passes down between the two heads of pronator teres and through a fibrous arch formed by flexor digitorum superficialis. The nerve may be involved at any of these sites. There is weakness of all the muscles innervated by the median nerve, including abductor pollicis brevis and the long finger flexors. There is also sensory impairment on the palm of the hand, which is spared in the carpal tunnel syndrome because the palmar cutaneous branch of the median nerve arises above the carpal tunnel and lies superficial to it.

The anterior interosseous nerve usually arises from the median nerve proximal to the site of compression in the pronator syndrome; it may be affected with the median nerve or by itself. Anterior interosseous nerve palsy may be due to external pressure, a form of Saturday night palsy, sometimes by tight grip in association with pronation without obvious cause. It may be a manifestation of neuralgic amyotrophy and tends to resolve spontaneously over several months. An anterior interosseous nerve palsy causes weakness of pinch grip due to involvement of flexor pollicis longus and flexor digitorum profundus to the index finger. Innervation of flexor digitorum profundus to the middle finger is rather variable, therefore this muscle may or may not be weak. The branches to these three muscles may arise separately from the median nerve, so that isolated weakness of the terminal phalanx to the thumb or index finger may occur. The pronator quadratus is also involved but is not clinically significant.

Carpal tunnel syndrome

This is the most common entrapment mononeuropathy and is caused by compression of the median nerve as it passes through the fibro-osseous tunnel beneath the flexor retinaculum. The carpal tunnel may be narrowed by arthritic changes in the wrist joint, particularly rheumatoid arthritis; soft tissue thickening as may occur in myxoedema and acromegaly; and with oedema and obesity including pregnancy. Normally the nerve slides smoothly in and out of the carpal tunnel with flexion and extension of the wrist; when the nerve is compressed there is an additional damage to the nerve with flexion and extension. The dominant hand is usually affected first, probably because this hand is used more frequently and more vigorously. There is wasting and weakness of abductor pollicis brevis and impairment of sensation in the thumb, index, middle and median side of the ring finger, but the palmar branch of the median nerve is spared since it does not pass through the carpal tunnel.

ULNAR NERVE

The ulnar nerve (**8**.370) arises from the medial cord (C8, T1) but, as described above (p. 1267), it often receives fibres from the ventral ramus of C7. It runs distally through the axilla medial to the axillary artery and between it and the vein, continuing distally medial to the brachial artery as far as midarm; here it pierces the medial intermuscular septum, inclining medially as it descends anterior to the medial head of the triceps to the interval between the medial epicondyle and the olecranon, with the superior ulnar collateral artery. At the elbow it is in a groove on the dorsum of the epicondyle. It enters the forearm between the two heads of the flexor carpi ulnaris superficial to the posterior and oblique parts of the ulnar collateral ligament. It descends the medial side of the forearm on the flexor digitorum profundus, covered proximally by the flexor carpi ulnaris; its lower half, covered by skin and fasciae, is lateral to this muscle. In the upper third of the forearm, it is distant from the ulnar artery but distal to this is close to its medial side (8.370). About 5 cm proximal to the wrist it gives off a dorsal branch which continues distally into the hand, anterior to the flexor retinaculum on the lateral side of the pisiform bone and posteromedial to the ulnar artery. It passes behind the superficial part of the retinaculum with the artery and divides into superficial and deep terminal branches. Its relation to the brachial artery and medial epicondyle makes it easy to map out in its proximal course; a line from the medial epicondyle to the lateral edge of pisiform represents its distal course (16.10).

Its branches are: articular, muscular, palmar cutaneous, dorsal, superficial terminal and deep terminal.

Articular branches. These branches to the elbow joint issue from the nerve between the medial epicondyle and olecranon. Others are described below.

Muscular branches. Usually two, these begin near the elbow; one supplies the flexor carpi ulnaris (p. 846), the other the medial half of the flexor digitorum profundus.

Palmar cutaneous branch. This arises about midforearm, descends on the ulnar artery (8.370), which it supplies, and perforates the deep fascia to end in the palmar skin, after communicating with the palmar branch of the median nerve. It sometimes supplies the palmaris brevis.

Dorsal branch. This arises about 5 cm proximal to the wrist, passes distally and backwards, deep to the flexor carpi ulnaris, perforates the deep fascia, descends along the medial side of the back of the wrist and hand and then divides into two, or often three, dorsal digital nerves. One supplies the medial side of the little finger, the second adjacent sides of the little and ring, while the third, when present, supplies adjoining sides of the ring and middle finger but may be replaced, wholly or partially, by a branch of the radial nerve, always communicating with it on the dorsum of the hand (8.373). In the little finger the dorsal digital nerves extend only to the base of the distal phalanx and in the ring finger to the base of the middle phalanx; most distal parts of these digits are supplied by dorsal branches of the proper digital branches of the ulnar and, on the lateral side of the ring finger, median nerves.

Superficial terminal branch. This supplies the palmaris brevis and the medial palmar skin, dividing into two palmar digital nerves, which can be palpated against the hook of the hamate bone (p. 649); one of these supplies the medial side of the little finger, the other (a *common* palmar digital nerve) sends a twig to the median nerve and divides into two *proper* digital nerves for the adjoining sides of little and ring fingers (8.370). The proper digital branches are distributed like those of the median nerve. Murakami (1969) has described articular branchlets from the superficial terminal branch of the ulnar nerve.

Deep terminal branch. With the deep branch of the ulnar artery, this passes between the abductor digiti minimi and flexor digiti minimi and then perforates the opponens digiti minimi to follow the deep palmar arch dorsal to the flexor tendons. At its origin it supplies the three short muscles of the little finger. As it crosses the hand, it supplies the interossei and the third and fourth lumbricals; it ends by supplying the adductor pollicis, the first palmar interosseous and usually (p. 859) the flexor pollicis brevis. It sends articular filaments to the wrist joint.

The medial part of the flexor digitorum profundus is supplied by the ulnar nerve, as are the third and fourth lumbricals which are connected with the tendons of this part of the muscle. Similarly, the lateral part of the flexor digitorum profundus and the first and second lumbricals are supplied by the median nerve. The third lumbrical is often supplied by both nerves. The deep terminal branch is said to give branches to some intercarpal, carpometacarpal and intermetacarpal joints, though, as with the median nerve, precise

details are uncertain. Vasomotor branches, arising in the forearm and hand, supply the ulnar and palmar arteries.

LESIONS OF THE ULNAR NERVE

Ulnar nerve lesions occur at four sites, behind the medial epicondyle, in the cubital tunnel, at the wrist and in the hand.

At the elbow. The ulnar nerve is in a vulnerable position as it lies between the median epicondyle and the olecranon: it lies on bone covered only by a thin layer of skin. It is easily damaged if the ulnar groove is shallow and the nerve may become more prominent than the medial epicondyle or the olecranon when the elbow is fully flexed. Sometimes the nerve may override the medial epicondyle in full flexion. Loss of the ulnar groove may be associated with arthritis of the elbow joint, often due to an old fracture, in which case there may be incomplete extension of the elbow with a wide carrying angle. The nerve is easily palpable and is often thickened. There is usually weakness of flexor digitorum profundus to the ring and little fingers, and if these muscles are involved the lesion must be at the elbow.

Cubital tunnel syndrome. This is an entrapment neuropathy of the ulnar nerve in the tunnel formed by the tendinous arch connecting the two heads of flexor carpi ulnaris at their humeral and ulnar attachments. The clinical features are precisely the same as a lesion in the ulnar groove and again, involvement of flexor digitorum profundus to the ring and little fingers is variable. Lesions at these two sites cannot be reliably distinguished neurophysiologically, but in the cubital tunnel syndrome the elbow joint is usually normal: elbow movements are full with a normal carrying angle; the ulnar nerve feels normal in the ulnar groove; it does not sublux; nor does it become superficial on elbow flexion.

At the wrist. The ulnar nerve may be compressed in Guyon's canal by a ganglion. There is preservation of flexor digitorum profundus to the ring and little fingers, but all the small hand muscles innervated by the ulnar nerve are involved. The dorsal cutaneous branch and the palmar branch of the ulnar nerve are both spared since the lesion is distal to their origin from the main trunk of the ulnar nerve in midforearm.

In the hand. The deep motor branch of the ulnar nerve may be compressed against the pisiform and hamate bones when the hand is used as a mallet, or if a vibrating tool or motorcycle handlebar is held in such a way that the hypothenar eminence is off the edge of the handle. The sensory branches are always spared and involvement of the hypothenar muscles is variable depending on the level at which branches to these muscles arise.

RADIAL NERVE

The radial nerve (8.371) arises from the posterior cord, C5, 6, 7, 8, (T1). The largest branch of the brachial plexus, it descends behind the third part of the axillary artery and the upper part of the brachial, anterior to the subscapularis and the tendons of the latissimus dorsi and teres major. With the arteria profunda brachii and, later, its radial collateral branch, it inclines dorsally between the long and medial heads of the triceps, after which it passes obliquely across the back of the humerus, first between the lateral and medial heads of the triceps, then in a shallow groove deep to the lateral head. On reaching the lateral side of the humerus it pierces the lateral intermuscular septum to enter the anterior compartment; it then descends deep in a furrow between the brachialis and proximally the brachioradialis, then more distally the extensor carpi radialis longus. Anterior to the lateral epicondyle it divides into superficial and deep terminal rami.

In the arm the radial nerve is indicated by a posterior line from the start of the brachial artery distally and laterally to the junction of the upper and middle thirds of a line between the lateral epicondyle and the deltoid tuberosity; the line is continued anteriorly as far as the lateral epicondyle, 1 cm or less lateral to the biceps tendon.

The branches of the radial nerve are: muscular, cutaneous, articular and superficial terminal and posterior interosseous.

Muscular branches. These supply the triceps, anconeus, brachioradialis, extensor carpi radialis longus and brachialis in *medial, posterior* and *lateral* groups. *Medial* muscular branches arise from the radial nerve on the medial side of the arm. They supply the medial and long heads of the triceps, the branch to the medial being a long, slender filament which, lying close to the ulnar nerve as far as the distal third of the arm, is often termed the *ulnar collateral* nerve. A large *posterior* muscular branch arises from the nerve as it lies in the humeral groove. It divides to supply the medial and lateral heads of the triceps and the anconeus, that for the latter being a long nerve which descends in the medial head of the triceps and partially supplies it; it is accompanied by the middle collateral branch of the arteria profunda brachii and passes behind the elbow joint to end in the anconeus. *Lateral* muscular branches arise in front of the lateral intermuscular septum; they supply the lateral part of the brachialis, brachioradialis and extensor carpi radialis longus.

Cutaneous branches. These are the posterior and lower lateral cutaneous nerves of the arm and the posterior cutaneous nerve of the forearm. The small *posterior cutaneous nerve* of the arm arises in the axilla and passes medially to supply the skin on the dorsal surface of the arm nearly as far as the olecranon. It crosses posterior to and communicates with the intercostobrachial nerve. The *lower lateral cutaneous nerve of the arm* perforates the lateral head of the triceps distal to the deltoid tuberosity, passes to the front of the elbow close to the cephalic vein and supplies the skin of the lateral part of the lower half of the arm (**8.372**). The *posterior cutaneous nerve of the forearm* arises with the preceding nerve. Perforating the lateral head of the triceps, it descends first lateral in the arm, then along the dorsum of the forearm to the wrist, supplying the skin in its course and joining, near its end, with dorsal branches of the lateral cutaneous nerve of the forearm (**8.373**).

Articular branches. These are distributed to the elbow joint.

Superficial terminal branch. This descends from the lateral epicondyle anterolaterally in the proximal two-thirds of the forearm, at first on the supinator, lateral to the radial artery and behind the brachioradialis; in the middle third of the forearm it is behind the brachioradialis, close to the lateral side of the artery, successively anterior to the pronator teres, the radial head of the flexor digitorum superficialis and the flexor pollicis longus. It leaves the artery about 7 cm proximal to the wrist, passes deep to the tendon of the brachioradialis, curves round the lateral side of the radius as it descends, pierces the deep fascia and divides into five, sometimes four, dorsal digital nerves. On the dorsum of the hand it usually communicates with the posterior and lateral cutaneous nerves of the forearm.

Dorsal digital nerves. There are usually four or five and they are small. The first supplies the skin of the radial side of the pollex and the adjoining thenar eminence, communicating with branches of the lateral cutaneous nerve of the forearm; the second supplies the medial side of the pollex; the third, the lateral side of the index; the fourth, the adjoining sides of the index and middle; the fifth communicates with a ramus of the dorsal branch of the ulnar nerve and supplies the adjoining sides of the middle and ring but is frequently replaced by the dorsal branch of the ulnar nerve. The pollicial digital nerves reach only to the root of the nail, those in the index midway along the middle phalanx, those to the medius and the lateral part of the ring finger not further than the proximal interphalangeal joints. The remaining distal dorsal areas of the skin in these digits are supplied by palmar digital branches of the median and ulnar nerves (**8.373**). The superficial terminal branch of the radial nerve may supply the whole dorsum of the hand; for variations consult Sayfi (1967).

Posterior interosseous nerve (**8.371**). This deep terminal branch reaches the back of the forearm round the lateral aspect of the radius and between the two planes of the fibres of the supinator. It supplies the extensor carpi radialis brevis and the supinator before entering it; as it traverses the muscle it supplies it with additional branches. The branch to the extensor carpi radialis brevis may arise from the beginning of the superficial branch of the radial nerve. As it emerges from the supinator posteriorly it gives off three short branches, to the extensor digitorum, extensor digiti minimi and extensor carpi ulnaris, and two longer branches, a *medial* to the extensor pollicis longus and extensor indicis and a *lateral*, supplying the abductor pollicis longus and ending in the extensor pollicis brevis. The nerve is at first between the superficial and deep extensor muscles; but at the distal border of the extensor pollicis brevis it passes deep to the extensor pollicis longus and, diminished to a fine thread, descends on the interosseous membrane to the dorsum of the carpus, where it presents a flattened and somewhat expanded termination or 'pseudoganglion', from which filaments supply the carpal ligaments and articulations (**8.371**).

Articular branches from the deep branch of the radial nerve supply the carpal, distal radio-ulnar and some intercarpal and intermetacarpal joints; digital branches supply the metacarpophalangeal and proximal interphalangeal joints.

LESIONS OF THE RADIAL NERVE

The two most common sites of radial nerve lesions are in the arm where the nerve lies against the humerus, and in the extensor muscle compartment of the forearm, when the posterior interosseous branch is affected.

Above the elbow

Lesions of the radial nerve at its origin from the posterior cord in the axilla may occur due to pressure from a long crutch (crutch palsy). Triceps is involved only with lesions at this level and is usually spared in the more common lesions of the radial nerve in the arm as it lies alongside the spiral groove, where the nerve is commonly affected by fractures of the humerus. Compression of the nerve against the humerus occurs if the arm is rested on a sharp edge such as the back of a chair, (Saturday night palsy). Both crutch palsy and Saturday night palsy cause weakness of brachioradialis with wasting and loss of the reflex. There is both wrist and finger drop due to weakness of wrist and finger extensors, as well as weakness of extensor pollicis longus and abductor pollicis longus. There may be sensory impairment or paraesthesiae in the distribution of the superficial radial nerve.

Posterior interosseous palsy

This is an entrapment neuropathy of the posterior interosseous nerve within the forearm extensor muscles. There is no sensory impairment since the superficial radial nerve arises above this level. Radial wrist extension and brachioradialis muscles are normal. Extensor carpi ulnaris is usually affected so that attempted wrist extension causes marked radial deviation. There is some variation in the level at which branches of the radial nerve arise from the main trunk in different subjects. Branches to extensor carpi radialis brevis and the supinator may arise from the main trunk of the radial nerve or from the proximal part of the posterior interosseous nerve, but almost invariably above the arcade of Frohse where entrapment occurs. There is weakness of finger extension and thumb extension and abduction.

The *superficial radial nerve* is purely sensory and supplies a variable area of skin over the lateral side of the dorsum of the hand. It lies superficially and relatively unprotected overlying the lateral aspect of the radius, where it is easily compressed by tight bracelets, watch straps and handcuffs.

THORACIC VENTRAL RAMI

There are twelve pairs of thoracic ventral rami (**8**.360, 374); all but the twelfth are between the ribs (*intercostal nerves*), the twelfth being below the last rib (*subcostal nerve*). Each is connected with an adjacent sympathetic ganglion by grey and white rami communicantes: the grey ramus joins the nerve proximal to the exit of the white ramus. Intercostal nerves are distributed chiefly to the thoracic and abdominal walls; the first two supply the upper limb in addition, the next four are limited to the thoracic wall, while the lower five supply the thoracic and abdominal walls (see below). The subcostal nerve supplies the abdominal wall and gluteal skin. Communicating branches link intercostal nerves posteriorly in the intercostal spaces; the lower five communicate freely in the abdominal wall (Davies et al 1932).

FIRST TO THE SIXTH THORACIC VENTRAL RAMI

The first thoracic ventral ramus divides unequally; a large branch ascends across the neck of the first rib, lateral to the superior intercostal artery, to enter the brachial plexus (see below). The smaller first intercostal nerve runs in the first intercostal space and ends as the first anterior cutaneous nerve of the thorax. A lateral cutaneous branch pierces the chest wall in front of the serratus anterior to supply the axillary skin; it may communicate with the intercostobrachial nerve and sometimes joins with the medial cutaneous nerve of the arm (Cave 1929). The first thoracic ramus often connects with the second across the neck of the second rib.

The second to sixth thoracic ventral rami proceed in their intercostal spaces below the intercostal vessels. Posteriorly they are between the pleura and posterior intercostal membranes but in most of their course run between the internal intercostals and the subcostales and intercostales intimi (**8**.360). Near the sternum, they cross anterior to the internal thoracic vessels and the transversus thoracis, pierce the internal intercostals, external intercostal membrane and pectoralis major, ending as the *anterior cutaneous nerves of the thorax*, which supply the skin on the front of the thorax. The second anterior cutaneous nerve may be connected to the medial supraclavicular nerves; twigs from the sixth supply abdominal skin in the upper part of the infrasternal angle.

Branches. Numerous muscular rami supply the intercostals, serratus posterior superior and transversus thoracis. Anteriorly some cross the costal cartilages from one intercostal space to another.

From each intercostal nerve a collateral and a lateral cutaneous branch leave before the main nerve reaches the costal angle. The *collateral branch* follows the inferior border of its space in the same intermuscular place as the main nerve, which it may rejoin before distribution as an additional anterior cutaneous nerve. The *lateral cutaneous* branch accompanies the main nerve a little way and then pierces the intercostal muscles obliquely; except for the first and second, each divides into anterior and posterior rami which pierce the serratus anterior. *Anterior branches* run forwards over the border of the pectoralis major to supply the overlying skin, the fifth and sixth also supplying twigs to a variable number of upper digitations of the obliquus abdominis externus. *Posterior branches* run back to supply the skin over the scapula and latissimus dorsi.

The second lateral cutaneous branch is the *intercostobrachial nerve* (**8**.370). It crosses the axilla to the medial side of the arm, joins with a branch of the medial cutaneous nerve of the arm, pierces the deep fascia and supplies the skin of the upper half of the posterior and medial aspects of the arm, connecting with the posterior cutaneous branch of the radial nerve. Its size is in inverse proportion to the size of the medial cutaneous nerve. A second intercostobrachial nerve often branches off from the anterior part of the third lateral cutaneous nerve supplying the axilla and the medial side of the arm.

SEVENTH TO THE TWELFTH THORACIC VENTRAL RAMI

These lower thoracic ventral rami continue anteriorly from the intercostal spaces into the abdominal wall. Approaching the anterior ends of their spaces, the seventh and eighth curve superomedially across the deep costal surface between the digitations of the transverse abdominis to reach the deep aspect of the posterior layer of the internal oblique aponeurosis. Piercing this they are posterior to the rectus abdominis and continue (**8**.375) for a short distance parallel with the costal margin. Both supply the rectus abdominis and, having traversed it near its lateral edge, pierce its anterior sheath to supply the skin. Both the seventh and eighth nerves cross the costal margin medial to the lateral border of the rectus abdominis and hence enter its sheath from behind.

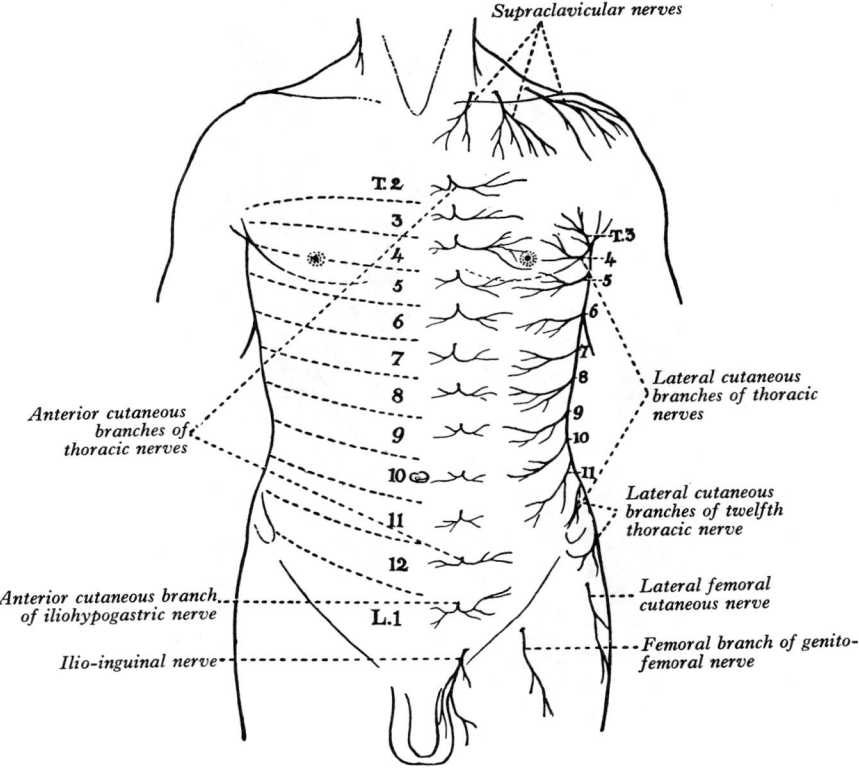

Supraclavicular nerves

T.2
3
4
5
6
7
8
9
10
11
12
L.1

T3
4
5
6
7
8
9
10
11

Anterior cutaneous branches of thoracic nerves

Lateral cutaneous branches of thoracic nerves

Lateral cutaneous branches of twelfth thoracic nerve

Anterior cutaneous branch of iliohypogastric nerve

Ilio-inguinal nerve

Lateral femoral cutaneous nerve

Femoral branch of genitofemoral nerve

8.374 The approximate segmental distribution of the cutaneous nerves on the front of the trunk. The contribution from the first thoracic spinal nerve is not shown and the considerable overlap which occurs between adjacent segments is not indicated. For the latter see **8**.367.

The ninth to eleventh intercostal nerves pass between digitations of the diaphragm and transversus abdominis to gain the interval between the transversus and the internal oblique. Here the ninth nerve runs forwards almost horizontally, while the tenth and eleventh pass inferomedially. At the lateral edge of the rectus abdominis they pierce the posterior layer of the internal oblique aponeurosis and pass behind the muscle, ending like the seventh and eighth intercostal nerves. The tenth supplies a band of skin which includes the umbilicus (8.367, 374).

These lower intercostal nerves supply intercostal, subcostal and abdominal muscles and the last three supply the serratus posterior inferior. They also provide sensory fibres to the costal parts of the diaphragm and related parietal pleura and peritoneum. Like the upper intercostal nerves they give off *collateral and lateral cutaneous branches* before they reach the costal angles. The collateral may rejoin its parent nerve but, if it does, it leaves it again near lateral border of the rectus abdominis to run forward below it (8.375), piercing the muscle and its anterior sheath near the linea alba to supply the skin. The lateral cutaneous branches pierce the intercostals and external oblique in the same line as the upper branches, dividing also into anterior and posterior rami, distributed to the skin of the abdomen and back; the anterior also supply digitations of the external oblique, extending antero-inferiorly nearly to the margin of the rectus abdominis; the posterior branches pass back to supply the skin over the latissimus dorsi. Each lateral cutaneous nerve descends as it pierces the external oblique and superficial fascia, reaching the skin on a level with the anterior and posterior cutaneous nerves of

the segment (p. 1263 and 8.375).

The ventral ramus of the *twelfth thoracic nerve* (subcostal nerve) is larger than the others; it connects with the first lumbar ventral ramus (*dorsolumbar nerve*). Like an intercostal nerve it has a collateral branch. It accompanies the subcostal vessels along the inferior border of the twelfth rib, passing behind the lateral arcuate ligament and kidney (13.37), anterior to the upper part of the quadratus lumborum, perforates the aponeurosis of the origin of the transversus and proceeds between the transversus and the internal oblique, to be distributed like the lower intercostal nerves. It connects with the iliohypogastric nerve and supplies the pyramidalis. Its *lateral cutaneous branch* pierces the internal and external oblique muscles, supplies the latter's lowest slip, crosses the iliac crest about 5 cm behind the anterior superior iliac spine (8.375) and supplies the anterior gluteal skin, some filaments reaching the greater trochanter of the femur.

Lesions of the intercostal nerves. In many conditions affecting spinal rami at or near their origins, pain is referred to their peripheral distributions. Thus, in tuberculosis of the lower thoracic vertebrae, pain is referred to the abdominal wall. When confined to a single pair of nerves the sensation is constrictive, as if a cord were tied round the abdomen. Where two or more nerves are involved, the pain is more diffused.

Subluxation of the interchondral joints between the lower costal cartilages may trap the intercostal nerves, causing referred abdominal pain. Abrahams (1976) has reviewed the literature on this subluxation or 'clicking rib syndrome'.

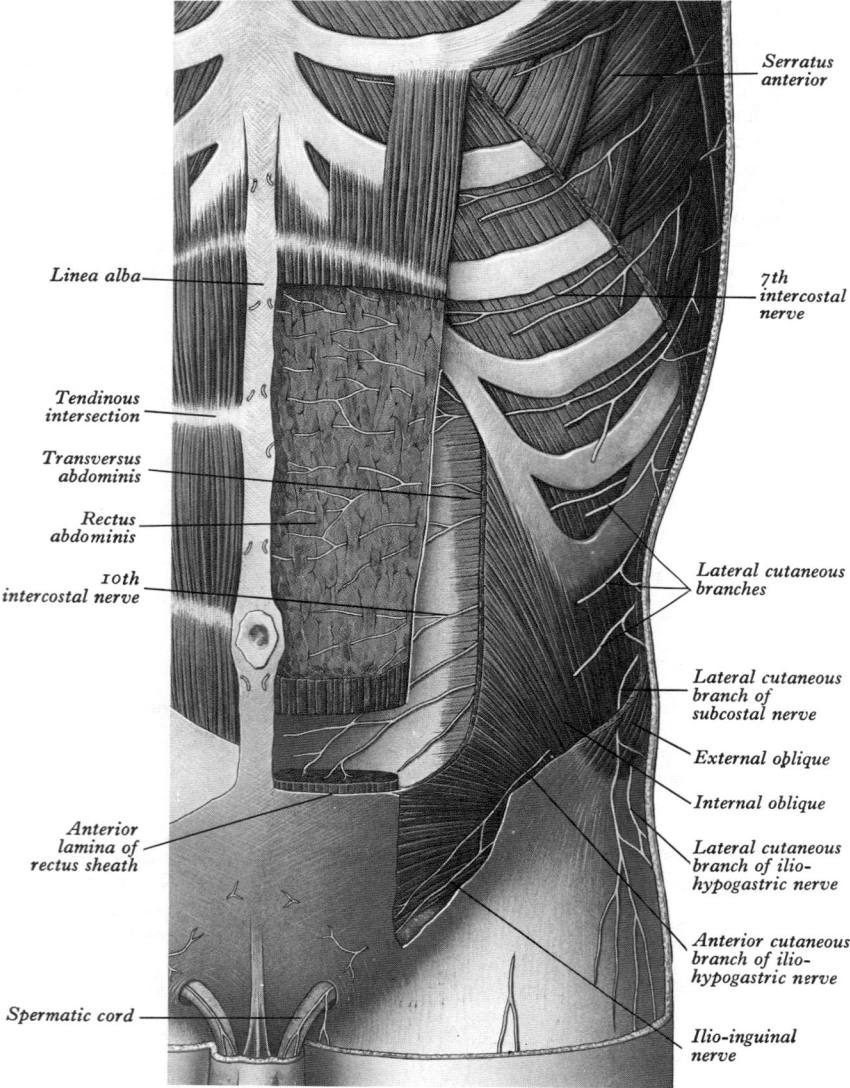

Linea alba

Tendinous intersection

Transversus abdominis

Rectus abdominis

10th intercostal nerve

Anterior lamina of rectus sheath

Spermatic cord

Serratus anterior

7th intercostal nerve

Lateral cutaneous branches

Lateral cutaneous branch of subcostal nerve

External oblique

Internal oblique

Lateral cutaneous branch of iliohypogastric nerve

Anterior cutaneous branch of iliohypogastric nerve

Ilio-inguinal nerve

8.375 The course of the lower intercostal and the cutaneous branches of some lumbar nerves. Portions of the muscles of the anterior abdominal wall have been removed, including most of the anterior layer of the rectus sheath and parts of the rectus abdominis.

The **dorsal** cutaneous branch of an intercostal nerve can become entrapped as it penetrates the fascia of the erector spinae muscles. This produces an area of numbness, usually with painful paraesthesiae, which extends from the midline laterally about 10 cm and the patch is usually about 10 cm in length (notalgia paraesthetica). Commonly the area between the medial edge of the scapula and the spine is affected.

The **anterior** cutaneous branches of the intercostal nerves can become entrapped as they penetrate the fascia of the rectus abdominus muscles and give rise to an area of numbness on the abdomen, usually with painful paraesthesiae, extending from the midline laterally 10 or 12 cm (rectus abdominus syndrome).

Nerves supplying the abdominal skin also supply the planes of underlying muscle, an important fact in protection of the abdominal viscera. A forceful blow will not injure the viscera if the muscles are contracted; but when a blow is unexpected, with the abdominal muscles relaxed, a force insufficient to damage the abdominal wall may rupture some of these viscera. Immediate reflex contraction is obviously important; the origin of the cutaneous and motor fibres from the same spinal segments accelerates the response.

Branches supplying abdominal muscles and skin, derived from the lower intercostal nerves, are intimately connected with the sympathetic nerves supplying the abdominal viscera through the lower thoracic ganglia, from which the splanchnic nerves are derived. Hence in injuries or acute infection of the abdominal viscera, the muscles of the abdominal wall become firmly contracted, resting and protecting the abdominal contents.

LUMBAR VENTRAL RAMI

Lumbar ventral rami increase in size from first to last and are joined, near their origins, by *grey rami communicantes* from the four lumbar sympathetic ganglia. These rami, long and slender, accompany the lumbar arteries round the sides of the vertebral bodies, behind the psoas major. Their arrangement is irregular: one ganglion may give rami to two lumbar nerves, one lumbar nerve may receive rami from the ganglia; rami often leave the sympathetic trunk between ganglia. The first and second, and sometimes the third, lumbar ventral rami are each connected with the lumbar sympathetic trunk by a *white ramus communicans*. The lumbar ventral rami descend laterally into the psoas major. The first three and most of the fourth form the lumbar plexus; the smaller moiety of the fourth joins the fifth as a *lumbosacral trunk*, which joins the sacral plexus. The fourth is often termed the *nervus furcalis*, being divided between the two plexuses; but the third is occasionally the nervus furcalis; or both third and fourth may be furcal nerves, when the plexus is termed *prefixed*. More frequently the fifth nerve is furcal, the plexus then being termed *postfixed*. These variations modify the sacral plexus. Piasecka-Kacperska and Gladyskowska-Rzeczycka (1972) have reviewed the variations in primates, including man.

LUMBAR PLEXUS

This plexus (**8.377, 378**) is in the posterior part of the psoas major, anterior to the lumbar transverse processes. It is formed by the first three lumbar ventral rami and most of the fourth; the first receives a branch from the last thoracic. The *paravertebral* part of psoas major has a *posterior* mass attached to the transverse processes and an *anterior* mass attached to the lips of the vertebral bodies, intervertebral discs and tendinous arches (p. 870); the lumbar plexus is between these masses and hence in 'line' with the intervertebral foramina.

In its usual arrangement the plexus is formed as follows: the first lumbar ramus, joined by a branch from the twelfth thoracic, bifurcates; the upper and larger part divides again into iliohypogastric and ilio-inguinal nerves; the lower unites with a second lumbar branch to form the genitofemoral nerve. The remainder of the second, third and the part of the fourth ramus joining the plexus divide into ventral and dorsal branches. Ventral branches of the second to fourth rami form the obturator nerve. Dorsal branches of the second and third rami each divide into smaller and larger parts; the smaller parts unite as the lateral femoral cutaneous nerve, the larger join with the dorsal branch of the fourth to form the femoral

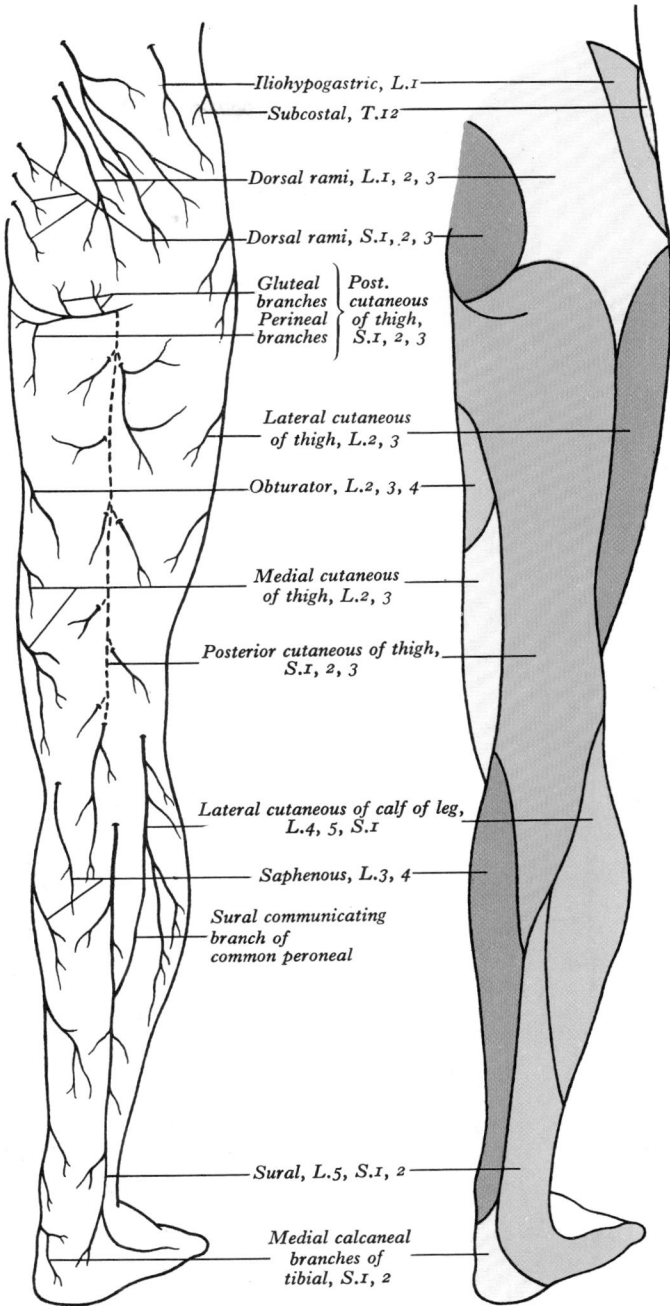

8.376 The cutaneous nerves of the right lower limb and their areas of distribution and segmental origins, viewed from the posterior aspect. The major part of the trunk of the posterior cutaneous nerve of the thigh lies deep to the deep fascia and is therefore shown by an interrupted line.

nerve. The accessory obturator, when it exists, arises from the third and fourth ventral branches. For details of the blood supply of the lumbar plexus see Day (1964).

The branches of the lumbar plexus are:

Muscular	T12, L1, 2, 3, 4
Iliohypogastric	L1
Ilio-inguinal	L1
Genitofemoral	L1, 2
	Dorsal divisions:
Lateral femoral cutaneous	L2, 3
Femoral	L2, 3, 4
	Ventral divisions:
Obturator	L2, 3, 4
Accessory obturator	L3, 4

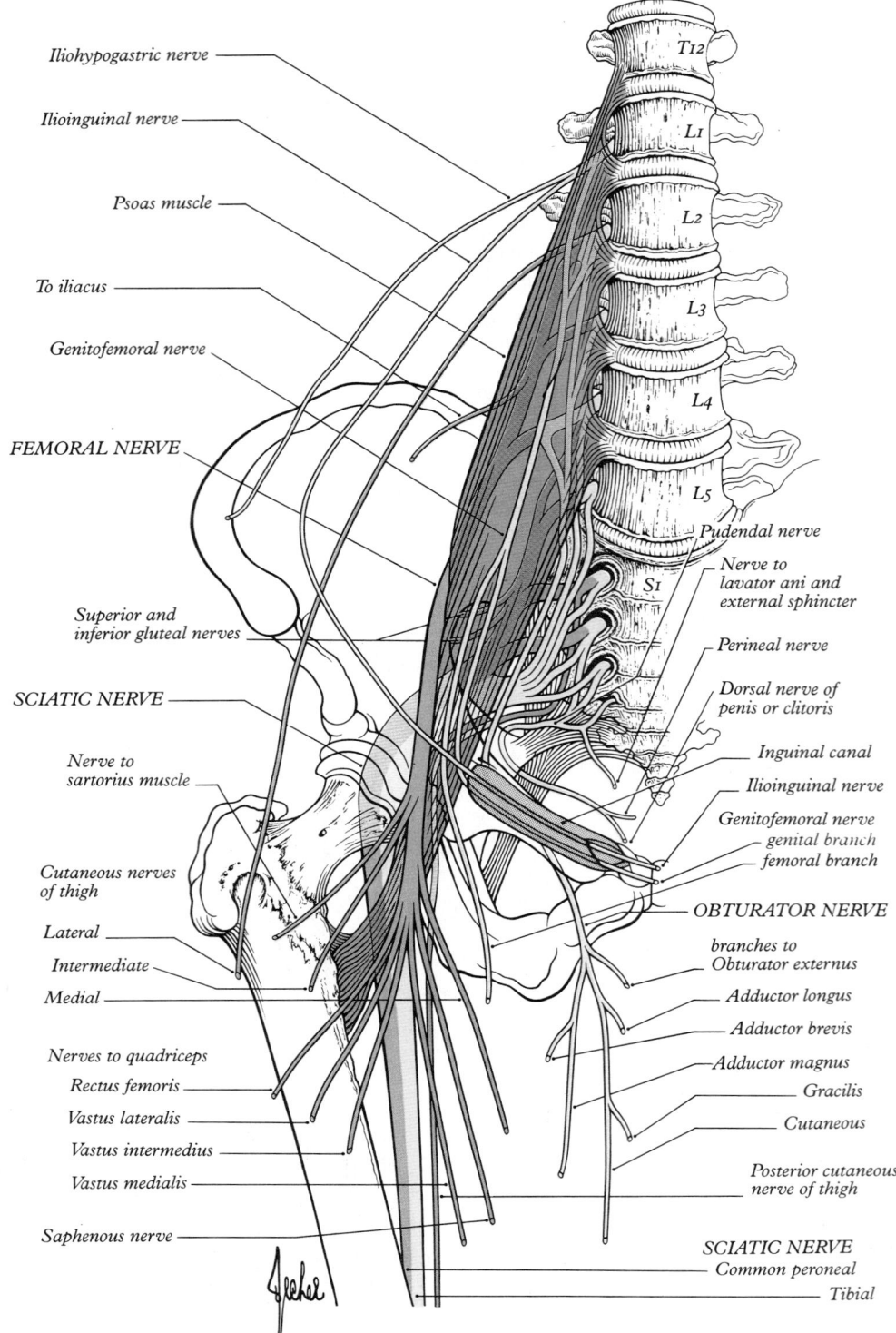

Iliohypogastric nerve

Ilioinguinal nerve

Psoas muscle

To iliacus

Genitofemoral nerve

FEMORAL NERVE

Superior and
inferior gluteal nerves

SCIATIC NERVE

Nerve to
sartorius muscle

Cutaneous nerves
of thigh

Lateral

Intermediate

Medial

Nerves to quadriceps

Rectus femoris

Vastus lateralis

Vastus intermedius

Vastus medialis

Saphenous nerve

T12

L1

L2

L3

L4

L5

Pudendal nerve

S1

Nerve to
lavator ani and
external sphincter

Perineal nerve

Dorsal nerve of
penis or clitoris

Inguinal canal

Ilioinguinal nerve

Genitofemoral nerve
genital branch
femoral branch

OBTURATOR NERVE

branches to
Obturator externus

Adductor longus

Adductor brevis

Adductor magnus

Gracilis

Cutaneous

Posterior cutaneous
nerve of thigh

SCIATIC NERVE
Common peroneal
Tibial

8.377   Diagram of the lumbosacral plexus, its branches and the muscles
which they supply.

Muscular branches. These supply the quadratus lumborum (T12, L1–4), psoas minor (L1), psoas major (L2, 3(4)) and iliacus (L2, 3).

Iliohypogastric nerve (L1). This emerges from the upper lateral border of the psoas major, crosses obliquely behind the lower renal pole and in front of the quadratus lumborum (**8.378**, **13.**4). Above the iliac crest it perforates the posterior part of the transversus abdominis, dividing between this and the internal oblique into lateral and anterior cutaneous branches, also supplying both muscles. The *lateral cutaneous branch* pierces the internal and external oblique muscles above the iliac crest a little behind the iliac branch of the twelfth thoracic nerve; it is distributed to the posterolateral gluteal skin. The *anterior cutaneous branch* (**8.375**) runs between and supplies the internal oblique and the transversus, pierces the internal oblique about 2 cm medial to the anterior superior iliac spine, and the external oblique aponeurosis about 3 cm above the superficial inguinal ring;

it is distributed to the suprapubic skin. The iliohypogastric nerve connects with the subcostal and ilio-inguinal nerves.

Ilio-inguinal nerve. Smaller than the iliohypogastric, this arises with it from the first lumbar ventral ramus (**8.377**), emerges from the lateral border of the psoas major, with or just caudal to the iliohypogastric, passes obliquely across the quadratus lumborum and the upper part of the iliacus and perforates the transversum abdominis near the anterior end of the iliac crest, sometimes connecting with the iliohypogastric. It then pierces the internal oblique, supplying it, traverses the inguinal canal below the spermatic cord, emerging with it from the superficial inguinal ring to supply the proximomedial skin of the thigh and either that over the penile root and upper part of the scrotum (**8.375**) or that covering the mons pubis and the adjoining labium majus.

The ilio-inguinal and iliohypogastric nerves are reciprocal in size.

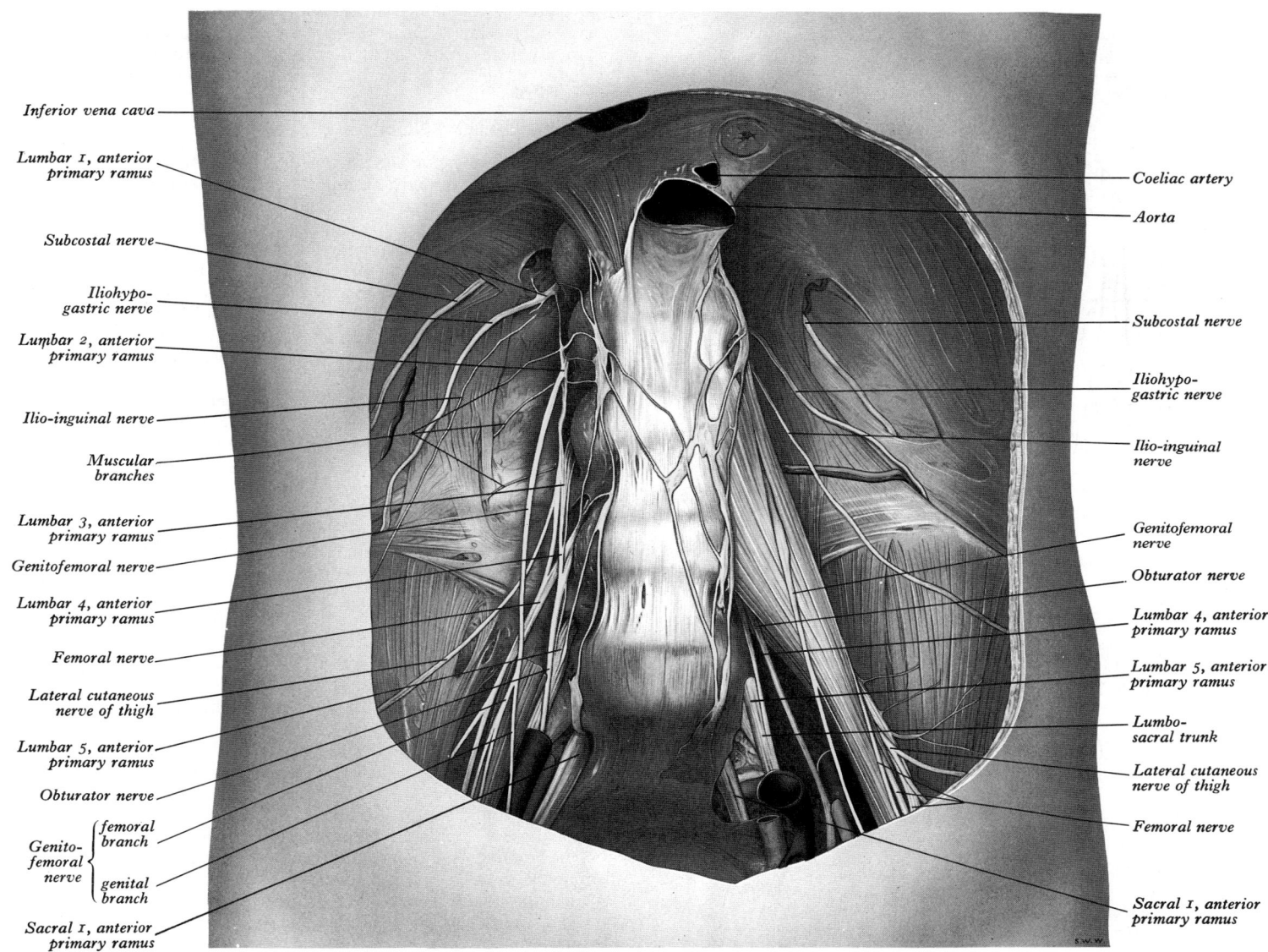

8.378 A dissection of the posterior abdominal wall to show the lumbar plexus and sympathetic trunks. The right psoas major has been removed.

The former is occasionally very small and ends by joining the iliohypogastric, a branch of the latter taking its place; or the ilio-inguinal may be absent. By analogy the ilio-inguinal may be regarded as the collateral branch of the first lumbar nerve (Davies 1935) and the iliohypogastric as the main trunk, providing the lateral cutaneous branch.

Genitofemoral nerve (L1, 2) (**8.377**). This descends obliquely forwards through the psoas major, emerging on the abdominal surface near its medial border, opposite the third or fourth lumbar vertebra; it descends subperitoneally on the psoas major, crosses obliquely behind the ureter, dividing variably above the inguinal ligament into genital and femoral branches. It often divides close to its origin, its branches then emerging separately from the psoas major. The *genital branch* crosses the lower part of the external iliac artery, enters the inguinal canal by its deep ring and supplies the cremaster and the scrotal skin. In females it accompanies the round ligament and ends in the skin of the mons pubis and labium majus. The *femoral branch* descends lateral to the external iliac artery, sending a few filaments round it; then crosses the deep circumflex iliac artery, passes behind the inguinal ligament, enters the femoral sheath lateral to the femoral artery, pierces the anterior layer of the femoral sheath and fascia lata and supplies the skin anterior to the upper part of the femoral triangle (**8.379**). It connects with the

femoral intermediate cutaneous nerve and supplies the femoral artery.

Injury to the iliohypogastric, ilio-inguinal or genitofemoral nerves. Damage to the iliohypogastric, ilio-inguinal or genitofemoral nerves is nearly always a result of direct injury, usually the result of surgery, particularly during inguinal herniorrhaphy or the exploration of a retrocaecal appendix.

Lateral femoral cutaneous nerve. This comes from the dorsal branches of the second and third lumbar ventral rami (**8.377**), and emerges from the lateral border of psoas major, crossing the iliacus obliquely towards the anterior superior iliac spine. It supplies the parietal peritoneum in the iliac fossa. The right nerve passes postero-lateral to the caecum, separated from it by the fascia iliaca and peritoneum; the left passes behind the lower part of the descending colon. Both pass behind or through the inguinal ligament, variably medial to the anterior superior iliac spine (commonly about 1 cm) and anterior to or through the sartorius into the thigh, dividing into anterior and posterior branches (**8.379**). The *anterior branch* becomes superficial about 10 cm distal to the anterior superior iliac spine, supplying the skin of the anterior and lateral thigh as far as the knee. It connects terminally with the cutaneous branches of the anterior division of the femoral nerve and the infrapatellar branch of the saphenous nerve, forming the *patellar plexus*. The *posterior*

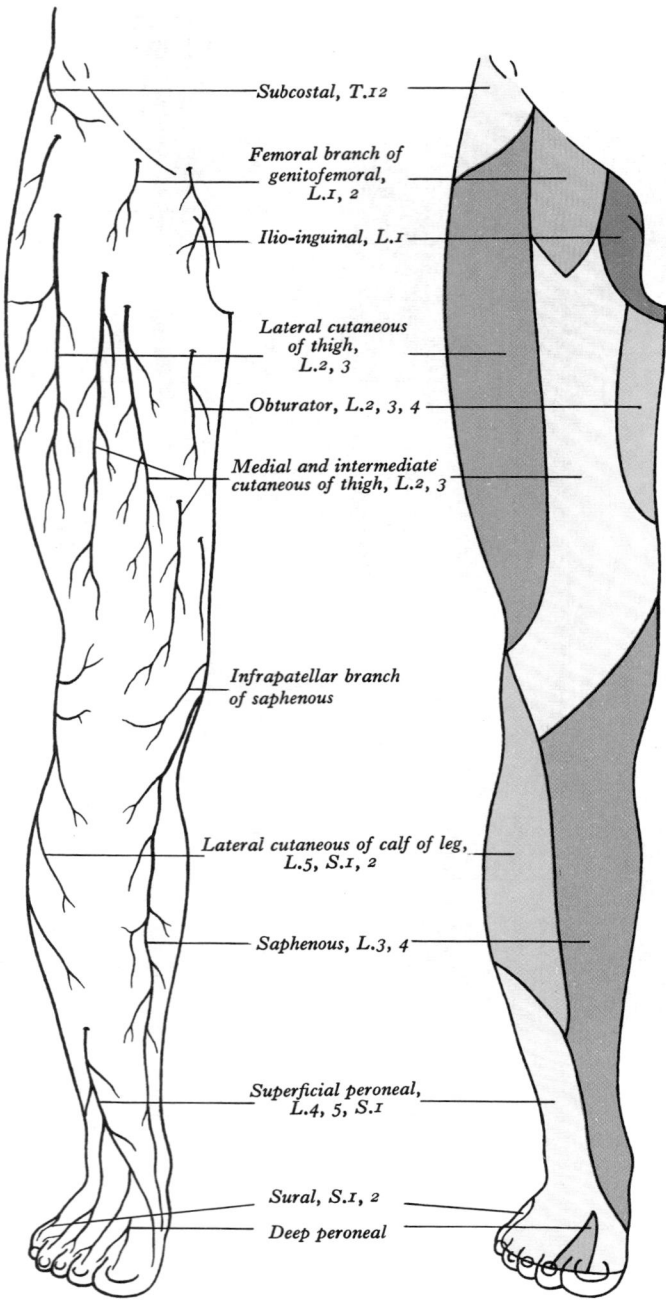

8.379 The cutaneous nerves of the right lower limb, their areas of distribution and segmental origins, viewed from the anterior aspect.

Labels on figure:
- Subcostal, T.12
- Femoral branch of genitofemoral, L.1, 2
- Ilio-inguinal, L.1
- Lateral cutaneous of thigh, L.2, 3
- Obturator, L.2, 3, 4
- Medial and intermediate cutaneous of thigh, L.2, 3
- Infrapatellar branch of saphenous
- Lateral cutaneous of calf of leg, L.5, S.1, 2
- Saphenous, L.3, 4
- Superficial peroneal, L.4, 5, S.1
- Sural, S.1, 2
- Deep peroneal

branch pierces the fascia lata higher than the anterior, dividing to supply the skin on the lateral surface from the greater trochanter to about midthigh. It may also supply the gluteal skin.

Lesions of the lateral cutaneous nerve of the thigh. This nerve is seldom involved in its retroperitoneal course through the pelvis. It leaves the pelvis just medial to the anterior superior iliac spine and either passes through or deep to the inguinal ligament, where it may become compressed. There is an area of impaired sensation, often with pain and paraesthesiae on the anterolateral aspect of the thigh (meralgia paraesthetica). The area involved is immensely variable, but is usually confined to the distal cutaneous distribution of the anterior branch of the lateral cutaneous nerve. This area does not extend across the midline anteriorly, it does not extend below the knee and it does not extend behind the hamstring tendons laterally. Exceptionally the posterior branch of the lateral cutaneous nerve of the thigh may be affected separately; this supplies a thin strip from

the greater trochanter of the femur down about two-thirds of the way to the knee. This branch leaves the main trunk of the nerve, usually distal to the inguinal ligament, and it then turns laterally to pierce the tensor fasciae latae muscle where it may become entrapped.

OBTURATOR NERVE

The obturator nerve arises from the ventral branches of the second to fourth lumbar ventral rami (**8.377, 378**), that from the third being the largest, the one from the second often very small. It descends in the psoas major, emerging from its medial border at the pelvic brim to pass behind the common iliac and lateral to the internal iliac vessels. It then descends forwards along the lesser pelvic lateral wall on the obturator internus, anterosuperior to the obturator vessels, to the obturator foramen, entering the thigh by its upper part. Near the foramen it divides into anterior and posterior branches, separated at first by part of the obturator externus, lower down by the adductor brevis.

The *anterior branch* (**8.380**) leaves the pelvis anterior to the obturator externus, descending in front of the adductor brevis, behind the pectineus and adductor longus; at the lower border of the latter it communicates with the medial cutaneous and saphenous branches of the femoral nerve, forming a *subsartorial plexus*, which supplies the skin on the medial side of the thigh (**8.379**). It descends on the femoral artery, which its termination supplies. Near the obturator foramen the anterior branch supplies the hip joint. Behind the pectineus it innervates the adductor longus, gracilis, usually the adductor brevis and often the pectineus; it connects with the accessory obturator nerve when present. Occasionally the communicating branch to the femoral medial cutaneous and saphenous branches continues as a cutaneous branch to the thigh and leg, emerging from behind the distal border of the adductor longus to descend along the posterior margin of the sartorius to the knee, where it pierces the deep fascia, connects with the saphenous nerve and supplies the skin halfway down the medial side of the leg. The *posterior branch* pierces the obturator externus anteriorly, supplies it and passes behind the adductor brevis to the front of the adductor magnus, dividing into branches to this and the adductor brevis when the latter is not supplied by the anterior division. It usually sends an *articular filament* to the knee joint which perforates the adductor magnus distally or traverses its opening with the femoral artery to enter the popliteal fossa. Here it descends on the popliteal artery to the back of the knee, pierces its oblique posterior ligament and supplies the articular capsule. It gives filaments to the popliteal artery.

Accessory obturator nerve (**8.377**). Occasionally present, this is small and arises from the ventral branches of the third and fourth lumbar ventral rami. It descends along the medial border of the psoas major, crosses the superior pubic ramus behind the pectineus and divides into branches, one entering the deep surface of the pectineus, another supplying the hip joint and a third connecting with the anterior branch of the obturator nerve; sometimes the accessory obturator nerve is very small and supplies only the pectineus. Any branch may be absent and others occur, one sometimes supplying the adductor longus. An accessory obturator nerve appeared in 69 of 800 dissections (p. 876, Woodburne 1960).

Lesions of the obturator nerve. Isolated lesions of the obturator nerve are extremely rare, but may occasionally occur as a result of direct trauma. The obturator nerves may be involved together with the femoral nerve in retroperitoneal lesions close to their origins from the lumbar plexus.

FEMORAL NERVE

The femoral nerve (**8.377, 378, 380, 16.**14), the largest branch of the lumbar plexus, arises from the dorsal branches of the second to fourth lumbar ventral rami. It descends through the psoas major, emerging low on its lateral border, and then passes between the psoas and iliacus, deep to the iliac fascia; passing behind the inguinal ligament into the thigh, it splits into anterior and posterior divisions. Behind the inguinal ligament it is separated from the femoral artery by part of the psoas major. In the abdomen the nerve supplies small branches to the iliacus and pectineus and a branch to the proximal part of the femoral artery; the latter branch may arise in the thigh.

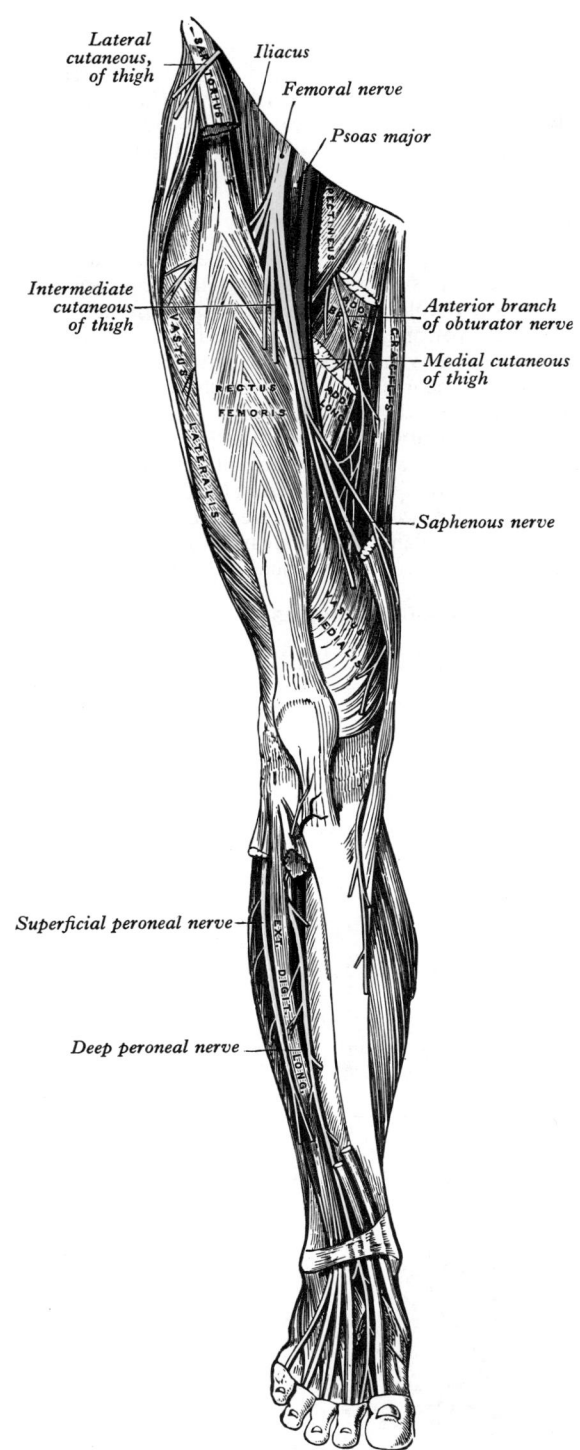

8.380 The nerves of the right lower limb, displayed from the anterior aspect.

the front of the thigh, supplying the skin as far as the knee and ending in the patellar plexus (p. 1279). The lateral branch of the intermediate cutaneous communicates with the femoral branch of the genitofemoral, frequently piercing the sartorius and sometimes supplying it.

Medial femoral cutaneous nerve. At first lateral to the femoral artery, this crosses anterior to it at the apex of the femoral triangle, dividing into anterior and posterior branches. Before this it sends a few rami through the fascia lata to supply the skin of the medial side of the thigh, near the long saphenous vein; one ramus emerges via the saphenous opening, another becomes subcutaneous about midthigh. The *anterior branch* descends on the sartorius, perforates the fascia lata beyond midthigh and divides into a branch supplying the skin as low as the medial side of the knee and another which crosses to the lateral side of the patella and connects with the infrapatellar branch of the saphenous nerve. The *posterior branch* descends along the posterior border of the sartorius to the knee, pierces the fascia lata, connects with the saphenous nerve and supplies several cutaneous rami, some as far as the medial side of the leg. Deep to the fascia lata, at the lower border of the adductor longus, it forms a *subsartorial plexus* with branches of the saphenous and obturator nerves. When the communicating branch of the obturator nerve is large and reaches the leg, the posterior branch of the medial cutaneous nerve is small, ending in the plexus and giving rise to a few cutaneous filaments.

Nerve to the sartorius. This arises in common with the intermediate femoral cutaneous nerve.

Posterior division

The posterior division of the femoral nerve supplies the saphenous nerve and branches to the quadriceps femoris and the knee joint.

Saphenous nerve (8.380). The largest femoral cutaneous branch, this descends lateral to the femoral artery into the adductor canal (p. 1564), where it crosses anteriorly to become medial to the artery. At the distal end of the canal it leaves the artery, emerging through the aponeurotic covering with the saphenous branch of the descending genicular artery. It proceeds vertically along the medial side of the knee behind the sartorius, pierces the fascia lata between the tendons of the sartorius and gracilis and becomes subcutaneous. Thence it descends the medial side of the leg with the long saphenous vein along the medial tibial border and divides distally into a branch continuing along the tibia to the ankle and into another passing anterior to the ankle to supply the skin on the medial side of the foot, often as far as the hallucial metatarsophalangeal joint; it connects with the medial branch of the superficial peroneal nerve. Near midthigh the saphenous nerve gives a branch to the subsartorial plexus. As it leaves the adductor canal an *infrapatellar* branch (8.379) pierces the sartorius and fascia lata to supply the prepatellar skin; proximal to the knee it connects with medial and intermediate femoral cutaneous nerves; distal to it, it connects with other branches of the saphenous nerve; laterally it connects with the lateral cutaneous femoral nerve, forming a *patellar plexus*.

Muscular branches. These branches of the posterior division of the femoral nerve supply the quadriceps femoris. A branch to the rectus femoris enters its proximal posterior surface, also supplying the hip joint. A larger branch to the vastus lateralis forms a neurovascular bundle with the descending branch of the lateral circumflex femoral artery in its distal part and also supplies the knee joint. A branch to the vastus medialis descends through the proximal part of the adductor canal, lateral to the saphenous nerve and femoral vessels; it enters the muscle at about its midpoint, sending a long articular filament distally along the muscle to the knee. Two or three branches to the vastus intermedius enter its anterior surface about midthigh; a branchlet from one descends through the muscle to the articularis genu and the knee joint.

Vascular branches. These branches of the femoral nerve supply the femoral artery and its branches (p. 1305).

Femoral neuropathy. The femoral nerve is not subject to an entrapment neuropathy, but may be compressed by retroperitoneal tumours, retroperitoneal haemorrhage in patients on anticoagulants or with a bleeding diathesis. A localized lesion of the femoral nerve may occur in diabetes mellitus (one of the forms of diabetic amyotrophy). The striking feature of femoral neuropathy is wasting and weakness of the quadriceps femoris muscles which cause con-

Nerve to the pectineus. This branches from the medial side of the femoral nerve near the inguinal ligament, passes behind the femoral sheath and enters the anterior aspect of the muscle.

Anterior division

The anterior division of the femoral nerve supplies intermediate and medial cutaneous femoral nerves (8.379, 380) and branches to the sartorius.

Intermediate femoral cutaneous nerve. This pierces the fascia lata about 8 cm below the inguinal ligament, either as two branches or as one trunk which quickly divides into two; these descend on

siderably difficulty in walking with a tendency for the leg to collapse. Pain and paraesthesiae may occur on the anterior and medial aspect of the thigh, extending down the medial aspect of the leg in the distribution of the saphenous branch of the femoral nerve. This branch may be the subject of an entrapment neuropathy as it leaves Hunter's canal.

SACRAL AND COCCYGEAL VENTRAL RAMI

The ventral rami of the sacral and coccygeal spinal nerves form the *sacral and coccygeal plexuses*. The upper four sacral ventral rami enter the pelvis by the anterior sacral foramina, the fifth between the sacrum and coccyx, while that of the coccygeal nerve curves forwards below the rudimentary transverse process of the first coccygeal segment. The first and second sacral ventral rami are large, the third to fifth diminish progressively and the coccygeal is the smallest. Each receives a *grey ramus communicans* from a corresponding sympathetic ganglion. *Visceral efferent rami* leave the second to fourth sacral rami as *pelvic splanchnic nerves* (8.381) containing parasympathetic fibres which reach minute ganglia in the walls of the pelvic viscera (p. 1297).

SACRAL PLEXUS

The sacral plexus (**8.**377, 382) is formed by the lumbosacral trunk, the first to third sacral ventral rami and part of the fourth, the remainder of the last joining the coccygeal plexus.

The lumbosacral trunk comprises part of the fourth and all the fifth lumbar ventral rami; it appears at the medial margin of the psoas major, descending over the pelvic brim anterior to the sacro-iliac joint to join the first sacral ramus. These rami converge to the greater sciatic foramen and unite with little intermingling to form upper and lower bands. The upper, larger one is the union of the lumbosacral trunk with the first, second and greater part of the third sacral rami; it becomes the *sciatic nerve*. The lower band, smaller and more plexiform, is mainly the junction of the smaller part of the third sacral ramus with part of the fourth; it becomes the *pudendal* nerve; it has a small contribution from the second sacral ramus. The sciatic comprises tibial and common peroneal nerves, which usually separate in the thigh but can be pulled apart to their origins, when it can be demonstrated that the tibial is formed by the union of the ventral divisions of the lumbosacral trunk and the first three sacral rami, while the common peroneal is formed by dorsal divisions of the lumbosacral trunk and the first two sacral rami. The sciatic nerve may, however, divide anywhere; when division is at the plexus the common peroneal nerve usually pierces the piriformis in the greater sciatic foramen. (For the blood supply of the sacral plexus see Day 1964.)

Relations of the sacral plexus

The sacral plexus adjoins the posterior pelvic wall anterior to the piriformis (**8.**383), posterior to the internal iliac vessels and ureter and to the sigmoid colon on the left and the terminal ileal coils on the right. The superior gluteal vessels lie between the lumbosacral trunk and first sacral ventral ramus or between the first and second sacral rami, while the inferior gluteal vessels lie between the first and second or second and third sacral rami.

Lesions of the lumbosacral plexus. Malignant infiltration is the most common cause of involvement of the lumbosacral plexus, usually due to spread of carcinoma from the cervix, uterus or rectum. The plexus may also be involved in the reticuloses or be affected by plexiform neuromas. Pain, which may be diffuse, is the most common feature, and there is clear involvement of several roots.

Branches of the sacral plexus

The branches of the sacral plexus are:

	Ventral divisions	Dorsal divisions
To quadratus femoris and gemellus inferior	L4, 5, S1	
To obturator internus and gemellus superior	L5, S1, 2	
To piriformis		S(1), 2
Superior gluteal		L4, 5, S1
Inferior gluteal		L5, S1, 2
Posterior femoral cutaneous	S2, 3	S1, 2
Tibial (sciatic)	L4, 5, S1, 2, 3	
Common peroneal (sciatic)		L4, 5, S1, 2
Perforating cutaneous		S2, 3
Pudendal	S2, 3, 4	
To levator ani, coccygeus and sphincter ani externus	S4	
Pelvic splanchnic	S2, 3, (4)	

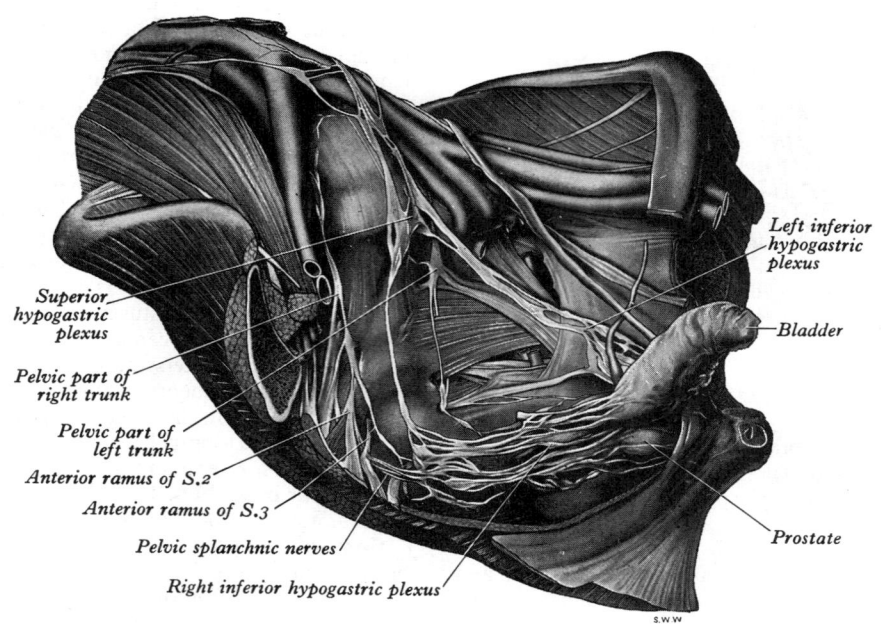

Superior hypogastric plexus

Pelvic part of right trunk

Pelvic part of left trunk

Anterior ramus of S.2

Anterior ramus of S.3

Pelvic splanchnic nerves

Right inferior hypogastric plexus

Left inferior hypogastric plexus

Bladder

Prostate

S.W.W.

8.381   The pelvic part of the sympathetic system, viewed from in front and from the right side, a large part of the right hip bone having been removed. The superior hypogastric plexus is seen to divide below into the right and left hypogastric nerves (which are not labelled), which run down to the inferior hypogastric plexuses. (Drawn from a dissection by the late G D Channell, Guy's Hospital Medical School, London.)

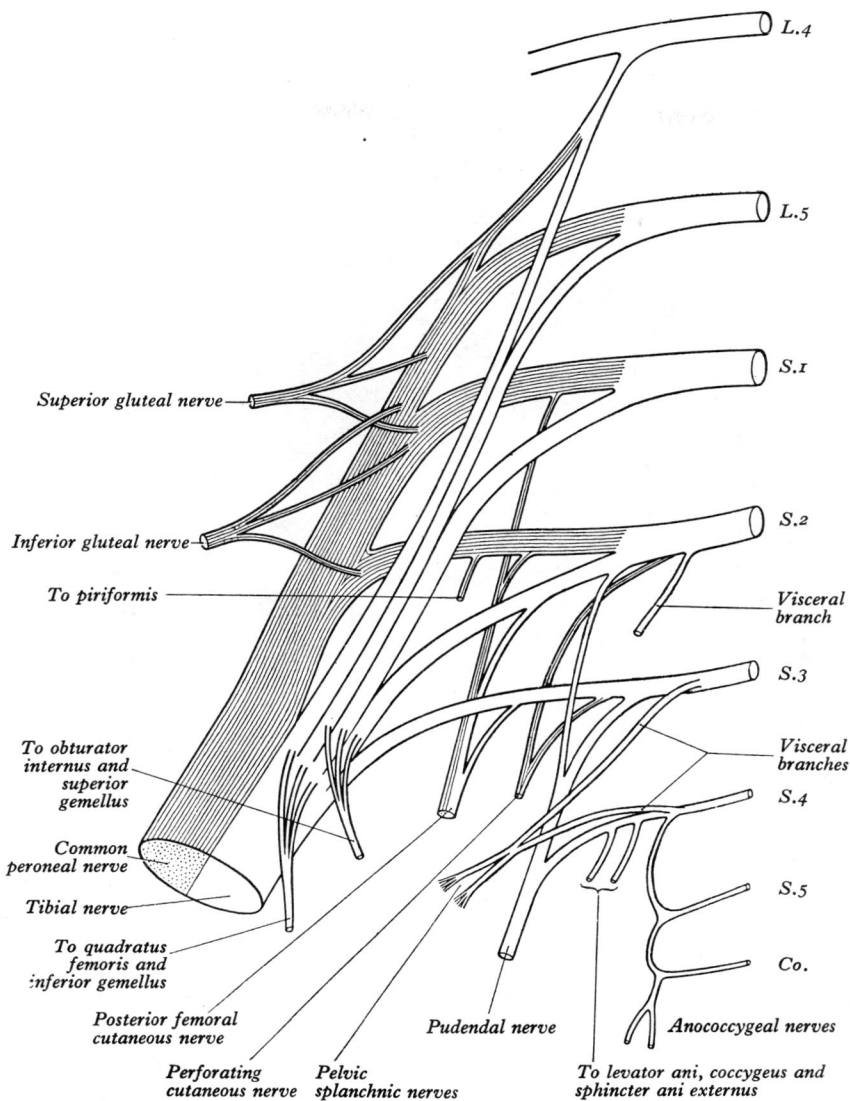

Superior gluteal nerve

Inferior gluteal nerve

To piriformis

To obturator internus and superior gemellus

Common peroneal nerve

Tibial nerve

To quadratus femoris and inferior gemellus

Posterior femoral cutaneous nerve

Perforating cutaneous nerve

Pelvic splanchnic nerves

Pudendal nerve

To levator ani, coccygeus and sphincter ani externus

Anococcygeal nerves

L.4

L.5

S.1

S.2

Visceral branch

S.3

Visceral branches

S.4

S.5

Co.

8.382 A plan of the sacral and coccygeal plexuses. L4–5, S1–5 and Co, indicate the *ventral rami* of these lumbar, sacral and coccygeal spinal nerves. The *ventral divisions* of these rami are unshaded, the *dorsal divisions*, and nerves derived from them, are shaded. The contribution from S2 to the pelvic splanchnic nerves is shown before joining those from 3 and 4.

Nerve to the quadratus femoris and gemellus inferior. This arises from the ventral branches of the fourth lumbar to the first sacral ventral rami (**8.382**), leaves the pelvis via the greater sciatic foramen below the piriformis, descends on the ischium deep to the sciatic nerve, gemelli and the tendon of the obturator internus and supplies the gemellus inferior, quadratus femoris and the hip joint.

Nerve to the obturator internus and gemellus superior. This arises from the ventral branches of the fifth lumbar and first and second sacral ventral rami (**8.382**), leaves the pelvis similarly to the above, supplies a branch to the upper posterior surface of the gemellus superior, crosses the ischial spine lateral to the internal pudendal vessels, re-enters the pelvis via the lesser sciatic foramen and enters the pelvic surface of the obturator internus.

Nerve to the piriformis. This usually arises from the dorsal branches of the first and second sacral ventral rami (sometimes only the second) and enters the anterior surface of the piriformis.

Superior gluteal nerve. This comes from the dorsal branches of the fourth and fifth lumbar and first sacral ventral rami (**8.382**), leaves the pelvis via the greater sciatic foramen above the piriformis with the superior gluteal vessels, and divides into superior and inferior branches. The *superior* branch accompanies the upper branch of the deep division of the superior gluteal artery to supply the gluteus medius and occasionally the gluteus minimus. The *inferior*

branch runs with the lower ramus of the deep division of the superior gluteal artery across the gluteus minimus, supplying the glutei medius and minimus and ending in the tensor fasciae latae.

Inferior gluteal nerve. This comes from the dorsal branches of the fifth lumbar and first and second sacral ventral rami, leaves the pelvis via the greater sciatic foramen below the piriformis, and divides into branches which enter the deep surface of the gluteus maximus.

The posterior femoral cutaneous nerve. This comes from the dorsal branches of the first and second and the ventral branches of the second and third sacral rami (**8.382**), issues via the greater sciatic foramen below the piriformis, descends under the gluteus maximus with the inferior gluteal vessels, lying posterior or medial to the sciatic nerve. It descends in the back of the thigh superficial to the long head of the biceps femoris, deep to the fascia lata; behind the knee it pierces the deep fascia and accompanies the short saphenous vein to midcalf, its terminal twigs connecting with the sural nerve. Its branches are all cutaneous, distributed to the gluteal region, perineum and the flexor aspect of the thigh and leg. Three or four *gluteal branches* curl round the lower border of the gluteus maximus to supply the skin over its inferolateral area. The *perineal branch* supplies the superomedial skin in the thigh, curves forwards across the hamstrings below the ischial tuberosity, pierces the fascia

1283

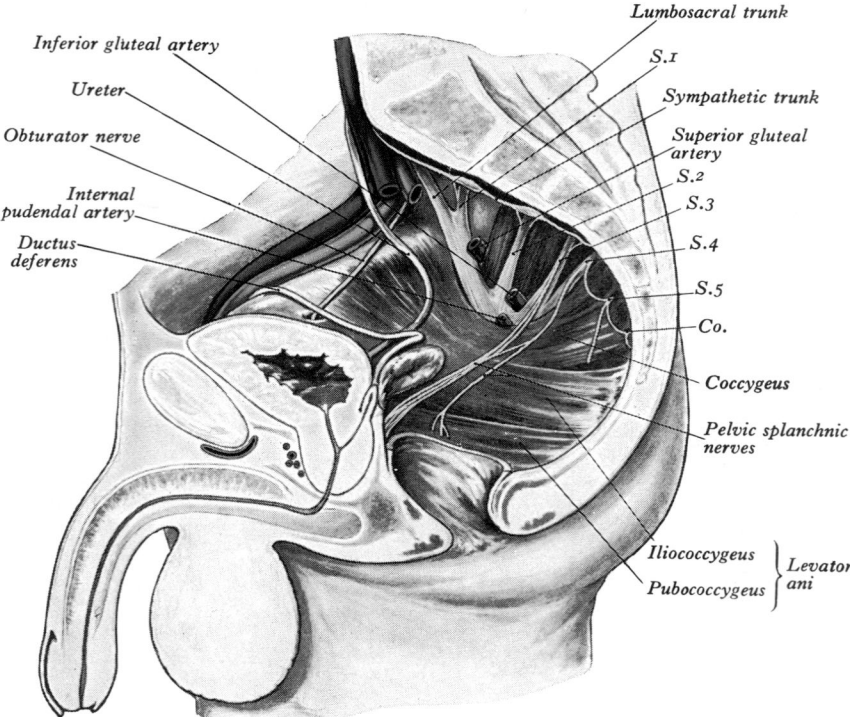

8.383 A dissection of the side wall of the pelvis, showing the sacral and coccygeal plexuses. S.1–5 indicate the ventral rami of the sacral spinal nerves; Co. indicates the ventral ramus of the coccygeal spinal nerve.

lata and runs in the superficial perineal fascia to the scrotal or labial skin, communicating with the inferior rectal and posterior scrotal branches of the perineal nerve. *Branches to the back of the thigh and leg* are numerous and from both sides of the posterior femoral cutaneous nerve; they supply the skin of the back and medial side of the thigh, the popliteal fossa and the proximal part of the back of the leg (**8.**376).

SCIATIC NERVE

The sciatic nerve (**8.**377, 384), 2 cm broad at its origin and the broadest nerve in the body, is the continuation of the upper band of the sacral plexus. It leaves the pelvis via the greater sciatic foramen below the piriformis and descends between the greater trochanter and ischial tuberosity, along the back of the thigh, dividing into the tibial and common peroneal (fibular) nerves, proximal to the knee. Superiorly it is deep to the gluteus maximus, resting first on the posterior ischial surface with the nerve to quadratus femoris between them; it then crosses posterior to the obturator internus and the gemelli, then on to the quadratus femoris, separated by it from obturator externus and the hip joint; it is accompanied medially by the posterior femoral cutaneous nerve and the inferior gluteal artery. More distally it is behind the adductor magnus and is crossed posteriorly by the long head of the biceps femoris. It corresponds to a line from just medial to the midpoint between the ischial tuberosity and greater trochanter to the apex of the popliteal fossa (see also **16.**8, 9).

Articular branches arise proximally to supply the hip joint through its posterior capsule; these are sometimes derived directly from the sacral plexus. *Muscular branches* are distributed to the biceps femoris, semitendinosus, semimembranosus and the ischial part of the adductor magnus (p. 877), as detailed below.

TIBIAL NERVE

The tibial nerve (**8.**384), the larger sciatic division (from the ventral branches of the fourth and fifth lumbar and first to third sacral ventral rami), descends along the back of the thigh and popliteal

fossa to the distal border of popliteus, passing anterior to the arch of soleus with the popliteal artery and continuing into the leg. In the thigh it is overlapped proximally by the hamstring muscles, but becomes more superficial in the popliteal fossa, where it is lateral to the popliteal vessels, becoming superficial to them at the knee and crossing to the medial side of the artery (**8.**385). Distally in the fossa it is overlapped by the junction of the two heads of gastrocnemius. Its surface projection (see also **16.**15) is a line in the midline of the limb, vertical from the apex of the popliteal fossa to the level of the fibular neck and thence to a point midway between the medial malleolus and calcanean tendon.

In the leg the tibial nerve descends with the posterior tibial vessels to lie between the heel and the medial malleolus, ending under the flexor retinaculum by dividing into medial and lateral plantar nerves. Proximally it is deep to the soleus and gastrocnemius, but in its distal third is covered only by skin and fasciae, overlapped sometimes by the flexor hallucis longus. At first medial to the posterior tibial vessels, it crosses behind them, descending lateral to them until it bifurcates. It lies on the tibialis posterior for most of its course, except distally, where it adjoins the posterior surface of the tibia.

Its branches are articular, muscular, sural, medial calcanean and medial and lateral plantar.

Articular branches. These accompany the superior, inferior medial and middle genicular arteries to the knee joint. The three form a plexus with an obturator branch, supplying the oblique posterior ligament; those with the superior and inferior genicular arteries supply the medial part of the capsule. Just before the tibial nerve bifurcates it supplies the ankle joint. Champetier and Déscours (1968) have surveyed these articular nerves. Gardner and Lenn (1977) assessed the ratios of myelinated to non-myelinated fibres in genual articular nerves in monkeys as about 4:1; they suggested that most are nociceptive.

Muscular branches. These arise between the heads of the gastrocnemius, and supply this, the plantaris, soleus and popliteus. The nerve to the soleus enters its superficial aspect; the branch to the popliteus descends obliquely across the popliteal vessels, curling round the distal border of the muscle to its anterior surface. It also supplies the tibialis posterior, the proximal tibiofibular joint, the

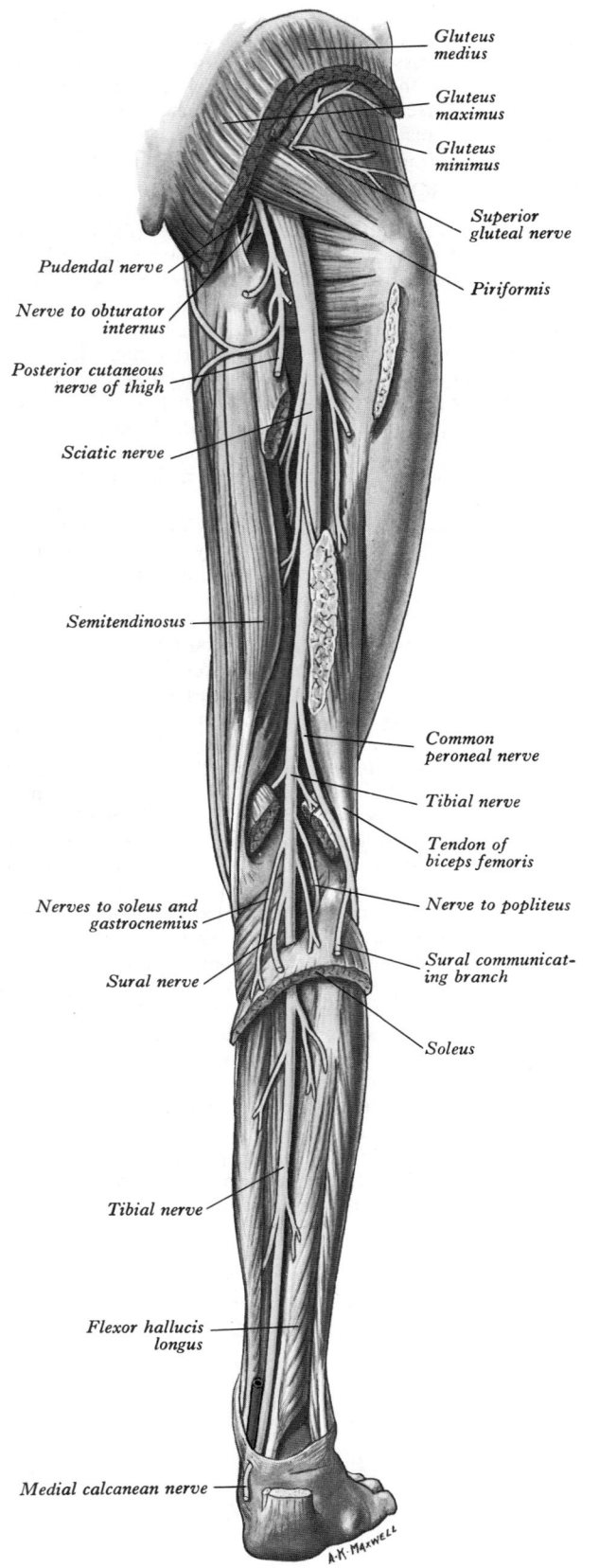

8.384   The nerves of the right lower limb: posterior aspect. Note that the gluteus maximus, the gluteus medius and the superficial muscles of the calf of the leg have been removed and the middle part of the long head of the biceps femoris has been excised.

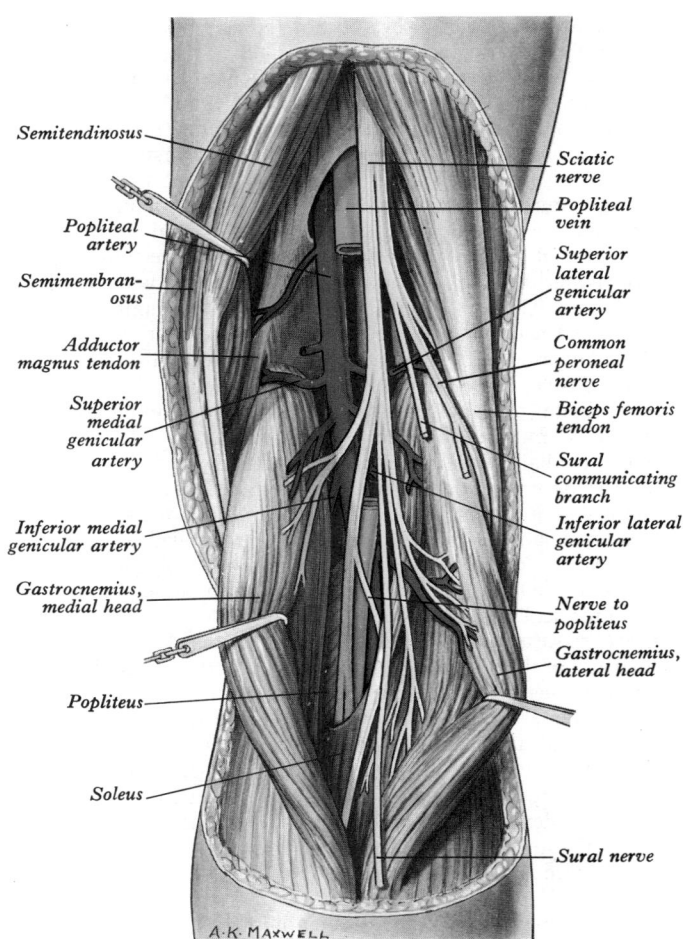

8.385   A dissection of the right popliteal fossa. The two heads of gastrocnemius and the semitendinosus and semimembranosus have been retracted in order to expose the contents of the fossa more fully.

tibia and an interosseous branch which descends near the fibula to reach the distal tibiofibular joint.

Muscular branches in the leg, independent or by a common trunk, supply the soleus (on its deep surface), the tibialis posterior, flexor digitorum longus and flexor hallucis longus, the branch to the last-named accompanying the peroneal vessels.

Sural nerve. This descends between the heads of the gastrocnemius, pierces the deep fascia proximally in the leg and is joined by a sural communicating branch of the common peroneal (**8.384**). It descends lateral to the tendo calcaneus, near the small saphenous vein, to the region between the lateral malleolus and the calcaneous; it supplies the posterior and lateral skin of the distal third of the leg, proceeding distal to the lateral malleolus along the lateral side of the foot and little toe; it connects on the dorsum of the foot with the superficial peroneal nerve, and in the leg with the posterior femoral cutaneous nerve. The fibre spectrum and ultrastructure of fetal sural nerves were described by Ochoa (1971) and in adults by Ochoa and Mair (1969a,b). The three-dimensional distribution of Schwann cells associated with unmyelinated nerve fibres in adult human sural nerves has been analysed by Carlsen and Behse (1980).

Medial calcanean branches. These perforate the flexor retinaculum to supply the skin of the heel and medial side of the sole.

Vascular branches. These supply arteries accompanying the tibial nerve and its branches (p. 1305).

Medial plantar nerve (**8.386**). The larger terminal division of the tibial nerve, this lies lateral to the medial plantar artery. From its origin under the flexor retinaculum it passes deep to the abductor hallucis, appears between it and the flexor digitorum brevis, gives off a medial proper digital nerve to the hallux and divides near the metatarsal bases into three common plantar digital nerves.

Cutaneous branches pierce the plantar aponeurosis between the abductor hallucis and the flexor digitorum brevis to supply the skin of the sole of the foot. *Muscular branches* supply the abductor hallucis, flexor digitorum brevis, flexor hallucis brevis and the first lumbrical; the first two arise near the origin of the nerve and enter the deep surfaces of the muscles; the branch to the flexor hallucis brevis is from the hallucial medial digital nerve, and that to the first lumbrical from the first common plantar digital nerve. *Articular branches* supply the joints of the tarsus and metatarsus.

Three common plantar digital nerves pass between the slips of the plantar aponeurosis, each dividing into two proper digital branches, the first supplying adjacent sides of the hallux and secundus, the second adjacent sides of the secundus and tertius, the third adjacent sides of the tertius and quartus and also connecting with the lateral plantar nerve. The first gives a branch to the first lumbrical. Each proper digital nerve has cutaneous and articular branches; near the distal phalanges a dorsal branch supplies structures around the nail; the end of each nerve supplies the ball of the toe. Note that the common digital branches of the medial plantar are **like those of the median nerve**; muscles supplied by both correspond closely. In the hand the median nerve supplies the abductor and flexor pollicis brevis, the opponens pollicis and the first and second lumbricals. The opponens is absent in the foot but the abductor hallucis, flexor hallucis brevis and the first lumbrical are all supplied by the medial plantar. Since the flexor digitorum brevis and flexor digitorum superficialis (median nerve) correspond, only the innervation of the second lumbrical differs.

Lateral plantar nerve (8.386). This supplies the skin of the digitus quintus, and of the lateral half of the quartus and most deep muscles, **like the ulnar nerve in the hand**. It passes laterally forwards with the lateral plantar artery lateral to it, towards the tubercle of the fifth metatarsal and then between the flexores digitorum brevis and accessorius, to end between the former and the abductor digiti minimi, dividing into superficial and deep branches. Before division it supplies the flexor digitorum accessorius and abductor digiti minimi and gives rise to small branches which pierce the plantar fascia to supply the skin of the lateral part of the sole (8.387). The *superficial branch* splits into two common plantar digital nerves: the lateral supplies the **lateral** side of the digitus quintus, flexor digiti minimi brevis and the two interossei in the fourth intermetatarsal space; the medial connects with the third common plantar digital branch of the medial plantar nerve, dividing into two to supply the adjoining sides of the digitus quartus and quintus. The *deep branch* accompanies

the lateral plantar artery deep to the flexor tendons and the adductor hallucis, supplying the second to fourth lumbricals, the adductor hallucis and all interossei (except those of the fourth intermetatarsal space); branches to the second and third lumbricals pass distally deep to the transverse head of the adductor hallucis, curling round its distal border to reach them (8.388).

COMMON PERONEAL NERVE

The common peroneal nerve (8.384), about half the size of the tibial, is derived from the dorsal branches of the fourth and fifth lumbar and first and second sacral ventral rami. It descends obliquely along the lateral side of the popliteal fossa to the fibular head, medial to the biceps femoris and lying between its tendon and the lateral head of the gastrocnemius. It curves lateral to the fibular neck deep to the peroneus longus and divides into superficial and deep peroneal nerves. Its course (see **16**.15) can be indicated by a line from the apex of the fossa, passing distally medial to the biceps tendon to the back of the head of the fibula, where the nerve can be rolled against the bone. Before division it gives off articular and cutaneous branches.

Of the three *articular branches* two accompany the superior and inferior lateral genicular arteries; they may arise in common. The third, termed the recurrent articular nerve, arises near the division of the common peroneal and ascends with the anterior recurrent tibial artery through the tibialis anterior to supply the anterolateral part of the genual capsule and the proximal tibiofibular joint. *Two cutaneous branches* (8.376), often from a common trunk, are the lateral sural and sural communicating nerves.

The *lateral sural nerve* (*lateral cutaneous nerve of the calf*) supplies the skin on the anterior, posterior and lateral surfaces of the proximal leg. The *sural communicating nerve* arises near the head of the fibula and crosses the lateral head of the gastrocnemius to join the sural nerve (p. 1285). It may descend separately as far as the heel.

Deep peroneal nerve (8.380). This begins at the common peroneal bifurcation, between the fibula and the proximal part of the peroneus longus and passes obliquely forwards deep to the extensor digitorum longus to the front of the interosseous membrane, reaching the anterior tibial artery in the proximal third of the leg; it descends with it to the ankle, dividing there into lateral and medial terminal branches. It is first lateral to the artery, then anterior and again lateral at the ankle. It supplies *muscular branches* to the tibialis anterior, extensor hallucis longus, extensor digitorum longus and peroneus tertius and an *articular branch* to the ankle joint.

The lateral *terminal branch* crosses the tarsus deep to the extensor digitorum brevis, enlarges as a pseudoganglion (cf. other sites p. 1270) and supplies the extensor digitorum brevis. From the enlargement three minute *interosseous branches* supply the tarsal and metatarsophalangeal joints of the middle three toes; the first branch supplies the second dorsal interosseous muscle.

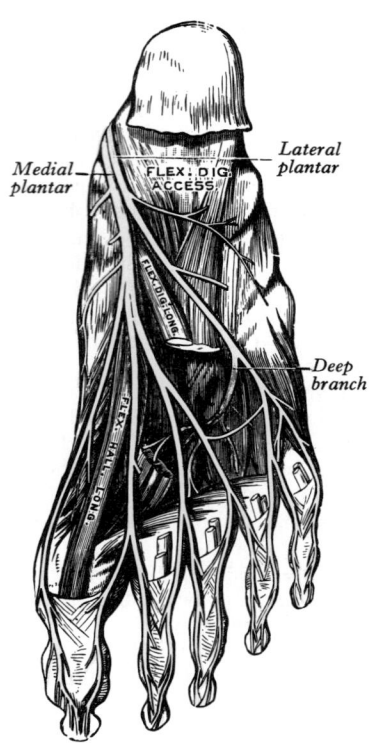

Medial plantar
Lateral plantar
FLEX: DIG: ACCESS
FLEX: DIG: LONG:
FLEX: HALL: LONG:
Deep branch

8.386   The plantar nerves of the right foot.

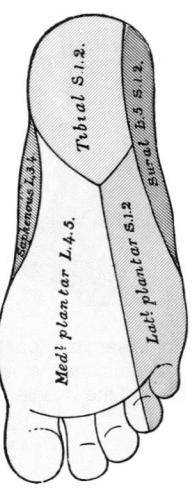

Saphenous L.3,4.
Tibial S.1,2.
Sural L.5 S.1,2.
Med: plantar L.4,5.
Lat: plantar S.1,2.

8.387   A diagram showing the distribution of the cutaneous nerves in the sole of the right foot.

Superficial peroneal branches supply the dorsal skin of all the toes except that of the lateral side of the fifth and adjoining sides of the great and second, the former being supplied by the sural, the latter by the medial terminal branch of the deep peroneal. Frequently some of the superficial peroneal lateral rami are absent and replaced by sural branches.

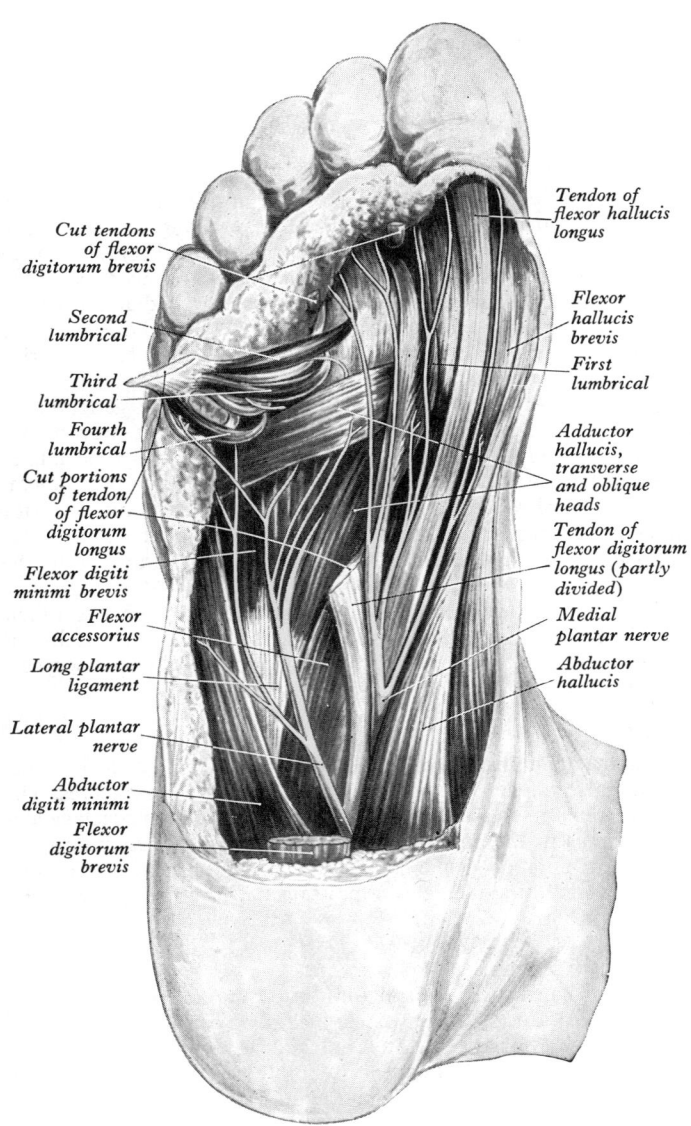

Cut tendons
of flexor
digitorum brevis

Second
lumbrical

Third
lumbrical

Fourth
lumbrical

Cut portions
of tendon
of flexor
digitorum
longus

Flexor digiti
minimi brevis

Flexor
accessorius

Long plantar
ligament

Lateral plantar
nerve

Abductor
digiti minimi

Flexor
digitorum
brevis

Tendon of
flexor hallucis
longus

Flexor
hallucis
brevis

First
lumbrical

Adductor
hallucis,
transverse
and oblique
heads

Tendon of
flexor digitorum
longus (partly
divided)

Medial
plantar nerve

Abductor
hallucis

8.388 A dissection of the lateral and medial plantar nerves of the right foot. Most of the flexor digitorum brevis has been removed. The flexor digitorum longus has been partially divided and its distal end has been displaced together with the second, third and fourth lumbricals.

The *medial terminal branch* runs distally on the dorsum of the foot lateral to the arteria dorsalis pedis, connecting at the first interosseous space with the medial branch of the superficial peroneal nerve and dividing into two dorsal digital nerves to supply adjacent sides of the great and second toes; before dividing it gives off an *interosseous branch* which supplies the hallucial metatarsophalangeal joint and the first dorsal interosseous. The deep peroneal nerve may end as three terminal branches (Geller & Barbato 1970).

Superficial peroneal nerve (8.380). This begins at the common peroneal bifurcation. It is at first deep to the peroneus longus, passing antero-inferiorly between the peronei and extensor digitorum longus to pierce the deep fascia in the distal third of the leg, where it divides into medial and lateral branches. Between the muscles it supplies the peroneus longus, peroneus brevis and the skin of the lower leg. The *medial branch* passes anterior to the ankle, dividing into two dorsal digital nerves, one supplying the medial side of the great and the other the adjacent sides of the second and third toes. It communicates with the saphenous nerve and deep peroneal nerves (8.379). The smaller *lateral branch* traverses the dorsum of the foot laterally, dividing into dorsal digital branches which supply the contiguous sides of the third to fifth toes, also supplying the skin of the lateral aspect of the ankle and connecting with the sural nerve (8.379).

LESIONS OF THE SCIATIC NERVE AND BRANCHES

The sciatic nerve supplies the knee flexors and all the muscles below the knee, so that a complete palsy of the sciatic nerve results in a flail foot and severe difficulty in walking. As the nerve leaves the pelvis it passes either behind the piriformis muscle or sometimes through the muscle and at that point it may become entrapped (the piriformis syndrome; this is a common anatomical variant but an extremely rare entrapment neuropathy). The sciatic nerve may be damaged in spontaneous retroperitoneal haematomas (as may the femoral nerve); misplaced therapeutic injections into gluteus maximus; by compression as it leaves the pelvis (in patients who lie immobile on a hard surface for a considerable length of time, a form of Saturday night palsy).

The *common peroneal nerve* is relatively unprotected as it traverses the lateral aspect of the head of the fibula and is easily compressed at this site. It may be damaged by stretching when the knee is in full flexion, particularly if it is tethered. The nerve may also become entrapped between the attachments of peroneus longus to the head and body of the fibula. Direct pressure in this site may occur from plaster casts and ganglia. Patients present with foot drop, which is usually painless, and examination shows weakness of ankle dorsiflexion, extensor hallucis longus and eversion of the foot, but inversion and plantar flexion are normal and the ankle reflex is preserved. Since the nerve divides at the fibular head into the superficial peroneal and the deep peroneal nerves, all lesions damaging the nerve at the fibular head may damage the main trunk of the nerve or either of its branches. A lesion of the superficial branch causes weakness of foot eversion with sensory loss on the lateral aspect of the leg extending onto the dorsum of the foot.

The *deep peroneal branch* supplies the muscles of the anterior tibial compartment and damage to this nerve results in weakness of ankle dorsiflexion and of extensor hallucis longus. Sensory impairment is confined to the first interdigital cleft. Extensor digitorum brevis is supplied by the deep branch in about 70% of patients.

Tarsal tunnel syndrome. This is an extremely rare entrapment neuropathy of the tibial nerve in the flexor retinaculum and is analogous to the carpal tunnel syndrome. The nerve is affected just as it divides into the medial calcanean branch and medial and lateral plantar nerves, so that one, two or all three branches may be affected.

REMAINING BRANCHES OF THE SACRAL PLEXUS

The perforating cutaneous nerve. Usually from the posterior aspects of the second and third sacral ventral spinal rami, this pierces the sacrotuberous ligament, curves round the inferior border of the gluteus maximus and supplies the skin over the inferomedial aspect of this muscle. The nerve may arise from the pudendal or, if absent, may be replaced by a branch from the posterior femoral cutaneous nerve or from the third and fourth or fourth and fifth sacral ventral rami.

Pudendal nerve (10.131). This is derived from the ventral divisions of the second, third and fourth sacral ventral rami (8.382). It leaves the pelvis via the greater sciatic foramen between the piriformis and coccygeous to enter the gluteal region, crossing the sacrospinous ligament close to the attachment to the ischial spine, sited medial to the internal pudendal vessels on the spine. It accompanies the internal pudendal artery through the lesser sciatic foramen into the pudendal canal (p. 1598) on the lateral wall of the ischiorectal fossa. In the posterior part of the canal it gives off the inferior rectal nerve, which divides into the perineal nerve and the dorsal nerve of the penis (or clitoris).

The *inferior rectal nerve* pierces the medial wall of the pudendal canal, crosses the ischiorectal fossa with the inferior rectal vessels and supplies the sphincter ani externus, the lining of the lower part of the anal canal and the circumanal skin. Its branches connect with the perineal branch of the posterior femoral cutaneous nerve and with the scrotal (or labial) nerves. It sometimes arises directly from the sacral plexus, may perforate the sacrospinous ligament (in 8 out of 40 dissections according to Roberts & Taylor 1973) and may reconnect with the pudendal nerve.

The *perineal nerve*, the inferior and larger terminal pudendal branch, runs forwards below the internal pudendal artery. It accompanies the perineal artery, dividing into posterior scrotal (labial) and muscular branches.

Posterior scrotal or *labial nerves*, medial and lateral, pierce or pass over the inferior fascia of the urogenital diaphragm and run forwards in the lateral part of the urethral triangle with the scrotal (or labial) branches of the perineal artery; they supply scrotal skin or that of the labius majus, connecting with the perineal branch of the posterior femoral cutaneous and inferior rectal nerve.

Muscular branches supply: the transversus perinei superficialis, bulbospongiosus, ischiocavernosus, transversus perinei profundus, sphincter urethrae and the anterior parts of the external sphincter and levator ani. In males a nerve to the *urethral bulb* leaves the nerve to the bulbospongiosus, piercing it to supply the corpus spongiosum penis; it ends in the urethral mucosa.

The *dorsal nerve of the penis* runs forwards in males above the internal pudendal artery along the ischial ramus and the margin of the inferior pubic ramus, deep to the inferior fascia of the urogenital diaphragm. It supplies the corpus cavernosum penis and, at the apex of the urogenital diaphragm, is lateral in the hiatus between this diaphragm and the inferior pubic ligament. It accompanies the dorsal penile artery between the layers of the suspensory ligament to the dorsum of the penis, ending in the glans. In females the homologous *dorsal nerve of the clitoris* is very small.

Clinical evidence indicates that the pudendal nerve supplies sensory branches to the lower part of the vagina, probably by fibres in the inferior rectal nerve and posterior labial branches of the perineal nerve. Pudendal nerves can be 'blocked' by infiltration with a local anaesthetic applied via a needle passed through the vaginal wall towards the ischial spine and sacrospinous ligament, both palpable per vaginam (Huntingford 1959; Nakanishi 1967).

Sacral visceral branches. These arise from the second to fourth sacral ventral rami to innervate the pelvic viscera; they are termed *pelvic splanchnic nerves* (p. 1297).

Sacral muscular branches. These come from the fourth sacral ventral ramus and supply the levator ani, coccygeus and sphincter ani externus (8.382). Those to the levator ani and coccygeus enter the pelvic surfaces of the muscles; the ramus to the sphincter ani externus (*perineal branch of the fourth sacral nerve*) reaches the ischiorectal fossa through the coccygeus or between that muscle and the levator ani, supplying the skin between the anus and coccyx via its cutaneous branches.

COCCYGEAL PLEXUS

The coccygeal plexus is formed by a small descending branch from the fourth sacral ramus and by the fifth sacral and coccygeal ventral rami (8.382). The fifth sacral ventral ramus emerges from the sacral hiatus, curving round the lateral margin of the sacrum below its cornu and piercing the coccygeus to reach its pelvic surface, where it is joined by a descending branch of the fourth sacral ventral ramus; the small trunk so formed descends on the pelvic surface of the coccygeus to join the minute coccygeal ventral ramus emerging from the sacral hiatus and curves round the lateral coccygeal margin to pierce the coccygeus and reach the pelvis. This small trunk is the

coccygeal plexus. *Anococcygeal nerves* arise from it, a few fine filaments piercing the sacrotuberous ligament to supply the adjacent skin.

MORPHOLOGY OF THE SPINAL NERVES AND LIMB PLEXUSES

Spinal nerves conforming to a more primitive arrangement are naturally located in segments largely retaining a metameric (segmental) structure, e.g. the thoracic region. Such typical spinal nerves show a common plan. The dorsal, epaxial ramus passes back lateral to the articular processes and divides into medial and lateral branches penetrating the deeper muscles of the back; both innervate the adjacent muscles and supply a band of skin from the posterior median line to the scapular line (see below). The ventral, hypaxial ramus is connected to a corresponding sympathetic ganglion by white and grey rami communicantes. It innervates the prevertebral muscles and curves round in the body wall supplying the lateral muscles of the trunk; near the midaxillary line it gives off a lateral branch which pierces the muscles to divide into anterior and posterior cutaneous branches. The main nerve advances in the body wall, supplying the ventral muscles and terminating in branches to the skin.

The arrangement of ventral rami in segments which have lost their obvious metamerism is greatly modified, especially by the union of adjacent nerves to form cervical, brachial, lumbosacral and coccygeal plexuses.

Cervical plexus

The cutaneous branches are homologous with the anterior terminal and lateral branches of ventral rami of typical spinal nerves. The cervical transverse cutaneous nerve and the medial supraclavicular nerves represent the anterior terminal branches; the lesser occipital and lateral supraclavicular represent lateral branches; the great auricular and intermediate supraclavicular probably represent elements of both.

Brachial plexus

Division of constituent ventral rami into ventral (anterior, flexor) and dorsal (posterior, extensor) branches occurs in both brachial and lumbosacral plexuses. In the brachial plexus division affects all three trunks (p. 1267) and conforms closely to the differentiation of the primitive musculature of the limb into ventral (flexor) and dorsal (extensor) groups. Branches of the ventral divisions largely supply **dorsal** skin in the limb, a discrepancy tentatively explained (Harris 1939) by assuming that each ventral ramus originally divided into ventral and dorsal branches and that, in human evolution, dorsal fibres entered the ventral branches of the **trunks**. As a result, fibres of the median and ulnar nerves have a wide dorsal area of supply in the hand.

The ventrolateral position of the limb buds and the arrangement of the first and second thoracic nerves support the view that the nerves of limb plexuses are only the **lateral** branches of typical ventral rami. The second thoracic ventral ramus gives off a lateral cutaneous branch which goes to the upper limb as the intercostobrachial nerve, its size inversely related to that of the **direct** contribution from the second thoracic to the brachial plexus. The second thoracic is otherwise typical. The first thoracic ventral ramus gives a large contribution to the brachial plexus and this could be homologous with a lateral branch; the remainder, despite its small size, is typical, but its anterior cutaneous branch is reduced and often absent.

Lumbosacral plexus

Division of constituent ventral rami into ventral and dorsal branches is not as clear here as in the brachial plexus, but anatomically the obturator and tibial nerves arise from ventral and the femoral and peroneal nerves from dorsal divisions. Lateral branches of the twelfth thoracic and first lumbar ventral rami are drawn into the gluteal skin but otherwise these nerves are typical. The second lumbar ramus is difficult to interpret; it not only contributes substantially to the lumbar plexus but also has an anterior terminal branch (genital branch of the genitofemoral) **and** a lateral cutaneous branch (lateral femoral cutaneous nerve and the femoral branch of the genitofemoral). Anterior terminal branches of the third to fifth lumbar and first sacral rami are suppressed but the corresponding parts of the second and third sacral rami supply the skin, etc., of the perineum. The posterior femoral cutaneous nerve poses an interesting problem: it arises from both ventral and dorsal divisions and supplies 'flexor' femoral skin **and** 'extensor' gluteal skin.

SEGMENTAL INNERVATION OF THE SKIN

The cutaneous area supplied by *one* spinal nerve, through both rami, is a *dermatome*; typically, dermatomes extend round the body from the posterior to the anterior median line (**8.367, 374**). Dermatomes of adjacent spinal nerves overlap markedly, particularly in the segments least affected by development of the limbs, i.e. the second thoracic to the first lumbar (**8.367, 374**).

In some regions, e.g. the upper anterior thoracic wall, cutaneous nerves supplying adjoining areas are *not* from consecutive spinal nerves and the overlap is minimal. When the second thoracic spinal ramus is severed, anaesthesia is sharply demarcated but some overlap for painful and thermal sensibility may exist. Likewise, after section of a peripheral nerve (e.g. the ulnar nerve at the wrist) the area of tactile loss is always greater than that for pain and thermal sensibilities. Hence the area of total anaesthesia and analgesia following section of peripheral nerves is always less than might be anticipated from their anatomical distribution (Foerster 1933; Wollard et al 1940).

Cutaneous innervation of the neck and upper limbs

The first cervical spinal nerve supplies no skin. The second cervical usually supplies the skin of the head from the vertex to the superior nuchal line, almost all of the lateral aspect of the ear and the skin over the mandibular angle and below the chin (**8.341**). The third cervical supplies an oblique band from the back of the scalp and upper neck, descending across the side of the neck and increasing in width, to the ventral median line from the hyoid bone to the first rib. The fourth cervical supplies the upper half of the back of the neck and an area widening down and forwards round the neck to the anterior thoracic aspect, supplying the skin over the clavicle, first intercostal space, acromion and the upper part of the deltoid. Each of these three areas is overlapped by the succeeding; the overlap is slight but greater for dorsal rami than for ventral.

The cutaneous distribution of those spinal nerves contributing to the brachial plexus is explained by the early development of the upper limbs. In human embryos at the fourth week the upper limb is a small, flattened ventrolateral elevation on the trunk, level with the lower four cervical and first thoracic segments; its ectoderm is continuous with that of the trunk, taking its supply from the nerves of corresponding segments; its mesoderm is also continuous with that in the same segments. Lower limb buds appear slightly later and always lag behind the upper limb buds until after the birth.

Limb buds have ventral and dorsal surfaces and *preaxial* (cranial) and *postaxial* (caudal) borders. In the upper limbs the *fifth cervical* ventral ramus supplies a strip of skin on the ventral and dorsal surfaces along the **pre**axial border; the *first thoracic nerve* has a similar distribution along the **post**axial border. Intervening nerves supply almost parallel strips on the ventral and dorsal surfaces. As the limb elongates, central nerves of the plexus (C6, 7 and 8) become buried proximally, reaching the skin only in distal parts; nerves of segments C4 and T2 and 3 are drawn in to supply proximal skin, i.e. at the root of the limb. During growth the lengthening limb is rotated laterally through about 90° and adducted to the trunk (p. 289). Hence the *preaxial border* runs distally on the lateral aspect of a supinated limb to the thumb, the *preaxial digit*, while the *postaxial border* runs along the medial aspect to the little finger, the *postaxial digit*. Therefore the cutaneous supply of the lateral aspect of adult limbs is from C4, drawn in at the root of the limb, then from C5 and C6; and its medial aspect is from T2, T1 and C8 (**8.389**). On the *front of the limb*, areas supplied by C5 and C6 adjoin those supplied by T2, T1 and C8; but at their frontier, the *ventral axial line*, overlap is minimal, for C7 is buried proximally and only reaches the skin a little proximal to the wrist (**8.389**). On the *back of the limb* the condition is similar; but C7 (in the posterior cutaneous nerves of the forearm) reaches the skin near the elbow, the *dorsal*

axial line ending at a more proximal level (**8.389**). Pronation of the forearm affects these lines (p. 288).

Cutaneous innervation of the trunk

The skin of the trunk is supplied by spinal nerves T1–L1, S2–4 and Co1 in consecutive, curved zones, the upper almost horizontal, the lower oblique. The upper half of each zone is supplemented by the nerve above, the lower half by the nerve below. No appreciable loss of sensibility follows section of any one spinal nerve. The zone including the subcostal angle is supplied by the seventh thoracic nerve; the umbilicus is in the upper part of a zone supplied by the tenth thoracic.

The area supplied by dorsal rami of these nerves is limited laterally by the dorsolateral line, descending laterally from the occiput to the medial end of the acromion, continued to the posterior aspect of the greater trochanter and curving medially to the coccyx. Cutaneous strips supplied by dorsal rami do not correspond exactly to those served by ventral rami, differing both in breadth and position.

On the upper ventral thoracic aspect, the third and fourth cervical areas adjoin the first and second thoracic areas (**8.367**) since the muscles and skin areas supplied by the intervening nerves have grown into the upper limb; a similar, less extensive posterior gap exists.

Similar arrangements exist in the lower trunk, but less obviously, due to approximation of the lower limbs, though apparent in the gluteal region. The first lumbar adjoins the second sacral area at the root of the penis and scrotum in the male and their homologues in the female (see p. 1876), intervening nerves having been drawn away into the lower limbs during development.

Cutaneous innervation of the lower limb

The skin in the lower limb is innervated by the nerves of its segments of origin, T12–S3 (**8.390, 391**). The arrangement developmentally begins like that in the upper limbs but its identification in adults is obscured by rotation of the lower limb in early development (p. 289). Initially the *preaxial border* follows the cranial border of the limb bud to the great toe, the *preaxial digit*; the *postaxial border* following its caudal margin to the little toe, the *postaxial* digit. The limb undergoes medial rotation, bringing the hallux to lie on the medial side of the foot. The tibia, though homologous with the radius, is also medial. Since rotation occurs at the hip, the gluteal region retains its dorsal (extensor) position.

The *preaxial* border starts near the midpoint of the thigh and descends to the knee; it then curves medially, descending to the medial malleolus and the medial side of the foot and hallux. The *postaxial* border commences in the gluteal region and descends to the centre of the popliteal fossa, deviating laterally to the lateral malleolus and the lateral side of the foot. *Ventral and dorsal axial lines* exhibit corresponding obliquity, the ventral starting proximally at the medial end of the inguinal ligament, descending the posteromedial aspect of the thigh and leg to end proximal to the heel; the dorsal axial line commences in the lateral gluteal region and descends posterolaterally in the thigh to the knee, inclining medially to end proximal to the ankle (**8.390, 391**). The segmental cutaneous distribution of the nerves to the lower limb is shown in **8.390, 391**.

Knowledge of the extent of individual dermatomes, especially in the limbs, is largely based on clinical evidence. Different authorities map variable areas for the same dermatomes, partly due to failure to adopt a common method in neurological examination and partly to individual differences in patients with similar lesions. There is more disagreement over dermatomes in the leg, perhaps because injuries to the brachial plexus are more frequent, affording greater opportunities of correlation between cutaneous defects and neural lesions. The figures for limb dermatomes inserted in **8.390, 391** are based on the Medical Research Council's *Report on Peripheral Nerve Lesions* 1942.

In using these figures it must be understood that **broken lines** indicate that the nerves on each side extend considerably beyond them, the overlap being difficult to define. But along ventral and dorsal axial lines, in **heavy black**, overlap is minimal; the nerves flanking a line are **not** derived from consecutive spinal nerves, the intervening nerve or nerves being buried in the limb and reaching the skin only at more distal points.

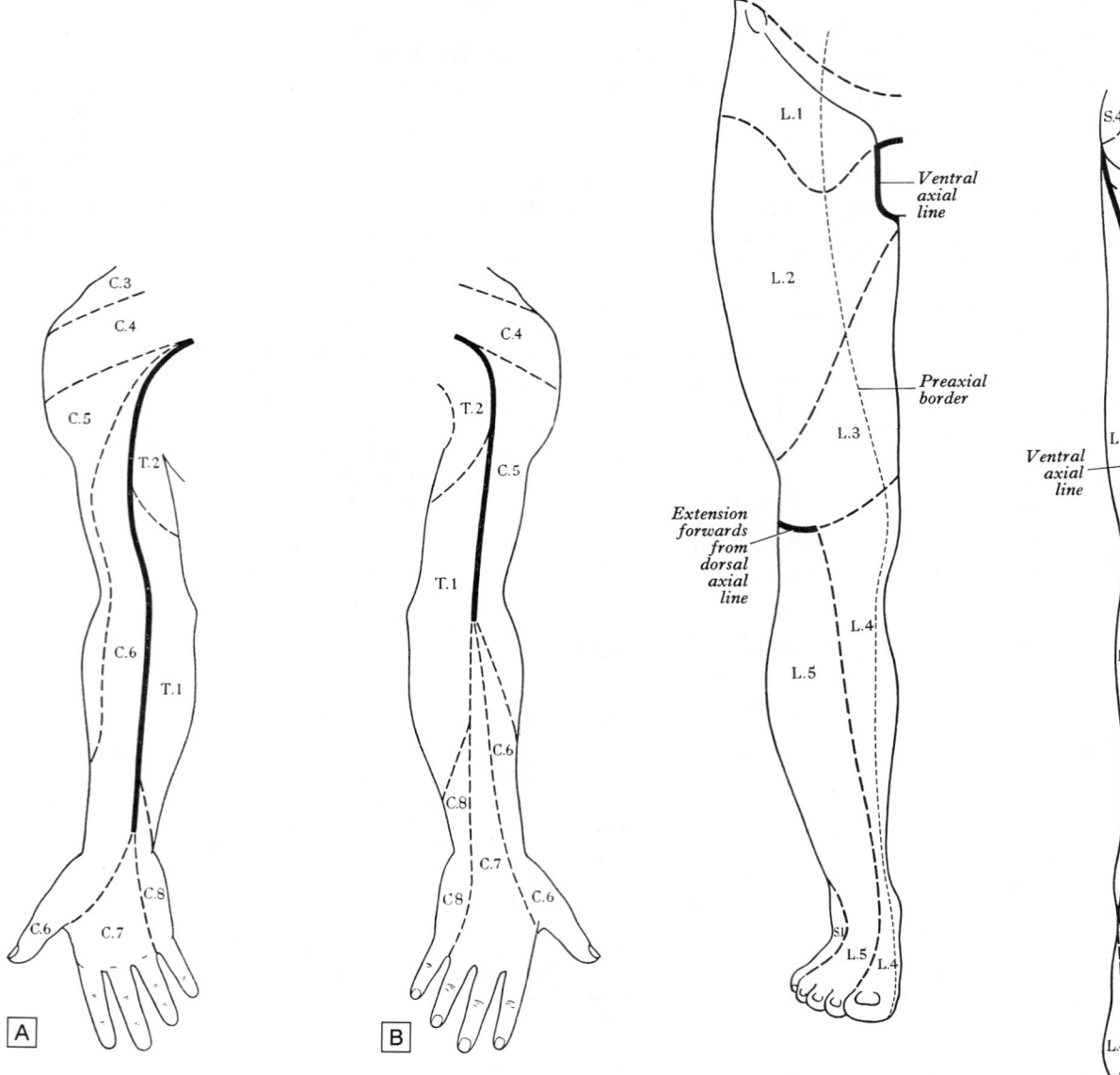

8.389A The arrangement of the dermatomes on the anterior aspect of the upper limb. The heavy black line represents the *ventral axial line* and the overlap across it is *minimal*. Across the interrupted lines, the overlap is considerable.

B The arrangement of the dermatomes on the posterior aspect of the upper limb. The heavy black line represents the *dorsal axial line* and the overlap across it is *minimal*. Across the interrupted lines the overlap may be, and often is, considerable.

8.390 (Left) The segmental distribution of the nerves of the lumbar and sacral plexuses to the skin of the anterior aspect of the lower limb.
8.391 (Right) The segmental distribution of the nerves of the lumbar and sacral plexuses to the skin of the posterior aspect of the lower limb. For the significance of the markings see caption to **8.389**.

Some (Keegan & Garrett 1948) maintain that during the embryonic development of dermatomes in limbs, the sensory nerves grow spirally from the dorsal surface of each limb bud around its preaxial and postaxial borders, to meet anteriorly along the ventral axial line; they deny the existence of a dorsal axial line. By plotting areas of hyposensitivity, particularly hypalgesia following damage to **individual** nerve roots, they have constructed charts of limb dermatomes, which show dermatomes as more continuous strips extending from the trunk along the limbs.

SEGMENTAL INNERVATION OF THE MUSCLES

Each spinal nerve originally supplies the musculature derived from its own myotome. Where myotomal derivatives remain entities they retain the original segmental supply; but when derivatives from adjoining myotomes fuse, the resulting muscles do not always retain a supply from each corresponding spinal nerve,

although they often do. Since muscles develop in situ in mesodermal cores of developing limbs, it is impossible to identify their original segments merely by a developmental study. The union of spinal nerves and branches in brachial and lumbosacral plexuses renders identification of segmental values impossible. The very concept of immutability of neuromuscular linkage, originally promoted by Furbinger (1873), has been criticized and exceptions recorded (Haines 1935; Minkoff 1974).

Segmental innervation of the muscles in limbs

Most muscles in limbs are innervated from more than one segment of the spinal cord; the segments involved for individual muscles are noted in Myology (p. 786). In Tables **8.6**, **8.7**, **8.8** below the **predominant segmental origin** of the nerve supply is stated; damage to these segments or their motor roots results in maximum paralysis. Data are based chiefly on clinical evidence (Bumke & Foerster 1936, Villiger 1946, Sharrard 1955) but opinion differs for some muscles and not all are included. Though evidence for some muscles is incontrovertible, it is scant and uncertain in many instances. An important example is provided by the intrinsic muscles of the hand, often regarded clinically as innervated solely by the first thoracic spinal segment, though the eighth cervical is also involved.

Anomalous branching and innervation

The text gives the usual anatomical arrangement but very considerable variations exist which may influence the clinical presentation. A peripheral branch to a group of muscles may arise as a single branch from the main trunk of the nerve, or individual muscles may be supplied by separate branches from the main trunk of a nerve, in which case injury to the nerve may result in less complete lesions than would be expected. Furthermore the intrafascicular segregation of fibres usually occurs well proximal to the site of branching. Lesions of a nerve proximally may only involve one fascicle and therefore mimic a lesion more distally. For example, compression of the sciatic nerve just below the buttock may only affect the fibres destined to form the common peroneal nerve. Since the fibres destined to become the tibial nerve are unaffected, such a lesion will therefore mimic a common peroneal palsy. Details of the different branching patterns that may occur, and of the differing levels at which main branches arise from peripheral nerves is given by Sunderland (1978).

Table 8.7   Lower limb muscles

L1	Psoas major, psoas minor
L2	Psoas major, iliacus, sartorius, gracilis, pectineus, adductor longus, adductor brevis
L3	Quadriceps, adductors (magnus, longus, brevis)
L4	Quadriceps, tensor fasciae latae, adductor magnus, obturator externus, tibialis anterior, tibialis posterior
L5	Gluteus medius, gluteus minimus, obturator internus, semimembranosus, semitendinosus, extensor hallucis longus, extensor digitorum longus, peroneus tertius, popliteus
S1	Gluteus maximus, obturator internus, piriformis, biceps femoris, semitendinosus, popliteus, gastrocnemius, soleus, peronei (longus and brevis), extensor digitorum brevis
S2	Piriformis, biceps femoris, gastrocnemius, soleus, flexor digitorum longus, flexor hallucis longus, some intrinsic foot muscles
S3	Some intrinsic foot muscles (except abductor hallucis, flexor hallucis brevis, flexor digitorum brevis, extensor digitorum brevis)

Table 8.6   Upper limb muscles

C3, 4	Trapezius, levator scapulae
C5	Rhomboids, deltoids, supraspinatus, infraspinatus, teres minor, biceps
C6	Serratus anterior, latissimus dorsi, subscapularis, teres major, pectoralis major (clavicular head), biceps, coracobrachialis, brachialis, brachioradialis, supinator, extensor carpi radialis longus
C7	Serratus anterior, latissimus dorsi, pectoralis major (sternal head), pectoralis minor, triceps, pronator teres, flexor carpi radialis, flexor digitorum superficialis, extensor carpi radialis longus, extensor carpi radialis brevis, extensor digitorum, extensor digiti minimi
C8	Pectoralis major (sternal head), pectoralis minor, triceps, flexor digitorum superficialis, flexor digitorum profundus, flexor pollicis longus, pronator quadratus, flexor carpi ulnaris, extensor carpi ulnaris, abductor pollicis longus, extensor pollicis longus, extensor pollicis brevis, extensor indicis, abductor pollicis brevis, flexor pollicis brevis, opponens pollicis
T1	Flexor digitorum profundus, intrinsic muscles of the hand (except abductor pollicis brevis, flexor pollicis brevis, opponens pollicis)

Table 8.8   Joint movements

In terms of movements of joints, segmental innervation of limb muscles may be expressed in general

Shoulder	Abductors and lateral rotators	C5
	Abductors and medial rotators	C6, 7, 8
Elbow	Flexors	C5, 6
	Extensors	C7, 8
Forearm	Supinators	C6
	Pronators	C7, 8
Wrist	Flexors and extensors	C6, 7
Digits	Long flexors and extensors	C7,8
Hand	Intrinsic muscles	C8, T1
Hip	Flexors, adductors, medial rotators	L1, 2, 3
	Extensors, abductors, lateral rotators	L5, S1
Knee	Extensors	L3, 4
	Flexors	L5, S1
Ankle	Dorsiflexors	L4, 5
	Plantar flexors	S1, 2
Foot	Invertors	L4, 5
	Evertors	L5, S1
	Intrinsic muscles	S2, 3

Determination of location of a lesion

In clinical practice it is only necessary to test a relatively small number of muscles in order to determine the location of a lesion. For example, abduction of the arm might be testing shoulder abduction, a C5 root lesion, the axillary nerve or the deltoid muscle.

A muscle should be chosen according to the following criteria:

- It should be visible, so that wasting or fasciculation can be observed and the muscle consistency with contraction can be felt.
- It should have an isolated action, so that its function can be tested separately.
- It should help to differentiate between lesions at different levels in the neuraxis and in the peripheral nerve, or between peripheral nerves.
- It should be tested in such a way that differentiates normal from abnormal so that slight weakness can be detected early with reliability.
- Some preference is given to muscles which have an easily elicitable reflex.

Table 8.9 gives a list of movements and muscles chosen according to these criteria. For example with an upper motor neuron lesion, shoulder abduction, elbow extension, wrist and finger extension and finger abduction are weaker than their opposing movements. Since this weakness may be more distal than proximal or vice versa, normal shoulder abduction and finger abduction excludes an upper motor neuron weakness of the arm. Similarly normal hip flexion and ankle dorsiflexion excludes an upper motor neuron weakness of the leg. Some muscles are difficult to test, but are included for special reasons. For example, the strength of brachioradialis is difficult to assess but it can be seen and felt, it is mostly innervated by

the C6 root and it has an easily elicitable reflex.

To determine the root level of a lesion, it is necessary to know an appropriate muscle to test for each root, preferably with an easily elicitable reflex. There is so much overlap in the leg that a series of muscles have to be tested to determine the level of the lesion.

The sequence of innervation of muscles from a peripheral nerve is very helpful in locating the level of the lesion (see diagrams). For example, with radial nerve

lesions, if triceps is involved then the lesion must be high in the axilla. If, as is usual, triceps is spared but brachioradialis, wrist extensors, finger extensors and the superficial radial nerve are involved, then the lesion is in the arm where the radial nerve is vulnerable to pressure against the humerus. If wrist extension is normal and the superficial radial nerve is not involved, but finger extension is weak, then the lesion is in the posterior interosseous branch of the radial nerve.

Table 8.9 Movements and muscles tested to determine the location of a lesion

Arm

Movement	Muscle	Upper motor neuron	Root	Reflex	Nerve
Shoulder abduction	Deltoid	+ +	C5		Axillary
Elbow flexion	Biceps		C5/6	+	Musculocutaneous
	Brachioradialis		C6	+	Radial
Elbow extension	Triceps	+	C7	+	Radial
Radial wrist extensors	Extensor carpii radialis longus	+	C6		Radial
Finger extensors	Extensor digitorum	+	C7	(+)	Posterior interosseous
Finger flexors	Flexor pollicis longus + Flexor digitorum profundus Index		C8	+	Anterior interosseous
	Flexor digitorum profundus Ring & Little				Ulnar
Finger abduction	1st Dorsal interosseous	+ +	T1		Ulnar
	Abductor pollicis brevis		T1		Median

Leg

Movement	Muscle	Upper motor neuron*	Root	Reflex	Nerve
Hip flexion	Iliopsoas	+ +	L1/2		Femoral
Hip adduction	Adductors		L2/3	(+)	Obturator
Hip extension	Gluteus maximus		L5/S1		Sciatic
Knee flexion	Hamstrings	+	S1		Sciatic
Knee extension	Quadriceps		L3/4	+ +	Femoral
Ankle dorsiflexion	Tibialis anterior	+ +	L4		Deep peroneal
Ankle eversion	Peroneii		L5/S1		Superficial peroneal
Ankle inversion	Tibialis posterior		L4/5		Tibial
Ankle plantar flexion	Gastrocnemius/soleus		S1/2	+ +	Tibial
Big toe extension	Extensor hallucis longus		L5	(Babinski reflex)	Deep peroneal

*The muscles listed in the column Upper motor neuron are those which are preferentially affected in upper motor neuron lesions. The root level is the principal supply to a muscle.

AUTONOMIC NERVOUS SYSTEM

GENERAL ORGANIZATION

The autonomic nervous system possesses both central and peripheral components, the latter being concerned with the innervation of the viscera, glands, blood vessels and non-striated (smooth) muscle. It therefore forms the visceral (splanchnic) component of the nervous system. The term 'autonomic' is a convenient rather than appropriate title. The **autonomy** of this part of the nervous system is illusory, since it is intimately responsive to changes in somatic activities. While its connections with somatic elements are not always structurally clear, the functional evidence for visceral reflexes stimulated by somatic events is abundant. (For general information consult

Langley 1921; Kuntz 1953; Mitchell 1953, 1956; Pick 1970; Gabella 1976; Björklund et al 1988; Bannister & Mathias 1992; Burnstock 1992–95.)

Visceral efferent paths differ from their somatic equivalents in being interrupted by peripheral synapses, at least two neurons being interposed between the central nervous connections and visceral effectors (8.392). The somata of the primary neurons are in the visceral efferent nuclei of cranial nerves and in the spinal lateral grey columns; their axons, variably but usually finely myelinated, traverse the cranial and spinal nerves to the peripheral ganglia, where they synapse with the dendrites of somata of secondary neurons. Axons of secondary, effector neurons are usually non-myelinated and supply non-striated muscle or glandular cells. These nerve fibres are also found close to adipocytes, mast cells, melanophores, interstitial cells, autonomic ganglia and motor end plates. There are therefore in peripheral efferent pathways *preganglionic* and *postganglionic neurons*, the latter being more numerous; one preganglionic neuron may synapse with 15–20 postganglionic neurons, permitting the wide diffusion of many autonomic effects. This disproportion between preganglionic and postganglionic neurons is said to be greater in the sympathetic than in parasympathetic parts of the autonomic nervous system. (In an investigation into human superior cervical ganglia, a ratio of preganglionic to postganglionic fibres of 1 to 196 was claimed; Ebbesson 1968.) Terminations of postganglionic neurons are described on page 959 and below. For the structure of sympathetic ganglia and details of other neuronal types, including interneurons, see page 1298 et seq.

Visceral afferent paths resemble somatic afferent paths; the cells of origin of their peripheral fibres are unipolar neurons in cranial and dorsal root ganglia. Peripheral processes are distributed through

autonomic ganglia or plexuses, or possibly through somatic nerves, without interruption. Their central processes (axons) accompany the somatic afferent fibres through dorsal spinal roots to the CNS (p. 1298).

The autonomic nervous system can be divided into three major parts, **parasympathetic**, **sympathetic** and **enteric**, which differ in structure and function. The broad anatomical organization of these subdivisions was summarized by Langley in 1921 and has been more or less retained since that time. Parasympathetic preganglionic efferent fibres emerge through certain cranial and sacral spinal nerves as a *craniosacral* outflow, while sympathetic preganglionic efferent fibres emerge through thoracic and upper lumbar spinal nerves as a *thoracolumbar outflow*. The somata of parasympathetic postganglionic neurons are peripheral, sited distant from the CNS either in discrete ganglia near to the structures innervated or often dispersed in the walls of viscera. The somata of sympathetic postganglionic neurons are located mostly in ganglia of the sympathetic trunk or ganglia in more peripheral plexuses but they are almost always

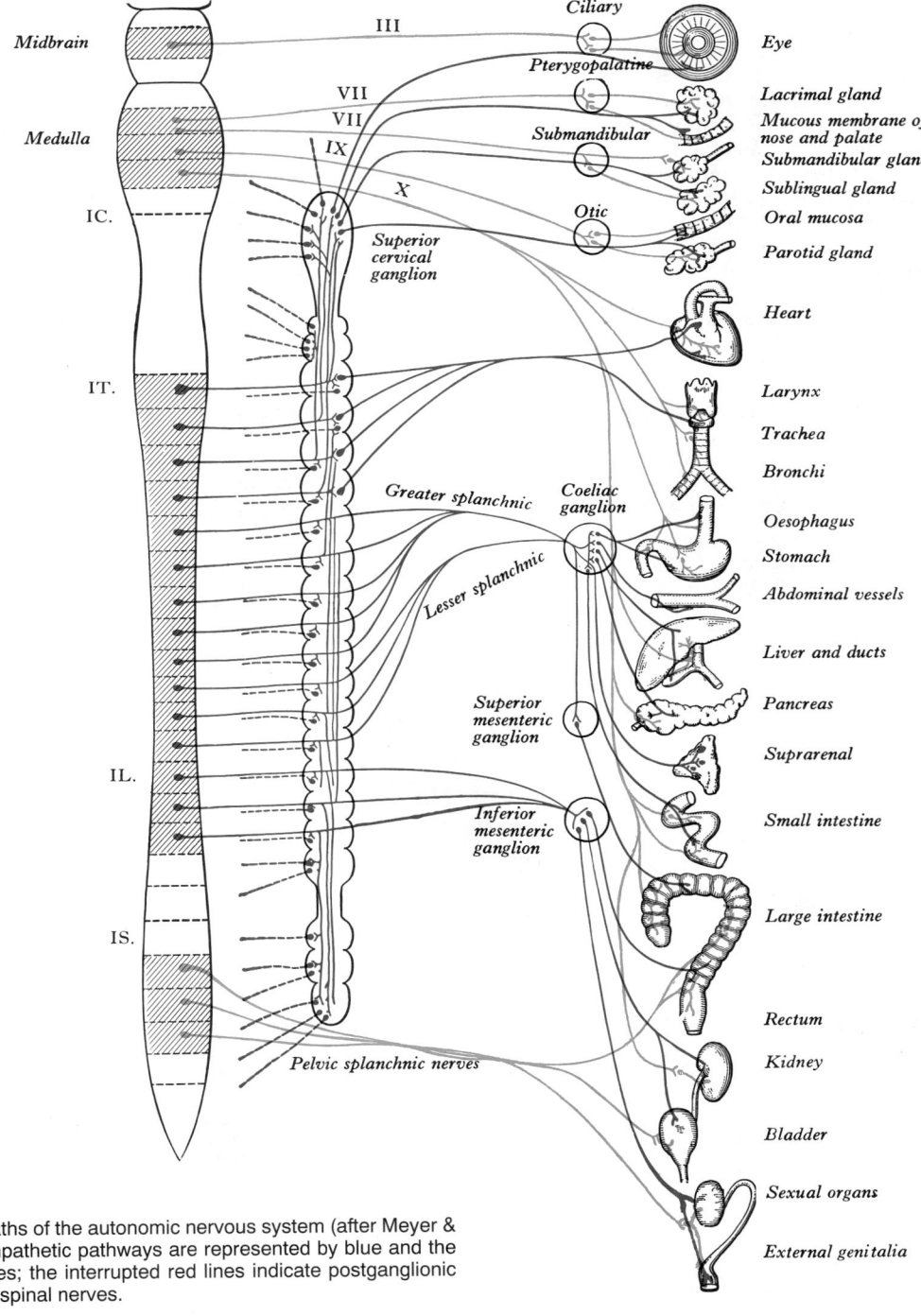

8.392   The efferent paths of the autonomic nervous system (after Meyer & Gottlieb). The parasympathetic pathways are represented by blue and the sympathetic by red lines; the interrupted red lines indicate postganglionic rami to the cranial and spinal nerves.

nearer to the spinal cord than to the effectors innervated, an exception being some of those innervating pelvic viscera. The enteric nervous system is comprised of ganglionated plexuses localized in the wall of the gastrointestinal tract (p. 1749). It contains reflex pathways through which the contractions of the muscular coats of the alimentary tract, the secretion of gastric acid, intestinal transport of water and electrolytes, mucosal blood flow and other functions are controlled. There are complex interactions between the enteric nervous system and extrinsic parasympathetic, sympathetic and sensory–motor nerves.

MECHANISM OF TRANSMISSION

It has been considered in the past that physiologically the parasympathetic and sympathetic systems differed in that parasympathetic reactions are generally localized, whereas sympathetic reactions are mass responses. However, even though widespread activation of the sympathetic nervous system may occur, for example in association with fear or rage, it is now recognized that the sympathetic nervous system is also capable of discrete activation, and many different patterns of activation of sympathetic nerves throughout the body occur in response to a wide variety of stimuli.

Parasympathetic activity results in cardiac slowing and an increase in intestinal glandular and peristaltic activities, which may be considered to conserve body energy stores. Sympathetic activity results, for example, in the general constriction of cutaneous arteries (increasing blood supply to the heart, muscles and brain), cardiac acceleration, increase in blood pressure, contraction of sphincters and depression of peristalsis, all of which mobilize body energy stores for dealing with increased activity (Macdonald 1992).

For many years the idea of antagonistic, parasympathetic cholinergic and sympathetic adrenergic control of most organs in visceral and cardiovascular systems formed the working basis of all studies. However, major advances have been made since the early 1960s that

make it necessary to revise this concept of the mechanism of autonomic transmission. These advances include:

NANC nerves. The discovery of non-adrenergic, non-cholinergic (NANC) nerves and the recognition of a multiplicity of neurotransmitter substances in autonomic nerves. Adenosine 5'-triphosphate (ATP) satisfied the criteria as a neurotransmitter in many of these NANC nerves and they were termed 'purinergic' (Burnstock 1972). Subsequently, it became clear that many other neuroactive substances, including many peptides, were present in autonomic nerves. Nitric oxide (NO) or a NO-related compound has recently been shown to play an important role as a primary messenger in transmitting information from nerves to smooth muscles in specific tissues (Bredt et al 1990; Rand 1992). The list of proposed neurotransmitters and neuromodulators in the autonomic nervous system thus includes monamines, purines, amino acids, a variety of peptides and NO (p. 935 and Table 8.1; Burnstock 1986).

Cotransmission. The concept of cotransmission that proposes that most, if not all, nerves release more than one transmitter (Burnstock 1976, 1990; Hökfelt et al 1986; Kupfermann 1991) and the 'chemical coding' of these nerves to establish the combinations of neurotransmitters contained in individual neurons whose projection and central connections are known. The principal neurotransmitters in most sympathetic nerves are ATP and neuropeptide Y (NPY), although NPY often acts as a neuromodulator. In parasympathetic nerves the principal cotransmitters are acetylcholine (ACh), and VIP, with subpopulations utilizing ATP and/or NO. In most sensory-motor nerves (p. 968), the neurotransmitters are substance P (SP) and calcitonin gene-related peptide (CGRP), with some utilizing ATP. Other neurotransmitters/neuromodulators are also sometimes colocalized with the principal transmitters in autonomic nerves (8.393). Although there are many different transmitter substances in the gut, most are involved in neurotransmission or neuromodulation at the ganglion level or may be trophic factors.

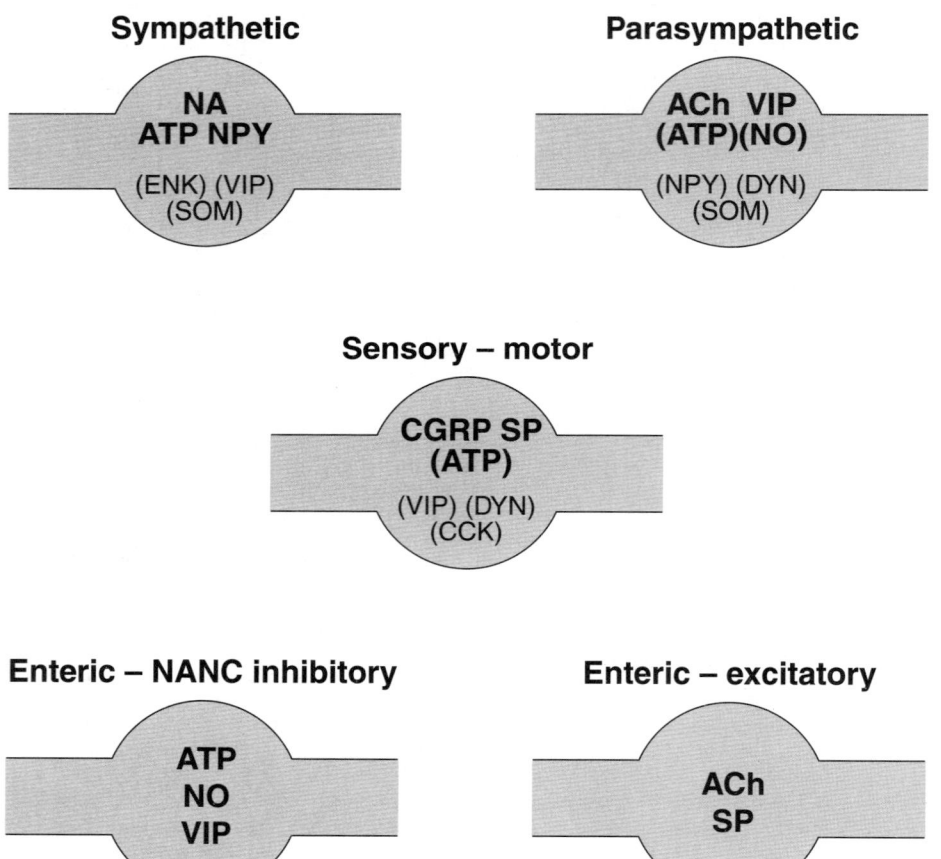

8.393 Schematic representation of chemical coding of neurotransmitters/neuromodulators colocalized in autonomic nerves (see text).

The number involved in neuromuscular transmission is more limited. Enteric NANC inhibitory nerves utilize, probably as cotransmitters, ATP, VIP, and NO whereas enteric excitatory nerves utilize ACh and SP (8.393).

Neuromodulation. The concept of neuromodulation where locally released agents can alter neurotranmission either by prejunctional modulation of the amount of transmitter released or by postjunctional modulation of the time course or intensity of action of the transmitter. The wide and variable cleft characteristic of autonomic neuroeffector junctions makes them particularly amenable to the mechanisms of neural control mentioned above. There are many different ways in which cotransmitters and neuromodulators interact to effect neurotransmission including:

- *Autoinhibition*, by which a transmitter, in addition to its postjunctional effects, modifies its own release, often inhibiting it which may in turn effect the release of cotransmitters;
- *Cross-talk*, by which a neuromodulator may act on closely juxtaposed terminals;
- *Synergism*, by which each of two transmitters, either from different nerve terminals or cotransmitters, have the same postjunctional effect so that there is a reinforcement of their individual effects;
- *Opposite actions*, which may result from a transmitter having opposite actions in different effector cells, or the response may depend on the tone of the effector cell;
- *Prolongation of effect*, by which a neuromodulator may act on degradative enzymes, for example peptidases responsible for removal of neuropeptides from the junctional cleft, to prolong the time course of their effect;
- *Trophic effects*, by which a neurotransmitter may effect the expression of another transmitter or receptor within a population of neurons (for example in ganglia) at the level of gene transcription.

All these mechanisms of control of neurotransmission reflect the versatility of the autonomic nervous system.

Sensory–motor nerves. The importance of sensory–motor nerve regulation in many organs is recognized (p. 667). These afferent nerves run in motor fibres with their cell bodies in cranial and dorsal root ganglia. While many such nerves are purely sensory, certain primary afferent nerve fibres have been termed sensory–motor since they release transmitter from their peripheral endings during the axon reflex and have a motor rather than sensory role (see p. 965) (Maggi 1991). For many years the status of the sensory nerve in the autonomic nervous system has been debated but it is now recognized that sensory–motor nerve regulation is an important feature of autonomic control in the gut, lungs, heart, ganglia and blood vessels.

Intrinsic circuitry. Recognition that many intrinsic ganglia contain integrative circuits and are capable of sustaining and modulating sophisticated local activities. Although the ability of the enteric nervous system to sustain local reflex activity independent of the CNS has been recognized for many years (Kosterlitz 1968), it has been generally assumed that the intrinsic ganglia in peripheral organs such as the heart, airways and bladder consisted of parasympathetic neurons that provided simple nicotinic relay stations. The high degree of electrophysiological specialization displayed by these intrinsic neurons suggests that they may act as sites of integration and/or modulation of the input from extrinsic nerves or permit some local control of aspects of visceral function by local reflex mechanisms (Allen & Burnstock 1990). Thus, since intrinsic neurons survive following section of the extrinsic sympathetic and parasympathetic nerves, transplanted organs are not denervated. Intrinsic neurons are derived from the neural crest, independent of sympathetic and parasympathetic nerves. Various combinations of transmitters have been shown to coexist in subpopulations of intrinsic neurons in atria, bladder and trachea and the chemical coding in the enteric nervous system has been studied extensively (Furness & Costa 1987, p. 1749).

Autonomic neuromuscular junction. Recognition that the autonomic neuromuscular junction differs in several important ways from the skeletal neuromuscular junction and from the synapses in the CNS and PNS (see Burnstock 1981). There is no fixed junction with well defined pre- and postjunctional specializations. Unmyelinated, highly branched, postganglionic autonomic nerve fibres reaching the effector smooth muscle become beaded or varicose (8.394). These varicosities are not static but are able to move along axons, consistent with the lack of postjunctional specialization. They are packed with mitochondria and vesicles containing neurotransmitters. The distance of the cleft between the varicosity and smooth muscle varies considerably depending on the tissue, from 20 nm in densely innervated structures such as the vas deferens to 1–2 μm in large elastic arteries. Neurotransmitter is released en passage from varicosities during conduction of an impulse along an autonomic axon; however, it is possible that a given impulse will evoke release from only some of the varicosities that it encounters.

Another important feature of the autonomic neuromuscular junction is that, unlike striated muscle, the effector tissue is a muscle bundle rather than a single cell and low resistance pathways between individual muscle cells allow electronic coupling and spread of activity within the effector bundle. These are represented by areas of close apposition between the plasma membranes of adjacent cells which can be identified under the electron microscope as gap junctions or nexuses (p. 958). Gap junctions vary in size from punctate junctions to junctional areas of more than 1 μm in diameter. Little is known about the quantity and arrangement of gap junctions in effector bundles relative to the density of autonomic innervation. Thus, within an effector muscle bundle only a certain percentage of cells are directly innervated, the remainder being coupled to these cells via gap junctions (Hillarp 1959; Burnstock 1986).

Plasticity. Recognition of the plasticity of the autonomic nervous system, not only in normal development and ageing, but also in changes in the expression of neurotransmitters and receptors in the mature adult in response to hormones and growth factors following trauma, surgery, chronic drug treatment and in a variety of disease situations (Burnstock 1990, p. 959).

PLASTICITY OF THE AUTONOMIC NERVOUS SYSTEM

Autonomic neuroeffector systems show a high degree of plasticity, even in mature adult animals (see Black et al 1988; Burnstock 1990; Hendry & Hill 1992). Changes in expression of transmitters and cotransmitters in autonomic nerves occur during developing and ageing, after chronic exposure to drugs, in a number of disease situations and in nerves that remain following trauma or surgery. Several different types of adaptive mechanisms appear to override the normal genetic programming of transmitter and receptor expression, for example alterations in availability to growth factors, levels of nerve activity, removal of inhibitory innervation and hormonal changes. Neurotrophins synthesized by target smooth muscle, of which *nerve growth factor* is the best-known example (Levi-Montalcini & Angeletti 1968; Thoenen 1991, p. 919), have long been recognized to have *trophic* influences on sympathetic and sensory nerves of the autonomic nervous system. There is growing evidence that several neurotransmitters, in particular the neuropeptides, which are involved in short-term communication between excitable cells, also have long-term trophic actions on autonomic nerves (Pincus et al 1992). Autonomic neurons are thus continually under the influence of the molecules of their environment, allowing for a considerable degree of plasticity following injury (Hendry & Hill 1992).

Degeneration in the autonomic nervous system resembles that in cerebrospinal nerves. Some evidence suggests that the rate of degeneration differs in different regions or different types of fibre. Regeneration of preganglionic fibres may vary with the site of lesion and, in postganglionic neurons, regeneration may be followed by reinnervation from neighbouring intact nerve fibres. As far as experimental evidence goes, the integrity of Schwann cell sheaths is essential in the regeneration of autonomic nerve fibres (Evans & Murray 1954; Kapeller & Mayor 1967; Williams 1971; King & Thomas 1971; Landon 1976). Some observations suggest that proximity of myelinated fibres is necessary for regeneration in non-myelinated fibres (Evans & Murray 1954; Williams 1971; Lisney 1989; consult Fawcett & Keynes 1990). It is pertinent to mention earlier experiments in which large experimental gaps in the sympathetic trunk, in monkeys and other mammals, have been filled by the growth of fibres, pre- or postganglionic (Tower & Richter 1931; Haxton 1954). Functional recoveries may sometimes be explained by incomplete interruption of the sympathetic supply or by alternative routes being overlooked.

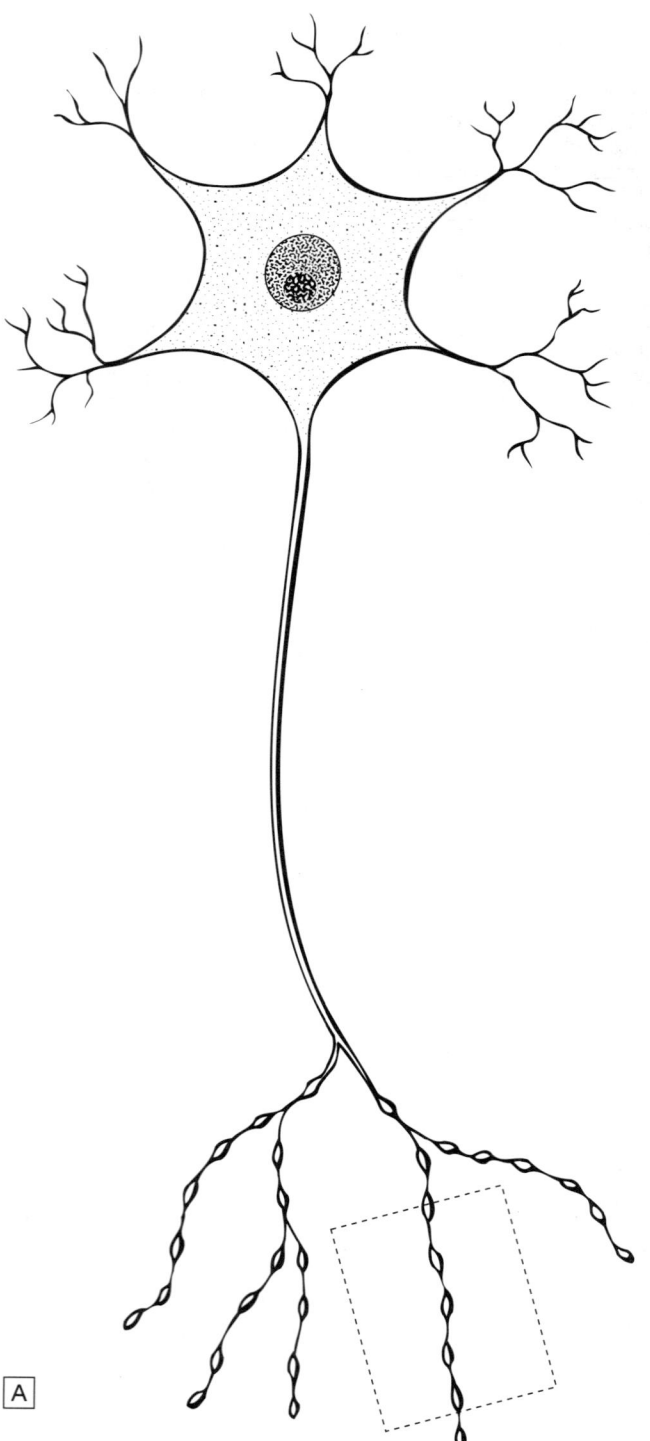

A

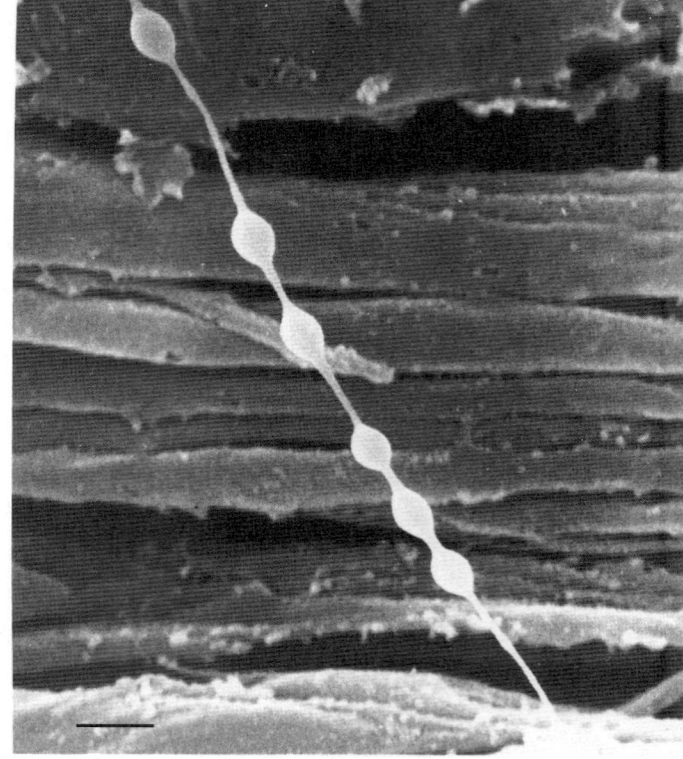

B

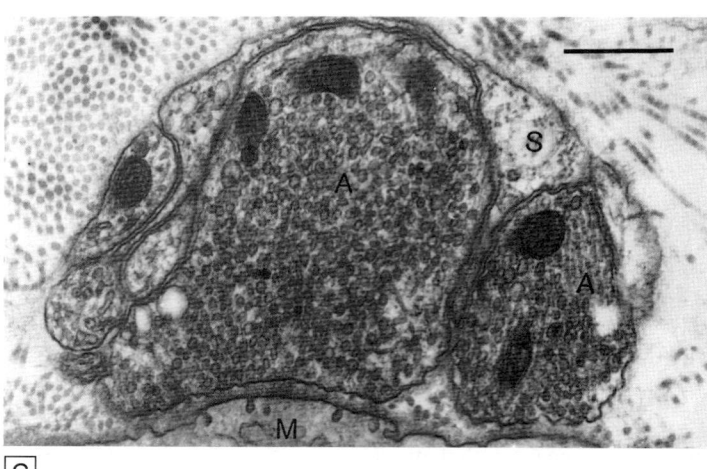

C

8.394 A. Schematic representation of an autonomic neuron becoming varicose as it reaches its smooth muscle target.

B. Scanning electron micrograph of single terminal varicose nerve fibre (enlargement of section within rectangle in A) lying over smooth muscle of small intestine of rat. Intestine was pretreated to remove connective tissue components by digestion with trypsin and hydrolysis with HCl. Bar = 3 μm. (From Hoyle and Burnstock 1989, with permission.)

C. Transmission electron micrograph of a section through varicosity profiles

(as seen in B). This shows the relationship of axons (A), Schwann cell cytoplasm (S) and smooth muscle (M) at the adventitial-medial border of the anterior cerebral artery of the rat. Basement membrane material is interposed between axonal and smooth muscle membranes. There are many synaptic vesicles and mitochondria in the terminal varicosities. Some small and large granular vesicles are also present. Note the absence of post-junctional specialization. Bar = 0.5 μm. (From Burnstock et al 1980, with permission.)

Surgical anatomy. Various autonomic nervous structures are divided or removed in treating several pathological conditions. In operations on the efferent sympathetic paths, ganglia on the sympathetic trunk are removed or preganglionic fibres cut, rather than postganglionic fibres, since the latter may regenerate. For example, the arteries of limbs may be denervated to alleviate vascular spasm (Raynaud's disease) and the parts removed are as described above

(pp. 1258, 1302). In the treatment of hypertension, more extensive sympathectomy has been performed, involving bilateral removal of the sympathetic trunks from the eighth thoracic to the first lumbar ganglia, including the greater and lesser thoracic splanchnic nerves. Sympathectomy is also performed to relieve pain, for example in severe angina pectoris (p. 1311). Division of the superior hypogastric plexus (presacral neurectomy) does not relieve all pain in disease of the pelvic organs, because many pain fibres traverse the pelvic splanchnic nerves. However uterine pain fibres pass in sympathetic nerves via the superior hypogastric plexus so that this division does relieve dysmenorrhoea. In males resection of the superior hypogastric plexus leads to loss of ejaculation and sterility, due to interruption of the sympathetic paths to the seminal vesicles, deferent ducts and

prostate. The routes of these nerves between the sympathetic ganglia and the superior hypogastric plexus are uncertain and may vary; but in some individuals an outflow from the first lumbar and possibly the twelfth thoracic ganglia is concerned and in others fibres from the third lumbar ganglion (White et al 1952).

PARASYMPATHETIC NERVOUS SYSTEM

EFFERENT PATHWAYS

Preganglionic parasympathetic axons are myelinated and occur in the oculomotor, facial, glossopharyngeal, vagal and accessory cranial nerves and in the second to fourth sacral spinal nerves. In the cranial part of the parasympathetic system there are four small peripheral ganglia: ciliary (p. 1228), pterygopalatine (p. 1235), submandibular (p. 1247) and otic (p. 1250), all described in this account with their cranial nerves. These are solely efferent parasympathetic ganglia, unlike the trigeminal, facial, glossopharyngeal and vagal ganglia, all of which are concerned exclusively with afferent impulses and contain the somata of sensory neurons only. The cranial parasympathetic ganglia are traversed by afferent fibres, postganglionic sympathetic fibres and, in the otic, even by branchial efferent fibres, but none of these are interrupted in the ganglia. Postganglionic parasympathetic fibres are usually non-myelinated and shorter than the sympathetic, since the ganglia in which they synapse are in or near the viscera they supply. Baumann and Gajisin (1975) have emphasized the occurrence of small subsidiary ganglia near those mentioned above, confirming reports by others; they also described minute ganglia at many other sites in fetal material, for example along the middle meningeal artery and in some petrosal nerves.

(1) *Oculomotor* preganglionic parasympathetic fibres commence in the midbrain at the accessory oculomotor (Edinger-Westphal) nuclei (p. 1227) and travel in the nerve in its branch to the inferior oblique to reach the ciliary ganglion. There they synapse, the postganglionic fibres leaving in the short ciliary nerves which pierce the sclera to run forwards in the perichoroidal space to the ciliary muscle (p. 1328) and the sphincter pupillae (p. 1331). These postganglionic axons are thinly myelinated.

(2) The *facial nerve* contains preganglionic parasympathetic axons of neurons with their somata in the superior salivatory nucleus (p. 1243), emerging from the medulla oblongata in the nervus intermedius. These fibres leave the main facial trunk above the stylomastoid foramen in the chorda tympani, which traverses the tympanic cavity to reach the lingual nerve (p. 1246). Thus they are conveyed to the submandibular ganglion, in which arise postganglionic secretomotor fibres for the submandibular salivary gland. Some preganglionic fibres may synapse around cells in the hilum of the gland (pp. 1693, 1698). Postganglionic secretomotor fibres for the sublingual gland continue in the lingual nerve from the submandibular ganglion (pp. 1247, 1693). Stimulation of chorda tympani dilates the arterioles in both glands in addition to having a direct secretomotor effect. The facial nerve is also usually said to contain efferent parasympathetic lacrimal secretomotor axons, which travel in its greater petrosal ramus and in the nerve of the pterygoid canal, relaying in the pterygopalatine ganglion. Postganglionic axons are said to travel by the zygomatic nerve to the lacrimal gland (p. 1235) and by ganglionic branches to the nasal and palatal glands. Evidence refuting the zygomatic route has been reported by Ruskell (1971), who favours direct lacrimal rami from a retro-orbital plexus of parasympathetic branches from the pterygopalatine ganglion. Clinical evidence suggests that some facial parasympathetic fibres reach the parotid gland (Diamant & Wiberg 1965 and p. 1243).

(3) The *glossopharyngeal nerve* contains preganglionic parasympathetic secretomotor fibres for the parotid gland. These start in the inferior salivatory nucleus (p. 1250) and travel in the glossopharyngeal nerve and its tympanic branch. They traverse the tympanic plexus and lesser petrosal nerve to reach the otic ganglion where they relay, the postganglionic fibres passing by communicating branches to the auriculotemporal nerve, which conveys them to the parotid gland. Stimulation of the lesser petrosal nerve produces vasodilator and secretomotor effects.

(4) The *vagus nerve* contains preganglionic parasympathetic fibres which arise in its dorsal nucleus (p. 1251) and travel in the nerve and its pulmonary, cardiac, oesophageal, gastric, intestinal and other branches. Some cardiac parasympathetic fibres may originate from neurons in or near the nucleus ambiguus (p. 1021). The proportion of efferent parasympathetic fibres in the vagus varies at different levels but is small relative to its sensory and sensory–motor content. Efferent fibres relay in minute ganglia in the visceral walls. The disproportion in the numbers of preganglionic to postganglionic fibres is greater in the vagus than in other cranial nerves; this cannot as yet be explained. Cardiac branches slow the cardiac cycle, joining the cardiac plexuses (p. 1306) and relaying in ganglia distributed freely over both atria in the subepicardial tissue (10.59), terminal fibres being distributed to the atria and the atrioventricular (AV) bundle and concentrated around the SA and (to a lesser extent) the AV nodes. It has been claimed in the past that only through the latter can the vagi influence ventricular muscle (Cullis & Tribe 1913), although there is a sparse postganglionic parasympathetic innervation of the ventricles (Higgins et al 1973). The smaller branches of the coronary arteries are innervated mainly via the vagus; larger arteries, with a dual innervation, are chiefly supplied by sympathetic fibres (Woollard 1926; Lundberg et al 1983; Owman 1988). Pulmonary branches are motor to the circular non-striated muscle fibres of the bronchi and bronchioles and are therefore bronchoconstrictor; synaptic relays occur in the ganglia of the pulmonary plexuses. Gastric branches are secretomotor and motor to the non-striated muscle of the stomach, with the exception of the pyloric sphincter, which they inhibit. Intestinal branches have a corresponding action in the small intestine, caecum, vermiform appendix, ascending colon, right colic flexure and most of the transverse colon; they are secretomotor to the glands, motor to the intestinal muscular coats but inhibitory to the ileocaecal sphincter. The synaptic relays are situated in the myenteric (Auerbach's) and the submucosal (Meissner's) plexuses (p. 1747).

(5) The anterior rami of the second, third and often fourth sacral spinal nerves issue pelvic splanchnic nerves (8.381) to the pelvic viscera. These nerves unite with branches of the sympathetic pelvic plexuses. Minute ganglia occur at the points of union and in the visceral walls. In these ganglia the sacral preganglionic parasympathetic fibres relay synaptically.

The pelvic splanchnic nerves are motor to the muscle of the rectum and bladder wall but inhibitory to the vesical sphincter, supply vasodilator fibres to the penile and clitoridic erectile tissue and are probably vasodilator to the testes and ovaries and vasodilator (and possibly inhibitory) to the uterine tubes and uterus (de Groat 1992). Filaments from the pelvic splanchnic nerves ascend in the hypogastric plexus to supply the sigmoid and descending colon, the left colic flexure and terminal transverse colon with visceromotor fibres (Telford & Stopford 1934; Mitchell 1935; Christensen et al 1984).

SYMPATHETIC NERVOUS SYSTEM

The sympathetic system includes the two ganglionated trunks and their branches, plexuses and subsidiary ganglia. It has a much wider distribution than the parasympathetic, for it innervates: all sweat glands, the arrectores pilorum, the muscular walls of many blood vessels, the heart, lungs and respiratory tree, the abdomino-pelvic viscera, the oesophagus, the muscles of the iris in the eye, and non-striated muscle of the urogenital tract, the eyelids and elsewhere.

There are differences in the pattern of sympathetic innervation of different effector tissues; for example, visceral smooth muscles such as the vas deferens and iris receive a dense varicose nerve plexus throughout with close, 20 nm neuromuscular separations, while most blood vessels receive an innervation which is confined to the adventitial–medial border with neuromuscular separations often greater than 80 nm (**8.395**).

EFFERENT PATHWAYS

The *preganglionic fibres* are axons of somata in the lateral grey column of all the thoracic and the upper two or three lumbar spinal segments, where they form intermediomedial and intermediolateral neuronal groups (p. 980). The axons are myelinated, with diameters of 1.5–4 μm, and emerge from the spinal cord through the ventral spinal roots, passing into the spinal nerves at the start of their ventral rami, which they soon leave in *white rami* communicantes, to join either the corresponding ganglia of the sympathetic trunks or their interganglionic segments. This outflow is confined to the thoracolumbar region, the white rami communicantes being restricted to these 14 pairs of spinal nerves, although a limited outflow in other spinal nerves has been suggested. Neurons like those in the lateral grey column exist at other levels of the cord above and below the thoracolumbar outflow (Mitchell 1953) and small numbers of their fibres issue in other ventral roots. Dorsal spinal roots may also contain vasodilator fibres. Reaching the sympathetic trunk, preganglionic fibres may behave in several ways (**8.396**): (1) They may synapse with neurons in the nearest ganglion. (2) They may traverse this, ascending or descending in the sympathetic chain to end in another ganglion; note however that preganglionic fibres do not divide into ascending and descending branches. A single preganglionic fibre may, through collateral and terminal branches, synapse with neurons in several ganglia or terminate in only one

ganglion. (3) They may traverse the nearest ganglion, ascend or descend and, without synapsing, emerge in one of the medially-directed branches of the sympathetic trunk to end at synapses in the ganglia of autonomic plexuses (mainly situated in the midline, for example around the coeliac and mesenteric arteries, p. 1307). Occasionally preganglionic fibres relay in ganglia situated proximal to the sympathetic trunks; these '*intermediate ganglia*' are most numerous on grey rami communicantes (see below) at cervical and lower lumbar levels; they may be of microscopic size and sometimes occur in spinal ventral roots or trunks. More than one preganglionic fibre may synapse with a single postganglionic neuron (see below).

The nervi terminales (p. 1225) may be rostral extensions of the sympathetic system, containing efferent postganglionic fibres distributed to the blood vessels and glands of the nasal cavity, although this view has been challenged (Bojsen-Møller 1975).

The *sympathetic ganglia* include collections of cells on the sympathetic trunks, in the autonomic plexuses and the 'intermediate' ganglia; some ganglionic cells are dispersed in the plexuses. Originally ganglia on the trunks correspond numerically to the ganglia on the dorsal spinal roots (p. 1261); but adjoining ganglia may fuse and in man there are rarely more than 22 or 23 and sometimes fewer. Subsidiary ganglia in the major autonomic plexuses (e.g. coeliac, superior mesenteric ganglion, etc.) are derivatives of the ganglia of the trunks. The functional properties of sympathetic ganglia have been investigated extensively over many decades, their peripheral location providing a valuable means of studying interneuronal communication, as well as other aspects of neurobiology (for reviews of the earlier literature, see p. 1292; more recent accounts are given by Gabella (1976), Eränkö (1978), Elfvin (1983) and Szurszewski and King (1989)).

Structure of sympathetic ganglia

The classic studies by Langley and his successors led to the view that the autonomic ganglia are relay stations, a concept largely corroborated by anatomical observation, although it was soon recognized that a minor fraction of the fibres traversed one or more ganglia without synapse, some being efferent fibres en route to another ganglion and others afferents from the viscera and glands. This concept remains substantially true but has been modified and extended by electron microscopy, neurohistochemistry and elec-

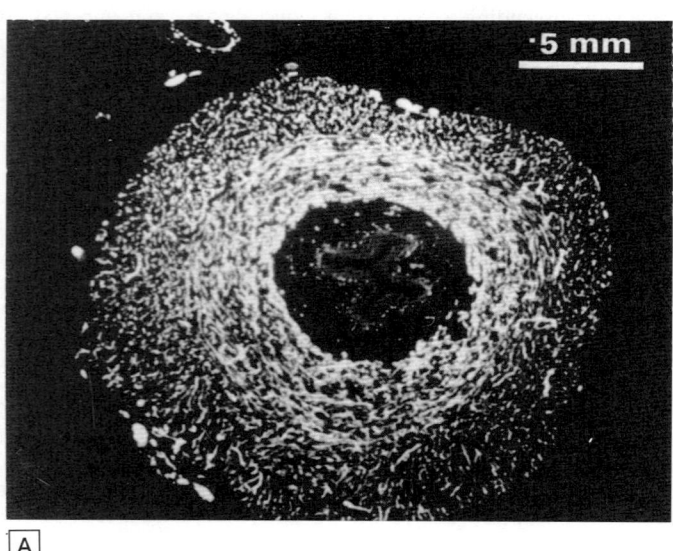

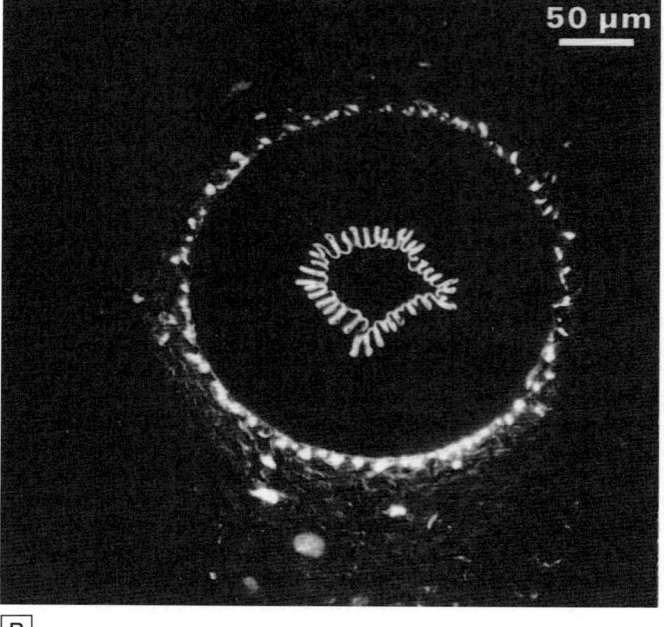

8.395 Fluorescence histochemical demonstration of a noradrenaline-containing nerve fibres in A. rat vas deferens (transverse section) and B. rabbit ear artery (transverse section). Note dense innervation of muscle coats in A compared to restriction of nerves fibres to adventitial-medial border in B. Bar = 0.5 mm in A and 50 μm in B. (From Burnstock & Bell 1974 and Burnstock et al 1972, respectively.)

Attempts to classify the neurons of the sympathetic (and parasympathetic) ganglia, often on inadequate criteria, have entailed disagreements and confusion. Most are multipolar, with somata ranging from 25–50 μm in mankind; a smaller type, of about 15–20 μm, less angular in shape and present in much smaller numbers, is often clustered in groups (De Castro & Herneros 1945) and probably corresponds to 'small intensely fluorescent' (SIF) cells (see below). Multipolar neurons display much more dendritic variation; according to McLachland (1974) they have (in guinea pigs) a mean of 13 dendrites per cell. The complexity of these dendrites, especially those ramifying in the capsular perikaryal space, is greater in human ganglion cells. Dendritic glomeruli have been observed in many ganglia. In general ultrastructure these glomeruli resemble others (p. 934); clusters of small, granular vesicles, adrenergic in type, are dispersed superficially in the perikaryon and also in the dendrites, probably representing the storage of catecholamines. Ganglionic neurons receive many axodendritic synapses from preganglionic nerve fibres, the axosomatic synapses being less numerous. Each preganglionic fibre forms several synapses with several separate dendrites, providing a mechanism for the dissemination and/or amplification of neural signals. Postganglionic fibres (see below) commonly arise from the initial stem of a large dendrite and produce few or no collateral neurites.

The existence of *interneurons* in sympathetic ganglia has been amply confirmed (Williams 1967; Williams & Palay 1969; Libet & Owman 1974), consisting of the SIF cells identified in sympathetic ganglia in many mammals, including man (Eränkö & Härkönen 1965; Jacobowitz 1970). Small chromaffin cells also occur in sympathetic ganglia, as recognized by Kohn in 1898. Coupland (1965) amongst other modern workers, has ascribed them to all ganglia of the sympathetic trunk and to other sites in human neonatal material. The distinction between SIF cells and chromaffin cells appears uncertain in many accounts. The supposed two types have been identified in ganglia by separate techniques (chromaffin reaction and formalin-induced fluorescence) which cannot be applied together to a single cell. In the sympathetic ganglia of rats (Santer et al 1975) SIF cells were found to be more numerous than chromaffin cells and their modes of distribution showed some differences. Both contain catecholamines, some possibly only enough to be revealed by the more sensitive formaldehyde-induced fluorescence technique (Falck-Hillarp), whereas others may have sufficient to produce a positive chromaffin reaction (Gabella 1976). Both types may be interneurons (Santer et al 1975; Gabella 1976) Greengard and Kebabian (1974) have suggested that the SIF cells release dopamine, which is then bound by dopamine receptors on ganglionic neurons causing hyperpolarization via a cyclic AMP-dependent 'second messenger' system. In the ganglia of some species, two types of SIF cell have been described (Williams et al 1975): a minority, with long processes, end near ganglionic neurons and hence can be regarded as interneurons (Type I), while the more numerous Type II cells have shorter processes ending near blood vessels. In bovine superior cervical sympathetic ganglia, 24% of SIF cells were described as Type I and 20% were so described in cats. Although the secretory granules in Type I cells may act directly on ganglionic neurons, some SIF cells, presumably Type II, may secrete into local blood vessels (Polóyni et al 1977), exerting more distant effects. The functions of SIF cells in neurotransmission in sympathetic ganglia have been reviewed by Eränkö (1978) and Szurszewski and King (1989), and quantification of numbers, dimensions and packing density of ganglionic neurons are reported by Gabella (1976).

The axons of the principal ganglionic cells are narrow, nonmyelinated *postganglionic fibres*, distributed to effector organs in various ways:

(1) Those from a ganglion of the sympathetic trunk may return to the spinal nerve of preganglionic origin through a *grey ramus communicans*, usually joining the nerve just proximal to the white ramus, to be distributed through ventral and dorsal spinal rami to blood vessels, sweat glands, hairs, etc. in their zone of supply. Segmental areas vary in extent and overlap considerably. The extent of innervation of different effector systems, for example vasomotor, sudomotor, etc., by a particular nerve may not be the same.

(2) Postganglionic fibres may pass in a medial branch of a ganglion direct to particular viscera.

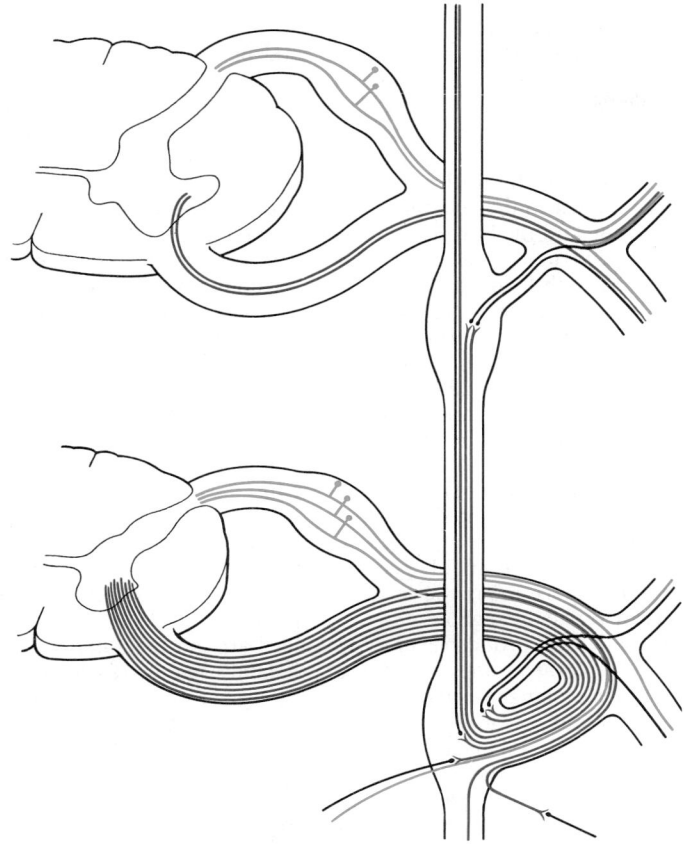

8.396 The constitution of a typical spinal nerve. In the upper part of the diagram the spinal nerve roots show the somatic components; in the lower part the spinal roots show the visceral components. Red = somatic and preganglionic visceral nerve fibres, blue = somatic and visceral afferent fibres, black = postganglionic afferent visceral fibres.

trophysiology, for example a considerable variation in the ratio between pre- and postganglionic fibres has been found (consult Skok 1973). The superior cervical sympathetic ganglion, the most extensively studied, has ratios varying from 1:28 to 1:176 in different mammalian species (Billingsley & Ranson 1918; Samuel 1953; Ebbeson 1968). It has long been accepted that preganglionic axons may synapse with many postganglionic neurons for the wide dissemination and perhaps amplification of sympathetic activity, a characteristic not shared to the same degree by parasympathetic ganglia. Dissemination may be achieved by:

- multiple synapses of preganglionic nerve fibres
- the mediation of interneurons
- the diffusion within the ganglion of transmitter substances locally produced (paracrine effect) or by a local response to a substance produced elsewhere (endocrine effect).

There is evidence that all of these mechanisms are involved. The connective tissue capsule of each ganglion, continuous with the epineurium of its connecting rami, also extends as septa into the ganglion, the surrounding groups of neurons and their fibres. More delicate extensions of this stroma spread amongst the cells, each of which is surrounded by a collagenous intercellular matrix containing a few fibroblasts and many small vessels including capillaries. Satellite cells (amphicytes) encapsulate the somata of ganglionic neurons and their processes. Externally this thin sheath of satellite cells has a continuous basal lamina and the two elements screen neurons from contact with the ganglionic extracellular matrix. Neurons thus have direct access only to the internal faces of satellite cells, the two being separated only by a narrow perineuronal space of 15–20 nm which is, however, linked to the extracapsular spaces by narrow channels between the satellite cells, providing possible routes for the movement of neurotransmitter and hormonal substances between the somata of neurons and the vascular compartment.

(3) They may innervate adjacent blood vessels or pass along them externally to their peripheral distribution.

(4) They may ascend or descend before leaving the sympathetic trunk as (1), (2) or (3). Many fibres are distributed along arteries and ducts as plexuses to distant effectors.

Fusion of grey and white rami may also occur, for example in the thoracic region; grey rami may also contain fasciculi of thick myelinated fibres which are somatic efferents using a grey ramus to reach the prevertebral muscles (see below), for example in the cervical region. For details of rami communicantes and their variations consult Winckler (1961).

Functional significance. Postganglionic fibres which return to the spinal nerves supply vasoconstrictor fibres to blood vessels, are secretomotor to sweat glands and motor to the arrectores pilorum in their dermatomes. Those which accompany the motor nerves to voluntary muscles are probably only vasodilatory. Most, if not all, peripheral nerves contain post-ganglionic sympathetic fibres. Those reaching the viscera are concerned with general vasoconstriction, bronchial and bronchiolar dilatation, modification of glandular secretion, pupillary dilatation, inhibition of alimentary muscle contraction, etc. A single preganglionic fibre probably synapses with the postganglionic neurons in only one effector system; hence effects such as sudomotor and vasomotor actions can be separate. This is not necessarily true of visceral *afferent* fibres.

Higher autonomic control. Peripheral autonomic activity is integrated at higher levels in the brainstem and cerebrum, including various nuclei of the brainstem reticular formation, thalamus and hypothalamus, the limbic lobe and prefrontal neocortex, together with the ascending and descending pathways which interconnect these regions (see details of these given earlier in this section). It is now recognized that central control of the cardiovascular system is exerted by a longitudinally arranged series of parallel pathways involving specific regions of the neuraxis extending from cerebral cortex to the spinal cord (Loewry & Spyer 1990).

The *sympathetic trunks* are two ganglionated, irregular nerve cords extending from the cranial base to the coccyx. In the neck each lies posterior to the carotid sheath and anterior to the cervical transverse processes; in the thorax each is anterior to the heads of the ribs, in the abdomen anterolateral to the lumbar vertebral bodies and in the pelvis anterior to the sacrum and medial to the anterior sacral foramina. Anterior to the coccyx the two trunks meet in the single, median, terminal *ganglion impar*.

Cervical sympathetic ganglia are usually reduced to three by fusion; from the cranial pole of the superior ganglion issues the internal carotid nerve, as a continuation of the sympathetic trunk, accompanying the internal carotid artery through its canal into the cranial cavity. There are from 10–12 (usually 11) thoracic ganglia, four lumbar and four or five in the sacral region.

CRANIAL PART OF THE SYMPATHETIC SYSTEM

This begins on each side as the *internal carotid nerve*, a branch of the superior cervical ganglion containing the postganglionic fibres of its neurons. Ascending behind the internal carotid artery it divides in the carotid canal into branches, one medial and the others lateral to the artery. The larger, *lateral branch* gives filaments to the internal carotid and forms the lateral part of the internal carotid plexus; the medial branch also gives filaments to the artery and, continuing on, forms the medial part of the internal carotid plexus.

Internal carotid plexus

This surrounds its artery and occasionally contains a small, medial *carotid ganglion*; elsewhere it has some scattered postganglionic neurons. Laterally the plexus communicates with the trigeminal and pterygopalatine ganglia, the abducent nerve and tympanic branch of the glossopharyngeal; it also distributes filaments to the wall of the internal carotid artery. One or two filaments join the abducent nerve as it lies on the lateral side of the internal carotid artery. The branch to the pterygopalatine ganglion is the *deep petrosal nerve*, which perforates the cartilage filling the foramen lacerum and forms with the greater petrosal nerve the *nerve of the pterygoid canal*, traversing the canal to the pterygopalatine ganglion. The communication with the tympanic branch of the glossopharyngeal nerve is effected by the

superior and *inferior caroticotympanic nerves* in the posterior wall of the carotid canal.

The medial part of the internal carotid plexus is inferomedial to the part of the internal carotid artery which indents the cavernous sinus lateral to the sella turcica; it gives branches to the artery and to the oculomotor, trochlear, ophthalmic and abducent nerves and the ciliary ganglion. It also sends vasomotor rami along branches of the internal carotid to the hypophysis cerebri (p. 1887).

The branch to the oculomotor nerve joins the nerve near its point of division and the branch to the trochlear joins it in the lateral wall of the cavernous sinus; filaments also connect with the medial side of the ophthalmic nerve and with the abducent. The filament to the ciliary ganglion, from the anterior part of the plexus, enters the orbit via the superior orbital fissure; this ramus may join the ciliary ganglion directly or unite with the communicating branch from the nasociliary nerve (p. 1228); or it may travel in the ophthalmic nerve and its nasociliary branch. Its fibres traverse the ganglion without synapsing and enter the short ciliary nerves to be distributed to the blood vessels of the eyeball. Fibres supplying the dilator pupillae usually travel via the ophthalmic, nasociliary and long ciliary nerves but occasionally via the short ciliary. Some fibres may also innervate the ciliaris muscle. The preganglionic fibres concerned leave the spinal cord predominantly in T1, pass to and through the cervicothoracic ganglion and ascend in the cervical sympathetic trunk to relay in the superior cervical ganglion.

The internal carotid plexus is prolonged around the anterior and middle cerebral arteries and the ophthalmic arteries, reaching the pia mater along the cerebral vessels; along the ophthalmic artery they pass into the orbit where the plexus accompanies each branch of that vessel. Filaments on the anterior communicating artery connect the sympathetic nerves of the right and left sides and may be associated with a small ganglion. Much of this detail depends on rather old observations; continued disagreement and discrepancy have been reviewed by Mitchell (1953) and Purves (1972). Electron microscopy shows that the sympathetic innervation of the cerebral arterial tree is like that of other vascular systems and the terminals of this rich perivascular plexus have been shown histochemically and immunohistochemically to contain NA and NPY in various mammals, including man (Iwayama 1970; Matsuyama et al 1985). The sources of these sympathetic vasoconstrictor nerve fibres are the internal carotid and vertebral plexuses. It should be noted that, in cerebral vessels, some NPY-containing fibres are of parasympathetic origin, and also contain ACh and VIP (Leblanc et al 1987; Uddman & Edvinsson 1989). NA-containing nerves present in some cerebral vessels after sympathectomy may be of central origin (Edvinsson 1991).

CERVICAL PART OF THE SYMPATHETIC SYSTEM

The cervical part of each sympathetic trunk contains three interconnected ganglia, the superior, middle and cervicothoracic (**8.397**), which send grey rami communicantes to all the cervical spinal nerves but receive no white rami communicantes from them; their spinal preganglionic fibres emerge in the white rami communicantes of the upper thoracic spinal nerves which enter the corresponding thoracic sympathetic ganglia, through which they ascend into the neck. In their course, the grey rami communicantes may pierce the longus capitis or the scalenus anterior. For details of the cervical grey rami see Potts (1925), Pick and Sheehan (1946), Sunderland and Bedbrook (1949).

Superior cervical ganglion

This is the largest of the three, adjoins the second and third cervical vertebrae and is probably formed from four fused ganglia corresponding to C1–4. Anterior to it is the internal carotid artery and sheath, while posterior to it is the longus capitis. The internal carotid nerve (see above) ascends from it into the cranial cavity; the lower end of the ganglion is united by a connecting trunk to the middle cervical ganglion. Its branches consist of lateral, medial and anterior groups.

The *lateral branches* are the grey rami communicantes to the upper four cervical spinal nerves and to some of the cranial nerves; delicate filaments pass to the inferior vagal ganglion and to the hypoglossal nerve; a branch, the *jugular nerve*, ascends to the cranial base and

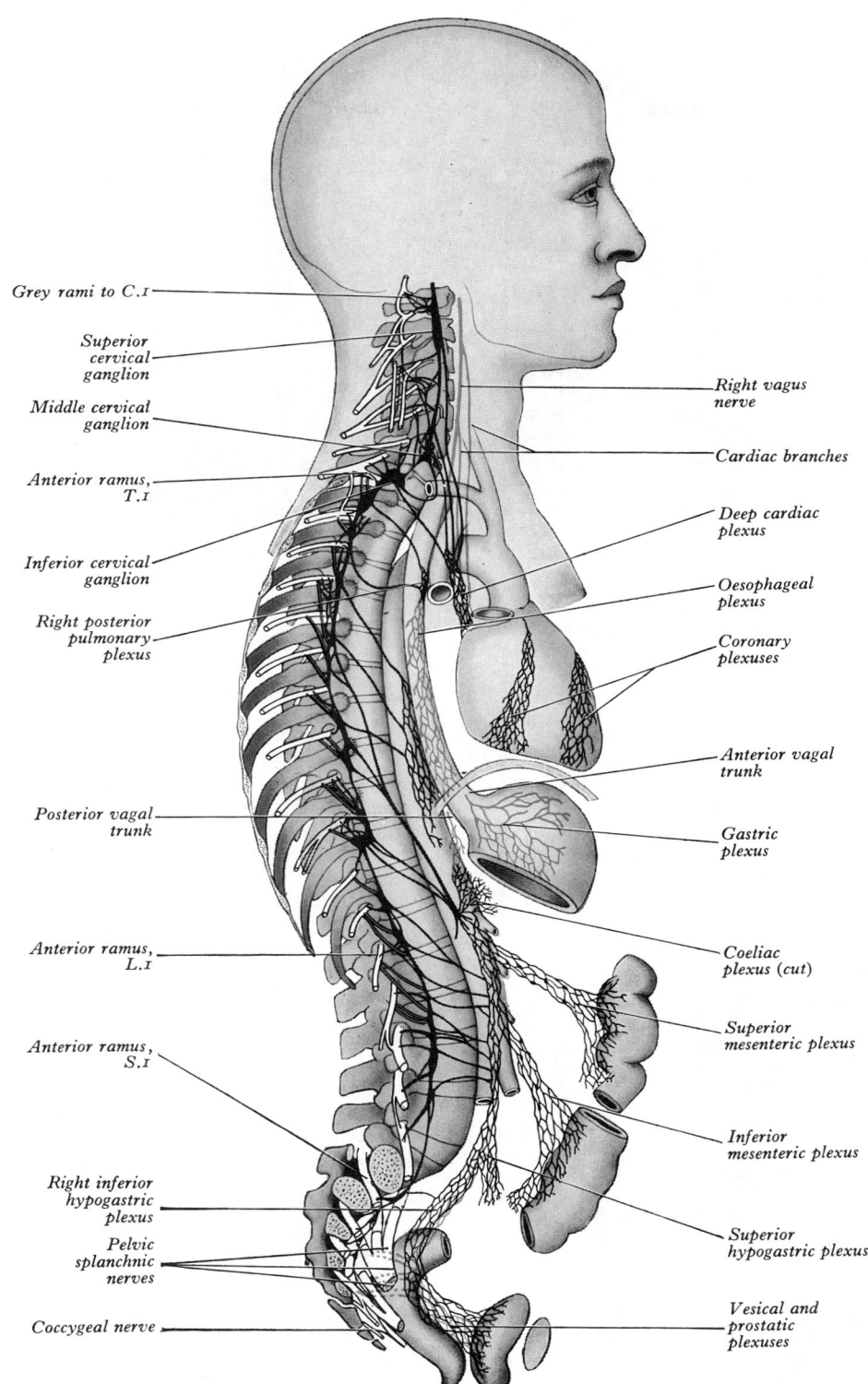

Grey rami to C.I

Superior cervical ganglion

Middle cervical ganglion

Anterior ramus, T.I

Inferior cervical ganglion

Right posterior pulmonary plexus

Posterior vagal trunk

Anterior ramus, L.I

Anterior ramus, S.I

Right inferior hypogastric plexus

Pelvic splanchnic nerves

Coccygeal nerve

Right vagus nerve

Cardiac branches

Deep cardiac plexus

Oesophageal plexus

Coronary plexuses

Anterior vagal trunk

Gastric plexus

Coeliac plexus (cut)

Superior mesenteric plexus

Inferior mesenteric plexus

Superior hypogastric plexus

Vesical and prostatic plexuses

8.397 The right sympathetic trunk and its connections with the thoracic, abdominal and pelvic plexuses. Blue = parasympathetic fibres, black = sympathetic trunk and branches, red = white rami communicantes.

divides into two, one part joining the inferior glossopharyngeal ganglion and the other the superior vagal ganglion; other twigs pass to the superior jugular bulb and associated jugular glomus or glomera and some to the meninges in the posterior cranial fossa.

The *medial branches* of the superior cervical ganglion are the laryngopharyngeal and cardiac. The *laryngopharyngeal branches* supply the carotid body and pass to the side of the pharynx, joining glossopharyngeal and vagal rami to form the pharyngeal plexus (p. 1252). A *cardiac branch* arises by two or more filaments from the

lower part of the superior cervical ganglion, occasionally receiving a twig from the trunk between the superior and middle cervical ganglia. It is thought to contain only efferent fibres, the preganglionic outflow being from the upper thoracic segments of the spinal cord, and to be devoid of pain fibres from the heart (p. 1306). It descends behind the common carotid artery, in front of the longus colli, crossing anterior to the inferior thyroid artery and recurrent laryngeal nerve. The courses on the two sides then differ. The *right cardiac branch* usually passes behind or sometimes in front of the subclavian artery

1301

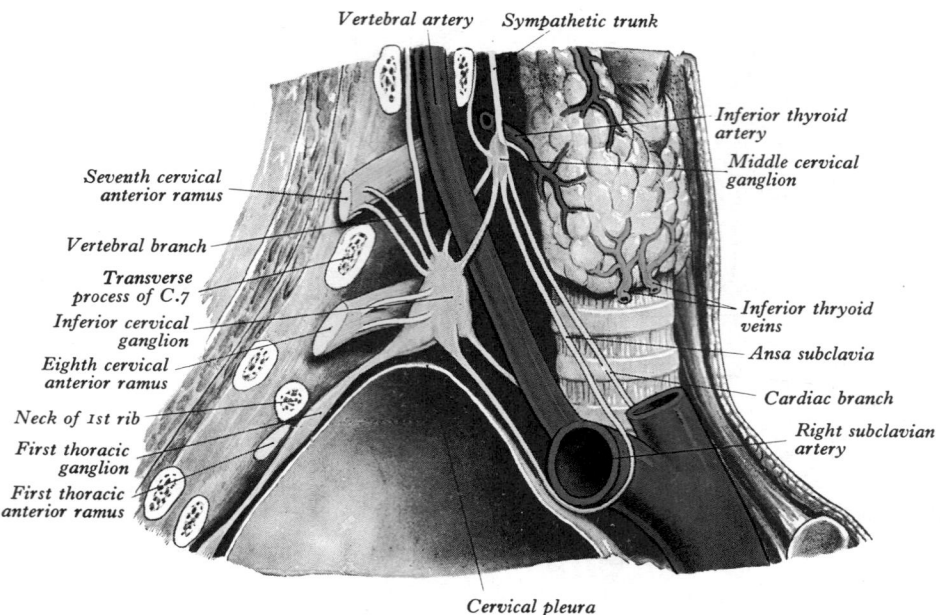

8.398 The middle and inferior cervical ganglia of the right side, viewed from the right. Note the proximity of the inferior cervical and first thoracic ganglia, usually fused to form a cervicothoracic (stellate) ganglion.

and posterolateral to the brachiocephalic trunk to the back of the aortic arch where it joins the deep (dorsal) part of the cardiac plexus. It has other sympathetic connections: about midneck it receives filaments from the external laryngeal nerve; inferiorly, one or two vagal cardiac branches join it; as it enters the thorax it is joined by a filament from the recurrent laryngeal nerve. Filaments from the

nerve also communicate with the thyroid branches of the middle cervical ganglion. The *left cardiac branch*, in the thorax, is anterior to the left common carotid artery and crosses in front of the left side of the aortic arch to reach the superficial (ventral) part of the cardiac plexus. Sometimes it descends on the right of the aorta to end in the deep (dorsal) part of the cardiac plexus. It communicates with the cardiac branches of the middle cervical and cervicothoracic sympathetic ganglia and sometimes with the inferior cervical cardiac branches of the left vagus; branches from these mixed nerves form a plexus on the ascending aorta.

The *anterior branches* of the superior cervical ganglion ramify on the common and external carotid arteries and the branches of the latter, forming a delicate plexus around each in which small ganglia are occasionally found. The plexus around the facial artery supplies a filament to the submandibular ganglion; the plexus on the middle meningeal artery sends one ramus to the otic ganglion and another, the *external petrosal nerve*, to the facial ganglion. Many of the fibres coursing along the external carotid and its branches ultimately leave them to travel to facial sweat glands via trigeminal nerve branches.

Middle cervical ganglion (8.398)

This is the smallest of the three. It is occasionally absent and may then be replaced by minute ganglia in the sympathetic trunk or may be fused with the superior ganglion. It is usually found at the sixth cervical vertebral level, anterior or just superior to the inferior thyroid artery, or it may adjoin the cervicothoracic ganglion (see below); it is probably a coalescence of the ganglia of the fifth and sixth cervical segments, judging by its postganglionic rami, which join the fifth and sixth cervical spinal nerves but sometimes also the fourth and seventh. The ganglion also has thyroid and cardiac branches. It is connected to the cervicothoracic ganglion by two or more very variable cords: the posterior usually splits to enclose the vertebral artery; the anterior loops down anterior to and then below the first part of the subclavian artery, medial to the origin of its internal thoracic branch, and supplies rami to it. This loop is the *ansa subclavia*; it is frequently multiple, lies closely in contact with the cervical pleura and generally connects with the phrenic nerve. Similar connections with the vagus nerve are of uncertain significance.

Thyroid branches accompany the inferior thyroid artery to the thyroid gland, communicating with the superior cardiac, external laryngeal and recurrent laryngeal nerves, and send branches to the parathyroid glands. Fibres to both glands are in part vasomotor but some reach the secretory cells (Raybuck 1952).

The *cardiac branch*, the largest sympathetic cardiac nerve, either

8.399 Anterior view of the same structures illustrated in **8.398**. Part of the vertebral artery has been excised to show the inferior cervical ganglion.

arises from the ganglion itself or more often from the sympathetic trunk cranial or caudal to it. On the **right side** it descends behind the common carotid artery, in front of or behind the subclavian, to the trachea where it receives a few filaments from the recurrent laryngeal nerve before joining the right half of the deep (dorsal) part of the cardiac plexus. In the neck, it connects with the superior cardiac and recurrent laryngeal nerves. On the **left side** the cardiac nerve enters the thorax between the left common carotid and subclavian arteries to join the left half of the deep (dorsal) part of the cardiac plexus. Fine branches from the middle cervical ganglion also pass to the trachea and oesophagus.

Cervicothoracic (stellate) ganglion

This is irregular in shape and much larger than the middle cervical ganglion. It is probably formed by a fusion of the lower two cervical and first thoracic segmental ganglia, sometimes including the second and even third and fourth thoracic ganglia. The first thoracic ganglion may be separate, leaving an *inferior cervical ganglion* above it (**8**.397). The sympathetic trunk turns backwards at the junction of the neck and thorax and so the long axis of the cervicothoracic ganglion becomes almost anteroposterior. The ganglion lies on or just lateral to the lateral border of the longus colli between the base of the seventh cervical transverse process and the neck of the first rib (which are posterior to it), the vertebral vessels being anterior. Below it is separated from the posterior aspect of the cervical pleura by the suprapleural membrane; the costocervical trunk branches near its lower pole. Lateral is the superior intercostal artery.

A small *vertebral ganglion* may be present on the sympathetic trunk anterior or anteromedial to the origin of the vertebral artery and directly above the subclavian. When present, it may provide the ansa subclavia and is also joined to the cervicothoracic ganglion by fibres enclosing the vertebral artery. It is usually regarded as a detached part of the middle cervical or cervicothoracic ganglion. Like the middle cervical ganglion it may supply grey rami communicantes to the fourth and fifth cervical spinal nerves. The cervicothoracic ganglion sends grey rami communicantes to the seventh and eighth cervical and first thoracic spinal nerves and gives off a cardiac branch, branches to nearby vessels and sometimes a branch to the vagus nerve.

The *grey rami communicantes* to the seventh cervical spinal nerve vary from one to five; two, the usual number, are shown in **8**.398, 399. A third often ascends medial to the vertebral artery in front of the seventh cervical transverse process, connects with the seventh cervical nerve and sends a filament upwards through the sixth cervical transverse foramen in company with the vertebral vessels to join the sixth cervical spinal nerve as it emerges from the intervertebral foramen. An inconstant ramus may traverse the seventh cervical transverse foramen. Grey rami to the eighth cervical spinal nerve vary from three to six in number.

The *cardiac branch* descends behind the subclavian artery and along the front of the trachea to the deep cardiac plexus. Behind the artery it connects with the recurrent laryngeal nerve and the cardiac branch of the middle cervical ganglion, the latter often being replaced by fine branches of the cervicothoracic ganglion and ansa subclavia.

Branches to blood vessels form plexuses on the subclavian artery and its branches. The subclavian supply is derived from the cervicothoracic ganglion and ansa subclavia, extending to the first part of the axillary artery; a few fibres may extend further. According to Pearson and Sauter (1971) an extension of the subclavian plexus to the internal thoracic artery is joined by a branch of the phrenic nerve (p. 1265). The vertebral plexus is derived mainly from a large branch of the cervicothoracic ganglion which ascends behind the vertebral artery to the sixth transverse foramen, reinforced by branches of the vertebral ganglion or the cervical sympathetic trunk which pass cranially on the ventral aspect of the artery; from this plexus *deep rami communicantes* join the ventral rami of the upper five or six cervical spinal nerves. The plexus contains some neuronal cell bodies and continues into the skull along the vertebral and basilar arteries and their branches as far as the posterior cerebral artery, where it meets a plexus from the internal carotid. Some consider the vertebral plexus to be the main intracranial extension of the sympathetic system (Lazorthes 1949; Mitchell 1952). The plexus on the inferior thyroid artery reaches the thyroid gland, connecting with recurrent and external laryngeal nerves, the cardiac branch of

the superior cervical ganglion, and the common carotid plexus.

The preganglionic fibres for the head and neck emerge from the spinal cord in the upper five thoracic spinal nerves (mainly the upper three), ascending in the sympathetic trunk to synapse in the cervical ganglia. The preganglionic fibres supplying the upper limb stem from upper thoracic segments, probably T2–6 (or 7), ascending via the sympathetic trunk to synapse mainly in its cervicothoracic ganglion, whence postganglionic fibres pass to the brachial plexus (mainly its lower trunk). Most of the vasoconstrictor fibres for the upper limb emerge in the second and third thoracic ventral roots; the arteries can thus be denervated by cutting the sympathetic trunk below the third thoracic ganglion, severing the rami communicantes connected with the second and third thoracic ganglia or by cutting the ventral roots of the second and third thoracic spinal nerves (intradurally). The white ramus to the cervicothoracic ganglion is not cut, partly because it does not convey many vasomotor or sudomotor fibres to the upper limb but mainly because it contains most of the preganglionic fibres for the head and neck; these ascend the trunk to the superior cervical ganglion, from which postganglionic branches supply vasoconstrictor and sudomotor nerves to the face and neck, secretory fibres to the salivary glands, dilator pupillae (and probably ciliaris oculi), non-striated muscle in the eyelids and the orbitalis. Destruction of this nerve would thus lead to meiosis, ptosis, enophthalmos and loss of sweating on the face and neck (*Horner's syndrome*) and possibly some disturbance of accommodation. For a review consult Haxton (1954) and Bannister and Mathias (1992).

Blood vessels of the upper limb beyond the first part of the axillary artery receive their sympathetic supply via branches of the brachial plexus adjacent to them, e.g. the median nerve supplies branches to the brachial artery and palmar arches, the ulnar nerve supplies the ulnar artery and palmar arches and the radial nerve supplies the radial artery.

The first and second (and occasionally the third) intercostal nerves may be interconnected anterior to the necks of the ribs by filaments containing postganglionic fibres from their grey rami; these fibres provide another path by which postganglionic nerves can pass from the upper thoracic ganglia to the brachial plexus.

THORACIC PART OF THE SYMPATHETIC SYSTEM

The thoracic sympathetic trunk (**8**.397, 400) contains ganglia almost equal in number to those of the thoracic spinal nerves (11 in more than 70%, occasionally 12, rarely 10 or 13). The first thoracic ganglion is usually fused with the inferior cervical, forming the cervicothoracic ganglion; Jit and Mukerjee (1960) found a fused ganglion in 80 out of 100 dissections. Rarely the middle cervical or second thoracic ganglion may be included. The succeeding ganglion is counted as the second in order to make the other ganglia correspond numerically with other segmental structures. Except for the lowest two or three, the thoracic ganglia lie against the costal heads, posterior to the costal pleura; the lowest two or three are lateral to the bodies of the corresponding vertebrae. Caudally, the thoracic sympathetic trunk passes dorsal to the medial arcuate ligament (or through the crus of the diaphragm) to become the lumbar sympathetic trunk. The ganglia are small and interconnected by intervening segments of the trunk. Two or more rami communicantes, white and grey, connect each ganglion with its corresponding spinal nerve, white rami joining the nerve distal to the grey. Sometimes a grey and a white ramus fuse to form a 'mixed' ramus (p. 1298).

The *medial branches from the upper five ganglia* are very small, supplying filaments to the thoracic aorta and its branches. On the aorta they form a fine *thoracic aortic plexus* with filaments from the greater splanchnic nerve. Rami of the second to fifth or sixth ganglia enter the posterior pulmonary plexus; others, from the second to fifth ganglia, pass to the deep (dorsal) part of the cardiac plexus. Small branches of these pulmonary and cardiac nerves pass to the oesophagus and trachea. The *medial branches from the lower seven ganglia* are large, supplying the aorta and uniting to form the greater, lesser and lowest splanchnic nerves, the last not always being identifiable.

The *greater splanchnic nerve*, consisting mainly of myelinated preganglionic efferent and visceral afferent fibres, is formed by branches from the fifth to ninth or tenth thoracic ganglia; but fibres in the upper branches may be traced to the first or second thoracic ganglion. Its roots vary from one to eight, four being the most usual number. It descends obliquely on the vertebral bodies, supplies branches to the descending thoracic aorta and perforates the ipsilateral crus of the diaphragm to end mainly in the coeliac ganglion but partly in the aorticorenal ganglion and suprarenal gland. A *splanchnic ganglion* exists on the nerve opposite the eleventh or twelfth thoracic vertebra in 17–68% of dissections (Jit & Mukerjee 1960); but Mitchell (1953) reported microscopic evidence that it is always present.

The *lesser splanchnic nerve*, formed by rami of the ninth and tenth (sometimes the tenth and eleventh) thoracic ganglia and the trunk between them, pierces the diaphragm with the greater splanchnic to join the aorticorenal ganglion.

The *lowest (least) splanchnic nerve* (or renal nerve) from the lowest thoracic ganglion enters the abdomen with the sympathetic trunk to end in the renal plexus.

Jit and Mukerjee (1960) described in great detail dissections of the thoracic sympathetic nerves in 50 cadavers and surveyed the previous findings. The incidence of the splanchnic nerves, according to seven observers, is as follows: greater—always present, lesser—94% (86–100%), least—56% (16–98%). A fourth (accessory) splanchnic nerve has been described by de Sousa (1955) but has not been confirmed.

LUMBAR PART OF THE SYMPATHETIC SYSTEM

The lumbar part of each sympathetic trunk (8.400, 401), usually containing four interconnected ganglia, runs in the extra-peritoneal connective tissue anterior to the vertebral column and along the medial margin of the psoas major. Superiorly it is continuous with the thoracic trunk posterior to the medial arcuate ligament; inferiorly, passing posterior to the common iliac artery, it becomes the pelvic trunk. On the right side it is overlapped by the inferior vena cava

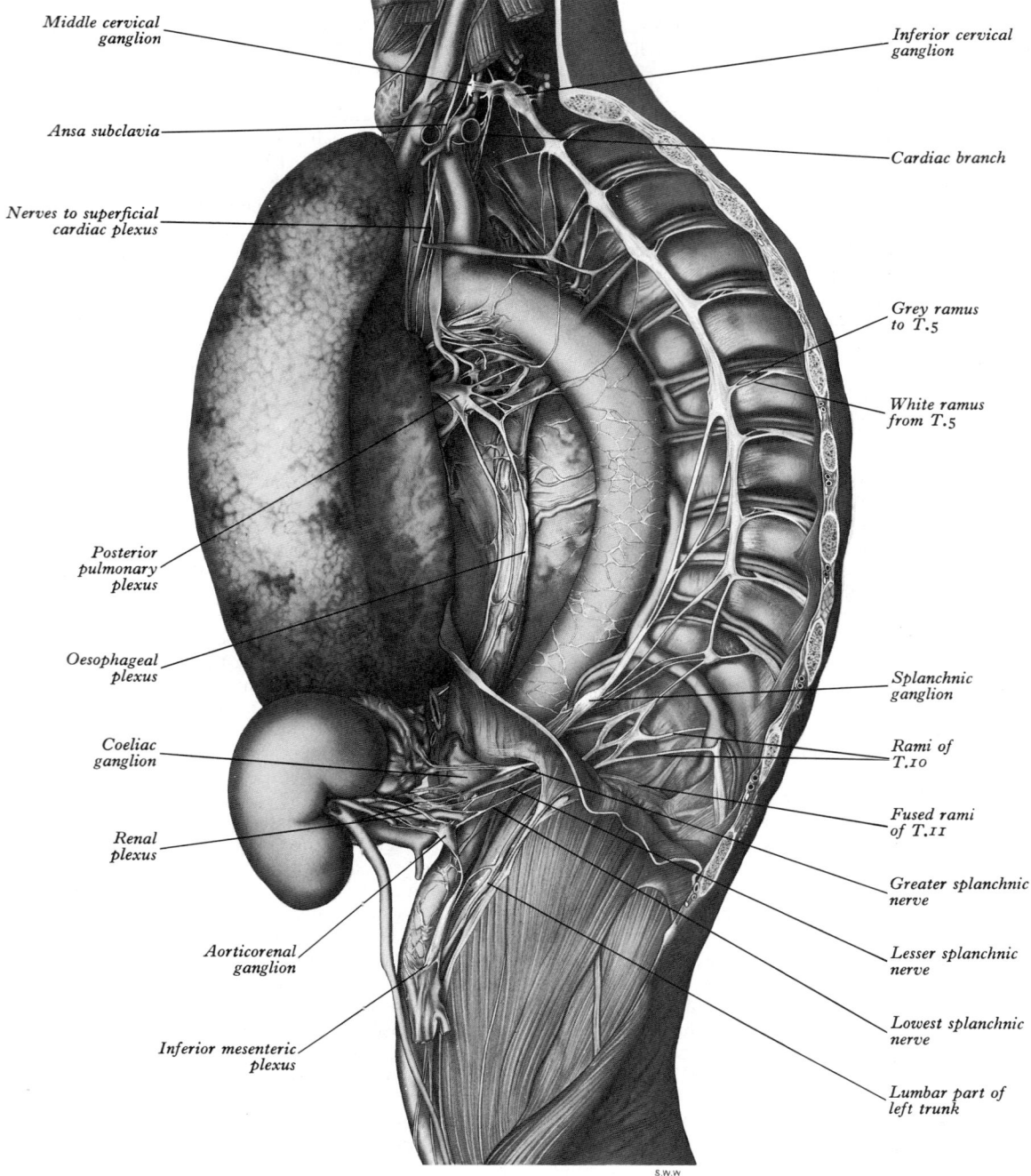

8.400 The thoracic part of the sympathetic system of the left side. Note that the diaphragm has been divided to its posterior attachment and the left lung and the left kidney have been drawn forwards and rotated to the right, so as to expose the posterior surface of the left kidney and suprarenal gland. (Drawn from a dissection by the late G D Channel, Guy's Hospital Medical School, London.)

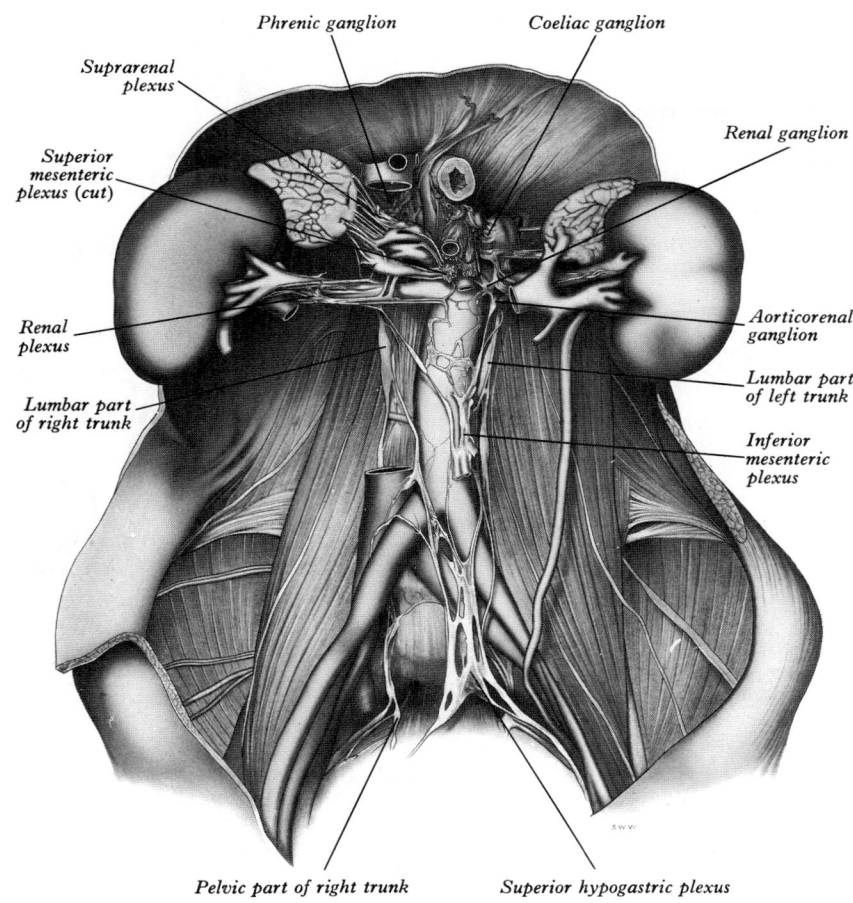

Phrenic ganglion

Coeliac ganglion

Suprarenal plexus

Renal ganglion

Superior mesenteric plexus (cut)

Renal plexus

Aorticorenal ganglion

Lumbar part of right trunk

Lumbar part of left trunk

Inferior mesenteric plexus

Pelvic part of right trunk

Superior hypogastric plexus

8.401 The abdominal part of the sympathetic system. (Drawn from a dissection by the late G D Channel, Guy's Hospital Medical School, London.)

and on the left by the lateral aortic lymph nodes. It is anterior to most of the lumbar vessels but may pass behind some lumbar veins.

The first, second and sometimes third lumbar ventral spinal rami send *white rami communicantes* to the corresponding ganglia. *Grey rami communicantes*, passing from all ganglia to the lumbar spinal nerves, are long and accompany the lumbar arteries round the sides of the vertebral bodies, medial to the fibrous arches to which the psoas major is attached.

Usually *four lumbar splanchnic nerves* pass from the ganglia to join the coeliac, intermesenteric (abdominal aortic) and superior hypogastric plexuses. The first lumbar splanchnic nerve, from the first ganglion, joins the coeliac, renal and intermesenteric plexuses. The second nerve, from the second and sometimes the third ganglion, joins the inferior part of the intermesenteric plexus; the third nerve issues from the third or fourth ganglion, passing anterior to the common iliac vessels to join the superior hypogastric plexus. The fourth lumbar splanchnic, from the lowest ganglion, passes dorsal to the common iliac vessels to join the lower part of the superior hypogastric plexus or the hypogastric 'nerve'.

Vascular branches from all lumbar ganglia join the intermesenteric (aortic) plexus. Fibres of the lower lumbar splanchnic nerves pass to the common iliac arteries, forming a plexus continued along the internal and external iliac arteries as far as the proximal part of the femoral artery. Many postganglionic fibres in the grey rami, connecting the lumbar ganglia to the spinal nerves, travel in the femoral nerve to its muscular, cutaneous and saphenous branches, supplying vasoconstrictor nerves to the femoral artery and its branches in the thigh. Other postganglionic fibres travel via the obturator nerve to the obturator artery. Considerable uncertainties persist regarding sympathetic supplies to the lower limb (Wilde 1951; Wyburn 1956; Pick 1970).

PELVIC PART OF THE SYMPATHETIC SYSTEM

The pelvic sympathetic trunk (**8**.400, 401) lies in the extraperitoneal tissue anterior to the sacrum, medial or anterior to the anterior sacral foramina, and has four or five interconnected ganglia. Above, it continues into the lumbar trunk; below, the two trunks converge to unite in the small *ganglion impar* anterior to the coccyx. *Grey rami communicantes* pass from the ganglia to sacral and coccygeal spinal nerves but white rami communicantes are absent. *Medial branches of distribution* connect across the midline; twigs from the first two ganglia join the inferior hypogastric plexus (pelvic plexus) or the hypogastric 'nerve'; others form a plexus on the median sacral artery. The glomus coccygeum is supplied from the loop between the two trunks. The hypogastric 'nerve', which is usually plexiform, is a redundant term for the right and left connections, between the superior and inferior hypogastric plexuses (p. 1308).

Vascular branches. Through the grey rami many postganglionic fibres pass to the roots of the sacral plexus, especially those forming the tibial nerve, to be conveyed to the popliteal artery and its branches in the leg and foot. Others are carried in the pudendal and superior and inferior gluteal nerves to the accompanying arteries. Branches to lymph nodes are also described (Woźniak 1966).

Preganglionic fibres for the lower limb are derived from the lower three thoracic and upper two or three lumbar spinal segments. They reach the lower thoracic and upper lumbar ganglia through white rami; some descend through the sympathetic trunk to synapse in the lumbar ganglia, whence postganglionic fibres join the femoral nerve to supply the femoral artery and its branches; other fibres descend to synapse in the upper two or three sacral ganglia, from which postganglionic axons join the tibial nerve to supply the popliteal artery and its branches in the leg and foot. Sympathetic denervation of vessels in the lower limb can thus be effected by removing the upper three lumbar ganglia and the intervening parts of the sympathetic trunk, all the preganglionic fibres to the lower limb thus being divided.

SEGMENTAL SYMPATHETIC SUPPLIES

Segmental sympathetic supplies are as follows:

Head and neck	T1–5
Upper limb	T2–5
Lower limb	T10–L2
Heart	T1–5
Bronchi and lung	T2–4
Oesophagus (caudal part)	T5–6
Stomach	T6–10
Small intestine	T9–10
Large intestine to splenic flexure	T11–L1
Splenic flexure to rectum	L1–2
Liver and gallbladder	T7–9
Spleen	T6–10
Pancreas	T6–10
Kidney	T10–L1
Ureter	T11–L2
Suprarenal	T8–L1
Testis and ovary	T10–11
Epididymis, ductus deferens, seminal vesicles	T11–12
Urinary bladder	T11–L2
Prostate and prostatic urethra	T11–L1
Uterus	T12–L1
Uterine tube	T10–L1

PLEXUSES IN THE THORACIC, ABDOMINAL AND PELVIC CAVITIES

The larger autonomic plexuses are aggregations of nerves and ganglia situated in the thoracic, abdominal and pelvic cavities. They are the cardiac, pulmonary, coeliac and hypogastric plexuses, supplying the thoracic, abdominal and pelvic viscera, respectively. Extensions of these major plexuses pass along most branches of the large vessels which they surround and are usually named after the artery along which they are distributed. This leads to a plethora of named plexuses, often separately described in detail which may overshadow their essential continuity.

CARDIAC PLEXUSES

The cardiac plexus (**8**.397, 400) at the base of the heart is divided into *superficial* (ventral) and *deep* (dorsal) *parts* which are closely connected. Several small ganglia lie within it, the most constant being the *cardiac ganglion* described below. Mizeres (1963) has emphasized the unity of the cardiac plexus, considering its division into two parts as an artefact of dissection; he was, however, prepared to allow regional names for its coronary, pulmonary, atrial and aortic extensions (**8**.402). Since major concentrations of the plexus are situated as described here, the terms superficial and deep have been retained.

Superficial (ventral) part of the cardiac plexus. This lies below the aortic arch and anterior to the right pulmonary artery. It is formed by the cardiac branch of the left superior cervical sympathetic ganglion and the lower of the two cervical cardiac branches of the left vagus. A *small cardiac ganglion* is usually present in this plexus immediately below the aortic arch, to the right of the ligamentum arteriosum. This part of the cardiac plexus connects with (1) the deep part, (2) the right coronary plexus, (3) the left anterior pulmonary plexus.

Deep (dorsal) part of the cardiac plexus. This is anterior to the tracheal bifurcation, above the point of division of the pulmonary trunk and posterior to the aortic arch. It is formed by the cardiac branches of the cervical and upper thoracic sympathetic ganglia and of the vagus and recurrent laryngeal nerves. The only cardiac nerves which do not join it are those joining the superficial part of the plexus.

Branches from the **right half** of the deep part of the cardiac plexus

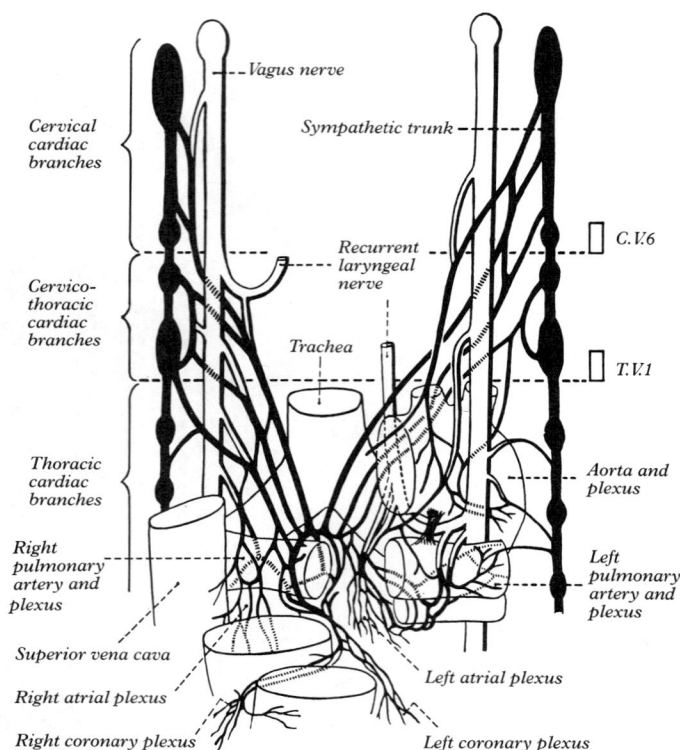

8.402   The human cardiac plexus, a semi-diagrammatic representation of its source from the cervical parts of the vagus nerves and sympathetic trunks and of its extensions, the pulmonary, atrial and coronary plexuses. Note the numerous junctions between sympathetic and parasympathetic (vagal) rami which form the plexus. Concerning the frequent variations, consult Mizeres 1963 (with permission of author and publisher).

pass in front of and behind the right pulmonary artery; those anterior to it, the more numerous, supply a few filaments to the right anterior pulmonary plexus and continue on to form part of the right coronary plexus; those behind the pulmonary artery supply a few filaments to the right atrium and then continue into the left coronary plexus. The **left half** of the deep part of the cardiac plexus is connected with the superficial, supplying filaments to the left atrium and left anterior pulmonary plexus and then continuing to form much of the left coronary plexus.

Left coronary plexus. This is larger than the right, and is formed chiefly by the prolongation of the left half of the deep part of the cardiac plexus and a few fibres from the right; it accompanies the left coronary artery to supply the left atrium and ventricle.

Right coronary plexus. This is formed from both superficial and deep parts of the cardiac plexus, and accompanies the right coronary artery to supply the right atrium and ventricle.

Atrial plexuses. Described by Mizeres (1963), these are derivatives of the right and left continuations of the cardiac plexus along the coronary arteries. Their fibres are distributed to the corresponding atria, overlapping those from the coronary plexuses.

All the cardiac branches of the vagus and sympathetic contain both afferent and efferent fibres, except the cardiac branch of the superior cervical sympathetic ganglion, which is purely efferent. The *efferent* preganglionic cardiac *sympathetic* fibres arise in the upper four or five thoracic spinal segments; they pass by white rami communicantes to synapse in the upper thoracic sympathetic ganglia, though many ascend to synapse in the cervical ganglia. Postganglionic fibres from the thoracic and cervical ganglia form the sympathetic cardiac nerves, which accelerate the heart and dilate the coronary arteries. Of the sympathetic fibres from the first four or five thoracic spinal segments, the upper pass to the ascending aorta, pulmonary trunk and ventricles, the lower to the atria.

The *efferent* cardiac *parasympathetic* fibres from the dorsal vagal nucleus and neurons near the nucleus ambiguus run in vagal cardiac branches to synapse in the cardiac plexuses and atrial walls. These vagal fibres slow the heart and cause constriction of the coronary arteries (p. 1500). In man (like most mammals) intrinsic cardiac neurons are limited to the atria and interatrial septum (Davies et al 1952; King & Coakley 1958); they are most numerous in the subepicardial connective tissue (**10**.59) near the SA and AV nodes. There is now evidence that these intrinsic ganglia are not simple nicotinic relays but may act as sites for integration of extrinsic nervous inputs and form complex circuits for the local neuronal control of the heart and perhaps even local reflexes (consult Saffrey et al 1992).

PULMONARY PLEXUSES

These are anterior and posterior to the other hilar structures of the lungs, the anterior plexus being much smaller. According to Mizeres (1963) they are extensions from the cardiac plexus along the right and left pulmonary arteries (**8**.402). They are formed by vagal and sympathetic branches. Efferent parasympathetic fibres arise from the dorsal vagal nucleus; efferent sympathetic fibres are postganglionic branches of the second to fifth thoracic sympathetic ganglia.

The *anterior pulmonary plexus* is formed by rami from vagal and cervical sympathetic cardiac nerves as well as direct branches from both sources; the *posterior pulmonary plexus* is formed by the rami of vagal cardiac branches from the second to fifth or sixth thoracic sympathetic ganglia, the left plexus also receiving branches from the left recurrent laryngeal nerve. The two plexuses are interconnected; from them nerves enter the lung as networks along branches of the bronchi and pulmonary and bronchial vessels extending as far as the visceral pleura. There are small ganglia within the tracheobronchial tree of the airways with which efferent vagal preganglionic fibres synapse (Coburn 1987). They may act as sites of integration and/or modulation of the input from extrinsic nerves or permit some local control of aspects of airway function by local reflex mechanisms (Allen & Burnstock 1990). In the small intestine interstitial cells have been described in terminal autonomic networks, but have not been seen in thoracic organs, apart perhaps from the oesophagus (Dijkstra 1969). Efferent vagal fibres are bronchoconstrictor, secretomotor to bronchial glands and vasodilator. Efferent sympathetic fibres are bronchodilator and vasoconstrictor.

COELIAC PLEXUS

The coeliac (**8**.397, 401), the largest major autonomic plexus, sited at the level of the last thoracic and first lumbar vertebrae, is a dense network uniting two large *coeliac ganglia*. It surrounds the coeliac artery and the root of the superior mesenteric artery. It is posterior to the stomach and omental bursa, anterior to the crura of the diaphragm and the commencement of the abdominal aorta and between the suprarenal glands. The plexus and ganglia are joined by the greater and lesser splanchnic nerves of both sides and branches from both the vagus and phrenic nerves. They extend as numerous secondary plexuses along adjacent arteries.

The *coeliac ganglia* are irregular masses, one on each side, between the suprarenal gland and the coeliac trunk and in front of the crura; the right one is behind the inferior vena cava, the left behind the splenic vessels. The upper part of each is joined by a greater splanchnic nerve; the lower part, more or less detached as the *aorticorenal ganglion*, receives the lesser splanchnic nerve and forms most of the renal plexus; its position is variable but near the origin of the renal artery from the aorta. (For details consult Norvell 1968). Secondary plexuses from or connected with the coeliac are: the phrenic, splenic, hepatic, left gastric, intermesenteric, suprarenal, renal, testicular or ovarian, superior mesenteric and inferior mesenteric.

Phrenic plexus. This accompanies the inferior phrenic artery to the diaphragm, with branches to the suprarenal gland. It arises near the upper end of the coeliac ganglion and is larger on the right. It receives one or two phrenic branches. At the junction of the right phrenic plexus with the phrenic nerve is a small *phrenic ganglion*, distributing branches to the inferior vena cava, suprarenal and hepatic plexuses.

Hepatic plexus. The largest coeliac derivative, this also receives filaments from the left and right vagi and right phrenic nerve. It accompanies the hepatic artery and portal vein and their branches into the liver, where its fibres are confined to the vicinity of the blood vessels. It follows all branches of the hepatic artery. Branches

to the gallbladder form a thin *cystic plexus*; bile ducts are also supplied. Branches accompanying the right gastric artery supply the pylorus. From the gastroduodenal extension of the plexus branches reach the pylorus and the first part of the duodenum. Many follow the right gastro-epiploic artery to supply the right side of the stomach and the greater curvature. The superior pancreaticoduodenal extension of the plexus supplies the descending part of the duodenum, the pancreatic head and the lower part of the bile duct. The hepatic plexus contains afferent and efferent sympathetic and parasympathetic fibres; the vagal constituents are said to be motor to the musculature of the gallbladder and bile ducts and inhibitory to the sphincter of the bile duct. Petkov (1968) identified a distinct nerve to the sphincter in 23 out of 25 human dissections.

Left gastric plexus. This accompanies its artery along the lesser curvature of the stomach, joining with the vagal gastric branches. Gastric sympathetic nerves are motor to the pyloric sphincter but inhibitory to the gastric mural musculature.

Splenic plexus. This is formed by branches of the coeliac plexus, left coeliac ganglion and right vagus, and accompanies its artery to the spleen, giving off subsidiary plexuses along arterial branches. The fibres are mainly, perhaps wholly, sympathetic and terminate in blood vessels and non-striated muscle of the splenic capsule and trabeculae.

Suprarenal plexus. This is formed by branches from the coeliac ganglion and plexus and greater splanchnic nerve. Relative to its size, the suprarenal gland has a larger autonomic supply than any other organ. Its fibres are commonly described as myelinated and preganglionic. In rats, however, non-myelinated fibres are ten times as numerous and are considered preganglionic; they end in synapses, often deeply invaginated, with large chromaffin cells, the phaeo-chromocytes, which are thus homologous with the postganglionic sympathetic neurons (p. 1905). A space of 150–200 nm separates the synaptic membranes, which often have electron-dense zones. Small and large vesicles with electron-dense granular contents occur in these endings. Only non-myelinated fibres appear to innervate chromaffin cells, all of which are related to one or more such terminals. Multi-polar neurons also occur in the adrenal medulla; some preganglionic non-myelinated fibres form axodendritic synapses with them. The destination of their axons is not known (Coupland 1965a). A preponderance of non-myelinated fibres has also been described in the human suprarenal plexus (Coupland 1965a,b; Grottel 1968).

Renal plexus. This is dense and formed by rami from the coeliac ganglion and plexus, aorticorenal ganglion, lowest thoracic splanchnic nerve, first lumbar splanchnic nerve and aortic plexus. Small ganglia occur in the renal plexus, the largest usually behind the start of the renal artery. The plexus continues into the kidney around the arterial branches to supply the vessels, renal glomeruli, and tubules, especially the cortical tubules (Norvell 1968). Renal nerves are mostly vasomotor. From the renal plexus branches supply ureteric and testicular (or ovarian) plexuses. The *ureteric plexus* receives, in its upper part, branches from the renal and aortic plexuses, in its intermediate part from the superior hypogastric plexus and hypogastric nerve and in its lower part from the hypogastric nerve and inferior hypogastric plexus. This supply influences the inherent motility of the ureter.

Testicular plexus. This accompanies the testicular artery to the testis. Its upper part receives branches from the renal and aortic plexuses. Distally it is reinforced from the superior and inferior hypogastric plexuses. Its rami pass to the epididymis and ductus deferens.

Ovarian plexus. This accompanies the ovarian artery to the ovary and uterine tube. The upper part is formed by branches from the renal and aortic plexuses; its lower part is reinforced from the superior and inferior hypogastric plexuses.

The nerves in the testicular and ovarian plexuses contain efferent and afferent sympathetic fibres; the efferents are vasomotor and derived from the tenth and eleventh thoracic spinal segments; the parasympathetic fibres, from the inferior hypogastric plexuses, are probably vasodilator.

Superior mesenteric plexus. This is a downward continuation of the coeliac, which receives a branch from the junction of the right vagus and coeliac plexus. It accompanies the superior mesenteric artery into the mesentery, dividing into secondary plexuses distributed to parts supplied by the artery: pancreatic, jejunal and ileal, ileocolic, right colic and middle colic. The *superior mesenteric ganglion* lies superior in the plexus, usually above the superior mesenteric artery's origin. Intestinal sympathetic nerves are motor to the ileocaecal sphincter but inhibitory to the mural musculature; some are vasoconstrictor.

Abdominal aortic plexus (intermesenteric plexus). This is formed by branches from the coeliac plexus and ganglia and receives rami from the first and second lumbar splanchnic nerves. It is on the sides and front of the aorta, between the origins of the superior and inferior mesenteric arteries. It consists of four to 12 intermesenteric nerves, connected by oblique branches. It is continuous above with the coeliac plexus and coeliac and aorticorenal ganglia, below with the superior hypogastric plexus. From it parts of testicular, inferior mesenteric, iliac and superior hypogastric plexuses arise; it also supplies the inferior vena cava.

Inferior mesenteric plexus. This is chiefly from the aortic plexus but also from the second and lumbar splanchnic nerves. It surrounds the inferior mesenteric artery and is distributed along its branches; thus a left colic plexus supplies the left part of the transverse colon, the descending and the sigmoid colon; a superior rectal plexus supplies the rectum. Near the origin of the inferior mesenteric artery an inferior mesenteric ganglion may occur but more often small ganglia are scattered around the origin of the artery in the proximal part of the plexus. In one study (Southam 1959) an *inferior mesenteric ganglion* occurred in all of 22 human stillborn infants. The colic sympathetic nerves are inhibitory to mural muscle in the colon and rectum. Branches from parasympathetic pelvic splanchnic nerves ascend occasionally through but usually near the superior hypogastric and inferior mesenteric plexuses to supply the large intestine from the left half of the transverse colon to the rectum (p. 1786 and see below); they are motor to the colic musculature. It is to be emphasized that the parasympathetic supply to the distal colon is largely by these direct branches of the pelvic splanchnic nerves, *not* via the hypogastric and inferior mesenteric plexuses (Mitchell 1935; Woodburne 1956).

SUPERIOR HYPOGASTRIC PLEXUS

The superior hypogastric plexus (**8.381, 401, 403**) is anterior to the aortic bifurcation, the left common iliac vein, medial sacral vessels, fifth lumbar vertebral body and sacral promontory and between the common iliac arteries. Often termed the *presacral nerve*, it is seldom a single nerve and is prelumbar rather than presacral. It lies in extraperitoneal connective tissue; the parietal peritoneum can easily be stripped off its anterior aspect. It varies in breadth and condensation of its constituent nerves and is often a little to one side of the midline (more often to the left); the attachment of the sigmoid mesocolon, containing superior rectal vessels, is to the left of the lower part of the plexus. Scattered neurons occur in it. The plexus is formed by branches from the aortic plexus and third and fourth lumbar splanchnic nerves. It divides into right and left hypogastric 'nerves' which descend to the two inferior hypogastric plexuses. The superior plexus supplies branches to the ureteric, testicular, ovarian and common iliac plexuses. In addition to sympathetic fibres, it may also contain parasympathetic fibres (from pelvic splanchnic nerves) which ascend from the inferior hypogastric plexus; but these fibres usually ascend to the left of the superior hypogastric plexus and across the sigmoid branches of left colic vessels. These parasympathetic fibres are distributed partly along the inferior mesenteric arterial branches and also as independent retroperitoneal nerves, to supply the left part of the transverse colon, left colic flexure, descending and sigmoid colon (p. 1298 and **8.401**).

INFERIOR HYPOGASTRIC PLEXUSES

The *superior hypogastric plexus* divides caudally into right and left *hypogastric* 'nerves', each descending in extraperitoneal connective tissue into the pelvis, medial to each internal iliac artery and its branches to become the *inferior hypogastric plexus* (**8.381**). Each nerve may be single or an elongated plexus of anastomosing filaments. (Hypogastric nerves can scarcely be distinguished from their continuations, the inferior hypogastric plexuses. The latter are joined by pelvic splanchnic nerves, a distinction minimized by the fact that both nerves and plexuses contain sympathetic and parasympathetic fibres. Some authorities prefer to describe a superior hypogastric plexus dividing into two inferior plexuses.) From each hypogastric nerve branches may pass to the testicular, ovarian and ureteric plexus or to the internal iliac plexuses and to the sigmoid colon; each nerve

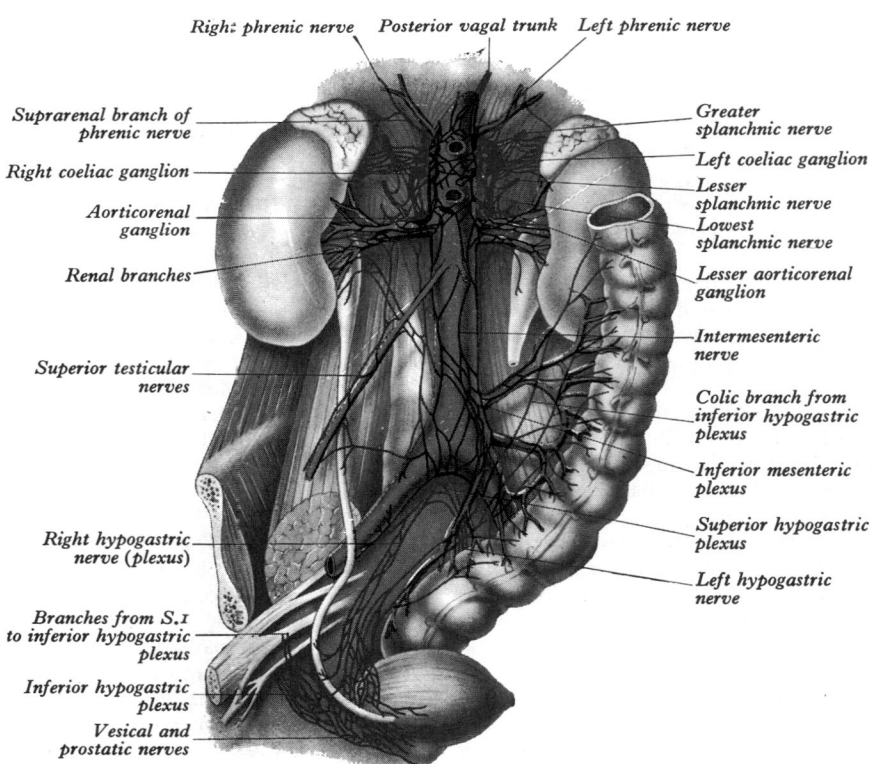

Right phrenic nerve   Posterior vagal trunk   Left phrenic nerve

Suprarenal branch of phrenic nerve

Right coeliac ganglion

Aorticorenal ganglion

Renal branches

Superior testicular nerves

Right hypogastric nerve (plexus)

Branches from S.1 to inferior hypogastric plexus

Inferior hypogastric plexus

Vesical and prostatic nerves

Greater splanchnic nerve

Left coeliac ganglion

Lesser splanchnic nerve

Lowest splanchnic nerve

Lesser aorticorenal ganglion

Intermesenteric nerve

Colic branch from inferior hypogastric plexus

Inferior mesenteric plexus

Superior hypogastric plexus

Left hypogastric nerve

8.403 Autonomic nerves and plexuses in the abdomen and pelvis. Note the ascending branches of the inferior hypogastric plexus passing up to supply the descending colon. The sympathetic trunks are not shown on the right side; note the upper, middle and lower ureteric nerves. (After Mitchell 1953, by courtesy of the author and the publishers.)

may be joined initially by the lowest lumbar splanchnic nerve from last lumbar sympathetic ganglion.

Inferior hypogastric (pelvic) plexus

This is in the extraperitoneal connective tissue. In males it is lateral to: the rectum, seminal vesicle, prostate and the posterior part of the urinary bladder. In females each plexus is lateral to: the rectum, uterine cervix, vaginal fornix and the posterior part of the urinary bladder, extending into the broad uterine ligament. Lateral to it are the internal iliac vessels and their branches and tributaries, the levator ani, coccygeus and obturator internus. Posterior are the sacral and coccygeal plexuses and above are the superior vesical and obliterated umbilical arteries. The plexuses contain numerous small ganglia. Each is formed by a hypogastric nerve, conveying most of the sympathetic fibres of the plexus, the remaining few arriving via branches from the ganglia. Parasympathetic fibres are derived from pelvic splanchnic nerves. Preganglionic efferent sympathetic fibres originate in the lower three thoracic and upper two lumbar spinal segments, some relaying in ganglia of the lumbar and sacral parts of the sympathetic trunk, others synapsing in the lower part of the aortic plexus and in the superior and inferior hypogastric plexuses. Preganglionic parasympathetic fibres originate in the second to fourth sacral spinal segments, reach the plexus in the pelvic splanchnic nerves and synapse in it or in walls of viscera supplied by its branches. Numerous branches are distributed to the pelvic and some abdominal viscera, either directly or along their arteries.

Parasympathetic fibres ascend in the hypogastric plexuses or as separate filaments to reach the inferior mesenteric plexus by way of the aortic plexus. By this route the descending and sigmoid parts of the colon receive parasympathetic innervation.

Middle rectal plexus

This is formed by fibres from the upper part of the inferior hypogastric plexus to the rectum passing directly or along the middle rectal artery. It connects above with the superior rectal plexus and extends below to the internal anal sphincter. The rectal and anal nerve supply is from:

- the superior rectal plexus
- the middle rectal plexus
- the inferior rectal (haemorrhoidal) nerves, branches of the pudendal nerve.

The parasympathetic preganglionic fibres from the rectal plexuses synapse with postganglionic neurons in the well-developed myenteric plexus, while sympathetic afferents pass through it without interruption. Efferent sympathetic fibres in the rectal plexuses inhibit the expulsive musculature and stimulate the sphincter. Pain impulses traverse the sympathetic and parasympathetic fibres but the parasympathetic afferent and efferent fibres are more active in normal defaecation. Inferior rectal nerves supply motor fibres to the striated external anal sphincter and sensory (somatic) fibres to the lower (ectodermal) part of the anal canal (p. 194).

Vesical plexus

Coming from the anterior part of the inferior hypogastric plexus, this comprises many filaments which pass along vesical arteries to the bladder. Branches supply the seminal vesicles and deferent ducts. Many small groups of neurons exist among the nerve fibres in the vesical muscular wall. Sympathetic preganglionic fibres in the plexus are from the lower two thoracic and upper two lumbar spinal segments, synapsing with neurons scattered in the superior and inferior hypogastric plexuses and vesical wall. The parasympathetic

preganglionic efferent fibres come from the second to fourth sacral spinal segments and synapse near or in the vesical wall with postganglionic neurons which stimulate its detrusor muscle and inhibit its sphincter. Efferent sympathetic nerves are motor to the sphincter and inhibitor to the detrusor muscle; but some maintain that they are mainly vasomotor and that vesical filling and emptying are controlled by parasympathetic nerves.

Prostatic plexus

Continued from the lower part of the inferior hypogastric plexus, this is composed of large nerves entering the base and sides of the prostate and contains neurons. It supplies: the prostate, seminal vesicles, prostatic urethra, ejaculatory ducts, corpora cavernosa, corpus spongiosum, membranous and penile urethra and bulbourethral glands. The nerves to the corpora cavernosa form two sets, the lesser and greater cavernous nerves, arising from the front of the plexus to join branches from the pudendal nerve and then passing below the pubic arch. The precise localization of the autonomic nerves from the pelvic plexus to the corpora cavernosa has been described by Lepor et al (1985) in the adult male pelvis. *Lesser cavernous nerves* pierce the fibrous penile sheath proximally to supply the erectile tissue of the corpus spongiosum and penile urethra. *Greater cavernous nerves* proceed on the dorsum penis, connect with the dorsal nerve and supply the erectile tissue, some filaments reaching the erectile tissue of the corpus spongiosum. Sympathetic supplies to the male genital organs produce vasoconstriction, the parasympathetic being vasodilator. Seminal vesicles are supplied from the vesical and prostatic plexuses and inferior hypogastric nerves; extensions pass to the ejaculatory and deferent ducts. Contraction of the seminal vesicles and ejaculation are considered to be due to the sympathetic supply, which also inhibits the vesical musculature and stimulates the sphincter during ejaculation, preventing reflux into the bladder. Others have suggested that contraction of the seminal vesicles is under parasympathetic control (Matthews & Raisman 1969).

Uterovaginal plexus

Uterine nerves arise from the inferior hypogastric plexus, mainly the part in the broad ligament, the uterovaginal plexus, from which branches descend with the vaginal arteries, while others pass directly to the cervix uteri or ascend with or near uterine arteries in the broad ligament. Nerves to the cervix form a plexus in which are small *paracervical ganglia*, one ganglion sometimes being larger and termed the *uterine cervical ganglion*. Nerves ascending with the uterine arteries supply the uterine body and tube, connecting with *tubal nerves* from the inferior hypogastric plexus and with the ovarian plexus. The uterine nerves ramify in the myometrium and endometrium, generally accompanying the vessels. Efferent preganglionic sympathetic fibres are from the last thoracic and first lumbar spinal segments; the sites of their postganglionic neurons are unknown. Preganglionic parasympathetic fibres arise in the second to fourth sacral spinal segments and relay in the paracervical ganglia. Sympathetic activity may produce uterine contraction and vasoconstriction and parasympathetic activity may produce uterine inhibition and vasodilatation, but these activities are complicated by hormonal control of uterine functions.

Vaginal nerves from the lower parts of the inferior hypogastric and uterovaginal plexuses follow the vaginal arteries to supply the vaginal walls, the erectile tissue of the vestibular bulbs and clitoris (cavernous nerves of the clitoris), the urethra and the greater vestibular glands. The nerves contain many parasympathetic fibres which are vasodilator to the erectile tissue.

Enteric nervous system

The enteric nervous system is defined as the system of neurons and their supporting cells that is found within the walls of the gastrointestinal tract, including the neurons within the pancreas and gallbladder; these neurons arise from neural crest tissue that is different from that giving rise to sympathetic and parasympathetic systems (for review consult Le Douarin 1982; Furness and Costa 1987; Le Douarin & Dulac 1992).

Organization of the enteric nervous system

The majority of nerve fibres which innervate the gut arise from the *intrinsic plexuses*. There are two main interconnecting ganglionated plexuses, the *myenteric (or Auerbach's) plexus*, which lies around the full circumference of the digestive tube between the external longitudinal and circular muscle coats, and the *submucous (or Meissner's and Henle's) plexus* which lies between the circular muscle and the muscularis mucosae. The myenteric plexus, a system of small interconnected ganglia, extends, uninterrupted, from the more oral part of the oesophagus to the margin of the internal anal sphincter. The submucous plexus extends from the stomach to the internal anal sphincter. The meshes of the submucous plexus are smaller than those of the myenteric plexus, the interconnecting strands are finer and the ganglia bigger. The ganglia often lie at two levels, one group being closer to the circular muscle, the other closer to the mucosa.

The total number of nerve cells in the myenteric and submucous plexuses is vast; it has been estimated that there are 10–100 million neurons in man (Furness & Costa 1980). The gallbladder also has a ganglionated plexus and ganglia are found in the pancreas.

Systems of nerve bundles connect the enteric ganglia and run from the ganglionated plexuses to form plexuses in the muscle layers, in the mucosa and around blood vessels. The different plexuses of nerve fibres are named by their location: the subserous, longitudinal muscle, circular muscle, mucosal and perivascular plexuses, and the plexus of the muscularis mucosae. Small ganglia are sometimes found in the subserous plexus, particularly in the stomach and near the mesenteric

attachment of the intestine and on the surface of the rectum (Furness & Costa 1987). Scanning and transmission-electron microscopic studies have shown that the organization of enteric ganglia is closer to that of the CNS than that of sympathetic or parasympathetic ganglia (Gabella 1972; Jessen & Burnstock 1982): glial cells and neurons are in close relationship and their processes form a dense neuropil; neither connective tissues nor blood vessels penetrate into the ganglia; and a blood–ganglion barrier analogous to the blood–brain barrier has been demonstrated. The myenteric plexus contains most of the intrinsic neurons of the gut. The intrinsic neurons either synapse with cells in the same or other ganglia or project to a range of effectors in the gut, including the smooth muscle of the outer longitudinal and inner circular muscle coats, the muscularis mucosae and the mucosa. They also connect with autonomic ganglia outside the walls of the gastrointestinal tract as well as sending afferents to the CNS. Some enteric neurons project from the intestine to innervate the mesenteric arteries and arterioles of the colon. The motor neurons for the circular muscle are located entirely in the myenteric plexus, whereas most for the mucosa are in the submucous plexus (Furness & Costa 1987). The normal motility and secretory functions of the intestine are thus dependent on the anatomical, chemical and functional integrity of this network of integrated plexuses that comprise the enteric nervous system.

The *extrinsic nerve supply* to the gut comprises postganglionic sympathetic fibres from the coeliac and superior and inferior mesenteric ganglia and preganglionic parasympathetic fibres running in the vagus and pelvic nerves. These nerves innervate all parts of the gut, including the nerve plexuses, muscle layers, blood vessels and epithelium. Many sympathetic nerves are associated with blood vessels and are probably related to vasomotor action. Sensory–motor nerves, with their cell bodies in spinal and vagal ganglia, also innervate nerve plexuses and blood vessels in the gut.

Autonomy of the enteric nervous system

The enteric nervous system is unusual in

that it retains many functions after all central connections are severed. Sympathetic and parasympathetic denervation have only transient effects on gut motility, highlighting the dominant role of the intrinsic plexuses which contain complete reflex pathways consisting of: enteric sensory neurons, which monitor such factors as intestinal wall tension and intestinal contents; interneurons, which form information links between enteric neurons; and motor neurons, which change the activity of the intestine (Furness & Costa 1987). The *peristalsis reflex* is thought to involve transfer of impulses from intrinsic sensory neurons, activated by stretching of the gut wall and from chemical stimulation of sensory endings in the mucosa, via interneurons to orally directed excitatory motor neurons and anally directed inhibitory motor neurons.

A multiplicity of substances have been revealed that are involved in neurotransmission in the enteric nervous system (see Cook & Burnstock 1976; Furness & Costa 1987; Gershon et al 1989; Hills & Jessen 1992). The rapid expansion of the list of proposed enteric neurotransmitters in recent years makes it likely that the list is still incomplete (pp. 1787, 1898). Enteric neurons have been identified containing up to six different neuropeptides in a single neuron. It is likely that many of these substances act as neuromodulators, enhancing or diminishing the release or actions of primary transmitters, and/or have trophic roles. The precise combinations of substances contained in individual enteric neurons and their projections and central connections, termed their 'chemical coding', has been defined in an elaborate series of surgical manipulations (Furness & Costa 1987; Furness et al 1992).

Intestinal smooth muscle is supplied by two types of intrinsic motor neurons, enteric excitatory neurons and enteric inhibitory neurons, which generally project orally and anally, respectively. *Enteric excitatory motor neurons* use ACh and SP as cotransmitters. There is much debate about the identity of the inhibitory transmitter(s) in the gut but it is currently thought that *enteric inhibitory motor neurons* use ATP, VIP and NO as cotransmitters, albeit in different proportions in different regions of the gut (**8.393**). ATP is the dominant cotransmitter in the small intestine and colon whereas VIP is the dominant transmitter in the stomach (Burnstock 1981; Hoyle & Burnstock 1989).

SENSORY AND SENSORY–MOTOR NERVES

Efferent autonomic fibres to the viscera and blood vessels are accompanied by their sensory counterparts, the *general visceral afferent* or *autonomic afferent* fibres. These are the peripheral processes of unipolar neurons in some cranial and spinal ganglia. While many nerves running in autonomic pathways are purely sensory, with terminals containing a few vesicles and a predominance of mitochondria, certain primary afferent nerve fibres also have an efferent function. Although the concept that antidromic impulses in sensory nerve collaterals form the basis of the 'axon reflex' vasodilatation of skin vessels was proposed many years ago (Lewis 1927), it was only after the discovery of the pharmacological properties of the sensory neurotoxin, capsaicin, that pharmacological studies on sensory neurons have focused on their efferent function (Maggi 1991). The efferent function of capsaicin-sensitive primary afferent nerves is produced through the release of transmitters, SP, CGRP and ATP, from their peripheral endings (Duckles & Buck 1982; Jahr & Jessel 1983; Lundberg et al 1985; Burnstock 1993). These substances act on target cells to produce several biological actions which include vasodilatation, increase in venular permeability, changes in smooth muscle contractility, degranulation of mast cells and a variety of effects on leucocytes and fibroblasts, a process collectively known as 'neurogenic inflammation' (Maggi & Meli 1988). There is also evidence that the local release of sensory neurotransmitters plays a long-term 'trophic' role in the maintenance of tissue integrity and repair in response to injury. It is now recognized that the efferent function of sensory nerves is widespread and that sensory–motor nerves are an important part of the autonomic nervous system, especially in the cardiovascular system, airways and gastrointestinal tract (consult Björklund et al 1988). The central axons of autonomic afferent fibres enter the CNS in the nerves concerned; their peripheral processes, myelinated or non-myelinated fibres of varying calibre, are distributed with pre- and postganglionic fibres of both autonomic divisions but do not synapse in their ganglia. Their terminals are described as knobs, loops, rings, tendrils and more elaborate encapsulated endings in the visceral and vascular walls, including the epithelia and serosae. Afferent impulses conducted by these neurons evoke visceral reflexes but usually do not obtrude on consciousness. They also probably mediate organic visceral sensations such as hunger, nausea, sexual excitement, vesical distension, etc. and visceral pain fibres may follow these routes. Although viscera are insensitive to cutting, crushing or burning, excessive tension in non-striated muscle and some pathological conditions produce visceral pain. It is not always easy to distinguish between what is pathological and mere exaggeration of normal activity. 'Abdominal' pain due to strong intestinal contraction is commonplace. In visceral disease vague pain may be felt near the viscus itself (visceral pain) or in a cutaneous area or other tissue whose somatic efferents enter spinal segments receiving afferents from the viscus; this is *referred pain*. If inflammation spreads from a diseased viscus to the adjacent parietal serosa (e.g. the peritoneum), somatic afferents will be stimulated, causing local somatic, commonly spasmodic, pain in this region. Referred pain is often associated with local cutaneous tenderness.

General visceral afferent fibres exist in vagal, glossopharyngeal and possibly other cranial nerves, in the second to fourth sacral nerves distributed with pelvic splanchnic nerves, and in thoracic and upper lumbar spinal nerves, distributed through rami communicantes and alongside the efferent sympathetic innervation of viscera and blood vessels.

The large vagal general visceral afferent components have their somata in the superior and inferior vagal ganglia, which appear predominantly sensory, despite contrary views regarding the inferior ganglion. Their central processes end in the dorsal vagal nucleus in the medulla oblongata or, according to some, the nucleus solitarius. Their peripheral processes are distributed to terminals in the pharyngeal and oesophageal walls, where with glossopharyngeal visceral afferents in the pharynx, they are concerned in swallowing reflexes. Vagal afferents are also ascribed to the thyroid and parathyroid glands. In the thorax some end in the heart, the walls of the great vessels, the aortic bodies and pressor receptors; in the last they are stimulated by raised intravascular pressure. Some reach the lungs through the pulmonary plexuses, being distributed to:

- bronchial mucosa, probably involved in cough reflexes
- bronchial muscle, where they encircle myocytes and end in tendrils sometimes regarded as 'muscle spindles', believed to be stimulated by change in the length of myocytes
- interalveolar connective tissue, where their knob-like endings, together with terminals on myocytes, may evoke Herring–Breuer reflexes
- adventitia of pulmonary arteries, where they may be pressor receptors, and the intima of pulmonary veins, where they may be chemoreceptors.

Antidromic activation of sensory–motor fibres can induce bronchoconstriction, protein extravasation and vasodilatation (Lundberg et al 1988). Afferent fibres from visceral pleura and bronchi may also travel with the pulmonary sympathetic supply, mediating nociceptive responses.

Vagal visceral afferent fibres also end in the gastric and intestinal walls, in digestive glands, and the kidney. Fibres ending in the gut and its ducts respond to stretch or contraction. Gastric impulses may evoke sensations of hunger and nausea.

Glossopharyngeal general visceral afferents innervate the posterior lingual region, tonsils and pharynx, whose epithelia are endodermal. Innervation of taste buds is not included; these have **special** visceral afferents (p. 914). Glossopharyngeal afferents also innervate the carotid sinus and body, receptors sensitive to tension and changes in chemical composition of the blood; impulses from these receptors are essential to circulatory and respiratory reflexes. Somata of the glossopharyngeal general visceral afferents are in the glossopharyngeal ganglia, their terminations in the medulla oblongata being probably like those of the vagal visceral afferents.

Sensory fibres in pelvic splanchnic nerves innervate pelvic viscera and the distal part of the colon. Vesical receptors are widespread; those in muscle strata are connected with thickly myelinated fibres reaching the spinal cord via pelvic splanchnic nerves and are believed to be stretch receptors, possibly activated by contraction. Pain fibres from the bladder and proximal urethra traverse both pelvic splanchnic nerves and the inferior hypogastric plexus, hypogastric nerves, superior hypogastric plexus and lumbar splanchnic nerves to reach their somata in ganglia on the lower thoracic and upper lumbar dorsal spinal roots. The significance of this dual sensory pathway is uncertain; lesions of the cauda equina abolish pain from vesical overdistension but hypogastric section is ineffective.

Though the fibres of pelvic splanchnic nerves, possible afferent, are described in the ovary, no supply from this source to the testis is known.

Pain fibres from the uterine body traverse the hypogastric plexus and lumbar splanchnic nerves to reach somata in the lowest thoracic and upper lumbar spinal ganglia; hypogastric division may relieve dysmenorrhoea. Afferents from the cervix, however, traverse the pelvic splanchnic nerves to somata in the upper sacral spinal ganglia. Stretch of the cervix uteri causes pain but cauterization and biopsy excisions do not.

Afferent fibres accompanying pre- and postganglionic sympathetic fibres have a generally segmental arrangement. They end in spinal cord segments from which preganglionic fibres innervate the region or viscus concerned (see below). General visceral afferents entering thoracic and upper lumbar spinal segments are largely concerned with pain. Nociceptive impulses from the pharynx, oesophagus, stomach, intestines, kidney, ureter, gallbladder and bile ducts seem to be carried in sympathetic pathways. Cardiac nociceptive impulses enter the spinal cord via the first to fifth thoracic spinal nerves, carried mainly in the middle and inferior cardiac nerves, but a few pass directly to the spinal nerves. There are no general visceral afferents in the superior cardiac nerves. Peripherally the fibres pass through the cardiac plexuses and along the coronary arteries. Myocardial anoxia may evoke symptoms of angina pectoris in which there is typically presternal pain, pain referred to much of the left chest, radiating to the left shoulder and the medial aspect of the left arm, along the left side of the neck to the jaw and occiput and down to the epigastrium; pain may be bilateral or even confined to the right. Sensory–motor reflex mechanisms may be an important link in a neurally-mediated metabolic regulation of local tissue (Owman

1311

1988). Cardiac afferents are also carried in vagal cardiac branches and are concerned with the reflex depression of cardiac activity. In some animals (e.g. rabbit) a separate depressor cardiac nerve is a branch of the vagus or superior laryngeal nerve. Human depressor fibres, however, run in branches of the superior or internal laryngeal nerves, cardiac branches of the vagus or the sympathetic. Ureteric pain fibres, also running with sympathetic fibres, are presumably concerned in the agonizing renal colic of obstruction by calculi. Afferent fibres from the testis and ovary run through the corresponding plexuses; their somata are in the tenth and eleventh thoracic dorsal spinal root ganglia.

It must be emphasized that autonomic reflexes are not initiated solely by general visceral afferent pathways; nor do impulses in these necessarily activate general visceral efferents. In most situations demanding general sympathetic activity for effect, the afferent element is usually somatic, either from special senses or the skin. Rises in blood pressure and pupillodilatation may result from the stimulation of somatic receptors in the skin and other tissues. Conversely, contraction of the rectus abdominis, a somatic structure, may result from irritation of abdominal viscera.

Denervation often has no obvious effect on the effector organs, non-striated muscle or glands innervated by autonomic fibres. Contraction may be unaffected by denervation and no structural changes ensue. This is variously attributed to the continued activity of local plexuses or the intrinsic activity of visceral muscle. The severance of preganglionic efferent fibres may result in the hypersensitivity of postganglionic neurons. Denervation does sometimes result in cessation of activity, e.g. in sweat glands, pilomotor muscle, orbital non-striated muscle and the suprarenal medulla (Pick 1970).

PERIPHERAL APPARATUS OF THE SPECIAL SENSES

In this chapter and the three following the detailed anatomy of the taste buds and the olfactory epithelium are considered together, as the sensory organs detecting changes in the chemical environment. Their anatomical positions are, of course, quite separate, but they play complementary roles in many respects.

GUSTATORY APPARATUS

The sense of taste is subserved by peripheral gustatory organs consisting of scattered groups of sensory cells contained in taste buds, situated in the oral cavity and pharynx. The perception of taste is difficult to separate from smell, however, because of the continuity between the oral and nasal cavities, and much of what is usually regarded as taste is in reality the result of airborne odorants from the oral cavity passing through the nasopharynx to the olfactory area above it. If this passage is blocked, it can be demonstrated that taste buds are able to detect only a rather restricted range of chemical substances in aqueous solution. However, such stimulation may have a profound effect on the feeding process, as it is related both to the selection of food and fluids with the tongue, or as monitors of and their suitability as nutrients once they have been taken into the oral cavity, and there are close neurological links to reflexes associated with alimentation.

Taste buds are sensory cells derived from the neighbouring epithelium, each linked by synapses at its base to one of the three cranial nerves: facial, glossopharyngeal and vagal. Whilst they can be regarded as essentially epithelial cells, they also have some physiological features found in neurons, for example synaptic transmission and action potential generation; they are therefore often referred to as *paraneurons*. In lower vertebrates taste buds are not confined to the anterior parts of the alimentary tract but are often widely distributed over the surface of the body including, in some fish, long sensory barbels which are used for hunting prey by external contact. In terrestrial vertebrates this ability is lost, although the tongue may be used to explore the chemical nature of the environment, as seen in its constant use in snakes (although this may also have olfactory connotations: see p. 1321). In mammals, taste buds are limited to the tongue, soft palate, palatoglossal arches, posterior surface of the epiglottis and the posterior wall of the oropharynx. It is also possible that scattered individual cells of the same type may be present throughout the lining of the alimentary tract, synaptically linked to the terminals of visceral afferents; if so, taste buds may be viewed as specialized concentrations of cells also widespread in the alimentary system.

In humans it has been estimated that lingual taste buds can total about 5000, although there is considerable individual variation, ranging from 500–20 000 (for reviews, see Finger & Silver 1987;

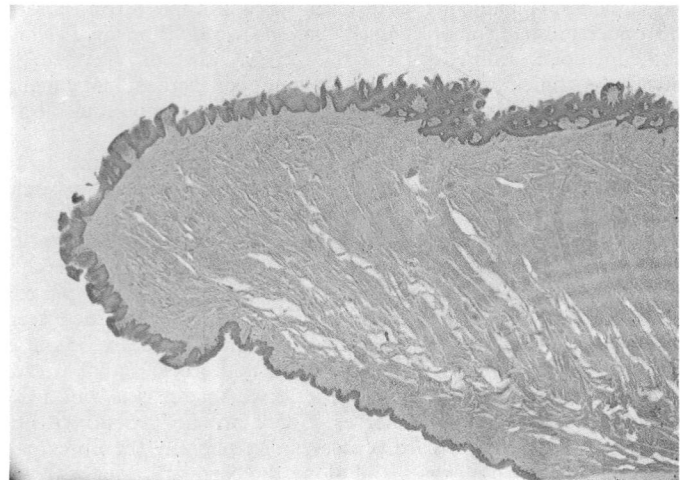

8.404 A low-power light micrograph of a sagittal section through the tip and anterior part of a human tongue, showing: muscle fibres orientated in three different directions; a delicate non-keratinized stratified squamous epithelium on the ventral surface; and a partly keratinized stratified epithelium on the dorsum. The latter is convoluted to produce filiform and fungiform papillae. Dermal papillae project into the deep surface of the epidermal irregularities, Haematoxylin and eosin. Magnification × 10.

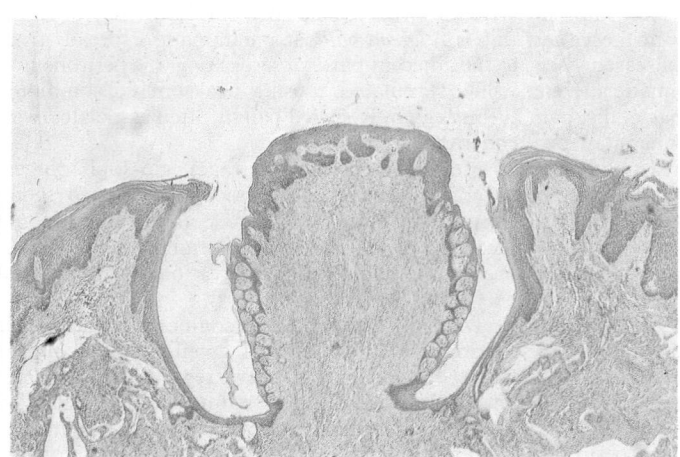

8.405 A light micrograph of a human vallate lingual papilla showing the numerous taste buds clustered along its lateral surfaces. A connective tissue papilla forms the core of the whole structure and serous glands, situated between the muscle blocks deep to the corium, open into the lateral recesses of the papilla. Haematoxylin and eosin. Magnification × 150.

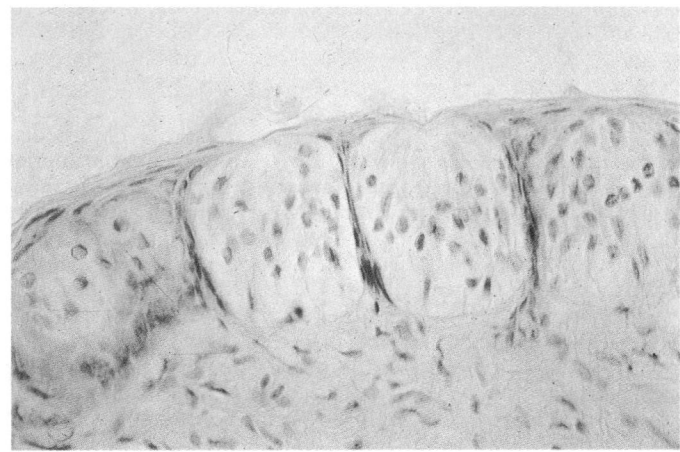

8.406   A light micrograph of a group of taste buds in a vallate lingual papilla, showing the apical cavity and various fusiform cells within the epithelial capsule. Haematoxylin and eosin. Magnification × 400.

Linden 1993). They are most frequent around the margins of the tongue, but virtually absent from the central part of its dorsum. Taste buds are concentrated on three type of lingual papillae, fungiform, vallate and foliate; they are absent from filiform papillae. Taste buds are most common on the posterior parts of the tongue, especially around the walls of the vallate papillae and their surrounding sulci (**8**.404, 405, 406), although fewer in the more peripheral wall than in that of the papilla itself; there are from 8–12 of these papillae, with an average of about 250 taste buds for each, although taste buds are also present in the epithelium between vallate papillae. Taste buds are abundant at the sides of the tongue over the more posterior folds of the two foliate papillae where they may total nearly 1200. On fungiform papillae they are sparsely and variably scattered, and sometimes absent, averaging 3 per papilla when they do occur, mainly on the anterior 2 cm of the tongue; these papillae number up to 250, providing a total of nearly 200 taste buds on these structures (Cheng & Robinson 1991). On the soft palate they have been reported clustered in islands of keratinized epithelium concentrated on its central part near the junction with the hard palate, each group up to 0.6 mm across and containing a maximum of 7 taste buds (Imfield & Schroeder 1992). Their distribution on the epiglottis and soft palate are not well documented but they are most numerous in fetal life and most of them disappear during postnatal development.

MICROSCOPIC STRUCTURE OF TASTE BUDS

Each taste bud (**8**.406, 407; caliculus or gemma gustatorius) is a barrel-shaped cluster of 50–150 fusiform cells lying within an oval cavity in the epithelium, converging apically on a small space opening by a *gustatory pore*, about 2 μm wide on to the mucosal surface. The whole structure is about 70 μm tall by 40 μm across. The group is separated by a basal lamina from the subjacent lamina propria and from this direction is penetrated by a small fasciculus of afferent nerve fibres which ramify and spiral around the contained sensory cells. A dense extracellular glycoprotein-rich material fills the apical space.

Reconstructions of taste buds from serial electron micrographs (Murray & Murray 1970) have shown at least five distinct types of epithelial cell to be present (designated in that paper Types I–V). Type I, which forms more than half of the total, is a densely staining cell, whereas Types II and III stain lightly; other light staining cells have also been reported (see Kinnamon et al 1985). Type IV is a rounded basal cell (**8**.407) and Type V cells form the boundary with the surrounding epithelium. However, the precise identities of the first three of these cell types is not certain, and it is possible that these categories reflect maturational processes accompanying the constant turnover of the taste bud cell population as well as functional classes. The dense Type I cells contain many dense vacuoles

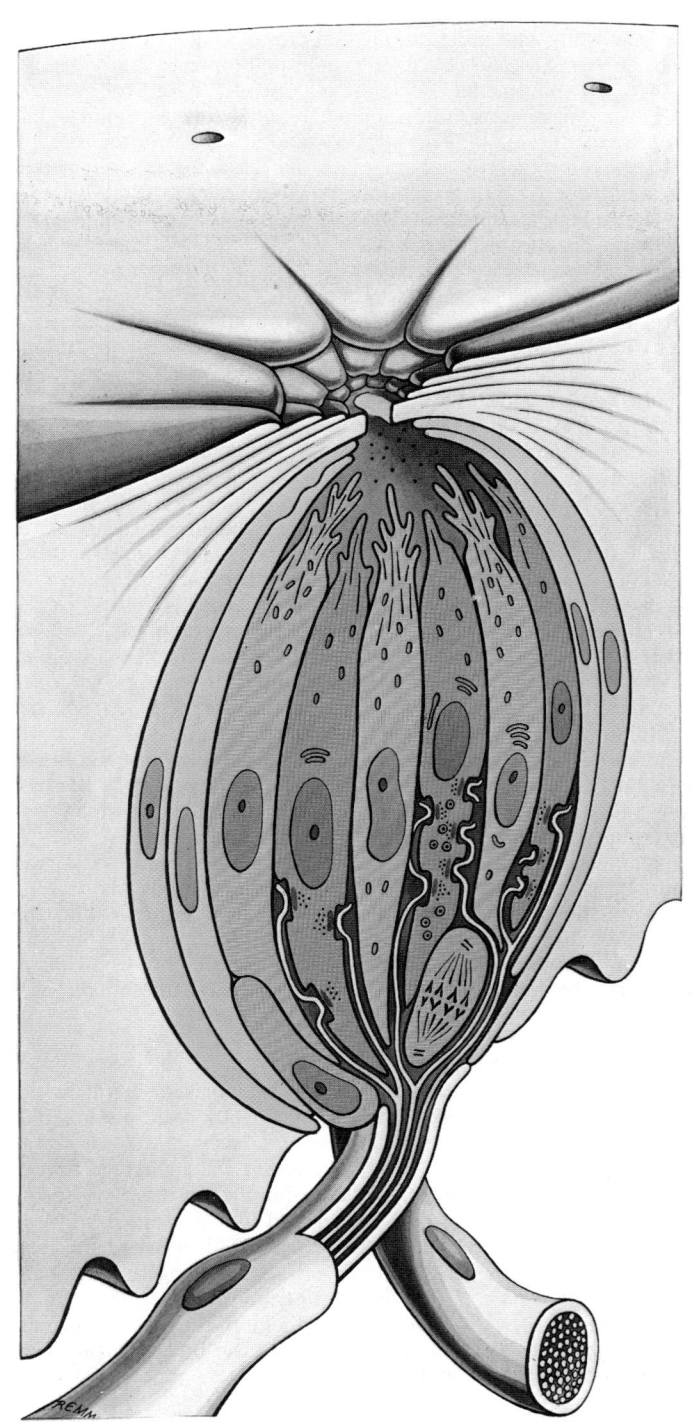

8.407   A schematic reconstruction of the structure of a taste bud, cut away to expose the various cell types. Presumed sensory cells of two types (one with dense-cored vesicles, the other without) are indicated in purple and their innervation in yellow. The supporting cells are indicated in magenta and basal cells in brick red. A dense mucosubstance is present in the apical cavity beneath the apical aperture.

in their apical regions which project into the apical space and bear short microvilli (Miller & Chaudry 1976); at least some of these cells ensheath Types II and III cells, and nerve fibres entering the base of the taste bud, and are therefore likely to be supporting cells. However, there is also evidence that cells of this description may be early stages in the turnover of receptor cells, and at least some of them have synaptic contacts with afferent fibres at their bases. The paler Types II and III or intermediate cells are also fusiform, the apices of Type III cells projecting further than those of Type II; both of them have synaptic contacts with nerve fibre terminals at their bases

1313

and sides, and are therefore considered to be receptor cells. However, it is interesting that recent studies of the neuron-specific adhesion molecule N-CAM shows this molecule to be present only around the Type III (intermediate) cell (see e.g. Nelson & Finger 1993).

The synaptic regions show a characteristic asymmetrical thickening and presynaptic small (50 nm), clear synaptic vesicles in the receptor cell, although these are less abundant than in many other synapses. Those of Type III cells contain dense-cored vesicles about 70 nm in diameter, identified in other sites as catecholamine vesicles. Type V cells form an encapsulating sheath for the bud, and may also be phagocytic. Type IV cells are located basally; these are rounded mitotically active stem cells which are the source of new cells for the taste bud, as demonstrated by appropriate labelling methods. Occluding junctions between the apices of various cells in the bud prevent the access of chemical stimuli to non-apical regions of the receptors (Akisada & Oda 1978).

Innervation. Each taste bud receives two distinct classes of fibres, one branching in the periphery of the bud to form a *perigemmal plexus*, the other within the bud itself (*intragemmal plexus*) which innervates the bases of the receptor cells. The perigemmal fibres contain various neuropeptides including calcitonin gene-related peptide (CGRP) and substance P, and appear to represent free sensory endings. Intragemmal fibres branch within the taste bud, and each forms a series of synapses with either a Type I or Types II and III cells. The analysis of this pattern is complicated by the turnover of receptor cells within taste buds, which must involve a progressive sequence beginning with the innervation of new receptor cells, maturation and degeneration, and has not yet been worked out fully.

Individual nerve fibres branch to give a complex distribution of taste bud innervation over the tongue's surface, as deduced by recordings from the proximal fasciculi of the chorda tympani and glossopharyngeal nerve. Each fibre may have many terminals, spreading to innervate widely separated taste buds and more than one sensory cell in each bud. Conversely, individual buds may receive the terminals of several different nerve fibres. Functionally, this cross-innervation may be of considerable importance (see below). No firm evidence has emerged concerning efferent terminals or inhibitory phenomena in the taste buds, although these have been claimed.

Replacement of cells in taste buds

The cells of taste buds resemble those in the adjacent epithelium in undergoing continual renewal (Farbman 1980). Isotopic labelling shows that none of the cells of taste buds survive for more than about 10 days, except the basal cells which are stem cells for the whole population. Experiments indicate that the sensitivity of sensory cells to particular chemicals is determined by the trophic influence of the nerve fibres rather than the reverse. If denervated the taste buds rapidly dedifferentiate and may disappear altogether, showing their dependence on a trophic influence from the nerve fibres. If the nerve terminals grow back into the epithelium, they can induce the formation of new, functionally competent taste buds. For a review of these topics, see Oakley (1991).

Taste discrimination

Gustatory receptors detect four main categories of tastants, customarily classified as salty, sweet, sour and bitter; other taste qualities have been suggested, including metallic, and *umami* (Japanese: 'delicious taste' typical of monosodium glutamate). Although it is commonly stated in textbooks that particular areas of the tongue are specialized to detect these different tastes, the electrophysiological evidence and indeed closer subjective examination indicates that all areas of the tongue are responsive to all tastants. Single unit recording from afferent nerves shows that each fibre is connected to widely separated taste buds and may respond to several different chemical stimuli. Some respond to all four classic categories, others to fewer or only one. Within a particular class of tastes, receptors are also differentially sensitive to a wide range of similar chemicals. It therefore seems that perceived sensations of taste are the results of analysis (presumably central) of a complex pattern of responses from particular areas of the tongue, so that even if there are only a few specific types of taste receptor, much more information about the chemical nature and intensity of a taste may be gained than if the innervation were simpler (Beidler & Smallman 1965; Beidler 1970; Pfaffman 1970).

GUSTATORY NERVES

Gustatory nerve fibres are the peripheral processes of unipolar neurons in the genicular ganglion of the facial nerve and the inferior ganglia of the glossopharyngeal and vagal nerves. Their central axons form the tractus solitarius (p. 1018), their terminals synapsing with neurons in the rostral third of the nucleus of that tract. Secondary gustatory axons cross the midline, many to ascend the brainstem in the dorsomedial part of the medial lemniscus to synapse with the most medial neurons of the thalamic nucleus ventralis posterior medialis (in a region sometimes termed the accessory arcuate nucleus). From the ventralis posterior medialis axons radiate through the internal capsule to the antero-inferior area of the sensorimotor cortex and the limen insulae. Electrophysiological recording from the ventralis posterior medialis and cortex largely confirms these anatomical pathways; some units react to one type of stimulus, others to several different stimuli. Other ascending paths have been described, ending in a number of the hypothalamic nuclei by which gustatory information may reach the limbic system (p. 1098) and allowing appropriate autonomic reactions to be made (p. 1295) (see Stewart & Shepherd 1985).

The gustatory nerve for the anterior part of the tongue, excluding the vallate papillae, is the chorda tympani (via the lingual nerve); in most individuals these fibres traverse the chorda tympani to the facial ganglion but in a few they diverge through connecting branches to the otic ganglion, proceeding thence in the greater petrosal nerve to the facial ganglion (Schwartz & Weddell 1938). Taste buds in the soft palate's inferior surface are also supplied mainly by the facial fibres, through the greater petrosal nerve distributing via the nerve of the pterygoid canal and middle and posterior palatine nerves; the glossopharyngeal also contributes to this region. Taste buds in the vallate papillae and the pharyngeal (postsulcal) part of the tongue and in the palatoglossal arches and the oropharynx are innervated by glossopharyngeal fibres, while those in the extreme pharyngeal part of the tongue and epiglottis receive fibres from the internal laryngeal branch of the vagus. (For older literature concerning gustatory paths consult Rollin 1979.) These supplies accord with the embryological development of the tongue (p. 280; see also p. 202).

GUSTATORY TRANSDUCTION AND NEUROTRANSMISSION

It has recently become possible to examine the responses of individual receptor cells by the patch clamp technique, and a clearer picture of their transduction mechanisms and electrical responses is emerging (see e.g. the reviews by Akabas 1990; Kinnamon & Cummings 1992). In general, chemical substances dissolving in the oral mucus diffuse through the taste pores of the buds and through the dense extracellular material within their apices to reach the taste receptor cell membranes. Here they cause membrane depolarization by a variety of mechanisms (see below) depending on the type of receptor, and this initiates an action potential within the receptor cell. In turn, the synapses at their bases are activated to initiate action potentials in the afferent terminals.

The different taste qualities are mediated by different transduction methods; salty tastes depend on the presence of monovalent cations, sour tastes (typifying acidic substances) on protons (H^+), sweet tastes by a number of different classes of compounds, including some carbohydrates and amino acids; bitter tastes are elicited by divalent cations, alkaloids, some amino acids and some other organic molecules. These initiate different responses in the sensory receptors specialized for their reception, involving either direct passage of ions through membranes or the reception by specific proteins followed by G-protein activation and second messenger-mediated ion gating (as in the olfactory receptors, see p. 1317). It is not certain whether individual cells have a mixture of these mechanisms, or if they are dedicated to a particular transduction method. Interactions between tastes certainly occur; for example, monovalent cation-mediated salty tastes are inhibited by large anions. Other types of interaction can also occur, for example between sweet and bitter substances, although central mechanisms are probably responsible for many of these.

The intensity of a taste is partly dependent on its solubility in saliva, and most tastants are readily soluble in water. Some classes, however, are more lipophilic; their solubility and carriage to the receptor may be enhanced by special carrier molecules such as the protein recently isolated from the specialized glands associated with vallate papillae (von Ebner gland protein; VEG: see the review by Spielman 1990).

OLFACTORY APPARATUS

The peripheral olfactory organs consist of bilateral areas of sensory epithelium lining the area olfactoria of the posterodorsal parts of the nasal cavities. The epithelium contains chemosensory receptor cells which can detect and discriminate between different airborne odorants; electrical signals encoding this information are sent back to the brain along their axons which together form the olfactory nerves (8.343). The olfactory epithelium is housed within the complex structure of the nose which determines the physiological environment controlling many of the activities of the sensory apparatus. The

detailed anatomy of the nasal structures is described with the respiratory system on pages 1627–1682.

MICROSTRUCTURE OF THE OLFACTORY MUCOSA

The olfactory mucosa occupies an area of about $10\,cm^2$ covering the posterior upper parts of the lateral nasal wall, including the back of the superior concha, the spheno-ethmoidal recess, the upper part of the perpendicular plate of the ethmoid and the roof of the nose arching between the septum and lateral wall, including the underside of the cribriform plate. This area has a yellowish brown colour due to the presence of pigment within the epithelium (see p. 1318). The mucosa consists of a pseudostratified *olfactory epithelium* in which the sensory receptors are situated, and an underlying *lamina propria* containing numerous olfactory nerve fascicles (fila olfactoria) and subepithelial olfactory glands (of Bowman) which secrete through ducts on to the epithelial surface. The mucus so secreted forms a thin layer in which are embedded the long trailing ends of sensory cilia and the interwoven microvilli of supporting cells (see below).

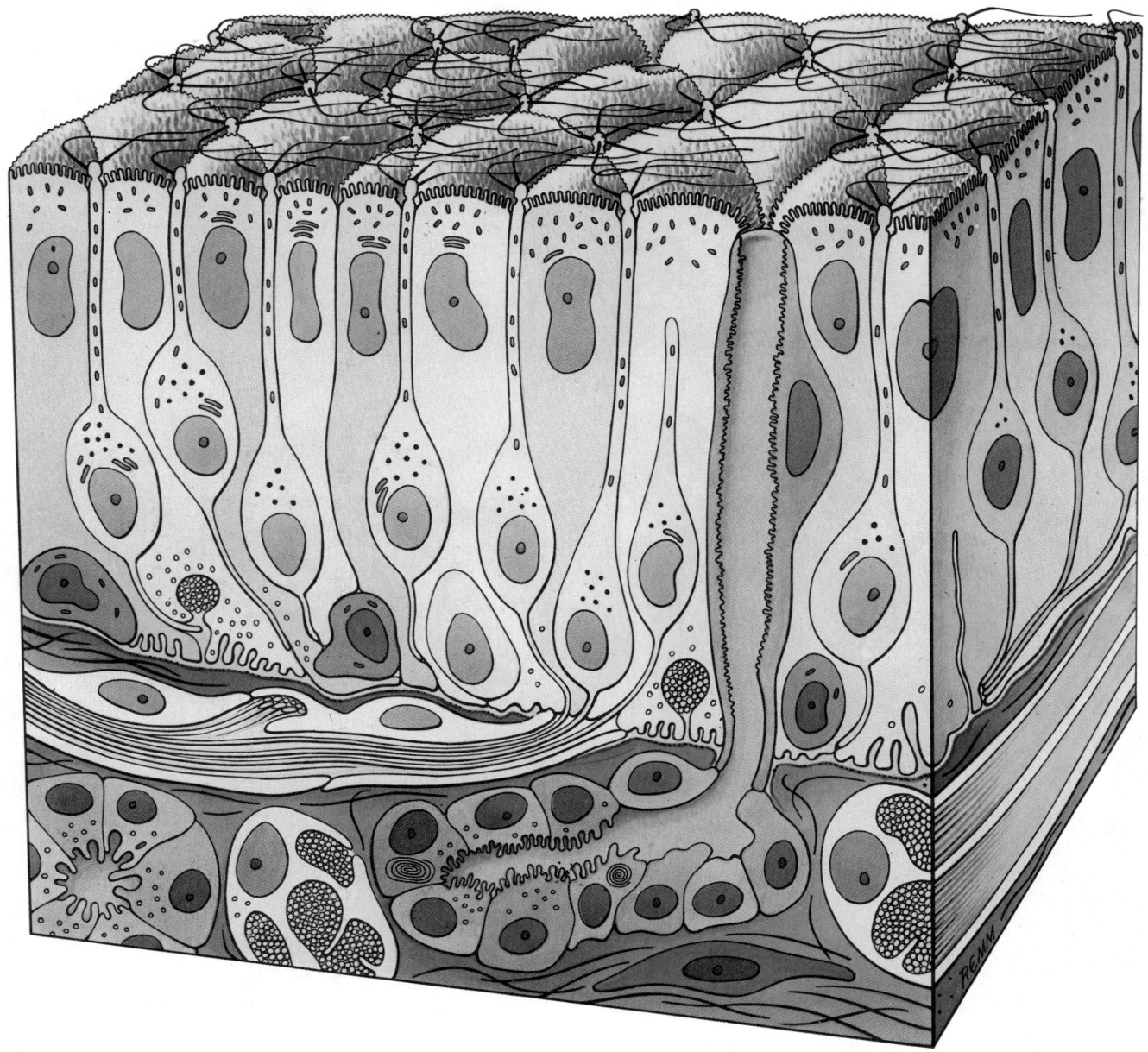

8.408 A schematic reconstruction showing the chief cytological features of the olfactory epithelium. Receptor cells (yellow) are situated among columnar supporting cells. The axons of the receptor cells emerge from the epithelium in groups ensheathed in Schwann cells. Observe the rounded basal epithelial cells and the subepithelial glands of Bowman with their intra-epithelial ducts. One of the basal cells is in process of differentiating into a receptor cell. At the surface are cilia of the receptor cells and microvilli of the supporting cells.

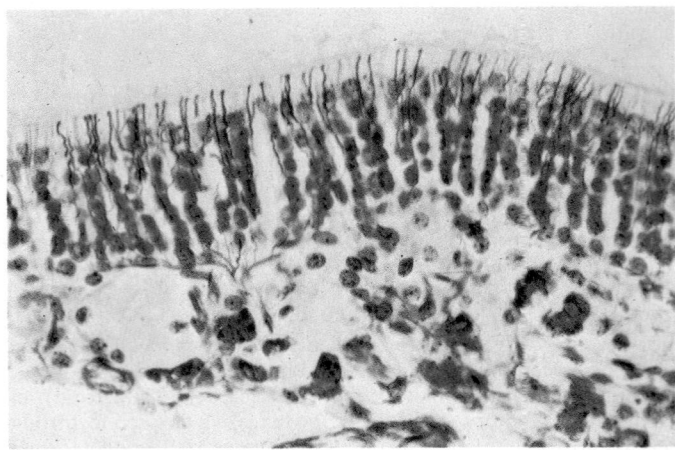

8.409 A vertical section through the olfactory epithelium of the mouse, stained with Holmes' silver method to show the olfactory dendrites and their terminal expansions (above). The nuclei of the receptor neurons are arranged in columns in this preparation; the fila olfactoria can also be seen emerging from the base of the epithelium (below). (Provided by A Cuschieri, University of Malta.)

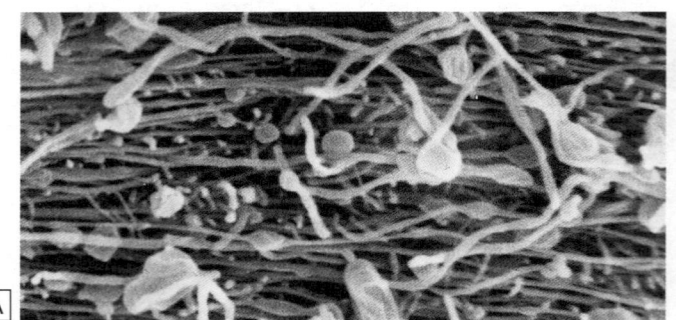

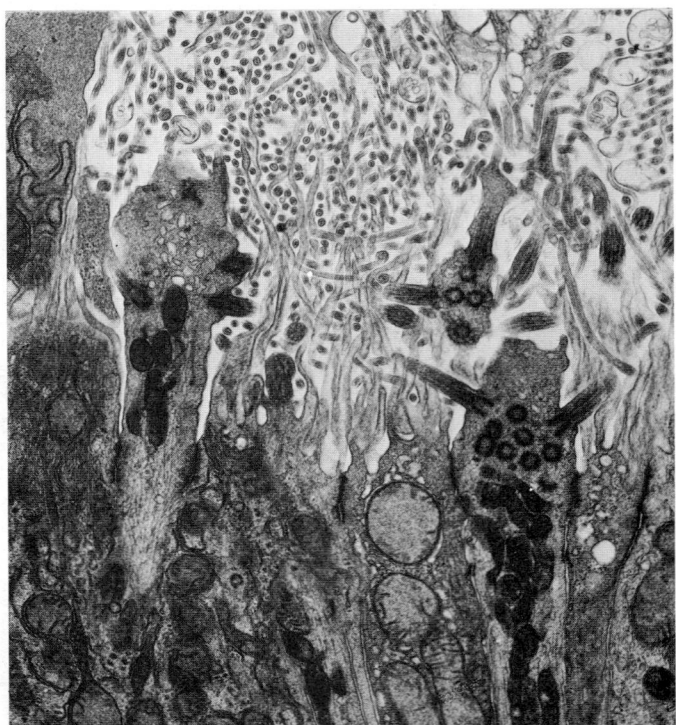

8.410 An electron micrograph showing receptor endings in the olfactory mucosa of a mouse. Note the presence of numerous cilia on the sensory terminals, interspersed by numerous microvilli on the surfaces of the supporting cells. Magnification × 10 000. (Provided by H C Dodson, Department of Anatomy, UMDS, Guy's Campus, London.)

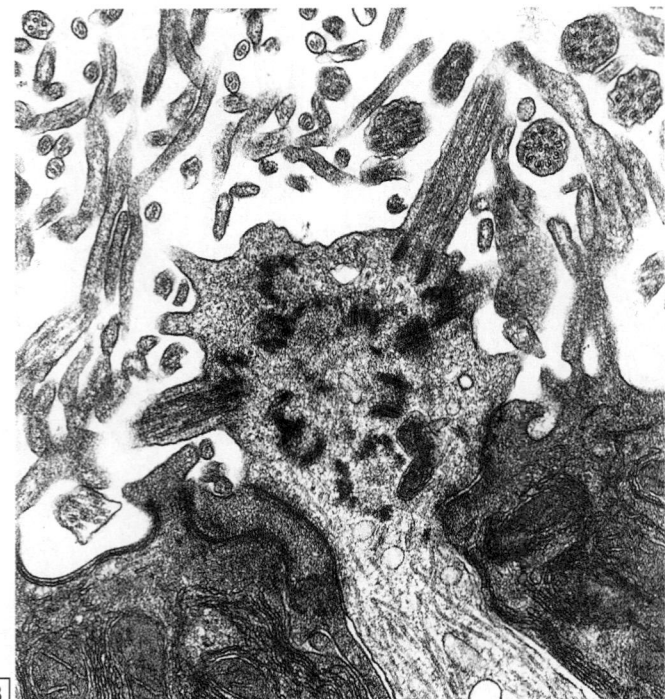

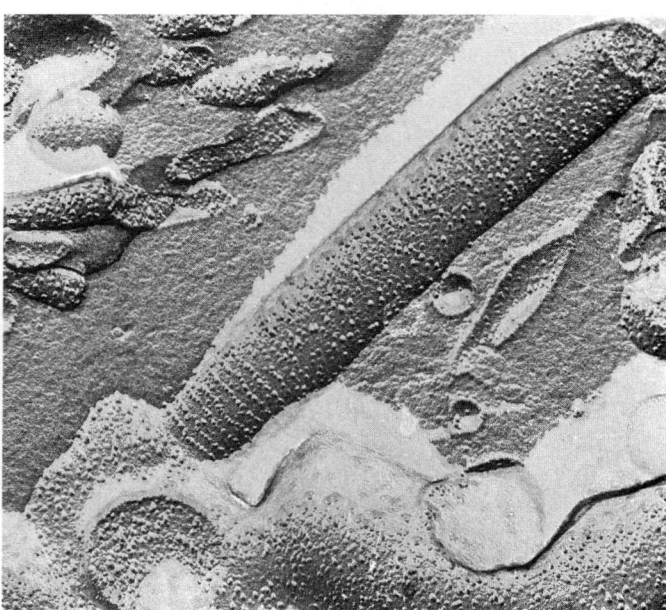

8.411 The surface of the olfactory epithelium (rat) showing the distribution of sensory and related structures.

A. Scanning electron micrograph of the olfactory surface (rat) showing the parallel trailing narrow segments of the olfactory cilia. Magnification × 25 000.
B. Transmission electron micrograph showing an olfactory ending, sensory and supporting cell microvilli in section. Magnification × 50 000.

8.412 An electron micrograph of an olfactory cilium (bovine) attached at its basal end to an olfactory dendrite terminal, freeze-fractured to expose the numerous intramembranous particles which are thought to be sites of odour reception. An extensive ciliary necklace is present at the base of the cilium and microvilli of a supporting cell are visible on the left. Magnification × 60 000. (Supplied by B Menco, University of Utrecht, Netherlands.)

OLFACTORY EPITHELIUM

The olfactory epithelium is considerably thicker (up to 100 μm) than the adjacent respiratory epithelium lining most of the nasal cavity. Within its thickness there are many layers of nuclei, although near the free surface there is a nucleus-free zone crossed by the apical processes of the receptors, supporting cells and ducts of the subepithelial glands. At the epithelial base is a narrow zone rich in a yellow-brown pigment similar to lipofuscin (see below). The epithelium is composed of four principal types of cell (**8**.408): *olfactory receptors*, *supporting cells* (sustentaculocytes) and two classes of basal cell—*basal cells proper* and *globose cells*. The nuclei of these various cells occupy specific zones within the epithelial thickness; there is a superficial stratum of supporting cell nuclei, then beneath this and occupying much of the epithelial thickness are several tiers of receptor cell bodies. The basal cells are situated between this middle zone and the basal lamina underlying the epithelium. Details of the cell types are as follows.

Olfactory receptor cells (8.409–414)

Olfactory receptor cells are bipolar cells, each with a cell body located in the midzone of the epithelium, an apical dendrite extending to the epithelial surface and a basally directed axon which passes out of the epithelium, into the olfactory nerve and eventually synapses with a second order neuron in the olfactory bulb. From this morphology it is clear that olfactory receptors are a specialized class of primary sensory neuron, a view supported by their physiology (see below). The location of the cell body very close to the sensory surface is unique among the neurons of vertebrates, although common in invertebrate phyla. Another unique feature is the continuous turnover in the olfactory cell population which occurs throughout life (see below).

The olfactory receptor cell has been extensively studied by electron microscopy in many species including humans (Morrison & Costanzo 1990); its main features are shown in **8**.408. From its ellipsoidal cell body a single unbranched apical dendrite about 2 μm across extends to the epithelial surface, projecting into the overlying mucus as an expanded cylindrical olfactory ending (rod, knob or vesicle, Reese 1965; Frisch 1967; Graziadei 1971, 1974; Menco 1983). From the circumference of each ending radiate many cilia (in humans from 10–23: Morrison & Costanzo 1990, 1992), extending for long distances parallel to the general epithelial surface. The cilia (pp. 1314–1316) have a short proximal segment 1–2 μm long and 0.25 μm in diameter which rapidly tapers to a much more extensive trailing portion about 0.1 μm across. Internally, the proximal part has the '9 plus 2' pattern of microtubules typical of motile cilia, whilst the distal trailing end contains only the central pair. The cilia lack dynein arms on the peripheral microtubule doublets (Lidow & Menco 1984) and in mammals are thought to be non-motile. The microtubular apparatus appears to be primarily an efficient way of maintaining a large area of sensory surface projecting from the surface and therefore more efficiently exposed to odorants.

The dendrite contains numerous mitochondria and other organelles typical of dendrites: microtubules, smooth and coated vesicles, agranular endoplasmic reticulum and some ribosomes; centrioles also often occur in or near the olfactory knob, especially in young animals. The cell body contains abundant granular and agranular endoplasmic reticulum, Golgi complexes and lysosomes, all indicating a high rate of organellar turnover. The nucleus is elliptical and heterochromatic. The exposed regions of olfactory dendrites and cilia are covered by plasma membrane containing high concentrations of intramembranous particles (**8**.412A,B) demonstrable by freeze-fracturing (Menco et al 1975; Kerjaschki & Horandner 1976; Menco 1984). These particles are thought to be the sites of olfactory reception and or ion channels related to sensory transduction; their large numbers accord with their ability to detect extremely low

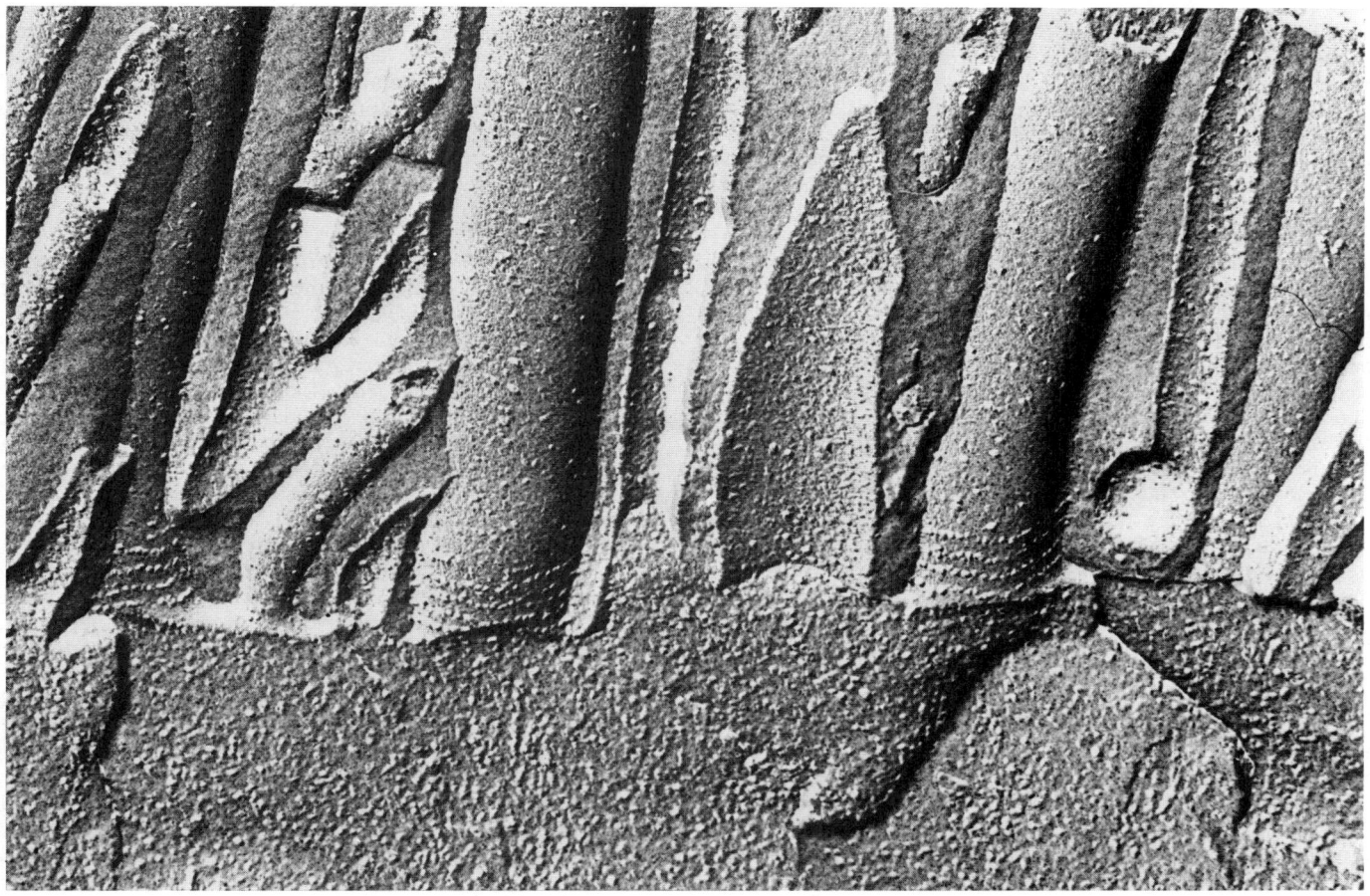

8.413 An electron micrograph of a group of non-sensory cilia from the respiratory epithelium of the nasal cavity (bovine), freeze-fractured to show the distribution of intramembranous particles. Note the presence of ciliary necklaces at the bases of cilia and the relative paucity of particles elsewhere on the cilia (compare with **8**.412). Magnification × 80 000. (Supplied by B Menco, University of Utrecht, Netherlands.)

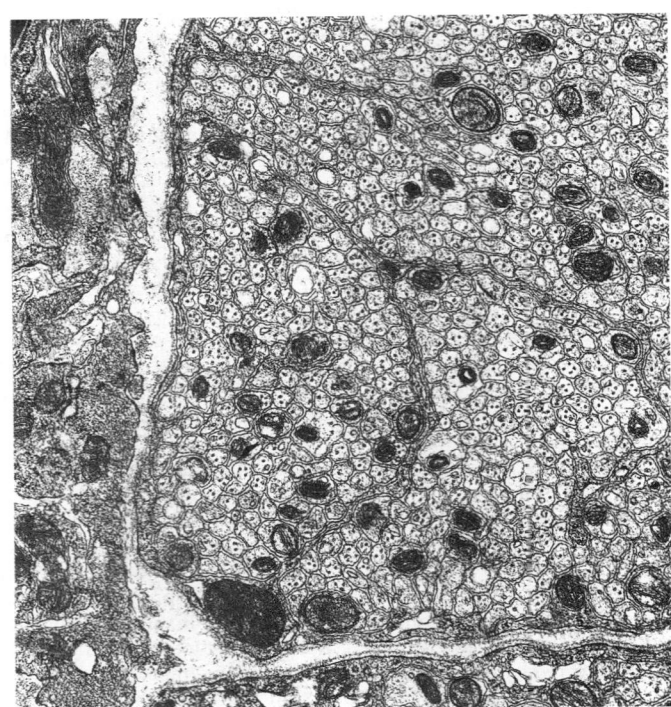

8.414A Electron micrograph of a section through olfactory axons in a fasciculus. Note the bundles of axons are ensheathed in thin processes of an olfactory glial cell. Rat.

8.414B Olfactory glial cell in tissue culture, immunostained to show glial fibrillar acidic protein. Magnification × 450. (Provided by Caroline Wigley, Department of Anatomy and Cell Biology, UMDS, Guy's Campus.)

concentrations of odorants (Menco 1976). In comparison non-olfactory cilia (8.413) have few particles in their investing membranes.

From the other pole of the cell a narrow non-myelinated axon passes towards the base of the epithelium, running close to others to form small intra-epithelial fascicles among the processes of supporting and basal cells, eventually penetrating the base of the epithelium, where each fascicle is immediately ensheathed by an olfactory glial cell (p. 1319). Many such fascicles or *fila olfactoria* join to form larger olfactory fasciculi which pass through the cribriform plate to enter the olfactory bulb, there synapsing in glomeruli with secondary sensory neurons (mitral cells, basket cells, periglomerular cells). Olfactory axons are amongst the most slender of nerve fibres, about 0.2 μm in diameter. Within the olfactory fila the axons are grouped in bundles of up to 50 or more with no intervening insulation (8.414A), each bundle virtually enclosed in a deep groove within a series of olfactory glial cells (Gasser 1956); the significance of this arrangement is not clear, but it may ensure that newly growing axons are entrained to the correct part of the olfactory bulb.

The receptor cells and their axons contain a number of characteristic proteins, among them a 19 kDa *olfactory marker protein* (Margolis 1982, 1988) and carnosine (Margolis et al 1985) which can be readily demonstrated immunohistochemically. They also express surface molecules which cross-react with the ABO blood group antigens, and carbohydrates which bind several lectins (Menco 1992), indicating specialized surface properties of use for experimental detection in studies of these cells.

Functional categories of receptor cells

Electrophysiology has shown that individual receptor cells are each tuned to a narrow range of odorants with particular chemical features in common (see below). The numbers of such odorant classes and corresponding receptor cell types have long been a matter of debate, and it has generally been considered that they are relatively few, since the subjective 'classes' of odorants with similar features (judged by the human nose) appear to be very limited, and therefore, can be classified according to these. Recently, a family of some hundreds of related genes has been isolated from olfactory receptor cells, coding for a set of proteins similar to the retinal-binding proteins of

photoreceptors (Buck & Axel 1991; Reed 1992). It has been possible to detect the sites of expression of some of these genes by means of in situ hybridization methods, and it appears that they are grouped in longitudinal zones stretching the whole length of the olfactory area (see e.g. Vassar et al 1993). Moreover, there is a tight demarcation of dorsally or ventrally expressing gene subfamilies. Some of these genes have now been transfected into non-neural cells in tissue culture, which are then able to respond to odorants, indicating that this gene family does indeed code for olfactory receptor protein molecules. The presence of such a large number of putative receptor genes is an unexpected development, and indicates that the olfactory system may be far more complex than, for example, the retina, which has just four primary receptor types, or the cutaneous somatosensory system with perhaps about 10. How the almost astronomical amounts of odorant information might be sorted and analysed centrally is hard to imagine, if this is indeed the case.

Supporting cells

Supporting cells (8.408, 410) are irregular columnar elements separating and partially ensheathing the receptors. Their large, vertically elongate, euchromatic nuclei form a layer superficial to the receptor perikarya. At the exposed surface of the epithelium, they send numerous long, somewhat irregular microvilli into the mucus layer, among the long trailing ends of olfactory cilia. Their cytoplasm contains many mitochondria, granular and, especially, much agranular endoplasmic reticulum. At their bases, abutting on to the basal lamina, they have expanded end-feet containing numerous lamellated dense bodies resembling the lipofuscin granules of neurons. These are remains of secondary lysosomes (residual bodies) formed as a result of their phagocytic activities, and are largely responsible for the pigmentation of the olfactory area; their numbers gradually accumulate with age, so that the pigmentation also increases in intensity, the cells being long-lived. A prominent Golgi apparatus and electron-lucent lysosomal structures including multivesicular bodies also exist in their apical parts. Near the epithelial surface fine microfilaments attached to desmosomes give mechanical coherence to the epithelium. Tight junctions also occur between the supporting cells and olfactory receptors at the level of the epithelial surface (Reese & Brightman 1970).

Numerous endocytic vesicles occur between the microvilli, and are responsible for the uptake of mucus and particulates from the surface (Bannister & Dodson 1992); the occurrence of high levels of cytochrome-P450 and other detoxifying enzymes demonstrated in these cells (Getchell et al 1993) suggests that the supporting cells play a part in ridding the epithelium of unwanted odorants which might otherwise swamp the olfactory sense. There is also structural and immunohistochemical evidence that more than one type of supporting cell may exist, although the significance of variations in form and antigenicity has yet to be determined.

Isotopic labelling experiments show that supporting cells are long-lived, and therefore constitute a stable population, contrasting with the rapid turnover of the receptor cells (see below). There is much evidence that the supporting cells have many important roles in the biology of olfaction; they insulate receptors from each other electrically, regulate the ionic environment of the receptors and their endings, remove debris, toxic substances and 'used' odorants from the epithelium and its surface, provide structural stability to the epithelium and anchorage for the receptors; moreover it is likely that they help to regulate receptor cell maturation and turnover, while the supporting cells themselves have only an exceedingly slow rate of replacement. It is interesting that their relation to the receptors resembles that of the radial glial cells of the embryonic neural tube, suggesting that like them, the supporting cells play an important role in assisting neurite migration and growth.

Basal cells

There are two types of basal cells, basal cells proper and globose basal cells (Graziadei & Monti Graziadei 1979; Yamagishi et al 1989; Suzuki & Takeda 1993). *Basal cells proper* are somewhat flat or angular, with condensed nuclei and darkly staining cytoplasm containing numerous intermediate filaments inserted into desmosomes contacting surrounding supporting cells; they lie in contact with the basal lamina. *Globose cells* (or blastema cells) have a quite different appearance, being rounded or elliptical in shape, with a pale staining, open face nucleus, and a pale cytoplasm rich in free ribosomes and clusters of centrioles; they form a distinct basal zone spaced slightly from the basal surface of the epithelium. Mitoses are found within this zone (Andres 1966), which is especially wide in young animals in which receptor formation is most active. Structurally the globose cells have many features similar to those of embryonic neuroblasts, and indeed it is clear that they are the immediate source of new olfactory receptor cells (see below).

Other cell types

Other cell types are much less frequent; microvillous cells are columnar and bear an apical array of long erect microvilli (Moran et al 1982a); whether these are receptor cells or a type of supporting cell has yet to be settled conclusively, although they do not contain olfactory marker protein, and, unlike the established olfactory receptors, do not degenerate when the olfactory nerve is transected. In addition to these cells there are the terminals of trigeminal nerve origin which penetrate the epithelium as free endings. At least some of them contain neuropeptides including SP and CGRP (p. 937) and are likely to be polymodal nociceptors stimulated when noxious chemicals are inhaled (see e.g. Silver et al 1991).

OLFACTORY NERVES

The anatomy of olfactory nerves is described elsewhere (p. 960); briefly, once the narrow (0.2 μm or less) olfactory axons have left the epithelium, they are enclosed in unmyelinated fibres in several bundles of 50 or more within individual large olfactory glial cells to form large but unmyelinated fibres. These are progressively grouped with similar fibres to form larger fasciculi (**8.414A**), passing back through the cribriform plate into the olfactory bulb.

Olfactory axons are among the smallest in the body, with very low conduction velocities (4 msec^{-1}); internally they contain a few microtubules with occasional neurofilaments and have intermittent swellings where mitochondria are housed. They terminate in the olfactory bulb in glomerular synapses with second order sensory neurons—mitral periglomerular and tufted cells (see p. 1118).

Olfactory glia. These resemble Schwann cells in their relations with the axons, but they possess distinctive features which show them to be a separate class of glia; they have a very distinctive morphology, bundling the olfactory axons in a quite unique manner, they are rich in glial fibrillary acidic protein (GFAP) intermediate filaments, have several different surface markers (Doucette 1990), and arise during early development from the olfactory placode rather than neural crest (Chuah & Au 1991). Olfactory glial cells ensheath the olfactory axons throughout their course to and even within the olfactory bulb, finally giving way to central glia just before they

make synaptic contact in the olfactory glomeruli. An olfactory glial cell in culture is shown in **8.414B**.

OLFACTORY GLANDS (OF BOWMAN)

The olfactory glands (**8.408**) are branched tubular structures lying beneath the olfactory epithelium, on to whose surface they secrete through narrow, vertical ducts. Their secretory cells are of two types, both containing dense secretory vesicles but one with denser cytoplasm. Their secretions include defensive substances: lysozyme, lactoferrin, IgA, as well as sulphated proteoglycans (Mellert et al 1992). Besides the inhibitory action on microbial flora and fauna, this fluid forms the environment of the receptor endings and their cilia. It must therefore regulate the presence and movements of ions for sensory transduction, and also form the environment for dissolving odorants and allowing their diffusion to the sensory receptor sites. In this respect, a set of odorant-binding proteins (OBPs) have been found in the olfactory and respiratory mucosal surface in many mammals; this is able to bind odorants quite strongly, and in some cases, with some specificity. OBPs are derived, at least in non-primate mammals, from glands in the walls of the anterior nasal chamber, and are carried to the olfactory area by the cilia of the respiratory epithelium. Their role in olfaction is uncertain: they may either help to present odorants to the receptors in enhanced concentrations, or may assist in the removal of odorants after they have been sensed. For further reading see Pelosi et al (1982), Pevsher et al (1990).

TURNOVER AND REGENERATION OF OLFACTORY RECEPTOR CELLS

Studies with nuclear labelling methods in different species of mammals show that there is a steady loss and replacement of receptor cells throughout life; stem cells situated near the base of the epithelium undergo periodic mitotic division throughout life, giving rise to new olfactory receptors which then grow a dendrite to the olfactory surface and an axon to the olfactory bulb. The cell bodies of these new receptors gradually move apically until they reach the region just below the supporting cell nuclei, after which they degenerate and are either shed from the epithelium or phagocytosed by supporting cells. During early life this recruitment is also needed for the epithelium to expand in area as the nasal cavity grows in size, but a slower, continuous addition of receptor cells occurs throughout life, balanced by the degeneration of existing cells, which (in rodents) may only last for 2 to 3 weeks (Moulton et al 1970; Graziadei 1973; Graziadei & Monti Graziadei 1979). A continuous turnover of olfactory receptors is an obvious advantage in such an exposed position, although studies with (^{3}[H] thymidine and bromodeoxyuridine (BDU) have shown that the kinetics are rather erratic and strongly subject to environmental influences. Individual receptor cells can occasionally stay alive for long periods, for example up to a year when an animal breathes filtered air to reduce the wear and tear at the olfactory surface. Section of the olfactory nerve leads to the death of all axotomized receptor cells, followed by a surge in mitosis in the basal globose cells which reconstitutes the receptor cell population (Carr & Farbman 1992). These and other relevant findings suggest that there is a cycle of replacement entailing a limited receptor cell life span, presumably limited by a timed or position-dependent receptor cell apoptosis, balanced by basal mitosis and differentiation, but that this can be considerably accelerated either by increasing local stresses, or by severing the axonal connection from sources of growth factors in the olfactory bulb (see Farbman 1992 for a review of this topic).

Regeneration of the epithelium can occur when it is damaged, for example experimentally with a zinc sulphate solution (Matulionis 1975), or as already noted, when the olfactory nerves are sectioned. In these cases the receptor cells rapidly die, and are in due course replaced by division of basally situated cells. Likewise, olfactory sensation lost after, for example influenza, may take months or even longer to return, although regrowth of axons may be prevented in some cases by the formation of scar tissue (see e.g. Douek et al 1975; Moran et al 1992). This ability to regenerate primary sensory neurons is unique in mammalian nervous systems, a phenomenon of much neurobiological interest. It is especially remarkable in that throughout life, newly formed axons are continually growing back to the olfactory bulb and making functionally correct connections, a process elsewhere found only in fetal development. This resemblance is also seen in many other fetal-like features of the adult olfactory organ, for example the occurrence of fetal tubulin, neural-cell adhesion molecules (N-CAMs) and intermediate filaments in olfactory receptors (for review see Miragall & Dermietzel 1992). It is also remarkable that after nerve section, new olfactory axons can innervate unusual targets if these are suitably presented, for example the frontal lobes of the brain (Graziadei et al 1978), although fully functional synapses do not appear to be formed in such cases.

DEVELOPMENT OF THE OLFACTORY EPITHELIUM

The cells of the olfactory epithelium develop from the embryonic olfactory placode, resembling the early ontogeny of the neural tube (p. 217). Although the cuboidal ectodermal cells of the placode gradually become taller they remain as a single layer throughout development. Mitosis occurs at first only near the placodal surface, the dividing cells rounding up and then re-extending to the epithelial base; but later mitoses appear deeper in the epithelium and are finally confined to the basal layers, where division persists throughout life (Smart 1971; Cuschieri & Bannister 1975a,b), many of the dividing cells being globose basal cells responsible for continued neurogenesis. Electron microscopy shows that receptor cells differentiate early, sprouting apical dendrites and basal axons with large growth cones which pierce the basal lamina and grow back to the olfactory bulb to synapse with the secondary neurons (see e.g. Hinds & Hinds 1972; Cuschieri & Bannister 1975b; Farbman & Gesteland 1975; Constanzo & Graziadei 1986; Farbman 1994). In the epithelium the dendrites grow apically, and on reaching the epithelial surface they protrude from it, forming rounded terminal expansions into which centrioles migrate from the receptor soma. These centrioles then become the bases of the olfactory cilia, which grow from them distally. Later the supporting cells, glands, basal and various other cells of the epithelium differentiate, the olfactory apparatus being functional at birth.

In addition to the cells of the epithelium, the placode gives rise to the olfactory glia which migrate basally as the olfactory axons grow out towards the olfactory bulb to ensheath them as far as the outer layer of that structure. From the placode also originate the respiratory parts of the nasal cavity, the vomeronasal organ. A recent most unexpected finding made in rodents has shown that some placodal cells migrate caudally from its medial part to enter the hypothalamus, populating the median eminence with luteinizing hormone-releasing hormone (LHRH)-secreting neuroendocrine cells. Such LHRH-positive cells are found too in the nervus intermedius. For further reading, see Schwanzel-Fukuda and Pfaff (1989).

The maturation and maintenance of the olfactory receptors are to a large extent dependent on synaptic contact with the olfactory bulb, and on complex interactions with the surrounding tissues. For an excellent review of this field, and of the olfactory organ in general, see Farbman (1992).

Effects of age on the olfactory epithelium

In old age the sense of smell is typically impaired, and histological studies show that there is an age-related tendency to lose olfactory receptor cells, the sensory surface being replaced by ciliated respiratory epithelium (see e.g. Paik et al 1992), a change related to the gradual loss of olfaction in senescence.

FUNCTION OF THE OLFACTORY RECEPTORS

The chemical sense served by the olfactory epithelium differs from the gustatory sense in discriminating between different airborne molecules, and can operate effectively even at very low odour concentrations. Although the human sense of smell is only moderate compared with that of macrosomatic species in whose behaviour odours play a dominant role, human olfaction may be more significant than imagined. As in all groups of vertebrates, mammals use specific scents or pheromones for chemical communication between individuals, to mark territories, attract mates, bond newborn offspring to their mothers, and many other social actions. How far this is true of humans is debatable, although there is good evidence that

apocrine glands of the axilla and other parts of the body (p. 406) may have had (or still have) such functions in human social behaviour. It is interesting that the central connections of the olfactory pathway are strongly linked with the limbic system, and thus with affective behaviour, as well as territorial, reproductive, and many other more complex aspects of existence.

Odour transduction

As a result of several recent important advances in olfactory research the mechanisms by which olfactory receptors detect odorants and pass appropriate information to the CNS are beginning to become clear. Briefly, the picture which is emerging is as follows. When an odorant reaches the olfactory area, it dissolves in the thin layer of mucus then diffuses to the exposed receptor membranes of the cilia and dendritic knobs, where the receptor sites are situated. There the interaction of odorant and receptor causes the activation within the cilium of one or more second messenger systems which entrain the opening of ion channels to sodium, calcium or other cations in the sensory membrane, causing a graded depolarization (receptor potential) in the receptor cell similar to that initiated in CNS neurons by excitatory neurotransmitters (p. 907). When the receptor cell is sufficiently depolarized, voltage sensitive ion channels at its base, i.e. in the most proximal part of its axon, open and an action potential (or a volley of action potentials) is initiated in the olfactory nerve. Under experimental conditions, the summated receptor potentials of many sensory cells simultaneously stimulated by an odorant summate as a wave or negative potential (the electro-olfactogram: Ottoson 1956) detectable with an extracellular electrode at the epithelial surface.

The details of these events are not yet fully known; the receptor molecules which bind odorants in the first phase of transduction have not yet been characterized sufficiently although the genes of several of the putative receptors have been sequenced and cloned, as noted above (Buck & Axel 1991; Reed 1992; Breer & Boekhoff 1992). Likewise the second messenger pathways have yet to be fully clarified; two distinct routes have been shown, one involving guanosine triphosphate (GTP)-dependent adenylate cyclase, and the other GTP-dependent phospholipase C (the phosphoinositide pathway). These pathways depend on a chain of molecular interactions, beginning with the receptor and its associated GTP-binding proteins (G-proteins), and involving amplification of the original signal. The olfactory-specific G-protein (G_{olf}) and its related (Type III) adenyl cyclase have been localized by immunoelectron microscopy to the distal segments of olfactory cilia (Menco et al 1992) which because of their great length present a relatively huge surface area for odorant reception. Whatever the final details, it is evident that complex biochemical events are responsible for the extreme sensitivity of the olfactory sense, and for its ability to discriminate between a great range of odorants.

As the receptor molecules have not yet been characterized (at the time of writing), it is not known how they might interact with odorants to initiate transduction, nor how different odours are discriminated. However from the gene sequences of the putative receptors recently discovered it is likely that they resemble neurotransmitter receptors with G-protein binding domains, and that different odorants initiate transduction in a similar manner, by some type of shape recognition. What molecular features are responsible for the subjective grouping of odorants into particular classes is at present unclear, although there are usually a number of resemblances in the shapes and chemical groups exposed at their surfaces. Classically only a fairly small number of odorant classes have been proposed. In the earlier attempts to relate the molecular shape to odorant qualities, it was postulated that there might be a simple basis for quality coding, with as few as perhaps seven or eight 'primary odours', analogous to primary colours (e.g. floral, fruity, minty, pungent, musky, urinous, etc.), with only a few corresponding receptor sites. Later studies have indicated a greater complexity than this, and the recent discovery in molecular genetics that the members of the putative receptor family are all expressed in the olfactory epithelium, make the situation very complex indeed. The receptor sites appear to be all on the surfaces of the olfactory receptor cells, and according to immunoelectron microscopic localization of olfactory G-proteins, predominantly on the distal segments of olfactory cilia (Menco et al 1994). Further studies at a cellular level are necessary for a fuller understanding of the general nature of olfaction, which in the past has been a somewhat neglected sense.

OTHER CHEMOSENSORY ENDINGS IN THE NASAL CAVITY

In humans, the olfactory area is probably the only part of the nasal cavity to possess primary sensory cells, but in most other mammals there are two other small accessory regions, the vomeronasal organ, and the septal organ (of Masera). In addition, the entire nasal epithelium including that of the olfactory area is innervated by sensory endings of the trigeminal nerve, and also receives innervation from the rather mysterious nervus terminalis.

Vomeronasal organ (of Jacobson)

Although generally considered to be non-functional in adult humans, the vomeronasal organ is found in various species of mammals including new world monkeys, carnivores, ungulates and rodents, as well as many lower vertebrates (see the review by Eisthen 1992; also Adams 1992). Recently it has been shown that in humans this organ develops to some extent during fetal life but usually degenerates, putative sensory cells being replaced by non-sensory epithelium when the organ persists into postnatal life (Boehm & Gasser 1993, Moran et al 1991). Typically it is a paired accessory olfactory organ situated in the base of the median nasal septum near its anterior end. Each is a tube enclosed in a bony or cartilaginous canal; in many mammals it opens at its anterior end directly into the nasal cavity, in some into the nasopalatine duct leading to the buccal cavity, or in others, into both spaces. Within the tubular organ, the sensory epithelium occupies the medial wall, the lateral surface of its lumen being composed of non-sensory ciliated cells lying on elastic, cavernous tissue. Mucus, with dissolved odorants, can be drawn into and expelled from the lumen by changes in blood pressure within the cavernous tissue, under autonomic nervous control (Meredith & O'Connell 1979).

The sensory epithelium resembles that of the main olfactory epithelium except that its receptors have much larger cell bodies, with copious agranular endoplasmic reticulum, and possess microvilli rather than cilia on their endings (Kolnberger 1971). They also lack globose basal cells, although cells with similar functions occur along the edges of the epithelium and can repopulate it with receptors if the vomeronasal nerve is sectioned (Barber & Raisman 1978). Electrical recordings show that vomeronasal receptors are physiologically similar to olfactory receptor cells, and respond similarly to odours, though possibly to a narrower range of substances. They have been shown to be important in sexual behaviour in several species, and may be especially concerned with detecting pheromones. In snakes and lizards they have large openings into the oral cavity, and odorants introduced into them by the sampling action of the forked tongue constitute an important aspect of chemosensation.

Septal olfactory organ (organ of Masera)

The septal olfactory organ is a small patch of olfactory epithelium situated ventrally in the posterior septum in some species of mammal (rodents, rabbit, marsupials: see Adams 1992). Apart from its isolation from the main olfactory area, its structure is very similar; it may serve as a monitor of odorants in the respiratory current during quiet respiration. It has not been found in humans.

Trigeminal endings

Other nasal chemoreceptors include terminals responsive to strong odours and noxious chemicals in aerial solution, for example ammonia and sulphur dioxide, even when the olfactory pathway has been destroyed by fracture of the cribriform plate or division of the olfactory tract. The major nerves possibly supplying nasal chemosensory endings include trigeminal fibres from ethmoidal branches of the ophthalmic nerve and various maxillary branches; small bundles of myelinated fibres from these were detected by Graziadei and Gagne (1973) in the basal olfactory epithelium, losing their sheaths as they penetrate amongst the supporting cells. Many of these terminals contain neuropeptides including substance P and calcitonin gene-related peptide (CGRP) (Finger et al 1990).

Nervus terminalis

Another possible chemosensory path is the nervus terminalis, whose functions are uncertain but which terminates widely in the nasal cavity in some species (see e.g. the account by Graziadei 1974). This nerve also has fibres belonging to luteinizing hormone releasing hormone (LHRH)-containing neurons with ganglia associated with the main nerve, and may in part represent a vestigial remnant of the embryonic migratory pathway of these neurons from the olfactory placode to the hypothalamus.

PERIPHERAL VISUAL APPARATUS

INTRODUCTION

The all-pervading nature of sunlight, the environment of almost all animal and plant life, makes a response to this form of electromagnetic radiation essential for animal survival. The photosynthetic processes in plants are paralleled by photochemical receptors occurring almost universally in the animal kingdom. Though the range of frequencies in solar radiation is much wider, the visible spectrum (400–760 nm) is the range within which most animal photoreceptors function. Some receptors react outside this range, either to ultraviolet or infra-red frequencies; in vertebrates some vipers and boas have facial pit organs responding to infra-red radiation. But in general *visual pigments*, the basis of photochemical response, display absorption maxima within the visible spectrum; for example human *rhodopsin* (visual purple), a retinal rod pigment, has a maximum at 497 nm. *Iodopsin*, a cone pigment, occurs in some avian species and several pigments exist in human cones, where differing absorption maxima may account for colour vision. The basis of the sensory response is a light-induced 'bleaching', the pigment changing to another form, with an accompanying electrical flux propagated by chemical transmission from photoreceptors to primary neurons. A rapid restoration of the pigment is obviously essential. Many visual pigments have been identified; further details may be obtained in monographs (e.g. Rushton 1962; Pirenne 1967; Davson 1976).

Next in the elaboration of visual organs is the introduction of a lens to concentrate light energy on photoreceptors and impart spatial discrimination. Many such adaptations have occurred in invertebrates, mostly in two forms: the eyes, as we may now call them, with many separate lens-photoreceptor units, the *compound eyes* familiar in insects and crustaceans; and a *single lens*, focusing light on an array of photoreceptors, as in snails and squids. The latter type is universal in vertebrates.

Such true eyes not only respond to varying **luminance**, a simple function of photoreceptors; by projecting a focused image on an array of receptors, each with neural pathways of some degree of specificity, a new modality appears, sensitivity to **form**. In both modes movement (always of great biological meaning) is detectable but the vertebrate type of focusing eye has potentialities for greater precision.

Primitively, vision is used for reception at a distance, to activate warning systems and to orientate the animal advantageously in light and shade. The paired eyes of most vertebrates, being lateral in position, permit an almost panoramic view. Such *panoramic vision*, with muscles which rotate the eyes reflexly towards anything of interest, especially movements (of prey, mate, or predator), is typical of mammals, in a few of which, and in some raptorial birds, the orbits have changed position so that two uniocular fields, each subtended by one eye, overlap to a greater or lesser extent. Part of the field in front of the animal is hence binocular. By gradual refinement of the control of ocular muscles, with constant retinal feedback, ocular movements become concerted enough to 'fuse' the two slightly dissimilar retinal images, leading finally to full *binocular vision*. This advance is usual in carnivorous mammals, who may track prey partly by smell but rely on accurate directional vision for the final attack. Primates also have binocular vision; the arboreal factor in their evolution is generally regarded as leading to not merely binocular, but *stereoscopic vision*, allowing a higher motor 'understanding' of three-dimensional space. Olfaction is less useful in trees; acquisition of the skill of not merely climbing but swinging or leaping from branch to branch could only evolve with stereoscopic vision (see also p. 7). An arboreal habitat also favoured the retention and elaboration of pentadactyl, grasping extremities. Though man, and perhaps his immediate ancestors, is not arboreal, the terrestrial specialization of feet has not afflicted his hands. Freed from locomotion by the adoption of a bipedal gait, human hands have formed a most significant partnership with the eyes. Added to this is the associated development of a large brain, able to process with increasing intricacy highly detailed information from the eyes and other senses and to co-ordinate the eyes and hands in increasingly skilful and subtle tasks, are surely the leading trio of factors in the extraordinary evolution of human abilities.

The eye, therefore, is not to be viewed in isolation. Its array of modalities—sensitivity to minute changes in luminosity, particularly in dark-adapted, *scotopic vision*, high discrimination of form, movement and colour in light-adapted, *photopic vision*—do not merely provide interesting information. The information is vital; a blind individual cannot long survive outside human society. The eyes continuously guide almost all that we do, especially in manual tasks. Visual communication has proved more useful and lasting than even auditory. The gradual evolution of visual signs, reacting with auditory communication, has led to language in all its permutations; and through language, with its potentialities for the exchange of increasingly precise information and conceptual influences, it becomes possible for generation after generation to profit from recorded knowledge in a unique extension of evolutionary progress. In human culture this now provides the mainstream of evolution. It is against this background that the structure of the visual apparatus should be studied.

ANATOMY OF THE EYE

The eyeball, the peripheral organ of vision, is situated in a skeletal cavity, the orbit, the walls of which help to protect it from injury; they also have a more fundamental role in the visual process itself in providing a rigid support and direction to the eye and in forming the sites of attachment to its external muscles. This setting permits the accurate positioning of the visual axis under neuromuscular control and determines the spatial relationship between the two eyes needed for binocular vision and conjugate eye movements. In the following account, the structure of the eyeball itself will first be considered, and then certain accessory structures, including extrinsic muscles, fasciae, eyebrows, eye-lids, conjunctiva and the lacrimal apparatus, will be described.

The eyeball is embedded in orbital fat, separated from it by a thin *fascial sheath* (capsule of Tenon) (p. 1359). The eyeball can be considered as being composed of the segments of two spheres of different radii. The anterior segment, part of the smaller sphere, is transparent and forms about one-sixth of the whole globe; it is more prominent than the posterior segment, which is part of a larger sphere and opaque, forming the remainder of the globe. The *anterior segment* is bounded by the cornea and the lens and is incompletely subdivided into *anterior* and *posterior chambers* by the iris, being continuous through its pupil. The anterior chamber's periphery is slightly overlapped by the sclera; thus the *angle* between the iris and cornea (p. 1325) forms an annulus of greater diameter than the *limbus*, the junction between the sclera and cornea. The difference between these two varies from 1 to 2 mm, the angle being deeper above and below than at the sides of the eyeball. The posterior chamber, between the posterior surface of the iris and the anterior aspect of the lens and its supporting ligament, the *zonule* (p. 1349), is triangular in section, the apex of the triangle being where the iris touches the lens; its base or zonular region is not the zonule itself,

since the posterior chamber extends among the zonule's collagenous bundles and even into a *retrozonular space* (canal of Petit) between the zonule and the vitreous humour in the posterior segment of the eyeball. The *posterior segment* consists of the parts of the eye posterior to the zonule and lens.

The *anterior pole* is the centre of the anterior (corneal) curvature, the *posterior pole* the centre of its posterior (scleral) curvature; a line joining these two points forms the *optic axis*. (By the same convention, the eye has an *equator*, equidistant between the poles; any circumferential line joining the poles is a *meridian*.) The optic axes of the two eyes, in their primary position, are parallel and do **not** correspond with the orbital axes which diverge anterolaterally at a marked angle to each other (see below). The optic nerves follow the orbital axes and are therefore not parallel; each enters its eye about 3 mm medial (nasal) to the posterior pole. The ocular vertical diameter (23.5 mm) is rather less than the transverse and anteroposterior diameters (24 mm); the anteroposterior diameter at birth is about 17.5 mm and at puberty 20–21 mm; it may vary considerably in *myopia* (c. 29 mm) and in *hypermetropia* (c. 20 mm). In females all diameters are on average slightly less than in the male (Stenström 1946; Sorsby & Sheridan 1960).

The eye has three *tunics* enclosing its contents. From without they are:

- a fibrous tunic consisting of the *sclera* behind and the *cornea* in front
- a vascular, pigmental tunic comprising from behind forwards the *choroid, ciliary body* and *iris*, collectively termed the *uveal tract*
- a neural layer, the *retina*.

OCULAR FIBROUS TUNIC

The fibrous layer of the eyeball (**8.415, 416**) has an opaque posterior *tunica sclera* and a transparent anterior *tunica cornea*. Together these form the protective enclosing capsule of the eye, a semi-elastic structure which when made turgid by intraocular pressure, determines with great precision the optical geometry of the visual apparatus. The scleral tunic also provides attachments to the extraocular muscles which rotate the eye, its smooth external surface translating easily on the adjacent tissues of the orbit. The cornea, besides admitting light with little hindrance, refracts it towards a retinal focus and is an important part of the eye's image-processing mechanism. For further details of the cornea and sclera, see Jakus (1964), Langham (1969) and Hogan et al (1971).

SCLERA (TUNICA SCLERA)

The sclera, so named from its relatively hard consistency, is a dense layer which, when distended by intraocular pressure, maintains the shape of the eyeball. It is thickest (about 1.1 mm) posteriorly, near the optic nerve's entry point, and is thinnest (0.4 mm) at the equator and at the attachments of the recti (p. 1354). Its *external surface* is white and smooth and is in contact with the inner surface of the fascial sheath of the eyeball (p. 1359).

Its anterior part is covered by conjunctiva reflected on to it from the deep surfaces of the eyelids. The scleral *internal surface* is attached to the choroid by a delicate fibrous layer, the *suprachoroid lamina* (*lamina fusca sclerae*), containing numerous fibroblasts and melanocytes. Anteriorly, it is attached to the ciliary body by the *lamina supraciliaris*. Posteriorly, the sclera is pierced by the optic nerve and is continuous with the nerve's fibrous sheath and hence with the dura mater. Where the nerve pierces the sclera, the latter has the appearance of a perforated plate, the *lamina cribrosa sclerae* (**8.443, 444**), the minute orifices in which transmit the optic nerve's fascicles. A larger, central aperture in this structure is traversed by the central retinal artery and vein. The lamina cribrosa is the weakest part of the sclera and bulges outwards in the condition of a cupped disc when intraocular pressure is raised chronically as in the condition of glaucoma. Numerous small apertures transmit the ciliary vessels and nerves through the sclera close to the perimeter of the cribriform plate. Just behind the equator four larger apertures tranmit the *venae vorticosae*.

Anteriorly, the sclera is directly continuous with the cornea at the

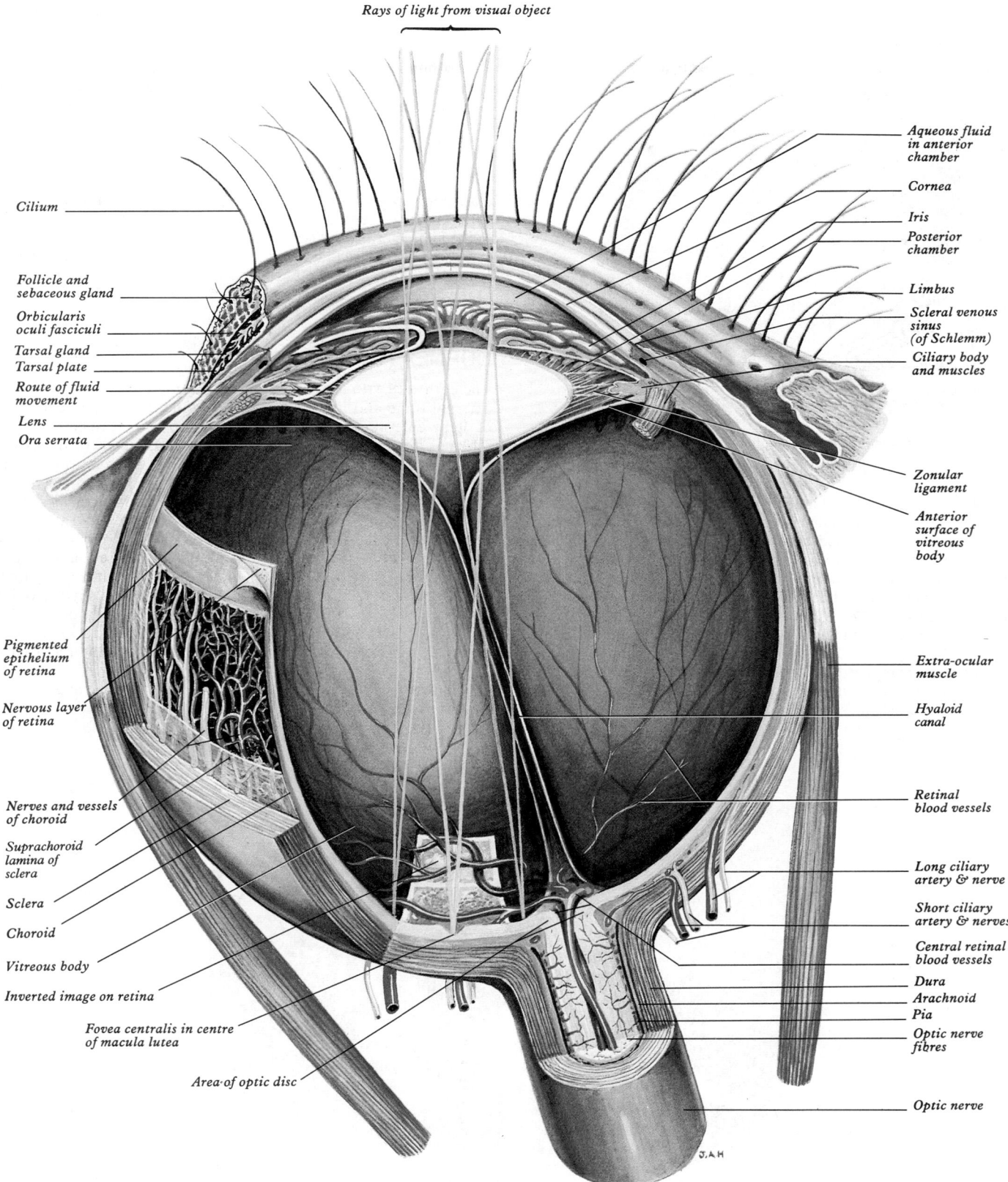

8.415   The organization of the eye, viewed from above. In this illustration the left eye and part of the lower eyelid are depicted in horizontal section and also cut away to show internal structure (compare **8.416**B).

corneoscleral junction (limbus; **8.415**). Near the internal surface of the sclera at this junction is an annular, endothelial canal, the sinus venosus sclerae (canal of Schlemm); in section this is an oval cleft, whose outer wall grooves the sclera. Posteriorly, this cleft extends as far as a rim of scleral tissue, the scleral spur, which is in section a

triangle with its apex directed forwards (**8.417**). The sinus may be double or multiple in part of its course. Its inner wall, adjoining the aqueous chamber, consists of loose trabecular tissue continuous anteriorly with the posterior limiting lamina and endothelium of the cornea; among its fibres are spaces through which aqueous humour

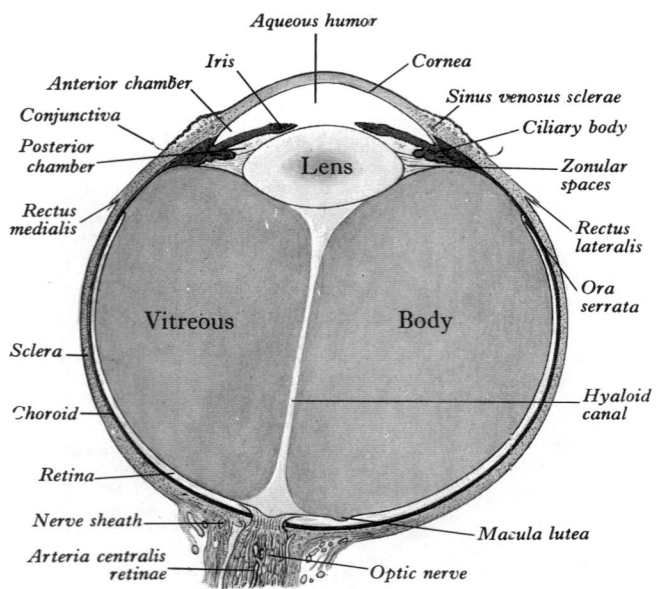

Aqueous humor
Iris
Cornea
Anterior chamber
Sinus venosus sclerae
Conjunctiva
Ciliary body
Posterior chamber
Lens
Zonular spaces
Rectus medialis
Rectus lateralis
Ora serrata
Vitreous
Body
Sclera
Choroid
Hyaloid canal
Retina
Nerve sheath
Macula lutea
Arteria centralis retinae
Optic nerve

8.416   A horizontal section through a right human eyeball: superior aspect.

ocular pressure (Gloster et al 1957), the collagen forming 75% of the dry scleral weight. Fibre bundles are arranged circumferentially around the optic disc, and around the orifices of the lamina cribrosa. Elsewhere on the external surface of the sclera, fibres are arranged mostly in a reticular manner and tendon fibres of the rectus muscles intersect scleral fibres at right angles at their attachments, then interlace deeper in the sclera (Thale & Tillmann 1993). Collagen fibres of the scleral spur are orientated circularly and the incidence of elastic fibres is increased here. Individual *scleral fibrils* vary in diameter from 28 to 280 nm with periodicities of 80 and 21 μm and, unlike those of the cornea, collagen fibrils of widely different diameters may occur in the same bundle. Type I and Type III collagen are present in the sclera generally and Type IV additionally in the lamina cribrosa (Tengroth et al 1985; Thale & Tillmann 1993).

Scleral vessels are few and mainly disposed in the episcleral lamina, especially close to the limbus; the sclera provides passage for nerves of the cornea and vascular autonomic nerves but its own innervation is sparse.

CORNEA (TUNICA CORNEA)

The cornea (8.418) is the anterior, projecting transparent part of the external tunic and its tear film cover is the major site of refraction of light entering the eye. Convex anteriorly, it projects from the sclera as a dome-shaped elevation forming about 7% of the external tunic's area. After the first year or so of life its curvature changes very little. Since it is more curved (radius (r) = 6.8–8.5 mm, averaging 7.8 mm) than the sclera (r = 11.5 mm), a slight *sulcus sclerae* marks the corneoscleral junction. Corneal thickness is about 1.0 mm at its periphery and 0.5–0.6 mm at its centre. Viewed from in front, the corneal perimeter is slightly elliptical, its transverse diameter being a little greater than its vertical; its posterior perimeter is circular and, because in section the corneoscleral junction is slightly oblique above and below, it is more extensive than the anterior surface in its vertical axis. The corneal diameter is about 11.7 mm on its posterior aspect; anteriorly it is 11.7 mm horizontally and 10.6 mm vertically.

Microscopically, the cornea consists of five layers arranged anteroposteriorly as follows:

filters from the anterior chamber to the sinus, thence draining peripherally to the anterior ciliary veins. To the scleral spur's anterior, external aspect are attached most of the fibres of the trabecular tissue mentioned above. Most of the remainder are continuous with meridional fibres of the ciliary muscle, some of which attach to the posterior internal aspect of the scleral spur. The anterior chamber's *iridocorneal angle* (8.417) is bordered anteriorly by the trabecular tissue and the scleral spur and posteriorly by the periphery of the iris.

The sclera is composed of dense collagenous tissue mixed with infrequent elastic fibres and interspersed with flat fibroblasts. It is a viscoelastic structure, a factor important in the regulation of intra-

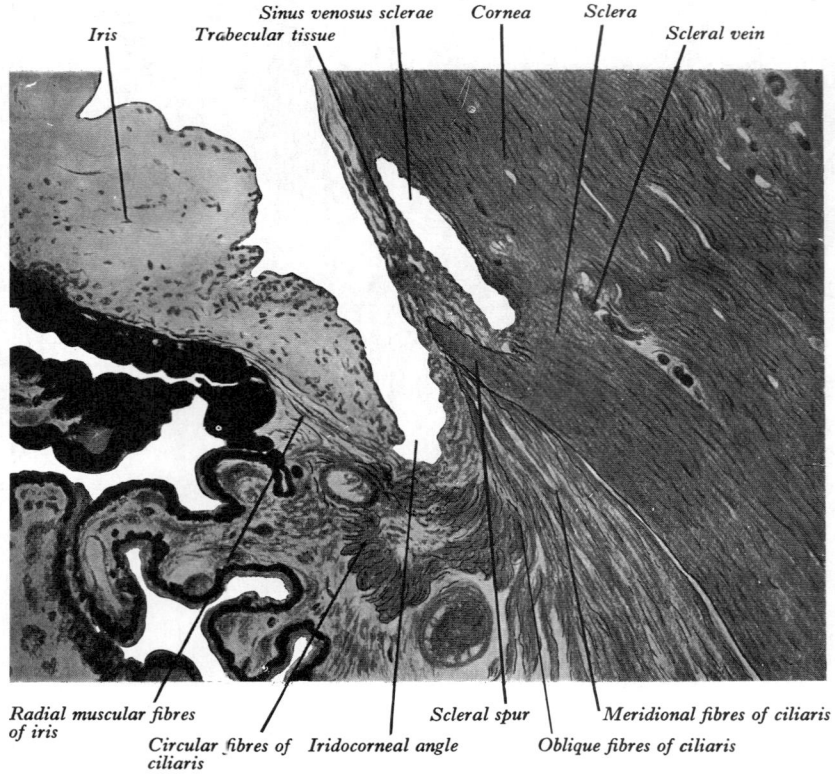

Iris
Sinus venosus sclerae
Cornea
Sclera
Trabecular tissue
Scleral vein

Radial muscular fibres of iris
Circular fibres of ciliaris
Iridocorneal angle
Scleral spur
Meridional fibres of ciliaris
Oblique fibres of ciliaris

8.417   A general view of a meridional section through the iridocorneal angle.

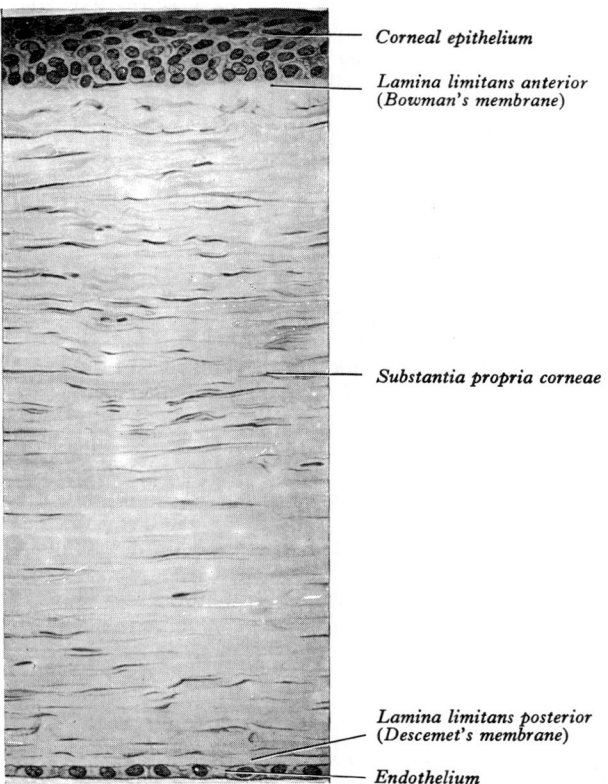

Corneal epithelium

*Lamina limitans anterior
(Bowman's membrane)*

Substantia propria corneae

*Lamina limitans posterior
(Descemet's membrane)*

Endothelium

8.418 Radial section through the human cornea. Magnification × 128.

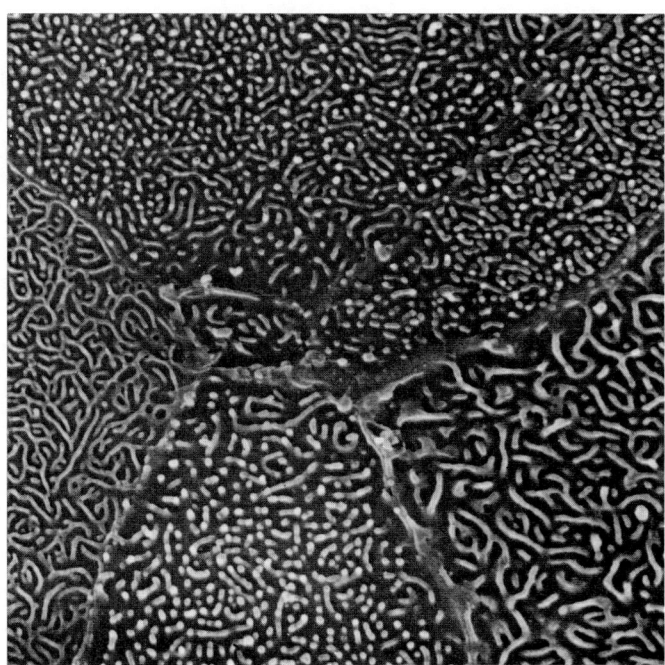

A

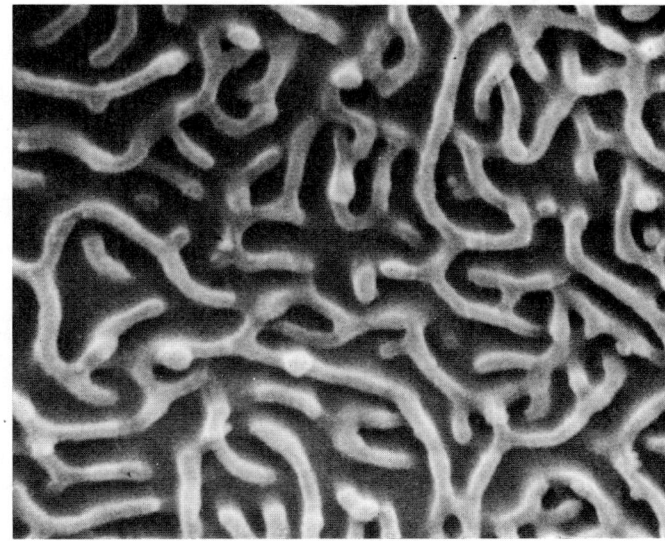

B

8.419 Scanning electrical micrographs of normal human corneal epithelial cells. In A Parts of the outlines of several cells are visible; in the upper and lower cells, microvilli predominate but some microplicae are seen. The cells at the right of the field display predominantly microplicae, with only a few microvilli. Magnification × 5000. In B A small number of microvilli are scattered amongst abundant microplicae. Magnification × 30 000. (By permission of Pfister & Burstein 1977.)

- the corneal epithelium, continuous with the conjunctival epithelium
- the anterior limiting lamina (of Bowman)
- the substantia propria
- the posterior limiting lamina (of Descemet) and
- the endothelium.

Corneal epithelium. This covers the anterior surface of the cornea and generally has five layers of cells. The deepest are columnar with flat bases and rounded apices, and large rounded or oval nuclei. Cells in the second layer are polyhedral, with oval nuclei; in the more superficial layers the cells become progressively flatter but, unlike those of the epidermis, they contain flat nuclei and are not normally keratinized. At medium light microscopic magnifications the cornea appears to have a smooth, optically perfect surface. Most corneal epitheliocytes are 'prickle' cells, like those in the epidermal stratum spinosum (p. 382). At the corneoscleral junction (limbus) the corneal epithelium merges with the limbal conjunctival epithelium which thickens (up to 12 cells) in most positions and soon loses the regular surface of the cornea. Scanning electron microscopy (**8.419**) presents a different appearance of the corneal surface cells: they are covered with small microvilli and more numerous sinuous, communicating ridges. Either one or the other of these projections predominates in different cells, some displaying microvilli and some microplicae, while others have both in varying proportions and a few have them only on their central surface. It is of clinical significance that the cornea does not appear to possess epithelial stem cells and consequently replenishment of this layer depends on centripetally migrating cells from the edges of the cornea, the progeny of mitotic limbal stem cells (Cotsarelis et al 1989).

The anterior limiting lamina (Bowman's membrane). Lying behind the corneal epithelium, it contains a dense mass of collagen fibrils set in a matrix similar to that of the substantia propria (see next paragraph). The lamina is 12 μm thick and is readily distinguishable from the substantia propria because it contains no fibroblasts and, with light microscopy, appears amorphous. Electron microscopy shows its collagen to be finer and more randomly arranged than in the substantia propria.

Substantia propria or stroma. Forming the bulk of the cornea, this is a compact and transparent layer, composed of 200–250 sequential lamellae, each made up of parallel collagen fibrils (Komai

and Ushiki 1991), mainly of Type I collagen, with smaller amounts of Types III, V and VI (Marshall et al 1993), interspersed with glycosaminoglycans (GAGs), glycoproteins and flat dendritic fibroblasts, interconnected to form a coarse mesh. Macrophages, neutrophils and lymphocytes may also enter the matrix. Alternate lamellae are typically orientated to each other at large angles (**8.420**). Each lamella is about 2 μm thick and of variable breadth (10–250 μm, or, rarely, more); all fibrils in a given lamella have similar diameters, being smaller in anterior lamellae than more posteriorly (a range of 21–65 nm). The dimensions of the fibrils are much smaller than the wavelength of light; this feature and the regularity of their spacing are principal factors determining the transparency of the cornea.

The posterior limiting lamina (Descemet's membrane). This

1325

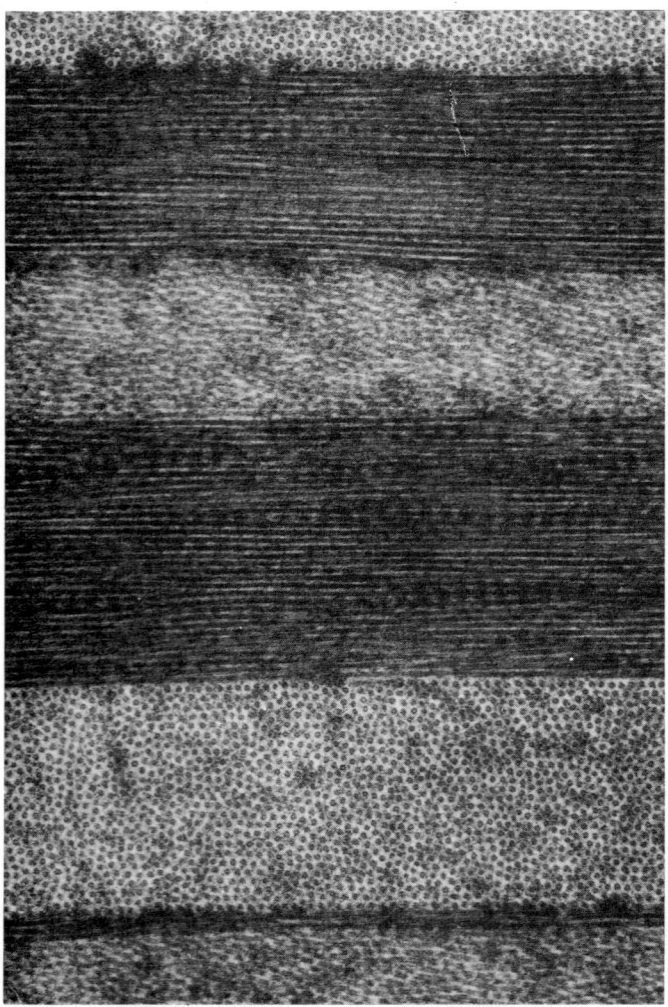

8.420 Transmission electron micrograph of the substantia propria of the human cornea; note the geometric precision of the alternation in direction of adjacent layers of collagen fibres. Magnification × 48 0000. (Preparation by John Marshall, Institute of Ophthalmology, London.)

covers the substantia propria posteriorly; it is thin and apparently homogeneous. Electron microscopy reveals a fibrillar structure anteriorly and a fine granular layer posteriorly, adjacent to the underlying endothelium. It is regarded as the basement membrane of the endothelium and is known to grow throughout life; with a thickness of 5 μm at birth, it may increase to 17 μm by the ninth decade, the growth being confined to the granular layer (Murphy et al 1984). At the limbus of the cornea it disperses into the fibres of trabecular tissue adjoining the inner wall of the scleral venous sinus (**8.417**); between these trabeculae are the *spaces of the iridocorneal angle*, connecting with the sinus venosus sclerae and with the anterior chamber (**8.421**). Some trabeculae join the scleral spur, others are continuous with the meridional fibres of the ciliary muscle. The iridocorneal angle is traversed at infrequent intervals by discrete strands of tissue joining the trabeculae and iris (the iris pillars), equivalent to the pectinate ligaments found in many non-primate mammals.

Aqueous humour drains from the eye through the iridocorneal angle. The trabecular spaces are interconnected and it is generally thought there is no impediment to flow from the anterior chamber to the inner wall of the sinus. The wall of the sinus is constructed of a continuous single thin endothelial layer and passage of aqueous to the sinus probably occurs through the frequent production of giant vacuoles formed on the inner face and discharging at the outer face into the sinus (Tripathi & Tripathi 1982). The further passage of aqueous humour is through a plexus of fine intrascleral vessels connecting the sinus with anterior ciliary veins. Normally the sinus

contains no blood; though the channels between the sinus and veins have no valves, pressure gradients prevent the reflux of blood. In venous congestion blood may indeed enter the sinus but the continuous endothelial outer wall of the trabeculae prevents further reflux.

Endothelium of the cornea (**8.418**). This covers the posterior surface of the cornea and lines the spaces of the iridocorneal angle. The endothelium is a layer of polygonal, flattened cells; at adjacent borders they have complex, interdigitating profiles. When seen by scanning electron microscopy their surfaces show only a few microvilli.

Vessels and nerves of the cornea. The cornea is non-vascular, the capillaries of the conjunctiva and sclera ending in loops near its periphery. Lymph vessels are also absent.

The *nerves* are numerous and arise as branches of the ophthalmic nerve. They form an *annular plexus* around the periphery of the cornea or pass directly from the sclera and enter the substantia propria radially as 70–80 small groups of fibres. Whether or not the cornea also has a sympathetic innervation is uncertain (Marfurt & Ellis 1993). Upon entering the cornea, nerves lose their myelin sheaths (present in a minority of fibres) and endoneurium (Matsuda 1968) to ramify throughout its matrix in a delicate reticulum. Their terminal filaments form an intricate *subepithelial plexus*, from which fine, varicose fibrils traverse the anterior limiting membrane to form an *intraepithelial plexus*. There are no specialized end organs and the epithelial nerve fibres are devoid of Schwann cells and they do not arborize.

OCULAR VASCULAR TUNIC

The vascular tunic, or *uveal tract*, comprises the choroid, ciliary body and iris (**8.416**), forming a continuous structure. The choroid covers the internal scleral surface, extending forwards to the ora serrata. The ciliary body continues from the anterior edge of the choroid to the circumference of the iris. The iris is a circular diaphragm behind the cornea, presenting an almost central aperture, the pupil.

CHOROID

The choroid is a thin, highly vascular, dark brown tissue which lines almost the posterior five-sixths of the eye; it is pierced behind by the optic nerve and is here firmly adherent to the sclera. Posteriorly it is thicker. Its external surface is loosely connected to the sclera by the *suprachoroid lamina* (lamina fusca); internally it is firmly attached to the retinal pigmented layer. At the optic disc it is continuous with the pia-arachnoid tissues around the optic nerve.

Structurally, the choroid consists largely of a dense capillary plexus, with its small arteries and veins of supply. The blood flow through the choroid is high, a feature probably associated with an intraocular pressure of 15–20 mmHg, requiring a venous pressure above 20 mmHg to maintain circulation. The cooling effect of the choroidal circulation on the retina may be important. Externally is the *suprachoroid lamina*, about 30 μm thick, composed of delicate non-vascular lamellae, each a network of fine collagen and elastic fibres with stellate cells containing dark brown granules. Ganglionic neurons and neural plexuses are enmeshed in the connective tissue.

Choroid proper (**8.422**). This lies internal to the suprachoroid lamina (which is partly scleral tissue) and has a number of layers. Although descriptions of these vary, those generally recognized are:

- an external *vascular lamina* of small arteries and veins and loose connective tissue, with scattered pigment cells
- an intermediate *capillary lamina* (choroidocapillaris)
- a thin, apparently structureless *basal lamina*.

The vascular lamina is sometimes subdivided on the basis of blood vessel calibre, which naturally decreases towards the capillary lamina; it also contains the terminals of short posterior ciliary arteries (**8.428**) which extend meridionally from their entry through the sclera near the optic disc. The veins are larger, converging spirally on to four or very occasionally more principal *vorticose veins*, which pierce the sclera to reach tributaries of the ophthalmic veins. The *capillary lamina*, separated from the retina only by the thin basal lamina of

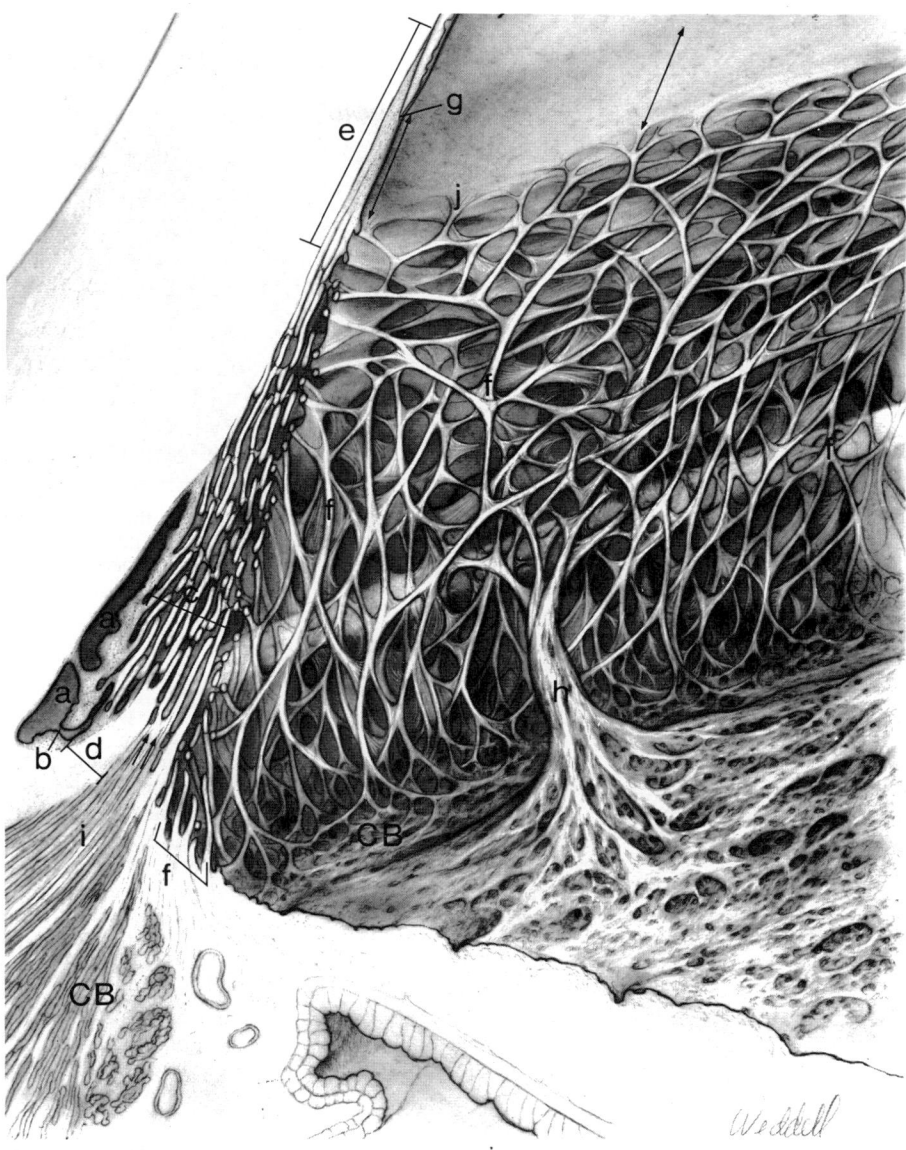

8.421 The iridocorneal angle and adjoining structures, showing the proximity of the scleral venous sinus (a) to the pectinate ligaments (f). The trabecular meshwork of the latter is partly uveal, being continuous with the iris (h) and ciliary body (CB) and muscle (i). Anterior to the scleral spur (d), scleral trabecular tissue (c) is even closer to the scleral venous sinus. Aqueous fluid percolates through this trabecular region, reaching the lumen of the sinus through small apertures (b). The pectinate ligament diminishes as it approaches the corneal limbus (e) and in this junctional zone the posterior limiting membrane (of Descemet) also terminates (g). The endothelium of the anterior chamber (posterior corneal epithelium) is continuous with the endothelium of the trabeculae (j) at the limbus. (From Hogan et al 1971, by permission of the authors, artist and publishers. **8**.424–427, 444 and 448A,B are from the same source.)

the choroid, provides a nutritive supply to the layers of the retina, at least in part. It constitutes a close meshwork of large vessels, but its meshes widen towards the ciliary body. The *basal lamina* (Bruch's membrane) is a glassy, homogeneous layer (lamina vitrea) under the light microscope, only 2–4 μm thick. Electron microscopy reveals that it has a more complex substructure. It has a middle stratum of elastic tissue between an internal and an external layer of collagenous tissue, united externally to the choroidocapillary basal lamina and internally to the basal lamina of the retinal pigment cell layer (Lerche 1965; Nakaizumi 1964). Its function is uncertain but is obviously related to the passage of fluid and solutes from the choroidal capillaries to the retina. It is also said to provide a smooth surface for the precise orientation of retinal pigment cells and receptors. It is formed by both the retina and the choroid (Takei & Ozanics 1955).

In advancing years, lipid may be deposited in the elastic part of this membrane, impairing the exchange of gases, nutrients and metabolites between the choroidal blood and the outer layers of the retina, causing degenerative disease in the photoreceptor lamina.

The functions of choroidal pigment cells are uncertain; they may prevent the passage of light through the sclera to the retina but more importantly may absorb light traversing the retina, preventing internal reflexion within the vitreous body. In many mammals, especially those of nocturnal habit, specialized choroidal cells form a reflecting *tapetum*, responsible for the greenish glare in their eyes at night (Walls 1963); its function is uncertain but it may be a mechanism of aggression or a means of augmenting the stimulation of retinal receptors under low light conditions.

While the vessels of the choroid have a rich sympathetic vasomotor supply, the sensory supply is at most very poor, although recent evidence indicates its presence. Crush lesions of the ophthalmic nerve (Bergmanson 1977) in simians yielded no evidence of any suprachoroidal fibres from ciliary nerves and no degenerating fibres were found terminating within the choroid.

CILIARY BODY (8.423–425)

The ciliary body is directly continuous with the choroid behind and with the iris in front; all these regions of the uveal tract have various features in common but also have regional differences related to

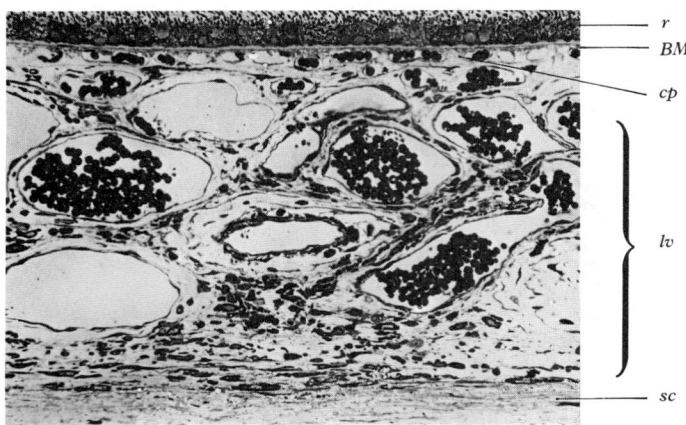

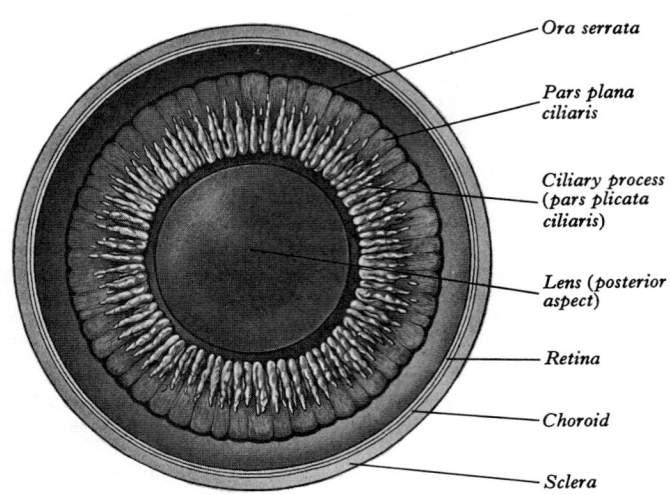

8.422 Light micrograph of a section of human eyeball showing full thickness of the choroid coat and adjacent parts of the retina (above) and inner edge of the sclera (below). Note, from above downwards: r = rod and cone processes projecting among pigment cells; Bm = the basal lamina (membrane of Bruch); cp = layer of capillaries (choriocapillaries); lv = layer of larger vessels and loose connective tissue merging into the sc = sclera. Numerous pigment cells are scattered throughout the choroid. Magnification × 350. (Provided by John Marshall, Institute of Ophthalmology, London.)

8.423 The interior aspect of the anterior half of the eyeball showing the postocular surface of the lens in position, with the surrounding ring of ciliary processes and or a serrata (compare **8**.424 and 428.).

variations in their function. The ciliary body is concerned with the suspension of the lens and with accommodation, related to the accumulation of muscle fibres which cause it to bulge internally (**8**.425). It is also a major source of aqueous fluid for the anterior segment of the eye, which its anterior aspect faces. Posteriorly it is contiguous with the vitreous humour and probably secretes some of the glycosaminoglycans (GAGs) of the vitreous body. The anterior and the long ciliary arteries meet in the ciliary body (**8**.427, 428), which is therefore a highly vascular region, involved not only in secretory and muscular activities but also in the blood supply to the iris and limbus. The ciliary body is traversed by the major nerves to all the anterior tissues of the eyeball.

Externally the ciliary body extends from a line about 1.5 mm posterior to the limbus of the cornea (corresponding also to the scleral spur) to a line about 7.5–8 mm posterior to this on the temporal side and 6.5–7 mm on the nasal. The ciliary body is thus slightly eccentric and projects posteriorly from the scleral spur which is its attachment, with a meridional width varying from 5.5 to 6.5 mm. Internally it shows a posteriorly crenated or scalloped periphery where it is continuous with the choroid and retina, termed the *ora serrata*. Anteriorly it is confluent with the periphery of the iris, externally to which it bounds the anterior chamber's iridocorneal angle. The ciliary body is brown, due to melanin in the deeper layer of its epithelium. It has an anterior plicated part, the *corona ciliaris* (pars plicata), surrounding the base of the iris and posterior to this is a smooth, annular *orbiculus ciliaris* (pars plana, ciliary ring). The orbiculus forms more than half of the meridional width of the ciliary body, being 3.5–4 mm across; its peripheral rim is the ora serrata, at which the *optical* or sensory part of the retina is suddenly reduced to two layers of epithelial cells, extending over the whole ciliary body as the *pars ciliaris retinae* and beyond this on to the posterior surface of the iris. The corona ciliaris, a smaller annular region within the orbiculus, is ridged meridionally by 70–80 *ciliary processes* radiating from the base of the iris to the orbiculus (**8**.423). Branching from the sides of these ridges into valleys between them are numerous minor ridges, the *ciliary plicae*, forming a complex pattern of intricate microscopic folds (**8**.424). Fibres of the *zonule* (the suspensory ligament of the lens) extend into the valleys, passing beyond the ciliary processes to fuse with the basement membrane of the superficial epithelial layer of the orbiculus ciliaris. Their sites of attachment are marked by striae passing back from the valleys of the corona across the orbiculus almost as far as the apices of the dentate processes of the ora serrata (**8**.424)

Ciliary epithelium. This is bilaminar, its two layers of simple epithelium being derived embryonically from the optic cup's two

layers. The *superficial lamina*, made up of columnar cells overlying the orbiculus and cuboidal cells over the ciliary processes, becomes irregular and more flattened between the processes. These cells, containing little or no pigment, are the sole anterior continuation of the *neural* layers of the retina, although its pigment epithelium is continuous with the *deeper layer* of the ciliary epithelium. The cells of the latter are also approximately cuboidal and are loaded with pigment. The two layers are firmly united, although pathologically fluid may separate them. A basement membrane exists between the two epithelia. Basally the superficial cells are much infolded, like other secretory epithelia. These superficial cells are connected by desmosomes; their cytoplasm contains many mitochondria and a well-developed endoplasmic reticulum, often stacked in perinuclear arrays. Lipid and melanin granules are often present but are not prominent.

The pigment layer is united to the stroma of the ciliary body by its basement membrane, which continues back into the basal lamina of the choroid (p. 1327). The cytoplasm of these cells contains abundant rounded melanin granules 0.6–0.8 μm in diameter. Cells are linked by a few lateral desmosomes, which are more numerous between the two epithelial strata, despite the intervention of a basement membrane.

Ciliary stroma. Composed largely of loose collagen fasciculi, this is aggregated into a considerable mass between the ciliary muscle and overlying processes, extending into both of them. In this inner stratum of connective tissue are numerous larger branches of the ciliary vessels, with a dense reticulum of large capillaries, most of them adjacent to the epithelium and especially concentrated in the ciliary processes, where they are chiefly of the fenestrated type. Numerous vessels also enter the ciliary muscle but its capillaries show far fewer fenestrations. Anteriorly, near the periphery of the iris, is the major arterial circle (**8**.426), formed chiefly by long posterior ciliary branches of the ophthalmic artery (p. 1526) which enter the eye some distance behind the ocular equator, passing between the choroid and sclera to the ciliary body. Ciliary veins, also draining the iris, pass posteriorly to join the vorticose veins of the choroid.

Ciliary muscle. This has been variously described, the differences being mainly in the subdivision of this small annular mass of smooth muscle. Most authors recognize three parts: *meridional, radial* or oblique and *circular* or sphincteric; but other views have been stated (Calasans 1953; Rohen 1964). Most, perhaps almost all, ciliary muscle fibres are attached to the scleral spur (**8**.425), spreading in several directions, upon which the somewhat arbitrary division of the muscle depends. The outermost fibres are meridional or

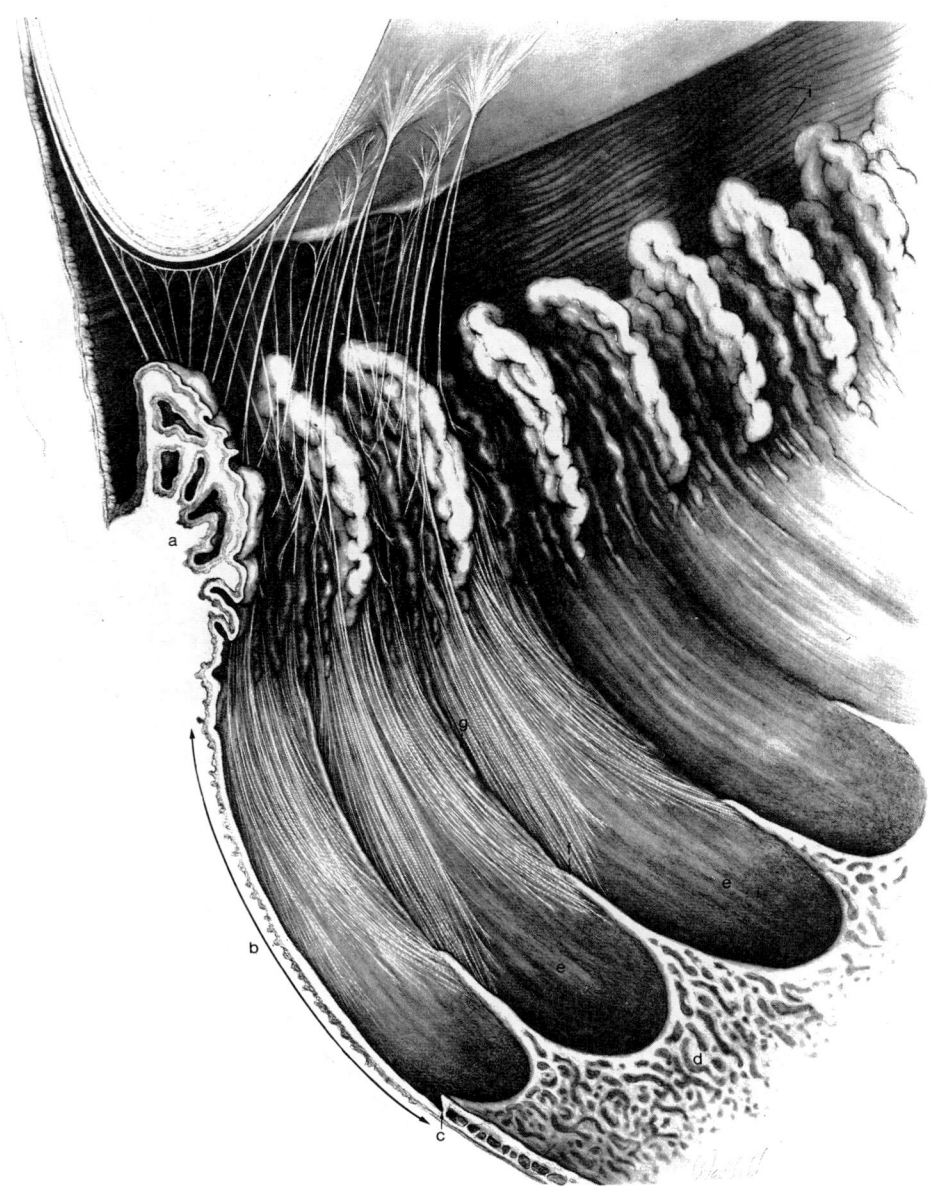

8.424 A magnified view of the ciliary region seen from the ocular interior. Above is the periphery of the lens, attached by the fibres of the *zonule* (suspensory ligament) to the processes of the *corona ciliaris* (pars plicata) of the ciliary body (a). The *orbiculus ciliaris* or pars plana ciliaris (b) has a scalloped boundary, the *ora serrata* (c), which separates it from the retina (d). Flanking the 'bays' (e) of this are the *dentate* processes (f), with which linear ridges or *striae* (g) are continuous. These striae extend forwards between the main ciliary processes, providing an attachment for the longer zonular fibres. The posterior aspect of the iris shows radial (h) and circumferential (i) sulci. (See **8.421** for acknowledgements.)

longitudinal, passing posteriorly into the stroma of the choroid, where many exhibit terminal branchings or *epichoroidal stars*. The innermost fibres swerve acutely from the spur (**8.425**) to run circumferentially as a sphincteric element near the periphery of the lens. Between these two muscular strata are obliquely interconnecting fibres, frequently forming an interweaving lattice, often referred to as *radial* in direction. In ultrastructure the ciliary muscle differs from other smooth muscle, the myocytes containing unusually abundant mitochondria and endoplasmic reticulum. A small bundle of fibres is usually surrounded by a common fibroblastic sheath to form units unlike those in any other types of smooth muscles. Gap junctions couple the myocytes electrically. Three types of nerve ending have been noted, the most common being an indirect contact of the presynaptic membranes with the interposed basal lamina; contact without the basal lamina also occurs; rarest are larger contacts in depressions in the surfaces of myocytes.

Myelinated and non-myelinated nerve fibres abound in the ciliary muscle and ciliary body, the latter being postganglionic parasympathetic axons from the ciliary ganglion, where they link with the oculomotor parasympathetic outflow; but some fibres appear to be sympathetic, according to much evidence. The parasympathetic supply stimulates the ciliary muscle to contract but the role of the sympathetic innervation is unsettled. Cervical sympathetic stimulation in experimental animals causes the lens to flatten, tantamount to the relaxation of accommodation, but the mechanism of this is uncertain; it may be due to an inhibition of the ciliary muscle or the ciliary body volume may be reduced by vasoconstriction, tensing the zonule and hence the periphery of the lens, the reverse of the slackening effects of the zonule in ciliary contraction (Morgan 1944; Alpern 1969). Electron microscopy of the ciliary autonomic plexus in rhesus monkeys reveals a cycle of degeneration and regeneration which becomes more marked in older animals (Townes Anderson & Raviola 1979).

IRIS (8.415, 416, 426)

The iris is an adjustable diaphragm around a central aperture (slightly medial to true centre), the *pupil*, which controls the amount of light entering the eye. Pupillary diameter varies from 1 to 8 mm at least and has an even wider range under the influence of drugs. This gives

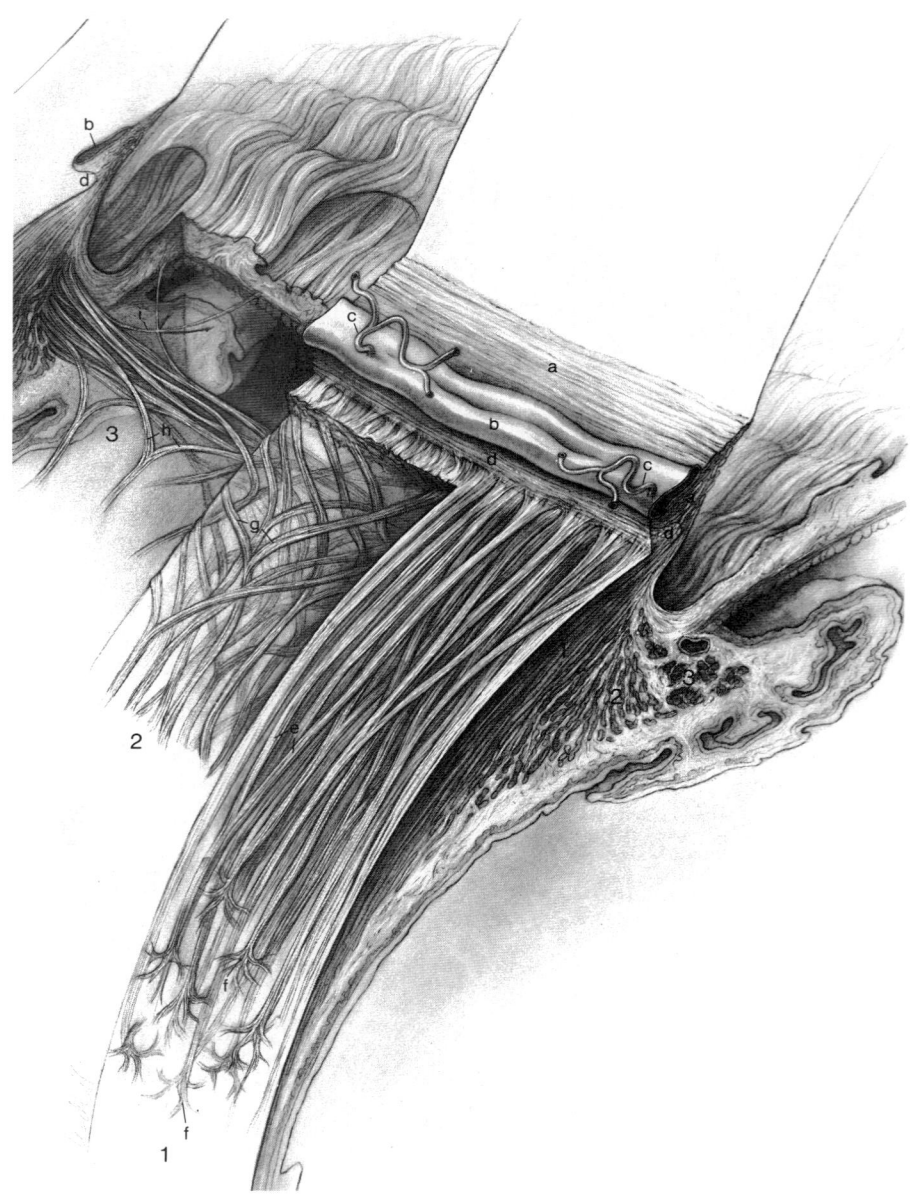

8.425 The ciliary muscle and its components. The meridional or longitudinal (1), radial or oblique (2), and circular or sphincteric (3) layers of muscle fibres are displayed by successive removal towards the ocular interior. The cornea and sclera have been removed, leaving the pectinate ligament (a), the scleral venous sinus (b), collecting venules (c) and scleral spur (d). The meridional fibres often display acutely angled junctions (e) and terminate in epichoroidal stars (f). The radial fibres meet at obtuse angles (g) and similar junctions, at even wider angles (h), occur in the circular stratum of the ciliaris. (See **8.421** for acknowledgements.)

an aperture range in excess of *f*20–*f*2.5, and a ratio of 32:1 in the amount of light permitted to enter the eye. While this is not enough to save the retina from the effects of intense illumination, it moderates the great range of luminosity encountered in ordinary use, preserving useful vision under highly variable conditions. (The pupillary diameters noted above and the average iridial diameter of about 12 mm are of course estimated through the cornea, introducing a magnification factor of about 12%.) Pupillary *constriction* and *dilatation* are self-explanatory terms, for which miosis and mydriasis are used clinically, though more properly reserved for the extreme limits of contraction and dilatation. The erudite surveys of the immense literature on the pupil and the iris by Loewenfeld (1958) and Loewenstein and Loewenfeld (1970) should be consulted for further information on this subject.

Though the iris is named after the rainbow, its range of colour extends only from light blue to very dark brown, often varying in the two eyes and even within the same iris. The colour is the combined effect of the iridial connective tissue and the pigment cells in selectively absorbing and reflecting different frequencies of light energy. When pigment is largely absent, as at birth, the colour is light blue; some pigment is necessary to confine light transmission to the pupil and central lens, where optical aberrations are least. The concentration of melanocytes is the main factor determining the hue of the iris, but the distribution of pigment is often irregular, producing a flecked or maculated appearance.

The iris is not a flat diaphragm; the lens causes it to bulge a little, so that it is more accurately a shallow cone, truncated by the pupillary aperture. Sited between the cornea and lens and immersed in *aqueous fluid*, it partially divides the *anterior segment* into an *anterior chamber*, enclosed by the cornea and iris (meeting at the *iridocorneal angle*) and a confusingly termed *posterior chamber*, between the iris and the lens (**8.416**). Into the latter, ciliary processes protrude from the periphery a little between the divisions of the zonular ligament of the lens; here most of the aqueous fluid is produced, traversing the pupil into the anterior chamber to its exit via the scleral venous sinus (p. 1324) at the iridocorneal angle: the 'filtration angle' in clinical parlance.

Microscopic structure

The microscopic structure of the iris includes several unusual features

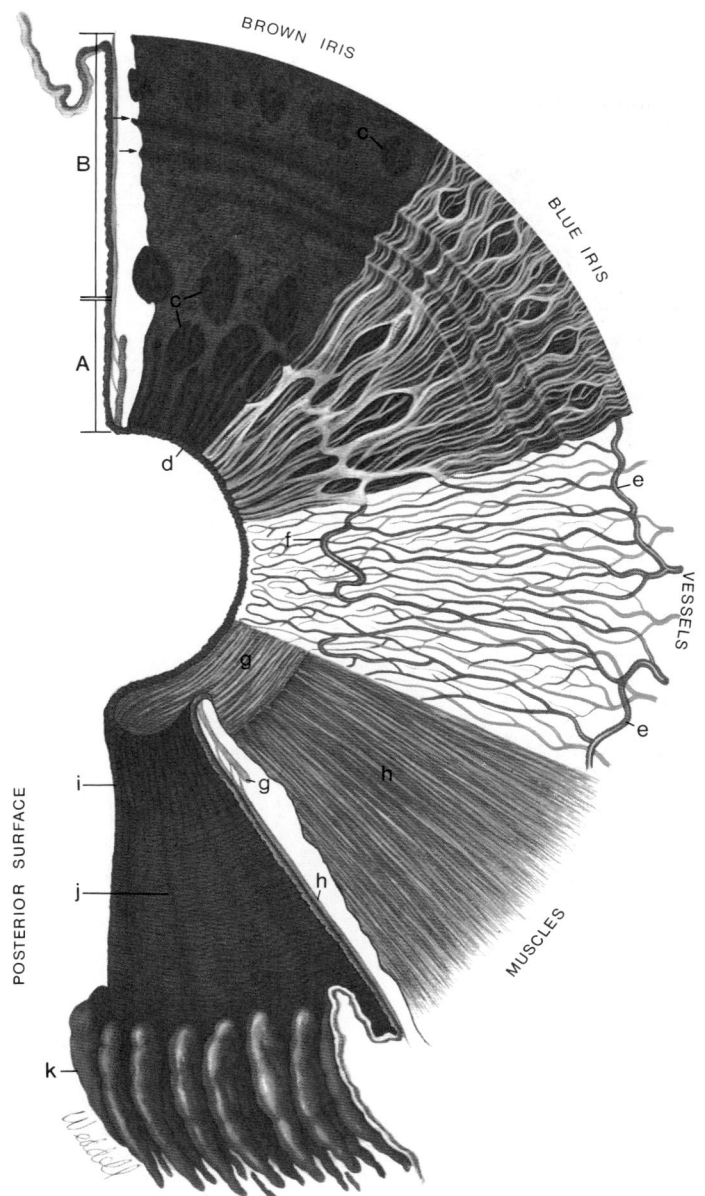

8.426 Composite view of the surfaces and internal strata of the iris. In a clockwise direction from above, the pupillary (A) and ciliary (B) zones are shown in successive segments. The first (brown iris) shows the anterior border layer and the openings of crypts (c). In the second segment (blue iris), the layer is much less prominent and the trabeculae of the stroma are more visible. The third segment shows the iridial vessels, including the major arterial circle (ee) and the incomplete minor arterial circle (f). The fourth segment shows the muscle stratum, including the sphincter (g) and dilatator (h) of the pupil. The everted 'pupillary ruff' of the epithelium on the posterior aspect of the iris (d) appears in all segments. The final segment, folded over for pictorial purposes, depicts this aspect of the iris, showing radial folds (i and j) and the adjoining ciliary processes (k). (See **8**.421 for acknowledgements.)

(8.417). Its anterior surface, forming the posterior boundary of the anterior chamber, possesses no distinct epithelium, despite statements to the contrary; this surface is merely a modified 'anterior border layer' of the general iridial *stroma*. This stroma contains the regional vessels and nerves and, near the pupillary rim, there is an aggregation of smooth muscle cells forming an annular contractile *sphincter pupillae*. The epithelial strata of the posterior aspect of the iris is a continuation of the bilaminar epithelium of the ciliary body representing the two layers of the optic cup. The pupil, through which this epithelium curves for a short distance on to the *anterior* iridial surface as the *pigment ruff* or 'border', therefore corresponds to the

opening of the optic cup. The deeper and hence on the back of the iris the posterior of these two epithelial layers is confusingly termed the *anterior epithelium*; although it is really *posterior* to its stroma. Its cells are pigmented, as are those of the same layer in the ciliary epithelium; from these arise the muscle fibre processes forming the dilatator pupillae, which like the sphincter has a most unusual embryological origin, from the neural ectoderm of the optic cup or, recent evidence indicates, the neural crest. Superficial (posterior) to this layer is a stratum of heavily pigmented cells, the so-called *posterior epithelium*, continuous with the internal *non-pigmented*, retinal layer of the ciliary epithelium.

The anterior iridial surface (anterior border layer) has been much studied at low magnification by slit-lamp microscopy; it then appears somewhat fluffy, except when heavily pigmented. *Crypts*, through which vessels may be visible in the stroma, and various radial and circular folds and striae can be observed (Vogt 1942). The constituents of this anterior border lamina are mainly dendritic fibroblasts and melanocytes, with no vestige of the endothelium which covers it at birth but rapidly disappears during the early postnatal years (Vrabec 1952). Electron microscopy confirms this (Tousimis & Fine 1959). Fibroblasts form an almost continuous surface monolayer; their branching processes form no actual junctions (Smelser & Ishikawa 1966). At the iridial periphery they blend with the trabecular connective tissue (pectinate ligament) of the iridocorneal angle. At the pupillary rim they meet the epithelium of the posterior iridial surface. Melanocytes are also intricately branched, again with no special junctions between them. Some capillaries invade the border layer. Naked sympathetic axons have also been found closely apposed to the melanocytes and fibroblasts, suggesting the release of transmitter substances into the anterior chamber (Ringvold 1975).

The *stroma of the iris* is, like the anterior border layer, derived most probably from neural crest between the developing lens and optic cup and is also formed of fibroblasts, melanocytes and a loose collagenous matrix. The intercellular spaces appear to communicate freely with the anterior chamber and interchange of fluid between the two may assist the large changes in thickness occurring during contraction and relaxation of the iris. The mesodermal stroma also contains not only abundant blood vessels and nerves but also the ectodermal sphincter and dilatator muscles. There is no elastic tissue. The elastic recoil sometimes attributed to the iris as a dilator force when the sphincter is relaxed must reside in other structures, if it exists at all. Collagen fibrils, about 60 nm in diameter, are loosely arranged, many describing incomplete circumferential loops around the pupil. 'Clump' cells, mast cells, macrophages and lymphocytes have also been described in the stroma.

Muscles of the iris

Sphincter pupillae. This is a flat annulus of smooth muscle about 0.75 mm wide and 0.15 mm thick. Its densely packed fusiform myocytes are often arranged in small bundles, as in the ciliary muscle, and pass circumferentially around the pupil. Collagenous connective tissue lies in front of and behind the muscle fibres and is very dense posteriorly, where it binds the sphincter to the pupillary end of the dilator muscle. Ultramicroscopy shows that muscle fascicles are well innervated, although muscle cells are also electrically coupled at gap junctions. Small nerves ramify in the connective tissue between bundles, most of their fibres being non-myelinated and often enclosed in common Schwann cell sheaths. They do not approach the surfaces of myocytes more closely than 0.1 μm.

Dilatator pupillae. A thin stratum lying immediately anterior to the epithelium of the posterior iridial surface, its fibres are in fact the muscular processes of the anterior layer of this epithelium, whose cells are therefore myoepithelial; their apical processes form the epithelium itself. Myofilaments appear in both parts of these cells but more abundantly in their fusiform basal muscular processes, which are about 4 μm thick, 7 μm wide and 60 μm in length; they form a stratum 3–5 elements thick through most of the iris, from its periphery to the outer perimeter of the sphincter which it slightly overlaps. Here the dilator thins out, sending spurs to blend with the sphincter; unlike the apical parts of the myocytes these have a basal lamina and are joined by gap junctions like those between the sphincteric myocytes. Myelinated nerve fibres appear near their muscular processes or 'fibres' and these terminate as unmyelinated fibres close (about 20 nm) to their surfaces.

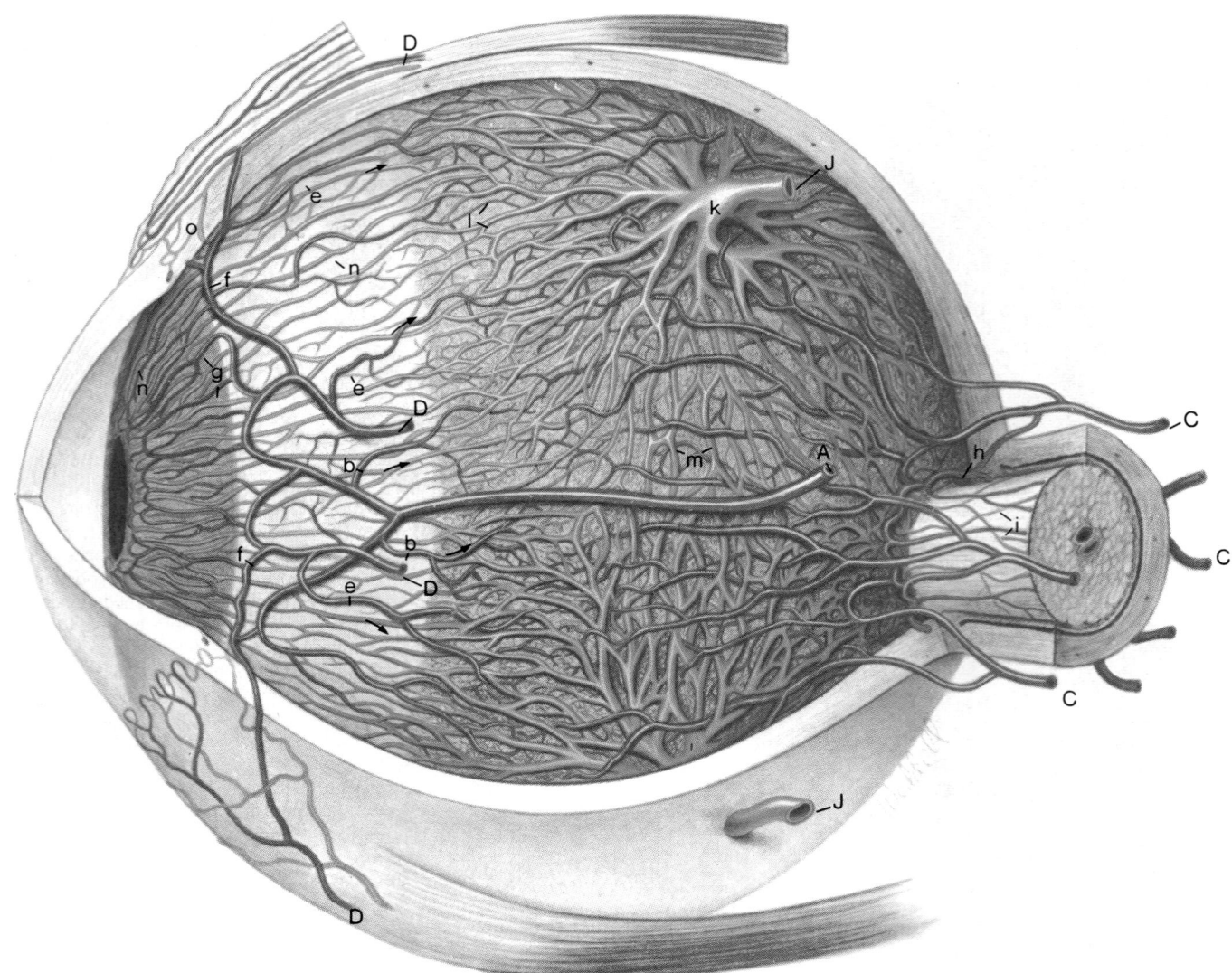

8.427 The vascular arrangements of the uveal tract. The long posterior ciliary arteries, one of which is visible (A), branch at the ora serrata (bb) and feed the capillaries of the anterior part of the choroid. Short posterior ciliary arteries (CC) divide rapidly to form the posterior part of the choriocapillaris. Anterior ciliary arteries (DD) send recurrent branches to the choriocapillaris (ee) and anterior rami to the major arterial circle (ff). Branches from the circle extend into the iris (g) and to the limbus. Branches of the short posterior ciliary arteries (CC) form an anastomotic circle (h) (of Zinn) round the optic disc, and twigs (i) from this join an arterial network on the optic nerve. The vorticose veins (JJ) are formed by the junctions (k) of supra-choroidal tributaries (l). Smaller tributaries are also shown (m, n). The veins draining the scleral venous sinus (o) join anterior ciliary veins and vorticose tributaries. (See **8.**421 for acknowledgement.)

Vessels of the iris (8.426–428)

The arteries arise from the long posterior and anterior ciliary arteries and from those in the ciliary processes. Both long ciliary arteries, on reaching the attached margin of the iris, divide into an upper and a lower branch anastomosing with corresponding arteries from the opposite side and with the anterior ciliary arteries, to form a vascular circle, the *circulus arteriosus major*. From this, vessels converge to the free margin of the iris, anastomosing to form a *circulus arteriosus minor*; this is incomplete and some regard its vessels as venous. The smaller arteries and veins are very similar in their structure and also share some peculiarities; they are often slightly helical, perhaps allowing them to adapt to changes in iridial shape as the pupil varies in size, which may also account for the peculiar structure of their vascular walls. All these vessels, including the capillaries, have a non-fenestrated endothelium and a prominent, often thick basal lamina. In the arteries and veins, there is no elastic lamina and myocytes are few, especially in the veins; connective tissue in the tunica media is loose and external to this a remarkably dense collagenous adventitia appears to form almost a separate tube. The loose stratum of the media has been regarded as a lymph space but this is improbable; it is about 7 μm in width and contains matrix probably derived from the endothelial basal lamina (Hogan et al 1971).

Nerves of the iris

As in the choroid, the nerves come chiefly from branches of the long ciliary rami of the nasociliary nerve and from the short ciliary rami of the ciliary ganglion, the latter providing postganglionic non-myelinated axons innervating the sphincter pupillae. The dilatator is supplied by non-myelinated postganglionic fibres from the superior sympathetic ganglion; their routes are not certain and may vary in different species and they may be multiple in man. The internal carotid sympathetic plexus is said to send a branch via the ciliary ganglion, reaching the eye in the short ciliary nerves; but some may travel in the long ciliary nerves. The innervation of iridial muscles, as also of the ciliaris, is probably more complex; both the sphincter and the dilatator may have a double autonomic supply. Histo-chemical stains for acetylcholinesterase and fluorescent techniques have demonstrated cholinergic and adrenergic activity in both muscles (Ehinger & Falck 1966; Lowenstein & Loewenfeld 1970). Though ganglion cells have been noted in the iris, almost all nerve fibres are probably postganglionic. They form a plexus around the

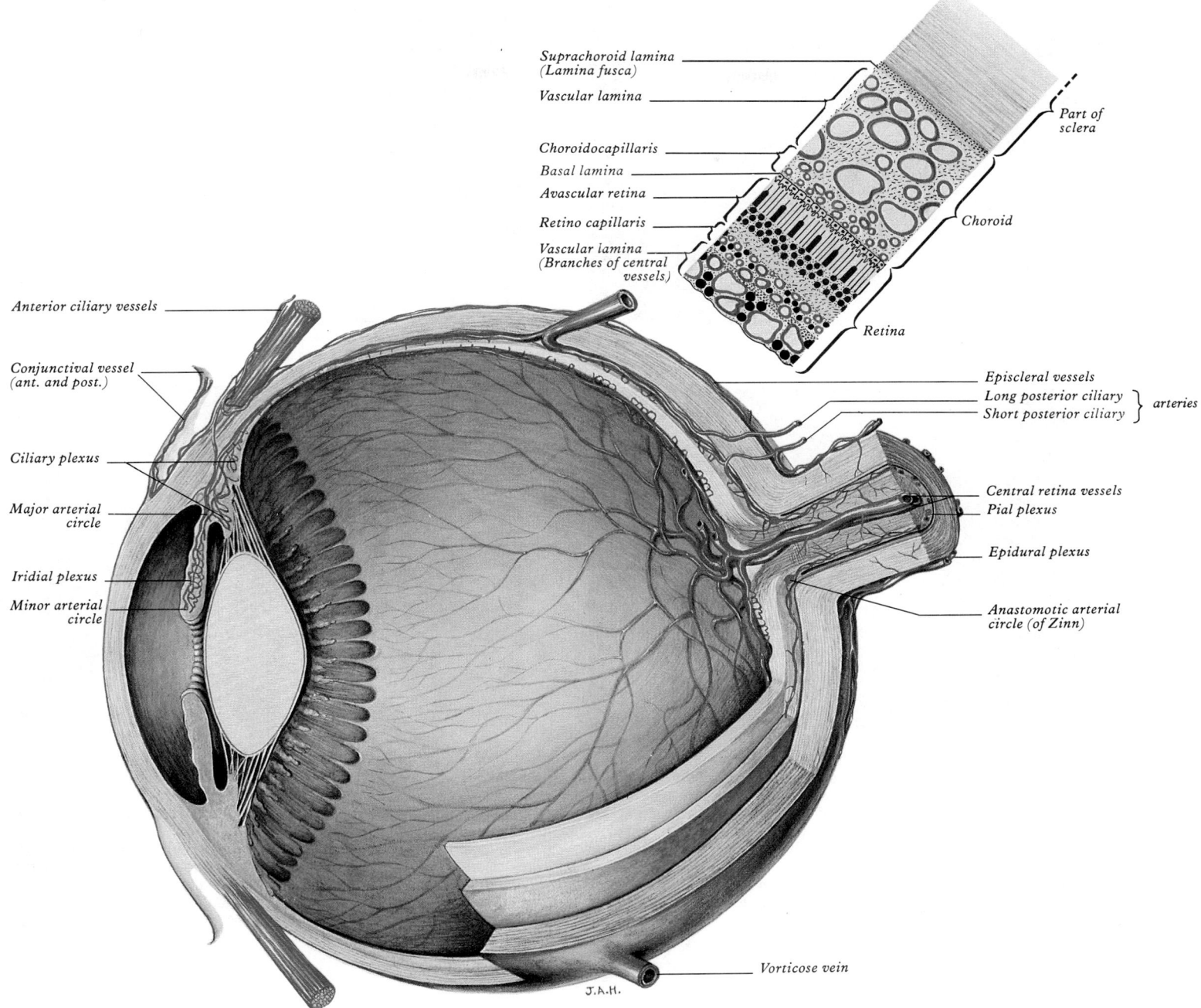

Suprachoroid lamina
(Lamina fusca)

Vascular lamina

Choroidocapillaris

Basal lamina

Avascular retina

Retino capillaris

Vascular lamina
(Branches of central
vessels)

Part of
sclera

Choroid

Retina

Anterior ciliary vessels

Conjunctival vessel
(ant. and post.)

Ciliary plexus

Major arterial
circle

Iridial plexus

Minor arterial
circle

Episcleral vessels

Long posterior ciliary
Short posterior ciliary   } arteries

Central retina vessels

Pial plexus

Epidural plexus

Anastomotic arterial
circle (of Zinn)

Vorticose vein

J.A.H.

8.428   The main features of the vascularity of the eye. The thickness of the sclera, cornea, choroid and neural retina are exaggerated, and the regional variations should be noted. The section of ocular wall at higher magnification is included for particular reference to the avascular zones of the retina (which contain the photoreceptors) and their dual relationship to the vascular laminae and capillary plexuses of the choroid and retina.

periphery of the iris, from which small nerves and fibres extend to the two muscles, to vessels, the anterior border layer and the anterior epithelium (though not the pigment layer) of the posterior layer of the iris. Some fibres may be afferent and some are vasomotor but little is known of either. (For distribution of non-myelinated autonomic nerve fibres in the choroid consult Ruskell 1971.) It is difficult to identify afferent nerve endings in the iris and ciliary body or to distinguish them from efferent autonomic endings, but such endings have been described in monkeys, using mitochondrial accumulations as a criterion (Bergmanson 1978; Cauna 1966; Macintosh 1974). Trigeminal (ophthalmic division) terminals and also autonomic endings in these sites are said to display this feature.

Pupillary membrane

In fetuses the pupil is closed by a thin, vascular *pupillary membrane* (p. 261). Its vessels are partly from those of the iridial margin and partly from those of the lens capsule; they end in loops near the membrane's centre, which is avascular. About the sixth month of gestation, the membrane begins absorption from the centre towards the periphery; at birth only scattered fragments remain but exceptionally it may persist and interfere with vision.

RETINA

MACROSCOPIC APPEARANCE

The retina (**8**.416, 428) is the neural, sensory stratum of the eyeball. It is thin, being thickest (0.56 mm) near the optic disc, diminishing to 0.1 mm anterior to the equator and continuing at this thickness to the ora serrata (**8**.428). It is even thinner at the optic disc and the fovea of the macula (Spence et al 1969). External to it is the choroid,

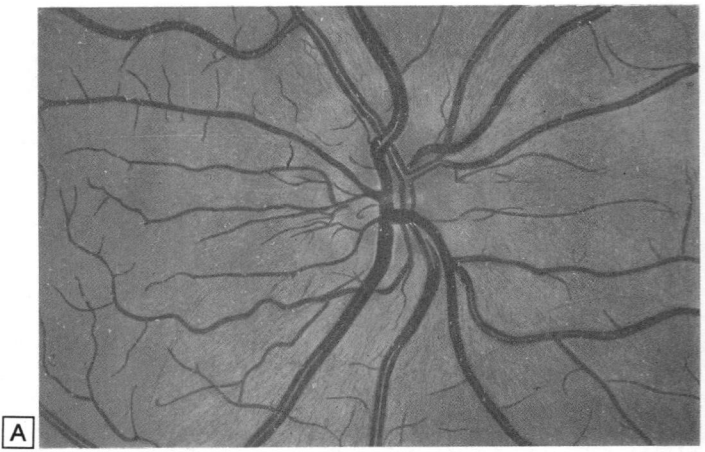

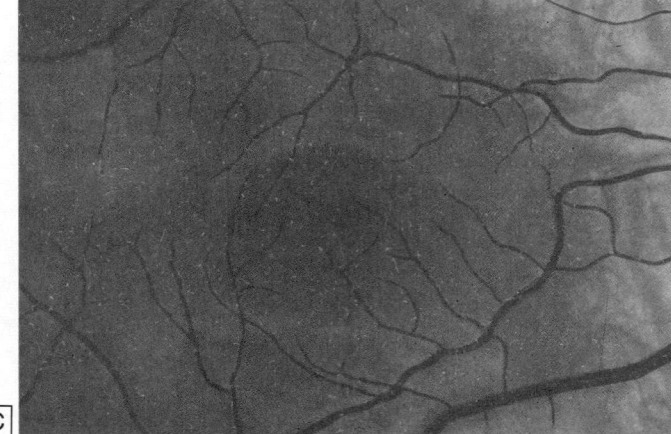

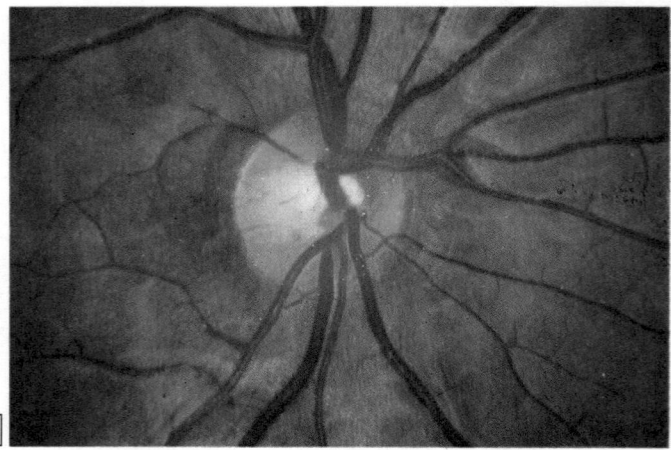

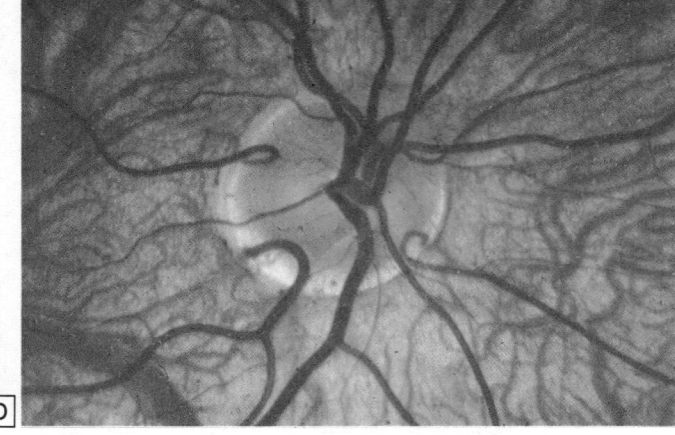

8.429   Ophthalmoscopic photographs of the right human retina.
A   Note dichotomous branching of vessels, arteries being brighter red and showing a more pronounced 'reflex' to light, as a pale stria along their length. The veins are also larger in calibre; more of them cross arteries superficially than is usual. The optic disc, around the entry of the vessels, is a light pink, with a surrounding zone of heavier pigmentation. Compare with **8.430**A from the same Caucasian adult.
B   Appearances in a heavily pigmented individual (Negroid adult), with a paler optic disc than in A. Note accentuation of the edge of the disc by retinal and choroidal pigmentation. The arteries cross the veins superficially in this retina.

C   Normal macula of a young Caucasian subject. Note the fovea, showing as a central, paler, circular area. The macular branches of the central retinal artery are approaching from the right. The macula is largely free of vessels of macroscopic size, but the capillaries here form a particularly close network, except at the fovea.
D   The region of the optic disc in an eye with poorly developed pigmentation. Three cilioretinal arteries are curving round the edge of the disc (two on the left, one on the right). Between the two cilioretinal arteries a single macular artery is apparent. Due to the depressed pigmentation choroidal vessels are also visible, especially veins; and on the left of the photograph two large vorticose venous tributaries can be seen.

internal to it the hyaloid membrane of the vitreous body. At the optic disc of the retina it is continuous with the optic nerve. Anteriorly, at the ora serrata (p. 1328), a thin, non-neural prolongation of the retina extends forwards over the ciliary processes and iris as the *ciliary* and *iridial parts of the retina*, which consist of retinal pigmented and columnar epithelial layers only (see above). From the optic disc to the ora serrata extends the *optic part of the retina*. This is soft, translucent and purple in the fresh, unbleached state, due to the presence of *rhodopsin* (*visual purple*) but soon becomes opaque and bleached when exposed to light. (It is hence difficult to demonstrate rhodopsin; in eyes preserved for dissection the *fixed* retina is cloudy white.) Near the centre of the retina is an oval, yellowish area, the *macula lutea* (**8.415**, 430c,D), which has a central depression, the *fovea centralis*, where visual resolution is highest. At the fovea, the retina is exceedingly thin, some of its layers being absent, and the dark choroid is distinctly visible through it. About 3 mm nasal to the macula lutea the optic nerve is continuous with the retina at the *optic disc*, about 1.5 mm in diameter. The circumference of the disc is slightly raised, while centrally it has a shallow depression, being pierced in this area by the central retinal vessels (**8.415**, 429, 430). The disc ('blind spot') is devoid of photoreceptors and therefore insensitive to light. By ophthalmoscopy it is

normally pink but it is much paler than the retina and may be grey or almost white. In optic atrophy the capillary vessels disappear and the disc is then white. The name 'optic papilla', often applied to the disc, is a misnomer; almost all of the normal disc is level with the retina and centrally *depressed*.

MICROSTRUCTURE OF THE RETINA

The retina is derived from the two layers of the invaginated optic vesicle (pp. 224, 259), the outer becoming the lamina of pigment cells, the inner developing into a complex multilaminar structure of sensory and neural cells. Anteriorly, as the retina approaches the ora serrata and merges into the ciliary body and iris, sensory and neural cells are absent (although in some non-mammalian forms this provides an area from which new photoreceptors and nerve cells can be recruited throughout life). These non-nervous regions have already been considered, and will not be described here.

The 'retina proper' contains a variety of cell types. They include the photoreceptors (rod and cone cells), their first order neurons (bipolar cells) and the somata and axons of the second order neurons (ganglion cells); also present are two major classes of interneurons arranged amongst the other cells, the horizontal and amacrine cells.

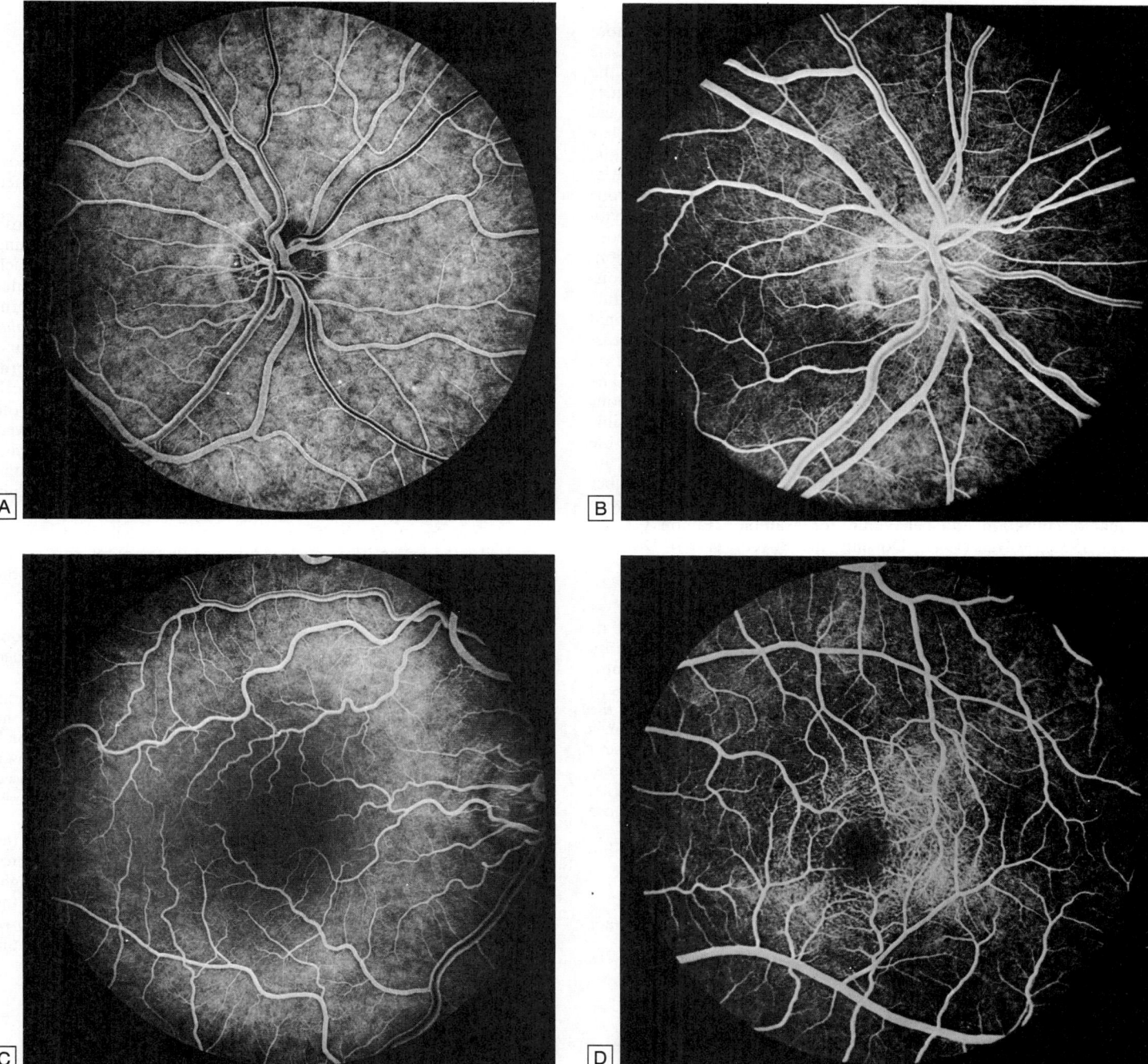

8.430 Fluorescence angiograms of the retina. These are produced by photography with a fundus camera at known periods of time following introduction of fluorescein into the circulation. (For details of the technique consult Rosen (1969) to whom we are indebted for all the colour photographs and angiograms in this illustration and **8.429**.)

A Angiogram of the same retina as that appearing in **8.429A** taken in 'mid-venous' phase. The arteries display an even fluorescence, but the veins appear striped, due to laminar flow. This appearance is the reverse of and not to be compared with the arterial 'reflex' which is seen in **8.429A**. The background mottling is due to fluorescence from the choroidal vessels.

B Angiogram of the left optic disc, showing the major arteries and veins and also their smaller branches. Note particularly the radial pattern in the retinal capillaries. The laminar flow in the veins is less obvious than in **8.430A**.

C Angiogram showing the macular region of a right eye. The main macular vessels are approaching from the right. The subject was an elderly person with considerable macular pigmentation, which masks fluorescence from the choroidal circulation. Compare with **8.430D**.

D Angiogram of the macula of a young subject (left eye) showing the macular capillaries in detail. Note the central avascular fovea. Compare with **8.430C**.

The retina also contains neuroglial elements and a rich vascular system, chiefly of capillaries, and is backed by specialized pigment epithelial cells.

Clearly, the retina is a most complex structure, and indeed is best viewed as a special area of the brain, from which it is derived by outgrowth from the diencephalon, dedicated to the detection and early analysis of visual information. In the present account the retina is dealt with separately from its central nervous connections. This is forced by practical considerations, but the organization of the retina can only really be appreciated if it is seen as an integrated part of the much larger apparatus of visual analysis present in the thalamus, cortex and other areas of the central nervous system (CNS). In the present account concentration will be on the structure and functions of the cells within the confines of the retina itself, and the reader is

1335

referred to the description of the central visual system for the rest of the story.

The modern period of retinal research has now spanned more than a century, inaugurated by the publication of Cajal's classic accounts of the retinal cells and their connections as seen with the recently perfected Golgi methods. Since then, many new techniques have become available for structural, physiological, biochemical and psychophysical research. In particular, electron microscopy has revolutionized our understanding of retinal organization, a technique enhanced in recent years by painstaking reconstruction from serial ultrathin sections. This approach has been accompanied by numerous other methods for studying the shapes, composition, connectivity and electrophysiological properties of retinal cells, so that a considerable body of knowledge exists about retinal form and function. Many of the earlier and, indeed, more recent studies were on various species of lower vertebrates and non-primate mammals, but it became apparent that while all vertebrates share a basic common retinal pattern, its details vary considerably even among mammals. Increasingly, research has concentrated on primates, and in recent years on human eyes from therapeutic enucleations or other sources. The picture at present is far from complete, and has many contradictions and uncertainties. For clarity, and to avoid as far as possible confusion over nomenclature, the present account will centre on the primate retina except where comparisons with other species are relevant. While the literature is very extensive, there are a number of classic reviews and more recent general accounts which deal with retinal organization and behaviour, for example, Ramón y Cajal (1893, 1933), Polyak (1941), Dowling and Boycott (1966), Dowling (1987), Wässle and Boycott (1991), and Kolb (1994).

Retinal layers

These are zones of the retina where distinctive components of its cells are clustered together or in register to form continuous strata (8.431, 433, 434). They extend uninterrupted throughout the photoreceptive retina except at the exit point of the optic nerve fibres at the optic disc, although certain strata are much reduced at the foveola where the photoreceptive elements predominate. The names given to the different strata reflect in part the components present within them, and also their position in the thickness of the retina. Conventionally, those structures furthest from the vitreous (i.e. towards the choroid) are designated as **outer** or external, and those towards the vitreous are **inner** or internal.

Customarily, 10 retinal layers are distinguished (8.431); beginning at the choroidal edge and passing towards the vitreous, these are:

(1) the retinal pigment epithelium
(2) the lamina of rods and cones (outer segments and inner segments)
(3) the external limiting lamina
(4) outer nuclear layer
(5) outer plexiform layer (OPL)
(6) inner nuclear layer (INL)
(7) inner plexiform layer (IPL)
(8) ganglion cell layer
(9) lamina of nerve fibres
(10) internal limiting lamina.

Some of these are subdivisible into substrata, and an innermost plexiform layer between layers 8 and 9 has also been demonstrated (see below).

The components of these layers belong to the retinal cells, i.e. rod and cone, bipolar, horizontal, ganglion and amacrine, intervening glial cells, and pigment epithelial cells. *Rod and cone cells* reach radially inwards from the rod and cone lamina through the outer nuclear layer, where they have their nuclei, to the outer plexiform layer in which they synapse with bipolar and horizontal cells. *Bipolar cells* possess dendrites in the outer plexiform layer, cell bodies and nuclei in the inner nuclear layer, and axons in the inner plexiform layer where they synapse with ganglion cell and amacrine cell dendrites. *Horizontal cells* have their dendrites and axons in the outer plexiform layer and their nuclei in the inner nuclear layer, while *ganglion cells* have their dendrites in the inner plexiform layer, their cell bodies in the ganglionic layer, and their axons in the lamina of nerve fibres (and optic nerve). *Amacrine cell* dendrites are mainly in the inner plexiform layer, although some (interplexiform cells) extend into the outer plexiform layer; amacrine cell dendrites are either situated in the inner nuclear layer or in the outer part of the ganglionic layer (displaced amacrines). Pigment cells lie behind the retina, and glial cells are distributed in distinctive locations among its different layers.

Before considering the retinal cell types and their connections further, the composition of the different retinal layers will be outlined briefly. These are as follows:

Layer 1: pigment epithelium. A layer of simple low cuboidal epithelium, it forms the back of the retina, and, therefore, the boundary with the choroid which is separated from it by a thick composite basement membrane (Bruch's membrane: see also below).

Layer 2: rod and cone processes. This is a lamina composed of the photoreceptive outer segments and the outer part of the inner segments of rod and cone cells.

Layer 3: external limiting lamina. A layer consisting of the junctional zones between radial glial (Müller) cells and photoreceptor processes, it appears as a stainable line (see also p. 1346) by light microscopy. Originally thought to be the outer boundary of the compact part of the neural retina, electron microscopy has shown that it consists of a stratum of intercellular junctions of the zonula

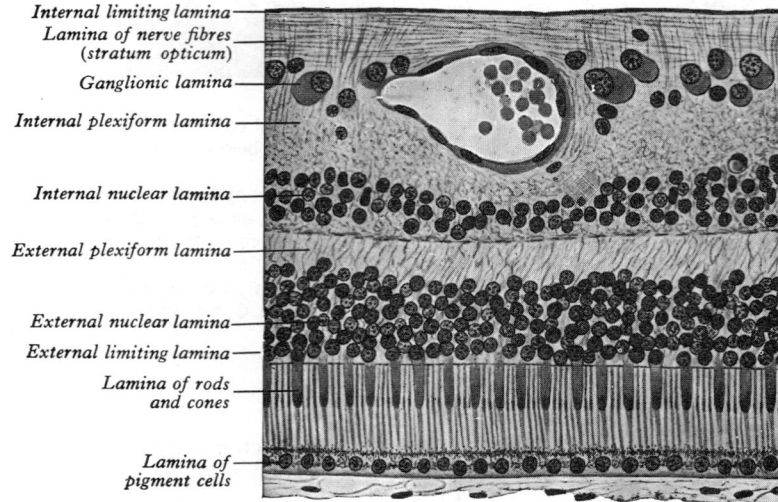

Internal limiting lamina
Lamina of nerve fibres (stratum opticum)
Ganglionic lamina
Internal plexiform lamina
Internal nuclear lamina
External plexiform lamina
External nuclear lamina
External limiting lamina
Lamina of rods and cones
Lamina of pigment cells

8.431 Section through the primate retina, from its vitreous aspect (above) to the choroid tunic (below), showing its layered structure some little distance from the macular region.

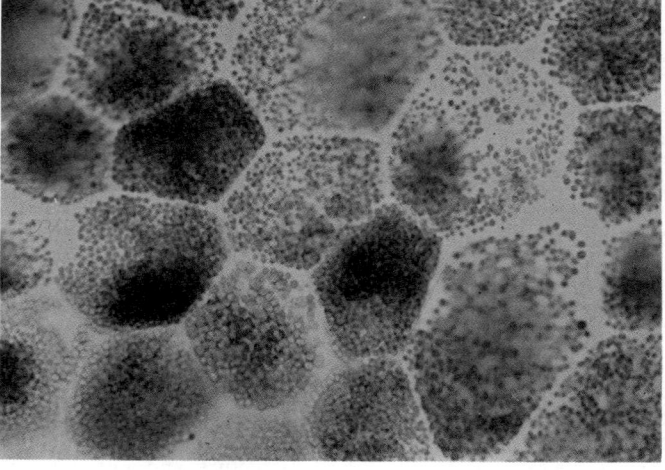

8.432 Colour photograph of unstained retinal pigment epithelium seen in surface view (human, aged 40 years). Magnification × 3500. (Preparation loaned by John Marshall, Institute of Ophthalmology, London.)

adherens type (p. 27) associated with dense cytoplasmic material within the radial processes of Müller cells (see also below).

Layer 4: outer nucleur layer. This comprises several tiers of rod and cone cell bodies with their nuclei. Mingled with these are the outer and inner fibres from the same cell bodies, directed outward to the bases of inner segments, and inwards towards the outer plexiform layer.

Layer 5: outer plexiform layer. A region of complex synaptic interactions between the processes of the cells whose cell bodies lie in the abutting laminae. As already noted, the outer plexiform layer has the synaptic processes of rod and cone cells, bipolar cells, horizontal cells, and some interplexiform cells (in this account grouped with the amacrines). It is sometimes subdivided into an outer stratum of synapses with rods and cones, and an inner stratum where interactions between other cells occur.

Layer 6: inner nuclear layer. This is composed of three nuclear strata: horizontal cell nuclei form the outermost zone, then in sequence inwards, the nuclei and cell bodies of bipolar cells, Müller cells and the outer set of amacrine cells, including interplexiform cells whose dendrites traverse this layer.

Layer 7: inner plexiform layer. This is divisible into three layers depending on the types of contact occurring: an outer *stratum a*, or 'OFF' stratum is where 'OFF' bipolar cells, ganglion cells and some amacrines synapse (see below); a middle *stratum b*, or 'ON' stratum contains synapses between the axons of 'ON' bipolars and the dendrites of ganglion cells and 'displaced' amacrines, and an inner 'rod' *stratum c* is where rod bipolars synapse with 'displaced' amacrines. Further details of these interactions are given later.

Layer 8: ganglion cell layer. This is really a misnomer because it also contains the nuclei of the 'displaced' amacrine cells, although its inner regions consist of the cell bodies, nuclei and initial segments of retinal ganglion cells of various classes.

Layer 9: nerve fibre layer. Containing the unmyelinated axons of retinal ganglion cells, this layer forms a zone of variable thickness over the retinal inner surface. It is the only component of the retina where the fibres pass into the nerve at the optic disc. Also present on the inner aspect of this layer are the nuclei and processes of astrocytes which, with those of Müller cells, ensheath the nerve fibres. Between the nerve fibre layer and the ganglion cells is another narrow *superficial plexiform layer* where neuronal processes make synaptic contact with the axon hillocks and initial segments of ganglion cells.

Layer 10: internal limiting lamina. A glial boundary between the retina and the vitreous body, formed by the end feet of Müller cells and astrocytes, it is separated by a basal lamina from the vitreous body (see also below).

The thicknesses of the different layers vary throughout the retina, being generally greatest in the central region and gradually diminishing peripherally. For example, the external nuclear lamina ranges from 27 μm in peripheral retina to 50 μm in the fovea, representing in the former a single row of cones with four of rod nuclei, and in the latter about 10 rows of cone nuclei. An exception to this is the foveola, which is almost totally made of cones, with fewer bipolar cells and ganglion cells; for further details of this region, see below (p. 1347).

CELLS OF THE RETINA

Cells of the retina are: retinal pigment cells; cone and rod cells; the neurons of the retina—bipolar, horizontal, ganglion and amacrine

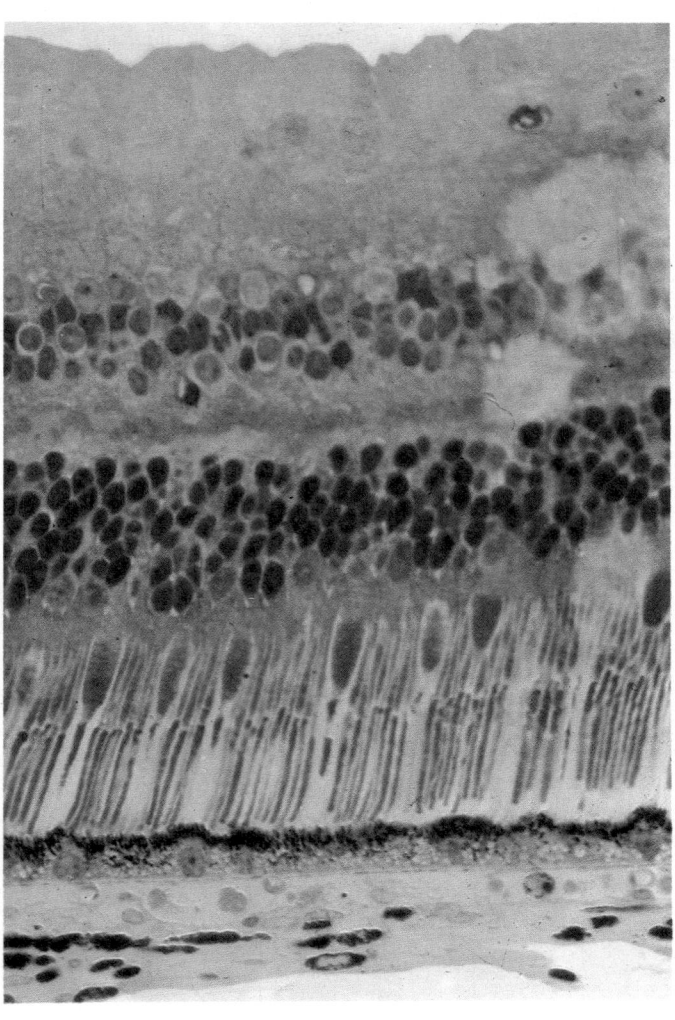

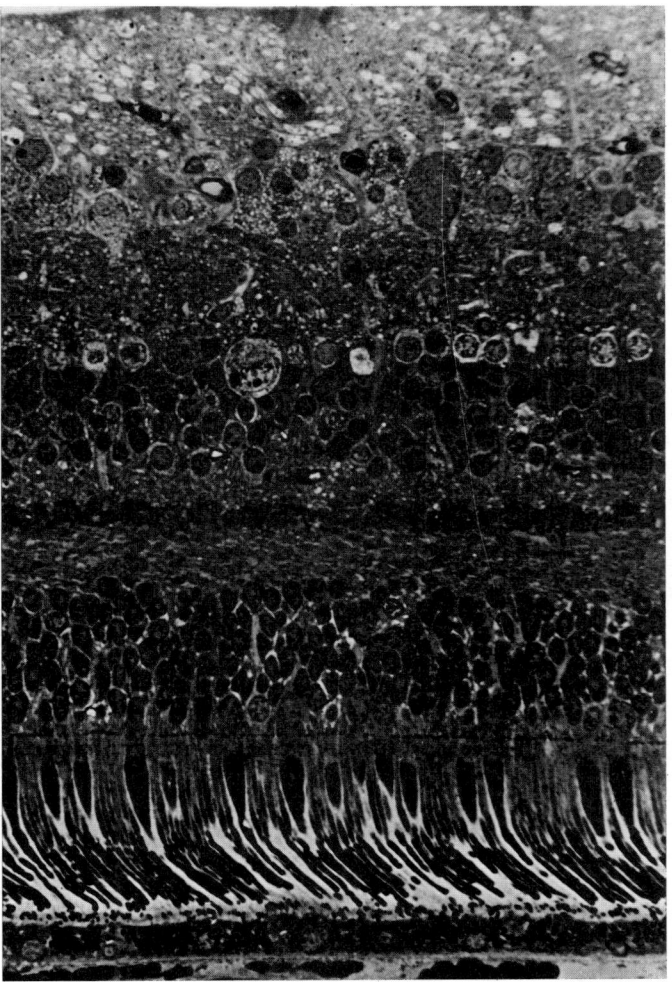

8.433   Thin section of simian retina in araldite-embedded material, stained by toluidine blue. Compare with 8.431. (Provided by N A Locket, Institute of Ophthalmology, London.)

8.434   Light micrograph of the retina of a 19-year-old male. Toluidine blue stain, resin-embedded. Magnification × 1750. (Preparation provided by John Marshall, Institute of Ophthalmology, London.)

cells; and neuroglial elements—radial glial (Müller) cells, astrocytes and microglial cells.

Retinal pigment epithelial cells (8.431–435)

The retinal pigment epithelial cells are low cuboidal cells which form a single continuous layer extending from the periphery of the optic disc to the ora serrata, then continuing from there into the ciliary epithelium (p. 1328). The cells are flat rectangles in radial section and hexagonal or pentagonal in surface view. They number about 4–6 million in the human retina. Near the macula they are about 10 by 14 μm in their radial and tangential dimensions respectively but are much flatter near the ora serrata (Ts'o & Friedman 1968; Watzke et al 1993). Their nuclei are basally placed, near the basal lamina of the choroid (p. 1326) and separated from it by their own basal lamina which is much infolded into grooves in the basal plasma membrane and joined to Bruch's membrane dividing the retina from the choriocapillaris (see p. 1327). Apically (towards the rods and cones) the cells bear long (5–7 μm) microvilli which contact or project between the outer ends of rod and cone processes. The tips of rod outer segments are deeply inserted into invaginations in the apical membrane. The cytoplasm contains numerous melanin granules and organelles associated with melanin synthesis, including arrays of granular and agranular endoplasmic reticulum, Golgi complexes, premelanosomes and melanosomes (Breathnach & Wylie 1966; Seyi 1967) and mitochondria. Also conspicuous are the phagocytosed ends of rods and cones and their remnants undergoing lysosomal destruction; the final products of this process are lipofuscin granules, which accumulate in these cells and add to their granular appearance. They also contain a cytoskeleton of actin filaments, microtubules and intermediate filaments of the vimentin type, although when proliferating they are also positive for a number of keratin types (Hunt and Davis 1990).

The lateral membranes of adjacent pigment cells do not interdigitate much, but form a zone of complex tight junctions around their apical ends (i.e. nearest the rods and cones), and, further basally, many gap junctions (Miki et al 1975). A viscous glycosaminoglycan (GAG)-rich substance fills the space between the pigment epithelium and the neural retina (Bishop et al 1993); this probably acts as a conducting medium for ionic currents as well as a glue attaching the neural retina to the pigment epithelium (and thence to the choroid).

Functions of pigment cells. These cells carry out a range of activities vital to vision (see the review by Bok 1993). Most intensively studied is their role in the turnover of rod and cone photoreceptive components. Autoradiography and ultramicroscopy (Young & Bok 1969; Spitznas & Hogan 1970; see also Bosch et al 1993) have shown that the terminal parts of the rods and cones are constantly being shed (see p. 1136) and phagocytosed by the pigment cells, then degraded within phagosomal vacuoles by lysosomal action as they pass deeper into the cells (Marshall & Ansell 1971; Bosch et al 1993; Deguchi et al 1994), the whole process being a vital part of the receptor membrane renewal cycle of photoreceptors. The failure of some part of this process may cause progressive loss of retinal function and eventual blindness, for example as when enzyme deficiencies cause the build-up of shed, but undegraded, photoreceptor components within the retina.

Secondly, the epithelium acts as an anti-reflection device, preventing the bouncing of light back into the photoreceptive layer with consequent loss of image sharpness. This process is complex, as the energy absorbed might be expected to be dissipated as heat or the production of free radicals, both potentially damaging products. Very intense light may indeed damage the pigment cells and may cause epithelial breakdown.

Thirdly, the epithelium forms an important *blood–retinal barrier* between the retina and the vascular system of the choroid by virtue of the zone of tight junctions between the pigment cells. These guard the special ionic environment of the retina, and inhibit the entry of leucocytes including lymphocytes into the immunologically sequestered compartment of the eye's interior. The epithelium may also

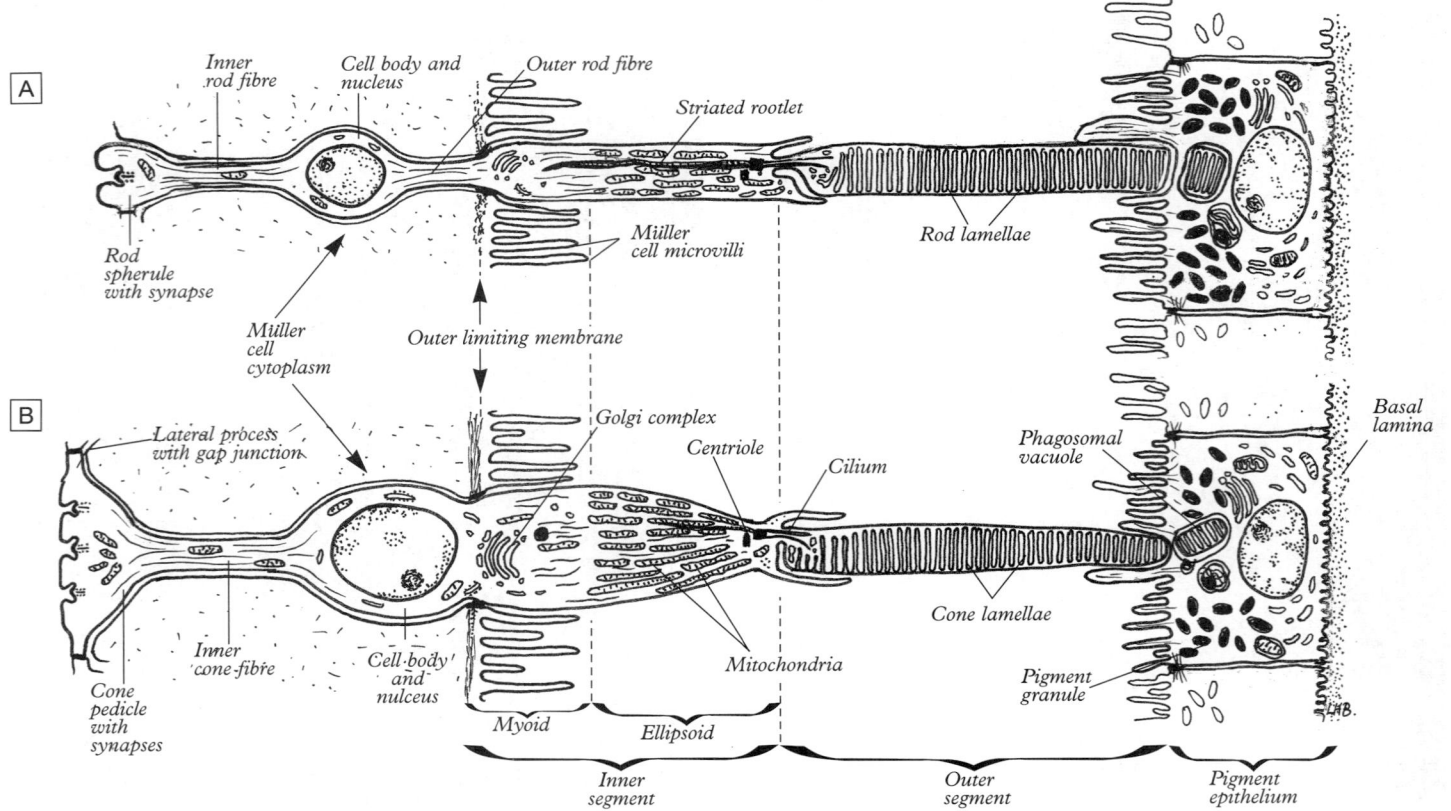

8.435 Diagrams depicting the major organizational features of (A) a retinal rod cell, and (B) a cone cell. Note that the relative size of the pigment epithelial cells has been exaggerated for descriptive purposes.

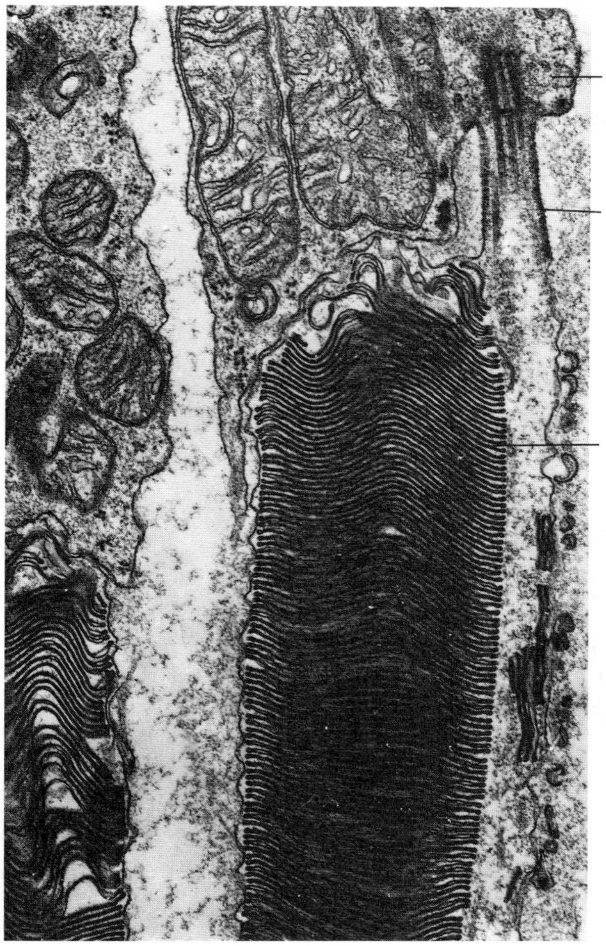

8.436 An electron micrograph of a section of a human retinal rod, showing the junction between the outer and inner segments. The outer segment is made up largely of photoreceptive lamellae (or discs), connected by a short cilium to the inner segment containing large mitochondria. Magnification × 50 000. (Provided by N A Locket, Institute of Ophthalmology, London.)

Inner segment

Cilium

Outer segment

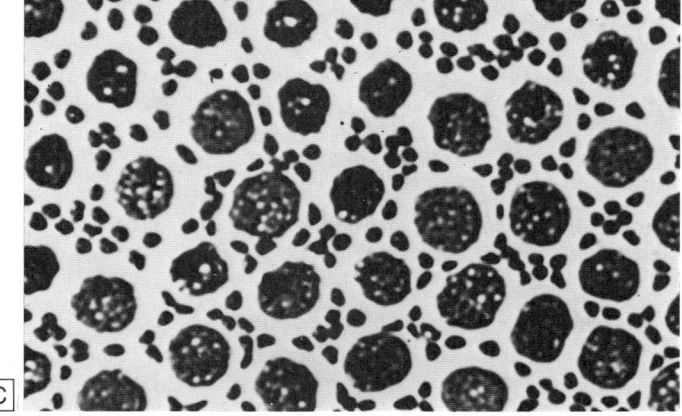

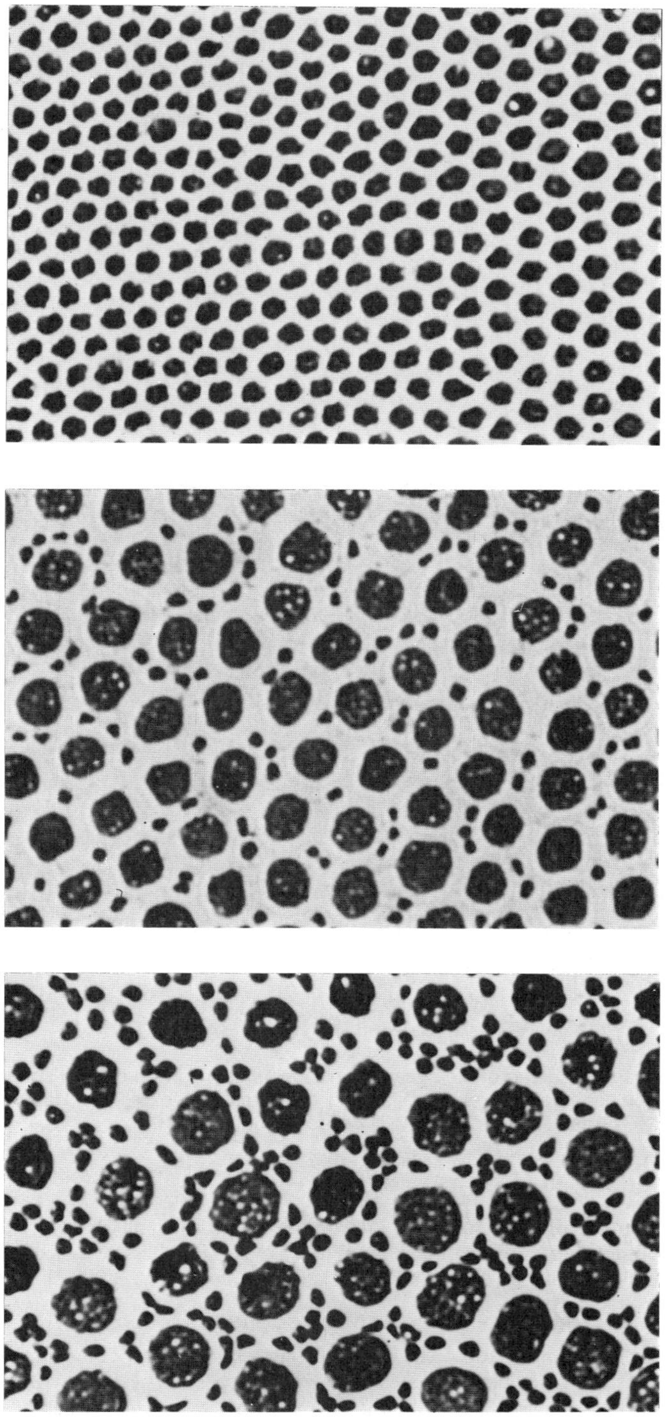

8.437 Tangential sections through the primate retina to show the variations in distribution of rod and cone processes in the foveola (A), fovea (B) and macula (C). Note the *small* cone processes in the foveola, from which rods are absent. The cones, which are elsewhere larger than the rods, predominate in the fovea, rods becoming more numerous towards the periphery. Magnification × 5000. (Preparations supplied by John Marshall, Institute of Ophthalmology, London.)

transport ions and secrete growth factors, among other poorly understood functions. If damaged, the epithelial cells can undergo limited repair by mitosis to reconstitute the blood–retina barrier (Heriot & Machemer 1992).

Cone and rod cells

The cone and rod cells are the retinal photoreceptor cells (**8.435**–437), long, radially orientated structures which have a cylindrical photoreceptive portion at one end (nearest the pigment epithelium) and synaptic contacts at the other end, within the outer plexiform lamina. Both types of cell have a similar organization, although details differ. From external (choroidal) end inwards, the parts of the cells are:

- *outer segment* and
- *inner segment*, together forming a *cone process* or a *rod process* (it should be noted that the terms cone and rod are also often loosely applied to the whole cell); the cone process is wider, but tapers (hence the name), whereas the rod cells are cylindrical. The outer and inner segments are connected by a short *cilium*. The inner segment is subdivided into an outer *ellipsoid* and an inner *myoid*;
- *external fibre* (variable depending on cell types and region of the retina), a narrow process connecting the rods and cones to
- the *cell body* or *soma* containing the nucleus;
- *inner fibre*, another narrow connecting process leading to
- either a *cone pedicle* or a *rod spherule* depending on cell type; this is an area of synaptic contact with adjacent bipolar and horizontal cells and with other cone or rod cells.

Cone cells are chiefly responsible for high spatial resolution and colour vision in good lighting conditions (photopic vision), while rod cells provide high monochromatic sensitivity to a much wider range of illumination down to much lower intensities (scotopic vision) although with relatively low spatial discrimination because of their different neural connections. Cone cells are of three types according to their maximum spectral sensitivities: red, green and blue (see below). Cone cells are highly concentrated in the centre of the retina (the fovea) where visual acuity is greatest, but they

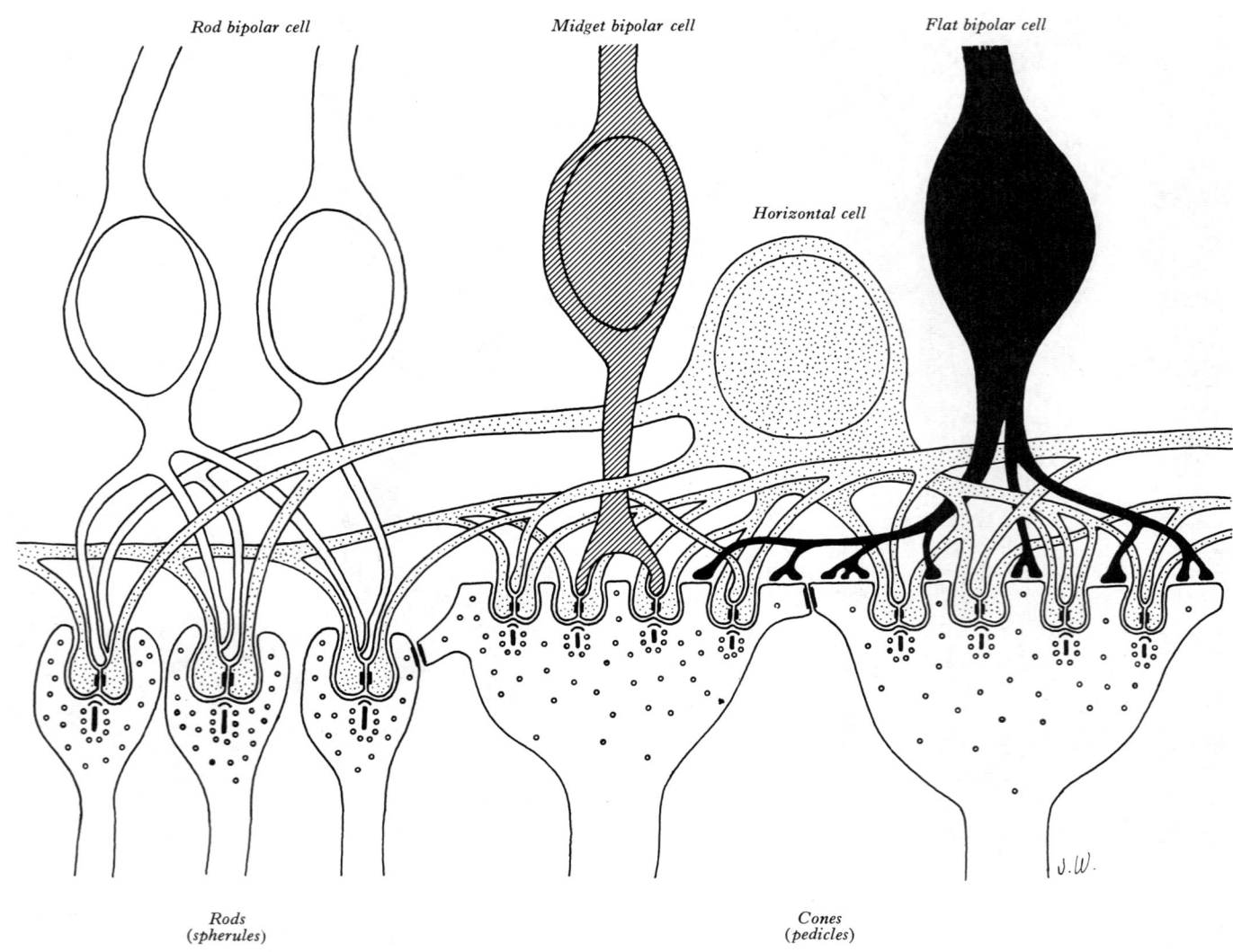

Rod bipolar cell

Midget bipolar cell

Flat bipolar cell

Horizontal cell

*Rods
(spherules)*

*Cones
(pedicles)*

J.W.

8.438 Scheme of the synaptic arrangements involving the rod spherules and cone pedicles of the retina. For details consult text. (From Hogan et al 1971, modified from Dowling & Boycott 1966.)

populate the whole retina, intermingled with rods, as far as its neural edge. Rods are excluded from the fovea. Further details of these distributions are given below.

Structure of cone and rod processes

By light microscopy, the external segments of both cones and rods are refractile, birefringent structures which stain weakly with eosin and are periodic acid-Schiff (PAS)-positive; inner segments stain deeply with eosin and are fibrillar in appearance. The combined outer and inner segments of a rod process measure about 100–120 μm long in freshly fixed human retinae, cone processes being about 65–75 μm (Eichner 1957); both diminish in length towards the ora serrata, especially cone processes. The latter are also much narrower at the fovea where they closely resemble rods in size (see **8**.437; also, e.g., Borwein 1983). The outer segments of rods contain the photoreceptive protein rhodopsin (visual purple); in cones (Rushton 1962) related photosensitive pigments with different absorption properties are present.

Outer segments of cones and rods. Ultrastructurally, cones and rods are broadly similar (Dowling 1965; Cohen 1965; Hogan et al 1971; Dowling 1987). The rod outer segment appears as a remarkably regular series of discoidal membranous sacs, stacked like thin coins and surrounded by a cell membrane, to the outer end of which are opposed the microvilli of pigmented epithelial cells (see above, p. 1338). These discs, numbering 600–1000 in rods of various species, are flat vesicles separated from each other by a less electron-dense intradisc space (**8**.436). In some vertebrates the discs are formed as

continuous infoldings of the lateral cell membrane but in human rods this continuity is lost. However, in cones, this connection persists even in mammals (Cohen 1970; Laties & Liebman 1970; Ripps & Weale 1976). In transverse section the discs of cones are circular, whereas those of rods have a scalloped profile (Cohen 1972). Cone discs are also flatter than those of rods but are more widely spaced, so that the numbers per unit length are similar at about 30 discs per micron.

Both types of disc are continually formed at the end closest to the soma and are progressively pushed away from this point towards the pigment epithelium as new discs are added (Steinberg et al 1980); thus the oldest discs are nearest to the pigment epithelial cells and they eventually break off and are phagocytosed by this epithelial layer (see above). Young (1971) has shown in rhesus monkeys that during 11 days nearly 1000 rod discs are generated proximally and an equal number removed peripherally. Since each pigment cell may interdigitate with 24–45 rod segments, it may engulf 2000–4000 discs per diem. This cycle of removal and renewal was established in various species by following the progression of radioactively labelled disc membranes along rod outer segments in autoradiographs of sectioned retinae (Droz 1968). Evidence for renewal in the outer processes of cones is less certain, although Hogan (1972) has described similar phagocytosis of cones of the human fovea; it may be that the open connections between cone discs and the plasma membrane (see above) allow the insertion of membrane components more randomly, although a proximal–distal progression of labelling also occurs (Eckmiller 1993). Such a rapid turnover of complex

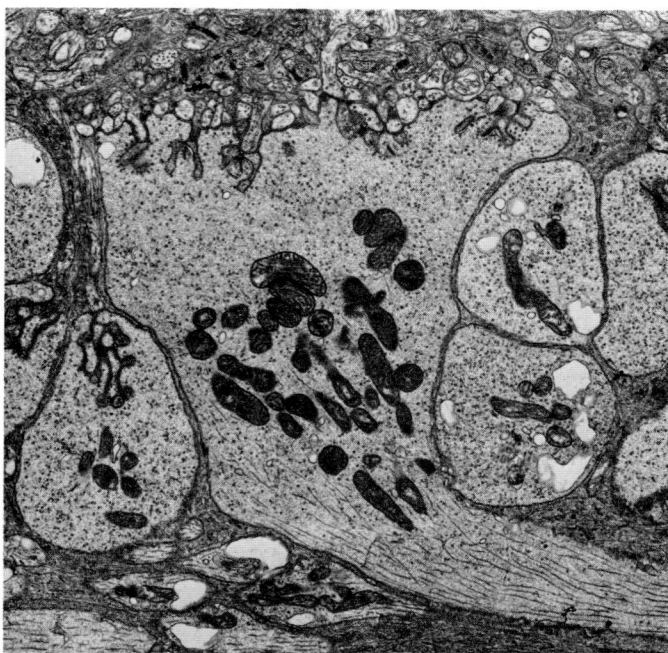

8.439 An electron micrograph of a part of the outer plexiform layer of the retina (monkey), showing synapses at the pedicle base of a cone (centre) and adjacent rod spherules. Note the presence of mitochondria and of synaptic ribbons surrounded by synaptic vesicles in the cone pedicle. The neuropil composed of interweaving dendritic processes of bipolar, horizontal and other cells is shown below. (Supplied by N A Locket, Institute of Ophthalmology, London.)

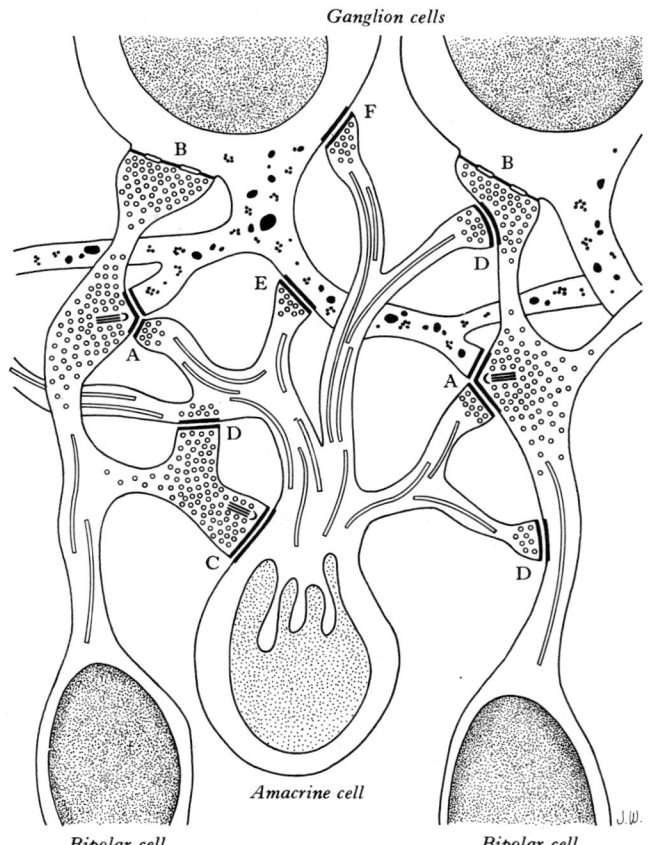

Ganglion cells

Amacrine cell

Bipolar cell   *Bipolar cell*

8.440 A scheme of the synaptic arrangements in the internal plexiform lamina of the retina. Note that bipolar axonal terminals of three types are shown: *axodendritic* (A) in *dyads* involving dendrites of amacrine and ganglion cells, *axosomatic* involving ganglion cells (B) and amacrine cells (C). Similarly the neurites of amacrine cells also make three types of contact: with the axons of bipolar neurons (D) and with the dendrites (E) and somata (F) of ganglion cells. (From Hogan et al 1971, modified from Dowling & Boycott 1966.)

intracellular structures is probably related to a limited lifespan in the photoreceptive molecular assemblies which may be degraded gradually by exposure to light and other environmental factors.

The rod disc membrane consists of a regular array of rhodopsin molecules embedded in a lipid bilayer (Schmidt 1938; Weale 1970), visible by freeze-fracture as densely packed intramembranous particles; each rhodopsin molecule consists of two closely associated components, a transmembrane glycoprotein (about 50 kDa) and the chromophore, 11-cis-retinal. There are also various other proteins within the outer segment cytosol, concerned with amplifying the light signal greatly. Similar, though chemically distinct, protein-chromophore complexes are present in the three colour subtypes of cone.

The molecular events of transduction in rods have been studied extensively, and are known to involve a series of second messenger steps which couple photoreception by rhodopsin to changes in ion conductance in the plasma membrane (see e.g. the review by Yarfitz & Hurley 1994). Briefly, when rhodopsin is activated by light, it catalyses the loading of a second protein, transducin (G-protein) with guanine nucleotide triphosphate (GTP). This then activates an enzyme, a cyclic guanine monophosphate phosphodiesterase (cGMP-PDE), which in turn depletes cyclic GMP within the cell. The final step is related to the permeability of the membrane to sodium ions; in the resting (dark) state there is a steady inward flow of ions through sodium channels in the membrane but to keep the channel open there must be sufficient cGMP available. When this is reduced by the enzyme activity described above, it causes the sodium gate to close and the electrical state of the cell changes, the outer segment becoming hyperpolarized. This change causes a hyperpolarizing current flow in the synaptic area, inhibiting the spontaneous release of neurotransmitter on to the next cell in the series (a bipolar cell) which occurs continuously in the dark. This system, though complex, ensures maximum multiplication of the signal because of its interactive cascade-like nature, so that, for example, a rod is able to detect as little as four photons.

Cilium (8.436). This is a short stalk about 300 nm in diameter connecting the outer and inner segments in rods and cones. It originates in a basal body in the inner segment and has nine microtubule doublets typical of other cilia although the central pair

of microtubules is absent (De Robertis 1960). It is the route by which molecules and organelles synthesized in the more proximal parts of the cell are conveyed to the outer segment, and it is possible that the microtubules are important in this motile activity. Recently actin and myosin have been located at the outer end of the cilium in the region where rod and cone discs are assembled, suggesting some form of motile function here (see Williams et al 1992).

Inner segments of cones and rods. These are longer and broader than the rod and cone outer segments and are particularly wide in cones. The outer part of the inner segment, or *ellipsoid*, contains numerous mitochondria, some glycogen and the base of the cilium, with which a centriole is also associated; the mitochondria are thought to provide much of the energy required for photo-transduction. The ellipsoid also has thin membranous extensions on its apical surface which partially enshroud the base of the outer segment.

The inner *myoid* part of the inner segment houses many membranous organelles associated with protein and lipid biosynthesis, including a Golgi complex, granular and agranular endoplasmic reticulum and free ribosomes; numerous microtubules are also present, providing motility for vesicular and other transport, and much glycogen, an energy store for these processes.

External fibre. A dendrite-like process connecting the inner segment to the soma, its length varies with retinal position both in rods and cones; it contains numerous microtubules and some mitochondria.

Soma. This region includes the nucleus which is smaller and its chromatin more condensed in rods than in cones. The cytoplasm forms a relatively narrow rim around the nucleus, enclosing various organelles in small numbers.

1341

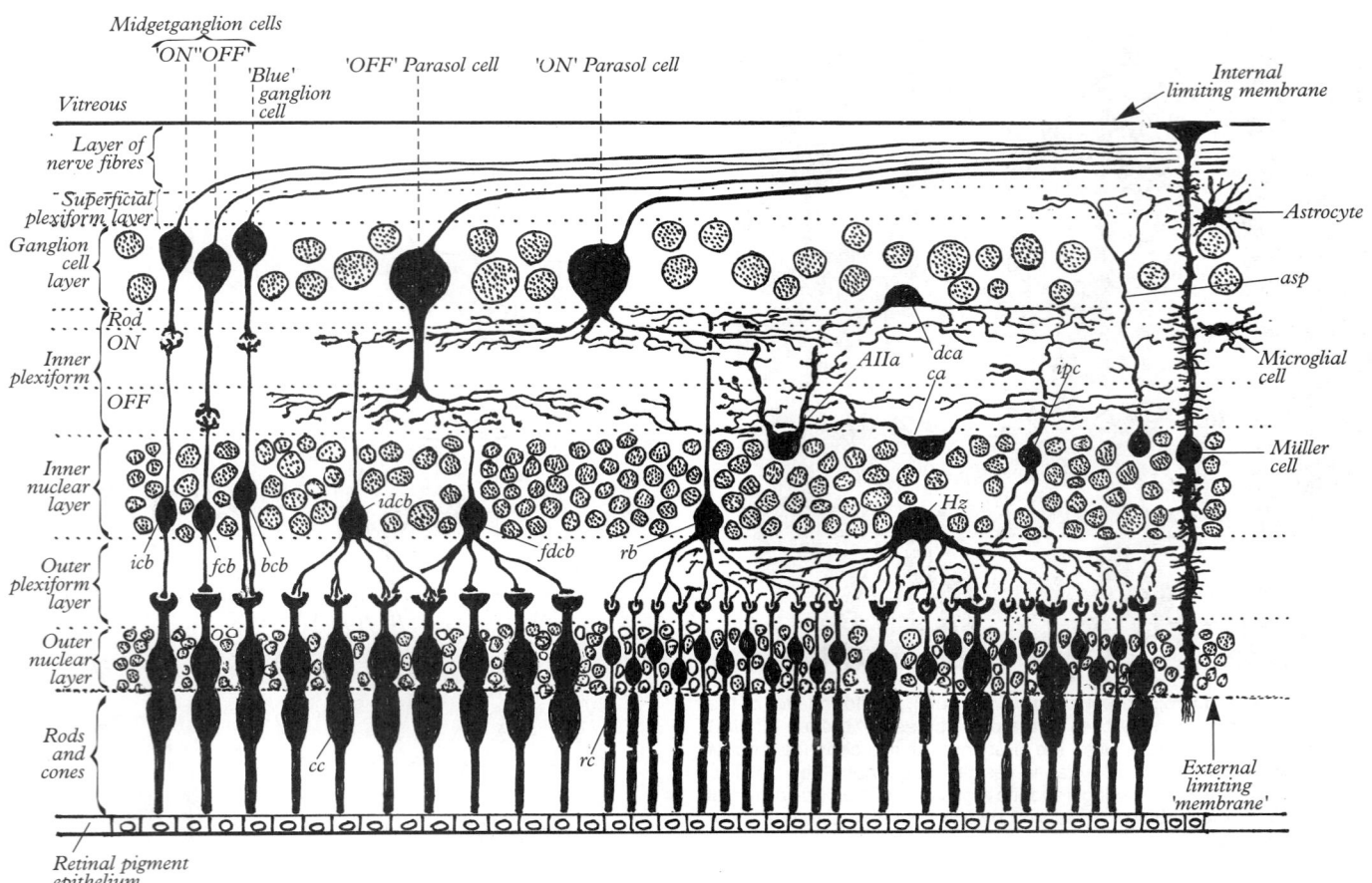

8.441   Diagram showing the appearances of various retinal neurons. All a = All amacrine cell; bcb = blue cone bipolar; ca = cholinergic amacrine cell; cc = cone cell; dca = displaced amacrine cell; fcb = flat cone bipolar; fdcb = flat diffuse cone bipolar; Hz = horizontal cell; idcb = invaginating diffuse cone bipolar; ipc = interplexiform cell; rb = rod bipolar; rc = rod cell.

Internal fibre. This resembles an axon, containing mitochondria, vesicles, free ribosomes, neurofilaments and microtubules. Rod axons are 1.5–2.5 μm in diameter and 10–60 μm or more in length, those of the cones being thicker and containing more microtubules. In the foveal region and around it, the internal fibres of cones have an oblique orientation, and at the sides of the foveola, an almost horizontal layering (fibres of Henle) as the bipolar (and ganglion cells) connected to them are displaced away from the foveolar centre (see p. 1347). Elsewhere the inner fibres become shorter and more perpendicular to the retinal surface.

Rod spherule and cone pedicle. Rod internal fibres (axons) end within the outer plexiform layer in pear-shaped or oval expansions termed *rod spherules*; cone axons end as *cone pedicles*, which are more extensive, flattened plates. Both types of ending form complex multiple junctions with bipolar and horizontal neurons, whose neurites approach from the internal nuclear layer and in many cases, deeply invaginate the base of spherules and cone pedicles (see below).

Rod spherule (**8.438, 439**). This forms synaptic junctions with three other components, namely bipolar and horizontal cell dendrites and, via gap junctions, the spherules or pedicles of other rods and cones. The base of the rod spherule is deeply invaginated, enclosing in its hollow a *triad*, a characteristic synaptic arrangement consisting of synaptic vesicles and a presynaptic ribbon directed at the combination of one or more central bipolar cell dendrites flanked by two HI horizontal cell axons. At the tip of the synaptic ribbon the membrane of the spherule has a small ridge with a dense undercoating (the presynaptic ridge and arciform density, respectively), presumably marking the site of vesicle fusion. Synaptic vesicles are also often present in the horizontal cell dendrites participating in a triad. This arrangement allows complex synaptic interactions to occur between the three types of cell, entailing an interplay of excitatory and inhibitory influences (see also p. 1344).

Cone pedicle (**8.438, 439**). This is more complex; in monkeys there

are 20–30 invaginations per pedicle each containing a typical triad of a central cone ('ON') bipolar and two flanking horizontal cell dendrites (Ahnelt et al 1990). In addition, there are numerous 'flat' (slightly invaginated) synaptic contacts on the pedicle's basal aspect with cone bipolar cells ('OFF' bipolars, see below), with vesicles clustered in the presynaptic (cone) cytoplasm (Boycott & Hopkins 1993). Each pedicle may be connected to two midget bipolar cells and up to 15 diffuse bipolars.

Lateral interreceptor contacts also occur between the peripheral surfaces of adjacent cone pedicles and rod spherules; these are gap junctions (electrical synapses, see pp. 28, 932; Raviola & Gilula 1973; Witkovsky et al 1974), each pedicle having six to twelve such contacts. They occur between foveal cones, and elsewhere are usually made between cone and rod cells which are increasingly towards the periphery. In view of the high resolution mediated by cones, such contacts have been only reluctantly accepted as synapses. They do, however, provide a route by which rods can signal through cone pathways (see below).

Distribution of rods and cones in the retina

The total number of rods in the human retina has been estimated at 110–125 million and of cones at 63–68 million (Österberg 1935). Their distribution differs; the cones are densest at the rod-free foveola (about 147 000 per mm²), where they achieve a minimum spacing of 2–3 μm centre to centre, being hexagonally packed (**8.437A**; see also Wässle & Boycott 1991) but diminish rapidly to a 10° circle round the macula, dropping to about 2000–5000/mm² at the periphery (Diaz-Arya et al 1993); a region of higher cone density (the cone streak) occurs in the human nasal retina. Rods are almost the reverse of this in their distribution, rising from zero at the foveola to a greater density than the cones at the 10° circle (160 000 per mm²), then diminishing again to the peripheral retina, where, however, there are still approximately 30 000 per mm², nearly ten times more

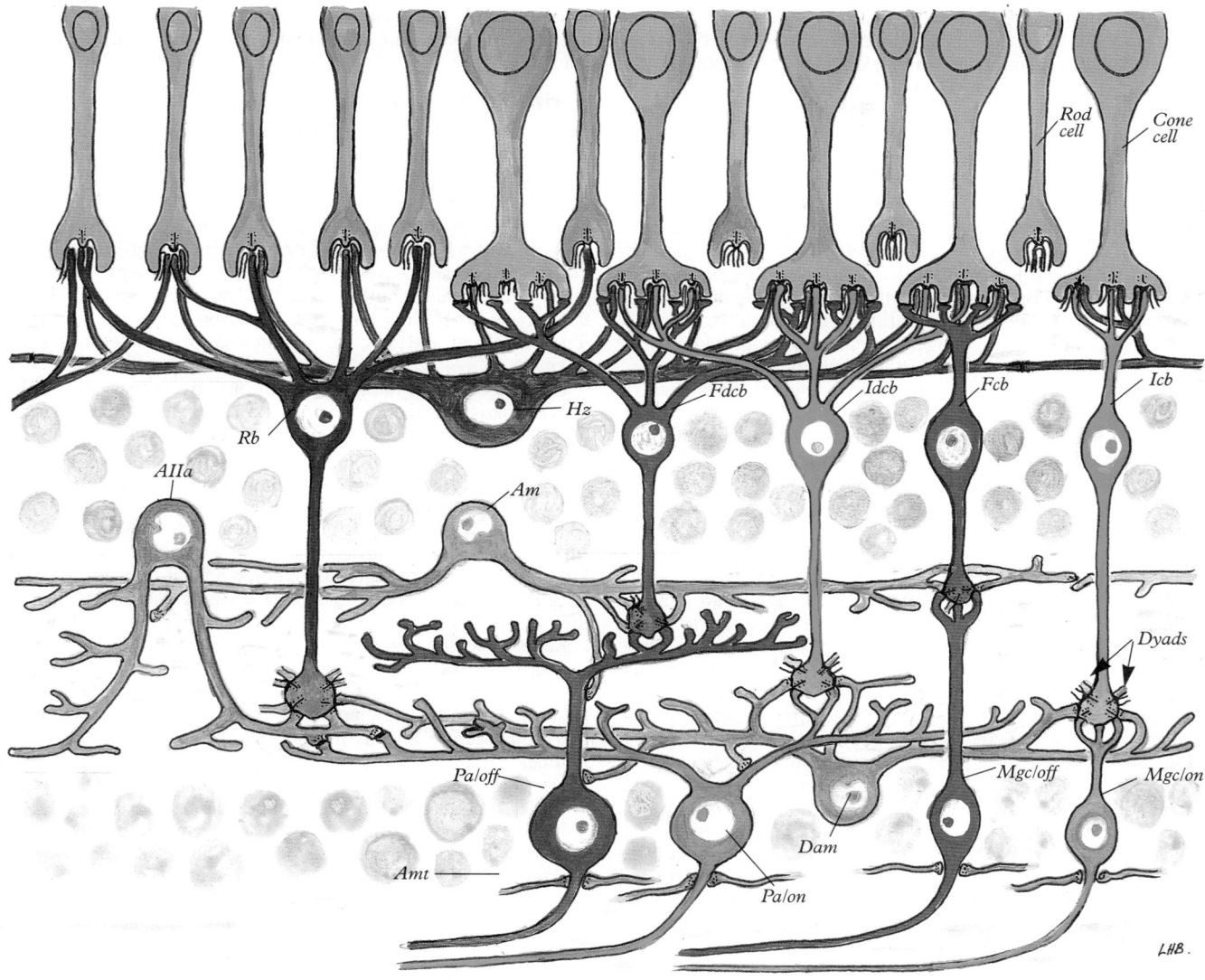

8.442 Schema showing the major features of the primate retina. (Modified from Dowling and Boycott 1966.) For abbreviations see **8**.441; also: Mgc/on = 'ON' midget ganglion cell; Mgc/off = 'OFF' midget ganglion cell;

Pa/on = 'ON' parasol cell; Pa/off = 'OFF' parasol cell; amt = amacrine terminal; Am = amacrine cell; Dam = displaced amacrine cell. Note that rod-rod and rod-cone contacts have been omitted.

numerous there than cones. This distribution accords well with the phenomena of photopic (cone) and scotopic (rod) vision in different parts of the retina. Retinal neurons are clearly seen to be less numerous than rod and cone cells; ganglion cells (see below), whose axons form the optic nerve, probably total about one million in each human retina. Hence large numbers of photoreceptive cells must activate single axonal paths in the optic nerve and beyond.

The distributions of cones detecting different colours have also been studied. Blue cones can be detected with antibodies directed against their photoreceptive proteins and by their ability to take up procion dyes selectively. Blue cones are seen to be slightly smaller than red and green cones, and to form less than a fifth of the total cone numbers (Shapiro et al 1985); they appear to be virtually absent from the fovea, but elsewhere form a regularly spaced hexagonal lattice (see e.g. Shapiro et al 1985). Red and green cones contain such closely similar pigments that antibodies distinguishing between them are not yet available; spectrophotometry in monkey (*Cercopithecus*) retinae indicate that they occur in equal numbers (Mollon & Bowmaker 1992).

Bipolar cells (8.438, 440–442)

The bipolar cells are radially orientated neurons, each with one or more dendrites synapsing with cones or rods and horizontal cells and interplexiform cells in the outer plexiform lamina; a soma is

located in the inner nuclear layer, and axonal branches in the inner plexiform layer synapsing with dendrites of ganglion cells or amacrine cells. They all have the form of typical neurons, with dendrites containing microtubules, mitochondria, ribosomes and other characteristic organelles. The soma is small and contains a euchromatic nucleus; its axon is short, branched and has terminals with presynaptic features: vesicles and presynaptic densities.

In primates there are at least nine categories of bipolar cells, differing in their connectivity, electrophysiological properties and immunochemical compositions (Boycott & Wässle 1991; Kolb et al 1992). They are customarily divided into two principal groups, rod and cone bipolars, according to their photoreceptive inputs.

Cone bipolars. Structurally, cone bipolars throughout the retina are of three major types: *midget*, *blue cone* and *diffuse* (**8**.442). Individual midget and blue cone bipolars are each connected to single cones, whereas diffuse bipolars are related to several or many.

Midget bipolars. As their name implies these are small cells, typically with a single main dendrite with a restricted dendritic field contacting the pedicle of only one cone. At the other pole of the cell their axons synapse in the inner plexiform layer with the dendrites of a single ganglion cell and with various classes of amacrine cells. Each cone pedicle is contacted by a pair of midget bipolars, one of them forming an invaginating triadic synapse, and the other a flat synaptic contact. There is now evidence that the invaginating contacts

1343

belong to 'ON' bipolars, and the flat contacts to 'OFF' bipolars (Boycott & Hopkins 1993) and their axons terminate respectively in the 'ON' and 'OFF' layers of the inner plexiform layer (Nelson et al 1978). 'ON' bipolars respond to the illumination of the cones they synapse with by depolarizing whereas 'OFF' bipolars hyperpolarize. It is useful experimentally that these cells have different immuno-reactivities, 'ON' bipolars being positive for cholecystokinin (CCK) and the 'OFF' bipolars for the protein recoverin (see Milam et al 1992; Wässle et al 1994a).

Because each midget bipolar is part of a single, one-to-one channel from a single cone to a single ganglion cell, they are thought to mediate high spatial resolution; further, peripherally in the retina these bipolar cells may contact more than one cone, an arrangement paralleling the loss of spatial discrimination at the retinal periphery. In primates including humans, midget bipolars are connected either to red- or green-sensitive cones, hence the alternative names L-cone and M-cone bipolars (L = long wavelength, M = medium wavelength) respectively.

Blue cone bipolars. (S-bipolars, where S = short wavelength). Although somewhat larger than midget bipolars, they form similar unitary channels between cones and ganglion cells (Kouyama & Marshak 1992). They form the third member of the colour-mediating bipolar cell family responsible for conveying trichromatic information vision with high visual acuity.

Diffuse cone bipolars. These are larger than midget bipolars, and each is connected apically to up to 10 or more cones regardless of colour specificity (Boycott & Wässle 1991; Wässle et al 1994b). Therefore, they are thought to signal luminosity rather than colour; because of their large receptive fields they have a lower spatial discrimination. Six morphologically distinct types have been described in primates (Boycott & Wässle 1991), three of them of the invaginating 'ON' type and the other three flat 'OFF' bipolars.

Rod bipolars. These receive direct photoreceptive inputs exclusively from rods, the branched dendrites of each neuron forming invaginating triad-like synapses with the bases of many photoreceptor cells (though involving more than three processes); conversely, each rod spherule may be contacted by four rod bipolar cells (in monkeys). Their axons do not contact ganglion cells directly, but terminate at dyads (see below) on amacrine AII cells which in turn contact the dendrites of large (parasol) ganglion cells and axon terminals of cone bipolars. They also receive synapses from other amacrine cells, including some which form reciprocal synapses with their axons (Grunert & Martin 1991). Rod bipolars are only of the 'ON' type.

Dyads. Distinctive combinations of synapses (**8.440**) between bipolar cells, ganglion cells and amacrine cells; they are found only in the inner plexiform layer. In each, the terminal (or preterminal) expansion of a bipolar axon makes synaptic contacts with a pair of closely apposed dendrites, one belonging to a ganglion cell, the other to an amacrine. The bipolar cell is presynaptic to both, at a ribbon synapse directed towards the midline between the two postsynaptic processes, but the amacrine cell also makes a reciprocal synapse of the symmetrical type (p. 928) back on to the bipolar cell terminal. This arrangement is thought to mediate lateral inhibition between neighbouring bipolar cells in contact with the same amacrine cell, so adding to the image 'sharpening' effects of the horizontal cells, and perhaps carrying out other types of lateral interactions, for example colour opponency between different chromatically coded cone bipolars.

Mechanisms of bipolar 'ON' and 'OFF' responses

The responses of the bipolar cells are determined by two factors: the way in which light modulates the release of neurotransmitter from rod spherules and cone pedicles, and the different effects of the neurotransmitter on the two types of bipolar cell (see Wässle & Boycott 1991). As mentioned above, neurotransmitter is maximally released from rod and cone cell synapses in the dark, and when illuminated this release is reduced or ceases. In the dark, the neuro-transmitter depolarizes 'OFF' bipolars, and hyperpolarizes 'ON' bipolars. When the photoreceptors are illuminated, neuro-transmission ceases or is reduced, causing hyperpolarization in the 'OFF' cell and depolarization in the 'ON' cell. Different receptor molecules in the postsynaptic membranes of the two cell types are coupled to different ion channels, although the details are not yet worked out. It should be added that depolarization of bipolar cells

causes them to release neurotransmitter at their own axon terminals in the inner plexiform layer, and that hyperpolarization stops this release.

Horizontal cells (8.438)

The horizontal cells are inhibitory interneurons whose dendrites and axons extend within the outer plexiform layer, making synaptic contacts with the bases of cones and rods, and via gap junctions at the tips of their dendrites, with each other (**8.438**). Their cell bodies lie in the outer part of the internal nuclear layer. They are of two classes, called HI and HII in primates including humans; HI cells are the larger and have higher numbers of synaptic contacts in a given retinal region; both are reported to contact rods and cones. A third type (HIII) has also been described recently in the human retina (Kolb et al 1992); the significance of these classes is not yet clarified.

Because of their interactions with photoreceptor cells and bipolar cells at triads (see above) horizontal cells create inhibitory surrounds: when illumination of a photoreceptor cluster with a point of light causes depolarization of synaptically connected 'ON' bipolars at its bright centre, horizontal cell dendrites cause inhibition at the edge of the illuminated area, thus sharpening contrast and maximizing spatial resolution. Colour opponency (e.g. red illumination inhibiting surrounding blue and green responses) is probably not mediated by horizontal cells in primates since these neurons do not appear to be selective in their cone connections (Wässle et al 1994b), although they are in lower vertebrates (and have been suggested to be so in humans by Kolb (1991), though this controversy has yet to be settled conclusively).

The receptive fields of both HI and HII cells vary with retinal position, being smallest and with fewest photoreceptor contacts in the retinal centre and as much as 1 mm across near its edge. The numbers of cones contacted increase likewise, for example for HI horizontal cells, only 6 cones in the centre to 46 more peripherally (Wässle & Boycott 1991). In primates the *axons* of HI cells contact only rod spherules; in the cat very extensive axon terminal branching systems exist, serving up to 3000 rods. There is strong evidence that horizontal cells use γ-aminobutyric acid (GABA) as a neuro-transmitter (p. 935). Ultrastructurally, their cytoplasm resembles that of bipolar cells but also contains a characteristic organelle rich in ribosomes (Kolmer's crystalloid).

Ganglion cells (8.440–442)

The ganglion cells are the final common pathway neurons of the retina, their dendrites being synaptically connected with processes of bipolar and amacrine neurons in the internal plexiform lamina and their axons to neurons in the CNS. Their axons form the lamina of nerve fibres on the inner surface of the retina; here they turn tangentially to the optic disc, by which they leave the eye as fibres of the optic nerve to be distributed to various parts of the brain including the lateral geniculate nucleus, the pretectal area and superior colliculus of the midbrain, the thalamic pulvinar and the accessory optic system (p. 1090). An interesting recent report with double labelling experiments in the rat indicates that in this species some ganglion cells send axons bilaterally to the lateral geniculate nuclei and superior colliculi on both sides of the brain (Kondo et al 1993).

Ganglion cell bodies form a single stratum in most of the retina but as the macula is approached they become progressively more numerous, and in the macular area they are ranked in about 10 rows, diminishing again towards the fovea, from which they are almost absent. They are multipolar neurons, varying from 10–30 μm or more in diameter, and have a large nucleus. Their dendrites are variable in number and branching patterns, and usually emerge opposite the axon. Numbers of ganglion cells in the human macular area reach 38 000/mm²; they are more numerous in the nasal retina than the temporal, and in the superior retina compared with the inferior, but vary considerably in different eyes (Curcio & Allen 1990).

Classes of ganglion cells (**8.441**, 442). According to their den-dritic patterns and their electrophysiological reactions to retinal illumination they have been classified into various types (see Ramón y Cajal 1911; Polyak 1941; Boycott & Dowling 1969, Boycott 1974; Kolb & Nelson 1984; Shapley & Perry 1986; Dowling 1987;

Watanabe & Rodiek 1989; Kolb & Dekorver 1991; Wässle & Boycott 1991; Dacey & Petersen 1992). The number of recognized classes has been steadily growing as new methods of labelling and recording are applied, and will doubtless increase further. Compounding the complexity (and the nomenclature), considerable species differences also exist. Here a simplified description based mainly on the primate retina will be used.

At the simplest level of subdivision, most are either *midget (β) cells* or the much larger *parasol (a) cells*. Through the optic nerve their axons connect with, respectively, the parvocellular and magnocellular parts of the lateral geniculate nucleus and are therefore also sometimes designated as P and M cells. They correspond to the X and Y ganglion cells of the cat retina physiology. Both of these have subclasses which respond respectively to the onset of illumination of their receptive field centres with a spot of light ('ON' cells) and those which respond when illumination ceases ('OFF' cells).

In addition there are cells which respond transiently to both the onset and the offset of illumination ('ON–OFF' cells), those which are activated by an illumination moving in a particular direction across the retina (directionally sensitive or DS cells), and various other categories (see below). The dendrites of 'ON' and 'OFF' ganglion cells spread and make synaptic contacts in the appropriate 'ON' and 'OFF' layers of the inner plexiform layer.

Midget (β) ganglion cells. These have a single apical process which branches into a small dendritic field making contact with a single midget cone bipolar cell (see Wässle & Boycott 1991). Because of this arrangement they become active (or inactive) when a single cone is illuminated, and can therefore mediate high resolution images as well as colour. Most of them can be divided according to their different chromatic responses, i.e. green or red, and also to their reaction to illumination, i.e. 'ON' and 'OFF' green and red midget ganglion cells. Blue cones connect through their own bipolars to their own distinctive class of (small bistratified) ganglion cell, as described later.

Midget ganglion cells are commonest in the macula, where they are twice as numerous as the densely packed cones to which they are connected, but they occur throughout the retina. These cells typically have brisk tonic responses; for example, 'ON' cells have a rapid onset with illumination and continue to fire when light levels are sustained. Serial reconstructions of human midget ganglion cells (Kolb & Dekorver 1991) show that each is connected to a single bipolar which makes up to 80 synaptic contacts, mainly at dyads, sharing these with an equal number of amacrine dendrites.

The dendritic fields of neighbouring midget ganglion cells form a non-overlapping mosaic over the retina; in the human central retina these form about 80–95% of all ganglion cells, and size measurements show their density corresponds well to the observed visual acuity (Dacey 1993).

Parasol. These only form about 10% of all ganglion cells (Peichl 1991) but are conspicuous because of their large size, being 3–10 times the diameter of midget bipolars in humans (Dacey & Petersen 1992); they receive the inputs of diffuse cone bipolars and, via amacrine II cells, of rod bipolars. They therefore have extensive receptive fields gathering signals from many photoreceptors. Parasol cells are phasic, adapting rapidly to sustained stimuli and, therefore, primarily signalling changes of illumination. Both 'ON' and 'OFF' parasol cells occur, their dendrites terminating in the appropriate inner plexiform strata with relevant bipolar cells; human 'ON'-centre parasol cells have diameters up to 50% larger than the 'OFF'-centre type (Dacey & Petersen 1992), and both cells have wider dendritic fields at the periphery of the retina than at its centre.

Other types of retinal ganglion cells. Various additional types of ganglion cells have been reported to occur in smaller numbers in primates and other mammalian groups on the basis of electro-physiological and structural data (see e.g. Rodieck & Watanabe 1993). *Bistratified ganglion cells* have dendrites which branch in both 'ON' and 'OFF' inner plexiform layer strata, and (at least in monkeys) connect to the parvocellular part of the lateral geniculate nucleus. They include small bistratified cells, like parasol cells but a little smaller, thought to be blue 'ON' cells (Dacey 1993). There is also evidence that others (at least in non-primates) are *directionally sensitive (DS) ganglion cells* which are 'ON–OFF' directional movement detectors (Famiglietti 1992). There are also some parasol-like cells with relatively huge dendritic fields, up to 850 μm diameter,

with axons projecting to the magnocellular part of the lateral geniculate.

It can be seen that apart from the small number of 'classic' cell types customarily described in elementary textbooks, there are many other structural categories of retinal ganglion cell. Some of these are undoubtedly part of the sophisticated apparatus proceeding via synapses in the lateral geniculate nucleus to the visual cortex, whereas others appear to be cells with CNS targets other than the lateral geniculate nucleus, each perhaps possessing its own characteristic set of retinal ganglion cells (Rodieck & Watanabe 1993).

Ganglion cell axons: the lamina of nerve fibres

The axons of ganglion cells converge on to the optic disc from the whole retina, forming the stratum opticum, which is consequently deepest (20–30 μm) at the disc's periphery. They converge in a simple radial pattern from the medial (nasal) half of the retina but the macular area, inferolateral to the optic disc, complicates the course of the lateral (temporal) axons. Those from the macula form a *papillomacular fasciculus* which passes almost straight to the disc; the more temporal fibres, being more peripheral, swerve circumferentially above and below to reach the disc.

Axons of ganglion cells are non-myelinated within the retina (in primates), an optical advantage since myelin is refractile. The myelin sheaths commence as the axons enter the optic disc to become the optic nerve. A few small myelinated fibres may appear in human retinae; myelination is usual in parts of the retina in many other mammals, for example the rabbit. The axons within the retina are surrounded by the processes of retinal gliocytes (Müller cells) and other retinal astrocytes (Wolter 1959). Like their somata, the axons of ganglionic neurons vary in size, ranging from 0.6–20 μm in diameter, with a typical axonal ultrastructure.

It has recently been shown that the ganglion cell bodies, their axon hillocks and initial segments also receive synapses mainly within the *superficial plexiform layer* which is now recognized to exist between the cell bodies of the ganglion cells and the layer of nerve fibres (Wieniawa-Narkiewicz & Hughes 1992). They are probably the GABA-ergic synaptic terminals of amacrine cells mainly of the symmetric type, and are likely to be inhibitory (Koontz 1993).

Centrifugal axons to the retina have often been described and almost as often denied (Bowin 1895; Mukai 1970). Their existence in the human retina is still an open issue. Various sources have been suggested including the lateral geniculate nucleus (p. 1090), superior colliculus, hypothalamus, etc. Such retinal efferents might be vaso-motor; but since efferent terminals have been described in relation to amacrine cells by Ramón y Cajal and others, it is tempting to assume in the visual pathway an analogue of the cortico–olivo–cochlear connections of the auditory system (p. 1394). The majority of such studies have been in birds (Cajal) or teleost fish (see Dowling 1987). Nevertheless, there is good evidence for a corticogeniculate pathway, modifying the activity of the afferent visual paths (p. 1090) and it is possible that such a connection reaches the retina. A recent account based on horseradish peroxidase (HRP) labelling of the distal ends of cut optic nerves in a number of mammalian species including monkeys describes neurons sending centrifugal axons to the retina from several regions of the brainstem and hypothalamus (Labandeira-Garcia et al 1990) suggesting that although few in number, the efferent pathways may be quite widespread, although this needs to be confirmed.

Amacrine cells

These neurons (8.440, 442) were so named by Cajal because they lack typical axons, and therefore did not fit in with the usual pattern propounded in the neuron theory. It has since been discovered that amacrine cell dendrites function both as axons and dendrites, and make both incoming and outgoing synapses; indeed, in larger ama-crines distant dendritic regions may be electrically independent of each other, and neighbouring afferent and efferent serial synapses may interact locally with little interference from more remote parts of the cell. For reviews, see Wässle and Boycott (1991) and Kolb (1994).

Each neuron has a cell body either in the inner nuclear layer, near its boundary with the inner plexiform layer, or on the outer aspect of the ganglion cell layer ('displaced' amacrine cells). From these, two to several primary dendrites arise, branching variably according to the cell type, of which there appear to be many. Their cell bodies typically contain an indented nucleus, much granular endoplasmic reticulum, ribosomes, microtubules and sometimes crystalline bodies and superficial smooth membraned cisternae; they also bear surface cilium, of unknown significance (Boycott & Hopkins 1984). The processes of amacrine neurons make scattered chemical synaptic contacts with the axons of bipolar cells, dendrites (and possibly axons) of ganglion cells, and the processes of other amacrine cells. Likewise, they also receive numerous synapses from bipolar and, in some cases, other amacrine cells. Some also form electrical synapses with bipolar cells (see below).

General activities of amacrine cells. Amacrine cells serve a number of important functions in vision. One class (amacrine II cells) transmits signals from rod bipolars on to ganglion cells and is therefore an essential element in the rod pathway. Others appear to be important modulators of photoreceptor signals, serving to adjust or maintain relative colour and luminosity inputs under changing light conditions, for example at different times of day, and in some cases probably being responsible for directional movement detection and other complex forms of image analysis known to be carried out within the retina.

Classes of amacrine cells. With the increased use of combined cell recording and labelling, and the use of immunochemical and fluorescent markers, the number of cell types recognized as amacrine or amacrine-like continues to increase steadily (see the reviews by Masland and Tauchi (1986) and Wässle and Boycott (1991). Most of them fall structurally into one of two broad categories, diffuse or stratified. *Diffuse amacrine cells* have dendrites which ramify at all levels of the inner plexiform layer, whereas *stratified amacrine cells* have a two-dimensional dendritic spread, each restricted to a specific narrow stratum in the inner plexiform layer. There are also a few cells with different dendritic distribution, for example interplexiform cells, as described below. Cells can also be classified according to their neurotransmitter content, as follows.

Glycinergic amacrine. These cells form about half of the diffuse cell population, and have a rather restricted spread of dendrites, which synapse with the various cells whose terminals occupy the three strata of the inner plexiform layer, i.e. the innermost layer of rod bipolar axons, the middle layer of 'ON' cone bipolars, and the outer stratum of 'OFF' bipolars. A well-studied member of this group is the amacrine AII (narrow field bistratified amacrine cell) which receives rod bipolar axon synapses in the innermost stratum and gives synaptic outputs to ganglion cell dendrites in that stratum. They also have gap junctions with 'ON' cone bipolars in the middle stratum and make synapses with 'OFF' bipolars in the outer stratum of the inner plexiform layer (see e.g. Strettoi et al 1992).

Cholinergic amacrine cells. Stratified in type, with cell bodies in either the inner nuclear layer or ganglion cell layer (displaced cholinergic amacrines), their dendrites spread in, respectively, the inner and outer strata of the inner plexiform layer. Seen in surface view these cells are spectacular in the sizes of their dendritic fields and their symmetry ('starburst cells'). They receive synaptic inputs from bipolar axons at dyads throughout their dendritic fields, but make efferent synapses only near their extremities with ganglion cell dendrites, including those of directionally sensitive (DS) ganglion cells (see e.g. Famiglietti 1991). They have been proposed as the major determinants of this directional response, but exactly how they may achieve this is not certain; the mechanism may entail an asymmetric pattern of conduction and connectivity which would switch a ganglion cell on at the leading edge of a spot of light, then off at its trailing edge. At least some of these cells contain GABA as well as acetylcholine (ACh), and may have various actions on postsynaptic cells depending on neurotransmitter receptor types, and even, perhaps, on local differences in neurotransmitter release from the same cell.

GABA-ergic amacrine cells. Forming about 30% of the total amacrine population, most of them are displaced amacrines with cell bodies in the ganglion cell layer. Their dendritic fields are exceedingly wide (up to 300 μm). Several subtypes have been described; they make reciprocal synapses with rod bipolars at dyads.

Somatostatin-positive amacrines. These neurons are also extraordinary in form; they are situated mainly in the ventral half of the retina, but have exceedingly long processes which extend some centimetres to the dorsal half of the retina. Functionally it has been

suggested that they act to balance the retinal sensitivity in the two halves, the lower part of the retina usually receiving greater illumination (from the sky) than the upper.

Interplexiform cells. Classed by some authors as amacrines, they have nuclei in the inner nuclear layer, but their dendrites extend from the inner plexiform layer, where they receive synaptic inputs from bipolar cells, to the outer plexiform layer to synapse with bipolar cell dendrites. At least some of these cells are dopaminergic.

Various other amacrine types, with different morphologies and neurotransmitter types (e.g. dopamine, vasoactive intestinal peptide; VIP) have also been described. As the reader will no doubt have appreciated from this account, it appears that the modulation of retinal output by amacrine cells is a most complex affair involving multiple synaptic interactions with a wide range of neuromediators.

Retinal glial cells

The retinal glial cells are of three types; radial retinal gliocytes (Müller cells), astrocytes and microglia. Müller cells form the predominant glial element of most of the retina, while retinal astrocytes are largely confined to the ganglion cell and nerve fibre layers; microglial cells are scattered throughout the neural part of the retina in small numbers. For reviews see Schnitzer (1985), Hollander et al (1991).

Müller cells. These are radially orientated glial cells which span the entire thickness of the neural retina. They ensheath and separate the various photoreceptive and neural cells of its different layers except at synaptic sites, forming the outer boundary of the solid retinal tissue at the level of the inner rod and cone segments, and the inner boundary at the internal limiting lamina (see e.g. Robinson & Dreher 1990; Hollander et al 1991).

Their nuclei lie within the inner nuclear layer, and from this region a single thick fibre ascends radially, giving off complex lateral lamellae which branch among the processes of the outer plexiform layer, and form basket-like calyces around the cell bodies of the different cell types. Apically the central process passes between the cone and rod cells to terminate in a surface from which microvilli project into the space between the rod and cone processes. Just beneath this area the Müller cells form a line of dense adhering zones (zonulae adherentes) with each other and with the inner segments, so forming the *external limiting lamina* (Spitznas 1970). The rods and cones thus have the appearance of having been thrust through the holes in a sieve formed by this dense layer of junctional material, and the whole arrangement suggests that it provides physical support to these delicate cell processes. On the inner aspect of the retina, the main Müller cell process expands in a terminal foot plate, contacting those of neighbouring Müller cells and astrocytes to form the internal limiting lamina (see below). Like other neuroglia they also contact blood vessels, especially capillaries; here their basal laminae fuse with those of vascular smooth muscle in the media of larger vessels or of the endothelia lining capillaries. These extensive neuroglial cells form much of the total retinal volume, almost totally filling the extracellular space between neural elements.

Their functions appear to be similar to those of astrocytes, i.e. maintaining the stability of the retinal extracellular environment by ionic transport, uptake of neurotransmitter, removal of debris, storage of glycogen, electrical insulation of receptors and neurons, and mechanical support of the neural retina, among other activities (Reichenbach et al 1992).

Retinal astrocytes. These resemble astrocytes of other parts of the brain; their cell bodies lie between the layer of nerve fibres and the internal limiting lamina, whilst their processes branch to form sheaths around ganglion cell axons (Distler et al 1993). Their expanded basal processes also participate (at least in the cat) with the Müller cells in forming the internal limiting lamina (Hollander et al 1991). In a number of species it has been shown that astrocytes are only present in regions of the retina which are vascularized, and are, for instance, excluded from the avascular part of the macula (Schnitzer 1987).

Retinal microglia. Scattered mainly within the inner plexiform layer but also extending into the outer (Boycott & Hopkins 1981), these cells resemble microglial cells in other parts of the CNS (see p. 942). They have radiating branched processes spreading mainly parallel to the retinal plane to give them a star-like appearance when viewed from the surface of the retina. They are approximately equally spaced without overlapping as though possessing their own individual territories (Schnitzer 1987). Apart from their phagocytic capacity (Roque & Caldwell 1993), seen especially when the retina is injured, they are likely to have immunological functions, and also to provide growth factors and cytokines important in the maintenance of the retinal cells.

Internal limiting lamina

Electron microscopy shows this to be a composite structure, composed of the expanded end-feet of Müller cells and astrocytes separated from the vitreous body by a complex, rather thick (0.5 μm) basal lamina, sinuously adapted to convoluted glial cell surface membrane on one side, but smooth on its external, vitreal aspect; the delicate collagen fibrils of the vitreous body blend with the glial basal lamina. The internal limiting lamina is involved in fluid exchange between the vitreous and the retina and, perhaps through the latter, with the choroid, and has various other functions including anchorage of retinal glial cells and inhibition of cell migration into the vitreous body.

Peculiarities of the macular area

The central retinal area is a region 5–6 mm in diameter, containing the *macula lutea*, an elliptical area about 2 mm horizontally and 1 mm vertically, its yellowish colour being due to the presence of xanthophyll or to a great reduction in the capillary bed or, perhaps, to other cell inclusions in bipolar and ganglion cells. The macula's central region, the *fovea centralis* or *foveola*, is a deep conical depression where all elements except cones are much reduced; its diameter is about 0.4 mm. The foveola is positioned about 4 mm lateral and 1 mm inferior to the centre of the optic disc (the latter corresponding to the 'blind spot' in the uniocular visual field). The minuteness of the foveola accounts for the accuracy with which the visual axes must be directed to achieve the most discriminative vision. The macula has been further divided into *peri-* and *parafoveal* areas, although these divisions are somewhat arbitrary, as there is a continuum of cell densities and sizes throughout the retina.

All the retinal layers are modified in the macular area and to a marked degree in the fovea, in the floor of which (the foveola, p. 1337) there are no rod cells but about 2500 close-packed elongated but very narrow cones; the cell bodies of even these small cone cells are displaced peripherally to the sloping foveal wall so that only the cone processes are present in the foveola. Despite this distorting effect, the foveolar cone processes are strictly perpendicular, i.e. radial in orientation, the only other element present (which light must traverse) being the fibrous cytoplasmic processes of the gliocytes, and their internal and external limiting laminae. At the rim of the conical wall of the foveolar pit other modifications appear. The fovea is largely devoid of rod cells or processes, which reach only to its periphery. Its rod-free central part contains approximately 35 000 cones and in the whole fovea (about 175 mm²) there are about 100 000 of these cells (**8.437**). Hence, in the fovea cones are most slender and most compacted and all other layers virtually absent, a condition which greatly favours photopic vision, and the high degree of spatial discrimination typical of foveal vision.

Because of the general displacement of the outer nuclear layer to the foveal periphery, the internal processes of the photoreceptors are stretched out tangentially in the external plexiform layer and hence no cone pedicles or rod spherules are present in the central fovea and foveola. The inner nuclear layer is also displaced to the edge of the foveal depression and the internal plexiform, ganglionic and nerve fibre laminae are almost absent from the whole fovea. Therefore, even on the foveal wall the retina is thinner and more transparent. Capillaries reach the foveal margin, invading only the ganglionic layer at its circumference. The fovea is thus normally devoid of all blood vessels.

In the *parafoveal region*, extending about 0.5 mm around the fovea (total diameter 1.5 mm), the retina is thickest, partly due to the accumulation of displaced bipolar and ganglionic neurons. Outside this is a *perifoveal* region in which the density of cones begins to diminish rapidly, the incidence of rods increasing. These divisions are, however, somewhat artificial, since there is a continuous gradation of cone densities and the boundaries cannot be distinguished on the basis of any sharp transition.

The fovea is the last part in the primate retina to attain full

development, which is not completed until about the fourth postnatal month in mankind. Prenatal development of the primate foveae has been chiefly studied in rhesus monkeys and the details are beyond the present scope of this section.

OPTIC DISC AND RETINAL BLOOD VESSELS

The retina is placed between two sets of arteries and veins—the ciliary vessels of the choroid and the branches of the central retinal vessels. It depends on both circulations, neither alone being sufficient to maintain full visual activity in the retina. The choroidal circulation (p. 1326) and the orbital and intraneural parts of the central retinal vessels are described elsewhere (pp. 1226, 1526). The central retinal vessels enter and leave the retina at the optic disc, which will be described before the vessels are considered.

Optic disc (8.443, 444)

This region, where retinal tissues meet the neural elements of the optic nerve (including astrocytes and oligodendrocytes) and also the connective tissues of the sclera and meninges, is a highly complex area. Besides being the exit point for the optic nerve fibres, it also provides a point of entry and exit for the retinal circulation and moreover is the only site of anastomoses with other arteries (the posterior ciliary arteries, see below). It is visible, by ophthalmoscopy (**8.428–430, 442, 443**), and is a region of much clinical importance since it is here that the central vessels can be inspected directly, the only vessels so accessible in the whole body. Oedema of the disc (papilloedema) may be the first sign of raised intracranial pressure, transmitted into the subarachnoid space around the optic nerve and compressing the central retinal vein where it crosses the space.

The optic disc, being superomedial to the posterior pole of the eye, lies away from the visual axis. It is round or oval, usually about 1.6 mm transversely and 1.8 mm in the vertical, and its appearance is very variable; for details see Duke-Elder & Wybar (1961). In light-skinned people the general retinal hue is a bright terracotta-red and the pale pink of the disc contrasts sharply with this; its central part is usually even paler and may be light grey. These differences are due to the degree of vascularization of the two regions, which is much less at the optic disc, and to a total absence of choroidal or retinal pigment cells, the retina being represented by little more than the internal limiting lamina. Even this does not pass far on to the disc, for the retinal gliocytes are replaced by the astrocytes of the optic nerve (Anderson & Hoyt 1969). In individuals with strongly melanized skins both retina and disc are darker (**8.429B**). The optic disc does not project at all in many eyes and rarely enough to justify the term *papilla*. It is usually a little elevated on its lateral side where the papillomacular nerve fibres turn into the optic nerve; where the retinal vessels traverse its centre there is usually a slight depression.

Central retinal vessels

The *central retinal artery* enters the optic nerve as a branch of the ophthalmic artery (**8.445**), about 1.2 cm behind the eyeball. It travels in the optic nerve to its head, where its fascicles (about 1000 in humans) traverse the lamina cribrosa. At this level, which is usually

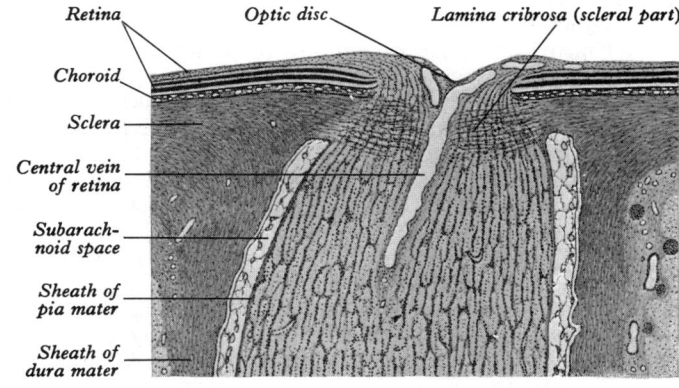

8.443 A horizontal section through the optic nerve at its point of exit from the human eyeball.

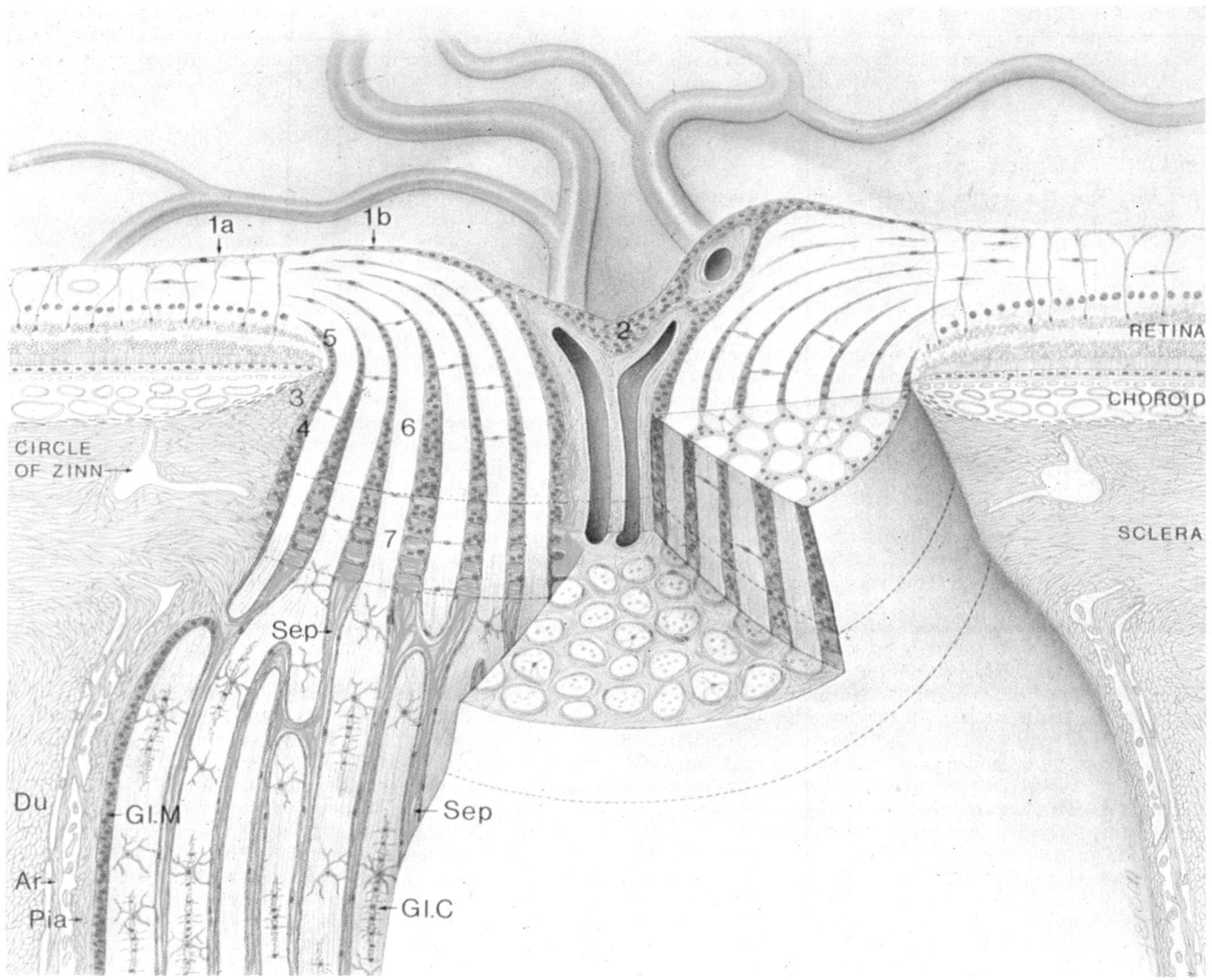

8.444 Schematic representation of the exit of the human optic nerve from the eyeball, showing the distribution of collagenous (blue) and neuroglial (magenta) tissues. Sep = septa of collagenous connective tissue carried into the nerve from the pia mater and dividing the nerve fibres into numerous fascicles; Gl.M = astrogical membrane separating nerve fibres from connective tissue; Gl.C = astrocytes and oligodendrocytes among the fibres in their fascicles; Du, Ar, Pia = dura, arachnoid and pia maters respectively. (1a) is the internal limiting lamina of the retina, which is continuous with an astroglial membrane (of Elschnig) covering the optic disc (1b). An accumulation of astrocytes forms a central meniscus of Kuhnt in the centre of the disc (2). The anterior or so-called 'choroidal part' of the lamina cribrosa (6) is separated from the choroid by a spur of collagenous tissue (3). The 'border tissue of Jacoby' (4), which is largely astroglia, frequently extends beyond the choroid (5) to separate much of the retina from the 'retinal part' of the optic nerve head. The posterior part of the lamina cribrosa (7) contains collagenous tissue derived from the optic nerve septa and fenestrated sheets of collagen fibres continuous with those of the sclera. (Reproduced by permission of Anderson & Hoyt 1969.)

not visible to ophthalmoscopy, the central artery divides into two equal branches: first into a superior and an inferior and again, after a few millimetres, into superior and inferior nasal and superior and inferior temporal branches. Each of these four supplies its own 'quadrant' of the retina, their territories being in fact much more than quadrants, since they ramify as far as the ora serrata. Corresponding retinal veins unite to form the *central retinal vein* but the courses of the venous and arterial vessels do not correspond exactly and arteries often cross veins, usually lying superficial to them. In severe hypertension the arteries may press on the veins and cause visible dilations distal to these crossings. Arterial pulsation is not visible by routine ophthalmoscopy without higher magnification.

The branching of the artery is usually dichotomous, equal rami diverging at angles of 45–60°; but smaller branches may leave singly and at right angles. Arteries and veins ramify in the nerve fibre layer, near the internal limiting membrane, accounting for their clarity when seen through an ophthalmoscope (**8.**429, 430A,B). Arterioles pass deeper into the retina and may penetrate to the internal nuclear lamina, from which venules return to larger superficial veins. A dense capillary bed extends between these vessels and is diffusely organized, showing no laminar pattern.

The structure of blood vessels resembles that of vessels elsewhere except that the internal elastic lamina is absent from the arteries and muscle cells may appear in their adventitia. Capillaries have a non-fenestrated endothelium and numerous mural *pericytes* are distributed along the vascular axis outside the endothelium, sharing the same basement membrane. (For the ultrastructure of retinal capillaries see Tominaga & Ikui 1964.)

Microcirculation. Microcirculatory studies of the human retina in flat preparations, stained after trypsin digestion, reveal many details of capillary arrangement resembling those in the renal glomeruli, a network of capillaries connecting individual arterioles and venules which are themselves devoid of anastomoses and arteriovenous shunts. Thus the territories of the arteries supplying a particular quadrant do not overlap, nor do the branches within a quadrant anastomose with each other. In consequence, a blockage

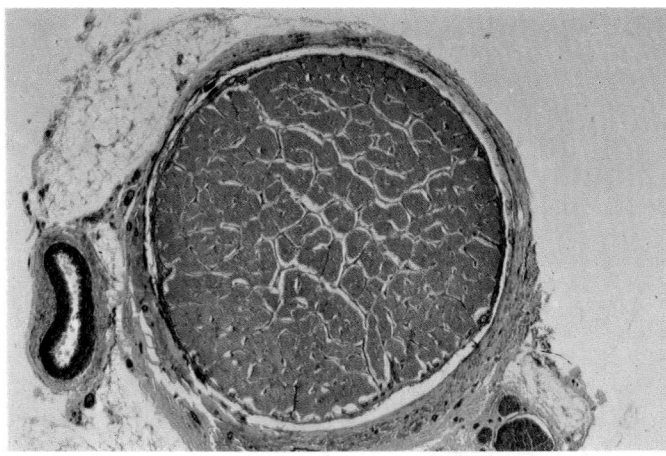

8.445 A transverse section of the optic nerve and its meningeal coverings. The ophthalmic artery is visible at the side of the nerve. The dural and pial sheaths are stained green, the subarachnoid pink. Note the fasciculation of the nerve. (Material stained by Masson's trichrome technique and provided by N A Locket, Institute of Ophthalmology, London.)

in a retinal artery causes loss of vision in the corresponding part of the visual field; the only exception to this end-arterial pattern is in the vicinity of the optic disc; the posterior ciliary arteries enter the eye near the disc (**8.415, 427, 428**) and, apart from supplying the adjacent choroid, their rami form an anastomotic circle (of Zinn) in the sclera around the head of the optic nerve (**8.444**). Branches from this ring join the pial arteries of the nerve (Hayreh 1969) and from any arteries in this region small *cilio-retinal arteries* may enter the eye to anastomose with a retinal artery (**8.429**); similarly, small retino-ciliary veins may sometimes also be present. For further details see Singh and Dass (1960), who have surveyed the anastomoses between the central retinal artery and pial branches of the ophthalmic artery in the optic nerve.

Retinal capillaries do not pass towards the external surface of the retina beyond the internal nuclear lamina; they show regional differences in density, being especially numerous in the macula but absent from the central fovea. They become less numerous in the peripheral retina and are altogether absent from a zone about 1.5 mm wide adjoining the ora serrata. The central artery is innervated by sympathetic fibres and also has a parasympathetic supply (Ruskell 1970).

OCULAR REFRACTIVE MEDIA

The components of the eye which transmit and refract light are the cornea, the aqueous humour, the lens and the vitreous body. Of these, only the refracting power of the lens can be varied.

AQUEOUS HUMOUR

The total quantity of aqueous humour is small, filling the anterior and posterior chambers. The ciliary processes are responsible for its production by diffusion from the capillaries and by active transport from the unpigmented ciliary epithelium. It enters the posterior chamber, passes into the anterior chamber through the pupil and drains from the eye to the anterior ciliary vein at the iridocorneal angle through the spaces of the trabecular tissue to the scleral venous sinus (canal of Schlemm). Any interference with its resorption into the sinus increases intraocular pressure leading to the condition of *glaucoma*; if this persists the optic disc becomes 'cupped' and retinal degeneration leads to blindness. Drug therapy may re-establish adequate flow through the trabeculae or surgical methods can be used to by-pass this tissue and facilitate drainage. The aqueous humour is an avenue for nutrients, and metabolic exchange for the avascular tissues of the cornea and lens, and it also maintains and regulates the intraocular pressure and hence the constancy of the

ocular dimensions of the eyeball. It carries glucose, amino acids and respiratory gases, and also many other minor constituents.

VITREOUS BODY

The vitreous body fills the vitreous chamber, occupying about four-fifths of the eyeball. It is hollowed in front as a deep concavity, the *hyaloid fossa*, which is adapted to the lens. It is colourless, consisting of approximately 99% water, and although apparently structureless, a sparse but organized cellular and fibrous content is present. At its perimeter it has a gel-like consistency and is firmly attached to the surrounding structures of the eye; nearer the centre it has a more liquid zone. Na-hyaluronate, in the form of long glycosaminoglycan (GAG) chains, fills the whole vitreous. Additionally the peripheral gel or cortex (100–300 μm thick) contains a random loose network of Type II collagen fibrils which are occasionally grouped into fibres (Balaz 1982). The cortex also contains scattered cells, the *hyalocytes*, with the characteristics of mononuclear phagocytes. They are responsible for the production of Na-hyaluronate and, whilst they are normally in a resting state, they also have the capacity to be actively phagocytic in inflammatory conditions. Hyalocytes are not present in the cortex bordering the lens. The liquid vitreous is absent at birth, appearing first at 4 or 5 years and increasing to occupy half the vitreous space by the seventh decade. The cortex is most dense at the pars plana of the ciliary body adjacent to the ora serrata where attachment is strongest, and this is often referred to as the base of the vitreous. In this region the vitreous is thickened into a mass of radial fibres forming the *suspensory ligament of the lens* (see also below). The zonular fibres are attached to the pars plana and pass between the ciliary processes on their way to the equator of the lens where they insert obliquely into the capsule. Others have their origin in the ciliary processes. Most of these fibres attach a little anterior to the equator, the remainder attaching to the posterior surface and a few to the equator itself (Farnsworth & Burke 1977). The fibres of the zonular ligament support the lens and provide the essential link between lens and ciliary muscle in the process of accommodation (p. 1359).

A narrow *hyaloid canal* (**8.416**) runs from the optic nerve head to the central posterior surface of the lens. In fetuses this contains the hyloid artery (p. 261) which normally disappears about 6 weeks before birth. It persists as a very delicate fibrous structure and is of no functional importance.

LENS

General structure (8.415, 416, 446, 449)

The lens (**8.446**) is a transparent, encapsulated, biconvex body, placed between the iris and the vitreous body. Posteriorly the lens abuts on to the hyaloid fossa of the vitreous body; anteriorly, it forms a ring of contact with the free border of the iris, but further away from the axis of the lens the gap between the two increases to form the posterior chamber of the eye (see p. 1322). The lens is encircled by the ciliary processes, to which it is attached by the *zonular fibres* (mainly from the pars plana of the ciliary body), collectively forming the *zonule* holding the lens in place and transmitting the forces stretching the lens except in visual accommodation. The zonular fibres are inserted into the *lens capsule*, a basement membrane completely enclosing the eye (see below).

The lens has a characteristic shape, its anterior convexity being less steep, with a greater radius of curvature than the posterior (**8.415**) which has a more parabolic shape. The central points of these surfaces are the *anterior* and *posterior poles*; a line connecting these is the *axis of the lens*. The marginal circumference of the lens is its *equator*. In fetuses the lens is nearly spherical, with a slight reddish tinge, and is soft, breaking up on the slightest pressure. A hyaloid artery from the central retinal artery traverses the vitreous body to the posterior pole of the lens, whence its branches spread as a plexus covering the posterior surface and continuous round the capsular circumference with the vessels of the pupillary membrane and iris. In adults the lens is avascular, colourless and transparent but still quite soft in texture. In old age, the anterior surface becomes a little more curved pushing the iris forward slightly. The lens becomes less clear, with an amber tinge, and its nucleus is denser.

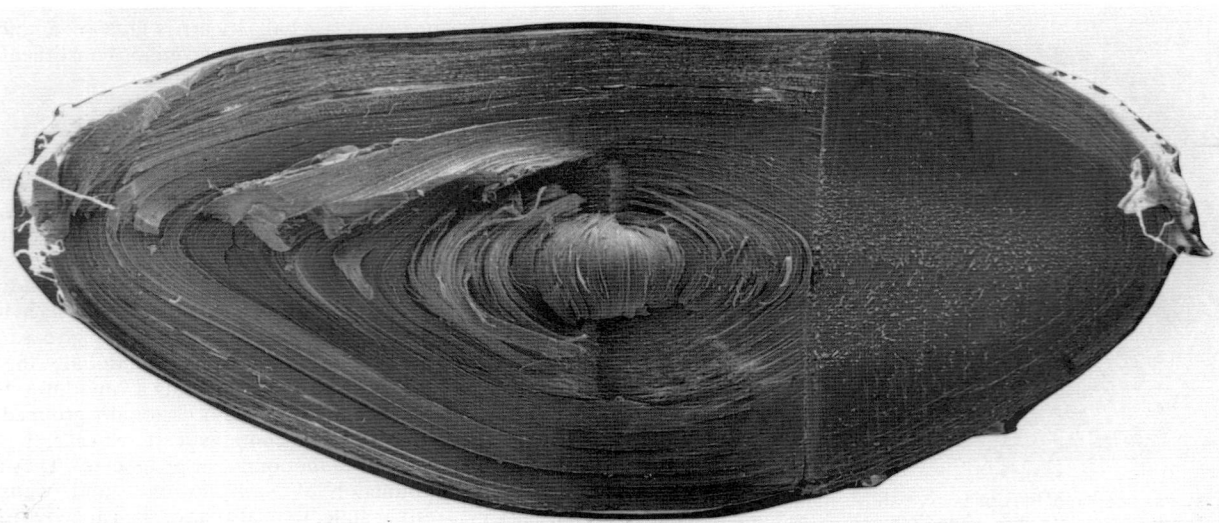

8.446 Scanning electron micrograph of an adult human lens, fractured across to reveal its lamellar structure. Note that the small central part with a different fibre orientation may represent the embryonic nucleus; the adult nucleus cannot be distinguished from the cortex. The more steeply curved surface (below) is posterior. The different texture of the lens in the right part of this picture is caused by cutting prior to the fracture procedure. Magnification × 15. (Provided by G. Vrensen and B. Willekens, Ophthalmic Research Institute of Amsterdam.)

In cataract the lens gradually becomes opaque and blindness ensues.

The **dimensions** of the lens are optically and clinically important, but they change with age as a consequence of continuous growth. Its equatorial diameter at birth is 6.5 mm, increasing rapidly at first, then more slowly to 9.0 mm at 15 and even more gradually to reach 9.5 mm in the ninth decade. Its axial dimension increases from 3.5–4.0 mm at birth to 4.75–5.0 mm at age 95. The radii of curvature reduce throughout life, the anterior surface showing the greater change as the lens thickens (Lowe & Clark 1973; Brown 1974). Average adult radii of the anterior and posterior surfaces are 10 mm and 6 mm respectively, the reduction during accommodation being mainly at the anterior surface.

Microstructure of the lens

The lens is derived from embryonic ectoderm (p. 259) and consists almost entirely of large numbers of stiff, very elongate, prismatic cells known as *lens fibres*, which are tightly packed together in a highly organized manner. The anterior surface of the eye as far as the equator is covered by a layer of *anterior lens cells*. Surrounding the whole structure is the *lens capsule* into which are inserted, around the equator, the *zonular fibres*. The lens is avascular and devoid of nerve fibres or other structures which might affect its transparency, and indeed its surface forms a very effective barrier against invasion by cells or agents of the immune system, creating within it an immunologically sequestered environment.

Lens fibres. Each fibre is up to 12 mm long, depending on age and position in the lens (related to their time of formation). Fibres near the surface at the equator are nucleated, the nuclei forming a short S-shaped bow extending inwards from the surface (8.447A–C), reflecting their sequence of formation from the superficial layer of anterior epithelial cells (see below); the deeper fibres lose their nuclei. In cross-section, individual fibres are flattened hexagons measuring about 10 μm by 2 μm. They are tightly packed, and adjacent fibres are firmly adherent and interlocked by innumerable junctions of various kinds, resembling ball-and-socket, tongue-and-groove joints and close-fitting angular processes (8.449) (Kuwabara 1975). Ball-and-socket junctions are plentiful in the outer, cortical fibres but infrequent in the lens nucleus, whereas tongue-and-groove junctions are characteristic of nuclear fibres but are absent from the cortex. Angle processes occur everywhere. Lens fibres are also in contact through desmosomes and numerous gap junctions including a modified form of these, the *square arrays* of intramembranous particles (Lo & Harding 1984; Vrensen et al 1992). For a review of lens fibre junctions, also see Zampighi et al (1992).

Internally, electron micrographs show the cells to be filled with a finely granular material in which are embedded a few organelles including scattered mitochondria and longitudinal microtubules in the more superficial fibres; all cells also contain a cytoskeleton of actin filaments around their margins (Rafferty & Goosens 1978), which perhaps helps to maintain the shape of the cells and may assist its elasticity, although it is unlikely to be actively involved in accommodation (Kibbelar et al 1980). The ubiquitous intracellular granular material just referred to appears to correspond to the dominant proteins of the lens, the *crystallins*, which are responsible for its transparency and refractile properties, and for much of its elasticity. At least two varieties coexist, α and β. These occur in very high concentrations, forming up to 60% of the lens fibre mass. The crystallins are responsible for the characteristic high refractive index on the lens, while variations in their concentration in different parts of the lens give rise to regional differences in refractive index, correcting for spherical and chromatic aberrations which might occur in a homogeneous lens.

Variations in lens fibre structure and composition make it possible to distinguish a softer *cortical zone* and a firmer central part, the *nucleus* (8.446). Where sheafs of lens fibres abut on each other at their ends, faint sutural lines are formed, radiating out from the poles towards the equator. In fetuses, the sutures on the anterior surface of the lens form a tri-radiate pattern (8.448A), centred on the anterior pole and resembling the limbs of an upright letter Y; posteriorly, a similar though inverted sutural configuration is present. In adults, the sutures increase in number and complexity because of lens growth and other changes in the arrangement of lens fibres (8.448B). These sutures represent the lines of linearly registered interlocking junctions between terminating lens fibres. When, after extraction, the lens is hardened with fixatives and broken open, the arrangement of lens fibres produces a striking, onion-like appearance, the fibres splitting into a series of concentric lamellae of varying thicknesses (8.446).

All lens fibres cross the equator (or the plane passing through it) where they are generated, and terminate on both an anterior and a posterior suture. Because of the curious growth pattern of the lens, fibres commencing near the central axis of the lens anteriorly terminate posteriorly on a suture near the periphery, and vice versa.

Anterior lens cells. These constitute a transparent layer of simple cuboidal epithelium over the anterior surface of the lens (8.447A–C); there they undergo mitosis and migrate back to the equator; they transform into lens fibres. In surface view anterior lens cells are polygonal; they are about 15 μm across and slightly less in height, while in the central area they may be flattened to a mere 6 μm. Towards the equator they are tall and thin, and mitosis is more frequent. Further peripherally, apposed lateral membranes become oblique and interdigitated. There are no tight junctions between adjacent anterior lens cells, but gap junctions are frequent, as are adherens junctions (see Zampighi et al 1992).

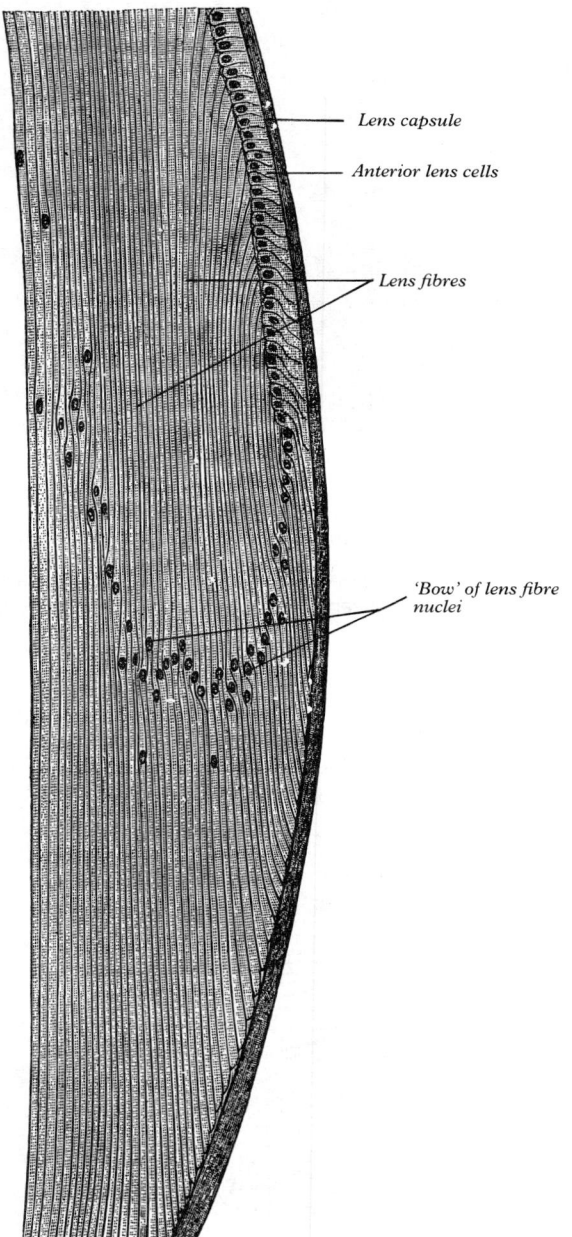

Lens capsule

Anterior lens cells

Lens fibres

'Bow' of lens fibre nuclei

A

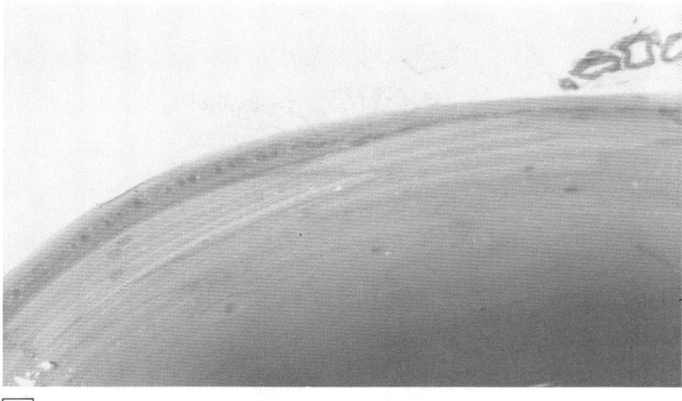

B

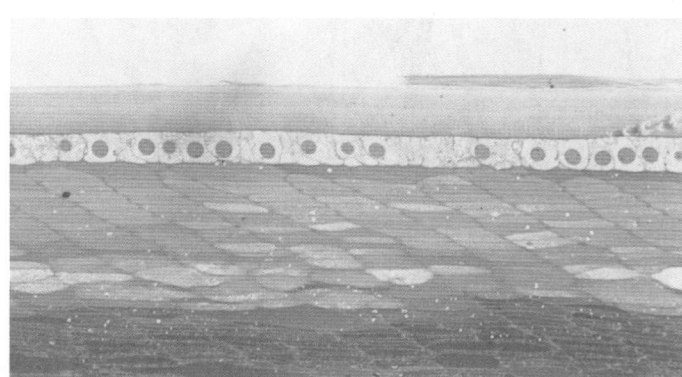

C

8.447A   Section through the edge of the lens equator, showing the transition of the epithelium of anterior lens cells into the lens fibres. Note that the lens cells retain their nuclei long after they have assumed the form of a fibre. The anterior direction is upward in this figure.

8.447B, C   Histological section through the margin of the lens equator (compare with 8.447A).

B   Medium power appearance showing the lightly stained lamina covering the single layer of epithelial cells in the capsule. Several lens fibres contain nuclei. Magnification × 50.

C is a more highly magnified micrograph showing the superficial nucleated precursors of the lens fibres and the overlying capsule. Toliudine blue, resin section. Magnification × 450. (Provided by G L Ruskell, Department of Optometry and Visual Science, The City University, London.)

Functionally these cells are of great importance; they are the precursors of the lens fibres, engaging in mitotic division, especially near the equator of the lens, and undergoing gradual differentiation there to synthesize the characteristic proteins and undergo the extreme elongation typical of the lens fibre. As other cells follow suit, the earlier cells come to occupy a deeper position in the lens and lose their nuclei as they are packed down by new recruits to the lens fibre population. This process can be traced clearly in sections through the lens equator (8.447A). Despite their very slow growth, the epithelial cells are relatively active; experimental injuries in mice heal completely within 3 days (Rafferty 1976).

Lens capsule and zonular fibres. The lens capsule is a thick basement membrane which covers the outer surface of the lens (8.447), including the anterior lens cell layer (Cohen 1965). It is thickest anteriorly (about 10 μm), becoming thinner posteriorly. In structure it resembles the posterior (Descemet's) membrane of the cornea, consisting of various classes of collagen fibres (I, III and IV: Marshall et al 1992) as well as a range of glycosaminoglycans and glycoproteins, for example fibronectin and laminin. Its chief source is probably the anterior lens cells and their fetal precursors. The capsule is elastic, and during the flattening of the lens can stretch considerably up to about 60% in circumference without tearing (Assia et al 1991).

Inserted into the capsule in the region of the equator are the zonular fibres. These are composed of thin (4–7 nm) fibrils with hollow centres, resembling fibrils associated with elastic connective tissue fibres (p. 80). The zonular fibres, too, have some elasticity, although this decreases with age.

Lens refraction

The dioptric power of the lens is much less than that of the cornea. All ocular optical media have a refractive index close to that of water but the corneal surface is in contact with air and most of the 58 dioptres of the eye's refractive power are effected here. The value of the lens is its ability to vary its dioptric power, depending on its capacity to change shape. It has a greater refractive index than the adjacent media, varying from 1.386 at its periphery to 1.406 at its core, and contributes about 17 dioptres to the total of the relaxed eye. Its **range in dioptric power** permits a further 12 dioptres in youth, but the available dioptric range decreases with age, being halved at 40 years and reduced to 1 dioptre or less at 60. Most young children show minor refractive errors (Sorsby et al 1961; Gwiazda et al 1993) modifying towards emmetropia in pre-school and later years. For further information on physiological optics consult Davson (1980) and Bennett and Rabetts (1984).

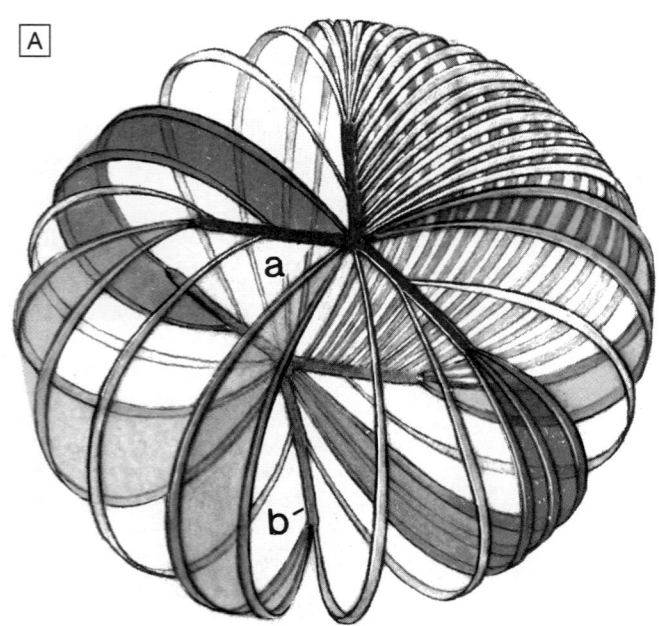

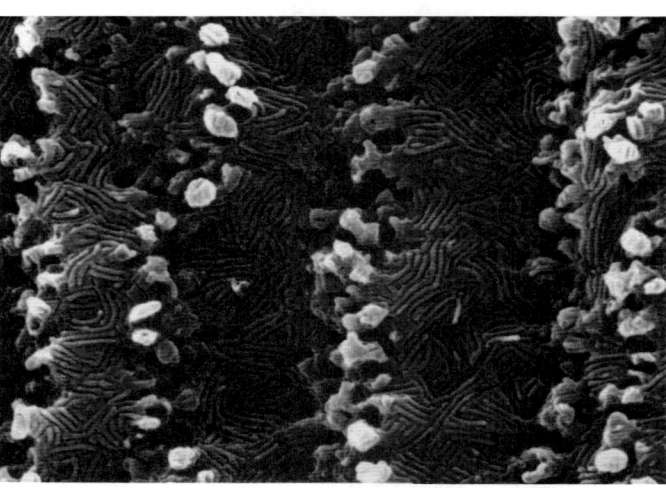

8.449   Freeze fracture preparation of lens fibre surfaces from the nucleus of an adult human lens. Ridges of tongue-and-groove joints forming small parallel groups cover the surfaces; the lighter knob-like structures are the interlocking angle processes. The small dark holes are the spaces vacated by the angle processes of the removed overlying fibres. Magnification × 5000. (Provided by G Vrensen and B Willekens, Ophthalmic Research Institute of Amsterdam.)

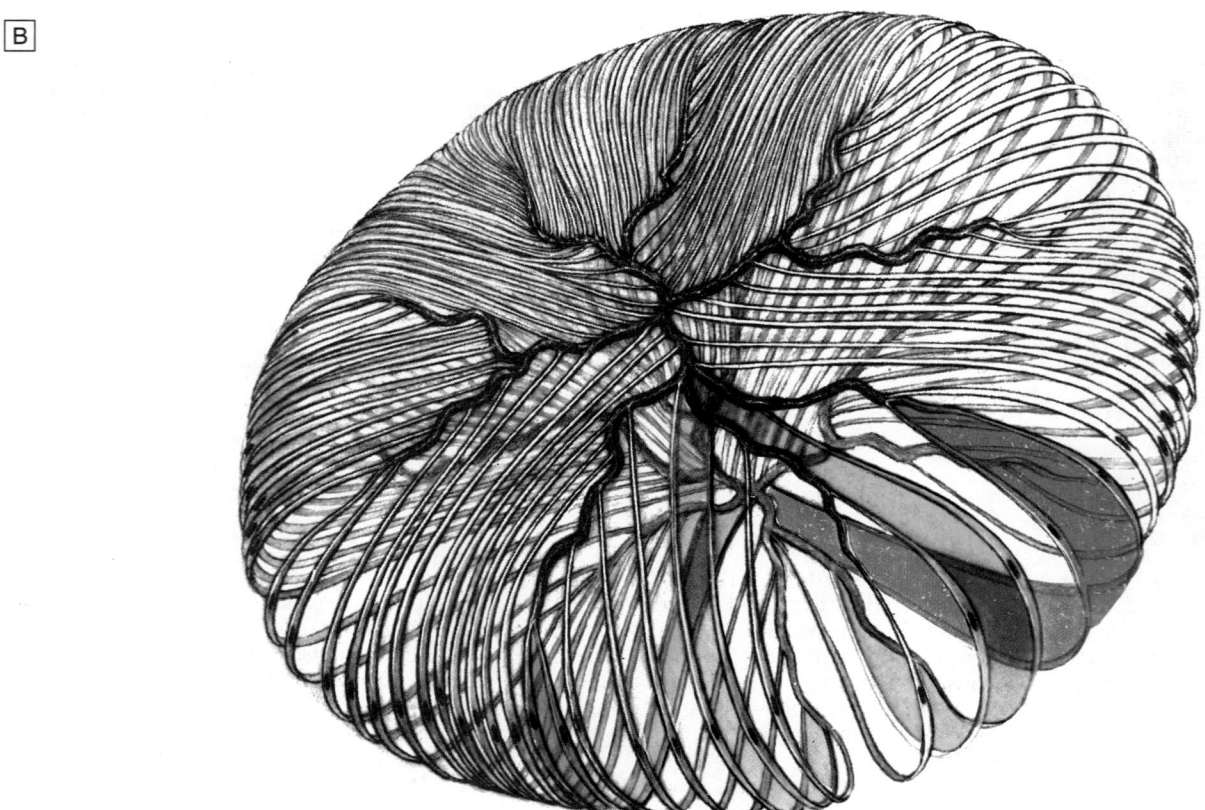

8.448   The structure of the fetal (A) and adult (B) human lens, showing the major details of arrangement of the lens cells or fibres. The anterior (a) and posterior (b) triradiate sutures are shown in the fetal lens and it is clear that fibres pass from the apex of an arm of one suture to the angle between two arms at the opposite pole, as shown in the coloured segments. Intermediate fibres show the same reciprocal behaviour, ending nearer to one pole, where they start further from the other, and so on. The suture pattern becomes much more complex as successive strata are added to the exterior of the growing lens, the original arms of each triradiate suture showing secondary and tertiary dichotomous branchings. (See **8**.421 for acknowledgement.)

ACCESSORY VISUAL APPARATUS

This includes the extraocular muscles, fasciae, eyebrows, eyelids, conjunctiva and lacrimal apparatus.

EXTRAOCULAR MUSCLES

There are seven extraocular or extrinsic muscles associated with the eye (8.450–456): *levator palpebrae superioris* is an elevator of the upper eyelid, while the other six are capable of moving the eye in almost any direction: *four recti* (*superior, inferior, medialis* and *lateralis*), and two *obliqui* (*superior* and *inferior*).

Also associated with the orbit, though not directly attached to the eyeball, are some minor muscles: *orbitalis* at the back of the orbit, and the *superior* and *inferior tarsal muscles*, small smooth muscle laminae inserted into the upper and lower eyelids; the superior tarsal is usually described as part of the levator palpebrae superioris, while the lower is related to the inferior rectus and inferior oblique. *Orbicularis oculi*, part of which runs within the upper and lower eyelids, and by its contraction closes the eye, is described elsewhere with the muscles of facial expression (p. 791).

The six muscles which move the eyeball are found in all vertebrates and are thus a phylogenetically ancient feature of this group of animals. The muscles of the eyelids are found only in tetrapods which are able to close their eyes (however not including snakes, which lack this ability); the levator palpebrae superioris appears to have arisen by the splitting of the superior rectus muscle.

In general structure the extraocular muscles resemble skeletal muscles elsewhere but they differ in some features, particularly in the details of their innervation, contraction and pharmacology (Spencer & Porter 1988). At least two types of muscle fibre are present: a slender (9–11 μm) slow-contracting 'non-twitch' form and a thicker (11–15 μm) 'twitch' type. The former have motor terminals of the 'en grappe' category (p. 1058), and the latter, motor end plates.

Levator palpebrae superioris (8.450, 455). This is a thin, triangular muscle; it arises from the inferior aspect of the lesser wing of the sphenoid, above and in front of the optic canal and separated from it by the attachment of rectus superior. It has a short narrow tendon at its posterior attachment, and broadens gradually then more sharply as it passes anteriorly above the eyeball. The muscle ends in front in a wide aponeurosis, some of its tendinous fibres passing straight into the upper eyelid to attach to the anterior surface of the tarsus, while the rest radiate, piercing the orbicularis oculi to pass to the eyelid skin.

The connective tissue coats of the adjoining surfaces of levator palpebrae superioris and rectus superior are fused; where the two muscles separate to reach their anterior attachments, the fascia between them forms a thick mass to which is attached the superior conjunctival fornix, usually described as an additional attachment of the levator palpebrae superioris. Traced laterally, the aponeurosis of the levator passes between the orbital and palpebral parts of the lacrimal gland to a tubercle on the zygomatic bone, just within the orbital margin (p. 552); traced medially it loses its tendinous nature as it passes closely over the reflected tendon of the obliquus superior, continuing on to the medial palpebral ligament as loose strands of connective tissue.

Levator palpebrae superioris raises the upper eyelid but during this process the lateral and medial parts of its aponeurosis are stretched and thus limit its action; the elevation is also said to be checked by the orbital septum (p. 1361). ('Check' mechanisms abound in the orbit but there is little direct evidence that connective tissue structures thus implicated do function in this manner. See also p. 1359.)

Minor muscles of the eyelids. Opposite the equator of the eye a thin lamella, the *superior tarsal muscle*, containing smooth muscle fibres, is attached to the inferior face of levator palpebrae superioris (Kuwabara et al 1975); a fibrous extension projects to the upper margin of the superior tarsus.

In the lower eyelid there is a corresponding *inferior tarsal muscle*, a less prominent smooth muscle stratum uniting the inferior tarsus to the fascial sheath of the inferior rectus and that muscle's expansion to the sheath of the inferior oblique. These muscles assist in the elevation of the upper and depression of the lower eyelids, and may adjust the size of the open eye aperture according to mood and other factors.

Orbitalis (*the orbital muscle of Müller*). This is another thin layer of smooth muscle, lying at the back of the orbit where it spans the inferior orbital fissure. Its functions are uncertain, but its contraction may possibly produce a slight forward protrusion of the eyeball; this certainly occurs in many other mammals, although in humans the muscle is almost vestigial in comparison. For a recent report, see Jordan 1992.

All three of these minor muscles, being composed of smooth muscle, receive a sympathetic innervation from the superior cervical

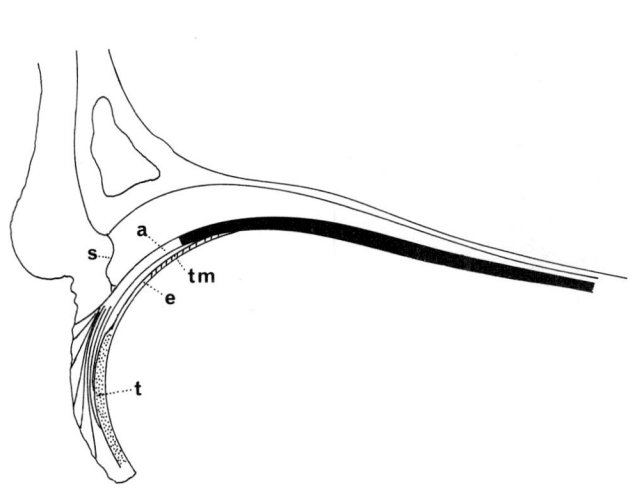

8.450 Diagram showing the components of levator palpebrae superioris and its connections. a = aponeurosis; tm = superior tarsal muscle (of Müller); e = tendinous extension of superior tarsal muscle; t = tarsus; s = orbital septum. (After Whitnall 1932. Provided by G L Ruskell, Department of Optometry and Visual Science, The City University, London.)

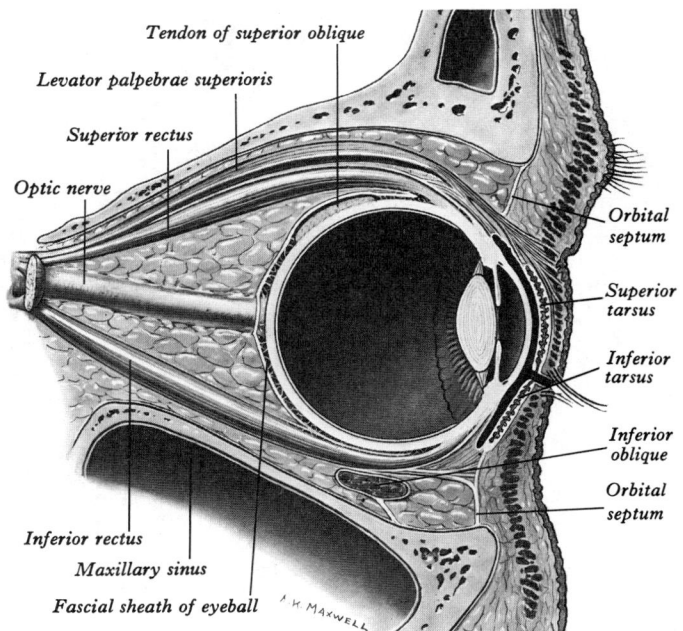

8.451 Sagittal section through the right orbital cavity.

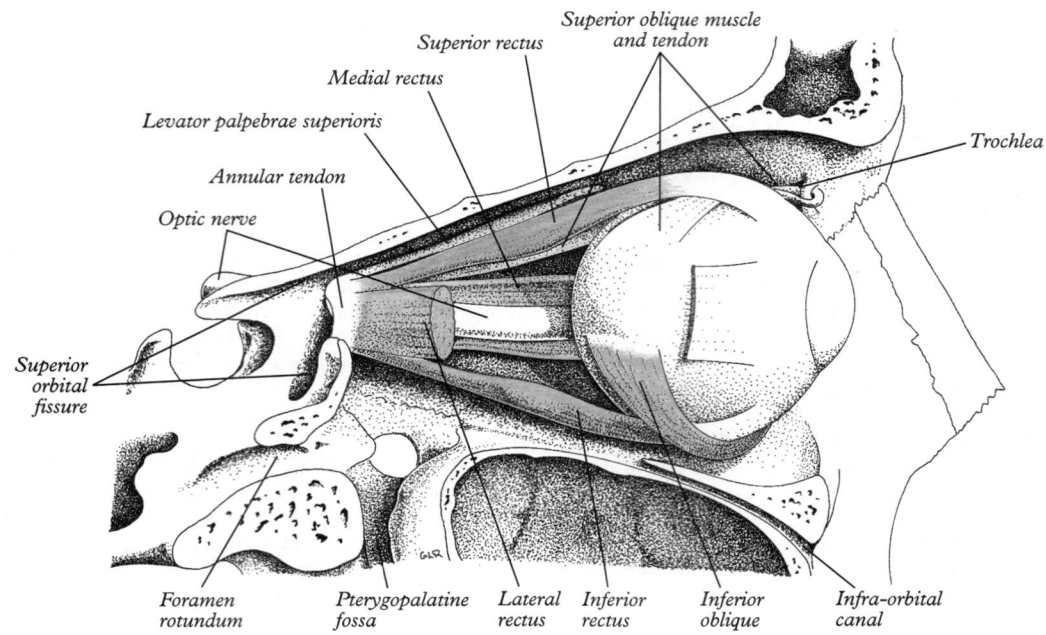

8.452   The muscles of the right orbit, lateral view. (Provided by G L Ruskell, Department of Optometry and Visual Science, The City University, London.)

ganglion via the carotid plexus; they are affected by dysfunction of the sympathetic innervation, for example as in Horner's syndrome which therefore causes the upper eyelid to droop (ptosis) as well as other less obvious changes to the eye.

The four recti (8.451–456). Each of these is approximately strap-shaped, with a thickened middle part thinning gradually to a tendon.

They are attached posteriorly to a *common annular tendon* around the superior, medial and inferior margins of the optic canal (8.455); this fibrous annulus continues laterally across the inferior and medial parts of the superior orbital fissure and is attached to a tubercle on the margin of the greater wing of the sphenoid. The tendon is closely adherent to the optic nerve's dural sheath and the surrounding

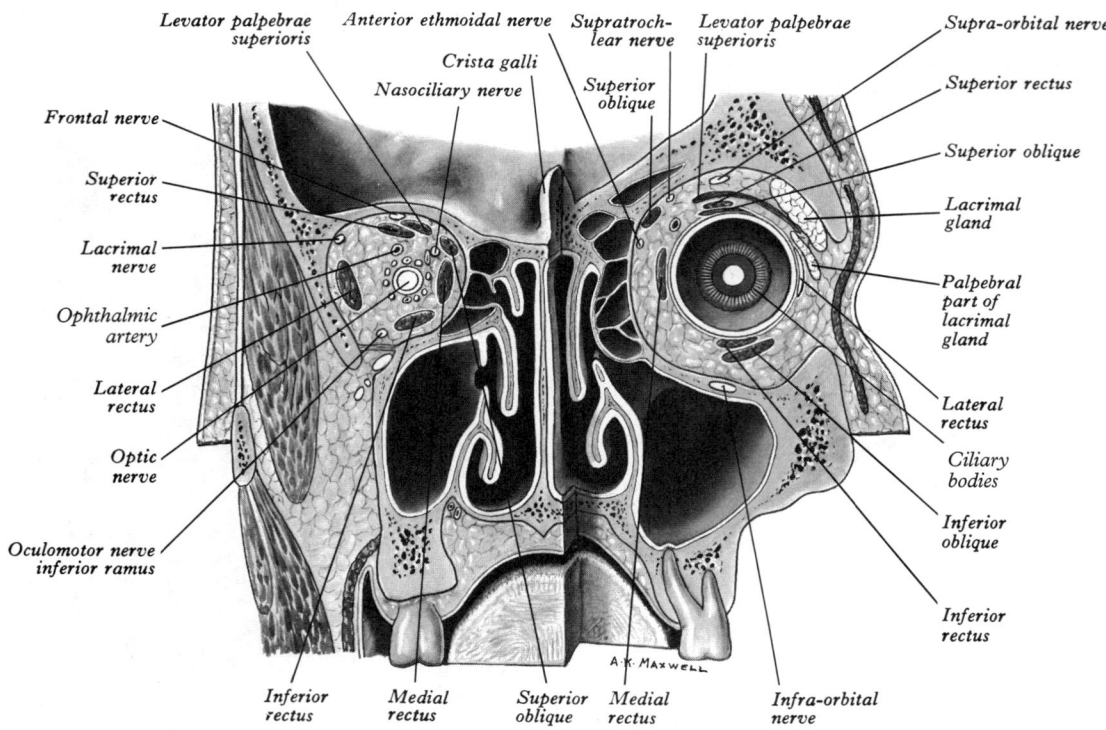

8.453   Coronal sections through the two orbits: posterior aspect. On the left side the plane of the section is more posterior and passes behind the eyeball.

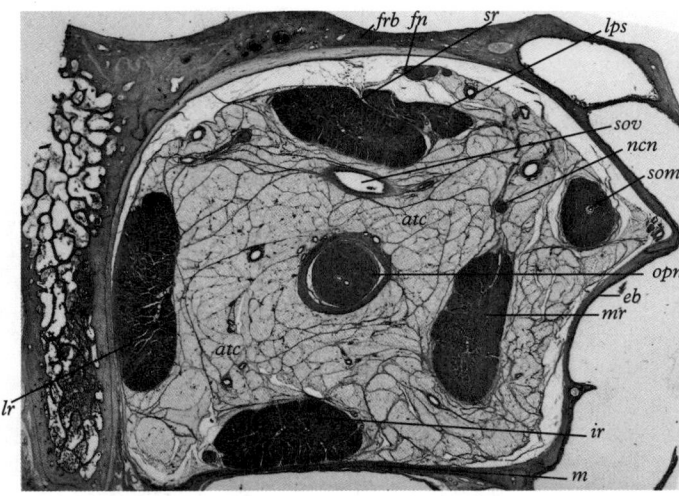

A

B

8.454 Two coronal sections through the right orbit (viewed from in front: left is lateral) cut through planes passing (A) 5 mm behind the posterior pole of the globe of the eye, and (B) 4.6 mm in front of its posterior pole (the lens which is visible, has been displaced backwards. Abbreviations: atc = adipose tissue compartments; eb = ethmoid bone; fn = frontal nerve; frb = frontal bone; iov = inferior orbital vein; ir = inferior rectus muscle; lb = lacrimal bone; lacg = lacrimal gland; lr = lateral rectus muscle; ls = lacrimal sac; m = maxilla (bone); ms = maxillary sinus; mr = medial rectus muscle; ncn = nasociliary nerve; oo = orbicularis oculi; opn = optic nerve; sb = sphenoid bone; lps = levator palpebrae superioris; som = superior oblique muscle; sov = superior ophthalmic vein; sr = superior rectus muscle; zyg = zygomatic bone. Approximate magnification × 2.5. (From Kornneef 1977, with permission. Compare with 8.53.)

periosteum. Two specialized parts of this ring may be discerned: a lower, to which are attached the rectus inferior, part of the rectus medialis and the lower fibres of the rectus lateralis; and an upper, providing attachment to the rectus superior, part of the rectus medialis and the upper fibres of the rectus lateralis; a second small tendinous slip of the rectus lateralis is attached to the orbital surface of the greater wing of the sphenoid, lateral to the annulus. Each muscle passes forwards, in the position implied by its name, to be attached anteriorly by a tendinous expansion into the sclera, posterior to the margin of the cornea, and at average distances from the latter as follows: medialis 5.5 mm; inferior 6.5 mm; lateralis 6.9 mm; superior 7.7 mm.

Obliquus superior (8.452, 454–456). This is fusiform and lies superomedial in the orbit; it arises from the body of the sphenoid superomedial to the optic canal and to the tendinous attachment of the rectus superior. Passing forwards it ends in a round tendon, which plays through a fibrocartilaginous loop, the *trochlea*, attached to the trochlear fossa of the frontal bone. Tendon and trochlea are separated by a delicate synovial sheath. After traversing the trochlea the tendon is deflected posterolaterally and inferior to the rectus superior to be attached to the sclera **behind** the equator in its superolateral posterior quadrant, between the recti superior and lateralis.

Obliquus inferior (8.452, 454–456). A thin, narrow muscle near the anterior margin of the floor of the orbit, it arises from the orbital surface of the maxilla lateral to the nasolacrimal groove. Ascending posterolaterally at first between the rectus inferior and the orbital floor and then between the eyeball and rectus lateralis, it is inserted into the lateral part of the sclera **behind** the equator of the eyeball in its inferolateral posterior quadrant between the rectus inferior and rectus lateralis, near to but slightly posterior to the attachment of the obliquus superior. The muscle broadens and thins, and, in contrast to the other extraocular muscles, it has a barely discernible tendon at its scleral attachment.

Nerve supply of extraocular muscles. The levator palpebrae superioris, obliquus inferior and recti superior, inferior and medialis are supplied by the oculomotor nerve, the obliquus superior by the trochlear and the rectus lateralis by the abducent nerve.

Structures enclosed by the tendinous ring (8.455). These are:

- the anterior aperture of the optic canal, transmitting the optic nerve and ophthalmic artery

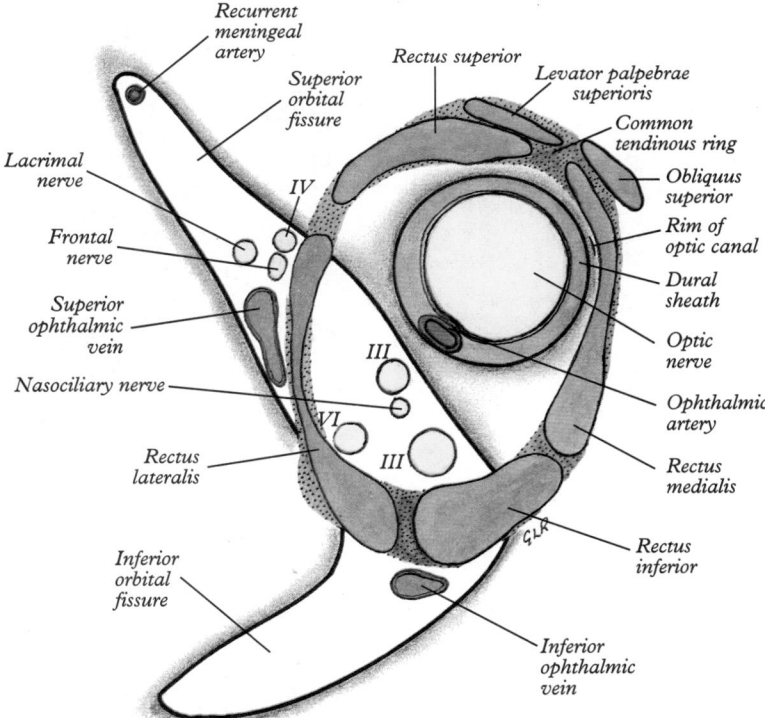

8.455 Schema showing the common tendinous ring with its muscle origins superimposed, and the relative positions of the nerves entering the orbital cavity through the superior orbital fissure and optic canal. Note that the attachments of levator palpebrae superioris and obliquus superior lie external to the common tendinous ring but are attached to it. The ophthalmic veins frequently pass through the ring. The recurrent meningeal artery, a branch of the ophthalmic artery, is often conducted from the orbit to the cranial cavity through its own foramen. Based mainly on the data of Whitnall (1932) and Koornneef (1977). (Provided by G L Ruskell, Department of Optometry and Visual Science, The City University, London.)

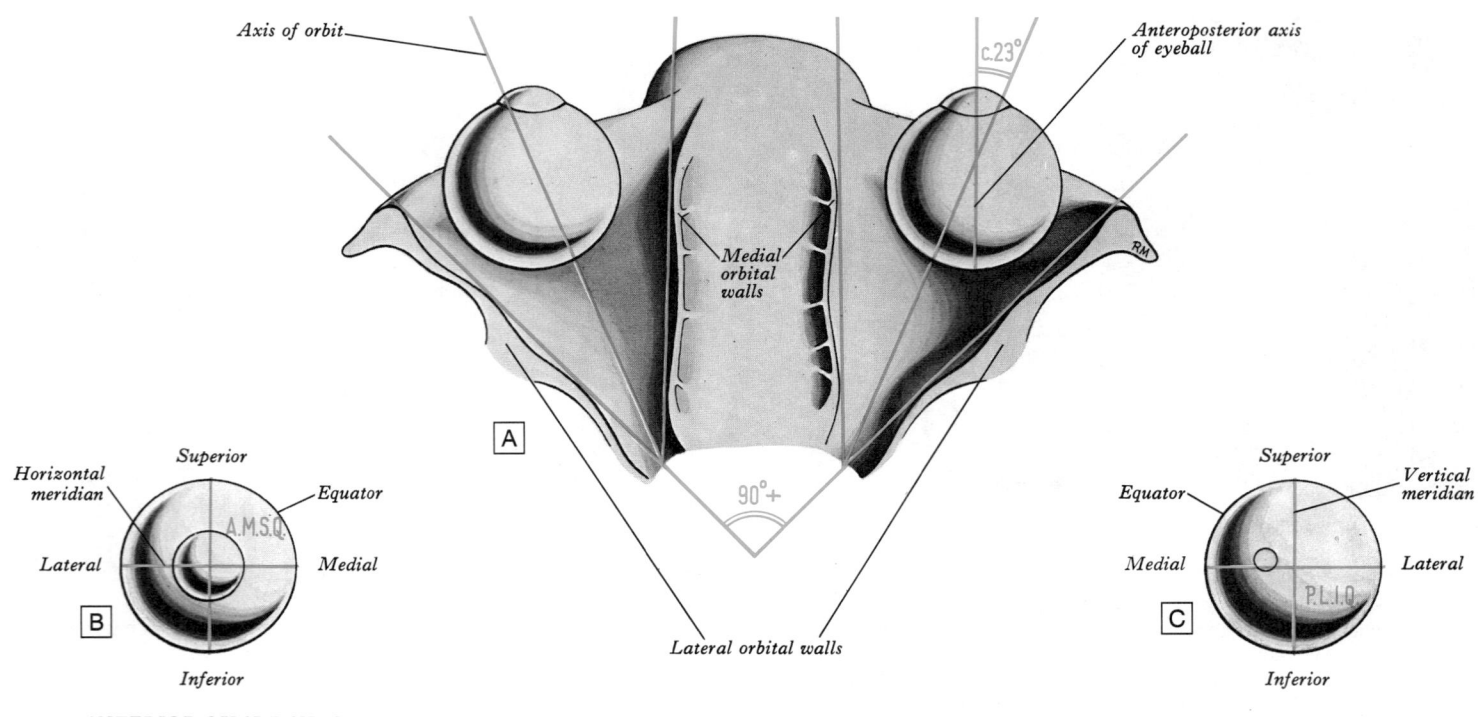

Axis of orbit

Anteroposterior axis of eyeball

c.23°

Medial orbital walls

A

90°+

Lateral orbital walls

Superior

Horizontal meridian

Equator

A.M.S.Q.

Lateral

Medial

B

Inferior

ANTERIOR QUADRANTS

Superior

Equator

Vertical meridian

Medial

Lateral

P.L.I.Q.

C

Inferior

POSTERIOR QUADRANTS

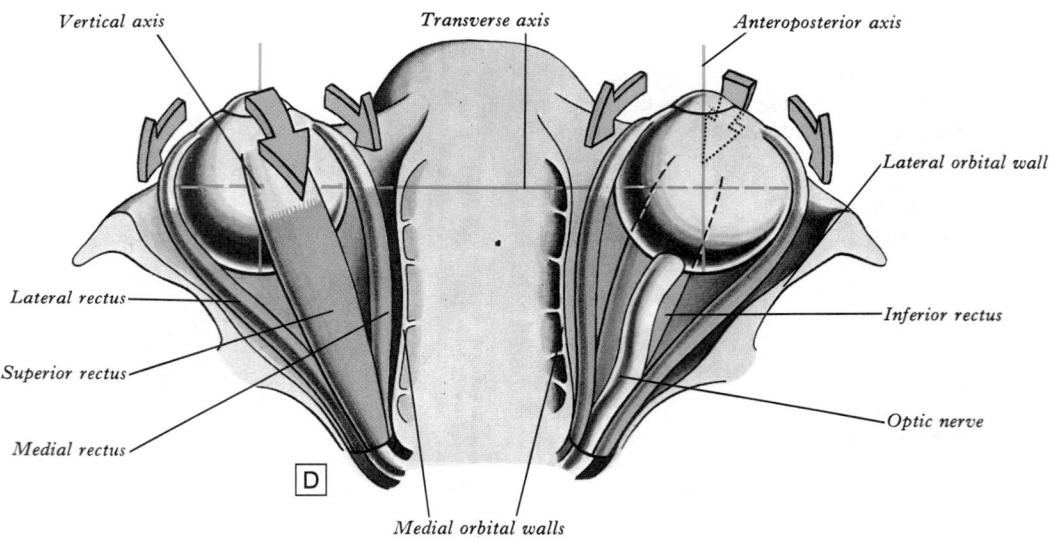

Vertical axis

Transverse axis

Anteroposterior axis

Lateral orbital wall

Lateral rectus

Superior rectus

Inferior rectus

Medial rectus

Optic nerve

D

Medial orbital walls

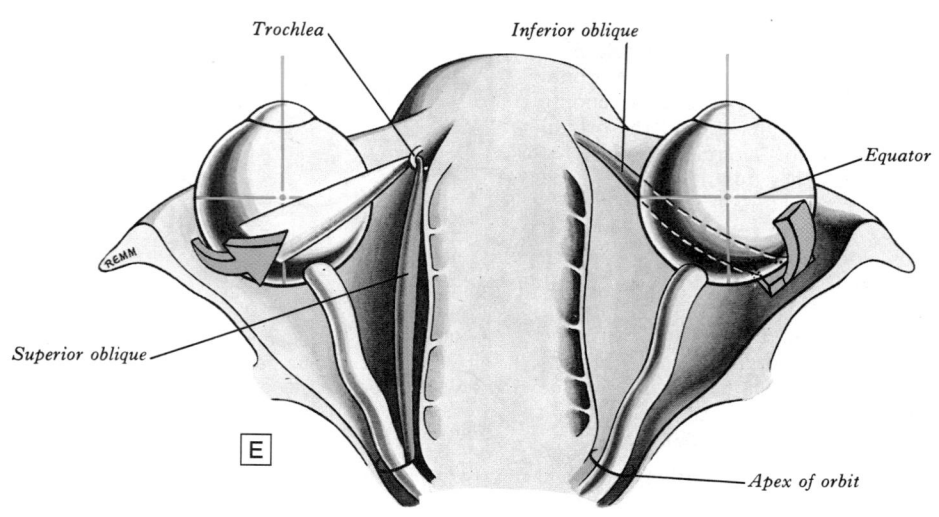

Trochlea

Inferior oblique

Equator

Superior oblique

E

Apex of orbit

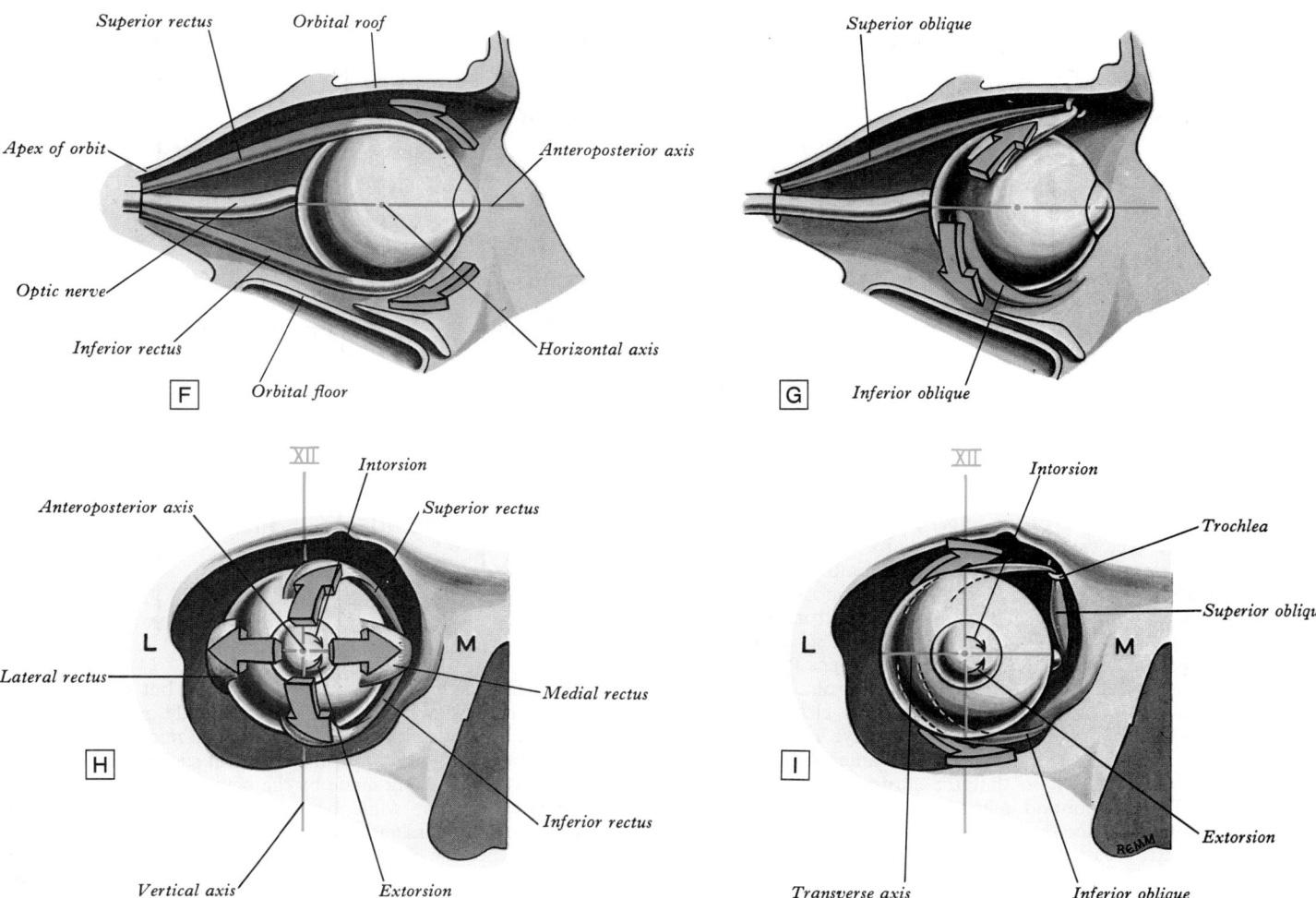

8.456 The geometrical basis of ocular movements.
A   The relationship between the orbital and ocular axes, with the eyes in the primary position of parallel visual axes.
B and C   The ocular globe in anterior and posterior views to show conventional geometry: meridia, equator, etc. A.M.S.Q = anterior medial superior quadrant; P.L.I.Q = posterior lateral inferior quadrant.
D   The orbits from above showing the medial and lateral recti and the superior rectus (left) and the inferior rectus (right), indicating turning moments primarily around the vertical axis.
E   Superior (left) and inferior (right) oblique muscles showing turning moments primarily around the vertical and also anteroposterior axes.
F   Lateral view to show the actions of the superior and inferior recti around the transverse axis.
G   Lateral view to show the action of the superior and inferior oblique muscles around the anteroposterior axis.
H   Anterior view to show the medial rotational movement of the superior and inferior recti around the vertical axis. Conventionally the 12 o'clock position indicated is said to be *intorted* (superior rectus) or *extorted* (inferior rectus) as indicated by the small arrows on the cornea.
I   Anterior view to show the torsional effects of the superior oblique (intorsion) and inferior oblique (extorsion) around the anteroposterior axis, as indicated by the small arrows on the cornea.

- the medial part of the superior orbital fissure transmitting the two divisions of the oculomotor and the nasociliary and abducent nerves.

The superior ophthalmic vein may pass within or above the annular tendon, the inferior ophthalmic vein within or below it.

Actions of extraocular muscles

Levator palpebrae superioris elevates the upper lid, its antagonist being the palpebral part of orbicularis oculi. The degree of elevation which, apart from blinking, is maintained for long periods during waking hours is a compromise between the adequate exposure of the optical media and the control of the amount of entering light, which in very bright sunshine can be reduced by lowering the upper lid, so limiting glare. Much is known of the physiology of blinking (Evinger et al 1991) and its significance in distributing lacrimal secretions. Electrically, the levator discharges steadily for a given fixation but with increasing rates with upward lid position, relaxing during closure of the palpebral fissure (Fuchs et al 1992). The role of the superior tarsal muscle is less clear, although its tonus is related to sympathetic nerve activity, as seen when impairment of the sympathetic supply of the head causes the eyelid to droop (ptosis), in Horner's syndrome.

The *six extraocular muscles* all **rotate** the eyeball in directions dependent upon the geometrical relation between their osseous and global attachments (**8.456**A,D,E), which are, of course, altered by the ocular movements themselves. Before considering their activities it must be recognized that **human** extraocular muscles are not generally accessible to inspection; consequently many opinions regarding them depend on deductions from malfunction due to disturbances of innervation the full extent of which is rarely possible to assess. It is also essential to appreciate that any movement of an eye alters the tension and/or length in **all six** muscles, though direct observation of this has rarely been attempted, even in experimental animals (Sherrington 1905; Szentágothai 1950). It is at least likely that all six muscles are continuously involved and it is therefore merely a preliminary but necessary exercise to consider each in isolation. Because they form more obvious groupings as antagonists or synergists, it is useful to consider the four recti and two obliques as separate groups, remembering always that they act in concert.

Of the four *recti*, the *medial* and *lateral* exert comparatively straightforward forces on the eyeball. Being approximately horizontal, when the visual axis is in its primary position, directed to the horizon, they rotate the eye medially (adduction) or laterally (abduction) about an imaginary vertical axis (**8.456**D). They are antagonists; by reciprocal adjustment of their lengths the visual axis can be swept through a horizontal arc. When both eyes are involved, as is usual, the four medial and lateral recti can either adjust both visual axes in a *conjugate* movement from point to point at infinity, their axes remaining parallel, or they can *converge* or *diverge* the axes to or from nearer or more distant objects of attention in the visual field. But since they do not rotate the eye around its transverse axis, the medial and lateral recti cannot effect the extremely frequent act of elevating or depressing the visual axes as gaze is transferred from nearer to more distant objects or the reverse. This is the contribution of the *superior* and *inferior recti* (aided, as will become apparent, by the two oblique muscles). However, the geometry of these two recti muscles is a little less simple; the key to the rotations which they effect is the obliquity of the orbit (**8.456A**), whose axis does not correspond with the visual axis in its primary position but diverges from it at an angle of approximately 23°, a value varying in different individuals, depending on the angle between the orbital axes and the median plane (**8.456A**). Hence, the simple rotation caused by an isolated *superior rectus*, analysed with reference to the three hypothetical ocular axes, appears to be complex, being primarily *elevation* (transverse axis), and secondarily a less powerful *medial rotation* (vertical axis) and slight *intorsion* (anteroposterior axis) in which the midpoint of the upper rim of the cornea (often referred to as '12 o'clock') is rotated medially towards the nose. These actions, compounded in fact as a single, simple rotation, are easily appreciated when it is seen that the direction of traction of the superior rectus runs in a *posteromedial* direction from its attachment in front, which is *anterior* to the equator and *superior* to the cornea, to its osseous attachment near the orbital apex (**8.456D,H**):

The *inferior rectus* pulls in a similar direction but rotates the visual axis **downwards** about the transverse axis. It is clear, from its comparable geometry, that it also rotates the eye **medially** on a vertical axis but that its action around the anteroposterior axis **extorts** the eye i.e. rotates it so that the corneal 12 o'clock point turns **laterally**. The superior and inferior recti, therefore, both rotate the eye medially and, since their effects around the transverse and anteroposterior axes are opposed, their combined, equal contractions could only rotate the eye medially. In binocular movements they thus assist the medial recti in converging the visual axes; and by reciprocal adjustment they can elevate or depress the visual axes. It must be added that, as the eye is rotated laterally, the lines of traction of the superior and inferior recti approach the plane of the anteroposterior ocular axis (**8.456I**); hence their rotational effects about this and the vertical ocular axis diminish. In abduction to about 23°, they become almost purely an elevator and depressor of the visual axis.

The *superior oblique* acts on the eye from the trochlea and, since the attachment of the *inferior oblique* is for practical purposes vertically below this, both muscles approach the eye at the same angle, being attached in approximately similar positions in the *superior* and *inferior posterolateral* ocular quadrants (**8.456H,I**). From this geometry it is easy to understand that the superior oblique elevates the **posterior** aspect of the eye, the inferior depressing it. Hence, the former rotates the visual axis **downwards** and the latter **upwards**, both movements being around the transverse axis. But the obliquity of both is such that their traction, when the eye is in the primary position, is in a direction **posterior** to the vertical axis; both therefore rotate the eye **laterally** around this axis. With regard to the anteroposterior axis it is not difficult to deduce that in isolation the superior oblique *intorts* the eye, the inferior oblique *extorting* it. Like the superior and inferior recti, therefore, the two obliques have a common turning movement around the vertical axis but are opposed forces in respect of the other two. Acting in concert they could therefore assist the lateral rectus in abducting the visual axis, as in *divergence* of the eyes in transferring attention from near to far. Again, like the superior and inferior recti, the directions of traction of the oblique muscles also vary with ocular position; they become more nearly a pure elevator and a depressor as the eye is adducted.

In a short analysis of this kind much must be omitted and nothing can be said of the defects of ocular movement. For further information refer to Whitnall (1932), Cogan (1956), Schlossman & Priestley (1966), Alpern (1969), Davson (1972) and Spencer and Porter (1988). For those requiring the barest data, the actions of extraocular muscles may be summarized in the following diagram:

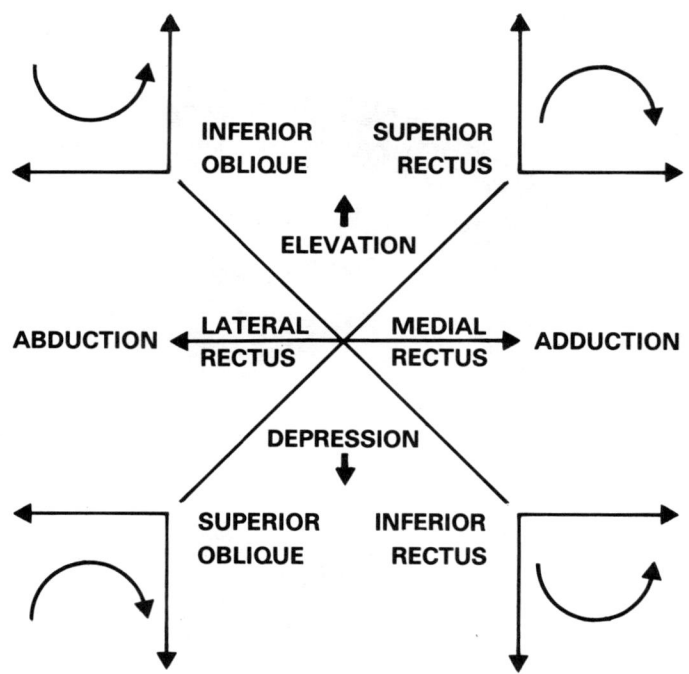

So far, head movements have been ignored but it is common observation that ocular movements are frequently, perhaps usually, accompanied by movements of the head, which might be likened to the **coarse** adjustment of an optical instrument such as a microscope, the **finer** adjustments being made by the ocular musculature.

It is interesting that while ocular rotations are clearly under voluntary control, **torsional** movements cannot be voluntarily initiated. But when the head is tilted in a frontal plane, reflex torsions occur. Any small lapse in the concerted adjustment of both eyes entails diplopia. It is indeed surprising that such a complex organization of extraocular, neck and other muscles is learnt so effectively early in life that diplopia is rarely experienced; but the prize, of course, *stereoscopic vision*, is a great one.

All binocular movements are either *conjugate* or *disjunctive*, the visual axes either being trained in parallel or inclined in convergence/divergence activity. While it is a necessary introductory simplification to analyse both forms of action in terms of static geometry, in reality both are dynamic and hence more complex than simple analysis suggests. In so-called 'fixation' of a focus of attention, whether uniocular or binocular, the visual axis is not 'fixed' in a perfectly steady manner but undergoes minute, but observable flicking (of a few minutes or even seconds of arc) across the true line of fixation. Such *microsaccades* are rapid and surprisingly complex (see Barlow 1952; Riggs et al 1960; etc.). The term *saccade* (a French word of obscure origin meaning a 'jerk on the reins') was introduced by Dodge in 1903 for similar but much larger swings of fixation observed in subjects reading a line of print. Amplitude, velocity and reaction time in saccadic movement were first studied in detail by Westheimer (1954) and Robinson (1964) and investigations carried even further by Childress & Jones (1967), Becker & Fuchs (1969), Hallett & Lightstone (1976) and others. In general, reaction times and movements are measured in microseconds; amplitude varies from seconds of arc to many degrees, with an accuracy of 0.2° or better, and the velocity of a large saccade may reach 500° per second. The speed of the saccades (an obvious survival factor) is assured by an initial contraction of the appropriate muscles which is slightly excessive (the 'pre-emphasis' of Robinson 1964), the necessary deceleration when the target is fixated being apparently due largely to the viscoelasticity of the extraocular muscles and orbital soft tissues, rather than to antagonistic muscular activity.

Clearly, saccadic activity is almost ever-present in human vision, and not merely in reading or the visual target practice of experimental laboratories. Not only are both visual axes endlessly and rapidly transferred to new points of interest in any part of the total visual field, but binocular gaze is very frequently made to travel routes of the most variable complexity in examining objects of some extent in the field; to this must be added the maintenance of **both** visual axes with sufficient accuracy to avoid diplopia. It is interesting to note in passing that binocular movements involving convergence are markedly slower than conjugate movements (Alpern & Wolter 1956), presumably due to the greater complexity of neural control (though the speed of contraction of the ciliaris must be a factor). Conjugate movements, indeed, might almost be 'programmed'; but most visual human activity concerns targets of regard near enough to demand convergence and hence a neuronal intermediation of greater flexibility. Since the prime purpose is clear perception of a 'target', it is not surprising that the visual input is itself utilized in continuous feedback to the correct aiming of visual axes.

In addition to these considerations, there is much evidence that the continual movements of the eye are actually essential for vision to occur at all; the retinal and more central neural networks appear to be designed primarily to detect transient events such as movements rather than static, maintained stimuli. Indeed, images which are essentially static, such as those due to retinal blood vessels, are not detectable unless the shadows they cast on photoreceptors are made to move, for example by shifting narrow-angle illumination with an ophthalmoscope. This finding may be related to the complex architecture of the retina and to the presence of circuits which are specifically used to detect movements, for example those involving cholinergic amacrine cells (p. 1346).

Since the recti exert a **posterior** traction while the obliques pull the eyeball to some degree **anteriorly**, it is sometimes suggested that they collectively position it in the orbital cavity, preventing anteroposterior movements of the eyeball, assisted perhaps by various 'check ligaments' (see below).

FASCIAL SHEATHS OF THE EYE AND ORBIT

A thin fascial membrane, the *vagina bulbi* (fascia bulbi or Tenon's capsule), envelops the eyeball from the optic nerve to the corneoscleral junction, separating it from the orbital fat and forming a socket (**8.457**A,B). Its ocular aspect is loosely attached to the sclera by delicate bands of episcleral connective tissue. Posteriorly the fascia is traversed by ciliary vessels and nerves; it fuses with the sclera and with the sheath of the optic nerve around its entrance to the eyeball. Attachment to the sclera is strongest in this position and also anteriorly, just behind the corneoscleral junction at the limbus. It is perforated by the tendons of the extraocular muscles and is reflected on to each as a tubular sheath, the *muscular fascia*. The sheath of the obliquus superior reaches this muscle's fibrous trochlea. The sheaths of the recti are very thick anteriorly but reduce posteriorly to a delicate perimysium, then shortly before they blend with the vagina bulbi, the thick sheaths of adjacent recti are confluent, forming a fascial ring. Expansions from the sheaths are important for the attachments they make; those from the recti medialis and lateralis are triangular and strong, and attached respectively to the lacrimal and zygomatic bones; as they may limit the actions of the two recti, they are termed the *medial* and *lateral check ligaments*. Other extraocular muscles have less substantial check ligaments but the capacity of any of them to actually limit movement has been questioned.

The sheath of the rectus inferior is thickened on its underside and blends with the sheath of the obliquus inferior. These two, in turn, are continuous with the fascial ring noted earlier and therefore with the sheaths of the recti medialis and lateralis. As the latter are attached to the orbital walls by check ligaments, a continuous fascial band is slung like a hammock below the eye, the *suspensory ligament of the eye* (Lockwood 1886). The thickened fused sheath of the rectus inferior and obliquus inferior also has an anterior expansion into the lower eyelid, where, augmented by the inferior tarsal muscle (p. 1361), it attaches to the inferior tarsus (Hawes & Dortzbach 1982); contraction of the rectus inferior in downward gaze therefore also draws the lid downward. The sheath of the levator palpebrae superioris also thickens anteriorly and just behind the aponeurosis it fuses inferiorly with the sheath of the rectus superior. It extends forward between the two muscles and attaches to the upper fornix of the conjunctiva.

Other extensions pass medially and laterally and attach to the orbital walls, forming the *transverse ligament of the eye* (Whitnall 1932). The transverse ligament is of uncertain significance but it presumably plays a part in drawing the fornix upwards in gaze elevation and it may act as a fulcrum for levator movements (Anderson & Dixon 1979). Other numerous finer fasciae form radial septa extending from the vagina bulbi and the muscle sheaths to the periorbita, providing compartments for orbital fat (Koornneeff 1977). The orbital septum (p. 1361) is the most anteriorly placed. Many of the fasciae contain smooth muscle cells. The ocular and orbital fasciae are arranged to assist in the location of the eye within the orbit without obstructing the activities of the extraocular muscles, except possibly in the extremes of rotation. They also prevent the gross displacement of orbital fat, for this could interfere with the accurate positioning of the two eyes in binocular vision.

The periosteum of the orbit, or *periorbita*, is only loosely attached to bone. Behind, it is united with the dura mater of the optic nerve and is continuous anteriorly with the periosteum of the orbital margin, where it gives off a stratum contributing to the orbital septum. One process of the periorbita attaches to the trochlea; another, the *lacrimal fascia*, forms the roof and lateral wall of the sulcus for the lacrimal sac (p. 1366). Lang (1975) has detailed the vascularization of the orbital periosteum and fascia.

VISUAL REFLEXES

The nerve impulses concerned with visual reflexes effecting movements of the eyes, head and neck in response to visual stimuli follow the optic nerves and tracts to the superior colliculi. Traversing complex connections there, they travel along the tectospinal and tectobulbar tracts to the motor neurons of spinal and cranial nerves (p. 1070).

Pupillary light reflex

Increased illumination causes reflex miosis (pupillary contraction), the impulses concerned travelling by the optic nerve and tract to the pretectal nuclei of both sides (p. 1226), whence short axons of secondary neurons run close to the central grey matter, conveying impulses to the accessory oculomotor (Edinger-Westphal) nuclei (p. 1227); from there, preganglionic axons reach the ciliary ganglia via the oculomotor nerves and their branches to the inferior oblique muscles. Postganglionic fibres from the ganglia traverse the short ciliary nerves to reach the pupillary sphincters. If only one eye is stimulated both pupils nevertheless contract (the *consensual pupillary light reflex*), because fibres from each optic tract pass to **both** pretectal nuclei, decussating in the posterior commissure.

The *dilatator pupillae* is supplied by fibres from the superior sympathetic cervical ganglion. The preganglionic fibres in this pathway arise from neurons in the lateral grey column of the first and second thoracic spinal segments, traversing the upper thoracic spinal nerves and their white rami communicantes to the sympathetic trunk, in which they ascend to the superior cervical ganglion (p. 1300).

Postganglionic fibres distribute to the carotid plexus, and thence chiefly through the long ciliary nerves (via the ophthalmic nerve) to the anterior part of the eye (for details see p. 1229).

Since pupillary size results from the *balanced action* of these two innervations, the pupil dilates when the parasympathetic stimulus ceases. The pupil dilates also in response to painful stimulation of almost any part of the body. Presumably fibres of sensory pathways connect with the sympathetic preganglionic neurons described above. Some believe, however, that reflex pupillodilatation is largely due to inhibition of the parasympathetic accessory oculomotor nuclei, though the paths involved are uncertain. One manifestation of this reflex is dilatation produced by pinching the skin of the neck, the *pupillary skin reflex*, a reminder that to the above, simplified account must be added other afferent influences, such as reticular connections with the superior collicular nuclei.

Accommodation reflexes

In accommodating for viewing near objects the eyes converge, the ciliary muscles contract to modify the shape of the lens and the pupils constrict to increase the depth of focus. Pathways for accommodation

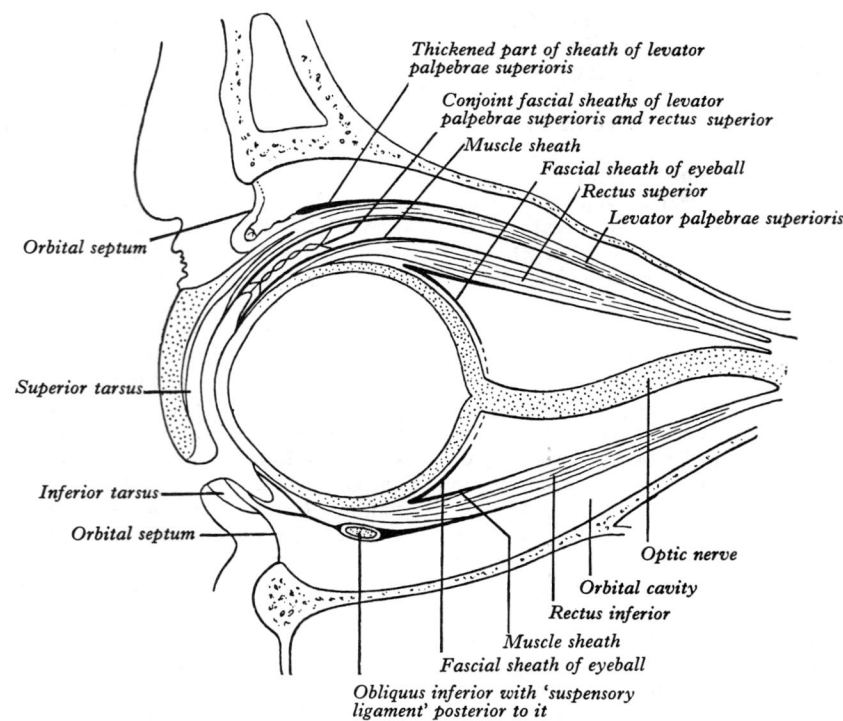

8.457A Scheme of the orbital fascia in sagittal section. (After Whitnall 1932.)

Labels on figure:
- Thickened part of sheath of levator palpebrae superioris
- Conjoint fascial sheaths of levator palpebrae superioris and rectus superior
- Muscle sheath
- Fascial sheath of eyeball
- Rectus superior
- Levator palpebrae superioris
- Orbital septum
- Superior tarsus
- Inferior tarsus
- Orbital septum
- Optic nerve
- Orbital cavity
- Rectus inferior
- Muscle sheath
- Fascial sheath of eyeball
- Obliquus inferior with 'suspensory ligament' posterior to it

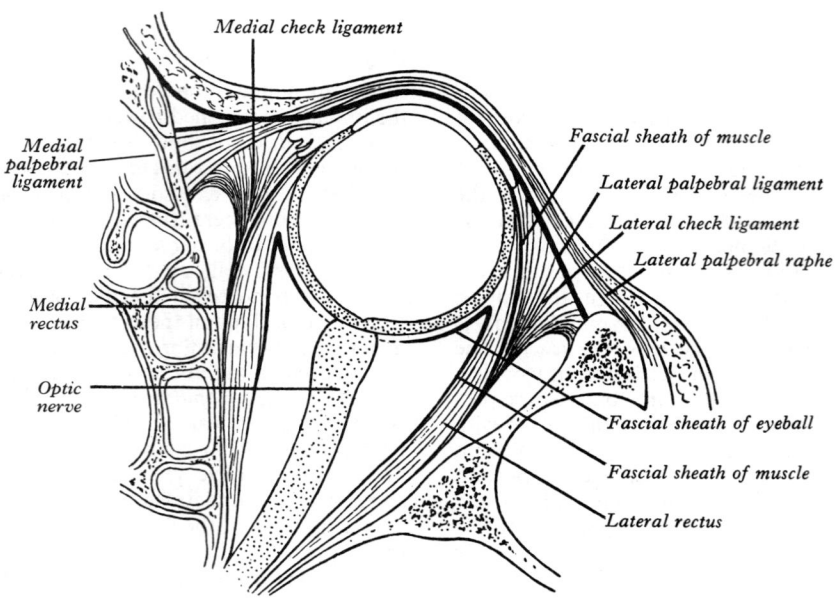

8.457B Scheme of the orbital fascia in horizontal section. (After Whitnall 1932.)

Labels on figure:
- Medial check ligament
- Medial palpebral ligament
- Medial rectus
- Optic nerve
- Fascial sheath of muscle
- Lateral palpebral ligament
- Lateral check ligament
- Lateral palpebral raphe
- Fascial sheath of eyeball
- Fascial sheath of muscle
- Lateral rectus

comprise the optic nerves and tracts, lateral geniculate bodies, optic radiations and the cortical visual areas, the latter probably being connected through the corticotectal tract to 'near response cells' in the pretectal region above and lateral to the oculomotor nucleus (Mays 1984; Judge & Cumming 1986). The pathway continues to the oculomotor nucleus and from there parasympathetic fibres pass to the ciliary muscle and sphincter pupillae after a relay in the ciliary ganglion. From the ventral part of the oculomotor nucleus (p.1227) fibres supply the medial recti and other muscles for the action of convergence (p. 1358). These routes have not been so clearly defined as those for the pupillary light reflex. In certain central nervous

diseases (e.g. tabes dorsalis) the pupillary light reflex may be lost but not pupilloconstriction as part of the accommodation reflex (the Argyll Robertson pupil). The site of a lesion producing such an effect is unclear, but may often involve the periaqueductal grey matter (p. 1088).

Conjunctival and corneal reflexes

Any stimulus to the conjunctiva or cornea excites blinking. Afferent impulses travel via the ophthalmic division of the trigeminal nerve and efferent impulses in branches of the facial nerve to orbicularis oculi.

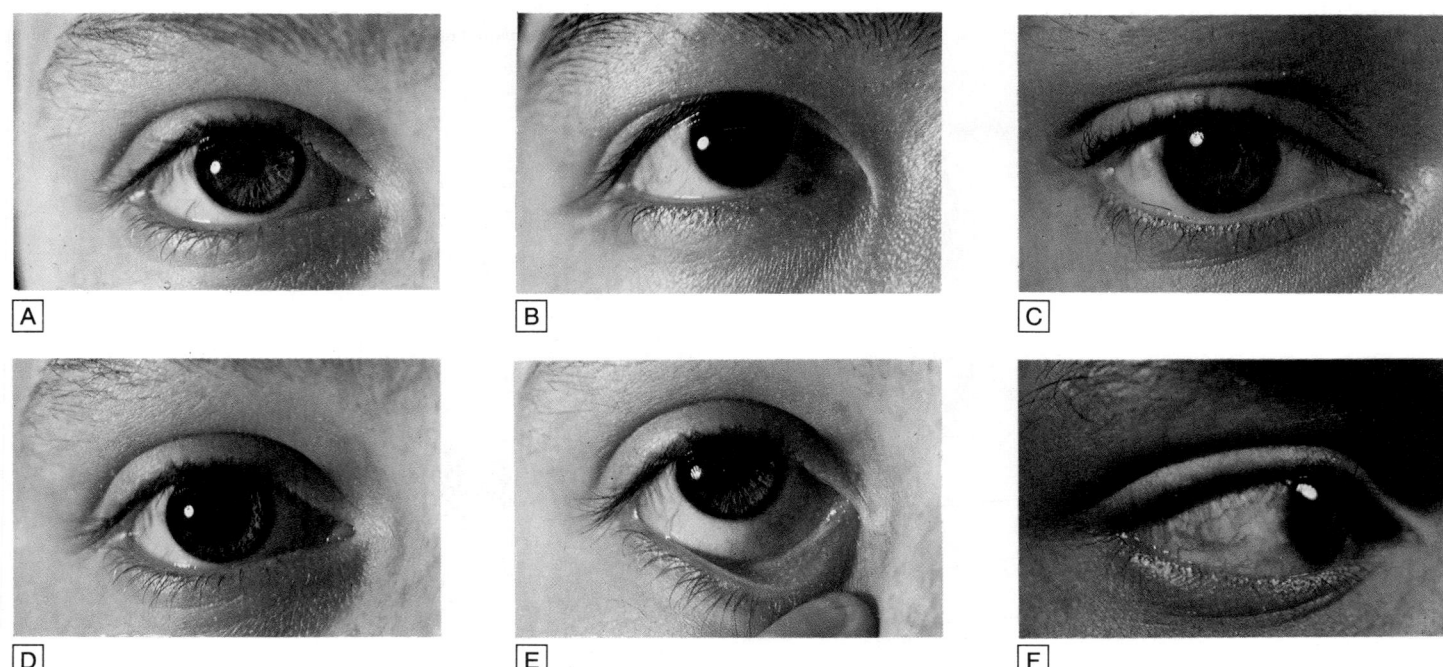

8.458   In the top row of photographs the typical appearances of the living eye are compared in a Caucasian female (A), a Mongoloid male (B) and a Negroid male (C). All subjects are about 20 years of age. Note the pale sclera and grey-blue iris in A, the epicanthus overlapping the medial end of the lower eyelid in B and the dark brown pigmentation of the iris in both B and C, rendering the pupil almost invisible. Compare the size of the pupil in the same eye, photographed under steady bright light in A and by sudden exposure to the same illumination after a period of dark adaptation in D. In E the lower eyelid had been everted somewhat to exhibit the lacrimal punctum and the rich subepithelial network of blood vessels. In F note the circumcorneal pigmentation and the conjunctival blood vessels, deep to which can be seen some details of the episcleral vessels. All photographs are of the right eye. (Photography by Kevin Fitzpatrick, Anatomy Department, Guy's Hospital Medical School, London.)

EYEBROWS AND EYELIDS

GENERAL STRUCTURE

The *eyebrows* are arched dermal eminences surmounting the orbits, with numerous short, thick hairs set obliquely in them. Fibres of the orbicularis oculi, corrugator and the frontal part of the occipitofrontalis are attached to the dermis of the eyebrows.

The *eyelids* or *palpebrae* are thin, movable folds, adapted to the front of the eyes and protecting them from injury, by rapid closure. The upper eyelid is larger and more mobile, being furnished with an elevator muscle, the levator palpebrae superioris (p. 1353). The two eyelids are united at their extremities, and when parted an elliptical space, the *palpebral fissure*, appears between their margins. The ends of the fissure are termed the *angles* or *canthi* of the eye.

The *lateral angle* of the eye or *lateral canthus* is more acute than the medial and is closely apposed to the eyeball. The *medial angle* or *medial canthus* is prolonged for a little towards the nose and is about 6 mm from the eyeball; the eyelids are here separated by a triangular space, the *lacus lacrimalis*, in which is a small reddish *caruncula lacrimalis* (**8.458**, 462, 463). On each palpebral margin, at the basal angles of the lacus, is a small, conical, *lacrimal papilla*, its apex pierced by the orifice of a *lacrimal canaliculus*, an aperture known as the *punctum lacrimale* (**8.463**). The puncta are turned towards the surface of the eye to receive tear fluid (p. 1367).

Eyelashes grow in the palpebral margins, their distribution extending from the lateral canthus to the lacrimal papillae. They are short, thick, curved hairs, arranged in double or triple rows; the upper, which are more numerous and longer, curve upwards while those in the lower lid curve down so that upper and lower lashes do not interlace when the lids are closed. Pairs of *ciliary sebaceous glands* and enlarged and modified sudoriferous *ciliary sweat glands* open into the eyelash follicles, or, sometimes in the case of the latter, on to the skin (p. 406).

MICROSTRUCTURE OF THE EYELIDS

From its facial surface inwards each eyelid consists of: skin, subcutaneous connective tissue, fibres of the palpebral part of orbicularis oculi, submuscular connective tissue, the tarsus with tarsal glands and orbital septum, and palpebral conjunctiva. The upper lid also contains the aponeurosis of the levator palpebrae superioris (**8.450**, 459–461). The *skin* is extremely thin and is continuous at the palpebral margins with the conjunctiva. The *subcutaneous connective tissue* is very lax and delicate, seldom containing any adipose tissue and without elastic fibres.

The *palpebral fibre bundles of orbicularis oculi* are thin and pale and run parallel with the palpebral fissure (Nelson & Blaivas 1991). Deep to them lies the *submuscular connective tissue*, a loose fibrous layer which in the upper lid is continuous with the scalp's subaponeurotic layer (p. 790); effusions of blood or pus at this level can pass down from the scalp into the upper eyelid. In this submuscular layer are the main nerves; local anaesthetics should hence be injected deep to orbicularis oculi.

The two *tarsi* (**8.459**, 460) are thin, elongated plates of firm, dense fibrous tissue about 2.5 cm long, one in each eyelid, providing support and determining eyelid form. The *superior tarsus*, the larger of the two, is semi-oval, about 10 mm in height centrally and narrowing towards its ends. Its inferior edge is parallel to, and about 2 mm from the lid margin. The deepest fibres of the aponeurosis of the levator palpebrae superioris are attached to its anterior surface, and the fibrous extension of the superior tarsal muscle to its upper margin (**8.450**, 461). The smaller *inferior tarsus* is narrower, about 4 mm in vertical height. The lower margin of the inferior tarsus and possibly part of the upper margin of the superior tarsus are attached to the orbital septum; in the latter case the central part is separated from the septum by the aponeurosis of the levator palpebrae superioris. Their lateral ends are attached by a band, the *lateral palpebral ligament*, to a tubercle on the zygomatic bone, just within the orbital margin (Gioia et al 1987). The medial ends of the tarsi are attached by a strong tendinous band, the *medial palpebral ligament*, to the upper part of the lacrimal bone's crest and to the adjoining frontal process of the maxilla in front of it; the lower edge of this ligament is separated from the lacrimal sac by some fibres of the orbicularis oculi which are attached to the ligament.

The *orbital septum* is a weak membranous sheet attached to the orbital rim, where it is continuous with the periosteum. In the upper lid it blends with the superficial lamella of the aponeurosis of levator

1361

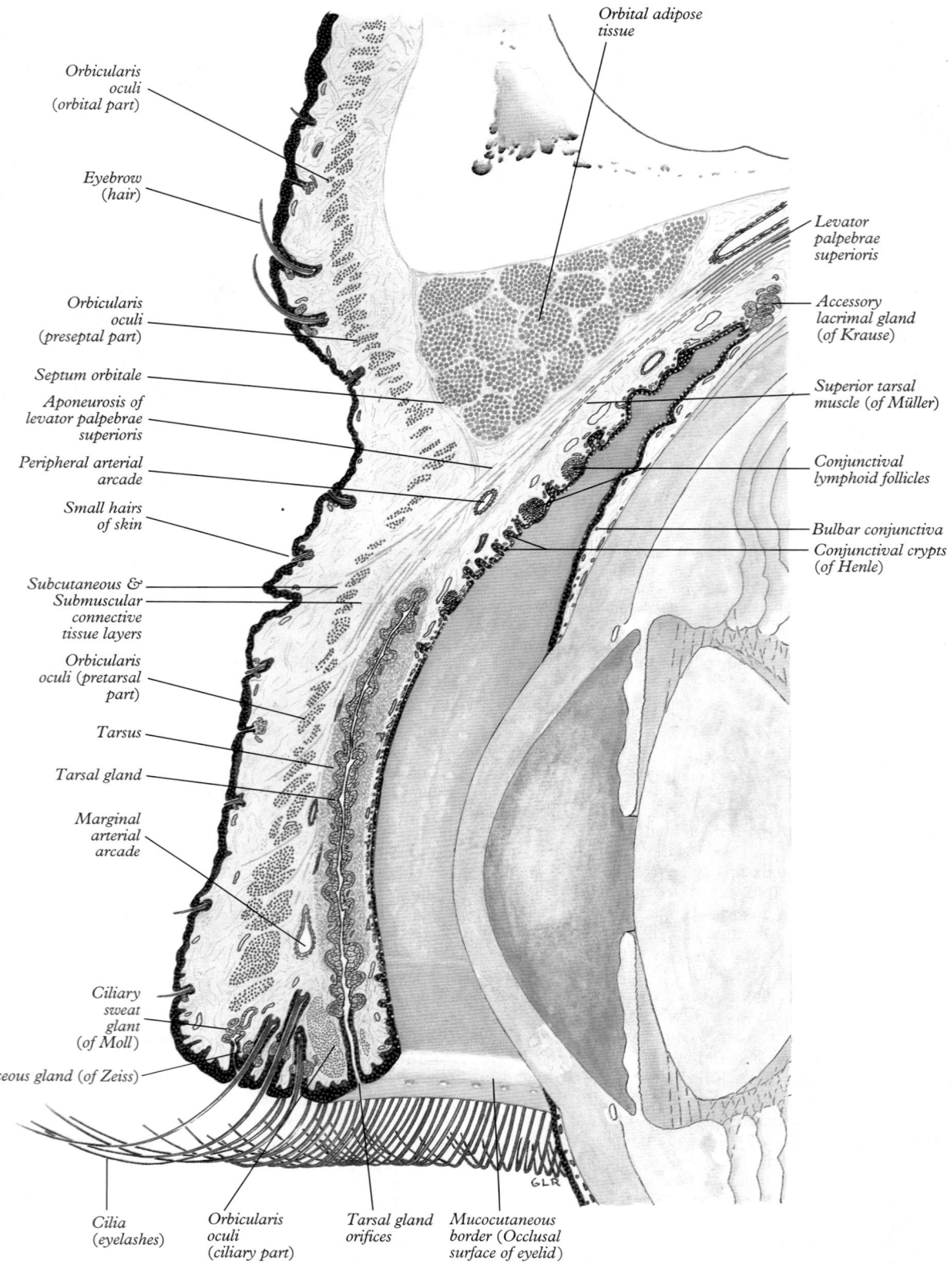

8.459 Illustration depicting the structure of the upper eyelid and anterior segment of the eye: sagittal section. (Provided by G L Ruskell, Department of Optometry and Visual Science, The City University, London.)

palpebrae superioris, and in the lower lid with the anterior tarsal surface and margin. It is perforated by vessels and nerves passing from the orbital cavity to the face and scalp.

The *tarsal glands* (**8**.459, 460, 462), embedded in the tarsi, may be visible through the conjunctiva when the eyelids are everted; they are yellow and arranged in a single row of about 25 in the upper lid

and fewer in the lower. They occupy the full tarsal height, being longer centrally where the tarsi are higher. Their ducts open by minute orifices on the free palpebral margins. They are modified sebaceous glands, each a straight tube with many lateral diverticula. They are enclosed by a basement membrane and lined at their orifices by stratified epithelium and elsewhere by a layer of polyhedral cells.

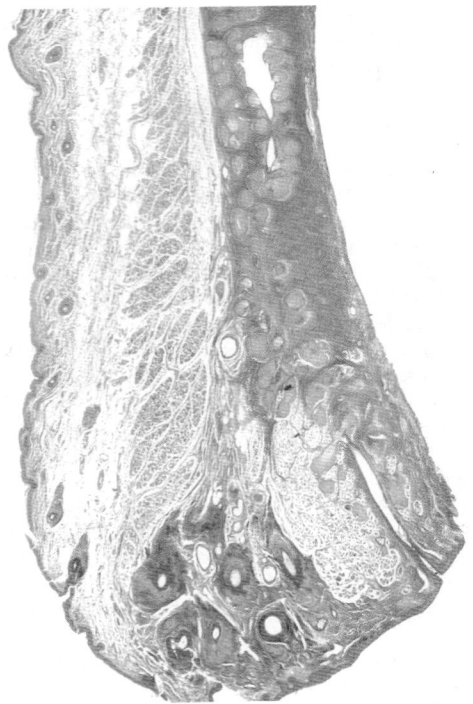

8.460 Low power micrograph of a sagittal section through part of an upper eyelid. Compare with **8.459**. Magnification × 30. (Provided by G L Ruskell, Department of Optometry and Visual Science, The City University, London.)

Their oily secretion spreads over the margins of the eyelids and an oily layer is drawn over the tear film as the fissure opens after a blink, reducing evaporation and contributing to tear film stability. The presence of the oily, hydrophobic secretions of tarsal glands along the margins of the eyelids also inhibits the spillage of tears on to the face.

CONJUNCTIVA

The conjunctiva, a transparent mucous membrane, covers the internal palpebral surfaces and folds on to the anterior sclera and cornea where it is continuous with the corneal epithelium; it is a *conjunction* between these structures.

The *palpebral conjunctiva* is very vascular with a dense subepithelial layer of capillaries, and contains mucosa-associated lymphoid tissue, including follicles, especially at the orbital edges of the tarsi; it is closely adherent to the tarsi. At the free palpebral margins the

conjunctiva is continuous with the skin, the lining epithelium of the ducts of the tarsal glands, and with the lacrimal canaliculi and lacrimal sac and hence the nasolacrimal duct and nasal mucosa (an important continuity in the spread of infection). The line of reflection of the conjunctiva from the lids to the eyeball is the *conjunctival fornix*, subdivided into *superior* and *inferior fornices*, the superior receiving the ducts of the lacrimal gland. Over the exposed sclera the *bulbar conjunctiva* is loosely connected to the eyeball; here it is thin and transparent, without papillae and slightly vascular. Reaching the cornea it continues as the corneal epithelium (p. 1325). The epithelium of the palpebral conjunctiva near the margin of the lids is non-keratinized stratified squamous; about 2 mm from each margin a subtarsal groove is often present in which foreign bodies frequently lodge and here the epithelium has two or three layers, consisting of columnar and flat surface cells; these persist through most palpebral conjunctiva but near the fornices in the *orbital conjunctiva* the cells are taller and a trilaminar conjunctival epithelium covers much of the anterior, exposed surface of the sclera. It thickens closer to the corneoscleral junction and then changes to stratified epithelium (p. 1325). Scattered in the conjunctival epithelium are mucus-secreting goblet cells, most frequent on each side of the fold but absent from the exposed surfaces of the bulbar conjunctiva and the corneoscleral junction (Kessing 1968) and also lymphoid tissue.

Vessels and nerves of the eyelids

Arteries. The eyelids receive their arteries from the medial palpebral branches of the ophthalmic artery and the lateral palpebral branches of the lacrimal artery, forming arcades (p. 1526).

Veins. Bulbar conjunctival veins pass to the orbital surfaces of the rectal muscles and join the superior or inferior ophthalmic vein; those from the palpebral conjunctiva join the facial vein. Lymph vessels of the eyelids and conjunctiva are described on page 1612.

Nerves. The bulbar conjunctiva is supplied by the ophthalmic division of the trigeminal nerve; the upper palpebral conjunctiva is supplied by the ophthalmic (branches of the supratrochlear, supraorbital, lacrimal and infratrochlear rami), the lower by the maxillary division. Several varieties of corpuscular and other nerve fibre endings are present in the eyelids (Munger & Halata 1984) and conjunctiva (Lawrenson & Ruskell 1991). Sympathetic and parasympathetic facial nerve fibres are probably all vasomotor in function.

Palpebral movements

The position of the lids depends on reciprocal tone in the orbicularis oculi and levator palpebrae superioris and on the degree of ocular protrusion. In the opened position the margin of the inferior eyelid usually crosses the eyeball level with the lower edge of the circumference of the iris, the upper covering about half of the width of the upper iris. The eyes are closed by movements of **both** lids, produced by the contraction of the palpebral part of orbicularis oculi and relaxation of the levator palpebrae superioris. In looking

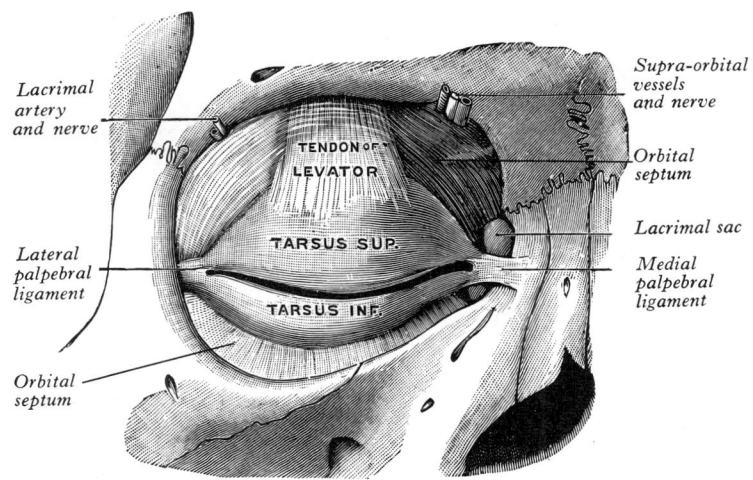

Lacrimal artery and nerve

Lateral palpebral ligament

Orbital septum

TENDON OF LEVATOR

TARSUS SUP.

TARSUS INF.

Supra-orbital vessels and nerve

Orbital septum

Lacrimal sac

Medial palpebral ligament

8.461 The tarsi and their ligaments: anterior aspect.

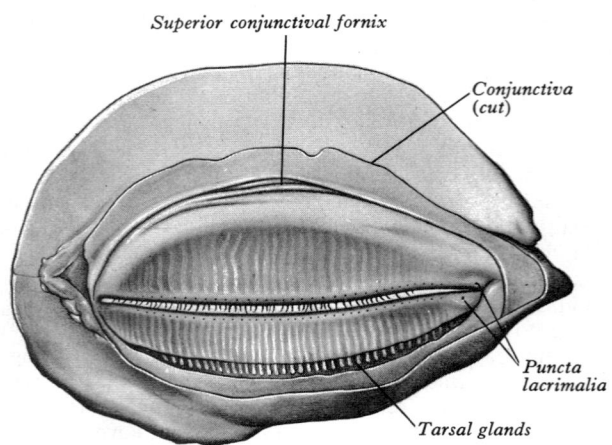

Superior conjunctival fornix

Conjunctiva (cut)

Puncta lacrimalia

Tarsal glands

8.462 The posterior surfaces of the upper and lower eyelids of the left side. The orifices of the tarsal glands can be seen on the free margins of the lids.

upwards, the levator contracts and the upper lid follows the ocular movement; at the same time, the eyebrows are also usually raised by the frontal parts of the occipitofrontalis to diminish their over-hang. The lower lid lags behind ocular movement, so that more sclera is exposed below the cornea and the lid is bulged a little by the lower part of the elevated eye. When the eye is depressed both lids move, the upper retaining its normal relation to the eyeball and still covering about a quarter of the iris. The lower lid is depressed by the pull on its tarsus by the extension of the thickened fascia of rectus inferior and obliquus inferior as the former contracts.

In states of fear or excitement the palpebral fissures are widened by contraction of the smooth muscle of the superior and inferior tarsal muscles, due to increased sympathetic activity. Lesions of the sympathetic supply result in drooping of the upper eyelid (ptosis), as seen in Horner's syndrome. For further comments on palpebral movement see page 1353.

LACRIMAL APPARATUS

The lacrimal apparatus (**8.463**–468) comprises the lacrimal gland, which secretes a complex fluid (tears) and whose excretory ducts convey fluid to the surface of the eye, the paired lacrimal canaliculi, the lacrimal sac and the nasolacrimal duct, by which the fluid is collected and conveyed into the nasal cavity.

LACRIMAL GLAND (8.463, 466, 467)

This is derived phylogenetically from serous secreting glands and those producing oily secretions. In primates the lacrimal (serous) element has migrated from its original position in the lower lid to the upper. The human lacrimal gland is superolateral in the orbit and has two parts: a large, upper orbital and smaller, lower palpebral part, the two being continuous posterolaterally around the concave lateral edge of the levator aponeurosis.

The *orbital part*, about the size and shape of an almond, lodges in the lacrimal fossa on the medial aspect of the zygomatic process of the frontal bone, just within the orbital margin. It lies above the levator palpebrae superioris and, laterally, above the lateral rectus; its inferior aspect is connected to the levator's sheath, its upper to the orbital periosteum; its anterior aspect adjoins the orbital septum and its posterior is attached to the orbital fat.

The *palpebral part*, about one-third the size of the orbital, has two or three lobules extending inferior to the levator aponeurosis into the lateral part of the upper lid, where it is attached to the superior conjunctival fornix. It is visible through the conjunctiva when the lid is everted.

Its ducts, about six in number, open into the superior fornix, those from the orbital part (four or five) penetrating the aponeurosis of levator palpebrae superioris to join those of the palpebral part. Thus excision of the palpebral part is functionally equivalent to the total removal of the gland.

Many small accessory lacrimal glands occur in or near the fornix; they are more numerous in the upper lid than in the lower. This may explain why the conjunctiva does not dry up after extirpation of the main lacrimal gland.

Microstructure of the lacrimal gland (8.466, 467)

The lacrimal gland is lobulated and tubulo-acinar in form (p. 73); its secretory units are acini resembling those of the salivary glands. The secretion is a watery fluid with an electrolyte content like that of plasma and containing, amongst other components, a bacteriocidal enzyme, *lysozyme*. Its glandular cells form two (Ito & Shibasaki 1964; Kühnel 1968), three (Ruskell 1975) or four (Hirsch-Hoffmann 1978) categories depending on which ultrastructural and his-tochemical criteria are considered to be significant. In rhesus monkeys, glandular cells with uniformly electron-dense secretory granules are described as *serous* and those with paler heterogeneous

Lacrimal gland

Aponeurosis of levator palpebrae superioris

Palpebral part of lacrimal gland

Conjunctiva

Lacrimal canaliculi

Lacrimal sac

Nasal septum

Middle nasal concha

Inferior nasal concha

Puncta lacrimalia

Nasolacrimal duct

Maxillary sinus

Inferior meatus of nasal cavity

8.463 The left lacrimal apparatus: anterior aspect.

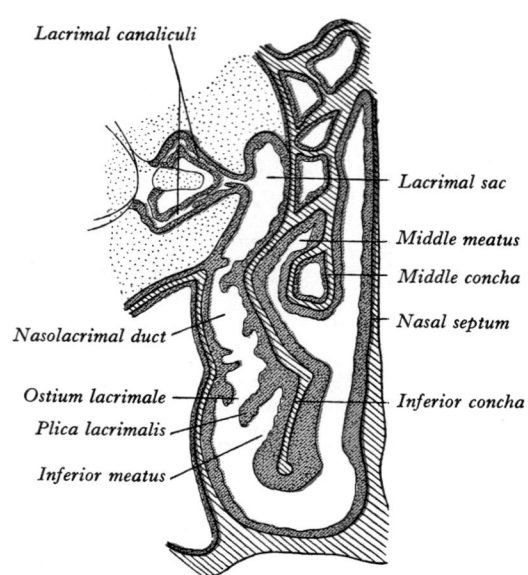

Lacrimal canaliculi

Lacrimal sac

Middle meatus

Middle concha

Nasal septum

Nasolacrimal duct

Ostium lacrimale

Plica lacrimalis

Inferior meatus

Inferior concha

8.464 Sketch from a coronal section through the right half of the nasal cavity (anterior aspect) to show the relation of the lacrimal passages to the maxillary and ethmoidal sinuses and the inferior nasal concha. The mucous membrane is coloured. (After Whitnall 1932.)

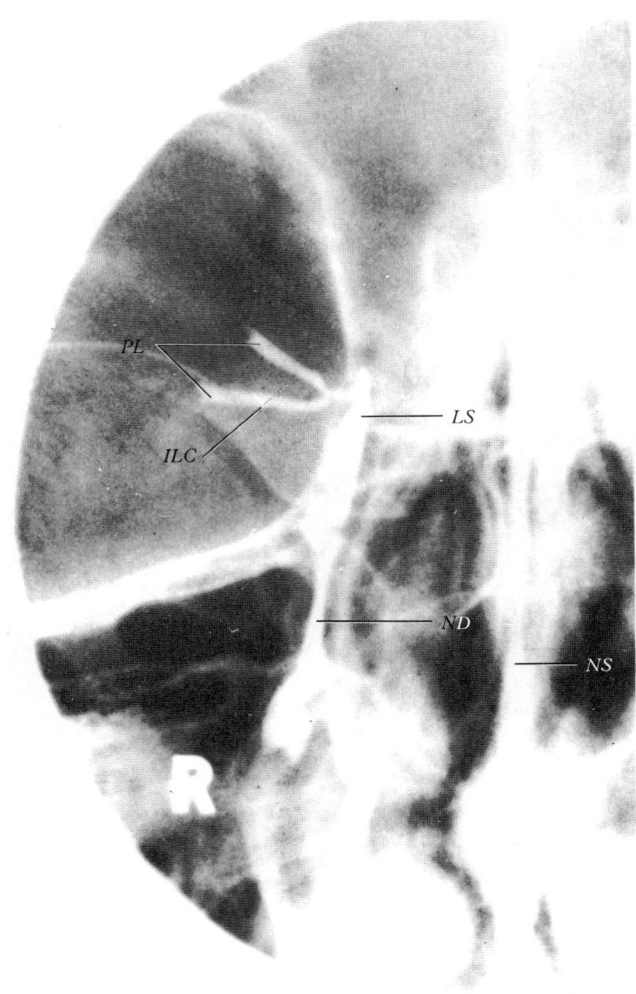

8.465 Radiograph of the lacrimal drainage pathway, demonstrated by the injection of radio-opaque tracer into the lacrimal duct. Note the following: PL = puncta lacrimalia; ILC = inferior lacrimal canaliculus; LS = lacrimal sac; ND = nasolacrimal duct; NS = nasal septum. (Provided by T D Hawkins, Addenbrooke's Hospital, Cambridge; photography by Sarah Smith.)

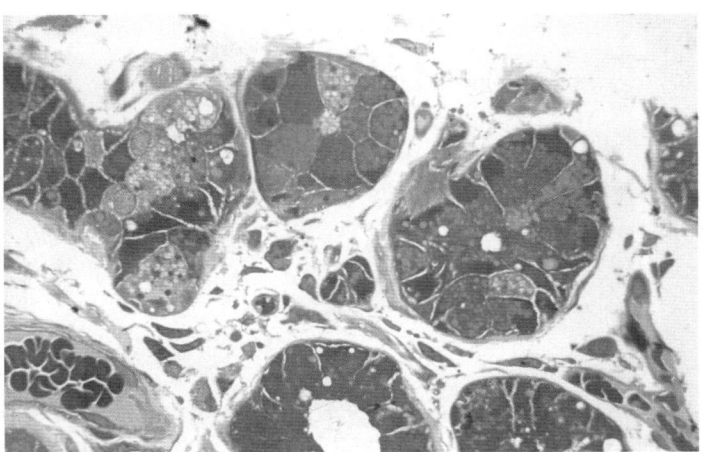

8.466 Section through a human lacrimal gland, showing secretory tissue. Note that the density of granules varies between single acinar cells. Toluidine blue, resin section. Magnification × 400. (Provided by G L Ruskell, Department of Optometry and Visual Science, The City University, London.)

granules *mucous* (Ruskell 1968). Ito & Shibasaki (1964) and Kühnel (1968) propose two distinct human types of cell: one, the K cell, contains small, electron-lucent granules and stains like a mucous cell; the other, termed the G cell, contains large, electron-dense granules and stains like a serous cell. According to Allen et al (1972) and Ruskell (1975) most glandular cells are mucous, a surprising report in view of the patently serous nature of tears. Ruskell (1975) distinguishes three categories of human glandular cell, arbitrarily grouping them into 'light', 'medium' and 'dark' according to the electron density of their secretory granules; acini contain either two or all three categories and are closely associated with lymphocytes and myoepitheliocytes. Hirsch-Hoffmann (1978) proposed **four** groups of human glandular cells, distinguishable by the number and electron density of the granules and surrounding cytoplasm; the largest group have pale cytoplasm and numerous granules of varying electron density; a second group, also pale, have fewer granules; a third have darker cytoplasm and numerous granules; the remainder, also dark, have fewer, uniformly electron-dense granules. Hirsch-Hoffmann has suggested that at least some may represent different stages in the secretory activity of one or two distinct types, an interpretation supported by Egebert & Jensen (1969) and Orzalesi et al (1971). If lacrimal cells differ in their secretory products, the biochemical evidence that mucin is one of them is weak (Thörig et al 1985). Other components of tears include the proteins lysozyme, lactoferrin, IgA, and tear-specific pre-albumen, as well as some major

serum proteins (IgM, IgG, transferrin and serum albumen; see e.g. Fullard & Snyder 1990). The concentrations of these vary considerably in the non-stimulated and stimulated states.

Innervation of lacrimal gland (8.467). The human lacrimal gland contains interstitial (epilemmal, p. 1698) and parenchymal (hypolemmal) nerve terminals (Ruskell 1975). The ultrastructure of most interstitial and all parenchymal terminals accords with cholinergic (parasympathetic) activity. A few interstitial terminals, containing small granular vesicles, may be adrenergic (sympathetic). Only 'dark' or 'serous' glandular cells have a parasympathetic, hypolemmal innervation (Ruskell 1975), as in rhesus monkeys (Ruskell 1969), in which ultrastructural changes after parasympathectomy suggested that serous cells are under parasympathetic control, mediated by hypolemmal terminals, while mucous cells may function autonomously. Similar parasympathetic terminals occur near the ducts and terminal tubules in the human lacrimal gland; the tubules connect secretory units and ducts, containing in their walls cells intermediate in form between glandular and ductal cells (Ruskell 1975); these cells of the terminal tubules are smaller than glandular cells and contain fewer granules. Most nerve terminals of ducts and tubules are near myoepitheliocytes, perhaps inducing myoepitheliocytic contraction and assisting secretory flow. Myoepitheliocytes in secretory units appear to have no direct, hypolemmal innervation; Ruskell (1975) suggests that nearby interstitial parasympathetic terminals may control them, releasing only sufficient transmitter to induce their contraction in hypersecretion. The role of the interstitial sympathetic terminals in the control of human lacrimal gland is undetermined, as are the ultrastructure and functions of its ducts. A number of peptides have been demonstrated in the lacrimal gland innervation, including calcitonin gene-related peptide (CGRP), substance P (SP), neuropeptide Y (NPY), vasoactive intestinal polypeptide (VIP) and acetylcholinesterase (AChE) (see p. 936; also Matsumoto et al 1992).

Lacrimal canaliculi

There is one lacrimal canaliculus in each lid, about 10 mm long; each commences at a *puncta lacrimalia* (8.462–464). The *superior canaliculus*, smaller and shorter than the inferior, first ascends and then curves acutely inferomedially to reach the lacrimal sac. The *inferior canaliculus* first descends and turns almost horizontally to the sac. At their angles they are dilated into *ampullae*. Their lining mucosa has a non-keratinized stratified squamous epithelium on a basement membrane, beyond which is a lamina propria rich in elastic fibres (the ducts therefore being easily dilated when probed) and a layer of skeletal muscle fibres continuous with the lacrimal part of

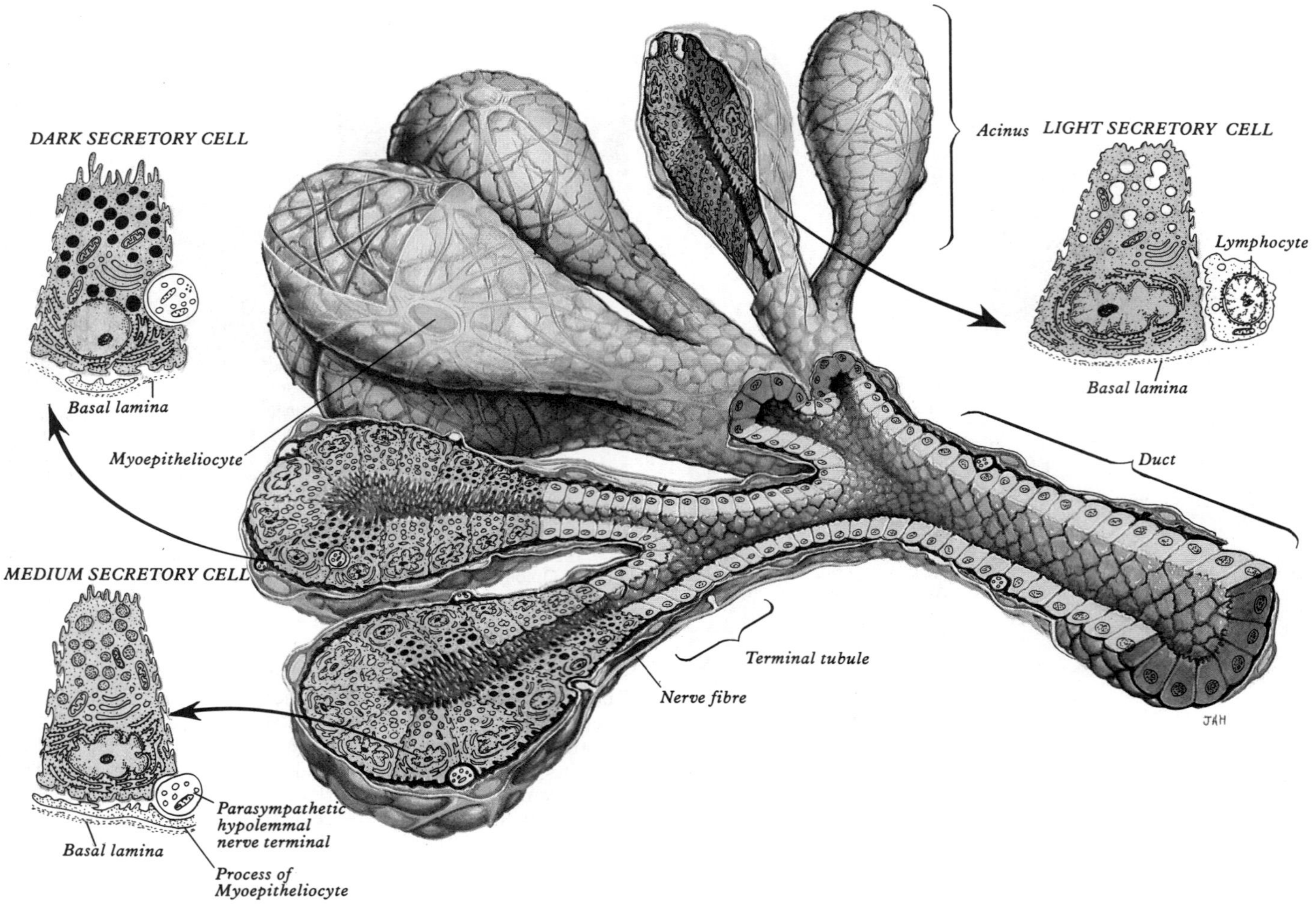

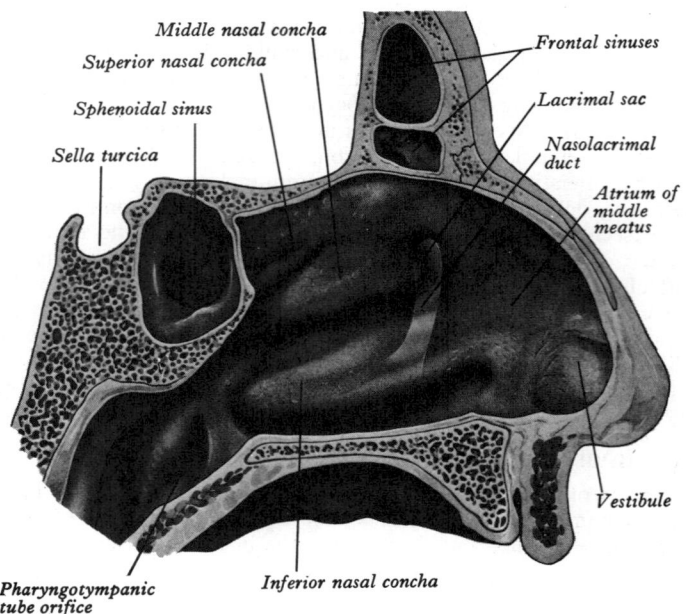

DARK SECRETORY CELL

Basal lamina

Myoepitheliocyte

MEDIUM SECRETORY CELL

Parasympathetic
hypolemmal
nerve terminal

Basal lamina

Process of
Myoepitheliocyte

Acinus LIGHT SECRETORY CELL

Lymphocyte

Basal lamina

Duct

Terminal tubule

Nerve fibre

8.467   The structure of the lacrimal gland, showing the organization of the secretory units.

the orbicularis oculi. At the base of each lacrimal papilla these fibres are sphincteric.

Lacrimal sac (8.463–465)

The closed upper end of the nasolacrimal duct lies in a fossa formed by the lacrimal bone, the frontal maxillary process and the lacrimal fascia. It is about 12 mm long; its closed upper end is laterally flattened and its lower part rounded and merging into the duct; the lacrimal canaliculi open into its lateral wall near its upper end.

A layer of *lacrimal fascia*, continuous with the orbital periosteum, passes between the lacrimal crest of the maxilla and the lacrimal bone, forming a roof and lateral wall to the lacrimal fossa; between the fascia and the lacrimal sac is a plexus of minute veins. The fascia separates the sac from the medial palpebral ligament in front and the lacrimal part of orbicularis oculi behind. The lower half of the lacrimal fossa is related medially to the anterior part of the nasal middle meatus; the upper half to the anterior ethmoidal sinuses. (In 100 skulls Whitnall, 1911, observed that in 14 the anterior ethmoidal sinuses were related only to the fossa's posterior wall; in 32 they reached the suture between the lacrimal bone and maxilla; in 54 one irregular sinus extended to the anterior lacrimal crest.)

The lacrimal sac has a fibro-elastic wall, lined internally by mucosa continuous through the lacrimal canaliculi with the conjunctiva and through the nasolacrimal duct with the nasal mucosa.

Nasolacrimal duct

The nasolacrimal duct (8.463–465), about 18 mm long, descends from the lacrimal sac to open anteriorly in the inferior meatus at an expanded orifice; a mucosal *lacrimal fold* forms an imperfect valve just above this opening. The duct runs down an osseous canal formed by the maxilla, lacrimal bone and inferior nasal concha; it is

Middle nasal concha

Superior nasal concha

Sphenoidal sinus

Sella turcica

Frontal sinuses

Lacrimal sac

Nasolacrimal duct

Atrium of middle meatus

Vestibule

Pharyngotympanic tube orifice

Inferior nasal concha

8.468   The left lateral wall of the nasal cavity medial aspect. The lacrimal sac and the nasolacrimal duct of the left side have been projected on to the lateral wall of the nasal cavity to show their positions relative to the middle nasal concha, the middle meatus and the inferior concha.

narrowest in the middle and directed down, back and a little laterally. The mucosa of the lacrimal sac and the nasolacrimal duct has a bilaminar columnar epithelium, ciliated in places. A surrounding plexus of veins, forming erectile tissue, may, when engorged, obstruct the duct.

Lacrimal fluid enters the conjunctival sac at its superolateral angle and, by capillarity and blinking, is carried across the eye to the lacus lacrimalis, mainly between the lower palpebral margin and the eyeball. From the lacus it enters the lacrimal canaliculi. Contraction of the orbicularis oculi presses the puncta lacrimalia more firmly into the lacus and capillary attraction draws the secretion into the lacrimal sac. Sudden dilatation of the sac, produced by the lacrimal part of the orbicularis oculi during blinking (p. 792), probably aids this. Normally the tarsal secretion prevents tear fluid from overflowing and also covers the capillary film of fluid on the cornea and sclera, perhaps delaying evaporation (Mishima & Maurice 1961; Wolff 1976).

AUDITORY AND VESTIBULAR APPARATUS

The *peripheral auditory apparatus* includes the various parts of the ear, but of particular functional importance is the *cochlear part* of its *membranous labyrinth*. Each ear is a *distance receptor* for the collection, conduction, modification, amplification and analysis of complex waves of sound reaching it. These are transduced into coded patterns of impulses in the afferent cochlear fibres of the vestibulocochlear nerve, for transmission and further analysis in the central auditory pathways of the brain (pp. 1024, 1026, 1071, 1090, 1110).

Sound waves consist of repetitive oscillations of the molecules constituting air; the waves vary in:

- the *direction* and *distance* or *location* of their source
- their *intensity* or *energy content*
- the mixture of *frequencies* in the train of waves
- the *phase* of their vibrations.

The structural and functional design of ears make them, within certain ranges, extremely sensitive to differences in frequency, intensity and phase and, when used binaurally, they are very effective range and direction finders. They are also most responsive to the *rate of change* in all these parameters. Frequencies are expressed as *cycles per second* or *Hertz* (c/s or Hz), which are subjectively appreciated as *pitch*, young adult ears responding to frequencies of about 20–20 000 Hz, although higher and lower values are not uncommon in youth. *Intensity* is expressed as the *quantity of energy* transmitted per *unit time* through a *unit area* perpendicular to the direction of propagation. The subjective appreciation of sound intensity is related to the logarithm of the absolute intensity as just defined but is also dependent on frequency, the human ear being most sensitive to sounds in the range of 1500–3000 Hz; above and below this the threshold rises sharply; for example, 10 000 times more energy is necessary for an equal perceptive effect at 15 000 Hz than at 2000 Hz. The ear's sensitivity is astounding; sounds may be discerned which involve pressure changes as small as 10^{10} atmospheres, a change equivalent to ascending or descending 1/30 000 of an inch! Because of the great variation in the intensity of sounds commonly experienced, the *decibel* has been introduced for convenience. It is defined as 10 times the logarithm of the ratio of the intensity of the sound, compared to an accepted reference level. In practice this reference level is defined as the Sound Pressure Level (SPL) and decibels are quoted as db SPL. A difference in intensity of about one decibel is usually just perceptible by the human auditory system.

The *quality* of a particular sound depends on the mixture of frequencies of which it is composed. Musical sounds usually consist of one or more fundamental frequencies each with its mathematically related series of *harmonics*. Mixtures of unrelated and *irregular* frequencies are regarded as 'noise'. Human speech has a marked content of noise. Moreover, consonants often involve higher frequencies than do vowels. Hence speech is easily obscured by concomitant noise and, with increasing age and consequent reduction of sensitivity at the high frequency range of the human ear, the elderly find speech less easy to interpret.

The elegant researches into the way in which the ear operates as a peripheral analyser of frequency and intensity and how intensity and phase differences impinging on the two ears are used in detecting the range and directions of the sound source, can merely be mentioned here. For details the reader must consult specialist accounts, for example Pickles (1992).

The human ear can be divided, according to phylogenetic, developmental, structural and functional criteria, into *external, middle* and *internal* parts. Associated topographically with the cochlear, auditory part of the labyrinth, are the sensory receptors of the other major region of the inner ear, consisting of specialized sensory areas of the utricle, saccule and ampullae of the semicircular ducts which, with their contained and surrounding fluids, bony cavities and the vestibular part of the eighth cranial nerve, constitute the *peripheral vestibular apparatus*. The latter provides the CNS with information concerning the static position of the head in space and of its linear or angular acceleration or deceleration.

The evolution of the auditory apparatus in land vertebrates has attracted an enormous literature which cannot be even considered here; for a recent survey consult Lombard and Bolt 1977.

EXTERNAL EAR

The external ear comprises the *auricle*, or *pinna*, and the *external acoustic meatus*. The auricle projects from the side of the head to collect sound waves, and the meatus leads inwards from the auricle to conduct vibrations to the tympanic membrane. These structures do not act merely as a simple ear-trumpet, for they are the first of a series of *stimulus modifiers* in the auditory apparatus, as will become apparent.

AURICLE

The lateral surface of the auricle or *pinna* (8.469) is irregularly concave, faces slightly forwards and displays numerous eminences

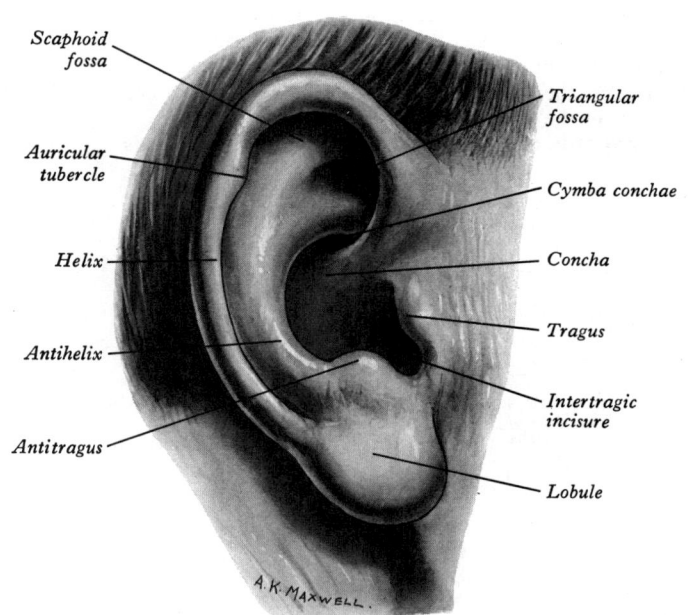

8.469   The right auricle: lateral aspect.

and depressions. Its prominent curved rim, or *helix*, usually bears posterosuperiorly a small *auricular tubercle* (of Darwin), a structure which is quite pronounced around the sixth month of intrauterine life, when the auricle closely resembles that of some adult monkeys. Another curved prominence, parallel and anterior to the posterior part of the helix, is the *antihelix*, dividing above into two *crura* flanking a depressed *triangular fossa*. The curved depression between the helix and antihelix is the *scaphoid fossa*. The antihelix encircles the deep, capacious *concha* of the auricle, which is incompletely divided by the *crus* or anterior end of the helix; the conchal area above this, the *cymba conchae*, overlies the supermeatal triangle of the temporal bone, which can be felt through it (pp. 560, 567), deep to which is the mastoid antrum. Below the crus of the helix and in front of the concha is a small curved flap, the *tragus*, which projects posteriorly, partly overlapping the meatal orifice. Opposite the tragus and separated from it by the *intertragic incisure*, is a small tubercle, the *antitragus*. Below this is the *lobule*; composed of fibrous and adipose tissues, this is soft, unlike the majority which, being supported by elastic cartilage, is firm. The cranial surface of the auricle presents elevations corresponding to the depressions on its lateral surface, after which they are named, for example the eminentia conchae, eminentia fossae triangularis, etc.

Though primarily acting as collecting 'trumpets' for sound waves, the auricles, by their asymmetry and variations in thickness, probably introduce *variable delay paths* in sound transmission, which may be important in the efficient binaural (and also the cruder monaural) localization of sources of sound.

In its structure the auricle is a thin plate of *elastic fibrocartilage* covered by skin and connected to the surrounding parts by ligaments and muscles; it is continuous with the cartilage of the external acoustic meatus, which is joined to the margins of the bony meatus by fibrous tissue. Its *skin* is thin, adherent to the cartilage and bears fine hairs furnished with sebaceous glands which are most numerous in the concha and scaphoid fossa. On the tragus, antitragus and intertragic incisure the hairs are strong and numerous, especially in elderly males. The skin is continuous with that of the external acoustic meatus.

Auricular cartilage (8.470). This is a single piece of elastic fibrocartilage, its surface moulded by eminences and depressions as described above; it is absent from the lobule and between the tragus and the crus of the helix, the gap being filled by dense fibrous tissue. Anteriorly, where the helix curves upwards, is a small cartilaginous projection, the *spine of the helix*, its other extremity being prolonged inferiorly as the *tail of the helix* and separated from the antihelix by the *fissura antitragohelicina*. The cartilage's cranial aspect bears the *eminentia conchae* and *eminentia triangularis*, corresponding to the depressions on the lateral surface. A transverse furrow, the *sulcus antihelicis transversus*, corresponding to the inferior crus of the antihelix on the lateral surface, separates the two eminences. The eminentia conchae is crossed by an oblique ridge, the *ponticulus*, for the attachment of the auricularis posterior muscle. There are two fissures in the auricular cartilage, one behind the crus helicis and another in the tragus.

Ligaments of the auricle. These consist of two sets:

- extrinsic, connecting it to the temporal bone
- intrinsic, interconnecting various parts of its cartilage.

There are two *extrinsic ligaments*, anterior and posterior, the *anterior* extending from the tragus and the spine of the helix to the root of the zygomatic process of the temporal bone and the *posterior ligament* passing from the posterior surface of the concha to the lateral surface of the mastoid process. The chief *intrinsic ligaments* are:

- a strong fibrous band from the tragus to the helix, completing the meatus anteriorly and forming part of the concha's boundary
- a band between the antihelix and the tail of the helix.

Less prominent bands also exist on the cranial aspect of the auricle.

Auricular muscles

These are two sets of auricular muscles: the *extrinsic*, connecting the auricle to the skull and scalp and moving the auricle as a whole; and the *intrinsic*, connecting the different parts of the auricle.

Extrinsic muscles. These are the auriculares anterior, superior and posterior. The *auricularis anterior*, the smallest of the three, is a thin fan of pale fibres, arising from the lateral edge of the epicranial aponeurosis, its fibres converging to insert into the spine of the helix. The *auricularis superior*, the largest of the three, is also thin and fan-shaped and converges from the epicranial aponeurosis via a thin, flat tendon to attach to the upper part of the cranial surface of the auricle. The *auricularis posterior* consists of two or three fleshy fasciculi arising by short aponeurotic fibres from the mastoid part of the temporal bone and inserted into the ponticulus on the eminentia conchae.

Nerve supply. The auriculares anterior and superior are supplied by temporal branches of the facial nerve and the auricularis posterior by the posterior auricular branch of the same nerve.

Actions. In man these muscles have very little obvious effect: the auricularis anterior draws the auricle forwards and upwards; the auricularis superior elevates it slightly; and the auricularis posterior draws it back. Despite the paucity of auricular movement, auditory stimuli may evoke patterned responses from these small muscles and electromyography can detect the 'crossed acoustic response' elicited by this means in investigative clinical neurology.

Intrinsic muscles. They are: helicis major and minor, tragicus, antitragicus, transversus auriculae and obliquus auriculae. They modify auricular shape minimally, if at all, in most human ears. Occasional individuals can, however, modify the shape and position of their external ears. *Helicis major* is a narrow vertical band on the anterior margin of the helix, passing from its spine to its anterior border, where the helix is about to curve back. *Helicis minor* is an oblique fasciculus, covering the crus helicis. *Tragicus* is a short, flattened, vertical band on the lateral aspect of the tragus. The *antitragicus* (muscle) passes from the outer part of the antitragus (prominence) to the tail of the helix and the antihelix. The *transversus auriculae*, on the cranial aspect of the auricle, consists of scattered fibres, partly tendinous, partly muscular, extending between the eminentia conchae and the eminentia scaphae. The *obliquus auriculae*, also on the cranial aspect of the auricle, comprises a few fibres extending from the upper and posterior parts of the eminentia conchae to the eminentia triangularis.

Nerve supply. On the lateral aspect this is from the temporal branches of the facial and to those on the cranial aspect from the facial's posterior auricular branch.

Vessels and nerves of the auricle

Arteries. These are:

- the posterior auricular branch of the external carotid, supplying three or four branches to its cranial surface; twigs from these reach the lateral surface, some through fissures in the cartilage, others round the margin of the helix
- the anterior auricular branches of the superficial temporal artery, distributed to the lateral surface
- a branch from the occipital artery.

Veins. These correspond to the arteries of the auricle. Arterio-venous anastomoses are numerous in the skin of the auricle.

Lymphatics. These drain into:

- the parotid lymph nodes, especially the node in front of the tragus

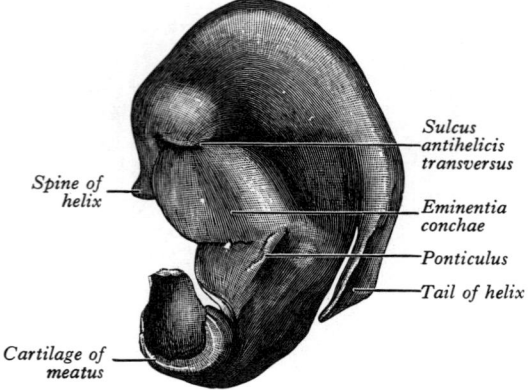

Spine of helix

Cartilage of meatus

Sulcus antihelicis transversus

Eminentia conchae

Ponticulus

Tail of helix

8.470   The medial surface of the right auricular cartilage.

- the upper deep cervical lymph nodes
- the mastoid lymph nodes.

Sensory nerves. These are:

- the great auricular nerve, supplying most of the cranial surface and the posterior part of the lateral surface (helix, antihelix, lobule)
- the lesser occipital nerve, supplying the upper part of the cranial surface
- the auricular branch of the vagus, supplying the concavity of the concha and posterior part of the eminentia
- the auriculotemporal nerve, supplying the tragus, crus of the helix and the adjacent part of the helix
- the facial nerve, which with the auricular branch of the vagus probably supplies small areas on both aspects of the auricle in the depression of the concha and over its eminence.

The details of the cutaneous innervation by the facial nerve and whether the facial fibres reach the external acoustic meatus and tympanic membrane require further clarification.

EXTERNAL ACOUSTIC MEATUS

The external acoustic meatus extends from the concha to the tympanic membrane (**8.471, 472, 474**). Its length, from the floor of the concha, is approximately 2.5 cm and from the tragus about 4 cm. It has two structurally different parts, the lateral third being *cartilaginous* and the medial two-thirds *osseous*. It forms an S-shaped curve, directed at first medially, anteriorly and slightly up (*pars externa*), then posteromedially and up (*pars media*) and lastly again anteromedially and slightly down (*pars interna*). It is oval in section, its greatest diameter being obliquely inclined postero-inferiorly at the external orifice but nearly horizontal at its medial end. There are two constrictions, one near the medial end of the cartilaginous part, the other, the *isthmus*, in the osseous part about 2 cm from the bottom of the concha. The tympanic membrane, which closes its medial end, is obliquely set and so the floor and the anterior wall of the meatus are longer than its roof and posterior wall.

The lateral, *cartilaginous part* is about 8 mm long: it is continuous with the auricular cartilage and attached by fibrous tissue to the circumference of the osseous part. This meatal cartilage is deficient posterosuperiorly, the gap being occupied by a sheet of collagen; two or three deep fissures exist in its anterior part.

The *osseous part* is about 16 mm long, and is narrower than the cartilaginous part. It is directed anteromedially and slightly downwards, with a slight posterosuperior convexity. Its medial end is smaller than the lateral end and terminates obliquely, the anterior

wall projecting medially about 4 mm beyond the posterior and marked, except above, by a narrow *tympanic sulcus*, to which the perimeter of the tympanic membrane is attached. Its lateral end is dilated and mostly rough for the attachment of the meatal cartilage.

The anterior, inferior and most of the posterior parts of the osseous meatus are formed by the tympanic element of the temporal bone, which in the fetus is only a *tympanic ring* (p. 592); the posterosuperior region is formed by the temporal squamous bone.

The skin of the auricle continues into the external acoustic meatus and covers the tympanic membrane's external surface. It is thin, with no dermal papillae, and is closely adherent to the cartilaginous and osseous parts of the tube; inflammation is very painful owing to increased tension in these tissues. In the thick subcutaneous tissue of the cartilaginous part of the meatus numerous *ceruminous glands* secrete ear wax or *cerumen*, their coiled tubular structure resembling that of sweat glands (p. 409). When active the secretory cells are columnar, but cuboidal when quiescent; they are covered externally by myoepithelial cells. Ducts open either on to the epithelial surface or into the nearby sebaceous gland of a hair follicle. Cerumen prevents the maceration of meatal skin by trapped water and may discourage invasion by insects. Over-production or accumulation of wax may completely block the meatus or obstruct the vibration of the tympanic membrane. Ceruminous glands and hair follicles are largely limited to the cartilaginous meatus, but a few small glands and fine hairs also occur in the roof of the lateral part of the osseous meatus. In addition to the protection given by the cerumen and meatal hairs, the warm humid environment of the relatively enclosed meatal air aids the mechanical responses of the tympanic membrane.

Relations of the meatus

The mandible's condyloid process lies anterior to the meatus and partially separated from its cartilaginous part by a small portion of the parotid gland. A blow on the chin may cause the condyle to break into the meatus. Mandibular movements affect the size of the cartilaginous lumen. The middle cranial fossa lies above the osseous meatus and the mastoid air cells are posterior to it, separated from the meatus by a thin layer of bone. Its deepest part is situated below the epitympanic recess (p. 1372) and antero-inferior to the mastoid antrum, the lamina of bone separating it from the antrum being only 1–2 mm thick and providing the 'transmeatal approach' of aural surgery.

Arteries. These are: the posterior auricular branch of the external carotid, the deep auricular branch of the maxillary and the auricular branches of the superficial temporal.

Veins. They drain into: the external jugular and maxillary veins and the pterygoid plexus.

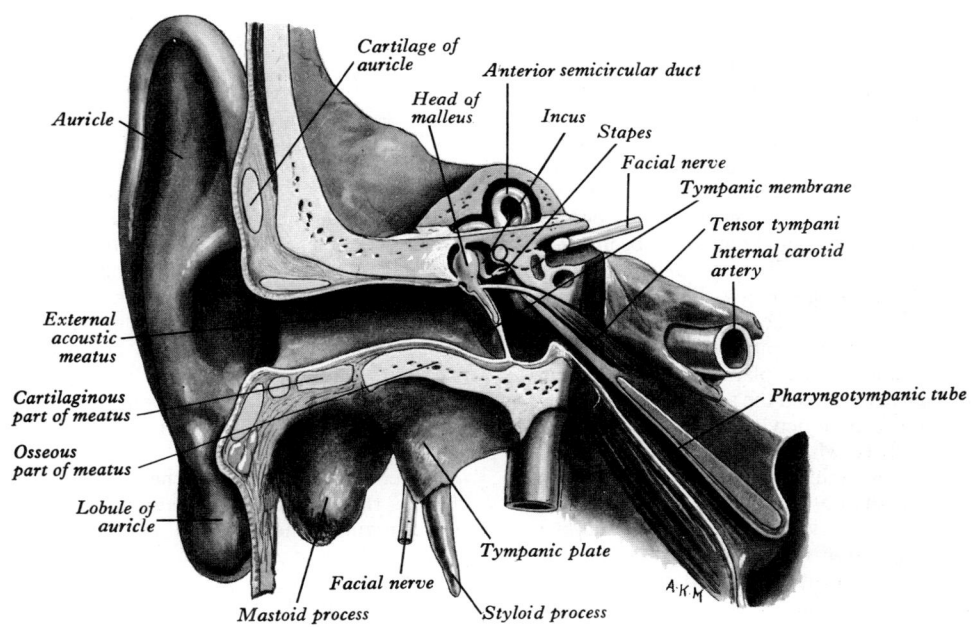

8.471 The external and middle regions of the right ear: anterior aspect.

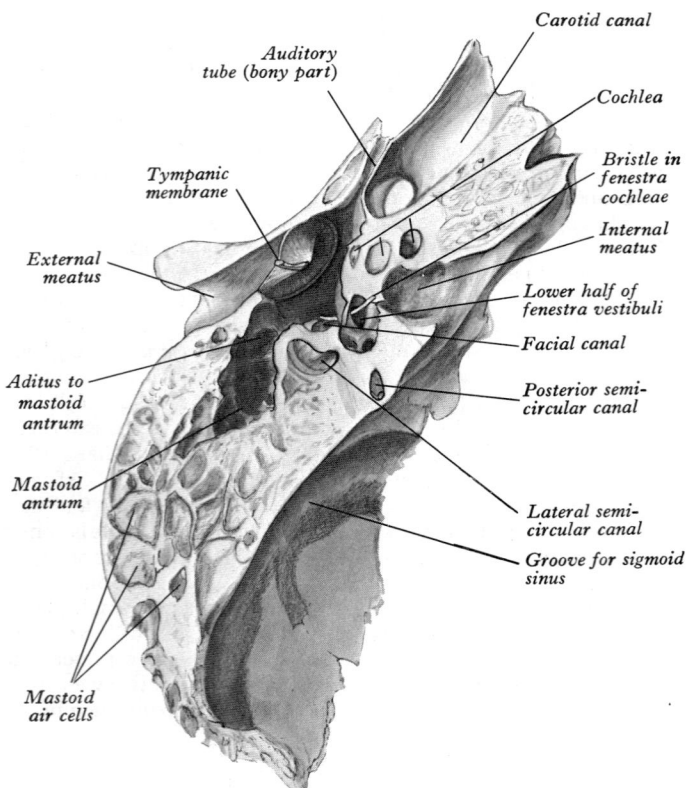

8.472 Oblique section through the left temporal bone viewed from above. Compare with 8.474 and 8.477. (From a section prepared by P F Milling.)

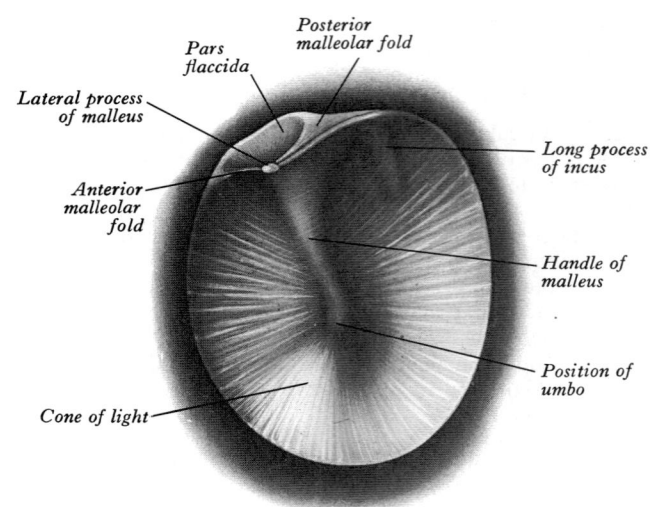

8.473 The left tympanic membrane: external aspect as seen through a speculum. (Anterior is towards the left.)

Lymphatics. These drain with those of the auricle (p. 1368).

Nerves. These are derived from the auriculotemporal branch of the mandibular, which supplies the anterior and superior walls of the meatus, and the auricular branch of the vagus, innervating the posterior and inferior walls.

Clinical examination of the meatus

To inspect the meatus and tympanic membrane satisfactorily with light reflected down a speculum, the sinuosity of the meatus can be to some extent straightened by pulling the auricle upwards, back and a little laterally. In this way, most of the meatus and tympanic membrane can be viewed.

At the junction of the osseous and cartilaginous parts the forward bend in the meatus constricts it, a point of importance in attempts to remove a foreign body lodged in the meatus. The shortness of the meatus in children also exposes the tympanic membrane to the danger of damage when an aural speculum is used. Even in adults a speculum should not be inserted beyond the constricted junction of the cartilaginous and osseous parts. Immediately anterolateral to the tympanic membrane is a depression on the meatal floor, bounded laterally by a prominent ridge, where foreign bodies may be impacted. Most of the tympanic membrane is visible through a speculum (8.473). It is pearly-grey and slightly glistening. Its external aspect faces forwards, laterally and downwards, i.e. it is placed at an acute angle of about 55° with the floor of the meatus and an obtuse angle with the roof. At birth it lies almost in the plane of the cranial base.

A reddish-yellow streak midway between the anterior and posterior margins extends from the centre obliquely upwards and forwards, marking the handle of the malleus, which is attached internally. At the upper part of this streak, near the roof of the meatus, a small, white round prominence marks the position of the lateral process of the malleus, projecting against the membrane. The tympanic membrane is not planar but is drawn in at its centre, or *umbo* (p. 1373), by the handle of the malleus. A bright reflected 'cone of light' appears in the antero-inferior quadrant. Anterior and posterior to the short process of the malleus, the variably prominent *anterior* and *posterior malleolar folds* appear, with the flaccid part of the membrane

(p. 1373) between them. Posterior and parallel to the upper part of the handle of the malleus, the long process of the incus is often visible as a whitish streak, sometimes ending below near a round spot, the head of the stapes. Also variably visible through the tympanic membrane are the chorda tympani, the recess of the round window, and the tympanic end of the pharyngotympanic tube, depending on the translucency of the tympanic membrane.

Clinical anatomy. Imperfect development of the external parts, a supernumerary auricle, preauricular cysts, fistulae and sinuses, or the absence of the meatus occasionally occur. In a child up to the age of 4 or 5 years a gap exists in the antero-inferior osseous wall of the meatus, the *foramen of Huschke* (pp. 593, 609) which is filled by a membrane; it may persist in the adult. The sources of the meatal innervation, which include the vagus, account for the occurrence of reflex coughing and sneezing when there is irritation of the meatus and for the vomiting which may follow syringing the ears in children, and also the occasional heart failure induced by this process in the elderly. The association of earache with toothache or with lingual carcinoma is due to the involvement of the mandibular branch of the trigeminal, which supplies the teeth and tongue as well as the meatus. The upper half of the tympanic membrane is more vascular: for this reason and to avoid the chorda tympani and ossicles, incisions of this membrane should be postero-inferior.

TYMPANIC CAVITY (TYMPANUM)

The tympanic cavity or *middle ear* (8.471–473, 475, 476) is an irregular, laterally compressed space in the temporal bone, lined by muco-periosteum (p. 1376) and containing air derived from the naso-pharynx via the pharyngotympanic tube. It contains a train of three movable ossicles, which connect the lateral to the medial wall to transmit vibrations of the tympanic membrane across the cavity of the middle ear to the cochlea; its essential function is to transfer energy efficiently from the relatively weak vibrations in the elastic, compressible **air** in the external acoustic meatus to overcome the inertia of the incompressible **fluids** around the delicate receptors in the cochlea. Mechanical coupling between the two systems must match their resistance to deformation or 'flow', i.e. their *impedance*, as closely as possible. Thus aerial waves of low amplitude and *low force* per unit area arrive at the tympanic membrane, which has 15–20 times the area of the *stapedial footplate* in contact with perilymph. In this manner, the force per unit area generated by the footplate is increased by a similar amount, while the amplitude of vibration is almost unchanged.

Protective mechanisms are also incorporated into the tympanic cavity's design, including the pharyngotympanic tube to equalize pressure on both sides of the delicate tympanic membrane, the

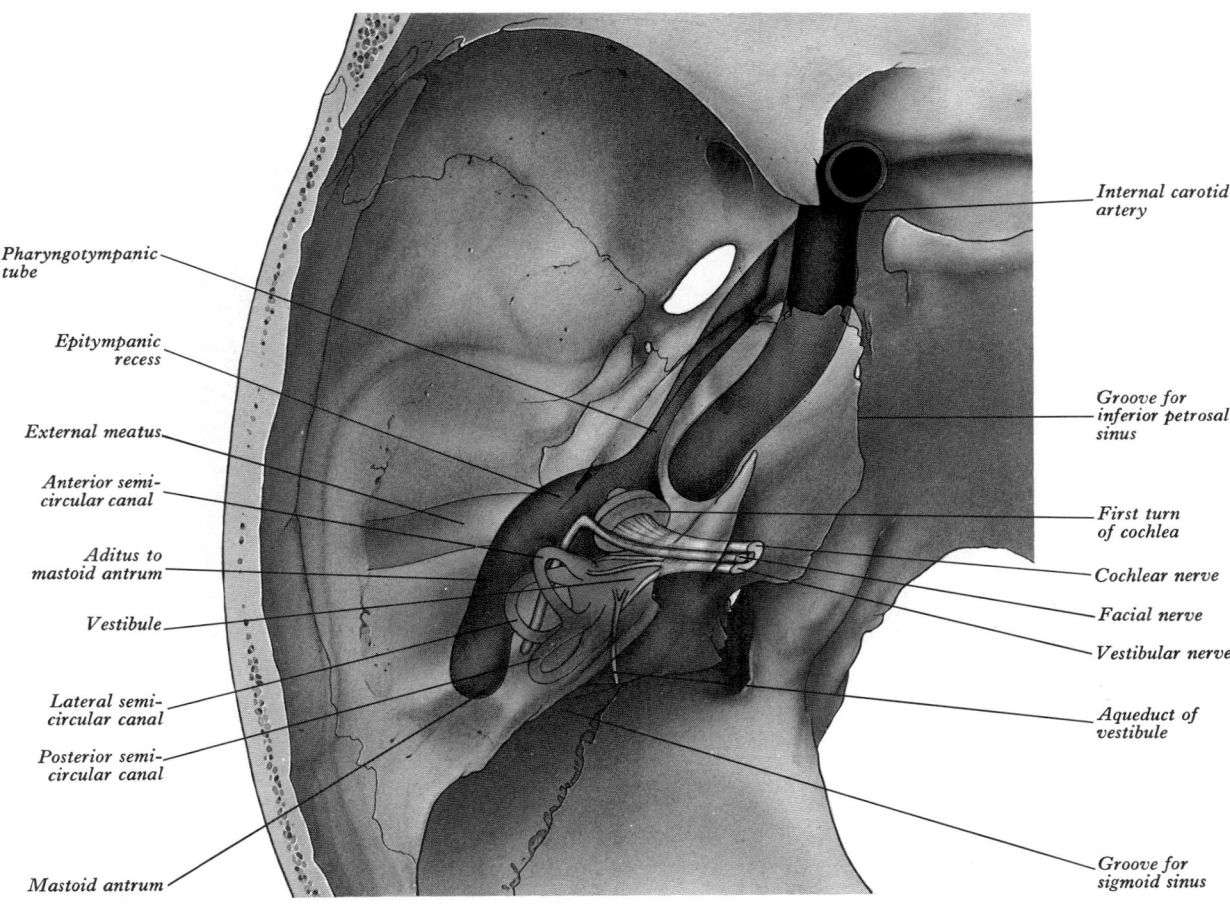

Pharyngotympanic
tube

Epitympanic
recess

External meatus

Anterior semi-
circular canal

Aditus to
mastoid antrum

Vestibule

Lateral semi-
circular canal

Posterior semi-
circular canal

Mastoid antrum

Internal carotid
artery

Groove for
inferior petrosal
sinus

First turn
of cochlea

Cochlear nerve

Facial nerve

Vestibular nerve

Aqueduct of
vestibule

Groove for
sigmoid sinus

8.474 Scheme showing the parts of the left auditory apparatus as if viewed through a semi-transparent temporal bone. Compare with **8.472** and **8.477**.

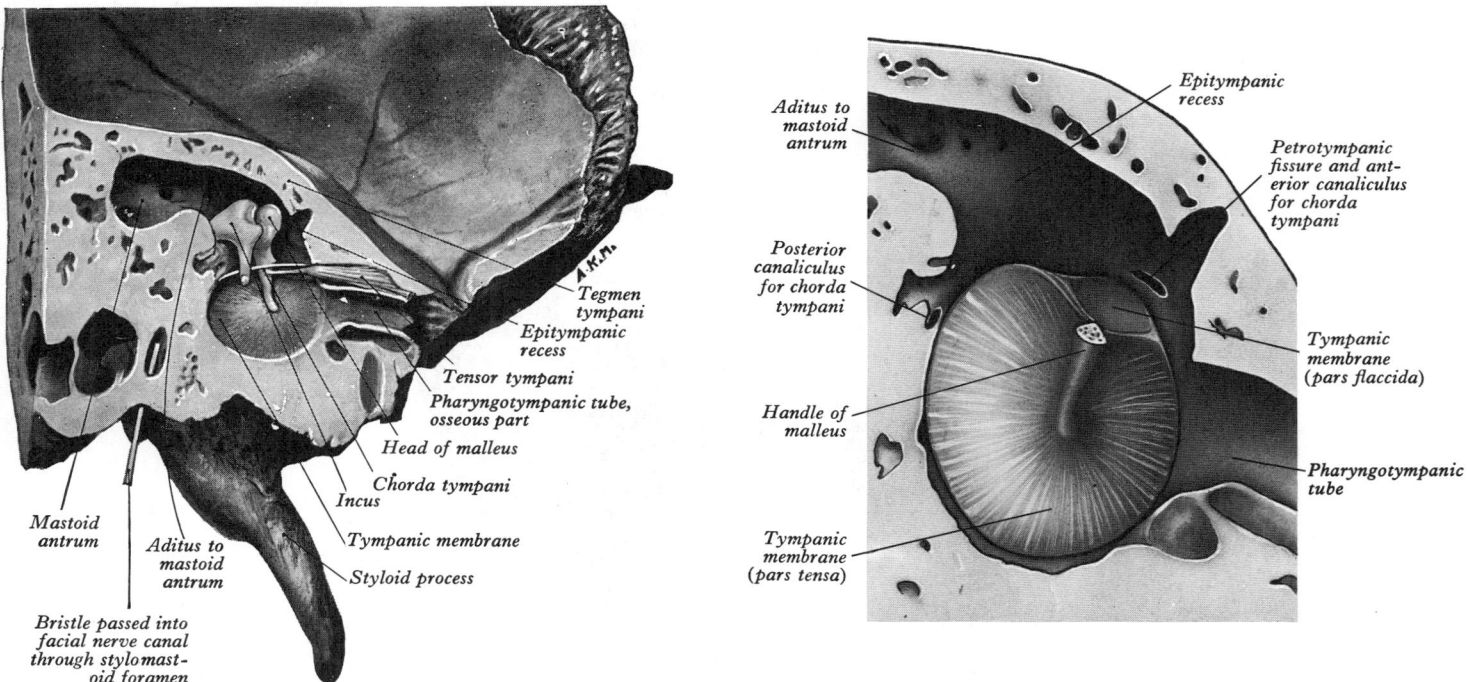

Tegmen
tympani

Epitympanic
recess

Tensor tympani

Pharyngotympanic tube,
osseous part

Head of malleus

Chorda tympani

Incus

Tympanic membrane

Styloid process

Mastoid
antrum

Aditus to
mastoid
antrum

Bristle passed into
facial nerve canal
through stylomast-
oid foramen

Aditus to
mastoid
antrum

Posterior
canaliculus
for chorda
tympani

Handle of
malleus

Tympanic
membrane
(pars tensa)

Epitympanic
recess

Petrotympanic
fissure and ant-
erior canaliculus
for chorda
tympani

Tympanic
membrane
(pars flaccida)

Pharyngotympanic
tube

8.475 Oblique vertical section through the left temporal bone, to show the lateral wall of the middle ear and the mastoid antrum.

8.476 The lateral wall of the left tympanic cavity.

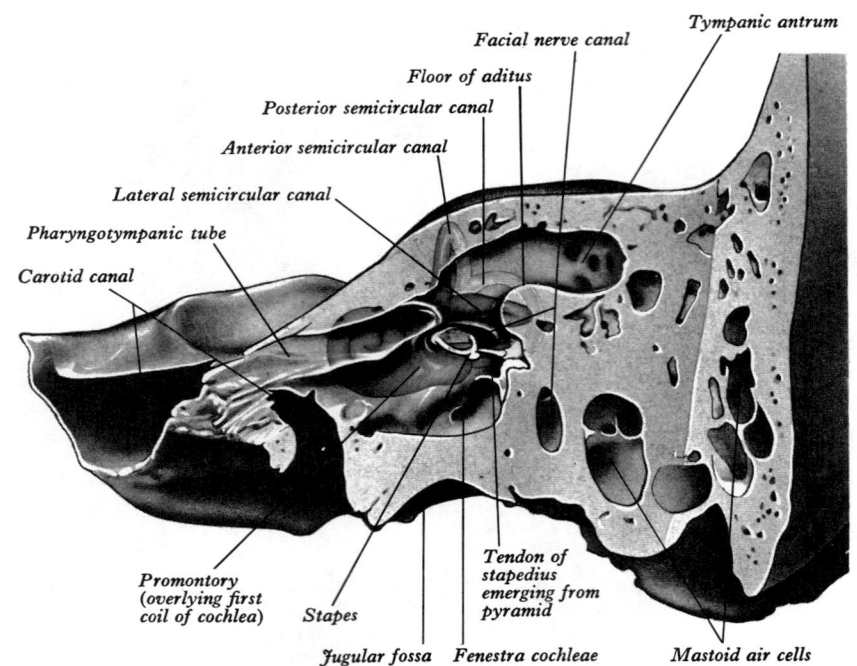

8.477 Oblique section through the left temporal bone, to show the medial wall of the middle ear. The cochlea and the semicircular canals are in blue. Note the relationship of the first coil of the cochlea to the promontory and the closeness of the facial nerve canal and the lateral semicircular canal to the medial wall of the aditus.

protective shape of articulations between the ossicles and the reflex contractions of the stapedius and tensor tympani muscles preventing damage due to sudden or excessive excursions of the ossicles.

The cavity has two parts: the *tympanic cavity proper*, opposite the membrane, and an *epitympanic recess*, above its level. The latter contains the upper half of the malleus and most of the incus. Including the recess, the vertical and anteroposterior diameters of the cavity are each about 15 mm; the transverse is about 6 mm above and 4 mm below but opposite the umbo it is only 2 mm. The cavity is bounded **laterally** by the tympanic membrane and **medially** by the lateral wall of the internal ear. It communicates posteriorly with the mastoid antrum and via this with the mastoid air cells; anteriorly it communicates with the pharyngotympanic tube (**8.**471, 474, 476, 477).

BOUNDARIES OF THE TYMPANIC CAVITY

The roof of the tympanic cavity (8.475–478)

A thin plate of compact bone, the *tegmen tympani*, separates the cranial and tympanic cavities, forming much of the anterior surface of the petrous temporal bone. The tegmen tympani is prolonged posteriorly to roof the mastoid antrum and anteriorly to cover the canal for the tensor tympani. In youth, the unossified petrosquamosal suture (p. 592) may allow the spread of infection from the tympanic cavity to the meninges. In adults, veins from the tympanic cavity traverse this suture to the superior petrosal or petrosquamous sinus (p.1587) and may also transmit infection to these structures.

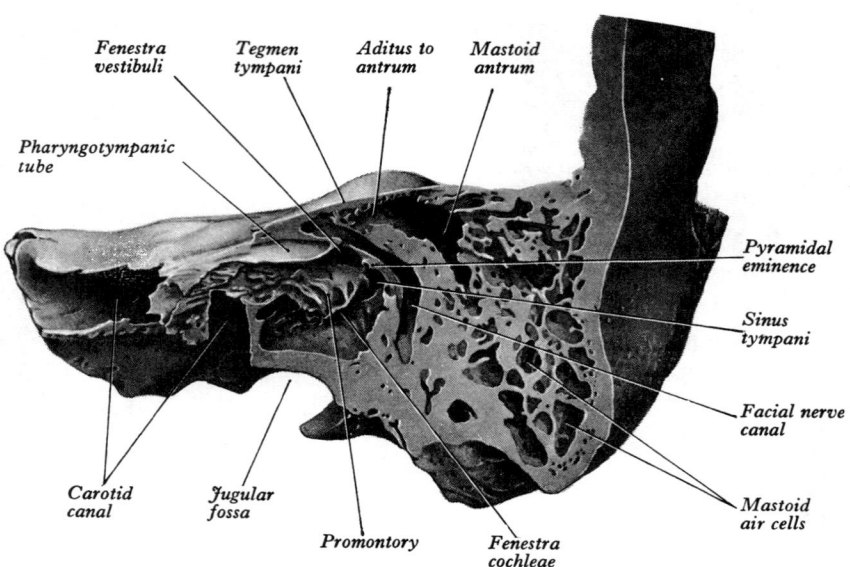

8.478 Oblique section through the left temporal bone, showing the medial wall of the middle ear. Compare with **8.**477.

The floor of the tympanic cavity (8.471, 477, 478)

The floor is a narrow, thin, convex plate of bone separating the cavity from the superior bulb of the internal jugular vein; bone may be patchily deficient here and the tympanic cavity and the vein are then separated only by mucous membrane and fibrous tissue. Near the medial wall is a small aperture for the tympanic branch of the glossopharyngeal nerve. The floor is sometimes thick and may contain some accessory mastoid air cells.

The lateral wall of the tympanic cavity (8.475, 476)

The lateral wall consists mainly of the tympanic membrane but is partly also composed of the ring of bone to which the membrane is attached. The ring is deficient or notched above and near this region are the openings of the anterior and posterior canaliculi for the chorda tympani and also the petrotympanic fissure.

The *posterior canaliculus for the chorda tympani nerve* is situated in the angle between the posterior and lateral walls of the tympanic cavity just behind the tympanic membrane and level with the upper end of the handle of the malleus; it leads into a minute canal which descends in front of the facial canal and ends in it about 6 mm above the stylomastoid foramen. Through it the chorda tympani nerve and a branch of the stylomastoid artery enter the tympanic cavity.

The *petrotympanic fissure* opens just above and in front of the ring of bone to which the tympanic membrane is attached; it is a mere slit about 2 mm in length, containing the anterior process and anterior ligament of the malleus and it transmits to the tympanic cavity the maxillary artery's anterior tympanic branch.

The *anterior canaliculus for the chorda tympani* opens at the medial end of the petrotympanic fissure; through it the chorda tympani leaves the tympanic cavity.

The tympanic membrane (8.471, 473, 476)

The tympanic membrane separates the tympanic cavity from the external meatus. It is thin and semi-transparent, almost oval, though somewhat broader above than below, and is placed at an angle of about 55° with the meatal floor. Its longest, antero-inferior diameter is from 9–10 mm and its shortest is from 8–9 mm. Most of its circumference is a thickened *fibrocartilaginous ring* attached to the *tympanic sulcus* at the medial end of the meatus; this sulcus is deficient superiorly and here, as noted above, the *anterior* and *posterior malleolar folds* pass to the lateral process of the malleus, leaving between them the triangular *pars flaccida*, a thin, lax part of the membrane; a small perforation may sometimes occur in this. The membrane is elsewhere taut, the *pars tensa*. The handle of the malleus is firmly attached to the membrane's internal surface as far as its centre, the *umbo*, which projects towards the tympanic cavity. Though this membrane as a whole is convex medially, its radiating fibres (see below) are curved with their concavities directed upwards.

Microstructure. Histologically, the tympanic membrane has three strata: an outer cuticular, an intermediate fibrous and an inner mucous. The *cuticular stratum* is continuous with the thin skin of the meatus and is keratinized, stratified squamous in type, devoid of dermal papillae and hairless. Its subepithelial tissue is vascularized and may develop a few peripheral papillae. The *fibrous stratum* has an external layer of radiating fibres diverging from the handle of the malleus and a deep layer of circular fibres, peripherally plentiful but sparse and scattered centrally in the membrane. Marginally and centrally a fine network of elastic fibres is said to be mixed with the collagen (but see below). The *mucous stratum* is a part of the mucosa of the tympanic cavity; it is thickest near the tympanic membrane's upper part and is covered, it has been claimed, by a layer of ciliated columnar epithelial cells. However, cilia occur only in patches or are entirely absent and are then replaced by a low cuboidal or simple squamous epithelium.

These appearances, based on light microscopy, have been much amplified by electron microscopy and other techniques: first in guinea-pigs (Johnson et al 1968), in which the **external** epithelium is approximately 10 cells thick and has two zones, a superficial of non-nucleated squames and a deep zone like the epidermal stratum spinosum, with numerous desmosomes between cells, the deepest of which lie on a continuous basal lamina but lack epithelial pegs and hemidesmosomes. The **internal** epithelium is a single layer of very flat cells, with overlapping interdigitating boundaries carrying desmo-

somes and tight junctions between cells. Their cytoplasm contains only a few organelles; the luminal surfaces of these apparently metabolically inert cells have a few irregular microvilli and are covered by an amorphous electron-dense material. Ciliated columnar cells are absent. Most interestingly the intermediate stratum contains filaments about 10 μm in diameter, with links between filaments at 25 nm intervals. The filaments are disposed in outer radial and inner non-radial zones, the former more numerous; neither resemble collagen or elastin. In amino acid composition, also, the filaments are distinctive and may consist of a protein peculiar to the tympanic membrane. McMinn and Taylor 1978, reporting on the development of the fibrillar component in guinea-pig and human embryos and fetuses, have confirmed the findings in guinea-pigs mentioned above, but in human fetuses small groups of collagen fibrils were apparent at 11 weeks in utero, with small bundles of elastin microfibrils. Older specimens showed more typically cross-banded collagen fibrils and the development of an amorphous elastin component. Large fibroblasts occur between the external radial fibres and basal lamina of the **external** epithelium, while blood capillaries and their basement membranes lie just deep to the basal lamina of the **internal** epithelium. In the pars flaccida the fibrous stratum is replaced by loose connective tissue.

Arteries of the tympanic membrane. They arise from: the maxillary artery's deep auricular branch (to the outer, cuticular stratum) and the stylomastoid branch of the occipital or the posterior auricular artery and the tympanic branch of the maxillary to the internal mucosa.

Veins of the tympanic membrane. The *superficial veins* drain to the external jugular; those in the *deep surface* drain partly to the transverse sinus and dural veins and partly to the venous plexus of the pharyngotympanic tube.

Nerve supply of the tympanic membrane. This is from: the auriculotemporal branch of the mandibular nerve, the auricular branch of the vagus, the tympanic branch of the glossopharyngeal and possibly from the facial nerve.

The medial wall of the tympanic cavity (8.471, 472, 477, 478)

The medial wall is also the lateral boundary of the internal ear. Its features are the promontory, fenestra vestibuli, fenestra cochleae and the facial prominence.

The rounded *promontory*, minutely grooved by the nerves of the tympanic plexus, overlies the lateral projection of the basal turn of the cochlea; a minute spicule of bone frequently connects the promontory to the pyramidal eminence of the posterior wall. Anterior to the promontory the apex of the cochlea lies near the medial wall of the tympanum. Behind the promontory the *sinus tympani* indicates the position of the ampulla of the posterior semicircular canal.

The *fenestra vestibuli* (*f. ovalis*) (8.482) is a kidney-shaped opening posterosuperior to the promontory, connecting the tympanic cavity to the vestibule; its long diameter is horizontal and its convex border directed superiorly. It is occupied by the base of the stapes, the circumference of which is attached to the fenestral margin by an annular ligament.

The *fenestra cochlea* (*f. rotunda*) (8.477, 482) is postero-inferior to the fenestra vestibuli and separated from it by the posterior part of the promontory. It lies completely under the overhanging edge of the promontory in a deep hollow or niche. It is placed very obliquely; in dried specimens it opens anterosuperiorly from the tympanic cavity into the scala tympani of the cochlea. It is closed by the *secondary tympanic membrane*, which is somewhat concave towards the tympanic cavity and convex towards the cochlea, the membrane being bent so that its posterosuperior one-third is at an angle to its antero-inferior two-thirds. The membrane has three layers: an external derived from the tympanic mucosa, an internal from the cochlear lining membrane and a middle, fibrous layer.

The *prominence of the facial nerve canal* indicates the position of the upper part of a bony canal for the facial nerve. The canal, its lateral wall sometimes being partly deficient, traverses the medial tympanic wall from before backwards, just above the fenestra vestibuli, then curves down into the posterior wall of the cavity.

The posterior wall of the tympanic cavity (8.472, 474)

Wider above than below, its main features are the aditus to the mastoid antrum, the pyramid and the fossa incudis.

The *aditus to the mastoid antrum*, a large irregular aperture, leads back from the epitympanic recess into the upper part of the *mastoid antrum*. On the medial wall of the aditus is a rounded eminence, above and behind the prominence of the facial nerve canal, due to the underlying lateral semicircular canal.

The *pyramidal eminence* is just behind the fenestra vestibuli and anterior to the vertical part of the facial nerve canal; it contains the stapedius muscle, its summit projecting towards the fenestra vestibuli; a small apical aperture transmits the muscle's tendon. Its cavity is prolonged down and back in front of the facial nerve canal and communicates with the latter by an aperture through which a small branch of the facial nerve passes to the stapedius (p. 1376).

The *fossa incudis*, a small depression low and posterior in the epitympanic recess, contains the short process of the incus, fixed to the fossa by ligamentous fibres.

The mastoid antrum (8.472, 474–478)

An air sinus in the petrous temporal bone, it has relations of considerable surgical importance, being often infected. In its upper **anterior wall** is an opening, the aditus to the mastoid antrum, leading back from the epitympanic recess, with the lateral semicircular canal medial to it. The antrum's **medial wall** is related to the posterior semicircular canal (**8.477**). **Posterior** is the sigmoid sinus; some mastoid air cells may intervene between this and the antrum. The roof, formed by the tegmen tympani, lies below the middle cranial fossa and temporal lobe of the brain. The floor has several openings communicating with the mastoid air cells. **Antero-inferior** is the descending part of the facial nerve canal. The **lateral wall** of the antrum, the usual surgical approach to the cavity, is formed by the postmeatal process of the squamous temporal bone. This is only 2 mm thick at birth but increases at a rate of approximately 1 mm a year to attain a final thickness of 12–15 mm. In adults the lateral wall of the antrum corresponds to the *suprameatal triangle* on the outer surface of the skull (pp. 560, 567), palpable through the cymba conchae (p. 1368). The triangle's superior side, the supramastoid crest, is level with the floor of the middle cranial fossa; the antero-inferior side, forming the posterosuperior margin of the external acoustic meatus, indicates approximately the position of the descending part of the facial nerve canal; and the posterior side, formed by a posterior vertical tangent to the posterior margin of the external acoustic meatus, is just anterior to the sigmoid sinus. The adult capacity of the antrum is about 1 ml and its general diameter about 10 mm. Unlike other air sinuses, it is present at birth and is indeed then almost adult in size, although it is at a higher level relative to the external acoustic meatus than in adults. In the very young, owing to the thinness of the lateral antral wall and the absence of the mastoid process, the stylomastoid foramen and emerging facial nerve are very superficially situated.

The mastoid air cells (8.472, 477, 478)

These air cells vary considerably in number, form and size. Usually they interconnect and are lined by a mucosa with squamous non-ciliated epithelium, continuous with that in the mastoid antrum and tympanic cavity. They may fill the mastoid process, even to its tip, and some may be separated from the sigmoid sinus and posterior cranial fossa only by extremely thin bone, which is occasionally deficient. Some may lie superficial to, or even behind the sigmoid sinus and others may occur in the posterior wall of the descending part of the facial nerve canal. Those in the squamous temporal bone may be separated from deeper cells in the petrous part by a plate of bone in the line of the squamomastoid suture. Sometimes they extend very little into the mastoid, this process consisting largely of dense bone or trabecular bone containing bone marrow. Varieties of the mastoid process occur (**6.176**) and three types are commonly described: *pneumatic*, with many air cells, *sclerotic*, with few or none, and *mixed*, containing both air cells and bone marrow. Pannoer (1970) proposed a more elaborate scheme, dependent on the degree of pneumatization and the relation of air cells to the lateral sinus; in a series of 100 mastoid processes, the cells most distant from the antrum were largest. Air cells may extend beyond the mastoid process into the squamous temporal bone above the supramastoid crest, into the posterior root of the zygomatic process of the temporal, into the osseous roof of the external acoustic meatus just below the middle cranial fossa and into the floor of the tympanic cavity very close to the superior jugular bulb. Rarely, a few may excavate the jugular process of the occipital bone. An important group may extend medially into the petrous temporal bone, even to its apex, related to the pharyngotympanic tube, carotid canal, labyrinth and abducent nerve; some investigators maintain that these are not continuous with the mastoid cells but grow independently from the tympanic cavity. The extensions of the mastoid air cells described above are pathologically important since infection may spread to the structures around them. Though the antrum is well developed at birth, the mastoid air cells are merely minute antral diverticula at this stage. As the mastoid develops in the second year, the cells gradually extend into it and by the fourth year they are well formed, although their greatest growth occurs at puberty. In about 20% of skulls the mastoid process has no air cells at all.

The anterior wall of the tympanic cavity (8.471, 472, 476–477)

Narrowed by the approximation of the medial and lateral walls of the cavity, its inferior, larger area is a thin lamina forming the posterior wall of the carotid canal, perforated by the superior and inferior caroticotympanic nerves and the tympanic branch or branches of the internal carotid. Opening above on the anterior wall are two parallel canals; superior is the *canal for the tensor tympani* and inferiorly the *osseous part of the pharyngotympanic tube*. These canals incline downwards and anteromedially to open in the angle between the squamous and petrous parts of the temporal bone; they are separated by a thin, osseous septum. The canal for the tensor tympani and the bony septum runs posterolaterally on the medial tympanic wall, ending immediately above the fenestra vestibuli, where the posterior end of the septum is curved laterally to form a pulley, the *processus trochleariformis* (*cochleariformis*), over which the tendon of the tensor tympani is turned laterally to its attachment on the upper part of the handle of the malleus.

PHARYNGOTYMPANIC (AUDITORY) TUBE

The pharyngotympanic or auditory tube (8.471, 472, 474, 477), connecting the tympanic cavity to the nasopharynx, allows the passage of air between these spaces to equalize the air pressure on both aspects of the tympanic membrane. It is about 36 mm long and descends anteromedially at an angle of about 45° with the sagittal plane and 30° with the horizontal. It is formed partly by bone and partly by cartilage and fibrous tissue.

The *bony* part, about 12 mm long, starts from the anterior tympanic wall and gradually narrows to end at the junction of the squamous and petrous parts of the temporal bone, where it has a jagged margin for the attachment of the cartilaginous part; the carotid canal lies medially. It is oblong in transverse section, with its greater dimension in the horizontal plane.

The *cartilaginous part*, about 24 mm long, is formed by a triangular plate of cartilage, the greater part being in the posteromedial wall of the tube. Its apex is attached by fibrous tissue to the circumference of the jagged rim of the bony part of the tube and its base is directly under the mucosa of the lateral nasopharyngeal wall, forming a *tubal elevation* behind the pharyngeal orifice of the tube. The cartilage's upper part is bent laterally and downwards, producing a broad *medial lamina* and narrow *lateral lamina*. In transverse section it is hook-like and incomplete below and laterally, where the canal is composed of fibrous tissue. The cartilage is fixed to the cranial base in the groove between the petrous temporal bone and the greater wing of the sphenoid, ending near the root of the medial pterygoid plate. The cartilaginous and bony parts of the tube are not in the same plane, the former descending a little more steeply than the latter. The diameter of the tube is greatest at the pharyngeal orifice, least at the junction of the two parts (the *isthmus*) and increases again towards the tympanic cavity.

The mucosa of the tube is continuous with the nasopharyngeal and tympanic mucosae; it is lined by a ciliated columnar epithelium and is thin in the osseous part but thickened by mucous glands in the cartilaginous part; near the pharyngeal orifice is a variable, but sometimes considerable, lymphoid mass, the *tubal tonsil*.

Relations of the pharyngotympanic tube

Anterolaterally the tensor veli palatini separates the tube from the otic ganglion, the mandibular nerve and its branches, the chorda tympani and the middle meningeal artery. Some fibres of the tensor are attached to the lateral lamina of the cartilage and to the fibrous part, forming the *dilatator tubae*. The salpingopharyngeus (p. 1732) is attached to the inferior part of the cartilaginous tube near its pharyngeal opening. **Posteromedially** are the petrous temporal bone and the levator veli palatini which arises partly from the medial lamina of the tube. The position and relations of the pharyngeal orifice are described with the nasopharynx (p. 1726).

The tube is opened during deglutition but the mechanism is uncertain. The dilatator tubae, aided by the salpinopharyngeus, may be responsible, though some deny the dilatator tubae's existence. The levator veli palatini, by elevating the cartilaginous part of the tube, might allow passive opening by releasing tension on the cartilage.

At birth the auditory tube is about half its adult length, its direction being more horizontal and its bony part relatively shorter but much wider. Its pharyngeal orifice is a narrow slit, level with the palate and without a tubal elevation.

Vessels and nerves

Arteries. These arise from the ascending pharyngeal branch of the external carotid and from two branches of the maxillary artery: the middle meningeal and the artery of the pterygoid canal.

Veins. These drain to the pterygoid venous plexus.

Nerves. These come from the tympanic plexus (p.1377) and from the pharyngeal branch of the pterygopalatine ganglion. The precise contribution from the nerves forming the plexus, i.e. the glossopharyngeal, the cervical sympathetic and possibly the facial, remains uncertain in man.

AUDITORY OSSICLES

A chain of three mobile ossicles, the *malleus*, *incus* and *stapes*, transfers sound waves across the tympanic cavity from its membrane to the fenestra vestibuli. The malleus is attached to the tympanic membrane and the base of the stapes to the rim of the fenestra vestibuli, while the incus is suspended between them, articulating with both bones.

Malleus (8.471, 475, 479). Shaped somewhat like a mallet, it is 8–9 mm long and is the largest of the ossicles; it has a head, neck, manubrium and anterior and lateral processes. The *head*, its enlarged, ovoid upper end, is situated in the epitympanic recess; it articulates posteriorly with the incus, being covered elsewhere by mucosa. The cartilaginous articular facet for the incus is narrowed near its middle and consists of a larger upper part and a smaller lower part, orientated almost at right angles to each other. Opposite the constriction the lower margin of the facet projects as the *spur* (*cog-tooth*) of the malleus. The *neck* is the narrowed part below the head and inferior to this is an enlargement from which the processes project.

The *manubrium mallei* (*handle of the malleus*) is connected by its lateral margin with the tympanic membrane (8.473, 475, 476). It descends posteromedially, diminishing towards its free end which curves slightly forwards and is transversely flat. High on its medial surface a small projection receives the tendon of the tensor tympani.

The *anterior process* is a delicate bony spicule, directed forwards from the enlargement below the neck and connected to the petrotympanic fissure by ligamentous fibres (see below); in fetal life this is the longest process of the malleus and is continuous in front with Meckel's cartilage (p. 277). The *lateral process*, a conical projection from the root of the manubrium, is directed laterally and is attached to the upper part of the tympanic membrane and via the anterior and posterior malleolar folds to the sides of the notch in the upper part of the tympanic sulcus (8.471).

Ossification. The cartilaginous precursor of the malleus originates as part of the dorsal end of Meckel's cartilage. Excepting its anterior process, it ossifies from a single endochondral centre which appears near the future neck of the bone in the fourth month in utero. The anterior process ossifies separately in dense connective tissue and joins the rest of the bone at about the sixth month of fetal life.

Incus (8.471, 475, 480). This is shaped less like an anvil (from which it is named) than a premolar tooth, with its two diverging roots. It has a body and two processes. The *body* is somewhat cubical but laterally compressed; it has an anterior, cartilage-covered, saddle-shaped facet for articulation with the head of the malleus. The *long process*, rather more than half the length of the handle of the malleus, descends almost vertically, behind and parallel to the handle; its lower end bends medially and ends in a rounded *lenticular process*, the medial surface of which is a cartilaginous facet for the head of the stapes. The *short process*, somewhat conical, projects posteriorly and is attached by ligamentous fibres to the fossa incudis in the postero-inferior part of the epitympanic recess (8.475).

Ossification. The incus has a cartilaginous precursor continuous with the dorsal extremity of Meckel's cartilage (p. 277). Ossification often spreads from a single centre in the upper part of its long process in the fourth fetal month; the lenticular process, however, may have a separate centre.

Stapes (8.471, 477, 481). Also known as the stirrup, it has a head, neck, two limbs and a base. The *head* (*caput*) is directed laterally and has a small cartilaginous facet for the lenticular process of the incus. To the constricted *neck* is attached posteriorly the tendon of the stapedius. The *limbs* (*crura*) curve away from the neck and merge with a flattened oval or reniform *base* forming the footplate of the stapes and attached to the margin of the fenestra vestibuli by a ring of fibres (*the annular ligament*). The anterior limb is shorter and less curved than the posterior (8.481).

Ossification. The stapes is preformed in the perforated dorsal moiety of the hyoid arch cartilage of the fetus. Ossification starts from a single endochondral centre, appearing in the base in the fourth fetal month and then gradually spreads through the limbs of the stapes to fuse in its body.

At birth the auditory ossicles have reached an advanced state of maturity.

Articulations of the auditory ossicles

The articulations are typical synovial joints. The incudomalleolar joint is saddle-shaped, the incudostapedial is a ball and socket articulation. Their articular surfaces are covered with articular cartilage and each joint is enveloped by a capsule containing much elastic tissue and lined by synovial membrane.

Ligaments of the auditory ossicles

The ossicles are connected to the tympanic walls by ligaments: three for the malleus and one each for the incus and stapes. Some of these are mere mucosal folds carrying blood vessels and nerves to and

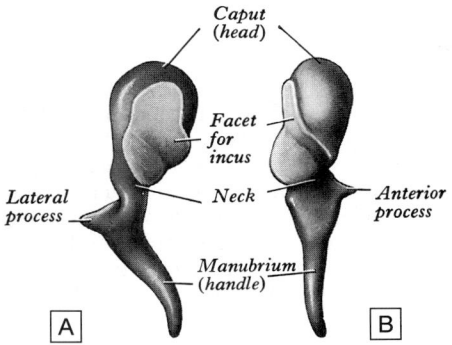

8.479   The left malleus: A. posterior aspect; B. medial aspect.

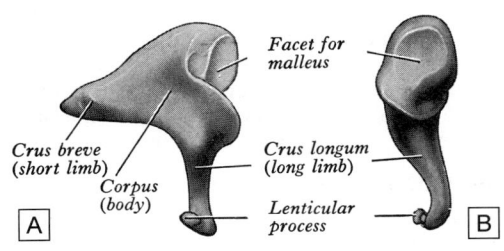

8.480   The left incus: A. medial aspect; B. anterior aspect.

1375

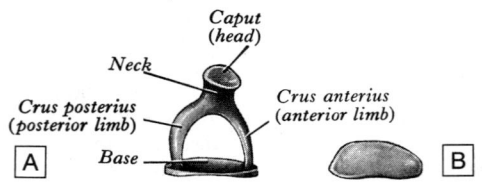

8.481 The left stapes: A. superior aspect; B. basal aspect.

from the ossicles and their articulations; others contain a central, strong band of collagen fibres.

The *anterior ligament of the malleus* stretches from the mallear neck, just above the anterior process, to the anterior wall of the tympanic cavity near the petrotympanic fissure, some of its collagen fibres traversing the fissure to reach the spine of the sphenoid; others continue into the sphenomandibular ligament which, like the anterior malleolar, is derived from the perichondrial sheath of Meckel's cartilage (p. 277). The ligament may contain muscle fibres (*laxator tympani* or *musculus externus mallei*).

The *lateral ligament of the malleus* is a triangular band stretching from the posterior part of the tympanic incisure's border to the head of the malleus. The *superior ligament of the malleus* connects the head of the malleus to the roof of the epitympanic recess. The *posterior ligament of the incus* connects the end of its short process to the fossa incudis. The *superior ligament of the incus* is little more than a mucosal fold passing from the body of the incus to the roof of the epitympanic recess.

The vestibular surface and rim of the stapedial base are covered with hyaline cartilage; the rim is attached to the margin of the fenestra vestibuli by an elastic *annular ligament of the base of the stapes*, parts of which are much narrower, acting as a kind of hinge on which the stapedial base moves when the stapedius muscle contracts and during acoustic oscillation (see below).

MUSCLES OF THE TYMPANIC CAVITY

Tensor tympani (8.471, 475). A long slender muscle, it occupies the bony canal above the osseous pharyngotympanic tube, from which it is separated by a thin bony septum. It arises from the cartilaginous part of the pharyngotympanic tube and the adjoining region of the greater wing of the sphenoid, as well as from its own canal. It passes back within its canal, ending in a slim tendon which bends laterally round the pulley-like processus trochleariformis and finally attaches to the handle of the malleus, near its root.

Nerve supply. This is a branch of the nerve to the medial pterygoid (a ramus of the mandibular nerve), traversing the otic ganglion without interruption (p. 1250). The muscle receives both motor and proprioceptive fibres (Candiollo 1965).

Stapedius extends from the wall of a conical cavity in the pyramidal eminence (and its continuation anterior to the descending part of the facial nerve canal, p. 1244), its minute tendon emerging from the orifice at the pyramid's apex to pass forwards to attach to the posterior surface of the neck of the stapes (8.477). The muscle is of an asymmetrical bipennate form, containing numerous small motor units, each of only six to nine muscle fibres. A few neuro-muscular spindles exist near the myotendinous junction.

Nerve supply. It is a branch of the facial nerve (for details see Blevins 1967).

Actions. The tensor tympani and stapedius usually contract together in reflex response to sounds of fairly high intensity, exerting a 'protective damping effect before vibrations reach the internal ear' (Hallpike 1935). The tensor pulls the tympanic membrane inwards to tense it and also pushes the stapes more tightly into the fenestra vestibuli. The strapedius muscle opposes the tensor in the latter action. Paralysis of the stapedius results in hyperacusis.

Movements of auditory ossicles

The malleolar manubrium faithfully follows all movements of the tympanic membrane, while the malleus and incus rotate together around an axis running from the short process and posterior ligament

of the incus to the anterior ligament of the malleus. When the tympanic membrane and manubrium move medially the long process of the incus moves in the same direction, pushing the stapedial base towards the labyrinth and perilymph. This causes a compensatory outward bulging of the secondary tympanic membrane of the fenestra cochleae. These events are reversed when the membrane moves outwards, but if its movement is large the incus does not follow the full outward excursion of the malleus, merely gliding on it at the incudomalleolar joint and thus preventing a dislocation of the stapedial base from the fenestra vestibuli. When the manubrium moves medially, the spur at the lower margin of the malleolar head locks the incudomalleolar joint, forcing a medial movement of the long process of the incus; the joint is unlocked again when the manubrium moves outwards. The three bones together act as a bent lever so that the stapedial base does not move in the fenestra vestibuli like a piston but rocks on a fulcrum at its antero-inferior border, where the annular ligament is thick. More complex stapedial movements have been described (Békésy 1960). The rocking movement around a vertical axis, which is like a swinging door, is said to occur only at moderate intensities of sound. With loud, low-pitched sounds, the axis becomes horizontal, the upper and lower margins of the stapedial base oscillating in opposite directions around this central axis, thus preventing excessive displacement of the perilymph.

Tympanic mucosa

The mucosa of the tympanic cavity is continuous with that of the pharynx, via the pharyngotympanic tube; it covers the ossicles, muscles and nerves in the cavity, forming the inner layer of the tympanic membrane and the outer layer of the secondary tympanic membrane; it also spreads into the mastoid antrum and air cells. It forms several vascular folds extending from the tympanic walls to the ossicles: of these, one descends from the roof of the cavity to the head of the malleus and the upper margin of the body of the incus and a second surrounds the stapedius, others investing the chorda tympani nerve and the tensor tympani muscle. These folds separate off saccular recesses and give the interior of the tympanic cavity a somewhat honeycombed appearance. One such *superior recess of the tympanic membrane* lies between the neck of the malleus and the pars flaccida. Two others, the *anterior* and *posterior recesses of the tympanic membrane*, are formed by the mucosa around the chorda tympani and lie, respectively, anterior and posterior to the manubrium of the malleus. The tympanic mucosa is pale, thin and slightly vascular. It has a ciliated columnar epithelium except over the posterior part of the medial wall, the posterior wall, often parts of the tympanic membrane and the auditory ossicles, the cells of these surfaces being flatter and non-ciliated. Near the pharyngo-tympanic tube, goblet cells are numerous; otherwise there are no mucous glands. The mastoid antrum and air cells are lined by flat, non-ciliated epithelium. Undoubtedly there are considerable mucosal variations in the middle ear, which include squamous, cuboidal, columnar and ciliated columnar epithelia. The epithelium is closely attached to periosteum (to form a mucoperiosteum) and has sur-factant on its surface.

It must be re-emphasized that the tympanic cavity and mastoid antrum, auditory ossicles and structures of the internal ear are almost fully developed at birth and subsequently alter little. In fetuses the cavity contains a gelatinous tissue which has practically disappeared by birth, when it is filled by a fluid which is absorbed when air enters via the auditory tube.

Vasculature of the tympanic cavity

Arteries. Six arteries supply the walls and contents of the tympanic cavity. Two are larger than the others: the *anterior tympanic* branch of the *maxillary*, supplying the tympanic membrane, and the *stylo-mastoid* branch of the *occipital* or *posterior auricular* arteries, supplying the posterior tympanic cavity and mastoid air cells. The smaller arteries include: the *petrosal* branch of the *middle meningeal*, entering through the hiatus for the greater petrosal nerve; the *superior tympanic* branch of the *middle meningeal*, traversing the canal for the tensor tympani; a branch from the *ascending pharyngeal* and from the *artery of the pterygoid canal*, accompanying the pharyngotympanic tube; and a *tympanic branch* or branches from the *internal carotid*, arising in the carotid canal and perforating the thin anterior wall of the tympanic cavity. In early fetal life a *stapedial artery* traverses the stapes (p. 314; a feature which persists in some other mammals).

Veins. These terminate in the pterygoid venous plexus and the superior petrosal sinus. From the mucosa of the mastoid antrum a small group of veins runs medially through the arch formed by the anterior semicircular canal, emerging on the posterior surface of the petrous temporal bone at the subarcuate fossa to drain into the superior petrosal sinus; these are the remains of the large *subarcuate veins* of childhood, a route for the spread of infection from the mastoid antrum to the meninges.

Lymph vessels. They are described on page 1613.

Nerves of the tympanic cavity

The nerves constitute the tympanic plexus, ramifying on the surface of the promontory. They arise from the tympanic branch of the glossopharyngeal nerve (**8.348**) and the caroticotympanic nerves of sympathetic origin (Arslan 1960). The former enters the cavity by the tympanic *canaliculus for the tympanic nerve*, ramifying to join the plexus; the *superior* and *inferior caroticotympanic nerves* (from the carotid sympathetic plexus) traverse the carotid canal's wall and also join the plexus. the tympanic plexus supplies:

- branches to the mucosa of the tympanic cavity, pharyngotympanic tube and mastoid air cells
- a branch traversing an opening anterior to the fenestra vestibuli and joining the greater petrosal nerve
- the *lesser petrosal nerve*, which may be regarded as the continuation of the tympanic branch of the glossopharyngeal nerve traversing the tympanic plexus.

The lesser petrosal nerve occupies a small canal below that for the tensor tympani; it runs past and receives a connecting branch from the facial nerve's genicular ganglion, emerges from the anterior surface of the temporal bone via a small opening lateral to the hiatus for the greater petrosal nerve and then traverses the foramen ovale or the small canaliculus innominatus to join the otic ganglion. Postganglionic secretomotor fibres leave this ganglion in the auriculotemporal nerve to supply the parotid gland.

The *chorda tympani* (**8.344**) leaves the facial nerve about 6 mm above the stylomastoid foramen and runs anterosuperiorly in a canal to enter the tympanic cavity via the *posterior canaliculus*. It then curves anteriorly in the substance of the tympanic membrane between its mucous and fibrous layers (p. 1373), crosses medial to the upper part of the manubrium of the malleus to the anterior wall, finally entering the *anterior canaliculus*. (For its further course see p. 1246.) The other nerves which are closely related topographically to the tympanic cavity include: the facial and its genicular ganglion and the stapedial and greater petrosal branches of this nerve; the auricular branch of the vagus; afferent and efferent terminals of the vestibulocochlear nerve; and the internal carotid sympathetic plexus (all detailed elsewhere in this section). The *meningeal branch* (p. 1237) of the mandibular nerve supplies branches to the mastoid air cells.

Clinical aspects of the middle ear. Fractures of the middle cranial fossa almost always involve the tympanic roof, accompanied by the rupture of the tympanic membrane or a fractured roof of the osseous external acoustic meatus. Such injuries usually entail prolonged bleeding from the ear, with escape of cerebrospinal fluid if the dura mater has been torn.

The tympanic cavity is a common site of infection, usually spreading to it from the nose and pharynx along the pharyngotympanic tube, which usually becomes occluded because of the inflammatory swelling of its mucosa. The products of inflammation, thus confined to the tympanic cavity, may spread into the mastoid antrum, their only escape then being by the rupture of the tympanic membrane, either spontaneous or surgically induced, followed by the free discharge of pus. If the swelling of the pharyngotympanic tube then subsides, normal drainage of the cavity returns and perforations in the tympanic membrane heal; but, if the tube is occluded by enlarged lymphatic tissue, pus may continue to gather and discharge through the perforations as a chronic otorrhoea. Intracranial complications may follow: an abscess may form between the bone and the dura mater, above the tympanic cavity, beneath the dura of the temporal lobe or between the deep aspect of the mastoid process and the sigmoid sinus, possibly extending widely and surrounding the sinus,

in which thrombosis may ensue; an infected clot may be detached into the general circulation, causing metastatic abscesses, for example in the lungs. Bone disease of the tympanic cavity or mastoid antrum may lead to severe and fatal septic meningitis or to the formation of brain abscesses, particularly in the temporal lobe of the cerebrum and the cerebellar hemisphere. In chronic bone disease in the tympanic cavity, the facial nerve may be exposed in its canal, its inflammation leading to facial paralysis of the infranuclear type (p. 1247).

INTERNAL EAR

The internal ear includes the *osseous labyrinth*, a complex series of cavities in the petrous temporal bone, and the contained *membranous labyrinth*, a corresponding complex set of interconnected membranous sacs and ducts.

OSSEOUS LABYRINTH

The osseous labyrinth (**8.474, 477, 482–484**) has three regions: the *vestibule, semicircular canals* and *cochlea*. These are all cavities within bone, lined by periosteum and containing a clear fluid, the *perilymph*, within which is the membranous labyrinth. The osseous labyrinth lies in denser, harder bone than that in other parts of the petrous bone; it is hence possible, particularly in young skulls, to dissect out the labyrinth from the petrous temporal.

Vestibule

The vestibule is the central part of the osseous labyrinth and lies medial to the tympanic cavity, posterior to the cochlea and anterior to the semicircular canals. Somewhat ovoid in shape but flattened transversely, it measures about 5 mm from front to back, the same from above to below and about 3 mm across. In its *lateral wall* is the opening of the fenestra vestibuli, closed in life by the stapedial base and its annular ligament. Anteriorly, on the *medial wall*, is a small *spherical recess* containing the *saccule* and perforated by several minute foramina, the *macula cribrosa media*; the recess adjoins the inferior vestibular area at the medial end of the internal acoustic meatus (**8.483**) and the foramina transmit twigs of the vestibular nerve to the saccule. Behind the recess is an oblique *vestibular crest*, its anterior end being the *vestibular pyramid*; this ridge divides below to enclose a small depression, the *cochlear recess*, perforated by vestibulocochlear fascicles passing to the cochlear duct's vestibular end. Posterosuperior to the vestibular crest, in the roof and medial wall of the vestibule, is the *elliptical recess* which contains the *utricle*. The pyramid and adjoining part of the elliptical recess are perforated by a number of foramina, forming the *macula cribrosa superior*; the

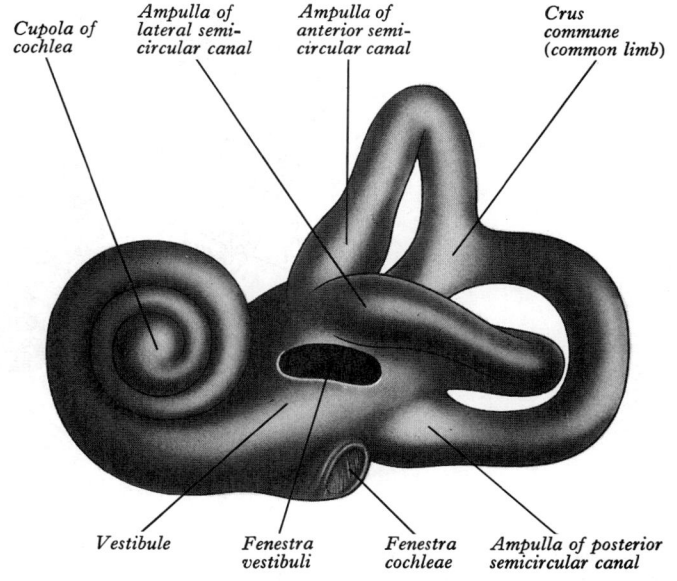

Cupola of cochlea

Ampulla of lateral semi-circular canal

Ampulla of anterior semi-circular canal

Crus commune (common limb)

Vestibule   *Fenestra vestibuli*   *Fenestra cochleae*   *Ampulla of posterior semicircular canal*

8.482   The left osseous labyrinth: lateral aspect.

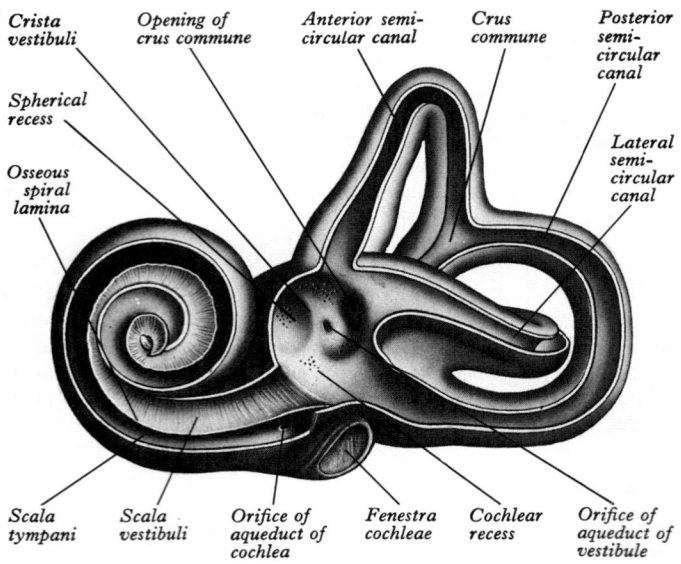

Crista vestibuli
Opening of crus commune
Anterior semi-circular canal
Crus commune
Posterior semi-circular canal

Spherical recess

Osseous spiral lamina

Lateral semi-circular canal

Scala tympani
Scala vestibuli
Orifice of aqueduct of cochlea
Fenestra cochleae
Cochlear recess
Orifice of aqueduct of vestibule

8.483   The interior of the left osseous labyrinth.

is almost twice the diameter of the canal. They open into the vestibule by five openings, one of which is shared by two of the canals.

The *anterior (superior) semicircular canal*, 15–20 mm in length, is vertical in orientation and placed transverse to the long axis of the petrous temporal bone, lying under the anterior surface of its arcuate eminence (p. 591). Some maintain, however, that the eminence does not accurately coincide with this semicircular canal, but is adapted to the occipitotemporal sulcus on the inferior surface of the temporal lobe of the brain. The canal's anterior end is ampullated, opening into the upper and lateral part of the vestibule; its other end unites with the posterior canal's upper end to form the *crus commune*, about 4 mm long, which opens into the medial part of the vestibule.

The *posterior semicircular canal*, also vertical, curves backwards almost parallel with the posterior surface of the petrous bone; it is 18–22 mm long; its ampullated end opens low in the vestibule, where the *macula cribrosa inferior* transmits nerves to the ampulla; this adjoins the *foramen singulare* in the internal acoustic meatus. The canal's upper end joins the crus commune.

The *lateral (horizontal) canal* is 12–15 mm long, its arch directed horizontally backwards and laterally. Its anterior, ampullated end opens into the upper and lateral angle of the vestibule, above the fenestra vestibuli and just below the superior canal's ampullated end; its posterior end opens below the orifice of the crus commune.

It is often said that the two lateral semicircular canals of the two ears are in the same plane and that the anterior canal of one side is almost parallel with the opposite posterior canal. Blanks et al (1975) measured the angular relations of the planes of the semicircular osseous canals in 10 human skulls. Although the planes of the three ipsilateral canals were almost perpendicular to each other, some variation was apparent, the angles being as follows: horizontal/anterior $111.76 \pm 7.55°$, anterior/posterior $86.16 \pm 4.72°$, posterior/horizontal $95.75 \pm 4.66°$. The planes of similarly orientated canals of the two sides showed marked departure from being parallel: left anterior/right posterior $24.50 \pm 7.19°$, left posterior/right anterior $23.73 \pm 6.71°$, left horizontal/right horizontal $19.82 \pm 14.93°$. The same observers (Curthoys et al 1977) have also measured the dimensions and radii of the canals; means for the radii of the osseous canals were as follows: horizontal 3.25 mm, anterior 3.74 mm, and posterior 3.79 mm. The functional implications of these data are still speculative. In diameter the osseous canals are about 1 mm (minor axis) and 1.4 mm (major axis). The membranous ducts within them are much smaller but are also elliptical in transverse section, with major and minor axes of 0.23 and 0.46 mm. Representative means for ampullary dimensions are as follows: length 1.94 mm, height

holes in the pyramid transmit the nerves to the utricle and those in the recess the nerves to the ampullae of the superior and lateral semicircular ducts. The region of the pyramid and elliptical recess corresponds to the superior vestibular area in the internal acoustic meatus (**8**.483). The opening of the vestibular *aqueduct* is below the elliptical recess; the aqueduct reaches the posterior surface of the petrous bone, containing one or more small veins and part of the membranous labyrinth, the *endolymphatic duct*. In the posterior part of the vestibule are the five *orifices of the semicircular canals*; in its anterior wall is an elliptical opening leading into the *scala vestibuli* of the cochlea.

Semicircular canals (8.474, 477, 482–484)

There are three semicircular canals: anterior (superior), posterior and lateral (horizontal); they lie posterosuperior to the vestibule. They are compressed from side to side and each describes about two-thirds of a circle; they are unequal in length but all are about 0.8 mm in diameter; each has a terminal swelling, an *ampulla*, which

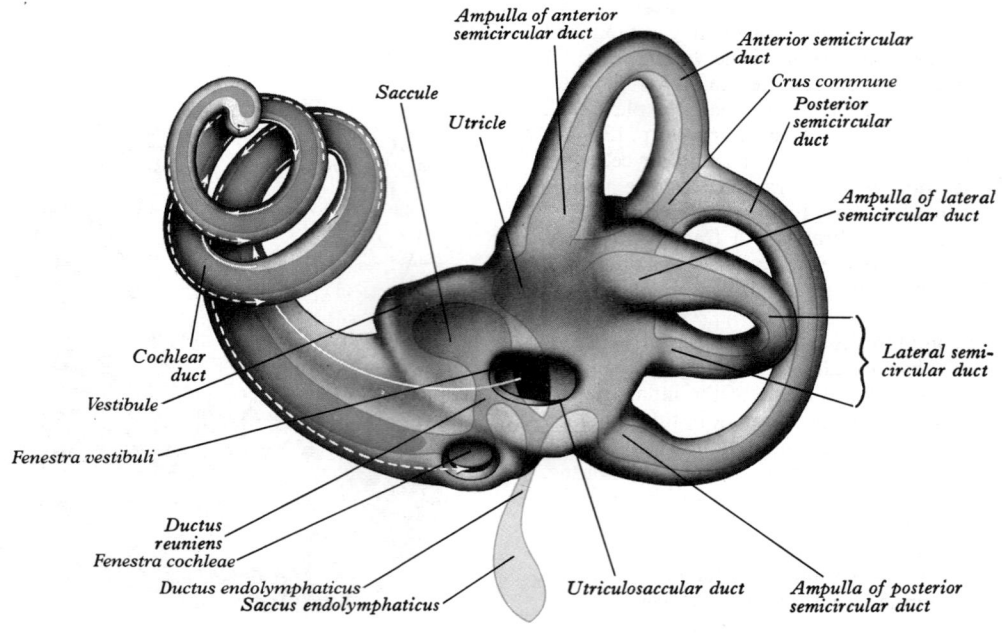

Ampulla of anterior semicircular duct
Anterior semicircular duct
Saccule
Crus commune
Posterior semicircular duct
Utricle
Ampulla of lateral semicircular duct
Cochlear duct
Lateral semi-circular duct
Vestibule
Fenestra vestibuli
Ductus reuniens
Fenestra cochleae
Ductus endolymphaticus
Saccus endolymphaticus
Utriculosaccular duct
Ampulla of posterior semicircular duct

8.484   Scheme of the membranous labyrinth (blue) projected on to the osseous labyrinth. The arrows indicate the direction of sound waves in the cochlea.

1.55 mm. Curthoys and collaborators have recorded many other labyrinthine dimensions. They attempt to equate the metrical data with theories of labyrinthine mechanics.

Cochlea

The cochlea (**8.474, 477, 482–484, 492**), shaped like a conical snail-shell, is the most anterior part of the labyrinth, lying anterior to the vestibule. It is about 5 mm from base to apex and 9 mm across its base. Its apex, or *cupula*, points towards the anterosuperior area of the medial wall of the tympanic cavity (**8.474, 492**). Its base faces the bottom of the internal acoustic meatus and is perforated by numerous apertures for the cochlear nerve. The cochlea has a central conical axis, the *modiolus*, with a spiral canal of about two and three-quarter turns around it; a delicate *osseous spiral lamina* projects from the modiolus, partially dividing the canal. Within this bony spiral lies the membranous cochlear duct, attached to the modiolus and to the outer cochlear wall by its other edge. There are thus formed three longitudinal channels within the cochlea, the middle one (the cochlear duct) being blind, ending at the apex of the cochlea and its flanking channels communicating with each other at the modiolar apex at a narrow slit, the *helicotrema*. The cochlear duct bears on one of its walls the sensory receptors responsible for audition (p. 1387). The perilymphatic channels on either side of it are the *scala vestibuli* and *scala tympani*. The former is in continuity with the vestibule and the latter is separated from the tympanic cavity by the secondary tympanic membrane at the fenestra cochleae.

Modiolus. The central cochlear pillar, this structure has a broad base near the lateral end of the internal acoustic meatus, where it corresponds to the *tractus spiralis foraminosus*, the multiple foramina of which transmit the fascicles of the cochlear nerve; those for the first $1\frac{1}{2}$ turns traverse the small foramina of the tractus spiralis, those for the apical turn traverse the *foramen centrale* in the tract's centre. Canals from the tractus traverse the modiolus and issue centrifugally in sequence into the base of the osseous spiral lamina. Here the small canals enlarge and fuse together to form the *spiral canal of the modiolus* (Rosenthal's canal) which follows the course of the osseous spiral lamina and contains the *spiral ganglion*. The foramen centrale continues as a canal through the modiolar centre to its apex.

Osseous cochlear canal. It spirals for about $2\frac{3}{4}$ turns around the modiolus; at its first turn, it bulges towards the tympanic cavity where it underlies the promontory (p. 1373). It is about 35 mm long, diminishing in diameter from the base to the summit and ending at the *cupula*, which forms the cochlea's apex; at its start the canal is about 3 mm in diameter. It has three openings at its base: the *fenestra cochleae* (round window) facing the tympanic cavity and closed by the *secondary tympanic membrane*; the *fenestra vestibuli* (oval window) occupied by the base of the stapes (p. 1373); and the *cochlear canaliculus*, a minute funnel-shaped canal opening on the inferior surface of the petrous temporal bone (p. 591), transmitting a small vein to the inferior petrosal sinus and connecting the subarachnoid space to the scala tympani (see above).

Osseous spiral lamina. This is a ledge projecting from the modiolus into the osseous canal like the thread of a screw (**8.494**). It reaches about halfway across the cochlear canal, in life forming an attachment to the cochlear duct. Its width decreases progressively towards its apex, ending in a hook-shaped *hamulus* partly bounding the *helicotrema*, through which the scalae are continuous. From the spiral modiolar canal many canaliculi radiate through the osseous lamina to its rim, carrying fasciculi of the cochlear nerve. In the lower part of the first turn a *secondary spiral lamina* projects **inwards** from the **outer** cochlear wall but does not reach the osseous spiral lamina, leaving a narrow *vestibular fissure* between them.

Microstructure of the osseous labyrinth

The space between the osseous and membranous labyrinths is filled with perilymph (see below; also **8.485**); lining the wall of the osseous labyrinth are fibroblast-like *perilymphatic* cells, with strands of extracellular fibres, the detailed form of the cells varying in different parts of the labyrinth. Where the perilymphatic space is narrow, the cells are essentially *reticular* or *stellate* in form, their sheet-like cytoplasmic extensions crossing and dividing this space into connected intercellular clefts of variable shape and size. This tissue and its spaces occupies the cochlear canaliculus; but where the space is wider, as in the scalae vestibuli and tympani of the cochlea and much of the

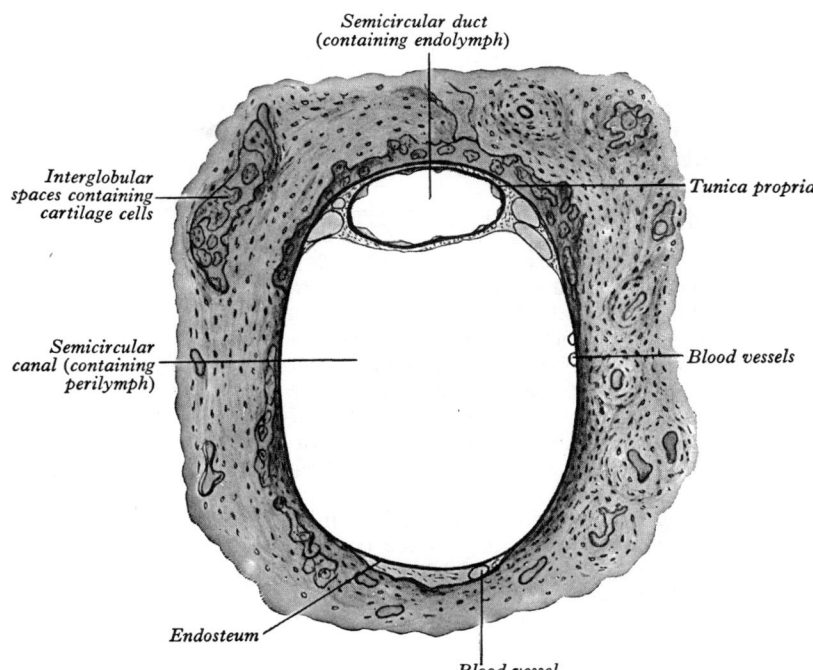

Semicircular duct (containing endolymph)

Interglobular spaces containing cartilage cells

Tunica propria

Semicircular canal (containing perilymph)

Blood vessels

Endosteum

Blood vessel

8.485 Transverse section through the left posterior semicircular canal and duct of an adult man. Magnification × 50. (After J K Milne Dickie.)

vestibule, the perilymphatic cells on the periosteum and the external surface of the membranous labyrinth are extremely flat, with a rather featureless cytoplasm. Apart from a few projections into the perilymph the arrangement approaches that of a true squamous epithelium. Elsewhere, on parts of the perilymphatic surface of the basilar membrane (p. 1386), the cells are cuboidal. Closely related to the periosteal and labyrinthine aspects of these cells are bundles of collagen fibres, which the cells may form. In some species fibres with a helical substructure, differing from collagen, have been described but their status in mankind is uncertain.

Perilymph. It resembles the cerebrospinal fluid in its composition but minor differences have been described (Ormerod 1960). Many regard it as an ultrafiltrate of plasma, with perhaps some addition from the cerebrospinal fluid. Its source, rate of production, circulation and absorption are as yet not fully known. The supposed connection between the perilymphatic and subarachnoid spaces via the *cochlear canaliculus* is controversial. The canaliculus was often described as containing a simple, epithelial duct connecting the two spaces, a view rejected by some (Waltner 1948; Mygind 1948; Young 1952, 1953), who surmised that the connective tissue blocked the canaliculus, thus separating the two fluid compartments. However, it seems likely that intercellular crevices persist in the canal; electron-dense tracers such as thorotrast, introduced into the subarachnoid space, readily appear in the perilymphatic spaces (Duvall & Quick 1969). Others (Silverstein et al 1969) point out that, in cats, even india ink or avian erythrocytes pass into the perilymphatic spaces via the cochlear canaliculus within 24 hours of their introduction into the subarachnoid space of the posterior cranial fossa. The latter authors regard perilymph as probably derived from:

- blood vessels surrounding the spaces
- fluid spaces surrounding the sheaths of the vestibulocochlear nerve fibres
- cerebrospinal fluid arriving along the cochlear canaliculus.

The mechanism of removal of perilymph is uncertain.

In summary, the organization of the perilymphatic spaces is as follows: the vestibular perilymphatic space connects posteriorly with that around the semicircular canals and opens anteriorly into the cochlear scala vestibuli, which in turn opens into the scala tympani via the helicotrema; the latter scala is separated from the tympanic cavity by the secondary tympanic membrane but is continuous with the subarachnoid space through the cochlear canaliculus (see above).

During development, the petrous bone adjoining the labyrinth is formed from the cartilaginous otic capsule by endochondral ossification; it is denser than the petrous bone elsewhere, with interglobular spaces containing cartilage cells (**8.**485). The cochlear modiolus, however, is formed from trabecular dermal bone (Fraser & Dickie 1914).

MEMBRANOUS LABYRINTH

The membranous labyrinth (**8.**483, 484) is a continuous system of ducts contained within the osseous labyrinth of the petrous temporal bone. It is filled with endolymph and separated from the periosteum by a space which contains perilymph and a web-like network of fine blood vessels; it can be divided into two major regions, the *vestibular apparatus* and the *cochlear duct*. The vestibular apparatus consists of three membranous *semicircular canals* communicating with the *utricle*, a membranous sac which in turn leads into another, smaller chamber, the *saccule* by *ductus utriculosaccularis*; this Y-shaped duct has a side branch to the *ductus endolymphaticus* which passes to the *saccus endolymphaticus*, a small but functionally important expansion situated under the dura of the petrous temporal bone. From the saccule, a narrow canal, the *ductus reuniens*, leads to the base of the *cochlear duct*. These various parts form a closed system of channels which communicate freely with one another.

VESTIBULAR APPARATUS

In the walls of the membranous labyrinth within the vestibular apparatus are five distinct areas of specialized sensory epithelium to which the terminal fibres of the vestibular nerve are distributed. These areas are the two *maculae* situated one each in the utricle and saccule, and the three *cristae* which are situated in the wall of expansions (*ampullae*) near the utricular openings of the three semicircular canals, one for each canal.

Utricle (8.484)

The utricle, the larger of the two major vestibular sacs, is an irregular, oblong, dilated sac which occupies the posterosuperior region of the osseous vestibule, in contact with the elliptical recess and the area inferior to it, the part of the utricle in the recess being a blind-ending pouch. A number of the labyrinthine ducts open into it, including, laterally, the ampullae of the lateral and anterior semicircular canals, and medially, the ampulla of the posterior canal, the crus communale (the conjoined medial ends of the anterior and posterior semicircular canals), and the posterior end of the lateral semicircular canal. The utriculosaccular duct originates from the utricle's anteromedial surface and follows a V-shaped course, from the middle of which arises the endolymphatic duct as a side branch.

Macula of the utricle. This is a specialized area of neurosensory epithelium lining the membranous wall; it is the largest of the vestibular sensory areas. It is triangular or shield-shaped in surface view (**8.**486, 488), lying horizontally with its long axis anteroposteriorly oriented and its sharp angle pointing posteriorly; it is flat except at the anterior edge which is gently folded on itself. It measures about 2.8 mm long by 2.2 mm wide. The mature form of the macula is attained early in development, but in the adult a bulge

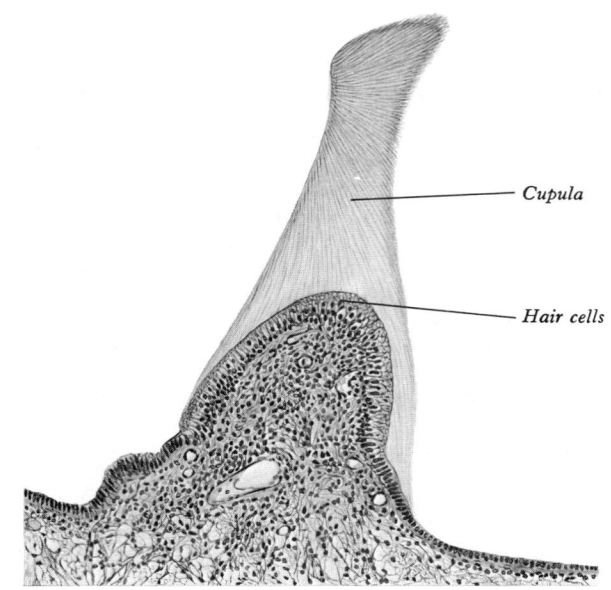

Cupula

Hair cells

8.487 Section of an ampullary crest of a six-month-old human fetus. Stained with haematoxylin and eosin. Magnification × 75. (From a section lent by E W Walls, Professor Emeritus, Middlesex Hospital Medical School, University of London.)

is often present on the anterolateral border and there is sometimes an incisure at the anteromedial border (Rosenhall 1972). Covering the epithelial surface is the *statoconial membrane* (or otolithic membrane), a gelatinous layer in which a multitude of crystals, the *otoconia* (otoliths, statoliths), are embedded. A curved median ridge runs along the lengths of the statoconial membrane, the 'snowdrift line', corresponding to a narrow crescentic area of underlying sensory epithelium termed the *striola*, approximately 0.13 μm wide. The density of sensory cells in this strip of epithelium is about 20% less than in the rest of the macula. The striola is convex laterally and runs from the medial aspect of the anterior margin in a posterior direction towards, but never reaching, the posterior pole. The part of the macula medial to the striola is designated the *pars interna* and is slightly larger than the *pars externa*, lateral to it. The structural and functional significance of this area is that the sensory cells are functionally and anatomically polarized towards it (Flock 1964; Lindeman 1969; see also below).

Saccule (8.484)

The saccule is a slightly elongated, globular sac lying in the spherical recess near the opening of the cochlea's scala vestibuli. As already noted, it is connected to the utricle and endolymphatic duct by the utriculosaccular duct, and to the cochlea by the ductus reuniens which leaves inferiorly to open into the base of the cochlear duct.

On the wall of the saccule is the *saccular macula*, an almost elliptical structure, 2.6 mm long and 1.2 mm at its widest point. Its long axis is orientated anteroposteriorly but, in contrast with that of the utricle, the saccular macula lies in a vertical plane on the saccule's side wall. Its elliptical shape is very slightly distorted by a small anterosuperior bulge. Like the utricular macula it is covered by statoconial membrane and possesses a striola, approximately 0.13 mm wide, which extends along its long axis as an S-shaped strip about which the sensory cells are also functionally orientated, though oppositely to those of the utricle (see below). The part of the macula superior to the striola is termed the *pars interna*, that inferior to it, the *pars externa*.

Semicircular ducts (8.483–48,5, 487)

The lateral, anterior and posterior semicircular ducts follow the course of their osseous canals (p. 1379). The ducts are about one-quarter of the diameter of their osseous canals but are similar in general shape; through most of their course, each membranous duct is securely attached by much of its circumference to the osseous wall (**8.**485).

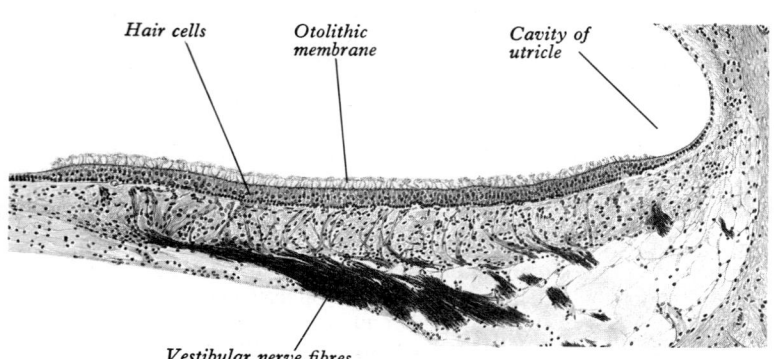

Hair cells   Otolithic membrane   Cavity of utricle

Vestibular nerve fibres

8.486 Section of the macula of the utricle of the cat. Weigert–Pal and iron haematoxylin stain. Magnification × 112. (For source see **8.**487.)

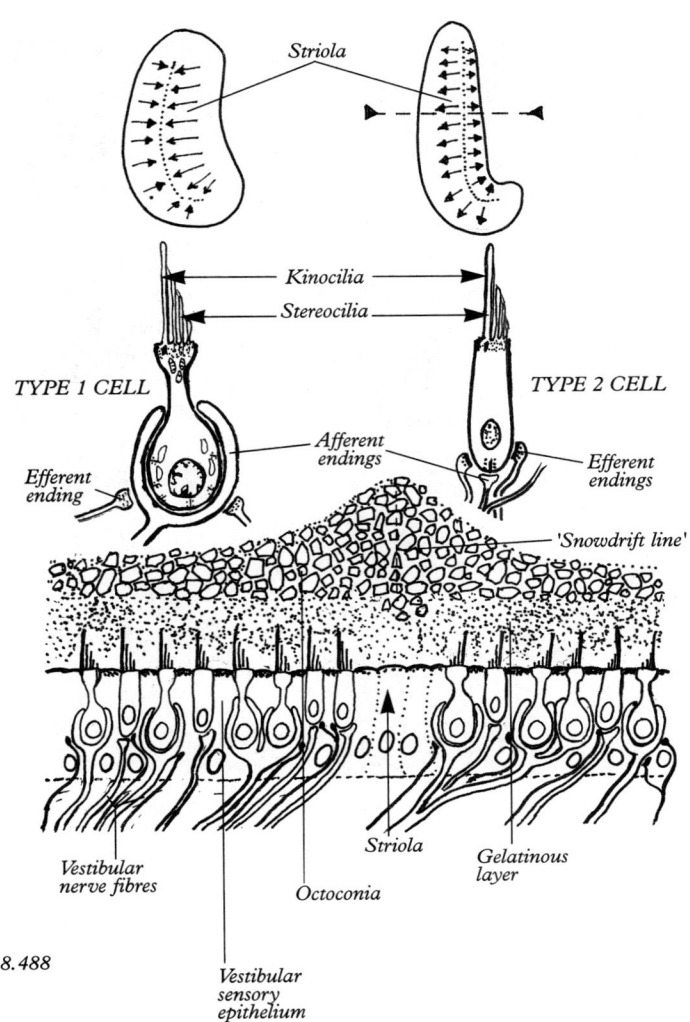

Striola

Kinocilia
Stereocilia

TYPE 1 CELL   TYPE 2 CELL

Afferent
endings

Efferent
ending

Efferent
endings

'Snowdrift line'

Vestibular
nerve fibres

Octoconia

Striola

Gelatinous
layer

Vestibular
sensory
epithelium

8.488

8.488 Diagrams of the morphological organization of the maculae of (A) the utricle, and (B) the saccule. Note the different shapes of the two maculae, and the different orientations of their stereocilia-kilocilium bundles; those of the utricle are orientated towards the striola, and those of the saccule, away from it. (After Lindeman 1969.)

The medial ends of the anterior and posterior canals fuse to form a single common duct, the *crus communale* before entering the utricle, while the lateral end of each canal is dilated to form an *ampulla* (lying within the ampulla of the osseous canal). The short segment of duct between the ampullae and utricle is the *crus ampullaris*. The membranous wall of each ampulla contains a transverse elevation (*septum transversum*) on the central region of which is a sensory area, the *crista* (*crista ampullaris*); this is a saddle-shaped ridge, also lying transversely across the duct, broadly concave on its free edge along most of its length and with a concave gutter (*planum semilunatum*) at either end between the ridge and the duct wall. Sectioned across the ridge, the cristae of the lateral and anterior semicircular canals have smoothly rounded corners, while the posterior crista is more angular. Attached along the free edge of the crista is a vertical plate of gelatinous extracellular material, the cupula (**8.487**). This projects far into the lumen of the ampulla, so that movements of endolymph within the duct readily deflect the cupula and therefore also the stereocilia of the sensory cells inserted into its base.

Microstructure of maculae and cristae

The maculae and cristae are specialized thickened regions of the

epithelial lining to the membranous labyrinth wall which detect the orientation of the head with respect to gravity and changes in head movement (p. 1384). The sensory epithelia consist of mechanoreceptive cells interspersed among non-sensory supporting cells, and in contact with afferent and efferent endings of vestibular nerve fibres by synapses at their bases.

Sensory cells. The sensory epithelia of the maculae and cristae are composed of neurosensory cells which form synapses at their bases with the terminals of the vestibular nerve. The sensory cells are of two categories, designated Types 1 and 2; interspersed with, and separating the sensory cells are *supporting cells* (see Gleeson et al 1990 for a description of the human macula). The whole epithelium lies on a bed of thick, fibrous connective tissue containing myelinated vestibular nerve fibres and blood vessels. The nerve fibres lose their myelin sheaths as they perforate the basal lamina of the sensory epithelium (Wersäll 1956; Ross 1986).

Type 1 vestibular sensory cells. In humans, these measure about 25 μm in length and present a surface of 6–7 μm in diameter (**8.489**A, **490**). The basal part of the cell does not reach the basal lamina of the epithelium. Each cell is typically bottle-shaped, with a narrow neck and a rather broad, rounded basal portion in which the nucleus is situated. Under the apical surface is a region of dense filamentous material, the cuticular plate, rich in actin filaments. From the apical surface project 30–50 *stereocilia* (large, regular microvilli about 0.25 μm across) and a single *kinocilium* with the typical '9 plus 2' arrangement of microtubules characteristic of true cilia. The kinocilium is considerably longer than the stereocilia, and may attain 40 μm, while the stereocilia are of graded lengths. They are characteristically arranged in regular rows behind the kinocilium in descending order of height, the longest being next to the kinocilium. Each stereocilium is narrow just above the cell apex and in this region contains a central dense rod or rootlet which is inserted into the dense material of the cuticular plate. For most of their length stereocilia are filled with regularly spaced parallel actin filaments. Each stereocilium is joined to adjacent stereocilia by filamentous material, and at its apex a proteinaceous thread ('tip link') joins it diagonally to the side of its taller neighbour.

The kinocilium emerges basally from a typical basal body situated in a gap in the apical cuticle, with a centriole immediately beneath it. The kinocilium is orientated with its central pair of microtubules positioned so that its plane of bending would be directly towards or away from the stereocilial rows (see p. 1391) along the axis of symmetry of the cuticular plate, a feature of much functional significance in vestibular sensory transduction (p. 1382).

The cytoplasm of the neck and supranuclear region of the cell contains many mitochondria, granular and agranular endoplasmic reticula, Golgi complexes, lysosomes and other inclusions distributed within a complicated structure of microtubules. The nucleus, 6–7 μm across, is rounded and contains both condensed and extended chromatin. The relatively small volume of infranuclear cytoplasm also contains mitochondria, membranous cisternae and microtubules.

Close to the inner surface of their basal two-thirds every cell contains numerous synaptic ribbons with associated synaptic vesicles (**8.36**). Opposite these is the postsynaptic surface of an afferent nerve ending, which takes the form of a cup (*chalice* or *calyx*) into which the cell is deeply inserted. This encloses the greater part of the sensory cell body. In some species of mammals a single nerve fibre may branch immediately before it terminates in calycial endings around more than one hair cell, or even enclose two adjacent cells in a single calyx.

Efferent nerve fibres make synapses with the external surface of the calyx rather than directly with the sensory cell.

Type 2 vestibular sensory cells. There is much greater variation in the sizes of Type 2 sensory cells (**8.489**B, **490**): some, up to 45 μm long, almost span the entire thickness of the sensory epithelium, while others are shorter than Type 1 cells. They are mostly cylindrical, but otherwise resemble Type 1 cells in their contents and the presence of a kinocilium and stereocilia apically. However, their kinocilia and stereocilia tend to be shorter and less variable in length. The most striking difference between these and the Type 1 cells is their efferent nerve terminals, Type 2 cells receiving multiple efferent nerve boutons around their bases as well as afferent endings, which are small expansions rather than chalices. The efferent endings contain a mixture of small clear and dense-core vesicles.

1381

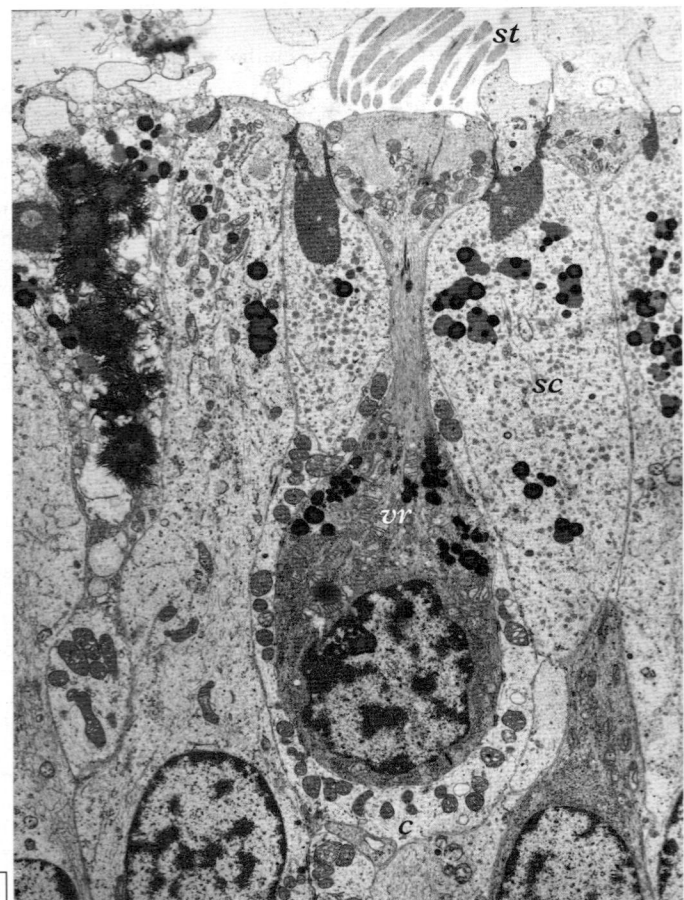

8.489A Transmission electron micrograph of human Type 1 vestibular sensory cell (vr) bearing apically a group of stereocilia (st) seen in vertical section through the macula. Note that the sensory cell is bottle-shaped, and that its greater part is enclosed in the calyceal ending (c) of an afferent nerve axon. Also visible are surrounded supporting cells (sc). Magnification × 6000. (Supplied by H Felix, M Gleeson and L-G Johnsson, ENT Department, University of Zurich and Guy's Hospital, London.)

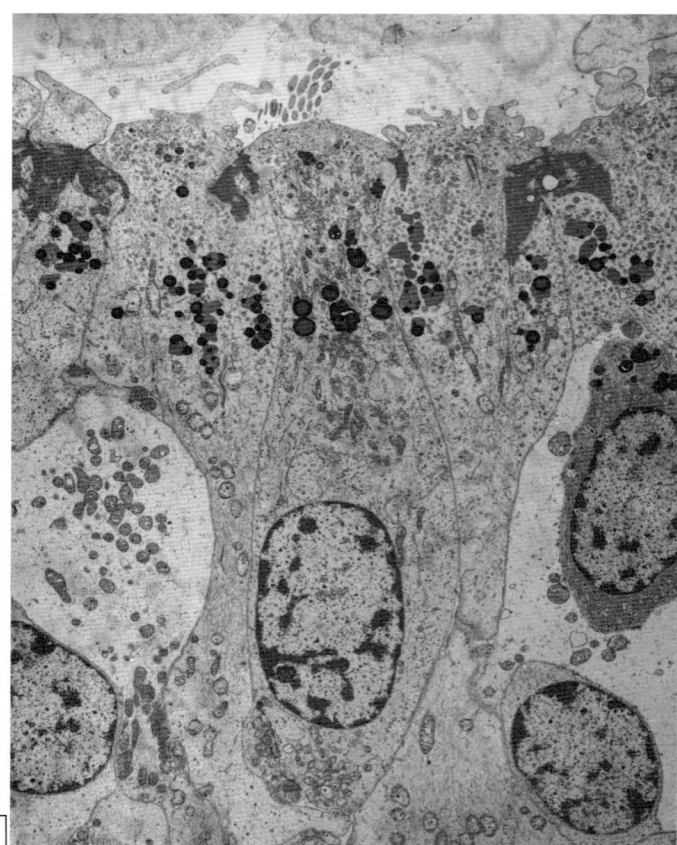

8.489B Transmission electron micrograph of human Type 2 vestibular sensory cell. The sensory cell is cylindrical, and a bouton-type afferent nerve terminal is in contact with the basal part. Magnification × 6000. (Supplied by H Felix, M Gleeson and L-G Johnsson, ENT Department, University of Zurich and Guy's Hospital, London.)

A glycocalyx about 40 nm thick invests the whole surface of the epithelium (Takumida et al 1989a,b,c). This carbohydrate-rich coat appears to be largely synthesized in the apical portion of the supporting cells, where it is visible within coated vesicles associated with the Golgi complex and within exocytic vesicles at the apical membrane. It probably plays an important part in transduction, regulating the kinetics of ionic movements, and helping to couple the stereocilia to each other mechanically to maintain their regular configuration (Ernstrom 1985).

Orientation of sensory cells. Because of the arrangement of the rows of stereocilia and the single kinocilium, each sensory cell is structurally polarized (Lowenstein & Wersäll 1959; Flock 1964; Spoendlin 1964; Lindeman 1969), and it has been shown by scanning electron microscopy that the hair cells also have specific orientations within each sensory organ. In the maculae, they are arranged symmetrically on either side of the striola, in the utricle the kinocilia being positioned on the side of the sensory cell nearest to the striola (**8.490**), and in the saccule, furthest from it. In the cristae the cells are orientated with their rows of stereocilia at right angles to the long axis of the semicircular duct: in the lateral crista the kinocilia are on the side towards the utricle whereas in the anterior and posterior cristae they are away from it (Lim 1969, 1971).

These different arrangements are important functionally, as the orientation of each cell determines its responses to directed mechanical stimuli (see p. 961).

Function of vestibular sensory cells. The mechanoreceptive functions of the receptor cells depend upon bending of the stereocilia/kinocilial bundle caused by movements either of the endolymph (cristae) or otoconial crystals (maculae). When the group is bent towards the kinocilium the cell becomes hyperpolarized, and depolarized when they are bent in the opposite direction. The core of each stereocilium contains numerous actin filaments (as many as 3000 in transverse sections), linked to each other and to the plasma membrane in a regular paracrystalline array. This arrangement imparts rigidity to the stereocilium allowing its main body to function like a stiff lever, its narrow basal neck being flexible (Tilney et al 1980; Hirokawa & Tilney 1982). This movement is thought to deform mechanically sensitive channels in the stereocilial membrane which, if the direction is appropriate, open to the diffusion of calcium ions, depolarizing the cell and causing the release of neurotransmitter at the afferent synapses with the vestibular nerve. If the bundle is bent in the opposite direction, the channels close and the cell becomes hyperpolarized. In the erect, resting position, a few channels remain open to give a moderate level of afferent synaptic activity, thus allowing the cell to detect movements in one direction or the other away from this baseline. The reason for this directionality appears to be the organization of the tip-link connections between stereocilia; these are obliquely placed so that if the stereocilia are bent in the direction of the shortest to the longest, the stereocilia pull on each other, thus stressing their membranes, whereas bending in the opposite direction will compress rather than stretch the links, releasing the tension on the membranes. This device is also found in the cochlear hair cells (see p. 1389).

Supporting cells. The Type 1 and 2 sensory cells are set within a matrix of supporting cells which reach from the base of the epithelium to its surface, and form rosettes around the sensory cells, as seen in surface view. Although their form is irregular they can easily be recognized by the position of their nuclei which tend to lie

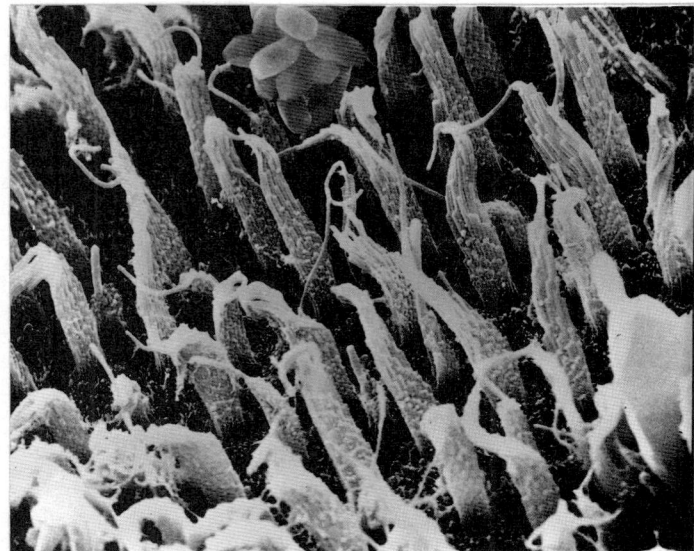

8.490 Scanning electron micrograph of the stereocilia-kinocilium bundles at the surface of a macula (guinea pig saccule). The sterocilia are grouped in tight conical bundles, from the apex of which the longer kinocilium emerges. Magnification × 2000. (Supplied by H Felix, M Gleeson and L-G Johnsson, ENT Department, University of Zurich and Guy's Hospital, London.)

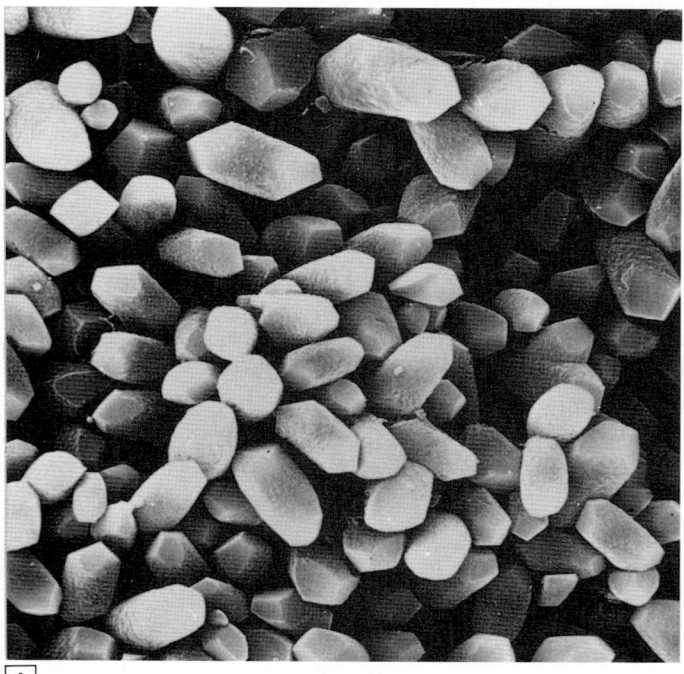

A

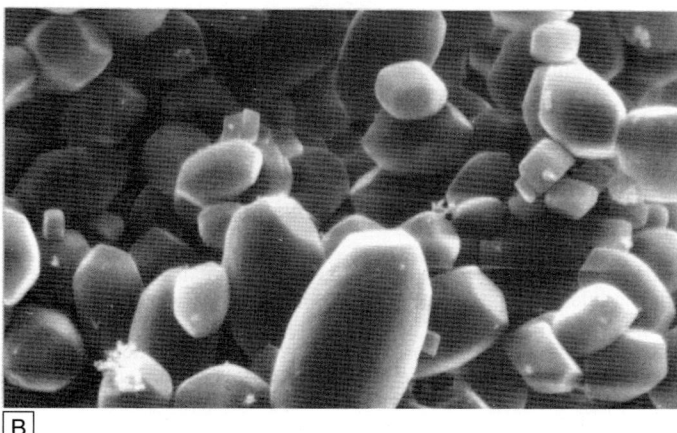

B

8.491 Scanning electron micrograph of otoconia overlying the saccular macula.
A.   This shows the arrangement in a guinea pig where the otoconia are all of similar sizes.
B.   Depicts human otoconia; note the great range of sizes of the otoconia. Magnification × 2500. (Supplied by H Felix, M Gleeson and L-G Johnsson, ENT Department, University of Zurich and Guy's Hospital, London.)

below the level of sensory cell nuclei and just above the basal lamina. Their cytoplasm contains many mitochondria, well-developed Golgi complexes and scattered lipofuscin granules. These cells lack stereocilia and a typical cuticular plate, although short microvilli are present, and the apex of the cell contains dense material around its margins, attached to the tight junctions with neighbouring cells. These dense areas contribute to the *reticular lamina*, a composite stratum formed by the apices of the sensory and supporting cells which constitutes a single mechanically stable plate necessary for accurate sensory transduction.

Statoconial (otolithic) membrane. This layer of extracellular material has a somewhat complex structure; it can be divided into two strata, an external one composed of a layer of *otoliths*—rounded crystals of calcium carbonate up to 30 μm long attached to a more basal *gelatinous layer*; the latter is subdivided into a superficial stratum and a deeper honeycomb layer which has vertical tubular areas of less dense material into which the stereocilia and kinocilia of the sensory cells are inserted. The gelatinous material consists largely of glycosaminoglycans associated with fibrous proteins. The otoconia are shaped like barrels with angular ends; in humans they are heterogeneous in size and distribution although much more regular in some mammals such as the guinea pig (see **8.491**A,B) (Lim 1973).

Microstructure of utricle, saccule and semicircular ducts

Throughout most of their extent these have a common organization, being composed of three major layers. The external layer is largely fibrous and vascular; its superficial fibres are often covered by flat perilymphatic cells and this outer surface sometimes blends with the labyrinthine periosteum. The middle layer, composed of more delicate vascular connective tissue, has on its internal surface a number of papilliform projections, especially in the semicircular ducts. The internal layer is usually a simple flat epithelium, its cells varying from squamous to cuboidal or polygonal; it is separated from the middle layer by a basal lamina.

The epithelial cells of such areas appear to be mainly non-specialized and only moderately active; they have elliptical or crenated heterochromatic nuclei, few mitochondria, occasional ribosomes and micropinocytotic vesicles and show a few microvilli on their luminal aspect. Junctional complexes occur near their luminal borders, with some interdigitation of the cell surfaces; the bases of these cells are flat. They appear to serve primarily as barriers preventing the intermixture of endolymph and perilymph. Among these cells are scattered another cell type, the dark cell, which is much more numerous around the edges of sensory areas (see below).

Transitional epithelium and dark cells. Where they border areas of sensory epithelium, the epithelial cells show a marked contrast with the unspecialized ductal cells, and here the underlying connective tissue layer is also thicker. In the maculae, the perimeter of the sensory epithelium is surrounded by a zone loosely termed 'transitional epithelium' (quite unrelated to urinary epithelium which is sometimes given this name); around the periphery of the transitional epithelium and to some extent also interspersed with its cells is a zone of 'dark' cells. In the cristae this arrangement is similar but differs slightly at each end of the ridge where the concavity (*planum semilunatum*) between the crest and the ampullary wall is covered by a layer of tall epithelium: the cells of this region are complexly interdigitated with each other and merge with the transitional epithelium.

The *transitional epithelium* lacks specialization, its cells being relatively small and with central nuclei. The *dark cells* abutting it vary much in size and shape, but can be recognized by their densely staining cytoplasm which contains numerous vacuoles, vesicles, free ribosomes and short elements of granular endoplasmic reticulum set in a densely staining cytosol. Apically they bear short microvilli and are joined to each other by junctional complexes. Their basal membranes are deeply pleated and have numerous mitochondria, an arrangement suggesting a role in ion transport, as also seen in the convoluted tubules of the kidney. In the maculae there is evidence that dark cells play a part in the turnover of otoconia too, as degenerate otoconia have been observed on the surface of these cells and their remnants appear to be internalized in vacuoles, indicating that dark cells play a part in otoconial metabolism (Nakai & Hilding 1968; Kimura 1969; LaFerriere et al 1974, Wright & Lee 1986, Kawamata et al 1986, Igarishi 1989). Melanocytes are present in the connective tissue beneath the dark cells and their elongated processes are closely associated with the basal infoldings.

Functions of the vestibular apparatus

The vestibular sensory pathways are concerned primarily with reflex movements governing the equilibrium of the body and the fixity of gaze. Functionally, the vestibular apparatus is customarily divided into two components, the *kinetic labyrinth* providing information about accelerations and decelerations of the head, and the *static labyrinth* which detects the orientation of the head in relation to the pull of gravity. In terms of structure, the kinetic labyrinth consists of the semicircular canals with their ampullary cristae, while the static labyrinth is comprised of the maculae of the utricle and saccule. However, the saccular macula also responds to head movements, and both maculae can be stimulated by low frequency sound, and may therefore have minor auditory functions.

Kinetic labyrinth. As already noted, angular accelerations and decelerations of the head cause a counterflow of endolymph in the semicircular canals, deflecting the cupola of each crista and bending the stereocilial/kinocilial bundles. This causes a change in the membrane potential of the receptor cell which is signalled to the brain as a change in the firing frequency of the vestibular nerve afferents, either an increase or a decrease of the basal resting discharge, depending on the direction of stimulation. When a steady velocity of head movement is reached, the endolymph rapidly adopts the same velocity as the surrounding structures because of friction with the canal walls, so that the cupula and receptor cells return to their resting state. Since the three semicircular canals are orientated at right angles to each other, all possible directions of acceleration can be detected. In addition, the labyrinths on both sides of the head provide complementary information which is integrated centrally.

Static labyrinth. In the maculae, the weight of the otoconial crystals creates a gravitational pull on the otoconial membrane and thus on the stereocilial bundles of the sensory cells inserted into its base. Because of this, they are able to detect the static orientation of the head with respect to gravity and also shifts in position according to how much the stereocilia are deflected from the perpendicular. As the two maculae are set at right angles to each other, and the cells of both maculae are orientated functionally in opposite directions across their striolar boundaries, this system is very sensitive to orientation. Moreover, because the otoconia have a collective inertia/momentum, linear accelerations and decelerations along the anteroposterior axis can be detected by the lag or overshoot of the otoconial membrane with respect to the epithelial surface, and so the saccular macula is able to signal such changes of velocity. Likewise, the macular receptors can be stimulated by low frequency sound which sets up vibratory movements in the otoconial membrane, although this appears to require relatively high sound levels. Efferent synapses on the afferent endings of the Type I sensory cells and the bases of Type II cells themselves receive inputs from the brainstem which appear to be inhibitory, serving to reduce the activity of the afferent fibres either indirectly, in the case of the Type I cells or directly, for the Type II.

The information gathered by these various detectors is signalled back to the CNS through the vestibular nerve via the afferent synapses to the vestibular nuclear complex for further processing, and thence to the motor nuclei of the brainstem and upper cord, the cerebellum and thalamus where it is relayed to the sensory cortex (for details of these pathways see pp. 1055, 1097). These pathways help to ensure that the motor activity of postural and locomotory muscles are adjusted to ensure either static equilibrium or effective

locomotion (see p. 1167). Another major function is the control of visual reflexes to allow the fixation of gaze on an object in spite of movements of the head, the visual axis being adjusted constantly through the movements of the eye, neck and upper trunk, chiefly through the medial longitudinal fasciculus (connecting the vestibular nuclear complex with the IIIrd, IVth and VIth cranial nerve nuclei, and upper spinal motor neurons) and the vestibulospinal tracts. Abnormal activity of the vestibular input or central connections have various effects on these reflexes, for example nystagmus, which can be elicited as a clinical test of vestibular function by syringing the external auditory meatus with water above or below body temperature, a procedure which appears to stimulate the crista of the lateral semi-circular canal directly.

Spontaneous high activity in the afferent fibres of the vestibular nerve are seen in Menière's disease in which those affected experience a range of disturbances including the sensation of dizziness and nausea, the latter reflecting the vestibular input to the vagal reflex pathway.

Endolymphatic duct and sac

Endolymphatic duct (8.484). This runs in the bony tunnel of the osseous vestibular aqueduct. It becomes dilated distally to form the endolymphatic sac, a structure of variable size which may extend through an aperture on the posterior surface of the petrous bone, to end between the two layers of the dura on the posterior surface of the petrous temporal bone near the sigmoid sinus (p. 591). Throughout the whole endolymphatic duct the surface cells resemble those lining the non-specialized parts of the membranous labyrinth, consisting of squamous or low cuboidal epithelium. Their cytoplasm contains relatively few ribosomes, lipid granules and sparse, but evenly distributed mitochondria. The epithelium has been described as 'leaky' on account of the paucity of tight junctions between the cells.

Endolymphatic sac. The epithelial lining and subepithelial connective tissue become more complex where the duct dilates to form the endolymphatic sac. Three parts of the sac are recognized in lower mammals, namely proximal, intermediate and distal. In humans, these subdivisions are less clear but distinction can be made between an intermediate or rugose part and a distal sac. In the intermediate segment, the epithelium consists of cylindrical cells which have been further categorized into two distinct types, light and dark cells. The *light cells* are regular in form, and have numerous long surface microvilli with endocytic invaginations between them, abundant ribosomes and mitochondria and large clear vesicles in their apical region; their bases are somewhat infolded, and their lateral margins have extensive interdigitations with adjacent cells. In contrast the dark cells are wedge-shaped with a narrow base, and large irregular nuclei; their apical surface has only a few microvilli and their cytoplasm is dense and fibrillar. Beneath the epithelium is a highly vascular connective tissue in which the capillaries come to lie very close to the epithelial layer (Lundquist et al 1984).

The endolymphatic sac has important roles in the maintenance of vestibular function; endolymph produced elsewhere in the labyrinth is absorbed in this region, and it is thought that the light cells are chiefly responsible for this. Damage to the sac or blockage of its connection to the rest of the labyrinth causes endolymph to accumulate, giving rise to the condition of hydrops which affects both vestibular and cochlear function. This region is also permeable to leucocytes including macrophages which can remove cellular debris from the endolymph, and to various cells of the immune system which contribute antibodies to this fluid.

Endolymph. The endolymph filling the membranous labyrinth contrasts in its composition with the perilymph outside it, the latter being rich in sodium but poor in potassium ions, closely resembling cerebrospinal fluid, with which it is in continuity through the vestibular aqueduct, while endolymph resembles intracellular fluid in its ionic composition being, in contrast, rich in potassium and poor in sodium ions. Endolymph is secreted from various sources in the membranous labyrinth although details are poorly understood. Structures involved in its production may include the dark cells of the utricle and semicircular ducts, the columnar cells of the planum semilunatum within the ampullae, and in the cochlear duct, the specialized epithelial cells of the stria vascularis (see below). Whatever their relative contributions, endolymph probably circulates in the labyrinth, entering the ductus endolymphaticus for removal by the specialized epithelium of its sac into the adjacent vascular plexus. Pinocytotic removal of fluid may also occur in other labyrinthine regions.

A unique positive electrical potential exists in the endolymphatic spaces, varying from +77 millivolts in the cochlear duct near the stria vascularis to about +44 millivolts in the utricle. This is additional to the normal resting potentials of the receptor cells, so that there is a very considerable potential difference across their membranes. This undoubtedly contributes to the extreme sensitivity of the labyrinth's sensory receptors to mechanical deformation.

COCHLEAR DUCT

The cochlear duct (**8**.484, 492–494) is a spiral tube running along the outer wall of the osseous cochlea. The osseous spiral lamina (p. 1379) projects for only part of the distance between the modiolus and the outer cochlear wall, the *basilar membrane* completing the roof of the scala tympani. The endosteum of the outer wall is thickened into a *spiral cochlear ligament* projecting inwards and attached to the outer edge of the basilar membrane. A second, thinner *vestibular membrane* (*Reissner's membrane*) extends from the thickened endosteum on the osseous spiral lamina to the outer wall, attached well above the outer edge of the basilar membrane. The canal thus enclosed, between the scala tympani below and the scala vestibuli above, is the *cochlear duct* (**8**.494). It is triangular in section, its roof the vestibular membrane, its outer wall the endosteum, its floor the basilar membrane and the outer part of the osseous spiral lamina. Its closed upper end, the *lagaena*, is attached to the cupula (p.1379). The duct's lower end turns medially, narrowing into the *ductus reuniens*, to connect with the saccule (**8**.484). The spiral organ (of Corti), comprising the sensory area of the cochlea, is set on the basilar membrane. The thin vestibular membrane is covered on both surfaces by flat epithelium. The endosteum of the outer wall is greatly thickened to form a *spiral ligament*, which projects inferiorly as a triangular *crista basilaris*, to which the rim of the basilar membrane is attached; immediately above this is a concavity, the *sulcus spiralis externus*, above which the thick, highly vascular periosteum projects as a *spiral prominence*, above which again is a specialized, thick epithelial layer, the *stria*

vascularis. (For ultrastructural details see Friedmann and Ballantyne (1984).)

Vestibular membrane (8.494, 495)

The vestibular membrane (of Reissner) has two layers of squamous epithelial cells separated by a basal lamina. The aspect facing the scala vestibuli bears perilymphatic cells, thick in their central perinuclear zone but elsewhere extremely thin; zonulae occludentes occur between them, creating a diffusion barrier. The endolymphatic aspect has typical squamous epithelial cells, also joined by zonulae occludentes and containing mitochondria and many vesicles; their basal surfaces are sometimes smooth but often complexly invaginated; the surface carries numerous, short, irregular microvilli. These cells may be involved in fluid transport.

Stria vascularis (8.498)

As noted above this is on the cochlear duct's outer wall above the spiral eminence. It has a special stratified epithelium continuing a dense *intraepithelial capillary plexus* and three cell types:

- superficial *marginal, dark* or *chromophil cells*
- *intermediate light*, or *chromophobe cells*
- *basal cells*.

The endolymphatic surface consists only of the apical aspects of marginal cells; the intermediate and basal cells are cytologically similar, differing in their position, their pale cytoplasm containing scattered mitochondria, many endocytic vesicles and some melanin granules; they send cytoplasmic processes towards the surface, insinuated between the deeper parts of the marginal cells. Marginal dark cells have dense granular cytoplasm with many mitochondria and endocytic vesicles. Their deep parts consist of long cytoplasmic processes separated by deep invaginations of plasmalemma, each containing many mitochondria. Intraepithelial capillaries are enveloped by the descending processes of dark cells and ascending processes from intermediate and basal cells. The stria vascularis is considered to be ion-transporting, assisting to maintain the unusual ionic composition of endolymph. But other regions of the membranous labyrinth may also be involved in this activity. Exploration

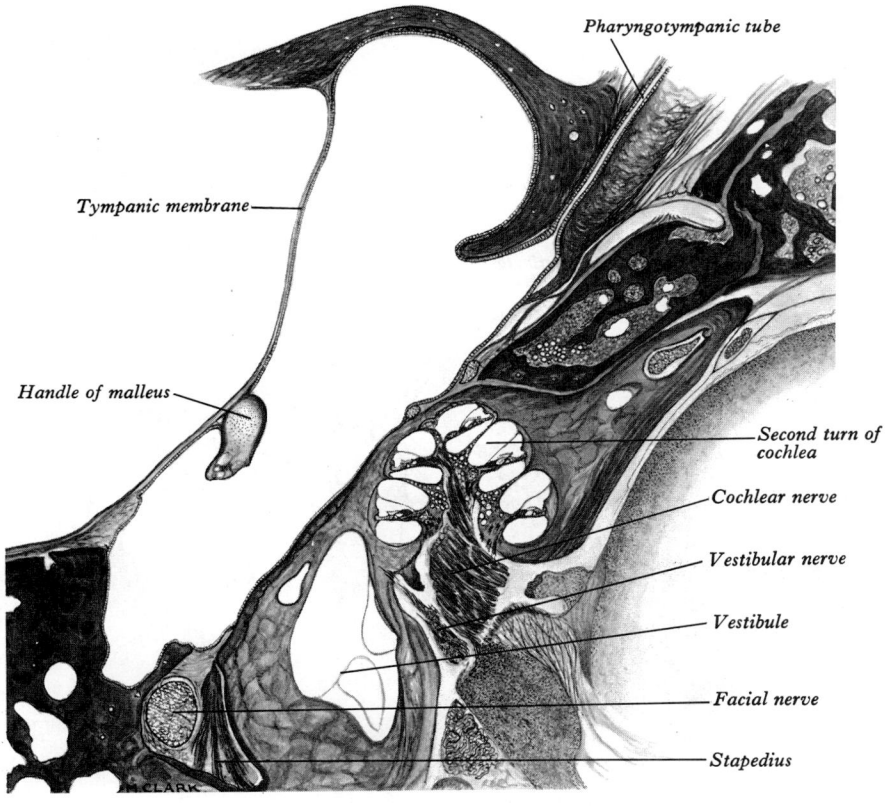

Pharyngotympanic tube

Tympanic membrane

Handle of malleus

Second turn of cochlea

Cochlear nerve

Vestibular nerve

Vestibule

Facial nerve

Stapedius

8.492 Horizontal section through the left temporal bone. (Drawn from a section prepared at the Ferens Institute and lent by the late J Kirk.)

Osseous spiral lamina

The osseous spiral lamina consists of two plates of bone, between which are canals for the cochlear nerve filaments. On the upper plate, within the duct of the cochlea, the periosteum is thickened as the *limbus laminae spiralis* (**8.494, 497**), ending externally in the *sulcus spiralis internus*, which in section is shaped like a C; its upper part, the overhanging limbic edge, is the *vestibular labium* and the lower tapering part is the *tympanic labium*, perforated by foramina (*habenula perforata*) for branches of the cochlear nerve. The upper surface of the vestibular labium is crossed at right angles by furrows, separated by numerous elevations, the *auditory teeth* (*dentes acoustici*) (**8.497, 498**). The limbus is covered by a layer appearing superficially as squamous epithelium, but only the cells over the 'teeth' are flat, those in the furrows being columnar (*interdental cells*) and occupying the intervals between the elevations. This epithelium is continuous with that in the sulcus spiralis internus and on the inferior surface of the vestibular membrane. It is considered by some that during development the interdental cells secrete material forming the tectorial membrane (see below).

Basilar membrane

The basilar membrane stretches from the tympanic lip of the osseous spiral lamina to the crista basilaris (**8.494, 498**). It consists of two zones, a thin *zona arcuata* stretching from the limbus spiralis to the bases of the outer rods and supporting the organ of Corti, and an outer thicker *zona pectinata*, commencing beneath the bases of the outer rods and attached laterally to the crista basilaris. The zona arcuata is composed of compact bundles of small collagenoid filaments 8–10 nm in diameter, mainly radial in orientation. In the zona pectinata the basilar membrane is trilaminar, its upper layer a homogeneous network of transverse fibres, the lower composed of compact bundles of longitudinal fibres with an intermediate structureless layer containing few cells. At its attachment to the crista basilaris the upper and lower layers fuse. The length of the basilar membrane is about 35 mm; its width **increases** from 0.21 mm basally to 0.36 mm at its apex, accompanied by corresponding narrowing of the osseous spiral lamina and a decrease in the thickness of the crista basilaris. Its inferior surface is covered by a layer of

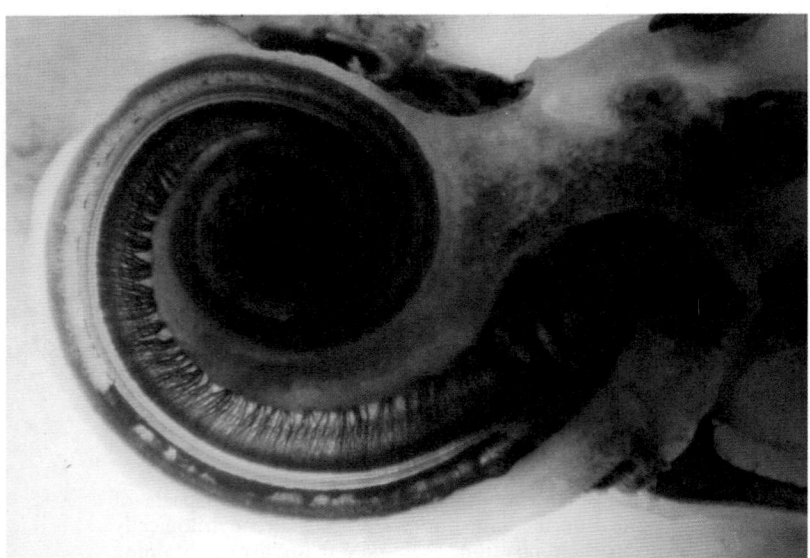

8.493 Whole mount preparation of the spiral organ from a human cochlea, stained with osmium to show the distribution of tissues including the myelinated nerve fibres. Magnification × 20. (Supplied by H Felix, M Gleeson and L-G Johnsson, ENT Department, University of Zurich and Guy's Hospital, London.)

of the stria by microelectrodes shows it to be the source of the large positive endocochlear electrical potential, the maintenance of which is directly dependent upon adequate oxygenation of the epithelial cells, provided by the intraepithelial capillary plexus.

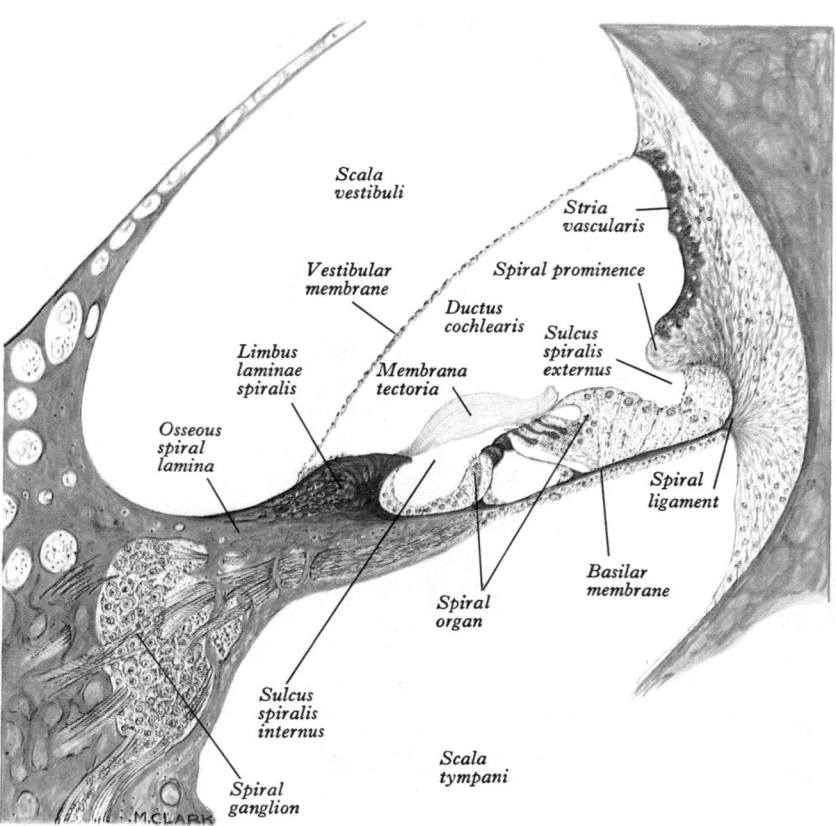

8.494 Section through the second turn of the cochlea indicated in the previous figure. The modiolus is to the left. Mallory's stain.

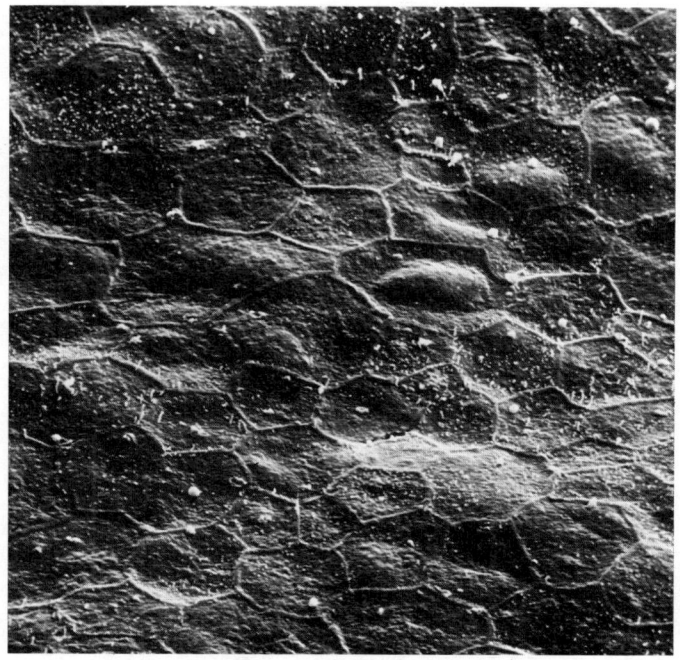

8.495 Scanning electron micrograph of the surface of Reissner's membrane, viewed from the cochlear duct aspect, showing the regular pattern of simple squamous epithelial cells (guinea pig). Magnification × 2500.

vascular connective tissue and elongated perilymphatic cells; one vessel is larger and termed the *vas spirale*; it lies immediately below the tunnel of Corti (*cuniculum internum*).

SPIRAL ORGAN OF CORTI (8.494–504)

The spiral organ (of Corti) (Engström & Wersäll 1958; Ades & Engström 1974) consists of a series of epithelial structures lying on the zona arcuata of the basilar membrane. The more central of these structures are two rows of cells, the *internal* and *external rod cells* (*of Corti*) or *pillar cells*. The bases or *foot plates* (*crura*) of the rod cells are expanded, resting contiguously on the basilar membrane but apically widely separated; the two rows incline to each other and come into contact above at the *heads of the pillars*, enclosing between them and the basilar membrane the *cuniculum internum* (tunnel of Corti) (**8**.496, 498), which has a triangular cross-section. Internal to the inner rods is a single row of *inner hair cells* and

external to the outer rods three or four rows of *outer hair cells*, with supporting cells, *phalangeal cells* (*of Deiters*) and *cellulae limitans externae* (cells of Hensen). The free ends of the external hair cells and apical processes of phalangeal cells form a regular mosaic termed collectively the *reticular lamina* or *reticular membrane*. The organ is covered by the *tectorial membrane*, a shelf of stiff gelatinous proteinaceous material; a narrow gap separates this from the reticular lamina except where the apical stereocilia of the outer hair cells project to make contact with it. In addition to the *inner tunnel* (*cuniculum internum* or tunnel of Corti), other intercommunicating spaces exist around the outer hair cells also connected with the inner tunnel, including an *outer tunnel* (*cuniculum externum*) between the outermost hair cells and inner cells (of Hensen), under the reticular lamina, and also a cuniculum medium (space of Nuel) between the outer pillar (of Corti) and the outer hair cells. The latter tunnel is continuous with the extracellular spaces around the apical two-thirds of the outer hair cells. This complex of intercommunicating spaces is filled with perilymph which diffuses into it through the matrix of the basilar membrane. The fluid in these spaces is also sometimes called the *cortilymph* and it is possible that minor alterations in perilymphatic composition occur within it, as it is exposed to the activities of synaptic endings and specialized excitable cells.

Pillar cells (rods of Corti) (**8**.497, 498). These have a base or *crus*, an elongated *scapus* (rod) and an upper end or *caput* (head); each crus and caput are in contact but the scapi are separated by the inner (Corti's) tunnel. The scapus is finely striated but an oval non-striated part of the caput stains deeply with carmine. Electron microscopy shows many microtubules 30 nm in diameter, arranged in linked parallel bundles of 2000 or more in the scapus and diverging above to terminate in superficial dense granular cytoplasm, the *cuticle*, in the head. Microtubules start in a wide area of limiting membrane in dense cytoplasmic material in the crus. In the rod transverse sections show microtubules arranged in a rectangular lattice with adjacent individuals linked to actin filaments lying parallel to them; many of them curve into the reticular lamina (see below) to end near the junctional complexes, with similar expansions from phalangeal cells (supporting cells of Deiters) and the subapical lateral surfaces of outer hair cells. Although the 'rod', as originally interpreted, corresponds only to the cytoskeletal structures and adjacent cytoplasmic densities, this term has now come to include the whole cell which forms these organelles. Their nuclei are situated in the foot-like expansion resting on the basal lamina.

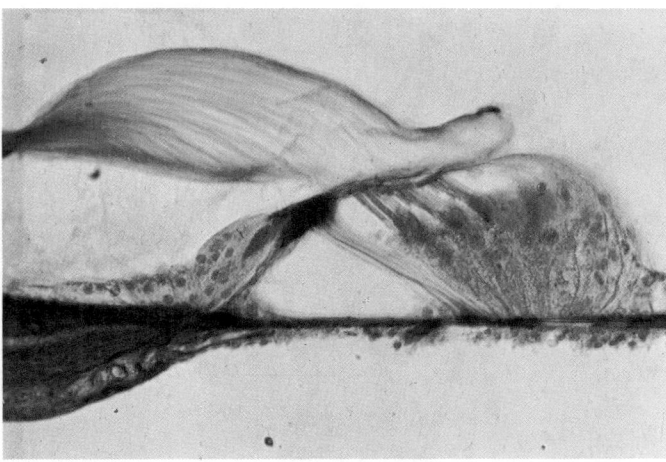

8.496 Transverse section of the spiral organ of Corti (cat), stained with the Mallory trichrome method to show the inner and outer hair cells (orange), the basilar membrane (dark blue) and tectorial membrane (light blue) and various supporting cells, including those surrounding the tunnel of Corti. Magnification × 400.

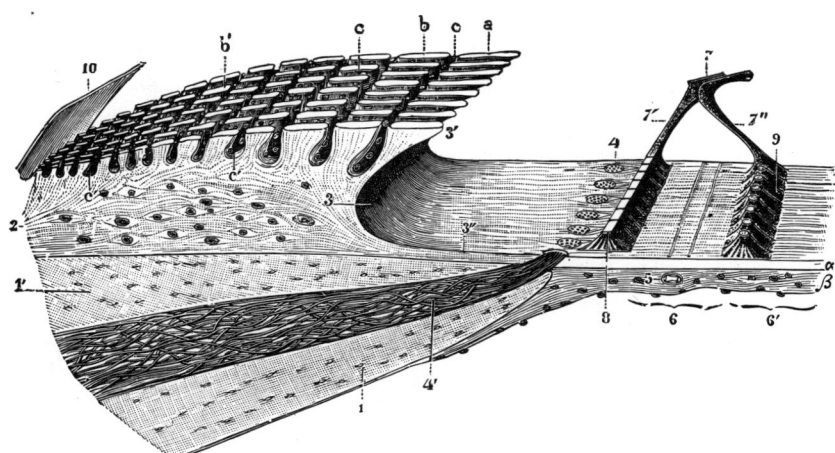

8.497 The limbus laminae spiralis and the basilar membrane (schematic, after Testut). 1, 1'. Lower and upper lamellae of the lamina spiralis ossea. 2. Limbus laminae spiralis, with a, the auditory teeth of the first row; b, b', the teeth of the other rows; c, c', the grooves between the auditory teeth and the cells which are lodged in them. 3. Sulcus spiralis internus, with 3', its labium vestibulare, and 3", its labium tympanicum. 4. Foramina nervosa, giving passage to the nerves from the spiral ganglion. 5. Vas spirale. 6. Zona arcuata. 6'. Zona pectinata of the basilar membrane, with α, its hyaline layer, β, its connective tissue layer. 7. Summit of the tunnel of Corti, with 7', its inner rod, and 7", its outer rod. 8. Bases of the inner rods, from which the cells are removed. 9. Bases of the outer rod. 10. Part of the vestibular membrane.

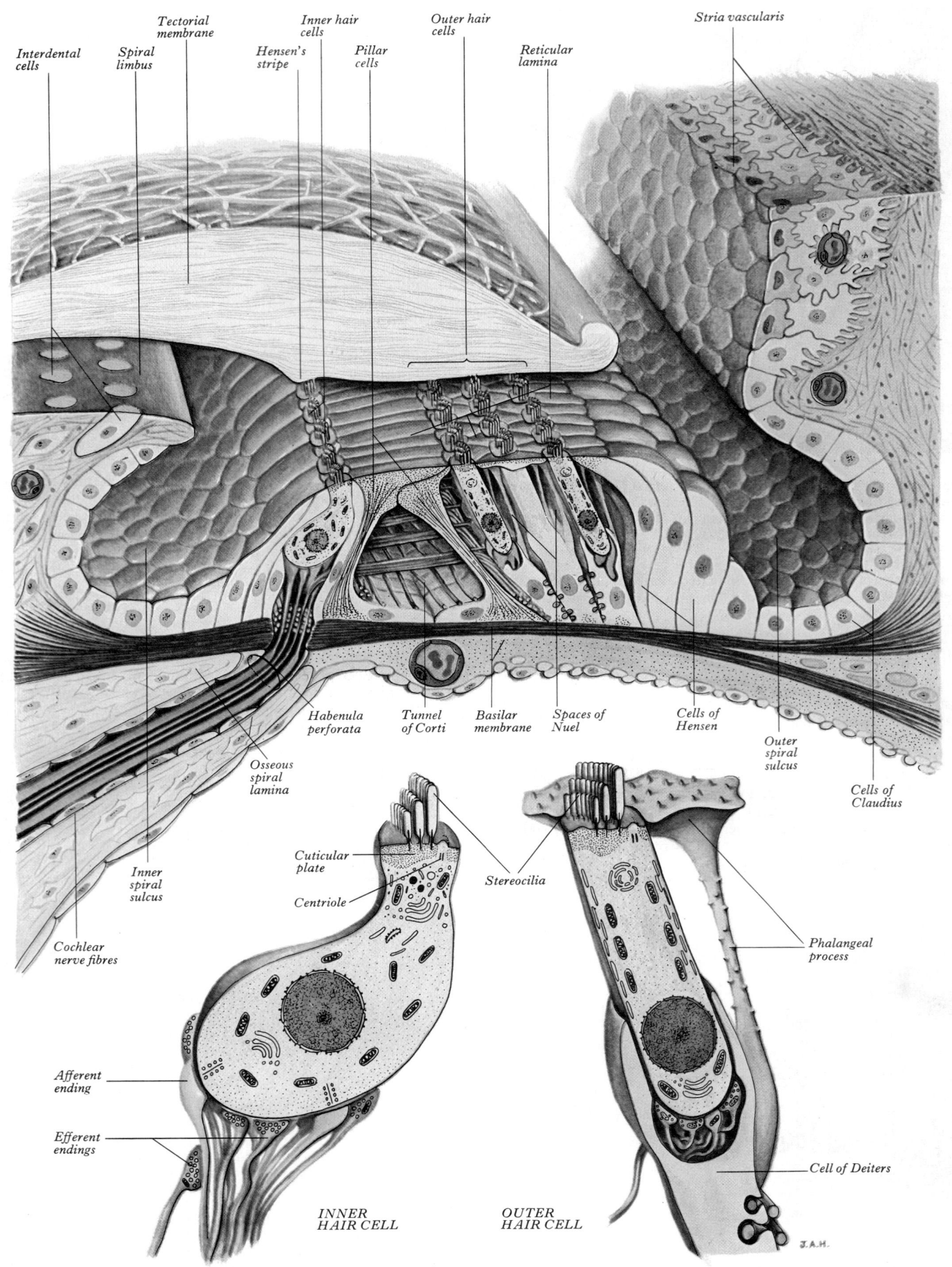

Interdental cells

Spiral limbus

Tectorial membrane

Hensen's stripe

Inner hair cells

Pillar cells

Outer hair cells

Reticular lamina

Stria vascularis

Habenula perforata

Tunnel of Corti

Basilar membrane

Spaces of Nuel

Cells of Hensen

Outer spiral sulcus

Cells of Claudius

Osseous spiral lamina

Inner spiral sulcus

Cochlear nerve fibres

Cuticular plate

Centriole

Stereocilia

Phalangeal process

Afferent ending

Efferent endings

Cell of Deiters

INNER HAIR CELL

OUTER HAIR CELL

J.A.H.

8.498 Three-dimensional schema of the structure of the cochlear spiral organ and stria vascularis, showing the arrangement of the various types of cell and their overall innervation. The organization of the inner and outer hair cells and their synaptic connections are depicted below. Sensory nerve terminals are coloured green and efferent fibres purple. See text for variant terminology.

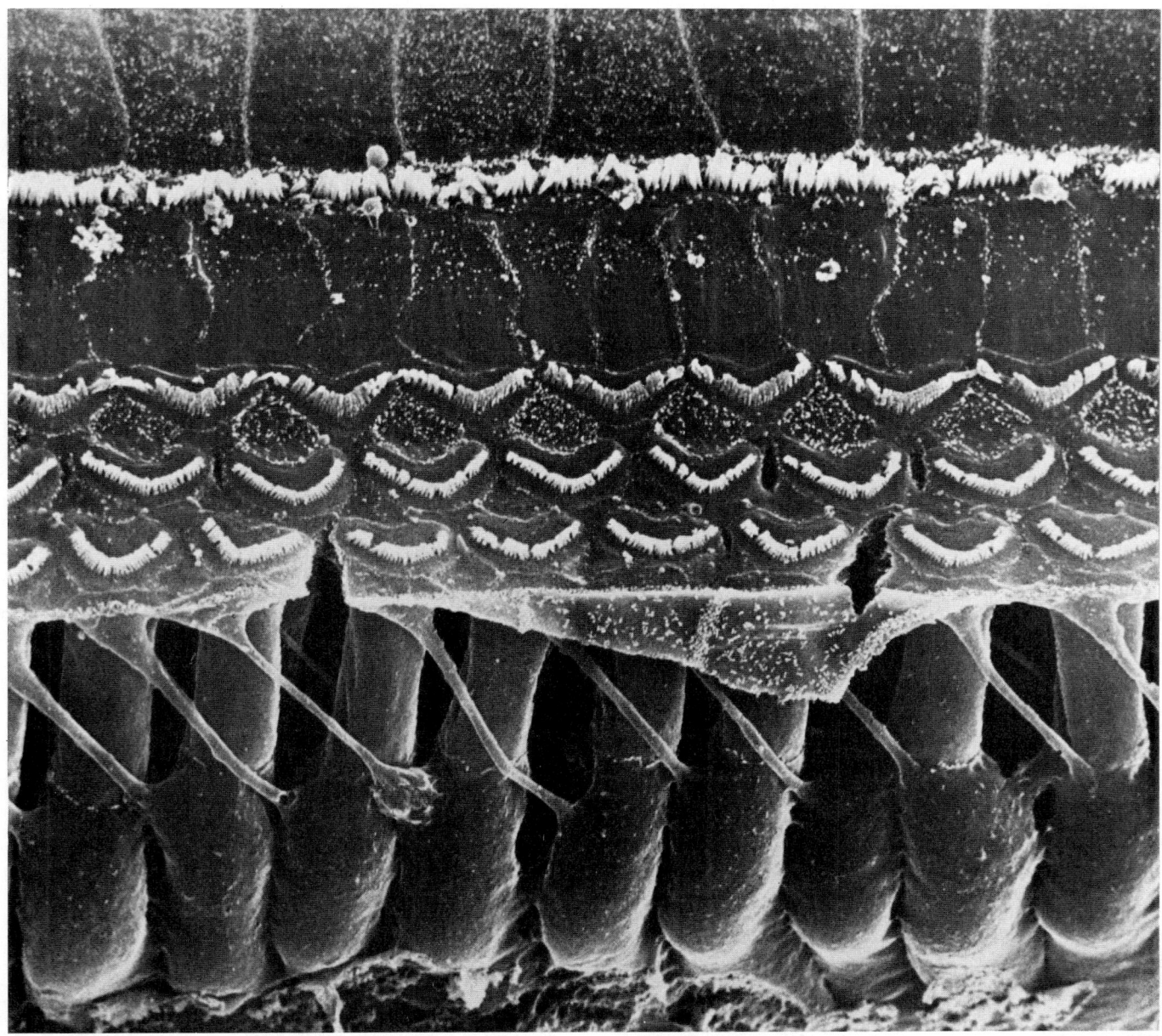

8.499 Scanning electron micrograph of a portion of the spiral organ of Corti (guinea pig) dissected to expose the outer row of outer hair cells and their attendant Deiters' cells with narrow phalangeal processes. The apices of three rows of outer hair cells with their stereocilia are visible in the foreground and behind them are the apices of the rod cells and a row of inner hair cells and their stereocilia. Magnification ×2500. (Supplied by Hilary C. Dodson, Institute of Otolaryngology, London.)

Internal pillar cells (rods). They number almost 6000, their bases resting on the basilar membrane near the tympanic lip of the sulcus spiralis internus. Their bodies form an angle of about 60° with the basilar membrane, their heads resembling the ulna's proximal end, with deep concavities for the heads of the outer pillar cells. Their heads overhang those of the latter.

External pillar cells (rods). Almost 4000 in number, they are longer and more oblique, forming with the basilar membrane an angle of only 40°. Their heads, convex internally, fit into the concavities on the heads of the inner pillar cells and project externally as thin, *phalangeal processes,* which unite with the phalangeal processes of the phalangeal (Deiters') cells to form the reticular lamina (see below).

The distances between the bases of the internal and external pillar cells increase from the cochlear base to its apex but the angles between them and the basilar membrane diminish.

Cochlear hair cells (8.498–504)

Hair cells (epitheliocyti pilosi) are the sensory transducers of the cochlea which collectively detect the amplitude and frequency of the sound waves entering it. All cochlear hair cells have a common pattern of organization, being vertically elongate cells with a group of regular microvilli, *stereocilia,* on their flat apical ends, which are level with the general surface of the spiral organ, and a group of synaptic contacts with cochlear nerve fibres at their rounded bases. They are surrounded to a greater or lesser extent by the processes of neighbouring supporting cells of various kinds, which also separate them from the basilar membrane beneath them. According to their position in the spiral organ they can be divided into *outer* and *inner hair cells* (the terms inner and outer refer to their position with respect to the modiolus, the central axis of the cochlea, inner being towards the axis and outer away from it). These two groups have distinctive roles in sound reception and the differences in their detailed structure reflect this functional divergence. The inner hair cells form a single row along the inner edge of inner pillar cells (and the spiral tunnel), whereas the outer hair cells are arranged in three, or in some regions of the human cochlea in four or even five rows, interspersed with supporting cells (8.504). Inner hair cells number

1389

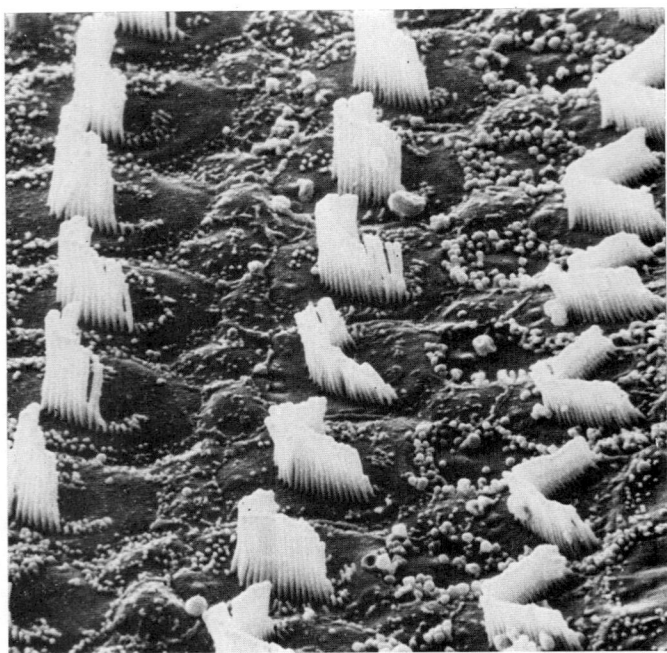

8.500 Scanning electron micrograph of a group of outer hair cells arranged in three rows, showing the arrangement of their stereocilia and related phalangeal processes of the Deiters' cells, collectively forming the reticular lamina (see text). Short microvilli are visible on the surfaces of the non-sensory cells (guinea pig). Magnification ×3000.

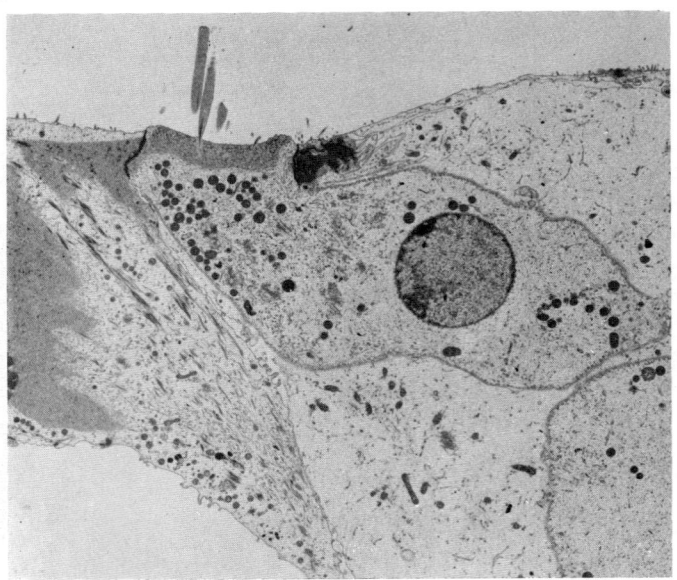

8.502 Electron micrograph of an inner hair cell (guinea pig) showing the apical stereocilia with bases embedded in the dense cuticular plate. Note the centrally placed nucleus and numerous cytoplasmic organelles. The apex of a rod cell is visible on the left and below it the cavity of the tunnel of Corti. Magnification ×3000. (Supplied by Hilary C. Dodson, Institute of Otolaryngology, London.)

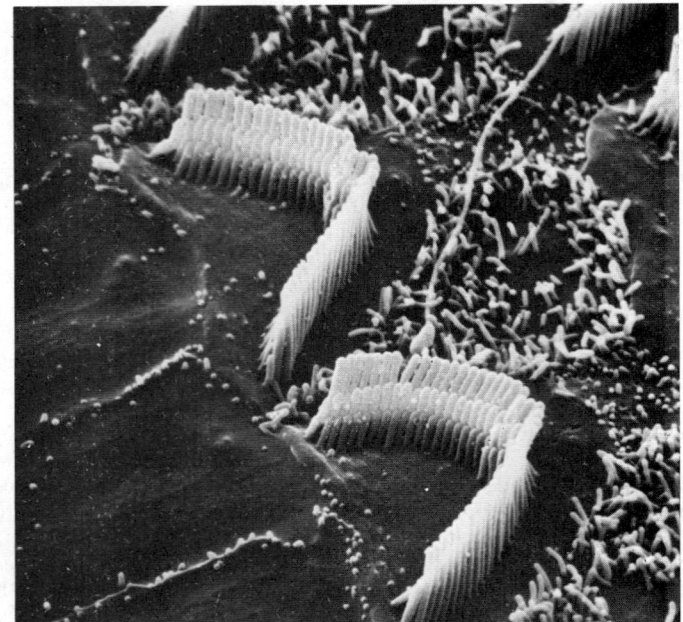

8.501 Scanning electron micrograph of the apices of two outer hair cells showing the different lengths of the stereocilia in the three ranks which constitute each group. Microvilli are also seen on the surface of the Deiters' cells (right). The innermost row of outer hair cells is shown; the tunnel of Corti, roofed by rod cell processes, is on the left. Magnification ×5000. (Supplied by Hilary C Dodson, Institute of Otolaryngology, London, photographed by Michael Crowder, Guy's Hospital Medical School, London.)

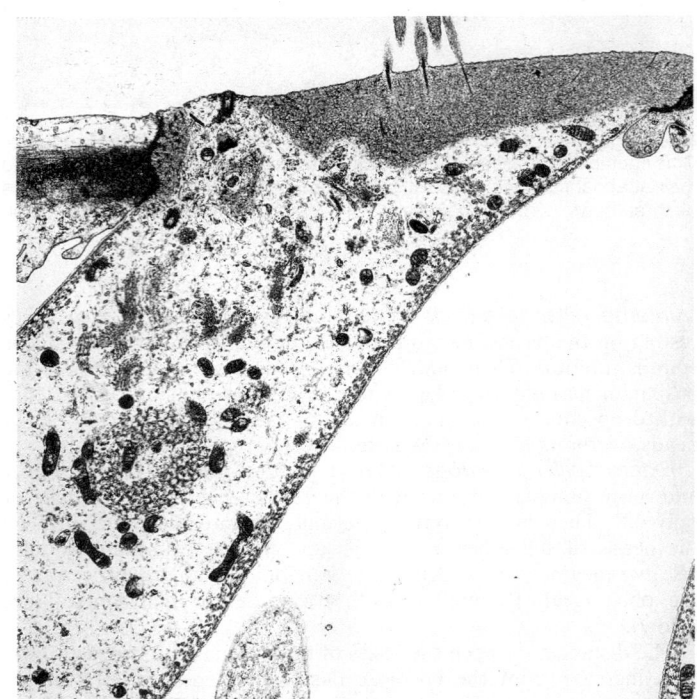

8.503 Transmission electron micrograph showing an outer hair cell apex (guinea pig). Magnification ×10 000. (Provided by H C Dodson, Institute of Otolaryngology, London.)

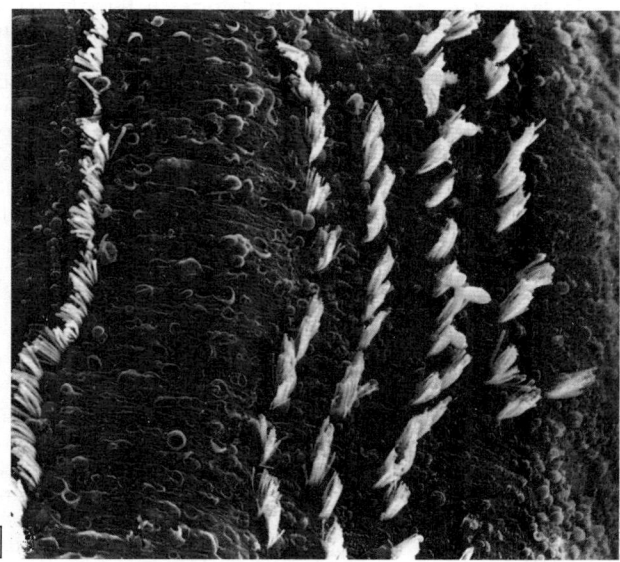

A

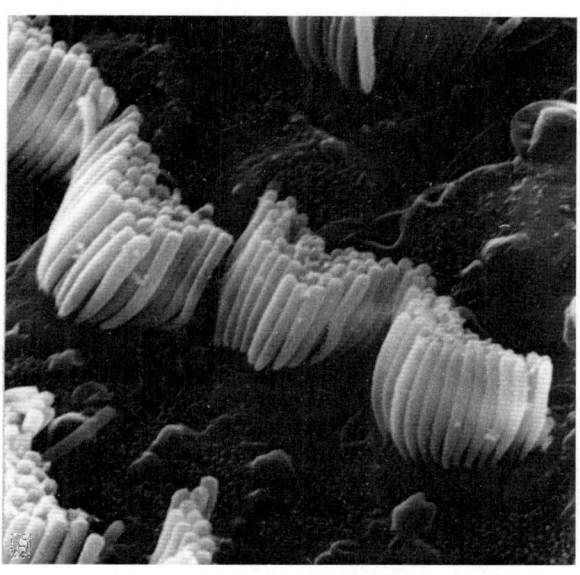

B

8.504 Scanning electron micrographs of the surface of a spiral organ from a human cochlea.
A is a low power view showing a single row of inner hair cells (left) and three rows of outer hair cells, with additional rows in places.

B is a higher magnification of stereocilial bundles of outer hair cells. (Supplied by H Felix, M Gleeson and L-G Johnsson, ENT Department, University of Zurich and Guy's Hospital, London.)

about 3500 and outer ones about 12 000. The two sets of hair cells lean towards each other apically at about the same angles as the neighbouring inner and outer pillar cells. The geometric arrangement of these cells is very precise, and this remarkable orderliness is closely related to the sensory performance of the cochlea (see below).

Inner hair cells. The inner hair cells are pear shaped and slightly curved, the narrower end directed towards the spiral organ's surface and the wider basal end positioned some distance above the inner end of the basilar membrane (8.498, 502). Inner hair cells are surrounded by supporting (inner phalangeal) cells, attached externally to the heads of the inner pillar cells. The flat apical surface is elliptical when viewed from above in whole mount preparations, its long axis directed in the direction of the row of hair cells; the breadth of the apex exceeds that of the inner pillar cells so that each inner hair cell is related to more than one of these. Immediately beneath the pillar cell's apical surface is a transverse lamina of dense fibrillar material, the *cuticular plate*, which spans the entire apex except at a small aperture in which a centriole is present (in early development a kinocilium is anchored here, a condition which persists in vestibular receptors). The apex bears 50–60 stereocilia, arranged in three ranks rather like rows of organ pipes of progressively ascending height, the tallest on the outer aspect. These are similar to the stereocilia of vestibular cells, containing regular arrays of actin filaments and actin-binding proteins and, near the narrow basal end, a dense central filament which is deeply inserted into the cuticular plate. The tips of the shorter rows are connected diagonally to the sides of the adjacent taller stereocilia by thin threads, *tip links*, and each stereocilium is also connected laterally to adjacent members by other less regular filamentous material. The length of stereocilial row varies in a regularly graded manner with cochlear region, being longest in the apical region of the cochlea and shortest at its base, a feature of some functional significance (see below).

The nucleus is rounded and euchromatic, and the cytoplasm contains an abundance of organelles, indicative of the high metabolic rate, including many mitochondria in the apical region, free poly-ribosome groups, agranular endoplasmic reticulum, various vesicles and lysosomes. Microtubules are abundant, and form regular, predictable patterns within the cell. At the base each inner hair cell forms ten or more synaptic contacts with afferent endings, each being marked by a presynaptic structure similar to the ribbon synapses of the retina, a plate or rod of dense material surrounded by synaptic vesicles being directed perpendicularly to the presynaptic membrane. Occasionally an efferent synapse makes direct contact with the hair cell base, but these are usually presynaptic to the

terminal expansions of afferent endings rather than the hair cell itself.

Outer hair cells (8.498–501, 504). These are long cylindrical cells nearly twice as tall as the inner hair cells, although there is a gradation of length, the outermost row being longest in any one cochlear region, and those of the cochlear apex being taller than those of the base. They are surrounded by the apical processes of phalangeal cells or, on the internal aspect of the inner row, by the heads of the outer pillar cells. The base is cupped in the concavity in the main part of a phalangeal cell, except for a gap where the axons of the cochlear nerve fibres make synapses. The stereocilia, which may number up to 100 per cell, are also arranged in three or more rows of graded heights, the longest being on the outer side, although the rows are pleated in the form of a V or W depending on cochlear region, the points of the angles directed externally (where a cuticle free gap and a centriole are also positioned in the cell's apex). The stereocilia are also graded in length according to cochlear region, those of the cochlear base being shortest. Like those of inner hair cells, the stereocilia possess tip links and other filamentous connections with their neighbours, and are inserted at their narrow bases into the cuticular plate. The tallest stereocilia are embedded in shallow impressions on the underside of the tectorial membrane.

The rounded, partly euchromatic nucleus is positioned near the base of the cell. The cytoplasm shows a general scarcity of organelles in comparison with inner hair cells; most of the inner region has an empty appearance except for a finely granular appearance in electron micrographs, although apically a core of filamentous material often protrudes from the base of the cuticular plate. Below the nucleus are numerous mitochondria, vesicles, lysosomes, microtubules and a few ribbon-like synapses associated with afferent endings of the cochlear nerve. Microtubules are also present in small numbers around the perimeter apically. Beneath the lateral walls of the cell lies a system of flat parallel membranous cisternae which stretches from near the basal pole of the cell to close to the cuticular membrane. Similar clusters of cisternae are also present more centrally (Hensen bodies) and may represent a stage in the assembly of these structures. The outermost layer of cisternae are connected to the plasma membrane by regularly placed, short filaments (pillars) inter-connected by a web of filaments running parallel to the cell surface. This intriguing apparatus has excited much speculation, but remains to be fully analysed. The proteins actin and fodrin have been demonstrated in this region by immunohistochemistry, but their precise location within the cortical zone is uncertain, although they are known to be richly represented in the cuticular plate and stereocilia. The plasma membrane of hair cells is also somewhat unusual in having a large protein content, visible in freeze-fracture preparations as clusters of spheroidal particles (see below).

The innervation of outer hair cells is both afferent and efferent. Afferent terminals are slightly expanded end-bulbs, each situated opposite a presynaptic ribbon or rod, as for inner hair cells. They are few in number compared with the large cluster of efferent boutons containing large numbers of small (50 nm) clear vesicles, contacting the base of the cell. A few larger dense-cored vesicles are also typically present. The neurotransmitter at the afferent synapse is probably glutamate, and that of the efferent endings acetylcholine (ACh), although other neurotransmitters or neuromodulators have also been demonstrated.

External phalangeal cells (of Deiters) (8.498, 499). These lie between the rows of outer hair cells, their expanded bases lying on the basilar membrane and their apical ends partially enveloping the bases of hair cells with a finger-like *phalangeal process* extending up diagonally between the hair cells to the reticular membrane, there forming a plate-like expansion completing the gaps between hair cell apices (see below). Their cytoplasm contains bundles of microtubules and actin filaments arising from the cell base and continuing up into the phalangeal process; other microtubules reinforce the cup supporting the base of the hair cell. External to them are five or six rows of columnar *supporting cells* (*of Hensen*) or *external limiting cells* (8.498), beyond which are the *external supporting cells* (of Claudius). Their surfaces bear microvilli.

Near the base of the cochlea, another group of small cells is present among the bases of the phalangeal cells; these are termed Böttcher's cells and their functions are unknown.

Reticular lamina (8.498). As seen by light microscopy, this is a delicate framework perforated by circular holes occupied by the apices of outer hair cells, extending from the heads of the external rods to the outer row of outer hair cells and completed by several rows of minute cuticular *phalanges*. The innermost row of phalanges are the phalangeal processes of external rods. Ultrastructurally the reticular lamina consists of the horizontal expansions of the outer rods and phalangeal cells carrying bundles of microtubules in an attenuated plate of dense cytoplasm. The expansions encircle the apical rims of the hair cells, where occluding zones and desmosomes are formed and the microtubules end. Between adjacent supporting cells are occluding junctions, most apically desmosomes and extensive gap junctions which couple them electrically. Under this delicate support the apical two-thirds of the lateral surfaces of the external hair cells are free and bathed by cortilymph (see below). The significance of this arrangement is twofold: the reticular lamina creates a highly impermeable barrier to the passage of ions except through cell membranes during sensory activity; it also forms a rigid support between the apices of the hair cells, coupling them mechanically to the movements of the underlying basilar membrane which causes lateral shearing movements between the cells and the overlying, static tectorial membrane.

If hair cells are lost through trauma, for example by excessive noise or ototoxic drugs, phalangeal processes rapidly fill the gap, disturbing the regular laminar pattern (*phalangeal scars*) but restoring its function.

TECTORIAL MEMBRANE

The tectorial membrane (membrana tectoria) (8.494, 496, 498), overlying the sulcus spiralis internus and spiral organ, is composed of a stiff, gelatinous plate of proteinaceous composition consisting ultrastructurally of fine (4 nm diameter) filaments embedded in a granular matrix (Iurato 1967; Steel 1978). Three classes of collagen are present (Types II, V and IX) interspersed with glycoproteins called *tectorins* which comprise about half of the total protein. In mice, at least seven tectorins with molecular weights of 173–231 kDa have been described, visible ultrastructurally as parallel inter-connected filaments 7–9 nm which form flat laminar stacks, enclosing collagen fibres to create a highly organized matrix with considerable mechanical coherence (see Richardson et al 1994).

In transverse section the tectorial membrane has a characteristic shape, the underside being nearly flat and the upper surface convex; it is thin on the modiolar side where it is attached to the vestibular lip of the limbus laminae spiralis, extending centrally as far as the vestibular membrane. Its outer part forms a thickened ridge, overhanging the edge of the reticular lamina. Scanning electron microscopy shows a network of fine ridges on the upper surface, the lower surface being relatively smooth, except where the stereocilia of the outer hair cells leave a pattern of W- or V-shaped impressions. Another feature, in some species, is a longitudinal ridge along its under surface near the inner tunnel, visible by light microscopy as Hensen's stripe. The interdental cells of the vestibular labium, to which the membrane is attached, have a well-developed Golgi apparatus, many mitochondria and free polysomes; they may secrete the membrane. The lips of the stereocilia of the outer hair cells are embedded in the membrane but this attachment is often broken during histological preparation.

VESTIBULOCOCHLEAR NERVE

The vestibulocochlear nerve emerges from the pontocerebellar angle and courses through the posterior cranial fossa to enter the petrous temporal bone via the internal acoustic meatus, in the deep recess of which it divides into an anterior trunk, the cochlear nerve, and a posterior one, the vestibular nerve (see p. 1248). Both consist of the centrally directed axons of bipolar neurons with cell bodies situated close to their peripheral terminals, together with a smaller number of efferent fibres arising from brainstem neurons, terminating on cochlear and vestibular sensory cells.

It should be noted that clinicians and anatomists differ in their use and meaning of the terms peripheral and central when referring to the vestibulocochlear nerve. In audiological practice, it is very important to distinguish between intratemporal and intracranial lesions but, unfortunately, this surgical distinction between auditory and vestibular systems fails to correlate with either strict anatomical definitions of peripheral and central or discriminant tests of the two. Hence the term 'peripheral auditory lesion' is used to describe lesions peripheral to the spiral ganglion, while the term 'peripheral vestibular disturbance' includes lesions of the vestibular ganglion and the whole vestibular nerve. Furthermore, the intratemporal portion of the vestibulocochlear nerve in humans consists of two histologically distinct portions, a central glial zone adjacent to the brainstem, and a peripheral or non-glial zone. In the glial zone the axons are supported by neuroglia whereas in the non-glial zone they are ensheathed instead by Schwann cells. Bridger and Farkashidy (1980) have shown that the non-glial zone extends into the cerebellopontine angle medial to the acoustic porus in over 50% of the nerves they examined.

The central pathways of the vestibular and cochlear nerves are described elsewhere in this Section (pp. 1248, 1249).

Intratemporal vestibular nerve

The maculae and cristae are innervated by dendrites arising from the bipolar neurons constituting the *vestibular* (*Scarpa's*) *ganglion* which is situated in the trunk of the nerve within the lateral end of the internal auditory meatus (8.506, 507).

The peripheral processes of the ganglion cells aggregate into definable nerves, each with a specific distribution. Thus the main nerve divides at and within the ganglion into a superior and inferior division connected by an isthmus. The *superior division*, which is the larger of the two, traverses the foramina in the superior vestibular area to supply the ampullary cristae of the lateral (horizontal) and the anterior (superior) semi-circular canals through the *lateral* and *anterior ampullary nerves*, respectively. A secondary branch of the lateral ampullary nerve supplies the macula of the utricle, but the greater part of this sensory area is innervated by a separate branch of the superior division, the *utricular nerve*. Another branch of the superior division, Voit's nerve, supplies part of the saccule.

The *inferior division* of the vestibular nerve passes through foramina in the inferior vestibular area to supply the remainder of the saccule and the posterior ampullary crista through its *saccular* and *singular* branches respectively, the latter passing through the foramen singulare (Bergstrom 1973). Occasionally a very small supplementary or accessory branch is present and this innervates the posterior crista. This branch is probably a vestigial remnant from the crista neglecta, an additional area of sensory epithelium found in some other mammals but seldom in man (Montandon et al 1970).

Afferent and efferent cochlear fibres are also present in the inferior division of the vestibular nerve but leave at the *anastomosis of Oort* to join the main cochlear nerve (Oort 1918; Rasmussen 1946). There is another anastomosis situated more centrally between the facial and vestibular nerves; at this, the *vestibulofacial anastomosis*, fibres originating in the nervus intermedius are conveyed in the vestibular nerve to the main trunk of the facial nerve.

There are approximately 20 000 fibres in the vestibular nerve, of which 12 000 travel in the superior division and 8000 in the inferior division. The fibre diameter distribution is bimodal, with peaks at 4 μm and 6.5 μm. The smaller fibres are distributed mainly to Type II vestibular sensory cells while the larger fibres tend to supply Type I. In addition to the afferent fibres, both efferent and autonomic elements have been identified. Efferent fibres synapse exclusively with the afferent calycial terminals around Type I cells and usually with the afferent boutons on Type II cells, although a few may terminate in direct contact with the Type II cell body. The autonomic fibres do not contact vestibular sensory cells but terminate beneath the sensory epithelia. Two distinct sympathetic components have been identified in the vestibular ganglion: a perivascular adrenergic system derived from the stellate ganglion and a blood vessel-independent system from the superior cervical ganglion.

Vestibular ganglion (8.506, 507). There is considerable variation in the size of the spheroidal or ellipsoidal bipolar cell bodies providing the afferent neurons of the vestibular nerve, their circumferences ranging (in humans) from 45–160 μm (Felix et al 1987). No topographically ordered distribution of these large or small ganglion cells has so far been found. Their perikarya are notable for the abundance of granular endoplasmic reticulum, which in places forms Nissl bodies together with prominent Golgi complexes. The central nucleus has several nucleoli, one of which tends to be more conspicuous. The human vestibular ganglion is distinct from all other species so far examined in that the perikarya are not myelinated, but are instead covered by a thin layer of satellite cells (Perre et al 1975; Felix & Baumgartner 1981; Ylikowski et al 1981; Ylikowski 1983). Often the ganglion cells are arranged in pairs, closely abutting each other with only a thin layer of endoneurium between adjacent coverings of satellite cells. This arrangement has led to speculation that ganglion cells may affect each other directly by electrotonic spread (ephaptic transmission: see Felix et al 1987).

Intratemporal cochlear nerve

The cochlear nerve connects the organ of Corti to the cochlear and related nuclei of the brainstem. The cochlear nerve lies inferior to the facial nerve throughout the internal acoustic meatus. It becomes intimately associated with the superior and inferior divisions of the vestibular nerve, which are situated in the posterior compartment of the canal, and exits the internal acoustic porus in a common fascicle (8.492).

There are approximately 30–40 000 nerve fibres in the human cochlear nerve (Rasmussen 1940; Spoendlin & Schrott 1990; Felix et al 1992). This compares with 24 000 fibres in the guinea pig, 30 000 in monkeys, 50 000 in the cat and 250 000 in the whale (Gacek & Rasmussen 1961; Hall 1966). The human nerve fibre diameter distribution is unimodal, ranging from 1–11 μm with a peak at 4–5 μm.

Functionally, it contains both afferent and efferent systems and also receives adrenergic sympathetic fibres which originate from the cervical sympathetic trunk.

Afferent cochlear innervation (8.511). This consists of myelinated nerve fibres whose bipolar cell bodies are located in the spiral ganglion of the modiolus (8.508, 509). Two types of ganglion cells have been found in all mammalian species that have been studied (Kellerhals et al 1967; Spoendlin 1975; Liberman 1982; Kiang et al 1984). Large, Type I ganglion cells predominate (90–95%), the remainder being smaller Type II cells. Type I cells contain a prominent spherical nucleus, abundant ribosomes and many mitochondria; in many mammals (though not generally in humans: see Ota & Kimura 1980) they are surrounded by myelin sheaths. In contrast, Type II cells are smaller, always unmyelinated, and have a lobulated nucleus. The cytoplasm of Type II cells is enriched with neurofilaments but has fewer mitochondria and ribosomes than Type I cells (Spoendlin 1985).

There is strong evidence that Type I ganglion cells are afferent to the inner hair cells and Type II to the outer hair cells. Each inner hair cell is in synaptic contact with the unbranched peripheral

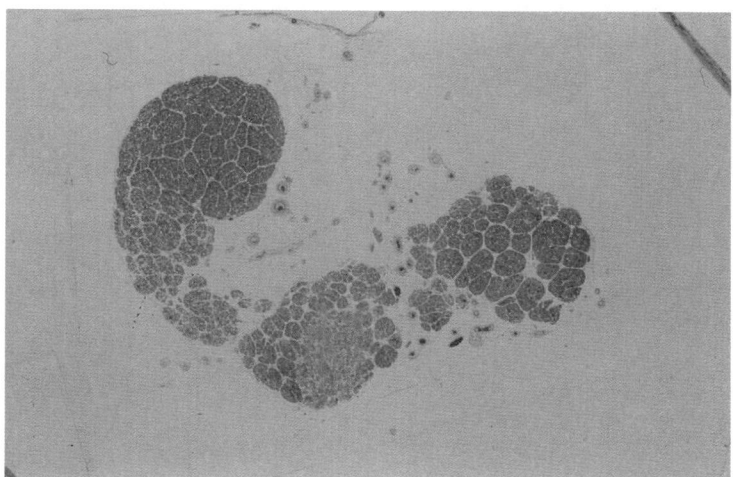

8.505 Human vestibulocochlear nerve, in transverse section. On the left, the cochlear nerve (seen as a comma-shaped profile) abuts the inferior division of the vestibular nerve (right). The singular nerve is a separate fascicle between the superior and inferior divisions of the vestibular nerve. (Magnification × 50.)

processes of approximately 10 Type I ganglion cells, while conversely those of Type II ganglion cells diverge within the spiral organ to innervate more than 10 outer hair cells (Spoendlin 1975, Liberman 1982). The peripheral and central processes of Type I ganglion cells are relatively large in diameter and myelinated whereas those of Type II are smaller and unmyelinated throughout. The peripheral processes of both radiate from the modiolus into the osseous spiral lamina where the Type I axons lose their myelin sheaths before entering the organ of Corti through the habenula perforata.

The distribution and course of the nerve fibres to inner and outer hair cells is complex, since once they have emerged from the habenula perforata many of them change course to run for variable distances along the longitudinal axis of the spiral organ before reaching their terminations. Three distinct groupings of afferent fibres have been identified: inner radial, basilar and outer spiral fibres.

Inner radial bundle. This consists of the majority of afferent fibres, running directly in a radial direction to the inner hair cells, each of which receives endings from several of these fibres, as already noted.

Basilar fibres. These are afferent to the outer hair cells; they take an independent spiral course, turning towards the cochlear apex near

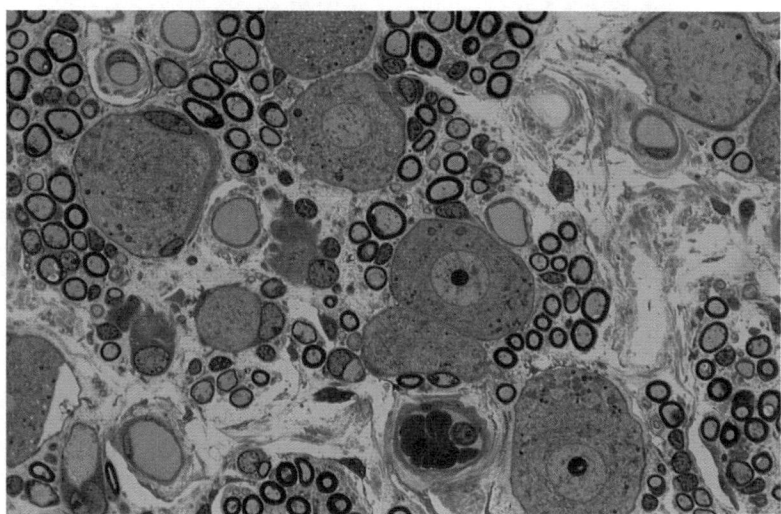

8.506 Micrograph showing part of a human vestibular ganglion, with ganglion cells and myelinated fibres. Toluidine blue stained resin section. Magnification × 200. (Supplied by H Felix, M Gleeson and L-G Johnsson, ENT Department, University of Zurich and Guy's Hospital, London.)

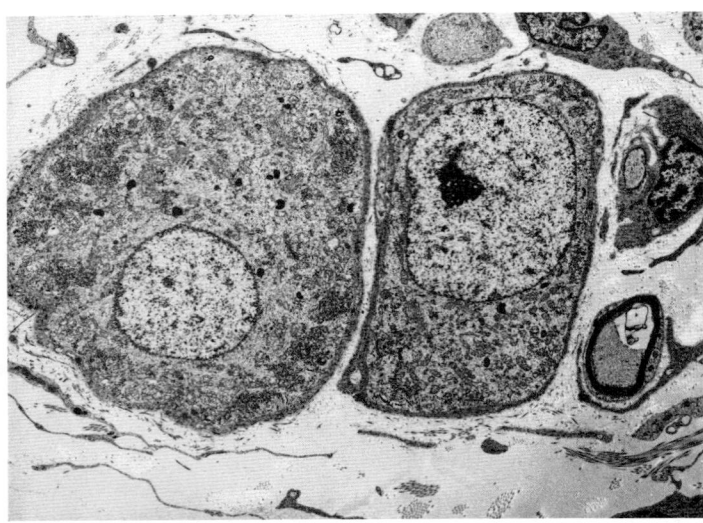

8.507 Transmission electron micrograph showing part of a vestibular ganglion (human). Two ganglion cells and myelinated nerve fibres are visible. Note the absence of myelin from the surrounding sheaths of the ganglion cells. Magnification × 2000. (Supplied by H Felix, M Gleeson and L-G Johnsson, ENT Department, University of Zurich and Guy's Hospital, London.)

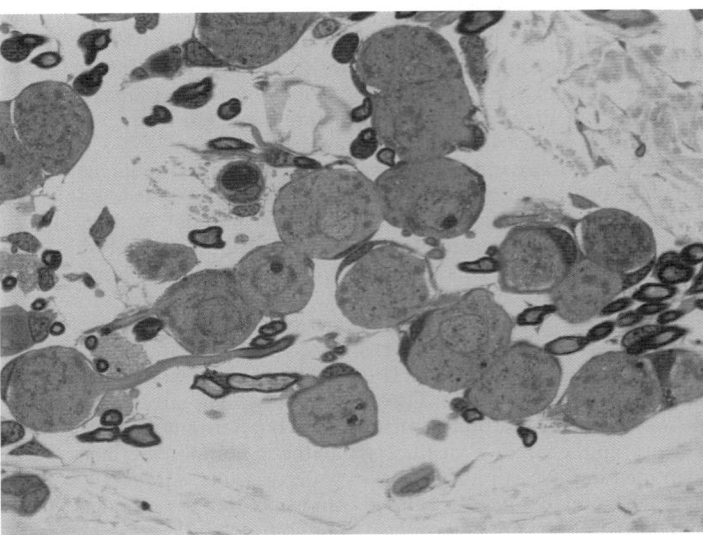

8.508 Micrograph showing part of a spiral ganglion from a human cochlea, with ganglion cells and myelinated fibres. Toluidine blue stained resin section. Magnification × 200. (Supplied by H Felix, M Gleeson and L-G Johnsson, ENT Department, University of Zurich and Guy's Hospital, London.)

the bases of the inner hair cells and running for a distance of about five of the pillar cells before turning radially again and crossing the floor of the tunnel of Corti, often diagonally, to form part of the outer spiral fibre group.

Outer spiral fibre group. It also contains efferent fibres (see below). The afferent fibres of this bundle course towards the basal part of

the cochlea, continually branching off en route to supply several outer hair cells.

Efferent cochlear neurons (8.510, 511). The efferent nerve fibres in the cochlear nerve are derived from the olivocochlear system (Rasmussen 1946; Spoendlin 1984). Within the modiolus, the efferent neurons form the intraganglionic spiral bundle which may be one or more discrete groups of fibres situated at the periphery of the spiral ganglion. It is now known that there are at least four different classes of efferent neuron, two each coming from the ipsilateral and contralateral sides of the brainstem respectively. Ipsilateral fibres derived from the medial and lateral components of the lateral superior olivary nucleus of the same side are organized into the inner spiral fibres before terminating on the afferent axons supplying the inner hair cells (p. 1391). From the contralateral side of the brainstem, other efferent fibres from the medial trapezoid body and periolivary nucleus innervate the outer hair cells. These efferent fibres cross the tunnel of Corti with the basilar fibres and synapse with the outer

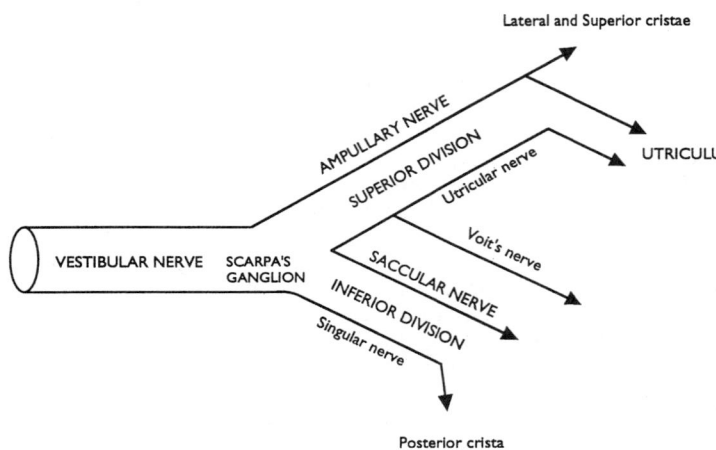

8.510 Diagram of the major branches of the vestibular nerve (see text for details). (Supplied by H Felix, M Gleeson and L-G Johnsson, ENT Department, University of Zurich and Guy's Hospital, London.)

8.509 Transmission electron micrograph showing part of a spiral ganglion (human). A number of (Type 2) ganglion cells and nerve fibres are visible. Note the absence of myelin from the surrounding sheaths of the ganglion cells. Magnification × 1500. (Supplied by H Felix, M Gleeson and L-G Johnsson, ENT Department, University of Zurich and Guy's Hospital, London.)

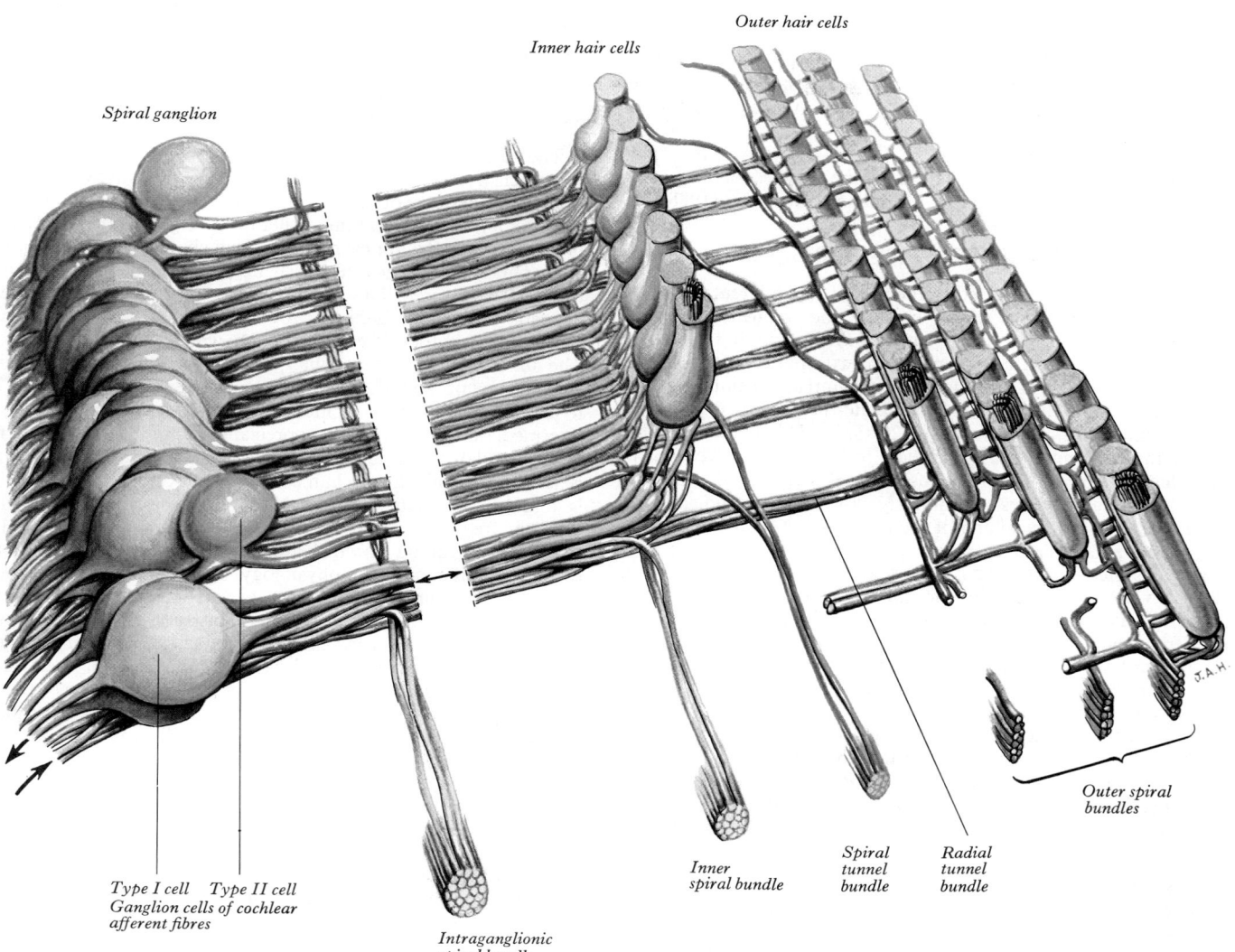

Outer hair cells

Inner hair cells

Spiral ganglion

Type I cell *Type II cell*
Ganglion cells of cochlear
afferent fibres

Intraganglionic
spiral bundle

Inner
spiral bundle

Spiral
tunnel
bundle

Radial
tunnel
bundle

Outer spiral
bundles

8.511 The innervation of the spiral organ, showing the distribution of afferent and efferent fibres. The ganglion cells of the sensory nerve fibres include those related to the inner hair cells (dark green) and others innervating the outer hair cells (light green). Efferent fibres are depicted in purple. Note the great contrast between the multiple, convergent afferent innervation of the inner hair cells (about 10 fibres to each cell) and the divergent supply of the outer hair cells (one afferent fibre to about 10 cells). This illustration is a very simplified view of the complex innervation of the spiral organ; for further details see the text.

hair cells mainly by direct contact with their bases, although a few synapse with the afferent terminals. The efferent innervation of the outer hair cells decreases along the spiral organ from cochlear base to apex, and from first (inner) row to the third. They use acetylcholine (ACh) as their chief neurotransmitter and are purely inhibitory, serving to hyperpolarize the outer hair cells which they contact.

The functions of this complex system of efferents are not yet clear. The efferents related to the inner hair cells appear to modify transmission through their inhibitory postsynaptic action on inner hair cell afferents, while those related to the outer hair cells are thought to modulate the micromechanics of the cochlea by altering the mechanical responses of the outer hair cells to sound, and therefore changing their contribution to frequency tuning (see below).

Autonomic cochlear innervation

Autonomic nerve endings have been observed but they appear to be entirely sympathetic (although any parasympathetic fibres would probably be indistinguishable from other cholinergic fibres). As in the vestibular system, there are two adrenergic systems within the cochlea, a perivascular plexus and a blood vessel-independent system, the former derived from the stellate ganglion and the latter from the superior cervical ganglion. Both systems would seem to be restricted to regions of the spiral organ on the modiolar side of the tunnel of Corti. Isolated sympathetic ganglion cells have occasionally been described in the cochlear nerve in various mammalian species.

Details of cochlear innervation are summarized in **8.510**.

VESSELS OF THE LABYRINTH

Arteries

These are:

- the labyrinthine artery (p. 1534), arising from the basilar artery, or sometimes the anterior inferior cerebellar artery.
- the stylomastoid branch of either the occipital artery or the posterior auricular artery (see p. 1519), supplying the semicircular canals.

The labyrinthine artery divides at the bottom of the internal auditory meatus into cochlear and vestibular branches. The cochlear branch divides into 12–14 twigs, traversing the canals in the modiolus and distributing as a capillary plexus to the lamina spiralis, basilar membrane, stria vascularis and other cochlear structures. Vestibular arterial branches supply the utricle, saccule and semicircular ducts (see also above).

Veins

The veins draining the vestibule and semicircular canals accompany the arteries; receiving the cochlear veins at the base of the modiolus, they form the labyrinthine vein, ending in the posterior part of the superior petrosal sinus or in the transverse sinus. A small vessel from the basal cochlear turn traverses the cochlear canaliculus to join the internal jugular vein (see p. 1379).

For details of the microvasculature of the cochlea of man and other mammals, see Axelsson (1968); Axelsson and Ryan (1988).

MECHANISM OF AUDITORY RECEPTION

Much research has been directed to the role of the different auditory components as analysers of sound intensity and frequency patterns and of the sources of the trains of sound waves impinging on them. Sound waves reaching the air column in the external acoustic meatus cause a comparable set of vibrations in the tympanic membrane and auditory ossicles. At the stapedial foot plate the force per unit area of the oscillating surface is increased 20 times. This overcomes the inertia of the perilymph, thus producing in it pressure waves which are conducted almost instantaneously to all parts of the basilar membrane. The latter varies continuously in width, mass and stiffness from the basal to the apical end of the cochlea; but its fibres are **not** under tension, as was once assumed. The behaviour of such a mechanical system as it reacts to periodic pressure waves in the perilymph varies with the frequency of the vibration. At very low frequencies, say 50 Hz, the whole membrane vibrates in phase at a similar frequency. As the frequency of the driving fluid pressure rises, different parts oscillate less rapidly and increasingly out of phase, from the basal to the apical end. *Travelling waves* hence progress along the membrane from the base to the apex. At intermediate frequencies, their *amplitude* rises slowly as they progress from the basal end to a maximum, after which the amplitude falls rapidly. With increasing frequency, the *locus* of *maximum amplitude* moves progressively from the apical to the basal end of the cochlea. Evidence for such a vibratory distribution in the basilar membrane comes from five main sources:

(1) observation of the membrane excited by sound stimuli in cadavers through drill holes in the cochlear bone, using stroboscopic illumination

(2) indirect biophysical measurements (e.g. by the Mossbauer effect) of vibrations with a probe placed in the (drained) perilymphatic space

(3) electrophysiological recording of *cochlear microphonic potential*, giving the total electrical activity in short sectors of the basilar membrane

(4) the effects of focal lesions at different loci in the membrane

(5) measurements of evoked otoacoustic emissions from the cochlea, combined with (3) and (4).

The pattern of vibrations in the basilar membrane thus varies with the intensity and frequency of the acoustic waves reaching the perilymph. Because of the arrangement of the hair cells on the basilar membrane, such oscillations generate a largely transverse shearing force between the outer hair cells which rest (indirectly) on the basilar membrane and the overlying tectorial membrane, in which the apices of stereocilia are embedded (see below). This movement depends on the mechanical properties of the whole spiral organ, including its cytoskeleton (see 8.512) which stiffens this structure. The inner hair cell stereocilia, which probably do not touch the tectorial membrane although they come very close to it, are likely to be stimulated by local movements of the endolymph. At most intermediate frequencies an appreciable sector of the basilar membrane oscillates and hence a specific group of auditory nerve fibres is activated. While the mechanical behaviour of the basilar membrane is mainly responsible for a rather broad discrimination between different frequencies (*passive tuning* see the review by Dallos 1992), the very fine tuning of which the cochlea is capable appears to be related to differences in physiology between individual hair cells which make them respond best to particular tones, even when experimentally isolated from the spiral organ. Such individual tuning of cells may be caused by differences in shape, stereocilia length or possibly variations in the molecular composition of their sensory membranes. To these factors may be added the activities of the outer hair cells, which are as yet not fully understood but may play an important part in regulating inner hair cell sensitivity at specific frequencies (*active tuning*). This is most dramatically seen in the ability of hair cells to change length when stimulated electrically, at frequencies of many thousands per second. The rapidity of such changes in length, and various other features, indicate a novel type of motile mechanism (see Holley & Ashmore 1988) possibly located in the plasma membrane itself (Kalinec et al 1992, Holley et al 1992). How such motility is used in hearing is not yet understood, but may be related to the need to adjust the mechanics of the spiral organ constantly, under the influence of the efferent pathway (see Brownell 1983; Kim 1985).

At a particular frequency an increase in the **intensity** of stimulus is signalled by an increase in the rate of discharge in individual cochlear nerve fibres, and at higher intensities, in the **number** of activated cochlear nerve fibres (recruitment). For discussion of these hypotheses consult Békésy (1960), Spoendlin (1968), Pickles (1985).

The roles of the two groups of hair cells have been much debated, particularly since differences in their innervation and physiological

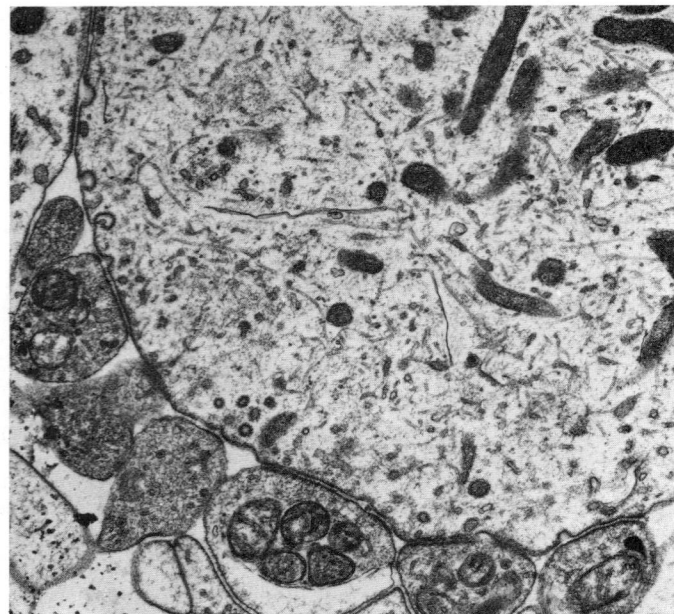

8.512 Electron micrograph of a group of efferent nerve endings at the base of an outer hair cell (guinea pig). Note the numerous mitochondria and vesicles within these endings and the cytoplasmic densities on both the pre- and postsynaptic membranes. Magnification × 10 000.

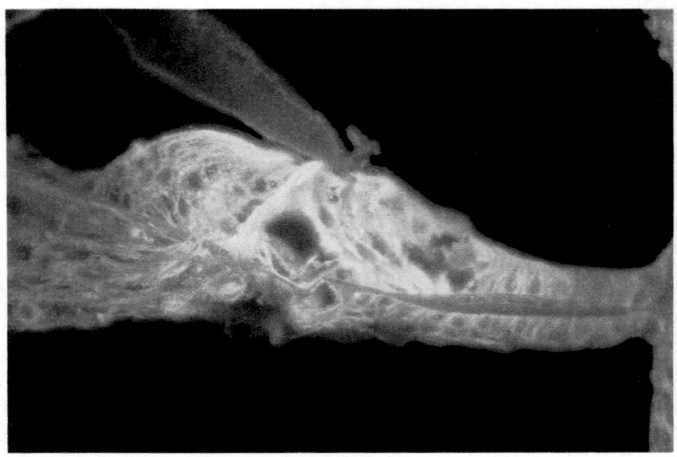

8.513 Section of the spiral organ, labelled by immunofluorescence to show the presence of tubulin, especially in the pillar and Dieters' cells. (Provided by Alun Thomas, UMDS, Guy's Campus, London.)

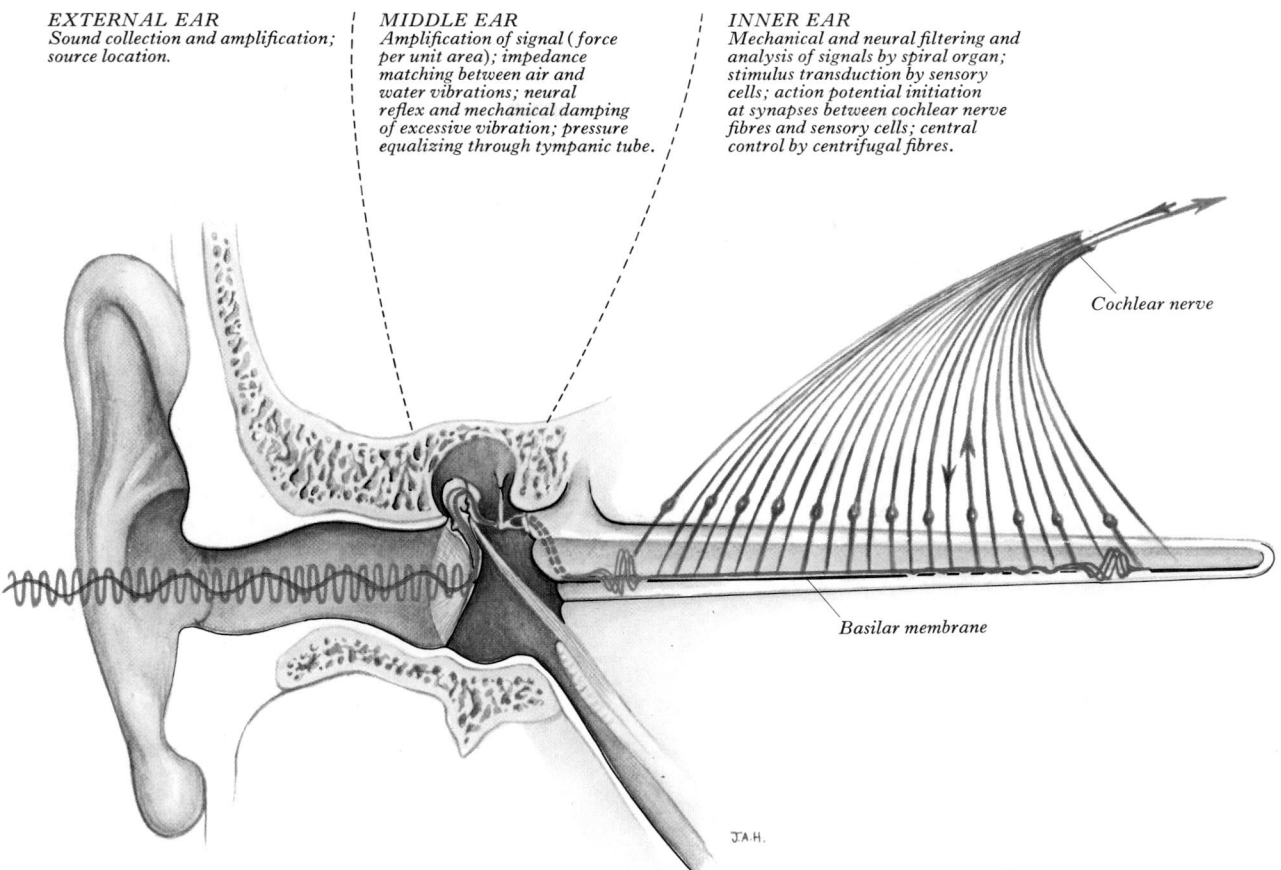

EXTERNAL EAR
Sound collection and amplification;
source location.

MIDDLE EAR
Amplification of signal (force per unit area); impedance matching between air and water vibrations; neural reflex and mechanical damping of excessive vibration; pressure equalizing through tympanic tube.

INNER EAR
Mechanical and neural filtering and analysis of signals by spiral organ; stimulus transduction by sensory cells; action potential initiation at synapses between cochlear nerve fibres and sensory cells; central control by centrifugal fibres.

Cochlear nerve

Basilar membrane

JA.H.

8.514 The principal activities of the peripheral auditory apparatus. For clarity the cochlea is depicted as though it had been uncoiled. The points of maximal stimulation of the basilar membrane by high frequency (blue) and low frequency (red) vibrations, together with their transmission pathways through the external and middle ear, are also indicated.

behaviour have become obvious. Because of their rich afferent supply internal hair cells have been favoured as the major source of auditory sensation, a view supported by much experimental and clinical evidence; for example animals treated with antibiotics specifically toxic to outer hair cells are still able to hear but discrimination is impaired (Harrison & Evans 1979).

Electrical responses of the cochlea are of considerable interest; extracellular potentials can be readily recorded with relatively crude electrode techniques (Evans 1974). The most significant is the *endolymphatic potential*, a steady potential recordable between the cochlear duct and the scala tymphani and caused by the different ionic compositions of their fluids. Since the resting potential of hair cells is about 70 mV (negative inside) and the endolymphatic potential is positive in the cochlear duct, a total transmembrane potential across the apices of hair cells is 150 mV, a higher resting potential than found anywhere else in the body.

Under stimulation by sound, a rapid oscillatory *cochlear microphonic* potential can be recorded, matching the frequency of the stimulus and movements of the basilar membrane precisely. This appears to depend on fluctuations in the conductance of hair cell membranes, probably that of the outer hair cells. At the same time an extracellular *summating potential* develops, a steady direct current shift related to the (intracellular) receptor potentials of hair cells. Cochlear nerve fibres then begin to respond with *action potentials* also recordable from the cochlea. Intracellular recording of auditory responses from inner hair cells (Russell & Sellick 1977; Oesterle & Dallos 1990) has shown that these cells resemble other receptors, their steady receptor potentials being related in size to the amplitude of the acoustic stimulus. At the same time, afferent nerve fibres are stimulated by synaptic action at the bases of the inner hair cells, firing more rapidly as vibration of the basilar membrane increases in amplitude.

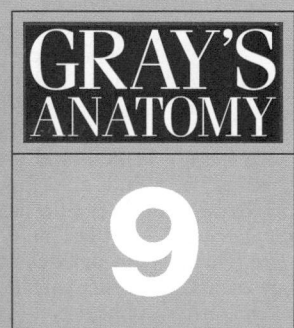

GRAY'S ANATOMY

9

HAEMOLYMPHOID SYSTEM

Section Editor: Lawrence Bannister

With contributions from Dr Philip Shepherd, the complete revision of lymphocyte biology; Professor Marion Kendall, extensive revision and illustration of thymus structure and function; Dr Marta Perry, the new section on the palatine tonsil; and Dr Niall Kirkpatrick, the new section on the nasopharyngeal tonsil.

INTRODUCTION

The haemolymphoid system is a complex array of cells and tissues which are closely interdependent in their origins and functions in the body. The **haemal** component, arising in the bone marrow, provides: *red cells* (*erythrocytes*) which carry oxygen and to a lesser extent carbon dioxide between the lungs and general tissues; a wide variety of defensive cells, *leucocytes*, including the *neutrophil*, *eosinophil* and *basophil granulocytes*, and *monocytes* (*macrophages*), engaged in a plethora of defensive activities, and *platelets* which assist in haemostasis. Of these cells, only two, erythrocytes and platelets, are generally confined to the blood vascular system once they have entered it from haemopoietic tissue. All leucocytes possess the ability to leave the circulation and enter the extravascular tissues, the numbers of cells so doing being greatly increased in local infections and other disease conditions. The **lymphoid** component includes cells which are formed both in the bone marrow and in many sites outside it: the thymus, lymph nodes, spleen and lymphoid tissue associated with the alimentary tract and bronchi (lymphoid nodules). These produce different varieties of *lymphocytes*, which in the blood are included among the leucocytes and like the others of this class are able to migrate into extravascular sites although, unlike haemal cells, lymphocytes may also be found within the channels of the lymphatic system. Lymphocytes are concerned with various types of defence and indeed are the main source of the body's ability to resist infections. Included in lymphoid tissue are various types of phagocytic cell which, with the monocytes in the blood and some other phagocytic cells in other tissues (e.g. macrophages), are often considered as a distinctive component of the body, the *mononuclear phagocyte system* (p. 1414).

HAEMAL BLOOD CELLS AND TISSUES

BLOOD

Blood is an opaque turbid fluid with a viscosity somewhat greater than that of water (mean relative viscosity 4.75 at 18°C), and a specific gravity of about 1.06 at 15°C. When oxygenated, as in the systemic arteries, it is bright scarlet and when deoxygenated, as in systemic veins, it is dark red to purple.

Blood is a heterogeneous fluid consisting of a clear liquid, *plasma*, and formed elements, *corpuscles*; because of this admixture it behaves hydrodynamically in a complex fashion and belongs to that class of fluids termed non-Newtonian. This characteristic has important consequences in the physical study of blood flow in vessels (haemorrheology).

Plasma

Plasma is a clear, slightly yellow fluid which contains many substances in solution or suspension; the *crystalloids* give a mean freezing-point depression of about 0.54°C. Plasma is rich in sodium and chloride ions and also contains potassium, calcium, magnesium, phosphate, bicarbonate and many other ions, glucose, amino acids, etc. The *colloids* include the high molecular weight plasma proteins, composed chiefly of those associated with clotting, particularly prothrombin, the immunoglobulins and complement proteins involved in immunological defence (p. 1418), glycoproteins, polypeptides and steroids concerned with hormonal activities and globulins engaged in the carriage of hormones, iron and numerous other blood-borne substances. Since most of the metabolic activities of the body are reflected in the composition of the plasma, routine chemical analysis of this fluid has become of great diagnostic importance and a considerable body of information on its chemistry is available.

The formation of clots by the precipitation of the protein fibrin from the plasma is initiated by the release of specific materials from damaged cells and blood platelets (p. 1406) in the presence of calcium ions. If blood or plasma samples are allowed to stand, clot formation occurs to leave a clear yellowish fluid, the *serum*. Removal of the available calcium ions by means of citrate, various organic calcium chelators (EDTA, EGTA) and oxalate prevents clot formation in vitro; heparin is also widely used as an anticlotting agent, its action interfering with another part of the complex series of chemical interactions leading to fibrin clot formation.

Blood as a tissue

Blood has many affinities with connective tissue, as, for example, in the mesenchymal origin of its cells, the free exchange of leucocytes with the connective tissues and the relatively low cell:matrix ratio. The plasma substances and cells, however, arise from more than one source and so blood is really a composite tissue pool.

Formed elements of blood

Blood contains three groups of formed elements: red and white blood cells and platelets. Some structural aspects of these elements are visible in fresh blood, but many others are seen only in fixed and stained specimens. The examination of blood cells is of considerable clinical importance since their numbers, proportions of different cell types and structure are valuable indicators of pathological changes in the body. Amongst other techniques, the Romanowsky methods of staining are particularly valuable and are widely used in clinical laboratories. These methods involve staining in aqueous solutions with methylene blue–eosin mixtures which colour both acidic dye binding and basic dye binding structures. The Giemsa and Leishman stains belong to this group. It should be noted that throughout this section, the figures given for cell dimensions and numbers are approximate ranges only. The data provided by different authorities vary somewhat; further, the dimensions of some cells when measured in the fresh state are substantially smaller than when measured in a dried smear; with erythrocytes the converse applies.

ERYTHROCYTES (9.1–3, 5A)

Erythrocytes (red blood cells, red blood corpuscles) form the greater proportion of the blood cells (99% of the total number), with a count of $4.1–6.0 \times 10^6/\mu l$ in adult males and $3.9–5.5 \times 10^6/\mu l$ in adult females. Each cell is a biconcave disc with a diameter in dried smear preparations of 6.3–7.9 μm (mean 7.1 μm) and a rim thickness of 1.9 μm; in wet preparations the mean diameter is 8.6 μm. Erythrocytes lack nuclei and are pale red by transmitted light, with paler centres because of their biconcavity. They show a tendency to adhere to one another by their rims to form loose piles of cells (*rouleaux*), a character determined by the properties of their cell coat. In normal

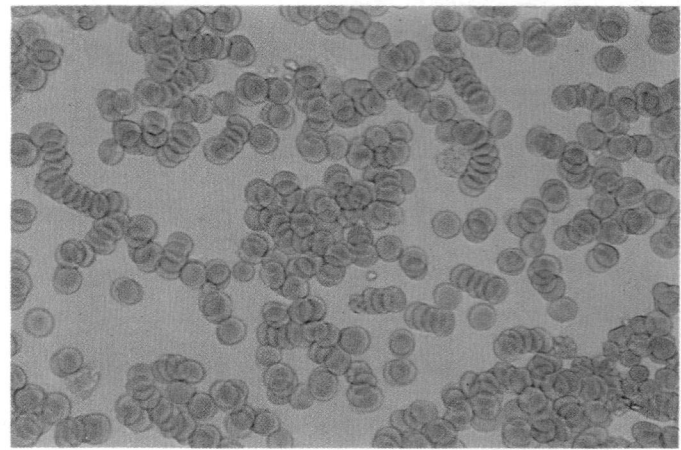

9.1 Fresh preparation of living erythrocytes showing rouleau formation and red pigmentation. Magnification × 500.

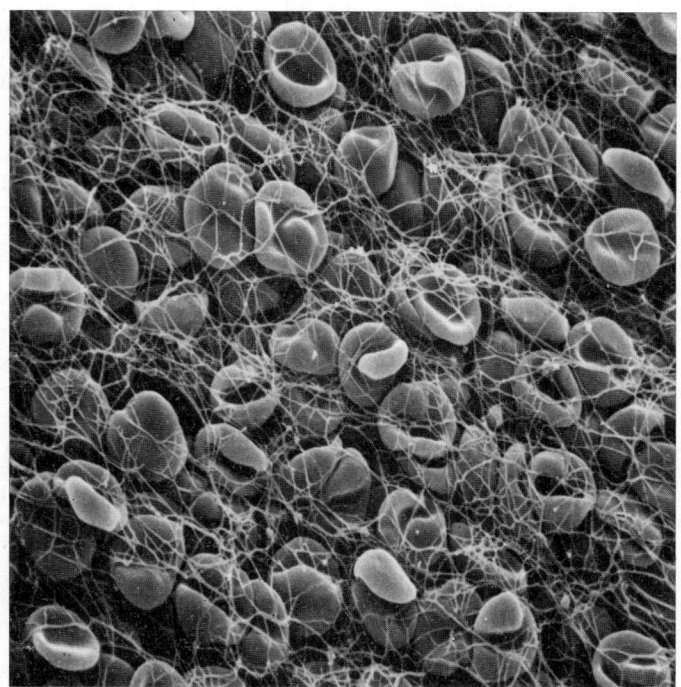

9.2 A scanning electron micrograph of erythrocytes, showing biconcave discoidal and other shapes; the filaments are fibrin resulting from clotting of the plasma after extravasation of blood. Magnification × 1500. (Photographed by Michael Crowder, Guy's Hospital, London.)

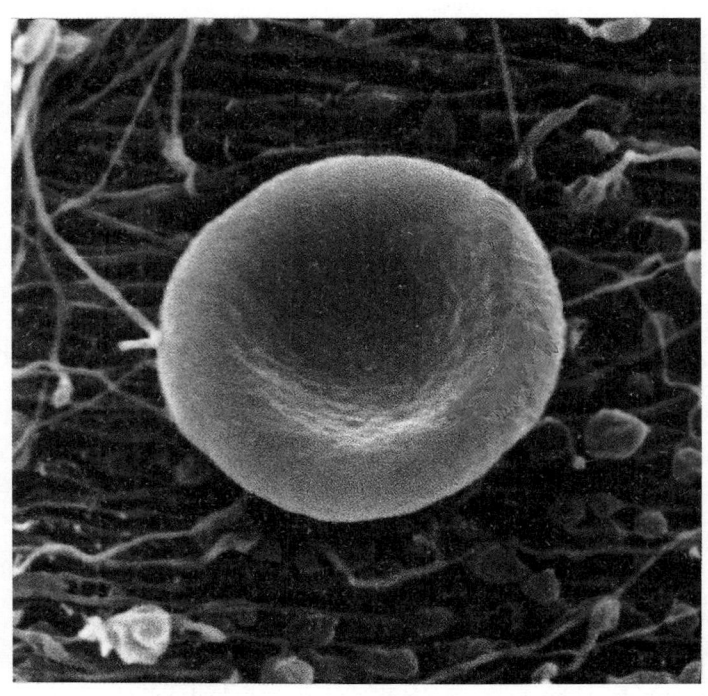

9.3 Scanning electron micrograph of an erythrocyte.

blood a few assume a shrunken star-like, *crenated* form, a shape which can be reproduced by placing normal biconcave erythrocytes in a hypertonic solution, which results in osmotic shrinkage. Such cells are called *echinocytes* (Bessis 1973). In hypotonic solutions erythrocytes take up water and become spherical and may eventually lyse to release their haemoglobin (*haemolysis*); they are then termed *red cell ghosts* (erythrocytic umbrae).

Erythrocytes are bounded by a plasma membrane and consist internally mainly of a single protein, haemoglobin. The plasma membrane of erythrocytes has received much attention because of the ease with which it can be obtained for analysis in quantity (Bretscher & Raff 1975). It is about 60% lipid and glycolipid and 40% protein and glycoprotein. More than 15 classes of protein are present, including two major types. Firstly, the glycoproteins *glycophorins A* and *B* (each with a molecular mass of about 50 kDa) span the membrane, and their negatively charged carbohydrate chains project from the outer surface of the cell, conferring most of the fixed charge on the cell exterior by virtue of their sialic acid groups. Secondly, comes the 'Band 2' protein which may bear some antigenic groups; 'Band 3' protein is also a transmembrane macromolecule, constituting the important chloride channels in the erythrocyte membrane; these proteins are probably mainly present in the form of dimers, which are visible as intramembranous particles in freeze-fractured erythrocyte membranes; the ABO antigens (p. 1406) are all glycolipids (Race & Sanger 1975). Other proteins include several enzyme systems, some concerned with ionic regulation, others with the addition of lipid to the cell membrane from serum lipid. (This is necessary because the cell does not possess its own synthetic apparatus.)

The shape of the eythrocyte is largely determined by the protein *spectrin* (a name which reflects its biochemical preparation from red cell 'ghosts') which is attached to integral membrane proteins (Band 3) on the inner surface of the cell membrane via short lengths of actin filaments and other proteins (e.g. 'Band 4.2' protein, and *ankyrin*), forming a stabilizing network. This considerably stiffens the membrane, an effect which is aided by the large amount of cholesterol in the membrane itself. Red cells can thus regain their shape and dimensions after passing through the lumina of the finest ramules of the blood-vascular system; microscopic examination has

shown that erythrocytes often pass through capillaries flattened face-first, buckling somewhat to a shield-like shape (Brånemark 1972) rather than rolling up, as might be expected.

Haemoglobin

Haemoglobin is a globular protein with a molecular mass of 67 kDa, consisting of *globulin* molecules bound to haem, an iron-containing *porphyrin* group (Purutz et al 1960). Each molecule is made up of four subunits, each in turn consisting of a coiled polypeptide chain with a cleft holding a single haem group. In normal blood, four types of polypeptide chain can occur, namely: α, β, γ and δ. Each haemoglobin molecule contains 2 α-chains and two others, so that several combinations and hence a number of different types of haemoglobin molecule are possible. Haemoglobin A (HbA), which is the major adult class, contains 2 α- and 2 β-chains. Haemoglobin A_2 (HbA2), a minor component in adults, is composed of 2 α- and 2 δ-chains. Haemoglobin F (HbF), found in fetal and early postnatal life, consists of 2 α- and 2 γ-chains. In the pathological condition *thalassaemia* only one type of chain is synthesized, so that a molecule may contain 4 α-chains (β-thalassaemia) or, more commonly, 4 β-chains (α-thalassaemia)—Haemoglobin H.

Each polypeptide chain is determined by a separate gene; a number of variant haemoglobins are known in which only one or a few amino acid residues are abnormal, reflecting slight alterations in the corresponding genes. In the Haemoglobin S of sickle-cell disease a single alteration in the β-chains (valine substituted for glutamine) causes a major alteration in the behaviour of the red cell and its oxygen-carrying capacity which, however, may confer some protection against malarial infection in areas where the disease is endemic. Other common variants include Haemoglobins C and D. The oxygen-binding power of haemoglobin is provided by the iron atoms of the haem groups, and these are always maintained in the ferrous (Fe^{++}) state by the presence of glutathione within the erythrocyte.

In addition to haemoglobin, erythrocytes possess a number of enzyme systems, notably those concerned with glycolysis and ionic transport, which together maintain low sodium levels within the cell against diffusion gradients, and thus create the appropriate conditions of pH and ionic strength for the normal functioning of haemoglobin. As intimated above, glutathione metabolism is also active. Although, of course, in the absence of a nucleus and ribosomes, no protein synthesis takes place in mature erythrocytes, lipid in the plasma membrane can be replaced to some extent from circulating serum lipids, by the activity of membrane enzyme systems synthesized and placed in the red cell membrane during formation in the bone marrow.

The iron-containing compound *ferritin* is also often present in newly formed erythrocytes, as are also persisting remnants of the apparatus of protein synthesis (ribosomal and other RNAs) from the stage of differentiation of the cell in the bone marrow. After Romanovsky staining, the residual RNA of young erythrocytes causes a slight bluish tinge; with the supravital stain brilliant cresyl blue it forms a reticulum, giving the name *reticulocyte* to this type of cell. Later in maturation such evidences of basophilia disappear. Other inclusions may be present in red cells, particularly in pathological conditions; amongst these are nuclear remnants (*Howell-Jolly bodies*) and altered haemoglobin (*Heinz-Ehrlich bodies*).

Life span and destruction

Erythrocytes which have been labelled radioactively or antigenically and then injected into the circulation, have been shown to last between 100 and 120 days before being destroyed (Berlin et al 1959). As erythrocytes age they become increasingly fragile and their surface charges decrease as their content of negatively charged membrane glycoproteins is progressively reduced (Marikovsky & Danon 1969). The lipid content of the membranes also lessens. Aged erythrocytes are eventually ingested by the macrophages of the spleen and liver sinusoids, without previous lysis, and are then hydrolysed. Here, the haemoglobin is broken into its globulin and porphyrin moieties; the globulin is then further degraded into its constituent amino acids which pass to the general amino-acid pool of the body. The iron is removed from the porphyrin and can be used either directly in the synthesis of new haemoglobin in the bone marrow, or stored in the liver as ferritin or haemosiderin; the remaining haem portion is converted in the liver to bilirubin and is then excreted in the bile. The recognition of the senescent erythrocytes by macrophages appears to depend, at least in part, on the exposure of normal inaccessible parts of the Band 3 molecules in their membranes, causing auto-antibodies in the plasma to bind to them and sensitizing the cells to macrophage removal. Such altered, antigenic sequences are referred to as erythrocyte senescence antigens.

Red cells are produced by the bone marrow and are destroyed at the rate of about 5×10^{11} cells a day.

Fetal erythrocytes up to the fourth month of gestation differ markedly from those of adults, in that they are larger ($10 \mu m$), are nucleated and contain a somewhat different type of haemoglobin (HbF). From this time they are progressively replaced by the adult type of cell.

LEUCOCYTES (9.4, 5)

Leucocytes (*white blood corpuscles* or *cells*) belong to at least five different categories, distinguishable by their size, nuclear shape and cytoplasmic inclusions (**9.5**). For practical convenience, these types of cell are often divided into two main groups, namely those with prominent stainable cytoplasmic granules, the granulocytes, and those without, the agranulocytes. However, in terms of their biology, this distinction is now known to be quite arbitrary.

Granulocytes. Also known as *granular leucocytes*, they all possess irregular or multilobed nuclei and are often termed *polymorphonuclear leucocytes* for this reason. This group is comprised of three types of cell, the granules of which give different staining reactions with the Romanovsky dyes: they are *eosinophil* leucocytes with granules which bind acidic dyes such as eosin, *basophil* leucocytes the granules of which bind basic dyes (methylene blue) strongly and *neutrophil* leucocytes whose granules stain weakly with both elements by a different type of reaction (see Wintrobe et al 1981; Zucker-Franklin et al 1981).

NEUTROPHIL LEUCOCYTES (9.4A, 5B)

Neutrophil polymorphonuclear leucocytes (*neutrophils, neutrophiles, heterophile leucocytes* or '*polymorphs*') form the largest proportion of the leucocytes (60–70% in adults, with a count of 3000–6000/μl). In dried smears, where the cells have flattened, they have a circular profile with a diameter of 10–15 μm. In the living state the cells may be spherical whilst passively circulating, but can flatten and become actively motile on contact with a suitable surface.

Within the cytoplasm the numerous granules give a variety of colour shades ranging from violet to pink when stained with Romanowsky stains such as Wright's and May-Grünwald-Giemsa, which are commonly employed in haematology. Under the electron microscope, too, the *granules* are heterogeneous in size, shape and content, but all are membrane-bound bodies containing hydrolytic and other enzymes. Two major categories can be distinguished according to their developmental origin and contents (Bainton et al 1971). Firstly, *non-specific* or *primary granules* which are formed early in neutrophil genesis (p. 1413); these are relatively large (0.5 μm) spheroidal lysosomes containing myeloperoxidase, acid phosphatase and several other enzymes. With light microscopy they stain strongly with neutral red and azure dyes and are thus said to be azurophilic. Secondly, *specific* or *secondary granules*, formed a little later, assume a wide range of shapes including spheres, ellipsoids and rods. These contain several substances with strong bactericidal actions, including alkaline phosphatase, aminopeptidase, lactoferrin and also collagenase, all of which are lacking in the primary granules. The secondary granules, however, lack peroxidase and acid phosphatase. Some enzymes such as lysozyme are present in both. The presence of these granules correlates well with the phagocytic activity of neutrophils.

In *mature neutrophil* granulocytes the nucleus is characteristically multilobate with up to six segments joined by narrow nuclear strands (the *segmented* stage). Less mature cells have fewer lobes, the earliest to be released under normal conditions being *juveniles* (*band* or *stab cells*) in which the nucleus is an unsegmented crescentic band. In certain clinical conditions, even earlier stages in neutrophil formation with indented or rounded nuclei (*metamyelocytes* or *myelocytes*, p. 1413) may be released from the bone marrow. In mature cells the edges of the nuclear lobes are often irregular; in females about 3% (range 1–17%) of the nuclei of neutrophils show a conspicuous 'drumstick' formation which represents the sex chromatin of the inactive X chromosome (*Barr body*; see also p. 63).

Mitochondria, a Golgi complex, a sparse endoplasmic reticulum and glycogen are present in the cytoplasm. A cytoskeleton of actin and myosin filaments is present, and a conspicuous array of microtubules is often seen between the 'arms' of the nucleus; it is interesting that locomotion of neutrophils is in the direction in which the free arms point. Neutrophil locomotion is dependent on actin–myosin interactions (see p. 739).

Neutrophils form an important element in the defence systems of the body; they can endocytose microbes and particles in the circulation and, after migrating between the endothelial cells lining capillaries or venules, can perform local phagocytosis in the extravascular tissues, wherever it is needed. The engulfing of foreign objects is followed by digestion through fusion of the phagocytic vacuole, first with the *specific* granules, the pH being reduced to 4.0 by active transport of protons, then with the *non*-specific (azurophilic, primary) granules, which finish the process of bacterial killing and digestion. The chemical reactions occurring in these events have been intensively studied and prove to be quite complex. They involve the oxidation and addition of halide (chloride and iodide) radicals to the engulfed materials by means of enzymic action (myeloperoxidase, etc.) which have the effects of denaturing their proteins and other macromolecules. Lysozyme and lactoferrin are also highly toxic to bacteria. These processes require atmospheric oxygen for successful completion, so that neutrophils active in defence have a high oxygen demand. Phagocytosis, or the release of granules, may be enhanced by the presence of antibodies attached to the surfaces of neutrophils which can bind specifically to target antigens, for example in a type of bacterium to which the body has previously been exposed. Opsonizing antibodies (*opsonins*, p. 1420) coating the antigenic target may also promote phagocytosis. The antibodies in both cases are secreted by lymphocytes (p. 1420), and the neutrophil granulocyte is just one in a series of defensive cells which form an interrelated system for the elimination of foreign materials from the tissues.

After phagocytosis, the neutrophil's cytoplasmic granules gradually become used up, so that a marked reduction in their number (degranulation) occurs. Granules may also be discharged from the surface of the cell when it is suitably stimulated, to damage or kill neighbouring organisms or cells. Inappropriate release of such enzymes is associated with various pathological conditions, for example rheumatoid arthritis, where tissue destruction and chronic inflammation may result.

The numbers of circulating neutrophils vary considerably, often rising during episodes of acute bacterial infection. They may circulate freely in the blood (the *circulatory pool*), or they may adhere to the walls of postcapillary venules and other vessels (the *marginal pool*) to re-enter the circulation when suitably recruited, for example during brief exercise or by exposure to noradrenaline. However, neutrophils are short-lived (half-life 7.5 hours); they may either be destroyed in the bloodstream, or pass through the endothelial walls

to the extravascular tissues, engaging in defence; alternatively, after entering various secretory ducts such as the bronchi, salivary gland ducts and the urinary tract, they are lost to the body. Their surfaces bear a number of well-characterized markers, including a number of adhesion molecules important in the migration of neutrophils through endothelia.

EOSINOPHIL LEUCOCYTES (9.4B, 5B)

Eosinophil leucocytes are similar in size, shape and motile capacity to neutrophils but are present only in small numbers in normal blood (100–400/ μl). Their cytoplasmic granules are uniformly large (0.5 μm) and give the living cell a slightly yellowish colour; with

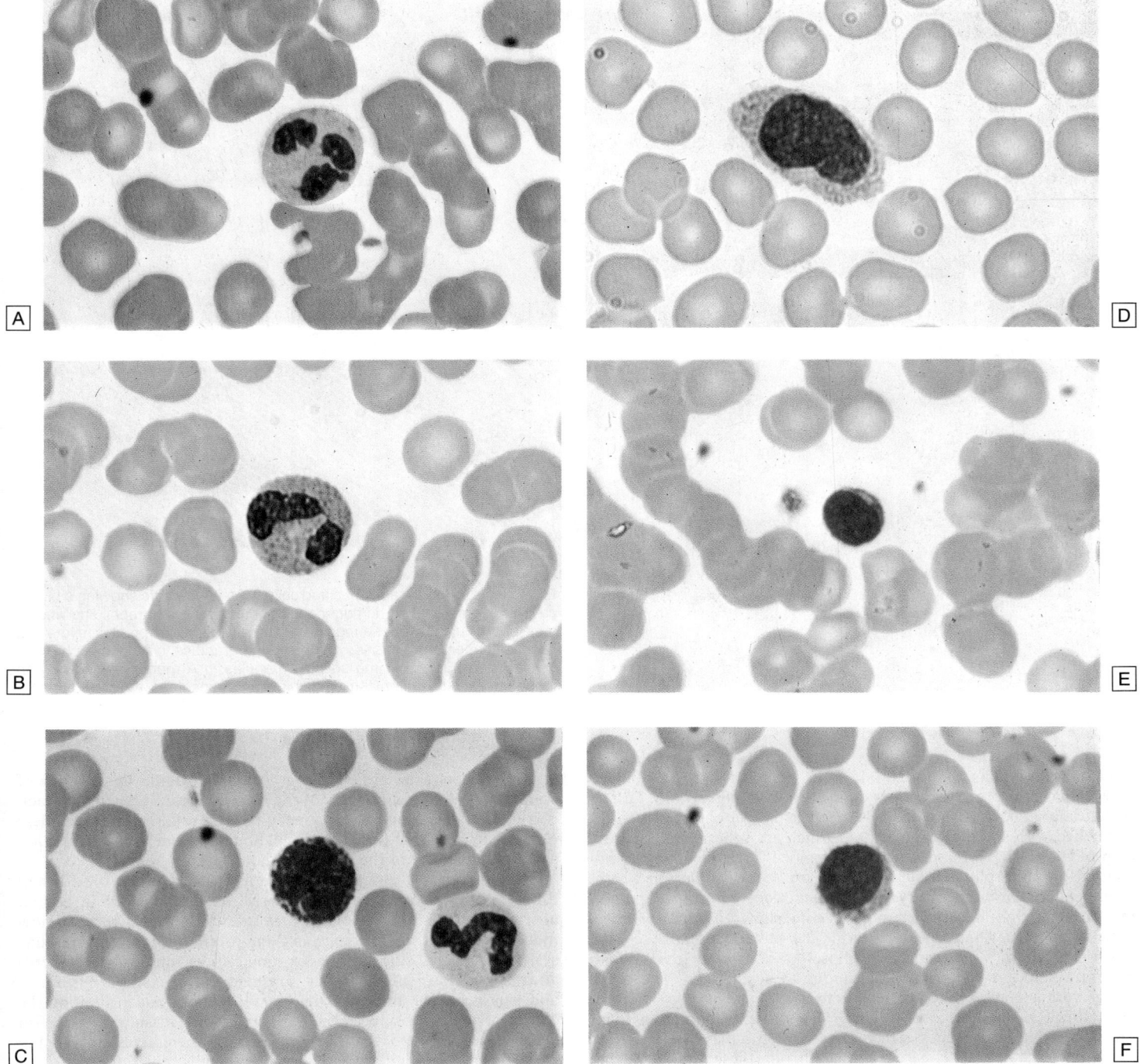

9.4 Blood cell types stained in smeared preparations by the Giemsa method. Erythrocytes are shown in all figures, which also demonstrate other cell types. A Neutrophil leucocyte and platelets. B Eosinophil leucocyte. C Basophil leucocyte with prominent densely staining cytoplasmic granules and neutrophil leucocyte. D Monocyte. E Small lymphocyte. F Medium-sized lymphocyte. (Material provided by J P Black, Department of Haematology, Guy's Hospital.)

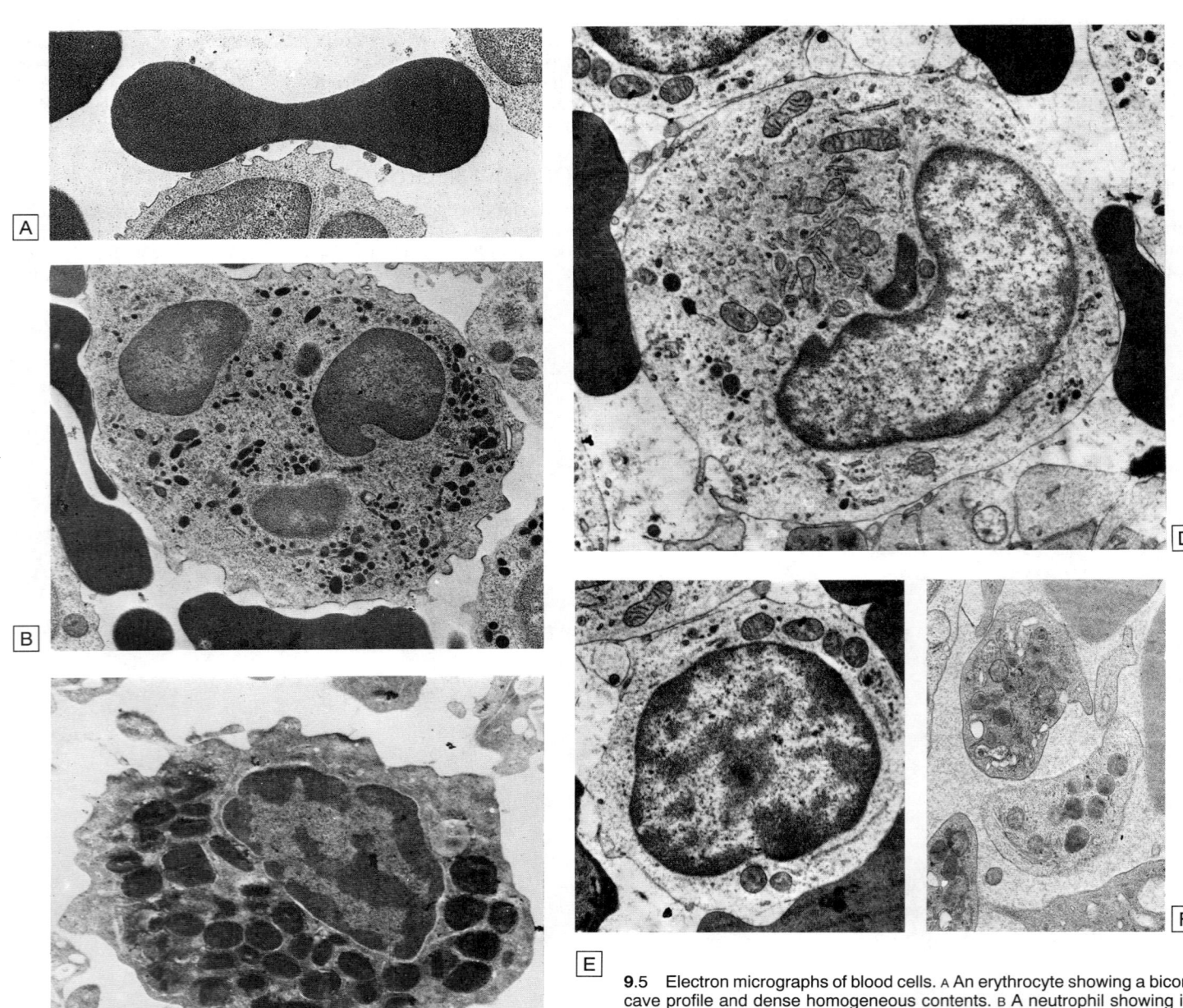

9.5 Electron micrographs of blood cells. A An erythrocyte showing a biconcave profile and dense homogeneous contents. B A neutrophil showing its multilobed nucleus appearing in section as separate profiles. Note the various shapes and densities of the specific granules. C An eosinophil, with crystalline inclusions in the specific granules. D A monocyte showing an indented nucleus, endoplasmic reticulum and lysosomes. E A small lymphocyte. F A group of platelets. (See text for further details.)

Romanowsky stains they are uniformly orange to red (**9.**4). The nucleus has two prominent lobes connected by a thin strand. Ultrastructurally (Zucker-Franklin 1980, 1985), the cytoplasm is seen to be packed with specific granules (**9.**5) which are spherical or slightly ellipsoidal. Each of these bodies is bounded by a membrane and contains an amorphous material (the *matrix* or *externum*) in which is embedded a prominent crystal (the *crystalline core* or *internum*); in human eosinophils the crystalline core shows a square lattice structure with a 4 nm repeat pattern. The matrix contains several lysosomal enzymes including acid phosphatase, ribonuclease, phospholipase and a myeloperoxidase unique to eosinophils. The crystalline core is composed of the characteristic *major basic protein*, of about 9.2 kDa in molecular weight. This protein contains a high ratio of arginine residues which give the granules their strong eosinophilic staining properties. Apart from these granules, the cytoplasmic organelles are similar to those of neutrophil granulocytes.

Like other leucocytes, eosinophils are able to pass into the extravascular tissues from the circulation when suitably stimulated. In small numbers they are typical constituents of the dermis and of connective tissue components of the bronchial tree, alimentary tract, uterus and vagina and thymic medulla. The total life span of these cells is a few days, of which about 30 hours is spent in the circulation and the remainder in the extravascular tissues.

The functions of eosinophils are not yet fully understood. Their ratio to other leucocytes rises greatly (an *eosinophilia*) in certain allergic disorders, and also in worm infestations, and there is now much evidence that they play an important part in the immune system, phagocytosing and inactivating antigen–antibody complexes and also various inflammatory substances, for example histamine and leukotrienes I and II so they may be important in limiting the effects of these substances on the surrounding tissues. It has also been shown in vitro that they can attach themselves to and kill parasitic schistosome larvae which invade the circulation.

BASOPHIL LEUCOCYTES (**9.**4c, 5c)

Like other granulocytes, these are 10–15 μm in diameter (**9.**4), but form only 0.5–2% of the total leucocyte population of normal blood, with a count of 25–200/μl. Their distinguishing feature is the presence of large, conspicuous basophilic granules (**9**.4c), varying in number from 10 to 100 per cell. The nucleus is somewhat irregular but not usually lobated, unlike those of the other granulocytes. Ultrastructurally, the basophilic granules are membrane-bound vesicles with densely stained contents showing a variety of crystalline, lamellar and granular inclusions. Heparin, histamine and several other inflammatory agents are contained in these granules, which closely resemble those of mast cells (p. 79). These substances are apparently associated with polysaccharides, since the granules are also positive to carbohydrate stains, for example periodic acid-Schiff (PAS) and Azure A, with which they are *metachromatic*, i.e. they stain a different colour from that of the dye. Their life span in the circulation is long (9–18 months in mice).

Although they resemble mast cells (Selye 1965) and, like these, are formed in the bone marrow, there is much evidence that many basophils represent a different, albeit closely related, cell line peculiar to the circulation, as shown by their reactions with monoclonal antibodies and differences in cell development (see also p. 1414). It is likely, however, that they include true mast cell precursors en route from the bone marrow to the extravascular tissues. Their functions in the circulatory system are at present rather obscure.

MONOCYTES (**9**.4D, 5D)

Monocytes are the largest of the agranular leucocytes (15–20 μm in diameter in smears) but they form only a small proportion of the total leucocytes (2–8% with a count of 100–700/μl of blood). The nucleus, which is euchromatic, is relatively large and has a characteristic indentation on one side. The cytoplasm forms a wide rim around the nucleus, near the indentation of which lies a prominent Golgi complex and vesicles stainable with neutral red. Ultrastructurally (Cawley & Hayhoe 1973; Zucker-Franklin et al 1981), many lysosomes are seen to be present, together with some peripheral rough endoplasmic reticulum. Mitochondria are quite abundant and the skeleton is well represented, reflecting the highly motile nature of the cell. Monocytes are actively phagocytic.

Their surfaces express Class II major histocompatibility complex (MHC) antigens and various CD44 markers which show that they belong to the mononuclear phagocyte family, and are indeed identical to macrophages. It would appear that monocytes are macrophages in the process of passing from the bone marrow, where they are formed, to the peripheral tissues via the bloodstream, these cells passing into extravascular sites through the walls of capillaries and venules. This topic is discussed further on pages 1414–1415.

LYMPHOCYTES (**9**.4E, F, 5E, 13–15)

Lymphocytes (**9**.4, 5) are the second most numerous type of leucocyte, forming 20–30% of their total number, i.e. 1500–2700/μl of blood. Like other leucocytes, they are also found in extravascular tissue, but they are remarkable in being formed in large numbers outside the bone marrow as well as within it. They therefore constitute a widely distributed *lymphoid* system (see p. 1417 for a fuller description).

Structural classification

Morphologically, in the blood, the term 'lymphocyte' refers to agranular leucocytes 5–15 μm in diameter. This size range represents a heterogeneous collection mainly of B and T lymphocytes in different stages of activity and maturity. About 85% of all circulating lymphocytes in normal blood are T cells. Included under the 'lymphocyte' heading are also a small percentage of cells ('null cells') which are not apparently true lymphocytes at all but either related cells (e.g. natural killer cells) or some other quite different form, such as circulating haemopoietic stem cells, antigen-presenting cells, and precursors of osteoclasts and chondroclasts in the process of passing from the bone marrow to other tissues. The various types and conditions of cells can now be at least partially separated by means of immunocytochemical techniques, involving the use of monoclonal antibodies (see p. 1420) raised against different components of their cytoplasm. Where these detect specific macromolecules exposed at the surface of lymphocytes, living cells can also

be separated into different classes by various techniques such as the fluorescence cell sorter.

In this account the B and T lymphocytes will form the main focus of description, except where otherwise stated. The terms B lymphocyte or T lymphocyte will all be used interchangeably with B cell and T cell respectively.

Small lymphocytes (both B and T cells) form the majority of lymphocytes in circulating blood. These are by definition within the size range 5–8 μm (some authorities extend this to 10 μm). Each cell contains a rounded densely staining nucleus, surrounded by a very narrow rim of cytoplasm. The nucleus contains dense, coarse bands of chromatin (a leptochromatic nucleus: *leptos* = a thread), and one or more small nucleoli. The cytoplasm stains slightly blue with Romanovsky dyes. Under the electron microscope (**9**.5E, 15), few organelles can be seen in the cytoplasm, apart from a small number of mitochondria, single ribosomes (monosomes), sparse profiles of endoplasmic reticulum and occasional lysosomes; these features indicate a low metabolic rate and such lymphocytes are said to be in the 'resting' phase. However, these cells are freely motile when they settle on to solid surfaces, and can pass between endothelial cells to exit from or enter the vascular system. They may make extensive migrations within the various tissues, including the epithelia, even passing into the body's secretions such as saliva.

Larger lymphocytes 9–15 μm in diameter, again belonging to both B and T cell classes, constitute within the circulation a mixture of very immature cells (lymphoblasts) capable of cell division to produce small lymphocytes, and maturing or mature cells which have become functionally active after stimulation by the immune system, for example in the presence of antigens (see p. 1407). Both lymphoblasts and maturing cells are actively engaged in synthesizing proteins, and thus contain a nucleus which is at least in part euchromatic, and a basophilic cytoplasm with numerous polyribosome clusters. The ultrastructure of these cells varies according to their class and will be described where appropriate (see below).

The life span of lymphocytes ranges from a few days to perhaps many years and so we can distinguish between *short-lived* and *long-lived* lymphocytes, the latter being of some significance in the mechanisms of *immunological memory* (but see p. 1421).

PLATELETS (**9**.6, 7)

Blood platelets, also known as *thrombocytes* (**9**.5, 6), are relatively small (2–4 μm across) irregular or oval discs present in large numbers (250 000–500 000/μl) in blood. In freshly taken blood samples they

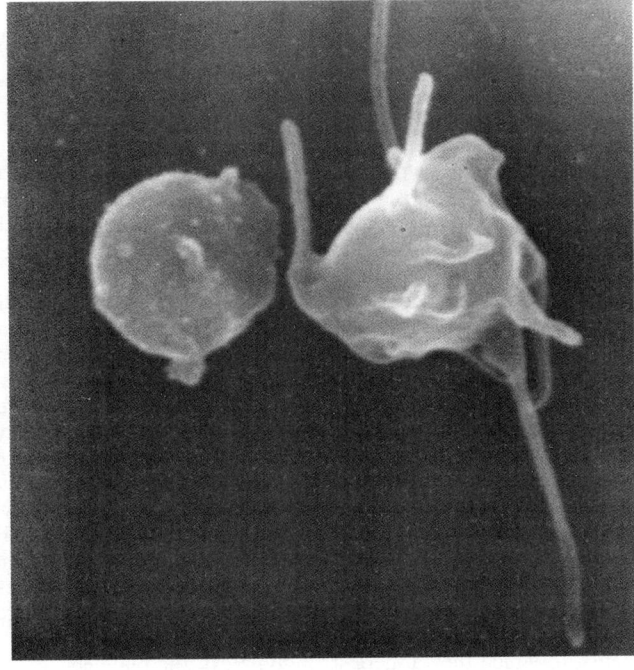

9.6   Scanning electron micrograph of a platelet with extended filopodia.

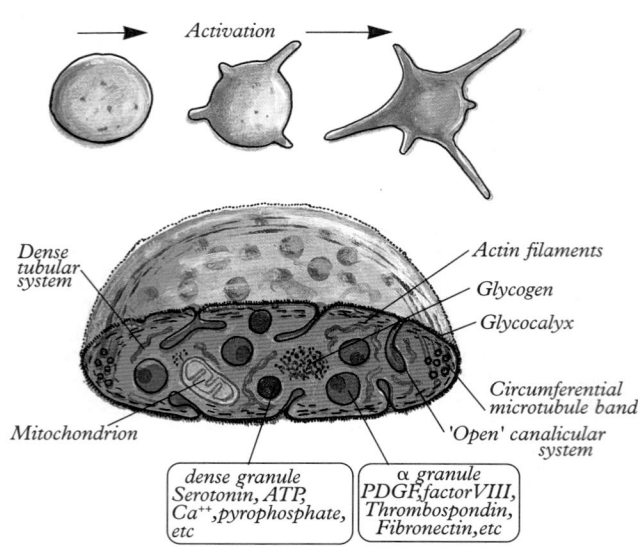

Activation

Dense tubular system

Mitochondrion

Actin filaments

Glycogen

Glycocalyx

Circumferential microtubule band

'Open' canalicular system

dense granule
Serotonin, ATP,
Ca⁺⁺, pyrophosphate,
etc

α granule
PDGF, factor VIII,
Thrombospondin,
Fibronectin, etc

9.7 Diagram of the internal organization of a platelet.

readily adhere to each other and to all available surfaces, unless the blood is treated with citrate or other substances which reduce the availability of calcium ions. In Romanowsky-stained preparations, platelets show an outer clear zone (*hyalomere*) and in inner basophilic (or azurophilic) granular region (*granulomere*). Ultrastructurally (Cawley & Hayhoe 1973; Zucker-Franklin et al 1981), each platelet is seen to be anucleate, unlike similar cells in submammalian vertebrates (for which the term *thrombocytes* is perhaps best reserved). Each platelet is surrounded by a plasma membrane bearing a thick glycoprotein-rich coat, responsible for the adhesive properties of platelets. Beneath the surface is a band of about 10 microtubules which runs around the perimeter of the cell and probably determines its shape. Associated with these are actin filaments, myosin and other proteins related to cell contraction. Within the cytoplasm are also mitochondria, glycogen, a few profiles of agranular endoplasmic reticulum, including some narrow tubular channels and tubular invaginations of the plasma membrane and various membrane-bounded vesicles. These vesicles include three major types, designated alpha, delta and lambda granules.

Alpha-granules are the most prominent, with diameters of up to 500 nm; they contain platelet-derived growth factor (PDGF), fibrinogen and other substances. In the smaller (300 nm) *delta*-granules are 5-hydroxytryptamine (serotonin), concentrated from the blood plasma by endocytosis; calcium ions, adenosine 5′-diphosphate (ADP), adenosine 5′-triphosphate (ATP) and pyrophosphate are also present. In the smaller (250 nm) *lambda* set, granules contain several lysosomal enzymes (Bentfield & Bainton 1975).

Platelets are important in haemostasis (the limiting of bleeding after injury to vessels) and a number of more general, systemic functions, which at present are rather poorly understood. When a blood vessel is damaged, platelets first aggregate at the site of injury, assisting to staunch the wound with a *platelet plug*. Adhesion between platelets (agglutination) and to other tissues is a function of the thick platelet coat and is promoted strongly by the release of ADP and calcium ions from the platelets as a response to vessel injury. Then, substances released from the alpha-granules, together with factors released from the damaged tissues, initiate a complex sequence of chemical reactions in the blood plasma, leading to the precipitation of insoluble *fibrin* filaments, generating a three-dimensional mesh-work, the *fibrin clot*, to which more platelets attach, inserting extensions of their surfaces (filopodia) deep into the spaces between the filaments, to which they adhere strongly. Next, the platelets contract (*clot retraction*) by actin–myosin interactions within their cytoplasm

(p. 45), concentrating the fibrin clot and pulling the adhering walls of the blood vessel together, limiting further any leakage of blood. Eventually, on repair of the vessel wall, *clot removal* occurs as a result of complicated enzymic activities, including those of *plasmin* formed by plasminogen activators in the plasma, and probably assisted by lysosomal enzymes derived from the small (lambda) granules of platelets.

Platelets may also be involved in various other biological activities; for example they have receptors for class IgE antibody molecules which enable them to adhere to and damage antibody-coated targets by means of their lysosomal secretions. PDGF is also a potent trophic substance in laboratory cell cultures and may also exert a similar effect elsewhere, for example in regenerating tissues after damage (see Longenecker 1985).

BLOOD GROUPS

Over 300 red cell antigens are recognizable with specific antisera, and the other cell types also carry many antigens of similar abundance. Antigens which are expressed by alleles at a simple locus or at loci which are closely linked are termed a *blood group system*.

Early attempts at transfusion of blood led to the discovery that erythrocytes bear antigens on their surface (see Race & Sanger 1975) which can interact with naturally occurring antibodies in the plasma of other individuals, causing agglutination and lysis of the erythrocytes. Such antigens, which are not shared with all members of a particular species, are termed *iso-antigens*; other iso-antigens are found amongst cells of other tissues (see below). Erythrocyte antigens are known as *agglutinogens* and the corresponding antibodies are *agglutinins*.

Erythrocytes from an individual can bear several different types of antigen, each type belonging to an antigenic system in which a number of alternative antigens are possible in different persons. So far 19 major groups have been identified, which vary in their frequency of distribution amongst the various races of mankind, including the ABO, Rhesus, MNS, Lutheran, Kell, Lewis, Duffy, Kidd, Diego, Cartwright, Colton, Sid, Scianna, Yt, Auberger, Ii, Xg, Indian and Dombrock systems. Clinically, only the ABO and Rhesus groups are of major importance. Red cells also bear various other minor antigens, some of them very infrequent. Some blood group antigens are also expressed in other tissues or secretions; for example olfactory receptors and salivary glands express the ABO antigens.

All of these antigens are determined by genes carried by autosomes, except Xg which is borne by the X chromosome. Within each group the antigens are determined by alleles and inheritance is in accordance with simple mendelian principles. Thus, in the ABO system the genome may be homozygous and carry the AA complement, the blood group being A, the BB complement giving blood group B; or it may carry neither (OO), the blood group consequently being O. In the heterozygous condition the following combinations can occur: A B (blood group AB), A O (blood group A) and B O (blood group B). In Caucasians and Negroes group O is the commonest, being present in about 50% of the population, followed in frequency by groups A, B and AB in that order (Mourant 1975). The ABO alleles are carried on chromosome 9. In West Africans the Duffy determinant (Fy) is almost always absent, a lack which confers resistance to *Plasmodium vivax* malaria (Miller & Carter 1976).

The plasma in each case carries naturally occurring antibodies specific to the antigens which are not present on the erythrocytes in the same blood, so that in group A blood, anti-B antibodies are found. Similarly, present in group B blood are anti-A antibodies, in Group O blood both anti-A and anti-B antibodies and in group AB blood there is neither type of antibody.

Transfusions succeed only if the recipient's antibodies do not correspond to the donor's antigens and cross-matching of blood antigens is therefore vitally important. Persons with group AB blood, lacking antibodies to both A and B antigens, can be transfused with blood of any group and are termed *universal recipients*; conversely, those with group O, *universal donors*, can give blood to any recipient, the donor's antibodies being diluted to insignificance. Normally, however, blood is only transfused between persons with precisely corresponding groups, since anomalous antibodies of the ABO system are occasionally found in blood and may cause agglutination or lysis.

Within the ABO system several subgroups exist (A_1, A_2, A_{1B}, etc.); the cross-matching of some of these is important in transfusions. The anti-ABO agglutinins, like all others (except those of the Rhesus system), belong to the immunoglobulin M (IgM) class and do not cross the placenta during pregnancy.

Rhesus antigen system

The Rhesus antigen system, so-called because of its presence also in the erythrocytes of the Rhesus monkey, is determined by three sets of alleles, namely Cc, Dd and Ee, the most important clinically being Dd; all are carried on chromosome 1. The commonest condition in the UK is CDe and about 83% of the population is Rhesus-positive. Inheritance of the Rh factor obeys simple mendelian laws and it is therefore possible for a Rhesus-negative mother to bear a Rhesus-positive child. Fetal Rh antigens can, under these circumstances, stimulate the production of anti-Rh antibodies by the mother and since these belong to the immunoglobulin G group of antibodies they are able to cross the placental barrier and cause agglutination of fetal erythrocytes. In the first of such pregnancies little damage is usually caused, but in subsequent Rh-positive ones massive destruction of fetal red cells may ensue, causing fetal or neonatal death. Sensitization of the mother's immune system can also result from abortion or miscarriage, or even occasionally amniocentesis, which may introduce fetal antigens into the mother's circulation (see Contreras & Hewitt 1989). Treatment is by exchange transfusion of the neonate infant or, prophylactically, by desensitizing the mother after the first Rh-positive pregnancy with Rh-immune serum, which appears to destroy the fetal Rh antigen in the maternal circulation before the processes of immunological memory can be entrained (see Clarke 1975).

Of the other antigenic systems known, some of which are occasionally of clinical importance, many are restricted to individual genic groups or even families; they can be of great value to anthropologists when tracing demographic relationships, as of course are the major systems described above (Mourant 1983).

Other antigenic systems such as MNS (shared with other tissues in the body) can be used in medicolegal investigations to establish identity of blood, or in parental identification. These antigens can remain intact long after death, and have been detected even in mummified tissues from Egypt over 4000 years old (Harrison et al 1969). The Lewis system is not synthesized by the red cell lineage itself, but is absorbed from the plasma; it is a secretory product of salivary and other glands.

The genetics of blood groups is complicated by gene linkage with other characters which may be of some clinical importance; for example duodenal ulcers show a higher incidence in those with group O blood than in the general population.

Leucocytes also bear antigens and about 12 such groups have so far been identified, 10 of them belonging to the same complex system. These are similar to the *histocompatibility antigens* involved in graft rejection. For further details of the blood groups, see Race and Sanger (1975); Mollison et al (1987); Contreras and Lubenko (1989).

HISTOCOMPATIBILITY ANTIGENS

Amongst important components exposed at the surfaces of most cells are the molecules which determine the individuality of tissues from different persons (the histocompatibility locus antigens) and which are intimately related to the functioning of the immune system. They also share the same region on one of the chromosomes, their genes being grouped together as the Major Histocompatibility Complex (MHC), expressed in the body as a number of distinctive proteins. This system has come into prominence because of its importance in tissue grafting and transplant surgery, and various other clinical approaches.

In humans, the MHC genes lie on the short arm of chromosome 6 and are grouped in a linear sequence close to each other; crossing over during meiosis rarely or never occurs in this sequence, due to either their proximity to each other or some other intrinsic resistance to this process. The MHC region expresses a number of distinctive classes of molecules in various cells of the body, the genes being, in order of sequence along the chromosome: the Class I, II and III

MHC genes. Class I consists of the histocompatibility locus antigen (HLA) genes, subdivided into A, B and C subregions, A and B being represented by a number of different alleles; these genes are capable of generating throughout the cells of the body a distinctive set of gene products, expressed at the surfaces of most cells. These appear to be different in all individuals, conferring a unique chemical identity which is the basis of the immune reactions in the body, since lymphocytes recognize and attack cells bearing alien antigens mainly when these are present alongside characteristic 'self'-HLA molecules. This enormous range of possible alternatives is a result of the substructure of the genes coding for them, which are subdivided into many smaller units; these can be spliced together in many different combinations, in a manner resembling the mechanisms for creating diversity amongst antibodies or T-cell receptors (pp. 1421, 1422), although of course there is a fundamental difference in the outcome, since only one HLA sequence out of a great possible range is selected during development. The HLA sequence also has interesting diagnostic aspects because of chromosomal linkage to sites affecting the frequencies of certain diseases (see below).

The genes for Class II MHC molecules include three sub-divisions termed DR, DQ and DP. Of their products, the MHC-DR molecules are best known; these occur on the surfaces of antigen presenting cells generally classed as macrophages (p. 1420) and including various dendritic cells of lymphoid tissue (e.g. follicular dendritic cells, interdigitating cells) and the epidermis (Langerhans cells). These molecules are anchored into the membrane and like the HLA antigens are highly polymorphic (i.e. have different chemical structures in different individuals). They can bind to alien antigens which the cells have phagocytosed and partially digested, and this combination is presented to helper or cytotoxic T cells where they temporarily bind to the CD 3 molecules (T-cell receptors) present on the lymphocyte surface to activate that cell (p. 1422). The genes for Class III MHC products are expressed in various components of the complement system, as well as some other, non-immune related proteins.

The HLA system has attracted much attention because of its importance in transplant surgery and, in a quite different way, because of the association between certain of its subgroups and some types of disease. For example, the subtype HLA-B27 is present in nearly all cases of ankylosing spondylitis; the condition of haemochromatosis, a disturbance of iron metabolism, is strongly associated with $HLA-A_3$ and rheumatoid arthritis with HL_4-D_4. Other conditions that display a statistical correlation with the HLA system include diabetes in juveniles, Hodgkin's disease and multiple sclerosis. The reasons for these associations are not clear, but are thought to represent some type of loose *genetic linkage* between the HLA determinants and other alleles predisposing the body to a range of diseases. In mice, where this system has been widely investigated, genes that apparently control the responsiveness of the immune system to infection (the Immune related, or Ir genes) are situated between those genes that determine the major histocompatibility (H2) factors.

HAEMOPOIESIS

EARLY DEVELOPMENT OF HAEMOPOIETIC TISSUE

The earliest sign of blood *vessel* formation in the human embryo is when, during the early primitive streak stage of development, angioblastic tissue differentiates almost simultaneously in various extraembryonic sites, namely, in the mesenchyme of the yolk sac wall and in similar tissue of the connecting stalk and chorion. The earliest formation of blood *cells* (**9.6**), however, is confined to the wall of the secondary yolk sac, where they differentiate from deeply placed mesenchymal cells which lie next to the yolk sac endoderm. Whilst a mesodermal or endodermal origin for these cells is still debated, they are unquestionably mesenchymal in character and differentiate into the primitive *stem cells* of the haemopoietic line, which give rise directly to fetal blood cells.

Beginning in the second month, a number of intraembryonic sites of haemopoiesis appear and slowly replace the earlier sites. These intraembryonic sites succeed but overlap each other in time, each site gradually increasing in importance and then waning. Initially,

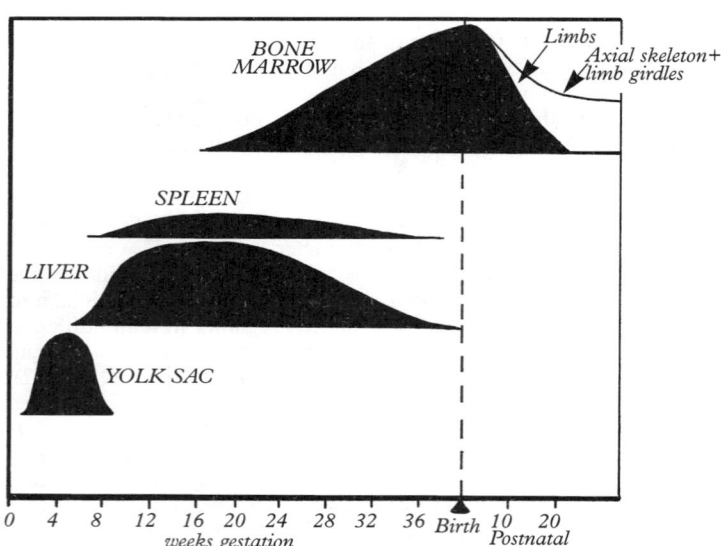

9.8 Diagram showing the sites of early haemopoiesis.

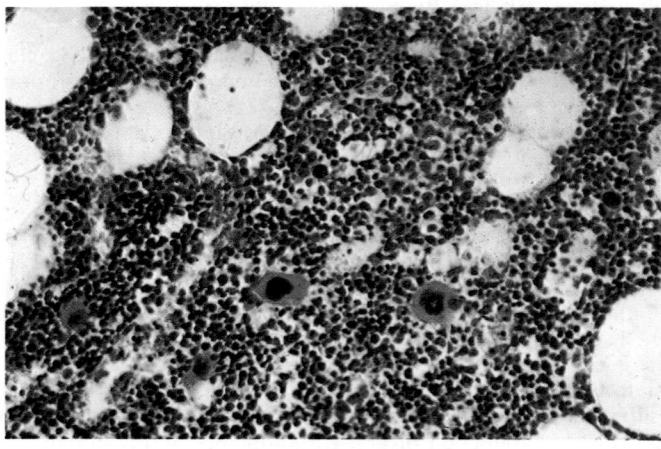

9.9 Photomicrograph of a section of bone marrow from a fetal human long bone. Note the heterogeneous collection of cell types including four large megakaryocytes. Magnification × 150.

the intraembryonic sites are broadly *intravascular*, but soon *extravascular* loci of haemopoiesis supervene. Rapidly the *liver* becomes the dominant organ of embryonic blood formation (the *hepatic phase*), its activities continuing until about the seventh month. Lagging somewhat behind the liver, the *spleen* is then added, its

haemopoiesis continuing from the third to sixth months. From late in the month, an additional source of blood cells emerges, namely the *bone marrow* (*myeloid tissue*) where **all** blood cell types are formed, and later the peripheral lymphoid tissues, where only lymphocytes are produced (lymphopoiesis). The *thymus* is an active lymphopoietic

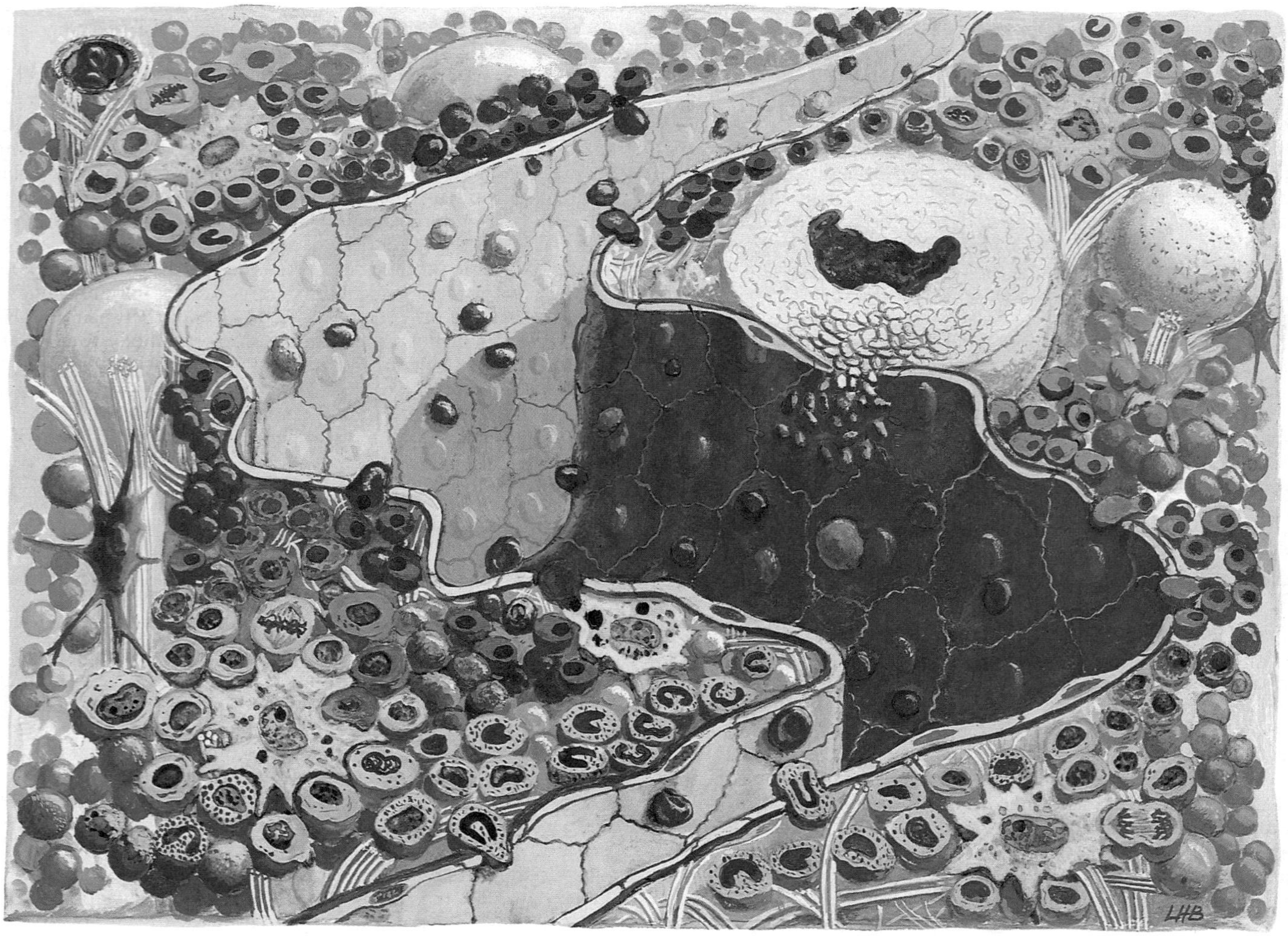

9.10 Microscopic organization of bone marrow depicting a sinusoid in section, showing haemopoietic islands centred on macrophages (yellow), forming erythrocytes (red), various classes of leucocytes (blue), megakaryocytes (beige), adipocytes (orange), fibroblasts (brown) and endothelial cells (dark blue-purple) flanked by a basal lamina and reticulin fibres (white). A group of platelets (white) and various other cellular types are shown passing through apertures in the endothelial linings of sinusoids. An arteriole is also depicted (top left).

organ from this stage (whilst initially it also has some general haemopoietic functions). The myeloid and lymphoid tissues become the dominant source of supply by the seventh month and shortly after birth all other sites have regressed completely. Occasionally, clumps of tissue capable of total haemopoiesis are found outside the bone marrow (*extramedullary tissue*) in paravertebral sites; in pathological cases, where there is more demand for haemopoiesis, and especially during early childhood, complete haemopoiesis may also occur in the liver, spleen and lymph nodes and infrequently also in the kidneys, adrenals, adipose tissue, general connective tissue and even in cartilage. In other species, such as mouse, haemopoietic sites may normally persist in small foci within extramyeloid tissues, for example the spleen and thymus.

BONE MARROW (9.9, 10, 13)

Bone marrow is a soft pulpy tissue which is found in the marrow cavities of all bones and even in the larger Haversian canal of lamellar bone. It differs in composition in different bones and at different ages and occurs in two forms, *yellow* and *red marrow.*

During fetal life and at birth there is red marrow throughout the skeleton. After about the fifth year the red marrow is gradually replaced in the long bones by yellow marrow. The replacement commences earlier and is more advanced in the more distal bones. Further, in each bone the replacement, in general, proceeds from the distal to the proximal end, though some maintain that it commences in the centre of the shaft and extends in both directions, but more rapidly in the distal. By 20–25 years of age the red marrow persists only in the vertebrae, sternum, ribs, clavicles, scapulae, pelvis, cranial bones and in the proximal ends of the femora and humeri. In old age the marrow of the cranial bones undergoes degeneration and is then termed *gelatinous marrow.*

Yellow marrow

The yellow marrow consists of a basis of connective tissue, supporting numerous blood vessels and cells, most of which are fat cells, although a small population of typical red marrow cells persists and may be reactivated when the demand for blood cells becomes sufficiently great, as noted above.

Red marrow (9.9, 10)

The red bone marrow consists of a network of loosely woven connective tissue, the *stroma*, supporting clusters of haemopoietic

cells (*haemopoietic cords* or *islands*) and a rich vascular supply in which large, thin-walled *sinusoids* are prominent (for reviews see Quesenberry & Levitt 1979; Tavasolli & Yoffey 1983; Weiss 1984; Golde & Takaku 1985). The stroma also contains a variable amount of fat, depending on age, site and the haematological conditions of the body; small patches of lymphoid tissue are additionally present. Thus, the marrow consists of two major compartments, one vascular and the other extravascular. The whole assembly is enclosed within a bony framework, from which it is separated by a thin layer of bone-lining cells (p. 459).

Stroma. This is composed of a delicate network of fine collagen (reticulin) fibres secreted by and adherent to highly branched *adventitial reticular cells* which appear to be a type of fibroblast and derived from embryonic mesenchyme. When haemopoiesis ceases, as in some limb bones in adult life, these adventitial cells become distended with fat globules, filling the marrow with yellow fatty tissue; but if there is a later demand for haemopoiesis, these cells can change back to their earlier stellate form. Also in the stroma are many *macrophages* attached to stromal fibres, some of them being embedded in the centres of haemopoietic cell clusters. These cells are actively phagocytic of cellular debris created by haemopoietic development, especially the extruded nuclei of erythroblasts and remnants of megakaryocytes, but they also have a major role in the control of haemopoietic cell differentiation, proliferation and maturation (see below).

Endothelial cells line the marrow sinusoids, the single layer of cells being supported by reticulin fibres on its basal surface. Endothelial cells are interconnected by tight junctions, which appear to be effective barriers between vascular and extravascular spaces. The passage of newly formed haemal cells from the haematopoietic compartment into the bloodstream occurs through temporary apertures (large fenestrae) formed in the endothelial cell cytoplasm, the migrating cell fitting tightly as it passes through, and the aperture closing immediately behind it.

Haemopoietic tissue. Cords and islands of haematogenous cells consist of clusters of immature haemal cells in various stages of development, typically several different cell lines being represented at each focal group. One or more macrophages of a dendritic shape lie at the core of each such group of cells, and may contain the iron-bearing molecules ferritin and haemosiderin. Besides the phagocytic functions already mentioned, there is evidence that such macrophages are important in transferring iron to developing erythroblasts for haemoglobin synthesis and may indeed exert control

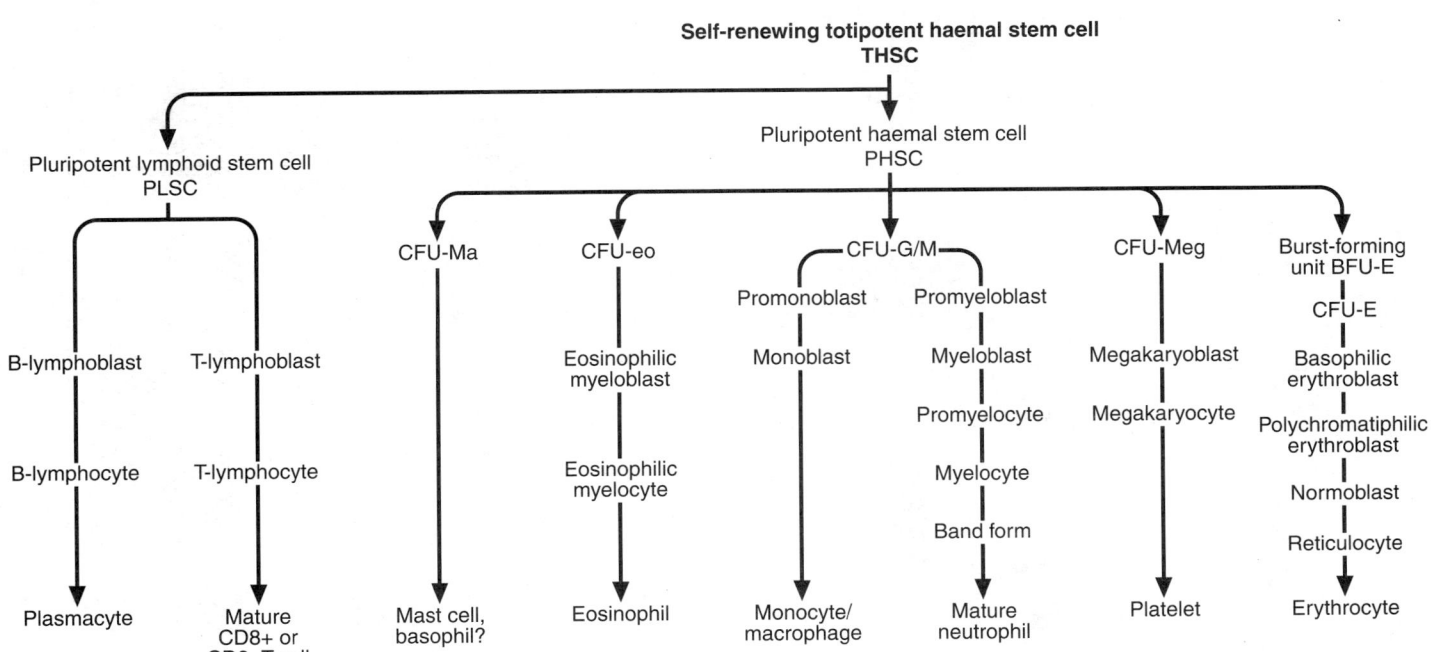

9.11 Diagram illustrating the process of cell division and differentiation during erythropoiesis.

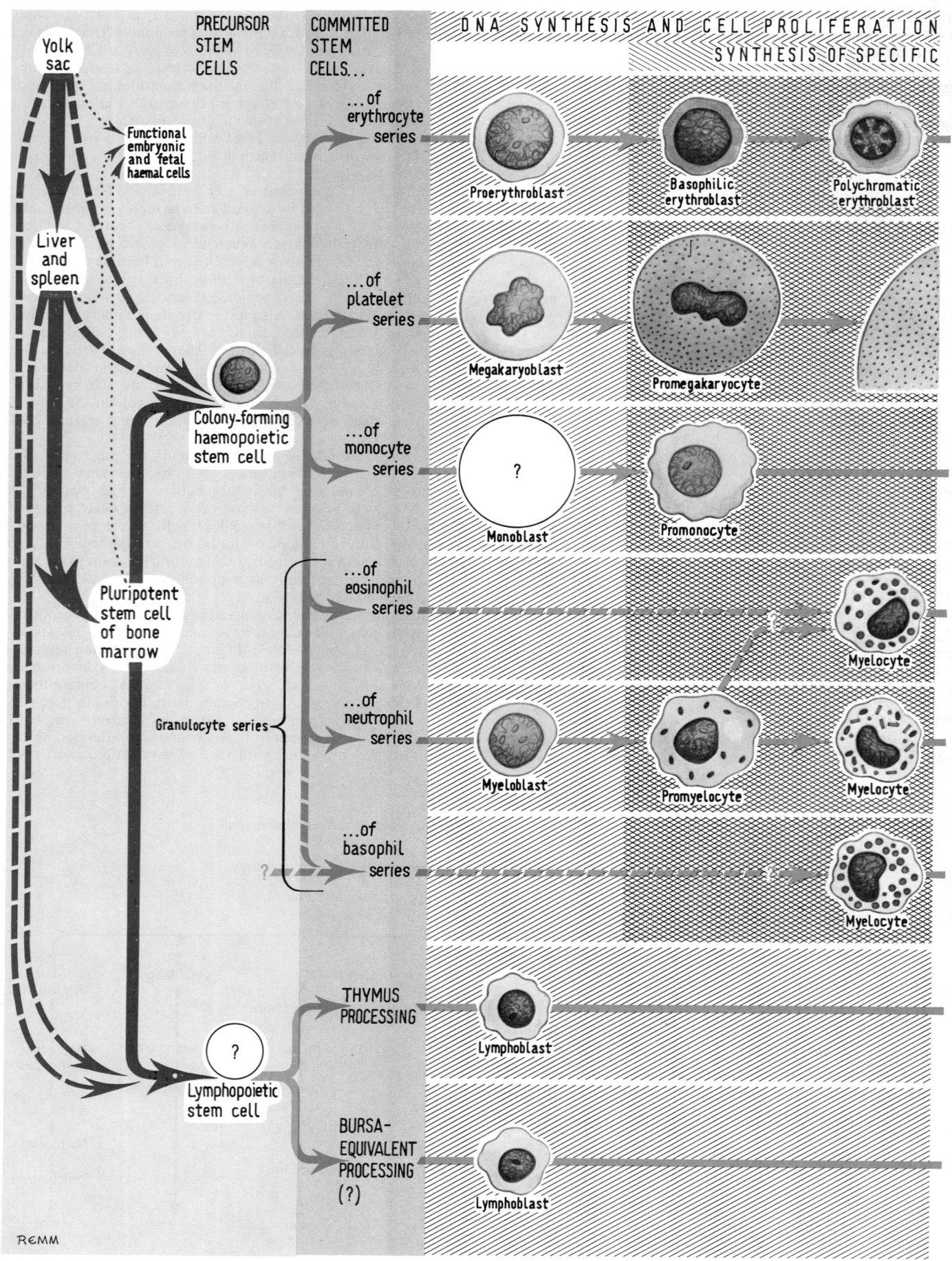

9.12 Haemopoiesis: a schema of the origins, developmental stages and fates of the different classes of haemal cells. Where details of development are uncertain, putative routes are shown in broken lines. Developmental pathways of the prenatal period are indicated (left) in red and different

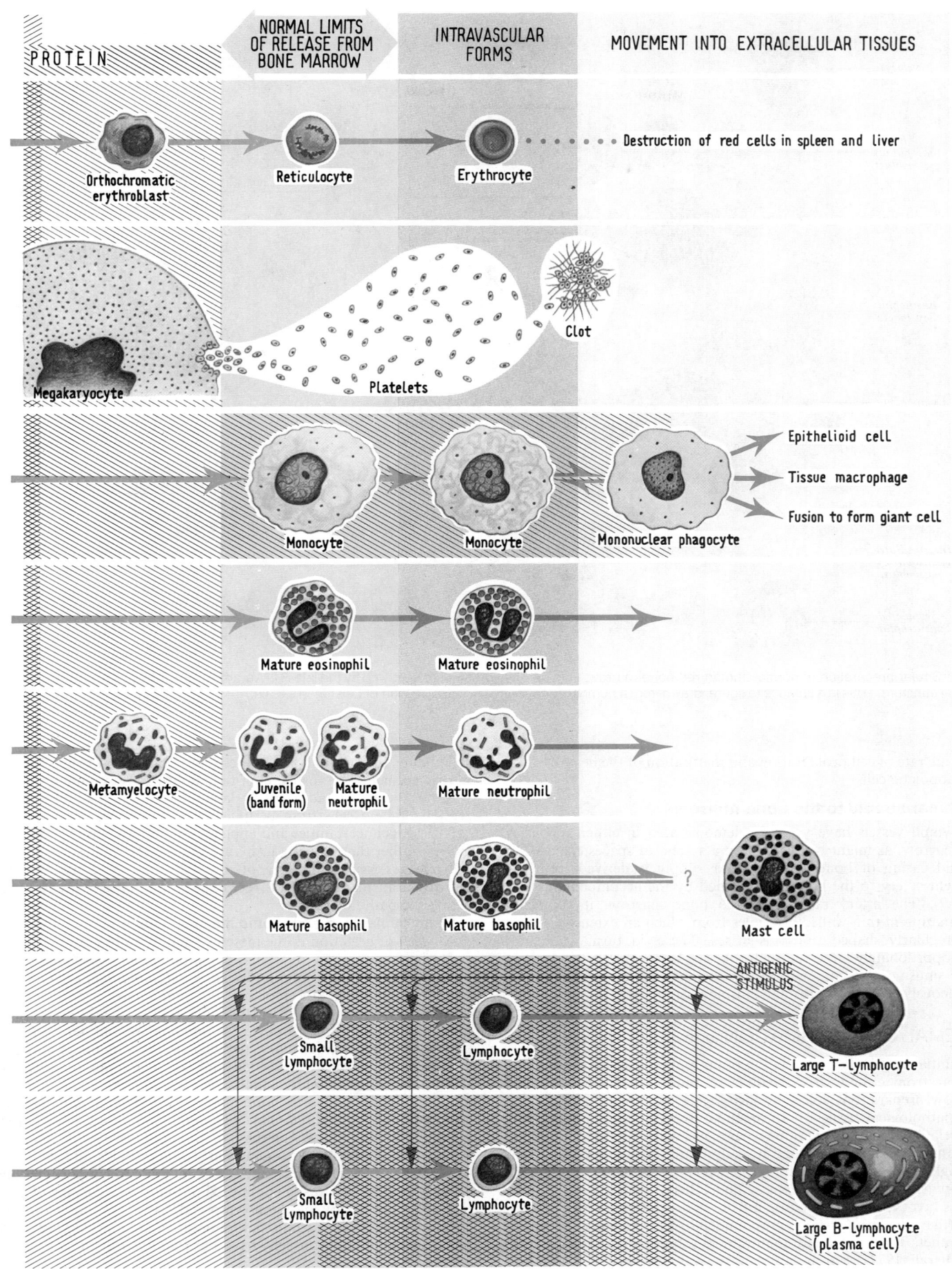

stages of cellular development are hatched diagonally according to the column headings. It should be noted also that there is evidence for macrophage proliferation in the extravascular tissues, a finding not indicated in this scheme.

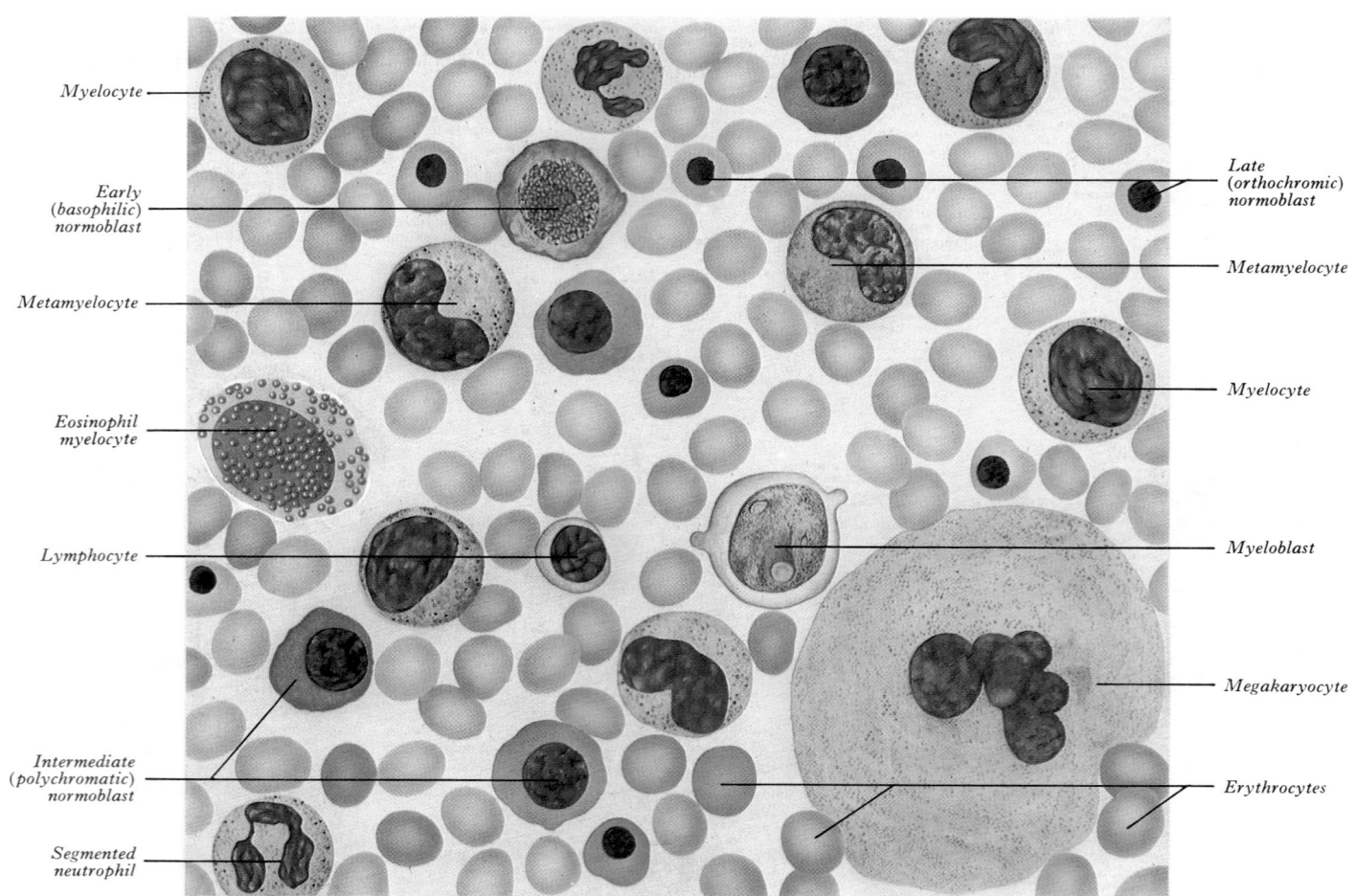

Myelocyte

Early
(basophilic)
normoblast

Metamyelocyte

Eosinophil
myelocyte

Lymphocyte

Intermediate
(polychromatic)
normoblast

Segmented
neutrophil

Late
(orthochromic)
normoblast

Metamyelocyte

Myelocyte

Myeloblast

Megakaryocyte

Erythrocytes

9.13   Smear preparation of normal human red bone marrow, obtained by sternal puncture. (This is a composite figure, drawn from a number of normal smears prepared by the late R L Waterfield, Guy's Hospital, and stained with a modification of Leishman's stain.)

over the rate of cell proliferation and maturation of the neighbouring haemopoietic cells.

Vascular supply to the bone marrow

No lymph vessels have yet been demonstrated in either yellow or red marrow, as might be expected in a system of spaces enclosed in a rigid casing of bone. The vascular supply is derived from the nutrient artery to the bone and drained by the accompanying vein (p. 469). The artery ramifies in the bone marrow, its branches terminating in thin-walled arterioles from which an extensive plexus of irregularly shaped sinusoids arises. These, in turn, drain into disproportionately large veins (Brookes & Harrison 1957). Many of these sinusoids are collapsed at any instant and are frequently but erroneously referred to as intersinusoidal capillaries.

HAEMAL CELL FORMATION (9.10–13)

The initial stages of differentiation of haemal cells in mature marrow are far from clear. Early attempts to trace cell lineages in bone marrow preparations solely by histological examination of normal and pathological tissue led to much controversy about the origins and relationships of the various types of cell which could be observed. Some investigators considered it likely that all cell lines arose from a single type of stem cell (*haemocytoblast*) in adult tissue (the *monophyletic theory* of Maximow and others), whereas other authorities favoured a multiple origin from many different types of stem cells (the *polyphyletic theory*, propounded by Ferrata and colleagues). Yet others have suggested compromise solutions (see Hardistry & Weatherall 1974). For many years it was also assumed that the lymphocytes arose exclusively in the peripheral lymphoid system and not in the bone marrow.

More recently, many experimental methods have been devised in

an attempt to settle this issue; these include cell and organ culture, the replacement or transfusion of radiation-inactivated bone marrow with genetically or radioactively labelled haemal cells and the separation of stem cells from peripheral blood. The picture emerging still presents uncertainties and applies mainly to rodent experimental models rather than directly to man, although the analysis of human cell lineages is a major area of research because of the need for marrow transplantation for the remedy of genetic diseases and neoplastic pathologies.

Haemopoiesis in embryonic life. This commences at about the third week of gestation in the mesenchymal *blood islands* of the yolk sac, where only giant nucleated erythroid cells, *megaloblasts*, are formed. But these are soon replaced by *nucleated fetal erythroblasts* and these, in turn, are replaced by moderately large *anucleate, biconcave fetal erythrocytes* by about the fourth month of gestation. The adult type of erythrocytes is present by full term. Megakaryocytes, then granulocytes, lymphocytes and monocytes appear in that order between the second and fourth months of gestation. During the earlier developmental stages, stem cells occur in the yolk sac, liver, spleen and early bone marrow (**9**.8) and these tissues can give rise to **all** *haemal cell lines*, including lymphocytic ones, if they are transplanted to adult spleens (i.e. they are haemally 'totipotent'). Meanwhile, the lymphoid organs start to be colonized by stem cells which under normal circumstances only give rise to lymphocytes and hence appear to be already committed to that particular line of cells. However, the ability of these lymphoid tissues to carry out full haemopoiesis under certain pathological conditions suggests that some uncommitted stem cells have been retained in these sites but are normally suppressed.

Haemopoietic stem cells

The cell lineages of haemopoietic tissue have not yet been entirely worked out, and there are a number of uncertainties, especially about the relation between the various stem cells. At the present time, the evidence suggests that within the adult marrow there is a very small number of *totipotent stem cells* capable of giving rise to all haemal cell types including lymphocytes. These differ from all other stem cells in one other respect, their ability to replicate themselves as well as produce lineage cells (therefore sometimes called *self-replicating stem cells*, SRTC, or *totipotent haemal stem cells*, THSC). The offspring of these cells, as well as maintaining the totipotent population, can give rise to lymphocytic stem cells of the T or B lines, or differentiate into pluripotent haemal stem cells which then divide into a series of stem cells for the different blood cells. The pluripotent haemal stem cell corresponds to the *colony forming unit stem cell* (CFU-S) of rodents, and its offspring to the precursors of each cell line, that is for the erythrocytic series, *burst forming units of the erythroid line* (BFU-E) for the monocyte/granulocyte line, *colony forming unit—granulocytes and macrophages* (CFU-G/M) giving rise to monocytes (and hence macrophages), eosinophils and possibly basophils; and for the megakaryocyte platelet line, *colony forming unit—megakarocyte* (CFU-Mk). Further differentiation along these lines is described below (see also **9.12**).

To generate a complete set of blood cells from a single totipotent cell takes a considerable period, up to some months, whereas the time is much shorter for the later stem cells to form their particular lineages, although because they are not self-renewing, grafts from these eventually fail as the cells they produce eventually age and die. This is of considerable importance in bone marrow replacement therapy, since the presence of totipotent stem cells in the donor's marrow is essential for success.

Next, we turn to the problem of the differentiation of such stem cells into the various cell lines of the blood. The early stages of these lines are difficult to distinguish since usually they cannot be recognized until well after they have begun to differentiate. In the cell line, however, a definite sequence of major stages can be recognized (or ascribed) (see **9.11, 12**). These stages are:

- the *final commitment* of a stem cell to a particular line of differentiation
- early cell *proliferation* to form a large pool of dividing cells
- *differentiation* as specific proteins characterizing the particular line are synthesized, accompanied by the gradual cessation of cell division
- final *maturation*, marked by the gradual closure of protein synthesis
- *release* of the cells from the bone marrow parenchyma into the circulation by passage through the endothelial linings of the sinuses.

In the case of some cell lines, cell division and protein synthesis may continue outside the bone marrow (e.g. monocytes or macrophages) and maturation may also be completed after release (e.g. erythrocytes).

The earliest 'committed' stages of each cell line are outwardly similar to the CFU-S, but at the next proliferative stage differences begin to emerge. In all, however, the initial picture is that of a rapidly dividing, relatively undifferentiated cell, in which the nucleus is large and euchromatic, with prominent nucleoli; the moderately basophilic cytoplasm contains unattached polyribosomes and the total cell size is large. As proliferation proceeds, the size of the cell usually diminishes as cell division outstrips cell growth. With continuing differentiation the ribosomes become numerous and the cytoplasmic basophilia increases as the specific messenger (m)RNAs begin to be synthesized, whilst the nucleus gradually becomes more heterochromatic and smaller, as DNA synthesis ceases; ultimately the nucleus becomes multilobed or pyknotic as protein synthesis terminates. The completed cell is then ready to be released, although the precise timing of its passage from the bone marrow varies with metabolic conditions and the 'demand' for more cells, so that relatively immature types of cell may be found in the circulating blood under abnormal conditions. This 'shift to the left' (a graphic convention of haematologists in which the cell is represented as maturing from the left to the right) is a useful concept in diagnostic haematology. These general features of development can be seen in several lines of haemal cells and underlie what appears at first sight to be a highly divergent series of progressions.

Erythropoiesis (9.11–13)

The earliest erythroid progenitor cells have not yet been identified, but the second stage includes cells which, after some delay, can multiply very rapidly to form numerous erythroblast cells; they have been named *burst-forming units of the erythroid line* BFU-E. Third in this lineage is a cell which is sensitive to the hormone erythropoietin, which induces it to further differentiation along the erythroid line. This is the *erythropoietin-dependent colony forming unit* (CFU-E).

The first readily identifiable cell of the erythroid series is the *proerythroblast (pronormoblast)*, a large (14–20 μm) cell with a large euchromatic nucleus and moderately basophilic cytoplasm. The latter already has small amounts of ferritin and bears some of the protein spectrin attached to its plasma membrane (p. 1401); both are characteristic of this cell line and can be detected by electron microscopy. Proerythroblasts proliferate, and haemoglobin-RNA synthesis begins, as the smaller (12–17 μm) *basophilic* or *early erythroblast (basophilic normoblast)* appears, rich in ribosomes. Shortly afterwards, haemoglobin synthesis commences so that the cytoplasm becomes partially eosinophilic (the *polychromatophilic* or *intermediate erythroblast/normoblast*) which has a diameter of 8–12 μm. At this stage, most of the cytoplasmic RNA is lost and the nucleus, becoming intensely pyknotic, is finally extruded from the cell, thus leaving an anucleate *reticulocyte*. At this point the cell is released into the circulation, losing its residual RNA in a few days to become a mature *erythrocyte*. The nucleus is phagocytosed by a macrophage. The whole process of erythropoiesis takes 5–9 days; after release, reticulocytes typically sojourn for up to 2 days in the marrow sinusoids and then for an equal time in the spleen, perhaps because of their particularly adhesive cell coat. During this period, the remaining ribosomes add a further small amount of haemoglobin to the cell; then all the organelles are finely dismantled by a soluble cytoplasmic enzyme system involving the protein ubiquitin.

The cell lineage of normal erythrocytes is often called the *normoblastic series* to distinguish it from abnormal erythroid lines; too few divisions of the early proliferative stages may give rise to abnormally large erythrocytes (*macrocytes*), whereas too many divisions, or insufficient early growth, can lead to the formation of abnormally small *microcytes*. Disturbances in haemoglobin synthesis can also give rise to a variety of anaemias and various other pathologies.

Granulocytopoesis (9.11–13)

The details of the processes by which the granulocytes are formed are best known for the *neutrophil*, which will be described in some detail. Initially, the putative stem cells transform into the large (10–20 μm) *myeloblasts* which are similar in general size and appearance, though not in internal details, to the proerythroblast (see above). These proliferative cells differentiate into the larger *promyelocytes*, in which the first group of specific proteins is synthesized in the granular endoplasmic reticulum and Golgi apparatus, both of these organelles being quite prominent. The proteins are stored in large (0.3 μm) *primary* ('*non-specific*') granules, large lysosomes containing acid phosphatase and having azurophilic staining properties (p. 1402). Next, in the smaller *myelocyte*—the last proliferative stage—the smaller *secondary* ('*specific*') granules, which contain a slightly different enzyme array, are formed in a similar manner, though described as being released into the cytoplasm from the '*cis*' side of the Golgi body, whereas the primary granules arise from the other ('*trans*') side (see p. 31). The nucleus is typically flattened on one side in myelocytes. Subsequently, in the *metamyelocyte* stage the cell size decreases further, the nucleus becomes heterochromatic and horseshoe shaped and protein synthesis practically ceases. Finally, as the neutrophil is released, the nucleus becomes heavily indented (the *juvenile* or '*stab*' form) and then partially divided into up to six lobes (the *segmented* or *mature neutrophil*). The whole process takes about 7 days to complete: the mitotic period about 3 days and maturation 4 days. They may then be stored in the medulla for a further 4 days, depending on demand, before final release into the circulation.

Eosinophils pass through a similar sequence except that their nuclei never become as irregular as that of the neutrophil, and only one set of lysosomal granules is synthesized. It is not certain whether the eosinophil differentiates from the same myeloblast (or promyelocyte) stock as the neutrophil, or whether it is distinct from the colony forming unit (CFU-G/M) stage, which at present seems more likely. In the case of *basophils*, it is not certain that they follow this general sequence at all; they may not even share this CFU as an ancestor.

Monocyte formation (9.11, 12)

Monocytes are also formed in the bone marrow. Monocytes and neutrophils appear to be closely related cells and arise from the same stem cell, the *colony forming unit for granulocytes and macrophages* (CFU-G/M) (the granulocytes in question being, of course, neutrophils). Subsequently they pass through a proliferative *monoblast* stage and then form differentiating *promonocytes* in which small lysosomes begin to be made (these may be demonstrated by neutral red staining). After further divisions, monocytes are released into the general circulation, and at least some are believed to pass to perivascular and extravascular sites, which they then populate as *mononuclear phagocytes* or *macrophages*.

Thrombocytopoiesis (9.11, 12)

Platelets, being fragments of cells, arise in a most unusual manner by the division of the cytoplasm of certain huge cells into many portions (Pennington 1979). The first detectable cell of this line is the highly *basophilic megakaryoblast* (15–50 μm); this is followed by a *promegakaryocyte* stage (20–80 μm) in which synthesis of granules begins; finally, the fully differentiated *megakaryocyte*, a giant cell (35–160 μm) with a large, dense, *polyploid*, *multilobate* nucleus, emerges. Once differentiation has commenced, mitoses proceed without cytoplasmic division and the chromosomes are retained within a single polyploid nucleus containing 8n, 16n or 32n chromosomes, depending upon how many nuclear mitoses finally occur. Under the electron microscope, the cytoplasm is distinguished by numerous centrioles and spindle microtubules, both of which reflect the repetitive mitotic activity. Meanwhile, differentiation proceeds in the cytoplasm with the production of free polysomes, smooth endoplasmic reticulum and fine basophilic granules. Cytomembranes within the cell fuse with one another and with invaginations of the plasma membrane to cut off portions of cytoplasm, which then break away from the parent cell to form platelets. The nucleus of the megakaryocyte eventually disintegrates. The release of platelets into the circulation has been described as involving first the protrusion of a long, narrow extension of the megakaryocyte cytoplasm through an aperture in the sinusoidal epithelium, which then separates at its end into individual platelets.

Control of haemopoiesis

The numbers of cells in the circulation are closely regulated in adult life, cell destruction being counterbalanced by cell replacement. How this system of control operates is known, at least in part, only for erythrocytes. Erythropoiesis is stimulated by a circulating protein *erythropoietin* synthesized by the tissues of the kidney and other parts of the body. The rate of erythropoietin synthesis is inversely proportional to the oxygen content of the tissues; hence low oxygen tensions, usually consequent upon lowered erythrocyte numbers, stimulate erythropoiesis whereas high oxygen tensions cause the withdrawal of the stimulus. At high altitude the lowering of the partial pressure of oxygen in the atmosphere leads to a raised erythrocyte count.

Many other factors also affect the rate of haemopoiesis, for example thyroid hormones, somatotrophic hormone androgenic steroids and other hormones. In recent years it has also become clear that many other factors affect haemopoiesis, including cytokines and growth factors released by T lymphocytes, macrophages, neutrophils and other cells. The numbers of cells in the blood show a *diurnal rhythm*, probably because of hormonal fluctuations. Infection, haemorrhage and other clinical disturbances also affect the pattern of cell production, as do cytotoxic chemicals and ionizing radiations, to which the dividing cells of the bone marrow are particularly susceptible.

MONONUCLEAR PHAGOCYTE SYSTEM

As noted above, the body deploys a range of defensive cells to perform many complex co-ordinated activities vital to survival in the face of immense pressure of attack from potentially pathogenic organisms. These cells include lymphocytes, to be considered later, and a range of phagocytes capable of ingesting and destroying micro-organisms. The phagocytic roles of neutrophil leucocytes have already been described (p. 1402). The other major types of phagocyte comprise a family of cells with related lineages and various molecular features in common, present in the vascular and extravascular tissues throughout the body. They constitute the *mononuclear phagocyte system*. Its members include the blood *monocytes*, *macrophages* of various kinds in extravascular tissues, and some mildly *phagocytic cells* which are extremely effective at stimulating immune responses in lymphocytes (antigen-presenting cells). They at all times express a characteristic group of surface molecules, the Class II major histocompatability complex (MHC) molecules (p. 1420) which enable them to select and stimulate lymphocytes appropriate to combating specific antigens. Recently it has become obvious that various other cells outside this system can also express MHC II molecules when suitably stimulated, but the mononuclear phagocytes appear to be the only cells to be permanently in this state. The term 'mononuclear phagocyte system' was originally proposed by Aschoff in 1924 to embrace different classes of phagocytic cells, most of which we now know to be macrophages, but this title has been extended more recently to cover various other related cells, as noted above. It is also in part equivalent to the *reticulo-endothelial system* of earlier times (a term that is still occasionally used, although generally superseded).

Although the phagocytic and antigen-presenting abilities of macrophages and related cells are of major importance, it has been discovered that these cells also engage in the synthesis and secretion of many *cytokines*—soluble proteins which regulate highly diverse aspects of cell biology such as growth, mitotic division and differentiation, tissue repair and modelling, as well as defence.

Mononuclear phagocytes can be divided into two groups: the macrophages, which are highly phagocytic ('professional phagocytes'), and the other antigen-presenting cells concerned primarily with lymphocyte activation.

MACROPHAGES

As a historical accident, the cells of this system were originally given different names according to their location. In connective tissue they are either *fixed* or *wandering macrophages* (histiocytes, clasmatocytes); in the liver they are called *littoral cells* of the sinusoids (von Kupffer cells); in the central nervous system, *microglial cells*; and in the meninges, *meningocytes*. They are known as *pleural*, *peritoneal*, *alveolar* and *splenic macrophages* in the sites denoted by these names, and in the synovial joints they are types *A* and *B synovial cells* (p. 497). In the blood they are represented by *monocytes*. In subserous tissue of the pleura and peritoneum, macrophages often aggregate as *milky spots*, near small lymphatic trunks. In the spleen they also occur in clusters (ellipsoids) around the exits of small (pencillar) arterioles (p. 1441) and diffusely throughout the splenic cords, while in the haemopoietic tissue of the bone marrow they are intimately associated with differentiating haemal cells (stromal macrophages).

Macrophages vary in structure depending on their location in the body. All are large cells (15–25 μm across) with a moderately basophilic cytoplasm containing some granular and agranular endoplasmic reticulum, an active Golgi complex, mitochondria, etc. and a large, euchromatic nucleus, signifying an active metabolism and continuing synthesis of lysosomal enzymes (unlike neutrophil granulocytes which virtually cease synthetic activity shortly after leaving the bone marrow). All cells have irregular surfaces with many filopodia and contain varying numbers of endocytic vesicles and lysosomes. Some macrophages are highly motile, whereas others tend to remain attached and sedentary (e.g. the littoral cells of hepatic and lymphoid sinuses).

Within the connective tissue, macrophages may fuse to form large syncytia (foreign body giant cells) around large particles which are too big to be phagocytosed, or when stimulated by the presence of infectious organisms, for example tubercle bacilli (epithelioid cells). As mentioned above, all of these cells express Class II MHC molecules on their surfaces; they are also positive for the characteristic (though not specific) molecular surface marker International

Cluster Determinant (CD)14 and the specific cytoplasmic granules marker CD68. Macrophages in certain localities express additional markers, for example CD33 in myeloid tissue and CD16 in pulmonary alveoli. Microglia also possess CD4 on their surfaces, as do T helper lymphocytes, a feature which unfortunately makes them susceptible to human immunodeficiency virus (HIV) infections, too.

Origins of macrophage cell lineages

There is now much evidence that macrophages arise in the bone marrow from stem cells concerned with the production of the neutrophil granulocyte-monocyte lineage (the colony forming unit—granulocytes and macrophages; CFU-G/M stem cell, see p. 1414), monocytes mostly representing blood-borne macrophages en route to their final extravascular tissue destinations. When the cells enter these tissues through the endothelial walls of capillaries and venules, they can undergo a limited number of rounds of mitosis before they die and are replaced from the bone marrow, although alveolar macrophages of the lung appear to be able to undergo many more mitotic divisions than those elsewhere. Some cells may remain quiescent for long periods of time, for example microglial cells in the central nervous system. Their mature morphology and activities appear to be largely determined by the tissues in which they reside, and cells appear to be seeded fairly randomly from the bone marrow.

Osteoclasts and chondroclasts may also be in some distant way related to these cells, since they have several structural and functional similarities and also arise from stem cells in the bone marrow; however, for various reasons including the existence of a number of distinctive molecular markers, it appears unlikely that they originate directly from the monocyte lineage (p. 459).

Macrophage functions

Macrophage functions include: phagocytosis, antigen presentation, cell and tissue regulation and remodelling in growth and repair, secretion of cytokines, and anti-tumour activity amongst a wide repertoire. In particular they are intimately involved in the mechanisms of innate and acquired immunity (see, for example, Lewis & McGee 1992; Gordon et al 1992).

Phagocytosis. The uptake of particulate material and organisms is carried out by macrophages in many locations. In general connective tissue they can dispatch invading micro-organisms and remove debris engendered by tissue damage, or engulf apoptotic cells in differentiating or remodelling tissue. In the lung, alveolar macrophages constantly patrol the surfaces of the air-filled cavities, into which they migrate from pulmonary connective tissue; there they engulf inhaled particles including bacteria, surfactant and debris and many enter the sputum (hence 'dust cells' and, in cardiac disease, 'heart failure cells' full of extravasated erythrocytes). Similar scavenger functions are performed in the pleural and peritoneal cavities. In lymph nodes they line the walls of sinusoids ('littoral macrophages') and remove particulate matter from the passing lymph as it percolates through their narrow sinuses. In the spleen and liver, macrophages carry out similar acts of particle removal but here they are also involved in the detection and destruction of aged or damaged erythrocytes, whose haemoglobin they begin to degrade preliminary to recycling iron and amino acids (see p. 1402). The phagocytic activities are greatly increased when the target has already been coated in antibody or complement (or both), since macrophages have Fraction crystalline (Fc) and complement component receptors on their surfaces, initiating endocytosis. Once phagocytosis has occurred, the vacuole bearing the ingested particle fuses with endosomal vesicles containing a wide range of lysosomal enzymes (over 100 have been described), including many hydrolases, and oxidative systems capable of rapid bacteriocidal action. These activities are much enhanced when macrophages are stimulated by various cytokines (activated macrophages), such as Interferon (IFN)-γ, secreted by other cells of the immune system, especially T lymphocytes. Lysosomal enzymes may also be secreted from the macrophage on to target microbial cells as part of the defensive mechanism.

Antigen presentation. The part which mononuclear phagocytes play in immune responses is complex and incompletely known. As mentioned elsewhere (p. 1420), they bear Class II MHC antigens at their surface, which enable them to stimulate different classes of T lymphocyte through close-range interactions: macrophages phagocytose alien antigens and partially digest them in their endosomal

systems, passing some of the antigenic remnants to the cell surface where they are bound by MHC molecules. This complex of alien antigen and MHC molecule is then presented to a T lymphocyte, which, if it possesses the appropriate receptor on its surface, is stimulated in various ways, depending on the type of T cell involved (p. 420). In turn, macrophages are also affected by activated T and B lymphocytes; and cytokines (including macrophage-activating factors, Interleukin II, etc.) secreted by certain T cells can determine their migration and degree of phagocytic activity (p. 1420). Under such influences the macrophages themselves can synthesize and secrete various other bioactive substances, for example Interleukin I which stimulates the proliferation and maturation of other lymphocytes, greatly amplifying the reaction of the immune system to foreign antigens. When activated by Interleukin II and other cytokines, macrophages synthesize and release many other bioactive molecules, including Tumour Necrosis Factor (TNF)-α which is able to kill neoplastic cells and appears to be a mechanism for the removal of small tumours which may appear in the body from time to time throughout life; it is interesting that TNF-α also depresses the anabolic activities of many cells in the body and this may be a major factor in cachexia (wasting) which typically accompanies more advanced cancers. Other macrophage products include plasminogen activator, promoting clot removal (p. 1406), and various lysosomal enzymes, several complement and clotting factors and lysozyme (an antibacterial protein). In pathogenesis, such substances may be 'erroneously' released to damage healthy tissues, for example in rheumatoid arthritis and various other inflammatory conditions. As noted above, because macrophages have receptors on their surfaces for the Fc ends of antibodies and for the C3 component of complement, and so can bind readily to and avidly phagocytose antibody-coated (opsonized) microbes and other 'alien' material. Such close antibody-mediated binding may also initiate the release of lysosomal enzymes on to the surfaces of the cellular targets to which the macrophages are bound (an example of Antibody-Dependent Cell-Mediated Cytotoxicity, ADCC, also shown by various other cells including neutrophils), particularly if these are too large to be phagocytosed (e.g. nematode worm parasites such as *Wuchereria bancrofti*). These reactions are much enhanced when macrophages are stimulated by cytokines.

Macrophages and related cells also produce several growth and differentiation factors with actions on other tissues. They release factors which stimulate haemopoiesis, including erythropoietin, and have complex metabolic actions through their production of prostaglandins, thromboxanes and other bioactive substances, including the stimulation of bone resorption by osteoclasts.

In summary, these various activities appear to be related to three quite distinct roles: the first associated with defence, the second with repair and regeneration of damaged tissues and the third with the ongoing maintenance of normal cell proliferation and differentiation in healthy tissues throughout the body. The full extent of macrophage-mediated effects has yet to be determined and some of them are quite unexpected; for example high levels of Interleukin I induce sleep, as found in some severe systemic infections. It seems that macrophages may be intricately connected with a vast array of cellular activities in a network of great complexity.

ANTIGEN-PRESENTING CELLS (9.14, 15)

Whilst macrophages are able to present antigens to lymphocytes, there is a category of mononuclear phagocytes which are perhaps a thousand times more effective at performing this function. These are all cells with a highly folded surface, often elongated into dendrites. They include the *interdigitating cells* and *follicular dendritic cells* of secondary lymphoid tissue, *Langerhans cells* of the epidermis (see, for example, Knight & Stagg 1993) and microfold and reticulated cells of the alimentary epithelium. These cells are mildly phagocytic, so that they are able to endocytose alien antigens, partially digest them, then present them on the surface in combination with Class II MHC molecules. Here they can bind to receptor molecules on the surfaces of lymphocytes to select and stimulate appropriate clones of these cells.

Interdigitating cells

Interdigitating cells are found in T-cell rich areas of secondary 1415

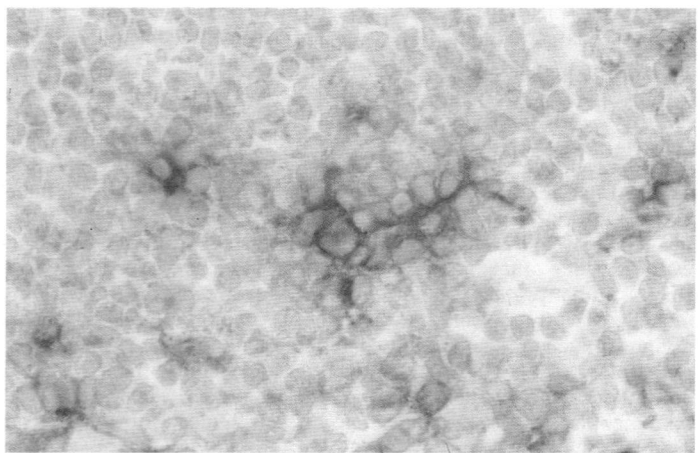

9.14 Follicular dendritic cells in the germinal centre of a palatine tonsil, (immunoperoxidase method). (Provided by M Perry, Division of Anatomy and Cell Biology, UMDS, Guy's Campus, London.)

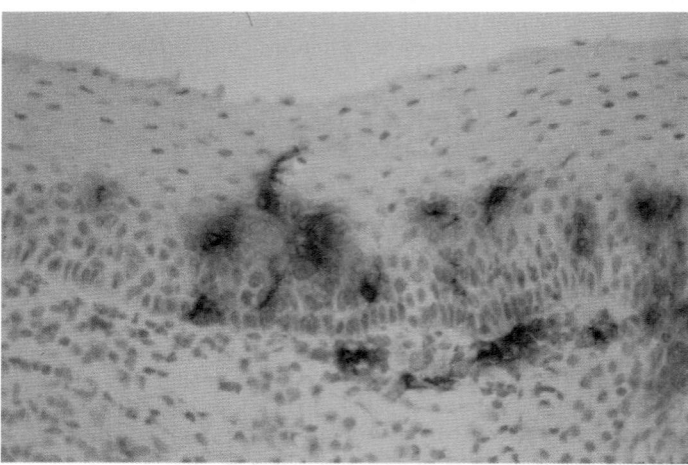

9.15 Langerhans' cells, in the epithelium overlying a palatine tonsil. Immunoperoxidase method. (Provided by M Perry, Division of Anatomy and Cell Biology, UMDS, Guy's Campus, London.)

lymphoid tissue (paracortical areas of lymph nodes, interfollicular areas of mucosa-associated lymphoid tissue (**9.52**), periarteriolar sheaths of splenic white pulp). The MHC II-antigen complexes on their surfaces bind specifically to the receptors on T-cell surfaces (T-cell receptors; TCR) accompanied by other adhesive and secretory interactions between these two cell types, activate appropriate T

cells to proliferate and prime them prior to carrying out their immunological activities. Only T cells with receptors corresponding to the specific antigen presented to them in combination with the MHC II molecules can be triggered in this way. The process is hence termed Class II MHC restriction.

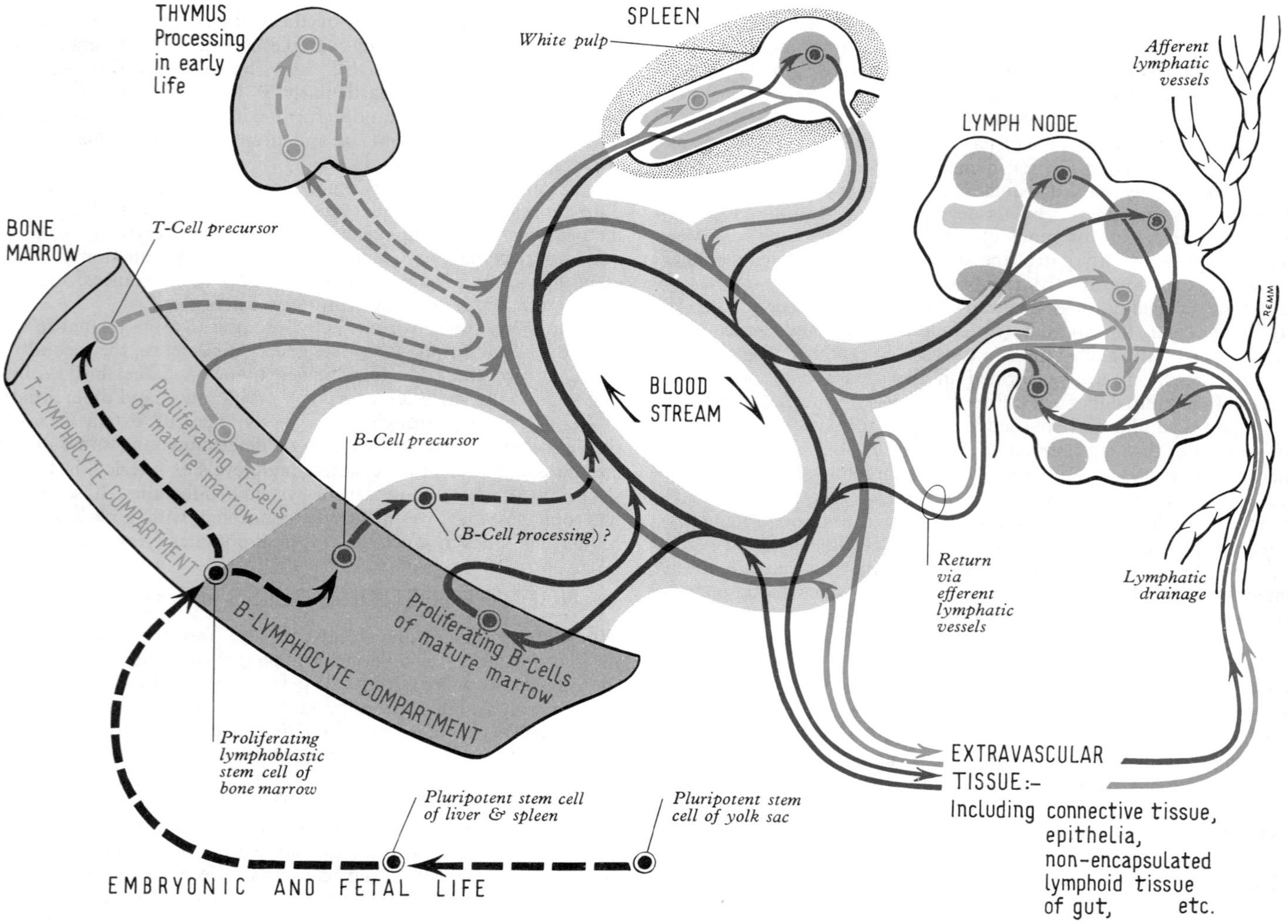

9.16 Diagram depicting the current views of the origins and circulation of the two major classes of lymphocyte from the bone marrow to the peripheral lymphoid tissues. Red = B lymphocytes; blue = T lymphocytes.

Follicular dendritic cells (9.15)

Follicular dendritic cells are similar cells, with long dendritic extensions, found in the follicles of secondary lymphoid tissues where they carry out similar antigen presentation to B cells. Only those B cells which possess appropriate receptors on their surfaces can be stimulated to divide and secrete antibody by this contact, so again these cells are part of the highly selective mechanism by which suitable immune responses are made to specific antigens.

Langerhans' cells

Langerhans' cells are similar dendritic cells present in the epidermis (5.11); they contain characteristic elongated membranous vesicles (Birbeck granules) of uncertain function, and appear to be involved in the immune responses of lymphocytes within the skin to antigens within the epidermis. Such cells (with the same curious granules) have also been found in lymph nodes and the thymic medulla, and it has been suggested that Langerhans' cells may migrate into these structures after they have picked up antigens, to stimulate the lymphocytes within them. The lymphocytes are then envisaged as passing back to the skin to carry out defensive actions there, or to populate regional lymph nodes to deal with any infectious agents which might pass into them from the lymphatic drainage of the area.

Reticulo-endothelial system

The concept of an interrelated system of mononuclear phagocytes has in recent years supplanted that of the reticulo-endothelial system, which at its inception was envisaged as a diffuse network of various phagocytic cells, mainly endothelial, lying in or in close proximity to the walls of certain blood vessels and lymphatics. It was found that these cells took up many particulate dyes and other substances infused into blood and lymph and thus seemed well fitted for the removal and destruction of particulate materials from these fluids. However, more detailed study showed that, in general, true endothelial cells are only mildly phagocytic, as indeed are many other tissue cells; the highly phagocytic cells are not endothelial cells at all, but types of macrophages of myeloid origin and, unlike endothelial cells, bear Class II MHC molecules at their surfaces.

LYMPHOID CELLS AND TISSUES

INTRODUCTION

As stated at the beginning of this section, the defence of the body against pathogens depends on the concerted efforts of a wide variety of cell types, present in vast numbers. The cells of the blood and mononuclear phagocytes can attack the alien organisms directly by phagocytosing them or liberating enzymes or other toxic substance on to their surfaces. In the lymphoid system, a battery of other defensive measures is provided against pathogenic organisms by several classes of lymphocytes. These have some remarkable properties: some of them (B lymphocytes or B cells) synthesize and secrete antibodies which can specifically recognize and neutralize a huge range of alien macromolecules (antigens) and prime various non-lymphocytic cells to engage in phagocytosis and other defensive manoeuvres. Other (T lymphocytes) can recognize and selectively kill virus-infected cells, or modulate the activities of other lymphocytes and phagocytes. Lymphocytes proliferate, differentiate and mature in specialized *lymphoid tissues*, collections of such cells and related antigen-presenting cells (APCs) which are situated in many sites within the body. Before considering these, the biology of the lymphocytes themselves will be briefly reviewed.

ORIGINS OF LYMPHOCYTES

Much of the knowledge of lymphocyte life history (9.16, 17) has come from experimental situations which include the tracing of radioactivity or genetically labelled cells, the latter involving transfusion of lymphocytes with chromosomal abnormalities into normal but inbred strains of laboratory animals. Other experiments have been based on the sensitivity of lymphocytes to ionizing radiation, the various components of the lymphocytic system being eliminated by selective irradiation, accompanied by appropriate transfusions or transplants of lymphopoietic tissue from bone marrow, lymph nodes, thymus and so forth. Thirdly, selective surgical removal of various lymphopoietic components and the removal of lymphocytes from the lymphatic channels has been carried out. In addition to these manoeuvres, a whole battery of immunological techniques has been brought to bear on the problem, including immunoassay, tissue culture methods, and techniques for the localization of antibodies by their reactions with antigens or antigen–antibody complexes previously labelled with fluorescent compounds or electron-dense substances (or enzymes), with subsequent examination by fluorescent and electron microscopy respectively.

Lymphocytes originate in the embryo from mesenchymal cells in the yolk sac initially, and later in the liver and spleen. These primitive lymphoid *stem cells* subsequently take up residence in the bone marrow, which becomes the only site of stem cell proliferation after birth (however, see p. 1412). When these stem cells divide, they give rise to further stem cells and to lymphoblasts which continue to divide, eventually becoming small lymphocytes. Some of these pass in the blood circulation to the thymus where they migrate into its cortex and divide repeatedly, undergoing a selection process to determine if they will be suitable members of the immune system's repertoire (p. 1427); the resulting small thymus-processed T lymphocytes then enter the bloodstream and migrate to the peripheral (secondary) lymphoid tissues of lymph nodes, spleen, alimentary, respiratory and urogenital tracts (Mucosa-Associated Lymphoid Tissue, MALT), and bone marrow. They enter these through the walls of postcapillary venules. Within these centres the T lymphocytes migrate to specific areas: in lymph nodes, the paracortex between the cortex and medulla; in the spleen, the periarteriolar sheaths; in MALT and bone marrow, the areas between or neighbouring the lymphoid follicles. From these, the lymphocytes can enter the efferent lymphatic drainage, returning to the bloodstream via the thoracic and right lymphatic ducts and the brachiocephalic veins, and so eventually back to the lymphoid tissues again; in the spleen they may also migrate directly into the bloodstream. This *circulation of lymphocytes*, first established by Gowans, is responsible for the large number of T lymphocytes found in the blood (9.16). When stimulated antigenically such lymphocytes enlarge and multiply, and their progeny are capable of a number of different defensive actions concerned with the regulation of immune responses and the elimination of virus-infected and other potentially pathogenic cells (see also below).

The *B lymphocytes* do not pass through the thymus, but undergo a phase of differentiation similar to that of the T lymphocytes, within the bone marrow itself. In birds, B lymphocytes are derived from a specialized diverticulum of the cloaca, called the *bursa of Fabricius* (giving this type of lymphocyte its title, the *bursa equivalent* or *B* lymphocyte, although subsequently it appears that such a prefix can be even more appropriately applied to denote the bone marrow origin of the B-cell class in mammals). Selected B lymphocytes then leave the bone marrow and migrate to peripheral lymphoid sites where they undergo yet another round of cell selection, but this time the major stimulus comes from antigen within the lymph nodes, presented to them by specialized *antigen-presenting cells*. On antigenic stimulation they multiply to form *germinal centres*; such lymphocytes can, while still within the lymphoid tissues or after further migration, mature into the large pyroninophilic (i.e. RNA-rich) plasma cell series, which produce antibodies in their extensive rough endoplasmic reticulum and secrete it into the adjacent tissues.

FUNCTIONING OF THE LYMPHOCYTIC SYSTEM

Lymphocytes, together with the phagocytes of the mononuclear phagocyte system, are responsible for the defensive reactions of the

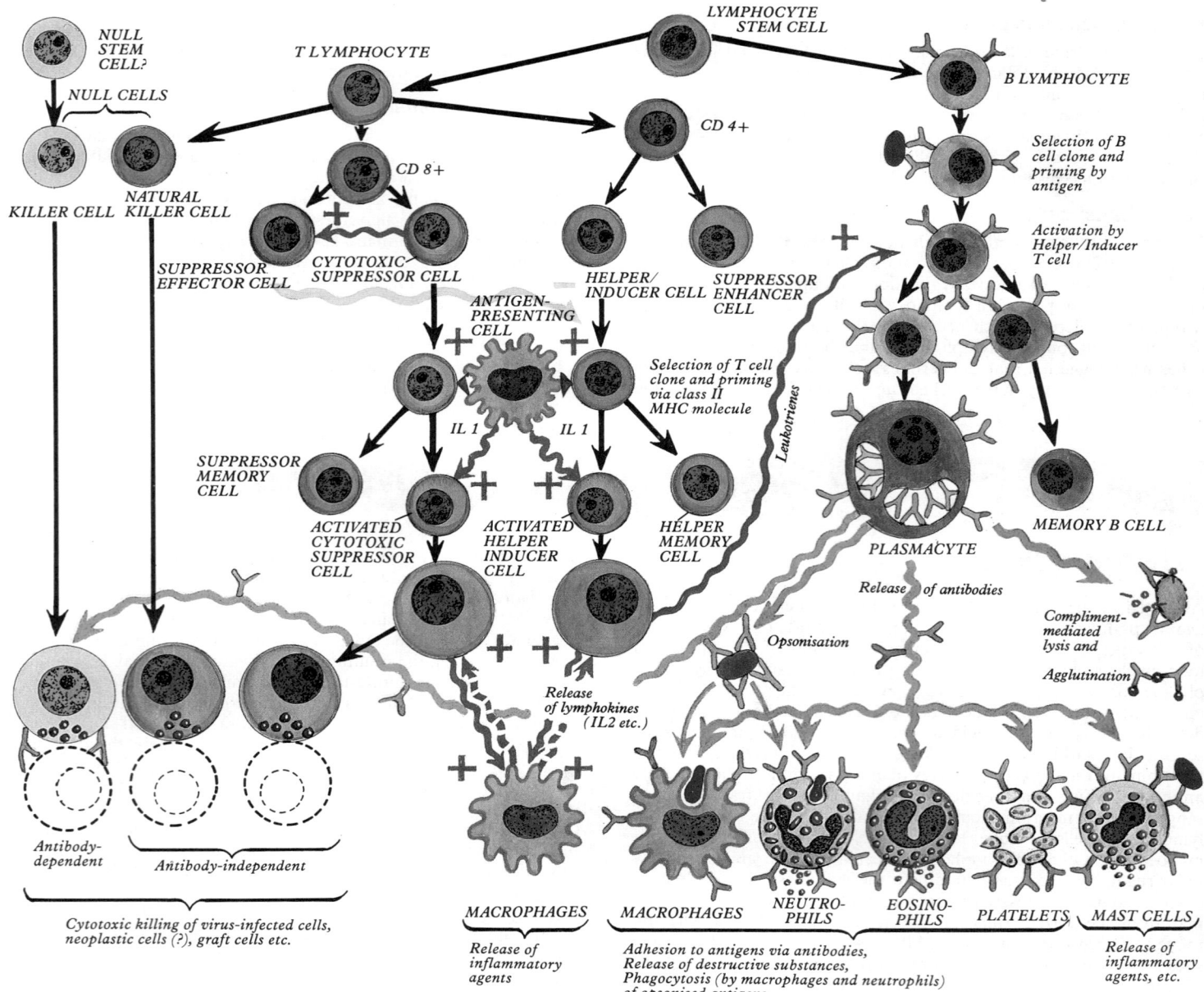

9.17 Schema of the origins and functional interactions by lymphocytes and other cells of the immune system.

body, the former by non-phagocyte interactions of various kinds, the latter mainly by phagocytosis (**9**.17, 18). These defences are directed against alien chemical substances (antigens) which can vary in size and composition from a few amino acids to large and complex antigenic systems such as those of bacteria, viruses, fungi, protozoa, helminth worms, etc. or their harmful metabolites (toxins). They also play a part in the removal of any unwanted or abnormal materials within the body such as foreign or altered proteins and effete, neoplastic or virally transformed cells (auto-antigens or self-antigens).

B lymphocytes (9.12, 17, 18A, B, D)

B lymphocytes can be antigenically stimulated by binding antigens via their B cell receptors (BCRs) after which they proliferate and their progeny transforms into larger B cells (*plasmacytes*) which synthesize and secrete *antibodies*; the latter chemically 'recognize' and bind specifically to their respective *antigens* to inactivate them or cause their destruction. Antibodies may circulate freely in the body fluids (*soluble antibodies*) or may be secondarily attached to a variety of defensive cells (*homocytotropic antibodies* or *cytophilic*

antibodies) to enhance their activities or to enable them to carry out a wider range of functions.

Chemically, *antibodies* (or immunoglobulins) are proteins with a molecular mass of 150–950 kDa. Each antibody molecule consists of at least one or more basic units of four polypeptide chains (150 kDa), comprising two *heavy chains* and two *light chains* held together by disulphide links between the two heavy chains and between the heavy and light chains. The whole molecule can be thought of as Y-shaped, with the arms of the Y being able to swing around a central hinge region. These molecules are bifunctional, i.e. with two interactive poles. The N terminal regions of the molecules have highly variable (*V*) regions in their amino-acid sequences and are responsible for specifically binding to antigens via their Fab (Fragment antigen binding) ends. There are vast numbers of B-cell types within the body ($1–2 \times 10^{12}$ in normal adults), each one representing a different antibody specificity capable of binding to a specific antigen at its Fab end in a manner closely analogous to a 'lock and key' system. The other end of the molecule (the C terminus), is much less variable in structure and is known as the Fc end or the *constant region*, and it is this constant region that defines the antibody *class*. There are

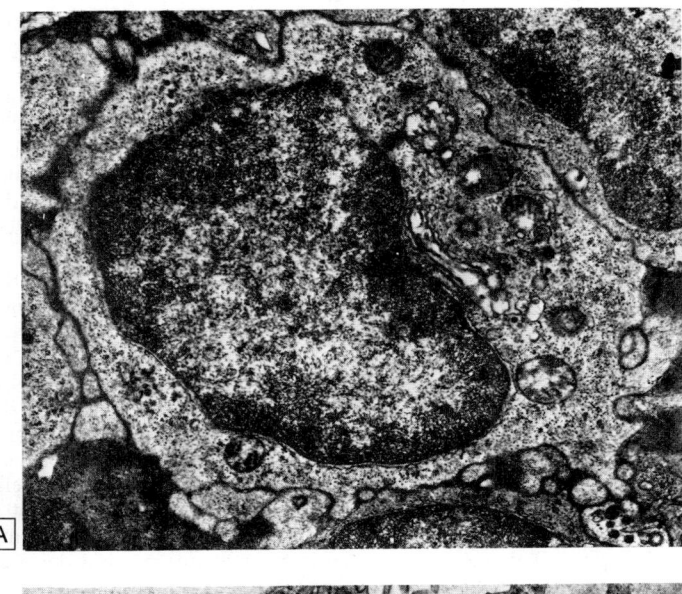

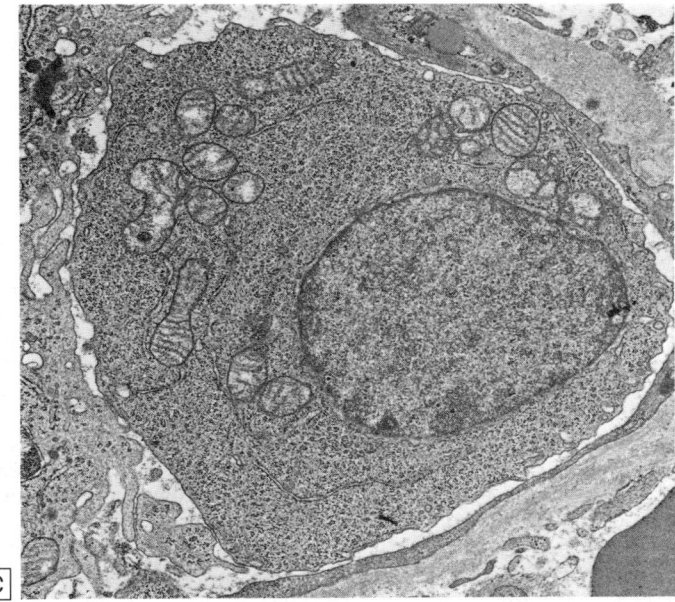

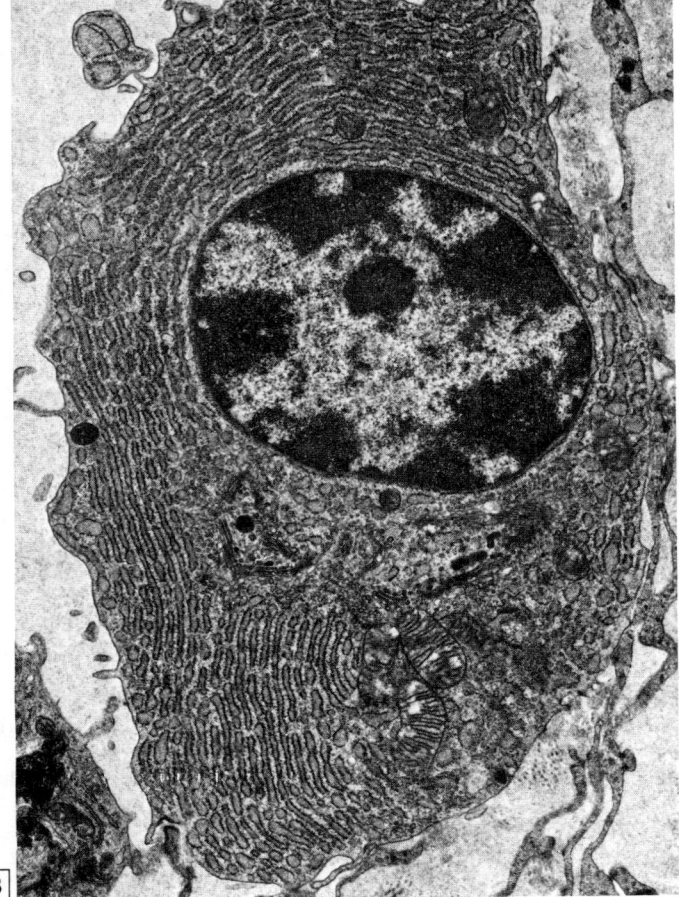

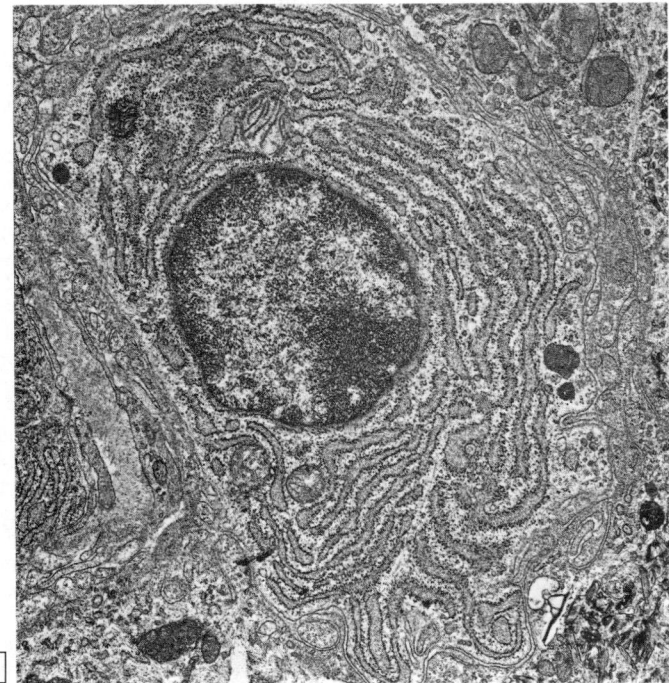

9.18   Electron micrograph of lymphocytes. A A small lymphocyte. Magnification ×6000. (Provided by D R Turner, Guy's Hospital Medical School, London.) B Electron micrograph of a plasmacyte in loose connective tissue. Magnification ×6000. C Transmission electron micrograph of a stimulated T lymphocyte in the spleen (monkey). Note the numerous free ribosomes and relative paucity of granular endoplasmic reticulum. Magnification ×10 000. D Transmission electron micrograph of a stimulated B lymphocyte (plasmacyte) in the spleen (monkey). Note the copious granular endoplasmic reticulum containing newly synthesized antibodies, seen here as finely granular material. Magnification ×10 000.

five classes (*isotypes*) of antibodies distinguishable in the blood plasma and interstitial fluids. These are:

(1) Immunoglobulin *G* (IgG), which forms the bulk of circulating antibodies and is subdivided into four subclasses ($\gamma 1$, $\gamma 2$, $\gamma 3$ and $\gamma 4$);

(2) Immunoglobulin *M* (IgM), which is normally synthesized early in immune responses and is secreted as a pentamer, the monomers being joined near their Fc ends into a starlike aggregate by a small polypeptide called the *J* chain (15 kDa);

(3) Immunoglobulin *A* (IgA), which has two subclasses α_1 and α_2; IgA is present in secretions of the body, particularly saliva and other fluids of the alimentary tract as a monomer or polymer containing J chains and another peptide called the *secretory piece* (70 kDa) which is synthesized by epithelial cells of the mucous membranes (see p. 69);

(4) Immunoglobulin *E* (IgE), which is a *cytophilic* antibody, found on the surface of mast cells and the basophil granulocytes in the blood;

(5) Immunoglobulin *D* (IgD), of uncertain significance, found

1419

together with IgM as a major membrane-bound immunoglobulin on mature immunocompetent B cells and thought to be important in the activation of these cells by antigen entering the immune system.

Certain tissue cells and leucocytes possess *isotype specific Fc receptors* for antibodies on their surfaces, conferring antigen-binding properties on these cells when they have bound antibodies, via their free Fab ends.

The defensive functions of antibodies are numerous. They can *agglutinate* antigens by forming cross-links between them, so rendering them inactive as infective agents (e.g. viruses and bacteria). After binding an antigen they may also activate the classical pathway of *complement* (a complex of at least 12 proteins in the plasma), which undergo a series of amplificatory reactions in a cascade manner similar to that of the blood coagulation system, finally causing the lysis of bacteria and other cells bound by antibody. If only parts of the complement proteins complex are bound (e.g. C3b), these can form bridges between antibody-coated target cells and phagocytic cells such as macrophages bearing C3b receptors on their surfaces, inducing their phagocytosis and ultimate destruction. Free antibodies may also bind to foreign antigens and then attach via their Fc ends to receptors on various defensive (effector) cells, which are then triggered to ingest or enzymatically damage the foreign antigens (*Fc receptor mediated endocytosis*); examples of such effector cells are macrophages and neutrophils and antibodies coating the antigens prior to endocytosis are termed *opsonizing antibodies* or *opsonins*. *Cytophilic antibodies* (i.e. those binding effector cells) may cause the activation of cells in other ways when they bind antigens. Thus, when IgE antibodies bound to mast cells encounter appropriate antigens, they trigger the release of histamine and other vasoactive agents (e.g. platelet-activating factors, leukotrienes, prostaglandins, etc.). This is an important mechanism in the host's defence against microbial invasion, but is also seen in an exaggerated form (hypersensitivity) in certain types of allergy, for example to the proteins of pollen, causing hay fever, asthma and other disorders.

B lymphocytes, themselves, can be activated to divide and differentiate into antibody-secreting *plasmacytes* by antigen–antibody complexes binding to Fc receptors on their surfaces. Activated T lymphocytes can also express Fc receptors and be induced to proliferate and secrete cytokines by this type of antibody-mediated mechanism. It should be emphasized that the antibody bound to these B and T lymphocytes or other cell types bearing the appropriate Fc receptors is derived from plasmacytes after passing into the tissue fluids or blood. Following antigen stimulation, some B lymphocytes are retained as a very long-lived pool of *memory* cells which are capable of responding to their specific antigens with a more rapid and higher antibody output and increased antibody affinity (a measure of the tightness of binding to antigen) compared with the primary response.

When circulating antibodies bind to antigens they form *immune complexes* which, if present in abnormal quantities, may cause pathological damage to the vascular system and other tissues, either, as in some types of glomerulonephritis, by interfering mechanically with membrane permeability to fluids, or alternatively, by causing local activation of the complement system to attack cell membranes, thus causing vascular disease. In pregnancy some maternal IgG is transferred across the placenta, conferring *passive immunity* on the fetus; but in the case of Rhesus factor incompatibility, it brings about the destruction of Rhesus-positive fetal erythrocytes and subsequent fetal anaemia and death if not treated (see p. 1407). In some mammals (oxen, sheep), antibodies are transferred to the offspring in the first formed milk (colostrum) after birth. In humans, maternal milk contains secretory immunoglobulins (IgA) which help to combat bacterial and viral organisms in the alimentary tract of the baby during the first few weeks, although it does not appear to be absorbed through the gut wall as it is in the mammals noted above.

T lymphocytes (9.12, 17, 18c)

T lymphocytes include a number of subclasses (see Marrack & Kappler 1986), all derived from stem lymphocytes originating in the bone marrow but later differentiating in the thymus (hence thymus-derived cell) and passing into various other lymphoid organs. They

carry out a wide variety of *cell-mediated* defensive actions which are not directly dependent on antibody activity and are therefore included under the heading of *cellular immunity*. T-lymphocyte responses can be loosely divided into *effector* and *controlling* actions. *Effector responses* are direct and indirect attacks against virus-infected tissue cells, fungi, some protozoal infections (e.g. trypanosomes), neoplastic cells and the cells of grafts from other individuals (allografts) when the tissue antigens of the donor and recipient are not sufficiently similar. *Controlling functions* are the induction or suppression of immune responses in other lymphocytes, namely B cells and T cells engaged in effector responses, as well as a variety of non-lymphocytic cells such as those derived from the bone marrow. The effector T cells can be divided into two major classes, those which are responsible for cytotoxic killing of virus-infected cells, etc. and those which give rise to a combination of defensive actions through the release of certain soluble proteins, *cytokines*, in delayed-type hypersensitivity reactions.

Cytoxic T cells. These cause the death of their targeted cells in a number of different ways, including the release of toxic lysosomal proteins ('perforins') able to lyse the cell membranes of other cells by forming large pores. Such actions occur at close range, the effector cell having contacted the target cell and recognized it as being pathological. This recognition step is of great interest and depends on the presence at the surface of the target cell of a foreign antigen (e.g. part of a vital antigen) in combination with the Class I MHC molecules that are expressed on the cell surfaces of all nucleated cells. Class I MHC molecules are highly polymorphic and, although very variable from person to person, are invariant within all the tissues of an individual (p. 1407). It is thought that during ontogeny and selection of T lymphocytes in the thymus of an individual person, only those cells that are able to recognize the MHC I molecules characteristic of that individual are retained. Thus a part of the *T-cell antigen receptor* (also variable, see p. 1422) binds to MHC I molecules on other cells, recognizes them as self-components and leaves them unmolested. If, however, the other cells also present a foreign antigen (peptide component) in association with the MHC I molecule, or in the case of transplants, a protein expressed by a different MHC I allele, then T cells mount an attack on those cells which bear these foreign antigens. In this way, intracellular pathogens, such as viruses lodged within cells and thus beyond the reach of antibodies, and also perhaps 'transformed' neoplastic cells, can be killed. Of course, the same applies to the foreign cells of an allograft. Other 'lymphocytes' which are larger in size and contain cytoplasmic granules containing cytotoxic substances (*large granular lymphocytes*) can kill 'target' cells through similar mechanisms, but do not have T-cell receptors and do not act in an MHC-restricted fashion. Natural killer cells (see below) have a similar appearance to those described above (see Hieberman 1985).

Delayed type hypersensitivity-related T cells. These lymphocytes also react to the presence of antigens by synthesizing and releasing *cytokines*, soluble proteins with a molecular mass of 20–80 kDa, which have a wide variety of actions on other cells. These include *chemotactic substances* which attract macrophages into the area of release (macrophage chemotactic factor) and then prevent them from migrating away (macrophage inhibitory factor). Other cytokines stimulate phagocytosis and the destructive activities of macrophages (see p. 1420), natural killer and other cells (macrophage activating factors and γ-interferon). Another important cytokine is *interleukin 2* (IL-2), which acts on B cells and other T cells to stimulate their proliferation and maturation; there are also many other actions of this complex group of secretions. The phenotype of T cells responsible for this cell mediated type inflammatory reaction is predominantly CD4 positive, although some CD8 positive cells are commonly found on the periphery of the mononuclear cell infiltrate of cells in these lesions.

Helper T cells (CD4 phenotype). These are vital to cell proliferation and secretion of antibodies by mature B lymphocytes. These processes are initiated by a foreign antigen being phagocytosed and partially digested by an antigen presenting cell (APC) (p. 1415). The products of this antigen processing pass via the endosomal pathway of the cell to the APC surface where they are presented on Class II MHC molecules (a family of cell surface molecules found mainly on dendritic cells, macrophages, B lymphocytes and other antigen-presenting cells with similar functions) expressed on the cell membrane. This combination of antigen and MHC II molecule is then presented at the cell surface to a helper T cell which recognizes the foreign peptide plus part of the Class II MHC molecule via its T-cell receptor. This interaction, together with secondary signals from cytokines released by the APC, and interactions with other cell adhesion molecules expressed on the two cells concerned, causes the activation and proliferation of the helper T cell. The T cell then activates B lymphocytes which are stimulated to differentiate into plasmacytes secreting antibody corresponding to the particular antigen involved in the APC–T-cell interaction. In this highly regulated way, clones of B cells that produce specific antibodies against an antigen can be stimulated to proliferate and secrete their products. Helper T cells are also required to supplement the activation of cytotoxic T cells, although a separate group of helper T cells is probably involved.

If such helper cell activities are destroyed or rendered non-functional (anergy), a state of immunodeficiency exists where potentially pathogenic organisms present in the body, but normally kept in check by the immune system, may proliferate, causing overt pathology and even death. A well-known example of this is the Acquired Immune Deficiency Syndrome (AIDS) where a virus (HIV I) specifically infects and kills predominantly helper T cells, but also a variety of antigen presenting cells. Similar secondary immunodeficiencies may result from other viral infections, from malnutrition, metabolic disorders, malignancies, drug therapies, radiotherapy and many other factors that suppress the cell-mediated immune system.

Suppression. There appear to be certain T cells which, when antigenically stimulated, release cytokines that actively suppress the defensive activities of B cells and of other T cells. The mechanism of their action is not well understood but may have features in common with both phenotypes of effector T cells (CD8 and CD4 phenotypes). The existence of both positive and negative controls in the immune system is of great significance, since for normal effective defence against infection, this system must be finely balanced to ensure destruction of foreign organisms without the body itself being damaged by the powerful agents released by the various defensive cells. Failure of this delicate control may be seen, at one extreme, in immunodeficiency states and, at the other, in responses to self-antigens such as in autoimmune diseases and in overactive responses called hypersensitivity reactions (e.g. allergic asthma, allergic dermatitis).

Structurally, T lymphocytes present different appearances depending on their type and state of activity. When 'resting' they are typical small lymphocytes morphologically indistinguishable from B lymphocytes; but when stimulated they become large (up to 15 μm), moderately basophilic cells with a partially euchromatic nucleus. In the cytoplasm are numerous free ribosomes, some agranular and granular endoplasmic reticula, a Golgi complex and a scattering of mitochondria (**9.18c**). Cytotoxic effector T cells also contain dense lysosome-like vacuoles used in cytotoxic killing (see above).

Natural killer cells. These constitute a pool of defensive elements which appear to have functional similarities to cytotoxic T cells, although they lack some typical lymphocyte features (see below). They normally form only a small percentage of all lymphocyte-like cells and are included technically in the 'large granular lymphocyte' category. Natural killer cells, when mature, have a mildly basophilic cytoplasm and a partially euchromatic nucleus. Ultrastructurally, the cytoplasm contains ribosomes, granular endoplasmic reticulum and dense, membrane-bound vesicles 200–500 nm in diameter with crystalline cores (Heiberman 1985). These contain some hydrolases, but the major active component is a protein, cytolysin, capable of inserting holes in the plasma membranes of other cells, so causing their death. Natural killer cells are activated to attach themselves to and kill target cells of various kinds by a number of factors, including IL-2 from T cells (see above). They represent a relatively non-specific means of attacking virus-infected cells, protozoa and other pathogenic cells (see also Henkart & Martz 1984).

T-cell classes: CD nomenclature

When monoclonal antibodies were raised against cell surface antigens of human lymphocytes, it was found that different classes of T lymphocytes could be grouped together according to the characteristic range of monoclonal antibodies they bound. When these cell surface molecules were finally identified by the determinants

recognized on them by monoclonal antibodies, they were given an International Cluster Determinant (CD) number. Nowadays, CD numbers define a very large number of cellular molecules which have been cloned and sequenced and whose biological functions are wholly or partially characterized (Singer et al 1994). All 'true' T cells express the CD3 molecular complex, which is responsible for signal transmission, mediated via the T-cell receptor (TCR) they also express either CD4 or CD8. Those which bear the CD4 molecule (CD4 +) include helper-inducer cells important in triggering antibody production from B lymphocytes, cytotoxic T cells, and T cells involved in delayed hypersensitivity reactions. Those bearing the CD8 molecule (CD8 +) comprise cytotoxic T cells and others with suppressor functions on other cell types. Natural killer cells are CD3 positive, but do not normally express CD4 or CD8 markers. This scheme of classification is by no means absolute in terms of relating T lymphocyte phenotypes to a particular function. At present the CD4 population has been subdivided into three subgroups (Th_0, Th_1, Th_2) based on the mix of cytokines released by these T cells following antigen stimulation. These CD molecular complexes are believed to act co-operatively with T-cell receptors, to mediate stimulus transduction and activation of a number of cellular functions. Both CD4 and CD8 molecules can be regarded as functioning as co-receptors to the TCR in the recognition of antigen, and are involved in the signal transduction from the cell surface to the nucleus to initiate 'helper' or other related activities, or in the case of CD8 to initiate cytotoxic activity, or 'suppressor' functions, etc. Although the plethora of activities carried out by lymphocytes seems highly complex, it is to be expected that the potent and wide-ranging defensive mechanisms of the body should be subject to multiple checks, controls and regulations. As yet, relatively little is understood about the manner in which the various parts of the whole system of cellular and chemical defences are **integrated**, but it is increasingly clear they must be viewed as a **single system** of great efficiency and elegance. When, however, such integration breaks down, the effects may be far reaching as, for example, in the wide variety of *autoimmune diseases* that occur in man, and in neoplasia of the immune system, such as myeloma.

Immunological memory

If after one antigenic response the body is again exposed to the same antigen, the second response is much more rapid and extensive, even after a period of years; this forms the basis of clinical immunization. This phenomenon implies the presence of some type of immunological 'memory'. It appears to be the result of a number of factors, which are at present not entirely clear, including the possible persistence of long-lived 'memory B and T cells'. However, there is growing evidence that it is the persistence of antigen in selected sites (e.g. follicular centres, associated by APCs) that is a major factor in immunological memory. Overreactivity of this system may be associated with various types of hypersensitivity, for example anaphylactic shock and delayed-type hypersensitivity.

The nature of antigenic response

The antibody–antigen reaction is **highly specific**, each antigen requiring its own antibody for binding to occur. In the life of an individual an enormous range of antigens impinges on the immunological system, requiring a correspondingly large number of antibody producing B lymphocytes and an equally large number of antigen-specific T lymphocytes to deal with them. Recent studies on the mechanisms of generating a wide variety of antibodies (antibody diversity) capable of recognizing any conceivable macromolecule which might challenge the body during infections, have indicated that control of this variability results from a number of different processes which operate during the formation and maturation of B lymphocytes. As already stated, antibody molecules consist of four polypeptide chain structures (two light and two heavy chains), and each of these has an antigen-binding end (Fab) of variable structure, as well as a constant (Fc) region. The constant and variable regions are coded for by separate genes, so that, for the IgG antibody, at least four genes are needed to code for a single molecule, two of which are variable and two constant. Different combinations from a limited number of variable region genes are, therefore, capable of producing a large number of different antibody specificities (antigen combining sites). In fact, there are families of variable (V) genes, and each member of the family is constructed from many subunits which can be spliced together in different combinations to give a vast range of possibilities. To produce the heavy chain V region a functional V gene is compiled from three gene segments, V, D and J (Variable, Diversity and Junctional), and for the light chain V region there are V and J segments. Each V region gene is then linked to a constant region gene thus creating two genes to produce one polypeptide chain. The antibody diversity in the V region is further increased by somatic mutations in the genes, particularly in the heavy chain D regions during B-cell development, and probably by other factors such as variations in the transcription of DNA into messenger (m)RNA. It has been calculated that from as few as 200 V region genes (and segments) it is possible to generate at least 10^9 different antibody specificities by random combinations of these different components. Similar considerations apply to the T-cell receptor molecules.

The T-cell receptor

The T-cell receptor molecule consists of two polypeptide chains, either $\alpha\beta$ or $\gamma\delta$, which like immunoglobulin heavy and light chains have an N-terminal variable region and a C-terminal constant region encoded by a cluster of variable region gene segments and four constant region genes. In the bone marrow and later on in the thymus these genes are rearranged to generate the wide variety of T-cell receptors encountered. T-cell receptor responses to antigen are said to be MHC-restricted because they will only recognize an antigen when it is presented to them on an autologous (self) MHC molecule (either Class I or Class II) on other cells. However, during T-lymphocyte ontogeny the cell selects either an $\alpha\beta$ chain complex or a $\gamma\delta$ combination from the four germ line genes coding for the constant regions of these molecules.

Clonal selection theory

When the great diversity of antibody and T-cell specificities became apparent, the mechanism by which the body is able to produce the appropriate T- and B-cell responses to neutralize a particular antigen came under scrutiny. It has been shown that the lymphocyte populations of the body include B cells which already have the capacity to make almost any antibody and all types of T-cell specificity which might be required in the life of the individual. It has also been demonstrated that an antigen causes those cells which possess antigen receptors able to bind it, to each proliferate into a series of identical cells (a *clone*) that all produce the same antibodies and, in the case of T cells, that all have the same T-cell receptors. As an extension of this, it was postulated that clones inappropriate to defence, for example those able to produce antibodies against the body's own substances (auto-antigens) are in some way suppressed, being either eliminated by induced cell death (apoptosis) or kept quiescent (anergy). Of the huge range of possible antibodies that a B cell might synthesize, it is found in practice that only one is expressed in a particular B cell (*allelic exclusion*), and that its progeny will all express exclusively the same antibody specificity for antigen. When suitably stimulated, such B cells proliferate and mature into plasmacytes synthesizing identical antibodies. However, during secondary immune responses B cells usually switch the class (isotype) of the immunoglobulin from IgM to IgG or to some other isotype (e.g. IgA or IgE) under the direction of T-helper (CD4) control, but the specificity for antigen (defined by the V region of the molecule) remains the same. This 'class' switching enables antibodies to perform different biological functions (via their Fc regions) while retaining the same antigen specificity. Besides its importance in immunology, this phenomenon forms the basis for modern monoclonal antibody technology.

Specific T-cell responses to antigens are controlled in a similar way, in that T-helper and cytotoxic T cells, and perhaps other types of lymphocyte, are activated by interaction with antigen-presenting cells. The specificity to a particular antigen is determined by the T-cell receptor (TCR). Thus, like B cells, a great variety of T cells exists, each with a specific T-cell receptor preselected to recognize almost any antigen that might enter the body and enable the host to launch an immune attack upon it (either by itself, or by helper actions in co-operation with other defensive cells). When the antigen-MHC II complex at the surface of the antigen presenting cell interacts with the T-cell receptor complex, signals are transduced to the T-

cell nucleus which lead to the proliferation of this clone and thus an amplification of the immune response. Cells not bearing the T-cell receptor corresponding to that antigen remain unresponsive. The existence of the same phenomenon in two cell types (B and T) is not accidental, since the control of most B-cell responses is regulated by helper T cells responding to the same antigen. B cells can also act as antigen presenting cells by taking in antigen via their surface antigen specific receptors and then processing it into small polypeptide pieces before presenting it on their cell surfaces in association with their Class II MHC molecules. T-cells then recognize this processed antigen via their specific T-cell receptors and respond by releasing an array of cytokines which act directly on the B cell, causing it to differentiate into a plasmacyte and secrete antibody.

Direct activation of B cells by antigen in the absence of T cells can also occur, but only by a narrow range of rather unusual antigens which can cross-link the B-cell receptors, for example by identical repeating epitopes on linear carbohydrate molecules such as pneumococcal polysaccharide, leading to the production of IgM rather than IgG antibody. This type of T-cell-independent response is of limited importance when compared to the main immune responses observed in vivo.

Immunological tolerance

Since lymphocytes react to foreign antigens and not usually to the proteins and carbohydrates of the body itself, there must be some mechanism which ensures the distinction of **self** from **non-self**, that is, an *immunological tolerance* to self. If a breakdown in self-tolerance occurs, the autoimmune sequelae may give rise to immunopathology such as autoimmune thyroiditis (Hashimoto's disease) where immune-mediated destruction of the thyroid gland occurs and the result is clinical hypothyroidism. Some evidence for such an immunological aetiology exists for a number of other chronic relapsing diseases, including disseminated sclerosis which causes demyelination of neurological tracts within the central nervous system. Self-tolerance is procured in man early on during fetal development, in the thymus and bone marrow (p. 1428) and continues throughout adult life in other peripheral lymphoid tissues and organs of the body in ways that are still not fully understood. Burnet widened the theory of selective antigenic response (see above) to attempt an explanation of the mechanism of self-tolerance (the *clonal theory*), suggesting that those lymphocytes capable of producing antibodies directed against the body's own tissues are suppressed in fetal life and are then no longer available to multiply at a later stage (see Burnet 1969; Edelman 1974). The reality, however, is that every individual has many B- and T-lymphocyte clones able to address a wide number of auto-antigens present in their immune repertoires, which in the majority of cases do not lead to overt disease and self-destruction. Therefore, there are several layers of carefully controlled regulatory mechanisms that keep in check immune responses directed against antigens, whether they be self-derived or from outside the body. These include:

(1) in the thymus (for T cells) and bone marrow (B cells), deletion of those lymphocytes that recognize 'self' peptides in association with 'self' MHC (see p. 1428);
(2) failure to provide the second signal necessary for lymphocyte stimulation following antigen recognition, for example lack of T-cell help for B cells, thus inducing a state of anergy on the 'self'-directed (autoreactive) cells;
(3) autoreactive cells that do not have the appropriate tissue-specific addressins to enable them to 'home' back to the organ or tissue which contains the relevant auto-antigen during lymphocyte recirculation (see p. 1423), and
(4) active suppression of autoreactive responses by T cells through their release of cytokines that down-regulate the expression of MHC molecules and receptors of other cytokines, for example IL-2 receptors.

Only when all these controls fail do auto-antigen-specific responses occur, and even then regulation can be partially restored, as seen in the chronic relapsing scenarios found in many of the so-called autoimmune diseases, for example rheumatoid arthritis, multiple sclerosis and autoimmune thyrotoxicosis (Grave's disease).

The principle of self-tolerance may also be put to clinical use when grafts of tissue between monozygotic twins or closely related individuals are exchanged. All tissues from within a particular species have antigenic classes similar to those expressed in man as *histocompatibility* (HLA) tissue antigens. The success or failure of *isologous grafts* (i.e. grafts between genetically dissimilar members of the same species) depends largely on the degree of matching of these antigens between donor and recipient.

LYMPHOID TISSUES

Lymphocytes are concentrated in many sites in the body, typically at strategic sites which are liable to infection, or in possible routes for the spread of pathogens. The main areas of lymphocyte proliferation can be classed as either primary or secondary lymphoid tissue. To understand these terms it is necessary to examine how lymphocytes are formed and distributed in the body.

Circulation of lymphocytes (9.16)

The pluripotent stem cells for both B and T lymphocytes are present in the bone marrow where they proliferate to produce the precursors of both of these cell lines. For their differentiation and maturation, T-lymphocyte precursors have to pass into the thymus, which they do through the circulation; there, a number of major differentiation stages are passed through before the T cells are ready to engage in immune defence. From the thymus, the T cells enter the circulation again and pass to various peripheral sites where they can further multiply under the control of antigen-presenting cells. Likewise, B cells have to undergo a series of differentiation steps before they can perform their defensive roles. It appears that this generally occurs within the bone marrow. The newly formed B cells leave the bone marrow through the circulation and, like the T cells, pass to peripheral sites. The thymus and bone marrow are therefore described as *primary* (or *central*) *lymphoid organs* because of their initial roles in lymphocyte generation. The secondary or peripheral lymphoid organs or tissues include lymph nodes, spleen, lymphoid tissue associated with epithelial surfaces, such as the palatine and nasopharyngeal tonsils, Peyer's patches in the small intestine and various lymphoid nodules in the respiratory and urinogenital systems, the skin and conjunctiva of the eye. The bone marrow also serves as secondary lymphoid tissue as well as being primary, as lymphocytes pass back into it through the circulatory system, to engage in further proliferation when needed. In all the secondary tissue there are specific areas where either B or T cells are concentrated; cells enter them by migration through the walls of capillaries or venules and, having proliferated, leave by the lymphatic system or, in the case of the spleen, also by the venous drainage. The lymphocytes are now ready for action, and may be distributed to many other sites in the body when the need arises.

In the present account the thymus will be described first, followed by examples of the secondary lymphoid tissues and organs and then the spleen. The bone marrow has already been described earlier in this section (p. 1409).

THYMUS (9.19–28)

The thymus (9.19) is one of the two primary lymphoid organs (the other being the bone marrow). It is responsible for the provision of thymus-processed lymphocytes (T lymphocytes) to the whole body. The thymus provides a unique microenvironment in which the T-cell precursors (thymocytes) undergo development, differentiation and clonal expansion; during this process, the exquisite specificity of T-cell responses is acquired, as also is their immune tolerance to the body's own components. These steps involve intimate interactions between thymocytes and other cells (mainly epithelial cells and antigen-presenting cells) and chemical factors of the thymic environment. The organ is also part of the neuroendocrine axis of the body, and it both influences and is influenced by the products of this axis. Its activity, therefore, varies throughout life under the influence of different physiological states, disease conditions and chemical insults such as drugs and pollutants.

THYMIC ANATOMY

The appearance of the thymus varies considerably with age. It is

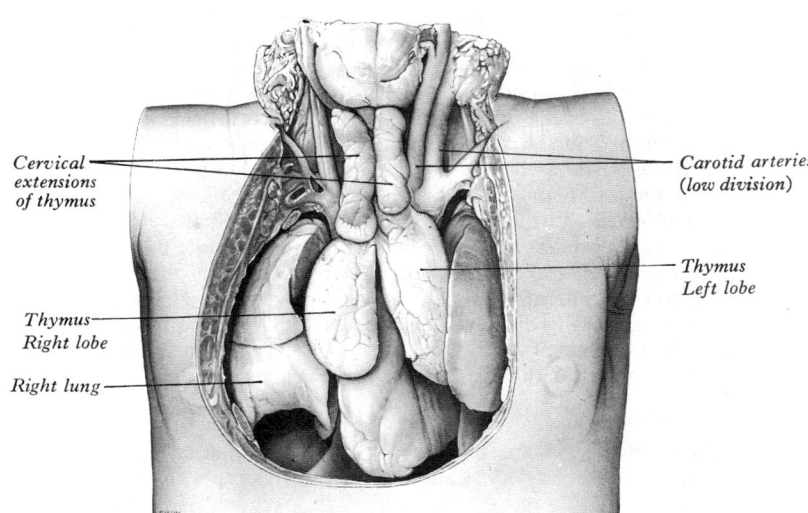

9.19   Dissection to display the neonatal thymus.

largest in the early part of life (9.19) up to the age of about 15, although it persists actively into old age (see p. 1429). It is a soft, bilobed organ, its two parts lying close together side by side, joined in the midline by connective tissue which merges with the capsule of each lobe. In children it is more pyramidal in shape and firmer than in later life, when its lymphoid content is reduced. In the fresh state (9.20) it is deep red due to its rich vascular supply; with age it becomes thinner and greyer before yellowing as adipose tissue infiltrates the organ, a process which is independent of obesity. Its weight also varies with age (see p. 1429); at birth it is 10–15 g and rapidly increases to about 20 g, then remains at that level thereafter, although the amount of lymphoid tissue gradually decreases (see 9.30, and below). Each of the two lobes is partially divided by the ingrowth of shallow septa so that superficially it appears lobulated; as fatty atrophy proceeds during ageing this lobulation becomes more distinct. The older thymus can be distinguished from the surrounding mediastinal fat only by the presence of its capsule, although even within greatly atrophied glands there are usually greyer areas around blood vessels, formed by persistent lymphoid tissue.

Position and relations

The greater part of the thymus lies in the superior and anterior inferior mediastinum, the lower border of the thymus reaching the level of the 4th costal cartilages. Superiorly, extensions into the neck

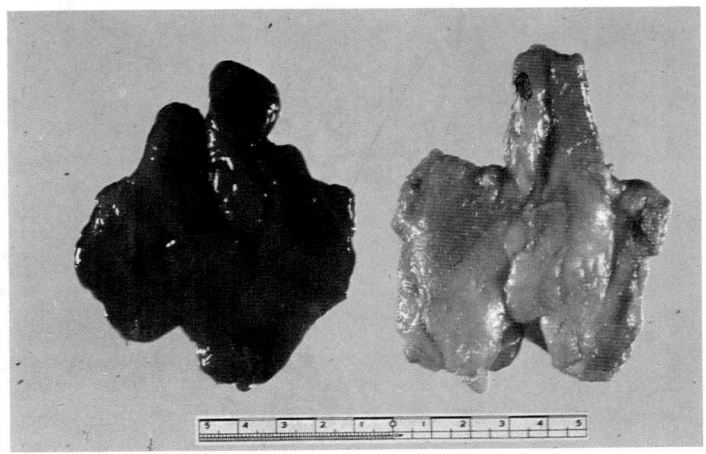

9.20   Human thymus from a 9-year-old girl (left) and an 80-year-old man (right). Note the fatty infiltration of the older thymus. (Provided by M Kendall, Department of Physiology, UMDS, St Thomas's Campus, London. Reproduced with permission from Kendall 1981.)

are common (**9**.19), reflecting the (bilateral) embryonic origins of the thymus from the third pharyngeal pouch (see p. 1428); it sometimes reaches the inferior poles of the thyroid gland or even higher. Its shape is largely moulded by the adjacent structures. **Anterior** are the sternum, adjacent parts of the upper four costal cartilages and the sternohyoid and sternothyroid muscles. **Posterior** are the pericardium and the aortic arch with its branches, the left brachiocephalic vein and the front and sides of the trachea. Ectopic thymic tissue is found in 25% of the population (Goldstein & MacKay 1969); small accessory nodules may occur in the neck representing portions which have become detached during their early descent, or the thymus may be found even more superiorly as thin strands along this path, reaching the thyroid cartilage or above. Connective tissue marking the line of descent during early development may, in some instances, run between the thymus and the parathyroids.

Vessels

Arteries. These are derived mainly from internal thoracic and inferior thyroid artery branches which also supply the surrounding mediastinal connective tissue, although a branch from the superior thyroid artery is also sometimes present. There is no main hilum but arterial branches pass either directly through the capsule or, more often, into the depths of the interlobar septa before entering the thymus at the junction of the cortex and medulla.

Veins. These drain to the left brachiocephalic, internal thoracic and inferior thyroid veins; one or more veins often emerge medially from each lobe of the thymus to form a common trunk opening into the left brachiocephalic vein.

Lymphatics. Afferent lymphatics are absent from the thymus but efferent lymphatics arising from the medulla and corticomedullary junction drain through the extravascular spaces in company with the arteries and veins entering and leaving the thymus. In rodents, large lymphatic vessels draining to perithymic lymph nodes are often found within the subcapsular cortex but these also receive lymph from other areas of the body; these lymph nodes drain in turn to

neighbouring regional nodes (Goldstein & MacKay 1969). Whether there is a similar perithymic lymphatic drainage in humans remains unknown.

Innervation

Thymic innervation is derived from the sympathetic chain via the cervicothoracic (stellate) ganglion (or from the ansa subclavia) and the vagus. Branches from the phrenic nerve and descendens cervicalis are distributed mainly to the capsule of the thymus. During development (Hammar 1935), vagal innervation of the thymus commences in the neck before its descent into the thorax. The two lobes are innervated separately through their dorsal, lateral and medial aspects and rich neural plexuses are formed in the medulla. After its descent, the thymus receives the sympathetic nerves along vascular routes, their terminals branching radially and forming with the vagal fibres a plexus at the corticomedullary junction. Innervation is complete by the onset of thymic function. While many of the autonomic nerves are doubtless vasomotor, many terminal branches also (at least in rodents) leave their perivascular pathways and pass among the cells of the thymus, particularly the medulla, suggesting that they may have other roles. The medulla also contains a variety of non-lymphoid cells, including cells positive for vasoactive intestinal polypeptide (VIP), acetylcholinesterase (AChE) large, non-myoid cells and cells containing oxytocin, vasopressin and neurophysin, with possible neural crest origin. Clearly, the roles of the nervous system and other neuroendocrine elements in the overall biology of the thymus are far from being understood and suggest many intriguing possibilities.

THYMIC MICROSTRUCTURE (**9**.21–31)

General architecture

To understand the cellular organization of the thymus it is helpful to consider its embryonic origins. The thymus is derived from a

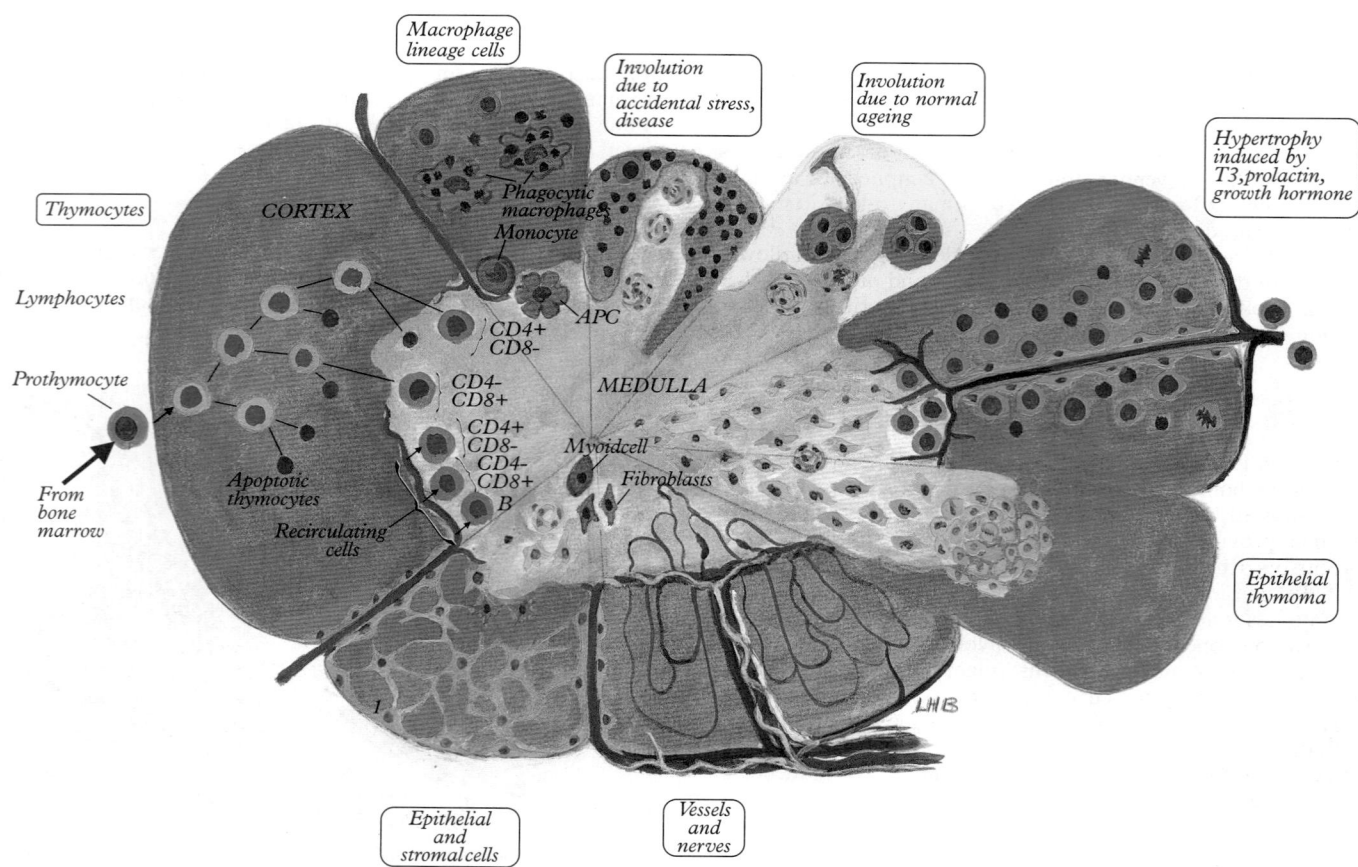

9.21 Schema illustrating the microscopic organization of the thymus at various stages of life and under different conditions.

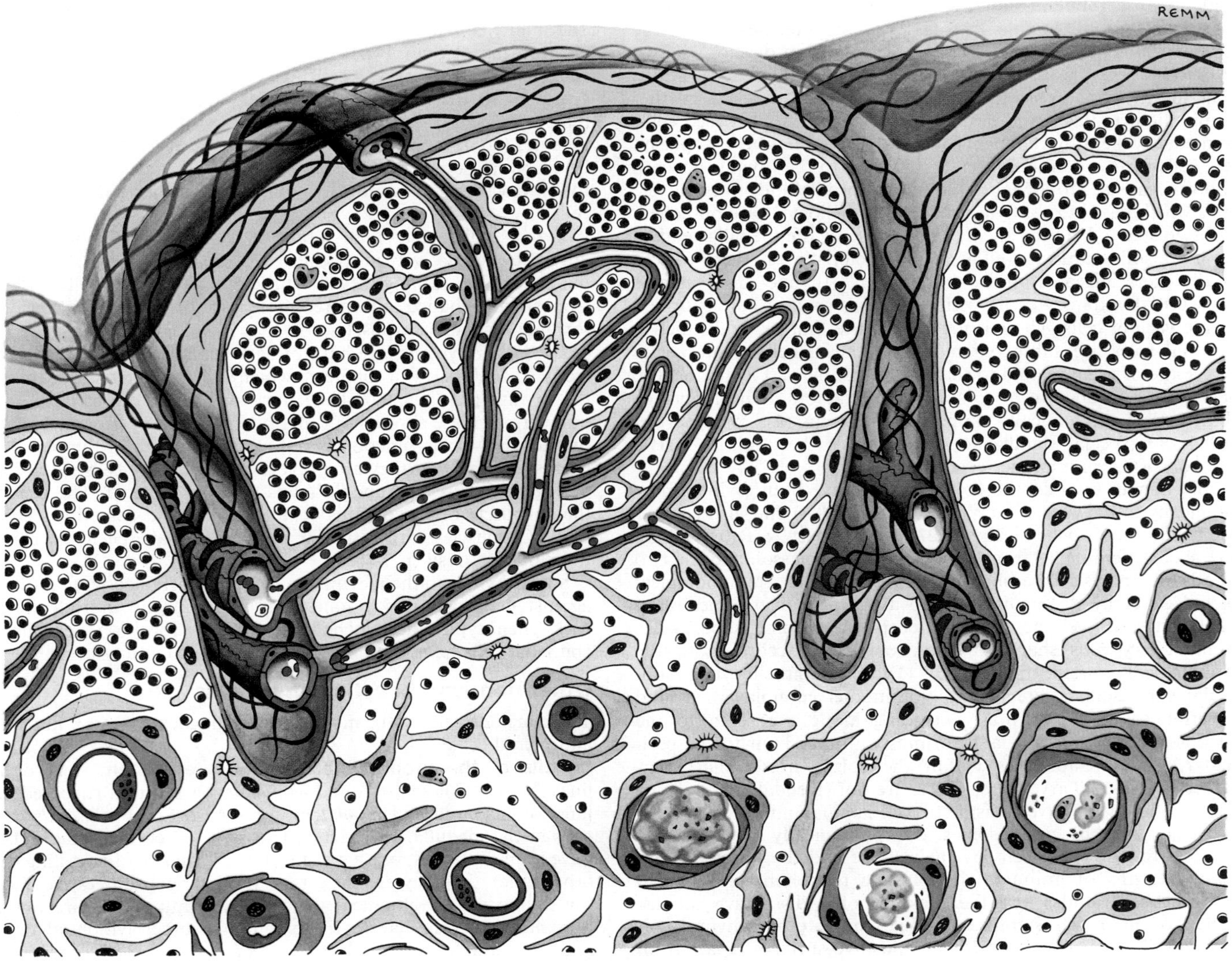

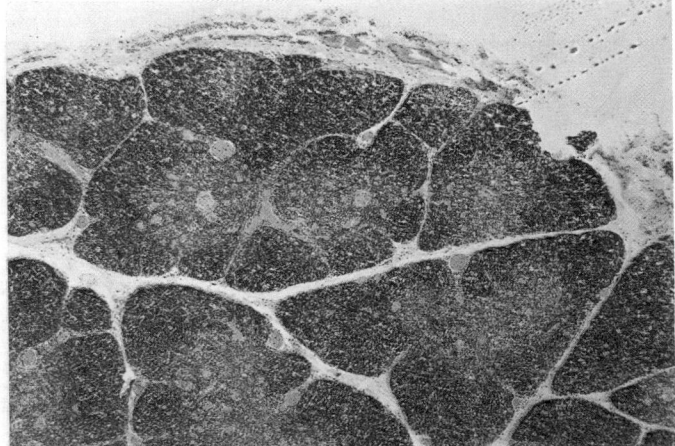

9.22 A scheme of thymic structure; the various elements are not drawn to scale to enable representation in a single diagram. Note the lobular outlines, capsule, delicate interlobular septa, cortical lymphocytes, the epithelial 'reticular' cells and their junctions and the medullary corpuscles of Hassall showing a graded series of increasing maturity; also the transcortical circulation. See text for further discussion.

9.23 Survey photograph of a neonatal human thymus stained with haematoxylin and eosin. The general lobular architecture is seen; each lobule contains a relatively pale medullary core surrounded by a densely cellular, dark, heavily stained cortex. (From a specimen prepared and provided by R O Weller, Department of Pathology, Guy's Hospital Medical School.)

number of sources, including epithelial derivatives of the pharyngeal wall, mesenchyme, haemolymphoid cells and vascular tissue. These form distinctive components within the mature thymus, interacting functionally to create its unique immunological properties.

When sectioned (**9.20–24**), the thymus is seen to consist of an outer *cortex* of densely packed cells mainly of the T-lymphocyte lineage, the *thymocytes*, and an inner *medulla* rich in connective tissue but with fewer lymphoid cells. Both lobes have a loose fibrous connective tissue capsule, from which septa penetrate to the junction of the cortex and medulla, to partially separate the irregular lobules, each 0.5–2.0 μm in diameter. A loose network of interconnected *thymic epithelial cells* permeates the cortex and medulla. In each lobule, the cortex has a superficial *outer cortical region* (subcapsular cortex) composed of a narrow band of cells immediately beneath the capsule, and the main cortex which is much more extensive. The central core of both thymic lobes is composed of a *medulla* which is continuous from one lobule to the next. The lobulations are partially separated from each other by connective tissue septa that form a route of entry and exit for blood vessels, efferent lymphatics and nerves. Most cells enter or leave the thymus by this route.

Epithelial framework (9.21–23, 25–27)

Unlike other lymphoid structures, where the supportive framework is chiefly collagenous reticular tissue, the thymus is permeated by a network of interconnected epithelial cells (*thymic epitheliocytes*) between which lodge lymphoid and other cells of the organ. There is only a little reticulin and few fibroblasts. By cell–cell contact and the release of soluble factors, the epitheliocytes create the microenvironments necessary for the thymocytes to develop.

Epitheliocytes vary in size and shape in the different positions within the thymus. Typically they have pale, oval nuclei, a rather eosinophilic cytoplasm and desmosomal attachments between cells. Intermediate (keratin) filament bundles lie within the cytoplasm. These cells form a continuous external lining to the thymus beneath its fibrous capsule, following its lobulated profile and investing the vessels which pass into it. Other cortical epitheliocytes are branched, with large spaces between them, while those of the medulla tend to form more solid cords as well as the characteristic whorls of (often) partially keratinized stratified epithelium (thymic or Hassall's corpuscles). Lymphocytes lie within the meshes and cords formed by these various cells. There is much evidence that many distinctive functional roles are subserved by the epithelial cells (Ritter et al 1985), some of them related to the differentiation of T lymphocytes, others to the production of soluble thymic factors or hormones or to barrier and mechanically supportive functions (see Wijngaert et al 1984). Of special significance, however, is their role in MHC restriction of T-cell immune responses.

In the human thymus, the epitheliocytes have been divided morphologically into Types 1–6 (Wijngaert et al 1984) and also characterized immunohistochemically (**9.27**A, B; Lampert & Ritter 1988). There is considerable heterogeneity within these classes, and the two methods of analysis give slightly different results. Immunological reagents generally distinguish subcapsular, cortical and medullary epitheliocytes as well as Hassall's corpuscles. Some subcapsular and medullary cells share the same epitopes. According to the morphological classification (**9.25**), Type 1 epitheliocytes (subcapsular-perivascular) create the continuous monolayer around the perimeter of the thymus, extending along the septa to the corticomedullary boundary and forming an outer limit to the perivascular spaces. Capillaries within the cortex are similarly ensheathed, but medullary blood vessels are not (Kendall 1989). Type 1 cells are flattened, have a distinct basal lamina and are connected to adjacent cells by desmosomes. Morphologically they are distinguished from Type 2 cells by their shape and the lower content of short lengths of granular endoplasmic reticulum, fewer small electron-dense granules and the presence of a distinctive tubular complex of unknown significance. Like most other thymic epitheliocytes, Type 1 cells have MCCII-positive surfaces, apart from their capsule-facing aspects which are MHCII-negative. Type 1 cells secrete factors (e.g. β2-microglobulin) that attract stem cells to the thymus (Dargemont et al 1989), and thymic hormones (Dardenne & Savino 1990).

Type 2 cells extend from the outer cortex towards the medulla forming a series of cells in contact with Types 3 and 4 epithelial cells. Types 2 and 3 cells are large, with long cytoplasmic extensions (sometimes extending 100 μm from the nucleus). They are active

cells with numerous cytoplasmic vesicles, several small Golgi bodies and many small electron-dense granules. Type 2 cells are more electron lucent than Type 3 cells which are, in turn, paler than the smaller very dense Type 4 cells. All cortical epitheliocytes are closely apposed to thymocytes, sometimes apparently engulfing them (emperiopoleisis). Large epitheliocytes with many associated thymocytes (50 or more) are called *thymic nurse cells* (TNC). These may be a special subset of Type 2 or 3 cells. They also contain mRNA for oxytocin and vasopressin, unlike most other cortical epithelial cells.

Type 5 cells are a small subset of medullary epithelial cells that appear to be relatively unspecialized. Type 6 cells are the commonest in the medulla, although several subsets may occur. Their forms range from spindle-shaped cells secreting thymic hormones to flattened cells forming Hassall's corpuscles.

Hassall's corpuscles are balls of flattened medullary epithelial cells from 30 to 100 μm in diameter which are characteristic features of the thymus (**9.25, 26, 29**). They start to form before birth and their numbers increase throughout life, often showing periods of increase or decrease. Their function is not clear, although in the past it has been suggested that they are graveyards for thymic cells (Blau 1969), or regions where immunoglobulins are concentrated. The centre of the corpuscle often contains cellular debris and sometimes eosinophils. Corpuscles with a similar appearance have been described in the palatine tonsil (p. 1444).

Some thymic epitheliocytes can be immunostained with antibodies against neuropeptides (Batanero et al 1992) and in rodents, cells with phenotypic and biochemical markers for both neurons and epithelial cells have been described in thymic cultures.

Other non-lymphocytic thymic cells

These include cells of the mononuclear phagocyte system, fibroblasts and myoid cells.

Cells of the mononuclear phagocyte system (macrophage lineage cells). These are found as *monocytes* at the corticomedullary junction, as *mature macrophages* in the cortex and as *interdigitating cells* in the medulla. In rodents, two types of cortical macrophages have been described, one a phagocytic cell capable of engulfing dying (apoptotic) thymocytes, the other producing proliferative factors for thymocyte development. The interdigitating cells are antigen-presenting cells similar to those found in other lymphoid organs, and are thought to be able to present antigens to the maturing T cells as they migrate from the cortex into the medulla, the medulla acting as a secondary lymphoid organ in this respect. Interdigitating cells are large, with characteristic infoldings of the plasma membrane, and do not generally contain phagocytic inclusions.

Fibroblasts. They are found in the capsule, perivascular spaces and medulla, but are infrequent in the cortex, except in involuted glands. Short-range or contact interactions between thymocytes, Class II MHC positive epitheliocytes and mesenchymal cells (or a

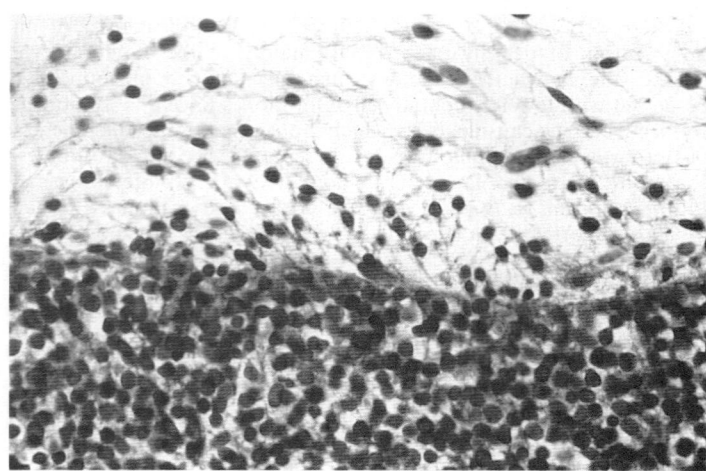

9.24 Prothymocytes entering the thymus rudiment through the capsule before blood vessels and nerves have invaded the epithelial cells. Haematoxylin and eosin. Magnification × 240. (Provided by M Kendall, Department of Physiology, UMDS, St Thomas's Campus, London.)

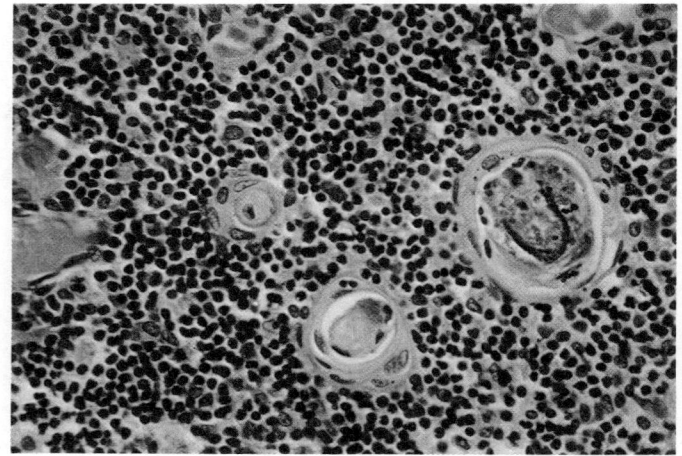

9.25 Neonatal thymus. A medullary field showing three concentric corpuscles of Hassall of varying degrees of maturity, surrounded by many closely packed lymphocytes and a number of reticular cells.

fibroblast cell line) have been found to be necessary for the in vitro development of thymocytes (Anderson et al 1993).

Myoid cells. These cells are situated mainly in the medulla and at the corticomedullar junction. They are large, rounded cells, with a central nucleus surrounded by irregularly arranged bundles of myofilaments. In lower vertebrates, where myoid cells are often more numerous, these cells are joined to neighbouring medullary epithelial cells by desmosomes. Their functions are unknown, although it has been suggested that their contractions might aid the movement of lymphoid cells across or out of the gland.

Lymphocytic population, thymocytes (9.21, 24–28)

In the cortex, massive numbers of densely packed small thymocytes (thymic lymphocytes) predominate, occupying the interstices of the epithelial reticulum, which in histological sections they largely obscure, and forming about 90% of the total weight of the thymus. A distinct subcapsular zone is present, housing the thymic stem cells, prothymocytes and lymphoblasts undergoing mitotic division. The first stem cells to enter the thymus in the embryo come from the yolk sac and liver during their haemopoietic phases, possibly, as in birds, being attracted by thymic chemotactic substances. During later periods it is probable that all thymic lymphocytes originate in the bone marrow, or at least have sojourned there, before passing in the bloodstream to the thymus.

The cortex has two rather ill-defined zones: an outer cortex with a framework of Types 1–3 epitheliocytes and a deep cortex where Type 4 cells occur. Thymocytes undergo mitosis in all cortical zones as the clones of differentiating T cells mature, gradually moving deeper in the cortex. In rodents, cell cycling times of 8 hours have been recorded in the outer cortex, but no estimates exist for the human thymus. The appropriate conditions for the proliferation and differentiation of thymocytes appear to be produced by their close proximity to neighbouring epitheliocytes (see Janossy et al 1986). Although the nature of these interactions is not clear, it may involve the release from the epitheliocytes of soluble mitogenic and differentiation factors as well as induction of changes through intercellular contact. During this process, thymocytes differentiate along the T-cell line, acquiring the CD3 + marker and T-cell receptors, and also switching into different subclasses of T cells (p. 1420). The great range of different T-cell receptor types, running into many millions, is also established here by the expression of variable genes and related mechanisms (p. 1420).

As time passes, the differentiating thymocytes enter the medulla, and migrate through the walls of venules and lymphatics to move into the circulation. Such cells (post-thymic thymocytes) are not immunocompetent within the cortex, and in general attain maturity only after entering the medulla or perhaps not until they reach their secondary lymphoid tissue destinations. However, the existence of antigen presenting cells and plasma cells in the medulla indicates

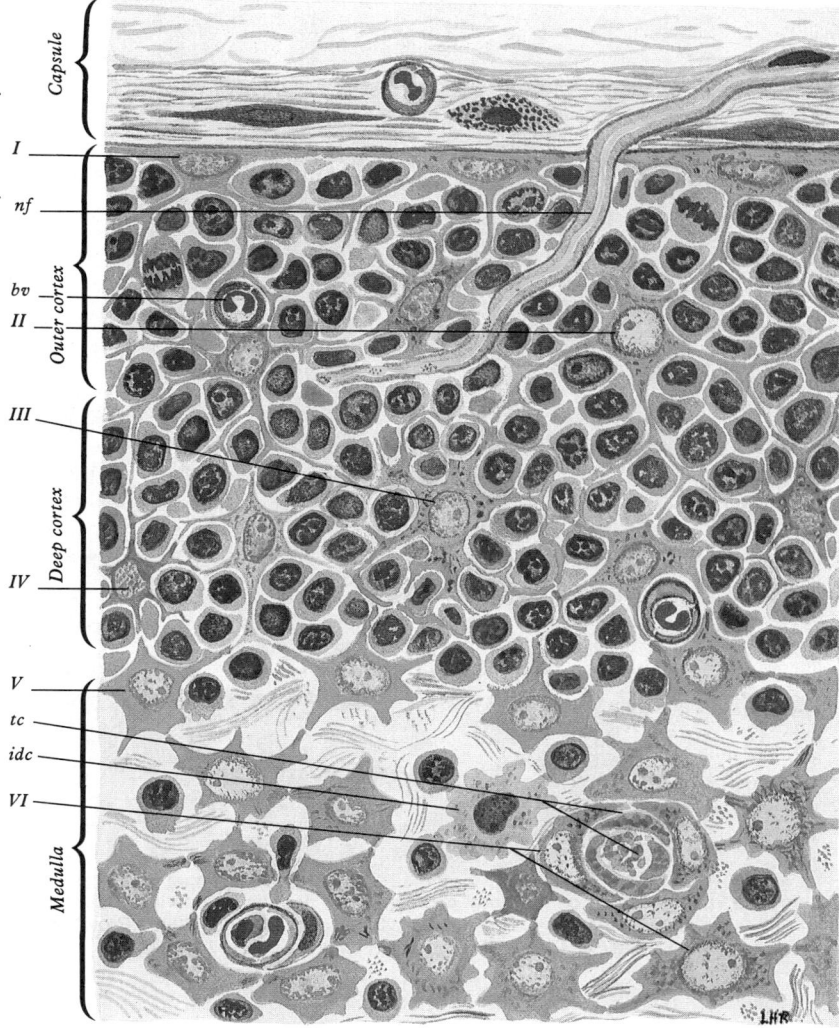

9.26   Cellular organization of the thymus showing thymocytes (blue) and epitheliocyte framework (green) of Types 1–6 cells. nf = nerve fibre; tc = thymic corpuscle; idc = interdigitating cell; bv = blood vessel.

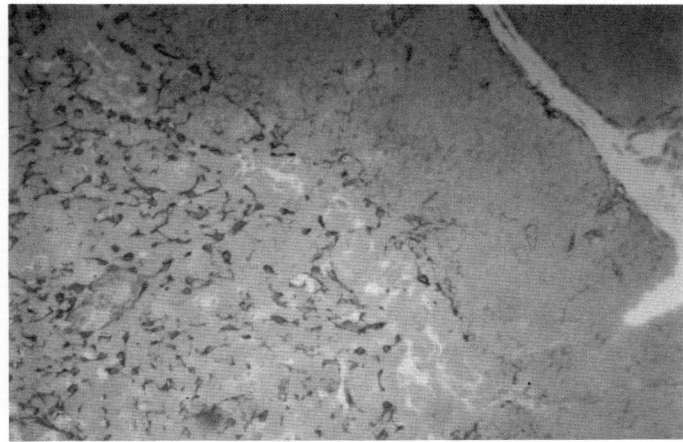

9.27A   Human pediatric thymus immunostained to show the distribution of the IL-4 receptor on Types 2 and 3 epithelial cells of the cortex. Peroxidase method. (Provided by Mary Ritter, Royal Postgraduate Medical School, London.)

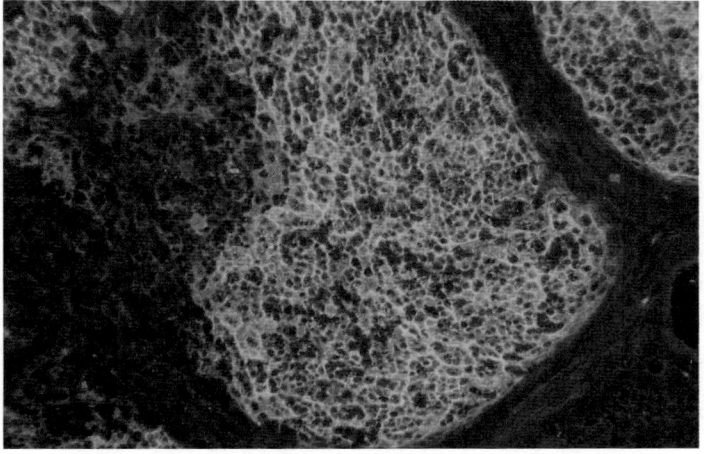

9.27B   Human pediatric thymus, near serial section corresponding approximately to 9.27A, immunostained to show thymulin-containing cells beneath the capsule (Type 1 epitheliocyte) and in the medulla (Type 6 epitheliocyte). Immunofluorescence (FITC) method. (Provided by Mary Ritter, Royal Postgraduate Medical School, London.)

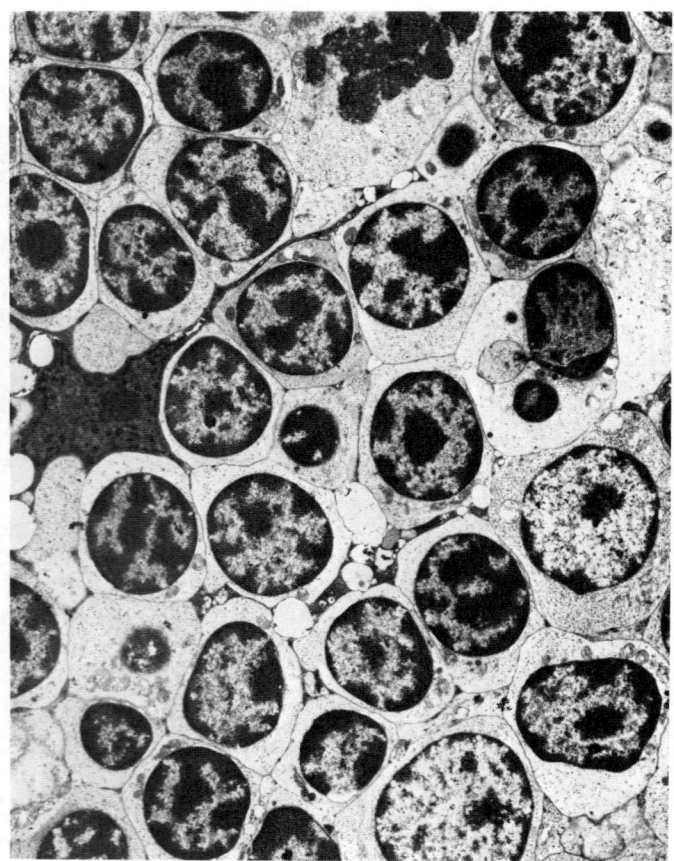

9.28 Transmission electron micrograph of the thymic cortex showing lymphocytes ensheathed in epitheliocytes. Magnification × 3000. (Provided by M D Kendall, UMDS, St Thomas's Campus, London.)

that T lymphocytes **can** be activated within the thymus, if not in large numbers.

Thymocyte classes. Four major lymphoid cell types are found in the thymic cortex, as determined by immunocytochemistry and flow cytometry; each of them has a different proportion of small, medium and large thymocytes. Firstly, there are cells which do not express the mature T-lymphocyte markers CD4 or CD8 (double negative cells) nor, initially, CD3. Most of these are large *blast cells*, which after undergoing mitosis become small, double negative thymocytes and begin to develop the T-cell receptor (TCR) complex and become CD3-positive. These blast cells are primarily located in the subcapsular cortex and around blood vessels, especially at the corticomedullary junction. During the development of the TCR the cells give a transient expression of γ/δ, followed by α/β and other TCR components (see p. 1421), and simultaneously become double positive for CD4 and CD8, as well as the histochemical marker TdT (terminal deoxynucleotidyl transferase), characteristic of thymocytes thereafter (see Janossy & Campaner 1989). The majority of these double-positive cells are small cortical thymocytes comprising 80–90% of the total thymocyte population. It is thought that the functional abilities of the T-cell repertoire is determined at this stage, with 'undesirable' lymphocytes dying in great numbers by apoptosis. The few that are rescued by the action of factors from the micro-environment (positive selection) become either CD4- or CD8-positive (i.e. single rather than double positives); these cells are found in the medulla and are slightly larger than cortical thymocytes.

Medullary single-positive thymocytes may either be cells about to be exported to the periphery where they will become fully immunocompetent, or recirculating activated T cells which have entered the medulla secondarily (Agus et al 1991). In addition, a few single positive cells represent early cortical cells that transiently express either CD4 or CD8 before becoming double-positive early thymocytes, as noted above.

In addition to these T-cell products, the thymus is also thought to be responsible for generating natural killer cell lineages.

The thymus often contains some immature B lymphocytes in the medulla or around blood vessels at the corticomedullary junction, and mature B cells (plasmacytes) throughout the thymus and in perivascular spaces. These cells are not formed in the thymus but arrive by immigration through the vasculature. The occurrence of occasional mature B lymphocytes and also, sometimes, germinal centres in the medulla (Middleton 1967) also supports the conclusion that at least part of the medulla is more like a secondary ('peripheral') as opposed to a primary ('central') lymphoid tissue, receiving previously differentiated lymphocytes capable of immune interactions.

Acquisition of self-tolerance

As indicated above, the great majority of thymocytes never leave the thymus. However, during their maturation, thymocytes acquire the ability to recognize the HLA (MHC) markers expressed by the unique genome of the individual they belong to, i.e. 'self-antigens', so that when they migrate to the peripheral lymphoid organs and other tissue sites, they and the clone of cells they give rise to can detect alien antigens when these are present in association with 'self'-MHC determinants (see p. 1407) and can mount an appropriate immune attack. It appears that the thymocyte's correctness of response to self-MHC antigens is in some way determined in the thymic cortex before release and that if they respond inappropriately, the thymocytes are deprived of appropriate growth factors and undergo apoptotic death. In this way the thymus selects only T cells which can recognize alien antigens in combination with self-MHC molecules (i.e. they become MHC-restricted, see p. 1407).

Embryonic origins of the thymus

Most embryological evidence at present favours the view that the thymic epithelium is derived from both the ectoderm and the endoderm of the third and often the fourth branchial clefts and pharyngeal pouches; these layers interact with the associated neural crest mesenchyme at about the 10 somite stage (day 23: see Hammar 1911; Weller 1933; Norris 1937; Hamilton et al 1972; Stark 1975) to initiate thymic development.

The first stages of thymic development are seen bilaterally in the third pharyngeal pouch towards the end of the 6th gestational week, when endodermal cells form a sacculation. As these cells move caudally and anterolaterally they become surrounded by mesenchymal and ectodermal cells (Norris 1938), attracting pro-thymocytes which enter through the surrounding mesenchymal capsule. By the 8th week the two advancing thymuses are united in the midline, and basophilic thymic stem cells and thymocytes come to lie between the epitheliocytes (von Gaudecker 1986), which are visibly differentiated. Myoid cells appear in the centre of the thymus.

With the descent of the thymus, vascularization begins, and nerve fibres from the vagus grow in along the blood vessels, following the inward growth of connective tissue septa which produce a lobulated form. By 10 weeks, over 95% of the cells belong to the T-cell lineage, with a few developing erythroblasts and B lymphocytes. Hassall's corpuscles are also present. By 12 weeks, the mesenchymal septa, blood vessels and nerves have reached the newly differentiating medulla, allowing the entry of macrophage lineage precursors, macrophages and interdigitating cells being first seen at 14 weeks. Granulopoiesis occurs in the perivascular spaces. The 17-week thymus appears fully differentiated, and after this time it produces the main type of thymocyte also present throughout life (designated TdT$^+$.

In the mutant mouse *nude*, where the ectodermal anlage for the thymus is deficient, the thymus is abnormal, cystic and does not support lymphopoiesis, although lymphocytes are still produced in the bone marrow (Pritchard & Micklem 1973; see also Cordier and Haumont 1980). Developmental abnormalities of neural crest derivative that also affect the development of the heart and peripheral neural ganglia also result in thymic deficiency, as seen in the Di George and Pierre Robin syndromes (Couly et al 1983).

Microcirculation and local innervation (9.21)

Vessels in the cortex. The pattern of blood flow differs in the cortex and medulla. Major blood vessels enter the gland at the corticomedullary junction and pass within each lobe giving off small capillaries to the cortex and larger vessels to the medulla. Most cortical capillaries loop around at different depths in the cortex and join venous vessels at the corticomedullary junction, but some continue through the cortex to exit from the thymus through the capsule and join larger veins running in the capsule. These smaller capillaries usually have a narrow perivascular space which sometimes contains pericytes and other cells, but rarely nerves.

There is a complete sheath of epithelial cells between the perivascular spaces and the cortex, an arrangement which has been called the blood–thymic barrier (Marshall & White 1961; Raviola & Karnovsky 1972). In the past it was assumed that thymocytes needed to be 'educated' in an antigenically pure environment. This was thought to be achieved in the cortex, since antigens in the blood would have to cross blood-vessel endothelium, the connective tissue of the perivascular space and an epithelial sheath in order to reach the lymphoid tissue of the cortex. More recently it has been shown that antigens can reach the cortex by a transcapsular route (Niewenhuis 1990). In the light of this finding it can be postulated that developing thymocytes are bathed in numerous antigens which could influence thymocyte education and subset formation (see below).

Vessels in the medulla. Medullary blood vessels are not so protected by epithelial cells, and those of the corticomedullary junction are only partially ensheathed (usually on their cortical aspect). Medullary vessels are surrounded by connective tissue and at certain times, for example in mid to late pregnancy (in rodents) the medulla may contain increased numbers of fibroblasts and connective tissue matrix. Medullary vessels are very variable in size, and some may have short lengths of high endothelium similar to those in lymph nodes and mucosa-associated lymphoid tissue.

Lymphatics. Efferent (though not afferent) lymphatics are also found in the perivascular spaces; they appear to begin in the medulla or at the corticomedullary junction.

Innervation. Most thymic nerves are seen near blood vessels, either in close apposition to them or forming complex ramifications in the tunica adventitia, or free in the perivascular spaces. Few nerves have been seen within the cortex or medulla in man. In rodents, however, subcapsular and corticomedullary nerve plexuses are present, and branches have been seen peeling off to enter the cortex to ramify between epithelial cells, macrophages and thymocytes (Felten & Felten 1989; Weihe et al 1989; Kendall & Al-Shawaf 1991). This has been disputed by other researchers (Novotny et al 1990).

Many nerve fibres in the major nerve bundles and plexuses are noradrenergic and therefore efferent sympathetic. Some nerves give a positive reaction with antibodies to vasoactive intestinal peptide (VIP), neuropeptide Y (NPY), substance P (SP) or calcitonin gene-related peptide (CGRP), and are presumably sensory or sensorimotor. Occasionally large neuronlike cells with either CGRP positively or acetylcholinesterase (AchE) activity have been reported in the medulla. The presence of cholinergic nerves is in dispute (Bulloch & Moore 1981; Nance et al 1987; Tollefson & Bulloch 1990), and therefore the vagal fibres may be afferents.

Thymic haemopoiesis

Haemopoietic cells are present in fetal life, when the thymus makes an important contribution to the formation of erythrocytes and leucocytes. Later haemopoietic cells are often present, possibly as a result of the reactivation of persistent fetal stem cells. Normoblasts have been found in the thymuses of many adult open-heart surgery patients, and immature eosinophils, neutrophils and mast cells have also been observed. Where present in adults, the erythropoietic foci are mainly in the subcapsular and outer cortex.

Thymic changes during postnatal life (9.21, 30)

The thymus is largest relative to body weight at birth. It was previously believed that it increased in size until puberty after which it declined dramatically (Bratton 1925; Young & Turnbull 1931; Boyd 1932). However, many of the studies giving rise to this conclusion were based on post-mortem findings after illnesses of varying durations, and several authors comment that the thymus weights recorded were, therefore, probably underestimates. Studies of thymus weight after sudden death (Kendall et al 1980; Steinmann 1986) have recorded a wide variation at all ages, but the general

pattern is that after the first year of life, when there is an increase, the mean weight is fairly constant at about 20 g until the 6th decade when a reduction occurs. Computed tomography and imaging studies of the thorax have given similar results (Stone et al 1980; Moore et al 1983).

Although the weight of the thymus may be fairly constant, it is increasingly infiltrated by adipose tissue and so the total amount of active lymphoid tissue becomes progressively smaller. At birth, individual adipocytes may be seen in connective tissue septa, and increased numbers are found within the cortex in the second and third decades. Fatty infiltration is usually complete by the fourth decade when only the medulla and small patches of associated cortex are spared. Thymic hormone-secreting cells in the medulla persist throughout life.

Because of these changes, the numbers of thymocytes present must be greatly reduced in old age, as has also been found in cultured tissue. However, thymocyte production and differentiation persist throughout life, and T cells from this source continue to populate the peripheral lymphoid tissue, blood and lymph (see Steinmann & Müller-Hermelink 1984b).

THYMIC HORMONES AND OTHER SECRETED FACTORS (9.31)

The well-characterized thymic hormones are principally thymulin, the thymosins, thymopentin and thymic humoral factor. Thymulin, originally called 'Facteur Thymique Sérique' (FTS) relies on zinc for its biological activity (Dardenne & Bach 1988). The thymosins are a large family isolated from thymosin fraction 5 (Goldstein et al 1977). The precursor of thymosin α1, prothymosin, is found in highest quantities in the thymus, but is also secreted elsewhere (Haritos et

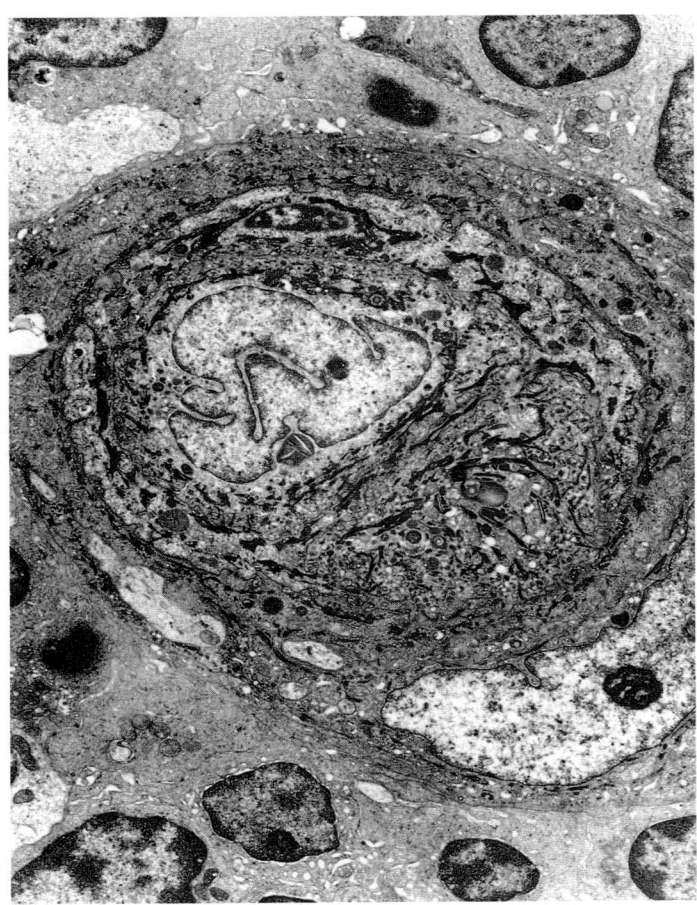

9.29 Electron micrograph of a section through thymic medullary epitheliocytes forming a Hassall's corpuscle. Rat. (Micrograph provided by M Kendall, Department of Physiology, UMDS, St Thomas's Campus, London.)

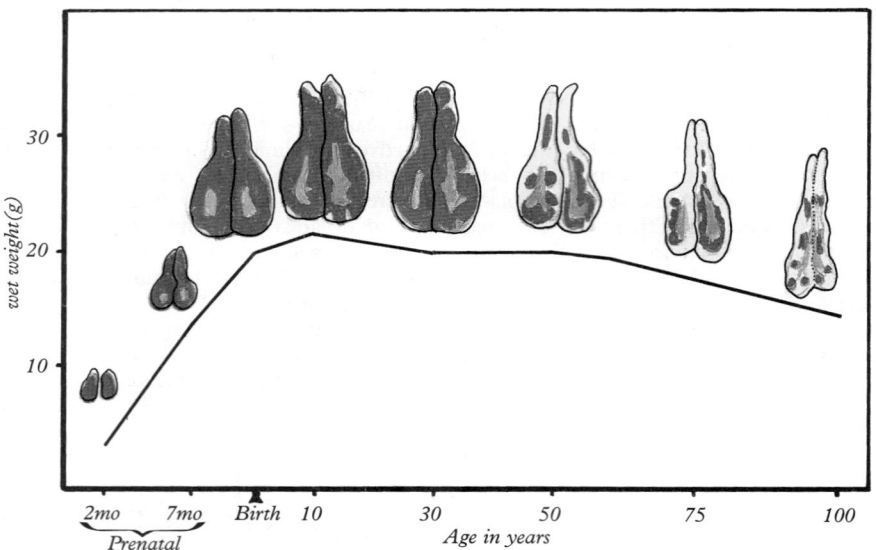

9.30 Diagram illustrating the age-related changes in thymic weight and composition. Pink = lymphoid medulla; red = the cortex, yellow = fatty infiltration. (After Kendall et al 1981 with permission.)

al 1984) as is parathymosin. Thymosin β1 is ubiquitin (Schlesinger et al 1975), and thymosins β4 and β10 have recently been shown to be sequestering components of connective tissue (Yu et al 1993). Thymopoietin, although originally studied for its neuromuscular effects, has its biological and immunological activity in residues 32–36 (thymopentin or TP5) (Goldstein et al 1979). Thymic humoral factor (THF) had also been sequenced (Burstein et al 1988) and no homology has been found between any of the thymic hormones.

The peptide hormones of the thymus have a range of immuno-modulatory effects on lymphocyte maturation within the thymus and in the periphery (reviewed in Trainin 1974; Dardenne & Bach 1988; Safieh-Garabedian et al 1992). Most will induce markers of early differentiation on lymphoid cells lacking such markers, and enhance various T-cell functions. The injection of most thymic hormones restores immunological competence to neonatally thymectomized mice, modulates surface epitopes in patients with immune deficiencies and improves immunocompetence in man and animals.

There are many other soluble factors in the thymic micro-environment, but cytokines have been shown (usually by in vitro methods) to be important singly or synergistically in thymocyte development. Their actions are very complex, and not yet fully understood. Interleukins IL-1, IL-2, IL-4 and IL-6 are secreted by thymocytes (as well as other cell types), and IL-1, IL-3, IL-4, IL-6 and IL-7 by the thymic epithelium. Cells bearing receptors for all of these cytokines, as well as for tumour necrosis factor a (TNFa), and colony stimulating factors for granulocytes and macrophages (GM-CSF, M-CSF or CSF-1) and γ-IFN, occur in the thymus.

NEUROENDOCRINE–THYMIC INTERACTIONS

All major hormones released from endocrine glands can influence thymic function and/or structure, and thymic factors often affect other endocrine organs. Many of these effects are mediated through the thymic microenvironment. Thymic epithelial cells have receptors for all of the sex steroid hormones (Grossman et al 1979; Pearce et al 1983), including a unique oestrogen receptor, corticosteroid receptors (Dardenne et al 1986), nuclear receptors for triiodothyronine (Villa Verde et al 1992) and low-affinity luteinizing hormone releasing hormone (LHRH) receptors. Receptors on thymocytes have been identified for growth hormone (Arrenbrecht 1974), corticosteroids (lower numbers than on epithelial cells), oxytocin (Elands et al 1990), and oestrogen (fewer than on epithelial cells) (Kawashima et al 1992).

Both gonadal steroids (except progesterone) and corticosteroids

are well documented as affecting the thymus. Oestrogens can increase vascular permeability and downregulate Class II MHC and increase macrophage numbers, all of which would alter the thymic micro-environment function (Moreno & Zapata 1991). The numbers of thymocytes in early and late stages of differentiation are increased by high levels of oestrogens (Screpanti et al 1989).

Man is considered to be 'resistant' to the action of corticosteroids in the thymus (rats are 'sensitive'). In general, high levels of corticosteroids preferentially kill cortical thymocytes by causing apoptosis (reviewed in Kendall 1990) but low levels have a potentiating thymopoietic effect in the embryo (Ritter 1977). Corticosteroids also

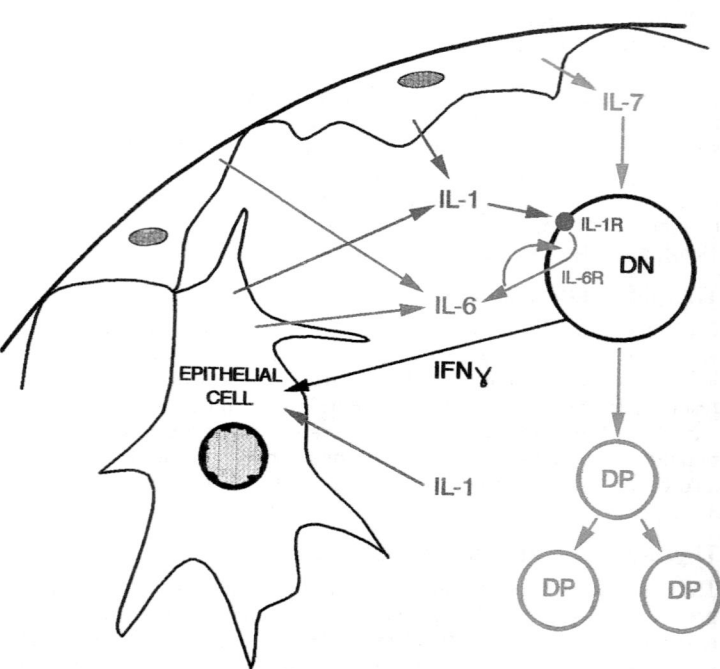

9.31 Schema illustrating the proposed cytokine interactions within the thymus between subcapsular epitheliocytes and prothymocytes. DN: CD4 –/CD8 – cells; DP: CD4 +/CD8 + cortical thymocytes. (Provided by M Kendall, Department of Physiology, UMDS, St Thomas's Campus, London.)

enhance the migration of prothymocytes into the thymus (Bomberger & Haar 1992). The weight of the thymus is increased by thyroid hormones, particularly exogenous T3, and in hyper-thyroidism, while hypothyroidism decreases thymic weight. In rats, perinatal hypothyroidism causes a rise in thymic oxytocin content, but not in hypothyroid adults with atrophied thymuses. Some cortical epithelial cells synthesize oxytocin and vasopressin, and contain neurophysin (Geenen et al 1991), but immunostaining for oxytocin gives different reactions in thymus and brain (Geenen et al 1991). Oxytocin levels in the thymus are very high (Argiolas et al 1990a,b; Jeremovic et al 1990) and can be increased with corticosteroids such as dexamethasone.

Any effect of hypothalamic factors on thymic function is probably mediated via the hypophysis except for LHRH where there is histological, and some functional evidence for a direct action (Marchetti et al 1989). *Thymosin fraction 5* stimulates the secretion of LHRH from the hypothalamus (Rebar et al 1981). LHRH agonists cause thymic enlargement in rats and increase the levels of thymosin α1 (Ataya et al 1989).

The hypophysis is a target for the thymic hormones. Not all of them act in the same way, but release of many pituitary hormones can be induced in vitro either directly or via an influence on the hypothalamus. Antibodies against adrenocorticotrophic hormone (ACTH), growth hormone (GH), prolactin (PRL), follicle stimulating hormone (FSH), β-FSH, luteinizing hormone (LH), β-LH and other anterior hypophyseal hormones, give positive reactions with thymic epithelial cells, especially those of the medulla (Batanero et al 1992). PRL, GH (probably via IGF-1), and thyrotrophin releasing hormone (TRH) (through T3 action) increase thymulin secretion. The reaction is pleiotrophic and quite slow (over days in vitro). It is also effected by met-enkephalin and β-endorphin as well as adrenal and sex steroids (reviewed in Dardenne & Savino 1990). A rapid release of thymulin, however, is achieved by elevated physiological levels of ACTH in vitro and in vivo and its action is potentiated by glu-cocorticoids (Buckingham et al 1992).

Oestrogen (or testosterone metabolized to oestrogen) inhibits the release of thymic serum factors. The treatment of mice with estradiol reduced the levels of thymosin α1 (Allen et al 1984). These findings, however, are in contrast to those of Stimson and Hunter (1980) where estradiol treatment caused the appearance of thymus-dependent factors in the serum. Progesterone and estradiol applied over several days induced thymulin release from cultured thymic epithelial cells (Savino et al 1988). Earlier work, however, had shown a very complex picture of thymulin release during adrenalectomy and gonadectomy. Conflicting results could be due, in part, to the concentrations of steroids used. It can be seen from this rather heterogeneous list of experimental data that neuroendocrine inter-actions with the thymus are complex and, at present, difficult to simplify into a clear picture. However, it is patent that there is considerable interchange, and that extreme modulation of thymic function must be important in the control of immune function in general, through direct effects on T-cell maturation, and indirect effects on more subtle activities of the thymus on the immune system of the body.

CLINICAL ASPECTS OF THE THYMUS

Congenital anomalies have been summarized by Gray and Skan-dalakis (1990). Undescended thymus, accessory thymic bodies and the rare cysts of the third branchial pouch are of no clinical significance (except where thymectomy is indicated). Patients with thymic agenesis, aplasia and hypoplasia, as in the Di George (Cri-du-chat) syndrome and severe combined immune deficiency disease, have reduced lymphocyte numbers, and early death from infection is common. Most cases are familial, with autosomal recessive genes.

In young children a large thymus may press on the trachea, causing attacks of respiratory stridor. Thymic tumours may also compress the trachea, oesophagus and large veins in the neck, causing hoarseness, cough, dysphagia and cyanosis. Thymomas may develop in one lobe of the thymus without affecting the other. Many of these patients have myasthenia gravis and other autoimmune conditions, too. Myasthenia gravis, a chronic autoimmune disease of adults (Castleman 1966), is a diminution in power of certain voluntary muscles for repetitive contraction. Although there may be more than

one condition with these signs, myasthenia gravis is essentially an autoimmune disease in which acetylcholine (ACh) receptor proteins of neuromuscular junctions are attacked by auto-antibodies. Muscles commonly involved are levator palpebrae superioris (leading to ptosis) and extraocular muscles (leading to diplopia). Others in the face, jaws, neck and limbs may be involved and in severe cases the respiratory muscles. About 10% of Caucasian myasthenia cases have a thymoma and 50% have medullary follicular hyperplasia. These are predominantly young females under 40 years of age who have a strong HLA-B8-DR3 expression. Thymectomy in this latter group often results in improvements in their symptoms. In the absence of a thymoma, the onset of myasthenia gravis occurs after 40 years of age in patients with a HLA-B7-DR2 phenotype, except for a group in which weaknesses are restricted to eye and eyelid movements (Willcox 1989).

As described above, during neonatal and early postnatal life, the thymus is essential to the normal development of lymphoid tissues. Thymectomy at this stage leads to a progressively fatal condition, with hypoplasia of the peripheral lymphoid organs, wasting and an inability to mount an effective immune response. By puberty, when the main lymphoid tissues are fully developed, thymectomy is less debilitating, but a reduction in effective responses to novel antigens ultimately ensues.

LYMPH NODES (9.32–38)

Lymph nodes are encapsulated centres of lymphocyte differentiation and proliferation, belonging to the class of *secondary* or *peripheral* lymphoid tissue. Structurally they are small, oval or reniform bodies, 0.1–2.5 cm long, lying in the course of the lymphatic vessels. Each usually has a slight indentation on one side, the *hilum*, through which blood vessels enter and leave; an *efferent lymphatic vessel* also emerges. Several *afferent lymphatic vessels* enter peripherally. Lymph nodes have a highly cellular *cortex* and a *medulla* containing numer-ous, poorly demarcated cavities which represent a network of minute lymphatic channels through which lymph from the afferent lym-phatics filters, to be collected at the hilum by the efferent lymphatic. The cortex is deficient at the hilum, where the medulla reaches the surface. Lymph nodes are particularly numerous in: the neck, mediastinum, posterior abdominal wall, abdominal mesenteries, pelvis and proximal regions of the limbs. By far the greatest number of these lie close to the viscera, especially in the mesenteries. Besides their immune functions in generating mature, primed B and T cells, lymph nodes add antibodies to the circulation, and also filter particles, including microbes from the lymph by the action of numerous phagocytic macrophages within their lymphatic spaces.

MICROSCOPIC STRUCTURE OF LYMPH NODES

A lymph node is essentially a continuous framework consisting of the capsule, trabeculae and the reticulum, with cells enmeshed in it.

Capsule and trabeculae. The capsule is composed mainly of collagen fibres, a few fibroblasts and elastin fibres, the latter being more numerous in the deeper layers. In some animals smooth myocytes occur but these are few in human nodes. From the capsule, trabeculae of dense connective tissue extend radially into the node's interior, continuous with the network of fine collagen (reticulin) fibres, the *reticulum*, which supports the lymphoid tissue. At the hilum, dense fibrous tissue may extend into the medulla, with an efferent lymphatic vessel embedded in it.

Reticulum. This network of fine collagen (reticulin) fibres and associated cells permeates the spaces enclosed in the capsule and trabeculae (**9.32, 33**) and supports the cell masses within them. Microscopically, the fibres are identifiable with reticulin stains (**9.34A, B**), which show how their bundles branch and interconnect, forming a very dense network in the cortex, although the germinal centres have fewer fibres. Bundles of these fibres, covered by endothe-liocytes, criss-cross the sinuses, providing attachment for various cells, mostly macrophages and lymphocytes. Reticulin fibres with an associated proteoglycan matrix are apparently formed by cells indistinguishable from the fibroblasts, though various names (e.g. 'reticular cells') have been applied in the past.

Lymphatic channels. Lymph nodes are permeated by channels

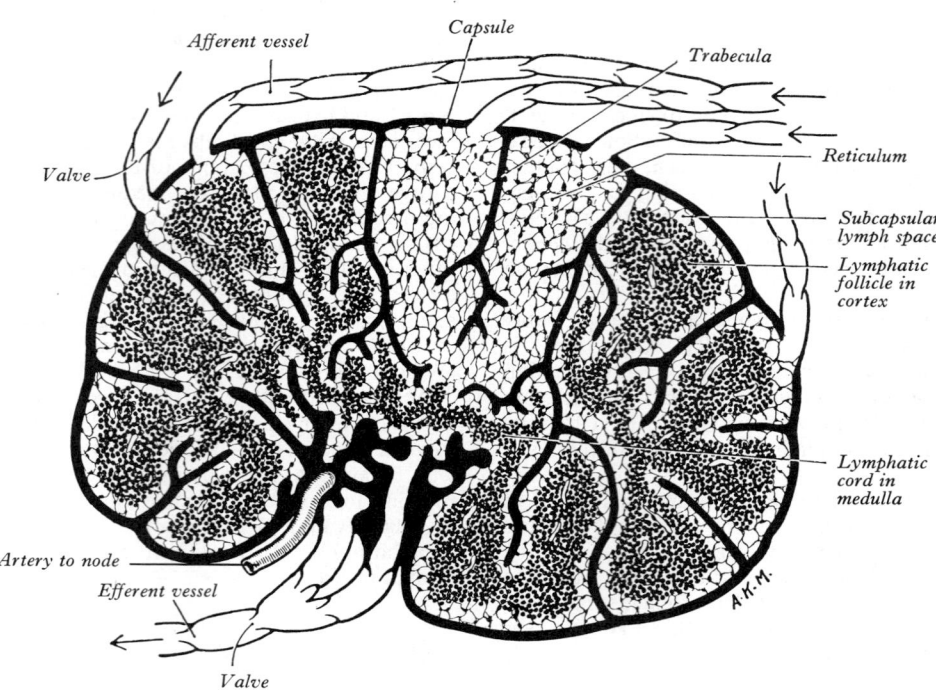

9.32   Diagram of a lymph node (modified from Maximow & Bloom). In part of the diagram, lymphocytes have been omitted to show the reticulum. This diagram from an earlier source has been retained for historical interest; greater detail and more modern concepts are displayed in **9.**33.

through which lymph percolates after its entry from the afferent vessels (**9.**37, 38A, C); because macrophages line channels or are entangled amongst the fibres crossing them, lymph is exposed to the action of these phagocytic cells, as well as to the activities of B and T lymphocytes adhering to endothelia.

Afferent vessels enter at many points on the periphery, branching to form a dense intracapsular plexus and then opening into the *subcapsular sinus*, a cavity peripheral to the whole cortex except at the hilum (**9.**33). From this sinus numerous radial *cortical sinuses* lead to the medulla, coalescing as larger *medullary sinuses*, which are in turn confluent at the hilum with the efferent vessel draining the node. All these spaces are lined by an endothelium which is continuous despite the constant passage of lymphocytes, macrophages and other cells through the walls of sinuses in both directions. Numerous trabeculae cross them, making their lumina almost labyrinthine and providing large areas for the attachment of various cell types in the spaces (Nopajaroonsri et al 1971; Luk et al 1973).

Lymphatic vasculature. Arteries and veins serving lymph nodes pass through the hilum, giving off straight branches which traverse the medulla and issue minor branches en route. On reaching the cortex, arteries form dense arcades of arterioles and capillaries in numerous anastomosing loops, eventually returning to highly branched venules and veins. Capillaries are especially profuse around the follicles, with fewer vessels within these structures (Herman et al 1973; Blau 1976); postcapillary venules are abundant in the paracortical zones, forming an important site of lymphatic migration (see below). The pattern of vascularization is altered when lymphocytes multiply in response to antigenic stimulation, and then the density of the capillary beds increases greatly (Herman et al 1972).

The structure of these blood vessels is normal except for the *postcapillary venules*, which are lined by tall cuboidal endothelial cells, between which colloids pass readily to perivascular spaces (Mikata & Niki 1970); they also allow extensive movement of lymphocytes from the bloodstream into the paracortex and probably also the reverse (Marchesi & Gowans 1964; Gowans & Knight 1964). The route of migration appears to be through tight junctions which part to allow the passage of cells (Schoefl 1972). Some veins may leave a node through its principal trabeculae and capsule, supplying these and the surrounding connective tissue.

Cells. Most of the cells in the reticulum are *B* and *T lymphocytes* but *macrophages* also occur, especially along the walls of sinuses and within germinal centres (see below). The distribution of lymphocytes

varies in different regions. In the sinuses are some cells which are swept into lymph as it circulates through the node; in the cortex, cells are densely packed and may form isolated *lymphoid follicles* (nodules **9.**35, 36). The number and isolation of follicles vary according to the prevailing antigenic stimulation. The follicular centre is composed of cells which are larger, less deeply staining and more rapidly dividing than those at its periphery. These areas are *germinal centres*, their cells being mainly *lymphoblasts* which, by prolific mitotic divisions, produce small lymphocytes which migrate outwards into the *mantle zones* surrounding the germinal centres. The cells pass from follicles into sinuses, which convey them across the medulla to the hilar efferent vessel.

In the medulla, lymphocytes are much less densely packed, forming irregular branching *medullary cords* between which the reticulum is easily seen. Entangled cells include some macrophages, more numerous in the medulla, plasmacytes and a few granulocytes. Under antigenic stimulation, for example, when the node drains a site of infection or an immunization, the whole node **reacts** by an increase in size and vascularity. The number and size of germinal centres also increases, as lymphocytes and macrophages proliferate, and differentiation of numerous plasma cells occurs in the sinuses. For further details of lymphocyte biology, see pages 1405, 1422.

CELL ZONES IN LYMPH NODES

As stated above, the cells of lymph nodes are arranged in regions of different packing densities and of distinct cell types. Nopajaroonsri et al (1971) have suggested the division of the cortex into three zones indicating the packing density of its cells (**9.**33):

- *Zone 1* is a region of loosely packed cells, predominantly small lymphocytes, macrophages and occasional plasmacytes around the extreme periphery of follicles and extending centrally into the medullary cords;
- *Zone 2* is a denser region internal to zone 1, limited to cortical and paracortical areas and composed mainly of small lymphocytes and macrophages;

9.33   (*opposite*) Schema of the general architecture and cellular organization of a lymph node. Particular reference is made to the differential distribution of lymphatic spaces and cell masses. Coloured arrows indicate the circulatory pathways of T and B lymphocytes. For details see text.

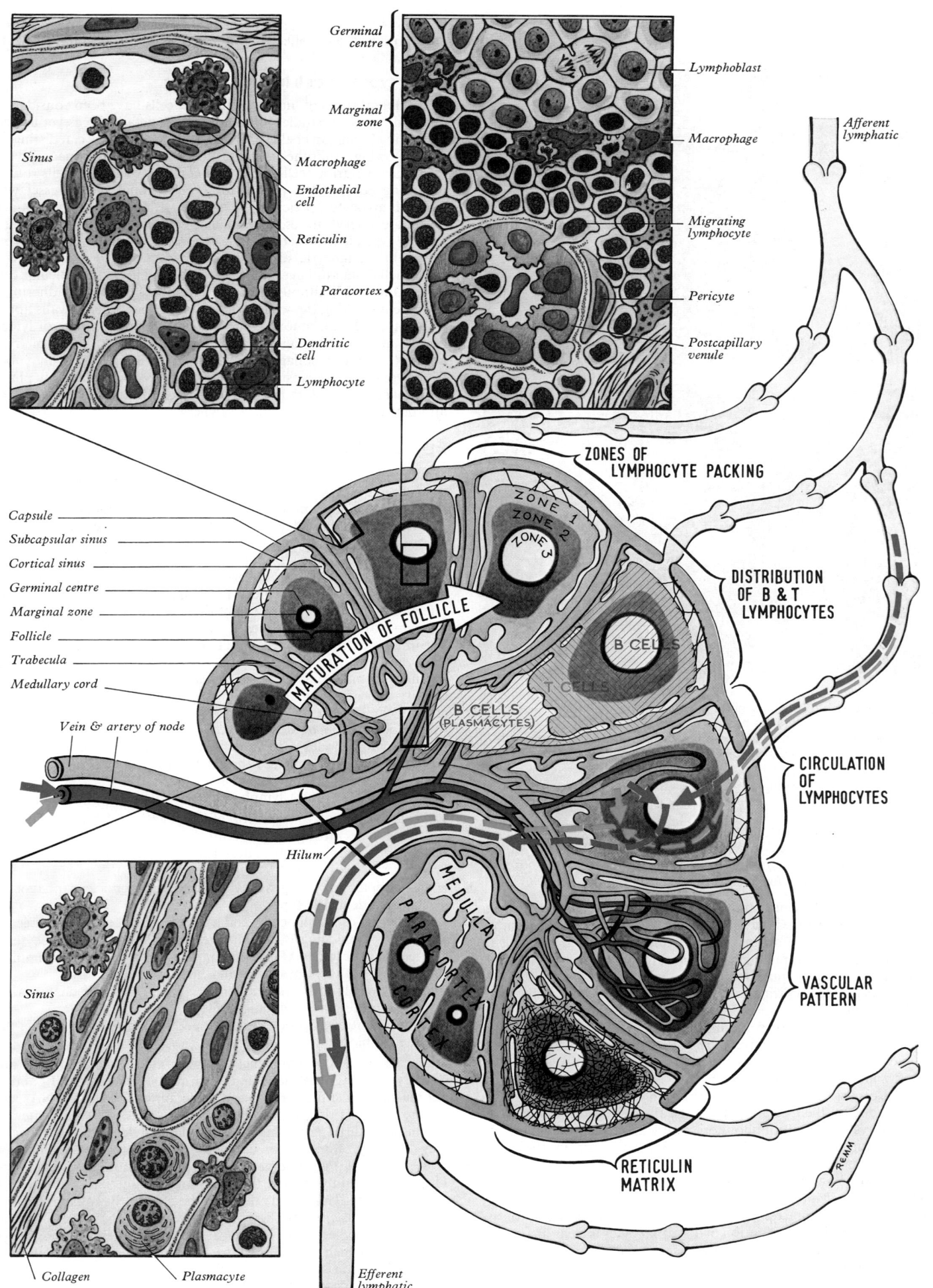

Germinal centre

Marginal zone

Macrophage

Endothelial cell

Reticulin

Paracortex

Dendritic cell

Lymphocyte

Sinus

Lymphoblast

Macrophage

Migrating lymphocyte

Pericyte

Postcapillary venule

Afferent lymphatic

ZONES OF LYMPHOCYTE PACKING

Capsule
Subcapsular sinus
Cortical sinus
Germinal centre
Marginal zone
Follicle
Trabecula
Medullary cord

ZONE 1
ZONE 2
ZONE 3

DISTRIBUTION OF B & T LYMPHOCYTES

B CELLS

T CELLS

MATURATION OF FOLLICLE

B CELLS (PLASMACYTES)

Vein & artery of node

Hilum

CIRCULATION OF LYMPHOCYTES

MEDULLA
PARACORTEX
CORTEX

VASCULAR PATTERN

Sinus

RETICULIN MATRIX

REMM

Collagen   *Plasmacyte*

Efferent lymphatic

1433

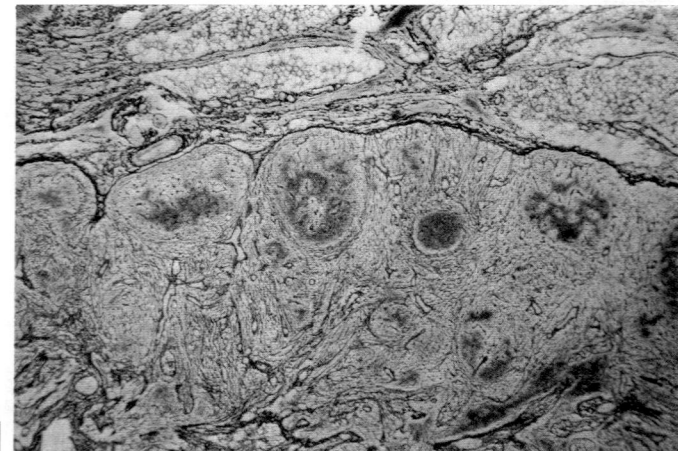

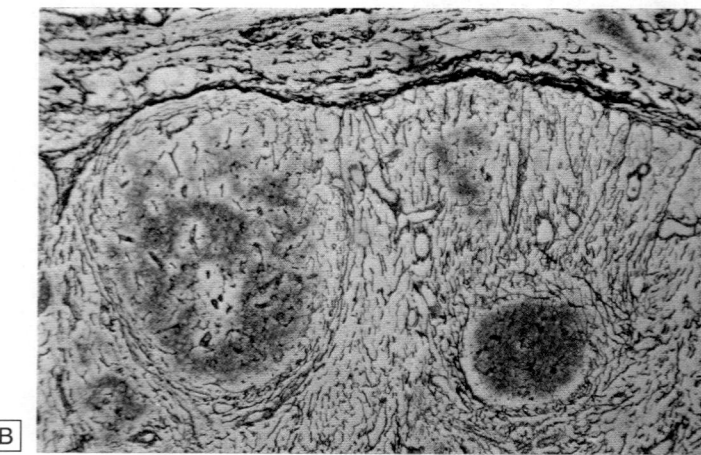

9.34A, B Sections of a lymph node stained by the method of Glees and Marsden for reticulin. Note the heavy concentration of fibres in the capsule and trabeculae. A fine network permeates the rest of the node, with a concentric accumulation surrounding the cortical lymphatic follicles.

- *Zone 3* comprises the germinal centres of follicles, which are particularly prominent in antigenically stimulated lymph nodes; its cells include large lymphoblasts, some in mitosis, together with dendritic cells and macrophages.

Fibroblasts, reticulin fibres and other cells, mentioned below, appear in all zones. These zones may form a maturational sequence, lymphocytes arising by division in germinal centres (zone 3), passing to the dense zone 2, becoming smaller and finally migrating to zone 1, from which they may traverse the endothelium into the sinuses. But the sequence is complicated by immigration of other cells from lymphatic and haemal sources, and the precise relation between overall cellular architecture and maturation is not clear. In any case, though helpful for descriptive purposes, purely structural schemes also have to note the different functional subclasses of lymphocytes in such zones.

It is also possible to map the distribution of B and T lymphocytes within nodes by their immunohistological reactions to monoclonal antibodies (**9.36A, B**). Immunofluorescent staining shows that they occupy distinct territories. Immature B cells occur in the more peripheral parts of follicles, whereas T cells lie mainly between the germinal centres and the medulla, i.e. in the *paracortex* or *thymus-dependent zone*. Mature B cells (plasmacytes) exist mainly in medullary cords and sinuses, while some are also peripheral to the cortical follicles. The distribution of T lymphocytes is clear in animals with a congenital absence of the thymus (e.g. *'nude'* mice), which fail to develop a paracortex. Whether germinal centres contain T or B cells or both is debatable; possibly also cytological markers for their

detection are only effective after the lymphocytes have left the germinal centres.

Other types of cell in lymph nodes

The different types of 'non-lymphocytic' cells have been considerably clarified by recent studies although certain details are as yet unclear. Following Steinman et al (1974) and other authors, we can distinguish the following: endothelial cells, fibroblasts, typical macrophages, follicular dendritic cells and paracortical dendritic cells ('interdigitating cells of the paracortex'); cells lining blood-vessel walls (smooth myocytes, pericytes) also occur, as do the terminals of non-myelinated nerve fibres. Endothelial cells lining the nodal sinuses appear typical in structure and, contrary to earlier views, do not show the phagocytic ability which had attracted terms such as 'endothelial macrophages', 'reticulo-endothelial cells', 'reticular cells' or 'littoral cells', although true macrophages do occur adhering to endothelium along the walls of sinuses. The endothelial walls appear to be of the discontinuous type, allowing the free passage of lymphocytes and macrophages. Fibroblasts ('reticular cells' of some authors) produce collagen including reticulin to form the nodal framework, i.e. the capsule, trabeculae and reticulum. Highly phagocytic macrophages (see p. 1415) are identifiable in the cortex within and between the follicles and elsewhere.

FUNCTIONS OF LYMPH NODES

Lymphatic capillaries and larger lymphatic vessels returning excess tissue fluid to the venous system carry particulate materials of various kinds to the lymph nodes scattered along their course. The nature of these materials will vary with the region drained; areas rich in microbial flora, for example the alimentary tract, are a major potential route of entry of pathogenic organisms and debris into the circulation and of course any area of the body may supply microbes and debris of various kinds, particularly after damage or local infections. In the respiratory tract there is the additional problem of the removal of inhaled particles from the alveoli, which is carried out in part by macrophages re-entering the tissues and passing into the lymphatic pathways. Lymph nodes form a major protection against such materials and organisms, removing them by phagocytic activity and exposing them to a wide variety of powerful defensive actions carried out by lymphocytes resident within them or added to the population of defensive cells circulating in the lymph and blood. Lymph nodes respond dynamically to the presence of such materials and can modulate their activities and structure according to the demands put upon them.

The essential roles of lymph nodes include:

- the provision of a labyrinth of channels, of large volume and surface area, through which lymph slowly percolates
- the exposure of foreign material in the lymph to macrophages in nodal sinuses
- the trapping of antigens by different mononuclear phagocytes including dendritic types
- production of lymphocytes and a pool of stem cells able to become antibody-producing B lymphocytes and mature T lymphocytes
- interaction between APCs and lymphocytes to produce an immune response, both cell-mediated and humoral
- re-entry of blood-borne lymphocytes into lymphatic channels and thence to the haemal circulation
- humoral antibody production and addition to lymph and, via that route, to blood.

There have been a number of important advances in this area recently, based on cell labelling with antibodies against T- and B-cell markers, in situ hydridization detection of specific mRNAs, and culture methods. It appears that when T and B cells first enter the lymph node through the high endothelial venules in the paracortex, they initially come into contact with interdigitating antigen-presenting cells and undergo a process of selection and stimulation. The T cells mainly stay in the same area or enter the sinusoids to pass out of the lymph node through the efferent lymphatic and thus into the general circulation. The primed B cells, however, pass into the follicles, where they displace the existing small lymphocyte population, which are pushed to the perimeter of the follicle to create its mantle zone. The B cells then come to lie amongst the reticular network formed by the follicular dendritic cells (an antigen-

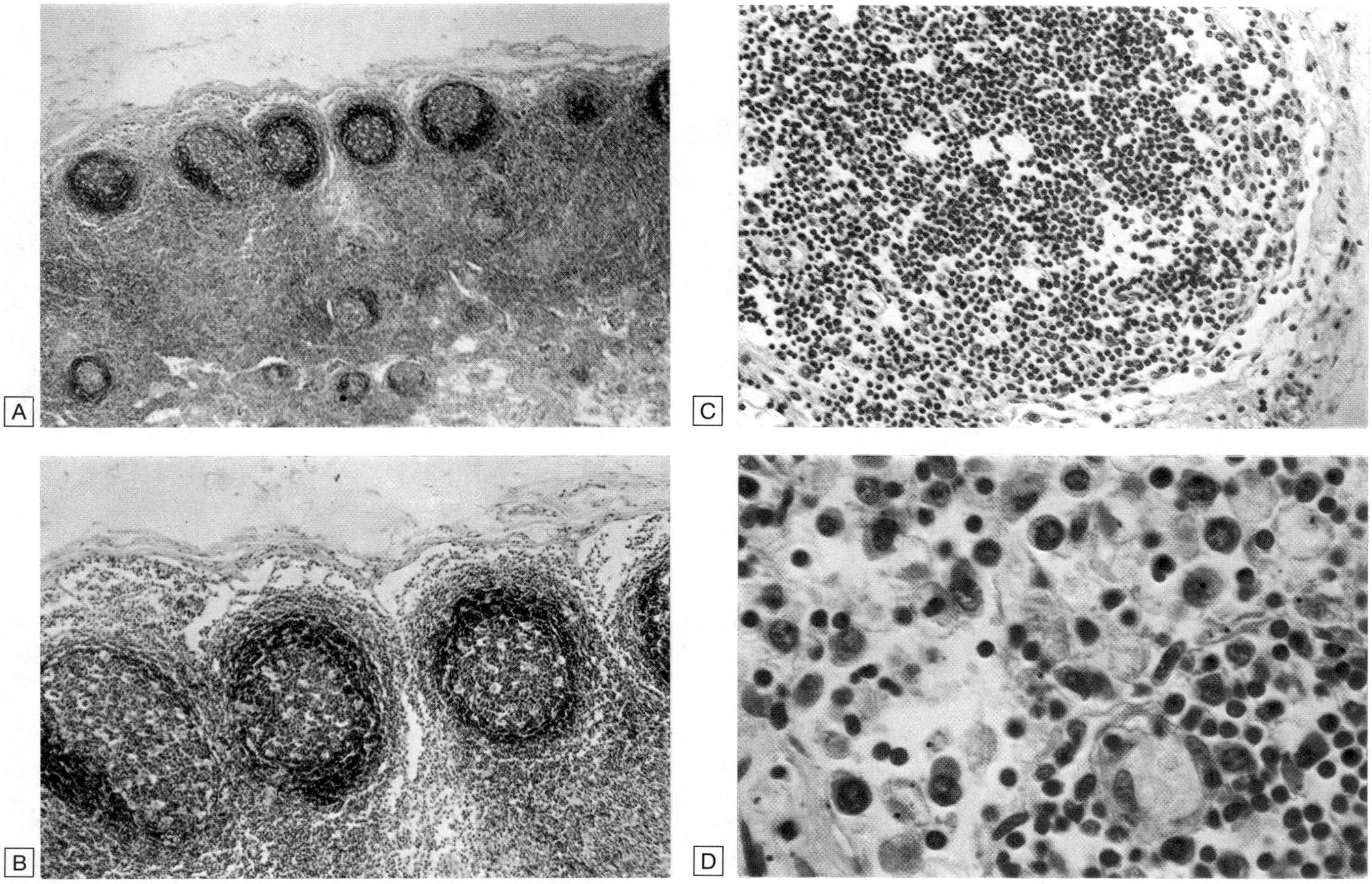

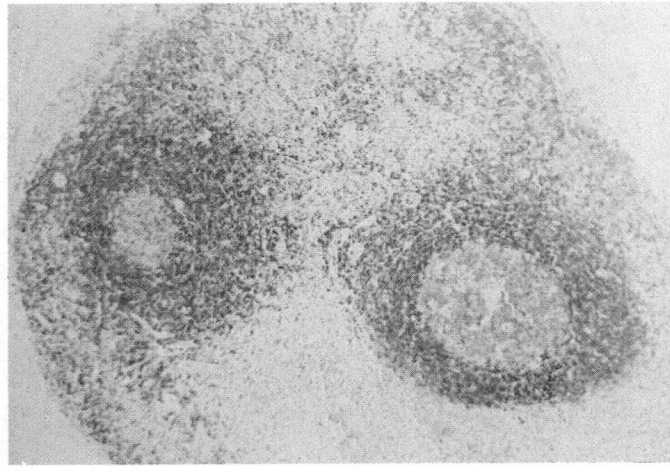

9.35A–D   Sections of lymph nodes stained with haematoxylin and eosin. A Note the round cortical lymphatic follicles with their dense, dark periphery and pale germinal centres and the irregular medullary tissue. Very low power survey micrograph. B Low-power view of germinal centres showing the variation in cell density. C Higher-power view of the peripheral zone of a follicle showing the densely packed small lymphocytes. D Higher-power view of the medulla showing a variety of cell types including small and large lymphocytes and prominent rounded plasmacytes.

presenting cell, APC) which possess antigen on their surfaces (probably having endocytosed this elsewhere before reaching the node via the same route as the lymphocytes). Contact between the antigen and the B-cell surface receptors selectively triggers intense cell division in the B cells (which are then first termed centroblasts, and subsequently centrocytes); only those B cells which are able to mount defensive responses to the relevant antigens are stimulated to divide, forming clones of B cells with identical responses (see p. 1422, clonal theory). These activated B lymphocytes then move to the edge of the follicle, where they may express IgM as an initial response to stimulation, then pass into the sinusoids in which they move to the medulla of the node and thence into the circulation, or they may

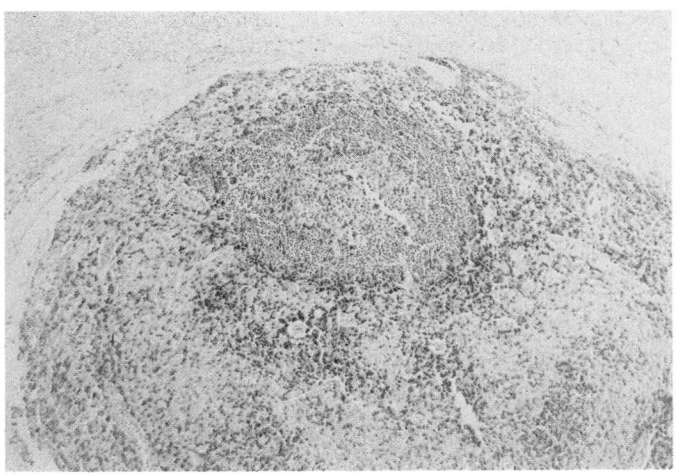

9.36A, B   Sections through lymph nodes showing different cells stained with the indirect antibody method (second antibody, HRP labelled). In A, lymphocytes of the B-cell class in two germinal centres are stained brown; in B, T cells are demonstrated chiefly in paracortical areas. (Provided by R Poston, Department of Histopathology, UMDS, Guy's Campus, London.)

1435

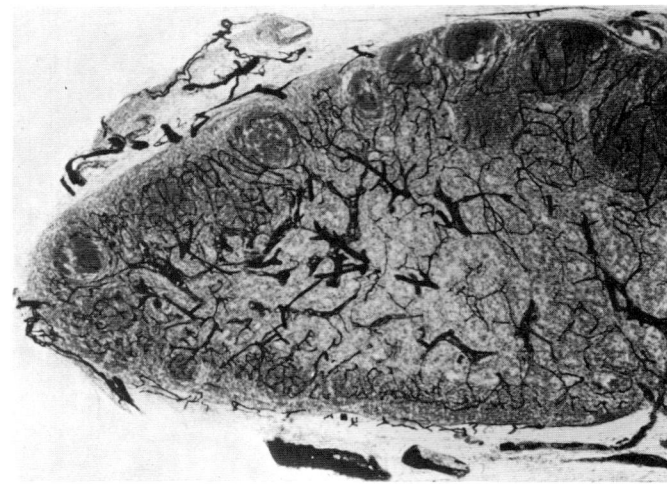

9.37 Lymph node (guinea-pig) in section, after blood vessels have been injected with indian ink. Note the large vessels in the medulla, ramifying to form a capillary plexus in the cortex. (Provided by N Blau, UMDS, Guy's Campus, London.)

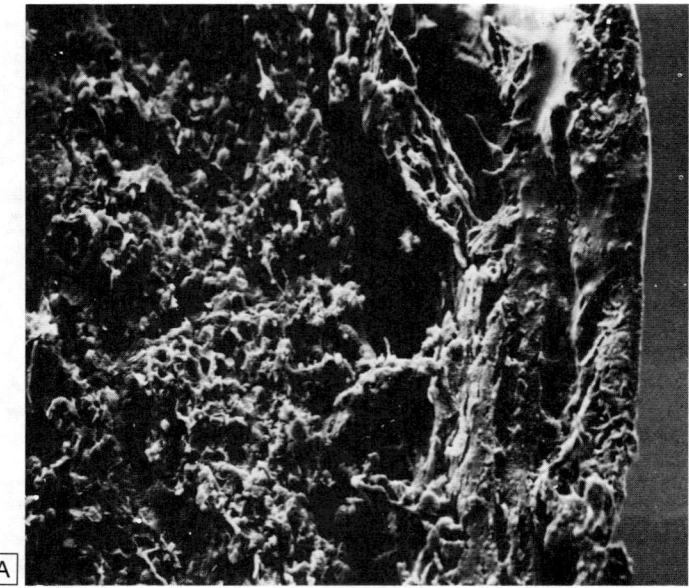

remain within the node as mature B cells (plasmacytes) secreting antibody. Those in the circulation can migrate out into the tissues through venules or capillary walls on demand, and also for normal immune surveillance.

Haemal nodes

In human lymph nodes, erythrocytes may sometimes be found within sinuses. In some animals, small encapsulated lymphoid bodies occur in relation to the abdominal and thoracic viscera, where the sinuses are typically filled with blood, giving the whole structure a red colour; these are termed *haemal nodes* and appear to be more closely related to the blood-vascular than to the lymphatic system, since they lack afferent lymphatics (although they have a single efferent lymphatic vessel). Their structure has been described in detail by Turner (1969), Nopajaroonsri et al (1974) and Hogg et al (1982).

Fast and slow routes of blood circulation have been reported, the former through arterioles, capillaries and venules, the latter through a tortuous sinusoidal system. Specialized postcapillary venules with a high endothelium occur as in ordinary nodes. It is possible that haemal nodes are intermediate between lymph nodes and spleen, and perhaps a basis from which both have evolved. Their human incidence remains uncertain. In some animals, *haemolymph nodes* have been described, with a structure intermediate between that of the lymphatic and haemal nodes and with both lymphatic **and** vascular connections. Some consider them stages in the transformation of lymph into haemal nodes; others deny the existence of such intermediary structures.

Clinical anatomy of lymph nodes. Lymphatic vessels and nodes draining infected areas are liable to inflammation, resulting in acute or chronic lymphangitis and lymphadenitis. Chronic lymphangitis, with blocking of vessels by the escaped ova of a minute parasitic worm, *Wuchereria bancrofti*, is the cause of elephantiasis (filariasis), typified by enormous thickening and reduplication of skin, frequently in the lower limbs and scrotum. Blockage of lymphatic vessels may also result from the spread of neoplasms or widespread surgical removal of nodes. Neoplastic cells may spread by minute emboli or may grow along lymphatic vessels in solid masses. Removals of tumours are therefore planned to take away **in one mass** the tumour,

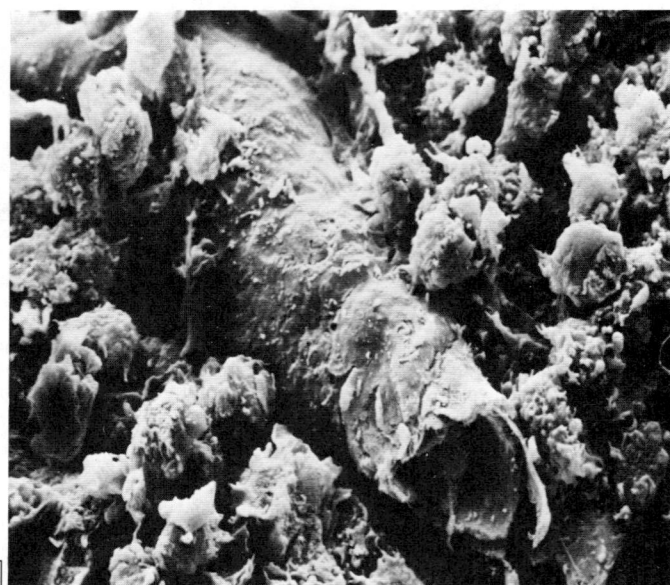

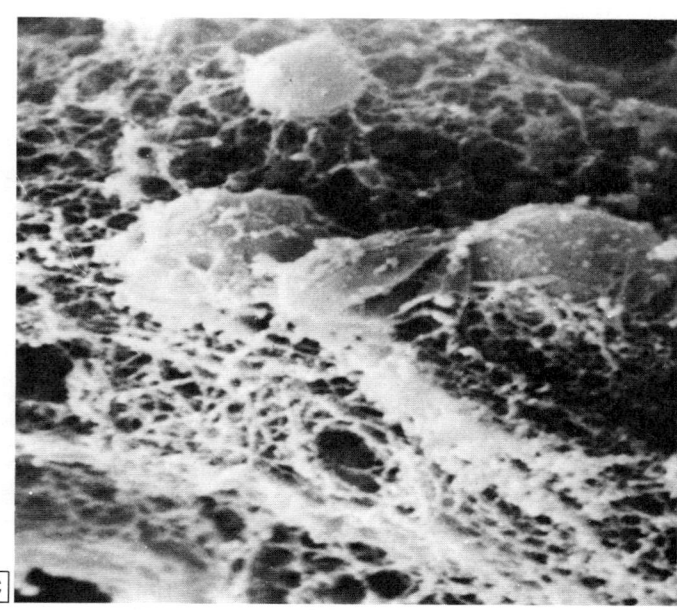

9.38A–C Scanning electron micrographs of the cut surface of a lymph node (guinea-pig). A Low-power micrograph of the outer cortex showing the capsule (right) together with the subcapsular sinus traversed by reticular fibres. Part of a germinal centre is visible on the left. Magnification ×400. B Medium-power micrograph of part of a germinal centre, showing lymphocytes clustered around a capillary. Magnification ×2000. C High-power micrograph of the wall of the subcapsular sinus, showing the fine network of reticular fibres with some attached cells. Magnification ×6000.

the intervening vessels and local nodes. It is important to note that lymphatic vessels from a region may not drain to the local lymph nodes, but to those more remote, often making operative removal difficult if not impractical.

SPLEEN (9.39–45)

INTRODUCTION

The spleen consists of a large encapsulated mass of vascular and lymphoid tissue situated in the upper left posterior region of the abdominal cavity between the fundus of the stomach and the diaphragm (**10**.114, **12**.77A, 97). After fixation in situ (**9**.39), its shape varies from a slightly curved wedge to a tetrahedron, depending on how much it was indented by the neighbouring colon at the time of death, the shape of the spleen being largely moulded by the surrounding structures. Its long axis lies approximately in the plane of the tenth rib, its posterior border being about 4 cm from the mid-dorsal line at the level of the tenth thoracic vertebral spine; its anterior border reaches the mid-axillary line.

The size and weight of the spleen vary with age, with the individual and in the same individual under different conditions. In the adult it is usually about 12 cm long, 7 cm broad and 3–4 cm wide. It tends to diminish in size and weight in older people. Its average adult weight is about 150 g (normal range: 80–300 g, largely reflecting its blood content).

The spleen has two major functions: the removal of particulate material including ageing erythrocytes from the circulation, and the provision of lymphocytes and antibodies as part of the body's system of secondary lymphoid tissues. Both of these activities are shared with other organs in the body, so the spleen is not essential to survival, although its removal diminishes the body's defence against disease.

TOPOGRAPHY AND RELATIONS OF THE SPLEEN

The spleen has diaphragmatic and visceral surfaces, superior and anterior borders and inferior and posterior extremities. The *diaphragmatic surface*, which is convex and smooth, faces posterosuperiorly and to the left, except at its posterior edge which faces slightly medial. It is related to the abdominal surface of the diaphragm which separates it from the lowest part of the left lung and pleura and the ninth to eleventh left ribs. The pleural costodiaphragmatic recess extends down as far as its inferior border. The *visceral surface* (**9**.39), facing the abdominal cavity, presents gastric, renal, pancreatic and colic impressions. The *gastric impression*, directed anteromedially and upwards, is broad and concave where the spleen abuts on to the posterior aspect of the stomach, from which it is separated by a recess of the greater sac. Near the inferior limit of the spleen is the hilum, a long fissure pierced by several irregular apertures through which vessels and nerves of the spleen enter and leave. The *renal impression*, which is slightly concave, is located on the lowest part of the visceral surface and is separated from the gastric impression above by a raised margin. It faces inferomedially and slightly backwards, being related to the upper and lateral area of the anterior surface of the left kidney and sometimes to the superior pole of the left suprarenal gland. The *colic impression*, at the extreme lateral end of the spleen, is usually flat and is related to the left colic flexure and phrenicocolic ligament (**12**.97). The *pancreatic impression*, small when present, is situated between the colic impression and the lateral part of the hilum; it is related to the tail of the pancreas which lies in the lienorenal ligament (**12**.77A).

The *superior border*, separating the diaphragmatic surface from the gastric impression, is usually convex and, near its lateral end, has one or two notches indicating the lobulated form of the spleen in early fetal life (p. 328). The *inferior border* separates the renal impression from the diaphragmatic surface and lies between the diaphragm and the upper part of the left kidney's lateral border. More blunt and rounded than the superior border, it corresponds in position to the eleventh rib's lower margin.

The *posterior extremity* usually faces the rounded vertebral column. The anterior extremity is more expanded and commonly forms a margin connecting the lateral ends of the upper and lower borders. It is related to the left colic flexure and to the phrenicocolic ligament.

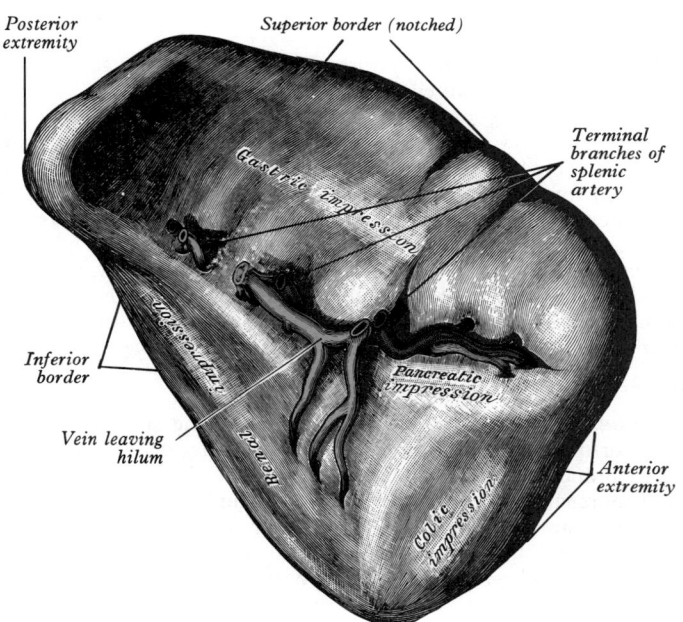

9.39 The visceral surface of the spleen.

The spleen is almost entirely covered by peritoneum, which adheres firmly to its capsule. Recesses of the greater sac separate it from the stomach and left kidney. It develops in the upper dorsal mesogastrium (**3**.76), remaining connected to the posterior abdominal wall and stomach by two folds of peritoneum, respectively the lienorenal ligament and the gastrosplenic ligament. The *lienorenal ligament* is derived from peritoneum where the wall of the general peritoneal cavity meets the omental bursa between the left kidney and spleen; the splenic vessels lie between its layers (**12**.77A). The *gastrosplenic ligament* also has two layers, formed by the meeting of the walls of the greater sac and the omental bursa between spleen and stomach (**12**.77A); the short gastric and left gastro-epiploic branches of the splenic artery pass between its layers. Most laterally the spleen is in contact with the phrenicocolic ligament.

The spleen is also covered externally by a series of connective tissue bars (trabeculae); they ramify throughout the whole structure to create a fibrous skeleton supporting its delicate tissues, which include both lymphoid tissues (white pulp) and extensive areas of

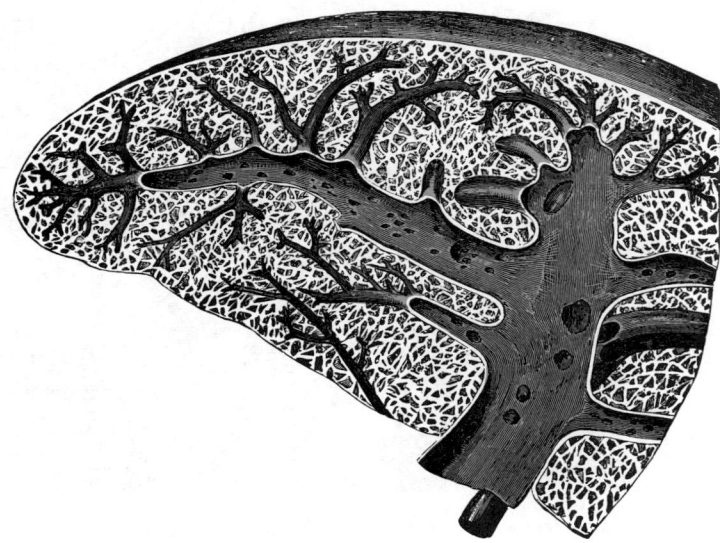

9.40 Transverse section through the spleen, showing the trabecular tissue and the splenic vein and its tributaries. From the first edition of *Gray's Anatomy* (1858).

1437

blood-filled tissue (red pulp). In the living the spleen is soft and friable, and is dark purple because of the considerable amount of blood within its substance.

Near the spleen, especially within the gastrosplenic ligament and greater omentum, small encapsulated nodules of splenic tissue may occur, isolated or connected to the spleen by thin bands of similar tissue. Such *accessory spleens* or *spleniculi* may be numerous and widely scattered in the abdomen. The spleen may retain its fetal lobulated form or show deep notches on its diaphragmatic surface and inferior border in addition to those usually present on its superior border.

Surface anatomy. The position of the spleen in the living can be assessed by percussion; the dull area extends over the ninth to eleventh ribs in vertical extent and should not go forward beyond the midaxillary line. The normal spleen is not palpable.

Vessels and nerves of the spleen

Arteries. The spleen receives its blood from the splenic artery, a large tortuous branch of the coeliac artery. After giving off various minor branches to the pancreas and stomach, this vessel divides in the lienorenal ligament shortly before reaching the spleen into two or three main branches from which four, five or more *segmental branches* enter the spleen's hilum to supply a territory within it termed a *splenic segment* (see below). Within each segment, the artery

ramifies in the trabeculae to supply the parenchyma and capsule of the spleen. The pathway of blood beyond this point is considered later (p. 1551).

Veins (9.40). The minor veins pass from the red pulp of the spleen into the trabeculae, and thence into segmental veins running alongside the segmental arteries. On leaving the hilum, they continue in company with the arterial branches, draining into the main splenic vein in the lienorenal ligament. After receiving venous tributaries from various sources, the splenic vein usually drains directly into the hepatic portal vein (p. 1603).

Lymphatics. These drain along the splenic trabeculae to pass out of the hilum into the lymphatic vessels accompanying the splenic artery and vein. They take splenic lymph to the pancreaticosplenic and coeliac nodes (p. 1618, 1619).

Nerves. The coeliac sympathetic plexus gives off nerve fibres which pass along the splenic artery and its branches as a surface plexus, to enter the hilum and run with the segmental arteries and their branches. These fibres appear to be mainly noradrenergic vasomotor, concerned with the regulation of blood flow through the spleen; adrenergic agonists inhibit the concentration of red cells in the splenic blood (plasma skimming, see below) indicating that sympathetic activity causes an increase in the 'fast' circulation of the spleen as opposed to slow filtration (Reilly 1985). The presence of other neural connections has not been demonstrated.

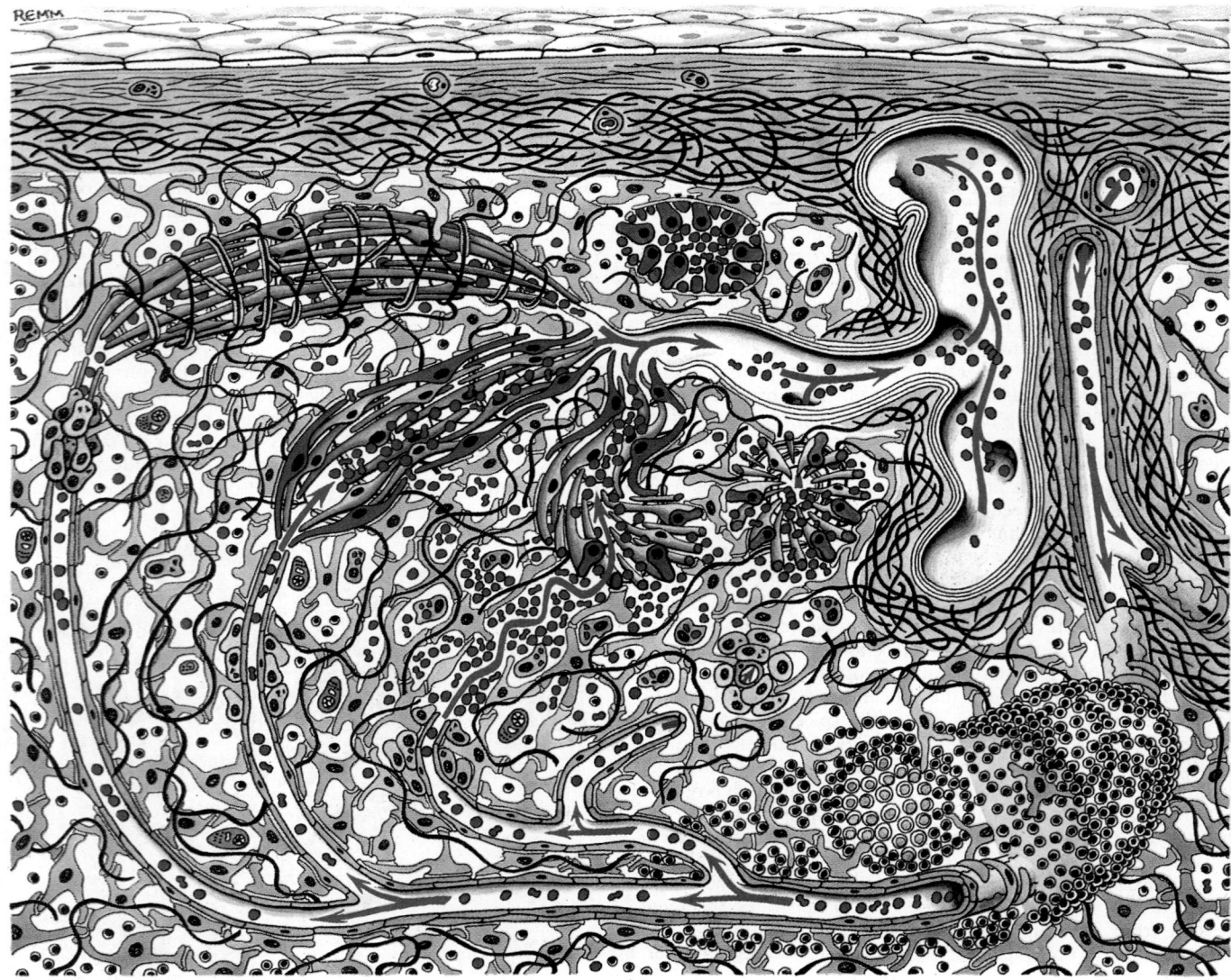

9.41 The main features of splenic structure; the various elements are not drawn to scale, to enable representation on a single diagram. Note the capsule, trabeculae, reticular fibres and cells, the perivascular lymphatic aggregation (white pulp), and the ellipsoids, cell cords and venous sinusoids of the red pulp. The 'open' and 'closed' theories of splenic circulation are illustrated. The venous sinusoids are shown in two states: (1) with their lining of 'stave' cells (bright blue) in close apposition, (2) with intercellular gaps (these have been over-emphasized for clarity). Consult text for further details.

Splenic vascular segmentation

There is evidence (Dreyer & Budtz-Olson 1952) that the human spleen, like that in other species, consists of separate 'segments' or 'compartments', each served by a hilar branch of the main splenic artery and splenic vein (Braithwaite & Adams 1957). Adjacent compartments, it is claimed, are connected by intersegmental veins; a congested compartment can thus pass excess blood to those adjacent (see below) but, when blood flow is not excessive, splenic segments may act as separate units. (For a review of splenic segmentation since first proposed by Kyber 1870, consult Gupta et al 1976; Treutner et al 1993.) Gupta et al studied corrosion casts of 50 adult human spleens. In 42 of these (84%) only two segments existed (superior and inferior); in 8 (16%) three segments (superior, intermediate and inferior) were demonstrated. There was no clear anastomosis between segments. A comparable segmental arrangement of splenic veins was described by Fuld and Irwin (1954). The occurrence of only two or three segments (arterial or venous) was supported by many investigators quoted by Gupta et al; but this does not accord with the usual description of splenic arteries dividing into five or more major branches in the lienorenal ligament before even entering the hilum: no explanation of this discrepancy is advanced by these authors.

SPLENIC MICROSTRUCTURE (9.41–45)

Microscopically, the internal mass (parenchyma) of the spleen consists of two major components, known as *white pulp* and *red pulp*, denoting their appearance when the freshly excised spleen is transected. The white pulp is composed of lymphoid tissue in which B and T lymphocytes can mature and proliferate under antigenic stimulation. The red pulp is a unique filtration device which enables macrophages in the spleen to extract particulates from the blood as it perfuses this organ. Red pulp is composed of a complex system of interconnected spaces inhabited by large numbers of phagocytic macrophages. These cells remove and dismantle effete red blood cells, micro-organisms, cellular debris and other particulates from the circulation. At the junction of white and red pulp is a narrow *marginal zone*, an area important in establishing immune responses and other aspects of splenic biology.

Fibrous framework of the spleen

The serosa of the peritoneum covers the entire organ except at its hilum and along the lines of reflexion of the lienorenal and gastrosplenic ligaments. Deep to this layer is the connective tissue *capsule*, a continuous layer about 1.5 mm thick, rich in collagen but also containing some elastin fibres. The capsule has an outer and an inner lamina in which the directions of collagen fibres differ (Faller 1985), presumably increasing its strength. From the capsule numerous trabeculae extend into the substance of the spleen, branching within it to form a supportive framework. The largest trabeculae enter at the hilum and ensheathe the splenic vessels and nerves, dividing into branches in the splenic pulp (9.40, 41). Like the capsule, trabeculae are composed of dense irregular connective fibres, rich in collagen and elastin. In many mammals, for example the cat or the horse, both capsule and trabeculae contain many smooth muscle cells which enable the spleen to contract on autonomic stimulation to expel its considerable quantity of stored blood into the general circulation. Such spleens are termed *storage spleens* (Weiss 1990). The human spleen lacks this potential, and its functions are related primarily to protection (a *defence spleen*); there is little smooth muscle, and the contraction and distension of the spleen are attributable to the effects of constriction or dilation of its inflow and outflow vessels which alter the volume of blood in the organ. An increase of intrasplenic blood pressure distends the spleen and stretches the elastic fibres, while contraction is due to their recoil when the pressure drops. Within the spleen, branching trabeculae are continuous with a delicate network of fine collagen (reticulin) fibres pervading both the white and red pulp, laid down by numerous fibroblasts which are present in its meshes (see also below).

White pulp

Within the spleen, the branches of the splenic artery radiate out from the hilum within trabeculae, ramifying a number of times and narrowing to arteriolar dimensions. In their terminal few millimetres, their connective tissue adventitia is replaced by a sheath of T lymphocytes, the *periarteriolar* (or *periarterial*) *lymphatic sheath*. This sheath is enlarged in places by *lymphoid follicles* (Malpighian bodies), aggregations of B lymphocytes visible to the naked eye on the freshly cut surface as white semi-opaque dots 0.25–1 mm in diameter, which contrast with the surrounding deep reddish-purple of the red pulp. Follicles are usually situated near the terminal branches of the arteriole, or at a larger branching point, and typically protrude to one side of the vessel. Like the periarteriolar sheaths, follicles are centres of lymphocyte proliferation as well as aggregation, and when antigenically stimulated, they develop germinal centres, as also in lymph nodes and nodules. The germinal centres regress when the infection subsides. Follicles also atrophy with increasing age and may be absent in the very old. The whole white pulp is supported by a network of fine collagen fibres interspersed with fibroblasts. Within the follicle, arterioles form a series of lateral terminal branches, often forming a series of parallel arterioles (called penicilli, alluding to their resemblance to the penicillium mould).

Red pulp (9.41, 43–45)

The red pulp constitutes the majority (about 75%) of the total splenic volume. Within it lie large numbers of venous sinuses draining into tributaries of the major splenic veins. The sinuses are separated from each other by a fibrocellular network, the *reticulum*, formed by numerous fibroblasts (*reticular cells*) and small bundles of delicate collagen fibres, in the meshes of which lie splenic macrophages. Seen in two-dimensional sections, these intersinusal regions appear as strips of tissue, *splenic cords* (of Billroth), alternating with splenic sinuses (9.41, 44, 45) although in reality they form a three-dimensional continuum around the venous spaces. To understand the organization of the red pulp some details of the sinuses and of the intersinusal reticulum are required, as follows.

Venous sinuses. These are elongated ovoid vessels about 50 μm in diameter, lined by a characteristic 'incomplete' endothelium unique to the spleen. The endothelial cells are long and narrow, aligned with the long axis of the venous sinus (for this reason they are often called *stave cells*, reminiscent of planks in a barrel (9.41, 44, 45)); along their length they are attached at intervals to their neighbours by short stretches of intercellular junctions (tight and adhering) which alternate with intercellular slits through which blood can pass. The luminal and external surfaces of the cells bear short irregular microvilli, and numerous endocytic/exocytic vesicles are formed at both surfaces. Internally the endothelial cells possess a well-organized cytoskeleton, with longitudinal bundles of vimentin and of actin and myosin which probably determine their elongated shape, and could actively modulate the form of the cell to alter the sizes of the slits in the sinus walls, thus regulating the passage of blood through the intercellular gaps (see Chen & Weiss 1972, 1973).

The endothelial cells are mildly phagocytic (as are others of this type elsewhere in the body) but do not appear to contribute strongly to the uptake of particles in the spleen. A perforated, discontinuous basal lamina is present on the aspect of the sinus facing away from the lumen. The presence of slits between the endothelial cells allows blood cells to slowly squeeze from the surrounding splenic cords into the lumen of the sinus, the cells distorting considerably in the process (see below). The sinuses are supported externally by circumferential and longitudinal reticulin fibres, which are connected to the fibrous reticulum of the splenic cordal tissue around them.

Reticular tissue of the splenic cords. Around the sinuses the network of collagen fibres bears a population of large, stellate fibroblasts, the reticular cells. The extensions of these cells are flattened and leaflike, and help to divide the reticular space into a series of defined loculi which contain macrophages. These cells synthesize the matrix components of the reticulum, including the collagen fibres and various proteoglycans. Blood released into the reticular space from the ends of capillaries trickles through these spaces, receiving the phagocytic attentions of macrophages which are able to remove particulates from blood. Under conditions of heavy loading, for example when there are many damaged erythrocytes in the circulation to be removed by splenic macrophages, the reticular cells proliferate and increase the size of the red pulp considerably, thus causing enlargement of the whole spleen, and in extreme cases, splenomegaly (see over).

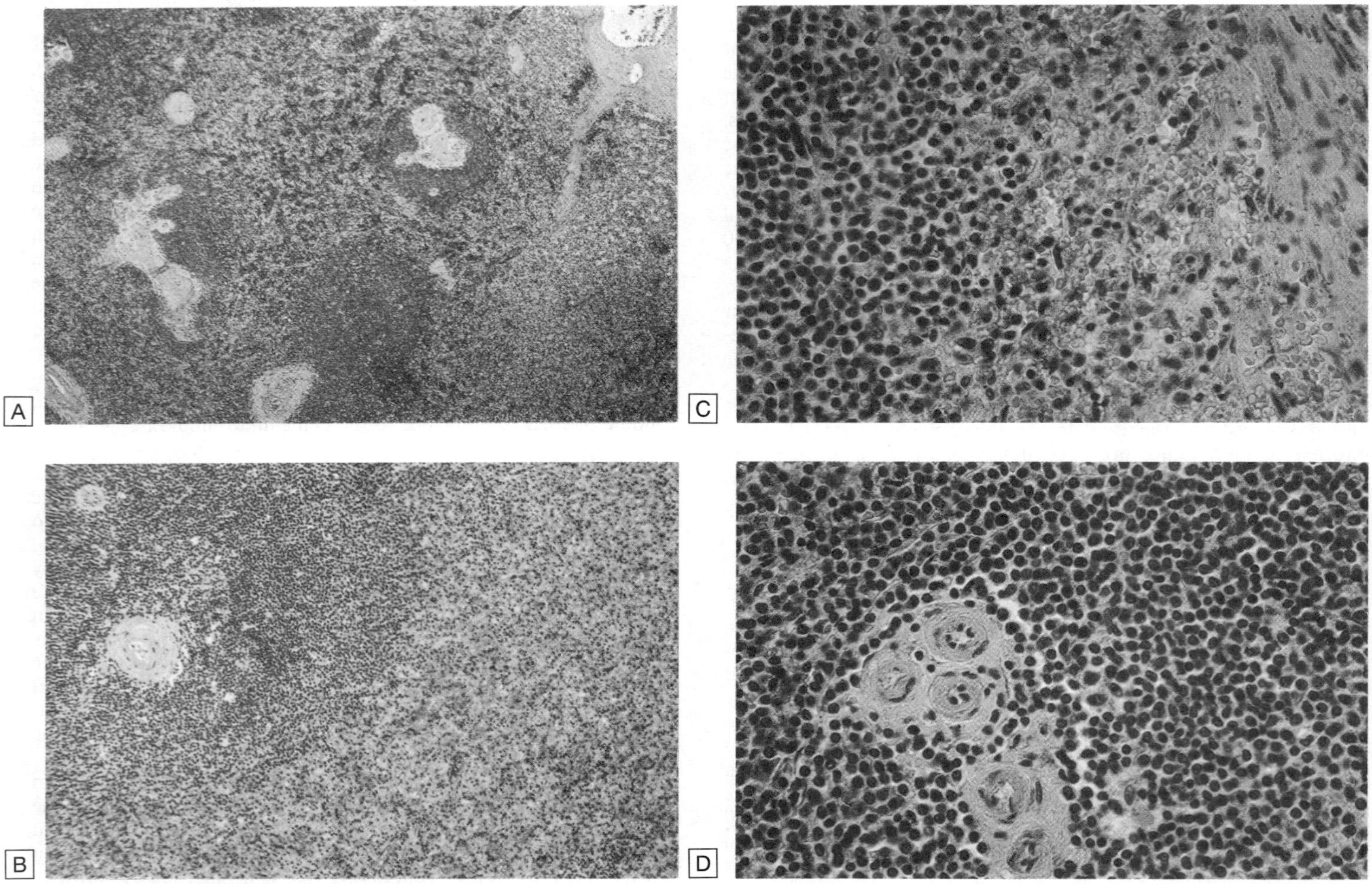

9.42 Sections of human spleen stained with haematoxylin and eosin. (Supplied by D R Turner of the Department of Pathology, Guy's Hospital Medical School.)
A, B Survey photographs at low power showing the general contrast between the white pulp (perivascular lymphatic aggregates, stained blue) and the red pulp (venous sinusoids and intervening cellular cords, stained reddish purple). C High-power view of the junctional (marginal) zone between the densely packed lymphocytes of the white pulp and the blood-filled sinusoids and cell cords of the red pulp. D A group of small (penicillar) arteries ensheathed by densely packed small lymphocytes.

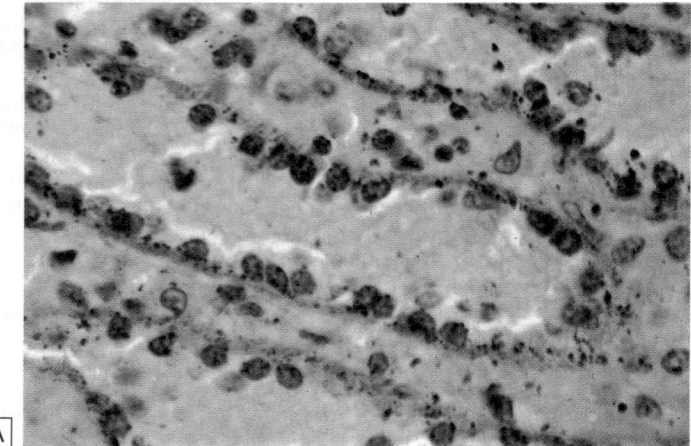

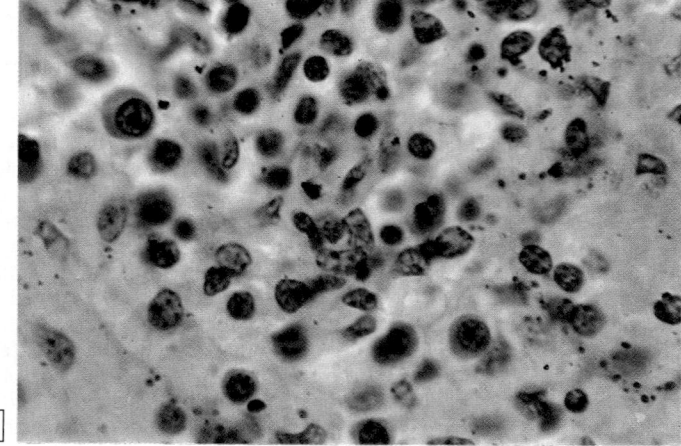

9.43 Section of monkey spleen following intravascular perfusion with a suspension of carbon particles followed later by perfusion fixation, stained by Weigert's haematoxylin and Van Gieson's stain.
A Showing empty, dilated venous sinusoids and intervening cell cords. The 'stave' cells lining the sinusoids are prominent. B High-power view of the cellular region between venous sinusoids. The cell types seen include reticular macrophages with carbon particles in their cytoplasm, small and large lymphocytes and a number of prominent rounded plasma cells.

Marginal zone

At the interface between the white and red pulp is the marginal zone, a region of great importance to the biology of the spleen. Here the lymphocytes are more loosely arranged than in the white pulp, and are held in a dense network of fine collagen fibres, intermingled with reticular cells. The arterioles leaving the white pulp often spread within the marginal zone before terminating, frequently bifurcating

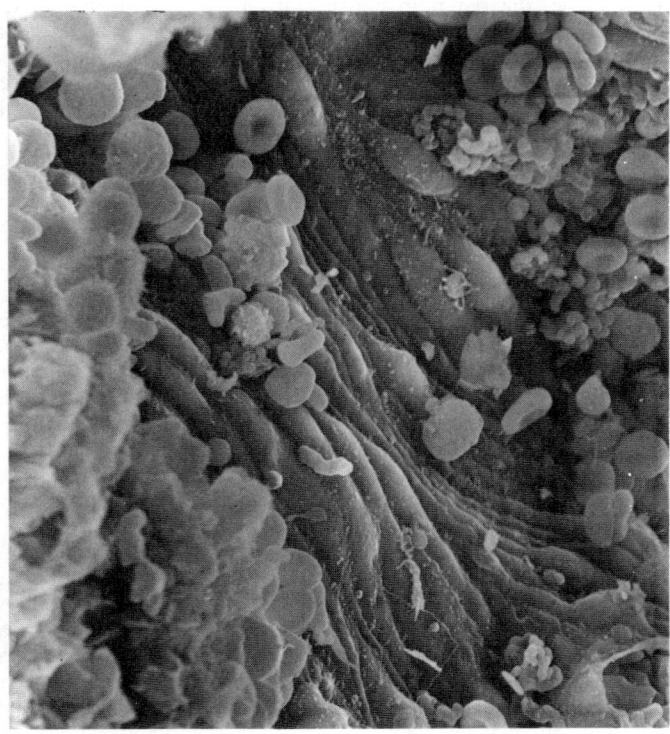

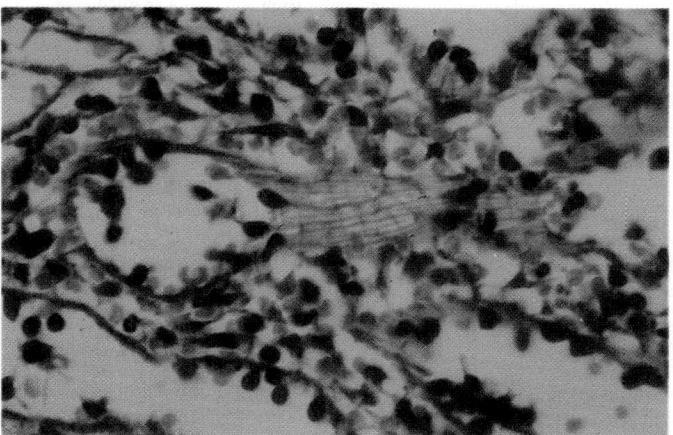

9.45   A splenic sinusoid sectioned tangentially to show parallel strap-like endotheliocytes and surrounding tissue. Gomori's method. Magnification × 600.

9.44   Scanning electron micrograph of a splenic sinusoid (monkey) to show endothelial cells and associated tissue. Magnification × 1000.

immediately before this point. Close to their ends, where the lumen is much narrowed, these vessels are surrounded by a small aggregation of macrophages, the *periarteriolar macrophage sheath* (of Schweigger-Seidel) or *ellipsoid*. Ellipsoids are well developed in some mammals, for example the pig, cat and dog, but not in humans. The marginal zone is a region where blood is delivered into the red pulp, and also where many lymphocytes leave the circulation to migrate into their respective T- and B-lymphocyte areas of the white pulp. In some species there is an extensive slitlike *marginal sinus* between the white pulp and marginal zone, into which many arterioles discharge, and which are in continuity with the venous sinuses. In humans this seems to be less conspicuous although arguably present (see Groom & Schmidt 1990).

Splenic microcirculation (9.41)

The circulation of blood within the spleen has long been a subject for dispute, partly because of the complexity of the vascular channels, but also because of conflicting experimental evidence in different species (Knisely 1936; MacKenzie et al 1941; Snook 1950; Peck & Hoerr 1951; Lewis 1957a; Wennberg & Weiss 1969; Chen & Weiss 1972, 1973). Before discussing the present consensus, it is necessary to clarify the vascular anatomy.

The large, tortuous splenic artery, before reaching the spleen, divides in the lienorenal ligament into as many as five or more rami entering the hilum to ramify in the trabeculae throughout the organ. Likewise, the splenic vein forms in the ligament from an equal number of tributaries emerging from the hilum. As already noted, small arteries tapering to arterioles pass through the white pulp then turn abruptly to form penicillar branches which, after a course of about 0.5 mm, pass out of the white pulp into the marginal zone and red pulp. The passage of blood through the vascular compartments between the arterioles and splenic veins is referred to collectively as the *intermediate circulation* of the spleen. By a number of routes (see below), blood is passed to the venous sinuses from which it enters venules leading to small veins (the latter running within trabeculae) and thence into larger veins draining the spleen at its hilum.

Open and closed splenic circulations. Two schools of thought arose from the 1930s onwards concerning whether blood passed from the arterioles (or their terminal capillaries) directly into the venous sinuses (a closed circulation) or was instead discharged into a network of spaces in the splenic cords before entering the sinuses through the minute slits in their walls (an open circulation). Recently, various observations using a number of complementary techniques (reviewed by Weiss 1990; Groom & Schmidt 1990) on human and animal spleens have helped to resolve this issue. Measurement of the transit time of isotopically labelled blood through the cat spleen has shown that there are three distinct velocity components, fast, intermediate and slow (see Levesque & Groom 1976). About 90% of the blood passes through very rapidly, in a few seconds, as might be expected of a closed circulation through a capillary bed. About 9.6% takes minutes to pass through, and a small amount (1.6%) takes an hour or more.

Microscopic visualization of the circulation in the transilluminated rat spleen (MacDonald et al 1987), and anatomical analysis based on electron microscopy and micro-corrosion casts of human and animal spleens indicate a likely structural basis for these three rates of flow (Groom & Schmidt 1990). The rapid transit probably occurs through a proportion of arterioles which connect directly to the ends of sinuses, i.e. a 'closed' circulation, presenting little resistance to the passage of blood. Also in this category may be blood which is discharged from arterioles or capillaries close to those sinuses which have open ends, for example in the perimarginal sinus, and thus present relatively little resistance to blood flow although appearing to be part of the anatomically 'open' circulation. The intermediate circulation appears to reflect the presence of an anatomically and physiologically **open** circulation, in which blood percolates slowly through the reticular tissue of the splenic cords and filters through slits in the sinus walls before joining the majority of the blood flow; this process exposes the blood to maximal contact with splenic macrophages and is likely to be the period when removal of particles and effete red cells occurs. Finally, the slow circulation is thought to involve temporary adhesive contacts between blood cells and splenic cordal cells, since the passage of plasma is not slowed in the same way. Red cells, leucocytes and platelets can be sequestered in the spleen by such actions, sometimes for considerable periods, and of course some of these adhesive events are preliminary to the removal of damaged or aged cells by macrophagic phagocytosis.

The total volume of blood in the intermediate and slow circulation greatly exceeds that of the fast transit because of the relatively much greater volume of the splenic cords compared with the blood in the arteries, sinusoids and veins. The retarding effect on blood cells exceeds that on the flow of plasma so that the concentration of red cells (the haematocrit) within the spleen is about twice that of the general circulation and the number of reticulocytes is especially high; numerous platelets are also sequestered, but can be released into the circulation on demand.

It must be added that these views of splenic circulation are not entirely agreed between investigators and further clarification is to be expected. It is also probable that the proportions of blood flow along these different routes vary with local changes in blood pressure within the spleen and in the general circulation.

FUNCTIONS OF THE SPLEEN

The spleen is essentially concerned with phagocytosis, immune responses, cytopoiesis and blood cell storage. In the fetus it is also an important site of haemopoiesis, and postnatally it may become haemopoietic in certain pathological conditions. However, although of great importance to the defence of the body, it is not absolutely essential since many of its functions can be assumed by the liver and by other lymphoid tissues if the spleen is removed.

Phagocytosis

Splenic macrophages constitute a large part of the mononuclear phagocytic system of the body (p. 1414). They are highly phagocytic cells distributed mainly in the splenic cords and marginal zones, where they are attached to reticulin fibres and neighbouring reticular cells. They can ingest particulate matter, micro-organisms and aged blood cells, especially erythrocytes and platelets. The processing of ageing or damaged red cells is especially important, as the spleen is the major site of their removal from the circulation. Within splenic macrophages, all stages of erythrophagocytosis, from disintegrating erythryocytes to granules of haemosiderin, can be discerned (Chen & Weiss 1972). Bilirubin, an end-product of haemoglobin catabolism, is conveyed in the bloodstream to the liver for excretion and the iron is largely re-used by bone marrow. Amino acids from the hydrolysis of globin are returned to the amino acid pool of the body. Splenic macrophages are also important in removing microbes and cellular debris from the circulation and their lysosomes possess many powerful enzymes which can hydrolyse or oxidize these bodies, particularly when the macrophages are activated by cytokines during immune responses (p. 1418) or the objects to be phagocytosed have been coated with antibodies.

How the macrophages recognize ageing red cells prior to phagocytic removal is an intriguing puzzle. Current evidence indicates that as erythrocytes get older, hitherto protected antigens in their surfaces become exposed to auto-antibodies in the circulation, and that the macrophages bind the antibodies which initiate phagocytosis (see also p. 1415).

Pitting of red cells

There is evidence that abnormal red cell inclusion such as Heinz bodies (intracellular masses of altered haemoglobin) can be removed from erythrocytes during their passage through the spleen without cell lysis. Exactly how this is done is not known. It has been suggested that such bodies might be squeezed out of the cell as it passes through the extremely narrow slits between sinusal stave cells, although how this could occur without red cell lysis is not clear.

Immune responses

Like other lymphoid organs, the spleen contains B and T lymphocytes in its white pulp and elsewhere, and also various antigen-presenting cells within the follicles and periarterial sheaths. It is, therefore, a site of antigen presentation by dendritic cells and the initiation of T- and B-cell activities involved in humoral and cellular immune responses (see also p. 1420). Some B lymphocytes mature into plasma cells particularly in the marginal zones, secreting antibodies into the circulating blood when stimulated. T lymphocytes carry out a wide range of defensive activities, described elsewhere in detail (p. 1420). Lymphocytes are also added to the general defence of the body by passing into the haemal circulation via venous sinuses and thus the spleen is an important source of these cells.

When antigenically stimulated, the white pulp increases in size as lymphocytes proliferate; the (primary) follicles become intensely active in B-cell proliferation, and gain the typical appearance of secondary follicles (germinal centres), as in lymph nodes (p. 1432). The presentation of antibody–antigen complexes by dendritic cells of the follicles and marginal zones are involved in these processes and in the generation of immunological 'memory' for future immune responses.

Cytopoiesis

In human fetuses, from the fourth month onwards, the spleen is

haemopoietic, the red pulp housing groups of myelocytes, erythroblasts and megakaryocytes. In some anaemias and myeloid leukaemia, stem cells persisting in red pulp may revert to haemopioesis. In the mature spleen lymphopoiesis in the white pulp contributes to a circulating reserve of immunologically competent T and B lymphocytes and also mononuclear phagocytes.

CLINICAL ASPECTS OF THE SPLEEN

Splenic hypertrophy

In individuals suffering chronic breakdown of erythrocytes, for example in malaria and other haemolytic diseases, the splenic tissues may be permanently hypertrophied and the spleen greatly enlarged (splenomegaly). These changes involve the distension of the reticular spaces of the red pulp with macrophages loaded with damaged red cells or their breakdown products, the proliferation of reticular cells, increases in macrophage numbers and hypertrophy of the fibrous framework. The spleen may increase to several times its normal size, and in children come to occupy much of the abdominal cavity. Similar events occur in various lipoidoses.

Splenectomy. Partial splenectomy is followed by rapid regeneration of lost tissue but even total splenectomy has few obvious effects, its functions being largely assumed by the liver. However, especially in the early years of life, splenectomy may entail a general reduction in the rapidity of immune responses and a consequent increased susceptibility to infection. Splenectomy in later life is followed by leucocytosis with increased lymphocytic, neutrophil, eosinophil and platelet counts in peripheral blood, interpreted as due to removal of humoral factors produced in the spleen which oppose the formation and release of cells from haemopoietic tissues. These effects fade and disappear within a few weeks.

Any massive immune response may be accompanied by splenic enlargement, also occurring in many reticuloses. In splenomegaly, the anterior border, anterior diaphragmatic surface and notched superior border become palpable below the left costal margin; the marginal notches are exaggerated and easily palpable. The transverse colon and left colic flexure are displaced downward, no area of colonic resonance remaining over the enlarged spleen, in contrast to a retroperitoneal tumour (e.g. renal), which does not displace the gut and, therefore, leaves an area of colonic resonance. There is no anastomosis between the smaller splenic arteries so that their obstruction leads to infarction. During splenectomy the tail of the pancreas is in danger.

EPITHELIUM-ASSOCIATED LYMPHOID TISSUE

In addition to the encapsulated peripheral lymphoid organs, lymph nodes and spleen, large amounts of unencapsulated lymphoid tissue exist in the walls of the alimentary, respiratory, reproductive and urinary tracts, and in the skin, termed collectively epithelio-lymphoid tissue. *Skin-associated lymphoid tissue (SALT)* also includes the lymphoid tissue of the breast; these are considered elsewhere with the integumental system (p. 424). The other types are usually referred to as *mucosa-associated lymphoid tissue (MALT)*, subdivided into those situated in the wall of the gut (*gut-associated lymphoid tissue; GALT*), the respiratory tract (*bronchial-associated lymphoid tissue; BALT*), and the less studied *genitourinary lymphoid tissue* (at present apparently devoid of acronyms). They have a similar structure, although regionally variable and functionally distinct in terms of their specific lymphocyte populations. The most intensively studied are those related to the alimentary tract, and emphasis will therefore be placed on these lymphoid structures, although the general principles apply to other groups (see 9.61).

MUCOSA-ASSOCIATED LYMPHOID TISSUE

Mucosa-associated lymphoid tissue includes an exceedingly large population of lymphocytes because of the extensive nature of the alimentary tract. The cell aggregations can be divided into two classes: the *organized mucosa-associated lymphoid tissue (O-MALT)* located in the lamina propria and sometimes the submucosa (also known as *lymphoid nodules*), and *diffuse mucosa-associated lymphoid tissue (D-MALT)*, consisting of numerous cells derived from the O-MALT, scattered throughout the lamina propria and the base of the epithelium. O-MALT includes the peripharyngeal lymphoid ring of tonsils (palatine, lingual, nasopharyngeal and tubal), oesophageal nodules and similar lymphoid tissue scattered throughout the alimentary tract from duodenum to anal canal, although, interestingly, absent from the stomach. There are especially prominent aggregations of nodules in the small intestine (Peyer's patches) and in the vermiform appendix. Bronchial-associated lymphoid tissue (BALT) is the equivalent lymphoid nodular tissue of the lower respiratory tract (of course derived embryonically from the alimentary tract).

ORGANIZED MUCOSA-ASSOCIATED LYMPHOID TISSUE

Although the detailed form of this tissue depends on its location, the basic organization is similar in all regions. Local variations are related to the type of epithelium which they are close to, and to the size of the lymphoid mass. In this account the general principles of their organization will first be described, and then the special features of large aggregations of particular clinical significance, namely the palatine and nasopharyngeal tonsils and Peyer's patches.

General features of O-MALT

Briefly, these are:

- the presence of proliferative centres for B- and T-lymphocyte production (follicles and parafollicular zones, respectively)
- proximity to an epithelial surface, the lymphoid tissue being essentially situated within the mucosal lamina propria
- the lack of a fibrous capsule
- the provision of high-endothelium venules (HEVs) for immigration of lymphocytes
- the presence of efferent lymphatics but virtual absence of afferents.

Follicles and parafollicular zones. B and T lymphocytes are to some extent segregated into distinctive territories within the lymphoid tissue. The B lymphocytes are mainly present in speroidal masses termed *follicles* where they proliferate and undergo maturation. T lymphocytes lie between the follicles in less well-defined *parafollicular zones*, where they also proliferate and begin maturation. The detailed arrangement of cells within these two areas closely resembles that of lymph nodes (see p. 1432 for details). The lymphoblasts (centroblasts) in each primary follicle undergo rapid mitosis to expand the clones of B lymphocytes which then migrate to the periphery of the follicle. The central dividing population and their newly arrived antecedents and newly formed progeny create a pale-staining *germinal centre* (*secondary follicle*) in the middle of the primary follicle. Each germinal centre is surrounded by a ring of closely packed small cells, which migrate predominantly towards the side of the follicle facing the overlying epithelium, to create a densely staining cap, the *mantle zone*. In the central region of the follicle there are follicular dendritic cells—antigen presenting cells (APCs) with long cytoplasmic extensions. Macrophages and a few T cells are also present.

Parafollicular zones. These are more uniform in appearance than the follicles, and consist of loosely packed T lymphocytes of various sizes, some of them mitotic but many small lymphocytes. Amongst these cells are *interdigitating cells*, another form of APC which is characteristic of T-cell areas, and *macrophages*. The parafollicular regions are rich in postcapillary venules with high endothelia, sites of lymphocytic immigration from the bloodstream (see below).

Follicle-associated epithelium (FAE). As noted above, the type of epithelium depends largely on the location of the lymphoid tissue. In the oropharynx and oesophagus it is stratified squamous, in the nasopharynx it is mainly ciliated pseudostratified and in the small and large intestine, simple columnar epithelium. The lymphoid tissue is often invaded by epithelial diverticula in the form of glands or crypts which create a larger area of contact between the two tissues. The FAE covering lymphoid tissue is unusual in possessing cells which are involved in sampling antigens present in the lumen and passing them to the underlying tissues. The main function of B lymphocytes is to produce IgA for secretion into the lumen of the tracts which they line, and so it is essential for lymphoid tissue to

'see' the antigen in order to produce the right antibodies to attack the organisms (and toxins) within the lumen on the other side of the epithelium. The epithelium is able to sample these antigens and translocate them to the antigen-presenting cells of the underlying lymphoid tissue so that appropriate clones of T and B cells can be selected and amplified prior to their migration into the surrounding mucosa. In the small and large intestine these epithelial cells have characteristic short microvilli on their luminal surface and are known as *microfold (M) cells* (pp. 1769, 1784). In the palatine tonsils they include modified stratified squamous *reticulated epithelial cells* (p. 1446).

Connective tissue framework. Lymphocyte populations are supported mechanically by a fine network of fine collagen (reticulin) fibres and associated fibroblasts, with coarser connective tissue trabeculae in the larger nodules, such as those in the pharyngeal tonsil. There is continuity between the nodules and surrounding tissues as, unlike the lymph nodes, there is no capsule; the lymphocytes can therefore migrate out into the neighbouring regions (although it is thought that they are mainly distributed through vascular channels, as described below).

Vascular routes of cell migration. Another important characteristic of O-MALT is that the lymphatic vessels of nodules are typically only efferent, draining into the lymphatic channels of the organ in which they are sited (although some instances of afferent lymphatics from local areas have also been described: see below).

Lymphocytes migrate into the lymphoid nodules through blood vessels from the surrounding connective tissue. These small arteries and arterioles branch to supply the parafollicular areas with capillary plexuses draining to specialized postcapillary venules whose walls are lined by high endothelium (high endothelium venules; HEVs). These endothelial cells possess adhesion molecules (e.g. vascular cell adhesion molecules; VCAM, see p. 1462) which bind ligands (selectins, p. 1461) on the lymphocyte surface to separate them from the flow of blood and initiate their migration through the vessel wall into the surrounding extravascular spaces of the lymphoid tissue. B and T lymphocytes migrate first into the parafollicular areas where interdigitating APCs also arrive from the bone marrow by the same route. As in the lymph node, T-cell clones are selected by APC–T-cell receptor contact, and the B cells are also activated in the same way. The B cells then migrate to the follicles where they form centroblasts and centrocytes, proliferating and eventually migrating out of the follicle as a primed B cell. Lymphocytes can leave the nodule mainly through the efferent lymphatic drainage and some by direct migration into the surrounding tissues. Some B lymphocytes around the periphery of the nodules mature into plasmacytes to provide IgA and IgG for local defence.

FUNCTIONS OF O-MALT

It can be concluded from the above account that organized mucosa-related lymphoid tissue nodules are secondary lymphoid organs seeded by B and T lymphocytes from primary lymphoid organs (thymus and bone marrow) via the bloodstream. Antigens derived from the neighbouring luminal surface of the neighbouring epithelium (and to some extent from the mucosa itself) are taken up by various APCs, processed and used to select clones of B and T lymphocytes for further proliferative expansion. The majority of lymphocytes resulting from these processes then migrate back into the circulation via the efferent lymphatic drainage, and home to various sites in the tissues related topographically to the nodules. Others may migrate directly into the surrounding tissues, while a few may remain within the nodule itself, to provide local defence. Because mature, antibody-synthesizing B cells (plasmacytes) form part of the latter population, IgA, IgG, IgM and IgE produced by these cells also pass into the efferent lymphatics and contribute to the circulating antibodies of the lymph and blood.

It has also been speculated that lymphoid nodules may contain primary lymphoid tissue responsible for the initial commitment and differentiation of B lymphocytes, in the same way that the thymus does for the T-cell lineage. This idea stems from the observation already noted (p. 1417) that in birds, a diverticulum of the hindgut proctodeum called the bursa of Fabricius houses primary B-cell lymphoid tissue (hence the 'B' of B lymphocytes, originally denoting *bursa equivalent*). This suggested that alimentary lymphoid tissues in mammals might have a similar function, but experiments have generally failed to support this idea. There is however some recent evidence suggesting that intestinal O-MALT may indeed contain primary B-cell lymphoid tissue during early development, although it is probably of relatively minor importance compared with the bone marrow in the total output of these cells.

DIFFUSE MUCOSA-ASSOCIATED LYMPHOID TISSUE

Diffuse mucosa-associated lymphoid tissue refers to the disseminated population of lymphocytes within the mucosal lamina propria and epithelial base. These have already been selected by APC action in lymphoid nodules and consist of T and B lymphocytes engaged in humoral and cellular immune responses, which have migrated to their final destinations within the circulation. These cells act co-operatively with each other, and also with the local macrophages and other surrounding tissue cells, especially the epithelium to:

(1) maintain the immune barrier functions at the mucosal surface by controlling potential pathogens on the external surface of the epithelium through antibody secretion, and also to eliminate tissue cells which may become infected with viruses or other pathogens (or perhaps have become neoplastic);

(2) engage in more aggressive defence if the epithelial barrier is broken and pathogens invade the lamina propria.

In these actions the lymphocytes are assisted and regulated by macrophages and the overlying epithelia, both of which can act as antigen-presenting, MHC II-positive cells under inflammatory conditions.

B lymphocytes. These are mainly involved in the synthesis of secretory antibodies of the IgA class occurring in alimentary secretions and in IgE (homocytotropic antibody mainly related to mast cell activities, see p. 79). These antibodies are secreted first by plasmacytes in the lamina propria and intercellular spaces of simple epithelia and in the vicinity of subepithelial glands. Antibodies are passed to certain glandular cells (although not goblet cells, at least in the gut) which possess characteristic polymeric IgA receptors on their basolateral surfaces, enabling them to endocytose IgA molecules and pass them into their secretory pathways. During this process the IgA is glycosylated to form *secretory IgA* (*sIgA*) which is then secreted with mucus into the lumen of the viscus they are located in. These antibodies are vital in eliminating pathogenic organisms, although other types of antibody (IgM and IgG), secreted by plasma cells of the lamina propria, are also essential to the destruction of any pathogens which breach the epithelium and infect the adjacent tissues. Some IgM and IgG is also secreted at the surface and can be found in many secretions, for example saliva, milk, etc.

T lymphocytes. These engage in the typical repertoire of this cell type (p. 78), CD4+ helper T cells stimulating B-cell activity, and CD8+ cytotoxic T cells engaging in the destruction of virus- and parasite-infected cells (especially those of the epithelium), and of neoplastic cells, as well as synthesizing various cytokines with complex actions on the lymphocyte population. The surveillance of the epithelium is of obvious importance, because it is a prime target for micro-organisms in the lumen of the gut and at other exposed surfaces, and many of the lymphocytes migrating within the intercellular spaces of the epithelia (see e.g. **12**.64) are T cells.

Lymphocyte homing. The delivery of lymphocytes formed in different types of MALT to their final destinations appears to be fairly specific, and so it seems that some mechanism must exist by which circulating lymphocytes can recognize the tissues or regions of the body they are appropriate for and then migrate into them to play their special part in the immune response. Although it is not certain exactly how specific this homing mechanism is, it appears that lymphocytes from Peyer's patches are seeded into the intestines, those from the BALT into the respiratory system, etc. This seems to be achieved by a system of variable adhesion molecules expressed on the surfaces of lymphocytes (homing receptors) and on the venular endothelium (vascular addressins) within different areas of lymphoid tissue.

PALATINE TONSIL (9.46–53)

Introduction

The topographical anatomy of the palatine tonsil is described with the alimentary tract on pages 1728, 1729. In brief, the palatine

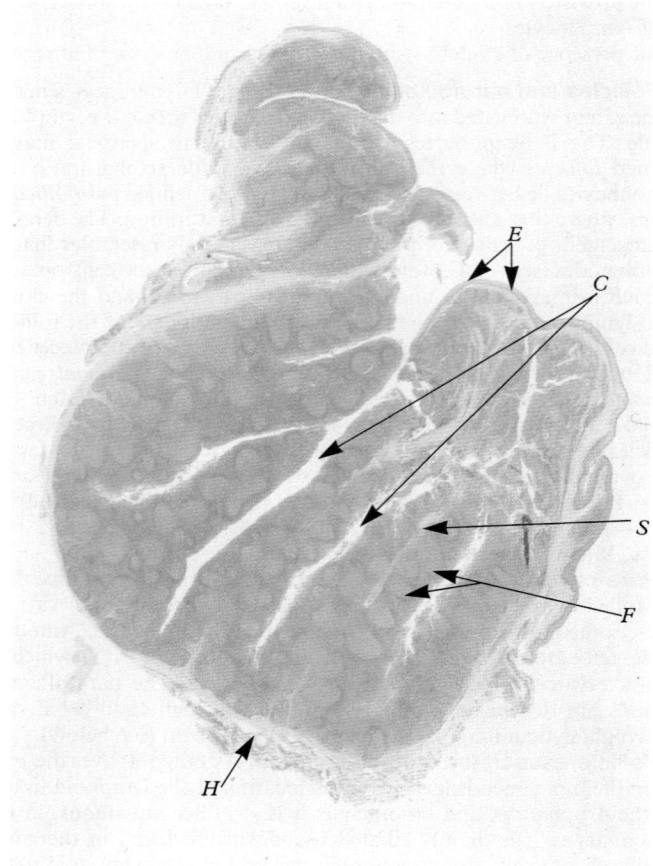

9.47 Transverse section through a whole palatine tonsil, showing many secondary follicles (F) arranged in parallel to the connective tissue septa (S); their dark-staining mantle zones are facing towards the tonsillar crypts (C). Also visible are the oropharyngeal surface epithelium (E) and the connective tissue hemicapsule (H). Haematoxylin and eosin. (Provided by M Perry and photographed by Sarah Smith, Division of Anatomy and Cell Biology, UMDS, Guy's Campus, London.)

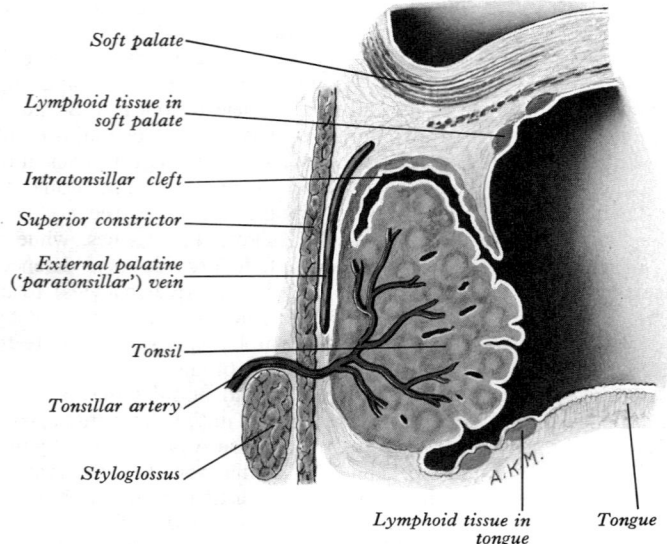

Soft palate

Lymphoid tissue in soft palate

Intratonsillar cleft

Superior constrictor

External palatine ('paratonsillar') vein

Tonsil

Tonsillar artery

Styloglossus

Lymphoid tissue in tongue   *Tongue*

A.K.M.

    9.46   Coronal section through the palatine tonsil.

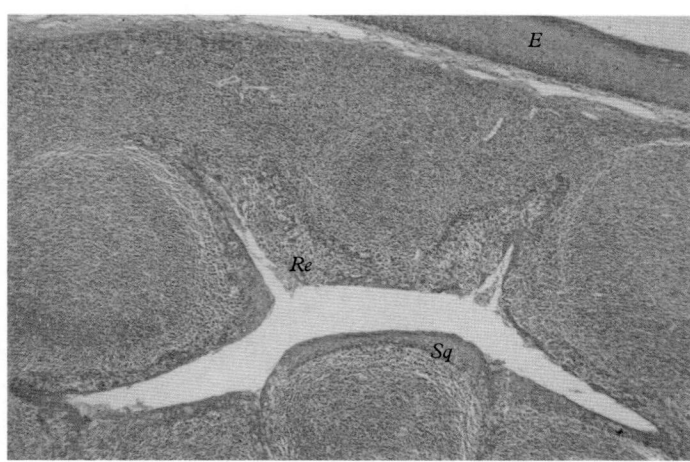

9.48   Palatine tonsil: transected tonsillar crypt lined with patches of stratified squamous (Sq) and reticulated (Re) epithelium, contrasting with the thick epithelial covering of the oropharyngeal surface (E). Haematoxylin and eosin. (Provided by M Perry and photographed by Sarah Smith, Division of Anatomy and Cell Biology, UMDS, Guy's Campus, London.)

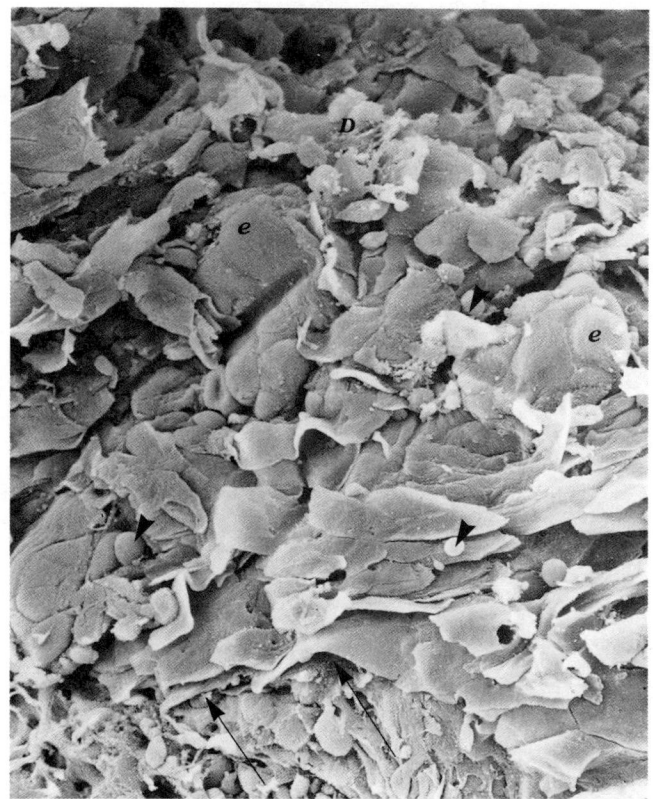

9.49   Scanning electron micrograph of the reticulated crypt epithelium (e) in a palatine tonsil, showing the tonsillar surface broken open to reveal the lymphocytes and other non-epithelial cells (arrowheads) within the cavities at the base of the attenuated stratified squamous epithelium. Also shown is cellular debris (D) within a crypt. (Provided by M Perry, Division of Anatomy and Cell Biology, UMDS, Guy's Campus, London.)

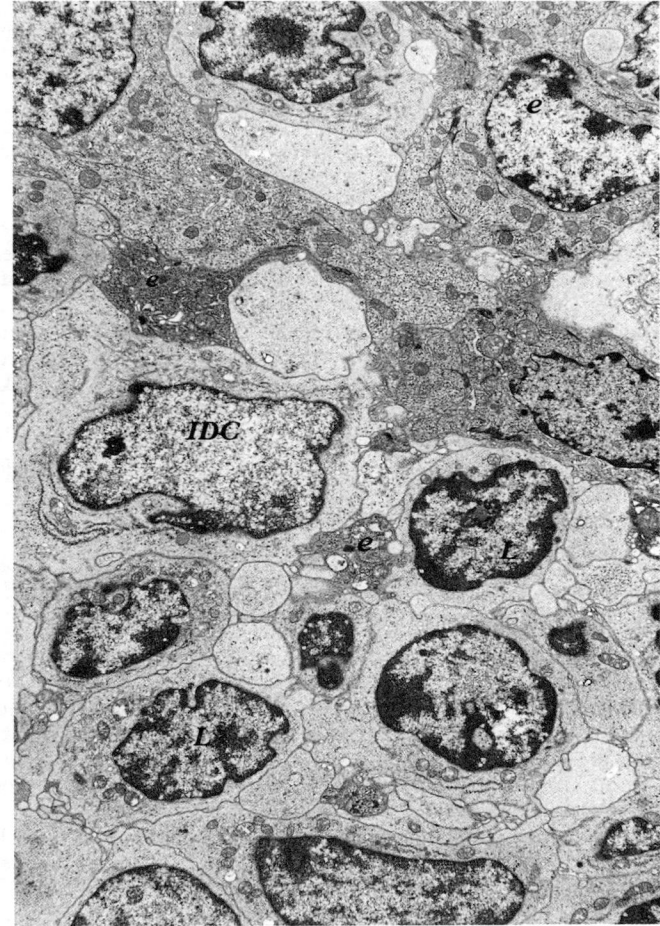

9.50   Transmission electron micrograph of a palatine tonsil through part of an interfollicular area showing interdigitating cells (IDC) and lymphocytes (L). The processes of a few epithelial cells (e) are also visible. (Provided by M Perry, Division of Anatomy and Cell Biology, UMDS, Guy's Campus, London.)

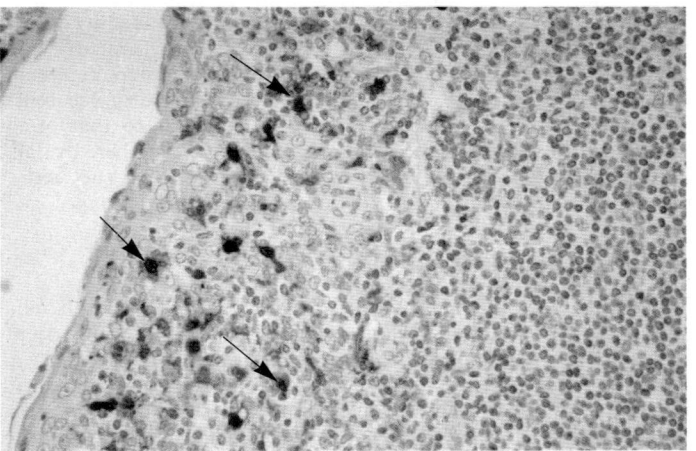

9.51   Reticulated epithelium from a crypt of a palatine tonsil, immuno-stained to show numerous interdigitating cells and macrophages, identified by their immunostaining for the S-100 antigen. Note the close contacts between these cells and infiltrating lymphocytes (arrows). Immuno-peroxidase stain on a paraffin section. (Provided by M Perry, Division of Anatomy and Cell Biology, UMDS, Guy's Campus, London.)

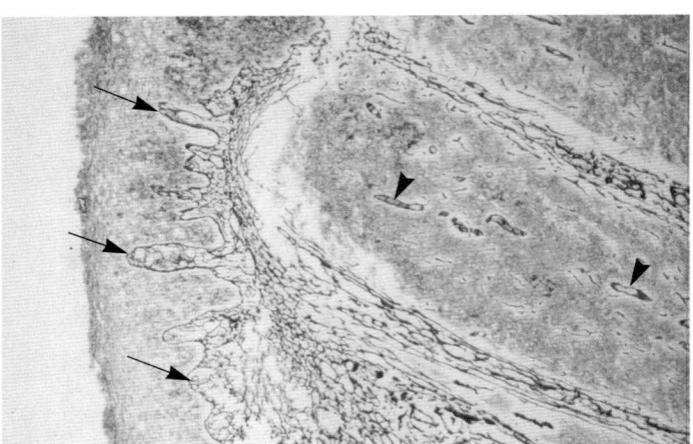

9.53 Palatine tonsil in section, stained with silver to demonstrate the fine reticulin network supporting the lymphoid tissue. Reticulin is seen to outline the undulating basement membrane of the non-keratinized stratified squamous epithelium covering the oropharyngeal surface (arrows). Reticulin also forms a lattice in the interfollicular areas, and also supports the tonsillar microvasculature including the follicular vessels (arrowheads). Gordon and Sweet silver method. (Provided by M Perry, Division of Anatomy and Cell Biology, UMDS, Guy's Campus, London.)

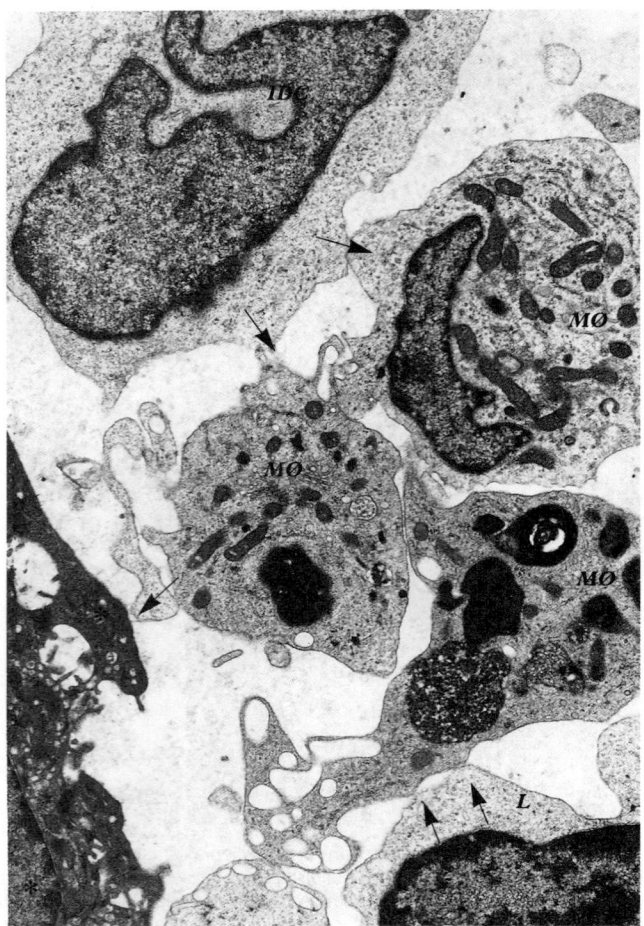

9.52 Transmission electron micrograph of an area of reticulated epithelium of a palatine tonsil, showing intimate contacts (arrows) between macrophages (Mφ), an interdigitating cell (asterisk) and a lymphocyte (L). (Provided by M Perry, Division of Anatomy and Cell Biology, UMDS, Guy's Campus, London.)

tonsils are bilateral almond-shaped masses (hence the Greek term *amygdala* = almond) situated in the oropharynx within the tonsilar recesses, between the palatoglossal and palatopharyngeal folds. Each is a mass of lymphoid tissue covered on its oropharyngeal aspect by non-keratinized stratified squamous epithelium. It is supported internally by connective tissue septa and a network of finer fibres, continuous with the hemicapsule of the tonsil which forms its lateral boundary with the oropharyngeal wall, and with the mucosa covering its free surface (**9.46**). 10–30 or more *crypts* are formed by the invagination of the latter surface. These are narrow tubular epithelial diverticula which often branch within the substance of the tonsil. The epithelium lining the crypts is in part similar to that of the general surface, i.e. stratified squamous in type, but there are also patches of *reticulated epithelium*, a much thinner tissue with a complex structure, and of great importance in the immunological function of the tonsil.

Reticulated epithelium

The reticulated epithelium (**9.47**, 48, 50–52) lacks the orderly laminar structure of the stratified squamous epithelium, its base being deeply invaginated in a complex manner, so that the epithelial cells, with their slender branched cytoplasmic processes, provide a mesh with large interspaces to accommodate the infiltrating lymphocytes and macrophages. The basal lamina of this epithelium is discontinuous. Although the oropharyngeal surface is unbroken, the epithelium may become exceedingly thin in places, with only a tenuous cytoplasmic lamina separating the pharyngeal lumen from the underlying lymphocytes. Epithelial cells are held together by small desmosomes, anchored into bundles of keratin filaments. Langerhans' cells and interdigitating APCs are also present within the reticulated epi-

thelium. The intimate association of epithelial cells and lymphocytes, often referred to as 'lympho-epithelial symbiosis' (Fioretti 1957), is particularly well designed for the direct transport of antigen from the external environment to the tonsillar lymphoid cells (Brandtzaeg 1988; Perry et al 1988) so that the reticulated epithelial cells are thought to be functionally similar to the microfold cells of the gut (p. 1769). The total surface area of the reticulated epithelium is very large because of the complex branched nature of the tonsillar crypts, estimated at 295 cm^2 for an average palatine tonsil (Slipka & Kotyza 1987). It is noteworthy that, in contrast, lymph nodes depend on indirect antigenic delivery through *afferent lymphatic vessels*, which are absent from the tonsil (although efferent lymphatics drain it, like other examples of MALT).

It is noteworthy that the crypts also often contain desquamated epithelial cells mixed with intact and degenerating lymphocytes, occasional erythrocytes, cellular debris and, sometimes, micro-organisms. The degeneration of epithelial cells is frequently accompanied by the formation of small spheroidal clusters of stratified squamous epithelium known as *tonsillar corpuscles*, especially in the narrower rami of the crypt system (Slipka & Kotyza 1987; Perry & Slipka 1993). These closely resemble thymic epithelial corpuscles (of Hassall, see p. 1426) and may represent sites of accidental separation of the pharyngeal epithelium from the tonsillar surface rather than any functional significant features of the tonsil.

Lymphoid tissue (9.49–52)

The tonsillar lymphoid tissue can be divided into four lymphoid compartments participating in immune responses (Brandtzaeg 1988). These are:

(1) lymphoid follicles with germinal centres, rounded cellular aggregations consisting mainly of B-lymphocytes and their precursors, scattered follicular dendritic cells and some macrophages with radiating extensions ('starry sky macrophages'). Germinal centres are arranged in rows roughly parallel to neighbouring connective tissue septa. Their size and cellular content varies in proportion to the immunological activity of the tonsil;

(2) the mantle zones of the lymphoid follicles, each with closely packed small lymphocytes forming a dense cap, always situated on the side of the follicle nearest to the mucosal surface. These cells are the products of B-lymphocyte proliferation within the germinal centres;

(3) extrafollicular, or T-lymphocyte areas containing specialized segments of microvasculature including high endothelial venules (HEVs), through which circulating lymphocytes enter the tonsillar parenchyma (Perry et al 1992a,b).

(4) the lymphoid tissue of the reticulated crypt epithelium containing predominantly IgG- and IgA-producing B lymphocytes (including some mature plasmacytes), T lymphocytes and antigen-presenting Langerhans cells. In this subsurface region there are also numerous capillary loops, and in some heavily reticulated areas, HEVs with transmigrating lymphocytes (Perry et al 1988, 1992b).

Connective tissue framework

The whole of the tonsil is supported by a delicate meshwork of fine collagen (reticulin) fibres secreted by their associated fibroblasts (9.53). The collagen fibres are condensed in places to form more robust connective tissue septa also containing elastin, creating a series of partitions within the tonsillar mass, the follicles being placed on either side of septa (9.46). The septa merge at their ends with the dense irregular fibrous hemicapsule on the deep aspect of the tonsil and with the lamina propria on the pharyngeal surface. Blood vessels, lymphatics and nerves branch or join within the connective tissue condensations.

Vascular systems

Blood vessels. These have been studied in detail in microcorrosion casts of the human tonsil by Ohtani et al (1989). Arteries enter the deep surface branch within the connective tissue septa, narrow to become arterioles and then give off capillary loops into the follicles, interfollicular areas and into the cavities within the base of the reticulated epithelium (see above). The capillaries rejoin to form venules, many with high endothelium, as already noted, and the veins return within the septal tissues to the hemicapsule as tributaries of the pharyngeal drainage. For further details of the macroscopic aspects of the vasculature, see page 1729.

Lymphatics. Efferent lymphatics arise in dense plexuses of fine capillaries surrounding each follicle. These join to form larger lymphatics which eventually exit through the connective tissue hemicapsule and thence through the adjacent superior constrictor to the nodes of the deep cervical lymphatic drainage (p. 1729).

Tonsillar functions

Like other mucosa-associated lymphoid masses, the major functions of the palatine tonsils are as follows (see Brandtzaeg 1988):

- to select clones of B and T cells relevant to the micro-organisms at the pharyngeal surface. To initiate this action it is envisaged that antigens cross the reticulated epithelium and are passed on to antigen-presenting cells which carry out T- and thus B-cell selection;
- to provide a site for the proliferative expansion of selected B- and T-lymphocyte clones destined for immune functions in neighbouring areas of the pharyngeal mucosa;
- to produce IgA and IgG for local secretion (apparently a minor function which may be primarily concerned with the immediate protection of the tonsil itself).

Palatine tonsils belong to the class of secondary lymphoid tissue, and the precursors of the proliferating B- and T-lymphocyte populations originate in the primary lymphoid tissues, i.e. the bone marrow and thymus, respectively. Entering the tonsils by migration across the walls of the HEVs, the two classes of lymphocytes move to their specific areas, and proliferate when suitably stimulated, under the influence of APCs and macrophages. After T-cell contact with an APC cell and B-cell stimulation, lymphocytes leave the tonsil in the efferent lymphatics, and probably also to some extent by direct peripheral migration into the mucosa of the surrounding pharynx. It is thought that those which leave by the lymphatic route and thus pass into the general circulation eventually migrate to the pharynx and adjacent areas of mucosa through venules and become important in local defence, including the secretion of IgA through mucoserous glands, immune surveillance and other related activities.

Tonsillar pathology

While the palatine tonsil is a substantial part of the pharyngeal immune system, it may itself become infected; in particular, pathogenic bacteria, for example streptococci, may invade the tonsillar crypts and proliferate within them, causing an inflammatory reaction including the migration of leucocytes into the cryptal spaces. Various

factors including the expansion of germinal centres cause swelling of the tonsillar mass, and the pus within the crypts is visible as yellowish spots on its inflamed surface. Tonsillectomy after repeated episodes of tonsillitis might be expected to cause considerable reduction of pharyngeal defence, but this usually does not appear to be the case, probably because other related lymphoid tissue masses, for example the lingual tonsil, increase their lymphocytic output.

NASOPHARYNGEAL TONSIL (ADENOIDS)

The nasopharyngeal tonsil is a median tonsillar mass, situated in the roof of the nasopharynx; it has many resemblances to the palatine tonsil in its cellular organization and functions, although there are also some differences, mainly because it is situated in the nasopharyngeal mucosa rather than that of the oropharynx. Its macroscopic anatomy is described with the alimentary tract (p. 1728), and the present account will be mainly restricted to its microstructure.

The nasopharyngeal tonsil at its maximal size (during the early years of life) is shaped like a truncated pyramid hanging from the nasopharyngeal roof. It consists of a mass of lymphoid tissue embedded in the mucosa of the nasopharynx (9.54), and is thus covered at its sides and below mainly by ciliated respiratory epithelium, although small patches of non-keratinized stratified squamous epithelium also occur. The superior surface is separated from the periosteum of the sphenoid and occipital bones by a connective tissue hemicapsule to which the fibrous framework of the tonsil is anchored. This forms what is described by Oláh (1978) as a three-dimensional labyrinth formed by supportive reticular fibres connected to both the basal lamina and the connective tissue hemicapsule, and filled with lymphoid parenchyma. The epithelium lines

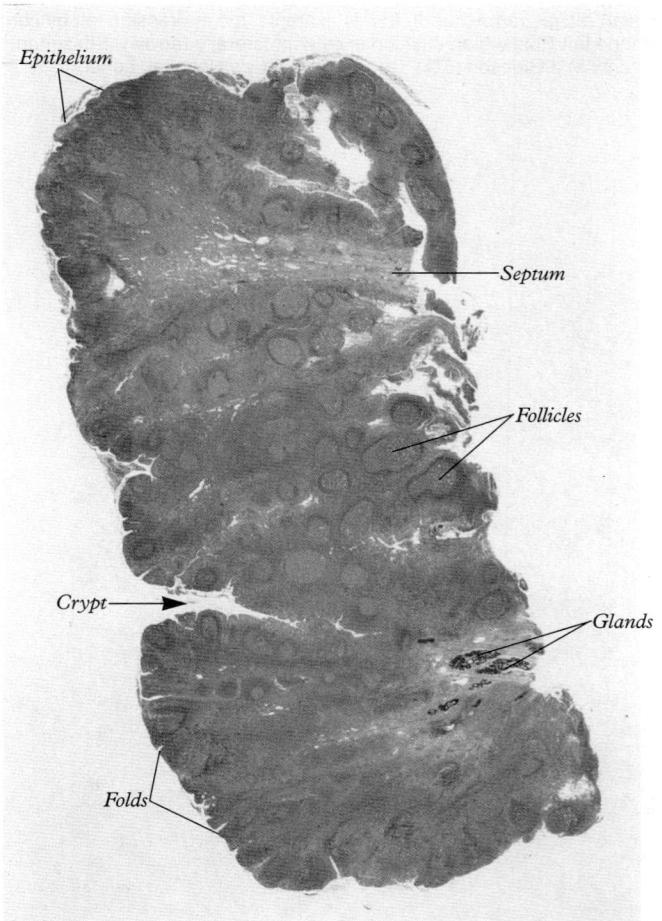

9.54 Transverse section of a nasopharyngeal tonsil. Note numerous lymphoid follicles (F); epithelium with folds (arrows) and the deep crypts (C). L = lacuna; S = scromucous gland; CT = connective tissue septa. Haematoxylin and eosin. Magnification × 9. Provided by N Kirkpatrick and photographed by Sarah Smith (Division of Anatomy and Cell Biology, UMDS, Guy's Campus, London).

a series of mucosal folds and crypts around which the lymphoid parenchyma is organized into follicles and extrafollicular areas.

The nasopharyngeal tonsil is subdivided into four to six lobes by connective tissue septa, which arise from the hemicapsule and penetrate into the lymphoid parenchyma (9.54). Located within this connective tissue are some seromucous glands with their ducts extending through the lymphoid tissue to the cryptal or nasopharyngeal surface (Barnes 1923; Eggston & Wolf 1947).

Tonsillar crypts (9.55–58). There has been a long standing debate on whether the nasopharyngeal tonsil really possesses true crypts

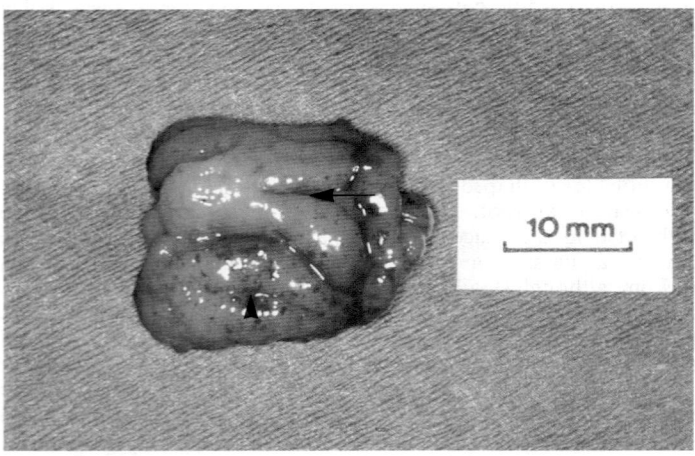

9.55 Appearance of a nasopharyngeal tonsil following adenoidectomy by curctage. Rostral surface is to the left; surface folds radiate forward from a median recess (arrowhead). In this example, the impression left by contact with the left Eustachian cushion is evident laterally (arrow). Specimen provided by M J Gleeson (ENT Department, Guy's Hospital, London).

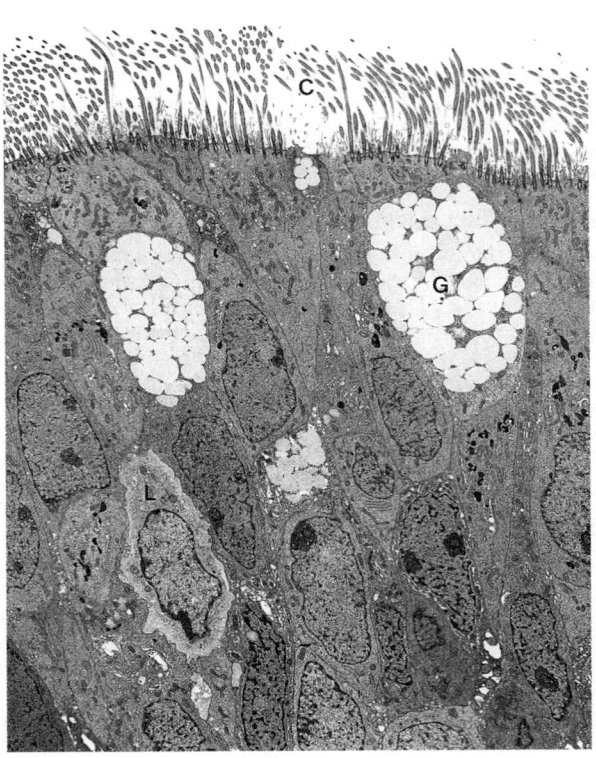

9.56 Transmission EM of a section through the surface of a nasopharyngeal tonsil, showing pseudostratified epithelial cells with cilia (C), a goblet cell (G), and an intraepithelial lymphocyte (L). Magnification × 4000. Specimen provided by N Kirkpatrick and photographed by Sarah Smith (Division of Anatomy and Cell Biology, UMDS, Guy's Campus, London).

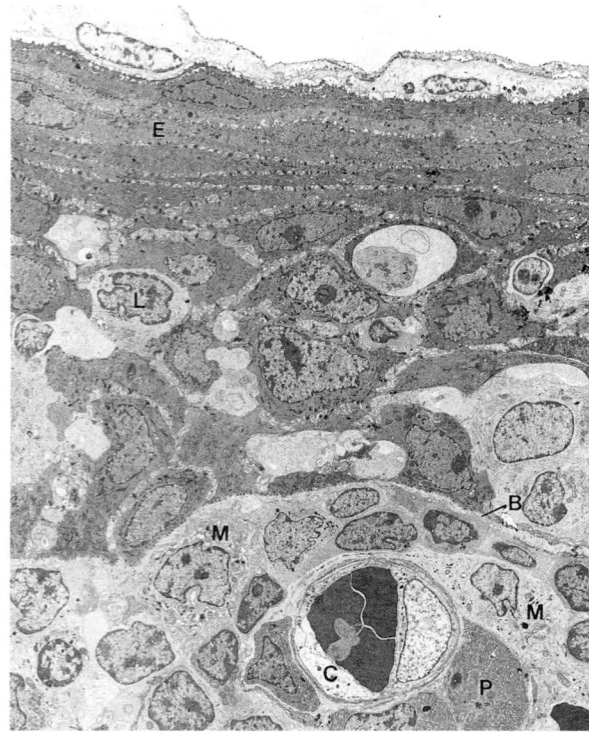

9.57 Transmission EM of stratified squamous epithelium at the nasopharyngeal surface, with macrophages (M), a capillary (C) and plasmacyte (P) in the lamina propria. Magnification × 2500. Specimen provided by N Kirkpatrick, and photographed by Sarah Smith (Division of Anatomy and Cell Biology, UMDS, Guy's Campus, London).

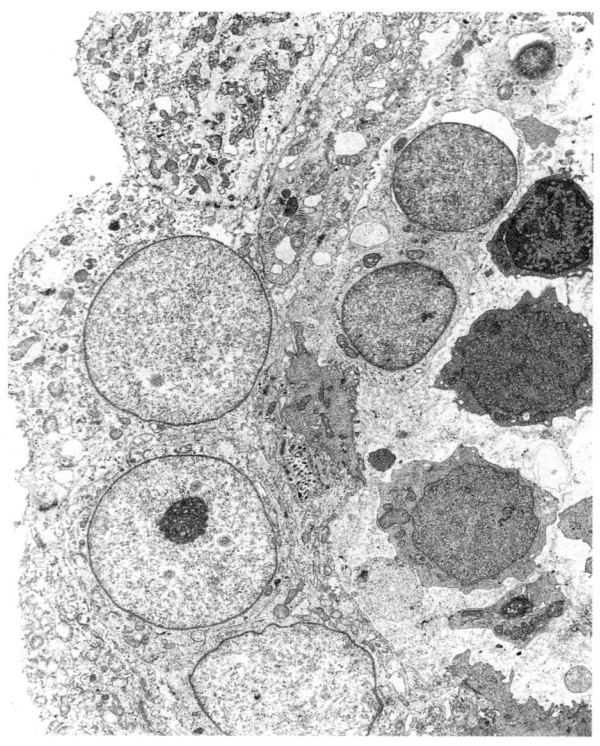

9.58 Transmission electron micrograph of the nasopharyngeal surface showing intermediate epithelium, with lymphocytes at its base. Magnification × 6500. Specimen provided by N Kirkpatrick, and photographed by Sarah Smith (Division of Anatomy and Cell Biology, UMDS, Guy's Campus, London).

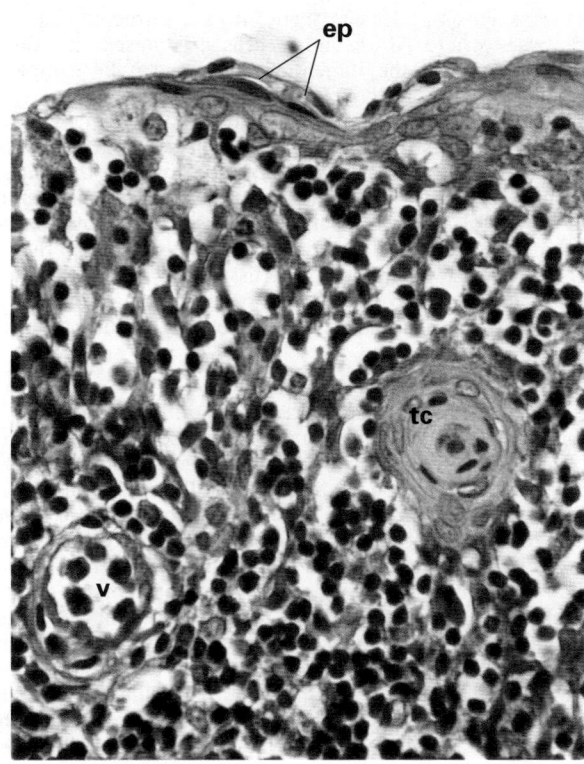

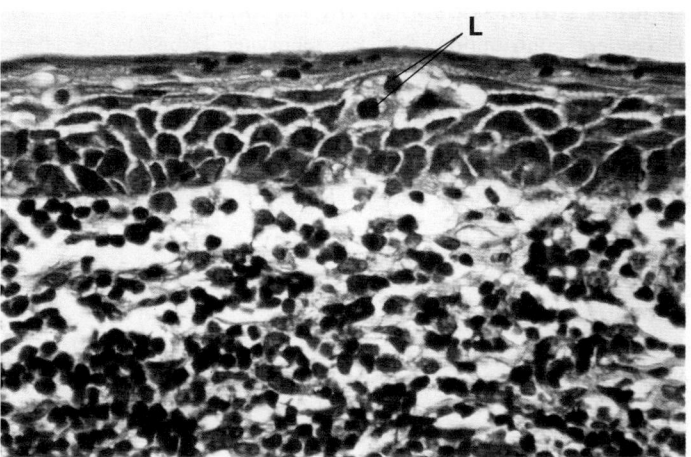

9.60 Section through surface of the nasopharyngeal epithelium showing a patch of stratified squamous epithelium with intraepithelial lymphocytes (L), subepithelial lymphocytes and capillaries. Movat's stain. Magnification × 250. Provided by N Kirkpatrick and photographed by Sarah Smith (Division of Anatomy and Cell Biology, UMDS, Guy's Campus, London).

9.59 Reticulated stratified squamous epithelium of a nasopharyngeal tonsil, with network of intraepithelial channels containing many non-epithelial cells. Note also: tonsillar corpuscle (tc) and an intraepithelial venule (v). PAS stain. Magnification × 640. Provided by N Kirkpatrick, and photographed by Sarah Smith (Division of Anatomy and Cell Biology, UMDS, Guy's Campus, London).

keratinized stratified squamous, and occasionally a simple cuboidal, epithelium in all locations. Pseudokeratinization occurs rarely in deep branching crypts. However, in all three of these types of epithelial cover there are patches of typical *reticulated epithelium* of variable size and depth, as in the palatine tonsil (see above, and 9.58–59). The degree of reticulation varies so that in some sites only a few lymphocytes and other non-epithelial cells infiltrate into the epithelial base, and in others there are dense cellular aggregates, resulting in the loss of the ordered epithelial architecture. This reticulated epithelium also frequently becomes vascularized (Kirkpatrick et al 1993).

The internal structure of the nasopharyngeal tonsil closely resembles that of the palatine tonsil, and the same lymphoid compartments can be discerned, i.e. follicles with germinal centres and mantle zones containing B lymphocytes, follicular dendritic cells and macrophages; extrafollicular areas with T lymphocytes and interdigitating cells; and the reticulated epithelium. HEVs also exist within the extrafollicular tissue, indicating similar routes of lymphocyte entry and dispersal (9.60).

like those of the palatine tonsil, or merely a deeply folded surface. Ali (1965a,b) and Kirkpatrick et al (1993) describe the presence of both numerous superficial folds and deep, sometimes branching crypts extending right through the nasopharyngeal tonsil almost to the connective tissue hemicapsule. The epithelium lining the folds and crypts, and that covering the nasopharyngeal surface is not uniform and there are patches of pseudostratified ciliated, non-

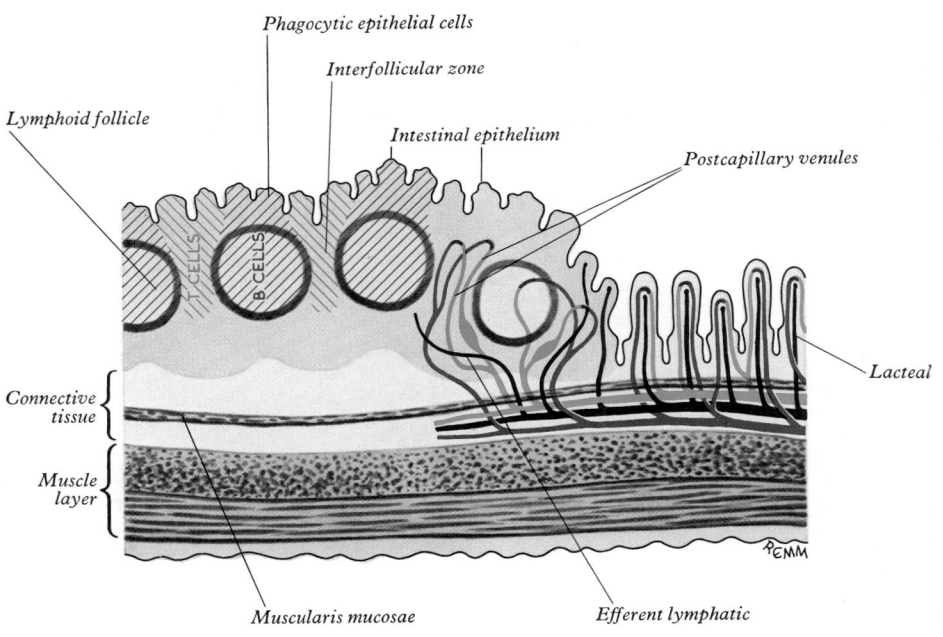

9.61 The organization of an epitheliolymphoid complex in the wall of the small intestine (a Peyer's patch), showing the distribution of B lymphocytes associated with the follicles and T lymphocytes in the interfollicular zones;

the arrangement of the vascular supply of the lymphoid tissue is also shown (right).

Functions of the nasopharyngeal tonsil

The general contribution of the nasopharyngeal tonsil to the defence of the upper respiratory tract is probably similar to that of the palatine tonsils and other parts of the circumpharyngeal lymphoid ring. The territories served by its lymphocytes are uncertain, but may include the nasal cavities, nasopharynx, pharyngotympanic tubes and the middle and inner ear which are topographically related areas. For clinical aspects, see page 1729.

PEYER'S PATCHES

Introduction

Peyer's patches are aggregations of O-MALT which form domelike elevations of the mucosa present throughout the small and large intestines. In the ileum they often form quite large areas of lymphoid tissue, up to 1 cm wide by 2 cm long (or sometimes larger), orientated with their long axes parallel to that of the intestine (**12**.111). The name Peyer's patch was originally given to the enlarged masses of lymphoid tissue found in the ileum during typhoid infections, but it is now usually applied to any group of lymphoid nodules in the wall of the small or large intestine including the appendix. The topography of a Peyer's patch is outlined on page 1771.

Microstructure of Peyer's patches (9.61)

In general plan Peyer's patches resemble other masses of O-MALT (see above) such as the tonsils.

Lymphoid tissue. This is contained mainly within the lamina propria, although large lymphoid masses can extend into submucosal tissues, but its presence causes the overlying epithelium to form a low convex elevation over the region. Within the lymphoid tissue are variable numbers of lymphoid follicles and parafollicular areas similar to those of the tonsil, including the presence of an epithelium-directed accumulation of small lymphocytes (mantle zone) on the follicle periphery, and, in active tissue, germinal centres. HEVs are also features of the parafollicular areas.

Follicle-associated epithelium. The domed surface is generally devoid of villi and crypts, but is covered by a unique epithelium of low columnar cells with short irregular microvilli, interspersed with characteristic *microfold* (*M*) *cells*. These are rather flat cells the bases of which are invaginated to form pockets which lymphocytes and APCs can enter in much the same way as in the reticulated epithelium of the tonsils. On their apical surfaces, M cells have many short ridges and stubby microvilli, and between these are deep endocytic pits and vesicles. The details of M cells and other epithelial covering cells vary with position (see Clark et al 1994). In the appendix the lymphoid tissue consists of a continuous layer around the narrow lumen, penetrated by numerous crypts (tubular intestinal glands).

M cells are highly endocytic, and can rapidly transfer material taken into vesicles at their luminal surface through the underlying tissues (transcytosis), releasing them into the intraepithelial pockets at their bases where APCs and T cells are present. In this way, antigenic material in the lumen of the gut can be sampled and presented via APCs to lymphocytes more deeply placed in the mucosa, where appropriate effector action can be taken. The M cells are particularly adhesive to carbohydrates of bacterial cell walls, and may indeed transport whole bacteria and viruses to the underlying tissues. Although this ability is no doubt a great advantage in eliciting powerful immune reactions against them, some pathogens unfortunately overpower the defensive mechanisms within the lymphoid tissue to spread within the body's tissues, for instance, poliovirus, which can gain access to the nervous system through enteric nerves, and *Salmonella typhi*, a bacterial pathogen of the gut wall tissues.

Immune functions

The result of normal antigen sampling and presentation is the selection and proliferation of suitable IgA-secreting B-cell clones which then disseminate through the efferent lymphatics and the systemic blood circulation to the D-MALT population in a much wider area of the alimentary mucosa. There the B cells secrete antibody for transport to the lumen. The antibody they secrete is IgA in the form of dimers which after release from the plasma cells can bind to polymeric IgA receptors on the basolateral surfaces of gland cells and enterocytes. These cells then endocytose the IgA dimers, and after attachment of the secretory component in the Golgi apparatuses of these cells, they are secreted into the lumen as secretory antibody, sIgA. This configuration of dimeric sIgA is highly resistant to enzymatic degradation, and is, therefore, very suitable for action within the hostile, protease-rich environment of the intestinal interior.

There are also various other routes for epithelium–lymphocyte interactions in the gut wall. The enterocytes themselves are MHC-II positive and can act as APCs to T lymphocytes, although these initiate suppressor activities, suggesting that the main importance of this pathway is to induce tolerance of epithelial antigens. Another possible entry point for antigens is the lymphatics. As elsewhere in O-MALT, these are primarily efferent and serve to take lymphocytes away from the lymphoid tissue. However, recent studies in various mammalian species indicate that afferent lymphatics arising in the villi and neighbouring parts of the lamina propria overlying the lymphoid tissue form a plexus of perifollicular sinuses and might, therefore, be involved in the passage of antigen from neighbouring tissues into the lymphoid structure (see Lowden & Heath 1992), although the functional significance of this arrangement is not known.

Because the surface area of the gut is greater than in all other areas of the body the total number of lymphocytes within its walls is substantial.

For further details of Peyer's patches, see the stimulating review by Kraehenbuhl and Neutra (1992).

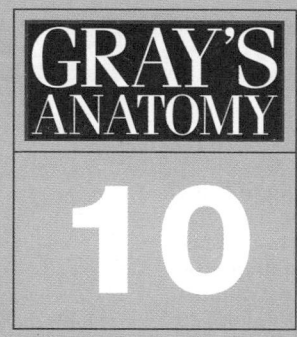

GRAY'S ANATOMY

10

CARDIOVASCULAR

Section Editor: Giorgio Gabella

With contributions from Professor Robert Anderson, MD, Mr Julian Dussek FRCS, Dr Susan Evans, PhD, Mr Adrian Marston, FRCS and Dr Marta Perry, MUDr, PhD, Professor Anderson was responsible for the revision of the Heart and contributed all the colour photographs of the heart and the diagrams 10.22, 43, 44, 57, 62, 63, 64. Dr Evans revised the General Introduction on the evolutionary aspects of cardiac morphology. The section on the pulse and central venous access were prepared by Mr Julian Dussek. Mr Marston advised on arteries and veins of the abdomen 10.116, 117, 120, 125–127, and Dr Perry wrote the essay on leucocyte-endothelial cell interaction.

BLOOD VESSELS

INTRODUCTION

Movement and exchange of materials in the watery medium of living tissues takes place by diffusion, most commonly along chemical gradients. A vital requirement in large and complex organisms, however, is a fast, widespread, high-capacity system for continuously transporting to and from every single part of the body a large number of specific components, ranging from ions and small molecules to whole cells. This is the main function served by the vascular or circulatory system.

- Blood (see section 9) is the vehicle which maintains a vast chemical traffic through the body, moving hormones, oxygen, nutrients, antibodies, catabolites, red and white blood cells, as well as infestants and toxic compounds. In addition, in ectotherms, blood redistributes and disperses heat, and, because of the pulse pressure, it also has mechanical effects, such as maintaining turgidity of tissues and counteracting certain effects of gravity.
- The circulatory system is fast and has high capacity, for several reasons: because of the rheological properties of blood, because of the large volume of blood, and because of the mechanical properties of the heart and muscular arteries.
- The circulatory system is made up of the heart—a central pump and the main motor of the system—and by a vast array of tubes which lead away from the heart (as arteries) and carry the blood to the 'periphery' of the body; at the periphery, that is within organs and tissues, the tubes loop back and (as veins) reach the heart again where the blood eventually returns.

Schematically, one can envisage the vascular system as made up of long loops which are centred on the heart (at which level both arteries and veins are largest) and are much reduced in size and extremely arborized at the periphery (capillaries) (**10**.1). There are, in fact, not one but two such loops, because the heart is a **pair** of muscular pumps, one feeding a minor loop (pulmonary circulation), which serves the lungs, the other feeding a major loop (systemic circulation), which serves all the rest of the body. The two loops are also referred to as the *greater* and *lesser circle*.

With limited exceptions, which will be discussed in due course, each loop is a closed system of tubes, so that blood per se does not usually leave the circulation. As William Harvey discovered in the seventeenth century, blood is pumped away from the heart but it all returns to the heart after circulation through the body. Arteries are the vessels that carry the blood away from the heart, and veins are the vessels that carry it back to the heart.

From the centre to the periphery, the vascular tree shows three main changes:

- The arteries increase in number by repeated division and by the issuing of side branches, in both the systemic and the pulmonary circulation.
- The arteries also decrease in diameter, although not to the same extent as they increase in number, so that a notional cross-section of all the vessels at a given distance will have the greatest area the furthest away it is from the heart. As a result, blood flow is faster near the heart than at the periphery.
- Among other structural changes, the wall of the arteries decreases in thickness, although this is not as substantial as the reduction of the vessel diameter. In consequence, in the smallest arteries (arterioles) the thickness of the wall represents about half the outer radius of the vessel, whereas in a large vessel it represents between one-fifteenth and one-fifth. For example, in the thoracic aorta the radius is about 17 mm and the wall thickness 1.1 mm (Wolinsky & Glagov 1967a). From a functional viewpoint, while **size** is a fundamental parameter of a blood vessel, **position** of the vessel in the body and **structure of the vessel wall** are also very important characteristics, which dictate the properties of the vessel. Furthermore, whereas microcirculation vessels are remarkably similar in animal species of very different body size, equivalent large vessels vary greatly not only in size but also in wall thickness in mammals of different body size—an important consideration when

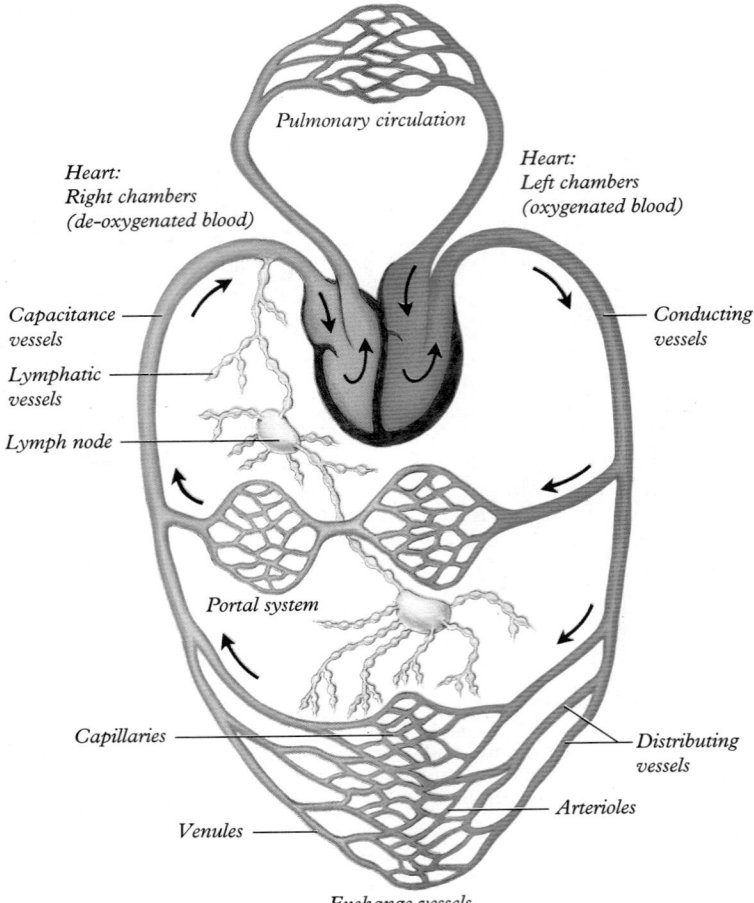

10.1 Diagrammatic drawing of the cardiovascular and lymphatic system. The nomenclature of the main vessel types is indicated; in red are the vessels carrying oxygenated blood, in blue those carrying un-oxygenated blood and in yellow the lymphatic structures.

data obtained on laboratory animals are extrapolated to man. As a first approximation, comparative studies show that in corresponding large arteries, the ratio between inner diameter and wall thickness is constant and is independent of body size (Caro et al 1978).

VASCULAR SYSTEM

VESSEL NUMBER

The aorta, the single systemic artery emerging from the heart, gives origin by successive branching to hundreds of arteries of progressively smaller calibre; by further branching these produce about 4×10^6 arterioles and four times as many capillaries. A similar number of venules converge onto each other forming a progressively smaller number of veins of increasingly larger size; eventually, two veins only, which are also the largest of the body, the superior and the inferior vena cava, open into the heart from the systemic circulation. A similar pattern is found in the pulmonary circulation (lesser circle). In the lesser circle, however, the vascular loop is shorter and has therefore fewer branching points; consequently, the number of vessels is smaller than in the greater circle.

VESSEL SIZE

At the emergence from the heart the aorta of an adult man has an outer diameter of about 30 mm (sectional area of nearly 7 cm²). The diameter decreases along the arterial tree until it is as little as 10 μm in arterioles (sectional area of about 80 μm²) (Rothe 1983). However, given the enormous number of arterioles, the total cross-sectional area at this level is about 150 cm², more than 200 times larger than at the level of the aorta (Wiedeman et al 1976); a further increase of the extent of the vascular bed takes place at the level of the capillaries and venules. In a 13-kg dog, the aorta had a cross-sectional area of 0.8 cm² and the capillaries (estimated at 1.2 × 10⁹) had a total cross-sectional area of 600 cm² (Green 1950). Veins leading back to the heart grow progressively larger and fewer in number. As with the arteries, a cross-sectional area of all veins at a given level is smaller the nearer this is to the heart. Veins are a little larger than the corresponding arteries. The reduction in diameter along the vascular tree occurs when a vessel divides or issues collateral branches; in the absence of branches, the shape of a segment of any vessel is not a truncated cone but a cylinder.

The size of the vessels increases during development, while there are substantial changes in the structure of their wall. In old age, vessels generally become enlarged. In animal species, the size of comparable vessels is related to body size; so, while in a mouse the ascending aorta measures less than 2 mm in diameter, the same vessel in a blue whale measures over 30 cm, large enough for a human baby to swim through. In spite of these enormous differences in size there are no qualitative differences in the structure of the constitutive materials: similar types of cell and of extracellular material are found in corresponding vessels ranging in linear size over more than three orders of magnitude.

BRANCHING PATTERNS

When an artery divides into two branches of roughly equal size, these are called terminal branches, as that artery ceases to exist at this point. Branches issued along the course of an artery, before its termination, are usually of smaller size than terminal branches and are called collateral (or side) branches.

The angle of branching is related to the calibre of the vessels and it conforms to theoretical predictions based on the principle of minimum work (namely, in this context, the highest efficiency in blood flow) or the minimum 'cost' of the bifurcation (Woldenberg & Horsfield 1986), although there are many exceptions.

The total cross-sectional area of the daughter vessels is invariably greater than the cross-sectional area of the parent vessel. For example, the terminal portion of the abdominal aorta has an internal diameter of 13.8 mm, while each of the common iliac arteries has an internal diameter of about 9.7 mm, so that the bifurcation produces a 1.5-fold increase in total cross-sectional area. It has been calculated that vessels arising by equal bifurcation have a diameter 0.76 of that of the parent vessel (Green 1950).

ANASTOMOSIS

Arteries can be joined to each other by anastomosis, which makes them able to feed each other's territory. An end-to-end anastomosis occurs when two arteries open directly into each other (for example, the vaginal and the ovarian artery, the right and the left gastroepiploic arteries, the ulnar artery and the superficial palmar branch of the radial artery). Anastomosis by convergence occurs when two arteries converge and merge, as in the case of the vertebral arteries forming the basilar artery. A transversal anastomosis occurs when a short arterial vessel links two large arteries transversely; examples are found in the anastomosis between the two anterior cerebral arteries, that between the posterior tibial artery and the peroneal artery, and that between radial and ulnar arteries at the wrist.

RELATIONS OF BLOOD VESSELS

Arteries are usually more deeply situated than veins, although there are several superficial or subcutaneous arteries, such as the occipital, temporal and frontal arteries and the epigastric artery.

In the proximity of the joints of limbs arteries are located on the flexor surface, but, characteristically, there are many transverse vessels which provide a collateral circulation over the lateral parts of the joint.

Arteries are usually separated from bones by muscles and fasciae. When they are in contact with bone tissue they leave an imprint or vascular groove, for example the subclavian artery on the first rib.

Large arteries (thoracic aorta, subclavian, axillary, femoral and popliteal) lie close to a single vein which drains the same territory supplied by the artery. The other arteries are usually accompanied by two veins, satellite veins (venae comitantes), lying on either side of the artery. Such venae comitantes flank an artery, with numerous cross-connections, the whole assembly being enclosed in a single connective tissue sheath. The artery and the two satellite veins are often associated with a nerve; when they are surrounded by a common connective tissue sheath they form a vasculo-nervous fascicle.

The close association between the larger arteries and veins in the limbs allows the counterflow exchange of heat to take place: this mechanism promotes heat transfer from arterial to venous blood, and thus helps to preserve body heat. Counterflow heat exchange apparatuses are found in other organs, for example in the testis, where the pampiniform plexus of veins surrounds the testicular artery: with this arrangement, not only is body heat conserved, but also the temperature of the testis is kept below average body temperature (Evans 1949; Grant & Wright 1971; see also p. 1854). Counterflow exchange mechanisms involving ions are found in the microcirculation, as exemplified by the arterial and venous sinusoids which exist in the vasa recta of the renal medulla where countercurrent exchange retains sodium ions at a high concentration in the medulla (p. 1824), efferent venous blood transferring sodium ions to the afferent arterial supply.

CLASSIFICATION OF VESSELS

Arteries and veins are identified and classified according to their anatomical position. A large part of this section (p. 1824) deals with the distribution, position and other systematic aspects of individual blood vessels. Furthermore, vessels can be classified anatomically according to their size and wall structure (**10**.2). Arteries can be divided into elastic and muscular: although muscle cells and elastic tissue are present in all arteries, while the relative amount of elastic material is largest in the largest vessels, the relative amount of musculature increases progressively towards the smallest arteries. Classifications of arteries are often presented or referred to; these classifications, however, are vague at best, because the changes of the structural and functional parameters are usually continuous rather than discrete. The gradual change of most parameters does not favour any firm classification, if one was needed. There is also considerable variability in vessel properties between individuals, based on heredity, individual history and age.

Functionally, arteries are often subdivided into conducting, distributing and resistance vessels. (In simplified functional terms some authors distinguish only three classes of vessels: resistance vessels, or arteries, exchange vessels, or microcirculation vessels, and capacitance vessels, or veins.)

Conducting vessels. The large arteries arising from the heart and their main branches, these are characterized by the predominantly elastic properties of the wall.

Distributing vessels. These are smaller arteries reaching the individual organs and branching into them, and their wall is characterized by a conspicuous muscular component.

Resistance vessels. Mainly arterioles; because of their small size and abundant musculature, these are the main source of the peripheral resistance to blood flow, and they cause a marked drop in the pressure of blood.

Exchange vessels. This is the collective term for capillaries, sinusoids and postcapillary venules. Their wall allows or favours exchange between blood and the tissue fluid surrounding the cells, the essential function of circulatory systems. The exchange includes oxygen, carbon dioxide, nutrients, water and inorganic ions, vitamins, hormones, metabolic products, antibodies and defensive cells of various kinds. Arterioles, capillaries and venules constitute the microvascular bed, the site of the microcirculation.

Capacitance or reservoir vessels. Larger venules and veins form a coextensive but variable, large-volume, low-pressure array of these vessels conveying blood back to the heart. The high capacitance of these vessels is due to the distensibility (compliance) of their wall, so that the content of blood is large even at low transmural pressures.

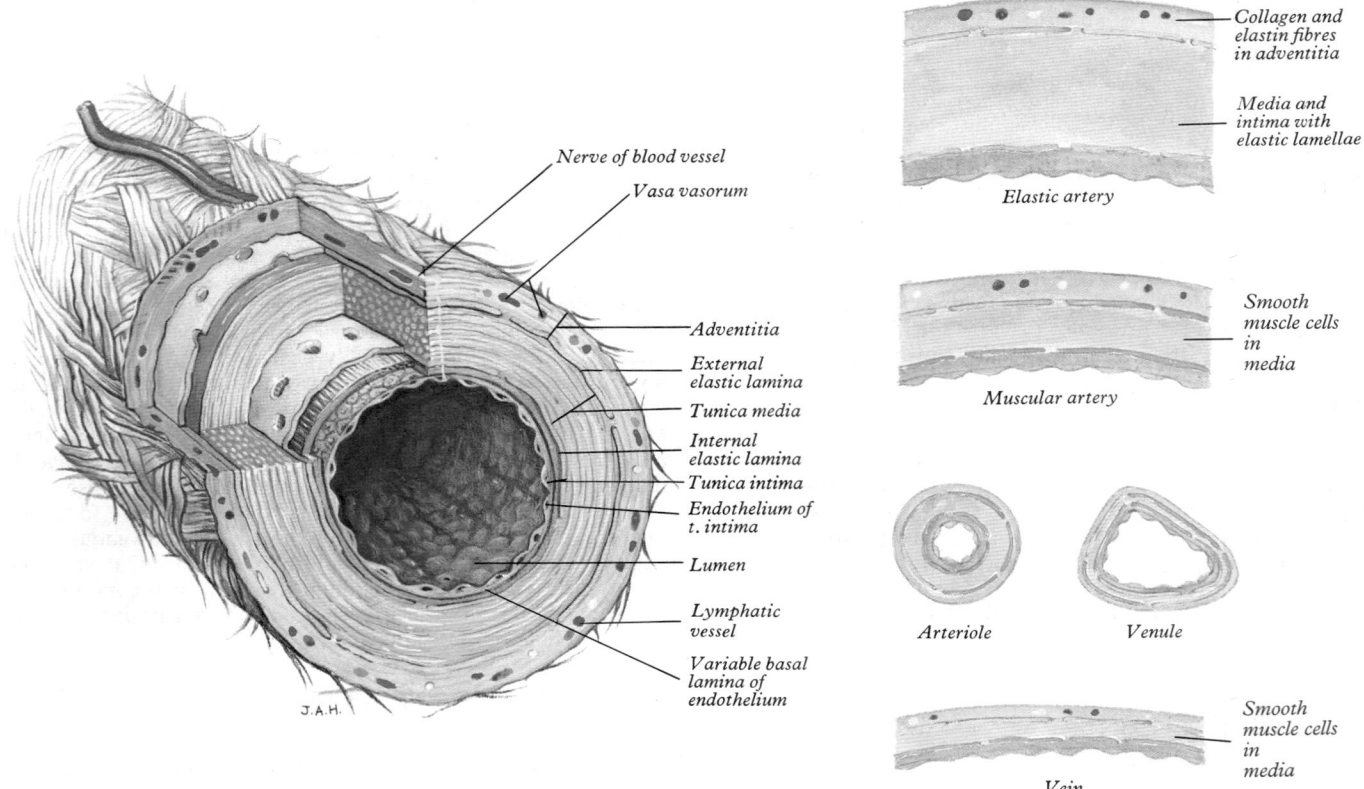

Nerve of blood vessel

Vasa vasorum

Adventitia

External elastic lamina

Tunica media

Internal elastic lamina

Tunica intima

Endothelium of t. intima

Lumen

Lymphatic vessel

Variable basal lamina of endothelium

J.A.H.

Collagen and elastin fibres in adventitia

Media and intima with elastic lamellae

Elastic artery

Smooth muscle cells in media

Muscular artery

Arteriole   Venule

Smooth muscle cells in media

Vein

10.2   Schematic drawing showing the principal structural features of the larger blood vessels. On the left the major layers and associated features of a muscular artery are depicted. On the right the particular features of an elastic artery, a muscular artery, an arteriole, a venule and a vein are shown, as they appear in transverse sections of these vessels.

Because of the large relative volume of veins, this part of the vascular bed contains the largest amount of blood.

BLOOD CIRCULATION

The cardiovascular or circulatory system provides a continuous circulation of the blood, in a system which is virtually closed. The heart itself is a large, muscular, valved vessel, and has four chambers: right atrium, left atrium, right ventricle and left ventricle. (These somewhat misleading names are discussed on p. 1474.) Each atrium leads into a corresponding ventricle, the right and left chambers being separated by septa. The right and left sides of the heart are thus twin pumps, topographically combined in a single organ but interposed in series in the vascular system, which through their connections they separate into a systemic and a pulmonary circulation (constituting the so-called double circulation typical of birds and mammals, see p. 1472). The course of blood from left ventricle through the body at large to the right atrium forms the systemic circulation, its passage from the right ventricle via the lungs to the left atrium being the pulmonary circulation. The relatively short pulmonary system offers much less peripheral resistance than the systemic circulation, as is reflected in the lower pressures in the pulmonary distribution vessels and in the thinner walls of the right ventricle (p. 1480). The average output volume of blood from the right and left sides of the heart must, of course, be the same. The superior and inferior venae cavae return to the right atrium blood which has become deoxygenated, has taken up carbon dioxide and been otherwise modified during circulation through the tissues of the body. This blood then enters the right ventricle, which expels it via the pulmonary trunk to the lungs. In the pulmonary capillaries blood is brought into close proximity to the inspired air, releasing some carbon dioxide and acquiring oxygen. This oxygenated blood, returned by the pulmonary veins to the left atrium, enters the left ventricle, which pumps it into the aorta for general distribution.

Blood traversing the spleen, pancreas, stomach and intestines is not carried back directly to the heart but passes through the portal vein to the liver. This vein divides like an artery, ending in the hepatic sinusoids intimately associated with the laminae of hepatocytes; the sinusoids are drained by the hepatic veins to the inferior vena cava, whence blood is conveyed to the right atrium. This route is the *portal circulation*; its essential feature is that the blood supplied to abdominal viscera, such as the spleen, pancreas, stomach and intestine traverses not one but **two** sets of capillaries before returning to the heart. One set of capillaries originates from the coeliac and mesenteric vascular bed and provides oxygenated blood to the above-mentioned organs. These are drained into the portal vein, which gives rise to the second set of capillaries, the hepatic sinusoids. The sinusoids carry through the liver unoxygenated blood rich in absorption products from the intestine. The conspicuous musculature of the hepatic portal vein helps to propel the blood through the second microvascular bed. Passage through these two sets of capillaries enables the blood to transfer the products of digestion directly from the alimentary canal to the cells of the liver. Another venous portal circulation connects the median eminence and infundibulum of the hypothalamus with the pars distalis of the adenohypophysis (p. 1884) (Akmayev 1971). A venous portal system is present in the kidney of non-mammalian vertebrates. In essence, a venous portal system is a capillary network that lies between two veins, instead of between an artery and a vein, as in standard circulation. In other situations a capillary network is interposed between two arteries, notably in the renal glomeruli (see p. 1826).

Another circulation in the body is provided by the system of lymphatic vessels and lymph nodes, which conduct the lymph from the interstitial spaces between cells to the large veins of the thorax. Other, more restricted, circulations are those of the cerebrospinal fluid (CSF), perilymph, various endocochlear fluids, ocular aqueous humour, synovial fluid and the fluids of the coelomic spaces, namely the pericardial, pleural and peritoneal cavities.

Dynamic aspects of circulation

Propulsive force is generated not only by the heart, but also by the musculature of arteries and veins, and by the compression of vessels, especially veins, exerted by contracting skeletal muscles and by taut fasciae and ligaments. Other factors influencing the mechanical behaviour of the system are the elasticity of arteries, the viscosity of blood, and the friction between blood and the surface of vessels. The last factor is the origin of laminar flow (or its disruption, as in turbulent flow).

There is a marked influence of gravity on the cardiovascular system, expressed as *hydrostatic pressure*, which, of course, is influenced by the position of the body, whether upright or lying down for example. (In contrast, gravity has very limited effect on the physiology of viscera.) The *hydraulic pressure* is that generated to overcome the resistance offered by the arteries and by the viscosity of blood.

Blood pressure and blood-flow velocity are not steady or constant but pulsatile. Approximately one-quarter of the blood resides in the lesser circulation and the rest in the greater circulation. Three-quarters of the total volume of blood is in veins, especially in small veins of less than 1 mm diameter.

The total cross-section of the vascular network varies with the distance from the heart. It is minimal in the aorta, and it is maximal (and about 4000 × larger) at the level of the venules. The blood pressure, generated to a greater extent by the cardiac musculature and to a lesser extent by vascular musculature, falls progressively but not linearly along the arterial tree. Major falls of pressure occur immediately beyond the arterioles, where the smooth musculature ends, and at the entry into the venules, because of the sudden expansion of the vessel size.

Tissue tethering: an isolated vein can fully collapse and expel the blood it contains, whereas a vessel in situ, especially a vein, a microvessel or a lymphatic, may never collapse completely even when compressed in vivo because of the restraints imposed by tissue tethering.

METHODS OF STUDY OF VESSEL STRUCTURE

The course of large and medium-sized blood vessels can be studied by dissection; injection of coloured tracers may help to identify the vessels. (It is salutary to remember how many centuries it took to work out the essence of the vascular system, even when the necessary means of observation were fully available.) Measurements of vessel size cannot normally be carried out on the cadaver. They can be carried out in vivo or in vessels fixed in situ by lumenal perfusion of the fixative at physiological pressure.

Vascular casts are prepared by injecting under pressure a fluid, coloured resin into the vascular bed of an organ, letting the resin polymerize and digesting away with acid all the tissue. The cast reproduces all the vascular spaces in the injected organ, and, in the case of the microcirculation, can be studied in a scanning electron microscope. The lumenal surface of the endothelium can be studied by scanning electron microscopy after covering it with an ultra-thin layer of metal (**10.**7A, 8A), while freeze-fracture preparations reveal the internal structure of the cell membrane (**10.**7B). To view intrinsic features of the vessel wall by scanning microscopy requires micro-dissection and chemical digestion of collagen and elastic materials, for example with collagenase or strong alkali (**10.**8B).

Histological sections are the method of choice to study the structure of vessel walls: transverse sections are orthogonal to the vessel's long axis, longitudinal sections are parallel to this axis and ideally should pass through the middle of the vessel. Since great structural distortion is produced by the collapse of the vessel, fixation under controlled conditions of distension or pressure is paramount for structural analysis.

HISTOLOGY OF THE VESSEL WALL

In cross-section a blood vessel has a circular profile and, with few exceptions, a wall of uniform thickness. Small but appreciable differences in wall thickness are found in very curved vessels such as the aorta arch: on the inner curve, where the wall stress is greater,

the wall is thicker than on the outer curve. The diameter of the vessel and thickness of the wall are greatly affected by contraction of the wall; great caution must be exerted in evaluating these parameters in histological sections, especially in postmortem material. On the other hand, these two structural parameters are essential to establish the mechanical properties of any vessel. For the structural analysis of blood vessels, irrespective of size, and with the exception of capillaries and venules, three concentric parts or layers (or tunicae) are recognized in the vessel wall (**10.**2):

- the intima (strictly speaking the tunica intima), or innermost layer, whose main component, the endothelium, lines the entire vascular tree.
- the media (tunica media), made of muscle tissue, elastic fibres and collagen; while it is by far the thickest layer in arteries, the media is absent in capillaries and is comparatively thin in veins.
- the adventitia (tunica adventitia), the outer wrapping of the vessel, made of connective tissue nerves and capillaries. The adventitia links the vessels to the surrounding tissues.

The main histological components of the vessel wall are therefore an endothelium, elastic tissue, muscle tissue, collagen and connective tissue (**10.**3). With the exception of the endothelium, the general features of the various tissues have already been described in sections 2 and 9.

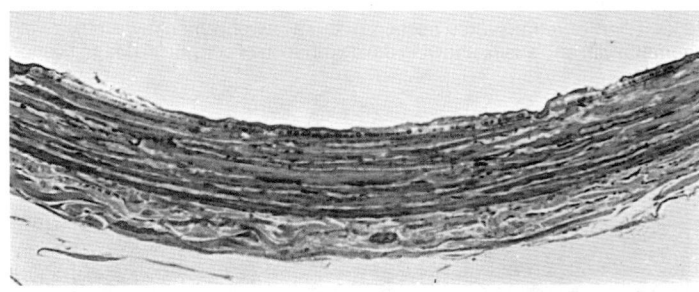

A

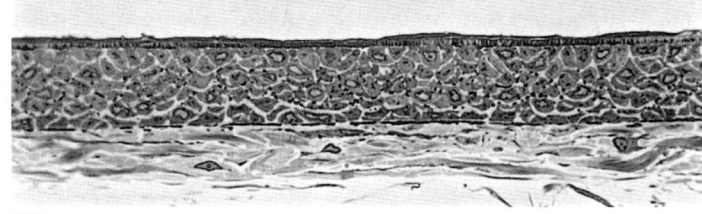

B

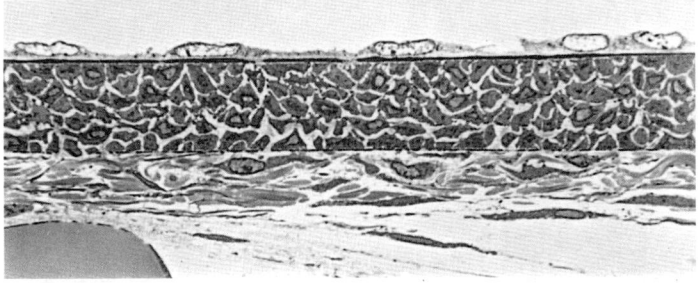

C

10.3 Histological sections of a muscular artery, fixed in situ in a condition of physiological distension. A. The artery is sectioned transversely, and the muscle cells of the media are cut longitudinally. Magnification × 510. B. The artery is sectioned longitudinally, and the muscle cells are cut transversely. Magnification × 510. C. At higher magnification, the endothelial cells can be seen, somewhat elongated in the direction of the blood flow; the dark line beneath the endothelium is the inner elastic lamina, which shows fenestration, and is straight in this preparation because it was fixed while distended. The tunica media is made of five or six arrays of muscle cells, which are transversely sectioned. The tunica adventitia displays collagen fibres and fibroblasts. Magnification × 510.

ENDOTHELIUM

The endothelium is a monolayer of flattened polygonal cells which extend continuously over the luminal surface of the entire vascular tree (**10**.4, 5, 6, 11). Its structure includes specific features in different

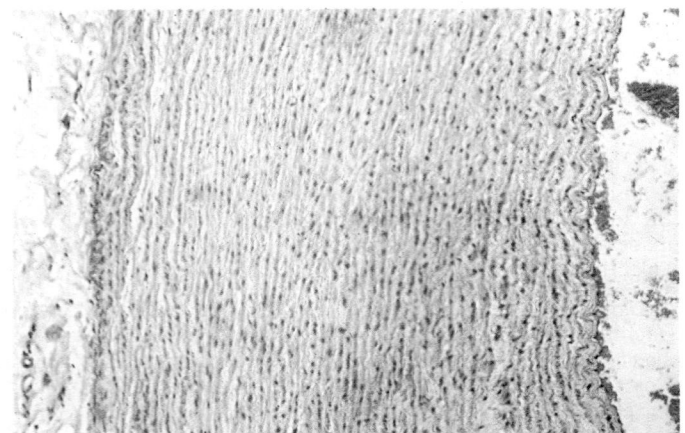

10.4A   Part of a transverse section of the aorta of a monkey, stained with haematoxylin and eosin, showing the distribution of cell nuclei. Magnification × 100.

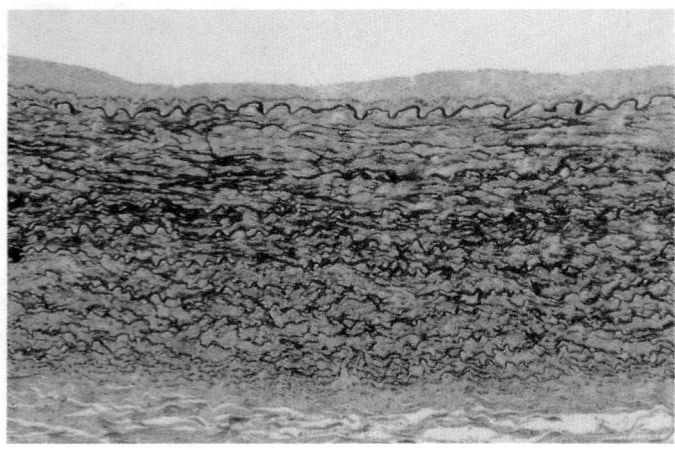

10.4B   Part of a transverse section of a young human aorta stained with Verhoeff's stain for elastin. Note the density of the concentric fenestrated elastic lamellae. Magnification × 100.

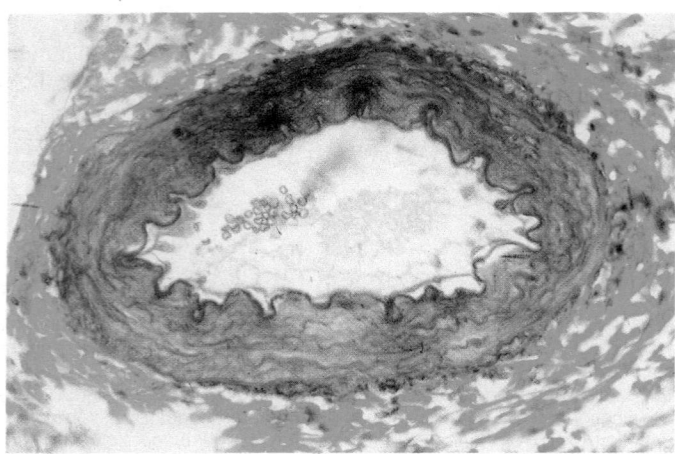

10.4C   Transverse section of a small muscular artery, stained with Verhoeff's stain for elastin and van Gieson stain for collagen. Note the prominent inner elastic lamina, which is heavily folded because the vessel was fixed postmortem when collapsed and virtually empty. Magnification × 200.

regions of the vascular bed. The endothelium is a key component of the vessel wall because it serves several major physiological roles, as listed below.

- Because of their position, endothelial cells influence blood flow.
- They regulate the diffusion of substances and of cells, out of and into the circulating blood, across cell junctions and through their cytoplasm.
- They participate in the process of coagulation (see p. 1400), by secreting clotting factors, and in the process of fibrinolysis.
- They have selective phagocytic activity and extract substances from the blood, and have other metabolic activities; for example, the endothelium of the pulmonary vessels removes and inactivates several polypeptides, biogenic amines, bradykinin, prostaglandins and lipids from the circulating blood. Endothelium Derived Relaxing Factor (Ryan & Ryan 1984).
- Endothelial cells secrete substances (endothelium derived relaxing factor or nitric oxide, and endothelins) which affect vasomotility, and probably also substances which promote the growth of the endothelium itself, such as Basic Fibroblastic Growth Factor (b-FGF) (Schweigerer et al 1987).
- They are sensitive to the transmural stretch imposed by the pulse, via stretch-sensitive ionic channels in the cell membrane, thus endowing the vessel wall with a sensor or a sensory element.
- They can synthesize (and at least they do so in in vitro cultures) fibronectin, laminin, collagen, elastin and other components of the subendothelium (Ryan & Ryan 1984).
- They are capable of proliferating to provide new cells during the period of increasing size of a blood vessel, to replace damaged or exfoliated endothelial cells, and also to provide growing solid cords of cells which are the forerunners of new blood vessels (see angiogenesis, p. 470).

Endothelial cells are wide and thin, tile-like and slightly curved to fit the curvature of the vessel. They are somewhat elongated in the direction of blood flow, especially in arteries (**10**.11). Endothelial cells firmly adhere to each other at their edges, so that the lining of the lumen presents no discontinuity (except in sinusoids, see p. 1466; **10**.4.) The thickness of endothelial cells is maximal at the level of their nucleus, where it can reach 2–3 μm, this part of the cell often bulging slightly into the lumen (**10**.3c). Elsewhere, the endothelial cell is thinner and laminar; in capillaries, these portions of the cell are very attenuated, often measuring as little as 0.2 μm in thickness (**10**.12).

The *luminal surface* of the endothelium is relatively smooth. However, it is common to find endothelial laminar projections into the lumen, especially near the cell junctions. The cell surface is pitted by the numerous caveolae (**10**.7B) and the membrane is coated by a prominent glycocalyx (Luft 1966; Ryan & Ryan 1984). The glycocalyx is a highly-charged, polysaccharide-rich felt of glycoproteins,

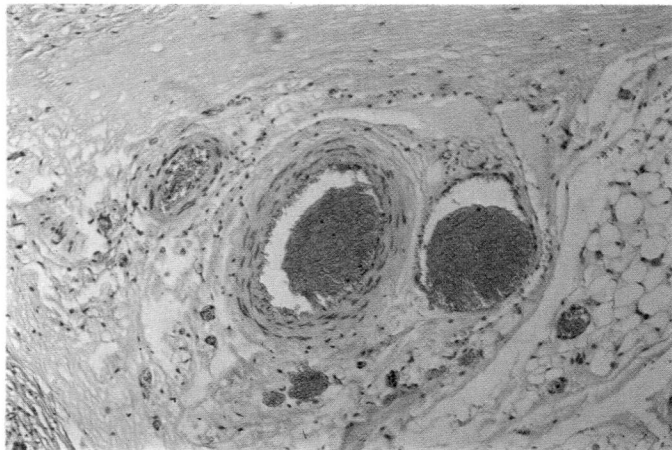

10.5   Transverse section of two small muscular arteries and a small vein, stained with haematoxylin and eosin. Numerous venules and capillaries are included but are indistinct at this magnification. (Supplied by D R Turner of the Department of Pathology, Guy's Hospital Medical School.)

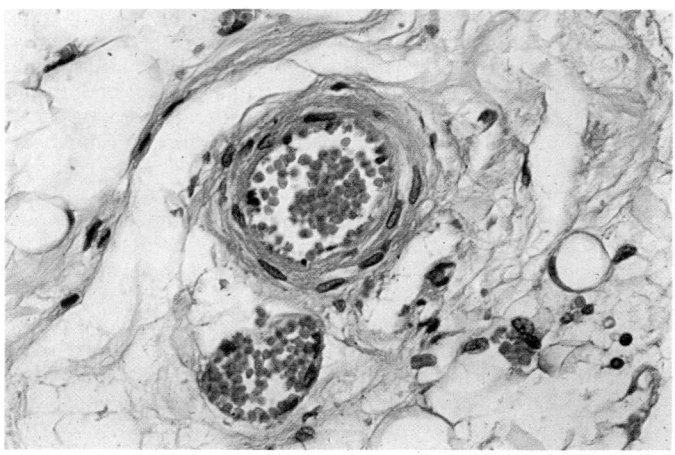

10.6   Transverse section of a large arteriole and venule in loose connective tissue, stained with haematoxylin and eosin. (Source as **10**.5.)

anchored to the cell membrane, which controls the transport of solutes and may mediate the mechanical effects of blood flow on the endothelial cells. Because of the high charge density the glycocalyx may contribute to the non-thrombogenic properties of the surface of the intact endothelium. The glycocalyx is not seen in standard electron micrographs of the endothelium, but can be visualized with electron-dense substances, such as ruthenium red, which bind specifically to glycoproteins. The abluminal surface is also pitted by caveolae and it rests over a basal lamina.

Caveolae are consistently observed in all endothelial cells. These invaginations of the cell membrane measure about 200 × 50 nm; their membrane is in continuity with the cell membrane proper and their cavity opens into the extracellular space through a narrow neck (**10**.7B, 12B). Their spatial density is of the order of several tens per square micron of cell surface; because of their large number, more than half of the plasma membrane at the cell surface is in the form of caveolae. Caveolae are regarded by several authors as manifestations of a process of transcytosis: the membrane is pinched in from **one surface** of the endothelial cell, and forms a caveola (which includes a tiny amount of extracellular fluid) that eventually detaches itself and becomes a free-moving spherical vesicle in the cytoplasm; the vesicle then merges with the membrane on the **other**

surface of the cell, again forming a caveola (and again releasing its tiny amount of fluid into the extracellular space). In this interpretation, a 'shuttle' system, caveola–vesicle–caveola, transports material across the endothelial cell, in both directions. It is a 'bulk' transport because it is relatively non-selective and it involves a sizeable amount of extracellular fluid. There have been strong doubts about this form of transendothelial transport, mainly because of its lack of selectivity. Studies of serial sections of endothelial cells of capillaries have shown that even those structures which appear as free-floating vesicles in a single section are actually connected with the extracellular space; true vesicles seem to be exceedingly rare and the caveolae are constantly open to the extracellular space (Frokjaer-Jensen 1984). In other cell types, such as smooth muscle cells, caveolae are known to be stable structures, not involved in endocytosis (unlike coated pits and coated vesicles).

Cytoplasmic organelles of endothelial cells include mitochondria, granular and agranular endoplasmic reticulum, some free ribosomes and occasionally a pair of centrioles. In spite of the evidence of chemical factors being released by endothelial cells, cytological signs of secretion are not prominent. Bundles of microfilaments and intermediate filaments are also found. The former are made of actin and the latter are usually vimentin filaments. Filaments contribute to maintaining a certain shape of the cell and impart mechanical stability, and presumably they play an important role when the cell changes shape or migrates. Characteristic organelles of endothelial cells are the *Weibel-Palade bodies*, which are cytoplasmic vesicles, elongated, 0.2 × 2–3 μm, containing regularly spaced tubular structures parallel to the long axis which give rise to a striation. These organelles produce and store a large glycoprotein known as von Willebrand protein (or factor VIII), which mediates the binding of platelets to the extracellular matrix of the subendothelium after vascular injury. Von Willebrand protein is also produced, in larger amounts, by megakaryocytes and is stored in platelets.

Seen from the lumen, endothelial cells usually have a polygonal contour. At their edge they adhere to adjacent cells through an area of apposition where junctions of the adherens, communicans and occludens types are found (the so-called junctional complex). The area of apposition can be a straight line covering the shortest distance between luminal and abluminal aspects of the endothelium. More commonly, there is an oblique or a tortuous line of apposition, sometimes with overlap or interdigitation between endothelial cells. Often a laminar process from the edge of an endothelial cell projects into the lumen and seems to guard the area of apposition of the endothelial cells. The role of these projections, however, is unknown. A tight junction forms a belt (zonula occludens) around the contour

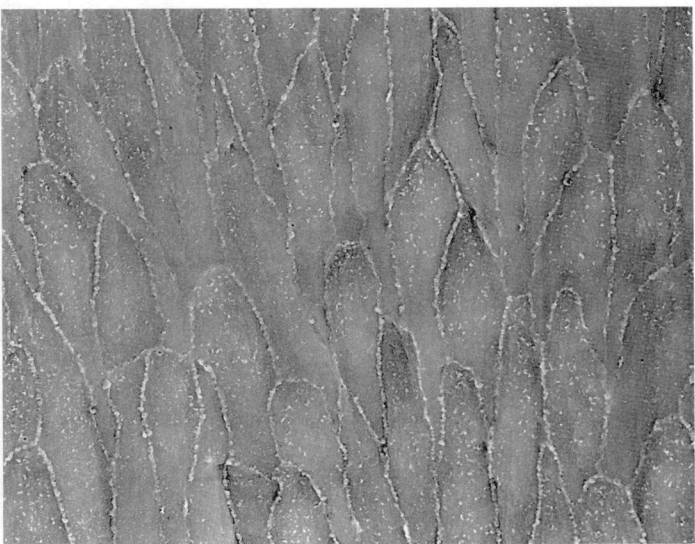

10.7A   Inner surface of the endothelium of a basilar artery, examined by scanning electron microscopy. The lumenal surface is tessellated by endothelial cells which are tightly packed and elongated in the direction of the blood flow. Magnification × 1250. (Supplied by Masoud Alian of University College London.)

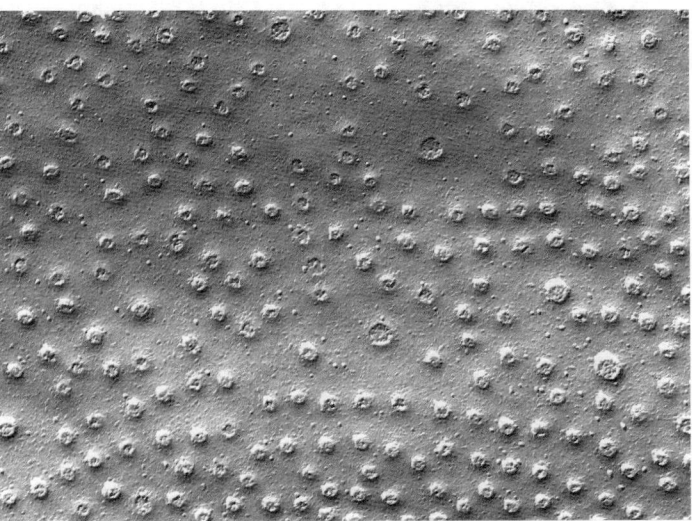

10.7B   Freeze-fracture preparation of the plasma membrane of an endothelial cell. The E-face of the membrane shows innumerable caveolae fractured at the level of their neck. Magnification × 40 000.

of an endothelial cell, involving all the cells that are directly adjacent. These tight junctions are best visualized by freeze-fracture, and they vary in extent in different vascular regions. They provide a seal which blocks or restricts movement of fluids through the intercellular gaps of the endothelium; they also limit the lateral diffusion of membrane proteins and lipid between the luminal and the abluminal domains of the cell membrane. Gap junctions and, occasionally, intermediate junctions accompany the tight junctions between endothelial cells (Hüttner et al 1973); they invariably reside further away from the lumen than the tight junctions. The gap junctions are likely to allow the bi-directional and non-selective diffusion of ions and small molecules between endothelial cells. Cell contacts between endothelial cells and muscle cells are common in arterioles, where the separation between endothelium and media is reduced and the inner elastic lamina is very thin or absent.

Endothelial cells can synthesize and secrete collagen; thus they are regarded as contributing to the formation of the inner elastic lamina.

SMOOTH MUSCLE

This is invariably of the smooth type (see p. 738), with the exception of small segments of the pulmonary veins (p. 738) which, in the portion nearest to the heart, have striated musculature of the cardiac type. Smooth muscle cells are the only cell type found in the media of most arteries of mammals (**10**.7A, 11). One function of smooth muscle in blood vessels is to reduce, with their contraction, the vessel's lumen and hence the flow through it, an action which has the effect of raising the pressure on the proximal side. This role is particularly effective in small resistance vessels where the thickness of the wall is great relative to the diameter of the vessel. Another function of smooth muscle is to alter the stiffness of the wall, causing no constriction (isometric contraction) but affecting the distensibility of the wall and the propagation of pulse. The mechanics of the musculature of the media is complex for several reasons: because the structures involved have a concentric arrangement; because the tissue is incompressible and therefore of constant volume; because the spatial arrangement of muscle cells and fibrous extracellular materials is variable and not well understood; because materials of different mechanical properties and different spatial arrangement are tightly linked together. Properties of distensibility, strength, self-support, elasticity, rigidity, concentric constriction, are interrelated and finely balanced in the various regions of the vascular bed.

Muscle cells are responsible for the active motility of the vessel wall. These cells also synthesize and secrete elastin, collagen, muco-polysaccharides and other extracellular components which bear directly on the mechanical properties of the vessel. The muscle cells of the arterial media have been rightly labelled multifunctional mesenchymal cells (Wissler 1968). After damage to the endothelium, muscle cells migrate into the intima and proliferate, forming bundles of longitudinally oriented muscle cells (neo-intima; Fishman et al 1975). In pathological conditions, muscle cells with their fatty degeneration participate in the formation of atheromatous plaques.

The vascular musculature is made of single, uninucleated muscle cells (vascular muscle cells) which have many common structural features with visceral muscle cells, but are also somewhat different (**10**.4A, 8, 11). The basic structural features of smooth muscles are described elsewhere (p. 771). In large arteries, where the blood pressure is high and the stress of the wall is high, the muscle cells are shorter (60–200 µm) and smaller in volume than in visceral muscles. The cell profile is very irregular and the cell membrane has many conspicuous dense bands where the contractile apparatus and the extracellular fibrous components are linked to each other. In arterioles and veins, smooth muscle cells resemble more closely visceral muscle cells.

The cells are packed with myofilaments and with elements of the cytoskeleton, including intermediate filaments. The latter, which are invariably of the desmin type in visceral smooth muscles, are made of vimentin or of vimentin and desmin in vascular muscle cells.

Cell-to-cell junctions are mainly of the adherens type and provide mechanical coupling between the cells (**10**.11). There is also a small number of gap junctions. Far more numerous than cell-to-cell junctions, especially in arteries, are the junctions between muscle cell and connective tissue matrix (*cell-to-stroma junctions*). Between adjacent muscle cells there are also interdigitations and extensive areas of apposition without apparent membrane specializations; they involve fusion or disappearance of the basal laminae and are likely to provide some adhesion between the two cells.

The orientation of muscle cells within the media has been the object of several investigations, and there is no conclusive account of this anatomical feature. In most arteries the orientation of the cells is approximately circumferential; over a wide range of vessel sizes the deviation from circumferential is minimal (Canham & Mullin 1978; Walmsley 1983), except for the occasional presence of a bundle of musculature of unexpected orientation within the media. In large vessels the musculature is divided into layers or into bundles and there are some variations even between adjacent lamellae. The circumferential arrangement appears more irregular when the vessel contracts and may be grossly disrupted in collapsed arteries. A helical orientation (as in a cylindrical spring) of muscle cells has

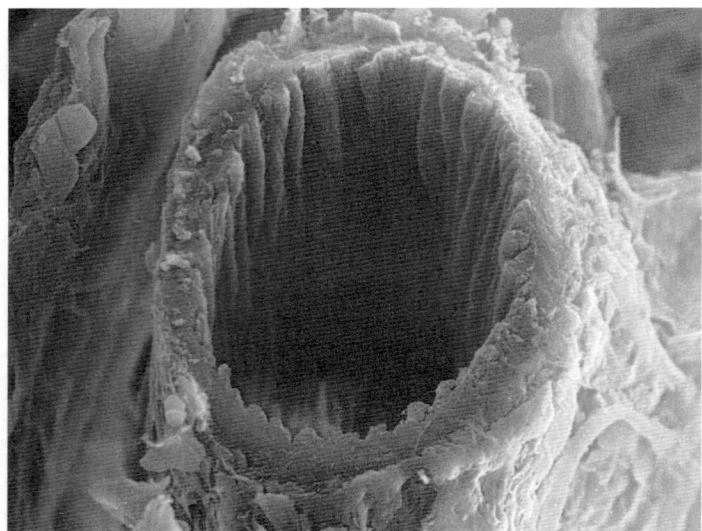

10.8A A small vessel approaching the surface of the brain, examined by scanning electron microscopy. The free surface of the endothelium is corrugated by the relief of the endothelial cells. Magnification × 750. (Source as **10**.7A.)

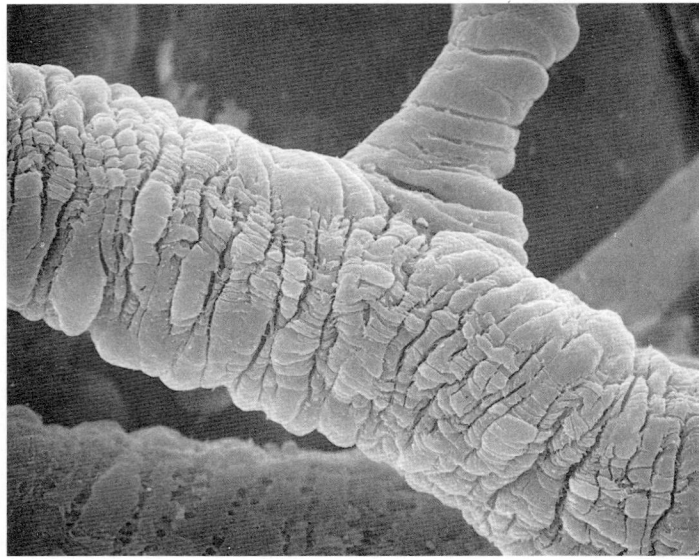

10.8B Arteriole isolated from the mesentery, freed of its adventitia by enzymatic digestion and examined by scanning electron microscopy. The muscle cells are contracted and are wound circumferentially in the vessel wall. Magnification × 1000. (Micrograph supplied by Professor Komuro, School of Human Sciences, Waseda University, Japan.)

been described in the lamellae of some large arteries. In the rat aorta, for example, where right- and left-handed helices may be present in successive lamellae (Rhodin 1962) has reported that the pitch increases during postnatal growth. In large elastic arteries, muscle cells often connect the elastic lamellae on either side, hence they have also a slightly spiral orientation (as in a two-dimensional spring, such as a watch spring). The spatial orientation of medial muscle cells is regarded as one of the anatomical factors affecting the mechanical properties of the vessel wall. It is possible, however, that the exact orientation of the muscle cells is not the most significant factor in this respect. Because of the cohesion of the media, the dense packing of cells and stroma, the vast number of cell-to-cell junctions and cell-to-stroma junctions and the lateral dislocation of volume when the cell shortens, a highly geometrical arrangement of the contracting cells is not a major requirement for an adequate functional performance.

In physiological conditions the intima of some large arteries contains a few smooth muscle cells, longitudinally arranged. In large arterioles some bundles of longitudinally oriented musculature are found near the adventitia. While in small arteries and arterioles the arrangement of the musculature becomes more regular and invariably circumferential (**10.**8B, 11), in veins the arrangement of the musculature is more variable (see p. 1466).

Even when they run circumferentially, muscle cells in the media of large arteries are only slightly curved, and many cell lengths are needed to make up the circumference of the vessel. In contrast, in arterioles the muscle cells are tightly coiled (see p. 1463).

COLLAGEN AND ELASTIC MATERIAL

A major constituent of the vessel wall are the extracellular materials, collectively known as the *stroma* or *matrix*. In large arteries and veins this constitutes more than half of the mass of the wall, and is mainly made of collagen and elastin (**10.**11). Other fibrous components, such as fibronectin microfibrils, and abundant amorphous or soluble materials are present in the extracellular spaces of the vessel wall.

Elastic material is found in all arteries and veins and it is especially abundant in elastic arteries (**10.**11A). Individual *elastic fibres* (0.1–$1.0\,\mu m$ in diameter) anastomose with each other forming net-like structures, which spread predominantly in a circumferential direction (**10.**8B). A more extensive degree of fusion produces lamellae of elastic material, which are usually perforated but separate layers of muscle cells, thus allowing the formation of lamellar 'units' (see p. 1463). A conspicuous elastic lamella occurs in arteries, between intima and media, the *inner elastic lamina*. This lamella is a tube of elastic material which allows the vessel to recoil after distension. When the intraluminar pressure falls below physiological limits, the inner elastic lamina is compressed sideways and it coils up into a regular corrugated shape (**10.**4C): in these conditions the lumen is much reduced but is not obliterated, and the profile of the artery remains circular. Fenestrations in the elastic lamina allow materials to diffuse between intima and media. An *outer elastic lamina*, similar in appearance but markedly less well developed than the inner elastic lamina, is situated at the outer aspect of the media at the boundary with the adventitia. Elastic fibres are less abundant in the adventitia.

Collagen fibrils (transversely banded cables of 30–50 nm diameter, see p. 81) are found in all three tunicae (**10.**11), and especially around the muscle cells of the media. Collagen is abundant in the adventitia where it forms large bundles of fibrils (*collagen fibres*) which increase in size from its innermost component near the media to its outermost component.

In general terms, collagen and elastic fibres in the media run parallel or at a small angle to those of the muscle cells, and therefore they are mainly circumferentially arranged. In contrast, the predominant arrangement of collagen fibres in the adventitia is longitudinal, and this imposes constraints on the elongation of large vessels under pressure. In large arteries, for example, the radial distension under the effect of the pulse far exceeds the longitudinal distension (Burton 1954). While the outer 'sheath' of collagen, i.e. that of the adventitia, limits the distensibility of the vessel, the collagen network of the media mainly provides attachment to the muscle cells and transmits force around the circumference of the vessel. While collagen fibres are inextensible, elastic fibres are very highly extensible. They provide ample attachment to the muscle cells, favouring a uniform spread of the muscle tension around the vessel wall; in a distended vessel, the elastic fibres store energy and, by recoiling, help to restore the resting length and calibre.

The extracellular material of the tunica media, including collagen and elastic fibres, is produced by the muscle cells during development. Its turnover is slow compared to that in other tissues, and this too is controlled by the muscle cells of the media. In the adventitia, collagen is synthesized and secreted by fibroblasts, as in other connective tissues. During development in postnatal life, while vessels increase in diameter and wall thickness, there is an increase in elastin and collagen content. Subsequent changes in vessel structure include an increase in the collagen-to-elastin ratio, with a reduction in vessel elasticity.

PERICYTES

In capillaries, where a proper adventitia is absent and where there are no muscle cells, other cells, the pericytes, are present at the outer surface of the vessel (**10.**12A). Pericytes, or cells of Rouget, are known under various other names and probably do not represent a uniform population of cells. They are elongated, have a bulging cell body and long laminar processes spread around the capillary endothelium. They do not form a continuous layer but their shape suggests a tight grip of the capillary and a mechanical supporting role. They (or some of them) may have a phagocytic role. It is possible that some pericytes are a source of new endothelial cells, to replace any which may become damaged in the endothelium, or of mesenchymal cells or of muscle cells. Their number and morphology are very variable. Because they contain some bundles of filaments, and they contain, as shown by immunohistochemistry, actin, myosin, tropomyosin and desmin (Uehara et al 1990), the pericytes are regarded by some authors as contractile cells (Rhodin 1962): the suggestion that they are a primitive type of muscle cell (Zimmermann 1923) is, however, purely speculative. Most pericytes have areas of close apposition with endothelial cells, occasionally forming adherens junctions (Forbes et al 1977). These are the only areas where a basal lamina does not coat the surface of the pericyte.

Leucocyte–endothelial cell interactions

INTRODUCTION

A remarkable feature of the immune system is the integration of functionally different organs and tissues by constant migration of lymphoid cells from one site to another along blood and lymphatic vessels. The migration of lymphocytes and the interactions of activated cells during immune responses are regulated by cell-surface molecules. Adhesive interactions between cells, and between cells and the extracellular matrix, are vital to all developmental processes and have a crucial role in a well-functioning immune system throughout life (Springer 1990).

Mature 'virgin' lymphocytes from the bone marrow and thymus, the sites of primary lymphoid organs, enter the blood circulation and reach secondary lymphoid organs such as lymph nodes, spleen, tonsils, Peyer's patches and appendix, as well as dispersed lymphoid tissues. The latter can be associated with skin ('skin associated lymphoid tissue' or SALT), or the mucosal surfaces of the gastrointestinal tract ('gut associated lymphoid tissue' or GALT), the respiratory tract ('bronchus associated lymphoid tissue' or BALT) and the urogenital tract (a part of the 'mucosa associated lymphoid tissue' or MALT). The secondary lymphoid organs and tissues guard the portals of entry for antigens and provide a favourable environment for the interactions of antigens with lymphocytes (Brandtzaeg 1984). Finally, using the efferent lymphatic drainage, both virgin and memory lymphocytes re-enter the venous limb of blood circulation via the lymphatic trunks and the thoracic duct and recirculate. This arrangement maximizes the probability of effective antigen–lymphocyte interaction throughout the body.

VASCULAR ENDOTHELIUM

The lumen of all blood vessels is lined by endothelial cells which maintain the fluidity of the blood, regulate the interactions of circulating cells and platelets with the vessel walls and form the interface between the bloodstream and extravascular tissues. Although the endothelium consists of a monolayer of cells it has, under normal conditions, two different surfaces that exhibit morphological as well as biochemical polarity: the luminal, non-thrombogenic surface, and the abluminal, adhesive surface (de Groot 1987). The abluminal surface faces the deeper layers of the vessel wall and is adhesive for platelets. In contrast, the luminal surface of endothelial cells can be considered blood cell-like, a haemocompatible interface. It represents a natural barrier capable of regulating the circulating levels of several vasoactive and platelet-active mediators and it does not support the adherence of leucocytes or platelets (Brown 1994). However, perturbation of endothelial cells induces the production of platelet-activation factor (PAF), which is a potent stimulus for platelet aggregation.

Many functions of human vascular endothelial cells are dynamic rather than fixed. For example, on endothelial injury, with the exposing of the subendothelial matrix, the nearby uninjured endothelial cells migrate across the denuded surface and can re-endothelialize a small defect within hours (Jarrell et al 1987).

LYMPHOCYTE CIRCULATION AND MIGRATION INTO LYMPHOID AND NON-LYMPHOID ORGANS

Under normal conditions there is a continuous flow of lymphocyte through secondary lymphoid organs. These organs are structurally analogous in that they all possess: first, a complex framework which provides ideal conditions for interactions between lymphocytes and antigen-presenting cells; second, separate domains which are more or less specific for T or B

cells; and third, specialized segments of vasculature supporting the extravasation of circulating lymphocytes, known as the postcapillary or high endothelial venules (HEVs) (**10.9**A).

The bulk of the lymphocyte traffic is thought to pass through HEVs located in the parafollicular areas of lymph nodes, palatine and nasopharyngeal tonsils, Peyer's patches, appendix and the mucosal lymphoid tissue aggregates of MALT. There are no HEVs in the spleen, yet more lymphocytes migrate through this organ than through all lymph nodes (Pabst & Binns 1989). Although it has been proposed that the marginal sinus lining cells may be responsible for the initial arrest of blood lymphocytes in the splenic marginal zones, little is known about the mechanism of lymphocyte traffic through the spleen (Stevens & Lowe 1992; Picker & Butcher 1992).

The HEVs are also absent from primary lymphoid organs (bone marrow and thymus) and, normally, they are not present in non-lymphoid organs and tissues in spite of a continuous lymphocytic migration through them, in the course of general surveillance. Here, migration may occur through capillaries, sinusoids and possibly low endothelial venules. Pabst and Binns (1989) studied the migration route of lymphocyte subsets in pigs and sheep using suspensions of in vitro fluorescein isothiocyanate (FITC) labelled peripheral blood lymphocytes. Within the first few minutes 40% of lymphocytes were found in the lungs and 14–21% in the liver. Thus, similar to spleen, the lungs and the liver are not only sites for capturing effete cells but these non-lymphoid organs actively participate in recirculation of lymphocytes.

Interestingly, HEV-like vessels have been found at many sites of chronic inflammation where they are believed to support the extravasation of large numbers of leucocytes. Neutrophils, lymphocytes and monocytes migrate into inflamed tissue sites with class-specific kinetics: the relatively nonspecific neutrophils appear within minutes of stimulation while the antigen-specific T and B cells and monocytes arrive within hours but may remain for days (Osborn 1990). One of the best-documented examples of this phenomenon is the rheumatoid synovium (Freemont et al 1983; Koch et al 1991).

Some lymphocytes move from one secondary lymphoid organ to another via the blood and lymphatic vessels while others stay resident in these organs for a variable period of time. For example, antigen-specific lymphocytes are preferentially retained in those lymph nodes which drain the source of the antigen (Picker & Butcher 1992). Moreover, there is evidence for carefully regulated, non-random migration of lymphocytes to particular anatomical sites, referred to as 'homing' (Rosen

1989; Springer 1990; Picker & Butcher 1992). Thus, lymphocytes which home to the gut are thought to be transported selectively across gut specific microvasculature, while other populations of lymphocytes home in a similar manner to different target organs, such as the tonsils or peripheral lymph nodes. This tissue specificity for lymphocyte homing is thought to be relative rather than absolute and may be determined by a combination of multiple factors rather than by a single specific factor (Shimizu et al 1992).

It has been now generally accepted that circulating lymphocytes are leaving the HEVs to home into the lymphoid compartments of secondary lymphoid organs and tissues, although in the past some researchers held the opposite view. In 1929 Ehrich proposed that in a lymph node 'small lymphocytes were immigrating into the vein lined with endothelium consisting of very high and crowded cells'. The physiological significance and the direction of transendothelial migration of lymphocytes had not been appreciated until the original autoradiographic experiments of Gowans and Knight (1964).

HIGH ENDOTHELIAL VENULES

High endothelial venules are found in most mammalian species and recognized by the conspicuous plump endothelial lining associated with numerous luminal mural and extramural lymphocytes (**10.9**A). These vessels are located within the T cell domains, between and around lymphoid follicles in all secondary lymphoid organs and tissues, with the exception of the spleen. In the human palatine tonsil HEVs were also seen in the lower parts of reticulated crypt epithelium (Perry et al 1992). On account of their position and diameter of 7–30 μm, HEVs are also referred to as post-capillary venules. They begin at a junction of flat-walled venous capillary limbs, receive venules draining the surrounding lymphoid follicles and end as tributaries to larger veins (Ohtani et al 1989).

The luminal aspect of HEVs presents a so-called 'cobblestones' appearance covered with a prominent glycocalyx (Anderson & Anderson, 1975). The single layer of high endothelial cells (HECs) rests on endothelial basement membrane which is intimately related to pericytes. The pericytes, in turn, are surrounded by their basement membrane and a small amount of connective tissue (**10.9**B). The HECs are linked by discontinuous macular junctions at their apical and basal aspects, which may be circumnavigated by migrating lymphocytes (Anderson & Anderson 1976).

Ultrastructurally, HECs have the characteristics of metabolically active secretory cells. They contain large, rounded euchromatic nuclei with one or two nucleoli, prominent Golgi regions,

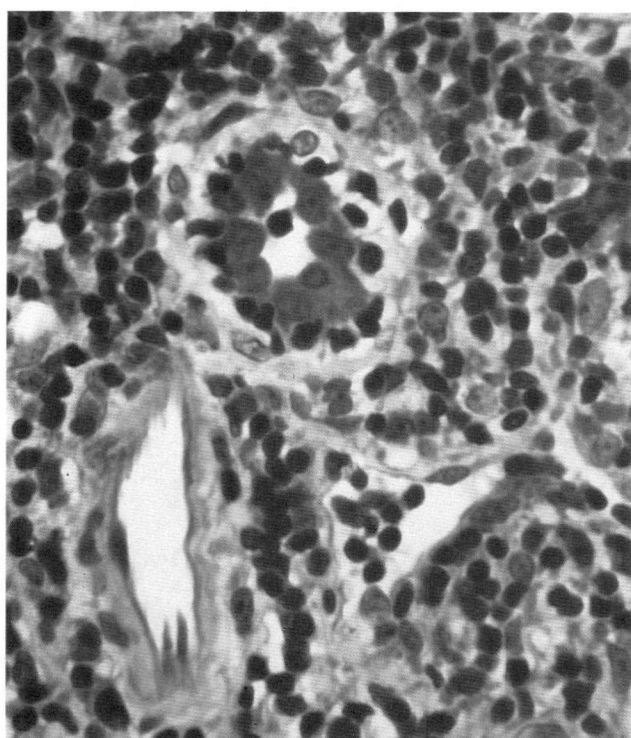

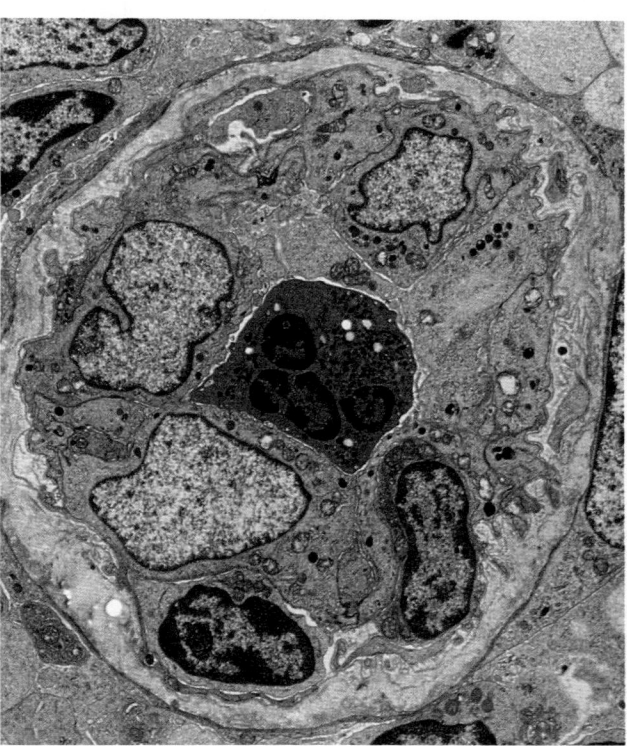

10.9A The height of the endothelium of transversely sectioned high endothelial venule (*HEV; upper field*), lined with columnar cells and associated with numerous dark blue stained lymphocytes, contrasts with the neighbouring low endothelial venule (*left lower field*) and lymphatic vessel (*right lower field*). Human palatine tonsil. Methylene blue/Azur II.

10.9B Transverse section of HEV in human palatine tonsil. The vessel lumen is occupied by a neutrophil completely surrounded by high endothelial cells. The electronlucent nuclei of three of these cells are present in the plane of this section. Pericyte (*right*) with its attenuated processes lies externally to the undulating endothelial basal lamina and a small amount of connective tissue. Note the position of the two mural (*right lower field*) and the extramural (*left upper field*) lymphocytes. TEM. Magnification × 3 000.

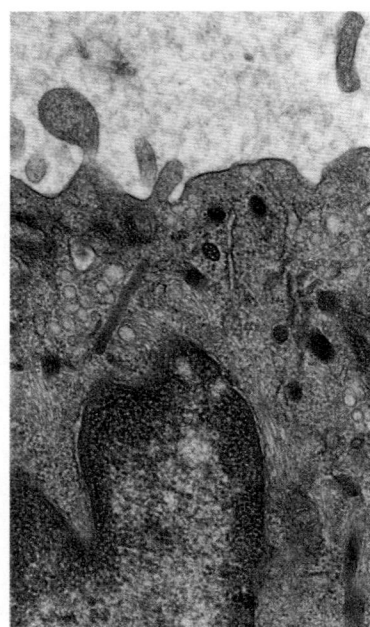

10.9C High endothelial cell in rheumatoid synovium containing many sectioned profiles of the microtubular Weibel-Palade bodies above and around the nucleus. TEM. Magnification × 20 000.

many mitochondria, ribosomes and pinocytotic vesicles. Typically, they also possess the microtubular Weibel-Palade bodies in which Factor VIII and P-selectin are stored (**10.9C**). Stimulation of the endothelium by thrombin, histamin or reactive oxygen species results in rapid translocation and redistribution of P-selectin to the endothelial surface (Hogg 1992; Cronstein & Weissmann 1993). The 10–12 μm high cuboidal or columnar cells protrude into the lumen and the rate of collision between circulating blood cells and vessel wall is increased. Subsequently collision attachment and migration of leucocytes can follow.

MOLECULAR BASIS OF HOMING LEUCOCYTES

Cell adhesion molecules (CAMs) is a collective term for cell surface glycoproteins regulating the adhesion between cells. Endothelial adhesion molecules facilitate the attachment of free circulating leucocytes to the vessel walls. A rapid transition between adherent and non-adherent states of leucocytes is essential for the maintenance of their dual function of immune surveillance and responsiveness. However, fundamental changes occur on endothelium in the vicinity of an inflammatory response when inflammatory mediators such as lipopolysaccharide, interleukin-1 (IL-1), tumour necrosis factor alfa (TNF-*a*) or gamma interferon (*γ*-IFN) increase the adhesion but reduce the selectivity of extravasating leucocytes (Shimizu et al 1992).

Many of the adhesion molecules that mediate interactions between blood leucocytes and HEVs or cytokine-activated endothelium have been identified. These molecules can be divided into three general categories: the selectin family, the integrin family and the immunoglobulin supergene family. The selectin and integrin molecules are expressed on leucocytes and mediate adhesion of circulating cells to the endothelium, whereas selectins and members of the immunoglobulin supergene family are expressed on the endothelium and provide the 'sticky' substrate to which leucocytes can adhere (Springer 1990; Cronstein & Weissmann 1993).

Selectins

Three molecules have been identified so

far as members of the selectin family of adhesive proteins. They are the L-selectin (also known as lymphocyte homing receptor, CD62L, Leu-8, Mel-14, LAM-1), E-selectin (CD62E, ELAM-1) and P-selectin (CD62P, GMP-140, PADGEM). Selectins have a characteristic amino-terminal lectin domain, an epidermal growth factor-like domain and a variable number of complement regulatory domains. The selectin molecules bind to specific sialyated carbohydrates, including sialyl Lewis X, which is a unique feature among adhesive proteins (Polley et al 1991).

The L-selectin is expressed on most leucocytes and its endothelial ligand has been termed recently GlyCAM-1 (Imai et al 1993). Importantly, L-selectin mediates homing of lymphocytes to peripheral lymph nodes as well as accumulation of neutrophils and monocytes at sites of inflammation.

The E-selectin is a molecule which is only transiently expressed on endothelium. It is an inducible adhesion molecule which was first described as mediating adhesion of neutrophils to inflammatory cytokine activated endothelium (Bevilacqua et al 1989).

The P-selectin is rapidly mobilized to the endothelial surface by fusion from storage in Weibel-Palade bodies following stimulation of the endothelium. Since P-selectin is quickly endocytosed by the endothelial cells its expression is only short lived. P-selectin binds to ligands expressed on neutrophils, platelets, and monocytes and, similar to E-selectin, it tethers leucocytes to endothelium at sites of inflammation (Zimmerman et al 1992).

Integrins

The integrins are a large family of molecules mediating cell-to-cell adhesion as well as interactions of cells with intercellular substances. They are therefore essential in regulating spatial orientation and cell movement. Integrins represent a group of related heterodimeric adhesion proteins and each molecule comprises an α- and a β-subunit ($\beta 1$, $\beta 2$ and $\beta 3$).

The $\beta 1$ integrins are a subfamily of six molecules known as 'very late antigens' (VLAs) which function mainly as receptors for components of extracellular matrix. The VLA-1 and VLA-2 adhesion molecules were found to be expressed on lymphocytes only 2 to 4 weeks after antigenic stimulation in vitro and they bind to the extracellular matrix (Keelan & Haskard 1992). On the other hand the VLA-4 integrin ($\alpha 4\beta 1$, CD49d/CD29), which is present on resting lymphocytes, monocytes and eosinophils, binds also to its ligand on activated endothelium, the vascular cell adhesion molecule 1 (VCAM-1 CD106).

In contrast to $\beta 1$ integrins the expression of $\beta 2$ integrins is limited to white blood cells. Although the leucocyte integrins are

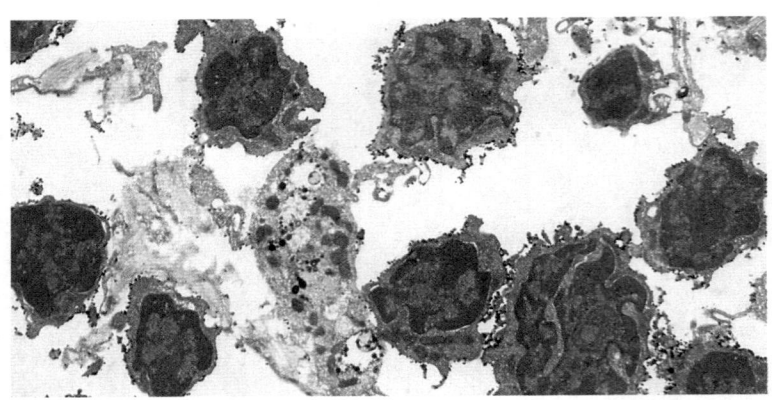

10.9D Lymphocytes in the interfollicular region of human palatine tonsil expressing LFA-1 (black dots) on their cellular membranes. Immunoelectron microscopy. Incubation with mAb to LFA-1. Magnification × 4 000.

not constitutively adhesive they become highly adhesive after cell activation and therefore play a key role in the events required for cell migration. The $\beta 2$ subfamily comprises three molecules with common $\beta 2$ subunit (CD18) and with chains of different molecular weight (CD11a, b, c) (Cronstein & Weissman 1993).

The CD11a/CD18 integrin molecule is known as the lymphocyte function-associated antigen 1 (LFA-1) and is present on the surface of all leucocytes (**10.9D**). The endothelial ligands for LFA-1 are the intercellular adhesion molecules 1 and 2 (ICAM-1 and ICAM-2) which belong to the immunoglobulin superfamily. The other two integrins of the $\beta 2$ subfamily are CD11b/CD18 (Mac-1, CR3) and the less well-characterized CD11c/CD18. These molecules have more limited distribution on neutrophils, monocytes and

natural killer cells and they mediate adhesion of leucocytes to endothelium by binding to ICAM-1. Recently, monoclonal antibodies directed against integrin-mediated adhesion have been administered in studies aimed to decrease inflammatory responses (Jasin et al 1992).

Immunoglobulin supergene family

Three members of this large family of proteins are involved in leucocyte-endothelial adhesion. They are the integrin counter-receptors ICAM-1 (CD54), ICAM-2 and VCAM-1, found on the endothelial cell membrane.

The ICAM-1 has five immunoglobulin-like domains and the ICAM-2 has only two. Both the ICAM-1 and ICAM-2 are constitutively expressed on endothelium and ICAM-1 is also present on activated B cells and follicular dendritic cells in germinal centres (Springer 1990). The

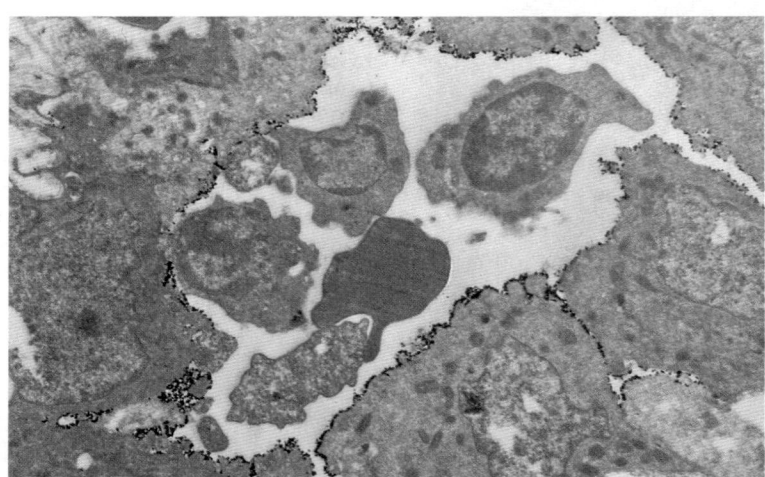

10.9E Transversely sectioned tonsillar HEV stained strongly with anti-ICAM-1 antibody on luminal and lateral (black dots), but not on the abluminal, surfaces of high endothelial cells. Immunoelectron microscopy. Incubation with mAb to ICAM-1. Magnification × 5 000.

known ligands for ICAM-1 are LFA-1 and Mac-1 integrins, whereas the ICAM-2 binds only to LFA-1. Furthermore, the expression of ICAM-1 is readily upregulated by inflammatory cytokines (**10**.9E) resulting in an increased binding of circulating lymphocytes and monocytes to the stimulated endothelium.

The last member of the immunoglobulin superfamily is the VCAM-1 molecule containing either six or seven immunoglobulin-like domains. Its ligand on the leucocytes is the VLA-4 integrin (Cronstein & Weissmann 1993). Although VCAM-1 is absent from resting endothelium its expression can be induced by cytokines. Thus, VCAM-1 is thought to promote an accumulation of mononuclear cells at sites of inflammation (Shimizu et al 1992; Picker & Butcher 1992).

In addition, the widely expressed cell surface molecule CD44 has been identified as a homing receptor of haematopoietic cells. The CD44 molecule is a highly glycosylated protein and the major receptor for hyaluronic acid. It has been proposed by Günther et al (1991), that CD44 isoforms may play an important role in organ specific recognition, cell motility and invasion mechanisms.

In summary, the process of adhesion of leucocytes to endothelium is believed to involve multiple receptor–counterreceptor (ligand) interactions. This 'adhesion cascade' requires a co-ordinated sequence of adhesion molecules expression on both the leucocytes and the endothelium, from the time of the initial attachment to the final step of extravasation into the surrounding tissue (Shimizu et al 1992; Tanaka et al 1993).

The first step in this cascade is the loose binding, 'rolling' or 'tethering' of leucocytes, which is initiated via P- or E-selectin. Coexpression of tethering and 'signalling' molecules on activated endothelial cells, such as P-selectin and PAF and E-selectin and IL-8, augments this initial interaction (Zimmerman et al 1992). The second step is referred to as 'triggering', in which a signal delivered to leucocytes converts the functionally inactive integrin molecules into active adhesive configurations. The third step represents the establishment of strong adhesion mediated by integrins expressed on leucocytes, binding to their endothelial ligands. The fourth and last step is the migration of leucocytes into the surrounding tissue. This step requires reduction in adhesion and 'shedding' of some molecules from the surface of leucocytes, followed by cell movement. The precise mechanisms involved in this process are as yet unknown (Hogg 1992; Shimizu et al 1992; Tanaka et al 1993).

An understanding of molecules that mediate cellular interactions in homing of recirculating lymphocytes and during the initial stages of inflammation may eventually lead to the development of a new generation of anti-inflammatory agents.

STRUCTURE OF BLOOD VESSELS

Sharp distinctions of blood vessels based on the structure of the wall are to some extent arbitrary, because the variations along the vascular tree are continuous. Nevertheless a few basic patterns can be identified, and are described here as different vessel types.

LARGE ELASTIC ARTERIES (**10**.4A, B, 11A)

The intima is made of an endothelium, resting on a basal lamina, and a subendothelial layer. The endothelial cells are flat, measuring between 1.0 and 0.2 μm in thickness, polygonal in outline and elongated with the long axis parallel to the direction of blood flow. The subendothelial layer is well developed, contains elastic fibres and collagen fibrils and small cells identified as muscle cells or muscle cell precursors and fibroblasts. The orientation of subendothelial cells is irregular but predominantly longitudinal.

In the human aorta at birth, the endothelium adheres to the internal elastic lamina. After birth the intima grows in thickness with the appearance of a subendothelial layer (subendothelial intima), composed of delicate elastic fibres and smooth muscle cells running longitudinally, intermingled with abundant ground substance, a small amount of collagen and occasional fibroblasts. Splitting of the inner elastic lamina is not uncommon. The thickening of the intima progresses with age and is more marked in distal than in the proximal segment of the aorta. The cells of the subendothelial layer are thought to migrate from the media across the inner elastic lamina.

Between the intima and the media lies a prominent inner elastic lamina. This lamina is smooth, measures about 1 μm in thickness, and is stretched under the effect of the pulse, recoiling elastically afterwards; it coils up into a serpentine outline when the vessel is completely emptied, a condition that does not normally occur in vivo. Even when empty a large elastic artery does not completely collapse.

The media has a markedly layered structure, being made of layers of elastic material (elastic lamellae) alternating with interlamellar zones made of muscle cells, collagen and elastic fibres. The arrangement is very regular and each elastic lamella with an adjacent interlamellar zone is regarded as a 'lamellar unit' of the media. In the human aorta there are approximately 52 lamellar units, measuring about 11 μm in thickness. A similar arrangement exists in all mammals, and the number of lamellar units is roughly proportional to the vessel diameter in different species and vessels (Wolinsky & Glagov 1967b). Number and thickness of lamellar units increases during development. At birth the aorta has about 40 lamellar units. However, the developmental increase in vessel diameter far exceeds the increase in number of lamellae and in the thickness of the wall.

In the media of the largest arteries such as the aorta some authors distinguish an internal layer of musculature, situated externally to the inner elastic lamina, with muscle cells of various orientations intermingled with elastic fibres running longitudinally.

The adventitia is well developed. In addition to collagen and elastic fibres, it contains fibroblasts (which are flattened and have extremely long and thin laminar processes), macrophages and mast cells. The vasa vasorum are usually confined to the adventitia, where there are also nerve bundles, which do not come close to muscle cells, and lymphatic vessels.

MUSCULAR ARTERIES

These include vessels of a large range of sizes, and they are characterized by the predominance of muscle in the media. The intima is made of an endothelium resting on a basal lamina (**10**.5, 11B). The inner elastic lamina is thin, and is occasionally absent. In the media about $\frac{3}{4}$ of the mass is represented by muscle cells. Therefore, the relative amount of extracellular space is less than in large arteries, but elastic fibres, running parallel to or at a very small angle with the muscle cells, remain prominent.

ARTERIOLES (**10**.10)

The endothelial cells are smaller than in large arteries; their nucleated portion is thicker and often projects markedly into the lumen. Even when fixed fully distended, the endothelium of arterioles has variable thickness and displays longitudinal grooves and ridges. The nuclei are elongated and oriented parallel to the vessel length and so is the long axis of the cell.

The abluminal surface of the endothelium is lined by a basal lamina, but an inner elastic lamina is absent or barely recognizable. When present, the elastic lamina is amply fenestrated and is traversed by cytoplasmic processes of muscle cells or of endothelial cells.

The muscle cells are larger in volume than those of large arteries and they form a layer one cell thick. They are arranged circumferentially and are tightly curved and wound around the endo-

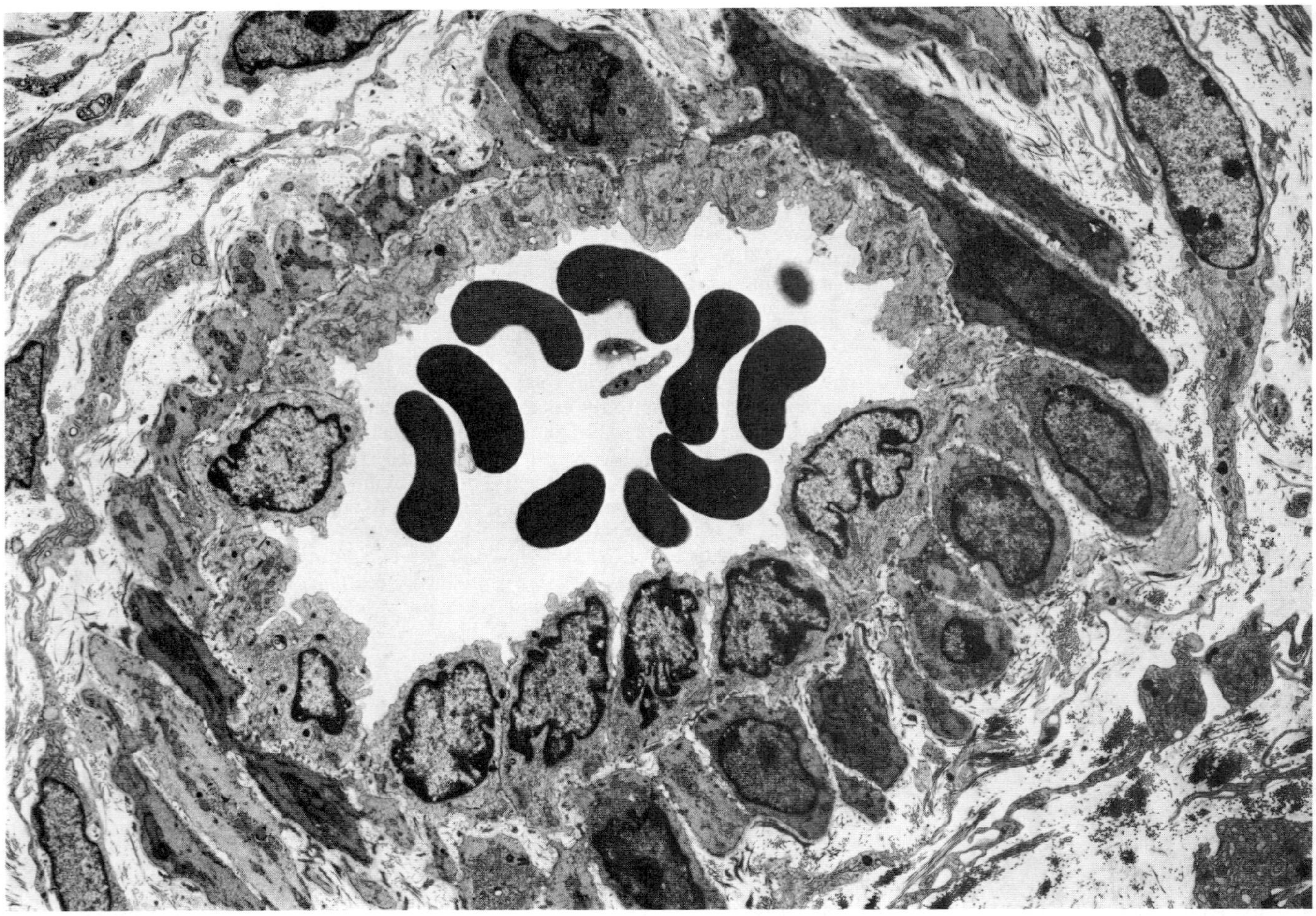

10.10   Transmission electron micrograph of a partially contracted small arteriole in transverse section, showing an outer zone of non-striated myocytes and an inner lining of endothelial cells. Erythrocytes are visible within the lumen. The specimen is from the uterus of a rat. Magnification × 4000. (Supplied by Dr Gail ter Haar.)

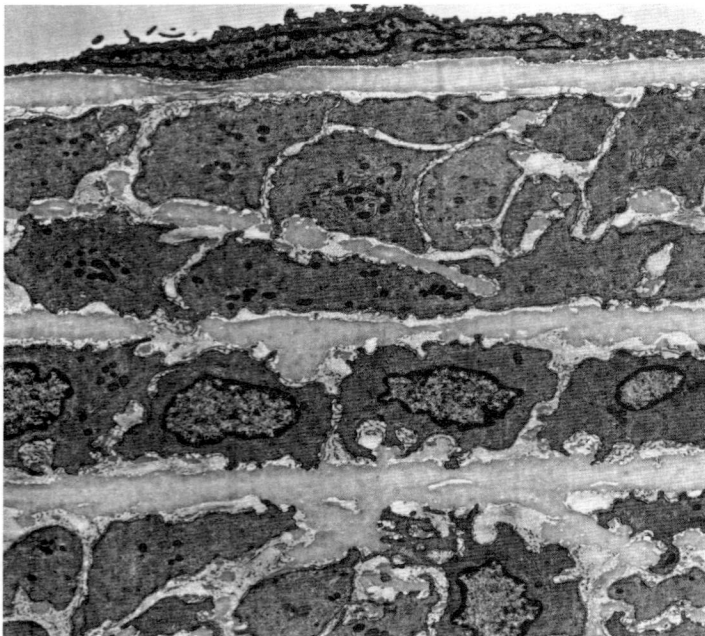

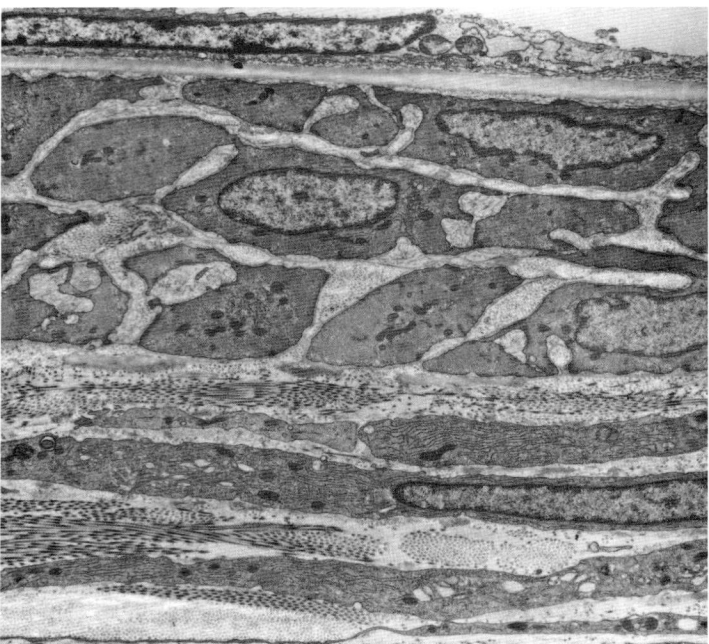

10.11A   Elastic artery sectioned longitudinally and examined by electron microscopy. Beneath the endothelium (*at top*) with the nucleated profile of a flat endothelial cell, is a thick inner elastic lamina. In the media (not shown in its full thickness) are several muscle cells profiles in transverse section, some nucleated, separated by large elastic fibres and elastic lamellae. Note the irregular, convoluted shape of the muscle cell surface. Magnification × 4500.

10.11B   Muscular artery sectioned longitudinally and examined by electron microscopy. Beneath the endothelium (*at top*) with the nucleated profile of a flat endothelial cell, is an inner elastic lamina. In the media are several muscle cells profiles in transverse section; they are closer to each other than in the elastic artery, and the intervening spaces are occupied by collagen fibrils. In the bottom part of the micrograph is the tunica adventitia with fibroblasts and collagen fibrils. Magnification × 4500.

thelium (**10**.8). In the smallest arterioles each cell makes several turns, producing extensive apposition between parts of the same cell. The muscle cell profiles are asymmetric in that the region of the cell membrane nearest the adventitia bears most of the dense bands, hence most of the insertions of myofilaments.

The *precapillary arteriole* (strictly speaking, however, all arterioles are pre-capillary), or *precapillary sphincter*, has been variously defined in the literature. The most acceptable definition is that the precapillary sphincter is that part of the arteriole where the most distal muscle cell is found, before the vessel opens into the capillary network (Wiedeman et al 1976). The functional interest in the precapillary sphincters is that they appear to be mainly under myogenic, rather than under nervous control. Because of their position they are regarded not so much as sites of regulation of peripheral resistance but rather as sites where the blood flow into the capillary network is monitored (Wiedeman et al 1976).

Arterioles are usually densely innervated by sympathetic fibres, via small nerve bundles containing axons expanded in varicosities and packed with axonal vesicles, mostly of the adrenergic type. The distance between axonal membrane and muscle cell membrane can be reduced to 50–100 nm and the gap is occupied by a single basal lamina. Ultrastructural studies with serial sections have shown that these contacts between adrenergic axons and muscle cells (autonomic neuromuscular junctions) are very common in arterioles (Luff et al 1987).

CAPILLARIES (**10**.12, 13)

The wall of capillaries is made of an endothelium and its basal lamina, plus a few isolated pericytes (see p. 1459). The capillaries are the vessels closest to the tissue they supply and their wall is in intimate relation with the tissue. Their structure varies in different locations. They measure 5–8 μm in diameter (and much more in the case of sinusoids) and are hundreds of microns long. Their lumen is just large enough to let blood cells through, one at a time and with considerable deformation of their shape. It has been pointed out, however, that the vascular lumen is not at its narrowest in capillaries: the true bottleneck of the circulatory system is at the level of the arterioles (Cliff 1976), where muscle contraction can obliterate the lumen.

Commonly, a single endothelial cell forms the outline of a capillary and then the junctional complex (see p. 1457) occurs between laminar extensions of the same cell. In some capillaries, usually near their venous end, there are 'seamless' endothelial cells, i.e. the lumen is a large membrane-bounded canal through the cytoplasm (Bär et al 1984): in this case the lumen probably originated by fusion of several intracellular vacuoles (Wolff et al 1975).

The structural characteristics of endothelial cells are discussed on page 1456. In capillaries the endothelium is at its thinnest: 2–3 μm at the level of the nucleus, and down to as little as one-fifth of a micron in certain regions. The endothelial cells of some capillaries have *fenestrations*, or pores, through their thinnest portions. Fenestrations are approximately circular, 50–100 nm in diameter, and at their edge the luminal and the abluminal membranes of the endothelial cell come into contact with each other. The fenestration, or fenestra, itself is usually occupied by a thin electron-dense diaphragm resembling in appearance a thin basal lamina. The chemical composition of endothelial fenestrae is still unknown. Permeability studies

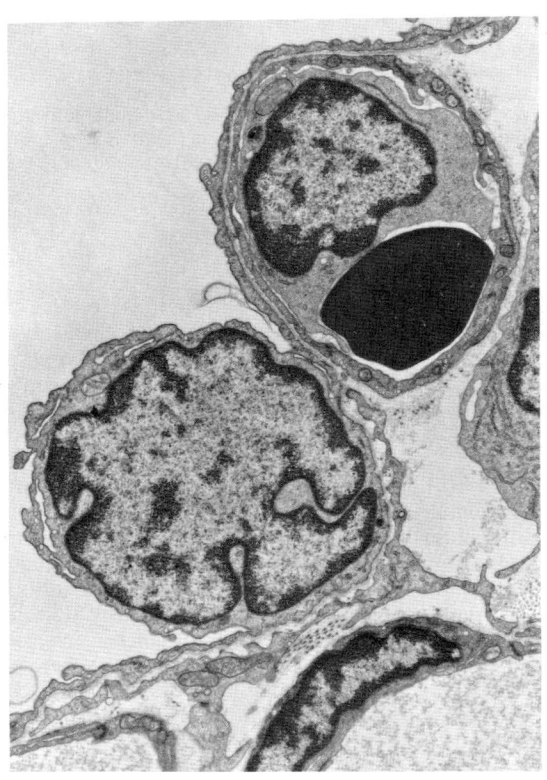

10.12A   To the right a blood capillary in the wall of a pulmonary alveolus. The lumen of the capillary is occupied by a red blood cell and a lymphocyte. Lower centre is a Type I pneumocyte with its nucleus and with slender cytoplasmic processes fully lining the lumen of the air-filled alveolus (*top left*). Two other capillaries are partially visible at the bottom; their lumen is occupied by plasma. Magnification × 8 000.

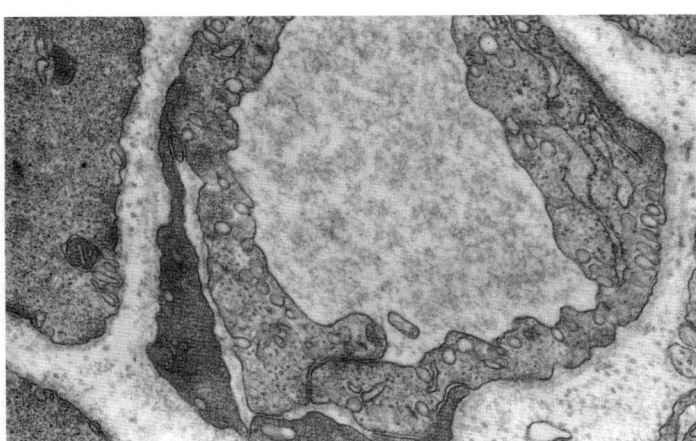

10.12B   Intramuscular blood capillary. The endothelial cell to the left shows the nucleus; at top and bottom are junctions with another endothelial cell. The lumen of the capillary is occupied by a red blood cell and plasma. On the outer surface is a basal lamina and (*at bottom*) a slim process of a pericyte. Magnification × 10 000.

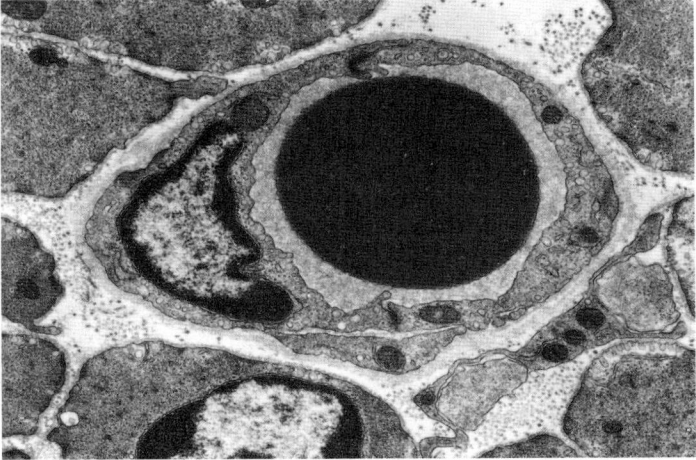

10.12C   Intramuscular blood capillary. Caveolae are visible on both the lumenal and the ablumenal surfaces of the endothelial cell, together with endoplasmic reticulum, microtubules and bundles of microfilaments. The edges of the cell are in contact with each other at the bottom, and they form specialized junctions. Magnification × 29 000.

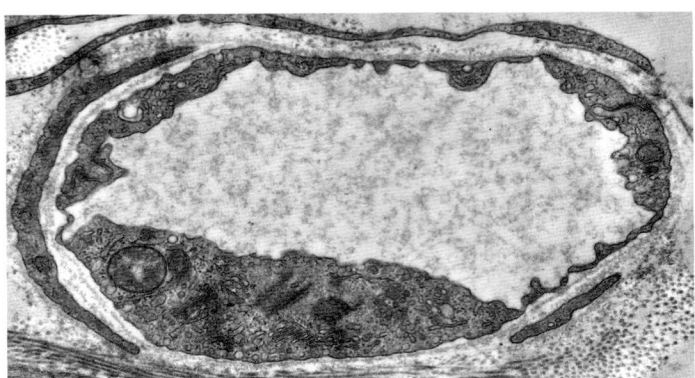

10.13A A fenestrated capillary, surrounded by a basal lamina, a laminar process of a pericyte (*left*) and collagen fibrils (*bottom*). The endothelial cell at top contains various organelles, including two centrioles, vesicles and Golgi complexes. Magnification × 18 000.

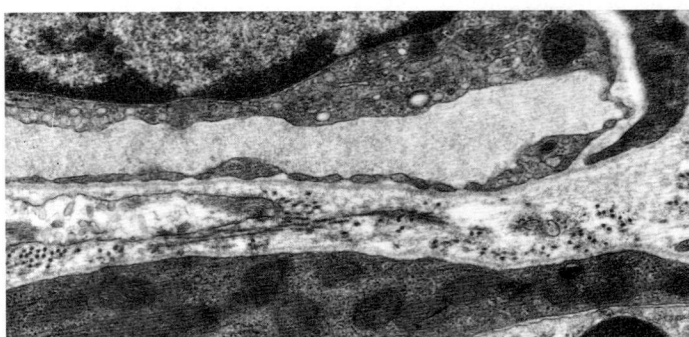

10.13B A fenestrated capillary in the intestinal mucosa. The fenestrations are close to the basal surface of the lining epithelium. Note the basal lamina on both the epithelial and the endothelial cell and the intervening collagen fibrils and fibroblastic process. Magnification × 30 000.

have shown that other components in addition to the diaphragm control the permeability of a fenestra (Levick & Smaje 1987). These capillaries are known as *fenestrated capillaries*, and they are found in renal glomeruli, in intestinal mucosa (**10.**13) and in endocrine and exocrine glands. Fenestrations are also almost invariably present in capillaries lying close to an epithelium, including skin (Imayama 1981).

Capillaries without fenestrations are known, somewhat inaccurately, as *continuous capillaries*. Capillaries in the brain, in striated and smooth muscles, in lung and in connective tissue are of this type. Capillary permeability varies greatly among tissues and can be correlated partly with the local type of endothelium. In tissues where large molecules pass easily (e.g. alimentary tract, endocrine glands) fenestrated endothelia exist, with numerous caveolae; intercellular junctions are either incomplete or 'leaky'. Where barriers to diffusion of large molecules occur (e.g. brain, thymic cortex and testis), endothelia are complete and not fenestrated, with efficient zonula junctions of the occludens type between cells; here, caveolae are somewhat fewer in number. Other tissues (e.g. skeletal muscle) show an intermediate condition.

Sinusoids. These are capillaries, large and irregular in shape, which have true discontinuities in their wall: blood can diffuse out of the circulation with only a minimal hindrance. A basal lamina may be found over these slits or holes in the endothelium, and other cell types may be found in the perisinusoidal space. Sinusoids occur in large numbers in the liver, spleen, bone marrow and adrenal medulla.

VENULES

Postcapillary venules are essentially tubes of flat, oval or polygonal endothelial cells supported by basal lamina and a delicate adventitia of collagen fibres mainly running longitudinally and fibroblasts (Rhodin 1968). They lack a distinct elastic lamina. Pericytes often accompany these venules. Postcapillary venules are sites of fluid exchange and leucocyte migration; in venules of lymphoid tissue of the gut and bronchi and in the lymph nodes and thymus, endothelial cells are taller and have intercellular junctions through which lymphocytes and other blood components can readily pass (see p. 1432). In other tissues these vessels are believed to be a major site of migration of neutrophils, macrophages and other leucocytes into extravascular spaces, and also a region of temporary endothelial attachment for neutrophils, forming marginated pools of these cells (see p. 1403).

The intracellular junctions of venules are sensitive to inflammatory agents which increase their permeability to fluids and defensive cells thus facilitating extravasation (see, e.g., Marchesi 1961, 1962). In general, the endothelium of venules has fewer tight junctions, and is more permeable. For example, in neurogenic inflammation venules are the primary site of extravasation of plasma.

When two or more capillaries converge the resulting vessel is larger (up to 30 μm), and is known as a *venule* (or a *postcapillary venule*). Venules do not acquire musculature until, after further convergence, they are about 30 μm in outer diameter, when they are known as *muscular venules* (**10.**14). The distinction is important because postcapillary venules are as permeable to solutes as capillaries, and are thus part of the microcirculatory bed. At the level of the postcapillary venule the cross-sectional area of the vascular tree is at its maximum, and there is a dramatic fall in pressure, from 25 mmHg in the capillary to about 5 mmHg (Rothe 1983). Muscular venules converge into *collecting venules* which lead to a series of veins of progressively larger diameter. Venules and veins are capacitance vessels (see p. 1453).

VEINS

Veins are characterized by a relatively thin wall in comparison with arteries of similar size and by a large capacitance. A small increase in lumenal pressure produces a large increase in volume, although the pressure–volume relation is not linear. The wall thickness is not exactly correlated to the size of the vein, but it varies in different districts: for example, the wall is thicker in veins of the leg than in veins of similar size in the arm (Kügelgen 1955).

The amount of muscle is considerably less than in arteries, while collagen and, in some veins, elastic fibres are the predominant components. In the cadaver the veins, even when collapsed, maintain their large diameter and they are more likely to be found full of blood than are the arteries. Furthermore, tethering of some veins to connective tissue fasciae and other surrounding tissues may prevent collapse of the vessel even with a negative transmural pressure.

Pressure within the venous system does not normally exceed 5 mmHg, it decreases centripetally as the veins grow larger and fewer in number, and it approaches zero in the proximity of the heart. Because of the small amount of musculature veins have limited influence on blood flow. However, during a sudden fall in blood pressure following a haemorrhage, elastic recoil and reflex constriction in veins compensate for the blood loss and tend to maintain venous return to the heart. Krogh (1959) stressed the importance of the active venous return by pointing to the fact that in man the heart is at a greater height above the feet than in any other mammal, except the elephant and the giraffe. Vasoconstriction in cutaneous veins in response to cooling is important in thermoregulation.

The structural plan of the wall is similar to that of other vessels, but the division into layers, especially media and adventitia, is often not clearly seen. The lumen is lined by an endothelium which lies over a basal lamina. A distinct inner elastic lamina is not found. The musculature is much thinner and has a more irregular distribution than in arteries. The orientation of muscle cells is not uniform and often variable and irregular. In most veins (for example those of the arm and leg) the musculature is arranged approximately circularly. Longitudinal musculature is present in the iliac vein,

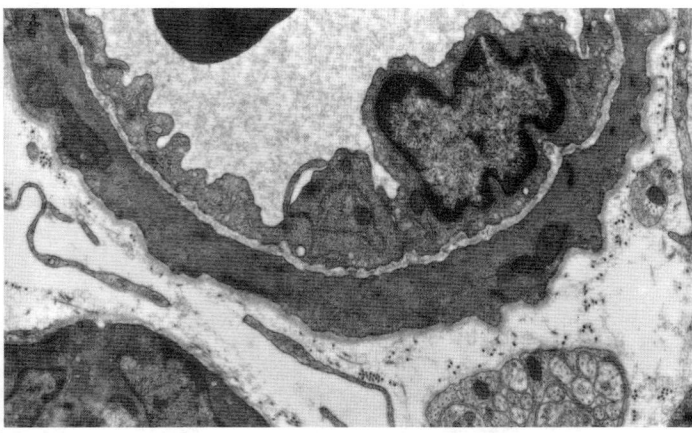

10.14 A venule transversely sectioned and examined by electron microscopy. One of the endothelial cell profiles is nucleated and the lumen contains an erythrocyte. The tunica media consists of a single layer of muscle cells running almost circumferentially. To the bottom right is a nerve bundle. Magnification × 11 000.

brachiocephalic vein, superior vena cava, inferior vena cava, portal vein and renal vein. In the renal vein and in parts of the inferior vena cava, virtually all the musculature is arranged longitudinally (Kügelgen 1955). Large veins entering the heart are encroached upon for a short distance by myocardial tissue, and in the coronary sinus this covering is complete (Coakley & King 1959); in the transition areas smooth and cardiac muscle lie side by side. Muscular tissue is absent in certain veins: the maternal placental veins, the dural venous sinuses and pial veins, the retinal veins, the veins of trabecular bone and the venous spaces of erectile tissue. Such veins consist of endothelium supported by variable amounts of connective tissue.

In the outer layer of connective tissue there are few nerve fibres, vasa vasorum and abundant elastic fibres. Overall, collagen is the main component of the venous wall in man, accounting for more than half its weight. Walls of the larger veins, like the arteries, are supplied by vasa vasorum but these in veins may penetrate the wall deeply, perhaps because of the lower oxygen tension. Postganglionic sympathetic efferent and primary afferent nerves are distributed to the veins, as in arteries, but less abundantly.

Most veins have valves to prevent reflux of blood (**10**.15). A valve is composed of an inward projection of the tunica intima, strengthened by collagen and elastic fibres and covered by endothelium differing in orientation on its two surfaces. Surface cells which are juxtamural are transversely arranged whereas on the luminal surface, over which the main stream of blood flows, cells are arranged longitudinally in the direction of the current. Most commonly, two such valves lie opposite one another, especially in smaller veins or in larger ones where smaller tributaries join; occasionally three valves lie in opposition, sometimes only one is present. The valves are semilunar (cusps) and attached by convex edges to the venous wall; their concave margins are directed with the current and apposed to the wall as long as flow is towards the heart, but when blood flow reverses the valves close. Centripetal to each valvular flap the wall is expanded into a sinus, which fills when blood flow is reversed against a closed valve, giving a 'knotted' appearance to the distended veins, if these have many valves. In the limbs, especially the legs where venous return is against gravity, such valves are of great importance to venous flow, as blood is moved towards the heart by the intermittent pressure produced by contractions of the surrounding muscles. Valves are absent in very small and in very large veins and in many tissues are rare or absent. Valves are absent in veins of the thorax and abdomen.

Special features are found in some veins such as the portal vein, where there is a prominent musculature made of a thick outer layer arranged longitudinally and mixed with abundant connective tissue (Ferraz de Carvalho & Rodrigues 1978) and a thin inner layer arranged as a low-pitched helix that is almost circular.

VASCULAR SHUNTS

These are communications between arteries and veins found in many regions of the body where the capillary circulation is bypassed by wider channels. They may be classified according to their dimensions, site and complexity as:

- preferential thoroughfare channels
- 'simple' arteriovenous anastomoses
- specialized arteriovenous anastomoses or *glomera*.

Preferential 'thoroughfare' channels

In many tissues true capillaries arise not only as direct side branches of terminal arterioles but also as side branches of a main or 'thoroughfare' channel connecting the terminal arteriole and the venule (Maggio 1965; Grant & Wright 1968, 1970; Zweifach 1973). This *thoroughfare channel* has a larger calibre than true capillaries and in ultrastructure resembles typical continuous capillaries, except that widely spaced smooth muscle cells spiral round the endothelium. Each capillary side branch has at its origin a precapillary sphincter. Such a channel and its capillaries form a functional *microcirculatory unit* (**10**.16). When functional demand is low, blood flow is largely limited to the bypass channel, with most precapillary sphincters closed. Periodic opening and closing of different sphincters may irrigate different parts of the capillary net. With increasing demand, blood flow may increase greatly following the opening of many sphincters. The size of the microcirculatory unit varies greatly, for example in skeletal muscle each channel gives rise to 20–30 true capillaries, but in some glandular tissues only one or two may be given off. Detailed investigations in the cremaster muscle and biceps femoris tendon of the rat (Grant & Wright 1968, 1970) have shown that in these sites, bypass channels are confined to perimuscular and peritendinous connective tissues and absent from the muscles itself. The form of the capillary net also varies with the tissue meshes being either round or elongated. Round or angular meshes are most common and prevail where networks are dense, as in the lungs, mucous membranes and skin. Elongated meshes occur in muscles and nerves, aligned parallel with their fibres. Sometimes capillaries are looped, as in the papillae of the skin and tongue. The number of capillaries and the size of their mesh determine the degree of vascularity; the smallest meshes occur in the lungs and the choroid of the eye.

Arteriovenous anastomoses (10.17)

Arteriovenous anastomoses are direct connections between smaller arteries and veins (Grant & Bland 1931; Popoff 1934; Clark 1938). Connecting vessels may be straight or coiled, often possessing a thick muscular tunic and a narrow lumen, about 10–30 μm across. Under sympathetic control through abundant non-myelinated fibres in its wall, the vessel is able to completely close, circulation being then via

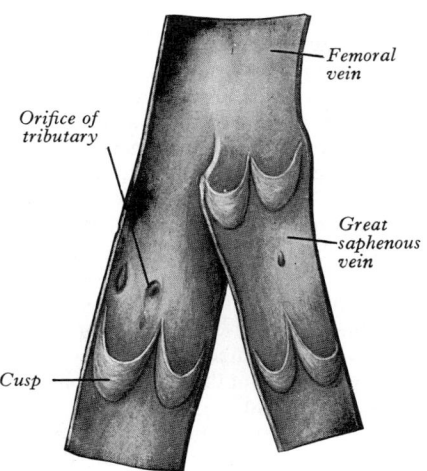

Femoral vein

Orifice of tributary

Great saphenous vein

Cusp

10.15 The upper portions of the femoral and great saphenous veins laid open to show the valves. About two-thirds of the natural size.

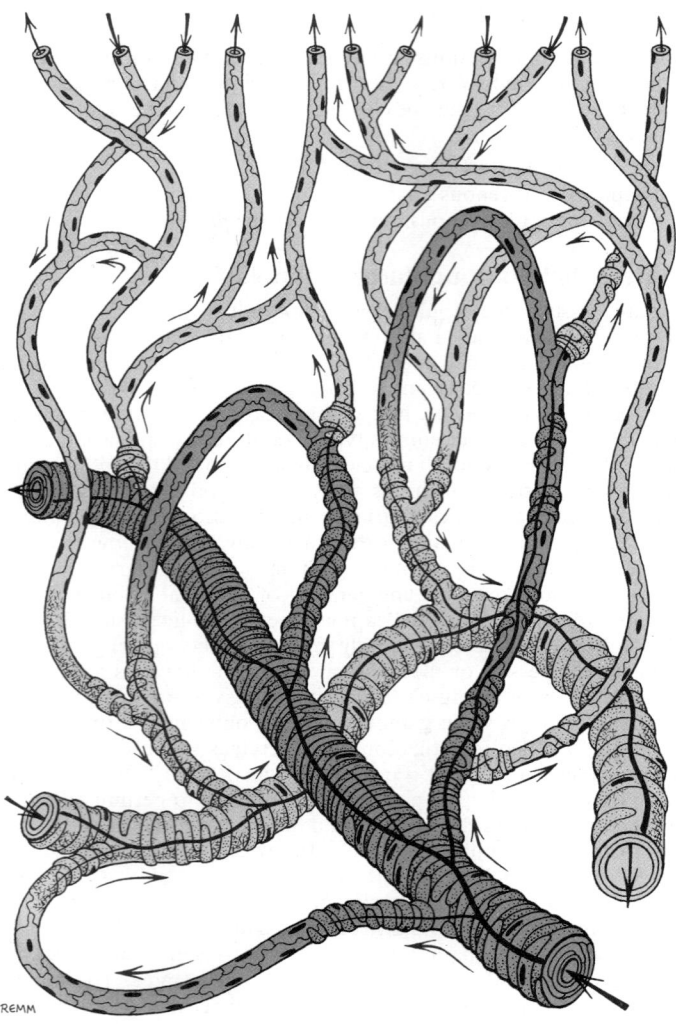

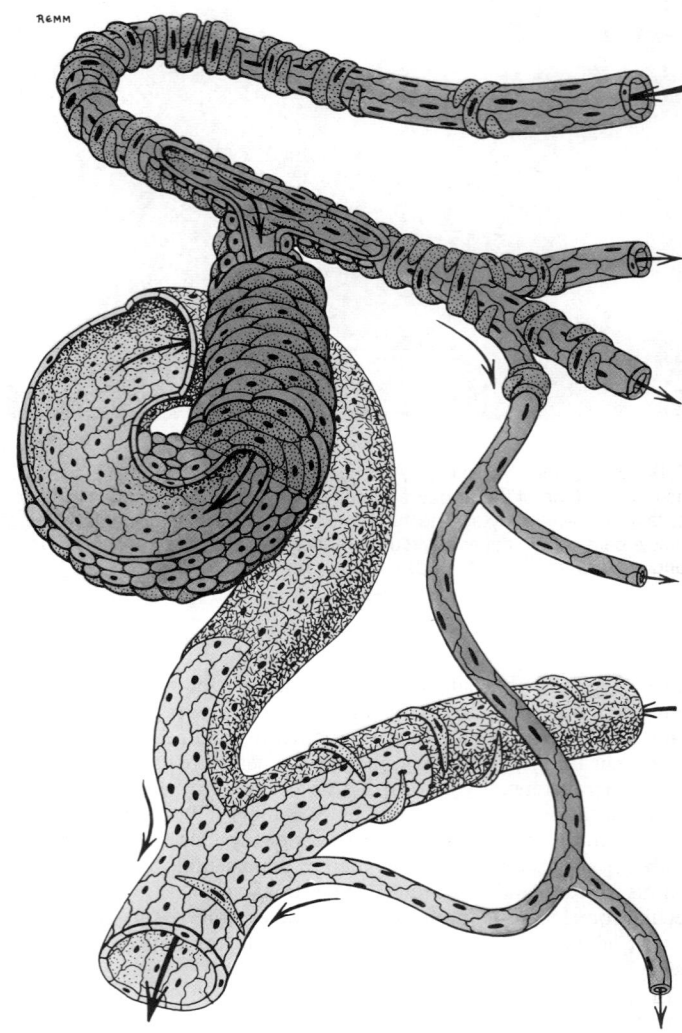

10.16   Diagram of a microcirculatory unit based upon descriptions in Zwei-fach (1959, 1961, 1973) and Reynolds and Zweifach (1959). Note the terminal arteriole, thoroughfare channels, capillaries and collecting venule. The distribution of smooth muscle cells and precapillary sphincters is shown.

10.17   Diagram of an arteriovenous anastomosis. Note the thick wall of the anastomotic channel composed of layers of modified smooth muscle cells.

the capillary bed. When patent, the vessel carries blood from artery to vein, partially or completely excluding the capillary bed from the circulation.

Arteriovenous anastomoses of relatively simple type occur in the nasal, labial and aural skin, nasal and alimentary mucous membranes, coccygeal body, erectile tissue, tongue, thyroid gland, sympathetic ganglia and probably elsewhere. Their ultrastructure has been investigated by Cauna (1970).

In the skin of the hands and feet (especially digital pads and nail beds) anastomoses form a large number of small units termed 'glomera'. They are deep in the corium and each 'glomus' has one or more afferent arteries, stemming from branches of cutaneous arteries approaching the surface (**10**.17, 18). These afferents arise at right angles from their parent vessels which then continue into the dermal papillary layer, ending in a capillary plexus. A short distance from its origin an afferent artery gives off a number of fine 'periglomeral' branches and then immediately enlarges, makes a sinuous curve and narrows again into a short funnel-shaped vein opening at right angles into a collecting vein. This vein commences on the deep aspect of the glomus, curving round its superficial surface, whence it retraces its course, receiving venules from the dermal papillary layer. Finally, it joins a deeper cutaneous vein.

In the newborn child arteriovenous anastomoses are generally few and poorly differentiated, but they develop rapidly during the early years of life. In old age they atrophy, sclerose and diminish in number.

The vessels concerned in digital arteriovenous anastomoses are

unusual (**10**.18). Where these enlarge the afferent artery has small luminal endotheliomuscular projections but proximal to this structure it is typical. The connecting vessel has an endothelium supported by fine collagenous fibres but no internal elastic lamina. Longitudinal and circular muscle layers are not sharply differentiated but the muscular wall is thick; in sections myocytes appear pale and swollen, with central nuclei, and hence described as 'epithelioid'. The efferent vein has a thin wall lacking muscle but containing many elastic fibres which pass into the tunica adventitia of the collecting vein.

The mechanisms by which arteriovenous anastomoses regulate local flow are poorly understood. Where they have circular muscle in their walls, epitheliocytes may help to narrow the lumen; where it is absent closure may be due to swelling of these epithelioid cells. Cutaneous arteriovenous anastomoses are essential to the control of general and local body temperature. When a rabbit's ear is raised above 40°C, muscle in the walls of the connecting vessels relax and increased blood flow at body temperature results, with a consequent cooling. When the local temperature is lowered below 15°C, the connecting vessels again relax and increased flow at body temperature then helps to raise local temperature, unless artificial cooling is intensified. When the animal's overall **body** temperature is raised experimentally, a general opening of all subcutaneous arteriovenous anastomoses results, with an increase in heat radiation and consequent drop in body temperature (Grant 1930). The cooling effect of panting in dogs also involves the opening of lingual arteriovenous anastomoses. The paucity and immaturity of arteriovenous anastomoses in the newborn and marked reduction in subcutaneous

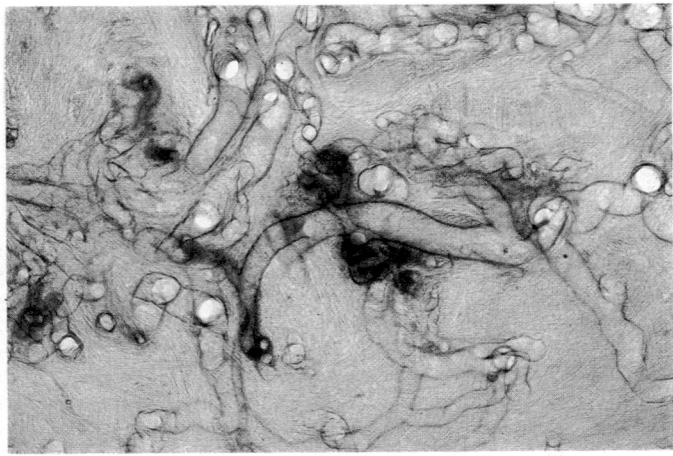

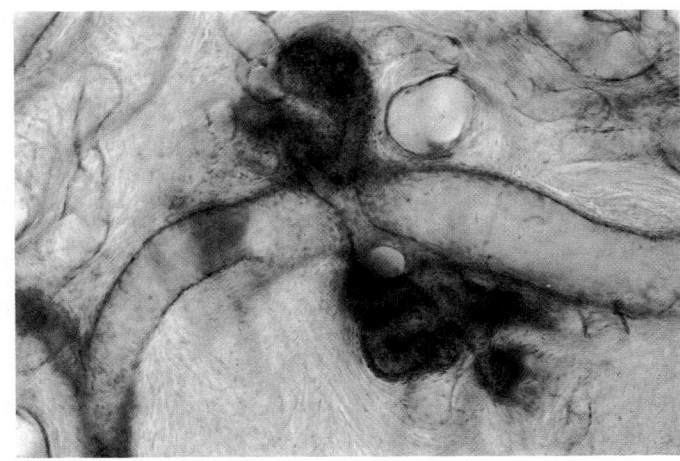

10.18 Human digital arteriovenous anastomoses prepared by intra-vascular perfusion of haematoxylin and subsequent clearing of a full thickness specimen of skin. The heavily stained, thick-walled, tortuous, anastomotic channels contrast with the central arterial stem and the thin-walled venous outflow channels. See text for further details. (The specimens were prepared and provided by R T Grant, Guy's Hospital Medical School.)

arteriovenous anastomoses with advancing years may be related to observed less efficient temperature regulation in these two extremes of age.

Arteriovenous anastomoses in alimentary mucous membranes fulfil a different function (Spanner 1932). An arteriole to a human villus has a direct connection with its corresponding venule and when absorption is in abeyance the connection is patent and helps to raise portal venous pressure; during alimentary absorption the anastomosis is closed and consequently blood traverses the capillary plexus.

Other suggested functions of arteriovenous anastomoses include regulation of blood pressure, secretion by epithelioid cells and pressor reception.

VASCULARIZATION OF BLOOD VESSELS

Some of the nourishment of the tissues of the vessel wall is provided by diffusion from the blood circulating in the vessel itself. In addition, large vessels have their own vascular supply, a network of small vessels, mainly microcirculatory vessels, the *vasa vasorum*. The wall thickness at which simple diffusion from the lumen becomes insufficient is about 1 mm (Kirk & Laursen 1955). The vasa vasorum originate from, and are drained into, adjacent vessels, which are peripheral branches of the vessel they supply. They are spread within the adventitia and, in the largest of arteries, penetrate into the outermost part of the media. The depth of penetration of capillaries into the media depends on the thickness of this tunica. Wolinsky and Glagov (1967b) in a comparative study of several mammals, found that only lamellar 'units' in excess of 29 are vascularized: if there are less than that number of units, the media remains avascular, and in the other cases the innermost 29 lamellae remain avascular.

INNERVATION OF BLOOD VESSELS

Blood vessels are innervated by efferent autonomic fibres, which regulate the contraction of the musculature, i.e. diameter and tone of the vessels, notably the arteries. In addition, most arteries also provide 'routes' along which nerves both travel to peripheral organs and arborize within them. These are *paravascular nerves* and they do not provide innervation to the vessel itself. They are parallel to the vessel but are situated at some distance from its adventitia and nerve and vessel are topographically but not physiologically related. In contrast, *perivascular nerves* run in the adventitia of the artery, where they branch and anastomose, forming a meshwork around the vessel. These nerves travel a long distance along the vessel, and they can provide innervation to its musculature. They are small bundles of axons, and the axons are almost invariably unmyelinated and typically *varicose*. Most of them are postganglionic fibres issuing from sympathetic ganglion neurons. However, some perivascular fibres originate from cranial parasympathetic ganglia and from ganglia of the enteric submucosal plexus, and some brain vessels are innervated by neurons of the central nervous system. The density of innervation varies in different vessels and in different areas of the body. The innervation is sparser in veins, where the musculature is consistently less well developed than in arteries, and the same is true of lymphatic vessels. But large veins with a conspicuous musculature, such as the portal vein, are richly supplied with nerves.

The principal site of action of nerves of blood vessels is on muscular artery and especially arterioles. The main effect of nerves is vasoconstriction and increase in vascular tone, and this role is particularly effective in arterioles, on account of their dense innervation and of the mechanical gain derived from the high ratio of wall thickness to vessel radius. *Adrenergic* fibres are vasoconstrictor and they act on adrenoceptors—of which several types are known—in the muscle cell membrane. Other substances are released with noradrenaline by the activated nerve endings, allowing for a complex regulation of the neurogenic control of vasomotility. The mechanical activity of vascular musculature is also under the influence of circulating factors such as hormones. In addition, there are factors, such as nitric oxide and endothelins, which are released from the endothelial cells and have a potent effect on vascular muscle cells. In this multiple control, while neurotransmitters reach the musculature from the adventitial surface of the media, the endothelial factors diffuse from its intimal surface. In some areas there are also sympathetic *cholinergic* fibres which inhibit muscle activity and induce vasodilatation. Afferent fibres from dorsal root ganglia are present in some vessels and can be identified either histochemically or with retrograde tracer studies. These afferent fibres usually end with a long chain of varicosities, but the physiology of their sensory transduction in the vessel wall is still obscure.

The terminal portions of the axons found in the vascular adventitia is varicose, i.e. it has a beaded appearance with expanded bulbous portions (up to 1.5 μm in diameter) and narrow intervaricose segments (about 0.2 μm in diameter). Varicosities contain mitochondria, microtubules, some neurofilaments and, above all, axonal vesicles, which transport and release the neurotransmitters. The intervaricose segments are occupied almost exclusively by a few microtubules.

All the perivascular fibres are confined to the adventitia of the vessel, where they run amid collagen fibres, fibroblasts and small vessels (lymphatics and vasa vasorum). Only in some large muscular arteries, small nerve fibres are occasionally found within the outermost layers of the musculature. As a general rule, nerve fibres do not penetrate into the media, and they are never found in the intima. (Nerve fibres are sometimes close to the wall of capillaries, and the possibility of a physiological interaction between nerve endings and endothelial cells cannot be ruled out.) Because of their location in the adventitia, nerve fibres run at a considerable distance even from the nearest muscle cell. In large muscular arteries many varicosities lie more than 1 μm away from the nearest muscle cell and any neuromuscular transmission requires diffusion of neurotransmitters over a considerable distance. In smaller vessels, such as arterioles, however, where the elastic and collagen material is less abundant, axonal varicosities lie within a few tens of nanometres from muscle cells. These points of close apposition are regarded as proper neuro-muscular junctions, and, when the tissue is examined in serial sections, they appear quite numerous (Luff et al 1987).

ANGIOGENESIS

Some tissues lack vascularization, for example cartilage, epithelia even when thick and stratified, the media of vessels themselves and elastic tissue in general. This may be partly due to an active inhibition of vascular growth by certain tissues.

Angiogenesis is the formation of new vessels starting from pre-existing vessels, during growth of an organ, both in development and in hypertrophy and also in pathological tissues as in tumours.

The existence of diffusible angiogenic factors is well documented and some angiogenic polypeptides have been isolated and sequenced, including some growth factors (Folkman & Klagsbrun 1987). One of the trophic factors that stimulates migration and division in endothelial cells is b-FGF (Tsuboi et al 1990). Interestingly, the endothelial cells themselves express the b-FGF gene and release b-FGF; this raises the possibility that endothelium regulates its own growth via this trophic factor (Schweigerer et al 1987).

New capillaries originate from sprouting of small venules (Ausprunk & Folkman 1977); there is a local disruption of the basal lamina followed by migration of endothelial cells. The sprout is initially solid, but then becomes partly canalized, while it grows by division of the endothelial cells, until it joins another sprout and blood flow begins.

The importance of angiogenesis in human pathology stems from the possible role of blood vessels in the growth of tumours. Tumours implanted into isolated perfused organs in vitro fail to grow beyond a few millimetres in diameter; the same tumours reimplanted into donor mice grow to more than 1 cm^3 and kill their hosts (Folkman & Klagsbrun 1987). Since only the reimplanted tumours become vas-cularized (Folkman & Klagsbrun 1987), the tumour growth seems to be linked to capillary growth.

THORACIC CAVITY AND HEART

The thoracic skeleton is described on pages 545–546. The volume enclosed within the thoracic cavity does not correspond with that enclosed by the osseous thorax because the lower part of the space surrounded by the bony elements is encroached upon by the diaphragm and the mobile and distensible organs within the upper abdomen. The capacity of the thoracic cavity also varies with posture and respiration, both affecting the position and relations of the thoracic organs. Its arbitrary upper limit is usually taken as the oblique plane of its inlet at the first rib, but the pulmonary apices and pleural cavities extend above this level into the neck, reaching the level of the **neck** of the rib.

UPPER OPENING (INLET) OF THORAX

The boundaries are formed by the skeleton described on page 545. The structures passing through the opening can be divided into two groups:

• those in or near the medial plane
• those on each side closely related to the cervical parts of the lungs.

Near the midline: behind the manubrium of the sternum, the lowest parts of the sternohyoid muscles enter the thorax, and behind them are the sternothyroid muscles along with vestiges of the thymus gland and the inferior thyroid veins passing down to empty into the brachiocephalic veins. In children, particularly, the left brachio-cephalic vein itself may be in the thoracic inlet. **Posteriorly**, the trachea and the oesophagus, with the left recurrent laryngeal nerves, pass through the median part of the opening. The thoracic duct also passes through the opening behind the left margin of the oesophagus. Anterior to the vertebral column are the prevertebral longus colli muscles and the anterior longitudinal ligament.

On each side: the upper part of the pleura and the pulmonary apex occupy the inlet. Between the pleura and neck of the first rib, mediolaterally, are found the sympathetic trunk, the superior intercostal artery and the ventral branch of the first thoracic nerve as it passes superolaterally to join the brachial plexus. Anteriorly, the internal thoracic artery enters the thorax between the pleura and the first costal cartilage while, medial to the artery, its vein leaves the thorax.

On the right (**10.**26): the brachiocephalic artery leaves the thorax between the trachea and pleura. The vagus nerve, having passed between subclavian artery and vein, is between the pleura and the brachiocephalic artery at the inlet. The right brachiocephalic vein enters the thorax anterolateral to its artery. The right phrenic

nerve crosses the internal thoracic artery and is lateral to the brachiocephalic vein behind the first costal cartilage.

On the left (**10.**26): the left common carotid and subclavian arteries leave the thorax between the pleura and trachea, the left vagus nerve descending lateral to the interval between them. Anterolateral to this is found the left brachiocephalic vein. The left phrenic nerve passing inferomedially crosses anterior to the internal thoracic artery at a higher level than the right. At the inlet, the left phrenic nerve is found between the left brachiocephalic vein anterolaterally and the subclavian and common carotid arteries posteromedially.

LOWER OPENING (OUTLET) OF THORAX

This extensive opening is wider transversely and slopes obliquely down and backwards, so that the vertical extent of the cavity is much longer posteriorly than it is anteriorly. The diaphragm (p. 815) closes the opening and forms a convex floor for the cavity. It is flatter centrally than at its peripheral attachments. It is higher on the right and, in cadavers, this side of the floor reaches the level of the upper border of the fifth costal cartilage. On the left, the diaphragm reaches only to the level of the sixth cartilage. (See p. 816 for further information on diaphragmatic shape and levels.) From the summit of each side, the diaphragm slopes abruptly down to its sternal, costal and vertebral attachments. The muscle is short anteriorly, progressively longer laterally, and it is longest and with a much more marked slope posteriorly, where the space between the diaphragm and the posterior thoracic wall narrows rapidly as it extends inferiorly.

DIVISIONS OF THORACIC CAVITY

The thoracic cavity is divided by the *mediastinum*, itself formed by the mass of structures between the lungs which extend from the sternum to the vertebral column and from the thoracic inlet to the diaphragm. The heart is in the mediastinum, enclosed by the *pericardium*. The lungs occupy the right and left regions of the thorax, each covered by a serosal membrane, the *pleura*, which also lines the corresponding half of the thorax and the lateral aspect of the mediastinum (**10.**21, 24).

For description, the mediastinum is arbitrarily divided into superior and inferior parts. The *superior part* extends from the thoracic inlet to an oblique (*transverse thoracic*) plane passing through the lower edge of the manubrium of the sternum and lower border of the fourth thoracic vertebra. The *inferior part*, below this plane, is subdivided into an *anterior* part in front of the pericardium, a *posterior* component behind this and the diaphragm, and a *middle* component, containing the pericardium and the heart together with the large vessels entering or leaving it. Detailed accounts of the mediastinal contents are included with descriptions of the respiratory organs (pp. 1636–1646); the heart (pp. 1474–1504); and the oesophagus (p. 1751).

PERICARDIUM

The pericardium contains the heart and the juxtacardiac parts of its great vessels. It consists of two components, the fibrous and the serosal pericardium. The *fibrous pericardium* is a sac made of tough connective tissue, fully surrounding the heart without being attached to it. This fibrous sac develops by a sequential process of cavitation of the embryonic body wall by expansion of the secondary pleural cavity (see p. 180); thus its lateral walls are clothed externally by *parietal mediastinal pleura*. The *serosal pericardium* consists of two sacs of serosal membrane, one inside the other, the inner (visceral) one adhering to the heart and forming its outer covering known as the *epicardium*, while the outer (parietal) one lines the internal surface of the fibrous pericardium. The two serosal surfaces are apposed and separated by a film of fluid, thus allowing movement of the inner membrane and the heart adhering to it, except at the arterial and venous areas of the pericardium where the two serosal membranes merge. The latter constitute two parietovisceral lines of serosal reflexion (see below). The separation of the two membranes of the serosal pericardium creates a narrow space, the *pericardial cavity*, which provides a complete cleavage between the heart and its surroundings thus allowing it some freedom to move and change shape.

Fibrous pericardium

The fibrous pericardium is roughly conical and clothes the heart. **Superiorly**, it is continuous exteriorly with the adventitia of the great vessels, while **inferiorly** it is attached to the central tendon of the diaphragm and a small muscular area of its left half. Above, the fibrous pericardium not only blends externally with the great vessels, but is continuous with the pretracheal fascia (p. 804). **Anteriorly** it is also attached to the posterior surface of the sternum by superior and inferior sternopericardial ligaments, although the extent of these 'ligaments' is extremely variable, the superior one often being undetectable. By these connections, the pericardium is securely anchored and maintains the general thoracic position of the heart, serving as the 'cardiac seat belt'.

Anteriorly, the fibrous pericardium is separated from the thoracic wall by the lungs and the pleural coverings. However, in a small area behind the lower left half of the body of the sternum and the sternal ends of left fourth and fifth costal cartilages, the pericardium is in direct contact with the thoracic wall. Until it regresses, the lower end of the thymus is also anterior to the upper pericardium. **Posteriorly** are the principal bronchi, the oesophagus, the oesophageal plexus, the descending thoracic aorta, and the posterior parts of the mediastinal surface of both lungs. **Laterally** are the pleural coverings of the mediastinal surface of the lungs. The phrenic nerve, with its accompanying vessels, descends between the fibrous pericardium and mediastinal pleura on each side. **Inferiorly**, the pericardium is separated by the diaphragm from the liver and fundus of the stomach.

Vessels receiving extensions of the fibrous pericardium are the aorta, the superior vena cava, the right and left pulmonary arteries and the four pulmonary veins. The inferior vena cava, traversing the central tendon, has no such covering.

Serosal pericardium

The serosal pericardium is a closed sac within the fibrous pericardium, having a visceral and a parietal layer (**10.22**). The visceral layer, or *epicardium*, covers the heart and great vessels and is reflected into the parietal layer, which lines the internal surface of the fibrous pericardium. The reflexions of the serosal layer are arranged as two complex 'tubes', the aorta and pulmonary trunk being enclosed in one and the superior and inferior venae cavae and the four pulmonary

veins in the other. The tube surrounding the veins has the shape of an inverted J (**10.19, 32**) and the cul-de-sac within its curve is behind the left atrium and is termed the *oblique sinus*. A passage between the two pericardial 'tubes' is the *transverse sinus* (**10.19**). This has the aorta and pulmonary trunk in front and the atria and great veins behind. The arrangement of the oblique and transverse sinuses, along with that of the main 'principal' cavity, is further affected by the development of complex three-dimensional pericardial recesses between adjacent structures. (For details, illustrations and bibliography see Vesely & Cahill 1986.) These recesses can be grouped according to the siting of their orifices or 'mouths'. From the principal pericardial cavity, the *postcaval recess* projects towards the left behind the atrial termination of the superior vena cava. It is limited above by the right pulmonary artery and below by the upper right pulmonary vein. Its mouth opens superolaterally to the right. The *right* and *left pulmonary venous recesses* each project medially and upwards on the back of the left atrium between the superior and inferior pulmonary veins on each side, indenting the side walls of the oblique sinus. The *superior aortic recess* extends from the transverse sinus. From its mouth, located inferiorly, it ascends posterior to, then right of, the ascending aorta to end at the level of the sternal angle. The *inferior aortic recess*, also extending from the transverse sinus, is a diverticulum descending from a superiorly located mouth to run between the lower ascending part of the aorta and the right atrium. The *left pulmonary recess*, mouth under the fold of the left vena cava, passes to the left between the inferior aspect of the left pulmonary artery and upper border of the superior left pulmonary vein. The *right pulmonary recess* lies between the lower surface of the proximal part of the right pulmonary artery and upper border of the left atrium.

A triangular fold of serosal pericardium is reflected from the left pulmonary artery to the subjacent upper left pulmonary vein as the *fold of the left superior vena cava*. It contains a fibrous ligament, a

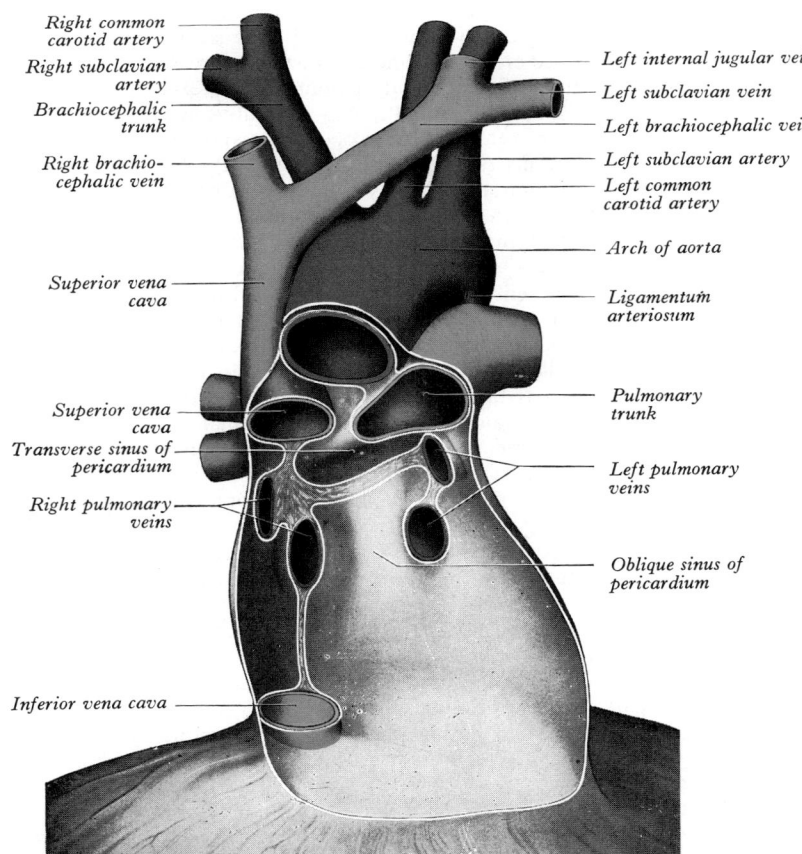

10.19 Interior of the serosal pericardial sac after section of the large vessels at their cardiac origin and removal of the heart (seen from the front). See text for additional named recesses of the general serosal pericardial cavity and its transverse sinus.

remnant of the obliterated *left common cardinal vein* (left duct of Cuvier, p. 302). This descends anterior to the left pulmonary hilum from the upper part of the left superior intercostal vein to the back of the left atrium, where it is continuous with the *oblique vein of the left atrium* (p. 1576). The left common cardinal vein may persist as a left superior vena cava which then replaces the oblique vein of the left atrium and empties into the coronary sinus. When both common cardinal veins persist as right and left superior venae cavae, the transverse anastomosis between them, normally forming the left brachiocephalic vein, may be small or absent. When there is a left superior vena cava, it is joined by the left superior intercostal vein.

Vessels and nerves. The arteries of the pericardium are derived from the internal thoracic and musculophrenic arteries and the descending thoracic aorta. The veins are tributaries of the azygos system. The nerve supply is from the vagus together with phrenic nerves and the sympathetic trunks.

Structure. The fibrous pericardium is compact collagenous fibrous tissue. The serosal pericardium is a single layer of flat cells on a thin subserosal layer of connective tissue which blends with the fibrous pericardium in the parietal membrane and with the interstitial myocardial tissue in the visceral membrane. On the cardiac side, the subserosal layer contains fat, this being greatest along the ventricular side of the atrioventricular groove, the inferior cardiac border and the interventricular grooves. The main coronary vessels and their larger branches are embedded in this fat, its amount being related to the general extent of body fat and gradually increasing with age.

Pericardial puncture

Pericardial puncture can be performed either in the fifth or sixth left intercostal space near the sternum to avoid the internal thoracic artery, or at the left costoxiphoid angle, passing up and backwards into the pericardial sac. The serosal pericardium extends on the pulmonary trunk, anterior to the transverse sinus, as far as the arterial ligament (p. 1504, see **10.66**).

HEART

GENERAL INTRODUCTION

All triploblastic organisms, including chordates, overcome the limitations of diffusion over long distances by circulating a fluid from regions of high-oxygen tension and high concentration of nutrient substances to mesodermal and other cells remote from the external environment. The fluid, and its mode of circulation, vary amongst invertebrate phyla, but the majority (for example, annelid worms, arthropods and molluscs) are coelomates with closed vascular systems and some localized means of propelling 'blood' in a true circulation. The most common pattern consists of a dorsal pulsatile vessel (which may be valved and respond to muscular pacemakers under the influence of nerves), and one or more accessory structures which show varying degrees of development. Gas exchange is generally across gills and/or skin, although alternative systems (such as the tracheae of insects and lung books of spiders) occur in terrestrial groups. Echinoderms (sea urchins, starfish, etc.), the invertebrate group closest to chordates, display a unique water vascular system which takes over much of the role of the blood vascular system—a specialization which makes comparisons difficult.

Chordates possess a single heart (although accessory pulsatile vessels may be present) and the circulation is closed, but chordates differ from other coelomates in that the heart is ventral and not dorsal to the gut. In the primitive urochordates (tunicates or 'sea squirts'), the capillary beds are essentially in series, and flow of blood through the heart is bi-directional. In cephalochordates (including *Branchiostoma*, the familiar amphioxus), capillary networks are largely in parallel and blood flows through the unvalved tubular 'heart' in one direction (Randall & Davie 1980). This forms the starting point for the development of the vertebrate heart.

In tracing cardiac phylogeny, especially in deriving the mammalian heart, no direct palaeontological evidence is available. Comparison of existing arrangements in extant vertebrate groups, therefore, is the only source of information. Such comparison can be misleading. Many older textbooks, dwelling only on the degree of septation, give the impression of an orthogenetic evolution of the mammalian four-chambered heart through a series of imperfect (yet surviving) intermediates. This overlooks the fact that, in all vertebrates, the structure of the heart is intimately related to the nature of surfaces for gas exchange, to locomotion and lifestyle, and to metabolism. Hearts must function early in embryonic life, throughout development, and then in greatly changed postnatal conditions.

In its simplest form the vertebrate heart is a single pump consisting of a succession of three or four enlarged segments. These are, first, a sinus venosus draining principal veins; second, a pulsatile but thin-walled atrium; third, a thick-walled muscular ventricle; and either a so-called bulbus cordis or conus, with cardiac muscle in its wall (primitive jawless vertebrates, elasmobranchs and lungfish) or a bulbus arteriosus (the swollen proximal end of the ventral aorta) consisting of smooth muscle and elastic tissue (teleost fish). The chambers are separated one from another by valves which maintain a unidirectional flow and permit increased pressures to develop at the arterial outlet. The conus, or bulbus arteriosus when present, opens into a ventral aorta from which arise a series of aortic arches that supply the gills before joining to form a median dorsal aorta. The heart has its own coronary circulation (except in primitive jawless vertebrates like lampreys and hagfish) and is contained in a pericardial coelom, a separated part of the general body cavity. The pericardial cavity is semi-rigid in some fish (for example, elasmobranchs) and lies dorsal to the pectoral girdle. The resultant constancy of volume aids atrial filling by suction as the ventricle empties. This effect is largely lost in tetrapods because of caudal 'migration' of the heart and less massive bony girdles. The pulsatile rhythm of vertebrate hearts is basically myogenic, but is co-ordinated with systemic demands by a supply of nerves. With increasing specialization from fishes to birds and mammals, nodes and tracts of cardiac muscle differentiate as focuses initiating contraction and as rapid conductors for the dissemination of cyclic stimuli (at particular sites the conduction is much slower, introducing physiologically imperative delays).

In most vertebrates, the cardiac tube outgrows the length of its pericardial sac, developing a sinuous bend. The venous end (sinus venosus and atrium) then becomes dorsal to the arterial end (ventricle and conus). Moreover, the heart becomes asymmetrical in position with the change from symmetrical cardinal veins to asymmetrical venae cavae. In the lungfish (Dipnoi), the venous sinus opens into the right of a partly divided atrium, a condition persisting in subsequent vertebrate classes. In frogs, most salamanders and all amniotes (reptiles, birds and mammals), this asymmetry is coupled with absorption of some of the venous sinus and its vestiges into the atrium. With complete separation of atria, a right-sided systemic venous return is established. At the arterial end, the bulbar segment of the embryo persists as the contractile bulbus cordis (conus) of the adult and, in elasmobranchs, commonly has serial valvar flaps. From these may be derived the spiral valves in the conus of lungfish and amphibians. This development is linked with the greatest era of transformation in cardiac evolution, the long series of adaptations which allowed vertebrates to spread from an aquatic to a terrestrial habitat.

It is thought that the ancestors of tetrapods were fish which were chiefly dependent on gills but could breathe air using a pharyngeal diverticulum, the so-called 'swim bladder' or, later, lungs. We have a living model for such a lifestyle in the Australian lungfish *Neoceratodus*, a facultative air-breather which relies mainly on gills and cutaneous gas exchange, but uses its lung when the oxygen concentration in the surrounding water falls (Burggren & Johansen 1986). The other two living dipnoan genera (*Protopterus* from Africa and *Lepidosiren* from South America) are more specialized and are fully dependent on air-breathing. An inherent duality is found in the circulation of dipnoans. They have a systemic 'portal' arterial circulation (through the gills) and also a parallel pulmonary 'portal' circulation (through the walls of the lung; the same system supplying the skin and the mucous membranes of the mouth and pharynx). The adoption of air-breathing, however, creates problems for the venous return. Blood leaving the lung capillaries lacks sufficient energy to perfuse the remaining body tissues effectively and must, therefore, be returned to the heart. If it simply joins the systemic venous return, there will be large-scale mixing of oxygenated and deoxygenated blood. Division of the atrial chamber, with pulmonary venous blood returning to a separate left atrium, is, therefore, a requirement for efficient air-breathing. Such circuits already return blood to discrete atria in dipnoans and, although the ventricle is only partly divided, perfusion studies have shown that obligate air-breathers have the ability to separate the different bloodstreams— partly by virtue of the highly trabecular internal ventricular surface. The ventricular output is divided into two streams by spiral valves in a large conus arteriosus. Oxygenated blood from the left side of the heart is directed preferentially to the head and dorsal aorta while blood from the right side is directed to the 'lungs' via the more caudal gill clefts (the passage through the gills being important for the removal of carbon dioxide).

The earliest tetrapods were in existence at least 360 million years ago in the Devonian Period of the Palaeozoic. From what we now know of them, it would seem that the first tetrapods were aquatic animals using, like the lungfish *Neoceratodus*, a combination of branchial, pulmonary and cutaneous gas exchange (Coates & Clack 1991). It may be, therefore, that no sudden change, either in structure or function, occurred in the slow adaptation from aquatic to terrestrial life. There was, instead, a change of balance between several coexistent modes of respiration. These respiratory changes, inseparable from cardiac circulatory modifications, were accompanied by changes in the locomotor system, with the evolution of limbs from fins, firstly as an aid to progression within an aquatic environment but then, with changes in the girdles and spine, to fully terrestrial locomotion.

In amphibians, the gills are usually lost at metamorphosis and the branchial capillary beds disappear. Gas exchange is mainly pulmonary and buccopharyngeal, with the skin becoming an important surface for the removal of carbon dioxide. In the heart, the atria are separate chambers (although the interatrial septum is perforated in most salamanders), but the ventricle is undivided (except in the salamanders *Siren* and *Necturus*). Despite this, perfusion studies have shown that several factors (a system of ventricular trabeculae, the spiral outlet valve, the position and volume of the returning blood) enable the streams of flow to be effectively separated when the animal is breathing. When the lungs are not in use, blood returning to the right atrium from the skin and buccopharyngeal region may contain more oxygen than the blood returning to the left atrium. The absence of the ventricular septum should not, therefore, be regarded as a primitive maladaptation but as a condition which permits an important flexibility in the cardiorespiratory pattern.

The earliest amniotes completed the transition to a terrestrial lifestyle with an egg that was capable of surviving out of water and a skin that was resistant to loss of water. Although some groups have returned to an aquatic or amphibious lifestyle, respiration is almost entirely pulmonary (some turtles and sea snakes are reported to use vascularized cloacal surfaces for limited gas exchange), and is linked with a complete interatrial septum and at least partial ventricular division.

The hearts of living reptiles are varied and complex and this is not a place for a detailed review (see references for further information). Reptilian hearts are unusual in having three incompletely separated ventricular compartments and a triple or quadruple arterial cardiac outflow with a pulmonary trunk, a right and a left aorta and, in turtles, a separate brachiocephalic trunk. The two aortae join dorsally to form a single median dorsal aorta. In lizards, snakes and turtles, all the outlet vessels arise from the right side of the heart (cavum venosum), although the pulmonary trunk issues from a more ventral compartment (cavum pulmonale). Blood from the left atrium flows into a left cavum arteriosum but no outflow vessels leave this compartment. The passages between the right and left ventricles, and between the two main compartments of the right ventricle, are at least partially separated one from another by valves which open and close in response to changes in pressure such that oxygenated and deoxygenated bloodstreams remain largely separated. As in amphibians the structure of the ventricle permits substantial right-to-left shunting (approaching pulmonary bypass) within the heart when the animal stops breathing (for example, when diving or, in the case of lizards, during sustained exercise—due perhaps to the disruptive effect of repeated lateral flexions of the body). In crocodiles, the arrangement is similar to that of lizards and snakes but there are two important differences. The first is the presence of a complete interventricular septum. The second is that, while the pulmonary trunk and left aorta arise from the right ventricle as usual, the right aorta leaves the left ventricle. An opening, the foramen of Panizza, permits a shunt from the right aorta into the left during breathing when little or no blood enters from the right ventricle. As in other reptiles, the system also permits a shunt in the opposite direction when the lungs are shut down in diving. Under these conditions, blood in the right ventricle passes preferentially into the left aorta due to the higher resistance of the pulmonary circuit.

The bird heart is closely similar to that of the crocodile except that degeneration of the left aortic arch (rarely present as a remnant), suppression of the interaortic septum and loss of the connection between the right ventricle and the aortic root has resulted in a fully divided heart with no possibility of right-to-left shunting. There is also a single right aortic arch. These changes probably occurred in the small, active bipedal dinosaurs which were ancestral to the first birds. In these animals, the upright posture and terrestrial lifestyle obviated the need for right-to-left shunts and permitted the continuous breathing required for a fully active lifestyle. Despite its four chambers, the bird heart differs from that of a mammal in several respects, most notably the retention of a right rather than left aortic arch and the presence of a flap-like muscular right atrioventricular valve which lacks either papillary muscles or tendinous chords (chordae tendineae).

Bird and mammal hearts have evolved independently to permit a lifestyle in which a high level of activity is maintained by a constant high metabolic rate, with all the demands that this makes on the system in terms of requirements for oxygen and energy supply. It is orthodox to derive mammals from 'reptiles', but it should be stressed that living reptiles are as far removed from such ancestral forms as are living mammals. Consequently, as we have seen, the hearts of living reptiles are specialized, and no extant reptile can provide a model for the ancestral mammalian heart. The earliest amniotes were derived from a lineage separate from that which gave rise to living amphibians. Similarly, the ancestors of mammals were primitive amniotes which separated at a very early stage (at least 300 million years ago) from the lineage which gave rise to modern reptiles and birds. We cannot easily predict, therefore, the structure of the heart in the amniotes which were ancestral to mammals. This heart seems likely to have shown full atrial and at least partial ventricular septation. Right-to-left shunting may have remained important until the limbs were brought under the body and lateral flexion of the trunk during walking no longer disrupted ventilation. The heart of the most 'primitive' living mammals, the egg-laying monotremes, is essentially mammalian, although there is reportedly some muscle within the right atrioventricular valve and its movements are regulated directly by papillary muscles without the intervention of tendinous cords.

In all mammals, including mankind, cardiac septation is complete but during embryonic life (p. 1501) stages occur that are rather like the final arrangements in some lower vertebrates. Abnormal development can lead to congenital defects resembling conditions in those forms. The resemblance is misleading because the heart must function effectively at all but its initial stages of development. The oval foramen, a feature of mammalian prenatal development, is a necessary shunt rather than an atavistic indication of earlier incomplete atrial septation. A persistently patent oval foramen, and other such cardiac abnormalities, are due to disturbed mammalian development rather than recapitulation. Equally, the functional fetal mammalian heart, with its elegant separation of blood flows within the right atrium by a combination of small valves, pressure differences and the positions of entry of the vessels, provides clear evidence that the absence of discrete septa does not necessarily render a heart inefficient. For further details consult Embryology in this volume and the following references and their bibliographies: Foxon (1955), Johansen and Burggren (1980) and Lawson (1979).

There is no entirely logical progression in describing the heart. Whatever standpoint is used, subsequent details are presumed. The sequence adopted here is a compromise. General organization precedes external features, surface anatomy and radiology, and is then followed by internal structure, including accounts of valves, myocardium, fibrous 'skeleton', specialized conducting tissues and the cardiac cycle.

GENERAL CARDIAC ORGANIZATION

The human heart is a pair of valved muscular pumps combined in a single organ (**10**.20, 24). But, while the fibromuscular framework and conduction tissues of these pumps are structurally interwoven, each pump (the so-called 'right' and 'left' hearts) is physiologically separate, being interposed in series at different points in the double circulation. Despite this functional disposition in series, the two pumps are usually described topographically in parallel.

Of the four cardiac chambers, the two atria receive venous blood as weakly contractile reservoirs for final filling of the two ventricles, which then provide the powerful expulsive contraction forcing blood into the main arterial trunks.

The **right heart** commences at the right atrium, and receives the superior and inferior venae cavae together with the main venous inflow from the heart itself via the coronary sinus. This systemic venous blood traverses the *right atrioventricular orifice*, guarded by the *tricuspid valve*, to enter the inlet component of the right ventricle. Contraction of the ventricle, particularly its apical trabecular component, closes the tricuspid valve and, with increasing pressure, ejects the blood through the muscular right ventricular outflow tract into the pulmonary trunk and thence to the pulmonary vascular bed, which has a relatively low resistance. Changes in pressure, time relations and valvar events are described below. Many structural features of the 'right heart', including its overall geometry, myocardial architecture and the construction and the relative strengths of the tricuspid and pulmonary valves, accord with this low resistance, being associated with comparatively low changes of pressure.

The **left heart** commences at the left atrium, which receives all the pulmonary inflow of oxygenated blood and some coronary venous inflow. It contracts to fill the left ventricle through the *left atrioventricular orifice* guarded by its *mitral valve*. The valve is the entry

to the inlet of the left ventricle. Ventricular contraction rapidly raises the pressure in the apical trabecular component, closing the mitral valve and opening the aortic valve so that the ventricle can eject via the left ventricular outflow tract into the aortic sinuses, ascending aorta and thence to the whole systemic arterial tree, including the coronary arteries. This vast vascular bed presents a high peripheral resistance which, with large metabolic demands, especially the sustained requirements of the cerebral tissues, explains the more massive structural organization of the 'left heart'. The ejectional phase of the left ventricle is shorter than that of the right, but its fluctuations of pressure are very much greater.

Because of its contrasting functional demands, the human heart is far from a simple pair of parallel pumps, structurally combined, even though the right and left ventricles must deliver more or less the same volume with each contraction. The heart has a complicated, spiralized, three-dimensional organization which is markedly skewed when compared with the planes of the body. Terms such as 'left' and 'right', 'anterior' and 'posterior', 'superior' and 'inferior', therefore, do not always assist the descriptions of cardiac anatomy. Another potential source of confusion is the usual study of isolated whole or dissected hearts, with the subsequent difficulty in relating details to the heart as it is positioned within the body. The following preliminary description emphasizes such difficulties so as to circumvent certain misconceptions before proceeding to an account of more detailed structure.

The principal features of cardiac anatomy can be illuminated by study of corrosion casts of normal hearts in which the two sides have been filled with resins of contrasting colours. Alternatively, similar information is obtained from horizontal mediastinal sections or scans taken at, or near, the seventh thoracic vertebral level (**10**.21, 25A, B).

The **right heart**, while forming the right aspect or 'border' (see p. 1476), follows a gentle curve and covers most of the anterior aspect of the left heart (except for a left-sided strip including the apex). Thus, the right heart forms the largest part of the **anterior** surface, its outflow tract ascending until it terminates on the **left** side of the outflow tract from the left ventricle. The sites of the tricuspid and pulmonary valves are widely separated and on different planes, the flat cavity of the right ventricle (crescentic in its section) splaying out between them. Conversely, the **left heart** (except the left-sided strip mentioned above) is largely **posterior** in position and is obscured when viewed from the front by the chambers of the right heart. The inlet to the left ventricle (containing the mitral valve) is very close to its outlet (the aortic valve), the two being embraced by the wide tract linking inlet and outlet components of the right ventricle. The

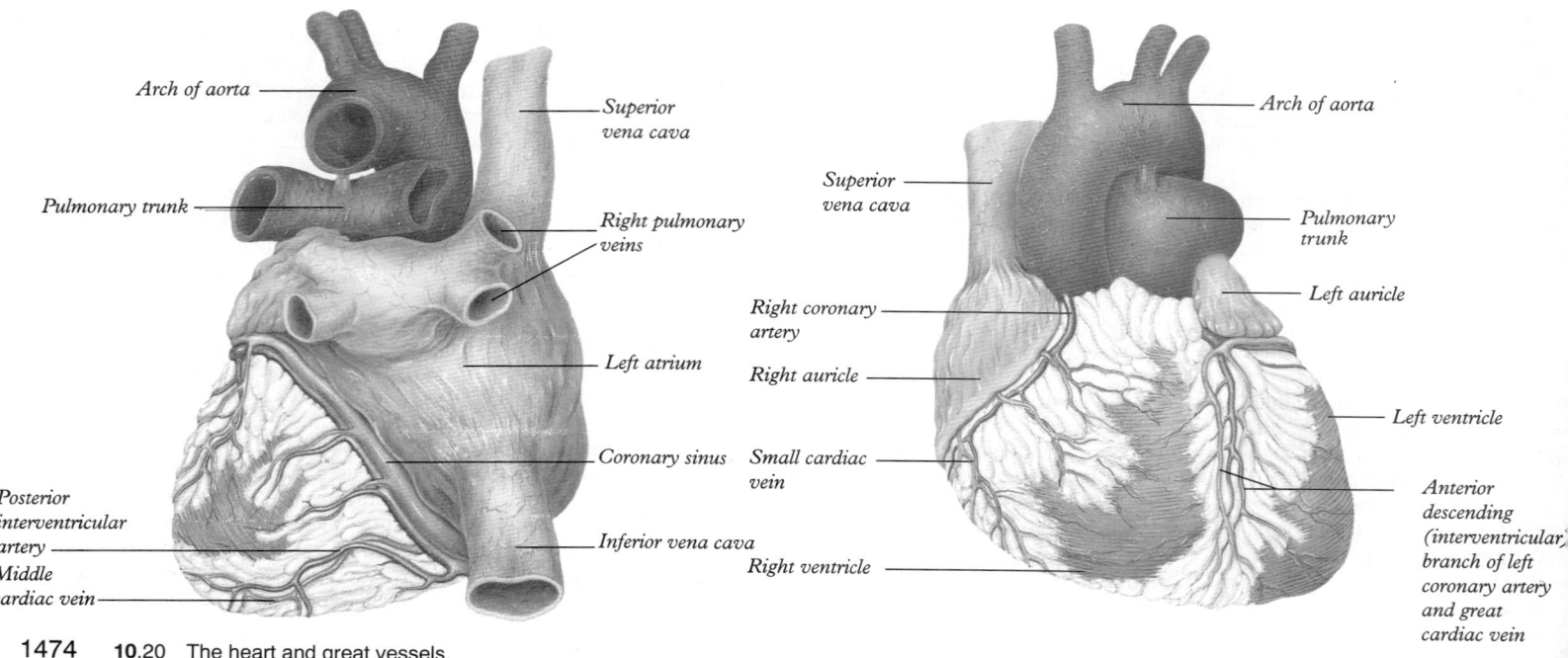

10.20 The heart and great vessels.

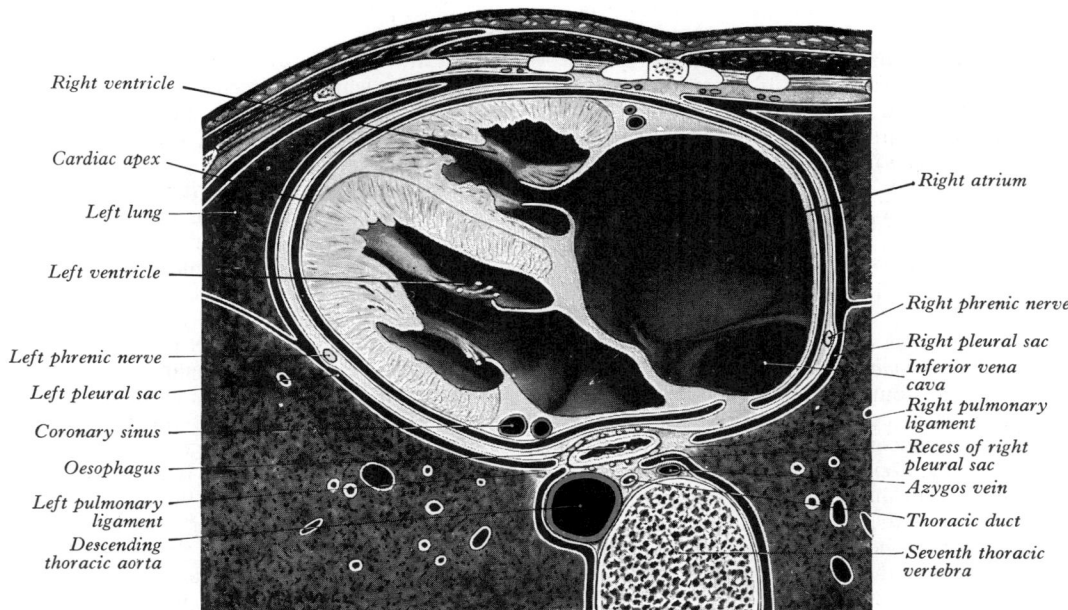

Right ventricle

Cardiac apex

Left lung

Left ventricle

Left phrenic nerve

Left pleural sac

Coronary sinus

Oesophagus

Left pulmonary ligament

Descending thoracic aorta

Right atrium

Right phrenic nerve

Right pleural sac

Inferior vena cava

Right pulmonary ligament

Recess of right pleural sac

Azygos vein

Thoracic duct

Seventh thoracic vertebra

10.21 Transverse section through the mediastinum at the level of the body of the seventh thoracic vertebra, viewed from above. Note the general disposition of cardiac cavities, their intervening septa (about 45° to sagittal and coronal planes) and, orthogonal to this, the plane of the atrioventricular valves. The oesophageal plexus of nerves is clear but not labelled.

planes of the left ventricular orifices, though relatively inclined, are more nearly coplanar than those of the right. The left ventricular cavity is narrow and conical, with its tip occupying the cardiac apex. Most of the base of the heart is made up of the left atrium.

The heart is placed **obliquely** in the thorax (**10.28**). The atrial and ventricular septal structures are virtually in line but inclined forwards and to the left at about 45° to a sagittal plane. The planes of the mitral and tricuspid valves, though vertical and not precisely coplanar, are broadly at right angles to the septal plane. The right atrium, therefore, is not only to the right but also anterior and inferior to the left atrium. It is also partly anterior to the left ventricle, an important atrioventricular septum intervening. The right ventricle forms most of the anterior aspect of the ventricular mass (**10.27**), only its inferior end being to the right of the left ventricle, its upper left extremity (pulmonary orifice) being to the left and superior relative to the aortic valve. The left atrium forms most of the posterior aspect of the heart, while the left ventricle is only prominent inferiorly, running along the left margin to reach the apex. The atria are essentially right of and posterior to their respective ventricles. These general dispositions are of the greatest importance in planning or interpreting radiographs, scans, angiocardiograms and echocardiograms.

CARDIAC SIZE, SHAPE AND EXTERNAL FEATURES

The heart is a hollow, fibromuscular organ of a somewhat conical or pyramidal form, with a base, apex and a series of surfaces and 'borders'. Enclosed in the pericardium (**10.**19, 21, 22), it occupies the middle mediastinum between the lungs and their pleural coverings. It is placed obliquely behind the body of the sternum and the adjoining costal cartilages and ribs (**10.**25A, B, 28). Approximately one-third of the mass lies to the right of the midline.

An average adult heart is about 12 cm from base to apex, 8–9 cm at its broadest transverse diameter and 6 cm anteroposteriorly. Its weight varies from 280–340 g (average 300 g) in males and from 230–280 g (average 250 g) in females. Cardiac weight is said to be about 0.45% of body weight in males and 0.40% in females (Hudson 1965). Adult weight is achieved between the ages of 17 and 20 years. The oblique position of the heart may be emphasized by comparing it to a rather deformed pyramid, with the base facing posteriorly and to

the right, and the apex anteriorly and to the left. A line from the apex to the approximate centre of the base, projected posterolaterally, emerges near the right midscapular line. Some surfaces of the cardiac 'pyramid' are flat, others more or less convex, these aspects merging along rather ill-defined 'borders'. Precise definition of surfaces and intervening 'borders' is, therefore, difficult. In the account which follows, official nomenclature (*Nomina Anatomica* 1989) and more generally used terms from clinical practice are given as alternatives. The heart is described as having a base and apex, its **surfaces** being designated as sternocostal (anterior); diaphragmatic (inferior); and right and left (pulmonary). Its borders are termed upper, inferior

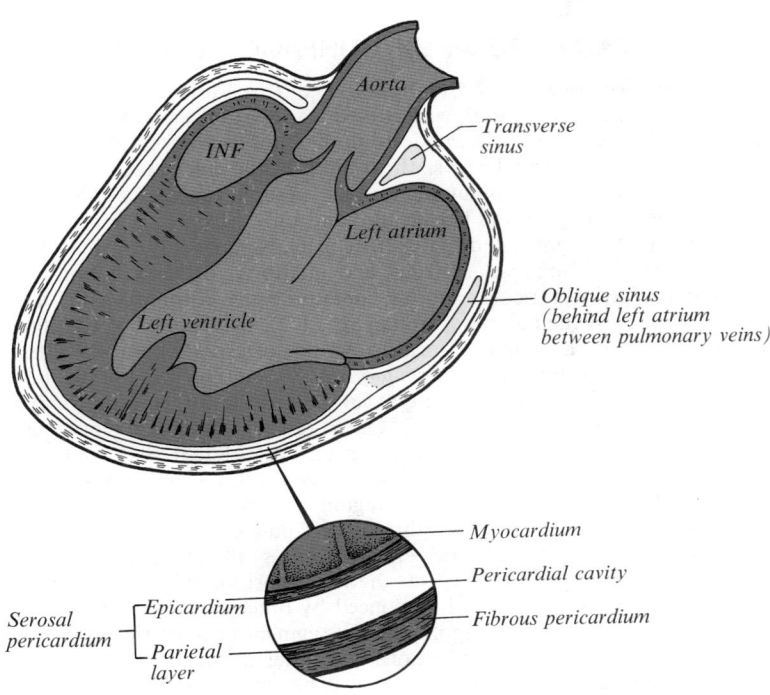

Aorta

Transverse sinus

INF

Left atrium

Oblique sinus (behind left atrium between pulmonary veins)

Left ventricle

Myocardium

Pericardial cavity

Epicardium

Serosal pericardium

Fibrous pericardium

Parietal layer

10.22 The arrangement of the layers of the pericardium, and the location of the two sinuses within the pericardial cavity.

('acute' margin or border) and left ('obtuse' margin or border). Some name the right surface a 'border', despite its extent. One avoidable source of confusion is the use of 'posterior', which can be replaced with the unambiguous term 'diaphragmatic'. If posterior is to be used for a cardiac surface, it should be reserved for the base. But, compounding this difficulty, there are a number of different usages of the term 'cardiac base' (see below).

GROOVES ON THE CARDIAC SURFACES

The division of the heart into four chambers produces boundaries visible externally as grooves or sulci. Some are deep and obvious and contain prominent structures. Others are less distinct, even barely perceptible, and are sometimes obscured, in part, by the major structures crossing them. The *coronary*, or *atrioventricular, groove* (or *sulcus*) separates the atria from the ventricles. This groove, containing the main trunks of the coronary arteries, is oblique. It descends to the right on the sternocostal surface (10.27), separating the right atrium (and its auricular appendage) from the oblique right margin of the right ventricle and its infundibulum. Its upper left part is obliterated where it is crossed by the pulmonary trunk and, behind this, the aorta from which originate the coronary arteries. Continuing to the left, the groove curves around the 'obtuse margin' and descends to the right, separating the atrial base from the diaphragmatic surface of the ventricles (10.32). This diaphragmatic part of the coronary groove then curves around the 'acute margin' at its lower right end to become confluent with the sternocostal part. Thus, the groove passes from high on the left to low on the right, with the diaphragmatic part being a little to the left of the sternocostal. A section which includes the coronary groove is at about 45° to the sagittal plane and at a greater but variable angle to the transverse and coronal planes. It approximately traverses the lines of attachment of the atrioventricular valves and (even less precisely) those of the aortic and pulmonary valves. A line at right angles to the centre of this plane will descend forwards and leftwards to the cardiac apex.

Internally, the ventricles are separated by the septum (pp. 1480, 1483), the mural margins of which correspond to the anterior and inferior (diaphragmatic) interventricular grooves. The anterior groove, seen on the sternocostal cardiac surface, is near and almost parallel to the left ventricular obtuse margin. On the diaphragmatic surface, in contrast, the groove is closer to the midpoint of the ventricular mass. The interventricular grooves extend from the coronary groove to the apical notch on the acute margin. This is a little to the right of the true cardiac apex.

CARDIAC BASE, APEX, SURFACES, BORDERS

Posterior aspect of the heart. The true *cardiac base*, this is somewhat quadrilateral, with curved lateral extensions. It faces back and to the right, separated from the thoracic vertebrae (fifth to eighth in the recumbent, sixth to ninth in the erect posture) by the pericardium, right pulmonary veins, oesophagus and aorta. It is formed mainly by the left atrium, and only partly by the posterior part of the right atrium (10.32). It extends superiorly to the bifurcation of the pulmonary trunk and inferiorly to the posterior part of the atrioventricular groove containing the coronary sinus and branches of the coronary arteries (p. 1477). It is limited to the right and left by the rounded surfaces of the corresponding atria. These are separated by the shallow *interatrial groove*. The point of junction of the atrioventricular, interatrial and posterior interventricular grooves is termed the *crux of the heart* (10.32). Two pulmonary veins on each side open into the left atrial part of the base, while the superior and the inferior vena cava open into the upper and lower parts of the right atrial basal region. The area of the left atrium between the openings of right and left pulmonary veins forms the anterior wall of the oblique pericardial sinus (10.19). This description of the anatomical base reflects the usual position of the heart in the thorax. Some confusion is produced by other current usages of the term 'base'. It is often applied to the segment of the atrioventricular and ventriculo-arterial junctions seen after dissections through the coronary groove (10.31). This area is better termed the base of the ventricles. In clinical practice, auscultation in or near the parasternal parts of the second intercostal spaces is often described as occurring at the *clinical 'base'*, to make the contrast with the *clinical 'apex'*.

Such descriptions, while less than perfect anatomically, will almost certainly persist.

Anatomical apex of the heart. This is the apex of the conical left ventricle, which is directed down, forwards and to the left. The left lung and pleura overlap it. It is located most commonly behind the fifth left intercostal space, near or a little medial to the midclavicular line.

Anterior, sternocostal surface of the heart (10.26, 27). Facing forwards and upwards, this has an acute right and a more gradual left convexity. It consists of an atrial area above and to the right, and a ventricular part below and to the left of the atrioventricular groove. The atrial area is occupied almost entirely by the right atrium. The left atrium is largely hidden by the ascending aorta and pulmonary trunk. Only a small part of the left appendage projects forwards to the left of the pulmonary trunk. Of the ventricular region, about one-third is made up by the left and two-thirds by the right ventricle. The site of the septum between them is indicated by the anterior interventricular groove. The sternocostal surface is separated by the pericardium from the body of the sternum, the sternocostal muscles and the third to the sixth costal cartilages. Owing to the bulge of the heart to the left, more of this surface is behind the left costal cartilages than behind the right ones. It is also covered by the pleural membranes and by the thin, anterior edges of the lungs, except for a triangular area at the cardiac incisure of the left lung. The lungs and their pleural coverings are variable in their degree of overlap of the heart.

Inferior, diaphragmatic surface of the heart (10.32). Largely horizontal, it slopes down and forwards a little towards the apex. It is formed by the ventricles (chiefly the left) and rests mainly upon the central tendon but also, apically, on a small area of the left muscular part of the diaphragm. It is separated from the anatomic base by the atrioventricular groove and is traversed obliquely by the posterior interventricular groove.

Left surface of the heart. Facing up, back and to the left, this consists almost entirely of the obtuse margin of the left ventricle, but has a small part of the left atrium and its auricle contributing superiorly. Convex and widest above, and crossed here by the atrioventricular groove, it narrows to the cardiac apex. It is separated by the pericardium from the left phrenic nerve and its accompanying vessels, and by the left pleura from the deep concavity of the left lung.

Right surface of the heart. A rounded surface is formed by the right atrial wall and is separated from the mediastinal aspect of the right lung by the pericardium and the pleural coverings. Its convexity merges below into the short intrathoracic part of the inferior vena cava and above into the superior vena cava. The *terminal groove* (*sulcus terminalis*) is a prominent landmark between the true atrial and the venous components of the right atrium, curving approximately along the junction of the sternocostal and right surfaces (10.29).

Upper border of the heart. This is atrial (mainly the left atrium). Anterior to it are the ascending aorta and the pulmonary trunk (10.19). At its extremity the superior vena cava enters the right atrium.

Right border of the heart. Corresponding to the right atrium, its profile is slightly convex to the right and it approaches the vertical.

Inferior border of the heart. Also known as the *acute margin* of the heart, it is sharp, thin and nearly horizontal. It extends from the lower limit of the right border to the apex and it is formed mainly by the right ventricle, with a small contribution from the left ventricle near the apex.

Left border of the heart. Also known as the *obtuse margin*, it separates the sternocostal and left surfaces. It is round and mainly formed by the left ventricle but, to a slight extent superiorly, is formed by the auricle of the left atrium. It descends obliquely, convex to the left, from the auricle to the cardiac apex.

CARDIAC CHAMBERS AND INTERNAL FEATURES

The right and left chambers of the heart will be described in sequence in terms of their general form, their walls and their internal features. The two sides have much in common, such as the structure of valvar leaflets, tendinous cords, and papillary muscles of atrioventricular (inlet) valves, and the architecture of the cusps of the pulmonary and aortic (outlet) valves. Repetition, as far as possible, will be kept to a minimum.

RIGHT ATRIUM

General and external features

The *interatrial septum* (or *atrial septum*) is oblique, so the right atrium is anterior as well as to the right of the left atrium (**10**.27, 32), also extending inferior to it. Its walls form the right upper sternocostal surface, the convex right (pulmonary surface) and a little of the right side of the anatomic base. The superior vena cava opens into its dome and the inferior vena cava into its lower posterior part (**10**.27). An extensive muscular pouch, the *auricle* or appendage, projects anteriorly to overlap the right side of the ascending aorta. The auricle is a broad, triangular structure and has a wide junction with the true atrial component of the atrium (**10**.23A, 29). The junction between the venous part (*sinus venarum*) and the atrium proper is marked externally by a shallow groove, the *sulcus terminalis*, extending between the right sides of the openings of the two venae cavae. The sulcus terminalis corresponds, internally, to the terminal crest (*crista terminalis*) which is the site of origin of the extensive pectinate muscles arising serially at right angles from the crest (**10**.33). Posteriorly, the vertical interatrial groove descends to the crux.

Anteriorly, the right atrium is related to the anterior part of the mediastinal surface of the right lung, separated from it by pleura and pericardium. **Laterally**, the atrium is also related to the mediastinal surface of the right lung, but anterior to its hilum and separated from it by the pleura, right phrenic nerve and pericardiacophrenic vessels and pericardium. **Posteriorly** and to the left (**10**.32, 35), the atrial septum and the surrounding infolded atrial walls separate the right from the left atrium (the mural infolding being indicated by the extensive interatrial groove). Posteriorly and to the right are the right pulmonary veins. **Medially** are the ascending aorta and, to a lesser extent, the root of the pulmonary trunk and its bifurcation.

Interior surface of the right atrium (**10**.24, 34). The interior surface can be divided into three regions: a smooth-walled venous component, posteriorly, leading, anteriorly, to the vestibule of the tricuspid valve and the auricle. The wall of the vestibule is smooth, but its junction with the auricle is ridged all around the atrioventricular junction. The smooth-walled part receives the opening of the venae cavae and the coronary sinus. It represents the venous component ('sinus venosus') of the developing heart (p. 303). The wall of the vestibule has a ridged surface and that of the auricle is trabeculated; both are derived from the embryonic atrium proper.

Opening into the venous component are the *superior vena cava* returning blood from head, neck and upper limb through an orifice which faces infero-anteriorly and has no valve, and the *inferior vena cava*. The latter vessel is larger than its superior counterpart and returns blood from the lower part of the body into the lowest part of the atrium near the septum. Anterior to its orifice is a flap-like valve, the *Eustachian valve* or valve of the inferior vena cava (**10**.33). Of varying size, this valve is found along the lateral, or right, margin of the vein. When traced inferiorly, it runs into the sinus septum (see below) where it is contiguous with the valve of the coronary sinus (*Thebesius' valve*, also known as the *Thebesian valve*). The lateral part of the Eustachian valve becomes continuous with the lower end of the terminal crest. The valve is a fold of endocardium enclosing a few muscular fibres. It is large during fetal life, when it serves to direct richly oxygenated blood from the placenta through the oval foramen of the atrial septum into the left atrium. The valve varies markedly in size in postnatal life, sometimes being cribriform or filamentous but often being absent. A particularly prominent recess is seen postero-inferiorly relative to the orifice of the coronary sinus (see below). This is the *postEustachian sinus*.

Also opening into the venous atrial component is the coronary sinus. This vessel returns the majority of blood from the heart itself, opening between the orifice or the inferior vena cava, the oval fossa and the vestibule of the atrioventricular opening (**10**.33). The coronary sinus is often guarded by a thin, semicircular valve which covers the lower part of the orifice (Thebesius' valve). The upper limb of this valve joins with the Eustachian valve and, from this commissure, a tendinous structure runs into the sinus septum (the septum between the coronary sinus and the oval fossa). The tendinous structure, called the *tendon of Todaro*, runs forwards to insert into the central fibrous body. It is one of the landmarks of the triangle of Koch (**10**.36 see below).

The orifice of the coronary sinus forms a prominent landmark in the right atrium (**10**.33). The sinus itself, however, lies within the left atrioventricular groove (**10**.32). It is the conduit for return of most of the venous blood from the heart, although some atrial veins drain directly to the right or left atrial chambers. The coronary sinus commences at the point where the oblique vein of the left atrium joins. The sinus receives the middle and small cardiac veins close to its junction with the right atrium.

Multiple small venous orifices, draining the minimal atrial veins, are found scattered around the atrial walls. They return a small

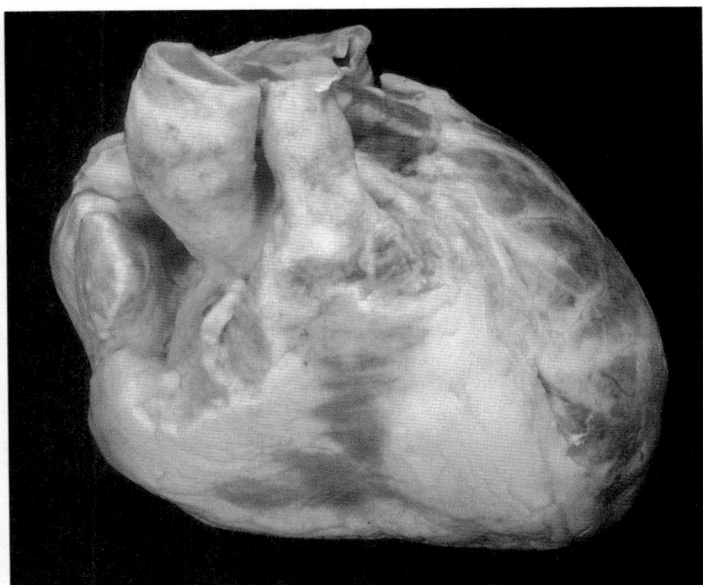

10.23A. The anterior surface of the removed heart oriented so that it lies, as far as possible, in its position within the body.

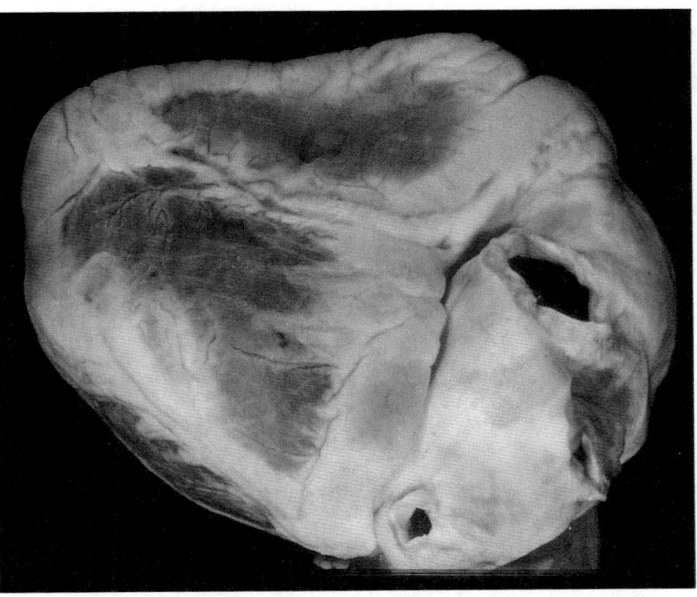

B. The posterior surface of the removed heart, oriented to take its position within the body.

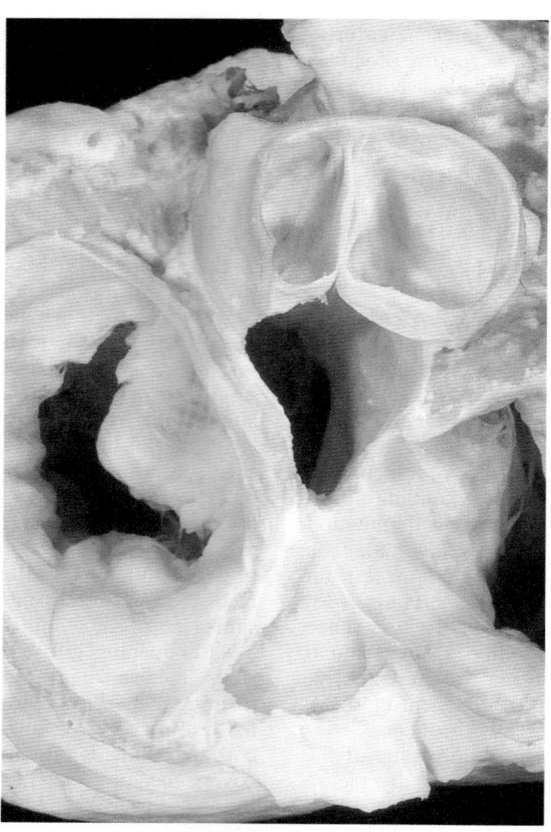

10.24 This dissection shows the crucial relation between subaortic outflow tract and ventricular inlet components, as shown in **10.**25. The non-coronary sinus of the aorta, with its corresponding aortic valvar cusp, has been removed.

fraction of blood from the heart (p. 1575), being most numerous on the septal aspect. The anterior cardiac veins and, sometimes, the right marginal vein may enter the atrium through larger orifices (p. 1576).

The atrium proper and the auricle are separated from the venous sinus by the *terminal crest* (*crista terminalis*). This smooth, muscular ridge begins on the upper part of the septal surface and, passing anterior to the orifice of the superior vena cava, skirts its right margin to reach the right side of the orifice of the inferior vena cava (**10.**33). It marks the site of the right venous valve of the embryonic heart (p. 303), and corresponds externally to the terminal groove

(p. 1477). Within the superior part of the groove, lateral to, and extending below, the orifice of the superior vena cava, is found the sinus node (p. 1496).

The *pectinate muscles* (*musculi pectinati*), almost parallel muscular ridges, extend anterolaterally from the terminal crest and reach into the auricle, where they form multiple trabeculations.

The septal wall presents the *oval fossa* (*fossa ovalis*), an oval depression found above and to the left of the orifice of the inferior vena cava. Its floor is the *primary atrial septum*, the '*septum primum*' (p. 303). The rim of the fossa is prominent and, although often said to represent the edge of the so-called '*septum secundum*' (p. 304), in

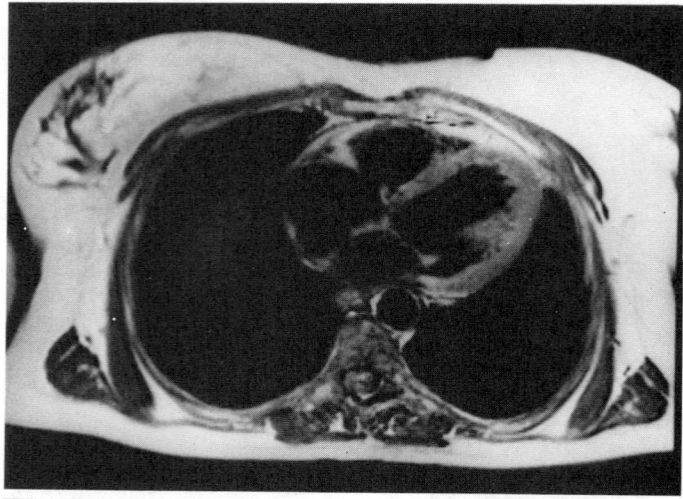

A

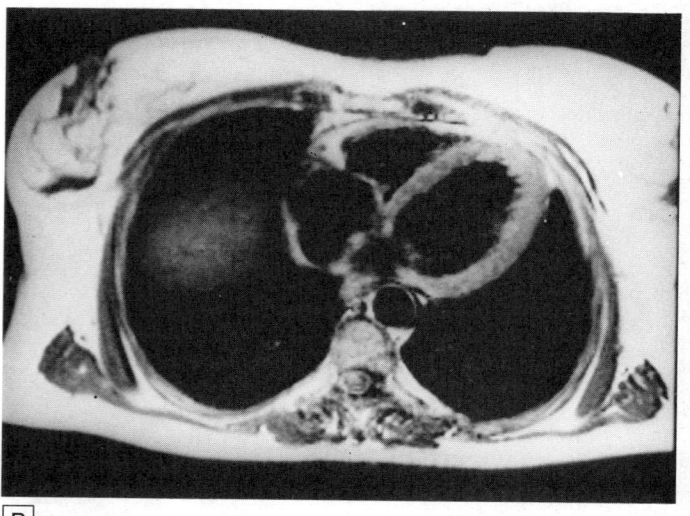

B

10.25 Computed tomograms of the thorax. A. Through the body of the seventh thoracic vertebra. B. Through the intervertebral disc between the seventh and eighth vertebrae. Note the overall disposition of the heart, its apex, base, oblique, interatrial and interventricular septa and, orthogonal to this, of the atrioventricular valves. Note also the atrioventricular septum, papillary muscles, trabeculae carneae, descending thoracic aorta and contrasting areas of right and left lungs and pleurae. (Provided by Shaun Gallagher, Guy's Hospital; photography by Sarah Smith.)

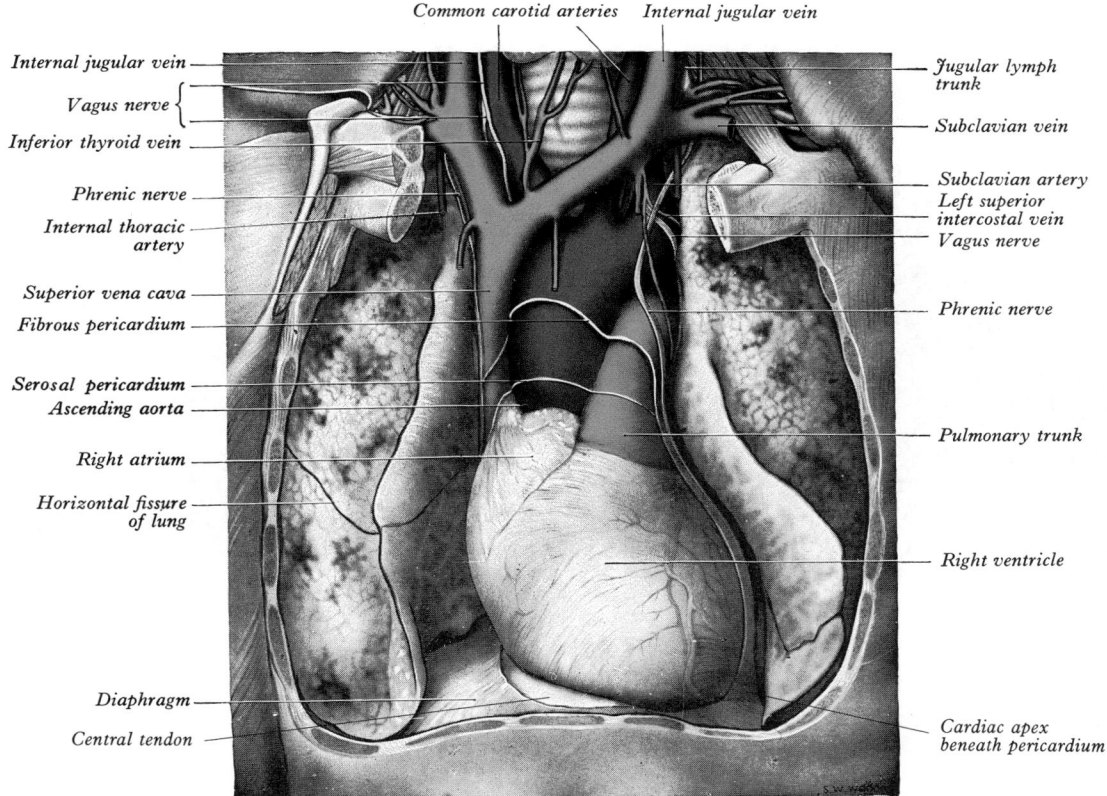

Common carotid arteries   *Internal jugular vein*

Internal jugular vein

Vagus nerve {

Inferior thyroid vein

Phrenic nerve

Internal thoracic artery

Superior vena cava

Fibrous pericardium

Serosal pericardium

Ascending aorta

Right atrium

Horizontal fissure of lung

Diaphragm

Central tendon

Jugular lymph trunk

Subclavian vein

Subclavian artery

Left superior intercostal vein

Vagus nerve

Phrenic nerve

Pulmonary trunk

Right ventricle

Cardiac apex beneath pericardium

10.26   Dissection which displays the heart, the great vessels and the lungs in situ. The sternum and the sternal ends of the costal cartilages, together with the parietal pleura on each side, have been excised and the mediastinal pleura and parietal layer of the pericardium over the sternocostal surface of the heart have been removed. The lungs have been displaced to expose the heart and the epicardium dissected off the heart and roots of the great vessels. On the right side, the inferior cardiac branch of the vagus nerve descends between the brachiocephalic artery and the right brachiocephalic vein. On the left side, a communication descends from the left superior intercostal vein and crosses the aortic arch and the left pulmonary artery to become continuous with the oblique vein of the left atrium.

reality it is merely the infolded walls of the atrial chambers. It is most distinct above and in front of the fossa, usually being deficient inferiorly. A small slit is sometimes found at the upper margin of the fossa, ascending beneath the rim to communicate with the left atrium. This represents failure of obliteration of the fetal oval foramen, which remains patent in up to one-third of all normal hearts.

Antero-inferior in the right atrium is the large, oval vestibule leading to the orifice of the tricuspid valve. A triangular zone (the *triangle of Koch*, **10.36**) is found between the attachment of the septal leaflet of the tricuspid valve, the anteromedial margin of the orifice of the coronary sinus, and the round, collagenous, palpable, sub-endocardial tendon of Todaro. The triangle is a landmark of particular surgical import, indicating the site of the atrioventricular node and its atrial connections (p. 1499). Anterosuperior to the insertion of the *tendon of Todaro*, the septal wall is the **atrioventricular** component of the *membranous septum*, intervening between the right atrium and subaortic outlet of the left ventricle (**10.36**). The atrial

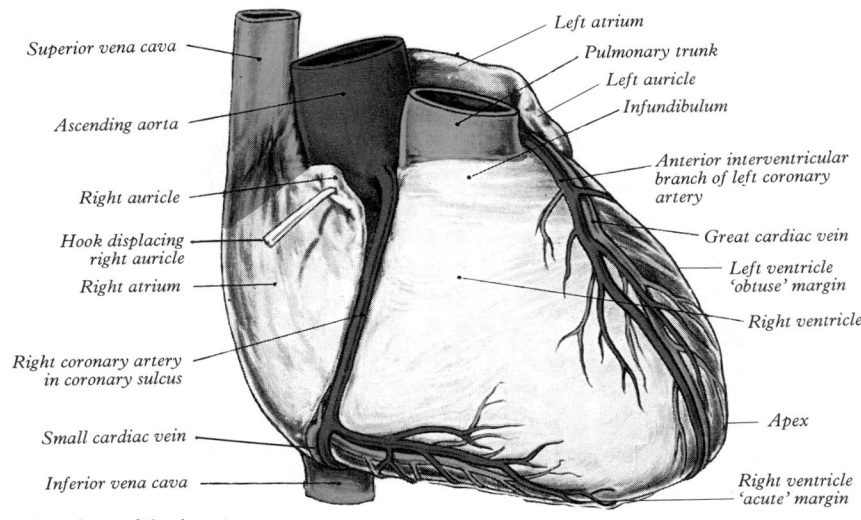

Superior vena cava

Ascending aorta

Right auricle

Hook displacing right auricle

Right atrium

Right coronary artery in coronary sulcus

Small cardiac vein

Inferior vena cava

Left atrium

Pulmonary trunk

Left auricle

Infundibulum

Anterior interventricular branch of left coronary artery

Great cardiac vein

Left ventricle 'obtuse' margin

Right ventricle

Apex

Right ventricle 'acute' margin

10.27   The anterior or sternocostal surface of the heart.

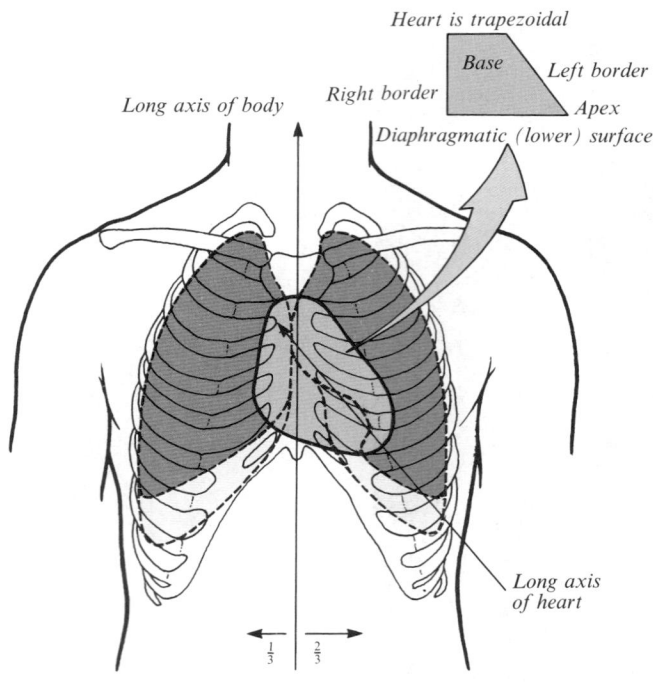

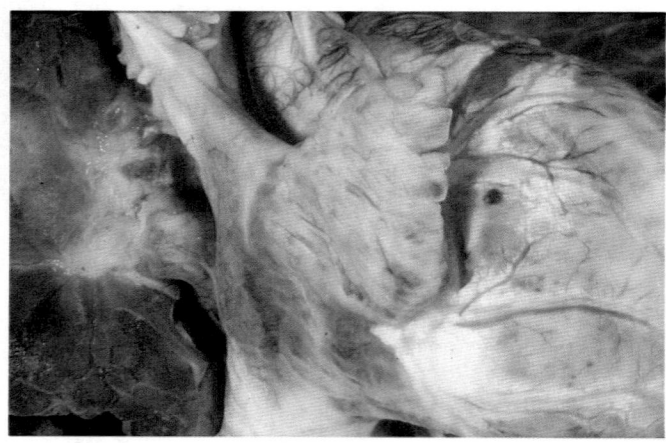

10.28 The front of the thorax, showing the surface relations of the bones, lungs (purple), pleurae (blue) and heart (red outline). Compare **10.46** for further cardiac detail.

10.29 Removal of the pericardium shows the right margin of the heart, made up mostly of the right atrium. Note the characteristic terminal groove (sulcus terminalis).

wall bulges anterosuperiorly above the membranous septum. This area is the aortic mound (*torus aorticus*) and marks the location of the non-coronary sinus of the aorta with its enclosed valvar cusp (p. 1488).

RIGHT VENTRICLE

The right ventricle extends from the right atrioventricular (tricuspid) orifice nearly to the cardiac apex. It then ascends to the left to become the *infundibulum*, or *conus arteriosus*, reaching the pulmonary orifice and supporting the cusps of the pulmonary valve. Topographically, the ventricle possesses: an inlet component, supporting and surrounding the tricuspid valve; a coarsely trabeculated apical component; and the muscular outlet or infundibulum surrounding the attachments of the cusps of the pulmonary valve (**10.37A**).

External features

The convex *anterosuperior surface* makes up a large part of the sternocostal aspect of the heart (**10.23A**), separated from the thoracic wall only by the pericardium. The left pleura and, to a lesser extent, the anterior margin of the left lung are interposed above and to the left. The *inferior surface* is flat and is related mainly, with the interposition of the pericardium, to the central tendon and a small adjoining muscular part of the diaphragm. The *left* and *posterior wall* is the ventricular septum. This is slightly curved and bulges into the right ventricle so that, in sections across the cardiac axis, the outline of the right ventricle is crescentic (**10.38**). A delicate collagenous band, the tendon of the infundibulum (conus ligament), is held by some to connect the pulmonary muscular infundibulum posteriorly to the root of the aorta. The wall of the right ventricle is significantly thinner (3–5 mm on average) than that of the left, the ratio usually being about 1 to 3.

Internal features

The inlet and outlet components of the ventricle, supporting and

surrounding the leaflets of the tricuspid and pulmonary valves respectively, are separated in the roof of the ventricle (**10.31**) by the prominent *supraventricular crest* (*crista supraventricularis*). The crest is a thick, muscular, highly arched structure, extending obliquely forwards and to the right from a *septal limb* high on the interventricular septal wall to a *mural* or *parietal limb* on the anterolateral right ventricular wall. The posterolateral aspect of the crest provides a principal attachment for the anterosuperior leaflet of the tricuspid valve (see below). The crest's septal limb may be continuous with, or embraced by, the septal limbs of the septomarginal trabecula (see below). The inlet and outlet regions extend apically into and from the prominent coarsely trabeculated component of the ventricle. The inlet component is itself also trabeculated, whereas the outlet component (or infundibulum) has predominantly smooth walls. The trabeculated appearance is due to myriad irregular muscular ridges and protrusions, which are known collectively as *trabeculae carnae*, and are lined by endocardium. These protrusions and intervening grooves impart great variation in wall thickness. Protrusions vary in extent from mere ridges to trabeculae which are fixed at both ends but free in-between. Other conspicuous protrusions are the papillary muscles, which are inserted at one end onto the ventricular wall and are continuous at the other end with collagenous cords, the chordae tendineae, inserted on the free edge and elsewhere on the free aspect of the atrioventricular valves (p. 148). One protrusion in the right ventricle, the *septomarginal trabecula* or septal band, is particularly prominent. It reinforces the septal surface where, at the base, it divides into limbs which embrace the supraventricular crest. Towards the apex, it supports the anterior papillary muscle of the tricuspid valve and, from this point, crosses to the parietal wall of the ventricle as the 'moderator band' (this alternative name records an old idea that the septomarginal trabecula prevents overdistension of the ventricle). A further series of prominent trabeculae extend from its anterior surface and run onto the parietal ventricular wall. These are the septoparietal trabeculations (**10.37A**). The smooth-walled *outflow tract*, or *infundibulum* (*conus arteriosus*), ascends to the left

above the septoparietal trabeculations and **below** the arch of the supraventricular crest to the pulmonary orifice.

TRICUSPID VALVE

The atrioventricular valvar complex, in both right and left ventricles, comprises the following:

- the orifice and its associated annulus
- the leaflets
- the supporting *tendinous cords* (*chordae tendineae*) of various types
- the papillary muscles.

Harmonious interplay of all these, together with the atrial and ventricular myocardial masses (p. 1494), depends on the conduction tissues (p. 1495) along with the mechanical cohesion provided by the fibro-elastic cardiac skeleton. All parts change substantially in position, shape, angulation and dimensions during a single cardiac cycle.

Tricuspid valvar orifice

The largest valvar orifice (circumference of around 11.4 cm in males and 10.8 cm in females according to Silver et al 1971), it is best seen from its atrial aspect (**10.31**). It has a clear line of transition from the atrial wall or septum to the lines of attachment of the valvar leaflets. Its margins are not precisely in a single plane; at a near approximation it is almost vertical but at about 45° to the sagittal plane and slightly inclined to the vertical, such that it 'faces' (on its ventricular aspect) anterolaterally to the left and somewhat inferiorly (**10.46**). Roughly triangular, its margins are described as antero-superior, inferior and septal, corresponding to the lines of attachment of the valvar leaflets.

The *annulus* of the tricuspid valve is an ill-defined term used without uniformity. Elementary accounts often describe all four valvar orifices as surrounded by uniform rings of collagenous tissue, the rings interconnected by dense masses of collagen which, in the mitral and tricuspid valves, are situated precisely at the atrioventricular junctions (presumed also to separate the atrial and ventricular myocardial masses). Only some of these assumptions are true. The connective tissues around the orifice of the atrioventricular valves, while serving to separate atrial and ventricular myocardial masses completely except at the point of penetration of the atrioventricular bundle, vary in density and disposition around the valvar circumference. Extending from the right fibrous trigone component of the central fibrous body are a pair of curved, tapered, subendocardial tendons, or 'prongs' (*fila coronaria*) which partly encircle the circumference; the latter is completed by more tenuous, deformable fibroblastic sulcar areolar tissue. The extent of fibrous tissue also varies with sex and age (Walmsley & Watson 1978). Nevertheless, the tissue within the atrioventricular junction around the tricuspid orifice is less robust than similar elements found at the attachments of the mitral valve (p. 1485). Furthermore, in the tricuspid valve, the topographical 'attachment' of the free valvar leaflets does not wholly correspond to the internal level of attachment of the fibrous core of the valve to the junctional atrioventricular connective tissue. It is the line of attachment of the leaflet which is best appreciated in the heart when examined grossly, and this feature is also more readily discerned clinically.

Tricuspid valve leaflets

It is usually possible to distinguish three leaflets in the tricuspid valve, hence the name. They are located septally, antero-superiorly and inferiorly, corresponding to the marginal sectors of the atrioventricular orifice so named. Each is a reduplication of endocardium enclosing a collagenous core, continuous marginally and on its ventricular aspect with diverging fascicles of tendinous cords (see below) and basally confluent with the annular connective tissue. All leaflets of the atrioventricular valves display, passing from the free margin to the inserted margin, *rough*, *clear* and *basal zones*. The rough zone is relatively thick, opaque and uneven on its ventricular aspect where most tendinous cords are attached. The atrial aspect of the rough zone makes contact with the comparable surface of the adjacent leaflets during full closure of the valve. The clear zone is smooth and translucent, receives few tendinous cords and has a thinner fibrous core. The basal zone, extending about 2–3 mm from

the circumferential attachment of the leaflets, is thicker, contains more connective tissue and is vascularized and innervated, containing the insertions of the atrial myocardium.

The *anterosuperior leaflet* is the largest component of the tricuspid valve (**10.37B**). It is attached chiefly to the atrioventricular junction on the posterolateral aspect of the supraventricular crest, but extends along its septal limb to the membranous septum, ending at the *anteroseptal commissure*. One or more notches often indent its free margin. The attachment of the *septal leaflet* passes from the *inferoseptal commissure* on the posterior ventricular wall across the muscular septum and then angles across the membranous septum to the anteroseptal commissure. The *inferior leaflet* is wholly mural in attachment and guards the diaphragmatic surface of the atrioventricular junction; its limits are the inferoseptal and *antero-inferior commissures*.

Tendinous cords (chordae tendineae)

The tendinous cords are fibrous collagenous structures supporting the leaflets of the atrioventricular valves. *False chordae* connecting papillary muscles to each other or to the ventricular wall including the septum, or passing directly between points on the wall (and/or septum), are irregular in numbers and dimensions in the right ventricle. The true chordae usually arise from small projections on the tips or margins of the apical thirds of papillary muscles, but sometimes from the bases of papillary muscles or directly from the ventricular walls and the septum. They are attached to various parts of the ventricular aspects or the free margins of the leaflets. They were classified by Tandler (1913) into first, second and third order chordae according to the distance of the attachment from the margins of the leaflets. Subsequent authors have usually followed this classification, although the scheme has little functional or morphological merit. According to their morphology, nonetheless, it is possible to distinguish several patterns (Lam et al 1970; Silver et al 1971).

Fan-shaped chordae have a short stem from which branches radiate to attach to the margins (or the ventricular aspect) of the zones of apposition between leaflets and to the ends of adjacent leaflets (**10.37A, B**). *Rough zone chordae* arise from a single stem which usually splits into three components which attach to the free margin, the ventricular aspect of the rough zone and to some intermediate point on the leaflet, respectively. *Free edge chordae* are single, threadlike and often long, passing from either the apex or the base of a papillary muscle into a marginal attachment, usually near the midpoint of a leaflet or one of its scallops. *Deep chordae*, also long, pass beyond the margins and, branching to various extents, reach the more peripheral rough zone or even the clear zone. *Basal chordae* are round chordae or flat ribbons, long and slender or short and muscular. They arise from the smooth or trabeculated ventricular wall and attach to the basal component of a leaflet.

Papillary muscles

The two major papillary muscles in the right ventricle are located in anterior and posterior positions; a third, smaller muscle has a medial position along with several smaller, and variable, muscles attached to the ventricular septum. The *anterior papillary muscle* is largest. Its base arises from the right anterolateral ventricular wall below the antero-inferior commissure of the inferior leaflet and it also blends with the right end of the septomarginal trabecula. The *posterior*, or *inferior*, *papillary muscle* arises from the myocardium below the inferoseptal commissure. It is frequently bifid or trifid. The *septal*, or *medial*, *papillary muscle* is small but typical, and arises from the posterior septal limb of the septomarginal trabecula. All the major papillary muscles supply chordae to **adjacent** components of the leaflets they support. A feature of the right ventricle, however, is that the septal leaflet is tethered by individual tendinous chordae directly to the ventricular septum. Such septal insertions are never seen in the left ventricle. When closed, the three leaflets fit snugly together, the pattern of the zones of apposition confirming the trifoliate arrangement of the tricuspid valve.

PULMONARY VALVE

The pulmonary valve, guarding the outflow from the right ventricle, surmounts the infundibulum and is situated at some distance from the other three cardiac valves (**10**.51, 52). Its general plane faces superiorly to the left and slightly posteriorly. It has three *semilunar leaflets* or *cusps* attached by convex edges partly to the infundibular wall of the right ventricle and partly to the commencement of the pulmonary trunk; the line of attachments is curved, rising at the periphery of each cusp near their zones of apposition (the *commissures*) and reaching the sinutubular ridge of the pulmonary trunk (**10**.43A). Removal of the cusps shows that the fibrous semilunar attachments enclose three crescents of infundibular musculature within the pulmonary sinuses, while three roughly triangular segments of arterial wall are incorporated within the ventricular outflow tract beneath the apex of each commissural attachment (**10**.43A). There is, thus, no proper circular 'annulus' supporting the leaflets of the valve, the *fibrous semilunar attachment* being an essential requisite for snug closure of the nodules and lunules of the cusps (see below) during ventricular diastole. It is difficult precisely to name the cusps and corresponding sinuses of the pulmonary valve and trunk according to the co-ordinates of the body since the valvar orifice is obliquely positioned. The official nomenclature (*Nomina Anatomica* 1989) refers to an *anterior*, a *posterior* and a *septal* cusp, based on their position in the fetus. The position changes with development and in the adult there are two *anterior* cusps, *right* and *left*, and a *posterior* one.

Each cusp is a fold of endocardium, with an intervening, and variably developed, fibrous core. The core is substantial along both the free edge and the semilunar attached border, and the latter is particularly thickened at the deepest central part (nadir) of the base of each cusp (thus never forming a simple complete fibrous ring). Central in the free margin of each cusp is a localized thickening of collagen, the *nodule of Arantius*. Perforations within the cusps close to the free margin and near the commissures are frequently present but of no functional significance. Each semilunar cusp is contained within one of the three sinuses of the pulmonary trunk. Except for differences in relations of timing and pressures, opening and closure of the pulmonary valve has much in common with that of the aortic valve (see p. 1487, **10**.55).

LEFT ATRIUM

Though smaller in volume than the right, the *left atrium* has thicker walls (3 mm on average). Its cavity and walls are largely formed by the proximal parts of the pulmonary veins, incorporated into the atrium during development (p. 303). The only clear derivative of the left part of the embryonic atrium is the auricle, along with the vestibule of the mitral valve. The left atrium is roughly cuboidal and extends behind the right atrium, separated from it by the obliquely positioned septum (**10**.25A, B). Thus, the right atrium is in front and anterolateral to the right part of the left atrium. The left part is concealed anteriorly by the initial segments of the pulmonary trunk and aorta, with part of the transverse pericardial sinus between it and these arterial trunks. Antero-inferiorly, and to the left, it adjoins the base of the left ventricle at the orifice of the mitral valve (see below). Its posterior aspect forms most of the anatomical base of the heart and is approximately quadrangular, receiving the terminations of (usually) two pulmonary veins from each lung. It forms the anterior wall of the oblique pericardial sinus (**10**.19). This surface ends at the shallow vertical interatrial groove that descends to the cardiac crux. The left atrial auricle is constricted at its atrial junction and all the pectinate muscles of the left atrium are contained within it. It is characteristically longer, narrower and more hooked than the right auricle, its margins being more deeply indented. It turns forwards to the left of the pulmonary trunk, overlapping its origin (**10**.30, 39).

Interiorly, the four *pulmonary veins* open into the upper posterolateral surfaces of the left atrium, two on each side. Their orifices are smooth and oval, the left pair frequently opening via a common channel. The *left atrioventricular orifice* is fully described below. Some minimal cardiac veins return blood directly from the myocardium to the cavity of the left atrium. The left atrial aspect of the septum has a characteristically rough appearance, bounded by a crescentic ridge, concave upwards, which marks the site of the oval foramen (p. 304).

LEFT VENTRICLE

General and external features

The left ventricle is constructed in accordance with its role as a powerful pump needed to sustain pulsatile flow in the high-pressured systemic arteries. Variously described as half-ellipsoid or cone-shaped, it is longer and narrower than the right ventricle, extending from its base in the plane of the coronary groove to the cardiac apex. Its long axis descends forwards and to the left. In transverse section, at right angles to the axis, its cavity is oval or nearly circular, with walls about three times thicker (8–12 mm) than those of the right ventricle. It forms part of the sternocostal, left and inferior (diaphragmatic) cardiac surfaces. Except where obscured by the aorta and pulmonary trunk, the base of the ventricular cone is superficially separated from the left atrium and atrial auricle by part of the atrioventricular groove, the coronary sinus running in the posterior aspect of the groove to reach the right atrium (**10**.30, 32). The anterior and posterior interventricular grooves indicate the lines of mural attachment of the ventricular septum and the limits of the left and right ventricular territories. The sternocostal surface of the ventricle curves bluntly into its left surface at the obtuse margin.

Internal features

Like the right, the left ventricle has an inlet region, guarded by the mitral valve (*ostium venosum*), an outlet region, guarded by the aortic valve (*ostium arteriosum*), and an apical trabecular component

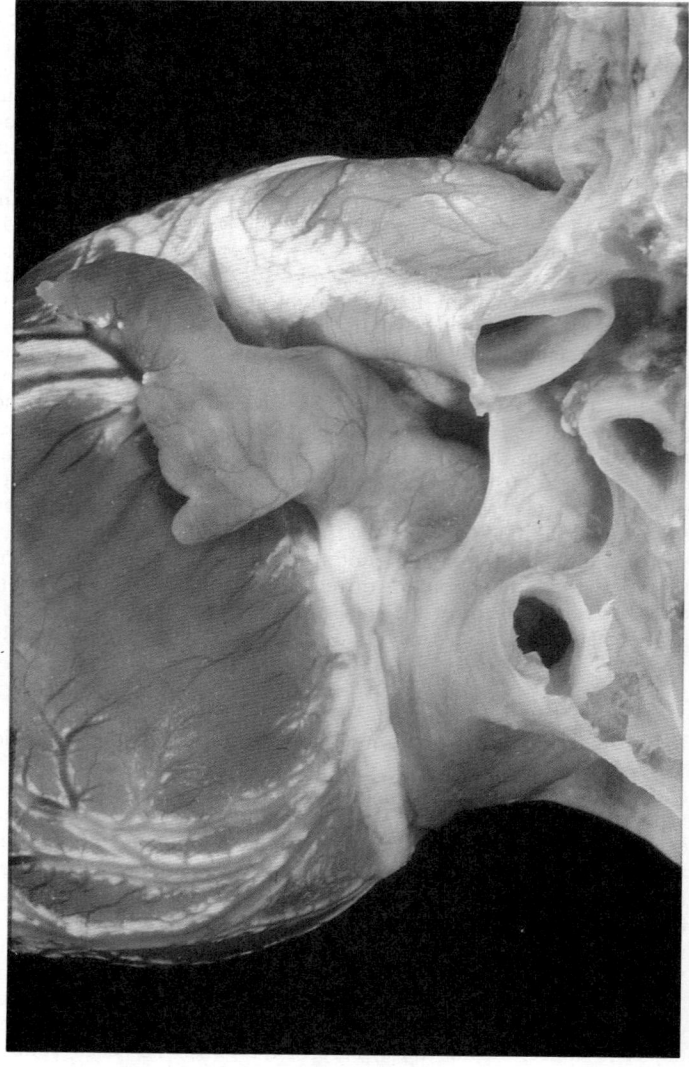

10.30   The characteristic morphology of the left atrial appendage (compare with **10**.29, the right appendage from the same heart).

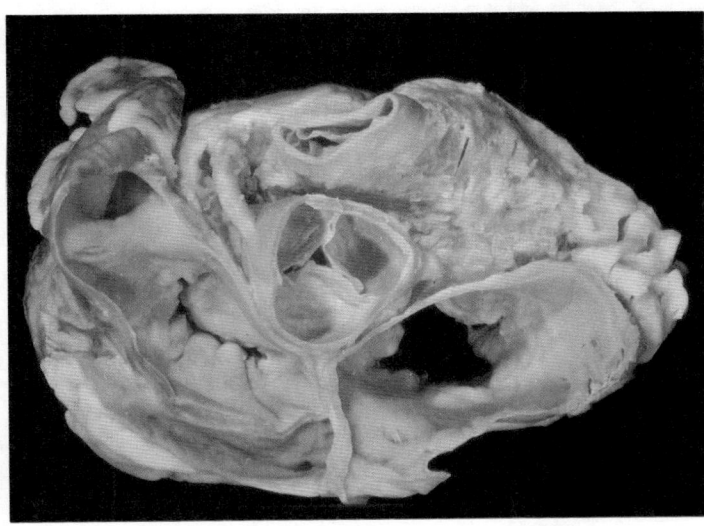

10.31 This section of the heart is taken to either side of the oblique atrioventricular groove, but is then laid horizontal and photographed from the atrial aspect. It shows the interrelationships of the four cardiac valves at the so-called base of the heart. Note the central location of the aorta.

(40A, B, C). The left atrioventricular orifice, with its mitral valve, admits atrial blood during diastole, flow being towards the cardiac apex. After closure of the mitral leaflets, and throughout the ejection phase of systole, blood is expelled from the apex through the aortic orifice. In contrast to the orifices within the right ventricle, those of the left ventricle are in close contact, with fibrous continuity between the leaflets of the aortic and mitral valves (the subaortic curtain; **10**.42). The inlet and outlet turn sharply round this fibrous curtain (**10**.40c, 51).

The anterolateral wall is the concavo-convex *ventricular septum*, a muscular wall whose convexity is the posteromedial profile of the right ventricle as seen in section. It thus completes the circular outline of the left ventricle. Towards the aortic orifice, the septum becomes the thin, collagenous interventricular component of the *membranous septum*, an oval or round area below and confluent with the fibrous triangle separating the right and the non-coronary cusps of the aortic valve (p. 1488).

Between the lower limits of the free margins of the leaflets of the mitral valve and the apex of the ventricle, the muscular walls are deeply trabeculated. These *trabeculae carneae* are finer and more intricate than those of the right ventricle, but similar in structure (p. 1480, **10**.40A, B). Trabeculation is characteristically well developed near the apex, whereas the upper reaches of the septal surface are smooth (**10**.42).

MITRAL VALVE

The general comments already made in respect to the tricuspid valve apply equally to the mitral. As expected, therefore, the valve has an orifice with its supporting annulus, leaflets, a variety of tendinous chordae and papillary muscles.

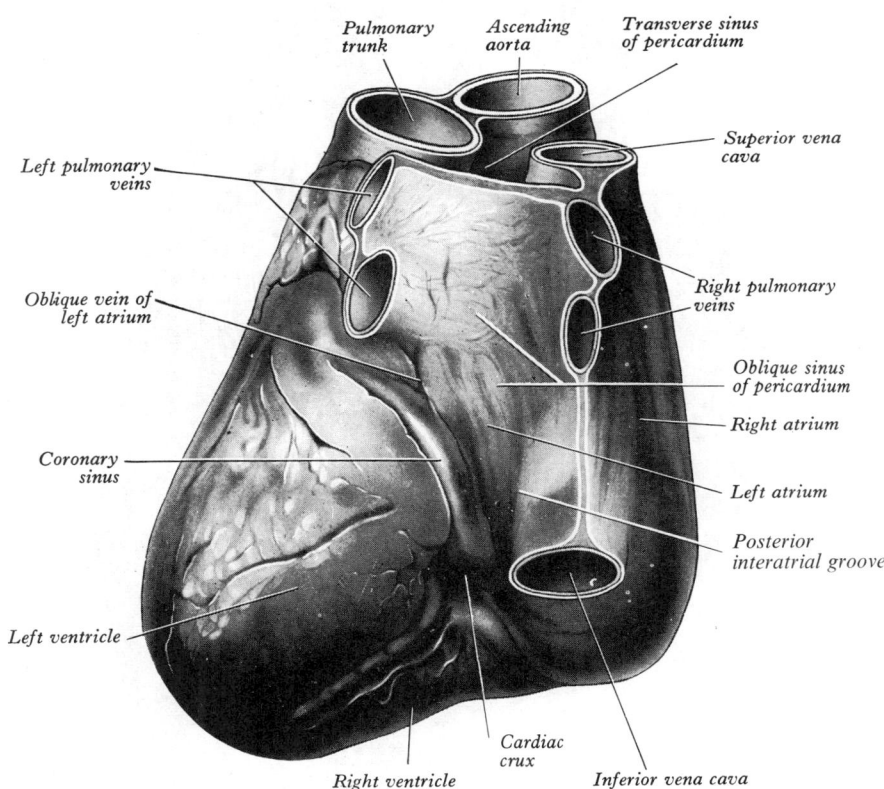

10.32 The base and the diaphragmatic surface of the heart. The serosal pericardium is in situ and its cut edge is seen around the great vessels; its disposition is highly schematic (recesses omitted). See text for additional details. The cardiac crux results from the confluence of the posterior interatrial groove, the posterior atrioventricular groove and the posterior interventricular groove.

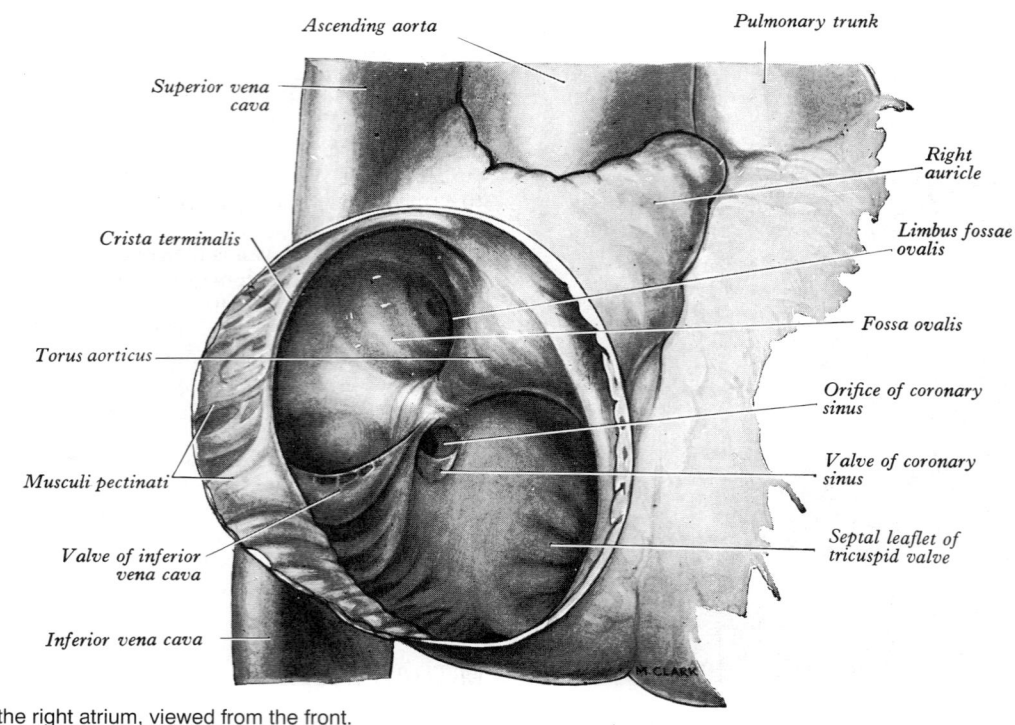

Ascending aorta

Pulmonary trunk

Superior vena cava

Right auricle

Crista terminalis

Limbus fossae ovalis

Torus aorticus

Fossa ovalis

Orifice of coronary sinus

Musculi pectinati

Valve of coronary sinus

Valve of inferior vena cava

Septal leaflet of tricuspid valve

Inferior vena cava

M. CLARK

10.33   The interior of the right atrium, viewed from the front.

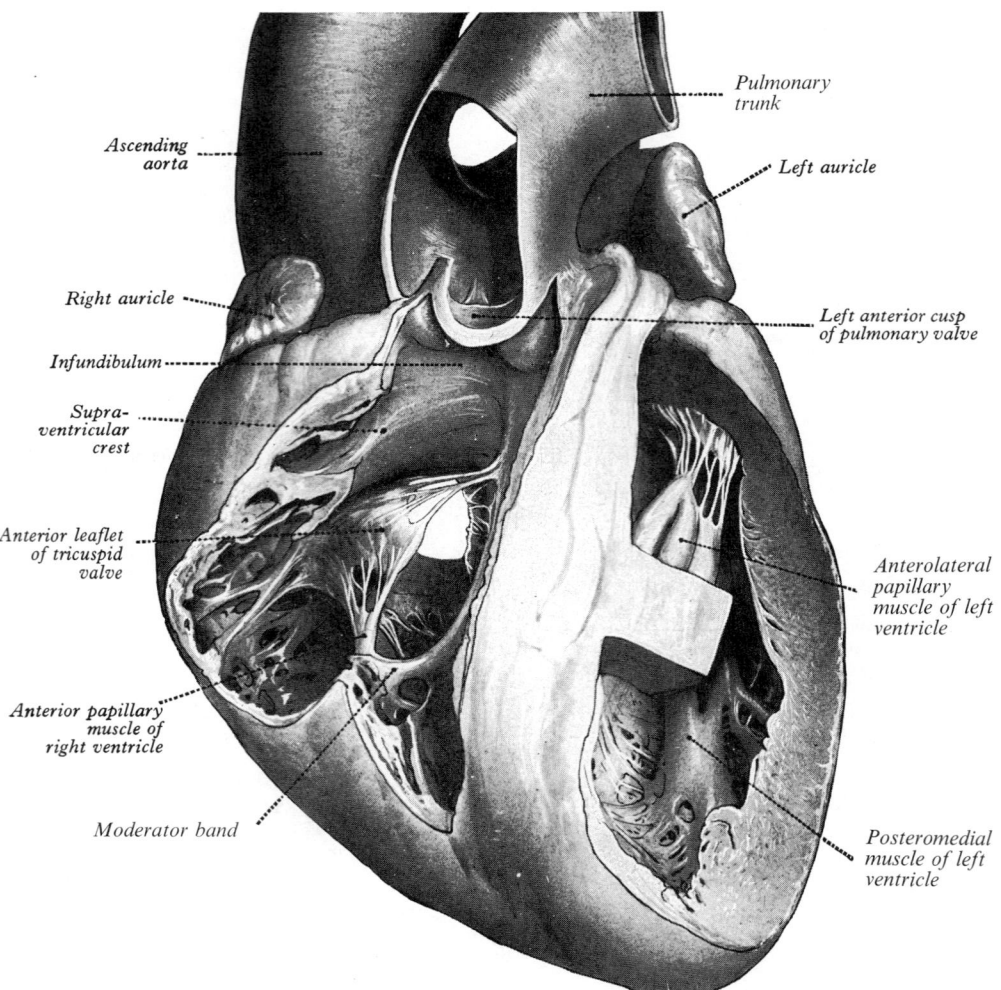

Pulmonary trunk

Ascending aorta

Left auricle

Right auricle

Left anterior cusp of pulmonary valve

Infundibulum

Supra-ventricular crest

Anterior leaflet of tricuspid valve

Anterolateral papillary muscle of left ventricle

Anterior papillary muscle of right ventricle

Moderator band

Posteromedial muscle of left ventricle

10.34   A dissection opening the ventricles, viewed from the front.

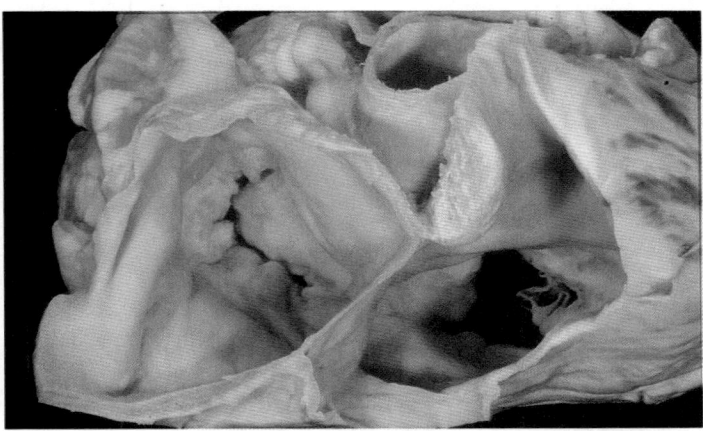

10.35   The surfaces of the right atrium are separated by the deep interatrial groove (Waterston's groove) from the left atrium. This groove forms the anterosuperior margin of the atrial septum (the oval fossa). Note the solitary line of coaptation of the leaflets of the mitral valve.

Mitral orifice

The mitral orifice is a well-defined transitional zone between the atrial wall and the bases of the leaflets (**10**.40B). It is smaller than the tricuspid orifice (mean circumference: 9.0 cm in males, 7.2 cm in females, according to Ranganathan et al 1970). The approximately circular orifice is almost vertical in diastole and at 45° to the sagittal plane but with a slight forward tilt. Its ventricular aspect faces anterolaterally to the left and a little inferiorly towards the left ventricular apex. It is almost coplanar with the tricuspid orifice but posterosuperior to it, whereas it is postero-inferior and slightly to the left of the aortic orifice. The mitral, tricuspid and aortic orifices are intimately connected centrally at the *central fibrous body* (p. 1493). When the leaflets of the mitral valve close, they form a single zone of coaptation, termed by some the *commissure* (**10**.35).

The *annulus* of the valve is not a simple fibrous ring, but comprises fibrocollagenous elements of varying consistency from which the fibrous core of the leaflets take origin. These variations allow major changes in the shape and dimensions of the annulus at different stages of the cardiac cycle and ensure optimal efficiency in valvar action.

The annulus is strongest at the internal aspects of the left and right fibrous trigones (**10**.51). Extending from these structures, the anterior and posterior coronary prongs (tapering, fibrous, sub-endocardial tendons) partly encircle the orifice at the atrioventricular junction (**10**.51, 52). Between the tips of the prongs, the atrial and ventricular myocardial masses are separated by a more tenuous sheet of deformable fibro-elastic connective tissue. Spanning anteriorly between the trigones, the fibrous core of the central part of the anterior aortic leaflet of the mitral valve is a continuation of the fibrous *subaortic curtain* which descends from the adjacent halves of the left and non-coronary cusps of the aortic valve (**10**.42).

Mitral valvar leaflets

Since the earliest descriptions, these leaflets have been described as paired structures. Hence, the name 'bicuspid valve' is more explicit, though erroneous (the leaflets are not cuspid, or peaked, in form) and surely less picturesque than the clinical term 'mitral'. Confusion, controversy and difficulties in quantitation have arisen, however, because small accessory leaflets are almost always found between

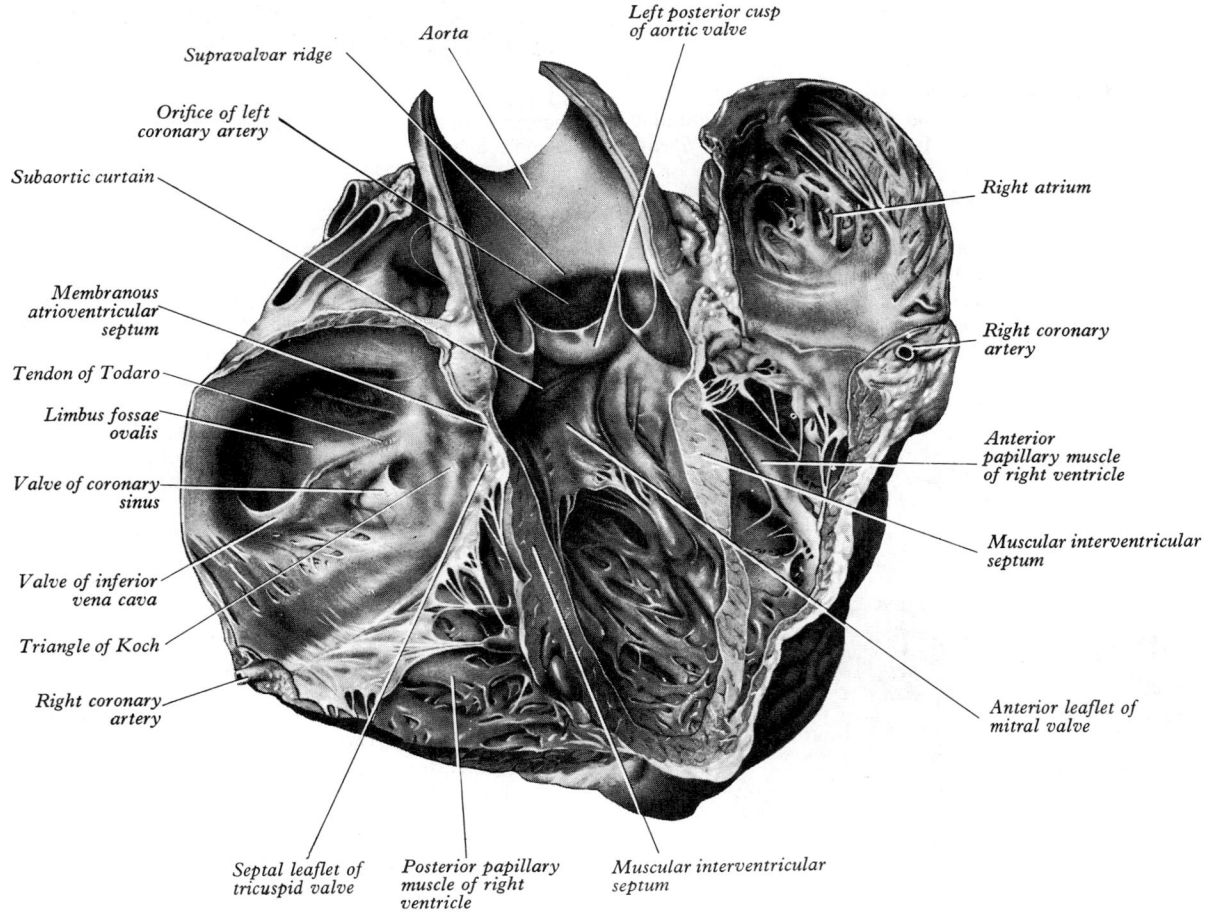

10.36   The interior of the heart revealed by incising it along its right and lower surfaces and excising the pulmonary trunk and infundibulum. The rest of the front of the heart has been turned over to the left.

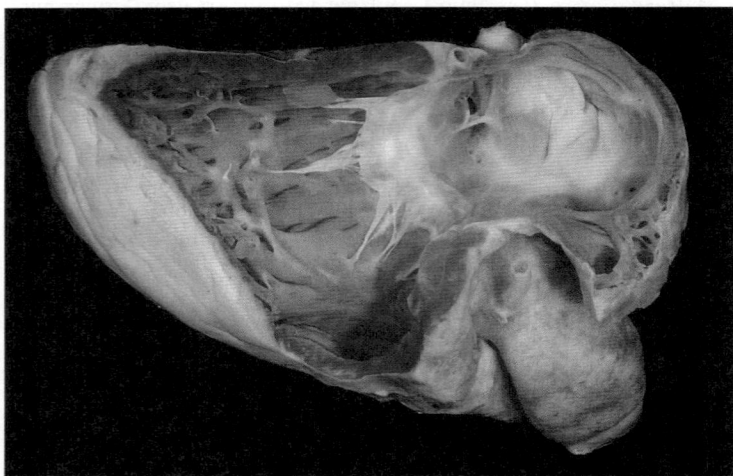

10.37A. Removal of the sternocostal parietal surface of the heart shows the components of the right ventricle. Note the supraventricular crest separating the attachments of the tricuspid and pulmonary valves.

the two major leaflets. These problems can be resolved if the mitral valve is described as consisting 'of a continuous veil attached around the entire circumference of the mitral orifice' (Harken et al 1952). Its free edge bears several indentations, two being sufficiently deep and regular to be nominated as the ends of a solitary and oblique zone of apposition, or *commissure* (**10.31, 35**). It is more usual, nonetheless, for these anteromedial and posterolateral extremities themselves to be designated as two commissures, each positionally named as indicated. The official names for these leaflets, anterior and posterior, though simple, are somewhat misleading because of the obliquity of the valve.

When the valve is laid open (**10.40B**), its *anterior leaflet* (aortic, septal, 'greater' or anteromedial) is seen to guard one-third of the circumference of the orifice and to be semicircular or triangular, with few or no marginal indentations. Its fibrous core (*lamina fibrosa*) is continuous on the outflow aspect, beyond the margins of the fibrous subaortic curtain, with the right and left fibrous trigones (**10.31, 36, 43B, 51**). Between these, it is continuous with the fibrous curtain itself and, beyond the trigones, with the roots of the annular fibrous prongs (**10.52**). The leaflet has a deep crescentic rough zone receiving various tendinous chordae (see below). The ridge limiting the outer margin of the rough zone indicates the maximal extent of

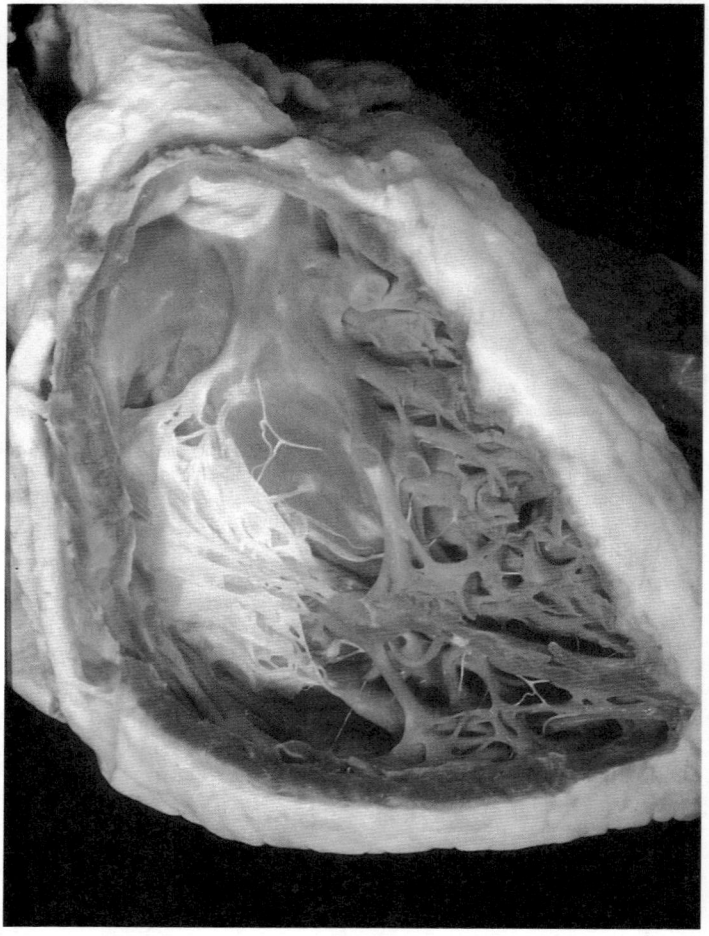

10.37B. This anterior view through a window into the right ventricle shows the extent of the supraventricular crest. Note the relatively smooth-walled infundibulum, the prominent spetomarginal trabecule and the extensive septoparietal trabeculation.

surface contact with the mural leaflet in full closure. A clear zone is seen between the rough zone and the valvar annulus which is devoid of attachments of chordae, though its fibrous core carries extensions from chordae attached in the rough zone. The anterior leaflet has no basal zone, continuing instead into the valvar curtain. Hinging on its annular attachment, and continuous with the subaortic curtain, it is critically placed between the inlet and the outlet of the ventricle. During passive ventricular filling and atrial systole, its smooth atrial surface is important in directing a smooth flow of blood towards the body and apex of the ventricle. After the onset of ventricular systole and closure of the mitral valve, the ventricular aspect of its clear zone merges into the smooth surface of the subaortic curtain which, with the remaining fibrous walls of the subvalvar aortic vestibule, forms the smooth boundaries of the ventricular outlet.

The *posterior leaflet* (mural, ventricular, 'smaller' or posterolateral) has usually two or more minor indentations. Lack of definition of major intervalvar commissures has previously led to disagreement and confusion concerning the territorial extent of this leaflet and the possible existence of accessory scallops. Examination of the valve in closed position, however, shows that the posterior leaflet can conveniently be regarded as all the valvar tissue posterior to the anterolateral and posteromedial ends of the major zone of apposition with the aortic leaflet. Thus defined, it has a wider attachment to the annulus than does the anterior leaflet, guarding two-thirds of the circumferential attachments. There are further indentations usually dividing the mural leaflet into a relatively large middle 'scallop' and smaller anterolateral and posteromedial commissural 'scallops'. Each scallop has a crescentic, opaque rough zone, receiving the attachment of the chords on its ventricular aspect which define the area of valvar apposition in full closure. From the rough zone to within 2–3 mm of its annular attachment is a membranous clear zone devoid of

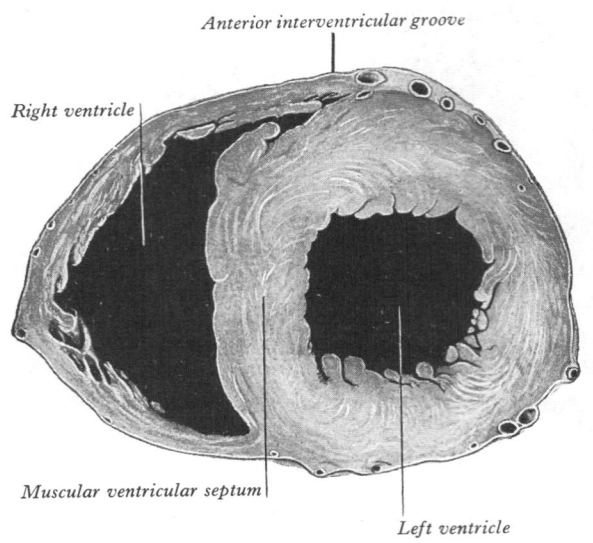

Anterior interventricular groove

Right ventricle

Muscular ventricular septum

Left ventricle

10.38 Transverse section through the ventricles of the isolated heart, viewed from below. Note that in this illustration the heart is not positioned as it would be in situ: in the latter position the crescentic 'right' ventricle overlaps most of the anterior surface of the 'left' ventricle.

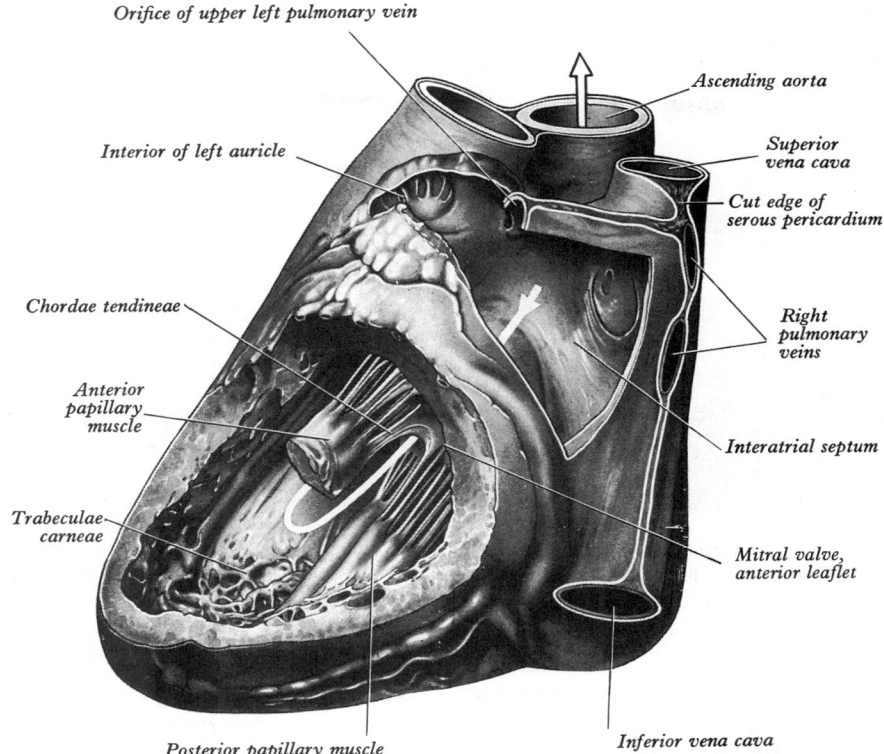

Orifice of upper left pulmonary vein

Ascending aorta

Superior vena cava

Interior of left auricle

Cut edge of serous pericardium

Chordae tendineae

Right pulmonary veins

Anterior papillary muscle

Trabeculae carneae

Interatrial septum

Mitral valve, anterior leaflet

Posterior papillary muscle

Inferior vena cava

10.39   Dissection showing the interior of the left side of the heart. The white arrow indicates the course of blood flow from the left atrium through the left ventricle to the aorta.

chordae. The basal 2–3 mm is thick and vascular, and receives basal chordae. The ratio of rough to clear zone in the anterior leaflet is about 0.6. In the middle 'scallop' of the posterior leaflet, it is 1.4. Thus, much more of the mural leaflet is in apposition with the aortic leaflet during closure of the mitral valve.

Mitral chordae tendineae (tendinous cords)

These cords resemble those supporting the tricuspid valve (**10**.40A, B). False chordae (trabeculae carneae **10**.39, 40A, B), are also irregularly distributed as in the right ventricle. They occur in about half of all human left ventricles and often cross the subaortic outflow. Many contain extensions from the ventricular conduction tissues. Such left ventricular bands can often be identified by cross-sectional echocardiography. Their role, if any, has still to be determined. True chordae of the mitral valve may be divided into interleaflet (or commissural) chordae, rough zone chordae, including the special strut chordae, so-called 'cleft' chordae, and basal chordae. Most true chordae divide into branches from a single stem soon after their origin from the apical third of a papillary muscle, or proceed as single chordae dividing into multiple branches near their attachment. Basal chordae, in contrast, are solitary structures passing from the ventricular wall to the mural leaflet.

There is such marked variation between the arrangement of the chordae in individual normal hearts that any detailed classification loses much of its clinical significance. Suffice it to say that, in the majority of hearts, the chordae support the entire free edges of the valvar leaflets together with varying degrees of their ventricular aspects and bases. There is some evidence to suggest that those valves with unsupported areas of the free edge become prone to prolapse in later life.

Papillary muscles

The two muscles supporting the leaflets of the mitral valve also vary in length and breadth and may be bifid. The *anterolateral muscle* arises from the sternocostal mural myocardium, the *posteromedial* from the diaphragmatic region. Tendinous chordae arise mostly from the tip and apical third of each muscle, but sometimes take origin near their base. The chordae from each papillary muscle diverge and

are attached to corresponding areas of closure on **both** valvar leaflets (**10**.40B).

Opening of the mitral valve

At the onset of diastole, opening is passive but rapid, the leaflets parting and projecting into the ventricle as left atrial pressure exceeds left ventricular diastolic pressure. Passive ventricular filling proceeds as atrial blood pours to the apex, directed by the pendant aortic leaflet of the valve. The leaflets begin to float passively together, hinging on their annular attachments, partially to occlude the ventricular inlet. Atrial systole now occurs, jetting blood apically and causing re-opening of the leaflets. As maximal filling is achieved, the leaflets again float rapidly together. Closure is followed by ventricular systole, which starts in the papillary muscles and continues rapidly as general contraction of the walls and septum. Co-ordinated contraction of the papillary muscles raises the tension in the chordae and promotes joining of the corresponding points on opposing leaflets, preventing their eversion. With general mural and septal excitation and contraction, left ventricular pressure rapidly rises (**10**.55). The leaflets 'balloon' towards the atrial cavity and the atrial aspects of the rough zones come into maximal contact. Precise papillary contraction, and increasing tension in the chordae, continues to prevent valvar eversion and maintains valvar competence.

The orifices and the leaflets of both atrioventricular valves undergo considerable changes in position, form and area during a cardiac cycle (**10**.50). Both valves move anteriorly and to the left during systole, and reverse their motion in diastole. The mitral valve reduces its orificial (annular) area by as much as 40% in systole. Its shape also changes from circular to crescentic at the height of systole, the annular attachment of its aortic leaflet being the concavity of the crescent. The attachment of its mural leaflet, although remaining convex, contracts towards the anterior wall of the heart.

AORTIC VALVE

The smooth left ventricular outflow tract, or aortic vestibule, ends at the leaflets of the aortic valve. Although stronger in construction, the aortic valve resembles the pulmonary (**10**.42, 43, 44, 45) in

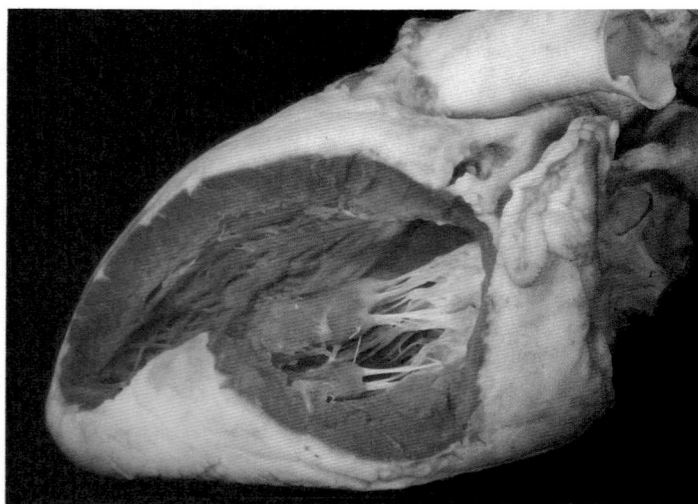

10.40A This dissection shows the papillary muscles of the left ventricle in their natural position. The cords from each muscle diverge to support the leaflets.

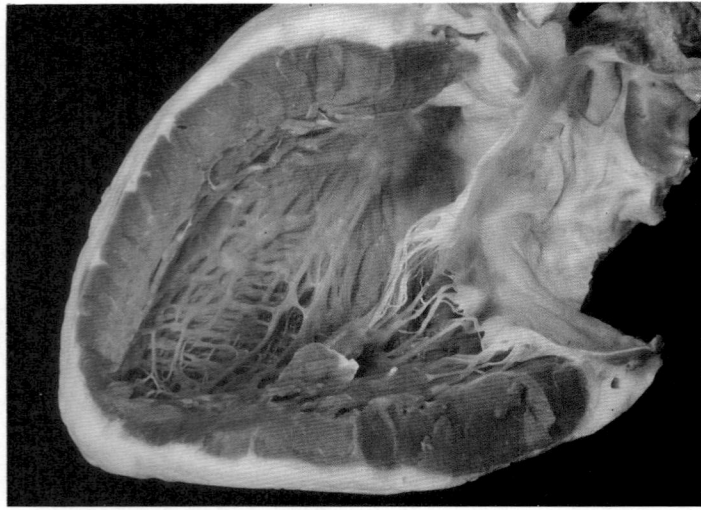

10.40B The left ventricle has been dissected by removing the obtuse margin so as to reveal its inlet, apical trabecular and outlet components.

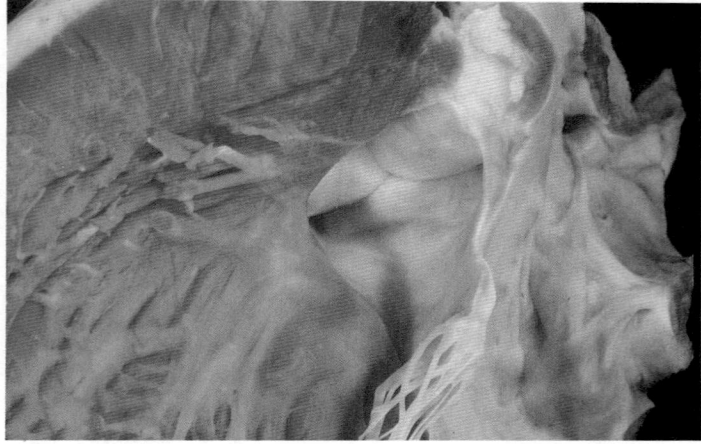

10.40C This detail of the heart shown in B emphasizes the area of fibrous continuity between the leaflets of the aortic and mitral valves.

possessing three semilunar leaflets, the *cusps*, supported within the three aortic sinuses of Valsalva. Although the aortic valve, like the pulmonary valve, is often described as possessing an annulus in continuity with the fibrous skeleton, there is no complete collagenous ring supporting the attachments of the leaflets. Instead, again as with the pulmonary valve, the anatomy of the aortic valve is dominated by the fibrous semilunar attachment of the cusps (**10.43B**).

Cusps

The cusps are, in part, attached to the aortic wall and in part to the supporting ventricular structures. The situation is more complicated than in the pulmonary valve, because parts of the cusps also take origin from the fibrous subaortic curtain, being continuous with the aortic leaflet of the mitral valve (**10.42**). This area of continuity is thickened at its two ends to form the right and left fibrous trigones (**10.51**). But, again as with the pulmonary valve (**10.43B**), the semilunar attachments incorporate segments of ventricular tissue within the base of each aortic sinus. These sinuses and leaflets are conveniently named as being *right*, *left* and *non-coronary* according to the origins of the coronary arteries (**10.43B**). The semilunar attachments also incorporate three triangular areas of aortic wall within the apex of the left ventricular outflow tract. Since these triangular areas are part of the aortic wall rather than the left ventricle, interposing between the bulbous aortic sinuses, they separate the cavity of the left ventricle from the pericardial space. Removal of the triangles in an otherwise intact heart is instructive in demonstrating the relationships of the aortic valve, which can justly be considered as the keystone of the heart. The base of the triangle between the non-coronary and the left coronary cusps is continuous inferiorly with the fibrous aortic-mitral curtain. The apex of this triangle 'points' into the transverse pericardial space. The triangle between right and non-coronary cusps has, as its base, the membranous components of the interventricular septum and thus 'faces' the right ventricle, whereas its apex 'points' towards the transverse pericardial space behind the origin of the right coronary artery. The third triangle, between the two coronary cusps, has its base on the muscular ventricular septum. Its apex 'points' to the plane of space found between the aortic wall and the free standing sleeve of right ventricular infundibular musculature which supports the cusps of the pulmonary valve. Although the basal attachments of each leaflet are thickened and collagenous at their ventricular origins, there is no continuous collagenous skeleton supporting, in circular fashion, all the attachments of the cusps of the aortic valve. Valvar function depends primarily upon the semilunar attachments of the cusps.

The cusps themselves are folds of endocardium with a central fibrous core. With the valve half-open, each equals slightly more than a quarter of a sphere, an approximate hemisphere being completed by the corresponding sinus. Each cusp has a thick basal border, deeply concave on its aortic aspect, and a horizontal free margin. The latter is only slightly thickened except at its midpoint where it has an aggregation of fibrous tissue, the valvar *nodule of Arantius*. Flanking each nodule, the fibrous core is tenuous, forming the *lunules* of translucent and occasionally fenestrated valvar tissue (**10.42**). Such fenestrations are of no functional significance. The aortic surface of each cusp is rougher than its ventricular aspect.

Three sets of names currently exist for the aortic cusps. Official terms in the *Nomina Anatomica* (1989) refer to presumed fetal positions before full cardiac rotation has occurred. They are *posterior*, *right* and *left*. Corresponding terms based on the approximate positions in maturity are *anterior*, *left posterior* and *right posterior*. But, as already indicated, widespread clinical terminology links both cusps and sinuses to the origins of the coronary arteries. Thus, the anterior is the *right coronary* structure, left posterior is *left coronary*, and right posterior is *non-coronary*. These clinical terms are preferable since they are simple and unambiguous.

Aortic sinuses (of Valsalva)

The aortic sinuses are more prominent than those in the pulmonary trunk. The upper limit of each sinus reaches considerably beyond the level of the free border of the cusp and forms a well-defined complete circumferential *sinutubular ridge* when viewed from the aortic aspect (**10.43B**). Coronary arteries usually open near this ridge within the upper part of the sinus, but are markedly variable in their origin. The walls of the sinuses are largely collagenous near the attachment of the cusps, but the amount of lamellated elastic tissue increases with distance from the zone of attachment. Strands of myocardium may enter this fibro-elastic wall. At the midlevel of each sinus, its wall is about half the thickness of the supravalvar aortic wall and less than one-quarter of the thickness of the sinu-tubular ridge. At this level, the mean luminal diameter of the beginning of the aortic root is almost double that of the ascending aorta. All such details are functionally significant in the mechanism of valvar motion.

The mechanism of valvar motion

During diastole, the closed aortic valve supports an aortic column of blood at high but slowly diminishing pressure. Each sinus and its cusp form a hemispherical chamber. The three nodules are apposed and the margins and lunular parts of adjacent cusps are tightly apposed on their ventricular aspects. From the aortic aspect, the closed valve is tri-radiate, three pairs of closely compressed lunules radiating from their nodules to their peripheral commissural attachments at the sinutubular junction (**10**.41, 45). As ventricular systolic pressure rises, it exceeds aortic pressure and the valve is passively opened. The fibrous wall of the sinuses nearest the aortic vestibule is almost inextensible but, in the upper parts of sinuses, the wall is fibro-elastic. Under left ventricular ejection pressure, the radius here increases about 16% in systole. Hence the commissures move apart, making the orifice triangular when fully open. The free margins of the cusps then become almost straight lines between peripheral attachments. But they do not flatten against the sinus walls, even at maximal systolic pressure, which is probably an important factor in subsequent closure. During ejection, most blood enters the ascending aorta, but some enters the sinuses, forming vortices which help to maintain the triangular 'midposition' of the cusp during ventricular systole and probably initiate their approximation with the end of systole. Tight and full closure ensues with the rapid drop of ventricular pressure in diastole.

Commissures narrow, nodules aggregate and the valve reassumes its triradiate form. Experiments indicate that about 4% of ejected blood regurgitates through a valve with normal sinuses, while 23% regurgitates through a valve without them (Bellhouse & Bellhouse 1968). The normal structure of the aortic sinuses also promotes non-turbulent flow into the coronary arteries.

Similar events occur in the pulmonary valve, albeit more leisurely, the pressure profiles being less extreme (**10**.55) and the valvar structure less substantial.

SURFACE ANATOMY OF THE HEART

The surface projections to be described below apply to an average

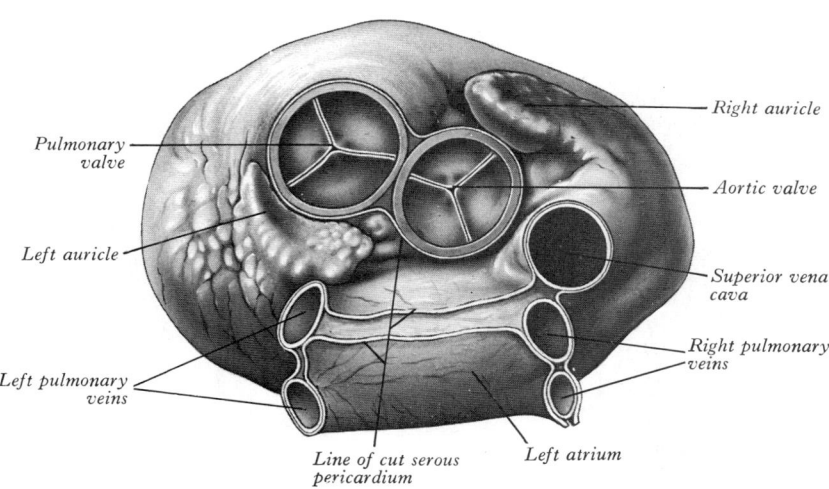

10.41 The heart viewed from above. The two continuous white lines which enclose the pulmonary trunk and aorta on the one hand and the pulmonary veins and the superior vena cava on the other, indicate the continuation of the parietal layer of the serous pericardium with the serous epicardium. The floor of the transverse sinus is seen from above, with the left coronary artery running in it. This diagram, from an earlier edition, has been retained for its pericardial details. However, in some respects it is misleading: the aortic and pulmonary valves are not, as shown, coplanar; the pulmonary valve is distinctly higher than the aortic valve; furthermore the planes of the valves 'face' approximately at right angles to each other.

adult. They are considerably modified by age, sex, stature and proportions, respiration and posture. The projections of the position of the valves to the surface are not the best sites for their auscultation (**10**.46). The cardiac apex almost corresponds to the apex beat, which is usually visible and always palpable in the fifth intercostal space, slightly medial to midclavicular line, about 9 cm from midline in average adult males. The apex beat is the most inferolateral point at which a pulsation can be felt. The true cardiac apex, however, is a short distance further inferolaterally. It does not contact the thoracic wall in systole.

The cardiac sternocostal surface, projected to the anterior thoracic wall, is a trapezoid (**10**.29, 46). Its right border corresponds to a line from the superior border of the right third costal cartilage, about 1 cm from the sternal margin, to the sixth costal cartilage. The line is convex to the right and is maximally distant from the midline (about 3–4 cm) in the fourth intercostal space. It represents the

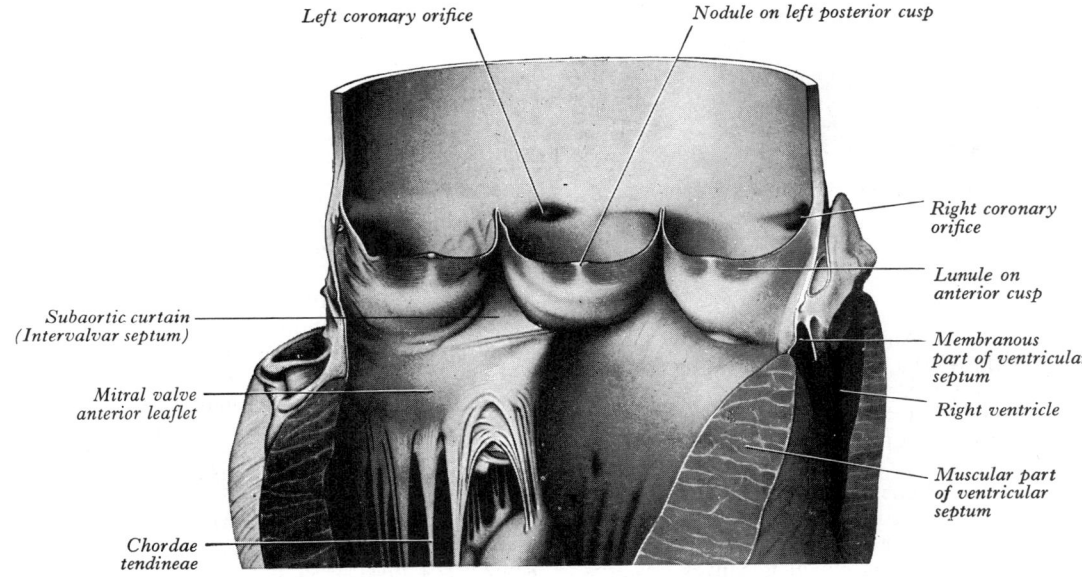

10.42 The aortic orifice opened from the front to show the cusps of the aortic valve, their nodules, lunules, commissures and the triple-scalloped line of annular attachment. Also shown is the continuity of the subaortic curtain with the mitral anterior leaflet (i.e. 'aortic baffle') and the coronary orifices.

1489

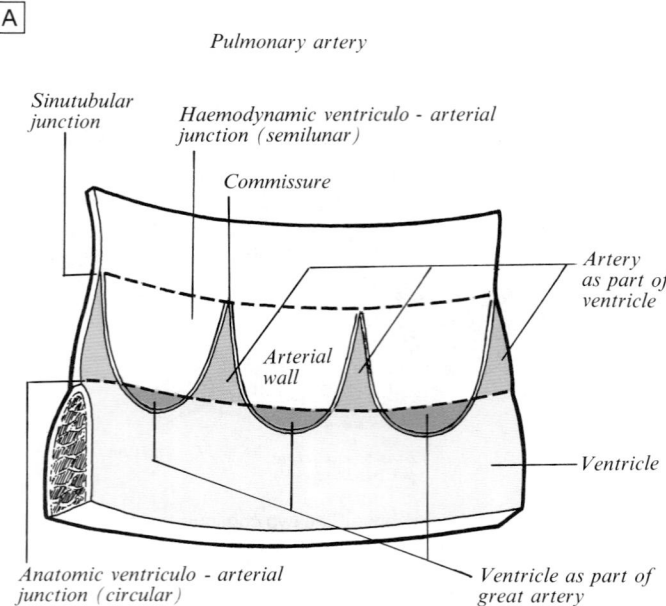

A

Pulmonary artery

Sinutubular junction

Haemodynamic ventriculo - arterial junction (semilunar)

Commissure

Artery as part of ventricle

Arterial wall

Ventricle

Anatomic ventriculo - arterial junction (circular)

Ventricle as part of great artery

10.43A. In this diagram of the aortic root (compare with B the cusps have been resected at the attachment to the aortic wall. Note the relation of the cusp insertions and the ventriculo-arterial junction.

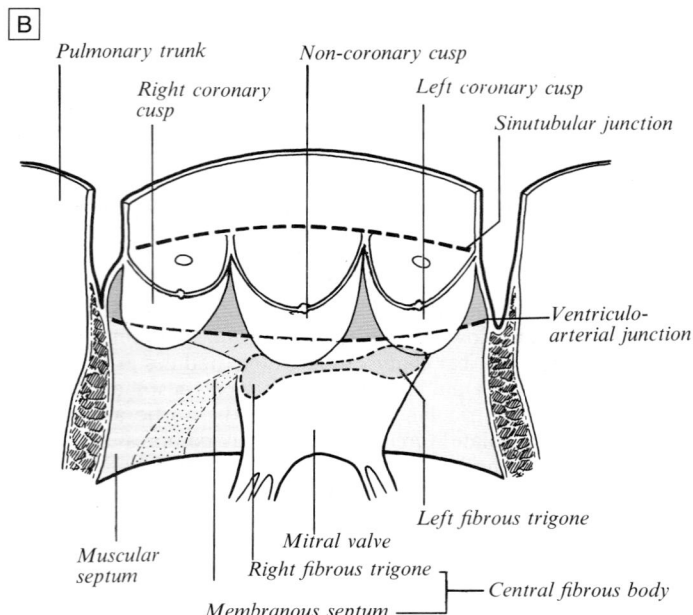

B

Pulmonary trunk

Non-coronary cusp

Right coronary cusp

Left coronary cusp

Sinutubular junction

Ventriculo-arterial junction

Muscular septum

Mitral valve

Left fibrous trigone

Right fibrous trigone

Central fibrous body

Membranous septum

10.43B. The root of the aorta cut open and distended, to show the insertion of the semilunar cusps. The diagram illustrates the structure of the zone of fibrous continuity between the cusps of the aortic valve and the leaflets of the mitral valve and their relation with the fibrous trigones. It also shows the semilunar attachment of the leaflets (compare with **10.43A**)

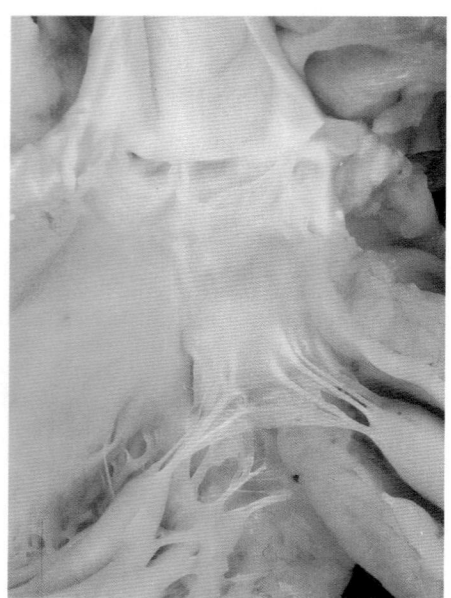

C

10.43C. A heart opened to show the aortic root as illustrated diagrammatically in figure **10.43A**.

lateral profile of the right atrium. An upward continuation of this line marks the right border of the superior vena cava while a downward continuation corresponds to the border of the inferior vena cava. The lower border of the surface projection is a line joining the lower end of the right border to the apex beat. Corresponding largely to the lower (acute) margin of the right ventricle, it crosses over the xiphisternal joint to include the apical part of the left ventricle. The left border of the heart is marked by a line from the apex beat to the lower border of the left second costal cartilage approximately 1 cm from the sternal margin. It is convex upwards and to the left, corresponding to the obtuse margin of the left ventricle and to the left atrial appendage above. The border is completed superiorly by a sloping line joining the upper ends of the

right and left borders, approximating to the upper limits of the atria. The left and right borders can be identified by heavy percussion.

The surface projection of the anterior part of the *atrioventricular groove* is an oblique line joining the sternal ends of the third left and sixth right costal cartilages. This line separates the atrial and ventricular areas. Although in different planes, the projections of the cardiac valves are also sited along or close to this line (**10.46**).

The *pulmonary orifice* is partly behind the superior border of the left third costal cartilage, and partly behind the left third of the sternum, being represented by a horizontal line, 2.5 cm long, crossing cartilage and sternum. Parallel lines from the ends of this line, up to the left second costal cartilage, indicate the site of the pulmonary trunk.

The *aortic orifice* is below and a little right of the pulmonary, marked by a line 2.5 cm long running from the medial end of the left third intercostal space downward to the right. Two parallel lines from the ends of this line, slanting up to the right half of the sternal angle, outline the location of the ascending aorta.

The *tricuspid valvar orifice* is represented by a line, 4 cm long, commencing near the midline just below the level of the fourth right costal cartilage and passing down and slightly to the right. The centre of this line should be level with the middle of the right fourth intercostal space.

The *mitral orifice* is behind the left half of the sternum opposite the fourth left costal cartilage and is represented by a line, 3 cm long, descending to the right.

Auscultation. As stated the foregoing are the approximate surface projections of the cardiac valves: they do **not** correspond to the sites for optimal auscultation of the contribution of each valve to the heart-sounds. To understand the latter an appreciation of the **position** and **plane** of each valve (the oscillator) must be combined with the geometry of its associated column of blood (in the ascending aorta, pulmonary trunk, right and left ventricles), which maximally carries the acoustic waveforms to the chest wall. Thus convenient sites to apply the stethoscope bell or diaphragm are:

- The *pulmonary area*, the sternal end of the second left intercostal space
- the *aortic area*, the sternal end of the second right intercostal space
- the *mitral* area, near the *cardiac apex*
- the *tricuspid area*, over the *centre* of the lower part of the *sternal body*, at the level of the fifth intercostal spaces.

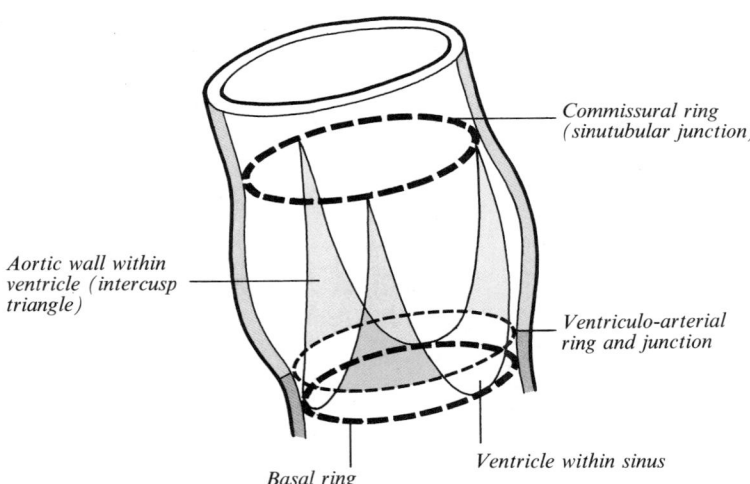

Commissural ring
(sinutubular junction)

Aortic wall within
ventricle (intercusp
triangle)

Ventriculo-arterial
ring and junction

Basal ring

Ventricle within sinus

10.44   Diagram showing how the structure of the aortic root is best conceptualized in terms of a three-pronged coronet. There are at least three rings within this coronet, but none support the entirety of the attachments of the valvar leaflets (see also **10**.43B).

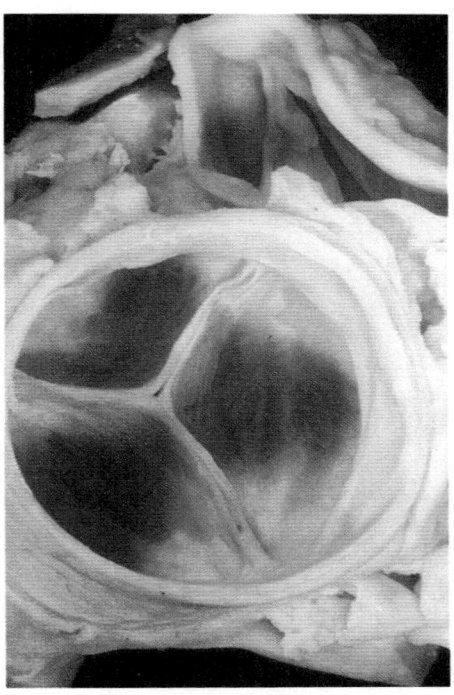

10.45   The arterial view of the aortic valve in its closed position shows the snug fit between its component leaflets.

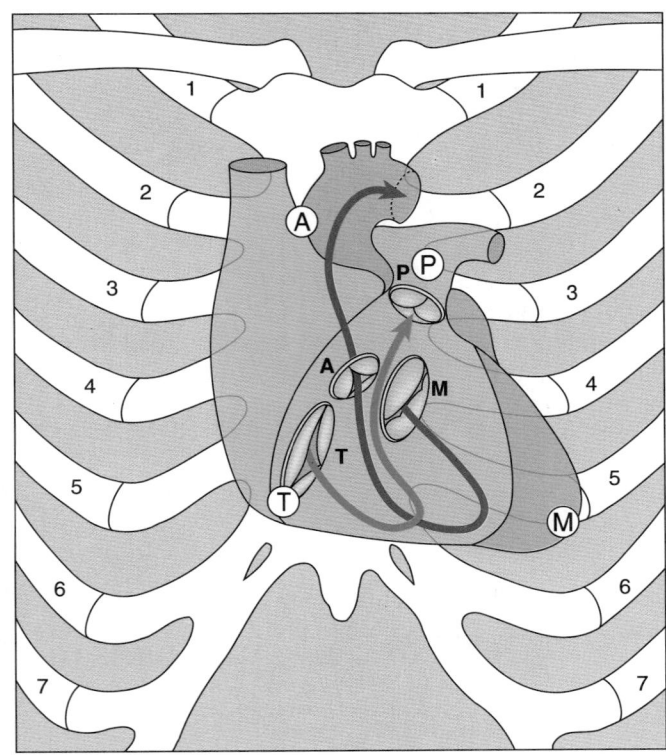

10.46   Diagram illustrating the relation of the sternocostal surface and valves of the heart to the thoracic cage. The right heart is blue, the arrow denoting the inflow and outflow channels of the right ventricle; the left heart is treated similarly in red. The positions, planes and relative sizes of the cardiac valves are shown. The position of the letters, A, P, T and M indicate the aortic, pulmonary, tricuspid and mitral auscultation areas of clinical practice. Note that, for purpose of illustration, the orifices of the aortic, mitral and tricuspid valves are shown with some separation between them. In reality, the leaflets of the three valves are in fibrous continuity (see **10**.52).

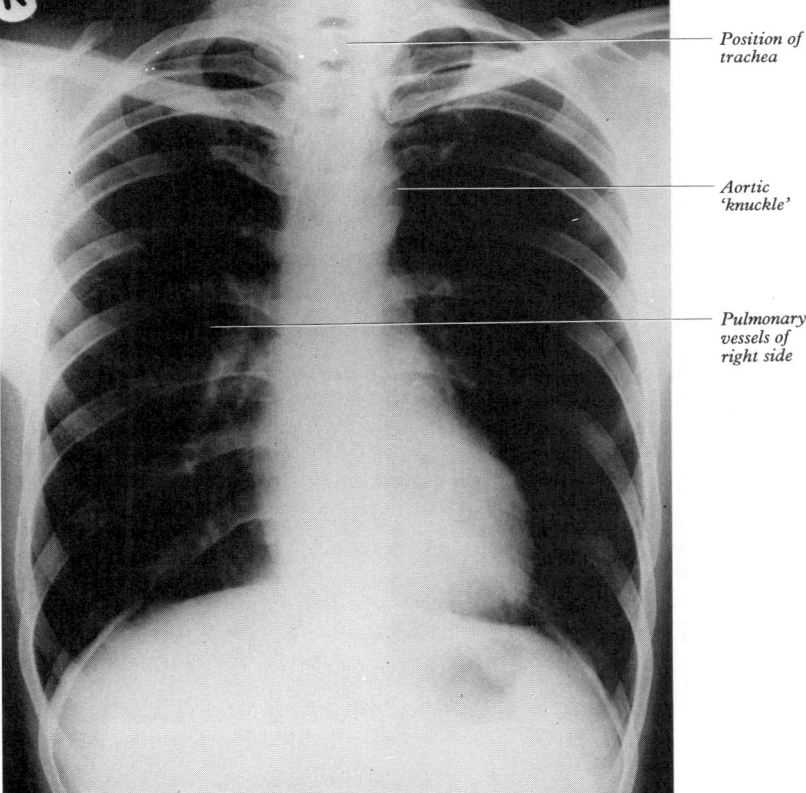

Position of
trachea

Aortic
'knuckle'

Pulmonary
vessels of
right side

10.47   Radiograph of chest, postero-anterior view, of adult male. Note the difference in level of the right and left halves of the diaphragm. (Supplied by Shaun Gallagher, Guy's Hospital.)

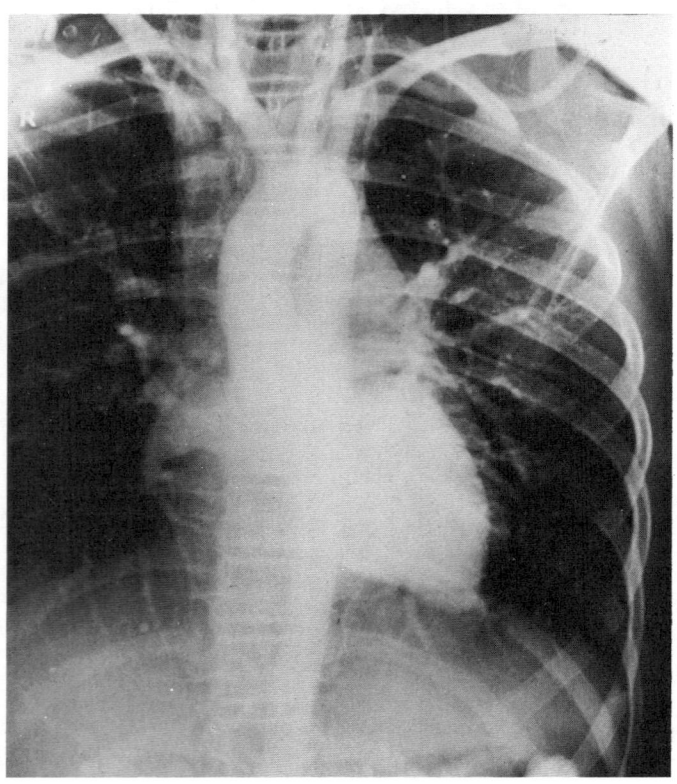

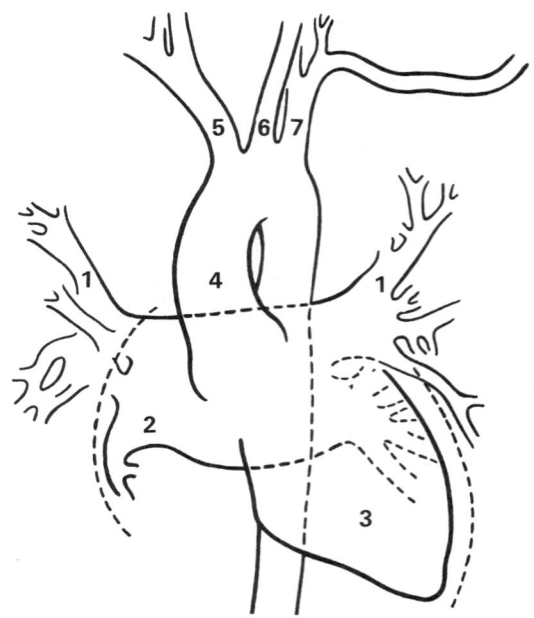

10.48 Angiocardiogram showing the left side of the heart in a child of 11 years; anteroposterior view. 1. Upper pulmonary vein. 2. Left atrium. (Note that owing to the great obliquity of the atrial septum, the left atrium extends to the right behind the right atrium). 3. Left ventricle. 4. Ascending aorta. 5. Brachiocephalic trunk. 6. Left common carotid artery. 7. Left subclavian artery. The arms of the patient are raised above the head and as a result the distal end of the artery passes upwards. (Provided by Frances Gardner.)

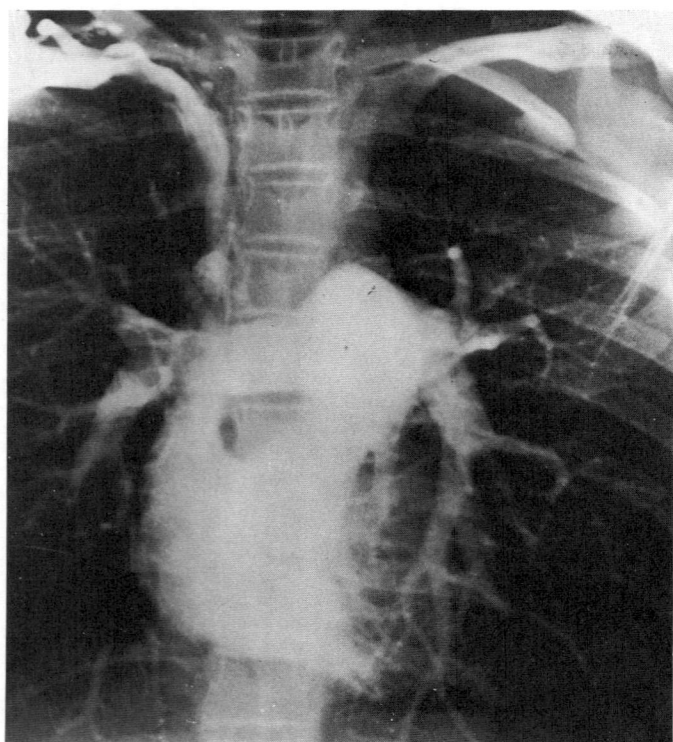

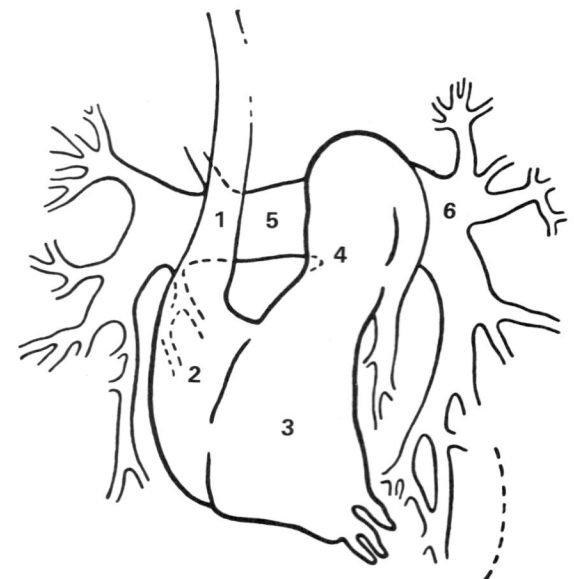

10.49 Angiocardiogram showing the right side of the heart in a child of 12 years; anteroposterior view. 1. Superior vena cava. 2. Right atrium. 3. Right ventricle. 4. Pulmonary trunk. 5. Right pulmonary artery. 6. Left pulmonary artery. (Provided by Frances Gardner.)

The area of superficial cardiac dullness as mapped out by light percussion is roughly triangular and corresponds to the area of the heart not covered by lung.

RADIOLOGICAL APPEARANCES OF THE HEART

The heart, being full of blood, casts a shadow, occupying the inferior mediastinum, which is in sharp contrast to those areas occupied by the air-filled lungs (**10.47**). In full inspiration, the apex is clear of the diaphragm, presenting a blurred outline in radiographs due to movement. The right border of the shadow is continuous with those of the venae cavae. Due to the attachment of the pericardium to the diaphragm, the heart elongates during inspiration and shortens during expiration. The cardiac shape also varies with stature and attitude (p. 1734). In lateral radiographs, the retrocardiac space is a translucent area between the heart and the vertebral column, occupied by the descending aorta and the oesophagus. Angiography was, and is, used routinely for detailed study of the cavities and larger

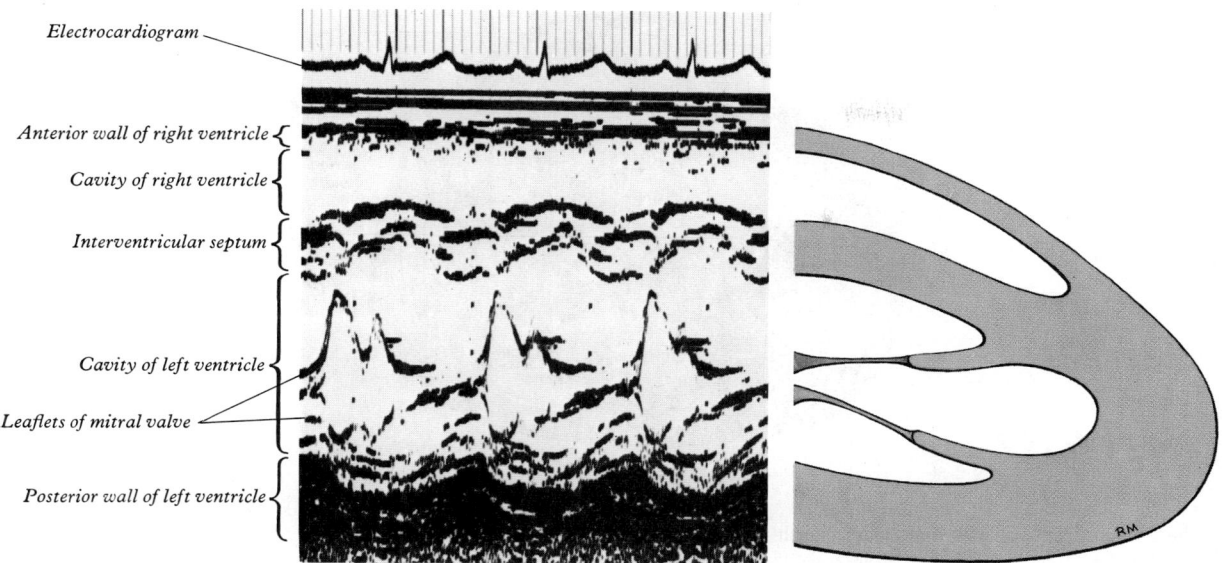

Electrocardiogram

Anterior wall of right ventricle

Cavity of right ventricle

Interventricular septum

Cavity of left ventricle

Leaflets of mitral valve

Posterior wall of left ventricle

10.50 A standard M (motion) mode echocardiogram recorded from the parasternal window. This technique, now supplemented in clinical practice by so-called 2-D formats, shows the movement of the parietal walls, ven- tricular septum and mitral valvar leaflets as indicated in the accompanying diagram. Note the biphasic nature of closure of the mitral valve.

vessels (**10**.48, 49). Nowadays, nonetheless, use of angiography is, in some centres, being supplemented, and sometimes replaced, by non-invasive studies such as computerized tomography (CT), echocardio-graphy (**10**.50), and magnetic resonance imaging (MRI). Interpret-ation of the images is unchanged and depends on knowledge of the location of the cardiac structures within the body.

CONNECTIVE TISSUES AND FIBROUS SKELETON OF THE HEART

From epicardium to endocardium, and from the orifices of the great veins to the roots of the arterial trunks, the intercellular spaces between contractile and conducting elements are everywhere per-meated by connective tissue. The amount varies greatly in arrange-ment and texture in different locations.

A fine layer of areolar tissue is found beneath the mesothelium of the serosal visceral epicardium over much of the heart (**10**.23). This accumulates *subepicardial fat*, the amount increasing with age, which becomes concentrated along the acute margin, the atrioventricular and interventricular grooves and their side channels. The coronary vessels and their main branches are embedded in this fat. The endocardium also lies on a fine areolar tissue, this time rich in elastic fibres. Fibrocellular components of these subepicardial and subendocardial layers blend on their mural aspects with the endo-mysial and perimysial connective tissue on the myocardium. Each cardiac myocyte is invested by delicate endomysium composed of fine reticular fibres, collagen and elastin fibres embedded in ground substance. This matrix is lacking only at desmosomal and gap junctional contacts of intercalated discs (p. 768). Similar arrange-ments apply to myocytes of the ventricular conduction tissues and their extensive contacts with the working myocardium. The con-nective tissue matrix itself is interconnected laterally to form bundles, strands or sheets of macroscopic proportions showing a complex geometric pattern (p. 1496). The larger myocardial bundles are sur-rounded by, and attached to, stronger perimysial condensations. The overall pattern is described in terms of struts and weaves.

The myocardial matrix, despite its importance, cannot be dissected grossly. Running at the ventricular base, nonetheless, and intimately related to atrioventricular valves and the aortic orifice, is a complex framework of dense collagen with membranous, tendinous and fibro-areolar extensions. The whole is sufficiently distinct to be termed the fibrous skeleton of the heart. (For detailed analyses see Zimmerman & Bailey 1962; Zimmerman 1966).

Although it is often stated that all four valves are contained within this skeleton, this is not the case. The cusps of the pulmonary valve are supported on a free-standing sleeve of right ventricular infundibulum which can easily be removed from the heart without disturbing either the fibrous skeleton or the left ventricle. The fibrous skeleton, rather, is strongest at the junction of aortic, mitral and tricuspid valves, the so-called *central fibrous body* (**10**.51, 52). Two pairs of curved, tapering, collagenous prongs (*fila coronaria*) extend from the central fibrous body, stronger on the left, passing partially around the mitral and tricuspid orifices, which are almost coplanar and incline to face the cardiac apex. The aortic valve, in contrast, faces up, right and slightly forwards. It is anterosuperior to and rightward of the mitral orifice. As already described, two of the cusps of the aortic valve are in fibrous continuity with the aortic leaflet of the mitral valve. This *aortic-mitral* or *subaortic curtain* (**10**.43B, 51) is also an integral part of the fibrous skeleton. The two ends of the curtain are strengthened as the *right* and *left fibrous trigones*, which are the strongest part of the skeleton. The *right trigone*, together with the membranous septum, then constitutes the *central fibrous body* (**10**.51). This important structure is penetrated by the mechanism for atrioventricular conduction (the bundle of His) while the membranous septum is crossed on its right aspect by the attachment of the tricuspid valve, dividing the septum into atrioventricular and interventricular components.

The functions of the fibrous skeleton are, first, to ensure elec-trophysiological discontinuity between the atrial and ventricular myocardial masses except at the site of penetration of the conduction tissue. Second, it functions as a stable but deformable base for the attachments of the fibrous cores of the atrioventricular valves.

The aortic root is central within the fibrous skeleton and, as discussed, is often described in terms of an 'annulus' integrated within the fibrous skeleton. As with the pulmonary valve, nonetheless, the structure of the aortic root corresponds to the triple fibrous semilunar attachments of its cusps. Within this complex circumferential zone are three crucially important triangular areas which separate, on the ventricular aspect, the aortic bulbous sinuses which house the valvar cusps. As a whole, these three triangles can be conceptualized in terms of a three-pointed coronet (**10**.44). These triangular areas were termed the *subaortic spans* by Zimmerman (1959), Zimmerman and Bailey (1962), but were originally described as the intervalvular spaces by Henle (1876). Their triangular apices correspond to the tips of the valvar commissures. Their walls, significantly thinner than the sinuses, variously consist of collagen or admixed muscle strands and fibro-elastic tissue. They form the subvalvar extensions of the aortic vestibule. The interval between the non-coronary and left coronary sinuses is filled with the deformable *subaortic curtain*. The span between the non-coronary and right coronary sinuses is continuous with the anterior surface of the *membranous septum*. The

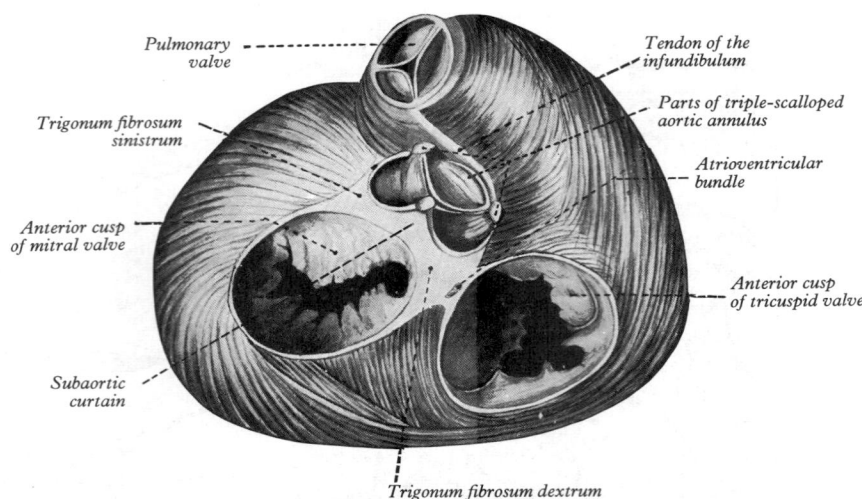

Pulmonary valve

Trigonum fibrosum sinistrum

Anterior cusp of mitral valve

Subaortic curtain

Tendon of the infundibulum

Parts of triple-scalloped aortic annulus

Atrioventricular bundle

Anterior cusp of tricuspid valve

Trigonum fibrosum dextrum

10.51 The base of the ventricles, after removal of the atria and the pericardium. Contrast the planes and positions of aortic and pulmonary valves. Contrast with **10**.52. (From Walmsley 1929.)

third subaortic span, namely that between the two coronary aortic sinuses, is filled with fibro-elastic tissue that separates the extension of the subaortic root from the wall of the free-standing subpulmonary infundibulum. Previously this was held to be the location of the *tendon of the infundibulum* (*conus ligament*). Similar fibrous triangles are found separating the sinuses of the pulmonary trunk, but these are significantly less robust.

The *mitral* and *tricuspid rings* (*annuli*) (pp. 1481, 1485), are also not simple and rigid collagenous structures but dynamic, deformable lines of valvar attachment that vary greatly at different peripheral points and change considerably with each phase of the cardiac cycle and with increasing age. The tricuspid attachments are even less robust than those of the mitral valve. At several sites it is only fibro-areolar tissue which separates the atrial and ventricular muscular masses.

ARCHITECTURE OF THE MYOCARDIUM

It has long been held that cardiac walls consist of 'fibres' transversely and longitudinally striated (p. 764) and intricately intermingled. They can be classed as atrial, ventricular, and conduction fibres (p. 1495). Atrial and ventricular muscle fibres are completely separated at the atrioventricular grooves, the only connection being via the axis of specialized myocardial cells responsible for atrioventricular conduction. The fibres of the working myocardium, atrial and ventricular, are aggregated by the fibrous matrix into well-organized rows and bundles (**10.53, 54**).

The *atrial fibres* are arranged in two layers: a superficial layer common to both atria and a deep layer proper to each. The *superficial fibres* are most distinct anteriorly where they cross the bases transversely as a thin, incomplete layer. Superiorly, the walls themselves are infolded to form the rim of the atrial septum. Deep fibres are looped and annular. The looped fibres pass over each atrium to its corresponding atrioventricular annulus, in front and behind, while annular fibres surround the appendages and encircle the openings of the venae cavae and the fossa ovalis. Further well-organized bundles are found within the terminal crest of the right atrium and its pectinate muscles.

The arrangement of the *ventricular fibres* within the ventricular mass is much more complicated, and has been the focus of many investigations over the years. Most of these have involved prior maceration or boiling of the hearts investigated, followed by dissection or tearing apart of the ventricular walls. Of necessity, these techniques are somewhat crude. Although they can produce remarkably photogenic specimens, they all suffer from the difficulty of distinguishing true tracts of fibres from artefactually induced pathways.

Combinations of dissections with study of orientations of fibres as measured in serial sections give a more accurate impression of the interrelationships of the musculature (Streeter et al 1969, 1979, 1980; Greenbaum et al 1981). These works have shown that earlier concepts, such as those espoused by MacCallum (1900) and Mall (1911), placed undue emphasis on the fibrous skeleton as the site of origin and insertion of the ventricular fibres. The heart is not to be compared with a skeletal muscle. Rather, it is a modified blood vessel. The myocardial fibres, in consequence, are attached to their neighbours and bound together by the fibrous matrix. The skeleton serves the purpose of anchoring the valves to the ventricular mass and, as discussed above, is significantly less well formed than is generally believed. Thus, concepts of the ventricular musculature being arranged in tracts which originate at the atrioventricular annulus and insert into the bases of the arterial trunks have little to support them in terms of anatomic fact. The dissections performed, which are backed up by histological studies, largely endorse the accounts of Pettigrew (1860, 1865).

The dissections show that the fibres can broadly be divided into subepicardial, middle, and subendocardial fibres. Simple inspection of the heart after the removal of the epicardium reveals the arrangement of the subepicardial fibres. By and large, these fibres run circumferentially around the right ventricle and longitudinally down the diaphragmatic surface of the left ventricle. Fibres cross over the posterior interventricular groove, and more complicated cross-over fibres are found at the anterior atrioventricular groove which continue into the free-standing subpulmonary infundibulum.

Superficial fibres also form vortices at the apices of both ventricles, turning in to form subendocardial fibres as well described by Mall (1911) (**10.53**). The middle fibres, arranged circumferentially, are confined to the left ventricle and the septum, the parietal wall of the right ventricle having only superficial subepicardial and deep subendocardial fibres. The greatest thickness of circumferential fibres is found at the base of the left ventricle, where they encircle the inlet and outlet components. This is the layer dubbed the '*bulbospiral*' *muscle* by earlier investigators. The subendocardial layers of both ventricles are continuous with the subepicardial fibres through the apical vortexes. These deep fibres form a thin layer in the left ventricle except where buttressed to form the papillary muscles. The fibres within the trabeculae run almost longitudinally, while those closer to the middle layer take an oblique course. The papillary muscles are less robust in the right ventricle. The septum belongs largely to the left ventricle, being formed for its greatest part by the circumferential layer of middle fibres (**10.38**). Since these circumferential fibres are lacking towards the ventricular apex, the apical septum is formed only by the co-apted subendocardial layers as they turn in from the ventricular apexes. There are major regional

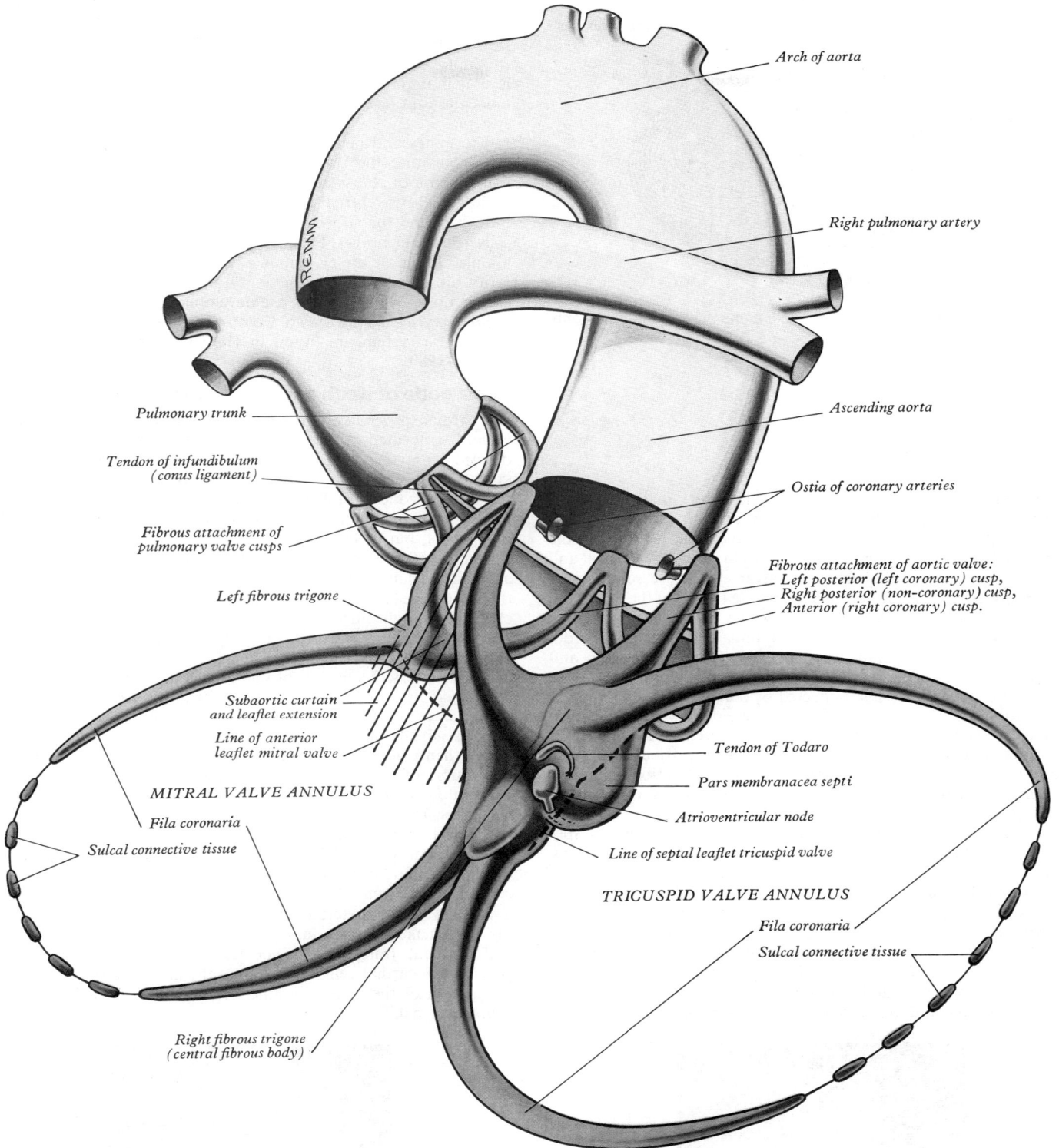

Arch of aorta

Right pulmonary artery

Pulmonary trunk

Tendon of infundibulum
(conus ligament)

Fibrous attachment of
pulmonary valve cusps

Left fibrous trigone

Subaortic curtain
and leaflet extension

Line of anterior
leaflet mitral valve

MITRAL VALVE ANNULUS

Fila coronaria

Sulcal connective tissue

Right fibrous trigone
(central fibrous body)

Ascending aorta

Ostia of coronary arteries

Fibrous attachment of aortic valve:
Left posterior (left coronary) cusp,
Right posterior (non-coronary) cusp,
Anterior (right coronary) cusp.

Tendon of Todaro

Pars membranacea septi

Atrioventricular node

Line of septal leaflet tricuspid valve

TRICUSPID VALVE ANNULUS

Fila coronaria

Sulcal connective tissue

10.52 Principal elements of the fibrous skeleton of the heart: red = mitral and aortic 'annuli', blue = tricuspid and pulmonary 'annuli', green = tendon of the infundibulum. For clarity the view is from the right posterosuperior aspect. Note that due to perspective the pulmonary annulus appears smaller than the aortic annulus, whereas in fact the reverse obtains. Based in part on the work of Zimmerman (1966). Consult text for an extended discussion.

variations in the arrangement of the fibres from heart to heart. Even greater departures from this variable 'norm' are found in hearts diseased due to dilatation, hypertrophy, coronary arterial disease, or congenital malformations. Much more work remains to be done before the true organization of the ventricular fibres is elucidated.

That which has been accomplished in recent years simply underlines the potential dangers inherent in imposing procrustean and oversimplified ideas on a complex biological structure (Greenbaum et al 1981).

CO-ORDINATION OF CARDIAC ACTIVITY: CONDUCTION SYSTEM

The human heart beats ceaselessly at about 70 or so cycles every minute for many decades, maintaining perfusion of pulmonary and systemic tissues. The rate and stroke volume fluctuate in accord with prevailing physiological demands. The principal events in a cardiac cycle, including the electrical events recorded in the electro-

1495

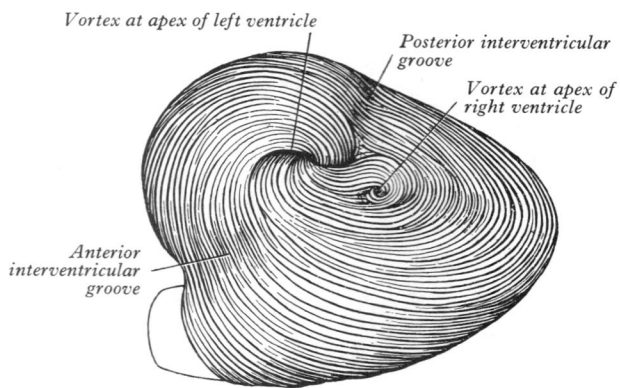

Vortex at apex of left ventricle

Posterior interventricular groove

Vortex at apex of right ventricle

Anterior interventricular groove

10.53   The two vortices in the myocardium at the apex of the heart (after Mall).

cardiogram (ECG), mechanical sequences of diastole, atrial systole, isovolumetric contraction, ejection and isovolumetric relax-ation in ventricular systole, the acoustic phenomena recorded in the phonocardiogram, pressure profiles of right and left hearts and arterial trunks and the sequences of valvar events are summarized in **10**.55. Cardiac efficiency depends on precise timing of the operation in interdependent structures. Passive diastolic filling of the atria and ventricles is followed by atrial systole, stimulated by discharge from the sinus node, which completes ventricular filling. Excitation and contraction of the atria must be synchronous and finish prior to ventricular contraction. This is effected by a **delay** in the conduction of excitation from atria to ventricles. Thereafter, ventricular con-traction proceeds in a precise manner, a specialized ventricular conduction system ensuring that closure of atrioventricular valves is followed rapidly by a wave of excitation and contraction spreading from the ventricular apices towards the outflow tracts and orifices, rapidly accelerating the blood during ejection.

Vertebrate cardiac contraction originates unequivocally in spe-cialized myocytes, but neural influences are important in adapting the intrinsic cardiac rhythm to functional demands from the whole body. All cardiac myocytes (p. 764) are excitable, with autonomous rhythmic depolarization and repolarization of the cell membrane, conduction of waves of excitation via gap junctions to adjacent myocytes, and excitation-contraction coupling to their actomyosin complexes (p. 774). These properties are developed to different degrees in different sites and in different types of myocyte. The rate of depolarization and repolarization is slowest in the ventricular

myocardium, intermediate in the atrial muscle, and fastest in the myocytes of the sinus node. The latter override those generating slower rhythms and, in the normal heart, are the locus for the rhythmic initiation of cardiac cycles. Conversely, conduction velocity is slow in nodal myocytes, intermediate in general 'working' cardiac myocytes and fastest in the myocytes of the ventricular conduction system.

The nodes and networks of the so-called specialized myocardial cells constitute the *cardiac conduction system* (**10**.56A, B, 57). The components of the system are the sinus node, the atrioventricular node, the atrioventricular bundle with its left and right bundle branches, and the subendocardial plexus of ventricular conduction cells (Purkinje fibres). Remnants of histologically specialized cells are also found at the insertions of right atrial myocardium into the atrioventricular junction. These are remnants of the more extensive conduction system found in the developing heart, and are described as *atrioventricular ring tissues*. Comprehensive accounts of the cardiac conduction system are found in Hudson (1965) and Anderson & Becker (1980).

Sinus node of Keith and Flack (1907)

The cardiac 'pacemaker', it initiates (in some of its cells) each cardiac cycle. It is located at the junction between parts of the right atrium derived from the embryonic venous sinus and the atrium proper (**10**.56A, 57). The node is distinctive histologically, with very short transitional zones peripherally. Nodal tissue does not occupy the full thickness of the right atrial wall from epicardium to endocardium in humans, but rather sits as a wedge of specialized tissue subepi-cardially within the terminal groove. The node is often covered by a plaque of subepicardial fat, making it visible in some instances to the naked eye. It extends between 1 and 2 cm on the right from the crest of the right auricle and runs postero-inferiorly into the upper part of the terminal groove. In a small proportion of cases, about one-tenth, it extends in horse-shoe fashion across the crest of the auricle. An obvious feature of the node is its *central artery*. This has a surprisingly large calibre and takes its origin from either the right or the circumflex coronary arteries. Usually originating from the initial segments of these arteries, it rarely takes a more distal origin which then places it at risk during routine opening of the atrium in the course of cardiac surgery. Its adventitia merges into a dense collagenous reticulum which permeates the node and surrounds its myocytes. Its small lateral branches supplying nodal tissue are few, the vessel continuing beyond the node to ramify in the atrial myocardium. The *nodal myocytes* themselves are slender and fusi-form. Such nodal myocytes themselves are confined to the nodal centre, circumferentially arranged around the nodal artery and more irregularly placed external to this. These cells are now considered the 'pacemakers'. They make functional contacts with each other and adjacent transitional myocytes, which are smaller than the general myocardial cells. There are only short transitional zones at the margin of the node, the junction with plain atrial myocardium being clear cut.

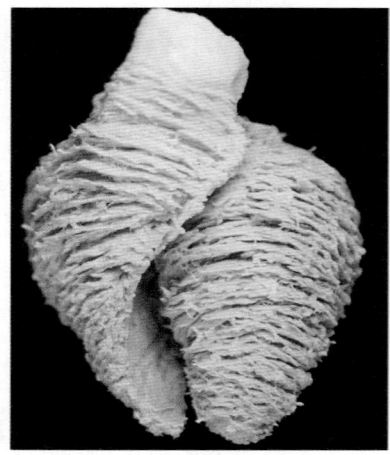

A

B

10.54A, B.   These standard dissections of the ventricular mass show the superficial layer of fibres extending over the anterior surface of both ven-tricles (A). In B further dissection reveals the important middle layer of circumferential fibres (the 'bulbospiral muscle') which is confined to the left ventricle. Dissection made by Professor Damian Sanchez-Quintana, Badajoz, Spain, and reproduced by kind permission.

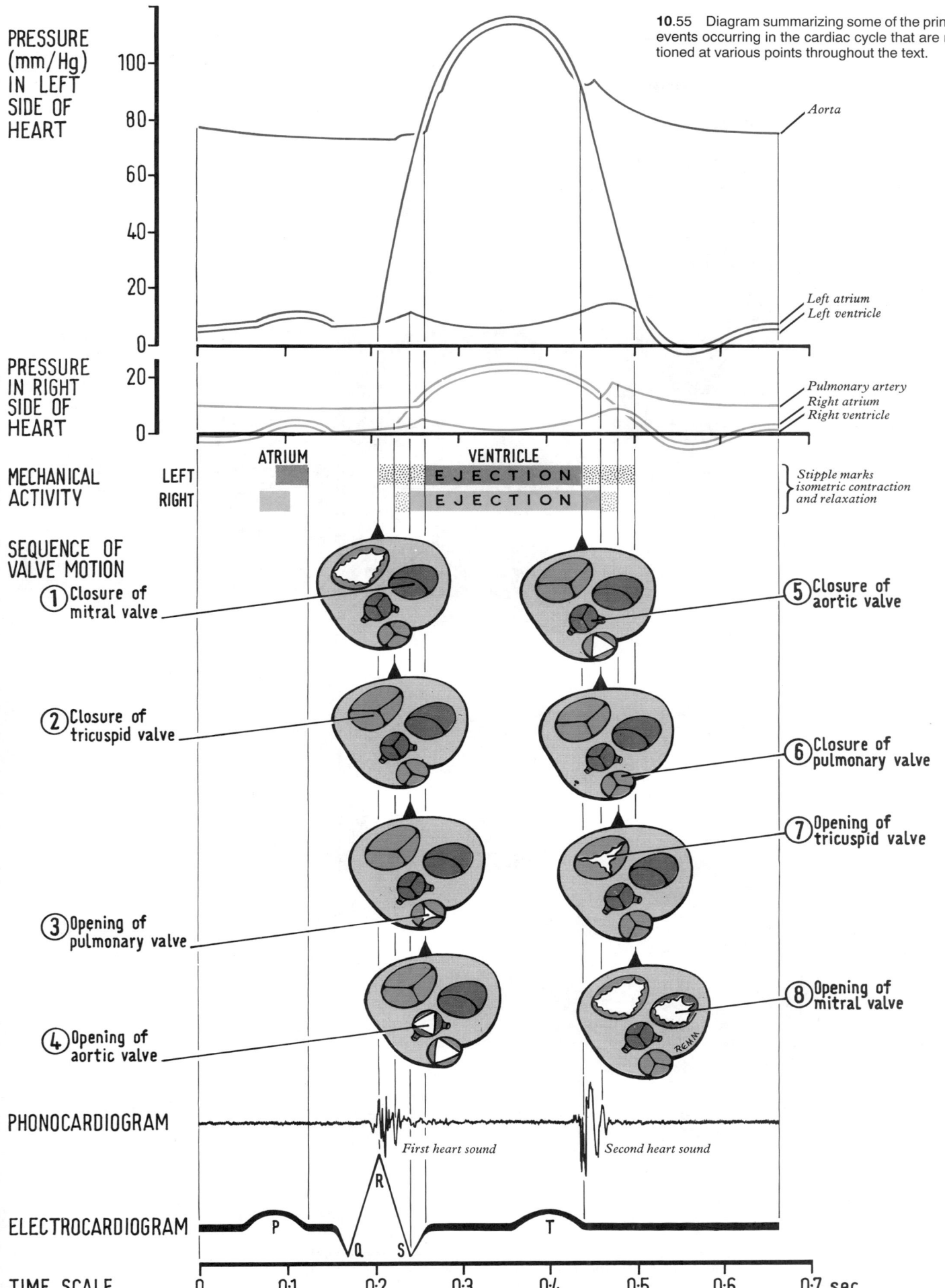

PRESSURE (mm/Hg) IN LEFT SIDE OF HEART

100
80
60
40
20
0

10.55 Diagram summarizing some of the principal events occurring in the cardiac cycle that are mentioned at various points throughout the text.

Aorta

Left atrium
Left ventricle

PRESSURE IN RIGHT SIDE OF HEART

20
0

Pulmonary artery
Right atrium
Right ventricle

MECHANICAL ACTIVITY

LEFT   ATRIUM   VENTRICLE
                         EJECTION
RIGHT   EJECTION

} *Stipple marks isometric contraction and relaxation*

SEQUENCE OF VALVE MOTION

① Closure of mitral valve

② Closure of tricuspid valve

③ Opening of pulmonary valve

④ Opening of aortic valve

⑤ Closure of aortic valve

⑥ Closure of pulmonary valve

⑦ Opening of tricuspid valve

⑧ Opening of mitral valve

REMN

PHONOCARDIOGRAM

First heart sound   *Second heart sound*

ELECTROCARDIOGRAM

R
P   T
  Q S

TIME SCALE

0   0.1   0.2   0.3   0.4   0.5   0.6   0.7 sec.

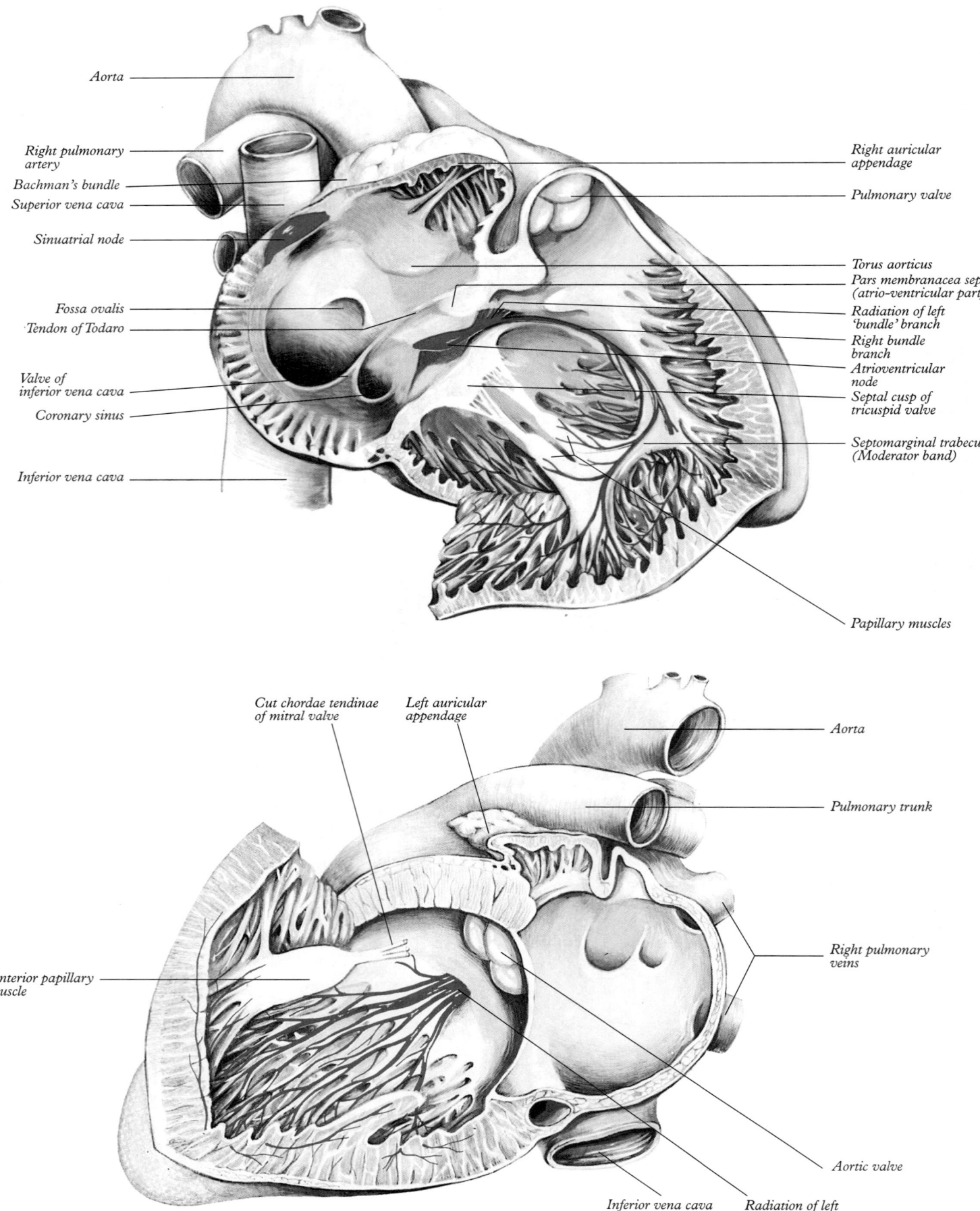

Aorta

Right pulmonary artery

Bachman's bundle

Superior vena cava

Sinuatrial node

Fossa ovalis

Tendon of Todaro

Valve of inferior vena cava

Coronary sinus

Inferior vena cava

Right auricular appendage

Pulmonary valve

Torus aorticus

Pars membranacea septi (atrio-ventricular part)

Radiation of left 'bundle' branch

Right bundle branch

Atrioventricular node

Septal cusp of tricuspid valve

Septomarginal trabecula (Moderator band)

Papillary muscles

Cut chordae tendinae of mitral valve

Left auricular appendage

Aorta

Pulmonary trunk

Right pulmonary veins

Anterior papillary muscle

Aortic valve

Inferior vena cava

Radiation of left 'bundle' branch

10.56 Diagrams of the conducting tissue of the heart as seen from the right (A) and left (B) aspects. The elements of the conducting system are shown in red. Note the conducting tissue accompanying fine trabeculae carneae and false chordae. Please note that in reality the radiation of the left bundle branch is directly related to the leaflets of the aortic valve.

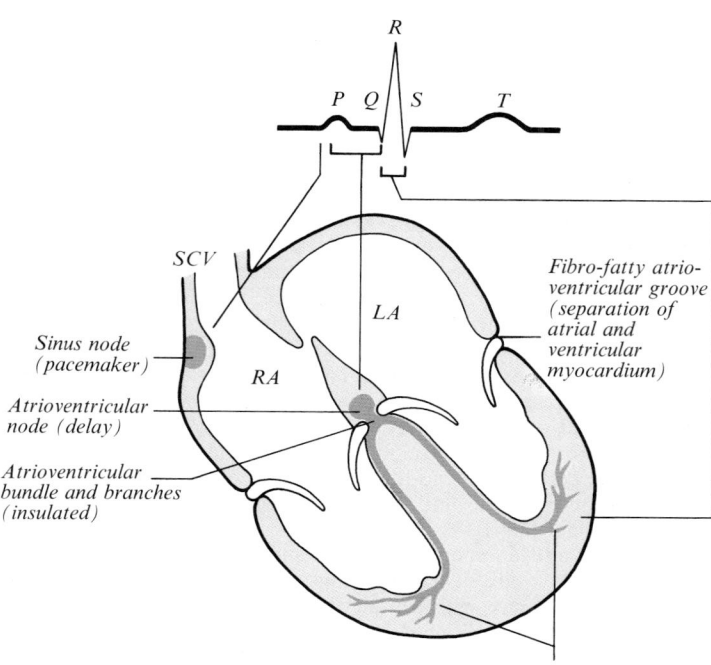

10.57 A diagram illustrating the basic structure of the conduction system, and showing the relationship with the electrocardiogram.

Atrioventricular node (Tawara 1906)

The atrioventricular node is an atrial structure which is at the root of an extensive tree of conduction tissue reaching the apex of the ventricles, the papillary muscles and other regions of the ventricles (**10.57**). The node, with its transitional zones, is located within the atrial component of the muscular atrioventricular septum, the anatomic landmarks being the boundaries of the triangle of Koch (**10.56A**). These are, inferiorly, the attachment of the septal leaflet of the tricuspid valve, basally the orifice of the coronary sinus and, superiorly, the tendon of Todaro. The compact node is a half oval set against the central fibrous body towards the apex of this triangle. Its atrial aspect is convex, being overlain by atrial myocardium. Its left margin is concave and abuts on the superior aspect of the central fibrous body. Its basal end projects into the atrial muscle while its antero-inferior end enters the central fibrous body to become the penetrating atrioventricular bundle. The node is pervaded by an irregular collagenous reticulum enmeshing the myocytes, but this is less dense than in the sinus node. Its arterial supply is from a characteristic vessel originating from the dominant coronary artery at the crux of the heart. The node has a well-formed compact zone made up of interlocking nodal cells which frequently show stratification. Superficially and posteriorly are found the transitional cell zones. The larger component of atrioventricular delay is probably produced in these transitional zones of the node.

Atrioventricular bundle

Originally described by His (1893) but clarified by Tawara (1906), the atrioventricular bundle is the direct continuation of the atrioventricular node, becoming oval, quadrangular or triangular in transverse sectional profile as it enters the central fibrous body (**10.56A**, p. 1493). Traversing the fibrous body, it branches on the crest of the muscular interventricular septum, the branching tract being sandwiched between the muscular and the membranous components of the septum. The *right branch* of the bundle (*crus dextrum*) is a narrow, discrete round group of fascicles which courses at first within the myocardium and then subendocardially towards the apex of the ventricle, entering the septomarginal trabecula to reach the anterior papillary muscle. It has few branches to the ventricular walls in its septal course, but, at the origin of the anterior papillary muscle, it divides profusely into fine subendocardial fascicles which diverge and embrace, first, the papillary muscle, then, recurving

subendocardially to the remaining ventricular walls. The *left branch* (*crus sinistrum*) arises as numerous fine intermingling fascicles which leave the left margin of the branching bundle through much of its course along the crest of the muscular ventricular septum (**10.56B**). These fascicles form a flattened sheet down the smooth left ventricular septal surface. The sheet diverges apically and subendocardially across the left aspect of the ventricular septum, separating into anterior, septal and posterior divisions. Fine branches leave the sheets, forming subendocardial networks, which first surround the papillary muscles and then curve back subendocardially to reach all parts of the ventricle.

The principal branches of the bundle are insulated from the surrounding myocardium by sheaths of connective tissue (**10.58**). Functional contacts between ventricular conduction and working myocytes become numerous only in the subendocardial terminal ramifications. Hence, papillary muscles contract first, followed by a wave of excitation and ensuing contraction travelling from the apex of the ventricle to the arterial outflow tract. And, because the Purkinje network is subendocardial, muscular excitation proceeds from the endocardial to the epicardial aspect. In the developing heart, it can be shown that the bundle responsible for atrioventricular conduction is a much more extensive structure (Wessels et al 1992). Recent work using immunohistochemical markers has shown that the precursor of the system is a ring of cells which surrounds the inlet and outlet components of the developing ventricular loop (see p. 308). With septation of the ventricles, this ring becomes modified so that it encircles the right atrioventricular orifice and the aortic outlet from the left ventricle. With subsequent growth, only the septal components of this 'figure of eight' persist as the atrioventricular conduction tract. Careful study, nonetheless, reveals that part of the aortic ring can persist as a 'dead-end tract' (Kurosawa & Becker 1985).

The components initially surrounding the tricuspid orifice also persist to varying degree, and can be found by careful study in most human hearts. These nodes of unequivocally specialized tissue are identical to the structures described and illustrated by Kent at the turn of the nineteenth century (1893, 1913). Kent was convinced that these structures were the substrates for normal atrioventricular conduction, which, he argued, occurred at multiple points around the atrioventricular junction. This contention is incorrect, and the remnants found as atrioventricular ring tissue are always sequestered by the fibrous insulation mechanism from the ventricular myocardium. Kent's findings, nonetheless, provided the stimulus for clinicians to explain the abnormal cardiac rhythm known as ventricular pre-excitation, specifically the variant known as the Wolff-Parkinson-White syndrome. It has now been shown that this syndrome is produced by abnormal small strands of otherwise unremarkable ventricular myocardium which connect the atrial and ventricular myocardial masses at some point around the atrioventricular junctions. Initially these muscular strands were described

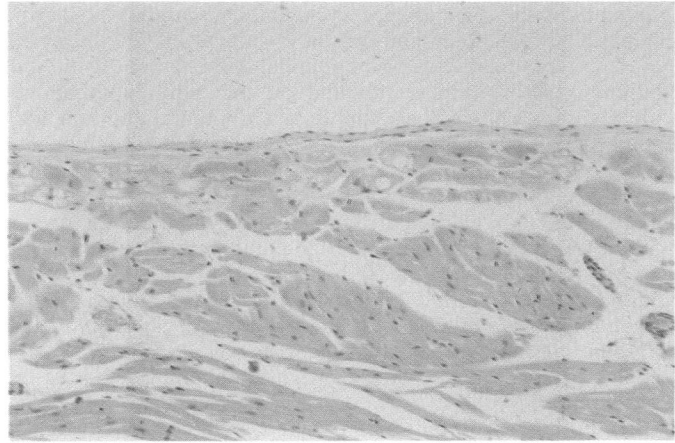

10.58 Section of conducting, Purkinje fibres in the left ventricular wall. Note the paler, enlarged cells beneath the endocardium among normal (or 'working') myocytes. Haematoxylin and eosin. Magnification × 500.

as 'bundles of Kent', the belief being that they represented the multiple connections postulated by Kent. When the connections were identified histologically, it was seen that they bore no resemblance to the remnants of atrioventricular ring tissue initially described by Kent. Instead, they were strands of working myocardium running through the fibro-areolar tissue of the atrioventricular groove.

Sinus node, atrioventricular node and atrioventricular bundle constitute a well-defined anatomical system; in it the main pacemaker rhythm of the heart is generated (sinus), is influenced by nerves (sinus and its innervation) and is transmitted specifically from atria to ventricles (atrioventricular node and bundle) and, within the ventricles, to all their musculature. The spread of excitation is very rapid but not instantaneous: different parts of the ventricles are excited at slightly different times, with important functional consequences. Failure of the conduction system will not block cardiac contraction, but this will become poorly co-ordinated or unco-ordinated; the rhythm will be slower as it then originates from a spontaneous (myogenic) activity in the working cardiac myocytes or in a subsidiary pacemaker in a more distal part of the diseased or disrupted conduction system.

One important question in this account of the role of the conduction system is: how does the excitation generated by the sinus reach the atrioventricular node? There has been considerable debate and controversy on this issue since the beginning of the century, when there were reports on the occurrence of bundles of specialized cardiac myocytes in the atria, connecting the sinus to the atrioventricular node and the right to the left atrium. Although only Thorel (1909) truly claimed to have distinguishd specialized tracts, two other tracts have been attributed to Wenckebach (1906) and Bachmann (1913). The latter workers, although describing tracts, made no claims concerning histological specialization. Furthermore, subsequent studies of the atrial walls have failed to show the existence of specialized muscle tissue, such as can be readily seen in the atrioventricular bundle. Modern authors, therefore, dismiss the occurrence of any specialized internodal and interatrial conduction pathways (Anderson et al 1974; Anderson 1975). In the absence of specialized internodal and interatrial conduction pathways, the excitation emanating from the sinus node spreads to the atrial musculature and to the atrioventricular node through ordinary atrial working myocardium. The studies of Spach and Kootsey (1983) have confirmed that there are no anatomically specialized pathways comparable with the ventricular system responsible for conduction. Instead, it is the packing and the geometric arrangement of fibres along well-organized atrial muscle bundles, such as the terminal crest and the rims of the oval fossa, which are responsible for conduction being marginally more rapid than elsewhere within the atrium. The muscle fibres responsible for such conduction, as far as can be judged with standard staining, are ordinary working atrial myocardial fibres (Janse & Anderson 1974).

NERVE SUPPLY TO THE HEART

Initiation of the cardiac cycle in vertebrates is myogenic, originating in the sinus node. The cardiac cycle initiated in this fashion is harmonized in rate, force and output by nerves of the autonomic nervous system operating on the nodal tissues and their prolongations, on coronary vessels and on the working atrial and ventricular musculature. This supply is autonomic, and has both efferent (sympathetic and parasympathetic) and afferent components. Parasympathetic fibres reach the heart through vagal branches (p. 1252), the sympathetic from the branches of the sympathetic trunk (p. 1303). Vagal preganglionic fibres proceed from origins within the brainstem, particularly the medulla, including the nucleus ambiguus (p. 1021), the reticular nuclei (p. 1073) and possibly the dorsal vagal nucleus (p. 1020). Preganglionic axons leave in the cardiac branches of both the right and the left vagus nerves to reach the cardiac plexus. Sympathetic preganglionic neurons are in the upper five or six segments of the intermediolateral column of the thoracic spinal cord (Kuntz 1953). These fibres end in the cervical and the third and fourth thoracic sympathetic ganglia (Mitchell 1953), from all of which postganglionic fibres proceed bilaterally to the heart (pp. 1252, 1306). (See also general comments and modern reservations concerning the simplification implicit in the terms pre- and postganglionic, p. 1293.)

The central connections of cardiac preganglionic neurons, parasympathetic and sympathetic, are described elsewhere (Reticular formation of the brainstem p. 1073, Hypothalamus p. 1141 and Cerebral cortex p. 1094). The existence and behaviour of these integrating influences can be deduced in terms of their function, but the precise locations of connecting pathways in the spinal cord, brainstem, and cerebrum are uncertain.

Nearing the heart, the autonomic nerves form a mixed cardiac plexus (p. 1306), usually described in terms of a superficial component found inferior to the aortic arch and between it and the pulmonary trunk, and a deep part between the aortic arch and tracheal bifurcation. These plexuses contain ganglion cells, with further ganglion cells found in the heart along the distribution of branches of the plexus (10.59). The branches of these cells are considered largely, if not exclusively, postganglionic and parasympathetic in nature. The advent of more reliable staining techniques for identification of cholinergic and adrenergic nerve cells and their ramifications has now helped clarify the distribution of cardiac autonomic components, although the discovery of additional neural transmitters which are neither truly cholinergic nor adrenergic has added a further complicating element (Corr 1992).

Cholinergic and adrenergic fibres, arising in or passing through the cardiac plexus, are distributed most profusely to the sinus and atrioventricular nodes, with a much less dense supply to the atrial and ventricular myocardium. Adrenergic fibres supply the coronary arteries and cardiac veins. Rich plexuses of nerves containing cholinesterase, adrenergic transmitters, and other peptides such as neuropeptide Y (NY) are found in the subendocardial regions of all chambers and in the leaflets of the valves. Complex endorgans have also been discovered in the subendocardium of the left atrium (Tranum-Jensen 1975).

Ganglion cells, the source of vagal postganglionic fibres, are confined to the atrial tissues in man, with a preponderance adjacent to the sinus node. Some ganglion cells in the atrium have now been shown to contain adrenergic transmitters, and they also contain small, intensely-fluorescent chromaffin cells (SIF-cells, see p. 1299).

VESSELS OF THE HEART

Arteries of cardiac supply, the aortic coronary branches, are described on pages 1495–1510, cardiac veins and the coronary sinus on pages 1575–1576 and lymphatic drainage on page 1625.

FETAL CIRCULATION

Fetal blood reaches the placenta via two umbilical arteries and

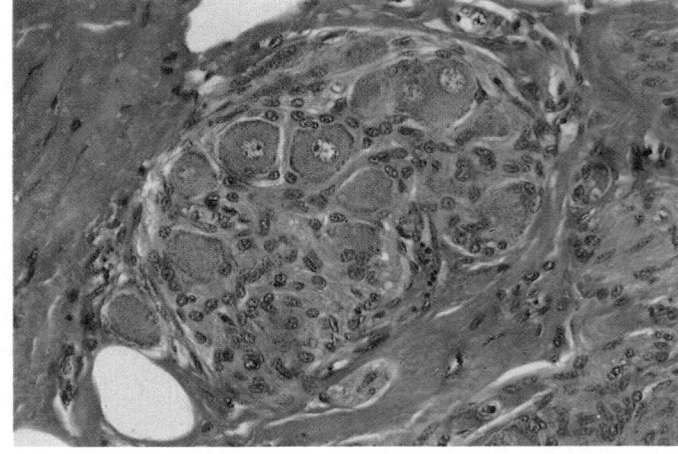

10.59 Small autonomic nerve ganglion in the wall of the left atrium (monkey). The ganglion lies within the atrial musculature; several ganglion neurons are grouped together, and each of them is surrounded by small satellite cells (glial cells). Masson trichrome stain. Magnification × 600.

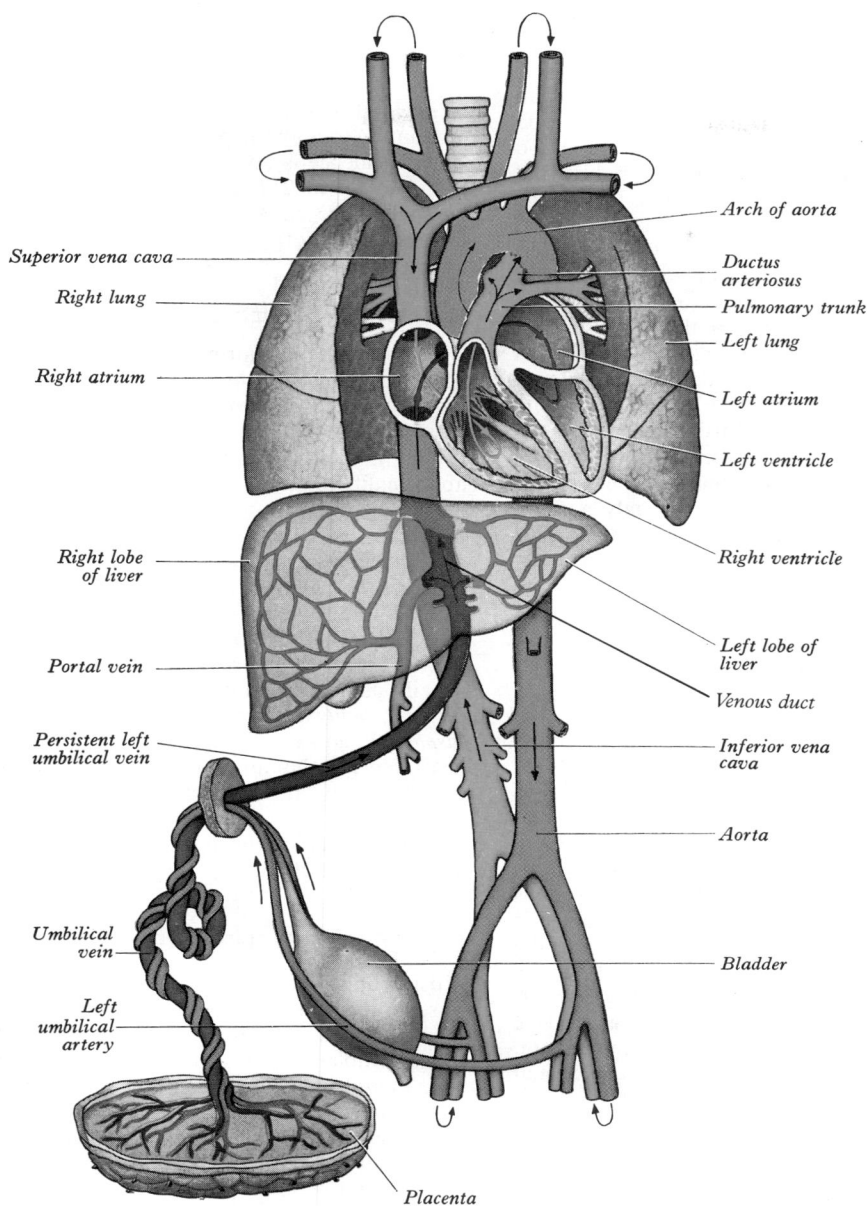

Superior vena cava

Right lung

Right atrium

Right lobe of liver

Portal vein

Persistent left umbilical vein

Umbilical vein

Left umbilical artery

Arch of aorta

Ductus arteriosus

Pulmonary trunk

Left lung

Left atrium

Left ventricle

Right ventricle

Left lobe of liver

Venous duct

Inferior vena cava

Aorta

Bladder

Placenta

10.60   Plan of the fetal circulation. The arrows indicate the direction of blood flow. The placenta is drawn to a greatly reduced scale.

returns in early fetal life by two umbilical veins (**10.60**). Later, the right one disappears (p. 324). The persisting left umbilical vein enters the abdomen at the umbilicus and traverses the edge of the falciform ligament to reach the hepatic surface of the liver. It then joins the left branch of the portal vein at the hepatic portal. Opposite the junction, a large vessel, the *venous duct (ductus venosus)*, arises and ascends posterior to the liver to join the left hepatic vein near its termination in the inferior vena cava. (For a detailed developmental account, with illustrations, of the circumhepatic veins see p. 321.) The portal vein is small in the fetus compared with the size of the umbilical vein. Parts of its left branch, proximal and distal to their junctions, function as branches of the portal vein, carrying oxygenated blood to the right and left parts of the liver. Hence, blood in the left umbilical vein reaches the inferior vena cava by three routes:

- Some enters the liver directly and reaches the vena cava via the hepatic veins
- A considerable quantity circulates through the liver with portal venous blood before also entering by the hepatic veins
- The remainder is bypassed into the inferior vena cava by the venous duct.

Blood from the venous duct and hepatic veins mixes in the inferior vena cava with blood from the lower limbs and abdominal wall. It enters the right atrium and, guided by the valve of the inferior vena cava, passes mostly through the oval foramen into the left atrium, where it mingles with the limited venous return from the pulmonary veins. Some blood returning via the inferior vena cava, instead of traversing the oval foramen, joins blood from the superior vena cava and passes through the right atrium to reach the right ventricle. From the left atrium, blood enters the left ventricle and thence the aorta, by which it is probably distributed almost entirely to the heart, head and upper limbs, little reaching the descending aorta. Blood from the head and upper limbs returns via the superior vena cava to the right atrium, all of which traverses the right atrioventricular orifice, along with the small amount returned via the inferior vena cava. From the right ventricle, this blood enters the pulmonary trunk. The fetal lungs are largely inactive, so only a little of the blood from the right ventricle traverses the right and left pulmonary arteries, and this returns by the pulmonary veins to the left atrium. The greater part of the outflow through the pulmonary trunk is carried by the *arterial duct (ductus arteriosus)* directly to the aorta, where it mixes with the small quantity of blood passed from the left ventricle into this part of the aorta. The mixture descends

1501

the aorta and is partly distributed to the lower limbs and the organs of the abdomen and pelvis. Most is returned via the umbilical arteries to the placenta.

In terms of function, it is the placenta which serves as the organ for fetal nutrition and excretion, receiving deoxygenated fetal blood and returning it oxygenated and detoxified. Most of the blood entering the left atrium comes from the right atrium, right atrial pressure being much higher than that in the left atrium. Hence, the flap-like valve of the primary septum (p. 304) is thrust to the left (3.168, 169, 170), allowing passage of blood from the right to the left atrium. The valve of the inferior vena cava is so placed as to direct nearly all the richly oxygenated blood from the umbilical vein to the oval foramen and left atrium, whereas most of the venous blood from the superior vena cava enters the right ventricle directly through the right atrioventricular orifice. The refreshed placental blood, therefore, mixed with blood from the portal vein and inferior vena cava, passes almost directly to the aorta for distribution to the head and upper limbs. In contrast, the blood which reaches the descending aorta through the ductus arteriosus is mostly the blood which has circulated through the head and upper limbs, with only a small amount coming from the pulmonary veins and left atrium. This blood is distributed to the abdomen and lower limbs, but principally returns to the placenta.

CHANGES IN THE VASCULAR SYSTEM AT BIRTH

At birth, as pulmonary respiration begins, increased amounts of blood from the pulmonary trunk traverse the pulmonary arteries to the lungs and return by the pulmonary veins to the left atrium. Consequently, pressure rises within the left atrium. A fall in pressure also occurs in the inferior vena cava due to reduction of venous return concomitant with occlusion of the umbilical vein and venous duct. Atrial pressures become equal and the valvar oval foramen is closed by apposition, and later fusion, of the primary septum to the rims of the foramen (p. 304). Contraction of the atrial septal muscle, synchronized with that in the superior vena cava, may assist this closure which occurs after functional closure of the ductus arteriosus. Sometimes fusion is incomplete, a potential atrial communication persisting throughout life. Almost always this has no functional effect, since the inequality of atrial pressures and the valve-like arrangement of the opening do not favour passage of blood. When the umbilical cord is ligated, arresting placental circulation, the umbilical vein thromboses, gradually becoming the ligamentum teres. Umbilical vessels are muscular but devoid of a nerve supply in their extra-abdominal course. They constrict in response to handling, stretching, cooling and altered tensions of oxygen and carbon dioxide. The venous duct (*ductus venosus*) shuts down by an unknown mechanism. It is already closed in about one-third of newborn infants (Rudolph et al 1961). Its fibrous remnant is the venous ligament (*ligamentum venosum*). After ligation of the umbilical cord, the umbilical (hypogastric) arteries also thrombose from the origin of their last branches (superior vesical arteries) to the umbilicus, subsequently becoming fibrous chordae (medial umbilical ligaments) in the extraperitoneal fat of the abdominal wall.

The ductus arteriosus contracts rapidly immediately after birth, although blood probably continues to flow intermittently through it for a week or so. Such flow, nonetheless, is reversed relative to that occurring in the fetal circulation. This is the consequence of the rise in systemic vascular resistance which results from exclusion of the placental circulation, and the fall in pulmonary resistance occurring with expansion of the lungs. Anatomic closure of the duct is due to endothelial proliferation but takes some months to complete. Initial constriction at birth has been attributed to raised oxygen tension. A neural factor may also be involved, the muscular wall having afferent and efferent nerve endings and responding to adrenaline and nor-adrenaline (Franklin 1939; Barcroft 1941; Barclay et al 1942). After closure, the duct becomes an impervious ligament connecting the left pulmonary artery (near its origin) with the aortic arch. (For morphological and biomechanical studies of the arterial ligament, consult Dohr et al 1986. For a general review of perinatal vascular changes, see Dawes 1969.)

CONGENITAL CARDIAC MALFORMATIONS

Congenital malformations of the heart are relatively common, amounting to about one-quarter of all developmental abnormalities. Their incidence is estimated at 8 per 1000 live births, but they are found in up to 2% of stillbirths. Only a small proportion of the anomalies are directly attributable to genetic or environmental factors, the majority being the result of multifactorial events.

ABNORMALITIES OF THE CARDIAC POSITION

The most severe abnormality of position is an extrathoracic heart, so-called *ectopia cordis*. The heart usually projects to the surface through the lower thoracic and upper abdominal wall, remaining covered in most instances by the fibrous pericardium. There is usually additional herniation of the abdominal contents. Another abnormality of position is for the heart to show a mirror-like reversal in shape and position, being found in the right hemithorax with its apex directed to the right instead of the left (*dextrocardia*). This arrangement may be part of a general mirror-like reversal (so-called general 'situs inversus'). More usually an abnormal location of the heart is found with an arrangement known as *isomerism*, in which both sides of the thorax, including the atrial appendages, retain features of either morphological rightness or leftness. This is also usually associated with anomalous arrangement of the abdominal organs, *right isomerism* associated with absence of the spleen (*asplenia*) and left isomerism with multiple spleens (*polysplenia*). The heart can also be abnormally located when the rest of the body is normal. Such an abnormal location usually indicates presence of additional lesions within the heart but can simply be the consequence of abnormality of the lungs, the abnormally located heart being anatomically normal.

DEFECTS OF THE CARDIAC SEPTATION

Most anomalies can be placed in this group, with simple deficiencies of septation affecting the atrial septum, the atrioventricular septum, the ventricular septum or the arterial pole of the developing heart. More complex forms with abnormal septation represent failure of, or inappropriate, connection of the atria to the ventricles. In this set can be placed anomalies such as double inlet ventricle; absence of one atrioventricular connection (tricuspid or mitral atresia); and discordant atrioventricular connections (congenitally corrected transposition).

Atrial septal defects

Defects within the oval fossa. A persistent communication between the atrial chambers within the oval fossa is common, resulting from failure of fusion of the primary atrial septum (the flap valve) with the infolded muscular rims of the fossa. When the flap valve is still able to overlap the rims, the communication is of no functional significance as long as left atrial pressure is higher than right, which is usually the case. In contrast, when the flap valve is smaller than the fossa, or when it is perforate, there is a true atrial septal defect (**10.61**).

Other atrial communications. In normal development, the free edge of the primary septum fuses with the atrioventricular endo-cardial cushions, permitting subsequent formation of the atrio-ventricular septum. When this process fails to occur, the entire atrioventricular junction is malformed, with an atrioventricular septal defect being part of the complex anomaly. This defect can be found when the leaflets of the atrioventricular valves are fused to the crest of the ventricular septum (**10.62**), producing an interatrial communication at the expected site of the atrioventricular septum. This so-called 'ostium primum' defect, therefore, is properly classed as an atrioventricular septal defect (see below). Other interatrial communications can be formed in the mouths of the venae cavae, most frequently the superior vena cava, and are usually associated with drainage of the right pulmonary veins into the cavo-atrial junction. Known as *sinus venosus defects* (**10.61**), their essential feature is a bi-atrial connection of the vena cava. An interatrial communication can also occur through the mouth of the coronary sinus when there is a deficiency or absence of the wall usually separating the sinus from the left atrium.

Atrioventricular septal defects

Atrioventricular septal defects result from failure of fusion of the endocardial atrioventricular cushions, leaving a common atrioventricular orifice and deficiencies of the adjacent septal structures (**10**.62). The common orifice is guarded by a basically common valve, with superior and inferior leaflets bridging the scooped-out ventricular septum to be tethered in both right and left ventricles. Although the left component of the valve thus formed is often interpreted as a 'cleft mitral valve', in reality it bears no resemblance to the normally structured mitral valve, having three leaflets and with the 'cleft' forming the zone of apposition between the left ventricular components of the bridging leaflets. The defects show marked variation according to the attachments of the bridging leaflets of the common valve to each other and to the adjacent atrial and ventricular septal structures. Two major subgroups are identified. The more frequent pattern has a common atrioventricular orifice and the potential for shunting through the septal defect at both atrial and ventricular levels (**10**.62, middle). The minority of cases have separate right and left atrioventricular orifices with shunting possible only at atrial level. Although the latter defect is often described as an *ostium primum atrial septal defect*, it is, in reality, an atrioventricular septal defect.

Ventricular septal defects

The commonest defect of the ventricular septum is found in the environs of the expected site of the membranous septum in the right wall of the aortic vestibule, below the commissure between the non-coronary and right coronary leaflets of the aortic valve (**10**.63). The defect is closely related to the septal leaflet of the tricuspid valve, but can extend to open into the ventricular outlet beneath the supraventricular crest (p. 1480). It results from incomplete closure of the ventricular septum by its membranous component, often being associated with overriding of the crest of the muscular septum by the aortic orifice, along with pulmonary stenosis or atresia and hypertrophy of the right ventricle (*Fallot's tetralogy*). Rarely the pulmonary trunk can be normal or even dilated with this combination, giving the so-called *Eisenmenger complex*. Such perimembranous defects, so called because they have the remnant of the membranous septum as part of their perimeter, can also be found with abnormal ventriculo-arterial connections (see below). It is then often the pulmonary trunk which overrides the muscular septum, giving the so-called *Taussig-Bing syndrome*. In perimembranous ventricular septal defects, the atrioventricular bundle and its right and left branches are always found along the *postero-inferior margin* of the defect (Latham & Anderson 1972).

Less commonly, a septal defect can be found in the ventricular outflow tracts roofed by the conjoined facing leaflets of the aortic and pulmonary valves. Such juxta-arterial defects are doubly committed in that they open beneath the orifices of both aortic and pulmonary valves. They are due to failure of formation of both the outlet component of the muscular ventricular septum and the free-standing subpulmonary muscular infundibulum, but with appropriate septation at the ventriculo-arterial junction. They usually have a muscular postero-inferior rim which protects the atrioventricular bundle, but can extend to become perimembranous.

The third type of ventricular septal defect is made up of those enclosed within the musculature of the septum. Such muscular defects can occur in all parts of the septum, and can be multiple, producing a so-called 'Swiss-Cheese' septum.

Defects within the inlet part of the septum are important because the atrioventricular bundle passes in their upper border, in contrast to perimembranous defects opening to the inlet of the right ventricle where the atrioventricular bundle is postero-inferiorly located.

Common arterial trunk

The essence of a common arterial trunk lesion is presence of an undivided arterial channel, guarded by a common arterial valve, positioned above and astride the free margin of the muscular ventricular septum (**10**.64). There is, therefore, a coexisting juxta-arterial deficiency of the ventricular septum. The right and left pulmonary arteries usually arise via a confluent segment but can take independent origin from the common arterial trunk, which continues as the ascending aorta. The common valve usually has three leaflets, but may have two, four, or more. The lesion is due to a failure of development of the aorticopulmonary septum, and is almost certainly linked to abnormal migration of cells into the heart from the neural crest.

ABNORMAL CONNECTIONS OF THE GREAT ARTERIES AND VEINS

Complete transposition is the condition in which the aorta arises from the right ventricle and the pulmonary trunk from the left. Better described as showing discordant ventriculo-arterial connections, such hearts can coexist with deficiencies of cardiac septation. They can also be found with discordant connections at the atrioventricular junction (congenitally corrected transposition). The developmental history of the discordant connections is still unknown.

Double outlet ventricle exists when the greater part of both arterial valves are attached within the same ventricle, almost always the right. For circulation to continue, it is then necessary for the ventricular septum to be deficient, although the septal defect can rarely close as a secondary event. The position of the septal defect serves for subclassification. It is usually beneath the aorta or the pulmonary trunk, but can be doubly committed or even non-committed.

Either the systemic or pulmonary veins can be anomalously connected. The commonest systemic anomaly is found when a persistent left superior vena cava drains into the right atrium through the enlarged orifice of the coronary sinus.

More rarely, the left vena cava may connect directly with the superior aspect of the left atrium, usually associated with unroofing of the coronary sinus, the orifice of the sinus then functioning as an interatrial communication. The commonest lesion of the inferior vena cava is for its abdominal course to be interrupted, with drainage to the heart via the azygos or hemiazygos venous system. This lesion is found most frequently with left isomerism.

The pulmonary veins can be connected to an anomalous site individually or in combination. Totally anomalous connection is of most significance. Usually the veins form a confluence behind the left atrium which then connects either to the superior vena cava, to the coronary sinus, or to the portal venous system having traversed the diaphragm.

A right aortic arch is found most frequently with tetralogy of Fallot or with common arterial trunk. It can also exist, together with a left arch, in various combinations known as arterial rings which compress the oesophagus, giving so-called dysphagia lusoria. Persistent patency of the ductus arteriosus (p. 1052) must be distinguished from delayed closure. The persistently patent duct can be an obligatory part of the circulation when associated with aortic or pulmonary atresia. Coarctation of the aorta can be found as an isolated lesion when the ductus arteriosus is closed, or with an open duct when it is more likely to be associated with additional lesions within the heart. Congenital cardiac malformations are often multiple and probably occur more frequently in siblings and in children of consanguineous marriages. There is a low correlation, however, among monozygotic twins. Ventricular septal defects are the commonest lesions, making up about 20% of all cases. This is followed by persistent patency of the ductus arteriosus, coarctation, pulmonary stenosis, Fallot's tetralogy, complete transposition, aortic stenosis, and hypoplastic left heart syndrome, each of these accounting for between 5% and 10% of all cases.

ARTERIAL SYSTEM

PULMONARY TRUNK

The pulmonary trunk, or pulmonary artery (**10**.65, 66, 68) conveys deoxygenated blood from the right ventricle to the lungs. About 5 cm in length and 3 cm in diameter, it is the most anterior of the cardiac vessels and it arises from the base of the right ventricle (from the pulmonary annulus surmounting the conus arteriosus) above and to the left of the supraventricular crest. It slopes up and back, at first in front of the ascending aorta, then to its left. Below the aortic arch it divides, level with the fifth thoracic vertebra and to the left of the midline, into the right and left pulmonary arteries of almost equal size. Thus the pulmonary trunk bifurcation lies **below**, **in front** and to the **left** of the tracheal bifurcation, which is also associated with the inferior tracheobronchial lymph nodes and the deep cardiac nerve plexus. In the fetus the pulmonary artery at the level of the bifurcation is connected to the aortic arch by the ductus arteriosus, which lies in the same direction as the pulmonary artery.

Relations

The artery is entirely within the pericardium, enclosed with the ascending aorta in a common tube of visceral pericardium; the fibrous pericardium gradually peters out in the adventitia of the pulmonary arteries. **Anteriorly** it is separated from the sternal end of the left second intercostal space by the pleura, left lung and pericardium. **Posterior** are at first the ascending aorta and left coronary artery, then the left atrium. The ascending aorta is finally on its right. An auricle and coronary artery are on each side of its origin. The superficial cardiac plexus is between the pulmonary bifurcation and the aortic arch; above, behind and right are the tracheal bifurcation, lymph nodes and nerves (see above).

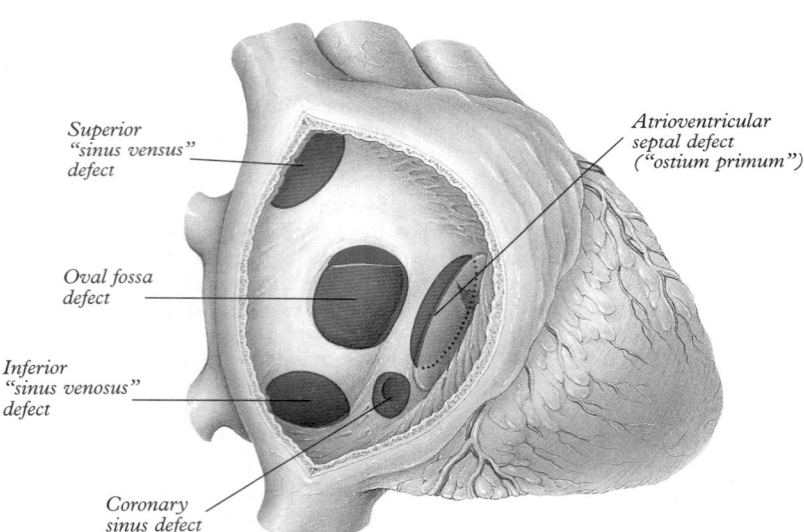

Superior
"sinus versus"
defect

Atrioventricular
septal defect
("ostium primum")

Oval fossa
defect

Inferior
"sinus venosus"
defect

Coronary
sinus defect

10.61   This drawing shows the location of the defects which produce an interatrial communication. Only defects within the oval fossa are true atrial septal defects.

During fetal life, when blood pressure is similar in the pulmonary artery and the aorta, the structure of the vessels is similar. After birth, with the expansion of the lungs and dilatation of pulmonary arterioles, pulmonary vascular resistance falls while blood flow increases; the systolic pressure in the pulmonary artery falls and this is accompanied by a structural remodelling of the wall. The elastic material, which has originally a lamellar structure, becomes aggregated into star-shaped units which are linked to many muscle cells. The amount of musculature grows extensively after birth and it exceeds that found in the aorta; in the latter, however, the thickness of the wall is about twice that in the pulmonary artery.

Right pulmonary artery. Slightly longer and larger than the left artery, it runs horizontally to the right, behind the ascending aorta, superior vena cava and upper right pulmonary vein, then in front and below the tracheal bifurcation (see above) and thence in front of the oesophagus and right main bronchus to the right pulmonary hilum. It divides as it emerges from behind the superior vena cava into two large branches. A lymph node usually occupies the bifurcation. The superior branch, which is the smaller of the two, goes to the superior lobe and it usually divides into two further branches which supply the majority of that lobe. The inferior branch descends anterior to the intermediate bronchus and immediately posterior to the superior pulmonary vein. It gives off a small recurrent branch to the superior lobe and, at the point where the horizontal fissure meets the oblique fissure, this branch of the pulmonary artery then gives off anteriorly the branch to the middle lobe and posteriorly the branch to the superior segment of the inferior lobe. It then continues a short distance before dividing to supply the rest of the inferior lobe segments.

Left pulmonary artery. Shorter and smaller than the right, it runs horizontally in front of the ascending aorta and the left principal bronchus to the left hilum. It emerges from within the concavity of the aortic arch and descends anterior to the descending aorta to enter the oblique fissure. The branches of the left pulmonary artery are extremely variable. Usually its first and largest branch is to the anterior segment of the left superior lobe. Prior to reaching the fissure it gives off a variable number of other branches to the superior lobe. As it enters the fissure it usually supplies a large branch to the superior segment of the inferior lobe. Lingular branches arise within the fissure and the rest of the lower lobe is supplied by many varied branching patterns. It was a surgical aphorism of the late Lord Brock that when performing a left upper lobectomy 'There was always one more branch of the pulmonary artery than you thought!'.

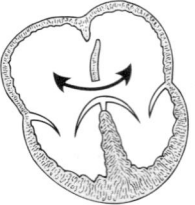 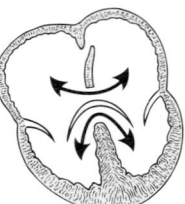 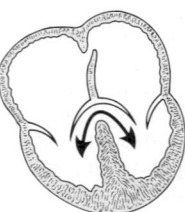

10.62   This drawing shows how, depending on the attachment of the bridging leaflets, shunting across an atrioventricular septal defect can be atrial, ventricular or both levels.

AORTA

The aorta, the trunk of the arterial tree conveying oxygenated blood to the body, begins at the aortic annulus (pp. 1488, 1493), part of the base of the left ventricle, where it is about 3 cm in diameter. Passing up and right for about 5 cm, it arches upwards, backwards

and to the left over the left pulmonary hilum and then descends in the thorax at first left of the vertebral column, then gradually inclining towards the midline, to enter the abdomen via the diaphragm's aortic hiatus. Diminished in size to about 1.75 cm, it ends a little left of the midline, level with the lower border of the fourth lumbar vertebra, dividing into the right and left common iliac arteries. For convenience it is described as arbitrarily divided into *ascending*, *arch* and *descending thoracic* and *abdominal* parts.

ASCENDING AORTA

The ascending aorta (**10**.23A, 26, 65, 66, 67), about 5 cm long, begins at the base of the left ventricle, level with the third left costal cartilage's lower border; it ascends obliquely, curving forwards and right, behind the left half of the sternum to the level of the second left costal cartilage's upper border. At its origin, close to the aortic annulus, the sectional profile is larger and not circular because of three almost hemispherical outward bulges (sinuses of Valsalva), one posterior (non-coronary), one left and one right, which correspond to the three cusps of the aortic valve (p. 1488). Distal to the aortic annulus are three aortic sinuses, beyond which the vessel's calibre is slightly increased by a bulging of its right wall; this aortic bulb gives the vessel an oval section.

Relations

The ascending aorta is within the fibrous pericardium, enclosed in a tube of serosal pericardium with the pulmonary trunk (**10**.19). Anterior to its lower part are the infundibulum (p. 1480), the initial segment of the pulmonary trunk, and the right auricle; superiorly, it is separated from the sternum by the pericardium, right pleura, anterior margin of the right lung, loose areolar tissue and thymic remains; posterior are the left atrium, right pulmonary artery and principal bronchus; right lateral are the superior vena cava and right atrium, the former partly posterior; left lateral are the left atrium and, at a higher level, the pulmonary trunk.

At least two structures (reminiscent of the carotid arterial chemoreceptors and baroreceptors, p. 971) lie between the ascending aorta and the pulmonary trunk. The inferior aorticopulmonary body is near the heart and anterior to the aorta; the middle aorticopulmonary body is near the right side of the ascending aorta (Boyd 1961).

Branches form the right and left coronary arteries (**10**.67A–E), supplying the heart itself.

CORONARY ARTERIES

The right and left coronary arteries issue from the ascending aorta in its anterior and left posterior sinuses (**10**.65, 67A–E). Variations are rare but the two may start, separately or in common, from the same sinus; three or even four coronary arteries have been observed; the most common variation concerns a right coronary branch, *arteria coni arteriosi* or 'conus artery', which is usually (64%) its first branch but often arises separately in the anterior sinus (36%), as a third coronary artery. The left coronary opening may be double, leading into major initial branches, usually the circumflex and anterior interventricular; one may lead into a stem common to one such branch and a diagonal ventricular ramus. The levels of coronary orifices are variable; Thebesius (1708) appears to have started a view that aortic cusps obstruct them when fully spread in systole; but the coronary orifices are at a higher level, at or above cuspal margins, though below in about 10% (right coronary) and 15% (left). (Further, as detailed on p. 1486 et seq, it is now established that, even at the

Doubly commited juxta-arterial defects
• *Beneath aortic and pulmonary values*

• *Can extend to become perimembranous*

Muscular defects
• *entirely enclosed in muscular septum*

• *can occur between inlet, apical trabecular or outlet ventricular*

Perimembranous defects

• *Abut on central fibrous body*

• *can extend to open between inlet, apical trabecular or outlet trabecular components, or can be confluent*

10.63 Diagram showing how, based on the structure of the anatomic borders seen from the right ventricle, ventricular septal defects can be placed into perimembranous, muscular or doubly committed groups.

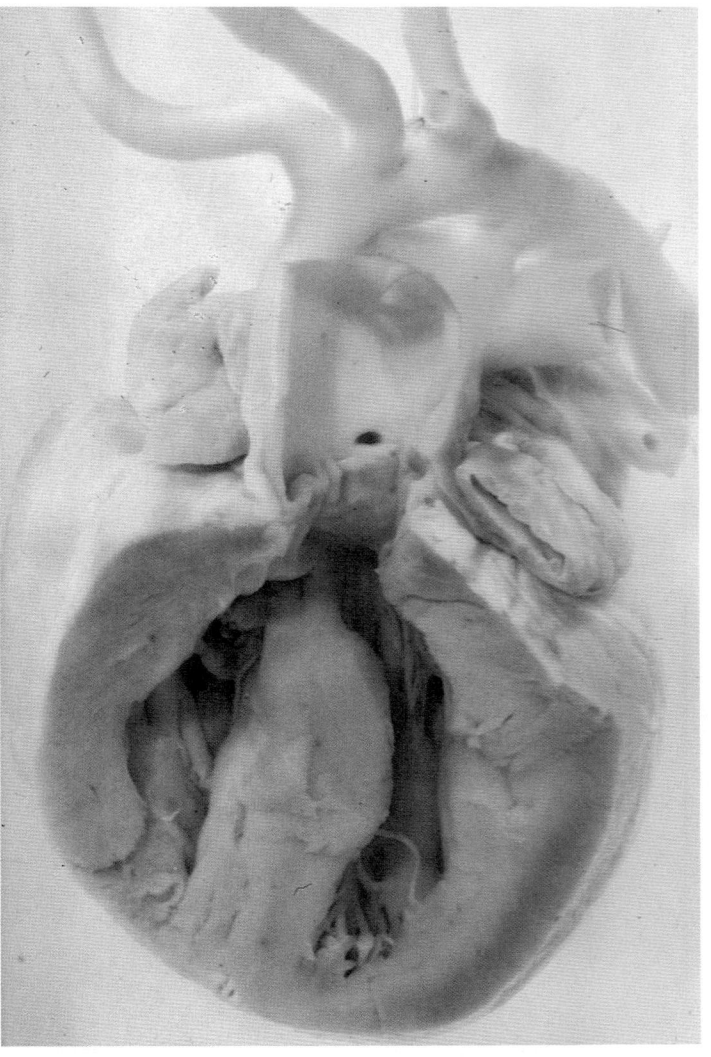

10.64 This heart possesses a common arterial trunk, with a common truncal valve overriding a juxta-arterial deficiency of the ventricular septum. It is due to failure of septation of the arterial pole of the developing heart. (Specimen prepared by Dr Leon M Gerlis.)

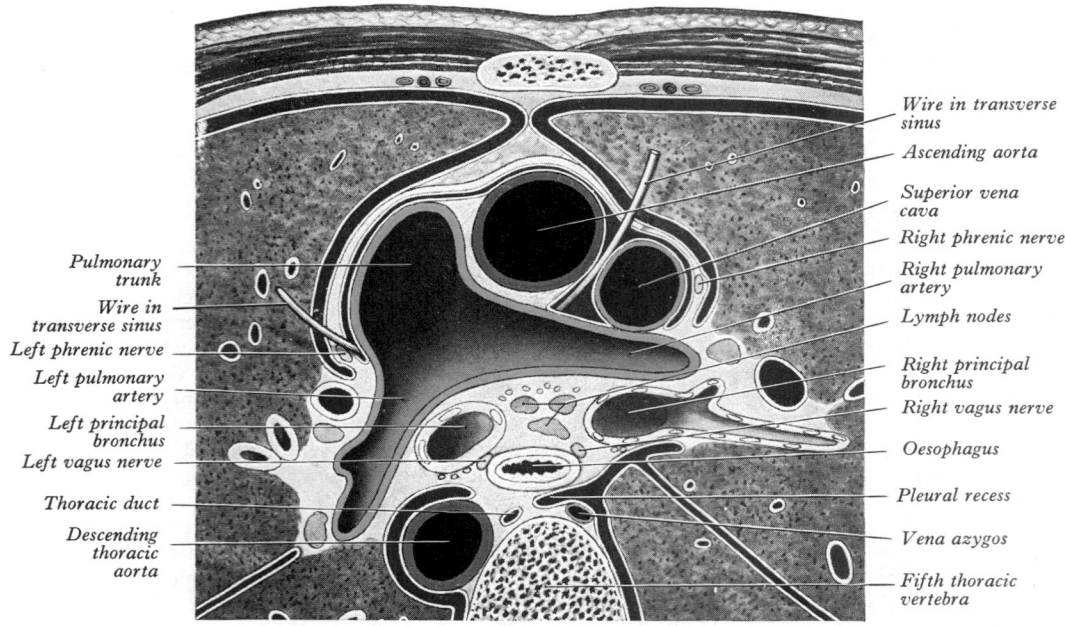

Pulmonary
trunk

Wire in
transverse sinus

Left phrenic nerve

Left pulmonary
artery

Left principal
bronchus

Left vagus nerve

Thoracic duct

Descending
thoracic
aorta

Wire in transverse
sinus

Ascending aorta

Superior vena
cava

Right phrenic nerve

Right pulmonary
artery

Lymph nodes

Right principal
bronchus

Right vagus nerve

Oesophagus

Pleural recess

Vena azygos

Fifth thoracic
vertebra

10.65 Transverse section through the mediastinum at the level of the upper border of the fifth thoracic vertebra: superior aspect. Note nerve fibres of the deep cardiac and posterior pulmonary plexuses, inferior tracheobronchial and hilar lymph nodes.

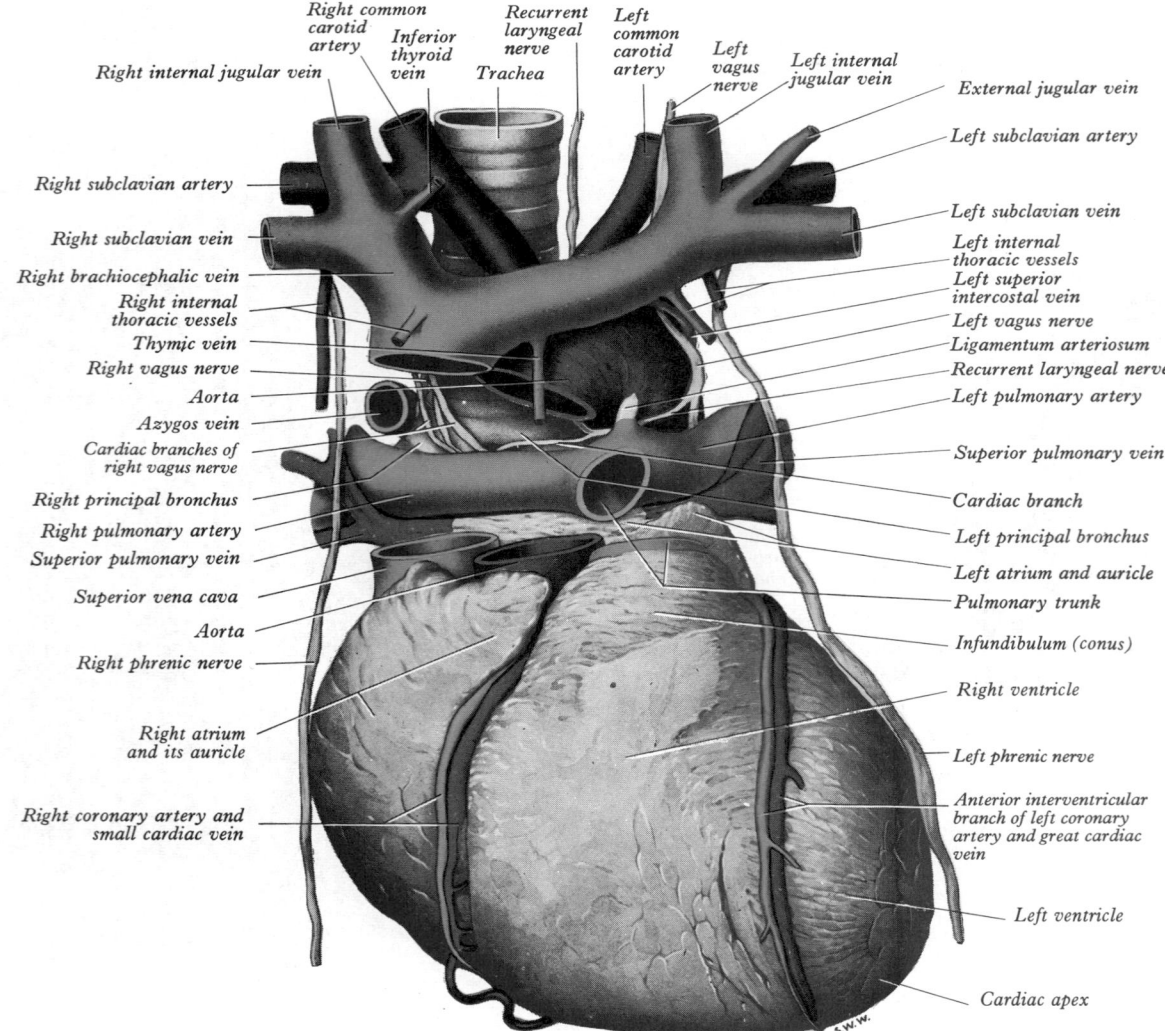

Right common
carotid
artery

Inferior
thyroid
vein

Recurrent
laryngeal
nerve

Trachea

Left
common
carotid
artery

Left
vagus
nerve

Left internal
jugular vein

Right internal jugular vein

Right subclavian artery

Right subclavian vein

Right brachiocephalic vein

Right internal
thoracic vessels

Thymic vein

Right vagus nerve

Aorta

Azygos vein

Cardiac branches of
right vagus nerve

Right principal bronchus

Right pulmonary artery

Superior pulmonary vein

Superior vena cava

Aorta

Right phrenic nerve

Right atrium
and its auricle

Right coronary artery and
small cardiac vein

External jugular vein

Left subclavian artery

Left subclavian vein

Left internal
thoracic vessels

Left superior
intercostal vein

Left vagus nerve

Ligamentum arteriosum

Recurrent laryngeal nerve

Left pulmonary artery

Superior pulmonary vein

Cardiac branch

Left principal bronchus

Left atrium and auricle

Pulmonary trunk

Infundibulum (conus)

Right ventricle

Left phrenic nerve

Anterior interventricular
branch of left coronary
artery and great cardiac
vein

Left ventricle

Cardiac apex

S.W.W.

10.66 The relations of the pulmonary arteries and primary bronchi seen from the front. Parts of the ascending aorta, pulmonary trunk and superior vena cava have been removed in the dissection. The right vagal trunk is uncoloured to avoid confusion.

height of the systole, the cusps do not 'flatten' against, i.e. co-apt to, the walls of their sinuses.)

The two arteries, as indicated by their name, form an oblique inverted crown, with an anastomotic circle in the atrioventricular sulcus connected by marginal and interventricular loops intersecting at the cardiac apex (**10.**67A–E). This is, of course, only an approximation; the degree of anastomosis is most variable and usually insignificant (see below). The main arteries and major rami are usually subepicardial but those in the atrioventricular and interventricular sulci are often deeply sited, occasionally hidden by overlapping myocardium or embedded in it. Myocardial strands may also cross atrial or ventricular branches; Póláček (1961) found them in more than 80% of ventricles; Bloor and Lowman (1963) have emphasized their importance in interpretation of coronary arteriograms.

The term 'dominant' is used to refer to the coronary artery which gives the posterior interventricular branch, supplying the posterior part of the ventricular septum and often part of the posterolateral wall of the left ventricle. In 70% of people this is the left coronary artery, which is also invariably the larger of the two vessels. In the remaining cases the posterior interventricular branch is either bilateral, issuing from both the right coronary artery and the left circumflex artery, or absent and replaced by a network of smaller vessels from both right and left coronaries. Anastomoses between right and left coronary arteries are abundant during fetal life but are much reduced by the end of the first year of life. Anastomoses providing collateral circulation may become prominent in conditions of hypoxia and in coronary artery diseases. An additional collateral circulation is provided by small branches from mediastinal, pericardial and bronchial vessels.

The diameters of coronary arteries, both main stems and larger branches, have often been recorded; such figures are of limited value, since technique is not always stated, physiological state often ignored and measurement of external or internal diameters not clearly distinguished. Calibre is usually the basis, most measurements being made on arterial casts or angiograms. The maximum ranges recorded in major studies are 1.5–5.5 mm for coronary arteries at their origins. Baroldi and Scomazzoni (1967) give means of 4.0 and 3.2 mm. The left exceed the right in about 60% of hearts, the right being larger in 17%, the vessels approximately equal in 23%. Vogelberg (1957) considered that coronary diameters increase up to the thirtieth year.

Right coronary artery

Arising from the anterior ('right coronary') aortic sinus, the artery passes at first anteriorly and slightly to the right between the right auricle and pulmonary trunk, where the sinus usually bulges. Reaching the atrioventricular (coronary) sulcus it descends in this almost vertically to the right (acute) cardiac border, curving around it into the posterior part of the sulcus, where it approaches its junction with both interatrial and interventricular grooves, a region appropriately termed the *crux of the heart*. In about 60% of subjects the artery reaches the crux and ends a little left of it by variable anastomosis with circumflex branch of the left coronary. In a minority, the right coronary artery ends near the right cardiac border (c. 10%) or between this and the crux (c. 10%); more often (c. 20%) it reaches the left border, replacing part of the circumflex artery.

Branches of the right coronary supply both right atrium and ventricle and, variably, parts of the **left** chambers and atrioventricular septum. The first branch (arising separately from the anterior aortic sinus in 36% of cases) is the *conus artery* (sometimes a 'third coronary'); since a similar vessel comes from the left coronary, this is more correctly named the *right conus artery*. It ramifies anteriorly on the lowest part of the pulmonary conus and upper part of right ventricle; it commonly anastomoses with a similar left coronary branch to form the '*annulus of Vieussens*', a tenuous anastomotic 'circle' around the pulmonary trunk. Descriptions of the conus artery vary (Baroldi & Scomazzoni 1967), some regarding the right conus artery of significance in coronary arterial disease; some consider it to be the right coronary's first ventricular branch, supplying a variable region from the conus to the apex.

Anterior atrial and ventricular rami diverge from the so-called *first segment of the right coronary*, extending from its origin to the right margin of the heart. Both groups diverge widely, approaching

a right angle in the case of ventricular arteries, in contrast to the more acute origins of the left coronary ventricular rami. The *right anterior ventricular rami*, usually two or three, ramify towards the cardiac apex, which they rarely reach unless the right marginal branch is included, as it is by some; this is then the largest right anterior ventricular ramus, greater in calibre and long enough to reach the apex in most hearts (93%; Baroldi & Scomazzoni 1967). When the right marginal artery is very large, the remaining anterior ventricular rami may be reduced to one, or may be absent. From the *second segment of the right coronary artery* (between the right border and crux) one to three small *right posterior ventricular rami*, commonly two, supply the diaphragmatic aspect of the right ventricle. Their size is inversely proportional to that of the right marginal artery, as in the anterior right ventricular supply, the right marginal usually extending to the cardiac diaphragmatic surface. Posterior right ventricular rami may be absent. As the right coronary approaches the crux, it produces one to three posterior interventricular rami but only one in the interventricular sulcus; this *posterior interventricular artery*, single in about 70%, is otherwise accompanied by parallel right coronary branches, to the right or left or on both sides of the sulcus. When these flanking vessels exist, branches of the posterior (descending) interventricular artery are small and sparse; when it exists alone it gives off a few branches, particularly to the right ventricle but also to the left. It is replaced in about 10% of cases by a left coronary branch.

The atrial rami of the right coronary artery are sometimes described as anterior, lateral (right or marginal) and posterior groups but are most frequently single, small vessels averaging 1 mm in diameter. The right anterior and lateral are occasionally double, very rarely triple, and supply chiefly the right atrium. The posterior ramus is usually single, distributed to the right and left atria; but in 40% or more a left posterior atrial branch of the right coronary exists. The artery of the sinuatrial node is an atrial branch, distributed largely to the myocardium of both atria, mainly the right. Its origin is variable: from the left coronary in about 35% (Hutchinson 1978), arising from its circumflex branch (see below); when it is a branch of the right coronary, it usually comes from its anterior stem, less often from its right lateral part, least often from its posterior atrioventricular part. This 'nodal' artery thus usually passes back in the sulcus between the right auricular appendage and aorta. Whatever its origin the artery usually branches around the superior vena cava's base, commonly as an arterial loop from which small rami supply the right atrium. A large '*ramus cristae terminalis*' (Spalteholtz 1924) traverses the sinuatrial node (**10.**67A–C); perhaps instead this ramus should be termed 'nodal artery', since most of the currently named vessel actually supplies the atria and is more appropriately named the 'main atrial branch' (Baroldi & Scomazzoni 1967).

Right coronary septal rami are relatively short, leaving its posterior interventricular ramus to supply the posterior interventricular septum. They are numerous but do not usually reach the apical septal parts (supplied by terminal septal branches of the anterior interventricular).

The largest posterior septal artery, usually the first, is commonly from the inverted loop said to characterize the right coronary artery at the crux, where its posterior interventricular branch arises; this large posterior septal artery usually supplies the atrioventricular node—in 80% of hearts, according to Hutchinson (1978).

DiDio et al (1967) described the atrioventricular rami of the right coronary artery as consisting of small recurrent branches from each ventricular artery crossing the atrioventricular sulcus to supply the adjoining atrial myocardium, or ventricular twigs from the atrial arteries.

Left coronary artery

The left coronary artery is the larger in calibre, supplying a greater volume of myocardium, including almost all the left ventricle and atrium, except in so-called 'right dominance' where the right coronary partly supplies a posterior region of the left ventricle (**10.**67A–C). The left coronary usually supplies most of the interventricular septum. Its initial stem, between its ostium in the left posterior ('left coronary') aortic sinus and its first branches, varies in length from a few millimetres to a few centimetres. It lies between the pulmonary trunk and the left auricular appendage, emerging into the atrioventricular sulcus, in which it turns left; this part is loosely embedded in

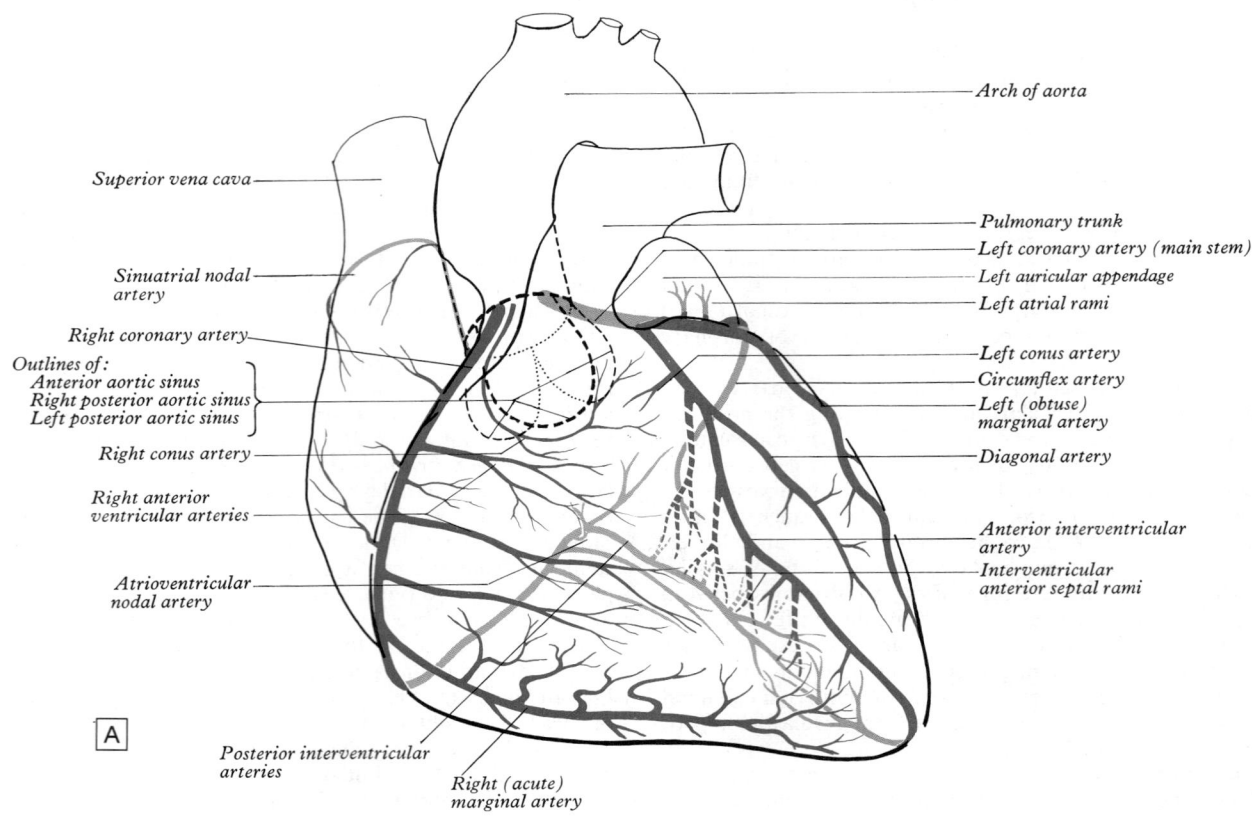

Arch of aorta

Superior vena cava

Pulmonary trunk
Left coronary artery (main stem)
Sinuatrial nodal
artery
Left auricular appendage
Left atrial rami

Right coronary artery
Left conus artery
Outlines of:
Anterior aortic sinus
Right posterior aortic sinus
Left posterior aortic sinus
Circumflex artery
Left (obtuse)
marginal artery

Right conus artery
Diagonal artery

Right anterior
ventricular arteries
Anterior interventricular
artery
Interventricular
anterior septal rami

Atrioventricular
nodal artery

Posterior interventricular
arteries

Right (acute)
marginal artery

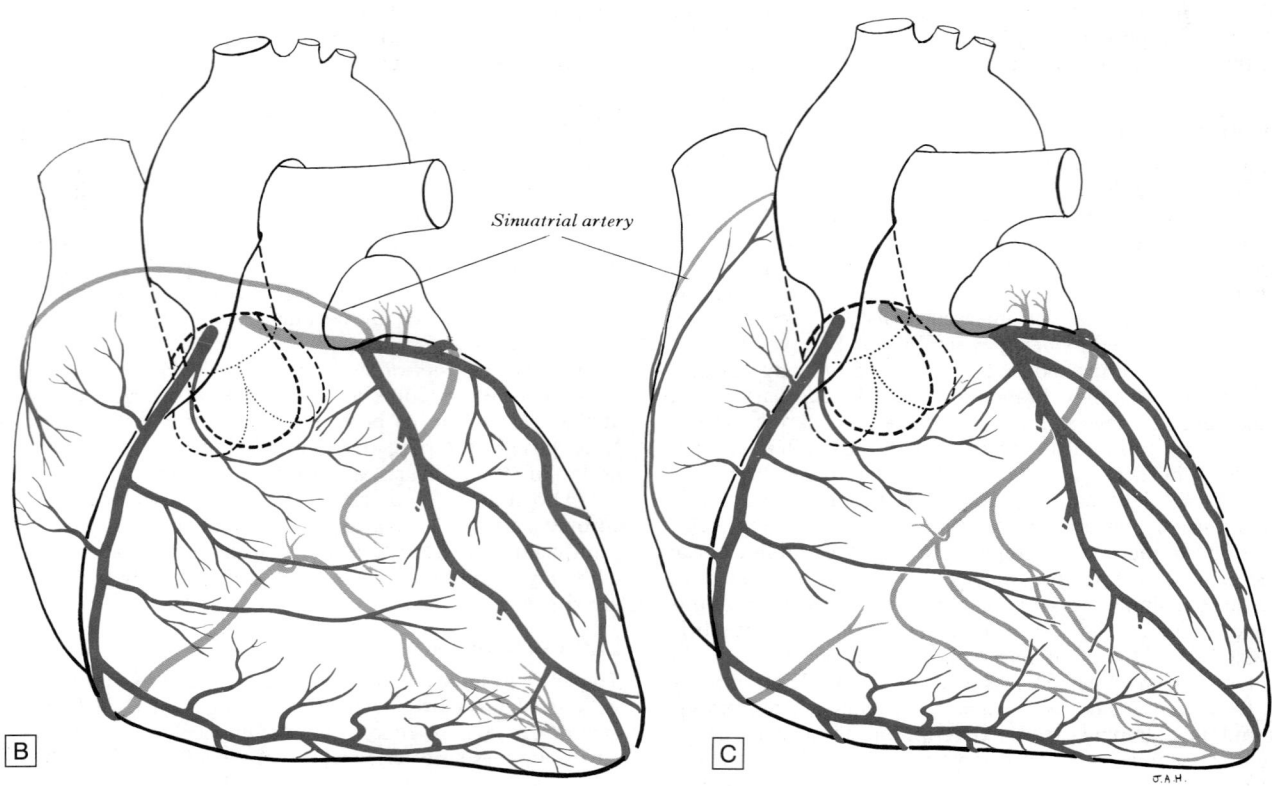

Sinuatrial artery

10.67A–C Anterior views of the coronary arterial system, with the principal variations.
A The commonest arrangement.
B A common variation in the origin of the sinuatrial nodal artery.
C An example of left 'dominance' by the left coronary artery, showing also an uncommon origin of the sinuatrial artery.
Note that in 10.67A–E the right coronary arterial tree is shown in magenta, the left in full red. In both cases posterior distribution is shown in a paler shade.

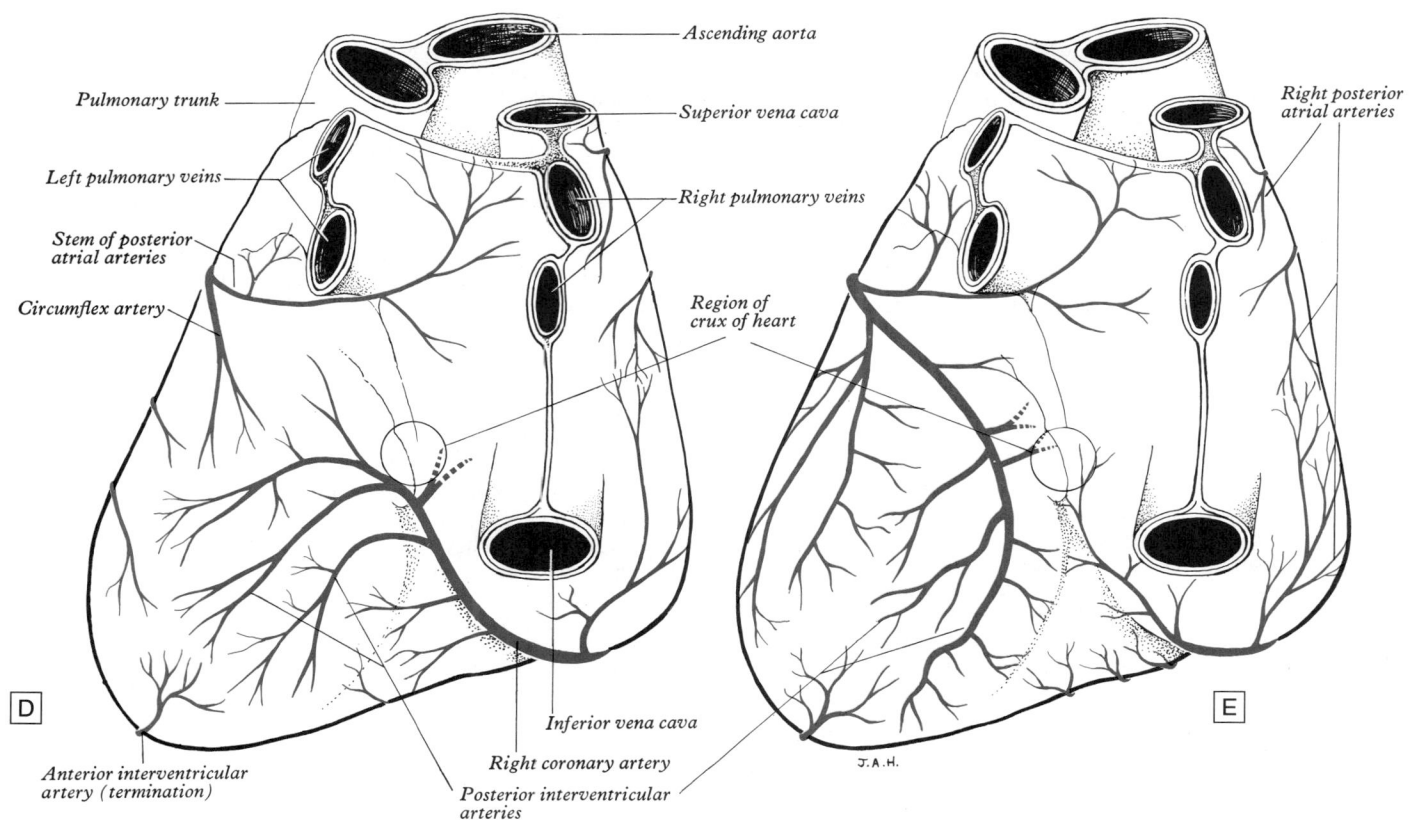

Pulmonary trunk

Left pulmonary veins

Stem of posterior
atrial arteries

Circumflex artery

Ascending aorta

Superior vena cava

Right pulmonary veins

Region of
crux of heart

Right posterior
atrial arteries

D

Anterior interventricular
artery (termination)

Inferior vena cava

Right coronary artery

Posterior interventricular
arteries

E

J.A.H.

10.67D, E   Postero-inferior views of the coronary arterial system.
D   An example of the more normal distribution in right 'dominance'.
E   A less common form of left 'dominance'.
N.B. In these 'posterior' views the diaphragmatic (inferior) surface of the
ventricular part of the heart has been artificially displaced and foreshortening
ignored to clarify the details of the so-called posterior (inferior) distribution
of the coronary arteries.

subepicardial fat and usually has no branches; but a small atrial
ramus may occur and, rarely, the sinuatrial nodal artery may arise
from the left coronary artery (James 1961); but when it is a ramus
of the left coronary it almost always comes from the circumflex
branch. Reaching the atrioventricular or coronary sulcus, the left
coronary divides into two or three main rami, its *anterior interventricular* (*descending*) *ramus* being commonly described as its continuation; this descends obliquely forward and left in the
interventricular sulcus, sometimes deeply embedded or crossed by
bridges of myocardial tissue and by the great cardiac vein and its
tributaries. It reaches the apex almost always, terminating there in
one-third of specimens, but more often turning round the apex into
the posterior interventricular sulcus, in which it traverses a third to
a half of its length, to meet the terminal twigs of the corresponding
right coronary ramus.

The *anterior interventricular artery* produces right and left anterior
ventricular, anterior septal and variable, corresponding posterior
rami. Right anterior ventricular rami are small and rarely number
more than one or two, the right ventricle being supplied almost
wholly by the right coronary artery.

From two to nine large left *anterior ventricular arteries* branch at
acute angles from the anterior interventricular to cross diagonally
the left ventricle's anterior aspect, larger terminals reaching the
rounded (obtuse) left border. One is often large and may arise
separately from the left coronary trunk (which then ends by
trifurcation); this left diagonal artery, reported in 33–50% or more
cases, is occasionally duplicated (20%). A small left conus artery
frequently leaves the anterior interventricular near its start, anastomosing on the conus with that of the right coronary and with the
vasa vasorum of the pulmonary artery and aorta. The anterior
septal rami leave the anterior interventricular almost perpendicularly,
passing back and down in the septum, of which they usually supply
about the ventral two-thirds. Small posterior septal rami from the
same source supply the posterior septal third for a variable distance
from the cardiac apex.

The *circumflex artery*, in calibre comparable to the anterior interventricular, curves left in the atrioventricular sulcus, continuing
round the left cardiac border into the posterior part of the sulcus
and ending left of the crux in most hearts, but sometimes continuing
as a posterior interventricular artery. Proximally the left auricular
appendage usually overlaps it. In about 90% a large ventricular
branch, the *left marginal artery*, arises perpendicularly from it to
ramify over the rounded 'obtuse' margin, supplying much of the
adjacent left ventricle, usually to the apex. Smaller anterior and
posterior rami of the circumflex artery also supply the left ventricle.
Anterior ventricular branches (1–5, commonly 2 or 3) course parallel
to the diagonal artery, when present, replacing it when absent.
Posterior ventricular branches are smaller and fewer, the left ventricle
being partly supplied by the posterior interventricular artery; when
this is small or absent, it is accompanied or replaced by an interventricular continuation of the circumflex. Such a *left posterior
interventricular artery* is frequently double or triple. Atrial rami,
anterior, lateral and posterior, from the circumflex, supply the left
atrium.

Inconstant branches of the circumflex artery require mention.
The *artery to the sinuatrial node* is a branch in about 35%
(Hutchinson 1978), usually from the anterior circumflex segment,
less often the circummarginal. It passes over and supplies the left
atrium, encircling the superior vena cava like a right coronary
nodal ramus. It sends a large branch to (and through) the node
but is predominantly atrial in distribution. The artery to the
atrioventricular node, the terminal ramus in 20%, arises near
the crux and then the circumflex usually supplies a posterior
interventricular ramus, an example of so-called 'left dominance'
(see below). *Kugel's anastomotic artery*, 'arteria anastomotica
auricularis magna,' was described by Kugel (1927) as a constant
circumflex branch, usually from its anterior part, traversing the
interatrial septum (near its ventricular border) to establish direct
or indirect anastomosis with the right coronary. This anastomosis
is controversial, apparently accepted by James (1978) but denied

1509

by Baroldi and Scomazzoni (1967). James considered it an auxiliary supply to the atrioventricular node.

Details of coronary distribution require integration into a concept of total cardiac supply. Most commonly the right coronary supplies all the right ventricle (except a small region right of the anterior interventricular sulcus), a variable part of the left ventricular diaphragmatic aspect, the postero-inferior third of the intraventricular septum, the right atrium and part of the left, and the conducting system as far as the proximal parts of the right and left crura. Left coronary distribution is, of course, reciprocal, including most of the left ventricle (see above), a narrow strip of right ventricle (see below), the anterior two-thirds of the interventricular septum and most of the left atrium. As noted, variations (**10**.67A–E) chiefly affect the diaphragmatic aspect of ventricles residing in relative 'dominance' of supply by the left or right coronary artery. The term is misleading, since the left artery almost always supplies a greater volume of tissue. In 'right dominance' the posterior interventricular artery is from the right coronary, in 'left dominance' from the left. In the so-called 'balanced' pattern, branches of both run in or near the sulcus. Less is known of variation in atrial supply; the small vessels involved are not easily preserved in corrosion casts. From Hutchinson's results (1978) it is apparent that in over 50% the right atrium is supplied only by the right coronary, the rest receiving a dual supply. More than 62% of left atria are largely supplied by the left and about 27% by the right coronary; but in each group a small accessory supply from the other coronary exists, 11% being supplied almost equally by both. Sinuatrial and atrioventricular supplies also vary. According to James (1961) right and left coronary arteries supply the sinuatrial node respectively in 55% and 45%, corresponding values from Baroldi and Scomazzoni's study (1967) being 51% and 41% (8% receiving bilateral supply), and from Hutchinson (1978) 65% and 35%. For the atrioventricular node James's values are 90% (right coronary) and 10% (left coronary), Hutchinson's 80% and 20% respectively; Baroldi and Scomazzoni merely note that right coronary supply is common and left supply rare.

Coronary anastomosis

Anastomoses between branches of coronary arteries, subepicardial or myocardial, and between these arteries and extracardiac vessels are of prime medical import. Clinical experience suggests that anastomoses cannot rapidly provide collateral routes sufficient to circumvent sudden coronary obstruction. It is hence traditional to regard coronary circulation as end-arterial. Nevertheless, anastomosis has long been established particularly between the finer subepicardial rami. According to Gross (1921) such anastomoses may improve during individual life. Those who have investigated coronary arteries by radio-opaque perfusants (Vastesaeger et al 1957 in postmortem hearts; Laurie & Woods 1958 by in vivo coronary radiography), by perfusion with calibrated spherules (Prinzmetal et al 1947) or by subsequent corrosion casts of plastic resins (Baroldi et al 1956, James 1961) have almost all described anastomoses, and in vessels up to 100–200 μm in calibre. Baroldi and Scomazzoni (1967) have tabulated all results reported since 1880; no study denying anastomoses has been recorded since 1957. Some describe anastomoses only between branches of individual coronary arteries but the majority record intercoronary anastomoses. James (1978) considers the evidence conclusive for anastomoses at all levels: subepicardial, myocardial, and subendocardial; the most frequent sites of extramural anastomoses are the apex, the anterior aspect of the right ventricle, posterior aspect of the left ventricle, crux, interatrial and interventricular sulci and between the sinuatrial nodal and other atrial vessels. The functional value of such anastomoses must vary but they appear to become more effective in slowly progressive pathological conditions. Their structure is uncertain; most observations depend on corrosion casts, which suggest that anastomotic vessels are relatively straight in normal hearts, but much coiled in hearts subject to coronary occlusion. Little has been recorded of their microscopic structure; they appear little more than endothelial tubes, without muscles or elastic tissue.

Extracardiac anastomoses may connect various coronary branches with other thoracic vessels via the pericardial arteries and arterial vasa vasorum of vessels linking the heart with systemic and pulmonary circulations. The classic study of Hudson et al (1932) showed that coronary injections of India ink could reach the diaphragm through the aortic vasa vasorum. Similar connections along pulmonary trunks reach the mediastinal and bronchial arteries and also exist along pulmonary veins and venae cavae. These results have been confirmed (Baroldi & Scomazzoni 1967) but the effectiveness of such connections as collateral routes in coronary occlusion is unpredictable.

Coronary arteriovenous anastomoses were reported by Nussbaum (1912). His evidence was indirect but Hirsch (1960) described glomeral structures with typical sphincteric appearances (p. 1468) in cardiac sulci; these must be regarded as at present unproven. Various other forms of 'arteriovenous' connections have been described; Wearn et al (1933) recorded numerous connections through the very thin-walled 'arterial' vessels between the coronary circulation and cardiac cavities, naming them 'myocardial sinusoids' and 'arterioluminal' vessels. They have been confirmed (Watanabe 1960) and indirect evidence of them, from perfusion experiments, dates back to Vieussens (1705). Their value in coronary disease is uncertain.

Histology of coronary arteries

The coronary arteries are highly muscular vessels, but rather variable in their structure, partly on account of their frequent branching and tortuous course. They differ in two respects from other vessels of similar size. The inner elastic lamina, discontinuous and poorly developed at birth, disappears during growth, and bundles of longitudinally oriented muscle are present in the outer part of the intima or the inner part of the media (a boundary between media and intima cannot be identified).

ARCH OF THE AORTA

The aortic arch (**10**.65, 70) continues the ascending aorta. Its origin, slightly to the right, is level with the upper border of the second right sternocostal joint. The arch first ascends diagonally back and to the left over the anterior surface of the trachea, then back across its left side and finally descends left of the fourth thoracic vertebral body, continuing as the descending thoracic aorta. Its end is level with the sternal end of the second, left costal cartilage (**10**.28). Thus, the aortic arch lies wholly in the superior mediastinum. It curves around the peduncle of the left lung, and extends upwards to the mid-level of the manubrium of the sternum. Its diameter at the origin is the same as in the ascending aorta, about 28 mm, but it is reduced to 20 mm at the end, after the issue of its large collateral branches. At the border with the thoracic aorta, a small stricture (aortic isthmus), followed by a dilatation, can be recognized. In fetal life the isthmus lies between the origin of the left subclavian artery and the opening of the ductus arteriosus.

Relations

Anteriorly and to the left is the left mediastinal pleura, deep to which it is crossed by four nerves: the left phrenic, left lower cervical vagal cardiac branch, left superior cervical sympathetic cardiac branch and left vagus, in anteroposterior order. As the left vagus crosses the arch its recurrent laryngeal branch hooks below the vessel left and behind (developmentally caudal to) the ligamentum arteriosum and then ascends on the arch's right. The left superior intercostal vein ascends obliquely forwards on the arch, superficial to the left vagus, deep to the left phrenic nerve (**10**.69). The left lung and pleura separate all these from the thoracic wall. Posterior to the right are the trachea and deep cardiac plexus, the left recurrent laryngeal nerve, oesophagus, thoracic duct and vertebral column. Above, the brachiocephalic, left common carotid and left subclavian arteries arise from its convexity, crossed anteriorly near their origins by the left brachiocephalic vein. Below are the pulmonary bifurcation, left principal bronchus, ligamentum arteriosum (p. 1467), superficial cardiac plexus and left recurrent laryngeal nerve. (Best viewed from the left, the concavity of the aortic arch is the upper curved limit through which structures gain access or exit through the hilum of the left lung.)

The fetal aortic lumen narrows between the origin of the left subclavian artery and the attachment of the ductus arteriosus, as the aortic isthmus; beyond the ductus arteriosus the vessel presents a fusiform aortic spindle, the junction of the two parts being marked inferiorly by an indentation; these features persist variably in adults.

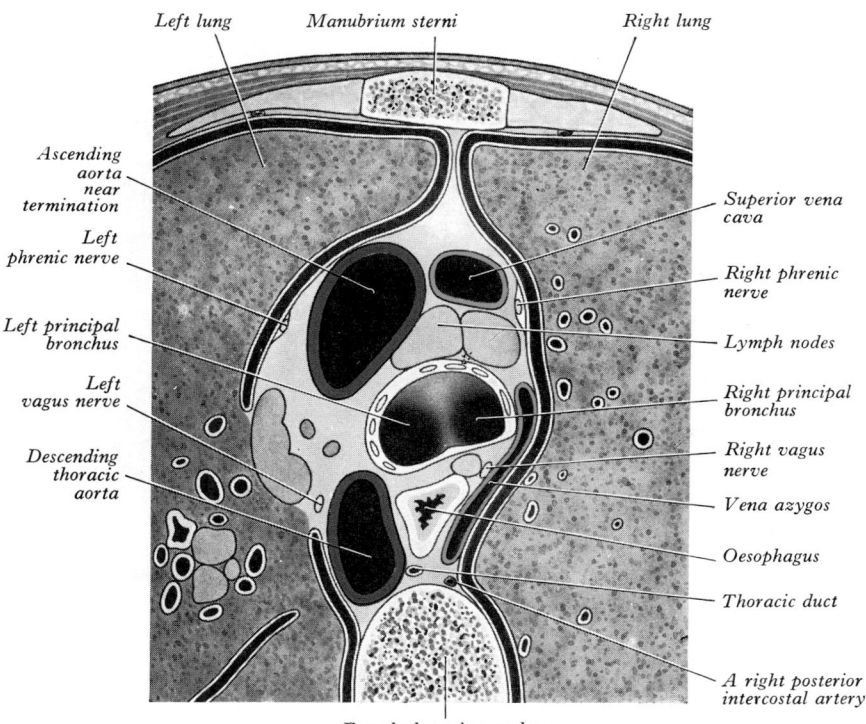

Left lung   Manubrium sterni   Right lung

Ascending aorta near termination

Left phrenic nerve

Left principal bronchus

Left vagus nerve

Descending thoracic aorta

Superior vena cava

Right phrenic nerve

Lymph nodes

Right principal bronchus

Right vagus nerve

Vena azygos

Oesophagus

Thoracic duct

A right posterior intercostal artery

Fourth thoracic vertebra

10.68   Transverse section through the mediastinum at the level of the lower part of the body of the fourth thoracic vertebra, viewed from above. The deep cardiac plexus of nerves is omitted.

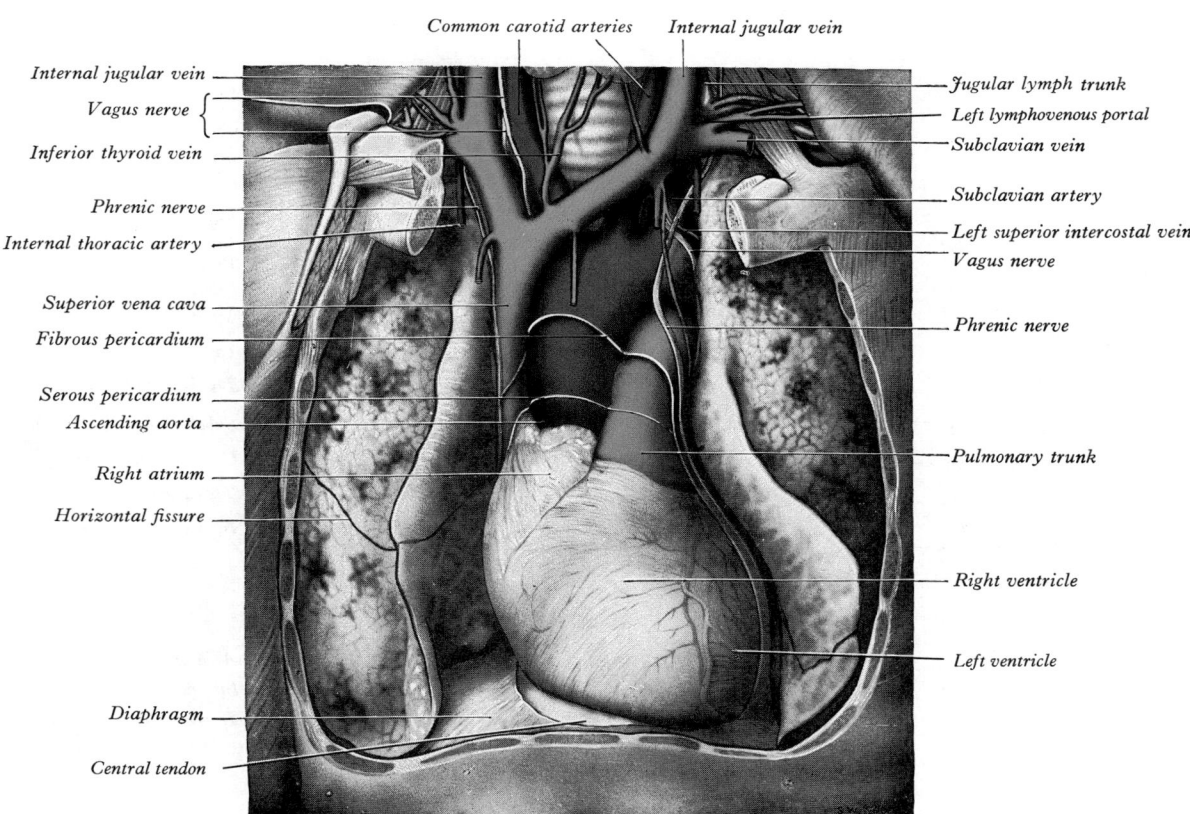

Common carotid arteries   Internal jugular vein

Internal jugular vein

Vagus nerve

Inferior thyroid vein

Phrenic nerve

Internal thoracic artery

Superior vena cava

Fibrous pericardium

Serous pericardium

Ascending aorta

Right atrium

Horizontal fissure

Diaphragm

Central tendon

Jugular lymph trunk

Left lymphovenous portal

Subclavian vein

Subclavian artery

Left superior intercostal vein

Vagus nerve

Phrenic nerve

Pulmonary trunk

Right ventricle

Left ventricle

10.69   Dissection to display the heart, great vessels and lungs in situ. The sternum and the sternal ends of the costal cartilages, together with the parietal pleura on each side, have been excised and the mediastinal pleura and parietal layer of the pericardium over the sternocostal surface of the heart have been removed. The lungs have been displaced to expose the heart and the epicardium dissected off the heart and the great vessels.

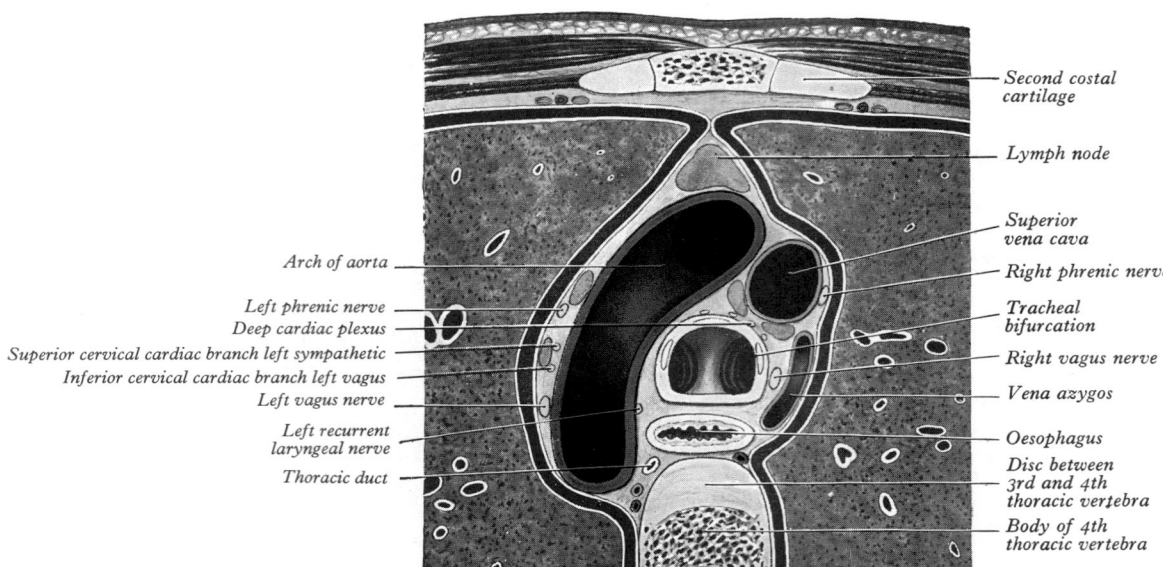

Second costal cartilage

Lymph node

Superior vena cava

Right phrenic nerve

Tracheal bifurcation

Right vagus nerve

Vena azygos

Oesophagus

Disc between 3rd and 4th thoracic vertebra

Body of 4th thoracic vertebra

Arch of aorta

Left phrenic nerve
Deep cardiac plexus
Superior cervical cardiac branch left sympathetic
Inferior cervical cardiac branch left vagus
Left vagus nerve

Left recurrent laryngeal nerve

Thoracic duct

10.70   Transverse section through the mediastinum at the level of the upper part of the body of the fourth thoracic vertebra, viewed from above.

Variations

The summit of the arch is usually about 2.5 cm below the superior sternal border but may diverge from this. In the infant it is closer to the upper border of the sternum; the same is often the case in old age, because of the dilatation of the vessel. Sometimes the aorta curves over the right pulmonary hilum descending right of the vertebral column, a condition normal in birds; there is usually transposition of thoracic and abdominal viscera. Less often, after arching over the right hilum, it passes behind the oesophagus to its usual position; this is not accompanied by visceral transposition.

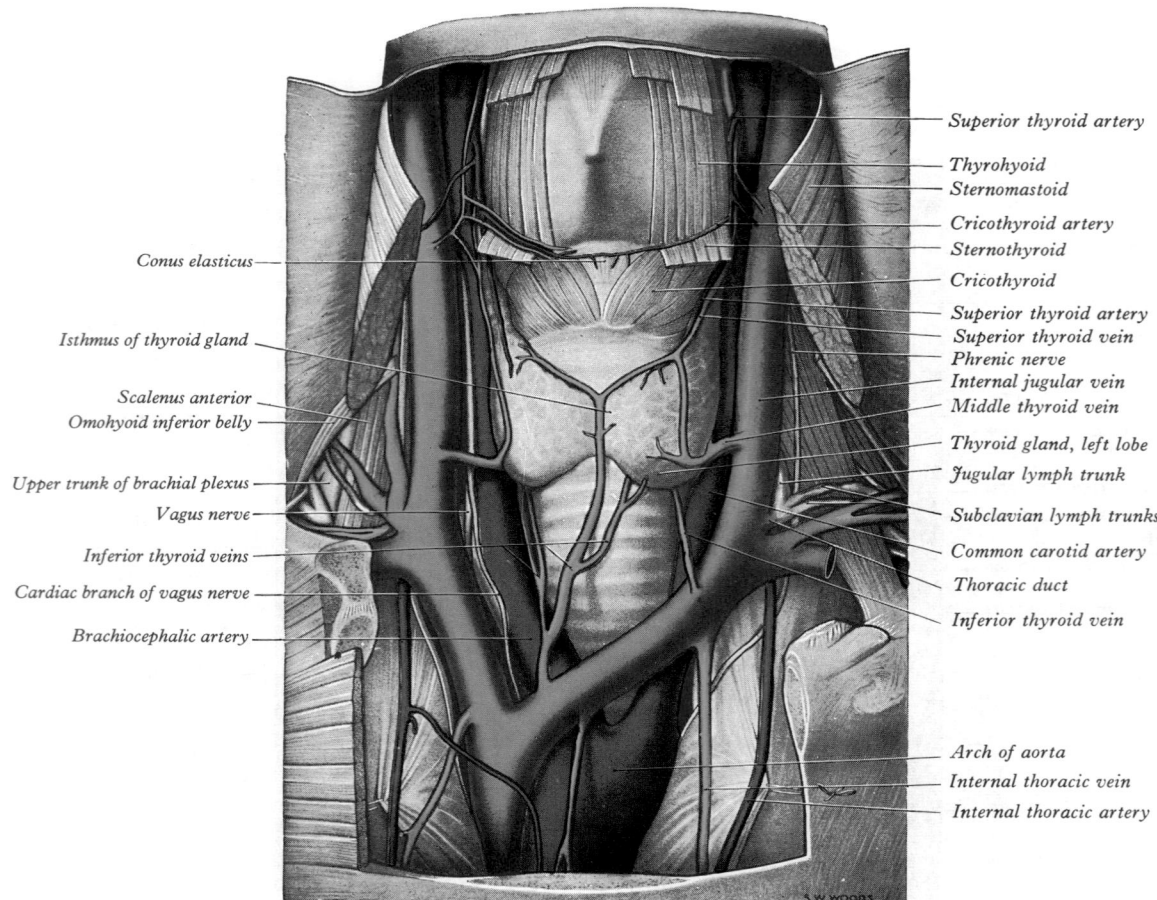

Superior thyroid artery

Thyrohyoid
Sternomastoid

Cricothyroid artery
Sternothyroid

Cricothyroid

Superior thyroid artery
Superior thyroid vein
Phrenic nerve
Internal jugular vein
Middle thyroid vein

Thyroid gland, left lobe
Jugular lymph trunk

Subclavian lymph trunks

Common carotid artery

Thoracic duct

Inferior thyroid vein

Arch of aorta
Internal thoracic vein
Internal thoracic artery

Conus elasticus

Isthmus of thyroid gland

Scalenus anterior
Omohyoid inferior belly

Upper trunk of brachial plexus
Vagus nerve
Inferior thyroid veins
Cardiac branch of vagus nerve
Brachiocephalic artery

S.W. WOODS

10.71   Dissection of the lower part of the front of the neck and of the superior mediastinum. The manubrium sterni and the sternal ends of the clavicles and the first costal cartilages have been removed and the pleural sac and lung have been retracted on each side. In this specimen each superior thyroid artery arose from the common carotid artery.

The aorta may divide, as in some quadrupeds, into ascending and descending trunks, the former dividing into three branches to supply the head and upper limbs. Sometimes it divides near its origin, the two branches soon reuniting; the oesophagus and trachea usually pass through the interval between them; this is the normal condition in reptilia and is due to the persistence of a part of the right dorsal aorta which usually disappears (p. 312).

Radiological appearances

The shadow of the arch is easily identified in anteroposterior radiographs (**10**.48, 49) and its left profile is sometimes called the 'aortic knuckle'. The arch may also be visible in left anterior oblique views enclosing a pale space, 'the aortic window', in which shadows of the pulmonary trunk and its left branch may be visible.

Branches (**10**.69, 71)

Three branches spring from the vessel's convex aspect: the brachiocephalic trunk, left common carotid and left subclavian arteries (**10**.69, 71). They may branch from the beginning of the arch or the upper part of the ascending aorta; the distance between these origins varies, the most frequent being approximation of the left common carotid artery to the brachiocephalic trunk (Wright 1969). Primary branches may be reduced to one, more commonly two, the left common carotid arising from the brachiocephalic trunk (7%), or (more rarely) the left common carotid and subclavian arteries arising from a left brachiocephalic or right common carotid and subclavian arising separately, in which case the latter more often branches from the left end of the arch and passes behind the oesophagus (p. 314). The left vertebral artery may arise between the left common carotid and the subclavian. Very rarely, external and internal carotid arteries arise separately, the common carotid being absent on one or both sides; or both carotids and one or both vertebrals may be separate branches. When a 'right aorta' occurs, the arrangement of its three branches is reversed. The common carotids may have a single trunk, the subclavians separate, the right arising from the left end of the arch. Other arteries may branch from it, most commonly one or both bronchial arteries and the arteria thyroidea ima.

An analysis of variation in branches from 1000 aortic arches (Anson 1963) showed in 65% the usual pattern; in 27% a left common carotid shared the brachiocephalic trunk (contrast percentage quoted above); in 2.5% the four large arteries branched separately. The remaining 5% showed a great variety of patterns, the commonest (1.2%) being symmetrical right and left brachiocephalic trunks.

BRACHIOCEPHALIC ARTERY

The brachiocephalic (innominate) artery, the largest branch of the aortic arch, is from 4–5 cm in length (**10**.66, 71, 72), arising from the arch's convexity posterior to the centre of the manubrium sterni; it ascends posterolaterally to the right, at first anterior to the trachea, then on its right. Level with the right sternoclavicular

joint's upper border it forks into the right common carotid and subclavian arteries.

Relations

Anterior are sternohyoid and sternothyroid, the remains of the thymus, left brachiocephalic and right inferior thyroid veins, crossing its root, and sometimes the right vagal cardiac branches, all separating it from the manubrium. Posterior are the trachea below, right pleura above, where the right vagus is posterolateral before passing lateral to the trachea; right lateral are the right brachiocephalic vein, the upper part of the superior vena cava and pleura; left lateral are the thymic remains, the origin of the left common carotid artery, the inferior thyroid veins and the trachea at a higher level.

Branches

The brachiocephalic artery usually has only terminal branches but occasionally an arteria thyroidea ima arises from it, sometimes a thymic or bronchial branch.

Arteria thyroidea ima, small and inconstant, ascends on the trachea to the thyroid isthmus, in which it ends. It may arise from the aorta, right common carotid, subclavian or internal thoracic arteries.

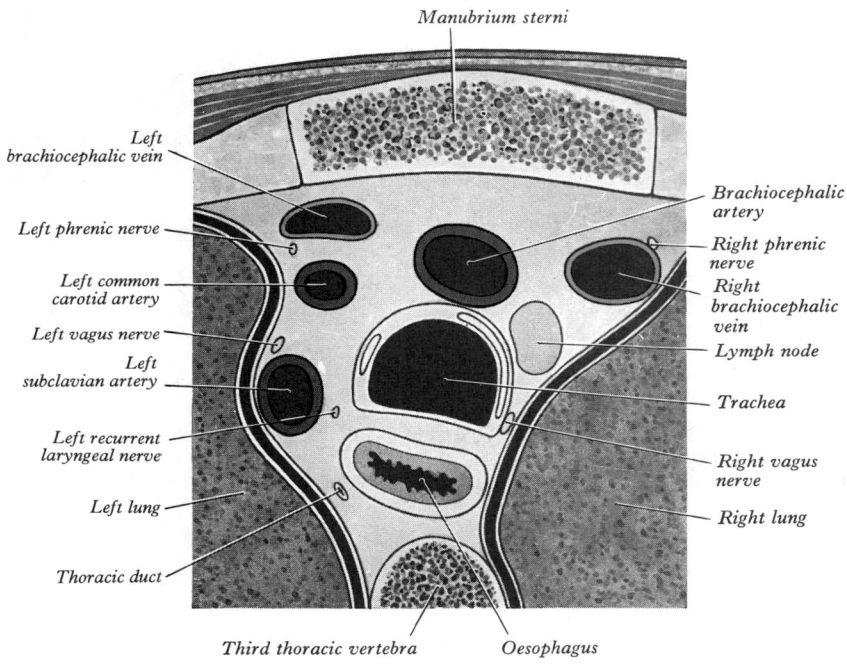

10.72 Transverse section through the superior mediastinum at the level of the body of the third thoracic vertebra, viewed from above.

CAROTID SYSTEM OF ARTERIES

The common carotid artery is a large bilateral vessel supplying head and neck; it ascends to just above the level of the thyroid cartilage's upper border, where it divides into an external carotid, supplying the exterior of the head, face and most of the neck, and an internal carotid, supplying the cranial and orbital contents.

The common and internal carotid arteries, with veins and nerves accompanying them, lie in a cleft bounded posteriorly by cervical transverse processes and attached muscles, medially by the trachea, oesophagus, thyroid gland, larynx and pharyngeal constrictors, anterolaterally by the sternocleidomastoid with, at different levels, omohyoid, sternohyoid, sternothyroid, digastric and stylohyoid muscles.

COMMON CAROTID ARTERIES

The right and left carotid arteries differ in length and origin. The **right** carotid, exclusively cervical, originates from the brachiocephalic trunk behind the right sternoclavicular joint. The **left** carotid originates directly from the aortic arch immediately posterolateral to the brachiocephalic trunk and therefore has both thoracic and cervical parts.

Thoracic part of the left common carotid artery (**10**.71, 72). This part ascends until level with the left sternoclavicular joint,

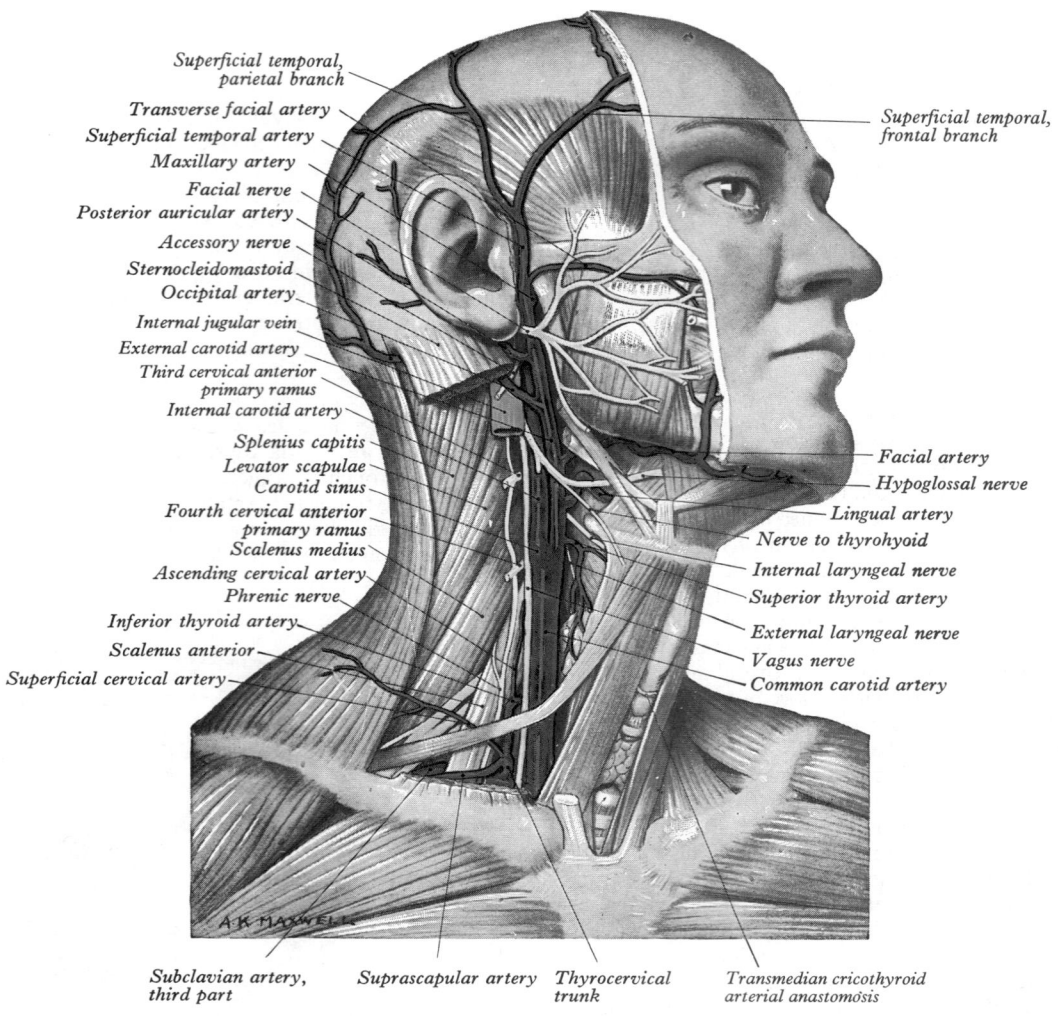

Superficial temporal,
parietal branch
Transverse facial artery
Superficial temporal artery
Maxillary artery
Facial nerve
Posterior auricular artery
Accessory nerve
Sternocleidomastoid
Occipital artery
Internal jugular vein
External carotid artery
Third cervical anterior
primary ramus
Internal carotid artery
Splenius capitis
Levator scapulae
Carotid sinus
Fourth cervical anterior
primary ramus
Scalenus medius
Ascending cervical artery
Phrenic nerve
Inferior thyroid artery
Scalenus anterior
Superficial cervical artery

Superficial temporal,
frontal branch

Facial artery
Hypoglossal nerve
Lingual artery
Nerve to thyrohyoid
Internal laryngeal nerve
Superior thyroid artery
External laryngeal nerve
Vagus nerve
Common carotid artery

A K MAXWELL

Subclavian artery,   Suprascapular artery   Thyrocervical   Transmedian cricothyroid
third part   trunk   arterial anastomosis

10.73   Dissection of the right side of the neck, showing the carotid and subclavian arteries and their branches. The parotid and submandibular glands have been removed together with the lower part of the internal jugular vein, most of the sternocleidomastoid and the upper parts of the stylohyoid and posterior belly of the digastric.

where it enters the neck. It is 20–25 mm long and it lies at first in front of the trachea, then it inclines to the left.

Relations. **Anterior** are the sternohyoid and sternothyroid, the anterior parts of the left pleura and lung, the left brachiocephalic vein and the thymic remnants, separating it from the manubrium; posterior are the trachea, left subclavian artery, left border of the oesophagus, left recurrent laryngeal nerve and thoracic duct. To the **right** are (below) the brachiocephalic trunk and (above) the trachea, inferior thyroid veins and thymic remains; to the **left** are the left vagus and phrenic nerves, left pleura and lung.

Cervical part of both common carotid arteries. Following a similar course (**10**.71–74), it ascends, diverging laterally from behind the sternoclavicular joint to the thyroid cartilage's upper border, where it divides into external and internal carotid arteries (**10**.73, 75). At its division the vessel has a dilatation, the *carotid sinus*, usually involving or restricted to the beginning of the internal carotid; the tunica·media is thinner here and the tunica adventitia, relatively thick, contains many receptor endings of the glossopharyngeal nerve (p. 1250). The sinus is responsive to changes in arterial blood pressure, leading to reflex haemodynamic modification. Its position on the main artery of the brain accounts for its role as a baroreceptor in control of intracranial pressure. The *carotid body*, behind the common carotid bifurcation, a small, reddish-brown structure, is a 'chemoreceptor'. (See Adams 1958 for a comparative account and p. 971 for modern views on its ultrastructure and function.)

In the lower neck the common carotids are separated by a narrow gap into which projects the trachea; above this the thyroid gland, larynx and pharynx project between them. Each is contained in a carotid sheath (p. 804), continuous with the deep cervical fascia and

of loose texture, though that actually around the artery is denser. This sheath encloses also the internal jugular vein and vagus nerve; the vein lies lateral to the artery, the nerve between them and posterior to both.

Relations. The artery is crossed **anterolaterally**, level with the cricoid cartilage, by the intermediate tendon (sometimes the superior belly) of the omohyoid. Below this muscle it is sited deeply, covered by skin, superficial fascia, platysma, deep cervical fascia, the sterno-cleidomastoid, sternohyoid and sternothyroid. Above the omohyoid it is more superficial, covered merely by skin, superficial fascia, platysma, deep cervical fascia and the medial margin of sterno-cleidomastoid and is crossed obliquely from its medial to lateral side by the sternocleidomastoid branch of the superior thyroid artery. In front of, or embedded in, the carotid sheath is the superior root of the ansa cervicalis, joined by its inferior root from the second and third cervical spinal nerves and crossing the vessel obliquely. The superior thyroid vein usually crosses near the artery's end, the middle thyroid vein a little below cricoid level; the anterior jugular vein crosses it above the clavicle, separated by sternohyoid and sterno-thyroid. **Posterior** are the fourth to sixth cervical transverse processes, and attached to them the longus colli and longus capitis and tendinous slips of scalenus anterior; the sympathetic trunk and ascending cervical artery are between the common carotid artery and the muscles. Below the level of the sixth cervical vertebra the artery is in an angle between the scalenus anterior and longus colli, anterior to the vertebral vessels, inferior thyroid and subclavian arteries, sympathetic trunk and, on the left, thoracic duct. **Medial** are the oesophagus, trachea, inferior thyroid artery and recurrent laryngeal nerve and, at a higher level, the larynx and pharynx; the thyroid gland overlaps it anteromedially. **Lateral** is the internal jugular vein, which in the lower neck is also anterior to the artery; posterolaterally in the angle between artery and vein is the vagus nerve.

On the right, low in the neck, the recurrent laryngeal nerve crosses obliquely behind the artery; the right internal jugular vein diverges from it below but the left vein approaches and often overlaps its artery.

Variations

In about 12% the right common carotid artery arises above the level of the sternoclavicular joint or it may be a separate branch from the aorta; again it may arise with its fellow. The left common carotid artery varies in origin more than the right; it may arise with the brachiocephalic (see also p. 1513). Division of the common carotid may occur higher, near the level of the hyoid bone, more rarely at a lower level alongside the larynx. Very rarely it ascends without division, either the external or internal carotid being absent. Rarely, also, it is replaced by separate external and internal carotid arteries arising directly from the aorta, on one side or bilaterally.

The common carotid artery usually has no branches but the vertebral, superior thyroid (**10**.71) or its laryngeal branch, ascending pharyngeal, inferior thyroid or occipital may be branches of it.

EXTERNAL CAROTID ARTERY

This artery (**10**.73–75) begins lateral to the thyroid cartilage's upper border, level with the disc between the third and fourth cervical vertebrae. A little curved, and with a gentle spiral, it first ascends slightly forwards and then inclines backwards and a little laterally, to pass midway between the mastoid tip and the mandibular angle where, in the substance of the parotid gland behind the mandible's neck, it divides into the superficial temporal and maxillary arteries. It diminishes rapidly in calibre due to its many large branches. In children it is smaller than the internal carotid but in adults the two are of almost equal size. At its origin, it is in the carotid triangle (p. 1521) and lies anteromedial to the internal carotid but becomes anterior, then lateral to this as it ascends. At mandibular levels the styloid process and its attached structures intervene between the vessels, the internal carotid being deep and the external carotid superficial to the styloid. A finger tip placed at the carotid triangle perceives a powerful arterial pulsation: beneath the finger lie the termination of the common carotid, the origins of external and internal carotids and the stems of the external carotid's initial branches.

Relations. Superficial to the artery in the carotid triangle are: the skin, superficial fascia, the loop between the facial nerve's cervical branch and the transverse cutaneous nerve of the neck, deep fascia and the anterior margin of sternocleidomastoid; it is crossed by the hypoglossal nerve and its vena comitans and by the lingual (common), facial and sometimes the superior thyroid veins. Leaving the triangle it is crossed by the posterior belly of the digastric and stylohyoid and ascends between this muscle and the posteromedial surface of the parotid gland, which it enters, lying medial to the facial nerve and the junction of the superficial temporal and maxillary veins. **Medial** to the artery are at first the pharyngeal wall, superior laryngeal nerve and ascending pharyngeal artery; at a higher level the internal carotid artery is separated from the external by the styloid process, styloglossus and stylopharyngeus, glossopharyngeal nerve, pharyngeal branch of vagus nerve and part of the parotid gland (**10**.74). The relation of the artery to the parotid gland is controversial, many clinicians asserting that it is often medial to it rather than in it. It seems that both relations occur at about equal frequency (Guffarth & Graumann 1975).

Branches (**10**.73, 74, 77). These are:

- Superior thyroid
- Ascending pharyngeal
- Lingual
- Facial
- Occipital
- Posterior auricular
- Superficial temporal
- Maxillary.

SUPERIOR THYROID ARTERY (**10**.73)

This arises from the front of the external carotid artery just below

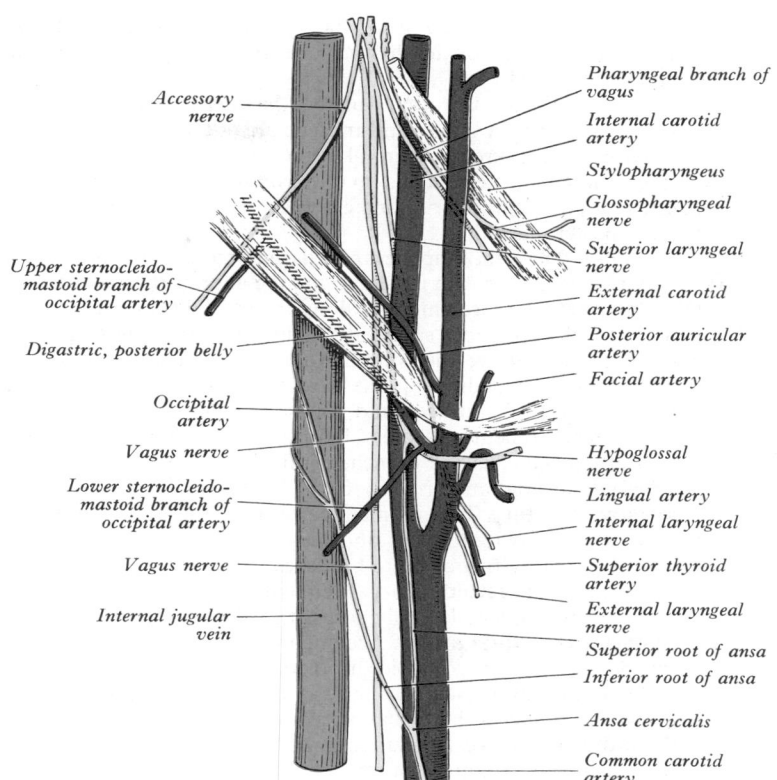

10.74   The structures crossing the internal jugular vein and carotid arteries and those intervening between the external and internal carotid arteries.

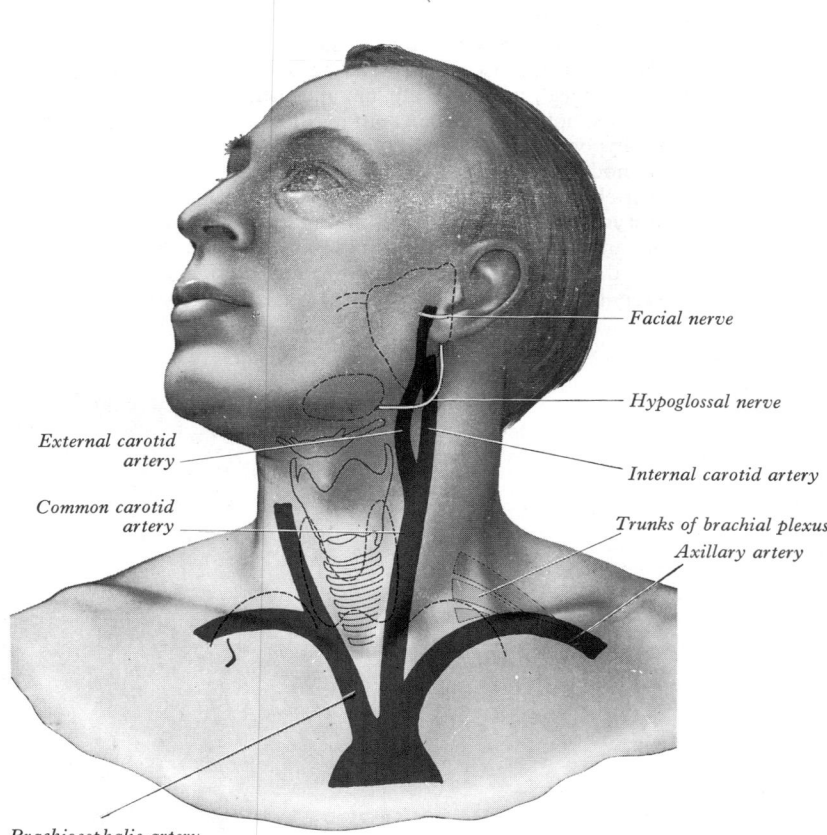

10.75   The surface projection of some of the larger structures in the face and neck. Note that the parotid gland and duct, and submandibular and thyroid glands and the apices of the lungs are shown as interrupted outlines; the hyoid bone and the thyroid, cricoid and tracheal cartilages are indicated by continuous outlines.

the level of the greater cornu of the hyoid, dividing into terminal branches at the apex of the thyroid lobe, but it may issue from the common carotid (**10.**71).

Relations. From an origin under the sternocleidomastoid it descends forwards in the carotid triangle along the lateral border of the thyrohyoid, covered by skin, platysma and fasciae and then deep to the omohyoid, sternohyoid and sternothyroid. Medial are the constrictor pharyngis inferior and external laryngeal nerve; the nerve is often posteromedial.

Branches. The artery supplies the adjacent muscles and the thyroid gland; it anastomoses with its fellow and the inferior thyroid arteries. Glandular branches are anterior, along the medial side of the upper pole of the lateral lobe, supplying mainly the anterior surface, a branch crossing above the isthmus to anastomose with its fellow; and posterior descending on the posterior border, supplying the medial and lateral surfaces and anastomosing with the inferior thyroid artery. Sometimes a lateral branch supplies the lateral surface. The artery also has named branches: infrahyoid, superior laryngeal, sternocleidomastoid and cricothyroid.

Infrahyoid artery. This is small, runs along the lower border of the hyoid deep to thyrohyoid and anastomoses with its fellow. It can be replaced by two or more branches.

Sternocleidomastoid artery. Frequently arising from the external carotid, it descends laterally across the carotid sheath.

Superior laryngeal artery. Accompanying the internal laryngeal nerve deep to the thyrohyoid, it pierces the lower part of the thyrohyoid membrane, supplies the larynx and anastomoses with its fellow and the inferior laryngeal branch of the inferior thyroid.

Cricothyroid artery. A small artery, it crosses high on the cricothyroid ligament, communicating with its fellow.

ASCENDING PHARYNGEAL ARTERY

This, the smallest branch of the external carotid, is a long, slender vessel, arising posteriorly near the external carotid's origin and ascending between the internal carotid artery and pharynx to the cranial base (**10.**84); it is crossed by the styloglossus and stylopharyngeus, with longus capitis posterior to it; it anastomoses with the facial artery's ascending palatine branch. Its named branches are: pharyngeal, inferior tympanic and meningeal. Numerous small branches supply the longus capiti and longus colli, the sympathetic trunk, hypoglossal, glossopharyngeal and vagus nerves and cervical lymph nodes, anastomosing with branches of the ascending cervical and vertebral arteries.

Pharyngeal arteries. Three or four supply the constrictors and stylopharyngeus. A variable ramus supplies the palate and may replace the facial's ascending palatine branch; it descends forwards between the superior border of the superior constrictor and the

levator veli palatini, accompanying the latter to the soft palate; it gives minute branches to the tonsil and one to the auditory tube.

Inferior tympanic artery. A small branch, it traverses the temporal canaliculus for the tympanic branch of the glossopharyngeal nerve to supply the tympanic cavity's medial wall.

Meningeal branches. These small vessels to the nerves, dura mater and adjacent bone enter the cranium through the foramen lacerum, jugular foramen and hypoglossal canal. They supply the nerves in these passages and their surrounding tissues. One of them, the *posterior meningeal artery*, which reaches the cerebellar fossa via the jugular foramen, is usually regarded as the terminal branch of the ascending pharyngeal artery.

LINGUAL ARTERY

This vessel, bringing the chief supply to the tongue and buccal floor of the mouth, arises anteromedially from the external carotid opposite the tip of the hyoid's greater cornu, between the superior thyroid and facial arteries (**10.**73, 74). Ascending medially at first, it loops down and forwards, passes medial to the posterior border of the hyoglossus and horizontally forwards deep to it and, ascending again almost vertically, courses sinuously forwards on the tongue's inferior surface as far as its tip (**10.**76). Its relation to the hyoglossus naturally divides the vessel into descriptive 'thirds'.

Relations. In its *first part* the lingual artery is in the carotid triangle; superficial to it are the skin, fascia and platysma; the middle pharyngeal constrictor is medial. It ascends a little medially, then descends to the level of the hyoid bone, its loop crossed externally by the hypoglossal nerve. Its *second part* passes along the hyoid's upper border, deep to the hyoglossus, the tendons of digastric and stylohyoid, the lower part of the submandibular gland and posterior part of the mylohyoid; the hyoglossus separates it from the hypoglossal nerve and its vena comitans; here its medial aspect adjoins the middle constrictor and crosses the stylohyoid ligament; it is accompanied by lingual veins (p. 1580). The *third part* is the *arteria profunda linguae*, which turns upward near the anterior border of the hyoglossus, passing forwards close to the inferior lingual surface near the frenulum, accompanied by the lingual nerve. Medial to it is the genioglossus, lateral to it the longitudinalis linguae inferior, below it the lingual mucous membrane. Near the lingual tip it anastomoses with its fellow. Its named branches are suprahyoid, dorsal lingual and sublingual.

The lingual artery often arises with the facial or, less often, with the superior thyroid artery. It may be replaced by a ramus of the maxillary artery.

Suprahyoid artery. This is very small and runs along the hyoid's upper border to anastomose with the contralateral artery.

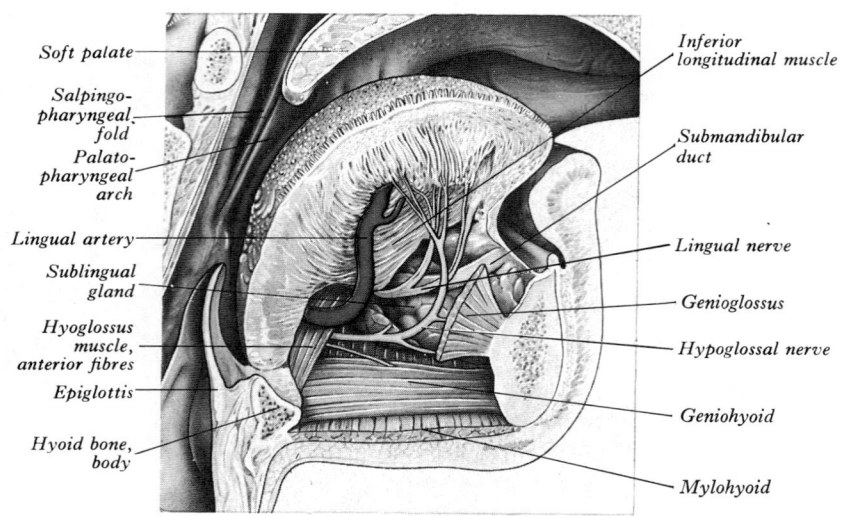

Soft palate —
Salpingo-pharyngeal fold —
Palato-pharyngeal arch —
Lingual artery —
Sublingual gland —
Hyoglossus muscle, anterior fibres —
Epiglottis —
Hyoid bone, body —

Inferior longitudinal muscle
Submandibular duct
Lingual nerve
Genioglossus
Hypoglossal nerve
Geniohyoid
Mylohyoid

10.76   Dissection of the left half of the tongue from the medial side, exposing the end of the second part and the beginning of the third part of the left lingual artery and adjoining structures, in an edentulous subject.

Dorsal lingual arteries. Usually two or three small vessels, these arise medial to the hyoglossus, and ascend to the posterior part of the lingual dorsum to supply its mucous membrane, palatoglossal arch, tonsil, soft palate and epiglottis; they anastomose with the opposite vessels.

Sublingual artery. Arising at the anterior margin of hyoglossus, it goes forward between the genioglossus and mylohyoid to the sublingual gland, supplying this, the mylohyoid and the buccal and gingival mucous membranes. One branch pierces the mylohyoid and joins the submental branches of the facial artery; another courses through the mandibular gingiva to anastomose with its fellow. From this anastomosis issues a single artery which enters the lingual foramen of the mandible, situated in the midline on the posterior aspect of the symphysis, immediately above the genial tuberculus (McDonnell et al 1994).

FACIAL ARTERY

This artery (also known as *external maxillary*) arises anteriorly from the external carotid in the carotid triangle above the lingual artery and immediately above the greater cornu of the hyoid bone (10.77, 84). Medial to the mandibular ramus it arches upwards and grooves the posterior aspect of the submandibular gland; it then turns down again between the gland and the medial pterygoid. Reaching the surface of the mandible it curves round its inferior border, anterior to the masseter, to enter the face. Here it ascends forwards across the mandible and buccinator to traverse a cleft in the modiolus (p. 796) near the buccal angle. It then ascends the side of the nose and ends at the medial palpebral commissure, supplying the lacrimal sac and joining the dorsal nasal branch of the ophthalmic artery. The artery is very sinuous throughout: in the neck perhaps to adapt to the movements of the pharynx during deglutition and on the face to movements of the mandible, lips and cheeks. Distal to its superior branch it is termed the *angular artery*. Facial artery pulsation is most palpable where it crosses the mandibular base and, between thumb and finger, near the buccal angle.

Relations. In the neck, at its origin, the artery is superficial, covered by the skin, platysma and fasciae and often crossed by the hypoglossal nerve. It runs up and forwards, deep to the digastric and the stylohyoid and posterior part of the submandibular gland. At first on the middle pharyngeal constrictor, it may reach the lateral surface of the styloglossus, separated there from the tonsil only by this muscle and the lingual fibres of the superior constrictor. Thence it descends to the lower border of the mandible in a lateral groove on the submandibular gland. In the face, where, as noted, its pulse can be felt as it crosses the mandible, it is superficial and at first just beneath the platysma. It is covered by skin, the fat of the cheek and near the buccal angle by superficial modiolar muscles (p. 796). Deep to it are the buccinator and levator anguli oris; it may pass over or through the levator labii superioris. Terminally it is embedded in the levator labii superioris alaeque nasi. The facial vein is posterior, in a more direct course across the face; at the anterior border of the masseter the two are in contact; in the neck the vein is superficial. Branches of the facial nerve cross forwards over the artery, which supplies the muscles and tissues of the face, submandibular gland, tonsil and soft palate. Its branches are cervical and facial.

Cervical branches

Ascending palatine artery (10.84). Starting near the facial's origin, it ascends between the styloglossus and stylopharyngeus to the side of the pharynx, along which it ascends between the superior constrictor and the medial pterygoid towards the cranial base. Near the levator veli palatini it bifurcates: one branch follows this muscle, winds over the upper border of the superior constrictor, supplies the soft palate and anastomoses with its fellow and the greater palatine branch of the maxillary artery; the other branch pierces the superior constrictor to supply the tonsil and pharyngotympanic tube, joining with tonsillar and ascending pharyngeal arteries.

Tonsillar artery. The main supply to the tonsil, it sometimes arises from the ascending palatine, though is usually separate; it ascends between the medial pterygoid and styloglossus and at the latter's upper border it perforates the superior constrictor and ramifies in the tonsil and posterior lingual musculature.

Glandular branches. Three or four large vessels, they supply the submandibular salivary gland and lymph nodes, adjacent muscles and skin.

Submental artery. The largest cervical branch, it arises as the facial separates from the submandibular gland, turning forwards on the mylohyoid (10.77) below the mandible. It supplies the surrounding muscles and anastomoses with a sublingual branch of the lingual and mylohyoid branch of the inferior alveolar arteries; at the chin it ascends the mandible, dividing into superficial and deep branches which anastomose with the inferior labial and mental arteries, supplying the chin and lower lip.

Facial branches

Inferior labial artery (10.77). Arising near the buccal angle, it passes up and forwards under the depressor anguli oris, penetrates the orbicularis oris and runs sinuously near the lower lip's margin between the muscle and the mucous membrane. It supplies the inferior labial glands, mucous membrane and muscles, anastomosing with its fellow and the mental branch of the inferior alveolar artery.

Superior labial artery (10.77). Larger and more tortuous than the inferior, it has a similar course along the superior labial margin between the mucous membrane and the orbicularis oris; it anastomoses with its fellow, supplying the upper lip, a septal branch, which ramifies antero-inferiorly in the nasal septum, and an alar branch.

Lateral nasal artery (10.77). Branching from the facial as it ascends the side of the nose, it supplies the nasal ala and dorsum, anastomosing with its fellow, the septal and alar branches of the superior labial, dorsal nasal ramus of the ophthalmic and infraorbital branch of the maxillary artery. It may be replaced by several small branches or arise from the superior labial, diverging from its septal branch (as in 10.77).

Facial anastomoses. These are numerous not only with corresponding contralateral branches but also: **in the neck**, with the sublingual branch of the lingual, ascending pharyngeal and palatine branch of the maxillary; **on the face**, with the mental branch of the inferior alveolar, transverse facial branch of the superficial temporal, infraorbital branch of the maxillary and dorsal nasal branch of the ophthalmic. The anastomoses in the lips are by main trunks, an important fact in labial injuries.

Variations. The facial artery may arise with the lingual, as a linguo-facial trunk. It varies in size and supply to the face: it may end as the submental artery and often extends only to the buccal angle. The deficiency is then filled by branches of neighbouring arteries. In 110 human fetuses a common linguo-facial trunk occurred in 43%; in 42% the facial did not reach the medial orbital angle, ending as a superior (20%) or inferior (22%) labial artery (Kozielec & Józwa 1977).

OCCIPITAL ARTERY

This artery arises posteriorly from the external carotid, about 2 cm from its origin; at first medial to the posterior belly of the digastric, it ends posteriorly in the scalp (10.78).

Course and relations. At its origin, the artery is crossed superficially by the hypoglossal nerve, winding round it from behind. It goes back, up and deep to the posterior digastric belly, crossing the internal carotid, internal jugular vein, hypoglossal, vagal and accessory nerves (10.78). Between the transverse process of the atlas and temporal mastoid process it reaches the lateral border of the rectus capitis lateralis. It then runs in the temporal bone's occipital groove, medial to the mastoid process and attachments of the sternocleidomastoid, splenius capitis, longissimus capitis and digastric, lying successively on the rectus capitis lateralis, obliquus superior and semispinalis capitis. Finally, accompanied by the greater occipital nerve, it turns up to pierce the fascia connecting the cranial attachments of the trapezius and sternocleidomastoid, ascends tortuously in the dense superficial fascia of the scalp and divides into many branches. Its branches are as follows.

Sternocleidomastoid branches. Two branches are usual, the **lower** arising near the origin of the occipital but sometimes directly from the external carotid. It descends backwards over the hypoglossal nerve and internal jugular vein, enters the sternocleidomastoid, and anastomoses with the sternocleidomastoid branch of the superior thyroid. The **upper** branch arises as the occipital crosses the accessory

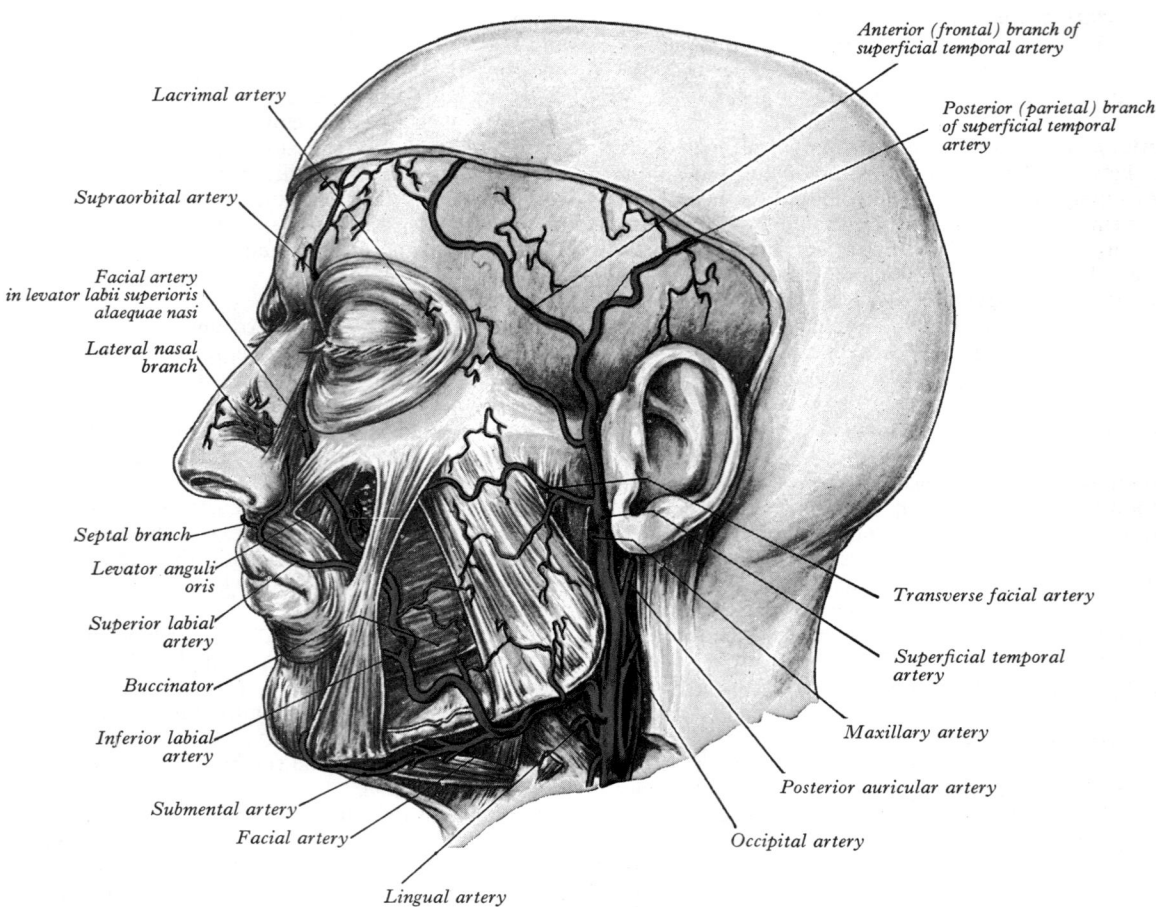

Anterior (frontal) branch of superficial temporal artery

Posterior (parietal) branch of superficial temporal artery

Lacrimal artery

Supraorbital artery

Facial artery in levator labii superioris alaequae nasi

Lateral nasal branch

Septal branch

Levator anguli oris

Superior labial artery

Buccinator

Inferior labial artery

Submental artery

Facial artery

Lingual artery

Transverse facial artery

Superficial temporal artery

Maxillary artery

Posterior auricular artery

Occipital artery

10.77 The arteries of the left side of the face and their main branches. Many of the postmodiolar muscles and part of the modiolus (through which the facial artery passes) have been resected. Note the less usual origin of lateral nasal branch in this specimen.

nerve, running down and backwards superficial to the internal jugular vein. It enters the deep surface of the sternocleidomastoid with the accessory nerve.

Mastoid artery. Small in size and sometimes absent, it enters the cranial cavity via the mastoid foramen, supplying the mastoid air cells and dura mater.

Stylomastoid artery. This branches from the occipital in two-thirds of subjects (p. 1520).

Auricular branch. It supplies the medial aspect of the auricle, anastomosing with the posterior auricular artery.

Muscular branches. These supply the digastric, stylohyoid, splenius, longissimus capitis and neighbouring muscles.

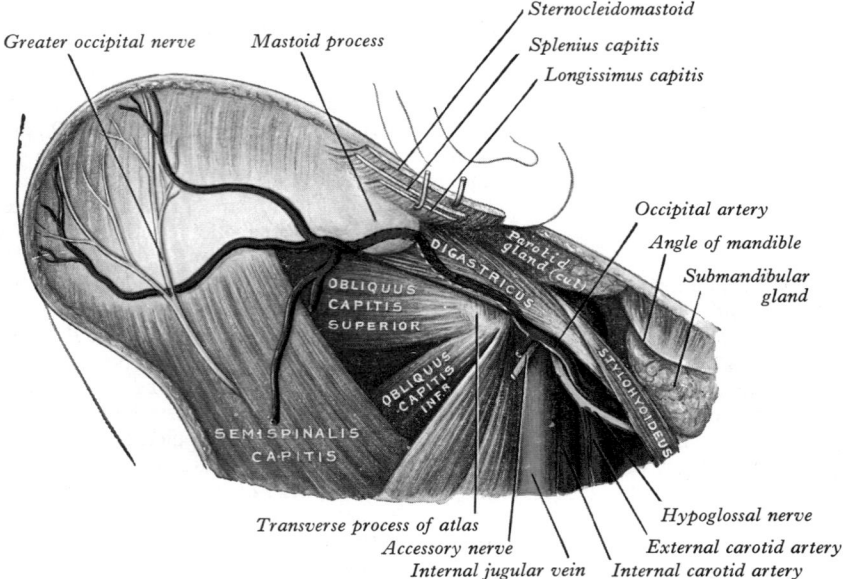

Greater occipital nerve

Mastoid process

Sternocleidomastoid

Splenius capitis

Longissimus capitis

Occipital artery

Angle of mandible

Submandibular gland

OBLIQUUS CAPITIS SUPERIOR

OBLIQUUS CAPITIS INFR.

SEMISPINALIS CAPITIS

DIGASTRICUS

Parotid gland (cut)

STYLOHYOIDEUS

Transverse process of atlas

Accessory nerve

Internal jugular vein

Hypoglossal nerve

External carotid artery

Internal carotid artery

10.78 Dissection to show the course of the occipital artery. The upper and lower sternocleidomastoid branches of the artery have been transected and are not labelled.

Descending branch (10.78). This arises where the occipital adjoins the obliquus superior, dividing into superficial and deep branches. The superficial ramus passes deep to the splenius, anastomosing with the superficial branch of the transverse cervical artery; the deep ramus descends between the semispinales capitis et cervicis, anastomosing with both the vertebral and the deep cervical artery (from the costocervical trunk) (10.84).

Meningeal branches. They enter the cranium via the jugular foramen and condylar canal to supply the dura mater and bone of the posterior cranial fossa and the caudal four cranial nerves.

Occipital branches. Tortuous terminal branches distributed to the scalp as far as the vertex, they run between the skin and the occipital belly of the occipitofrontalis, anastomosing with the opposite occipital, posterior auricular and temporal arteries and supplying the occipital belly of the occipitofrontalis, skin and pericranium. There may be a meningeal lateral branch, traversing the parietal foramen.

POSTERIOR AURICULAR ARTERY

This small vessel branches posteriorly from the external carotid just above the digastric and stylohyoid (10.77). It ascends between the parotid gland and the styloid process to the groove between the auricular cartilage and mastoid process, dividing into auricular and occipital branches. As well as supplying the digastric, stylohyoid, sternocleidomastoid, and parotid gland, the posterior auricular artery has three named branches.

Stylomastoid artery. An indirect branch of the posterior auricular in about a third of subjects (Blunt 1954), it enters the stylomastoid foramen to supply the facial nerve, tympanic cavity, mastoid antrum and air cells, and semicircular canals. In the young its posterior tympanic ramus forms a circular anastomosis with the anterior tympanic artery (see below).

Auricular branch. Ascending deep to auricularis posterior, it ramifies on the cranial aspect of the auricle; some branches pierce this, others curve round it to supply its lateral aspect.

Occipital branch. It passes laterally across the mastoid process, turning back over the sternocleidomastoid to supply the occipital belly of the occipitofrontalis and scalp above and behind the ear; it anastomoses with the occipital artery.

SUPERFICIAL TEMPORAL ARTERY

This, the smaller terminal branch of the external carotid, begins in the parotid gland behind the mandible's neck, crosses the posterior root of the zygomatic process of the temporal bone and about 5 cm above this divides into anterior and posterior branches (10.73).

Relations. As it crosses the zygoma it is covered by the auricularis anterior; in the parotid gland temporal and zygomatic branches of the facial nerve cross it; in the scalp it is accompanied by corresponding veins, and just posterior to it lies the auriculotemporal nerve.

Branches. The superficial temporal supplies the parotid gland, temporomandibular joint and masseter and it also has several named branches.

Transverse facial artery (10.77). Arising before the superficial temporal emerges from the parotid gland, it traverses the gland, crosses the masseter between the parotid duct and the zygomatic arch, accompanied by one or two facial nerve branches, and divides into numerous branches supplying the parotid gland and duct, masseter and skin, anastomosing with the facial, masseteric, buccal, lacrimal and infraorbital arteries.

Anterior auricular branches. These are distributed to the lobule and anterior part of the auricle and the external acoustic meatus.

Zygomatico-orbital artery. Sometimes from the middle temporal, it skirts the upper border of the zygomatic arch between two layers of temporal fascia to the lateral orbital angle. It supplies the orbicularis oculi, and anastomoses with the lacrimal and palpebral branches of the ophthalmic artery.

Middle temporal artery. This branches just above the zygomatic arch, perforates the temporal fascia, supplies the temporalis and anastomoses with the deep temporal branches of the maxillary.

Frontal (anterior) branch. Meandering towards the frontal tuberosity, it supplies muscles, skin and pericranium in this region. It anastomoses with its fellow and the supraorbital and supratrochlear arteries.

Parietal (posterior) branch. Larger than the frontal, it curves up and back, superficial to the temporal fascia, anastomosing with its fellow and the posterior auricular and occipital arteries.

Variation

Variation in the superficial temporal artery is largely in the relative sizes of the frontal, parietal and transverse facial branches; the first two may be absent, the transverse facial may replace a shortened facial artery. Variations in fetal material have been described by Kozielec and Józwa (1976).

Clinical anatomy

Crossing the zygomatic process the artery is palpable through skin and fascia and is easily compressed here to control temporal haemorrhage. This vessel and other arteries supplying the scalp from below are well protected by dense tissue. Rarely are all implicated in a scalping injury and its branches anastomose so freely that a partially detached scalp may be replaced with reasonable hope of success as long as one vessel is intact. In craniotomy, incisions should be convex upwards to include the superficial temporal artery in the flap. In carotid angiograms branches of the superficial temporal and middle meningeal arteries are superimposed, but are distinguishable by the straighter course, lack of anastomoses and narrower calibre in the meningeal branches (Dominić-Stošić & Jeličić 1974).

MAXILLARY (INTERNAL MAXILLARY) ARTERY

This, the larger terminal branch of the external carotid, arises behind the mandibular neck, at first embedded in the parotid gland; it then passes medial to the mandibular neck and superficial or deep to the lower head of the lateral pterygoid to reach the pterygopalatine fossa, usually passing between the two heads of the lateral pterygoid (10.79). It has mandibular, pterygoid and pterygopalatine segments, related sequentially to bone, muscle and bone, a useful indication of its branches.

The **first, mandibular, part** is horizontal and passes between the mandible's neck and the sphenomandibular ligament, parallel with and slightly below the auriculotemporal nerve; it crosses the inferior alveolar nerve and skirts the lower border of the lateral pterygoid.

The **second, pterygoid, part** ascends obliquely forwards medial to the temporalis and superficial to the lower head of the lateral pterygoid; it is often deep to the latter, lying between it and branches of the mandibular nerve and it may then project as a lateral loop between the two parts of the lateral pterygoid.

The **third, pterygopalatine, part** passes between the heads of the lateral pterygoid and through the pterygomaxillary fissure into the pterygopalatine fossa, where it is situated anterior to the pterygopalatine ganglion.

Branches. The artery is distributed to the mandible, maxilla, teeth, muscles of mastication, palate, nose and cranial dura mater. Its branches form three groups, corresponding with its parts.

Branches of the first part (10.79)

Deep auricular artery. Often arising with the anterior tympanic, it ascends in the parotid gland behind the temporomandibular joint, pierces the cartilaginous or osseous wall of the external acoustic meatus and supplies its cuticular lining, the exterior of the tympanic membrane and the joint.

Anterior tympanic artery. Ascending behind the temporomandibular joint, it enters the tympanic cavity through the petrotympanic fissure and ramifies on the interior of the tympanic membrane, forming a vascular circle around it with the posterior tympanic branch of the stylomastoid; it anastomoses with twigs of the artery of the pterygoid canal and caroticotympanic branches of the internal carotid artery in the mucosa of the tympanic cavity.

Middle meningeal artery. Largest of the meningeal arteries, it ascends between the sphenomandibular ligament and lateral pterygoid, passes between the roots of the auriculotemporal nerve and may lie lateral to the tensor veli palatini before entering the cranial cavity through the foramen spinosum. It then runs in an anterolateral groove on the squamous part of the temporal bone, dividing into frontal and parietal branches. The *frontal (anterior) branch,* the

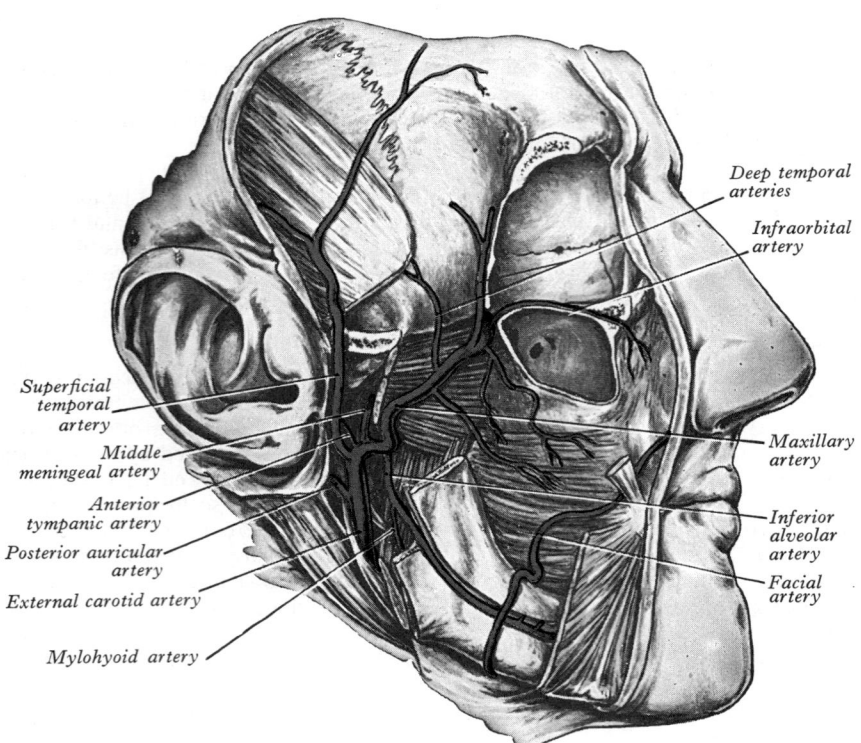

10.79 The right maxillary artery. An extensive dissection has been carried out, involving the removal of the parotid gland, the zygomatic arch, part of the ramus of the mandible, the lateral walls of the orbit and maxillary sinus and the orbital contents.

larger, crosses the greater wing of the sphenoid, reaches a groove or canal in the parietal's sphenoidal angle and divides into branches between the dura mater and cranium, some ascending to the vertex, others to the occipital region. One ascending branch grooves the parietal bone about 15 mm behind the coronal suture, corresponding approximately to the precentral sulcus. The *parietal* (*posterior*) *branch* curves back on the squamous temporal bone, reaching the lower border of the parietal anterior to its mastoid angle and dividing to supply the posterior parts of the dura mater and cranium. These branches anastomose with their fellows and with the anterior and posterior meningeal arteries.

In the cranial cavity the artery has the following branches:

- Numerous *ganglionic branches* supply the trigeminal ganglion and roots.
- A *petrosal branch* enters the hiatus for the greater petrosal nerve and supplies the facial nerve, ganglion and tympanic cavity, anastomosing with the stylomastoid artery (p. 1519).
- A *superior tympanic artery* runs in the canal for the tensor tympani, supplying both muscle and the mucosa lining the canal.
- *Temporal branches* traverse minute foramina in the sphenoid's greater wing and anastomose with deep temporal arteries.
- An *anastomotic branch* (p. 1526) enters the orbit lateral in the superior orbital fissure, anastomosing with a recurrent branch of the lacrimal artery; enlargement of this anastomosis explains an occasional origin of the lacrimal from the middle meningeal artery.

Apart from these and a supply to the dura mater, the middle meningeal artery is predominantly periosteal, supplying bone and red bone marrow.

Surface anatomy (**10.79**). The middle meningeal artery enters the skull medial to the zygoma's midpoint, dividing 2 cm above this. From here the frontal branch runs first up and forwards to the pterion and then up and back towards a point midway between the inion and nasion. The parietal branch runs up and back towards the lambda.

Clinical anatomy. The middle meningeal artery may be torn in temporal fractures or by injuries separating the dura mater from the bone, followed by haemorrhage between them. Trephining may be necessary to reduce cerebral compression.

Accessory meningeal artery. This may arise from the maxillary or the middle meningeal. It enters the cranial cavity through the foramen ovale, supplying the trigeminal ganglion, dura mater and bone, but its main distribution is extracranial (Baumel & Beard 1961), principally the medial pterygoid, lateral pterygoid (upper head), tensor veli palatini, sphenoid bone (greater wing and pterygoid processes), mandibular nerve and otic ganglion. It is sometimes replaced by separate small arteries.

Inferior alveolar (dental) artery. Descending posterior to the inferior alveolar nerve, to the mandibular foramen, here it is between bone laterally and the sphenomandibular ligament medially. Before entering the foramen it has a mylohyoid branch, which pierces the sphenomandibular ligament to descend with the mylohyoid nerve in its groove on the mandibular ramus; it ramifies superficially on the muscle and anastomoses with the facial's submental branch. The inferior alveolar artery then traverses the mandibular canal with the inferior alveolar nerve and divides into the incisor and mental branches near the first premolar. The incisor branch continues below the incisor teeth to the midline, where it anastomoses with its fellow. In the canal the arteries supply the mandible, tooth sockets and teeth with branches entering the minute hole at the apex of the root to supply the pulp. The mental branch leaves the mental foramen, supplies the chin and anastomoses with the submental and inferior labial arteries. Near its origin the inferior alveolar artery has a lingual branch, which descends with the lingual nerve to supply the buccal mucous membrane.

Branches of the second part (10.79)

Deep temporal branches. Anterior and posterior, these branches ascend between the temporalis and bone, supplying mainly the former. They anastomose with the middle temporal artery. The anterior connects with the lacrimal by small branches perforating the zygomatic bone and greater wing of the sphenoid.

Pterygoid branches. Irregular in number and origin, these supply the pterygoid muscles.

Masseteric artery. This is small and with the masseteric nerve passes behind the tendon of temporalis through the mandibular incisure (notch) to the deep surface of masseter, in which it anastomoses with the masseteric branches of the facial and transverse facial arteries.

Buccal artery. Running obliquely forwards with the buccal nerve between the medial pterygoid and the attachment of the temporalis it supplies the external surface of the buccinator (and through it the mucosa), anastomosing with branches of the facial and infraorbital arteries.

Branches of the third part

Posterior superior alveolar (dental) artery. Leaving the maxillary artery as it enters the pterygopalatine fossa, it descends on the maxilla's infratemporal surface. It then divides, some branches entering the alveolar canals to supply molar and premolar teeth and the maxillary sinus, others continuing over the alveolar process to supply the gingivae.

Infraorbital artery. Often arising with the posterior superior alveolar, it enters the orbit posteriorly through the inferior orbital fissure, to run in the infraorbital groove and canal with the infraorbital nerve, both emerging on the face via the infraorbital foramen, deep to the levator labii superioris. In the canal it has:

- *orbital branches*, which supply the rectus inferior, obliquus inferior and lacrimal sac
- *anterior superior alveolar* (*dental*) *branches*, which descend via the anterior alveolar canals to supply the upper incisor and canine teeth and the mucous membrane in the maxillary sinus.

On the face some branches ascend to the medial canthus and lacrimal sac, anastomosing with the terminal branches of the facial; others anastomose with a dorsal nasal branch of the ophthalmic artery and some descend between the levator labii superioris and levator anguli oris, anastomosing with the facial, transverse facial and buccal arteries.

The remaining branches arise in the pterygopalatine fossa.

Greater (or descending) palatine artery. This artery and nerve descend in their palatine canal; the artery gives off two or three lesser palatine arteries, transmitted through lesser palatine canals to supply the soft palate and tonsil, anastomosing with the ascending palatine. The main vessel emerges on the palate's oral surface by the greater palatine foramen and runs in a curved groove near the alveolar border of the hard palate to the incisive canal; it ascends this canal and anastomoses with a branch of the sphenopalatine artery. It supplies the gingivae, palatine glands and mucous membrane.

Pharyngeal artery. Very small, runs back through the pharyngeal (palatovaginal) canal with the pharyngeal branch of the pterygopalatine ganglion; it supplies the mucosa of the nasal roof, the nasopharynx, sphenoidal air sinus and auditory tube.

Artery of the pterygoid canal. Frequently from the greater palatine, it passes back in the pterygoid canal with the corresponding nerve, supplying its walls and contents and the mucous membrane of the upper pharynx, pharyngotympanic tube and tympanic cavity.

Relations. The pharyngeal artery is medial, that of the pterygoid canal lateral and the trunk of the maxillary artery passes anterior to the pterygopalatine ganglion.

Sphenopalatine artery. The termination of the maxillary, it traverses the sphenopalatine foramen into the walls of the nasal cavity posterior in the superior meatus. Here its *posterior lateral nasal branches* ramify over the conchae and meatuses, anastomosing with the ethmoidal arteries and nasal branches of the greater palatine, supplying the frontal, maxillary, ethmoidal and sphenoidal sinuses. Crossing anteriorly on the inferior sphenoid surface, the artery ends on the nasal septum as the *posterior septal branches*, which anastomose with the ethmoidal arteries; one branch descends on the vomer to the incisive canal to join the end of the greater palatine artery and septal branch of the superior labial.

Collateral circulation

Collateral circulation, after interruption of one common carotid, is often established by the connections across the midline between the carotids, intra- and extracranial, and by enlargement of the subclavian branches. Chief extracranial connections are between superior and inferior thyroid arteries, the deep cervical and the descending branch of the occipital; the vertebral artery substitutes for the internal carotid in the cranium. Nevertheless symptoms of cerebral disturbance supervene in about 25% of cases.

After interruption of the *external* carotid, circulation is maintained by anastomoses between most of its large branches (facial, lingual, superior thyroid, occipital) and their fellows, by their anastomoses with branches of the internal carotid and of the occipital with branches of the subclavian, etc.

Triangles of the neck

Anterolaterally the neck (**10.80, 81**) presents a somewhat quadrilateral area, limited **above** by the base of the mandible and a line continued from its angle to the mastoid process, **below** by the clavicle's upper border, **in front** by the anterior median line, **behind** by the anterior margin of trapezius. This region is divided by the sternocleidomastoid, ascending obliquely from the sternum and clavicle to the mastoid process and occipital bone. The area anterior to this is the *anterior triangle* and that behind it the *posterior triangle*. While these triangles and their subdivisions are emphasized by some as being purely arbitrary because many major structures (arteries, veins, lymphatics, nerves, some viscera) transgress their boundaries without interruption, nevertheless they have a topographical value in description. However, two further points should be made. Some of their subdivisions are easily identified by inspection and palpation and provide invaluable assistance in surface anatomical and clinical examination (see below). As the neck has a roughly cylindrical form, crossed obliquely by the sternocleidomastoid, the

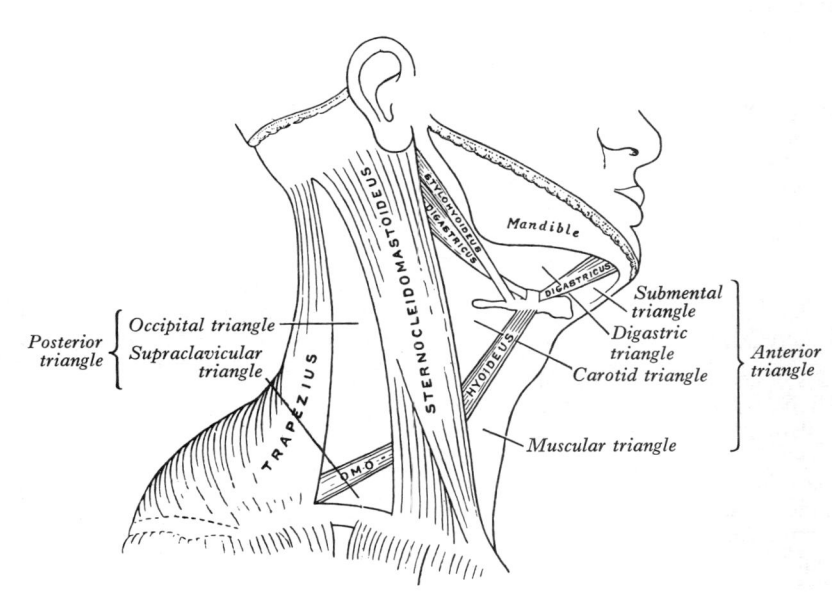

10.80   The triangles of the right side of the neck: a highly schematic two dimensional representation of what in reality are non-planar trigones distributed over a waisted column. Submandibular would be an alternative name for digastric.

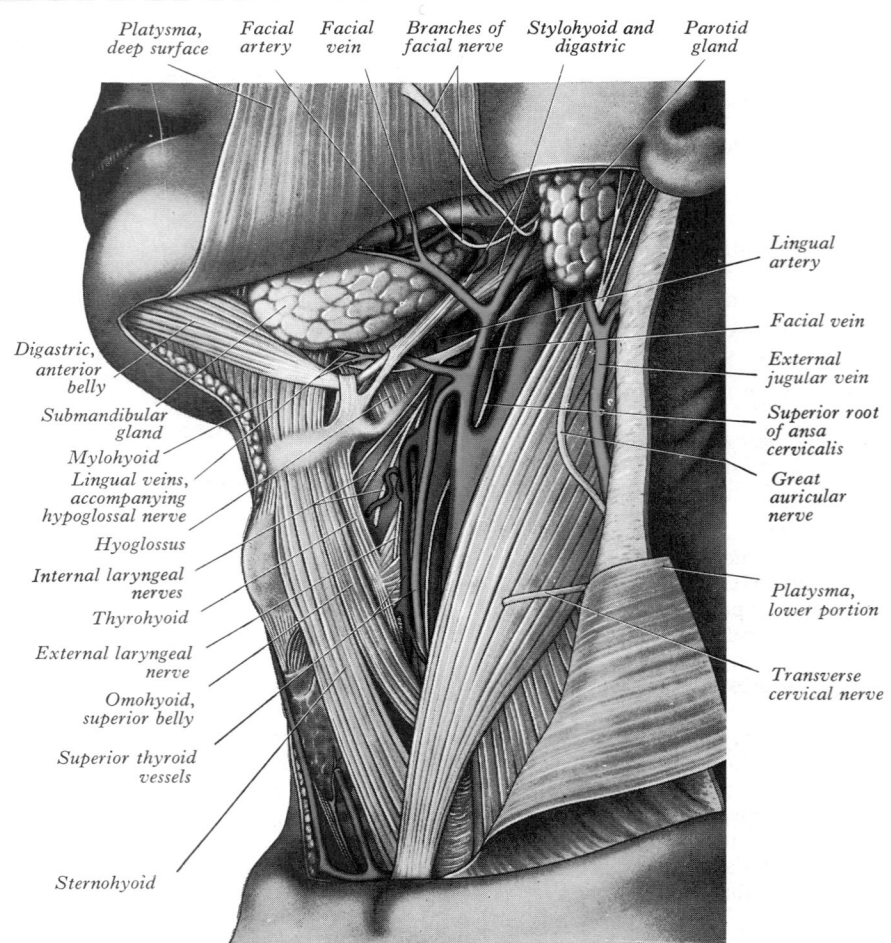

Platysma, deep surface — Facial artery — Facial vein — Branches of facial nerve — Stylohyoid and digastric — Parotid gland

Digastric, anterior belly
Submandibular gland
Mylohyoid
Lingual veins, accompanying hypoglossal nerve
Hyoglossus
Internal laryngeal nerves
Thyrohyoid
External laryngeal nerve
Omohyoid, superior belly
Superior thyroid vessels
Sternohyoid

Lingual artery
Facial vein
External jugular vein
Superior root of ansa cervicalis
Great auricular nerve
Platysma, lower portion
Transverse cervical nerve

10.81 Dissection of the left anterior triangle. The platysma has been divided transversely; its upper part has been turned upwards on to the face, its lower part turned backwards, exposing the lower part of the sternocleidomastoid. Dominating the centre of the illustration is the carotid triangle, with many of its contents and surrounding structures.

names anterior and posterior are not particularly apt; the triangles are not plane (and coplanar as represented in a two-dimensional diagram such as **10**.80) but both are spiralized regions (trigones) on the surface of the column.

ANTERIOR CERVICAL TRIANGLE

This is bounded anteriorly by the median line, and posteriorly by the anterior margin of the sternocleidomastoid, its base being the inferior mandibular border and its mastoid extension noted above; its apex is at the manubrium. It may be subdivided into muscular, carotid, digastric and submental triangles.

Muscular triangle

The muscular triangle is bounded by the median line from the hyoid bone to the sternum, inferoposteriorly by the anterior margin of the sternocleidomastoid and posterosuperiorly by the superior belly of the omohyoid.

Carotid triangle

The carotid triangle is limited posteriorly by the sternocleidomastoid, anteroinferiorly by the superior belly of the omohyoid and superiorly by the stylohyoid and posterior belly of the digastric; in the living, except the obese, the triangle is usually a small visible triangular depression, sometimes best seen with the head and cervical vertebral column slightly extended and the head contralaterally rotated. Often the latter position is quite unnecessary; judicious oblique lighting (window or lamp) throws the hollow into relief.

It is covered by the skin, superficial fascia, platysma and deep fascia containing branches of facial and cutaneous cervical nerves. The hyoid bone forms its anterior angle and adjacent floor; its position can be located immediately on simple inspection, verified by palpation. Parts of thyrohyoid, hyoglossus and inferior and middle pharyngeal constrictors form its floor. It contains the upper part of the common carotid and its division into external and internal carotid

arteries, overlapped by the anterior margin of the sternocleidomastoid; the external carotid is first anteromedial, then anterior to the internal. Branches of the external carotid are also encountered: the superior thyroid runs antero-inferiorly, the lingual anteriorly with its upward loop, the facial anterosuperiorly, the occipital posterosuperiorly and the ascending pharyngeal medial to the internal carotid. Massive arterial pulsation greets the examining finger. The veins correspond to the branches of the external carotid artery: superior thyroid, lingual, facial, ascending pharyngeal and sometimes the occipital, all ending in the internal jugular vein. The hypoglossal nerve crosses both carotid arteries, curving round the origin of the lower sternocleidomastoid branch of the occipital, where the superior root of the ansa cervicalis leaves it, descending anteriorly in the carotid sheath. Medial to the external carotid, below the hyoid bone, is the internal laryngeal nerve and, below this, the external laryngeal. Many structures in this region, such as all or part of the internal jugular vein, associated deep cervical lymph nodes, vagus nerve, etc., may be variably obscured by the sterno-cleidomastoid and, pedantically, are thus 'outside the triangle'; much more import-antly, their location is obvious during clinical examination.

Digastric triangle

The digastric triangle is bordered above by the base of the mandible (and its pro-jection to the mastoid process), postero-inferiorly by the posterior belly of the digastric and stylohyoid and antero-inferiorly by the anterior belly of digastric. It is covered by the skin, superficial fascia, platysma and deep fascia, in which are branches of facial and transverse cutaneous cervical nerves. Its floor is formed by the mylohyoid and hyoglossus. Its anterior region contains the sub-mandibular gland, superficial to which is the facial vein and deep to it the facial artery, crossing the lower border of the mandible at the anterior edge of the mas-seter; on the mylohyoid are the submental artery and mylohyoid artery and nerve. Variably related to the submandibular gland are the submandibular lymph nodes (p. 1612). Its posterior region contains the lower part of the parotid gland; the exter-nal carotid, passing deep to the stylohyoid, curves above the muscle and overlaps its superficial surface where it ascends deep to the parotid gland to enter it. The external carotid, which is superficial to the internal carotid, crosses it posterolaterally; deeper and separated from the external carotid by styloglossus, stylopharyngeus and the glossopharyngeal nerve, are the internal carotid artery, internal jugular vein and vagus nerve.

Submental triangle

The submental triangle, unpaired, is demarcated by both digastric muscles (anterior bellies); its apex is at the chin, its base the body of the hyoid and its floor the mylohyoid muscles. It contains lymph nodes and small veins uniting to form the anterior jugular.

POSTERIOR CERVICAL TRIANGLE

The posterior triangle is delimited anteriorly by the sternocleidomastoid, posteriorly by the anterior edge of tra-pezius, inferiorly by the middle third of the clavicle; its apex is between the attach-ments of the sternocleidomastoid and tra-pezius to the occiput and is often blunted, the 'triangle' becoming quadrilateral. It is crossed, about 2.5 cm above the clavicle, by the inferior belly of the omohyoid, which divides it into occipital and supra-clavicular triangles.

Occipital triangle

The occipital triangle, the upper, larger part of the posterior triangle, has the same borders, except below where its limit is the omohyoid. Its floor is, from above down: splenius capitis, levator scapulae, and scaleni medius and posterior. (Sometimes semispinalis capitis appears at the apex.) It is covered by the skin, superficial and deep fasciae and below by the platysma. The accessory nerve pierces the sternocleidomastoid and crosses on the levator scapulae obliquely down and back to the deep surface of the trapezius; cutaneous and muscular branches of the cervical plexus emerge at the posterior border of the sternocleidomastoid; below, supraclavicular nerves, transverse cervical vessels and the uppermost part of the brachial plexus cross the triangle. Lymph nodes are arranged along the posterior border of the cleidomastoid from the mastoid process to the root of the neck.

Supraclavicular triangle

The supraclavicular triangle, the lower, smaller division, is bounded like the pos-terior triangle, except above where the omohyoid limits it. It corresponds in the living neck with the lower part of the deep, prominent hollow, the greater supra-clavicular fossa (colloquially 'the salt cellar'). Its floor contains the first rib, scalenus medius and the first slip of ser-ratus anterior. Its size varies with the extent of the clavicular attachments of the sternocleidomastoid and trapezius and also the level of the inferior belly of the omohyoid. The triangle is covered by the skin, superficial and deep fasciae and plat-ysma and crossed by the supraclavicular nerves. Just above clavicular level the third part of the subclavian artery curves infero-laterally from the lateral margin of the scalenus anterior, across the first rib to the axilla. The subclavian vein is behind the clavicle and is not usually in the tri-angle; but it may rise as high as the artery and even accompany it behind scalenus anterior. The brachial plexus is partly above, partly behind the artery and closely related to it. The trunks of the brachial may easily be palpated here, the neck being contralaterally flexed and the exam-ining finger drawn across the trunks at right angles to their length. With the musculature relaxed, pulsation of the sub-clavian artery may be felt or the arterial flow controlled by retroclavicular com-pression against the first rib. The supra-scapular vessels pass transversely behind the clavicle; at a higher level are the trans-verse cervical artery and vein. The external jugular vein descends behind the posterior border of the sternocleidomastoid to end in the subclavian vein; it receives the trans-verse cervical and suprascapular veins, which form a plexus in front of the third part of the subclavian artery; occasionally it is joined by a small vein crossing the clavicle anteriorly from the cephalic vein. The nerve to the subclavius also crosses this triangle and some lymph nodes are contained in it.

INTERNAL CAROTID ARTERY

The internal carotid artery (10.82–89) supplies most of the ipsilateral cerebral hemisphere, eye and accessory organs, forehead and, in part, the nose. From the carotid bifurcation, where it usually has a carotid sinus (p. 1514), it ascends to the cranial base, enters the cranial cavity by the carotid canal and turns anteriorly through the cavernous sinus in the carotid groove on the side of the sphenoid body, ending below the anterior perforated substance by division into the anterior and middle cerebral arteries.

It may be divided conveniently into cervical, petrous, cavernous and cerebral parts. In the broadest outline its course is:

- **vertically upwards** in the neck
- curving **horizontally forwards** and **medially** in the petrous carotid canal
- **upwards** in the upper foramen lacerum
- **horizontally forwards** in the cavernous sinus
- **vertically upwards** medial to the anterior clinoid process
- looping a short distance **backwards** and **upwards** to its terminal division.

Cervical part

This section begins at the carotid bifurcation and ascends in front of the upper three cervical transverse processes to the inferior aperture of the carotid canal in the petrous temporal bone. It is superficial at first in the carotid triangle, then passes deeper, medial to the posterior belly of the digastric. Except near the skull, the internal jugular vein and vagus nerve are lateral; the external carotid is first anteromedial but then curves back to become superficial. The artery has many other relations. **Posteriorly** it adjoins the longus capitis, with the superior cervical sympathetic ganglion between them and the superior laryngeal nerve crossing obliquely behind it. **Medial** is the pharyngeal wall separated by fat and pharyngeal veins from the ascending pharyngeal artery and superior laryngeal nerve. **Antero-laterally** the artery is covered by the sternocleidomastoid; **below** the digastric, the hypoglossal nerve and superior root of the ansa cervicalis and the lingual and facial veins are superficial. **At the level of** the digastric it is crossed by the stylohyoid muscle and the occipital and posterior auricular arteries. **Above** the digastric it is separated from the external carotid by the styloid process, styloglossus and stylopharyngeus, glossopharyngeal nerve, vagal pharyngeal branch

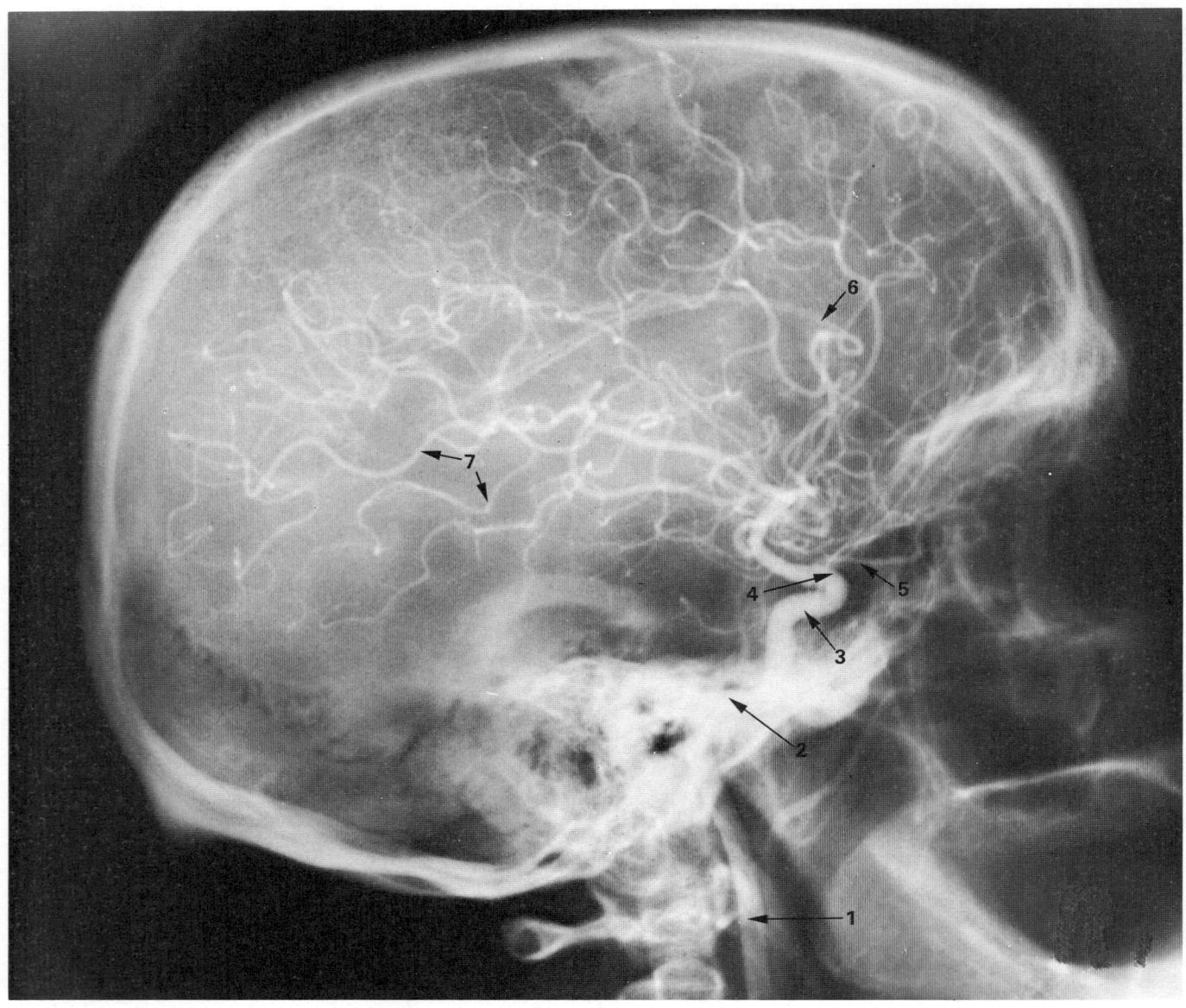

10.82 Internal carotid arteriogram (right): lateral view, in adult male of 33 years. The following can be identified: parts of the internal carotid artery (and individual vessels): 1. Cervical. 2. Intrapetrous. 3. Cavernous. 4. Terminal. 5. Ophthalmic artery. 6. Anterior cerebral artery. 7. Branches of middle cerebral artery. Note the absence of radio-opaque injectant from the cerebellar vessels.

and the deeper part of the parotid gland. **At the base of the skull** the glossopharyngeal, vagus, accessory and hypoglossal nerves are between the internal carotid artery and the internal jugular vein, which here has become posterior.

Petrous part

The artery at first ascends in the carotid canal, curves anteromedially and then superomedially above the cartilage filling the foramen lacerum, to enter the cranial cavity, passing between the lingula and petrosal process. It is at first anterior to the cochlea and tympanic cavity, separated from the latter and the pharyngotympanic tube by a thin, bony lamella, cribriform in the young, partly absorbed in old age; anterior to this it is separated from the trigeminal ganglion by the thin roof of the carotid canal, often deficient. The artery is surrounded by a venous plexus and the carotid autonomic plexus derived from the internal carotid branch of the superior cervical ganglion.

Cavernous part

In the cavernous sinus the artery is covered by lining endothelium of the veins. It ascends to the posterior clinoid process, turns

anteriorly to the side of the sphenoid and again curves up medial to the anterior clinoid process, emerging through the dural roof of the sinus; occasionally the two clinoid processes form a ring round the artery, which is also surrounded by a sympathetic plexus; the oculomotor, trochlear, ophthalmic and abducens nerves are lateral to it.

Cerebral part

Having traversed the dura mater the artery turns back below the optic nerve, passing between this and the oculomotor nerve to the anterior perforated substance at the medial end of the lateral cerebral sulcus, where it divides into anterior and middle cerebral arteries.

Variations. The length of the artery varies with the length of the neck and the point of carotid bifurcation. It may arise from the aortic arch and then be medial to the external carotid as far as the larynx but there crossing behind it. Its cervical part is normally straight but on occasion may be very tortuous, being nearer to the pharynx than usual and very near the tonsil. Its absence has also been recorded.

Surface anatomy. The internal carotid corresponds in position to a broad line from the termination of the common carotid to the back of the mandibular neck (**10**.75).

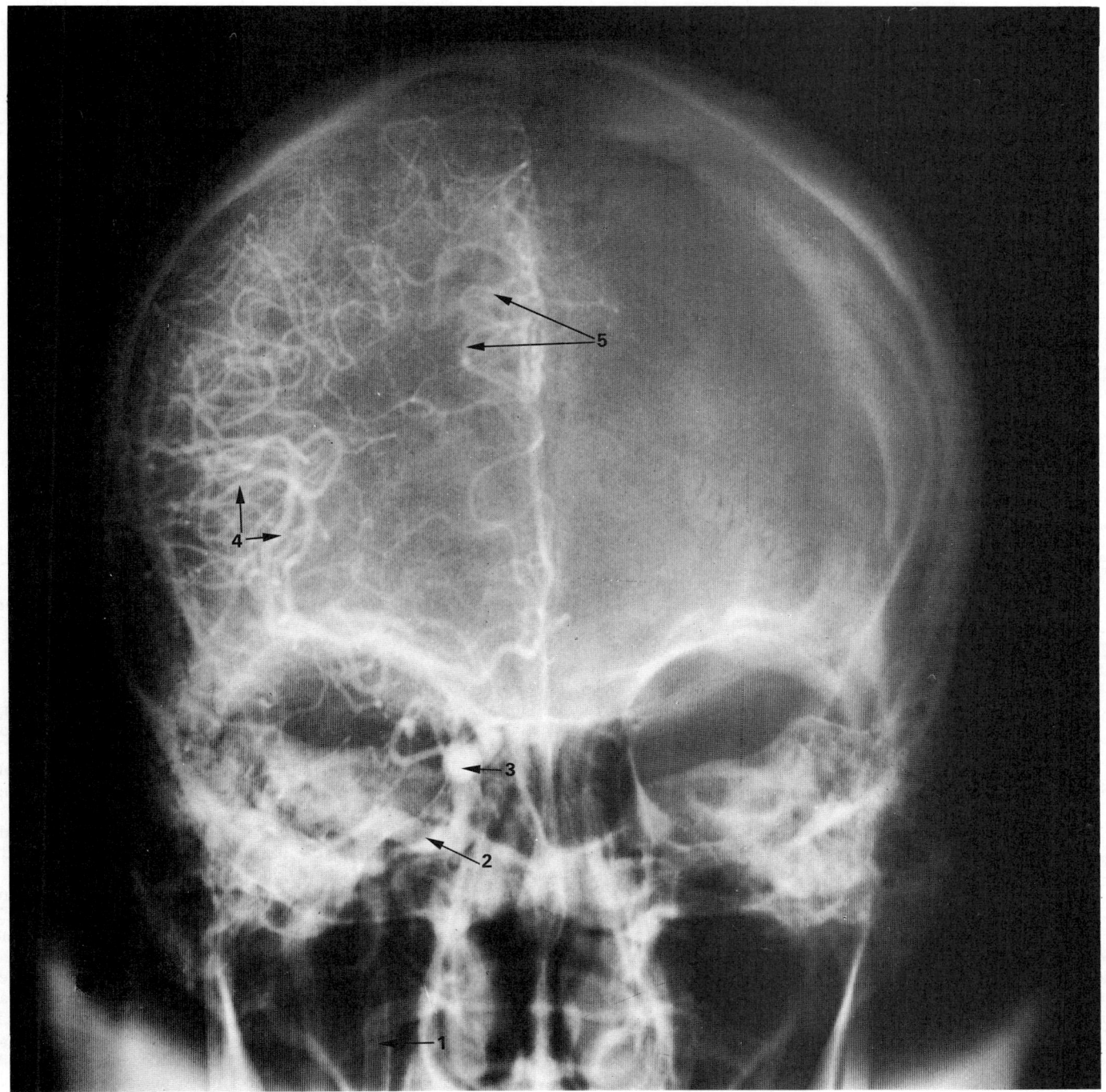

10.83 Internal carotid arteriogram (right): anteroposterior view of same subject as 10.82. Parts of the internal carotid artery: 1. Cervical. 2. Intra-petrous. 3. Cavernous. 4. Branches of middle cerebral artery. 5. Branches of anterior cerebral artery. Note the lack of contrast medium on the left side.

Branches. The cervical part has no branches. Those from the other parts are:

From the petrous part

- Caroticotympanic
- Pterygoid

From the cavernous part

- Cavernous
- Hypophyseal
- Meningeal

From the cerebral part

- Ophthalmic
- Anterior cerebral
- Middle cerebral
- Posterior communicating
- Anterior choroid.

Caroticotympanic artery. Small, occasionally double, it enters the tympanic cavity by a foramen in the carotid canal, anastomosing with the anterior tympanic branch of the maxillary artery and the stylomastoid artery.

Pterygoid artery. Inconstant, it enters the pterygoid canal with the nerve of the same name, anastomosing with a (recurrent) branch of the greater palatine artery.

Cavernous branches. Numbers of these small vessels supply the trigeminal ganglion, walls of the cavernous and inferior petrosal sinuses and contained nerves. Some anastomose with middle meningeal branches.

Hypophyseal branches. Small but numerous, they are important vessels (for details see p. 1887).

1525

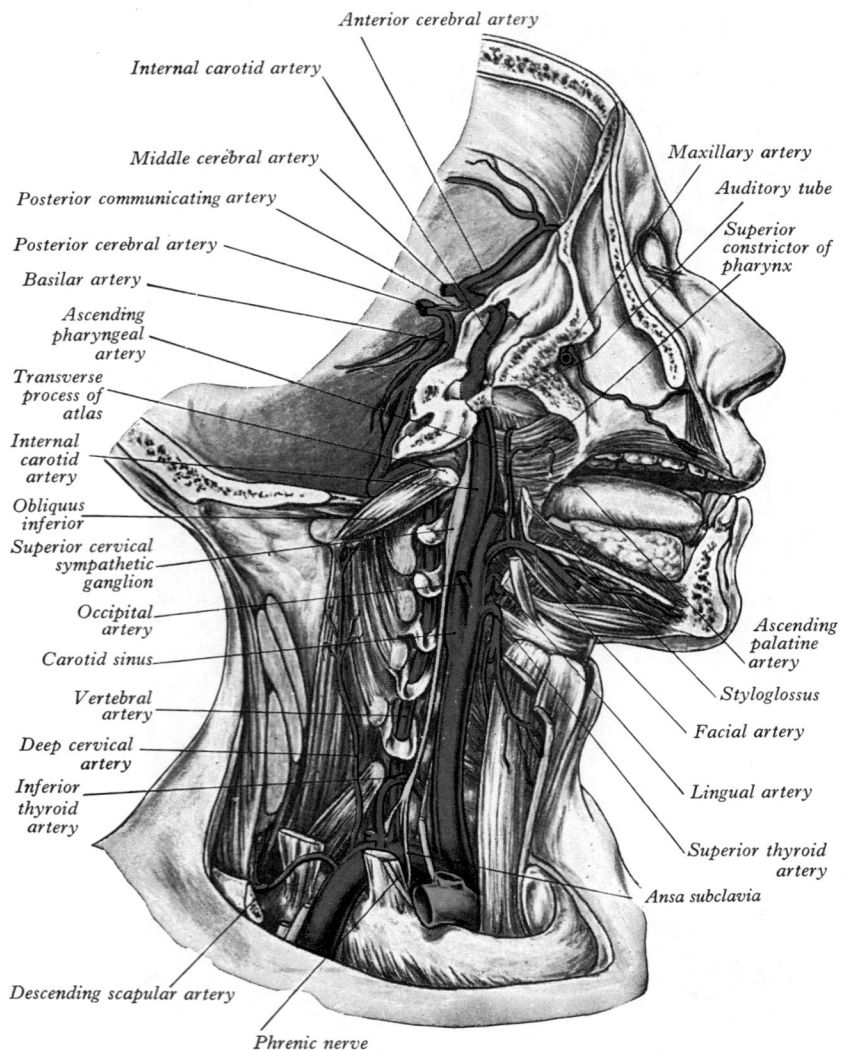

10.84 Dissection to show the course of the right vertebral and internal carotid arteries and some of their branches.

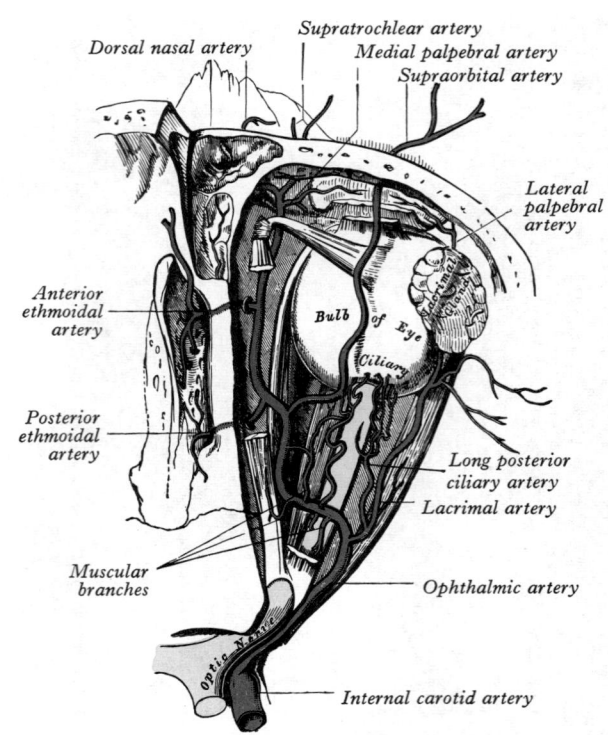

10.85 The ophthalmic artery and its branches in the right orbit, as seen from above.

Meningeal branch. This is minute and passes over the lesser sphenoid wing to supply the dura mater and bone in the anterior cranial fossa; it anastomoses with a meningeal branch of the posterior ethmoidal artery.

Ophthalmic artery (10.85). It leaves the internal carotid as it quits the cavernous sinus medial to the anterior clinoid process; it enters the orbit by the optic canal, inferolateral to the optic nerve; for a short distance it is then lateral to the nerve, medial to the oculomotor and abducens nerves, ciliary ganglion and rectus lateralis. It crosses between the optic nerve and rectus superior to the medial orbital wall, runs between the obliquus superior and the rectus medialis to the medial end of the upper eyelid, dividing into *supratrochlear* and *dorsal nasal branches*. As it crosses the optic nerve with the nasociliary nerve it is separated from the frontal nerve by the rectus superior and levator palpebrae superioris; its terminal branch accompanies the infratrochlear nerve. In about 15% of subjects the ophthalmic artery is below the optic nerve. Its branches are as follows:

Central artery of the retina. A first and small branch, it begins below the optic nerve. For a short distance it is in the nerve's dural sheath; about 1.25 cm behind the eye it enters the nerve's inferomedial surface and runs to the retina along its axis. Its distribution is described on page 1347.

Lacrimal artery. Leaving the ophthalmic near its exit from the optic canal, it is a large branch, sometimes arising before the ophthalmic enters the orbit; a branch of the middle meningeal artery (p. 1520) may replace it. It accompanies the lacrimal nerve along the upper border of the rectus lateralis, supplying the lacrimal gland, after traversing which it ends in the eyelids and conjunctiva as *lateral*

palpebral arteries running medially in the upper and lower lids to anastomose with the medial palpebral arteries. The lacrimal artery gives off one or two *zygomatic branches*: one reaches the temporal fossa via the zygomaticotemporal foramen, anastomosing with the deep temporal arteries; another reaches the cheek by the zygomaticofacial foramen, anastomosing with transverse facial and zygomatico-orbital arteries. A *recurrent meningeal branch* passes back via the lateral part of the superior orbital fissure to anastomose with a middle meningeal branch; enlargement of this anastomosis may provide an alternative lacrimal artery.

Muscular branches. These frequently spring from a common trunk but form superior and inferior groups, most accompanying branches of the oculomotor nerve. The inferior, more constant, contains most of the anterior ciliary arteries. Other muscular vessels branch from the lacrimal and supraorbital or the trunk of the ophthalmic artery.

Ciliary arteries. They are divisible into three groups: long and short posterior and anterior. *Long posterior ciliary arteries*, usually two, pierce the sclera near the optic nerve (p. 1132). About seven *short posterior ciliary arteries* pass around the optic nerve to the eyeball; dividing into 15–20 branches, they pierce the sclera around the optic nerve to supply the choroid and the ciliary processes. At the optic disc they anastomose with twigs of the central retinal artery and at the ora serrata with the long posterior and anterior ciliary arteries. *Anterior ciliary arteries* arise from muscular branches of the ophthalmic; reaching the eyeball on tendons of the recti to form a circumcorneal subconjunctival vascular zone, they pierce the sclera near the sclerocorneal junction and end in the greater arterial circle of the iris (p. 1132).

Supraorbital artery. Leaving the ophthalmic where it crosses the optic nerve, it ascends medial to the rectus superior and levator palpebrae superioris, meets the supraorbital nerve and runs with it between the periosteum and levator palpebrae superioris to the supraorbital foramen or notch; traversing this it divides into superficial and deep branches, supplying the skin, muscles and frontal periosteum, anastomosing with the supratrochlear artery, frontal branch of the superficial temporal and its fellow. It supplies the rectus superior and levator palpebrae and sends a branch across the trochlea to the medial canthus. At the supraorbital margin it often sends a branch to the diploe of the frontal bone and may also supply the mucoperiosteum in the frontal sinus.

Posterior ethmoidal artery. Entering the posterior ethmoidal canal,

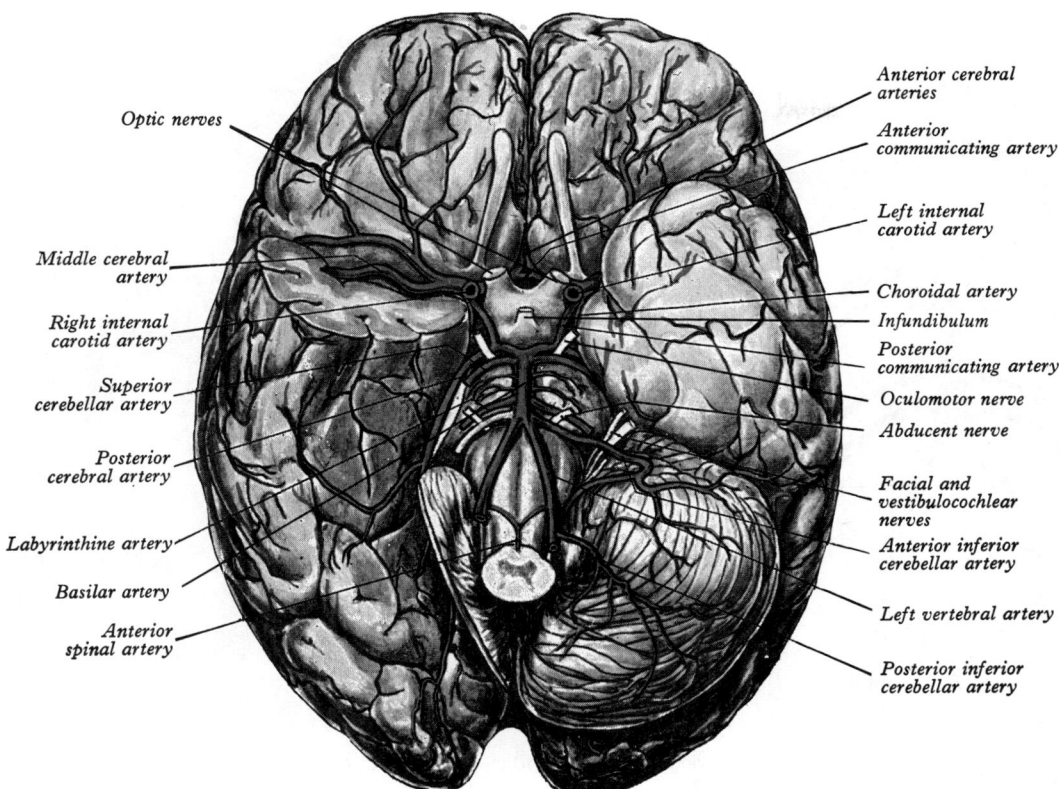

Optic nerves

Middle cerebral artery

Right internal carotid artery

Superior cerebellar artery

Posterior cerebral artery

Labyrinthine artery

Basilar artery

Anterior spinal artery

Anterior cerebral arteries

Anterior communicating artery

Left internal carotid artery

Choroidal artery

Infundibulum

Posterior communicating artery

Oculomotor nerve

Abducent nerve

Facial and vestibulocochlear nerves

Anterior inferior cerebellar artery

Left vertebral artery

Posterior inferior cerebellar artery

10.86 The arteries at the base of the brain. The right temporal pole and most of the right hemisphere of the cerebellum have been removed. Variations in the pattern of these vessels are common.

it supplies the posterior ethmoidal air sinuses, enters the cranium, sends a meningeal branch to the dura mater and nasal branches descending into the nasal cavity via the cribriform plate, to anastomose with the sphenopalatine branches supplying bone.

Anterior ethmoidal artery. Together, artery and nerve traverse their canal, the artery supplying anterior and middle ethmoidal and frontal air sinuses and, entering the cranium, giving a meningeal branch to the dura mater and nasal branches descending into the nasal cavity with the anterior ethmoidal nerve; they run in a groove on the deep surface of the nasal bone to supply the lateral nasal wall and septum; a terminal branch appears on the nose between the nasal bone and the upper nasal cartilage. Angiographic studies (Kuru 1967) show the meningeal branch extending to the falx; Müller (1977) has confirmed this in fetal and adult material; he also derives such *'falciate arteries'* from the recurrent meningeal branch of the lacrimal artery.

Meningeal branch. A small artery passing back by the superior orbital fissure to the middle cranial fossa, it anastomoses with the

middle and accessory meningeal arteries, supplying bone.

Medial palpebral arteries. Superior and inferior, they leave the ophthalmic below the trochlea, descending behind the lacrimal sac to enter the lids, where each divides into two branches coursing laterally along the tarsal edges, to form the superior and inferior arches, completed by anastomoses with branches of the supraorbital and zygomatico-orbital (superior arch) and palpebral branches of the lacrimal (both arches); the inferior arch also links with the facial artery, thus supplying the mucosa of the nasolacrimal duct.

Supratrochlear artery. A terminal branch of the ophthalmic, it leaves the orbit superomedially with the supratrochlear nerve, ascending on the forehead to supply the skin, muscles and pericranium, anastomosing with the supraorbital artery and with its fellow.

Dorsal nasal artery. The other terminal branch, it emerges from the orbit between the trochlea and medial palpebral ligament, gives a branch to the upper lacrimal sac and divides; one branch joins the terminal part of the facial artery, the other runs along the dorsum

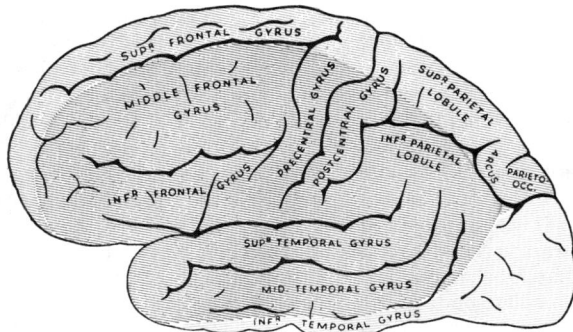

10.87A The lateral surface of the left cerebral hemisphere, showing the areas supplied by the cerebral arteries. In this and the next figure the area supplied by the anterior cerebral artery is coloured blue, that by the middle cerebral artery pink and that by the posterior cerebral artery is yellow.

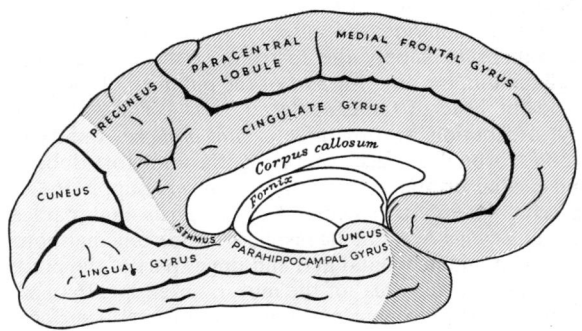

10.87B The medial surface of the left cerebral hemisphere, showing the areas supplied by the cerebral arteries (see description of **10.86**).

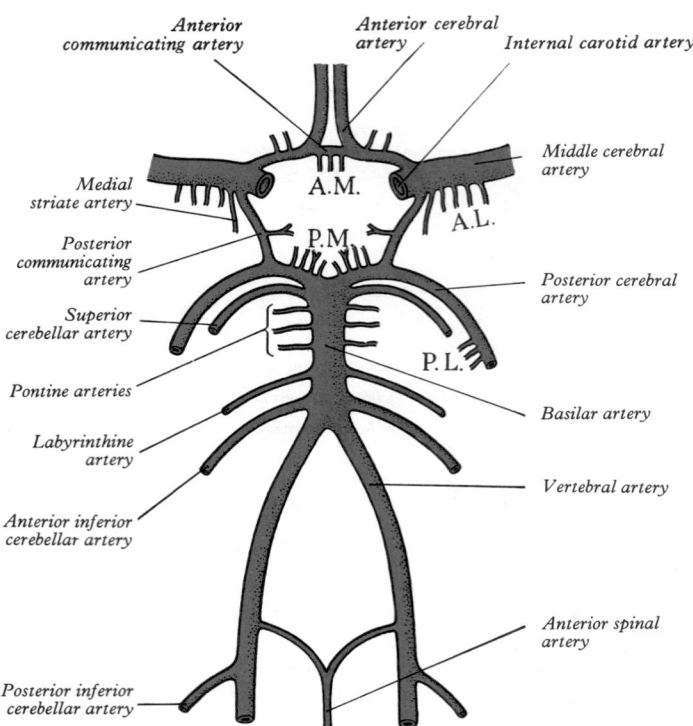

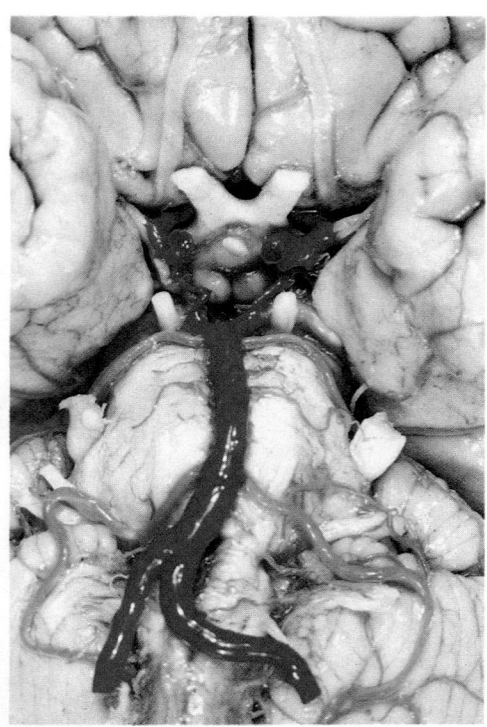

10.88 Diagram of the arteries at the base of the brain, showing the constitution of the arterial circle. The arteries constituting this so-called arterial 'circle' are commonly asymmetrical and sometimes a constituent vessel is missing. AL = anterolateral central branches; AM = anteromedial central branches; PL = posterolateral central branches; PM = posteromedial central branches.

10.89 Resin cast of the arteries at the base of the brain, showing the components of the arterial circle. (Cast prepared by M C E Hutchinson and photographed by Kevin Fitzpatrick, Department of Anatomy, UMDS, Guy's Campus, London.)

of the nose supplying its exterior and joining its fellow and lateral nasal branch of the facial.

Anterior cerebral artery (10.86–89). The smaller terminal branch of the internal carotid, it starts at the medial end of the stem of the lateral cerebral sulcus and passes anteromedially above the optic nerve to the longitudinal fissure, where it connects with its fellow by a short transverse anterior communicating artery. The two arteries thence travel together in the fissure, curving round the genu of the corpus callosum and back along its upper surface to its posterior end, where they anastomose with posterior cerebral arteries. Occasionally they are a single vessel. There are central and cortical branches.

Anterior communicating artery. With an average length of 4 mm, it connects anterior cerebral arteries across the anterior end of the longitudinal fissure; it may be double. It has a few anteromedial central branches. According to Crowell and Morawetz (1977) its branches, from three to 13, supply the optic chiasma, lamina terminalis, hypothalamus, paraolfactory areas, fornix (anterior columns) and cingulate gyrus.

Central branches. These arise from the commencement of the anterior cerebral, entering the anterior perforated substance and lamina terminalis to supply the rostrum of the corpus callosum, septum pellucidum, the anterior part of the putamen of the lentiform nucleus and the head of the caudate nucleus. *Cortical branches* are named by distribution: two or three *orbital branches* ramify on the frontal lobe's orbital surface, supplying the olfactory lobe, gyrus rectus and medial orbital gyrus; *frontal branches* supply the corpus callosum, cingulate gyrus, medial frontal gyrus and paracentral lobule, sending twigs over the hemisphere's superomedial border to the superior and middle frontal gyri and upper part of the precentral gyrus (including the 'leg area' of the motor cortex, p. 1164); *parietal branches* supply the precuneus and the adjacent lateral surface.

Middle cerebral artery (10.86–89). The larger terminal branch of the internal carotid, it runs first in the lateral cerebral sulcus, then posterosuperiorly on the insula, dividing into branches distributed to this and the adjacent lateral cerebral surface. Its *central branches* are small and from its commencement they enter the anterior

perforated substance, arranged in two sets: *medial striate arteries* ascend through the lentiform nucleus to supply it, the caudate nucleus and the internal capsule; *lateral striate arteries* ascend over the lower lateral aspect of the lentiform nucleus (in the external capsule) and turn medially to traverse it and the internal capsule to supply the caudate nucleus. One lateral branch, usually the largest, was termed by Charcot the 'artery of cerebral haemorrhage'. *Cortical branches* supply orbital branches to the inferior frontal gyrus and the lateral orbital surface of the frontal lobe; frontal branches supply the precentral, middle and inferior frontal gyri; two *parietal branches* are distributed to the postcentral gyrus, the lower part of the superior parietal lobule and the whole inferior parietal lobule. Two or three *temporal branches* supply the lateral surface of the temporal lobe. Cortical branches of the middle cerebral thus supply all the motor area (excluding the leg), the corresponding somaesthetic area (p. 1116) and the auditory area (p. 1204).

Posterior communicating artery (10.86, 88, 89). This runs back from the internal carotid above the oculomotor nerve, anastomosing with the posterior cerebral, a basilar branch. It is usually small but sometimes so large that the posterior cerebral appears to come from the internal carotid rather than basilar artery. It is often larger on one side. From its posterior half several small branches pierce the posterior perforated substance with others from the posterior cerebral to supply the medial thalamic surface and walls of the third ventricle (p. 1203).

Anterior choroidal artery. Small but constant, it leaves the internal carotid near its posterior communicating branch (Abbie 1933, 1934), passing back above the medial part of the uncus to cross inferior to the optic tract and reach and supply the crus cerebri. Turning laterally, it recrosses the optic tract, arrives lateral to the lateral geniculate body and supplies it with several branches. Finally it enters the inferior cornu of the lateral ventricle via the choroidal fissure to end in the choroidal plexus. It supplies: the globus pallidus, caudate nucleus and amygdaloid body, hypothalamus, tuber cinereum, red nucleus, substantia nigra, posterior limb of the internal capsule, the optic radiation, optic tract, hippocampus and the fimbria of the fornix.

Circle of Willis

Much of the brain is supplied by the two internal carotid arteries (p. 1523), and a central anastomosis, the Circle of Willis (also known as *circulus arteriosus*), exists between these and the two vertebral arteries (p. 1530) that supply the remainder. This 'circle', more polygonal than circular, is in the cisterna interpeduncularis, surrounding the optic chiasma, the neural infundibular stem of the hypophysis cerebri and other related neural structures in the interpendicular fossa (**10.**88, 89). **Anteriorly** the anterior cerebral arteries (from the carotids) are joined by the anterior communicating artery; **posteriorly** the basilar artery (p. 1534) divides into two posterior cerebral arteries, each joined to the ipsilateral internal carotid by a posterior communicating artery (**10.**88).

Vessels of this 'circle' vary in calibre, being often partially developed, sometimes even absent. About 60% of circles display 'anomalies'; the above description applies to a minority.

Variations

Variations have been much studied, from Windle's account in 1888 of 200 specimens to that of Puchades-Orts et al (1976) in 62 dissections, the largest series being the 700 dissections of Fawcett and Blachford (1906) and Riggs and Rupp's (1963) 994 dissections. Fields et al (1965) have summarized such studies. Cerebral and communicating arteries, anterior and posterior, may all be absent, variably hypoplastic, double or even triple. In about 90% there is, nevertheless, a complete 'circular' channel but in most one vessel is sufficiently narrowed to reduce its role as a collateral route. The haemodynamic 'balance' is usually disturbed by variation in the calibre of communicating arteries, often with variation in the segments of anterior and posterior cerebral arteries extending from their origins to their junctions with the corresponding communicating arteries. This is especially true in the case of the posterior cerebral artery and its anastomosis with the posterior communicating artery. Commonly the precommunicating part of the posterior cerebral artery has a diameter larger than the posterior communicating artery; in this case the blood supply to the occipital lobes is mainly from the vertebrobasilar system. Less commonly the diameter of the precommunicating part of the posterior cerebral artery is smaller than that of the posterior communicating artery, in which case the blood supply to the occipital lobes is mainly from the internal carotids via the posterior communicating arteries (Van Overbeeke et al 1991). The latter arrangement, whose frequency ranges according to different studies from 6% (McCormick 1969) to 40% (Zeal and Rhoton 1978), is sometimes referred to as the 'embryonic configuration' (as opposed to the standard 'adult configuration'), and according to Abbie (1933), Williams (1936) and Kaplan (1956) is accounted for by the ontogenetic and phylogenetic association of posterior cerebral and internal carotid arteries. However, a recent study has shown that the 'embryonic configuration' is not more common in human fetuses than in adults (Van Overbeeke et al 1991). Anterior in the arterial circle, agenesis or hypoplasia of the initial anterior cerebral segment is more frequent than anomalies in the anterior communicating, and hence a commoner cause of defective circulation. Angiographic evidence indicates such defective or absent circulation in about a third of individuals (Sedzmir 1959); existence of an effective arterial circle can never be assumed and surgical procedures involving its 'feeders' must be preceded by angiography. Radio-opaque substances may be injected into the internal carotid or vertebral arteries in the neck for radiography of the condition of their intracranial branches (**10.**82, 83, 93, 94).

Further details of the distribution of cerebral arteries and veins appear on pages 1218 to 1220 and of intracranial venous sinuses on pages 1582 to 1589.

SUBCLAVIAN SYSTEM OF ARTERIES

The stem artery of the upper limb is single as far as the elbow, but its name changes in the regions traversed. From its origin to the outer border of the first rib it is *subclavian*; thence to the tendon of teres major it is *axillary*; and from this to its division at the elbow it is *brachial*.

SUBCLAVIAN ARTERY

The right subclavian arises from the brachiocephalic trunk, the left from the aortic arch. For description, each is divided into a *first part*, from its origin to the medial border of the scalenus anterior, a *second part* behind this muscle and a *third part* from the muscle's lateral margin to the first rib's outer border, where the artery becomes axillary. Each subclavian artery arches over the cervical pleura and pulmonary apex. Their first parts differ, the second and third parts are almost identical.

First part of right subclavian artery

The right subclavian, branching from the brachiocephalic trunk behind the upper border of the right sternoclavicular joint, passes superolaterally to the medial margin of the scalenus anterior (**10.**66, 84, 90). It ascends about 2 cm above the clavicle but this varies.

Relations. The artery is deep to the skin, superficial fascia, platysma, anterior supraclavicular nerves, deep fascia, clavicular attachment of the sternocleidomastoid, sternohyoid and sternothyroid. It is at first behind the right common carotid's origin; more laterally it is crossed by the vagus nerve, the cardiac branches of the vagus and the sympathetic chain and by internal jugular and vertebral veins; the subclavian sympathetic loop encircles it. The anterior jugular vein diverges laterally in front of it, separated by the sternohyoid and sternothyroid. Below and behind the artery are the pleura and pulmonary apex but separated by the suprapleural membrane (p. 1663), the ansa subclavia, an accessory vertebral vein (p. 1580) and the right recurrent laryngeal nerve (curving round inferoposterior to the vessel).

First part of left subclavian artery

This springs from the aortic arch, behind the left common carotid, level with the disc between the third and fourth thoracic vertebrae; it ascends into the neck, then arches laterally to the medial border of the scalenus anterior (**10.**48, 66, 91).

Relations. In the *thorax* it is related, **anteriorly** to the left common carotid artery and left brachiocephalic vein, separated by the left vagus, cardiac (p. 1253) and phrenic nerves. Superficial to these the anterior pulmonary margin, pleura, sternothyroid and sternohyoid are between the vessel and the upper left area of the manubrium sterni. **Posterior** are the left side of the oesophagus, the thoracic duct and longus colli; it is in contact posterolaterally with the left lung and pleura. **Medial** are the trachea, the left recurrent laryngeal nerve, oesophagus and thoracic duct. **Laterally** the artery grooves the mediastinal surface of the left lung and pleura which also encroach on its anterior and posterior aspects.

In the neck, near the medial border of the scalenus anterior, the artery is crossed anteriorly by the left phrenic nerve and the termination of the thoracic duct. Otherwise anterior relations are as

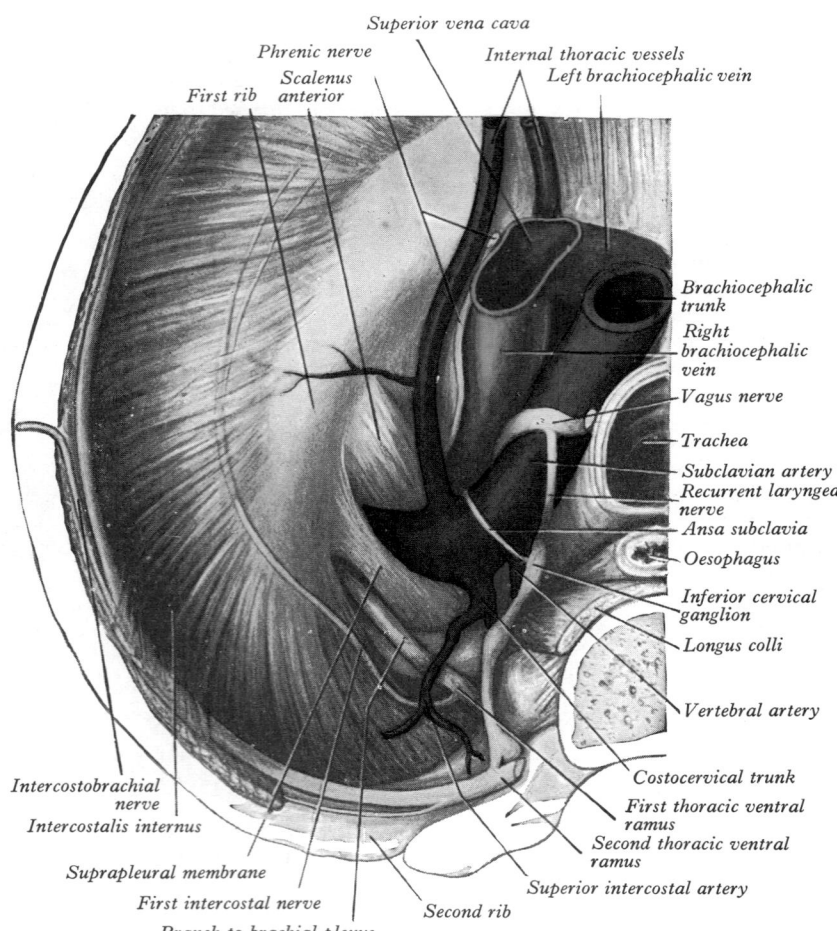

10.90   Structures related to the right cervical pleura, as seen from below.

previously described for the first part of the right subclavian artery. Posteriorly and inferiorly, the relations of both vessels are identical but the left recurrent laryngeal nerve, medial to the left subclavian artery in the thorax, is not directly related to its cervical part.

Second part of subclavian artery

This is behind the scalenus anterior; it is short and the highest part of the vessel (**10**.73, 92).

Relations. Anterior are the skin, superficial fascia, platysma, deep cervical fascia, sternocleidomastoid and scalenus anterior; the right phrenic nerve is often described as separated from the second part by the scalenus anterior, but crossing the first part on the left; Qvist (1977) stated that both nerves are anterior to the muscle. Postero-inferior are the suprapleural membrane, pleura and lung and the lower trunk of the brachial plexus; superior are the upper and middle trunks of the plexus; the subclavian vein is antero-inferior, separated by the scalenus anterior (**10**.92).

Third part of subclavian artery

This descends laterally from the lateral margin of the scalenus anterior to the outer border of the first rib, where it becomes axillary; it is the most superficial part of the artery and lies partly in the supraclavicular triangle (p. 1523), where its pulsations may be felt and it may be compressed.

Relations. Anterior are the skin, superficial fascia, platysma, supraclavicular nerves and deep cervical fascia (**10**.68, 92). The external jugular vein crosses its medial end and here receives the suprascapular, transverse cervical and anterior jugular veins, together often forming a venous plexus. The nerve to the subclavius descends between the veins and the artery; the latter is terminally behind the clavicle and subclavius, where it is crossed by the suprascapular vessels. The subclavian vein is antero-inferior and the lower trunk of the brachial plexus is postero-inferior, between the artery and the

scalenus medius (and on the first rib). Superolateral are the upper and middle trunks of the brachial plexus (palpable here) and the inferior belly of the omohyoid. Inferior is the first rib.

Surface anatomy. The subclavian artery describes a broad line, convex superiorly, from the sternoclavicular joint to the midpoint of the clavicle (**10**.75).

Variations. The right subclavian may arise above or below sterno-clavicular level; it may be a separate aortic branch and be the first or last branch of the arch; when first, it is in the position of a brachiocephalic trunk and when last it arises from the arch's left end, ascending obliquely to the right behind the trachea, oesophagus and right common carotid to the first rib. In this case the proximal part of the artery represents a persistent part of the right dorsal aorta, the right fourth aortic arch taking no part in its formation (p. 1510); hence the right recurrent laryngeal nerve hooks round the common carotid, derived from the third arch. Sometimes, when the right subclavian is the last aortic branch, it passes between trachea and oesophagus. It may perforate the scalenus anterior; very rarely it passes anterior to it. Sometimes the subclavian vein accompanies the artery behind the scalenus anterior. The artery may ascend as high as 4 cm above the clavicle or it may reach only its upper border. The left subclavian is occasionally combined at its origin with the left common carotid.

Clinical anatomy. The third part of the subclavian artery is the most accessible. Since the line of the posterior border of the sterno-cleidomastoid approximates to the (deeper) lateral border of the scalenus anterior, the artery is just lateral to the former and, as noted, can be felt in the antero-inferior angle of the posterior triangle. It can only be effectively compressed against the first rib; with shoulder depressed, pressure is exerted down, back and medially in the angle between the sternocleidomastoid and clavicle. The palpable trunks of the brachial plexus may be injected with local anaesthetic allowing major surgical procedures to the arm.

BRANCHES OF THE SUBCLAVIAN ARTERY

These branches are:

1. Vertebral
2. Internal thoracic
3. Thyrocervical
4. Costocervical
5. Dorsal scapular.

On the left all branches except the dorsal scapular arise from the first part; on the right the costocervical trunk usually springs from the second part. The origins of branches proceeding into the posterior triangle are variable but distributions are relatively constant.

1. Vertebral artery

This artery arises from the superoposterior aspect of the subclavian, passes through the foramina of all cervical transverse processes except the seventh, curves medially behind the lateral mass of the atlas and then enters the cranium via the foramen magnum. At the lower pontine border it joins its fellow to form the basilar artery. Occasionally it may enter the bone at the fifth, fourth or seventh cervical transverse foramen (**10**.83, 86, 88, 89, 90, 93, 94, 154; p. 1510).

Relations. The *first part* ascends back between the longus colli and scalenus anterior, behind the common carotid artery and ver-tebral vein, and crossed by the inferior thyroid artery, and on the left also by the thoracic duct. **Posterior** are the seventh cervical transverse process, the stellate ganglion (**10**.86, 89, 90, 91) and ventral rami of the seventh and eighth cervical spinal nerves. The *second part* ascends through the transverse foramina, with a large branch from the stellate ganglion and a plexus of veins which form the vertebral vein low in the neck. It is anterior to the ventral rami of the cervical spinal nerves (C.2–C.6), ascending almost vertically to the transverse process of the axis, through which it turns laterally to the transverse foramen of the atlas; from here the *third part* issues medial to the rectus capitis lateralis, curving back and medially behind the lateral mass, the first cervical ventral spinal ramus being medial. It is then in a groove on the upper surface of the posterior arch of the atlas, entering the vertebral canal below the inferior border of the posterior atlanto-occipital membrane. This part,

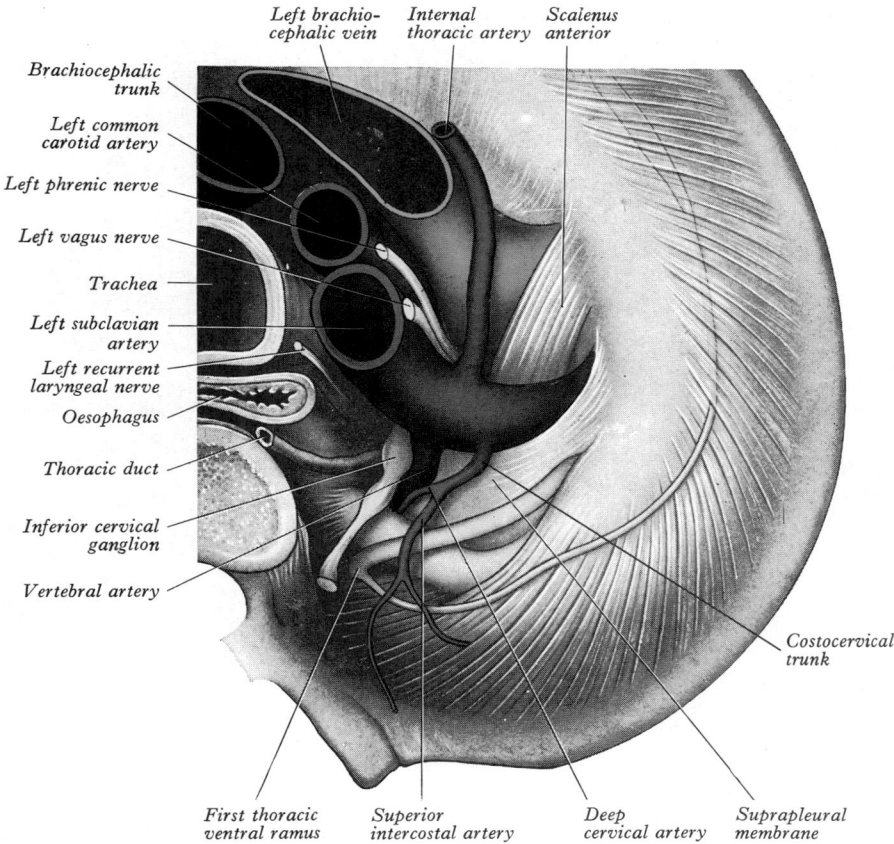

Left brachio-cephalic vein

Internal thoracic artery

Scalenus anterior

Brachiocephalic trunk

Left common carotid artery

Left phrenic nerve

Left vagus nerve

Trachea

Left subclavian artery

Left recurrent laryngeal nerve

Oesophagus

Thoracic duct

Inferior cervical ganglion

Vertebral artery

Costocervical trunk

First thoracic ventral ramus

Superior intercostal artery

Deep cervical artery

Suprapleural membrane

10.91   Structures related to the left cervical pleura, as seen from below.

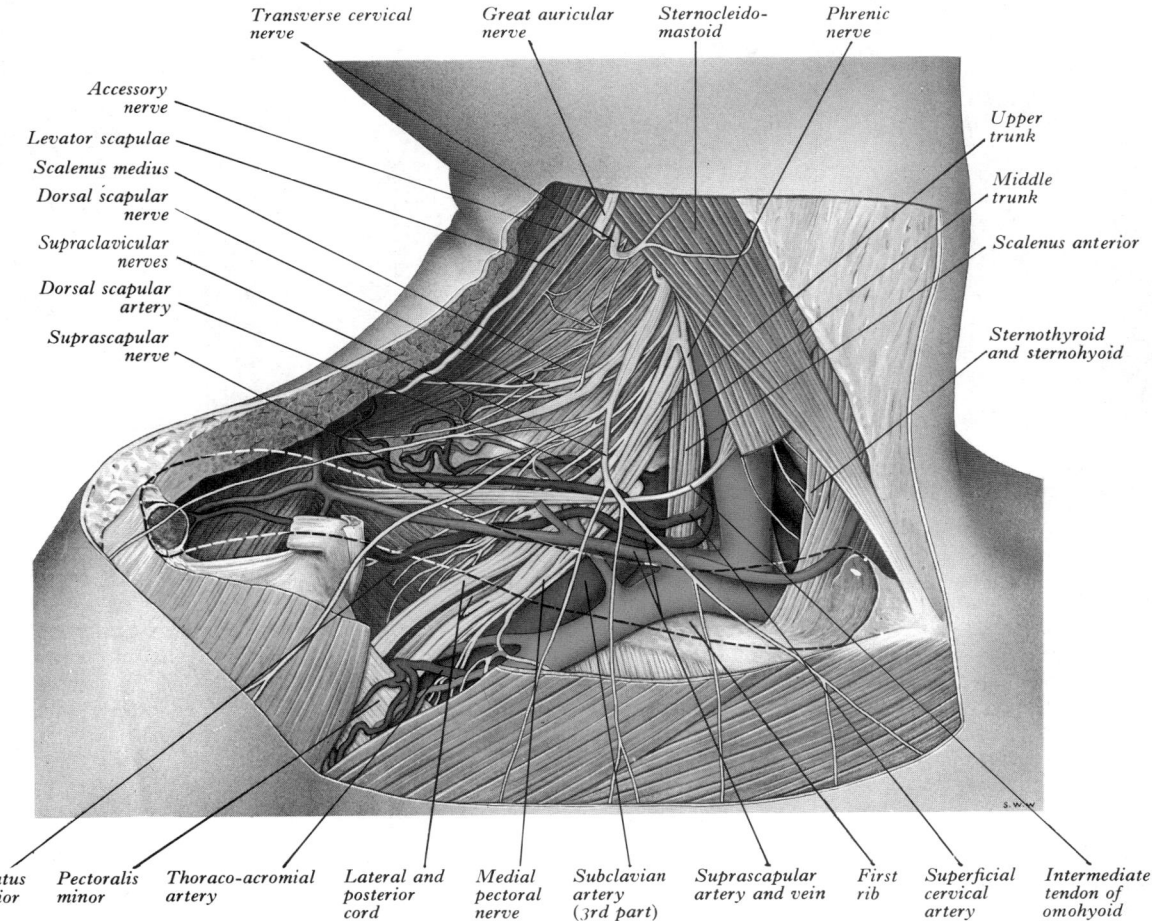

Transverse cervical nerve

Great auricular nerve

Sternocleido-mastoid

Phrenic nerve

Accessory nerve

Levator scapulae

Scalenus medius

Dorsal scapular nerve

Supraclavicular nerves

Dorsal scapular artery

Suprascapular nerve

Upper trunk

Middle trunk

Scalenus anterior

Sternothyroid and sternohyoid

Serratus anterior

Pectoralis minor

Thoraco-acromial artery

Lateral and posterior cord

Medial pectoral nerve

Subclavian artery (3rd part)

Suprascapular artery and vein

First rib

Superficial cervical artery

Intermediate tendon of omohyoid

10.92   The lower part of the posterior triangle showing the relations of the third part of the right subclavian artery. Note the clavicle has been removed but its outline is indicated by a dashed line; the middle trunk of the brachial plexus gives an unusual contribution to the medial cord.

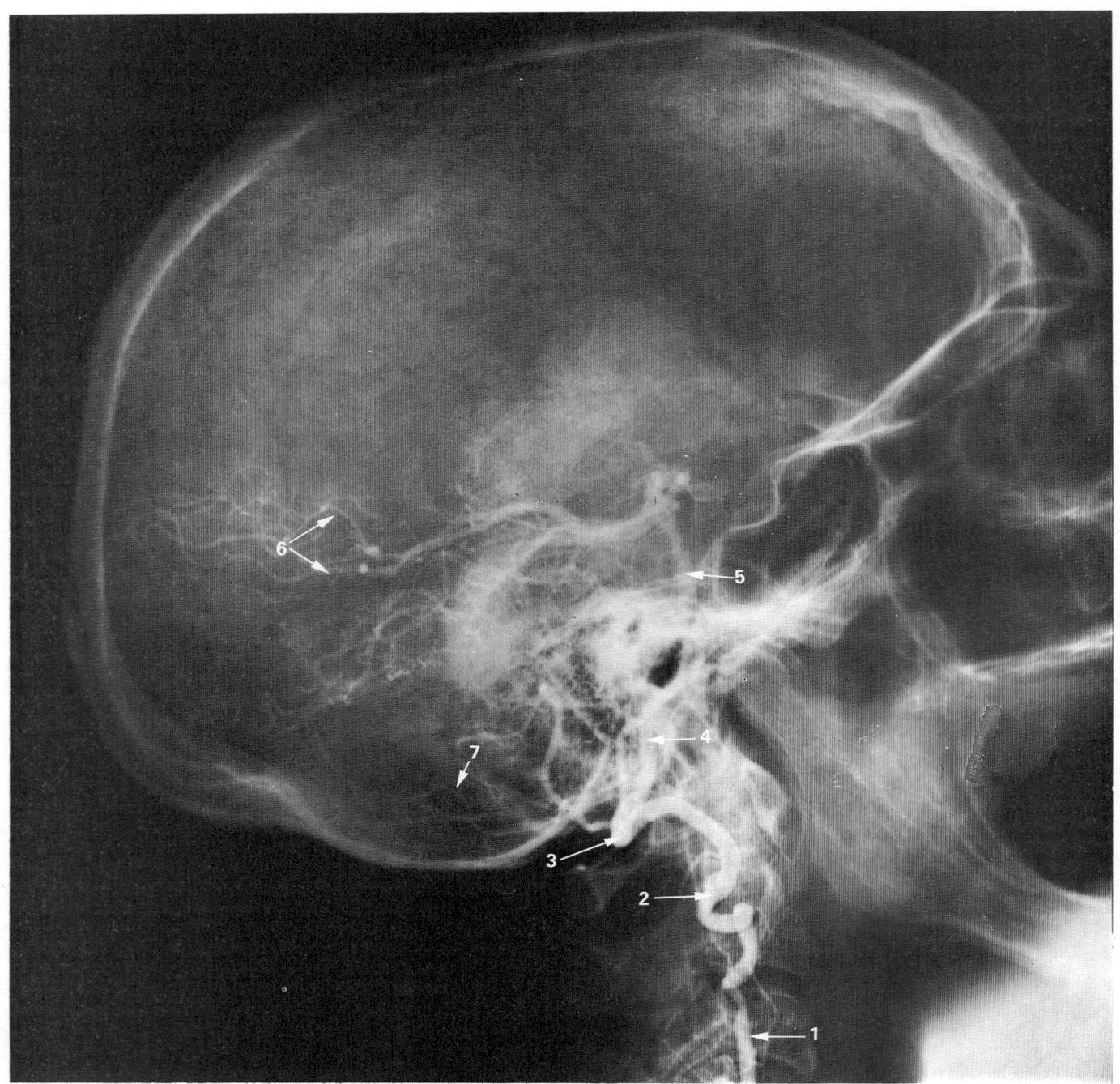

10.93 Vertebral arteriogram (left): lateral view. 1. Vertebral artery, ascending part. 2. Loop between transverse foramina of axis and atlas. 3. Sub-occipital part. 4. Intracranial part. 5. Basilar artery. 6. Posterior cerebral branches. 7. Inferior cerebellar branches.

covered by the semispinalis capitis, is in the suboccipital triangle. The first cervical dorsal spinal ramus is between the artery and the posterior arch. The *fourth part* pierces the dura and arachnoid mater, ascends anterior to the hypoglossal roots (p. 1256) inclining anterior to the medulla oblongata where, at the lower pontine border, it unites with its fellow to form the midline basilar artery (**10**.88, 89).

Winckler (1972) has described variation in elastic and muscular tissue in the vertebral artery; in its first and third parts it appears adapted by increased elasticity to the greater mobility and lack of support in these regions.

Cervical branches of the vertebral artery

Spinal branches. These small branches enter the vertebral canal by the intervertebral foramina, supplying branches to the spinal cord and its membranes. They anastomose with other spinal arteries, which fork into ascending and descending rami, to unite with those above and below, forming two lateral anastomotic chains on the

posterior surfaces of the vertebral bodies near the attachment of their pedicles. From these chains branches supply the periosteum and vertebral bodies, while others communicate with similar branches across the midline; from these connections small rami join similar ones above and below, forming a median anastomotic chain on the posterior surfaces of the vertebral bodies.

Muscular branches. Arising from the vertebral artery as it curves round the lateral mass of the atlas, they supply the deep muscles of this region and anastomose with the occipital, ascending and deep cervical arteries.

Cranial branches of the vertebral artery

Meningeal branches. One or two of these branches from the vertebral artery near the foramen magnum ramify between the bone and dura mater in the cerebellar fossa, supplying bone, diploë and the falx cerebelli.

Posterior spinal artery. This may arise from the vertebral near

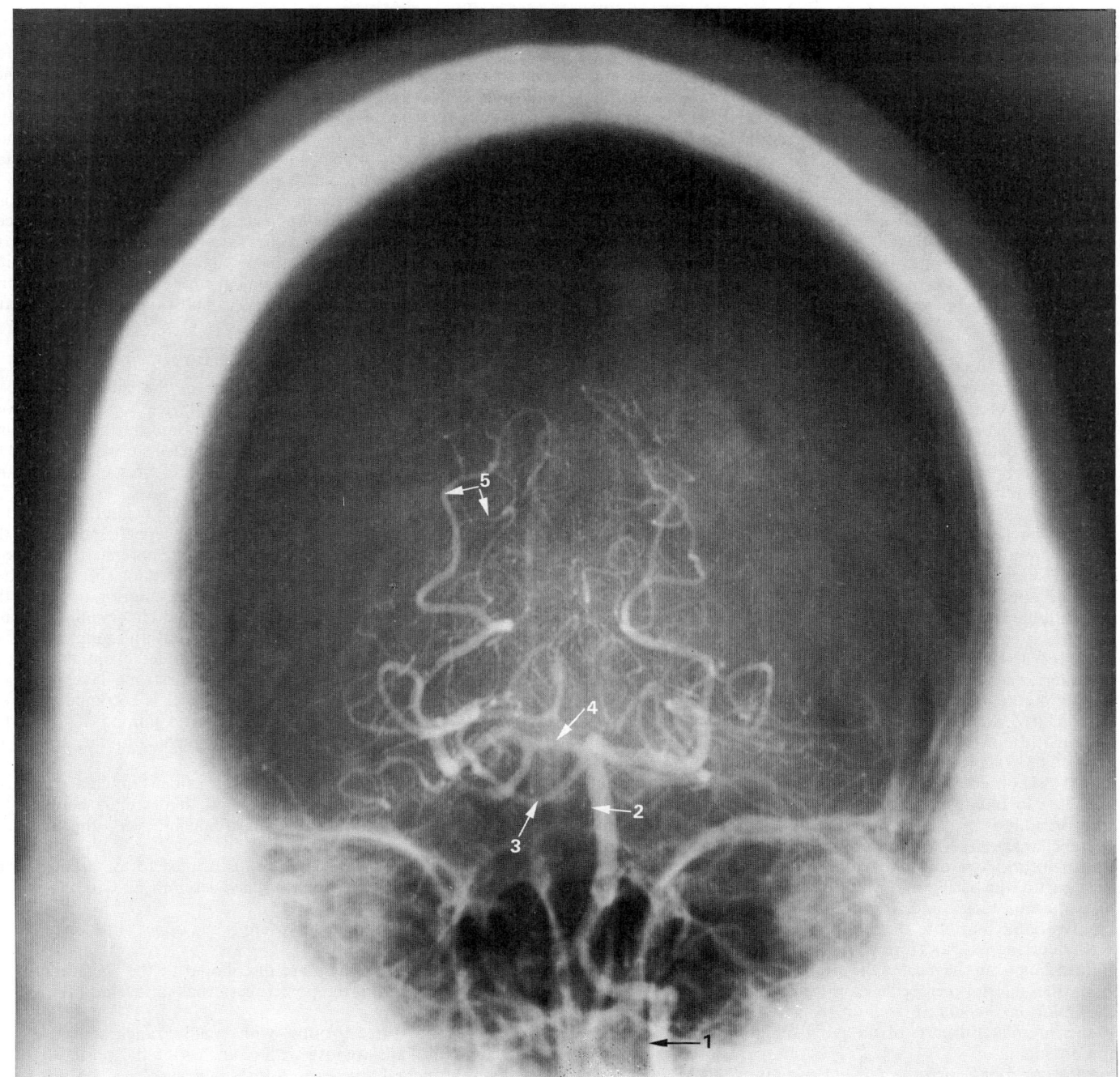

10.94 Vertebral arteriogram (left): anteroposterior view. 1. Left vertebral artery. 2. Basilar artery. 3. Right superior cerebellar artery. 4. Right posterior cerebral artery. 5. Branches of right posterior cerebral artery.

the medulla oblongata but most frequently from its posterior inferior cerebellar branch (see below). It passes posteriorly, descending as two branches, anterior and posterior, to the dorsal roots of the spinal nerves; these are reinforced by spinal twigs from the vertebral, ascending cervical, posterior intercostal and first lumbar arteries, which reach the vertebral canal by the intervertebral foramina, sustaining the posterior spinal arteries to the lower spinal levels (8.329).

Anterior spinal artery. A small branch arising near the vertebral's end, it descends anterior to the medulla oblongata and unites with its fellow at midmedullary level. The single trunk then descends on the ventral midline of the spinal cord, reinforced by a succession of small spinal rami entering the vertebral canal through the intervertebral foramina from the vertebral, ascending cervical, posterior intercostal and first lumbar arteries. They unite by ascending and descending branches as a single anterior median artery, which reaches

the lower spinal cord and filum terminale. This median artery is encased in the pia mater along the anterior median fissure; it supplies the spinal cord and inferiorly the cauda equina. Branches from the anterior spinal arteries and beginning of their common trunk pass into the medulla oblongata, with a central distribution sharply limited dorsally by the trigonum hypoglossi (p. 1218, 8.329).

Posterior inferior cerebellar artery (10.46). The largest branch, it is sometimes absent. Arising near the lower end of the olive, it curves back around it to ascend behind glossopharyngeal and vagal roots to the inferior border of the pons, where it curves and descends along the inferolateral border of the fourth ventricle. Finally it turns laterally into the cerebellar vallecula, dividing into medial and lateral branches. The *medial branch* runs back between the cerebellar hemisphere and inferior vermis, supplying both; the *lateral branch* supplies the inferior cerebellar surface as far as its lateral border, anastomosing with the anterior inferior and superior cerebellar

1533

arteries (from the basilar artery). Its trunk supplies the medulla oblongata and choroid plexus of the fourth ventricle, sending up a branch lateral to the (cerebellar) tonsil to supply the dentate nucleus. The medullary area supplied is dorsal to the olivary nucleus and lateral to the hypoglossal nucleus and its emerging fila.

Clinical anatomy. The posterior inferior cerebellar artery supplies the lateral medulla. Thrombosis therefore causes loss of function ('lateral medullary syndrome') in the nucleus ambiguus, nucleus of the tractus solitarius, vestibular and cochlear nuclei, spinocerebellar tracts, the lateral spinothalamic tract, trigeminal spinal nucleus and tract. The anterior spinal artery supplies the medial medulla; thrombosis of it ('medial medullary syndrome') affects the hypoglossal nucleus and nerve, medial lemniscus and corticospinal tract.

Medullary arteries. These are minute vessels from the vertebral and its branches, distributed to the medulla oblongata.

Basilar artery

This median vessel, formed by the junction of the vertebral arteries, extends from the lower to the upper pontine borders in the cisterna pontis (**10**.86, 88). It adjoins a shallow, median groove on the ventral pontine surface, between the abducent nerves at the lower pontine border and the oculomotor at the upper pontine border, where it divides into two posterior cerebral arteries.

Pontine branches. These are numerous and leave the front and sides of the basilar to supply the pons and adjacent parts.

Labyrinthine (internal auditory) artery. Long and slender, it may branch from the lower part of the basilar but more often from the anterior inferior cerebellar artery (see below); it accompanies facial and vestibulocochlear nerves into the internal acoustic meatus and is distributed to the internal ear (p.1376). In a radiographic study of this artery Wende et al (1975) identified the origins of 238. Only 38 (16%) were from the basilar; 108 (45%) were from the anterior inferior cerebellar. The superior cerebellar artery accounted for 58 (25%), the posterior inferior cerebellar for 13 (5%). The remaining 21 (9%) were reduplicated and were branches of the basilar and one or other of the cerebellar arteries. They found a unilateral artery in 24 of 316 subjects. Others have recorded different incidences. Cavatori (1908) observed a basilar origin for the labyrinthine artery in about 70% in Italians; Stopford (1916) and Adachi and Hasche (1928) recorded it as most often from a trunk common to it and one of the cerebellar arteries. Gillilan (1972) has indicated racial variation.

Anterior inferior cerebellar artery (**10**.86). This branches from the lower part of the basilar and runs posterolaterally usually ventral to the abducent, facial and vestibulocochlear nerves, commonly forming a variable loop into the internal acoustic meatus below the nerves (Sunderland 1945a), from which the labyrinthine artery often arises. Emerging from the meatus the artery supplies the anterolateral region of the inferior cerebellar surface, anastomosing with the posterior inferior cerebellar branch of the vertebral. A few branches supply the inferolateral parts of the pons and sometimes the upper medulla oblongata.

Superior cerebellar artery (**10**.86). Arising near the basilar's end, it passes laterally below the oculomotor nerve which separates it from the posterior cerebral artery and curves round the cerebral peduncle below the trochlear nerve; arriving at the superior cerebellar surface, it divides into branches ramifying in the pia mater to supply this cerebellar aspect and anastomose with branches of inferior cerebellar arteries. It also supplies the pons, pineal body, superior medullary velum and tela choroidea of the third ventricle.

Posterior cerebral artery (**10**.86, 88, 89). Frequently double, this is larger than the superior cerebellar, from which it is separated near its origin by the oculomotor nerve and, lateral to the midbrain, by the trochlear nerve. Passing laterally, parallel with the superior cerebellar, it receives the posterior communicating artery, winds round the cerebral peduncle and reaches the tentorial cerebral surface, where it supplies the temporal and occipital lobes. Its branches are central and cortical.

Central branches. Several small *posteromedial central branches* (**10**.88) from the beginning of the posterior cerebral, with similar branches from the posterior communicating artery, pierce the posterior perforated substance to supply the anterior thalamus, lateral wall of the third ventricle and the globus pallidus. *Posterior choroidal branches* vary (Abbie 1933); one or more course over the lateral geniculate body and supply it before entering the posterior part of

the inferior cornu of the lateral ventricle via the lower part of the choroidal fissure. Others curl round the posterior end of the thalamus and traverse the transverse fissure, some going to the third ventricle's tela choroidea, some to traverse the upper choroidal fissure; they supply the choroid plexuses of the third and lateral ventricles and the fornix (Percheron 1977, p.1220). Small posterolateral central branches arise from the posterior cerebral artery beyond the cerebral peduncle; they supply this and the posterior thalamus, colliculi, pineal gland and medial geniculate body.

Cortical branches. The temporal branches, usually two, are distributed to the uncus, parahippocampal, medial and lateral occipitotemporal gyri; occipital branches supply the cuneus, lingual gyrus and posterolateral surface of the occipital lobe; parieto-occipital branches supply the cuneus and precuneus. The posterior cerebral artery supplies the visual area (p.1220) and other structures in the visual pathway.

2. Internal thoracic (mammary) artery

This arises inferiorly from the first part of the subclavian artery, about 2 cm above the sternal end of the clavicle, opposite the root of the thyrocervical trunk (**10**.90, 91, 95). It descends behind the first six costal cartilages about 1 cm from the lateral sternal border; level with the sixth intercostal space it divides into musculophrenic and superior epigastric branches.

Relations. At first it descends anteromedially behind the clavicle's sternal end, the internal jugular and brachiocephalic veins and the first costal cartilage. As it enters the thorax, the phrenic nerve crosses it obliquely from its lateral side, usually in front. The artery then descends almost vertically to its bifurcation; anterior to it are the pectoralis major, the first six costal cartilages and intervening external intercostal membranes and internal intercostals and terminations of the upper six intercostal nerves. It is separated from the pleura, down to the second or third cartilage, by a strong layer of fascia and below this by the transversus thoracis. It is accompanied by a chain of lymph nodes and venae comitantes uniting at about the third costal cartilage into a single vein medial to the artery. Its intermediate branches are as follows:

Pericardiacophrenic artery. A long, slender branch accompanying the phrenic nerve to the diaphragm, it descends between the pleura and pericardium, finally anastomosing with the musculophrenic and phrenic arteries.

Mediastinal arteries. These are distributed to the areolar tissue and lymph nodes in the anterior mediastinum and to the thymic vestiges.

Pericardial branches. These supply the upper anterior region of the pericardium.

Sternal branches. These are distributed to the transversus thoracis, the periosteum of the posterior sternal surface and the sternal red bone marrow.

The foregoing three groups, with small branches of the pericardiacophrenic, anastomose with branches of the posterior intercostal and bronchial arteries to form a *subpleural mediastinal plexus*.

Anterior intercostal branches. Distributed to the upper six intercostal spaces, two in each space, they pass laterally along the borders of the space to anastomose with the posterior intercostal arteries (and their collateral branches). They lie at first between the pleura and the internal intercostals, then between the intercostales intimi and the internal intercostals. They supply the intercostal muscles and send branches through them to the pectoral muscles, breast and skin.

Perforating branches. They traverse the upper five or six intercostal spaces with anterior cutaneous branches of the corresponding intercostal nerves. They enter the pectoralis major and, curving laterally, supply the muscle and skin. In the female the second to fourth branches supply the breast; during lactation they are enlarged.

Musculophrenic artery. This passes inferolaterally behind the seventh to ninth costal cartilages, traverses the diaphragm near the ninth and ends near the last intercostal space. It anastomoses with the inferior phrenic and the lower two posterior intercostal and ascending branches of the deep circumflex iliac arteries. Two anterior intercostal arteries branch from it for each of the seventh to ninth intercostal spaces, distributed like those in other spaces. The musculophrenic also supplies the lower part of the pericardium and the abdominal muscles.

Superior epigastric artery. It descends between the costal and xiphoid slips of the diaphragm, anterior to the lower fibres of the transversus thoracis and the upper fibres of the transversus abdominis. Entering the rectus sheath, at first behind the muscle and then perforating and supplying it, it anastomoses with the inferior epigastric branch of the external iliac. Branches perforate the sheath to supply the abdominal skin; a branch anterior to the xiphoid process anastomoses with its fellow. The artery supplies the diaphragm; on the right small branches reach the falciform ligament to anastomose with the hepatic artery.

3. Thyrocervical trunk

This short, wide artery, from the front of the subclavian's first part near the medial border of the scalenus anterior, divides almost at once into the inferior thyroid, suprascapular and superficial cervical arteries (**10**.73, 154).

Inferior thyroid artery. This is looped; first it **ascends** anterior to the medial border of the scalenus anterior, turns **medially** just below the sixth cervical transverse process, passing anterior to the vertebral vessels and posterior to the carotid sheath and its contents and usually the sympathetic trunk, whose middle cervical ganglion usually adjoins the vessel. It finally **descends** on the longus colli to the lower border of the thyroid gland. As it approaches this, its relation to the recurrent laryngeal nerve is surgically important (p. 1252). Nearing the gland the artery usually passes behind the nerve, but nearer the gland, on the right, the nerve is with equal frequency anterior or posterior to or amongst the branches of the artery; the left nerve is usually posterior. Relations between the terminal branches of artery and nerve are very variable (Bowden 1955). On the left, near its origin, the artery is crossed anteriorly by the thoracic duct, curving inferolaterally to its end.

Muscular branches. These supply the infrahyoid muscles, longus colli, scalenus anterior and the inferior pharyngeal constrictor.

Ascending cervical artery. A small branch, it arises as the inferior thyroid turns medially behind the carotid sheath and ascends on the anterior tubercles of the cervical transverse processes between the scalenus anterior and the longus capitis. It supplies the adjacent muscles and has one or two spinal branches which enter the vertebral canal through the intervertebral foramina to supply the spinal cord and membranes and vertebral bodies, as do the spinal branches of the vertebral artery. The ascending cervical artery anastomoses with the vertebral, ascending pharyngeal, occipital and deep cervical arteries.

Inferior laryngeal artery. It ascends on the trachea with the recurrent laryngeal nerve, enters the larynx at the inferior constrictor's lower border and supplies the laryngeal muscles and mucosa, anastomosing also with its contralateral fellow, and with the superior laryngeal branch of the superior thyroid artery.

Pharyngeal branches. These supply the lower pharynx: *tracheal branches* the trachea (anastomosing with the bronchial arteries), and *oesophageal branches* the oesophagus (anastomosing with the oesophageal branches of thoracic aorta). Inferior and ascending *glandular branches* supply the posterior and inferior regions of the thyroid gland, anastomosing with the opposite inferior and ipsilateral superior thyroid arteries. The ascending branch also supplies the parathyroid glands.

Suprascapular artery (10.92). This first descends laterally across the scalenus anterior and phrenic nerve, posterior to the internal jugular vein and sternocleidomastoid; it then crosses anterior to the subclavian artery and brachial plexus, posterior and parallel to the clavicle and subclavius and the inferior belly of the omohyoid, to reach the superior scapular border. Here it passes above (sometimes under) the superior transverse ligament, separating it from the suprascapular nerve, to enter the supraspinous fossa (**10**.96), where it lies on the bone, supplying the supraspinatus. It descends behind the scapular neck, through the great scapular notch deep to the inferior transverse ligament to the deep surface of the infraspinatus, where it anastomoses with the circumflex scapular and deep branch of the transverse cervical artery. Besides supplying the sternocleidomastoid, subclavius and infraspinatus, it has a *suprasternal branch* which crosses the sternal end of the clavicle to the skin of the upper thorax and an *acromial branch* which pierces the trapezius to supply the skin over the shoulder, anastomosing with the thoracoacromial and posterior circumflex humeral arteries. As the supra-

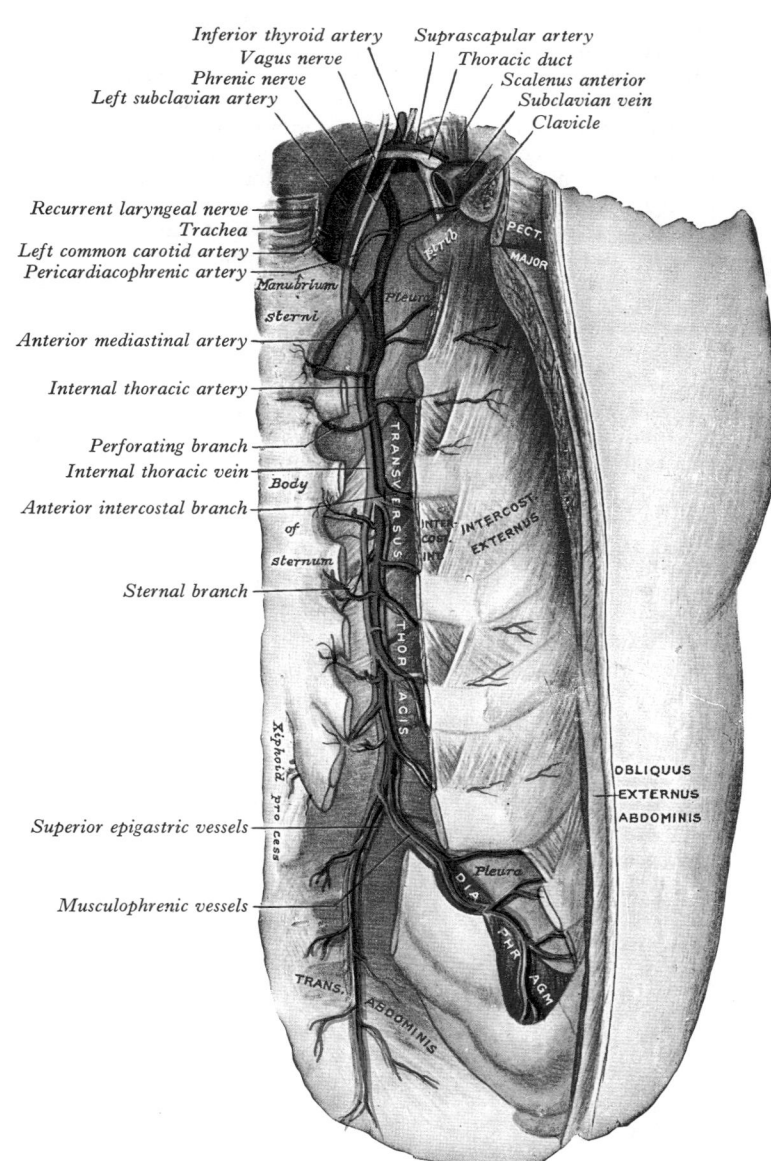

10.95 The left internal thoracic artery and vein and their main branches. The lateral end of the resected clavicle has been artificially elevated.

scapular artery passes the superior transverse ligament, a branch of it enters the subscapular fossa beneath the subscapularis; this anastomoses with the subscapular artery and the deep branch of the transverse cervical. It also supplies the acromioclavicular and glenohumeral joints, the clavicle and scapula. It may arise from the third part of the subclavian artery.

Superficial cervical artery (10.92). At a higher level than the suprascapular, it crosses anterior to the phrenic nerve, the scalenus anterior and brachial plexus and is covered by the internal jugular vein, sternocleidomastoid and platysma. It crosses the posterior triangle's floor to the anterior margin of the levator scapulae, ascending deep to the anterior part of the trapezius, supplying it, the adjoining muscles and the cervical lymph nodes. It anastomoses with the superficial ramus of the descending branch of the occipital artery. (See also p. 1536: variations of superficial cervical and dorsal scapular arteries.)

4. Costocervical trunk

On the right, this short vessel arises posteriorly from the second part of the subclavian artery, and, on the left, from its first part (**10**.91, 92). It arches back above the cervical pleura to the first rib's neck, dividing here into superior intercostal and deep cervical branches.

Superior intercostal artery. It descends between the pleura and necks of the first and second ribs to anastomose with the third posterior intercostal artery (**10.91**). Crossing the neck of the first rib it is medial to the ventral branch of the first thoracic spinal nerve, which it crosses at a lower level, and lateral to the stellate ganglion. In the first space it provides the first posterior intercostal artery, similar in distribution to the lower posterior intercostals. It descends to become the second posterior intercostal artery, usually joining a branch from the third; it is not constant, and is more common on the right; when absent, it is replaced by a direct aortic branch.

Deep cervical artery (**10.84**). Usually arising from the costo-cervical trunk, it is analogous in its first segment to a posterior branch of a posterior intercostal artery: occasionally it is a separate branch of the subclavian. Passing back above the eighth cervical spinal nerve between the seventh cervical transverse process and the neck of the first rib (sometimes between the sixth and seventh cervical transverse processes), it then ascends between the semispinales capitis and cervicis to the second cervical level. It supplies adjacent muscles and anastomoses with the deep branch of the descending branch of the occipital artery (p. 1519) and branches of the vertebral. A spinal branch enters the vertebral canal between the seventh cervical and first thoracic vertebrae.

5. Dorsal scapular artery

This arises from the third or less often second part of the subclavian, passing laterally through the brachial plexus in front of the scalenus medius and then deep to the levator scapulae to the superior scapular angle; here it descends with the dorsal scapular nerve under the rhomboids along the medial scapular border to the inferior angle (**10.92**, 96). It supplies the rhomboids, latissimus dorsi and trapezius and anastomoses with the suprascapular, subscapular and posterior branches of some posterior intercostal arteries. It has a small branch, sometimes arising directly from the subclavian, for the scalenus anterior.

Variations. About a third of the superficial cervical and dorsal

scapular arteries arise in common from the thyrocervical trunk as a *transverse cervical artery*, with a superficial (*superficial cervical artery*) and a deep branch (*dorsal scapular artery*); the latter passes laterally anterior to the brachial plexus and then posterior to the levator scapulae.

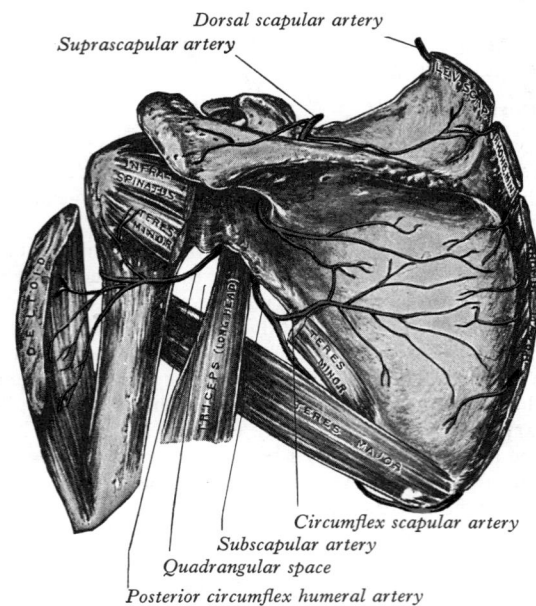

10.96 Scapular anastomoses of the left side: dorsal aspect.

Axilla

The axilla is a pyramidal region between the upper thoracic wall and the arm. Its blunt **apex** continues into the root of the neck (*cervico-axillary canal*) between the external border of the first rib, superior scapular border, posterior surface of the clavicle and the medial aspect of the cora-coid process; through it pass the axillary vessels and nerves. Its imaginary **base**, facing down, is broad at the chest, narrow at the arm and corresponds to the skin and a thick layer of *axillary fascia*, between the inferior borders of the pectoralis major in front and the latissimus dorsi behind. It is of course convex up, conforming to the armpit's concavity. The *anterior wall* is formed by the pectorales major et minor, the former covering the whole wall, the latter its intermediate part. The interval between the upper border of the pectoralis minor and clavicle is occupied by the clavipectoral fascia. The *posterior wall* is formed by the subscapularis above, teres major and latissimus dorsi below. **Medial** are the first four ribs with their intercostal muscles and the upper part of serratus anterior; this 'wall' is convex laterally. **Laterally** anterior and posterior walls converge, the 'wall' being narrow, consisting of the humeral intertubercular sulcus; the lateral angle lodges the coracobrachialis and biceps.

The axilla contains axillary vessels, the infraclavicular part of the brachial plexus and its branches, lateral branches of some intercostal nerves, many lymph nodes and vessels, loose adipose areolar tissue and in many instances the 'axillary tail' of the breast. The axillary vessels and brachial plexus run from the apex to the base along the lateral wall and nearer to the anterior wall, the axillary vein being anteromedial to the artery. Owing to the obliquity of the upper ribs, the neurovascular bundle, emerging from behind the clavicle, crosses the first intercostal space; its relations are therefore different at upper and lower levels. Thoracic branches of the axillary artery are in contact with the pectoral muscles; along the lateral margin of the pectoralis minor the lateral thoracic artery reaches the thoracic wall. Subscapular vessels descend on the posterior wall at the lower margin of the subscapularis, and subscapular and thoracodorsal nerves cross the anterior surface of the latissimus dorsi at different inclinations; circumflex scapular vessels wind round the lateral scapular border; posterior circumflex humeral vessels and the axillary nerve curve back and laterally around the humeral surgical neck. No large vessel lies on the medial 'wall', which is crossed proximally only by small branches of the superior thoracic artery. The long thoracic nerve descends on the serratus anterior and the intercostobrachial nerve perforates the upper anterior part of this wall,

crossing the axilla to its lateral 'wall'. The position and arrangement of lymph nodes are described on page 1613, nerves on page 1266 et seq.

Clinical Anatomy. When axillary suppuration occurs, fascial arrangement affects the spread of pus. As described on page 839, the clavipectoral fascia, between the clavicle and superomedial border of the pectoralis minor, splits to enclose the muscle, blending at its lateral border with the axillary fascia in the anterior axillary fold. Suppuration may be superficial or deep to this layer, either between the pectoral muscles or behind the pectoralis minor; in the former an abscess would appear at the edge of the anterior axillary fold or the groove between the deltoid and pectoralis major; in the latter, pus would tend to surround vessels and nerves and ascend into the neck, the direction of least resistance; pus may also track along vessels into the arm. When an axillary abscess is incised, a knife should enter the axillary 'base', midway between the anterior and posterior margins and near the thoracic side to avoid the lateral thoracic, subscapular and axillary vessels on the anterior, posterior and lateral walls. Relations of vessels and nerves in the axilla are important when lymph nodes are removed from the axilla in operations for mammary carcinoma; the positions of major structures in the lateral wall must be remembered.

AXILLARY ARTERY

The axillary artery (**10**.97), a continuation of the subclavian, begins at the first rib's outer border, ending nominally at the interior border of the teres major where it becomes brachial. Its direction varies with the limb's position: thus it is almost straight when the arm is raised at right angles, concave up when the arm is elevated above this and convex up and laterally with the arm pendent. At first deep, it becomes superficial, covered only by the skin and fasciae. The pectoralis minor crosses it and divides it into **three parts**: proximal, posterior and distal to the muscle.

Relations of the first part. **Anterior** are the skin, superficial fascia, platysma, supraclavicular nerves, deep fascia, clavicular fibres of the pectoralis major and the clavipectoral fascia. This part is crossed anteriorly by the lateral pectoral nerve, the loop of communication between it and the medial pectoral nerve, and by the thoraco-acromial and cephalic veins. **Posterior** are the first intercostal space and external intercostal, the first and second digitations of the serratus anterior, the long thoracic and medial pectoral nerves and the medial cord of the brachial plexus. **Lateral** is the posterior cord of the brachial plexus. **Anteromedial** is the axillary vein. The first part is enclosed with the axillary vein and brachial plexus in a fibrous *axillary sheath*, continuous with the prevertebral layer of the deep cervical fascia.

Relations of the second part. **Anterior** are the skin, superficial and deep fascia, pectoralis major and minor. Posterior are the posterior cord of the brachial plexus and the areolar tissue between it and the subscapularis. **Medial** is the axillary vein, separated from it by the medial cord of the brachial plexus and medial pectoral nerve. **Lateral** is the lateral cord of the brachial plexus, separating it from the coracobrachialis. The cords of the brachial plexus thus surround the second part on three sides, with the dispositions implied by their names, and separate it from the vein and adjacent muscles.

Relations of the third part. **Anterior** are pectoralis major, distal to this skin and fasciae. **Posterior** are the lower part of the subscapularis and tendons of the latissimus dorsi and teres major. **Lateral** is the coracobrachialis. **Medial** is the axillary vein. Branches of the brachial plexus are arranged as follows: **laterally** the lateral root and then trunk of the median nerve and, for a short distance, the musculocutaneous nerve; **medially** the medial cutaneous nerve of the forearm between the axillary artery and vein anteriorly, between them posteriorly the ulnar nerve; the medial cutaneous nerve of upper arm is medial to the vein; anterior is the medial root of the median nerve and posterior are radial and axillary nerves, the latter only to the distal border of the subscapularis.

BRANCHES OF THE AXILLARY ARTERY

The artery's branches are superior thoracic, thoraco-acromial, lateral thoracic, subscapular, anterior and posterior circumflex humeral.

Superior thoracic artery (**10**.97). A small vessel from the first part of the axillary near the lower border of the subclavius (sometimes from the thoraco-acromial), it runs anteromedially above the medial border of the pectoralis minor, then passes between it and the pectoralis major to the thoracic wall. It supplies these muscles and the thoracic wall, anastomosing with the internal thoracic and upper intercostal arteries.

Thoraco-acromial (acromio-thoracic) artery (**10**.92, 97). A short branch from the second part, it is at first overlapped by the pectoralis minor; skirting its medial border, it pierces the clavipectoral fascia and divides into the pectoral, acromial, clavicular and deltoid branches.

Pectoral branch. This descends between the pectoral muscles, is distributed to them and the breast and anastomoses with the intercostal branches of the internal thoracic and lateral thoracic arteries.

Acromial branch. It crosses the coracoid process under the deltoid,

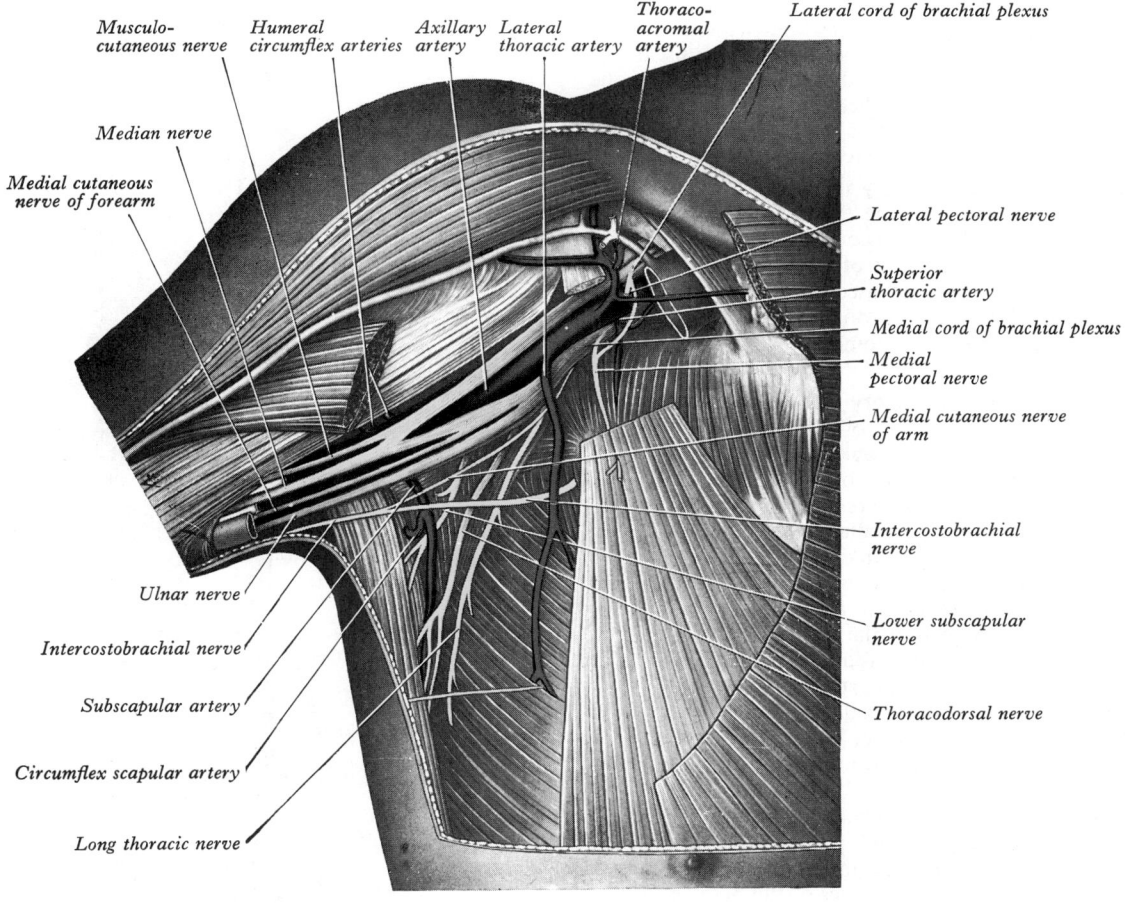

Musculo-cutaneous nerve — Humeral circumflex arteries — Axillary artery — Lateral thoracic artery — Thoraco-acromial artery — Lateral cord of brachial plexus

Median nerve

Medial cutaneous nerve of forearm

Lateral pectoral nerve

Superior thoracic artery

Medial cord of brachial plexus

Medial pectoral nerve

Medial cutaneous nerve of arm

Intercostobrachial nerve

Ulnar nerve

Intercostobrachial nerve

Subscapular artery

Lower subscapular nerve

Circumflex scapular artery

Thoracodorsal nerve

Long thoracic nerve

10.97   The right axillary and its branches. The pectoralis major and part of the pectoralis minor have been removed. Prominent but unlabelled features are the medial and lateral roots of the median nerve.

which it supplies, pierces the muscle and ends on the acromion, anastomosing with rami of the suprascapular, deltoid branch of the thoraco-acromial and posterior circumflex humeral arteries.

Clavicular branch. Ascending medially between the clavicular part of the pectoralis major and clavipectoral fascia, it supplies the sternoclavicular joint and subclavius.

Deltoid branch. It often arises with the acromial, crossing the pectoralis minor to accompany the cephalic vein between the pectoralis major and deltoid, supplying both.

Lateral thoracic artery (10.97). Following the lateral border of the pectoralis minor to the thoracic wall, it supplies the serratus anterior and pectoral muscles, the axillary lymph nodes and subscapularis; it anastomoses with the internal thoracic, subscapular, and intercostal arteries and the pectoral branch of the thoracoacromial artery. In females it is large and has lateral mammary branches which curve round the lateral border of the pectoralis major to the mammary gland.

Subscapular artery (10.96, 97). The largest branch of the axillary, it usually arises at the distal (inferior) border of the subscapularis which it follows to the inferior scapular angle, where it anastomoses with the lateral thoracic and intercostal arteries and the deep branch of the transverse cervical. It supplies adjacent muscles and the thoracic wall. It is accompanied distally by the nerve to the latissimus dorsi; about 4 cm from its origin it divides into the circumflex scapular artery and the thoracodorsal artery. The *circumflex scapular artery*, the larger of the two, curves backwards around the lateral scapular border, traversing a *triangular space* between subscapularis above and teres major below and the long head of the triceps laterally. It enters the infraspinous fossa under the teres minor and then divides. One branch (*infrascapular*) enters the subscapular fossa deep to the subscapularis, anastomosing with the suprascapular and dorsal scapular arteries (or deep branch of the transverse cervical); the other continues along the lateral scapular border between the teres major and minor and, dorsal to the inferior angle, anastomoses with the deep branch of the transverse cervical artery. Small branches supply the posterior part of the deltoid and the long head of the triceps, anastomosing with an ascending branch of the arteria profunda brachii. The other terminal branch of the subscapular artery, the *thoracodorsal artery*, follows the lateral margin of the scapula, posterior to the lateral thoracic, between the latissimus dorsi and serratus anterior. It supplies these two muscles and teres major and intercostales, anastomosing with intercostal arteries.

Anterior circumflex humeral artery (10.97). Arising from the lateral side of the axillary artery at the distal border of the subscapularis, runs horizontally behind coracobrachialis and short head of biceps, anterior to the surgical neck of the humerus. Reaching the intertubercular sulcus, it sends an ascending branch to supply the humeral head and shoulder joint. It continues laterally under the long head of biceps and deltoid, anastomosing with the posterior circumflex humeral artery.

Posterior circumflex humeral artery (10.96). Larger than the anterior, it branches from the third part of the axillary at the distal border of the subscapularis and runs back with the axillary nerve through a *quadrangular space*, bounded by the subscapularis, the capsule of the shoulder joint and the teres minor above, the teres major below, the long head of triceps medially and the surgical neck of the humerus laterally. It curves round the humeral neck and supplies the shoulder joint, deltoid, teres major and minor, and long and lateral heads of triceps, giving off a descending branch to anastomose with the deltoid branch of the arteria profunda brachii and with the anterior circumflex humeral and acromial branches of the suprascapular and thoraco-acromial arteries.

Surface anatomy. Pulsation of the axillary artery can be felt against the axillary lateral wall. Its upper segment can be mapped out, when the arm is raised, by a line from this to the midpoint of the clavicle.

Variations. Branches vary considerably; an alar thoracic, often from the second part, may supply fat and lymph nodes in the axilla. Occasionally the subscapular, circumflex humeral and arteria profunda arise in common and then branches of the brachial plexus surround this instead of the axillary artery. The posterior circumflex humeral artery may be from the arteria profunda brachii, passing back below the teres major instead of traversing the quadrangular

space. Sometimes (anomalous 'high division') the axillary divides into radial and ulnar arteries and is occasionally the source of the anterior interosseous artery.

Clinical anatomy. Axillary compression is most effective against the humerus. Except for the popliteal, the axillary artery is more frequently lacerated by violence than any other, being most susceptible when diseased. It has been ruptured in attempts to reduce old dislocations, especially when the artery is adherent to the articular capsule.

BRACHIAL ARTERY

The brachial artery (10.98, 102), a continuation of the axillary, begins at the distal (inferior) border of the tendon of teres major and ends about a centimetre distal to the elbow joint (at the level of the neck of the radius) by dividing into radial and ulnar arteries. At first it is medial to the humerus, but gradually spirals anterior to it until it lies midway between the humeral epicondyles. Its pulsation can be felt throughout.

Relations. The artery is wholly superficial, covered **anteriorly** only by skin and superficial and deep fasciae; the bicipital aponeurosis crosses it anteriorly at the elbow, separating it from the median cubital vein; the median nerve crosses it **lateromedially** near the distal attachment of coracobrachialis. **Posterior** are the long head of triceps, separated by the radial nerve and arteria profunda brachii and then successively by: the medial head of triceps, the attachment of coracobrachialis and the brachialis. **Lateral** are: proximally the median nerve and coracobrachialis and distally the biceps and the muscles overlapping the artery. **Medial** are: proximally the medial cutaneous nerve of forearm and ulnar nerve, distally the median nerve and basilic vein (separated distally by the deep fascia). With

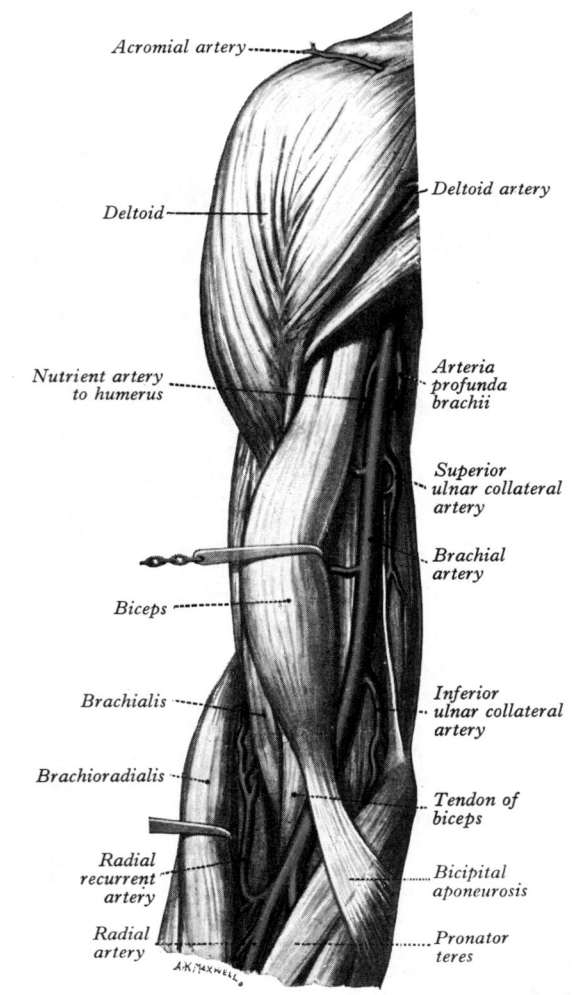

Acromial artery

Deltoid

Nutrient artery
to humerus

Biceps

Brachialis

Brachioradialis

Radial
recurrent
artery

Radial
artery

Deltoid artery

Arteria
profunda
brachii

Superior
ulnar collateral
artery

Brachial
artery

Inferior
ulnar collateral
artery

Tendon of
biceps

Bicipital
aponeurosis

Pronator
teres

A.K.MAXWELL

10.98 The right brachial artery and its branches.

the artery are two venae comitantes, connected by transverse and oblique branches.

At the elbow the brachial artery sinks deeply into the triangular intermuscular cubital fossa. The fossa's base is an inter-epicondylar line, the sides being the medial edge of the brachioradialis and the lateral margin of pronator teres; the 'floor' consists of brachialis and supinator. The fossa contains the tendon of the biceps, the terminal part of the brachial artery and accompanying veins, the commencement of the radial and ulnar arteries and parts of the median and radial nerves. The brachial artery is central and it divides near the neck of the radius into its terminal branches, the radial and ulnar arteries. **Anterior** to it are the skin, superficial fascia and median cubital vein, separated by the bicipital aponeurosis. **Posteriorly** the brachialis separates it from the elbow joint. The median nerve is **medial** proximally but is separated from the ulnar artery by the ulnar head of the pronator teres. **Lateral** are the tendon of biceps and the radial nerve, the latter concealed between supinator and brachioradialis.

Variations. The brachial artery, with the median nerve, may diverge from the medial border of the biceps, descending towards the medial humeral epicondyle, usually behind a *supracondylar process* from which a fibrous arch crosses the artery, and which then runs behind or through the pronator teres to the elbow. This resembles the normal arrangement in some carnivores (p. 626). Occasionally the artery divides proximally into two trunks which reunite. Frequently it divides more proximally than usual into radial, ulnar and common interosseous arteries. Most often the radial branches arise proximally, leaving a common trunk for the ulnar and common interosseous; sometimes the ulnar arises proximally, the radial and common interosseous forming the other division; the common interosseous may also arise proximally. Sometimes slender *vasa aberrantia* connect the brachial to the axillary artery or to one of the forearm arteries, usually the radial. The brachial artery may be crossed by muscular or tendinous slips from the coracobrachialis, biceps, brachialis or pronator teres.

Branches. These are arteria profunda brachii, nutrient, superior and inferior ulnar collateral, muscular, radial and ulnar arteries.

Arteria profunda brachii (10.98, 99, 102). A large branch from the posteromedial aspect of the brachial, distal to the teres major, follows the radial nerve closely, at first back between the long and medial heads of the triceps, then in the nerve's groove covered by the lateral head of triceps; here it divides into terminal branches (10.102). Apart from the muscular branches, it supplies the following: the nutrient, deltoid, middle collateral and radial collateral arteries.

Nutrient artery. This enters the humerus posterior to the deltoid tuberosity but may be absent.

Deltoid (ascending) branch. Ascending between the lateral and long heads of triceps, it anastomoses with a descending branch of the posterior humeral circumflex artery.

Middle collateral (posterior descending) branch. The larger terminal vessel, it arises behind the humerus and descends in the medial head of the triceps to the elbow (10.100), anastomosing with the interosseous recurrent artery behind the lateral epicondyle; it often has a small branch which accompanies the nerve to the anconeus.

Radial collateral. The other terminal branch, this is the artery's continuation (10.101). It accompanies the radial nerve through the lateral intermuscular septum, descending between the brachialis and brachioradialis anterior to the lateral epicondyle, anastomosing with the radial recurrent artery.

Nutrient artery of the humerus. This arises near the mid-level of the upper arm, and enters the nutrient canal near the attachment of coracobrachialis; it is directed distally.

Superior ulnar collateral artery (10.98, 100, 102). It arises a little distal to the upper arm's mid-level, often as a branch from the arteria profunda brachii. It accompanies the ulnar nerve, piercing the medial intermuscular septum to descend between the medial epicondyle and olecranon, ending deep to flexor carpi ulnaris by anastomosing with the posterior ulnar recurrent and inferior collateral arteries; sometimes a branch of it passing anterior to the medial epicondyle anastomoses with the anterior ulnar recurrent artery.

Inferior ulnar collateral (supratrochlear) artery (10.98, 102, 103). It begins about 5 cm proximal to the elbow, passes medially between the median nerve and brachialis and, piercing the medial inter-

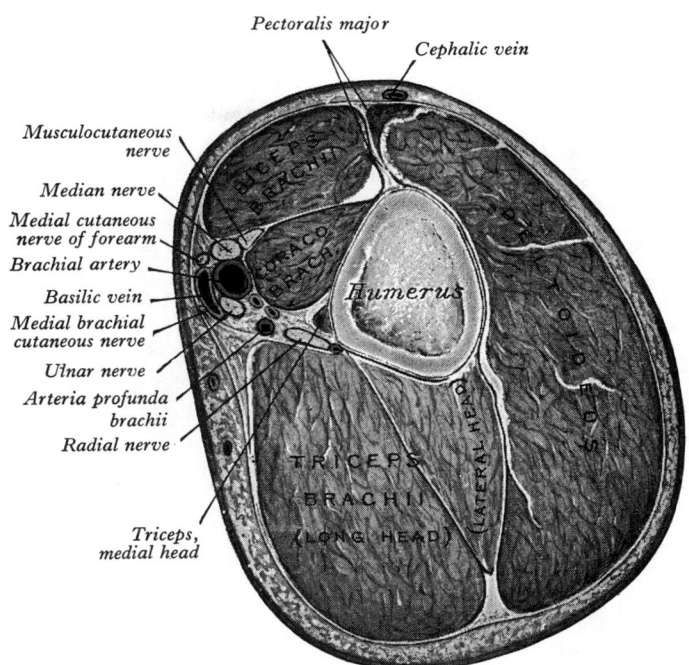

10.99 Transverse section through the right arm at the junction of the proximal and middle thirds of the humerus: proximal aspect.

muscular septum, curls round the humerus between the triceps and bone, forming, by its junction with the middle collateral branch of arteria profunda brachii, an arch proximal to the olecranon fossa. As it lies on brachialis it has branches descending anterior to the medial epicondyle to anastomose with the anterior ulnar recurrent artery. Behind the epicondyle a branch anastomoses with the superior ulnar collateral and posterior ulnar recurrent arteries.

Muscular arteries from the brachial. These are distributed to the coracobrachialis, biceps and brachialis.

Clinical anatomy

Compression of the brachial artery may be effected at almost any level; if proximal, it should be directed laterally, if distal, backwards. The most favourable site is about midway, where the artery is on the tendon of the coracobrachialis and still medial to the humerus; pressure should be exerted slightly posterolaterally.

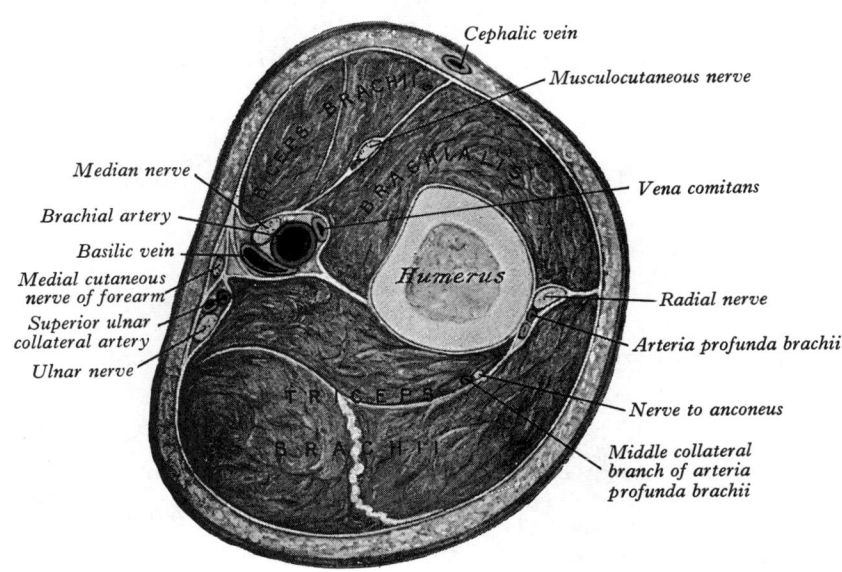

10.100 Transverse section through the right arm, a little below the middle of the shaft of the humerus: proximal aspect.

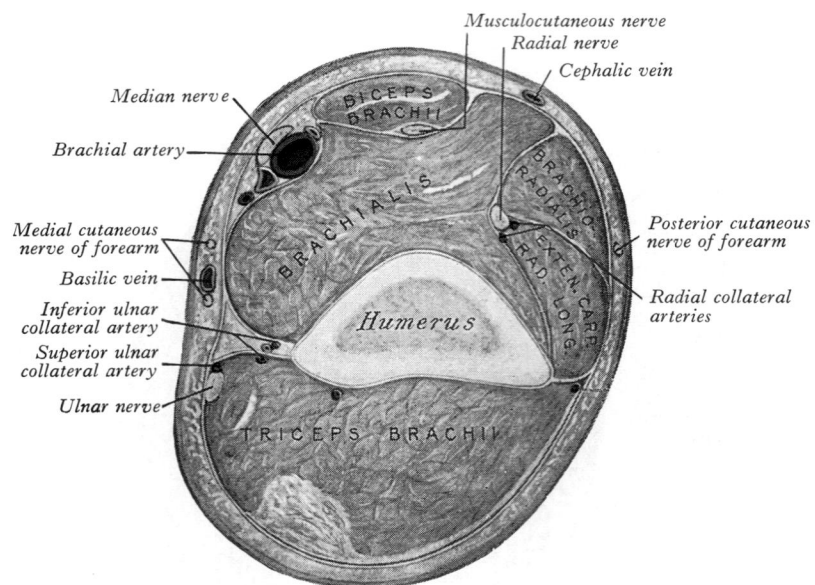

10.101   Transverse section through the right arm, 2 cm above the medial epicondyle of the humerus: proximal aspect.

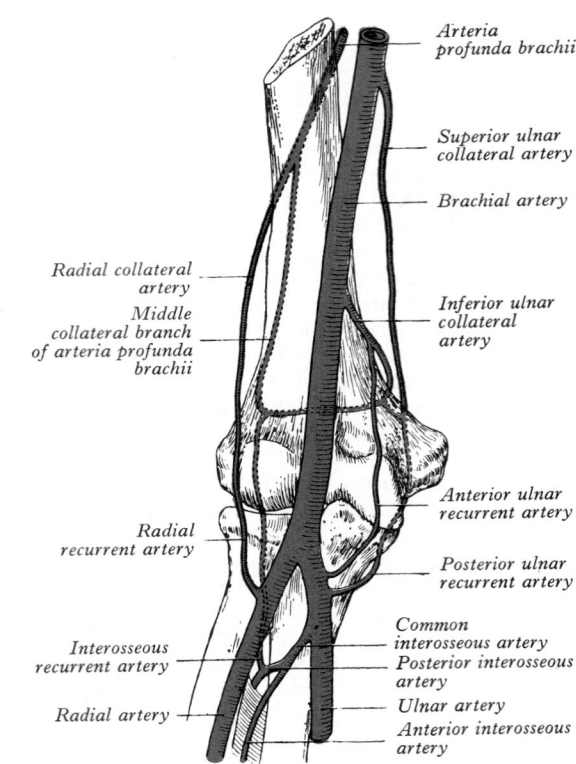

10.102   The arterial anastomoses around the (right) elbow joint. Anterior side seen from the front.

RADIAL ARTERY

The radial artery (**10.**103–105), though smaller than the ulnar, appears a more direct continuation of the brachial. It begins about 1 cm distal to the bend of the elbow (level of the neck of the radius, **10.**102), then descends along the lateral side of the forearm to the wrist, where it is palpable between the flexor carpi radialis medially and the salient anterior border of the radius. It then curls postero-laterally round the carpus, beneath the tendons of abductor pollicis longus and extensor pollicis brevis and longus, to the proximal end of the first intermetacarpal space, swerving medially between the heads of the first dorsal interosseous into the palm and then crossing medially to form the deep palmar arch with the deep branch of the ulnar artery. The radial artery is thus divisible into parts: in the forearm, wrist and hand.

In the forearm (**10.**103–106) the artery extends from the medial side of the neck of the radius to the front of its styloid process, being medial to the radial shaft proximally, but anterior to it distally. Proximally it is overlapped anteriorly by the belly of brachioradialis, whereas the rest is covered only by the skin, superficial and deep fasciae. Posterior are successively: the tendon of biceps, supinator, the distal attachment of pronator teres, radial head of flexor digitorum superficialis, flexor pollicis longus, pronator quadratus and the lower end of the radius (where its pulsation is most accessible). Proximally pronator teres is medial, brachioradialis lateral; distally the tendon of flexor carpi radialis is medial, that of brachioradialis lateral. The superficial branch of the radial nerve is lateral in the vessel's middle third, and filaments of the lateral cutaneous nerve of the forearm run along its distal part as it curves round the carpus. The vessel is accompanied by paired venae comitantes.

At the wrist (**10.**107, 108) the radial artery passes on to the dorsal aspect of the carpus between the lateral carpal ligament and tendons of abductor pollicis longus and extensor pollicis brevis. It crosses the scaphoid bone and trapezium (in the 'anatomical snuff-box'), where again its pulsation is obvious, and as it passes between heads of the first dorsal interosseous it is crossed by the tendon of extensor pollicis longus. Between the thumb extensors it is crossed by the beginning of the cephalic vein and the digital branches of the radial nerve supplying the thumb and index.

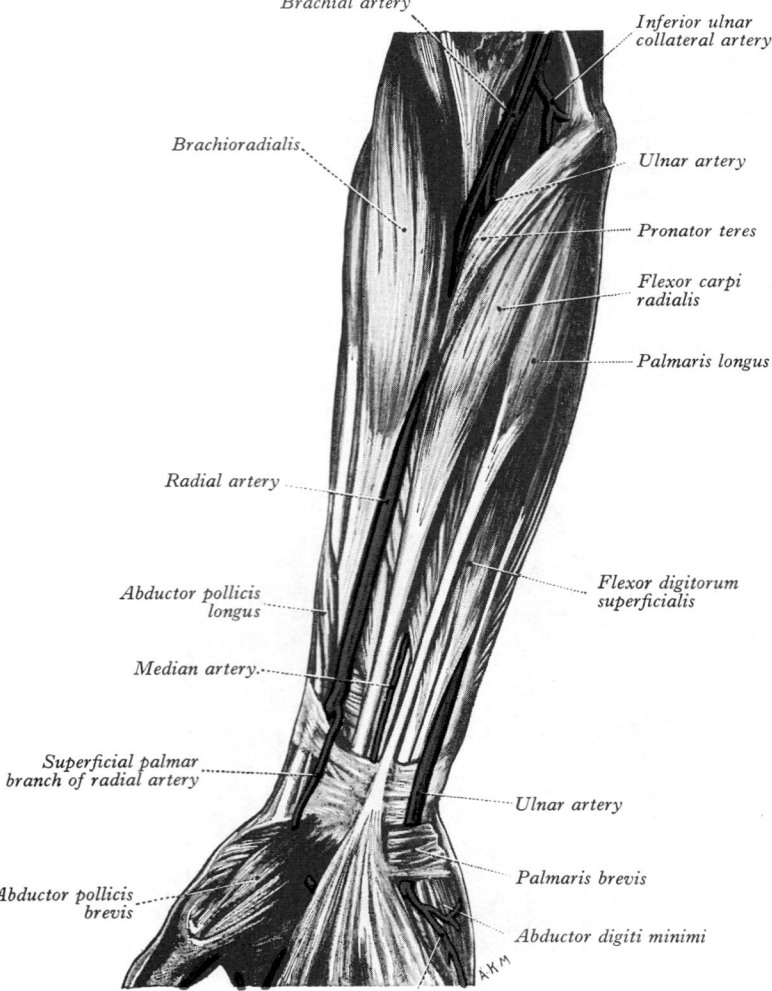

10.103   The right radial and ulnar arteries, superficial dissection.

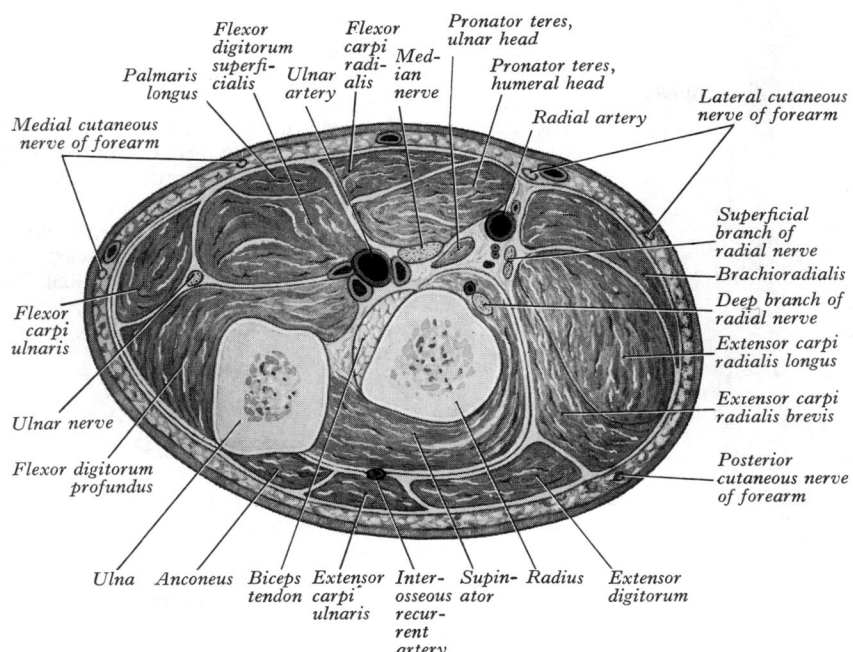

10.104   Transverse section through the right forearm at the level of the radial tuberosity: distal aspect.

In the hand (**10**.109) the radial artery, having traversed the first interosseous space between the heads of the first dorsal interosseous, crosses the palm, at first deep to the oblique head of adductor pollicis and then between its oblique and transverse heads or through the transverse head. At the fifth metacarpal base it anastomoses with the deep branch of the ulnar artery, completing the *deep palmar arch* (**10**.105).

Variations. Sometimes the radial artery arises proximally, usually from the axillary or beginning of the brachial artery. In the forearm it is sometimes superficial to the deep fascia and occasionally superficial to the thumb extensor tendons (see also under 'Variations of the Brachial Artery', above).

Radial recurrent artery (**10**.102, 105). This arises just distal to the elbow, passing between superficial and deep branches of the radial nerve to ascend behind the brachioradialis, anterior to the supinator and brachialis; it supplies these muscles and the elbow joint, anastomosing with the radial collateral branch of the arteria profunda brachii.

Muscular branches. These are distributed to muscles on the radial side of the forearm.

Palmar carpal branch (**10**.105). A small vessel, it arises near the distal border of pronator quadratus and crosses the anterior surface of the distal end of the radius, near the palmar carpal surface, passing medially to anastomose behind the long flexor tendons with the palmar carpal branch of the ulnar; this transverse anastomosis is joined by longitudinal branches from the anterior interosseous and recurrent branches from the deep palmar arch, forming a *cruciate palmar carpal arch*, which, by descending branches, supplies the carpal articulations and bones. (Although so named this is usually sited near the wrist joint on the distal forearm bones.)

Superficial palmar branch (**10**.109). Arising from the radial artery just before it curves round the carpus, it passes through and occasionally over the thenar muscles, which it supplies, sometimes anastomosing with the end of the ulnar artery to complete a superficial palmar arch.

Dorsal carpal branch. This arises deep to the pollicial extensor tendons, runs medially across the dorsal carpal surface under them and anastomoses with the ulnar dorsal carpal branch and also with the anterior and posterior interosseous arteries to form a *dorsal carpal arch*. The carpal arches are both close to bone and supply the distal epiphyseal parts of the radius and ulna. From the dorsal arch three *dorsal metacarpal arteries* descend on the second to fourth dorsal interosseous muscles and bifurcate into the *dorsal digital*

branches for the adjacent sides of all four fingers; they anastomose with the palmar digital branches from the superficial palmar arch; near their origins they also anastomose with the deep palmar arch by the *proximal perforating arteries* and, near their bifurcation, with the palmar digital rami of the superficial palmar arch by *distal perforating arteries*.

First dorsal metacarpal artery (**10**.108). A branch of the radial just before it passes between the heads of the first dorsal interosseous, it divides almost at once into two branches supplying the adjacent sides of the pollex and index; the radial side of the pollex receives a branch direct from the radial artery itself (see below).

Arteria princeps pollicis (**10**.105). This arises from the radial as it turns into the palm, and descends on the palmar aspect of the first metacarpal under the oblique head of adductor pollicis lateral to the first palmar interosseous. At the base of the proximal phalanx, deep to the tendon of flexor pollicis longus, it divides into two branches, appearing between the medial and lateral attachments of the oblique head of adductor pollicis to run along both sides of the pollex, forming, on the palmar surface of its distal phalanx, a pollicial arch supplying the skin and subcutaneous tissue. The arterial princeps pollicis is the usual nutrient of supply to the first metacarpal bone.

Arteria radialis indicis (**10**.105, 109). Often a proximal branch of the arteria princeps pollicis, it descends between the first dorsal interosseous and transverse head of adductor pollicis, and along the lateral side of the index finger to its end; it anastomoses with the indicial medial digital artery. At the distal border of the transverse head of the adductor pollicis it anastomoses with the arteria princeps pollicis and links with the superficial palmar arch.

The arteriae princeps pollicis et radialis indicis may be combined as the *first palmar metacarpal artery*.

Deep palmar arch

This is formed by anastomosis of the end of the radial with the deep palmar branch of the ulnar artery (**10**.105). It crosses the bases of the metacarpal bones and interossei, covered by the oblique head of adductor pollicis, the digital flexor tendons and lumbricals. In its concavity, running laterally, is the deep branch of the ulnar nerve. The arch was incomplete in six of 200 arches (Coleman & Anson 1961). Variation is chiefly in the size of contribution from the ulnar artery.

Surface anatomy. The deep palmar arch is indicated by a horizontal line about 4 cm long from a point just distal to the hamate's hook (**10**.110). It is about 1 cm proximal to the superficial arch. 1541

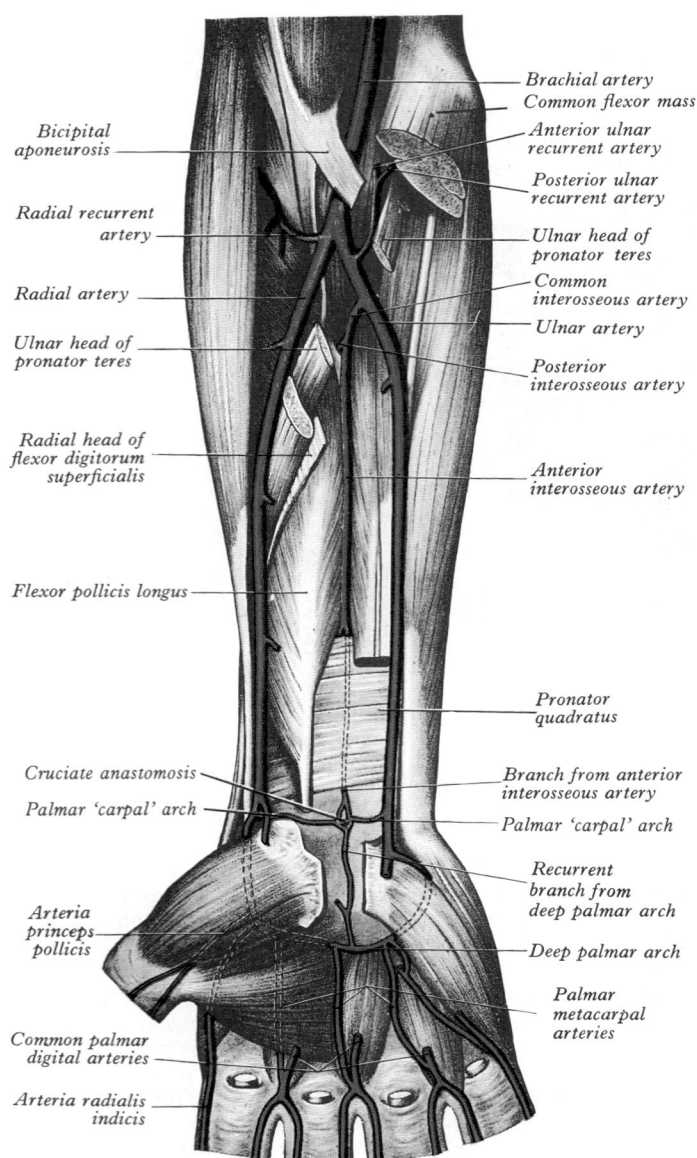

10.105   The arteries of the right forearm and hand: deep dissection. The palmar 'carpal' arch lies across forearm bones.

Branches of the deep palmar arch are the palmar metacarpal, perforating and recurrent.

Palmar metacarpal arteries (**10**.105). The three arteries run distally from the convexity of the arch on the interosseous muscles of the second to fourth spaces; at the digital clefts they join the *common digital branches* of the superficial arch. They supply nutrient branches to the medial four metacarpals.

Perforating branches. These three branches from the deep palmar arch traverse the second to fourth interosseous spaces between the heads of the corresponding dorsal interossei to anastomose with the dorsal metacarpal arteries.

Recurrent branches (**10**.105). They ascend proximally from the deep palmar arch anterior to the carpus to supply the carpal bones and intercarpal articulations, ending in the palmar carpal arch (mentioned above).

ULNAR ARTERY

The ulnar artery (**10**.102–109), the larger terminal branch of the brachial, begins just distal to the bend of the elbow. It reaches the medial side of the forearm midway between elbow and wrist, which it passes vertically, crossing the flexor retinaculum lateral to the ulnar nerve and pisiform bone; distal to this it has a deep branch and then continues across the palm as the superficial palmar arch.

Relations. In the forearm the **proximal half** of the artery (**10**.103–106) passes posterior to the pronator teres, flexor carpi radialis, palmaris longus and flexor digitorum superficialis; medially it is overlapped in its middle third by flexor carpi ulnaris; it lies in front of the brachialis and flexor digitorum profundus. Distal to the elbow the median nerve is medial for about 2.5 cm and then crosses it but is separated by the ulnar head of pronator teres. The artery's **distal half** (**10**.103, 105, 109) lies on the flexor digitorum profundus, covered by the skin, superficial and deep fasciae, between the flexor carpi ulnaris and flexor digitorum superficialis. It is accompanied by venae comitantes; the ulnar nerve lies medial to its distal two-thirds and its palmar cutaneous branch descends along it to the hand.

At the wrist (**10**.105, 107, 109) the artery is covered by skin, fasciae and palmaris brevis, and it lies between the superficial and main parts of the flexor retinaculum (p. 852); the ulnar nerve and pisiform bone are medial.

Surface anatomy. A line from a point in the limb's midline just distal to the elbow's fold descends medially to meet a line stretching from the medial epicondyle to the pisiform bone, from the junction of its upper and middle thirds. Together these represent the artery's upper third and distal two-thirds respectively.

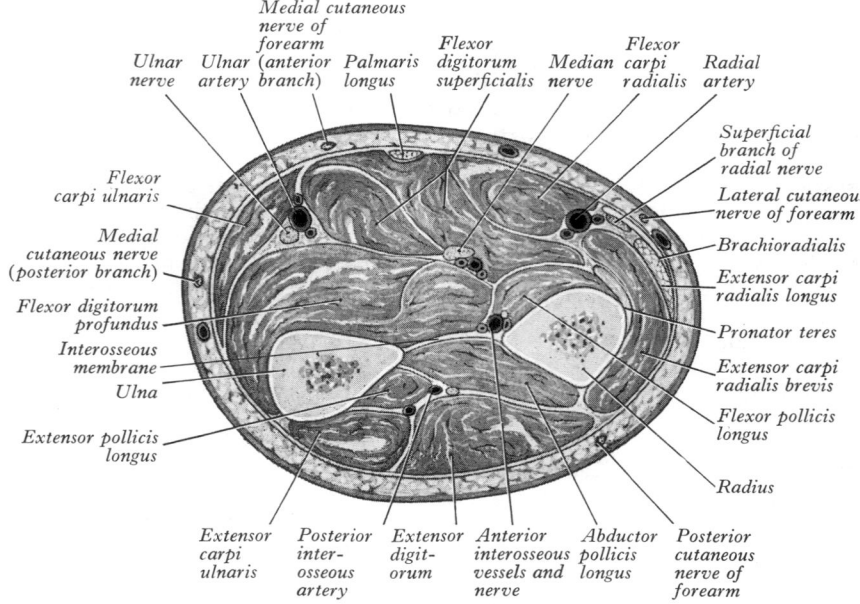

10.106   Transverse section through the middle of the left forearm: proximal aspect.

Variations. The ulnar artery may arise proximal to the elbow, the brachial being more often its source than the axillary artery; it is then usually superficial to the forearm flexors, commonly under the deep fascia, and is rarely subcutaneous; the brachial artery then supplies the common interosseous and this the ulnar recurrent arteries.

Branches. The artery supplies medial muscles in the forearm and hand, the common flexor synovial sheath and ulnar nerve (Blunt 1959), including the following named branches:

Anterior ulnar recurrent artery (10.102, 105)**. This arises just distal to the elbow, ascends between the brachialis and pronator teres, supplies them and anastomoses with the inferior ulnar collateral artery anterior to the medial epicondyle.

Posterior ulnar recurrent artery (10.102, 105)**. A larger artery, it arises distal to the anterior recurrent, and passes dorsomedially between the flexores digitorum profundus and superficialis, ascending behind the medial epicondyle; between this and the olecranon it is deep to the flexor carpi ulnaris, ascending between its heads with the ulnar nerve. Supplying adjacent muscles, nerve, bone and elbow joint, it anastomoses with the ulnar collateral and interosseous recurrent arteries (**10**.102).

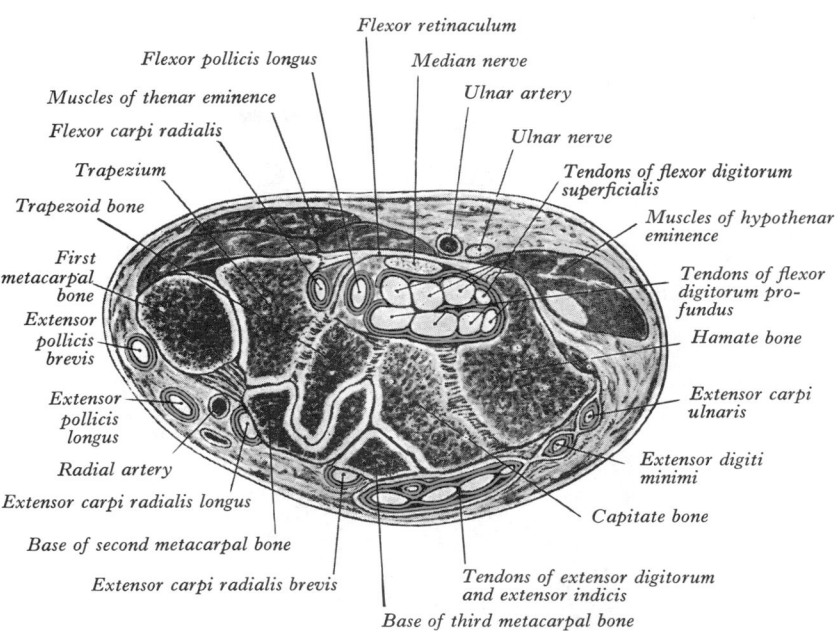

10.107   Transverse section through the left wrist: proximal aspect. The section is slightly oblique and divides the distal row of the carpus and the bases of the first, second and third metacarpal bones. The arrangement of the tendons of the flexors of the fingers shown in the figure represents the actual condition in the specimen. Observe that the carpometacarpal joint of the thumb is separate from the joint between the trapezium and the base of the second metacarpal bone.

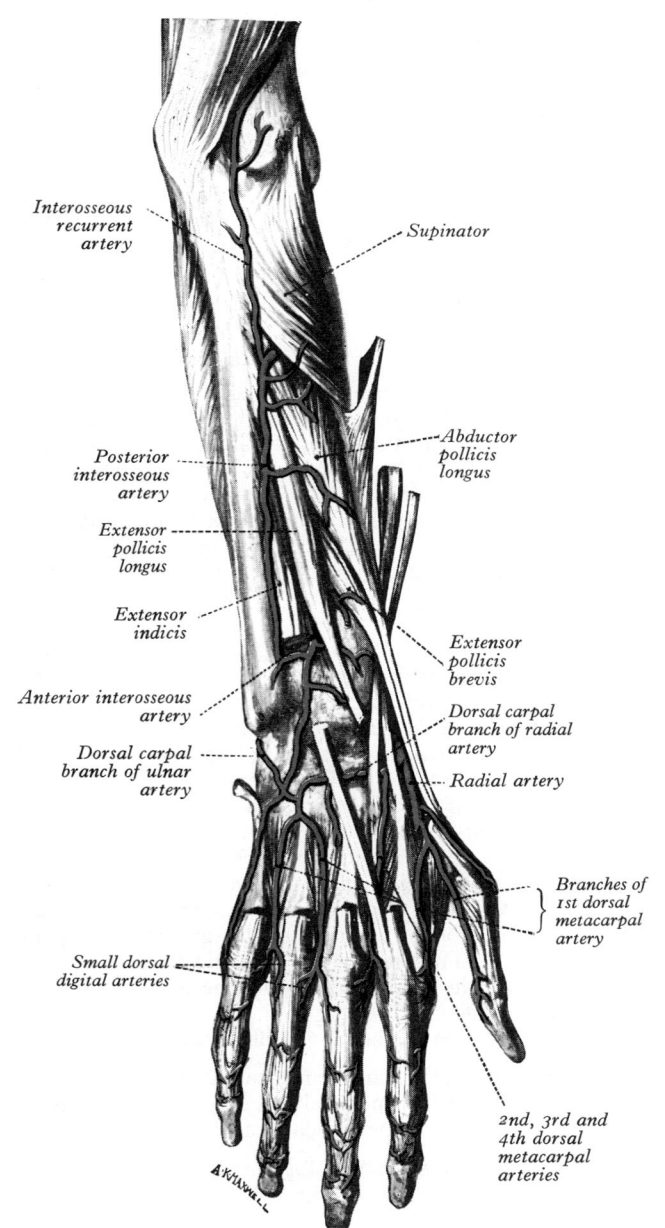

10.108   The arteries of the posterior surface of the right forearm and hand.

Common interosseous artery (10.102, 105)**. A short branch of the ulnar, just distal to the radial tuberosity, it passes back to the proximal border of the interosseous membrane, dividing into the *anterior* and *posterior interosseous arteries.*

Anterior interosseous artery (10.102, 105)**. Descending on the anterior aspect of the interosseous membrane with the median nerve's anterior interosseous branch, it is overlapped by contiguous sides of flexor digitorum profundus and flexor pollicis longus; it has *muscular branches* and *nutrient branches* for the radius and ulna. On the membrane, branches leave to pierce it and supply deep extensor muscles. Proximal to pronator quadratus its continuation also traverses the membrane to the back of the forearm where it anastomoses with its own posterior interosseous branch, descending over the carpal dorsum to join the dorsal carpal arch. It is in the extensor retinacular compartment with the tendons of digital extensors. Before it pierces the interosseous membrane, a branch descends behind the pronator quadratus to the anterior 'carpal' arch. (Strictly, as mentioned, the latter is **proximal** to the line of the wrist joint.) The slender *median artery*, from the start of the anterior interosseous, accompanies and supplies the median nerve; it often arises from the common interosseous, sometimes much enlarged, reaching the palm with the nerve (p. 319), where it may join the superficial palmar arch or end as one or two palmar digital arteries.

Posterior interosseous artery (10.105, 108)**. Usually smaller than the anterior, it passes dorsally between the oblique cord and proximal border of the interosseous membrane and then between supinator and abductor pollicis longus, descending deep to the superficial extensors, which it supplies. On abductor pollicis longus it accompanies the deep branch of the radial nerve. Distally it anastomoses with the end of the anterior interosseous and dorsal carpal arch. Near its origin the *interosseous recurrent artery* leaves it to ascend between the lateral epicondyle and olecranon, either on or through the supinator but deep to anconeus, to anastomose with the middle collateral branch of the arteria profunda brachii, posterior ulnar recurrent and ulnar collateral arteries.

Muscular branches.   These arise directly from the main vessel and distribute to muscles in the ulnar region.

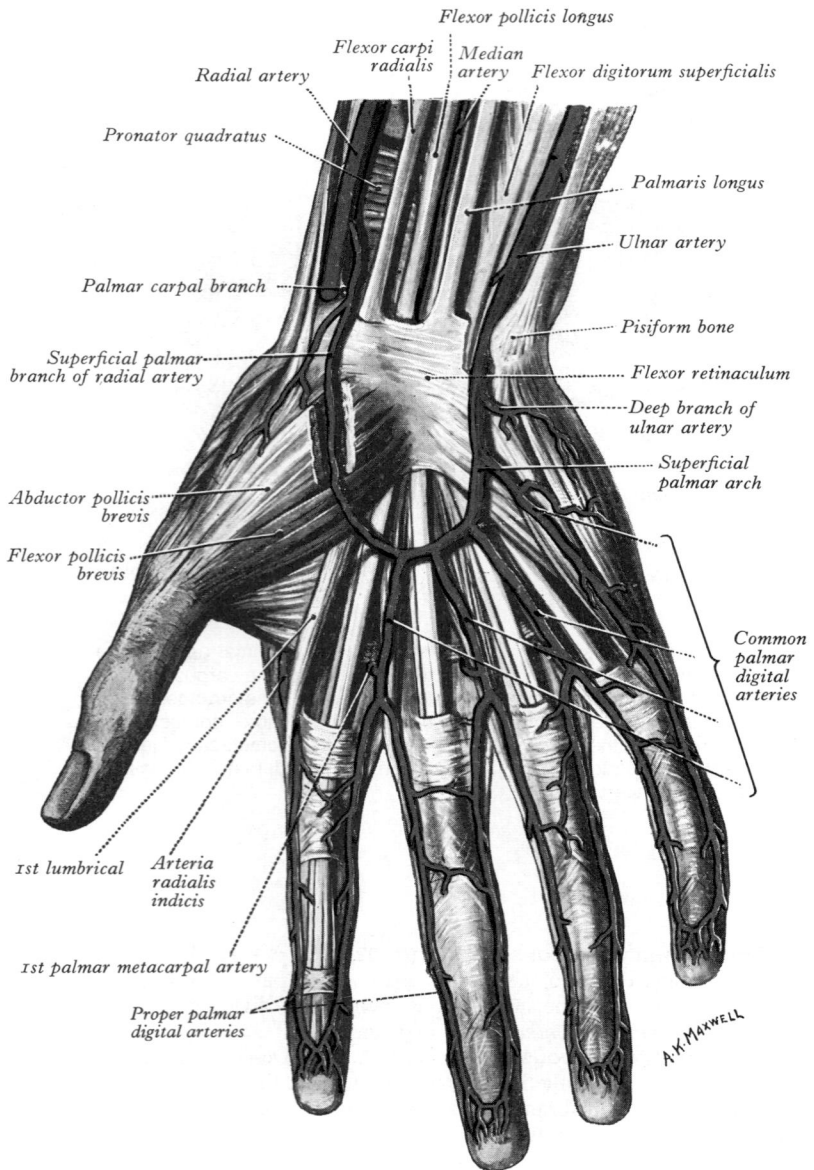

10.109 The superficial palmar arch and its branches in the right hand. A part of the abductor pollicis brevis has been excised to expose the superficial palmar branch of the radial artery.

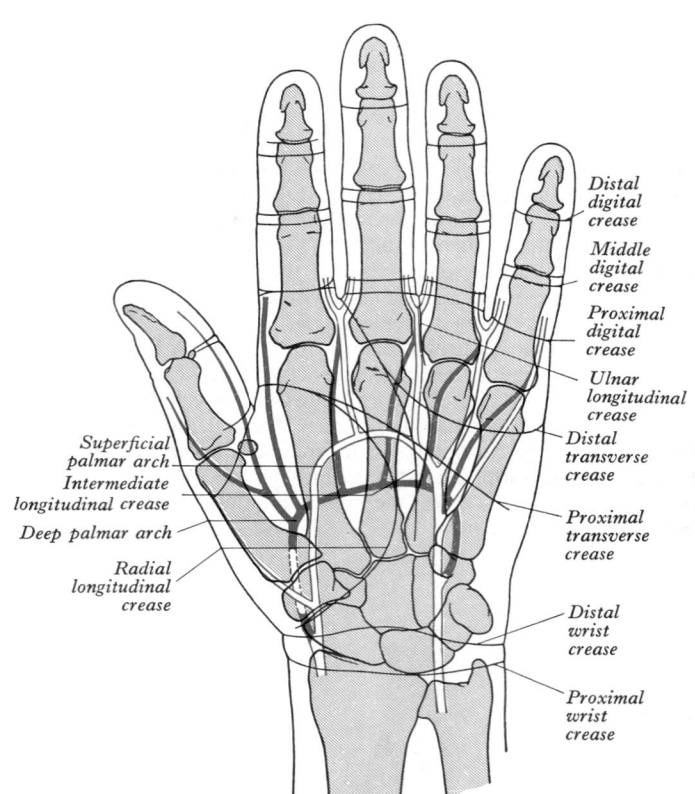

10.110 The relation of the skin flexure lines and palmar arterial arches to the bones of the left hand (simplified).

Palmar carpal branch (10.105). A small vessel, it crosses the distal ulna behind the tendons of flexor digitorum profundus; it anastomoses with a palmar carpal branch of the radial to make a so-called palmar carpal arch (p. 1541).

Dorsal carpal branch (10.108). Arising just proximal to the pisiform bone, it curves deep to the tendon of flexor carpi ulnaris to the carpal dorsum to pass laterally across it under the extensor tendons, anastomosing with the radial dorsal carpal branch to complete the dorsal carpal arch (p. 1541). Near its origin it sends a small digital branch along the ulnar side of the fifth metacarpal to supply the medial side of the dorsal surface of the fifth finger.

Deep palmar branch (10.105, 109). Often double, it passes between the abductor and flexor digiti minimi, through or deep to the opponens digiti minimi; it anastomoses with the radial, completing the deep palmar arch, accompanied by the deep branch of the ulnar nerve.

Superficial palmar arch (10.109, 110)

This anastomosis is fed mainly by the ulnar artery, entering the palm with the ulnar nerve, anterior to the flexor retinaculum and lateral

to the pisiform, passing medial to the hamate's hook, then curving laterally to form an arch, convex distally and level with a transverse line through the distal border of the fully extended pollicial base. About a third of the superficial palmar arches are formed by the ulnar alone; a further third are completed by the superficial palmar branch of the radial and a third either by the arteria radialis indicis, a branch of arteria princeps pollicis or by the median artery (Coleman & Anson 1961). It is covered by the palmaris brevis and palmar aponeurosis and it is superficial to the flexor digiti minimi, branches of the median nerve and to the long flexor tendons and lumbrical muscles.

Branches. Three common palmar digital arteries (10.109) from the convexity of the superficial palmar arch proceed distally on the second to fourth lumbricals, each joined by a corresponding palmar metacarpal artery from the deep palmar arch and dividing into two *proper palmar digital arteries.* These run along the contiguous sides of all four fingers, dorsal to the digital nerves, anastomosing in the subcutaneous tissue of the finger tips and near the interphalangeal joints. Each digital artery has two *dorsal branches* anastomosing with the *dorsal digital arteries* and supplying the soft parts dorsal to the middle and distal phalanges, including the matrices of the nails. The *palmar digital artery* for the medial side of minimus leaves the arch under the palmaris brevis. Palmar digital arteries supply metacarpophalangeal and interphalangeal joints and nutrient rami to the phalanges. They are the main digital supply, the dorsal digital arteries (p. 1541) being minute.

Anastomoses between the radial and ulnar arteries occur:

- at the wrist by the palmar and dorsal carpal arches
- in the hand through the superficial and deep palmar arches
- between their digital and metacarpal branches.

Wounds of the palmar arches. Ligature of **one** forearm artery may be ineffective in wounds of the palmar arches; simultaneous tying of both proximal to the carpus may also fail, because of interosseo–carpal anastomoses. If local pressure fails the brachial artery may be compressed (p. 1538) as a temporary expedient.

ARTERIES OF THE TRUNK

THORACIC AORTA

The thoracic aorta (**10.**111) is the segment of *descending aorta* confined to the posterior mediastinum. It begins level with the fourth thoracic vertebra's lower border, continuous with the aortic arch, ending anterior to the twelfth thoracic's lower border in the diaphragmatic aortic aperture. At its origin it is left of the vertebral column; as it descends it approaches the midline and at its termination is directly anterior to it.

Relations. **Anterior**, from above down, are the left pulmonary hilum, the pericardium separating it from the left atrium, oesophagus and diaphragm; **posterior** are the vertebral column and hemiazygos veins; **right lateral** are the azygos and thoracic duct and below, the right pleura and lung; **left lateral** are the pleura and lung. The oesophagus, with its plexus of nerves, is right lateral above but becomes anterior in the lower thorax; close to the diaphragm it is **left anterolateral**. Thus, to a limited degree, the descending aorta and oesphagus are mutually spiralized.

Surface anatomy. The vessel is projected as a band 2.5 cm broad from the sternal end of the second left costal cartilage to a median position about 2 cm above the transpyloric plane (p. 1733).

Branches. The thoracic aorta provides visceral branches to the pericardium, lungs, bronchi, oesophagus and parietal branches to the thoracic wall.

Pericardial branches. A few small vessels: they are distributed to the posterior pericardial aspect.

Bronchial arteries. These vary in number, size and origin. Usually one *right bronchial artery*, from the third posterior intercostal or upper left bronchial artery, runs posteriorly on the right bronchus and its branches, supplying them, the pulmonary areolar tissue and the bronchopulmonary lymph nodes, pericardium and oesophagus. The *left bronchial arteries*, usually two, arise from the thoracic aorta, the upper near the fifth thoracic vertebra, the lower below the left bronchus. They run posteriorly to the left bronchus and are distributed as on the right. Cauldwell et al (1948) found this arrangement in 40% of 150 cadavers; less frequent (at about 20% each) were two left and two right bronchial arteries or one on each side, all direct branches of the thoracic aorta, arising near the third and fourth intercostal arteries. In about 10%, one left and two right bronchial arteries existed. Complex variations consisted chiefly of more numerous aortic branches. Very rarely a bronchial artery arose from the aortic arch.

Oesophageal arteries. These are four or five, which arise anteriorly from the aorta and descend obliquely to the oesophagus, forming a vascular chain on it which anastomoses above with the oesophageal branches of the inferior thyroid arteries and below with the ascending branches from the left phrenic and gastric.

Mediastinal branches. These are numerous small vessels supplying lymph nodes and areolar tissue in the posterior mediastinum.

Phrenic branches. These arise from the lower thoracic aorta and are distributed posteriorly to the superior diaphragmatic surface and anastomose with the musculophrenic and pericardiacophrenic arteries.

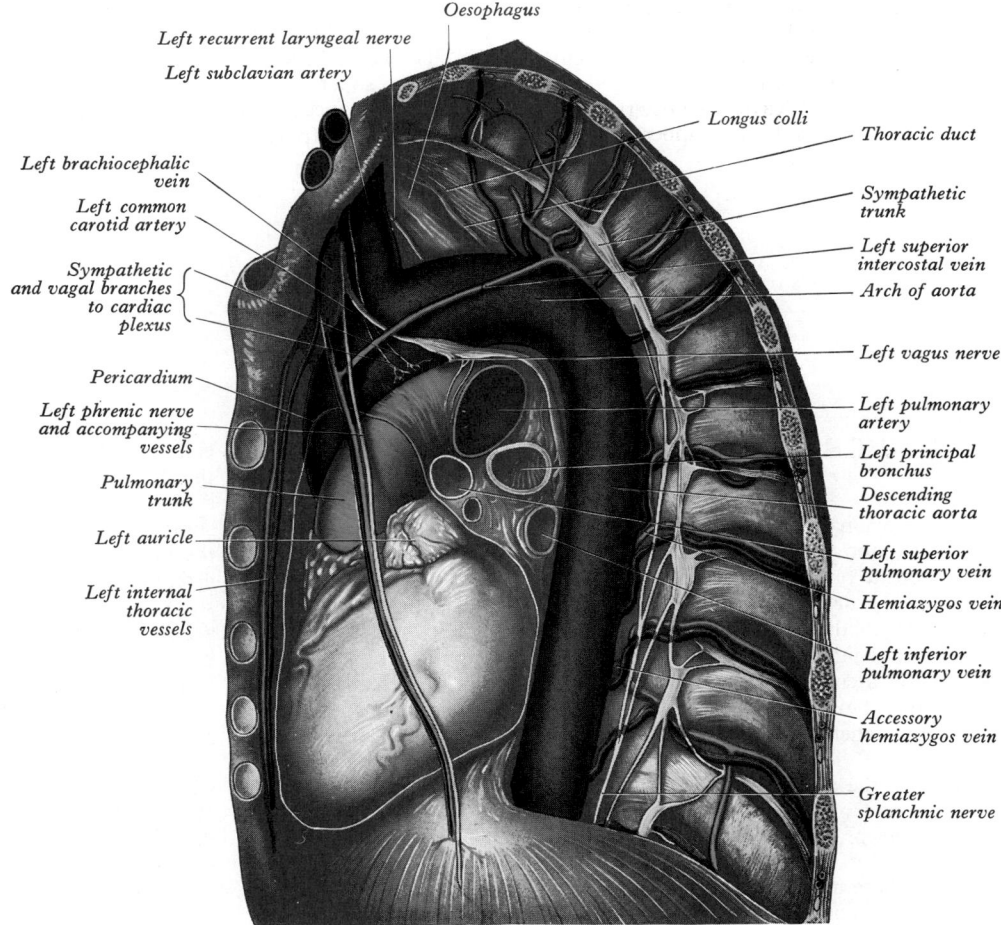

10.111   The left aspect of the mediastinum. The left lung and pleura have been removed and an extensive opening has been made into the pericardial sac to expose the heart. Note the oblique orientation of the thoracic inlet, and the forward inclination of the longus colli, upper oesophagus and thoracic duct.

Posterior intercostal arteries

Usually nine pairs of posterior intercostal arteries derive from the posterior aspect of the descending thoracic aorta. They are distributed to the lower nine intercostal spaces, the first and second being supplied by the superior intercostal artery (p. 1535). *Right posterior intercostal arteries* are longer, due to aortic deviation to the left; they cross the vertebral bodies behind the oesophagus, thoracic duct and azygos vein, right lung and pleura. *Left posterior intercostal arteries* turn backwards on the vertebral bodies in contact with the left lung and pleura, the upper two crossed by the left superior intercostal vein, the lower by the hemiazygos and accessory hemiazygos veins. Their further course is the same on both sides. Anterior to the heads of the ribs the sympathetic trunk descends in front of them and additionally the splanchnic nerves in front of the lower arteries.

Each artery crosses its intercostal space obliquely towards the angle of the rib above and continues forward in its costal groove (**10**.111). At first between the pleura and internal (posterior) intercostal membrane as far as the costal angle, it passes between the intercostalis internus and intercostalis intimus muscles (p. 815), anastomosing with an anterior intercostal branch from an internal thoracic or musculophrenic artery. It has a vein above and a nerve below, except in the upper spaces where the nerve is at first above the artery. The third anastomoses with the superior intercostal artery and may largely supply the second space. The lower two arteries continue anteriorly into the abdominal wall to anastomose with the subcostal, superior epigastric and lumbar arteries. Each posterior intercostal artery has dorsal, collateral, muscular and cutaneous branches.

Dorsal branch. This runs dorsally between the necks of adjoining ribs, with a vertebral body and a superior costotransverse ligament lying medial and lateral, respectively. It has a spinal branch entering the vertebral canal by the intervertebral foramen to supply vertebrae, spinal cord and meninges; it anastomoses with the spinal arteries above and below and with its fellow. It then crosses a transverse process with the dorsal branch of a thoracic spinal nerve to supply the dorsal muscles; a cutaneous twig accompanies the cutaneous branch of the spinal nerve's dorsal ramus.

Collateral intercostal branch. It leaves its posterior intercostal near the costal angle and descends to the upper border of the subjacent rib, along which it courses to anastomose with an anterior intercostal branch of the internal thoracic or musculophrenic artery.

Muscular branches. These supply intercostal and pectoral muscles and the serratus anterior, anastomosing with the superior and lateral thoracic branches of the axillary artery. Lateral cutaneous branches accompany the same branches of the thoracic spinal nerves. Mammary branches from the vessels in the second to fourth spaces supply the pectoral muscles, skin and mammary tissue; they enlarge during lactation.

Unnamed branches. They supply all other tissues constituting the thoracic wall, e.g. costal periosteum, bone and bone marrow of ribs, tissues of synovial and synarthrodial joints and parietal pleura.

Right bronchial artery. It may arise from the right third posterior intercostal artery (see above).

Clinical anatomy. A thoracic puncture needle should not be introduced posteriorly medial to the costal angles, as the intercostal artery (and vein) crosses its space medial to this. Laterally, however, it is in the upper part of its intercostal space; therefore puncture should be through the **lateral** chest wall in the *lower* half of a space.

Subcostal arteries. The last paired branches of the thoracic aorta, in series with the posterior intercostal arteries, they are below the twelfth ribs. Each runs laterally anterior to the twelfth thoracic vertebral body and posterior to the splanchnic nerves, sympathetic trunk, pleura and diaphragm; the right is also posterior to the thoracic duct and azygos vein, the left to the accessory hemiazygos vein. Each then enters the abdomen posterior to the lateral arcuate ligament with the twelfth thoracic (subcostal) nerve at the lower border of the twelfth rib, anterior to quadratus lumborum and posterior to the kidney. The right artery courses posterior to the ascending colon, the left to its descending part. Piercing the aponeurosis of the transversus abdominis each proceeds between this and the obliquus internus, anastomosing with the superior epigastric, lower posterior intercostal and lumbar arteries. Each has a dorsal branch, distributed like those of the posterior intercostal arteries.

Aberrant artery. A small artery sometimes leaves the thoracic aorta on its right near the right bronchial. It ascends to the right behind the trachea and oesophagus and may anastomose with the right superior intercostal. It is a vestige of the right dorsal aorta (p. 316); occasionally it is enlarged as the first part of a right subclavian (p. 1530).

VARIATIONS OF THORACIC AORTA

The aortic lumen is occasionally partly or completely obliterated, above (preductal or infantile type), opposite or just beyond (postductal or adult type) the entry of the ductus arteriosus. The condition, *coarctation of the aorta*, is congenital; the ductus arteriosus may remain patent, but rarely compensates, systemic blood pressure being usually much higher than pulmonary.

In the *preductal* type, the coarctation's length is variable and may involve the left subclavian and even the brachiocephalic artery, with little scope for the development of an effective collateral circulation to regions distal to the stenosis. Many cases are incompatible with survival for more than a few months and surgical problems are great. However, coarctation may be restricted to a short segment between the brachiocephalic and left subclavian arteries, pressures in the left arm being lower than in the right; a collateral circulation may develop through branches of the brachiocephalic.

The *postductal* type of coarctation has been attributed to abnormal extension of the ductal tissue into the aortic wall, stenosing both vessels as the duct contracts after birth. This form can permit many years of normal life, allowing the development of an extensive collateral circulation to the aorta distal to the stenosis. High vascularity of the thoracic wall is important and clinically characteristic; many arteries arising indirectly from the aorta, proximal to the coarctation segment, anastomose with vessels connected with it distal to the block; these become greatly enlarged. In the anterior thoracic wall the thoraco-acromial, lateral thoracic and subscapular arteries from the axillary, the suprascapular from the subclavian and the first and second posterior intercostal arteries from the costocervical trunk anastomose with other posterior intercostal arteries; the internal thoracic artery and its terminal branches anastomose with the lower posterior intercostal and inferior epigastric arteries. Posterior intercostal arteries are always involved, and enlargement of their dorsal branches may eventually groove ('notch') the inferior margins of the ribs. The radiograph shadow of the enlarged left subclavian artery is also increased. Enlargement of the scapular vessels and anastomoses may lead to widespread interscapular pulsation (easily appreciated with the palm of the hand, and sometimes heard on auscultation).

ABDOMINAL AORTA

The abdominal aorta (**10**.112, 113, 115, 128) begins at the median, aortic hiatus of the diaphragm, anterior to the twelfth thoracic vertebra's inferior border and the thoracolumbar intervertebral symphysis ('disk'), descending anterior to the vertebrae to end at the fourth lumbar, a little left of the midline, by dividing into two common iliac arteries. It diminishes rapidly in calibre, since its branches are large. Measurements of casts of the abdominal aorta in 100 individuals, from 16–70 years, showed a widening with age. In males superior and inferior ends measured 9.8–14.1 mm and 8.1–14.6 mm; in females luminal diameters were 9.7–15.7 mm and 9.1–14.6 mm (Aleksandrowicz et al 1974). These values conflict with radiological observation of 61 adults (17–41 years) by Leithner et al (1975), who recorded 26 mm and 19 mm (averages) for both ends of the abdominal aorta; they also gave a mean value of 37 for the angle of aortic bifurcation. Dimensions are of interest in attempts to estimate a suspected hydrodynamic ('haemodynamic') factor in the genesis of atherosclerosis (Newman et al 1971; Lallemand & Newman 1973). Theoretically, the pressure pulse wave in arteries is reflected at any junction, at certain values of combined arterial luminal areas of the branch or branches relative to that of the parent vessel; this is the area ratio of a junction. At an equal bifurcation, such as the aortic, with an area ratio of 1:1.5, reflection of the pressure pulse wave is near to zero; the vessels are said to be 'matched'. Oscillations and possibly turbulence set up by 'mismatching' (at other ratios), perhaps also influenced by asymmetry of bifurcation, may cause intimal damage, predisposing to aortic atheroma. Luminal and other dimensions of the bifurcation may assume special significance, as may changes in these during life. Measurement of aortico–iliac junctions in humans, dogs and domestic fowls (free from vascular disease) has shown area ratios usually close to the theoretical value for 'matching' and independent of age in dog and fowl (Gosling et al 1971). However, the human aortic bifurcation appears to be 'matched' only in infancy; it is 1.11 ± 0.02 at birth, diminishing with advancing age to a value of about 0.7 in the fifth decade, at which theory predicts a 'mismatch' reflecting pulse pressure wave at about one-third of its amplitude. These studies give special interest to a study of the geometry of aortic bifurcation by Shah et al (1978), containing the most extensive data so far recorded, including diameters and angles of deviation, iliac lengths and curvatures and dorsal angulations of these vessels as they enter the pelvis. Unfortunately, diameters were external and only on a small series of cadavers at autopsy, and cannot be compared with those cited above. These interesting observations should be carried further with improved techniques and greater cohesion between different groups involved.

Relations. The abdominal aorta has at first **anterior** to it the coeliac trunk and its branches, with the coeliac plexus and the lesser sac (omental bursa) which intervenes between it and the hepatic papillary process and lesser omentum. Below this the superior mesenteric artery leaves the aorta, crossing anterior to the left renal vein. The body of the pancreas, with splenic vein applied posteriorly, extends obliquely up and left across the abdominal aorta, separated from it by the superior mesenteric artery and left renal vein. Below the pancreas, the proximal parts of its testicular (or ovarian) arteries, and the horizontal part of the duodenum are anterior. In its lowest part it is covered by the posterior parietal peritoneum and crossed by the oblique parietal attachment of the mesentery.

Posterior to the abdominal aorta are the thoracolumbar intervertebral 'disk', the upper four lumbar vertebrae, intervening intervertebral discs and the anterior longitudinal ligament. Lumbar arteries, arising from its dorsal aspect, and the third and fourth (sometimes second) left lumbar veins, crossing behind it to reach the inferior vena cava, separate it from the ligament. It may overlap the anterior border of the left psoas major.

On the right the aorta is related above to the cisterna chyli and thoracic duct, azygos vein and right crus of diaphragm, which overlaps and separates it from the inferior vena cava and right coeliac ganglion. Below the second lumbar vertebra it adjoins the inferior vena cava.

On the left it is related above to the left diaphragmatic crus and left coeliac ganglion. Level with the second lumbar vertebra are the duodenojejunal flexure and sympathetic trunk descending, at its left side, and the ascending duodenum and inferior mesenteric vessels.

Surface anatomy. The vessel is indicated by a band about 2 cm wide from a median level 2.5 cm above the transpyloric plane to one about 1 cm below and left of the umbilicus. When the abdominal wall

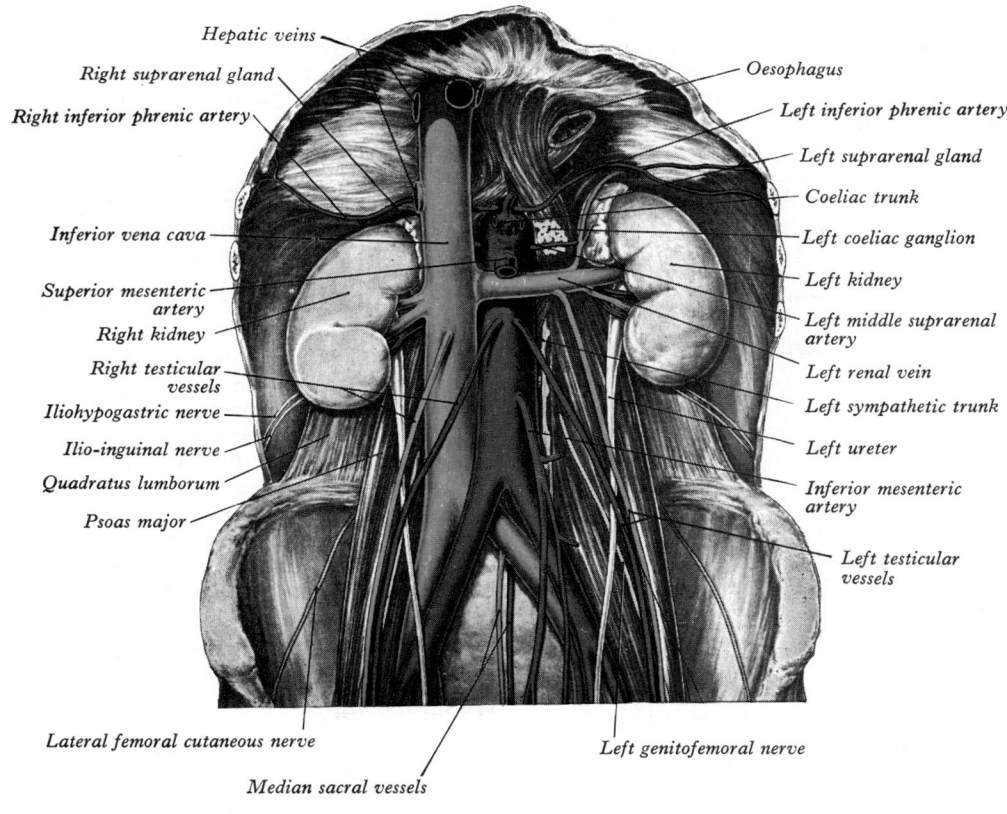

Hepatic veins

Right suprarenal gland

Right inferior phrenic artery

Inferior vena cava

Superior mesenteric artery

Right kidney

Right testicular vessels

Iliohypogastric nerve

Ilio-inguinal nerve

Quadratus lumborum

Psoas major

Oesophagus

Left inferior phrenic artery

Left suprarenal gland

Coeliac trunk

Left coeliac ganglion

Left kidney

Left middle suprarenal artery

Left renal vein

Left sympathetic trunk

Left ureter

Inferior mesenteric artery

Left testicular vessels

Lateral femoral cutaneous nerve

Median sacral vessels

Left genitofemoral nerve

10.112   The abdominal aorta and its branches in the male.

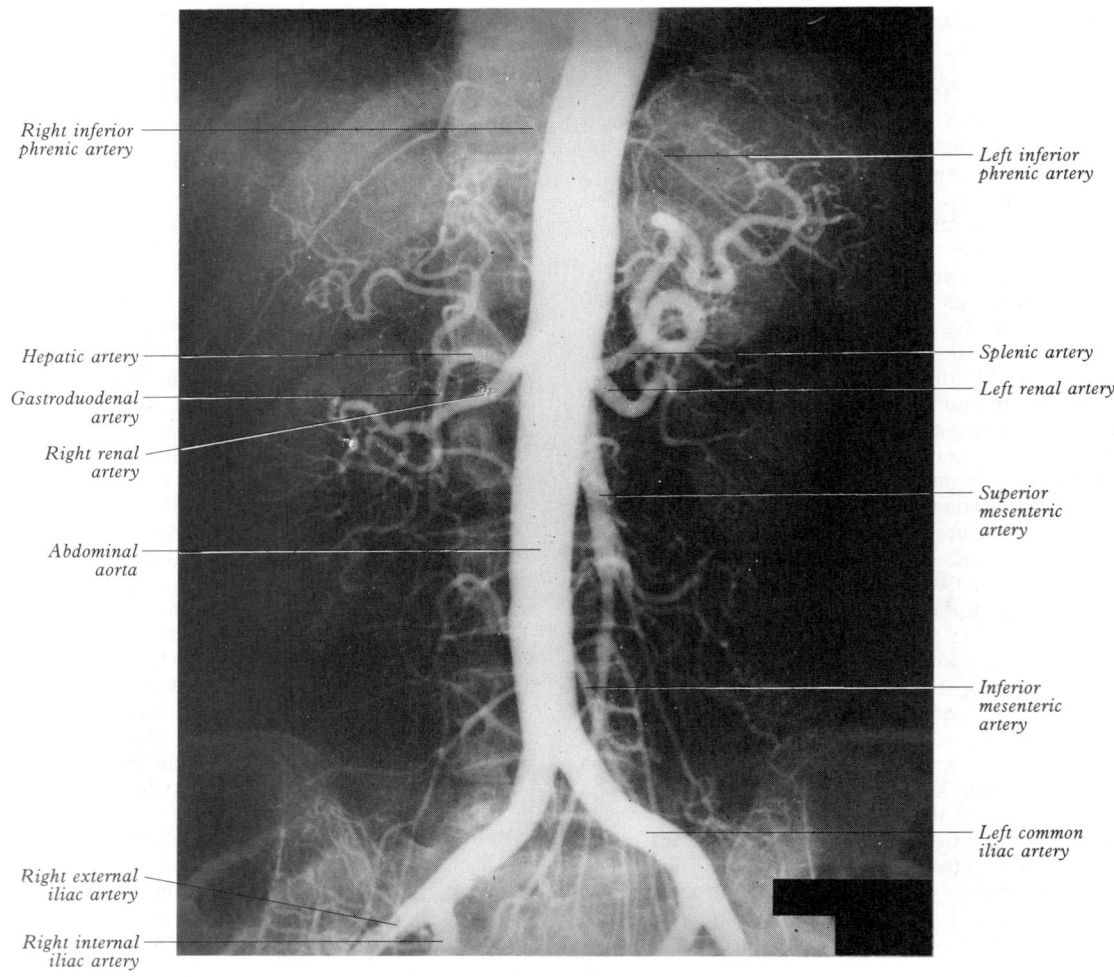

Right inferior phrenic artery

Left inferior phrenic artery

Hepatic artery

Splenic artery

Gastroduodenal artery

Left renal artery

Right renal artery

Abdominal aorta

Superior mesenteric artery

Inferior mesenteric artery

Left common iliac artery

Right external iliac artery

Right internal iliac artery

10.113   Aorto-iliac angiogram. (Supplied by Shaun Gallagher, Guy's Hospital; photography by Sarah Smith.)

is relaxed the aorta may be felt pulsating just above its bifurcation and its pulsation may be visible. This is frequently the case in thin subjects. An easily palpable aorta in someone who is obese should raise the suspicion of an aneurysm, to be checked by ultrasound scan.

Branches (**10**.112, 113)**.** These may be described as ventral, lateral, dorsal and terminal; ventral and lateral are distributed to the viscera, the dorsal branches supplying the body wall, vertebral column, canal and its contents:

Ventral: Coeliac, superior and inferior mesenteric
Dorsal: Lumbar and median sacral
Lateral: Inferior phrenic, middle suprarenal, renal, ovarian or testicular
Terminal: Common iliac.

COELIAC TRUNK

The coeliac trunk (**10**.114–117), a wide ventral branch, about 1.25 cm long, just below the aortic hiatus, passes almost horizontally forwards and slightly right above the pancreas and splenic vein, dividing into:

- *left gastric*
- *common hepatic*
- *splenic arteries.*

It may also give off one or both inferior phrenic arteries. The superior mesenteric may arise with the coeliac trunk, or the latter's usual branches may be direct independent branches of the aorta.

Relations. **Anterior** is the omental bursa (lesser sac); the coeliac plexus surrounds the trunk, sending extensions along its branches.

Right lateral are the right coeliac ganglion, right crus and hepatic caudate process; **left lateral** are the left coeliac ganglion, left crus and cardiac end of the stomach. The right crus may compress the origin of the coeliac trunk, giving the appearance of a stricture. Symptoms have been attributed to this (the 'coeliac axis compression syndrome'), and operations designed to relieve it, but the concept is of doubtful validity. **Inferior** are the pancreas and splenic vein. The duodenum's suspensory muscle (p. 1763) may encircle the coeliac artery but is usually on its left.

Left gastric artery

The left gastric artery, the smallest coeliac branch, ascends to the left, posterior to the omental bursa, to the cardiac end of the stomach (**10**.114, 115). It is near the left inferior phrenic artery and medial or anterior to the left suprarenal gland. Near the stomach two or three *oesophageal branches* ascend through the oesophageal opening to anastomose with the aortic oesophageal branches; others supply the cardiac part of the stomach and anastomose with the splenic branches. The artery then turns antero-inferiorly into the left gastro-pancreatic fold to run (often doubled) curving to the right near the gastric lesser curvature to the pylorus between layers of the lesser omentum; it supplies both gastric surfaces and anastomoses with the right gastric artery. An *accessory left gastric* artery may arise from the left branch of the hepatic, also reaching the lesser curvature through the lesser omentum.

Hepatic artery

The hepatic artery is intermediate in size between the left gastric and splenic arteries; but in **later** fetal and early postnatal life it is the largest coeliac branch (**10**.114–116, 118). Accompanied by the hepatic autonomic plexus it first passes forwards and right, below the epiploic

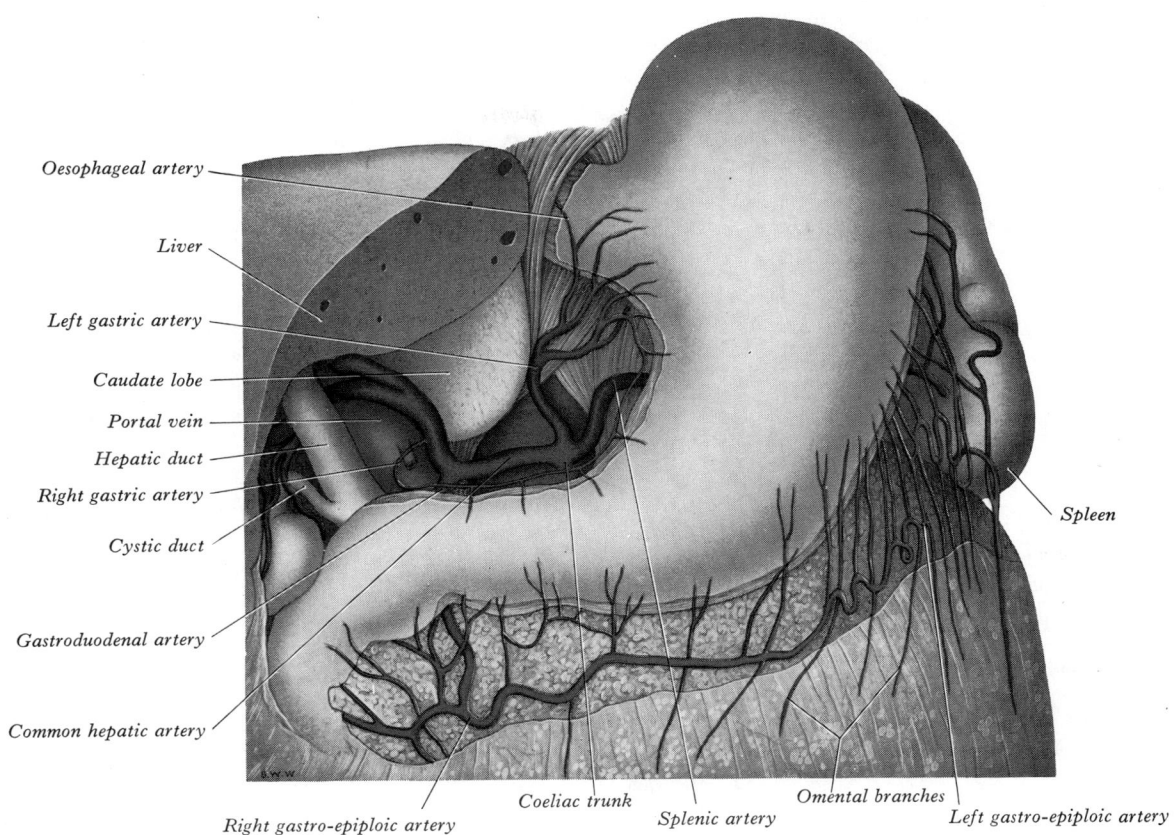

Oesophageal artery

Liver

Left gastric artery

Caudate lobe

Portal vein

Hepatic duct

Right gastric artery

Cystic duct

Gastroduodenal artery

Common hepatic artery

Spleen

Right gastro-epiploic artery

Coeliac trunk

Splenic artery

Omental branches

Left gastro-epiploic artery

10.114   The coeliac trunk and its branches. Part of the liver and all the lesser omentum have been removed, as well as the posterior wall of the omental bursa and part of the anterior layer of the greater omentum.

foramen to the upper aspect of the superior part of the duodenum (**10**.114). Crossing the portal vein, it ascends between layers of the lesser omentum, anterior to the epiploic foramen, to the porta hepatis, where it divides into right and left branches to the hepatic lobes, accompanying the ramifications of the portal vein and hepatic ducts. In the lesser omentum it is anterior to the portal vein and left of the bile duct, its right branch crossing posterior (occasionally anterior) to the common hepatic duct (**10**.115). The artery may be subdivided into:

- the *common hepatic artery*, from the coeliac trunk to the origin of the gastroduodenal artery
- the *hepatic artery proper*, from that point to its bifurcation.

In embryonic and early fetal life, the hepatic artery arises from the left gastric (in 67% of 56 individuals; Godlewski et al 1975). This condition rarely persists, but the hepatic may arise from the superior mesenteric, or the hepatic's right or left branches may be from other vessels; the former from the superior mesenteric, the latter from the left gastric. For other variations consult Quain (1865, 1899) and Woodburne (1962) (see also pp. 1550, 1810). The hepatic artery has right gastric, gastroduodenal and cystic branches, branches to the bile duct from the right hepatic and sometimes the supraduodenal artery (see below).

Right gastric artery (**10**.114). It arises above the duodenum's superior part, usually before, or sometimes beyond the gastro-duodenal, descending in the lesser omentum to the pyloric end of the stomach; it passes left along the lesser gastric curvature, supplying the upper parts of the anterior and posterior gastric surfaces. It ends by anastomosing with the left gastric; the supraduodenal artery may be a branch (see below).

Gastroduodenal artery (**10**.114–116). Arising behind, sometimes above, the superior part of the duodenum, it is short and wide. It descends between the duodenum and the neck of the pancreas, immediately to the right of the peritoneal reflection from the posterior duodenal surface. It is usually left of the bile duct but sometimes anterior. At the lower border of the duodenum's superior part it divides into the *right gastro-epiploic* and *superior pancreaticoduodenal* arteries, after supplying small branches to the pyloric end of the stomach and to the pancreas, retroduodenal branches to the superior part of the duodenum, and sometimes providing the supraduodenal artery (see below). The first branch of the common hepatic artery is usually the gastroduodenal artery, but this may come from the superior mesenteric, coeliac trunk or an aberrant right hepatic artery (p. 1552); its most invariable feature is its intermediate position between the **neck** of the pancreas and the duodenum, this being clinically important due to its frequent involvement in duodenal ulceration (Bradley 1973).

The *supraduodenal artery*, sometimes double, is variable; it may arise from the gastroduodenal, hepatic (common, proper or the latter's branches) or from the right gastric artery. It supplies the superior half circumference of the proximal half or more of the duodenum's superior part; but the duodenum is often invaded proximally by branches of the right gastric artery (p. 1765).

Right gastro-epiploic artery (**10**.114, 115, 118). The larger terminal branch of the gastroduodenal, it skirts the right margin of the omental bursa and then turns left along the greater curvature, between the (anterior two) layers of the greater omentum. It ends in direct anastomosis with the left gastro-epiploic branch of the splenic. Except at the pylorus, where it adjoins the stomach, it is about 2 cm from the greater curvature. Of its many branches some ascend to both gastric surfaces, others descend into the greater omentum. It also supplies the inferior aspect of the duodenum's superior part.

Superior pancreaticoduodenal arteries (**10**.115). These are usually double: the *anterior* descends anteriorly between the duodenum and head of the pancreas. It supplies both, and anastomoses with the anterior division of the inferior pancreaticoduodenal branch of the superior mesenteric. The *posterior superior pancreaticoduodenal artery*, which is usually a separate branch of the gastroduodenal arising at the upper border of the superior part of the duodenum, descends to the right, anterior to the portal vein and bile duct and

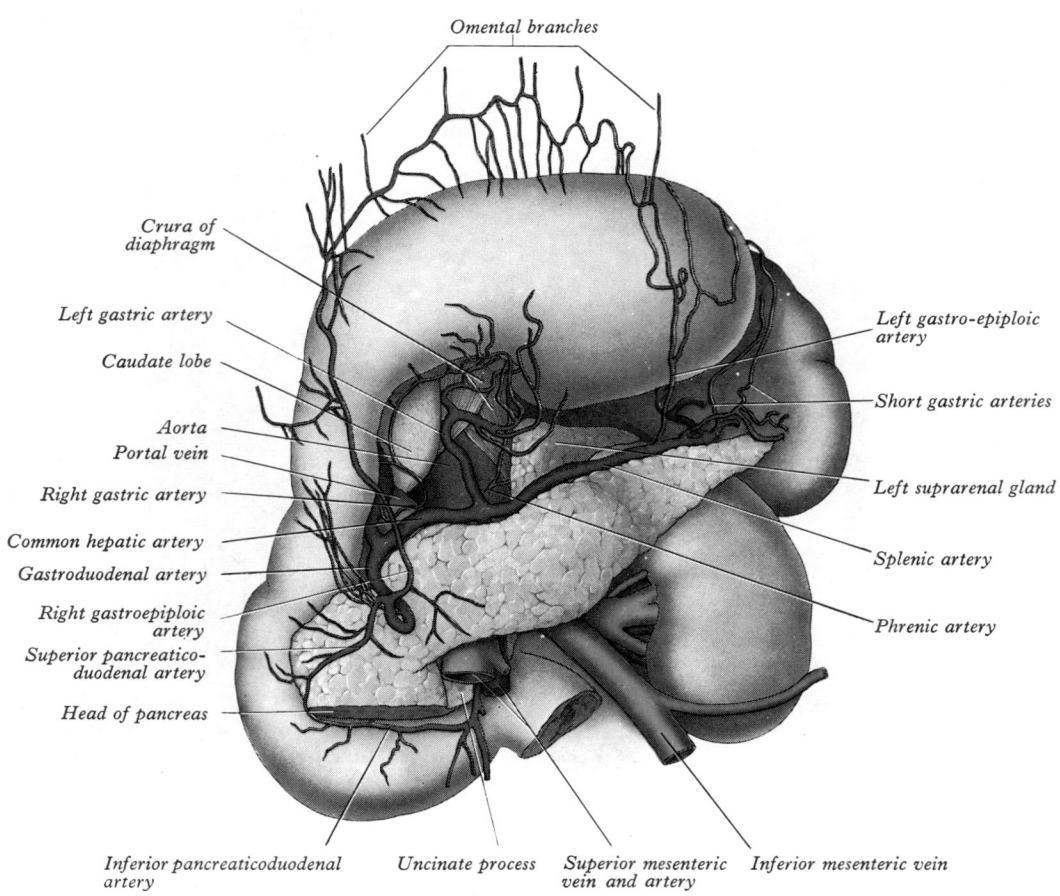

Omental branches

Crura of diaphragm

Left gastric artery

Caudate lobe

Aorta
Portal vein
Right gastric artery

Common hepatic artery
Gastroduodenal artery

Right gastroepiploic artery
Superior pancreatico-duodenal artery

Head of pancreas

Left gastro-epiploic artery

Short gastric arteries

Left suprarenal gland

Splenic artery

Phrenic artery

Inferior pancreaticoduodenal artery   Uncinate process   Superior mesenteric vein and artery   Inferior mesenteric vein

10.115   The coeliac trunk and its branches exposed by turning the stomach upwards and removing the peritoneum on the posterior abdominal wall.

then posterior to the head of the pancreas, supplying branches to it and the duodenum; it crosses posterior to the bile duct, piercing the duodenal wall to end by anastomosing with the posterior division of the inferior pancreaticoduodenal artery. The artery supplies several branches to the lower part of the common bile duct (p. 1810).

Cystic artery (10.118). Usually from the right branch of the hepatic proper, it passes behind the common hepatic and over the cystic duct to the superior aspect of the gallbladder's neck, on which it descends to divide into *superficial* and *deep* branches. The former ramifies on the inferior, the latter on the superior aspect. The cystic artery may arise from the hepatic artery itself (rarely from the gastroduodenal), crossing anterior or posterior to the bile or common hepatic duct to reach the gallbladder. Direct origin from the hepatic artery varies from its beginning to its bifurcation. An *accessory cystic artery* may arise from the common hepatic or one of its branches. The cystic artery supplies the hepatic ducts and upper part of the common bile duct (p. 1810). A comparative study of its distribution in various reptilian, avian and mammalian species included 74 injected and cleared human gallbladders (Gordon 1967). The cystic artery in man reaches the gallbladder at its neck but is not in contact with the cystic duct.

Anteriorly, two to five ascending vessels arise from the retro-duodenal branch of the gastroduodenal artery, as it crosses the anterior surface of the duct at the upper border of the duodenum. Three or four descending branches of the right hepatic and cystic arteries arise from them as these vessels pass close to the lower common hepatic duct. These ascending and descending arteries form long narrow anastomotic channels along the length of the duct, which are roughly disposed into medial and lateral trunks which some authors have described as 'three o'clock and nine o'clock' vessels. From the point of view of applied anatomy, the surgeon should dissect very carefully this area, and should keep the vessels under close endoscopic control.

Posteriorly, the 'retroportal artery' arises from the coeliac axis or superior mesenteric artery (or one of their major branches) close to the origin from the aorta, and runs upwards on the back of the portal vein. It can end in two different ways. In 20% of cases it passes up behind the bile duct to join the right hepatic artery, but in the majority it ends by joining the retroduodenal artery close to

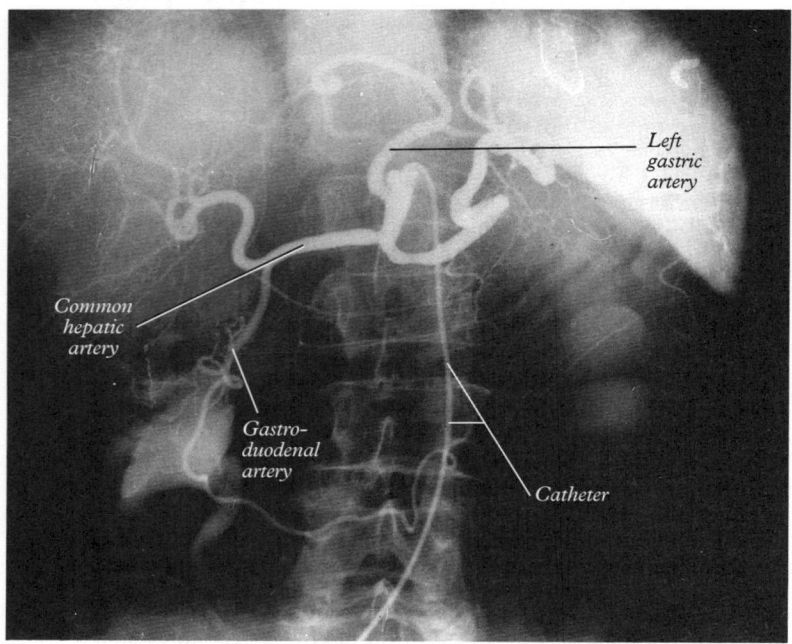

Left gastric artery

Common hepatic artery

Gastro-duodenal artery

Catheter

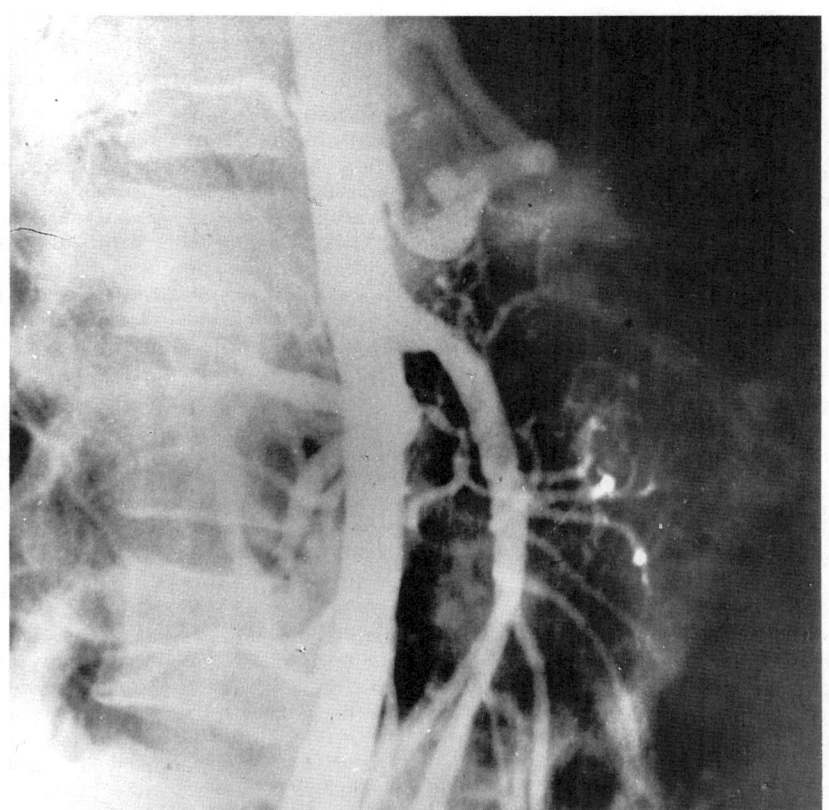

10.117   The origin of the coeliac trunk is compressed by the median arcuate ligament of the diaphragm, formed by the right crus.

the lower end of the supraduodenal bile duct. When present, the retroportal artery plays a definite role in the blood supply of the supraduodenal duct system.

Terminal, intrahepatic branches. These display a pattern of branching relatively constant in its major details (p. 1797), which justifies a segmental description of the liver; it is the result, as in other organs, of growth and branching of an epithelial blastema, its pattern accompanied by vascular branches and nerve trunks. Arterial hepatic segmentation is described on page 1798. Consult also Woodburne (1962).

Splenic artery

The largest branch of the coeliac axis, the splenic is remarkably tortuous (**10**.114–116). Surrounded by a splenic nerve plexus and accompanied by the straight splenic vein, it ascends to the left, behind the stomach and omental bursa, along the superior border of the pancreas; it is anterior to the left suprarenal gland and upper part of the left kidney and enters the lienorenal ligament. Nearing the spleen it divides into five or more *segmental* branches which enter its hilum (p. 1438).

Branches of the splenic artery are as follows:

Pancreatic branches (**10**.115). Numerous and small, they supply the neck, body and tail of the pancreas, leaving the splenic artery as it runs along its superior border. A *dorsal branch* (sometimes from the superior mesenteric, middle colic, hepatic or, more rarely, coeliac artery) descends posterior to the pancreas, dividing into right and left branches. The former, usually double, runs between the neck and uncinate process to form a *prepancreatic arterial arch* with a branch from the anterior superior pancreaticoduodenal; the left branch runs along the inferior border to the pancreatic tail; it anastomoses with branches (*arteria pancreatica magna* and *arteria caudae pancreatis*) from the splenic artery which supply the left part of the body and the tail.

Short gastric arteries (**10**.115). Five to seven, these arise terminally from the splenic and its final divisions or from the left gastro-epiploic artery. They pass between layers of the gastrosplenic

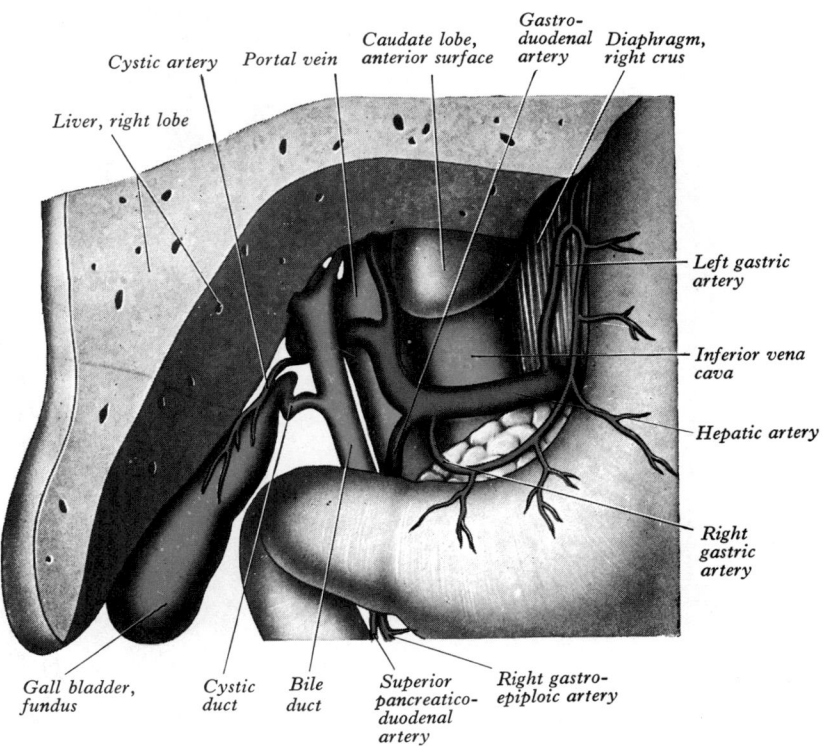

10.118   The relations of the hepatic artery, bile duct and portal vein exposed by removal of the lesser omentum and the peritoneum on the posterior abdominal wall.

ligament to supply the gastric fundus, anastomosing with branches of the left gastric and gastro-epiploic arteries.

Posterior gastric artery. This arises from any part of the splenic but most commonly its middle section; it has been described by many authorities (e.g. Quain 1844) but many subsequent texts have omitted it. Susuki et al (1978), also surveying reports on it, found it present in 38 (62.3%) of 61 adult cadavers; the incidence from 14 reports (1904–1968) varied from 12.7 to 77%, with an average of 58% in a total of 870 cadavers. They described the vessel as ascending behind the peritoneum of the omental bursa towards the gastric fundus to reach the posterior gastric wall in the gastrophrenic fold; it was usually about 2 mm in diameter.

Left gastro-epiploic artery (10.114, 115). The splenic's largest branch, it arises near the splenic hilum and runs antero-inferiorly and right, sending branches through the gastrosplenic ligament to supply the proximal third of the greater curvature; these are necessarily longer than the gastric branches of the right gastro-epiploic artery and may be 8–10 cm long. A large terminal omental branch descends to the right in the greater omentum. The main vessel curves forwards at a higher level to join the right gastro-epiploic. This loop leaves part of the greater curvature devoid of branches. At partial gastrectomy the greater omentum is divided below the right gastro-epiploic artery, cutting all omental branches; the greater omentum survives because its supply from this large omental branch of left gastro-epiploic usually escapes damage (Horton 1952). Vessels supplying the greater omentum are epiploic (omental) branches of the right and left gastro-epiploic arteries. The right, middle and left colic arteries do not supply the greater omentum; the transverse mesocolon, though usually adherent to the greater omentum, is separable from it (p. 1743).

Terminal splenic branches. These enter the hilum in the lieno-renal ligament. Their distribution is described with the spleen (p. 1439).

Variations of the splenic and hepatic arteries

Variations in the arrangement of these arteries and their branches are common and surgically important. They include:

- the origin of the common hepatic from the superior mesenteric or, less often, from the aorta; it usually passes behind the portal vein to enter the lesser omentum
- an *accessory left hepatic artery* most often from the left gastric artery passing right in the lesser omentum to the porta hepatis, and easily damaged during partial gastrectomy
- an *accessory right hepatic artery* most often from the superior mesenteric, usually running behind the portal vein and bile duct in the lesser omentum to the porta hepatis.

Accessory left or right hepatic arteries may also arise from the gastroduodenal or aorta. They may be combined with 'normal' branches of the hepatic artery or replace them as the sole supply to parts of the liver, being called '*aberrant replacing arteries*'.

Clinical anatomy

Collateral circulation after hepatic ligature or obstruction: although blockage of the hepatic artery may lead to necrosis, this is by no means inevitable, because some two-thirds of the oxygen demands of the liver are met by the portal vein. The effect will depend on the site of the block. Occlusion of the common hepatic artery, proximal to the origin of the right gastric, allows collateral circulation to the liver through the left and right gastric, left and right gastro-epiploic, pancreaticoduodenal and gastroduodenal arteries, and so necrosis is unlikely. If, however, an obstruction of the hepatic artery proper occurs beyond the origin of the gastroduodenal artery, any collateral circulation is limited to the small inferior phrenic arteries (p. 1558).

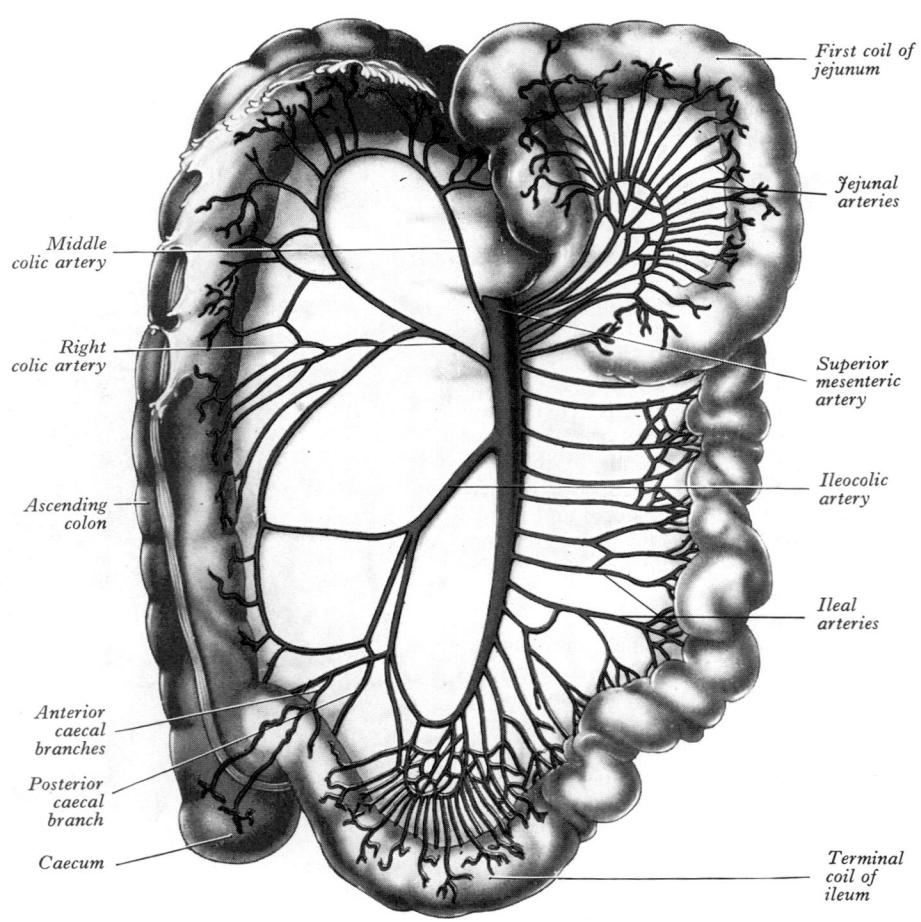

First coil of jejunum

Jejunal arteries

Middle colic artery

Right colic artery

Superior mesenteric artery

Ileocolic artery

Ascending colon

Ileal arteries

Anterior caecal branches

Posterior caecal branch

Caecum

Terminal coil of ileum

10.119 The superior mesenteric artery and its branches. The first coil of the jejunum and the terminal coil of the ileum have been spread out to show the arrangement of their arteries.

If, of course, the portal vein has been compromised as a result of thrombosis or of surgery, then the liver is entirely dependent on the hepatic artery for its survival.

SUPERIOR MESENTERIC ARTERY

The superior mesenteric artery (**10**.119–121) is by far the most important of the arteries to the alimentary tract, as it supplies the whole of the small intestine from the superior part of the duodenum to the midtransverse colon, and is functionally an end artery. It leaves the front of the aorta about 1 cm below the coeliac trunk, at the level of the L1–L2 vertebral disk, and is crossed anteriorly by the splenic vein and the body of the pancreas, separated from the aorta by the left renal vein. It runs downwards and forwards, anterior to the uncinate process, and passes in front of the transverse part of the duodenum. This can sometimes be seen on a radiograph as an area of translucency, running across the duodenum, and was at one time thought to represent a sphincter (the sphincter of Ochsner) to which all manner of symptoms were attributed. Endoscopy has disproved this concept. As it descends in the root of the small bowel mesentery, the artery crosses in front of the inferior vena cava, the right ureter, and psoas major, becoming steadily narrower in its course, and eventually joins its own ileocolic branch. It is accompanied by the superior mesenteric vein and is surrounded by a plexus of nerves. A fibrous strand from the region of its last branch runs to the umbilicus, and represents a vestige of the embryonic artery which originally connected it to the yolk sac.

Inferior pancreaticoduodenal artery (**10**.115). It leaves the superior mesenteric, or its first jejunal branch, near the superior border of the horizontal part of the duodenum, usually dividing at once into anterior and posterior branches. The *anterior branch* passes to the right, anterior to the head of the pancreas, and ascends to anastomose with the anterior superior pancreaticoduodenal artery. The *posterior branch* ascends to the right, posterior to the head of the pancreas, which it sometimes traverses, and then anastomoses with the posterior superior pancreaticoduodenal artery. Both branches supply the pancreatic head, its uncinate process and the adjoining duodenum.

Jejunal and ileal branches (**10**.119, 120). These arise from the left side of the superior mesenteric; usually 12–15 are distributed to the jejunum and ileum, except in the latter's terminal part, which is supplied by the ileocolic artery. They run almost parallel in the mesentery, each dividing to unite with adjacent branches in a series of arches (**10**.119). Branches from these unite to form a second series and this may be repeated three or four times. In the short, upper part of the mesentery one set of arches exists but, as the mesentery increases in depth, a second, third, fourth and even fifth series appear. From the terminal arches numerous *straight* vessels supply

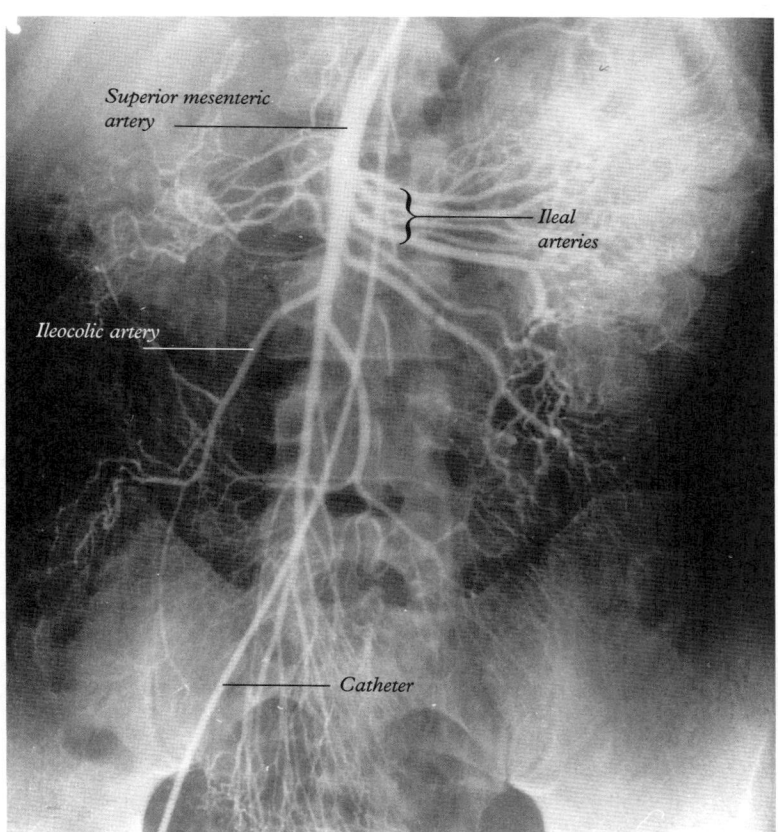

10.120 A superior mesenteric arteriogram with filling of ileal arteries (including several small branches) and of the ileocolic artery.

the intestine, distributed alternately to opposite aspects of its wall. Adjacent branches do not anastomose. Jejunal arteries are longer and fewer in number. Small twigs supply regional lymph nodes and other structures in the mesentery.

Ileocolic artery (**10**.119). The last branch from the right side of the superior mesenteric, it descends to the right under the parietal peritoneum to the right iliac fossa, where it divides; its *superior branch* anastomoses with the right colic, the inferior with the end of the superior mesenteric. The ileocolic artery crosses anterior to the right ureter, testicular or ovarian vessels and psoas major. Its *inferior branch* approaches the superior border of the ileocolic junction and branches as follows (**10**.119, 122):

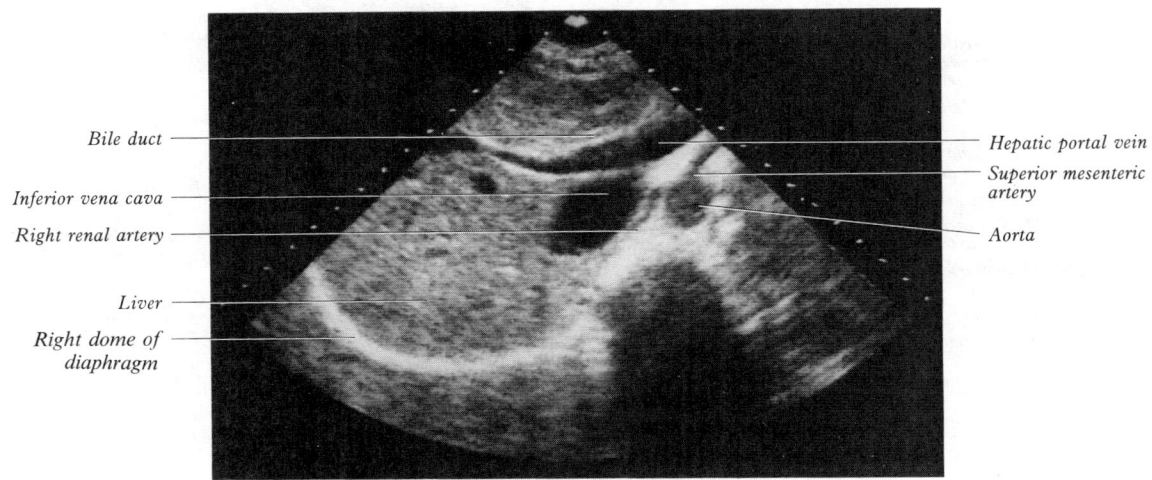

10.121 Ultrasonogram through the origin of the superior mesenteric artery. (Provided by Shaun Gallagher, Guy's Hospital; photography by Sarah Smith.)

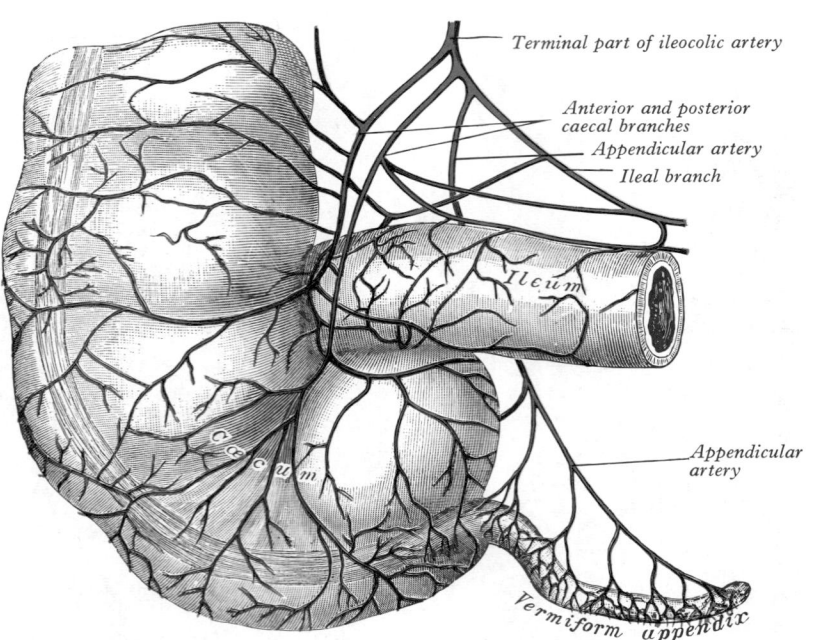

10.122   The arteries of the caecum and vermiform appendix.

* *ascending* (*colic*) passing up on the ascending colon
* *anterior* and *posterior caecal*
* an *appendicular artery*, descending behind the terminal ileum to enter the mesoappendix; after giving off a recurrent branch anastomosing with one from the posterior caecal artery, it runs

close to and then in the edge of the mesoappendix, its terminal part being in actual contact with the appendix

* an *ileal* branch ascending to the left on the lower ileum, supplying it and anastomosing with a terminal twig of the superior mesenteric artery.

Right colic artery (**10**.119). This is a small vessel and it may be absent. It arises near the middle of the superior mesenteric, or in common with the ileocolic and passes to the right behind the parietal peritoneum and anterior to the right ovarian or testicular artery and vein, right ureter and psoas major, towards the ascending colon. Sometimes it is higher and crosses the descending duodenum and right inferior renal pole. Near the colon it divides into a descending branch, which anastomoses with the ileocolic, and an ascending branch anastomosing with the middle colic. These form arches, from which vessels are distributed to the ascending colon, supplying its upper two-thirds and the right colic flexure.

Middle colic artery (**10**.119). It leaves the superior mesenteric just inferior to the pancreas; descending in the transverse mesocolon it divides into a right and left branch; the former anastomoses with the right colic artery, the latter with the left, a branch of *inferior* mesenteric. Arches thus formed are 3 or 4 cm from the transverse colon, which they supply.

Variations

The superior mesenteric artery may be the source of the common hepatic, gastroduodenal, accessory right hepatic, accessory pancreatic or splenic arteries. It may arise from a common coeliaco–mesenteric trunk (Mangoushi 1975).

INFERIOR MESENTERIC ARTERY

The inferior mesenteric artery (**10**.123–127) supplies the left third of the transverse colon, all the descending colon, sigmoid colon and most of the rectum. It is smaller than the superior mesenteric, arising

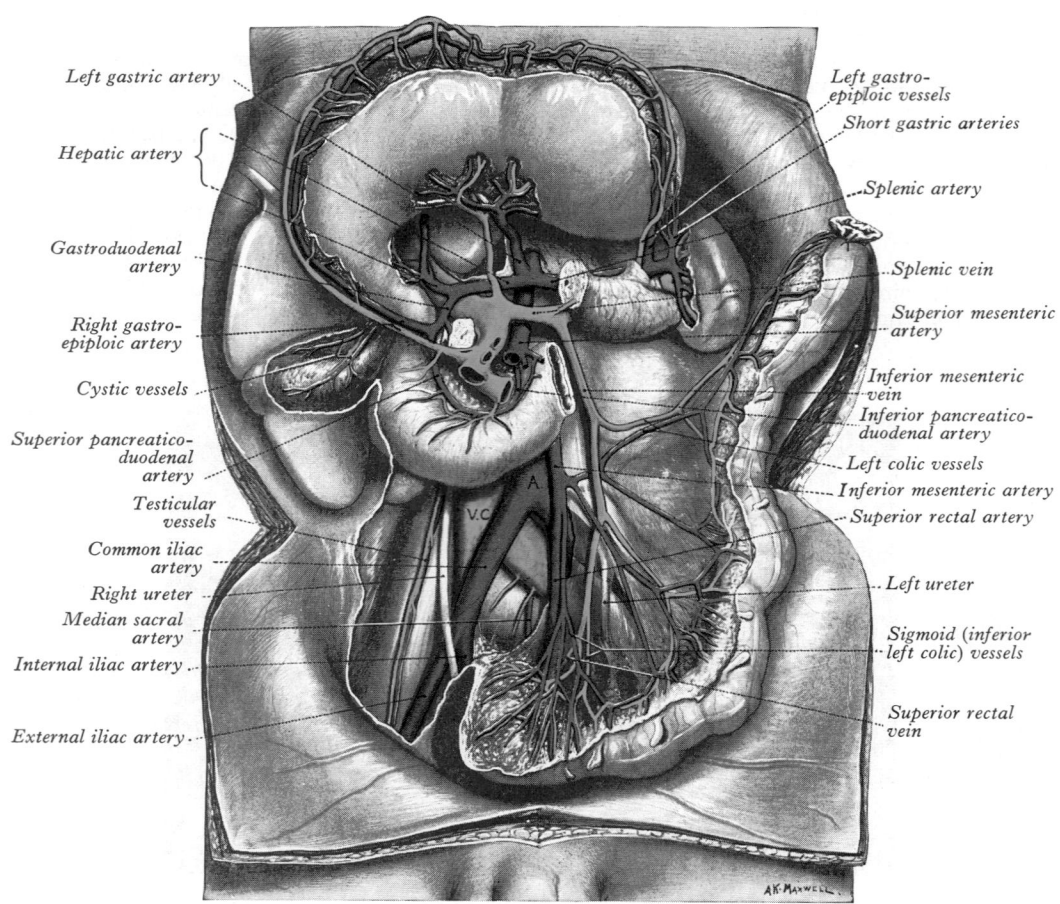

    10.123   The inferior mesenteric vessels and their branches (male subject). Note the stomach has been turned upwards and the whole of the jejunum and ileum, the caecum, ascending colon and transverse colon have been removed, together with part of the pancreas.

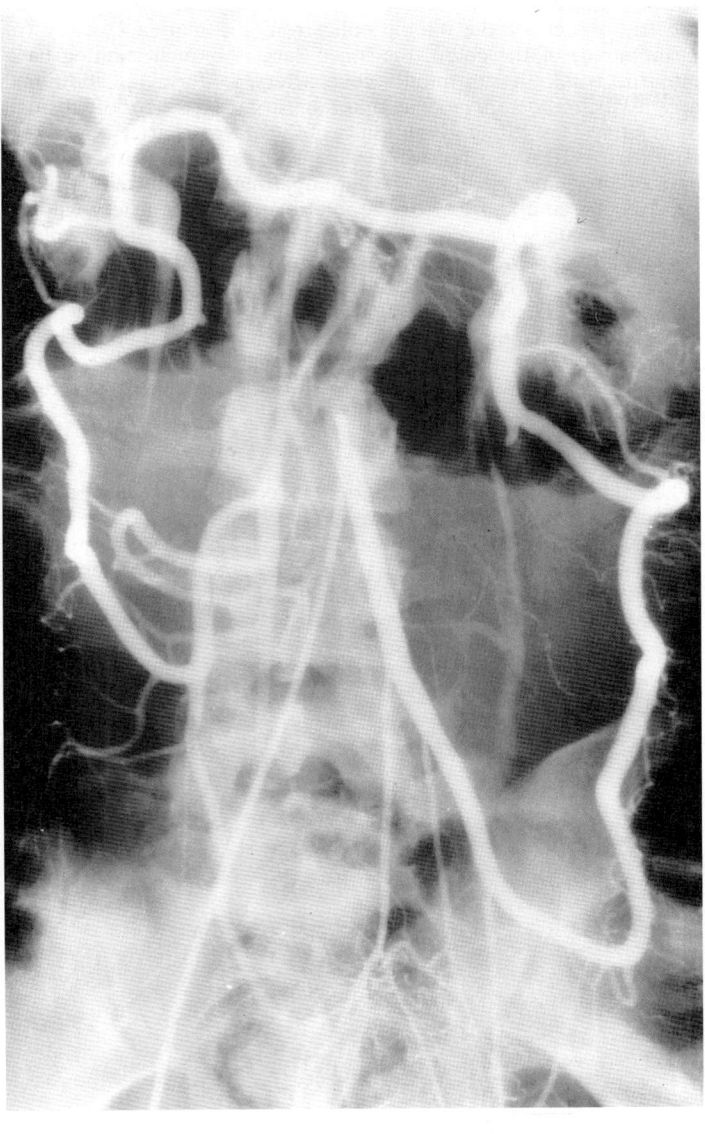

10.124 Inferior mesenteric arteriogram. When the superior mesenteric artery is blocked, the marginal artery to the colon enlarges and the inferior mesenteric artery then becomes the blood supply to the midgut.

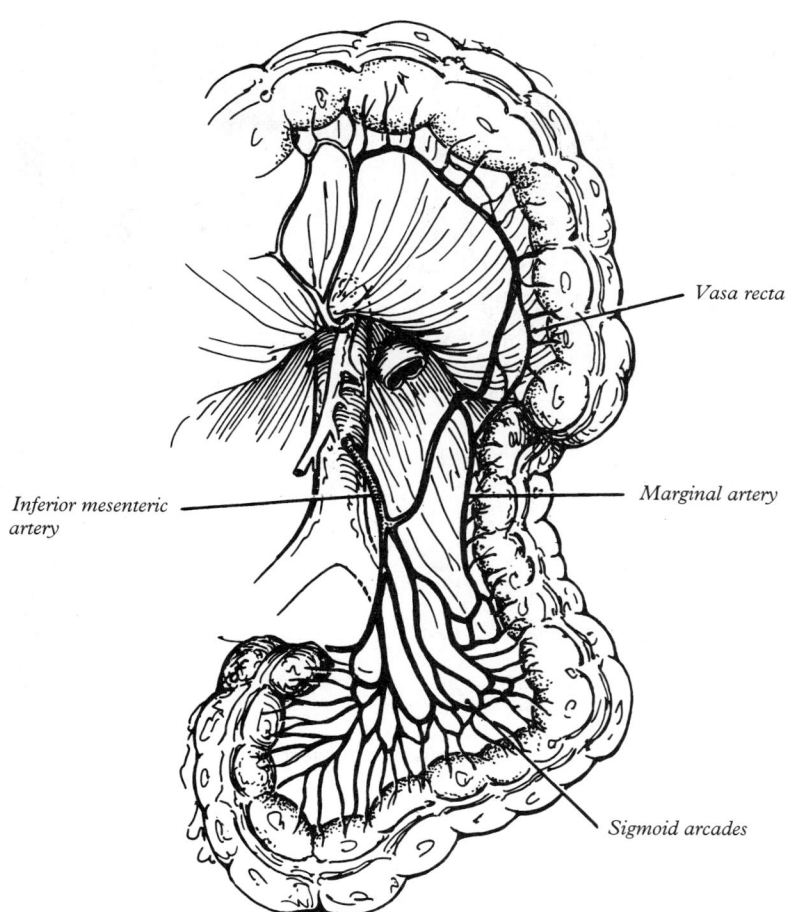

10.125 Sigmoid colon and rectum, showing the distribution of the branches of the inferior mesenteric artery and their anastomoses.

3 or 4cm above the aortic bifurcation, posterior to the horizontal part of the duodenum. It descends behind the peritoneum, at first anterior to the aorta, then on its left, crosses the left common iliac artery medial to the left ureter and then enters and continues in the sigmoid mesocolon into the lesser pelvis as the *superior rectal artery*. Distally the inferior mesenteric vein is lateral. The artery has left colic, sigmoid and superior rectal branches.

Left colic artery (10.123–127). It ascends subperitoneally to the left, anterior to the psoas major, and divides into ascending and descending branches. The trunk and its branches cross the left ureter and ovarian or testicular vessels. The ascending branch passes anterior to the left kidney into the transverse mesocolon, where it anastomoses with the middle colic artery; the descending branch anastomoses with the highest sigmoid artery. From arches thus formed, branches supply the left half of the transverse and the descending colon. Territories of supply by middle and left colic arteries show reciprocal variation; the left branch of the middle colic may take over the supply of the splenic flexure (in 19 of 100 cadavers, according to Sierociński 1975).

Sigmoid (inferior left colic) arteries (10.123–127). Two or three in number, they descend obliquely to the left under the peritoneum anterior to the left psoas major, ureter and testicular or ovarian vessels. Branches supply the lower descending colon and sigmoid colon, anastomosing above with the left colic artery, below with the superior rectal artery.

Superior rectal artery (10.123–126). A continuation of the inferior mesenteric, it descends into the pelvis in the sigmoid mesocolon, crossing the left common iliac vessels. It divides, near the third sacral vertebra, into two branches descending one on each side of the rectum; about halfway they divide into smaller branches, which pierce the muscular rectal wall to descend vertically, at submucosal level, to the sphincter ani internus; here, by mutual anastomoses, they form loops around the lower rectum, communicating with the middle rectal artery, a branch of the internal iliac, and with the inferior rectal from the internal pudendal (p. 1561).

Marginal artery of the colon. This is formed by the union of the three main colonic branches described above, which arise from the right side of the superior mesenteric artery and then continue around the splenic flexure to join the upward running left colic branch of the inferior mesenteric artery. This is an important vessel from the clinical point of view, because in the event of an occlusion of the two upper vessels (the coeliac trunk and the superior mesenteric artery) it represents the only surviving route of supply to the alimentary tract, flow proceeding retrograde from the inferior mesenteric artery to the superior mesenteric artery (see 10.124–126). The arrangement of vessels along the right colon is fairly constant, there being one marginal artery giving off *vasa recta* and *vasa brevia*, which occasionally communicate, although the anastomoses are less well developed than they are in the small bowel. It is at the point of junction of the superior and inferior mesenteric system (at the splenic flexure) that confusion and variability occur.

Relations

The inferior mesenteric artery divides into two or three branches, the uppermost of which (the left colic) almost always reaches the 1555

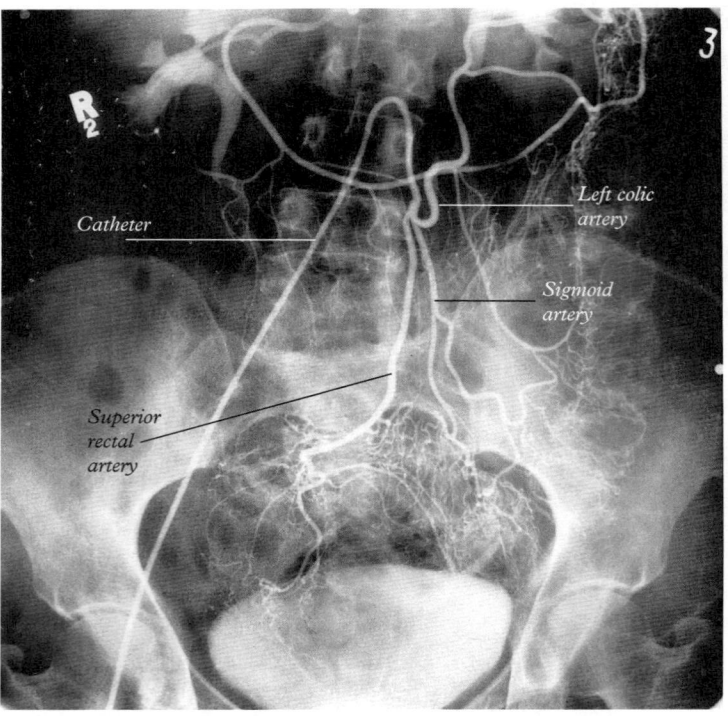

10.126   Arteriogram of the inferior mesenteric.

splenic flexure. Here it bifurcates, the slender outer branch joining the left branch of the middle colic from the marginal artery (of Drummond) of the colon, the inner (larger) branch running back into the trunk of the middle colic artery to form an additional arcade, the *arc of Riolan*. The outer anastomosis is here often small or incomplete, so that the continuity of the marginal artery is broken. If the arc of Riolan is not well developed, then there exists a critical area of anastomotic supply, so that impairment of flow either in the superior mesenteric artery or the inferior mesenteric artery will not be compensated, and ischaemic damage may ensue. This explains the relative frequency of ischaemic lesions in the region of the splenic flexure. It used to be taught that there was a critical point (of Sudek) between the last sigmoid branch and the first rectal branch of the superior haemorrhoidal artery, but that is now known not to be the case. The arterial anastomosis here is well-developed (see **10**.127) and if a critical point exists at all then it is at the splenic flexure, as already described.

Clinical anatomy

When the superior mesenteric artery is completely occluded, then the marginal artery to the colon may become enormously dilated (see **10**.124) as it is required to supply the whole of the midgut loop. Alternatively, occlusion of the aorta or common iliac arteries may result in a similar dilatation of the marginal artery, which then becomes an important source of collateral supply to the legs.

ANTEROLATERAL VISCERAL ARTERIES

Middle suprarenal arteries

These two small vessels arise laterally from each side of the aorta, level with the superior mesenteric, ascending slightly over the crura

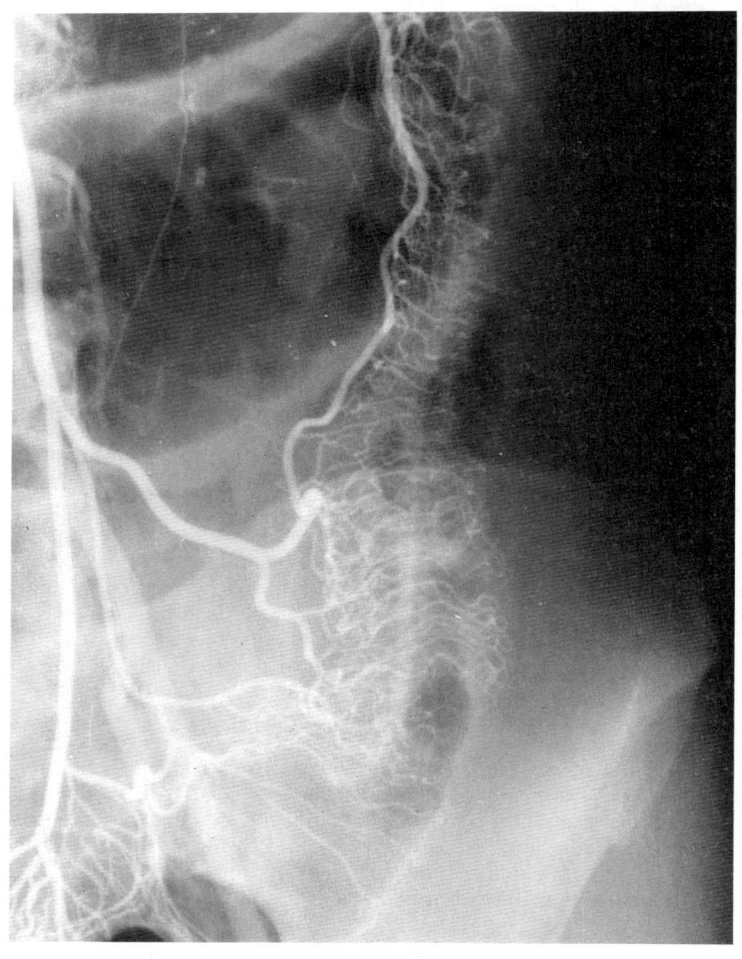

10.127   An inferior mesenteric arteriogram showing details of the intramural colonic circulation and the occurrence of good anastomotic connections around Sudek's point.

of the diaphragm to the suprarenal glands, where each anastomoses with the suprarenal branches of the phrenic and renal arteries. The right passes behind the inferior vena cava and near the right coeliac ganglion; the left is related to the left coeliac ganglion, splenic artery and superior border of the pancreas.

Renal arteries

These two large vessels branch laterally from the aorta just below the inferior mesenteric; both cross the corresponding crus at right angles to the aorta (**10**.112, 113, 128). The **right** is longer and often higher, passing posterior to the inferior vena cava, right renal vein, head of the pancreas and descending part of the duodenum. The **left** is a little lower; it passes behind the left renal vein, the body of the pancreas and splenic vein and may be crossed anteriorly by the inferior mesenteric vein. Nearing its renal hilum, each divides into four or five branches, most between the renal vein and ureteric pelvis, the vein being anterior, the pelvis posterior, but one or more usually behind the pelvis. Each renal artery supplies small *inferior suprarenal branches* (p. 204) and also the ureter, surrounding cellular tissue and muscles. The distribution of the renal arteries is described on page 1826.

Surface anatomy. The renal arteries can be projected as broad lines running laterally for 4 cm from the aorta (**10**.112) just inferior to the transpyloric plane; the left inclines across the plane.

Variations. One or two *accessory renal arteries* frequently occur, especially on the left, usually from the aorta above or below the main artery, the former slightly more often. They usually enter above or below the renal hilum; if below, the vessel crosses anterior to the ureter and, on the right, usually also anterior to the inferior vena cava.

Testicular arteries

These two long, slender vessels arise anteriorly from the aorta a little inferior to the renal arteries (**10**.112, 113, 128). Each passes inferolaterally under the parietal peritoneum on the psoas major; the *right* lies anterior to the inferior vena cava and posterior to the horizontal part of the duodenum, right colic and ileocolic arteries, root of the mesentery and terminal ileum; the *left* testicular artery lies posterior to the inferior mesenteric vein, left colic artery and lower part of the descending colon. Each crosses anterior to the genitofemoral nerve, ureter and the lower part of the external iliac artery, passing to the deep inguinal ring to enter the spermatic cord with other constituents, via which the vessel traverses the inguinal canal to the scrotum. At the posterosuperior aspect of the testis it divides into two branches on its medial and lateral surfaces, which pass through its tunica albuginea to ramify in the tunica vasculosa. Terminal branches enter the testis over its surface. Some pass into the mediastinum testis and loop back before reaching their distribution (Harrison & Barclay 1948). In the abdomen the testicular artery supplies perirenal fat, ureter and iliac lymph nodes; in the inguinal canal it supplies the cremaster.

Sometimes the right testicular artery passes **posterior** to the inferior vena cava. Both arteries represent persistent lateral splanchnic aortic branches (p. 318) which enter the mesonephros and cross ventral to the supracardinal but dorsal to the subcardinal vein. Normally the lateral splanchnic artery which persists as the *right* testicular passes **caudal** to the suprasubcardinal anastomosis forming part of the inferior vena cava (p. 318). When it passes **cranial** to this, the right testicular artery is behind the inferior vena cava.

Clinical anatomy. The testicular artery is not the sole supply to the testis, which also receives some blood from the cremasteric branch of the inferior epigastric artery (see p. 1563). Thus interference with the testicular artery high in the abdomen usually leaves the testis unharmed, whereas interruption in the region of the spermatic cord involves both sets of vessels and leads to infarction.

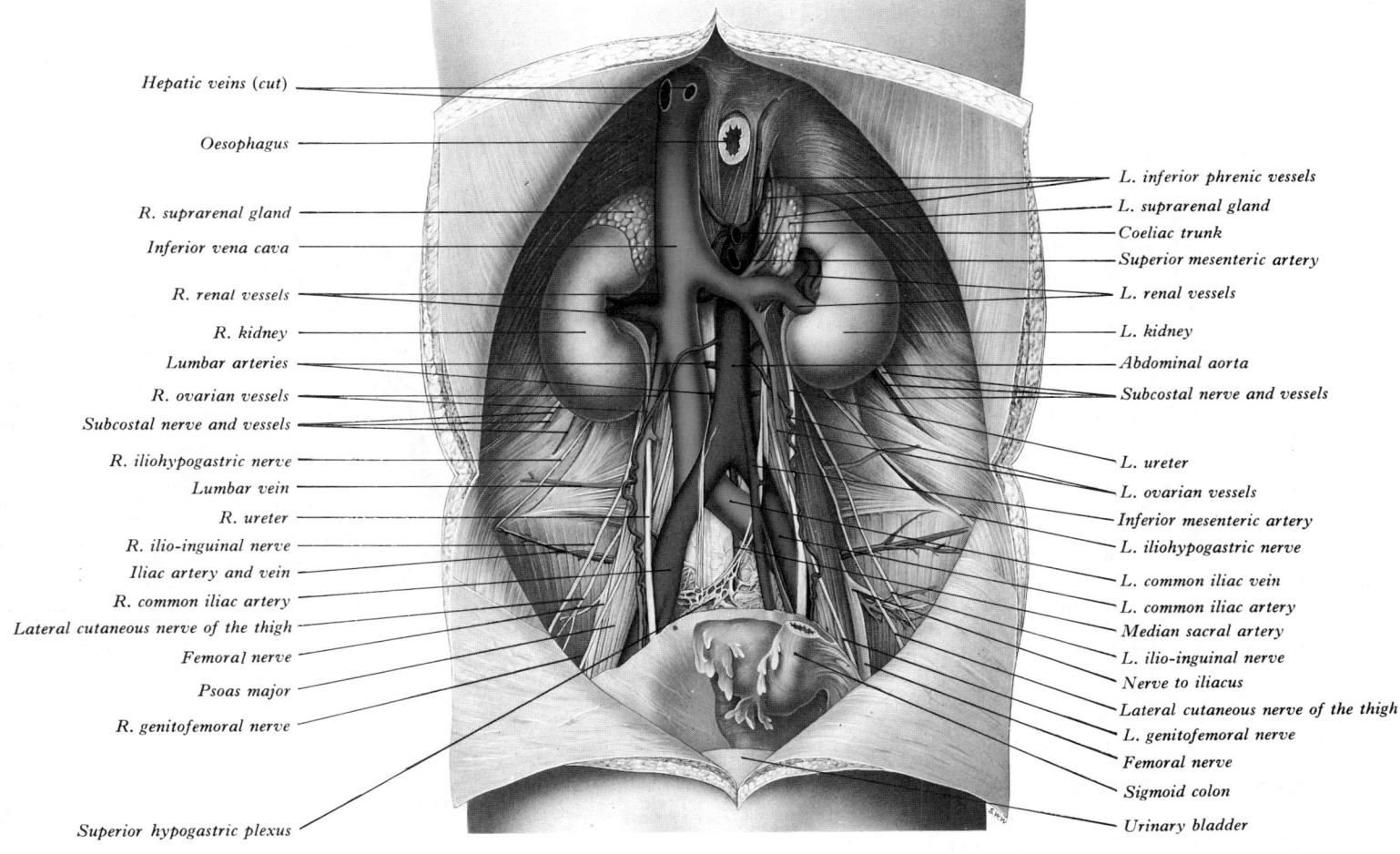

Hepatic veins (cut)
Oesophagus
R. suprarenal gland
Inferior vena cava
R. renal vessels
R. kidney
Lumbar arteries
R. ovarian vessels
Subcostal nerve and vessels
R. iliohypogastric nerve
Lumbar vein
R. ureter
R. ilio-inguinal nerve
Iliac artery and vein
R. common iliac artery
Lateral cutaneous nerve of the thigh
Femoral nerve
Psoas major
R. genitofemoral nerve
Superior hypogastric plexus

L. inferior phrenic vessels
L. suprarenal gland
Coeliac trunk
Superior mesenteric artery
L. renal vessels
L. kidney
Abdominal aorta
Subcostal nerve and vessels
L. ureter
L. ovarian vessels
Inferior mesenteric artery
L. iliohypogastric nerve
L. common iliac vein
L. common iliac artery
Median sacral artery
L. ilio-inguinal nerve
Nerve to iliacus
Lateral cutaneous nerve of the thigh
L. genitofemoral nerve
Femoral nerve
Sigmoid colon
Urinary bladder

10.128 Dissection to show the relations of structures on the posterior abdominal wall (female subject).

Ovarian arteries

These correspond to the testicular arteries but enter the pelvis to supply the ovaries (**10**.132). Initially they resemble the testicular arteries but at the brim of the lesser pelvis each crosses the lower external iliac artery and vein to enter the true pelvic cavity, turning medially in the ovarian suspensory ligament to continue into the uterine broad ligament, below the uterine tube. At ovarian level it passes back in the mesovarium and divides into branches to the ovary. Small branches supply the ureter and uterine tube and one passes to the side of the uterus to unite with the uterine artery. Others accompany the round ligament through the inguinal canal to the skin of the labium majus and the inguinal region.

Early in intrauterine life, when testes or ovaries flank the vertebral column inferior to the kidneys, the testicular and ovarian arteries are relatively short; but with descent of the gonads into the pelvis and beyond, they gradually lengthen.

(Inferior) phrenic arteries

These two small vessels help to supply the diaphragm (**10**.112, 113, 128), They may arise separately from the aorta, just above its coeliac trunk, by a common aortic stem or from the coeliac trunk; sometimes one is from the aorta, the other from a renal artery. Each artery ascends laterally anterior to a crus of the diaphragm, near the medial border of the suprarenal gland. The **left** passes behind the oesophagus and forwards on the left side of its diaphragmatic opening. The **right** phrenic passes posterior to the inferior vena cava then along the right of its opening. Near the posterior border of the diaphragm's central tendon each divides into medial and lateral branches. The medial curves forwards to anastomose with its fellow in front of the central tendon and with the musculophrenic and pericardiacophrenic arteries; the lateral approaches the thoracic wall, anastomosing with the lower posterior intercostal and musculophrenic arteries. The lateral branch of the right artery supplies the inferior vena cava while the left sends ascending branches to the oesophagus. Each has two or three small *superior suprarenal branches.* The liver (p. 1556) and spleen also receive small branches from the phrenic arteries.

Lumbar arteries

These are in series with the posterior intercostal arteries (**10**.128). Usually four on each side, they arise posterolaterally from the aorta, opposite the lumbar vertebrae. A fifth, smaller pair occasionally arise from the median sacral artery but lumbar branches of the iliolumbar arteries usually take their place. The lumbar arteries run posterolaterally on the four upper lumbar vertebral bodies, behind the sympathetic trunks, to intervals between the lumbar transverse processes and continue into the abdominal wall. The right arteries pass posterior to the inferior vena cava; the upper two right and first left are also posterior to the corresponding crus. Arteries of both sides pass under tendinous arches (which span the lateral concavities of the vertebral bodies, p. 870) for attachment of psoas major, proceeding posterior to the muscle and the lumbar plexus. They then cross the quadratus lumborum, the upper three posterior, the last usually anterior to it. At its lateral border they pierce the posterior aponeurosis of the transversus abdominis, advancing between it and the internal oblique. They anastomose with one another and the lower posterior intercostal, subcostal, iliolumbar, deep circumflex iliac and inferior epigastric arteries.

Branches. Each lumbar artery has a *dorsal branch* passing back between the adjacent transverse processes to supply the dorsal muscles, joints and skin; this also has a spinal branch entering the vertebral canal to supply its contents and adjacent vertebra, anastomosing with the arteries above and below it and across the midline. The *spinal branch* of the first lumbar supplies the terminal spinal cord itself; the remainder supply the cauda equina, meninges and vertebral canal. Branches of the lumbar arteries and their dorsal branches supply the adjacent muscles, fasciae, bones, red marrow, ligaments and joints (symphyses, syndesmoses and synovial joints).

Median sacral artery

This small posterior branch leaves the aorta a little above its bifurcation (**10**.112, 113, 128). It descends in the midline, anterior to the fourth and fifth lumbar vertebrae, sacrum and coccyx, ending in the coccygeal body. At fifth lumbar level it is crossed by the left

common iliac vein and often gives off a small lumbar artery (*arteria lumbalis ima*), minute branches of which reach the rectum. Anterior to the last lumbar vertebra the median sacral anastomoses with a lumbar branch of the iliolumbar; anterior to the sacrum it anastomoses with the lateral sacral arteries and sends branches into the anterior sacral foramina.

COMMON ILIAC ARTERIES

The abdominal aorta bifurcates, anterolateral to the **left** side of the **fourth** lumbar vertebral body, into the right and left common iliac arteries (**10**.112, 113, 128, 129). These diverge as they descend to divide near the level of the lumbosacral intervertebral disc (between the last lumbar and first sacral vertebrae) into external and internal iliac arteries; the former supplies most of the lower limb, the latter the pelvic viscera and walls, perineum and gluteal region. The division of the common iliac is anterior to its sacro-iliac joint.

A collateral circulation may be established, in young adults, after ligature of the common iliac artery; when arterial walls degenerate in older patients it is unlikely to supply the leg adequately.

Right common iliac artery

This is about 5 cm long and passes obliquely across part of the fourth and the fifth lumbar vertebral body (**10**.112, 113, 128, 129). **Anteriorly**, it is crossed by the sympathetic rami to the pelvic plexus and, at its division, by the ureter; it is covered by the parietal peritoneum, which separates it from the coils of the small intestine. **Posteriorly**, it is separated from the fourth and fifth lumbar vertebral bodies and their intervening disc by the sympathetic trunk, the terminal parts of the common iliac veins and the commencement of the inferior vena cava; the obturator nerve, lumbosacral trunk and iliolumbar artery are also posterior, traversing fatty tissue between

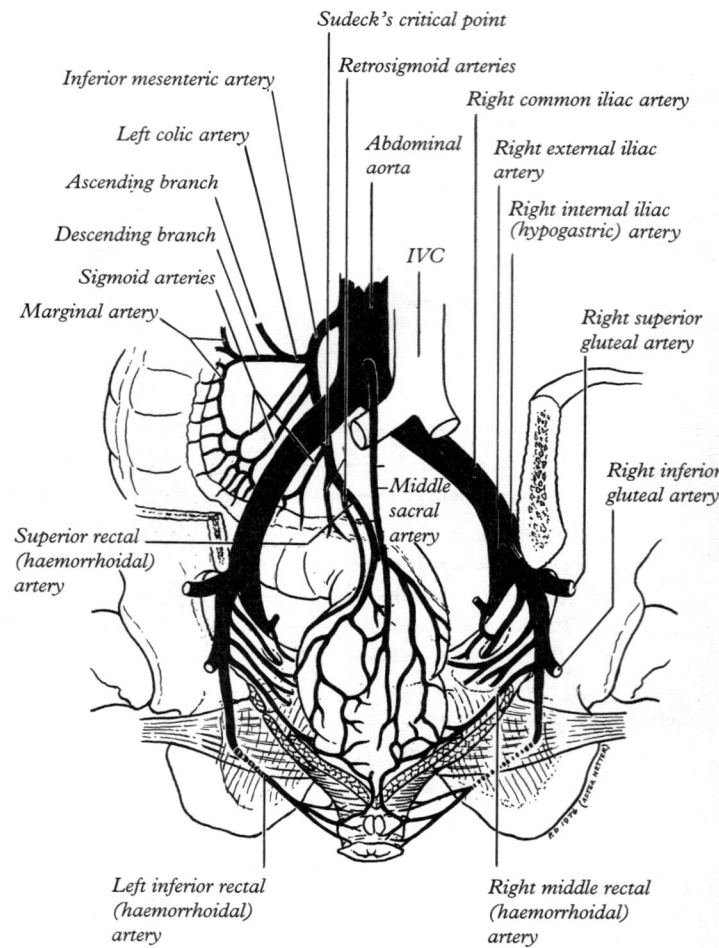

10.129 Schematic representation of the main vessels in the pelvic cavity, seen from the back (after Netter).

the fifth lumbar vertebra and the psoas major. **Lateral** to its upper part are the inferior vena cava and the right common iliac vein to which it has a surgically important relationship (see above); lateral to its lower part is the right psoas major; **medial** to its upper part is the left common iliac vein.

Left common iliac artery

The artery is about 4 cm long (**10**.112, 113, 128, 129). **Anterior** are the peritoneum, ileum, the sympathetic rami to the pelvic plexus, the superior rectal artery and, at its terminal bifurcation, the ureter. Posterior are the sympathetic trunk, fourth and fifth lumbar vertebral bodies and intervening disc; the obturator nerve, lumbosacral trunk and iliolumbar artery are more posterior (i.e. deeply situated). The left common iliac vein is partly **medial**, partly **posterior** to the artery; **lateral** and closely related is the left psoas major.

Surface anatomy. The vessel corresponds to the superior third of a broad line from the aortic bifurcation (p. 1547) to a point midway between the anterior superior iliac spine and the pubic symphysis. The *external iliac artery* corresponds to the inferior two-thirds of this line, which is laterally slightly convex.

Branches. In addition to the terminal branches, each common iliac artery gives small branches to the peritoneum, psoas major, ureter, adjacent nerves and surrounding areolar tissue; occasionally it has the iliolumbar and accessory renal arteries as branches.

INTERNAL ILIAC ARTERIES

Each internal iliac artery (**10**.130, 131), about 4 cm long, begins at the common iliac bifurcation, level with the lumbosacral intervertebral disc and anterior to the sacro-iliac joint; it descends posteriorly to the superior margin of the greater sciatic foramen, dividing here into: an *anterior trunk*, which continues in the same line towards the ischial spine; and a *posterior trunk*, passing back to the foramen (Braithwaite 1952). **Anterior** are the ureter and, in females, the ovary and fimbriated end of the uterine tube; **posterior** are the internal iliac vein, lumbosacral trunk and sacro-iliac joint; **lateral** is the external iliac vein, between the artery and the psoas major and inferior to this the obturator nerve; **medial** is the parietal

peritoneum, separating it from the terminal ileum on the right and the sigmoid colon on the left, and tributaries of the internal iliac vein.

In the fetus the internal iliac artery is twice the size of the external and is the direct continuation of the common iliac. It ascends on the anterior abdominal wall to the umbilicus, converging on its fellow. Having traversed the opening, the two arteries, now umbilical, enter the umbilical cord, coil round the umbilical vein and ultimately ramify in the placenta. At birth, when placental circulation ceases, only the pelvic segment remains patent as the internal iliac artery and part of the superior vesical, the remainder becoming a fibrous *medial umbilical ligament* raising the peritoneal *medial umbilical fold* from the pelvis to the umbilicus. In males, the patent part usually gives off an artery to the ductus deferens (see below).

BRANCHES OF ANTERIOR TRUNK OF INTERNAL ILIAC ARTERY

Superior vesical artery (**10**.130, 131). This supplies many branches to the vesical fundus (Braithwaite 1951); from one the *artery to the ductus deferens* occasionally starts and accompanies the ductus to the testis, anastomosing with the testicular artery. Others supply the ureter. The beginning of the superior vesical artery is the proximal, patent section of the fetal umbilical artery (see above).

Inferior vesical artery (**10**.130, 131). Often arising with the middle rectal, it supplies the vesical fundus, prostate, seminal vesicles and lower ureter. Prostatic branches communicate across the midline. The inferior vesical may sometimes provide the artery to the ductus deferens.

Middle rectal artery (**10**.125, 130). It usually arises with the inferior vesical. It vascularizes muscular tissue in the lower rectum, anastomosing with the superior and inferior rectal arteries. It supplies the seminal vesicles and prostate by branches which join those of the inferior vesical.

Uterine artery (**10**.132). This runs medially on the levator ani to the cervix uteri; about 2 cm from this it crosses above the *ureter*, to which it supplies a small branch, and above the *lateral vaginal fornix*. It ascends tortuously lateral to the uterus in its broad ligament to the junction of the uterine tube and uterus, turning laterally towards

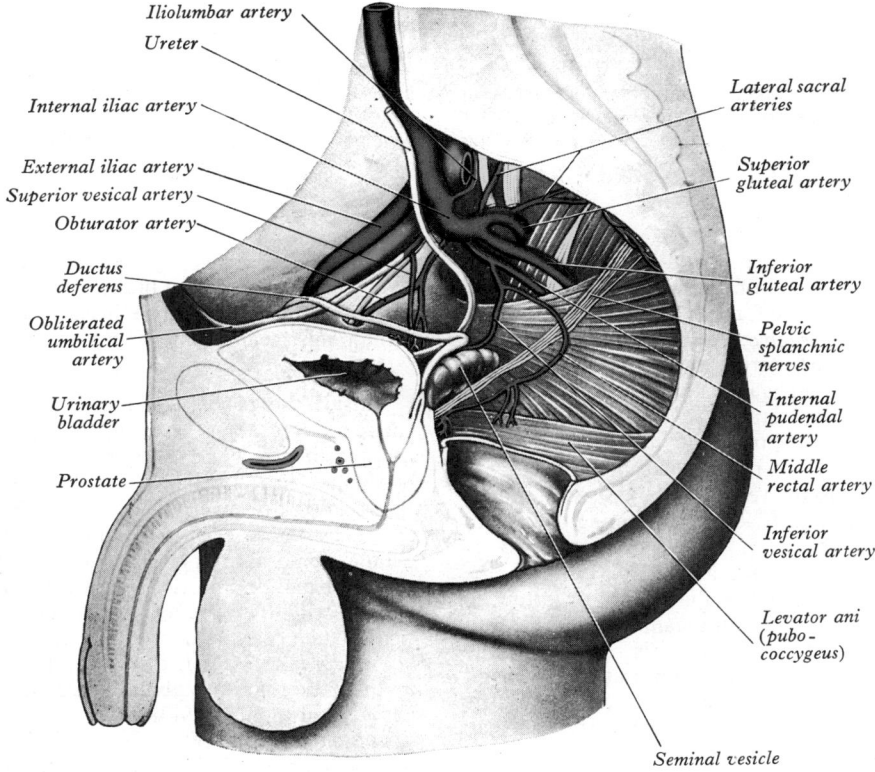

Iliolumbar artery
Ureter
Internal iliac artery
External iliac artery
Superior vesical artery
Obturator artery
Ductus deferens
Obliterated umbilical artery
Urinary bladder
Prostate
Lateral sacral arteries
Superior gluteal artery
Inferior gluteal artery
Pelvic splanchnic nerves
Internal pudendal artery
Middle rectal artery
Inferior vesical artery
Levator ani (pubo-coccygeus)
Seminal vesicle

10.130   The arteries of the male pelvis (right side). The internal iliac vein and its tributaries have been removed; the rectum has been divided just above the anal canal and its upper part has been taken away.

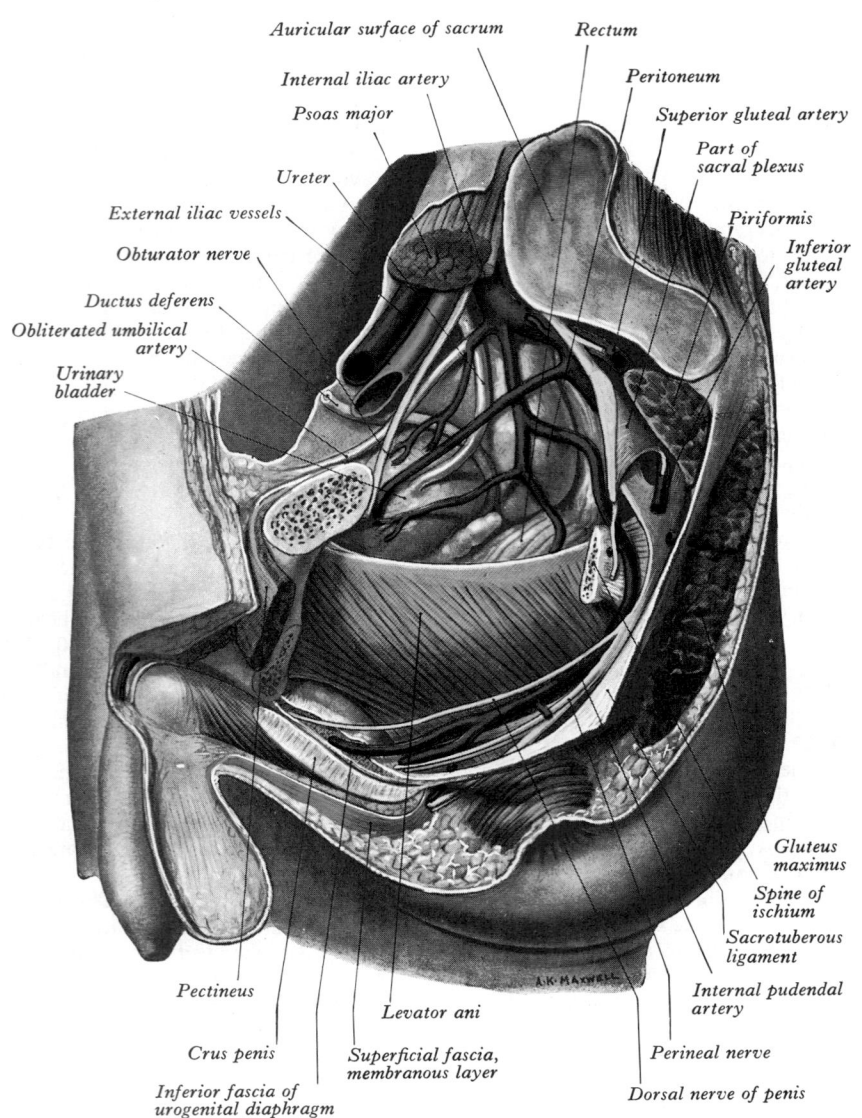

Auricular surface of sacrum
Rectum
Internal iliac artery
Peritoneum
Psoas major
Superior gluteal artery
Ureter
Part of sacral plexus
External iliac vessels
Piriformis
Obturator nerve
Inferior gluteal artery
Ductus deferens
Obliterated umbilical artery
Urinary bladder
Gluteus maximus
Spine of ischium
Sacrotuberous ligament
Pectineus
Internal pudendal artery
Levator ani
Crus penis
Perineal nerve
Superficial fascia, membranous layer
Inferior fascia of urogenital diaphragm
Dorsal nerve of penis

10.131   Structures of the male pelvic contents from the left side. Most of the left innominate bone has been removed together with the obturator internus. The sciatic nerve has been cut away close to its origin from the sacral plexus. All the vessels and nerves exposed are those of the left side. Note the superior vesical, obturator, inferior vesical and middle rectal arteries which are, for technical reasons, unlabelled.

the ovarian hilum, and ends by joining the ovarian artery. It supplies the cervix uteri and branches descend on the vagina, anastomosing with branches of the vaginal arteries to form two median longitudinal vessels, the *azygos arteries of the vagina*; one descends anterior, the other posterior, to the vagina. The uterine artery supplies the body of the uterus, uterine tube and round ligament of the uterus. Terminal branches in the uterine muscle are tortuous *helicine arteries*.

Vaginal artery. Often double or triple, it corresponds to the inferior vesical in males; it descends on the vagina, supplying mucous membrane, and sends branches to the vestibular bulb, vesical fundus and the adjacent part of the rectum. It assists in forming the azygos arteries of the vagina (see above).

Obturator artery (**10**.130). It inclines antero-inferiorly on the lateral pelvic wall to the upper part of the obturator foramen. Leaving the pelvic cavity by the obturator canal, it divides into anterior and posterior branches. In the pelvis it is related laterally to the obturator fascia, separating it from the obturator internus; it is crossed medially by the ureter and the ductus deferens, separating it from the parietal peritoneum. In the nullipara the ovary is medial. The obturator nerve is above, the vein below.

Branches. In the pelvis, the obturator artery provides:

- *iliac branches* to the iliac fossa, supplying the bone and iliacus and anastomosing with the iliolumbar artery

- a *vesical branch* passing medially to the bladder, sometimes replacing the inferior vesical branch of the internal iliac
- a *pubic branch* just before it leaves the pelvis, which ascends over the pubis to anastomose with its fellow and the pubic branch of the inferior epigastric.

Outside the pelvis its anterior, and posterior terminal branches encircle the foramen between the obturator externus and the obturator membrane. The *anterior branch* curves forwards on the membrane and then down along its anterior margin, supplying branches to the obturator externus, pectineus, femoral adductors and gracilis and anastomosing with the posterior branch and the medial circumflex femoral artery. The *posterior branch* follows the foramen's posterior margin and turns forwards on the ischial branch to anastomose with the anterior. It supplies the muscles attached to the ischial tuberosity and anastomoses with the inferior gluteal. An *acetabular branch* enters the hip joint at the acetabular notch, ramifies in the fat of the acetabular fossa and sends a branch along the ligament of the femoral head.

Variations. In 20–30% of subjects the obturator artery is replaced by an enlarged pubic branch of the inferior epigastric (p. 1563); this descends almost vertically to the obturator foramen. Such an abnormal obturator artery is usually near the external iliac vein, lateral to the femoral ring, and is then safe in herniotomy. Sometimes

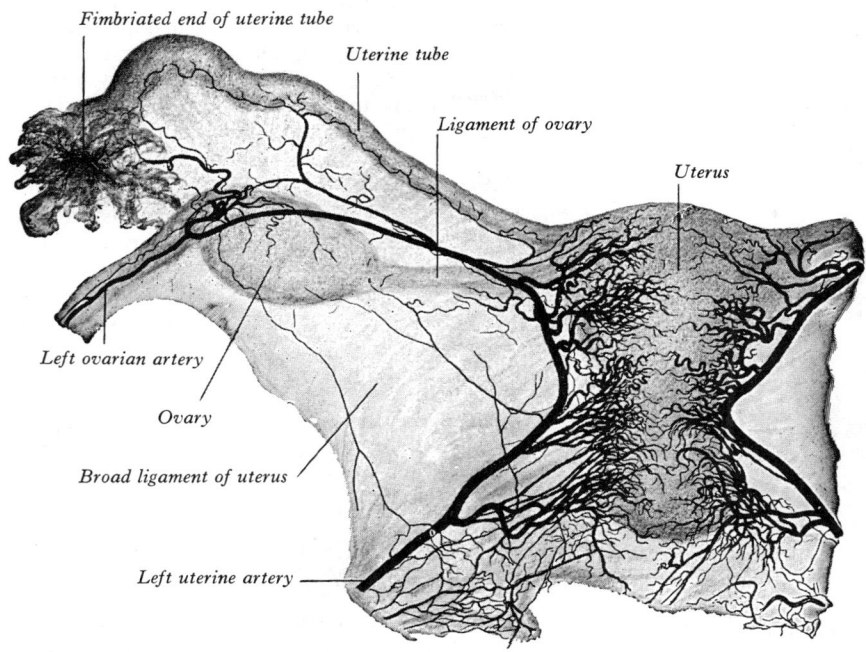

10.132   The left uterine and ovarian arteries of a nullipara of 17½ years: posterior aspect. (From a preparation by Hamilton Drummond.)

it curves along the edge of the lacunar part of the inguinal ligament, partly encircling the neck of a hernial sac, and may be inadvertently cut during enlargement of the femoral ring in reducing a femoral hernia.

Internal pudendal artery in the male (10.130, 131, 133, 134)

The artery descends laterally to the inferior rim of the greater sciatic foramen, where it leaves the pelvis between piriformis and coccygeus and enters the *gluteal region*; then curving around the dorsum of the ischial spine to enter the perineum by the lesser sciatic foramen, it traverses the pudendal canal in the lateral wall of the *ischiorectal fossa*, medial to the obturator internus, about 4 cm above the ischial tuberosity's lower limit. Approaching the margin of the ischial branch, it proceeds above or below the inferior fascia of the urogenital diaphragm along the medial margin of the inferior pubic ramus and ends behind the inferior pubic ligament, dividing into the *deep* and *dorsal arteries of the penis*. It may descend through the inferior fascia before its division. (The internal pudendal distal to its perineal branch has been named *artery of the penis*, appropriately in view of its distribution; see below.)

Relations. In the pelvis the internal pudendal artery crosses anterior to the piriformis, sacral plexus and inferior gluteal artery. Behind the ischial spine it is covered by the gluteus maximus, with the pudendal nerve medial and the nerve to obturator internus lateral. In the pudendal canal (p. 832) it travels at first with companion veins and the pudendal nerve; beyond this the dorsal nerve of the penis is above, the perineal nerve below.

Muscular branches (10.133, 134). These leave the artery in the pelvis and gluteal region to supply the adjacent muscles and nerves.

Inferior rectal artery. This arises above the ischial tuberosity. Escaping from the pudendal canal (p. 832), it divides into two or three branches crossing the ischiorectal fossa medially to supply the anal skin and musculature. Small branches skirt the lower edge of the gluteus maximus to supply the gluteal skin. The inferior rectal anastomoses with its fellow, and with the superior, middle rectal and perineal arteries.

Perineal artery (10.133). It leaves the internal pudendal near the anterior end of its canal, turns down through the inferior fascia of the urogenital diaphragm (p. 834) and approaches the scrotum in the superficial perineal region, between the bulbospongiosus and ischiocavernosus. Beyond the diaphragm, and near its base, a small *transverse branch* passes medially inferior to the superficial transverse perineal muscle to anastomose with its fellow and the posterior

scrotal and inferior rectal arteries, supplying tissues between the anus and the penile bulb. The posterior *scrotal arteries*, distributed to the scrotal skin and dartos muscle, are usually terminals of the perineal but may also arise from its transverse branch; they also supply the perineal muscles.

Artery of the bulb of the penis. Short but wide, it runs medially through the deep transverse perineal muscle and inferior urogenital fascia to the penile bulb. Penetrating this, it supplies the posterior part of the corpus spongiosum and the bulbo-urethral gland.

Urethral artery. This traverses the urogenital diaphragm's inferior fascia and enters the corpus spongiosum, reaching the glans penis. It supplies the urethra and erectile tissue around it.

Deep artery of the penis. A terminal branch of the internal

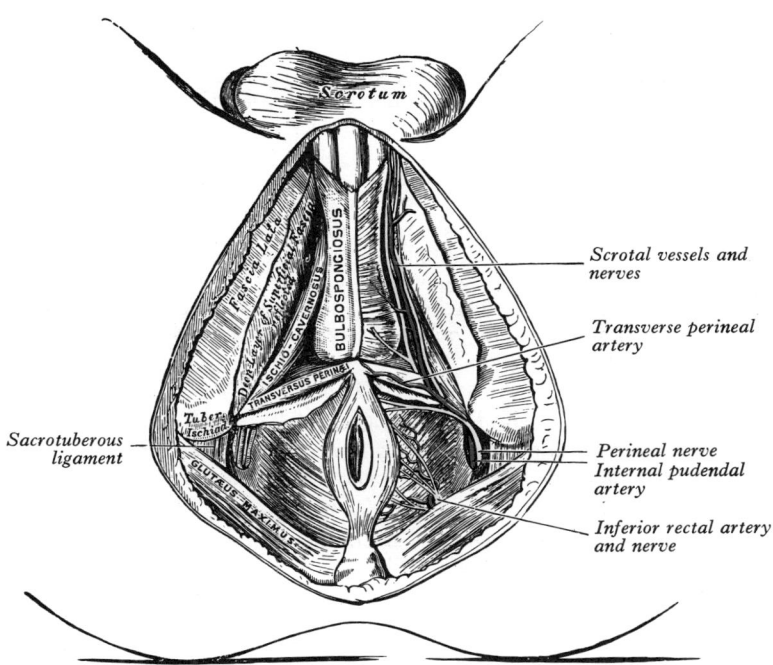

10.133   The superficial branches of the internal pudendal artery, in the male.

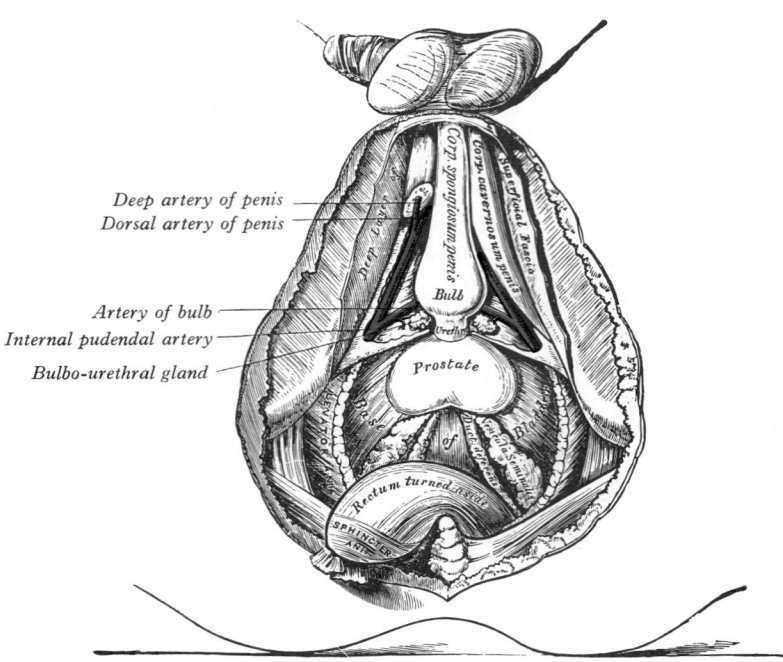

10.134 The deeper branches of the internal pudendal artery, in the male.

pudendal, it passes through the inferior fascia of the urogenital diaphragm to enter the crus penis. It traverses the corpus cavernosum and supplies its erectile tissue.

Dorsal artery of the penis. The other terminal branch of the internal pudendal, it leaves the inferior aspect of the urogenital diaphragm, **ascends** between the crus penis and pubic symphysis, and traverses the suspensory ligament of the penis to run along its dorsum to the glans, where it forks into branches to the glans and prepuce. In the penis it lies between its dorsal nerve and deep dorsal vein, the latter being most medial. It supplies penile skin and the fibrous sheath of the corpus cavernosum, anastomosing through the sheath with the deep penile artery.

Inferior gluteal artery

The larger terminal branch of the anterior internal iliac trunk, it chiefly supplies the buttock and thigh. It descends anterior to the sacral plexus and piriformis, posterior to the internal pudendal artery (**10.**129, 135). Passing between the first and second or second and third sacral anterior spinal nerve rami, then between the piriformis and coccygeus, it traverses the lower part of the greater sciatic foramen to reach the gluteal region. Descending between the greater trochanter and ischial tuberosity with the sciatic and posterior femoral cutaneous nerves, deep to the gluteus maximus, it continues down the thigh, supplying the skin and anastomosing with branches of the perforating arteries. The inferior gluteal and internal pudendal arteries are often a common stem from the internal iliac, sometimes including the superior gluteal artery.

Surface anatomy. The inferior gluteal artery leaves the pelvis near the midpoint of a line joining the posterior superior iliac spine and the ischial tuberosity.

Branches. Inside the pelvis there are branches to the following:

- the piriformis, coccygeus and levator ani
- the perirectal fat, occasionally replacing the middle rectal artery
- the vesical fundus, seminal vesicles and prostate.

Outside the pelvis muscular branches supply the gluteus maximus, obturator internus, gemelli, quadratus femoris and the proximal parts of the hamstring muscles, anastomosing with the superior gluteal, internal pudendal, obturator and medial circumflex femoral arteries. *Coccygeal branches* run medially through the sacrotuberous ligament to supply the gluteus maximus and the structures attached to the coccyx. The *artery to the sciatic nerve* runs on the nerve for a short distance, then descends in it to the lower thigh. An *anastomotic branch* descends obliquely across obturator internus, gemelli and

quadratus femoris, to join the *cruciate anastomosis* (p. 1567) linking with the first perforating and medial and lateral circumflex femoral arteries. This may become an important route of collateral supply in cases of occlusion of the aorto-iliac system. An *articular branch*, usually from the anastomotic, is distributed to the hip joint. *Cutaneous branches* supply the buttock and back of the thigh.

Internal pudendal artery in the female

The internal pudendal in the female is naturally smaller but its origin, course and branches are similar, including the *posterior labial branches*, the *artery of the bulb* (distributed to the erectile tissue of the vestibular bulb and vagina), *deep artery of the clitoris*, supplying the corpus cavernosum, and a *dorsal artery* to the glans and prepuce of the clitoris.

Variations

Branches of the internal pudendal are sometimes derived from an *accessory pudendal*, usually a branch of the pudendal before its exit from the pelvis.

BRANCHES OF POSTERIOR TRUNK OF INTERNAL ILIAC ARTERY

Iliolumbar artery (**10.**130). This ascends laterally **anterior** to the sacro-iliac joint and lumbosacral trunk, **posterior** to the obturator nerve and external iliac vessels, to reach the medial border of psoas major, dividing behind it into the lumbar and iliac branches. The *lumbar branch* supplies the psoas major and quadratus lumborum, anastomoses with the fourth lumbar artery and sends a small *spinal branch* through the intervertebral foramen between the fifth lumbar and first sacral vertebrae, which supplies the cauda equina. The *iliac branch* supplies the iliacus; between the muscle and bone it anastomoses with the iliac branches of the obturator. A large nutrient branch enters an oblique canal in the ilium; others skirt the iliac crest, supplying the gluteal and abdominal muscles and anastomosing with the superior gluteal, circumflex iliac and lateral circumflex femoral arteries.

Lateral sacral arteries (**10.**130). These are from the posterior trunk of the internal iliac, usually as a superior and an inferior branch. The *superior* and larger passes medially into the first or second anterior sacral foramen, supplies the sacral vertebrae and contents of the sacral canal and escapes via the corresponding dorsal foramen to supply the skin and muscles dorsal to the sacrum. The *inferior lateral sacral artery* crosses obliquely anterior to the piriformis and the sacral anterior spinal rami, then descends lateral to the sympathetic trunk to anastomose with its fellow and the median sacral artery anterior to the coccyx. Its branches enter the anterior sacral foramina, distributed like those of the superior artery.

Superior gluteal artery (**10.**129, 130, 135). The largest branch of the internal iliac and the continuation of its posterior trunk, it runs back between the lumbosacral spinal trunk and the first sacral ramus or between the first and second rami, leaving the pelvis by the greater sciatic foramen above the piriformis and dividing into *superficial* and *deep branches*. In the pelvis it supplies the piriformis, obturator internus and an innominate nutrient artery. The superficial branch enters the deep surface of the gluteus maximus; its numerous branches supply the muscle and anastomose with the inferior gluteal, others perforating its tendinous medial attachment to supply the skin over the sacrum, anastomosing with the posterior branches of the lateral sacral arteries. The deep branch is between the gluteus medius and the bone, soon dividing into superior and inferior branches. The *superior* skirts the superior border of the gluteus minimus to the anterior superior iliac spine, anastomosing with the deep circumflex iliac artery and the ascending branch of the lateral circumflex femoral. The *inferior branch* traverses the gluteus minimus obliquely and supplies it and also the gluteus medius, anastomosing with the lateral circumflex femoral; a branch enters the trochanteric fossa to join the inferior gluteal and ascending branch of the medial circumflex femoral; other branches pierce the gluteus minimus to supply the hip joint.

The superior gluteal artery may arise from the internal iliac with the inferior gluteal and sometimes the internal pudendal.

Surface anatomy. The artery's pelvic exit corresponds to the

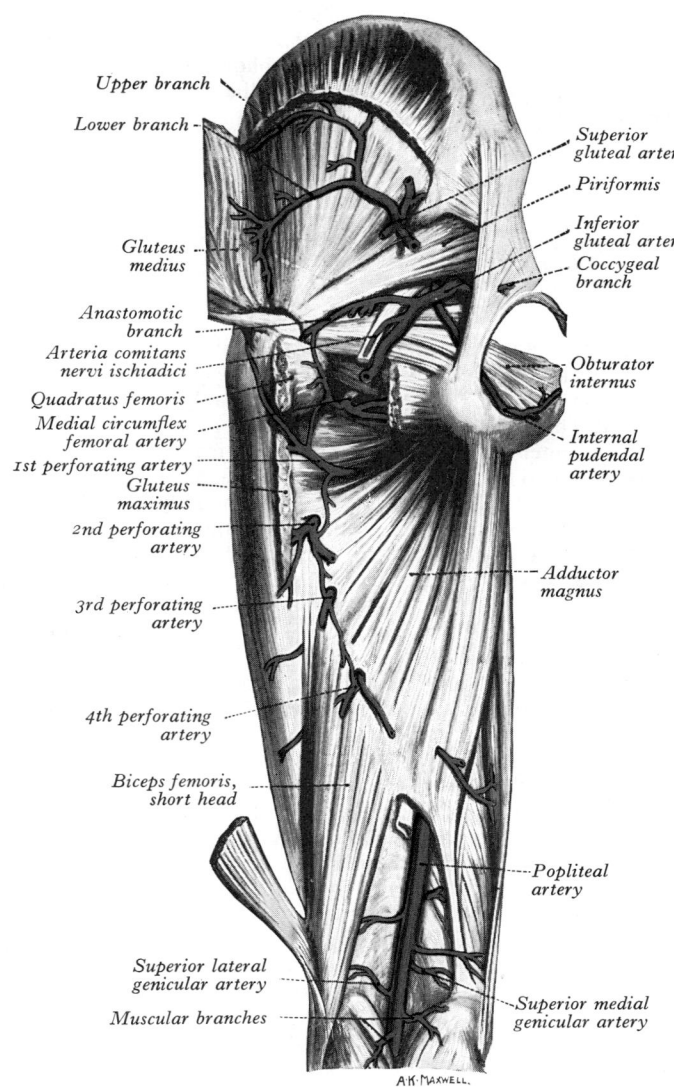

Upper branch
Lower branch
Gluteus medius
Anastomotic branch
Arteria comitans nervi ischiadici
Quadratus femoris
Medial circumflex femoral artery
1st perforating artery
Gluteus maximus
2nd perforating artery
3rd perforating artery
4th perforating artery
Biceps femoris, short head
Superior lateral genicular artery
Muscular branches

Superior gluteal artery
Piriformis
Inferior gluteal artery
Coccygeal branch
Obturator internus
Internal pudendal artery
Adductor magnus
Popliteal artery
Superior medial genicular artery

A·K·MAXWELL.

10.135 The arteries of the left gluteal and posterior femoral regions.

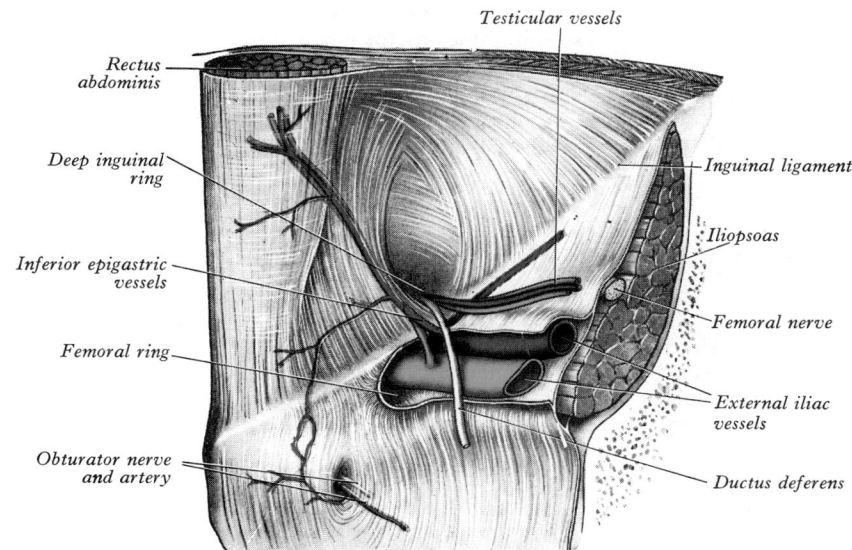

Rectus abdominis
Deep inguinal ring
Inferior epigastric vessels
Femoral ring
Obturator nerve and artery

Testicular vessels
Inguinal ligament
Iliopsoas
Femoral nerve
External iliac vessels
Ductus deferens

10.136   Dissection of the deep aspect of the lower part of the abdominal wall of the right side with the thinner posterior wall of the rectus sheath. The femoral and deep inguinal rings are displayed together with the vessels and other structures in relation to them and also the opening into the obturator canal.

junction of the upper and middle thirds of a line joining the posterior superior iliac spine to the apex of the greater trochanter.

EXTERNAL ILIAC ARTERIES

The external iliac arteries (**10**.129–131, 136) are larger than the internal. Each descends laterally along the medial border of the psoas major from the common iliac bifurcation (anterior to the sacro-iliac joint at lumbosacral disc level) to a point midway between the anterior superior iliac spine and the symphysis pubis, entering the thigh posterior to the inguinal ligament to become the femoral artery.

Anteromedially the artery is related to the parietal peritoneum and extraperitoneal tissue, separating the right from the terminal ileum and often the appendix, the left from the sigmoid colon and coils of the small intestine. At its origin the artery may be crossed by the ureter, in females by ovarian vessels. Testicular vessels are anterior for some distance near its distal end, and it is crossed here by the genital branch of the genitofemoral nerve, the deep circumflex iliac vein and the ductus deferens or round ligament. **Posteriorly** the iliac fascia separates it from the medial border of the psoas major. The external iliac vein is partly posterior to its upper part, medial to it below. **Laterally** it is related to the psoas major, the iliac fascia lying between them. Numerous lymph vessels and nodes lie on its front and sides.

Branches. Apart from very small vessels to the psoas major and neighbouring lymph nodes, the artery has no branches until the inferior epigastric and deep circumflex iliac arise near to its termination. Besides supplying the psoas major and neighbouring lymph nodes, the artery has inferior epigastric and deep circumflex iliac branches.

Inferior epigastric artery (**7**.84, **10**.136). This leaves the external iliac just proximal to the inguinal ligament, curves forwards in extraperitoneal tissue, ascends obliquely along the medial margin of the deep inguinal ring, continues up to pierce the transversalis fascia and the attenuated part of the rectus sheath (p. 825) and ascends between the rectus abdominis and the posterior lamina of its sheath. It divides into numerous branches, which anastomose with those of the superior epigastric and lower posterior intercostal arteries. The artery thus skirts the deep inguinal ring inferomedially, passing posterior to the spermatic cord but separated from it by the transversalis fascia. It raises the parietal peritoneum of the anterior abdominal wall as the *lateral umbilical fold* (p. 1737). The ductus deferens, or round ligament, winds laterally round it. It supplies the following branches:

- The *cremasteric artery* (see above) accompanies the spermatic cord, supplies the cremaster and other coverings of the cord and anastomoses with the testicular artery. In females it is small and accompanies the round ligament.
- A *pubic branch*, near the femoral ring, descends posterior to the pubis and anastomoses with the pubic branch of the obturator. In 20–30% of subjects, the pubic branches of the inferior epigastric are larger than, and replace, those of the obturator artery (p. 1560).
- *Muscular branches* supply the abdominal muscles and peritoneum, anastomosing with the circumflex iliac and lumbar arteries.
- *Cutaneous branches* perforate the aponeurosis of the external oblique, supply the skin and anastomose with branches of the superficial epigastric artery.

Variations. The artery may arise from the femoral and then ascend, anterior to the femoral vein, to the abdomen. It often arises from the external iliac artery in common with an abnormal obturator and, rarely, directly from the obturator artery.

Clinical anatomy. The inferior epigastric artery is a main route, through anastomosis with the internal thoracic, for collateral circulation after ligature of either the common or the external iliac arteries. It is **medial** to the neck of an oblique inguinal hernia but **lateral** to that of a direct inguinal hernia (p. 1560).

Deep circumflex iliac artery. This branches laterally from the external iliac almost opposite the inferior epigastric. It ascends   1563 laterally to the anterior superior iliac spine posterior to the inguinal ligament in a sheath formed by the junction of the transversalis and iliac fasciae. There it anastomoses with the ascending branch of the lateral circumflex femoral artery, pierces the transversalis fascia and skirts the internal lip of the iliac crest; about halfway it perforates the transversus abdominis and runs between this and the internal

oblique to anastomose with the iliolumbar and superior gluteal arteries. At the anterior superior iliac spine it has a large *ascending branch*, which runs between the internal oblique and the transversus, supplying them and anastomosing with the lumbar and inferior epigastric arteries.

ARTERIES OF THE LOWER LIMBS

The main artery of the thigh is the continuation of the external iliac, extending from the inguinal ligament to the distal border of the popliteus, where it divides into the anterior and the posterior tibial artery. Its proximal section, the femoral artery, lies among the knee extensor muscles; its continuation, the popliteal artery, is among the knee flexors.

FEMORAL ARTERY

The femoral artery (**10.**137–142), a continuation of the external iliac, begins behind the inguinal ligament, midway between the anterior superior iliac spine and the pubic symphysis, descends along the anteromedial part of the thigh in the femoral triangle and becomes the popliteal as it passes through the adductor canal, an opening in the adductor magnus near the junction of the middle and distal thirds of the thigh. Its first 3 or 4 cm are enclosed, with its vein, in the femoral sheath.

FEMORAL SHEATH

Distal prolongations, behind the inguinal ligament, of the transversalis fascia, anterior to the femoral vessels, and of the iliac fascia, posterior, together form a short funnel, wider proximally, its distal end fusing with the vascular fascia 3 or 4 cm distal to the ligament (**10.**137). At birth the sheath is shorter, elongating when extension at the hips becomes habitual. Its vertical lateral wall is perforated by the femoral branch of the genitofemoral nerve; the medial wall slopes laterally and is pierced by the great (long) saphenous vein and lymphatic vessels. Like the carotid sheath, the femoral sheath encloses a mass of connective tissue in which the vessels are embedded. Three compartments are described: a lateral one containing the

femoral artery; an intermediate one for the femoral vein; medial and smallest is the femoral canal, containing the lymph vessels and a lymph node embedded in areolar tissue, probably to allow the vein to distend. This canal is conical, about 1.25 cm in length; its proximal end is the outer femoral ring, bounded in front by the inguinal ligament, behind by the pectineus and its fascia, medially by the crescentic edge of the lacunar ligament and laterally by the femoral vein (p. 1789). The spermatic cord, or the round ligament, is just above its anterior margin; the inferior epigastric vessels are near its anterolateral rim. It is larger in women than in men due partly to the greater breadth of the pelvis, partly to the smaller size of the femoral vessels, in women. The ring is filled by condensed extraperitoneal tissue, the femoral septum, covered by the parietal peritoneum (p. 1788). The femoral septum is traversed by numerous lymph vessels connecting the deep inguinal to the external iliac lymph nodes.

Femoral triangle (10.138–140)

The femoral triangle is a depressed area of the thigh lying distal to the inguinal fold. Its apex is distal, its limits being laterally the medial margin of sartorius, medially the medial margin of adductor longus; proximally (the base) is the inguinal ligament. Its floor is provided laterally by iliacus and psoas major, medially by pectineus and adductor longus. The femoral vessels, passing from midbase to apex, are in the deepest part of the triangle. Lateral to the artery the femoral nerve divides. The triangle also contains fat and lymph nodes.

Relations of the femoral artery in the femoral triangle (**10.**140). **Anterior** to the artery are the skin, superficial fascia, superficial inguinal lymph nodes, fascia lata, femoral sheath, superficial circumflex iliac vein (crossing in the superficial fascia) and the femoral branch of the genitofemoral nerve (at first lateral then anterior). Near the apex the medial femoral cutaneous nerve crosses the artery from the lateral to the medial side. **Posterior** are the femoral sheath and the tendons of psoas, pectineus and adductor longus. The artery is separated from the hip joint by the tendon of psoas major, from the pectineus by the femoral vein and profunda vessels and from the adductor longus by the femoral vein. Proximally, the nerve to the pectineus passes medially behind the artery; **lateral** to it is the femoral nerve. The femoral vein is **medial** in the proximal part of the triangle, becoming posterior near its apex, distally.

Adductor canal (**10.**138–140). It is an aponeurotic tunnel in the middle third of the thigh, from the apex of the femoral triangle to the opening in adductor magnus, through which femoral vessels reach the popliteal fossa. Triangular in section, it is bounded **anterolaterally** by vastus medialis, **posteriorly** by adductor longus, distally by adductor magnus and **anteromedially** by a strong aponeurosis extending between the adductors across the vessels to vastus medialis. The sartorius is anterior. The canal contains the femoral artery and vein, the saphenous nerve, and the nerve to vastus medialis until it enters its muscle.

Relations of the femoral artery in the adductor canal (**10.**139–141). **Anterior** to the artery are the skin, superficial and deep fasciae, sartorius and fibrous roof of the canal. The saphenous nerve is first lateral, then anterior and finally medial. **Posterior** are the adductor longus and adductor magnus; the femoral vein is also posterior proximally, but becoming lateral distally. Anterolateral are the vastus medialis and its nerve.

Surface anatomy. The artery corresponds to the proximal two-thirds of a line drawn from the midpoint between the anterior–superior iliac spine and the pubic symphysis to the adductor tubercle

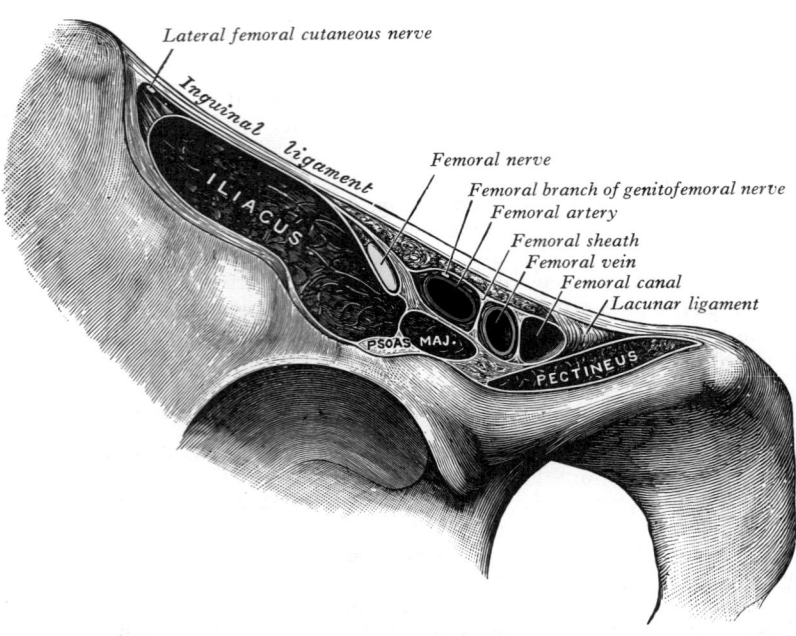

10.137 The structures passing posterior to the right lacunar ligament: inferior (distal) aspect. Note the lacuna musculorum and the lacuna vasorum.

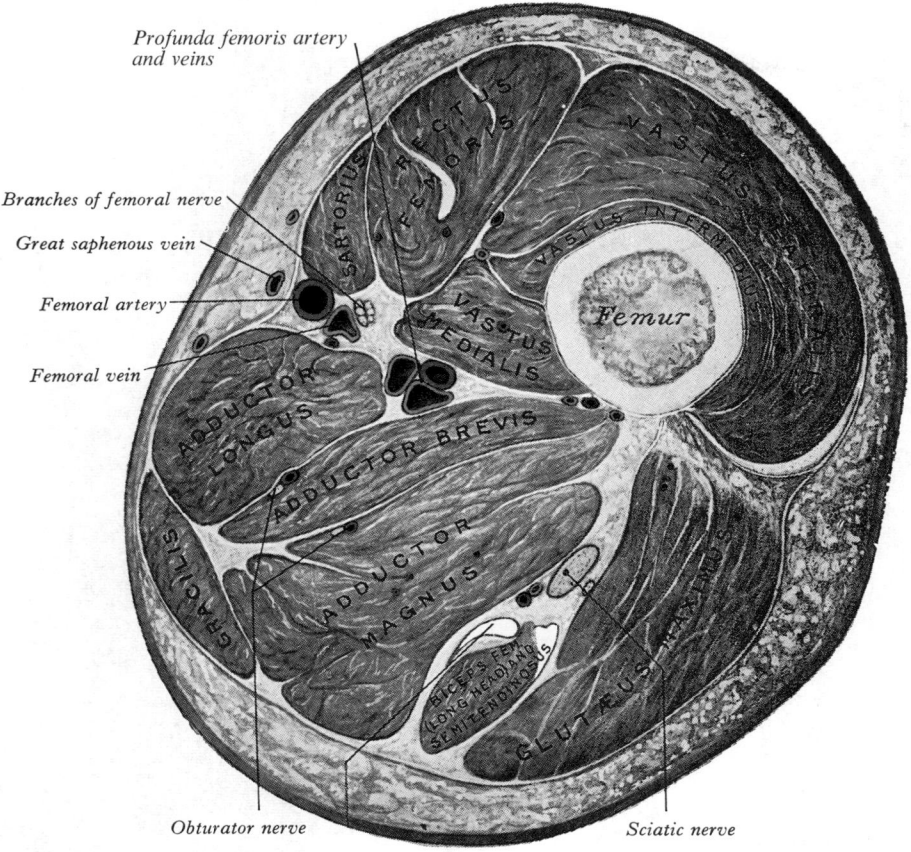

Profunda femoris artery
and veins

Branches of femoral nerve

Great saphenous vein

Femoral artery

Femoral vein

RECTUS FEMORIS

SARTORIUS

VASTUS INTERMEDIUS

Femur

VASTUS MEDIALIS

ADDUCTOR LONGUS

ADDUCTOR BREVIS

ADDUCTOR MAGNUS

GRACILIS

BICEPS FEMORIS
LONG HEAD AND
SEMITENDINOSUS

GLUTAEUS MAXIMUS

Obturator nerve

Sciatic nerve

10.138 Transverse section through the right thigh at the level of the apex
of the femoral triangle: superior (proximal) aspect. About three-fifths of the
natural size. The cutaneous nerves are omitted.

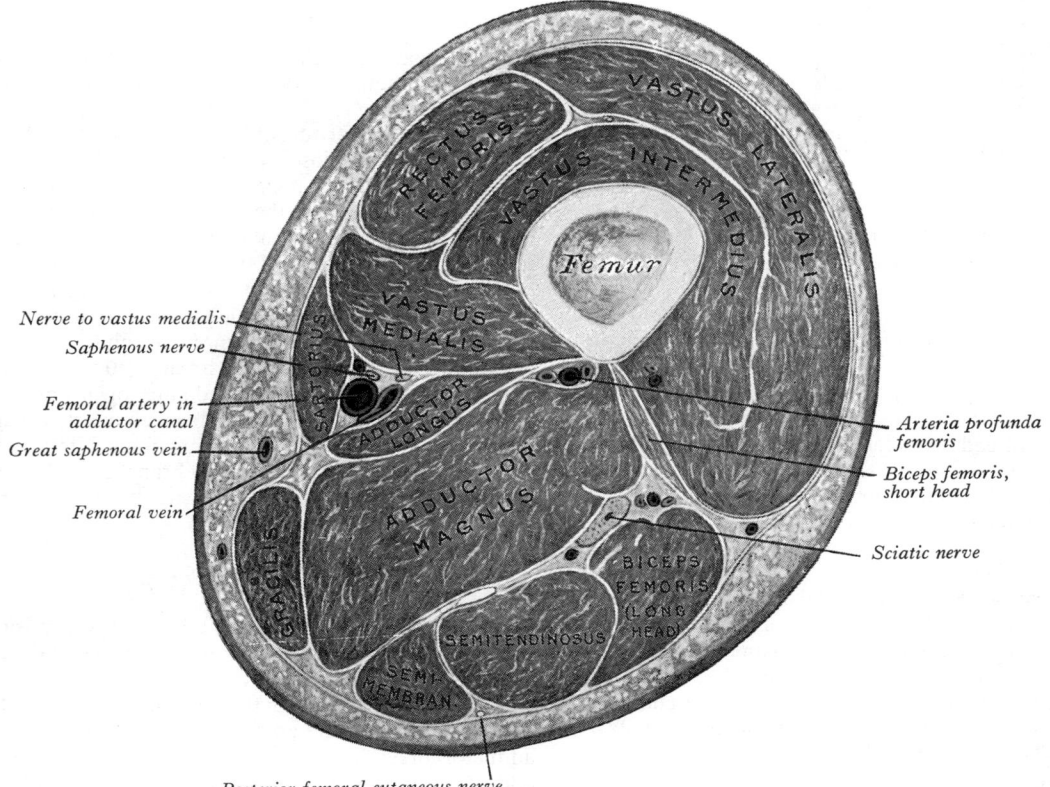

RECTUS FEMORIS

VASTUS LATERALIS

VASTUS INTERMEDIUS

VASTUS MEDIALIS

Femur

Nerve to vastus medialis

Saphenous nerve

Femoral artery in
adductor canal

Great saphenous vein

Femoral vein

SARTORIUS

ADDUCTOR LONGUS

ADDUCTOR MAGNUS

GRACILIS

SEMITENDINOSUS

SEMI-
MEMBRAN

Arteria profunda
femoris

Biceps femoris,
short head

Sciatic nerve

BICEPS
FEMORIS
(LONG
HEAD)

Posterior femoral cutaneous nerve

10.139 Transverse section through the middle of the right thigh: superior
(proximal) aspect. About three-fifths of the natural size.

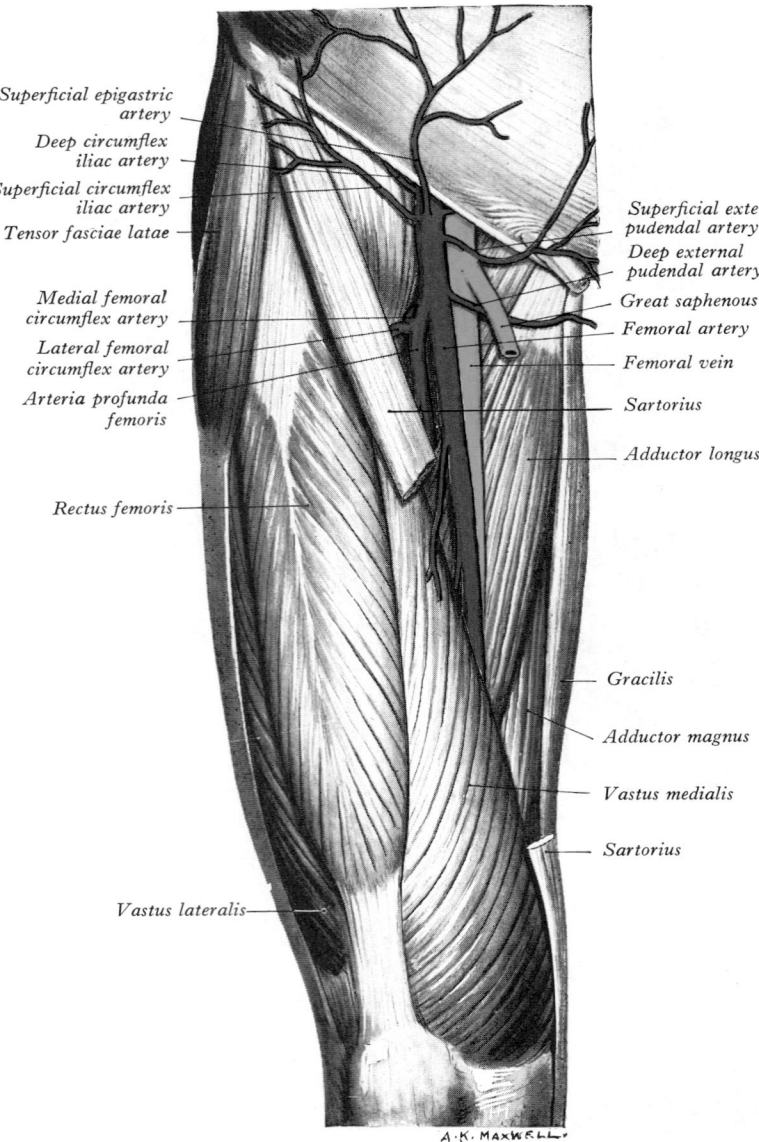

Superficial epigastric artery
Deep circumflex iliac artery
Superficial circumflex iliac artery
Tensor fasciae latae
Medial femoral circumflex artery
Lateral femoral circumflex artery
Arteria profunda femoris
Rectus femoris
Vastus lateralis

Superficial external pudendal artery
Deep external pudendal artery
Great saphenous vein
Femoral artery
Femoral vein
Sartorius
Adductor longus
Gracilis
Adductor magnus
Vastus medialis
Sartorius

A·K·MAXWELL·

10.140   The right femoral vessels and some of their branches.

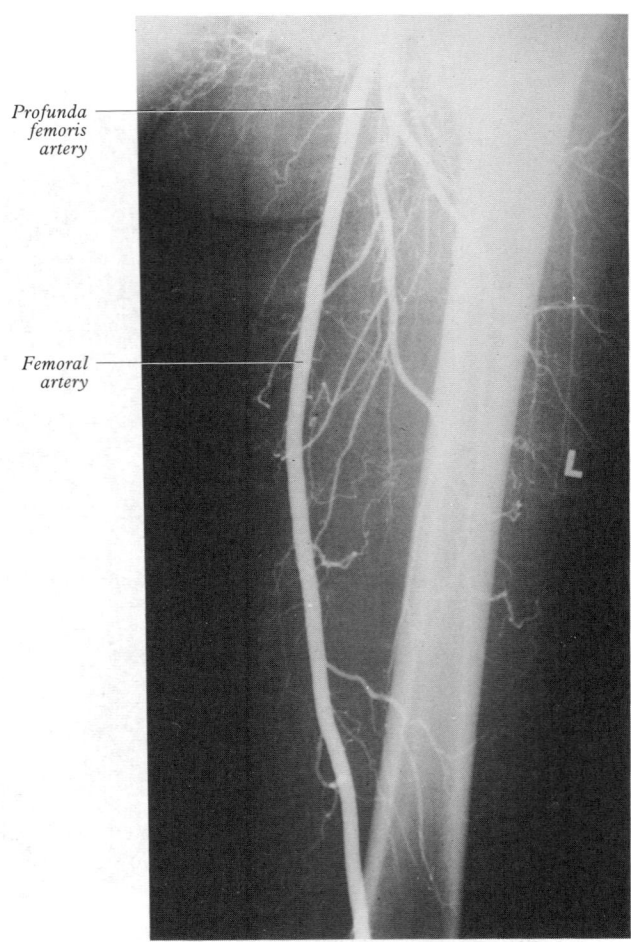

Profunda femoris artery
Femoral artery

10.141   Femoral arteriogram. (Supplied by Shaun Gallagher, Guy's Hospital; photography by Sarah Smith.)

above the medial condyle of the femur, with the thigh semiflexed, abducted and laterally rotated. Its pulsation is easily palpable in its proximal course.

Variations. Rarely, the femoral artery divides, distal to the origin of the arteria profunda femoris, into two trunks reuniting near the adductor opening. It may be replaced by the inferior gluteal artery, accompanying the sciatic nerve to the popliteal fossa and representing a proximal persistence of the original axial artery (p. 318); the external iliac is then small, ending as the arteria profunda femoris.

Clinical anatomy. Compression of the femoral artery is most effective just distal to the inguinal ligament, where it is superficial and separated from the bone (iliopubic eminence) only by the psoas tendon.

Branches. These are as follows:

Superficial epigastric artery (**10**.140). Arising anteriorly from the femoral about 1 cm distal to the inguinal ligament, it traverses the cribriform fascia to ascend anterior to the ligament and run in the abdominal superficial fascia almost to the umbilicus. It supplies the superficial inguinal lymph nodes and superficial fascia and skin, anastomosing with branches of the inferior epigastric and its fellow.

Superficial circumflex iliac artery (**10**.140). This is the smallest superficial branch of the femoral; it arises near or with the superficial epigastric. Usually emerging through the fascia lata, lateral to the saphenous opening, it turns laterally distal to the inguinal ligament towards the anterior–superior iliac spine; it supplies the skin, super-

ficial fascia and superficial inguinal lymph nodes, anastomosing with the deep circumflex iliac, superior gluteal and lateral circumflex femoral arteries.

Superficial external pudendal artery (**10**.140). It arises medially from the femoral, close to the preceding branches. Emerging from the cribriform fascia, it passes medially, usually deep to the great saphenous vein, across the spermatic cord (or round ligament) to supply the lower abdominal, penile, scrotal or labial skin, anastomosing with branches of the internal pudendal.

Veins accompanying the superficial epigastric, superficial circumflex iliac and external pudendal arteries join the great saphenous vein before it enters the saphenous opening.

Deep external pudendal artery (**10**.140). This artery passes medially across the pectineus and anterior or posterior to the adductor longus, covered by fascia lata, piercing it to supply the skin of the perineum and scrotum or labium majus; its branches anastomose with the posterior scrotal or labial branches of the internal pudendal.

Muscular branches. These supply the sartorius, the vastus medialis and the adductors.

ARTERIA PROFUNDA FEMORIS

The arteria profunda femoris is a large branch arising laterally from the femoral about 3.5 cm distal to the inguinal ligament (**10**.139–142). At first lateral to the femoral artery, it spirals posterior to this and the femoral vein to the medial side of the femur; it passes between pectineus and adductor longus, then between the latter and adductor brevis and then descends between adductor longus and adductor magnus to finally pierce the latter and anastomose with the upper muscular branches of the popliteal. This terminal part is sometimes named the *fourth perforating artery*.

The deep femoral artery is the main supply to the adductor,

extensor and flexor muscles; it also anastomoses with the internal and external iliac arteries above and the popliteal artery below.

Relations. Posterior, in proximodistal order, are: the iliacus, pectineus, adductor brevis and adductor magnus. Anterior are the femoral and profunda veins and distally the adductor longus, separating it from the femoral artery. Laterally vastus medialis separates its proximal part from the femur.

Variations. Its origin is sometimes medial, or rarely posterior on the femoral artery; if the former, it may cross anterior to the femoral vein and then pass backwards around its medial side.

Branches. These are as follows:

Lateral circumflex femoral artery (10.142). A lateral branch near the root of the profunda, it inclines laterally between divisions of the femoral nerve, posterior to sartorius and rectus femoris, dividing into ascending, transverse and descending branches. It may arise from the femoral. The *ascending branch* ascends along the intertrochanteric line, under the tensor fasciae latae, lateral to the hip joint; it anastomoses with the superior gluteal and deep circumflex iliac arteries, supplying the greater trochanter, and forms an anastomotic ring round the femoral neck with branches of the medial circumflex femoral; from this ring the femoral neck and head are supplied. The *descending branch*, sometimes direct from the profunda or the femoral, descends posterior to the rectus femoris, along the anterior border of the vastus lateralis, which it supplies: a long ramus descends in vastus lateralis to the knee, anastomosing with the lateral superior genicular branch of the popliteal, accompanied by the nerve to vastus lateralis. The *transverse branch*, the smallest, passes laterally anterior to vastus intermedius, pierces vastus lateralis to wind round the femur, just distal to the greater trochanter, anastomosing with the medial circumflex, inferior gluteal and first perforating arteries (cruciate anastomosis).

Medial circumflex femoral artery (10.142). Originating usually from the posteromedial aspect of the profunda but often the femoral artery, this artery supplies the adductor muscles and curves medially round the femur between pectineus and psoas major and then obturator externus and adductor brevis, finally appearing between quadratus femoris and upper border of adductor magnus, dividing into transverse and ascending branches. The *transverse branch* takes part in the cruciate anastomosis. The *ascending branch* ascends on the tendon of the obturator externus, anterior to the quadratus femoris, to the trochanteric fossa, where it anastomoses with branches of the gluteal and lateral circumflex femoral arteries. An acetabular branch at the proximal edge of the adductor brevis enters the hip joint under the transverse acetabular ligament with one from the obturator artery; it supplies the fat in the fossa, and reaches the femoral head along its ligament. For blood supply of the proximal end of the femur consult Crock (1965).

Perforating arteries (10.135). Usually three, they perforate the attachment of adductor magnus to reach the thigh's flexor aspect. They pass close to the linea aspera under small tendinous arches and issue muscular, cutaneous and anastomotic branches. Diminished, they pass deep to the short head of biceps femoris (the first usually through the attachment of gluteus maximus), traverse the lateral intermuscular septum and enter vastus lateralis. The first arises proximal to the adductor brevis, the second anterior and the third distal. The *first perforating artery* passes back between the pectineus and adductor brevis (sometimes through the latter), piercing the adductor magnus near the linea aspera to supply adductor brevis, adductor magnus, biceps femoris and gluteus maximus, anastomosing with the inferior gluteal, medial and lateral circumflex femoral and second perforating arteries. The larger *second perforating artery*, often arising with the first, pierces the attachments of adductor brevis and magnus, divides into the ascending and descending branches supplying the posterior femoral muscles and anastomoses with the first and third perforating arteries. The *femoral nutrient artery* usually arises from it; when two nutrient arteries exist, they usually come from the first and third. The *third perforating artery* starts distal to adductor brevis, pierces the attachment of adductor magnus and divides into branches to the posterior femoral muscles; it anastomoses proximally with the perforating arteries, distally with the end of the profunda and muscular branches of the popliteal. The femoral nutrient artery may arise from it. Side branches of the diaphyseal nutrient and other branches of the profunda also provide subsidiary cortical arteries (Crock 1967).

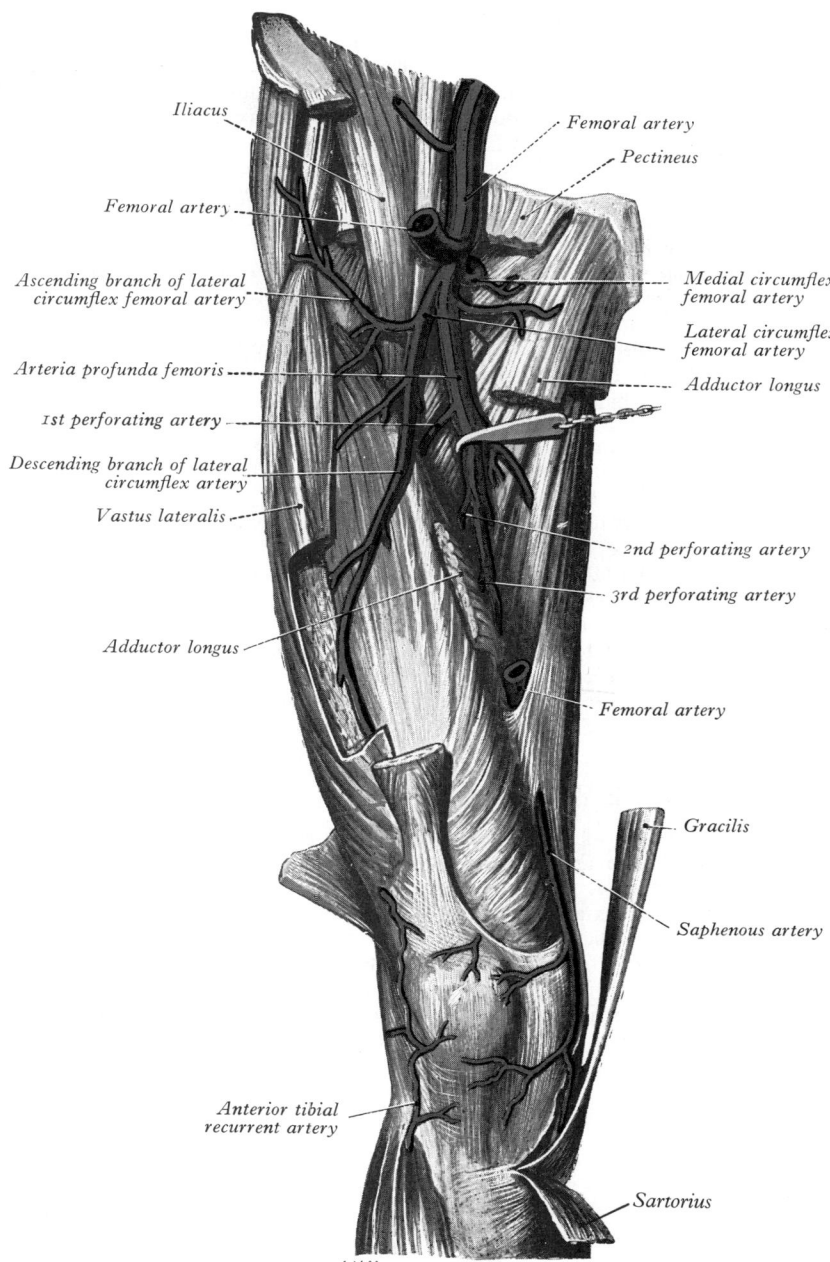

Iliacus

Femoral artery

Pectineus

Femoral artery

Ascending branch of lateral circumflex femoral artery

Medial circumflex femoral artery

Lateral circumflex femoral artery

Arteria profunda femoris

Adductor longus

1st perforating artery

Descending branch of lateral circumflex artery

Vastus lateralis

2nd perforating artery

3rd perforating artery

Adductor longus

Femoral artery

Gracilis

Saphenous artery

Anterior tibial recurrent artery

Sartorius

A.K.MAXWELL.

10.142 The right profunda femoris artery and its branches.

The end of arteria profunda femoris is the *fourth perforating artery*. The perforating arteries form a double chain of anastomoses:

(1) in the adductor muscles
(2) near the linea aspera.

Muscular branches. These are numerous and arise from the arteria profunda femoris; some end in the adductors, others pierce adductor magnus, supply the flexors and anastomose with the medial circumflex femoral artery and superior muscular branches of the popliteal. The profunda is thus the **main** supply to the femoral muscles.

Anastomosis on the back of the thigh. This important chain of anastomoses stretches from the gluteal region to the popliteal fossa, formed in proximodistal order by anastomoses between:

- gluteal arteries and terminals of the medial circumflex femoral
- circumflex femoral arteries and the first perforating artery
- perforating arteries and each other
- the fourth perforating artery and the superior muscular branches of the popliteal.

Descending genicular artery (**10**.146). It arises from the femoral just proximal to the adductor opening, at once supplying a saphenous branch and then descending in the vastus medialis, anterior to the tendon of adductor magnus, to the medial side of the knee, anastomosing with the medial superior genicular artery. Muscular branches supply vastus medialis and adductor magnus and have articular branches, which anastomose round the knee joint. One articular branch crosses above the femoral patellar surface, forming an arch with the lateral superior genicular artery and supplying the knee joint. The saphenous branch emerges distally through the roof of the adductor canal to accompany the saphenous nerve to the medial side of the knee. Passing between sartorius and gracilis it supplies the skin of the proximomedial area of the leg, anastomosing with the medial inferior genicular artery.

Collateral circulation. After ligation of the femoral artery proximal to the origin of the arteria profunda femoris, the main anastomotic channels available are:

- superior and inferior gluteal branches of the internal iliac with the medial and lateral circumflex femoral and the first perforating branch of the arteria profunda femoris
- the obturator branch of the internal iliac with the medial circumflex femoral of the arteria profunda femoris
- the internal pudendal branch of the internal iliac with superficial and deep external pudendal branches of the femoral
- a deep circumflex iliac branch of the external iliac with the lateral circumflex femoral branch of the arteria profunda femoris and the superficial circumflex iliac branch of the femoral
- the inferior gluteal branch of the internal iliac with perforating branches of the arteria profunda femoris

POPLITEAL FOSSA

The popliteal fossa is a rhomboidal region posterior to the knee joint, more apparent when disturbed by dissection (**7**.136, **8**.384, **8**.385, **10**.144). **Lateral** are proximally the biceps femoris and distally the plantaris and lateral head of gastrocnemius; **medial** and proximally are the semitendinosus and semimembranosus, and distally the medial head of the gastrocnemius; **anterior** are the femoral popliteal surface, oblique popliteal ligament, back of the proximal end of the tibia and the fascia covering the popliteus, collectively forming a so-called floor. The fossa is covered **posteriorly** by the popliteal fascia. (Note that 'popliteal fascia' refers to part of the general investing layer of deep fascia that forms a 'roof' for the fossa; to be carefully distinguished from the 'fascia of popliteus' which forms part of the floor.)

Contents (**8**.260, **10**.144). Until disturbed, the popliteal fossa is about 2.5 cm wide and its contents are largely hidden, especially in its distal part, where the heads of gastrocnemius are in contact. When its boundaries are separated its contents are seen to be the popliteal vessels, the tibial and common peroneal nerves, the small saphenous vein, posterior femoral cutaneous nerve, an obturator articular branch, lymph nodes and fat. The tibial nerve descends centrally immediately anterior to the popliteal fascia, crossing the vessels posteriorly from lateral to medial. The common peroneal nerve descends laterally near the tendon of biceps femoris. Popliteal vessels are deep on the floor, the vein superficial to the artery, and united by dense areolar tissue. The vein is thick-walled, proximally lateral to the artery, and crossing to its medial side distally; sometimes it is double with the artery between the veins, the latter usually being interconnected. An articular branch from the obturator nerve descends on the artery to the knee. Six or seven popliteal lymph nodes are embedded in the fat, one under the popliteal fascia near the end of the small saphenous vein, one between the popliteal artery and knee joint, others around the popliteal vessels.

POPLITEAL ARTERY

The popliteal artery (**10**.143–145), continuing the femoral, traverses the popliteal fossa; from the opening in adductor magnus it descends laterally to the intercondylar fossa, inclining obliquely to the distal border of the popliteus, where it divides into the *anterior* and *posterior tibial arteries* (**10**.144). This division is at the proximal end of the crural interosseous space (which is asymmetrical) between the wide tibial metaphysis and the slender fibular metaphysis. Thus the popliteal artery extends from the medial border of the femur to the laterally placed interosseous space, accounting for its oblique descent (**10**.145).

Relations. **Anterior**, proximodistally, is fat covering the femoral popliteal surface, the capsule of the knee joint, and the fascia of popliteus. **Posterior** are, proximally, the semimembranosus and, distally, the gastrocnemius and plantaris. At intermediate level the artery is separated from the skin and fasciae by fat and crossed from

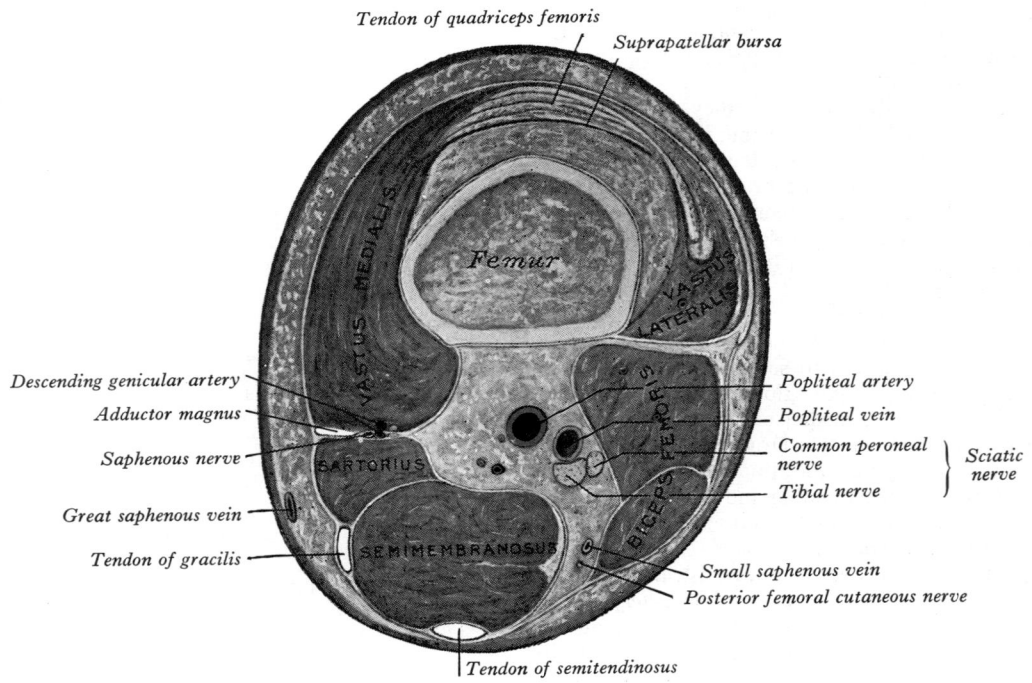

Tendon of quadriceps femoris

Suprapatellar bursa

Femur

Descending genicular artery

Adductor magnus

Saphenous nerve

Great saphenous vein

Tendon of gracilis

Popliteal artery

Popliteal vein

Common peroneal nerve ⎫ *Sciatic*

Tibial nerve ⎬ *nerve*

Small saphenous vein

Posterior femoral cutaneous nerve

Tendon of semitendinosus

10.143 Transverse section through the right thigh, 4 cm above the adductor tubercle of the femur: superior (proximal) aspect. About three-fifths of the natural size.

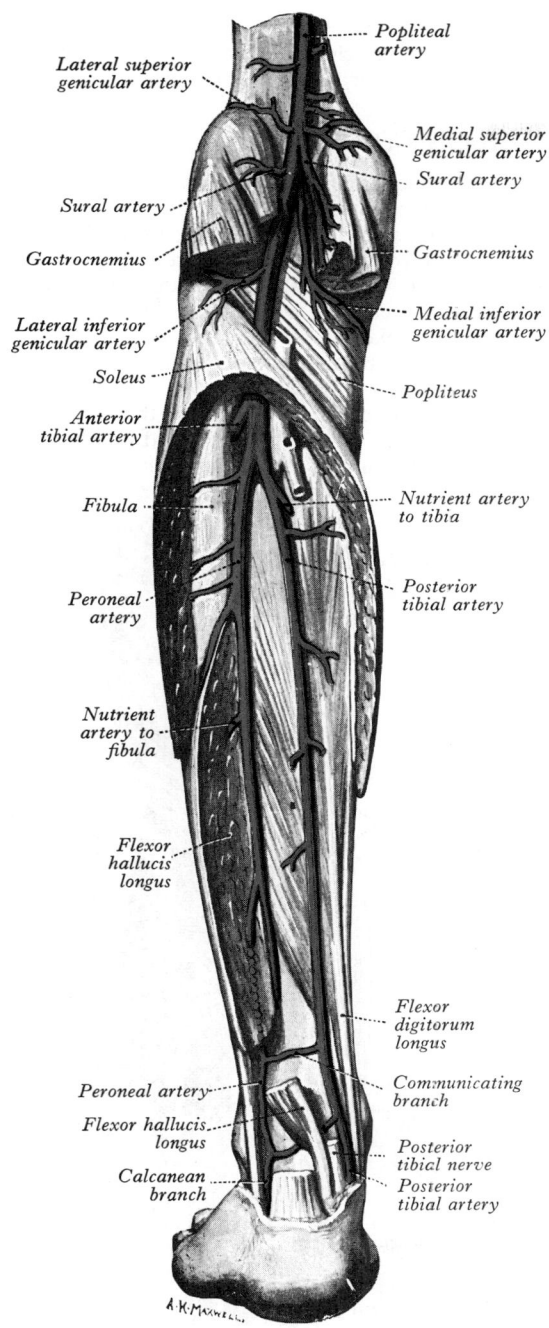

10.144   The left popliteal, posterior tibial and peroneal arteries: dorsal aspect.

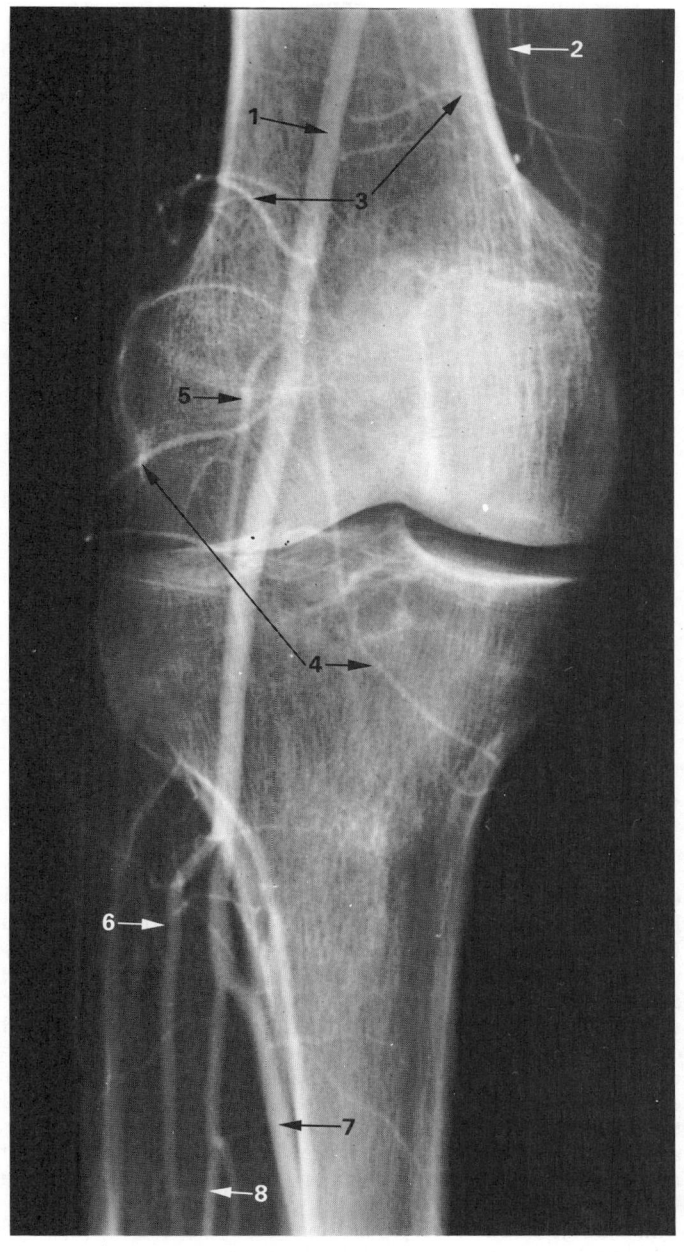

10.145   Popliteal arteriogram: anteroposterior view of adult male of 63 years. The following arteries can be identified: 1. popliteal; 2. descending genicular; 3. superior medial and lateral genicular; 4. inferior medial and lateral genicular; 5. middle genicular; 6. anterior tibial; 7. posterior tibial; 8. peroneal. Note the (normal) obliquity of the popliteal artery.

lateral to medial by the tibial nerve and popliteal vein, the vein veing between the nerve and artery and adherent to the latter. **Lateral** are proximally the biceps femoris, tibial nerve, popliteal vein and lateral femoral condyle and distally the plantaris and lateral head of gastrocnemius. **Medial** are the semimembranosus and medial femoral condyle and distally the tibial nerve, popliteal vein and medial head of gastrocnemius. Relations of the popliteal lymph nodes are described on page 1616.

Variations. The artery may divide into terminal branches **proximal** to the popliteus, the anterior tibial artery then descending **anterior** to the muscle. Sometimes it divides into the anterior tibial and peroneal arteries, the posterior tibial being absent or rudimentary; it may divide into the anterior and posterior tibial and peroneal.

Surface anatomy. The popliteal artery is approximately represented as extending from the junction of the middle and lower thirds of the thigh, 2.5 cm medial to its posterior midline, to the

midpoint between the femoral condyles, continuing inferolaterally to the level of the tibial tuberosity, medial to the fibular neck.

Branches. These are the cutaneous, muscular and genicular branches which reach the tibiofibular interosseous gap.

Cutaneous branches. They leave the popliteal or its side branches, descend between the heads of gastrocnemius and perforate the deep fascia to supply the skin on the back of the leg; one usually accompanies the small saphenous vein.

Superior muscular branches. Two or three in number, they arise proximally and pass to the adductor magnus and femoral flexors, anastomosing with the termination of the arteria profunda femoris.

Sural arteries. Two in number, these are large and arise behind the knee joint to supply gastrocnemius, soleus and plantaris.

Superior genicular arteries (**10**.144, 146)**.** They diverge from the popliteal, curving round proximal to both femoral condyles, to the anterior aspect of the knee. The *medial superior genicular artery* lies

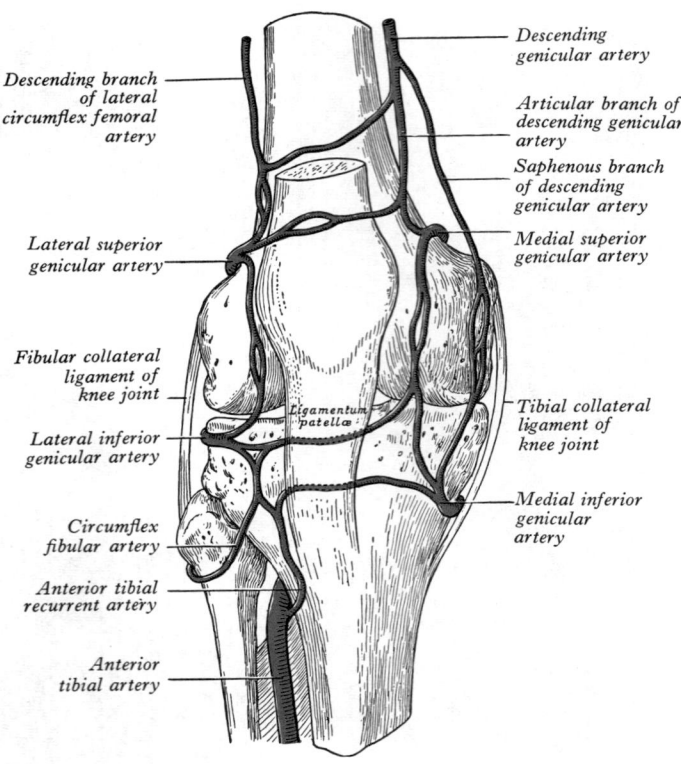

10.146   The arterial anastomosis around the knee joint (schematic).

under semimembranosus and semitendinosus, proximal to the medial head of gastrocnemius and deep to the tendon of adductor magnus. It divides into a branch to the vastus medialis which anastomoses with the descending genicular and medial inferior genicular arteries, and one ramifying on the femur and anastomosing with the lateral superior genicular artery. Its size varies inversely with that of the descending genicular. The *lateral superior genicular artery* passes under the tendon of biceps femoris, dividing into superficial and deep branches; the superficial supplies the vastus lateralis, anastomosing with the descending branch of the lateral circumflex femoral and lateral inferior genicular; the deep branch anastomoses with the medial superior genicular, forming an anterior arch across the femur with the descending genicular.

Middle genicular artery. This small artery arises from the popliteal near the posterior centre of the knee joint; it pierces the oblique popliteal ligament to supply the cruciate ligaments and synovial membrane.

Inferior genicular arteries (**10**.144, 146). They arise from the popliteal deep to the gastrocnemius. The medial is deep to its medial head, descending along the proximal margin of the popliteus, which it supplies, and passing inferior to the medial tibial condyle and under the tibial collateral ligament, at the anterior border of which it ascends anteromedial to the joint; it supplies this and the tibia, anastomosing with the lateral inferior and medial superior genicular arteries and also with the anterior tibial recurrent artery and saphenous branch of the descending genicular. The lateral inferior genicular artery runs laterally across the popliteus and forwards over the fibula's head to the front of the knee joint, passing under the lateral head of gastrocnemius, the fibular collateral ligament and tendon of biceps femoris. Its branches anastomose with the medial inferior and lateral superior genicular, anterior and posterior tibial recurrent and circumflex fibular arteries.

Genicular anastomosis

Around the patella and femoral and tibial condyles an intricate anastomosis exists. A superficial network spreads between the fascia and skin around the patella and in the fat deep to the ligamentum patellae. A deep network lies on the femur and tibia near the adjoining articular surfaces, supplying the bone and marrow, the articular capsule and synovial membrane. The vessels involved are

the medial and lateral genicular, descending genicular, the descending branch of the lateral circumflex femoral, circumflex fibular and the anterior and posterior tibial recurrent arteries.

ANTERIOR TIBIAL ARTERY

The anterior tibial artery is the terminal branch of the popliteal and arises at the distal border of the popliteus (**10**.144–148). At first in the flexor compartment, it passes between the heads of tibialis posterior and through the oval aperture in the proximal part of the interosseous membrane (p. 712) to the extensor region, passing medial to the fibular neck. Descending anteriorly on the membrane it approaches the tibia and, distally, lies anterior to it (**10**.149). At the ankle it is midway between the malleoli, continuing on the dorsum of the foot as the *arteria dorsalis pedis*.

Relations. In its proximal two-thirds the artery descends on the interosseous membrane, in its distal third anterior to the tibia and ankle joint. Proximally it is between tibialis anterior and extensor

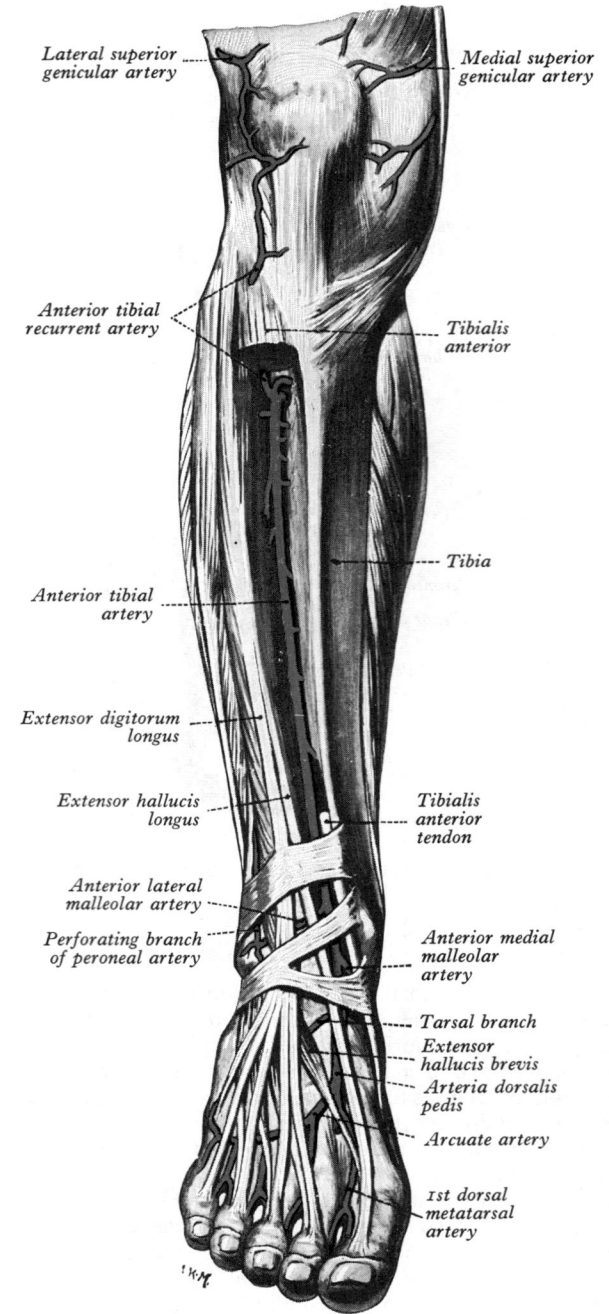

10.147   The right anterior tibial and dorsalis pedis arteries. A large part of the tibialis anterior has been excised and the extensor hallucis longus retracted laterally to expose the anterior tibial artery.

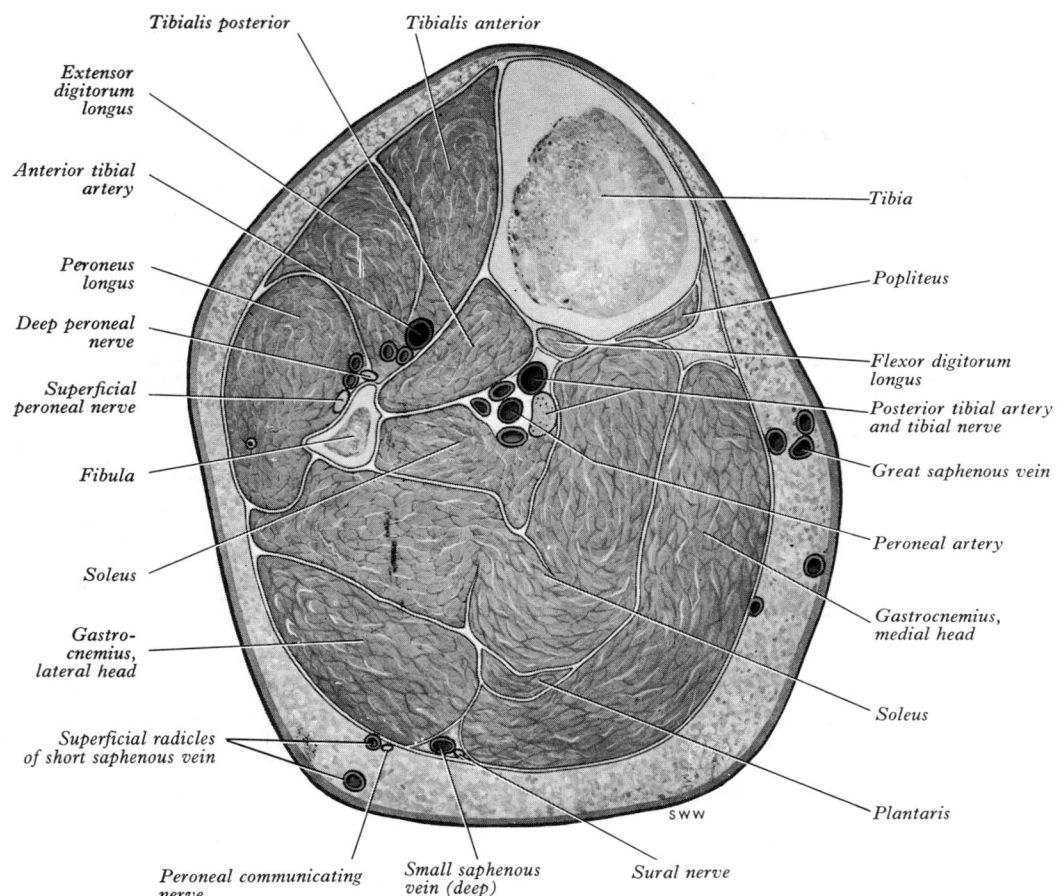

10.148 Transverse section through the right leg, about 10 cm below the knee joint: inferior (distal) aspect. At a slightly lower level the flexor digitorum longus intervenes between the soleus and the fascia on the posterior surface of the tibialis posterior.

digitorum longus, then between tibialis anterior and extensor hallucis longus. At the ankle it is crossed superficially from the lateral side by the tendon of extensor hallucis longus and is then between this and the first tendon of the extensor digitorum longus. Its proximal two-thirds are covered by adjoining muscles and deep fascia, its distal third by the skin, fasciae and extensor retinacula. Venae comitantes accompany it. The deep peroneal nerve, curling laterally round the fibular neck, reaches the lateral side of the artery where it enters the extensor region but in the middle third of the leg becomes anterior to it and distally again becomes lateral.

Surface anatomy. Surface projection of the anterior tibial artery begins 2.5 cm distal to the medial side of the fibular head and ends midway between the malleoli. It can be felt pulsating lateral to the tendon of extensor hallucis longus.

Variations. This vessel may be small or even absent, replaced by perforating branches from the posterior tibial or the perforating branch of the peroneal. It occasionally deviates laterally, regaining its usual position at the ankle.

Branches. These are the anterior and posterior tibial recurrent; muscular; and anterior medial and lateral malleolar.

Posterior tibial recurrent artery. It is an inconstant branch, which arises before the anterior tibial reaches the extensor compartment, ascending anterior to the popliteus with the muscle's recurrent nerve, anastomosing with the inferior genicular branches of the popliteal. It supplies the superior tibiofibular joint.

Anterior tibial recurrent artery (10.147). Arising near the preceding vessel, it ascends in tibialis anterior, ramifies on the front and sides of the knee joint and joins the patellar network, anastomosing with the genicular branches of the popliteal and circumflex fibular arteries.

Muscular branches. These numerous branches supply the adjacent muscles; some pierce the deep fascia to supply the skin, others traverse the interosseous membrane to anastomose with branches of the posterior tibial and peroneal arteries.

Anterior medial malleolar artery (10.147, 150). It arises about 5 cm proximal to the ankle, passing posterior to the tendons of extensor hallucis longus and tibialis anterior medial to the joint, where it joins branches of the posterior tibial and medial plantar arteries.

Anterior lateral malleolar artery (10.147, 150). This artery pro-

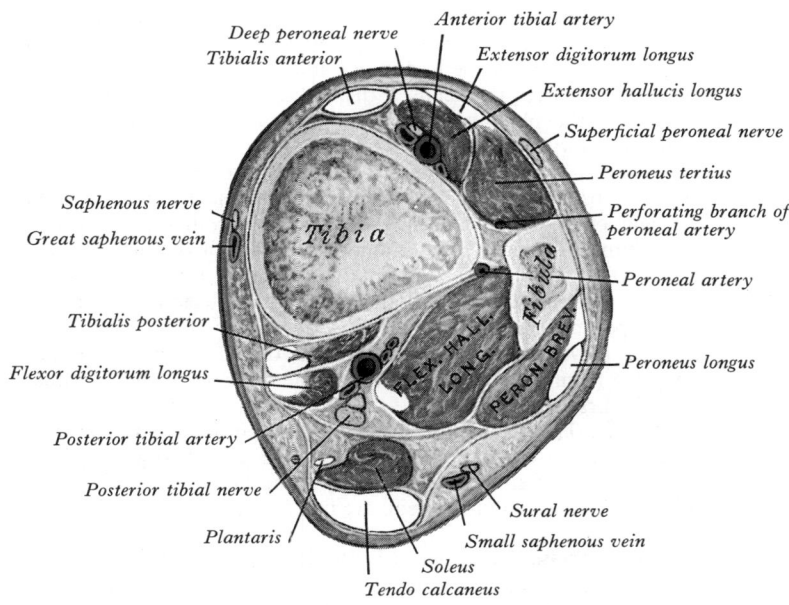

10.149 Transverse section through the right leg, about 6 cm above the tip of the medial malleolus: superior (proximal) aspect.

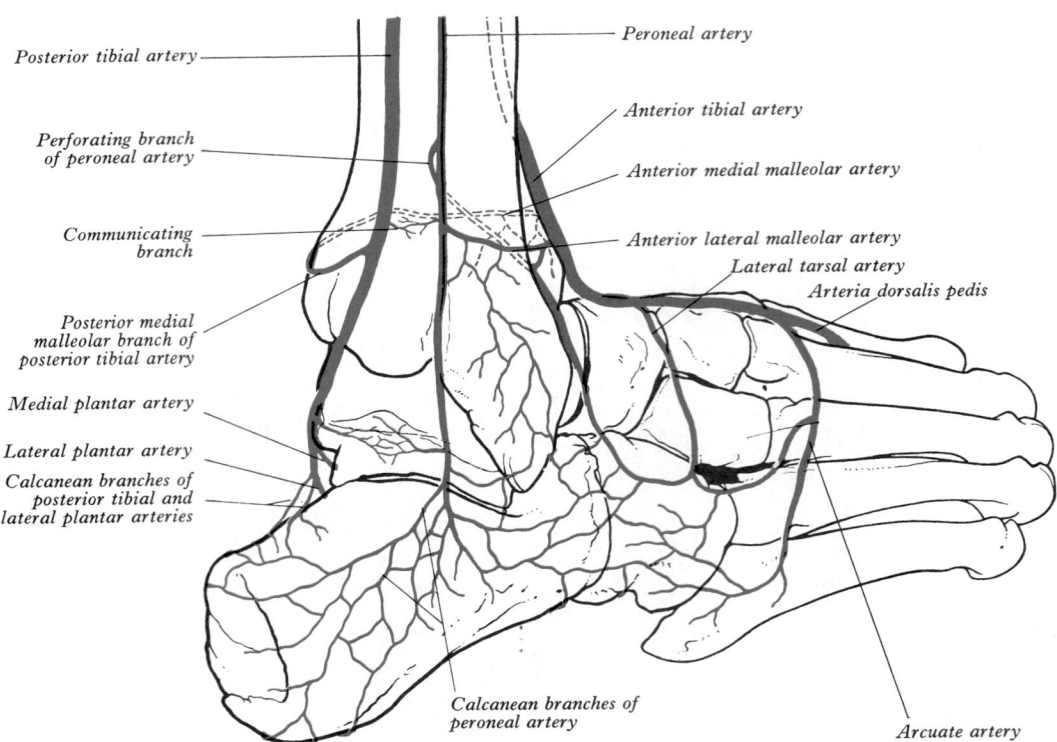

Posterior tibial artery

Perforating branch
of peroneal artery

Communicating
branch

Posterior medial
malleolar branch of
posterior tibial artery

Medial plantar artery

Lateral plantar artery

Calcanean branches of
posterior tibial and
lateral plantar arteries

Peroneal artery

Anterior tibial artery

Anterior medial malleolar artery

Anterior lateral malleolar artery

Lateral tarsal artery

Arteria dorsalis pedis

Calcanean branches of
peroneal artery

Arcuate artery

10.150   The arterial anastomoses of the ankle, tarsus and metatarsus.

ceeds posterior to the tendons of extensor digitorum longus and
peroneus tertius to the lateral side of the ankle, anastomosing with
the perforating branch of the peroneal and ascending branches of
the lateral tarsal artery.

Anastomosis at the ankle joint (**10**.150). This consists of vascular
networks around the malleoli. The *medial malleolar network* is formed
by the anterior medial malleolar branch of the anterior tibial, the
medial tarsal branches of the arteria dorsalis pedis, the malleolar
and calcaneal branches of the posterior tibial and branches of the
medial plantar artery. The *lateral malleolar network* is formed by the
anterior lateral malleolar branch of the anterior tibial, lateral tarsal
branch of arteria dorsalis pedis, the perforating and calcaneal branches of the peroneal and side branches of the lateral plantar artery.

Arteria dorsalis pedis

The dorsal artery of the foot (**10**.147), it is the continuation of the
anterior tibial distal to the ankle. It passes medially along the dorsum
to the proximal end of the first intermetatarsal space, where it turns
into the sole between the heads of the first dorsal interosseous muscle
to complete the plantar arch, where it provides the first plantar
metatarsal artery.

Relations. The dorsal artery successively crosses the talocrural
articular capsule, talus, navicular and intermediate cuneiform and
their ligaments; **superficial** are the skin, fasciae, inferior extensor
retinaculum and, near its termination, extensor hallucis brevis.
Medial is the tendon of extensor hallucis longus, **lateral** the medial
tendon of extensor digitorum longus and medial terminal branch of
the deep peroneal nerve.

Surface anatomy. The pulsation of the dorsal artery of the foot
is palpable from the midpoint between the malleoli to the proximal
end of the first intermetatarsal space.

Variations. The artery may be larger to compensate for a small
lateral plantar artery or replaced by a large perforating branch of
the peroneal. It often diverges laterally from its usual route.

Branches. These are the tarsal, arcuate and first dorsal metatarsal
arteries.

Tarsal arteries. These two arteries, lateral and medial (**10**.147),
arise as the arteria dorsalis pedis crosses the navicular; the former
runs laterally under the extensor digitorum brevis; it supplies this
and the tarsal articulations, anastomosing with branches of the
arcuate, anterior lateral malleolar, lateral plantar and the perforating

branch of the peroneal. Two or three medial tarsal arteries ramify
on the foot's medial border and join the medial malleolar network.

Arcuate artery (**10**.147). It arises near the medial cuneiform,
passing laterally over the metatarsal bases, deep to the tendons of
the digital extensors, and anastomosing with the lateral tarsal and
plantar arteries. It supplies the *second* to *fourth dorsal metatarsal
arteries*, running distally superficial to the corresponding dorsal
interosseous muscles; in the interdigital clefts each divides into two
dorsal digital branches for the adjoining toes. Proximally, in the
interosseous spaces, they receive *proximal perforating branches* from
the plantar arch and distally are joined by the *distal perforating
branches* from the plantar metatarsal arteries. The fourth dorsal
metatarsal sends a branch to the lateral side of the fifth toe.

First dorsal metatarsal artery (**10**.147). It arises just before the
arteria dorsalis pedis enters the sole; it runs distally on the first
dorsal interosseous; at the cleft between the first and second toes it
divides, one branch passing under the tendon of extensor hallucis
longus and supplying the medial side of the hallux and one bifurcating
to supply the adjoining sides of hallux and the second toe.

POSTERIOR TIBIAL ARTERY

The posterior tibial artery begins at the distal border of the popliteus,
between tibia and fibula, descending medially in the flexor compartment to divide midway between the medial malleolus and the
medial tubercle of calcaneus, under abductor hallucis, into the medial
and lateral plantar arteries (**10**.144, 145, 148).

Relations. The artery is successively **posterior** to tibialis posterior,
flexor digitorum longus, tibia and ankle joint. Proximally, gastrocnemius, soleus and the deep transverse fascia of the leg are **superficial**
and distally only the skin and fascia. It is parallel with and about
2.5 cm anterior to the medial border of the tendo calcaneus; terminally it is **deep** to the flexor retinaculum and abductor hallucis. It
is accompanied by two veins and the tibial nerve, the latter first
medial, but soon crossing posterior, and then largely posterolateral.
The arrangement of structures passing from the leg to the sole is
described on page 890.

Surface anatomy. The posterior tibial artery corresponds to a line
joining a point 1–2 cm lateral to the calf's midline at the fibular
neck's level, extending downwards and medially to the midpoint
between the medial malleolus and the heel (medial calcaneal tubercle).

Branches. These are circumflex fibular, peroneal, nutrient, medial and lateral plantar.

Circumflex fibular artery. This artery, which sometimes arises from the anterior tibial artery, passes laterally round the fibula's neck through the soleus to anastomose with the lateral inferior genicular, medial genicular and anterior tibial recurrent arteries. It supplies bone and articular structures.

Peroneal artery (10.144, 148, 149). It arises about 2.5 cm distal to popliteus, and passes obliquely to the fibula, descending along its medial crest in a fibrous canal between tibialis posterior and flexor hallucis longus or in the latter. Reaching the inferior tibiofibular syndesmosis, it divides into the calcaneal branches, ramifying on the lateral and posterior surfaces of the calcaneus. **Proximally** it is covered by the soleus and deep transverse fascia, between this and the deep muscles; **distally** it is overlapped by flexor hallucis longus.

Variations. The artery may spring earlier from the posterior tibial, or even the popliteal, sometimes 7 or 8 cm **distal** to popliteus. It is more often enlarged and either joins and reinforces the posterior tibial artery or replaces it in the distal leg and foot.

Muscular branches. These supply soleus, tibialis posterior, flexor hallucis longus and peronei.

Nutrient artery. This runs proximally into the fibula.

Perforating branch. It traverses the interosseous membrane about 5 cm proximal to the lateral malleolus to enter the extensor compartment, where it anastomoses with the anterior lateral malleolar artery; descending anterior to the inferior tibiofibular syndesmosis, it supplies the tarsus, anastomosing with the lateral tarsal artery. This branch is sometimes enlarged and may replace the arteria dorsalis pedis. A *communicating branch* connects it about 5 cm proximal to the ankle to a *communicating branch* of the posterior tibial. The calcaneal or terminal branches anastomose with the anterior lateral malleolar and calcaneal branches of the posterior tibial artery.

Nutrient artery of the tibia. It arises from the posterior tibial near its origin; supplying a few muscular branches it descends into the bone immediately distal to the soleal line. It is one of the largest of the nutrient arteries.

Muscular branches. These are distributed to the soleus and deep flexors of the leg.

Communicating branch of the posterior tibia. This runs posteriorly across the tibia about 5 cm above its distal end, deep to flexor hallucis longus, to join a communicating branch of the peroneal.

Medial malleolar branches. These pass round the tibial malleolus to the medial malleolar network.

Calcaneal branches. They arise just proximal to the terminal division of the posterior tibial; they pierce the flexor retinaculum to supply the fat and skin behind the tendo calcaneus and in the heel and muscles on the tibial side of the sole; they anastomose with medial malleolar arteries and calcaneal branches of the peroneal.

Medial plantar artery (10.151A, B). It is the smaller terminal branch of the posterior tibial, which passes distally along the medial side of the foot with the medial plantar nerve lateral to it. At first deep to abductor hallucis, it runs distally between this and flexor digitorum brevis, supplying both. Near the first metatarsal base, its calibre, diminished by muscular branches, is further diminished by a superficial stem and it then passes to reach the medial border of the hallux where it anastomoses with a branch of the first plantar metatarsal artery (see below). Its superficial stem trifurcates and supplies three superficial digital branches accompanying the digital branches of the medial plantar nerve to join the first to third plantar metatarsal arteries.

Surface anatomy. The trunk of the artery begins midway between the medial malleolus and heel (medial calcaneal tubercle) extending towards the first interdigital cleft as far as the navicular bone.

Lateral plantar artery (10.151A, B). The larger terminal branch of the posterior tibial passes distally and laterally to the fifth metatarsal base, the lateral plantar nerve medial to it. (Note that the plantar nerves lie between the plantar arteries.) Turning medially, with the nerve's deep branch, to the interval between the first and second metatarsal bases, it unites with the arteria dorsalis pedis to complete the plantar arch. As it passes laterally, it is first between the calcaneus and abductor hallucis, then between flexor digitorum brevis and flexor accessorius; running distally to the fifth metatarsal base it passes between flexor digitorum brevis and abductor digiti minimi

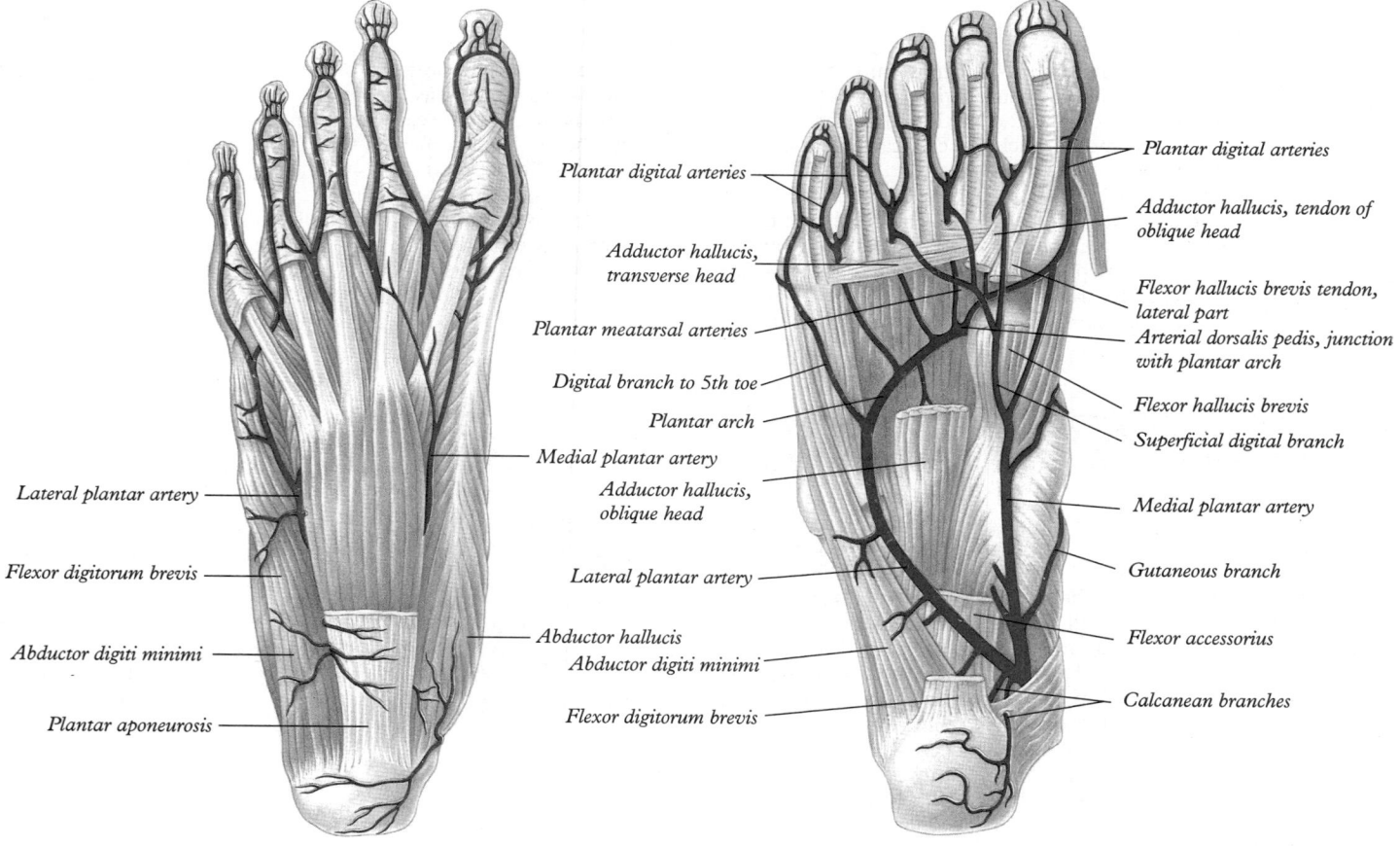

Plantar digital arteries

Adductor hallucis, transverse head

Plantar meatarsal arteries

Digital branch to 5th toe

Plantar arch

Medial plantar artery

Adductor hallucis, oblique head

Lateral plantar artery

Abductor hallucis
Abductor digiti minimi

Flexor digitorum brevis

Lateral plantar artery

Flexor digitorum brevis

Abductor digiti minimi

Plantar aponeurosis

Plantar digital arteries

Adductor hallucis, tendon of oblique head

Flexor hallucis brevis tendon, lateral part

Arterial dorsalis pedis, junction with plantar arch

Flexor hallucis brevis

Superficial digital branch

Medial plantar artery

Gutaneous branch

Flexor accessorius

Calcanean branches

10.151A The plantar arteries of the right foot: superficial dissection.

10.151B The plantar arteries of the right foot: deep dissection.

and is covered by the plantar aponeurosis, superficial fascia and skin.

Branches. Muscular branches supply the adjoining muscles; *superficial branches* emerge along the lateral intermuscular septum to supply the skin and subcutaneous tissue lateral in the sole; *anastomotic branches* run to the lateral border, joining branches of the lateral tarsal and arcuate arteries. Sometimes a *calcaneal branch* pierces abductor hallucis to supply the skin of the heel.

PLANTAR ARCH

The plantar arch is deeply situated, extending from the fifth metatarsal base to the proximal end of the first interosseous space. Convex distally, it is plantar to the bases of the second to fourth metatarsal bones and corresponding interossei but dorsal to the oblique part of adductor hallucis.

Branches. Three perforating and four plantar metatarsal branches, and numerous branches supply the skin, fasciae and muscles in the sole. Three *perforating branches* ascend through the proximal ends of the second to fourth intermetatarsal spaces, between the heads of the dorsal interosseous muscles, anastomosing with the dorsal metatarsal arteries. Four *plantar metatarsal arteries* (**10**.151B) extend distally between the metatarsal bones in contact with the interossei. Each divides into two *plantar digital arteries*, supplying the adjacent digital aspects. Near its division each plantar metatarsal sends dorsally a *distal perforating branch* to join a dorsal metatarsal artery. The *first plantar metatarsal artery* springs from the junction between the lateral plantar and dorsalis pedis arteries, sending a digital branch to the medial side of the hallux. The lateral digital branch for the fifth toe arises directly from the lateral plantar artery near the fifth metatarsal base.

Surface anatomy. Beginning between the heel and medial malleolus, the lateral plantar artery crosses obliquely to a point 2.5 cm medial to the fifth metatarsal's tuberosity and with a slight distal convexity reaches the proximal end of the first intermetatarsal space.

Clinical anatomy. Haemorrhage from the plantar arch is difficult to stem, due to the depth of the vessel and its important close relations. It must be treated like the palmar arches (p. 1544).

PULSE

Palpating the pulse must surely be one of the most important aspects of the physical examination of a patient, giving information about both the state of the circulation and the rhythm of the heart. Prior to modern diagnostic techniques such as echocardiography and cardiac catheterization, feeling the pulse was (and still is in many circumstances) extremely helpful in diagnosing and assessing the state of diseased cardiac valves. The pulse is usually felt in the upper part of the body to assess the state of the circulation or cardiac output, and in the lower part of the body to evaluate the vascular tree with special reference to arteriosclerotic disease. The following are the commonly felt and most useful pulses in clinical practice.

Most of them are found where an artery is superficial and overlying bone.

Superficial temporal pulse (**10**.73). This pulse is of special value to anaesthetists as their access to patients is frequently restricted to the head. It is palpable anterior to the tragus of the ear as it crosses the zygomatic process of the temporal bone. The artery may be thickened and tender when involved by an arteritis.

Carotid pulse (**10**.75). This important pulse is palpable at the carotid bifurcation which usually lies at the level of the upper border of the thyroid cartilage just lateral to it. The pulse that one feels is formed by a complex of vessels: the common, internal and external carotid arteries plus the roots of the initial branches of the external carotid at that site. The carotid and femoral pulses are the ones usually sought in cases of suspected cardiac arrest.

Brachial pulse (**10**.98). Usually easily felt, it is in the cubital fossa lying medial to the tendon of biceps before disappearing under the bicipital aponeurosis. Many feel that this is the ideal site at which to assess the quality of the cardiac output. This is also a useful site at which to pass an arterial catheter for coronary angiography or cardiac catheterization.

Radial pulse (**10**.109). This is the most accessible pulse for palpation under normal clinical circumstances and it is usually of sufficient calibre to enable good quality information to be derived from it. Because of the palmar arches it is a safe site for cannulation for blood pressure monitoring and arterial blood sampling, as thrombosis there will not normally jeopardise the circulation of the hand. It is most easily felt on the ventral aspect of the wrist between the tendon of flexor carpi radialis and the lower lateral aspect of the radius.

Femoral pulse (**10**.140). Like the carotid pulse the femoral is of great value in assessing whether there is any significant cardiac output in cases of circulatory collapse. However, as with the other lower limb pulses, it may be reduced or obliterated by arteriosclerotic disease. It is a common site for coronary angiography and cardiac catheterization and is also a useful site for arterial puncture for blood gas analysis. It can usually be felt in the femoral triangle just below the inguinal ligament half way between the symphysis pubis and the anterior superior iliac spine.

Popliteal pulse (**10**.144). Lying deep in the popliteal fossa this is the most difficult of the peripheral pulses to feel. It is important, however, when assessing the state of the arterial supply to the lower limb especially in the presence of peripheral vascular disease, most commonly arteriosclerosis. The pulse is best felt with the knee flexed to relax the popliteal fascia when it may then be felt in the midline against the popliteal surface of the lower end of the femur.

Posterior tibial pulse (**10**.144). This may be felt behind and below the medial malleolus at the ankle between the tendons of flexor hallucis longus and flexor digitorum longus.

Dorsalis pedis pulse (**10**.147). Like the posterior tibial pulse, the dorsalis pedis may frequently be obliterated by peripheral vascular disease. It is normally palpable lateral to the tendon of extensor hallucis longus as it overlies the tarsal bones.

VENOUS SYSTEM

The veins as a whole form three main systems: pulmonary, systemic and portal. The *pulmonary veins* carry oxygenated blood from the lungs to the heart. The *systemic veins* return venous blood to the heart from much of the rest of the body. *Superficial veins* are located in the superficial fascia, especially in the limbs, and are variable in disposition. *Deep veins* lie beneath the deep fascia and are usually enclosed in connective tissue sheaths with accompanying arteries, the latter assisting venous return (p. 1468). Smaller arteries are accompanied by paired veins flanking them (*venae comitantes*); larger arteries are usually associated with single veins, although some run separately. Veins are usually more variable, in course and structure, than arteries. In many regions, such as the pelvis and vertebral column, veins form extensive plexuses devoid of valves. These plexuses are the basis of anastomosis between the veins of the trunk; they may also act as blood reservoirs of variable capacity. At many

points, such as the junctional regions between the trunk and limbs and near joints, valved *connecting veins* join superficial and deep systemic veins.

The *portal vein* receives tributaries draining venous blood from the subdiaphragmatic part of the oesophagus, the small intestine and the large intestine, the pancreas and the spleen: the blood from this vast area passes through the liver (hepatic circulation) before returning to a general systemic vein, the inferior vena cava.

PULMONARY VEINS

The pulmonary veins return oxygenated blood to the left atrium. Usually four, two from each lung, and devoid of valves, they originate from capillary networks in the alveolar walls. By repeated junctions tributary veins finally form a single trunk in each lobe, i.e. three in the right lung, and two in the left. The right middle and superior lobar veins usually join so that two veins, superior and inferior, leave each lung; they perforate the fibrous pericardium and open separately in the posterosuperior aspect of the left atrium (**10**.32, 39, 56B). Occasionally the three right lobar veins remain separate. Sometimes the two left pulmonary veins form a single trunk. Occasionally the two left pulmonary veins form a single trunk. Occasionally the two left pulmonary veins, each draining a lobe, may be augmented by an accessory lobar vein from each lobe and these may unite to form a third left pulmonary vein (Cory & Valentine 1959).

In the pulmonary hilum (pp. 1659, 1674) the superior pulmonary vein is antero-inferior to the pulmonary artery, the inferior being the most inferior hilar structure and also slightly posterior. The principle bronchus is posterior to the pulmonary artery. On the right the superior pulmonary vein passes posterior to the superior vena cava, the inferior behind the right atrium. On the left both pass anterior to the descending thoracic aorta. In the pericardium, they are partly covered by serous pericardium. Between the terminations of the right, and left veins is, centrally, the oblique pericardial sinus and, laterally, directed medially and upwards, smaller and variable pulmonary venous pericardial recesses (p. 1471).

SYSTEMIC VEINS

In the following description the systemic veins are divided into six groups: cardiac veins, which drain directly into the heart; veins of the head and neck; veins of the upper limbs and veins of the thorax, all three groups draining into the superior vena cava; and veins of the lower limbs and veins of the abdomen and pelvis, both groups draining into the inferior vena cava.

CARDIAC VEINS

Veins draining the heart can be grouped as:

- the *coronary sinus* and *tributaries*, returning blood to the right atrium from the whole heart (including its septa) except the anterior region of the right ventricle and small, variable parts of both atria and left ventricle
- the *anterior cardiac veins* draining an anterior region of the right ventricle and a region around the right cardiac border when the right marginal vein joins this group, ending principally in the right atrium
- the *venae cordis minimae* (Thebesius' veins), opening into the right atrium and ventricle and, to a lesser extent, the left atrium and sometimes left ventricle.

CORONARY SINUS

The large majority of cardiac veins drain into the wide coronary sinus, about 2 or 3 cm long, lying posterior in the coronary sulcus (atrioventricular groove) between the left atrium and ventricle (**10**.32, 152). The sinus opens into the right atrium between the opening of the inferior vena cava and the right atrioventricular orifice, and its opening is guarded by an endocardial fold (*semilunar valve of the coronary sinus*; **10**.33). Its tributaries are the great, small and middle cardiac veins, the posterior vein of the left ventricle and the oblique vein of the left atrium, all except the last having valves at their orifices.

Great cardiac vein (**10**.152)**.** It begins at the cardiac apex, ascends in the anterior interventricular sulcus to the coronary sulcus and follows this to the left and round posterior to the heart to enter the coronary sinus at its origin. It receives tributaries from the left atrium and both ventricles, including the large *left marginal vein* ascending the left aspect ('obtuse border') of the heart.

Small cardiac vein (**10**.152)**.** This lies posterior in the coronary

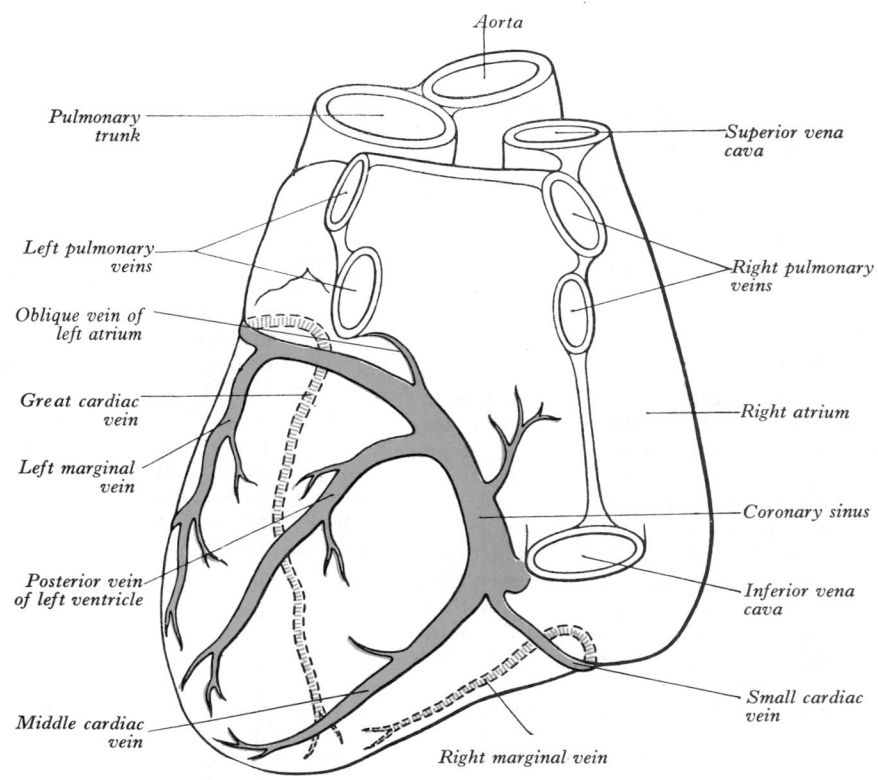

Aorta

Pulmonary trunk

Left pulmonary veins

Oblique vein of left atrium

Great cardiac vein

Left marginal vein

Posterior vein of left ventricle

Middle cardiac vein

Superior vena cava

Right pulmonary veins

Right atrium

Coronary sinus

Inferior vena cava

Small cardiac vein

Right marginal vein

10.152   The principal veins of the heart.

sulcus between the right atrium and ventricle and opens into the coronary sinus near its atrial end. It receives blood from the back of the right atrium and ventricle; the *right marginal vein* passes right, along the inferior cardiac margin ('acute border'), and may join the small cardiac vein in the coronary sulcus but more often opens directly into the right atrium.

Middle cardiac vein (10.152). Beginning at the cardiac apex, it runs back in the posterior interventricular groove to end in the coronary sinus near its atrial end.

Posterior vein of the left ventricle (10.152). Found on the diaphragmatic surface of the left ventricle a little left of the middle cardiac vein, it usually opens into the centre of the coronary sinus but sometimes into the great cardiac vein.

Oblique vein of the left atrium. This small vessel descends obliquely on the back of the left atrium to join the coronary sinus near its end; it is continuous above with the *ligament of the left vena cava* (p. 1472); the two structures are remnants of the left common cardinal vein.

ANTERIOR CARDIAC VEINS

The anterior cardiac veins drain the anterior part of the right ventricle. Usually two or three, sometimes even five (Baroldi & Scomazzoni 1967), they ascend in subepicardial tissue to cross the right part of the atrioventricular sulcus, passing deep or superficial to the right coronary artery. They end in the right atrium, near the sulcus, separately or in variable combinations. A subendocardial collecting channel, into which all may open, has been described (James 1961). The right marginal vein courses along the inferior ('acute') cardiac margin, draining adjacent parts of the right ventricle, and usually opens separately into the right atrium but may join the anterior cardiac veins or, less often, the coronary sinus. Because it is commonly independent it is often grouped with the venae cordis minimae but, since it is larger in calibre, it is comparable with the anterior cardiac veins or even wider. It is perhaps better considered one of the latter, which also sometimes drain with it into the coronary sinus. Mechanik (1934) described all cardiac veins as draining into the coronary sinus in the early fetal period.

VENAE CORDIS MINIMAE

The existence of venae cordis minimae, opening into all cardiac cavities, has been confirmed by many subsequent to their first recording by Thebesius (1708); they are more difficult to demonstrate than larger cardiac vessels. Their numbers and size are highly variable. Aho (1950) demonstrated 'minimal' veins of up to 2 mm in diameter opening into the right atrium and of about 0.5 mm into the right ventricle. He found venae minimae numerous in the right atrium and ventricle, occasional in and often absent from the left atrium, and rare in the left ventricle. Grant and Regnier (1926) considered venae minimae as derived from the intertrabecular spaces of the developing heart.

Cardiac venous anastomoses

There are widespread anastomoses at all levels of cardiac venous circulation, on a scale exceeding that of the arteries and amounting to a veritable venous plexus, according to some investigators (Baroldi & Scomazzoni 1967). Not only are adjacent veins often connected but connections also exist between tributaries of the coronary sinus and those of the anterior cardiac veins (Mierzwa & Kozielec 1975). Regions of abundant anastomoses are the apex and its anterior and posterior aspects. Like coronary arteries (p. 1505) cardiac veins connect with extracardiac vessels, chiefly the vasa vasorum of the large vessels continuous with the heart.

Variation in cardiac veins

Attempts to categorize variations in cardiac venous circulation (Aho 1950) into 'types' have not produced any accepted pattern. Major variations concern the general directions of drainage. The coronary sinus may receive all cardiac veins (except the venae minimae), including the anterior cardiac veins (33%), which may be reduced by diversion of some into the small cardiac vein and then to the coronary sinus (28%); the remainder (39%) represent the 'normal' pattern, as described above. Baroldi and Scomazzoni (1967) distinguished two major variants: a majority (70%) in which the small cardiac vein is independent, small or absent and a less frequent pattern (30%) in which this vein, though variable in size, connects with both coronary and anterior cardiac 'systems'.

VEINS OF THE HEAD AND NECK

The veins of the head and neck can be subdivided into three groups:

- veins of the exterior of the head and face
- cervical veins
- diploic, meningeal, intracranial veins and dural venous sinuses.

This classification is particularly significant at cranial level, where veins, like arteries, are arranged as a three-layered system:

- vessels of the scalp
- dural vessels
- cerebral and cerebellar vessels.

By comparison with the corresponding arteries, the veins of the scalp and dura are very variable and usually intercommunicate more extensively (emissary veins, p. 1589). Dural or meningeal arteries, on the other hand, are independent of cerebral and cerebellar arteries, the latter being derived from the internal carotid, whereas dural venous sinuses share a drainage to the internal jugular vein which is also common to veins of the cerebrum and cerebellum. The diploic veins constitute a hypothetical fourth venous tier; however, since these drain into dural veins, they are here grouped with them, following Browder and Kaplan (1976). It is to be noted that intracranial veins communicate at many points with extracranial vessels via the emissary and other veins (p. 1589).

Developmentally the venous sinuses emerge as venous plexuses; and it is clear, from angiographic studies and corrosion casts, that most sinuses preserve a plexiform arrangement to a variable degree, rather than being simple vessels with a single lumen. Browder and Kaplan (1976), examining human venous sinuses in hundreds of

corrosion casts, have observed vascular plexuses adjoining, in particular, the superior and inferior sagittal and straight sinuses and, with a lesser incidence, the transverse sinuses. Details show much individual variation; departures from 'average' patterns are frequent in earlier years; for example, the falx cerebelli may in infancy contain large plexiform channels and venous lacunae, augmenting the occipital sinus. Such variations cannot be detailed in a general text; in any case they must be established for the individual by angiography when clinical necessity arises; but the wide variation possible in the structure of cranial venous sinuses, with their plexiform nature and wide connections with cerebral and cerebellar veins, must be emphasized. Another kind of connection may be noted here; experiment shows (Rowbotham & Little 1962; Browder & Kaplan 1976) that parts of sinuses (and even diploic veins) can be filled by forcible internal carotid injection, suggesting the existence of arteriovenous shunts. Browder and Kaplan, by injection of the middle meningeal arteries, established a connection between these and the superior sagittal sinus at sites still unknown.

EXTERNAL VEINS OF THE HEAD AND FACE

As with most superficial veins these are subject to variations, far too numerous to illustrate. Some major features are, however, relatively constant; a common pattern is shown in (10.153).

Supratrochlear vein. This starts on the forehead from a venous network connected to the frontal tributaries of the superficial tem-

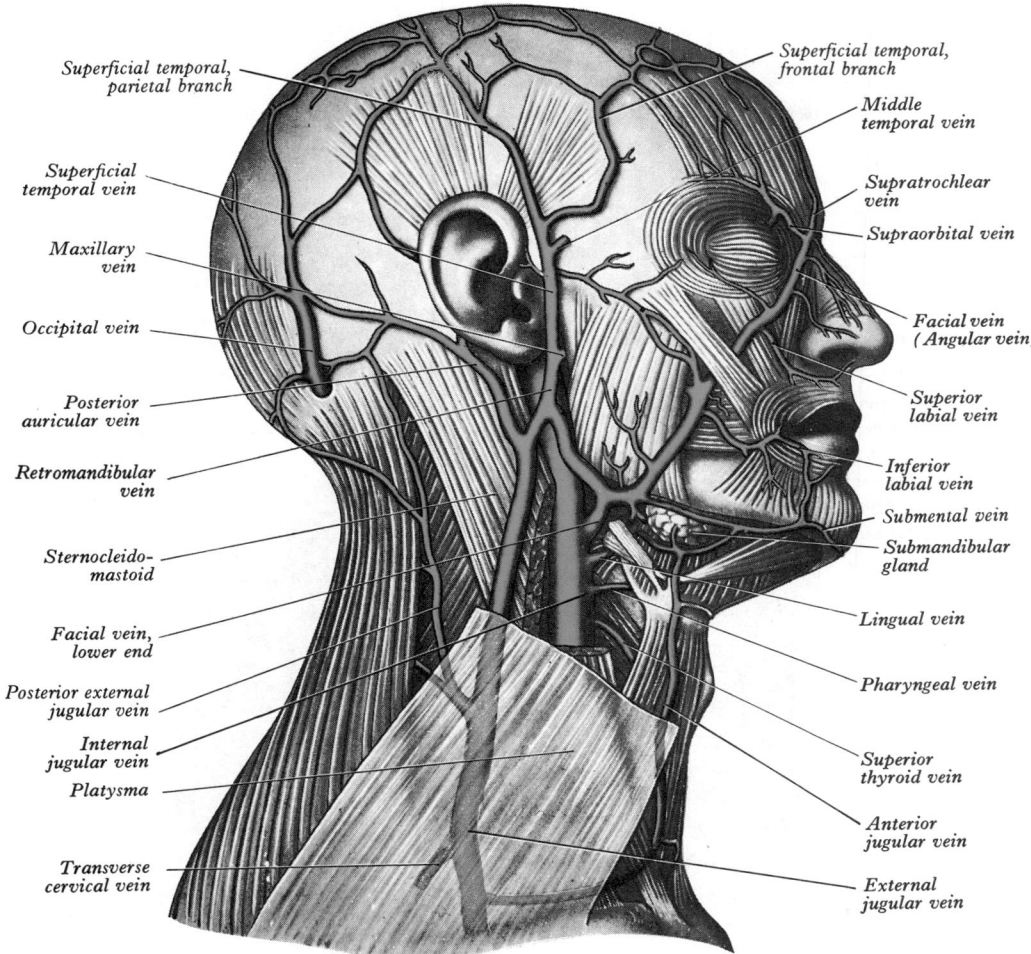

10.153   The veins of the right side of the head and neck. Parts of the right sternocleidomastoid and platysma have been excised to expose the trunk of the internal jugular vein. The external jugular vein is visible through the lower part of the platysma.

poral vein. Veins from this form a single trunk, descending near the midline parallel with its fellow to the radix nasi, across which they are joined by a nasal arch draining the dorsum nasi. The veins then diverge, each joining a supraorbital vein to form the facial vein near the medial canthus. Supratrochlear veins may join, dividing again on the radix nasi to form the two facial veins.

Supraorbital vein. It begins near the zygomatic process of the frontal bone, connecting with radicles of the superficial and middle temporal veins. Passing medially above the orbital opening under orbicularis oculi, it pierces this to form the facial vein by joining the supratrochlear near the medial canthus. A branch through the supraorbital notch joins the superior ophthalmic vein, receiving in the notch veins from the frontal sinus and frontal diploë.

Facial vein. After receiving the supratrochlear and supraorbital veins, this vessel descends obliquely near the side of the radix nasi, receding from the ala, and then turns posterolaterally below the orbital opening, passing downwards and backwards behind the facial artery, being less tortuous. It passes under zygomaticus major, risorius and platysma and then descends on to the anterior border and then the surface of the masseter, crosses the body of the mandible and runs obliquely back under the platysma but superficial to the submandibular gland, digastric and stylohyoid. A little antero-inferior to the mandibular angle it is joined by the anterior division of the retromandibular vein; descending superficial to the lingual artery's loop, the hypoglossal nerve and external and internal carotid arteries, it enters the internal jugular near the greater cornu of the hyoid bone (i.e. in the upper angle of the carotid triangle). Near its end a large branch often descends along the anterior border of sternocleidomastoid to the anterior jugular vein. Its uppermost segment, above its junction with the superior labial vein (see below), is often termed the *angular vein*.

Tributaries. Near its beginning the facial vein connects with the superior ophthalmic directly and via the supraorbital; it is thus connected to the cavernous sinus. It receives veins of the ala nasi and, lower, a large deep facial vein from the pterygoid venous plexus and also the inferior palpebral, superior and inferior labial, buccinator, parotid and masseteric veins. Below the mandible, submental, tonsillar, external palatine (paratonsillar) and submandibular veins join it and sometimes the vena comitans of the hypoglossal nerve, and the pharyngeal and superior thyroid veins.

Clinical anatomy. The facial vein has no valves. It connects, as noted, with the cavernous sinus by two routes: through the ophthalmic vein or its supraorbital tributary, or by the *deep facial vein* to the pterygoid plexus and hence the cavernous sinus. Infection may thus spread from the face to the intracranial venous sinuses.

Superficial temporal vein (**10**.153). This begins in a widespread network joined across the scalp to the contralateral vein and to the ipsilateral supratrochlear, supraorbital, posterior auricular and occipital veins, all draining the same network. Anterior and posterior tributaries unite above the zygoma to form the superficial temporal, joined here by the *middle temporal vein*. It crosses the posterior root of the zygoma and enters the parotid gland to join the maxillary vein, to form the *retromandibular vein*.

Tributaries. These are the parotid veins, rami for the temporomandibular joint, anterior auricular veins, and transverse facial vein. The middle temporal vein, after receiving the orbital vein which is formed by the lateral palpebral veins, passes back between layers of temporal fascia, piercing this to join the superficial temporal vein.

Pterygoid venous plexus. It is found partly between temporalis and the lateral pterygoid, and partly between the pterygoids. Sphenopalatine, deep temporal, pterygoid, masseteric, buccal, dental, greater palatine and middle meningeal veins and a branch or branches from

1577

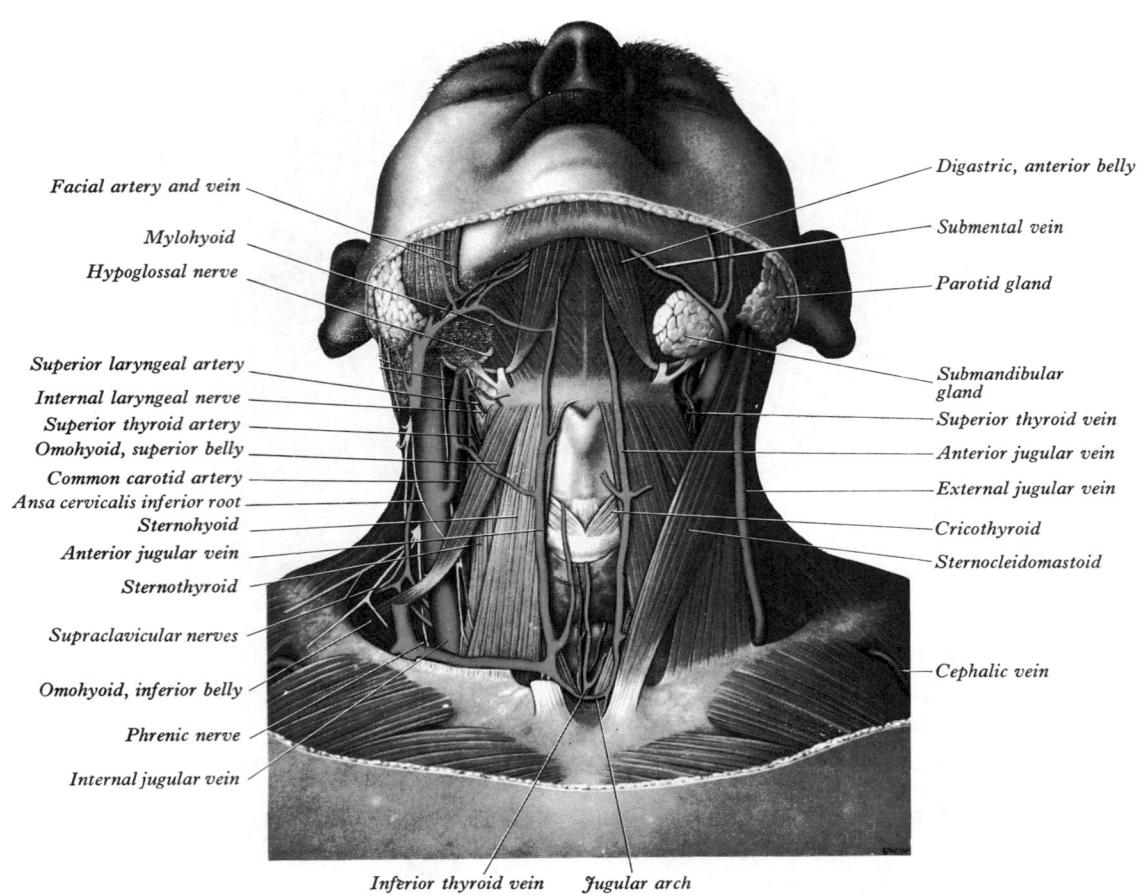

Facial artery and vein
Mylohyoid
Hypoglossal nerve

Superior laryngeal artery
Internal laryngeal nerve
Superior thyroid artery
Omohyoid, superior belly
Common carotid artery
Ansa cervicalis inferior root
Sternohyoid
Anterior jugular vein
Sternothyroid

Supraclavicular nerves

Omohyoid, inferior belly

Phrenic nerve

Internal jugular vein

Digastric, anterior belly
Submental vein
Parotid gland

Submandibular gland
Superior thyroid vein
Anterior jugular vein
External jugular vein
Cricothyroid
Sternocleidomastoid

Cephalic vein

Inferior thyroid vein   Jugular arch

10.154   Anterior view of the veins of the neck.

the inferior ophthalmic are all tributaries. The plexus connects by the *deep facial vein* with the facial and with the cavernous sinus through the sphenoidal emissary foramen, foramen ovale and foramen lacerum. Its deep temporal tributaries often connect with tributaries of the anterior diploic (p. 1580) and thus with the middle meningeal veins.

Maxillary vein. This short trunk accompanies the first part of the maxillary artery; it derives from the confluence of veins from the pterygoid plexus, passing back between the sphenomandibular ligament and mandibular neck, uniting with the superficial temporal to form the retromandibular vein.

Retromandibular vein. It descends in the parotid gland, between the external carotid artery and, superficially, the facial nerve. It divides into an anterior branch going forwards to join the facial and a posterior branch, joining the posterior auricular to form the *external jugular vein*. Occasionally it is not connected to the external jugular, which is then small, the anterior jugular often being enlarged.

Posterior auricular vein (10.153). Beginning in a parieto-occipital network, it also drains into tributaries of the occipital and superficial temporal veins. It descends behind the auricle to join the posterior division of the retromandibular vein in or just below the parotid gland, to form the external jugular. It receives a stylomastoid vein and tributaries from the cranial surface of the auricle.

Occipital vein (10.153). It begins in a posterior network in the scalp, pierces the cranial attachment of trapezius, turns into the suboccipital triangle and joins the deep cervical and vertebral veins. It may follow the occipital artery to end in the internal jugular; sometimes it joins the posterior auricular and hence the external jugular vein. Parietal and mastoid emissary veins link it with the superior sagittal and transverse sinuses. The occipital diploic vein sometimes joins it (see above).

VEINS OF THE NECK

1578   Veins of the neck are superficial or deep to the deep fascia but

they are not entirely separate (**10**.153, 154, 170). *Superficial veins*, tributaries (some with specific names, given below) of the external jugular, drain a much smaller volume of tissue than the *deep veins*, which drain all but the subcutaneous structures, mostly into the internal jugular vein (but some into the vertebral veins).

External jugular vein (10.153). This largely drains the scalp and face but also some deeper parts. The union of the posterior division of the retromandibular and posterior auricular veins begins near the mandibular angle just below or in the parotid gland, descending from the angle to the midclavicle. It crosses obliquely, superficial to sternocleidomastoid, to the subclavian triangle, where it traverses the deep fascia to end in the subclavian vein, lateral or anterior to scalenus anterior. Its wall is adherent to the rim of the fascial opening. It is covered by platysma, superficial fascia and skin, separated from sternocleidomastoid by deep cervical fascia; it crosses the transverse cervical nerve and is parallel with the great auricular nerve, ascending posterior to its upper half. In size the vein is inversely proportional to other veins in the neck; it is occasionally double. It has valves at its entrance into the subclavian vein and about 4 cm above the clavicle, between which it is often dilated, is a so-called sinus. The valves do not prevent regurgitation.

Tributaries. In addition to formative tributaries, the external jugular receives the posterior external jugular and, near its end, transverse cervical, suprascapular and anterior jugular veins; in the parotid gland it is often joined by a branch from the internal jugular. The occipital vein occasionally joins it.

Posterior external jugular vein. It begins in the occipital scalp and drains the skin and the superficial muscles posterosuperior in the neck. It usually joins the middle part of the external jugular.

Anterior jugular vein (10.153, 154). This vein starts near the hyoid bone by the confluence of the superficial submandibular veins. It descends between the midline and the anterior border of sterno-cleidomastoid; turning laterally, low in the neck, posterior (deep) to the muscle but superficial to the hyoid depressors, it joins the end of the external jugular vein or the subclavian vein directly. In size it is usually inverse to the external jugular. It communicates with the

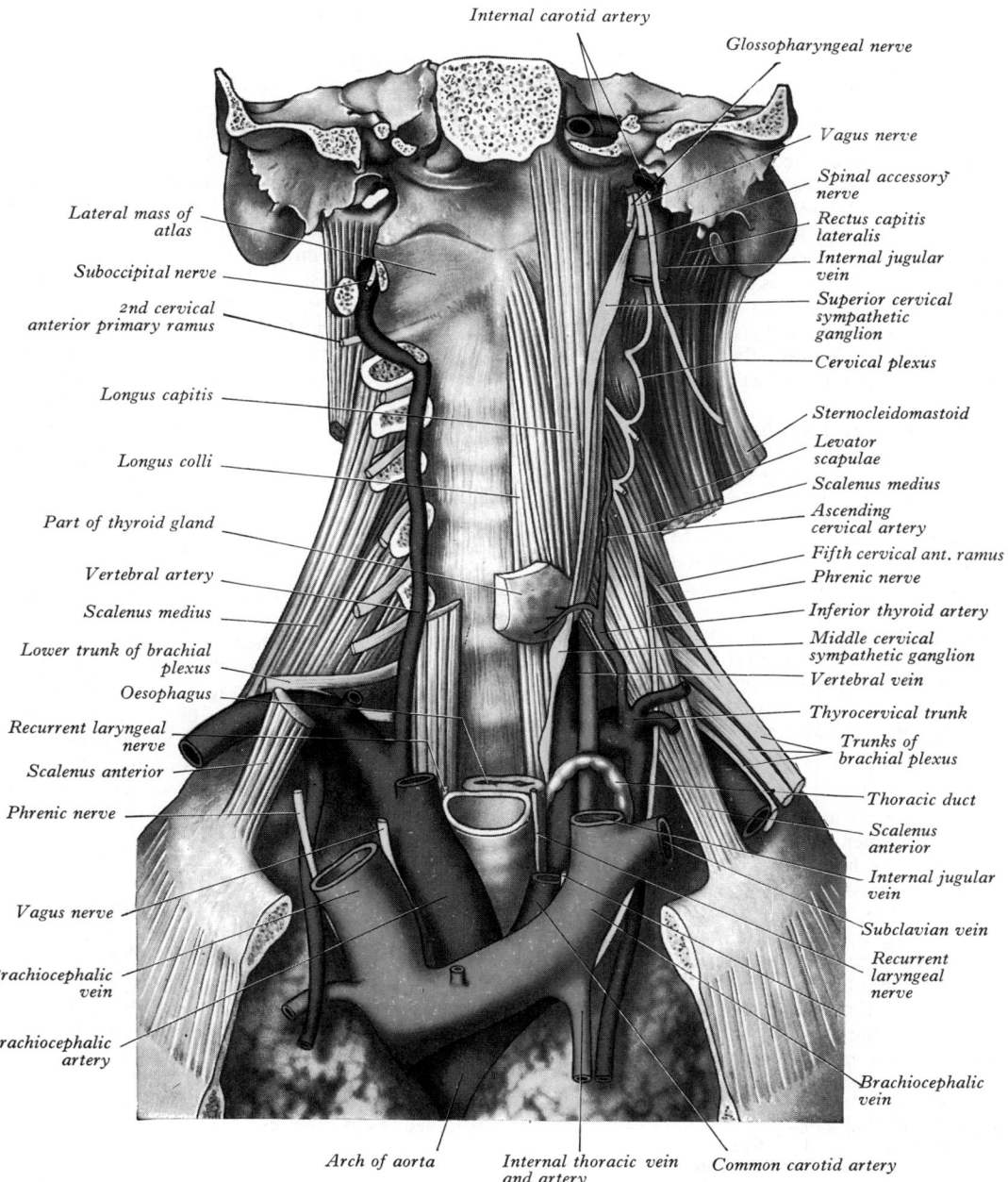

Internal carotid artery

Glossopharyngeal nerve

Vagus nerve

Spinal accessory nerve

Lateral mass of atlas

Rectus capitis lateralis

Internal jugular vein

Suboccipital nerve

Superior cervical sympathetic ganglion

2nd cervical anterior primary ramus

Cervical plexus

Sternocleidomastoid

Longus capitis

Levator scapulae

Scalenus medius

Longus colli

Ascending cervical artery

Part of thyroid gland

Fifth cervical ant. ramus

Phrenic nerve

Vertebral artery

Inferior thyroid artery

Scalenus medius

Middle cervical sympathetic ganglion

Lower trunk of brachial plexus

Vertebral vein

Oesophagus

Thyrocervical trunk

Recurrent laryngeal nerve

Trunks of brachial plexus

Scalenus anterior

Thoracic duct

Phrenic nerve

Scalenus anterior

Internal jugular vein

Vagus nerve

Subclavian vein

Brachiocephalic vein

Recurrent laryngeal nerve

Brachiocephalic artery

Brachiocephalic vein

Arch of aorta   *Internal thoracic vein and artery*   *Common carotid artery*

10.155 A dissection to show the prevertebral region and the superior mediastinum. On the right the costal elements of the upper six cervical vertebrae have been removed to expose the cervical part of the vertebral artery. On the left most of the deep relations of the common carotid artery and the internal jugular vein are exposed. Details of the terminal parts of the left lymphatic trunks have been omitted.

internal jugular, receiving the laryngeal veins and sometimes a small thyroid vein. There are usually two anterior jugular veins, united just above the manubrium by a large transverse jugular arch, receiving the inferior thyroid tributaries. They have no valves and may be replaced by a midline trunk.

Surface anatomy. Usually the external jugular vein is visible where it crosses the sternocleidomastoid; it can be distended and made more visible by expiring against resistance (Valsalva's manoeuvre) or by gentle supraclavicular digital pressure. Similarly, the anterior jugular vein can often be made visible in the upper two-thirds of the neck. The end of the facial vein runs from a point where the anterior border of the masseter meets the inferior mandibular border, to the greater hyoid cornu.

Internal jugular vein (**10**.153, 154). This large vein collects blood from the skull, brain, superficial parts of face and much of the neck. It begins at the cranial base in the posterior compartment of the jugular foramen, continuous with the sigmoid sinus. At its origin is its *superior bulb*, which is below the posterior part of the tympanic floor. The vein descends in the carotid sheath (p. 804), uniting with

the subclavian, posterior to the sternal end of the clavicle, to form the brachiocephalic vein. It is also dilated near its end as its *inferior bulb*, above which it contains a pair of valves. **Posterior** to the vein, from above, are: the rectus capitis lateralis, transverse process of atlas, levator scapulae, scalenus medius and cervical plexus, scalenus anterior, phrenic nerve, thyrocervical trunk, vertebral vein and first part of subclavian artery; on the left it also crosses anterior to the thoracic duct (**10**.155). **Medial** to the vein are the internal and common carotid arteries and the vagus nerve between vein and arteries but posterior to them. **Superficially** the vein is overlapped above, then covered below by sternocleidomastoid and crossed by the posterior belly of the digastric and the superior belly of omohyoid. Superior to the digastric, the parotid gland and styloid process are superficial, the accessory nerve, posterior auricular and occipital arteries crossing the vein. Between the digastric and the omohyoid, the sternocleidomastoid arteries and inferior root of the ansa cervicalis cross it, but the nerve often passes between the vein and the common carotid. Below the omohyoid, it is covered by the infrahyoid muscles and the sternocleidomastoid and it is crossed by the anterior jugular vein. Deep cervical lymph nodes lie along the vein, mainly on its superficial aspect. At the root of the neck the right internal jugular is separated from the common carotid, but the left usually overlaps its artery. At the base of the skull the internal carotid artery is **anterior**, separated from the vein by the *ninth* to *twelfth cranial nerves*.

Clinical anatomy. The vein is represented in surface projection by a broad band from the ear's lobule to the medial end of the clavicle; its inferior bulb is in the depression between the sternal and clavicular heads of the sternocleidomastoid, the lesser supraclavicular fossa, where a needle can be inserted with precision in the living subject.

Tributaries. These are: the inferior petrosal sinus, facial, lingual, pharyngeal, superior and middle thyroid veins, sometimes the occipital. The internal jugular vein may communicate with the external. The thoracic duct opens near the union of the left subclavian and internal jugular veins; the right lymphatic duct is at the same site on the right.

Inferior petrosal sinus. It leaves through the anterior part of the jugular foramen, crosses lateral or medial to the ninth to eleventh cranial nerves and joins the superior jugular bulb.

Lingual veins. These veins follow two routes:

- *Dorsal lingual veins* drain the dorsum and sides of the tongue and join the lingual veins accompanying the lingual artery between hyoglossus and genioglossus. Near the greater cornu of the hyoid bone they join the internal jugular.
- The *deep lingual vein* begins near the tip and runs back near the mucous membrane on the tongue's inferior surface. Near the anterior border of hyoglossus it joins a *sublingual vein*, from the salivary gland, to form the *vena comitans nervi hypoglossi* which runs back between the mylohyoid and hyoglossus with the hypoglossal nerve to join the facial, internal jugular or lingual vein.

Pharyngeal veins. These begin in a pharyngeal plexus external to the pharynx. After receiving meningeal veins and a vein from the pterygoid canal, they end in the internal jugular but sometimes in the facial, lingual or superior thyroid vein.

Superior thyroid vein (10.153,154). Formed by deep and superficial tributaries corresponding to the arterial branches, this vein accompanies the artery and receives the *superior laryngeal* and *cricothyroid veins*, ending in the internal jugular or facial vein.

Middle thyroid vein (10.154). It drains the lower part of the gland and also receives veins from the larynx and trachea. It crosses anterior to the common carotid artery to join the internal jugular vein behind the superior belly of omohyoid.

Facial and occipital veins. These are described on pages 1577–1578.

Inferior thyroid veins. See page 10.142.

Vertebral vein. In the suboccipital triangle many small tributaries from internal vertebral plexuses leave the vertebral canal above the posterior atlantal arch and join small veins from local deep muscles making a vessel which enters the foramen in the atlantal transverse process and forms a plexus around the vertebral artery, descending through successive transverse foramina. This ends as the vertebral vein, emerging from the sixth cervical transverse foramen, whence it descends, at first anterior then anterolateral to the vertebral artery, to open superoposteriorly into the brachiocephalic vein; the opening has a paired valve. The vertebral vein descends behind the internal jugular, passing in front of the first part of the subclavian artery (10.155). A small accessory vertebral vein usually descends from the vertebral plexus, traverses the seventh cervical transverse foramen and turns forwards between the subclavian artery and the cervical pleura to join the brachiocephalic vein.

Tributaries. The vein connects with the sigmoid sinus by a vessel in the posterior condylar canal, when this exists. It also receives branches from the occipital vein, prevertebral muscles, internal and external vertebral plexuses. It is joined by anterior vertebral and deep cervical veins (see below) and sometimes near its end by the first intercostal vein.

Anterior vertebral vein. Starting in a plexus around the upper cervical transverse processes, it descends near the ascending cervical artery between attachments of scalenus anterior and longus capitis and opens into the end of the vertebral vein.

Deep cervical vein. It accompanies its artery between the semispinales capitis et cervicis. It begins in the suboccipital region from communicating branches of the occipital and veins from suboccipital muscles and also from plexuses around the cervical spines. It passes forwards between the seventh cervical transverse process and the neck of the first rib to end in the lower part of the vertebral vein.

Clinical anatomy

When the superior jugular bulb thromboses (e.g. in otitis media), the glossopharyngeal, vagus and accessory nerves may be affected. The internal jugular vein may be endangered during removal of tuberculous or neoplastic lymph nodes.

Venous pulsation may be visible in the external jugular at the root of the neck. There are no valves in the brachiocephalic veins or the superior vena cava; hence the right atrial systole causes a wave of distension up these vessels, which may appear as a feeble flicker over the external jugular vein. This atrial systolic impulse is much increased when the right atrium is abnormally distended or hypertrophied, as in diseases of the mitral valve.

CRANIAL AND INTRACRANIAL VEINS

DIPLOIC VEINS

Diploic veins occupy channels in the diploë of some cranial bones (10.156) and are devoid of valves. They are large, with dilatations at irregular intervals; their thin walls are merely endothelium supported by elastic tissue. Radiographically they may appear as relatively transparent bands 3 or 4 mm wide. Absent at birth, they begin to develop with the diploë at about 2 years. They communicate with meningeal veins, dural sinuses and pericranial veins. Recognizably regular channels are:

- a *frontal diploic vein*, emerging from bone in the supraorbital foramen to join the supraorbital vein
- an *anterior temporal (parietal) diploic vein*, confined chiefly to the frontal bone, which pierces the greater wing of the sphenoid to end in the sphenoparietal sinus or anterior deep temporal vein
- a *posterior temporal (parietal) diploic vein*, in the parietal bones, descending to the parietal mastoid angle to join the transverse sinus through a foramen at the angle or mastoid foramen
- an *occipital diploic vein*, the largest, confined to the occipital bone, opening into occipital veins or the transverse sinus near the confluence of sinuses or into an occipital emissary vein.

Numerous small diploic veins emerge near the superior sagittal sinus to end in its venous lacunae (p. 1583).

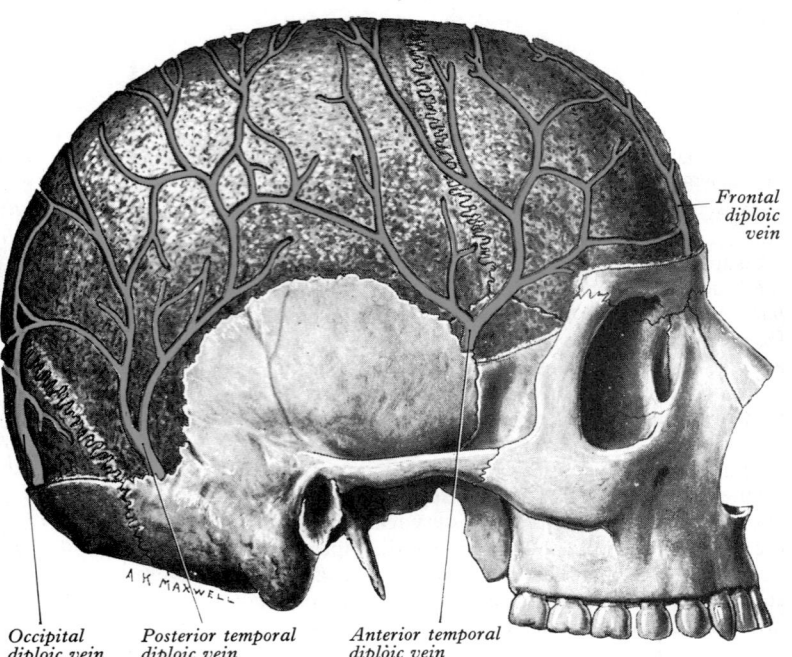

Frontal diploic vein

Occipital diploic vein   *Posterior temporal diploic vein*   *Anterior temporal diploic vein*

10.156   The veins of the diploë, displayed by the removal of the outer table of the skull.

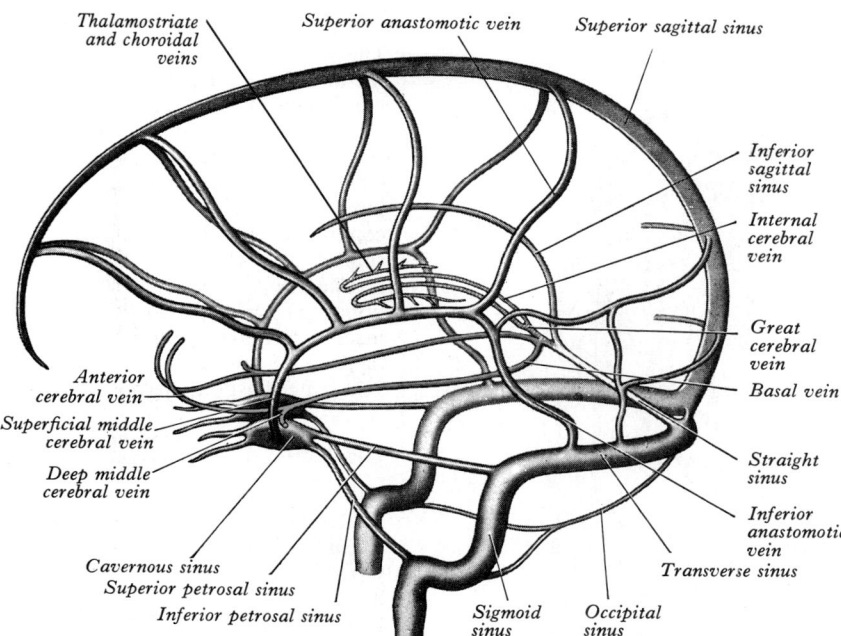

Labels in figure: Thalamostriate and choroidal veins; Superior anastomotic vein; Superior sagittal sinus; Inferior sagittal sinus; Internal cerebral vein; Great cerebral vein; Basal vein; Straight sinus; Inferior anastomotic vein; Transverse sinus; Anterior cerebral vein; Superficial middle cerebral vein; Deep middle cerebral vein; Cavernous sinus; Superior petrosal sinus; Inferior petrosal sinus; Sigmoid sinus; Occipital sinus

10.157 Schema of the venous sinuses of the dura mater and their connections with the cerebral vein: left side. The more deeply placed cerebral veins are shown in blue and those inside the brain are shown in interrupted blue.

MENINGEAL VEINS

Meningeal veins begin from plexiform vessels in the dura mater and drain into efferent vessels in the outer dural layer which connect with lacunae of the superior sagittal sinus and with other cranial sinuses, including those accompanying the middle meningeal arteries (p. 1519), and with diploic veins.

CEREBRAL AND CEREBELLAR VEINS

The veins of the brain (p. 1220) have no valves; their thin walls have no muscular tissue. They pierce the arachnoid mater and the inner dural layer to open into the cranial venous sinuses. They comprise cerebral and cerebellar veins and veins of the brainstem.

The cerebral veins (**10.157**), external and internal, drain the surfaces and the interior of the hemispheres.

External cerebral veins (**10.157**)

The external cerebral veins form superior, middle and inferior groups.

Superior cerebral veins. Eight to twelve to each hemisphere, they drain their superolateral and medial surfaces and mainly follow the sulci, though some cross the gyri. Ascending to the superomedial border, they receive small veins from the medial surface and open into the superior sagittal sinus; *anterior veins* open almost at right angles; the larger, *posterior veins* are directed obliquely forwards against the current in the sinus. This may resist the collapse of thin-walled cerebral veins which might result from a rise of intracranial pressure; but another factor is the backward growth of the cerebral hemispheres and the consequent displacement of vessels during development.

Superficial middle cerebral vein. It begins on the lateral surface, following the posterior ramus and stem of the lateral sulcus to end in the cavernous sinus. A superior anastomotic vein runs posterosuperiorly between the middle cerebral vein and the superior sagittal sinus, thus connecting the superior sagittal and cavernous sinuses. An *inferior anastomotic vein* courses over the temporal lobe, connecting the middle cerebral vein to the transverse sinus.

Inferior cerebral veins. Those on the frontal orbital surface join the superior cerebral veins and thus drain to the superior sagittal sinus; those on the temporal lobe anastomose with basal and middle cerebral veins, draining to the cavernous, superior petrosal and transverse sinuses.

Basal vein. It begins at the anterior perforated substance by the union of:

- a small *anterior cerebral vein*, accompanying the anterior cerebral artery
- a *deep middle cerebral vein* receiving tributaries from the insula and neighbouring gyri and running in the lateral cerebral sulcus
- *striate veins* emerging from the anterior perforated substance.

The basal vein passes back round the cerebral peduncle to the great cerebral vein (**10.157**), receiving tributaries from the interpeduncular fossa, inferior cornu of the lateral ventricle, parahippocampal gyrus and midbrain.

Internal cerebral vein (**10.157**)

The internal cerebral vein is formed near the interventricular foramen primarily by the thalamostriate and choroid veins; it drains the deep parts of its hemisphere. Numerous smaller veins from surrounding structures also converge here; each runs back parallel to its fellow between the layers of the tela choroidea of the third ventricle and below the splenium, where they join to form the median great cerebral vein.

Thalamostriate vein. Running anteriorly between the caudate nucleus and thalamus, this vein receives many veins from both and unites behind the anterior column of the fornix with the choroid vein to form the internal cerebral.

Choroid vein. This runs along (curves or 'spirals' along) the whole choroid plexus, receiving veins from the hippocampus, fornix, corpus callosum and adjacent structures.

Great cerebral vein

The great cerebral vein starts by union of the two internal cerebral veins as a short median vessel curving sharply up around the splenium to open into the anterior end of the straight sinus, after receiving the right and left basal veins.

Cerebellar veins

The cerebellar veins course on the cerebellar surface, and comprise superior and inferior sets.

Superior cerebellar veins. Some run anteromedially across the superior vermis to the straight sinus or great cerebral vein; others run laterally to the transverse and superior petrosal sinuses.

Inferior cerebellar veins. They include a small median vessel running backwards on the inferior vermis to enter the straight or (either) sigmoid sinus; laterally coursing vessels join the inferior petrosal and occipital sinuses.

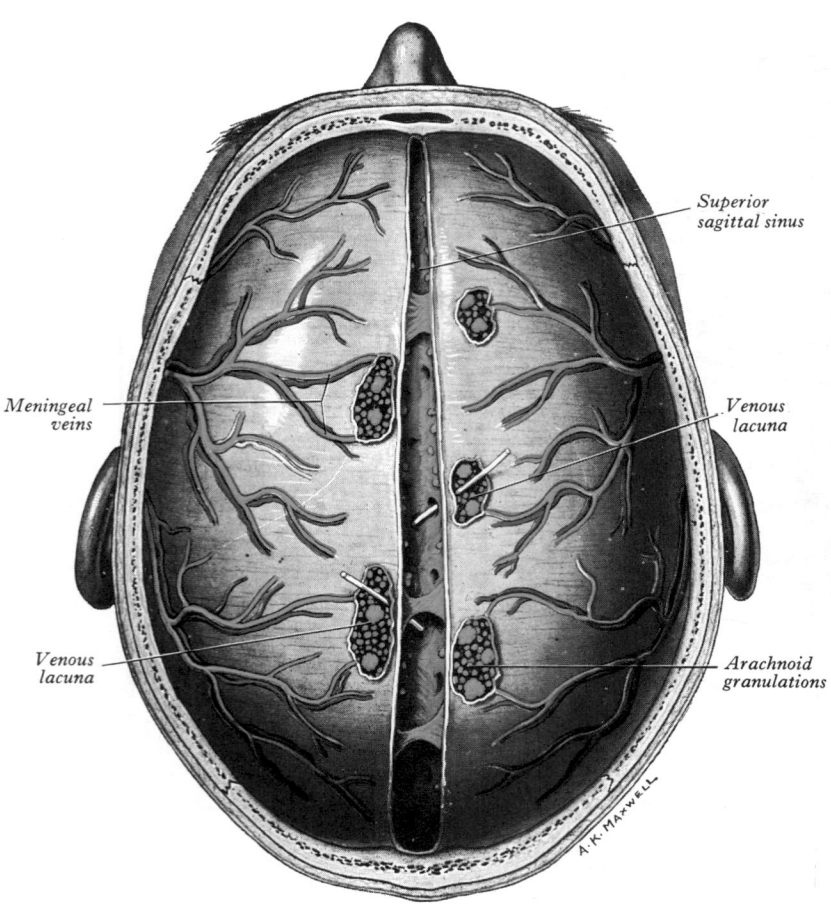

10.158 The superior sagittal sinus laid open after removal of the cranial vault. Some of the fibrous bands which cross the sinus are clearly seen; from two of the venous lacunae, bristles are passed into the sinus.

Veins of the brainstem

The veins of the brainstem form a superficial venous plexus deep to the arteries. Veins of the midbrain may reach the great cerebral or basal vein. Over the pons they tend to form a lateral vein on each side which, with upper medullary veins, may enter the petrosal sinuses, transverse sinus, cerebellar veins or the venous plexus of the (sphenoidal) foramen ovale. A median pontine vein may exist and join one of the basal veins. Veins of the inferior medulla oblongata communicate with spinal veins and drain into the adjacent venous sinuses or along variable radicular veins following the last four cranial nerves to the inferior petrosal or occipital sinuses or the upper part of the internal jugular vein. Anterior and posterior median medullary veins may run along the anterior medial fissure or posterior median sulcus and are then continuous with the spinal veins in corresponding positions (p. 1220).

CRANIAL DURAL VENOUS SINUSES

Dural sinuses are venous channels, draining blood from the brain and cranial bones, and lying between two layers of dura mater. They are lined by endothelium, they have no valves, and their wall is devoid of muscular tissue. Although most accounts describe sinuses as largely simple, smooth channels, a complex 'cavernous' or plexiform nature has been emphasized by Browder and Kaplan (1976), at least in some sites (p. 1585). They may be divided into:

● a posterosuperior group
● an antero-inferior group on the cranial base.

Posterosuperior group of venous sinuses

The posterosuperior group comprises the superior and inferior sagittal, straight, transverse, petrosquamous, sigmoid and occipital sinuses.

Superior sagittal sinus (10.157–159). It runs in the attached, convex margin of the falx cerebri. It is said to begin near the crista galli by receiving a vein from the nasal cavity when the foramen caecum is patent; but Kaplan et al (1973) found no such tributary in 201 specimens; in only 9% did the sinus extend as far as the

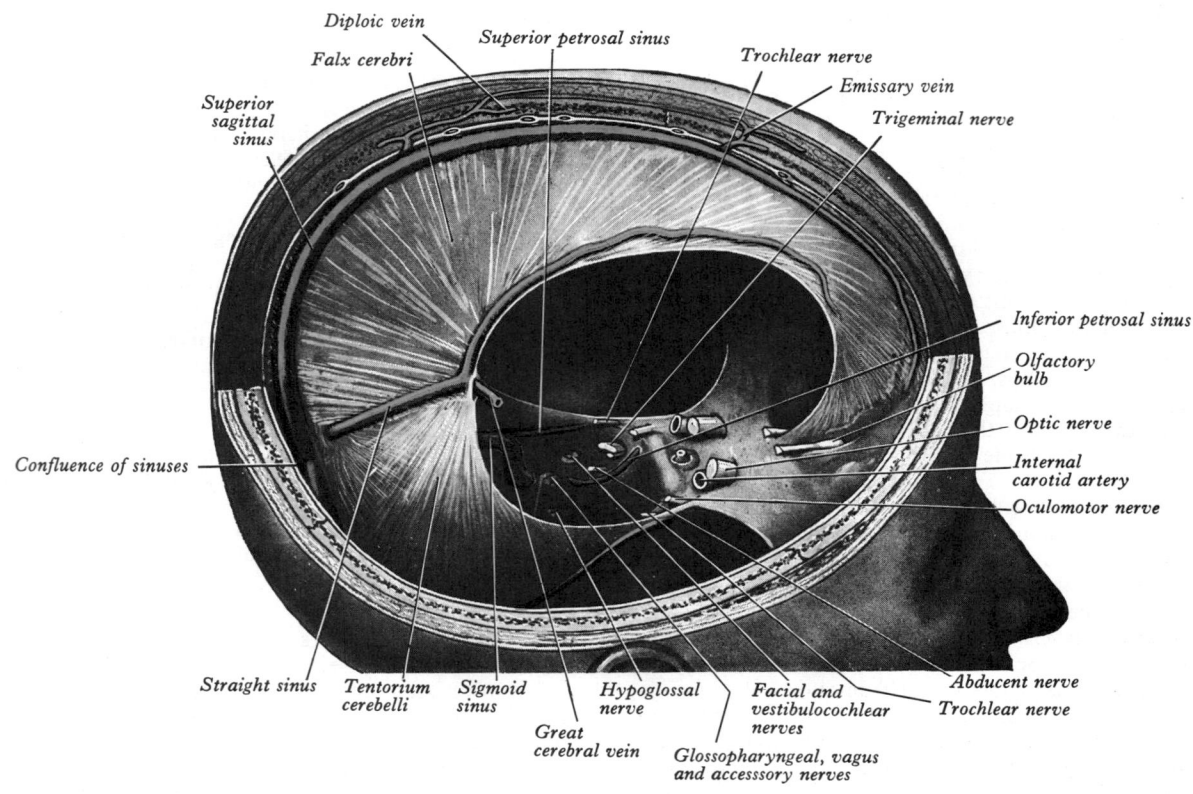

10.159 The dura mater, its processes and venous sinuses: right aspect. The cavernous and sphenoparietal sinuses are not represented.

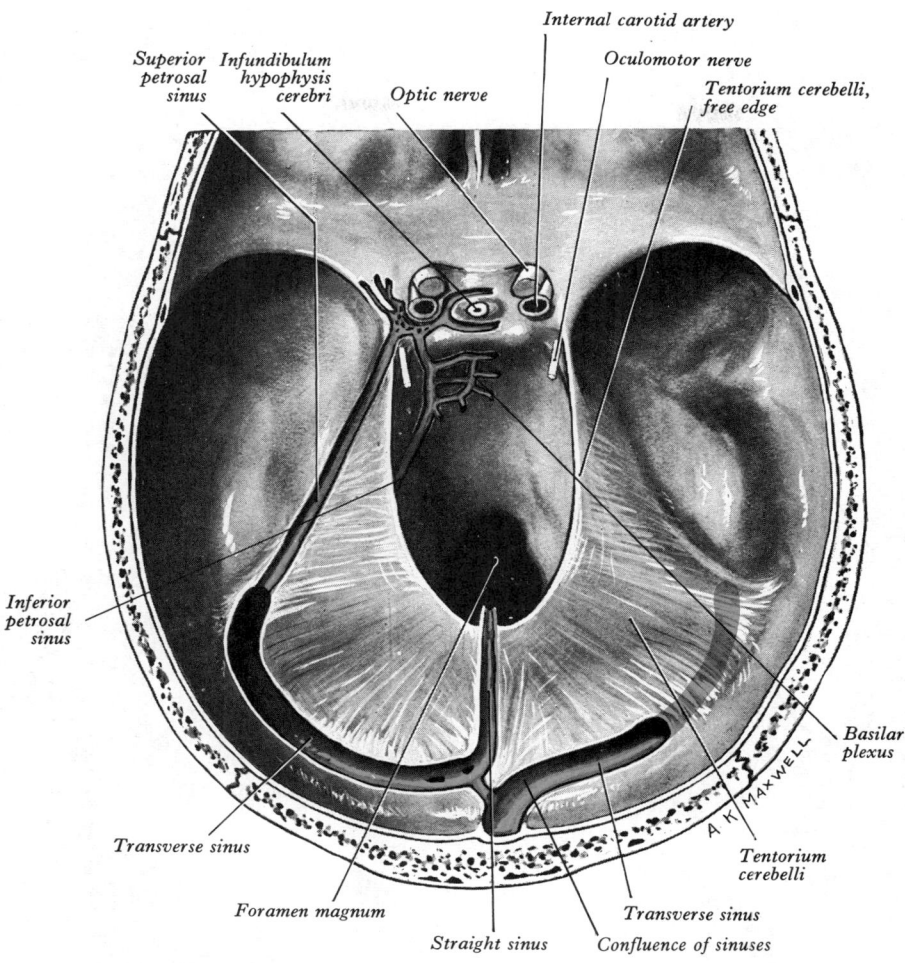

Superior petrosal sinus

Infundibulum hypophysis cerebri

Optic nerve

Internal carotid artery

Oculomotor nerve

Tentorium cerebelli, free edge

Inferior petrosal sinus

Transverse sinus

Foramen magnum

Straight sinus

Confluence of sinuses

Transverse sinus

Tentorium cerebelli

Basilar plexus

10.160   The tentorium cerebelli and venous sinuses: superior aspect. Representation of the cavernous sinuses (or 'plexuses', see text) and their extensions is greatly simplified.

foramen; the first tributaries were cortical veins from the frontal lobes, the *ascending frontal veins* of Kravenbuhl (1967). The sinus usually begins a few millimetres posterior to the foramen caecum and runs back, grooving the internal surface of the frontal bone, the adjacent margins of the two parietal bones and the squamous occipital bone. Near the internal occipital protuberance it deviates, usually to the right, continuing as a transverse sinus. Triangular in cross-section, it gradually enlarges backwards. Its interior shows the openings of superior cerebral veins, projecting arachnoid granulations, and many fibrous bands across its inferior angle; it also communicates by small orifices with irregular *venous lacunae*, situated in the dura mater near the sinus, usually three on each side: a small frontal, a large parietal and an occipital intermediate in size. In the elderly, lacunae tend to become confluent as one elongated lacuna on each side. Fine fibrous bands cross them and numerous arachnoid granulations project into them. The superior sagittal sinus receives the superior cerebral veins and, near the posterior end of the sagittal suture, veins from the pericranium passing through the parietal foramina; the lacunae drain the diploic and meningeal veins.

The complexity of these lateral lacunae and of the sinus itself has been obscured by over-simplification in general texts; but this complexity has often been emphasized (Clark 1920; Baló 1950) and studies of corrosion casts (Browder & Kaplan 1976) and cerebral angiography have revived earlier descriptions. Lateral lacunae are often so complex as to be almost plexiform and rarely the simple venous spaces usually depicted. All more recent observers have described plexiform arrays of small veins adjoining the sagittal, transverse and straight sinuses. Clark and Baló regarded these masses as cavernous tissue, which commonly adjoin all sinuses intercommunicating at their confluence. Ridges of such 'spongy' venous tissue often project into the lumina of the superior sagittal

and transverse sinuses. Their function can only be conjectured (p. 1214). The superior sagittal sinus is also invaded, in its intermediate third, by variable bands and projections from its dural walls, even extending as horizontal shelves dividing its lumen into superior and inferior channels. Such variable features make it impossible to give a simple description of this or other venous sinuses, whose variations have been detailed by Browder and Kaplan (1976) in a large series of corrosion casts; individual variations can only be shown by angiography.

Confluence of the sinuses (10.160). This term refers to the dilated posterior end of the superior sagittal sinus, situated to one side (usually right) of the internal occipital protuberance, where it turns to become a transverse sinus. It also connects with the occipital and contralateral transverse sinus. The size and degree of communication of the channels meeting at the confluence are variable (Browder & Kaplan 1976). In more than half of the specimens all venous channels converging towards the occiput do interconnect, including straight and occipital sinuses. In many instances, however, communication is absent or tenuous. Any sinus involved may be duplicated, narrowed or widened near the confluence. Variation is too great for useful description.

Clinical anatomy. Connections between the superior sagittal sinus and veins of the nose, scalp and diploë explain the occasional spread of infective thrombosis in these parts.

Inferior sagittal sinus. Located in the posterior half or two-thirds of the free margin of the falx cerebri, it increases in size posteriorly, ending in the straight sinus. It receives veins from the falx and sometimes from the medial cerebral surfaces.

Straight sinus (10.159, 160, 161). It lies in the junction of the falx cerebri with the tentorium cerebelli. Triangular in cross-section, it has a few transverse bands. It runs **postero-inferiorly**, continuing the

1583

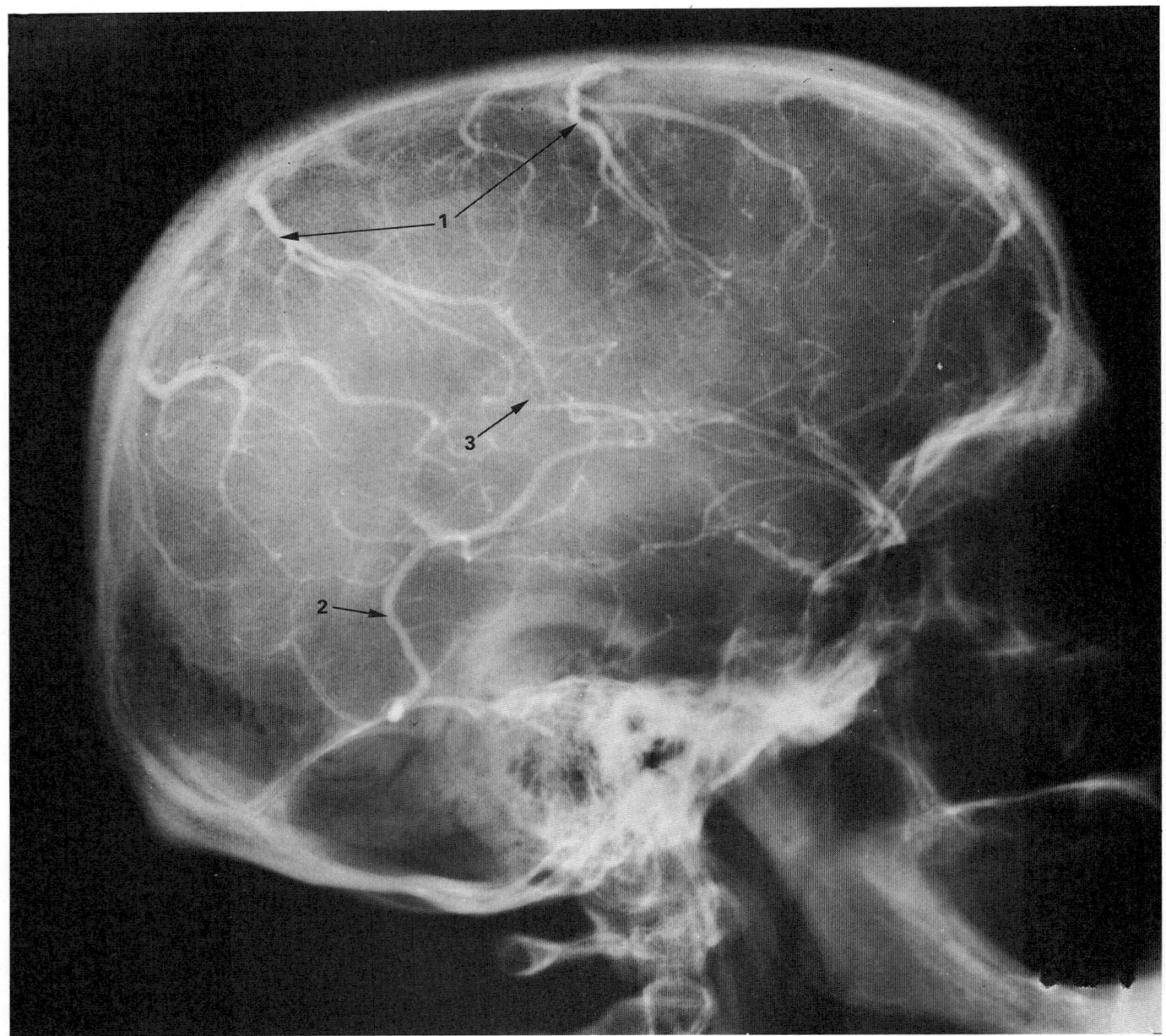

10.161 Internal carotid arteriogram (right), venous phase: lateral view. (Same subject as in **10**.81 and **10**.82, pp. 1522, 1524.) 1. Superior cerebral veins. Note the anterior course at entry into the superior sagittal sinus.

2. An inferior cerebral vein ending in the straight sinus. 3. Region of venous anastomoses.

inferior sagittal sinus into that transverse sinus which is not, or only tenuously, continuous with the superior sagittal sinus. It may communicate terminally, but quite variably, at the confluence. Its tributaries include some superior cerebellar veins and the great cerebral; the site of the latter's opening is marked by a dilatation. A small body projects into the floor of the sinus at its junction with the great cerebral vein. This contains a sinusoidal plexus of vessels; it may become engorged and act as a valve controlling outflow from the great cerebral vein, affecting the secretion of cerebrospinal fluid in the lateral ventricles. As noted, other masses of cavernous tissue are related to other dural sinuses; engorgement possibly influences their blood flow but structural data make this unlikely (see above).

Transverse sinuses (10.160, 162**).** They begin at the internal occipital protuberance, one (right) directly continuous with the superior sagittal sinus, the other with the straight sinus. Each curves anterolaterally to the posterolateral part of the petrous temporal bone, where it turns down as a sigmoid sinus. It is in the attached margin of the tentorium cerebelli, first on the occipital's squama, then on the parietal's mastoid angle. It has a gentle curve, convex upwards, and increases in size as it proceeds forwards. Transverse sinuses are triangular in section and usually unequal in size, the one

draining the superior sagittal sinus being the larger. Where they continue as sigmoid sinuses, they are joined by the superior petrosal sinuses; they receive the inferior cerebral, inferior cerebellar, diploic and inferior anastomotic veins (p. 1581).

Petrosquamous sinus. It runs back in a groove, which sometimes becomes a canal posteriorly, along the junction of the squamous and petrous parts of the temporal bone, opening behind into the transverse sinus. Anteriorly it connects with the retromandibular vein through a postglenoid or squamous foramen (pp. 589, 590). The sinus may be absent; it may drain entirely into the retromandibular vein.

Sigmoid sinuses (10.162, 163**).** They are continuations of the transverse sinuses, beginning where these leave the tentorium cerebelli. Each sigmoid sinus curves inferomedially in a groove on the mastoid temporal bone, crosses the occipital's jugular process and turns forwards to the superior jugular bulb, lying posterior in the jugular foramen. Anteriorly, a thin plate of bone alone separates its upper part from the mastoid antrum and air cells. It connects with pericranial veins via mastoid and condylar emissary veins.

Occipital sinus (10.162**).** The smallest of the sinuses, it lies in the attached margin of the falx cerebelli, occasionally paired. It commences near the foramen magnum in several small channels, one

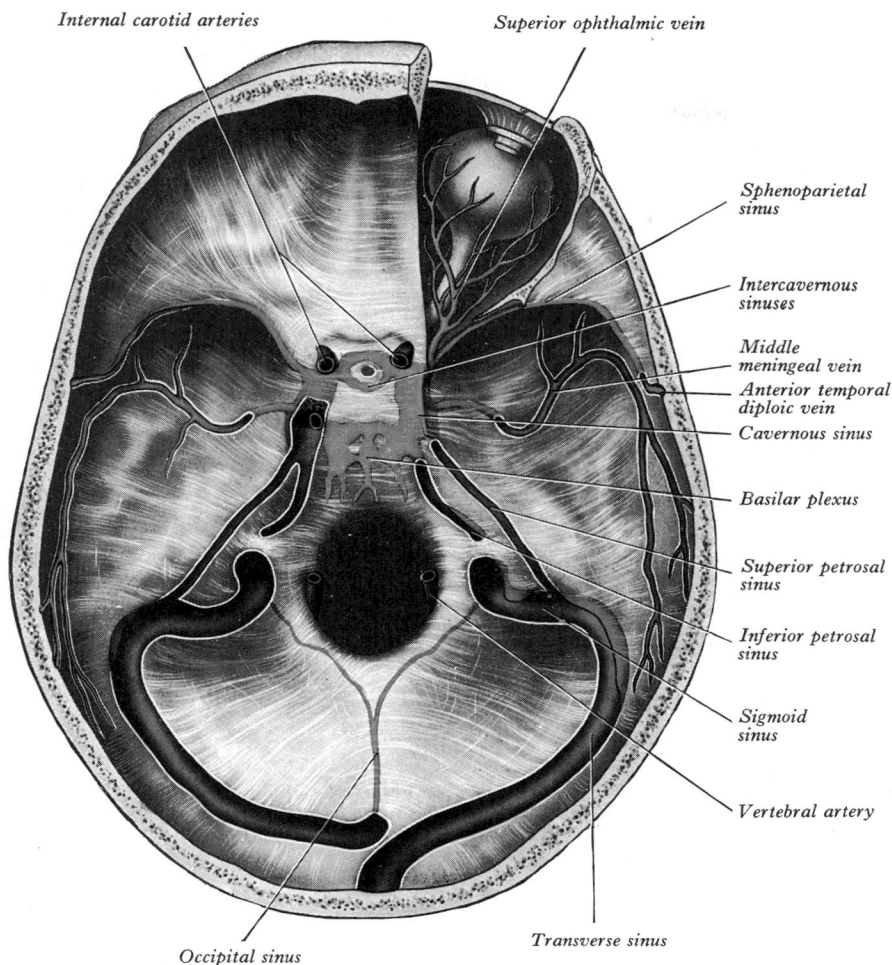

Internal carotid arteries

Superior ophthalmic vein

Sphenoparietal sinus

Intercavernous sinuses

Middle meningeal vein

Anterior temporal diploic vein

Cavernous sinus

Basilar plexus

Superior petrosal sinus

Inferior petrosal sinus

Sigmoid sinus

Vertebral artery

Occipital sinus

Transverse sinus

10.162   The sinuses at the base of the skull. The sinuses coloured dark blue have been opened up. See text and **10**.165, 166 for alternative views on the construction of the cavernous sinuses.

joining the end of the sigmoid sinus; it connects with the internal vertebral plexuses and ends in the confluence of sinuses.

Antero-inferior group of venous sinuses

The antero-inferior group includes: cavernous, intercavernous, inferior petrosal, sphenoparietal, superior petrosal and basilar sinuses and middle meningeal 'veins'.

Cavernous sinuses (**10**.158, 163–166). They lie on the sides of the body of the sphenoid bone; their name refers to their internal structure. It has been asserted that a distended adult sinus contains a few trabeculae, mostly in its periphery near the entry of its tributaries, and that these are incorporations of plexiform tributaries during developmental expansion. When the sinus is collapsed, as is usual in cadavers, its cavity is encroached upon by the nerves and arachnoid granulations in its wall, creating a spurious resemblance to cavernous tissue (Butler 1957). From corrosion casts, however, Parkinson (1973) concluded that the sinus is usually a plexus (as it is during development), a finding in accord with some earlier descriptions; Pernkopf (1963) depicted the 'sinus' as a venous plexus (see **10**.165, 166). Browder and Kaplan (1976), from examination of many casts prepared in cadavers, described the sinus as 'reticulated'. It is not clear whether they meant plexiform or cavernous. The sinus extends from the superior orbital fissure to the apex of the petrous temporal bone, with an average length of 2 cm and width of 1 cm. The internal carotid artery, with a sympathetic plexus, passes forwards through the sinus, as does the abducent nerve, inferolateral to the artery; the oculomotor and trochlear nerves and ophthalmic and maxillary divisions of the trigeminal (**10**.164) are usually said to be in the thickness of its lateral wall; but they are of such diameters that they project into the sinus; while they may be surrounded by

dural connective tissue, they are usually covered medially by little more than endothelium (McGrath 1977). The sphenoidal air sinus and hypophysis cerebri are medial; the trigeminal cave is near the inferoposterior part of its lateral wall, extending posteriorly beyond it and enclosing the trigeminal ganglion. The uncus is also lateral.

Tributaries. These are: the superior ophthalmic vein, a branch from the inferior ophthalmic vein (or the whole vessel), the superficial middle cerebral vein, inferior cerebral veins and sphenoparietal sinus; the central retinal vein and frontal tributary of the middle meningeal sometimes drain to it. The sinus drains to the transverse sinus via the superior petrosal sinus, to the internal jugular via the inferior petrosal sinus and a plexus of veins on the internal carotid, to the pterygoid plexus by veins traversing the emissary sphenoidal foramen, foramen ovale and foramen lacerum and to the facial vein via the superior ophthalmic. The two sinuses are connected by anterior and posterior intercavernous sinuses and the basilar plexus. All connections are valveless; the direction of flow in them is reversible.

Propulsion of blood in the sinus is partly due to pulsation of the internal carotid artery. It is also influenced by gravity and hence by the position of the head.

Clinical anatomy. An arteriovenous leak may occur between the cavernous sinus and internal carotid artery, causing a pulsating orbital swelling. Ligation of the internal or common carotid artery has sometimes alleviated the condition. Suppuration in the upper nasal cavities and paranasal sinuses or near the medial canthus may lead to septic thrombosis of the cavernous sinuses.

Ophthalmic veins (**10**.163, 167). There is a superior and an inferior, devoid of valves, linking the facial and intracranial veins. The *superior ophthalmic vein* forms posteromedial to the upper

1585

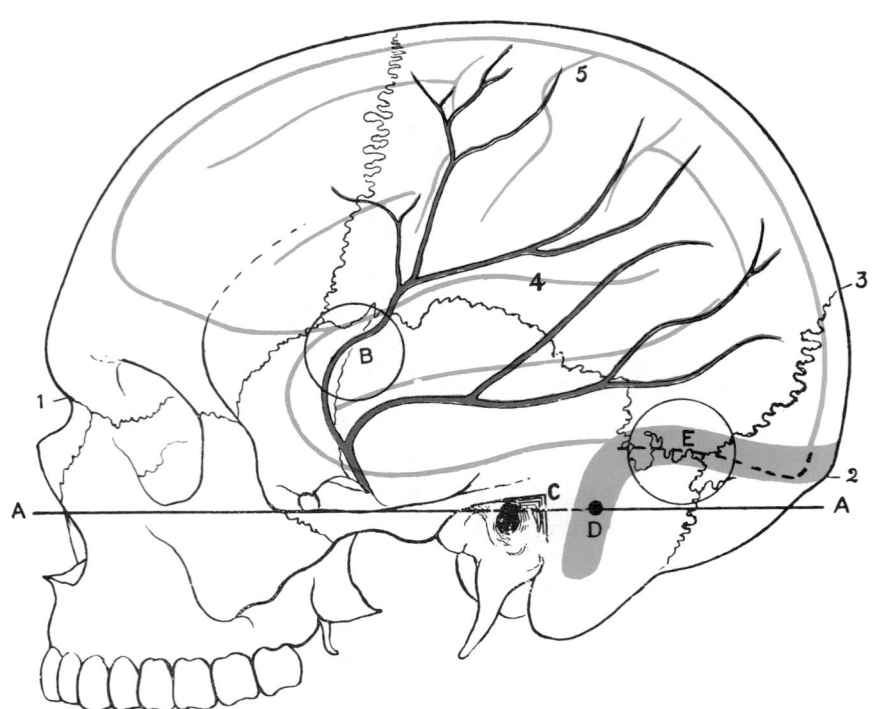

10.163 The relations of the brain, the middle meningeal artery and the transverse and sigmoid sinuses to the surface of the skull. 1. Nasion. 2. Inion. 3. Lambda. 4. Lateral cerebral sulcus. 5. Central sulcus. AA = Frankfurt plane, which traverses the lower margin of the orbital opening and the upper margin of the external acoustic meatus; B = area (including the pterion) for trephining over the frontal branch of the middle meningeal artery and the cerebral Sylvian point; C = suprameatal triangle; D = sigmoid sinus; E = area for trephining over the transverse sinus, exposing the dura mater of both cerebrum and cerebellum. The outline of the cerebral hemisphere and its major sulci are indicated in blue; the course of the middle meningeal artery is in red.

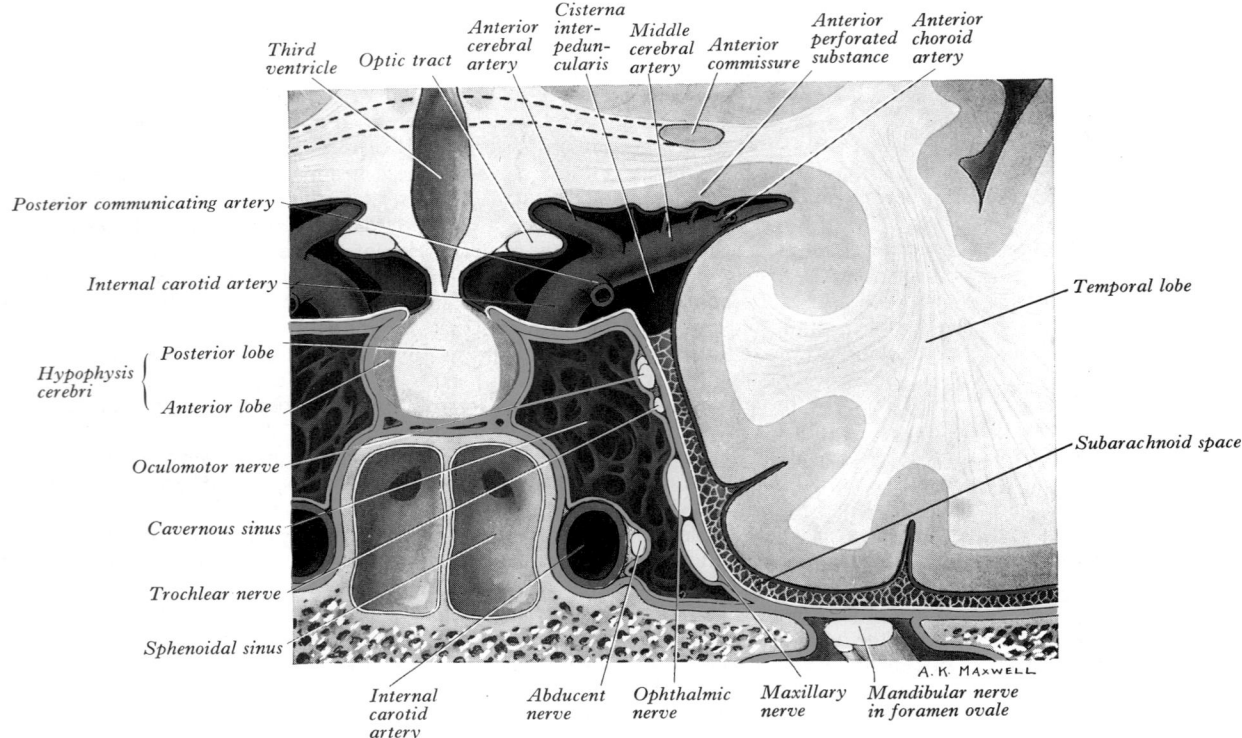

10.164 Coronal, slightly oblique section through the middle cranial fossa, showing the cavernous and cerebral portions of the internal carotid artery and the cavernous sinus: mauve = pia mater; white = arachnoid mater; green = layers of dura mater (the mesothelium of the dura mater is not indicated); blue = endothelium of cavernous sinus.

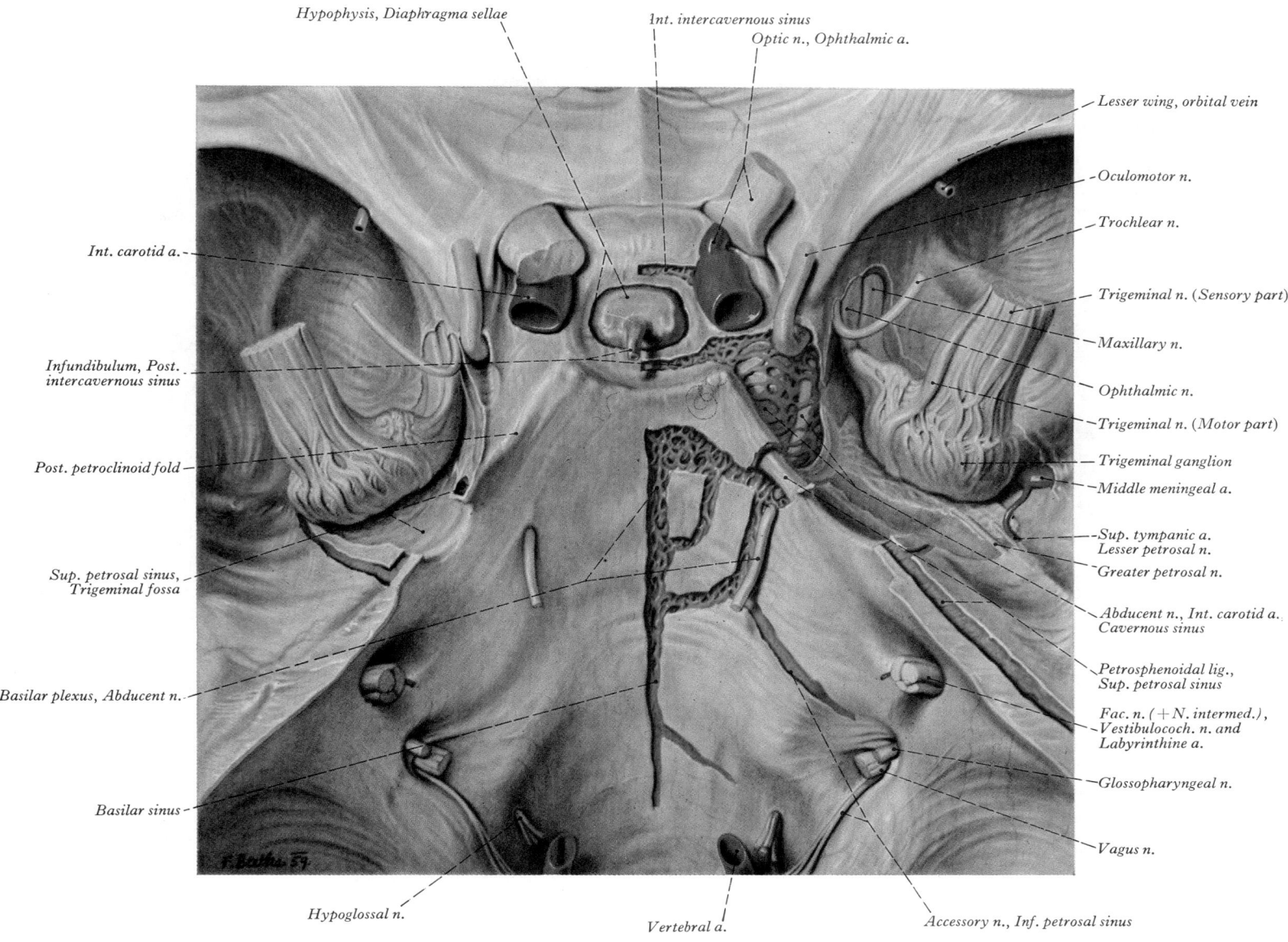

10.165   The middle cranial fossa, viewed from above to show the termination of the internal carotid artery, its branches and the cavernous sinus. Note the plexiform nature of the 'sinus', which communicates with similar venous plexuses in the hypophyseal fossa and over the clivus. These have been exposed by partial removal of the dura mater. (See also **10.**166.)

lid from two tributaries connecting anteriorly with the facial and supraorbital veins (p. 1577). It runs with the ophthalmic artery, receiving corresponding tributaries, and traverses the superior orbital fissure to end in the cavernous sinus. The *inferior ophthalmic vein* begins in a network near the anterior region of the orbital floor and medial wall, receiving veins from the rectus inferior, obliquus inferior, lacrimal sac and eyelids; it runs back above the rectus inferior and often joins the superior ophthalmic vein but may reach the cavernous sinus. It connects with the pterygoid venous plexus by small rami through the inferior orbital fissure.

Central retinal vein. This vein first traverses the optic nerve then it leaves it to pursue a long course in the subarachnoid space before entering the cavernous sinus or the superior ophthalmic vein. It receives a *central vein* which drains the nerve while still within it.

Sphenoparietal sinuses (**10.**163). They are located below the periosteum of the lesser wings of the sphenoid bone, near their posterior edges. Each receives small veins from the adjacent dura mater and sometimes the frontal ramus of the middle meningeal vein; curving medially it opens into the anterior part of the cavernous sinus. It often receives connecting rami, in its middle course, from the superficial middle cerebral vein, sometimes veins from the temporal lobe and the anterior temporal diploic vein. When these connections are well developed it is a large channel.

Intercavernous sinuses. These two sinuses, anterior and posterior, interconnect the cavernous sinuses in the anterior and posterior attached borders of the diaphragma sellae; they thus complete a venous circular sinus (**10.**163). Small, irregular sinuses inferior to the hypophysis cerebri drain into them. Such *inferior intercavernous sinuses* were studied by Kaplan et al (1976), who emphasized their size and plexiform nature, features important in a surgical transnasal approach to the hypophysis.

Superior petrosal sinuses (**10.**163). These small and narrow sinuses drain the cavernous to the transverse sinuses. Leaving the posterosuperior part of the cavernous sinus, each runs posterolaterally in the attached margin of the tentorium cerebelli, crossing above the trigeminal nerve to a groove on the superior border of the petrous temporal bone; each ends by joining a transverse sinus where this curves down to become the sigmoid. It receives *cerebellar*, *inferior cerebral* and *tympanic veins*. It connects with the inferior petrosal sinus and basilar plexus.

Inferior petrosal sinuses. They drain the cavernous sinuses to the internal jugular veins. Each (**10.**163) begins postero-inferiorly at its cavernous sinus and runs back in a groove between the petrous temporal and basilar occipital bones. Traversing the anterior part of the jugular foramen it ends in the superior jugular bulb. It receives labyrinthine veins via the cochlear canaliculus and the vestibular

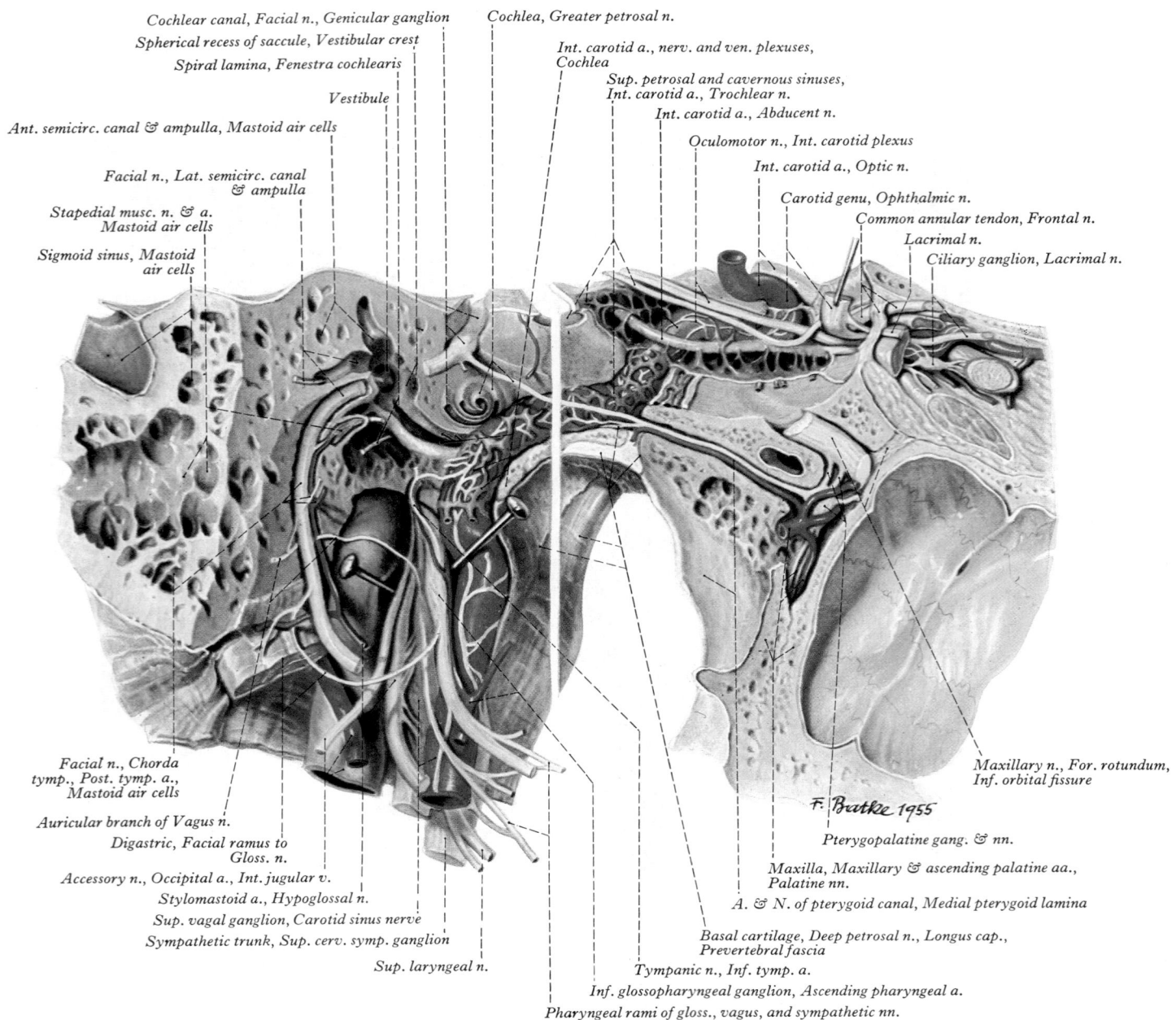

Cochlear canal, Facial n., Genicular ganglion
Spherical recess of saccule, Vestibular crest
Spiral lamina, Fenestra cochlearis
Vestibule
Ant. semicirc. canal & ampulla, Mastoid air cells
Facial n., Lat. semicirc. canal & ampulla
Stapedial musc. n. & a. Mastoid air cells
Sigmoid sinus, Mastoid air cells

Cochlea, Greater petrosal n.
Int. carotid a., nerv. and ven. plexuses, Cochlea
Sup. petrosal and cavernous sinuses, Int. carotid a., Trochlear n.
Int. carotid a., Abducent n.
Oculomotor n., Int. carotid plexus
Int. carotid a., Optic n.
Carotid genu, Ophthalmic n.
Common annular tendon, Frontal n.
Lacrimal n.
Ciliary ganglion, Lacrimal n.

F. Batke 1955

Facial n., Chorda tymp., Post. tymp. a., Mastoid air cells
Auricular branch of Vagus n.
Digastric, Facial ramus to Gloss. n.
Accessory n., Occipital a., Int. jugular v.
Stylomastoid a., Hypoglossal n.
Sup. vagal ganglion, Carotid sinus nerve
Sympathetic trunk, Sup. cerv. symp. ganglion
Sup. laryngeal n.

Maxillary n., For. rotundum, Inf. orbital fissure
Pterygopalatine gang. & nn.
Maxilla, Maxillary & ascending palatine aa., Palatine nn.
A. & N. of pterygoid canal, Medial pterygoid lamina
Basal cartilage, Deep petrosal n., Longus cap., Prevertebral fascia
Tympanic n., Inf. tymp. a.
Inf. glossopharyngeal ganglion, Ascending pharyngeal a.
Pharyngeal rami of gloss., vagus, and sympathetic nn.

10.166   An oblique vertical section through the cranial base to display in lateral view the right internal carotid artery and the continuity of the venous plexus around the intraosseous and cavernous parts of the artery. (**10**.165 and 166 are from Pernkopf 1963, by permission of W B Saunders and Urban & Schwarzenberg.)

aqueduct and tributaries from the medulla oblongata, pons and inferior cerebellar surface. According to Browder and Kaplan (1976) the sinus is more often a plexus and sometimes drains by a vein in the hypoglossal canal to the suboccipital vertebral plexus.

Relations of structures in the jugular foramen. These are as follows: the inferior petrosal sinus is anteromedial with a meningeal branch of the ascending pharyngeal artery, and the sinus descends obliquely backwards; the sigmoid sinus is situated at the lateral and posterior part of the foramen with a meningeal branch of the occipital artery; between the sinuses are in succession, posterolaterally: the glossopharyngeal, vagus and accessory nerves (p. 1254).

Basilar venous plexus (**10**.163). It consists of interconnecting channels between layers of dura mater on the clivus; it interconnects the inferior petrosal sinuses and joins with the internal vertebral venous plexus. It also usually connects with the cavernous and superior petrosal sinuses at its anterior end. When marginal sinuses (p. 1589) are large they communicate anteriorly with the plexus; an almost complete circular venous channel may then surround the foramen magnum, connecting the basilar plexus intracranially to the

inferior petrosal, sigmoid and occipital sinuses and to variable extracranial vertebral plexuses in the suboccipital region.

Middle meningeal veins (or sinuses) (**10**.163). They communicate above with the superior sagittal sinus through its venous lacunae; below they converge and unite as frontal and parietal trunks, which accompany branches of the middle meningeal arteries in grooves on the internal parietal surfaces; but the veins are closer to bone and sometimes occupy separate grooves. The veins' situation has been said to make them liable to tears in fractures (Jones 1911). Their termination is variable. The parietal trunk may traverse the foramen spinosum to the pterygoid venous plexus; the frontal may also reach the plexus via the foramen ovale or may end in the sphenoparietal or cavernous sinus. Besides meningeal tributaries they receive small inferior cerebral veins and connect with the diploic and superficial middle cerebral veins. Browder and Kaplan (1976) state that middle meningeal 'veins' are histologically sinuses, in places almost surrounding the middle meningeal arteries; they also report frequent arachnoid granulations in them.

Surface anatomy. The superior sagittal sinus runs from the glabella

(p. 554) to the inion (**6.168A**). Narrow anteriorly, it widens to about 1 cm. The transverse sinus begins at the inion and runs laterally, with slight upward convexity, to the base of the mastoid process, from which the sigmoid sinus passes down just anterior to the posterior mastoid border to a point about 1 cm above its tip.

EMISSARY VEINS

Emissary veins traverse cranial apertures and make connections between venous sinuses and extracranial veins. Some are constant, others sometimes absent:

- A *mastoid emissary vein* in the mastoid foramen unites the sigmoid sinus with the posterior auricular or occipital vein.
- A *Perietal emissary vein* traverses the parietal foramen to connect the superior sagittal sinus with the veins of the scalp.
- The *venous plexus of the hypoglossal canal*, occasionally a single vein, connects the sigmoid sinus to the internal jugular vein.
- A *posterior condylar emissary vein* connects the sigmoid sinus with veins in the suboccipital triangle via the condylar canal.
- A plexus of emissary veins (*venous plexus of foramen ovale*) links the cavernous sinus to the pterygoid plexus via the foramen ovale.
- Two or three small veins traverse the foramen lacerum connecting the cavernous sinus with the pharyngeal veins and pterygoid plexus.
- A vein in the emissary sphenoidal foramen (of Vesalius) connects the same vessels.
- The *internal carotid venous plexus*, passing through the carotid canal, connects the cavernous sinus to the internal jugular vein.
- The petrosquamous sinus (p. 1584) connects the transverse sinus with the external jugular vein.
- A vein may traverse the foramen caecum (patent in about 1% of adult skulls) connecting nasal veins with the superior sagittal sinus.
- An *occipital emissary vein* usually connects the confluence of sinuses with the occipital vein through the occipital protuberance, receiving also the occipital diploic vein.
- The occipital sinus connects with variably developed veins around

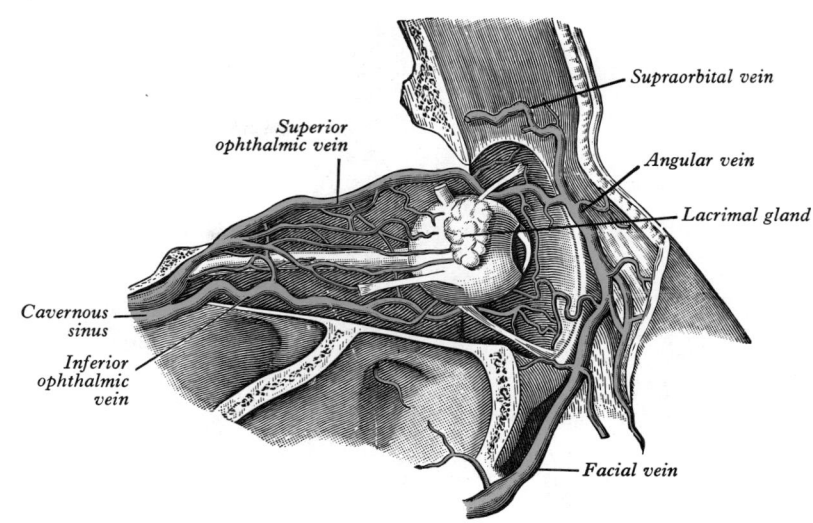

10.167   The veins of the right orbit: lateral aspect.

the foramen magnum (so-called *marginal sinuses*) and thus with the vertebral venous plexuses, an alternative venous drainage when the jugular vein is blocked or tied.

- The ophthalmic veins are potentially emissary, since they connect intracranial to extracranial veins; but parietal emissary veins, included here, are usually minute and do not appear to connect with veins of the scalp in corrosion casts.

These connections are significant in the spread of infection from extracranial foci to venous sinuses. The success of a ligature of the internal jugular vein, to limit the spread of some oral and pharyngeal pathologies, depends on the adequacy of the collateral drainage.

VEINS OF THE UPPER LIMBS

Veins are conveniently grouped as *superficial* and *deep* but these are widely interconnected. The superficial veins are subcutaneous in the superficial fascia; deep veins accompany arteries between the muscles of the limb. Both groups have valves, which are more numerous in deep veins.

SUPERFICIAL VEINS OF THE UPPER LIMB

Superficial veins (**10.168, 169**) include the cephalic, basilic, median cubital and additional antebrachial veins and their tributaries.

Dorsal digital veins pass along the sides of the fingers, joined by oblique branches; they unite from the adjacent sides of digits into three dorsal metacarpal veins (**10.168**), which form a *dorsal venous network* over the metacarpus; this is joined laterally by a dorsal digital vein from the radial side of the index finger and both dorsal digital veins of the thumb and is prolonged proximally as the cephalic vein. Medially a dorsal digital vein from the ulnar side of minimus joins the network, which drains proximally into the basilic vein. A vein often connects the central parts of the network to the cephalic near midforearm.

Palmar digital veins connect to the dorsal by oblique intercapitular veins passing between metacarpal heads; they also drain to a plexus superficial to the palmar aponeurosis, extending over both thenar and hypothenar regions.

Cephalic vein (**10.168, 169**). Commonly formed over the 'anatomical snuff box', it curves proximally from the radial end of the dorsal plexus round the forearm's radial side to its ventral aspect, receiving veins from both aspects. Distal to the elbow a branch, the *median cubital vein*, joined by a branch from the deep veins, diverges

proximomedially to reach the basilic vein. The cephalic ascends in front of the elbow superficial to a groove between the brachioradialis and biceps, crosses superficial to the lateral cutaneous nerve of the forearm, ascends lateral to the biceps and between pectoralis major and the deltoid, where it adjoins the deltoid branch of the thoraco-acromial artery. Entering the infraclavicular fossa to pass behind the clavicular head of pectoralis major, it pierces the clavipectoral fascia, crosses the axillary artery and joins the axillary vein just below clavicular level. It may connect with the external jugular by a branch anterior to the clavicle. Sometimes the median cubital vein is large, transferring most blood from the cephalic to the basilic vein, the proximal cephalic vein then being absent or much diminished.

Accessory cephalic vein. Arising in a dorsal forearm plexus or from the ulnar side of the dorsal venous network in the hand, this joins the cephalic distal to the elbow. It may spring from the cephalic proximal to the carpus and rejoin it later. A large oblique vein often connects the basilic and cephalic veins dorsally in the forearm.

Basilic vein (**10.169**). Beginning medially in the hand's dorsal venous network, it ascends posteromedially in the forearm inclining forwards to the anterior surface distal to the elbow. Joined by the median cubital vein, it ascends superficially to and between biceps and pronator teres; filaments of the medial cutaneous nerve of the forearm pass here, in front and behind it. It ascends medial to biceps and perforates the deep fascia about midway in the arm, continuing medial to the brachial artery to the lower border of teres major, there becoming the axillary vein. (Its relation to the brachial veins is variable; see p. 1590.)

Median vein of the forearm (**10.169**). It drains the superficial palmar venous plexus. It ascends anterior in the forearm to join the

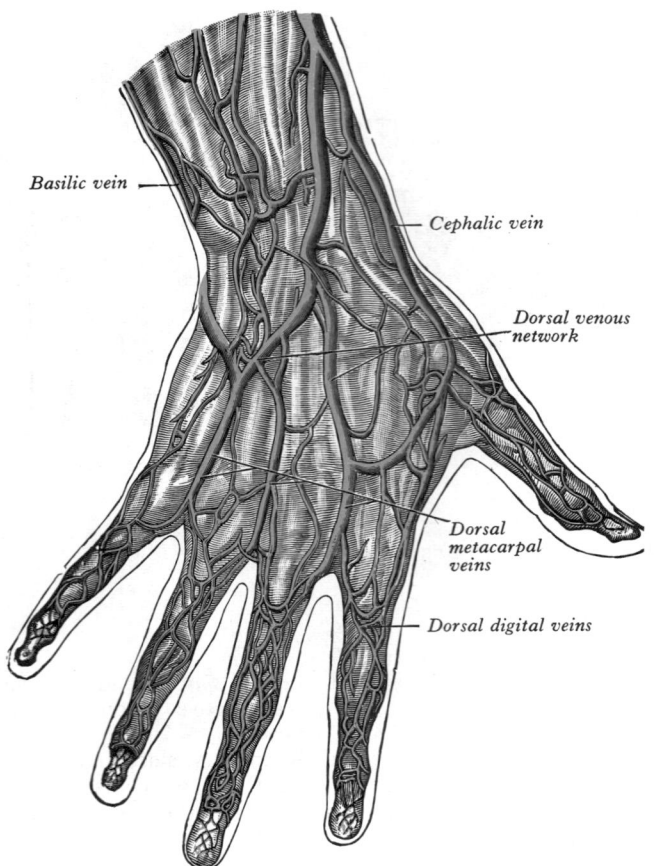

Basilic vein

Cephalic vein

Dorsal venous network

Dorsal metacarpal veins

Dorsal digital veins

10.168　The veins of the dorsum of the hand.

basilic or median cubital vein; it may divide distal to the elbow to join both.

Surface anatomy

Superficial veins are usually visible until they pierce the deep fascia. Larger ones are obvious when the limb is dependent and its muscles contracted, driving blood from the deep to the superficial veins.

Clinical anatomy

Blood sampling, blood transfusion and intravenous injection are commonly done near the elbow or more distally in the forearm; the largest vein is usually the median cubital. The cubital veins are also used for cardiac catheterization for many purposes. Equally useful for such procedures is the cephalic vein where it is superficial to the distal end of the radius in the 'anatomical snuffbox'. The cephalic vein, a little proximal to the snuff box, is the site with many advantages for an indwelling cannula or fine tube when a lengthy period is contemplated; the position of the arm, forearm and hand is optimal for this purpose.

DEEP VEINS OF THE UPPER LIMB

Deep veins (venae comitantes) accompany arteries, usually in pairs, flanking the artery and connected by short transverse links. Since much blood from the upper limb is returned by the superficial veins, the deep ones are relatively small.

Deep veins of the hand. Superficial and deep palmar arterial arches are accompanied by superficial and deep palmar venous arches, receiving the corresponding branches. Thus common palmar digital veins join the superficial arch and palmar metacarpal veins join the deep arch. Deep veins accompanying the dorsal metacarpal arteries first receive perforating branches from the palmar metacarpal veins and then end in the radial veins and the dorsal venous network.

Deep veins of the forearm. Running with the radial and ulnar arteries they drain respectively the deep and superficial palmar venous arches; they unite near the elbow as paired *brachial veins*.

The radial veins are smaller, receiving the deep dorsal veins of the hand; ulnar veins drain the deep palmar venous arch, connecting with superficial veins near the wrist; near the elbow they receive the anterior and posterior interosseous artery companion veins; a large branch connects them to the *median cubital vein*.

Brachial veins. They flank the brachial artery, with tributaries similar to the arterial branches; near the lower margin of subscapularis they join the axillary vein, the medial one, however, often joining the basilic before it becomes the axillary.

These deep veins have numerous anastomoses with each other and with the superficial veins.

Axillary vein. This large vein is the continuation of the basilic; it begins at the lower border of teres major, and ascends to the outer border of the first rib, where it becomes the subclavian. Near subscapularis the brachial vein joins it and, near its costal end, the cephalic; other tributaries follow the axillary arterial branches. It is

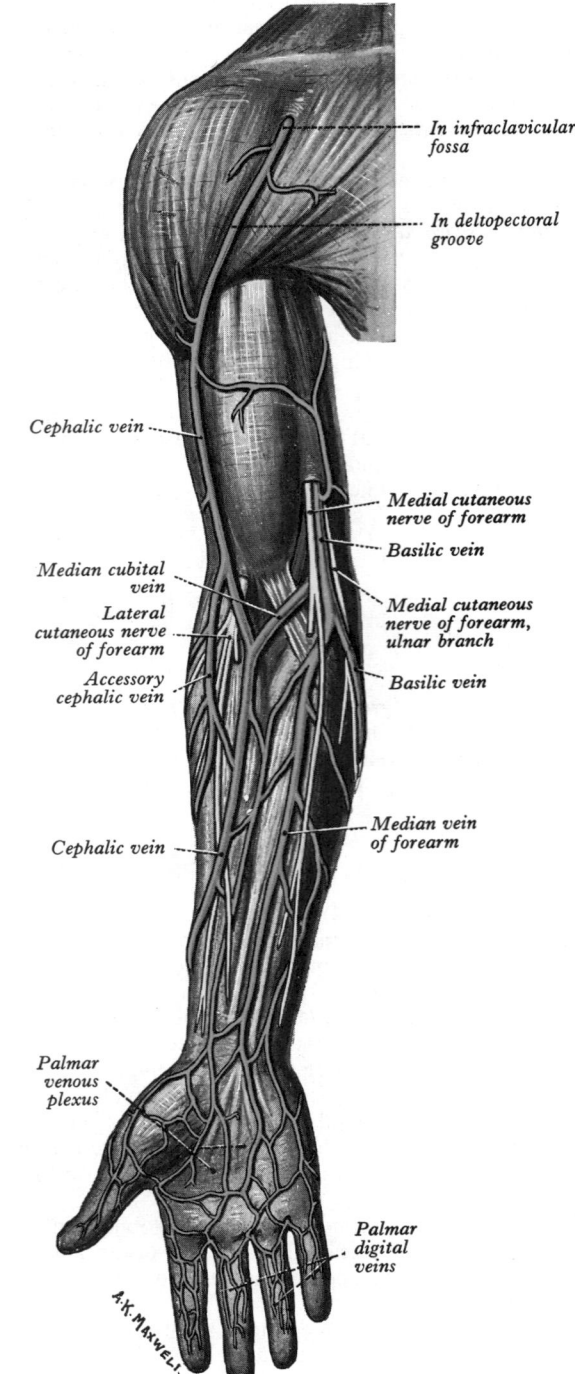

In infraclavicular fossa

In deltopectoral groove

Cephalic vein

Medial cutaneous nerve of forearm

Basilic vein

Median cubital vein

Lateral cutaneous nerve of forearm

Medial cutaneous nerve of forearm, ulnar branch

Accessory cephalic vein

Basilic vein

Cephalic vein

Median vein of forearm

Palmar venous plexus

Palmar digital veins

10.169　The superficial veins of the right upper extremity: anterior aspect.

medial to the axillary artery, which it partly overlaps; between them are the medial pectoral nerve, medial cord of the brachial plexus, the ulnar nerve and the medial cutaneous nerve of the forearm. The medial cutaneous nerve of the arm is medial to the vein; the lateral group of axillary lymph nodes is posteromedial. It has a pair of valves near its distal end; valves also occur near the ends of the cephalic and subscapular veins.

Subclavian vein (10.92). Continuing the axillary, this vein extends from the outer border of the first rib to the medial border of scalenus anterior, where it joins the internal jugular to form the brachiocephalic vein. **Anterior** are the clavicle and subclavius, **posterosuperior** the subclavian artery, separated by the scalenus

anterior and phrenic nerve; **inferior** are the first rib and pleura. The vein usually has a pair of valves about 2 cm from its end. Its tributaries are the external jugular, dorsal scapular and sometimes the anterior jugular; occasionally a small branch ascends in front of the clavicle from the cephalic vein. At its junction with the internal jugular the left subclavian receives the thoracic duct, the right subclavian vein and the right lymphatic duct.

Surface anatomy

The vein can be projected as a broad band, convex upwards, from just medial to the midclavicular point to the medial edge of the clavicular attachment of sternocleidomastoid.

VEINS OF THE THORAX

Brachiocephalic veins

The brachiocephalic (innominate) veins, two large vessels at the junction of the neck and thorax, are the united trunks of the internal jugular and subclavian veins. Both are devoid of valves.

Right brachiocephalic vein (10.170). About 2.5 cm long, it begins posterior to the sternal end of the right clavicle, and descends almost vertically to join the left brachiocephalic forming the superior vena cava posterior to the lower border of the first right costal cartilage, near the right sternal border. It is anterolateral to the brachiocephalic artery and right vagus nerve. The right pleura, phrenic nerve and internal thoracic artery are posterior to it above, becoming lateral below. Its tributaries are the right vertebral, internal thoracic, inferior thyroid and sometimes the first right posterior intercostal veins.

Left brachiocephalic vein (10.170). Some 6 cm long, it begins posterior to the sternal end of the left clavicle, anterior to the cervical

pleura. It descends obliquely to the right, posterior to the upper half of the manubrium sterni, to the sternal end of the first right costal cartilage, uniting here with the right brachiocephalic to form the superior vena cava. It is separated from the left sternoclavicular joint and manubrium by the sternohyoid and sternothyroid, the thymus or its remains and areolar tissue; terminally it is overlapped by the right pleura. It crosses anterior to the left internal thoracic, subclavian and common arteries, left phrenic and vagus nerves, trachea and brachiocephalic artery. The aortic arch is inferior to it. The vein's tributaries are the left vertebral, internal thoracic, inferior thyroid, superior intercostal, sometimes the first left posterior intercostal, thymic and pericardial veins.

Surface anatomy. The brachiocephalic veins can be projected as broad bands 1.5 cm wide from the sternal ends of the clavicles to the parasternal lower border of the first right costal cartilage.

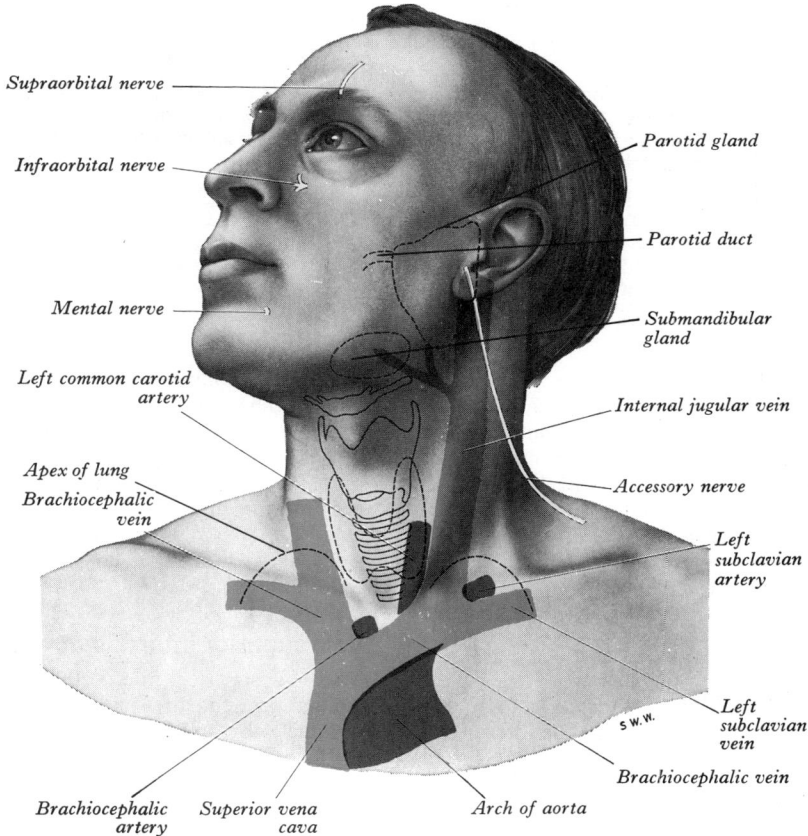

Supraorbital nerve

Infraorbital nerve

Mental nerve

Left common carotid artery

Apex of lung

Brachiocephalic vein

Brachiocephalic artery

Superior vena cava

Arch of aorta

Parotid gland

Parotid duct

Submandibular gland

Internal jugular vein

Accessory nerve

Left subclavian artery

Left subclavian vein

Brachiocephalic vein

S.W.W.

10.170 The surface projections of some of the important structures in the face, neck and upper part of the thorax. The apices of the lungs, the thyroid, submandibular and parotid glands and the parotid duct are indicated in interrupted dotted outline; the hyoid bone, the thyroid and cricoid cartilages and the rings of the trachea are shown in continuous outline.

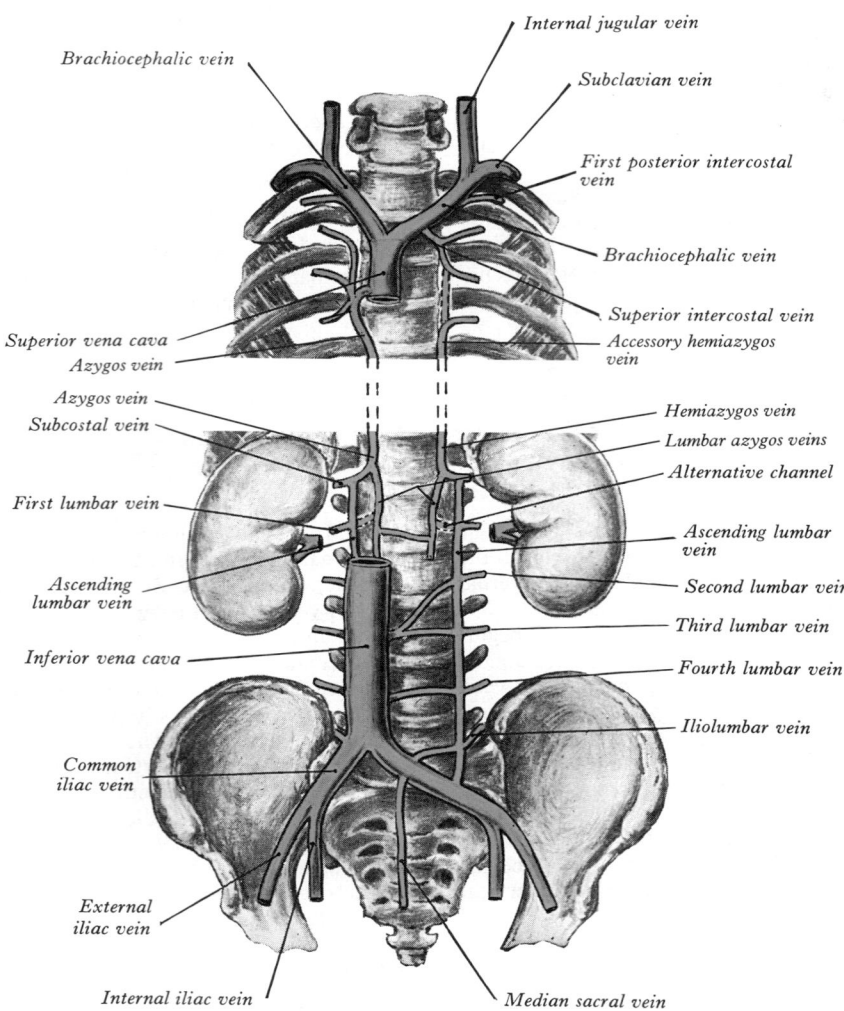

Internal jugular vein

Brachiocephalic vein

Subclavian vein

First posterior intercostal vein

Brachiocephalic vein

Superior intercostal vein

Accessory hemiazygos vein

Superior vena cava

Azygos vein

Azygos vein

Subcostal vein

Hemiazygos vein

Lumbar azygos veins

Alternative channel

First lumbar vein

Ascending lumbar vein

Second lumbar vein

Ascending lumbar vein

Third lumbar vein

Inferior vena cava

Fourth lumbar vein

Iliolumbar vein

Common iliac vein

External iliac vein

Internal iliac vein

Median sacral vein

10.171 Schema showing the superior and inferior extremities of the azygos system of veins and their principal associated veins. The intervening parts have been omitted because schemata of this region are often topographically misleading. Much variation occurs in the transthoracic parts of the azygos and hemiazygos veins, in terms of numbers of radicles, levels of transmedian crossing, etc. Schemata are usually misleading. That depicted by painting in **10**.172 is the most common condition.

Variations. The brachiocephalic veins may enter the right atrium separately, the right vein descending like a normal superior vena cava; a left superior vena cava may have a slender connection with the right and then cross the left side of the aortic arch to pass anterior to the left pulmonary hilum before turning to enter the right atrium. It replaces the oblique atrial vein and coronary sinus and receives all the latter's tributaries. This abnormality, due to persistence of an early fetal condition, is normal in birds and some mammals. The left brachiocephalic vein sometimes projects above the manubrium (more frequently in childhood), crossing the suprasternal fossa in front of the trachea.

Internal thoracic (mammary) veins

The internal thoracic veins are venae comitantes to the inferior half of the internal thoracic artery; they have several valves. Near the third costal cartilages the veins unite to ascend medial to the artery, ending in their brachiocephalic vein (**10**.71, 95). Tributaries correspond to branches of the artery (p. 1534), and include a pericardiophrenic vein.

Inferior thyroid veins

The inferior thyroid veins arise in a glandular venous plexus,

which also connects with the middle and superior thyroid veins (**10**.71). These veins form a *pretracheal plexus* from which the left inferior vein descends to join the left brachiocephalic, the right descending obliquely across the brachiocephalic artery to the right brachiocephalic vein, at its junction with the superior vena cava; the inferior thyroid veins often open in common into the vena cava or left brachiocephalic vein. They drain the oesophageal, tracheal and inferior laryngeal veins and have valves at their terminations.

Left superior intercostal vein

The left superior intercostal vein drains the second and third (sometimes fourth) left posterior intercostal veins, ascending obliquely forwards across the left aspect of the aortic arch, lateral to the left vagus, medial to the left phrenic nerve, to open into the left brachiocephalic vein (**10**.71). It usually receives the left bronchial veins, sometimes the left pericardiacophrenic; it connects inferiorly with the accessory hemiazygos vein.

Superior vena cava

The superior vena cava is about 7 cm in length, formed by the junction of the brachiocephalic veins, and has no valves. It returns to the heart blood from the superior half of the body. It begins behind the lower border of the first right costal cartilage near the sternum, descends vertically behind the first and second intercostal spaces, ending in the upper right atrium behind the third right costal cartilage; its inferior half is within the fibrous pericardium, which it pierces level with the second costal cartilage. Covered anterolaterally by serous pericardium from which projects a *retrocaval recess*, it is slightly convex to the right (**10**.66, 68–71).

Relations. Anterior are the anterior margins of the right lung and pleura, the pericardium intervening below; these separate the vein from the internal thoracic artery and first and second intercostal spaces, and second and third costal cartilages; posteromedial are the trachea and right vagus nerves and posterolateral the right lung and pleura; posterior is the right pulmonary hilum. Right lateral are the right phrenic nerve and pleura, left lateral the brachiocephalic artery and ascending aorta, the latter overlapping it.

Surface anatomy. The superior vena cava, 2 cm wide, is partly behind but projects well beyond the right sternal margin, from the lower border of the first to the lower border of the third right costal cartilage. Its lateral border is visible in anteroposterior radiographs.

Tributaries. These are: the azygos vein and small veins from the pericardium and other mediastinal structures.

Azygos vein (**10**.171–173).

An origin from the posterior aspect of the inferior vena cava, at or below the level of the renal veins, is to be expected from its development but it is not constant (Gladstone 1929). Such a lumbar azygos vein frequently occurs, ascending anterior to the upper lumbar vertebrae. The vein may pass behind the right crus of the diaphragm or pierce it. It may traverse the aortic opening on the right of the cisterna chyli. Anterior to the twelfth thoracic vertebral body it is joined by a large vessel formed by the right ascending lumbar and right subcostal veins, which passes forward and right of the twelfth thoracic vertebra behind the right crus. This common trunk may, in the absence of a lumbar azygos, form the azygos itself. Whatever its origin, the azygos vein ascends in the posterior mediastinum to the fourth thoracic vertebra, arching forward above the right pulmonary hilum to end in the superior vena cava, before the latter pierces the pericardium. It is **anterior** to the lower eight thoracic vertebral bodies (see below), anterior longitudinal ligament and right posterior intercostal arteries. **Right lateral** are the right greater splanchnic nerve, lung and pleura; **left lateral** in most of its course are the thoracic duct and aorta and, where it arches forward, the oesophagus, trachea and right vagus. In the lower thorax it is covered anteriorly by a recess of the right pleural sac and oesophagus, emerging from behind the latter to ascend behind the right hilum (**10**.173). Because of the closeness of the azygos vein to the right posterolateral aspect of the descending thoracic aorta, aortic pulsations may assist venous return in azygos and hemiazygos veins.

Tributaries. The azygos vein drains: the right posterior intercostal veins except the first, the veins from the second to fourth intercostal spaces usually via a right superior intercostal vein, the hemiazygos and accessory hemiazygos veins, oesophageal, mediastinal and pericardial veins and, near its end, right bronchial veins. When it begins as a lumbar azygos, the common trunk formed by the right ascending lumbar and subcostal veins is its largest tributary. Imperfect valves occur in the azygos vein, some tributaries having complete valves.

Hemiazygos vein. It starts on the left like the azygos; ascending anterior to the vertebral column to the eighth thoracic level, it crosses the column posterior to the aorta, oesophagus and thoracic duct to end in the azygos vein. Its tributaries are the lower three posterior intercostal veins, a common trunk formed by the left ascending lumbar and subcostal veins and oesophageal and mediastinal rami. Its lower end often connects with the left renal vein.

Accessory hemiazygos vein. It descends to the left of the vertebral column, receiving veins from the fourth (or fifth) to eighth intercostal spaces and sometimes the left bronchial veins. It crosses the seventh thoracic vertebra to join the azygos vein. It sometimes joins the hemiazygos, their common trunk opening into the azygos vein.

Variations of the azygos veins. They vary much in their mode of origin, course, tributaries, anastomoses and termination. For a survey consult Grzybiak et al (1975), who consider the accessory

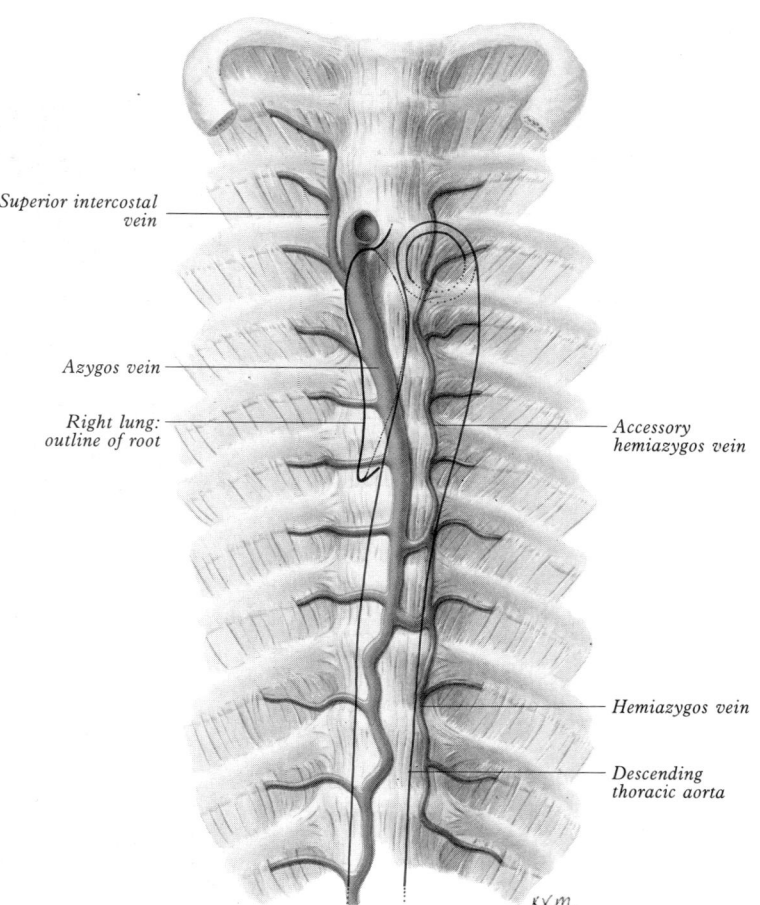

10.172 A frequent (perhaps the commonest) course followed by the intra-thoracic azygos, hemiazygos and accessory hemiazygos veins. Outlines of the root of the right lung and descending thoracic aorta are included. (Dissection by M C E Hutchinson, Guy's Hospital Medical School, London.)

Superior intercostal vein

Azygos vein

Right lung: outline of root

Accessory hemiazygos vein

Hemiazygos vein

Descending thoracic aorta

hemiazygos most variable, draining into the left brachiocephalic, azygos or hemiazygos. The arrangement shown in **10**.172 represents a common pattern. In about 1 or 2% of subjects according to Anson (1963) there are left and right independent azygos veins (the early embryonic form) and occasionally a single azygos without hemiazygos tributaries, in a midline position. In more than 95% a main 'right-sided' azygos and at least some representative of hemiazygos veins exist. The latter vary, one or the other being absent or poorly developed. Retro-aortic transvertebral connections from hemiazygos and accessory hemiazygos veins to the azygos are also extremely variable; there may be from one to five, or more; when either hemiazygos is absent, intercostal veins involved cross vertebral bodies to end in the azygos. These transvertebral routes are often very short, since the azygos vein is more commonly anterior to the vertebral column (Anson 1963) and often passes left of the midline in part of its course.

Posterior intercostal veins

The posterior intercostal veins accompany their arteries in eleven pairs. Approaching the vertebral column each vein receives a posterior tributary returning blood from the dorsal muscles and skin and vertebral venous plexuses (**10**.111, 173). On both sides the first posterior intercostal vein ascends anterior to the first rib's neck, arching forward above the pleural dome to end in the ipsilateral brachiocephalic or vertebral vein. On the right the second, third and often fourth, form a right superior intercostal vein joining the arch of the azygos vein. Veins from the lower spaces drain directly to it. On the left the second and third (sometimes fourth) form a left superior intercostal vein (p. 1592). Veins from the fourth (or fifth) to eighth spaces end in the accessory hemiazygos vein, veins from the lower three spaces in the hemiazygos.

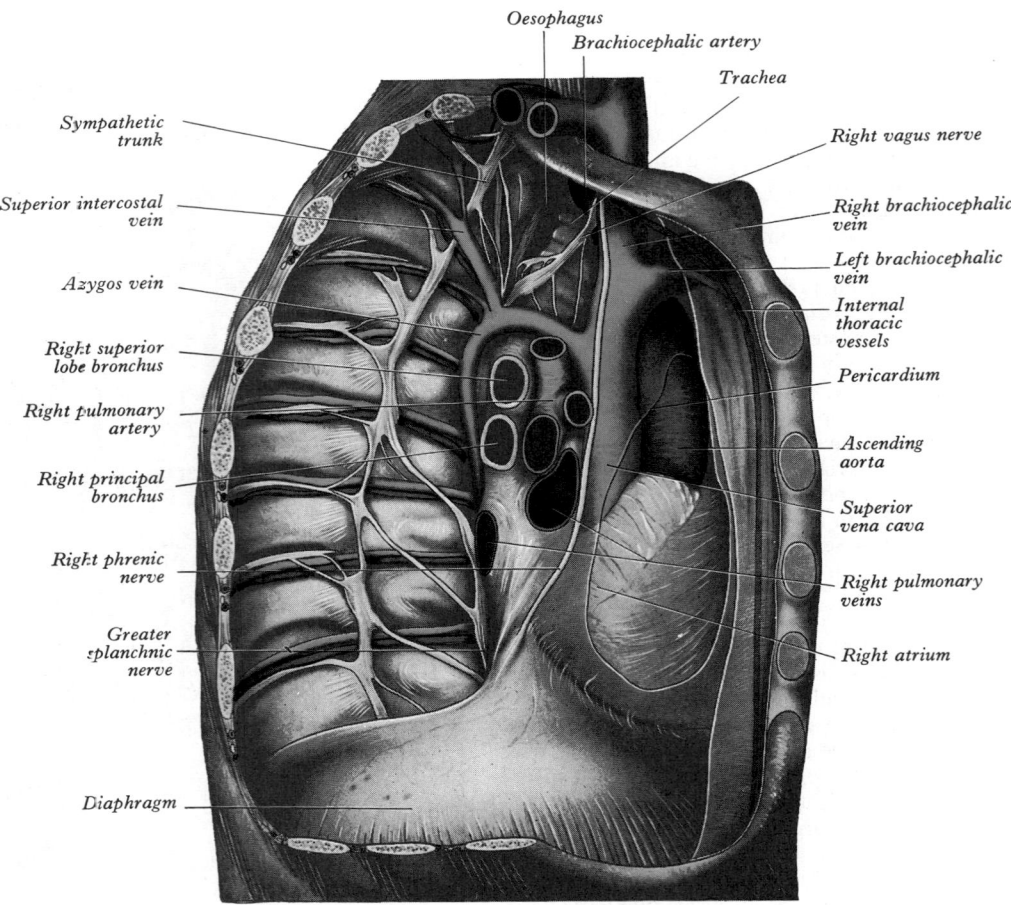

10.173   The right aspect of the mediastinum. The right lung and most of the right pleura have been removed and a large opening made into the pericardial sac to expose the heart. In this specimen the fourth right posterior intercostal vein did not join the superior intercostal vein.

Posterior intercostal veins are so called to distinguish them from small *anterior intercostal veins* which are tributaries of the internal thoracic and musculophrenic veins.

Clinical anatomy. In obstruction of the upper inferior vena cava, the azygos and hemiazygos veins and vertebral venous plexuses are the main collateral channels maintaining venous circulation, by connecting superior and inferior venae cavae and communicating with the common iliac by ascending lumbar veins and with many tributaries of the inferior vena cava.

Bronchial veins

Usually two on each side, the bronchial veins drain blood from larger bronchi and from hilar structures. The right bronchial veins join the end of the azygos, the left join the left superior intercostal or hemiazygos vein. Some blood carried to the lungs by bronchial arteries returns via the pulmonary veins (see p. 1674).

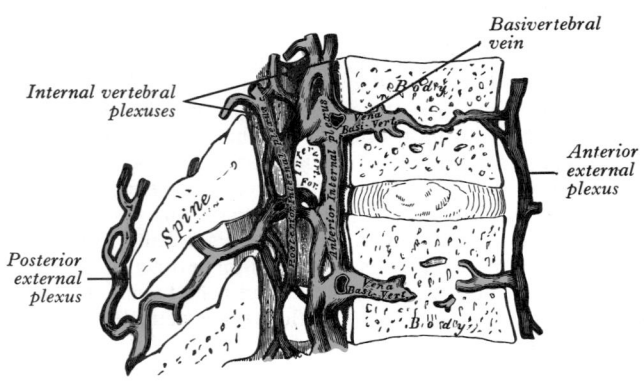

10.174   Transverse section through the body of a thoracic vertebra showing the vertebral venous plexuses and basivertebral veins.

10.175   Median sagittal section through two thoracic vertebrae showing the vertebral venous plexuses and basivertebral veins.

VEINS OF THE VERTEBRAL COLUMN

Veins of the vertebral column form intricate plexuses along the entire column, external and internal to the vertebral canal. Both groups are devoid of valves, anastomose freely with each other and join the intervertebral veins (**10**.174, 175). Interconnections are widely established between these plexuses and longitudinal veins early in fetal life (Loginova 1972).

External vertebral venous plexuses

The external vertebral venous plexuses are anterior and posterior, anastomosing freely, and are most developed in the cervical region. *Anterior external plexuses* are anterior to the vertebral bodies, communicating with basivertebral and intervertebral veins and receiving tributaries from vertebral bodies. *Posterior external plexuses* lie posterior to vertebral laminae and around spines, transverse and articular processes. They anastomose with the internal plexuses and join the vertebral, posterior intercostal and lumbar veins.

Internal vertebral venous plexuses

The internal vertebral venous plexuses occur between the dura mater and vertebrae, receiving tributaries from the bones, red bone marrow and spinal cord. They form a denser network than the external plexuses and are arranged vertically as four interconnecting longitudinal vessels, two in front, two behind.

The *anterior internal plexuses* are large plexiform veins on the posterior surfaces of vertebral bodies and intervertebral discs, flanking the posterior longitudinal ligament; under this they are connected by transverse branches, into which the large basivertebral veins open. The *posterior internal plexuses*, on each side in front of the vertebral arches and ligamenta flava, anastomose with the posterior external plexuses by veins passing through and between the ligaments. The internal plexuses interconnect by venous rings near each vertebra. Around the foramen magnum they form a dense network connecting with: vertebral veins, occipital and sigmoid sinuses, basilar plexus, venous plexus of the hypoglossal canal and the condylar emissary veins.

Basivertebral veins

The basivertebral veins emerge from the posterior foramina of vertebral bodies. They are large and tortuous channels in bone, like those in cranial diploë. The trabecular bone in vertebral bodies contains much haemopoietic tissue. The basivertebral veins also drain into the anterior external vertebral plexuses through small openings in the vertebral bodies. Posteriorly they form one or two short trunks opening into the transverse branches uniting anterior internal vertebral plexuses. They enlarge in advanced age.

Intervertebral veins

The intervertebral veins accompany the spinal nerves through intervertebral foramina, draining the spinal cord and internal and external vertebral plexuses, and ending in the vertebral, posterior intercostal, lumbar and lateral sacral veins. Whether the basivertebral or intervertebral veins contain effective valves is uncertain but experiment strongly suggests that their blood flow can be reversed (Batson 1957). This may explain how pelvic neoplasms, in particular, may metastasize in vertebral bodies, the cells spreading into the internal vertebral plexuses by connections with the pelvic veins when blood flow is temporarily reversed by raised intra-abdominal pressure or postural alterations.

Veins of the spinal cord

The veins of the spinal cord lie in the pia mater, forming a tortuous venous plexus. In this there are:

- two *median longitudinal veins*, one near the anterior median fissure, the other behind the posterior median septum
- two *anterolateral* and two *posterolateral longitudinal veins* respectively behind the ventral and dorsal spinal nerve roots.

They drain to internal vertebral plexuses, and thence to intervertebral veins. Near the skull they unite into two or three small veins joined to the vertebral veins and ending in inferior cerebellar veins or the inferior petrosal sinuses.

VEINS OF THE LOWER LIMBS

Veins of the lower limbs can be subdivided, like those of the upper, into *superficial* and *deep* groups, the superficial being subcutaneous in the superficial fascia, the deep veins (beneath the deep fascia) accompanying major arteries. Both have valves, more numerous in deep veins and also more numerous than in the upper limb.

SUPERFICIAL VEINS OF THE LOWER LIMBS

The principal named superficial veins are the great and small saphenous; their numerous tributaries are mostly (but not wholly) unnamed; named vessels will be noted (**10**.176, 177). (For variations consult Kosinski 1926.) As in the upper limb the vessels will be described centripetally from peripheral to major drainage channels.

Dorsal digital veins receive, in the clefts between the toes, rami from the plantar digital veins and then join to form dorsal metatarsal veins, which are united across the proximal parts of the metatarsal bones in a *dorsal venous arch*. Proximal to this is an irregular *dorsal venous network* receiving tributaries from deep veins and continuous proximally with a venous network in the leg. At each side of the foot this network connects with *medial* and *lateral marginal veins*, both formed mainly by veins from more superficial parts of the sole. In the sole superficial veins form a *plantar cutaneous arch* across the roots of the toes and also drain into the medial and lateral marginal veins. Proximal to the plantar arch is a *plantar cutaneous venous plexus*, especially dense in the fat of the heel; this connects with the plantar cutaneous venous arch and other deep veins, but drains mainly into the marginal veins.

Great (long) saphenous vein

The great saphenous vein starts inferiorly (below) as a continuation of the medial marginal vein and ends in the femoral vein a short distance distal to the inguinal ligament (see below), being thus the body's longest vein (**10**.176). It ascends about 2.5–3 cm anterior to the tibial malleolus, crosses the distal third of the medial surface of the tibia obliquely to its medial border, then ascends a little behind the border to the knee; proximally it is posteromedial to the medial tibial and femoral condyles, then ascends the medial aspect of the thigh; after traversing the saphenous opening (p. 873) it finally opens into the femoral vein. The so-called 'centre' of the opening is often said to be 2.5–3.5 cm inferolateral to the pubic tubercle; and the vein is then held to be represented by a line drawn from this to the femoral adductor tubercle. However, the saphenous opening, as noted elsewhere, varies greatly in size and disposition and its imagined centre has proved a poor indicator of the saphenofemoral junction.

In its course through the thigh the great saphenous vein has branches of the medial femoral cutaneous nerve accompanying it: at the knee the saphenous branch of the descending genicular artery and, in the leg and foot, the saphenous nerve, are anterior to it. The vein is often duplicated, especially distal to the knee. It has from 10 to 20 valves, which are more numerous in the leg than the thigh. One is present just before it pierces the cribriform fascia, another at its junction with the femoral vein. In almost its entire extent the vein lies in superficial fascia, but it has many connections with the deep veins, especially in the leg (see below).

Clinical anatomy. Royle and Eisher (1981) made a careful quantitative study in 167 flush ligations in 136 subjects noting, in particular, the relative positions of the pubic tubercle, the venous junction and the inguinal skin crease. They concluded that a correctly placed incision for flush saphenofemoral ligation should be made

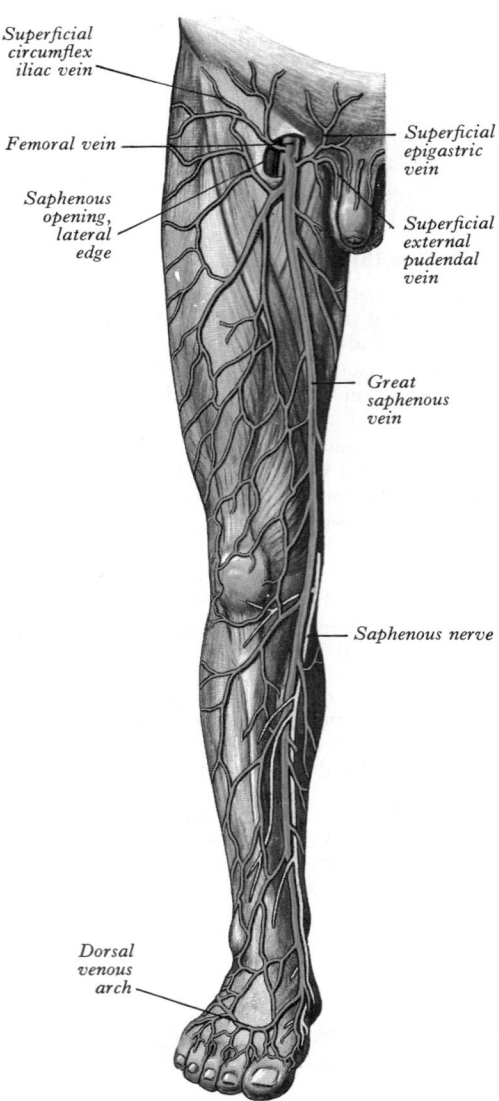

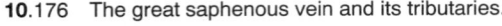

10.176   The great saphenous vein and its tributaries.

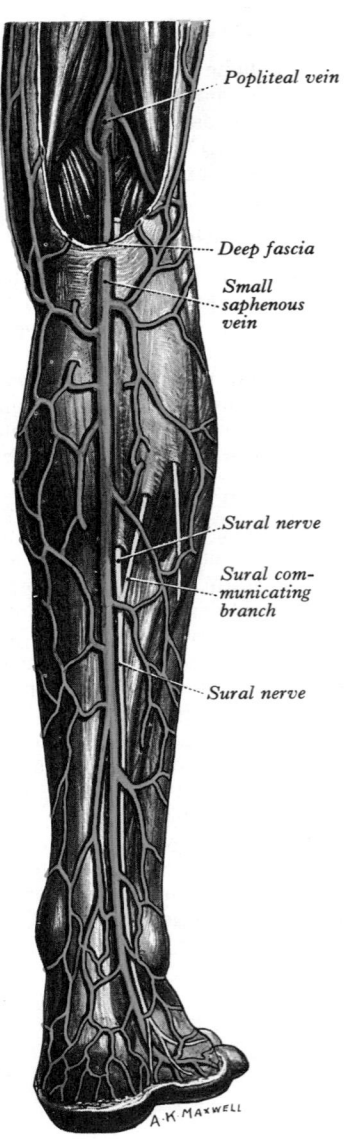

10.177   The small saphenous vein and its tributaries.

1 cm above, and parallel to, the inguinal skin crease, centring the incision at a point 4 cm lateral to and level with the pubic tubercle.

Tributaries. At the ankle the great saphenous drains the sole by medial marginal veins. In the leg it often connects with the small saphenous vein and with deep veins through *perforating veins*. Just distal to the knee it usually has three large tributaries: one from the front of the leg, a second from the tibial malleolar region (connecting with some of the 'perforating' veins) and a third from the calf (communicating with the small saphenous vein). The second of these forms below in a fine network or 'corona' of delicate veins over the medial malleolus and then ascends the medial aspect of the calf as the '*posterior arch vein*' of Dodd and Cockett (1976); the clinical importance of its connections with posterior tibial venae comitantes by a series of perforating (communicating) veins was emphasized by Platz and Adelmann (1976), who proposed the term '*vena arcuata cruris posterior*'. The clinical significance of the latter should be reaffirmed, with relevant points concerning other venous channels in the leg. Although Platz and Adelmann (1976) mentioned 3–6 perforating veins, it has been indicated that three are most usual, being equally spaced between the medial malleolus and the midcalf; more than three was termed 'most uncommon' and an arch vein perforator above midcalf 'extremely rare'. The posterior crural arch vein was first illustrated by Leonardo da Vinci and his name is often applied to the vein in some surgical circles.

Above the posterior crural arch vein, perforating veins join the great saphenous or one of its main tributaries at two main sites. The

first is at a level in the upper calf indicated by its name, the *tibial tubercle perforator* (*Boyd's perforator*); the second is in the lower/intermediate third of the thigh where it perforates the deep fascial roof of the subsartorial canal to join the femoral vein (*Hunterian perforator*).

In the thigh the great saphenous vein receives many tributaries; some open independently, whilst others converge to form large named channels that frequently pass towards the basal half of the femoral triangle before joining the great saphenous near its termination. These may be grouped thus: one or more large post-eromedial tributaries, one or more large anterolateral tributaries, four or more peri-inguinal veins. The *posteromedial vein of the thigh*, large and sometimes double, drains a large superficial region indicated by its name: it has (as have the other tributaries) radio-logical and surgical significance. One of its lower radicles is often continuous with the small saphenous vein. The posteromedial vein is sometimes (perhaps unhelpfully) named the *accessory saphenous vein* with greater emphasis on its variability of form and level of junction with the great saphenous. Some restrict the term accessory to a lower (more distal) posteromedial branch when two (or more) are present. Another large vessel, the *anterolateral vein of the thigh* (*anterior femoral cutaneous vein*), usually commences from an anterior network of veins in the distal thigh and crosses the apex and distal half of the femoral triangle to reach the great saphenous vein. As the latter traverses its saphenous opening (**10**.176), it is joined by the superficial epigastric, superficial circumflex iliac and superficial external pudendal veins. Their mode of union varies. Superficial epigastric and circumflex iliac veins drain the inferior abdominal wall, the latter also receiving tributaries from the proximolateral region of the thigh; superficial external pudendal veins drain part of the scrotum, one being joined by the superficial dorsal vein of the penis. The deep external pudendal vein joins the great saphenous in its opening.

A *thoraco-epigastric vein* lies along the anterolateral aspect of the trunk and connects the superficial epigastric or femoral vein to the lateral thoracic veins, thus connecting femoral and axillary veins and hence the superior and inferior vena caval fields of drainage. It is held to be in line with the primitive mammary ('milk') ridge which extends from the axilla to the pubic region (p. 296).

Small (short) saphenous vein (10.177)

The small saphenous vein begins posterior to the lateral malleolus, as a continuation of the lateral marginal vein. In the lower third of the calf it ascends lateral to the tendo calcaneus, lying on the deep fascia and covered only by superficial fascia and skin. Inclining medially to the midline of the calf it penetrates into the deep fascia within which it ascends on the gastrocnemius, only emerging between the deep fascia and gastrocnemius gradually at about the junction of the intermediate and proximal thirds of the calf (usually well below the lower limit of the popliteal fossa). Continuing its ascent it passes between the heads of the gastrocnemius, then proceeds to its termination in the popliteal vein, 3–7.5 cm above the knee joint in the popliteal fossa.

Tributaries. The small saphenous vein connects with deep veins on the dorsum of the foot, receives many cutaneous tributaries in the leg and sends several rami proximally and medially to join the great saphenous vein. Sometimes a communicating branch from it ascends medially to the accessory saphenous vein (see above); this may be the main continuation of the small saphenous. In the leg the small saphenous lies near the sural nerve. It has 7–13 valves, one near its termination. Its mode of ending is variable; it may join the great saphenous vein in the proximal thigh or it may bifurcate, one branch joining the great saphenous, the other the popliteal or deep posterior femoral veins; sometimes it ends distal to the knee in the great saphenous or deep sural muscular veins.

Clinical anatomy. In a standing position, venous return from the lower limb depends largely on muscular activity (p. 1466), especially contraction of the calf muscles, known as the 'calf pump', whose efficiency is aided by the tight sleeve of deep fascia. 'Perforating' veins have been noted that connect the great saphenous with the deep veins, particularly near the ankle, distal calf and knee regions. In these channels valves are arranged to prevent flow of blood from deep to superficial veins. At rest, pressure in a superficial vein is equal to the height of the column of blood extending therefrom to the heart. When calf muscles contract, blood is pumped proximally in the deep veins but is normally prevented from flowing into superficial veins by the valves in the perforating veins; during relaxation blood can be aspirated from superficial into deep veins. If the valves in the perforating veins become incompetent, these veins become 'high pressure leaks' during muscular contraction; this transmission of high pressure in deep veins to superficial veins results in dilatation and blood stagnation in the latter, producing varicosities, anoxia of tissues and ultimately varicose ulceration. In operative treatment of severe varicose veins and ulcers, perforating veins must be ligatured. Similar perforating connections occur in the anterolateral region and varicosities may also occur here (Cockett 1956; Green et al 1958). Veins connecting the great saphenous to the femoral vein, in the adductor canal, may also become varicose (Dodd & Cockett 1956; Dodd 1959).

DEEP VEINS OF THE LOWER LIMBS

Deep veins of the lower limbs accompany the arteries and their branches; they have numerous valves (10.178). *Plantar digital veins* arise from plexuses in the plantar regions of the toes, connecting with dorsal digital veins and uniting into four *plantar metatarsal veins*; these run in the intermetatarsal spaces and connect by perforating veins with dorsal veins, then continue to form the *deep plantar venous arch*, accompanying the plantar arterial arch. From this *medial* and *lateral plantar veins* run near the corresponding

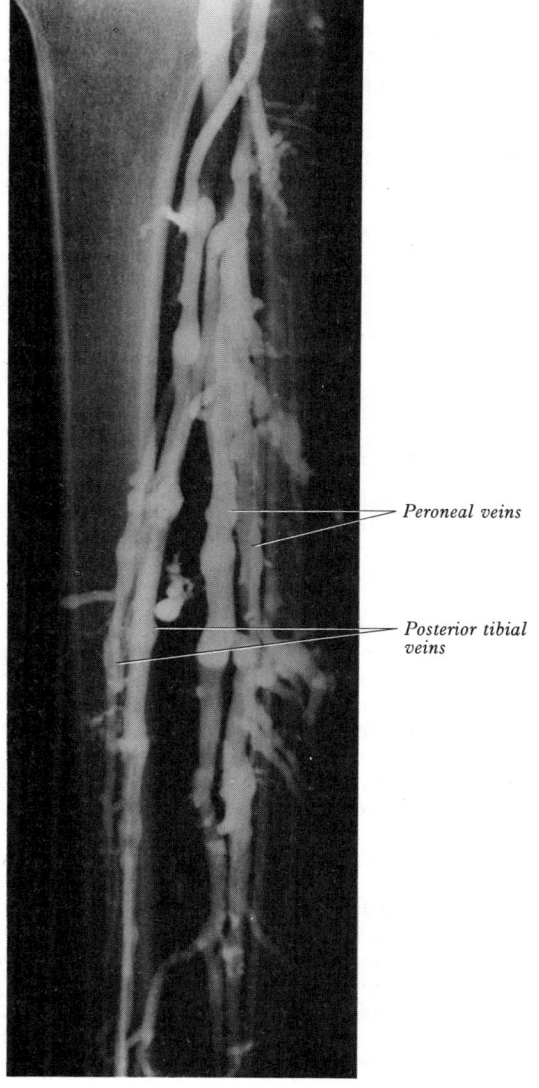

Peroneal veins

Posterior tibial veins

10.178 Venogram of the leg to show the deep veins; the valves are clearly demonstrated. (Supplied by Shaun Gallagher, Guy's Hospital; photography by Sarah Smith.)

arteries and, after communicating with the great and small saphenous veins, form behind the medial malleolus the posterior tibial veins.

Posterior tibial veins. They accompany the posterior tibial artery, receiving veins from sural muscles, especially the venous plexus in the soleus, connections from superficial veins and the *peroneal veins*. The latter, running with their artery, receive rami from the soleus and superficial veins.

Anterior tibial veins. Continuations of the venous companions of the dorsal pedal artery, they leave the extensor region between the tibia and fibula, pass through the proximal end of the interosseous membrane, and unite with the posterior tibial veins to form the *popliteal vein* at the distal border of the popliteus.

Popliteal vein. Ascending through the popliteal fossa to an aperture in adductor magnus, it becomes the femoral vein. Distally it is medial to the artery; between the heads of gastrocnemius it is superficial (dorsal) to it; proximal to the knee joint it is posterolateral. Its tributaries are: the small saphenous vein, veins corresponding to branches of the popliteal artery and muscular veins, including a large one from each head of gastrocnemius. There are usually four valves in the popliteal vein.

Femoral vein. It accompanies its artery, beginning at the adductor opening as the continuation of the popliteal, and ending posterior to the inguinal ligament as the external iliac. In the distal adductor canal, it is posterolateral to the femoral artery; more proximally in the canal, and in the distal femoral triangle (i.e. its apex), it is posterior to it; at the triangle's base it is medial (10.137, 140). The vein occupies the middle compartment of the femoral sheath, between the femoral artery and canal, fat in the latter allowing expansion of the vein. It has many muscular tributaries: about 4–12 cm distal to the inguinal ligament the *vena profunda femoris* joins it posteriorly and then the great saphenous vein, which enters anteriorly. Lateral and medial circumflex femoral veins are usually tributaries. There

are usually four or five valves in the femoral vein, the most constant being one just distal to the entry of the profunda femoris and one near the inguinal ligament.

Vena profunda femoris. It is anterior to its artery, its tributaries corresponding; through these it connects distally with the popliteal and proximally inferior gluteal veins. It sometimes drains medial and lateral circumflex femoral veins. It has a valve just before its end.

VEINS OF THE ABDOMEN AND PELVIS

EXTERNAL ILIAC VEIN

The proximal continuation of the femoral vein is the external iliac: it thus begins posterior to the inguinal ligament, ascends the pelvic brim and ends anterior to the sacro-iliac joint by joining the internal iliac to form the common iliac vein. On the right, it is first medial to the external iliac artery, gradually inclining behind it as it ascends; on the left, it is wholly medial. This is a point of great surgical importance. Disease of the external iliac artery may cause it to adhere closely to the vein at the point where it is in contact, and (especially on the right side) the walls of the vessels may become fused. Dissection in this area risks producing severe venous haemorrhage which may be difficult to control. Medially the external iliac vein is crossed by the ureter and internal iliac artery, and is elsewhere covered by parietal peritoneum. In males it is crossed by the ductus deferens, in females by the round ligament and ovarian vessels. Lateral is psoas major, except where the artery intervenes. The vein is usually valveless, but may contain a single valve.

Tributaries. These are: the inferior epigastric, deep circumflex iliac and pubic veins.

Inferior epigastric vein. It derives from the union of the venae comitantes of the inferior epigastric artery, which connect above with the superior epigastric veins; it joins the external iliac about 1 cm proximal to the inguinal ligament.

Deep circumflex iliac vein. It is formed from venae comitantes of the corresponding artery; it joins the external iliac about 2 cm proximal to the inguinal ligament after crossing anterior to the external iliac artery.

Pubic vein. Connecting the external iliac with the obturator vein in the obturator foramen, it ascends on the pelvic surface of the pubis with the pubic branch of the inferior epigastric artery. It sometimes replaces the normal obturator vein.

INTERNAL ILIAC VEIN

Veins converge superiorly in the great sciatic foramen to form the internal iliac vein, which ascends posteromedial to the internal iliac artery to join the external iliac vein, forming the common iliac at the pelvic brim, anterior to the lower part of the sacro-iliac joint. It is covered anteromedially by parietal peritoneum.

Tributaries. These are:

- gluteal, internal pudendal and obturator veins, with origins outside the pelvis
- lateral sacral veins, anterior to the sacrum
- middle rectal, vesical, uterine and vaginal veins, originating in the venous plexuses of pelvic viscera.

The superior gluteal veins, venae comitantes of the superior gluteal artery, receive rami corresponding to branches of the artery; entering the pelvis via the greater sciatic foramen, above piriformis, they join the internal iliac vein, frequently as a single trunk.

Clinical anatomy. The venous drainage of the leg is frequently blocked by thrombosis, usually originating in the soleal sinusoids, but frequently extending up into the external iliac systems and the inferior vena cava. Under these circumstances, the pelvic veins enlarge and provide a major avenue of venous return from the femoral system. Surgical interference with these veins (as for example

in hysterectomy) may seriously compromise venous drainage and precipitate oedema of one or both legs.

Inferior gluteal veins. These venae comitantes of the inferior gluteal artery begin proximally and posterior in the thigh, where they anastomose with the medial circumflex femoral and first perforating veins; they enter the pelvis low in the greater sciatic foramen, joining to form a vessel opening into the distal (lower) part of the internal iliac vein. They connect with the superficial gluteal veins by perforating veins (Doyle 1970) similar to those in the calf (p. 1596). These *gluteal perforating veins* are, indeed, even more numerous than the sural ones. In addition to a probable venous 'pumping' role, they provide collaterals between the femoral and internal iliac veins.

Internal pudendal veins. These venae comitantes of the internal pudendal artery begin in the prostatic venous plexus (p. 1599), accompany the artery and unite as a single vessel ending in the internal iliac vein. They receive veins from the penile bulb and the scrotal (or labial) and inferior rectal veins. The deep dorsal vein of the penis connects with the internal pudendal but ends mainly in the prostatic plexus.

Obturator vein. This begins in the proximal adductor region, enters the pelvis superiorly in the obturator foramen, and runs back and up on the lateral pelvic wall below the obturator artery covered by peritoneum; it then passes between the ureter and internal iliac artery to end in the internal iliac vein. Sometimes it is replaced by an enlarged pubic vein, which joins the external iliac (see above).

Lateral sacral veins. They accompany the lateral sacral arteries, being interconnected by a sacral venous plexus.

Middle rectal vein. It begins in the rectal venous plexus, with tributaries from bladder, prostate and seminal vesicle; it is variable in size and runs laterally on the pelvic surface of levator ani to end in the internal iliac vein.

Rectal venous plexus. This plexus surrounds the rectum, connecting anteriorly with the vesical plexus in males and the uterovaginal plexus in females. It consists of an **internal** part beneath the rectal and anal epithelium and an **external** part outside the muscular stratum. In the anal canal the internal plexus has longitudinal dilatations, connected by transverse branches in circles immediately above the anal valves. The dilatations are most prominent in the left lateral, right anterolateral and right posterolateral sectors. The internal plexus drains mainly to the superior rectal vein but connects widely with the external plexus. The external plexus is drained inferiorly by the inferior rectal vein into the internal pudendal, its middle part by a middle rectal vein into the internal iliac, its superior part by the superior rectal vein, which is the commencement of the inferior mesenteric (a tributary of the portal vein). Communication between portal and systemic venous systems is thus established in the rectal plexus.

Clinical anatomy. Veins of the internal rectal plexus are apt to become varicose. The vessels lie in very loose areolar tissue, less supported by surrounding structures than most veins, and are less able to resist increased blood pressure; the superior rectal vein and the portal vein have no valves; rectal veins pass through muscular tissue and are liable to compression, especially during defecation; they are affected by every form of portal obstruction. A clear distinction cannot be made between rectal varices and haemorrhoids. *Varices* occur as a result of portal hypertension: they are dilated venous channels structurally similar to oesophageal varices, and caused by the same mechanism. *Internal haemorrhoids* are engorged arteriovenous cushions, which are thought to arise as a result of

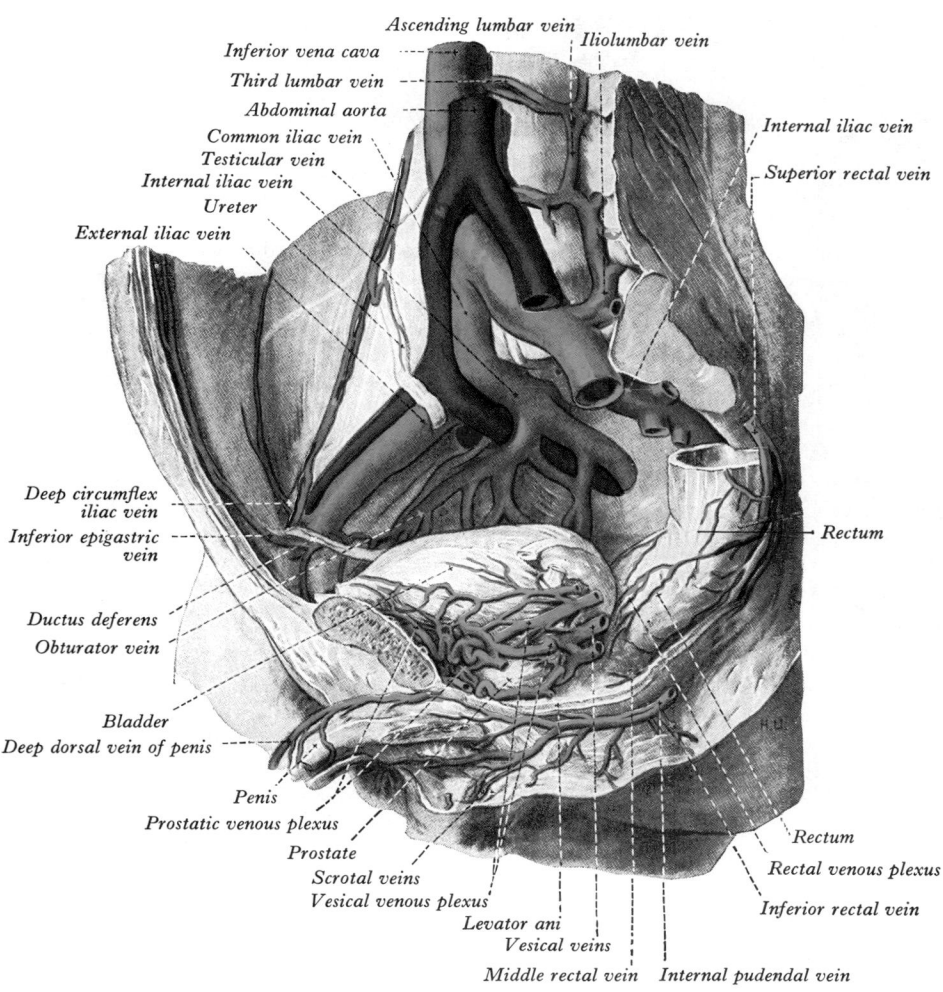

Ascending lumbar vein
Inferior vena cava
Third lumbar vein
Abdominal aorta
Common iliac vein
Testicular vein
Internal iliac vein
Ureter
External iliac vein

Iliolumbar vein
Internal iliac vein
Superior rectal vein

Deep circumflex iliac vein
Inferior epigastric vein

Ductus deferens
Obturator vein

Rectum

Bladder
Deep dorsal vein of penis

Penis
Prostatic venous plexus
Prostate
Scrotal veins
Vesical venous plexus
Levator ani
Vesical veins
Middle rectal vein

Rectum
Rectal venous plexus
Inferior rectal vein

Internal pudendal vein

10.179   The veins of the right half of the male pelvis (after Spalteholz).

faecal pressure against an abnormally resistant sphincter. They originate above the dentate line and are covered by rectal (columnar) epithelium. The term *external haemorrhoid* is probably a misnomer and refers to thrombosis or rupture of one of the veins in the subcutaneous part of the external plexus.

Prostatic venous plexus. It is posterior to the arcuate pubic ligament and lower part of symphysis pubis, anterior to the bladder and prostate (**10**.179). Its chief tributary is the deep dorsal vein of the penis; it also receives anterior vesical and prostatic rami, connecting with the vesical plexus and internal pudendal vein. It drains into vesical and internal iliac veins. The plexus is embedded in the lateral fascial prostatic sheath (p. 1859).

Vesical plexus. It envelops the lower bladder and, in males, the prostatic base, communicating with the prostatic plexus in males and the vaginal plexus in females. It is drained by several vesical veins which usually unite to enter the internal iliac vein.

Dorsal veins of the penis. They are unpaired, and are superficial and deep: the *superficial dorsal vein* drains the prepuce and penile skin; running back in subcutaneous tissue it inclines right or left, and opens into one of the external pudendal veins. The *deep dorsal vein* is inside the fibrous penile sheath; it receives blood from the glans penis and corpora cavernosa penis, coursing back in the midline between the paired dorsal arteries; near the radix penis it passes deep to the suspensory ligament and through a gap between the arcuate pubic ligament and anterior margin of the perineal membrane (inferior fascia of the urogenital diaphragm), dividing into right and left branches which enter the prostatic plexus after connecting below the symphysis pubis with the internal pudendal veins. The *dorsal vein of the clitoris*, after a similar course, ends in the vesical plexus.

Uterine plexuses. They extend lateral to the uterus in the broad

ligaments, communicating with the ovarian and vaginal plexuses. They are drained by two uterine veins on each side, arising inferiorly in the plexuses, level with the external os and draining to the internal iliac veins.

Vaginal plexuses. Flanking the vagina, they connect with uterine, vesical and rectal plexuses and are drained by vaginal veins, one each side, to the internal iliac veins. The uterine and vaginal plexuses may provide collateral venous drainage to the lower limb (see above).

Common iliac veins (**10**.180). They result from the union of external and internal iliac veins, anterior to the sacro-iliac joints. They ascend obliquely to end at the right side of the fifth lumbar vertebra, uniting at an acute angle to form the inferior vena cava. The *right common iliac vein*, the shorter, is nearly vertical, ascending posterior, then lateral to its artery. The right obturator nerve passes posterior, descending forward to its foramen. The *left common iliac vein*, longer and more oblique, is first medial to its artery, then posterior. It is crossed anteriorly by the attachment of the sigmoid mesocolon and superior rectal vessels. In the rest of its course it is covered only by peritoneum. Each vein receives iliolumbar and sometimes lateral sacral veins; the left common iliac drains the median sacral vein. There are no valves in these veins.

Variations. The left common iliac vein occasionally ascends left of the aorta to the level of the kidney where, receiving the left renal vein, it crosses anterior to the aorta to join the inferior vena cava. This vessel represents the persistent caudal half of the left postcardinal or supracardinal vein (p. 324).

Median sacral veins. These veins accompany the corresponding artery anterior to the sacrum, joining into a single vein usually ending in the left common iliac but sometimes at the common iliac junction.

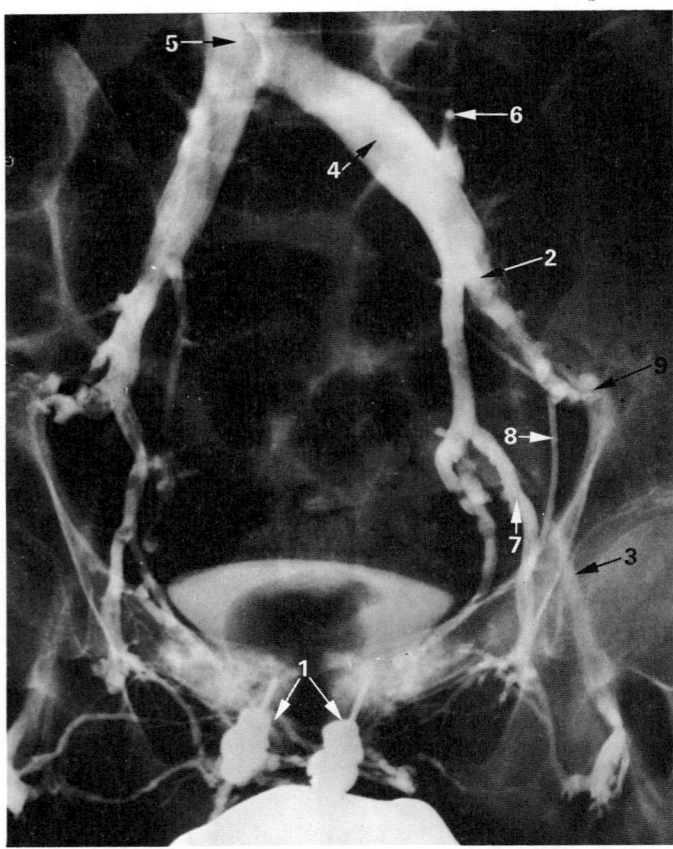

10.180 Venogram showing the veins of the pelvis and groin. The contrast medium has been injected into the bodies of the pubic bones. 1. Injected contrast medium in pubic bones. 2. Internal iliac vein. 3. External iliac vein (faintly outlined). 4. Common iliac vein. 5. Inferior vena cava. 6. Ascending lumbar vein. 7. Obturator vein. 8. Internal pudendal vein. 9. Gluteal vein. (Radiograph supplied by M Lea Thomas.)

INFERIOR VENA CAVA

The inferior vena cava conveys blood to the right atrium from all structures below the diaphragm (**10**.112, 179, 181). It is formed by the junction of the common iliac veins anterior to the fifth lumbar vertebral body, a little to its right. It ascends anterior to the vertebral column, to the right of the aorta. Reaching the liver, it is contained in a deep groove on its posterior surface or sometimes in a tunnel completed by a band of liver tissue. It perforates the tendinous part of the diaphragm between its median and right 'leaves' and inclines slightly anteromedially. Passing through the fibrous pericardium and through a posterior inflexion of the serous pericardium it opens into the inferoposterior part of the right atrium. Anterior and left of its atrial orifice is a *semilunar valve of the inferior vena cava*, relatively less prominent in adults, but large and overtly functional in the fetus (p. 1501). The vessel is otherwise devoid of valves.

Relations of the abdominal part. **Anteriorly** the inferior vena cava is overlapped at its commencement by the right common iliac artery and covered, below the horizontal part of the duodenum, by the posterior parietal peritoneum. It is crossed obliquely by the root of the mesentery and its contained vessels and nerves and by the right testicular or ovarian artery. It ascends behind the head of the pancreas and then the superior part of the duodenum, separated from it by the common bile duct and portal vein. Above the duodenum it is again covered by peritoneum of the posterior wall of the epiploic foramen (**12**.65), separating it from the right free border of the lesser omentum and its contents. Above this the liver is anterior.

Posterior are the lower three lumbar vertebral bodies, their intervening 'discs' and the anterior longitudinal ligament, the right psoas major, right sympathetic trunk, and third and fourth right lumbar

arteries; superior to these are the right crus (partially separated by the medial part of the right suprarenal gland and the right coeliac ganglion) and the right renal, suprarenal and inferior phrenic arteries.

Right lateral are the right ureter, the descending part of the duodenum, the medial border of the right kidney and right lobe of the liver. **Left lateral** are the aorta and above this the right crus and caudate lobe.

Relations of the thoracic part. This part of the inferior vena cava is very short, partly inside and partly outside the pericardial sac. The extrapericardial part is separated from the right pleura and lung by the right phrenic nerve. The intrapericardial part is covered, except posteriorly, by inflected serous pericardium.

Surface anatomy. The vein begins in, or just below, the transtubercular plane, its centre 2.5 cm right of the midline; about 2.5 cm wide, it ends behind the sternal end of the sixth right costal cartilage. A band from its lower end to a part of the inguinal ligament centred at a point 1 cm medial to the midinguinal point indicates the common and external iliac veins on each side.

Variations. Numerous anomalies occur and are attributable to arrests or errors in its complex formation. It is sometimes replaced, below the level of the renal veins, by two more or less symmetrical vessels, often associated with the failure of interconnection between the common iliac veins, and due to persistence on the left of a longitudinal channel (usually supra- or subcardinal) which normally disappears in early fetal life (p. 324). In complete visceral transposition, the inferior vena cava is left of the aorta.

Clinical anatomy. Thrombosis of the inferior vena cava leads to oedema of the legs and back, without ascites. Collateral venous circulation is soon established by enlargement of either the superficial or deep veins, or both; the epigastric, circumflex iliac, lateral thoracic, thoraco-epigastric (p. 1597), internal thoracic, posterior intercostal, external pudendal and lumbovertebral anastomotic veins connect it with the superior vena cava; deep connections are made through the azygos, hemiazygos and lumbar veins. Vertebral venous plexuses may also provide effective collateral circulation between the venae cavae (Batson 1957).

Tributaries. These are the common iliac, lumbar, right testicular or ovarian, renal, right suprarenal, inferior phrenic and hepatic veins.

Lumbar veins. Four pairs of lumbar veins collect blood by dorsal tributaries from lumbar muscles and skin, and by abdominal tributaries from the walls of the abdomen, where they connect with the epigastric veins. Near the vertebral column they drain the vertebral plexuses and are connected by the ascending lumbar vein, a longitudinal vessel anterior to the roots of the lumbar transverse processes. The third and fourth lumbar veins pass forward on the sides of the corresponding vertebral bodies to enter the posterior aspect of the inferior vena cava; the left veins pass behind the abdominal aorta and are therefore longer. First and second lumbar veins may join the inferior vena cava, ascending lumbar, or lumbar azygos veins; the first does not usually enter the inferior vena cava; it may turn down to join the second and so open into it indirectly, but more often it ends in the ascending lumbar vein or passes forward over the first lumbar vertebral body to the lumbar azygos vein (p. 1593). The second lumbar vein may join the inferior vena cava at or near the level of the renal veins; sometimes it joins the third lumbar vein or may end in the ascending lumbar. First and second lumbar veins are often connected to each other, to contralateral veins and to right and left lumbar azygos veins by a plexus on the upper lumbar vertebral bodies.

Ascending lumbar vein. It connects the common iliac, iliolumbar and lumbar veins. It lies between psoas major and roots of the lumbar transverse processes. Superiorly it joins the subcostal vein and the vessel so formed turns forward over the twelfth thoracic vertebral body and, passing deep to the crus, ascends as the azygos vein on the right and as the hemiazygos on the left. There is an angle on the vessel as it turns up; it is usually joined here by a small vessel from the back of the inferior vena cava (or left renal vein on the left). This little vein represents the azygos line (p. 325), already described as the lumbar azygos vein (p. 1593). Sometimes the ascending lumbar vein ends in the first lumbar, which then skirts the first lumbar vertebra with the first lumbar artery to join the lumbar azygos vein, the subcostal vein then joining the azygos vein on the right and the hemiazygos on the left.

Testicular veins (10.112). They emerge posteriorly from the testis,

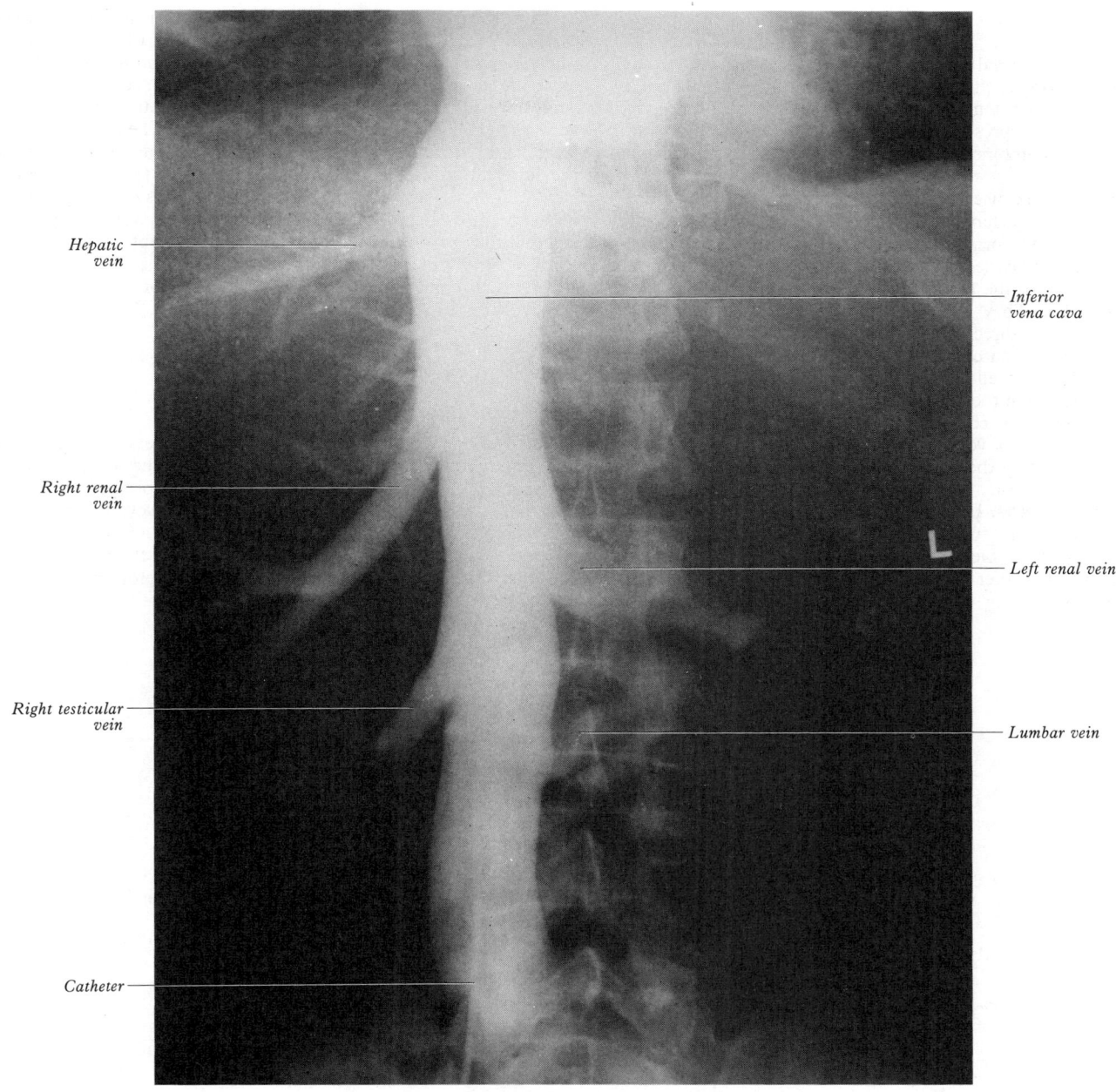

10.181 Inferior vena cavogram in an adult male while performing the Valsalva manoeuvre. (Supplied by Shaun Gallagher, Guy's Hospital; photography by Sarah Smith.)

drain the epididymis and unite to form the pampiniform plexus, a chief component of the spermatic cord, ascending anterior to the ductus deferens. Distal to the superficial inguinal ring the plexus is drained by three or four veins traversing the inguinal canal to the abdomen through the deep inguinal ring; they coalesce into two veins, which ascend anterior to psoas major and ureter, behind the peritoneum, on each side of the testicular artery. These veins join and open into the inferior vena cava on the right at an acute angle just inferior to the level of the renal veins; the left testicular vein opens into the left renal vein at a right angle. The testicular veins contain valves; the left passes behind the lower descending colon and inferior margin of the pancreas and is crossed by the left colic vessels; the right passes behind the terminal ileum and horizontal part of the duodenum and is crossed by the root of the mesentery, ileocolic and right colic vessels.

Clinical anatomy. The testicular veins are frequently varicose; varicocele, which is almost always on the left, is perhaps due to the orthogonal junction of the left testicular and renal veins. There is evidence that the presence of a varicocele raises testicular temperature

and impairs fertility, which is why an operation to correct it is often advised. After removal of a varicocele, venous return is by the small veins of the ductus deferens, cremaster and scrotal tissues.

Ovarian veins. Each of them forms a plexus in the broad ligament near the ovary and uterine tube, communicating with the uterine plexus. Two veins issue from this and ascend across the external iliac artery with the ovarian artery. Their further course is like that of the testicular veins. Valves may occur in them. Like the uterine veins, they are much enlarged in pregnancy.

Renal veins. These large veins lie anterior to the renal arteries and open into the inferior vena cava almost at right angles. The left is three times the right in length (7.5 cm and 2.5 cm); it crosses the posterior abdominal wall posterior to the splenic vein and body of pancreas and, near its end, is anterior to the aorta, just below the origin of the superior mesenteric artery. The left testicular or ovarian vein enters it from below and the left suprarenal vein, usually receiving one of the left inferior phrenic veins, enters it above but nearer the midline. The left renal vein enters the inferior vena cava a little superior to the right. The right renal vein is behind the

1601

descending duodenum and sometimes the lateral part of the head of the pancreas.

Variations. The left renal vein may be double, one vein passing posterior, one anterior to the aorta to join the inferior vena cava, a condition named persistence of the 'renal collar' (p. 325); the anterior may be absent, representing persistence of the posterior limb of the renal collar combined with absence of an intersubcardinal anastomosis.

Clinical anatomy. Because of its close relationship with the aorta, the left renal vein may have to be ligated in the course of, for example, an operation for aneurysm. This seldom results in any harm to the kidney, provided that the ligature is placed to the right of the point of entry of the testicular and suprarenal veins.

Suprarenal veins. They issue from each suprarenal hilum. The right is short, passing directly and horizontally into the posterior aspect of the inferior vena cava; the left descends medially anterior to lateral to the left coeliac ganglion, to pass posterior to the pancreatic body to reach the left renal vein. Whereas the suprarenal glands have a multiple arterial supply from the aorta, phrenic and renal arteries (see p. 1557), venous drainage is by one single drainage on each side. Damage to the suprarenal vein is thus likely to cause an infarction of the gland.

Inferior phrenic veins. Following the corresponding arteries on the inferior diaphragmatic surface, the right ends in the inferior vena cava; the left is often double, one branch ending in the left renal or suprarenal vein, the other passing anterior to the oesophageal opening to join the inferior vena cava.

Hepatic veins. They drain the liver, commencing as *intralobular veins*, draining the sinusoids of liver lobules (p. 1802); these lead to *sublobular veins*, which eventually unite into *hepatic veins*, emerging from the posterior hepatic surface to open at once into the inferior vena cava in its groove on the posterior hepatic surface. Hepatic veins are arranged in upper and lower groups. The **upper** are usually large veins, right, left and middle, the last from the caudate lobe; the **lower**, varying in number, are small and from the right and caudate lobes. The hepatic veins are contiguous with hepatic tissue and have no valves. Large 'accessory' hepatic veins of the lower group, draining a variable volume of the right lobe, have been studied in 93 adult livers by corrosion casts; they are usually single, occasionally double, with an incidence of 15% (Sledzinski & Tyszkiewicz 1975).

HEPATIC PORTAL SYSTEM

The portal system (**10**.182, 183) includes all the veins draining the abdominal part of the digestive tube (except the lower anal canal but including the abdominal part of the oesophagus) and spleen, pancreas and gallbladder. The portal vein conveys the blood from these viscera to the liver, where it ramifies like an artery, ending in the sinusoids, from which vessels again converge to reach the inferior vena cava via the hepatic veins. The blood therefore passes through two sets of 'exchange' vessels:

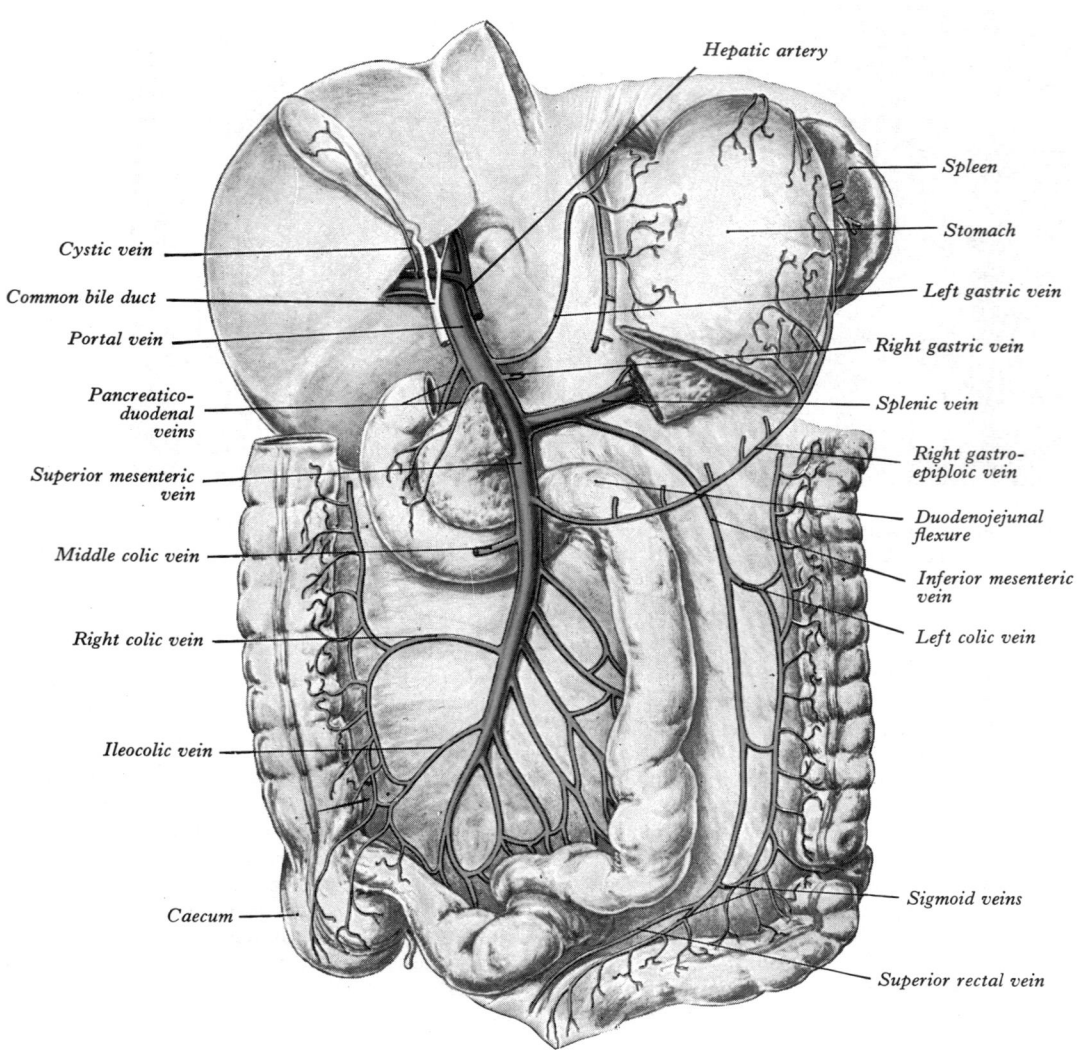

Hepatic artery

Spleen

Stomach

Left gastric vein

Cystic vein

Common bile duct

Portal vein

Right gastric vein

Splenic vein

Pancreatico-duodenal veins

Right gastro-epiploic vein

Superior mesenteric vein

Duodenojejunal flexure

Inferior mesenteric vein

Middle colic vein

Left colic vein

Right colic vein

Ileocolic vein

Sigmoid veins

Caecum

Superior rectal vein

10.182   The portal vein and its tributaries (semi-diagrammatic). Portions of the stomach, pancreas and left lobe of the liver and the transverse colon have been removed.

- capillaries of the digestive tube, spleen, pancreas and gallbladder
- hepatic sinusoids.

In adults, the portal vein and its tributaries have no valves; in fetal life and for a short postnatal period valves are demonstrable in its tributaries; usually they atrophy but some may persist in atrophic form.

Portal vein

About 8 cm long, the portal vein begins at the second lumbar vertebral level from the convergence of superior mesenteric and splenic veins, anterior to the inferior vena cava, posterior to the neck of the pancreas (**10**.182). It inclines slightly right as it ascends behind the superior part of the duodenum, bile duct and gastroduodenal artery and is here directly anterior to the inferior vena cava; however, it enters the right border of the lesser omentum, ascending anterior to the epiploic foramen to the right end of the porta hepatis, dividing into right and left stems, which accompany the corresponding branches of the hepatic artery into the liver. In the lesser omentum it is posterior to both bile duct and hepatic artery, the former being to the right; it is surrounded by the hepatic nerve plexus and accompanied by many lymph vessels and some lymph nodes. The right branch enters the right hepatic lobe but usually first receives the cystic vein. The left branch, longer but of smaller calibre, branches into caudate, quadrate and left lobes. (See a discussion of hepatic lobation and lobulation, pp. 1796, 1797.) As it enters the left lobe it is joined by para-umbilical veins (p. 1604) and the *ligamentum teres*, which contains the functionless and partly obliterated left umbilical vein. It is connected to the inferior vena cava by the *ligamentum venosum*, a vestige of an obliterated ductus venosus, ascending in a fissure on the liver's posterior aspect (p. 1501). The small extrahepatic section of the left branch, from which veins to the quadrate and left lobes arise, is a persistent part of the left umbilical vein.

Tributaries. These are: splenic, superior mesenteric, left gastric, right gastric, para-umbilical and cystic veins.

Splenic vein

Large and **not** tortuous, the splenic vein is formed by five or six tributaries from the spleen (**10**.182, 183). It traverses the lienorenal ligament with the splenic artery and tail of the pancreas, and descends to the right, across the posterior abdominal wall inferior to its artery and posterior to the body of the pancreas (which it grooves), receiving numerous short rami from the gland. It crosses anterior to the left kidney and its hilar structures (or lower pole of the left suprarenal gland), separated from the left sympathetic trunk and crus by the left renal vessels and from the abdominal aorta by the superior mesenteric artery and left renal vein. It ends behind (lodged in) the neck of the pancreas, where it joins the superior mesenteric vein at a right angle to form the portal vein.

Tributaries. These are: short gastric, left gastro-epiploic, pancreatic and inferior mesenteric veins.

Short gastric veins. Four or five of these veins drain the gastric fundus and the left part of its greater curvature, traversing the gastrosplenic ligament to reach the splenic vein or one of its large tributaries.

Left gastro-epiploic vein. This drains both gastric surfaces and the adjacent greater omentum; it runs from right to left along the greater curvature, between the anterior two omental layers, ending in or near the beginning of the splenic vein.

Pancreatic veins. They drain the body and tail of the pancreas. They may be small and many or large and few. The former empty more or less directly into the splenic vein; in the latter case, superior and inferior arcades receive these larger veins, their ultimate drainage being into the splenic (Sow et al 1975, and p. 1795).

Inferior mesenteric vein (**10**.182). It drains the rectum, and sigmoid and descending parts of the colon. It begins as the superior rectal vein, from the rectal plexus (p. 1598), through which it connects with middle and inferior rectal veins. The superior rectal vein leaves the pelvis and crosses the left common iliac vessels medial to the left ureter with the superior rectal artery, continuing up as the inferior mesenteric vein. This is left of its artery, ascending behind the peritoneum anterior to the left psoas major; it may cross the testicular or ovarian vessels or be medial to them and then passes above, or behind, the duodenojejunal flexure, opening into the splenic vein posterior to the body of the pancreas; sometimes it ends at the union of the splenic and superior mesenteric veins. If a duodenal or paraduodenal fossa exists, the vein is usually in its anterior wall

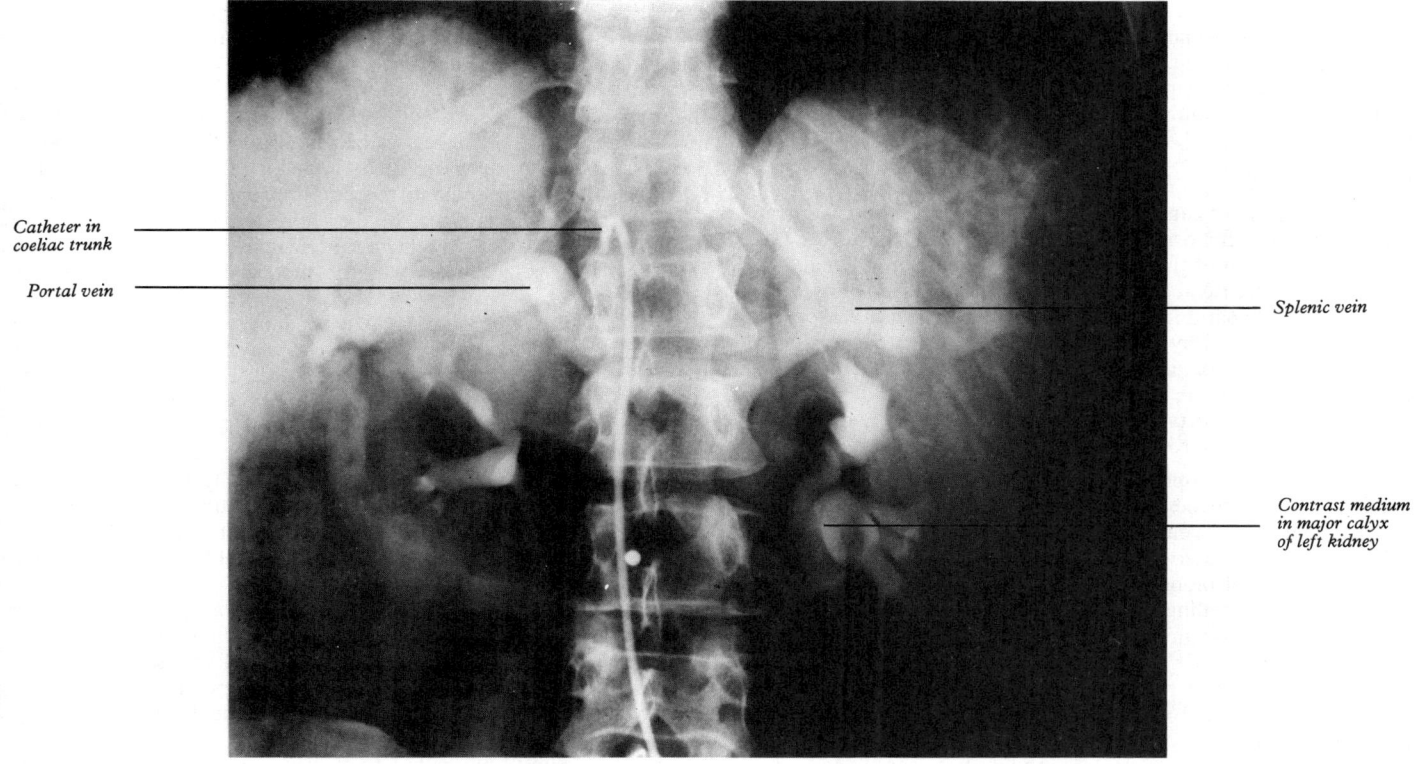

Catheter in coeliac trunk

Portal vein

Splenic vein

Contrast medium in major calyx of left kidney

10.183   Venous phase showing the splenic and portal veins after injection of contrast medium into the coeliac trunk.

(p. 1744). Its tributaries are sigmoid veins from the sigmoid colon and the left colic vein from the descending colon and the left colic flexure.

Superior mesenteric vein

The superior mesenteric vein drains the small intestine, caecum and ascending and transverse parts of the colon (10.182). Beginning in the right iliac fossa by the union of tributaries from the terminal ileum, caecum and vermiform appendix, it ascends in the mesentery on the right of the superior mesenteric artery, passing anterior to the right ureter, inferior vena cava, the horizontal part of the duodenum and uncinate process of the pancreas, joining the splenic vein behind its neck to form the portal vein (10.182, 183).

Tributaries. These are: jejunal, ileal, ileocolic, right and middle colic, right gastro-epiploic and pancreaticoduodenal veins.

Right gastro-epiploic vein. This drains the greater omentum and distal part of the stomach, passing right on the gastric greater curvature between the anterior layers of the greater omentum to join the superior mesenteric vein below the neck of the pancreas.

Pancreaticoduodenal veins. They accompany their corresponding arteries: the inferior often joins the right gastro-epiploic vein; the superior usually ascends to the left behind the bile duct to end in the portal vein. Sow et al (1975) have observed anterior intraglandular and posterior venous arcades between the superior and inferior pancreaticoduodenal veins in about 70% of 157 pancreatic corrosion preparations.

Left gastric vein. It drains both gastric surfaces, ascending the lesser curvature to the left in the lesser omentum, to the oesophageal opening, where it receives the oesophageal veins. It then curves back down and to the right behind the omental bursa to end in the portal vein at the upper border of the superior part of the duodenum.

Right gastric vein. This is small and runs to the right along the pyloric section of the lesser curvature in the lesser omentum, ending in the portal vein. It is joined by a prepyloric vein ascending anterior to the pylorus (a surgical guide to the pyloric opening).

Para-umbilical veins. Connecting veins of the anterior abdominal wall and portal vein, they extend along the ligamentum teres and median umbilical ligament (p. 1838). Best developed is one beginning at the umbilicus and running in or on (the hepatic) ligamentum teres in the falciform fold to end in the left branch of the portal vein.

Cystic veins. These veins which drain the gallbladder vary. Those from its superior surface are in areolar tissue between the gallbladder and liver, usually entering the liver through the vesical fossa to join the hepatic veins. The remainder form one or two cystic veins which commonly also enter the liver either directly or after joining the veins draining the hepatic ducts and upper bile duct. Only rarely does a single or double cystic vein drain into the right portal branch.

Clinical anatomy

Portal obstruction may cause ascites, whether obstruction is intra- or extrahepatic. In cirrhosis, radicles of the portal vein are compressed by contraction of the fibrous tissue in their portal canals. In valvular cardiac disease, back-pressure on the hepatic veins, and thus on the whole hepatic circulation, has similar effects. The portal vein may be compressed by hepatic tumours, enlarged lymph nodes in the lesser omentum or carcinoma of the pancreatic head. Portal thrombosis may complicate various conditions. In portal obstruction anastomoses between portal and systemic circulations, which may offer effective collateral circulation, are as follows:

- On the abdominal oesophagus tributaries of the left gastric vein (portal) connect with oesophageal tributaries of the azygos and accessory hemiazygos veins (systemic). Enlargement of these may result in varicosity (oesophageal varices) and even fatal haematemesis (vomiting of blood).
- In the rectal wall opening up of connections between the inferior and middle rectal (systemic) and superior rectal (portal) veins may result in varicosity.
- At the umbilicus, veins running on the ligamentum teres to the left portal branch (p. 1603) connect with the epigastric veins (systemic); enlargement of these connections may produce varicosities of veins radiating from the umbilicus, the caput Medusae.
- Retroperitoneal veins communicate directly with venous radicles of the colon and bare area of the liver.

- Very rarely a patent ductus venosus connects the left branch of the portal vein to the inferior vena cava.

Portal obstruction and variceal haemorrhage were formerly treated by surgical anastomosis between the portal and systemic beds (portocaval or splenorenal anastomosis), but these shunts give rise to severe side-effects due to by-passing the hepatic circulation. They are nowadays best treated by introducing portosystemic connections into the liver substance, by means of an intravascular probe.

CENTRAL VENOUS ACCESS

In clinical practice access is frequently required to the superior vena cava and the right side of the heart. This may be for monitoring of central venous, intracardiac and pulmonary artery pressures, for long-term feeding, the safe administration of powerful drugs or for passing a cardiac pacing catheter or biopsy forceps. The first successful placement of a central venous catheter was via a peripheral vein but now it is common practice to use one of the larger and more central veins in the upper part of the body, the internal jugular and the subclavian being the most popular. The main advantage of cannulating one of the large central veins lies in the fact that they are almost constant in their position and are available when peripheral veins are thrombosed or collapsed. The following are some of the common venous sites of access.

Cephalic vein. At the wrist this is situated over the dorsolateral aspect of the lower end of the radius (10.168) just proximal to the anatomical snuffbox. This is one of the few constantly sited peripheral veins. However, it is sometimes difficult to negotiate a long catheter past the elbow, and in particular through the clavipectoral fascia where the cephalic vein turns almost through a right angle to join the axillary vein.

Median cubital and basilic veins. These may be identified in the cubital fossa (10.168, 169). They are, however, frequently covered by fat, especially in the female, which makes them difficult to see but they are usually palpable especially if the venous return is occluded proximally by a tourniquet. A catheter passed from this site will not always enter the intrathoracic veins though, and may turn upwards into the neck.

Subclavian vein. This is the second most commonly used vein for central venous cannulation, the internal jugular being the most common. There are two percutaneous approaches to the subclavian vein, the supraclavicular and the infraclavicular, though the infraclavicular is more popular.

Infraclavicular approach (10.92). With the patient lying supine and slightly head down to distend the vein, the catheterizing needle is inserted at a point 1 cm below the midpoint of the clavicle. Some prefer a point slightly more medial to this. The needle is initially introduced at a right angle to the skin, but once through is directed towards the posterior aspect of the suprasternal notch which may be made more obvious by placing a finger in it. The needle should enter the vein as it arches over the first rib anterior to scalenus anterior.

Supraclavicular approach (10.92). The most popular skin puncture site is immediately posterior to the clavicle at the lateral edge of the clavicular head of sternocleidomastoid. The needle is initially advanced caudally but then directed medially such that its proximal end (the portion outside the skin) bisects the angle between the clavicle and sternocleidomastoid. The advancing needle is also angled 10° anteriorly towards the retromanubrial area at the level of the sternal angle. Complications arising from attempted subclavian vein cannulation include damage to the brachial plexus, subclavian artery, thoracic duct and, not infrequently, pneumothorax. Fatalities have occurred.

Internal jugular vein (10.154). Percutaneous puncture of the internal jugular vein has become the most popular route for central venous access and it has the advantage of being very safe even when performed by relatively inexperienced operators. It is of particular value when seeking venous access in the patient with circulatory collapse.

There are many approaches to this vein and they may be categorized as high or low, medial, central or lateral. The high approach is at or above the level of the thyroid cartilage, while the low is about

1 cm above the clavicle. The terms medial, central and lateral refer to the puncture site relative to sternocleidomastoid. The high approach is popular because it is very unlikely to cause a pneumothorax.

Most commonly a high, right-sided, medial approach is used in which case the patient should be placed supine and tilted slightly head down to distend the neck veins. The head is turned to the left and the puncture site made just lateral to the upper border of the thyroid cartilage. Some operators like to place one finger on the carotid artery and another on the medial border of sterno-cleidomastoid and to introduce their needle between those two fingers. The needle is then advanced at 45° to the skin aiming at a point three to four fingers' breadth from the right lateral edge of the sternum until venous blood can be aspirated freely.

Femoral vein (10.176). While femoral venous puncture is relatively easy and supplies ready access to the right atrium, the use of this approach is relatively unpopular for long-term cannulation because of a higher incidence of thrombosis and sepsis. It is, however, a useful site for venous sampling in a patient with collapsed veins. For femoral venous cannulation the skin puncture site is approximately 1 cm medial to the femoral artery and just below the inguinal ligament. After skin puncture the needle is advanced with the syringe at an angle of 30° to the skin aiming cephalad.

LYMPHATIC SYSTEM

INTRODUCTION

Dispersed widely in the body are the tissues, fluids and cells concerned in a variety of interrelated functions, including the drainage of tissue fluid formed in the interstitial spaces, the removal by phagocytes of cell debris and foreign matter (p. 1414) and the immune responses of the lymphocytes (p. 1405) and other cells. In part these activities overlap and have a common cellular base with those of the blood vascular system. It is important to distinguish between *lymphatic vessels* or 'lymphatics' which are tubes of endothelial cells, lined externally by some connective tissue, and *lymphoid tissue*, consisting of large aggregates of lymphocytes and associated cells. These cells are in many instances intimately connected with the lymphatic channels, and process or add to their fluid and cellular contents, for example, in lymph nodes and lymphoid nodules. In other cases, lymphoid tissue may be quite separate from lymphatics, for example the spleen, which is concerned with modifying the blood, and the bone marrow and thymus, which produce lymphocytes and other cells to populate the lymphoid tissue elsewhere, with immunologically active cells of different classes. As stated elsewhere, most tissue fluid formed at the arterial ends of capillaries returns to the circulation via their venous ends, but 10–20% of such fluid passes instead into blind-ending lymphatic capillaries, then traverses one or more lymph nodes before returning to the venous system and thus the blood circulation. Before considering the detailed **topography** of lymphatic vessels and lymph nodes, we will consider the **general structure** of lymphatic vessels, lymph nodes, lymphatic nodules, the spleen and the thymus.

LYMPHATIC VESSELS

Lymphatic capillaries form plexuses in tissue spaces which have wider meshes than those of the adjacent blood capillaries. They often begin as dilated tubes with closed ends; the calibres are larger and cross-sectional appearances are less regular than those of blood capillaries, and they lack a basal lamina, though they have numerous vesicles within their cytoplasm, a typical endothelial feature. (See Leak 1984 for a review of lymphatic structure and physiology.) Their endothelium is generally quite permeable to much larger molecules (Allen 1967) and, unlike most blood capillaries, they are readily permeable to colloidal material and larger particles such as cell debris and micro-organisms from tissue spaces, and to cells. When lymph vessels are obstructed, the surrounding tissues become oedematous, i.e. distended with fluid containing much protein. Experiments suggest that the observed absorption of macromolecules and particles is via gaps between endothelial cells or by micropinocytosis through them. Lymph from most tissues is clear and colourless. In contrast, the lymph from the small intestine is dense and milky, due to the presence of lipid globules (*chylomicrons*) derived from fat absorbed by the mucosal epithelium; the terminal vessels in the mucosa of the small intestine are thus known as *lacteals* and the lymph as *chyle*. Lymphatic capillaries, though present in many tissues, are absent from avascular structures (epidermis, hair, nails, cornea, cartilages), and from central nervous tissue and bone

marrow; there are very few in the endomysium of skeletal muscles.

Lymphatic capillaries join into larger vessels which pass to local or sometimes more remote lymph nodes. These are arranged largely in *regional groups*, sufficiently regular in position to be named. Each has its region of drainage but a local group is often bypassed. Nodes within a group are often interconnected (Kubik 1974). In general, lymph traverses a series of nodes before reaching a major collecting duct. There are exceptions to this: lymph vessels of the thyroid gland and oesophagus and of the coronary and triangular ligaments of the liver drain directly to the thoracic duct without passing through lymph nodes (Rusznyák et al 1960). The superficial lymphatics of skin adjoin the deep fascia and accompany superficial veins, but some run independently; they have few connections with deep lymphatics. Deep lymphatic trunks usually accompany arteries or veins, almost all reaching either the thoracic duct or the right lymphatic duct (p. 1609), which join the left and right brachiocephalic veins respectively at the root of the neck. Some observers have also reported additional entry points into the venous system through the inferior vena cava and the renal, suprarenal, azygos and iliac veins. As the lymphatic vessels are closely associated with veins in their development (p. 327), such additional connections would not be surprising, although they are likely to be variable. Most lymphatic vessels anastomose freely and across the midline; larger ones have their own plexiform vasa vasorum and nerve fibres. If their walls are acutely infected (lymphangitis) this plexus is congested, marking the paths of superficial vessels by red lines, visible through the skin and tender to the touch.

Lymphatic vessels repair easily and new vessels readily form after damage; these are at first solid cellular sprouts from the endothelial cells of persisting vessels, which later canalize.

Microscopic structure of lymphatic vessels

The wall of lymphatic capillaries consists of a single layer of endothelium, as in haemal capillaries. A continuous basal lamina is often lacking, and specialized intercellular junctions are few. Fenestrae have been demonstrated in subserosal lymphatics, though they are absent in well-fixed subcutaneous lymphatic vessels, except after trauma. Filopodia are frequent on the luminal surfaces and in lacteals similar projections may exist on their external surface. Bundles of extracellular filaments, lymphatic anchoring filaments, 5–10 nm in diameter, extend from the abluminal surface of the endothelial cells to the surrounding stroma. Pericytes are absent (Fraley & Weiss 1961). There is extensive structural variation between lymphatic capillaries in different tissues (Allen 1967; Leak & Burke 1968). As they unite into larger vessels, a thin external connective tissue coat supports the endothelium. Larger collecting trunks (>200 μm) have three layers, similar to those of small veins, although the lumen is considerably larger, relative to wall thickness, than in veins. The tunica intima consists of an endothelium with a thin subendothelial layer of fibrous tissue. The tunica media contains some smooth muscle cells, mostly arranged circumferentially; the tunica adventitia is mainly fibrous connective tissue, with collagen and elastic fibres and occasional nerve fibres (Boggon & Palfrey 1973). Elastic fibres are sparse in the tunica intima, but sufficient to form an external elastic lamina in the tunica adventitia. Lymphatics differ from small veins in having many more valves, which are semilunar, generally paired and each composed of an extension of the intima. Their edges point in the direction of the current and the vessel wall downstream is expanded into a sinus, giving the vessels a beaded appearance when distended. Valves are important in preventing the backflow of lymph.

The thoracic duct is structurally similar to a medium-sized vein, but the smooth muscle in the tunica media is more prominent and pulsatile movements have been described (see below and p. 1609).

Satiukova and Rassokhina-Volkova (1972) have studied regeneration of lymphatic capillaries in dogs after autotransplantations of hindlegs and lungs; they observed early formation of buds from severed lymphatics in junctional scar tissue, concluding that lymph flow was largely restored.

Movement of lymph

Several factors aid the propulsion of lymph from tissue spaces to lymph nodes and the venous bloodstream:

- 'Filtration pressure' in tissue spaces is generated by filtration of fluid under pressure from blood capillaries.
- Contraction of neighbouring muscles compresses lymph vessels, moving lymph in the directions determined by their valves; extremely little lymph flows in an immobilized limb, whereas flow is increased by either active or passive movements. This fact has been used clinically to diminish dissemination of toxins from infected tissues by immobilization of the relevant regions. Conversely, massage aids the flow of lymph from oedematous regions.
- The pulsation of neighbouring arteries probably compresses adjacent lymphatic vessels, assisting flow in them.
- Respiratory movements and the negative blood pressure in the brachiocephalic veins also promote flow of lymph.
- Smooth musculature in the wall of the lymphatic trunks contracts when sympathetic nerves are stimulated, resulting in reduction of the lumen. Pulsatile contractions in the thoracic duct also occur (Kinmonth 1982) and, because of the numerous valves along this structure, lymph is forced unidirectionally by this muscular action. However, in markedly dilated vessels valves may become incompetent, allowing retrograde flow, perhaps explaining the observed retrograde spread of some malignant tumours.

Methods of study

Infective material and neoplastic cells often spread from an affected site along lymphatics, and so the details of their pathways from different regions and organs are clinically important. Dissection is not a suitable method for the tracing of these routes because lymphatic vessels are slender and difficult to see. More reliable information has been obtained as follows:

- Experimental injection of substances into organs or tissues of living or dead animals, including man. These enter the lymphatics draining the site of injection and render them and their related lymph nodes visible. The materials most commonly used for this purpose are suspensions of India ink, Neoprene latex or Prussian blue, the latter employed by Jamieson and Dobson (1907–1908, 1910, 1920) in extensive studies of human pathways. In living animals methylene blue and radio-opaque substances, such as lipiodol, have been injected, the latter requiring radiography. Lymphangiography in human subjects, following the injection of lipiodol into the appropriate peripheral lymphatic channels has much increased our knowledge of their routes and is much used diagnostically (Kinmonth 1964; Kinmonth & Taylor 1964).
- Clinical observation of lymph nodes involved in the spread of known inflammatory or malignant disease. However, it must be cautioned that retrograde spread of tumour cells after blockage of a channel limits the reliability of such observations by altering the normal directions of flow.

SPLEEN

(Although part of the cardiovascular system, the spleen is essentially concerned with immune functions and a filtering of blood. Its structure is dealt with on pages 1437–1442 in the Haemolymphoid system, Section 9.)

TOPOGRAPHY OF LYMPH NODES AND VESSELS

The detailed architecture of lymph nodes and lymphatic vessels is discussed on pages 1431–1432. The structure of lymph nodes is described on pages 1605–1626, that of the spleen on page 1439, and that of the thymus on pages 1424–1429. Lymph nodes occupy fairly well-defined topographical sites, specifically named, each with its area of drainage, interconnections with other nodes or groups and a predominant destination of its efferent vessels. A more detailed consideration of these matters is the concern of the remainder of this chapter; this must be prefaced by a summary, or sometimes a reiteration, of a few general principles. Lymphatic anatomy often appears an almost impossible plethora of topographical names for trunks, groups and subgroups of nodes and their connections. However, an elemental knowledge of general anatomy and a recognition of which of the general principles apply to the major organ systems make many of the difficulties evaporate. It is particularly useful to appreciate the overall pattern present in a particular organ, whole organ system or whole body segment. (Good examples are: the whole subdiaphragmatic alimentary tract, the foregut, the stomach, the tracheobronchopulmonary system, the similarities and contrasting features of the arm and leg and the head and neck as a whole.) These encompass all the main patterns and principles, include all the main terminal lymph trunks whereby lymph is returned to the venous system. The principal groups of lymph nodes towards which lymph converges from wide tissue areas (often through one or more subgroups) and knowledge of which, for many, is mandatory, are clarified. Thereafter, many (but not all) the lesser subgroups, in relation to their formal topographical names, assume a diminished importance in terms of mental retention; nevertheless, their distribution can usually be predicted with confidence. The criteria for the topographical naming of nodes will be mentioned below. Certain general names applied to nodes, although not universally used, often prove useful. Lymph circulating in lymphatic capillaries may be returned to the venous system (ignoring intralymphoidal venular events on a microscopic scale, p. 1432) almost entirely at bilateral sites at or near the junctions between internal jugular and subclavian veins forming right and left brachiocephalic veins; however, their routes vary enormously in length and complexity. In certain exceptional sites (thyroid, oesophagus, dorsal hepatic 'bare areas', p. 1800) the capillaries drain via a radicle of the thoracic duct with no intervening lymph node (an anodal route). In some, a single node provides uninodal routes; the majority of routes are multinodal with sometimes many nodes forming irregular cross-connected chains. In such a chain, the node or group nearest the tissue drained is termed *primary* (outlying, or peripheral), and the last group of the chain, whose efferents form a final uninterrupted principal lymph trunk, is termed *terminal*. Between its primary peripheral and its terminal groups intervening nodes are often segregated into *intermediary* groups; some use the collective term *regional lymph nodes* to include all three groups; others, peripheral and intermediary only. The significance of multinodal pathways is by no means clear; it should be noted that classifications may impose an artificial simplicity on a potentially highly complex monitoring and reacting system. Thus, briefly, a particular node is not one element in a simple chain but, receiving multiple afferent vessels, may, for example, be the primary node for various loci, number three in the chain for other loci, number five for others and so forth. Such considerations, of course, apply to other members of the chain and, summating for the whole chain, there emerges the notion of a system of lymphatic channels and lymphoid stations of great three-dimensional complexity. Differential lymphangiography amply confirms this complexity. This prompts the question: are lymph nodes in general roughly equivalent in their ranges of receptivity (monitoring) and reactivity or do they vary? If variation exists, to what degree? An extreme (and fanciful) extension of this is the possibility of individual nodes, or even sectors of nodes, being unique in their properties, as they unquestionably are in their locations and connections.

TOPOGRAPHICAL NAMING OF LYMPH NODES

Topographical naming of lymph nodes has not followed a single rigid classification; four main frames of reference have been found convenient, and sufficiently clear. These are:

- superficial or deep position
- related vasculature
- related organ's name and architecture
- general topographical location.

Superficial and deep position

Superficial and deep refer to the location of the nodes with respect to the deep fascia. As noted below, many superficial nodes are closely applied to prominent superficial veins. An interesting but unexplained fact is that the upper limb has few superficial nodes and its superficial lymphatic drainage mostly passes directly to deep axillary nodes; in contrast, in the leg the superficial lymphatic drainage passes, almost exclusively, to the large superficial inguinal nodes before continuing to the external iliac nodes.

Relation to vasculature

The majority of nodes and node groups are clustered around or abut a prominent blood vessel or one of its branches; from this (with many notable exceptions) the name of the group is derived. The association assists in recalling the location of the group and in many instances is a strong pointer to the main region of lymph drainage. Examples of superficial nodes associated with veins are: buccal nodes (facial vein), superficial cervical nodes (external jugular vein), anterior cervical nodes (anterior jugular vein), infraclavicular nodes (cephalic vein), supratrochlear nodes (basilic vein), superficial inguinal nodes (great saphenous vein). Deep nodes associated with vessels are so numerous that only a few illustrative examples can be given. The abdominal aorta and common, internal and external iliac arteries are surrounded by nodes. The whole consists of massive chains of nodes, interconnected by lymphatic vessels, predominantly vertically but also obliquely and transversely. Thus, the main groups are named with their vessels: external, internal and common iliac and circumaortic. The latter (often grouped with neighbouring nodes particularly scattered over the inferior vena cava as lumbar nodes) are divided, on sound developmental and lymphodynamic grounds, into a large median ventral aortic group, prominent right and left lateral aortic groups and a sparse retro-aortic group. Details are given in subsequent pages, but a few examples with comments and one possible synthetic approach to study are outlined here. The ventral aortic group aggregates around the three large subdiaphragmatic ventral splanchnic arteries (p. 1548) as coeliac, superior mesenteric and inferior mesenteric groups of nodes, which drain the subdiaphragmatic foregut, midgut and hindgut (and their derivatives), respectively. The foregut provides an excellent framework with respect to its extent and parts (terminal oesophagus, stomach, proximal duodenum); its derivatives (liver, gallbladder and biliary ducts, pancreas and the closely associated spleen); and the mutual disposition of the foregoing and their peritoneal reflexions, omenta and the lesser sac. To this is added the position of the upper abdominal aorta, the coeliac artery, its trifurcation into common hepatic, left gastric and splenic arteries and the courses and main branches of these. Groups of nodes named in relation to these are, for example, left gastric, right gastro-epiploic, hepatic and pancreaticosplenic; other related groups have visceral names, for example paracardial and pyloric (stomach), cystic (gallbladder), 'anterior border of epiploic foramen' (bile duct). The general (interconnected) areas of drainage of these groups are evident and their efferents discharge into the coeliac nodes. The latter also receive the efferents of the superior and inferior mesenteric groups, each of which has received the efferents from systematically named groups, aggregated along their branches, or scattered in the mesentery. The coeliac nodes are thus the terminal group for the whole subdiaphragmatic gut down to midrectal level and for most of the liver, the gallbladder and biliary ducts, pancreas and spleen. Their efferents join to form wide right and left intestinal lymph trunks; these coalesce and also join the right and left lumbar lymph trunks (see below) to form the morphologically variable *abdominal confluence of lymph trunks*, the cranial end of which is the entry to the thoracic duct. Briefly (details p. 1621), the lateral aortic groups drain the tissues supplied by the lateral splanchnic and dorsolateral somatic intersegmental aortic branches; caudally they receive the profuse efferents from the common iliac groups which in turn receive the efferents from the internal and external iliac groups, each with their extensive areas of drainage and further associated outlying groups of nodes. The cranial members of the lateral aortic groups are the terminal nodes for all these tissues; their efferents converge to form the bilateral lumbar lymph trunks which are the other main avenues forming the abdominal confluence of lymph trunks and thence the initial (caudal) end of the thoracic duct. Mention may be made of the nodes associated with drainage of the leg, often misrepresented. Some drainage first involves a limited outlying group of popliteal nodes (near their vessels), then traverses the superficial or deep inguinal nodes which are *intermediary* (**not** terminal) groups at the limb's root; thereafter the lymph node ascends the chains just described, i.e. via the external and common iliac, the lateral aortic to its upper terminal nodes, then the lumbar lymph trunk, confluence and thoracic duct. (Some deep gluteal lymph follows the internal iliac path to the same destination.) Prominent nodes in the thorax named in relation to vessels are the brachiocephalic group.

Relation to viscera

The names of the visceral lymph nodes are self-evident. Examples already mentioned are the paracardial and pyloric, gastric groups; others are the *superficial* and *deep parotid*, *submandibular* and *paracolic*. The best examples are concerned with, primarily, the drainage of the lower respiratory tract. Passing from the periphery these are named: *pulmonary* (at major bronchial divisions within the lung), *bronchopulmonary* (or simply 'hilar'), *inferior* and *superior tracheobronchial* (p. 1625) and paratracheal. Their ascending efferents are joined by some from the ipsilateral parasternal, brachiocephalic and posterior mediastinal nodes, forming the right and left bronchomediastinal lymph trunks; these incline over the trachea, then to the ventral aspect of their jugulosubclavian venous junctions. At or in either great vein, near the junction, the trunks usually open independently, but in about one-fifth of individuals the right trunk may join a right lymphatic duct; the left may join the thoracic duct or both may occur.

Names related to general topography

The groups of nodes most easily accessible to clinical palpation have widely used general positional names, which vary considerably in their precision. The relation of many (but not all) their subgroups to prominent blood vessels and their branches is close and this provides a more accurate reference system; in some notable sites this is seldom adopted.

Leg. Outlying *popliteal nodes*—here the name is used indiscriminately with respect to the vessels or the fossa; their palpation is by finger tips probing the fossa along the line of the popliteal vessels with the passively supported limb gradually moved from extension to semiflexion. *Inguinal nodes*: superficial and deep—here inguinal simply implies that they are 'related to the groin'. The deep nodes are few and applied to the medial aspect of the femoral vein; the superficial nodes comprise a lower vertical group clothing the upper great saphenous vein; an upper group parallel to but below the inguinal ligament (related to the superficial circumflex iliac and superficial external pudendal vessels). Palpation is done with the supported limb slightly flexed, abducted and laterally rotated, along a strip 1 cm below the inguinal ligament and a strip 1 cm medial to the central apicobasal line of the femoral triangle.

Arm. Outlying *supratrochlear nodes* (more aptly supra-epicondylar) are adjacent to the basilic vein. Palpation is done along the line of the vein a few centimetres above the elbow joint; many approaches are satisfactory: facing the subject, an elegant approach is to cup the back of the supracubital arm with the appropriate palm; the semi-flexed fingers encircle the medial aspect and their aligned tips effortlessly probe along the vein. The *axillary nodes* have subgroups with alternative names; one system applies to their topographical positioning with respect to the 'walls' of the axilla, the second system to their disposition close to the axillary vessels and their branches (especially the veins). These are detailed on page 1613 and will not be pursued here. Palpation demands a systematic approach, exploring each wall of the axilla and any attendant vessels and nodes as separate manoeuvres. The supported arm is slightly abducted, the examiner facing the lateral aspect of the shoulder; each fold of the axilla is examined with the appropriate hand, semiflexed fingertips invaginating the axillary floor while the thumb grips the fold externally. The fingertips of one or both hands next probe deeply, then down and laterally along the axillary vessels. Finally, the fingers of the pronated hand, inserted deeply, are drawn down the medial wall, i.e. the resistant thoracic wall and serratus anterior. It should be noted that most of the axillary groups are intermediary, with their wide areas of drainage, and the central group is preterminal; only the *apical group* is *terminal*. The latter's efferents form the *subclavian lymph trunk* which approaches and, with variable final morphology, opens at or near its jugulosubclavian junction. The trunk and its opening are on the anterior aspect of the venous walls.

Head and neck. Apart from a few retrovisceral nodes and some deep to the sternocleidomastoid, members of all the nodal groups in the head and neck are clinically palpable when enlarged and all receive regional topographical names. Many of the latter are appropriate and helpful; in the neck, however, the major groups have only the most generalized names, despite their principal relationship to large vessels. (Alternative names based on this merit consideration.) The various groups are detailed elsewhere (p. 1612); thus a simplified overall plan for the head and neck will be mentioned and some group names added to a suggested approach to their clinical examination. The relationship of craniocervical nodes to the deep fascia is discussed subsequently but in some important cases is implied in their names. At the junction of the head with the neck an encircling band extends bilaterally from the chin to the external occipital protuberance, the pericraniocervical ring (often shortened to 'pericervical ring'). Throughout, this encompasses topographically named regional groups with outlying nodes in the face; sequentially the groups are: submental, submandibular (with outlying buccal nodes), retromandibular (outlying parotid), retro-auricular (or mastoid) and occipital. As noted, verbal descriptions of their sites and areas of drainage are given (p. 1612) but in general are obvious from their names. Palpation is carried out from behind the seated subject, using both hands simultaneously, their fingers semiflexed and adducted and thumbs in partial opposition; the fingers explore systematically: the submental triangle, the submandibular glands and triangles (thumbs probing over buccinators), the retromandibular depressions (thumbs over parotids), the upper attachment of sternocleidomastoid and the occipital attachment of trapezius. Palpation now continues along the approximately vertical chains of cervical nodes, superficial and deep. The superficial chains of relatively few, small nodes are associated with the external jugular and anterior jugular veins, the superficial cervical and anterior cervical groups respectively; both drain finally into deep nodes. (These, and unqualified 'deep cervical' are indifferent, non-specific, unhelpful names; the relative precision of vascular or visceral names is preferable.) The main chain of deep cervical nodes is ranged along and embedded in, or in areolar tissue near, the carotid sheath but particularly those aspects surrounding the internal jugular vein. Customarily divided into upper and lower groups, they receive, in addition to their direct areas of drainage, all the efferents from the pericraniocervical ring, efferents from the superficial cervical nodes and efferents from other paravisceral deep nodes (e.g. *retropharyngeal*, *infrahyoid*, *prelaryngeal*, *pretracheal*, *paratracheal* and *subclavian*). All the lymph from the head and neck finally traverses its ipsilateral *lower deep cervical group*, which is the terminal group. Efferents from the latter converge, forming (right and left) jugular lymph trunks; each descends on its vein to its termination at the jugulosubclavian venous junction.

Lymph node numbers: regional distribution

Accurate, large statistical surveys are not available; the following are pooled data from many limited sources; nevertheless, the overall approximations allow interesting speculation. A normal young adult body contains some 400–450 lymph nodes. Of these the limbs and associated superficial body wall are least well served. The arm and superficial thoraco-abdominal wall (down to the umbilicus) contain about 30 nodes, the leg and superficial buttock, infra-umbilical abdominal wall and perineum only about 20 nodes. (This does not include the iliac and lateral aortic groups which have numerous additional intra-abdominal afferents.) The head and neck carry some 60–70 nodes. The remainder (about 330) is divided between the

thorax (deep walls and contents, some 100 nodes or less), and the abdomen and pelvis (deep walls and contents, some 230 nodes or more). Most richly served by nodes is the gastrointestinal tract; also profusely served is the tracheobronchopulmonary tract.

CERVICAL LYMPHOVENOUS PORTALS

Lymph is returned to the venous blood circulation via the right and left lymphovenous portals which are sited at, or near, the junctions of the large internal jugular and subclavian veins forming the even larger right and left brachiocephalic veins. On the right, **three** main lymph trunks converge towards their venous junction; on the left **four** main trunks (three corresponding to the right-sided trunks, but additionally the largest trunk, the thoracic duct). The morphology of the venous termination of these trunks is subject to much variation and the account frequently given in textbooks is a fairly uncommon occurrence, hence the introduction of the generalized term lymphovenous portal.

On the right. The three trunks converging here are:

(1) The *right jugular trunk* which extends along the ventrolateral aspect of the internal jugular vein from the terminal lower deep cervical nodes and conveys all the lymph from the right half of the head and neck.

(2) The *right subclavian trunk* from the terminal apical axillary group extending along the axillary and subclavian veins and conveying lymph from the right upper limb and superficial tissues of the right half of the thoraco-abdominal wall down to the umbilicus anteriorly and iliac crest posteriorly (and including much of the mammary gland).

(3) The *right bronchomediastinal trunk* (p. 1625), which ascends over the trachea towards the portal and conveys lymph from the thoracic walls, the right cupola of the diaphragm and subjacent liver, the right lung, bronchi and trachea, the greater part of the 'right heart' (of clinical parlance, not the geometric right half, see p. 1625) and a proportionately small drainage from the thoracic oesophagus.

The *right venous termination* of the three lymphatic trunks is subject to great variation. In the great majority of subjects (80%) they open independently, their orifices clustered on the ventral aspect of the jugulosubclavian junction or in the nearby wall of either of the great veins. In a proportion of these one or more of the trunks may bifurcate (or even trifurcate) preterminally and then have multiple orifices. In one-fifth of subjects only, the three trunks fuse to form a short (1 cm) single right lymphatic duct that inclines across the medial border of scalenus anterior to the ventral aspect of the venous junction, where its orifice is preceded by a bicuspid semilunar valve. An incomplete right lymphatic duct may be present following fusion of, usually, the subclavian and jugular trunks, or any combination of their terminals when divided. In such cases the bronchomediastinal trunk almost invariably opens separately.

Summary. The **right** lymphovenous portal, whatever the final morphology of its trunks, receives lymph from: the right half of the head and neck, the thorax and its contents and superficial tissues of the abdomen and trunk down to the umbilicus and iliac crest, part of the right cupola of the diaphragm and convex surface (only) of the underlying liver and the whole of the right arm. The **left** portal receives much the greater volume of lymph from all the remainder of the body.

On the left. The four trunks converging here on the lymphovenous portal are:

(1) The left jugular trunk, mirroring its right fellow;
(2) the left subclavian trunk, also with a disposition corresponding to its contralateral fellow;
(3) the left bronchomediastinal trunk, similar to the right trunk, but draining more of the heart (the 'left' and part of the 'right hearts' of clinical parlance, p. 1474) and more of the oesophagus;
(4) the thoracic duct, which drains all the extensive remaining regions of the body. At its caudal origin as a continuation of the abdominal confluence of lymphatic trunks (see below), throughout its course and at its cervical venous termination, it is subject to considerable variation.

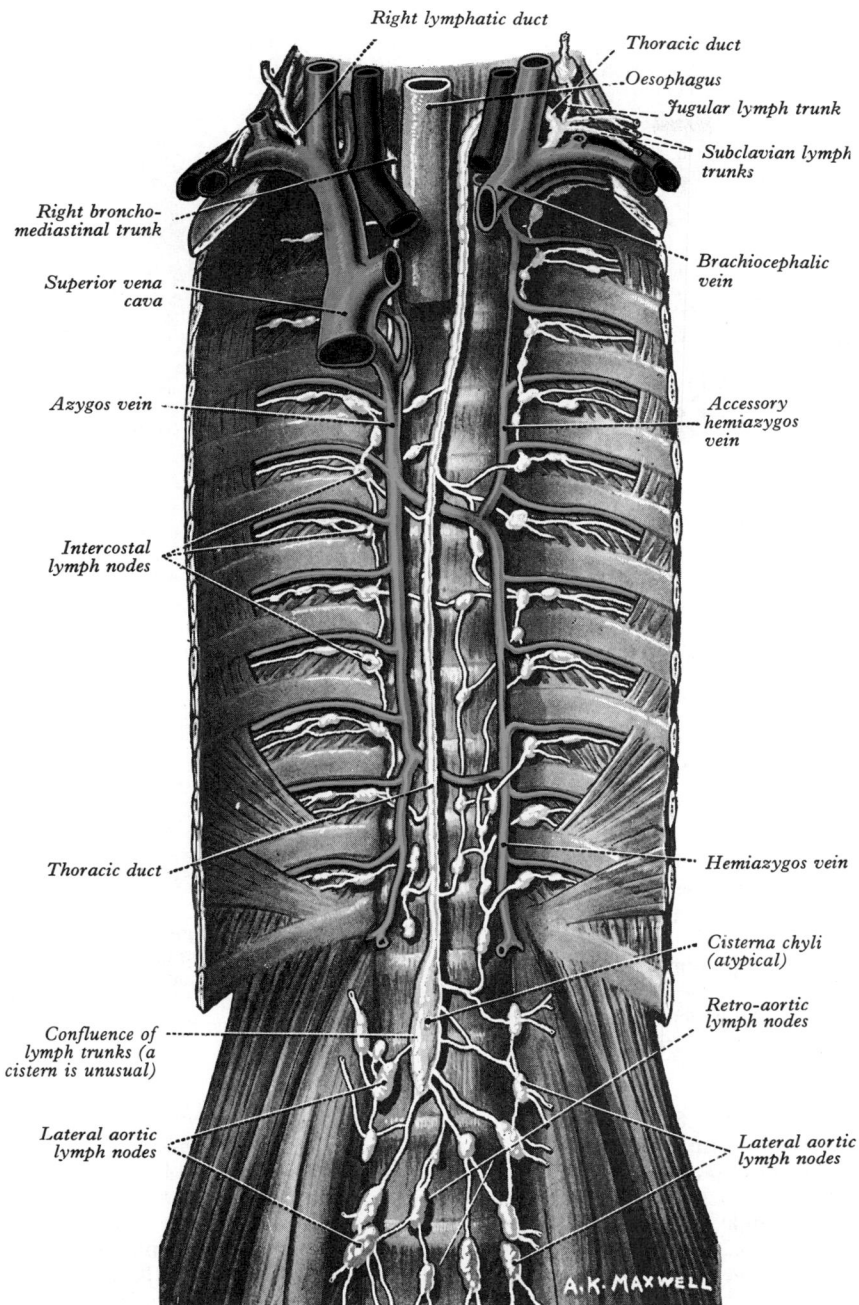

Right lymphatic duct

Thoracic duct

Oesophagus

Jugular lymph trunk

Subclavian lymph trunks

Right broncho-mediastinal trunk

Brachiocephalic vein

Superior vena cava

Azygos vein

Accessory hemiazygos vein

Intercostal lymph nodes

Thoracic duct

Hemiazygos vein

Cisterna chyli (atypical)

Retro-aortic lymph nodes

Confluence of lymph trunks (a cistern is unusual)

Lateral aortic lymph nodes

Lateral aortic lymph nodes

A.K. MAXWELL

10.184   The thoracic and right lymphatic ducts. The accessory hemiazygos vein is crossing the median plane lower and the hemiazygos higher than usual. Note also the comments concerning the more common course of the azygos vein made in illustration **10**.171 and on page 1593. Two features are also uncommon: a single right lymphatic duct (usually two or more trunks open independently); a simple cisterna chyli is infrequent (it is usually a confluence of lymph trunks of varying morphology, page 1610).

THORACIC DUCT (**10**.184–186)

In adults the thoracic duct including the confluence of lymph trunks (or the cisterna chyli in the small proportion in whom the latter is saccular) is 38–45 cm in length, extending from the second lumbar vertebra to the base of the neck. Starting from the superior pole of the confluence near the lower border of the twelfth thoracic vertebra, it traverses the diaphragm's aortic aperture, then ascends the posterior mediastinum, right of the midline, between the descending thoracic aorta (on its left) and the azygos vein (on its right). **Posterior** to it is the vertebral column (vertebral bodies, symphyses, anterior longitudinal ligament), the right aortic intercostal arteries and terminal segments of the hemiazygos and accessory hemiazygos veins. **Anterior** to it are the diaphragm and oesophagus; a recess of the right pleural cavity may separate the duct and oesophagus. Reaching the level of the fifth thoracic vertebral body it gradually inclines to the left, enters the superior mediastinum and then ascends to the thoracic inlet along the left border of the oesophagus. In this part of its course the duct is first crossed anteriorly by the aortic arch and it then runs posterior to the left subclavian artery's initial segment, in close contact with the left mediastinal pleura. Passing into the neck it arches laterally at the level of the seventh cervical vertebral transverse process. Its arch rises 3 or 4 cm above the clavicle and curves anterior to the vertebral artery and vein, the left sympathetic trunk, thyrocervical artery or its branches and the left phrenic nerve and medial border of scalenus anterior (but is separated from the nerve and muscle by the prevertebral fascia). The arch passes posterior to: the left common carotid artery, vagus nerve and internal jugular vein. Finally, the duct descends anterior to the arched cervical 'first part' of the left subclavian artery and ends by opening into the junction of the left subclavian and internal jugular veins. However, the duct may open into either of the great veins,

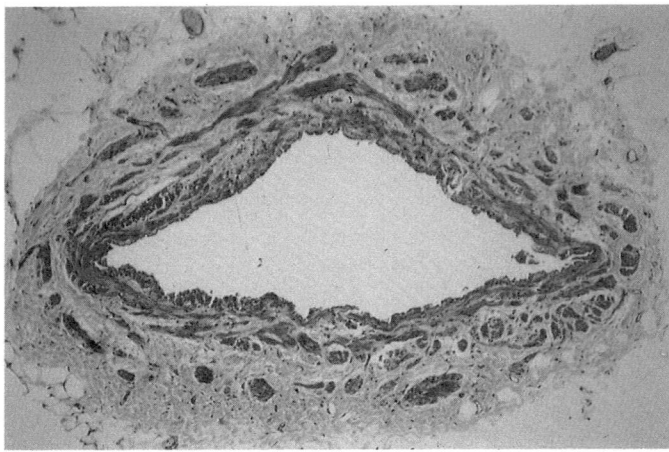

10.185 Transverse section of the thoracic duct showing the fibro-muscular coat (see text). Stained with haematoxylin and eosin. Magnification × 80. (Preparation by Millie Harrison, Department of Anatomy, UMDS, Guy's Campus, London.)

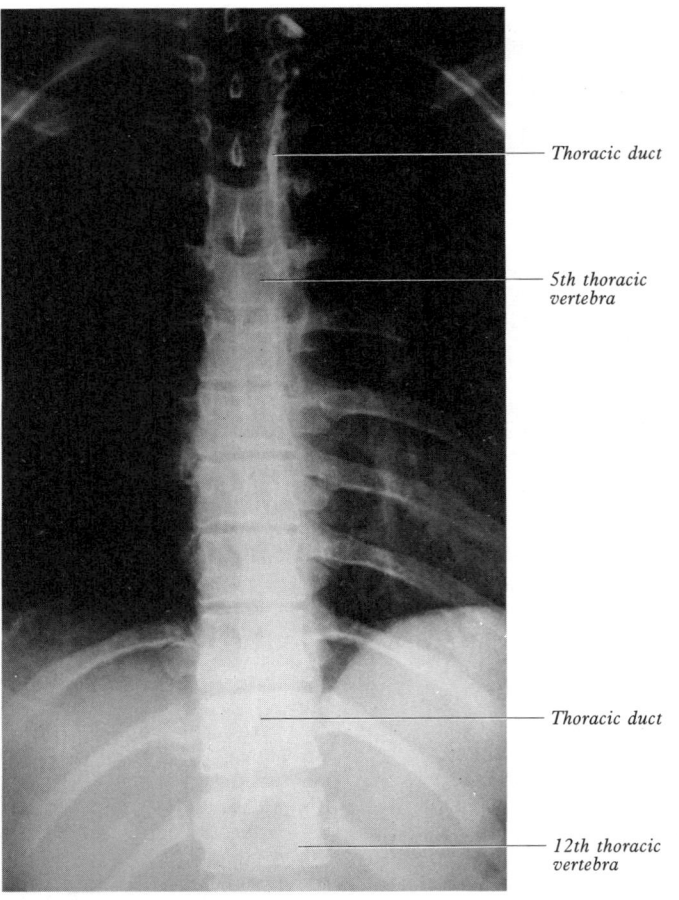

Thoracic duct

5th thoracic vertebra

Thoracic duct

12th thoracic vertebra

10.186 Lymphangiogram showing the entire length of the thoracic duct, approximately 24 hours after injection of lipiodol into a lymphatic vessel on the dorsum of each foot; the cisterna chyli is not evident. (Supplied by G I Verney, Addenbrooke's Hospital, Cambridge; photography by Sarah Smith, Department of Anatomy, UMDS, Guy's Campus, London.)

near the junction, or it may divide into a number of smaller vessels before terminating (see below).

At its abdominal origin the thoracic duct is about 5 mm in diameter but diminishes in calibre at mid-thoracic levels, then in about 50% of subjects is again slightly dilated before its termination. It is slightly sinuous, constricted at intervals and appears varicose. It may divide in its midcourse into two unequal vessels which soon reunite, or into several small branches which form a plexus before continuing as a single duct. At a higher level it occasionally bifurcates, the left branch ending as usual, the right branch diverging to join one of the right lymph trunks or, when present, a right lymphatic duct; the combined vessel usually opens into the right subclavian vein. The thoracic duct has several valves corresponding to sites exposed to pressure. At its termination a bicuspid valve faces into the vein to prevent or reduce reflux of blood. (After death blood regurgitates freely into the duct, which then looks like a vein.)

Termination

Kinnaert (1973) has collected accounts of 529 dissections (49 his own) of the thoracic duct's termination. In 0–4.5% of subjects no thoracic duct appeared on the left. Multiple terminal openings were frequent (10–40%, according to different observers). In Kinnaert's series the preterminal duct was multiple in 66%, but in only 21% were actual terminal openings multiple. Patterns varied greatly in different studies but, in the two largest by Jdanov (1959) and Kinnaert (1973), sites of termination were respectively 48% and 36% internal jugular vein, 9% and 17% subclavian vein, 35% and 34% jugulosubclavian junction. Termination in the left brachiocephalic (innominate) vein occurred in 8% of Jdanov's series, but never in Kinnaert's.

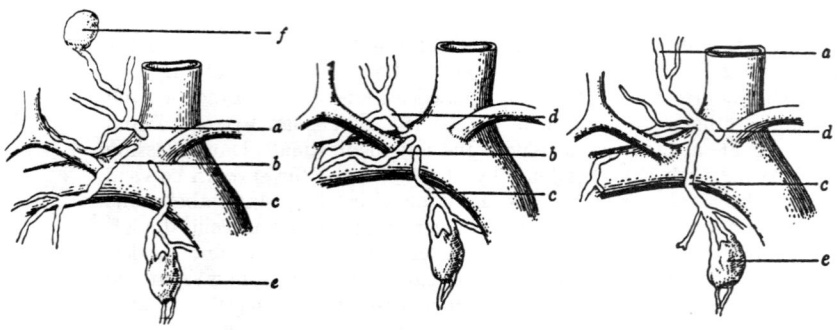

10.187 Variations in the terminal lymph trunks of the right side. a = jugular trunk; b = subclavian trunk; c = bronchomediastinal trunk; d = right lymphatic duct; e = lymph node of parasternal chain; f = lymph node of deep cervical chain. (After Poirier & Charpy.)

Origin and tributaries

The abdominal origin of the thoracic duct proper is, as stated, situated to the right of the midline at the level of the lower border of the twelfth thoracic vertebral body or the thoracolumbar intervertebral disc. It is the recipient of all the lymph delivered by the four main abdominal lymph trunks, which converge to an elongated arrangement of channels of variable morphology here given the generalized name, *abdominal confluence of lymph trunks.* This may be a simple duct-like extension or be duplicated, triplicated or plexiform; when it is wider than the thoracic duct its interior is sometimes irregular and bilocular or trilocular and may surround intercalated lymph nodes. Only in a small proportion of instances is it a simple, fusiform, saccular dilatation, and the widely-used name *cisterna chyli* should be reserved for these. A published thorough statistical study of the origin of the thoracic duct in mankind appears lacking. Anson (1963) depicted variations: in many a cisterna was absent; when present it was usually multilocular or plexiform; no statistics of incidence were given. Kubik (personal communication 1978) observed a 'cisterna' in 14 of 70 dissections. In only six was it single; it was double in five specimens and trilocular in three. In 56 dissections no cisterna was observed; in half of these collecting trunks formed a direct extension of the thoracic duct; in the other half intercalated nodes (also depicted by Anson 1963) simulated the profiles of cisternae.

The abdominal confluence extends from the caudal beginning of the thoracic duct, vertically, for 5–7 cm anterolateral to the right of the first and second lumbar vertebral bodies (and their intervening disc), and immediately to the right of the abdominal aorta. (Thus its site is overlapped by territories containing upper right lateral aortic lymph nodes and right-sided members of the coeliac and superior mesenteric pre-aortic groups.) The upper two right lumbar arteries and the right lumbar azygos vein (p. 1593) are between the confluence and the vertebral column. Anterior to it is the medial edge of the right diaphragmatic crus. As mentioned, the confluence (and thence the thoracic duct) receives the right and left lumbar and intestinal lymph trunks. In summary:

(1) The *lumbar trunks* are formed by efferents from lateral aortic lymph nodes. Thus, either directly or after traversing intermediary groups, they carry lymph from: the lower limbs, the full thickness of the pelvic, perineal and infra-umbilical abdominal walls, the deep tissues of most of the supra-umbilical abdominal walls, the pelvic viscera, testes or ovaries, kidneys and suprarenals.

(2) The *intestinal lymph trunks* receive efferents from the coeliac nodes (terminal ventral aortic group) which, after traversing intermediary groups, drain the stomach, intestines (to midrectal levels), pancreas, spleen and the (greater) antero-inferior part of the liver.

Tributaries of the thoracic duct proper (10.187). In summary these are:

- the *confluence of lymph trunks*, just described, the whole outflow of which enters the origin of the thoracic duct
- the bilateral *descending thoracic lymph trunks* from intercostal lymph nodes of the lower six or seven intercostal spaces of both sides which traverse the aortic orifice and join the lateral aspects of the thoracic duct in the abdomen immediately after its origin
- the bilateral *ascending lumbar lymph trunks* from the upper lateral aortic nodes which ascend and pierce their corresponding diaphragmatic crus, then join the the thoracic duct at a variable level within the thorax
- the *upper intercostal trunks* draining the intercostal nodes in the upper five or six left intercostal spaces
- the *mediastinal trunks* draining various nodal groups noted below and providing (amongst other tissues) paths to the thoracic duct

from the convex diaphragmatic aspect of the liver, the diaphragm, the pericardium, heart and oesophagus
- the *left subclavian trunk* which usually joins the thoracic duct, but may open independently into the left subclavian vein
- the *left jugular trunk* which usually joins the thoracic duct, but may open independently into the left internal jugular vein
- the *left bronchomediastinal trunk* which occasionally joins the thoracic duct, usually having an independent venous opening.

Many of the trunks listed above are described as possessing terminal bicuspid valves which possibly prevent reflux of lymph. However, Sapin and Borziak (1974) studied the behaviour of radio-opaque masses in thoracic ducts of 180 cadavers; they found that reflux into several groups of mediastinal and paravertebral groups was usual (under these conditions!).

LYMPHATIC DRAINAGE OF HEAD AND NECK

Nodes in the head and neck comprise a terminal (collecting) group and intermediary, outlying groups. The terminal group is related to the carotid sheath and is named deep cervical. All lymph vessels of the head and neck drain into this, directly from tissues or indirectly through nodes in outlying groups. Efferents of the deep cervical nodes form the *jugular trunk*, which on the right may end in the jugulosubclavian junction or right lymphatic duct; on the left it usually enters the thoracic duct but may join the internal jugular or subclavian vein. In lymphatic drainage the tissues of the head and neck, like other regions, can conveniently be considered as superficial and deep. (See also the generalized arrangement of a pericraniocervical ring and vertical cervical chains, p. 1608.)

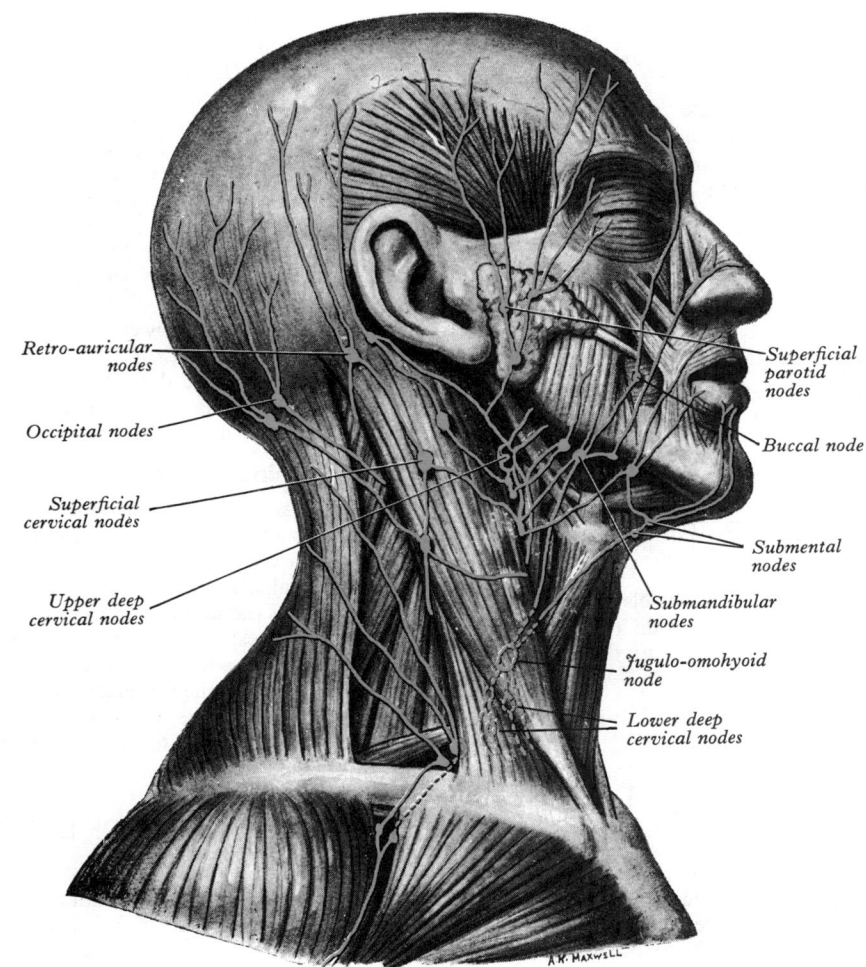

Retro-auricular nodes

Occipital nodes

Superficial cervical nodes

Upper deep cervical nodes

Superficial parotid nodes

Buccal node

Submental nodes

Submandibular nodes

Jugulo-omohyoid node

Lower deep cervical nodes

10.188 The superficial lymph nodes and lymph vessels of the head and neck.

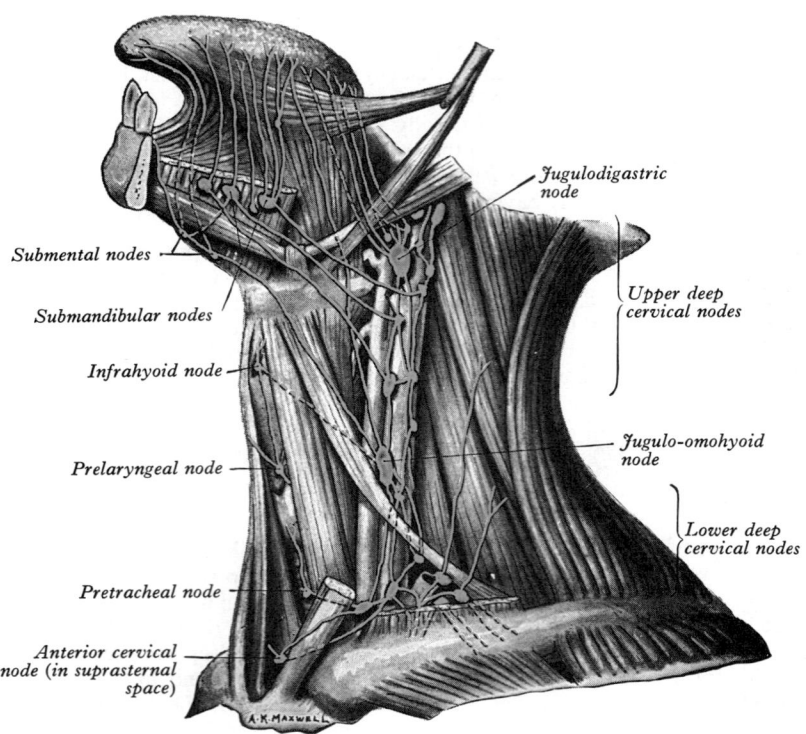

Jugulodigastric node

Submental nodes

Submandibular nodes

Infrahyoid node

Upper deep cervical nodes

Prelaryngeal node

Jugulo-omohyoid node

Lower deep cervical nodes

Pretracheal node

Anterior cervical node (in suprasternal space)

A. K. MAXWELL

10.189 The lymphatic drainage of the tongue. Removal of the sterno-cleidomastoid has exposed the whole chain of deep cervical lymph nodes. (After Jamieson & Dobson.)

DEEP CERVICAL LYMPHATIC NODES

The deep cervical lymphatic nodes are alongside the carotid sheath; they form superior and inferior groups.

Superior deep cervical nodes (**10**.188)**.** These adjoin the upper internal jugular vein. Most are deep to the sternocleidomastoid; a few extend beyond it. One subgroup, of one large and several small nodes, is in a triangular region bounded by the posterior belly of the digastric and the facial and internal jugular veins; this jugulodigastric group is concerned specially with lingual drainage. Efferents from the upper deep cervical nodes drain to the lower group or direct to the jugular trunk.

Inferior deep cervical nodes. They are partly deep to the sterno-cleidomastoid, particularly related to the lower internal jugular vein but some, extending also into the subclavian triangle, are closely related to the brachial plexus and subclavian vessels. One node is on or just above the intermediate tendon of omohyoid, the *jugulo-omohyoid node*, and is concerned especially with the tongue (p. 1613). Efferents from this lower group join the jugular lymph trunk.

LYMPHATIC DRAINAGE OF SUPERFICIAL TISSUES OF HEAD AND NECK

Most superficial tissues in the region drain by vessels afferent to local groups of nodes, and efferents from these drain to the deep cervical nodes; but some structures drain directly to deep nodes (**10**.188). Groups concerned in superficial drainage are:

• in the *head*: occipital, retro-auricular (mastoid), parotid, buccal (facial)
• in the *neck*: submandibular, submental, anterior cervical, super-ficial cervical.

Lymphatic drainage of scalp and ear

Vessels from the frontal region above the root of the nose drain to the submandibular nodes (**10**.188) and are considered with the face. Vessels from the rest of the forehead, temporal region, upper half of the lateral auricular aspect and anterior wall of the external acoustic meatus drain to the superficial parotid nodes, just anterior to the tragus, on or deep to the parotid fascia. These also drain lateral

vessels from the eyelids and skin of the zygomatic region. Their efferent vessels pass to the upper deep cervical nodes. A strip of scalp above the auricle, the upper half of the auricle's cranial aspect and margin and the posterior wall of the external acoustic meatus all drain to the upper deep cervical and retro-auricular nodes.

The *retro-auricular nodes* (**10**.188), superficial to the mastoid attachment of sternocleidomastoid and deep to auricularis posterior, drain to the upper deep cervical nodes. The auricular lobule, floor of the meatus and skin over the mandibular angle and lower parotid region are drained to the superficial cervical or upper deep cervical nodes. *Superficial cervical nodes* spread along the external jugular vein superficial to sternocleidomastoid, some efferents passing round the anterior border of sternocleidomastoid to the upper deep cervical nodes; others follow the external jugular vein to the lower deep cervical nodes in the subclavian triangle.

The occipital scalp is drained partly to the occipital nodes, partly by a vessel along the posterior border of sternocleidomastoid to the lower deep cervical nodes. Occipital nodes are occasionally in the superior angle of the posterior triangle but commonly superficial to the upper attachment of trapezius.

Lymphatic drainage of face

Lymph vessels draining the eyelids and conjunctiva commence in a subcutaneous plexus and a deep plexus around the tarsal plates; these communicate and medial and lateral vessels drain from them. Lateral vessels drain the whole thickness of both lids, except their medial parts and all the conjunctiva. They pass from the lateral commissure to the superficial parotid nodes and deep nodes embed-ded in the parotid gland, also receiving lymph from the middle ear (see below). The medial palpebral vessels drain the whole thickness of the medial parts of the lids and caruncula lacrimalis. Following the facial vein, they end in submandibular nodes.

There are usually three *submandibular nodes* (**10**.188, 189), internal to the deep cervical fascia in the submandibular triangle. There is one at the anterior pole of the submandibular gland, and two flanking the facial artery as it reaches the mandible. Other nodes are often embedded in the gland or deep to it. Submandibular nodes drain a wide area, including vessels from the submental, buccal and lingual groups of nodes; their efferents pass to the upper and lower deep cervical nodes. The external nose, cheeks, upper lip and lateral parts of the lower lip drain directly to the submandibular nodes; the afferent vessels may have a few *buccal nodes* along their course and near the facial vein. The mucous membrane of lips and cheeks also drains to the submandibular nodes. The lateral part of the cheek drains to the parotid nodes. The skin over the nasal radix and central forehead drains partly to the parotid nodes, partly to the submandibular.

The central part of the lower lip, buccal floor and lingual apex drain to the *submental nodes*, which are on the mylohyoid between the anterior bellies of the digastric muscles (**10**.189). They receive afferents from **both** sides, some decussating across the chin; their efferents pass to the submandibular and jugulo-omohyoid nodes.

Lymphatic drainage of neck

Many vessels draining the superficial cervical tissues skirt the borders of sternocleidomastoid to the superior or inferior deep cervical nodes; but some pass over sternocleidomastoid and the posterior triangle to the superficial cervical and occipital nodes. Lymph from the superior region of the anterior triangle drains to the submandibular and submental nodes; vessels from the anterior cervical skin inferior to the hyoid bone pass to the anterior cervical lymph nodes near the anterior jugular veins; their efferents go to the deep cervical nodes of both sides, including the infrahyoid, prelaryngeal and pretracheal groups (see below). An anterior cervical node often occupies the suprasternal space (p. 804).

LYMPHATIC DRAINAGE OF DEEP TISSUES OF HEAD AND NECK

Tissues of the head and neck internal to the deep fascia drain to the deep cervical nodes directly or through outlying groups which include, in addition to those named above: the retropharyngeal, paratracheal, lingual, infrahyoid, prelaryngeal and pretracheal groups.

Retropharyngeal nodes. These comprise a median and two lateral groups, the latter anterior to the lateral atlantal masses along the lateral borders of the longi capitis. All lie between the pharyngeal and prevertebral fasciae, receiving afferents from the nasopharynx, pharyngotympanic tube and atlanto-occipital and atlanto-axial joints. They drain to the upper deep cervical nodes.

Paratracheal nodes. They flank both trachea and oesophagus along the recurrent laryngeal nerves. Efferents pass to the corresponding deep cervical nodes.

Infrahyoid, prelaryngeal and pretracheal nodes. Found beneath the deep cervical fascia, they drain afferents from the anterior cervical nodes, their efferents joining the deep cervical nodes. The infrahyoid nodes are anterior to the thyrohyoid membrane, prelaryngeal on the conus elasticus and cricovocal membrane, pretracheal anterior to the trachea near the inferior thyroid veins.

Lingual nodes. Small and inconstant, they are situated on the external surface of hyoglossus and also between the genioglossi. They drain to the upper deep cervical nodes.

Lymphatic drainage of nasal cavity, nasopharynx and middle ear

Lymphatics of the nasal cavity can be injected from the subarachnoid space, via communications along the olfactory nerves. Lymph vessels from its anterior region pass superficially to join those of the external nasal skin, ending in the submandibular nodes. The rest of the cavity, paranasal sinuses, nasopharynx and pharyngeal end of the auditory tube drain to the upper deep cervical nodes, directly or through the retropharyngeal nodes. The posterior nasal floor probably drains to the parotid nodes.

Lymphatic vessels of the tympanic and antral mucosae drain to the parotid or upper deep cervical lymph nodes; vessels of the tympanic end of the auditory tube probably end in the deep cervical nodes; its vessels have been identified in the submucosa by injection and electron microscopy (Pulec et al 1975).

Lymphatic drainage of larynx, trachea and thyroid gland

Laryngeal lymphatic vessels form superior and inferior groups; on the lateral wall they are distinct, their division being at the level of the vocal fold; the two sets anastomose on the posterior wall. Superior vessels pierce the thyrohyoid membrane to accompany the superior laryngeal vessels, ending in the superior deep cervical nodes; inferior vessels pass between the cricoid cartilage and the first tracheal ring to the inferior deep cervical lymph nodes, or pierce the cricovocal membrane to reach the pretracheal and prelaryngeal nodes.

A dense network of lymph vessels exists in the tracheal wall; its cervical part drains to the pretracheal and paratracheal nodes, or directly to the inferior deep cervical nodes.

Thyroid lymphatic vessels communicate with the tracheal plexus, passing to the prelaryngeal nodes just above the thyroid isthmus and to the pretracheal and paratracheal nodes; some may drain into the brachiocephalic nodes, related to the thymus in the superior mediastinum. Laterally, the gland is drained by vessels along the superior thyroid veins to the deep cervical nodes. Some thyroid lymphatics may drain directly, with no intervening node, to the thoracic duct (p. 1609).

Lymphatic drainage of mouth, teeth, tonsil and tongue

Mouth. Gingival vessels drain to the submandibular nodes; those of the hard palate continue anteriorly into the superior gingival channels but also run back to pierce the superior constrictor, ending in the superior deep cervical and retropharyngeal nodes; from the soft palate they pass posterolaterally partly to the retropharyngeal, partly to the superior deep cervical nodes. The anterior part of the floor of the mouth drains to the lower nodes of the upper deep cervical group, either directly or via the submental nodes; vessels from the remainder of the floor drain to the submandibular and superior deep cervical nodes.

Teeth. Dental lymphatics pass to the submandibular and deep cervical nodes.

Tonsil. Vessels from the tonsil pierce the buccopharyngeal fascia and superior constrictor to pass between the stylohyoid muscle and the internal jugular vein to the superior deep cervical nodes. Most end in the jugulodigastric nodes; occasionally one or two vessels run

to the small nodes on the lateral aspect of the internal jugular vein, deep or medial to sternocleidomastoid.

Tongue (10.189). A lymphatic plexus in the lingual mucosa is continuous with an intramuscular plexus. The anterior lingual region drains into the marginal and central vessels and behind the vallate papillae into the dorsal lymph vessels.

Vessels. These are divided into marginal, central and dorsal.

Marginal vessels. They come from the lingual apex and frenular region and descend under the mucosa to widely distributed nodes:

- Some pierce the mylohyoid in contact with the mandibular periosteum to enter the submental nodes and also pass anterior to the hyoid bone to the jugulo-omohyoid node. Vessels arising in the plexus on one side may cross under the frenulum to end in the contralateral nodes; efferent vessels of submental nodes, which are median, pass to both sides.
- Some vessels pierce the mylohyoid to enter the anterior or middle submandibular node.
- Some pass inferior to the sublingual gland and, accompanying the companion vein of the hypoglossal nerve, end in jugulodigastric nodes; one often descends further, superficial or deep to the intermediate tendon of the digastric, to reach the jugulo-omohyoid node.
- Some vessels from the lateral lingual margin cross the sublingual gland, pierce the mylohyoid and end in the submandibular nodes; others end in the jugulodigastric or jugulo-omohyoid nodes. Vessels from the posterior part of the lingual margin traverse the pharyngeal wall to the jugulodigastric lymph nodes.

Central vessels. The regions of the lingual surface draining into the marginal or central vessels are not distinct. Central vessels descend between the genioglossi, some turning laterally through the muscles; but most pass between them and diverge to the right or left, following the lingual veins to the deep cervical nodes, especially the jugulodigastric and jugulo-omohyoid. Some pierce the mylohyoid to enter the submandibular nodes.

Dorsal vessels. Vessels draining the region of the vallate papillae and behind them run postero-inferiorly, some near the median plane to both sides. They turn laterally to join the marginal vessels; all pierce the pharyngeal wall, passing around the external carotid arteries to reach the jugulodigastric and jugulo-omohyoid lymph nodes. One may descend posterior to the hyoid bone, perforating the thyrohyoid membrane to end in the jugulo-omohyoid node.

Lymphatic drainage of pharynx and cervical part of the oesophagus

Collecting vessels from the pharynx and cervical oesophagus pass to the deep cervical nodes, either directly or through the retropharyngeal or paratracheal nodes. From the epiglottic region lymph vessels run to the infrahyoid nodes.

LYMPHATIC DRAINAGE OF UPPER LIMBS

All lymphatic vessels from the upper limb (and superficial tissues of a wide area of the side of the trunk) drain to the axillary nodes, either directly or (a few) through a more peripheral group. Vessels internal to the deep fascia follow the principal vascular bundles; superficial vessels, except in the hand and dorsum of the forearm, converge towards the superficial veins, which they accompany.

Axillary nodes

Axillary nodes drain the whole upper limb and areas of the trunk indicated, are large, vary from 20 to 30 in number, and may be divided into five not wholly distinct groups (10.191, 193). Four of these groups are intermediary; only the apical group is terminal.

(1) A *lateral group* (10.190, 191, 193) of four to six nodes is posteromedial to the axillary vein, its afferents draining the whole limb except the vessels accompanying the cephalic vein. Efferent vessels pass partly to the central and apical axillary groups, partly to the inferior deep cervical nodes.

(2) An *anterior* or *pectoral group* of four or five nodes spreads along the inferior border of pectoralis minor near the lateral thoracic

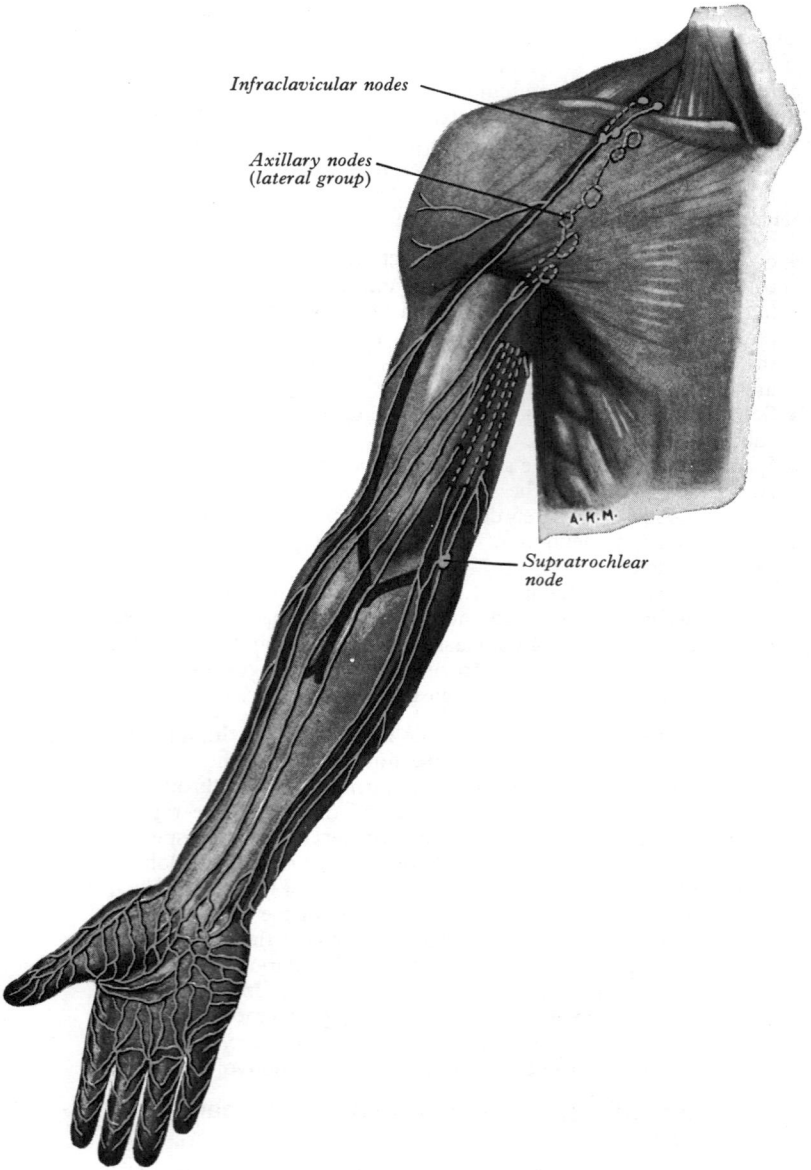

Infraclavicular nodes

Axillary nodes (lateral group)

Supratrochlear node

A.K.M.

10.190   The lymphatic drainage of the superficial tissues of the upper limb: anterior aspect (semi-diagrammatic).

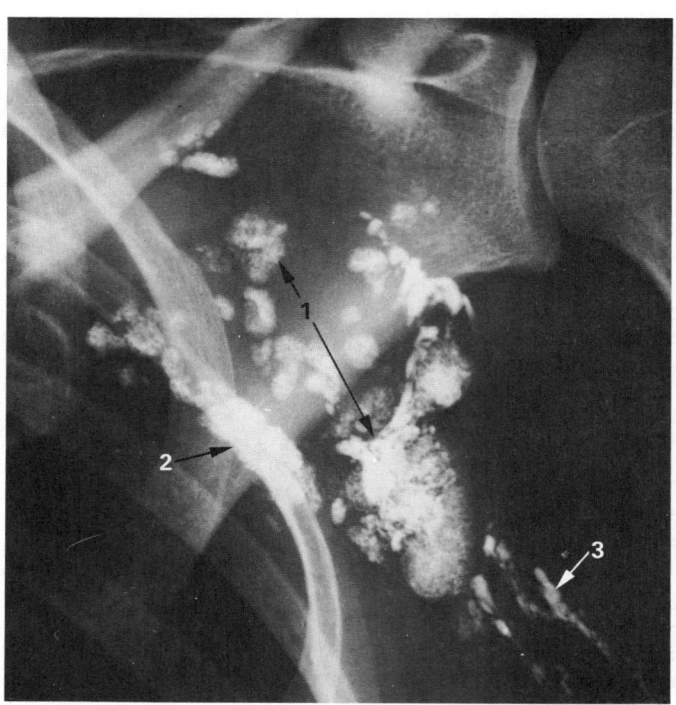

10.191   Normal axillary lymphangiogram, four days after injection of ultrafluid lipiodol into a lymph vessel on the dorsum of the hand. 1 = lateral group of lymph nodes; 2 = pectoral group of lymph nodes; 3 = brachial lymph vessels. (Supplied by J B Kinmonth.)

vessels. Its afferents drain the skin and muscles of the supra-umbilical anterolateral body wall and mammary gland (centrolateral part, p. 1615); efferents pass partly to the central and partly to the apical axillary nodes.

(3) A *posterior* or *subscapular group* of six or seven nodes is deployed on the posterior axillary wall's inferior margin, along the subscapular vessels. Afferents drain the skin and superficial muscles of the inferior posterior region of the neck and the dorsal aspect of the trunk down to the iliac crest; efferents pass to the apical and central axillary nodes.

(4) A *central group* of three or four large nodes embedded in axillary fat receives afferents from all preceding groups: its efferents drain to the apical nodes.

(5) An *apical group* of six to twelve nodes is partly posterior to the superior part of pectoralis minor and partly above its superior border, extending to the axilla's apex medial to the axillary vein. The only direct territorial afferents are those with the cephalic vein and some draining the mammary gland (upper peripheral region); but the group drains all other axillary nodes. Its efferents unite as the subclavian trunk, draining directly to the jugulosubclavian venous junction, the subclavian vein, or to the jugular lymphatic trunk or on occasion to a right lymphatic duct; the left trunk usually ends in

the thoracic duct. A few efferents from apical nodes usually reach the inferior deep cervical nodes.

Extra-axillary outlying groups in the upper limb are few, comprising: supratrochlear, infraclavicular (both interposed in superficial routes) and isolated nodes occasionally appearing along principal blood vessels.

(1) *Supratrochlear nodes*, only one or two, are superficial to the deep fascia proximal to the medial epicondyle and medial to the basilic vein; their efferents accompany the vein to join the deep lymph vessels.

(2) *Infraclavicular nodes* appear beside the cephalic vein, one or two in the groove between the pectoralis major and deltoid, just inferior to the clavicle; efferents pass through the clavipectoral fascia to apical axillary nodes; more rarely some pass anterior to the clavicle to reach the inferior deep cervical (supraclavicular) nodes.

(3) Small isolated nodes sometimes occur along the radial, ulnar and interosseous vessels, in the cubital fossa near the bifurcation of the brachial artery, or in the arm medial to the brachial vessels.

Lymphatic drainage of superficial tissues

Superficial lymphatic vessels in the upper limb begin in the cutaneous plexuses. In the hand, the palmar plexus is denser. Digital plexuses are drained along the digital borders to their webs, where they join the distal palmar vessels which pass back to the hand's dorsal aspect (10.190, 192). The proximal palm drains towards the carpus, medially by vessels along its ulnar border and laterally to join those of the thumb. Several vessels from the central palmar plexus form a trunk winding round the second metacarpal bone to join the dorsal vessels from the index and thumb. In the forearm and arm, superficial vessels run with superficial veins. Collecting vessels from the hand pass into the forearm on all carpal aspects. Dorsal vessels, after running proximally in parallel, curve successively round the borders of the limb to join the ventral vessels (10.192). Anterior carpal vessels traverse the forearm parallel with the median vein of the forearm to the cubital region, proximal to which they follow the medial border of the biceps, then pierce the deep fascia at the anterior axillary fold and end in the lateral axillary lymph nodes.

Vessels which are lateral in the forearm follow the cephalic vein to the level of the tendon of the deltoid, where most incline medially to reach the lateral axillary nodes; a few, however, continue with the vein to the infraclavicular nodes. These lateral vessels receive those curving round the lateral border from the limb's dorsal aspect. Vessels which are medial in the forearm follow the basilic vein. Proximal to the elbow some end in supratrochlear lymph nodes, whose efferents, with the medial vessels which have bypassed them, pierce the deep fascia with the basilic vein to end in the lateral axillary nodes or deep lymphatic vessels. They are joined by vessels curving round the medial border of the limb.

Collecting vessels from the deltoid region pass round the anterior and posterior axillary fold to end in the axillary nodes. The scapular skin drains either to subscapular axillary nodes or by channels following the transverse cervical vessels to the inferior deep cervical nodes.

Lymphatic drainage of deep tissues of upper limb

Deep lymph vessels follow the main neurovascular bundles (radial, ulnar, interosseous and brachial) to the lateral axillary nodes. They are less numerous than the superficial vessels, communicating with them at intervals. A few lymph nodes occur along them. Scapular muscles drain mainly to the subscapular axillary nodes and pectoral muscles to the pectoral, central and apical nodes.

Mammary lymphatic drainage

Lymph vessels of the mammary gland start in a plexus in the interlobular connective tissue and walls of the lactiferous ducts, communicating with a cutaneous subareolar plexus around the nipple (**10**.193). The gland is also said to connect with a plexus of minute vessels on the subjacent deep fascia; this connection plays little part in normal lymphatic drainage nor in early spread of carcinoma (Turner-Warwick 1959). It offers an alternative route when the usual pathways are obstructed. Efferent vessels directly from the gland pass round the anterior axillary border through the axillary fascia to the pectoral lymph nodes; some may pass directly to the subscapular nodes. From the gland's superior region a few vessels pass to the apical axillary nodes, sometimes interrupted in the infraclavicular nodes or in small, inconstant interpectoral nodes. Axillary nodes receive more than 75% of lymph from the gland, the remainder largely draining to parasternal nodes from the medial and lateral parts of the organ; these vessels accompany perforating branches of the internal thoracic artery. Lymphatic vessels occasionally follow lateral cutaneous branches of the posterior intercostal arteries to the intercostal nodes. Cutaneous lymphatic drainage is described on page 1624.

Clinical anatomy

Enlargement of the axillary nodes is frequent in malignant disease and infective processes affecting the upper back and shoulder, the front of the chest and mammary gland, upper anterolateral abdominal wall or upper limb (palpation, see p. 1607). In operations for mammary carcinoma, pectoralis major, its deep fascia and surrounding muscles are usually removed en bloc because of the wide ramifications of its lymphatics. Axillary nodes, the sternocostal head of pectoralis major and frequently pectoralis minor are also removed, to ensure complete removal of the affected lymphatics and nodes. (Some surgeons, relying on more effective diagnostic techniques, now advocate less radical extirpation.)

LYMPHATIC DRAINAGE OF LOWER LIMBS

Most lymph from the lower limb traverses a large intermediary inguinal group of nodes; some may first traverse a few more peripheral intermediary nodes, however, these are less numerous in the lower limb than elsewhere. The inguinal nodes are superficial and deep to the deep fascia. Although commonly stated as such, the inguinal nodes are not the terminal group for the lower limb; from them the lymph traverses the external and common iliac groups, followed by the lateral aortic group. Deep gluteal lymph reaches the same group through the internal and common iliac chains. The upper lateral aortic nodes are terminal, forming bilateral lumbar

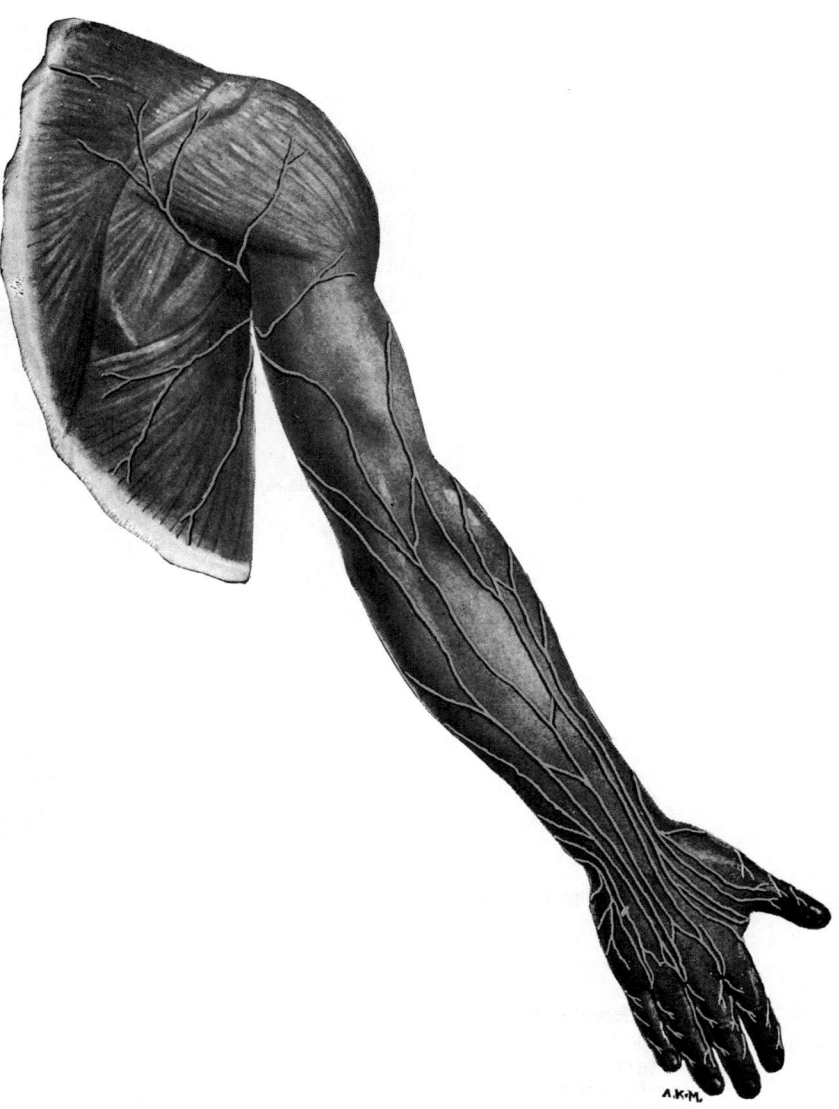

10.192   The lymphatic drainage of the superficial tissues of the upper limb: posterior aspect (semi-diagrammatic).

trunks which discharge lymph into the confluence of trunks (p. 1611) and thence the thoracic duct.

Superficial inguinal nodes

The superficial inguinal nodes form proximal and distal groups (**10**.194A, 195–197). The proximal is usually of five or six nodes just distal to the inguinal ligament. Its lateral members receive afferent vessels from the gluteal region and adjoining infra-umbilical anterior abdominal wall. Medial members receive superficial vessels from: the external genitalia (including the inferior vagina), inferior anal canal and perianal region, adjoining abdominal wall, umbilicus and the uterine vessels accompanying the round ligament. The distal group, usually four or five, along the termination of the great saphenous vein, receives all superficial vessels of the lower limb, except those from the calf's posterolateral region. All superficial inguinal nodes drain to the external iliac nodes, some via the femoral canal and others anterior or lateral to the femoral vessels. Numerous vessels interconnect individual nodes.

Deep inguinal nodes

The deep inguinal nodes vary from one to three, situated medial to the femoral vein. One is just distal to the saphenofemoral junction, one in the femoral canal; the most proximal one lies laterally in the femoral ring; the middle node is the most inconstant and the proximal node is often absent. All receive deep lymphatics accompanying the femoral vessels, lymph vessels from the glans penis (or clitoris) and

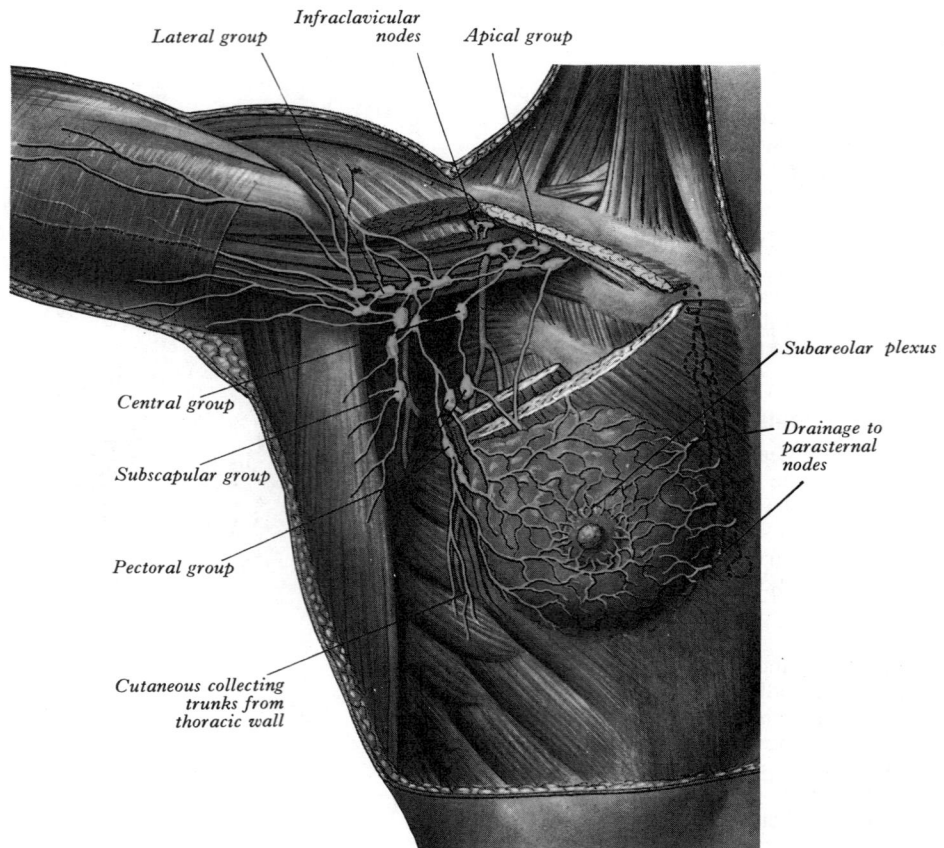

Lateral group   Infraclavicular nodes   Apical group

Subareolar plexus

Drainage to parasternal nodes

Central group

Subscapular group

Pectoral group

Cutaneous collecting trunks from thoracic wall

10.193   Lymph vessels of the mammary gland and the axillary lymph nodes.

a few efferents from the superficial inguinal nodes; their own efferents traverse the femoral canal to the external iliac nodes.

Peripheral nodes are few and are all deeply sited. Except for one sometimes proximal on the interosseous membrane near the anterior tibial vessels, they occur only in the popliteal fossa.

Popliteal lymph nodes

The small popliteal lymph nodes, usually six, are embedded in popliteal fat (**10.**194B). One, near the end of the small saphenous vein, drains the superficial region served by the vein. Another is between popliteal artery and posterior aspect of the knee joint, receiving direct vessels from the knee joint and those accompanying the genicular arteries. The remainder flank the popliteal vessels, receiving trunks accompanying the anterior and posterior tibial vessels. Popliteal efferents ascend close to the femoral vessels to reach the deep inguinal nodes but some may accompany the great saphenous vein to the superficial inguinal nodes.

Clinical anatomy. Inflammation of the popliteal nodes is often due to lateral lesions of the heel. Superficial inguinal nodes are frequently enlarged in disease or injury in their region of drainage (palpation, see p. 1607). Thus in malignant or infective disease of the prepuce, penis, labia majora, scrotum, abscess in the perineum, anus and lower vagina or in diseases affecting skin and superficial structures in these regions, or the infra-umbilical part of the abdominal wall, the gluteal region: in all these the proximal inguinal nodes are almost invariably affected, the distal group being implicated only in disease or injury of the limb.

Lymphatic drainage of superficial tissues in lower limbs

The superficial lymph vessels begin in subcutaneous plexuses. Collecting vessels leave the foot medially, along the great saphenous vein and, laterally, with the small saphenous.

Medial vessels are larger, more numerous and begin on the tibial side of the foot's dorsum, some ascending anterior and others posterior to the medial malleolus; thereafter both converge on the

great saphenous vein and accompany it to the distal superficial inguinal nodes. *Lateral vessels* begin on the fibular side, some crossing anteriorly in the leg to join the medial vessels and so to the distal superficial inguinal lymph nodes; others accompany the small saphenous vein to the popliteal nodes. Superficial lymph vessels of the gluteal region circle anteriorly to the proximal superficial inguinal nodes.

Lymphatic drainage of deeper tissues in lower limbs

The deep vessels accompany the main blood vessels: anterior and posterior tibial, peroneal, popliteal and femoral. The deep vessels from the foot and leg are interrupted by popliteal nodes; those from the thigh pass to the deep inguinal nodes.

The deep lymph vessels of the gluteal and ischial regions follow their corresponding blood vessels. Those with the former end in a node near the intrapelvic part of the superior gluteal artery, near the superior border of the greater sciatic foramen; those which follow the inferior gluteal vessels traverse one or two of the small nodes below the piriformis and pass to the internal iliac nodes.

LYMPHATIC DRAINAGE OF ABDOMEN AND PELVIS

Lymph from most of the abdominal wall and all abdominal viscera (except a small hepatic region) is returned via the thoracic duct. Lymphatic vessels run with their corresponding arteries, the lymphatic nodes forming a large number of intermediary groups along the arteries concerned and a few terminal groups near the abdominal aorta. Although referred to as illustrative examples in the introductory paragraphs, they are summarized here with numerous additions.

Lumbar nodes

The lumbar nodes include three terminal groups, each of which although interconnected has its own large area of drainage, a number

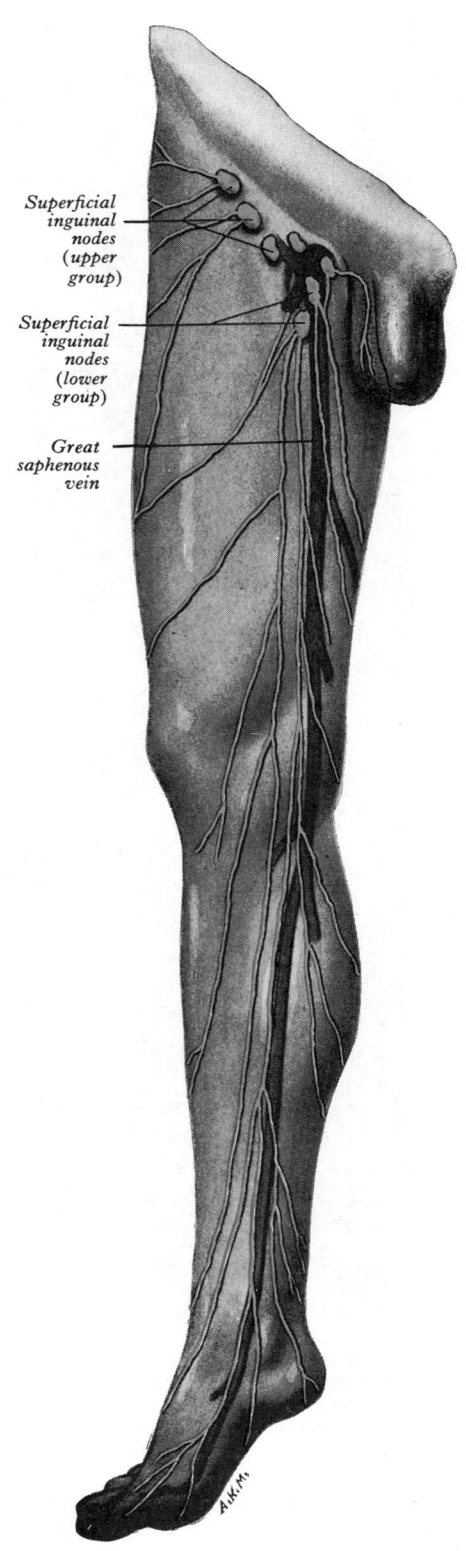

Superficial inguinal nodes (upper group)

Superficial inguinal nodes (lower group)

Great saphenous vein

A

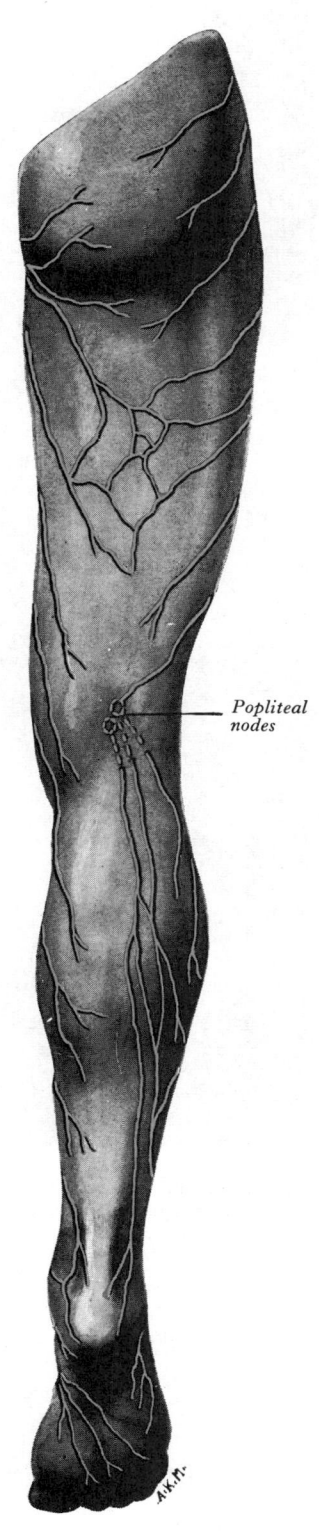

Popliteal nodes

B

10.194A   The lymphatic drainage of the superficial tissues of the lower limb: anteromedial aspect (semi-diagrammatic).

10.194B   The lymphatic drainage of the superficial tissues of the lower limb: posterior aspect (semi-diagrammatic).

of intermediary groups and one 'subsidiary' group (**10.196, 197**). These groups are pre-aortic, lateral aortic (right and left) and retro-aortic.

The pre-aortic group. It drains viscera supplied by the ventral splanchnic aortic branches, i.e. the abdominal part of the alimentary canal (down to midrectum) and its derivatives.

The lateral aortic groups. They drain viscera and other structures supplied by the lateral splanchnic and dorsolateral somatic aortic branches, receiving efferents from the large intermediary groups associated with the iliac vessels; their upper members are therefore

terminal groups for suprarenal glands, kidneys, ureters, testes, ovaries, pelvic viscera (apart from the gut) and the deeper tissues of the posterior abdominal wall, the full thickness of the subumbilical abdominal, pelvic and perineal walls and the whole of the lower limbs.

The retroaortic group. This has no special area of drainage; though it may have been primarily associated with drainage of the posterior abdominal wall, it may be regarded as comprising peripheral nodes of the lateral aortic groups and interconnecting surrounding groups.

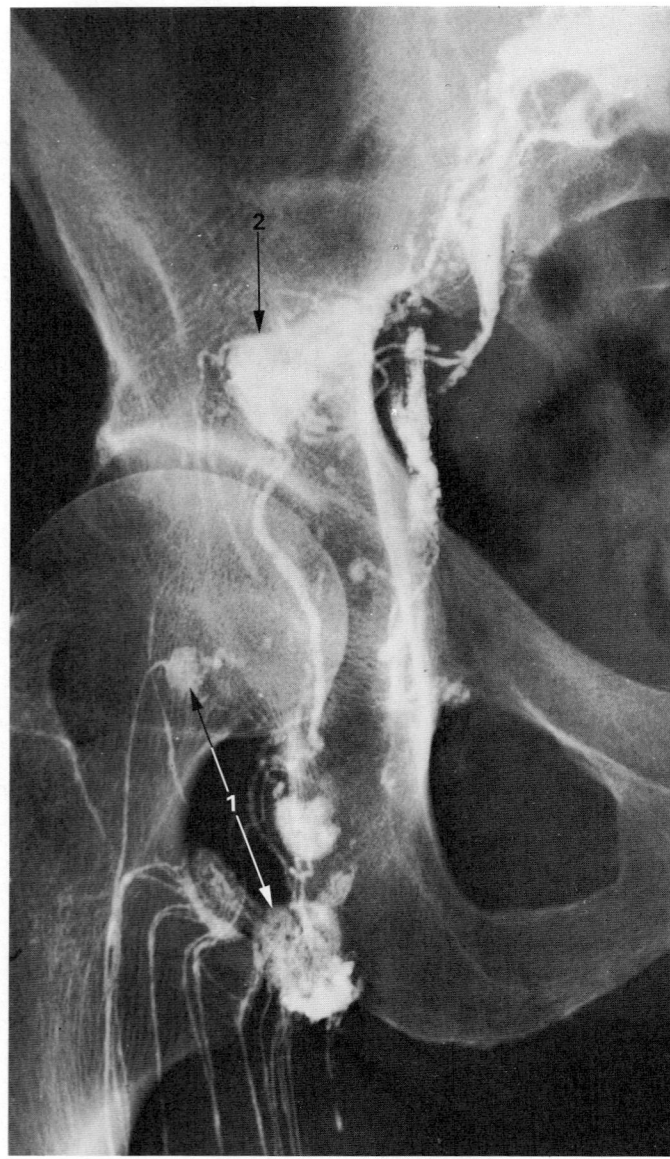

10.195 Lymphangiogram showing the inguinal lymph vessels and nodes taken immediately following injection of ultrafluid lipiodol into a lymph vessel on the dorsum of the foot. 1. Inguinal lymph nodes. 2. External iliac lymph node. (Supplied by J B Kinmonth.)

Lateral aortic nodes

Common iliac nodes

External iliac nodes

Pre-aortic node

10.196 Lymphangiogram showing the lateral aortic and proximal iliac lymph nodes, approximately 24 hours after the injection of lipiodol into a lymphatic vessel on the dorsum of each foot. Intravenous contrast was given to show the kidneys and ureters. (Supplied and photographed as in **10**.191.)

PRE-AORTIC LYMPH NODES

Pre-aortic lymph nodes are anterior to the abdominal aorta; they receive lymph from the regional nodes associated with the subdiaphragmatic part of the alimentary canal, pancreas, liver and spleen. Their cranial efferents form intestinal trunks entering the abdominal confluence of lymph trunks (p. 839). They are divisible into coeliac, superior mesenteric and inferior mesenteric groups, being near the origins of these arteries.

In the alimentary canal, lymph vessels begin as minute subepithelial radicles, blind at one end and opening into a *periglandular plexus.* In the small intestine each villus has a central vessel, known as a *lacteal* from its milky appearance. From the periglandular plexuses vessels pierce the muscularis mucosae to join a submucosal plexus, efferents from which traverse the muscularis, where they connect with or bypass the vessels draining it. The submucosal plexus is also joined by vessels from the lymph spaces at the bases of solitary

lymphatic follicles. Lymphatics of intestinal muscle drain into a plexus mainly between the longitudinal and circular layers. Collecting vessels leave the gut through the muscle to enter the larger vessels following their mesenteric arteries. Collecting vessels from the alimentary canal pass through local nodes before reaching the pre-aortic group.

Coeliac nodes

Coeliac nodes lie anterior to the abdominal aorta around the origin of the coeliac artery. They are a terminal group, their efferents forming right and left intestinal lymph trunks. Their afferents are from the regional nodes along branches of the coeliac artery, forming three main groups: gastric, hepatic and pancreaticosplenic; and they also come from the lower pre-aortic groups.

Gastric nodes (**10**.198, 199). They comprise the left gastric, right gastro-epiploic and pyloric groups. *Left gastric nodes*, along the left gastric artery, are divisible into subgroups: **superior** on the artery's stem and **inferior** with descending branches along the cardiac half of the lesser curvature in the lesser omentum and paracardial, a chain around the cardiac orifice. They receive lymph both from the stomach and the abdominal part of the oesophagus; their efferents pass to the coeliac group of pre-aortic nodes. *Right gastro-epiploic lymph nodes*, four to seven, lying in the greater omentum along the pyloric half of the greater curvature, receive afferents from the stomach; their efferents mostly pass to the *pyloric* nodes. Four or five pyloric lymph nodes are near the gastroduodenal artery's bifurcation, in the angle between the superior and the descending parts of the duodenum; an outlying node is sometimes sited above the duodenum near the right gastric artery. These nodes drain the pyloric part of the stomach, the first part of the duodenum and finally the right gastro-epiploic nodes; their efferents end in coeliac nodes.

Hepatic nodes (10.198). These extend in the lesser omentum along the hepatic arteries and bile duct. They vary in number and site but almost constant are: one at the junction of the cystic and common hepatic ducts, the cystic node; and another alongside the upper bile duct, the node of the anterior border of the epiploic foramen. Hepatic nodes drain the stomach, duodenum, liver, gallbladder, bile ducts and pancreas; they drain to the coeliac nodes and thence to the intestinal trunks. Enlarged hepatic nodes may press on and obstruct the portal vein.

Pancreaticosplenic nodes (10.199). They accompany the splenic artery, near the posterior surface and superior border of the pancreas; one or two are in the gastrosplenic ligament. Their afferents are from the stomach, spleen and pancreas; their afferents join the coeliac nodes.

Lymphatic drainage of stomach and duodenum. Gastric lymphatics (10.198, 199) are continuous at the cardiac orifice with the oesophageal vessels and at the pylorus with the duodenal channels. They largely follow blood vessels and form four groups: vessels of the first group accompany branches of the left gastric artery, receive from a large area on both gastric surfaces and end in the left gastric lymph nodes; a second group drains the gastric fundus and body left of a vertical from the oesophagus, accompanying the short gastric and left gastro-epiploic vessels to end in the pancreaticosplenic nodes; the third group drains the right half of the greater curvature as far as the pylorus, ending in the right gastro-epiploic nodes which drain to pyloric nodes; the fourth group drains the pyloric part of the stomach and drains to the hepatic, pyloric and left gastric nodes. Although these vessels communicate, their valves direct lymph from the right part of the stomach to the lesser curvature and from the left part to the greater curvature.

Duodenal lymphatics run anteriorly and posteriorly into the small pyloric lymph nodes, lying in the anterior and posterior grooves between the pancreatic head and the duodenum. They drain up to the hepatic and down to the pre-aortic nodes around the origin of the superior mesenteric artery.

Lymphatic drainage of liver. Hepatic collecting vessels are divisible into superficial and deep systems.

Superficial hepatic vessels. These run in subserosal areolar tissue over the whole surface of the organ, draining in four directions:

(1) From the middle part of its posterior surface, the caudate lobe, the posterior part of the convex surfaces of both lobes near the hepatic attachment of the falciform ligament, the posterior part of the inferior surface of the right lobe, vessels accompany the inferior vena cava to nodes around its terminal part. Vessels in the coronary and right triangular ligaments may directly enter the thoracic duct without any intervening node.

(2) Vessels from the rest of the inferior surface and anterior part of the convex surfaces of both lobes near the attachment of the falciform ligament all converge to the porta hepatis to end in the hepatic nodes.

(3) From the posterior region of the left lobe a few vessels pass towards the oesophageal opening to end in the paracardial nodes.

(4) From the remaining convex surface of the right lobe one or two trunks accompany the inferior phrenic artery across the right crus to the coeliac nodes.

Deep hepatic lymphatics. They form the ascending and descending trunks; the ascending trunks accompany the hepatic veins and pass through the vena caval opening to end in the nodes round the end

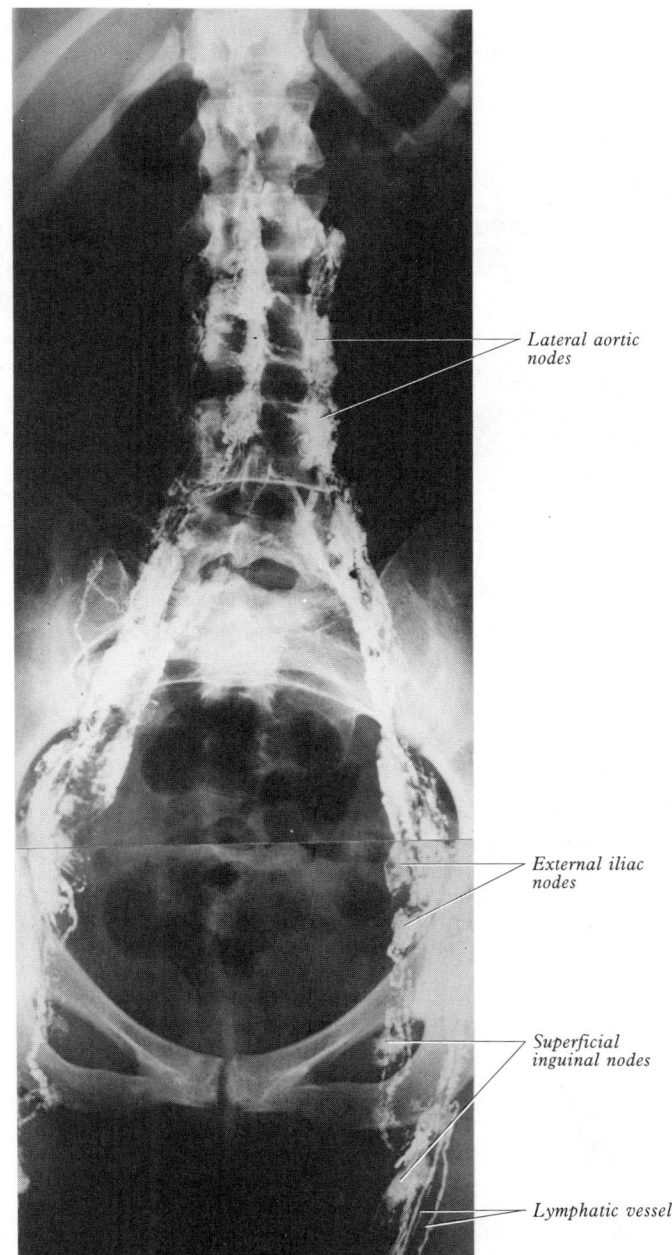

Lateral aortic nodes

External iliac nodes

Superficial inguinal nodes

Lymphatic vessels

10.197 Lymphangiogram showing the lymphatic vessels and nodes of the iliac and lateral aortic regions taken approximately 3 hours after the injection of lipiodol into a lymphatic vessel on the dorsum of each foot. (Supplied by G I Verney, Addenbrooke's Hospital, Cambridge; photographs prepared by Sarah Smith and K Fitzpatrick, Guy's Hospital.)

of the inferior vena cava; the descending trunks emerge from the porta hepatis to end in the hepatic nodes (p. 1802).

Lymphatic drainage of gallbladder and bile ducts. Numerous vessels run from the submucosal and subserosal plexuses on all aspects of the gallbladder and cystic duct, those on the former's hepatic aspect connecting sparsely with the hepatic vessels. They pass to the hepatic nodes, especially the cystic node and node of the anterior epiploic border (see above). Hepatic nodes also collect from vessels accompanying the hepatic ducts and the upper part of the bile duct, those of its lower part draining into the inferior hepatic and upper pancreaticosplenic nodes.

Lymphatic drainage of pancreas. Lymph capillaries commence around the acini and their continuations, following the blood vessels; there are no lymphatics in the pancreatic islets. Most vessels end in the pancreaticosplenic nodes, some in nodes along the pancreaticoduodenal vessels and others in the superior mesenteric pre-aortic nodes.

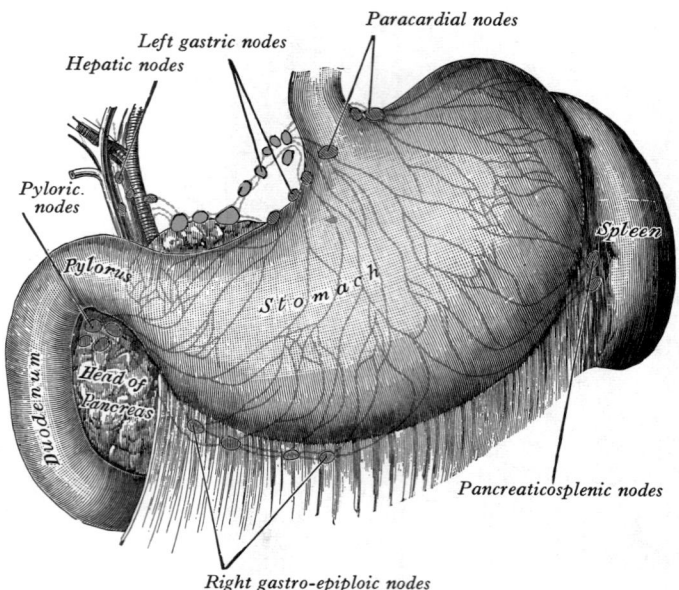

10.198 The lymphatic drainage of the stomach and duodenum. (After Jamieson & Dobson.)

Lymphatic drainage of spleen. Collecting vessels from the capsule end in the pancreaticosplenic lymph nodes.

Superior and inferior mesenteric nodes

Located anterior to the aorta near the origins of these arteries, the superior and inferior mesenteric nodes are preterminal groups for the alimentary canal from the duodenojejunal flexure to the upper anal canal and collect from outlying groups, including the mesenteric,

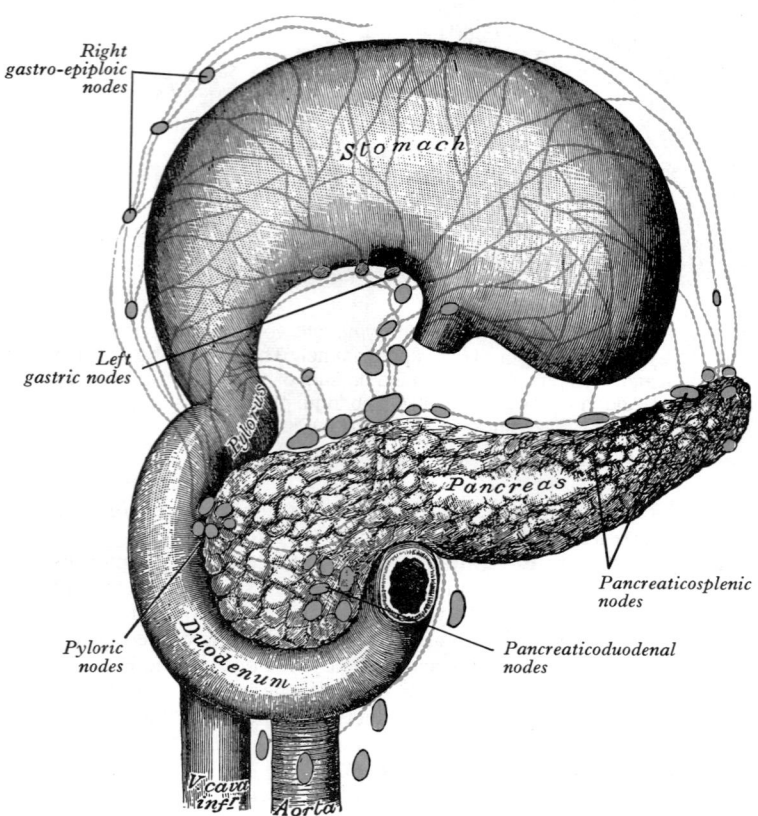

10.199 The lymph vessels and nodes of the stomach, duodenum and pancreas. The stomach has been turned upwards. (After Jamieson & Dobson.)

ileocolic, colonic and pararectal nodes. They discharge into the coeliac nodes and thence intestinal trunks, confluence and thoracic duct.

Mesenteric nodes. Numbering 100–150, the mesenteric nodes comprise three series: one close to the intestinal wall among the terminal rami of the jejunal and ileal arteries (mural); a second is among the loops and primary branches of the vessels (intermediate); and a third is along the upper trunk of the superior mesenteric artery (juxta-arterial). Vessels from the terminal centimetres of the ileum follow the ileal branch of the ileocolic artery to the ileocolic nodes.

Clinical anatomy. Enlargement of the mesenteric nodes occurs in many intestinal diseases, especially typhoid fever, tuberculous ulceration and malignant tumours. Enlarged nodes can often be palpated through the abdominal wall.

Ileocolic nodes (10.200, 201). They form a chain of 10–20 around the ileocolic artery but tend to form two groups: near the duodenum and along the artery's terminal part. The chain divides with the artery, into:

- *ileal nodes* close to the ileal branch;
- *anterior ileocolic nodes* (usually 3) in the ileocaecal fold, near the caecal wall;
- *posterior ileocolic nodes*, mostly in the angle between ileum and colon but partly behind the caecum at its junction with the ascending colon;
- an *appendicular node* in the mesoappendix.

Colic nodes. They form four groups: epicolic, paracolic, intermediate colic and preterminal colic.

Epicolic nodes. They are merely minute nodules on the colonic wall, sometimes in the appendices epiploicae.

Paracolic nodes. These lie along the medial borders of the ascending and descending colon and along the mesenteric borders of the transverse and sigmoid colon.

Intermediate colic nodes. They lie along the right, middle and left colic arteries.

Preterminal colic nodes. Adjoining the main trunks of the superior and inferior mesenteric arteries, they are near their corresponding pre-aortic nodes.

Pararectal nodes. These nodes, in contact with the rectal muscular wall, drain to an intermediate group around the superior rectal artery and thence to nodes near the origin of the inferior mesenteric. Others drain to nodes at the bifurcation of the common iliac artery.

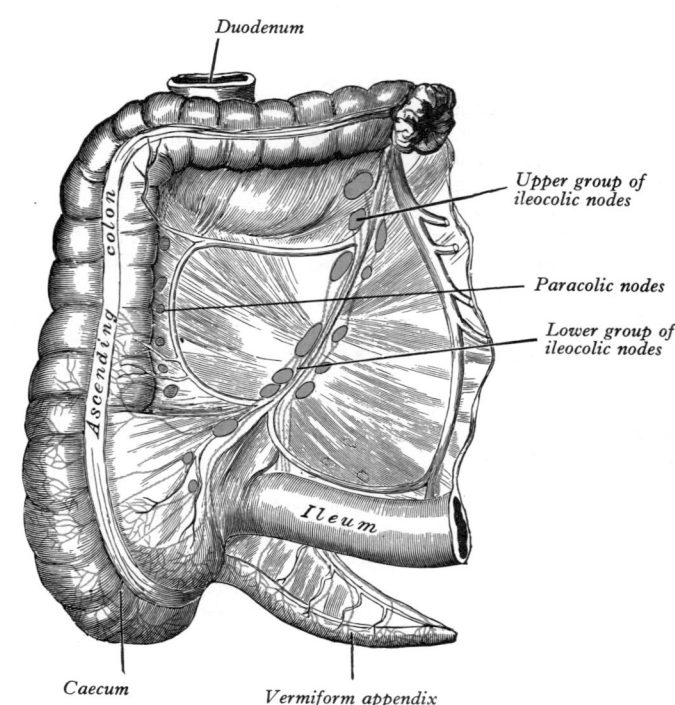

10.200 The lymph vessels and nodes of the caecum and vermiform appendix: anterior aspect. (After Jamieson & Dobson.)

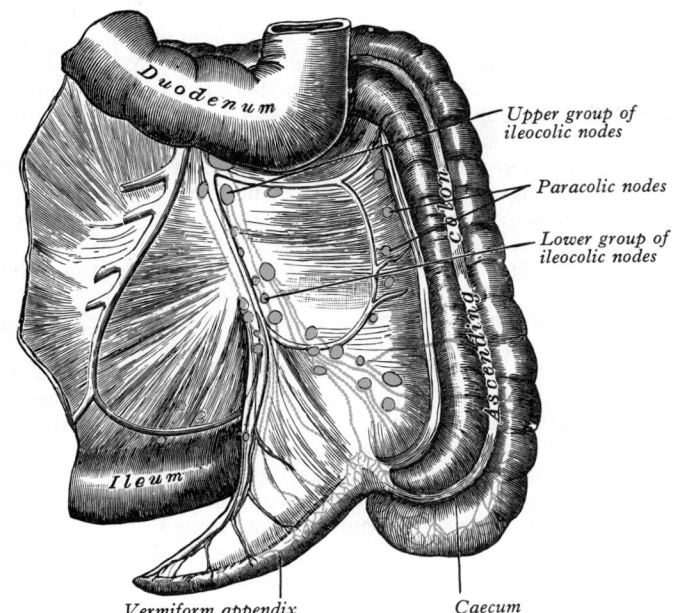

10.201   The lymph vessels and nodes of the caecum and vermiform appendix: posterior aspect. (After Jamieson & Dobson.)

Lymphatic drainage of jejunum and ileum. Lacteals pass between layers of the mesentery but, before reaching the superior mesenteric nodes, the lymph traverses the mesenteric nodes.

Lymphatic drainage of vermiform appendix and caecum (**10**.200, 201). Lymphatic vessels are numerous, since lymphoid tissue abounds in their walls. From the body and apex of the appendix 8–15 vessels ascend in the mesoappendix, a few interrupted by one or more nodes in it. They unite to form three or four larger vessels, ending in the inferior and superior nodes of the ileocolic chain.

Vessels from the root of the appendix and caecum are anterior and posterior. Anterior vessels pass in front of the caecum to the anterior ileocolic nodes and nodes of the ileocolic chain; posterior vessels ascend behind the caecum to the posterior and inferior ileocolic nodes.

Lymphatic drainage of colon (**10**.200–203). Lymphatic vessels of ascending and transverse parts of the colon end in the superior mesenteric nodes, after traversing nodes along the right and middle colic arteries and their branches. Those of the descending and sigmoid parts are interrupted by small nodes on branches of the left colic arteries, ending in the pre-aortic nodes around the origin of the inferior mesenteric artery.

Lymphatic drainage of rectum and anal canal. From the upper half, or more, of the rectum vessels emerge from its wall to ascend with the superior rectal vessels through the pararectal nodes to nodes in the lower sigmoid mesocolon and along the inferior mesenteric artery. From the lower half of the rectum and the anal canal, above its mucocutaneous junction, lymph vessels ascend through the wall to accompany the middle rectal vessels to the internal iliac nodes. Some are said to traverse the levator ani into the ischiorectal fossa, to accompany the inferior rectal and internal pudendal vessels to the internal iliac nodes. Lymphatics of the anal canal below the mucocutaneous junction descend to the anal margin, curving laterally to reach the most medial superficial inguinal nodes.

LATERAL AORTIC NODES

The lateral aortic nodes flank the abdominal aorta anterior to the medial margins of the psoas major muscles, diaphragmatic crura and sympathetic trunks (**10**.196, 197). On the right, some are lateral to the inferior vena cava and anterior to it near the end of the right renal vein. Afferents reach these nodes from structures supplied by the lateral splanchnic and dorsolateral somatic aortic branches and from outlying nodes near the iliac arteries and their branches. Efferents form a *lumbar trunk* on each side, both terminating in the confluence of lymph trunks (occasionally a cisterna chyli, p. 1610); a few may pass to the pre-aortic and retro-aortic nodes. Some of the efferents of the right lumbar lymph trunk and its nodes may

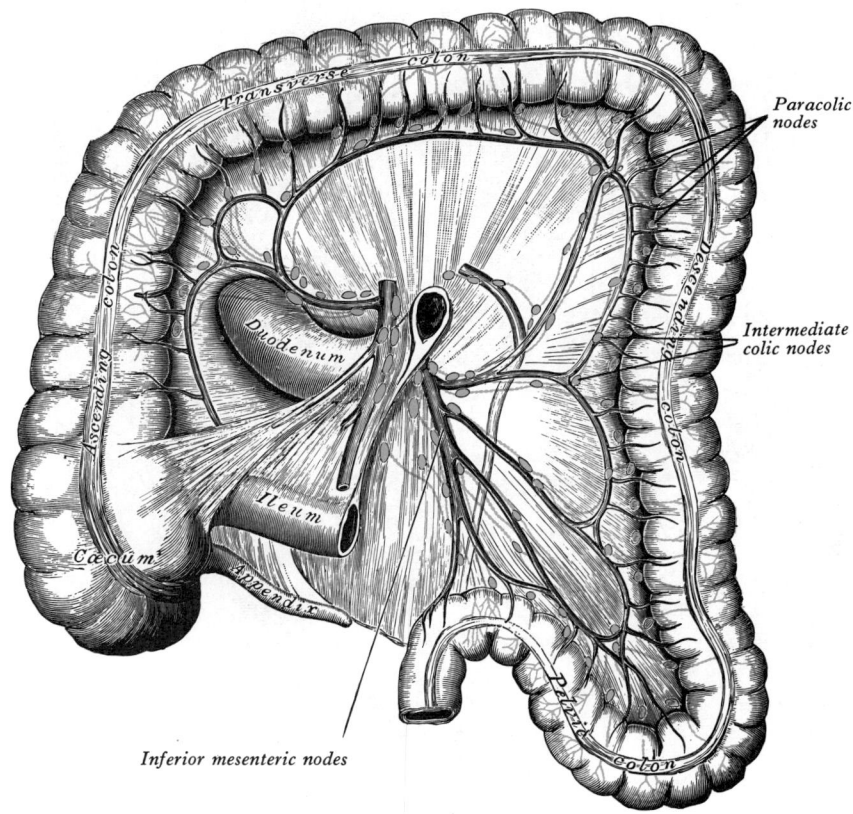

10.202   The lymph vessels and nodes of the colon. (After Jamieson & Dobson.)

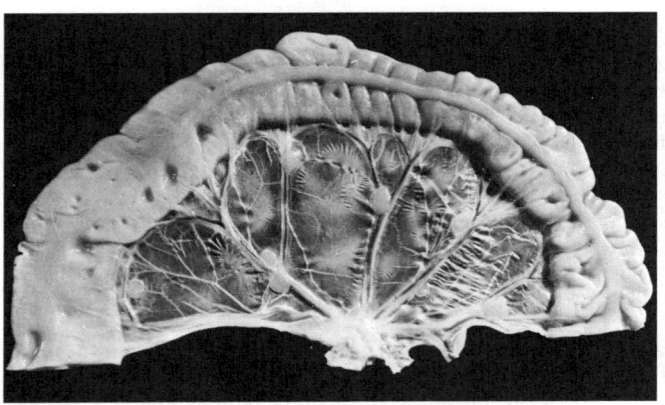

10.203   Preparation of the human colon and mesocolon displaying arterial arcades, neurovascular bundles, lymphatics and paracolic and intermediate lymph nodes. (Provided by S Kubic, University of Zürich.)

cross to their left counterparts; or both trunks may divide forming a loose plexus.

Lymphatic vessels from the kidney, suprarenal gland, abdominal ureter, posterior abdominal wall, testis and ovary, uterine tube and upper part of the uterus all pass directly to the lateral aortic nodes. Lymphatics from the pelvis, most pelvic viscera and the anterolateral abdominal wall pass first to regional nodes largely related to the internal iliac arteries and their branches. These include the following groups: common, external, internal and circumflex iliac, inferior epigastric and sacral. It must also be emphasized that the external iliac group receives the efferents from the inguinal nodes and the internal iliac group receives deep gluteal lymph; thus the lateral aortic groups ultimately drain the whole of both lower limbs.

Common iliac nodes. The 4–6 nodes are grouped around the artery, one or two inferior to the aortic bifurcation and anterior to the fifth lumbar vertebra or sacral promontory (**10.204**). They drain the external and internal iliac nodes and send efferents to the lateral aortic nodes. They are usually in medial, lateral and intermediate (anterior) chains, the lateral being the main route.

External iliac nodes (**10.**196, 197, 204). These 8–10 nodes usually form three subgroups, lateral, medial and anterior to the external iliac vessels; the anterior is inconstant. The medial nodes are considered the main channel of drainage, collecting from: the *inguinal nodes* (p. 1615), the deeper layers of the infra-umbilical abdominal wall, the adductor region of the thigh, the glans penis or clitoris, the membranous urethra, prostate, vesical fundus, cervix uteri and upper vagina. Their efferents pass to the common iliac nodes.

Inferior epigastric and circumflex iliac nodes. They are associated with their vessels and drain the corresponding areas, being outlying members of the external iliac group and inconstant in number.

Internal iliac nodes (**10.**204–206). Surrounding the vessels, they receive afferents from all the pelvic viscera, deeper parts of the perineum and gluteal and posterior femoral muscles. Efferents pass to the common iliac nodes.

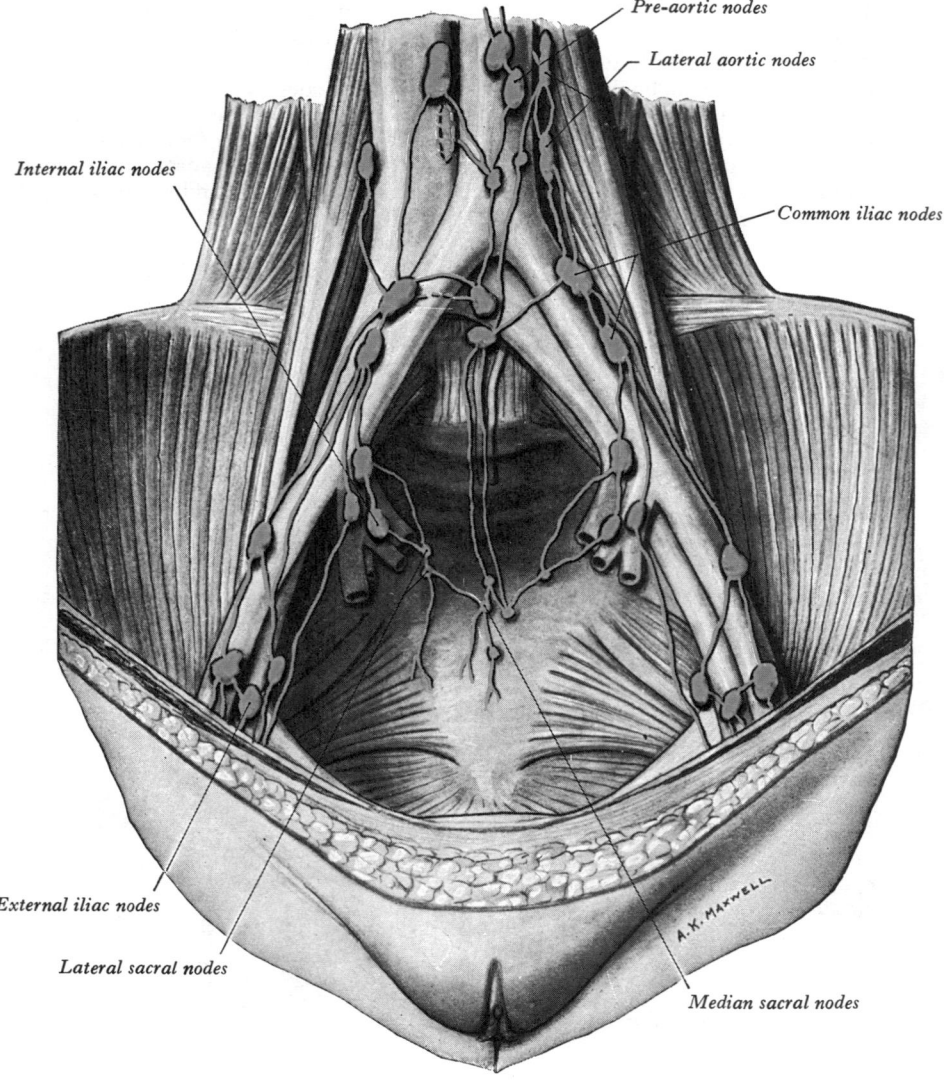

Sacral nodes. Found along the median and lateral sacral vessels and an obturator node, sometimes occurring in the obturator canal, they are outlying members of the internal iliac group. There is considerable bypassing in the iliac groups of lymph nodes. Lymphangiographic studies have demonstrated the connections between the right and left groups.

Lymphatic drainage of urinary tract

Renal. Renal lymphatic vessels begin in three plexuses: one around the renal tubules, a second under the renal capsule and a third in the perirenal fat connecting freely with the second plexus. Collecting vessels from the intrarenal plexus form four or five trunks following the renal vein to end in the lateral aortic nodes; as they leave the hilum they are joined by the subcapsular collecting vessels. The perirenal plexus drains directly into the same nodes.

Ureteric. Vessels begin in submucosal, intramuscular and adventitial plexuses which intercommunicate. Collecting vessels from the upper ureter may join the renal collecting vessels or pass directly to the lateral aortic nodes near the origin of the gonadal artery; those from its lower abdominal part go to the common iliac nodes; those from its pelvic part end in the common, external or internal iliac nodes.

Vesical. Lymphatics (10.205) begin in the mucosal, intermuscular and serosal plexuses. Collecting vessels, nearly all ending in the external iliac nodes, are in three sets:

- vessels from the trigone emerge on the vesical exterior to run superolaterally;
- those from the superior surface converge to the posterolateral angle and pass superolaterally across the lateral umbilical ligament to the external iliac nodes (one may go to the internal or common iliac group);
- those from the inferolateral surface ascend to join those from the superior surface.

Minute nodules of lymphoid tissue may occur along the vesical lymph vessels.

Urethral. These are of two sorts:

- Vessels from the prostatic and membranous urethra in males and the whole female urethra pass mainly to the internal iliac nodes; a few may end in the external iliac nodes. Vessels from the membranous urethra accompany the internal pudendal artery.
- Vessels of the male spongiose urethra accompany those of the glans penis, ending in the deep inguinal nodes. Some may end in superficial nodes, others may traverse the inguinal canal to the external iliac nodes.

Lymphatic drainage of male reproductive organs

Testis. Testicular vessels commence in a superficial plexus, under the tunica vaginalis, and a deep plexus in the substance of the testis and the epididymis. Four to eight collecting trunks ascend in the spermatic cord and accompany the testicular vessels on the psoas major, ending in the lateral aortic and pre-aortic nodes.

Ductus deferens, seminal vesicle and prostate gland. Collecting vessels from the ductus end in the external iliac nodes, while those from the seminal vesicle go to the internal and external iliac nodes. Prostatic vessels end mainly in internal iliac and sacral nodes; a vessel from the posterior surface accompanies the vesical vessels to the external iliac nodes and one from the anterior surface gains the internal iliac group by joining vessels of the membranous urethra.

Scrotum and penis. The skin of these parts is drained by vessels which, with those of all perineal skin, accompany the external pudendal blood vessels to the superficial inguinal nodes. Lymph vessels of the glans penis pass to the deep inguinal and external iliac nodes, from the erectile tissue and penile urethra to the internal iliac lymph nodes.

Lymphatic drainage of female reproductive organs
(10.206)

Ovary. The vessels, like the testicular, ascend along the ovarian artery to the lateral aortic and pre-aortic nodes.

Uterus and uterine tube. Uterine lymphatics are superficial (or subperitoneal) and deep in the uterine wall. Collecting vessels from the cervix pass laterally in the parametrium to the external iliac

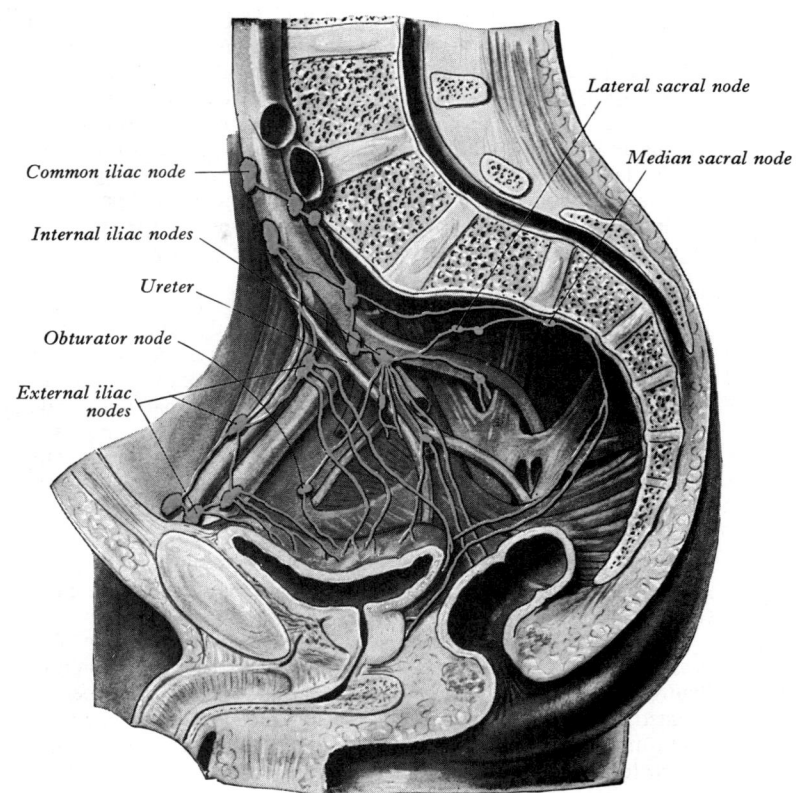

10.205 The lymphatic drainage of the urinary bladder (semidiagrammatic).

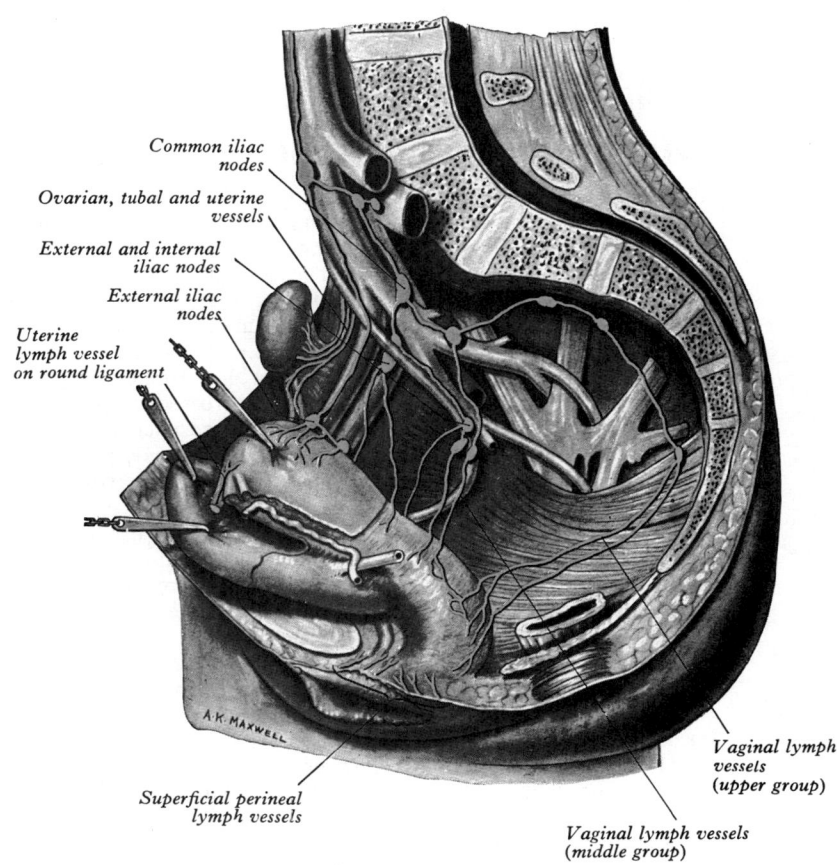

10.206 The lymphatic drainage of the female reproductive organs (semidiagrammatic). (After Cunéo & Marcille.)

nodes, posterolaterally to the internal iliac nodes and posteriorly in the sacrogenital fold to the rectal and sacral nodes. Some cervical efferents may reach the obturator or gluteal nodes. Vessels from the lower part of the uterine body pass mostly to the external iliac nodes, with those from the cervix. From the upper part of the body, the fundus and the uterine tubes, vessels accompany those of the ovaries to the lateral aortic and pre-aortic nodes, a few passing to the external iliac nodes. The region surrounding the isthmic part of the uterine tube is drained along the round ligament to the superficial inguinal nodes. Uterine lymph vessels enlarge greatly during pregnancy.

Vagina. Vaginal lymphatic vessels link with those of the cervix uteri, rectum and vulva. They form three groups but the regions drained are not sharply demarcated. Upper vessels accompany the uterine artery to the internal and external iliac nodes, intermediate vessels accompany the vaginal artery to the internal iliac nodes; vaginal vessels below the hymen, from the vulva and perineal skin, pass to the superficial inguinal nodes but the clitoris and labia minora drain to the deep inguinal nodes and direct clitoridial efferents may pass to the internal iliac nodes (Kubik 1967).

Lymphatic drainage of abdominal wall

The lymphatic vessels here are either superficial or deep to the deep fascia.

Superficial vessels. These accompany the subcutaneous blood vessels. Lumbar and gluteal vessels run with the superficial circumflex iliac vessels, those from the infra-umbilical skin with the superficial epigastric vessels. Both drain into the superficial inguinal nodes. The supra-umbilical region is drained by vessels running obliquely up to the pectoral and subscapular axillary nodes, a few to the parasternal nodes.

Deep vessels. They accompany the deep arteries, the posterior passing without interruption with the lumbar arteries to the lateral aortic and retro-aortic nodes; those from the upper anterior abdominal wall run with the superior epigastric vessels to the parasternal nodes; those of its lower part end in the circumflex iliac, inferior epigastric and external iliac nodes. Vessels of the pelvic wall follow the internal iliac artery and its parietal branches to end in the iliac or lateral aortic nodes.

LYMPHATIC DRAINAGE OF THORAX

LYMPHATIC DRAINAGE OF THORACIC WALLS

Superficial lymphatic vessels of the thoracic wall ramify subcutaneously and converge on the axillary nodes. Those superficial to the trapezius and latissimus dorsi unite to form 10 or 12 trunks ending in the subscapular nodes. Those in the pectoral region, including vessels from the skin covering the periphery of the mammary gland and its subareolar plexus, run back, collecting those superficial to serratus anterior, to reach the pectoral nodes. Vessels near the lateral sternal margin pass between the costal cartilages to the parasternal nodes but also anastomose across the sternum. A few vessels from the upper pectoral region ascend over the clavicle to the inferior deep cervical nodes. Lymph vessels from deeper tissues of the thoracic walls drain mainly to the parasternal, intercostal and diaphragmatic lymphatic nodes.

Parasternal (internal thoracic) nodes. Four or five on each side, they are at the anterior ends of the intercostal spaces, along each internal thoracic artery. They drain afferents from the mammary gland, deeper structures of the supra-umbilical anterior abdominal wall, the superior hepatic surface through a small group of nodes behind the xiphoid process and deeper parts of the anterior thoracic wall. Their efferents usually unite with those from the tracheobronchial and brachiocephalic nodes to form the bronchomediastinal trunk; this may open, on either side, directly into the jugulosubclavian junction into either great vein near the junction or may join the right subclavian trunk, the right lymphatic duct or, on the left, the thoracic duct.

Intercostal nodes. These occupy the intercostal spaces near the heads and necks of the ribs. They receive deep lymph vessels from the posterolateral aspects of the chest and the mammary gland; some are interrupted by small lateral intercostal nodes. Efferents of nodes

in the lower four to seven spaces unite into a trunk descending to the abdominal confluence of lymph trunks or to the commencement of the thoracic duct (p. 1610). Efferents of nodes in the left upper spaces end in the thoracic duct, those of the right upper spaces end in one of the right lymph trunks.

Diaphragmatic nodes. Located on the thoracic surface of the diaphragm, they comprise: anterior, right and left lateral and posterior groups.

The anterior group. This consists of two or three small nodes behind the base of the xiphoid process, draining the convex hepatic surface, and one or two nodes on each side near the junction of the seventh rib and cartilage, which receive anterior lymph vessels from the diaphragm. The anterior group drains to the parasternal nodes.

The lateral groups. They each contain two or three nodes, close to the entry of the phrenic nerves into the diaphragm. On the right some nodes lie within the fibrous pericardium anterior to the intrathoracic end of the inferior vena cava. Their afferents are from the central diaphragm, the right also draining the convex surface of the liver. Their efferents pass to the posterior mediastinal, parasternal and brachiocephalic nodes.

The posterior group. It contains a few nodes on the back of the crura, connected with the lateral aortic and posterior mediastinal nodes.

Lymphatic drainage of deeper tissues

Collecting vessels of the deeper thoracic tissues include the following:

- Lymphatics of muscles attached to the ribs: most end in axillary nodes, some from pectoralis major in the parasternal nodes.
- Intercostal vessels draining the intercostal muscles and parietal pleura; those from the anterior thoracic wall and pleura end in the parasternal nodes, the posterior in intercostal nodes.
- Vessels of the diaphragm form two plexuses, thoracic and abdominal, anastomosing freely and best marked in areas covered respectively by pleurae and peritoneum. The thoracic plexus unites with lymph vessels of the costal and mediastinal pleura, its efferents being: *anterior*, passing to the anterior diaphragmatic nodes near the junctions of the seventh ribs and cartilages; *middle*, to nodes on the oesophagus and around the end of the inferior vena cava; *posterior*, to nodes around the aorta where it leaves the thorax. The abdominal plexus anastomoses with the hepatic lymphatics and peripherally with those of the subperitoneal tissue. Efferents from its right half end partly in a group of nodes on the inferior phrenic artery, others in the right lateral aortic nodes. Those from the left half of the abdominal diaphragmatic plexus pass to the pre-aortic and lateral aortic nodes and nodes near the terminal oesophagus.

LYMPHATIC DRAINAGE OF THORACIC CONTENTS

Lymph from thoracic viscera traverses one or other of three groups of nodes, brachiocephalic, posterior mediastinal or tracheobronchial, before entering the thoracic duct, the right lymphatic duct or some other lymph trunk entering one of the great veins at the root of the neck.

Brachiocephalic nodes. These are in the superior mediastinum, anterior to the brachiocephalic veins and large arterial trunks springing from the aortic arch. They drain the thymus and thyroid glands, pericardium, heart and lateral diaphragmatic nodes; their efferents unite with those of the tracheobronchial nodes to form the right and left bronchomediastinal trunks.

Posterior mediastinal nodes. Behind the pericardium, near the oesophagus and the descending thoracic aorta, their afferents are from: the oesophagus, posterior pericardium, diaphragm, lateral and posterior diaphragmatic nodes and sometimes the left lobe of the liver. They drain chiefly to the thoracic duct but some join the tracheobronchial nodes.

Tracheobronchial nodes (10.207). They are in five main groups (Naruke et al 1978), including some of the largest nodes:

- *paratracheal*, in front and to the sides of the thoracic portion of the trachea but continuous above with the cervical paratracheal nodes
- *superior tracheobronchial*, in the angles between the trachea and the bronchi

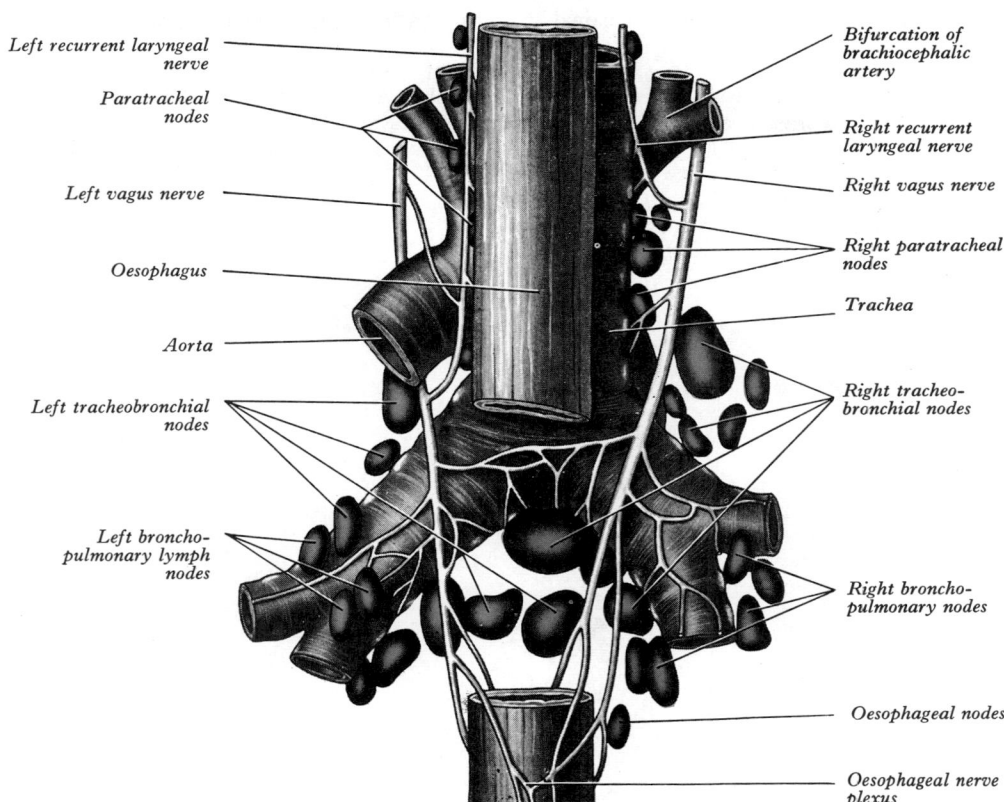

Left recurrent laryngeal nerve

Paratracheal nodes

Left vagus nerve

Oesophagus

Aorta

Left tracheobronchial nodes

Left broncho-pulmonary lymph nodes

Bifurcation of brachiocephalic artery

Right recurrent laryngeal nerve

Right vagus nerve

Right paratracheal nodes

Trachea

Right tracheo-bronchial nodes

Right broncho-pulmonary nodes

Oesophageal nodes

Oesophageal nerve plexus

10.207   The lymph nodes of the trachea, bronchi and lungs. Note the large 'carinate' node lodged between the bifurcation of the principal bronchi.

- *inferior tracheobronchial* or *subcarenal nodes*, in the angle between the bronchi
- *bronchopulmonary* or *hilar nodes*, in the hilum of each lung around the main bronchi
- *pulmonary* or *intralobar*, in the lung substance on larger branches of the principal bronchi.

These groups are not sharply demarcated; pulmonary nodes become continuous with the bronchopulmonary and they in turn with the inferior and superior tracheobronchial nodes, continuous with the paratracheal group. Afferents of tracheobronchial nodes drain the lungs and bronchi, thoracic trachea, heart and some efferents of the posterior mediastinal nodes. Their efferent vessels ascend on the trachea to unite with efferents of the parasternal and brachiocephalic nodes as the right and left bronchomediastinal trunks; the right trunk may occasionally join a right lymphatic duct or another right-sided lymph trunk and on the left the thoracic duct; but more often they open independently in or near the jugulo-subclavian junction on their own side.

Clinical anatomy. In all town dwellers large quantities of dust and carbonaceous pigment may be freely inhaled and are continually swept into these nodes from the bronchi and alveoli.

Lymphatic drainage of heart

Cardiac lymphatic vessels form subendocardial, myocardial and subepicardial plexuses, the first two draining into the third, efferents of which form the left and right cardiac collecting trunks. Two or three left trunks ascend the anterior interventricular sulcus, receiving vessels from both ventricles; reaching the coronary sulcus, they are joined by a large vessel from the diaphragmatic surface of the left ventricle, which first ascends in the posterior interventricular sulcus and then turns left along the coronary sulcus. The vessel formed by the union of these two ascends between the pulmonary artery and the left atrium, usually ending in an inferior tracheobronchial node. The right trunk receives afferents from the right atrium and right border and diaphragmatic surface of the right ventricle. It ascends in the coronary sulcus, near the right coronary artery, and then

anterior to the ascending aorta to end in a brachiocephalic node, usually on the left.

Lymphatic drainage of lungs and pleurae

Pulmonary lymphatic vessels originate in a superficial subpleural plexus and a deep plexus accompanies the branches of pulmonary vessels and bronchi. In larger bronchi the deep plexus has submucosal and peribronchial parts; in smaller bronchi a single plexus extends to the bronchioles but not to the alveoli, whose walls have no lymphatic vessels. Superficial efferents turn round borders and the margins of fissures to converge in the bronchopulmonary nodes; deep efferents reach the hilum along the pulmonary vessels and bronchi, ending mainly in the same nodes. There is little anastomosis between the superficial and deep lymphatics, except in the hilar regions. In peripheral parts of the lungs small channels connect superficial and deep lymphatic vessels, capable of dilatation to direct lymph from the deep to the superficial channels when outflow from deep vessels is obstructed by pulmonary disease. Deep in the fissures, lymphatic vessels of adjoining lobes connect; hence, though there is a tendency for vessels from the upper lobes to pass to the superior tracheobronchial nodes and those from lower lobes to the inferior tracheobronchial group, these connections are not exclusive. At the level of pulmonary lobation the arrangement of lymphatic vessels follows with the central artery of a lobule and its peripheral veins (Kubik 1970), confirming the findings of Celtis and Porter (1952). Policard (1950) has described lymphoid aggregations, non-follicular in appearance, in peribronchial sites and in 'placoid' formations adjoining pulmonary pleura.

Pleural lymphatic vessels exist in visceral and parietal layers, those of the visceral pleura draining to the superficial pulmonary efferents, forming a plexus beneath the pulmonary pleura (see above). Those of the parietal pleura end in three ways:

- those from the costal region join vessels of the internal intercostal muscles to reach the parasternal nodes;
- those of the diaphragmatic pleura form a plexus on its thoracic surface (p. 1624);

1625

- those of the mediastinal pleura end in the posterior mediastinal nodes.

Lymphatic drainage of thymus

Thymic lymphatic vessels end in the brachiocephalic, tracheo-bronchial and parasternal nodes.

Lymphatic drainage of oesophagus

Efferent vessels from the cervical oesophagus drain to the deep cervical nodes, those from its thoracic part to the posterior mediastinal nodes and those from its abdominal part to the left gastric lymph nodes. Some may pass directly to the thoracic duct (p. 1610).

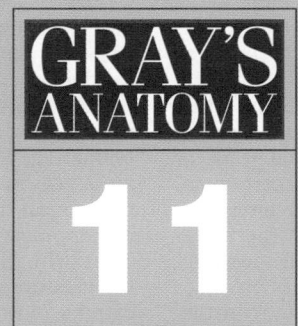

GRAY'S ANATOMY

11

RESPIRATORY SYSTEM

Section Editor: Lawrence Bannister

Contributors: Roger Parker for revision of structure and clinical aspects of the larynx, Professor J Joseph for essay on Anatomy of speech, Julian Dussek for essay on Clinical examination of the chest and for revision of bronchial vasculature and various clinical aspects of the thorax and MRI sections, Mary Dyson for contributions to pulmonary microstructure and pulmonary response to acute injury and Professor Giorgio Gabella for various contributions to pulmonary microstructure.

INTRODUCTION

The respiratory system consists of the respiratory surfaces of the lungs, and the air passages provided by the nose, phraynx (in part), larynx and respiratory tree. Associated with the nasal cavities are a series of bony sacs, the paranasal sinuses, which are uncertain in function but included here with the respiratory tract. The lungs are enclosed by the membranes of the pleurae, and between the lungs are a number of major thoracic structures which, with their investing tissue, form the mediastinum; for convenience these topics are also incorporated in this section although only partly respiratory in the strict sense.

Before proceeding to describe the anatomy of the respiratory system, its functional organization will be briefly reviewed. Besides its primary respiratory role in gaseous exchange and ventilation, a number of accessory activities are performed by the respiratory system as a whole, examples being: the production of sounds (phonation) by the larynx and related structures, odorant sampling by olfactory sensors in the nasal chambers, mechanical stabilization of the thorax during mechanical exertion, and various biochemical operations concerned with blood-borne molecules.

Gaseous exchange

Because most of the energy production in the body requires the use of molecular oxygen, the passage of oxygen into its cells largely determines the rate of activity in the body as a whole. Conversely, carbon dioxide, the mildly toxic waste product of these and some other chemical reactions, has constantly to be removed to allow metabolism to continue. In very small, especially single-celled, organisms the two-way exchange of oxygen and carbon dioxide is achieved by simple diffusion across their surfaces, but this puts a size limitation on active cells because the rates of gaseous diffusion depend on the surface area, whereas oxygen use and carbon dioxide production are related to cell volume; as an animal increases in size, its diffusional area increases by the square, whereas its volume enlarges by the cube of the linear dimension. This problem has been solved by two complementary developments: a large respiratory area at the body surface in contact with the outside environment, and an efficient circulatory system to convey gases to and from the tissues, which can then be remote from the surface. It is interesting that different groups of animals have made structurally diverse but functionally similar arrangements for respiratory exchange and transport. Many aquatic invertebrates and some vertebrates have extensive projections of the body surface—gills—which create large areas for gaseous exchange, perfused with blood through capillary plexuses, and often ventilated in some way to improve the efficiency of exchange. In terrestrial creatures, however, external gills are generally impractical, mainly because of dehydration, and instead we find internalized, protected exchange surfaces: in insects these take the form of small tubular invaginations of the epidermis (tracheae and tracheoles) which penetrate deeply into the tissues themselves, the circulatory system then lacking much respiratory transport function. Amongst vertebrates, the wall of the alimentary tract is often used for direct respiratory exchange with the air; in lungfish (Dipnoans) and all tetrapods, lungs are formed as large, thin-walled and highly vascular extensions of the foregut. In lungfish and amphibia the lungs are relatively simple, paired (usually), partially divided sacs opening together into the pharynx through a sphincteric aperture, the glottis, whereas in reptiles, birds and mammals the lungs are much more highly divided into minute alveoli which create a relatively huge surface area for respiratory exchange, connected to the pharynx by a system of branching tubes converging on a single pipe, the trachea, which again opens through a glottis. Ventilatory mechanisms involving muscular actions used to inflate the lungs are relatively simple in lower tetrapods, mainly using the pharyngeal muscles to force air from the buccal cavity into the lungs, the elastic recoil of the lungs returning the air to the pharynx. In reptiles, birds and mammals, ventilatory movements involve much more muscular action by the muscles and skeleton of the trunk (including movable ribs), which, in mammals becomes divided into a thorax and abdomen by the development of a muscular diaphragm. This arrangement effectively separates respiratory and alimentary functions, and greatly enhances the efficiency of ventilation; birds achieve the same result by increasing the complexity of the respiratory passages to ensure a very effective tidal flow, essential for the very high metabolic rate needed for flying.

Besides ensuring gaseous exchange, the respiratory system engages in a number of secondary functions, the most important of which is phonation; in addition it facilitates olfactory sampling of inhaled air, assists in the venous return of blood to the heart and has various mechanical actions on other parts of the body due to changes in intrathoracic pressure which can also be transmitted to the abdomen. Thus, with the glottis closed, thoracic muscles can be used to increase the pressure within the thorax, to give it mechanical stability during extreme muscular effort, to increase abdominal pressure in defecation and parturition, and, when suddenly released, to clear the respiratory tract of obstructions by coughing.

Phonation

In humans the development of a phonatory larynx has been part of a system for auditory communication which has had considerable significance for the evolution of the brain, social behaviour and general intelligence. Although the larynx still houses a sphincteric glottis controlling the passage of air (and ultimately preventing the inhalation of substances other than air by its reflex closure), the development of vocal cords, articulating cartilages and delicately controllable muscles driven by a complex nervous system has allowed the generation of speech, a process with exceedingly subtle features, which has affected the morphology of much of the head and neck, as well as other body regions. Speech, which must of course be heard and interpreted but may also be expressed in visible, written form, has led to the increasingly complex symbolism of language (with which mathematical and musical notation may be coupled, as well as the types of communication exampled by the present text). In this development, which is unparalleled in any other animal, very high levels of integration between the nervous system and locomotor structures are attained. The elaboration of laryngeal musculature and its neural control, integrating laryngeal sound production with movements of respiratory, pharyngeal, palatal, lingual and labial muscles during the complex articulation of speech, provide mankind with a unique ability. All other tetrapods do, however, engage in some form of sound production; in the birds this has been raised to a high degree of complexity, using structures rather different from the mammalian larynx, including bronchial specializations and a larynx-like structure, the syrinx, at the base of the trachea.

Olfactory sampling

In the human respiratory system, a portion of the inspiratory air current drawn through the nose contacts the olfactory epithelium on a part of the roof, septum and walls of the nasal cavity, where olfactory receptor cells can detect and discriminate between a wide variety of air-borne molecules (odorants) for transmission to the brain. The precise arrangement of this mechanism has changed somewhat during evolutionary history.

In the tetrapods the nasal cavity, which in most fishes is a separate blind-ending sac separate from the mouth, is integrated into the respiratory system with the development of the nostrils, partially separating the respiratory from the alimentary pathway. In amphibia and many reptiles the nasal aperture leads almost directly into the oral cavity, but in mammals the development of a secondary palate makes a more extensive separation of a nasal cavity which communicates posteriorly via the nasopharynx with the shared portion (the oropharynx) of the alimentary and respiratory passages. The detachment of respiratory and olfactory functions from the mouth allows predatory mammals to breathe while the mouth is obstructed by prey, and herbivores to sense warning odours when feeding. In aquatic vertebrates, such as crocodiles, dolphins and whales, a spout-like elongation of the larynx can project into the nasopharynx, largely separating the airway, so that respiration can continue at the surface with the mouth submerged, open and ready for prey.

Mechanical stabilization of the thorax

When the entrance to the lower respiratory tract through the glottis is closed with the lungs full of air, contraction of the intercostal and diaphragmatic muscles causes the intrathoracic pressure to rise and the wall of the thorax to become more rigid. Limb muscles attached to the thorax can then distribute their reactive force most efficiently

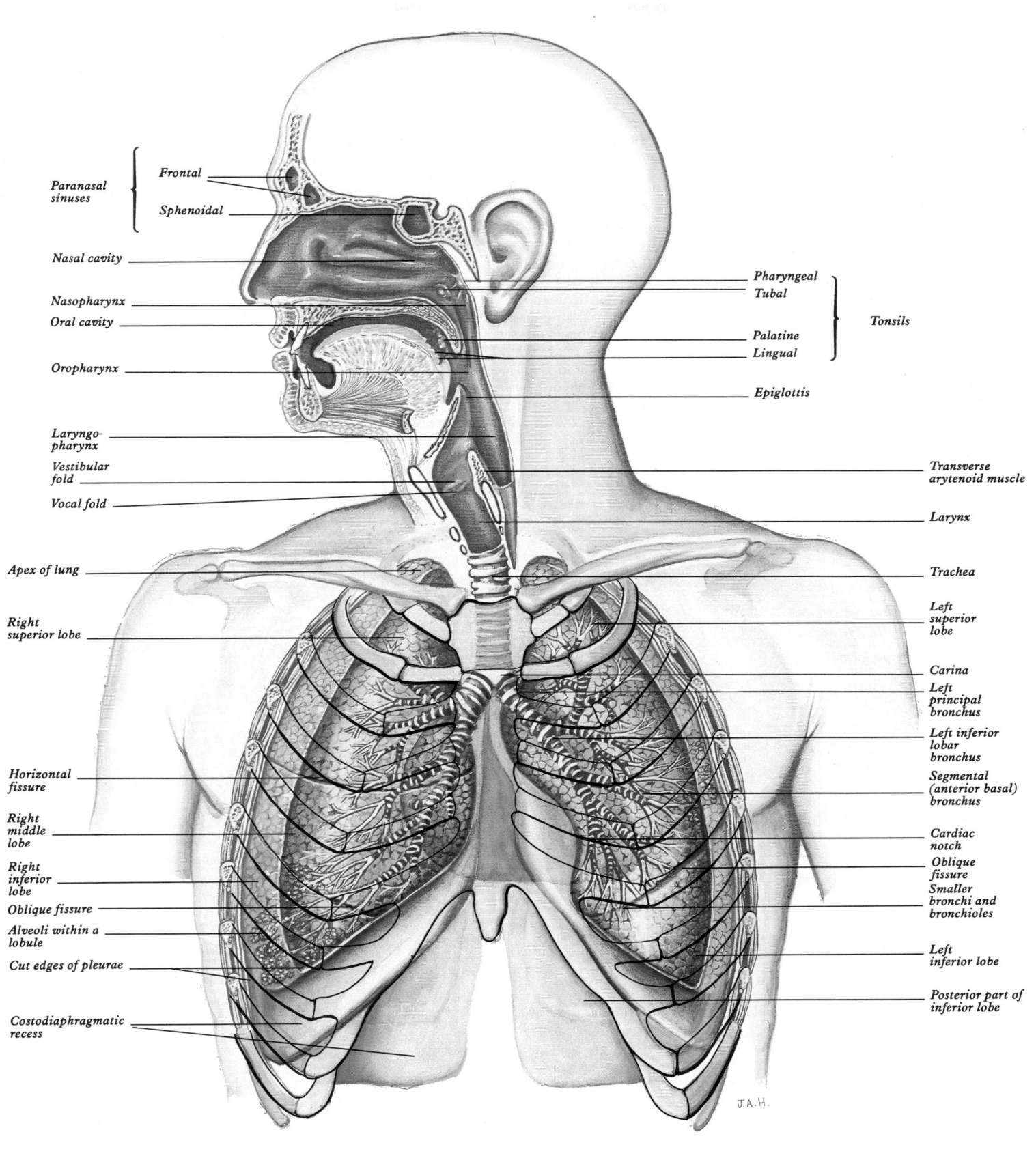

Paranasal sinuses
Frontal
Sphenoidal
Nasal cavity
Nasopharynx
Oral cavity
Oropharynx
Laryngo-pharynx
Vestibular fold
Vocal fold
Apex of lung
Right superior lobe
Horizontal fissure
Right middle lobe
Right inferior lobe
Oblique fissure
Alveoli within a lobule
Cut edges of pleurae
Costodiaphragmatic recess

Pharyngeal
Tubal
Palatine
Lingual
Tonsils
Epiglottis
Transverse arytenoid muscle
Larynx
Trachea
Left superior lobe
Carina
Left principal bronchus
Left inferior lobar bronchus
Segmental (anterior basal) bronchus
Cardiac notch
Oblique fissure
Smaller bronchi and bronchioles
Left inferior lobe
Posterior part of inferior lobe

J.A.H.

11.1 Diagrammatic representation of the respiratory tract. Those parts of the tract in the head and upper neck are shown in sagittal section, in the lower neck turned anteriorly and, in the remainder of the tract, from the anterior aspect.

1629

on the trunk, so that in strenuous pulling or pushing, for example, more power can be exerted. Likewise, if the thoracic pressure is high and the diaphragm relaxed, the lungs can be used to push against the abdominal compartment to increase its internal pressure, so for example, assisting the processes of defecation and childbirth.

Biochemical functions

The vascular channels within the lung present a huge surface area between the blood and endothelial linings of the vessels. The endothelium of the lungs engages in various biochemical interactions with the bloodstream, such as the conversion of angiotensin I to angiotensin II, a process concerned with the regulation of the body's blood pressure.

Structural features of the respiratory system

The human respiratory system has general design features which can be related to a number of important activities. Essentially, of course, it consists of a *respiratory surface* and branched *conducting passages* forming the respiratory tree. The respiratory surface is very large, as much as 200 m², and forms a very thin, moist barrier between the air and blood capillaries around the perimeters of the many millions of blind-ending sacs (alveoli), constituting much of the lung's mass. Because of their delicate structure these respiratory surfaces are very vulnerable to mechanical damage from inhaled particles, and also to infectious organisms. Protecting the surface area against dehydration, heat loss and abrasive particles, the conducting passages form a series of moist, warm, adhesive (to dust) channels between the alveoli

and the pharynx; in addition to mucus secreted on to these surfaces, these tubes are lined by cilia which beat towards the pharynx, so continually removing most inhaled particles from the respiratory system (the *mucociliary clearance current*). The nasal cavity has similar protective features. Particles which because of their minute size do reach the alveoli are immediately phagocytosed by macrophages which wander over their internal surfaces, and these can either move into the mucociliary current or migrate back into the tissues where they may deposit their load and where they will do no damage. Against microbial infections, there is a battery of defensive devices: bacteriostatic substances and immunoglobulins are secreted with the mucus into the respiratory passages, and the alveoli also have a range of antimicrobial chemicals (see p. 1673). Lymphoid tissue scattered along the walls of the respiratory passages (bronchial-associated lymphoid tissue; BALT; see p. 1673) provides lymphocytic defence against bacteria, fungal organisms, viruses and other microbes.

The passage of air is controlled by variations in the rate of ventilatory movements, and also by modulation of the diameters of the air passages of the lower respiratory tract, which are enwrapped with bronchial smooth muscle fasciculi whose tonus is controlled largely by the autonomic nervous system. These arrangements allow the respiratory system to respond to metabolic demand while minimizing the loss of water and heat from the lungs, by adjusting air flow to a suitable level. This is an important feature, also related to the mechanics of ventilation, since it determines the transmission of pressure changes within the thorax during breathing. During

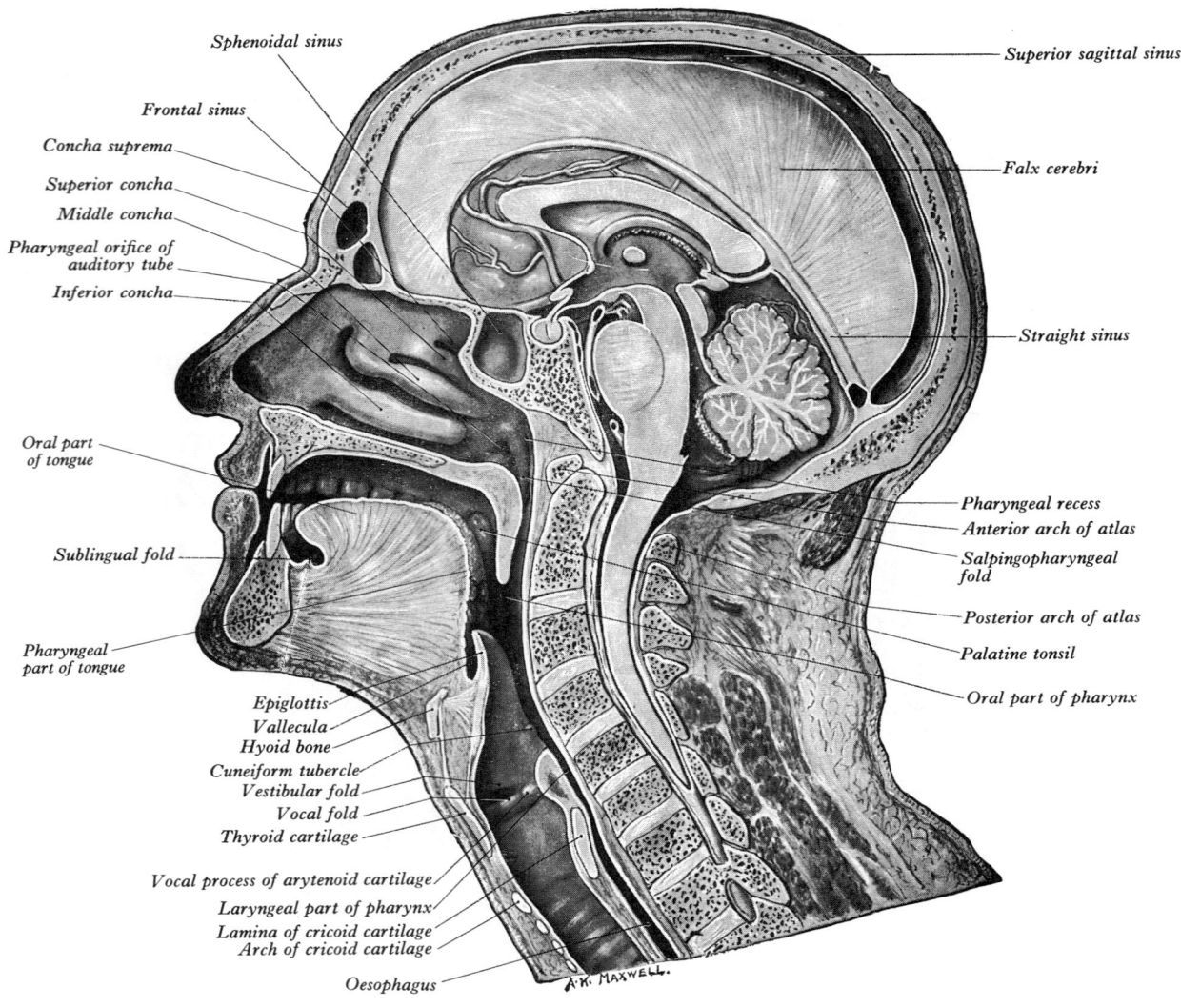

11.2   Median sagittal section showing the position of the upper respiratory tract, larynx and the first part of the cervical trachea in relation to other structures of the head and neck.

inspiration, when the volume of the thorax increases the intrathoracic pressure decreases so that air flows through the respiratory passages into the enlarging alveoli, and in expiration the reverse processes occur. The rate of flow is affected by airway diameter, so the time course of the pressure changes also varies with the tonus of the bronchial smooth muscle. In the larger air passages these fluctuations in intrathoracic pressure tend to cause overinflation or collapse, and these are prevented by the presence of semi-rigid cartilage rings encircling them entirely (in bronchi) or partially (in the trachea). Pressure differentials such as these do not operate across the walls of the smaller vessels, and these are devoid of cartilage. The lower respiratory tract is also provided with much elastic tissue which allows it to stretch and store energy during inspiration, and to recoil during expiration.

Divisions of the respiratory system (11.1, 2).

The division of the respiratory system into an upper and lower respiratory tract is in reality a clinical convenience related largely to the spread of infection rather than any fundamental anatomical concept. The *upper respiratory tract* can be defined as those parts of the air passages which lie above the inlet to the larynx, namely the nasal cavities, nasopharynx and oropharynx. The *lower respiratory tract* comprises the larynx, trachea, bronchi and the rest of the respiratory tree and respiratory surfaces of the lungs.

Parts of the upper respiratory tract are shared with the alimentary system, or are anatomically closely related to it in organization and continuity, and the nasopharynx and oropharynx are described with the laryngopharynx in the 'Alimentary System', Section 12 (p. 1683) of this book. The olfactory organ is described with the other special sense organs in the 'Nervous System', Section 8 (p. 901), but the rest of the nasal cavity and paranasal sinuses are described with the respiratory system, a departure from previous editions. After this, the larynx is considered, followed by the rest of the respiratory tree and lungs. The pleurae are then examined, and the mediastinal structures briefly considered. Finally, these structures are related to the clinical examination of the chest.

NOSE, NASAL CAVITY AND PARANASAL SINUSES

The first part of the upper respiratory tract consists of the paired nasal cavities divided from each other sagittally by a septum. In the lateral walls of these cavities, and in communication with them, are a series of air-filled expansions, the paranasal sinuses. These nasal cavities are housed in a bony framework which extends anteriorly as the external nose. This apparatus serves to warm, humidify and to some extent filter particles from the inhaled air, and by virtue of the olfactory epithelium which lies at its upper and posterior recesses, to sense and discriminate between airborne chemicals.

EXTERNAL NOSE (11.3, 4)

Externally the nose is pyramidal in shape, its upper angle or root being continuous with the forehead, and its free tip forming the *apex*. Inferiorly are two ellipsoidal apertures, the *external nares* or *nostrils*, separated by the nasal septum. The lateral surfaces of the nose form by their union in the median plane the *dorsum nasi*, the shape of which varies greatly between individuals; the upper part of the external nose is kept patent by the nasal bones and the frontal processes of the maxillae; below this the cartilages form the walls. The lateral surfaces end below in the rounded *alae nasi*.

Skeleton of the external nose

The supporting framework (11.3, 4) is composed of bone and hyaline cartilages. The *bony framework*, supporting the upper part of the nose, consists of the nasal bones, the frontal processes of the maxillae and the nasal part of the frontal bone; the *cartilaginous framework* consists of the septal, lateral and major and minor alar nasal cartilages (11.3, 4), connected to each other and to nearby bones by the continuity of the perichondrium and periosteum. These junctions, though of much interest, have attracted little attention; the cartilages with their intervening connective tissue, which collectively surround the nares, may be regarded as a valve controlling the intake of air (Cottle 1960; Galindo et al 1977).

Septal cartilage (11.3, 4). Almost quadrilateral in side view, this is thicker around its perimeter than at its centre. It forms almost the whole of the septum between the anterior parts of the nasal cavity. Its anterosuperior margin is connected above to the posterior border of the internasal suture; the middle part is continuous with the lateral cartilages, and its lowest part is attached to these cartilages by perichondrium. Its antero-inferior border is connected on each side

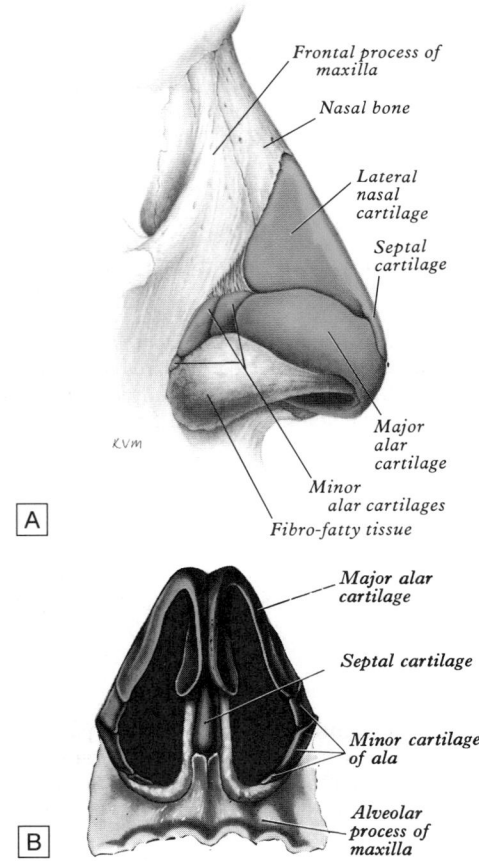

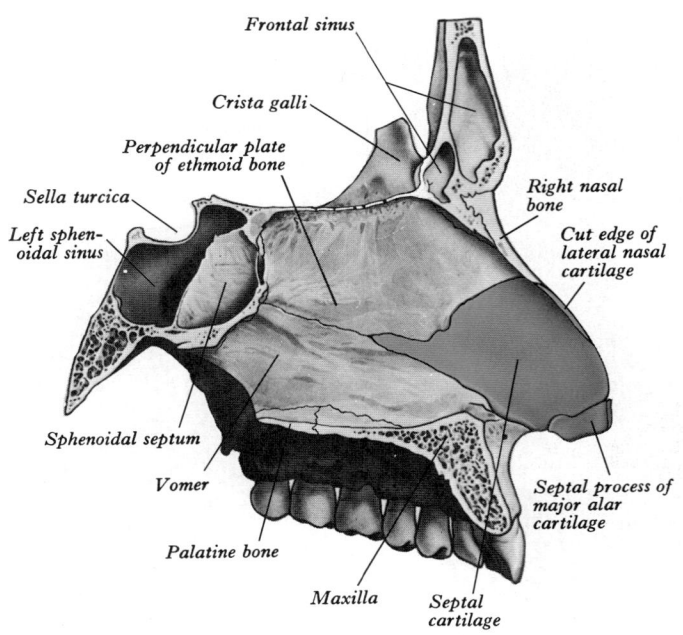

11.3 A The cartilages of the right side of the nose: lateral aspect. B The cartilages of the nose: inferior aspect. Note changes in terminology.

11.4 The right side of the septum of the nose, showing its constituent bones and cartilages. Note the changes in terminology.

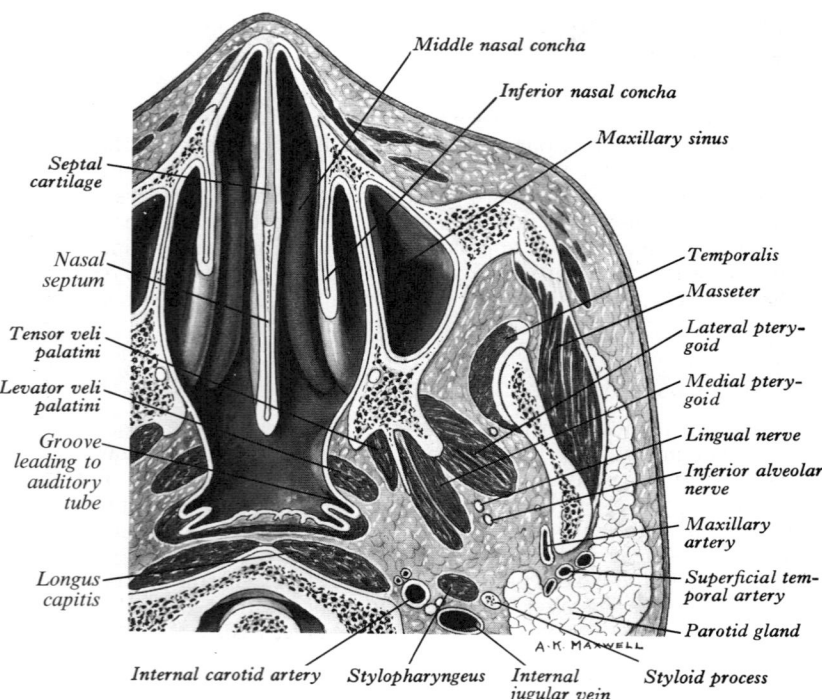

11.5 A transverse section through the anterior part of the head at a level just inferior to the apex of the odontoid process: inferior aspect.

with the septal process of the major alar cartilage. Galindo et al 1977 suggest that the two lateral and septal cartilages should be regarded as a unit, the *septodorsal cartilage*, an older term used in the Jena *Nomina Anatomica*.) Its posterosuperior border joins the perpendicular plate of the ethmoid; its postero-inferior border is attached to the vomer and to the nasal crest and anterior nasal spine of the maxilla. The septal cartilage may extend back (especially in children) as a narrow *sphenoidal process* for some distance between the vomer and the perpendicular plate of the ethmoid. The antero-inferior part of the nasal septum between the nares is freely movable and, therefore, named the *septum mobile nasi*; it is formed by the septal processes of the major alar cartilages and skin and not by the main septal cartilage.

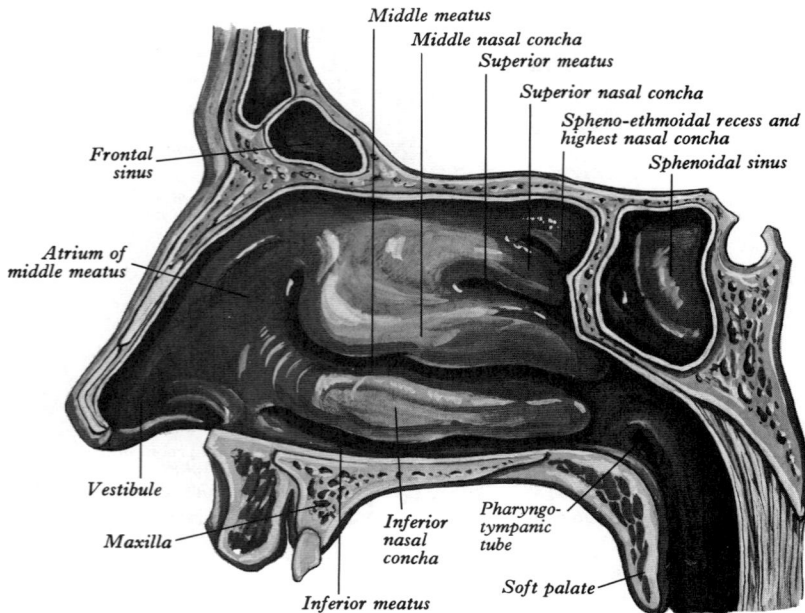

1632   **11.6**   The lateral wall of the right half of the nasal cavity: internal aspect.

Lateral (superior) nasal cartilage (**11**.3, 4). This plate of cartilage is triangular, its anterior margin being thicker than the posterior. Its upper part is continuous with the septal cartilage, but lower, more anteriorly, it is separated from it by a narrow fissure; its superior margin is attached to the nasal bone and frontal process of the maxilla and its inferior margin is connected by fibrous tissue to the major alar cartilage.

Major alar (inferior) cartilage (**11**.2, 3). A thin flexible plate lying below the lateral cartilage, it is curved acutely around the anterior part of its naris. Its medial part, the narrow *medial crus* (septal process), is loosely connected by fibrous tissue to its contralateral fellow and to the antero-inferior part of the septal cartilage, thus forming part of the septum mobile nasi. The *lateral crus*, situated lateral to the naris, is little more than the inferior border of the major alar cartilage. The upper border of the lateral part of the major alar cartilage is attached by fibrous tissue to the lower border of the lateral nasal cartilage. Its narrow posterior end is connected to the frontal process of the maxilla by a tough fibrous membrane containing three or four **minor cartilages of the ala** (**11**.2, 3). According to Drumheller (1969) the junction between the major alar and the lateral cartilages is variable; the two edges may abut or overlap, the lateral cartilage being then the more lateral at the junction. The lower edge (lateral crus) of the major cartilage is shorter than the lateral margin of the naris, the lower part of the ala nasi being fibro-adipose tissue covered by skin. In front, the major alar cartilages are separated by a notch palpable at the tip of the nose. The muscles acting on the external nose are described on page 792.

Nasal skin

The skin covering the nose is thin and loosely connected to the underlying structures. Over the apex and alae it is thicker and more adherent and bears numerous large sebaceous glands, their orifices usually being very distinct.

Vessels and nerves of the external nose

The **arteries** of the nose are the alar and septal branches of the facial artery, supplying the alae and lower septum; the dorsal nasal branch of the ophthalmic artery and infraorbital branch of the maxillary artery supply the lateral aspects and the dorsum.

The **veins** end in the facial and ophthalmic veins.

The **nerves**: motor nerves for the nasal muscles are buccal branches of the facial nerve (p. 1243); the skin receives sensory branches from the ophthalmic nerve through the infratrochlear and external nasal branches of the nasociliary nerve (p. 1233) and from the nasal branch of the infraorbital ramus of the maxillary nerve.

NASAL CAVITY

The nasal cavity is divided sagittally into right and left halves by the nasal septum (**11**.5, 9). These two halves open on the face through the nares and are continuous posteriorly with the nasopharynx through the posterior nasal apertures. The *nares* are ellipsoid or piriform, narrower in front; each one measures 1.5–2 cm antero-posteriorly and 0.5–1 cm transversely. The *posterior nasal apertures* (*choanae*) are two oval openings, each about 2.5 cm in vertical height and 1.3 cm transversely (**12**.65).

For details of nasal skeletal structures, see page 574. Each half of the nasal cavity has a *floor*, *roof* and a *lateral* and *medial* (*septal*) *wall*. It is divisible into three regions: the nasal vestibule anteriorly, the respiratory region and the (chemosensory) olfactory area; the vestibule forms the beginning of the nasal cavity anteriorly; the respiratory region constitutes the majority of the nasal cavity, while the limited and variable olfactory area is confined mainly to its posterosuperior parts.

Nasal vestibule

The nasal vestibule is a slightly expanded anterior part of the air passage just inside the naris (**11**.6, 7), bounded laterally by the ala and lateral part of the lower nasal cartilage, and medially by the septal process of this cartilage; the vestibule extends as a small recess towards the apex of the nose. Its lumen is lined with skin, the inferior region bearing sebaceous and sweat glands, and coarse hairs (vibrissae) curving towards the naris and helping to arrest the passage of particles in inspired air. In males, after middle age, these hairs

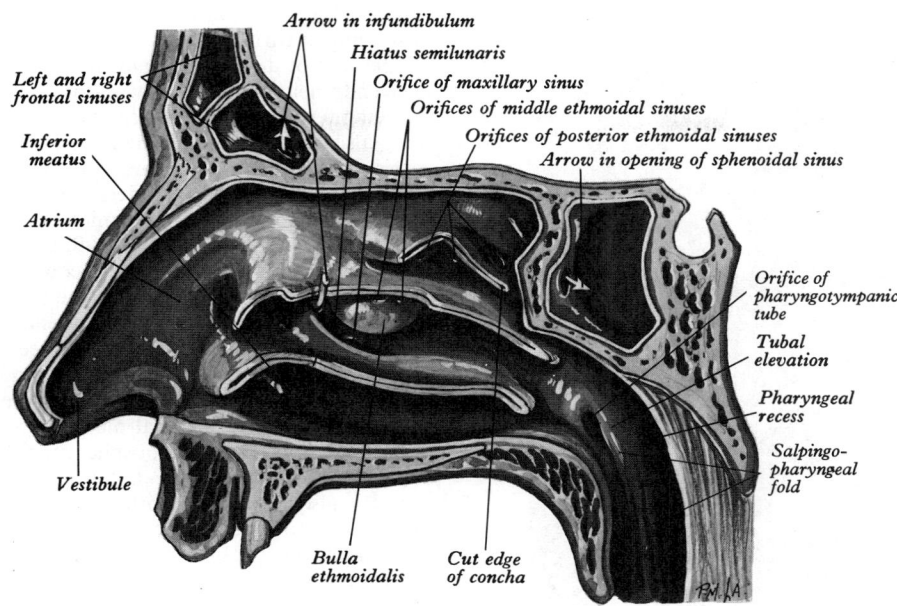

11.7 The lateral wall of the right half of the nasal cavity; the three nasal conchae have been partially removed.

increase considerably in size. The vestibule is limited above and behind by a curved ridge, the *limen nasi*, corresponding to the upper margin of the major alar cartilage; at this demarcation, the skin of the vestibule is continuous with the nasal mucosa.

Respiratory region

Lateral wall (**11.6, 7**). This wall of the main nasal cavity shows three elevations: the *superior, middle* and *inferior nasal conchae*, inferolateral to each being a corresponding passage or *meatus*. Above the superior concha the triangular *spheno-ethmoidal recess* bears the opening of the sphenoidal sinus; sometimes a fourth concha, the *highest nasal concha*, appears on the lateral wall of this recess (**11.6**), the passage immediately beneath it then being termed the *supreme nasal meatus*, sometimes displaying an opening of a posterior ethmoidal sinus. The *superior meatus* is a short oblique passage extending about halfway along the upper border of the middle concha; the posterior ethmoidal sinuses open, usually by one aperture, into its anterior part. The *middle meatus*, which is deeper in front than behind, lies below and lateral to the middle concha and continues anteriorly into a shallow fossa above the vestibule, termed the *atrium of the middle meatus*.

Above the atrium an ill-defined curved ridge, the *agger nasi* (p. 600), slopes downwards and forwards from the upper end of the anterior free border of the middle concha; it is better developed in the newborn than in adults. The middle concha must be displaced to display the lateral wall of the middle meatus fully. The main features of this wall are a rounded elevation, the *bulla ethmoidalis*, and below it and extending up in front of it, a curved cleft, the *hiatus semilunaris*. The bulla ethmoidalis is formed by the expansion of the middle ethmoidal sinuses, which open on or just above it, its size varying with the contained sinuses. The hiatus semilunaris, bounded inferiorly by a sharp concave ridge produced by the ethmoid bone's uncinate process, leads forwards and up into a curved channel, the *ethmoidal infundibulum*; the anterior ethmoidal sinuses open into it and in 50% or more of subjects it is continuous with the *frontonasal duct* from the frontal sinus; otherwise the infundibulum ends blindly in front in one or more anterior ethmoidal sinuses (*infundibular sinuses*) and the frontonasal duct then opens directly into the anterior end of the middle meatus. The *opening of the maxillary sinus* lies below the bulla, usually hidden by the flange-like lower edge of the hiatus; this opening is near the roof of the sinus (**11.9**); an accessory opening of the maxillary sinus frequently exists inferoposterior to the hiatus. The *inferior meatus*, below and lateral to the inferior concha, contains the opening of the nasolacrimal duct under cover of the anterior end of the inferior concha.

Medial wall or nasal septum (**11.4**). It is often deflected from the midline, making the nasal chambers unequal in size; ridges or spurs of bone sometimes project from the septum on either side. Above the incisive canals at the lower edge of the septal cartilage there is sometimes a depression which points down and forwards, occupying the position of the nasopalatine canal, connecting the nasal and buccal cavities in early fetal life. On each side of the septum near this recess a minute orifice may be seen leading back into a blind tubule, 2–6 mm long, the vestigial *vomeronasal organ* (p. 1321), supported by a vomeronasal cartilage; it is lined by a single layer of tall columnar cells and contains many glands. It is a prominent sensory organ in amphibians and reptiles, moderately developed in most mammals including New World monkeys but is vestigial in adult primates (Graziadei 1974); in species having a functional vomeronasal organ, it is a chemosensory structure similar to the olfactory epithelium, being connected to the accessory olfactory bulb by the vomeronasal nerve (see p. 1321).

Nasal roof. Narrow transversely, except posteriorly, from behind forwards it can be divided into *sphenoidal, ethmoidal* and *frontonasal* regions (pp. 280, 554), corresponding to the bones participating in its formation. The ethmoidal part is almost horizontal, the frontonasal part slopes down and forwards, and the sphenoidal portion is inclined downwards and backwards. The nasal cavity is therefore deepest under the cribriform plate of the ethmoid.

Nasal floor. It is transversely concave, anteroposteriorly flat and almost horizontal; its anterior three-quarters is formed by the palatine process of the maxilla and the rest, behind, by the horizontal part of the palatine bone. About 2 cm behind its anterior end a slight depression in the mucosa marks the position of the underlying incisive canals.

Nasal conchae. These add greatly to the surface area of the nasal cavity, which increases the turbulence of inhaled air, perhaps improving olfaction by slowing the passage of air past the area olfactoria. Humidification and warming of the inhaled air are also augmented by the increased mucosal area and turbulence, even in a microsomatic mammal such as man (Cole 1954). Swirling currents also aid the trapping of particles by mucous secretion. In many mammals the conchae are large and highly elaborate structures and the olfactory area spreads over much of their superior and medial surfaces, producing a highly developed olfactory system (Negus 1958; see also p. 1634).

Olfactory area. This is limited to the superior nasal concha, the opposed part of the septum and the intervening roof. It contains the sensory terminals of the olfactory nerve (see below and p. 1315).

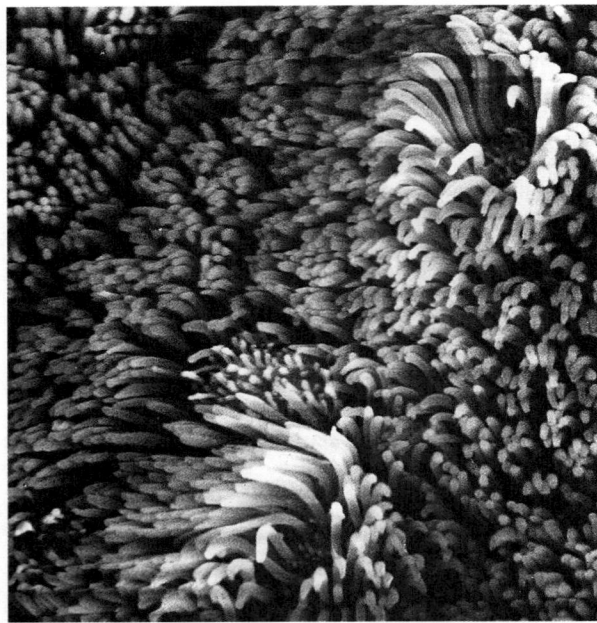

11.8 Scanning electron micrograph of the ciliated surface of the respiratory nasal epithelium. Rat; magnification × 5000.

MICROSTRUCTURE OF THE NASAL LINING

The lining of the anterior part of the nasal cavity and vestibule is continuous with the skin, consisting of keratinized stratified squamous epithelium overlying a connective tissue lamina propria. Further posteriorly, at the limen nasi, this grades into a mucosa lined at first by non-keratinizing stratified squamous epithelium, then by pseudostratified ciliated (respiratory) epithelium which forms most of the surface of the nasal cavity, i.e. the conchae, meatuses, floor and roof, except where the olfactory epithelium is present. The latter occupies the olfactory region over the upper 1 cm or so of the upper posterior part of the septum and superior concha, with the lateral wall above it; here the mucosa has a distinctive yellowish colour, and the epithelium contains the olfactory receptor cells which give rise to the olfactory nerves.

The nasal mucosa has numerous underlying glands within its lamina propria, and is adherent to the periosteum or perichondrium of the neighbouring skeletal structures. The respiratory mucosa is continuous with the following: the nasopharyngeal mucosa through posterior nasal apertures, the conjunctiva through the nasolacrimal duct and lacrimal canaliculi and the mucosae of the sphenoidal, ethmoidal, frontal and maxillary sinuses through their openings. The mucosa is thickest and most vascular over the conchae, especially at their extremities, and also on the nasal septum, but is very thin in the meatuses, on the floor and in the sinuses. Its thickness reduces materially the volume of the nasal cavity and its apertures.

Respiratory epithelium (11.8)

As already indicated, most of the non-olfactory regions of the nasal cavity are covered by pseudostratified epithelium consisting of ciliated columnar or cuboidal epithelial cells interspersed with goblet cells, non-ciliated columnar cells with microvilli, and basal cells (Mygind 1975, 1978), collectively termed the respiratory epithelium (Negus 1958). This epithelium also extends through the apertures of the paranasal sinuses to form their linings. In some areas cells may be low columnar or cuboidal, and the proportion of ciliated to non-ciliated cells is variable. The epithelium lies on a thin basal lamina, and beneath this are clustered groups of serous and mucous glands of variable cytological detail and secretory contents, many of them opening by confluent ducts on to the epithelial surface. Within the lamina propria, cavernous vascular tissue with large venous sinusoids is generally extensive (see below) and local vascular changes, for example, due to vasomotor autonomic innervation, can alter the

thickness and contours of the mucosal surfaces, a change visible as a swelling or shrinkage of the nasal lining, and resulting in alterations in the rate of airflow through the passages which the mucosa lines. The endothelium in these cavernous regions is particularly interesting in being fenestrated; the muscular walls of their supplying arterioles may also be under endocrine as well as neural control, providing a basis for cyclical fluctuations in their blood pressure and degree of enlargement (Cauna & Hinderer 1969; Cauna et al 1972). Beneath the epithelium and its basal lamina is a fibrous layer infiltrated with lymphocytes which often form diffuse lymphoid tissue, under which is a nearly continuous layer of mucous and serous glands, their ducts traversing the lymphoid layer to the surface. Abundant mucus from glands and goblet cells makes the surface sticky and dust in the inspired air is deposited on the surface, while the air is humidified and warmed. The mucous film is continually moved by ciliary action backwards into the nasopharynx at a rate of about 6 mm per minute (Proctor et al 1978). Palatal movements transfer the mucus and its entrapped particles to the oropharynx for swallowing, but some also enters the nasal vestibule anteriorly. The secretions of the nasal mucosa also serve many other functions, as they contain the bacteriocides lysozyme and lactoferrin, and also immunoglobulins (IgA), to inhibit the proliferation of microbes in this very susceptible environment. The mucus may also play a part in olfactory sensation; it has been shown in several species of mammals that groups of glands situated anteriorly in the nasal cavity secrete mucus containing distinctive odorant-binding proteins which are thought to be important in presenting odours to the receptors in the area olfactoria. In the walls of the sinuses the epithelium is closely bound to the underlying periosteum to form a combined mucoperiosteum.

Olfactory epithelium

The area olfactoria is covered with a sensory epithelium much thicker than that of the respiratory mucosa, containing the cell bodies of bipolar olfactory receptor cells, interspersed with non-sensory supporting cells. The apical dendrite of each receptor cell reaches the epithelial surface where it bears a group of long cilia; the trailing ends of these form a complex meshwork in the surface mucus and present a relatively enormous area of sensory membrane for the detection of odorants. Each receptor gives off a basal axon, and these collect together in the connective tissue beneath the epithelium as fasciculi of the olfactory nerve; mucus-secreting subepithelial glands (of Bowman) are also present in this layer. Further details of these structures are given on pages 1320 et seq.

VESSELS AND NERVES OF THE NASAL CAVITY

Vessels

Arteries. These arise as branches of the ophthalmic, maxillary and facial which supply different territories within its walls, floor and roof, and ramify to form anastomotic plexuses within and deep to the nasal mucosa; anastomoses also occur between some larger arterial branches. Their principal distributions are as follows:

- The anterior and posterior ethmoidal branches of the ophthalmic artery supply the ethmoidal and frontal sinuses and nasal roof.
- The sphenopalatine branch of the maxillary artery supplies the mucosa of the conchae, meatuses and septum.
- The terminal part of the greater palatine artery (from the maxillary artery) ascends through the incisive canal to anastomose with a branch of the sphenopalatine artery (p. 1521).
- The septal branch of the superior labial ramus of the facial artery supplies the septum in the region of the vestibule, and anastomoses with the sphenopalatine artery; this is a common site of bleeding from the nose (epistaxis).
- The infraorbital, superior anterior and posterior alveolar branches of the maxillary artery supply the mucosa of the maxillary sinus.
- The pharyngeal branch of the maxillary artery distributes to the sphenoidal sinus.

Veins. These form a rich submucosal cavernous plexus which is especially dense in the lower part of the septum and in the middle and inferior conchae; arteriovenous anastomoses also occur (Harper 1947). Venous drainage is into the sphenopalatine vein, facial vein

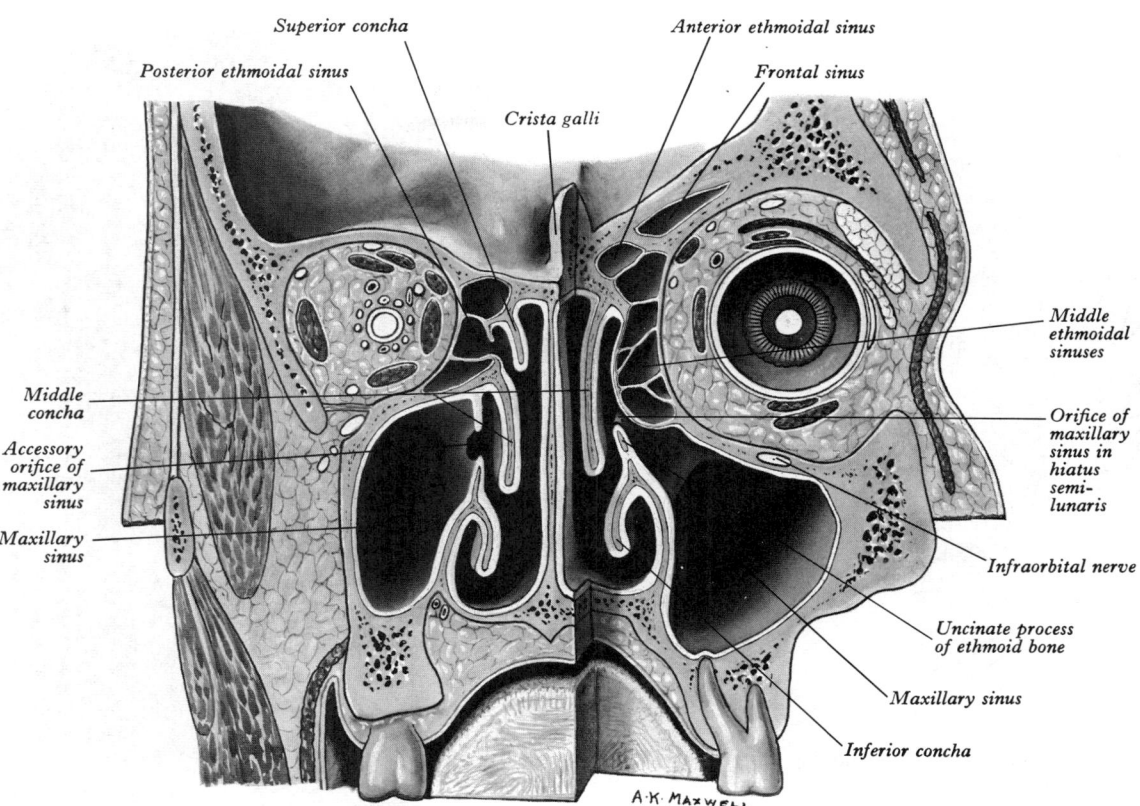

Superior concha

Posterior ethmoidal sinus

Crista galli

Anterior ethmoidal sinus

Frontal sinus

Middle concha

Accessory orifice of maxillary sinus

Maxillary sinus

Middle ethmoidal sinuses

Orifice of maxillary sinus in hiatus semi-lunaris

Infraorbital nerve

Uncinate process of ethmoid bone

Maxillary sinus

Inferior concha

A·K· MAXWELL

11.9 A coronal section through the nasal cavity, viewed from the posterior aspect. On the right side the plane of the section is more anterior. The normal orifice of the maxillary sinus is shown on the right side and the not uncommon accessory orifice on the left side.

and the ophthalmic veins (accompanying the ethmoidal arteries en route); a few veins pass through the cribriform plate to connect with those on the orbital surface of the brain's frontal lobes. When the foramen caecum is patent it transmits a vein from the nasal cavity to the superior sagittal sinus.

Lymphatic vessels. These are described on page 1612.

Innervation

The nerves include sensory branches of the trigeminal and olfactory nerves and autonomic vasomotor and secretomotor fasciculi.

Nerves of ordinary sensation (8.334). These are all derived from the maxillary nerve, except for a contribution from the nasociliary branch of the ophthalmic nerve. They are:

- the anterior ethmoidal branch of the nasociliary nerve, supplying the anterior and upper parts of the septum, the anterior part of the roof, the anterior parts of the middle and inferior conchae with the lateral wall anterior to these;
- the infraorbital nerve, supplying the nasal vestibule;
- the anterior superior alveolar nerve, supplying part of the septum and the floor near the anterior nasal spine and the anterior part of the lateral wall as high as the opening of the maxillary sinus;
- the lateral posterior superior nasal and medial posterior superior nasal nerves (including the nasopalatine nerve) which are branches from the pterygopalatine ganglion, and the posterior inferior nasal branches of the anterior palatine nerve, together supplying the posterior three-quarters of the lateral wall, roof, floor and septum;
- branches from the nerve of the pterygoid canal to the upper and posterior part of the roof and septum.

These various branches mediate the sensations of touch, pain and temperature but also include trigeminal fibres, close to and within the epithelial layer, sensitive to noxious chemicals, for example, ammonia and sulphur dioxide, which may therefore be perceived even when the olfactory nerves have been lost.

Olfactory nerves. Arising from the sensory cells of the area olfactoria, they form a meshwork of unmyelinated fasciculi, giving the appearance of a plexus within the mucosa; they then ascend in grooves or canals within the ethmoid bone, and pass into the cranial cavity through the foramina of the cribriform plate to unite with the inferior surface of the olfactory bulb (see p. 1317). Closely associated with the olfactory nerves are the *nervi terminales* (p. 1321).

Autonomic nerves. These accompany the sensory innervation. They include *sympathetic postganglionic vasomotor fibres* to the nasal blood vessels, and *postganglionic parasympathetic fibres* from the pterygopalatine ganglion, providing the secretomotor supply to the nasal glands.

PARANASAL SINUSES (11.5, 6, 8–11)

Paranasal sinuses include the bilaterally paired *frontal, ethmoidal, sphenoidal* and *maxillary sinuses*, housed within the bones from which they are named. The ethmoidal sinuses differ from the others in being formed of small multiple cavities, divisible into *anterior, middle and posterior groups*. All sinuses open into the lateral wall of the nasal cavity by small apertures which allow the equilibration of air and movement of mucus; the detailed position of these apertures, and indeed of the precise form and sizes of the sinuses, vary between individuals. Their mucosa is continuous with that of the nasal cavity (a feature unfortunately favouring the spread of infections), and is similar histologically although thinner, less vascular and less adherent to bone. Mucus is secreted by glands within their mucosa and is swept through their apertures into the nose by cilia; these are not uniformly distributed but are always present near the apertures of the sinuses. Most sinuses are rudimentary or absent at birth; they enlarge appreciably during the eruption of the permanent teeth and after puberty, markedly altering the size and shape of the face at these times.

Frontal sinuses

The paired frontal sinuses, situated posterior to the superciliary arches, lie between the outer and inner tables of the frontal bone. Each usually underlies a triangular area on the surface, its angles formed by the nasion, a point 3 cm above the nasion and the junction of the medial third and lateral two-thirds of the supraorbital margin

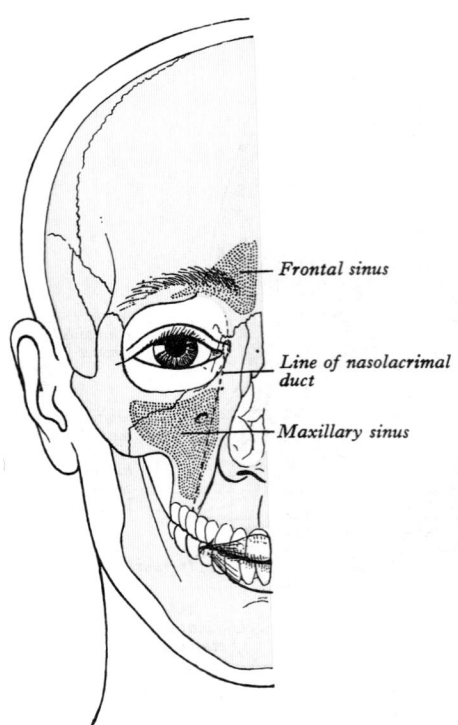

11.10 An outline of the bones of the face, showing the positions of the frontal and maxillary sinuses.

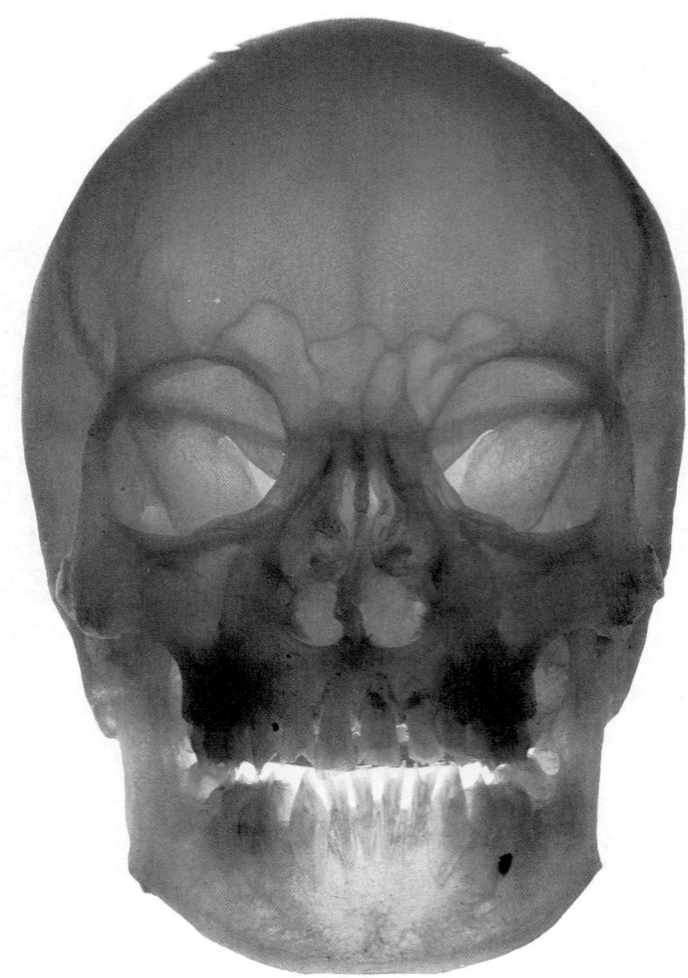

11.11 The skull of an adult woman which has been decalcified and then cleared in methyl salicylate; the specimen was transilluminated and then photographed from the ventral aspect. Note particularly the profiles of the frontal and maxillary paranasal air sinuses, the orbits and superior orbital fissures and the nasal cavities and conchae. (The specimen was prepared by D. H. Tompsett of the Royal College of Surgeons of England.)

(**6**.152, **11**.9–11). The two sinuses are rarely symmetrical, the septum between them usually deviating from the median plane. Their average measurements are: height 3.2 cm; breadth 2.6 cm; depth 1.8 cm. Each extends upwards above the medial part of the eyebrow and back into the medial part of the roof of the orbit. The frontal sinus is sometimes divided into a number of communicating recesses by incomplete bony septa. Rarely, one or both sinuses may be absent, but the prominence of the superciliary arches is no indication of presence or size of the frontal sinuses. The part of the sinus extending upwards in the frontal bone may be small and the orbital part large, or vice versa. Sometimes one sinus may overlap in front of the other. A sinus may extend posteriorly as far as the lesser wing of the sphenoid bone but does not invade it.

The *aperture* of each frontal sinus opens into the anterior part of the corresponding nasal middle meatus by the *ethmoidal infundibulum* or through the *frontonasal duct*, traversing the anterior part of the ethmoid labyrinth (see also p. 597). Rudimentary or absent at birth, the frontal sinuses are generally well developed between the seventh and eighth years but reach full size only after puberty (p. 595). They are more prominent in males, giving the forehead an obliquity contrasting with the vertical or convex profile typical of children and females.

Vessels and nerve supply. Their **arterial supply** is from the supraorbital and anterior ethmoidal arteries and their **venous drainage** is into the anastomotic vein in the supraorbital notch connecting the supraorbital and superior ophthalmic veins. **Lymphatic drainage** is to the submandibular nodes. The **nerve supply** is from the supraorbital nerve.

Ethmoidal sinuses (11.8; see also 6.139, 180B, 182A)

Ethmoidal sinuses are small, thin-walled cavities in the ethmoidal labyrinth, completed by the frontal, maxillary, lacrimal, sphenoid and palatine bones (see pp. 585, 603). They range from three large to 18 small sinuses on each side, and their openings into the nasal cavity are also very variable in position. They lie between the upper part of the nasal cavity and the orbit, separated from the latter by the paper-thin orbital plate of the ethmoid, a poor barrier to infection which may spread into the orbit to give orbital cellulitis. The ethmoidal sinuses consist of *anterior*, *middle* and *posterior* groups on each side. (Some anatomists recognize only an anterior and a

posterior group, the anterior including those described here as anterior and middle.) The groups are not sharply delimited from each other, and one may encroach on territory usually occupied by another. They are, however, distinguished by their sites of communication with the nasal cavity. In each group the sinuses are only partially separated by incomplete bony septa.

Anterior group (the infundibular sinuses). These number up to 11 and open into the ethmoidal infundibulum or the frontonasal duct by one or more orifices; one sinus often lies in the agger nasi while the most anterior ethmoidal sinus may encroach on the frontal sinus.

Middle group (bullar sinuses). Usually three in number, they open into the middle meatus by one or more orifices on or above the ethmoidal bulla.

Posterior group. Varying from one to seven, they usually open by a single orifice into the superior meatus inferior to the superior concha, though one may open into the highest meatus (when present) and one or more into the sphenoidal sinus. The posterior group lies very close to the optic canal and optic nerve. The ethmoidal sinuses are small though of clinical importance at birth, and grow rapidly between 6 and 8 years and after puberty.

Vessels and nerves. The **arterial supply** is from the spheno-palatine artery (p. 1521) and the anterior and posterior ethmoidal arteries; their **venous drainage** is by the corresponding veins. The **lymphatics** of the anterior and middle groups drain to the submandibular nodes, and those of the posterior group to the retro-pharyngeal nodes.

The **innervation** is from the anterior and posterior ethmoidal nerves (sensory supply), and from orbital branches of the pterygopalatine ganglion (parasympathetic secretomotor fibres).

Sphenoidal sinuses (11.7; see also 6.171, 183)

The paired sphenoidal sinuses (p. 586) are sited posterior to the upper part of the nasal cavity, within the body of the sphenoid bone. They are related above to the optic chiasma and hypophysis cerebri and on each side to the internal carotid artery and cavernous sinus. If the sinuses are small, they lie anterior to the hypophysis cerebri. They vary in size and shape and are rarely symmetrical, one often being much larger and extending across the median plane behind the other; occasionally one overlaps above and, rarely, they intercommunicate. One or both may approach closely to the optic canal or even partly encircle it. Their average measurements are: vertical height 2 cm; transverse breadth 1.8 cm; anteroposterior depth 2.1 cm. They may extend, if exceptionally large, into the roots of the pterygoid processes or the greater wings of the sphenoid, and they may invade the basilar part of the occipital bone. Gaps in their osseous walls may occasionally leave their mucosa in contact with the overlying dura mater. Bony ridges, produced by the internal carotid artery or pterygoid canal, may project into the sinuses from their lateral walls and floor respectively. A posterior ethmoidal sinus may invade the sphenoid and largely replace a sphenoidal sinus. The aperture of each sphenoidal sinus opens into the corresponding spheno-ethmoidal recess high in its anterior wall.

Vessels and nerve supply. At birth the sinuses are minute cavities, and their main development occurs after puberty. Their **arterial supply** is via the posterior ethmoidal artery and **venous drainage** through the corresponding vein; **lymph drainage** is to the retropharyngeal nodes and the **nerve supply** arises from the posterior ethmoidal nerves (sensory) and orbital branches of the pterygopalatine ganglion (parasympathetic secretomotor).

Maxillary sinuses (11.5, 7, 9–11; see also 6.186)

The paired maxillary sinuses, occupying most of the bodies of the maxillae are the largest accessory air sinuses of the nose. Pyramidal in shape, they have a base formed by the lateral wall of the nasal cavity, and the apex extends laterally into the zygomatic process of the maxilla. The roof is the floor of the orbit, frequently ridged by the overlying infraorbital canal; the floor is formed by the maxilla's alveolar process and is usually about 1.5 cm below the level of the nasal floor, on a line drawn laterally from the lower border of the ala. Several conical elevations corresponding to the roots of the first and second molar teeth project into the floor, which they sometimes perforate. The roots of the first and second premolars and third molar, and occasionally the canine root, may also project into the sinus (p. 1719). The size of the sinus varies, even on the two sides of an individual skull; when large, its apex may invade the zygomatic bone. Average measurements are: vertical height opposite the first molar 3.5 cm; transverse breadth 2.5 cm; anteroposterior depth 3.2 cm. The sinus opens into the lowest part of the hiatus semilunaris by an aperture in the anterosuperior part of the sinus' base (11.7); a second orifice is frequently present in or just below the hiatus. Both are nearer the roof than the floor of the sinus. During early development, the sinus appears as a mere groove on the medial surface of the maxilla in the fourth prenatal month, and only reaches its full size after the eruption of all the permanent teeth.

Vessels and nerve supply. The **blood vessels** are the facial, infraorbital and greater palatine arteries and veins; **lymph drainage** is to the submandibular nodes and the **nerve supply** is derived from the infraorbital and the anterior, middle and posterior superior alveolar nerves.

Functions of the sinuses

The functions of the sinuses are uncertain and a matter of some speculation; they have been thought to add some resonance to the voice, and also to allow the enlargement of local areas of the skull whilst minimizing a corresponding increase in bony mass. It is likely that such growth-related changes serve to strengthen particular regions, for example the alveolar process of the maxilla when the secondary dentition erupts, but they may also have an important function in contouring the head to provide visual signals indicating the individual's status in a social context, for example gender, sexual maturity and group identity.

For details of the human and comparative anatomy of the paranasal sinuses consult Negus (1958).

RADIOLOGICAL APPEARANCES OF PARANASAL SINUSES

Normal sinuses are radiolucent, whereas when they are diseased they show varying degrees of opacity. In *anteroposterior views* (6.134B, 171) most of the sinuses are visible. The frontal sinuses appear above the nasal cavity and the medial part of the orbits; their asymmetry, vertical extent and the position of their septa can be assessed. The ethmoidal sinuses are superimposed on each other and on the sphenoidal sinuses in this view, lying between the orbits below the cribriform plate. The sphenoidal sinuses are obscured in this view. Each maxillary sinus is a pyramidal radiolucent area below the orbit and lateral to the lower part of the nasal cavity, extending inferiorly into the alveolar process of the maxilla. In *lateral views* (6.134A, 143B, 187), the extent of the frontal sinus both upwards into the frontal bone and back into the orbital roof can be assessed. The ethmoidal sinuses are seen to extend back from the frontal process of the maxilla as far as the sphenoidal sinus, which is clearly visible below and in front of the hypophyseal fossa, although the two sphenoidal sinuses appear superimposed; the individual sphenoidal sinuses are seen better from above. The maxillary sinus is clearly seen in a lateral view; it lies below the orbit and its relation to the roots of the teeth is obvious. Maxillary and frontal sinuses can also be transilluminated. In a dark room, a light is placed in the mouth, for the maxillary sinus or, for the frontal sinus, against the superomedial angle of the orbital opening. A red glow normally appears in the region of these sinuses, but may be absent when the sinuses are diseased. Both the frontal and maxillary sinuses show well in cleared preparations of the skull (11.9).

CLINICAL ANATOMY OF THE NOSE AND SINUSES

Congenital nasal deformities can occur, for example a complete absence of the external nose, with only an aperture existing, or else suppression or malformation on one side. The nasal septum may be displaced by injury or by some congenital defect; sometimes the deviation may be so great as to bring the septum and one lateral wall into contact, causing complete unilateral nasal obstruction.

Suppuration in the paranasal sinuses occurs frequently and pus from the frontal or anterior ethmoidal sinuses may run via the hiatus semilunaris into the maxillary sinus, which thus becomes a secondary reservoir for pus. All paranasal sinuses can be infected from the nasal cavity but a maxillary sinus infection may also spread from the teeth (p. 1719) and this sinus is most often chronically infected, resulting in the loss of mucosal cilia and an impaired flow of mucus. Because its opening is high above its floor, the natural drainage of the maxillary sinus is hindered but may be effected by puncture in the lateral wall of the inferior nasal meatus or through the canine fossa on the anterior surface of the maxilla, which is nearer to its floor.

LARYNX (11.2, 12–32)

The larynx, which is an air passage, a sphincteric device and an organ of phonation, extends from the tongue to the trachea (Terracol et al 1965; Fink & Demarest 1978). It projects ventrally between the great vessels of the neck and is covered anteriorly by skin, fasciae and the hyoid depressor muscles (11.19). Above, it opens into the laryngopharynx and forms its anterior wall; below, it continues into the trachea. In adult males it lies opposite the third to sixth cervical vertebrae, although it is somewhat higher in children and adult females. In infants between 6 and 12 months, the tip of the epiglottis (the highest part of the larynx) is a little above the junction of the dens and body of the axis vertebra. Its average measurements in European adults are:

	In males	In females
Length	44 mm	36 mm
Transverse diameter	43 mm	41 mm
Sagittal diameter	36 mm	26 mm

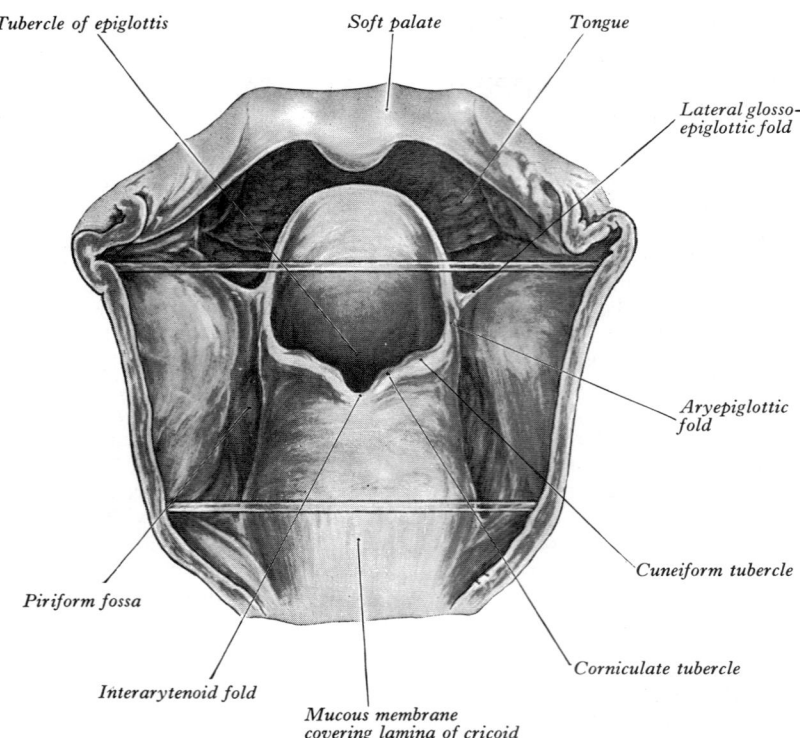

Tubercle of epiglottis

Soft palate

Tongue

Lateral glosso-
epiglottic fold

Aryepiglottic
fold

Cuneiform tubercle

Piriform fossa

Corniculate tubercle

Interarytenoid fold

Mucous membrane
covering lamina of cricoid

11.12 The inlet of the larynx, viewed from the posterior aspect. The posterior wall of the pharynx has been divided in the median plane and two glass rods have been inserted to keep the cut portions apart.

These figures are, of course, a rough indication of the general dimensions; for a much more extensive set of measurements, see Eckel et al 1994.

Until puberty the male and female larynges are similar in size, but afterwards the male larynx enlarges considerably in comparison with the female, all the cartilages increasing in size and the thyroid cartilage projecting in the anterior midline of the neck, while its sagittal diameter nearly doubles during this process. In males, the thyroid cartilage continues to increase in size until 40 years of age, after which no further growth occurs (Harjeet & Jit 1992).

SKELETON OF THE LARYNX (11.13–18)

Cartilages form the skeletal framework of the larynx. They are interconnected by ligaments and fibrous membranes, and moved by a number of muscles. The hyoid bone (p. 582) is also intimately associated with the larynx, although it is usually regarded as a separate structure with distinctive functional roles.

LARYNGEAL CARTILAGES

The laryngeal cartilages comprise the single cricoid, thyroid and epiglottic cartilages, and the paired arytenoid, cuneiform and corniculate cartilages. Also related to the larynx are the paired tritiate cartilages in the thyrohyoid ligaments on either side.

Cricoid cartilage

The cricoid cartilage (**11**.13–16, 20, 25) can be regarded as the skeletal foundation of the larynx, attached below to the trachea, and articulated by synovial joints to the thyroid cartilage and the two arytenoids. It forms a complete ring around the airway, the only laryngeal cartilage to do so. The cricoid is smaller but thicker and stronger than the thyroid cartilage and shaped like a signet ring (hence its name), with a narrow curved anterior *arch*, and a broad, flatter posterior *lamina*. Together these form the inferior parts of the anterior and lateral walls of the larynx and most of its posterior wall.

Cricoid lamina. This is approximately quadrilateral in outline, 2–3 cm in vertical dimension. It has a posterior median vertical ridge, to the upper part of which the two fasciculi of the longitudinal layer of oesophageal muscle fibres (muscularis externa) are attached by a

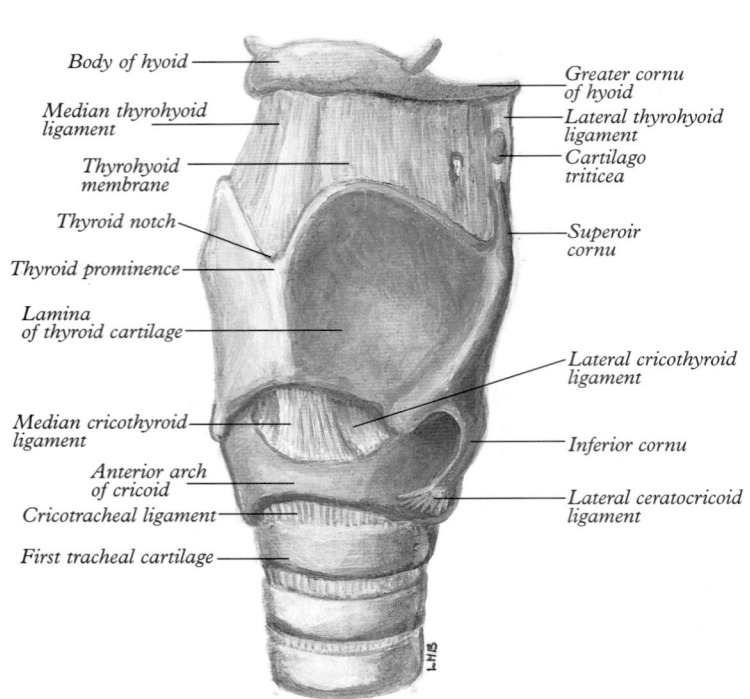

Body of hyoid

Median thyrohyoid
ligament

Thyrohyoid
membrane

Thyroid notch

Thyroid prominence

Lamina
of thyroid cartilage

Median cricothyroid
ligament

Anterior arch
of cricoid

Cricotracheal ligament

First tracheal cartilage

Greater cornu
of hyoid

Lateral thyrohyoid
ligament

Cartilago
triticea

Superoir
cornu

Lateral cricothyroid
ligament

Inferior cornu

Lateral ceratocricoid
ligament

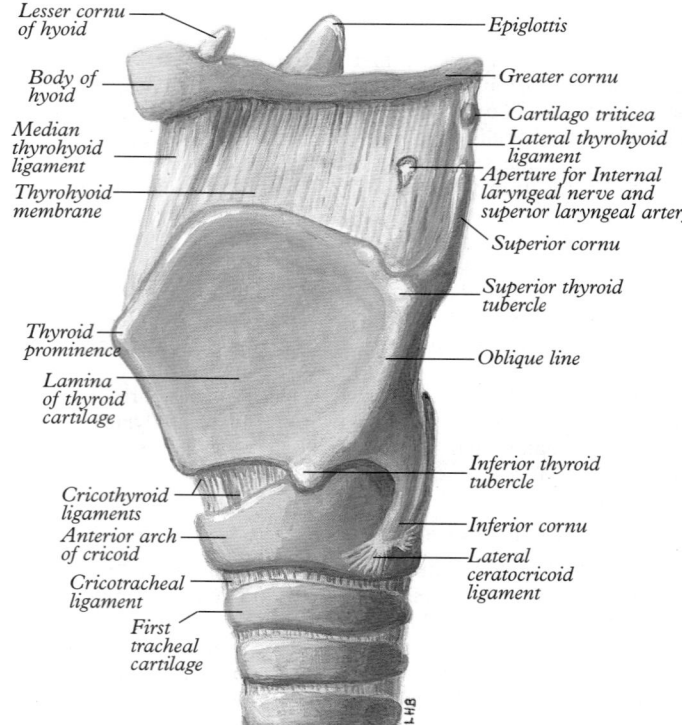

Lesser cornu
of hyoid

Body of
hyoid

Median
thyrohyoid
ligament

Thyrohyoid
membrane

Thyroid
prominence

Lamina
of thyroid
cartilage

Cricothyroid
ligaments

Anterior arch
of cricoid

Cricotracheal
ligament

First
tracheal
cartilage

Epiglottis

Greater cornu

Cartilago triticea

Lateral thyrohyoid
ligament

Aperture for Internal
laryngeal nerve and
superior laryngeal artery

Superior cornu

Superior thyroid
tubercle

Oblique line

Inferior thyroid
tubercle

Inferior cornu

Lateral
ceratocricoid
ligament

11.13A Anterolateral view of the laryngeal cartilages and ligaments.

11.13B Lateral view of the laryngeal cartilages and ligaments.

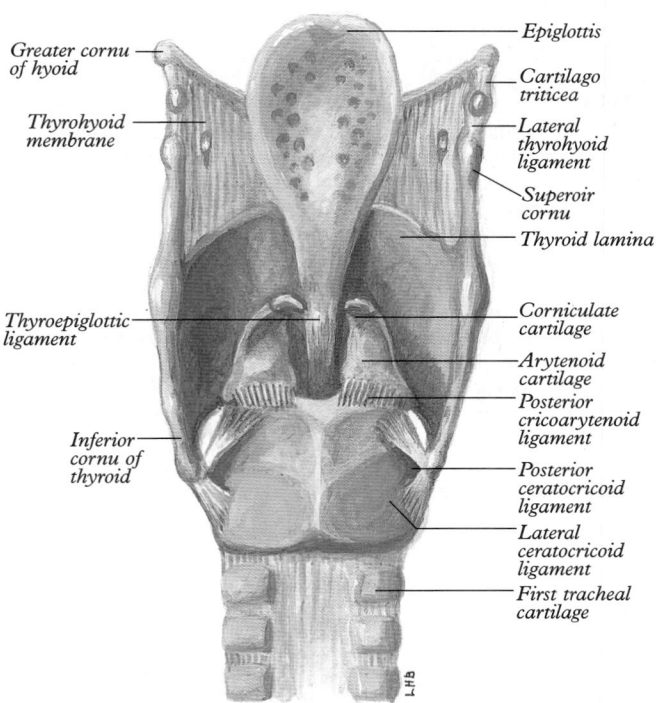

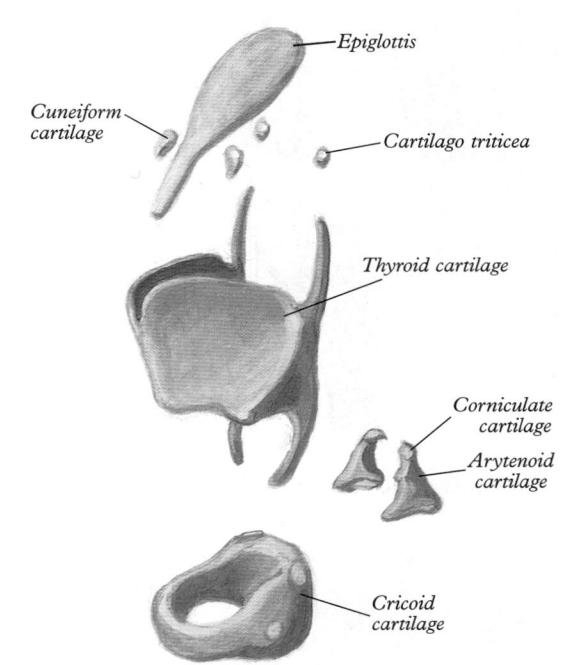

11.14 Posterior view of the cartilages and ligaments of the larynx.

11.15 Exploded view of the different cartilages of the larynx.

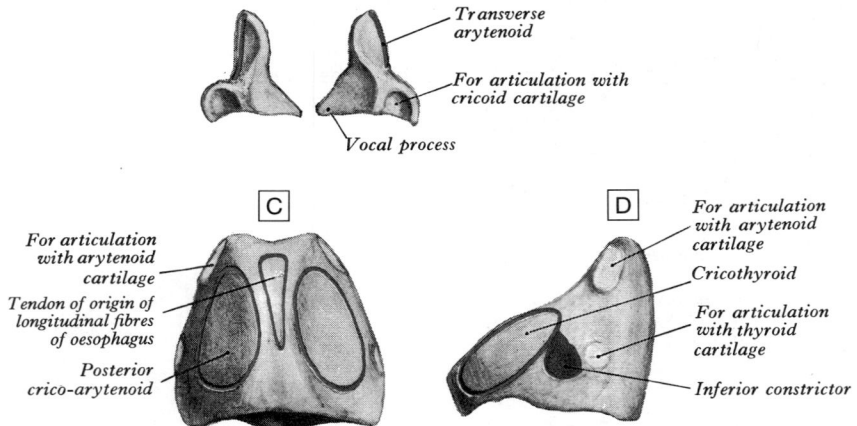

11.16 The arytenoid and cricoid cartilages. A The left arytenoid cartilage: medial aspect. B The right arytenoid cartilage: medial aspect. C The cricoid cartilage: posterior aspect. D The cricoid cartilage: left lateral aspect. Red = muscle attachments.

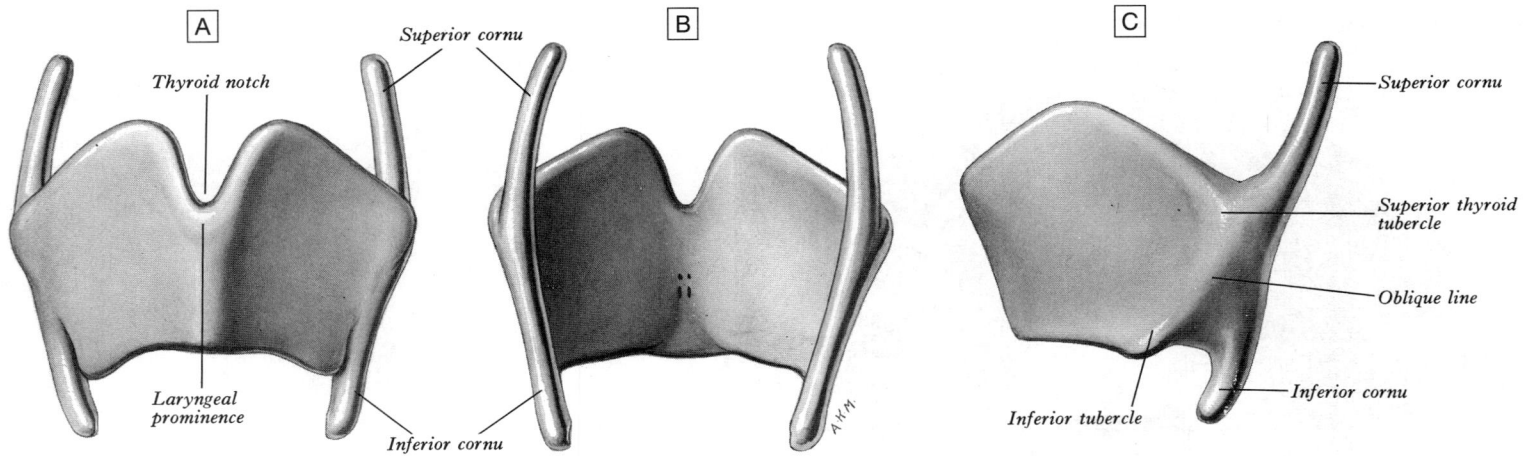

11.17 The thyroid cartilage. The attachments of the vestibular ligaments (above) and the vocal ligaments (below) are shown in B. A Anterior aspect. B Posterior aspect. C Lateral aspect.

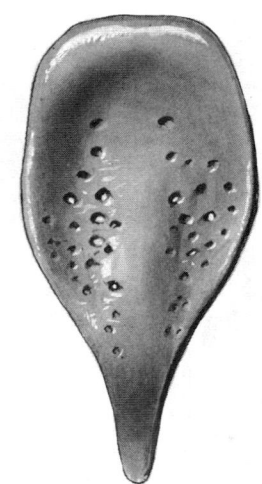

11.18   The epiglottis: posterior aspect. Note its pitted surface.

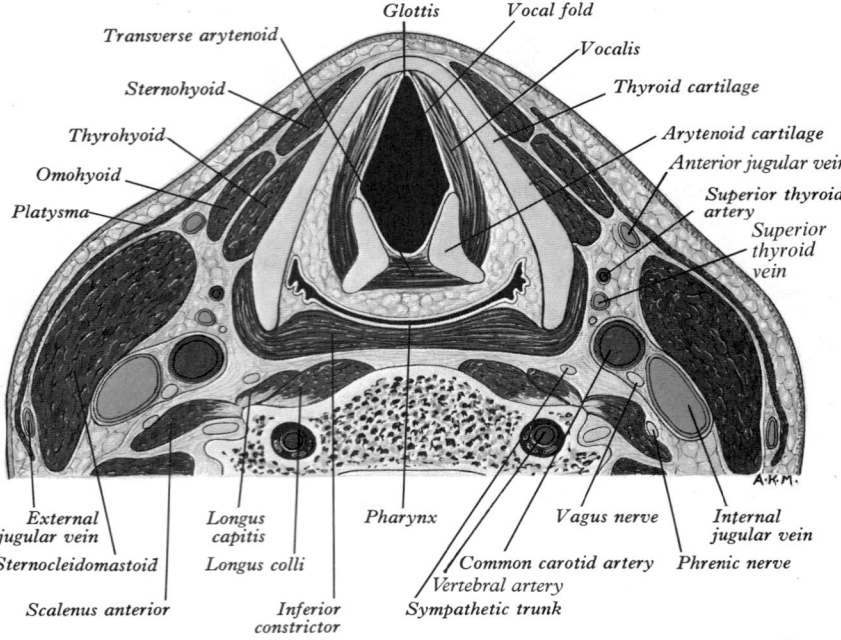

11.19   Transverse section across the ventral region of the neck at the level of the vocal folds: superior aspect.

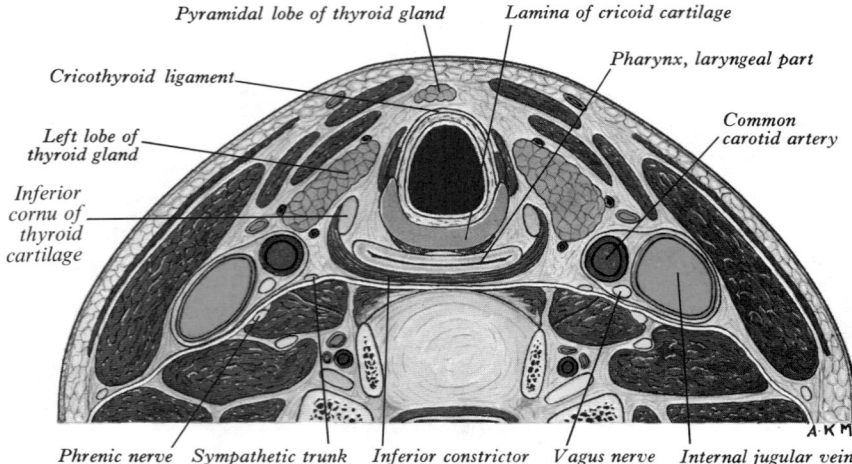

11.20   Transverse section through the ventral region of the neck, between the fifth and sixth cervical vertebrae: superior aspect (semi-diagrammatic).

tendon. Lateral to this are two shallow depressions for the fibres of the posterior crico-arytenoid muscle.

Cricoid arch. Vertically narrow in front (5–7 mm in height), it widens posteriorly towards the lamina. To the external aspect of its front and sides are attached the cricothyroid muscle and behind this, the cricopharyngeus part of the inferior pharyngeal constrictor. The arch is palpable below the laryngeal prominence, from which it is separated by a depression containing the resilient conus elasticus.

On each side of the cricoid, at the junction of the lamina and arch, a prominent circular synovial facet, facing posterolaterally, articulates with the inferior thyroid cornu. The *inferior border* of the cricoid is horizontal, and joined to the first tracheal cartilage by the *cricotracheal ligament*. The *superior border* of the cricoid runs obliquely up and back, giving attachment anteriorly to the thick median part of the cricothyroid ligament, and laterally to the membranous lateral parts of the cricothyroid ligament; here the lateral crico-arytenoid muscles are also attached. Posteriorly, this superior aspect of the lamina presents a shallow median notch, on each side of which is a smooth, oval, convex facet, directed upwards and laterally, articulating with the base of an arytenoid cartilage (see, however, Sellars & Keen 1978).

The *internal surface* of the cricoid cartilage is smooth and lined by mucosa.

Thyroid cartilage

The thyroid cartilage (**11**.10, 12, 13) is the largest of the laryngeal cartilages. It consists of two quadrilateral *laminae* whose anterior borders fuse along their inferior two-thirds at a median angle, forming the subcutaneous *laryngeal prominence* ('Adam's apple'). This projection is most distinct at its upper end, and is well marked in men but scarcely visible in women. Above, the laminae are separated by a V-shaped superior *thyroid notch* or *incisure*; posteriorly they diverge, the posterior borders of each being prolonged as slender horns, the *superior* and *inferior cornua*. On the external surface of each lamina a shallow ridge, the *oblique line*, curves downwards and forwards, running from the *superior thyroid tubercle* lying a little anterior to the root of the superior cornu, to the *inferior thyroid*

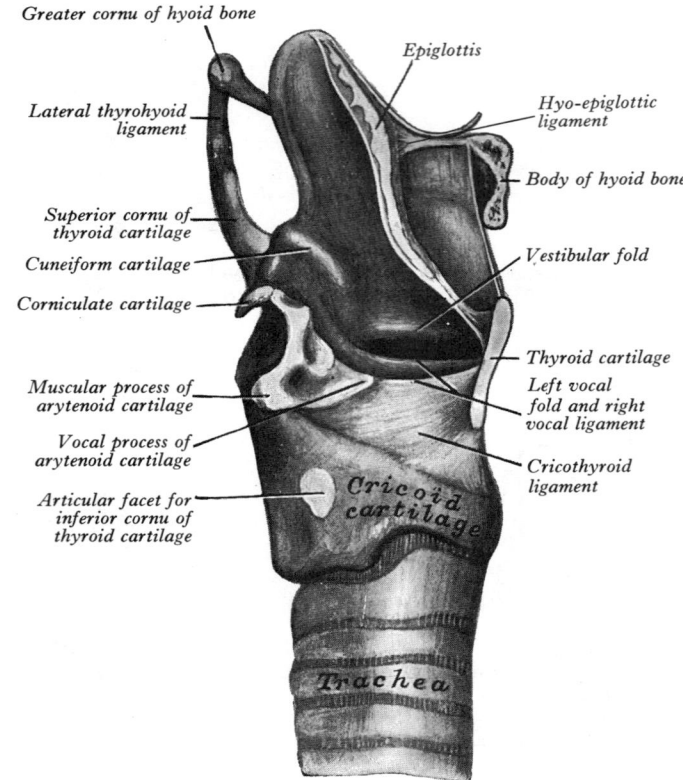

11.21   Dissection to show the right half of the cricothyroid ligament. The right lamina of the thyroid cartilage and the subjacent muscles have been removed.

tubercle on the inferior border of the lamina. To this line are attached the sternothyroid and thyrohyoid muscles, and the thyropharyngeus part of the inferior pharyngeal constrictor.

The *internal surface* of the lamina is smooth; above and behind, it is slightly concave and covered by mucosa. In the upper part of the angle between the laminae, the thyro-epiglottic ligament is attached; below this, near the midline, the paired vestibular and vocal ligaments and the thyro-arytenoid, thyro-epiglottic and vocal muscles are attached. The *superior border* of each lamina is concave behind and convex in front; the thyrohyoid membrane is attached along this edge. The *inferior border* of each is concave behind and nearly straight in front, the two parts separated by the *inferior thyroid tubercle*. In and on either side of the midline anteriorly, the thyroid cartilage is connected to the cricoid cartilage by the anterior (median) cricothyroid ligament (see p. 1642).

The *anterior border* of each lamina fuses with its partner at an angle of about 90° in men and about 120° in women. This shallower angle in men is associated with the larger laryngeal prominence, the greater length of the vocal folds and the resultant deeper pitch of voice. The *posterior border* is thick and rounded; it receives the fibres of stylopharyngeus and palatopharyngeus. The *superior cornu*, which is long and narrow, curves upwards, backwards and medially, ending in a conical apex to which the lateral thyrohyoid ligament is attached. The *inferior cornu*, short and thick, curves down and slightly antero-medially; on the medial surface of its lower end, a small oval facet articulates with the side of the cricoid cartilage. Some fibres of palatopharyngeus, stylopharyngeus and salpingopharyngeus are inserted into the posterior surface of the lamina and cornua.

During infancy a narrow, rhomboidal, flexible strip, the *intra-thyroid cartilage*, lies between the two laminae and is joined to them by fibrous tissue.

Arytenoid cartilages

The paired arytenoid cartilages (**11**.15, 16, 19, 22) are placed on the lateral part of the cricoid lamina's superior border at the back of the larynx. Each is pyramidal, with three surfaces, two processes, a base and an apex. The *posterior surface*, which is triangular, smooth

and concave, is covered by the transverse arytenoid muscle. The *anterolateral surface* is convex and rough; on it, near the apex of the cartilage, is an elevation from which a crest curves back, down and then forwards to the vocal process. The lower part of this crest separates two depressions (foveae), the upper being triangular, the lower oblong; to the upper is attached the vestibular ligament, to the lower the vocalis and lateral crico-arytenoid muscles. The *medial surface* is narrow, smooth, and flat; it is covered by mucosa and its lower edge forms the lateral boundary of the intercartilaginous part of the rima glottidis (p. 1643). The *base* is concave, with a smooth surface for articulation with the lateral part of the upper border of the cricoid lamina. Its round, prominent lateral angle, or *muscular process*, projects backwards and laterally, giving attachment to the posterior crico-arytenoid muscle behind and the lateral crico-arytenoid in front. To its pointed anterior angle (the *vocal process*), projecting horizontally forward, is attached the vocal ligament. The *apex* curves backwards and medially to articulate with the corniculate cartilage.

Corniculate cartilages (**11**.15, 22, 23)

The corniculate cartilages are two conical nodules of elastic fibro-cartilage which articulate with the apices of the arytenoid cartilages, prolonging them posteromedially. They lie in the posterior parts of the aryepiglottic mucosal folds, and are sometimes fused with the arytenoid cartilages.

Cuneiform cartilages (**11**.22, 23)

These cuneiform cartilages are two small elongated, club-like nodules of elastic fibrocartilage, one in each aryepiglottic fold anterosuperior to the corniculate cartilages and visible as whitish elevations through the mucosa.

Epiglottic cartilage (**11**.18, 22, 23, 29)

The epiglottic cartilage is a thin leaf-like plate of elastic fibrocartilage, projecting obliquely upwards behind the tongue and hyoid body, and in front of the laryngeal inlet. Its free end, which is broad and round, is directed upwards; its attached part, or stalk (*petiolus*) is long and narrow, and is connected by the elastic *thyro-epiglottic ligament* to the back of the laryngeal prominence just below the thyroid notch. Its sides are attached to the arytenoid cartilages by aryepiglottic folds (see above). Its free upper *anterior surface* is covered by mucosa (the epithelium is non-keratinized stratified

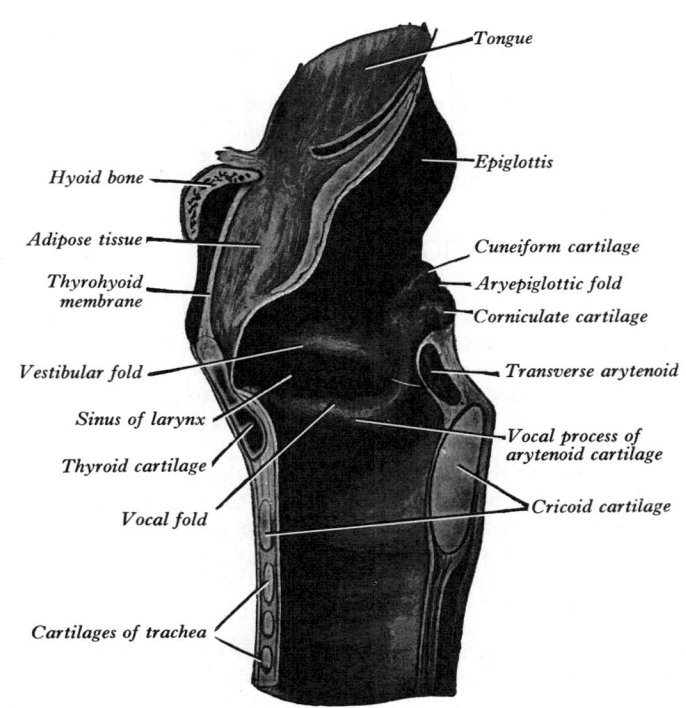

11.22 Superior view of laryngeal cartilages together with cricothyroid, quadrangular, and related ligaments and membranes.

11.23 Sagittal section showing the medial aspect of the right half of the larynx.

squamous), reflected on to the pharyngeal aspect of the tongue and the lateral pharyngeal walls as a *median glosso-epiglottic* and two *lateral glosso-epiglottic folds*. On each side of the median fold is a depression, the *vallecula*. The lower part of the anterior surface, behind the hyoid bone and thyrohyoid membrane, is connected to the upper border of the former by an elastic *hyo-epiglottic ligament*, and separated from the thyrohyoid membrane by adipose tissue. The smooth *posterior surface* is transversely concave and vertically concavo-convex; it is covered by ciliated respiratory mucosa; its lower projecting part is called the *tubercle*. The cartilage is posteriorly pitted by small mucous glands and perforated by branches of the internal laryngeal nerve.

Functions of the epiglottis. During deglutition (p. 1732) the epiglottis moves upwards and forwards and is squeezed between the base of the tongue and the rest of the larynx; the bolus slips over its anterior surface as it bends back over the laryngeal inlet. In humans it is somewhat degenerate in function and is well separated from the soft palate; it is not essential to swallowing, which occurs normally even if the epiglottis is destroyed by disease, nor is it essential for respiration or phonation.

Some mammals which are keen-scented even when the mouth is open for feeding have a large epiglottis which projects into the nasopharynx above the soft palate; when eating, it is drawn down and forward by the hyo-epiglottic muscle (in man a mere ligament) against the upper surface of the soft palate, keeping the nasal airway clear and the buccal airway closed, thus permitting olfaction even when the mouth is open.

Tritiate cartilages (Cartilago triticea) (11.15)

The tritiate cartilages are two small nodules of elastic cartilage situated one on either side above the larynx within the posterior free edge of the thyrohyoid membrane, about halfway between the superior cornu of the thyroid cartilage and the tip of the hyoid's greater cornu. Their functions are unknown, although they may serve to strengthen this connection.

Microstructure of laryngeal cartilages

The corniculate, cuneiform, tritiate and epiglottic cartilages (**11.**31) and the apices of the arytenoids are composed of elastic fibrocartilage with little tendency to ossify or calcify. The thyroid, cricoid and greater part of the arytenoids consist of hyaline cartilage and may undergo mottled calcification or ossification as age advances, commencing about the twenty-fifth year in the thyroid cartilage and somewhat later in the cricoid and arytenoids; by the sixty-fifth year these cartilages commonly appear patchily dense in radiographs (**11.**32).

During prenatal development laryngeal cartilages begin chondrification at about 50 days' gestation, and all the major skeletal components of the larynx are visible as cartilaginous masses by the third gestational month (Doménech-Mateu & Sañudo 1990).

LARYNGEAL ARTICULATIONS

The joints between the inferior cornua of the thyroid cartilage and the sides of the cricoid cartilage are synovial, each enveloped with a capsular ligament strengthened posteriorly by a fibrous band. At these joints the cricoid rotates on the inferior cornua around a transverse axis passing transversely through both joints; to a limited extent the cricoid also glides in different directions on the thyroid cornua.

A pair of synovial joints exists between the facets on the lateral part of the upper border of the lamina of the cricoid cartilage and the bases of the arytenoids, each joint being enclosed by a capsular ligament; a strong posterior crico-arytenoid ligament connects the cricoid to the posterior and medial part of the base of the arytenoid. These joints permit two movements:

- arytenoid rotation about an oblique axis (dorsomediocranial to ventrolaterocaudal), (Frable 1961), by which each vocal process swings laterally or medially, increasing or decreasing the width of the rima glottidis;
- a gliding movement, by which the arytenoids approach or recede from one another, the direction and slope of their articular surfaces

imposing a forward and downward movement on lateral gliding. The movements of gliding and rotation are associated: medial gliding with medial rotation and lateral gliding with lateral rotation (von Leden & Moore 1961). The posterior crico-arytenoid ligaments limit forward movements of the arytenoid cartilages on the cricoid. (For details consult Sonesson 1959 and Sellars & Keen 1978.) Sometimes the synchondrosis between the apex of the arytenoid cartilage and the corresponding corniculate cartilage is replaced by a synovial joint.

Numerous lamellated (Pacinian) corpuscles, some Ruffini and some free nerve endings occur in the capsules of the laryngeal joints. In cats these respond to mechanical stimuli and are involved in the normal co-ordination of laryngeal muscles during respiration and phonation (Kirchner & Wyke 1965). The human articular supply is chiefly from branches of the recurrent laryngeal nerves, arising independently or from branches of the nerve to the laryngeal muscles (Pšenicka 1966).

LARYNGEAL LIGAMENTS AND MEMBRANES

Extrinsic ligaments

Thyrohyoid membrane (11.13–17). This is a broad, fibro-elastic layer, attached below to the superior border of the thyroid cartilage lamina and the front of its superior cornua; above, it is attached to the *superior* margin of the hyoid bone's body and greater cornua. It thus ascends **behind** the concave posterior surface of the hyoid, separated from its body by a bursa which facilitates the ascent of the larynx during swallowing. Its thicker part is the *median thyrohyoid ligament*; the more lateral, thinner parts are pierced by the superior laryngeal vessels and internal laryngeal nerves. Externally it is in contact with the thyrohyoid, sternohyoid and omohyoid muscles and the hyoid body. Its inner surface is related to the epiglottis and pharyngeal piriform fossae. The round, cord-like, elastic *lateral thyrohyoid ligaments* form the posterior borders of the thyrohyoid membrane, connecting the tips of the superior thyroid cornua to the posterior ends of the greater hyoid cornua. A small *cartilago triticea* occurs frequently in each ligament.

The epiglottis is attached to the hyoid bone and thyroid cartilage by the extrinsic *hyo-epiglottic* and intrinsic *thyro-epiglottic ligaments* respectively (p. 1641). The *cricotracheal ligament* unites the lower cricoid border to the first tracheal cartilage, being thus continuous with the tracheal perichondrium.

Intrinsic ligaments

Within the cartilage encasement, beneath the laryngeal mucosa, is the *fibro-elastic membrane of the larynx*, a fibrous sheet containing many elastic fibres; it is interrupted on both sides of the larynx by the horizontal cleft between the vestibular and vocal ligaments. Its upper part, the *quadrangular membrane* (often an ill-defined structure), extends between the arytenoid cartilages and the sides of the epiglottis; its lower part forms the well-marked *cricothyroid ligament* (*cricovocal membrane*), connecting the thyroid, cricoid and arytenoid cartilages. The articular ligaments between cartilages are described above.

Cricothyroid ligament (11.22, 23). Comprising the inferior, larger part of the laryngeal membrane, this ligament is composed mainly of elastic tissue; it has distinct anterior and lateral parts. The single thick *anterior* (*median*) *cricothyroid ligament*, which is broad below and narrower above, connects the adjacent margins of the cricoid and thyroid cartilages. An anastomosis between the cricothyroid arteries crosses it and supplies perforating branches to the larynx. The paired smaller *lateral cricothyroid ligaments* (*cricothyroid* or *cricovocal membranes*) are thinner; they are covered internally by mucosa and externally by the lateral crico-arytenoid and thyro-arytenoid muscles. From the internal rim of the superior border of the cricoid the three ligaments ascend and converge; their superior edges form the basis of the vocal folds, extending back horizontally from the dorsal aspect of the angle of the thyroid cartilage (just below its midpoint) to the apices of the arytenoid vocal processes (11.22). The thickened edges of the cricothyroid ligament complex are the *vocal ligaments* (11.22). The term *cornus elasticus* is commonly applied to the entire complex but sometimes only its anterior part.

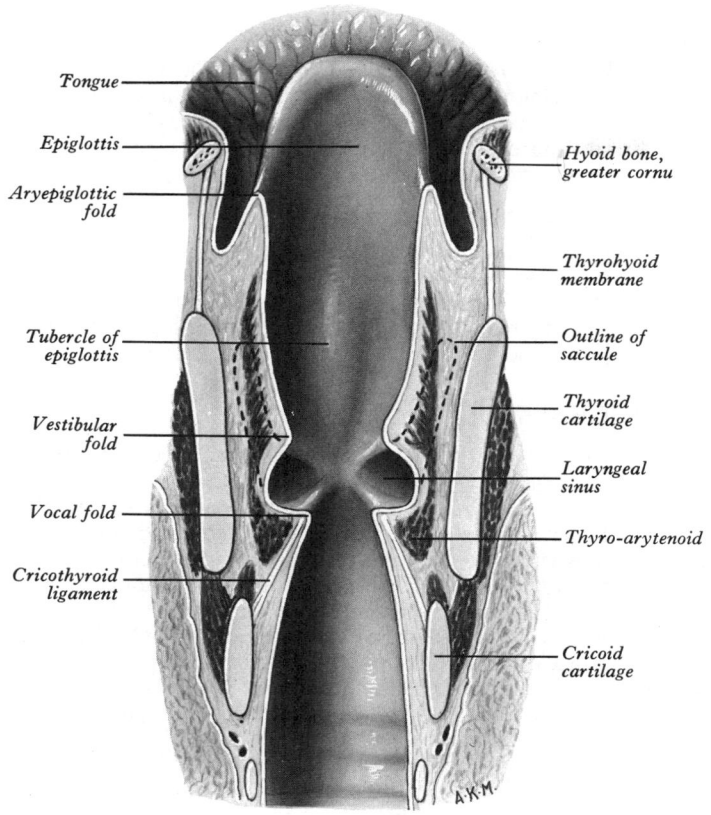

Tongue

Epiglottis

Aryepiglottic fold

Hyoid bone, greater cornu

Thyrohyoid membrane

Tubercle of epiglottis

Outline of saccule

Thyroid cartilage

Vestibular fold

Laryngeal sinus

Vocal fold

Thyro-arytenoid

Cricothyroid ligament

Cricoid cartilage

A.K.M.

11.24 Coronal section through the larynx and the cranial end of the trachea: posterior aspect.

LARYNGEAL CAVITY

The laryngeal cavity space extends from the laryngeal inlet from the pharynx, down to the cricoid cartilage's lower border where it continues into the trachea (**11**.23, 24). It is partially divided into upper and lower parts by paired upper and lower mucosal folds projecting into its lumen, with a middle part between the two sets of folds. The upper folds are the *vestibular folds*, the median aperture which they guard being the *rima vestibuli*; the lower pair are the *vocal folds*, the fissure between the latter being the *rima glottidis* or *glottis*. The vocal folds are the primary source of phonation, whereas the vestibular folds do not contribute directly to sound production.

Upper part of the laryngeal cavity

The upper part of the laryngeal cavity is entered by the *laryngeal inlet* or '*aditus laryngis*' (**11**.12, 23), the aperture between the larynx and pharynx, which faces back and somewhat upwards, the anterior wall of the larynx being much longer than the posterior and sloping downwards and forwards in its upper part because of the oblique inclination of the epiglottis which forms this region. The inlet is bounded anteriorly by the upper edge of the epiglottis, posteriorly by the transverse mucosal fold between the two arytenoids and on each side by the edge of a mucosal ridge (the *aryepiglottic fold*) between the side of the epiglottis and the apex of the arytenoid. The aryepiglottic fold contains ligamentous and muscular fibres; the posterior part of its margin has two oval swellings, one above and in front, the other behind and below; these mark, respectively, the positions of the underlying cuneiform and corniculate cartilages, separated by a shallow vertical furrow which continues below with the opening of the laryngeal sinus (see below).

The *laryngeal vestibule* (**11**.23, 24) is the space between the laryngeal inlet and vestibular folds; it is wide above, narrow below and higher anteriorly than posteriorly. Its anterior wall is formed by the posterior epiglottic surface, the lower part of which (the epiglottic tubercle) bulges backwards a little. Its lateral walls which are higher in front and shallow behind, are the medial surfaces of the aryepiglottic folds; its posterior wall is the interarytenoid mucosa, above the vestibular folds.

Middle part of the laryngeal cavity

The middle part of the laryngeal cavity is the smallest, extending from the rima vestibuli above to the rima glottidis below. On each side it opens by a slit between vestibular and vocal folds into the *laryngeal sinus* **ventricle** (**11**.23, 24), a fusiform recess opening between the folds and extending upwards into the laryngeal wall lateral to

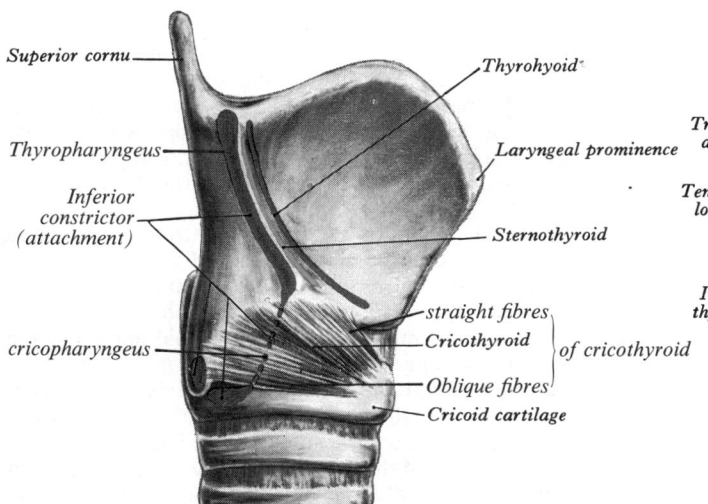

Superior cornu

Thyrohyoid

Thyropharyngeus

Laryngeal prominence

Inferior constrictor (attachment)

Sternothyroid

cricopharyngeus

straight fibres
Cricothyroid } *of cricothyroid*
Oblique fibres

Cricoid cartilage

11.25 Lateral view of the larynx, showing the muscular attachments and cricothyroid muscle fibres.

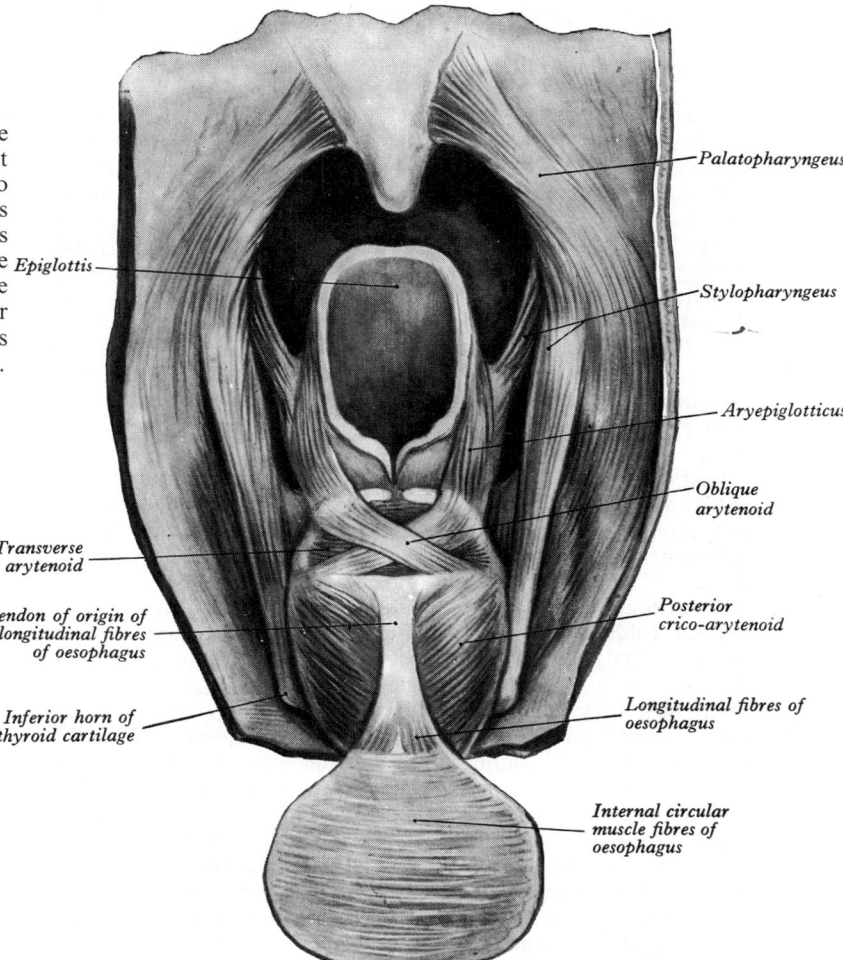

Palatopharyngeus

Epiglottis

Stylopharyngeus

Aryepiglotticus

Oblique arytenoid

Transverse arytenoid

Tendon of origin of longitudinal fibres of oesophagus

Posterior crico-arytenoid

Inferior horn of thyroid cartilage

Longitudinal fibres of oesophagus

Internal circular muscle fibres of oesophagus

11.26 The muscles of the larynx: posterior aspect.

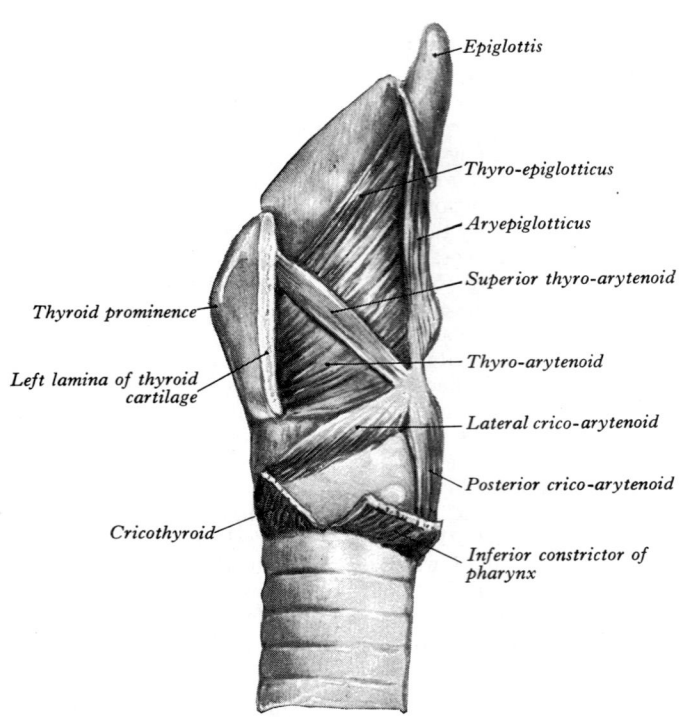

11.27 The muscles of the larynx (most of the left lamina of the thyroid cartilage has been removed): left lateral aspect.

Labels on figure: Epiglottis; Thyro-epiglotticus; Aryepiglotticus; Superior thyro-arytenoid; Thyroid prominence; Thyro-arytenoid; Left lamina of thyroid cartilage; Lateral crico-arytenoid; Posterior crico-arytenoid; Cricothyroid; Inferior constrictor of pharynx

the vestibular fold. It is lined by mucosa and covered externally by the thyro-arytenoid muscle. Anteriorly on each side, the sinus opens into a *laryngeal saccule* (**11.24**), a pouch ascending forwards from the sinus between the vestibular fold and thyroid cartilage, occasionally reaching the cartilage's upper border; it is conical, curving slightly backwards. On its luminal surface open 60–70 mucous glands, sited in the submucosa. The saccule has a fibrous capsule, continuous below with the vestibular ligament, and is covered medially by a few muscular fasciculi from the apex of the arytenoid cartilage which pass forwards between the saccule and vestibular mucosa into the aryepiglottic fold. Laterally the saccule is separated from the thyroid cartilage by thyro-epiglottic muscles, which compress it, expressing its secretion on to the vocal folds (which lack glands) to protect them against desiccation and infection. Saccules occasionally protrude through the thyrohyoid membrane.

In some apes the saccules form air sacs, which may extend into superficial cervical and even axillary tissues; they aid resonance, often spectacularly, as in howler monkeys which may project their voices up to a distance of 5 miles.

Vestibular folds and ligaments. The pink mucosa of each vestibular fold (**11.22–24**) covers a narrow vestibular ligament, fixed in front to the thyroid angle below the epiglottic cartilage and behind to the anterolateral surface of the arytenoid cartilage above its vocal process. Like the whole interior of the larynx (except the vocal folds) the epithelium is ciliated pseudostratified, respiratory in type.

Vocal folds and ligaments. The vocal folds are white mucosal elevations (**11.22–24, 30, 31**) which stretch back on either side from the midlevel of the thyroid angle to the vocal processes of the arytenoids. They form the anterolateral edges of the rima glottidis and, as already noted, are concerned with sound production. They are covered by non-keratinized stratified squamous epithelium which is closely bound to the vocal ligaments which run beneath; since a submucosa and blood vessels are absent, the folds are pearly white. Each vocal ligament is continuous below with the lateral part of the cricothyroid ligament (see above), and is composed of a band of yellow elastic tissue related laterally to the vocalis muscle (see below).

The *rima glottidis* or *glottis* (**11.24**), the fissure between the vocal folds anteriorly and the arytenoid cartilages posteriorly, is bounded behind by the mucosa passing between the arytenoid cartilages, at the level of the vocal folds. The rima glottidis is customarily divided into two regions, an anterior *intermembranous part*, comprising

about three-fifths of its anteroposterior length, and a posterior *intercartilaginous part* between the arytenoids. The average sagittal diameter of the glottis in adult males is 23 mm and in adult females 17 mm. It is the narrowest part of the larynx. Its width and shape vary with the movements of the vocal folds and arytenoid cartilages during respiration and phonation (see below).

Lower part of the laryngeal cavity

The lower part of the laryngeal cavity extends from the vocal folds to the lower border of the cricoid. In transverse section it is elliptical above and wider and circular below; it is continuous with the trachea. Lined by respiratory mucosa, its walls are supported by the cricothyroid ligament above and the cricoid cartilage below.

LARYNGEAL MUSCULATURE (11.25–27)

The muscles of the larynx are divisible into extrinsic and intrinsic groups. The *extrinsic muscles* connect the larynx to neighbouring structures and are responsible for moving it vertically during phonation and swallowing; they include the thyrohyoid and thyrosternoid muscles, and the thyropharyngeus and cricopharyngeus components of the inferior pharyngeal constrictor, although muscles attached to the hyoid may also move the larynx indirectly because of the hyoid's strong connections to the larynx (p. 582). The three small pharyngeal muscles (stylo-, palato- and salpingopharyngeus) are, however, connected directly to the thyroid cartilage, mainly to the posterior aspects of the thyroid lamina and cornua. These muscles are considered in detail elsewhere in this text.

The *intrinsic muscles* are confined to the larynx in their attachments. They are: the cricothyroid, posterior and lateral cricoarytenoid, transverse and oblique arytenoid, aryepiglotticus, thyroarytenoid and its subsidiary part, vocalis, and thyro-epiglotticus. All but the transverse arytenoid are paired.

Cricothyroid (**11.25**). As its name implies, this muscle runs between the cricoid and thyroid cartilages. It is attached anteriorly to the external aspect of the cricoid cartilage's arch. Its fibres pass backwards, diverging into two groups, a lower 'oblique' part which slants backwards and laterally to the anterior border of the thyroid's inferior cornu, and a superior 'straight' part ascending more steeply backwards to the posterior part of the lower border of the thyroid lamina. The medial borders of the paired cricothyroids are separated anteriorly by a triangular gap occupied by the conus elasticus.

Posterior crico-arytenoid (**11.26**). This muscle arises from the posterior surface of the cricoid lamina, its attachment being on the inferomedial area of the depression on the same side of the midline. Ascending laterally its fibres converge to insert on the back of the muscular process of the arytenoid of the same side. The highest fibres run almost horizontally, the middle obliquely; the lowest are almost vertical, and some of these reach the anterolateral surface of the arytenoid.

Lateral crico-arytenoid (**11.27**). Smaller than the preceding muscle, it is attached anteriorly to the upper border of the cricoid arch and ascends obliquely backwards to the front of the muscular process of the arytenoid cartilage of the same side.

Transverse arytenoid (**11.26**). A single, unpaired muscle which bridges the gap at the back of the larynx between the two arytenoid cartilages and fills their posterior concave surfaces, it is attached to the back of the muscular process and adjacent lateral border of both arytenoids.

Oblique arytenoid (**11.26**). Lying superficial to the transverse arytenoid, the paired muscles cross each other obliquely at the back of the larynx, each extending from the back of the muscular process of one arytenoid cartilage to the apex of the opposite one. Some fibres of each continue laterally round the arytenoid apex into the aryepiglottic fold, so forming the *aryepiglottic muscle*.

Thyro-arytenoid and vocalis (**11.27**). This is a broad but thin muscle, lying near the internal wall of the larynx lateral to the vocal fold, cricothyroid ligament, laryngeal sinus and saccule. It is attached anteriorly to the lower half of the thyroid cartilage's angle, and from the cricothyroid ligament. Its fibres pass backwards, laterally and upwards to the anterolateral surface of the arytenoid cartilage. Its lower and deeper fibres form a band which in coronal section appears as a triangular bundle, and is attached to the lateral surface of the vocal process and to the inferior impression on the anterolateral surface of the arytenoid cartilage. This bundle, the *vocalis muscle*, is parallel with and just lateral to the vocal ligament; it is said to be thicker behind than in front, because many deeper fibres start from the vocal ligament and so do not extend to the thyroid cartilage. Others consider that all its fibres loop and intertwine as they pass from the thyroid to the arytenoid (Tautz & Rohen 1967). Many of the thyro-arytenoid fibres are prolonged into the aryepiglottic fold, where some terminate, others continuing to the epiglottic margin as the *thyro-epiglotticus*. A few fibres extend along the wall of the sinus from the lateral arytenoid margin to the side of the epiglottis. The *superior thyro-arytenoid* (**11.27**), a small muscle not always present, lies on the lateral surface of the main mass of the thyro-arytenoid, extending obliquely from the thyroid angle to the muscular process of the arytenoid.

Actions

The intrinsic laryngeal muscles may be placed in three groups according to their main actions (Negus 1947):

- those which vary the rima glottidis—the posterior and lateral crico-arytenoids and oblique and transverse arytenoids
- those regulating the tension of the vocal ligaments—the crico-thyroids, posterior crico-arytenoids (again), thyro-arytenoids and vocales
- those which modify the laryngeal inlet—the oblique arytenoids, aryepiglottici and thyro-epiglottici (**11.26, 27**).

Bilateral pairs of muscles usually act in concert with each other. Details of these are as given below.

Varying the rima glottidis. The *posterior crico-arytenoids* are the only laryngeal muscles which open the glottis, rotating the arytenoid cartilages laterally around an axis passing through the crico-arytenoid joints (p. 1644), thus separating the vocal processes and the attached vocal folds. They also pull the arytenoids backwards, assisting the cricothyroids to tense the vocal folds. The most lateral fibres draw the arytenoids laterally, so the rima glottidis becomes triangular when the posterior crico-arytenoid muscles contract.

The *lateral crico-arytenoids* close the glottis by rotating the arytenoids medially, to approximate their vocal processes. The *transverse arytenoid* pulls the arytenoid cartilages towards each other, closing the posterior (intercartilaginous) part of the rima glottidis.

Regulating tension in the vocal ligaments. The *cricothyroids* stretch the vocal ligaments by tilting the thyroid cartilage forwards and downwards on the cricoid. Because the arytenoid cartilages are anchored to the cricoid lamina, the sagittally directed rotation of the thyroid cartilage increases the distance between their vocal processes and the anterior angle of the thyroid, so lengthening the vocal ligaments. The cricoid is usually held immovably against the vertebral column by the cricopharyngeus during phonation so that under these conditions it is the thyroid cartilage which moves. During swallowing, however, the cricopharyngeus relaxes, allowing the cricoid to tilt forwards during laryngeal closure.

The *thyro-arytenoids* draw the arytenoids towards the thyroid cartilage, shortening and relaxing the vocal ligaments. At the same time, they rotate the arytenoids medially to approximate the vocal folds. Their deeper fibres, the vocales, relax the posterior parts of the vocal ligaments, their anterior parts remaining tense and thus raising the vocal pitch. For details of arytenoid movements consult Sellars (1978).

Modifying the laryngeal inlet. The *oblique arytenoids* and *ary-epiglottici* act as a sphincter of the laryngeal inlet by adducting the aryepiglottic folds and approximating the arytenoid cartilages to the tubercle of the epiglottis. The *thyro-epiglottic muscles* widen the inlet by their action on the aryepiglottic folds.

Summary. Neuromuscular spindles have been found in all human laryngeal muscles (Keene 1961), the maximum number (23) being in the transverse arytenoid (Voss 1966). The control of phonation requires very considerable neuromuscular co-ordination and effective proprioception would appear to be essential to this capacity.

Movements of the vocal folds (11.28)

In quiet respiration the anterior, intermembranous part of the rima glottidis is triangular when viewed from above, its apex being in

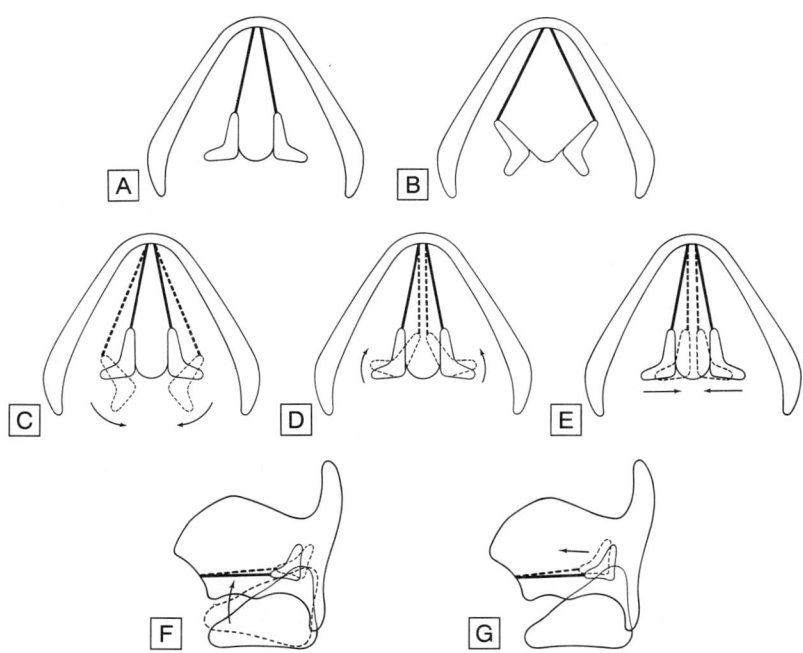

11.28 Different positions of the vocal folds and arytenoid cartilages.

A Position of rest in quiet respiration. The intermembranous part of the rima glottidis is triangular and the intercartilaginous part is rectangular in shape.

B Forced inspiration. Both parts of the rima glottidis are triangular in shape.

C Abduction of the vocal folds. The arrows indicate the lines of pull of the posterior crico-arytenoid muscles. The abducted vocal folds and the abducted, retracted and laterally rotated arytenoid cartilages are shown in dotted outline. Both parts of the rima glottidis are triangular.

D Adduction of the vocal folds. The arrows indicate the lines of pull of the

lateral crico-arytenoid muscles. The adducted vocal folds and the medially rotated arytenoid cartilages are shown in dotted outlines.

E Closure of the rima glottidis. The arrows indicate the line of pull of the transverse arytenoid muscle. Both the vocal folds and the arytenoid cartilages are adducted, but there is no rotation of the latter.

F Tension of the vocal folds, produced by the action of the cricothyroid muscles which tilt the anterior part of the cricoid cartilage cranially and so carry the arytenoid cartilages dorsally.

G Relaxation of the vocal folds, produced by the action of the thyroarytenoid muscles, which draw the arytenoid cartilages ventrally.

front and its base behind, represented by a line (about 8 mm long), connecting the anterior ends of the arytenoid vocal processes; the intercartilaginous part is rectangular, between the medial surfaces of the arytenoids which lie parallel to each other. In forced inspiration the vocal folds are fully abducted; the arytenoid cartilages rotate laterally, their vocal processes moving apart. The glottis is then rhomboid, its intermembranous and intercartilaginous parts being both triangular, the greatest width being opposite the attachments of the folds to the vocal processes.

Movements of the vocal folds during phonation have been studied by high-speed cinematography (Pressman 1942). Preparatory to phonation, the intermembranous and intercartilaginous parts of the glottis are reduced to a linear chink by adduction of the vocal folds and by adduction and medial rotation of the arytenoids. The folds then tense, the degree of tension determining sound pitch (frequency). To raise the pitch, tension is increased; the folds may lengthen by 50% in the highest tones. Photographs suggest that this lengthening affects both ends of the folds as the cricothyroid muscles tilt the thyroid cartilage down and forwards. In whispering the inter-membranous glottis is closed, but the intercartilaginous part remains widely patent, so that air escapes freely.

Fink (1975, 1978) considered that 'laryngeal biomechanics' depend much on the behaviour of the various laryngeal folds which project into the laryngeal cavity to highly variable degrees dependent upon respiration, physical effort and phonation. In addition to the vocal, vestibular and aryepiglottic folds mentioned above, he identified *median thyrohyoid and interarytenoid folds*. The latter consists of the transverse arytenoid muscle and its covering mucous membrane which **folds** into the larynx when the muscle adducts the arytenoids.

(thus aiding obliteration of the intercartilaginous part of the rima glottidis). The median thyrohyoid fold is more complex: as shown in **11**.15, the lower part of the epiglottic cartilage is attached to the hyoid bone and thyroid cartilage by elastic ligaments (hyo-epiglottic and thyro-epiglottic, pp. 1641, 1642), separated from the median thyrohyoid ligament by adipose tissue, anterior to which is the elastic anterior part of the thyrohyoid membrane including the median thyrohyoid ligament. During swallowing (p.1732) the thyroid cartilage and hyoid bone are approximated (in addition to general elevation of the pharynx, larynx and trachea). This causes the structures defined above to bulge posteriorly into the laryngeal inlet as a transverse fold and narrow it during swallowing. The reverse occurs during inspiration, all folds being reduced to a minimum. Intrusion of **all** the folds is important in phonation, since the vocal cavity (see below) is thereby altered, modifying its resonant properties. (The median thyrohyoid fold contains the so-called '*pre-epiglottic space*' of laryngeal surgery, an important region in the spread of supra-epiglottic tumours (see Maguire & Dayal 1974).

The movements of the larynx during deglutition are described on page 1732.

MICROSTRUCTURE OF THE LARYNGEAL MUCOSA

The laryngeal mucosa is continuous with that of the pharynx above and the trachea below. It lines the entire inner surface of the larynx including the sinus and saccule, being thickened over the vestibular folds of which it is the chief component, but thin over the vocal folds, where it is firmly attached to the underlying vocal ligaments. It is loosely adherent to the anterior surface of the epiglottis, but firmly attached to its anterior surface and the floor of the valleculae. On the aryepiglottic folds it is reinforced by a considerable amount of fibrous connective tissue, and adheres closely to the laryngeal surfaces of the cuneiform and arytenoid cartilages.

The *laryngeal epithelium* is mainly ciliated pseudostratified (i.e. respiratory) where it covers the inner aspects of the larynx, including the posterior surface of the epiglottis, providing a ciliary clearance mechanism shared with most of the respiratory tract. However, over the vocal folds it is non-keratinized stratified squamous, an important variation which protects the tissue from the effects of the considerable mechanical stresses acting on the surfaces of the vocal folds. The exterior surfaces of the larynx which merge with the laryngopharynx and oropharynx (including the anterior surface of the epiglottis), and are subject to the abrasive effects of alimentation, are also non-keratinized stratified squamous.

The laryngeal mucosa has numerous *mucous glands*, especially over the epiglottis, where they pit the cartilage, and along the margins of the aryepiglottic folds anterior to the arytenoid cartilages, where they are termed the *arytenoid glands*. Many large glands in the

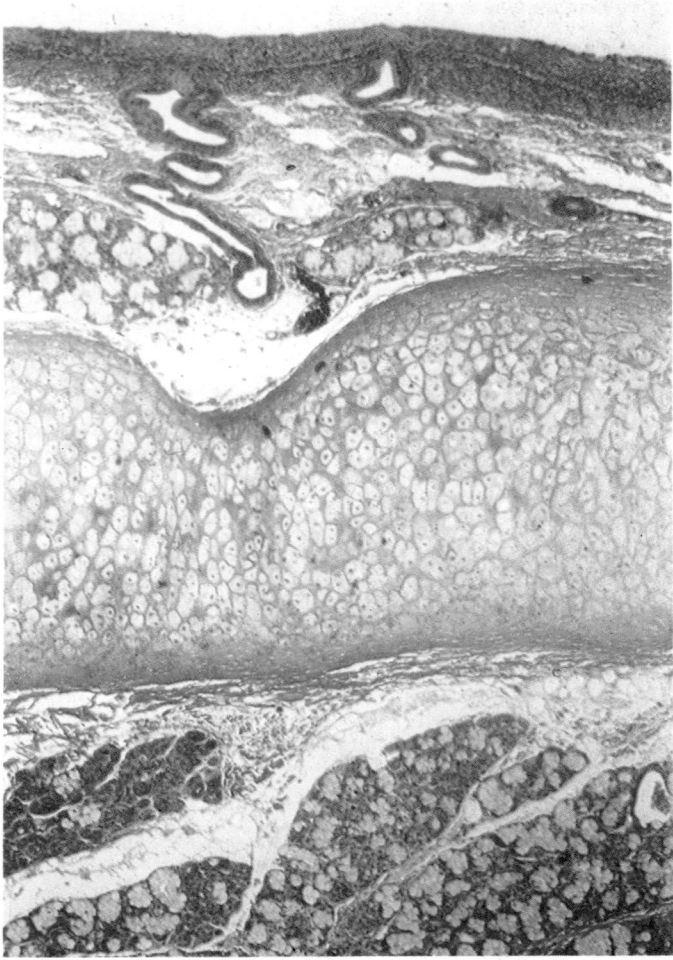

11.29 A low magnification light micrograph of a transverse section of the epiglottis, showing stratified squamous epithelium covering the anterior surface, mucous glands and fibro-elastic cartilage. Mallory's trichrome stain. (Prepared by David Ristow; photography by Marina Morris, Department of Anatomy, Guy's Hospital Medical School, London.)

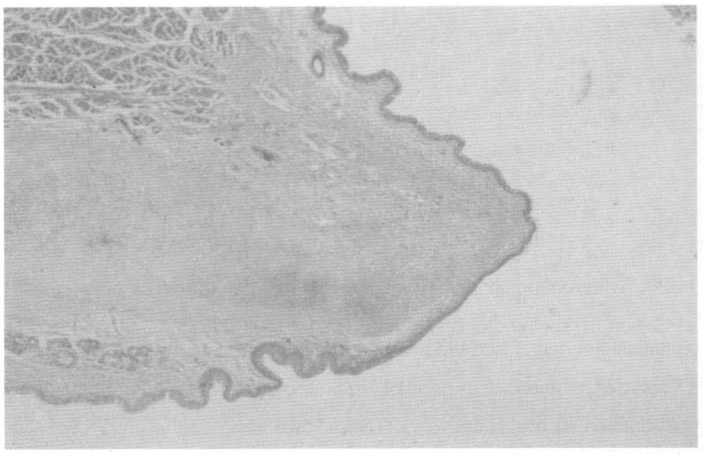

11.30A Coronal section through the vocal fold showing distribution of the mucosa and underlying connective tissue. Haematoxylin and eosin. Magnification × 50.

saccules of the larynx secrete periodically over the vocal folds during phonation; the free edges of these folds are devoid of glands, their stratified epithelium thus being vulnerable to drying and requiring the secretions of neighbouring glands. Hoarseness due to excessive speaking is due to partial temporary failure of this secretion. Scanning electron microscopy demonstrates microvilli and microplicae on the surface epithelial cells of the vocal folds and elsewhere in the larynx (Andrews 1975, Tillmann et al 1977), features common to other epithelia subjected to drying (e.g. corneal epithelium). Microplicae are regarded as aiding the retention of surface secretions.

Taste buds, like those in the tongue, occur on the posterior epiglottic surface, aryepiglottic folds and less often in other laryngeal regions (p. 1312). Their centripetal pathway is via the vagus nerve.

LARYNGEAL VESSELS AND NERVES (10.81)

Vessels

The chief **arteries** of the larynx are branches of the superior and inferior thyroid arteries; their accompanying **veins** join both the superior thyroid vein, opening into the internal jugular, and the inferior thyroid vein, draining into the left brachiocephalic. **Lymph vessels** form groups above and below the vocal folds; the superior accompany the superior laryngeal artery, traverse the thyrohyoid membrane and end in the deep cervical lymph nodes near the bifurcation of the common carotid artery; some of the inferior group of lymphatics pierce the cricothyroid ligament to reach a lymph node in front of the ligament or the upper trachea; others pass below the cricoid cartilage to the deep cervical lymph nodes and to nodes along the inferior thyroid artery

Nerves

The **nerve supply** is from the internal and external branches of the superior laryngeal and from the recurrent laryngeal and sympathetic nerves. The *internal laryngeal nerve* is probably entirely sensory and autonomic, although special visceral motor fibres to the transverse arytenoid have been reported (Williams 1951). This nerve enters postero-inferiorly through the thyrohyoid membrane above the superior laryngeal artery; its branches supply both epiglottic surfaces, the aryepiglottic fold and the laryngeal interior as far as the vocal folds. The *external laryngeal nerve* (p. 1253) supplies the cricothyroid muscle, which it enters via its external surface. Terminally the *recurrent laryngeal nerve* (with the laryngeal branch of the inferior thyroid artery) ascends medial to the lower border of the inferior pharyngeal constrictor immediately behind the cricothyroid joint, supplying all the intrinsic laryngeal muscles except the cricothyroid and innervating the mucosa below the vocal folds. Before entering the larynx this nerve usually divides into motor and sensory rami, not 'adductor' and 'abductor' rami as is sometimes asserted (Williams 1954). Motor units in such skilled musculature might be expected to be small: a ratio of 30 muscle fibres to each motor neuron has been estimated (English & Blevins 1969).

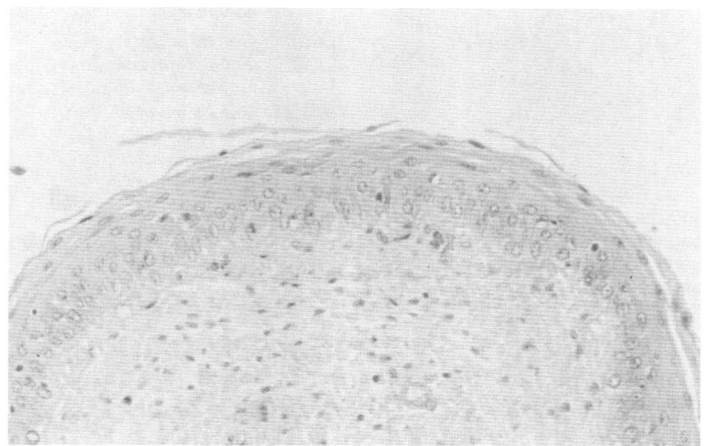

11.30B Detail of **11.30A** showing the non-keratinized stratified squamous epithelium lining the vocal fold. Haematoxylin and eosin; magnification × 400.

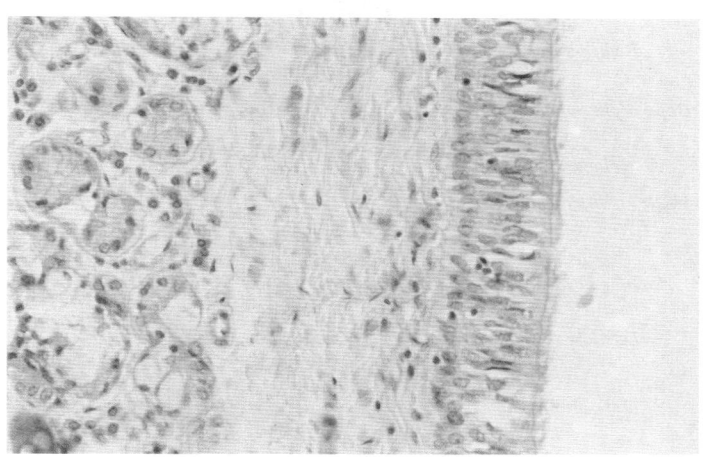

11.30c Mucosal surface of the subglottal larynx showing the ciliated respiratory epithelium lining this structure and muco-serous glands in the lamina propria. Haematoxylin and eosin; magnificiation × 400.

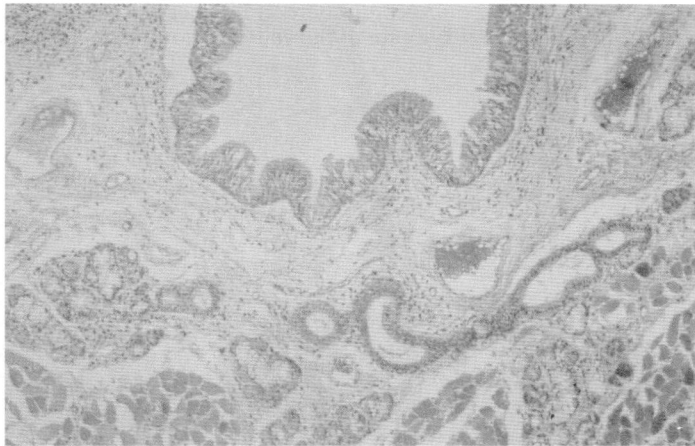

11.30D Coronal section through the laryngeal sinus showing mucosa and glands including prominent ducts (below). Haematoxylin and eosin; magnification × 150.

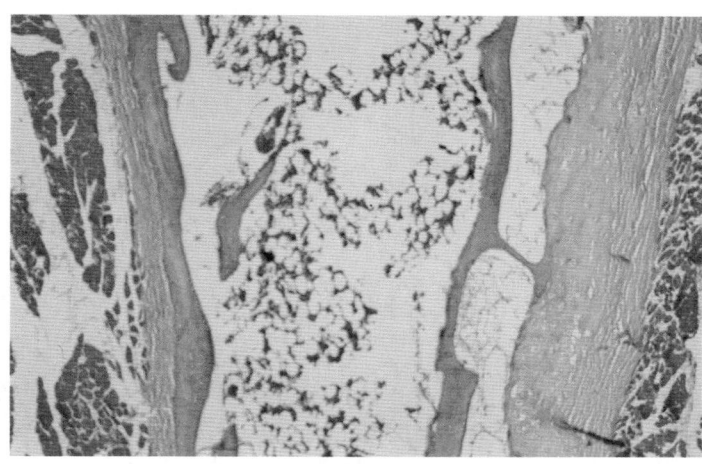

11.30E Coronal section of the thyroid cartilage from an aged person, showing ossification and medullary, haemopoietic tissue within its wall of hyaline cartilage. Haematoxylin and eosin; magnification × 150.

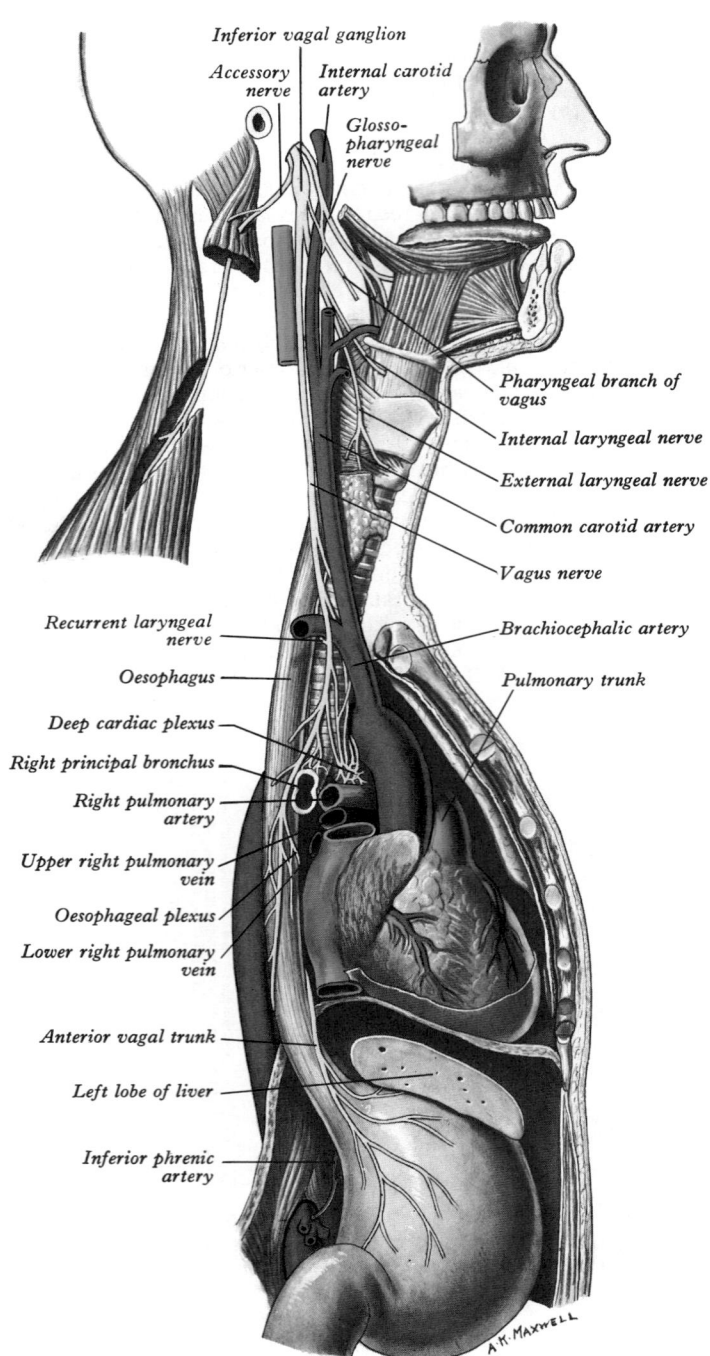

Inferior vagal ganglion

Accessory nerve

Internal carotid artery

Glosso-pharyngeal nerve

Pharyngeal branch of vagus

Internal laryngeal nerve

External laryngeal nerve

Common carotid artery

Vagus nerve

Recurrent laryngeal nerve

Brachiocephalic artery

Oesophagus

Pulmonary trunk

Deep cardiac plexus

Right principal bronchus

Right pulmonary artery

Upper right pulmonary vein

Oesophageal plexus

Lower right pulmonary vein

Anterior vagal trunk

Left lobe of liver

Inferior phrenic artery

A.K.MAXWELL

11.30F   The course and distribution of the glossopharyngeal, vagus and accessory nerves.

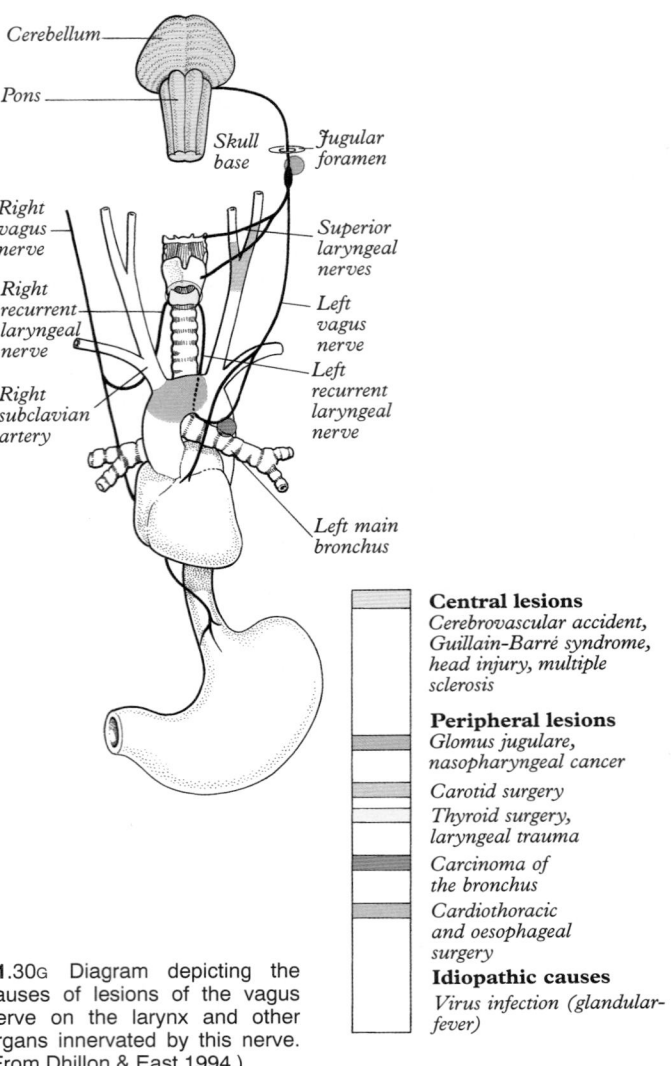

Cerebellum

Pons

Skull base

Jugular foramen

Right vagus nerve

Superior laryngeal nerves

Right recurrent laryngeal nerve

Left vagus nerve

Right subclavian artery

Left recurrent laryngeal nerve

Left main bronchus

Central lesions
Cerebrovascular accident, Guillain-Barré syndrome, head injury, multiple sclerosis

Peripheral lesions
Glomus jugulare, nasopharyngeal cancer

Carotid surgery

Thyroid surgery, laryngeal trauma

Carcinoma of the bronchus

Cardiothoracic and oesophageal surgery

Idiopathic causes
Virus infection (glandular-fever)

11.30G Diagram depicting the causes of lesions of the vagus nerve on the larynx and other organs innervated by this nerve. (From Dhillon & East 1994.)

EFFECTS OF VAGAL NERVE LESIONS ON THE LARYNX AND OTHER STRUCTURES

Acute damage to the proximal vagus nerve (**11**.30G) may lead to palpitation, vomiting, and a feeling of suffocation associated with tachycardia and tachypnoea. In normal subjects bilateral anaesthesia of the glossopharyngeal and vagus nerves in the neck results in temporary hypertension, tachycardia and an increase in muscle and skin sympathetic activity presumably as a result of blocking both baroreceptor and chemoreceptor afferents (Guz et al 1966; Fagius et al 1985). The patient is aware of difficulty swallowing liquids and

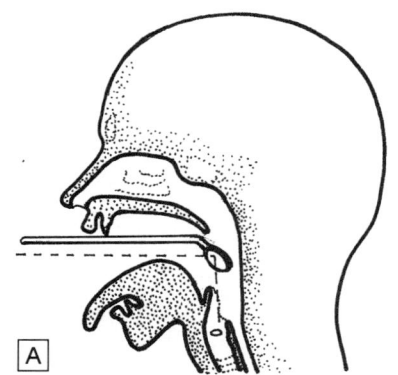

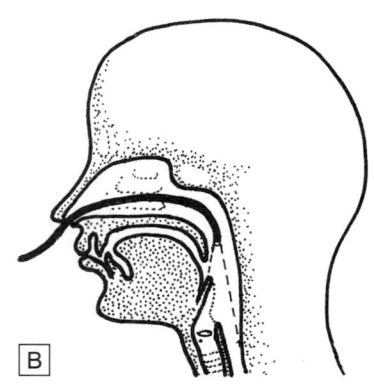

11.31A, B   Laryngoscopic approaches. A shows the oral and B the naso-pharyngeal approaches to the visualization of the larynx.

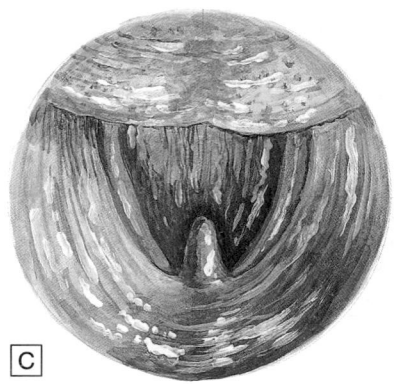

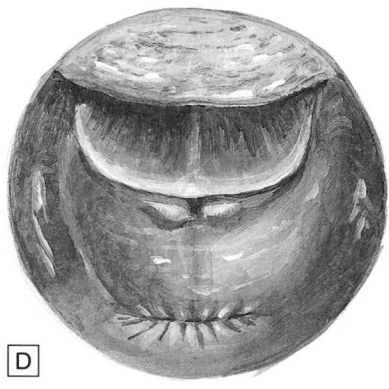

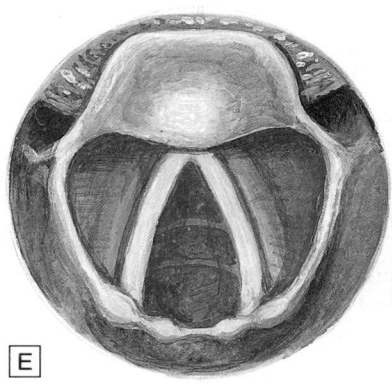

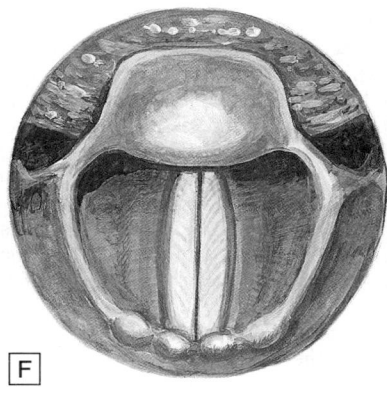

11.31c–f Different views of the oropharynx, epiglottis and larynx seen during the insertion of a laryngoscope. c shows the back of the tongue and soft palate, D the epiglottis, pharyngeal surface of the larynx, and laryngopharynx, E the open glottis, with the vocal folds abducted; F the closed larynx with the white vocal folds adducted. (From originals provided by R. Parker, Division of Anatomy and Cell Biology, UMDS, Guy's Campus, London.)

solids, a hoarse or nasal voice and an inability to cough adequately. Complete interruption of the vagus nerve proximally leads to unilateral paralysis of the soft palate, pharynx and larynx. Effects may be variable as a result of bilateral supranuclear representation. The arch of the soft palate is lowered on the ipsilateral side. On phonation the soft palate fails to elevate, the uvula deviates to the unaffected side and the posterior and lateral wall of the pharynx tend to move medially to the unaffected side like a curtain (signe de rideau) because of the unopposed action of the contralateral superior constrictor. There is ipsilateral loss of the pharyngeal (gag) reflex, in which touching the posterior wall of the pharynx evokes its constriction and elevation, and of the palatal reflex in which touching the soft palate evokes an upward movement. Both these reflexes are mediated by an afferent limb in the glossopharygeal nerve and an efferent limb in the vagus.

Selective involvement of the pharyngeal branches causes a nasal voice and nasal regurgitation of liquids. Bilateral lesions give rise to severe dysphagia.

Unilateral complete palsy of the recurrent layngeal nerve (more commonly on the left side) leads to isolated paralysis of all the laryngeal muscles with the exception of the cricothyroid (superior laryngeal nerve). The patient may be asymptomatic or have a transiently hoarse voice. The affected vocal cord lies paralysed in an adducted, paramedian position but the cricothyroid is able to act as a tensor of the cord. As a consequence of acute bilateral complete palsies the cords usually lie in close apposition leading to preservation of the voice but causing severe stridor and dyspnoea due to limitation of the airway. Such acute lesions may necessitate tracheostomy. With chronic lesions the cords lie more widely separated leading to a weakened voice but a more secure upper airway. With partial lesions of the recurrent laryngeal nerve movements of abduction are affected more than those of adduction (Semon's law) and the cords eventually come to lie at a lower level and in the midline. The mechanism of this effect is unclear. Involvement of the superior laryngeal nerve in addition to the recurrent laryngeal nerve suggests a lesion proximal to the nodose ganglion. This results in paralysis of all laryngeal musculature (including the cricothyroid). The affected cord is paralysed and lies in the cadaveric position halfway between abduction and adduction. If the lesion is unilateral the voice is weak and hoarse but if it is bilateral phonation is almost absent, the vocal pitch cannot be altered and the cough is weak and ineffective. The relative frequency of dysphagia and aspiration in patients with unilateral hemispheric stroke suggests that there may be significant lateralization of supranuclear control of swallowing mechanisms.

LARYNGOSCOPIC EXAMINATION (**11.**31A, B)

The laryngeal inlet, the structures around it and the cavity of the larynx can be inspected by suitable optics, for example a laryngoscopic mirror. The epiglottis is seen foreshortened, but its tubercle is visible. From the epiglottic margins the aryepiglottic folds can be traced posteromedially and the cuneiform and corniculate elevations recognized. The pink vestibular folds and pearly white vocal folds are visible and, when the rima glottidis is wide open, the tracheal mucosa and cartilages may be seen. The piriform fossae can also be inspected. A sequence of views visible at different stages of insertion of the laryngoscope is illustrated in **11.**31B–E.

RADIOGRAPHY

In lateral cervical radiographs (**11.**32) the epiglottis, aryepiglottic folds, arytenoid, corniculate and sometimes cuneiform cartilages and laryngeal sinus are all visible, as well as ossification in the cartilages.

SURFACE ANATOMY OF THE LARYNX AND RELATED STRUCTURES

Around the midline of the neck the following structures can be identified (**7.**62). The laryngeal prominence where the two laminae of the thyroid cartilage meet is visible in men, but not always in women, and the superior borders of the thyroid laminae and the thyroid notch are palpable. (Note that the vocal folds are nearly level with the midpoint of the prominence.) Above the thyroid cartilage, the U-shaped hyoid arch consisting of the median body and more lateral greater cornua can be felt, though less easily, the latter most convincingly when the throat at this level is gripped

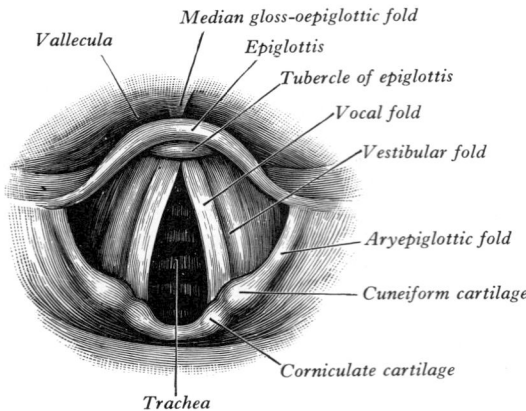

Vallecula

Median gloss-oepiglottic fold

Epiglottis

Tubercle of epiglottis

Vocal fold

Vestibular fold

Aryepiglottic fold

Cuneiform cartilage

Corniculate cartilage

Trachea

11.31G Laryngoscopic view of the interior of the larynx, with the vocal folds abducted during breathing.

between finger and thumb. The thyrohyoid membrane can be palpated in the depression between the thyroid cartilage and the hyoid bone.

Below the thyroid cartilage, the arch of the cricoid can be felt; it is level with the lower part of the cricoid lamina and the body of the sixth cervical vertebra. In the midline between the cricoid and thyroid cartilage is a small interval occupied by the cricothyroid ligament. Below the cricoid is the first tracheal cartilage; the trachea is variably palpated below depending on the amount of superficial tissue, and on either side of the lower half of the larynx and upper trachea can be felt the soft thyroid gland, which rises with the whole laryngeal framework on swallowing. For further details of surface anatomy see page 1914.

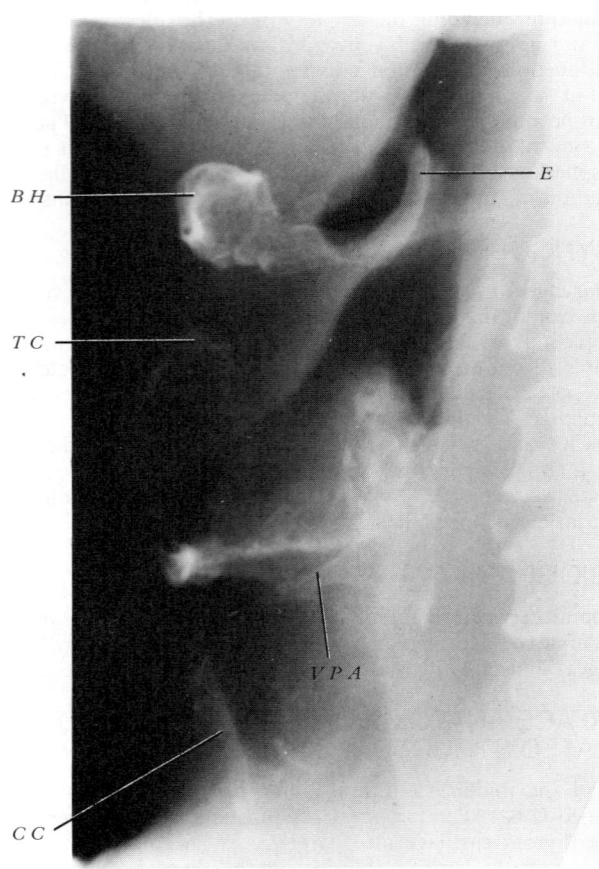

B H

E

T C

V P A

C C

11.32 Lateral soft tissue radiograph of the larynx and adjacent structures in a young adult. BH = body of hyoid bone; CC = cricoid cartilage; E = epiglottis; TC = thyroid cartilage; VPA = vocal process of arytenoid cartilage. (Supplied by Shaun Gallagher, Guy's Hospital; photographed by Sarah Smith, UMDS, Guy's Campus, London.)

CLINICAL ANATOMY OF THE LARYNX

Laryngeal obstruction and trauma

Large foreign bodies may obstruct the laryngeal inlet or rima glottidis and suffocation may ensue, while smaller ones can enter the trachea or bronchi, or lodge in the laryngeal sinus and cause reflex closure of the glottis with consequent suffocation. Inflammation of the upper larynx may swell the mucosa by effusion of fluid into the abundant, loose submucous tissue (oedema of the glottis). The effusion does not involve or extend below the vocal folds, since the mucosa adheres directly to the vocal ligaments without the intervention of submucous tissue. Laryngotomy below the vocal folds through the cricothyroid ligament or tracheotomy may be necessary to restore a free airway (see below). The mucosa of the upper larynx is highly sensitive, and contact with foreign bodies excites immediate coughing.

Suicidal wounds are usually made through the thyrohyoid membrane, damaging the epiglottis, superior thyroid vessels, external and internal carotid arteries and internal jugular veins; less frequently they are above the hyoid with damage to the lingual muscles and lingual and facial vessels.

Recurrent (inferior) laryngeal nerve palsy

If the recurrent nerve is functionless the only laryngeal activity on the affected side is from the cricothyroid muscle, supplied by the external branch of the superior laryngeal nerve. On vocalization, lengthening and tensing of both vocal folds can, therefore, still occur, but there is no thickening of the vocal fold on the affected side by vocalis. On indirect laryngoscopy the arytenoid of the innervated side passes medially below the paralysed cord, due to the action of the innervated vocalis, effectively putting the two vibrating vocal folds at different levels.

Vocal cord nodes

The mucous membrane is loosely attached throughout the larynx and can permit considerable swelling which may compromise the airway in acute infections. At the edge of the true vocal folds the mucosal covering is tightly bound to the underlying cricovocal ligament so that oedema fluid does not pass between upper and lower compartments of the vocal fold mucosa. Any ensuing tissue swelling above the vocal fold exaggerates the potential space deep to the mucosa (Reincke's space) and is seen in vocal abuse. Vocal cord changes for this reason commonly take place at the junction between its posterior third and more anterior two-thirds, at a point where the vocalis fibres of the thyro-arytenoid muscle insert into the vocal fold. This arrangement produces a relatively sharp transition between regions of differing vibration amplitudes so that excessive trauma may produce subepithelial haemorrhage or bruising, and subsequent pathological changes ('singer's nodes', or 'clergyman's nodes').

Tracheostomy

The anatomy of tracheostomy conventionally requires an entry into the trachea at the second to third tracheal ring: a higher tracheostomy, just below the cricoid or at the first tracheal ring (the subglottic area), can lead to fibrosis and stenosis in a region that is already relatively narrow. The surface anatomy for the conventional tracheostomy site is halfway between the thyroid and suprasternal notch; a vertical incision at this point facilitates a rapid and easy access to the airway, although a horizontal incision leaves less scarring by virtue of the direction of the cleavage lines of the dermis. Unless these superficial tissues contain an anterior jugular venous arch at this point, then deep to the deep fascia is found the thyroid gland isthmus embedded in the pretracheal fascia which when divided or retracted exposes the tracheal rings. The second and third rings can be identified by palpating down from the cricoid and even visually by identifying the common abnormal feature of the first ring. A window can then be made about the second to third rings: any lower entry finds the tracheostomy site lower than the skin incision, with the tracheal lumen passing postero-inferiorly behind the great vessels which in the child may even be at risk surgically because the left brachiocephalic vein may rise posteriorly above the sternum.

Another commonly used site for an emergency airway entry is through the midline of the cricothyroid membrane which enters the laryngeal lumen just below the vocal folds before passing down through the cricoid ring into the lower airway. This form of entry requires no formal surgical exposure, for the area is identified by palpation. The skin and laryngeal entry is performed with a sharp knife and dilating instrument that allows a tube to be guided into the airway.

Anatomy of speech

In addition to the sphincteric functions of the larynx for the protection and control of respiratory activities, already mentioned, the larynx has developed during its evolution a complex mechanism of skeletal structures and neuromuscular control which allows it to modify the expiratory stream to produce highly complex patterns of sound with varying loudness, frequency and duration. A phonatory larynx is present in many animals and is used for communication between members of the same species for a wide variety of behavioural purposes, for example breeding, nuture of the young, group co-ordination and the creation of social hierarchies, intimidation, hunting, defence, territorial behaviour, and so forth. In the mammals it is most highly developed among the primates (see the reviews by Negus 1962; Bluck 1992), where social behaviour is generally most advanced. There is, however, an enormous gap between human speech as a form of communication and the type of purposive sound produced by any other animal. Speech and other aspects of language with all their complexities have played a large part in producing the human pre-eminence in the animal kingdom. These complexities, however, depend largely on the cerebral hemispheres many parts of which are involved in the motor aspects of language such as speech and writing, and its sensory manifestations such as reading and understanding what is heard. Language in all its forms, because of its importance and ramifications, has developed its own sciences such as phonetics, phonology, linguistics and semiotics. The purpose of this section is limited to the description of the way in which the larynx functions in producing speech and the role played by the pharynx, palate and oral and nasal cavities.

The physics of speech production. The production of any sound as, for example, that produced by a musical instrument, requires a source of energy (*initiation*), a structure or structures which can oscillate (*phonation*) and a resonator. In the case of the human voice the source of energy is the momentum of the expired air. In speech the force exerted is of the order of 7 cm H_2O, with a range of about 5–35 cm H_2O in singing. Variation in the force exerted can produce variation in the loudness and pitch of the sound, and periodic interruption of expiration is used in the phrasing of speech. The velopharyngeal impairment in subjects with repaired cleft palate results in difficulty in producing the adequate pulmonic pressure required for certain consonants. Warner et al (1992) suggest that these subjects can make adequate adjustment to their expiratory airstream to overcome their problem. Oscillation is due primarily to the activity of the vocal folds. Resonance occurs in the air in the larynx above the vocal folds and in the pharynx, mouth and nasal cavity.

Muscular control of the airstream. The expiratory force used in speech is produced by the controlled relaxation of the expiratory muscles mainly the diaphragm. These muscles can affect not only the pitch but also the loudness and phrasing of speech. The anterior abdominal muscles which are used in prolonged and forced expiration, and in some subjects at the end of quiet respiration, may be involved in speech especially in shouting and attempts to speak without the interruption necessary for inspiration.

Although the pulmonic airstream is the source of energy in normal speech, after removal of the larynx patients can be taught to swallow air and use this as a source of energy (*oesophageal speech*). Speech in these circumstances tends to have a somewhat belching quality and is badly phrased. It has been shown radiologically that the swallowed air remains in the oesophagus. Other methods have been used for the production of an egressive airstream involving prostheses and surgical shunts (Rovira et al 1991; Brasnu 1991; Van Weissenbruch & Albers 1992).

Modulation of the voice. The way in which the vocal folds act together as an oscillator is very complex. As in a vibrating string their length, tension and mass affect the pitch of the voice, but the range of frequencies of the human voice cannot be explained by assuming that the vocal folds act only in this way. The range of frequencies characteristic of human speech vary from 60–500 Hz with an average of about 120 Hz in males, 225 Hz in females and 265 Hz in children. A normal vocal fold can be increased about 50% in length by means of the cricothyroid and posterior cricoarytenoid muscles (p. 1644) but that cannot account for the normal variations in the pitch of the human voice, especially in singing. The breaking of the voice in males at puberty, due to changes mainly in the thyroid cartilage which produce a lengthening of the vocal folds, is an obvious example of the effect of changes in their length.

Changes in mass can affect the pitch of the voice and this is probably produced by the vocalis part of the thyroarytenoid muscle (p. 1644). Because of its attachment to the vocal ligament the vocalis muscle can also affect the length and tension of the vocal fold. The hoarse voice of swollen vocal folds due to inflammation is an example of the effect of changes in mass. Changes in tension of the vocal folds are produced by the same muscles as cause their lengthening, the cricothyroid and posterior crico-arytenoid as well as the vocalis muscle. Paralysis of both cricothyroid muscles, an unusual but possible complication of thyroidectomy, results in permanent hoarseness.

High-speed cinemaphotography has shown that the pitch of the voice is basically varied by the siren-like effect of the vocal folds interrupting the airstream in expiration. At the beginning of phonation the intermembranous and intercartilaginous parts of the glottis (p. 1644) are closed by both rotation and gliding at the crico-arytenoid joints due to the contraction of the lateral crico-arytenoid (rotation) and transverse arytenoid (gliding) muscles (p. 1644). The closure of the glottis results in an increase in the air pressure below the vocal folds sufficient to separate them. The fall in pressure due to their separation and the elasticity of the vocal folds result in closure of the glottis. This is assisted by the suction effect of the fall in pressure (Bernoulli effect). During the opening and closing of the glottis the vocal folds exhibit longitudinal and transverse waves due to their structure, as described by Sataloff (1992). These add to the harmonics of the fundamental frequency of the tone produced.

The sound produced by the mechanism described is transmitted to the column of air extending from the vocal folds to the exterior mainly through the oral opening, but a significant element also usually passes through the nasal cavities. This column of air acts as a *selective resonator* but unlike, for example an organ pipe, it is variable in its axis, shape and size, all of which can be altered by the muscles of the pharynx, soft palate, fauces, tongue oral diaphragm, cheeks and lips. In addition the tension of the walls of the column can be altered. The result is that the fundamental frequency (pitch) and harmonics produced by the passage of air through the adducted glottis are modified by changes in the harmonics. These may be added to, dampened or enhanced. The fundamental frequency and its associated harmonics may also be raised or lowered by appropriate elevation or depression of both hyoid and larynx together by the selective actions of many of the muscle complexes mentioned above, including the infrahyoid, pharyngeal and hyoid-associated muscles. Effectively, these movements shorten or lengthen the resonating column, and also alter the geometry of the walls of the air passages to some extent. Analysis of a particular sound produced by the human voice shows that for all fundamental frequencies the sound has a very similar pattern of harmonics, determined by the vocal tract acting as a selective filter and resonator. This is necessary for the maintenance of a constant quality of voice without which intelligibility would be lost, so that, for example, recorded speech played back without its harmonics is completely unintelligible.

Frequency characteristics of speech. Each vowel sound has its own higher characteristic frequency components or harmonics (*frequency spectrum*) due to the pharynx and oral cavity acting as resonators to reinforce and absorb different frequencies. These frequencies are always higher than that of the fundamental one and are called *formants*; each vowel sound has its own characteristic formants. Just as each musical instrument has its own frequency spectrum, so the human voice is recognizable as a human voice because of its special characteristics. It has even been suggested that each individual voice has its own frequency spectrum so that an analysis of an individual's voice could be used for personal identification.

Articulation. The next basic component of speech sounds is *articulation* in which the sound is given a specific quality by the articulatory organs which include the tongue, palate, teeth, lips and nasal cavity. In order to analyse the way in which these organs are used in different speech sounds, words are broken down into units called *phonemes* which may be defined as the minimal sequential contrastive units used in any language (Catford 1992). The discipline of *phonetics* primarily deals with the way in which speech sounds are produced, and consequently with the analysis of phonemes in terms of their mode of production by the vocal apparatus. But before outlining the phonemes of English it is important to realize that not all languages have the same phonemes and that within the same language the phonemes can vary in different parts of the same country and in other countries where that language is also spoken.

Phonation of vowels. For the analysis of the phonemes in the English language, it is customary to use what is called *received pronunciation* (R.P.) (for a short history of this somewhat controversial term see Gimson 1981). This is said to be the pronunciation used by the educated people in London and south-east England and for many years by the BBC newsreaders. Phonemes are divided into *vowels* and *consonants* and in the R.P. system there are 5 long and 7 short vowels and 8 diphthongs.

Anatomically, the sounds of the different vowels are mainly determined by the shapes and sizes of the resonating chambers of the mouth and pharynx as determined by the positions of the tongue and lips. The tongue may be placed high or low (*close* and *open vowels*) or further forwards or back (*front* and *back vowels*) and the lips *rounded* or *unrounded*. For example, in articulating the long vowel in *bean* the front of the tongue is high and the lips unrounded, in *boon* the back of the tongue is high and the lips are rounded. The short vowel in *pat* is articulated with the front part of the tongue in a lower position as compared with the position of the tongue for the vowel in *pit* in which the tongue is high. *Diphthongs* are vowels in which one vowel changes into another in the same syllable, for example *pay*, *out*, *ice*.

Phonation of consonants. *Consonants* may be defined as speech sounds which are determined by the closure or narrowing of some part of the vocal tract. If the consonant is sounded without vibration of the vocal folds they are defined as *voiceless*, while if the vocal folds are involved, they are *voiced*. Consonants are more precisely classified according to the parts and positions of the speech organs involved – lips, tongue, teeth and palate. For this purpose, these organs can be subdivided into a number of regions; for example, the tongue can be divided into a tip, an anterior edge, a front part of dorsum (lamina), two parts of the remaining dorsum and a most posterior part (radix).

The classification of consonants has become very complex. The most widely accepted grouping is as follows:

(1) 6 plosives (also called *stops*):
    p, b, t, d, c (*can*), g (*good*)
(2) 2 affricates:
    ch (*chain*), j (*join*)
(3) 9 fricatives:
    f, v, th (*think*), th (*this*), s (*sole*), z (*zeal*), sh, s (*leisure*, h (*how*)
(4) 3 nasals:
    m, n, ng (*hang*)
(5) 1 lateral: l
(6) 3 approximants (semivowels):
    r (*rule*), w (*wet*), y (*yet*).

It is not proposed to deal in detail with the way in which the speech organs are used in producing the different consonants but some comments may be made. Many of the consonants form pairs of voiceless and voiced using the same parts of the speech organs – p and b, t and d, k and g, the two ths, f and v, s and z, ch and j, sh and s (as in *leisure*). Each pair can be named in terms of the anatomical structures or part of the structures involved, for example, p and b are *bilabial*, f and v are *labiodental*. An *affricate* is defined as a plosive followed by a fricative and a *fricative* as a rustling of the breath due to a considerable narrowing of the oral cavity by, for example, an approximation of the tongue to the palate or upper teeth, without complete closure.

There is considerable variation in the phonemes of different dialects in English, especially in the vowel sounds. The partially trilled *r* and the voiceless fricative as in *loch* of Scotland are not found among the consonants R.P. Analysis of the phonemes of different languages illustrates that although the vocal apparatus is the same or similar in all human beings there are marked differences in how often the various parts of the vocal tract are used. Several languages, for example Arabic, have three or more pharyngeal and glottal consonants as compared with only one in English. This shows that the phonemes of R.P. cannot be the same as those of English as spoken in the United States or as those of any of the world's languages. Recent studies of stops by Henton et al (1992) and Keating and Lahiri (1993) involve the analysis of these speech sounds in a number of languages.

For some time the concept of the phonemes as the unit of speech has been questioned since it was found that the same phoneme was not always produced by the same articulatory movements. Emphasis has shifted to the role of the central nervous system in determining the way in which the articulatory organs function in the production of speech sounds. For a review of the control of orofacial movements in speech and of different schools of thought concerned with the analysis of speech production, see Smith 1992.

Phonology. It should be emphasized that the above analysis of speech sounds deals in a limited way with what may be termed the units from which the words of a language are built. This is an important part of the subject of *phonology*, which may be defined as the study of the way in which speech sounds are organized into systems and utilized in language. Phonology must include phonetics in order to understand the way in which individual speech sounds are formed. Folkins and Bleille (1990) suggest that phonology has a variety of meanings for different people. The broadest definition would include all aspects of the study of speech sounds, including the central and peripheral mechanisms of both speech production and speech perception. It is suggested that the anatomy of speech as outlined above is an essential part of the study of language.

TRACHEA AND BRONCHI

TRACHEA

The trachea is a tube formed of cartilage and fibromuscular membrane, lined internally by mucosa. It is about 10–11 cm long, descends from the larynx (11.33, 34), extending from the level of the sixth cervical to the upper border of the fifth thoracic vertebra, where it divides into right and left principal (pulmonary) bronchi. It lies approximately in the sagittal plane but its point of bifurcation is usually a little to the right. The trachea is mobile and can rapidly alter in length; during deep inspiration the bifurcation may descend to the sixth thoracic vertebral level. Its cylindrical shape is flattened posteriorly so that in transverse section it is shaped, with some individual variation, like a letter D (11.59). Its external transverse diameter is about 2 cm in adult males, and 1.5 cm in adult females. In children it is smaller, more deeply placed and more mobile. The lumen in live adults is about 12 mm in transverse diameter, although this increases after death due to relaxation in the smooth muscle at its posterior aspect. In the first postnatal year, the tracheal diameter does not exceed 3 mm while during later childhood its diameter in millimetres is about equal to age in years. The transverse shape of the lumen is variable, especially in later decades, being round, lunate or flattened (Campbell & Liddelow 1967). Wang and Tai (1965) have studied tracheobronchial dimensions extensively; in Chinese subjects (presumably cadavers) the tracheal lumen averaged 16.17 mm (range 9.5–22.0 mm).

Relations of the trachea

Cervical part of the trachea (11.19, 20, **15**.12).
Anterior relations. The cervical trachea is crossed by skin and by the superficial and deep fasciae. It is also crossed by the jugular arch and overlapped by the sternohyoid and sternothyroid muscles. The second to fourth tracheal cartilages are crossed by the isthmus of the thyroid gland, above which an anastomotic artery connects the bilateral superior thyroid arteries; below this and in front are the pretracheal fascia, inferior thyroid veins, thymic remnants and the arteria thyroidea ima (when it exists). In children the brachiocephalic artery crosses obliquely in front of the trachea at or a little above the upper border of the manubrium; the left brachiocephalic vein may also rise a little above this level.

Posterior relations. Behind the cervical trachea is the oesophagus, running between the trachea and the vertebral column; the recurrent laryngeal nerves ascend on each side, in or near the grooves between the sides of the trachea and oesophagus.

Lateral relations. These are the paired lobes of the thyroid gland descending to the fifth or sixth tracheal cartilage, and the common carotid and inferior thyroid arteries.

Thoracic part of the trachea (11.33–35, 59, 60).
Anterior relations. As it descends through the superior mediastinum, the thoracic trachea lies behind the following: the manubrium sterni, the attachments of the sternohyoid and sternothyroid muscles, the thymic remnants, the inferior thyroid and left brachiocephalic veins, the aortic arch, the brachiocephalic and left common carotid arteries, deep cardiac plexus and some lymph nodes; the brachiocephalic and left common carotid arteries come to lie respectively right and left of the trachea as they diverge upwards into the neck.

Posterior relations. Behind the trachea is the oesophagus, separating it from the vertebral column.

Lateral relations. On the **right** are: the right lung and pleura, right brachiocephalic vein, superior vena cava, right vagus nerve and the azygos vein; on the **left**: the arch of the aorta, left common carotid and left subclavian arteries.

The left recurrent laryngeal nerve is at first situated between the trachea and aortic arch, then in or just in front of the groove between the trachea and the oesophagus.

RIGHT PRINCIPAL BRONCHUS AND ITS BRANCHES

The right principal bronchus (11.33–35, 61, 62) is wider, shorter and more vertical than the left, being about 2.5 cm long. It gives rise to its first branch, the *superior lobar bronchus*, then enters the right lung opposite the fifth thoracic vertebra. The greater width and more vertical course of the right principal bronchus explain why foreign bodies enter it more often than the left. The azygos vein arches over it and the right pulmonary artery lies at first inferior, then anterior to it. After giving off the superior lobar bronchus, which arises posterosuperior to the right pulmonary artery, it crosses the posterior aspect of this artery to enter the pulmonary hilum postero-inferior to the artery, where it divides into a *middle* and an *inferior lobar bronchus*.

The right superior lobar bronchus. This branch arises from the lateral aspect of the parent bronchus and runs superolaterally to enter the hilum. About 1 cm from its origin it divides into three segmental bronchi: the *apical segmental bronchus* continues superolaterally towards the apex of the lung, which it supplies, dividing near its origin into apical and anterior branches; the *posterior segmental bronchus* serves the postero-inferior part of the superior lobe, passing posterolaterally and slightly superiorly and soon dividing into a lateral and a posterior branch; the *anterior segmental bronchus* runs antero-inferiorly to supply the rest of the superior lobe; it divides near its origin into a lateral and an anterior branch of equal size.

The middle lobar bronchus. It starts about 2 cm below the superior, from the front of the parent trunk, descends anterolaterally and soon divides into a *lateral* and a *medial segmental bronchus* passing to the lateral and medial parts of the middle lobe, respectively.

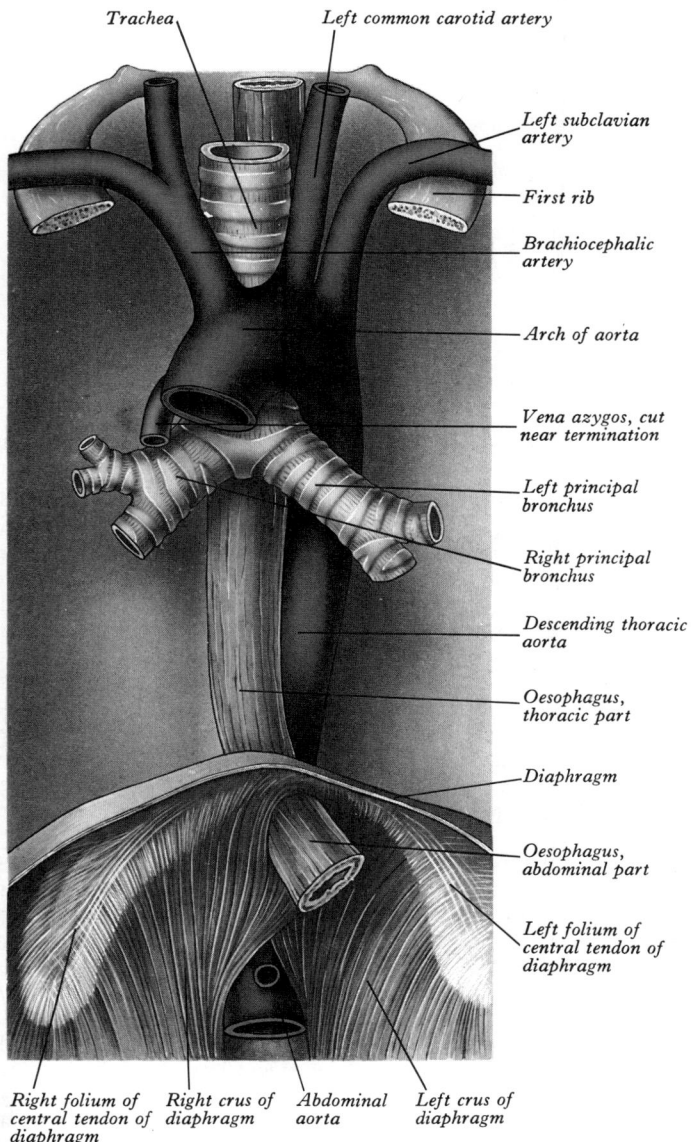

Trachea

Left common carotid artery

Left subclavian artery

First rib

Brachiocephalic artery

Arch of aorta

Vena azygos, cut near termination

Left principal bronchus

Right principal bronchus

Descending thoracic aorta

Oesophagus, thoracic part

Diaphragm

Oesophagus, abdominal part

Left folium of central tendon of diaphragm

Right folium of central tendon of diaphragm   *Right crus of diaphragm*   *Abdominal aorta*   *Left crus of diaphragm*

11.33 Dissection to show the bifurcation of the trachea and the principal bronchi, viewed from the front.

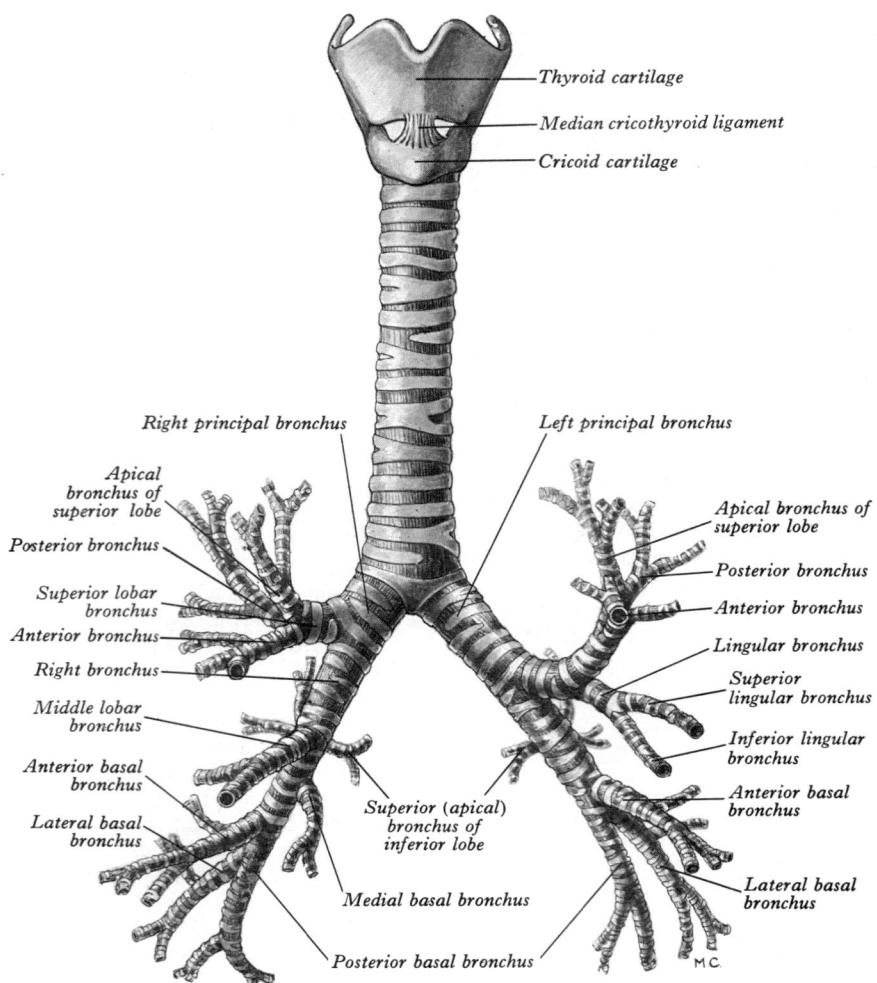

Thyroid cartilage

Median cricothyroid ligament

Cricoid cartilage

Right principal bronchus

Left principal bronchus

Apical bronchus of superior lobe

Posterior bronchus

Superior lobar bronchus

Anterior bronchus

Right bronchus

Middle lobar bronchus

Anterior basal bronchus

Lateral basal bronchus

Apical bronchus of superior lobe

Posterior bronchus

Anterior bronchus

Lingular bronchus

Superior lingular bronchus

Inferior lingular bronchus

Anterior basal bronchus

Superior (apical) bronchus of inferior lobe

Lateral basal bronchus

Medial basal bronchus

Posterior basal bronchus

M.C.

11.34 The cartilages of the larynx, trachea and bronchi: anterior aspect. (Drawn from a metal cast made by the late Lord Russell Brock, Guy's Hospital, London.)

The right inferior lobar bronchus. This is the continuation of the principal bronchus beyond the origin of the middle lobar bronchus. At or a little below its origin from the principal bronchus, it gives off posteriorly a large *superior* (apical) *segmental bronchus*. This runs posteriorly to the upper part of the inferior lobe, subsequently dividing into medial, superior and lateral branches, the first two usually arising from a common stem. After giving off the superior segmental branch, the continuing right inferior lobar bronchus descends posterolaterally. The *medial basal segmental bronchus* branches from its anteromedial aspect, running inferomedially to serve a small region below the hilum; the inferior lobar bronchus continues downwards then divides into an *anterior basal segmental bronchus*, which descends anteriorly, and a trunk which soon divides into a *lateral basal segmental bronchus* descending laterally and a *posterior basal segmental bronchus* descending posteriorly. In more than half of all right lungs a *subsuperior* (subapical) *segmental bronchus* arises posteriorly from the right inferior lobar bronchus 1–3 cm below the superior segmental bronchus. This is distributed to the region of lung between the superior and posterior basal segments.

LEFT PRINCIPAL BRONCHUS AND ITS BRANCHES
(11.33, 34, 40A, 61)

The left principal bronchus which is narrower and less vertical than the right, is nearly 5 cm long, and enters the hilum of the left lung level with the sixth thoracic vertebra. Passing left inferior to the aortic arch, it crosses anterior to the oesophagus, thoracic duct and descending aorta; the left pulmonary artery is at first anterior and then superior to it. Having entered the hilum it divides into a superior and an inferior lobar bronchus.

The left superior lobar bronchus. Arising from the antero-lateral aspect of its parent stem, this bronchus curves laterally and soon divides into two bronchi. These correspond to the branches of the right principal bronchus supplying the right superior and middle lobes, but on the left both are distributed to the left *superior* lobe, there being no separate middle lobe. The *superior division* ascends about 1 cm, gives off an *anterior segmental bronchus*, then continues a further 1 cm as the *apicoposterior segmental bronchus* before dividing into apical and posterior branches. The apical, posterior and anterior segmental bronchi are largely distributed as in the right superior lobe. The inferior division descends antero-laterally to the antero-inferior part of the left superior lobe (the lingula) forming the *lingular bronchus* which divides into *superior* and *inferior lingular segmental bronchi*, unlike the pattern in the right middle lobe where the corresponding distribution is superior and inferior.

The left inferior lobar bronchus. This branch descends postero-laterally for 1 cm and then the *superior* (apical) *segmental bronchus* arises from it posteriorly and is distributed in essentially the same manner as in the right lung. After a further 1–2 cm the inferior lobar bronchus divides into an anteromedial and a posterolateral stem. The former divides into *medial basal* and *anterior basal segmental bronchi*; the latter into *lateral* and *posterior basal segmental bronchi*. The territories supplied resemble those on the right. The medial basal segmental bronchus is an independent branch of the inferior lobar bronchus in about 10% of lungs; this fact, and the similarity of its territory to that on the right, supports its recognition as a separate segmental bronchus. A *subsuperior* (subapical) *segmental bronchus* arises posteriorly from the left inferior lobar bronchus in 30% of lungs.

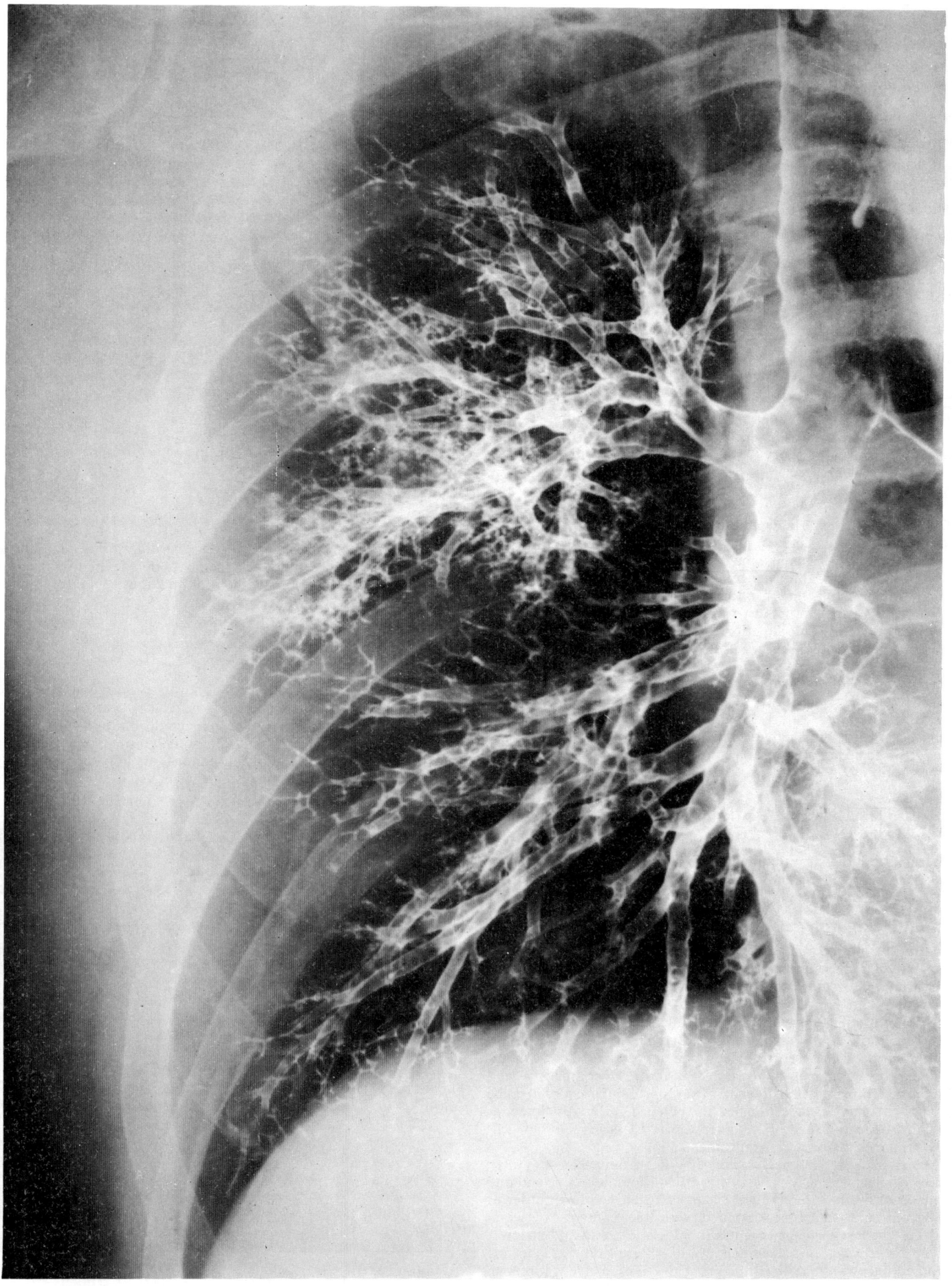

11.35 Bronchogram showing the branching pattern of the trachea and bronchi of the right lung, in slightly oblique anteroposterior view. In this procedure, a radio-opaque contrast medium has been introduced into the respiratory tract, to coat the walls of the respiratory passages. For identification of the major branches, compare with **11.40**A.

BRONCHOPULMONARY SEGMENTATION

Primary branches of the right and left *lobar bronchi* are termed *segmental bronchi* because each ramifies in a structurally separate, functionally independent unit of lung tissue called a *broncho-pulmonary segment* (**11.34, 40, 41**). The main segments are **named** and **numbered** as follows:

Right lung

Superior lobe:	(1) apical, (2) posterior, (3) anterior
Middle lobe:	(4) lateral, (5) medial
Inferior lobe:	(6) superior (apical), (7) medial basal, (8) anterior basal, (9) lateral basal, (10) posterior basal

Left lung

Superior lobe:	(1) apical, (2) posterior, (3) anterior, (4) superior lingular, (5) inferior lingular
Inferior lobe:	(6) superior (apical), (7) medial basal, (8) anterior basal, (9) lateral basal, (10) posterior basal

Each segment is surrounded by connective tissue continuous with the visceral pleura, and is a separate respiratory unit. The vascular and lymphatic arrangements of the segments are described on pages 1624, 1672. (For further details of segmentation consult Brock 1942, 1943, 1944, 1954; Boyden 1955; Bloomer et al 1960; Volpe et al 1969.)

Clinical anatomy. While pathological conditions such as bronchi-ectasis and some infections may be restricted to one or more bronchopulmonary segments, malignant neoplasms and tuberculosis are not so confined. A knowledge of bronchial branching is essential during bronchoscopy and for the correct interpretation of bronchograms. It is also determinative in the postural drainage of infected pulmonary regions. The superior (apical) segment of the inferior lobe is a common site of abscess following aspiration of material by supine patients. Inhaled foreign bodies may obstruct a main, lobar, segmental or smaller bronchus according to their size. The interpretation of their effects and the design of surgical treatment inevitably involve considerations of bronchial branching patterns. Resection of a single segment is practicable, while more extensive procedures may include the removal of several segments, lobectomy or a complete pneumonectomy.

MICROSTRUCTURE OF THE TRACHEA AND MAJOR BRONCHI (11.36, 37)

The trachea and extrapulmonary bronchi have a framework of incomplete rings of hyaline cartilage (**11.34, 36**), united by fibrous tissue and smooth muscle (11.35) and lined internally by mucosa.

Cartilage skeleton (11.34, 36)

Tracheal cartilages. These vary from 16 to 20 in number, each an imperfect 'ring' surrounding approximately the anterior two-thirds of the tracheal circumference; behind, where they are deficient, the tube is flat and is completed by fibro-elastic tissue and smooth muscle. The cartilages are horizontally stacked, separated by narrow intervals and are about 4 mm vertically and 1 mm in thickness; their external surfaces are vertically flat, their internal surfaces convex. Two or more cartilages often unite, partially or completely, and sometimes bifurcate at their ends. They are composed of hyaline cartilage but may become calcified in the aged. In extrapulmonary bronchi, cartilages are shorter, narrower and less regular but generally similar in shape and arrangement.

The first and last tracheal cartilages differ from the rest (**11.34**); the **first cartilage** is the broadest. It is often bifurcate at one end and is connected by the cricotracheal ligament to the inferior border of the cricoid and sometimes blended with the cricoid or second cartilage. The **last cartilage** is centrally thick and broad and its lower border, the *carina*, is a triangular hook-shaped process, curving down and backwards between the bronchi. On each side it forms an imperfect ring, enclosing the start of a principal bronchus. The penultimate cartilage is centrally broader than the others.

Bronchial cartilages. The irregularity of the cartilaginous plates

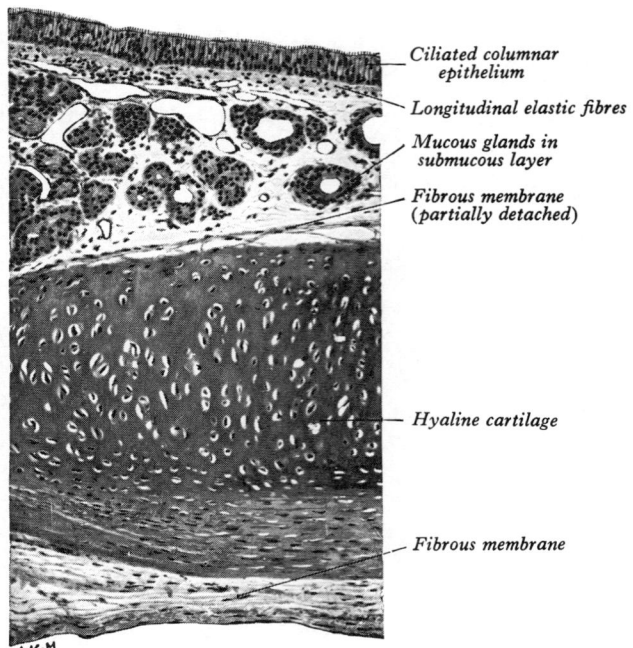

11.36 Transverse section through a part of the wall of a human trachea.

Ciliated columnar epithelium
Longitudinal elastic fibres
Mucous glands in submucous layer
Fibrous membrane (partially detached)
Hyaline cartilage
Fibrous membrane

in the extrapulmonary bronchi increases distally; as the major bronchi approach their lungs and lobes, the plates invade their dorsal aspects but never quite encompass their bifurcations. In intrapulmonary bronchi, plates of cartilage progressively form less and less of the bronchial wall, disappearing where the bronchioles begin (**11.47**; Reid 1976).

Fibrous membrane (11.36)

Each cartilage is enclosed in perichondrium, continuous with a dense fibrous membrane situated between the adjacent cartilages, and filling in the back of the trachea. The perichondrium and membrane are mainly composed of collagen with some elastin fibres; fibres cross each other diagonally, allowing changes in luminal diameter, the elastic component providing some recoil from stretching. Smooth

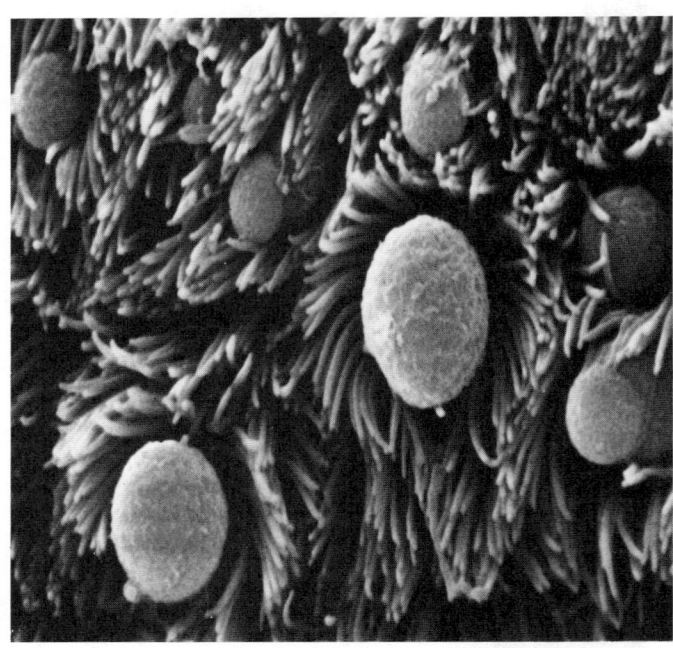

11.37 Surface view of the ciliated epithelium of the trachea (rat). Mucus-secreting goblet cells occur between the ciliated cells. Magnification × 5100. (Prepared by Michael Crowder, Department of Anatomy, Guy's Hospital Medical School, London.)

muscle fibres occur in the membrane posteriorly; most are transverse, being attached to the perichondrium at the ends of the cartilages and forming a transverse sheet between them. Contraction, therefore, alters the cross-sectional area of the trachea and bronchi. A few external longitudinal fibres also occur. Smooth muscle in the intrapulmonary bronchi is not attached to cartilages and, where the latter begin to disappear, i.e. in smaller bronchi, contraction may actually obliterate the lumen (Reid 1976).

Mucosa (Tunica mucosa)

The mucosa is continuous with and closely resembles that of the larynx above and the intrapulmonary bronchi below, being a layer of pseudostratified ciliated columnar epithelium interspersed with goblet cells (Dalen 1983), both lying on a basal lamina (**11**.36, 37). Some pseudostratified cells possess unusually large nuclei and may be polytene in chromosomal content. Numerous lymphocytes usually occur deep in the epithelium. The cilia impel mucus towards the laryngeal inlet (aditus). Deep to the basal lamina are a lamina propria with abundant longitudinal elastic fibres and a submucosa of loose connective tissue, containing larger blood vessels, nerves and most of the tubular (tracheal) seromucous glands and lymphoid nodules; external to the submucosa are the perichondrium and the fibrous membrane. Most external of all is the deep fascia, merging with the fascial planes of the surrounding muscles, oesophagus and associated structures.

Vessels and nerves

The trachea is supplied with blood mainly by the inferior thyroid **arteries**, while its thoracic end is also supplied by the bronchial arteries, whose branches ascend to anastomose with the former; all the vessels also supply the oesophagus. **Veins** draining the trachea end in the inferior thyroid venous plexus. The **lymph vessels** pass to the pretracheal and paratracheal lymph nodes. The **nerve supply** is from the tracheal branches of the vagi, recurrent laryngeal nerves and the sympathetic trunks and is distributed to the tracheal muscle and mucosa. Sympathetic nerve endings evoke bronchodilatation by releasing catecholamines; they may also exert a direct aminergic effect on glandular acini in the bronchi (Pack & Richardson 1984). Parasympathetic activity which is cholinergic causes broncho-constriction. Many small postsynaptic ganglia occur in the autonomic plexuses of the tracheal and bronchial walls (Feyler 1965). In cats, paraganglia composed of chromaffin cells and arteriovenous anastomoses appear in the bronchial wall (Muratori 1965). Afferent fibres include those with sensorimotor functions and can mediate local inflammatory influences by means of their collateral terminae which can release neuropeptides to trigger mast cell degranulation. For a quantitative technique for assessing amounts and distribution of the tissues in the bronchial walls, normal or pathological, see Hale et al (1968).

Surface anatomy. The *trachea* is about 2 cm wide and extends almost vertically in the midline from the cricoid cartilage to the sternal angle, inclining slightly to the right. The *right principal bronchus* runs from the trachea down to the right for 2.5 cm to the right hilum behind the sternal end of the right third costal cartilage. The *left principal bronchus* runs for 5 cm more obliquely to its left and down to the hilum behind the left third costal cartilage, 3.5 cm from midline. The trachea may be opened by median vertical incision above the thyroid isthmus (high tracheotomy) or below it (low tracheotomy), the latter being more difficult because the trachea recedes as it descends and has hazardous anterior relations (p. 1653). The trachea may be compressed by pathological enlargements of the thyroid gland, thymus and aortic arch. The radiological appearances of the trachea, bronchi and lungs are dealt with on page 1675.

Bronchoscopy. By means of a bronchoscope passed through the mouth and larynx under local anaesthesia, the interior of the larynx, trachea and bronchi, with the openings of the main segmental branches, may all be examined and biopsies taken; foreign bodies or accumulations of fluid may also be removed.

LUNGS (11.1, 38–41, 64–9)

The lungs are the essential organs of respiration. They are situated on either side of the heart and other mediastinal contents (**11**.1, 38–41, 64–9). Each lung is free in its pleural cavity, except for its attachment to the heart and trachea at the hilum and pulmonary ligament. When removed, a lung, being spongy, can float in water and crepitates when handled, due to the air within its alveoli. It is also highly elastic and retracts when removed from the thorax. Its surface is smooth, shiny and separated by fine, dark lines into numerous small polyhedral domains, each crossed by numerous finer lines, indicating the areas of contact between its most peripheral lobules and the pleural surface.

At birth the lungs are pink, in adults a dark grey and patchily mottled; as age advances this maculation becomes black, due to granules of inhaled carbonaceous material deposited in loose connective tissue near the surface; this darkening increases as age advances, often more markedly in men than women, and more in those who have dwelt in industrial areas or in smokers. The posterior pulmonary border is usually darker than the anterior. In the upper, less movable parts of the lung, this surface pigmentation tends to be concentrated opposite the intercostal spaces. Lungs from fetuses or stillborn infants who have not respired differ from those of infants who have, being firm, non-crepitant and unable to float in water.

The adult right lung usually weighs about 625 g, and the left 565 g, but they vary greatly. Their weight also depends on the amount of blood or serous fluid. In proportion to body stature, the lungs are heavier in men than women.

PULMONARY SURFACE FEATURES

Each lung has an apex, base, three borders and two surfaces (**11**.38, 39, 41). In shape each lung approximates to half a cone.

Apex. This rounded upper extremity protrudes above the thoracic inlet where it contacts the cervical pleura, covered in turn by the suprapleural membrane. Owing to the inlet's obliquity (p. 545), the apex rises 3–4 cm above the level of the first costal cartilage although level posteriorly with the neck of the first rib. Its summit is about 2.5 cm above the medial third of the clavicle; the apex is therefore in the root of the neck (**11**.1, 42, 43). It has been asserted that because the apex does not rise above the neck of the first rib it is really intrathoracic, and that it is the anterior surface which ascends highest in inspiration (Andreassi 1967), but this requires confirmation. Over the suprapleural membrane, the subclavian artery arches up and laterally, grooving the anterior surface of the apex near its summit and separating it from scalenus anterior. Posterior to the apex are the cervicothoracic (stellate) sympathetic ganglion, the ventral ramus of the first thoracic spinal nerve and the superior intercostal artery (**10**.91). Scalenus medius is lateral and the brachiocephalic artery, right brachiocephalic vein and trachea are on the right, while the left subclavian artery and left brachiocephalic vein are on the left.

Base. This is semilunar and concave, resting upon the superior surface of the diaphragm, which separates the right lung from the right lobe of the liver and the left lung from the left lobe of the liver, the gastric fundus and spleen. Since the diaphragm extends higher on the right than on the left, the concavity is deeper on the base of the right lung. Posterolaterally, the base has a sharp margin which projects a little into the costodiaphragmatic recess (p. 1664).

The costal surface. This aspect of the lung is smooth and convex, its shape adapted to that of the thoracic wall which is vertically deeper posteriorly. It is in contact with the costal pleura and exhibits, in specimens preserved in situ, grooves corresponding with the overlying ribs.

The medial surface. This has two parts: a posterior *vertebral* and anterior *mediastinal* part. The vertebral part lies in contact with the sides of the thoracic vertebrae and intervertebral discs, the posterior intercostal vessels and the splanchnic nerves. The mediastinal area is deeply concave, as it is adapted to the heart at the *cardiac impression*, which is much larger and deeper on the left lung as the heart projects more to the left of the median plane. Posterosuperior to this concavity is the somewhat triangular *hilum*, where various structures (p. 1659) enter and leave the lung, collectively surrounded by a sleeve of pleura which also extends below the hilum and behind the cardiac impression as the *pulmonary ligament*.

Other impressions of the lung surface

In addition to these pulmonary features, preserved lungs show a number of other impressions which indicate their relations with

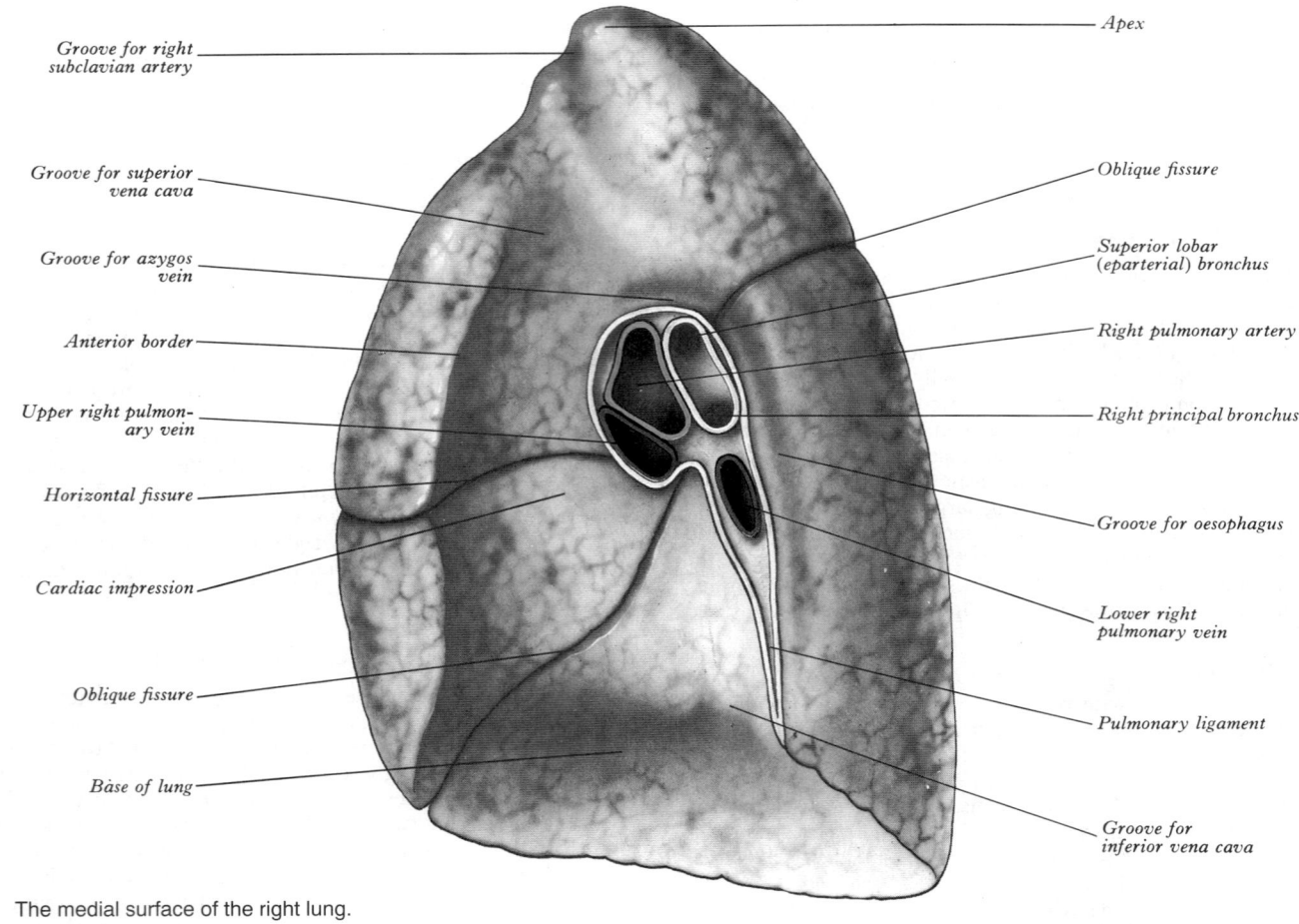

Groove for right
subclavian artery

Groove for superior
vena cava

Groove for azygos
vein

Anterior border

Upper right pulmon-
ary vein

Horizontal fissure

Cardiac impression

Oblique fissure

Base of lung

Apex

Oblique fissure

Superior lobar
(eparterial) bronchus

Right pulmonary artery

Right principal bronchus

Groove for oesophagus

Lower right
pulmonary vein

Pulmonary ligament

Groove for
inferior vena cava

11.38   The medial surface of the right lung.

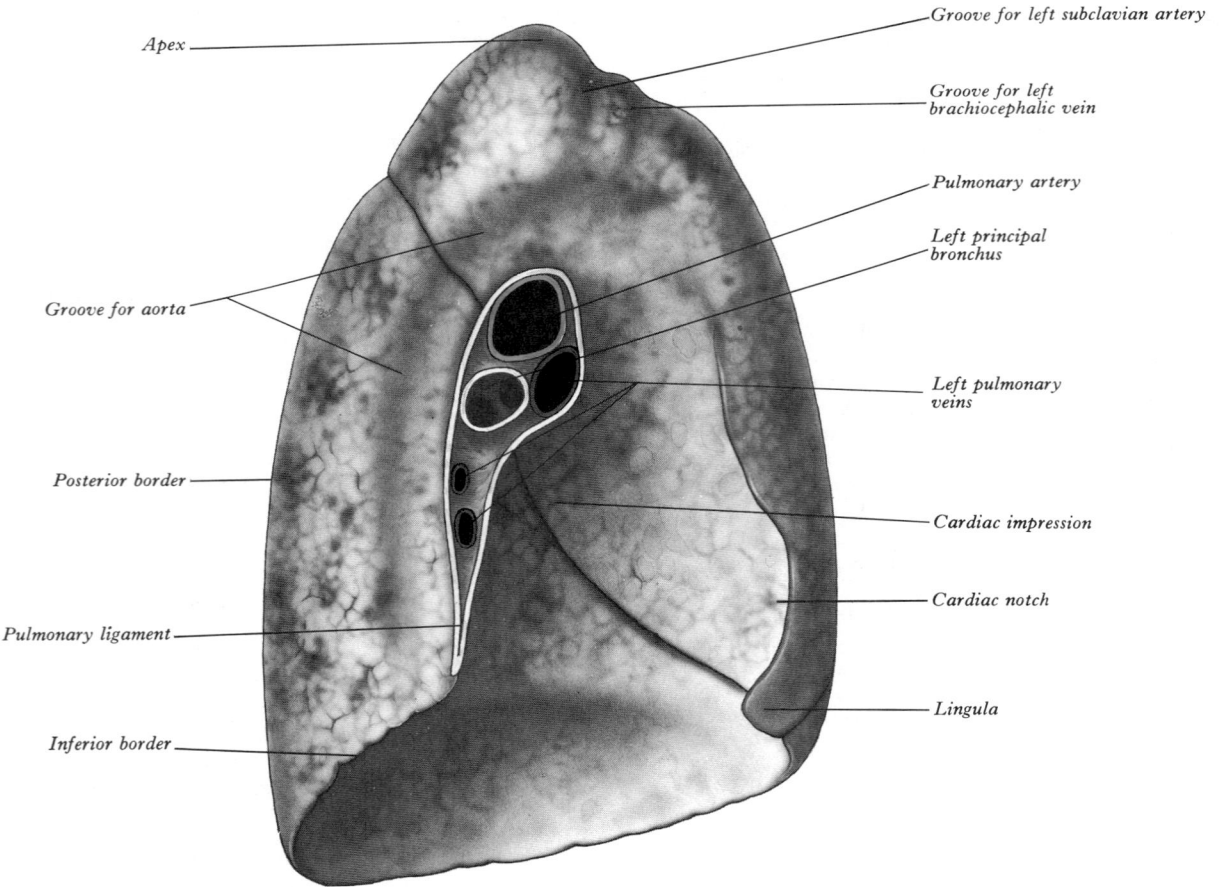

Apex

Groove for aorta

Posterior border

Pulmonary ligament

Inferior border

Groove for left subclavian artery

Groove for left
brachiocephalic vein

Pulmonary artery

Left principal
bronchus

Left pulmonary
veins

Cardiac impression

Cardiac notch

Lingula

11.39   The medial surface of the left lung.

surrounding structures (**11**.38, 39, 57, 58). On the **right lung** the cardiac impression is related to the anterior surface of the right auricle, the anterolateral surface of the right atrium and partially to the anterior surface of the right ventricle. The impression ascends anterior to the hilum as a wide groove for the superior vena cava and the end of the right brachiocephalic vein (**11**.38). Posteriorly this groove is joined by a deep sulcus arching forwards above the hilum and occupied by the azygos vein. The right side of the oesophagus makes a shallow vertical groove behind the hilum and the pulmonary ligament; nearing the diaphragm it inclines left and leaves the right lung; the groove, therefore, does not reach the lower limit of this surface. Postero-inferiorly the cardiac impression is confluent with a short wide groove adapted to the inferior vena cava. Between the apex and azygos groove the trachea and right vagus are close to the lung, but do not mark it.

On the **left lung** (**11**.39) the cardiac impression is related to the anterior and left surfaces of the left ventricle and auricle and the anterior infundibular surface and adjoining part of the right ventricle; it ascends in front of the hilum to accommodate the pulmonary trunk. A large groove arches over the hilum, descending behind it and the pulmonary ligament, corresponding to the aortic arch and descending aorta; from its summit a narrower groove ascends to the apex for the left subclavian artery. Behind this, above the aortic groove, the lung contacts the thoracic duct and oesophagus. In front of the subclavian groove is a faint linear depression for the left brachiocephalic vein. Inferiorly, the oesophagus may mould the surface in front of the lower end of the pulmonary ligament.

Pulmonary borders

The *inferior border* is thin and sharp where it separates the base from the costal surface and extends into the costodiaphragmatic recess; medially, where it divides the base from the mediastinal surface, it is rounded. It corresponds, in quiet respiration, to a line drawn from the lowest point of the anterior border (see below) passing to the sixth rib at about the midclavicular line, then to the eighth rib in the midaxillary line (nearly 10 cm above the costal margin), continued posteriorly, medially and slightly up to a point 2 cm lateral to the tenth thoracic *spine* (**11**.42–44). The *posterior border* separates the costal surface from the mediastinal, corresponding to the heads of the ribs. It has no recognizable markings and is really a rounded junction of costal and vertebral (medial) surfaces. The thin, sharp, *anterior border* overlaps the pericardium; on the **right** it corresponds closely to the costomediastinal line of pleural reflexion, being almost vertical; on the **left** it approaches the same line above, but below the fourth costal cartilage it shows a variable *cardiac notch*, the edge of which passes laterally for about 3.5 cm before curving down and medially to the sixth costal cartilage about 4 cm from midline. It thus does not reach the line of pleural reflexion here (**11**.1, 42, 43), leaving the pericardium covered by a double layer of pleura (area of superficial cardiac dullness, p. 1492). However, surgical experience suggests that the line of pleural reflexion, the anterior pulmonary margin and the costomediastinal pleural recess are all most variable.

PULMONARY FISSURES AND LOBES

The **right lung** is divided into superior, middle and inferior lobes by two fissures, an oblique and a horizontal (**11**.38). The upper, *oblique fissure*, separates the inferior from the middle and upper lobes, and corresponds closely to the left oblique fissure although it is less vertical, crossing the inferior border of the lung about 7.5 cm behind its anterior end. On the posterior border it is level with the spine of the fourth thoracic vertebra or slightly lower. It descends across the fifth intercostal space and follows the sixth rib to the sixth costochondral junction. The short *horizontal fissure* separates the superior and middle lobes, passing from the oblique fissure, near the midaxillary line, horizontally forwards to the anterior border of the lung, level with the sternal end of the fourth costal cartilage; on the mediastinal surface it passes backwards to the hilum. The small *middle lobe* is thus cuneiform and includes some of the costal surface, the lower part of the anterior border and the anterior part of the base of the lung. Sometimes the medial part of the upper lobe is partially separated by a fissure of variable depth containing the terminal part of the azygos vein, enclosed in the free margin of a

mesentery derived from the mediastinal pleura, so forming the '*lobe of the azygos vein*'. This varies in size and sometimes includes the apex of the lung; it is always supplied by one or more branches of the apical bronchus. Radiographically, pleural effusion may be limited to the azygos fissure.

The **left lung** is divided into a superior and an inferior lobe by an *oblique fissure* (**11**.39), extending from the costal to the medial surfaces of the lung both above and below the hilum. Superficially this fissure begins on the medial surface at the posterosuperior part of the hilum and ascends obliquely back to cross the posterior border of the lung about 6 cm below the apex. It then descends forwards across the costal surface, reaching the lower border almost at its anterior end. It finally ascends on the medial surface to the lower part of the hilum. At the posterior border of the lung the fissure lies opposite a surface point 2 cm to the side of the midline between the spines of the third and fourth thoracic vertebrae, but may be above or below this level. Traced around the chest, the fissure reaches the fifth intercostal space (at or near the midaxillary line) and follows this to intersect the inferior border of the lung close to or just below the sixth costochondral junction (7.5 cm from the midline). The left oblique fissure is usually more vertical than the right, and is indicated approximately by the medial border of the scapula when the arm is fully abducted above the shoulder. The *superior lobe*, which lies anterosuperior to this fissure, includes the apex, anterior border, much of the costal and most of the medial surfaces of the lung. At the lower end of the cardiac notch a small process, the *lingula*, is usually present. The larger, *inferior lobe* lies behind and below the fissure; it comprises almost the whole of the *base*, much of the costal surface and most of the posterior border of the lung. (See p. 1656 for details of bronchopulmonary segmentation.)

Attempts to equate the lobation in the two lungs, particularly the right middle lobe and lingula, are not supported by developmental data (p. 178). For discussion and bibliography consult Yokoh (1977).

Since the diaphragm rises higher on the right to accommodate the liver, the right lung is vertically shorter (by 2.5 cm) than the left, but due to cardiac asymmetry the right is broader, and in capacity and weight greater, than the left.

Bronchopulmonary segments

These subdivisions of the pulmonary lobes are described above with the segmental bronchi, and are illustrated in **11**.40 and 41.

PULMONARY HILA AND ROOTS

The pulmonary root (**11**.38, 39, 57, 58) connects the medial surface of the lung to the heart and trachea and is formed by a group of structures entering or leaving the hilum. These are: the principal bronchus, pulmonary artery, two pulmonary veins, bronchial arteries and veins, a pulmonary autonomic plexus, lymph vessels, bronchopulmonary lymph nodes and loose connective tissue, all enveloped by pleura. The pulmonary roots, or pedicles, lie opposite the bodies of the fifth to seventh thoracic vertebrae. The **right root** is situated behind the superior vena cava and right atrium and below the terminal part of the azygos vein. The **left root** lies below the aortic arch and in front of the descending thoracic aorta. Common relations of both are: **anterior**, the phrenic nerve, pericardiacophrenic artery and vein, and anterior pulmonary plexus; **posterior**, the vagus nerve and posterior pulmonary plexus; **inferior**, the pulmonary ligament.

The major structures in both roots are similarly arranged, as follows: the upper of the two pulmonary veins are in front, the pulmonary artery and principal bronchus are behind, and the bronchial vessels most posterior. Their vertical arrangement differs slightly on the two sides. On the **right**, from above downwards, the sequence is: superior lobar bronchus, pulmonary artery, principal bronchus, lower pulmonary vein; on the **left**: pulmonary artery, principal bronchus, the lower pulmonary vein. The lower left pulmonary vein is inferior to the principal bronchus which is the lowest hilar structure (**11**.38, 39).

The different pulmonary regions do not all move equally in respiration. In quiet respiration the juxtahilar part of the lung scarcely moves and the middle region only slightly. The superficial parts of the lung expand the most, while the mediastinal surface, posterior border and apex move less, being related to less movable

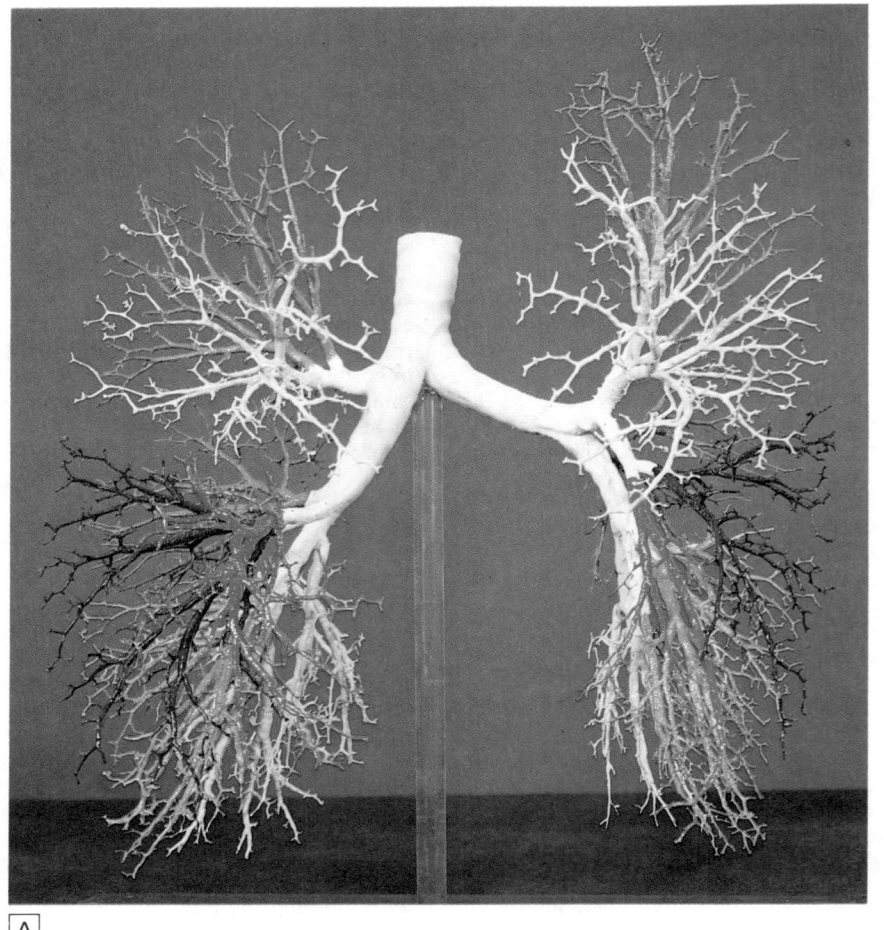

A

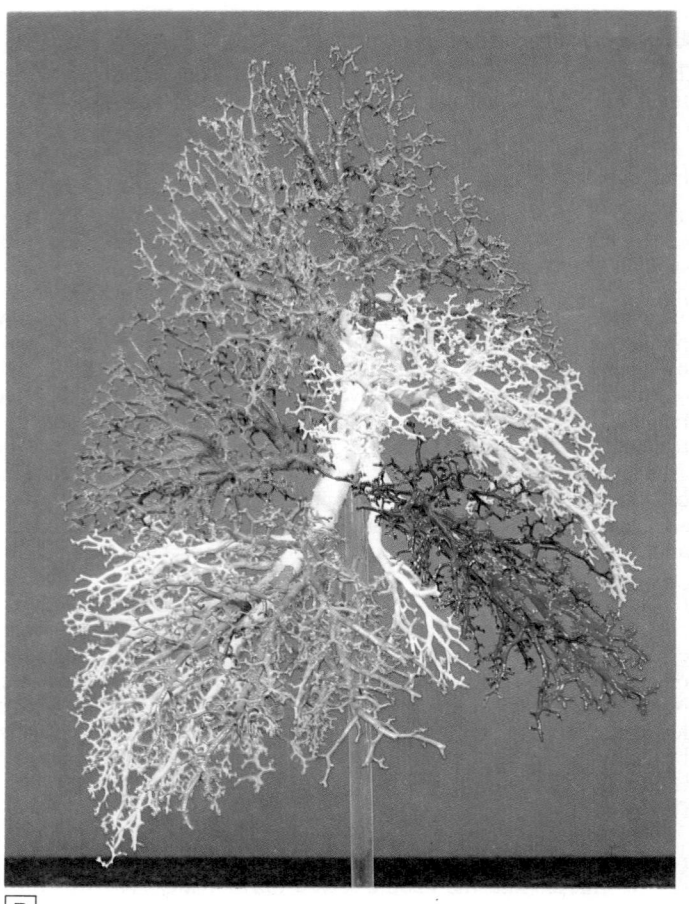

B

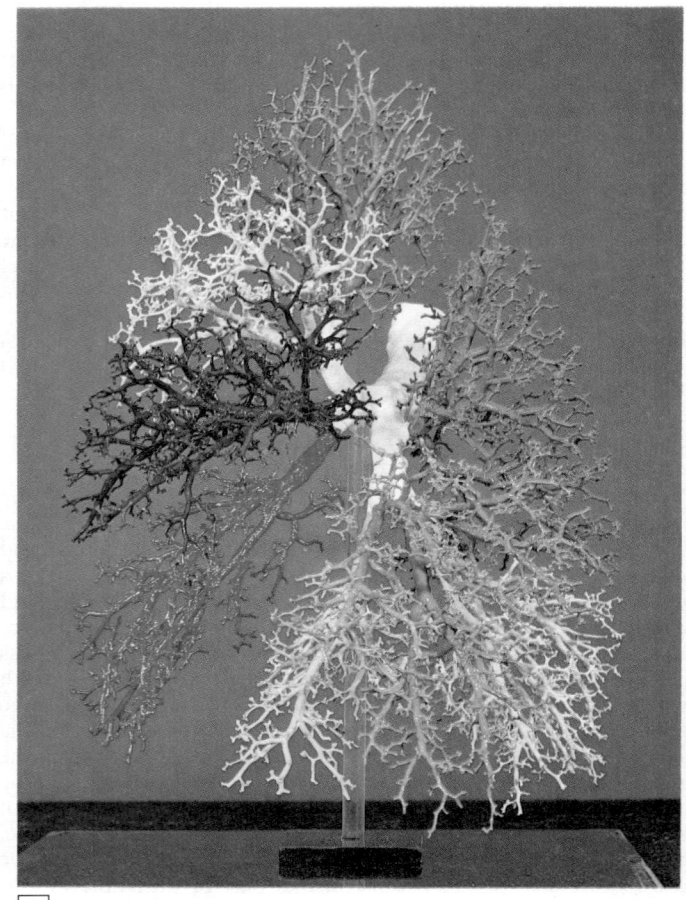

C

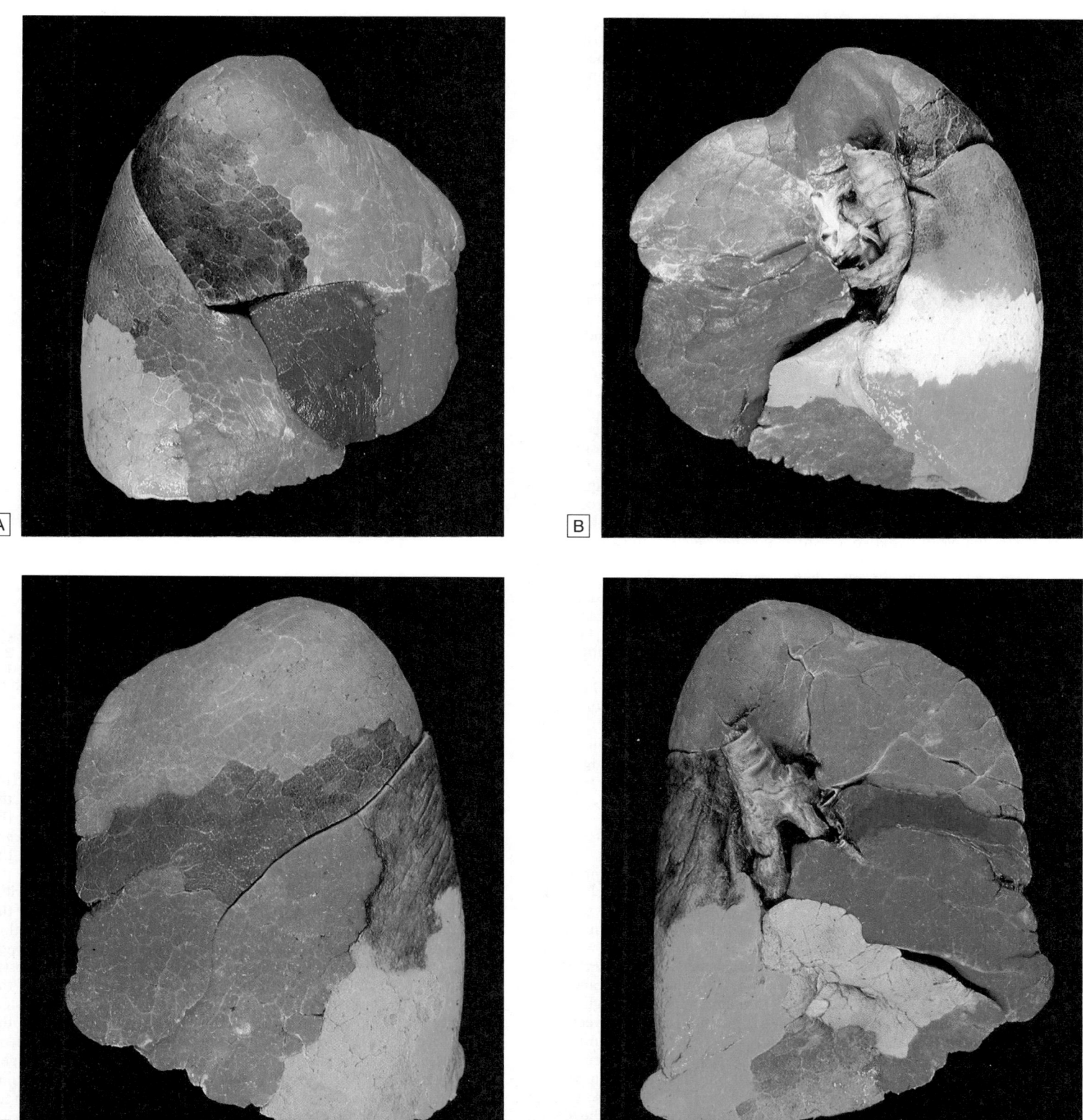

11.40 (opposite) A   A resin corrosion cast of the adult human lower trachea and bronchial tree photographed from the anterior aspect. The segmental bronchi and their main branches have been coloured: brown = apical; grey/blue = posterior; pink = anterior; dark blue = lateral (middle lobe) and superior lingular; red = medial (middle lobe) and inferior lingular; dark green = superior (apical) of inferior lobe; yellow = medial basal; orange = anterior basal; blue = lateral basal; light green = posterior basal.

11.40B   Corrosion cast of the bronchial tree of the right lung, colour coded as in B to indicate the territories supplied by different segmental bronchi.

11.40C   Corrosion cast of the bronchial tree of the left lung, colour coded as in A. Note that in this and other preparations shown in **11.**40 many of the finer bronchial branches have been trimmed away to reveal the larger bronchi. (All specimens were prepared by M. C. E. Hutchinson and photo-

graphed by Kevin Fitzpatrick, Anatomy Department, Guy's Hospital Medical School, London.)

11.41 (Above)   Bronchopulmonary segments of the right and left lungs, coloured to indicate the different territories as in **11.**40, except that in the right lung, the medial view shows a subsuperior segment which is painted white. A shows the costal surface of the right lung, and B the mediastinal surface of the right lung. C depicts the costal surface of the left lung; D shows the left lung's mediastinal surface. The lungs were prepared by injecting individual bronchial trees with appropriate pigments in gelatin, followed by formalin fixation. (All specimens were prepared by M. C. E. Hutchinson and photographed by Kevin Fitzpatrick, Anatomy Department, Guy's Hospital Medical School, London.)

structures. The diaphragmatic and costomediastinal regions expand most of all (see 'Movements of respiration', p. 818). Most of the lung's volumetric change during respiration occurs in the alveoli, which number more than 20 million in a neonatal lung, increasing to 300 million or more during childhood. An alveolus varies from 200–300 μm in diameter and numerous capillary segments (1800 is suggested) may contact each alveolus. The air–epithelium–blood interface is enormous even in childhood. Figures of 70–100 m² have been estimated (Peters 1969; Fishman & Pietra 1974) and even higher values have been suggested (Gehr et al 1978).

RESPIRATORY PASSAGES AND SPACES

The 'lower' respiratory tract includes the larynx, trachea, extra-pulmonary bronchi (see below) and various orders of intrapulmonary tubes which repeatedly dichotomize. Whilst the *primary bronchi* each supply a lung, the *secondary (lobar) bronchi* each supply a lung lobe; *tertiary* (or *quaternary*), *segmental bronchi* supply bronchopulmonary segments; further subdivisions branch repeatedly within segments, becoming increasingly narrow. All intrapulmonary bronchi are kept patent by cartilaginous plates which decline in size and number and disappear from tubes less than 1 mm in diameter, termed bronchioles. After repeated branching, one *lobular bronchiole* enters each lobule, dividing at once into about six *terminal bronchioles*; these subdivide into one to three generations of *respiratory bronchioles* (Spencer 1977). Terminal bronchioles are the most distal air passages to be lined solely by simple columnar epithelium. Respiratory bronchioles in contrast have a few small alveoli arising directly from their walls and finally end in two or three *alveolar ducts*, thin-walled tubes expanding terminally into atria, which lead into *alveolar sacs*. The thin walls of the alveolar ducts, atria and sacs are studded with *alveoli* or acini, separated from adjacent alveoli by thin interalveolar septa of epithelium, connective tissue and capillary plexuses. The above arrangement, shown diagrammatically in **11**.46 and **11**.47, 50, is normal in adults, although there are variations during active growth in childhood (see Engel 1947).

N.B. The terminology used here for the orders of branches is not universally agreed and confusion persists in the naming of conducting passages smaller than bronchi. For example, some authors define a terminal bronchiole as serving a lobule (often of unspecified type) and others adopt a simpler view of the passages leading to the alveoli.

PLEURAE (11.1, 42–45)

Each lung is covered by *pleura*, a serous membrane arranged as a closed invaginated sac. Part of the pleura adheres closely to the pulmonary surface and its interlobar fissures as the *visceral* or *pulmonary pleura*. Its continuation lines the corresponding half of the thoracic wall and covers much of the diaphragm and structures occupying the middle region of the thorax; this is the *parietal pleura*. The pulmonary and parietal pleurae are continuous with each other around the hilar structures. They remain in close though sliding contact at all phases of respiration, the potential space between them being the *pleural cavity*. When air or fluid collects between the two layers, the pleural cavity expands. The right and left pleural sacs form separate compartments and touch only behind the upper half of the sternal body (**11.42, 43**), although they are also close to each other behind the oesophagus at the midthoracic level. The region between them is the *mediastinum* (interpleural space). The left pleural cavity is the smaller of the two because the heart extends further to the left. The upper and lower limits of the pleurae are about the same on the two sides, but the left sometimes descends lower in the midaxillary line.

Pulmonary pleura

The pulmonary pleura is inseparably adherent to the lung over all its surfaces including those in the fissures, but absent from an area where the root of the lung enters, and along a line descending from this, marking the attachment of the pulmonary ligament (**11**.38, 39).

Parietal pleura

Different regions of parietal pleura are customarily distinguished by

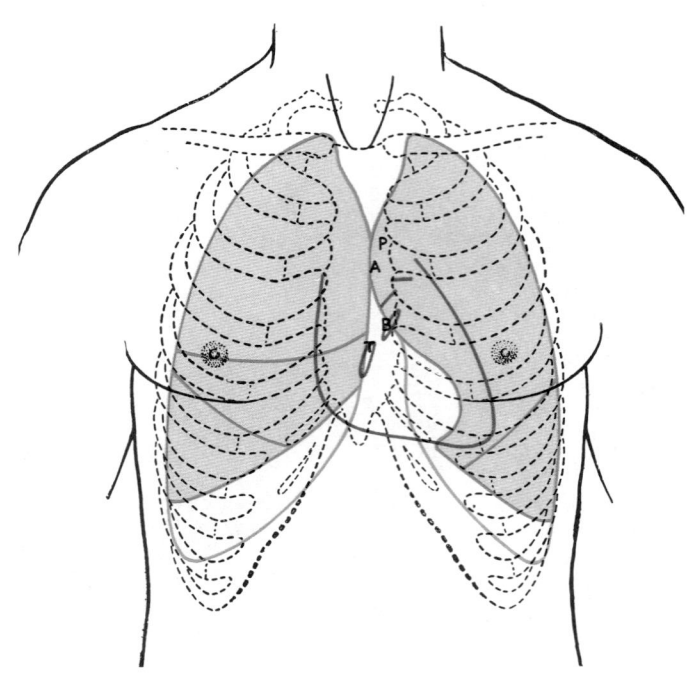

11.42 Ventral aspect of the thorax, showing surface projections: purple = pulmonary; blue = pleural; red outline = cardiac. A = orifice of aorta; B = left atrioventricular (mitral) orifice; P = orifice of pulmonary trunk; T = right atrioventricular (tricuspid) orifice. Skeletal structures are indicated by broken lines.

name; that lining the internal surface of the thoracic wall (p. 813) and the vertebral bodies is the *costovertebral pleura*, that on the thoracic surface of the diaphragm is the *diaphragmatic pleura*, the part over the pulmonary apices (in the neck) is the *cervical pleura* (*domes of the pleura*) and that applied to the structures between the lungs is the *mediastinal pleura*.

Costovertebral (costal) pleura. This lines the sternum, ribs, transversus thoracis and intercostal muscles and the sides of the vertebral bodies; it is easily separated from them. Outside it is a thin loose connective tissue layer of *endothoracic fascia*; this corresponds to the transversalis fascia of the abdominal wall. In front, the costal pleura begins behind the sternum where it is continuous with the mediastinal pleura, at a junction extending from behind the sternoclavicular joint down and medially to the midline behind the sternal angle. From here, the right and left costal pleurae descend in contact with each other to the level of the fourth costal cartilages, below which the two lines of junction differ. On the right the line descends to the back of the xiphisternal joint. The left line diverges laterally and descends at a distance of 2–25 mm from the sternal margin (Woodburne 1947) to the sixth costal cartilage. On each side the costal pleura sweeps laterally, lining the internal surfaces of the costal cartilages, ribs, transversus thoracis and intercostal muscles; posteriorly it passes over the sympathetic trunk and branches and to the sides of the vertebral bodies, where it is again continuous with the mediastinal pleura. The costal pleura is continuous with the cervical pleura at the inner margin of the first rib and below it becomes continuous with the diaphragmatic pleura along a line differing slightly on the two sides. On the right this *line of costo-diaphragmatic reflexion* begins behind the xiphoid process, passes behind the seventh costal cartilage to reach the eighth rib in the midclavicular line, the tenth rib in the midaxillary line and, ascending slightly, crosses the twelfth rib level with the upper border of the twelfth thoracic spine (**11**.42–44). On the left the line follows at first

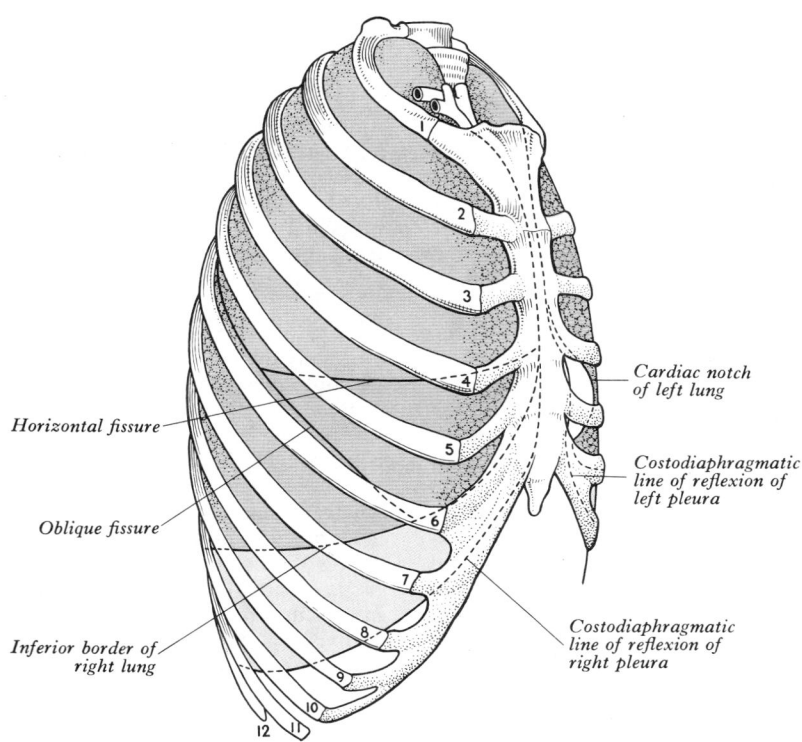

11.43   The relations of the pleurae and lungs to the chest wall: right lateral aspect. Purple = lungs, covered with the pleural sacs; Blue = pleural sac, with no underlying lung.

Labels on figure: *Horizontal fissure* — *Oblique fissure* — *Inferior border of right lung* — *Cardiac notch of left lung* — *Costodiaphragmatic line of reflexion of left pleura* — *Costodiaphragmatic line of reflexion of right pleura*

the ascending part of the sixth costal cartilage, but then follows a course similar to that on the right, although it may be slightly lower.

Diaphragmatic pleura. A thin pleura, it covers most of the upper surface of its own half of the diaphragm. Its circumference is largely the line described above, along which it is continuous with the costal pleura; it is continuous with the mediastinal pleura along the line of attachment of the pericardium to the diaphragm.

Cervical pleura. The continuation of the costal pleura over the pulmonary apex (**10**.91), it ascends medially from the first rib's internal border to the apex of the lung, as high as the lower edge of the neck of the first rib, descending lateral to the trachea to become the mediastinal pleura. Due to the rib's obliquity, the cervical pleura extends 3–4 cm above the first costal cartilage but not above the neck of the first rib. The cervical pleura is strengthened by a fascial *suprapleural membrane*, attached in front to the first rib's internal border, behind to the anterior border of the seventh cervical transverse process. It contains a few muscular fibres, spreading from the scaleni (p. 808). A *scalenus minimus* muscle often extends from the anterior border of the seventh cervical transverse process to the inner border of the first rib behind its subclavian groove, spreading also into the pleural dome, which it therefore tenses. Some regard the suprapleural membrane as the tendon of this muscle. The cervical pleura (like the pulmonary apex) reaches the level of the seventh cervical spine 2.5 cm from the midline. Its projection is a curved line from the sternoclavicular joint to the junction of the medial and middle thirds of the clavicle, its summit being 2.5 cm above it. The subclavian artery ascends laterally in a furrow below the summit of the cervical pleura, the relations of which are like those of the apex of the lung (p. 1657, and **10**.91).

Mediastinal pleura. The lateral boundary of the mediastinum (p. 1676), it forms a continuous surface above the hilum of the lung from sternum to vertebral column. On the right it covers: the right brachiocephalic vein, the upper part of the superior vena cava, the terminal part of the azygos vein, the right phrenic and vagus nerves, the trachea and oesophagus; and on the left, the aortic arch, left phrenic and vagus nerves, left brachiocephalic and superior inter-

costal veins, left common carotid and subclavian arteries, thoracic duct and oesophagus. At the hilum it turns laterally to form a tube enclosing the hilar structures and continuous with the pulmonary pleura. Below the hilum the mediastinal pleura extends as a double layer from the lateral surface of the oesophagus to the mediastinal

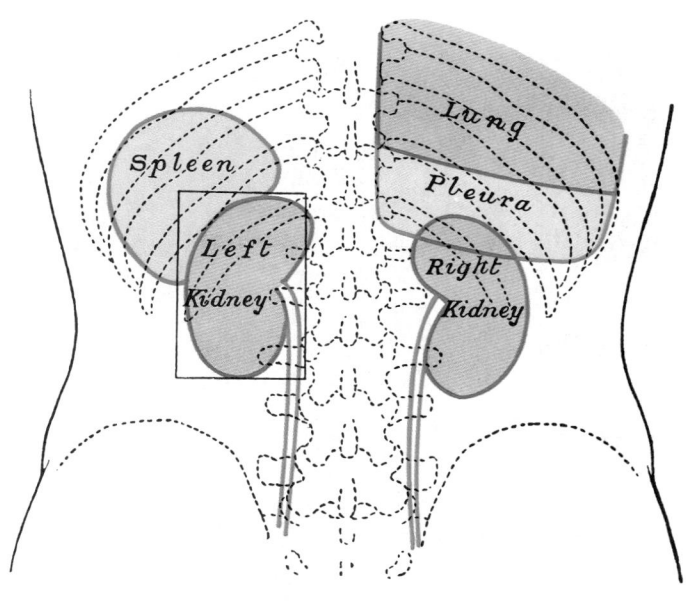

Labels on figure: *Spleen* — *Left Kidney* — *Lung* — *Pleura* — *Right Kidney*

11.44   The lower limits of the lung and pleura: posterior view. The lower portions of the lung and pleura are shown on the right side.

surface of the lung, where it is continuous with the pulmonary pleura; this double layer is the *pulmonary ligament* (**11**.38, 39), continuous above with the pleura around the hilar structures; below it ends in a free sickle-shaped border.

The pleura extends considerably beyond the inferior border of the lung but not to the diaphragm's attachments. Hence, below the line of pleural reflexion from the thoracic wall to the diaphragm the latter is in contact with the costal cartilages and intercostal muscles. In quiet inspiration the lung's inferior margin does not reach this reflexion, the costal and diaphragmatic pleurae being separated merely by a narrow slit, the *costodiaphragmatic recess*. In quiet inspiration the lower limit of the lung is about 5 cm above the lower pleural limit. A similar *costomediastinal recess* exists behind the sternum and the costal cartilages, where the thin anterior margin of the lung falls short of the line of pleural reflexion. The extent of this recess, the anterior costomediastinal line of pleural reflexion and the position of the anterior margin of the lung all vary individually.

Pleural microstructure

The pleural surface is smooth, moistened by serous fluid, and consists of a single layer of flat mesothelial cells on a basal lamina beneath which is a lamina propria of loose connective tissue (p. 75). The deeper layers of fibrous tissue are continuous with tissue around the pulmonary lobules. Blood and lymph vessels and nerves are distributed in the pleura. In ultrastructural details pleural mesothelial cells are like those of the peritoneum (p. 1734). Material from human biopsies (de Gasperis & Miani 1969) shows that their basal lamina has a lamina densa 30–40 nm thick, but their highly folded basal plasma membranes are separated from it by a lamina lucida 20–30 nm. Adjacent cell surfaces interdigitate and are joined by desmosomes. Their luminal surfaces bear numerous microvilli and some cilia (see **11**.45). Micropinocytotic vesicles are common in their cytoplasm. Structural squamous variants are recognized, one probably being a stem cell.

Vessels and nerves

The parietal and visceral pleurae are developed respectively from somatopleural and splanchnopleural layers of the lateral plate mesoderm (p. 180). The *parietal pleura* is therefore supplied by **arteries** from somatic sources (intercostal, internal thoracic and musculophrenic arteries); its **veins** join systemic veins in the thoracic wall; its **lymphatics** also join those in the wall, draining into intercostal, parasternal, posterior mediastinal and diaphragmatic nodes.

Innervation is from spinal sources. The costal and peripheral

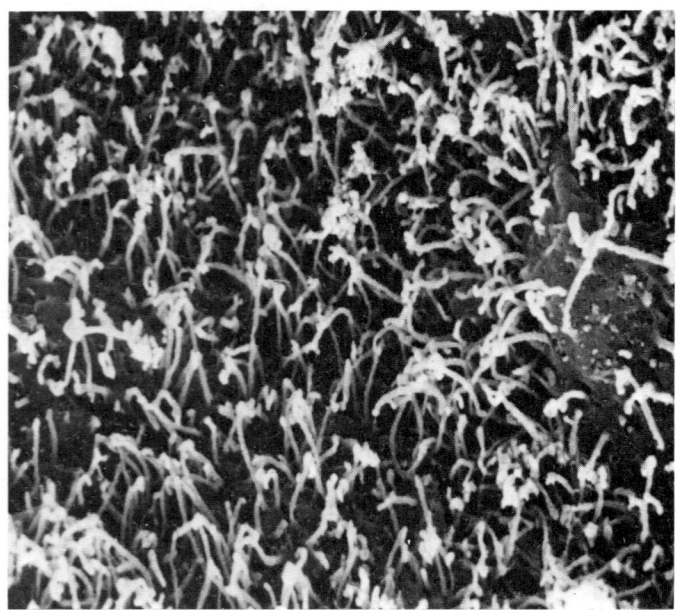

11.45 The surface of the pleura viewed by scanning electron microscopy, showing the numerous processes of the mesothelial cells lining this structure (murine).

diaphragmatic pleurae are supplied by intercostal nerves, and the mediastinal and central diaphragmatic pleurae by the phrenic. Irritation of the former results in pain referred along intercostal nerves to the thoracic or abdominal wall; irritation of the latter causes pain referred to the lower neck and shoulder tip, i.e. to the area of skin supplied by the same spinal segments as the phrenic nerve (C 3, 4, 5).

The *visceral pleura* forms an integral part of the lung; accordingly its **arterial supply** and **venous drainage** are provided by the bronchial vessels; its **lymphatics** join those of the lung (for details see Pennell 1966). Its **innervation** is autonomic, reaching the visceral pleura along bronchial vessels supplying it. Whereas tactile or thermal stimuli to the parietal pleura elicit pain, these stimuli are inadequate when applied to the visceral pleura (cf. peritoneum).

Clinical anatomy of the pleurae

Normally the visceral pleura glides on the parietal during respiration without detectable sound or pain, but when the pleura is inflamed, characteristic friction sounds can be auscultated. If fluid then distends the pleural cavity, the sounds disappear and the lung gradually collapses, the heart and mediastinum being displaced towards the opposite side of the thorax. Air in the pleural cavity (pneumothorax), whether admitted by a penetrating wound, rupture of the lung or as a therapeutic measure (e.g. to rest the lung in tuberculosis), also entails the collapse of the lung, caused by the recoil of its elastic tissue. Normally such extreme recoil is prevented by a negative intrapleural pressure and the cohesion between the opposed parietal and visceral pleura.

In the surgical posterior approach to the kidney the relation of the costal pleura to the twelfth rib is a hazard; usually the pleura crosses the rib at the lateral border of the erector spinae, so that the kidney's medial region is above the pleural reflexion (**11**.44). If this rib does not project beyond this muscle, the eleventh may be mistaken for the twelfth in palpation, and an incision prolonged to this level will damage the pleura. Whether the lowest palpable rib is the eleventh or twelfth can be ascertained by counting from the second rib (identified at its junction with the sternal angle).

MICROSTRUCTURE OF THE LOWER RESPIRATORY TRACT

General organization (**11**.46, 47)

The trachea and lungs are epithelial–mesenchymal outgrowths of the anterior foregut (pp. 178, 179), forming tubes which branch dichotomously as they increase in size. During early development (p. 180), these growing masses protruding into the anterior coelomic cavity (later the pleural cavities), are covered externally by coelomic mesothelium which eventually becomes the lining of the pulmonary pleurae, and are surfaced internally by epithelium of enteric origin. Within each lung the larger proximal tubes become *conducting airways* (from the larynx to the terminal bronchioles); the more distal conduits and cavities form the *areas of respiratory exchange* between the atmosphere and adjacent capillaries (respiratory bronchioles, alveolar ducts and sacs and alveoli).

The conducting passages are lined internally by airway epithelium lying on a thin connective tissue lamina propria. External to this is a submucosa, also composed of connective tissue, in which are embedded airway smooth muscle, glands, cartilage plates (depending on the level in the respiratory tree), vessels, lymphoid tissue and nerves. Cartilage is present from the trachea to the smallest bronchi but is absent (by definition) from bronchioles.

Air passage epithelium

The epithelia of the trachea, extrapulmonary and intrapulmonary bronchi and bronchioles are in general similar to each other, with graded variations in the numbers of different cell types (Collet et al 1967). In the larger intrapulmonary passages it is pseudostratified and largely ciliated; in terminal and respiratory bronchioles there are fewer cilia, and the cells are reduced in height to low columnar or cuboidal. The epithelium of smaller bronchi and bronchioles is folded into conspicuous longitudinal ridges which allow for changes in luminal diameter (**11**.46, 47). In the respiratory bronchioles it

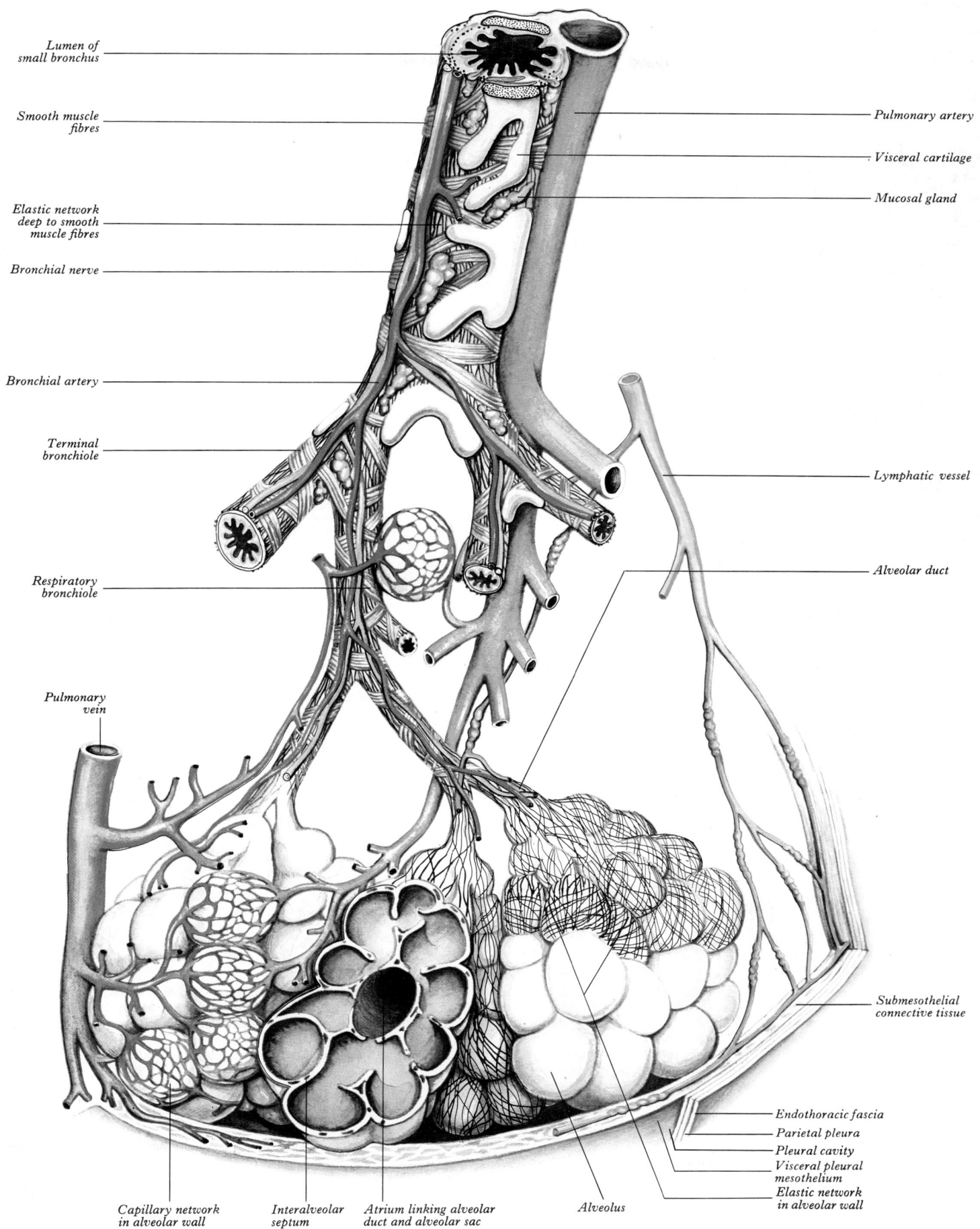

Lumen of
small bronchus

Smooth muscle
fibres

Elastic network
deep to smooth
muscle fibres

Bronchial nerve

Bronchial artery

Terminal
bronchiole

Respiratory
bronchiole

Pulmonary
vein

Pulmonary artery

Visceral cartilage

Mucosal gland

Lymphatic vessel

Alveolar duct

Submesothelial
connective tissue

Endothoracic fascia

Parietal pleura

Pleural cavity

Visceral pleural
mesothelium

Elastic network
in alveolar wall

Capillary network
in alveolar wall

Interalveolar
septum

Atrium linking alveolar
duct and alveolar sac

Alveolus

11.46 Diagram of the detailed structure of the respiratory tree and its blood supply and drainage, lymphatic drainage and nerve supply. Blue = vessels which contain de-oxygenated blood; red = vessels which contain oxygenated blood.

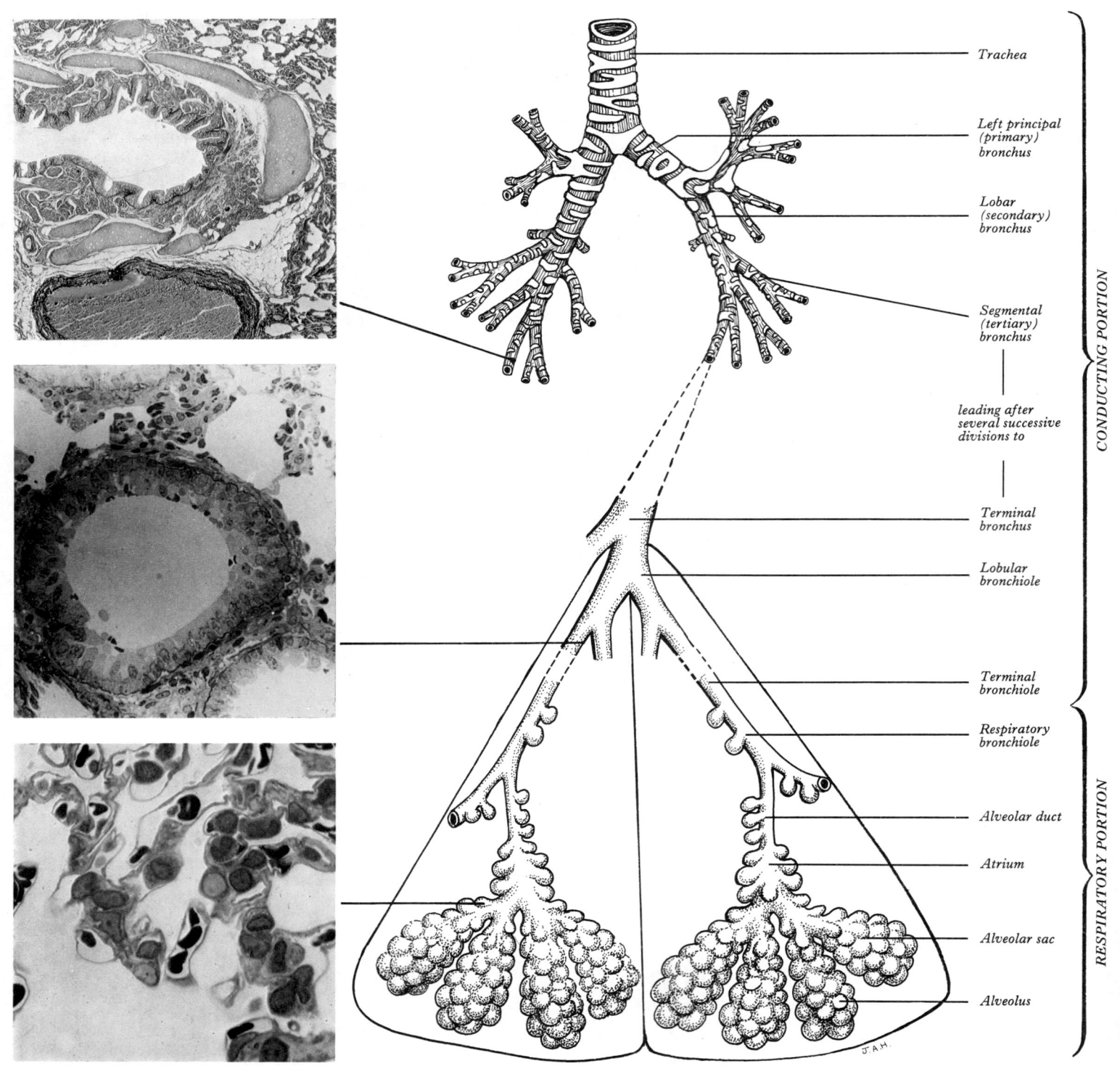

11.47 Bronchopulmonary structure. The diagram on the right shows the gross architecture of the conducting and respiratory parts of the trachea and lungs at segmental levels. On the left are three sections at the levels indicated. Top: a small bronchus lined by highly convoluted epithelium, surrounded by plates of hyaline cartilage. A pulmonary arteriole is visible below. Middle: a bronchiole. Note absence of cartilage and conspicuous smooth muscle external to the epithelium. (Epoxy resin section prepared by Susan Smith; photographed by Marina Morris, Guy's Hospital Medical School, London.) Bottom: An interalveolar septum. Note capillaries containing erythrocytes (dark blue) separated from air species by thin alveolar epithelial cells. Epoxy resin section stained by toluidine blue.

progressively thins towards the alveolar termination, eventually being composed of cuboidal, non-ciliated cells; the lateral pouches are lined with squamous cells, providing an accessory respiratory surface.

Cell types. Eight types of epithelial cell have been described in humans and other mammals; also present within the epithelium are two other classes of cells which migrate into the epithelium from the underlying connective tissue. (For an ultrastructural review of human lung, see Jeffery 1990.) The epithelial cell types are: ciliated columnar,

goblet, Clara, dense-core granule, serous, brush, basal and intermediate. The migratory cells include lymphocytes and mast cells (histaminocytes). In non-human mammals, there is much species variation in the appearances, numbers and, in some instances, the types of these cells.

Ciliated cells (**11.48**). These are the driving force of the ciliary clearance current in the bronchial tree. They vary from low to tall columnar, and have electron-lucent cytoplasm containing numerous

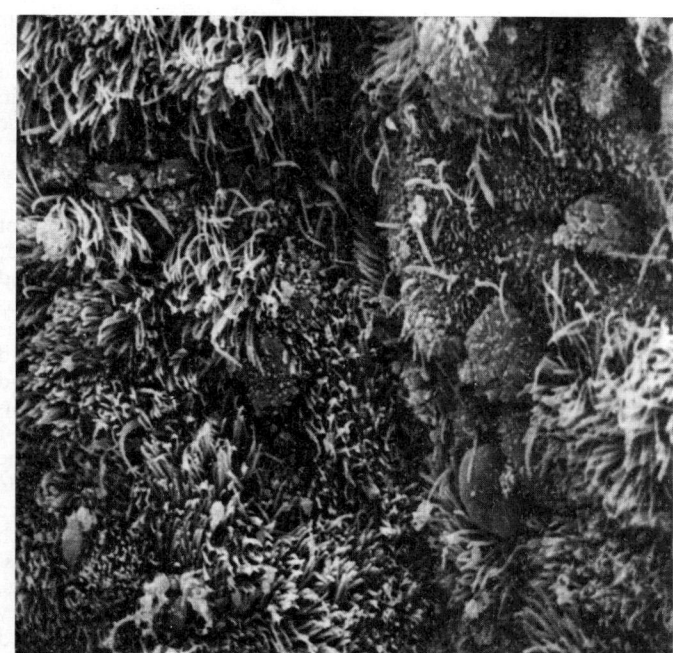

11.48 Electron micrograph showing the epithelium lining the bronchus of a rat. Clustered between the ciliated cells are a variety of non-ciliated cells, including goblet cells and Clara cells. Magnification × 1800. Magnification × 90 000. (Preparations by Michael Crowder, Department of Anatomy, Guy's Hospital Medical School, London.)

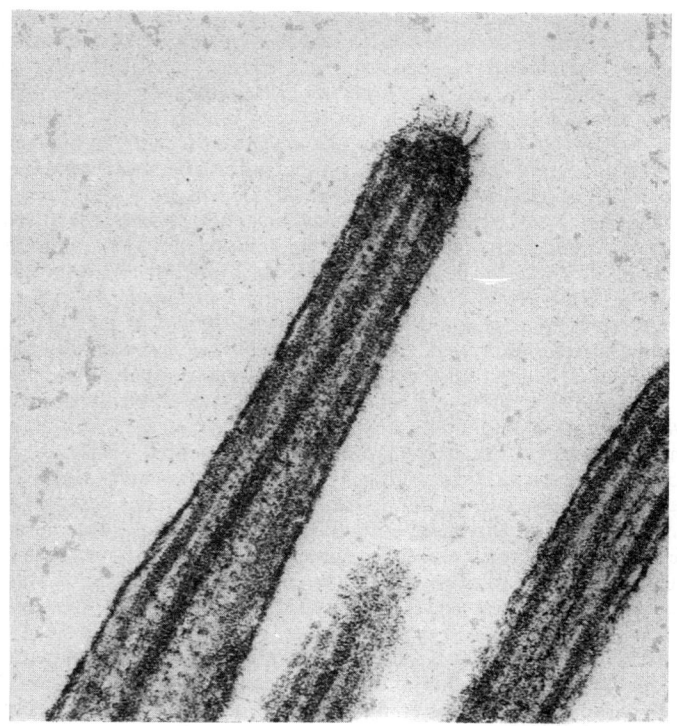

11.49 Claw-like projections at the apex of a cilium of a bronchial epithelial cell (rat). Magnification × 90 000. (Preparations by Michael Crowder, Department of Anatomy, Guy's Hospital Medical School, London.)

mitochondria, especially near the ciliated surface, and a euchromatic nucleus. Each possesses up to 300 cilia at its surface, interspersed with long irregular microvilli; the cilia vary in length from about 6 μm in the trachea to about 4 μm in the terminal bronchioles. Respiratory cilia are blunt-ended, and their tips bear a number of projecting filaments (hooklets: Jeffrey & Reid 1975; see 11.49). The cilia extend into a low-viscosity liquid thought to be largely the secretions of submucosal glands (see below), but their tips are in contact with a more superficial zone of thicker mucus (Van As & Webster 1972) secreted by goblet cells and mucous cells in the submucosal glands. Only the ciliary tips contact this mucus, which they 'claw' along towards the larynx (Sleigh 1977). The rate of ciliary beating is usually about 12–16 per second, although mechanical stimulation of the epithelial surface, and inflammatory mediators increase the rate. In addition to tight junctions which seal the intercellular gaps around the apical ends of these and other cells of the epithelium, the ciliated cells are coupled by gap junctions which allow the rate increase to spread from stimulated cells to their neighbours so that their metachronal co-ordination remains intact; this effect appears to be mediated by a calcium influx (Dirksen & Sanderson 1990). However, the actual spread of the metachronal wave itself is due to mechanical coupling between individual cilia through viscous interactions with the mucus. Ciliated cells are numerous throughout the respiratory tract, although there are few in the respiratory bronchioles (see Jeffery 1990).

Goblet cells. These cells are present from the trachea (where they number from 6000–7000 per mm²: Ellefsen & Tos 1972) down to the smaller bronchi, but are generally absent from bronchioles. These cells contain an apical region full of large, dense, secretory vacuoles rich in mucins rich in acidic glycosaminoglycans (AGAGs) (Spicer et al 1983); the composition of these varies in pathological conditions, and the numbers of goblet cells also increase when the epithelium is irritated, for example, by tobacco smoke. Goblet cells are able to divide mitotically, and under certain conditions can give rise to other types of epithelial cell (Ayers & Jeffery 1988).

Serous cells. These are also columnar glandular cells; they have an irregular nucleus, copious granular endoplasmic reticulum and electron-dense supranuclear granules about 600 nm across. These cells are uncommon in the human surface epithelium except in fetal life. In some other mammals, for example the rat, they form about one-fifth of all the epithelial cells. Similar cells exist in human bronchial submucosal glands (see below). They are able to divide mitotically (Ayers & Jeffery 1988). Their functions are uncertain, but they may be a source of secretory antibody (IgA) as well as contributing to the low-viscosity circumciliary fluid.

Clara cells (bronchiolar non-ciliated cells). In humans these cells are restricted mainly to the terminal and respiratory bronchioles, although in other species they also occur at higher levels of the respiratory tract, and even in the nasal mucosa (Matulionis & Parks 1973). They are cuboidal non-ciliated cells, with apices which bulge from the luminal surface (Clara 1937); they contain numerous irregular electron-dense secretory granules about 500–600 μm across, and many lysosomes; in the rat they also possess much agranular endoplasmic reticulum (Spencer 1977). Various studies have shown them to be an important source of surfactant (Niden & Yamada 1966), including its lipidic component (Etherton & Conning 1971), and surfactant proteins (Voorhout et al 1992). These cells therefore have functional similarities to the Type II alveolar cell of pulmonary alveoli (see below) although their secretory granules differ in fine structure; their abundance in the narrowest portions of the respiratory tree (respiratory bronchioles), where mucous glands are excluded, suggests that they are important in maintaining the patency of these channels, where mucus might clog the restricted space. It is also interesting that, like Type II alveolar cells, they also give rise to other epithelial cells in epithelial regeneration after damage.

Undifferentiated basal cells. Present in parts of the airway lined by pseudostratified epithelium, they are mitotic stem cells for other epithelial cell types (Blenkinsopp 1967). They are rounded or elliptical cells with relatively little cytoplasm and few organelles although they do contain cytokeratin intermediate filaments. They are most frequent in the larger conducting passages, a feature which may be related to the relatively greater occurrence of carcinoma in the upper parts of the bronchial tree (Baldwin 1994).

Intermediate epitheliocytes. Present in the trachea and bronchi, (Rhodin & Dalhamn 1956; Rhodin 1966; Jeffery & Reid 1975), these cells are columnar in shape but generally lack cilia; they have an electron-dense cytoplasm lacking secretory granules. They are generally considered to be immature forms of ciliated or secretory cells which have been formed from stem cells.

Brush cells. These have a characteristic set of long, stiff apical

1667

microvilli from which they are named (see Meyrick & Reid 1968). Within their apical cytoplasm are numerous endocytic vesicles formed between the microvilli, suggesting a specialization for absorption. These cells are infrequent; in the tracheal epithelium (of rats) they are more numerous, forming about 1% of all epithelial cells, although probably much fewer than this in humans. They are present throughout all other parts of the air passages including the nasal epithelium (p. 1634), and cells resembling these also occur in the alimentary tract. These cells have been variously suggested to be sensory cells (like taste buds), or antigen processing components of the immune system; however, firm evidence for either function is at present lacking.

Dense-core granulated cells (DCGCs; Kulchitsky cells). Also termed *Feyrter cells*, *P cells*, or *neuroendocrine cells*, these rather infrequent cells are rounded or elliptical in shape, situated mainly in the basal part of the epithelium, although with apical processes which reach the luminal surface (Bensch et al 1965). Basal to their nuclei they contain numerous small dense-cored vesicles about 150 nm across, although other types of granule have also been described (Capella et al 1978). They are generally considered to be neuroendocrine cells, similar to the entero-endocrine (argentaffin) cells of the alimentary tract (Ericson et al 1972), and should thus be included in the diffuse endocrine system of amine precursor uptake and decarboxylation (APUD) cells (Pearse & Polak 1972; Hage 1973).

Data on the immunocytochemical localization of putative neuro-transmitters, and of other antigen markers have been compiled for the pulmonary dense-core granule cells by Polak et al (1993); possible neurotransmitters include serotonin, substance P, calcitonin gene-related peptide (CGRP), somatostatin, calcitonin and bombesin/gastrin-releasing factor. Among the rather heterogeneous collection of other antigens for which they are positive are protein gene product 9.5 and neuron-specific enolase (as also are alimentary enteroendocrine cells) and chromogranin (a synapse-related protein suggesting neuroendocrine affinities). Innervated groups of similar cells form *neuroepithelial bodies* (neurite-receptor complexes) in human bronchial and bronchiolar mucosa (Lauweryns & Peuskens 1972), and have been found in rodents to be clustered around the openings of bronchioles into alveolar ducts.

Suggested functions of DCGCs include regulation of bronchial secretion, smooth muscle contraction, lobular growth (Rosan & Lauweryns 1971), ciliary activity and chemoreception (Lauweryns et al 1972). The dense-core granule cells discharge their granules in response to hypoxia (Moosavi et al 1973; Lauweryns & Cokelaere 1973), suggesting that they play a part in regulating the responses of the airway to changes in oxygen tension (e.g. blood flow, muscle tone).

DCGCs are much more numerous in fetal lungs, so that there is a widely held belief that their most important role is related to fetal pulmonary development and, perhaps, the transition from fetal to neonatal life. After birth they decrease greatly, although they may proliferate in certain pulmonary diseases. After this early reduction, there appears to be little change in their frequency, as shown by Gosney (1993) in a postmortem study of the lungs of 40 subjects from childhood to the ninth decade, their numbers remaining steady within the range 2.9–4.2 per 10 000 epithelial cells.

Lymphocytes. Small lymphocytes occur within the epithelium of all the conducting tissues, although they are most numerous in the extrapulmonary portion. They are chiefly typically T cells derived from bronchus-associated lymphoid tissue in the walls of the passages, and are probably concerned with the immune surveillance of the epithelium and the destruction of virus-infected cells, etc. In places, clusters of lymphocytes lie basally to thin, irregular non-ciliated epithelial cells to form a *lympho-epithelium* (McDermott et al 1982) resembling that of the nasopharyngeal tonsil (p. 1447), the epithelial cells being of the microfold (M-cell) type. Such assemblages are likely to have similar functions in presenting lumen antigens to the underlying defensive cells to initiate immune responses as in other instances of mucosa-associated lymphoid tissue.

Mast cells (histaminocytes). These are also present within the basal regions of the epithelium, where they have a structure similar to that of connective tissue mast cells (p. 79), although they may represent a subtype specifically associated with epithelium (Enerback 1986). They contain numerous large electron-dense vesicles rich in

histamine and various other inflammatory substances. In rodents another type of cell with some resemblance to mast cells also occurs, termed a 'globule leucocyte', but it is apparently not found in humans. This name is given to a type of rounded cell situated in the basal region of the epithelium, possessing large electron-dense granules resembling those of mast cells (Murray et al 1968).

Submucosal glands

Tubulo-acinar, mucoserous glands are present in the submucosa of the trachea and bronchi and, to a lesser extent, in the larger bronchioles. These contain separate mucous and serous cells, and are an important source of the different components of the mucous layer at the surface of the ciliated respiratory epithelium. Their secretions include mucins, the bacteriostatic substances lysozyme and lactoferrin (Bowes et al 1981), secretory antibodies, mainly IgA, and a protease inhibitor (Kramps et al 1981) important for the neutralizing of leucocyte-derived proteases in the respiratory tract.

The glands are composed of four components. Furthest from the epithelial surface are acini composed of serous cells, which secrete into tubular regions lined by mucous cells; these are the source of secretory IgA, derived from the numerous plasmacytes which congregate around the glands. These acini lead into tubular mucus-secreting regions, which in turn open into wide collecting ducts, then, via narrower ciliated ducts, on to the surface of the respiratory passage. In some instances, combined ducts open into larger ciliated diverticula of the epithelial surface. The secretory parts of the glands are enclosed in myoepithelial cells, innervated by autonomic fibres (Meyrick & Reid 1970).

Connective tissue and muscle (11.46, 47)

The epithelium of the trachea, bronchi and bronchioles rests on a basement membrane about 1 μm thick in normal lungs, composed of a typical thin basal lamina and a thicker reticular lamina. Beneath this is the connective tissue lamina propria, grading into a rather more loosely fibred submucosa; in the latter, broad, longitudinal bands of elastin follow the course of the respiratory tree, branching at bifurcations and spiralling and forming rings around alveolar ducts to finally spread into the elastin networks of the interalveolar septa. This elastic framework is a vital mechanical element, responsible for much elastic recoil during expiration, although in respiratory regions surface tension may be more important (see below, and Peters 1969).

Airway smooth muscle. As noted elsewhere, in the trachea (p. 1653) and extrapulmonary bronchi the smooth muscle is mainly confined to the posterior, non-cartilaginous part of the tracheal tube. Along the entire intrapulmonary bronchial tree smooth muscle forms two opposed helical tracts, becoming thinner and finally absent at the alveolar bases (Stephens & Kroeger 1980). The tonus of these muscle fibres is under nervous and hormonal control; many gap junctions couple groups of muscle cells to spread excitation within blocks of muscle. Muscle cell contraction narrows the airway, while their relaxation permits bronchodilatation. Normally, there is some tone in the muscular bands, which relax slightly during inspiration and contract during expiration, assisting the tidal flow of air. Abnormal contraction may be caused by circulating smooth muscle stimulants or by local release of excitants such as serotonin, histamine and leukotrienes, producing bronchospasm. Numerous mast cells are present in the connective tissue of the respiratory tree, and increase considerably as its passages are followed towards the bronchioles.

Serous tunic and associated connective tissue

The *tunica serosa* forms the visceral pleura, a thin, transparent layer composed of a single stratum of mesothelium covering a thin lamina propria of connective tissue, inseparably attached to the various structures of the lung, which it invests except at the hilum. Deep to the serosal layer, loose connective tissue covers the entire pulmonary surface and extends along the conducting tubes and blood vessels from the hilum to finally delineate the numerous small lung lobules. Each *lobule* is a small polyhedral mass receiving a lobular bronchiole and the terminal rami of arterioles, venules, lymphatics and nerves. Lobules vary in size, the superficial ones being large and pyramidal, their bases visible as polygonal areas about 5–15 mm across separated by thin layers of connective tissue. Internal lobules are smaller and

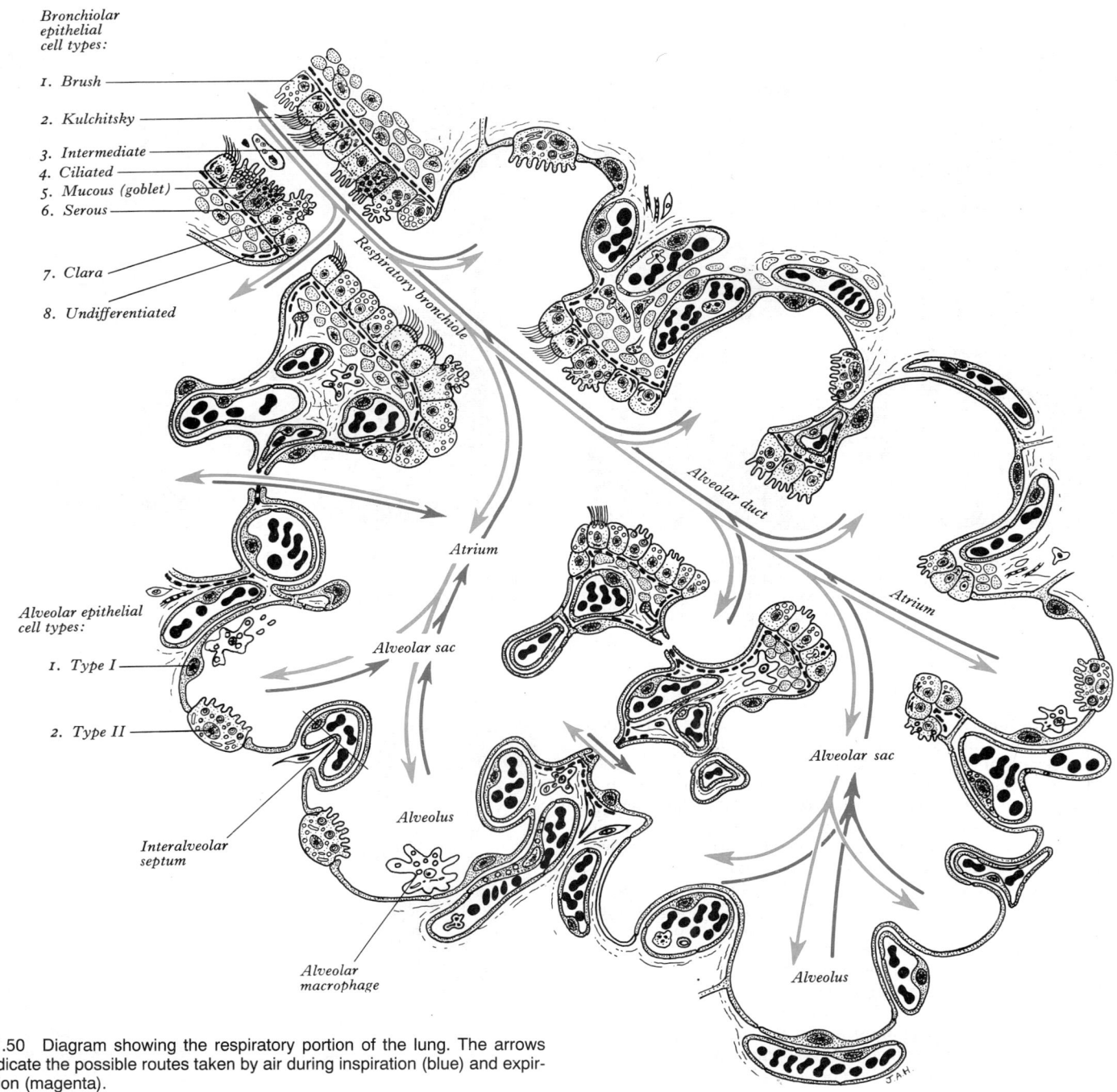

Bronchiolar epithelial cell types:

1. Brush

2. Kulchitsky

3. Intermediate
4. Ciliated
5. Mucous (goblet)
6. Serous

7. Clara

8. Undifferentiated

Respiratory bronchiole

Alveolar duct

Atrium

Atrium

Alveolar sac

Alveolar epithelial cell types:

1. Type I

2. Type II

Alveolar sac

Interalveolar septum

Alveolus

Alveolus

Alveolar macrophage

11.50   Diagram showing the respiratory portion of the lung. The arrows indicate the possible routes taken by air during inspiration (blue) and expiration (magenta).

vary in shape. In structure the lung resembles a lobulated gland, consisting of terminal lobules for respiratory exchange and extra-lobular ducts for ventilation (Miller 1947; von Hayek 1960; Engel 1962; Krahl 1964). The terminal lobules are also called secondary lobules, delineated on the surface by substantial septa enclosing areas of 1–2 cm, and subdivided by delicate septa into areas of about 1 mm, the surfaces of the primary lobules.

Alveolar structure (11.46, 50–55)

The alveoli are thin-walled pouches which collectively provide the respiratory surface for gaseous exchange. The cellular lining of this surface is exceedingly thin, presenting a minimal barrier to gaseous exchange between the atmosphere and the blood within capillaries lining the alveolar walls (Karrer 1956; Klika & Petrick 1965; Collet et al 1967). The surface is composed of two types of epithelial cell (pneumocytes), covering a layer of connective tissue in which the exchange capillaries spread. Adjacent alveoli frequently abut on to one another, the connective tissue and blood vessels of each then

being sandwiched between the two layers of lining epithelium; the combined layers of tissue between the two alveolar cavities is then termed the *interalveolar septum*. Migratory alveolar macrophages are present within the alveolar lumen, wandering on the epithelium surface.

Alveolar epithelium. This varies in thickness, but extensive areas of it are as little as $0.05\,\mu m$ thick. The epithelium lies on a thin basal lamina which is in places fused with that of the adjacent capillaries. It forms a continuous layer about $0.1\,\mu m$ thick; the thickness of the capillary endothelium is about $0.05\,\mu m$, so that the total barrier to diffusion between air and blood may be as little as $0.2\,\mu m$ (Collet et al 1967). However, because of variations in the alveolar wall components, the mean barrier thickness is $2.2\,\mu m$ in the normal human lung (Gehr et al 1978), much exceeding the range of 0.6–$1.5\,\mu m$ in other mammals (Meban 1980). The reasons for this difference are uncertain; Wang and Ying (1977) have suggested that the large human lung needs more fibrous tissue to support the weight of the contained blood. This cannot be the full explanation, for the

1669

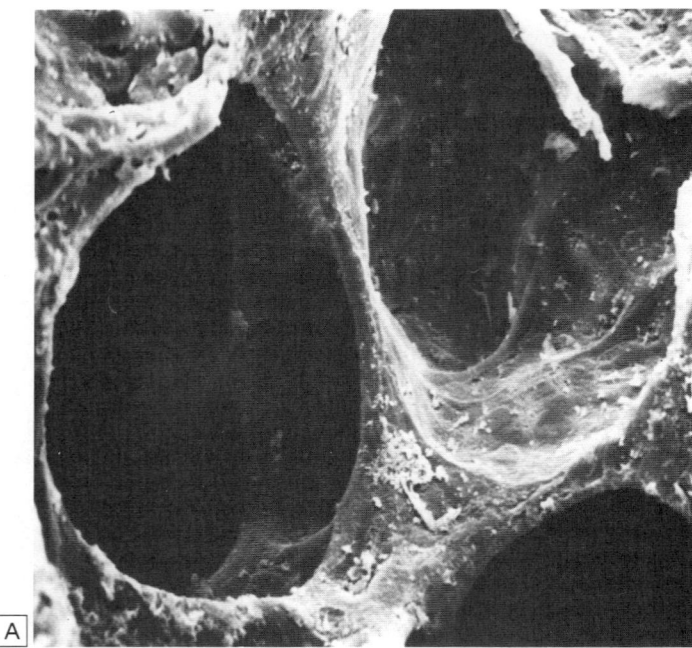

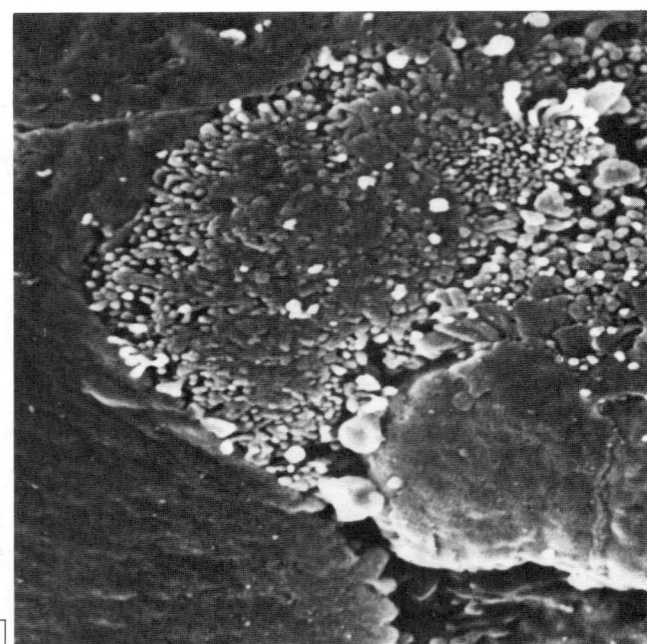

11.51A Scanning electron micrograph showing adjacent interalveolar septa in section and the lining epithelium of several alveoli in surface view. Magnification × 900. B   Scanning electron micrograph showing the surface of a Type II alveolar epithelial cell surrounded by several Type I alveolar epithelial cells. Magnification × 7000. (Specimens prepared and photographed by Michael Crowder, Department of Anatomy, Guy's Hospital Medical School, London.)

barrier is much thinner in the still larger lungs of cattle and horses (Gehr et al 1978), although the erect posture of humans may present different mechanical factors. Capillaries tend to be closely related to only one side of the interalveolar septum, so that other connective tissue components may separate them from the epithelium on the opposite side. There are also other areas in the septum which contain connective tissue elements: proteoglycans, collagen and elastic fibres, fixed and migratory cells and free tissue fluid (**11**.50).

Alveolar area. An extensive stereological evaluation by Gehr et al 1978 of normal human alveoli from electron micrographs (based on samples from 8 pairs of lungs) gave a mean total alveolar surface area value of $143\,m^2$ for the adult respiratory system. The same study indicated a total capillary surface area and volume of $126\,m^2$ and 231 ml respectively. There are about 300 million alveoli on average per adult respiratory system; their inflated diameter (approximately $250\,\mu m$) varies with lung position, being greater in the upper regions than the lower because of the increased gravitational pressure at the lung base. There is, of course, also considerable variation between normal individuals and because of common degenerative changes due to age.

Alveolar epithelial cells (pneumocytes or pneumonocytes). The alveolar epithelium is a mosaic of two cell types, Types I and II alveolar cells. Type I cells form over 90% of the alveolar area although the smaller Type II cells are more numerous.

Type I alveolar cells. These are simple squamous epithelial cells which have a central nucleus and a highly attenuated cytoplasm about 0.05–$0.2\,\mu m$ thick, extending from a thicker perinuclear region. As noted above, the thinness of the cytoplasm facilitates gaseous diffusion between the lumen of the alveolus and its capillaries. While individual cells are mostly confined to the surface of a single alveolus, some extensions of their bases occasionally traverse the interalveolar septum and expand as part of the lining of a neighbouring alveolus (Weibel 1971: see also **11**.50). In view of this intricate arrangement, it is perhaps not surprising that these cells do not undergo mitotic division (see below).

The attenuated cytoplasm of Type I cells contains endocytic and exocytic vesicles which, like those of endothelial cells (transcytotic vesicles), are thought to allow the shuttling of selected macromolecules across the epithelial lining. The perinuclear cytoplasm contains a few mitochondria, a little agranular endoplasmic reticulum

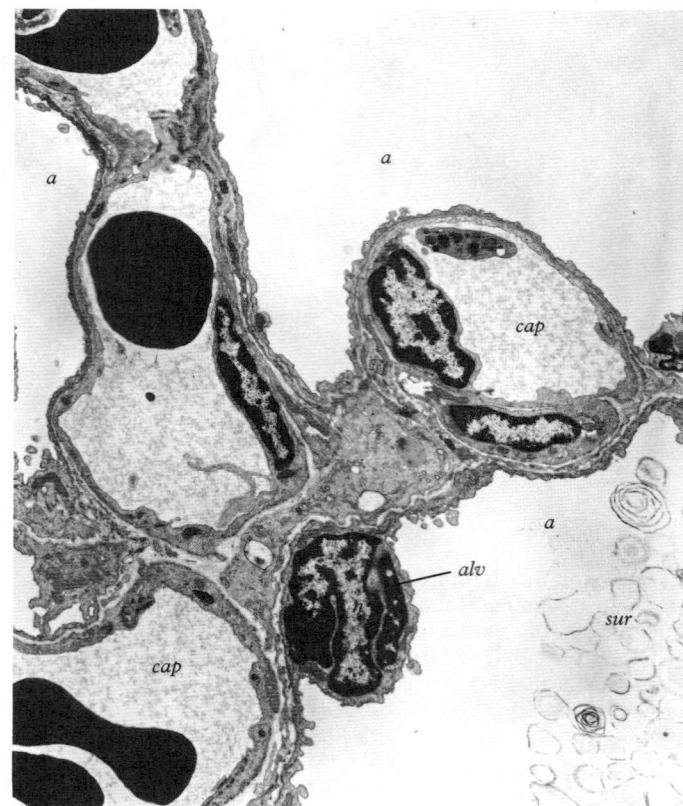

11.52   Electron micrograph of part of an interalveolar septum showing portions of three adjacent alveoli, and four sectioned capillaries (cap), three of them containing erythrocytes (dense profiles). The alveoli are lined by Type I alveolar cells (alv), one sectioned through its nuclear region (n). Note the close proximity of the air spaces (a) and the capillary contents, with minimal distance for gaseous diffusion. Some myelin-like surfactant bodies are also visible (sur). Ovine lung. (Provided by G. Gabella, Department of Anatomy and Developmental Biology, University College, London.)

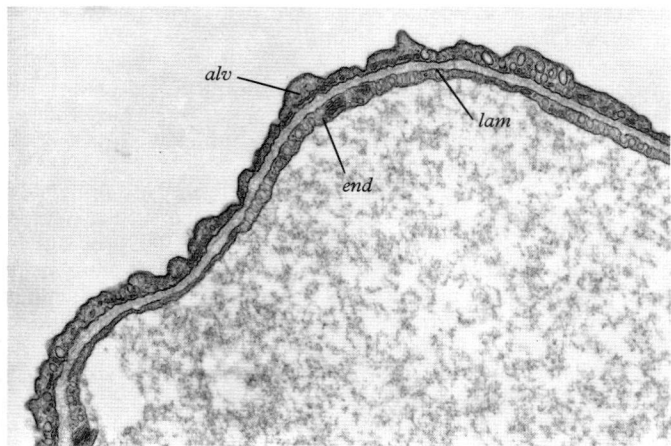

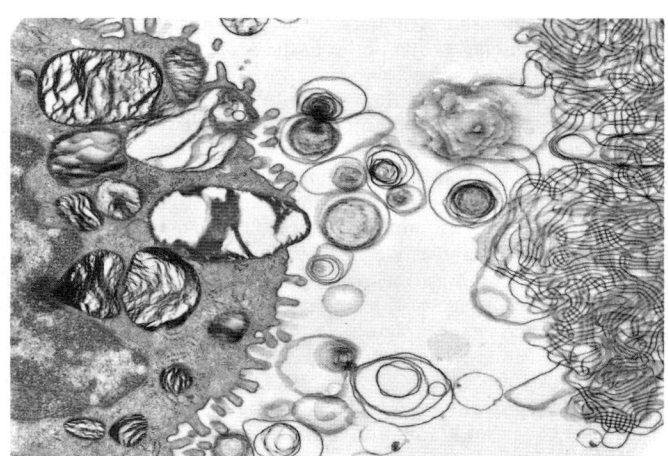

11.53 Electron micrograph of part of an alveolar wall, showing the triple structure formed by the flattened cytoplasm of a Type I alveolar cell (alv), an endothelial cell (end) and the fused basal lamina of the two cells (lam). The flocculent material within the capillary lumen represents fixed plasma proteins. Note the small distance between the air and blood. Also visible are numerous endocytic vesicles in the cytoplasm of both cell types. Ovine lung. (Provided by G. Gabella, Department of Anatomy and Developmental Biology, University College, London.)

11.55 Electron micrograph of the apex of a Type II alveolar cell (left) in the process of secreting pulmonary surfactant, which in the right is seen to form complex sacular vesicles superimposed on each other to give a grid-like pattern, in section. Ovine lung. (Provided by G. Gabella, Department of Anatomy and Developmental Biology, University College, London.)

and occasional lysosomes. The edges of adjacent cells overlap, and are joined by tight junctions which create a strict diffusion barrier preventing diffusion between the alveolar surface and underlying tissues, a vital feature, which with a similar endothelial barrier, limits the movement of fluid from blood and intercellular spaces into the alveolar lumen (the *blood–air barrier*: see, e.g., Simionescu 1985). If damaged, the Type I cells are replaced by the multiplication of Type II cells which may later differentiate into Type I (Spencer 1977).

Type II alveolar epithelial cells. These cells were first described by Reinhardt in 1847. They are much less extensive, rounded cells which protrude from the alveolar surface, particularly at the angles between the curved alveolar profiles, seen in section. Their free surfaces bear short microvilli; their cytoplasm contains abundant mitochondria, granular endoplasmic reticulum, lysosomes and numerous characteristic secretory multilamellar vesicles which contain the precursors of alveolar surfactant (see below) (Gil & Weibel 1969; King & Clements 1972; Gil & Reiss 1973). They are more numerous than Type I cells, but because of their lesser size, they form only about 3% of the total alveolar surface. In the human lung they are often associated with alveolar septal pores (of Köhn) (Takaro et al 1987). The ultrastructure of the multilamellar bodies has been described in detail by Stratton (1976): freeze-fracture preparations have shown that the lamellae are without membrane particles, and that they are arranged in cup-shaped layers of lipid bilayers around a core (Weibel et al 1976). Recent studies indicate that in addition to secreting surfactant components these cells also endocytose and degrade or recycle it.

Interalveolar pores (of Kohn). Reconstructions from serial sections have confirmed the existence of small apertures lined by epithelium (usually Type II alveolar cells) through interalveolar septa to link adjacent alveolar cavities. These small passages may allow the flow or air even in the event of blockage of one of the alveolar ducts, although it has also been suggested, on the basis of electron microscopy of frozen hydrated lung tissue, that (at least in rodents) they are normally closed by surfactant and are principally routes of migration for alveolar macrophages or storage of surfactant (Bastacky & Goerke 1992). Up to 7 pores occur per alveolus in humans, ranging in size from 2–13 µm (see Jeffery 1990).

Alveolar macrophages (dust cells). Like macrophages in other sites in the body (p. 78), these cells or their precursors are derived from haemopoietic tissue in the bone marrow and form part of the mononuclear phagocyte system of the body (see p. 1414); they migrate into the lumen of the alveoli from adjacent blood vessels (circulating in the bloodstream as monocytes) and from adjacent connective tissue, and wander about on the epithelial surfaces (Collet & Normand-Reuet 1967). These phagocytes clear the respiratory spaces of inhaled particles small enough to reach the alveoli, then most of them pass with their phagocytosed load to the bronchioles where they are swept into the mucociliary current and removed from the lung: others migrate instead through the epithelium

11.54 Electron micrograph of part of a Type II alveolar cell, showing lamellar vacuoles (v) containing pulmonary surfactant. Part of the nucleus (n) is also visible. Ovine lung. (Provided by G. Gabella, Department of Anatomy and Developmental Biology, University College, London.)

of the alveoli into the lymphatics, draining the lung tissue, and thence into the patches of lymphoid tissue around the lobules. Under normal conditions these cells have a granular cytoplasm because of the phagocytosed particles they contain; in smokers these have a characteristic appearance ('tar bodies'). Alveolar macrophages can be recovered from sputum, and are of diagnostic importance if they are abnormal in appearance; for instance, whenever erythrocytes escape from pulmonary capillaries, the macrophages become brick-red due to engulfed cells, and are detectable in 'rusty' sputum. Such cells are typical of congestive heart failure and are often termed 'heart-failure cells'. Those macrophages which have migrated back into the connective tissue of the lung settle in patches or lines, clearly visible beneath the visceral pleura, so that, for example, carbon-filled cells cause the lungs to assume a mottled appearance. However, if inhaled particles are abrasive, or chemically active, they may elude macrophagic removal, and damage the respiratory surface, with consequent fibrosis and reduction in the respiratory area. This occurs in many industrial diseases, such as pneumoconiosis, which is due to coal dust, and asbestosis, where the long thin fibres of asbestos can cause considerable damage and may trigger fatal mesothelioma in the pleural lining. When engaged in phagocytosis, macrophages release proteases, and these may also damage the lung if antiproteases normally present in the alveolar lining are deficient.

Alveolar macrophages also perform many other functions within the alveoli and other parts of the lung. They engage in the turnover of surfactant (see below) and can secrete various enzymes if suitably stimulated, for example both a collagenase and a collagenase inhibitor (Welgus et al 1985). They may thus produce a profound effect on the connective tissue matrix of the lung and on any scar tissue produced in response to damage to the alveolar surface.

In pathological conditions other cells may enter the alveoli and other parts of the respiratory tree, for example neutrophil leucocytes and lymphocytes in infections, giving the sputum a characteristic yellow appearance.

Cells of the interalveolar interstitium. As noted above, the interstitium between the two layers of alveolar epithelium is composed of connective tissue rich in capillaries, matrix including collagen and elastin fibres and a number of cell types. These include fibroblast-like cells, and various migratory forms, i.e. macrophages, mast cells, neutrophils, as well as endothelial cells and pericytes. Fibroblast-like cells include typical fibroblasts which are the source of the matrix fibres and proteoglycans, and other cells (myofibroblasts) which are closely associated with capillaries, and are thought to be contractile, perhaps helping to regulate blood flow through the vascular bed. The latter cells have actin and myosin filaments, but interestingly their structure and immunohisto-chemistry suggest similarities with the perisinusoidal (Ito) cells of the liver.

Conditions or treatments such as assisted ventilation with positive end-expiratory airway pressure in which alveolar pressure is raised can increase the possibility of invasion of the interstitial spaces of the interalveolar septa by leucocytes. It has been shown that the resulting compression of the alveolar capillaries and reduced pulmonary blood flow can produce an increased entrapment of neutrophils and lymphocytes in the pulmonary vasculature (Loick et al 1993), increasing the possibility of these leucocytes leaving the vessels and entering the interstitial spaces.

Alveolar surfactant. The alveolar surface is normally covered by a film of pulmonary surfactant composed of a complex mixture of phospholipid: dipalmitoylphosphatidylcholine (DPPC): 50%; cholesterol: 10% and protein (Gil & Reiss 1973; Golde 1985; Bourbon & Rieutort 1987). They are derived from multilamellar bodies secreted by the Type II alveolar cells, although the Clara cells of the bronchiolar epithelium appear to carry out similar functions.

Ultrastructurally (**11.55**), pulmonary surfactant appears in sections after suitable fixation (e.g. in tannic acid-glutaraldehyde) as a complex laminated meshwork. The layers typical of human surfactant are:

- recently secreted multilamellar bodies nearest to the alveolar epithelium
- paired lamellae expanded and re-arranged as tubules
- mature tubular myelin-like surfactant
- a surfactant–air interface, usually a single lipid bilayer

- degraded surfactant, consisting of lipid bilaminar spheres formed at the air interface (Stratton 1978).

Alveolar macrophages remove degraded surfactant, leaving some areas denuded of this covering until it is replaced by further secretion of multilamellar bodies. Localized lack of surfactant is part of the normal cycle of secretion and degradation.

The surfactant has a number of interesting properties. Principally, it acts as a reducer of surface tension at the alveolar surface (Goerke 1974; King 1974; Tierney 1974; Kikkawa & Smith 1983). Because of the minute sizes of the alveoli, the surface tension forces are incipiently very high, opposing expansion during inspiration, and tending to collapse the alveoli in expiration. The detergent-like properties of the pulmonary surfactant greatly reduce the surface tension, and make ventilation of the alveoli much more efficient (Macklin 1954; Stratton 1978; Shimura et al 1986).

The main component of pulmonary surfactant responsible for reducing alveolar surface tension is the phospholipid DPPC; (Goerke 1974). However, in addition to DPPC, pulmonary surfactant also contains considerable amounts of polyunsaturated phospholipid species which appear to play an essential role in normal surfactant function, acting as liquefiers and helping DPPC to spread at the air–water interface at body temperature (Bangham 1987). These polyunsaturated phospholipids are subjected to strongly oxidizing conditions within the alveolus; they are exposed directly to oxidative air pollutants, and also to hydrogen peroxide and reactive oxygen species produced by activated neutrophils and macrophages (Weiss & Lobuglio 1982; Test & Weiss 1984). Oxidation leads to degradation of the polyunsaturated phospholipids and a loss of surfactant function, without a decrease in DPPC. Furthermore, lipid peroxidation products inhibit the synthesis and secretion of new surfactant (Crim & Simon 1988). Antioxidative protection of the surfactant is thus literally vital, and is provided by lipophilic antioxidants such as vitamins A and E which are secreted by Type II pneumocytes as a component of the surfactant (Rustow et al 1993).

Specific pulmonary surfactant proteins are also important in surfactant function (Cochrane & Revak 1991; Lacaze-Mastmonteil 1993). Representing approximately 5% of the total surfactant, they include the glycoprotein surfactant protein SP-A which contains both collagen-like and lectin-like domains (Weaver & Whitsett 1991), the low-molecular weight hydrophobic surfactant protein SP-B and hydrophobic surfactant protein SP-C. SP-A collaborates with SP-B in promoting the structural transformation of intracellular surfactant, stored within multilamellar bodies, into extracellular mature tubular 'myelin' surfactant, and with both SP-B and SP-C in spreading and stabilizing the phospholipid layer at the alveolar surface. It apparently also limits the influx of serum proteins into the alveolar space and prevents the inhibitory effect on surfactant function of various compounds which can accumulate in this space after injury (Hallman et al 1991). Ex vivo experiments suggest that SP-A may have a defensive role by increasing phagocytosis by alveolar macrophages (Van Iwardeen et al 1990) and is involved in enhancing the uptake and inhibiting the secretion of phospholipids by Type II pneumocytes, but these functions have not yet been confirmed in vivo (Lacaze-Mastmonteil 1993). SP-B, in addition to collaborating with SP-A, has the most potentially significant effect in reducing surface tension to a very low value by squeezing polyunsaturated phospholipids from the monolayer at the surfactant–air interface (Sarin et al 1990).

Considerable progress has been made in analysing the regulation of gene expression of surfactant proteins, and it is anticipated that continued progress will provide new tools for gene therapy of genetic defects involving surfactant production by the lung epithelium (Lacaze-Mastmonteil 1993). cDNAs and promoters of the genes involved have already been cloned from a number of species (Glasser et al 1991; Lacaze-Mastmonteil et al 1992; Qing et al 1992). When driven by an appropriate promoter these cDNAs may allow the synthesis of functional peptides in suitable cells. Clinical applications of these developments are awaited with considerable interest.

Pulmonary endothelial cells In addition to a respiratory role, pulmonary endothelial cells have other activities: they can clear up emboli and thrombi (Heinemann & Fishman 1969), assist in the metabolism of chylomicrons (Schoefl & French 1968), convert angiotensin I to angiotensin II, produce thromboplastin (Zeldis et al

1972), process hormones and prohormones arriving via the circulation (Vane 1969), synthesize prostaglandins and related substances (Ryan & Ryan 1977), inactivate serotinin and carry out a wide range of other metabolic activities. Their microanatomy and ultrastructure accord with these functions. The capillary endothelium is a simple continuous layer of squamous cells (Smith & Ryan 1973), whose particular features are abundant transcytotic vesicles (Smith & Ryan 1970; Simionescu 1985), extreme thinness (less than 0.1 μm in some areas) and an extensive array of luminal projections, thus presenting a huge surface area to blood, an area which in man must be many times greater (Ryan & Ryan 1977) than the commonly quoted 70 m^2 (Fishman & Pietra 1974). According to Ryan and Ryan (1977) the adult human lung may have 3×10^8 alveoli, each with a thousand or more capillary segments in its walls; the pulmonary capillary bed may measure 1500 miles or more, 1.0 ml of blood occupying 10 miles of capillaries. The capillaries are enclosed in alveolar walls or interalveolar septa and course through the interstitial space, interlacing with connective tissue fibres and bulging alternatively into one or other of the alveoli on either side of each interalveolar septum. Thus, while on one side the capillary endothelium is separated by connective tissue fibres from the alveolar epithelium, on the opposite aspect their fused basal laminae are a minimal barrier, on about half the capillary surface, to gas and other solutes in blood, as already noted above. Where the endothelium is closely apposed to an epithelial cell, the endothelial wall is particularly thin (as little as 35 nm) and devoid of vesicles (Simionescu 1985).

PULMONARY DEFENSIVE MECHANISMS

The problems associated with the protection and maintenance of the respiratory tract are great. Such a huge exposed area is vulnerable to desiccation, microbial invasion and the mechanical and chemical effects of inhaled particles. Inhaled air is humidified chiefly in the upper respiratory tract where it passes, with some turbulence, over the nasal and buccopharyngeal mucosae. Secretions of the various glands of the bronchial tree also help to prevent desiccation. The composition of these secretions is hence important. Goblet cells secrete sulphated acid mucosubstances, whereas cells in mucous glands beneath the epithelial surface contain mainly carboxylated mucosubstances, particularly those associated with sialic acid, though sulphated groups also occur (de Haller 1969). In contrast, cells of serous glands contain neutral mucosubstances. Goblet cells respond mainly to local irritation and tubular glands, both mucous and serous, to neural and hormonal control. Excessive or altered secretions may obstruct the flow of air. In addition to mucosubstances secreted by bronchial glands, antibacterial and antiviral substances also appear in the secreted fluid, for example lysozyme, antibodies of the IgA type and possibly interferon (Havez et al 1966).

Another defence against inhaled particles is the ciliary rejection current; cilia sweep the fluid overlying the surfaces of bronchioles, bronchi and trachea upwards at about 1 cm/minute and much inhaled matter trapped in the viscous fluid may be thus removed. However, particles small enough to reach the alveoli may be removed by alveolar phagocytes (see above). Alveolar epithelium has limited powers of regeneration but normally is continually replaced. The lifespan of alveolar squamous cells is about 3 weeks, that of alveolar phagocytes about 4 days (Bertalanffy 1966). Finally, numerous lymphoid nodules (bronchus-associated lymphoid tissue; BALT, see p. 1630) occur in the bronchial lining, providing foci for the production of lymphocytes and giving local immunological protection against infection both by cell mediated (T cell) activities and the production of immunoglobulins (mainly IgA) from B cells to be passed on to gland cells for secretion to the epithelial surface.

In addition to these cellular mechanisms, coughing to clear pulmonary obstructions is, of course, essential. Initiation of such muscular responses to irritation involves stimulation of sensory endings. The identity of these afferent terminals is still somewhat uncertain except at the laryngeal aditus, where epithelial receptors similar to taste buds are considered responsible. However, at least some of the 'brush cells' of the respiratory epithelium appear to have neural contacts and may represent sensory cells with basal synaptic outputs.

PULMONARY RESPONSE TO ACUTE INJURY

Acute pulmonary injury is potentially lethal, with less than 50% of affected patients surviving (Pontoppidan et al 1985). Exposure of the pulmonary mucosa to noxious environmental or endogenous agents produces a dramatic inflammatory response (Schraufstatter et al 1984). This exacerbates pulmonary tissue destruction, reducing the area available for efficient gaseous exchange, but is generally of short duration, as in other forms of acute injury (p. 412). However, during this process a fibroproliferative response is initiated within the interalveolar septa, leading to extensive granulation tissue formation, a process which reduces the intra-alveolar air spaces and thus diminishes further the area over which gaseous exchange can occur. The granulation tissue formed is rich in mesenchymal cells, fibroblasts and endothelial cells. Although it persists up to death in many patients, in survivors it is resolved and the damaged lung remodelled, a process leading to the reconstruction of the gas exchange system. Growth factors involved in the promotion of pulmonary fibroproliferation include two unique forms of platelet-derived growth factor (PDGF), an angiogenesis factor and basic fibroblast growth factor isoforms (Snyder et al 1991; Henke et al 1991). At a later stage, peptides capable of inducing mesenchymal, fibroblast and endothelial cell death appear at the air–lung interface, only the actively proliferating cells of the granulation tissue being affected by these agents. Such cell death is an important factor in the remodelling which occurs within the granulation tissue at the site of injury (Polunovsky et al 1993), leading to the re-establishment of a functioning, adequate gas exchange system within the lung.

PERINATAL PULMONARY DEVELOPMENT

Histologically the lung changes much during development, which is divisible for description into three phases: glandular, canalicular and alveolar (Engel 1947; de Reuck & Porter 1967; Emery 1969; Reid 1976). In the *glandular period*, during the first 16 weeks (approximately) of embryonic development, the tubular epithelial outgrowth ducts of the pulmonary rudiments are lined by tall columnar epithelial cells rich in glycogen, the cells almost obliterating the ductal lumina; between these tubes are closely packed mesenchymal cells and vascular tissue, the whole lung bud being a concentrated mass of cells resembling glandular tissue. At about the sixteenth week a *canalicular period* commences, marked by a rapid proliferation of the ducts, which branch profusely and become canalized as many cells become cuboid and often ciliated. Some cells become squamous and begin to associate with capillaries, a change predominant in the *alveolar period*, which lasts from about 24 weeks onwards to birth, during which alveoli and the bronchial tree finally differentiate. Expansion of the future respiratory spaces is associated with the passage of fluid from lung tissue into their lumina, although incipient respiratory movements, causing inhalation of amniotic fluid, may also aid expansion. By full term and indeed some time before, the lungs are able to support normal respiration once fluid is expelled by expiration in air. After birth minor structural changes continue, alveolar surfaces becoming more complex and alveoli more numerous with increase in body size. Alveolar surfactant is synthesized late and premature births, particularly, may give rise to difficulties in expanding the lungs (respiratory distress syndrome); this can usually be corrected by glucocorticoid administration, which stimulates the synthesis of surfactant. For further details of lung development see page 349.

PULMONARY VASCULATURE AND INNERVATION

Vessels

The lungs have two functionally distinctive circulatory pathways, provided by:

(1) the *pulmonary vessels* which convey deoxygenated blood to the alveolar walls and drain oxygenated blood back to the left side of the heart
(2) the much smaller bronchial vessels which perfuse those parts of the heart with oxygenated blood, to provide the needs of lung

tissues which do not have close access to atmospheric oxygen, for example those of the bronchi and larger bronchioles.

The **pulmonary artery**: After bifurcating from the pulmonary trunk, the right and left pulmonary arteries pass to the hila of the lungs to enter them, and both then divide into branches which accompany segmental and subsegmental bronchi and lie mostly dorsolateral to them. For details of lung development see page 349. They end in the dense capillary networks in the walls of alveolar sacs and alveoli (**11.146, 149**). The arteries of neighbouring segments are independent. Elliot and Reid (1965) have demonstrated a fairly constant relation between the luminal and mural dimensions in the pulmonary arterial tree, this ratio (total diameter : wall thickness) being less than in most systemic arteries, as might be expected from the pressure differences. No regional differences have been detected (Simons & Reid 1969), despite evidence suggesting a large difference between blood flow in the upper and lower pulmonary regions. (See Van Meurs-Van Woezik et al 1987 for changes in the internal diameters in the pulmonary arterial tree with increasing age in infants and children.)

The **pulmonary capillaries** form plexuses immediately outside the epithelium in the walls and septa of alveoli and alveolar sacs. In interalveolar septa the network is a single layer, with meshes smaller than the capillaries, whose walls are exceedingly thin (see above and Suarez 1979). The pulmonary capillaries vary in width but are generally very narrow. In human lungs 38% are narrower than the mean diameter of neutrophils, which deform from a spherical to an ellipsoid shape as they pass through these capillaries (Doerschuk et al 1993). It has been suggested that neutrophils are sequestered in the capillary bed of the lung because their size relative to the capillaries is such that their transport through the capillaries is delayed (Hogg 1987). They are also less deformable than erythrocytes (Chien 1985) and so are delayed more than the latter. The observed concentration of neutrophils in pulmonary capillaries may be due to variation in the width of these vessels. According to this view, the narrower vessels restrict the passage of neutrophils, while the wider vessels provide pathways through which erythrocytes can be diverted, thus avoiding those capillaries in which slower moving neutrophils are located. One consequence of delay in the transport of neutrophils through the pulmonary capillary network is that neutrophil margination occurs more readily than in other organs where the capillaries are broader and less variable in width.

Arteriovenous shunts have been demonstrated in human lungs near the terminal bronchioles. Experiments show that such shunts may pass particles of 500 μm diameter; the functional implications of this are not clear (Tobin 1966).

Pulmonary veins, two from each lung, drain the pulmonary capillaries, the radicles coalescing into larger branches which traverse the lung independently of the pulmonary arteries and bronchi (see below). Communicating freely they form large vessels, which ultimately accompany the arteries and bronchial tubes to the pulmonary hilum, the bronchi often separating the dorsolateral artery and the ventromedial vein. The pulmonary veins open into the left atrium, conveying oxygenated blood for systemic distribution by the left ventricle.

At the hilum the pulmonary arteries and veins accompany the main bronchial divisions but peripheral to this, in the bronchopulmonary segments, relations change (pp. 1656–1661). In general a bronchus and its branches in a segment are central and accompanied by branching arteries but many tributaries of the pulmonary veins run **between** segments, serving adjacent segments, which drain into more than one vein. Some veins also lie beneath the visceral pleura, including that in the interlobar fissures. Thus a bronchopulmonary segment is not a complete vascular unit, with an individual bronchus, artery **and** vein. In the resection of segments it is obvious that the planes between them are not avascular but crossed by pulmonary veins and sometimes by branches of arteries. This pattern of bronchi, arteries and veins varies much, the veins being the most variable and arteries more variable than bronchi (Brock 1942, 1943, 1944, 1954; Boyden 1955; Cory & Valentine 1959; Bloomer et al 1960; Volpe et al 1969). Therefore the following general account requires amplification by reference to the above classic and to later reports.

Arteries of the right lung. The right pulmonary artery (p. 1504) divides as it emerges behind the superior vena cava into two large branches. A lymph node usually occupies the bifurcation. The superior branch, which is the smaller of the two, goes to the superior lobe and usually divides into two further branches which supply the majority of that lobe. The inferior branch descends anterior to the intermediate bronchus and immediately posterior to the superior pulmonary vein. It provides a small recurrent branch to the superior lobe, then at the point where the horizontal fissure meets the oblique fissure it gives off anteriorly the branch to the middle lobe and posteriorly the branch to the superior segment of the inferior lobe. It then continues a short distance before dividing to supply the rest of the inferior lobe segments.

Arteries of the left lung. The left pulmonary artery (p. 1504) emerges from within the concavity of the aortic arch and descends anterior to the descending aorta to enter the oblique fissure. The branches of the left pulmonary artery are extremely variable. Usually its first and largest branch is to the anterior segment of the left superior lobe. Prior to reaching the fissure it gives off a variable number of other branches to the superior lobe. As it enters the fissure it usually supplies a large branch to the superior segment of the inferior lobe. Lingular branches arise within the fissure and the rest of the lower lobe is supplied by many varied branching patterns. It was a surgical aphorism of the late Lord Brock that when performing a left upper lobectomy 'there was always one more branch of the pulmonary artery than you thought!'

Variations. Although the pulmonary arteries rarely depart from the above mode of primary (lobar) branching, segmental branches vary much in their sites of origin and numbers, reduplication being frequent. From observations at 521 partial pneumonectomies, Cory and Valentine (1959) recorded many variations: the right and left upper lobes showed the greatest range of variation, with 14 types of pattern in 152 right-sided operations, and 29 types in 107 on the left; other lobes displayed less variation, the patterns noted being five in the right middle, six in the right lower and four in the left lower lobe.

Veins of the right lung (see also p. 1575). In the hilum the superior right pulmonary vein is formed by the union of apical, anterior and posterior veins (upper lobe) with a middle lobar vein (formed by lateral and medial tributaries). The inferior right pulmonary vein is formed by the hilar union of superior (apical) and common basal veins from the lower lobe, the common basal being formed by the union of superior and inferior basal tributaries.

Veins of the left lung (p. 1575). In the hilum the superior left pulmonary vein, which drains the upper lobe, is formed by the union of apicoposterior (draining the apical and posterior segments), anterior and lingular veins, the last-named consisting of an upper and a lower part. The inferior left pulmonary vein, which drains the lower lobe, is formed by the hilar union of two veins, superior (apical) and common basal, the latter formed by the union of a superior and an inferior basal vein.

All the main tributaries of the pulmonary veins receive smaller tributaries, some intrasegmental and others intersegmental (see above).

Bronchial arteries. These supply oxygenated blood to maintain the pulmonary tissues. They are derived from the descending thoracic aorta directly or indirectly; the right is usually a branch of the third posterior intercostal artery, whilst there are normally two left bronchial arteries (upper and lower) which branch separately from the thoracic aorta. The bronchial arteries accompany the bronchial tree and supply bronchial glands and the walls of the bronchial tubes and larger pulmonary vessels. The bronchial branches form, in the muscular tunic of the air passages, a capillary plexus supporting a second, mucosal plexus which communicates with branches of the pulmonary artery and drains into the pulmonary veins. Other arterial branches ramify in interlobular loose connective tissue and end partly in deep and partly in superficial, bronchial veins. Some also ramify on the surface of the lung, forming subpleural capillary plexuses. Bronchial arteries supply the bronchial wall as far as the respiratory bronchioles. They anastomose with branches of the pulmonary arteries in the walls of the smaller bronchi and in the visceral pleura. Such bronchopulmonary anastomoses may be more numerous in the newborn, and then later obliterated to a marked degree (Wagenvoort & Wagenvoort 1967). In addition to the main bronchial arteries, smaller bronchial branches arise from the descending thoracic aorta; one of these may lie in the pulmonary ligament and may cause bleeding during inferior lobectomy.

Bronchial veins. These form two distinct systems (Marchand et al

1950). *Deep bronchial veins* commence as intrapulmonary bronchiolar plexuses, communicating freely with the pulmonary veins and eventually joining a single trunk which ends in a main pulmonary vein or in the left atrium. *Superficial bronchial veins* drain extrapulmonary bronchi, visceral pleura and the hilar lymph nodes; they also communicate with the pulmonary veins and end on the right in the azygos vein and on the left in the left superior intercostal or the accessory hemiazygos veins. Bronchial veins do not receive all the blood conveyed by bronchial arteries; some enters the pulmonary veins. The main bronchial arteries and veins run on the dorsal aspect of the extrapulmonary bronchi.

Pulmonary lymph vessels. These are described on page 1625. For reconstructions of the bronchial lymphatic networks consult Bastianini (1967, 1968). Major ultrastructural features of pulmonary lymphatics include a thin basal lamina and abundant vesicles in the cytoplasm of the endothelial cells, with other evidence of pinocytosis, suggesting considerable passage of fluid across the lymphatic wall (Lauweryns & Boussaw 1967).

Pulmonary innervation

The anterior and posterior pulmonary plexuses are largely formed by sympathetic and vagal branches. Rami from these accompany the bronchial tubes, carrying efferent fibres to the bronchial muscles and glands and afferent fibres from the bronchial mucous membrane and alveoli. Small ganglia occur along these nerves. It is generally accepted that bronchoconstrictors are supplied by the vagus (pp. 1251, 1297), the sympathetic supply being inhibitory and relaxing the bronchial smooth muscle, as does also the withdrawal or reduction of parasympathetic (vagal) stimulation. The actual stimulus for bronchodilatation is the pressure of inspired air. The innervation of the alveolar walls in the human lung has been studied at the ultrastructural level by Fox et al (1980).

Radiology. The trachea, because of its content of air, is more radiotranslucent than neighbouring structures and hence visible in

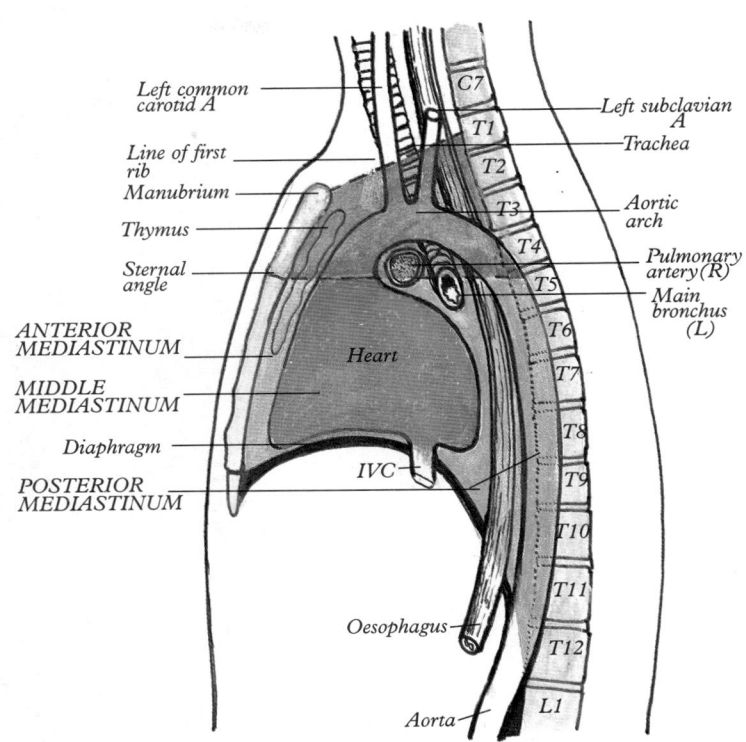

11.56   Diagram indicating the major divisions of the mediastinum (see text for further details). Note that not all mediastinal contents are depicted.

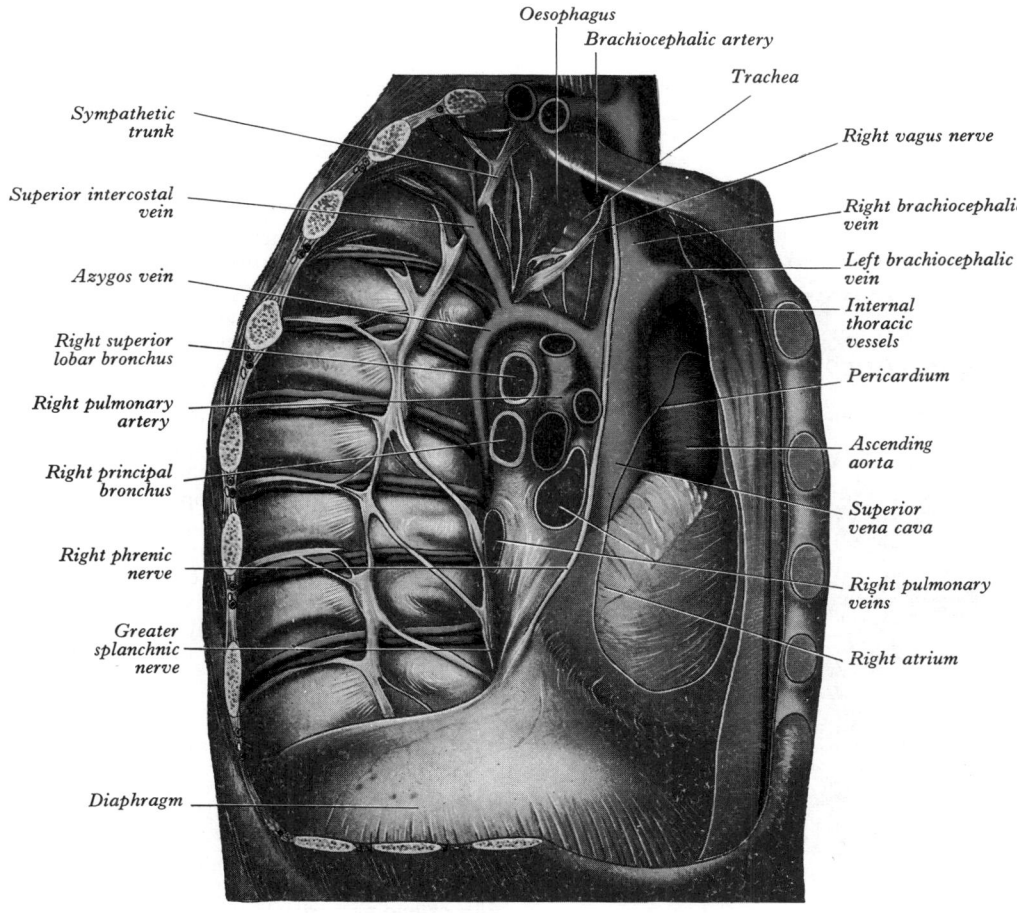

11.57   The mediastinum: right lateral aspect. A part of the pericardial sac has been removed to expose the lateral surface of the right atrium.

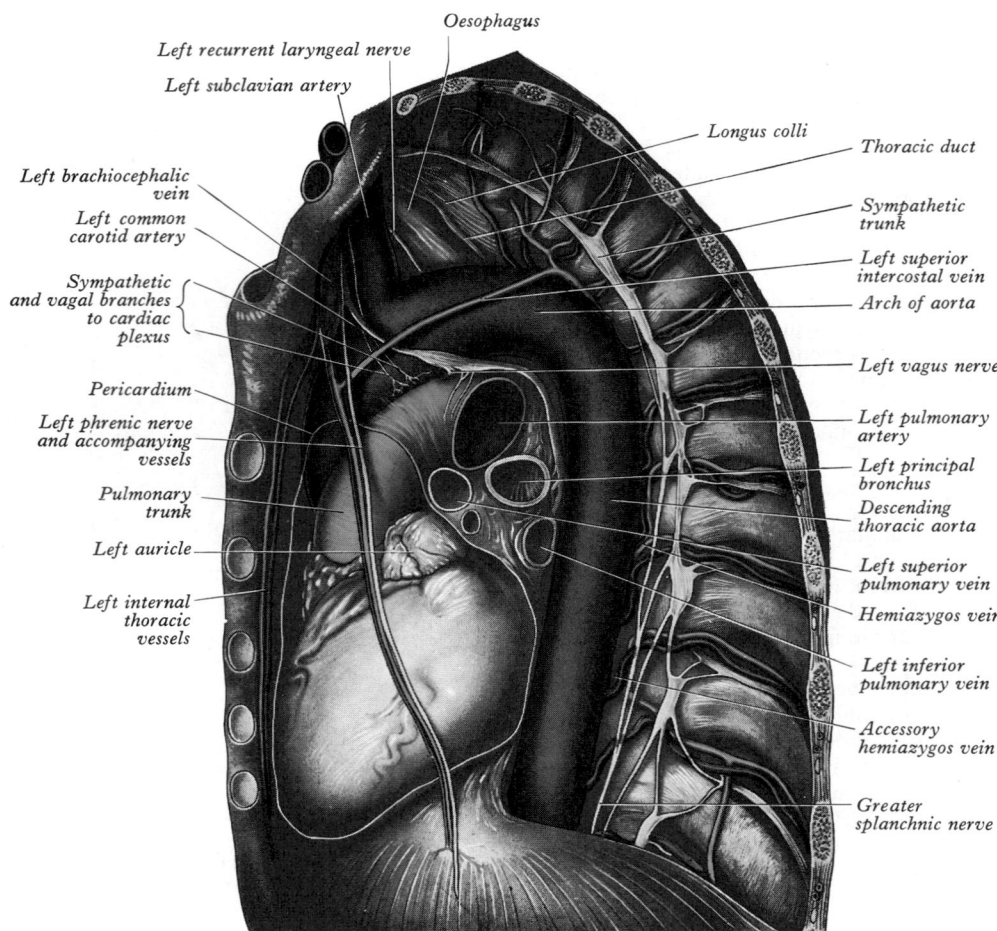

11.58   The mediastinum: left lateral aspect.

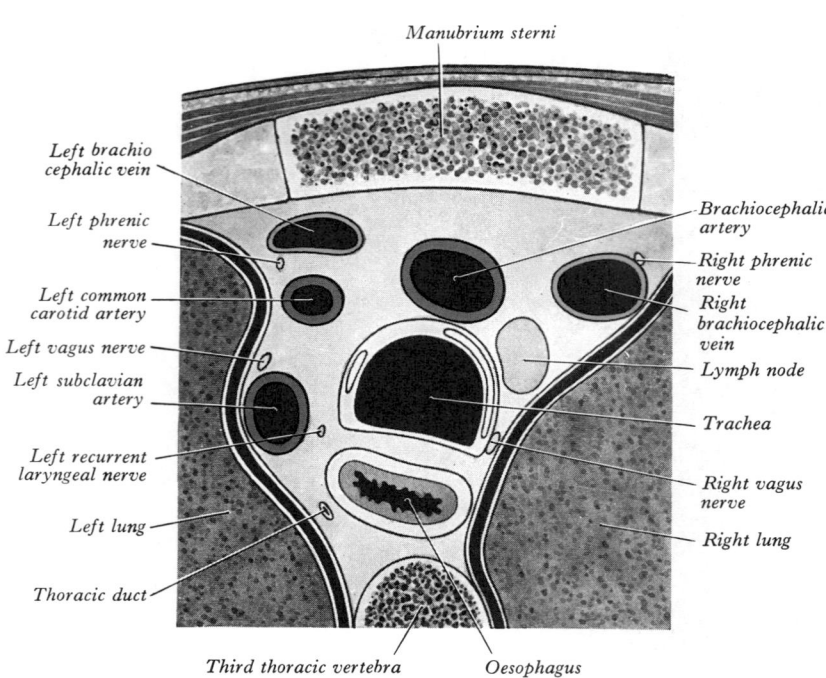

11.59   Transverse section through the mediastinum at the level of the body
of the third thoracic vertebra: superior aspect.

lateral and anteroposterior radiograms of the neck and upper thorax
as a dark area in negatives (light in positive prints, 4.000). Similarly,
the lungs appear as dark areas in the thorax, flanking the central
mediastinal opacity; they also appear darker at the end of inspiration
and in diseased conditions in which the alveoli are permanently
distended (emphysema), but are more radio-opaque in pathological
states which reduce the air in them (e.g. pneumonia). Pulmonary
shadows have superimposed on them the light shadows of pulmonary
blood vessels branching from the hilum (see **11.70** and Lodge 1946).
These are sometimes mistaken for bronchi but the latter (because of
contained air) obviously appear dark. Where a blood vessel is
photographed end-on, it appears as a white circle, a bronchus
appearing as a dark circle surrounded by a white line (its wall). Hilar
lymph nodes, if enlarged or calcified, appear as mottled areas near
the mediastinum. The lumina of bronchi and bronchioles can be
made radiologically visible by injecting a suitable radio-opaque oil
into the trachea. Effusions of fluid into pleural cavities appear
opaque in radiograms.

MEDIASTINUM (11.56–69)

The mediastinum is, strictly, the partition between the lungs and
includes the mediastinal pleura, although it is commonly applied to
the region between the two pleural sacs. It is bounded anteriorly by
the sternum and posteriorly by the thoracic vertebral column (**11.56–
58**), extending vertically from the thoracic inlet to the diaphragm.
For descriptive purposes it is divided into a superior and an inferior
mediastinum, the latter being subdivided into anterior, middle and

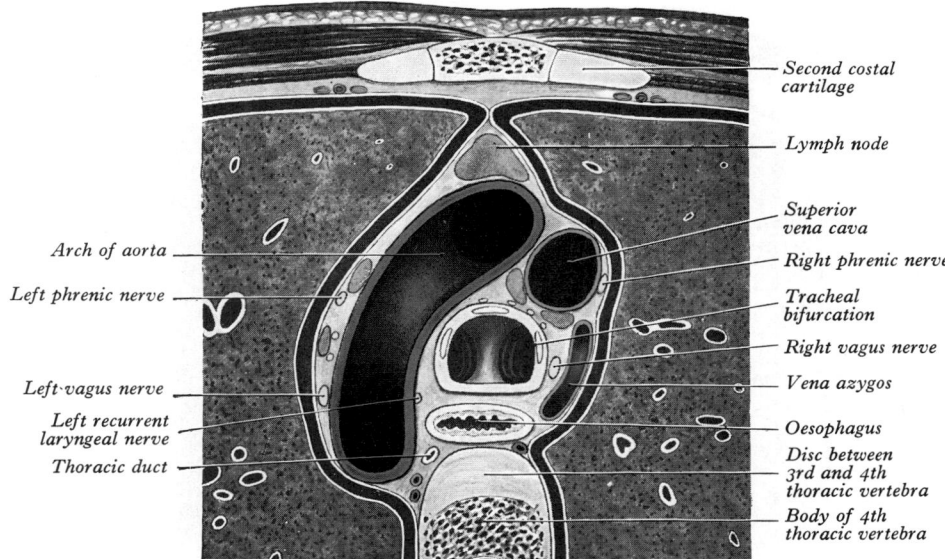

Second costal
cartilage

Lymph node

Superior
vena cava

Right phrenic nerve

Tracheal
bifurcation

Right vagus nerve

Vena azygos

Oesophagus

Disc between
3rd and 4th
thoracic vertebra

Body of 4th
thoracic vertebra

Arch of aorta

Left phrenic nerve

Left·vagus nerve

Left recurrent
laryngeal nerve

Thoracic duct

11.60   Transverse section through the mediastinum at the level of the upper
part of the body of the fourth thoracic vertebra: superior aspect.

posterior parts. The plane of division into upper and lower mediastina
traverses the manubriosternal joint and the lower surface of the
fourth thoracic vertebra (**11.56**).

Superior mediastinum (**11.59, 60, 64–69**). This lies between the
manubrium sterni and the upper four thoracic vertebrae. It is
bounded below by the sternal plane, above by the plane of the
thoracic inlet and laterally by the mediastinal pleurae. It contains
the lower ends of the sternohyoid, sternothyroid and longus colli
muscles, thymic remnants, internal thoracic arteries and veins,
brachiocephalic veins and upper half of the superior vena cava, the
aortic arch, the brachiocephalic artery, left common carotid and
subclavian arteries, the left superior intercostal vein, the vagus,
cardiac, phrenic and left recurrent laryngeal nerves, the trachea,
oesophagus, the superficial part of the cardiac plexus and thoracic
duct. Associated with their named structures are also the paratracheal, brachiocephalic and tracheobronchial lymph nodes.

Anterior mediastinum (**11.61–63**). Lying between the sternal body

and pericardium, this region narrows above the fourth costal
cartilages, where the pleural sacs come close to each other. It contains loose connective tissue, the sternopericardial ligaments, a few
lymph nodes and the mediastinal branches of the internal thoracic
artery and sometimes part of the thymus gland or its degenerated
remains.

Middle mediastinum (**11.57, 58, 61–63**). The broadest part of the
inferior mediastinum, it contains: the pericardium, heart, ascending
aorta, the lower half of the superior vena cava, the terminal azygos
vein, tracheal bifurcation and both main bronchi, the pulmonary
trunk dividing into right and left pulmonary arteries, both pulmonary
veins, the phrenic nerves, the deep part of the cardiac plexus and
the tracheobronchial lymph nodes.

Posterior mediastinum (**11.57, 58, 61–63**). This region is bounded:
in front by the tracheal bifurcation, pulmonary vessels, pericardium
and the posterior part of the upper surface of the diaphragm; **behind**
by the vertebral column, from the lower border of the fourth thoracic

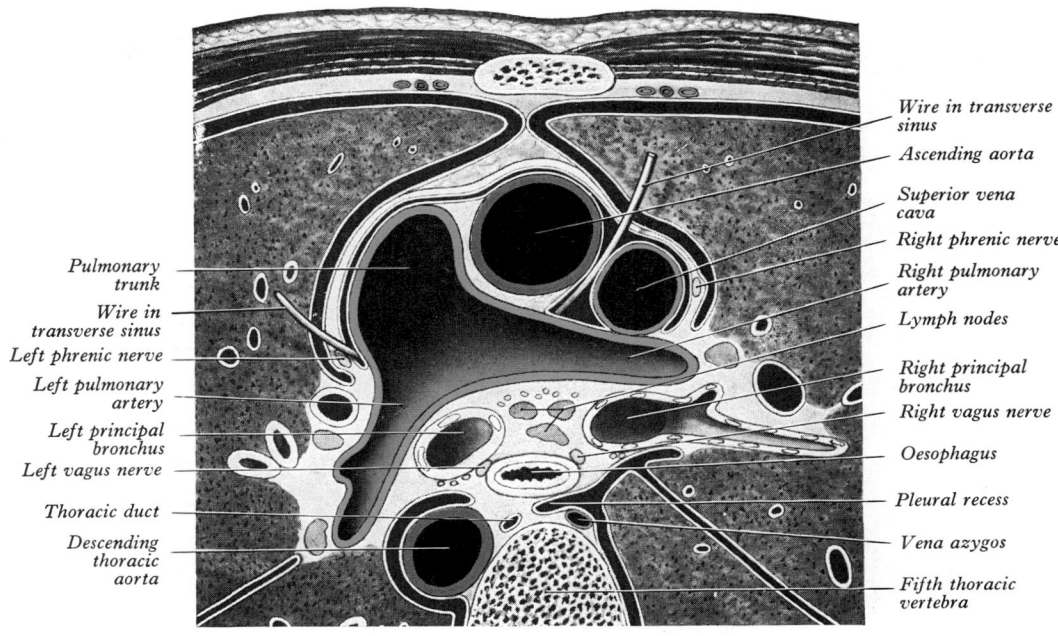

Wire in transverse
sinus

Ascending aorta

Superior vena
cava

Right phrenic nerve

Right pulmonary
artery

Lymph nodes

Right principal
bronchus

Right vagus nerve

Oesophagus

Pleural recess

Vena azygos

Fifth thoracic
vertebra

Pulmonary
trunk

Wire in
transverse sinus

Left phrenic nerve

Left pulmonary
artery

Left principal
bronchus

Left vagus nerve

Thoracic duct

Descending
thoracic
aorta

11.61   Transverse section of the mediastinum at the level of the lower part
of the body of the fifth thoracic vertebra: superior aspect.

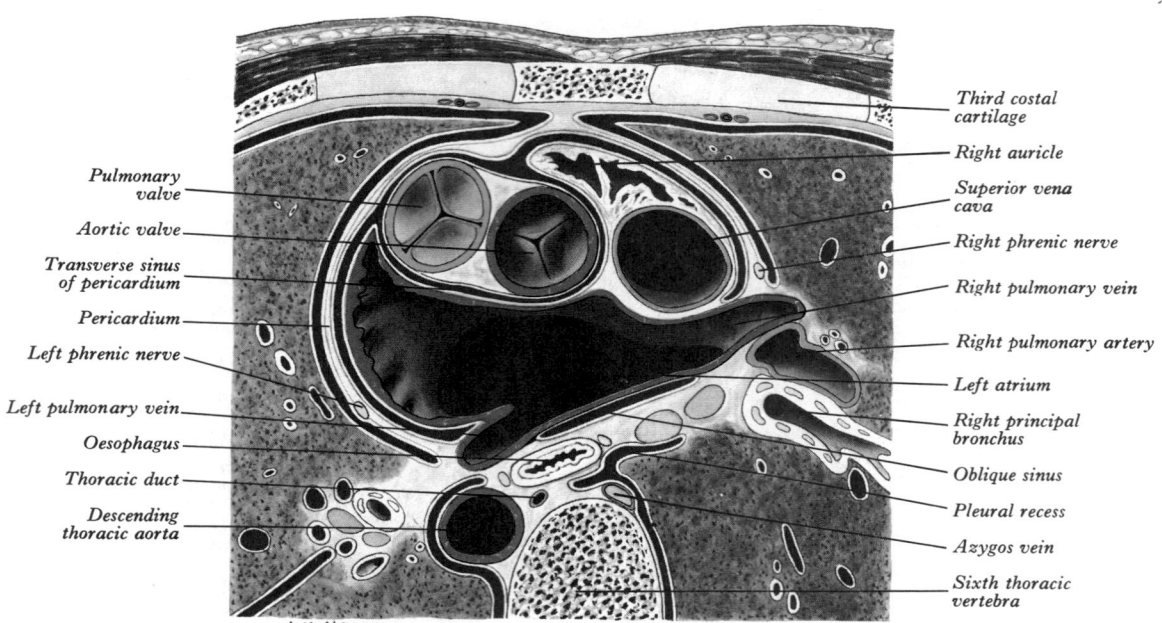

Third costal
cartilage

Right auricle

Superior vena
cava

Right phrenic nerve

Right pulmonary vein

Right pulmonary artery

Left atrium

Right principal
bronchus

Oblique sinus

Pleural recess

Azygos vein

Sixth thoracic
vertebra

Pulmonary
valve

Aortic valve

Transverse sinus
of pericardium

Pericardium

Left phrenic nerve

Left pulmonary vein

Oesophagus

Thoracic duct

Descending
thoracic aorta

A.K. MAXWELL

11.62 Transverse section of the mediastinum at the level of the body of the sixth thoracic vertebra: superior aspect.

vertebra to the twelfth, and on each side by the mediastinal pleura. It contains: the descending thoracic aorta, the azygos, hemiazygos and accessory azygos veins, the vagus and splanchnic nerves, the oesophagus, thoracic duct and the posterior mediastinal lymph nodes.

Sections obtained by magnetic resonance imaging (Mk1) depicting six different levels of the thorax are shown in **11.64–69** (compare with **11.56**).

Mediastinal radiology (10.47–49, 11.70)

Viewed in anteroposterior radiograms (10.43) the heart and large blood vessels appear as the 'mediastinal shadow'. Forming its *left border* from above down, are: the left subclavian artery, aortic arch ('aortic knuckle'), left auricle and left ventricle. Below the arch the right ventricle's infundibulum or the pulmonary trunk may be

recognizable. On the *right border* are the right brachiocephalic vein, superior vena cava, right atrium and thoracic inferior vena cava. Enlargements or displacements of any of these structures accentuate the normal bulges on the borders of the mediastinal shadow. On both sides opacities due to pulmonary vessels associated with the roots of the lungs form *hilar shadows*. In the upper thorax the less dense shadow of the trachea is visible in the median plane.

In lateral or oblique views the cardiac shadow is above the anterior part of the diaphragm. In front of it is the retrosternal space (anterior mediastinum); behind is the retrocardiac space (posterior mediastinum) containing the oesophagus, which can be visualized with a barium swallow (**12.86**), and the descending thoracic aorta. Above, the less dense trachea and bronchi are recognizable; the aortic arch and large vessels produce faint shadows in the superior mediastinum.

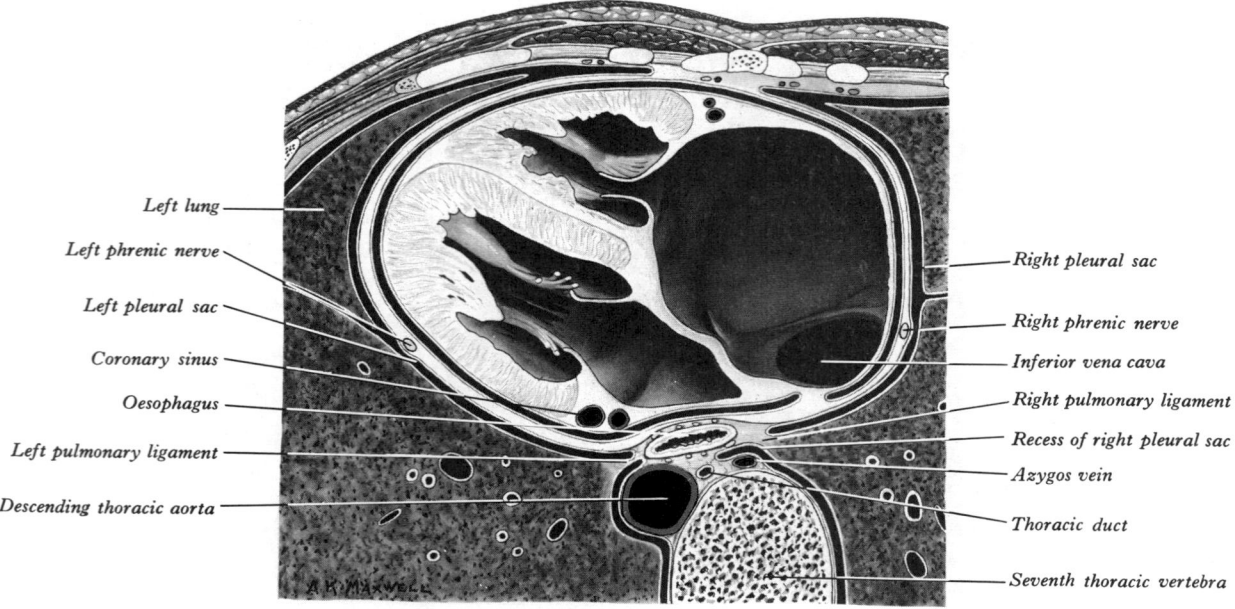

Left lung

Left phrenic nerve

Left pleural sac

Coronary sinus

Oesophagus

Left pulmonary ligament

Descending thoracic aorta

Right pleural sac

Right phrenic nerve

Inferior vena cava

Right pulmonary ligament

Recess of right pleural sac

Azygos vein

Thoracic duct

Seventh thoracic vertebra

A.K. MAXWELL

11.63 Transverse section through the mediastinum at the level of the body of the seventh thoracic vertebra: superior aspect.

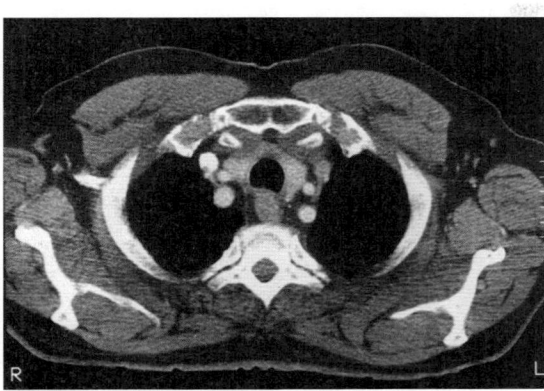

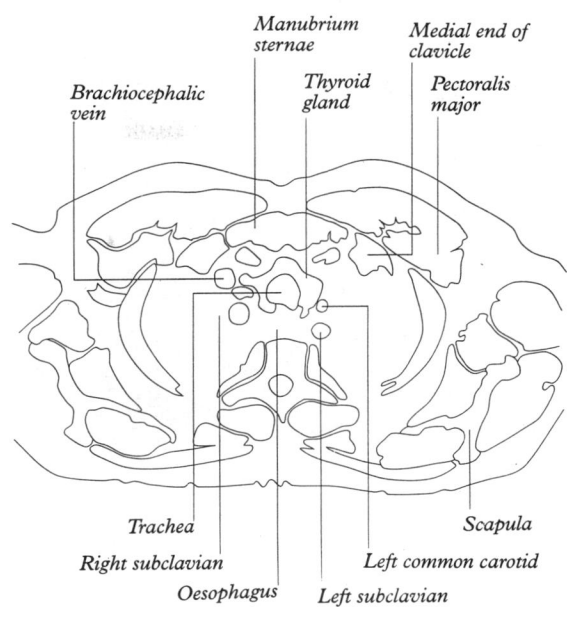

11.64 Transverse section of thorax at the level of the junction of the first rib with the manubrium sternae seen by MRI, as also in **11.**65–69. (Supplied by J Dussek, Dept of Surgery, Guy's Hospital, London.)

Brachiocephalic vein
Manubrium sternae
Thyroid gland
Medial end of clavicle
Pectoralis major

Trachea
Right subclavian
Oesophagus
Left subclavian
Left common carotid
Scapula

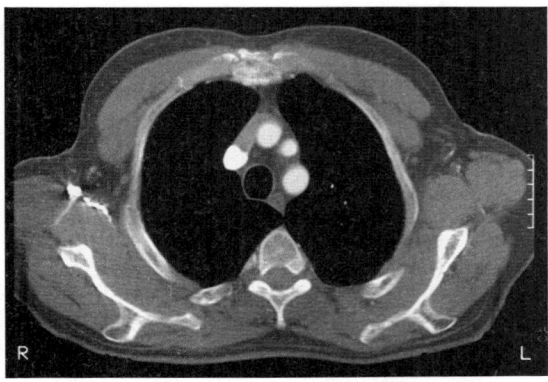

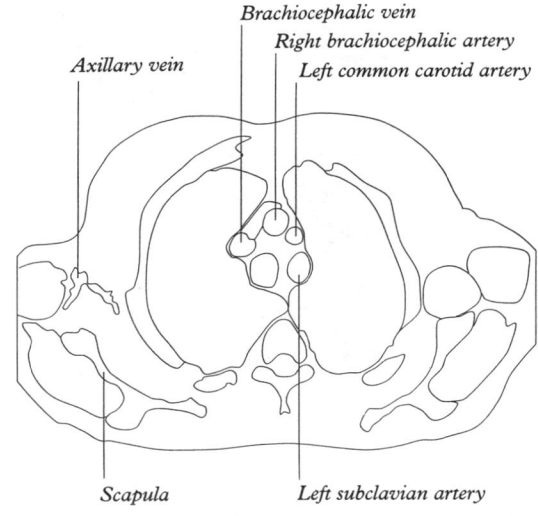

11.65 Transverse section of thorax through the lower portion of the third thoracic vertebra.

Axillary vein
Brachiocephalic vein
Right brachiocephalic artery
Left common carotid artery

Scapula
Left subclavian artery

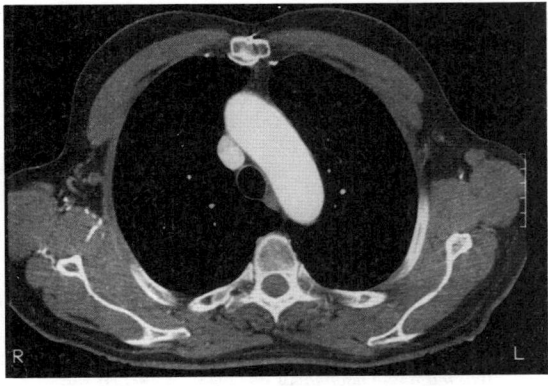

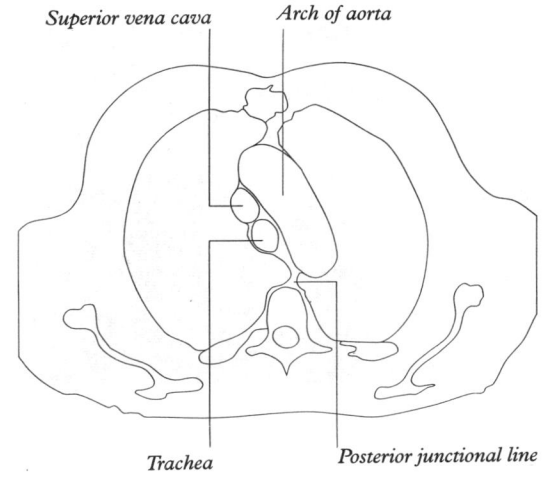

11.66 Transverse section of thorax through the middle of the fourth thoracic vertebra and aortic arch.

Superior vena cava
Arch of aorta

Trachea
Posterior junctional line

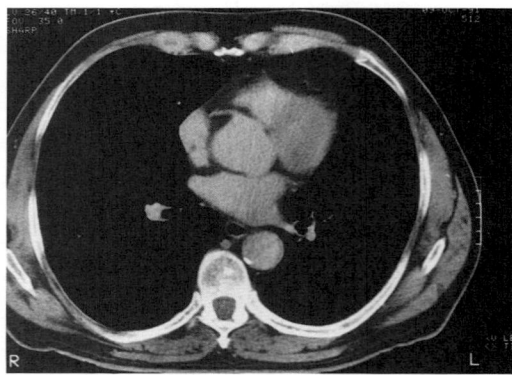

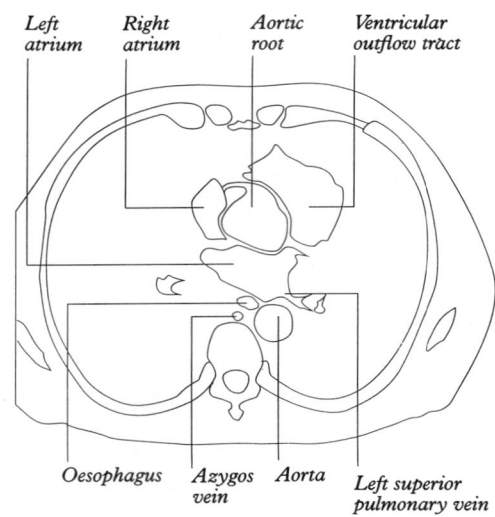

11.67 Transverse section of thorax at the level of the lower border of the fourth thoracic vertebra, just at the level of the tracheal bifurcation.

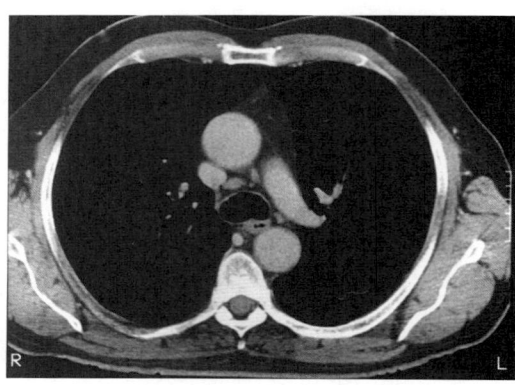

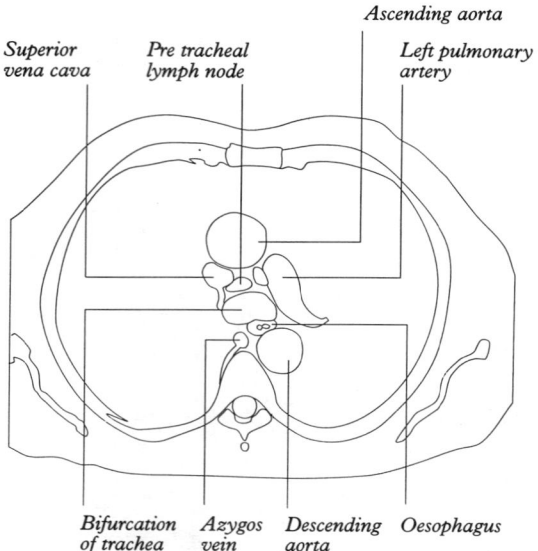

11.68 Transverse section of thorax at upper border of the sixth thoracic vertebra, below the carina at the level of the pulmonary trunk and right main pulmonary artery.

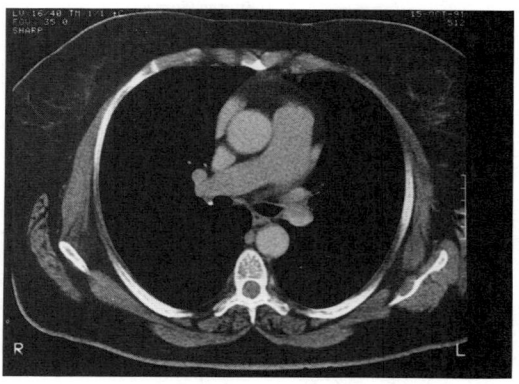

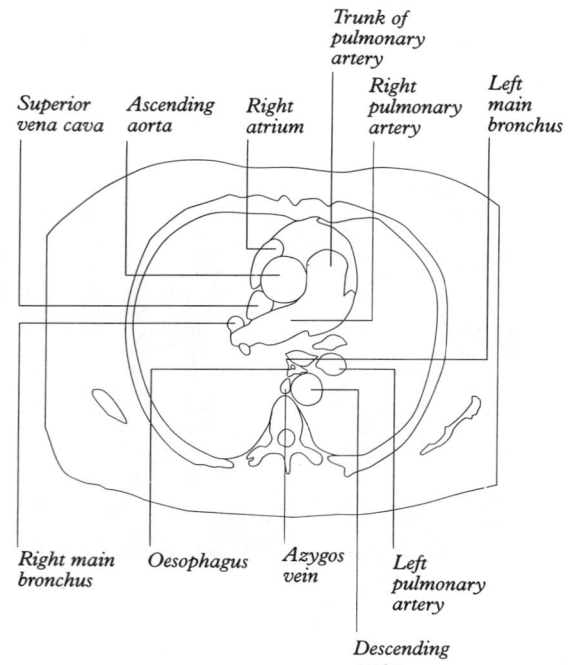

11.69 Transverse section of thorax through lower portion of seventh thoracic vertebra, passing through the aortic root.

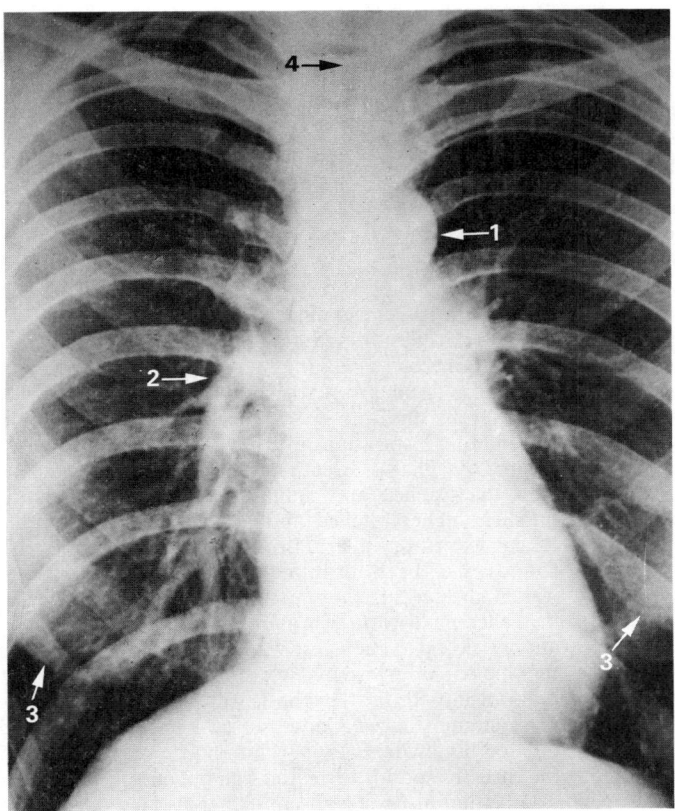

11.70 Radiograph of chest: postero-anterior view of adult female. Note the difference in level of the right and left halves of the diaphragm. 1. Aortic 'knuckle'. 2. Pulmonary vessels of right side. 3. Edge of shadow caused by breast. 4. Position of trachea.

Clinical examination of the chest

Although modern radiological techniques (see p. 1678) have revolutionized the diagnosis of chest diseases, the physical examination of the thorax is a necessary and valuable art for all clinicians. The classical quartet of inspection, palpation, percussion and auscultation form the basis of a systematic examination of the chest just as they do in the abdomen (see p. 1746). However, one should not commence examining the thorax until a careful history has been obtained and the extremities and overall appearance of the subject have been assessed. By the time the examiner approaches the chest, a working diagnosis may well have been established and much more information will thus be derived from the examination.

Such observation may, for example, reveal the blue plethoric appearance of a patient with cor pulmonale and emphysema, a malar flush from mitral stenosis, a spinal deformity from old tuberculosis or the anatomical abnormalities of a collagen disorder such as Marfan's syndrome. Examination of the hands is often particularly helpful, revealing perhaps the nicotine stained and clubbed fingers of a subject with carcinoma of the bronchus,

or the tattooing of the skin by coal dust in a miner with pneumoconiosis. The pulse may reveal evidence of a cardiac disorder, for example, the slow rising pulse of aortic stenosis or the collapsing pulse of aortic regurgitation. Examination of the supraclavicular fossa may reveal enlarged nodes from an intrathoracic malignancy.

Inspection

The subject should be examined lying back supported by pillows at an angle of 45° in a warm room and in a good light. From the front the general shape and size of the thorax are noted, together with the condition of the skin, adipose tissue, musculature and, particularly in the female, the breasts. Note should be taken of the vessels of the chest wall which may, for example, be dilated, as with superior vena caval obstruction. Abnormalities of the musculature may be congenital or acquired, for example a congenitally absent pectoralis major muscle, or there may be use of accessory muscles and intercostal recession in laboured breathing. The bony structure may not be easily visible in plump subjects but congenital abnormalities of the sternum are usually appar-

ent even in the obese, for example a pectus excavatum or carinatum.

The nipples in the male and the breasts of the female should be inspected. Accessory nipples are not infrequent and carcinoma of the breast, the most common carcinoma of females in the United Kingdom, may produce visible abnormalities. Normal chest expansion is symmetrical. The subject should be observed breathing normally and taking deep breaths. A stiff or shrunken lung, or pleural disease will impair expansion on that side. The cardiac apex beat may just be visible in thin subjects and abnormal cardiac impulses should be noted. The size of the chest should also be noted. It may, for example, be barrel shaped with increase in the anteroposterior diameter when the lungs are over inflated as in emphysema.

From behind, with the subject sitting forward the thoracic spine should be inspected, again looking for congenital or acquired abnormalities.

Palpation

Many of the observations of inspection can be confirmed or extended by palpation. The position of the mediastinum is assessed by feeling the position of the trachea and the apex beat. The trachea is normally palpable in the midline within the suprasternal notch and may be felt either with one finger rolled over its convex surface or with two fingers, one either side of it. Shift to one side indicates that the mediastinum is either pulled over by loss of lung volume or pushed over, for example, by a large pneumothorax or pleural effusion. The position of the apex beat should be confirmed and, using the flat of the hand on the anterior chest wall, the cardiac impulse should be assessed. It may be exaggerated by ventricular hypertrophy or by the heart being pushed anteriorly by an enlarged left atrium. Thrills caused by turbulent blood flow may be felt. Expansion of the chest is assessed by placing the palms of the hands on the anterior chest wall with the fingers gripping laterally and the thumbs in the midline. The subject should take deep even breaths and the symmetry of expansion should be noted. A pleural friction rub may be felt occasionally in cases of pleural disease.

The angle of Louis (see p. 1916) and the male nipple are useful fixed reference points. Abnormalities of bony structure or tenderness may be defined and special attention should be paid to feeling the supraclavicular fossa and axillae for enlarged lymph nodes.

Percussion

The technique of percussion is important if useful information is to be obtained. The percussed finger must lie in firm apposition to the chest wall. The percussing movement should be done loosely from the wrist and the strike should be short and decisive, the percussing finger being withdrawn immediately the blow is struck. The percussion note is resonant over the air-containing lungs, but flat or dull over solid structures such as the heart and liver. Pathological dullness may be elicited over consolidated lung or pleural fluid. Percussion over a gas-filled gastric fundus will produce a tympanitic note hyperresonance and the normal dullness over the liver and heart may be lost if the lungs are hyperinflated as in emphysema.

Auscultation

By the time the examiner has come to listen to the chest he/she should have some expectation of what might be heard. Normal (vesicular) breath sounds emanating from the lungs are soft, heard throughout inspiration and have a short expiratory phase. Breath sounds heard over the trachea and main bronchi are harsher, higher pitched and have a prolonged expiratory phase. Bronchial breath sounds may be transmitted to the chest wall if the lung is more solid than usual or if there is distortion bringing the major airway closer to the chest wall. Similarly, the spoken or whispered word may also be transmitted to the chest wall under these circumstances. Conversely, a hyperinflated lung will result in a diminution of the breath sounds. Breath sounds may also be diminished or absent if there is air or fluid between the lung and the chest wall. The examiner should listen to all areas of the lung and compare one side with the other. Added sounds which are not normally present include wheezes and crackles. Wheezes which occur mostly on expiration may be polyphonic when there is narrowing of many bronchi (as in asthma) or monophonic when there is narrowing of a single and usually larger bronchus (as in endobronchial carcinoma). Crackles on inspiration are usually alveolar in origin and coarse ones are usually due to secretions in the bronchi.

When auscultating the heart the examiner will be listening for the normal heart sounds of valve closure and for additional clicks and murmurs. The first heart sound is due to closure of the atrioventricular valves and the second heart sound to aortic and pulmonary valve closure. Characteristically, the second heart sound is split, the aortic component being heard first. This splitting varies with respiration but may, for example, be fixed and widely split with an atrial septal defect (due to a conduction defect). The intensity and frequency of the individual valve sounds should be noted. Additional sounds may be heard, for example the midsystolic click of mitral valve prolapse. The aortic valve is best heard at the angle of Louis to the right of the midline, the pulmonary valve in the second intercostal space at the left border of the sternum, the tricuspid valve just above the xiphisternum and the mitral valve at the apex of the heart (10.46). It should be noted that these are the sites where the valves are best heard, and not their site of maximum intensity. The timing of any murmur should be noted as well as the direction in which it radiates. For example, the diastolic murmur of mitral stenosis is soft, low pitched and radiates to the apex, often being best heard with the patient tilted to the left. The diastolic murmur of aortic regurgitation, however, is clearest at the left sternal edge at the end of expiration and with the patient sitting up and leaning forward. The rhythm of the heart should be noted and correlated with both a peripheral arterial pulse and the jugular venous pulse, if visible.

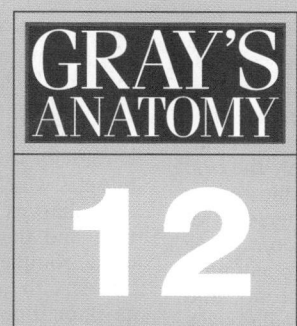

GRAY'S ANATOMY

12

ALIMENTARY SYSTEM

Section Editor: Lawrence H. Bannister

The text on the oral cavity and teeth was extensively revised by Douglas Luke. Contributions on the comparative anatomy of the teeth was by Moya Meredith Smith and on oesophageal structure by Bill Owen. Donald Low provided advice on the structure of the gastro-oesophageal orifice. The essay on liver transplantation was provided by P. McMaster, on pancreatic transplantation by Robert Sells and on hernia and clinical examination by Harold Ellis. My editorial colleagues Giorgio Gabella and Mary Dyson contributed advice and additional material on the enteric microstructure and pancreatic and hepatic anatomy respectively.

INTRODUCTION

This section deals sequentially with the anatomy of the different regions of the human alimentary tract and associated glands. After a consideration of the general features of the tract as a whole, details are given of the initial, rather specialized structures, namely the oral cavity, palatine musculature, salivary glands and teeth, followed by the tongue and pharynx. Next, for convenience, the arrangement of the abdomen and its peritoneal lining are described, before continuing with the oesophagus, stomach, small intestine (duodenum, jejunum, ileum), large intestine (caecum and appendix, colon, rectum), and the anal canal and musculature. Finally, the major abdominal glands, the pancreas and liver (with the gallbladder), are considered. The microscopic anatomy of these structures and relevant aspects of clinical anatomy are described at appropriate points in the text.

General features of the alimentary system

The alimentary system, also described as the digestive or gastro-intestinal tract, is by definition primarily concerned with the intake, digestion and absorption of nutrients (alimentation), although it has a number of important accessory functions, e.g. in its upper part it also possesses some respiratory features, since the mouth and parts of the pharynx are shared alimentary and respiratory pathways. Two of its glands, the pancreas and liver, also play more general systemic roles in the body. The anatomical organization of the alimentary system reflects these various activities closely both at the topographic and microscopic levels of organization.

The functions of the alimentary tract, in the context of the process of digestion, are multiple:

- it provides a space for the storage and processing of ingesta, and the elimination of its unabsorbed components (faeces)
- it secretes enzymes and lubricants which process and facilitate the passage of the ingesta
- it absorbs nutrients and other materials and passes them into the body
- it propels material within it by muscular action
- it has defensive, especially immunological, properties
- it houses microorganisms
- its epithelial lining forms a thin but strong barrier between its lumen (a space open to the outside) and the interstitium or true interior of the body.

These functions, together with the structural organization, vascularization, innervation and evolution of the alimentary tract, will be briefly reviewed in this introductory section.

Essentially, the alimentary tract is an epithelium-lined muscular tube capable of selecting then propelling ingested material through a series of different physiological environments created by its secretory and absorptive epithelia. In these compartments, food already broken down mechanically by the teeth is exposed to digestive enzymes which reduce the large biomolecules to components small enough to pass through selective channels in epithelial cell membranes, and thence into the intercellular spaces of the gut wall. Such molecules are then taken into the vascular system for distribution to the body. The undigested remnants within the alimentary lumen are finally eliminated through the anus. As the interior surface of the alimentary tract is continuous at the mouth and anus with the external surface of the body, material within its lumen can be regarded as external to the body, actually entering it only when in the form of small molecules and ions it traverses the cells lining its wall into the surrounding tissues.

The *glands* lining the tract provide the water, enzymes, ionic environments and other attributes required for these purposes. All alimentary glands are epithelial–mesenchymal derivatives; they include large populations of microscopic invaginations of the luminal surface, confined to the alimentary wall. A few are much larger and located mainly outside the tract; these are formed as major diverticula of the tract's epithelial lining, retaining connections in the form of secretory ducts. They comprise the three pairs of major oral salivary glands (parotid, submandibular and sublingual), and the pancreas and liver. The latter two organs have additional functions related to general metabolism as well as to alimentation; the pancreas secretes hormones from specialized endocrine islet cells and the liver carries

out a wide range of synthetic and metabolic functions (and in fetal life, haemopoiesis, see p. 187). The control of secretion is carried out by a combination of autonomic nervous, hormonal and local chemical regulation (see p. 1794).

The *motility* of the alimentary canal depends on muscle fasciculi within its wall and, in some regions, also on specialized external muscles which assist or oppose the passage of ingesta. In the mouth and pharynx and at the anus these muscles are largely skeletal in type and under voluntary motor control. Their actions are often quite complex and are precisely co-ordinated; in the mouth and pharynx they are also employed for non-alimentary purposes such as phonation. Throughout most of its extent the alimentary wall contains smooth muscle and is regulated by the autonomic nervous system. In much of the tract the co-ordinated actions of circular and longitudinal muscle layers propel the contents caudally by peristalsis, lubricated by the secretions of the glands in the walls of the tract which also protect the lining against excessive abrasion. Specialized areas of circular muscle form a number of sphincters regulating the passage of substances from one region of the gut to the next; these include the two oesophageal sphincters (upper and lower), and the pyloric and anal sphincters. The control of motility is complex and depends on regional monitoring, in part by sensory nerves connected synaptically to a network of ganglion calls and local motor neurons within the alimentary wall, forming the *enteric nervous system* (p. 1749). Another major controlling influence is the *enteroendocrine system* (p. 1787), a scattered population of peptidergic cells within the lining epithelium which can secrete various peptide hormones from their bases into the subjacent tissues when suitably stimulated by the alimentary contents. Motility is influenced too by circulating hormones, e.g. noradrenalin, products of defensive cells and by extrinsic nervous action, the presiding efferent nerves for most of the tract being the vagus and branches of the thoracolumbar sympathetic system (see pp. 1303–1304).

Alimentation. The breakdown of solid ingested material is begun in the mouth by the mechanical action of the teeth (mastication), the tongue and various neighbouring muscles. These actions greatly increase the surface area of the ingesta and mix them with the secretions of the salivary glands (insalivation). The secretions begin to dissolve soluble substances, promoting their access to taste buds and beginning the digestion of polysaccharides by the action of salivary amylase from the parotid glands. After swallowing (deglutition) by the concerted actions of the tongue, palatine muscles and pharynx, and the rapid transport to the stomach via the oesophagus, gastric digestion proceeds by the action of acidic, protease-rich secretions of multitudes of small gastric glands, which also release intrinsic factor needed for the absorption of iron, and protective mucus. Passing through the pylorus into the first part of the small intestine, the duodenum, the semi-fluid products of gastric digestion encounter alkaline bile from the liver and gallbladder (entering via the bile duct), and pancreatic enzymes from the pancreatic duct. Bile salts physically disrupt liquid masses by detergent action, and the pancreatic secretions contain a wide variety of enzymes capable of hydrolysing many classes of biomolecules. Digestion proceeds throughout the considerable length (up to 6 m) of the small intestine, accompanied by absorption of the resulting small molecules: amino acids, monosaccharides, triglycerides, nucleotides, and of vitamins, etc. by the specialized epithelial cells (enterocytes) lining the small intestine. Enterocytes transport these molecules into the intercellular spaces of the intestinal walls to diffuse into the vascular plexuses lining the alimentary tract. The rate of such movements depends on the surface area of absorptive membrane bordering the intestinal lumen, an area which is quite enormous due to a combination of intestinal length, the considerable folding of its wall and the presence of numerous microvilli on the apices of the absorptive epithelial cells.

The alimentary tract also transports water and electrolytes across its wall; as the enzymes and lubricants are all in aqueous, ionically defined suspensions, large quantities of water and ions, especially sodium and chloride, are released into the tract. These are selectively resorbed (and, in certain cases, exchanged for other ions) through specialized absorptive epithelial cells which are especially numerous in the more caudal parts of the small intestine, the colon and rectum (pp. 1767, 1782). Absorptive cells in the small and large intestines also salvage bile salts and other secreted materials, and absorb vitamins produced by the symbiotic bacteria in the colon. The large intestine is rich in mucous glands which lubricate the passage of the increasingly solidified faecal material moving through it. Finally, faeces are stored and expelled under voluntary control via the colon, rectum and anal canal, a complex system of sphincters under autonomic and somatomotor control regulating these processes (p. 1781).

Protection of the tract against infection is of course vital because its interior provides an excellent habitat for a diverse bacterial and fungal flora. Although most resident organisms are non-pathogenic if confined to the lumen, and some are important to the body because of their ability to synthesize vitamins, they may cause disease or threaten life if they pass into or through the tract wall. Such populations are normally kept at a harmless level by the secretion of bacteriostatic substances (e.g. lysozyme and lactoferrin) and antibodies (mainly IgA) from glands in its wall. The antibodies are synthesized by congregations of lymphocytes (mucosa-associated lymphoid tissue, MALT: see p. 1442) situated beneath its lining epithelium, and are passed to the epithelial glands for secretion. Other types of lymphocyte and co-operative defensive cells are also numerous within the walls and can combat infectious agents and their toxic products penetrating its lining. Lymphoid tissue is particularly well developed at a number of strategic sites: around the upper end of the pharynx (Waldeyer's ring, p. 1729), at the gastro-oesophageal junction, and in the small intestine (Peyer's patches, pp. 1450, 1771) and appendix; these masses furnish large populations of primed T and B lymphocytes which migrate to and within the surrounding regions.

Barrier functions. Although immunological defence is important, a vital feature of the tract's lining is that it forms a physical barrier to the passage of microorganisms and many potentially harmful substances. The barrier consists of the specialized epithelia lining its lumen. Where considerable abrasion may occur, in the oral cavity, pharynx, oesophagus and anal canal, the epithelia are stratified squamous in type, providing a mechanically protective layer many cells thick. Elsewhere, the epithelium is only one cell thick, but has junctional complexes with tight junctions between cells (p. 1747), preventing diffusion from the lumen into the tissues beneath. The barrier is aided by mucus overlying the epithelium, and by the rapid turnover of epithelial cells which have only a limited lifespan, ensuring that damaged, leaky cells are soon replaced from mitotic stem cells.

Vascular supply and drainage of the alimentary tract

The general pattern of vascularization has already been described in Section 3. Details of the enteric blood system are given in Section 10, and will be reviewed only briefly here. Essentially, the *arterial supply* at both ends of the tract is shared with that of the surrounding regional structures, i.e. in the head and neck, the branches of the external carotid (oral cavity, pharynx), and thyrocervical trunk (cervical oesophagus); in the thorax, it is supplied by segmental arteries from the descending aorta (thoracic oesophagus); most caudally, by branches of the internal iliac (middle rectal artery, inferior rectal branch of the internal pudendal artery) and median sacral artery, which provide blood to the lower two-thirds of the rectum and anal canal. Between these regions, i.e. in the abdomen and pelvic basin, forming the great majority of the tract, there is a very rich blood supply, as might be expected from its secretory and absorptive capabilities. Here, three major median branches from the abdominal aorta serve the three embryonic subdivisions of the gut:

- the coeliac artery to the abdominal part of the foregut (abdominal oesophagus, stomach, and the duodenum as far as the opening(s) of the bile and pancreatic duct)
- the superior mesenteric artery to the midgut (remainder of small intestine and large intestine as far as a point two-thirds along the tranverse colon)
- the inferior mesenteric artery to the hindgut (the rest of the colon and upper third of the rectum).

In the non-abdominal regions of the tract, the *venous drainage* has some similarities with the arterial supply. The alimentary tract in the head and neck are drained by tributaries of the internal jugular vein; in the thorax, the azygos, hemi- and accessory azygos veins, and most caudally, tributaries of the inferior parts of the rectum

and anal canal to the internal iliac veins (middle rectal vein; inferior rectal branch of the internal pudendal veins). The majority of the abdominal and pelvic tract has quite a different venous drainage, constituting the hepatic portal system by which nutrients absorbed by the capillary plexuses of the intestines are taken directly to the liver where the veins ramify as a second set of exchange vessels. The main collecting channels of this region are the superior and inferior mesenteric and splenic veins which conjoin as the hepatic portal vein, bifurcating as the paired hepatic veins just before entering the liver. Venous blood from the abdominal oesophagus, stomach, pancreas and gallbladder also drains into this system.

The *lymphatic drainage* of the tract follows similar rules: its parts in the head and neck drain regionally (into the internal jugular lymph trunks); the thoracic oesophagus drains via posterior mediastinal lymph nodes into the thoracic duct, bronchomediastinal trunks and right lymphatic duct (p. 1609). Within the abdomen, the intestine has a rich lymphatic drainage which forms an accessory transport system for the distribution of lipids from their sites of absorption. Lymph is conveyed from the stomach, small and large intestines along lymphatic vessels running parallel with their arteries, to the confluence of abdominal lymphatics and thence to the thoracic duct. This passes the flow of lymph through the thorax to the enter the venous system at the junctions of the left subclavian and internal jugular veins with the left brachiocephalic. Associated with this drainage system are large numbers of mesenteric and related para-aortic lymph nodes (p. 1431), an important line of defence against microorganisms which might enter the circulation by this route.

Nervous supply of the alimentary tract

Motor control of the voluntary skeletal muscles of the oral cavity and pharynx is by the segmental cranial nerves: branchiomotor to most of the musculature (trigeminal, facial, glossopharyngeal, vagal and cranial accessory), and somatomotor to the tongue (hypoglossal). Voluntary muscle of the anal canal is innervated by the somatomotor sacral branches, forming the pudendal nerve. Throughout the tract smooth muscle is regulated by a combination of autonomic efferents:

- parasympathetic via the splanchnic branch of the vagus nerve (all parts of the fore- and mid-gut below the pharynx) and pelvic splanchnic nerves (hindgut)
- sympathetic through the segmental outflow of the thoracolumbar spinal cord (p. 1303) distributed via the sympathetic trunks.

These autonomic inputs are co-ordinated and effected by the enteric nervous system within the wall of the tract (see above, and p. 1749) and receive reflex-mediating afferent branches from the visceral sensory nerves.

The glands of the oral cavity and pharynx are controlled by autonomic nerves, the parasympathetic innervation arising from three cranial nerves: the facial via the pterygopalatine ganglion (all minor glands of the palate) and submandibular ganglion (submandibular and sublingual salivary glands; lingual and buccal glands; possibly a component also to the parotid gland, see p. 1691); the glossopharyngeal via the otic ganglion (mainly the parotid gland); and the vagus (oropharynx, laryngopharynx, pharyngotympanic tube).

The sensory supply of the oral cavity and pharynx comes from general visceral components of cranial nerves V, VII, IX and X; these include chemosensory fibres to the mucosal taste buds of the oral cavity and pharynx, and general sensation to the mucosa. Caudally, the most inferior part of the anal canal is supplied by the sensory nerves of the surrounding structures, that is by the inferior rectal branch of the pudendal nerve, of segmental sacral origin. For the large part of the tract, visceral sensory nerves, chiefly of local segmental origin running with autonomic efferent fibres, monitor the state of the tract, its motility and its mechanical and chemical stresses, perceived consciously mainly as pain, fullness or emptiness, rather imprecisely localized but referred to the particular body segments served by its spinal nerves.

Evolutionary development of the tract

The course of evolution in the alimentary tract can be traced tentatively from comparative vertebrate anatomy and the fossil record. Such studies indicate a common pattern achieved early in the chordate lineage, and which is still clearly visible in the embryonic development of the human tract and to some extent expressed in its pattern of blood supply and innervation. Throughout chordate evolution the anterior part of the alimentary tract has been associated with the respiratory system (see p. 1628); in the primary aquatic era the two functions appear to have been intimately connected, as they are in extant representatives such as larval lampreys (e.g. *Lampetra*). In such primitive forms, dissolved oxygen and suspended particulate matter are obtained by filtration from the same stream of water, entering through a single opening, the mouth, and sieved through clefts in the walls of the pharynx between branchial arches, the filtered food being passed to a gastrointestinal tract for digestion and absorption. This filter-feeding phase was probably soon superseded by more complex forms of feeding, associated with specialized jaws, teeth and cranial muscles, and the filtering arches were converted into jaws and gills; in such forms, e.g. all modern fishes, the respiratory stream still shares the mouth and pharynx with food. In tetrapods these functions became partially separated with the development of lungs which replaced gills as the major respiratory surfaces, and the system of branchial arches and clefts was converted into a complete buccopharyngeal wall, although the cleft and arch arrangement is still transiently visible in human embryonic development, and its segmental pattern is reflected in the distribution of a number of cranial nerves. The pharyngotympanic tube and middle ear cavity are also relics of a cleft, converted to auditory rather than respiratory purposes in all tetrapods.

In reptiles the separation of the buccal cavity by a partial transverse secondary palatal shelf into a respiratory (nasal) chamber and a true oral cavity allowed a more effective division of the respiratory and alimentary tracts, taken to extremes in the Crocodilia in which the extensive bony secondary palate and a raised larynx allow complete separation of breathing and feeding. A definitive division was achieved in mammals by the growth of horizontal plates from the maxilla and palatine bones to create a rigid hard palate, continuous posteriorly with a movable soft palate capable of sealing off the nasal cavity during swallowing. Some species, e.g. the dog, can elevate the laryngeal opening into the nasopharynx whilst feeding, and this also occurs to some extent during suckling in human infants. In the Cetacea (whales) the position is more extreme, the larynx being permanently inserted into the nasopharynx and quite separate from the alimentary pathway.

The development of hinged jaws and of teeth greatly improved the selection, diminution and ingestion of a wide variety of foodstuffs. It is possible to trace in fossil and modern mammals the elaboration of a complex dentition, and the reduction of the mandibular bones to a single strong tooth-bearing plate articulating with the temporal bone instead of the reptilian quadrate bone, with the incorporation of the latter and some mandibular bones into the auditory apparatus of the middle ear (see p. 1370). Indeed, much of the evolution of the human skull is to be understood in this context, and it can also be speculated that the increased efficiency of food acquisition (and of digestion and assimilation) were prerequisites for many other features needing much chemical energy, for example, the high metabolic rate and homeothermy typical of mammals, and the elaboration of a large brain (neurons having a high demand for circulatory glucose which they are unable to store).

In other parts of the alimentary tract it is also possible to discern evolutionary trends. Its subdivision into an oesophagus, stomach, small and large intestines, with an attendant liver, gallbladder and pancreas appears to be a primitive chordate pattern. Superimposed on this simple arrangement are many variations, often related to specialized diets; for example, in herbivores the breakdown of cellulose requires extensive digestive and absorptive action, assisted by symbiotic organisms within the gut; the stomach is sometimes very elaborate (as in ruminants) and the intestine extensive, frequently having major diverticula. The caecum and vermiform appendix in humans appear to be relics of such a herbivorous past, although now functionless in this respect. The most caudal parts of the alimentary tract have also undergone major changes during evolutionary development. In primitive chordates, alimentary, urinary and genital systems share a common cloacal aperture to the exterior, a condition reflected in human embryonic development (p. 191). The division of the cloaca into separate anal and urinogenital regions, each with its own opening, was probably an adaptation to terrestrial life, occurring first in reptiles; failure to complete this separation during human development is seen in congenital abnormalities such as rectovaginal fistulae.

One other aspect of the alimentary tract must be remarked upon: the origin of important endocrine and defensive structures now quite separate from this structure, but owing an embryonic origin to its epithelial lining. Endocrine derivatives include the thyroid and parathyroid glands and the adenohypophysis; defensive components are the thymus and Waldeyer's ring of lymphoid tissue (p. 1729) comprising the palatine, nasopharyngeal, lingual and tubal tonsils. All of these structures arise during ontogeny from either the buccal cavity or pharynx (p. 176). Their evolutionary origins appear to be from specialized epithelia in the pharynx of lower vertebrates, migrating to a separate site and losing any direct connection to that cavity. In support of this view, among other data, the thyroid of the primitive chordate *Amphioxus* is a specialized patch of epithelial cells on the pharyngeal floor, and in some primitive bony fishes (e.g. *Erpetoichthys*) the adenohypophysis is an open diverticulum of the buccal roof. It can be speculated that the wall of the alimentary tract is an important interface with the outside world which favoured the development of specialized epithelial endocrine and immune control systems.

ORAL CAVITY AND RELATED STRUCTURES

ORAL CAVITY

The oral or buccal cavity, the 'mouth', consists of a narrow *vestibule* outside the teeth, and an inner, larger *oral cavity proper*. The vestibule is bounded externally by the lips and cheeks and internally by gums and teeth, communicating with the exterior by the oral fissure. Above and below, the vestibule is limited by the reflexion of the mucosa from the lips and cheeks on to the gums, forming a horseshoe-shaped trough (the *fornix*). When the teeth are apposed, the vestibule is continuous with the oral cavity proper behind the third molar teeth and by minute clefts between adjacent teeth. The part of the vestibule adjacent to the lips is the *labial sulcus* and the remainder, related to the cheeks, is the *buccal sulcus*. The oral cavity proper (**12**.1) is bounded at the front and laterally by the alveolar arches, teeth and gums; behind, it communicates with the pharynx at the oropharyngeal isthmus (the space between the palatoglossal folds). Its roof is formed by the hard and soft palates; its floor mainly by the anterior region of the tongue, and the remainder by the mucosa lying on mylohyoid anteriorly and laterally between the base of the tongue and the internal surface of the mandible, on to which it is reflected. The inferior surface of the tongue is connected to the floor of the mouth anteriorly by the lingual frenulum, a crescentic median mucosal fold reinforced by connective tissue. On each side of the lower edge of the frenulum, anteriorly, a small sublingual papilla bears the orifice of the duct of the submandibular salivary gland. From this papilla a ridge extends posterolaterally in the floor, produced by the subjacent sublingual salivary gland and hence termed the sublingual fold. Minute openings of the sublingual gland ducts appear on the edge of the fold.

ORAL MUCOSA

The oral mucosa is continuous with the skin at the labial margins and with the pharyngeal mucosa at the oropharyngeal isthmus. It varies in structure, function and appearance in different regions of the oral cavity and is traditionally divided into three major types:

the lining, masticatory and specialized mucosae. The *lining mucosa*, red in colour, covers the soft palate, ventral surface of the tongue, floor of the mouth, alveolar processes excluding the gingivae and the internal surfaces of the lips and cheeks. It has a non-keratinized epithelium overlying a loosely fibrous lamina propria, and the submucosa contains some fat deposits and collections of minor mucous glands. The *masticatory mucosa*, roseate-pink, covers the hard palate and gingivae; it is normally orthokeratinized. A submucosa is absent from the gingivae and the midline palatine raphe, but is present over the rest of the hard palate; it is thick posterolaterally where it contains mucous salivary glands, and also the greater palatine nerves and vessels. The masticatory mucosa is bound firmly to underlying bone or to the necks of the teeth, forming in the gingivae and palatine raphe a *mucoperiosteum*. Where a substantial thickness of submucosa exists in the palate, longitudinal collagenous septa orientated anteroposteriorly anchor the mucosa to the periosteum of the maxillae and palatine bones. The third type of mucosa is the *specialized mucosa* covering the anterior two-thirds of the tongue's dorsum: its surface is orthokeratinized and bears the four types of lingual papillae (p. 1724), all of them carrying taste buds except for the filiform papillae. The richly collagenous lamina propria binds the mucosa of the tongue to the underlying muscles.

The surface of the oral mucosa can have various histological characteristics: it may be orthokeratinized, parakeratinized, or non-keratinized, depending upon its location. These designations are based primarily on the appearance of the epithelium in histological sections, a rather crude reflection of more subtle differences detectable with immunohistological and molecular techniques.

Orthokeratinized epithelium (often referred to as 'keratinized', see p. 71) resembles the epidermis of skin, its most superficial layer consisting of flattened, anucleate epithelial cells which are bright pink in sections stained with haematoxylin and eosin because of the strongly eosinophilic nature of the keratin within them; these superficial squames are sharply demarcated from the underlying granular layer rich in basophilic keratohyalin granules.

Parakeratinized epithelium also has a superficial keratinized layer which is likewise eosinophilic but retains many shrunken nuclei within its flattened cells. Furthermore, the underlying granular layer is usually less distinct than in orthokeratinized epithelium. Occasionally the orthokeratin on the surface of healthy gingivae is replaced by parakeratin. This is assumed to occur when mild inflammation increases the rate of transit of epithelial cells from the basal layer to the surface, thereby compromising their complete differentiation.

Non-keratinized epithelium lacks an eosinophilic surface layer, and its cells all contain well-defined nuclei. Together with the absence of a subjacent granular layer, this means that there is no clear stratification in the superficial region of non-keratinized epithelium (see also p. 72).

LIPS

The lips are two fleshy folds surrounding the oral orifice (**12**.1). They are lined externally by skin and internally by mucosa, these two layers enclosing the orbicularis oris, labial vessels and nerves, fibroadipose connective tissue and numerous small labial salivary glands secreting into the vestibule. The skin is continuous with the mucosa

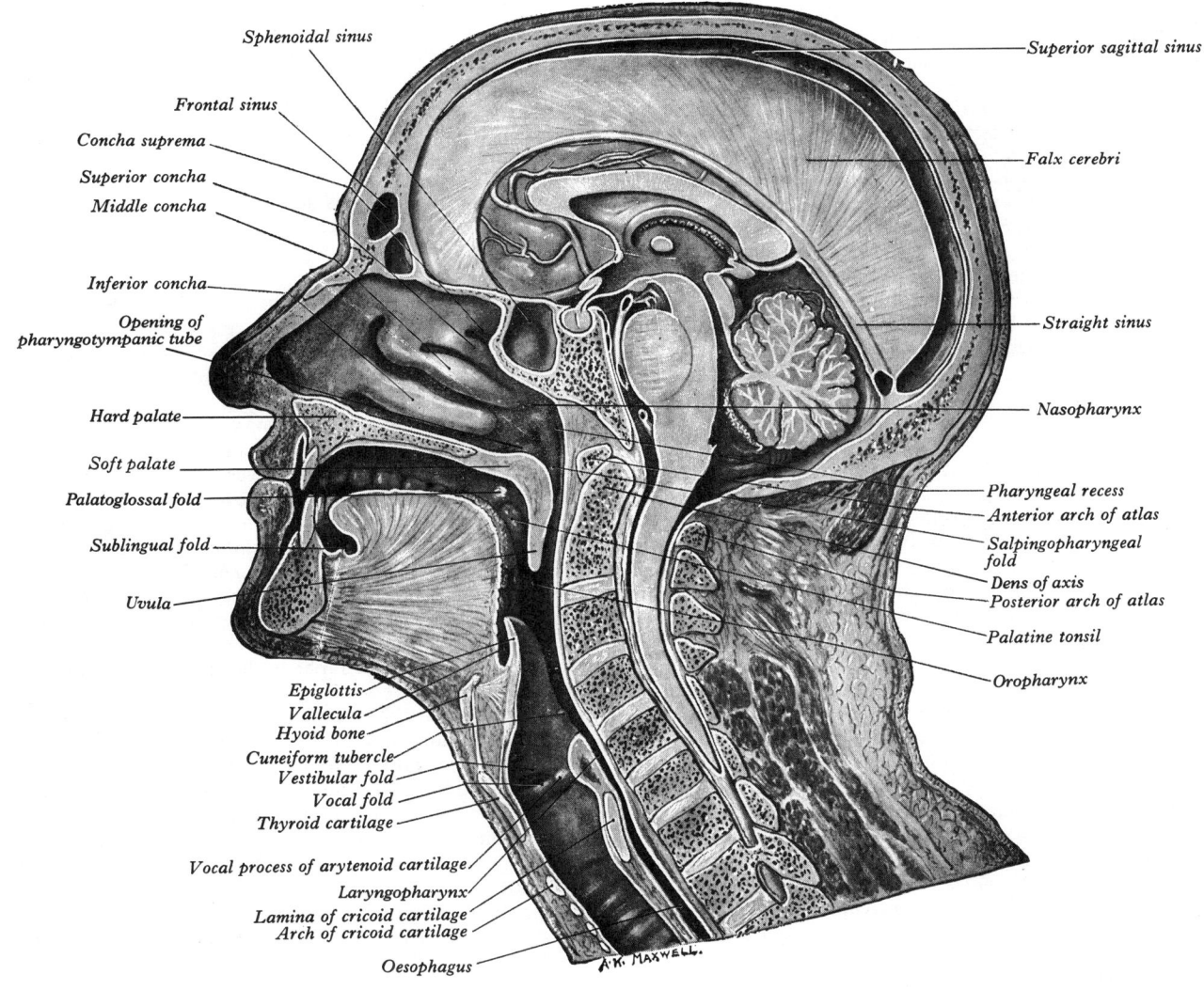

Sphenoidal sinus
Frontal sinus
Concha suprema
Superior concha
Middle concha
Inferior concha
Opening of pharyngotympanic tube
Hard palate
Soft palate
Palatoglossal fold
Sublingual fold
Uvula
Epiglottis
Vallecula
Hyoid bone
Cuneiform tubercle
Vestibular fold
Vocal fold
Thyroid cartilage
Vocal process of arytenoid cartilage
Laryngopharynx
Lamina of cricoid cartilage
Arch of cricoid cartilage
Oesophagus

Superior sagittal sinus
Falx cerebri
Straight sinus
Nasopharynx
Pharyngeal recess
Anterior arch of atlas
Salpingopharyngeal fold
Dens of axis
Posterior arch of atlas
Palatine tonsil
Oropharynx

A.K. MAXWELL.

12.1 Median sagittal section through the head and neck. Where it passes through the brain, the section passes slightly to the left of the median plane but, below the base of the skull including the nasal cavity, it passes slightly to the right of the median plane.

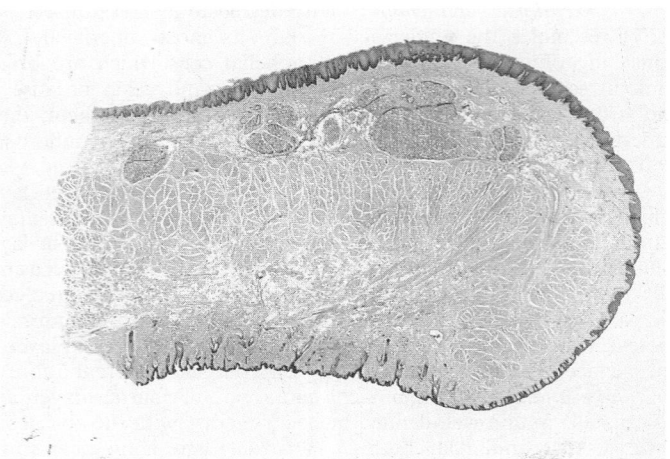

12.2 Sagittal section through the lower lip of a neonate, showing thin non-hairy skin of the vermilion border (above) grading into thicker stratified squamous epithelium of the vestibule, with mucosal labial glands (right). Small fasciculi of circumoral muscles are also visible. Haematoxylin and eosin. (Provided by A Hayward; photography: Sarah Smith.)

at the *transitional* or *vermilion border*, a reddish zone (depending upon the degree of melanization) covered by thin keratinized epithelium with connective tissue papillae approaching close to the surface between rete pegs (**12**.2). The colour of this region is due to the proximity of blood vessels to the epithelial surface. The transitional zone is devoid of salivary glands but in the upper lip, and rarely in the lower, it often contains sebaceous glands. The line of contact between the lips (the *oral fissure*) lies just above the cutting edges of the superior incisor teeth; on each side a *labial commissure* forms the *angle of the mouth*, usually near the first premolar tooth. Externally central in the upper lip is a shallow vertical groove, the *philtrum*, ending below in a slight *tubercle* and limited by lateral ridges. Internally each lip is connected to the gum by a *median labial frenulum*, that of the upper lip being the larger. Lateral frenula, of variable number and height, cross the fornix of the vestibule in the region of the canine or premolar teeth. The *labial glands*, situated between the mucosa and orbicularis oris, are about the size of small peas and in structure resemble mucous salivary glands elsewhere (p. 1691).

CHEEKS

The cheeks are continuous in front with the lips, the junction being indicated externally by the *nasolabial sulcus* and lateral to it the *nasolabial fold*, which descends from the side of the nose to each oral angle. Each cheek contains a stratum of skeletal muscle and a variable but usually considerable amount of adipose tissue often encapsulated to form a biconcave mass, the *buccal fat pad* (of Bichat), particularly evident in infants. Also present in the walls of the cheek are fibrous connective tissue, vessels, nerves and numerous small buccal mucous (salivary) glands. The cheek is covered on the inner surface by mucosa, and on the outer surface by skin. The mucosa lining the interior of the cheek is reflected via the vestibule on to the external surfaces of the maxilla and mandible and thence to the gums; it is continuous behind with the palatal mucosa. On the cheek's internal surface, opposite the crown of the second molar, a small papilla bears the opening of the parotid duct which reaches this point by piercing the buccinator muscle. The small *buccal mucous glands* lie mainly between the mucosa and buccinator; four or five of the largest of these glands (*molar glands*) lie external to buccinator around the parotid duct, their ducts piercing buccinator to open near the last molar tooth. Sebaceous glands also occur in the buccal mucosa, often in large numbers, and can be seen as yellowish maculae (*Fordyce spots*), especially if the cheek is stretched; their numbers increase at puberty and during later life (Miles 1958). The principal muscle of the cheek is buccinator, but others are also involved, e.g. zygomaticus major, risorius and platysma (see p. 796).

GUMS (GINGIVAE)

The gums are composed of dense, vascular fibrous tissue, and are normally covered by orthokeratinized stratified squamous epithelium. They are firmly attached to the cement at the necks of the teeth and to the bone of the adjacent alveolar process (**12**.4). The anchoring collagen fibres produce small depressions in the mucosal surface, giving it a stippled appearance. The part of the gum associated with the necks of the teeth (*marginal gingiva*) is not stippled; in young individuals it is partly attached to the enamel via a basal lamina produced by the epithelial cells. The extreme edge of the marginal gingiva is not attached to the enamel but forms the outer lining of a normally shallow gingival crevice around each tooth (see p. 1712). In older individuals the epithelial attachment often migrates on to the cement. The gingival epithelium, like that of the skin, contains melanocytes in its basal layer but these produce melanosomes (and therefore pigmentation) only in the more pigmented races. Langerhans cells, the most peripheral outpost of the immune system (p. 392), occur in the more superficial layers of the mucosal epithelium. The incidence of these last two types of cell has been assessed (Barker 1967).

Nerves of the gums. They come from the maxillary nerve via its greater palatine, nasopalatine and anterior, middle and posterior superior alveolar branches. The mandibular nerve innervates the lower gum by its inferior alveolar, lingual and buccal branches; the buccal branch supplies the external surface of the lower gum as far forward as the mental foramen. The lingual nerve can be palpated where it lies against the alveolar process of the mandible close to its upper margin at the inner aspect of the lower third molar tooth, and here the nerve is at risk during the surgical removal of the tooth.

Vessels in the gums. These usually accompany the nerves. Lymphatics of the upper gum drain to the submandibular nodes; those from the anterior part of the lower gum pass to the submental nodes and from its posterior part to the submandibular nodes.

For a detailed study of the oral cavity, consult DuBrul 1988.

PALATE

The palate, or oral roof, is divisible into two regions: the *hard palate* in front and *soft palate* behind.

Hard palate

The hard palate is formed by the palatine processes of the maxillae and the horizontal plates of the palatine bones (**12**.1, 24). It is bounded in front and at the sides by the superior and inferior arches of the alveolar processes and gums, and is continuous posteriorly with the soft palate. The hard palate is covered by a thick mucosa bound tightly to the underlying periosteum, its more lateral regions also possessing a submucosa containing mucous glands and (anteriorly) adipose tissue. Its covering of stratified squamous epithelium is orthokeratinized, but shows regional variations.

The periphery of the hard palate consists of gingiva, and a zone similarly lacking submucosa runs anteroposteriorly in the midline as a narrow, low ridge, the *palatine raphe*. At the anterior extremity of the raphe an oval prominence, the *incisive papilla*, covers the incisive fossa at the oral opening of the incisive canal (p. 602), also marking the position of the fetal nasopalatine canal (p. 280). Radiating outwards from the palatine raphe in the anterior half of the hard palate are irregular transverse ridges or *rugae*, each containing a core of dense connective tissue. In long-jawed mammals, prominent rugae occur throughout the hard palate and are believed to assist the backwards transport of food during mastication. This function is less important in the human, although the rugae may still have a role in suckling by infants. Their vestigial nature is associated with a considerable variation in form; indeed, each individual may have a virtually unique pattern of rugae, a point of forensic interest.

The submucosa beneath the rugae contains adipose tissue but in the posterior half of the hard palate there are small *mucous palatine salivary glands*. These secrete through numerous small ducts, although bilaterally a larger duct collecting from many of these glands often opens at the paired *palatine foveae*, two sagittally elongated depressions, sometimes a few millimetres deep, which flank the midline raphe at the posterior border of the hard palate. The upper surface of the hard palate is the floor of the nasal cavity and is covered by ciliated respiratory epithelium.

Soft palate

The soft palate is a mobile flap suspended from the posterior border of the hard palate, sloping down and back between the oral and nasal parts of the pharynx (**12**.1). It is a thick fold of mucosa enclosing an aponeurosis, muscular tissue, vessels, nerves, lymphoid tissue and mucous glands. In its usual position, relaxed and pendant, its anterior (oral) surface is concave, with a median raphe; its posterior aspect is convex and continuous with the nasal floor. Its anterosuperior border is attached to the hard palate's posterior margin, its sides blend with the pharyngeal wall and its inferior border is free, hanging between the mouth and pharynx.

A median conical process, the *uvula*, projects downwards from its posterior border; the palatal arches, two curved folds of mucosa containing muscle, descend laterally from each side of the soft palate (**12**.54, 56). The anterior of these, the *palatoglossal arch*, contains the palatoglossus muscle and descends to the side of the tongue at the junction of its oral and pharyngeal parts, forming the lateral limits of the oropharyngeal isthmus. The posterior *palatopharyngeal arch* contains the palatopharyngeus muscle, and descends on the lateral wall of the oropharynx (p. 1728). The *isthmus of the fauces* is the aperture between the oral cavity and oropharynx guarded on either side by the palatoglossal folds.

Just behind and medial to each upper alveolar process, in the lateral region of the anterior part of the soft palate, a small bony prominence can be felt. This is produced by the pterygoid hamulus, an extension of the medial pterygoid plate (p. 566). The ptery-gomandibular raphe (p. 816), a tendinous band interposed between buccinator and the superior constrictor muscle, passes downwards and outwards from the hamulus to the posterior end of the mylohyoid line. When the mouth is opened wide, this raphe elevates a fold of mucosa which marks internally the posterior boundary of the cheek.

The oral surface of the soft palate is covered with non-keratinized, stratified squamous epithelium. On its upper nasopharyngeal surface and near the orifices of the auditory tubes it is lined by pseudo-stratified ciliated ('respiratory') epithelium. Deep to the mucosa on both surfaces are palatine mucous glands; they are most abundant around the uvula and on the oral aspect of the soft palate, where taste buds also occur.

Vessels

The arteries of the palate are the greater palatine branch of the maxillary artery, the ascending palatine branch of the facial artery and the palatine branch of the ascending pharyngeal artery. The veins drain largely to the pterygoid and tonsillar plexuses. The lymph vessels pass to the deep cervical lymph nodes.

Nerves

The *sensory nerves* issue from the greater and lesser palatine, and nasopalatine branches of the maxillary nerve, and also the glos-sopharyngeal nerve (posteriorly). The lesser palatine nerve also contains taste fibres of facial nerve (greater petrosal) origin supplying taste buds in the oral surface of the soft palate. *Parasympathetic postganglionic secretomotor* fibres arising from the facial nerve via the pterygopalatine ganglion run with these nerves to the palatine mucous glands; it is also possible that some parasympathetic fibres pass to the posterior parts of the soft palate from the glos-sopharyngeal nerve, perhaps synapsing in the otic ganglion. *Sym-pathetic fibres* run from the carotid plexus along arterial branches supplying this region.

Palatine aponeurosis

A thin, fibrous *palatine aponeurosis* supports the muscles and streng-thens the soft palate; it is attached to the posterior border and inferior surface of the hard palate behind the palatine crest (p. 563). It is thick in the anterior two-thirds of the soft palate but very thin further back. It is composed of the expanded tendons of the tensores veli palatini; near the midline it encloses the musculus uvulae. All the other palatine muscles are attached to it. The anterior third of the soft palate contains little muscle, consisting mainly of the palatine aponeurosis, inferior to which are many mucous glands; this region

is less mobile and more horizontal than the rest of the soft palate and is the chief area acted upon by the tensores veli palatini.

Palatine musculature

The palatine muscles (**12**.3, 61, 67–69) include levator veli palatini, tensor veli palatini, palatoglossus, palatopharyngeus and musculus uvulae. For their activities in swallowing and speech see page 1732. Their nerve supply is summarized on page 1691.

Levator veli palatini (**12**.3, 61, 67–69). This muscle is cylindrical and lies lateral to the posterior nasal aperture. According to Rohan & Turner (1956) it is attached:

- by a small tendon to a rough area on the inferior surface of the petrous temporal bone in front of the lower opening of the carotid canal
- by muscle fibres to a sheet of fascia descending from the vaginal process of the tympanic bone to form the upper part of the carotid sheath
- by a few fibres to the inferior aspect of the cartilaginous part of the pharyngotympanic tube.

At its origin the muscle is inferior rather than medial to the pharyngotympanic tube and only crosses medial to it at the level of the medial pterygoid plate. Passing medial to the upper margin of the superior constrictor and in front of salpingopharyngeus, its fibres spread in the medial third of the soft palate between the two strands of the palatopharyngeus, its fibres being attached to the upper surface of the palatine aponeurosis as far as the midline where they interlace with those of the contralateral muscle. Thus the two levator muscles form a sling above and just behind the palatine aponeurosis.

Actions. The primary role of the levator veli palatini is to elevate the almost vertical posterior part of the soft palate and pull it slightly backwards. During swallowing, the soft palate is at the same time made rigid by the contraction of the tensores veli palatini and touches the posterior wall of the pharynx, thus separating the

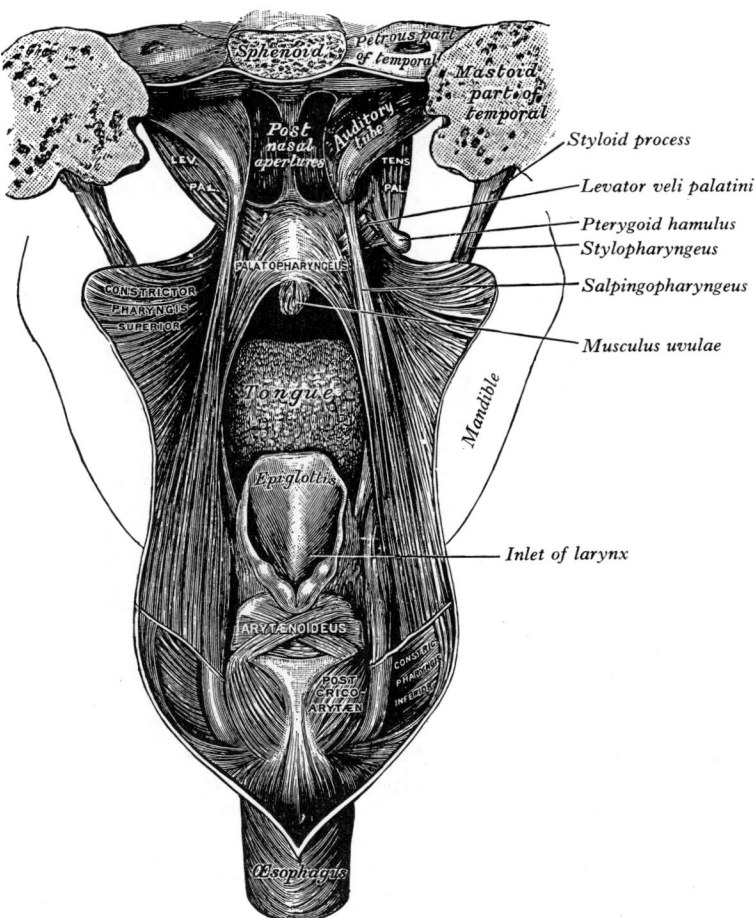

12.3　The muscles of the palate, exposed from the posterior aspect.

nasopharynx from the oropharynx. By additionally pulling on the lateral walls of the nasopharynx posteriorly and medially, the muscles also narrow that space (Honjo et al 1976). The levator veli palatini has little or no effect on the pharyngotympanic tube.

Tensor veli palatini (**12**.3, 61, 67–69). This is a thin, triangular muscle, lateral to the medial pterygoid plate, pharyngotympanic tube and levator veli palatini. Its lateral surface contacts the upper and anterior part of the medial pterygoid muscle, the mandibular, auriculotemporal and chorda tympani nerves, the otic ganglion and the middle meningeal artery. It is attached to the scaphoid fossa of the pterygoid process and posteriorly to the medial aspect of the spine of the sphenoid; between these two sites it is attached to the anterolateral membranous wall of the pharyngotympanic tube, including its narrow isthmus where the cartilaginous medial two-thirds meets the bony lateral one-third. Some fibres may be continuous with the tensor tympani muscle (Rood & Doyle 1978). Inferiorly, the fibres converge on a delicate tendon which turns medially around the pterygoid hamulus to pass through the attachment of buccinator to the palatine aponeurosis and the osseous surface behind the palatine crest on the horizontal plate of the palatine bone. Between the tendon and the pterygoid hamulus is a small bursa.

Actions. Acting together the tensores tauten the soft palate, principally its anterior part, depressing it by flattening its arch. Alone, the muscle pulls the soft palate to one side. Although contraction of the tensores will slightly depress the anterior part of the soft palate, it is often assumed that the increased rigidity aids palatopharyngeal closure. However, it is now believed that the primary role of the tensor is to open the pharyngotympanic tube, for example during deglutition and yawning, thereby equalizing air pressure with the middle ear and nasopharynx (Maue-Dickson & Dickson 1980).

Musculus uvulae. A bilateral structure, this arises from the posterior nasal spine of the palatine bone and the dorsal surface of the palatine aponeurosis, between the two laminae of which the uvular muscles lie; it runs posteriorly above the levator sling to insert beneath the mucosa of the uvula. A paired structure at its anterior and posterior attachments, for most of its length the two sides are united.

Actions. Elevation and retraction of the uvula; by retracting the uvular mass and thickening the middle third of the soft palate, it aids the levatores in palatopharyngeal closure. Running at right angles to each other, contraction of the levatores and musculi uvuli raises a 'levator eminence' which seals off the nasopharynx 'like a cork in a bottle' (DuBrul 1988).

Palatoglossus (**12**.67). This is a small fasciculus narrower at its middle than at its ends and forming, with the mucosa overlying it, the palatoglossal arch or fold (**12**.4, 56, 67). It arises from the oral surface of the palatine aponeurosis about half-way along the soft palate where it is continuous with its fellow and extends forwards, downwards and laterally in front of the palatine tonsil to the side of the tongue; some of its fibres spread over the dorsum of the tongue, others passing deeply into its substance to intermingle with the transversus linguae.

Actions. Palatoglossus elevates the root of the tongue and approximates the palatoglossal arch to its fellow, thus shutting off the oral cavity from the oropharynx.

Palatopharyngeus (**12**.3, 67). This forms, with its overlying mucosa, the palatopharyngeal arch (**12**.55). Within the soft palate it is composed of two fasciculi which are attached to the upper surface of the palatine aponeurosis in the same plane but separated from each other by levator veli palatini. The thicker anterior fasciculus is attached to the posterior border of the hard palate as well as to the aponeurosis where some fibres interdigitate across the midline. The posterior fasciculus is in contact with the mucosa of the pharyngeal aspect of the palate; it joins the posterior band of the opposite muscle in the midline. At the soft palate's posterolateral border the two layers unite and are joined by fibres of salpingopharyngeus (p. 1727). Passing laterally and downwards behind the tonsil, palatopharyngeus descends posteromedial to and in close contact with stylopharyngeus, to be attached with it to the posterior border of the thyroid cartilage; some fibres end on the side of the pharynx, attached to pharyngeal fibrous tissue and others cross the midline posteriorly, decussating with those of the opposite muscle. The palatopharyngeus thus forms an incomplete internal longitudinal muscular layer in the wall of the pharynx.

Actions. Together, the palatopharyngei pull the pharynx up, forwards and medially, thus shortening it during swallowing. They also approximate the palatopharyngeal arches and draw them forwards.

Summary of soft palate muscle attachments

In the soft palate the muscles are arranged as follows: the palatine aponeurosis (tendon of the tensores veli palatini) is an intermediate

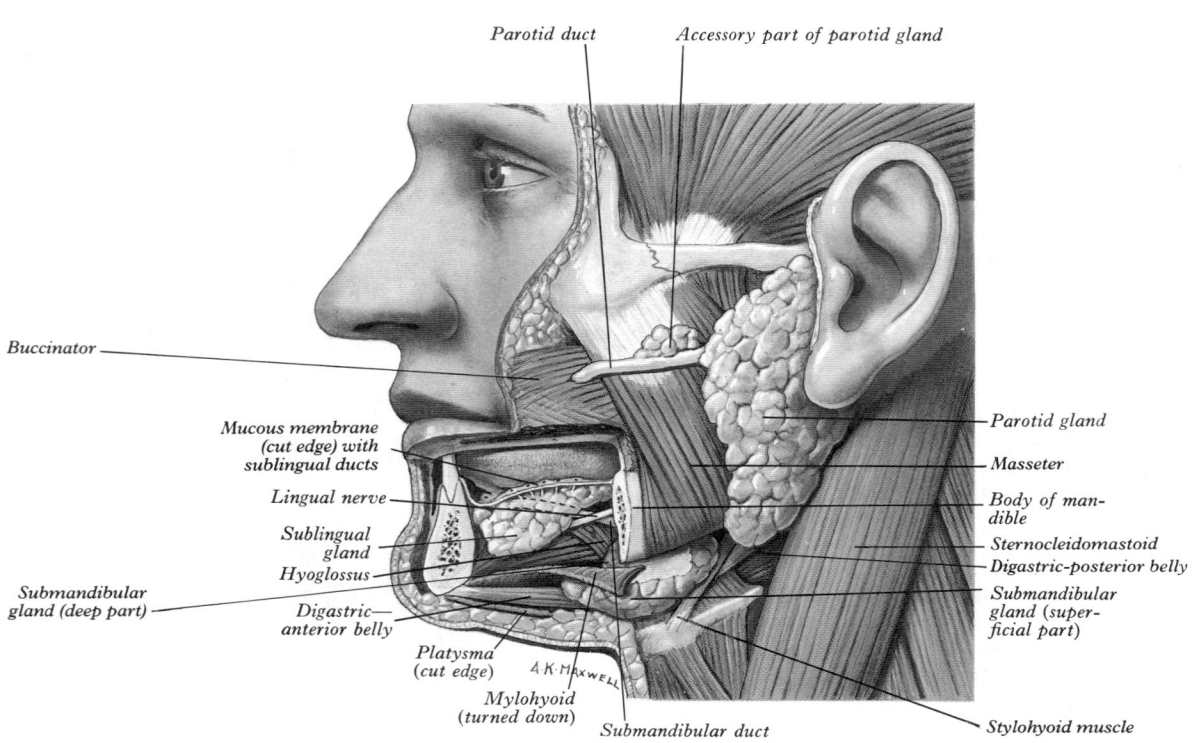

Parotid duct

Accessory part of parotid gland

Buccinator

Mucous membrane (cut edge) with sublingual ducts

Lingual nerve

Sublingual gland

Hyoglossus

Submandibular gland (deep part)

Digastric—anterior belly

Platysma (cut edge)

A.K. MAXWELL

Mylohyoid (turned down)

Submandibular duct

Parotid gland

Masseter

Body of mandible

Sternocleidomastoid

Digastric-posterior belly

Submandibular gland (superficial part)

Stylohyoid muscle

12.4 Dissection showing the salivary glands of the left side. The cranial region of the superficial part of the submandibular gland has been excised and the cut mylohyoid has been turned down to expose a portion of the deep part of the gland.

sheet, enclosing the uvular muscles near the midline; the levatores veli palatini and the palatopharyngi are attached to its upper surface, the two fasciculi of the latter lying in the same plane, one in front of and the other behind levator veli palatini. The palatoglossi are inserted into the inferior surface of the aponeurosis. (For a description of the palatopharyngeal sphincter, see p. 1730.)

Nerve supply of palatine muscles

Except for tensor veli palatini, which is innervated by the mandibular nerve (p. 1237), all the palatine muscles are supplied by nerve fibres which leave the medulla in the cranial part of the accessory nerve and reach the pharyngeal plexus via the vagus nerve and possibly the glossopharyngeal. More controversially, several investigators have suggested that levator veli palatini is also supplied by the facial nerve. Ibuki et al (1978) report electromyographic evidence that in monkeys this motor route involves the greater petrosal nerve, pterygopalatine ganglion and lesser palatine nerves. In contrast, Keller at al (1984), using retrograde axonal transport in cats, found levator veli palatini motor neurons in the nucleus ambiguus but not in the facial nucleus. These authors also confirmed that tensor veli palatini motor neurons are situated in the trigeminal motor nucleus.

Defects of the palate

The condition of congenital cleft palate has been noted already as a developmental defect (p. 284). Rarely, palatopharyngeal incompetence may be due to muscle hypoplasia, particularly of the musculus uvulae; submucous clefts resulting from this may be revealed clinically as a V-shaped notch in the midline of the soft palate during function. Paralysis of the soft palate may follow diphtheria due to the action of the toxin on the nerve cells of the medulla oblongata; in this state, the voice becomes nasal and fluids regurgitate into the nose during swallowing; the palate is visibly flaccid and motionless and also anaesthetic. Other pathological processes involving the glossopharyngeal, vagus and accessory nerves or their nuclei in the medulla oblongata also cause palatal paralysis.

SALIVARY GLANDS

A salivary gland is any cell or organ discharging a secretion into the oral cavity. Distinction is customarily made between the *major salivary glands*, located at some distance from the oral mucosa, with which they connect by extraglandular ducts, and the *minor salivary glands* which lie in the mucosa or submucosa, opening directly through the mucosa or indirectly via many short ducts. In humans the major salivary glands comprise the paired parotid, submandibular and sublingual glands; the minor salivary group includes those in the tongue, the anterior lingual glands and numerous small lingual (including von Ebner's) glands of the lingual mucosa (see p. 1724). Elsewhere in the oral cavity are the small labial, buccal and palatal glands (p. 1688). Their functions include: lubrication of food to assist deglutition, moistening the buccal mucosa (important for speech), provision of an aqueous solvent necessary for taste and as a fluid seal for sucking and suckling, secretion of digestive enzymes such as salivary amylase and of hormones and other compounds, such as a glucagon-like protein (Lawrence et al 1977) and possibly serotonin (Feyrter 1961), and secretion of antimicrobial agents (including IgA, lysozyme and lactoferrin). An illustration of the position of the major salivary glands and their ducts is shown in **12**.4.

PAROTID GLANDS

The paired parotid glands (**12**.4–8) are the largest of the salivary glands; each has an average weight of about 25 g and is an irregular, lobulated, yellowish mass, lying largely below the external acoustic meatus between the mandible and sternocleidomastoid. The gland also projects forwards on the surface of the masseter, where a small, usually detached part lies between the zygomatic arch above and the parotid duct below, the *pars accessoria* or *socia parotidis*. The parotid consists almost entirely of serous glandular tissue (see p. 74).

The *capsule* of the gland is derived from the deep cervical fascia; its superficial layer is dense, closely adherent and sends fibrous septa into the gland, it is attached to the zygomatic arch. Medial to the gland it is firmly attached to the styloid process, mandible and tympanic plate, blending with the fibrous sheaths of related muscles. The fascia extending from the styloid process to the mandibular angle forms the stylomandibular ligament, which intervenes between the parotid and submandibular glands. The parotid gland is like an inverted, flat, three-sided pyramid, presenting a small superior surface, and superficial, anteromedial and posteromedial surfaces; it tapers inferiorly to a blunt apex.

The concave *superior surface* is related to the cartilaginous part of the external acoustic meatus and posterior aspect of the temporomandibular joint; here the auriculotemporal nerve curves round the neck of the mandible, embedded in the gland's capsule. The *apex* overlaps the posterior belly of the digastric and the carotid triangle to a variable extent.

The *superficial surface* is covered by skin and superficial fascia, which contains the facial branches of the great auricular nerve, superficial parotid lymph nodes and the posterior border of platysma. It extends upwards to the zygomatic arch, back to overlap the sternocleidomastoid, down to its apex postero-inferior to the mandibular angle and forwards superficial to the masseter below the parotid duct (**12**.4, 7).

The *anteromedial surface* is grooved by the posterior border of the mandibular ramus. It covers the postero-inferior part of the masseter, the lateral aspect of the temporomandibular joint and the adjoining part of the mandibular ramus, passing forwards medial to the ramus to reach the medial pterygoid. Branches of the facial nerve emerge on the face from the anterior margin of this surface.

The *posteromedial surface* is moulded to the mastoid process, sternocleidomastoid, posterior belly of the digastric and the styloid process and its muscles. The external carotid artery grooves this surface before entering the gland. The internal carotid artery and internal jugular vein are separated from the gland by the styloid process and its muscles (**12**.7). The anteromedial and posteromedial surfaces meet at a medial margin which may project so deeply as to be in contact with the lateral wall of the pharynx.

Several structures traverse the gland partly or wholly and even branch within it. The external carotid artery enters the posteromedial surface, dividing into the maxillary artery, which emerges from the anteromedial surface, and the superficial temporal artery which gives off its transverse facial branch in the gland and ascends to leave its upper limit (**12**.6, 7). The posterior auricular artery may also branch from the external carotid within the gland, leaving by its posteromedial surface. The retromandibular vein (p. 1578), formed by the union of the maxillary and superficial temporal veins (which enter near the points of exit of the corresponding arteries), is superficial to the external carotid artery and emerges behind the gland's apex to join the posterior auricular vein, forming the external jugular; it has a communicating branch which leaves anterior to the apex to join the facial vein. Most superficial is the facial nerve, entering high on the posteromedial surface (**12**.7) and passing forwards and down behind the mandibular ramus in two main divisions, from which its terminal branches diverge to leave by the anteromedial surface, passing medial to its anterior margin.*

The parotid gland develops as an outgrowth from the buccal cavity (p. 175), spreading back towards the ear and covering the facial nerve; prolongations of the gland penetrate medially between the branches of the nerve to form its deeper part, the largest part being between the nerve's main temporal and cervical divisions (Bailey 1947, McKenzie 1948). These processes finally engulf the nerve and its branches, which are sometimes considered to divide the gland into a superficial and a deep lobe.

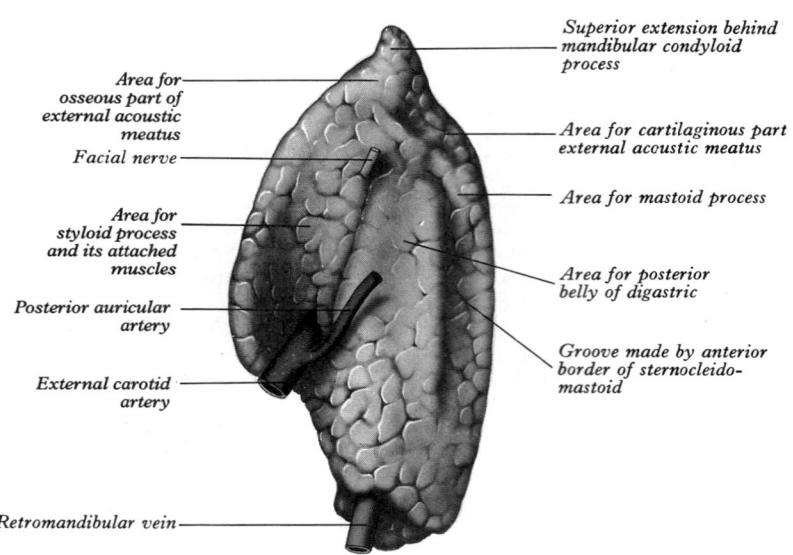

Superior extension behind mandibular condyloid process

Area for osseous part of external acoustic meatus

Facial nerve

Area for cartilaginous part of external acoustic meatus

Area for styloid process and its attached muscles

Area for mastoid process

Posterior auricular artery

Area for posterior belly of digastric

External carotid artery

Groove made by anterior border of sternocleido-mastoid

Retromandibular vein

12.5   The right parotid gland: posteromedial aspect.

Parotid duct (12.4, 16A).

About 5 cm long, this begins by the confluence of two main tributaries within the anterior part of the gland (p. 1699), then crosses the masseter and at its anterior border turns medially at almost a right angle, traversing the corpus adiposum (suctorial pad of infants) and the buccinator. It then runs obliquely forwards for a short distance between the buccinator and the oral mucosa to open upon a small papilla opposite the second upper molar crown. While crossing the masseter it receives the accessory parotid duct and here lies between the upper and lower buccal branches of the facial nerve; the accessory part of the gland and the transverse facial artery are above it. The buccal branch of the mandibular nerve, emerging from beneath the temporalis and masseter, is just below the duct at the masseter's anterior border.

The wall of the parotid duct is thick, with an external fibrous layer containing smooth muscle and a mucosa lined by low columnar epithelium (see below). Its calibre is about 3 mm, although smaller at its oral orifice.

Surface anatomy

The parotid duct can be felt on the face or more easily in the vestibule of the mouth, and rolled on the anterior border of the masseter, by pressing the finger **backwards** on it (with teeth clenched

to make the muscle tense). The anterior border of the parotid gland is represented by a line descending from the mandibular condyle to a point just above the middle of the masseter and then to a point about 2 cm below and behind the mandibular angle. Its concave upper border corresponds to a curve traced from the mandibular condyle across the ear's lobule to the mastoid process. The posterior border is indicated by a straight line drawn between the posterior ends of the anterior and upper borders. The parotid duct corresponds to the middle third of a line drawn from the lower border of the tragus to a point midway between the nasal ala and upper labial margin.

Vessels and nerves

The parotid **arterial supply** is from the external carotid and its branches within and near the gland. The **veins** drain to the external jugular, through local tributaries. The **lymph vessels** end in the superficial and deep cervical lymph nodes, interrupted by two or three nodes lying on and within the gland. The **efferent innervation** is autonomic, consisting of sympathetic fibres from the external carotid plexus and parasympathetic fibres which reach it via the tympanic branch of the glossopharyngeal nerve relaying in the otic ganglion and then travelling along the auriculotemporal nerve. Clinical observations suggest that in humans the gland also receives secretomotor fibres through the chorda tympani (Reichert & Poth 1933, Diamant & Wiberg 1965). Holmberg (1972) has shown that in **dogs** secretomotor fibres pass to the parotid gland from the maxillary plexus and the facial and auriculotemporal nerves, a supply unconfirmed in man. The termination of these supplies is still controversial. Studies in **cats** suggest that both parasympathetic and sympathetic fibres end in relation to glandular cells (Génis-Gálvez et al 1966, and see below).

SUBMANDIBULAR GLANDS

The paired submandibular glands (**10.**81, **12.**4, 7) are irregular in shape and about the size of walnuts. Each consists of a large superficial and a smaller deep part, continuous with each other around the posterior border of the mylohyoid. They are seromucous (but predominantly serous) glands.

The *superficial part*, situated in the digastric triangle, reaches forward to the anterior belly of the digastric and back to the stylomandibular ligament, which separates it from the parotid gland. Above, it extends medial to the mandible's body; below, it usually overlaps the intermediate tendon of the digastric muscle and the hyoidean attachment of stylohyoid. It has an inferior, a lateral and a medial surface and is partially enclosed between two layers of deep cervical fascia extending from the hyoid's greater cornu; one layer passes to the mandible's lower border, covering the gland's inferior surface, the other passes to the mylohyoid line on the medial surface of the mandible and covers the gland's medial surface.

The *inferior surface*, covered by skin, platysma and deep fascia, is crossed by the facial vein and the facial nerve's cervical branch; near the mandible the submandibular lymph nodes are in contact with the gland and some may be embedded in it (p. 1612).

The *lateral surface* is in relation with the submandibular fossa (on the medial surface of the mandibular body) and the mandibular attachment of the medial pterygoid; the facial artery grooves its posterosuperior part, lying at first deep to the gland and then emerging between its lateral surface and the mandibular attachment of the medial pterygoid to reach the mandible's lower border.

The *medial surface* is related anteriorly to mylohyoid, separated from it by the mylohyoid nerve and vessels and branches of the submental vessels. More posteriorly, it is related to styloglossus, the stylohyoid ligament and the glossopharyngeal nerve, which separate it from the pharynx; in its intermediate part the medial surface is related to hyoglossus, separated from it by styloglossus, the lingual nerve, submandibular ganglion, hypoglossal nerve and deep lingual vein (sequentially from above down). Below, the medial surface is related to stylohyoid and the posterior belly of digastric.

The *deep part* of the gland extends forwards to the posterior end of the sublingual gland and lies between mylohyoid inferolaterally and hyoglossus and styloglossus medially; above it runs the lingual nerve and, below it, the hypoglossal nerve and deep lingual vein.

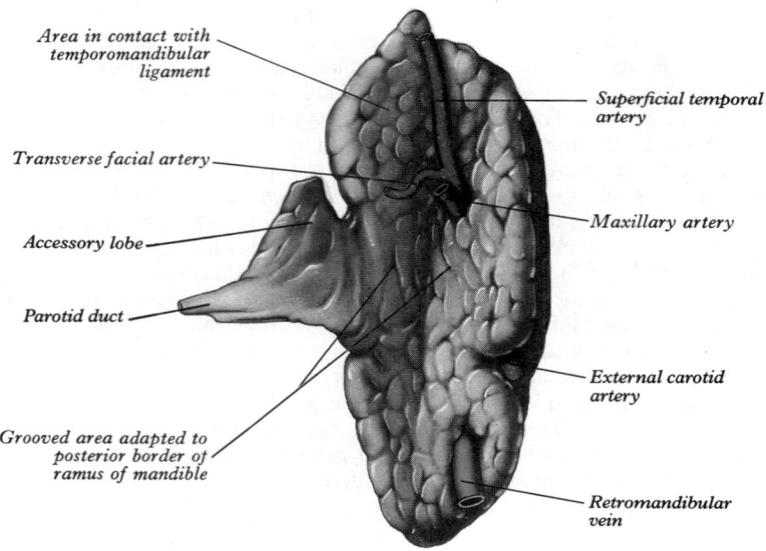

Area in contact with temporomandibular ligament

Superficial temporal artery

Transverse facial artery

Maxillary artery

Accessory lobe

Parotid duct

External carotid artery

Grooved area adapted to posterior border of ramus of mandible

Retromandibular vein

12.6   The right parotid gland: anteromedial aspect.

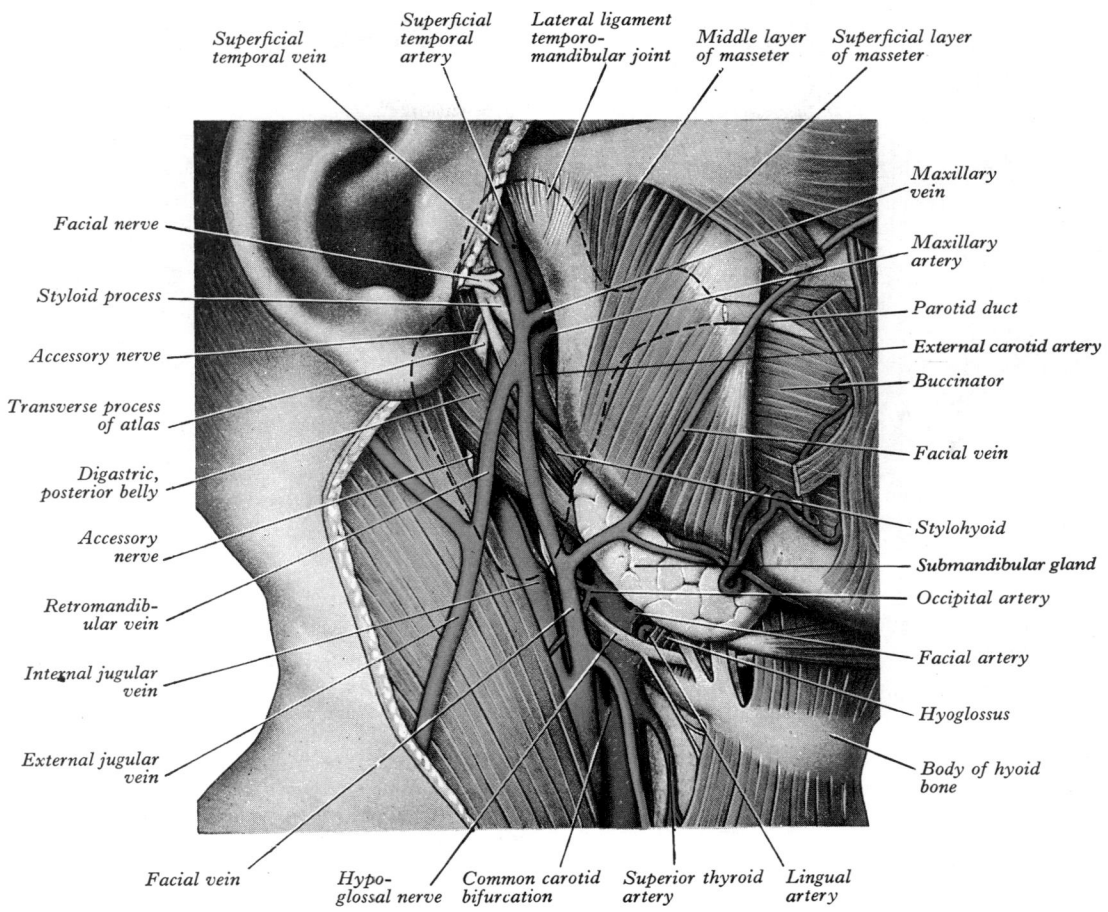

Superficial temporal vein
Superficial temporal artery
Lateral ligament temporo-mandibular joint
Middle layer of masseter
Superficial layer of masseter

Facial nerve

Styloid process

Accessory nerve

Transverse process of atlas

Digastric, posterior belly

Accessory nerve

Retromandib-ular vein

Internal jugular vein

External jugular vein

Maxillary vein

Maxillary artery

Parotid duct

External carotid artery

Buccinator

Facial vein

Stylohyoid

Submandibular gland

Occipital artery

Facial artery

Hyoglossus

Body of hyoid bone

Facial vein
Hypo-glossal nerve
Common carotid bifurcation
Superior thyroid artery
Lingual artery

12.7 Drawing of a dissection to show the principal immediate deep relations of the parotid gland. The outline of the parotid gland is indicated by the interrupted black line.

The gland is palpable between an index finger placed on the floor of the mouth and a thumb placed below the floor, anteromedial to the angle of the mandible.

Submandibular duct (12.16B, 60).

About 5 cm long, this has a thinner wall than the parotid duct. It begins from numerous tributaries in the superficial part of the gland and emerges from the medial surface of this part of the gland behind the posterior border of mylohyoid; it traverses the deep part, passing at first up and slightly back for 4 or 5 mm and then forwards between mylohyoid and hyoglossus. Passing between the sublingual gland and genioglossus it opens in the floor of the mouth on the summit of the sublingual papilla at the side of the frenulum of the tongue (12.55). On hyoglossus it lies between the lingual and hypoglossal nerves, but at the muscle's anterior border it is crossed laterally by the lingual nerve, terminal branches of which ascend on its medial side (12.60). As it traverses the gland's deep part it receives small tributaries draining this part of the gland. Salivary calculi occasionally occur in the submandibular duct; they are radio-opaque and may be palpable.

Vessels and nerves

The arteries supplying the submandibular gland are branches of the facial and lingual arteries; the veins correspond. The lymph vessels drain into the deep cervical group of lymph nodes, particularly the jugulo-omohyoid node, interrupted by the submandibular nodes, some of which are in close relation with the anterior end and medial aspect of the superficial part of the gland and may be embedded in it. The nerves are derived from the submandibular ganglion, through which it receives fibres from the chorda tympani (parasympathetic), the lingual branch of the mandibular nerve (sensory) and the sympathetic trunk. In dogs and cats the gland receives its nerve supply

through the subsidiary ganglion of Langley (p. 1297), but in humans the parasympathetic nerve supply (chorda tympani) relays mainly in the submandibular ganglion. Small parasympathetic ganglia may occur in the gland's hilum and in the branches of the submandibular ganglion passing to it. Garrett and Kemplay (1977), using catecholamine fluorescence and electron micrography, observed that in cats all adrenergic fibres are derived from the superior cervical sympathetic ganglion.

SUBLINGUAL GLANDS

The paired sublingual glands (**12**.4), the smallest of the main salivary glands, lie beneath the oral mucosa, each in contact with the sublingual fossa on the lingual aspect of the mandible, close to the symphysis. Each is narrow, flat, shaped like an almond, and weighs 3–4 g. The sublingual glands are mucous in type (p. 74).

Above the gland is the mucosa of the oral floor, raised as a sublingual fold; **below** is mylohyoid; **in front** is the anterior end of its fellow; **behind** lies the deep part of the submandibular gland; **lateral** is the mandible above the anterior part of the mylohyoid line, and **medial** is genioglossus, separated from it by the lingual nerve and submandibular duct. It has 8–20 excretory ducts; of the *smaller sublingual ducts* most open separately on the summit of the sublingual fold and a few sometimes into the submandibular duct. From the anterior part of the gland small rami sometimes form a *major sublingual duct*, opening with or near to the orifice of the submandibular duct.

Vessels and nerves

The arterial supply is from the sublingual and submental arteries. The veins correspond to the arteries. Innervation is by the lingual

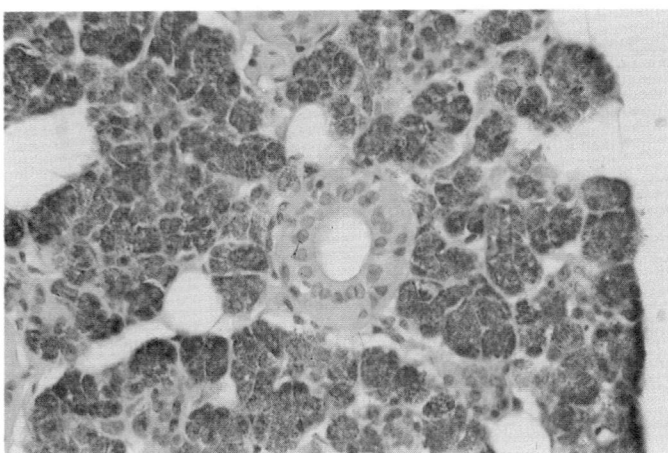

12.8 Section through the parotid gland, stained with haematoxylin and eosin. Magnification × 350.

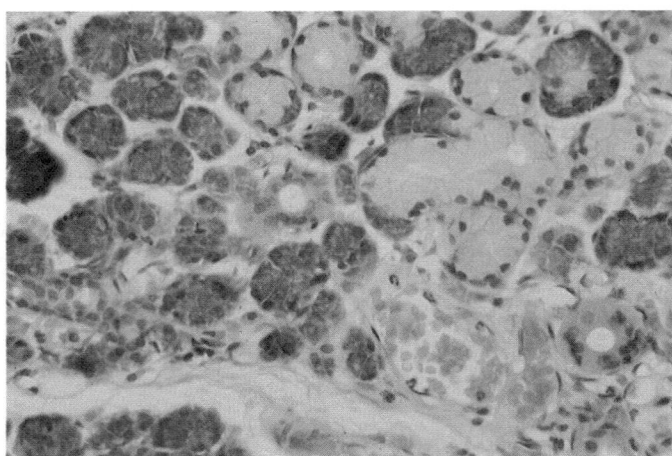

12.9 Section of the submandibular gland, stained with haematoxylin and eosin. Magnification × 350.

nerve, chorda tympani and sympathetic fibres. The parasympathetic relay is in the submandibular ganglion; neurons may occur among its distal fibres to the lingual nerve forming a distinct sublingual ganglion. The precise terminations of the nerve supply are not fully known (see below).

MICROSTRUCTURE OF MAJOR SALIVARY GLANDS

These glands are compound racemose in type (12.9–13) and have numerous lobes composed of lobules linked by dense connective tissue containing excretory (collecting) ducts, blood vessels, lymph vessels, nerve fibres and small ganglia. Each lobule has a single duct, whose branches begin as dilated secretory 'endpieces' or acini. Their primary secretion is modified as it traverses intercalated, striated and excretory ducts into one or more main ducts which discharge saliva into the oral cavity (see below).

Salivary acini or 'endpieces' (12.13)

The variety of different terms used to describe the form and cytology of secretory acini or endpieces has caused much confusion. Garrett (1976) and Young and van Lennep (1978) have appraised the problems involved. (The official term is *portio terminalis*—of acinar, alveolar or tubulo-alveolar types—inelegantly translated as 'endpiece'.)

In the following description a secretory 'endpiece' is termed an *acinus* if approximately spheroidal, a *tubule* if elongate; *tubuloacini* are intermediate in shape. The secretory cells of acini are pyramidal, with narrow luminal apices and broad bases; those of tubules are more cylindrical. Such cells, the main producers of salivary protein and glycoprotein, are usually described according to their appearance as *serous, seromucuous* or *mucous*, though unfortunately without unanimity in use. A serous secretion of low viscosity, and a highly viscous mucus were correlated initially with serous and mucous cells distinguished by simple histological staining methods. Improved techniques later identified a range for seromucous secretions. It is now established that the products of these cells form an almost continuous series, from serous secretions with negligible amounts of acidic proteoglycans to mucous secretions rich in them. Applying the criteria of Young and van Lennep (1978) glandular cells are here dubbed: *serous* if the granules are small, discrete, homogeneous, generally eosinophilic and electron-dense; *mucous* if their granules are larger, close-packed and ill-defined, with low eosinophilia and a homogeneous, fairly electron-translucent matrix; or *seromucous* if they are intermediate in appearance, with granules either close-packed, eosinophilic and homogeneous, or more discrete, larger and heterogeneous. A gland or secretory acinus with only one type of cell is described as *homocrine*, while one containing more than one type is *heterocrine*.

The secretory 'endpieces' of the human **parotid gland** are mainly seromucous (or serous) acini (12.8); mucous acini are rare. In the

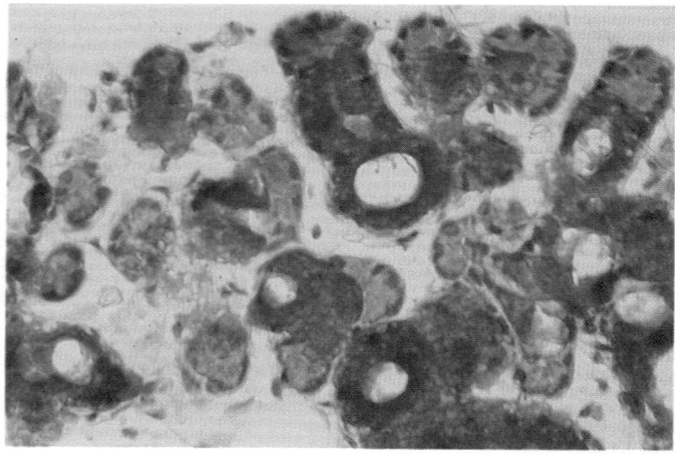

12.10 Section through the submandibular gland, stained with haematoxylin and alcian blue. Mucous cells are stained blue, the serous glands only with haematoxylin and eosin. Magnification × 350.

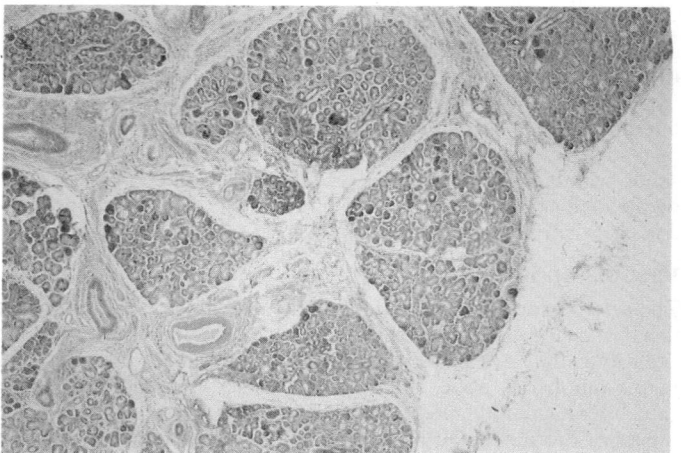

12.11 Section through the sublingual gland, stained with haematoxylin and eosin. Magnification × 80.

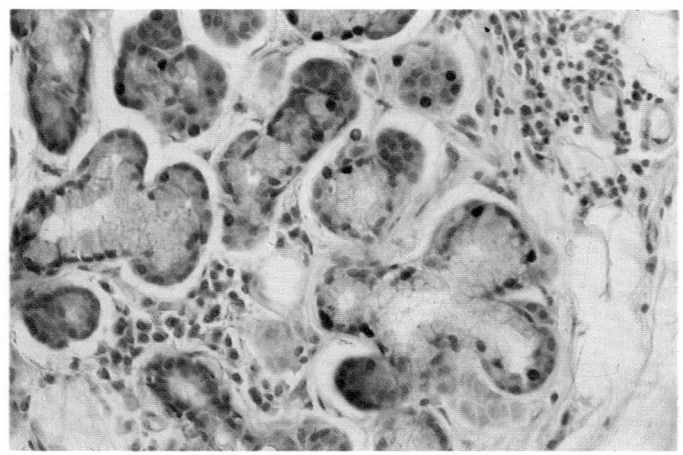

12.12   Section through the sublingual gland, stained with haematoxylin and eosin. Magnification × 350.

submandibular gland acini are usually seromucous, with some mucous ones. (**12**.9, 10) In the **sublingual gland** (**12**.11, 12) they are typically mucous tubules, but seromucous cells also occur, frequently as acini or as *demilunes* (Young & van Lennep 1978). Seromucous demilunes, which also exist in submandibular glands of many mammalian species, are crescentic groups of glandular cells found at the bases of some mucous endpieces (**12**.13); sited between the mucous cells and basal lamina, they apparently communicate with the lumen by fine canaliculi which pass between the mucous cells. Using the criteria described above all the major human salivary glands are thus heterocrine.

The ultrastructure of these glandular cells is shown diagrammatically in **12**.13. *Seromucous* (and *serous*) *cells* are roughly pyramidal. The basal plasmalemma is usually smooth, while the lateral is plicated and interdigitates with that of the adjacent cells. The apical (luminal) surface bears microvilli, between which are often endocytic vesicles. Discrete, secretory canaliculi lie between the cells; limited basilaterally by junctional complexes, they open into the lumen of the 'endpiece'; their zonulae occludentes are often assumed to form a continuous seal around each cell but freeze-fracture micrographs of parotid 'endpiece' tight junctions in rats (de Camilli et al 1976) suggest that the 'seals' may be incomplete. Nuclei vary in shape and position, but are more spheroidal and less basal than in mucous cells. Apically the cytoplasm is filled by secretory granules of variable form (Tandler 1972; Riva & Testa-Riva 1973); a conspicuous feature of the infranuclear cytoplasm is an abundant granular endoplasmic reticulum arranged in stacks of parallel, flat cisternae. Golgi complexes are supranuclear with adjacent small coated and smooth vesicles. Elongated mitochondria, lysosomes, microfilaments and occasional large lipid droplets also occur.

Mucous cells are cylindrical; their luminal plasma membrane is smoother and secretory canaliculi between the cells are rare. The supranuclear cytoplasm is typically packed with large, electron-translucent, frequently fused secretory droplets. Granular endoplasmic reticulum and Golgi complexes resemble those of serous and seromucous cells, but the nucleus is flatter and more basal.

Ducts of salivary glands (12.13)

Leading consecutively from the secretory 'endpieces' are *intercalated, striated* and *excretory ducts*.

In *intercalated ducts*, the lining cells are cuboidal or flat. Their cytoplasm contains long mitochondria, a few cisternae of granular endoplasmic reticulum, juxtanuclear Golgi complexes, lysosomes and secretory granules. While this suggests little participation in protein synthesis, it does not preclude involvement in the addition of water and electrolytes to saliva; the cells responsible for this, in either 'endpiece' or duct, are unknown but, although this function is often assigned to glandular cells, the intercalated ducts may also be involved.

In *striated ducts* (**12**.13) the lining cells are basally striated, 'like a thick lawn' according to Pfluger (1866). Ultrastructurally, these striations are seen to be regions of highly folded basal plasmalemma, between which are columns of packed mitochondria. These folds are also interdigitated laterally with those of adjacent cells, often linked by desmosomes. This folding and local abundance of mitochondria is typical of many epithelial cells engaged in electrolyte transport, as these cells certainly are; they transport potassium into saliva and by reabsorbing sodium ions in excess of water they render saliva hypotonic (Thaysen et al 1954). The lateral plasmalemmae of cells lining striated ducts are linked by 'leaky' junctional complexes (Garrett & Parsons 1974). The luminal plasmalemma bears microvilli and their cytoplasm often extends into the lumen as apical blebs which may be shed into the saliva (apocrine secretion: p. 74; see also Takano 1969, Garrett 1976). As well as modifying electrolyte composition, striated ducts secrete immunoglobulin A (Kraus & Mestecky 1971), lysozyme (Kraus & Mestecky 1971) and kallikrein (Garrett & Kidd 1975). Immunoglobulin A is produced by subepithelial plasma cells.

For excretory ducts few ultrastructural details have been recorded; in rats they are lined by simple columnar or pseudostratified epithelium, mainly of tall columnar cells with basal striations containing packed, elongate mitochondria (Tamarin & Sreebny 1965). These striations, and their more intimate relation to capillaries than elsewhere in the ductal system, suggest that excretory ducts are more than passive conduits; an involvement in electrolyte transport is possible (Young & van Lennep 1978).

Myoepitheliocytes of salivary glands (12.13–15)

These contractile cells are associated with intercalated ducts and secretory endpieces, lying between the basal lamina and the epithelial cells proper, and also with intra- and extralobular ducts (Chaudhry et al 1987). Garrett and Emmelin (1979) summarized the effects of myoepithelial contraction as follows: the outflow of saliva is accelerated, luminal volume of intercalated ducts and endpieces is reduced, secretory pressure is aided, the underlying parenchyma supported, salivary flow is helped to overcome peripheral resistance and, in certain circumstances, discharge from the actual secretory cells is also assisted.

The shape of salivary myoepitheliocytes depends on their location: in endpieces they are stellate, dendritic, with long overlapping processes ('basket cells') which, with those of other such cells, form a reticulum around each endpiece. Those in the walls of ducts are fusiform, with fewer branches, and extend along the intercalated ducts longitudinally. 'Endpiece' myoepitheliocytes have a central perikaryon with four to eight radial processes, each with two or more successions of branches which cross but do not fuse or extend on to the ducts. In contrast, myoepitheliocytic processes in intercalated ducts seldom branch and often overlap with those of the endpieces.

Myoepitheliocytic cytoplasm (**12**.15) may be divided into filamentous and non-filamentous compartments, the latter containing the nucleus, juxtanuclear Golgi complexes, lysosomal bodies and mitochondria. Globules of neutral fat may occur in human cells (Garrett 1963). The filaments, conspicuous in the processes and their rami resemble the myofilaments of smooth muscle cells (p. 738). Both thin (4 nm) and thick (10 nm) filaments are described, the former arranged longitudinally in processes, with the less numerous thick filaments scattered amongst them. Filaments often pass to attachment plaques on the basal plasmalemma, causing indentations. Basal lamina opposite the plaques appears thicker and may be linked to the cells at these sites. Bannerjee et al (1977) have shown that the basal lamina strengthens and supports the adjacent epithelium. When myoepitheliocytes contract, the basal lamina is probably tensed at the attachment plaques (Garrett & Emmelin 1979). Numerous caveolae are commonly associated with the stromal plasmalemma, but less frequently so with the plasmalemma adjacent to the epithelial cells. Myoepitheliocytes are linked to secretory and ductal cells by desmosomes and occasional cilia extend from them into indentations of the adjacent epithelial cells. Cilia were first observed by Tandler (1965) in myoepitheliocytes of human submandibular glands and subsequently described in other human salivary glands (Tandler et al 1970) and in glands of other species (Cutler & Chaudhry 1973, Kidd 1978). Garrett and Emmelin (1979) suggest that there may be a cilium on each salivary myoepitheliocyte, as proposed by Stirling and Chandler (1976) for human mammary myoepitheliocytes

1695

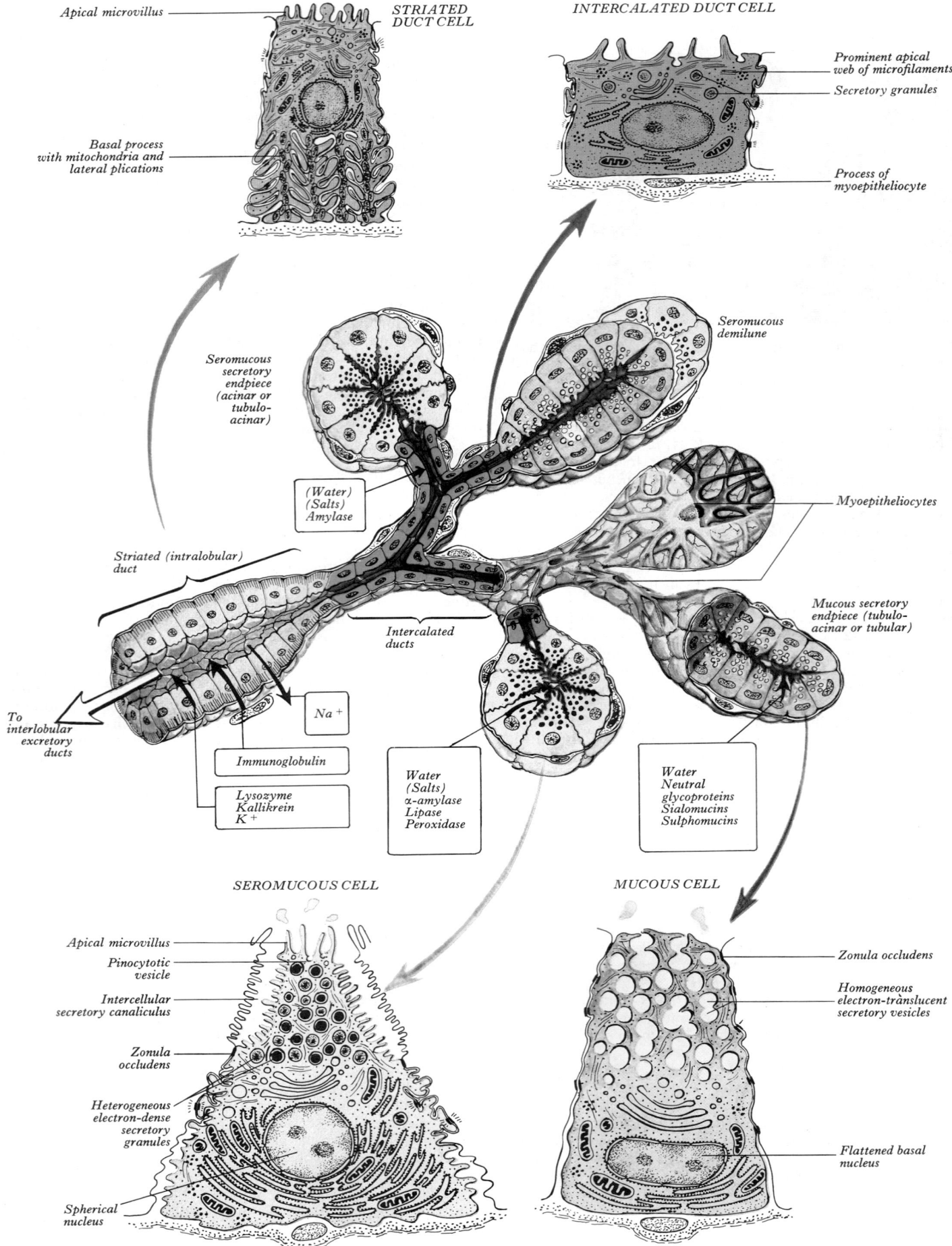

Apical microvillus

STRIATED
DUCT CELL

INTERCALATED DUCT CELL

*Prominent apical
web of microfilaments*

Secretory granules

*Basal process
with mitochondria and
lateral plications*

*Process of
myoepitheliocyte*

*Seromucous
secretory
endpiece
(acinar or
tubulo-
acinar)*

*Seromucous
demilune*

(Water)
(Salts)
Amylase

Myoepitheliocytes

*Striated (intralobular)
duct*

*Intercalated
ducts*

*Mucous secretory
endpiece (tubulo-
acinar or tubular)*

*To
interlobular
excretory
ducts*

Na^+

Immunoglobulin

*Lysozyme
Kallikrein
K^+*

Water
(Salts)
α-amylase
Lipase
Peroxidase

Water
Neutral
glycoproteins
Sialomucins
Sulphomucins

SEROMUCOUS CELL

MUCOUS CELL

Apical microvillus

*Pinocytotic
vesicle*

*Intercellular
secretory canaliculus*

*Zonula
occludens*

*Heterogeneous
electron-dense
secretory
granules*

*Spherical
nucleus*

Zonula occludens

*Homogeneous
electron-translucent
secretory vesicles*

*Flattened basal
nucleus*

12.13 Diagram of the architecture of a generalized salivary gland including ultrastructural details. Solid and outlined black arrows indicate direction of saliva transport.

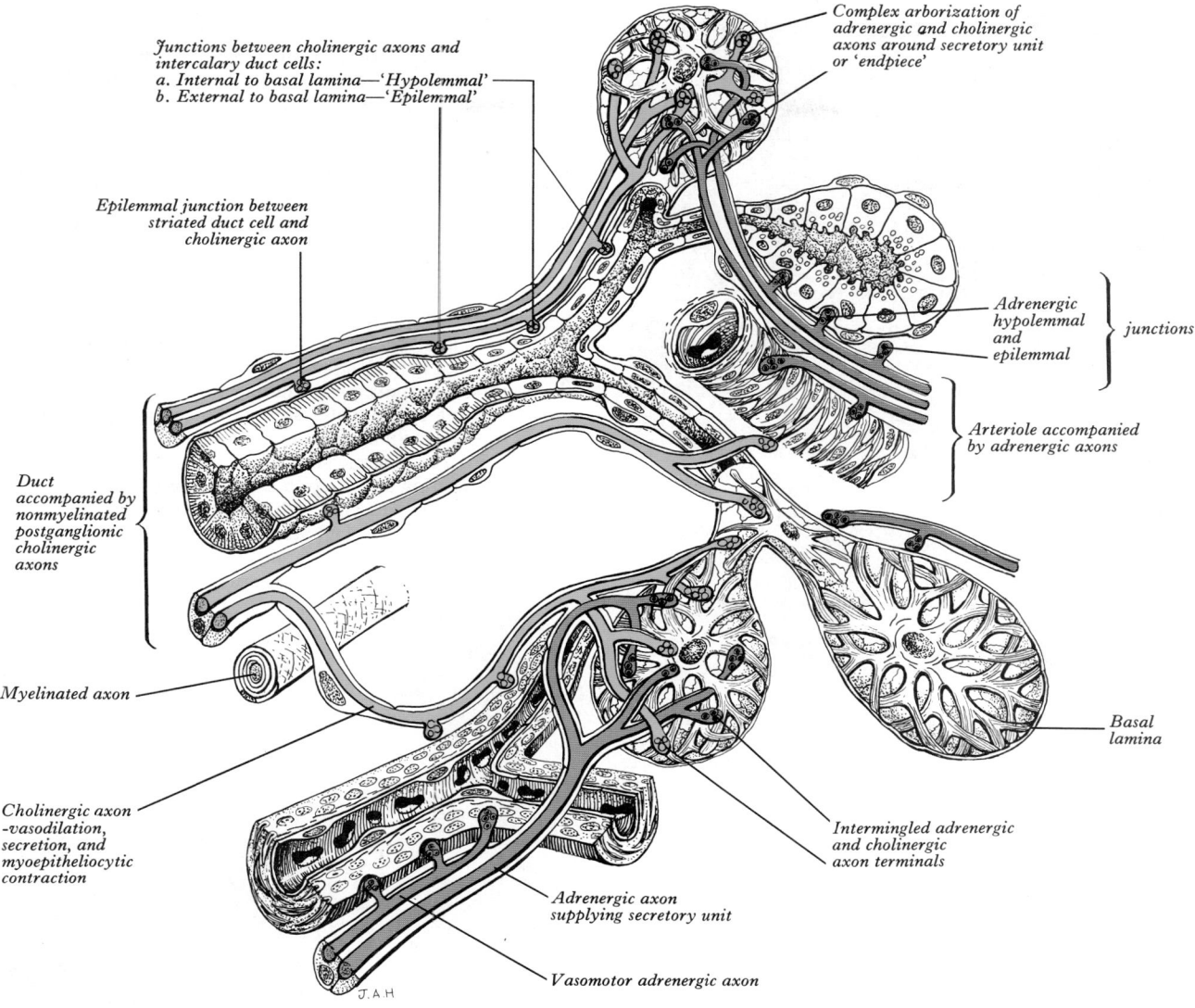

12.14   The innervation of the ducts, secretory units and arterioles in a generalized salivary gland.

(p. 423). The cilia may have a chemoreceptive and/or mechano-receptive role.

Salivary myoepitheliocytes appear to have both sympathetic and parasympathetic innervation (Garrett 1972, 1976), with several axons of either type, or jointly, supplying a single cell. In the sublingual gland of the rat, myoepitheliocytes may have only cholinergic inner-vation (Templeton & Thulin 1978). Stimulation by sympathetic or by parasympathetic nerves may result in myoepitheliocyte contraction (Garrett & Emmelin 1979). For further details of these cells, see p. 71.

CONTROL OF SALIVARY GLAND ACTIVITY

The observed wide and rapid variation in the composition, quantity and rate of salivary secretion in response to various stimuli suggests an elaborate control mechanism (Emmelin 1972). In some glands salivary secretion is spontaneous; in others secretion follows different types of sensory stimulation: gustatory, nociceptive, olfactory and tactile. Secretion may be continuous, but at a low resting level, and may be in part spontaneous, although it is mainly a response to the drying of the oral and pharyngeal mucosae. A rapid increase can be superimposed on the resting level, e.g. during mastication or when stimulated by the autonomic innervation. The controlled variation in the activity of the many types of salivary effector cells (serous, as

well as seromucous and mucous secretory cells, myoepitheliocytes, epithelial cells of all the ductal elements and the smooth muscle of local blood vessels) affects the quantity and quality of saliva. The control of these is both hormonal and neural.

Hormonal control

The effects of circulating hormones upon salivary secretion were reviewed by Blair-West et al (1967). There is no clear evidence that they evoke secretion directly at physiological levels, but they may alter the response of glandular cells to neural stimuli. Local hor-mones, however, have profound effects in feline submandibular glands; e.g. vasodilatation, though neurally initiated, is maintained by plasma-kinins formed locally when kallikrein is released from secretory cells stimulated by sympathetic amines (Gautvik et al 1972).

Neural control

Most salivary glands, except those secreting spontaneously, depend on autonomic nerves to evoke secretion, and in all of them salivary flow is mainly under nervous control. The nerves involved are cholinergic (parasympathetic) and adrenergic (sympathetic) (Garrett 1976).

The typical pattern of innervation is shown in **12**.14, but details vary in different glands and species (Garrett 1972); differences may also occur with age (Yohro 1971). Only the more constant features are illustrated and described here. Cholinergic nerves often accompany ducts and arborize freely around secretory endpieces,

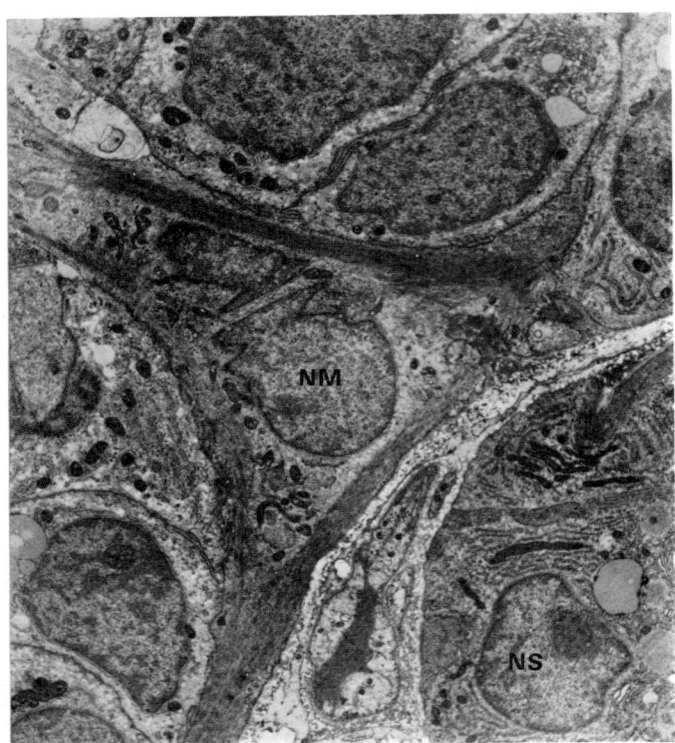

12.15 Transmission electron micrograph of a myoepitheliocyte of a salivary gland. The superficial filamentous and juxtanuclear non-filamentous compartments of the cytoplasm can be seen. NM = nucleus of myoepitheliocyte; NS = nucleus of secretory cell. (Provided by R M Palmer, UMDS, Guy's Campus, London.)

but adrenergic nerves usually enter glands along arteries and ramify with them. The main secretomotor nerves contain largely non-myelinated axons, but a few myelinated axons occur, presumably either preganglionic efferent or afferent. Postganglionic efferent axons, like those elsewhere (Norberg 1967), show periodic dilatations containing mitochondria and vesicles, the latter electron-lucent in cholinergic axons and with electron-dense cores in adrenergic axons. Within the glands the nerve fibres intermingle, cholinergic and adrenergic axons often lying in adjacent invaginations of one Schwann cell (Eneroth et al 1969, Garrett 1972, 1976).

At *neuroeffector junctions* (**12**.14) the synaptic regions of axons and the effector cells they supply are functionally related, the axonal surfaces closest to the effector cells being free of Schwann cell covering. Where effector cells are epithelial, the junctions may be *epilemmal* or *hypolemmal* (Garrett 1975), terms introduced by Arnstein (1889, 1895). At epilemmal sites, the axonal and effector surfaces are separated by about 100 nm, with the basal lamina intervening. At hypolemmal sites the axon penetrates the basal lamina and is separated from the effector cell by only 20 nm. One axon may supply several effector cells directly and many more indirectly through electrical coupling of adjacent cells (Lowenstein & Kanno 1964); group activity thus occurs. One effector cell may also receive several axons, both cholinergic and/or adrenergic. Single axons may act on several types of effector. Although there are separate sympathetic axons for secretion and vasoconstriction (Emmelin & Engström 1960), the former may also induce myo-epitheliocyte contraction and a single parasympathetic axon may, through serial neuro-effector junctions of the *en passant* type (p. 1297), induce vasodilatation, secretion and myoepitheliocytic contraction (Emmelin 1972).

Secretory endpieces usually have the most innervation, cholinergic and adrenergic, individual cells often having both. Cholinergic axons have long been accepted as the secretomotor innervation; however, in 1974 it was shown that in the parotid gland of the rat, at least, sympathetic nerves are also secretomotor (Harrop & Garrett 1974, Hodgson & Spiers 1974). Adrenergically evoked saliva differs in quantity and composition but by what mechanism is uncertain. In

heterocrine glands adrenergic and cholinergic nerves might activate different types of cell but in homocrine glands (p. 1694), where all cells appear similar, they presumably affect the same cells differently (Garrett 1972). In some situations sympathetic activity may modify saliva produced in response to parasympathetic stimulation, rather than directly inducing flow.

The ductal elements of salivary glands can markedly modify the composition of saliva (p. 1695) and, though less intensely innervated than secretory endpieces, their activity is also under neural influences, in part at least. In 1958 Lundberg showed that cells, assumed to be ductal, in the feline submaxillary gland, responded electrically to both parasympathetic **and** sympathetic stimulation. Cholinergic fibres lie adjacent to the striated ducts of most species, occasionally hypolemmal in position, but more commonly so in intercalated ducts. In some species, including mankind, adrenergic nerves are also associated with striated ducts (Garrett 1967). The main excretory ducts appear to have only cholinergic nerves but Schneyer (1976) observed that sympathetic stimulation alters electrolyte transport across the epithelium of the submaxillary main duct in the rat, suggesting an adrenergic supply.

The innervation of myoepitheliocytes adjoining secretory endpieces and intercalated ducts is physiologically obscure, but electron microscopy suggests a sympathetic and parasympathetic hypolemmal supply (Kagayama & Nishiyama 1972). Myoepitheliocytes are stimulated to contract by adrenergic axons; they may respond to a single

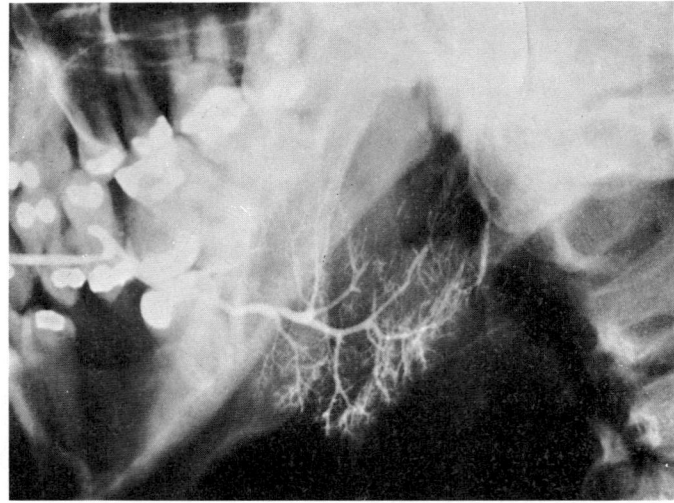

A

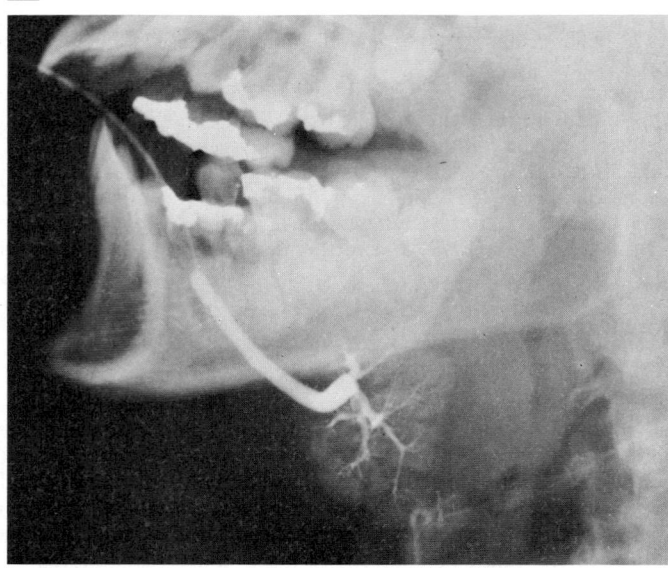

B

12.16A, B A. Parotid sialogram; B. Submandibular sialogram. In each case the shadow of the cannula used to introduce the radio-opaque medium into the duct of the gland is visible. See text for description.

impulse, suggesting high sensitivity. The role of cholinergic axons is less certain, but they also may cause contraction (Garrett 1975), thus aiding salivation.

Structural evidence shows that salivary arterioles are innervated by both adrenergic and cholinergic axons (Young & van Lennep 1978). The former, the more numerous, maintain vasoconstrictor tone; the latter may induce vasodilatation but this is maintained by local plasma kinins (see above).

Little information is available on the afferent nerves of salivary glands. Pain due to obstruction of salivary ducts and sialography suggests a nociceptive function, but this awaits anatomical investigation. Sensory endings occur in the main ducts and presumably elsewhere in the glands. Afferent axons are postulated to occur in the main parasympathetic and sympathetic nerve trunks to the glands. Increasing pressure in the submandibular ducts in dogs enhances afferent activity in the chorda tympani (Garrett 1975); intraglandular baroceptors are presumed to be involved in this response. Detailed studies of salivary sensory innervation are clearly needed.

ACCESSORY SALIVARY GLANDS

Besides the main salivary glands many others exist: some in the tongue (p. 1721), others around and in the palatine tonsil between its crypts, with large numbers in the soft palate, the posterior part of the hard palate, the lips and cheeks. These are similar in structure to larger salivary glands and are mainly of the mucous type.

SIALOGRAPHY

Cannulae can be introduced into the parotid and submandibular ducts and used to inject radio-opaque substances (e.g. lipiodol) to outline the ramifications of the ductual systems of these glands, showing their patterns and calibres. The *parotid duct*, as seen in lateral sialograms, is formed near the centre of the posterior border of the mandibular ramus by the union of two ducts which respectively ascend and descend at right angles to the main duct (**12.**16A). As it crosses the face, it also receives from above five or six ductules from the accessory parotid gland; as it curves round the anterior border of the masseter it is often compressed, its shadow being attenuated here. The intraglandular part of the main duct receives an alternating series of descending and ascending tributaries, each formed from an arborization of fine ductules receiving acini. The acini usually do not show as dilatations in sialograms but are represented by the 'free' endings of the smallest ducts. The *submandibular duct* starts from that gland's lowest part, below the mandible in lateral views, ascends vertically above the mandible's lower border and turns sharply forwards, gradually ascending to its opening. The duct's vertical part receives anterior and posterior tributaries and, as it turns sharply forwards, it receives a large tributary from the posterior region (**12.**16B). Each tributary is formed from ductules (with their terminal acini) visualized as in the parotid gland. Contrast medium injected into the submandibular duct may also enter the major sublingual duct, revealing the ductules of the anterior part of the sublingual gland.

TEETH

INTRODUCTION

Except in mankind, teeth are necessary for survival in most mammals and other vertebrates, and longevity is related to the endurance of the dentition under the abrasive process of mastication. In non-mammalian vertebrates, teeth are constantly replaced, a condition known as *polyphyodonty*, related to the need for successively larger teeth in animals which grow throughout life. In mammals, where skeletal growth is typically limited to an early period of life, there are generally two dentitions, the first deciduous and the other permanent, the condition of *diphyodonty*; in some mammalian species, e.g. the rat, there is only one set (*monophyodonty*), there being continuous growth of individual teeth. The emergence and success of diphyodonty was probably related to the evolution of occlusion during mastication. In non-mammalian vertebrates, the jaw joint is formed between the quadrate bone of the upper jaw and the articular bone of the lower one, structures homologous respectively with the incus and malleus of mammalian skulls; the lower teeth are also set on a curve so far inside the upper tooth row that, due also to restricted lateral movement, they cannot meet the upper teeth. The evolution of mammals was associated with the posterosuperior growth of the dentary bone (one of several lower jaw elements existing in all non-mammalian vertebrates towards the squamosal, a bone homologous with the squamous temporal in most mammals. In accord with these skeletal changes, the jaw muscles were also rearranged to move the mandible (now formed entirely by the dentary) transversely. Together with these trends there was a change in the shape of the teeth; from the simple conical structures of reptilian ancestors, mammals evolved teeth with complex shearing planes. Lateral movements of the mandible were now possible, allowing the lower teeth to grind across the upper to produce a more effective trituration. Although the deficiencies in the fossil record make some details of this evolutionary process uncertain, the principal stages are known and the cusps of human molars can be homologized with those of early mammals (**12.**17).

After a few months of active use, the newly erupted teeth in mammals are worn to produce precisely matching upper and lower shearing edges. A continued eruption of new teeth would constantly

disrupt this relationship and therefore be disadvantageous. However, because of the need to accommodate teeth in small, young jaws, a deciduous dentition is an almost universal requirement in mammals. With this reduction of replacement, dental tissues evolved to minimize the effects of wear. Thus a harder, thicker enamel emerged in mammals, with a prismatic structure which evolved and diversified into a variety of complex and distinctive patterns (Boyde 1976) to resist wear and breakage through fracture, and produce sharp cutting edges.

The teeth in reptiles, apart from some, e.g. the Crocodilia, are firmly attached by bone to the jaws, but in mammals each is suspended in a socket by a periodontal ligament. This flexible system allows adaptive movements of teeth under masticatory loads, and a degree of further eruption (occlusal drift) to compensate for wear; the latter is even more remarkable in species which possess teeth of continuous growth or extended crowns. This suspension also acts as a shock absorber, moderating the effects of transient loads due to mastication on the surrounding bone. Finally, it provides the environment for a rich, spatially ordered periodontal innervation mediating a comprehensive flow of proprioceptive data to nervous centres concerned with control of masticatory patterns.

The introduction of refined carbohydrates in the human diet has made human teeth susceptible to caries and periodontal disease. Outside human culture such dental impairment would probably have led to extinction, but this problem has to some extent been overcome by breaking down, softening or in a sense predigesting food by cooking and other types of culinary preparation. Nevertheless, chewing does facilitate the digestion of most foods, including cooked meat and vegetables (Farrell 1956) and the natural dentition comminutes food much more efficiently than an artificial replacement (Lucas et al 1986). However, teeth are no longer vital to survival and therefore selective pressure leading to further evolutionary change in the human detition will probably be limited.

Because they are the hardest and most stable of tissues, teeth are selectively preserved and fossilized, providing by far the best evolutionary record. Hence teeth are excellent models for studying the relations between ontogeny and phylogeny. In modern societies, the durability of teeth to fire and bacterial decomposition makes

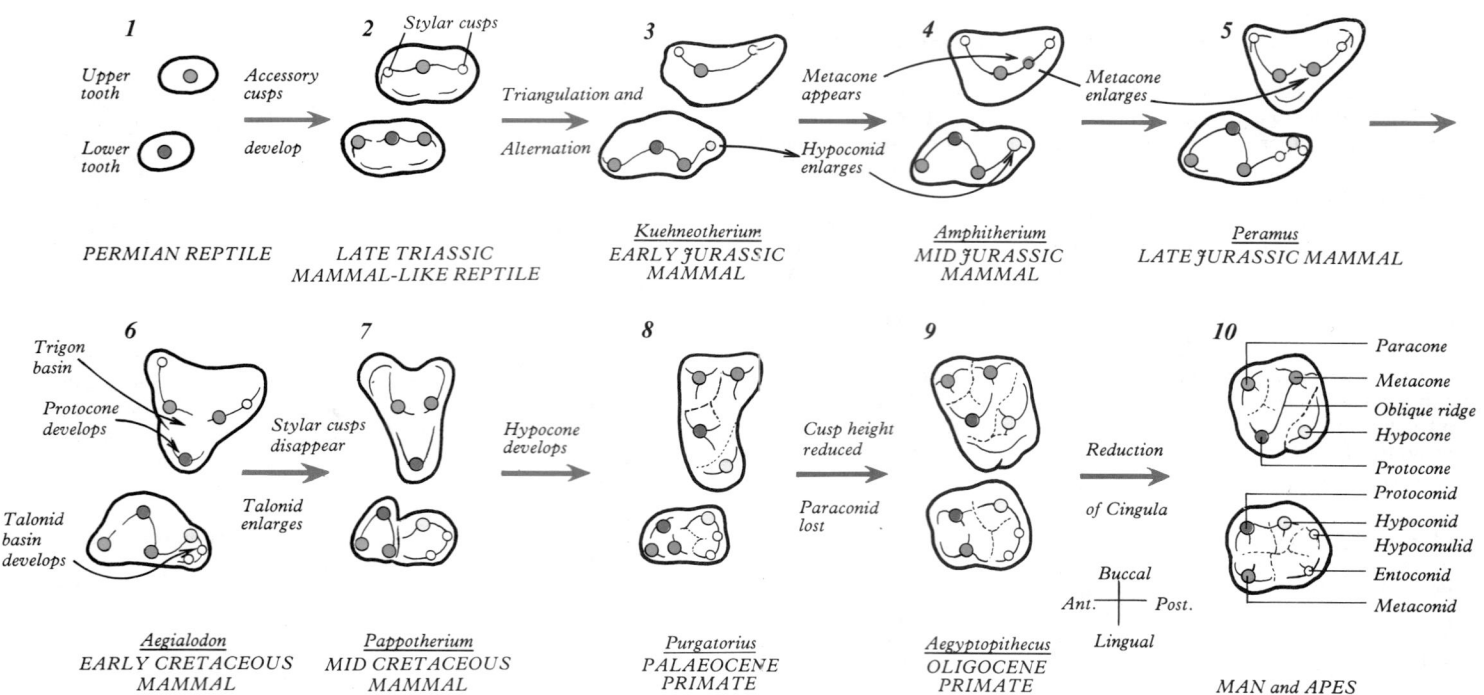

PERMIAN REPTILE   *LATE TRIASSIC*   Kuehneotherium   Amphitherium   Peramus
                     MAMMAL-LIKE REPTILE   *EARLY JURASSIC*   *MID JURASSIC*   *LATE JURASSIC MAMMAL*
                                             MAMMAL   *MAMMAL*

Aegialodon   Pappotherium   Purgatorius   Aegyptopithecus
EARLY CRETACEOUS   *MID CRETACEOUS*   *PALAEOCENE*   *OLIGOCENE*   *MAN and APES*
MAMMAL   *MAMMAL*   *PRIMATE*   *PRIMATE*

KEY • PARACONE (upper tooth) PARACONID (lower tooth)
     • METACONE (upper tooth) METACONID (lower tooth)
     • PROTOCONE (upper tooth) PROTOCONID (lower tooth)
     ◦ HYPOCONE (upper tooth) HYPOCONID (lower tooth)

12.17 Occlusal views of the left upper and right lower teeth showing a series of steps in the evolution of complex molar occlusion. Large cusps (coloured) and smaller cusps are joined together by raised cutting edges.

The cutting edges of opposing teeth pass each other during occlusion and certain cusps (e.g. the protocone and hypoconid) then crush into opposing basins (e.g. talonid and trigon basins).

them invaluable in identification of otherwise unrecognizable bodies, a point of great forensic importance (see p. 1720).

General arrangement of dental tissues

A tooth (**12**.18–20) consists of a crown, covered by very hard translucent *enamel* and a root covered by yellowish bone-like *cement*. These meet at the neck or *cervical margin*. A longitudinal section (**12**.19, 20) reveals that a tooth is mostly *dentine* (ivory) with an enamel covering about 1.5 mm thick, while the cement is usually much thinner. The dentine contains a central *pulp cavity*, expanded at its coronal end into a *pulp chamber* and narrowed in the root as a *pulp canal*, opening at or near its tip by an *apical foramen*, occasionally multiple. The root is surrounded by *alveolar bone*, its cement separated from the osseous socket (*alveolus*) by the soft *periodontal ligament*, about 0.2 mm thick. Coarse bundles of collagen fibres, embedded at one end in cement, cross the periodontal ligament to enter the osseous alveolar wall. In most non-mammalian vertebrates (see above) teeth are rigidly connected (ankylosed) directly to bone, a rather brittle attachment. Only in mammals (and Crocodilia) does a periodontal ligament provide an independent, tough suspension for each tooth. Near the cervical margin, the tooth, periodontal ligament and adjacent bone are covered by the *gingiva* (gum), clearly recognizable in health by its pale pink, stippled appearance (**12**.21). This is continuous at the *mucogingival junction* with the red, smooth oral mucosa lining much of the oral cavity and is adherent to the tooth near the cervical margin by an *epithelial attachment*. The pulp is a connective tissue, continuous with the periodontal ligament via the apical foramen. It contains vessels for the support of the dentine and sensory nerves.

DENTAL MORPHOLOGY

The curvature of the dental arches renders the terms of descriptive anatomy, such as anterior and posterior, inappropriate. The aspect of teeth adjacent to lips or cheeks is therefore termed *labial* or *buccal*,

that adjacent to the tongue being *lingual* or *palatal*. Labial and lingual surfaces of an incisor meet medially at a *mesial* surface and laterally at a *distal* surface, terms also used to describe the equivalent surfaces of premolar and molar (*postcanine*) teeth (**12**.24, 25). Mesial surfaces of postcanine teeth are, of course, directed anteriorly and distal surfaces posteriorly. Thus the point of contact between the central incisors is the datum point for mesial and distal. The biting or *occlusal* surfaces of postcanine teeth are tuberculated by *cusps* separated by *fissures* forming a pattern characteristic of each tooth. The biting surface of an incisor is the *incisal edge*.

PERMANENT TEETH (**12**.22, 24, 25, 39)

The names for teeth in all mammals are based on the appearance, function or position of the equivalent human teeth: they are the *incisors*, *canines*, *premolars* and *molars*.

There are two incisors, a central and a lateral in each half jaw or *quadrant*. In labial view, the crowns are trapezoid, the maxillary incisor, particularly the central, being larger than the mandibular. The biting or *incisal edges* originally have three tubercles or *mammelons* which are rapidly removed by wear. In mesial or distal view their labial profiles are convex; their lingual surfaces are concavo-convex (ogival); the convexity near the cervical margin is due to a low ridge or *cingulum*, prominent only on upper incisors. The roots of incisors are single and rounded in maxillary teeth, but flattened mesiodistally in mandibular teeth.

Distal to each lateral incisor is a rather larger *canine* with a single cusp (hence the American term *cuspid*) instead of an incisal edge. The lingual cingulum is more prominent in the maxillary than in the mandibular canine. The canine root, which is the longest of any tooth, produces a bulge (*canine eminence*) on the bone externally, particularly in the upper jaw. Although canines usually have single roots, that of the lower may sometimes be bifid (Kraus et al 1969).

Distal to the canines are two *premolars*, each with a buccal and lingual cusp (hence the term *bicuspid*). The occlusal surfaces of the upper premolars are oval (the long axis is buccopalatal) with a

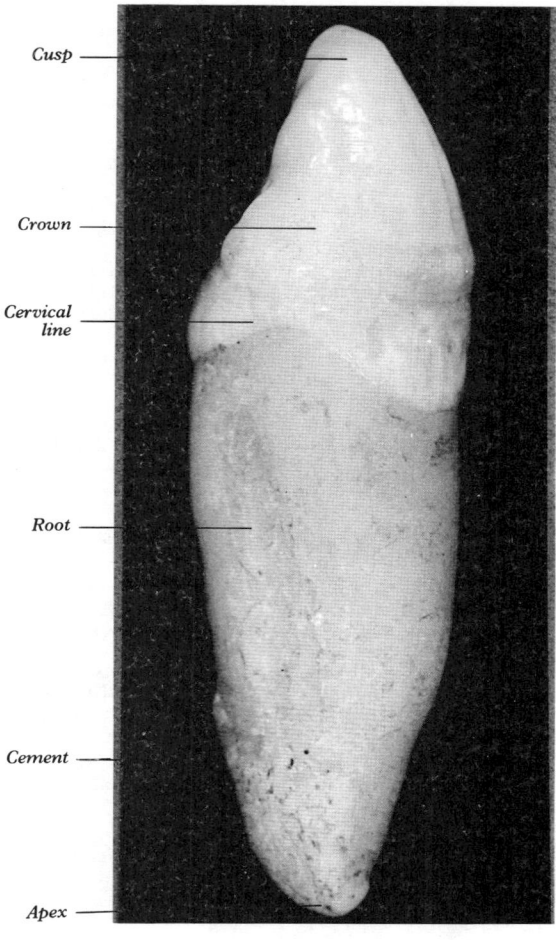

Cusp

Crown

Cervical
line

Root

Cement

Apex

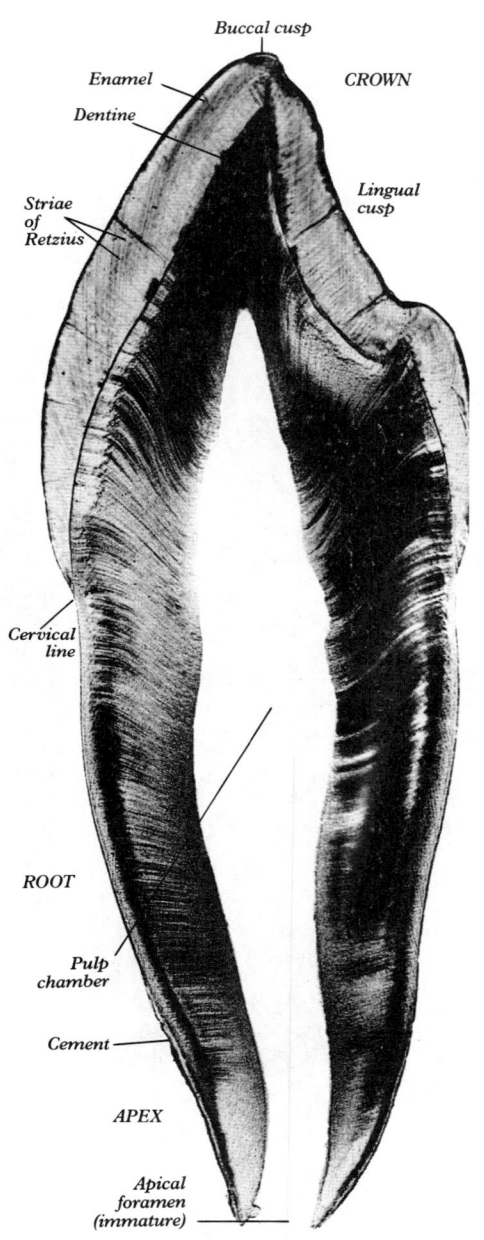

Buccal cusp

Enamel

Dentine

CROWN

Striae
of
Retzius

Lingual
cusp

Cervical
line

ROOT

Pulp
chamber

Cement

APEX

Apical
foramen
(immature)

12.18 An extracted upper right canine tooth viewed from its mesial aspect, showing its principal parts. Note the root covered by cement (partially removed), and the curved cervical margin, convex towards the cusp of the tooth (as also on the distal side of the tooth, not visible here).

12.19 A ground section of a young (permanent) lower first premolar tooth sectioned in the bucco-lingual longitudinal plane, photographed with transmitted light. The coarse dark lines perpendicular to the enamel surface are artefactual cracks caused during grinding of the section; the thinner lines in the enamel running parallel to these cracks indicated the long axes of the enamel prisms. The lines of Retzius are incremental lines of enamel growth (compare with **12.33**). Within the dentine the lines of the dentinal tubules are visible, forming S-shaped curves in the apical region but straighter in the root. The thin layer of cement covering the dentine has been partially removed except where indicated.

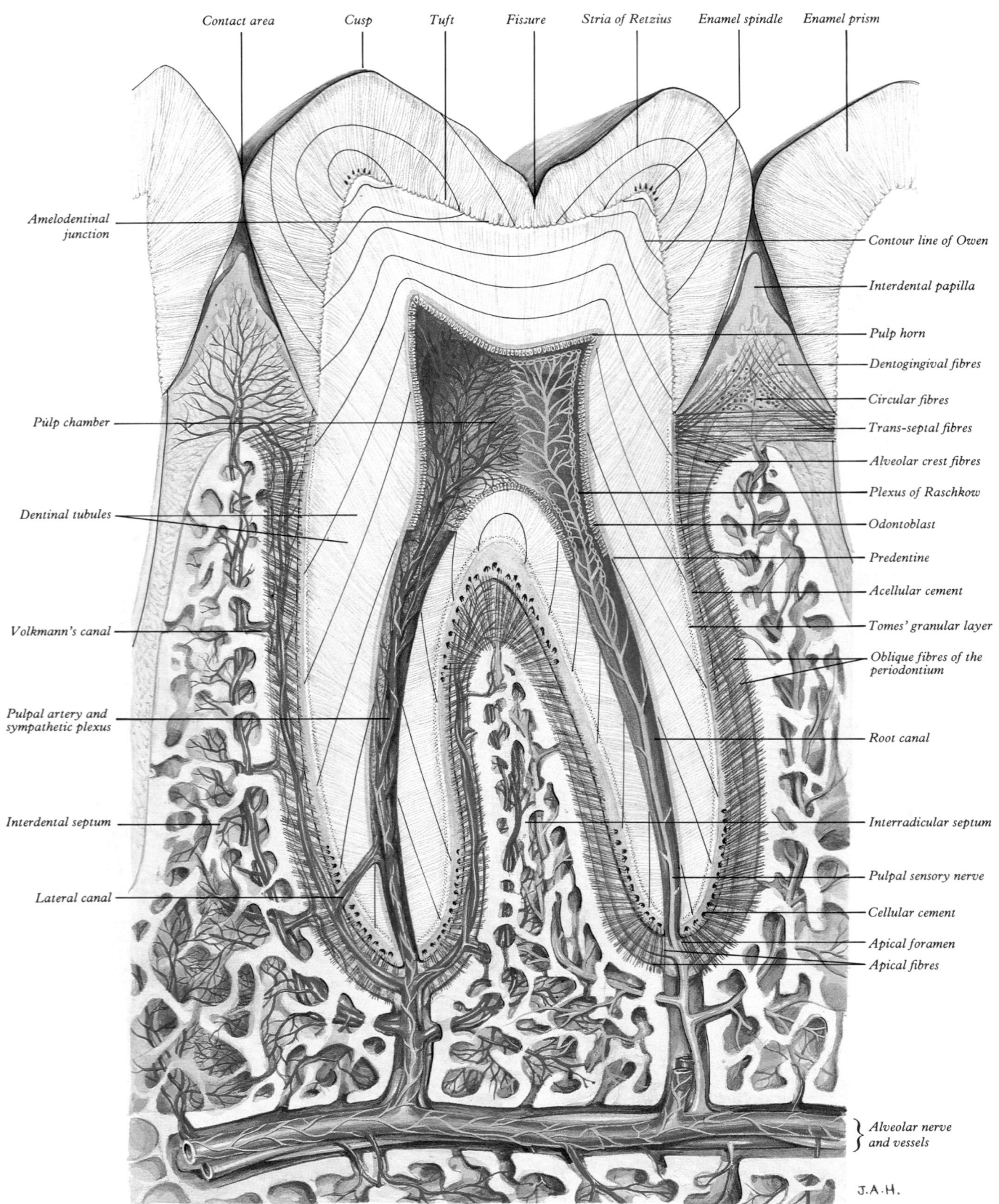

Contact area   Cusp   Tuft   Fissure   Stria of Retzius   Enamel spindle   Enamel prism

Ameloduntinal junction

Contour line of Owen

Interdental papilla

Pulp horn

Dentogingival fibres

Circular fibres

Trans-septal fibres

Alveolar crest fibres

Pulp chamber

Plexus of Raschkow

Odontoblast

Predentine

Dentinal tubules

Acellular cement

Tomes' granular layer

Oblique fibres of the periodontium

Volkmann's canal

Root canal

Pulpal artery and sympathetic plexus

Interradicular septum

Interdental septum

Pulpal sensory nerve

Cellular cement

Lateral canal

Apical foramen

Apical fibres

Alveolar nerve and vessels

J.A.H.

12.20   Diagram of a longitudinal section of a tooth and its environs.

mesiodistal fissure separating the two cusps. In buccal view, premolars resemble the canines but are smaller. The *upper first premolar* usually has two roots (one buccal, one palatal) but may have one and very rarely three roots (two buccal and one palatal). The upper second premolar usually has one root. The occlusal surfaces of the

lower premolars are more circular or square than those of the uppers. The buccal cusp of the lower first premolar towers above the lingual cusp to which it is connected by a ridge separating the mesial and distal occlusal pits. In the lower second premolar a mesiodistal fissure usually separates a buccal from two smaller lingual cusps. Each

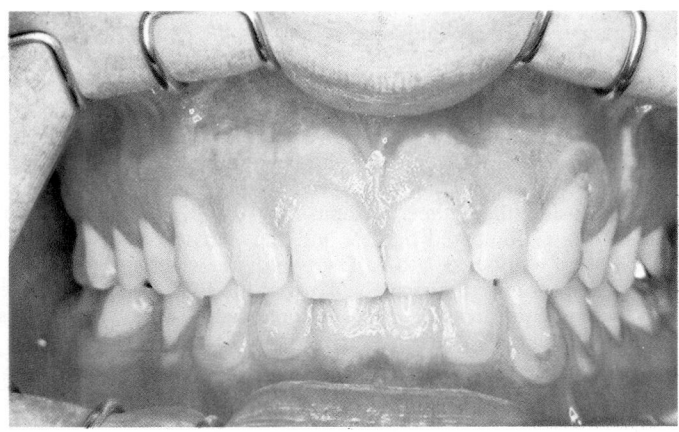

12.21   Anterior view of the dentition in centric occlusion, with the lips retracted. Note the pale pink, stippled gingivae and the red, shiny, smooth alveolar mucosa. The degree of overbite is rather pronounced and the gingiva and its epithelial attachment have receded on to the root of the upper left canine.

lower premolar has one root, but very rarely the root of the first is bifid. Lower second premolars fail to develop in about 2% of individuals (Garn & Lewis 1962).

Posterior to the premolars are three *molars* whose size decreases distally; each has a large rhomboid (upper jaw) or rectangular (lower jaw) occlusal surface with four or five cusps. The upper first molar has a cusp at each corner of its occlusal surface and the mesiopalatal cusp is connected to the distobuccal by an oblique ridge, a primitive feature shared with many lower primates. A fifth cusp, the *cusp of Carabelli*, may appear on the mesiopalatal aspect, most commonly in caucasian races (Kraus 1959; Alvesalo et al 1975). The tooth has three widely separated roots, two buccal and one palatal. The smaller *upper second molar* has a reduced or occasionally absent distopalatal cusp; its three roots are divergent and two of them may be fused. The *upper third molar*, the smallest, usually has three cusps (the distopalatal being absent) and commonly one root. The *lower first molar* has three buccal and two lingual cusps on its rectangular occlusal surface, the smallest being distobuccal. The cusps of this tooth are all separated by fissures; it has two widely separated roots, one mesial and one distal. The smaller *lower second molar* is like the first but usually lacks the distobuccal cusp and its (two) roots are closer together. The *lower third molar* is smaller still and like the upper third molar it is variable in form. Its crown may resemble that of the lower first or second molar and its roots are frequently fused. Because it erupts anterosuperiorly it is often impacted against the second molar whereas the upper third molar erupts postero-inferiorly and is rarely impacted. In various populations one or more third molars, upper or lower, fail to develop in 0.2–25% of individuals (Brothwell et al 1963). In general, absence of third molars is commoner in mongoloid and caucasian than in negroid races.

DECIDUOUS TEETH (**12**.23, 48)

The incisors, canine and premolars of the permanent dentition replace two deciduous incisors, a deciduous canine and two deciduous molars in each jaw quadrant (**12**.23). The deciduous incisors and canine are shaped like their successors but are smaller and whiter

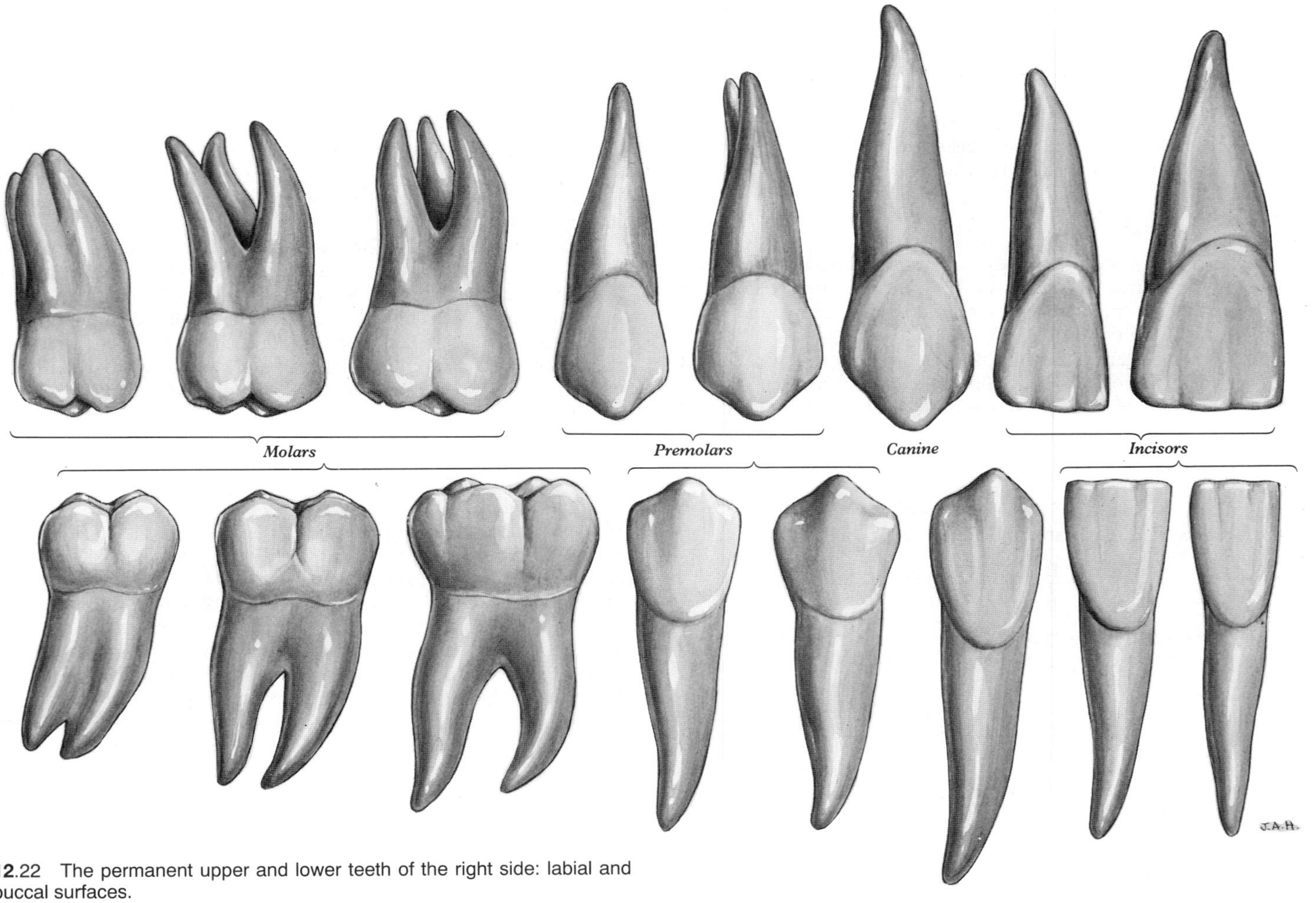

Molars   *Premolars*   *Canine*   *Incisors*

12.22   The permanent upper and lower teeth of the right side: labial and buccal surfaces.

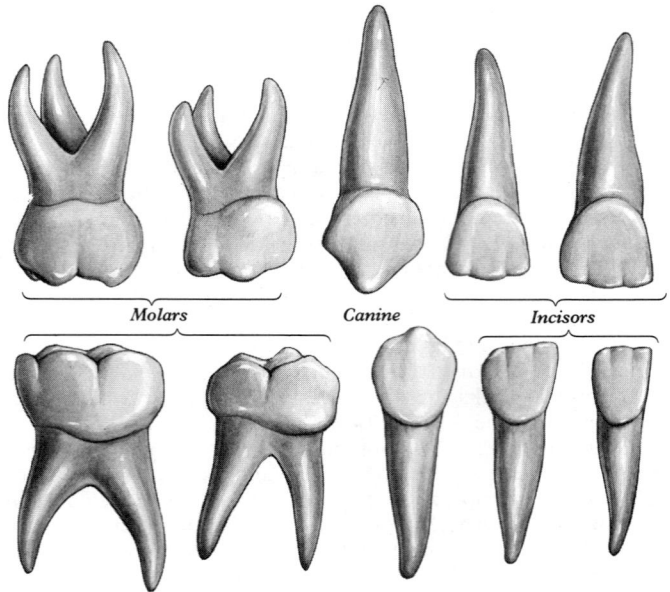

12.23 The deciduous upper and lower teeth of the right side: labial and buccal surfaces.

and become extremely worn in older children. The deciduous molars resemble permanent ones rather than their successors, the premolars. Each second deciduous molar has a crown almost identical to that of the posteriorly adjacent first permanent molar. The *upper first deciduous molar* has a triangular occlusal surface (its rounded 'apex' being palatal) and a fissure separates a double buccal cusp from the palatal cusp. The *lower first deciduous molar* is long and narrow; its two buccal cusps are separated from the two lingual cusps by a zigzagging mesiodistal fissure. Like permanent molars, upper deciduous molars have three roots and lower deciduous molars have two roots; these diverge more than those of permanent teeth since each developing premolar is accommodated directly under the crown of its deciduous predecessor. The roots of deciduous teeth are progressively resorbed by osteoclasts prior to being shed. An extracted deciduous tooth may thus have very short roots.

TOOTH DESIGNATION

Communication between clinicians, often nowadays using computer technology, requires a simple method of indicating each tooth. Unfortunately, no single system is internationally accepted and three methods are currently in use.

The Palmer System uses a horizontal line and a vertical line to partition the dentition into four qudrants and then assigns a number from 1 to 8 to the teeth in each quadrant, beginning with the central incisor:

Right $\dfrac{8\ 7\ 6\ 5\ 4\ 3\ 2\ 1\ \big|\ 1\ 2\ 3\ 4\ 5\ 6\ 7\ 8}{8\ 7\ 6\ 5\ 4\ 3\ 2\ 1\ \big|\ 1\ 2\ 3\ 4\ 5\ 6\ 7\ 8}$ Left

Deciduous teeth are indicated by capital letters A–E:

$$\dfrac{E\ \ D\ \ C\ \ B\ \ A\ \big|\ A\ \ B\ \ C\ \ D\ \ E}{E\ \ D\ \ C\ \ B\ \ A\ \big|\ A\ \ B\ \ C\ \ D\ \ E}$$

The Universal System, popular in the USA, assigns a unique number to each tooth, beginning with the upper right third permanent molar:

1	2	3	4	5	6	7	8	9	10	11	12	13	14	15	16
32	31	30	29	28	27	26	25	24	23	22	21	20	19	18	17

In the universal system, deciduous teeth are indicated by capital letters, beginning with the upper right second deciduous molar (A) and ending with the lower right second deciduous molar (T).

While the universal system is compatible with information storage and transmission using computer technology, its major disadvantage

is the need to memorise a different number or letter for each of the 32 permanent or 20 deciduous teeth. This led the Federation Dentaire Internationale to introduce the Two Digit System. Each tooth is designated by two numbers. The first number indicates the quadrant in which the tooth is situated. In the permanent dentition, the quadrants are numbered 1 to 4 in a clockwise direction when the dentition is viewed from in front and beginning with the upper right quadrant. The second number specifies the individual teeth in a quadrant using the Palmer system. For the deciduous dentition, quadrants are numbered 5 to 8 and the individual teeth in each quadrant are numbered 1 to 5. The two digits which designate each tooth are pronounced separately. Thus in the FDI system the upper right permanent canine is 13 (one-three) and the lower left first deciduous molar is 74 (seven-four).

VARIATIONS IN TOOTH NUMBER, SIZE AND FORM

Variation in number and form, the incidence of which is often related to race, is rare in deciduous teeth but not uncommon in the permanent dentition. One or more teeth may fail to develop, a condition known as *hypodontia*; conversely, additional or *supernumerary* teeth may form, producing *hyperdontia*. The third permanent molar is the most frequently missing tooth: Brothwell et al (1963) found that one or more third molars failed to form in 32% of Chinese mongoloids, 24% of English caucasians and 2.5% of West African negroids. Other missing teeth are, in declining order of incidence, maxillary lateral incisors, maxillary or mandibular second premolars, mandibular central incisors and maxillary first premolars.

Hyperdontia affects the maxillary arch much more commonly than the mandibular dentition (Stafne 1932): the extra teeth are usually situated on the palatal aspect of the permanent incisors or distal to the molars. More rarely, additional premolars develop. Although supernumerary teeth in the incisor region are often small with simple conical crowns, they may impede the eruption of the permanent incisors. A supernumerary tooth situated between the central incisors is known as a *mesiodens*. Teeth may be unusually large (*macrodontia*) or small (*microdontia*). For example, the crowns of maxillary central incisors may be abnormally wide mesiodistally; in contrast, a common variant of the maxillary lateral incisor has a small, peg-shaped crown.

Epidemiological studies reveal that hyperdontia tends to be associated with macrodontia and hypodontia with microdontia, the most severely affected individuals representing the extremes of a continuum of variation. Together with family studies, this indicates that the causation is multifactorial, combining polygenic and environmental influences (Brook 1984).

Some variations in the form of teeth, being characteristic of race, are of anthropological and forensic interest. Mongoloid dentitions tend to have shovel-shaped maxillary incisors with enlarged palatal marginal ridges. The additional cusp of Carabelli is commonly found on the mesiopalatal aspect of maxillary first permanent or second deciduous molars in caucasian but rarely in mongoloid dentitions (Kraus 1959). In negroid races the mandibular second permanent molar often has five rather than four cusps.

DENTAL OCCLUSION

It is possible to bring the jaws together so that the teeth meet or *occlude* in many positions (Kraus et al 1969). When opposing occlusal surfaces meet with maximal 'intercuspation' (i.e. maximum contact), the teeth are said to be in *centric occlusion* (**12**.26, 27). In this position the lower teeth are normally opposed symmetrically and lingually with respect to the upper. Some important features of centric occlusion in a normal dentition must be noted. Each lower postcanine tooth is slightly in front of its upper equivalent and the lower canine is in front of the upper. Buccal cusps of the lower postcanine teeth lie between the buccal and palatal cusps of the upper teeth. Thus the lower postcanine teeth are slightly lingual and mesial to their upper equivalents. Lower incisors bite against the lingual surfaces of upper incisors, the latter normally obscuring about one-third of the crowns of the lower. This vertical overlap of incisors in centric occlusion is the *overbite*. The extent to which upper incisors are anterior to lowers is the *overjet*. In the most habitual jaw position, the *resting posture*, the teeth are slightly apart, the gap between being the *free-way space* or *interocclusal clearance*.

Each dental arch is approximately *catenary*, the form of a chain suspended at both ends (MacConaill & Scher 1949), the lower arch being slightly narrower (**12**.24, 25). Viewed from the side, a line joining the buccal cusps of the upper postcanine teeth is curved (*curve of Spee*), concave upwards. The lower molar teeth are tilted slightly lingually so that a line joining the buccal and lingual cusps of the left and right lower first molars is curved (*curve of Monson*), concave upwards. These curvatures accord with movements of the mandible during mastication and are important in the construction of dentures.

DENTAL BLOOD AND LYMPHATIC VESSELS

The *inferior alveolar artery*, a branch of the maxillary artery, enters the mandibular foramen and travels forwards in its canal to divide into *incisive* and *mental* branches to supply the lower teeth, their supporting structures and the mandibular body, including its cortical bone (Saunders and Röckert 1967). About eight to 12 main rami and variable finer ones supply alveolar bone and teeth (Castelli 1963). Few anastomotic vessels cross the symphysis (Howkins 1935). Veins from alveolar bone and teeth collect either into larger vessels in the interdental septa or into plexuses around the dental apices and thence into several *inferior alveolar veins*; some of these drain through the mental foramen to the facial vein, others via the mandibular foramen to the pterygoid venous plexus (Cohen 1959).

The upper jaw is supplied by *anterior* and *posterior superior alveolar arteries*. The *posterior superior alveolar artery*, from the maxillary artery, gives off branches over the maxillary tuberosity, supplying alveolar bone, mucosa and teeth in the molar region and adjacent buccal mucosa, where they anastomose with the penetrating branches of the facial artery. Other rami supply the lateral wall of the maxillary sinus. The *anterior superior alveolar artery*, a branch of the infraorbital, curves through the *canalis sinuosus* (Jones 1939), which swerves laterally from the infraorbital canal and inferomedially below it in the wall of the maxillary sinus, following the rim of the anterior nasal aperture, between the alveoli of canine and incisor teeth and the nasal cavity; it ends near the nasal septum where its terminal branch emerges. The canal may be up to 55 mm long. Occasionally a small *middle superior alveolar artery* forms anastomotic arcades with the anterior and posterior vessels. On the palatal aspect of the upper teeth, the *greater palatine artery* supplies the palatal gingiva, and its terminal branch ascends through the incisive canal to anastomose with septal branches of the nasopalatine artery. Veins accompanying the superior alveolar arteries drain anteriorly into the facial vein, or posteriorly into the pterygoid venous plexus.

The periodontal ligaments are supplied by *dental branches* of alveolar arteries. One branch enters the alveolus apically and, of its small rami, two or three pass into the dental pulp through the apical foramen, others ascending in the periodontal ligament. *Interdental arteries* ascend in the interdental septa, sending branches at right angles into the ligament, and terminate by communicating with gingival vessels. Thus the ligament receives its blood from three sources: from the apical region, ascending interdental arteries and descending vessels from the gingiva; all anastomose with each other. Veins drain the periodontal ligament either into the *interdental veins* or into the *periapical plexus*. Longer vessels seen in the ligament are probably veins rather than anastomosing arteries (Folke & Stallard 1967).

Lymphatic drainage of human jaws and teeth is uncertain (Saunders & Röckert 1967). Injection techniques in monkeys (MacGregor 1936) suggest that the upper jaw drains mainly to the submandibular and thence to supraclavicular lymph nodes, the lower to submental and on to the paratracheal nodes. Many dental abscesses lead to enlargement of the submandibular and upper deep cervical lymph nodes, indicating a common path for lymphatic drainage of the upper and lower teeth. Buccal lymph nodes may be affected by infection of the upper teeth. Lower incisors drain to the submental nodes and thence either to the submandibular or lower

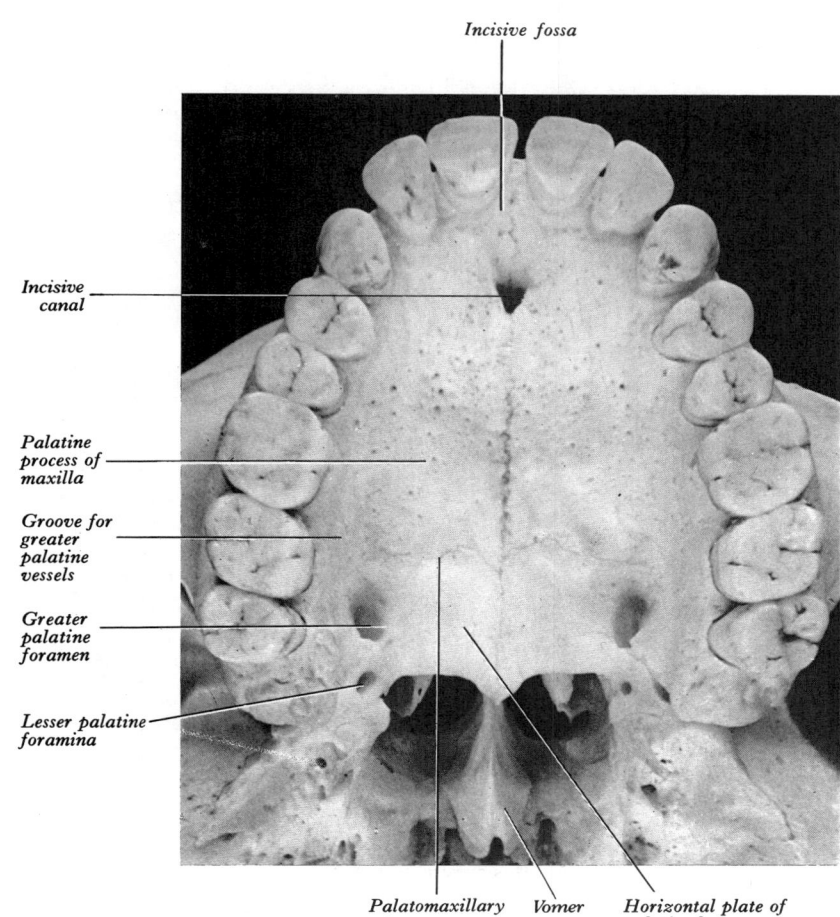

12.24 The permanent teeth of the upper dental arch: inferior aspect.

Incisive fossa

Incisive canal

Palatine process of maxilla

Groove for greater palatine vessels

Greater palatine foramen

Lesser palatine foramina

Palatomaxillary suture   *Vomer*   *Horizontal plate of palatine bone*

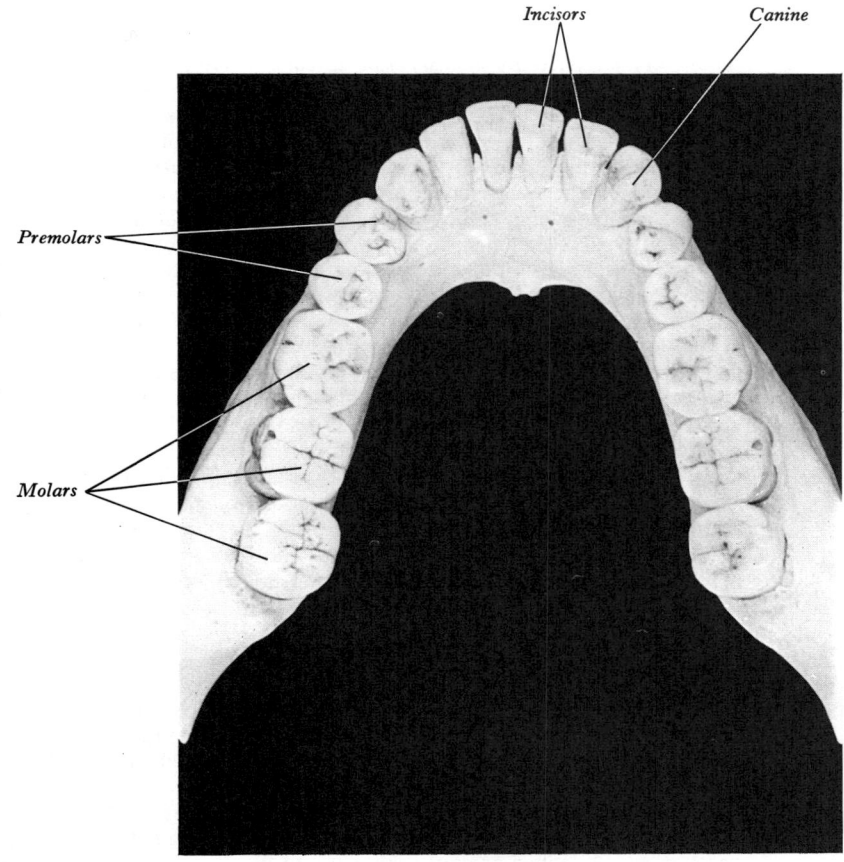

12.25 The permanent teeth of the lower dental arch: superior aspect.

Incisors   *Canine*

Premolars

Molars

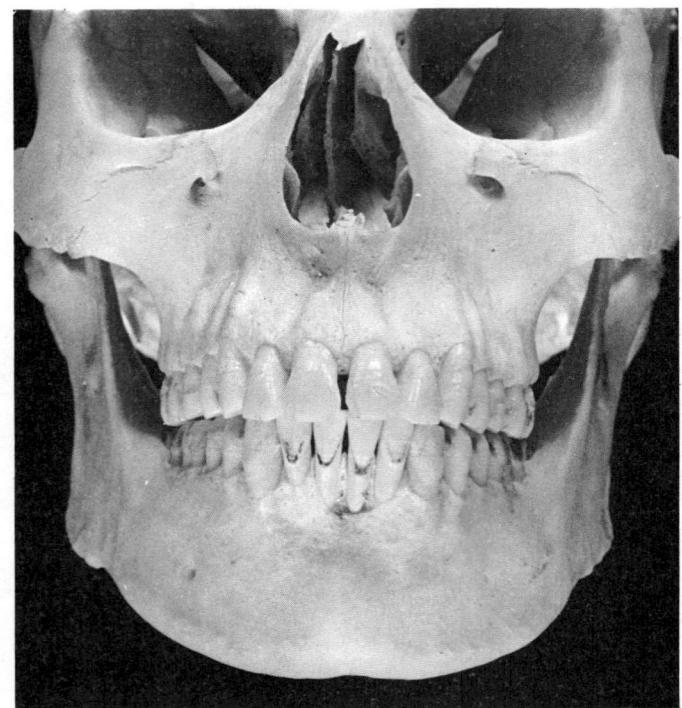

12.26 Anterior view of the dentition in centric occlusion. There has been some resorption of bone around the lower incisors.

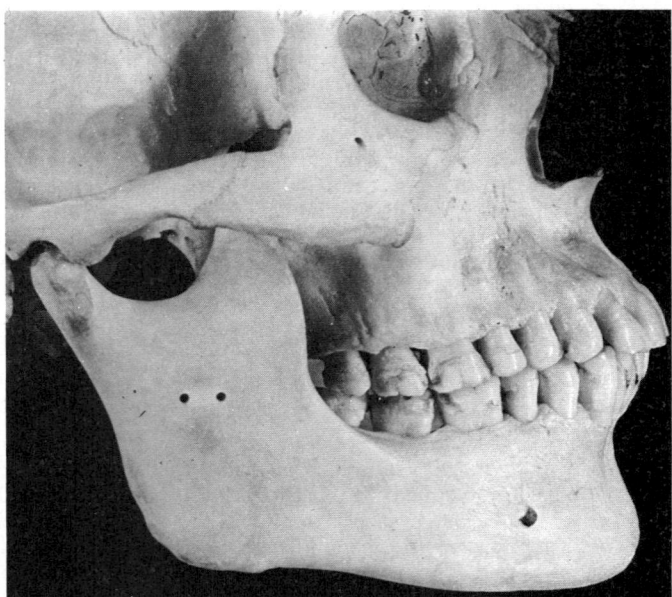

12.27 Lateral view of the dentition in centric occlusion.

deep cervical nodes. It is presumed that the alveolar bone, periodontal ligament and gingiva share the same route.

DENTAL INNERVATION

Upper teeth

These are supplied by the *superior alveolar nerves*, *anterior* and *posterior*; in 80% of individuals a *middle* nerve is also present (Fitzgerald & Scott 1958). These nerves supply a plexus lying above the apices of the teeth, partly on the posterior surface of the maxilla and partly within canals in the lateral and anterior surfaces of the bone (**12.20**). The *buccal nerve* provides a variable contribution to the buccal molar gingiva; the *greater palatine* and *nasopalatine* nerves pass to the palatal gingiva, overlapping in the region of the canine tooth. Surgical division of the nasopalatine nerve causes no obvious sensory deficit in the anterior palate, suggesting that the territory of the greater palatine nerve reaches as far forwards as the gingiva lingual to the incisor teeth (Langford 1989).

The *posterior superior alveolar nerves* are two or three trunks from the postorbital section of the maxillary nerve (**8.339**). They divide into several rami within the periosteum and enter widely scattered foramina on the maxilla's posterior surface. Higher branches descend outside the antral mucosa to meet lower branches passing forwards above the teeth. The variable *middle alveolar nerve*, which may branch anywhere along the orbital part of the maxillary nerve, runs down the antral wall; the *anterior alveolar nerve* occupies the *canalis sinuosus* (p. 1705). The bony canals of the superior alveolar nerves also contain corresponding arteries forming the *superior alveolar neurovascular bundles*.

Lower jaw and its alveolar bone

These are largely supplied by the *inferior alveolar nerve*, with branches of the *buccal nerve* to the buccal gingiva of the molar and premolar teeth and branches of the *lingual nerve* to the lingual gingiva of all the lower teeth.

In its commonest form (six out of eight mandibles studied by Carter & Keen 1971), the inferior alveolar nerve is single, travelling through a well-defined osseous canal close to the dental roots (**12.28**, 39), supplying individual branches to these and the interdental septa.

Between the premolar teeth the mental nerve, often multiple, leaves via the mental foramen. Intraosseous *incisive nerves* continue to supply the first premolar, canine and incisor teeth. Branches leave the mental nerve at its origin to form an *incisor plexus* labial to the teeth, probably supplying their labial periodontium and gingiva. From this plexus and the dental branches, rami turn down and then lingually to emerge on the lingual surface of the mandible on the posterior aspect of the symphysis or opposite the premolar teeth, probably communicating with the lingual or mylohyoid nerve.

Less commonly (two out of eight mandibles in the above study), the inferior alveolar nerve was close to the lower border of the mandible, well below the roots of the teeth (**12.28**) with a variable number of large rami passing anterosuperiorly towards the roots before dividing to supply the teeth and interdental septa.

In three out of eight dissected mandibles nerves passed from the temporal muscle to enter the mandible through the retromolar fossa, communicating with branches of the inferior alveolar nerve. Foramina occur in about 10% of retromolar fossae (Azaz &

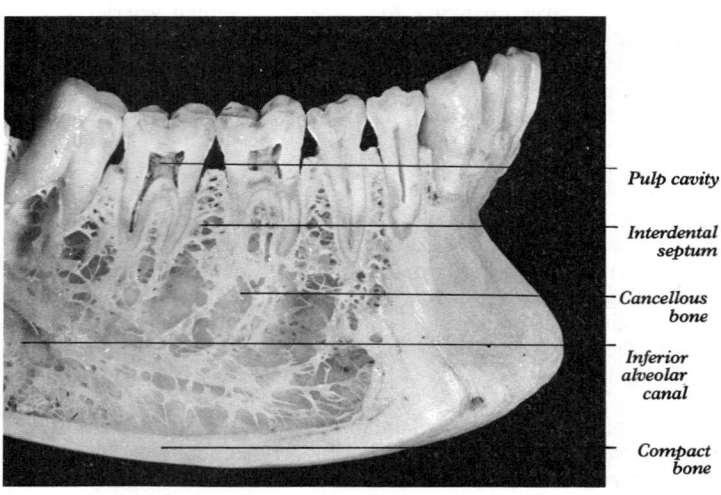

Pulp cavity

Interdental septum

Cancellous bone

Inferior alveolar canal

Compact bone

12.28 Anterior part of the right mandible, with the superficial bone removed on the buccal side to show the roots of a number of teeth, some of which have also been sectioned vertically. Note: the cortical plate of compact bone lining the sockets of the teeth (the lamina dura of radiographs: see **12.50–53**), and the flat table of bone surmounting the interdental bone septa. In this specimen the inferior alveolar canal is widely separated from the roots of the teeth, a variable condition.

Lustmann 1973) and infiltration in this region can abolish sensation, occasionally remaining after an inferior alveolar nerve block. Similarly, branches from the buccal, mylohyoid and lingual nerves which enter the mandible may provide additional routes of sensory transmission from the teeth.

The lower central incisor teeth receive a bilateral innervation, fibres probably crossing the midline within the periosteum to re-enter the bone via numerous canals in the labial cortical plate (Rood 1977).

Local and regional analgesia

For restorative procedures, it is sufficient to block conduction in nerves supplying the pulp of a tooth; but for surgical operations on the jaws, such as the extraction of teeth, it is also necessary to obtain analgesia of their supporting tissues: the alveolar bone, gingiva and periodontal ligament. In the upper jaw, where the outer alveolar bone is thin, analgesia of teeth as well as the labial and buccal periodontium is achieved by local infiltration of an anaesthetic solution into the submucosa of the sulcus adjacent to the root apices. In extracting maxillary teeth, analgesia of palatal alveolar bone and gingiva requires a submucosal infiltration next to the tooth on its palatal aspect or blockage of the greater palatine or nasopalatine nerves near the foramina where they enter the oral cavity.

Pulpal analgesia of mandibular incisors and canines can be obtained by submucosal infiltration in the labial sulcus; an infiltration on the lingual aspect will complete analgesia of the supporting tissues when extracting these teeth. Because the alveolar bone supporting the mandibular premolars and molars is thick, particularly on the buccal aspect, local infiltration is not effective in producing pulpal analgesia and a regional block of the inferior alveolar nerve is required. With the mouth wide open and the syringe directed from the region of the contralateral premolar teeth, the needle penetrates the mucosa and buccinator muscle immediately anterior to the stretched pterygomandibular raphe, and anaesthetic solution is deposited around the inferior alveolar nerve just above the mandibular foramen. An aspirating syringe is recommended to prevent accidental injection into nearby blood vessels. In the majority of cases, such a regional block will produce pulpal analgesia of all mandibular teeth on the injected side of the jaw, apart from the central mandibular incisor which is usually partly supplied by fibres from the contralateral nerve. However, because of individual variations in the nerve supply of teeth (see above), buccal and lingual infiltrations adjacent to the operative site may be needed to obtain full pulpal analgesia. For tooth extraction, when analgesia of the lingual alveolar bone and mucosa is essential, the lingual nerve can be blocked as it runs anteromedial to the inferior alveolar nerve. Additionally, an injection is required in the buccal sulcus to prevent conduction in the buccal nerve.

DENTAL HISTOLOGY

DENTINE (12.18–20, 29–31, 33, 34, 39)

Dentine is yellowish avascular tissue forming the bulk of the tooth. It is a tough (work of fracture, $Wf = 270$–550 J/m^2) and compliant (stiffness $= 12 \text{ GN/m}^2$) composite material, about 70% by weight mineral (largely crystalline hydroxyapatite and fluorapatite but some calcium carbonate) and 20% organic matrix (type I collagen fibres, glycosaminoglycans and phosphoprotein, Weinstock & Leblond 1973). Its conspicuous feature is the regular pattern of microscopic dentinal tubules, about 1–2 μm in diameter, extending from the pulpal surface (about 50 000 tubules per 1 sq mm cross-sectional area) to the enamel–dentine junction (about 20 000 per sq mm). Tubules have a single sinuous primary curvature (12.19) oriented apically and more pronounced in the crown. A spiral secondary curvature, less regular, has a periodicity and amplitude of a few microns. Near the enamel–dentine junction tubules bifurcate, some with short extensions into enamel. Abundant lateral branches interconnect adjacent tubules (12.29). Each tubule encloses a single cytoplasmic process of an odontoblast, containing microtubules, microfilaments but few ribosomes or mitochondria. Odontoblast cell bodies are in a pseudostratified layer lining the pulpal surface. In newly erupted teeth, processes are believed to extend the full thickness

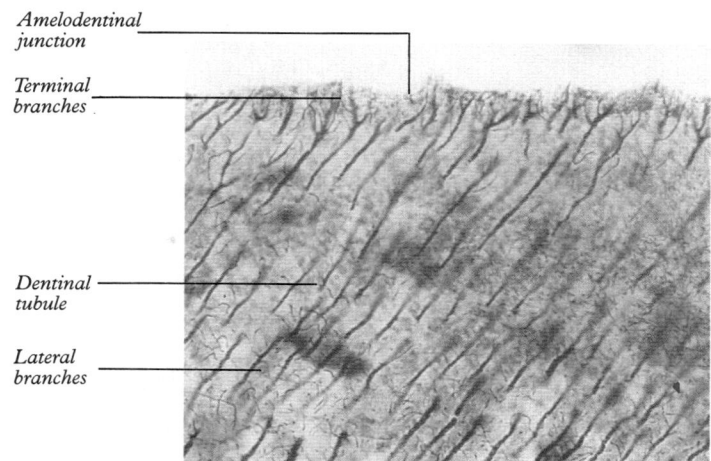

12.29   A demineralized section of dentine, cut in the plane of the dentinal tubules, showing their lateral and, near the ameloddentinal junction, terminal branching. Magnification × 600. (Provided by D. Luke, Department of Anatomy and Cell Biology, UMDS, Guy's Campus, London.)

of dentine (Sigal et al 1984; Holland 1985) but in older teeth may be partly withdrawn so as to occupy only the pulpal third, the outer regions containing extracellular fluid (Thomas 1979). Lining most tubules is a heavily mineralized cylinder of peritubular dentine, devoid of collagen fibres, separated from the plasma membrane of the process by a glycosaminoglycan-rich lamina limitans (Thomas & Carella 1983). It is uncertain whether the process directly abuts the lamina limitans or whether there is a fluid-filled periodontoblastic space separating them.

Between the odontoblasts and the dentine is a layer of non-mineralized matrix, the *predentine* (12.30, 31). The predentine–dentine border is irregularly scalloped (12.30) because dentine mineralizes as microscopic spherical aggregates of crystals (calcospherites). The enamel–dentine junction is more regularly scalloped, with convexities towards the dentine, a pattern unrelated to mineralization. Next to the enamel–dentine junction is a 30–40 μm layer (mantle dentine) which is less mineralized and has collagen fibres arranged parallel to the tubules. In the remaining circumpulpal dentine, fine collagen fibres are perpendicular to and interwoven around the tubules.

Dentine, like enamel is deposited incrementally and is not remodelled. Both tissues carry a permanent record of changing shape, rhythmical formation and disturbances during development. The nomenclature of the resulting pattern of lines seen in sections of dentine has been revised by Dean et al (1993) and is used here. Fine *incremental lines of von Ebner*, 2–5 μm apart in the bulk of dentine, record diurnal alterations in the orientation of collagen fibres and

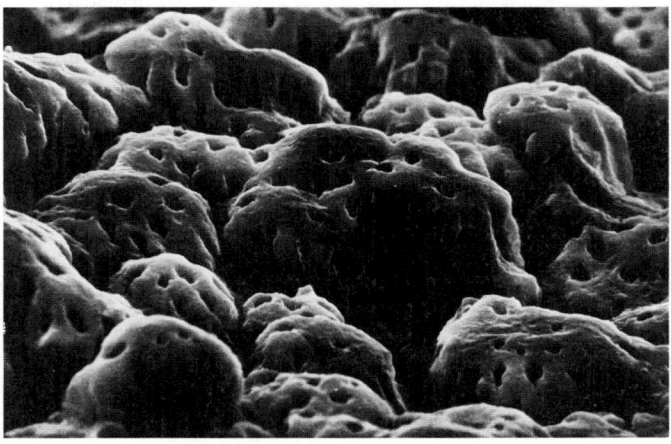

12.30   Surfaces of calcospherites. The holes (about 1 μm wide) are dentinal tubules. (Provided by D Whittaker, The Dental School, University of Wales, Cardiff.)

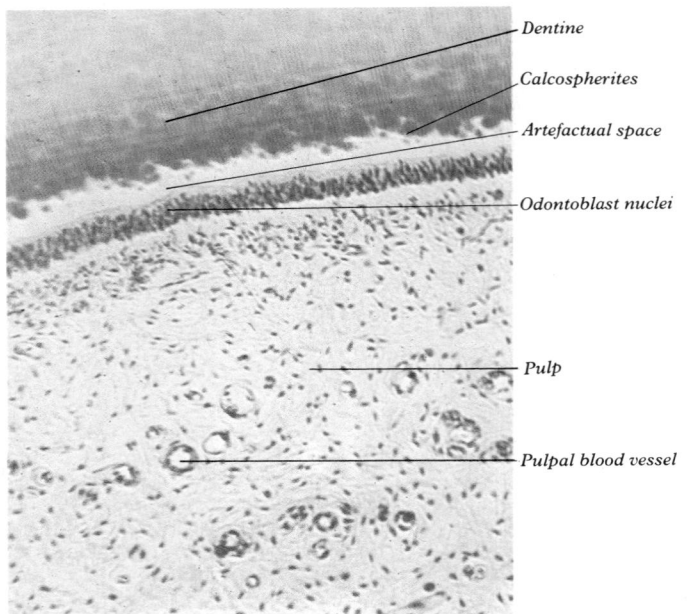

12.31 Section of a demineralized tooth showing the junctional region between the pulp and dentine, sectioned parallel to the plane of the dentinal tubules. Haematoxylin and eosin. For details see text.

levels of mineralization. Longer periodicity lines, 15–30 μm apart, occur at intervals of 6 to 10 days. These are now referred to as *Andresen lines* and are equivalent to the Retzius lines in enamel. A third type, at irregularly spaced intervals, is due to the coincidence of slight variations in direction of the dentinal tubules. These *contour lines of Owen* do not represent incremental growth but probably reflect minor disturbances in tooth formation due to illness or malnutrition. As in enamel, a prominent feature is formed in dentine where mineralization spans birth (all deciduous teeth and usually the first permanent molars); this is the *neonatal line*, a result of the associated abrupt changes in environment and nutrition. During dentinal development, failure of fusion of calcospherites produces interglobular areas. Often regarded as evidence of defective dentinogenesis, they are so common in a region 100–300 μm from the enamel–dentine junction that they must be considered normal.

The outermost 10 μm of root dentine, the hyaline layer (Owens 1972), may incorporate enamel matrix proteins secreted by the epithelial root sheath (Schonfeld & Slavkin 1977). Internal to this is the granular layer of Tomes (**12**.32), whose granularity may be due to minute interglobular areas or to small terminal expansions and anastomoses of adjacent odontoblast processes (Ten Cate 1972).

Primary dentine formation proceeds at a steady but declining rate as first the crown and then the root is completed. Further reduction in the size of the pulp chamber continues throughout life with the very slow and intermittent deposition of secondary dentine, sometimes distinguished from primary dentine by an Owen line and by a sudden change in direction of dentinal tubules. If dentine receives a severe stimulus (e.g. rapidly advancing caries or wear, tooth breakage) the odontoblasts of the affected region die, leaving a dead tract. This is sealed pulpally by a thin zone of sclerosed dentine and the deposition by newly differentiated pulp cells of reparative dentine, a poorly mineralized and sporadically formed tissue with few and irregular tubules. A less severe stimulus results in the odontoblasts increasing the deposition of peritubular dentine so as to fill the tubules. In ground sections this dentine appears translucent because it has assumed a near-uniform refractive index. Translucent dentine also develops with age near the root apices.

DENTAL PULP (**12**.20, 31, 33, 34, 39)

The pulp is a well-vascularized volume of loose connective tissue, enclosed by dentine (Frank & Nalbandian 1989). It is continuous with the periodontal ligament via the apical and accessory foramina.

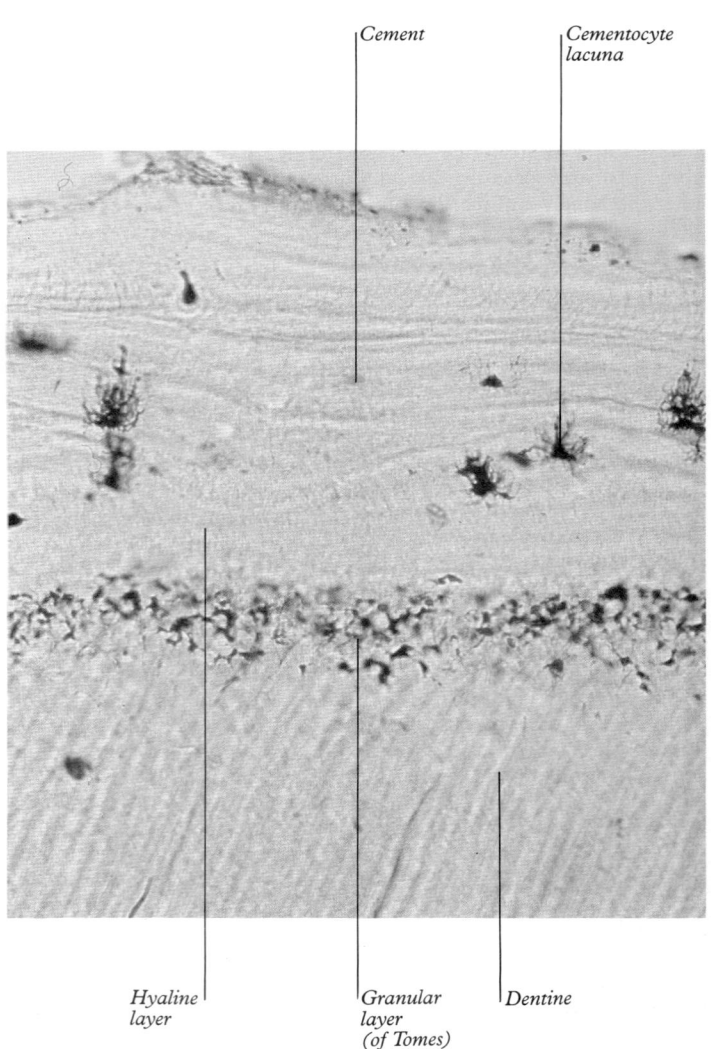

12.32 Ground, unstained longitudinal section of the root of a tooth, showing the cementum and superficial dentine. Note in the cementum the dark lacunae with projecting canaliculi, originally occupied by cementocytes and their processes. Magnification × 800. (Provided by D. Luke, Department of Anatomy and Cell Biology, UMDS, Guy's Campus, London.)

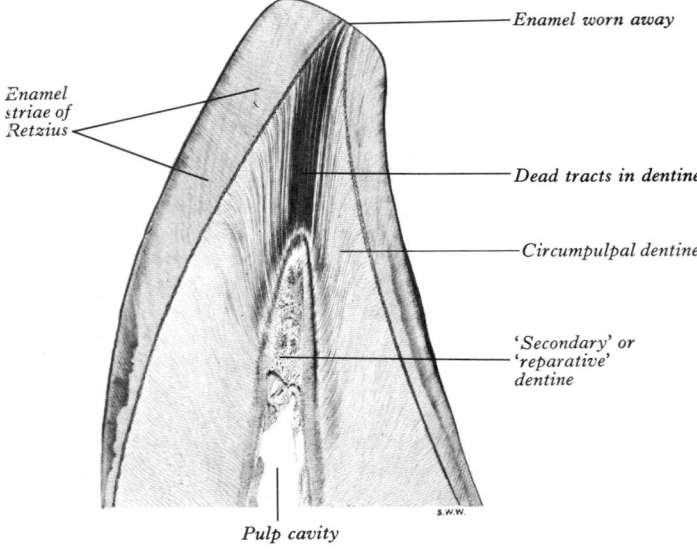

12.33 Longitudinal ground section of an incisor tooth. Compare the brown striae labelled on this section with those visible on **12**.19.

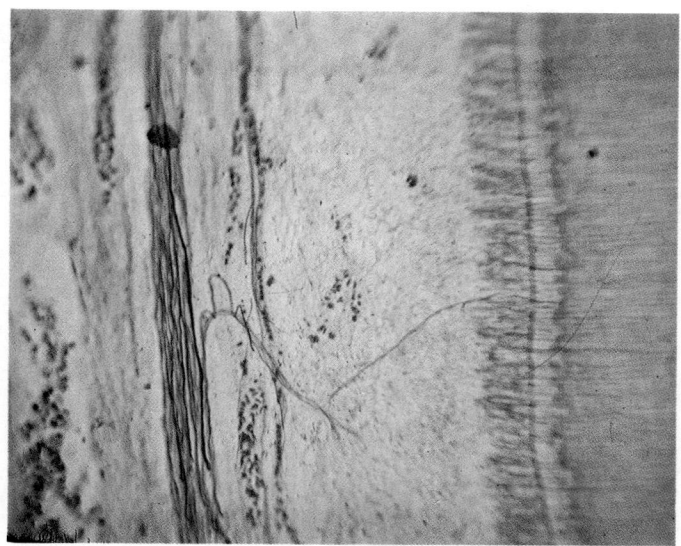

12.34 Longitudinal demineralized section of a tooth stained with a silver impregnation technique. Note the vertical nerve trunk (left of centre) within the pulp, with fine nerve fibres, one of which crosses transversely to pass between the odontoblasts lining the surface of the predentine (the pale-staining vertical layer, right of centre).

Several thin-walled arterioles enter by the apical foramen to run longitudinally, giving branches to an extensive subodontoblastic plexus (Takahashi et al 1982). Capillary loops may also occur in the odontoblast layer. Blood flow, in terms of rate per unit volume, is greater in the pulp than in other oral tissues (Kim 1990). Micropuncture measurements of interstitial fluid pressure (5–8 mmHg) indicate that it is much lower than hitherto supposed (Tonder & Kvinnsland 1983). Several small veins and lymphatic vessels (Bernick & Patek 1969) emerge from the pulp. Unmyelinated postganglionic sympathetic nerve fibres from the superior cervical ganglion enter the pulp with the arterioles. Myelinated (Aδ) and unmyelinated (C) sensory nerve fibres from the trigeminal ganglion traverse the pulp longitudinally (**12.**34) giving branches to ramify in the *plexus of Raschkow* (Scheinin & Light 1969) in the cell-rich parietal zone. Here fibres lose their myelin sheaths and continue into the odontoblast layer, some entering the dentinal tubules. Intratubular nerves are distinguishable from odontoblast processes

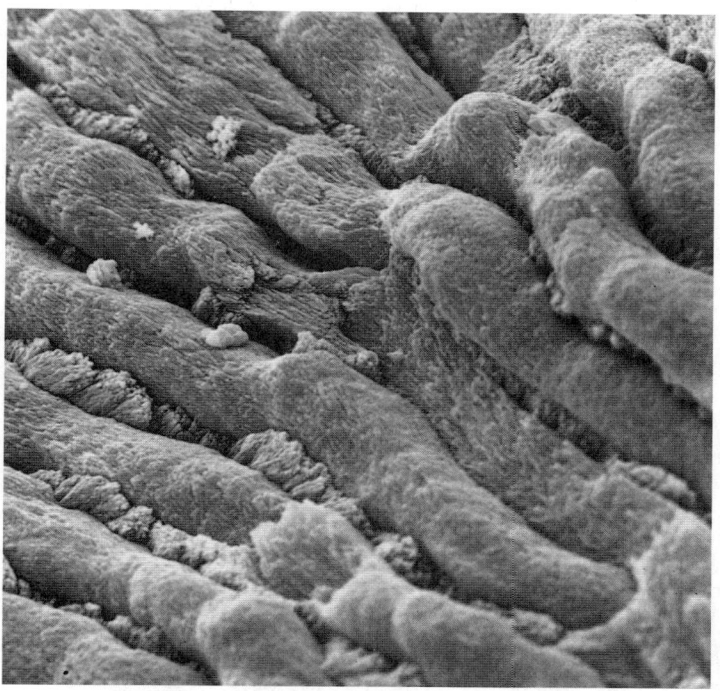

12.35B Scanning electron micrograph of the surface of fractured enamel at a higher magnification than **12.**35A. The rope-like prisms run approximately parallel to each other and show periodic variations in thickness, representing daily growth increments. Abrupt alterations in the direction of individual prisms are responsible for the appearance of the striae of Retzius. (Provided by D Luke, Department of Anatomy and Cell Biology, UMDS, Guy's Campus, London.)

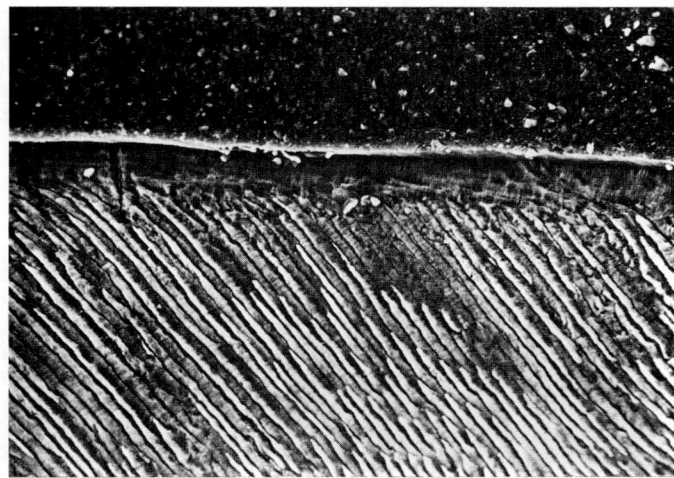

12.35A Scanning electron micrograph of enamel prisms. Each prism is about 5 μm wide and separated from adjacent prisms by interprismatic material which has been removed from this specimen by acid etching. A thick structureless surface layer is present. (Provided by D Whittaker, The Dental School, University of Wales, Cardiff).

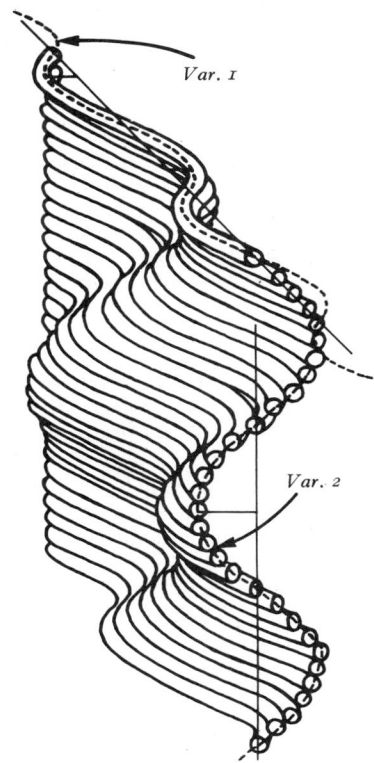

12.36 Diagram illustrating the relationships existing between a vertical stack of enamel prisms. Each prism undulates in the transverse plane of the tooth but its undulations are out of phase with those of vertically adjacent prisms. Hence, when a section is viewed by reflected light, the undulations are responsible for the characteristic alternation of dark and light bands which cross the prisms obliquely (the Hunter-Schreger bands). Var. 1 and 2 indicate the sine-wave undulations in the transverse and vertical planes, which vary in amplitude and periodicity in the enamel of different species. (From Osborn 1973 with permission of the author and publishers, Springer.)

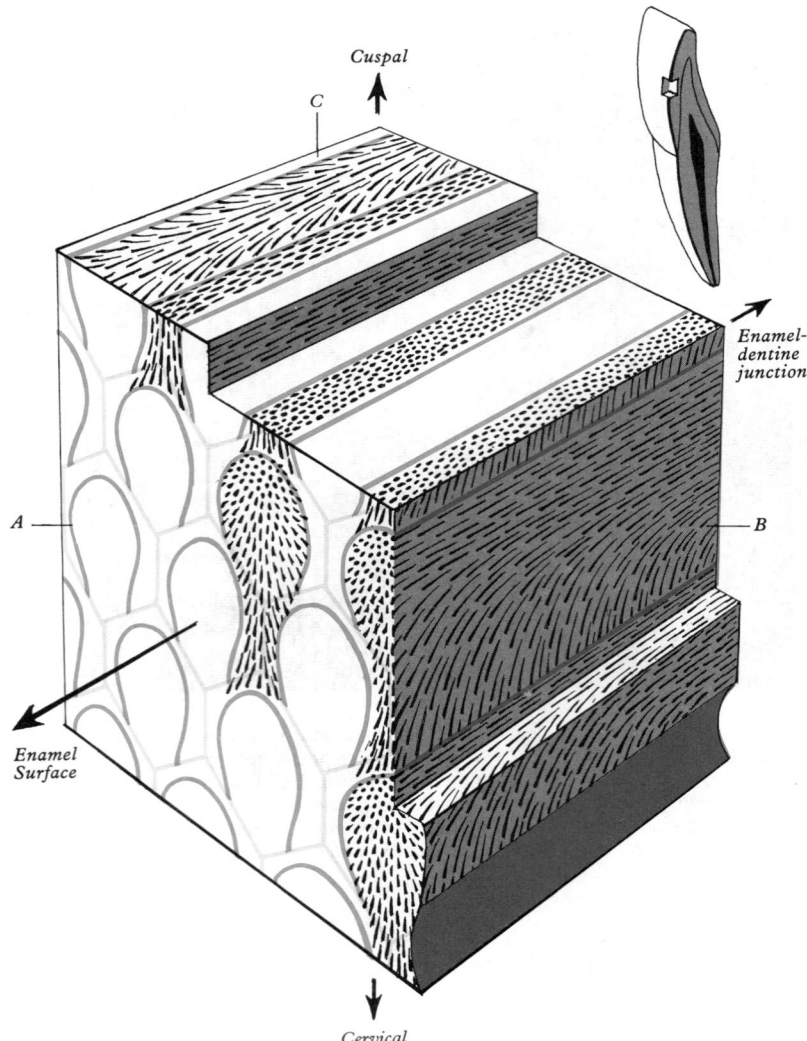

Cuspal

C

A

Enamel Surface

Enamel–dentine junction

B

Cervical

12.37 Diagram of a block of enamel showing how the orientation of the crystallites determines their appearance when the prisms are cut transversely (face A), longitudinally (face B) or at right angles to both these planes (face C). Prism boundaries or sheaths (blue) are formed wherever crystallites meet at highly discordant angles. Superimposed on the transversely cut face (A) are cross-sectional outlines of the ameloblasts (yellow).

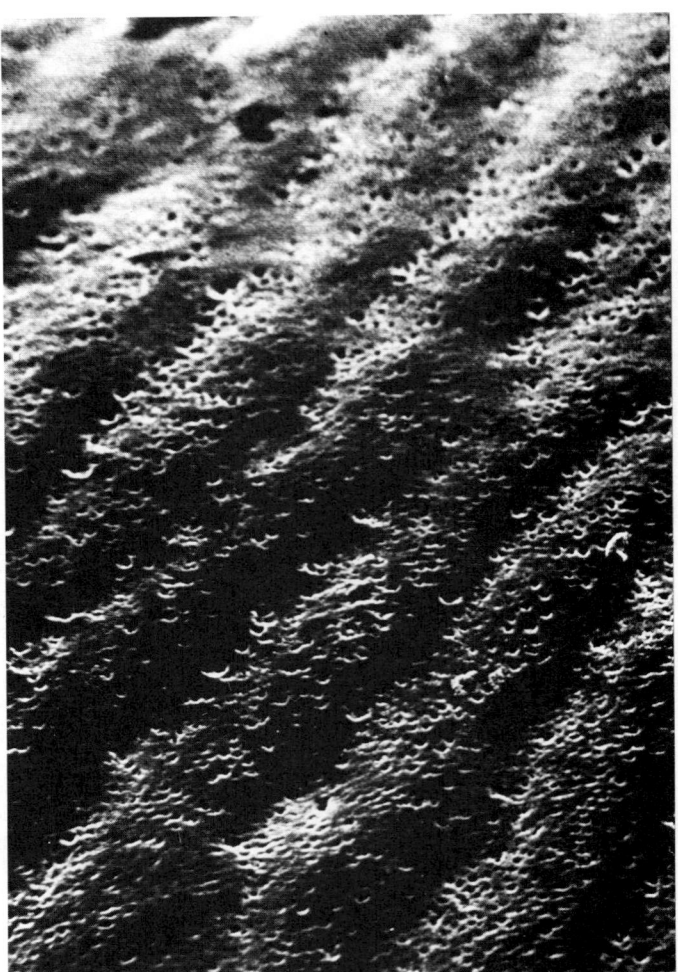

12.38 Scanning electron micrograph of the enamel surface showing perikymata. The holes (about 4 μm wide) were occupied by Tomes' processes of ameloblasts when the development of the enamel was completed. (Provided by D Whittaker, The Dental School, University of Wales, Cardiff.)

because the former contain many mitochondria (Frank 1968); they are more numerous beneath the cusps (where one in four tubules is occupied) than elsewhere (Lilja 1979). Ultrastructrual studies have failed to show nerve fibres beyond 100 μm into human dentine but autoradiography of rats' teeth following injection of tritiated proline into the trigeminal ganglion and axonal transport of labelled proteins has revealed innervation in dentinal tubules near the enamel–dentine junction (Pimendis & Hinds 1977).

Stimulation of dentine, whether by thermal, mechanical or osmotic means, evokes a pain response. The mechanism of stimulus transduction is unknown but is unlikely to involve the direct stimulation of nerve endings in dentine. Newly erupted teeth are sensitive yet do not have a plexus of Raschkow, although, in contrast to earlier studies, some nerve fibres have been found in dentinal tubules before tooth eruption (Byers 1984). Pain-producing chemicals and local anaesthetics show little ability to stimulate or anaesthetize exposed dentine. One possibility is that the odontoblast process can propagate some kind of impulse and excite nerve endings in contact with the proximal part of the process or the cell body. But neither synapses nor gap junctions have been definitely identified between nerves and odontoblasts; although their cell membranes occasionally come into close approximation, the nature and functional significance of such junctions are unknown (Sessle 1987). An alternative hypothesis suggests that stimuli generate movement of intracellular fluid or

extracellular fluid along the dentinal tubules, causing in turn a local distortion of the pulp, sensed by free nerve endings in the plexus (Brännström 1963; Anderson et al 1970). Evidence that odontoblasts are joined together by continuous tight junctions (Bishop 1985) suggests that the odontoblast may be directly involved in relaying intratubular fluid movements to nerve endings. This 'hydrodynamic' theory would explain the ineffectiveness of neuroactive agents and why pain is produced by drying and by solutions of high osmotic pressure. Solutions equally effective in producing pain, however, create very different rates of flow (Anderson & Matthews 1967; Horiuchi & Matthews 1973).

ENAMEL (12.19, 20, 33, 35–38)

Enamel (Osborn 1973; Boyde 1989) is an extremely hard (Knoop number = 300+) and rigid (stiffness = 40–80 GN/m^2) material covering the crowns of teeth. It is a heavily mineralized cell secretion, containing 95–96% by weight crystalline apatites (88% by volume) and less than 1% organic matrix. Since its formative cells are lost from the surface (**12.38**) during eruption, it is incapable of further growth; repair is limited to the remineralization of minute incipient carious lesions. It reaches a maximum thickness of 2.5 mm over cusps and thins to knife edge at the cervical margins. Enamel is composed of closely packed enamel *prisms* (or rods), U-shaped in cross section (**12.37**), extending from close to the enamel–dentine junction to within 6–12 μm of the surface. Each prism is partially delineated by a matrix-rich *prism sheath*, 70 nm thick, and is separated from neighbouring prisms by a continuous *interprismatic region*. Prisms are about 3–4 μm wide in inner enamel, increasing to about

6 μm near the surface. Prisms are packed with flattened hexagonal hydroxyapatite crystallites, 26 nm × 68 nm in cross-section (Daculsi & Kerebel 1978). Hexagonal transverse profiles of ribbon-like crystallites are randomly oriented. In the cuspal region of a prism (plane C in **12**.37) these are almost parallel to the prism's long axis and may be as long as the enamel is thick (i.e. up to 2.5 mm); but in the cervical region of a prism (plane B in **12**.37) and in interprismatic regions, the crystallites have a pronounced cervical inclination and end at the cervically-adjacent prism sheath. A sudden change always exists between crystallite orientation on the two sides of a prism sheath. In surface enamel, crystallites are packed with their long axes parallel so that prism sheaths do not form.

At intervals of about 4 μm along its length, each prism is crossed by a dark *striation*, the light microscope manifestation of a rhythmic swelling and shrinking of prism diameter during one day's growth. Higher order incremental lines in enamel are *striae of Retzius* (**12**.20), passing from the enamel–dentine junction obliquely to the surface where they end in shallow furrows, *perikymata*, visible on newly erupted teeth (**12**.38). Each stria represents a period of 7–8 days' enamel growth (Bromage & Dean 1985). Striae are produced by a sudden double right-angle translocation of the prisms in the longitudinal plane and may be clear or brown in transmitted light. Tyndall scattering of short wavelengths is due to accumulations of matrix in the prism translocations. A prominent stria, the *neonatal line* (Whittaker & Richards 1978), is formed in teeth whose mineralization spans birth. Neonatal lines in enamel and dentine are of forensic importance, indicating that an infant has survived for a few days.

Each prism is sinuous in the tooth's transverse plane with a wavelength of about 1.5 mm, undulations of one prism being matched by those lateral to it but slightly (2°) out of phase with those above or below (**12**.37). Prism sheaths are comparatively weak interfaces in enamel (work of fracture, Wf = 200 J/m² perpendicular to prisms but only 13 J/m² parallel to prisms; Waters 1980). Decussation of prisms in the tooth's longitudinal plane is an adaptation which increases the toughness of enamel by enlarging the surface area of potential cracks between prisms in that plane. Similar regular undulations over cusps produce the appearance of gnarled enamel in sections.

Prism sheaths in the inner enamel are considerably thickened to form tuft-like projections from the enamel–dentine junction, extending for a considerable distance in the longitudinal plane of the tooth. Longitudinal sheets of organic material penetrating the full thickness of enamel are *enamel lamellae*. Extensions into the enamel of dentinal tubules are *enamel spindles*, prominent over cusps.

CEMENT (**12**.18–20, 32, 40)

Cement is a bone-like tissue covering the dental roots, about 50% by weight hydroxyapatite and amorphous calcium phosphates (Selvig 1964; Frank & Steuer 1977). In newly erupted teeth, the cement generally overlaps the enamel slightly but may just meet the cervical margin or fall short, leaving dentine exposed at the periodontal ligament. All three situations may prevail around the neck of a single tooth. In older teeth, when the root becomes exposed in the mouth through occlusal drift and gingival recession, cement is often worn away and dentine revealed.

Cement is perforated by *Sharpey's fibres*, attachment bundles of periodontal ligament collagen fibres (extrinsic fibres). New layers of cement are deposited incrementally throughout life to compensate for tooth movements, incorporating new Sharpey's fibres. Incremental lines (of Salter) are irregularly spaced.

The first formed cement is thin (up to 200 μm), acellular and contains only extrinsic fibres; but cement formed later is produced more rapidly and contains cementocytes in lacunae joined by canaliculi mainly directed towards the periodontal ligament. This cement contains both extrinsic fibres and matrix (intrinsic) fibres of cementoblastic origin. With increasing age cellular cement may reach a thickness of a millimetre or more around the apices and at the furcations of the roots, where it compensates for the loss of the periodontal attachment area through occlusal drift. Cement is not usually remodelled but will repair both small areas of resorption and fractures of the dentine. Cement deposition within the apical foramen is a cause of vascular strangulation of the pulp which progresses with age.

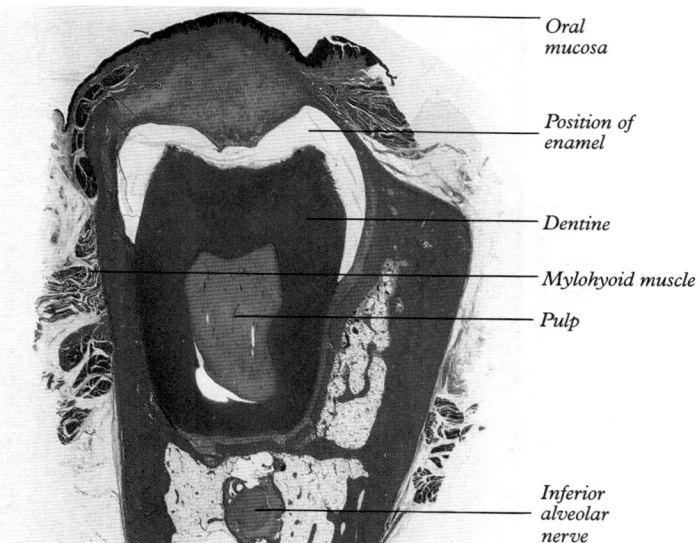

Oral mucosa

Position of enamel

Dentine

Mylohyoid muscle

Pulp

Inferior alveolar nerve

12.39   Section through the body of the mandible and associated soft tissue, demineralized and cut in the coronal plane. An unerupted third permanent molar tooth is visible in this section. The buccal side is to the right. Note that decalcification prior to sectioning has removed the enamel, whose position is represented by an empty space outlined by the juxtaposed tissues. Magnification × 3.5. (Provided by D. Luke, Department of Anatomy and Cell Biology, UMDS, Guy's Campus, London.)

PERIODONTAL LIGAMENT (MEMBRANE) (**12**.20, 39)

The periodontal ligament (Berkovitz et al 1982) is a dense connective tissue (50% dry weight is collagen types I and III) between 0.15 and 0.3 mm wide. It contains cells typical of connective tissue with the addition of a network of epithelial cells, the *epithelial debris of Malassez*, remnants of the root sheath. These have no evident function but may produce commonly occurring *dental cysts*.

The principal functions of the periodontal ligament are to anchor the teeth in their sockets and to provide sensory information about tooth movements (Anderson et al 1970). The majority of collagen fibres are arranged in a number of *principal groups* which connect alveolar bone and cement. *Horizontal fibres* at the alveolar crest and near the apex restrict tilt; between these groups are the *oblique fibres*, restricting intrusive movement. Radiating from the apex are *apical fibres*, resisting extrusive movement. *Gingival fibres* pass from the cervical region of the root and from the osseous alveolar crest into the gingival lamina propria, anchoring it firmly to the tooth, aided by a *circular group* arranged concentrically around the neck. The collagen fibres compartmentalize the proteoglycan-rich hydrophilic ground substance (Sloan 1978) which provides a compressive viscoelastic support (Melcher & Walker 1976). Hydrodynamic damping, as blood is squeezed through the numerous vascular channels in the socket wall, also contributes to the dissipation of impact loads during mastication (Picton 1990).

Each periodontal ligament has a nerve supply from several sources (see above); the chief role of the innervation seems to be proprioception. Various endings have been described: irregularly branched, knob-like, Meissner's corpuscle-like, Ruffini-like and spindle-shaped. Structural variations of the mechanoreceptors appear to be less important than their spatial arrangement in determining the response (Hannam 1976; Linden 1990). Impulses from such endings probably provide an input to many brainstem centres and the cerebellum, where masticatory cycles may, in part, be integrated.

Turnover of collagen in periodontal ligaments is remarkably rapid. Fibroblasts are involved in both fibre synthesis and degradation, processes which may occur simultaneously within the same individual cell (Ten Cate & Deporter 1975).

GINGIVAE (GUMS)

The gingiva is a specialized region of the oral mucosa surrounding the necks of the teeth (Squier et al 1976). In a healthy mouth it is distinguished from the oral mucosa by its pale pink, stippled appearance (**12**.21, 40), the adjacent alveolar mucosa being red, shiny and

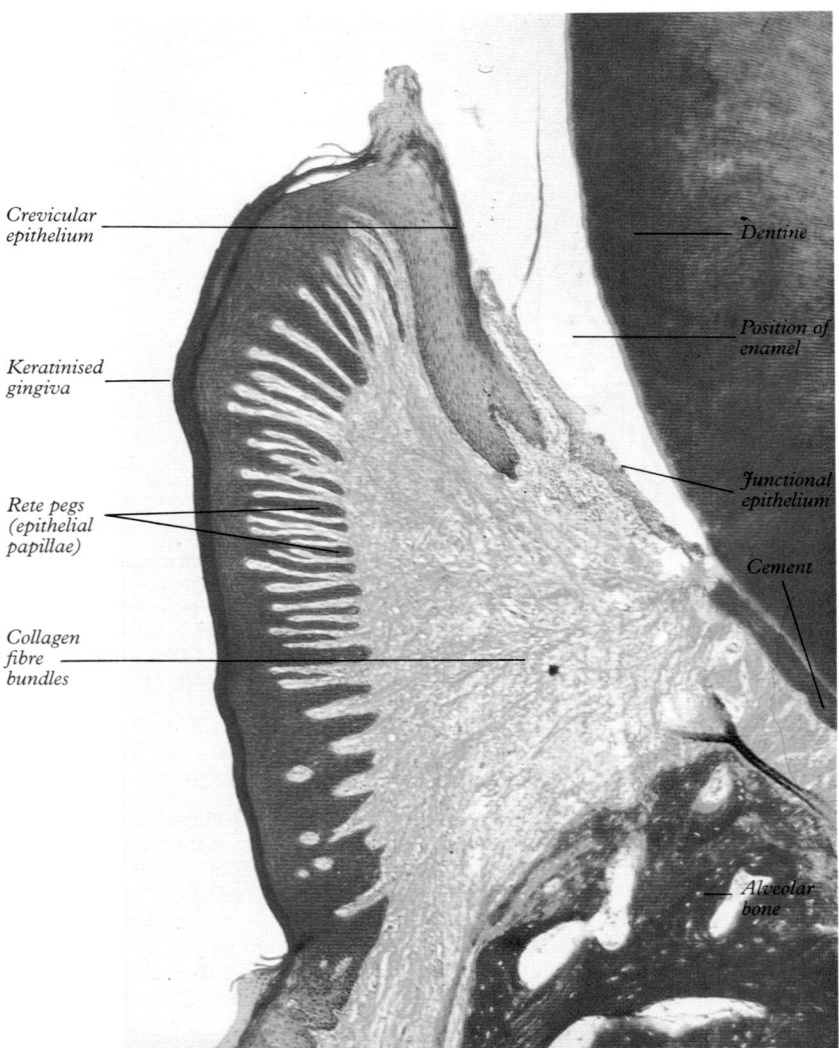

Crevicular
epithelium

Keratinised
gingiva

Rete pegs
(epithelial
papillae)

Collagen
fibre
bundles

Dentine

Position of
enamel

Junctional
epithelium

Cement

Alveolar
bone

12.40 Vertical demineralized section through the neck of a tooth and related gingiva (non-human primate). The enamel has been removed by the decalcification process, as indicated. In life, the junctional epithelium is adherent to the surface of the enamel. Magnification × 30.

smooth; gingival, palatal and dorsal lingual epithelia are keratinized (or parakeratinized), while alveolar epithelium is non-keratinized. Gingival lamina propria is firmly connected to the underlying alveolar bone, forming a virtually immovable mucoperiosteum.

At the gingival crest, the epithelium is reflected towards the root

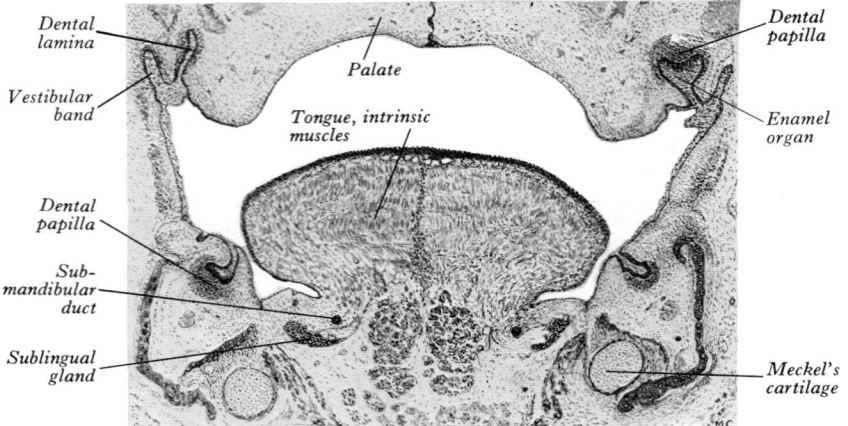

Dental
lamina

Vestibular
band

Dental
papilla

Sub-
mandibular
duct

Sublingual
gland

Palate

Tongue, intrinsic
muscles

Dental
papilla

Enamel
organ

Meckel's
cartilage

12.41 Coronal section of the head of a human embryo (CR length 34 mm), showing developing teeth. The pointer line to Meckel's cartilage passes through the developing mandible.

so that its outer surface is attached to the tooth, forming the *epithelial attachment*. Surrounding the tooth there may be a shallow *gingival sulcus* between tooth and gingiva, its floor being the epithelial attachment. The epithelium attached to the tooth is termed the *junctional epithelium*, that lining the sulcus is the *sulcular epithelium*. Junctional epithelium is non-keratinized, has wide intercellular spaces, few cytokeratin filaments and few desmosomes (Schroeder & Listgarten 1971); it is permeable, weakly cohesive and easily ruptured. Its superficial cells (equivalent to the prickle cells of normal keratinized epithelium) adhere tightly by hemidesmosomes to an outer basal lamina covering the adjoining dental surface (Listgarten 1970) to which they are firmly bonded; this is enamel in newly erupted teeth but in older individuals the junctional epithelium extends onto the cement. Junctional epithelial cells have a very high turnover and move rapidly up the dental surface, whence they are shed into the sulcus.

TOOTH DEVELOPMENT

DECIDUOUS TEETH (12.41–48)

At the 9 mm embryonic stage primitive oral epithelium (**12.**42A) begins to bulge into the underlying mesenchyme where teeth will form (**12.**41, 45). From these separate ingrowths and the mesenchyme associated with them, the four anterior deciduous teeth (central and lateral incisors, canine and first molar) will arise (Ooé 1957; Nery et al 1970). In amphibian embryos, odontogenic mesenchyme originates from the mesencephalic levels of the cranial neural crests, migratory ectomesenchyme entering and expanding the branchial arches (de Beer 1947; Chibon 1967) under the inductive influence of oral epithelium (Wagner 1955; Henzen 1957). The tooth inductive potency of mandibular arch ectoderm on cranial neural crest cells has been demonstrated in the mouse embryo (Lumsden 1987).

At about the 20 mm stage the ingrown epithelial dental laminae have expanded into knob-like swellings (Ooé 1956), each surrounded by a dense aggregate of vascular mesenchyme (Gaunt 1959). The combined organ rudiment is the *tooth bud*. Ectoderm starts to grow around the mesenchymal aggregate; the ectodermal part is now an *enamel organ*, the mesenchymal part a *dental papilla*. Peripheral cuboidal cells of the enamel organ are soon distinguished from central polygonal cells. At this stage (48 mm) the bud of the second deciduous molar appears on the posteriorly growing dental lamina.

The spherical dental papilla enlarges but the encircling edge of the enamel organ (the *cervical loop*) continues to surround more of its periphery until it sits on the papilla like a cap, the *cap stage* of development (**12.**42C). Meanwhile the central polygonal cells of the enamel organ have been secreting glycosaminoglycans into intercellular spaces which attract water, swelling the enamel organ and compressing the cells. Since desmosomal connections persist, the central cells become stellar, forming a *stellate reticulum* (**12.**42E, 43). The originally cuboidal cells adjacent to the dental papilla lengthen to form the columnar cells of the *inner enamel epithelium* (**12.**42E, 43). Cells forming the outer surface of the enamel organ are the *outer (external) enamel epithelium* (**12.**42E, 43, 45), continuous via the dental lamina with the oral epithelium. By continued growth the cervical loop surrounds about three-quarters of the enlarging dental papilla, the *bell stage* of tooth development. Now a layer of flatter cells develops between the inner enamel epithelium and the stellate reticulum; this *stratum intermedium* derives from the original polygonal cells of the enamel organ (the *enamel knot*). Tissue interactions between the peripheral cells of the dental papilla and the adjacent cells of the inner enamel epithelium (Thesleff et al 1989) result in the differentiation of odontoblasts from the former and of ameloblasts from the latter.

The development of a nerve supply to deciduous teeth has attracted little attention. Alveolar nerves enter into maxillary and mandibular processes during the fifth week, before the dental laminae form (Pearson 1977). A close association has been noted between peripheral nerve branches and the sites of prospective tooth development in the mouse (Kollar & Lumsden 1979) but initiation of tooth development does not appear to depend on innervation (Lumsden & Buchanan 1986). At cap and bell stages bundles of nerve fibres have entered the dense mesenchyme of dental papillae and follicles.

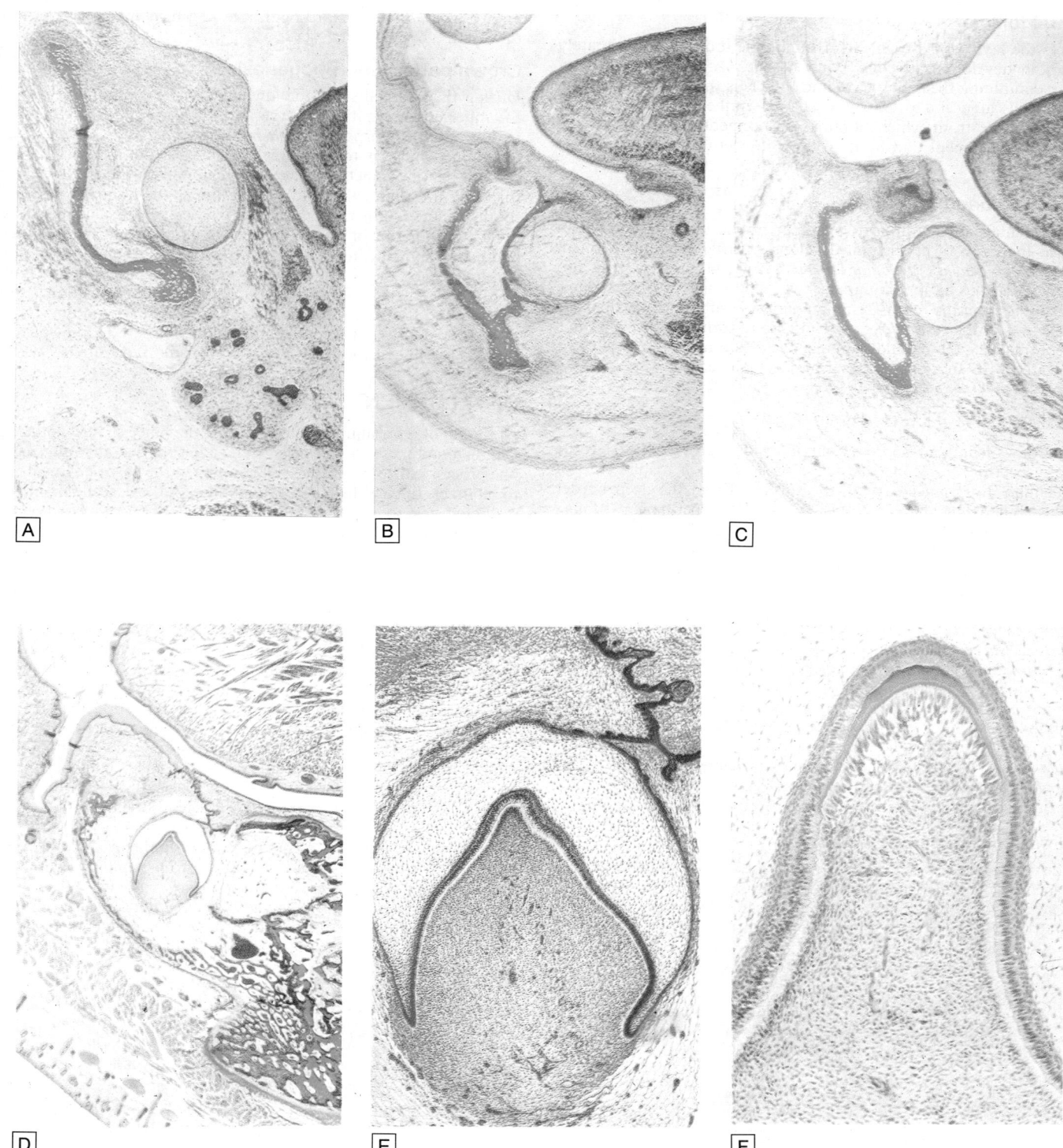

12.42A–F   A series of stages illustrating the early development of teeth. These are all coronal sections through the right half of the body of the mandible, showing the tongue in the top right-hand corner. The mandible is mineralizing to the left of the circular profile of Meckel's cartilage.

A. The stage of development before the ingrowth of the dental lamina from the oral epithelium.

B. The dental lamina is growing between the buccal and lingual plates of the ossifying mandible.

C. The cap stage of development. The enamel organ is growing from the dental lamina around the condensation of cells which forms the dental papilla.
Slightly later stages in tooth development than shown in **12**.42A–C.

D. The bell stage of development. The external enamel epithelium of the enamel organ is connected to the oral mucosa by an irregularly-stranded dental lamina. Lateral to the buccal plate of the mandible the vestibular band

has atrophied centrally to initiate the oral vestibule. The tooth germ is separated from the bone by the tooth follicle.

E. A photograph at higher magnification of the bell stage. Note from above downwards: (1) the degenerating dental lamina, top right; (2) the fibrous tooth follicle surrounding the developing tooth; (3) the external enamel epithelium; (4) the delicate stippled appearance produced by the nuclei of the stellate reticulum; (5) the darkly stained, somewhat flattened cells of the stratum intermedium, which is seen more clearly in F; (6) the columnar cells of the internal enamel epithelium; (7) the more closely packed cells of the dental papilla which extend outside the cervical loop; (8) the capillaries of the pulp and tooth follicle.

F. Dentine formation beginning at the cuspal tip. From above downwards note: (1) the loose stellate reticulum; (2) the stratum intermedium; (3) a layer of columnar ameloblasts; (4) a thin strip of enamel matrix (mauve); (5) mineralized dentine (pink); (6) predentine (pale blue); (7) a layer of odontoblasts.

1713

Dental follicle

This is the layer of cells which surrounds the tooth germ ultimately to adjoin developing alveolar bone (12.42D, 42E, 43, 45); the bony cavity containing the tooth germ and follicle is the *dental crypt*. The follicle cells adjacent to the outer enamel epithelium form a dense *investing layer* from which develops the cement of the root. The periodontal ligament and bone develop respectively from the loose intermediate layer and outer osteogenic layer of the follicle.

Vestibular band

As the dental laminae appear, a similar but continuous horseshoe-shaped ingrowth of epithelium develops external (buccal) to them. This *vestibular band (vestibular lamina)* (12.41, 44) grows deeply into the mesenchyme of the primitive jaws, separating prospective lips and cheeks from the tooth-forming regions. It subsequently thickens and cleaves at the *vestibular groove* (12.44) to form the *oral vestibule*. In contrast to the dental lamina, the vestibular lamina is not associated with an aggregation of mesenchyme cells.

PERMANENT TEETH (12.39, 46, 47)

As the jaws lengthen the dental lamina grows posteriorly from the distal aspect of the second deciduous molar germ as a solid cord of epithelium, not connected with the surface. From the deep border of this 'burrowing' lamina, buds for the three permanent molars develop in mesiodistal sequence, the first molar bud appearing in the 16-week fetus, the second at about 1 year and the third at 5 years. Each bud is initiated in the ramus of the lower jaw but, with progressive resorption of the anterior border of the coronoid process, they come to occupy the body of the mandible.

From each deciduous tooth germ at its bell stage (about 16 weeks) a lingual *successional lamina* grows from the site of continuity between outer enamel epithelium and dental lamina. Each grows down into mesenchyme lingual to a deciduous tooth and from its end a bud develops for a permanent successor which becomes surrounded by its own follicle and crypt. The follicle maintains fibrous continuity with the lamina propria of oral mucosa by *gubernacular cords*, whose original positions are visible in young skulls as *gubernacular canals*. The gubernacular canals are said to guide erupting permanent teeth into their correct positions (Scott 1967).

The fate of the dental laminae

As dentine and enamel start to develop, the dental laminae begin to degenerate (12.42E), separating into clumps, many with a whorled appearance over developing deciduous teeth. These persist as epithelial rests but may sometimes proliferate to form cystic cavities,

known as *eruption cysts*, recognizable as bluish swellings over erupting teeth.

Crown pattern morphogenesis

During the late bell stage the amelodentinal membrane, formed by the inner enamel epithelium, the peripheral cell layer of the dental papilla and the interposed basement membrane, folds in a genetically determined pattern to assume the definitive outline of the future enamel–dentine junction. Because regional variations in enamel thickness are slight, this folding determines the ultimate shape of a tooth, i.e. the number and positions of cusps. Cap stage incisor and molar tooth germs of mouse embryos separated into their epithelial and mesenchymal components and reciprocally recombined in organ culture develop the morphology expected of the mesenchyme (Kollar 1972). How the dental papilla mesenchyme acquires positional specification and how the information for shape is encoded and relayed to the apparently indifferent enamel epithelium are unknown. For a further account of tooth development consult Ten Cate (1994).

DEVELOPMENT OF DENTINE

At the tip of a presumptive cusp, cells of the inner enamel epithelium lengthen and mesenchyme cells of the adjacent dental papilla extend fine processes through the reticular lamina of the basement membrane to contact the epithelial basal lamina. An extracellular matrix-mediated cell to cell interaction (Thesleff 1977) induces the mesenchyme cells to differentiate into odontoblasts, which will lay down dentine (12.42F, 46, 47). Newly differentiated odontoblasts, with well-developed endoplasmic reticulum and Golgi apparatus, secrete dentine matrix into the space between the basal ends of the inner enamel cells and their own secreting ends. Collagenase-containing vesicles in this early matrix (Sorgente et al 1977) may be involved in digestion of the epithelial basal lamina which permits the odontoblast processes to push up between the inner enamel epithelial cells where they may form direct cell contacts, mediating the differentiation of ameloblasts. Accumulating matrix pushes the odontoblasts back, their processes lengthening as their perikarya recede, becoming enclosed within tubules of the matrix. As soon as a few microns of matrix are formed, the matrix adjacent to the inner enamel epithelium begins to mineralize (Silva & Kailis 1972), possibly with the agency of alkaline phosphatase-rich matrix vesicles (Bernard 1972, see also p. 472).

From this region, the summit of a presumptive dentine cusp, a wave of differentiation of odontoblasts from papillary cells slowly spreads to the growing cervical loop. As soon as each differentiates, the matrix is formed, pushing the layer of odontoblasts, united by desmosomes, into the papilla. The layer of unmineralized matrix

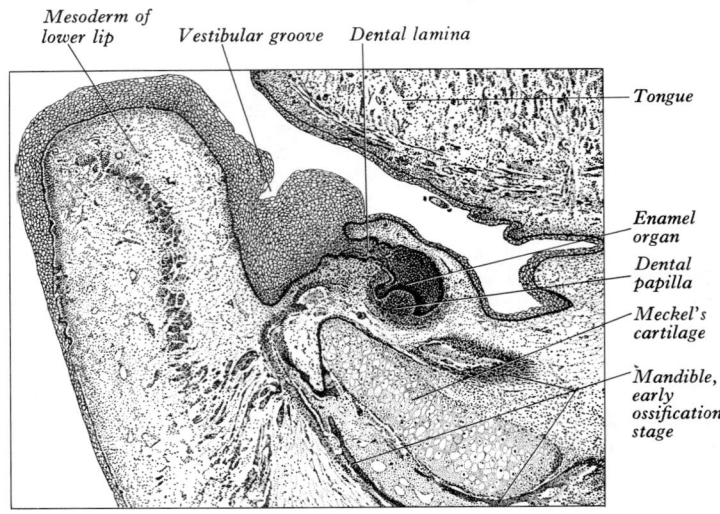

12.44 Part of a sagittal section through the head of a human embryo (CR length 60 mm), passing through the right lower central incisor tooth germ. Magnification × 12. (Drawn from a photomicrograph given by C H Tonge, Department of Oral Biology, University of Newcastle-upon-Tyne. Stained with haematoxylin and eosin.)

12.43 Simplified diagram of a developing tooth to show the approximate arrangement of its principal components. Compare with 12.42F.

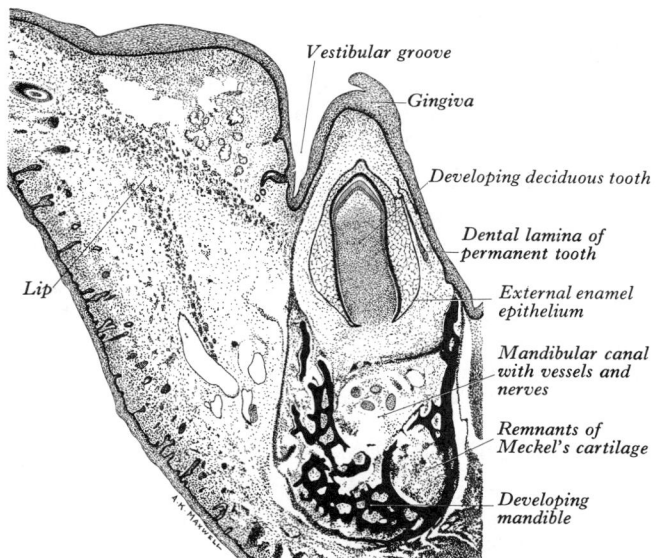

12.45 Developing tooth with mandible and lip in situ. (Drawn from a photograph by F Harrison, Dental Department, University of Sheffield, and reproduced from Pedley & Harrison with permission from Blackie.)

adjacent to the odontoblasts is termed predentine (**12**.47). First-formed collagen fibres lie parallel to the odontoblast processes; after this thin layer of *mantle dentine* (see above) is formed, fine collagen fibres of *circumpulpal dentine* are elaborated, interlacing at right angles to the processes. In mantle dentine each odontoblast has two or more processes but, as it recedes from the enamel–dentine junction, its processes unite into a single main process. This accounts for the bifurcation of the tubules near the junction. During circumpulpal dentinogenesis odontoblasts constantly extend short lateral processes at the base of the main process; these are later embedded by

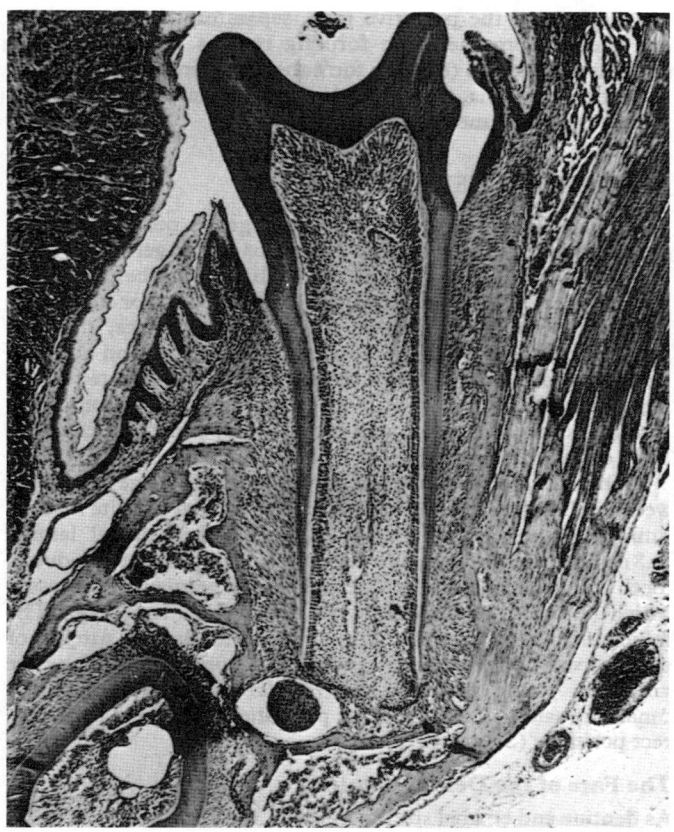

12.46 A longitudinally sectioned developing tooth showing advanced root formation. See text for further details.

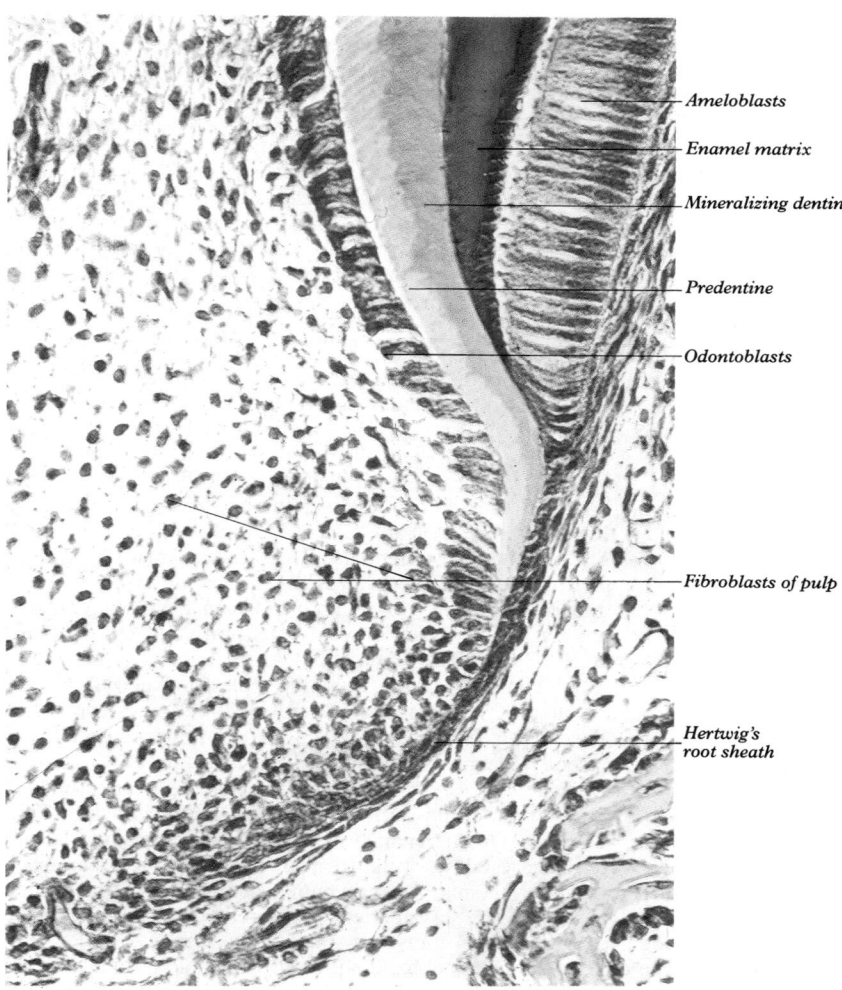

12.47 Vertical section through the neck of a developing tooth, with part of the crown above, and the developing root below. The layer of columnar ameloblasts terminate at the tooth neck where the latter is continuous with the developing root. Magnification × 600.

mineralized dentine to become fine lateral tubules. Dentinal tubules are much thinner in mineralized dentine than in predentine; this constriction starts at the level where predentine mineralization is beginning and is due to the deposition of a highly mineralized cylinder of *peritubular dentine* around the inside of the tubule, progressively reducing its lumen. It does not develop in interglobular areas (see above) where the tubule is walled by unmineralized intertubular dentine matrix.

DEVELOPMENT OF ENAMEL

Ameloblasts differentiate from cells of the inner enamel epithelium under the inductive influence of newly differentiated odontoblasts; the interaction between these cells is thought to involve direct cell contacts and/or the extracellular matrix. The first signs of differentiation are the manufacture of organelles required for enamel matrix production and the reversal of cell polarity; ameloblasts secrete from their original basal ends. Mitochondria, originally dispersed throughout the cytoplasm, congregate at the non-secreting pole where they cluster around the nucleus. The Golgi apparatus is located centrally; cisternae of the extensive endoplasmic reticulum are stacked in rows parallel to the cell's long axis. The mature cell is about 40 μm long and about 5 μm wide. In cross-section ameloblasts are regular hexagons, accounting for the classic honeycomb appearance, and are interconnected by junctional complexes at both secreting and non-secreting poles. Their non-secreting poles are attached by desmosomes to the stratum intermedium cells, which may

1715

elaborate and transport materials to the ameloblasts (Kurahashi & Yoshiki 1972). Alkaline phosphatase, found in other hard-tissue forming cells, exists in the stratum intermedium but not in secretory ameloblasts.

Enamel matrix is secreted between mineralizing dentine and ameloblasts; a rise or potential rise in hydrostatic pressure produced by the accumulation of enamel matrix in this enclosed region probably provides the force to push ameloblasts away from the enamel–dentine junction (Osborn 1973). Since ameloblast differentiation depends on and shortly follows odontoblast differentiation, developing enamel spreads down the sides of the presumptive enamel–dentine junction in the same way as developing dentine, just behind it (**12**.47).

At the start of amelogenesis, in each region of the tooth germ, adjacent stellate reticulum seems to collapse, the enamel organ being progressively reduced in thickness until it has only three layers (outer enamel epithelium, stratum intermedium and ameloblast layer). It is widely assumed that this brings the ameloblasts, inside an avascular enamel organ, closer to the capillaries which have invaded the investing layer of the follicle adjacent to the external enamel epithelium. Meanwhile, cells of the latter, originally cuboidal, become squamous, throwing the outer surface of the enamel organ into microscopic folds to increase the area for diffusion.

When ameloblasts have moved about 10 μm from the enamel–dentine junction they develop conical extensions into the accumulating enamel. These *Tomes' processes*, whose bases are limited by the junctional complex at the secreting pole of the cell, bear a peripheral collar of microvilli (see Reith 1970). Tomes' processes give the developing front of enamel a pitted appearance (Boyde 1969); adjacent to each is an unmineralized layer about 50–100 nm thick, the *enamel matrix*. This is stippled under the electron microscope and similar material is seen in membrane-bound vesicles within Tomes' processes. On the enamel side of this stippled material are long ribbon-like crystallites. First-formed enamel is non-prismatic or contains irregular prisms. At the enamel–dentine junction, enamel (recognized by long crystallites) is intermixed with dentine (recognized by collagen fibres and small crystallites).

The mineralizing enamel front shows little change until nearly the full thickness of enamel has been secreted. This is immature enamel, containing narrow crystallites about 3 nm × 29 nm in cross-section, and has a composition of about 40% mineral by weight. As ameloblasts approach the final surface, deeper crystallites thicken by accretion of ions from the surrounding matrix. Diminishing calcium-rich matrix is replenished by ameloblasts, water and protein being resorbed. The matrix can travel long distances through the developing enamel. Ultimately the crystallites can widen no more, no further space being available between them. Theoretical analysis suggests that about 12% by volume of unmineralized enamel matrix and water would thus remain (Carlström 1964), according well with the observation that mature enamel is 96% by weight mineral (i.e. 88% by volume). No new crystallites appear to be added to the enamel except at the mineralizing front (Ronnholm 1962); crystals therefore grow in length as the enamel is deposited and achieve their final length as maturation begins. As secretion ends the ameloblast shortens, withdraws its previously conical Tomes' process and forms a ruffled membrane with numerous microvilli which endocytose the matrix (Reith 1967a,b). The maturative ameloblast contains numerous lysosomes. Over some of the enamel surface developed at this time, crystallites are parallel and prism sheaths are not formed (see above). This non-prismatic surface layer is about 6–12 μm deep (Gwinnett 1967; Osborn 1973) and is about 1% by weight more mineralized than the rest, possibly because of closer packing of crystallites permitted by parallel orientation.

ROOT DEVELOPMENT

As enamel maturation proceeds towards completion of the tooth crown, the cervical loop of the enamel organ starts to recede from the cervical margin as a double-layered cylinder, Hertwig's root sheath, around the lengthening dental papilla. The outer layer of this sheath is continuous with the outer enamel epithelium (**12**.46, 47). The inner layer, like the inner enamel epithelium with which it is continuous, induces the differentiation of odontoblasts from contiguous mesenchyme cells. Odontoblasts now deposit a layer of

dentine against the basal surface of the epithelium (**12**.46, 47). The sheath continues to grow, outlining the final shape of the roots and inducing differentiation of odontoblasts, surrounding vessels and nerves supplying the dental papilla. These vessels remain and it is because of them, particularly those located centrally near the future apex, that the foramina open through canals in the dentine into the pulp of a fully developed tooth.

During crown development the capillaries are most numerous beneath the cuspal growth centres. The papilla grows more rapidly near the capillaries, and less rapidly elsewhere. In the latter regions a growing tip of root sheath is able to penetrate under the papilla to meet a growing tip from the other side, separating the two roots. They may, however, just fail to meet, in which case a single flattened root is formed with two root canals. Thus the principal cusps of a multicusped tooth are each supported by a root, which is either separate or incompletely separated from its neighbours.

DEVELOPMENT OF CEMENT

Shortly after initial dentinogenesis in the root, the adjacent root sheath epithelium becomes fenestrated (see below), exposing the unmineralized exterior of the dentine to the vascularized follicular mesenchyme, from whose investing layer cementoblasts are differentiated. These early cementoblasts do not synthesize collagen but secrete ground substance onto the dentine matrix and around bundles of collagen fibres developed in the follicle which have fanned out on the dentine surface. This composite matrix (which may also include epithelial cell secretions, see above) is mineralized under the influence of cementoblasts (Owens 1975). The collagen fibre bundles are about 6 μm wide and their cores mineralize more rapidly than their peripheries. Because it is unmineralized at the time of its formation, the junction between dentine and cement has crystalline continuity and is hence not easy to define in electron micrographs.

First-formed cement, containing only extrinsic collagen fibres, develops while the tooth is erupting and is therefore present on the cervical third of the root dentine. Cementoblasts differentiate over the remainder of the root and, in all later cement, contribute collagen fibres to the matrix (Jones & Boyde 1972). This mixed fibre cement therefore contains both *extrinsic* (Sharpey's) *fibres* of periodontal origin and *intrinsic fibres* from cementoblasts, the former being perpendicular to the developing surface, the latter parallel. Intrinsic fibres are mineralized first. Sharpey's fibres are then mineralized around their peripheries, while the cores are unmineralized. In later or more rapid cementogenesis, the cementoblasts are frequently trapped within the matrix; cellular cement is most commonly formed around the apical two-thirds of the root surface.

DEVELOPMENT OF THE PERIODONTIUM

During the cap and bell stages of tooth development some cells of the dental papilla are displaced by the growing cervical loop to lie adjoining the outer enamel epithelium. Cementoblasts and fibroblasts of the tooth-related periodontal ligament are probably derived from these cells (Ten Cate 1975; Palmer & Lumsden 1987). It has even been suggested that they give rise to osteoblasts of the alveolar bone, but this remains to be definitely demonstrated (Lubbock 1993).

The principal oblique fibre group of the ligament becomes organized at the time of root development and eruption, with an orientation which is visible first as an oblique array of fibroblasts. Once formed, their oblique orientation is maintained as the tooth moves relative to the alveolar bone. Based on its appearance in sections, it was formerly considered that the principal fibres were formed, broken and reformed at an intermediate plexus in the central zone of the ligament (Hindle 1967). However, autoradiographic studies following tritiated proline uptake have not confirmed that collagen turnover is faster in the central zone than elsewhere (Rippin 1976).

The epithelial debris of Malassez is formed by the remains of Hertwig's root sheath which, following its fenestration and the translocation of presumptive cementoblasts from the follicle to the dentine surface, moves away from cement into the tooth-related periodontal ligament.

DENTAL ERUPTION

When the deciduous dentition is initiated, the five tooth germs in

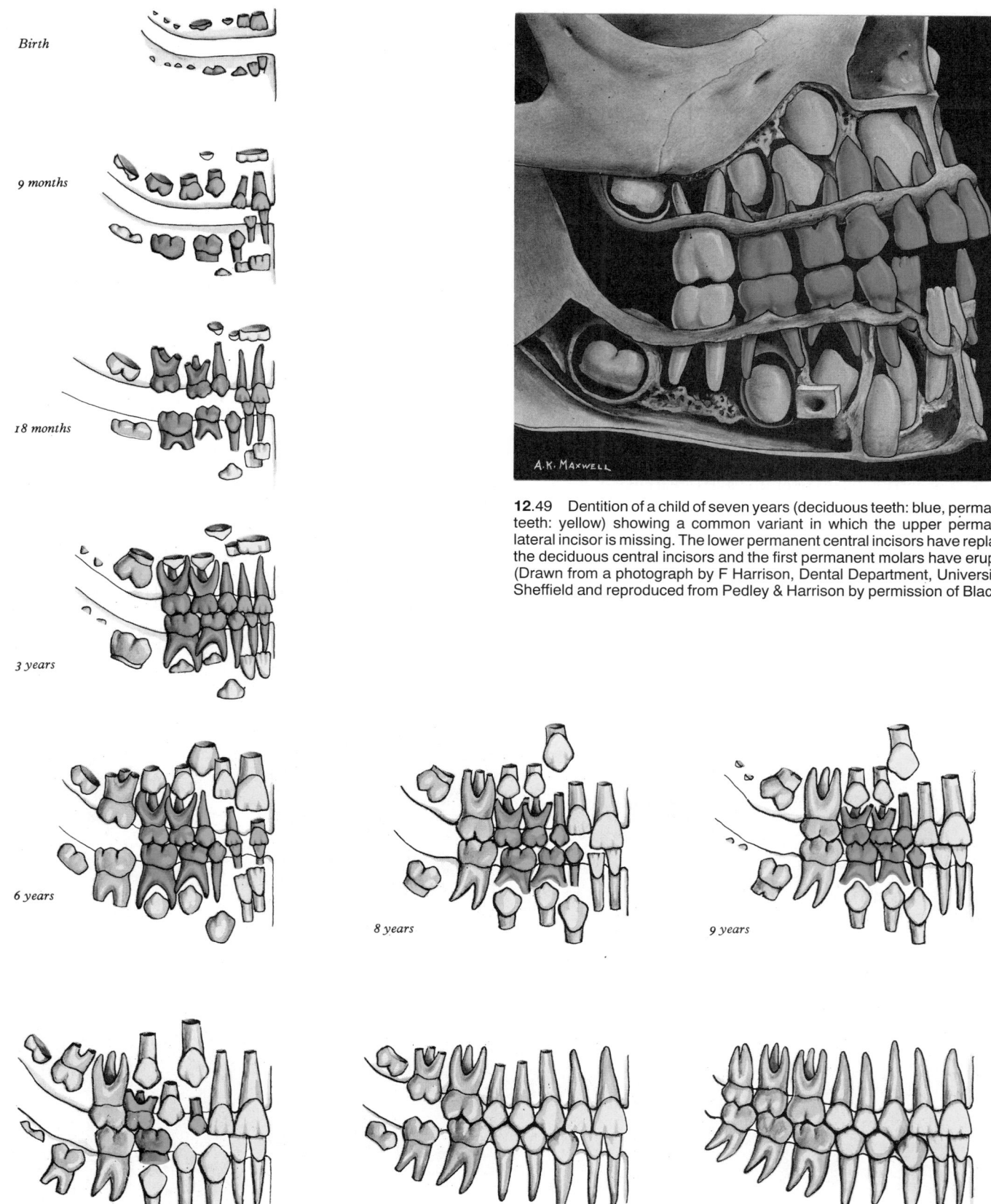

Birth

9 months

18 months

3 years

6 years

8 years

9 years

10 years

12 years

21 years

12.49　Dentition of a child of seven years (deciduous teeth: blue, permanent teeth: yellow) showing a common variant in which the upper permanent lateral incisor is missing. The lower permanent central incisors have replaced the deciduous central incisors and the first permanent molars have erupted. (Drawn from a photograph by F Harrison, Dental Department, University of Sheffield and reproduced from Pedley & Harrison by permission of Blackie.)

12.48　Development of the deciduous (blue) and permanent (yellow) dentitions from birth to maturity. Modified from Schour & Massler (1941).

each quadrant occupy jaws which are about 1 mm long. By the time the teeth have erupted into the oral cavity they occupy 3 or 4 cm of jaw; during development the teeth have migrated apart. It is not known how this movement is brought about.

Very soon after root formation starts, the teeth begin to move towards the oral cavity (Darling & Levers 1976). The origin of the forces which move teeth is not certainly known. A tooth could be **pushed** by growth of its root, proliferation of cells in the pulp or by tissue hydrostatic pressure. In support of the latter, the eruption rate can be experimentally altered by cervical sympathectomy or the administration of vasoactive drugs (Moxham 1979). But as Burn-Murdoch (1990) points out, such experiments do not prove that tissue fluid pressure is the cause of eruption because changes in blood flow could affect several possible eruptive mechanisms. Alternatively, a tooth could be **pulled** out of its socket by shrinkage of the obliquely placed collagen fibres (Thomas 1976) or by the movement of fibroblasts within the periodontal ligament (Beertsen et al 1974). It has also been suggested that the remodelling of alveolar bone may cause eruption (Marks & Cahill 1984). In reality, several of the above factors are likely to co-operate in the eruptive process (Moxham & Berkovitz 1983).

The permanent incisors and canines initially develop lingual to their predecessors (**12.**48, **49**) but erupt along labially-inclined paths. This movement is associated with the intermittent but progressive osteoclastic resorption of the roots of deciduous teeth (Furseth 1968). In periods of quiescence, the resorbed tissues are temporarily repaired by the deposition of cement.

Early in its development, each premolar moves directly deep to its predecessor to become lodged between widely-divergent roots (**12.**23, **49**). As the premolar erupts it induces resorption of the deciduous molar. The enamel of the underlying permanent tooth is protected from resorption by its *reduced enamel epithelium* (see p. 1715).

Eruption times of teeth

Information on the development of teeth and their emergence ('eruption') into the oral cavity is important in clinical practice and also in forensic medicine and archaeology. The tabulated data

provided in Table **12.**1 are largely based on European-derived populations (see also **12.**48, **49**). The developmental stages of initial calcification and crown completion are less affected by environmental influences than eruption, the timing of which may be modified by several factors such as caries, tooth loss and severe malnutrition.

ALVEOLAR DEVELOPMENT

Jaws begin to develop when the dental lamina is forming. In the mandible the growing margin of membrane bone lateral to Meckel's cartilage passes back caudal to the inferior alveolar nerve; from it lateral and medial plates grow upwards (Dixon 1958). Developing teeth thus appear to descend between the plates (**12.**45). An osseous horizontal partition divides the teeth from the inferior alveolar nerve and vertical septa later isolate each tooth in its own crypt. Bone does not develop over deciduous teeth and in skeletonized neonatal jaws teeth are usually lost. A similar process is involved in the development of maxillary crypts.

When the teeth start to move towards the oral cavity, their sockets also grow, deepening the crypts and increasing the height of the jaw. The rate of eruption outstrips the rate of upward bone growth until the teeth meet their opponents. Developing roots have wide open apices but these later close around nerves and vessels to form foramina. The lengthening of osseous sockets for the teeth much increases the depth of the face up to and during puberty (Scott 1967).

CUTICLES AND EPITHELIAL ATTACHMENT

At the end of amelogenesis, the cells of the enamel organ revert to a squamous shape, becoming a thin stratified layer covering the whole surface of the enamel. This is referred to as the *reduced enamel epithelium*. During eruption it fuses with the oral epithelium to provide an epithelium-lined path for the tooth. The reduced enamel epithelium is rapidly worn away from the exposed surface of the tooth except at the neck where it forms the *epithelial attachment* (**12.**41, **46**) at the dentogingival junction. The reduced enamel epi-

Table 12.1	Chronology of the human dentition				
Dentition	**Tooth**	**First evidence of calcification (weeks in utero for deciduous teeth)**	**Crown completed (months)**	**Eruption (months)**	**Root completed (years)**
Deciduous upper	i1	14	$1\frac{1}{2}$	10 (8–12)	$1\frac{1}{2}$
	i2	16	$2\frac{1}{2}$	11 (9–13)	2
	C	17	9	19 (16–22)	$3\frac{1}{4}$
	m1	$15\frac{1}{2}$	6	16 (13–19)	$2\frac{1}{2}$
	m2	19	11	29 (25–33)	3
Deciduous lower	i1	14	$2\frac{1}{2}$	8 (6–10)	$1\frac{1}{2}$
	i2	16	3	13 (10–16)	$1\frac{1}{2}$
	C	17	9	20 (17–23)	$3\frac{1}{4}$
	m1	$15\frac{1}{2}$	$5\frac{1}{2}$	16 (14–18)	$2\frac{1}{4}$
	m2	18	10	27 (23–31)	3
Permanent upper	I1	3–4 month	4–5 yr	7–8 yr	10
	I2	10–12 month	4–5 yr	8–9 yr	11
	C	4–5 month	6–7 yr	11–12 yr	13–15
	P1	$1\frac{1}{2}$–$1\frac{3}{4}$ yr	5–6 yr	10–11 yr	12–13
	P2	2–$2\frac{1}{4}$ yr	6–7 yr	10–12 yr	12–14
	M1	at birth	$2\frac{1}{2}$–3 yr	6–7 yr	9–10
	M2	$2\frac{1}{2}$–3 yr	7–8 yr	12–13 yr	14–16
	M3	7–9 yr	12–16 yr	17–21 yr	18–25
Permanent lower	I1	3–4 month	4–5 yr	6–7 yr	9
	I2	3–4 month	4–5 yr	7–8 yr	10
	C	4–5 month	6–7 yr	9–10 yr	12–14
	P1	$1\frac{3}{4}$–2 yr	5–6 yr	10–12 yr	12–13
	P2	$2\frac{1}{4}$–$2\frac{1}{2}$ yr	6–7 yr	11–12 yr	13–14
	M1	at birth	$2\frac{1}{2}$–3 yr	6–7 yr	9–10
	M2	$2\frac{1}{2}$–3 yr	7–8 yr	11–13 yr	14–15
	M3	8–10 yr	12–16 yr	17–21 yr	18–25

From Ash M M 1993 Dental anatomy, physiology and occlusion W B Saunders Co, Philadelphia (slightly modified).

thelium is separated from the enamel surface by a structureless layer, the *primary enamel cuticle*, about 1 μm thick, which may be the final, unmineralized product of ameloblasts. This cuticle together with the reduced enamel epithelium is called *Nasmyth's membrane*. A form of cement known as *afibrillar cement* has been observed over the enamel around the necks of teeth (Listgarten 1966). Afibrillar cement is only about 100 nm thick, contains no banded collagen and is probably produced by cementoblasts following premature disruption of part of the reduced enamel epithelium. Occasionally a cuticle about 4 μm thick is found between the epithelial attachment and the tooth. This is the *secondary enamel cuticle*. It may be a product of the epithelial cells or it may be the remains of blood which has leaked through the epithelial attachment following some slight trauma (Hodson 1966). Finally, salivary protein and carbohydrate form an adherent film on tooth surfaces. This is known as the *pellicle* and is the foundation of *dental plaque*.

CLINICAL ASPECTS

The cortical plate of bone in each jaw is continuous over the alveolar crest with the cortical plate lining the tooth socket (the *cribriform plate* or *lamina dura* of radiographs). On the labial and buccal aspects of *upper teeth*, these two cortical plates usually fuse with very little trabecular bone between them, except where the buccal bone thickens over the molar teeth near the root of the zygomatic arch (DuBrul 1988). It is easier and more convenient to extract upper teeth by fracturing the buccal than the palatal plate. Anteriorly in the *lower jaw*, labial and lingual plates are thin but in the molar region the buccal plate is thickened as the external oblique line. Near the lower third molar, the lingual bone is much thinner than the buccal and it is mechanically easier to remove this tooth, when impacted, via the lingual plate. However, the lingual nerve is here exposed to damage.

Abscesses developing in relation to the apices of roots ultimately penetrate the surrounding bone where it is thinnest. The position of the resultant swelling in the soft tissues is largely determined by the relationship between muscle attachments and the sinus (the path taken by the infected material) in the bone. Thus, in the lower incisor region, because the labial bone is thin, abscesses generally appear as a swelling in the labial sulcus, above the attachment of the mentalis. But the abscess may open below the mentalis and point beneath the chin. If an abscess from a lower postcanine tooth opens below the attachment of the buccinator, the swelling is in the neck; if it opens above, the swelling is in the buccal sulcus. If an abscess opens lingually above the mylohyoid, the swelling is in the lingual sulcus; if it is below, the swelling is in the neck. Because the mylohyoid ascends posteriorly, third molar abscesses tend to track into the neck rather than the mouth.

Apart from canine teeth, which have long roots, abscesses on upper teeth usually open buccally below, rather than above, the attachment of buccinator. Because its root apex is occasionally curved towards the palate, abscesses of the upper lateral incisors may track into the palatal submucosa. Abscesses of upper canines often open facially just below the orbit. Here the swelling may obstruct drainage in the angular part of the facial vein (p. 1577) which has no valves; it is therefore possible for infected material to travel via the angular and ophthalmic veins into the cavernous sinus. Abscesses on the palatal roots of upper molars usually open on the palate.

Upper second premolars and first and second molars are related to the maxillary sinus. When this is large, the root apices of these teeth may be separated from its cavity solely by the lining mucosa. Sinus infections may stimulate the nerves entering the teeth, simulating toothache. Upper first premolars and third molars may be closely related to the maxillary sinus.

With loss of teeth, alveolar bone is extensively resorbed. Thus in the edentulous mandible the mental nerve, originally inferior to premolar roots, may lie near the crest of the bone. In the edentulous maxilla, its sinus may enlarge to approach the bone's oral surface.

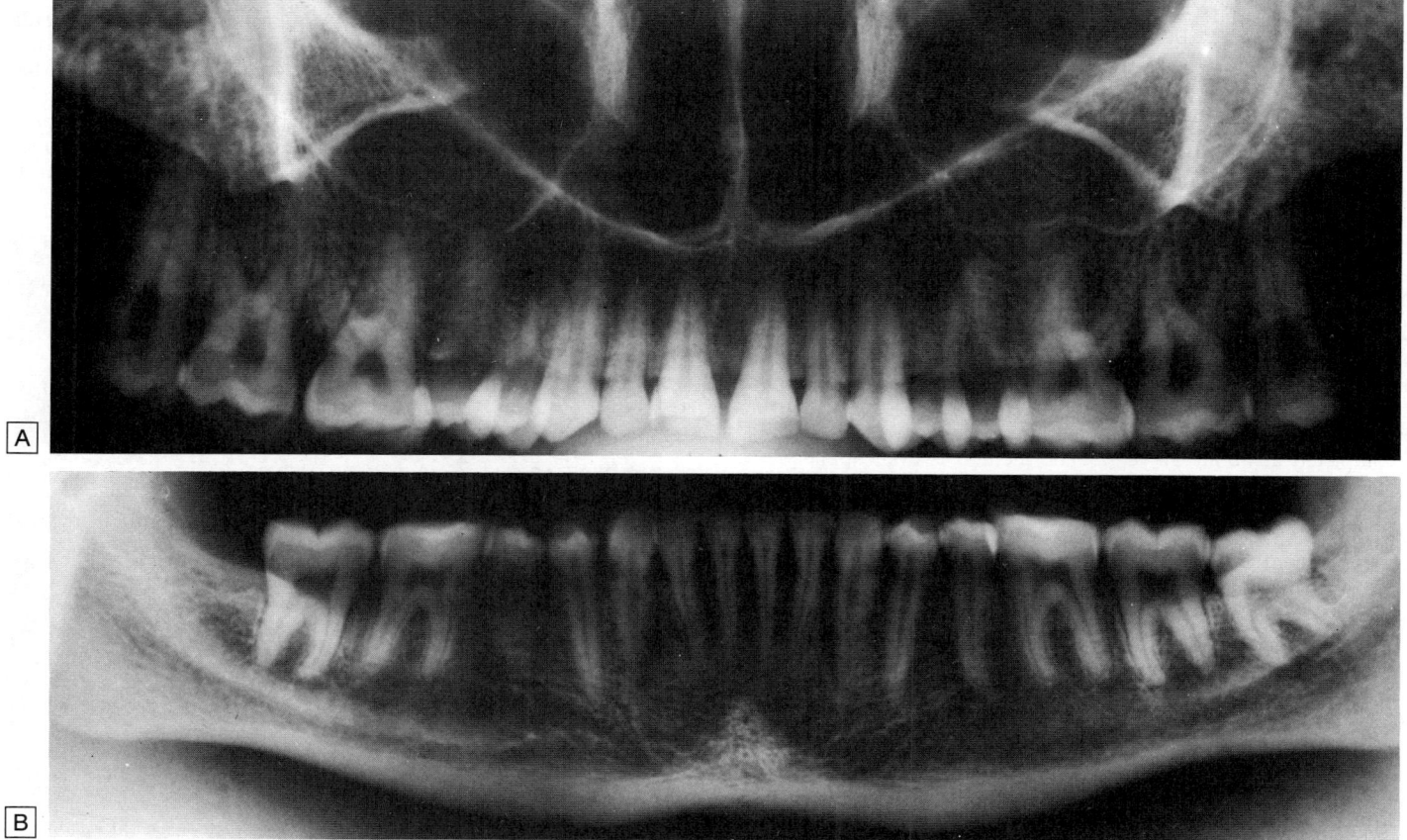

12.50A, B Pan-oral radiographs of the whole dentition of A the upper and B lower jaws of a mature human skull. Note the right lower third molar is missing. To achieve these radiographs, an X-ray source is introduced into the buccal cavity, directed towards the palate for the upper jaw and towards the floor of the cavity for the lower jaw. The X-ray beam is deflected magnetically to disperse anterolaterally and the film is wrapped around the external aspect of the jaws. The clarity of the radiographs is much greater than that possible during clinical radiography of the living head. (The radiographs were prepared by D White of the X-ray Department of the Royal Dental Hospital, London.)

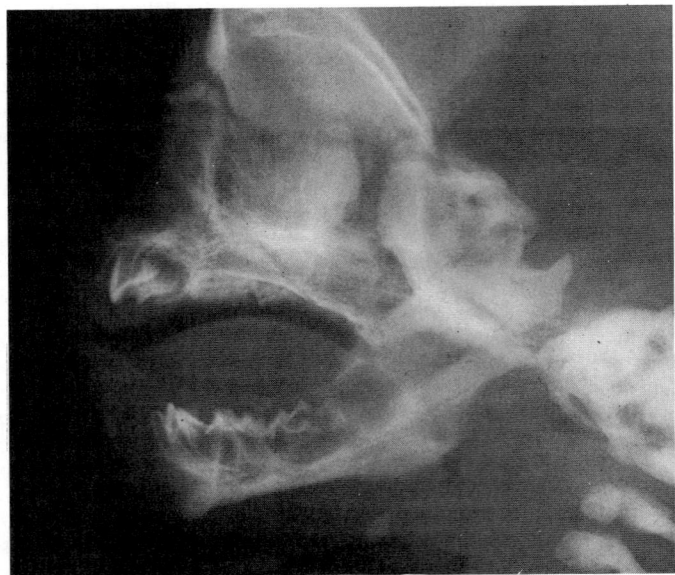

12.51   A lateral radiograph of the jaws of a newborn child. Note the state of development of the jaws and teeth.

Floor of maxillary sinus

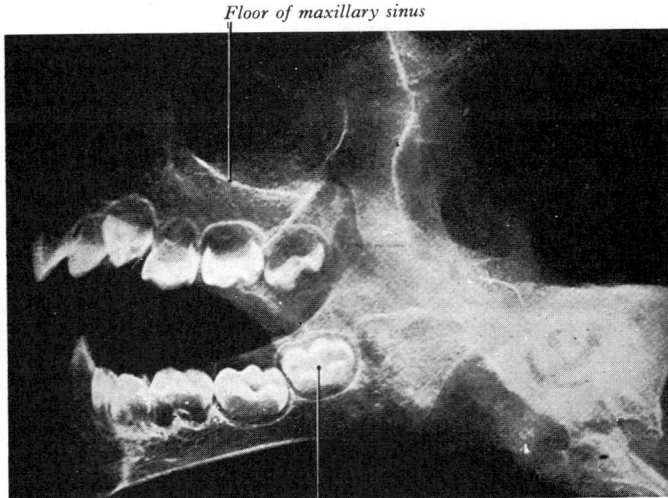

First permanent molar

12.52   Radiograph of the jaws of an infant, nine months old (from Symington & Rankin *Atlas of Skiagrams*). Only the lower central incisor has erupted; the roots of the first lower deciduous molar are just beginning to form; the crown of the first lower permanent molar faces inwards.

Lingual to the lower premolars or molars, the upper molars and in the midline of the palate, there are occasional bony prominences termed the *torus mandibularis*, *torus maxillaris* and *torus palatinus* (p. 563). They may need surgical removal before satisfactory dentures can be fitted.

Severe systemic infections during the time the teeth are developing may lead to faults in enamel, visible as horizontal lines (cf. Harris's growth lines p. 441).

FORENSIC APPLICATIONS

Dental evidence is valuable in three areas of forensic medicine:

* identification of individuals, especially following mass disasters
* estimation of age at death of skeletonized remains
* cases of criminal injury by biting.

If some teeth have been repaired, extracted or replaced by a denture, an individual will have a virtually unique dentition and the dentist will have recorded it in the form of charts, radiographs or plaster casts. Being the most indestructible bodily structures, teeth can provide an identification when trauma or fire has rendered the face unrecognizable. Estimating age may also of course help to establish a body's identity. The chronology of crown development, eruption and root formation can be used to estimate age until the third molar is completed at about 21 years. The method is even applicable to the fetus: Stack (1964) has shown that the weight of mineralized tissue in teeth is closely related to age from about 22 weeks' gestation until birth. Parturition is indicated in the deciduous dentition and first permanent molars by a neonatal line, identifiable in ground sections of teeth or by electron microscopy and which can serve as a marker in estimating the age of an infant by counting the subsequent incremental striae of Retzius formed at intervals of 7–8 days. Since structural changes occur throughout life in all dental tissues, teeth can be used to determine the age of an adult. The features used for this purpose include wear of the crown, reduction in size of the pulp and increase in thickness of cement in the apical half of the root. But the most useful single characteristic is the amount of sclerotic or translucent dentine in the root. This begins to form at the apex and progresses cervically, its linear extent as seen in longitudinally sectioned teeth being proportional to age. Such estimations are within 5–7 years of the chronological age (Whittaker 1992) and likely to be closer to the true age than those derived from skeletal changes.

Photographs of dermal bite marks can be compared with casts of a suspect's dentition: unusual irregularities in form or arrangement of teeth will aid in the culprit's identification. Saliva obtained from bite marks may be even more useful: in most people it contains blood group agglutinogens in very high concentrations. But saliva also contains cells and hence a precise biochemical identification by DNA 'fingerprinting' may be possible.

DENTAL RADIOLOGY

Due to dense mineralization, the enamel and dentine are radio-opaque whereas pulp appears as a radiolucent region (**12**.50, 51, 52, 53). Caries, which attacks teeth through the enamel or root surface, is easily diagnosed by intraoral radiographs because it demineralizes teeth. The root of a tooth is separated from cortical bone (*lamina dura*) by the radiolucent periodontal ligament. Chronic infections of the pulp spread into this ligament, leading to resorption of the

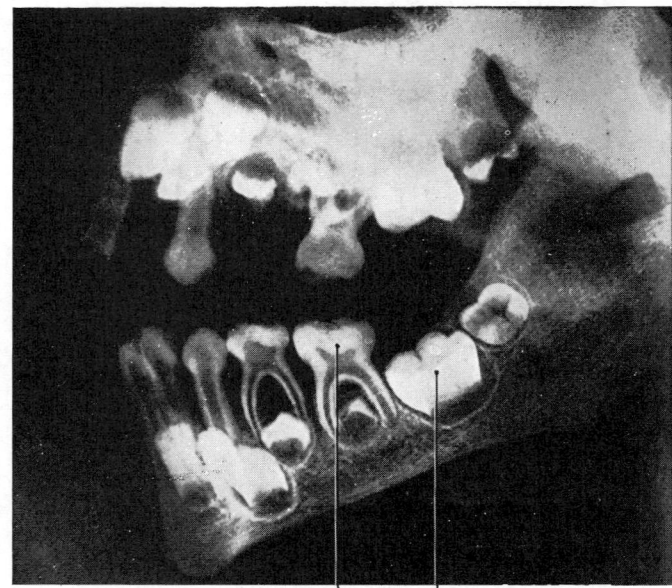

Second deciduous molar   *First permanent molar*

12.53   Radiograph of the teeth of a boy, aged five years (from Symington & Rankin *Atlas of Skiagrams*). In the maxilla the lateral deciduous incisor and the first deciduous molar have been lost, but all the deciduous teeth are present in the mandible. No absorption of the roots of the deciduous teeth has occurred. No permanent teeth have erupted.

lamina dura around the dental apex. Thus continuity of the lamina dura around the apex of a tooth usually indicates a healthy apical region, except in acute infections where resorption of bone has not yet begun.

Anteriorly, interdental septa form sharp crests between the teeth; between molariform teeth they form tables. In periodontal disease, the eventual sequel to gingival disease, bony crests or tables are resorbed and the extent of the condition can therefore be determined radiographically.

Radiographs are commonly used to estimate separation between the roots of maxillary teeth and the maxillary sinus; roots of the

second premolar and first and second molar often project into the sinus. Mandibular third molars are commonly prevented from erupting by impaction against the second molars and radiographs are indispensable in assessing the degree of difficulty in extracting such teeth. Superior to the mental spines (genial tubercles), many mandibles exhibit a well-defined pit ending in a canal, presumably containing a median blood vessel or perhaps penetrating collagen fibres connected to the lingual frenulum. This pit, together with a radio-opaque ring of compact bone, can usually be seen in radiographs of incisors and is a useful median landmark in an edentulous mandible.

TONGUE AND PHARYNX

TONGUE

The tongue (**12**.54, 55, 56) is a highly muscular organ of deglutition, taste and speech. It is partly oral and partly pharyngeal in position, and is attached by its muscles to the hyoid bone, mandible, styloid processes, soft palate and the pharyngeal wall. It has a *root*, an *apex*, a curved *dorsum* and an *inferior surface*. Its mucosa is normally pink and moist, and is attached closely to the underlying muscles. The *root of the tongue* (**12**.55) is attached to the hyoid bone and mandible; between these it is in contact inferiorly with the geniohyoid and mylohyoid muscles. The *dorsum* (posterosuperior surface) is generally convex in all directions at rest. It is divided by the V-shaped *sulcus terminalis* into an *anterior*, *oral* or *presulcal part* facing upwards and a *posterior*, *pharyngeal* or *postsulcal part* facing posteriorly, the anterior part forming about two-thirds of the tongue's length. The two limbs of the sulcus terminalis run anterolaterally to the palatoglossal arches from a median depression, the *foramen caecum* (**12**.54), the site of the upper end of the embryonic thyroid diverticulum (p. 175). The oral and pharyngeal parts of the tongue differ in their mucosa, nerve supply and developmental origins (p. 1714).

Oral (presulcal) part (**12**.54, 55). Located in the floor of the oral cavity, this has an *apex* touching the incisor teeth; a *margin* in contact with the gums and teeth; and a *superior surface* (dorsum) related to the hard and soft palates. On each side, in front of the palatoglossal arch, are four or five vertical folds, the *foliate papillae* (**12**.54). The dorsal mucosa has a longitudinal *median sulcus* (**12**.54), and is papillated. The inferior mucosa is smooth, purplish and reflected on to the oral floor and gums, being connected to the former anteriorly by the median mucosal fold, the *frenulum linguae* (**12**.55); lateral to this on either side, the deep lingual vein is visible, and lateral to the vein is a fringed mucosal ridge, the *plica fimbriata*, directed anteromedially towards the lingual apex. The oral part of the tongue develops from the lingual swellings of the mandibular arch and from the tuberculum impar (p. 175). Its general sensory nerve is the lingual branch of the mandibular, whilst the chorda tympani branch of the facial mediates taste. (For the origin of lingual musculature see p. 274.)

Pharyngeal (postsulcal) part (**12**.54). Forming the base of the tongue, it lies posterior to the palatoglossal arches within the oropharynx, forming its anterior wall. Its mucosa is reflected laterally on to the palatine tonsils and pharyngeal wall and posteriorly on to the epiglottic folds. Devoid of papillae, it has low elevations, due to lymphoid nodules embedded in the submucosa, collectively termed the *lingual tonsil*. The ducts of small seromucous glands open on the

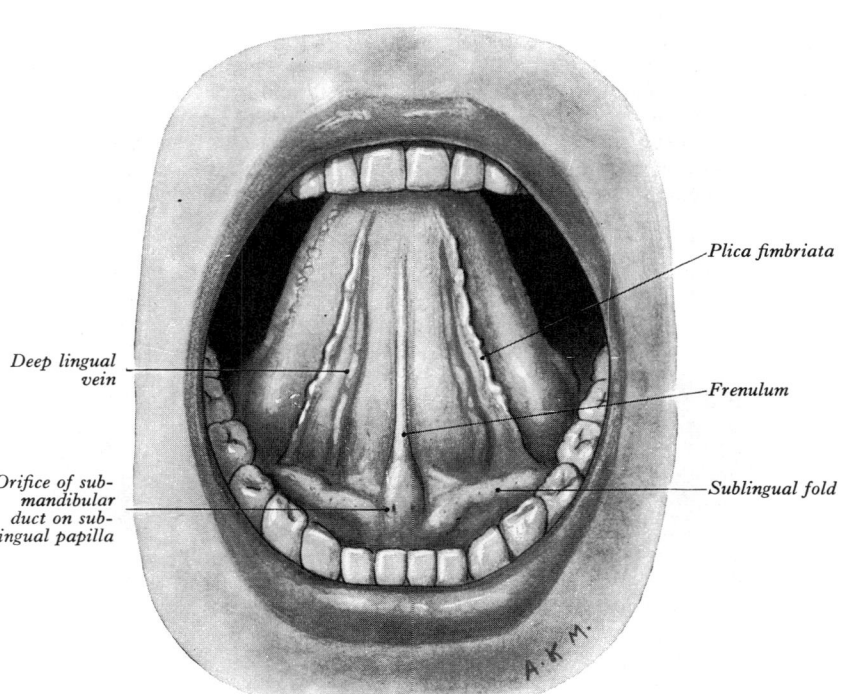

12.54 The dorsum of the tongue, with adjoining palatoglossal and palatopharyngeal arches, and epiglottis. Note the palatine tonsils in the tonsillar recesses on either side.

12.55 The cavity of the mouth. The tip of the tongue is turned upwards. In the person from whom the drawing was made the two sublingual papillae formed a single median elevation.

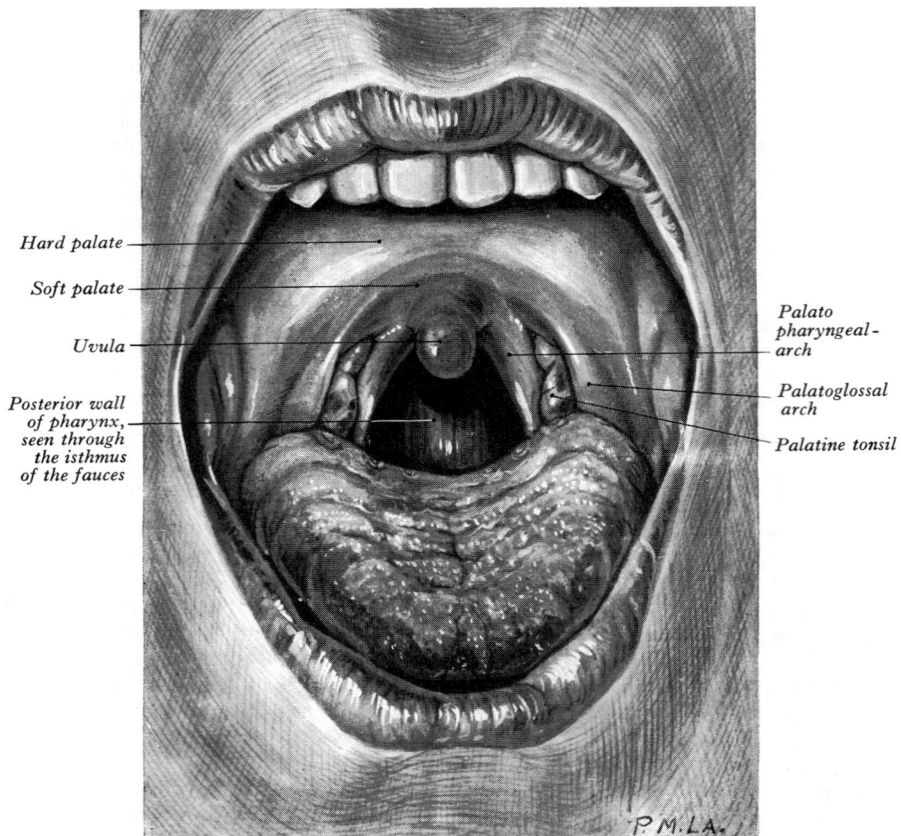

12.56   The cavity of the mouth with the tongue depressed, showing the oral cavity and also the oropharyngeal isthmus between the palatoglossal folds.

apices of these elevations. The postsulcal tongue develops from the hypobranchial eminence (p. 175). Its sensory nerve, including general sensation and taste, is the glossopharyngeal, whose rami also extend to a narrow strip of mucosa anterior to the sulcus terminalis to supply the taste buds of the vallate papillae, an arrangement explained by the embryonic extension of the hypobranchial eminence (derived from the third pharyngeal arch) anteriorly over the posterior part of the lingual swellings (p. 175). Rarely the thyroid gland fails to migrate away from the tongue during development, and then forms a lingual thyroid gland.

Lingual papillae (**12**.54). These are projections of mucosa from the dorsum of the tongue. (See also p. 1687.) They are numerous but limited to the presulcal part of the dorsum, producing its charac-

teristic roughness; there are four principal types: *filiform, fungiform, foliate* and *vallate papillae*. All except the filiform papillae bear taste buds. These projections are modifications of mucous membrane which increase the area of contact between the tongue and the contents of the mouth, and in some cases are also gustatory structures. *Taste buds* (see p. 1312) are microscopic barrel-shaped epithelial structures which contain chemosensory cells in synaptic contact with the terminals of gustatory nerves; they are not restricted to the papillae, being scattered over the entire lingual dorsum and sides, epiglottis and lingual aspect of the soft palate. They are innervated by the appropriate gustatory nerves (facial, glossopharyngeal or vagal according to their position). The papillae are more visible in the living when the tongue is dry.

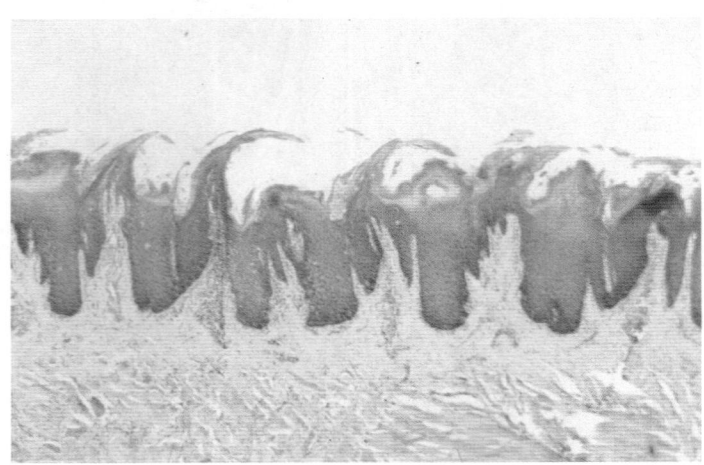

12.57   Section through filiform papillae from the anterior part of the tongue, showing keratinized stratified squamous epithelial covering and connective tissue papillae. Haematoxylin and eosin. Magnification × 300.

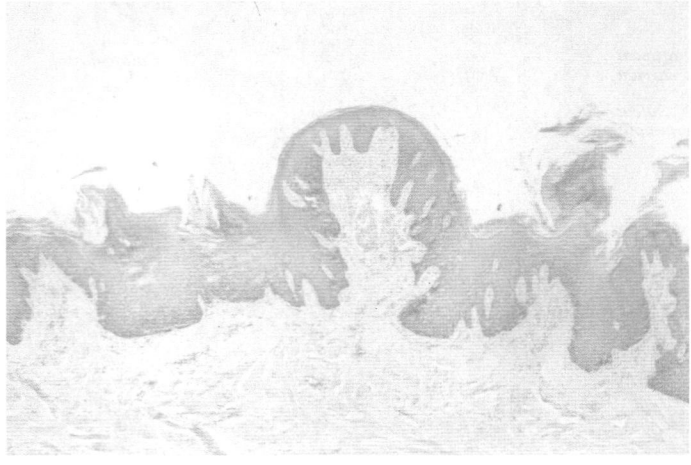

12.58   Vertical section through a fungiform papilla, stained with haematoxylin and eosin (primate). Magnification × 300.

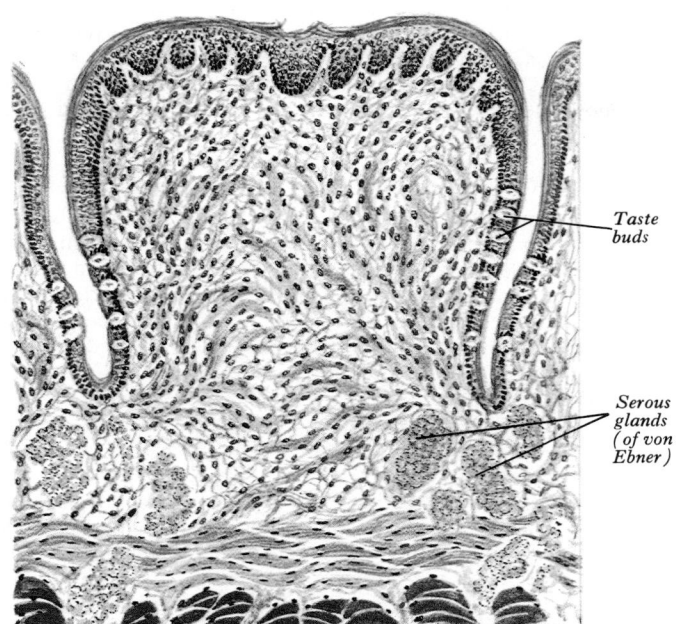

12.59 Section through a vallate papilla (after Sobotta). Stained with haematoxylin and eosin. Magnification × 32.

Taste buds

Serous glands (of von Ebner)

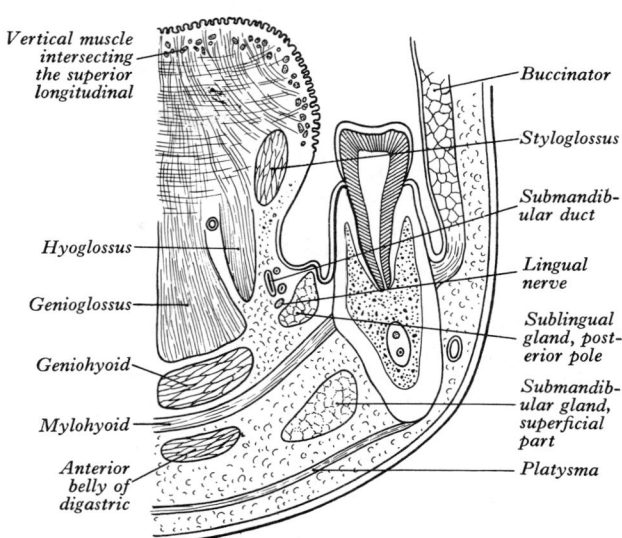

Vertical muscle intersecting the superior longitudinal

Buccinator

Styloglossus

Submandibular duct

Hyoglossus

Genioglossus

Lingual nerve

Geniohyoid

Sublingual gland, posterior pole

Mylohyoid

Submandibular gland, superficial part

Anterior belly of digastric

Platysma

12.60 Diagram of a coronal section through the tongue, the mouth and the body of the mandible opposite the first molar tooth.

Filiform papillae (**12**.57). Covering most of the presulcal dorsal area (Kullaa-Mikkonen et al 1987), they are minute, conical or cylindrical and arranged in diagonal rows directed anterolaterally, parallel with the sulcus terminalis, except at the lingual apex where they are transverse. They have irregular cores of connective tissue ('secondary papillae'), and their epithelium, which is keratinized, may split into fine processes, each being the apex of a secondary papilla; these processes are whitish, owing to a thickened epithelium, the elongated cells being keratinized. The role of these papillae appears to be to increase the friction between the tongue and food, facilitating the movement of particles by the tongue within the oral cavity.

Fungiform papillae (**12**.54, 58). These are more frequent than vallate; they occur mainly on the lingual margin but also irregularly on the dorsum, where they may occasionally be numerous. They differ from filiform papillae by their larger size, rounded shape and deep red colour; each usually bears one or more taste buds on its apical surface.

Foliate papillae (**12**.54) (folia linguae). Lying bilaterally, these are two zones, each formed by a series of red, leaf-like mucosal ridges at the sides of the tongue near the sulcus terminalis; they bear numerous taste buds.

Vallate papillae (**12**.54). Large cylindrical structures, varying in number from 8 to 12 on the dorsum of the tongue; they form a V-shaped row immediately in front of the sulcus terminalis. Each papilla, 1–2 mm in diameter, is encompassed by a slight circular elevation (vallum or wall) in the mucosa separated from the papilla by a circular sulcus (**12**.59). The papilla is narrower at its base than its apex. The entire structure is covered with stratified squamous epithelium; taste buds (p. 1312) abound in both walls of the sulcus, and small mucoserous glands (of von Ebner) open into the sulcal base.

Other papillae. The epithelium of the tongue has a highly folded interface with the underlying connective tissue, a condition similar to that of the epidermis (**12**.57). The connective tissue papillae are sometimes termed *papillae simplices*; they are present beneath the entire tongue surface including the mucosal papillae described above and this arrangement serves to increase the anchorage of the epithelium to the underlying tissues.

LINGUAL MUSCULATURE

The tongue is divided by a median fibrous septum, attached to the body of the hyoid bone. In each half are both the extrinsic and intrinsic muscles, the former extending outside the tongue, the latter wholly within it.

Extrinsic muscles (**12**.60, 61, 67)

These (**12**.94B) include the *genioglossus, hyoglossus, styloglossus, chondroglossus* and *palatoglossus* muscles.

Genioglossus. This is triangular in sagittal section, lying near and parallel to the midline; it arises from a short tendon attached to the superior genial tubercle behind the mandibular symphysis, above the origin of the geniohyoid. From this point it fans out backwards and upwards. The inferior fibres of genioglossus are attached by a thin aponeurosis to the upper anterior surface of the hyoid body near the midline, a few fasciculi passing between hyoglossus and chondroglossus to blend with the pharyngeal middle constrictor; intermediate fibres pass backwards into the posterior tongue, and superior fibres ascend forwards to enter the whole length of the ventral surface of the tongue from root to apex, intermingling with the intrinsic lingual muscles. The muscles of opposite sides are separated posteriorly by the lingual septum (p. 1724); anteriorly they are variably blended by decussation of fasciculi across the midline. Doran & Baggett (1972) considered that no fibres reach the lingual apex in man or other mammals.

Actions. Genioglossus brings about the forward traction of the tongue to protrude its apex from the mouth. Acting bilaterally, the two muscles depress the central part of the tongue, making it concave from side to side. Acting unilaterally, the tongue diverges to the opposite side.

Hyoglossus. Thin and quadrilateral, this muscle is attached to the whole length of the greater cornu and the front of the body of the hyoid bone, passing almost vertically up to enter the side of the tongue between styloglossus laterally and the inferior longitudinal muscle medially. Fibres arising from the hyoid body overlap those from the greater cornu.

Relations. Hyoglossus is related at its *superficial surface* with: the digastric tendon, stylohyoid, styloglossus and mylohyoid, the lingual nerve and submandibular ganglion, the sublingual gland, the deep part of the submandibular gland and duct, the hypoglossal nerve and the deep lingual vein. By its *deep surface* it is related with: the stylohyoid ligament, genioglossus, inferior longitudinal muscle, lingual artery and glossopharyngeal nerve. Postero-inferiorly it is separated from the middle constrictor by the lingual artery; this part of the muscle is in the lateral wall of the pharynx, below the palatine tonsil. Passing deep to the muscle's posterior border are, in descending order: the glossopharyngeal nerve, stylohyoid ligament and lingual artery.

Action. The hyoglossus depresses the tongue.

Chondroglossus. Sometimes described as a part of hyoglossus,

1723

it is separated from it by some fibres of genioglossus which pass to the side of the pharynx. It is about 2 cm long, arising from the medial side and base of the lesser cornu and the adjoining part of the hyoid body and ascending to merge into the intrinsic musculature between the hyoglossus and genioglossus. A small slip occasionally springs from the cartilago triticea and enters the tongue with the posterior fibres of hyoglossus.

Action. Chondroglossus assists hyoglossus in depressing the tongue.

Styloglossus. The shortest and smallest of the three styloid muscles, it arises from the anterolateral aspect of the styloid process near its apex, and from the styloid end of the stylomandibular ligament. Passing down and forwards, it divides at the side of the tongue into a longitudinal part, which enters the tongue dorso-laterally to blend with the inferior longitudinal muscle in front of the hyoglossus, and an oblique part, overlapping the hyoglossus and decussating with it.

Action. Styloglossus draws the tongue up and backwards.

Nerve supply. Excepting palatoglossus, which is innervated by the cranial accessory/vagal component of the pharyngeal plexus (p. 1252), all extrinsic lingual muscles are supplied by the hypoglossal nerve.

Palatoglossus. This muscle is closely associated with the soft palate in function and innervation, and is described with the other palatal muscles (p. 1690).

Intrinsic muscles (12.60)

These are the bilateral superior and inferior longitudinal, the transverse and the vertical lingual muscles.

Superior longitudinal muscle. A thin stratum of oblique and longitudinal fibres lying beneath the dorsal lingual mucosa, this muscle extends forwards from the submucous fibrous tissue near the epiglottis and from the median lingual septum to the lingual margins, some fibres being inserted into the mucous membrane.

Inferior longitudinal muscle. A narrow band close to the inferior lingual surface between genioglossus and hyoglossus, this extends from the lingual root to the apex, some of its posterior fibres being connected to the body of the hyoid bone; anteriorly it blends with the styloglossus.

Transverse muscle. It passes laterally from the median fibrous septum to the submucous fibrous tissue at the lingual margin, blending with palatopharyngeus (p. 1690).

Vertical muscle. This extends from the dorsal to the ventral aspects of the tongue in the borders of its anterior part.

Nerve supply. All intrinsic lingual muscles are supplied by the hypoglossal nerve.

Actions. The intrinsic muscles alter the shape of the tongue; thus, the superior and inferior longitudinal muscles tend to shorten it; but the former also turns the apex and sides upwards to make the dorsum concave, while the latter pulls the apex down to make the dorsum convex. The transverse muscle narrows and elongates the tongue; the vertical muscle makes it flatter and wider. Acting alone or in pairs and in endless combination, they give the tongue precise and highly varied mobility, important not only in alimentary function but also in speech (p. 1651).

MICROSTRUCTURE OF THE TONGUE

The tongue consists largely of skeletal muscle, partly invested by mucosa. The *lingual mucosa* of the inferior surface is thin, smooth and like that in much of the rest of the oral cavity. The mucosa of the pharyngeal part of the dorsum contains many lymphoid follicles, each follicle forming a rounded eminence, central in which is the minute orifice of a funnel-shaped recess. Many round or oval lymphoid nodules, each encapsulated by submucous fibrous tissue, surround each recess, which receives the ducts of mucous glands in its floor. In the oral part the dorsal mucosa is somewhat thicker than ventrally and laterally; it is adherent to muscular tissue, and covered by numerous *papillae* (p. 396). It consists of connective tissue (*lamina propria*) and stratified squamous epithelium, which also covers each papilla. The lamina propria is a dense fibrous connective tissue, with numerous elastic fibres, united to similar tissue which spreads between the lingual muscle fasciculi. It contains the ramifications of numerous vessels and nerves from which the papillae are supplied, and also large lymph plexuses and lingual glands. The epithelium varies from parakeratinized stratified squamous epithelium posteriorly, to fully keratinized epithelium overlying the filiform papillae more anteriorly; these features appear to be related to the fact that the apex of the tongue is subject to greater dehydration than the posterior and ventral parts and is more abraded during mastication.

Lingual glands

These are of mucous, serous and mixed types. The *mucous glands* are like the labial and buccal glands in structure; they are numerous in the postsulcal region but are also present at the apex and margins. The *anterior lingual salivary glands* lie at the ventral surface of the apex (**12**.62), one on each side of the frenulum, where they are covered by mucosa and a muscular fasciculus derived from the styloglossus and inferior longitudinal muscles. From 12 mm to 20 mm long and about 8 mm broad, each has mucous and serous alveoli and opens by three or four ducts on the inferior surface of the lingual apex. The fine structure of the human *deep posterior lingual glands* has been described in detail by Testa Riva et al (1985).

The *serous glands* (of von Ebner, **12**.59) occur near the taste buds, their ducts opening mostly into the sulci of vallate papillae. They are racemose, the main duct dividing into several channels ending in acini. Their secretion is watery, probably assisting in gustation by spreading substances over the taste area and then washing them away afterwards. The pyramidal shape and ultrastructure of the secretory cells of the acini are similar to those of serous cells elsewhere (see also Testa Riva et al 1985).

The *lingual septum* is a median fibrous partition extending through the length of the tongue but it does not quite reach the dorsum. It is an attachment of the transverse lingual muscles and appears prominently in coronal sections. Posteriorly it extends laterally to form the *hyoglossal membrane*, connecting the lingual root to the hyoid bone, and the inferior fibres of the genioglossi are attached to it.

LINGUAL VESSELS AND NERVES (12.62)

Vessels

The main **artery** is the lingual branch of the external carotid (p. 1516, **10**.76) but the tonsillar and ascending palatine branches of the facial and ascending pharyngeal arteries also supply the lingual root. In the vallecula (p. 1642) epiglottic branches of the superior laryngeal artery anastomose with the inferior dorsal branches of the lingual artery. Lingual muscles are supplied from this rich anastomotic network and there is a very dense submucosal plexus (Combelles 1974). The **veins** are described on p. 1580 and **lymph vessels** on p. 1613.

Nerves

The *sensory nerves* are:

- the lingual branch of the mandibular nerve for general sensation in the presulcal region (p. 1247, **8**.339, 357);
- the chorda tympani branch of the facial nerve (p. 1246), running in the sheath of the lingual nerve, for gustation in the presulcal region exclusive of the vallate papillae (p. 1313); its sensory fibres are derived from the nervus intermedius (p. 1243);
- the lingual branch of the glossopharyngeal nerve (p. 1249), distributed to the postsulcal mucosa of the lingual base and sides and to the vallate papillae and mediating general and gustatory sensation;
- the superior laryngeal nerve (vagus) (p. 1253), which sends fine branches to the root immediately in front of the epiglottis.

The problem of proprioception in the tongue has been reviewed by Fitzgerald and Sachithanadan (1979). Muscle spindles occur in monkeys (Bowman 1968) and in mankind (e.g. Nakayama 1944; Cooper 1953; Kubota et al 1975), as also confirmed in extensive simian material by the above reviewers. The peripheral route from these undoubted receptors is not clear, though it is perhaps in the lingual or hypoglossal nerves and by cervical spinal nerves communicating with the latter. In monkeys Fitzgerald and Sachithanadan presented strong evidence indicating the hypoglossal nerve as the main proprioceptor route for the intrinsic and extrinsic musculature, many fibres leaving it to enter the second and third cervical anterior primary spinal rami.

The *motor innervation* to all tongue muscles except palatoglossus is from the hypoglossal nerve (p. 1256); palatoglossus receives its supply from the pharyngeal plexus (vagus and cranial accessory, see p. 1252).

The *parasympathetic innervation* of the various glands of the tongue is from the chorda tympani branch of the facial nerve, synapsing in the submandibular ganglion and distributing to the tongue mucosa via the lingual nerve branches. The *sympathetic supply* to lingual glands and vessels enters the tongue through plexuses around its arteries, arising from the carotid plexus (p. 1300). In the postsulcal region, isolated nerve cells have been observed, perhaps postganglionic parasympathetic neurons, **probably** innervating glandular tissue and perhaps vascular smooth muscle (Chu 1968).

CONGENITAL ABNORMALITIES OF THE TONGUE

Congenital cysts and fistulae may develop from the persistent remains of the thyroglossal duct (p. 176). Failure of the thyroid gland to migrate out of the tongue may result in its retention as a lingual

thyroid in the posterior, postsulcal region. The attachment of the genioglossi to the genial tubercles behind the mandibular symphysis prevents the tongue from sinking back and obstructing respiration; therefore, anaesthetists pull forward the mandible to obtain the full benefit of this connection.

OROPHARYNGEAL ISTHMUS

The aperture of communication between the mouth and pharynx, the *oropharyngeal isthmus* (**12**.56) is situated between the soft palate and the lingual dorsum, bounded at the sides by the palatoglossal arches. Each *palatoglossal arch* runs down, laterally and forwards, from the soft palate to the side of the tongue; it is formed by the projecting palatoglossus (p. 1690) with its covering mucous membrane. The approximation of the arches, to shut off the mouth from the oropharynx, is essential to deglutition (p. 1730).

PHARYNX (12.1, 3, 63–69)

The pharynx, situated behind the nasal cavities, mouth and larynx,

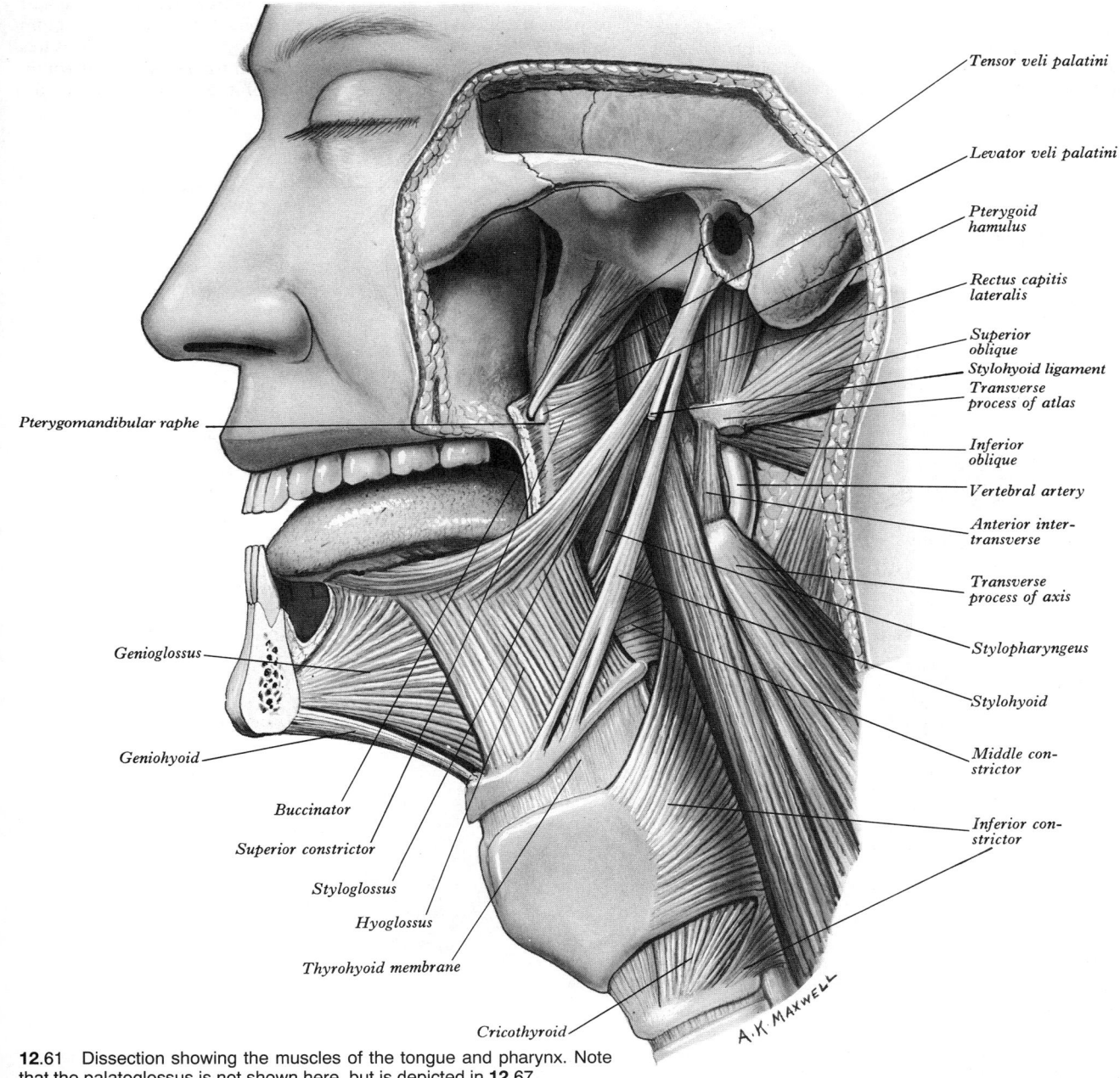

12.61 Dissection showing the muscles of the tongue and pharynx. Note that the palatoglossus is not shown here, but is depicted in **12.67**.

Labels (clockwise from top right):
- Tensor veli palatini
- Levator veli palatini
- Pterygoid hamulus
- Rectus capitis lateralis
- Superior oblique
- Stylohyoid ligament
- Transverse process of atlas
- Inferior oblique
- Vertebral artery
- Anterior inter-transverse
- Transverse process of axis
- Stylopharyngeus
- Stylohyoid
- Middle con-strictor
- Inferior con-strictor
- Cricothyroid
- Thyrohyoid membrane
- Hyoglossus
- Styloglossus
- Superior constrictor
- Buccinator
- Geniohyoid
- Genioglossus
- Pterygomandibular raphe

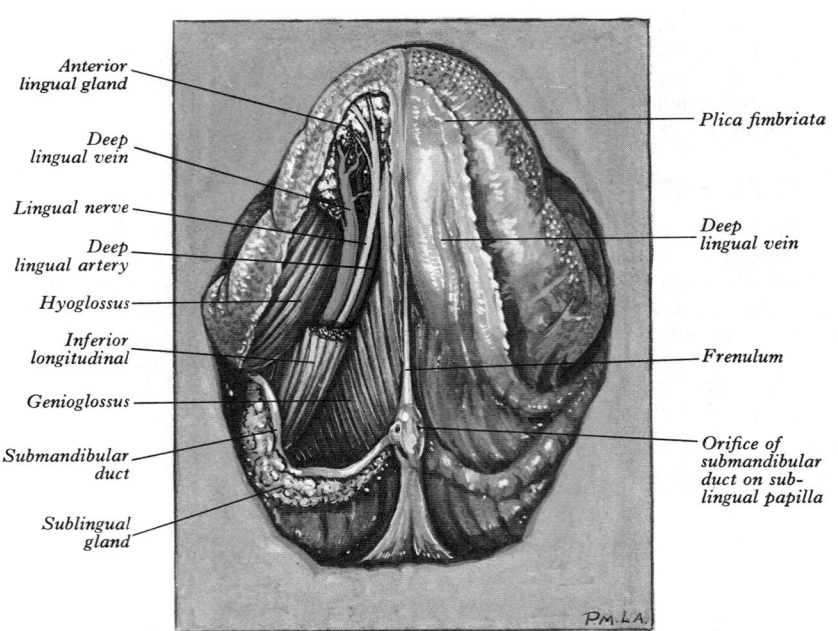

12.62 Dissection of the inferior surface of the tongue, also showing the sublingual glands and submandibular duct openings. On the right side (left side of figure) the mucous membrane has been removed and the inferior longitudinal muscle has been divided and partially resected.

Labels (figure 12.62):
Anterior lingual gland
Deep lingual vein
Lingual nerve
Deep lingual artery
Hyoglossus
Inferior longitudinal
Genioglossus
Submandibular duct
Sublingual gland
Plica fimbriata
Deep lingual vein
Frenulum
Orifice of submandibular duct on sublingual papilla

is a musculomembranous tube, 12–14 cm long, extending from the cranial base to the level of the sixth cervical vertebra and the lower border of the cricoid cartilage where it is continuous with the oesophagus. Its width is greatest superiorly, measuring 3.5 cm; at its junction with the oesophagus it is reduced to about 1.5 cm, this being the narrowest part of the alimentary canal (except for the vermiform appendix). It is limited **above** by the posterior part of the sphenoid body and the basilar part of the occipital bone; **below**, it is continuous with the oesophagus; **behind**, loose connective tissue separates it from the cervical part of the vertebral column and prevertebral fascia covering longus colli and capitis; **in front**, it opens into the nasal cavity, mouth and larynx, its anterior wall being therefore incomplete. It is attached, from above downwards on each side to: the medial pterygoid plate, pterygomandibular raphe, mandible, tongue, hyoid bone, thyroid and cricoid cartilages; **laterally**, it communicates with the tympanic cavities via the pharyngotympanic (auditory) tubes and is related to the styloid processes and their muscles, the common, internal and external carotid arteries, and some of the branches of the last named. The pharynx has three parts: nasal, oral and laryngeal (**12**.63).

NASAL PART OF THE PHARYNX (NASOPHARYNX)

The nasopharynx (**12**.63, 65, 67) lies above the soft palate and behind the *posterior nares (choanae)* which allow free respiratory passage between the nasal cavities and the nasopharynx. The nasal septum separates the two posterior nares (**12**.65), each of which measures approximately 25 mm vertically and 12 mm transversely. Just within these openings lie the posterior ends of the inferior and middle

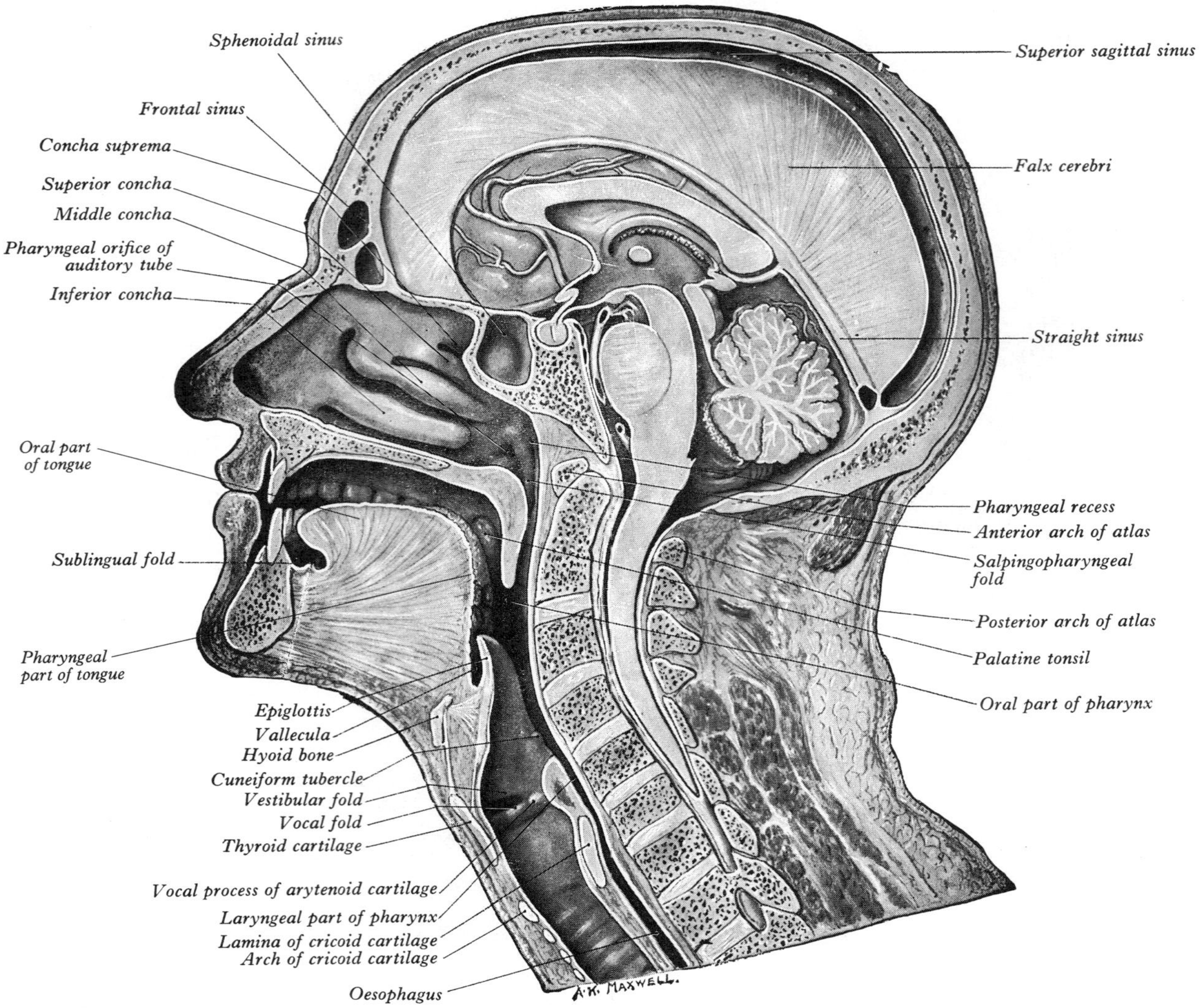

Labels (figure 12.63):
Sphenoidal sinus
Frontal sinus
Concha suprema
Superior concha
Middle concha
Pharyngeal orifice of auditory tube
Inferior concha
Oral part of tongue
Sublingual fold
Pharyngeal part of tongue
Epiglottis
Vallecula
Hyoid bone
Cuneiform tubercle
Vestibular fold
Vocal fold
Thyroid cartilage
Vocal process of arytenoid cartilage
Laryngeal part of pharynx
Lamina of cricoid cartilage
Arch of cricoid cartilage
Oesophagus
Superior sagittal sinus
Falx cerebri
Straight sinus
Pharyngeal recess
Anterior arch of atlas
Salpingopharyngeal fold
Posterior arch of atlas
Palatine tonsil
Oral part of pharynx

12.63 Sagittal section through the nose, mouth, pharynx and larynx. Where it divides the skull and the brain, the section passes slightly to the left of the median plane but, below the base of the skull, it passes slightly to the right of the median plane.

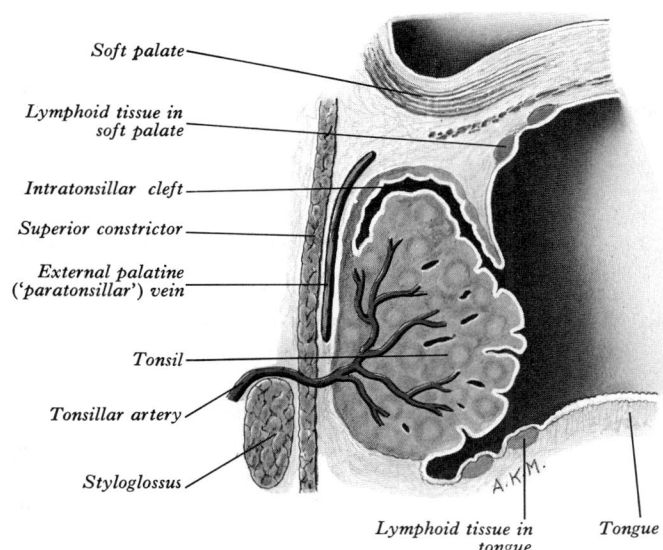

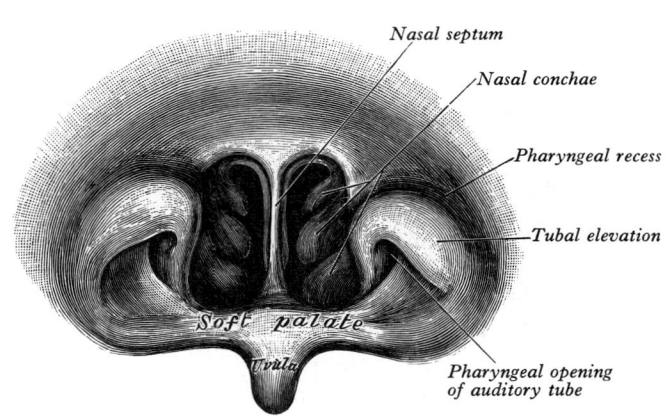

12.65   Ventral boundary of the nasal part of the pharynx, as seen in posterior rhinoscopy.

12.64   Coronal section through the palatine tonsil.

turbinates (**12.64**). Except for the soft palate the walls of the naso-pharynx are static and its cavity is never obliterated, in which respect it differs from the oral and laryngeal parts and resembles the nasal cavities. Between the posterior border of the soft palate and the posterior pharyngeal wall the nasal and oral parts of the pharynx communicate through the *pharyngeal isthmus*, which is closed during swallowing by the elevation of the soft palate and constriction of the palatopharyngeal sphincter (p. 1730). The nasopharynx has a roof, a posterior wall, two lateral walls and a floor.

The *roof* and *posterior wall* together form a continuous, concave slope leading down from the nasal septum to the oropharynx, bounded above by mucosa overlying the posterior part of the body of the sphenoid and further back by the basilar part of the occipital bone as far as the pharyngeal tubercle. Following the posterior wall further downwards, the mucosa overlies the pharyngobasilar fascia and the upper fibres of the superior constrictor, and behind these, the anterior arch of the atlas. A lymphoid mass, the *nasopharygeal tonsil*, lies in the mucosa of the upper part of the roof and posterior wall in the midline (see below; also p. 1374).

The *lateral walls* of the nasopharynx have a number of important surface features. On either side each receives the opening of the *pharyngotympanic tube* (also termed the auditory or Eustachian tube), situated 10–12 mm behind and a little below the level of the inferior nasal turbinate's posterior end (**12.63, 65, 67**). The tubal aperture is approximately triangular in shape, bounded above and behind by the *tubal elevation* consisting of mucosa overlying the protruding pharyngeal end of the tubal cartilage (p. 1374); the prominent posterior margin of this elevation facilitates the intro-duction of catheters passed along the floor of the nasal cavity for the intubation of the pharyngotympanic tube.

Behind the tubal opening, a vertical *salpingopharyngeal fold* of mucosa descends from the tubal elevation, covering the salp-ingopharyngeus muscle in the wall of the pharynx. In front of the aperture, a smaller *salpingopalatine fold* extends from the antero-superior angle of the tubal elevation to the soft palate. The levator veli palatini, entering the soft palate, produces an elevation of the mucosa immediately below the tubal opening (**12.63, 67**). In the mucosa immediately posterior to the opening of the pharyn-gotympanic tube is a small mass of lymphoid tissue, the (bilateral) *tubal tonsils*. Further behind the tubal elevation the lateral wall has a variable depression, the *pharyngeal recess* or *fossa of Rosenmüller* (extensively surveyed by Khoo et al 1969). The *floor* of the naso-pharynx is formed by the upper surface of the soft palate.

Nasopharyngeal tonsil

The nasopharyngeal or pharyngeal tonsil is defined as a collection of lymphoid tissue in the mucosa of the nasopharyngeal roof and posterior wall (see above). Like other components of the lymphoid

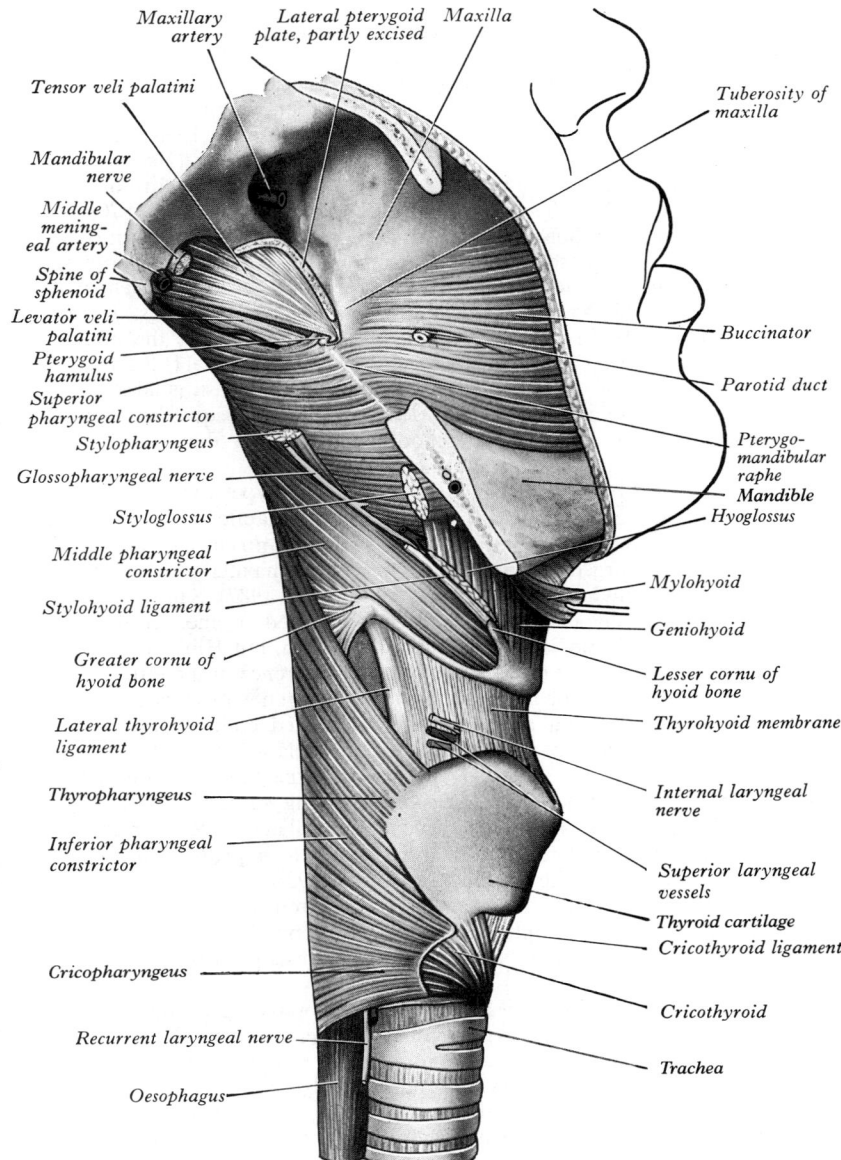

12.66   The buccinator and the muscles of the pharynx.

tissue annulus encircling the pharynx (Waldeyer's ring, p. 1729), it belongs to the category of mucosa-associated lymphoid tissue (MALT: see p. 1442, and below). When the nasopharyngeal tonsil is enlarged, it is commonly referred to as the adenoid or adenoids (Beasley 1987), and in the past, Luschka's tonsil (Bershof et al 1987; p. 1447).

The nasopharyngeal tonsil hangs from the roof of the nasopharynx. In surface view it is an oblong, truncated pyramid, its apex pointing towards the nasal septum and its base at the junction of the roof and posterior wall of the nasopharynx. The anterior border is vertical, parallel to the posterior nares, while the posterior border gradually merges into the posterior pharyngeal wall. The lateral borders slope downwards and medially. The free surface is marked by folds radiating forwards and laterally from a median blind recess extending backwards and up, the *pharyngeal bursa* (bursa of Luschka), developmentally the rostral end of the notochord. The number and position of the folds and of the deep fissures separating them vary. A median fold may pass forwards from the pharyngeal bursa towards the nasal septum, or instead a fissure may extend forwards from the bursa, dividing the nasopharyngeal tonsil into two distinct halves (reflecting its paired developmental origins, p. 176). The fissures passing forwards are often curved with their convexity directed outwards, while those near the base of the tonsil are generally straight and nearly transverse (Symington 1914). The size of the nasopharyngeal tonsil is variable according to age (see below), individuality and changes involving hypertrophy and inflammation.

Postnatal development. The prenatal origins and growth of the nasopharyngeal tonsil are described on page 176. After birth the nasopharyngeal tonsil increases rapidly in size in the first few years of life, but there is no unanimous opinion on the time course of its postnatal progression. Its developmental peak has been suggested by various authors to be the second or third year (Hollender & Szanto 1945), the fifth year (Linder-Aronson 1983), the fifth or sixth year (Lion 1950), between the fifth and tenth year (Meyer 1870) and the tenth year (Suarez 1980). All authors describe the involution or atrophy of the nasopharyngeal tonsil at puberty, although hypoplasia may still occur in adults up to the seventh decade (Hollender & Szanto 1945; Yeh 1962). Using lateral skull radiographs, Linder-Aronson (1983) observed two peaks in its size, one, the greater, occurring at 5 years, and the second between 10 and 11. Relative to the volume of the nasopharynx, the size of the tonsil is largest at 5 years, a finding which could account for the frequency of nasal breathing problems in preschool children, and the incidence of adenoidectomy in this age group.

In the literature, nasopharyngeal tonsil hypertrophy has been commonly associated with maxillary growth abnormalities leading to discrepancies in dental occlusion. However, no causal relationship between enlarged nasopharyngeal tonsils and maxillary abnormalities has been convincingly demonstrated (Hibbert 1987). Similarly, nasopharyngeal hypertrophy has been implicated in the aetiology of chronic otitis media with effusion in children, but Hibbert and Stell (1982) found no statistically significant difference in the radiological size of the nasopharyngeal tonsil in children with this condition compared with an age and gender matched control group. Furthermore, Gates et al (1989) found no relationship between preoperative nasopharyngeal tonsil size and the rate of resolution of chronic otitis media with effusion following surgery. Nevertheless, surgical removal of the nasopharyngeal tonsil in children with chronic otitis media with effusion has been shown to improve resolution of this disease in children (Maw & Parker 1993).

Microstructure. The nasopharyngeal tonsil is composed of a rather modified nasopharyngeal epithelium overlying mucosa-associated lymphoid tissue. Details of its microscopic organization are given on page 1448.

Vessels. *The arterial supply* of the nasopharyngeal tonsil derives from branches of the external carotid artery, namely the ascending pharyngeal artery, the ascending palatine artery, the tonsillar branches of the facial artery, the pharyngeal branch of the maxillary artery and the artery of the pterygoid canal. In addition, a nutrient or emissary vessel to the neighbouring bone, the *basisphenoid artery*, a branch of the inferior hypophysial arteries, supplies the bed of the nasopharyngeal tonsil and is a possible cause of persistent postadenoidectomy haemorrhage in some patients (Duncan 1963).

Numerous communicating veins drain the nasopharyngeal tonsil into the internal submucous and external pharyngeal venous plexuses (p. 1580).

Lymphatics. As with other types of mucosa-associated lymphoid tissue, there are no afferent lymphatics. Efferent lymphatics commence in a closed plexus around each lymphoid follicle, pass into the connective tissue septa, pierce the hemicapsule and drain to the upper deep cervical lymph nodes directly, or indirectly through the retropharyngeal lymph nodes.

Innervation. The nasopharynx is innervated by the pharyngeal plexus (p. 1252) situated mainly in the buccopharyngeal fascia. In addition, a small part of the nasopharynx behind the opening of the pharyngotympanic tube receives a sensory supply from the pharyngeal branch of the maxillary nerve.

ORAL PART OF THE PHARYNX (12.56, 63)

The *oropharynx* extends from the soft palate to the upper border of the epiglottis. It opens into the mouth through the oropharyngeal isthmus, demarcated by the palatoglossal arch, and faces the pharyngeal aspect of the tongue. Its lateral wall consists of the palatopharyngeal arch and palatine tonsil. Posteriorly, it is level with the body of the second and upper part of the third cervical vertebrae. The *palatopharyngeal arch* lies behind the *palatoglossal arch*, projecting more medially than the latter, and descends posterolaterally from the uvula to the lateral wall of the pharynx as a fold of mucosa covering palatopharyngeus (p. 1690). On each side of the oropharynx, between the diverging palatopharyngeal and palatoglossal arches, lies the triangular *tonsillar fossa* or *tonsillar sinus* containing the *palatine tonsil*.

Palatine tonsils

The palatine tonsil (tonsilla palatina) (**12.**54, 56, 63, 64) is a bilaterally paired mass of lymphoid tissue situated in the lateral wall of the oropharynx and forming part of a protective annulus of lymphoid tissue, the *Waldeyer's ring* (see p. 1729).

The shape of the palatine tonsil is ovoid and its size is variable according to age, individuality and tissue changes leading to hypertrophy and/or inflammation. It is therefore difficult to define its normal appearance. For the first 5 or 6 years of life the tonsils increase rapidly in size, reaching a maximum at puberty when they average 20–25 mm in vertical and 10–15 mm in transverse diameter, projecting conspicuously into the oropharynx (Symington 1914; McNab Jones 1979). Tonsillar involution begins at puberty when the reactive lymphoid tissue starts to undergo atrophic changes, and by old age only a little tonsillar lymphoid tissue remains.

The long axis of the tonsil is directed from above, downwards and backwards. Its *medial* or *free surface* usually presents a pitted appearance. These *pits*, 10–15 in number, lead to a system of blind-ending, often highly branching *crypts*, which extend through the whole thickness of the tonsil and almost reach the connective tissue hemicapsule (Kassaz & Sandor 1962). In a healthy tonsil the openings of the crypts are fissure-like and the walls of the crypt lumina are collapsed and in contact with each other. The human tonsil is a polycryptic structure, unlike the monocryptic tonsil of some other mammals, e.g. rabbit and sheep (Oláh 1978). The branching crypt system reaches its maximum size and complexity during childhood (Fioretti 1957). In the upper part of the medial surface of the tonsil is the mouth of a deep *intratonsillar cleft*, or *recessus palatinus* (Killian 1898), often erroneously termed the *supratonsillar fossa*. It is **not** situated above the tonsil but within its substance (**12.**63), and the mouth of the cleft is semilunar in shape, curving parallel to the convex dorsum of the tongue in the parasagittal plane. The upper wall of this recess contains lymphoid tissue extending into the soft palate as the *pars palatina of the palatine tonsil* (Hett & Butterfield 1910). After the age of 5 years this embedded part of the tonsil diminishes in size; from the age of 14, there is a tendency for the whole tonsil to retrogress, and for the tonsillar bed to flatten out (Hett 1913). During young adult life a mucosal fold termed the *plica triangularis* (for developmental aspects see p. 176), stretching back from the palatoglossal arch down to the tongue, is infiltrated by lymphoid tissue and frequently represents the most prominent (antero-inferior) portion of the tonsil. However, it rarely persists into middle age.

The *lateral* or *deep surface* of the tonsil spreads downwards, upwards and forwards. Inferiorly, it invades the dorsum of the tongue, superiorly, the soft palate, and, anteriorly, it may extend for some distance under the palatoglossal arch. This deep, lateral aspect is covered by a layer of fibrous tissue, the *tonsillar hemicapsule*, separable with ease for most of its extent from the underlying muscular walls of the pharynx which is formed here by the superior constrictor, with the styloglossus on its lateral side (**12**.63, 66). Antero-inferiorly the hemicapsule adheres to the side of the tongue and to the palatoglossus and palatopharyngeus muscles. In this region the tonsillar artery, a branch of the facial, pierces the superior constrictor to enter the tonsil, accompanied by venae comitantes. An important and sometimes large vein (the external palatine or paratonsillar vein) descends from the soft palate lateral to the tonsillar hemicapsule before piercing the pharyngeal wall (**12**.63); haemorrhage from this vessel, from the upper angle of the tonsillar fossa, may complicate tonsillectomy (Browne 1928). The muscular wall of the tonsillar fossa separates the tonsil from the ascending palatine artery, and, occasionally, from the tortuous facial artery itself (p. 1517) which may be near the pharyngeal wall at the lower tonsillar level. The internal carotid artery lies about 25 mm behind and lateral to the tonsil.

Surface anatomy. The palatine tonsil is too deeply placed to be felt externally, even when enlarged. When the mouth is closed the medial surface of the tonsil touches the dorsum of the tongue. In this position the surface marking of the palatine tonsil on the exterior of the face corresponds to an oval area over the lower part of the masseter muscle, a little above and in front of the angle of the mandible and behind the third lower molar tooth.

Microstructure. The basic structure of the palatine tonsil is that of an accumulation of mucosa-associated lymphoid tissue covered by stratified squamous non-keratinizing epithelium on its oropharyngeal surface, and supported by connective tissue septa arising from the hemicapsule. On the medial, oropharyngeal surface the tonsillar epithelium is deeply invaginated to form 10–30 or more crypts. Like other neighbouring masses of mucosa-associated lymphoid tissue forming Waldeyer's ring (see below), the palatine tonsil is a major source of T and B lymphocytes for local mucosal defence. Further details of its immunological functions and microstructure are given on page 1446.

Blood vessels. The **arterial blood supply** to the palatine tonsil derives from branches of the external carotid artery. The principal artery is the *tonsillar artery*, which is a branch of the facial or sometimes the ascending palatine artery. The tonsillar artery and its venae comitantes often lie within the palatoglossal fold; hence a haemorrhage may be caused by interference with this fold during an operation. Additional small tonsillar branches may derive from the following: the ascending pharyngeal artery; the dorsales linguae, branches of the lingual artery, supplying the lower part of the palatine tonsil; the greater palatine artery (a branch of the maxillary artery) supplying the upper part of the tonsil; and the ascending palatine artery, a branch of the facial artery.

The **tonsillar veins** are numerous and emerge from the deep, lateral surface of the tonsil as the *paratonsillar veins*. They pierce the superior constrictor either to join the pharyngeal venous plexus, or to unite to form a single vessel which enters the facial vein.

Lymphatics. Unlike lymph nodes, the tonsils do not possess afferent lymphatics or lymph sinuses (p. 1432), but dense plexuses of fine lymphatic vessels surround each follicle, forming *efferent lymphatics* which pass towards the hemicapsule, pierce the superior constrictor and drain to the upper deep cervical lymph nodes, especially the *jugulodigastric nodes* (p. 1613). Typically, the latter are enlarged in tonsillitis; they then project beyond the anterior border of the sternocleidomastoid muscle and are palpable superficially 1–2 cm below the angle of the mandible. They represent the most common swelling in the neck.

Nerves. The tonsillar region receives its nerve supply through *tonsillar branches of the trigeminal (maxillary)* and the *glossopharyngeal nerves*. The maxillary nerve fibres passing through (though not synapsing in) the pterygopalatine ganglion and are distributed through the lesser palatine nerves (p. 1235), which, together with the tonsillar branches of the glossopharyngeal nerve (p. 1249), form a plexus around the tonsil. From this plexus, termed the 'circulus tonsillaris' (Barnes 1923), nerve fibres are also distributed

to the soft palate and the region of the oropharyngeal isthmus. The glossopharyngeal nerve additionally supplies, through its tympanic branch, the mucous membrane lining the tympanic cavity. Hence, tonsillitis may be accompanied by pain referred to the ear. The nerve supply to the tonsil is so diffuse that tonsillectomy under local anaesthesia is performed successfully by local infiltration rather than by blocking the main nerves.

WALDEYER'S RING

This annulus of mucosa-associated lymphoid tissue surrounds the openings into the digestive and respiratory tracts and consists antero-inferiorly of the lingual tonsil, laterally the palatine and tubal tonsils, posterosuperiorly the nasopharyngeal tonsil (p. 1728) and smaller collections of lymphoid tissue in the intertonsillar intervals (Waldeyer 1884; Graney 1986).

LARYNGEAL PART OF THE PHARYNX (**12**.63, **11**.1)

The laryngeal part of the pharynx (*laryngopharynx*) extends from the superior border of the epiglottis to the inferior border of the cricoid cartilage, where it becomes continuous with the oesophagus. In its incomplete anterior wall is the laryngeal inlet (p. 1643) and below this the posterior surfaces of the arytenoid and cricoid cartilages.

A small *piriform fossa* on each side of the inlet is bounded medially by the aryepiglottic fold and laterally by the thyroid cartilage and thyrohyoid membrane. Beneath its mucous membrane are the branches of the internal laryngeal nerve which have pierced the thyrohyoid membrane. Foreign bodies may lodge in the fossa and, if the mucous membrane is pierced during their removal, the nerve may be damaged, with consequent anaesthesia of the region. Posteriorly the laryngopharynx extends from the lower part of the third cervical vertebral body to the upper part of the sixth.

MICROSTRUCTURE OF THE PHARYNX

The pharynx wall has, from within outwards, mucous, fibrous and muscular layers, and finally a thin buccopharyngeal fascia external to the constrictor muscles and passing forwards over the pterygomandibular raphe on to the buccinator.

The *mucosa* is continuous with that lining the pharyngotympanic tubes, nasal cavity, mouth and larynx. The nasopharyngeal epithelium is anteriorly ciliated, pseudostratified 'respiratory' in type, with goblet cells and receiving the ducts of mucosal and submucosal seromucous glands. There is a transition in the posterior region of the nasopharynx to non-keratinized stratified squamous epithelium which continues to cover the surfaces of the oropharynx and laryngopharynx. Between the two types of epithelium there is a transitional zone of columnar epithelium with short microvilli instead of cilia. Superiorly this zone adjoins the nasal septum; laterally it passes over the orifice of the pharyngotympanic tube and turns posteriorly at the union of the soft palate and the lateral wall (pp. 1689, 1730). Mucous glands are numerous around the tubal orifices.

The mucosa is supported by an intermediate *fibrous layer*. This is thick above (the *pharyngobasilar fascia*) where muscle fibres are absent, and is firmly connected to the basilar part of the occipital and petrous temporal bones medial to the pharyngotympanic tube and forwards to the posterior border of the medial pterygoid plate and pterygomandibular raphe. As it descends it diminishes in thickness but is strengthened posteriorly by a fibrous band attached to the pharyngeal tubercle of the occipital bone and descending as the median *pharyngeal raphe* of the constrictors. This fibrous layer is really the thick, deep epimysial covering of the muscles and their aponeurotic attachment to the base of the skull; the thinner external part of the epimysium is then the *buccopharyngeal fascia* (p. 796). The muscular coat is described below.

PHARYNGEAL MUSCULATURE (**12**.66–69)

This consists of: three *constrictor* muscles, superior, middle and inferior, and a trio of muscles descending from the styloid process, the cartilaginous torus of the pharyngotympanic tube, and the soft palate, respectively the *stylo-*, *salpingo-* and *palatopharyngei*, all of which pass obliquely into the muscular wall (**12**.67).

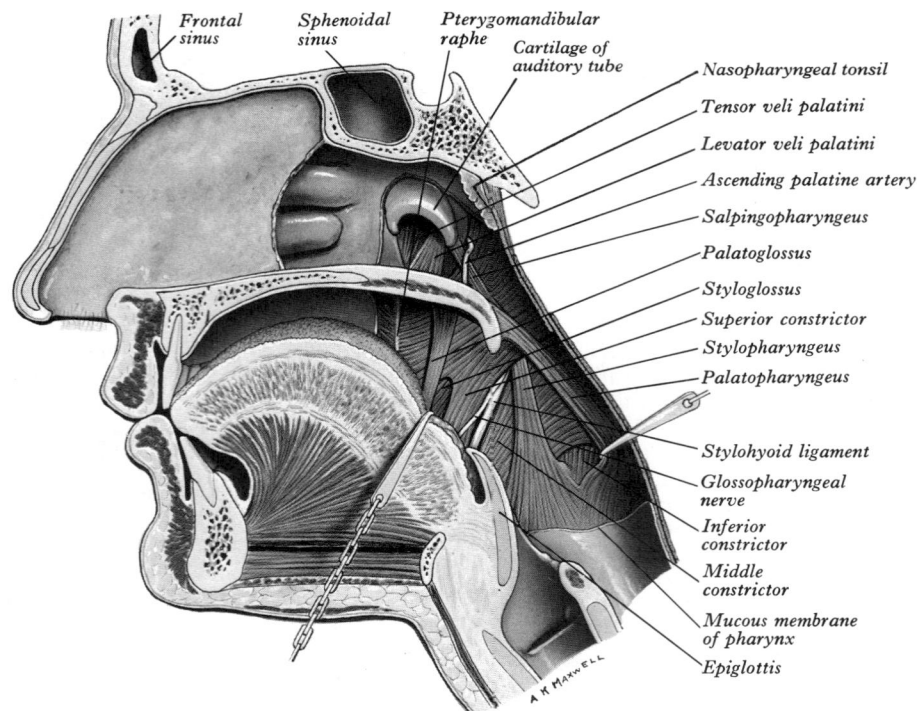

Frontal sinus Sphenoidal sinus Pterygomandibular raphe Cartilage of auditory tube

Nasopharyngeal tonsil

Tensor veli palatini

Levator veli palatini

Ascending palatine artery

Salpingopharyngeus

Palatoglossus

Styloglossus

Superior constrictor

Stylopharyngeus

Palatopharyngeus

Stylohyoid ligament

Glossopharyngeal nerve

Inferior constrictor

Middle constrictor

Mucous membrane of pharynx

Epiglottis

12.67   Median sagittal section of the head, showing a dissection of the interior of the pharynx, after the removal of the mucous membrane. The bodies of the cervical vertebrae have been removed and the cut posterior wall of the pharynx then retracted dorsolaterally. The palatopharyngeus is drawn dorsally to show the cranial fibres of the inferior constrictor; the dorsum of the tongue is drawn ventrally to display a part of the styloglossus in the angular interval between the mandibular and the lingual fibres of origin of the superior constrictor.

Superior constrictor. This is a quadrilateral sheet of muscle, thinner and paler than the other two constrictors. It is attached anteriorly to the pterygoid hamulus (and sometimes to the adjoining posterior margin of the medial pterygoid plate), the pterygomandibular raphe, and below to the posterior end of the mylohyoid line of the mandible and by a few fibres to the side of the tongue (**12**.66). These attachments define, respectively, the *pterygopharyngeal, buccopharyngeal, mylopharyngeal* and *glossopharyngeal* parts of the superior constrictor. Its fibres curve back into the median pharyngeal raphe; some are also prolonged by an aponeurosis to the pharyngeal tubercle on the basilar part of the occipital bone, the superior fibres curving under levator veli palatini and the pharyngotympanic tube and leaving an interval below the cranial base for passage of the pharyngotympanic tube. This interval is limited anteriorly by the medial pterygoid plate and closed by the pharyngobasilar fascia (p. 1729).

A constant band of muscle sweeps backwards from the anterolateral part of the upper surface of the palatine aponeurosis, lateral to levator veli palatini, to blend internally with the superior constrictor near its superior border (**12**.69). This band is the *palatopharyngeal sphincter*; it ridges the pharyngeal wall (*ridge of Passavant*) visibly when the soft palate is elevated (Whillis 1930). It is hypertrophied in cases of complete cleft palate. The change from columnar, ciliated, 'respiratory' epithelium to stratified, squamous epithelium on the superior palatal aspect occurs at the attachment of the palatopharyngeal sphincter to the palate.

Relations. External to the superior constrictor are the prevertebral fascia and muscles, the ascending pharyngeal artery and the pharyngeal venous plexus, glossopharyngeal and lingual nerves, styloglossus, middle constrictor, medial pterygoid, stylohyoid ligament and stylopharyngeus; the internal carotid artery, sympathetic trunk, hypoglossal nerve, internal jugular vein and styloid process are more distant relations. **Internal** are palatopharyngeus, the tonsillar capsule and pharyngobasilar fascia. **Superiorly** it is separated from the cranial base by a crescentic interval containing levator veli palatini, tensor veli palatini and the pharyngotympanic tube. **Inferiorly** its border is separated from the middle constrictor by stylopharyngeus and the glossopharyngeal nerve. **Anteriorly** it is separated from buccinator by the pterygomandibular raphe.

Middle constrictor (**12**.66, 68). This is a fan-shaped sheet attached anteriorly to the lesser cornu of the hyoid and the lower part of the stylohyoid ligament (the *chondropharyngeal* part of the muscle) and to the whole upper border of the greater cornu of the hyoid (the *ceratopharyngeal* part). The lower fibres descend deep to the inferior constrictor to the lower end of the pharynx, the middle fibres pass transversely and the superior fibres ascend and overlap the superior constrictor. It is inserted posteriorly into the median pharyngeal raphe with its opposite fellow.

Relations. Through the small gap between the middle and superior constrictors pass the glossopharyngeal nerve and the stylopharyngeus muscle; between the middle and inferior constrictors pass the internal laryngeal nerve and laryngeal branch of the superior thyroid artery. **Posterior** are the prevertebral fascia, longus colli and longus capitis; **lateral** are the carotid vessels, pharyngeal plexus of nerves and some lymph nodes. Near its hyoid attachment the constrictor is deep to hyoglossus, the lingual artery lying between them. **Internal** are the superior constrictors, stylopharyngeus, palatopharyngeus and the fibrous lamina.

Inferior constrictor. The thickest of the constrictors, this has two parts, cricopharyngeus and thyropharyngeus (**12**.66, 68). It is attached to (**12**.65) the side of the cricoid cartilage between the attachment of cricothyroid and, posteriorly, the articular facet for the inferior thyroid cornu (*cricopharyngeus*). It also arises from:

* the oblique line of the thyroid lamina
* a strip of the lamina behind this
* a fine tendinous band crossing cricothyroid from the inferior thyroid tubercle to the cricoid cartilage
* the inferior cornu (*thyropharyngeus*) by a small slip.

Both parts spread posteromedially to join the opposite muscle in the median pharyngeal raphe. The inferior fibres, which are horizontal, blend with the circular oesophageal fibres round the narrowest part of the pharynx; the rest ascend obliquely and overlap the middle constrictor. During swallowing the cricopharyngeus is 'sphincteric' (Fuller et al 1959) and the thyropharyngeus 'propulsive'; failure of relaxation of the cricopharyngeus may cause posterior mucosal herniation between the two parts of the muscle (Killian's dehiscence).

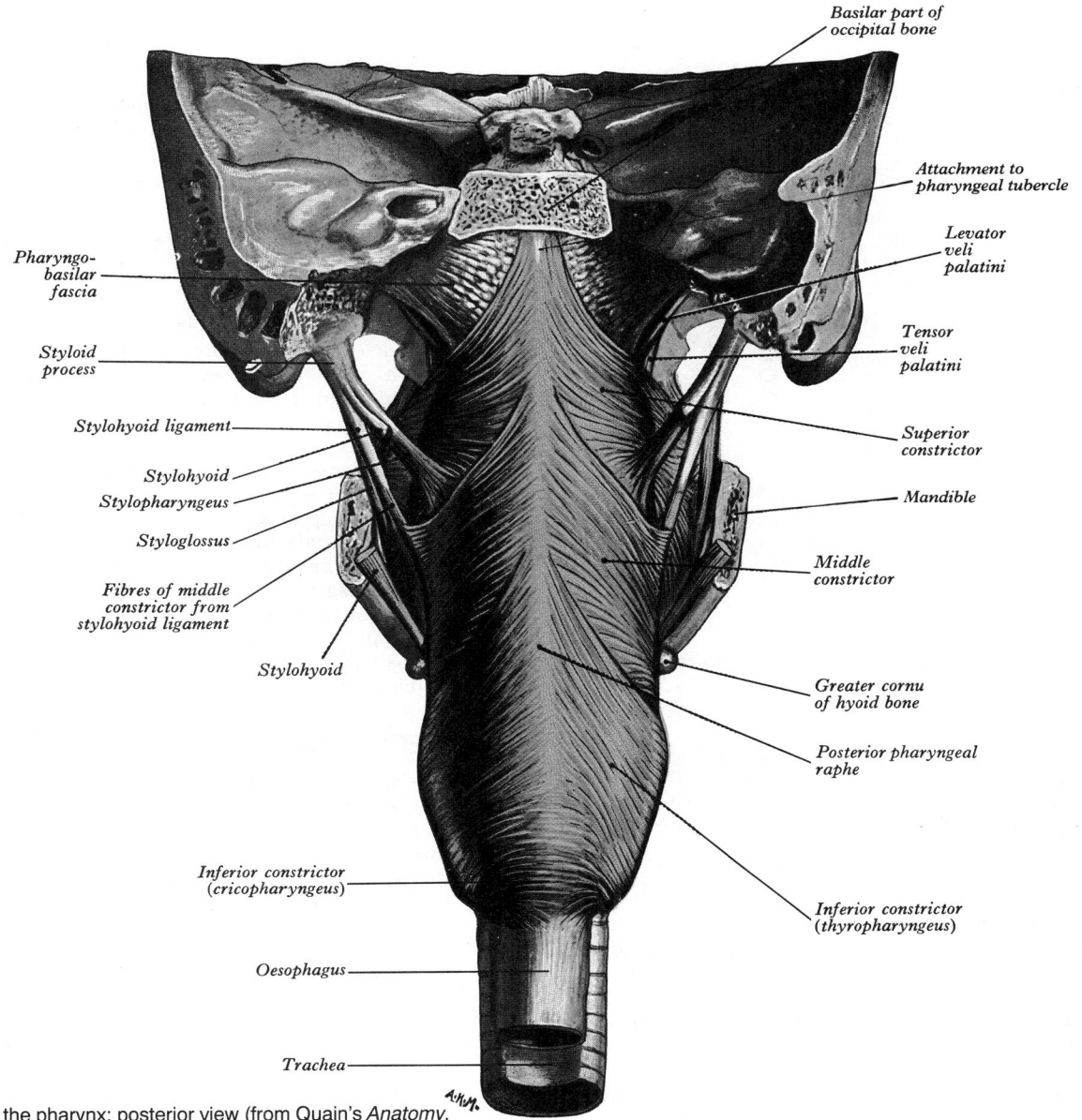

Basilar part of occipital bone

Attachment to pharyngeal tubercle

Levator veli palatini

Tensor veli palatini

Superior constrictor

Mandible

Middle constrictor

Greater cornu of hyoid bone

Posterior pharyngeal raphe

Inferior constrictor (thyropharyngeus)

Pharyngo-basilar fascia

Styloid process

Stylohyoid ligament

Stylohyoid

Stylopharyngeus

Styloglossus

Fibres of middle constrictor from stylohyoid ligament

Stylohyoid

Inferior constrictor (cricopharyngeus)

Oesophagus

Trachea

12.68 The muscles of the pharynx: posterior view (from Quain's *Anatomy*, 11th edn).

Relations. The buccopharyngeal fascia is external to the inferior constrictor. **Posterior** are the prevertebral fascia and muscles, **lateral** the thyroid gland, common carotid artery and the sternothyroid, **internal** are the middle constrictor, stylopharyngeus, palatopharyngeus and the fibrous lamina. The internal laryngeal nerve and laryngeal branch of the superior thyroid artery reach the thyrohyoid membrane between the inferior and middle constrictors. The external laryngeal nerve descends on the superficial surface of the muscle, just behind its thyroid attachment and piercing its lower part. The recurrent laryngeal nerve and the laryngeal branch of the inferior thyroid artery ascend internal to its lower border to enter the larynx.

Nerve supply of the constrictors

The constrictors are supplied by the *pharyngeal plexus* (p. 1252), the inferior constrictor also by rami of the external and recurrent laryngeal nerves. The pharynx is largely a branchial derivative (p. 175), hence its motor and sensory supply is through the trigeminal, glossopharyngeal, vagus nerves and cranial accessory. Additionally, glandular tissue in the pharyngeal mucosa and vascular smooth muscle receive an autonomic supply through the pharyngeal plexus. Postganglionic sympathetic fibres reach this plexus from the superior cervical ganglion via special rami; the preganglionic parasympathetic supply issues from the medulla oblongata, chiefly in the glossopharyngeal nerve, which also contains afferents from the oral and

laryngeal mucosae, the nasal mucosa being trigeminal territory. The vagus nerve carries branchial efferent fibres for pharyngeal striated musculature but most of these fibres probably emerge from the brainstem in the cranial, bulbar part of the accessory nerve.

The pharyngeal rami of the glossopharyngeal and vagus nerves and of the superior cervical ganglion form a plexus in the connective tissue external to the constrictors, particularly the intermediate muscle (Hovelacque 1927). From the plexus, in which autonomic (sympathetic and parasympathetic) and branchial (efferent and afferent) fibres intermingle, mixed rami ascend and descend exterior to the superior and inferior constrictors, branching into the muscular layer and mucosa. This pattern is common to most primates (Sprague 1944), including mankind; but in some lower primates the plexus is absent or simplified and may lack glossopharyngeal or vagal components. In other mammals arrangements vary; in many there is no plexus, but precise information on the main rami of supply and their exact brainstem sources is lacking. The marked development of the plexus in man and some other primates has been ascribed to phonation; perhaps this is too facile a view, considering the lack of factual evidence.

Actions of constrictors

The constrictors exercise a general sphincteric and peristaltic action in swallowing. For details, see below.

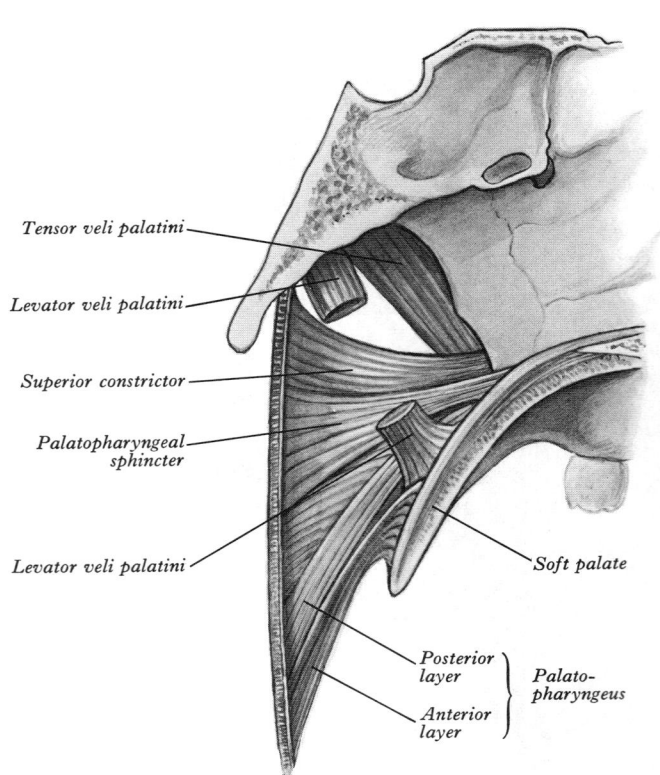

12.69 The muscles of the left half of the soft palate and adjoining part of the pharyngeal wall in sagittal section. Part of the levator veli palatini has been removed to reveal the palatopharyngeal sphincter. The soft palate is cut sagittally. (Dissection by the late James Whillis, Department of Anatomy, Guy's Hospital Medical School, London.)

Stylopharyngeus (12.1, 66–68). A long slender muscle, cylindrical above and flat below, it arises from the medial side of the base of the styloid process, descending along the side of the pharynx and passing between the superior and middle constrictors to spread out beneath the mucous membrane. Some fibres merge into the constrictors and the lateral glosso-epiglottic fold, others are attached with palatopharyngeus to the posterior border of the thyroid cartilage. The glossopharyngeal nerve curves round the posterior border and the lateral side of stylopharyngeus, passing between the superior and middle constrictors to the tongue.

Nerve supply. A branch of the glossopharyngeal nerve.

Action. Elevation of the pharynx in swallowing and speech (see below).

Salpingopharyngeus (12.3, 67). This muscle arises from the inferior part of the cartilage of the pharyngotympanic tube near the tube's pharyngeal opening to pass downwards and blend with palatopharyngeus.

Nerve supply. The pharyngeal plexus.

Action. Elevation of the upper lateral wall of the pharynx, i.e. the part above the attachment of stylopharyngeus. For its role in swallowing, see below.

Palatopharyngeus (12.67, 69). This is described with the other muscles on page 1690.

Vessels

The **pharyngeal arterial supply** is from the ascending pharyngeal, ascending palatine and tonsillar branches of the facial artery, branches of the maxillary artery (greater palatine, pharyngeal and artery of the pterygoid canal) and dorsal lingual branches of the lingual artery. The **veins** form a plexus connected above with the pterygoid plexus and draining below into the internal jugular and facial veins.

The **lymph vessels** are described on pages 1612, 1623.

Nerves

Innervation is derived mainly from the pharyngeal plexus (p. 1252). The principal **motor** element is the cranial part of the accessory

nerve, which, through vagal branches, supplies all pharyngeal and palatal muscles except stylopharyngeus (glossopharyngeal nerve) and tensor veli palatini (mandibular nerve). The main **sensory** nerves are the glossopharyngeal and vagal; much nasopharyngeal mucosa is supplied by the maxillary nerve (via the pterygopalatine ganglion); the mucosa of the soft palate and tonsil is supplied by the lesser palatine and glossopharyngeal nerves. Proprioceptor endings have not been convincingly identified in the pharynx (Bossy & Vidić 1967).

PALATINE MOVEMENTS

Movements of the palate are essential to swallowing, blowing and speech; all require variable degrees of closure of the pharyngeal isthmus (p. 1730). Closure is maximal in blowing out through the mouth, when the prevention of escape of air through the nose is needed. In deglutition, closure prevents regurgitation into the nasopharynx. In speech, closure is maximal in the production of explosive consonants (e.g. *b, p*). Closure of the isthmus is effected as follows: the levatores veli palatini pull the soft palate up and back towards the posterior pharyngeal wall, while simultaneously the palatopharyngeal sphincter raises the wall to meet the palatine nasopharyngeal surface over a wide area. (It is at the upper limit of this contact area that the epithelium on the upper surface of the soft palate changes from respiratory to stratified squamous.)

The palatal tensors are active in deglutition rather than speech; by producing a localized anterior depression in the soft palate (p. 1689) they squeeze the bolus against the tongue, aiding its descent in the oropharynx.

MECHANISM OF DEGLUTITION

The *first stage* of swallowing is *voluntary*: the anterior part of the tongue is raised and pressed against the hard palate, the movement commencing at the lingual apex and spreading rapidly back. A bolus, formed behind the apex, is thus pushed posteriorly. At the end of this stage the soft palate descends on to the lingual dorsum, helping to grip the bolus. Lingual movements are effected by the intrinsic muscles, especially the superior longitudinal and transverse. Simultaneously the hyoid bone is moved up and forwards by the geniohyoid, mylohyoid, digastric and stylohyoid. The postsulcal part of the tongue is drawn up and back by the styloglossi and the palatoglossal arches are approximated by the palatoglossi, pushing the bolus through the oropharyngeal isthmus into the oropharynx, where the second, *involuntary*, stage begins. In swallowing fluids, the intrinsic lingual muscles squirt liquid backwards in the mouth, after which mylohyoid contraction bulges the lingual base into the oropharynx. In swallowing solids only the mylohyoid action is needed, except in cleansing the mouth of saliva and debris after a bolus is swallowed (Whillis 1946). Hiiemae et al (1978) analysed lingual and hyoid activity in swallowing, using the cat and the opossum as models. By cineradiography and electromyography (EMG) they described the cyclic activities of hyoid muscles, delineating 'envelopes' of movement. They regard lingual movements as largely transportive, the precise combination of lingual and hyoid movements depending on the nature of the ingested material. The extension of these studies to primates is awaited with interest.

In the **second stage**, the soft palate is elevated (by levator muscles), tightened (tensor muscles) and firmly approximated to the posterior pharyngeal wall by the palatopharyngeal sphincter (p. 1690) and the upper part of the superior constrictor. The pharyngeal isthmus closes tightly to prevent food from ascending into the nasopharynx. Meanwhile the larynx and the pharynx are drawn up, behind the hyoid bone, by stylopharyngeus, salpingopharyngeus, thyrohyoid and palatopharyngeus. Simultaneously the aryepiglottic folds are approximated and the arytenoid cartilages drawn up and forwards by the aryepiglottic, oblique arytenoid and thyroarytenoid muscles, excluding the bolus from the larynx. Partly by gravity and partly by successive contractions of the superior and middle constrictors, the bolus slips over the epiglottis (now bent back on to the laryngeal aditus), the closed laryngeal inlet and posterior arytenoid surfaces into the lowest part of the pharynx. Its passage is facilitated by the palatopharyngei, which shorten the pharynx by elevating it; on contraction, they make the posterior pharyngeal wall into an inclined plane directed postero-inferiorly, and under this the bolus descends. The aryepiglottic folds provide lateral channels leading from the sides of the epiglottis through the piriform fossae into the oesophagus. They are kept tense and vertical by the backward pull of the posterior crico-arytenoids on the arytenoid cartilages and by the muscles (aryepiglottic and thyroepiglottic) within them, assisted by the cuneiform cartilages which act as passive props. In paralysis of these muscles (which are supplied by the recurrent laryngeal nerves) the laryngeal inlet is not closed in swallowing, the folds sink medially and fluids tend to enter the larynx.

The **last stage** in swallowing is the expulsion, by the inferior constrictors, of the now compressed bolus into the oesophagus (p. 1751). The pump-like action of the pharyngeal muscles in this activity has been described by Buthpitiya et al (1987).

These stages follow on each other, but it is easy to ascertain by palpation of the hyoid bone and laryngeal prominence that, during swallowing, elevation and forward movement of the hyoid precede laryngeal elevation. Note that the thyroid cartilage, and hence the whole larynx, ascends also **relative** to the hyoid, shortening the larynx and causing structures between the hyoid bone and thyroid

cartilage to bulge posteriorly into the larynx above the vestibular folds. This also increases the curvature of the epiglottis, especially in its lower part, aiding stenosis of the laryngeal aditus during swallowing (see Fink & Martin 1977).

The evidence for the foregoing analysis comes from various sources: radiological studies, the effects of known paralyses, EMG, ultrasound analysis (Shawker et al 1984) and cineradiography. Swallowing is, however, a highly complex process, depending on highly patterned neural control, and it is not surprising that some disagreement over its detail still persists. For full critiques of the literature consult Bosma (1957), Doty (1968), Hiiemae (1978), and Buthpitiya et al (1987).

OESOPHAGUS

This tubular part of the alimentary tract, continuing from the pharynx, passes through the neck and thorax to the abdominal cavity. It is described with the abdominal alimentary tract on page 1751.

ABDOMEN: GENERAL ORGANIZATION

Abdominal boundaries

The abdomen extends from the diaphragm to the base of the pelvis (**12**.70, 71), comprising the *abdomen proper* and the *lesser pelvis*, continuous with each other at the plane of the inlet into the lesser pelvis, which is bounded by the sacral promontory, arcuate lines of the innominate bones, pubic crests and the upper border of the symphysis pubis. The abdomen is largely enclosed by muscles, its shape and size varying with the degrees of distension of the contained hollow organs and the phases of respiration. Muscular tone is a large factor in maintaining the positions of the abdominal and pelvic viscera (pp. 826, 832).

Abdomen proper. This is bounded: **in front** by the rectus abdominis muscles, the pyramidales and the aponeurotic parts of the obliqui externus, internus and transversus abdominis; **laterally** by the fleshy parts of these flat muscles, the iliacus muscles and iliac bones, **behind** by the lumbar vertebral column, diaphragmatic crura, paired psoas and quadratus lumborum muscles and the posterior parts of the iliac bones; **above** by the diaphragm, while **below** it is continuous with the lesser pelvis through its superior aperture (p. 670). Since the diaphragm, the domed roof of the abdominal cavity, is convex upwards, part of the cavity lies within the skeletal framework of the thorax (pp. 815–816). The abdomen proper contains most of the digestive tube, liver, pancreas, spleen, kidneys, ureters (in part), suprarenal glands and numerous blood and lymph vessels, lymph nodes and nerves.

Lesser pelvis. Approximately funnel-shaped, like an inverted, truncated cone, this region extends postero-inferiorly from the abdominal cavity proper (**12**.73, 74) and is bounded: **anterolaterally** by the innominate (hip) bones below their pubic crests and arcuate lines, and by the obturatores interni; **posterosuperiorly** by the sacrum, coccyx, piriformes and coccygei; **inferiorly** by the levatores ani which, with their covering fasciae, form the pelvic diaphragm (p. 829), and by the transversi perinei profundi and sphincter urethrae which, with **their** fascial coverings, constitute the urogenital diaphragm. The lesser pelvis contains: the urinary bladder, terminal parts of the ureters, the sigmoid colon, rectum, some ileal coils, internal genitalia, blood and lymph vessels, lymph nodes and nerves.

The abdominal and pelvic muscles are ensheathed in fascia, which receives regional names from adjacent structures, e.g. on the internal surface of transversus abdominis is the *transversalis fascia* (p. 829), inferior to the diaphragm is the *diaphragmatic fascia*, covering the psoas and iliacus is the *iliac fascia* (p. 870); anterior to the quadratus lumborum is the *anterior layer of the thoracolumbar fascia* (p. 809) and over the muscles in the pelvis is the *pelvic fascia* (p. 830). Most abdominal and pelvic organs are largely covered by a serous membrane, the *visceral peritoneum* (pp. 1734–1746) whereas the walls of the abdomen are lined by *parietal peritoneum*.

Abdominal regions

For the location of viscera in clinical practice, the abdomen is divided into nine regions by imaginary planes, two horizontal and two parasagittal, their edges indicated by lines projected to the surface of the body (**12**.70). The upper, horizontal, *transpyloric plane* (of Addison) is indicated by a line encircling the body midway between the suprasternal notch and the symphysis pubis (or midway between the umbilicus and inferior end of the sternal *body* or a hand's breadth below the xiphisternal joint); it intersects the first lumbar vertebral body near its lower border and meets the costal margins at the tips of the ninth costal cartilages. The lower horizontal, *transtubercular plane* corresponds to a line round the trunk level with the iliac tubercles (**12**.70, p. 671); it cuts the front of the fifth lumbar vertebral body near its upper border. The abdomen is thus divided into three arbitrary zones; each is further subdivided into three by the *right* and *left lateral planes*, indicated on the surface by vertical lines through points midway between the anterior superior iliac spines and the symphysis pubis (these lines are also called 'mid-clavicular' or 'mammary' lines).

The median upper *epigastric* is flanked by *right* and *left hypochondriac* regions; the median region of the middle zone is the *umbilical* region, flanked by *right* and *left lumbar*, or *lateral*, regions. The lower median *hypogastric* or *pubic* region is between the *right* and *left iliac* or *inguinal regions* (**12**.70) (see Addison 1899–1901). A third horizontal plane, often used in abdominal topography, the *subcostal plane*, corresponds to a line level with the lowest limits of the tenth costal cartilages. It cuts the front of the third lumbar vertebral body nears its upper border. It often replaces the transpyloric plane in descriptions of abdominal regions.

The *umbilicus* is variable in position, being usually level with the disc between the third and fourth lumbar vertebrae in young adults but, as age advances and in conditions of deficient abdominal tone, it sinks lower. It is also lower in children because of the underdeveloped condition of the pelvic region.

On the body's posterior surface a transverse line between the highest points on the iliac crests and level with the fourth lumbar vertebral spinous process delineates a *supracristal plane*. The fourth spine is a useful landmark in identifying other vertebral spinous processes. After removal of the anterior abdominal wall (**12**.70), the viscera are partly displayed as follows: above and right is the liver, largely in the shelter of the lower right ribs and cartilages, extending across the midline, where it descends to the transpyloric plane. The stomach is partly exposed in the angle between the left costal margin and the lower hepatic border; from its lower border an apron-like peritoneal fold, the *greater omentum*, descends for a varying distance anterior to the other viscera. Below this, however, some coils of the small intestine are usually visible. In the right iliac region the caecum and, in the left iliac region, the lower part of the descending colon are partly exposed (p. 1777). The urinary bladder, in the anterior part of the pelvis, ascends above the symphysis pubis into the hypogastric region when distended; the rectum is in the sacral concavity, usually hidden by coils of the small intestine. The sigmoid colon may appear between the rectum and the bladder.

Followed to the right, the stomach is continuous with the *duodenum*, their junction being marked by a thick, palpable *pyloric sphincter*. The duodenum reaches the liver and curves down under its cover. If, however, the great omentum and the transverse colon behind it are turned up over the chest, the horizontal part of the duodenum can be seen crossing the vertebral column from right to left. The duodenum then ascends to the second lumbar vertebra to become continuous with the coils of the *jejunum* and *ileum*, which are about 6 metres long (p. 1765) and form the rest of the small intestine. Followed inferiorly, the ileum ends in the right iliac region, opening into the colon at the junction of the *caecum* and *ascending colon*. From the caecum the colon ascends on the right, then loops to the left across the median plane below the liver and stomach and turns downwards; thus it is composed of *ascending, transverse* and *descending* parts. In the pelvis it forms a loop, the *sigmoid colon*, ending in the rectum. The *spleen* is posterolateral to the stomach in the left hypochondriac region and is partly exposed by displacing the stomach to the right.

The sheen on the surfaces of the abdominal wall and exposed viscera is due to their covering of *peritoneum*, a serous membrane.

The relations of the organs described here obtain in the recumbent position, but visceral relations depend on posture, respiratory movements and the degree of distension of the hollow organs. The shapes of chest, abdomen and pelvis also vary, as do organs in the same individual and at different times, depending on physiological activity and mobility. Therefore the surface outlines of viscera, particularly the hollow organs described here, must be regarded as highly variable within wide limits.

In physique, individuals have been classified into two extremes: *hypersthenic* (pyknic) and *asthenic* (leptosomatic) with intermediate grades, *sthenic* and *hyposthenic* (Mills 1917, 1922). In the hypersthenic, with massive physique, the thorax is wide and short and the subcostal angle very obtuse, so that the heart and lungs are wide transversely; the abdomen is widest superiorly and the stomach less elongated vertically, with the pylorus relatively high; while the transverse colon is more truly transverse. In the asthenic type, with a light and slender physique, the thorax is long and narrow and the subcostal angle acute, so that the heart and lungs are long and narrow; the abdomen is widest inferiorly, the stomach being long with a relatively low pylorus and the colon long with a V-shaped transverse colon descending to the pelvis. Varieties of physique (somatotypes) have also been classified as endomorphic (massive), mesomorphic (intermediate) and ectomorphic (slender) with intermediate grades, each reputed to have predominant psychological characteristics (Sheldon et al 1940; Sheldon & Stevens 1942; see current physical anthropology monographs for details).

PERITONEUM (12.72–81)

The peritoneum (Brizon et al 1956), the largest and most complexly arranged of the serous membranes, is an empty and intricately folded sac, lining the abdomen and reflected over the viscera. In males it is a closed sac; in females the lateral ends of the uterine tubes open into the sac's potential cavity. Where it lines the abdominal wall (parieties) it is named the *parietal* peritoneum and is reflected over the viscera as the *visceral* peritoneum. Its free surface is covered by a layer of *mesothelium*, kept moist and smooth by a film of serous fluid. Hence mobile viscera glide freely on the abdominal wall and each other within limits dictated by their attachments. Sessile organs are covered by peritoneum wherever they are in contact with mobile viscera.

The peritoneal cavity is a *coelom* (p. 192)—a discontinuity in the mesoderm lined by an epithelium-like single layer of cells (mesothelium) which maintains the surface. Loss of this mesothelium leads to the adherence of underlying tissues and interference with visceral function, which may be serious and even lethal (p. 1745), providing convincing evidence of an essential function of the serosa,

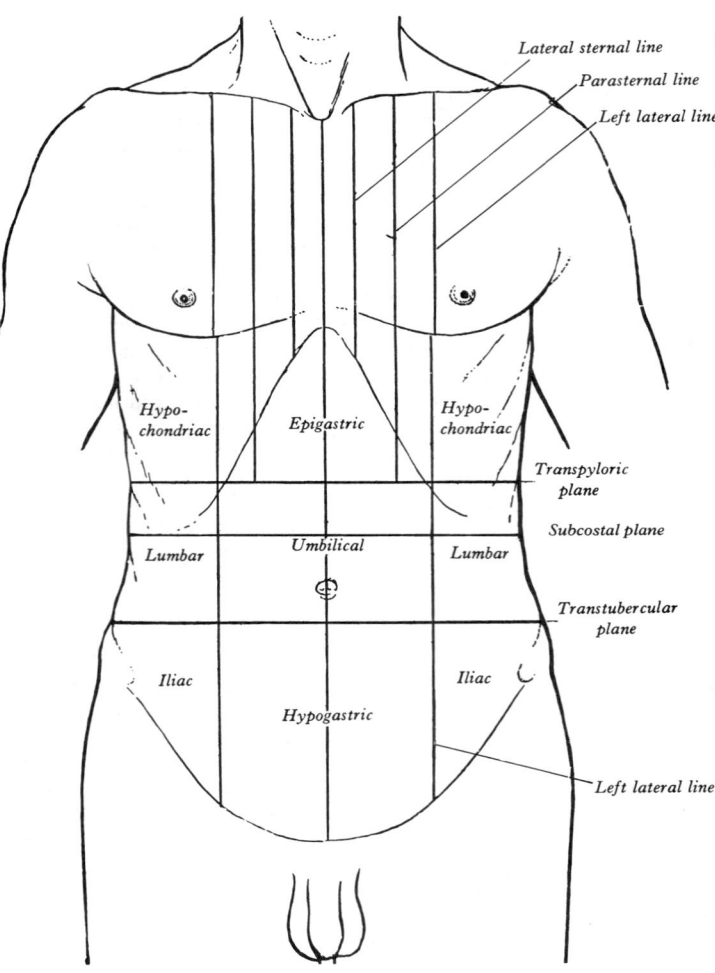

12.70   Reference lines on the anterior aspect of the thorax and abdomen for use in delineating surface projections.

the separation of the viscera sufficiently for unimpeded activity.

Many functions are served by coelomic spaces in invertebrates and vertebrates (Jones 1913; Romer 1970). Excretory organs such as nephridia drain fluid and excretory products from a general coelom, and vertebrate nephric systems are partly derived from it. As animals evolved to greater size, a coiled gut became essential but such coiling could not evolve and develop without the emergence of a coelom. In some lower vertebrates the gametes are extruded from the gonads into a coelom in both sexes, persisting in the females of more advanced forms, including mankind. Special ducts have evolved to connect the kidneys and testes to the cloaca (and its derivatives) and are in part formed from coelomic epithelium, which is also involved in formation of the gonads themselves (p. 199).

GENERAL STRUCTURE

A considerable amount of *extraperitoneal connective tissue* separates the parietal peritoneum from the muscular strata of the abdominal walls, blending with their fascial lining. Its thickness and content of fat vary in different regions. While parietal peritoneum is generally attached only loosely by this tissue to the abdominal and pelvic walls and so is easily stripped from them, the tissue is denser on the inferior surface of the diaphragm and behind the linea alba, the parietal peritoneum being here more firmly adherent. Its attachment is especially loose in some places, allowing the alteration in size of certain organs; e.g. in the pelvis and the adjoining anterior abdominal wall it allows the urinary bladder to distend upwards behind the

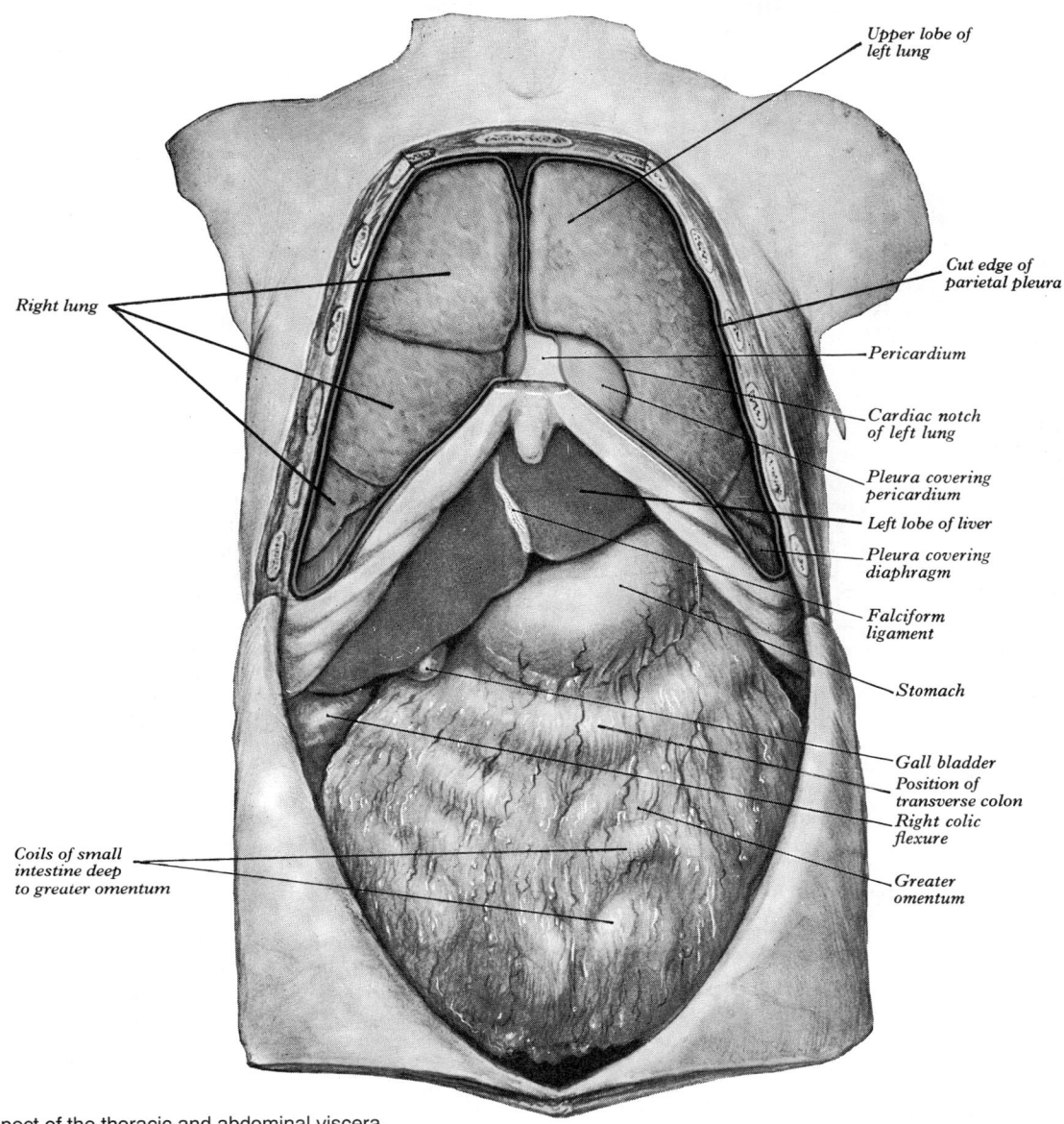

12.71 Anterior aspect of the thoracic and abdominal viscera.

Upper lobe of left lung

Cut edge of parietal pleura

Pericardium

Cardiac notch of left lung

Pleura covering pericardium

Left lobe of liver

Pleura covering diaphragm

Falciform ligament

Stomach

Gall bladder

Position of transverse colon

Right colic flexure

Greater omentum

Right lung

Coils of small intestine deep to greater omentum

wall, from which it temporarily strips the peritoneum as it ascends. There is usually much perinephric extraperitoneal fat on the posterior abdominal wall. The visceral peritoneum, in contrast, is firmly united to the underlying tissues and cannot be easily detached; its connective tissue layer (*tela subserosa*) is continuous with the fibrous matrix of the visceral wall; and the visceral peritoneum must therefore be considered as part of its viscus, a concept of significance in pathology.

PERITONEAL CAVITY

The parietal and visceral layers of peritoneum are in sliding contact, the potential space between them being the *peritoneal cavity*. This consists of:

- a main region, the *greater sac*
- a diverticulum, the *omental bursa* or *lesser sac* behind the stomach and adjoining structures.

The two communicate via the *epiploic foramen (aditus to the lesser sac)*.

The complex arrangement of the peritoneum can best be rationalized by the study of alimentary development (pp. 181–186) and by examination in cadavers before they are made unnaturally rigid by preservative fluids. To trace the peritoneum from one viscus to

another and from viscera to parieties, it is useful to follow its continuity in vertical and horizontal directions and simpler to describe the greater and lesser sacs separately.

VERTICAL DISPOSITION OF THE PERITONEUM

The ensuing descriptions will be more clearly comprehended by making frequent reference to the development of the alimentary tract (pp. 181–186) and to the illustrations in this section.

It is convenient to commence tracing the arrangement of the greater sac in the vertical plane (**12.**75) from the anterior abdominal wall at the umbilical level. A fibrous *ligamentum teres (obliterated left umbilical vein*, p. 1502) ascends from this point to the inferior surface of the liver. It inclines slightly to the right, and recedes from the anterior abdominal wall as it ascends, to raise a triangular *falciform ligament of the liver (***12.**72, 139); this is composed of two layers of parietal peritoneum (right and left) with connective tissue between, continuous with the anterior body wall in front, and the inferior surface of the diaphragm above. This develops from the most ventral part of the embryonic mesogastrium. The falciform ligament has right and left peritoneal layers with intervening connective tissue (**12.**77A, B). Its juxta-umbilical region has a posterior free border from the umbilicus to the inferior hepatic surface,

1735

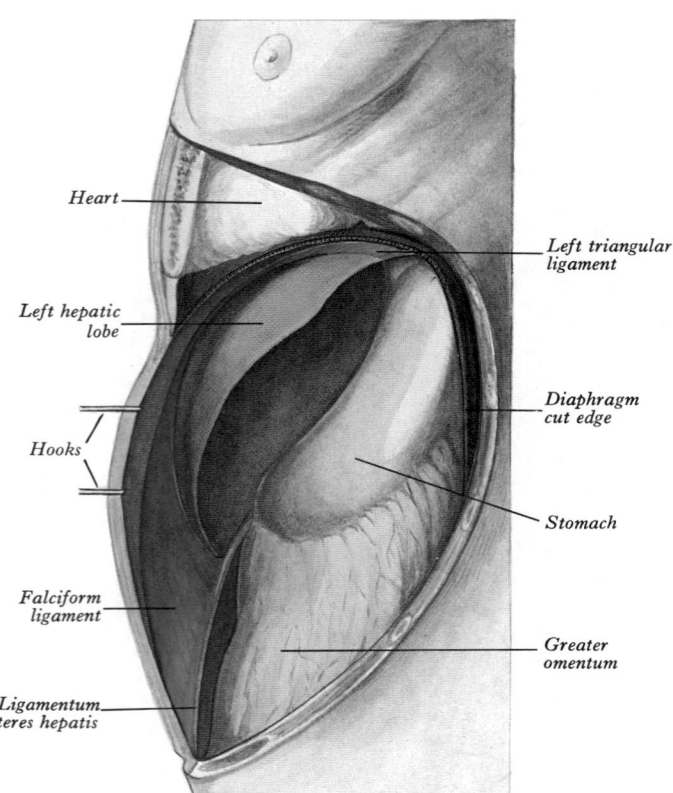

12.72   Dissection to expose the left side of the falciform fold or ligament of the liver.

containing the *ligamentum teres*. Superiorly the falciform ligament extends from the diaphragm to become continuous with the visceral peritoneum on the anterosuperior surface of the liver (**12**.72). At the site of reflexion from the diaphragm to the liver, the two layers diverge (**12**.113, 139–141), the right passing transversely to the right as the *superior layer of the hepatic coronary ligament* (from the diaphragm to the upper surface of the right hepatic lobe), the left layer passing left as the *anterior layer of the left hepatic triangular ligament* (from the diaphragm to the upper surface of the left hepatic lobe).

The visceral peritoneum on the anterosuperior surface of the liver continues down and round the sharp inferior hepatic border to the inferior (visceral) surface, where it is arranged as follows: right of the gallbladder it covers the inferior surface of the right lobe of the liver and is reflected posteriorly to the right suprarenal gland and the upper pole of the right kidney, forming the *inferior layer of the coronary ligament*; it often passes direct from the liver to the kidney as the *hepatorenal ligament*. From the right kidney it descends to the front of the first part of the duodenum and right colic flexure; it also passes medially in front of a short segment of the inferior vena cava (between the duodenum and liver), continuing on to the posterior wall of the omental bursa (**12**.75, 76). Between the two layers of the coronary ligament is a large, triangular, posterior area on the right hepatic lobe devoid of peritoneal covering, the *bare area of the liver*, where the liver is attached to the diaphragm by loose connective tissue.

Near the right hepatic margin, layers of the coronary ligament converge, fusing to form the *right triangular ligament* which connects the right hepatic lobe to the diaphragm (**12**.76, 139, 140) and forms the apex of the bare area, the base being the *groove for the inferior vena cava.*

Visceral peritoneum covers the inferior aspect and sides of the gallbladder, the inferior surfaces of the quadrate lobe of the liver as far back as the anterior margin of the porta hepatis and of the left lobe, from whose posterior surface it reaches the diaphragm as the *posterior layer of the left triangular ligament*. Along the anterior margin of the porta hepatis the peritoneum is continuous at its right end with the peritoneum of the omental bursa, the latter being

reflected from the posterior margin of the porta hepatis (**12**.140). The visceral peritoneum plunges into the fissure for the ligamentum venosum, (**12**.141), between the caudate and left hepatic lobes, in two layers, anterior and posterior. The anterior layer merges with peritoneum reflected from the anterior portal margin (**12**.140, 141). From this L-shaped line, formed by the left margin of the fissure for the ligamentum venosum and the anterior margin of the porta hepatis, peritoneum is reflected to the gastric lesser curvature and approximately the first 2 cm of the duodenum, as the *anterior layer of the lesser omentum.*

The region of lesser omentum connecting liver to stomach is the *hepatogastric ligament*, the part passing from the liver to the duodenum being the *hepatoduodenal ligament*. The anterior layer, traced to the right, passes anterior to the hepatic artery, bile duct and portal vein, turning round their right side to continue behind them into the posterior omental layer, which here forms the anterior surface of the bursa. Thus the lesser omentum has a free right border, in which lie the hepatic artery, bile duct and portal vein; behind this border is the *epiploic foramen* (foramen of Winslow) (**12**.75, 77A). The anterior layer of the lesser omentum is continuous below with the visceral peritoneum of the anterior gastric surface and the first 2 cm of the duodenum. This layer then descends from the greater curvature and neighbouring duodenum to become the *most anterior layer of the greater omentum*. Reaching the lower edge of this large fold, it ascends as the greater omentum's *most posterior layer*, running to the anterosuperior aspect of the transverse colon (at the *taenia omentalis*). It then turns back, adherent to but separable from the **upper** layer of the transverse mesocolon, to the anterior aspect of the pancreatic head and the anterior border of the body of the pancreas; it leaves the latter as the upper layer of the transverse mesocolon (**12**.75), passing to the posterior surface of the transverse colon (at the *taenia mesocolica*) and covering all but its posterior aspect, returning thence to the pancreatic head and body as the **inferior** layer of the transverse mesocolon. It then descends over the pancreas to the front of the horizontal and ascending parts of the duodenum, from there turning downwards on the posterior abdominal wall. It is also carried forward on the superior mesenteric vessels to the jejunum and ileum as the *right layer of the mesentery*. It invests them and reaches the posterior abdominal wall as the *left layer of the mesentery*, descending over the abdominal aorta, inferior vena cava, ureters and psoas major muscles into the lesser pelvis. Reflected from the posterior pelvic wall as the *anterior layer of the sigmoid mesocolon*, it encloses the sigmoid colon and returns to the pelvic wall as the *posterior layer* of that mesocolon, descending then to cover the front and sides of the rectum's upper third and the front of its middle third.

In males, the peritoneum leaves the junction of the middle and lower thirds of the rectum, passing forwards to the upper poles of the seminal vesicles and superior aspect of the bladder. Between the rectum and bladder it forms the *rectovesical pouch*, descending slightly below the upper seminal poles to a level about 7.5 cm from the anal orifice. From the apex of the bladder it returns along the median and medial umbilical ligaments (**12**.73) to the anterior abdominal wall and umbilicus. When the bladder distends, the peritoneum is lifted from the lower anterior abdominal wall so that part of the bladder's anterior surface is in **direct** contact with the wall (p. 1838). Instruments can then be passed through the wall into the bladder without traversing the peritoneum.

In females, the peritoneum passes from the rectum to the posterior vaginal fornix and then to the back of the uterine cervix and body, as the *recto-uterine fold*, which descends to form the *recto-uterine pouch* (of Douglas), the base of which is only 5.5 cm from the anal orifice. The peritoneum spreads over the uterine fundus to its anterior (vesical) surface as far as the junction of the body and cervix, from which it is reflected forwards to the upper surface of the bladder, forming a shallow *vesico-uterine pouch*. Peritoneum on the anterior and posterior uterine surfaces leaves the organ to reach the lateral pelvic walls as the *broad ligaments of the uterus*, each consisting of antero-inferior and posterosuperior layers continuous at the upper border of the ligament; between them at this border is the uterine tube. Behind the broad ligament a double fold of peritoneum passes back to the ovary and blends with its covering (see p. 1869). Peritoneum is reflected from the bladder to the anterior abdominal wall as in males.

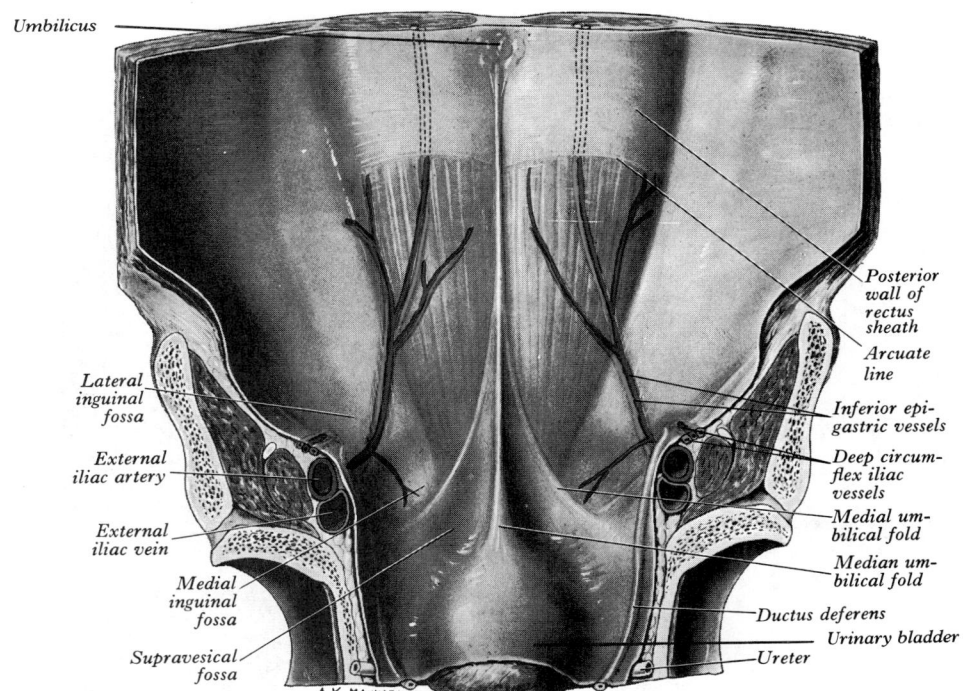

Umbilicus

Lateral inguinal fossa

External iliac artery

External iliac vein

Medial inguinal fossa

Supravesical fossa

A K MAXWELL

Posterior wall of rectus sheath

Arcuate line

Inferior epigastric vessels

Deep circumflex iliac vessels

Medial umbilical fold

Median umbilical fold

Ductus deferens

Urinary bladder

Ureter

12.73   The infra-umbilical part of the anterior abdominal wall of a male subject: posterior surface, with the peritoneum in situ. Note the pelvic bones flanking the wide greater pelvis (middle) and narrower lesser pelvis (below) containing the bladder.

HORIZONTAL DISPOSITION OF THE PERITONEUM

Below the transverse colon the arrangement is simple, but differs at pelvic, lower abdominal and upper abdominal levels.

In the lesser pelvis

The peritoneum follows the surfaces of the pelvic viscera and walls, with differences in the sexes. **In males (12.**73, 74) it almost encircles the sigmoid colon, passing to the posterior pelvic wall as the *sigmoid mesocolon*. It leaves the sides and finally the front of the rectum, continuing over the upper poles of the seminal vesicles to the bladder; lateral to the rectum it forms right and left *pararectal fossae*, varying with rectal distension, and anteriorly a *rectovesical pouch*, limited laterally by peritoneal folds reading from the sides of the bladder posteriorly to the anterior aspect of the sacrum, the *sacrogenital folds*, each lateral to its pararectal fossa. Anteriorly peritoneum covers the superior surface of the bladder, forming on each side a *paravesical fossa*, limited laterally by a ridge containing the ductus deferens. The size of these fossae depends on the state of the bladder; when it is empty, a variable *transverse vesical* fold bisects each fossa, and the anterior ends of the sacrogenital folds may sometimes be joined by a ridge separating a *middle fossa* from the main rectovesical pouch (**12.**73). Between the paravesical and pararectal fossae the only elevations are due to the ureters and internal iliac vessels.

In females, pararectal and paravesical fossae also appear, the lateral limit of the latter being the peritoneum investing the round ligament of the uterus. The rectovesical pouch is, of course, divided by the uterus and vagina into a small, anterior, vesico-uterine and a deep, posterior, recto-uterine pouch (**14.**15). Marginal recto-uterine folds of the latter correspond to the sacrogenital folds in males and pass back to the sacrum from the sides of the cervix lateral to the rectum. The *broad ligaments* extend from the sides of the uterus to the lateral pelvic walls, with the uterine tubes contained in their free superior margins and the ovaries attached to their posterior layers. Below, they are continuous with the lateral pelvic parietal peritoneum. Between the elevations over the obliterated umbilical artery and the ureter on the lateral pelvic wall is a shallow *ovarian fossa* containing the ovary in nulliparous females. It lies behind the lateral attachment of the broad ligament.

In the lower abdomen

The peritoneum of the lower anterior abdominal wall is raised into five ridges converging upwards (**12.**73). A *median umbilical fold* extends from the apex of the bladder to the umbilicus. It contains the urachus (p. 1838). On each side of it the obliterated umbilical artery raises a *medial umbilical fold*, ascending from pelvis to umbilicus. Between these three folds are the two *supravesical fossae*. Further laterally each inferior epigastric artery raises a *lateral umbilical fold*, below its entry into the rectus sheath. *Medial inguinal fossae* exist between the lateral and medial umbilical folds. A *lateral inguinal fossa* over the deep inguinal ring is lateral to the lateral umbilical fold and indicates the site of descent of the processus vaginalis and testis into the anterior abdominal wall. A *femoral fossa*, inferomedial to the lateral inguinal and separated from it by the medial end of the inguinal ligament, overlies the femoral ring (p. 1564).

From the linea alba, caudal to the level of the transverse colon, the peritoneum, followed horizontally to the right, lines the abdominal wall almost to the lateral border of quadratus lumborum; it is reflected over the sides and front of the ascending colon, enclosing the caecum and vermiform appendix and passing medially over the duodenum, psoas major and inferior vena cava towards the median plane, whence it passes along the superior mesenteric vessels to invest the small intestine and back again to the large vessels anterior to the vertebral column, forming the *mesentery* (**12.**75, 76). This encloses: the jejunum, the ileum, superior mesenteric blood vessels, nerves, lacteals and lymph nodes. The peritoneum then continues left across the abdominal aorta and left psoas major, covering the sides and front of the descending colon, and then returns round the abdominal wall to the midline.

In the upper abdomen (**12.**75, 76, 77A, 88, 89)

Above the transverse colon, the arrangement of the peritoneum in the greater sac is more complex. From the front of the inferior vena cava, just above the first part of the duodenum, it passes **left** behind the epiploic foramen to form the posterior wall of the omental bursa (**12.**77A); it passes **right** over the front of the right suprarenal gland and the upper pole of the right kidney to the anterolateral abdominal wall. From the anterior median line a double fold, the *falciform ligament*, passes back to the right around the liver. To the left the

1737

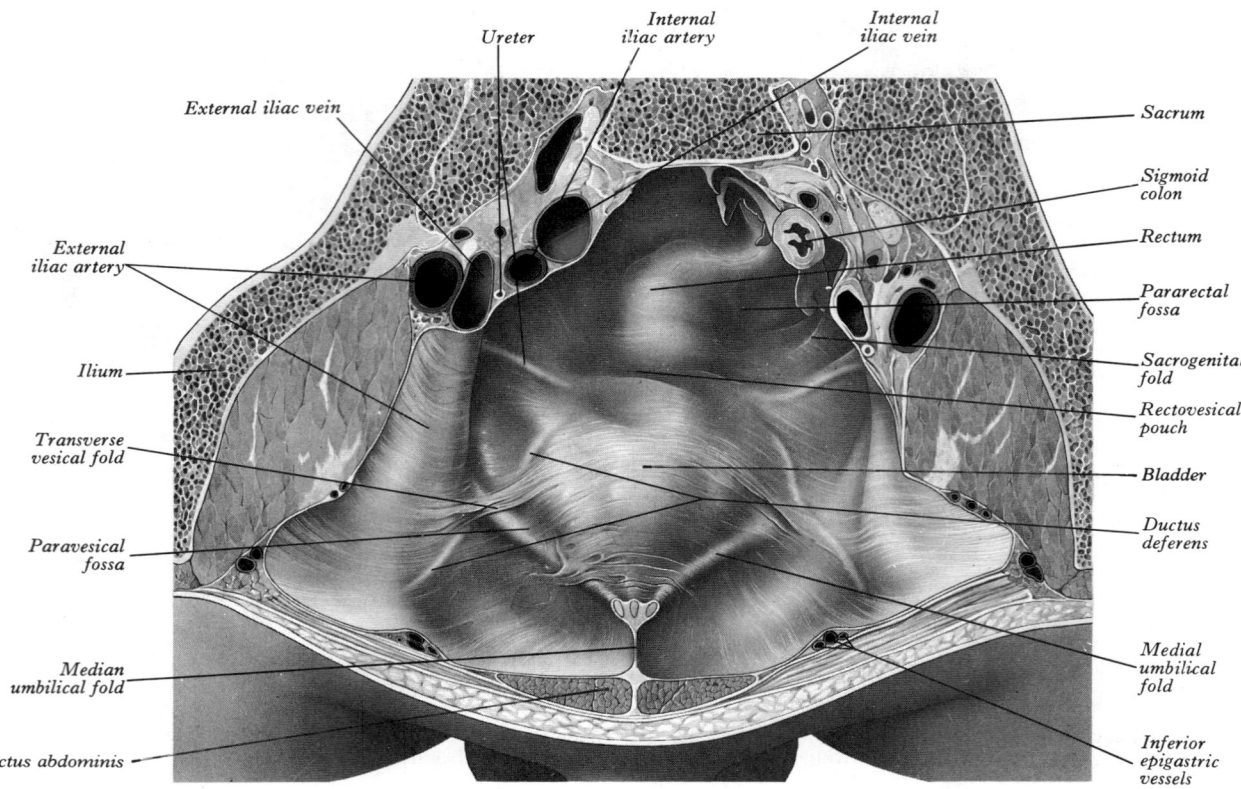

12.74   The peritoneum of the male pelvis: anterosuperior view. The median umbilical fold contains both the unpaired median and the paired medial umbilical ligaments in the plane of section in this subject.

peritoneum lines the anterolateral abdominal wall, covers the lateral part of the left kidney and passes to the splenic hilum as the posterior (lateral) layer of the *splenicorenal* (lienorenal) or *phrenicolienal ligament* (**12**.77A). It then invests the spleen, returning to the front of its hilum and thence to the cardiac end of the greater curvature as the left layer of the *gastrosplenic ligament*. Covering the anterosuperior gastric surface and adjacent duodenum, it ascends from the lesser curvature to the liver as the anterior layer of the lesser omentum, whose right free border has been described (p. 1736); this anterior layer of the lesser omentum (peritoneum of the greater sac) continues as the posterior layer of the omental bursa (peritoneum of the omental bursa).

OMENTAL BURSA (LESSER SAC)

The omental bursa or lesser sac is a large, irregular, potential recess behind the stomach and beyond its limits. Its name is related to the concept that it forms a bursa (p. 781) facilitating movements of the posterior aspect of the stomach. However, it is not closed; its connection with the greater sac is narrowed by embryological rather than functional factors. The stomach expands or contracts just as freely in vertebrates with no special narrow-necked diverticulum. (In any case movements of the *anterior aspect* of the stomach also occur.) The extensive anterior and posterior walls of the 'bursa' are limited by variable borders (right, left, inferior and superior). It is separated from the greater sac except at its upper *right border* where they communicate by a vertical slit, the *epiploic foramen*. Its upper posterior wall is a single peritoneal layer closely applied to the posterior abdominal wall (**12**.75) but below the pancreas its potential cavity projects into the greater omentum, whose posterior wall is formed by two layers which, above the transverse colon, blend with the transverse mesocolon (**12**.75). The greater omentum is traditionally described as having **four** peritoneal layers; but it must be understood that the mesothelial peritoneum is lost, except where a true surface persists. Where two separate 'folds' of peritoneum adhere and blend, the opposed mesothelia disappear but recognizable layers of subepithelial connective tissue often remain.

Epiploic foramen

The epiploic foramen (foramen of Winslow, aditus to the lesser sac) is a short, vertical slit of about 3 cm, leading from the upper part of the right border of the lesser sac into the greater sac, this border forming the foramen's *anterior margin* and containing between its layers the bile duct (on the right), portal vein (posterior) and hepatic artery (left) (**12**.77A). Superiorly the two layers separate, the posterior covering the caudate process of the liver in the *roof* of the foramen (**12**.78) and descending anterior to the inferior vena cava as the foramen's *posterior margin*. At the upper border of the first duodenal segment this layer passes forwards from the inferior vena cava, above the head of the pancreas, into the posterior layer of the lesser omentum, forming the foramen's *floor* which is medially continued down into the right border of the lesser sac (**12**.87). Passing forwards below the medial end of this floor the hepatic artery passes between the two layers of the lesser omentum (**12**.77A). A narrow passage, the *vestibule* of the omental bursa, is left of the foramen between the caudate process and the first part of the duodenum. To the right the rim of the foramen is continuous with the peritoneum of the greater sac: the roof is continuous with the peritoneum on the inferior surface of the right hepatic lobe (**12**.139–141); the posterior wall with the peritoneum on the right suprarenal gland (**12**.88); its anterior wall with the anterior layer of the lesser omentum round the portal vein and bile duct (**12**.77A), the floor with the peritoneum on the lower part of the right suprarenal gland and on adjacent parts of the duodenum and right kidney. Anterior and posterior walls of the foramen are normally apposed.

Omental bursa

The omental bursa has an anterior wall formed by three peritoneal components which are continuous with each other, as follows: (1) peritoneum over the postero-inferior aspect of the stomach and about the first 2 cm of the duodenum; this layer descends to become the posterior of the anterior two layers of (2) the greater omentum, and then ascends to the right to leave the lesser gastric curvature and duodenum at its upper border, becoming (3) the posterior layer

Figure labels:
- Ureter
- Internal iliac artery
- Internal iliac vein
- External iliac vein
- Sacrum
- Sigmoid colon
- Rectum
- Pararectal fossa
- External iliac artery
- Ilium
- Sacrogenital fold
- Rectovesical pouch
- Transverse vesical fold
- Bladder
- Paravesical fossa
- Ductus deferens
- Median umbilical fold
- Medial umbilical fold
- Rectus abdominis
- Inferior epigastric vessels

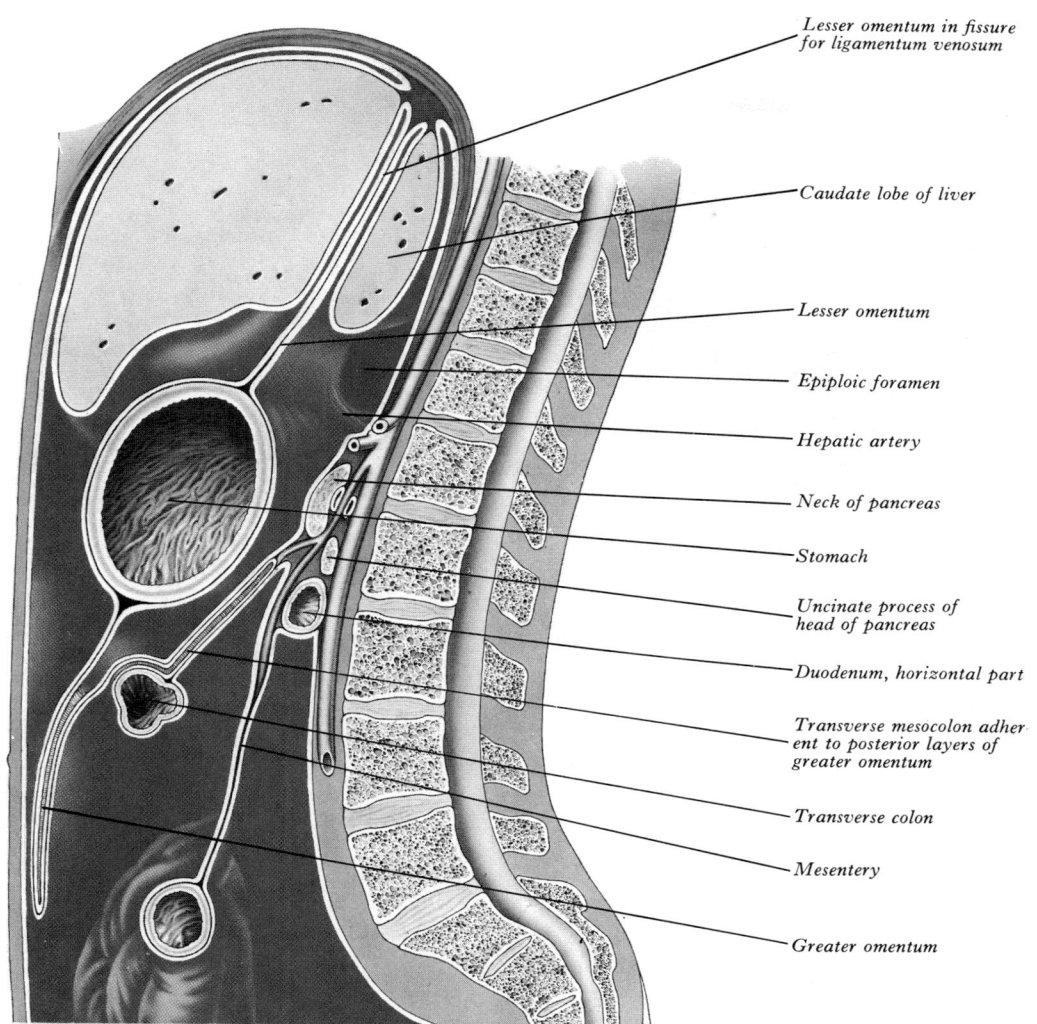

Lesser omentum in fissure
for ligamentum venosum

Caudate lobe of liver

Lesser omentum

Epiploic foramen

Hepatic artery

Neck of pancreas

Stomach

Uncinate process of
head of pancreas

Duodenum, horizontal part

Transverse mesocolon adherent to posterior layers of
greater omentum

Transverse colon

Mesentery

Greater omentum

12.75   Sagittal section through the abdomen, approximately in the median plane. Compare with **12.76**. The section cuts the posterior abdominal wall along the line YY in **12.76**. The peritoneum is shown in blue except along its cut edges, which are left white.

of the lesser omentum. The bursa is often described as ascending behind the caudate lobe, but this projects into the bursa from its right border and is covered by peritoneum on both anterior and posterior surfaces (**12.75, 139–141**).

The *posterior wall* is formed by the anterior of two posterior layers of the greater omentum. Above, the posterior of these is fused, but not inseparably, with the upper peritoneum of the transverse colon and mesocolon. Surgical separation of the greater omentum from these provides posterior access to the stomach through the posterior wall of the greater omentum. Dissection where the omentum and transverse colon meet opens up an embryological 'bloodless plane' between vessels of the greater omentum (from the gastro-epiploic) and the middle colic vessels in the transverse mesocolon (Freder 1905; Lardennois & Okinczyc 1913; Grégoire 1922; Ogilvie 1935). There are no anastomoses across this plane. Above the anterior pancreatic border the posterior bursal peritoneum covers the posterior abdominal wall, a small part of the head and the whole neck and body of the pancreas, part of the anterior aspect of the left kidney, most of the left suprarenal gland, the commencement of the abdominal aorta and coeliac artery and part of the diaphragm. The inferior phrenic, splenic, left gastric and hepatic arteries lie partly behind the bursa (**12.75–77A, 96**).

The *limits of the bursa* are the lines where its posterior peritoneal wall is reflected to be continuous with its anterior; their positions vary somewhat. The *inferior border* is, developmentally (p. 185), the lower limit of the greater omentum; but partial fusion of the latter's layers usually occurs after birth, so that the bursa's *cavity* in adults does not usually extend very far below the transverse colon. The

internally apposed peritoneal surfaces lose their mesothelium. The narrow *upper border* is between the right side of the oesophagus and the upper end of the fissure for the ligamentum venosum (**12.141**). Here peritoneum of the posterior omental wall is reflected anteriorly from the diaphragm to join the posterior layer of the lesser omentum.

The *right border* corresponds, below, to that of the greater omentum; above, its upper part is formed by reflexion of the peritoneum from the pancreatic neck and head on to the inferior aspect of the beginning of the duodenum; the line of this reflexion ascends to the left, along the medial side of the gastroduodenal artery. Near the upper duodenal margin the right border joins the floor of the epiploic foramen round the hepatic artery proper (**12.76**). Above this interruption the border is formed by the reflexion of peritoneum from the diaphragm to the right margin of the liver's caudate lobe and along the left side of the inferior vena cava (**12.76**).

The *left border* again corresponds, below, to that of the greater omentum. Above the root of the transverse mesocolon (**12.76**) the border broadens and is formed by the *splenico- (lieno-) renal* and *gastrosplenic ligaments* (**12.77A**), both formed from a part of the original dorsal mesogastrium (p. 183). The splenicorenal ligament extends from the front of the left kidney to the splenic hilum as a bilaminar fold, enclosing the splenic vessels and pancreatic tail (**12.75, 77A**). From the hilum these two layers proceed to the greater curvature of the stomach as the gastrosplenic ligament. The inner (right) layer of the splenicorenal ligament joins the corresponding layer of the gastrosplenic; but its outer (left) layer joins the peritoneum covering the spleen at the back of the hilum. The latter is reflected from the front of the hilum, as the outer (left) layer of the

1739

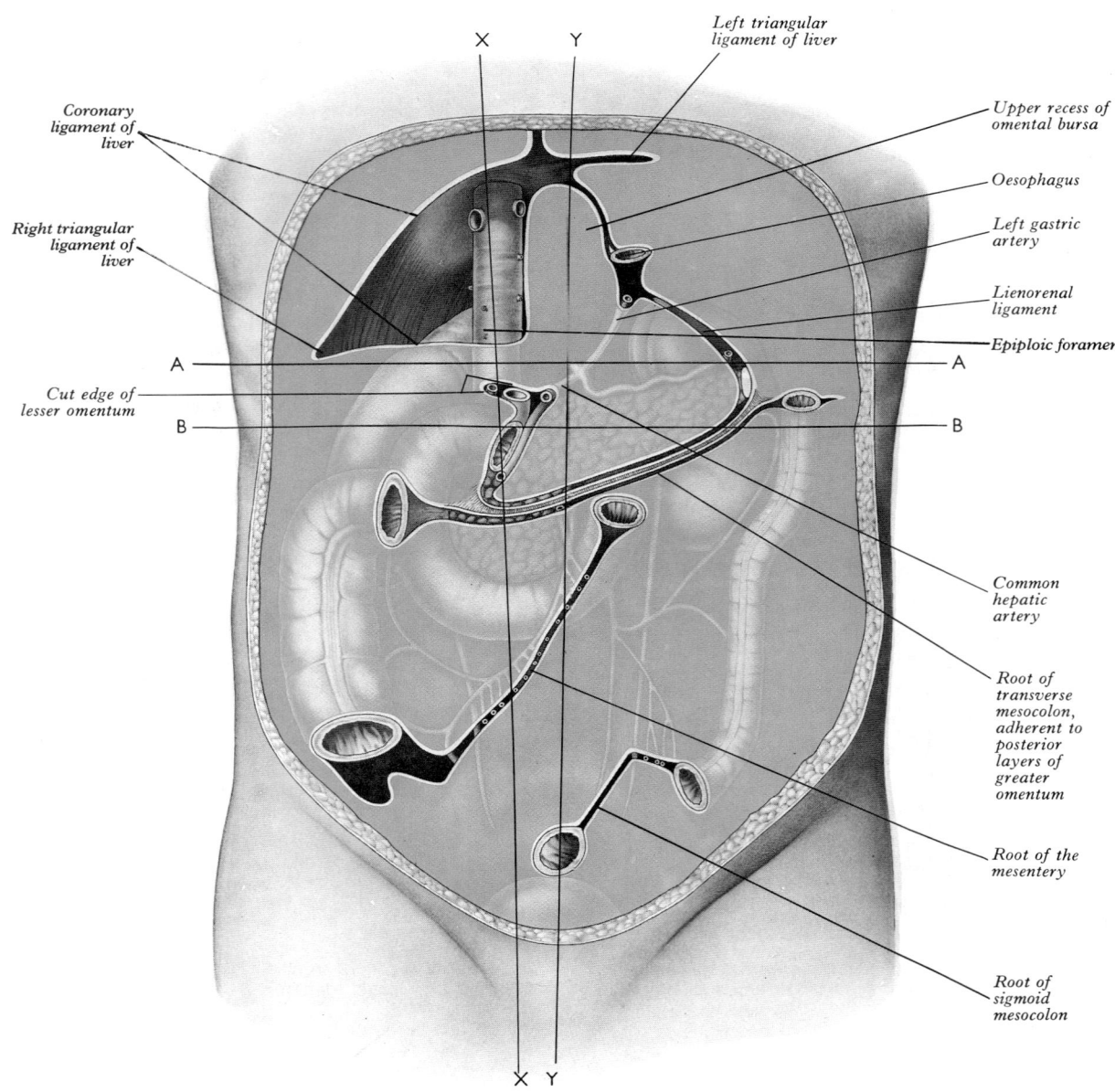

12.76 The posterior abdominal wall, showing the lines of peritoneal reflexion, after removal of the liver, spleen, stomach, jejunum, ileum, caecum, transverse colon and sigmoid colon. The various sessile (retroperitoneal) organs are seen shining through the posterior parietal peritoneum. Note: the ascending and descending colon, duodenum, kidneys, suprarenals, pancreas and inferior vena cava. Line YY represents the plane of **12.75**. Line AA represents the plane of **12.77A**. Line XX represents the plane of **12.77B**.

gastrosplenic ligament. The spleen thus projects left into the greater sac (**12.77A**). The part of the bursa projecting towards it, between the splenic ligaments, is the *splenic recess*. Superiorly the two ligaments merge into a short *gastrophrenic ligament*, passing forwards from the diaphragm to the posterior aspect of the fundus of the stomach. Its two layers diverge near the oesophagus, leaving part of the posterior gastric surface devoid of peritoneum. The upper end of the left border is continuous with the left end of the roof; the left gastric artery turns forwards here into the lesser omentum. (Many peritoneal **folds** are misleadingly termed 'ligaments'. With little in common in structure or function with skeletal ligaments, they are more often neurovascular pedicles of organs which **must** be covered by peritoneum. Some may have a supportive function, but the evidence for this is usually tenuous.)

The omental bursa is narrowed by two crescentic peritoneal folds drawn into the lesser sac by the hepatic and left gastric arteries. The *left gastropancreatic fold* transmits the left gastric artery from the posterior abdominal wall to the lesser curvature of the stomach; the *right gastropancreatic fold*, at a lower level, transmits the hepatic artery from the posterior abdominal wall to the lesser omentum

(**12.76**). The folds vary much in size, but when well marked they constrict the lesser sac to form a *foramen bursae omenti majoris*. The *superior recess* of the omental bursa is above this constriction, communicating through it to the *inferior recess* (representing the embryonic pancreatico-enteric recess, p. 183). The superior recess thus lies posterior to the lesser omentum and liver, the inferior behind the stomach and in the fold of the greater omentum.

During much of fetal life the transverse colon is attached to the posterior abdominal wall by its own mesentery, the posterior two layers of the greater omentum passing in front of the colon, a condition which may persist (see **12.75**); usually, however, the mesentery of the transverse colon and posterior omental layer adhere; even so, these layers are separable in adults, especially in the living (pp. 1742, 1743), though their mesothelial elements disappear where the layers have fused. In its final form the omental bursa separates the stomach from structures which form the 'stomach bed' (p. 1757) and therefore facilitates movements of the stomach over these structures.

Peritoneal folds between various organs, or connecting them to the abdominal and pelvic walls, enclose the vessels and nerves

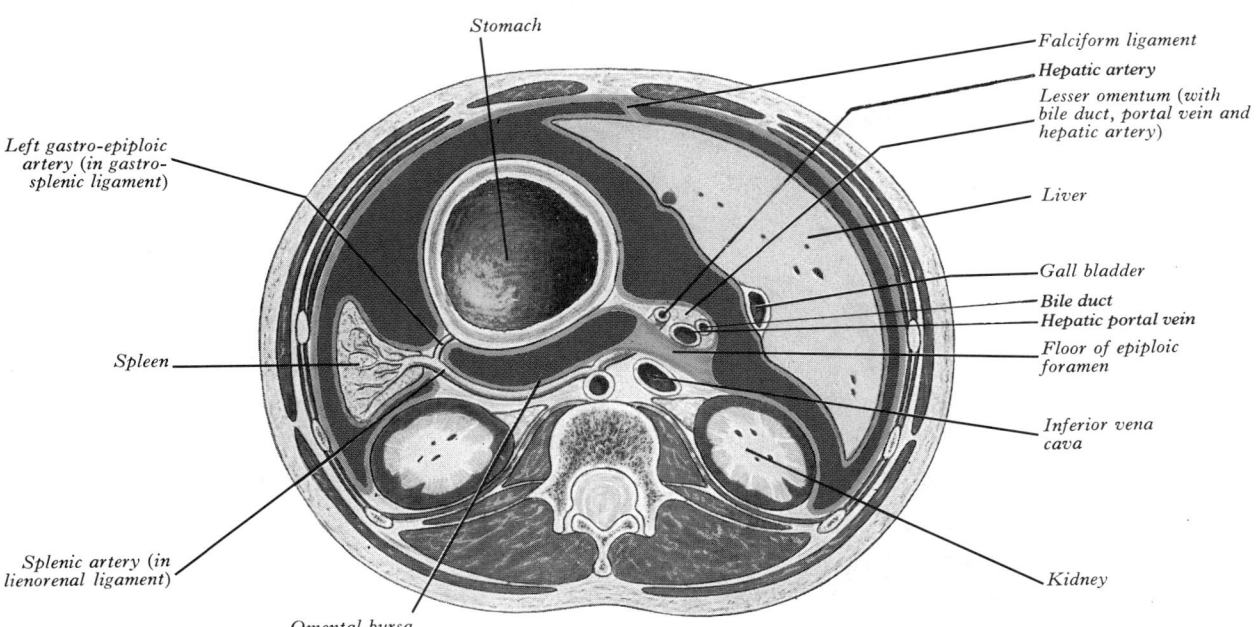

12.77A Transverse section through the abdomen, at the level of line AA in **12.76**, viewed from above. The peritoneal cavity is shown in dark blue; the peritoneum and its cut edges in lighter blue.

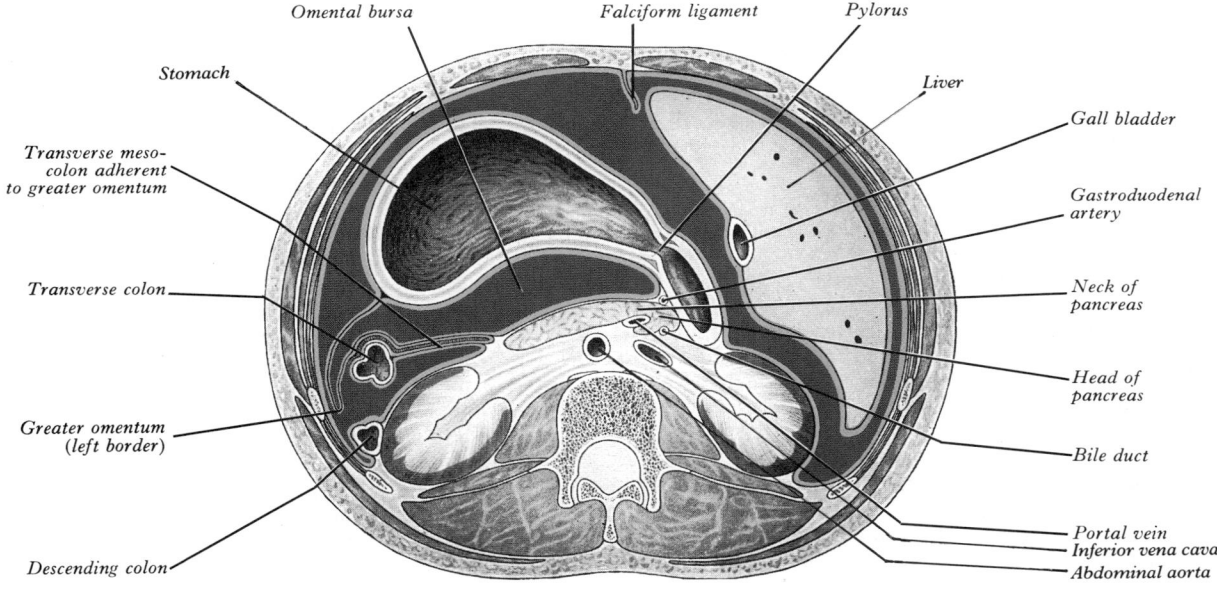

12.77B Transverse section through the abdomen at the level of the line BB in **12.76**, viewed from above. Colours as in **12.77A**.

proceeding to the viscera; though clearly not designed to sustain much weight, they may help to retain certain viscera in contact with each other. They are named ligaments, omenta and mesenteries. (The inappropriate nature of the term 'ligament' has been alluded to above.) An 'omentum' is a cover; the word may have been used to denote an apron and is thus suitable for the greater omentum, but is less suitably extended to other gastric peritoneal folds. The peritoneal 'ligaments' will be described with their respective organs.

OMENTA

Lesser omentum

The lesser omentum is the fold of peritoneum that extends to the liver from the lesser gastric curvature and the commencement of the duodenum; it develops from the embryonic ventral mesogastrium (p. 183). It is continuous with the two layers covering the antero-

superior and postero-inferior gastric surfaces and about the first 2 cm of the duodenum. From the lower part of the lesser curvature and upper border of the duodenum these two layers ascend as a double fold to the porta hepatis; from the upper part of the lesser curvature they pass to the bed of the fissure for the ligamentum venosum. This hepatic attachment is J-shaped, with a hook-like limb corresponding to the margins of the porta hepatis and a vertical ascending along the roof of the fissure (**12.140, 141**), at the superior limit of which the lesser omentum reaches the diaphragm where its two layers separate around the abdominal part of the oesophagus. At the right omental border the two layers are continuous and this free margin is anterior to the epiploic foramen. (The omentum may be described as consisting of *hepatogastric ligament* between the liver and stomach, and a *hepatoduodenal ligament* between the liver and duodenum, although these are continuous and essentially form a single entity.) Close to its right free margin the two omental layers enclose the hepatic artery, portal vein and bile duct, a few lymph

1741

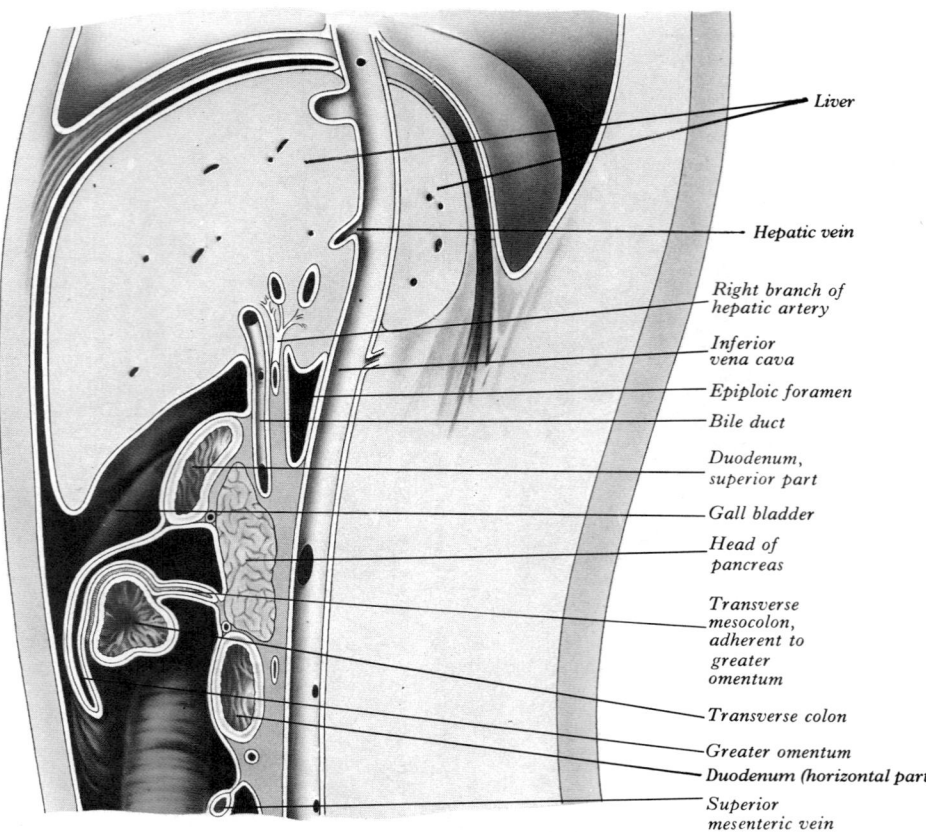

12.78   Section through the upper part of the abdominal cavity, along the line XX in (**12**.76). The boundaries of the epiploic foramen are shown and a small recess of the omental bursa is displayed in front of the head of the pancreas. Note that the tranverse colon and its mesocolon are adherent to the posterior two layers of the greater omentum.

nodes and lymph vessels and the hepatic plexus of nerves, all ensheathed in a *perivascular fibrous capsule* (**12**.77A). The right and left gastric vessels, branches of the gastric (vagus) nerves (p. 1253), and some of the left gastric lymph nodes and their lymph vessels are all contained between the two layers near their gastric attachment. The lesser omentum is thinner on the left and may be fenestrated. This variation in thickness is dependent upon the amount of connective tissue, especially fat.

Greater omentum

The greater omentum, the largest of the peritoneal folds (**12**.71, 72, 75, 78), is a double sheet, folded on itself to make four layers. The anterior double-layered fold descends from the greater curvature of the stomach and first part of the duodenum in front of the succeeding

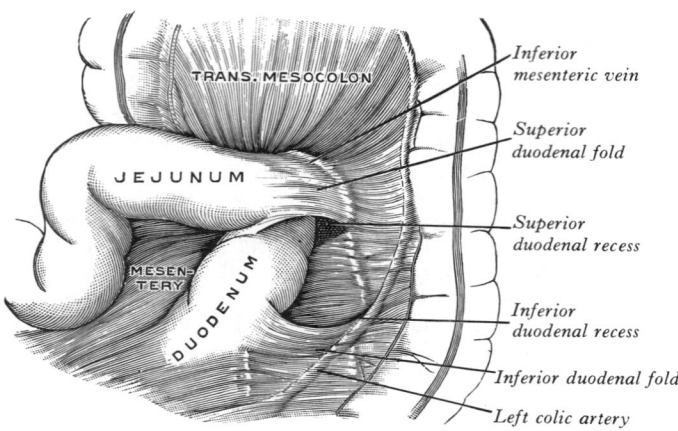

12.79   The superior and inferior duodenal recesses. The transverse colon and jejunum have been displaced (after Jonnesco, from Poirier & Charpy *Traité d'Anatomie humaine*. Masson et Cie).

part of the small intestine for a variable distance and ascends behind itself as far as the transverse colon (opposite the taenia omentalis). It adheres to, though it is separable from, the peritoneum on the superior surface of the transverse colon and mesocolon (p. 1740). The left border is continuous above with the gastrosplenic ligament; the right border extends to the commencement of the duodenum. (It must be emphasized that the greater omentum and gastrosplenic ligament are not merely continuous but the same structure, separated only by descriptive convenience and terminology. Their continuity has been further obscured by **changes** in terminology; the gastrosplenic *ligament* was formerly an *omentum* but is now officially the gastro-*lienal* ligament (an inadvisable use of the stem 'lien', the spleen, in a region where all else is 'splenic'!). The greater omentum is usually thin and cribriform but it always contains some adipose tissue, which in the obese may be massive in amount. Between the two layers of its anterior fold, close to the greater curvature of the stomach, the right and left gastro-epiploic vessels form a wide anastomotic arc. Variations in distribution and anastomoses of arteries in the omentum were recorded by Jiang Dian-fu (1978).

Apart from storing fat, the greater omentum may limit peritoneal infection. When the abdomen is opened without disturbance it is frequently found wrapped about the organs in the upper abdomen; it is rarely evenly dependent anterior to the intestines. It is less absorptive than the general peritoneum. It may be congenitally absent and may be removed without apparent ill effect and is hence not physiologically vital. It contains numerous fixed macrophages which are easily mobilized. These may accumulate into dense, oval or round visible 'milky-spots'. Similar spots may occur on other serous membranes (pleura p. 1662), pericardium and sometimes the leptomeninges.

MESENTERIES

Peritoneal folds, designated mesenteries, include the mesentery of the small intestine (the mesentery proper), the mesoappendix, transverse mesocolon, sigmoid mesocolon, (sometimes) an ascending or descending mesocolon and occasionally a mesentery for the gallbladder. They attach these viscera to the posterior body wall, allowing some degree of movement and providing access to vessels and nerves.

Mesentery (of the small intestine)

A broad, fan-shaped fold, it connects the coils of the jejunum and ileum to the posterior abdominal wall. The attached, parietal border is the *root of the mesentery* (**12**.76) about 15 cm (6 in.) long and directed obliquely down from the duodenojejunal flexure (left of the second lumbar vertebra) to the upper part of the right sacro-iliac joint. (Schmidt 1974 measured the mesenteric 'root' in 44 cadavers, finding a mean length of 13.9 cm, with extremes of 7.4 and 19.3 cm.) It passes successively in front of the horizontal part of the duodenum (where the superior mesenteric vessels enter it), the abdominal aorta, inferior vena cava, right ureter and right psoas major. The intestinal border is about 6 m (20 ft) long and compactly plicated. (For variations in length, see p. 1763.) The plication diminishes towards the posterior abdominal wall where the attachment is almost along a straight line. The central part is longest (measured from its root to the intestinal border), attaining a maximum of about 20 cm (8 in.); it shortens towards each end. The mesentery consists of two layers of peritoneum, a right and a left, enclosing the jejunal and ileal branches of the superior mesenteric vessels, with their accompanying neural plexuses, lymph vessels (here called *lacteals*), mesenteric lymph nodes, loose connective and adipose tissue. Fat is most abundant in its lower part and here extends from the root to the intestinal border; the upper mesentery contains less fat, with a tendency to accumulate near the root, leaving rounded, translucent, fat-free areas adjoining the upper jejunum. At the intestinal border, the layers separate to enclose the gut, as its visceral peritoneum. At the mesenteric root the right layer is reflected in its lower part to the posterior abdominal wall and ascending colon and in its upper part to become continuous with the inferior layer of the transverse mesocolon; the left layer passes to the posterior abdominal wall and descending colon. (This arrangement helps to distinguish between the proximal and distal coils of the small intestine when in situ.)

Mesoappendix (12.81)

This is a triangular fold of peritoneum around the vermiform appendix, attached to the back of the lower end of the mesentery close to the ileocaecal junction. It usually reaches the tip of the appendix but sometimes fails to reach the distal third, being then represented by a low peritoneal ridge containing fat. It encloses the blood vessels, nerves and lymph vessels of the vermiform appendix, together with a lymph node (p. 1620).

Transverse mesocolon

A broad fold connecting the transverse colon to the posterior abdominal wall, its two layers pass from the anterior aspect of the head and anterior border of the body of the pancreas to the posterior aspect of the transverse colon (opposite the *taenia mesocolica*), where they separate to surround it. The upper layer is adherent to, but separable from, the greater omentum (pp. 1739, 1740). Posteriorly, the inferior layer covers the inferior aspect of the pancreas and passes in front of the horizontal and ascending parts of the duodenum. Between its layers are the blood vessels, nerves and lymphatics of the transverse colon. The middle colic artery descends to the right, leaving a large avascular area to its left and a smaller one to its right.

Sigmoid mesocolon

This is a peritoneal fold attaching the sigmoid colon to the pelvic wall, the attachment being an inverted V with an apex near the division of the left common iliac artery (**12**.76); the left limb descends medial to the left psoas major and the right passes into the pelvis to end in the midline at the level of the third sacral vertebra. Sigmoid and superior rectal vessels run between its layers and the left ureter descends into the pelvis behind its apex.

Other mesenteric structures

Peritoneum usually covers only the front and sides of the ascending and descending parts of the colon, but sometimes these are virtually surrounded by peritoneum and attached to the posterior abdominal

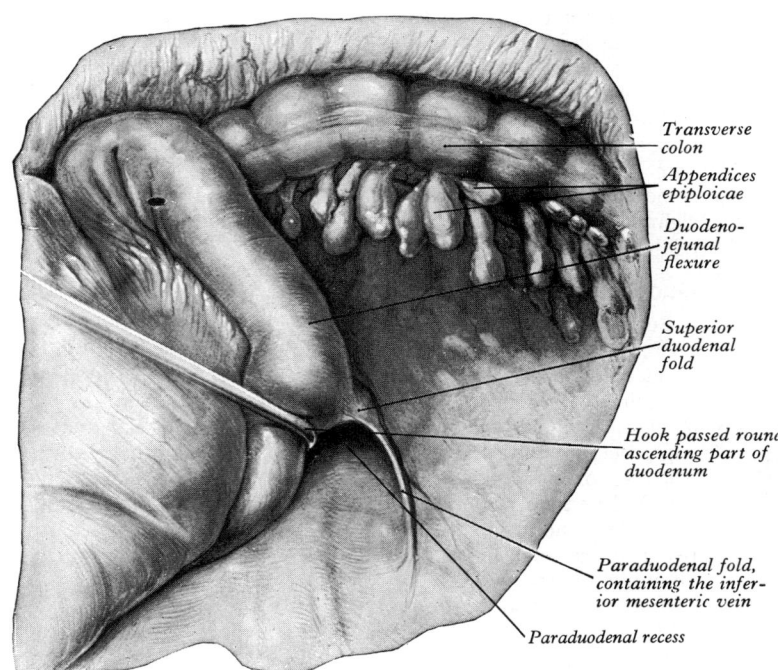

12.80   The paraduodenal recess.

wall by an ascending and descending mesocolon respectively. The *phrenicocolic ligament* is a peritoneal fold extending from the left colic flexure to the diaphragm level with the tenth and eleventh ribs; it has an anterior edge and passes inferolateral to the lateral end of the spleen, sometimes being misleadingly named the *sustentaculum lienis* or 'splenic shelf', implying a hypothetical supportive role.

Appendices epiploicae are small peritoneal appendages filled with adipose connective tissue and situated along the colon; they are most conspicuous on the transverse (**12**.80) and sigmoid parts, absent from the rectum and rudimentary on the caecum and appendix. Many contain a small arteriole from the wall of the gut. In the colon they are most numerous along the line of the *taenia libera* (p. 1784).

PERITONEAL RECESSES

Peritoneal folds may create fossae or recesses of the peritoneal cavity.

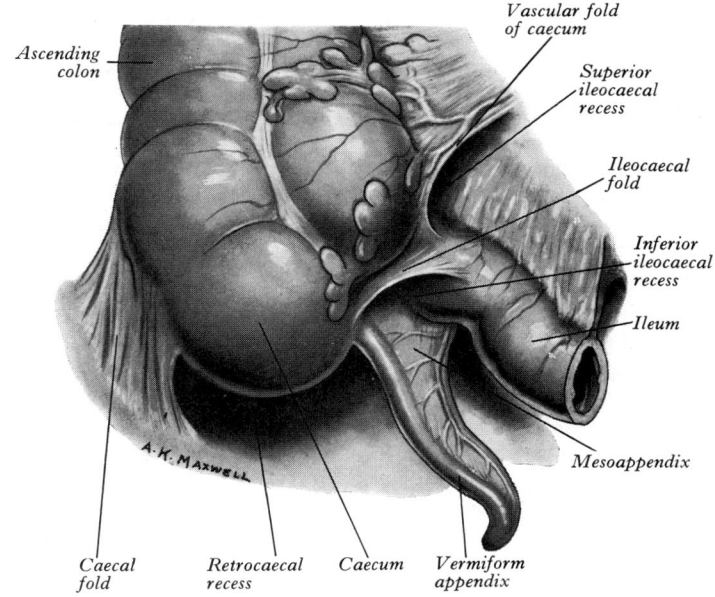

12.81   The peritoneal folds and recesses in the caecal region.

These are of clinical interest because a segment of intestine may enter one and be constricted by the fold at the entrance to the recess and may be a site of a kind of 'internal' hernia. Since the entrance to a recess may need to be cut to relieve strangulation and to withdraw the gut, the degree of vascularization of the fold becomes important. Surgically the omental bursa belongs to this category, with its opening at the epiploic foramen. Much smaller recesses sometimes occur, sometimes related to the duodenum, caecum and sigmoid mesocolon. For a discussion of the developmental origins of these recesses, see pages 193–194.

Duodenal recesses

Superior duodenal recess (12.79). Present in about 50% of people, this may exist alone but usually occurs with an inferior duodenal recess. It is to the left of the distal end of the duodenum, opposite the second lumbar vertebra, behind a crescentic *superior duodenal fold* (*duodenojejunal fold*), which has a semilunar free lower edge, merging on the left with peritoneum anterior to the left kidney. The inferior mesenteric vein is behind the junction of the left end of this fold and the posterior parietal peritoneum. The recess is about 2 cm deep, admitting a fingertip; it opens downwards, its orifice being in the angle formed by the left renal vein as it crosses the abdominal aorta.

Inferior duodenal recess (12.79). This is present in about 75% of subjects, usually associated with a superior recess with which it may share an orifice; it lies left of the distal end of the duodenum, opposite the third lumbar vertebra, behind a non-vascular, triangular *inferior duodenal fold* (*duodenomesocolic fold*), which has a sharp upper edge. It is about 3 cm deep, admits one or two fingers and opens upwards towards the superior duodenal recess. It sometimes extends behind the ascending part of the duodenum and to the left, in front of the ascending branch of the left colic artery and inferior mesenteric vein. This large fossa is liable to become the site of an internal hernia.

Paraduodenal recess (12.80). It may occur with the superior and inferior duodenal recesses. It is more frequent in the fetus and newborn than in adults, in whom it occurs in about 2%. It is a little to the left of the ascending part of the duodenum, behind a falciform *paraduodenal fold*, the free right edge of which contains the inferior mesenteric vein and ascending branch of the left colic artery, the fold being their mesentery. Its free edge lies in front of the wide orifice of the recess, which faces right.

Retroduodenal recess. Rarely present, it is the largest of the duodenal recesses, and lies behind the horizontal and ascending parts of the duodenum in front of the abdominal aorta. It ascends nearly to the duodenojejunal junction, being about 8–10 cm deep and bounded on both sides by *duodenoparietal folds*; its orifice faces down to the left.

Duodenojejunal or mesocolic recess. Present in about 20% and rarely or never accompanied by any other duodenal recess, it is about 3 cm deep and lies on the left side of the abdominal aorta, between the duodenojejunal junction and the root of the transverse mesocolon. Bounded above by the pancreas, on the left by the kidney, and below by the left renal vein, it has a circular opening between two peritoneal folds, which faces down to the right.

Mesentericoparietal recess (of Waldeyer). This is more frequent in the fetus and newborn, occurring in only about 1% of adults. It lies just below the horizontal part of the duodenum, invaginating the upper part of the mesentery towards the right. Its orifice is large and faces left behind a fold of mesentery raised by the superior mesenteric artery.

Caecal recesses

Superior ileocaecal recess (12.81). Usually present and best developed in children, it is often reduced and absent in the aged, especially the obese. It is formed by the *vascular fold of the caecum*, which arches over the anterior caecal artery, supplying the anterior part of the ileocaecal junction, and its accompanying vein. It is a narrow slit bounded in front by the vascular fold, behind by the ileal mesentery, below by the terminal ileum and on the right by the ileocaecal junction. Its orifice opens downwards to the left.

Inferior ileocaecal recess (12.81) It is well marked in youth but frequently obliterated by fat in later years. It is produced by the *ileocaecal fold*, extending from the antero-inferior aspect of the

terminal ileum to the front of the mesoappendix (or to the appendix or caecum). It is also known as the '*bloodless fold of Treves*', although it sometimes contains blood vessels; if inflamed, especially when the appendix and its mesentery are retrocaecal, it may be mistaken for the mesoappendix. (For the source of vessels in this fold, see Cabanie & Javelle 1966.) The recess is bounded in front by the ileocaecal fold, above by the posterior ileal surface and its mesentery, to the right by the caecum, and behind by the upper mesoappendix. Its orifice opens downwards to the left.

Retrocaecal recess (12.81). Behind the caecum, it varies in size and extent and ascends behind the ascending colon, being large enough to admit an entire finger. It is bounded in front by the caecum (and sometimes the lower ascending colon), behind by the parietal peritoneum and on each side by *caecal folds* (parietocolic folds) passing from the caecum to the posterior abdominal wall. The vermiform appendix frequently occupies this recess (pp. 1775–1776).

Intersigmoid recess

This recess is constant in fetal life and infancy, but may later disappear. It lies behind the apex of the V-shaped parietal attachment of the sigmoid mesocolon, is funnel-shaped and directed upwards and opens downwards. It varies in size from a dimple to a fossa admitting the fifth finger. Its posterior wall of posterior parietal peritoneum covers the left ureter as this crosses the bifurcation of the left common iliac artery. Occasionally the recess is within the layers of the sigmoid mesocolon nearer the gut than its root. Its presence is due to an imperfect blending of the mesocolon with the posterior parietal peritoneum.

ANOMALOUS PERITONEAL FOLDS

Certain other folds, bands or ligaments sometimes occur in the abdomen. Some are considered to cause obstruction by pulling on or kinking sections of intestine; others may limit the spread of peritoneal effusions. Their exact modes of origin are doubtful; they have been attributed to errors in development, previous inflammation (peritonitis), mechanical traction by the gut and even (and improbably) linked with the evolution of upright posture. These anomalous folds must be distinguished from pathological adhesions definitely due to peritonitis; also, when coils of intestine are pulled out of normal position during examination they may be artificially kinked, with resultant simulation of bands. Anomalous folds are only clinically important if proved to interfere with normal function; their presence should not halt a search for other possible causes of the symptoms. The commonest anomalous folds encountered are as follows:

- Occasionally the lesser omentum is prolonged to the right of the usual site of the epiploic foramen by a peritoneal fold extending from the gallbladder to the superior part of the duodenum (*cystoduodenal ligament*), or in front of the superior part of the duodenum to the greater omentum or right colic flexure, or from the inferior surface of the right hepatic lobe to the right colic flexure (*hepatocolic ligament*).

- The duodenojejunal junction is sometimes joined to the transverse mesocolon by a peritoneal band.

- The greater omentum may be attached to the front of the ascending colon or extend over it to the lateral abdominal wall. A thin sheet of peritoneum (*Jackson's membrane*), containing small blood vessels, may spread from the front of the ascending colon and caecum to the posterolateral abdominal wall and may merge on the left with the greater omentum. Occasionally a band passes from the right side of the ascending colon to the lateral abdominal wall near the level of the iliac crest. Sometimes termed a 'sustentaculum hepatis', it is closely related to the liver only in fetal and early postnatal life, when the liver is relatively larger. Other folds between the ascending colon and posterolateral abdominal wall may divide the right lateral paracolic gutter (between the ascending colon and posterior abdominal wall) into several small recesses.

- The ascending and less frequently the descending colon may have a mesentery.

- Proximal and distal ends of the sigmoid colon may be tied together by a fibrous band.
- Frequently a fan-shaped *presplenic fold* extends from the front of the gastrosplenic ligament (near the greater gastric curvature), below the inferolateral pole of the spleen, to blend with the phrenicocolic ligament; it may adhere to the spleen or diaphragm and contain rami of the splenic or the left gastro-epiploic artery; the omental bursa may enter it. It is more obvious in the fetus, often appearing as just part of the phrenicocolic ligament in adults. It may limit peritoneal effusions in the left supracolic space (see below), and, if adherent to the spleen or diaphragm, it may form a vascular obstruction in splenectomy.
- A fibrous band, described as passing from the terminal ileum to the posterior abdominal wall, and a similar one from the proximal sigmoid colon to the same wall, were once thought to be causes of partial obstruction by kinking of these parts of the gut, but this view is no longer popular.

SPECIAL PERITONEAL REGIONS

Regarding the spread of pathological collections of fluid, certain potential peritoneal spaces or recesses, normally in communication with each other, must be mentioned because they may be sealed off by pathological adhesions. These are as follows:

Supracolic space (subphrenic region). Between the diaphragm and the transverse colon and mesocolon, it is subdivided into the following:

Right subphrenic space. This is between the diaphragm and the anterior, superior and right lateral surfaces of the right lobe of the liver, bounded on the left side by the falciform ligament and behind by the coronary ligament's upper layer.

Left subphrenic space. Between the diaphragm, the anterior and superior surfaces of the left hepatic lobe, the anterosuperior surface of the stomach and the diaphragmatic surface of the spleen, it is limited to the right by the falciform ligament and behind by the left triangular ligament's anterior layer.

Right subhepatic space (hepatorenal recess, or Morison's pouch). Bounded above and in front by the inferior surface of the right hepatic lobe and gallbladder, below and behind by the right suprarenal gland, the upper part of the right kidney, the descending part of the duodenum, right colic flexure, transverse mesocolon and part of the head of the pancreas, above and behind, it extends between the right kidney and the liver as far as the inferior layer of the coronary ligament and right triangular ligament.

Left subhepatic space. i.e. the omental bursa.

Right infracolic space. This lies postero-inferior to the transverse colon and mesocolon and to the right of the mesentery, whose obliquity narrows the lower part of the space. The vermiform appendix is often in the lower part of this space.

Left infracolic space. This is below and behind the transverse colon and mesocolon and left of the mesentery; it is widest below, continuing into the pelvis.

Pelvic cavity. (See p. 829.)

Paracolic gutters. These are alongside the ascending and descending colon (which are normally sessile), where the peritoneum turns dorsally on the medial and lateral aspects of the gut. *Medial and lateral paracolic gutters* flank both left and right parts of the colon. Of commonest clinical interest is the *right lateral paracolic gutter*, which skirts the superolateral aspect of the hepatic flexure of the colon and continues into the hepatorenal pouch (of Morison) and, through the epiploic foramen, into the omental bursa and its superior recess. Inferiorly, around the caecum it curves over the pelvic brim into the *rectovesical pouch* (male) or *recto-uterine pouch* of Douglas (female). Related to this gutter, and its superior extension, are the vermiform appendix, right kidney, gallbladder, lesser gastric curvature and the first and second parts of the duodenum; all are common sites of acute abdominal disease. Seepage of infected fluid along this channel, from place to place, may cause puzzling symptoms and signs and errors in diagnosis. In supine patients infected fluid in the right lateral gutter may **ascend** to, enter and accumulate in the superior recess of the omental bursa, with grave consequences, because of its inaccessibility and nearness to the pleural and pericardial cavities. In patients nursed in a sitting posture, fluid **descends** to the relatively accessible rectovesical pouch or to the recto-uterine

pouch, approachable surgically through the rectum or vagina.

Two extraperitoneal subphrenic regions. These may become infected:

- the *right extraperitoneal space*, between the two layers of the coronary ligament, i.e. the 'bare area' of the liver and the diaphragm
- the *left extraperitoneal space*, which contains extraperitoneal connective tissue around the left suprarenal gland and upper pole of left kidney.

PERITONEAL MICROSTRUCTURE

The peritoneum is composed of a single layer of flat mesothelial cells lying on a layer of loose connective tissue. The mesothelium usually forms a continuous surface, adjacent cells being joined by junctional complexes but probably allowing the passage of macrophages, just as leucocytes pass between endothelial cell junctions. In some areas, e.g. the greater omentum, the peritoneum may be discontinuous, having fenestrations which are sometimes visible to the unaided eye; but mesothelium continues over the trabeculae of connective tissue interlacing around such fenestrae.

Submesothelial connective tissue contains cells typical of loose connective tissue (p. 75) but macrophages, lymphocytes and in some regions adipocytes are particularly numerous. Macrophages and lymphocytes may aggregate as submesothelial 'milky spots'. Mesothelial cells may also transform into fibroblasts; the fusion between layers of fibroblasts of mesothelial origin may cause macroscopic adhesions between the peritoneal surfaces, interfering with intestinal motility or even leading to complete obstruction of the gut.

The mesothelium resembles vascular endothelium in being a dialysing membrane which fluids and small molecules may traverse. Numerous endocytic vesicles occur near the cell surfaces, the remaining cytoplasm being poor in organelles, indicating low metabolic activity (Tesi & Forssmann 1970). Normally the volumes of fluid transmitted by peritoneal surfaces are small, but large volumes may be administered via the intraperitoneal route; conversely, substances such as urea can be dialysed from blood into fluid circulated through the peritoneal cavity.

PERITONEAL FLUID

The fluid covering the peritoneal surfaces contains water, electrolytes and other solutes derived from interstitial fluid in the adjacent tissues and from the plasma of local vessels. It also contains proteins and cells (Carr 1967), the latter varying in number, structure and type in different diseases; hence it is of diagnostic importance. Normally they are mesothelial desquamated elements, nomadic peritoneal macrophages, mast cells, fibroblasts, lymphocytes and some other leucocytes. Some, particularly macrophages, migrate freely between the peritoneal cavity and the surrounding connective tissue; intraperitoneally injected particles are ingested by them and transported to various tissue sites. Lymphocytes provide both cellular and humoral immunological defence mechanisms.

Absorption

Substances in **solution** are probably absorbed into the capillaries, whereas suspended matter is thought to pass into the lymph vessels, aided by macrophages. After abdominal or pelvic operations, it has been customary to prop up patients to encourage intraperitoneal effusions to gravitate into the pelvis. One reason for this was the belief that the subphrenic peritoneum was more absorptive than elsewhere and hence inflammatory products would enter the circulation more rapidly here. It was supposed that gaps or (peritoneal stomata) between the mesothelial cells of the subphrenic peritoneum and similar gaps (endothelial stigmata) between the endothelial cells of lymph vessels greatly facilitated absorption. Such gaps have been often considered to be histological artefacts, but scanning electron microscopy supports the existence of slit-like orifices. However, absorption is believed to be much the same in all parts of the peritoneum. Greater absorption in the upper abdomen may be due to the larger subphrenic peritoneal area and to respiratory movements.

PERITONEAL VESSELS AND NERVES

The parietal and visceral peritoneum are developed from, respectively, the somatopleural and splanchnopleural layers of lateral plate mesoderm (p.155). Parietal peritoneum is therefore supplied by somatic blood vessels of the abdominal and pelvic walls; its lymphatics join those in the body wall and drain to parietal lymph nodes; its nerve supply is derived from nerves supplying the muscles and skin of the parietes. Visceral peritoneum, however, as an integral part of the viscera, derives its blood vessels from those supplying viscera. Its lymphatics join the visceral vessels and its nerve supply is autonomic or visceral afferent. Differences in the sensibility of the two layers correlate with their innervations. Whereas pain is elicited by mechanical, thermal or chemical stimulation of the parietal peritoneum, the visceral peritoneum and viscera are not affected; e.g. the liver, stomach or intestine can be injured without evoking pain, insensibility extending from the mid-oesophagus to the junction of endoderm and ectoderm in the anal canal. However, tension *does* evoke pain when applied to viscera or visceral peritoneum by overdistension or traction on mesenteries, stretching various neural elements in the visceral walls or mesenteries. Also effective are spasms of visceral muscle and ischaemia. Somatic nerves of the parietal peritoneum also supply the corresponding segmental areas of skin and muscles and, when the parietal peritoneum is irritated, muscles are reflexly contracted, causing rigidity of the abdominal wall. The parietal peritoneum on the underside of the diaphragm is supplied with afferent fibres centrally by the phrenic nerves and peripherally by the lower six intercostal and subcostal nerves. Hence peripheral irritation may result in pain, tenderness and muscular rigidity in the distribution of the lower thoracic spinal nerves, while central irritation may result in pain in the cutaneous distribution of the third to fifth cervical spinal nerves, i.e. the shoulder region.

Examination of the Abdomen

Clinical examination of the abdomen is nothing more than an exercise in applied anatomy. As each part of the abdomen is viewed or felt, the underlying anatomical structures must be in the mind's eye of the observer. The subject is placed supine with a single pillow behind the head and shoulders. Systematic examination comprises the classical quartet of inspection, palpation, percussion and auscultation.

Inspection

Inspection reveals useful information about the build of the subject. The superficial fatty layer of the abdomen is normally 1 to 2 cm in thickness. This is reduced to millimetres in the cachectic and increased to 5 or more centimetres in the obese. The umbilicus is normally situated half way between the tip of the xiphoid process and the top of the symphysis pubis. It is displaced upwards by swellings which arise in the pelvis, for example the pregnant uterus, and displaced downwards in gross obesity and ascites.

When the muscles of the anterior abdominal wall are contracted by raising the head and shoulders from the couch, the midline linea alba and the linea semilunaris on either side can be seen, demarcating the rectus abdominis muscle. In a well-built subject, the transverse ridges of its muscle intersections can also be seen.

Palpation

Palpation is performed using the flat of the hand, the palpating agent being the flexor surfaces of the fingers used collectively. Relaxation of the abdomen is vital so the subject is reassured and asked to breathe quietly through the mouth. The pulsations of the aorta can be felt in the midline by firm pressure on the anterior abdominal wall, against the lumbar spine. The aorta terminates in front of the fourth lumbar vertebra. This corresponds with the supracristal plane, which is the line joining the uppermost part of the iliac crest on each side. In the normal subject, this corresponds to a point about 3 cm distal to the umbilicus. In most normal subjects, no other intra-abdominal viscus is palpable and any mass which is detected requires careful further elucidation. However, in healthy, well-relaxed thin subjects, especially female, the following structures may be palpated:

- The lower pole of the right kidney may just be felt on full inspiration by bimanual palpation, in which the fingers of one hand rest on the anterior abdominal wall and the other hand presses firmly forwards in the right flank.
- The lower margin of the liver may be palpable immediately below the right costal margin on full inspiration.
- The sigmoid colon may be felt in the left iliac fossa, particularly if loaded with faeces.

Percussion

The normal abdomen is universally resonant because of the gas-containing gut which lies in front of the solid retroperitoneal organs and the fact that the normal pelvic viscera lie entirely within the true bony pelvis. However, the liver gives a dull note to percussion throughout its extent from the level of the right fifth rib anteriorly to the right costal margin.

Percussion over a palpable mass is useful in determining whether the mass is solid or fluid-filled (dull to percussion) or contains gas (resonant). The clinical presence of free fluid in the abdomen is revealed by dullness in the flanks which moves as the patient rolls from side to side (shifting dullness). However, it requires the presence of a litre or more of fluid before this can be detected by physical examination—more so in the obese subject.

Auscultation

Stethoscopic examination of the normal abdomen reveals low-pitched gurgles of intestinal peristalsis. These sounds are increased, both in volume and in pitch, in organic intestinal obstruction and are absent in paralytic ileus and peritonitis. The presence of a bruit within the abdomen, as elsewhere, signifies turbulent flow in an artery, for example, in a patient with stenosis of the common iliac artery.

It should be noted that examination of the abdomen is not complete without inspection and palpation of the hernial orifices and the external genitalia and examination of the supraclavicular lymph nodes, the last for clinical evidence of metastatic lymphatic spread from intra-abdominal malignant disease.

ALIMENTARY SYSTEM FROM OESOPHAGUS TO ANUS

INTRODUCTION

Despite structural variations along the alimentary tract, there is a common basic plan which is best appreciated by reference to its development (p.174). Much of the alimentary canal originates as a tube of endoderm enveloped in the splanchnopleuric mesoderm, its external surface facing the intraembryonic coelom. The endodermal lining forms the epithelium of the tract and also the secretory and ductal cells of various glands secreting into the lumen, including the pancreas and liver. The surrounding splanchnopleuric mesoderm forms the connective tissue, muscle layers, blood vessels and lymphatics of the wall, its external surface becoming visceral mesothelium; this is of course absent throughout the neck and thorax and where the hindgut traverses the pelvic floor. The disposition and development of the dorsal and ventral mesenteries of the subdiaphragmatic foregut and of the dorsal mesentery of the midgut and hindgut are described elsewhere (pp. 186, 188, 191). Associated neural elements invade the gut from neighbouring neural crest tissue (p. 220). Cranially, the skeletal muscle of branchial arch origin and caudally of less certain origin, contribute to the musculature of the gut's extremities. An outline of the alimentary organization is depicted in **12**.82.

GENERAL MICROSTRUCTURE

MATURE GUT WALL (12.82A)

This has a laminated structure in which four main layers (or tunicae) are readily distinguishable; although the layers are firmly attached to each other, the boundaries are clear cut. The innermost layer is the *mucosa* (tunica mucosa, or mucous membrane); this is subdivided into three strata, from inside outwards:

- the lining *epithelium*,
- the *lamina propria*, a layer of loose connective tissue immediately beneath it, where many of the glands are also found,
- the *muscularis mucosae*, a thin layer of smooth muscle.

Beneath the mucosa is the *submucosa* (tunica submucosa), a strong and highly vascularized layer of connective tissue which in some regions also contains glands. External to the submucosa is the *muscularis* (tunica muscularis), also referred to as the *muscularis externa* or muscle coat to distinguish it from the much thinner muscularis mucosae; in most regions this has an inner circular layer and an outer longitudinal, but in the stomach a third, oblique layer is added to the inner surface of the circular layer. Finally, the external surface is bounded by a serosa or adventitia, depending on its position within the body.

Mucosal layers

Epithelium. This is a protective barrier and the site of secretion and absorption (i.e. of selective entry into the body of chemicals derived from the food). The protective function against mechanical (abrasive), thermal and chemical injury is well in evidence in the oesophagus and in the terminal part of the rectum, where the epithelium is thick and stratified, and is covered in mucus which acts as a protective lubricant, as also in the oral cavity and pharynx. Elsewhere in the gut the epithelium is simple, either cuboidal or columnar, and includes cells for absorption and various types of secretory cells. The barrier function and selectivity of absorption is assisted by the presence of tight junctions (p. 27) over the entire epithelium. The amount of secretion and absorption depends on the number of relevant cells present, and on their individual surface areas; these are related to the surface area of the lumen which is increased by the presence of mucosal folds and pits, by crypts, by villi and by glands, while microvilli on the surfaces of individual absorptive cells considerably magnify the area of plasma membranes presented to the contents of the gut. Some glands lie in the lamina propria, some in the submucosa, and some (namely the liver and pancreas) completely outside the wall of the gut. All glands drain into the lumen of the gut through individual ducts. There are also scattered enteroendocrine cells within the epithelial lining.

Lamina propria. Made of compact connective tissue, often rich in elastin fibres, this supports and moulds the shape of the surface epithelium, providing nutrient vessels and lymphatics and immune defence: lymphoid follicles are present in many regions of the gut, including some prominent masses in the appendix, and small intestine (Peyer's patches). It is also the source of various growth factors which regulate cell turnover, differentiation and repair in the overlying epithelium.

Muscularis mucosae. This is well developed in the oesophagus and in the large intestine, especially in the terminal part of the rectum. In spite of its thinness, an inner circular and an outer longitudinal component can usually be distinguished, the latter

thicker than the former. In addition, single muscle cells emanating from the muscularis mucosae are found inside the villi or between the columnar glands of the stomach and large intestine. By its contraction, the muscularis mucosae can alter the surface configuration of the mucosa locally, allowing it to adapt to the shapes and mechanical forces imposed by the contents of the lumen, and in the case of intestinal villi, promoting vascular exchange.

Submucosa

The submucosa is the strongest layer of the gut wall, as it contains large bundles of collagen, but it is also pliable and deformable so that it adjusts to changes in length and diameter of the gut. In the oesophagus and rectum the submucosa enters into the folds that project into the lumen; it also enters into the rugae of the gastric wall, and the plicae circulares (valves of Kerkring) of the small intestine, but not into the villi. The submucosa also contains the largest arterial network of the wall, which feeds both the mucosa and the muscle coat.

Muscularis externa

This coat usually consists of distinct inner circular and outer longitudinal layers, the antagonistic activities of which create waves of peristalsis responsible for movement of ingested material through the lumen of the gut. In the stomach, where movements are more complex, there is a partial oblique layer, internal to the other two layers. The muscularis externa is chiefly smooth in type, except in the upper oesophagus where skeletal muscle blends with it; here, the musculature resembles that of the pharynx except that it is entirely under involuntary control. For most of its length the smooth muscle of the tract is made of ill-defined bundles of cells, arranged in layers. The smooth muscle cells are typically visceral in type, being somewhat larger than vascular smooth muscle cells; they have a smooth surface, and are about 500 μm long (regardless of body size), and are electrically and mechanically coupled. Their fasciculi lack a perimysium but have sharp boundaries. The layer of circular muscle is invariably thicker than the more external longitudinal coat, except in the colon where the longitudinal muscle is gathered into three cords (taeniae).

Because of the arrangement of the musculature a segment of gut can change extensively not only its diameter (down to a virtual occlusion of the lumen) but also its length; elongation is limited by the insertion of the mesentery. The co-ordinated activity of the two muscle layers and the pattern of activity along the length of the gut produces a characteristic motor behaviour, mainly a propulsive motor activity directed anally (peristalsis) and a non-propulsive motor activity which mixes the luminal contents, as in the stomach, or segments them, e.g. the pyloric sphincter. An important property which bears on the mechanics of the muscle is that it maintains constant volume, so that its shortening is accompanied by an increase in muscle girth. The muscularis externa is traversed by connective tissue septa which pick up the mechanical activity of the muscle, in the manner of minute intramuscular tendons, and discharge it on the submucosa.

Some controversy has existed over the direction of fibres in the layers of the muscularis externa, one suggestion being that the inner circular muscle is a tight helix and the longitudinal one an open spiral (Carey 1921). Other observations (Elsen & Arey 1966) on various mammals, including man, indicated that, despite some deviations from precisely circular and longitudinal directions and some exchange of fasciculi between adjacent circular muscle rings and layers, their fibres do not follow spiral pathways (Schofield 1968).

Interstitial cells (of Cajal). Originally described by Ramon y Cajal in 1893, these cells are thin, flat, and somewhat branched, forming strata associated with the enteric neural plexuses and related smooth muscle of the muscularis externa. At the light microscopic level they can be demonstrated with methylene blue staining and Zinc-iodide-osmium impregnation but whether they are muscle or some other (e.g. neural) cell type was a controversy for many years. The recent application of electron microscopy, immunocytochemistry and electrophysiology has to a large degree clarified their nature (see e.g. Berezin et al 1988; Thuneberg 1989; Rumessen 1992; Faussonne-Pellegrini 1992). In general the cells resemble smooth muscle cells in that they contain actin and myosin filaments (Torihashi et al 1993), dense bodies, caveolae and numerous mitochondria, and are linked

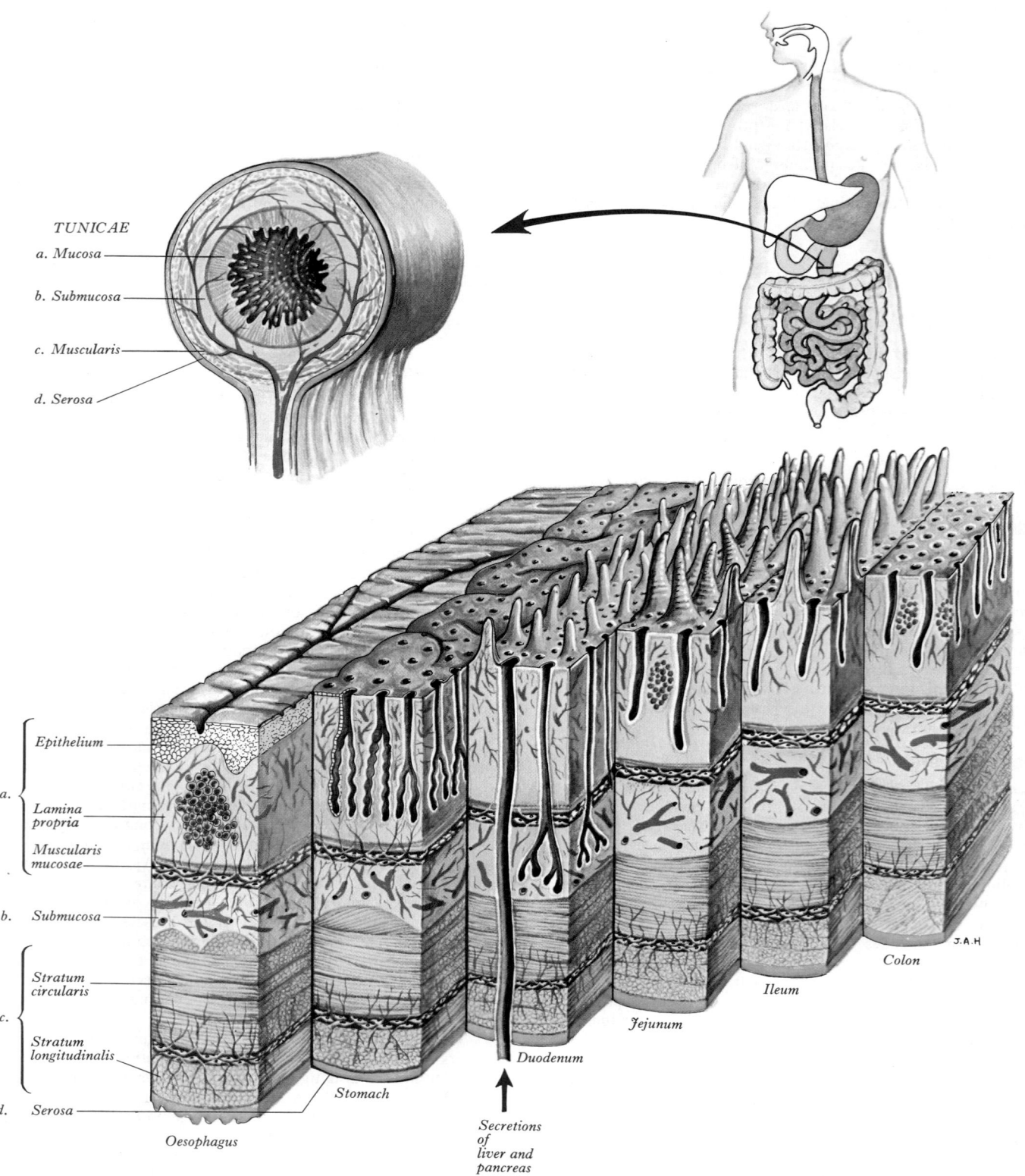

TUNICAE

a. *Mucosa*

b. *Submucosa*

c. *Muscularis*

d. *Serosa*

Epithelium

a.

Lamina propria

Muscularis mucosae

b. *Submucosa*

Stratum circularis

c.

Stratum longitudinalis

d. *Serosa*

Oesophagus

Stomach

Secretions of liver and pancreas

Duodenum

Jejunum

Ileum

Colon

J.A.H

12.82A The general arrangement of the alimentary canal, its mural tunicae and (below) the general histology at the levels indicated (highly diagrammatic). The transverse colon (above right) has been displaced downwards to reveal the duodenum.

by gap junctions to typical smooth muscle elements. However there are also differences, for example in the presence of a characteristic flattened, branched smooth endoplasmic reticulum, small ovoid mitochondria and a discontinuous basal lamina, and intermediate filaments of the vimentin type rather than the desmin typical of muscle cells (Torihashi et al 1993). The interstitial cells are in close apposition to the varicose nerve endings of at least two types, one with small (50 nm) round clear vesicles, the other with flat discoidal (70 nm

diameter) vesicles (Zhou & Komoro 1992). The neurotransmitters have yet to be identified with certainty, although they may include VIP. Electrophysiology indicates that these cells act as pacemakers for the myogenic contraction of the muscularis externa smooth muscle (Barajas-Lopez et al 1989), and receive modulatory inputs from the enteric nervous system and extrinsic innervation of the gut.

The positions of the interstitial cell strata vary regionally (Faussonne-Pellegrini 1992). In general they lie in the same layers as

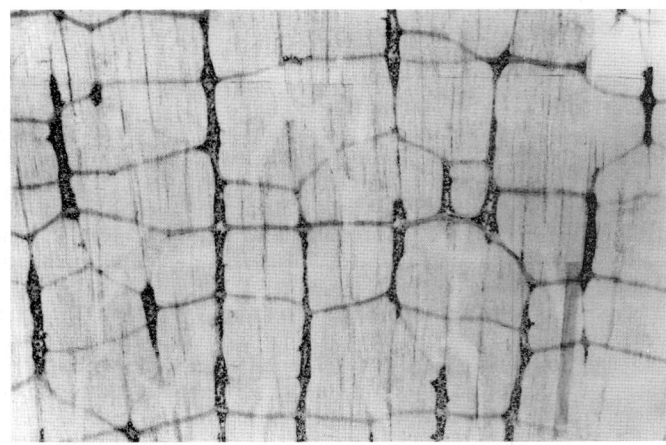

12.82B Myenteric plexus in the small intestine, visualised by selective staining in a whole mount preparation, as seen in a micrographic montage. Note the presence of polygonal areas of ganglion cells interconnected by thinner fasciculi. The smooth muscle fibres run transversely in this illustration. Magnification × 200. (Provided by G. Gabella, Department of Anatomy and Embryology, University College, London.)

the enteric plexuses, i.e. in the small intestine close to the myenteric plexus between circular and longitudinal muscle, and between the inner and outer layers of circular smooth muscle (the deep muscle plexus of Schabadasch, see p. 1750). In the oesophagus and stomach they have also been described as scattered among the cells of the circular layer (which is not separated into deep and superficial parts as in the small intestine), and in the large intestine they colocalize with the myenteric plexus and the single layer of the submucosal plexus on the luminal side of the circular component of the muscularis externa. These differences must reflect differing patterns of innervation and muscular activity in the different gut regions, although these remain to be worked out in detail.

Serosa and adventitia

Outside the muscularis externa is a layer of connective tissue of variable thickness, in many places the site of adipose tissue deposition. Where the tract is attached to the body wall by mesentery within the abdominal cavity, i.e. covered in visceral peritoneum, it is lined by *serosa* (serous membrane) consisting of a thin connective tissue layer and an external coat of mesothelium. Elsewhere the connective tissue blends with the surrounding fascial planes of connective tissue and is then termed the *adventitia*. Where the alimentary tract is retroperitoneal (e.g. much of the duodenum) the surface facing the abdominal cavity is lined by serosa, and other parts by adventitia.

Neural and vascular plexuses

Neuronal cell bodies of the enteric nervous system (p. 1310 and see below) are present between the circular and longitudinal components of the muscularis externa (the *myenteric (Auerbach's) plexus*) and in the submucosa (*submucosal (Meissner's) plexus*), providing the intrinsic sensory and motor supply of the gut wall. Extrinsic sensory, motor and sensorimotor nerves from cranial or spinal sources are connected with the enteric nervous system (see below). Vascular plexuses are also present at various levels of the wall especially in the submucosa and mucosa. These plexuses connect with vessels of the surrounding tissues or those entering through the mesentery, and accompany the ducts of outlying glands.

Sources of innervation. The gut is densely innervated by the autonomic nervous system.

Extrinsic innervation. This originates from neurons outside the gut, with functional components from the sympathetic, parasympathetic and visceral sensory divisions of the peripheral nervous system (PNS). Visceral afferent nerves come from sensory ganglion cells situated in the nodose ganglion of the vagus and spinal dorsal root ganglia; parasympathetic efferent neurons originate from the vagal dorsal motor nucleus in the medulla oblongata, and sym-

pathetic efferent neurons arise from the thoracic and lumbar spinal cord, via the prevertebral sympathetic (coeliac, mesenteric and pelvic) ganglia.

Intrinsic innervation. Consisting of neurons located entirely within the gut wall (the intramural ganglionated plexuses), this is so well developed and so complex in its organization that since Langley (1921) it is known as the *enteric nervous system*, a division that is connected with but distinct from, the sympathetic and parasympathetic divisions. Further details are given on p. 1310.

ENTERIC NERVOUS SYSTEM

Introduction

Within the wall of gastrointestinal tract from the oesophagus to anal canal lies a series of ganglionated plexuses. Collectively these form the enteric nervous system, a highly organized neural assemblage with some remarkable features similar to those of the central nervous system (CNS). Because of the intrinsic sensory, motor and interneuronal microcircuitry of the enteric nervous system (ENS) the gut can make complex reflex responses to local stimulation even when, experimentally, all connections to the CNS have been severed. In normal life the ENS governs many activities of the alimentary system, both motor and sensory. It regulates and directs peristaltic contractions of the muscularis externa and movements of the muscularis mucosae, and it governs secretion by mucosal and submucosal glands, local vasoconstriction and vasodilatation, water absorption and electrolyte exchange, and other less well-understood functions including local neuro-immunological and neurotrophic modulations of surrounding tissues. From the vagus and other autonomic nerves the plexuses also receive the preganglionic axons of the parasympathetic system and the postganglionic axons of the sympathetic system which exert external regulatory influences upon the ENS. Sensory information is also relayed to the CNS through visceral afferents, although the relation of these with the ENS is not yet clear. Recent reviews of the ENS have been given by Furness and Costa (1987); see also Hoyle and Burnstock (1989); Timmermans et al (1992); Gershon and Wade (1993).

Locations of enteric plexuses

The cell bodies of the enteric neurons are located in three (or more) ganglionated plexuses situated within the gut wall; they give off numerous axons and other processes which branch and interweave to form non-ganglionated plexuses and ramifications among the surrounding tissues. Ganglia are located at two main levels in the wall thickness, namely:

- within the muscularis externa (the *myenteric ganglionated plexus*) between the circular and longitudinal strata
- the submucosa (two or more *submucosal ganglionated plexuses*).

The non-ganglionated nerve plexuses lie at various levels in the wall, notably in the lamina propria (mucosal plexus), at the interface between the submucosa and muscularis externa (*plexus entericus (submucosus) extremis*), between the circular and longitudinal muscles (the non-ganglionated part of the myenteric plexus), and within the serosa (*serosal plexus*). In the small intestine an extra non-ganglionated plexus lies between the internal and external components of the circular muscle (*plexus entericus profundus*). Fibres, often in groups, also penetrate all tissues of the gut wall including the epithelium.

Ganglion cell types and microcircuitry

The details of ENS microcircuitry have not yet been thoroughly worked out, although recent studies using electrophysiological recording combined with dye injection, immunohistochemistry and lesioning experiments have begun to reveal what appears to be quite a complex and regionally variable organization (see e.g. Furness & Costa 1987; Gershon & Wade 1993). Major species differences in immunohistochemistry also occur even between closely related mammals, making it difficult to draw general conclusions about neurotransmitters and the chemical identities of cell types.

In a classic study with intravital methylene blue staining, Dogiel (1899) distinguished four types of enteric ganglion neurons on the basis of their size and neurite patterns, as follows:

- *Type I cells* are relatively large, with short, stubby irregular paddle-shaped dendrites and a single axon, usually directed orally and therefore perhaps associated with orally-directed peristalsis. They occur only in the myenteric plexus; some of them contain substance P (SP).
- *Type II cells* are smaller with several axon-like processes directed circumferentially and radially. They may represent interneurons or possibly primary sensory cells. They are CGRP-positive in humans, and calbindin positive in guinea pigs.
- *Type III cells* possess a number of branched dendrites and a single axon, often directed anally, and therefore a possible mediator of anally-directed peristaltic waves. They are mostly immunoreactive for 5-HT and calbindin, and some are enkephalin positive. In more recent years Stach (1989) has added to this list other cells with various morphologies.
- *Dendritic (filamentous) Type II cells* which have a number of short as well as long neurites; *Types IV* and *V cells* and *microneurons* (minineurons) which contain various neuromodulatory peptides including vasoactive intestinal polypeptide (VIP), galanin (GAL), substance P (SP) and neuromodulator U (NMU).

The relationships of the different cell types to the large number of known neurotransmitters or neuromodulators (see the list on p. 937) have yet to be satisfactorily worked out. It should however be mentioned that enteric neurons often contain more than one of these chemicals, underlining the functional complexity of the ENS. An interesting recent finding is that some groups of cells are positive for nicotineamide adenine dinucleotide (NADH) diaphorase, identical with nitric oxide synthase, and are therefore probably agents of the nitric oxide-mediated smooth muscle relaxation important in peristalsis and the opening of sphincters (see the review by Sanders & Ward 1992). There is evidence that this role is shared with some other neuromodulators including VIP and ATP.

Ganglionated plexuses

For convenience, in this description the transmitter/neuromodulators reported for porcine enteric plexuses by Timmermans et al 1992 will be followed, although as stated above, other species may show different chemicals and chemical combinations.

Myenteric (Auerbach's) plexus (12.82B). This lies between the circular and longitudinal layers of the muscularis externa, consisting of groups of motor neurons and interneurons. It is composed predominantly of Type I cells containing (in pigs) substance P (SP), Type II cells reactive for CGRP and VIP, Type III cells for 5-HT, ENK and calbindin, and microneurons for VIP and GAL (Timmermans et al 1992). The myenteric plexus serves the muscles around it (i.e. the deep part of the circular muscle and the longitudinal layer of the muscularis externa).

Submucosal plexus. This is divisible into a *deep submucosal plexus (of Schabadasch or of Henle*: see Hoyle & Burnstock 1989) adjacent to the submucosal surface of the muscularis externa, and a *superficial submucosal plexus* (of *Meissner*) near the submucosal surface of the muscularis mucosae. In the colon other ganglia are present throughout the considerable thickness of the submucosa, and may constitute an additional intermediate plexus, although its cells resemble those of Meissner's plexus in size and immunoreactivity (Hoyle & Burnstock 1989). Neural processes extend from all these ganglia into adjacent structures: the *deep submucosal plexus.*

Deep submucosal plexus. Composed of cells innervating the circular layer of the muscularis externa (among other functions), these contain Type II cells with calcitonin gene-related peptide (CGRP), VIP, SP and DYN, and Type III cells immunoreactive as in the myenteric plexus; microneurons are positive for VIP and GAL.

Superficial submucosal plexus. Supplying the surrounding submucosa, muscularis mucosae, lamina propria and epithelial base, this is thought to contain sensory cells reactive to mucosal stimulation as well as secretomotor neurons and interneurons. Its cells are mainly Type II ganglion cells containing CGRP, SP, GAL and NMU.

Electrical activity of enteric neurons

Electrophysiologically (see e.g. Gershon & Wade 1993), most ganglion cells fall into two categories, designated 1/S and 2/AH types on the basis of their electrical activity (e.g. action potentials of 2/AH

cells differ from the 1/S in having a calcium conductance in their falling phase and showing a prolonged after-hyperpolarisation, hence the designation AH). The experimental evidence points to the 2/AH cells being interneurons, at least some of them within the Type II category, with synaptic inputs and, in some cases cholinergic synaptic outputs on to (1/S) motor neurons innervating smooth muscle. Another set of 2/AH-like cells in the submucosal ganglia are thought to be primary sensory neurons with dendrites reaching the base of the epithelium. However, they may only be the second cell in the sensory pathway, as they are stimulated strongly by 5-HT, and the primary receptors may therefore be 5-HT-releasing enteroendocrine cells in the gut epithelium.

The 1/S cells include putative motor neurons, but other functional classes may also show these physiological characteristics. Further research is expected to clarify the relation between the rather simple electrophysiological classification and the undoubtedly complex morphological and functional natures of enteric neurons.

Enteric plexuses and gut motility

Axons from the enteric plexuses pass in various directions: circumferentially around the gut, radially into its different mural layers, and longitudinally into adjacent segments of the alimentary tract. The longitudinal organization is of considerable importance since peristalsis in most of the gut occurs mainly unidirectionally from the oral towards the anal end, and individual peristaltic waves only move for a limited distance along the gut.

Each peristaltic wave of the gut must have an initiation site and as it moves along, must be preceded by a wave of circular muscle relaxation to allow the propulsion of the bolus along the gut. Behind the peristaltic wave the longitudinal muscle is then activated to restore the gut to its resting shape and prepare for the next peristaltic wave. Although visceral smooth muscle is spontaneously contractile, its co-ordination depends on the ENS, coupled with pacemaker activity in specialized smooth muscle cells (see Interstitial cells of Cajal, p. 155) which can spread excitation through gap junctions to many smooth muscle cells. However, other types of motile behaviour can occur; peristalsis in the the ascending and transverse colon, and in the small intestine can undergo reversals of direction during normal alimentation, and static constrictions of circular smooth muscle may also periodically constrict the small and large intestines into segments (segmentation); these activities are thought to promote the mixing of the luminal contents. Movements of these kinds imply a longitudinal and circumferential pattern of co-ordination, involving the organization of smooth muscle cell connectivity, neuronal microcircuitry and appropriate neurochemical control.

In emphasizing the role of the enteric nervous system in these activities one should not, of course, lose sight of the controlling influence of the extrinsic neural connections. As described elsewhere, the cholinergic terminals of parasympathetic fibres act via the enteric plexuses and also directly on smooth muscle to cause increased motility (and secretory activity in the alimentary glands). Postganglionic fibres of the sympathetic system release noradrenalin on to the smooth muscle, causing hyperpolarization and decreased motility. Feedback systems from visceral afferent fibres are involved in the reflex regulation of such effector actions, although the precise routes of peripheral and central nervous interactions accompanying these activities are rather obscure.

Enteric glia. Associated with all layers are enteric glial cells which ensheath neurons and their processes in the same way that Schwann cells do in other parts of the peripheral nervous system (PNS). However, they have some features which mark them as special cells of considerable biological interest because of their similarity to central nervous glial cells. Like the latter cells (and unlike Schwann cells), they contain intermediate filaments composed of glial fibrillary acidic protein (GFAP). Further details are given on p. 939.

Enteric nervous system disease

Much of alimentary pharmacology is concerned directly or indirectly with malfunctions of the enteric nervous system, as affected by microbial infections and other harmful agents which cause increased or decreased gut motility, abnormalities of secretion and other dysfunctions. Apart from the actions of neurotoxins and inflammatory chemicals on the ganglion cells, they can be damaged or killed by invasive organisms, with ensuing alimentary stasis, constipation and various other complications. This is seen, e.g. in Chagas' disease, a tropical infection of the viscera by the flagellate *Trypanosoma cruzi*, and after the prolonged intake of certain chemical substances such as chlorpromazine and senna. The numbers of ganglion cells also diminish in old age, a factor which could contribute to alimentary dysfunction in the elderly (de Souza et al 1993). In Hirschsprung's disease there is a congenital absence of enteric ganglion cells due to embryonic non-migration of neural and glial precursors from the neural crest from which they are derived (p. 220). Typically only part, often only a small sector of the gut, is affected (usually somewhere between the midjejunum and the anal canal, and most often the rectum: see e.g. Kamm 1994). Large defects tend to be fatal during early development or childhood. Biopsies diagnostically show a local absence of ganglion cells from affected regions.

OESOPHAGUS (12.1, 3, 68, 83, 87–89)

The oesophagus is a muscular tube about 25 cm (10 in) long, connecting the pharynx to the stomach. It begins in the neck, level with the lower border of the cricoid cartilage and the sixth cervical vertebra; descending largely anterior to the vertebral column through the superior and posterior mediastina. It traverses the diaphragm, level with the tenth thoracic vertebra, and ends at the gastric cardiac orifice level with the eleventh thoracic vertebra. Generally vertical in its course, it has two shallow curves. At its beginning it is median but inclines to the left as far as the root of the neck, gradually returns to the median plane near the fifth thoracic vertebra, and at the seventh deviates left again, finally turning anterior to traverse the diaphragm at the tenth. The tube also bends in an anteroposterior plane to follow the cervical and thoracic curvatures of the vertebral column. It is the narrowest part of the alimentary tract, except for the vermiform appendix, and is constricted:

- at its commencement, 15 cm (6 in) from the incisor teeth
- where crossed by the aortic arch, 22.5 cm (9 in) from the incisor teeth
- where crossed by the left principal bronchus, 27.5 cm (11 in) from the incisors
- as it traverses the diaphragm, 40 cm (16 in) from the incisors.

These data are important clinically with regard to the passage of instruments along the oesophagus.

Cervical part (12.1, 68)

This is posterior to the trachea and attached to it by loose connective tissue; the recurrent laryngeal nerves ascend on each side in or near the groove between the trachea and the oesophagus; **posterior** are the vertebral column, longus colli and prevertebral layer of deep cervical fascia; **lateral** on each side are the common carotid artery and posterior part of the thyroid gland. In the lower neck, where the oesophagus deviates left, it is closer to the left carotid sheath and thyroid gland than it is on the right. The thoracic duct ascends for a short distance along its left side.

Thoracic part (12.83, 11.59, 60, 46)

At first situated a little to the left in the *superior mediastinum* between the trachea and the vertebral column, this passes behind and to the right of the aortic arch to descend in the posterior mediastinum along the right side of the descending thoracic aorta. Below, as it inclines left, it crosses anterior to the aorta to enter the abdomen through the diaphragm at the level of the tenth thoracic vertebra.

Anterior (from above downwards) are: the trachea, right pulmonary artery, left principal bronchus, pericardium (separating it from the left atrium) and the diaphragm; **posterior** are the vertebral column, longus colli muscles, right posterior (aortic) intercostal arteries, thoracic duct, azygos vein and the terminal parts of the hemiazygos and accessory hemiazygos veins and, near the diaphragm, the aorta. In the posterior mediastinum there is a long recess of the right pleural sac between the oesophagus in front and the vena azygos and vertebral column behind.

Left lateral, in the superior mediastinum, are the terminal part of the aortic arch, the left subclavian artery, thoracic duct, the left pleura and the recurrent laryngeal nerve which ascends in or near

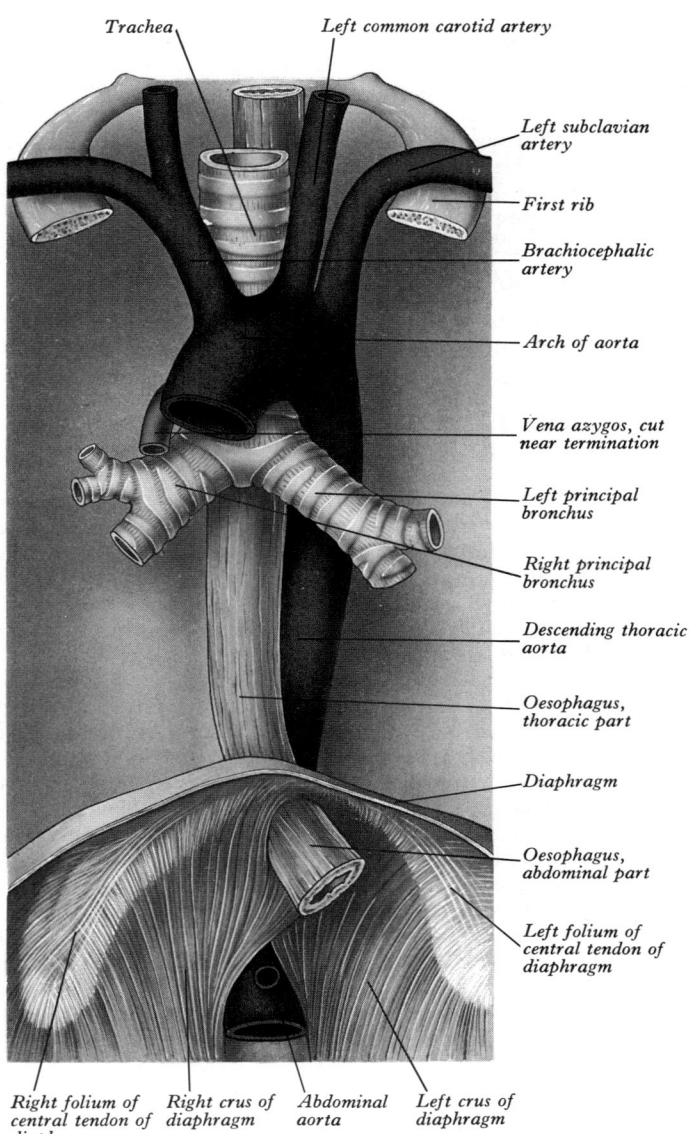

Trachea — *Left common carotid artery*

Left subclavian artery

First rib

Brachiocephalic artery

Arch of aorta

Vena azygos, cut near termination

Left principal bronchus

Right principal bronchus

Descending thoracic aorta

Oesophagus, thoracic part

Diaphragm

Oesophagus, abdominal part

Left folium of central tendon of diaphragm

Right folium of central tendon of diaphragm   *Right crus of diaphragm*   *Abdominal aorta*   *Left crus of diaphragm*

12.83 Dissection to expose the oesophagus in the posterior mediastinum and in the abdomen, and its relation to the trachea and aorta in the thorax.

the groove between the oesophagus and trachea. In the *posterior mediastinum* the oesophagus is related to the descending thoracic aorta and left pleura. *Right lateral* it is related to the right pleura, with the azygos vein intervening as it arches forwards above the right principal bronchus to join the superior vena cava. Below the pulmonary roots the vagus nerves descend in contact with the oesophagus, the right chiefly behind and the left in front, uniting to form an oesophageal plexus around it (p. 1253). Low in the posterior mediastinum the thoracic duct is behind and to the right; higher, it is posterior, crossing to the left at about the level of the fifth thoracic vertebra and then ascending on the left. On the right of the oesophagus, just above the diaphragm, a small serous *infracardiac bursa* may occur, representing the detached apex of the right pneumato-enteric recess.

Abdominal part (12.87–89)

This emerges from the right diaphragmatic crus (p. 816), slightly left of the midline and level with the tenth thoracic vertebra, grooving the posterior surface of the left lobe of the liver. It forms a truncated cone, about 1 cm long, curving sharply left, its base continuous with the cardiac orifice of the stomach; its right side continues smoothly into the lesser curvature, while the left is separated from the gastric fundus by the cardiac notch. Covered by peritoneum on its front and left side, it is contained in the upper left part of the lesser

1751

omentum; the peritoneum reflected from its posterior surface to the diaphragm is part of the gastrophrenic ligament (p. 1739), through which oesophageal branches of the left gastric vessels reach it. Posterior are the left crus and left inferior phrenic artery. The relations of the vagus nerves vary as the oesophagus traverses the diaphragm (Doubilet et al 1948). Usually the *left* vagus is composed of two or three trunks firmly applied to the anterior aspect of the oesophagus; the *right* vagus is usually single, a thick cord some distance from the posterior aspect of the oesophagus.

OESOPHAGEAL MICROSTRUCTURE (**12**.82, 84, 85)

The organization of tissues within the oesophageal wall follows the general pattern outlined above, namely (from lumen outwards), the mucosa consisting of epithelium, lamina propria, and muscularis mucosae; then the submucosa, muscularis externa, and adventitia, or, below the level of the diaphragm, serosa instead of adventitia.

Mucosa

The mucosa is thick and, in the living, pink above but pale below. At its lowermost end, at the gastro-oesophageal junction, there is an abrupt transition, the crenated boundary line separating the greyish-pink, smooth, oesophageal mucosa from the red, mamillated, gastric mucosa. Throughout its length, the oesophageal lumen is marked by deep longitudinal grooves and ridges which disappear when the lumen is distended but obliterate the lumen at all other times.

Epithelium. Non-keratinized stratified squamous in type, it is continuous with that of the pharynx. In humans this protective layer is quite thick (300–500 μm: see **12**.84, a property not affected by oesophageal distension. At the gastro-oesophageal junction the stratified squamous epithelium is abruptly succeeded by simple columnar epithelium with gastric pits and glands (p. 1758). The boundary between the general oesophageal epithelium and the lamina propria undulates and tall connective tissue papillae invaginate the epithelial base (**12**.85, 86) assisting in the anchorage of the epithelium to the underlying tissues. These papillae are permanent structures, unaffected by oesophageal distension; they are rich in blood vessels and nerve fibres. At the base of the epithelium is a basal lamina, to which epithelial cells are attached by hemidesomes, as in the oral mucosa. Similar to other stratified replacing epithelial, the oesophageal epithelium can be divided into:

- a basal, proliferative layer
- a parabasal layer of cells undergoing terminal differentiation
- a flattened layer of superficial cells or squames (sometimes termed the stratum corneum although its cells are nucleated).

The deepest cells are attached basally to the underlying basal lamina, and the parabasal cells to each other by numerous desmosomes. Between these cells the narrow spaces are filled with proteoglycans which are stainable with alcian blue or demonstrable by electron microscopy after tannic acid fixation (Hopwood et al 1994). Cytokeratins similar to those of the oral mucosa are present in the epithelium, their precise immunochemical identity changing as the cells migrate apically. The most superficial strata of cells also contain a few keratohyalin granules in addition to cytokeratin filaments and nuclei. For further ultrastructural details see Hopwood et al 1978.

The epithelial cell population is constantly renewed by mitosis of the cuboidal basal cells and the deepest of the parabasal cells. As they migrate towards the lumen they become progressively polygonal then more flattened, eventually being desquamated at the epithelial surface. This sequence of events normally takes 2–3 weeks, and is markedly slower than in the stomach and intestine (MacDonald et al 1964; Bell et al 1967); however, it is greatly affected by the mechanical conditions at the luminal surface. In rodents, where the oesophageal epithelium is keratinized, the renewal rate of these epithelial cells is faster than in man, and the cells migrate through the thickness of the epithelium in about 1 week (Marques-Pereira & Leblond 1965).

Barrier functions. Although it appears to lack tight junctions between its cells, the oesophageal epithelium is a considerable permeability barrier. Tracers such as horseradish peroxidase (HRP) placed in the lumen fail to penetrate its surface, while if introduced into the lamina propria, the tracer diffuses superficially to about two-thirds the thickness of the epithelium but is then stopped

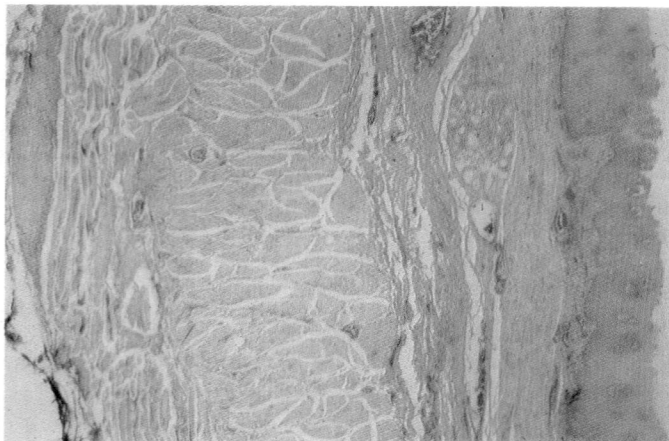

12.84 A low-power micrograph of a vertical section through the wall of a human oesophagus taken in the upper thorax. Visible in this section are: the epithelium (blue-grey on the right), the lamina propria, muscularis mucosae, submucosa with a group of mucous glands, the external muscle with the circular fibres more deeply placed and the longitudinal fibres placed externally. See text for further description. Mallory's triple stain. Magnification × 6. (Prepared by W Owen, Department of Anatomy, Guy's Hospital Medical School, London.)

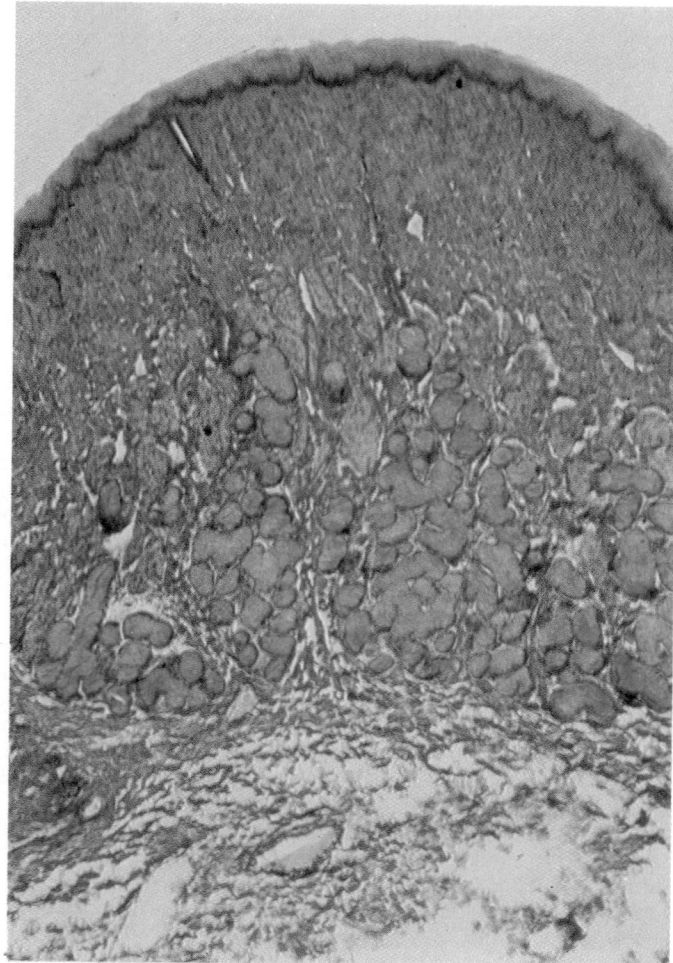

12.85 Low magnification light micrograph of a section of the oesophagus showing the stratified squamous non-keratinized epithelium lining it and mucous glands (stained turquoise) of the submucosa. Weigert and Van Gieson, with alcian blue. (Prepared by David Ristow; photographed by Marina Morris, Department of Anatomy, Guy's Hospital Medical School, London.)

(Orlando et al 1982). The nature of this barrier is not certain, but it is likely that the proteoglycans between the cells play an important part. Because of its thickness and the presence of mucus at its surface, the epithelium is also a good protection against mechanical injury. However, it is only a limited protection if exposed repeatedly to the very acid, protease-rich secretions of the stomach, as occurs abnormally during reflux. Normally the lower oesophageal sphincter prevents such an occurrence (see below), but if it does occur, ulceration and fibrosis of the oesophageal wall accompanied by considerable pain and difficulties in swallowing may ensue. Exposure to acid may also cause an epithelial redifferentiation to a gastric-like mucosa (Barrett's mucosa), or to more overt neoplastic changes (Hamilton 1990).

Langerhans cells. Besides replacing epithelial cells, *Langerhans cells* also occur in the oesophageal epithelium (Al Yassin & Toner 1976; Geboes et al 1983). These dendritic cells resemble those of the epidermis, and are thought to carry out similar antigen-presenting activities which are important in the immune defence of the mucosa and surrounding tissues (see p. 1415).

Lamina propria. This has already been referred to. In addition to its supportive functions, it contains scattered groups of lymphoid follicles which are especially prominent near the gastro-oesophageal junction. Small tubular mucous glands also occur in this region and in the upper part of the oesophagus close to the pharynx.

Muscularis mucosae. Composed of bundles of mainly longitudinal smooth muscle, this forms a sheet near the epithelium whose undulations it closely follows. At the pharyngeal end of the oesophagus it may be absent or represented merely by sparse, scattered bundles; below this it becomes progressively thicker. The longitudinal orientation of its cells changes to a more plexiform arrangement near the gastro-oesophageal junction.

Submucosa

The submucosa loosely connects the mucosa and the muscularis externa, and invades the longitudinal ridges of the oesophageal mucosa. It contains larger blood vessels, nerves and mucous glands. Its elastic fibres are also important in the reclosure of the oesophageal lumen after peristaltic dilatation.

Oesophageal glands. These are small compound tubulo-acinar glands lying in the submucosa, each group sending a single long duct through the intervening layers of the gut wall to the surface. They contain mainly mucous cells, although serous cells have also been described (Hopwood et al 1986). In the region close to the pharynx and at the lower end close to the stomach, the glands are simpler in form and restricted to the lamina propria: those of the abdominal oesophagus closely resemble the gastric cardiac glands (Johns 1952) and are termed *oesophageal cardiac glands*.

Muscularis externa

The muscularis externa is up to 300 μm thick; it has the usual outer longitudinal and inner circular layers. The longitudinal fibres form a continuous coat around almost the whole length of the oesophagus; but posterosuperiorly, 3–4 cm below the cricoid cartilage, they diverge as two fascicles ascending obliquely to the front of the tube. Here they pass deep to the lower border of the inferior constrictor, and finally they end in a tendon attached to the upper part of the ridge on the back of the cricoid lamina (12.3). The V-shaped interval between these fascicles is filled by circular fibres of the oesophagus, thinly covered below by some decussating longitudinal fibres and above by the overlapping inferior constrictor. The longitudinal layer is generally thicker than the circular. Accessory slips of smooth muscle sometimes pass between the oesophagus and left pleura or the root of the left principal bronchus, trachea, pericardium or aorta. These are sometimes considered to fix the oesophagus to these structures.

Superiorly the circular fibres are continuous behind with the inferior pharyngeal constrictor; in front, the uppermost are attached to the lateral margins of the tendon of the two longitudinal fasciculi of the oesophagus. Inferiorly, the circular muscle is continuous in the stomach wall with the oblique layer of its muscle fibres. As an approximation, skeletal muscle is limited to the upper two-thirds of the muscularis externa in the human oesophagus; the lower third contains only smooth muscle. In the upper quarter both layers are skeletal; in the second quarter smooth muscle appears, at first

internally and below this it gradually replaces the skeletal muscle. Whitmore (1982), using primate (including human) material, has identified 'fast' and 'slow' twitch fibres in oesophageal skeletal muscle; he also observed that the striated musculature gave way to smooth muscle more gradually and proximally in primates than in rodents.

Lower oesophageal sphincter

Radiological studies show that swallowed food stops momentarily in the gastric end of the oesophagus, before entering the stomach (**12.**86) suggesting the presence of a sphincter at this point. In the past there was much controversy about the reason for this behaviour (see e.g. DiDio & Anderson 1968; Code 1968), since only slight thickening of the muscle coat has been found in humans (although sphincteric muscle with a rich innervation has been described in macaque monkeys: Vaithilingham et al 1984). There is now ample physiological and clinical evidence that closure depends on two major mechanisms operating at the lower end of the oesophagus. The most important of these is the *lower oesophageal sphincter*, a specialized zone of circular smooth muscle surrounding the oesophagus at its transit through the diaphragm and for much of its short abdominal course. This region of the oesophagus is maintained under tonic contraction, except during swallowing when it relaxes briefly to admit ingesta to the stomach (Fyke et al 1956; Zaninotto et al 1988), and during vomiting. It is controlled by the intramural plexuses of the enteric nervous system, the neural release of nitric oxide contributing to its relaxation. The second mechanism is a functional *external sphincter* provided by the crural diaphragm, usually the right crus (p. 816) which encircles the oesophagus as it passes into the abdomen and is attached to it by the phreno-oesophageal ligament (Bombeck et al 1966). Radiological, electromyographic and manometric analyses have shown that its muscular fibres contract around the oesophagus during inspiration and when intra-abdominal pressure is raised, thus helping to prevent gastro-oesophageal reflux, even when the lower oesophageal sphincter is inhibited experimentally with atropine (see the review by Ferrarini et al 1993). The relative importance of these two agents in the prevention of oesophageal reflux is still being debated; clinically, there is a good correlation of this condition with lower oesophageal sphincter dysfunction in some cases, whilst in others failure of the diaphragmatic component, as seen in hiatus hernia, appears to be a major factor. The anatomical configuration of the gastro-oesophageal orifice may also play some part in these processes (see below). For recent reviews of this topic, see Ferrarini et al (1993) and Kahrilas (1993).

STOMACH (12.71, 88–95)

The stomach (ventriculus or preferably *gaster*) is the most dilated part of the alimentary canal and is situated between the oesophagus and the small intestine; it lies in the epigastric, umbilical and left hypochondriac areas of the abdomen, occupying a recess bounded by the upper abdominal viscera and completed above and anterolaterally by the anterior abdominal wall and diaphragm. Its shape and position are modified by changes within itself and by the surrounding viscera. Its mean capacity varies from about 30 ml at birth, increasing to 1000 ml at puberty and about 1500 ml in adults. It has two openings and is described as if it had two borders or curvatures and two surfaces. In reality its external surface is a continuum and not divided by perceptible 'borders'. However, since its peritoneal surface is interrupted by the attachments of the greater and lesser omenta along profiles which define the gastric radiographic shadow, these curvatures may be conveniently regarded as 'borders' separating the surfaces.

GASTRIC ORIFICES

The opening from the oesophagus into the stomach is the *cardiac orifice* situated to the left of the midline behind the seventh costal cartilage, 2.5 cm (1 in) from its sternal junction at the level of the eleventh thoracic vertebra. It is about 10 cm (4 in) from the anterior abdominal wall and 40 cm (16 in) from the incisor teeth. The short abdominal part of the oesophagus, shaped like a truncated cone, curves sharply left as it descends, the base of the cone being

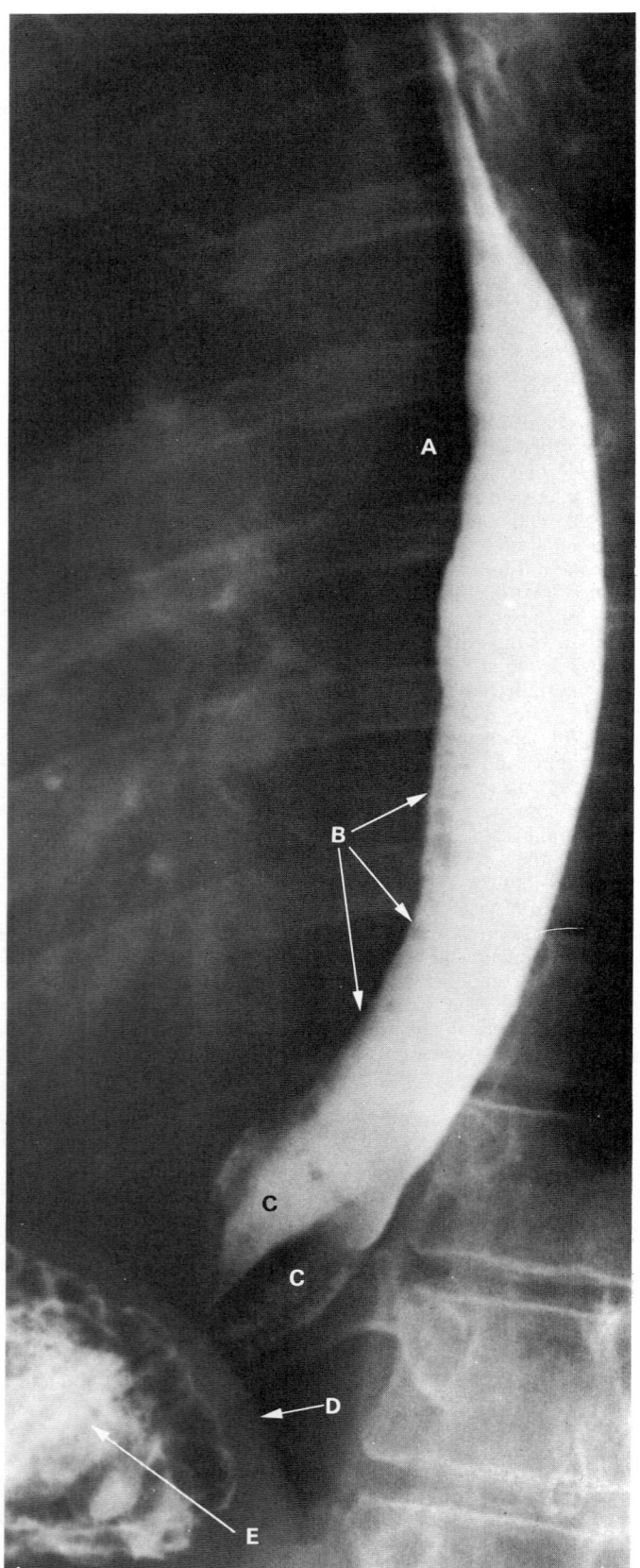

12.86 An oblique radiograph of the thorax during the oesophageal transit of part of a 'meal' of barium sulphate paste. At [A] the translucency of the air-containing right principal bronchus is visible. The concave ventral aspect of the oesophagus [B] is topographically related to the pericardium covering the left atrium of the heart. Longitudinal mucosal folds are visible [C] immediately proximal to the soft tissue shadow of the diaphragm [D]. Some barium sulphate is already admixed with the gastric contents [E]. The oesophagus in the lower thorax curves ventrally away from the vertebral column to reach the oesophageal orifice in the diaphragm.

continuous with the cardiac orifice. The right side of the oesophagus is continued as the *lesser curvature*, while its left side joins the *greater curvature* at an acute angle, the *cardiac notch* or *incisure*. The *cardia* is the region immediately adjacent to the cardiac orifice. The part of the stomach above the level of the cardiac orifice is the *fundus*, an inappropriate term, but it is the **bottom** of the stomach, when entered surgically from below.

The *pyloric orifice*, the opening into the duodenum, is usually indicated (**12**.87, 88, 90, 91) by a circular *pyloric constriction* on the surface of the organ, indicating the pyloric sphincter; it can be identified by the prepyloric vein crossing its anterior surface vertically. The pyloric orifice is about 1.2 cm (0.5 in) to the right of the midline in the transpyloric plane (level of the lower border of the first lumbar vertebra), with the body supine and the stomach empty.

GASTRIC CURVATURES (**12**.87, 88)

Lesser curvature. Extending between the cardiac and pyloric orifices, this is the right (posterosuperior) border of the stomach. It descends from the right side of the oesophagus in front of the decussating fibres of the right crus, curving to the right below the omental tuberosity of the pancreas to end at the pylorus. In the most dependent part there is typically a notch, or *incisura angularis (angular incisure)*, its position varying with gastric distension; it is sometimes used to define the right and left parts of the stomach. The lesser omentum is attached to the lesser curvature and contains the right and left gastric vessels adjacent to the line of the curvature.

Greater curvature. This is directed antero-inferiorly and is four or five times as long as the lesser; it starts from the cardiac incisure and arches upwards posterolaterally and to the left; its highest convexity, the fundus, is level with the left fifth intercostal space just below the left nipple in males, though varying with respiration (pp. 818–819). From this level it sweeps down and forwards, slightly convex to the left, almost as far as the tenth costal cartilage in the supine body; it finally turns right to end at the pylorus. Opposite the angular incisure of the lesser curvature, the greater curvature presents a bulge, taken as the left limit of the *pyloric part* of the stomach, its right limit being a slight groove (*sulcus intermedius*) indicating subdivision into the *pyloric antrum* and *canal*, the latter only 2–3 cm in length and terminating at the pyloric constriction. The start of the greater curvature is covered by peritoneum continuous with that anterior to the stomach. Left of the fundus and the adjoining body of the stomach the greater curvature gives attachment to the gastrosplenic ligament and beyond this to the greater omentum, the two layers of which are separated by the gastro-epiploic vessels. The gastrosplenic ligament and the greater omentum (with the gastrophrenic and lienorenal ligaments, see p. 1738, **12**.77A) are continuous parts of the original dorsal mesogastrium (p. 183). The names merely indicate regions of the same fold.

GASTRIC SURFACES

When the stomach is empty and contracted, its surfaces are almost superior and inferior; but in distension they become anterior and posterior respectively, and are therefore described here as anterosuperior and postero-inferior surfaces.

Anterosuperior surface. The left part of this surface is posterior to the left costal margin and in contact with the diaphragm which separates it from the left pleura, the base of the left lung, the pericardium and the left sixth to ninth ribs and intercostal spaces. It is related to the costal attachments of the upper fibres of the transversus abdominis, which separate it from the seventh to ninth costal cartilages. The upper and left part of this surface becomes posterolateral and is in contact with the spleen's gastric surface. The right half of the anterosuperior surface is related to the left and quadrate lobes of the liver and the anterior abdominal wall. When the stomach is empty, the transverse colon may lie on its anterior surface. The whole surface is covered by peritoneum and part of the greater sac separates it from the above structures.

Postero-inferior surface. This is related to the diaphragm, the left suprarenal gland, upper part of the front of the left kidney, the splenic artery, anterior pancreatic surface, left colic flexure and the transverse mesocolon (upper layer), which together form the shallow

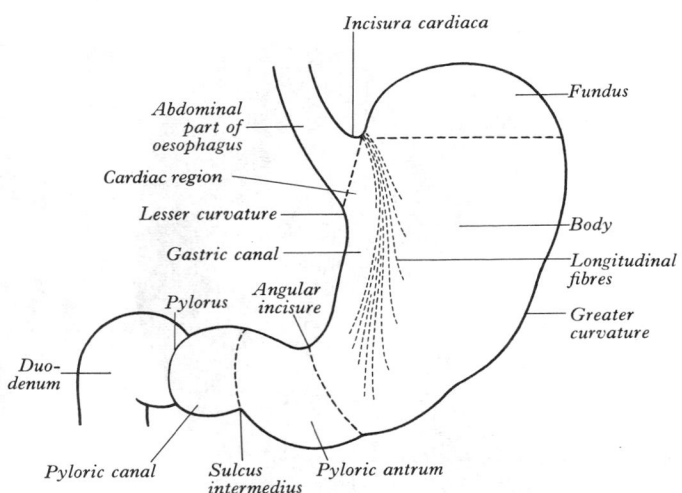

12.87   The parts of the stomach.

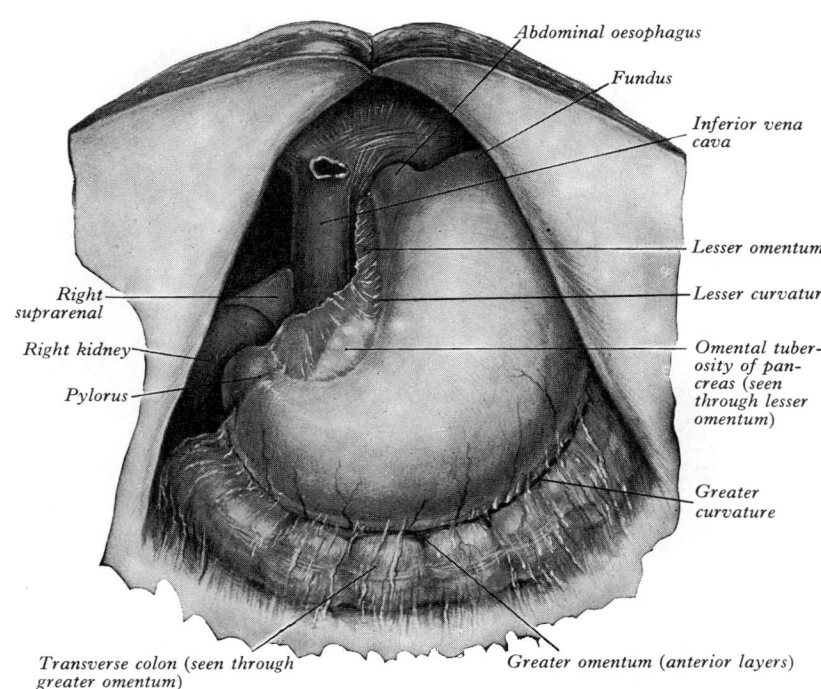

12.88   The stomach in situ, after removal of the liver.

stomach bed (**12.89**), over which the stomach slides, due to the intervening lesser sac. The spleen's gastric surface is usually included in the stomach bed, though separated from the stomach by part of the greater sac. The greater omentum and the transverse mesocolon separate the stomach from the duodenojejunal flexure and small intestine. The postero-inferior surface is covered by peritoneum, except near the cardiac orifice, where a small, triangular area contacts the left diaphragmatic crus and sometimes the left suprarenal gland. The left gastric vessels reach the lesser curvature at the right extremity of this area in the left gastropancreatic fold (p. 1740); from its left side the *gastrophrenic ligament*, continuous below with the splenicorenal and gastrosplenic ligaments, passes to the diaphragm's inferior surface.

A plane passing through the angular incisure of the lesser curvature and the left limit of the opposed bulge on the greater curvature arbitrarily divides the stomach into a large *body* (left) and a smaller *pyloric part* (right).

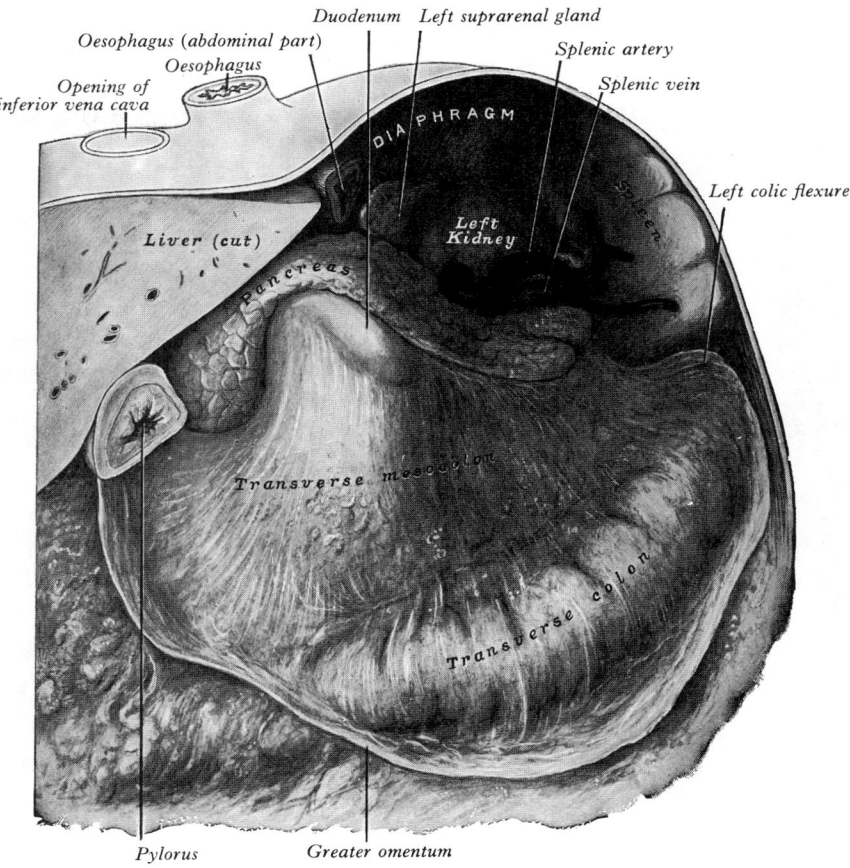

12.89   The stomach bed: a dissection in which the stomach has been removed to show its posterior relations.

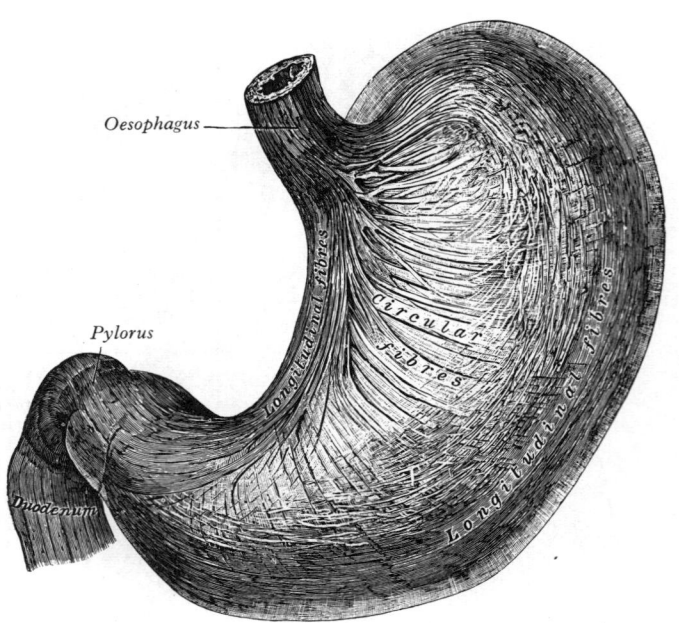

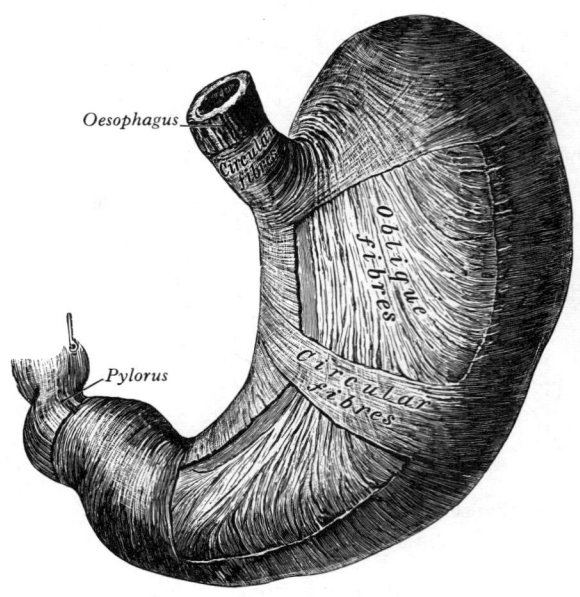

12.90A The longitudinal and circular gastric muscular fibres: antero-superior aspect (Spalteholz).

12.90B The oblique muscular fibres of the stomach, shown by partial dissection of its wall: anterosuperior aspect (Spalteholz).

RADIOLOGY

The form and position of the stomach can be studied after swallowing a suitable 'meal' containing barium sulphate (**12**.91, 92). During digestion it is divided by a muscular constriction in its body into a large, dilated, left region and a narrow, contracted, tubular right one. The constriction in the body follows no anatomical landmarks but moves gradually left as digestion progresses. The position of the stomach varies with posture, contents and the state of the intestines, on which it rests; it is also influenced by the tone of the abdominal wall and gastric musculature and by the individual's build. Most commonly the empty organ is J-shaped and, in the erect posture, the pylorus descends to the level of the second or the third lumbar vertebra, its most dependent part being subumbilical. The fundus usually contains gas. Variation in content mainly affects the body, the pyloric part remaining contracted during digestion. As the stomach fills it expands forwards and downwards but, when the colon or intestines are distended, the fundus presses on the liver and diaphragm and may evoke discomfort. When hardened in situ the contracted stomach is crescentic, the fundus directed backwards.

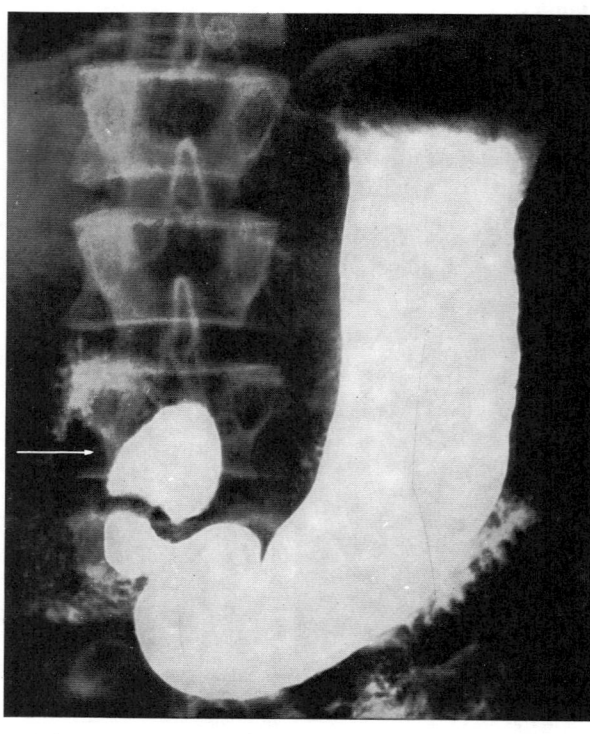

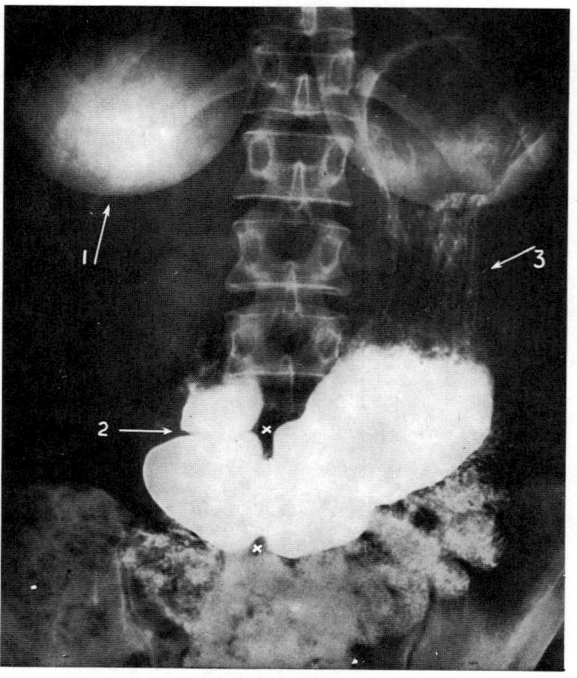

12.91 Radiograph of a normal stomach after a barium meal. The tone of the muscular wall is good and supports the weight of the column in the body of the organ. The arrow points to the duodenal cap, below which a gap in the barium indicates the position of the pylorus.

12.92 Radiograph of an atonic stomach after a barium meal. Note that this stomach contains the same amount of barium suspension as the stomach in **12**.91. Arrow 1 points to the shadow of the right breast, arrow 2 to the pylorus, arrow 3 to the upper part of the body of the stomach, where longitudinal folds can be seen in the mucous membrane. XX marks a wave of peristalsis.

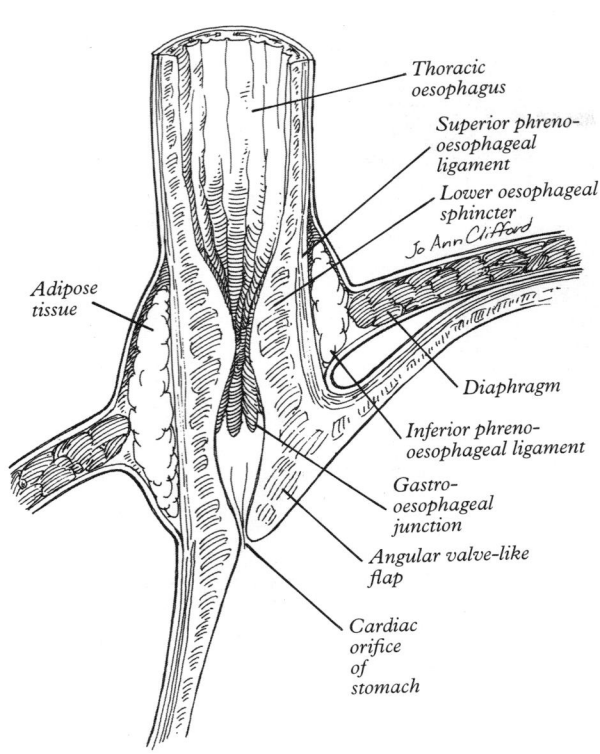

12.93A Diagram showing the valve-like structure formed by the cardiac angle wall at the cardiac orifice. (Provided by Donald E Low, Department of Surgery, Virginia Mason, Seattle, USA.)

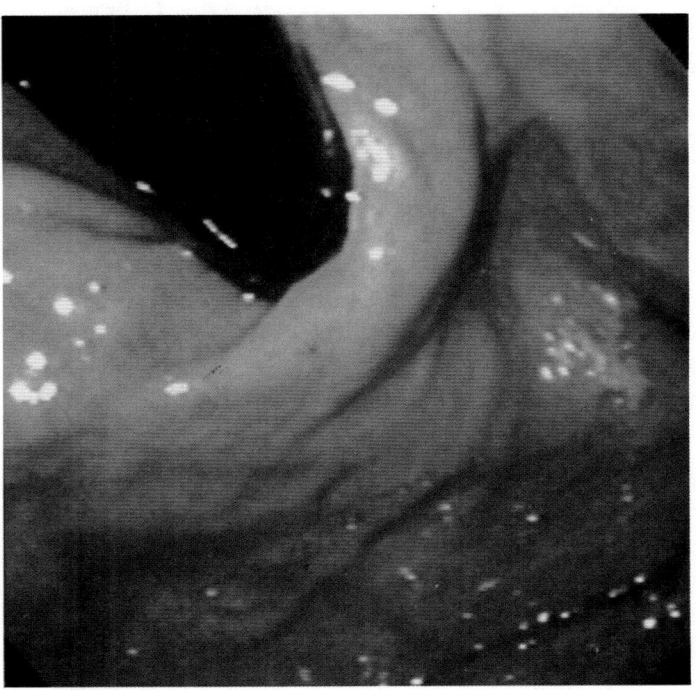

12.93B Endoscopic view of the cardiac orifice from below, showing the valve-like fold illustrated in **12.93A**. The black rod inserted in the orifice is the stem of the endoscope. (Provided by Donald E Low, Department of Surgery, Virginia Mason, Seattle, USA.)

Surfaces are superior and inferior, the former sloping gradually to the right, the greater curvature being anterior to and at a slightly higher level than the lesser.

The position of the full stomach varies. When the intestines are empty the fundus expands vertically and forwards, the pylorus is displaced right and the whole organ becomes oblique. Its surfaces are then directed more forwards and backwards, the lowest part being the pyloric antrum which extends below the umbilicus. When intestinal distention interferes with downward expansion of the fundus, the stomach retains the horizontal position characteristic of the contracted viscus. Less commonly it may lie almost transversely, even in the erect posture, as the '*steer-horn*' type. Intermediate types of stomach, between J-shaped and 'steer-horn', also occur (Barclay 1936).

INTERIOR OF THE STOMACH

After death the stomach is usually fixed at some stage of the digestive process, commonly as shown in **12.94**). When it is laid open after section along the plane of its curvatures, it shows two segments:

- a large globular left part
- a narrow tubular right part

The transition is gradual, so their division is arbitrary. The cardiac incisure lies to the left of the abdominal part of the oesophagus and its projection into the cavity increases as the organ distends, supposedly acting as a valve preventing oesophageal regurgitation. The elevation opposite the angular incisure is at the beginning, and the circular thickening of the pyloric sphincter at the end, of the pyloric region.

Modelling of human fetal gastric epithelium (Lewis 1912) has shown that a *gastric canal* extends along the lesser curvature from the cardiac orifice to the angular incisure (**12.87**). Jefferson (1915) demonstrated such a canal radiologically in adults, and examination during the act of swallowing radio-opaque fluid showed that it was first confined to the region adjacent to the lesser curvature, suggesting that contraction of oblique muscle fibres causes temporary separation of a canal along the lesser curvature.

Pyloric sphincter. This is a muscular ring formed by a marked thickening of the circular gastric muscle, some longitudinal fibres also interlacing with it (DiDio & Anderson 1968.)

Cardiac sphincter. This sphincter is sometimes described as being formed from the circular fibres of the gastric wall. However, closure of the gastro-oesophageal junction appears to be performed by the tonic contraction of the lower oesophagus (see p. 1753).

Gastro-oesophageal junction. The transition between the oesophagus and stomach is difficult to define, as the gastric mucosa extends some distance up the tube of the abdominal oeso-phagus, forming a zig-zag squamo-columnar epithelial junction. The external muscle layers of the two organs also blend, except that a sling of longitudinal gastric muscle forms a loop on the superior, left side of .the junction between the oesophagus and the lesser curvature, and this is often taken as the boundary for practical purposes.

The acute angle between the oesophagus and the upper part of the cardia (the angle of His or cardiac incisure) is extended within the lumen as a large fold. Because it is suitably positioned to act as a valvular flap (**12.93A, B**) which with raised intragastric pressure is likely to close the oesophageal entrance, it has been proposed as a mechanism additional to the lower oesophageal sphincter (p. 1753), limiting oesophageal reflux of gastric fluids by occluding the entrance to the oesophagus when intragastric pressure is raised. The acute oesophagogastric angle and thus the valve disappear in hiatus hernia and, when patients have symptoms and complications of gastro-oesophageal reflux which cannot be controlled with medicines, they will often undergo surgery to re-establish an antireflux barrier. The various operations which are currently utilized in these patients accomplish this goal by reducing any hiatal hernia which is present back into the abdominal cavity and rebuilding a functional flap valve mechanism.

GASTRIC MICROSTRUCTURE (12.94, 95)

The gastric wall consists of the major layers found elsewhere in the gut, i.e. mucosa, submucosa, muscularis externa and serosa, together

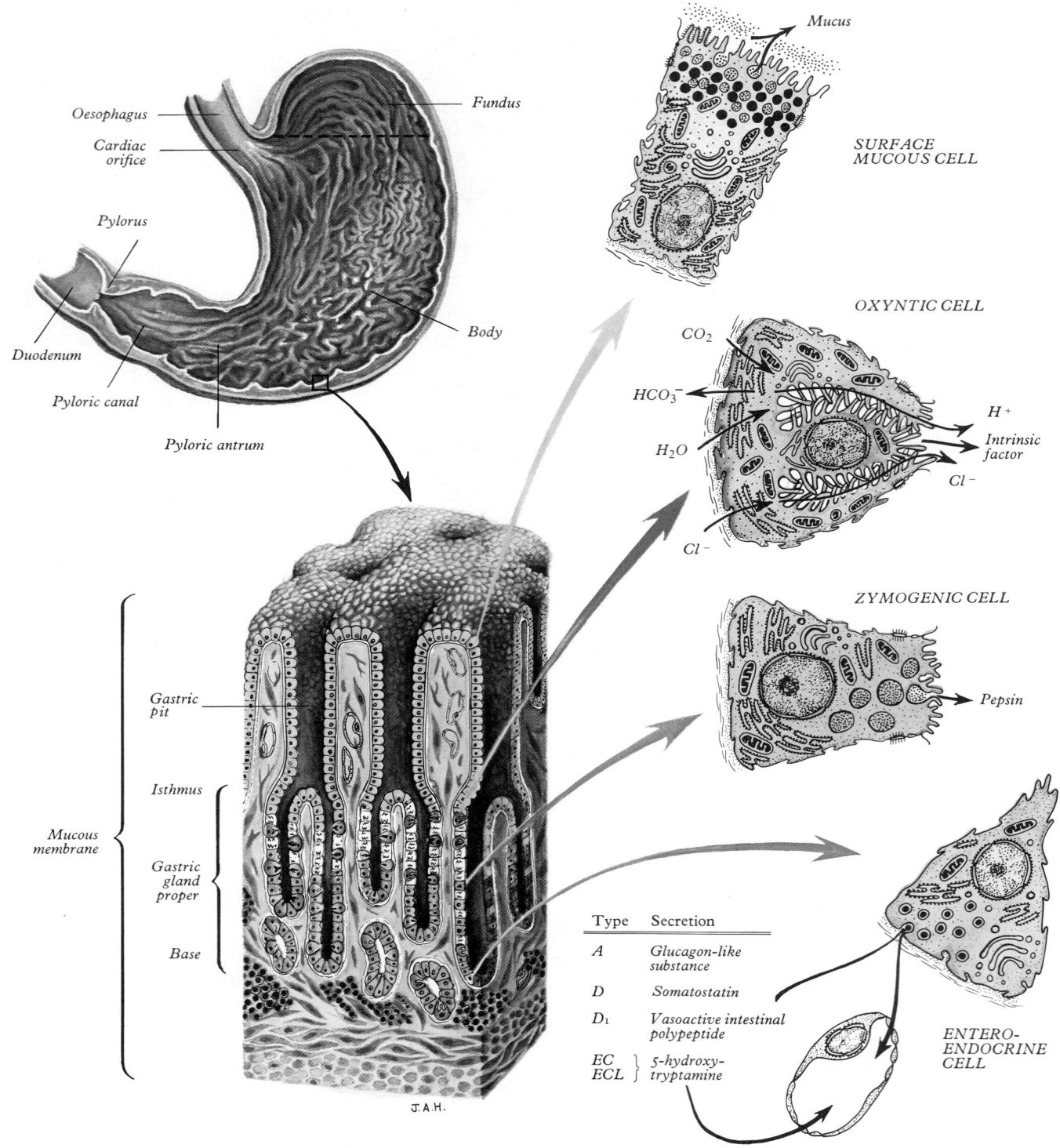

12.94 Diagram showing the principal regions of the interior of the stomach and the histology and ultrastructure of its mucous membrane.

Undifferentiated, dividing cells are shown in white.

with gastric vessels and nerves. The microstructure of these reflects the functions of the stomach as an expandable, muscular sac lined by secretory epithelium, although there are local structural and functional variations in this pattern.

Mucosa

The mucosa is a thick layer, its surface smooth, soft, velvety and, over most of its surface, reddish brown in life; it is pink in the pyloric region. In the contracted stomach the mucosa is folded into numerous folds or *rugae*, most of which are longitudinal; they are most marked towards the pyloric end and along the greater curvature

(**12.93**). The rugae represent large folds in the submucosal connective tissue (see below) rather than variations in the thickness of the mucosa covering them, and they are obliterated when the wall is stretched in gastric distension. As elsewhere in the gut, the mucosa is composed of a surface epithelium, lamina propria and muscularis mucosae.

Epithelium. When viewed microscopically at low magnification, the internal surface of the stomach wall (**12.95**A, B, D) appears honeycombed by small somewhat irregular *gastric pits* (foveolae), polygonal or slit-like funnel-shaped depressions about 0.2 mm in diameter. The base of each gastric pit receives several long tubular

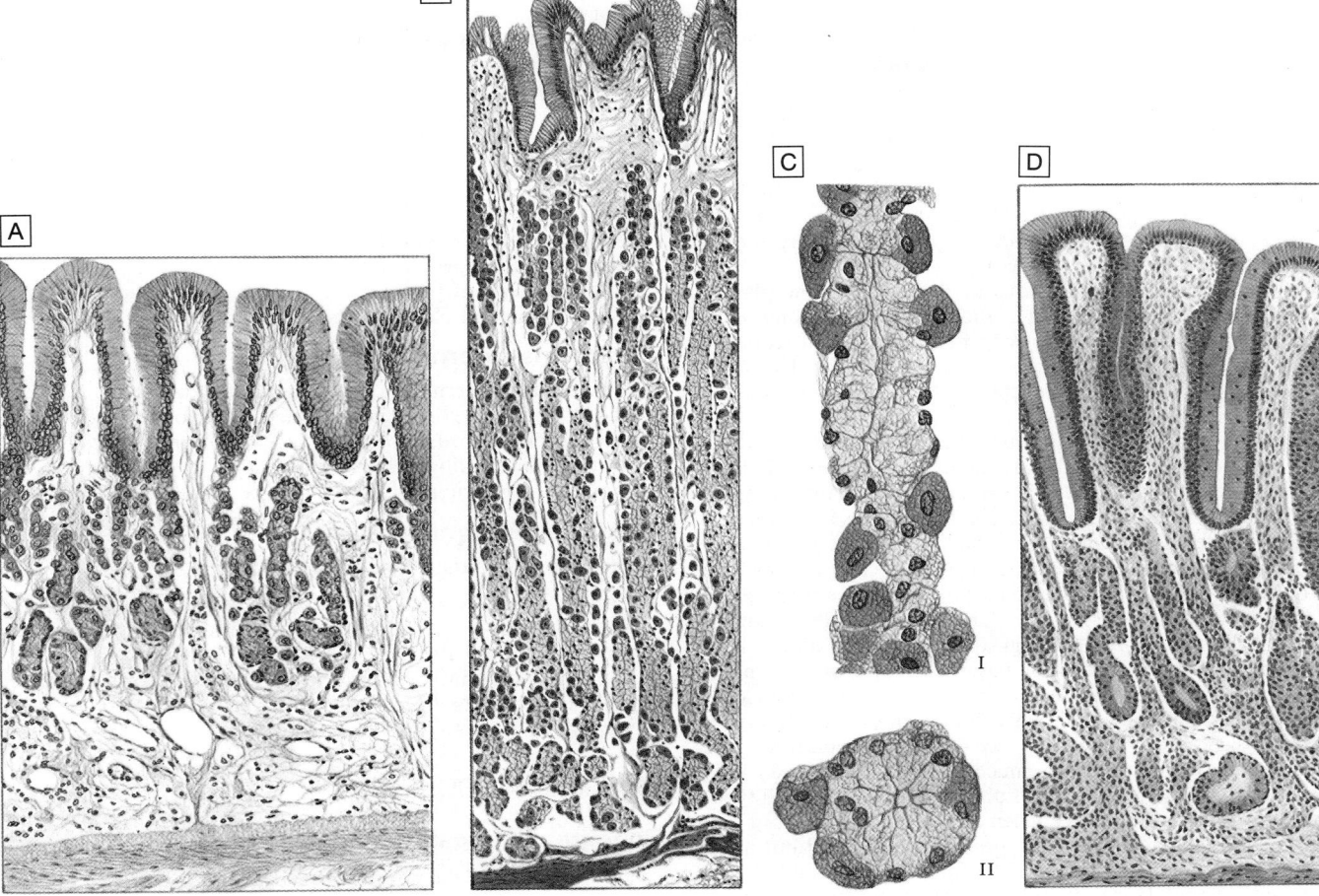

12.95[A]   Vertical section through the mucous membrane of the cardiac part of the stomach (human). Stained with haematoxylin and eosin. Magnification c. × 150.

12.95[B]   Vertical section through the mucous membrane of the fundus of the stomach (cat). Note the beaded appearance given by the oxyntic cells. Stained with haematoxylin and eosin. Magnification c. × 100.

12.95[C]   (I) Gland from the fundus of the stomach (cat). (II) Lower part

of the gland cut transversely. Stained with haematoxylin and eosin. The peripherally placed cells staining deeply with eosin are the oxyntic cells. Magnification c. × 530.

12.95[D]   Vertical section through the mucous membrane of the pyloric part of the stomach (cat). Stained with haematoxylin and eosin. Magnification c. × 75.

gastric glands which extend deep into the lamina propria as far as the muscularis mucosae. Simple columnar mucus-secreting epithelium covers the entire luminal surface including the gastric pits, composed of a continuous layer of *surface mucous cells* which liberate gastric mucus from their apices to form a thick protective, lubricant layer over the gastric wall (see below). This epithelium commences abruptly at the cardiac orifice, where there is a sudden transition from the oesophageal stratified epithelium.

Gastric glands. Although all are tubular, they vary in form and cellular composition in different parts of the stomach. They can be divided into the following categories (see Ito & Winchester 1963):

- cardiac
- principal (in the body and fundus)
- pyloric glands.

All are tubular, sometimes branched structures. The most highly differentiated are the principal glands, and these will be described first.

Principal gastric glands. These are found in the body and fundus, three to seven opening into each gastric pit; (**12.94**, 95A, B). Their confluence with the base of the pit is termed the *isthmus* of the gland and immediately basal to this is the *neck*, the remainder being the *base*. In the walls of the gland are at least five distinct cell types: chief, parietal, mucous neck, stem and enteroendocrine, as follows:

- The *chief (peptic or zymogenic) cells* (**12.94**, 95) are the source of the digestive enzymes pepsin and renin. They are usually basal in

position, their shape being cuboidal and their nuclei rounded and open-faced. They contain secretory granules and because of the abundant cytoplasmic RNA they are strongly basophilic. Ultrastructurally they show typical features of active protein secretors, namely a copious granular endoplasmic reticulum, well-developed Golgi apparatus, large dense rounded secretory vesicles (containing pepsinogen), and interspersed lysosomes. At their lumen they bear short microvilli.

- The *parietal (oxyntic) cells* are the source of gastric acid and of intrinsic factor. They are large, oval and strongly eosinophilic, with centrally placed nuclei; they are mainly sited in the more apical half of the gland, reaching as far as the isthmus. They occur only at intervals along the walls, and bulge laterally into the encircling connective tissue, giving the glands a beaded appearance (**12.95**B, C). At the luminal surface of the gland they appear recessed between neighbouring cells. Parietal cells have a unique ultrastructure clearly related to their remarkable ability to secrete hydrochloric acid. The luminal side of the cell is deeply and tortuously invaginated to form a series of deep blind-ending channels (*canaliculi*) furnished with numerous irregular microvilli. Within the cytoplasm facing these channels are myriads of fine membranous tubules (the *tubulo-vesicular system*) directed towards the canalicular surface. Abundant mitochondria are interspersed among these organelles. The membranes lining the microvilli have a high concentration of H^+/K^+ATPase antiporter channels which actively secrete hydrogen ions into the lumen, chloride ions following along the electrogenic gradient. The precise structure of the cell varies with its secretory phase: when stimulated to secrete the numbers and surface areas of the microvilli increase up to five-fold, an event thought to be caused by the addition of membrane by rapid fusion of the tubulo-vesicular system with the plasma membrane, accompanied by polymerization of g-actin into actin filaments supporting the microvilli. At the end of stimulated secretion, this process is reversed, the excess membrane retreating back into the tubulo-alveolar system and the microvilli being erased. Parietal cells also contain a prominent Golgi body and a modicum of granular endoplasmic reticulum, which amongst other functions, must be responsible for the synthesis and secretion of *intrinsic factor*, a glycoprotein necessary for the absorption of vitamin B_{12} (Hoedemseker et al 1966).

- *Mucous ('neck') cells* are numerous at the necks of the glands, and also scattered along the walls of the more basal regions. They are typical mucus-secreting cells, with numerous apical secretory vesicles containing mucins, and basally displaced nuclei. However, their products are distinct histochemically from those of the superficial mucous cells.
- *Stem cells* are relatively undifferentiated mitotic cells from which the other types of gland cell already mentioned are derived. They are relatively few in number, and are situated in the isthmus region of the gland and bases of the gastric pits. These calls are columnar in form, with a few short apical microvilli; internally their organelles are typical of stem cells in general, with a central open-face nucleus, large nucleolus and scattered polyribosomes with sparse granular endoplasmic reticulum. They periodically undergo mitosis, the cells they produce migrating apically to differentiate into new surface mucous cells, or basally to form mucous neck, parietal and chief cells, and also possibly the enteroendocrine cells (see p. 1787). All of these cells have limited lifespans, especially the mucus-secreting types, and need constant replacing. The replacement period for surface mucous cells is about 3 days; mucous neck cells are replaced after about 1 week. Other cell types appear to live much longer (see Chen & Le Blond 1965).
- *Enteroendocrine cells* occur in all types of gastric gland but more frequently in the body and fundus. They are situated mainly in the deeper parts of the glands, among the zymogenic cells. They are columnar cells with irregular nuclei surrounded by granular cytoplasm which can be stained strongly with silver salts (hence the older term, *argentaffin cells*). Ultrastructurally their luminal surface bears short microvilli, whilst at their base, facing the lamina propria and intervening basal lamina, they have clusters of large (0.3 μm) secretory granules synthesized in the granular endoplasmic reticulum and infranuclear Golgi apparatus for release into the surrounding tissues. These cells secrete a number of biogenic amines and polypeptides important in the control of motility and glandular secretion. In the stomach they include cells designated as G-cells secreting gastrin, D cells (somatostatin), and EC cells (see p. 1787). They form part of the enteroendocrine system of the alimentary tract and related organs, described further on p. 1787.

Cardiac glands. These are confined to a small area near the cardiac orifice (**12.**95A); some are simple tubular glands, others are compound branched tubular. Mucus-secreting cells predominate and parietal and zymogenic cells are few, although present.

Pyloric glands. Pyloric glands enter as groups of two or three short convoluted tubes into the bases of the deep gastric pits of the pyloric antrum which occupy about two-thirds of the mucosal depth (**12.**94). Pyloric glands are mostly furnished with mucus-secreting cells, parietal cells being few and chief cells mainly absent. Enteroendocrine cells are numerous however, especially G-cells secreting gastrin when activated by appropriate mechanical stimulation, causing increased gastric motility and secretion of gastric juices (see also p. 1787). Although parietal cells are few in pyloric glands, they are always present in fetal and postnatal material; in adults they may also appear in the duodenal mucosa but only proximally, near the pylorus (Leela & Kanagasuntheram 1968).

Lamina propria. Found between the glands, this forms a connective tissue framework and contains lymphoid tissue which, especially in early life, collects in small masses, termed gastric lymphatic follicles, resembling solitary intestinal follicles. A complex periglandular vascular plexus is also present and is thought to be important in the maintenance of the mucosal environment, including

the removal of bicarbonate produced in the tissues as a counterpart to acid secretion. Neural plexuses are also present; these are both sensory and motor terminals (see p. 1307).

Muscularis mucosae. This is a thin stratum of smooth muscle fibres lying external to the layer of glands. Its fibres are arranged as inner circular and outer longitudinal layers, with a third external, circular layer in places. The inner layer sends strands of smooth muscle cells between the glands, contraction probably aiding their emptying.

Submucosae

The submucosa is a variable layer of loose connective tissue containing thick collagen bundles and numerous elastin fibres; blood vessels and nervous plexuses are also present including the ganglionated submucosal plexus of the stomach.

Muscularis externa

The muscularis externa is a coat immediately under the serosa, with which it is closely connected by subserous loose connective tissue. From within outwards it has *oblique, circular* and *longitudinal* layers of smooth muscle fibres. Further details of the macroscopic organization of the gastric muscle are given below.

Serosa or visceral peritoneum

The serosa covers the entire surface except:

- along the greater and lesser curvatures at the attachment of the greater and lesser omenta, where the peritoneal layers leave space for vessels and nerves
- a small postero-inferior area, near the cardiac orifice, where the stomach contacts the diaphragm at the reflexions of the gastrophrenic and left gastropancreatic folds.

GASTRIC MUSCLE

Topographic organization of layers

The three layers of the muscularis externa form distinct tracts which can be demonstrated by dissection (**12.**90, 91). Viewed from outside, the *oblique fibres* are deepest; they are limited in distribution to the gastric body and are most developed near the cardiac orifice. They sweep down from the cardiac incisure more or less parallel with the lesser curvature, near which they present a free and well-defined margin; on the left they blend with the circular fibres nearer the greater curvature. *Circular fibres* form a uniform layer over the whole stomach external to the oblique fibres. At the pylorus they are most abundant, aggregated into the annular pyloric sphincter; they are also continuous above with the circular fibres of the oesophagus but sharply separated from those of the duodenum by a septum of connective tissue. *Longitudinal fibres* are the most external; they are arranged in two groups. The first set is continuous with the longitudinal oesophageal fibres; radiating from the cardiac orifice, they are best developed near the curvatures and end proximal to the pyloric region. The fibres of the second group commence in the body and pass to the right, becoming thicker as they approach the pylorus; some superficial fibres pass to the duodenum, deeper ones turning inwards to interlace with the fibres of the pyloric sphincter.

Gastric muscle action

The gastric musculature can be divided functionally into:

- an upper region comprising the fundus, cardia and the superior part of the body of the stomach which form an area of storage;
- a lower region made up of the lower part of the gastric body and the pyloric antrum, which has a pump-like action mixing the stomach contents and delivering the semi-fluid chyme to the duodenum through the pyloric canal.

The muscle of the upper region exerts a maintained moderate tonic contraction on the stomach contents, whereas the lower muscle is much more motile, repeated peristaltic waves passing along this part of the stomach towards the pylorus when stimulated by the presence of food. The pyloric sphincter, which is open in the resting state, contracts as each peristaltic wave advances, narrowing it so that only finely divided material and fluids can pass through its aperture, larger material being forced back into the pyloric antrum for further digestion and diminution.

GASTRIC VESSELS

Arteries

The arterial supply comes from the left gastric artery (directly from the coeliac artery), right gastric and right gastro-epiploic (from the common hepatic) and the left gastro-epiploic and short gastric (from the splenic) artery. These vessels not only anastomose extensively on the serosal aspect of the stomach (p. 1548) but also form anastomotic networks within its walls at intramuscular, submucosal and mucosal levels; a true plexus of small arteries and arterioles is present in the submucosa. This *submucosal plexus*, from which the mucosa is supplied, shows considerable regional variation both in the gastric wall and also in the proximal duodenum.

In view of a possible vascular factor in the genesis of peptic ulcers, the local details of angioarchitecture are of interest. For a review of the older literature see the study by Piasecki (1974, 1977), who studied the arterial supply in fetal, neonatal and adult human stomachs, using India ink injections of fresh post mortem specimens (**12.96**A). From anastomotic arcades along the greater and lesser curvatures, formed by the main arteries of supply described above, many *anterior* and *posterior gastric arteries* pass to the anterior and posterior aspects of the stomach, approximately transverse to the organ's long axis. Smaller rami, often paired, also pass directly to parts of the gastric wall subjacent to the omental attachments.

All these vessels ramify on the external surface and penetrate the muscular layers to reach the submucosa and mucosa, forming subserosal, intramuscular and submucosal plexuses, the second of these being the best developed (**12.96**A, B). This muscular plexus is supplied by branches from the subserous and submucosal plexuses; the muscular vessels vary in their direction in different muscular laminae, perhaps adapting to directions of contraction. Submucosal arteries anastomose freely, but the incidence of anastomoses varies. Counts by Piasecki (1974) showed that while anastomoses along, e.g. the lesser curvature, increased in **number** from cardia to pylorus; the mean **calibre** of anastomosing arteries showed a reverse tendency. Mucosal arteries, which fill the capillary networks supplying the epithelium and its glands, are mainly from the submucosal plexus; but along both curvatures a few mucosal arteries come directly from subserosal sources, traversing the muscular layers and submucosa, often without lateral junctions with submucosal arteries; their frequency apparently increases from the cardiac to the pyloric regions; the capillary networks supplied by them are largely independent of those fed by adjacent submucosal arteries and the patch of mucosa supplied by such a vessel is perhaps more vulnerable to vascular obstruction.

Piasecki also showed a different pattern of supply in the pyloric canal and sphincter. 'Pyloric arteries', rami of the right gastric and gastro-epiploic arteries, pierce the duodenum distal to the sphincter around its entire circumference, passing through the muscular layer to the submucosa where each divides into two or three rami, which turn into the pyloric canal, internal to the sphincter; they traverse the submucosa to the end of the pyloric antrum (**12.96**B), supplying the whole mucosa of the pyloric canal. Branches of these pyloric submucosal arteries may anastomose at their commencement with the duodenal submucosal arteries and, by their terminal rami, with corresponding gastric arteries. The pyloric sphincter is supplied by the gastric and pyloric arteries, whose rami leave their parent vessels in the subserosal and submucosal levels to penetrate the sphincter. In a more recent study, Piasecki (1986) has described arrangements in a large number of animals, including rodents, swine, cats, dogs and monkeys, with little modification from the pattern he found earlier in primates.

Veins

These commence as straight vessels between the mucosal glands and drain into the submucosal veins. Their further arrangement has not received as much attention as that of the corresponding arteries; but the larger veins generally accompany main arteries to their ultimate drainage into the splenic and superior mesenteric veins, while some pass directly to the portal vein.

Lymphatic vessels

These smaller vessels are said to resemble the veins in distribution. Regional lymph nodes and their drainage are described on p. 1619.

Microvasculature of the gastric mucosa

Functionally the microvessels of the mucosa are thought to be important in protecting its cells against the extremely acid conditions of the gastric lumen (see Gannon et al 1984, Raschke et al 1987, Gannon 1990 for studies and reviews of this subject). The mucosa has a rich blood supply, its pattern varying in different regions of the stomach, although there is some difference of opinion as to its detailed organization. It is generally accepted that arterioles from the submucosal arterial plexus penetrate into the mucosa and branch to form rich capillary beds around the gastric glands, anastomizing laterally with each other, and conveying blood towards the mucosal surface where they drain into rather sparsely scattered venules leading back to the submucosal venous plexus. It has been proposed that the rich lumen-directed flow of blood enables bicarbonate generated basally by parietal cells as a counterpart of their secretion of acid, to be carried into the apical parts of the mucosa so as to protect its cells against acid damage. It is also interesting that the capillaries in this area are fenestrated, a feature likely to facilitate the delivery of bicarbonate to the surface regions of the mucosa. In the gastric antrum where there are few or no bicarbonate-secreting parietal cells, the capillary beds and their blood supply are even richer, and the apical and basal regions of the mucosa receive separate arteriolar supplies (Gannon et al 1984), perhaps to increase the perfusional removal of acid. For further review of the microvasculature, and of disagreements about its details, see Gannon (1990).

The extent of lateral anastomosis between arteriolar territories in the mucosa is a matter of some debate; Piasecki et al (1989) found that in guinea pigs, ligation of single mucosal arterioles led to full thickness ulceration, indicating that they are end-arterioles, although this condition has not yet been confirmed in humans. These considerations are of course relevant to the formation and growth of gastric ulcers. The dynamic behaviour of the microvasculature is regulated by various neural and paracrine factors which increase mucosal perfusion with the intake of food into the stomach, due to vagal stimulation and the release of different local regulatory factors such as prostanoids, nitric oxide, sensory neuropeptides (e.g. CGRP, SP; see Whittle & Tepperman 1990). Inhibition of endogenous vasodilators, especially the prostanoids e.g. by aspirin, may lead to local ischaemia, ulceration and haemorrhage (Whittle 1986).

GASTRIC NERVES

Innervation arises from several sources (Kyösola et al 1980). The *sympathetic supply* is mainly from the coeliac plexus through its extensions around the gastric and gastro-epiploic arteries. Some rami from the hepatic plexus reach the lesser curvature between the layers of the hepatogastric ligament (p. 1741). Branches from the left phrenic plexus pass to the cardiac end of the stomach, as does one from the left phrenic branch to the right crus of the diaphragm. Inconstant gastric branches come from the left thoracic splanchnic nerves and the thoracic and lumbar sympathetic trunks.

The *parasympathetic supply* is from the vagus nerves (Mackay & Andrews 1983) (p. 1253). Usually one or two rami branch on the anterior and posterior aspects of the gastro-oesophageal junction; the anterior nerves are mostly from the left vagus and the posterior from the right vagus, emerging from the oesophageal plexus. The anterior nerves supply filaments to the cardiac orifice and divide near the oesophageal end of the lesser curvature into branches:

- The *gastric branches* (4–10) radiate on the anterior surface of the body and fundus; one, larger than the others, lies in the lesser omentum near the lesser curvature (*greater anterior gastric nerve*).
- The *pyloric branches*, generally two, one of which traverses the lesser omentum almost horizontally to the right, towards its free edge, then turns down on the left side of the hepatic artery to reach the pylorus, while the other, usually arising from the greater anterior gastric nerve, passes obliquely to the pyloric antrum.

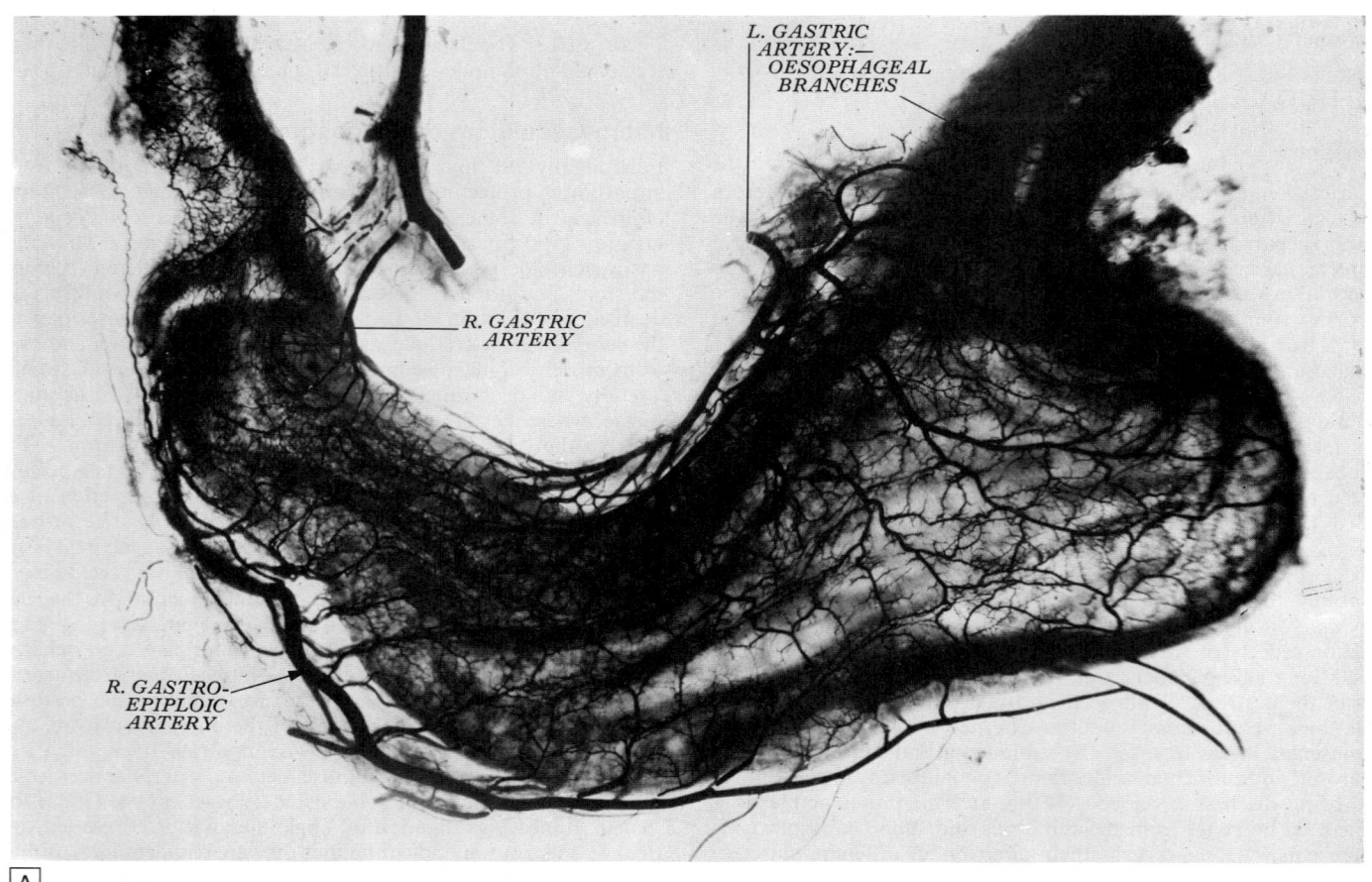

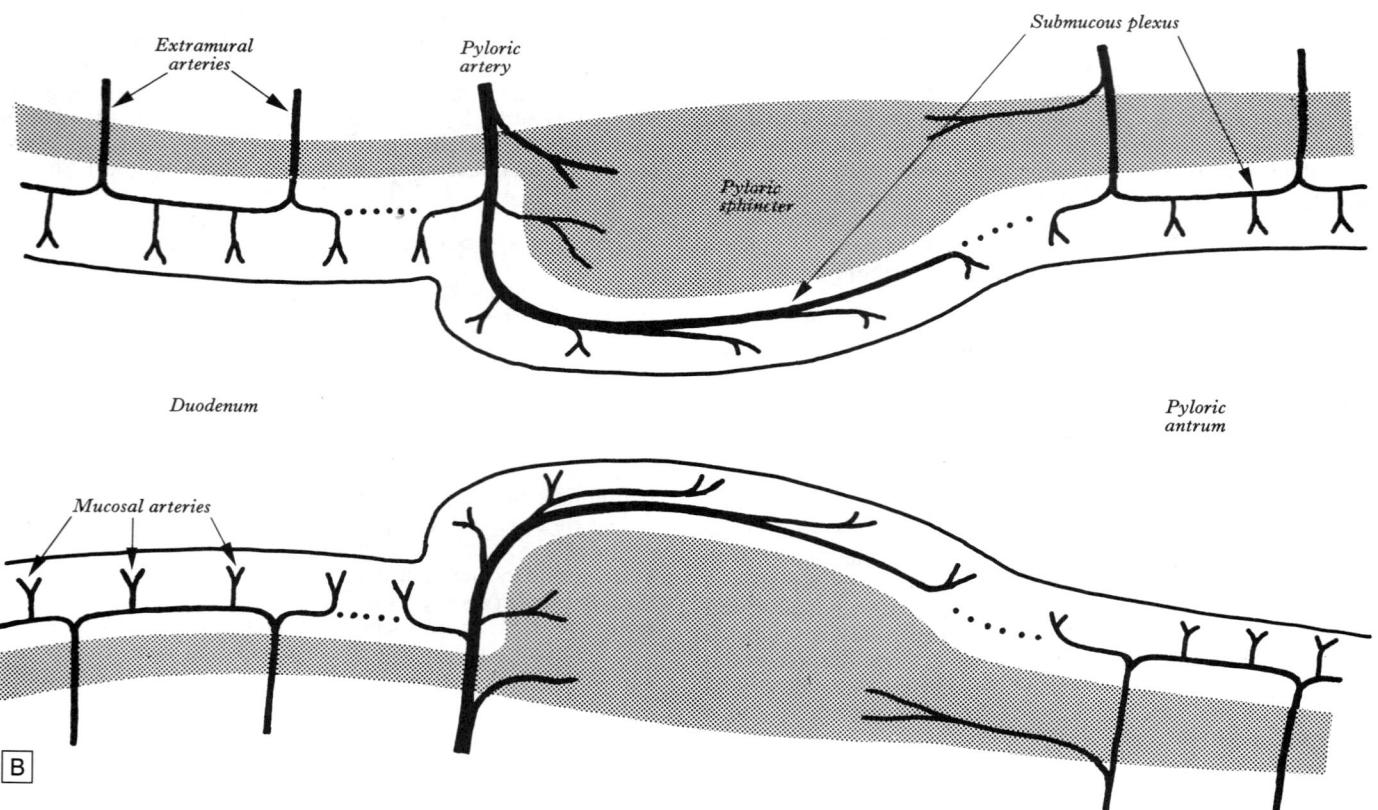

12.96 Blood supply of the stomach and the proximal duodenum. A. Arterial system in a fetal human stomach. The muscle layer has been removed. Note double arcade along the lesser curvature. The arteries have been injected with a mixture of 2% gelatin and India ink and subsequently cleared by the Spalteholz technique. Magnification ×6. B. A scheme of arterial arrangements at the gastroduodenal junction. Dotted lines indicate sites where the submucous plexus may be deficient in continuity. Shaded areas represent the muscular layer of the visceral wall. By courtesy of C Piasecki, Department of Anatomy, Royal Free Hospital School of Medicine, London and the *Journal of Anatomy*.

The posterior nerves produce two groups of branches, gastric and coeliac:

- *Gastric branches* radiate over the posterior surface of the body and fundus and extend to the pyloric antrum but do not reach the pyloric sphincter; the largest (*greater posterior gastric nerve*) passes posteriorly along the lesser curvature, giving branches to the *coeliac plexus*.
- *Coeliac branches*, larger than the gastric, pass in the lesser omentum to the coeliac plexus.

No true plexuses occur on either the anterior or posterior gastric surfaces, but they do in the submucosa and between the layers of the muscularis externa. The latter corresponds to the myenteric (Auerbach's) plexus and contains many neurons. They distribute many axons containing a variety of neurotransmitters and neuro-modulators (Burnstock 1986) and also sensory and sensorimotor fibres to the muscular tissue and the mucosa.

The vagus has both secretory and motor effects on the stomach; vagal stimulation evokes a secretion rich in pepsin and increases gastric motility; after vagotomy the stomach is flaccid and empties only slowly. The sympathetic nerve supply is vasomotor to the gastric blood vessels and visceral sensory fibres running within sympathetic nerve trunks provide the main pathway for gastric pain.

SMALL INTESTINE

The small intestine, a coiled tube, extends from the pylorus to the ileocaecal valve, where it joins the large intestine. It is usually said to be 6–7 m long, gradually diminishing in diameter towards its termination. However, it is longer after death owing to the loss of muscle tone; its average length in living adults is perhaps about 5 m (see below). In 109 adult subjects shortly after death it ranged from 3.35–7.16 m in women and from 4.88–7.85 m in men, the average being 5.92 m in women and 6.37 m in men (Underhill 1955). Length was correlated with the height of the individual but was independent of age; the large intestine was much more constant in length. Jit and Grewal (1975), reviewing the topic, reported findings in 137 Indian subjects confirming these associations with height and noting lack of a correlation with weight. They observed that fixation in formalin caused contraction which sometimes reached 44%. Various observers have also passed flexible tubes through the alimentary tract, recording total lengths of 2.7–4.5 m (see Jit & Grewal 1975).

The small intestine occupies the central and lower parts of the abdominal cavity, usually within the colonic loop; it is related in front to the greater omentum and abdominal wall; a portion may reach the pelvis in front of the rectum. It consists of a short, curved sessile section, the *duodenum*, and a long, greatly coiled part attached to the posterior abdominal wall by the mesentery (p. 1743), the proximal two-fifths being the *jejunum*, the distal three-fifths the *ileum*.

DUODENUM (12.97–99)

The duodenum is 20–25 cm long (12 in, hence the name) and is the shortest, widest and most sessile part of the small intestine. It has no mesentery, and is thus only partially covered by peritoneum. It is constantly curved in an incomplete circle, enclosing the head of the pancreas. It is situated entirely above the level of the umbilicus. Arising from the pylorus, it passes backwards, up and to the right for about 5 cm, inferior to the posterior part of the quadrate lobe, to the neck of the gallbladder; its direction varies slightly according to the distension of the stomach. It then curves abruptly (*superior duodenal flexure*) to descend about 7.5 cm anterior to the medial part of the right kidney, usually to the level of the lower border of the third lumbar vertebral body, just medial to the lateral plane (**12.98**). At a second bend (*inferior duodenal flexure*), it turns horizontally left across the vertebral column for about 5–10 cm, just above the umbilical level, with a slight upward slope; it then ascends in front and to the left of the abdominal aorta for about 2.5 cm, ending opposite the second lumbar vertebra in the jejunum. At this union it turns abruptly forwards; this *duodenojejunal flexure* is about 2.5 cm left of the midline and 1 cm below the transpyloric plane. For descriptive purposes it is hence divided into parts: first (superior), second (descending), third (horizontal) and fourth (ascending).

Duodenal relations

Superior (first) part. About 5 cm long, it is the most mobile section, extending from the pylorus to the neck of the gallbladder. Peritoneum covers its anterior aspect but it is bare of this posteriorly, except for about 2.5 cm near the pylorus where it takes a small part in the formation of the anterior wall of the omental bursa; here the lesser omentum is attached to its upper border and the greater omentum to its lower (proximal half). It is related above and in front with the quadrate lobe of the liver and gallbladder and more posteriorly above with the epiploic foramen, behind with the gastroduodenal artery, bile duct and portal vein and posteroinferiorly with the head and neck of the pancreas. It is usually stained by leakage of bile after death especially on its anterior surface where it is related to the gallbladder.

Descending (second) part. From 8–10 cm long, it descends from the neck of the gallbladder along the right side of the vertebral column to the lower border of the third lumbar vertebral body. Crossed by the transverse colon, it is connected to it by some loose connective tissue and above and below this attachment it is covered in front with peritoneum. It is related in front, from above down-wards: to the right lobe of the liver, transverse colon and the root of its mesocolon and to the jejunum; behind it is variably related to the right kidney near its hilum (being connected to it by loose connective tissue) to the right renal vessels, the edge of the inferior vena cava and psoas major. Medial to it are the head of the pancreas and bile duct, while lateral is the right colic flexure. A small part of the pancreatic head is sometimes embedded in the duodenal wall. The bile and pancreatic ducts come into contact at its medial side, entering its wall obliquely and uniting to form the *hepatopancreatic ampulla* (p. 1810). The narrow, distal end of this opens on the summit of the *major duodenal papilla*, sited posteromedially in the descending duodenum (**12.99, 134**), 8–10 cm distal to the pylorus. An accessory pancreatic duct may open about 2 cm above to the major papilla on a *minor duodenal papilla*.

Horizontal (inferior or third) part. About 10 cm long, this passes from the right of the lower border of the third lumbar vertebra, sloping slightly up and to the left across the inferior vena cava, to end in the fourth part in front of the abdominal aorta. Its anterior surface is crossed with peritoneum, except in the median plane where it is crossed by the superior mesenteric vessels and mesenteric root. Its posterior surface is covered by peritoneum only at its left end, where the left layer of the mesentery sometimes covers it. The posterior surface rests upon: the right ureter, right psoas major, right testicular (or ovarian) vessels, the inferior vena cava and the abdominal aorta (with the origin of the inferior mesenteric artery). Its superior aspect is related to the head of the pancreas, its inferior to coils of the jejunum.

Ascending (fourth) part. About 2.5 cm long, it ascends on or immediately to the left of the aorta, to the level of the upper border of the second lumbar vertebra, where it turns forwards into the jejunum at the *duodenojejunal flexure*; it is anterior to the left sympathetic trunk, left psoas major, left renal and gonadal vessels and the inferior mesenteric vein. To the right it gives attachment to the upper part of the root of the mesentery, its left layer being continued over the duodenum's anterior surface and left side. To its left are the left kidney and ureter; above is the body of the pancreas; in front are the transverse colon and transverse mesocolon, the latter separating the duodenojejunal flexure from the omental bursa and stomach.

Peritoneal attachments

The superior part of the duodenum is slightly mobile, while the rest is almost fixed, being sessile upon neighbouring structures. Radiologically, after a barium meal, the superior part appears as a triangular, homogeneous shadow, the 'duodenal cap' (**12.92, 93**).

The terminal part and the duodenojejunal flexure are said to be positioned by the '*suspensory muscle of the duodenum*' (suspensory muscle, or ligament, of Treitz), often described as being in two parts:

- a slip of *skeletal* muscle derived from the diaphragm near its oesophageal opening, ending in connective tissue near the coeliac artery
- a fibromuscular band of *smooth* muscle, passing from the

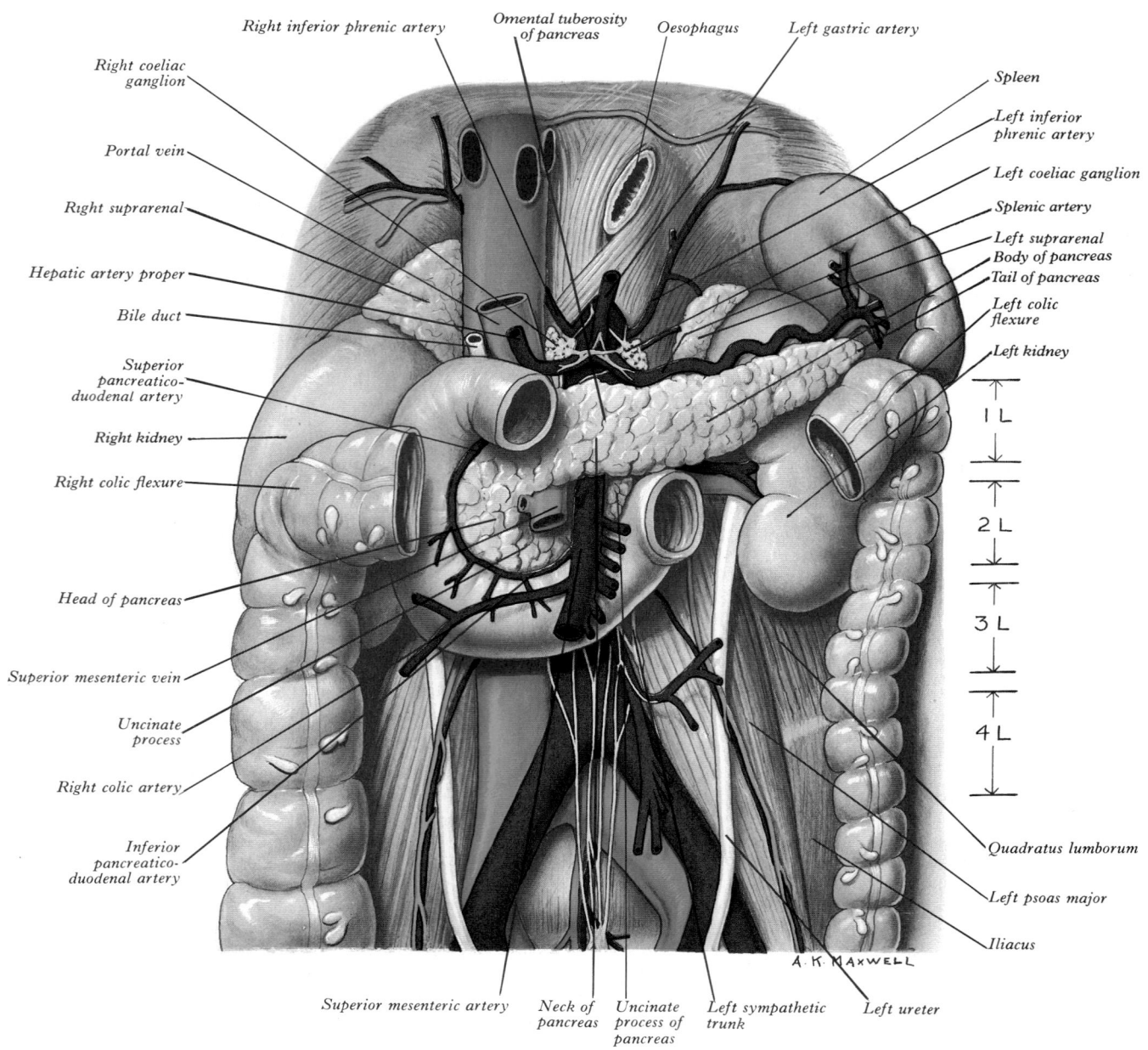

Right inferior phrenic artery
Omental tuberosity of pancreas
Oesophagus
Left gastric artery

Right coeliac ganglion
Portal vein
Right suprarenal
Hepatic artery proper
Bile duct
Superior pancreatico-duodenal artery
Right kidney
Right colic flexure

Head of pancreas

Superior mesenteric vein
Uncinate process
Right colic artery
Inferior pancreatico-duodenal artery

Spleen
Left inferior phrenic artery
Left coeliac ganglion
Splenic artery
Left suprarenal
Body of pancreas
Tail of pancreas
Left colic flexure
Left kidney

1 L
2 L
3 L
4 L

Quadratus lumborum
Left psoas major
Iliacus

A. K. MAXWELL

Superior mesenteric artery
Neck of pancreas
Uncinate process of pancreas
Left sympathetic trunk
Left ureter

12.97 Dissection to show the duodenum, pancreas, major arterial trunks of the gastrointestinal tract and surrounding structures. The right and left hepatic veins have been cut away at their points of entry into the inferior vena cava. The superior hypogastric plexus is shown in front of the sacral promontory and the sympathetic nerves which form it are seen descending across the bifurcation of the aorta, the left common iliac vein and the body of the fifth lumbar vertebra. (In this specimen the left renal artery is situated anterior to the left renal vein at the hilum of the kidney.)

duodenum (third and fourth parts and duodenojejunal flexure) to blend with the same pericoeliac connective tissue.

Treitz (1853) described both entities, naming the former *der Hilfsmuskel* (the accessory muscle). Subsequent authorities (Low 1907) regarded them as a digastric muscle, naming the whole the suspensory **muscle** of Treitz, a misnomer perpetuated in most textbooks. Confusion was increased by Haley & Peden (1943), who derived the 'suspensory muscle' from the right crus, and by Argème et al (1970), who described an intermediate tendon but regarded this as part of a 'false' digastric muscle. Jit (1952, 1977) has persistently repeated the dual nature of the original description by Treitz, supporting it by embryological and histological evidence. The diaphragmatic slip (Hilfsmuskel) has no satisfactory official name. It is supplied, according to Jit, by myelinated nerve fibres probably from the phrenic nerve (pp. 816, 1265) and is sometimes considered an aberrant part of iliocostalis thoracis. The suspensory muscle proper (smooth muscle) is supplied by autonomic fibres from the coeliac and superior

mesenteric plexuses (Jit & Grewal 1977). Descriptions of the duodenal attachments of the muscle vary; none of these accounts contain a convincing view of its function, the usual suggestion being that it augments duodenojejunal flexure, acting like a valve.

Vessels and nerves

Arteries supplying the duodenum. Arising from the right gastric, supraduodenal, right gastro-epiploic and superior and inferior pancreaticoduodenal arteries (pp. 1549, 1553) the first (superior) part receives two leashes of small rami, one from the hepatic artery proper and one from the gastroduodenal artery. These branches also supply the adjacent pyloric canal, with some anastomosis in the muscular layer across the pyloroduodenal junction.

Veins. These end in the splenic, superior mesenteric and portal veins.

Microvasculature. The mucosa has a rich supply of microvessels, arranged so as to enhance the accumulation of bicarbonate near the mucosal surface, and so protect it against gastric acid by bicarbonate

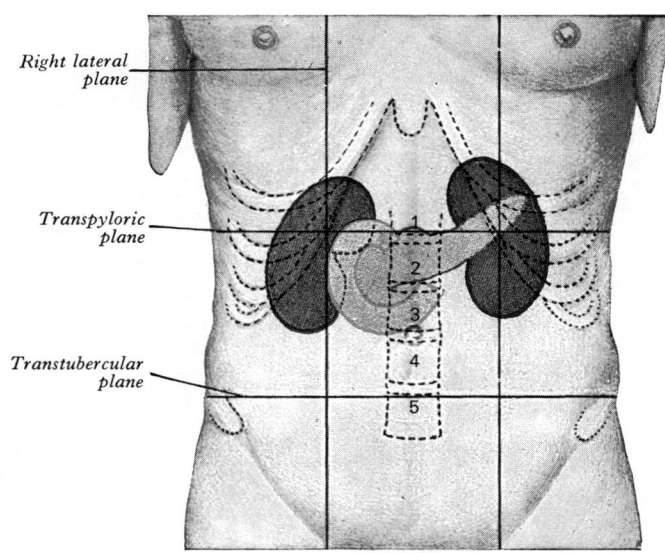

12.98 Surface projection of the duodenum, pancreas and kidneys on the anterior wall of the trunk. The lumbar vertebrae are numbered.

Right lateral plane

Transpyloric plane

Transtubercular plane

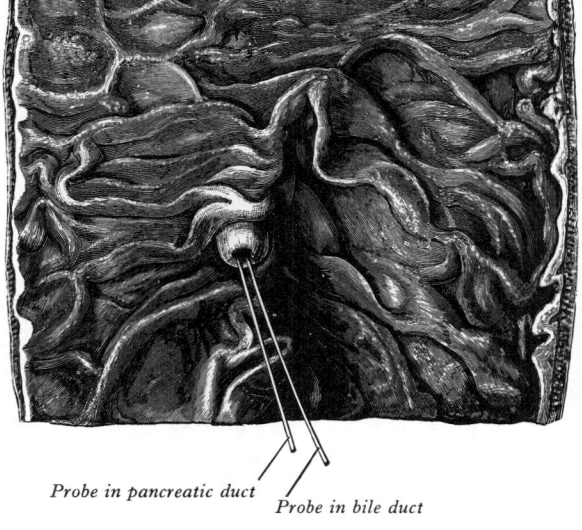

Probe in pancreatic duct *Probe in bile duct*

12.99 Interior of the descending (second) part of the duodenum, showing the major duodenal papilla.

secretion from the surface epithelium. For details of microvasculature see Gannon 1990.

Nerves. They come from the coeliac plexus.

JEJUNUM AND ILEUM

The rest of the small intestine extends from the duodenojejunal flexure to the ileocaecal valve, ending at the junction of the caecum and ascending colon. It is arranged in a series of coils attached to the posterior abdominal wall by the mesentery. It is completely covered by peritoneum, except along its mesenteric border where the two mesenteric layers diverge to enclose it. Its proximal two-fifths is the *jejunum*, the rest the *ileum*; the division is arbitrary, as the character of the intestine changes only gradually, but samples from these two 'parts' show characteristic differences.

Jejunum

The jejunum, with a diameter of about 4 cm, is thicker walled, redder in life and more vascular. Its circular mucosal folds (see below) are large and frequent and its villi larger. Aggregated lymphatic follicles (p. 1771) are almost absent from the proximal (upper) jejunum; distally they are still fewer and smaller than in the ileum and are often discoidal. The circular folds can be felt through its wall and, since they are absent from the distal ileum, palpation allows a crude distinction between upper and lower intestinal levels. The jejunum lies largely in the umbilical region but may extend into surrounding areas. The first coil occupies a recess between the left part of the transverse mesocolon and the left kidney.

Ileum

The ileum has a diameter of 3.5 cm; its wall is thinner than in the jejunum. A few circular folds occur proximally but these are small and disappear almost entirely in its distal part. Aggregated lymphatic follicles are, however, larger and more numerous than in the jejunum. The ileum is mainly in the hypogastric (pubic) and pelvic regions. Its terminal part usually lies in the pelvis, from which it ascends over the right psoas major and right iliac vessels to end in the right iliac fossa, opening into the medial side of the junction between the caecum and colon.

The fan-like mesenteric attachment of the jejunum and ileum to the posterior abdominal wall allows free movement, each coil adapting to changes in form and position.

The mesentery

The mesentery (p. 1742), like a complex fan, has a root, about 15 cm long, attached to the posterior abdominal wall along a line running diagonally from the left side of the second lumbar vertebral body to the right sacro-iliac joint, crossing successively: the horizontal part of the duodenum, aorta, inferior vena cava, right ureter and right psoas major (**12**.76). Its average breadth from its root to the intestinal border is about 20 cm, but is greater at intermediate levels. Its two peritoneal layers contain: the jejunum, ileum, jejunal and ileal branches of the superior mesenteric vessels, nerves, lacteals and lymph nodes, together with a variable amount of fat.

Ileal diverticulum

The ileal diverticulum (of Meckel) projects from the antimesenteric border of the distal ileum in about 3% of subjects, its average position being about 1 m above the ileocaecal valve and its average length about 5 cm. Its calibre is like that of the ileum, its blind extremity being free or connected with the abdominal wall or some other part of the intestine by a fibrous band. It represents the vitelline (yolk) duct's persistent proximal part; its mucosa is ileal in type but small areas may have a gastric structure, with oxyntic cells secreting acid. Sometimes heterotopic areas of pancreatic or other tissues occur in its wall. In a study of 1816 late fetal and neonatal cadavers Miyabara et al (1974) found a diverticulum in 61 individuals (3.4%). Of these, gastric mucosa was present in 11, jejunal mucosa in two, colonic mucosa in two and pancreatic tissue in one.

MICROSTRUCTURE OF SMALL INTESTINE

The intestinal wall has the usual layers of mucosa, submucosa, muscularis externa and serosa or adventitia (**12**.82, 100, 102–109). The mucosa is thick and very vascular in the proximal small intestine, but thinner and less vascular in the distal. In part of its course it is ridged by the underlying submucosa to form *circular folds*, and the whole surface is covered by mucosal finger- or leaf-like *intestinal villi*. Between the bases of the villi are numerous simple tubular *intestinal glands*, while in the duodenum there are also *submucosal glands*.

Circular folds (plicae circulares or 'valves' of Kerkring (**12**.101). These are large, crescentic folds of mucosa which project into the intestinal lumen transversely or slightly obliquely to the long axis. Unlike gastric folds they are not obliterated by distension of the intestine. Most extend round half or two-thirds of the luminal circumference; some are complete circles, some bifurcate and join adjacent folds, some are spiral but extend little more than once round the lumen, though occasionally two or three times. Larger folds are about 8 mm deep at their broadest, but most are smaller than this, and larger folds often alternate with smaller ones. Plicae begin to appear about 2.5–5 cm beyond the pylorus. Distal to the major duodenal papilla they are large and close together, as they

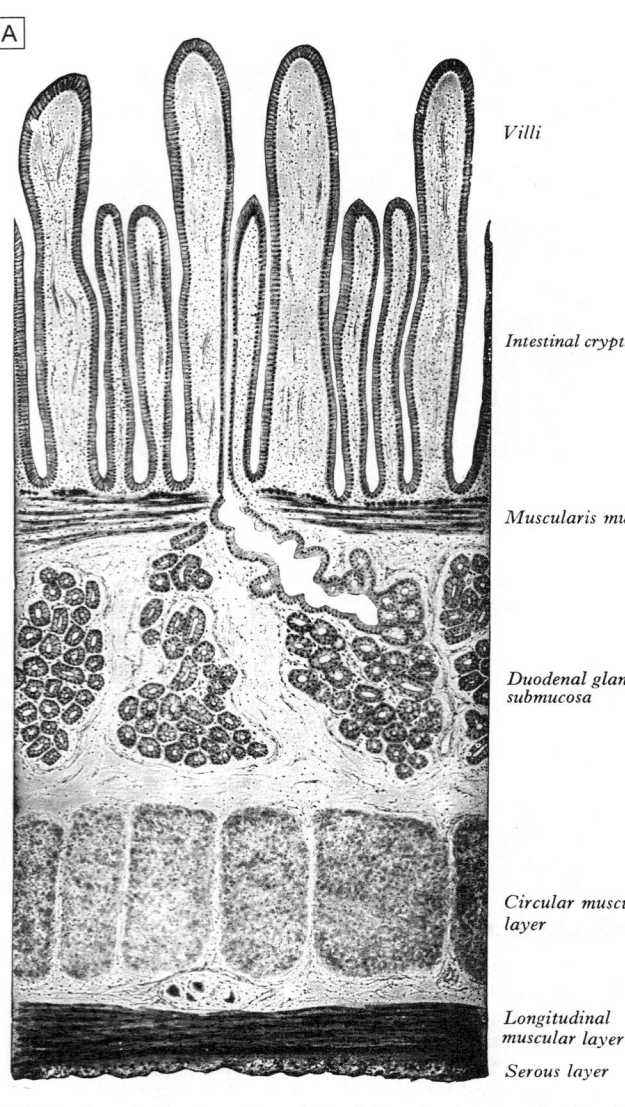

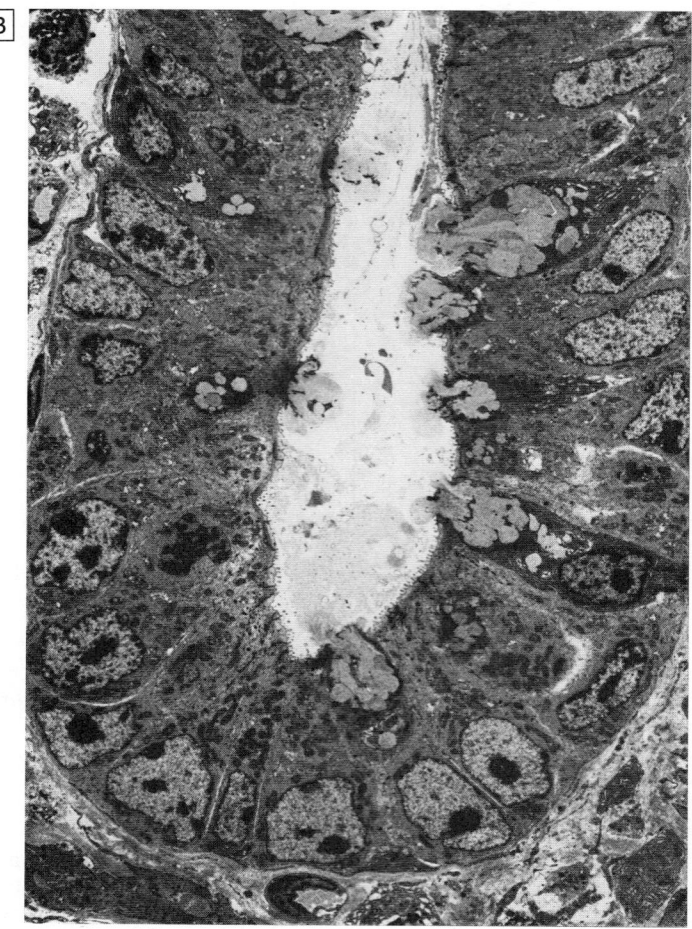

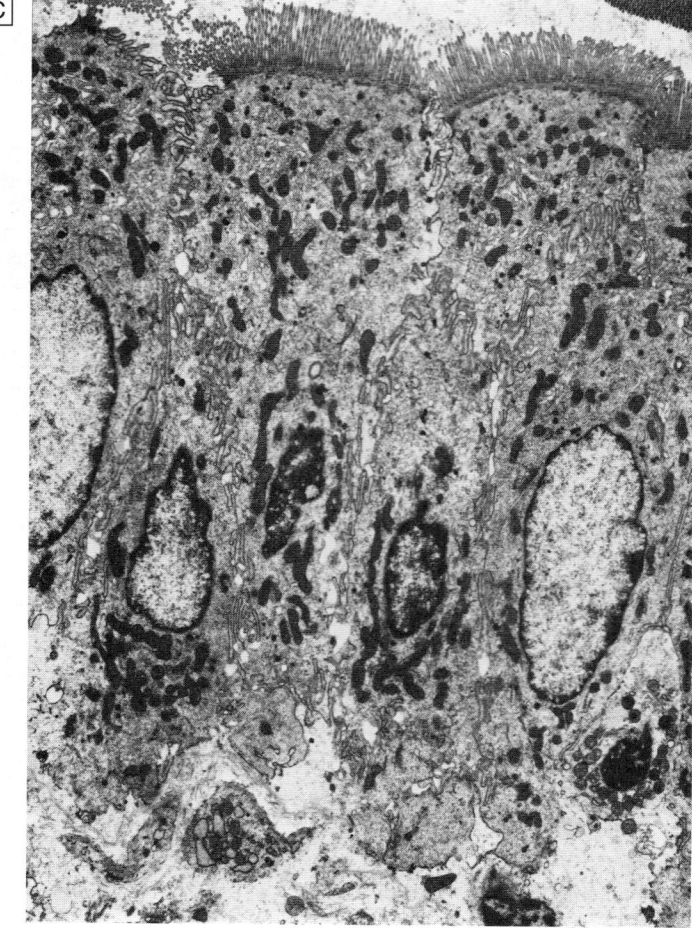

Villi

Intestinal crypts

Muscularis mucosae

Duodenal glands in submucosa

Circular muscular layer

Longitudinal muscular layer

Serous layer

12.100A Longitudinal section of the feline duodenal wall. Magnification c. × 60. B Electron micrograph of the base of a duodenal crypt showing absorptive columnar epithelial cells interspersed with mucus-secreting goblet cells (rat). Magnification × 1700. C. Electron micrograph showing absorptive columnar epithelial cells of a duodenal villus (rat). Magnification × 3700. (Specimens B and C prepared and photographed by Susan Smith, Department of Anatomy, Guy's Hospital Medical School, London.)

also are in the proximal half of the jejunum; but from here to midway along the ileum they diminish, disappearing almost wholly in the distal ileum, hence the thinness of this part of the intestinal wall. The circular folds slow the passage of the intestinal contents and increase the absorptive surface; they are visible in radiographs after a barium meal (**12**.109, 110).

Intestinal villi (**12**.82, 102–106). Highly vascular processes just visible to the naked eye, they project from the entire intestinal mucosa, giving it a velvety texture. Large and numerous in the duodenum and jejunum, they are smaller and fewer in the ileum. In the first part of the duodenum they are broad ridges, changing to tall foliate villi in the distal duodenum and proximal jejunum, beyond which they gradually shorten to a finger-like form in the distal jejunum and ileum (Verzar & McDougall 1936; McMinn & Mitchell 1954). They vary in density from 10–40 per square millimetre and from about 0.5–1.0 mm in height. They increase the surface area about eightfold.

Mucosa

The mucosa (**12**.82, 103) has three layers: epithelium, lamina propria and muscularis mucosae.

Epithelium (**12**.104–107). This covers the intestinal villi and also

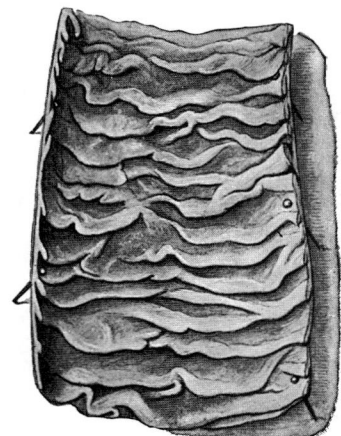

12.101   Internal aspect of a representative sample of the proximal jejunum, showing circular folds.

the intestinal glands (crypts) which discharge their contents between the bases of villi. Covering the surfaces of the villi are two types of cell, *enterocytes* and *goblet* cells. In localized areas covering lymphoid tissues, another type, the *microfold cell* (*M cell*) is also present in smaller numbers.

These various cell types rest on a basal lamina to which they adhere. Although this is too thin to be resolved by light microscopy, its position is marked by a thicker, periodic acid–Schiff (PAS) stainable layer, mostly of connective tissue matrix, the basement membrane (see p. 87).

Enterocytes. These are absorptive columnar cells, prismatic in shape and about 20 μm tall (**2.00**, **12**.100c, 108, 109). They are much the more numerous class of cell in the intestinal lining, and are the site of nutrient absorption. Their surfaces bear up to 3000 microvilli which are collectively though not individually visible by light microscopy as a striated border about 1 μm thick (p. 40). (**2**.24, **12**.108). By light microscopy the cytoplasm appears rather granular, and the vertically elongate nucleus is quite euchromatic, and placed a little below the centre of the cell. Electron microscopy shows enterocytes to be rich in organelles, as might be expected of such active cells.

Because of its importance in nutrition, and the relative ease with which it can be isolated for experiments, the striated border has been the subject of considerable research. Electron microscopy shows it to be composed of multitudes of parallel cylindrical microvilli, each about 1 μm long and 0.1 μm broad. On the external surface of the microvillar plasma membrane is a thick glycocalyx (p. 24) composed of fine perpendicular filaments, the glycosylated terminals of membrane proteins. These are particularly long at the tips of microvilli, and collectively form a thick (up to 0.5 μm) stratum over the surface of the striated border. The glycocalyx is resistant to protease attack and is thought to protect the underlying epithelium against pancreatic enzymes in the intestinal lumen. It also serves to adsorb a number of such enzymes so that there is a zone of digestion of food close to the site of absorption. In the cytoplasmic core of each microvillus are fine actin filaments basally continuous with a plexiform sheet of similar filaments, the terminal web, lying across the cell's apical cytoplasm (**2**.23, **12**.109). Myosin I and other actin-binding proteins also participate in forming these arrays, serving to form a firm anchorage, and perhaps to institute changes in cell shape under some circumstances (see below). The ultrastructural details of microvillar organization are further described on page 40.

Within the general cytoplasm, rod-shaped mitochondria are numerous, indicating that absorption requires much chemical energy on the part of the enterocyte. There is also copious agranular endoplasmic reticulum which, amongst other functions, bears enzymes for synthesizing lipid from the fatty acids and glycerol absorbed by the striated border. There are also some granular endoplasmic reticulum and free ribosomes; the Golgi apparatus is supranuclear and the apical region, beneath the terminal web, con-

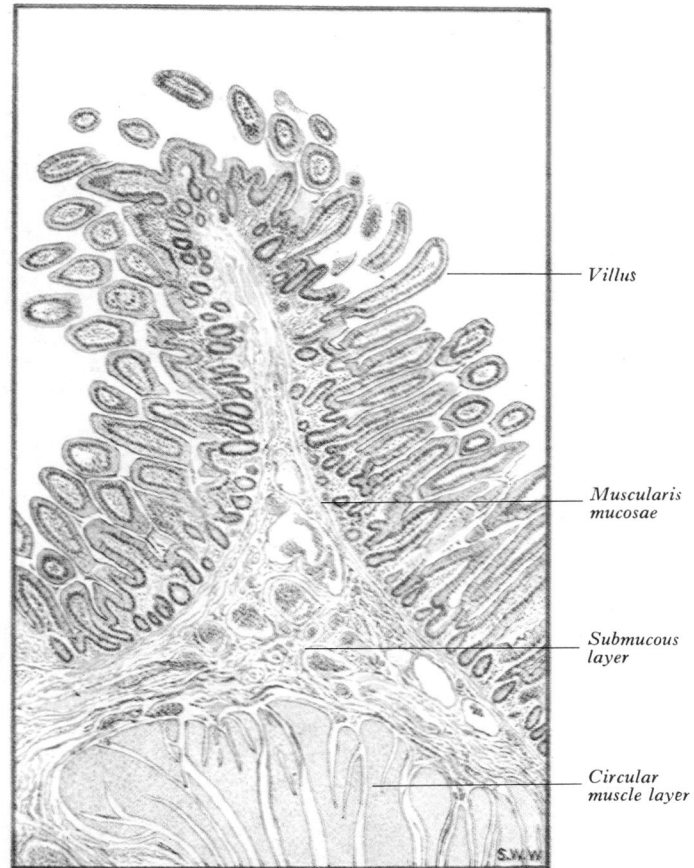

— *Villus*

— *Muscularis mucosae*

— *Submucous layer*

— *Circular muscle layer*

12.102   Section through a circular fold from the human small intestine. Stained with haematoxylin and eosin. Magnification × 19.

tains numerous lysosomes and endocytic vesicles as well as microtubules and a centriole pair (p. 43).

Enterocyte structure varies with their position on the villus, reflecting the stage in the cycle of differentiation and replacement by stem cell mitosis (see below). At the summits of intestinal villi they undergo programmed, apoptotic cell death, during which process their cytoplasm becomes darkly stained and their microvilli stunted and degenerate before the cell finally disintegrates. Changes in the microvillous surface area have also been shown to occur during the reproductive cycle (in female rats) and during ageing (Penzes & Regius 1985).

The luminal surface is an important barrier to diffusion, so that nutrients generally have to pass through enterocytes (*transcellular absorption*) before they can reach the underlying tissues. Classical junctional complexes (p. 28) surround the polygonal apices of enterocytes, their tight junctions forming an effective diffusion barrier. However, when some nutrients, e.g. glucose, are in high luminal concentrations, extensive leakage may occur through intercellular junctions (*paracellular absorption*), perhaps assisted by contraction of the cell web; this may also be a route for transepithelial absorption of antibodies in certain cases, e.g. in premature babies. Further basally, the lateral walls of enterocytes are highly folded, interdigitating with each other to form complicated intercellular boundaries, anchored periodically by desmosomes and making contact at gap junctions.

The roles of these cells in digestion and absorption have attracted much attention. The absorption of amino acids and simple carbohydrates is probably facilitated by diffusion across cell membranes, materials traversing the cells to subjacent capillary arrays in the lamina propria. Lipid absorption appears to be by diffusion of small molecules (fatty acids, etc.) through the luminal membrane, the lipid accumulating in vacuoles in the apical cytoplasm, before being discharged into the lateral and basal intercellular spaces and thence to the subjacent lymphatics. Examination of striated borders isolated

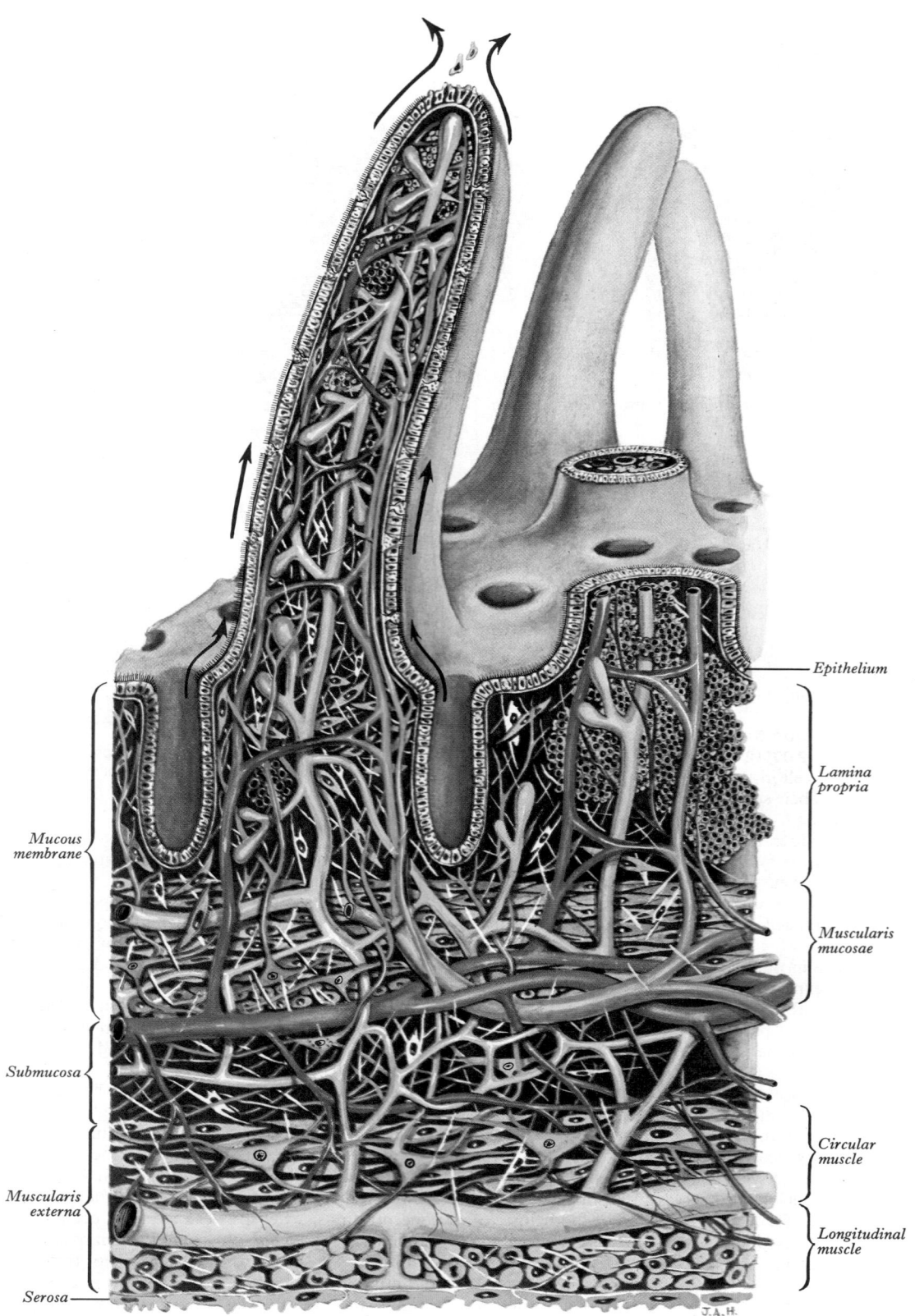

Epithelium

Lamina propria

Mucous membrane

Muscularis mucosae

Submucosa

Circular muscle

Muscularis externa

Longitudinal muscle

Serosa

12.103 A three-dimensional reconstruction of the architecture of the intestinal villi and subjacent wall (the principal layers of the latter are indicated): arteries and arterioles (red), veins and venules (blue), central lacteals and other lymphatic channels (orange), aggregations of lymphocytes (yellow), neural elements (green), non-striated muscle fibres (magenta), fibroblasts (white). Note the orifices of the intestinal crypts (of Lieberkühn). Types of cells in the epithelium include absorptive cells, goblet cells and enteroendocrine cells. Arrows indicate the direction of cell migration. The various layers are not drawn to scale.

by fractionation and centrifugation has shown that enzymes such as disaccharidases are bound to their surfaces, where much intestinal digestion may occur, perhaps in the cell coat in close proximity to the site of absorption. Although most of these enzymes are derived from the pancreas, some disaccharidases are synthesized by the enterocytes themselves, as shown by the demonstration of mRNA for this enzyme by in situ hybridization.

Mucous (goblet) cells. These have elongated, basal nuclei and an

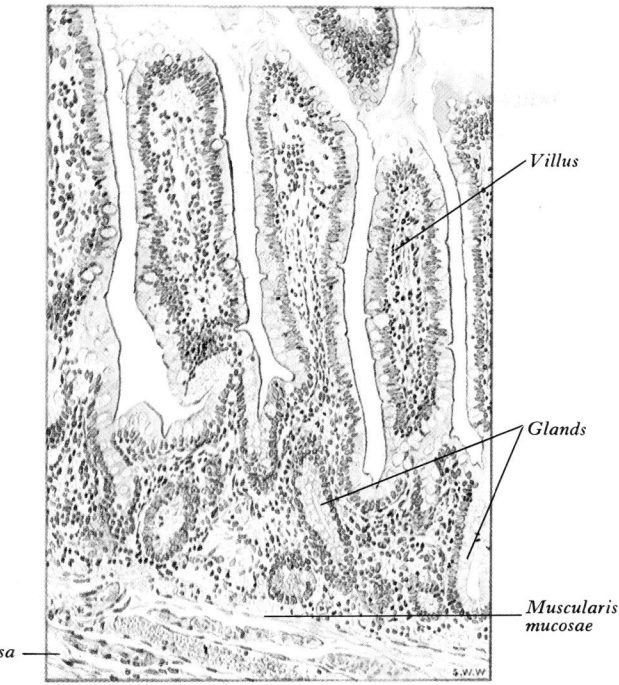

12.104   Intestinal glands and villi in the human small intestine. Stained with haematoxylin and eosin. Magnification × 120.

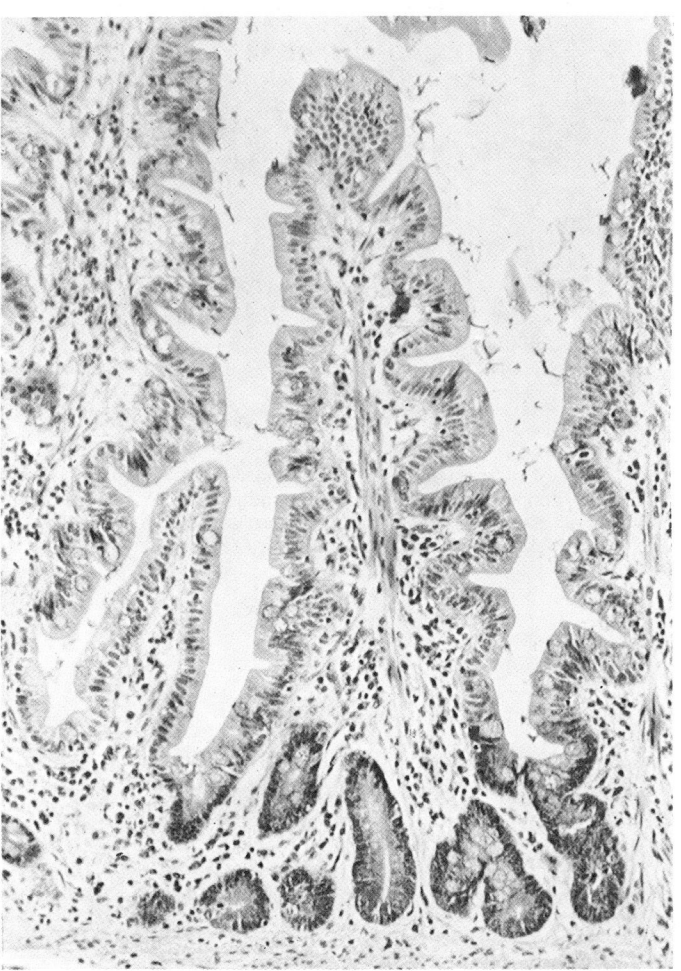

12.105   Light micrograph of part of the mucosa of the murine small intestine, showing a villus in longitudinal section. Non-striated myocytes (pink) can be seen in the lamina propria of the villus. Their contraction has caused the villus to shorten, so that its surface is folded into a series of ridges and grooves (compare **12.**106). Stained with haematoxylin, eosin, and periodic acid/Schiff. Magnification × 250. (Prepared and photographed by Stephen Sitch, Department of Anatomy, Guy's Hospital Medical School, London.)

apical region containing many membrane-bound mucin granules (**12.**108A). When tissues are fixed in formalin, and also many other fixatives, these granules swell rapidly to produce the characteristic but artefactual goblet-like shape. When fixed more rapidly, e.g. by quick freezing, they are more columnar or conical in form. Their apical surface bears a few short microvilli, and in the supranuclear region there is a prominent Golgi apparatus, with granular endoplasmic reticulum more basally situated. Their secretions are important in the chemical and mechanical protection and lubrication of the intestinal wall, and also in its immune defence, since class IgA antibodies are also secreted; at their bases and sides the goblet cells endocytose IgA originally secreted by B lymphocytes present in the underlying lamina propria, and this provides a major source of protection against microbial organisms in the gut lumen.

Microfold cells. They are present where the epithelium covers masses of lymphoid tissue in the intestinal wall. They have long, rather widely spaced microvilli between which are numerous endocytic vesicles. They are thought to transfer antigens from the lumen of the intestine to the underlying tissues, acting as a sampling system to enable the lymphoid tissue to produce appropriate antibodies for secretion (Owen & Nemanic 1978). Further details are given on page 78.

Lymphocytes. These are also present between the basal regions of the epithelial cells (**12.**108). They are migratory cells derived from the underlying lymphoid tissue and constitute an important means of defence against viral attack, and against the proliferation of cancerous cells (see p. 1423 et seq).

Intestinal glands or intestinal crypts (of Lieberkühn). Numerous throughout the intestinal mucosa (**12.**82, 100A, 103, 104, 106), they are tubular, perpendicular pits, opening at small circular apertures between the bases of the villi. Their thin walls consist of columnar epithelium bounded externally by a basement membrane, associated with which is a rich capillary plexus. The epithelium consists of mucous cells, Paneth cells, stem cells and enteroendocrine cells.

Mucous cells. These are similar to the goblet cells of the villi.

Paneth cells. Numerous in the deeper parts of the intestinal crypts, particularly in the duodenum, they are rich in zinc and contain large acidophilic granules (**12.**107) staining with, e.g. eosin, and phosphotungstic haematoxylin. Electron microscopy shows irregular apical microvilli and prominent membrane-bound vacuoles containing a granular matrix with crystalline inclusions in the

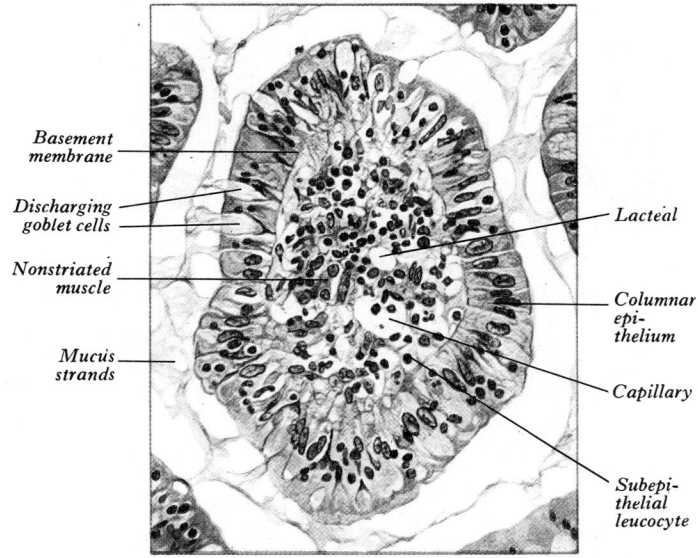

12.106   Transverse section through a villus in the human jejunum. Stained with haematoxylin and eosin. Magnification × 380.

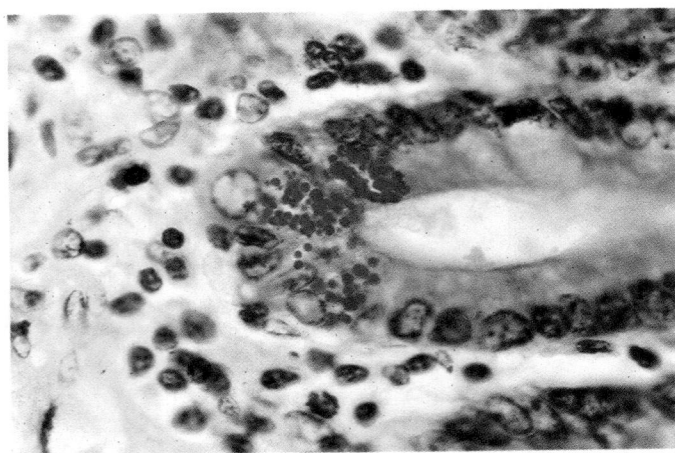

12.107 Part of a transverse section of the ileum, showing zymogenic (Paneth) cells containing orange-stained zymogen granules at the base of an intestinal gland. 'Undifferentiated' epithelial cells are also visible. Mallory's azan stain. Magnification × 400.

supranuclear cytoplasm. These vacuoles are PAS positive and they contain some carbohydrate. Scattered mitochondria, lysosomes and much granular endoplasmic reticulum are present, especially in the basal region. The functions of these cells are not certain, but there is evidence that they secrete lysozyme, an antibacterial substance, and also that they can phagocytose luminal particles. For further details see Rodning et al (1982).

Stem cells. The most numerous cells; they occur in a zone occupying the middle region of the crypts, and provide the source of most of the cell types of the intestinal epithelium. They proliferate by mitotic division, their progeny ascending out of the intestinal glands along the sides of the villi, where they differentiate into columnar or goblet cells; eventually they reach the apices of villi and are shed or die and disintegrate in situ as a result of apoptosis. Thus the villous epithelium is continually renewed. The apical surfaces of these cells, when not dividing, have fewer and more irregular microvilli than do the columnar cells, with occasional pseudopodia. Their lateral plasma membranes are smooth, but intercellular junctions are similar in both types of cell. Their nuclei are basal and the terminal webs poorly developed. Membrane-bound secretory granules are believed to be discharged by both apocrine and merocrine methods. These cells multiply at the rate of 1 cell per 100 per hour, one of the most rapid proliferation rates in the body (Lipkin et al 1963; MacDonald et al 1964).

Enteroendocrine cells. Scattered among the walls of the intestinal glands, and less commonly over the villi, they are of several types, secreting bioactive peptides and bioamines at their bases into the surrounding lamina propria. For further details see page 1787.

Lamina propria. This is composed of connective tissue, providing

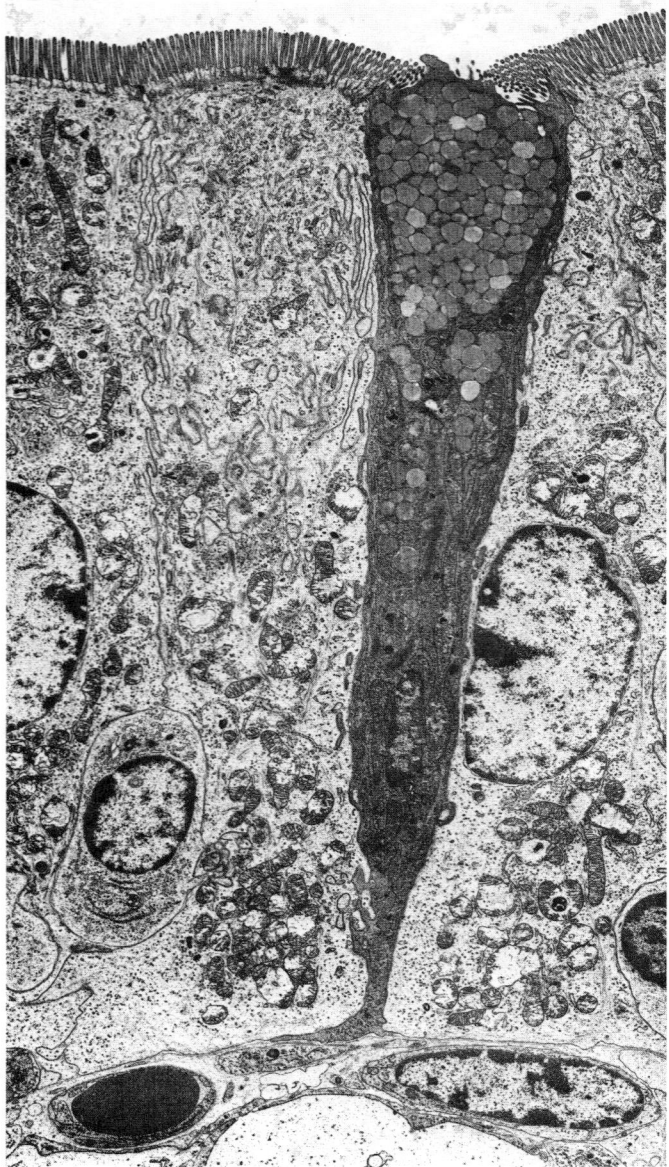

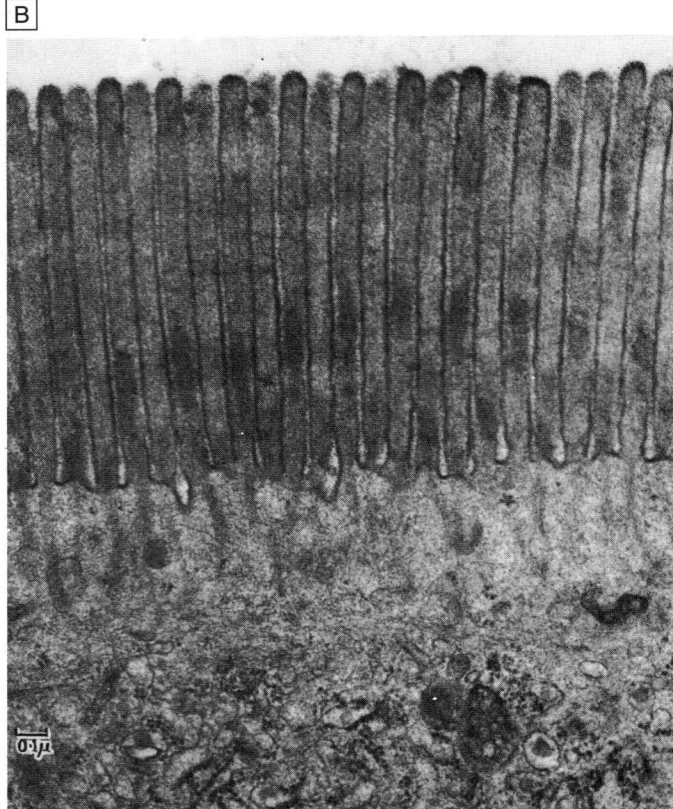

12.108A Transmission electron micrograph of the columnar epithelium lining the murine small intestine, showing a mucus-secreting goblet cell between two absorptive cells which bear microvilli. The cells rest on a delicate basal lamina deep to which is the vascular lamina propria. Magnification × 4800. (Prepared and photographed by Derrick J Lovell, Department of Anatomy, Guy's Hospital Medical School, London.)

12.108B Electron micrograph of the apical region in a columnar cell from the jejunum (rat) showing the regular series of microvilli which constitutes the striated border of light microscopy. Microfilaments can be seen passing from the microvilli to the terminal web. Magnification *c.* × 32 500.

mechanical support for the epithelium: it has a rich vascular plexus, receiving absorbed nutrients from the enterocytes, and forms the cores of the villi. It also contains lymphoid tissue, fibroblasts and connective tissue fibres, smooth muscle cells, eosinophilic leucocytes, macrophages, mast cells, capillaries, lymphatic vessels and non-myelinated nerve fibres. Plasma cells are numerous and lymphocytes in many regions are clustered in solitary and aggregated lymphatic follicles (Peyer's patches), some extending through the muscularis mucosae into the submucosa (see below).

Muscularis mucosae. The muscularis mucosae forms the base of the mucosa, with external longitudinal and internal circular layers of smooth muscle cells; it follows the surface profiles of the circular folds and sends slips of smooth muscle cells into the cores of villi.

Structure of intestinal villi. A villus has a core of delicate connective tissue containing a large blind-ending lymphatic vessel (lacteal), blood vessels, nerves and smooth muscle cells, covered by columnar epithelium on a basement membrane (**12**.103, 104, 105, 108). The lacteal, which is usually single but occasionally double, starts in a closed, dilated extremity near the villous summit and descends to empty into a narrower lymphatic plexus in the lamina propria. Its wall is a single layer of endothelial cells. Smooth muscle cells derived from the muscularis mucosae cluster around the lacteal from the base to the summit of the villus, some being attached to both the basement membrane of the epithelium and the lacteal. Contraction of these myocytes therefore 'milks' the lacteals, forcing its contents into the underlying lymphatic plexus. Blood vessels form a capillary plexus in the lamina propria, enclosed in fine-fibred connective tissue. These capillaries are lined by fenestrated endothelium, probably to ensure the rapid intake of nutrients diffusing from epithelium (Clementi & Palade 1969).

Mucosa-associated lymphoid tissue. This includes masses of lymphoid tissue situated mainly in the lamina propria, but sometimes expanding into the submucosa. They are the source of B and T lymphocytes and other related cells for the immune defence of the gut wall (for details see p. 1444). Essentially they are comprised of one or more lymphoid *follicles* (centres of B lymphocyte proliferation) and attendant clusters of T-lymphocytes and antigen presenting cells. In the epithelium overlying these structures there are a few specialized microfold (M) cells (see above) which are thought to provide a route for sampling the antigens of the gut lumen. The lymphoid follicles have a rich blood supply, and are the source of efferent lymphatics. Villi are small or absent over the larger of the follicular groups. They can be classified as *solitary* and *aggregated lymphoid follicles*. *Solitary lymphoid follicles* are scattered along the length of the intestinal mucosa, being most numerous in the distal ileum. *Aggregated lymphoid follicles* (*Peyer's patches*, **12**.111) are circular or oval masses containing 10–260 follicles, and varying in length from 2 to 10 cm. Like other masses of mucosa-associated lymphoid tissue (except lymph nodes), solitary and aggregated lymphoid follicles are most prominent around the age of puberty, when they may number up to 300, thereafter diminishing in number and size although many persist into old age (Cornes 1965). Aggregated follicles are largest and most numerous in the ileum, whilst in the distal jejunum they are small, circular and few, and only occasional in the duodenum. They are usually situated in the wall opposite the mesenteric attachment. In typhoid fever follicles may ulcerate, such ulcers being oval, their long axes lying along the gut; hence subsequent fibrosis does not constrict the intestine.

Submucosa

The submucosa is composed of loose connective tissue carrying blood vessels, lymphatics and nerves. Its ridged elevations form the cores of the plicae circulares, and, more generally, the obliquely crossing geometry of its collagen fibres, together with elastin fibres, permits the considerable changes in transverse and longitudinal dimensions which accompany peristalsis, whilst still providing adequate support, elasticity and strength (Gabella 1987).

Submucosal (duodenal) glands (of Brunner). As their name implies, these are limited to the submucosa of the duodenum (**12**.82, 100A, B), their ducts traversing the muscularis mucosae to enter the bases of the mucosal crypts. They are largest and most numerous near the pylorus, and form an almost complete layer in the superior part and proximal half of the descending duodenum. Thereafter they gradually diminish in number and disappear at the duodenojejunal

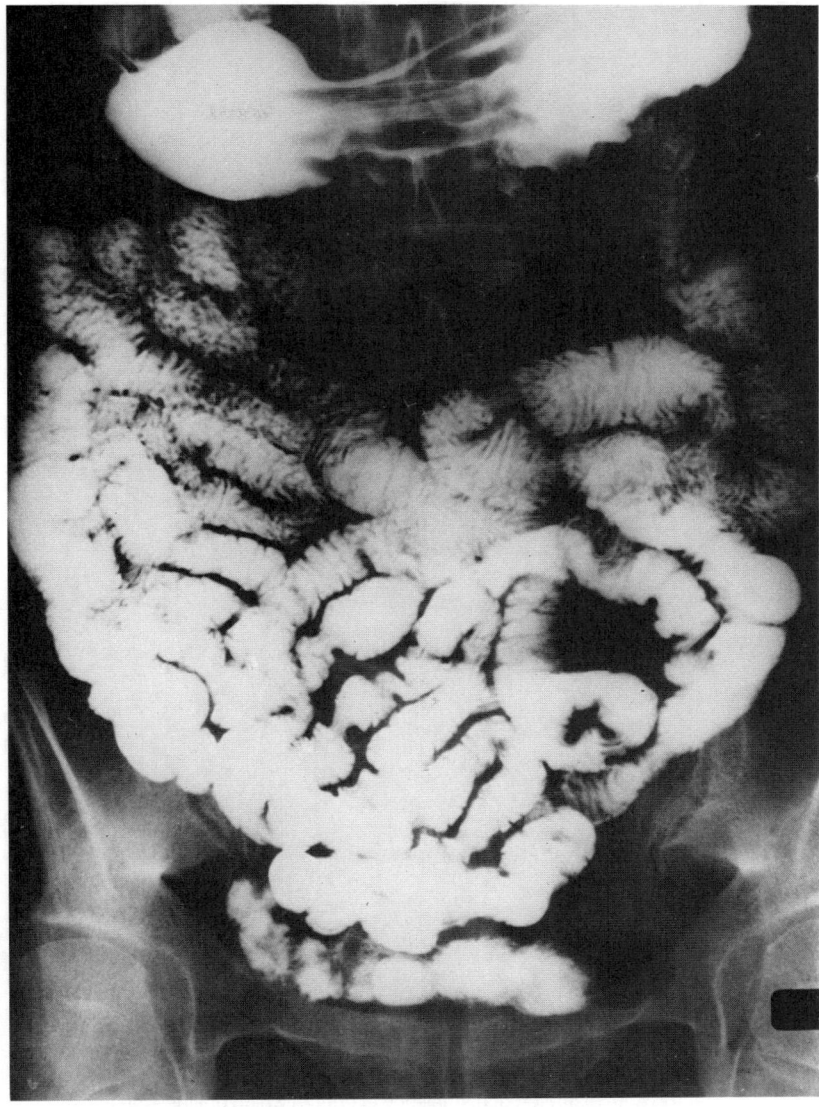

12.109 Radiograph showing the small intestine, taken during a barium follow-through. The feathery appearance of the profile of the small intestine is due to the plicae circulares; constrictions due to peristalsis can also be seen. (Provided by Shaun Gallagher; photography by Sarah Smith, UMDS, Guy's Hospital Campus, London.)

junction. They are small, branched compound acino-tubular glands, each having several acini lined by short columnar epithelial cells and apparently (in humans) containing a single type of mucous secretory cell. The small, basal nuclei of these cells vary during the secretory cycle. The Golgi apparatus is extensive and mucin droplets numerous. Many enteroendocrine cells (see above) are present among the mucinogenic cells. These glands secrete a watery fluid rich in bicarbonate, which helps to neutralize the acid secretions of the stomach as the food enters the duodenum. The cells may also secrete a trypsinogen-activating factor which converts this enzyme to trypsin after secretion from the pancreas.

Muscularis externa

The muscularis externa is thicker in the proximal intestine, consisting of a thin external longitudinal and a thick internal circular layer of smooth muscle cells. For details, see Gabella (1988).

Serosa

The serosa is visceral peritoneum consisting of a subserous stratum of loose connective tissue covered by mesothelium. Where the duodenum becomes retroperitoneal it is mainly covered by a connective tissue adventitia rather than serosa.

Enteric plexuses. These are present in the wall of the small intestine, as elsewhere in the tract, consisting of two ganglionated strata, the myenteric (Auerbach's) plexus between the two layers of external muscle, and the submucosal (Meissner's) plexus on the submucosal surface of the circular layer of muscle. Numerous axons extend from these to all parts of the wall, providing its motor, sensory and sensorimotor supply (see p. 1749).

Vessels

Jejunal and ileal arteries (12.112). These stem from the superior mesenteric, branches of which, reaching the mesenteric border, extend between the serosal and muscular layers. From these, numerous branches traverse the muscle, supplying it and forming an intricate submucosal plexus from which minute vessels pass to glands and villi (see p. 1771). Anastomoses between the terminal intestinal arteries are few and alternate vessels are often distributed to opposite sides of the gut. The **veins** follow the arteries. (For a detailed investigation of the distribution and variations in coeliac and superior mesenteric arteries consult Nesebar et al 1969.)

Lymph vessels (lacteals). They are arranged at two levels, one mucosal, the other in the muscular coat. Lymph vessels of villi commence, as described on p. 1771, form an intricate plexus in mucosa and submucosa, are joined by vessels from lymph spaces at the bases of solitary follicles and drain to larger vessels at the mesenteric aspect of the gut. The lymph vessels of the muscular tunic form a close plexus running mostly between the two muscle layers; they communicate freely with mucosal vessels and open like them into the lacteal drainage at the attached border of the gut.

Nerves

These are supplied from the vagi and thoracic splanchnic nerves through the coeliac ganglia and superior mesenteric plexuses. Fibres pass to the *myenteric plexus* (p. 1749) of nerves and ganglia between the circular and longitudinal layers of the muscularis externa, which they supply. From this a secondary, *submucous plexus* is derived, formed by branches perforating the circular muscular layer; it also contains ganglionic neurons from which fibres pass to the muscularis mucosae and the rest of the mucosa. Nerve bundles in the submucous plexus are finer. Ganglion cells in both plexuses are essentially parasympathetic (vagal). An old controversy on the source of postganglionic neurons in the enteric ganglia was renewed by Andrew (1971); endodermal and mesodermal origins have been suggested, but the evidence now indicates the neural crest as their source (see p. 235). In general the sympathetic system inhibits peristalsis but stimulates the sphincters and muscularis mucosae. The parasympathetic generally augments peristalsis and inhibits the sphincters, the results of parasympathetic stimulation depending on the state of contraction or relaxation of the organ at the time of stimulation. The parasympathetic also augments intestinal secretion.

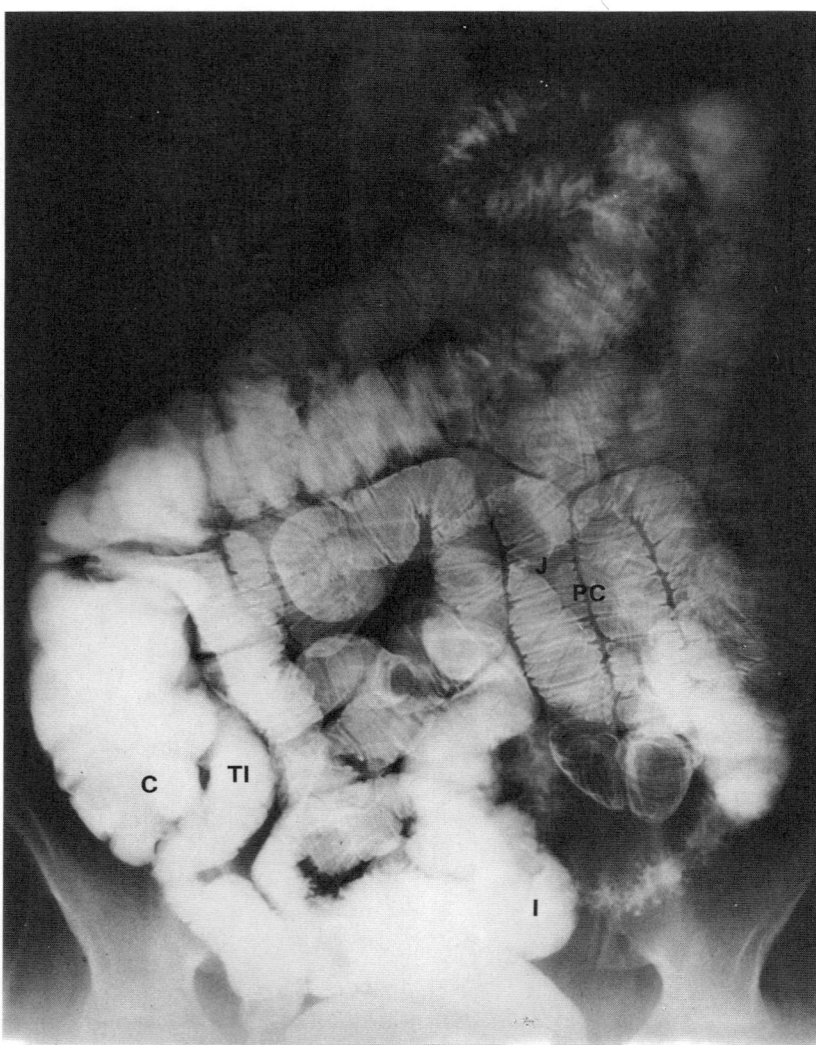

12.110 Radiograph showing part of the small and large intestine, taken after the administration of a small bowel enema which outlines the intestine, followed by methyl cellulose which distends it and produces a double contrast image. The plicae circulares are clearly demonstrated by this technique. C = caecum; I = ileum; J = jejunum; PC = plicae circulares; TI = terminal part of ileum. (Supplied by Shaun Gallagher; photography by Sarah Smith, UMDS, Guy's Hospital Campus, London.)

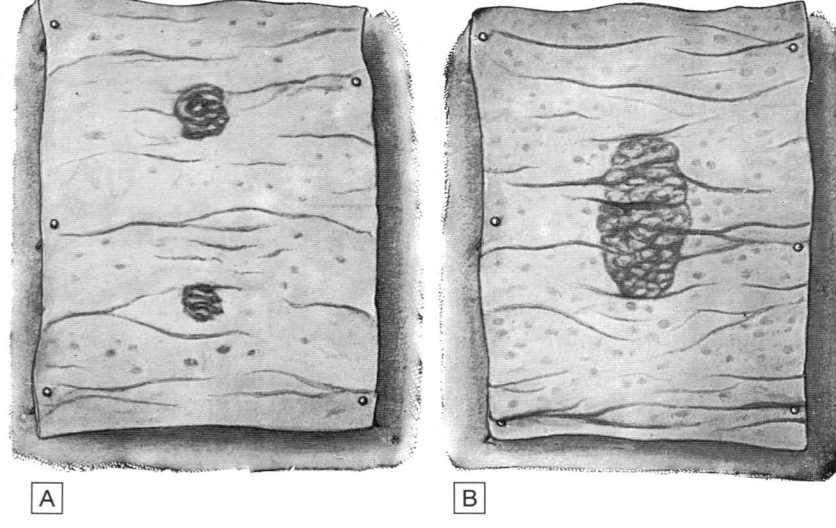

12.111A, B Aggregated lymphatic follicles in the proximal (A) and distal (B) parts of the ileum.

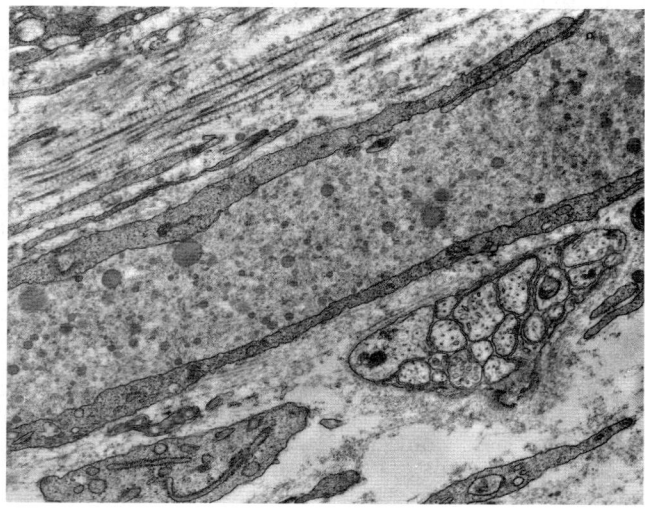

12.111C Electron micrograph of a section through a lymphatic vessel from the small intestine (rat) showing numerous fat droplets (chylomicrons) within the vessel lumen; also visible is a bundle of enteric plexus axons (lower right). (Provided by G Gabella, Department of Anatomy and Embryology, University College London.)

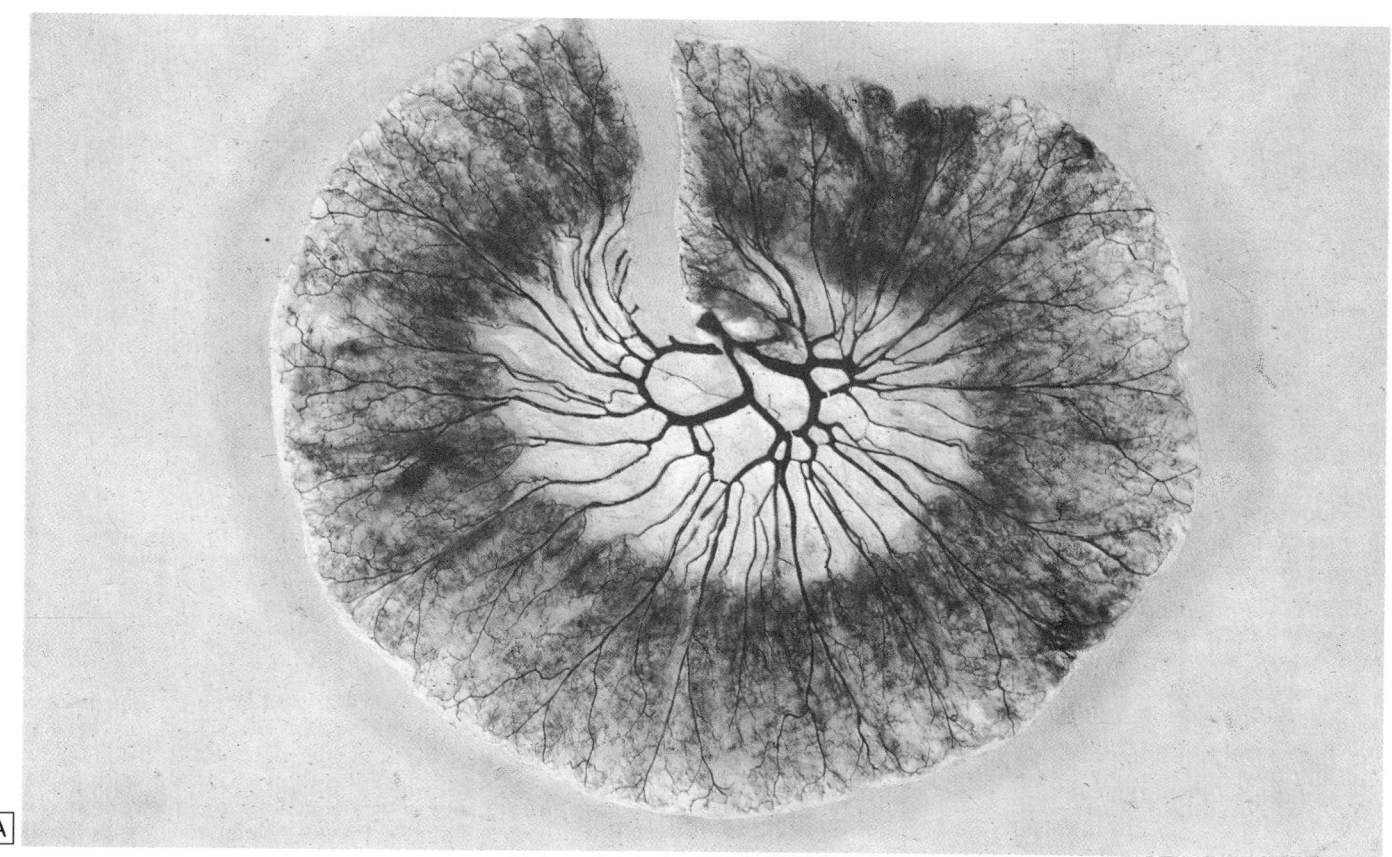

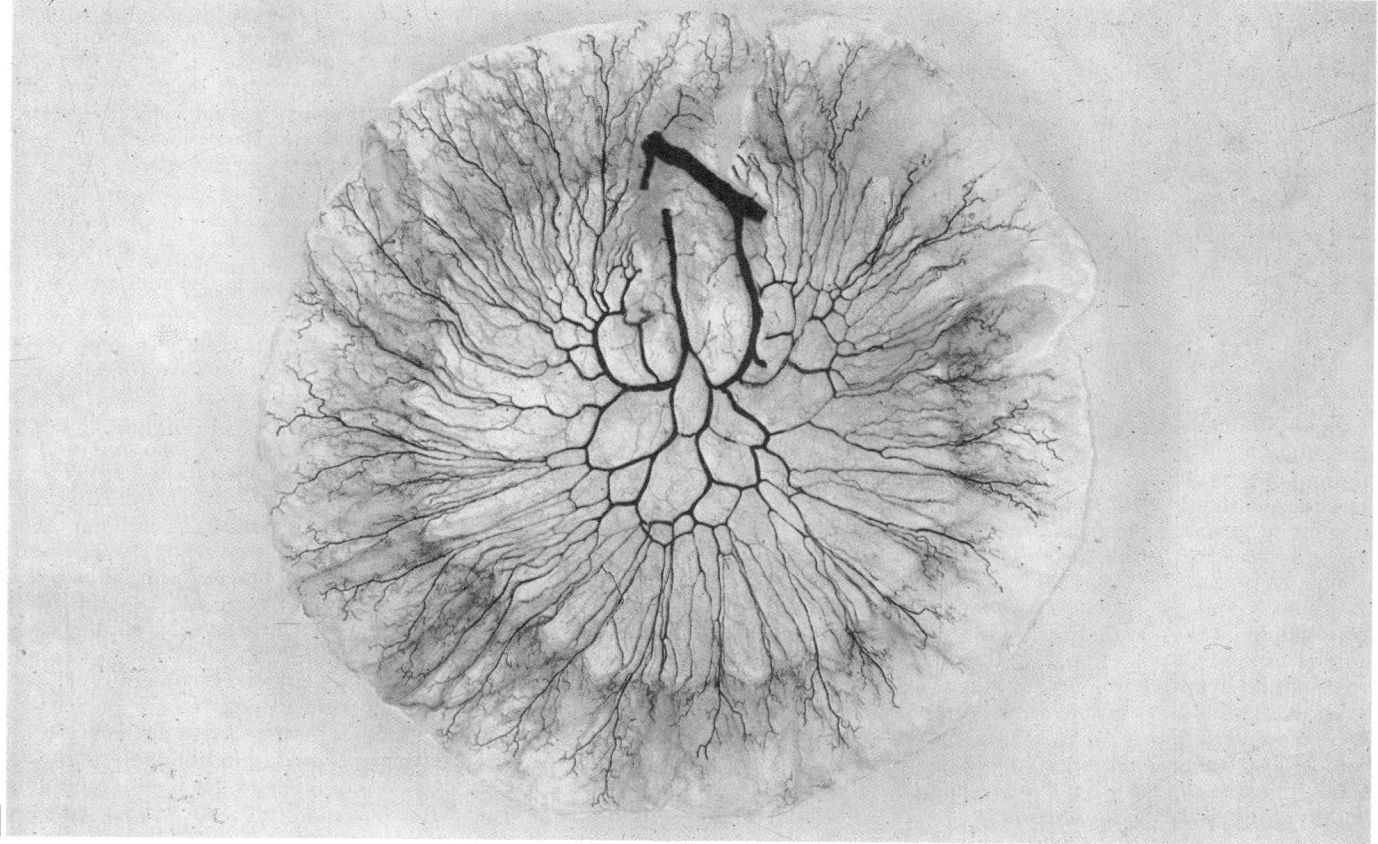

12.112   Specimens of the jejunum (A) and ileum (B) from a subject in whom the superior mesenteric artery was injected with a red coloured mass of gelatin before fixation. Subsequently the specimens were dehydrated and then cleared in benzene followed by methyl salicylate. The largest vessels present are the jejunal and ileal branches of the superior mesenteric artery and these are succeeded by anastomotic arterial arcades, which are rela-tively few in number (1–3) in the jejunum, becoming more numerous (5–6) in the ileum. From the arcades, straight arteries pass towards the gut wall; frequently, successive straight arteries are distributed to opposite sides of the gut. Note the denser vascularity of the jejunal wall. (Specimens prepared by Michael C E Hutchinson and photographed by K Fitzpatrick, Department of Anatomy, Guy's Hospital Medical School, London.)

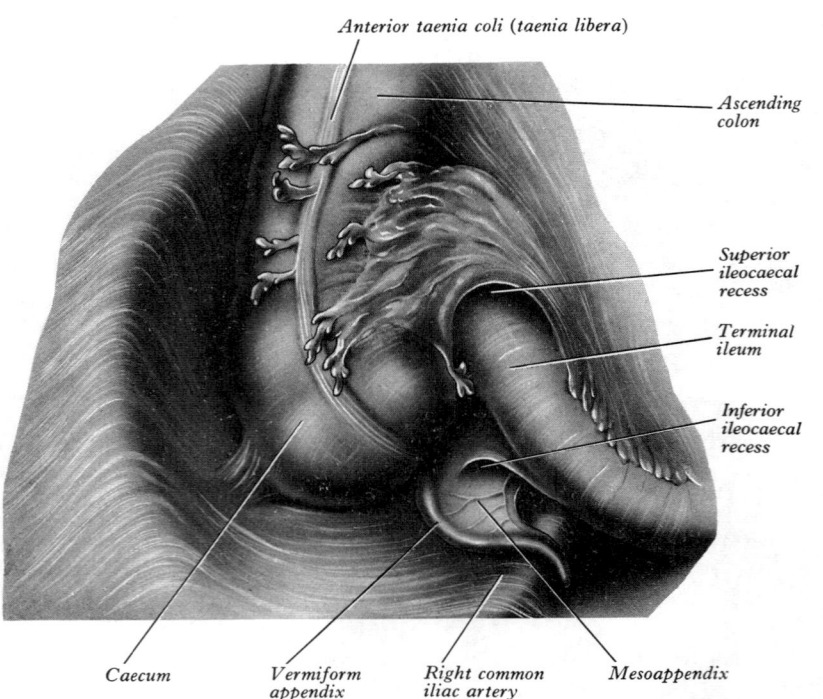

12.113 The terminal ileum, caecum and vermiform appendix: anterior aspect.

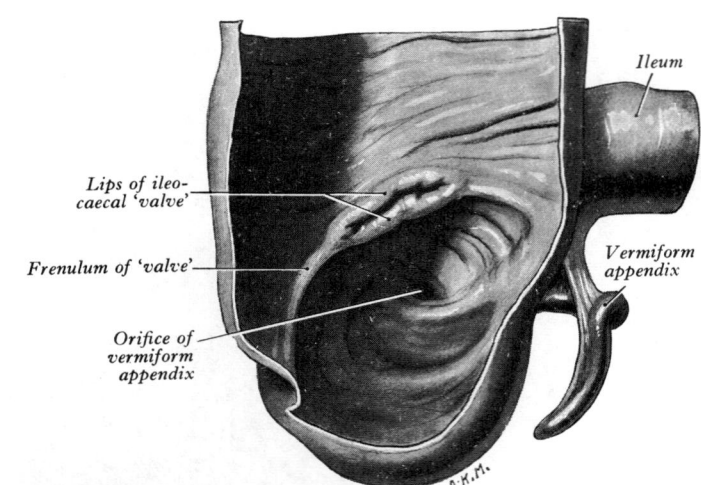

12.114 The interior of the caecum and commencement of the ascending colon, showing the ileocaecal 'valve'. See text for discussion.

LARGE INTESTINE (12.113–127)

The large intestine, extending from the distal end of the ileum to the anus, is about 1.5 m long; its calibre is greatest near the caecum and gradually diminishes to the rectum, where it enlarges just above the anal canal. Its function is chiefly absorption of fluid and solutes, and it differs in structure, size and arrangement from the small intestine in the following ways:

- it has a greater calibre
- it is for the most part more fixed in position
- its longitudinal muscle, though a *complete* layer, is concentrated into three longitudinal *taeniae coli*
- the colonic wall is puckered into *sacculations* (*haustrations*) by the taeniae (so it is said) but sacculation is probably not thus fully explained (p. 1784; see also Hamilton 1946; Pace 1968).

Small adipose projections, *appendices epiploicae*, are scattered over the free surface of the whole colon, but are absent from the caecum, vermiform appendix and rectum.

The large intestine (**12.**117, 118) curves around the coils of the small intestine, commencing in the right iliac region as a dilated *caecum* (*intestinum crassum caecum*). (The term *caecum*, like rectum, duodenum, etc. is an adjective, used by linguistic abbreviation as a noun.) The caecum leads to the *vermiform appendix* and *colon*, the latter ascending in the right lumbar and hypochondriac regions to the inferior aspect of the liver; here it bends (*right colic flexure*) to the left and, with an antero-inferior convexity, loops across the abdomen as the *transverse colon* to the left hypochondriac region, where it curves again (*left colic flexure*) to descend through the left lumbar and iliac regions to the lesser pelvis. Here it forms a sinuous loop, the *sigmoid colon* (**12.**119), continuing along the lower posterior pelvic wall as the *rectum* and *anal canal*.

CAECUM (12.113, 114)

The caecum (**12.**113, 114) lies in the right iliac fossa; its surface projection occupies the triangular area between the right lateral and transtubercular planes and the inguinal ligament. It is a large cul-de-sac continuous with the ascending colon at the level of the ileal opening on the medial side and below this with the vermiform

appendix. Its average axial length is about 6 cm and its breadth about 7.5 cm. It is superior to the lateral half of the inguinal ligament, resting posteriorly on the right iliacus (with the lateral cutaneous nerve of the thigh interposed) and psoas major, separated from both by covering fasciae and peritoneum. Posterior to it is the *retrocaecal recess* (p. 1744), frequently containing the vermiform appendix. Anteriorly, it usually contacts the anterior abdominal wall, but the greater omentum and, when it is empty, some coils of the small intestine may intervene. Usually it is entirely covered by peritoneum, but sometimes incompletely, when the upper part of the posterior surface is sessile and connected to the iliac fascia by loose connective tissue. Commonly, however, the caecum is mobile, and may even herniate through the right inguinal canal. It can also usually be delivered through an appropriate incision in the anterior abdominal wall at appendicectomy.

Caecal variations

The caecum has been classified into four types (Treves 1885). In early fetal life it is short, conical and broad at the base, with an apex turned superomedially towards the ileocaecal junction. As the fetus grows, the caecum increases more in length than breadth, to form a longer tube with a narrower base but retaining the same inclination. Distal growth later ceases, but the proximal part continues to grow in breadth, so that at birth a narrow vermiform appendix extends from the apex of a conical caecum. This *infantile form* persists throughout life in about 2%, regarded by Treves as the *first type*; the three taeniae coli (p. 1784) start from the appendix and are equidistant from each other. In the *second type*, the conical caecum becomes quadrate by outgrowth of a saccule on each side of the anterior taenia; these saccules are of equal size and the appendix arises from the depression between them instead of from the apex of a cone. This type occurs in about 3%. In the *third type* (normal in humans) the two saccules grow at unequal rates, the right more rapidly, forming a new 'apex'; the original apex, with the appendix attached, is pushed towards the ileocaecal junction; the taeniae still start from the appendicular base but are not equidistant, the growth of the right saccule pushing between the anterior and posterolateral taeniae. This type occurs in about 90%. The *fourth type* is merely an exaggeration of the third, the right saccule growing still further and the left atrophying so that the original caecal apex and appendix are near the ileocaecal junction, the anterior taenia also turning medially to it. This type occurs in about 4%. In a more recent study (Pavlov & Pétrov 1968) of 82 males and 44 females (adolescent and adult), the third type was designated *ampullary*, accounting for 78%. An *infundibular* type, approximating to the infantile conical category, occurred in 13%; 9% were intermediate. The caecum was mobile 20% more often in females. (For further analyses consult Balthazar & Gade 1976.)

ILEOCAECAL VALVE

The ileum opens into the posteromedial aspect of the large intestine, at the junction of the caecum and colon (**12**.114). A surface marking of this structure is the intersection of the right lateral and transtubercular planes; about 2 cm below this the vermiform appendix opens into the caecum. The ileocaecal orifice has a so-called 'valve', consisting of two flaps projecting into the lumen of the large intestine (Decarvalho et al 1987). In the distended, fixed caecum the flaps are semilunar. The upper, approximately horizontal, is attached to the junction of the ileum and colon, the lower, longer and more concave, to the junction of the ileum and caecum. At their ends the flaps coalesce, continuing as narrow membranous ridges, the *frenula* of the valve. The anterior or left end of the aperture is rounded, the right or posterior is narrow and pointed. In the natural state the valvular lips project as thick folds into the caecal lumen, the orifice appearing like a slit or oval. Circular and longitudinal muscle layers of the terminal ileum continue into the valve to form a sphincter. However, direct observation of the living ileocaecal 'valve' does not corroborate this description (Rosenberg & DiDio 1969); in nine cases, studied by caecostomy, the ileal projection was papillary in shape. Radiological evidence also contradicts the concept of an effective ileocaecal valve at this junction.

Accumulations of circular fibres, sometimes described as sphincters, have been observed at various levels in all parts of the colon (DiDio & Anderson 1968; Rosenberg & DiDio 1969). The functional reality of most of these remains doubtful. Such sphincteric mechanisms must, of course, be balanced by antagonistic, dilatatory actions.

The margin of the ileocaecal valve is a reduplication of the intestinal mucosa and *circular* muscle; longitudinal muscle fibres are partly reduplicated as they enter the valve (Jit & Singh 1956), but the more superficial fibres and the peritoneum continue uninterruptedly from the small to the large intestine. The ileal valvular surfaces are covered with villi and have the structure of the mucosa of the small intestine; their caecal aspects display no villi but numerous orifices of tubular glands peculiar to the colonic mucosa. It is usually said that the valve not only prevents reflux from the caecum to the ileum but is probably also a sphincter regulating the passage of ileal contents into the caecum; the valve is kept in tonic contraction by sympathetic innervation. Entry of food into the stomach initiates contraction of the small intestine, expelling ileal contents into the large intestine (the gastro-ileal reflex).

VERMIFORM APPENDIX

The vermiform appendix (**12**.113–116) is a narrow, vermian (worm-shaped) tube, arising from the posteromedial caecal wall, 2 cm or less below the end of the ileum. It may occupy one of several positions (**12**.115):

- behind the caecum and lower ascending colon (*retrocaecal* and *retrocolic*);
- dependent over the pelvic brim (*pelvic* or *descending*), in females in close relation to the right uterine tube and ovary;
- lying below the caecum (*subcaecal*);
- in front of the terminal ileum when it may be in contact with the anterior abdominal wall;
- behind the terminal ileum.

In 10,000 subjects (Wakeley 1933) the vermiform appendix was retrocaecal and retrocolic (65.28%), pelvic (31.01%), subcaecal (2.26%), pre-ileal (1.0%) and postileal (0.4%). Subsequent literature, anatomical and surgical, shows much contradiction of this classic study. Buschard and Kjaeldgaard (1973), reporting a short series (234 autopsies), compared the results of several studies dating from 1885–1973, Wakeley's remaining by far the largest. They classified all positions as either *anterior* (pelvic and ileocaecal) or *posterior* (retrocaecal and subcaecal). All but three of 11 series quoted found anterior positions more frequent. Like Wakeley they observed posterior positions more commonly in their own Danish series; in German autopsies the finding was reversed. Collins (1932), in the second largest series (4680), returned percentages the reverse of Wakeley's, the ratio of anterior to posterior being 78.5% to 21.5% (Collins) and 32.4% to 67.6% (Wakeley). In view of these dis-

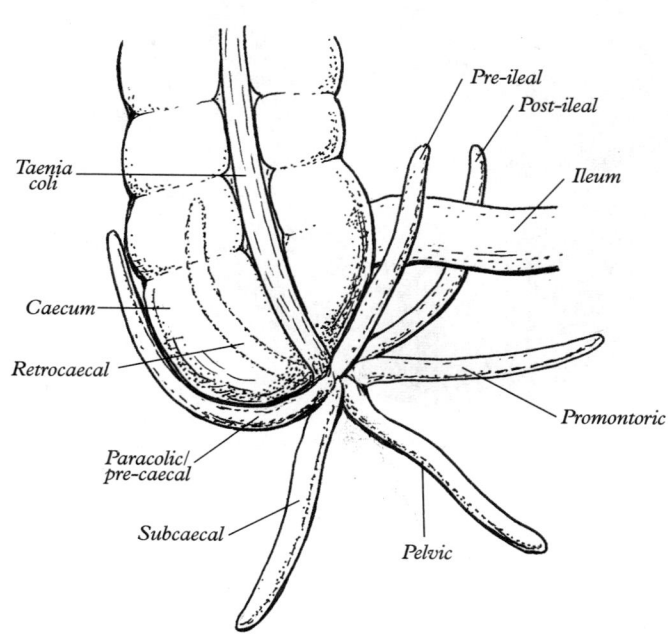

12.115 Diagram illustrating the major positions of the appendix encountered at surgery or post-mortem.

agreements, such figures are of dubious value. Perhaps observers have used differing criteria or possibly there are demographic variations. For the present, however, such percentages remain unreliable.

The usual *surface marking* for the appendicular base is the junction of the lateral and middle thirds of the line joining the right anterior superior iliac spine to the umbilicus (*McBurney's point*); but this is merely a useful surgical approximation, with considerable variation. The three taeniae coli on the ascending colon and caecum converge on the base of the appendix, merging into its longitudinal muscle. The anterior caecal taenia is usually distinct and traceable to the appendix, affording a guide to it. The appendix varies from 2–20 cm in length, the average being about 9 cm. It is longer in children and may atrophy or diminish after mid-adult life. It is connected by a short *mesoappendix* to the lower part of the ileal mesentery. This fold is usually triangular, extending almost to the appendicular tip along the whole tube.

The main *appendicular artery*, a branch from the lower division of the ileocolic (p. 1554), runs behind the terminal ileum to enter the mesoappendix a short distance from the appendicular base. Here it gives off a recurrent branch which anastomoses at the base of the appendix with a branch of the posterior caecal artery, the anastomosis sometimes being large. The main appendicular artery approaches the tip of the organ, at first near to and then in the edge of the mesoappendix. The terminal part of the artery, however, lies on the wall of the appendix and may be thrombosed in appendicitis, resulting in distal gangrene or necrosis. The arterial supply of the appendix may vary considerably. Accessory arteries are common; in 80% of subjects there are two or more arteries of supply (Solanke 1968).

The canal of the appendix is small and opens into the caecum by an orifice lying below and a little behind the ileocaecal opening. The orifice is sometimes guarded by a semilunar mucosal fold forming a valve. The lumen may be partially or wholly obliterated in the later decades of life. In view of its rich vascularity and histological differentiation, the appendix is probably a specialized rather than a degenerate or vestigial structure. The caecum and appendix in man and anthropoid apes is considered to be less primitive than in monkeys. A comparative study of the primate vermiform appendix has been made by Scott (1980).

1775

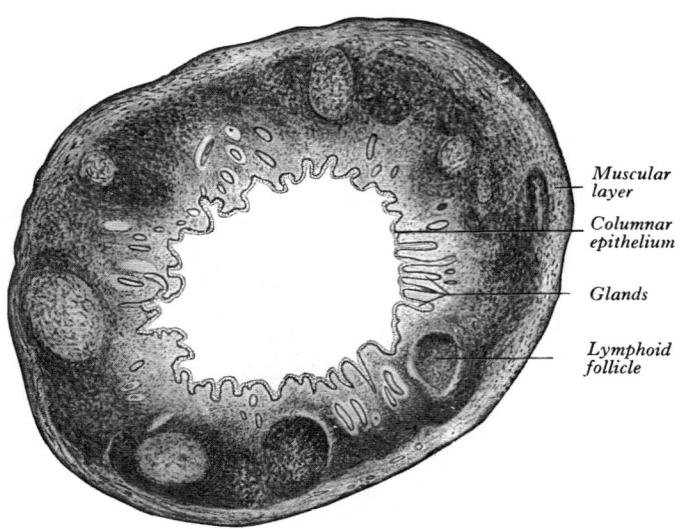

12.116   Transverse section of human vermiform appendix. Magnification × 20.

Labels on figure:
- Muscular layer
- Columnar epithelium
- Glands
- Lymphoid follicle

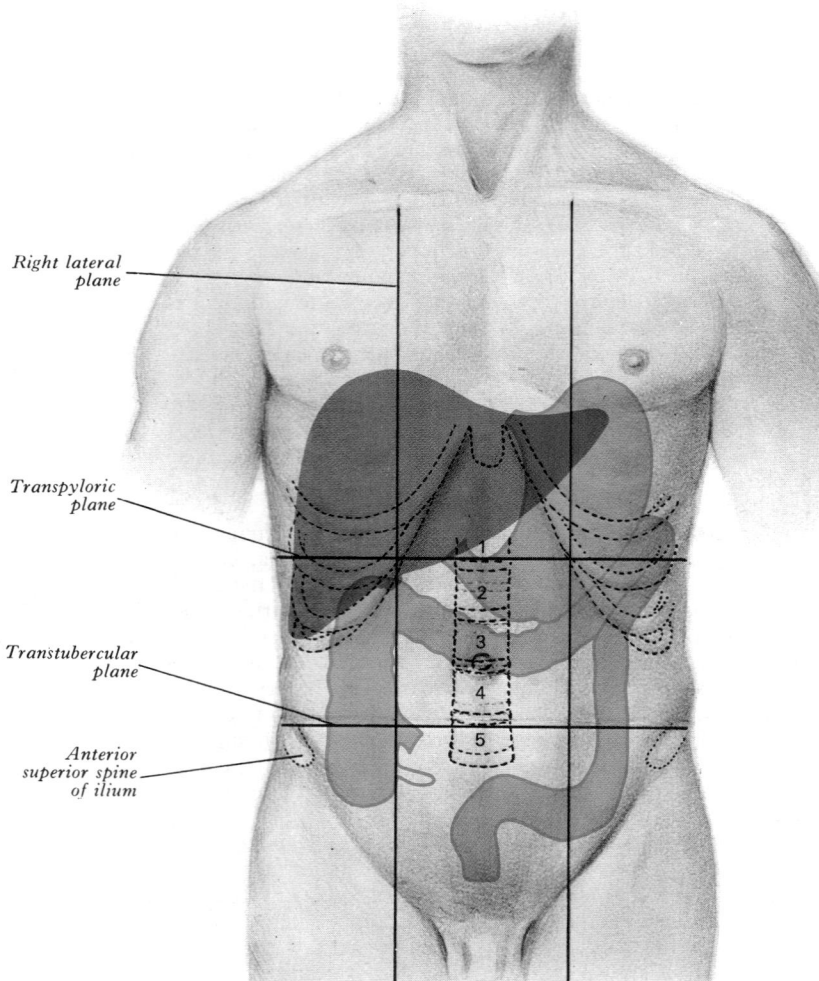

12.117   Surface projection of the stomach, liver and colon. The outlines of the lumbar vertebral bodies and intervertebral discs, lower ribs, xiphoid process and parts of the iliac crests are indicated.

Labels on figure:
- Right lateral plane
- Transpyloric plane
- Transtubercular plane
- Anterior superior spine of ilium

Microstructure of the appendix

The layers of the appendix wall are essentially as in the rest of the large intestine. The *serosa* is a complete investment, except along the mesenteric attachment; there is a subserous layer of connective tissue. The *longitudinal muscular fibres* form a complete, uniformly thick layer, except over a few small areas where both muscular layers are deficient, leaving the serosa and submucosa in contact. At the base the longitudinal muscle thickens to form rudimentary taeniae continuous with those of the caecum and colon. The *circular muscular fibres* form a thicker layer separated from the longitudinal by connective tissue. The *submucosa* is well developed, containing many lymphoid masses which cause the mucosa to bulge into the lumen, narrowing it irregularly. The *mucosa* is covered by columnar epitheliocytes and attenuated antigen-transporting 'M' cells (Owen & Nemanic 1978). Glands (crypts similar to those of the colon) are few and penetrate deeply into the lymphoid tissue (**12**.116), which in the normal human appendix is situated primarily in the lamina propria and extends into the submucosa; follicular and parafollicular zones containing B- and T-lymphocytes (p. 1417) can be distinguished; clustered lymphocytes also appear between the epithelial cells, where some may possibly differentiate into plasma cells (Gorgollón 1978). Lymphoid tissue in the lamina propria contains many plasma cells, with lymphocytes, eosinophils and other leucocytes, mast cells and macrophages embedded in a fibrocellular reticulum. The submucosal follicles (germinal centres) are organized like those of other examples of gut-associated lymphoid tissue (p. 1417; see also Kaiserling et al 1974). The *lymphoid masses* are a local defence against infection; it has also been suggested that they may be a homologue of the avian *bursa of Fabricius* concerned in the acquisition of immunological competence by certain lymphocytes. However, experimental evidence argues against this function (p. 1417). In many mammals, particularly herbivores, the caecum and appendix are large and constitute a highly important site of digestion of cellulose by symbiotic bacteria.

COLON (**12**.117, 118, 123)

The colon is conveniently considered in four parts: ascending, transverse, descending and sigmoid.

Ascending colon. About 15 cm long and narrower than the caecum, it ascends to the inferior surface of the right lobe of the liver, on which it makes a shallow depression; here it turns abruptly forwards and to the left, at the *right colic flexure* (**12**.95). In surface projection it ascends lateral to the right lateral plane (**12**.117) from the transtubercular to midway between the subcostal and transpyloric planes. It is covered by peritoneum except where its posterior surface is connected by loose connective tissue to the iliac fascia, and to the iliolumbar ligament, quadratus lumborum, aponeurosis of transversus abdominis and the perirenal fascia on the front of the inferolateral area of the right kidney. Crossing behnd it are the lateral femoral cutaneous nerve, usually the fourth lumbar artery, and sometimes the ilio-inguinal and iliohypogastric nerves. Sometimes it possesses a distinct but narrow mesocolon. In a series of 100 subjects, 52% had neither an ascending nor descending mesocolon, 14% had both, 12% an ascending and 22% a descending mesocolon (Treves 1885). Anteriorly it is in contact with the coils of the ileum, the greater omentum and the anterior abdominal wall.

Right colic flexure. This is found at the junction of the ascending and transverse colon; the latter turns down, forwards and to the left. Posterior is the inferolateral part of the anterior surface of the right kidney; above and anterolaterally is the right lobe of the liver; anteromedially are the descending part of the duodenum and fundus of the gallbladder. Its posterior aspect is not covered by peritoneum and is in direct contact with renal fascia. It is not so acute as the left colic flexure.

Transverse colon (**12**.88, 89, 117, 118). About 50 cm long, it extends from the right colic flexure in the right lumbar region, across into the left hypochondriac region, here curving sharply down and backwards below the spleen as the *left colic flexure*. The transverse colon describes an arch, its concavity usually directed back and up; near its splenic end an abrupt U-shaped curve may descend lower than the main arch. Its surface projection (**12**.117) extends from a point situated just lateral to the right lateral plane, and midway between the subcostal and transpyloric planes, to the umbilicus and

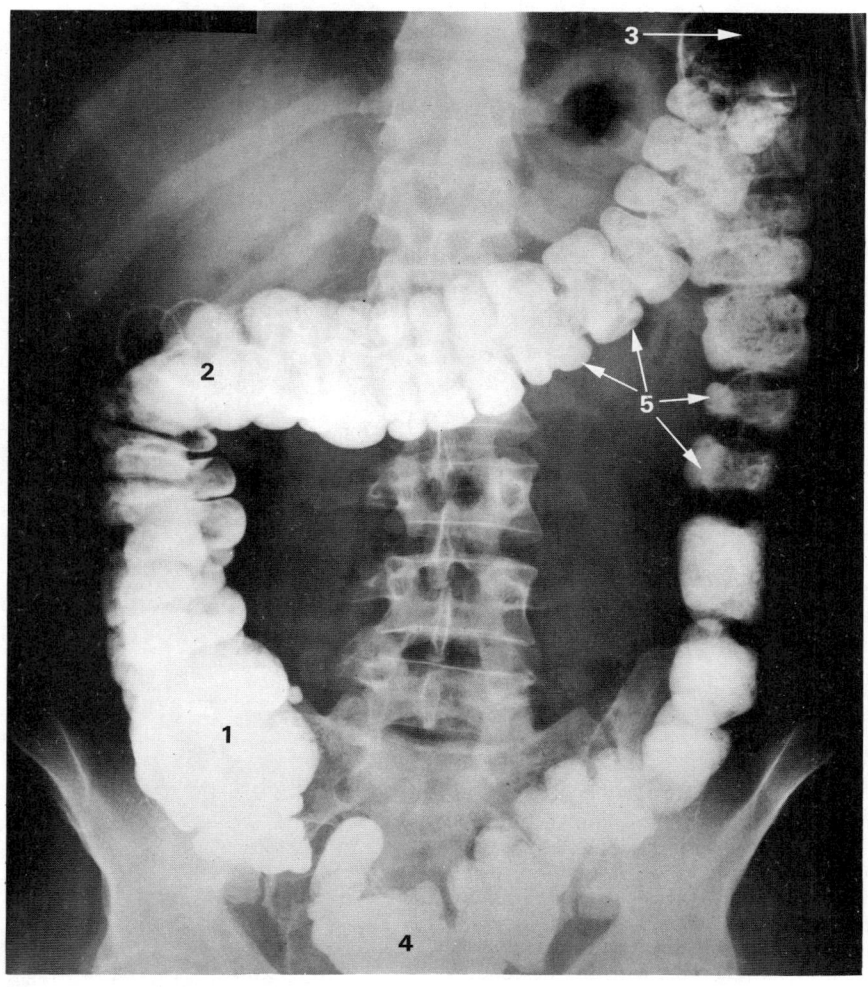

12.118   A radiograph of the abdomen after the administration of a barium enema which has filled the whole of the large intestine as far as the caecum and ileocaecal valve. (1) the caecum; (2) the right or hepatic flexure of the colon, which is much inferior to (3) the left or splenic flexure of the colon; (4) the sigmoid colon; (5) the sacculations, or haustrations, which are clearly visible throughout most of the colon.

then up and left to a point just superolateral to the intersection of the left lateral and transpyloric planes. A precise projection is difficult to define, varying much even in the same individual. Commonly it is in the lower umbilical or upper hypogastric region. It frequently descends in a V-shaped manner, the apex being well below the level of the iliac crests (p. 1734). In a radiological assessment in the upright position, its lowest level in 1000 young adults was found to vary much, even reaching the true pelvis; levels varied as much as 17 cm in the same individual between upright and recumbent positions (Moody 1927).

The posterior surface at its right end is devoid of peritoneum and is attached by loose connective tissue to the front of the descending part of the duodenum and the head of the pancreas; but from the latter to the left colic flexure it is almost completely invested by peritoneum, connecting it to the anterior border of the body of the pancreas by the *transverse mesocolon*. Above the transverse colon are the liver and gallbladder, the greater gastric curvature and the lateral end of the spleen; below is the small intestine, in front are the posterior layers of the greater omentum and behind are the descending part of the duodenum, the head of the pancreas, the upper end of the mesentery, the duodenojejunal flexure and coils of the jejunum and ileum.

Left colic flexure (12.96). This is the junction of the transverse colon and descending colon in the left hypochondriac region; it is related to the lower part of the spleen and pancreatic tail above and medially with the front of the left kidney. It is so acute that the end of the transverse colon usually overlaps the front of the descending colon. The left flexure is above and on a more posterior plane than the right flexure and is attached to the diaphragm level with the

tenth and eleventh ribs by the *phrenicocolic ligament*, which lies below the anterolateral pole of the spleen (p. 1743).

Descending colon (12.96). About 25 cm long, it descends through the left hypochondriac and lumbar regions, at first following the lower part of the lateral border of the left kidney and then descending in the angle between the psoas major and quadratus lumborum to the iliac crest; it then curves downwards and medially in front of the iliacus and psoas major to end in the sigmoid colon at the inlet of the lesser pelvis. (It is sometimes described as ending at the iliac crest, the part between this and the pelvic inlet being named the *iliac colon*.) In surface projection (**12.**117) it descends just lateral to the left lateral plane, from a little above and left of the intersection of the transpyloric and left lateral planes as far as the inguinal ligament. Peritoneum covers all but its posterior surface, which is connected by loose connective tissue to fascia over the inferolateral region of the left kidney, the aponeurosis of transversus abdominis, the quadratus lumborum, iliacus and psoas major (**12.**96). Crossing behind it are the following left structures: subcostal vessels and nerve, iliohypogastric and ilio-inguinal nerves, fourth lumbar artery (usually), the lateral femoral cutaneous, femoral and genitofemoral nerves, the testicular (or ovarian) vessels and the external iliac artery. The descending colon is smaller in calibre, more deeply placed, and more frequently covered behind by peritoneum than the ascending colon (p. 1776). Anteriorly are the coils of the jejunum, except for its lower part which is palpable when the abdominal muscles are relaxed.

Sigmoid colon (pelvic colon) (12.119). It begins at the pelvic inlet, continuing in the descending part; it forms a variable loop of about 40 cm and is normally in the lesser pelvis. The loop first descends in contact with the left pelvic wall, then crosses the pelvic

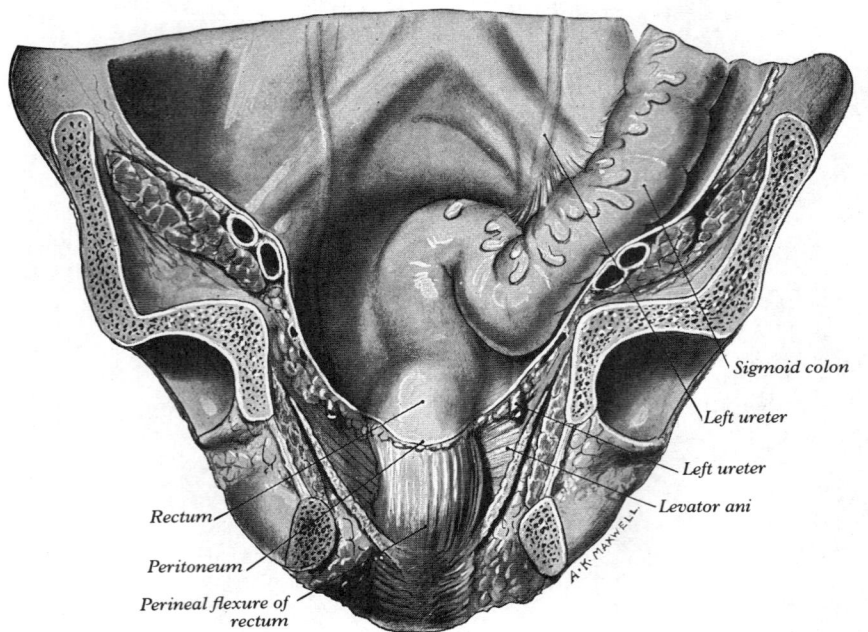

12.119   Oblique coronal section through the pelvis to expose the anterior aspect of the rectum.

cavity between the rectum and bladder in males, and rectum and uterus in females, and may reach the right pelvic wall; finally it turns back to the midline level with the third piece of the sacrum, where it bends downwards and ends in the rectum. It is closely surrounded by peritoneum, forming a mesentery, the *sigmoid mesocolon* (p. 1743), which diminishes in length from the centre towards its ends, where it disappears; the loop is fixed at its junctions with the descending colon and rectum but quite mobile between them. Its relations are therefore variable. **Laterally** are: the left external iliac vessels, the obturator nerve, ovary or ductus deferens and the lateral pelvic wall; **posteriorly** the left internal iliac vessels, ureter, piriformis and sacral plexus; **inferiorly** the bladder in males or uterus and bladder in females; **superiorly** and to the **right** it is in contact with terminal coils of the ileum.

The position and shape of the sigmoid colon vary much, depending on:

- its length
- the length and mobility of its mesocolon
- the degree of distension (when distended it rises into the abdominal cavity, sinking again into the lesser pelvis when empty)
- the condition of the rectum, bladder and uterus (when these are distended the sigmoid colon tends to rise and to fall when they are empty).

Racial variation has been noted (Lisowski 1969): in some groups, particularly Ethiopians, the incidence of a suprapelvic loop, perhaps conducive to volvulus, is particularly high.

RECTUM

The rectum (**12.**119, 120, 121) is continuous with the sigmoid colon at the level of the third sacral vertebra, the junction being at the lower end of the sigmoid mesocolon. The rectum descends along the sacrococcygeal concavity, with an anteroposterior curve, the *sacral flexure* of the rectum. It thus curves down and back, then downwards, and finally down and forwards to join the anal canal by passing through the pelvic diaphragm (p. 830). The *anorectal junction* is 2–3 cm in front of and slightly below the tip of the coccyx; from this level (in males opposite the apex of the prostate) the anal canal passes down and backwards from the lower end of the rectum, this backward bend of the gut being termed the *perineal flexure* of the rectum. The rectum also deviates in three lateral curves: the upper is convex to the right, the middle (the most prominent) bulges to the

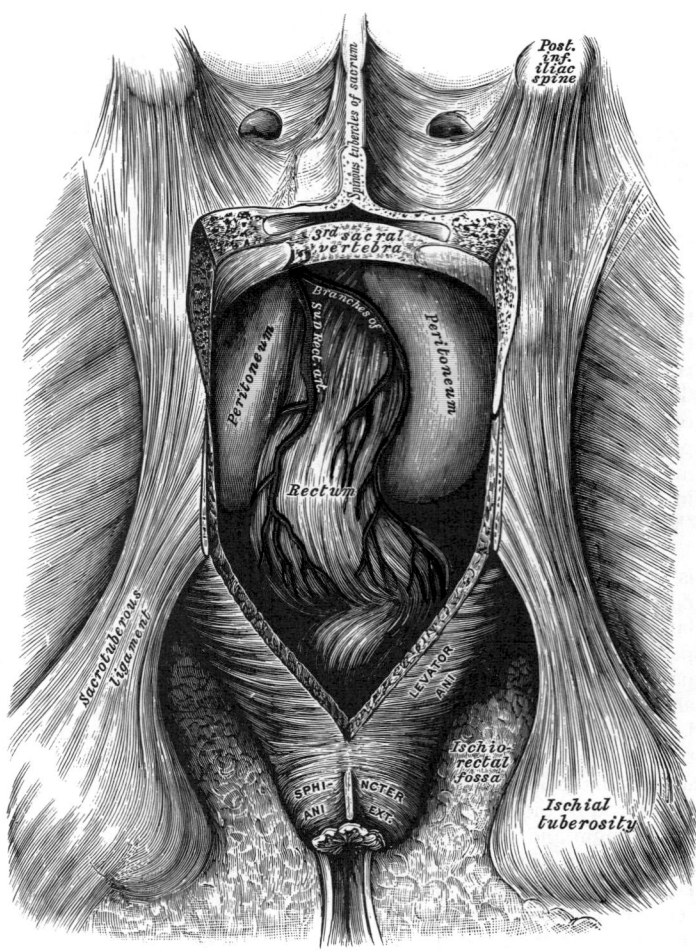

12.120   Posterior aspect of the rectum exposed by removal of the lower part of the sacrum and coccyx. Note the superior rectal artery (red) and peritoneum of the pararectal fossae (blue).

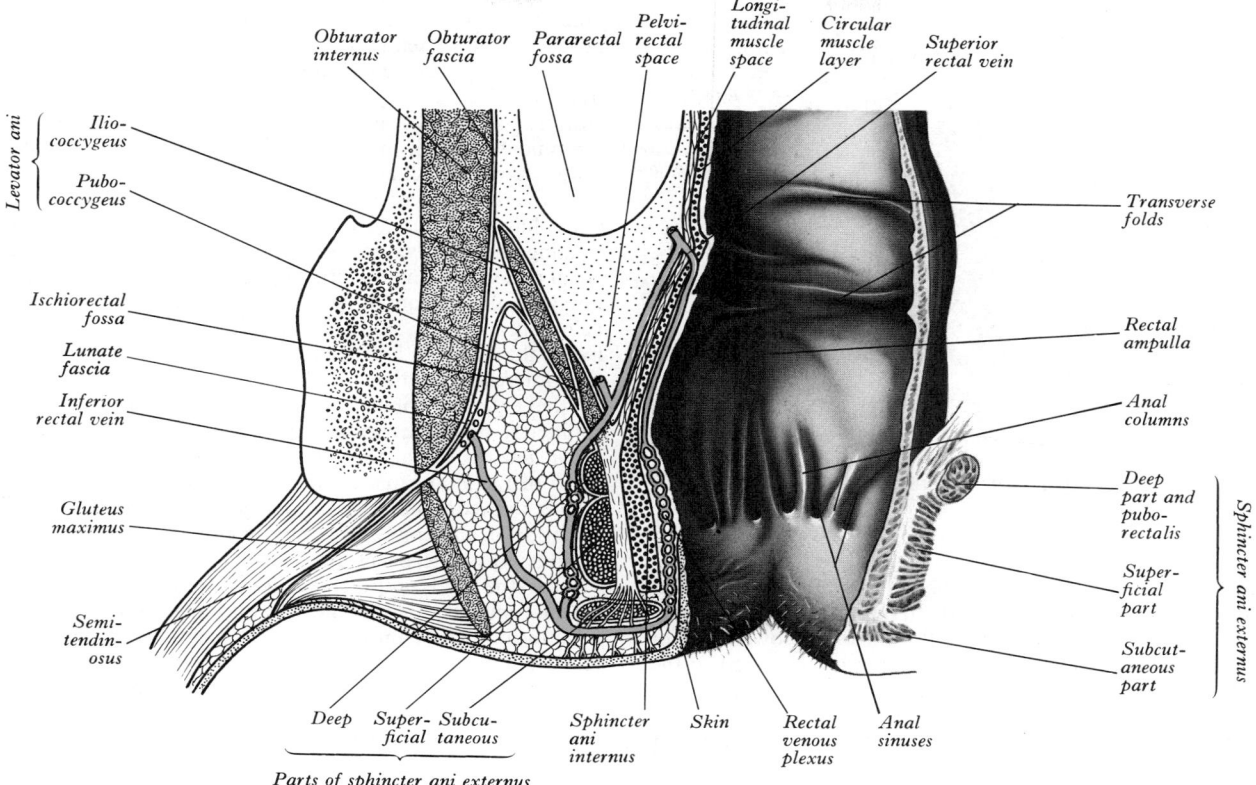

12.121 Diagram of a coronal section of the rectum and anal canal and the adjacent structures (adapted from Rauber-Kopsch, *Lehrbuch und Atlas der Anatomie des Menschen*, 1919). The internal pudendal vessels, the dorsal nerve of the penis and the perineal nerve are shown transected in the lateral wall of the ischiorectal fossa, where they are traversing the 'lunate fascia' (pudendal canal).

left and the lower is convex to the right. Both ends of the rectum are in the median plane.

The rectum is about 12 cm long, with the same diameter as the sigmoid colon above (about 4 cm in the empty state), but its lower part is dilated as the *rectal ampulla*. The rectum differs from the sigmoid colon in having no sacculations, appendices epiploicae or mesentery; the taeniae blend about 5 cm above the rectosigmoid junction, forming two wide muscular bands which descend, anterior and posterior, in the rectal wall. The peritoneum is related only to the upper two-thirds, covering its front and sides above, and lower down only its front, from which it is reflected on to the bladder in males, forming the rectovesical pouch, and on to the posterior vaginal wall in females, forming the recto-uterine pouch. The level of this reflexion is higher in males, the rectovesical pouch being about 7.5 cm (about the length of the index finger) from the anus; in females the recto-uterine pouch is about 5.5 cm from the anus. In the male fetus, peritoneum extends on to the front of the rectum as far as the lower limit of the prostate (p. 1859). On the sigmoid colon, peritoneum is firmly attached to the muscle layer by fibrous connective tissue but as it descends on to the rectum it is more loosely attached by fatty connective tissue, allowing for considerable expansion.

In the empty rectum, the mucosa in its lower part presents a number of longitudinal folds which become effaced during distension. There are also permanent semilunar *transverse* or *horizontal folds*, most marked in rectal distension. Two forms of horizontal fold have been recognized (Jit 1961); one consists of the mucosa, a circular muscle layer and part of the longitudinal muscle, and an indentation on the rectal exterior; the other is devoid of longitudinal muscle and has no external marking. Their number is variable but there are commonly three folds. An upper one, near the beginning of the rectum, may be either on the left or right; occasionally it encircles the gut, constricting its lumen. The middle fold is largest and most constant; it lies immediately above the ampulla, projecting from the anterior and right wall just below the level of the anterior peritoneal reflexion; the circular muscle is more marked in this fold than in the

others. The lowest fold, inconstant and on the left, is about 2.5 cm below the middle fold. Sometimes a fourth occurs on the left about 2.5 cm above the middle fold.

It has been suggested (Paterson 1912) that the rectum consists of two functional parts, above and below the middle fold, the upper containing faeces and being free to distend into the peritoneal cavity, the lower more confined, enclosed in a tube of condensed extraperitoneal tissue and (except during defaecation) normally empty; in chronic constipation or after death it may contain faeces. (Note that the rectum above the middle fold is considered to develop from the hindgut and the part below, with the upper anal canal, to originate from the cloaca or postallantoic gut.) Others (O'Beirne 1833; Hurst 1919) have considered the sigmoid colon a faecal reservoir, the rectum being normally empty and the entry of faeces into it exciting defaecation. Experimental distension of the rectum and anal canal results in the desire to defaecate and causes the relaxation of the anal sphincters (Denny-Brown & Robertson 1935).

Relations of the rectum

Posterior to the rectum in the median plane are: the lower three sacral vertebrae, coccyx, median sacral vessels, ganglion impar and branches of the superior rectal vessels; while on each side, particularly on the left, are: the piriformis, the anterior rami of the lower three sacral and coccygeal nerves, sympathetic trunk, lower lateral sacral vessels, the coccygei and the levatores ani. The rectum is attached to the sacrum along the lines of the anterior sacral foramina by fibrous connective tissue enclosing: the sacral nerves and the pelvic splanchnic nerves from the anterior rami of the second to fourth sacral nerves, which join the pelvic plexuses on the rectal wall; rami of the superior rectal vessels, lymphatic vessels, lymph nodes; and loose perirectal fat. **Anterior in males** above the site of the peritoneal reflexion from the rectum are the upper parts of the base of the bladder and of the seminal vesicles, the rectovesical pouch and its contents (terminal coils of the ileum and sigmoid colon); below the reflexion are: the lower parts of the base of the bladder and of the seminal vesicles, deferent ducts, terminal parts of the ureters and

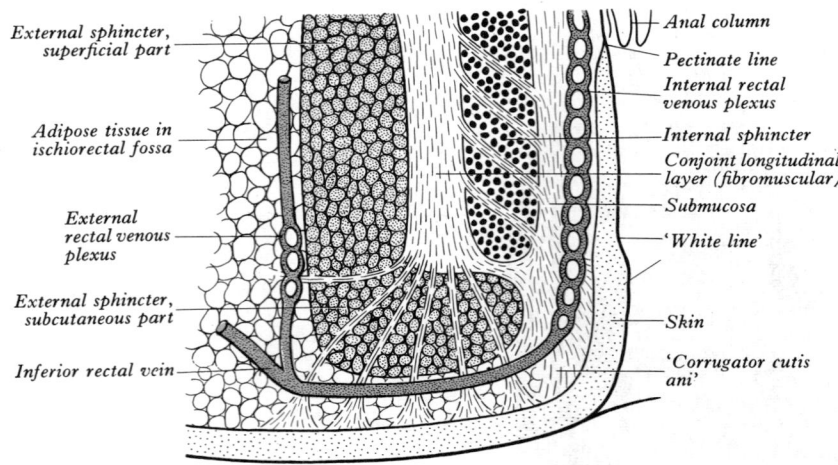

External sphincter, superficial part

Adipose tissue in ischiorectal fossa

External rectal venous plexus

External sphincter, subcutaneous part

Inferior rectal vein

Anal column

Pectinate line

Internal rectal venous plexus

Internal sphincter

Conjoint longitudinal layer (fibromuscular)

Submucosa

'White line'

Skin

'Corrugator cutis ani'

12.122   Part of **12**.121 enlarged to show greater detail.

the prostate. **In females**, above the reflexion are: the uterus, upper vagina, recto-uterine pouch and contents (terminal coils of the ileum and sigmoid colon), while below the reflexion is the lower part of the vagina. **Laterally**, the upper part of the rectum is related to the pararectal fossa and contents (sigmoid colon or lower ileum), while below the peritoneal reflexion laterally are the pelvic sympathetic plexuses, coccygei and levatores ani and branches of the superior rectal vessels.

ANAL CANAL (**12**.121–123)

The anal canal (Milligan et al 1937; Gabriel 1945; Wilde 1949; Goligher et al 1955; Fowler 1957) begins where the rectal ampulla suddenly narrows, passing down and backwards to the anus (**12**.121, 122). It is about 4 cm long in adults, its anterior wall being slightly shorter than its posterior. When empty its lumen is a sagittal or triradiate longitudinal slit. **Posterior** is a mass of fibromuscular tissue, the *anococcygeal ligament*, separating it from the tip of the coccyx; **anteriorly** it is separated by the *perineal body* (p. 833) from the membranous urethra and penile bulb or from the lower vagina; **laterally** are the ischiorectal fossae. Over its whole length it is surrounded by sphincters which normally keep it closed.

Lining of the anal canal

The lining of the anal canal varies along its course. The mucosa of the lower part of the rectum is pale pink and semitransparent, the branching pattern of the superior rectal vessels being visible through it. The upper half (15 mm) of the anal canal is also lined by mucosa, plum-red in colour due to blood in the subjacent internal rectal venous plexus. The epithelium is variable. In the upper part it is similar to that of the rectum, consisting of simple columnar cells, some secretory and others absorptive, with numerous tubular glands or crypts. In the lower half, this gives way to non-keratinized stratified squamous epithelium of the perianal epidermis (Walls 1958). In this part of the canal are 6–10 vertical folds, the *anal columns*, well marked in children but sometimes less defined in adults (**12**.121). Each column contains a terminal radicle of the superior rectal artery and vein, these radicles being largest in the left-lateral, right-posterior and right-anterior quadrants of the wall of the canal; enlargements of venous radicles in these three sites constitute primary internal haemorrhoids. The lower ends of the columns are linked by small crescentic mucous folds, the *anal valves*, above each of which is a small recess or *anal sinus*. The sinuses, deepest in the posterior wall, may retain faecal matter and become infected, leading to abscess formation in the anal canal wall; anal valves may be torn by hard faeces, producing an anal fissure (p. 1782). Anal valves are situated along the *pectinate line*, opposite the middle of the sphincter ani internus and commonly considered to be the site of the anal membrane in early fetal life, thus representing the junction of the endodermal (cloacal) and ectodermal (proctodeal) parts of the canal. Small epithelial anal papillae may occur on the edges of the anal

valves, perhaps remnants of the anal membrane. However, the junction of ectodermal and endodermal parts may be at the lower border of the pecten (Johnson 1914).

The anal canal extends about 15 mm below the anal valves, as the *transitional zone* or *pecten*, whose epithelium is non-keratinized, stratified squamous and intermediate in thickness between that of the mucosa of the upper part of the canal and the epidermis in its lowest part; only the latter contains sweat glands. The transitional zone overlies part of the internal rectal venous plexus and is shiny and bluish. Its submucosa contains dense connective tissue, contrasting with the lax connective tissue in the upper half of the anal canal and suggesting the firm support and anchorage of the pectineal lining to the surrounding anal muscle. The transitional zone ends below at a narrow sinuous zone, the *'white line'* (of Hilton). In the living this 'line' is bluish pink and rarely visible (Ewing 1954), its only interest being that it is at a level between the subcutaneous part of the external sphincter and the lower border of the internal sphincter; digital examination in the living reveals an *anal intersphincteric groove* at this site. Below the white line, the final 8 mm or so of the anal canal is lined by true skin, dull white or brown in colour and containing sweat and sebaceous glands. There is much variation in the epithelial zones described above and frequently the various types interpenetrate, the zones being poorly defined.

Near the anal sinuses, *anal glands* (Fowler 1957; McColl 1967) extend upwards or downwards into the submucosa, occasionally penetrating deeply into the internal sphincter. Each consists of one to six spiral or straight tubules, sometimes branched, and lined by two or three layers of mucous secretory cells. The duct of each gland, lined by stratified columnar epithelium, opens into a small depression, an *anal crypt*. The glands are surrounded by lymphocytes in a form similar to lymphatic follicles and the submucosal smooth muscle is thick in their vicinity. Occasionally the termination of a duct is not canalized and secretions may then form a cyst. The glands are sometimes infected, producing an abscess or fistula. They vary widely in number and depth of penetration, even extending into the submucosa above the anorectal junction. For details of comparative anatomy and pathology see McColl 1967. In this study, 50 normal anal canals were examined; half had anal glands passing right through the internal sphincter; the average number of such extensions was four but the range extended up to 16. McColl considered that these human glands were not homologous with the *anal scent glands* of some other mammals.

ANAL MUSCULATURE (**12**.121, 122)

The anal walls are surrounded by a complex tube of sphincters which tightly occlude the anal canal except during defaecation. The muscular components are divisible into the internal and external anal sphincters (*sphincter ani internus* and *sphincter ani externus*) and the *puborectalis* muscle which is part of levator ani (p. 831). There are also longitudinal muscle components forming the *conjoint longitudinal coat*.

Sphincter ani internus (internal sphincter)

The sphincter ani internus is a thickened (5–8 mm wall) tube of circular smooth muscle representing a thickening of the rectal muscularis externa. It encloses the upper three-quarters (30 mm) of the anal canal, extending from the anorectal junction down to the white line which marks its lower border.

Sphincter ani externus (external sphincter)

The sphincter ani externus is a tube of skeletal muscle situated externally to the muscularis externa and surrounding the whole anal canal (**12**.121). It is usually described as consisting of three parts. These are, from superior to inferior, the *deep, superficial* and *subcutaneous* parts. However, a clear threefold separation has also been denied (Goligher et al 1955). In females according to Oh and Kark (1972) and Wendell-Smith and Wilson (1991) the muscle forms a single band anteriorly. In the present account we will follow the classical description.

Deep part. This is a thick annular band around the upper part of the internal sphincter; its deeper fibres blend inseparably with the puborectalis muscle (p. 831); anterior to the anal canal many of its fibres decussate into the superficial transverse perineal muscles, especially in females. Some posterior fibres are usually attached to the anococcygeal raphe.

Superficial part. This lies above the subcutaneous part and surrounds the lower part of the internal sphincter. Viewed from above it is elliptical, being attached anteriorly to the perineal body, and posteriorly to the coccyx (the posterior surface of its last segment) via the median anococcygeal raphe, and hence being the only part of the external sphincter attached to bone.

Subcutaneous part. This is a flat band, about 15 mm broad, circumscribing the lower anal canal; it lies horizontally below the lower border of the internal sphincter and superficial part of the external sphincter; it is deep to the skin at the anal orifice and inferior to the white line. Anteriorly a few fibres join the perineal body (or the superficial transverse perineal muscles); posteriorly some fibres are usually attached to the anococcygeal ligament.

Muscle fibre types. Histochemically the external sphincter is composed mainly of Type I (slow twitch) skeletal muscle fibres, which are well suited to prolonged contraction (p. 739), although there are more fast twitch (type II) fibres in children (Lierse et al 1993).

Puborectalis

The puborectalis, the most medial portion of levator ani (histologically skeletal muscle), a band of muscle which loops posteriorly around the anorectal junction, slinging it forwards towards the pubis; some of its fibres mingle with those of the deep part of the external sphincter while others join the longitudinal (smooth) muscle of the anal canal to form the conjoint longitudinal coat (see below). Some of its fibres also pass in front of the anorectal junction, although these are relatively few so that the muscular ring around the anorectal junction is thinner at the front than posteriorly.

The conjoint longitudinal coat

The conjoint longitudinal coat is a fibromuscular layer surrounding the anal canal and situated between the internal and external sphincters. It is formed at the anorectal junction by the fusion of the pubococcygeal fibres of levator ani with the longitudinal layer of the rectal muscularis externa (**12**.122). Distally, this layer is increasingly fibro-elastic; at the white line it breaks up into 9–12 circumferential septa which radiate outwards mainly through the subcutaneous part of the external sphincter to become attached to the dermis of the circumanal skin. These septa are composed largely of elastic fibres; the most peripheral of the septa extend between the subcutaneous and superficial parts of the external sphincter into the ischiorectal fat. The most central (juxta-anal) septum is said to pass between the internal sphincter and the subcutaneous part of the external sphincter to reach the anal lining at the white line as the *anal intermuscular septum*, producing an anal *intersphincteric groove*. Wilde (1949), Goligher et al (1955) and Fowler (1957), however, considered that the longitudinal fibres in this position (compared with those penetrating the subcutaneous part of the external sphincter) were too scanty to warrant a name, maintaining that the groove is due to the muscle masses of the internal sphincter above and the subcutaneous part of the external sphincter below and to the contraction of the latter.

Other fibromuscular structures of the anal canal

In the anal submucosa, inferior to the anal sinuses, is a layer composed of smooth muscle, yellow elastic fibres and collagenous connective tissue, derived mainly from strands of the conjoint longitudinal coat, which descends inwards between the fascicles of the internal sphincter (**12**.121, 122). Some of the strands end by turning outwards around the lower edge of the internal sphincter to rejoin the main longitudinal layer, but most continue obliquely downwards and inwards, then superficial to the subcutaneous part of the external sphincter, inserting into the dermis from the white line to well beyond the anus. These attachments corrugate the region so that the name *corrugator cutis ani* muscle has been attributed to it. However, there is some dispute about whether it is indeed a muscle: Wilde (1949) considered its fibres to be exclusively elastic, but Goligher et al (1955) noted smooth muscle fibres among them. Fowler (1957), finding no muscle fibres here, ascribed puckering of the perianal skin to the combined effects of levator ani and the subcutaneous part of the external sphincter.

The radiating elastic septa end in a network dividing the narrow cleft between the subcutaneous part of the external sphincter and the skin into a compact honeycomb-like arrangement of fibres, which may explain the severe pain produced by pus or blood collecting here, and the localization of a haemorrhage following the rupture of a vein from the external rectal plexus (p. 1309).

A *muscularis mucosae* has also been described in the anal canal immediately above the pectinate line and possibly extending below it (Jit 1974).

Actions of anal muscles in anal closure

Muscle tone in both internal and external sphincters keeps the canal and anus closed except during defaecation, their contraction increasing when the intra-abdominal pressure rises, e.g. in forced expiration, muscular straining, coughing, parturition, etc.

The external sphincter can also be voluntarily contracted to occlude the anus more firmly. It is likely that the external sphincter is more effective at closure than the internal, which appears unable to seal off the anal canal completely (Lestar et al 1992). Puborectalis, forming a sling around the posterior aspect of the deep sphincter, pulls the upper part of the canal forward to form the anorectal angle, thus assisting its closure.

In resting conditions the anal sphincters undergo periodic increased contractions at the rate of about 15 per minute, with some reversal of peristaltic action, presumably helping to prevent leakage, and returning faecal debris to the rectum.

Defaecation

During defaecation a number of co-ordinated actions occur in the muscles of the pelvic floor including the internal and external sphincters, levator ani, and other perineal muscles (Wendell-Smith & Wilson 1991). These have been studied using various imaging techniques including radiography, ultrasonography and magnetic resonance imaging (MRI) (see e.g. Kruyt et al 1991).

Prior to defaecation, faeces move from the colon by peristaltic action into the rectum (from which they are usually excluded except during this process), initiating the desire to defaecate; faeces as far proximally as the splenic flexure may be moved to the rectum in one defaecatory event. When defaecation itself commences, the anorectal (perineal) angle becomes less acute or straight as the puborectal muscle sling (p. 831) normally pulling it forward relaxes, facilitating the passage of faeces into the anal canal. A sitting posture also assists the reduction of the anorectal angle. The muscles of the pelvic floor including the external sphincter now relax, too, so that pelvic floor descends a little, and the muscles of the anterior abdominal wall and diaphragm contract to raise the intra-abdominal pressure. The internal and external anal sphincters then relax, and at the same time the anal canal shortens and widens (see Shafik 1986) due to the contraction of the longitudinal muscle of the conjoint longitudinal tract and recoil of related elastic tissue. Because of this shortening the lower end of the anal canal becomes everted so that during the peak of defaecation the lower border of the internal sphincter and thus the intersphincteric groove come to lie at the anal orifice, with the subcutaneous external sphincter now situated radially lateral to it. The internal surface of the canal also becomes everted so that its epithelial lining below the white line is presented at the body surface.

At the end of defaecation, the external and internal sphincters, puborectalis and perineal muscles contract again (the closing reflex), and these arrangements are reversed to restore the original length and shape of the anal canal, the anorectal angle and the closure of the anal orifice.

Innervation of anal muscles

The *internal sphincter* has an autonomic supply from sympathetic fibres running in the plexuses around the superior rectal artery and the hypogastric plexus; parasympathetic fibres enter from the pelvic splanchnic nerves (S2, 3, 4) (see also pp. 1282, 1297).

The motor supply of the *external sphincter* is from the inferior rectal branch of the pudendal nerve (S2, 3) and the perineal branch of the fourth sacral nerve (S4) (see also pp. 1282, 1288). *Puborectalis* has the same supply as the rest of levator ani, i.e. somatic motor axons from the fourth sacral nerve and the inferior rectal branch of the pudendal nerve (S2, 3, 4).

The conjoint longitudinal coat, being derived from the rectal smooth muscle and surrounding sphincters, shares their innervation.

The muscle co-ordination required for these complex activities depends on reflex control involving, for the smooth muscle of the internal sphincter, the enteric plexus and associated autonomic and visceral sensory nerves; for the skeletal muscle of the external sphincter, puborectalis and associated perineal muscles, regulation is partly reflex, and partly voluntary through the visceral and somatic afferents and somatic efferent nerves. Essential for all of these purposes are the rich sensory innervation of the rectal and anal canal linings, and proprioceptive fibres in the muscle and surrounding tissues (see p. 1781). Neural integration of these sensory inputs and appropriate motor control are performed at many levels in the nervous system including the spinal cord, brainstem, thalamus and cortex. These operations not only monitor and regulate the actual process of defaecation, but also engage in more subtle behaviours within the rectum and anal canal, e.g. in the separation of faeces from rectal gas, local adjustments to faecal consistency and quantities, self-cleansing movements in the rectum and anal canal and co-ordination with other actions of the perineal and abdominal muscles.

Dual embryonic origin of the anal canal

The anal canal is derived embryonically from two sources. The region above the anal valves arises from the endodermally-lined cloaca, whilst below this boundary it comes from the proctodeum, covered with ectoderm (see p. 191).

The cloacal part (above) is innervated by autonomic nerves; the arterial supply (Griffiths 1961) is mainly from the superior and middle rectal arteries, while the venous drainage is to the superior rectal vein, a tributary (via the inferior mesenteric vein) of the portal venous system. The lymphatics drain with those of the rectum (p. 1621).

The proctodeal part (below) is covered mainly by skin, and is hence innervated by spinal nerves (the inferior rectal), and its vasculature is also that of the body wall, namely the inferior rectal artery and vein, branches and tributaries of, respectively, the internal pudendal artery and vein. Likewise, the lymphatic drainage of this region joins that of the perianal skin and passes to the superficial inguinal lymph nodes.

The differing nerve supply of the two parts is apparent in the condition of haemorrhoids, which may be covered by skin inferiorly and mucosa superiorly; to thrombose these varicose veins by injection, a needle is inserted into the insensitive upper mucosal part rather than the lower part which is well endowed with pain fibres. Fissure in ano (tearing of anal valves) is very painful because it involves this lower part of the anal canal. In portal obstruction, the collateral circulation opened up by anastomosis between portal and system veins in the anal canal may cause these veins to dilate, predisposing to haemorrhage.

RECTAL EXAMINATION

On inserting the index finger through the anal orifice in rectal examination, the finger is first resisted by the subcutaneous external sphincter and then by the internal sphincter, superficial and deep parts of the external sphincter and the puborectalis; beyond this it may reach the inferior (or even middle) transverse rectal fold. Many structures related to the canal and lower rectum may be palpated.

In males through the anterior rectal wall (see **13**.32), the penile bulb and (particularly with a catheter in the urethra) the membranous urethra are first identified; about 4 cm from the anus the prostate can be felt and beyond this the seminal vesicles (if enlarged) and the base of the bladder (especially if distended). Posteriorly, pelvic surfaces of the lower sacrum and coccyx are palpable and laterally the ischial spines and tuberosities and (if enlarged) the internal iliac lymph nodes. Pathological thickening of the ureters, swellings in the ischiorectal fossa and abnormal contents of the rectovesical recess may also be detected.

In **females** the uterine cervix is palpable through the anterior rectal wall (see **14**.15A); its degree of dilatation during parturition may be assessed in this manner. Pathological conditions causing tenderness or changes in the shape, size, consistency or position of the ovaries, uterine tubes, broad ligaments and recto-uterine pouch may be detected.

In both sexes, tenderness of an inflamed vermiform appendix (if pelvic) can also be elicited.

RECTAL FASCIAE AND 'SPACES'

Parts of the pararectal pelvic fascia are composed of loose connective tissue, whilst others are denser, with particular orientations and attachments; the latter are often considered to be rectal 'supports' requiring surgical division to mobilize the organ. From the lower sacrum's anterior surface a strong avascular condensation proceeds to the posterior aspect of the anorectal junction (*fascia of Waldeyer*). Around the middle rectal vessels fascia extends from the posterolateral pelvic wall (level with the third sacral vertebra) to the rectum as the *lateral rectal ligaments*. Anteriorly, between the rectum and the seminal vesicles and prostate, the *rectovesical fascia* (p. 1859) is more loosely attached to the seminal vesicles and prostate than to the rectum and in rectal excision it must be separated from them.

In addition to the ischiorectal fossae (p. 832) several '*spaces*' of surgical importance are related to the rectum and anal canal. The *pelvirectal space* comprises the loose extraperitoneal connective tissue above the levator ani; it is divided into anterior and posterior regions by the *lateral rectal ligaments*. The *submucous space* of the anal canal is between the mucosa (above the white line) and the internal sphincter; it contains the superior part of the internal rectal venous plexus and lymphatics; above, it is continuous with the rectal submucosa, below with the *perianal space*, the lateral part of which is bounded above by the most lateral elastic septum traversing the subcutaneous part of the external sphincter. The septum divides the ischiorectal fossa into a superior part containing coarsely lobulated fat and a smaller, lower, perianal space containing fine, compact fat. The perianal space contains the subcutaneous part of the external sphincter, the external rectal venous plexus and terminal rami of the inferior rectal vessels and nerves. The radiating septa traversing the subcutaneous part of the external sphincter tend to divert pus in the perianal space to the anal canal at the white line or to the surface of the perianal skin, rather than to the main ischiorectal fossa. Since the perianal space surrounds the lower anal canal, pus on one side may spread around it.

MICROSTRUCTURE OF THE LARGE INTESTINE

The layers of mural tissue in the large intestine (**12**.82, 123) resemble those in the small intestine (p. 1767), except that villi are absent. The microscopic appearance of the anal canal is described on p. 1780.

Mucosa

The mucosa is pale, smooth, and, in the colon, raised into numerous crescentic folds between the sacculi; in the rectum it is thicker, darker, more vascular, and more loosely attached to the submucosa.

Epithelium of the caecum, colon and upper rectum (**12**.123–127). This consists of the following at the luminal surface: columnar cells, mucous (goblet) cells, and occasional microfold cells (p. 1443) overlying lymphoid follicles. Columnar and mucous cells are also present in the intestinal glands which additionally contain stem and enteroendocrine cells (see below). Ultrastructural details of these cell types have been described by Pittman and Pittman (1966), Lorenzonn & Trier (1968) and Altmann (1989), and may be summarized briefly as follows.

Columnar cells (vacuolar absorptive cells). These are the most numerous of the epithelial cell types; they are responsible for ionic exchange and other transepithelial transport activities in the colon, including ionic regulation and water resorption. Although there is some variation in their structure, they all bear apical microvilli, somewhat shorter and less regular than on small intestinal enterocytes, but otherwise similar in structural organization. Many of these cells also contain secretory granules in their apical cytoplasm; their secretion appears to be largely mucins, but is also rich in antibodies of the IgA type. All cells have typical junctional complexes around their apices, limiting extracellular diffusion from the lumen into the intestine wall.

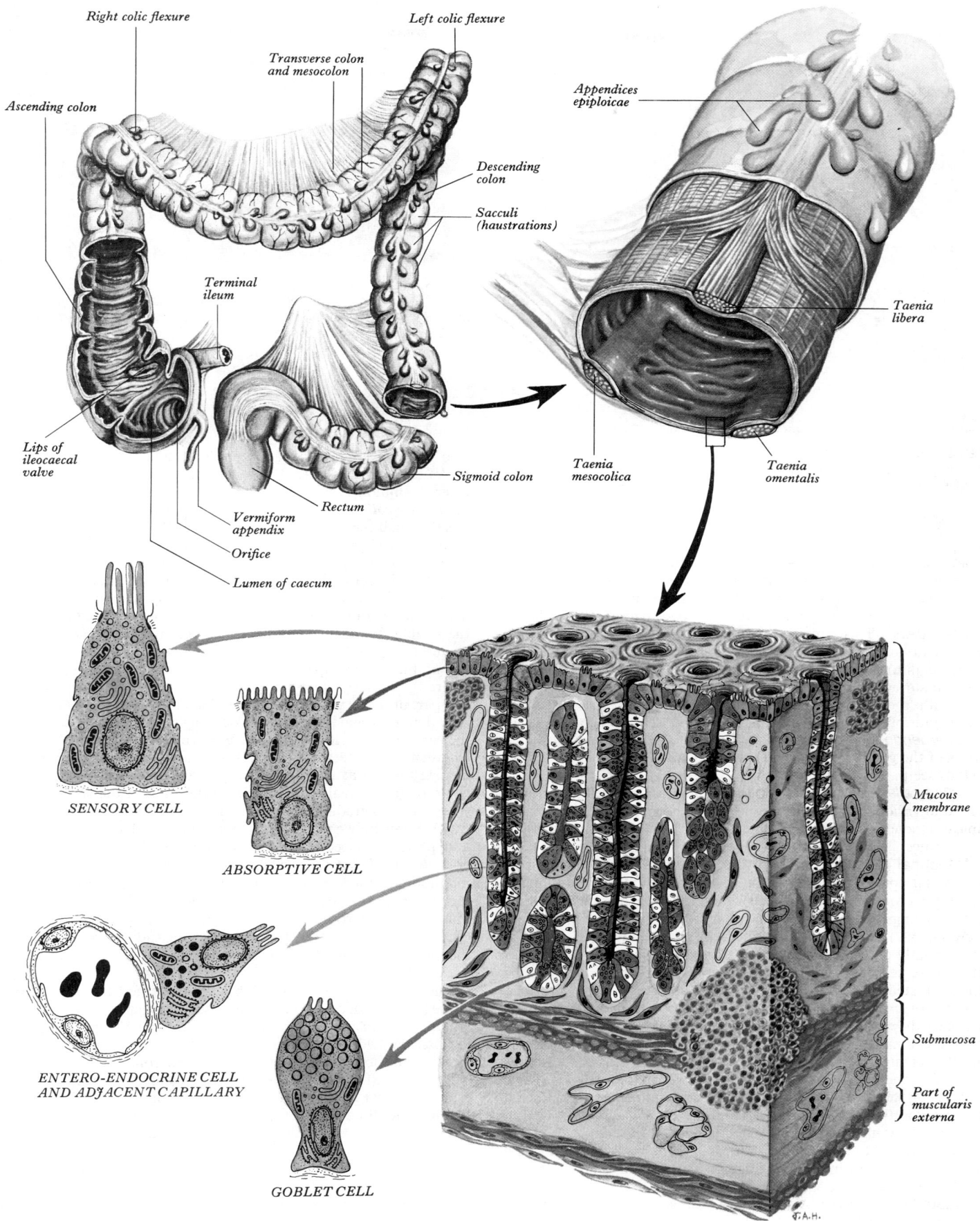

12.123 Diagrams of the disposition of the major regions of the large intestine, the micro-architecture and histology of the colonic wall and the ultrastructure of its epithelial cells. Note the aggregations of lymphocytes (shown in yellow) and undifferentiated epithelial cells (shown in white).

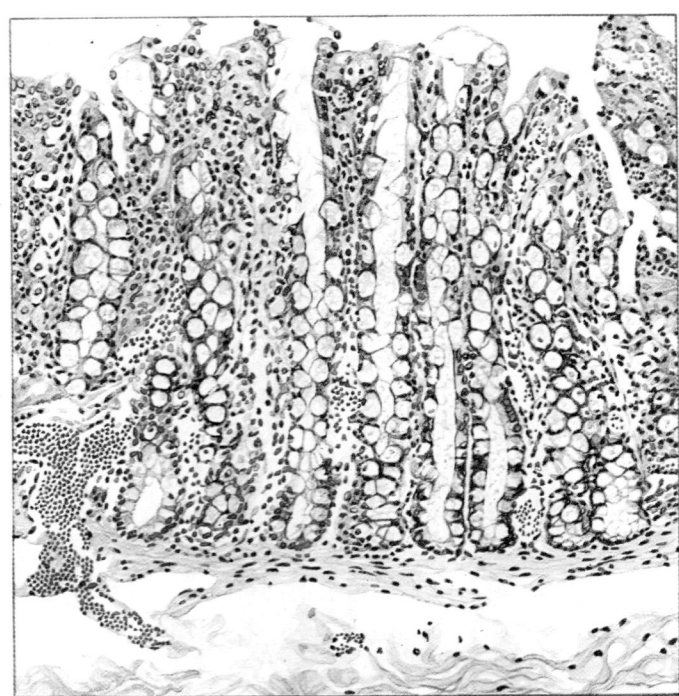

12.124 Section of the mucous membrane of the feline large intestine. Note the presence of large numbers of goblet cells and the vascularity of the mucosa. Stained with haematoxylin and eosin. Magnification c. × 100.

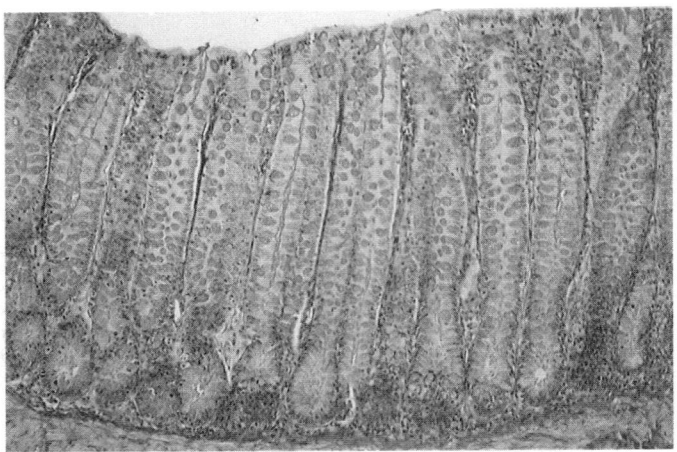

12.125 Medium-power light micrograph of the rectal mucosa showing crypts containing goblet cells. Stained with alcian blue/light green. Magnification × 80. (Material provided by D Ristow, Department of Anatomy, UMDS, Guy's Campus, London.)

Mucous cells (goblet cells). They resemble those of the small intestine, and they have a similar structure.

Microfold cells. Also similar to those of the small intestine, they consist of cells with long microvilli, lying over lymphoid follicles.

Stem cells. The source of the other epithelial cell types, they are located at or near the bases of the intestinal glands, undergoing periodic mitosis to give a stream of cells that migrate on to the luminal surface of the intestine and are shed (or otherwise disposed of) at the boundaries between individual glands (*extrusion zones*) (for details of kinetics, see Chang & Leblond 1971; Potten et al 1990)

Enteroendocrine cells (**12**.129). These are situated mainly at the bases of the glands, and secrete into the lamina propria. For further details see p. 1787.

Brush cells. An infrequent type of columnar epithelial cell, also found in various other mucosal sites in the body, these cells have an apical bundle of long, straight microvilli giving them a characteristic appearance. Their functions are unknown (see also p. 69).

Intestinal glands (crypts) of the large intestine. Narrow perpendicular epithelial tubules of mucosal epithelium, they are longer, more numerous and closer together than those of the small intestine; their openings give a cribriform appearance to the mucosa in surface view (**12**.127). The glands are lined by short columnar epithelial cells, mainly goblet cells (**12**.123–125), between which are columnar absorptive cells and enteroendocrine cells, and at their bases, the epithelial stem cells (Lorenzonn & Trier 1968).

Lamina propria. This is composed of connective tissue which supports the epithelium. Surrounding the glands is a specialized zone of connective tissue forming a fibrous sheath around each; here the fibroblasts migrate apically alongside the epithelial cells as they move from the zone of cell proliferation in the bases of the glands (Kaye et al 1968); they are thought to have directive influences on epithelial cell proliferation and migration. Solitary *lymphoid follicles* within the lamina propria are most abundant in the caecum, vermiform appendix (p. 1776) and rectum, but are also present scattered along the rest of the large intestine (Langman & Rowland 1986). They are similar to those of the small intestine (p. 1771).

Muscular mucosae. Also resembling that of the small intestine, it has prominent longitudinal and circular layers, and some slips of muscle pass towards the intestinal lumen between the glands.

Submucosa. This too is like that of the small intestine.

Muscularis externa

The muscularis externa has outer longitudinal and inner circular layers of smooth muscle. The longitudinal fibres form a continuous layer (Hamilton 1946) but are also aggregated as longitudinal bands or *taeniae coli* (**12**.96, 123), between which the longitudinal layer is less than half the circular layer in thickness. In the caecum and colon three taeniae appear, each varying from 6 to 12 mm in width. The *taenia libera* is anterior in the caecum, the ascending, descending and sigmoid colon, but inferior in the transverse colon. The *taenia mesocolica* is posteromedial in the caecum, the ascending, descending and sigmoid colon, but posterior in the transverse, being located at the attachment of the transverse mesocolon. The *taenia omentalis* is posterolateral in the caecum, the ascending, descending and sigmoid colon, but anterosuperior in the transverse colon, being located where the posterior (ascending) layers of the greater omentum meet this part of the large intestine. These bands are said to be shorter than the other intestinal layers, thus producing puckering or haustration of the caecum and colon into sacculi. When they are removed, the tube lengthens and loses its sacculation. In the descending colon the taeniae thicken at the expense of the rest of the longitudinal layer, while there is a real increase in its total bulk in the sigmoid colon, where the longitudinal fibres are more scattered. They form a layer which completely encircles the rectum, but are thicker on its anterior and posterior aspects, producing recognizable broad *anterior* and *posterior bands*. At the rectal ampulla a few strands of the anterior longitudinal fibres pass forwards to the perineal body (p. 833), as the *musculus recto-urethralis*. In addition, two fasciculi of smooth muscle pass antero-inferiorly from the front of the second and third coccygeal vertebrae to blend with the longitudinal muscle fibres on the posterior wall of the anal canal, forming the *rectococcygeal muscles* (Wesson 1951).

The circular fibres form a thin layer over the caecum and colon, aggregated particularly in the intervals between the sacculi; in the rectum they are a thick layer; in the anal canal they form the *sphincter ani internus*. Older observations of an interchange of fascicles between circular and longitudinal layers have been confirmed in a study of 112 cadavers (from early fetal life to 88 years); interchanges of fibres, especially near the taenia coli, are commonplace. Deviation of longitudinal fibres from the taeniae to the circular layer may, in some instances, explain the haustration of the colon (Pace 1968).

Serosa

The serosa or visceral peritoneum is variable in extent. Along the colon the peritoneum forms small fat-filled *appendices epiploicae*, (**12**.80, 96, 123) most numerous on the sigmoid and transverse colon but generally absent from the rectum. Subserous loose connective tissue attaches the peritoneum to the muscularis externa.

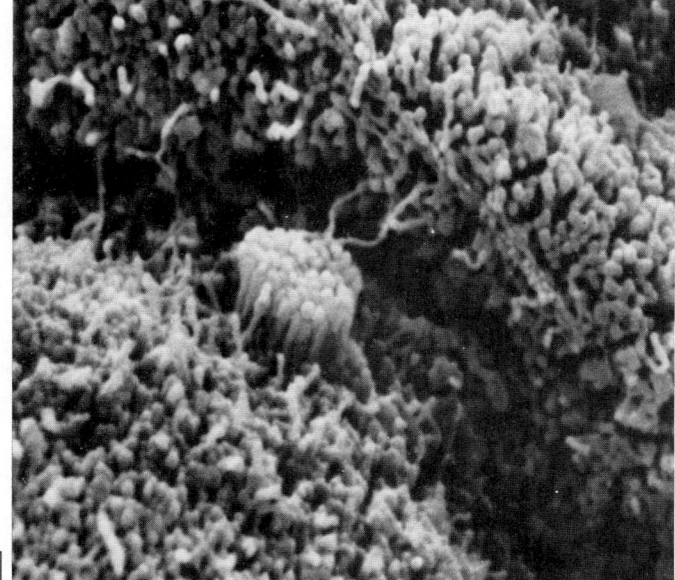

A

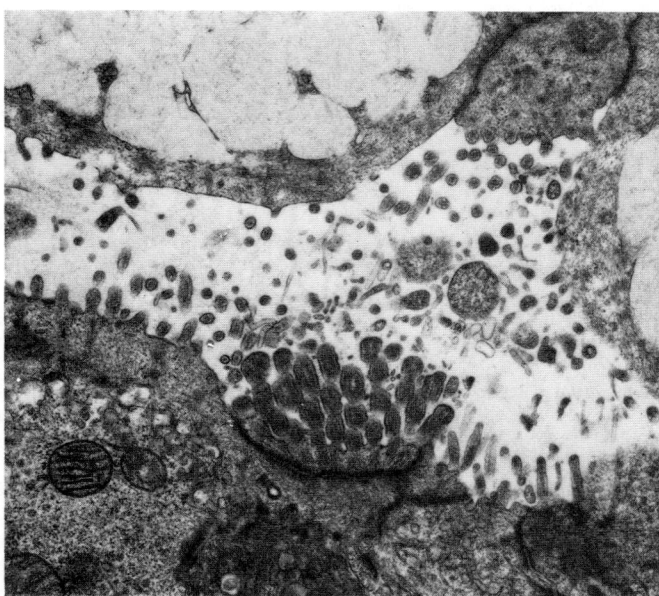

B

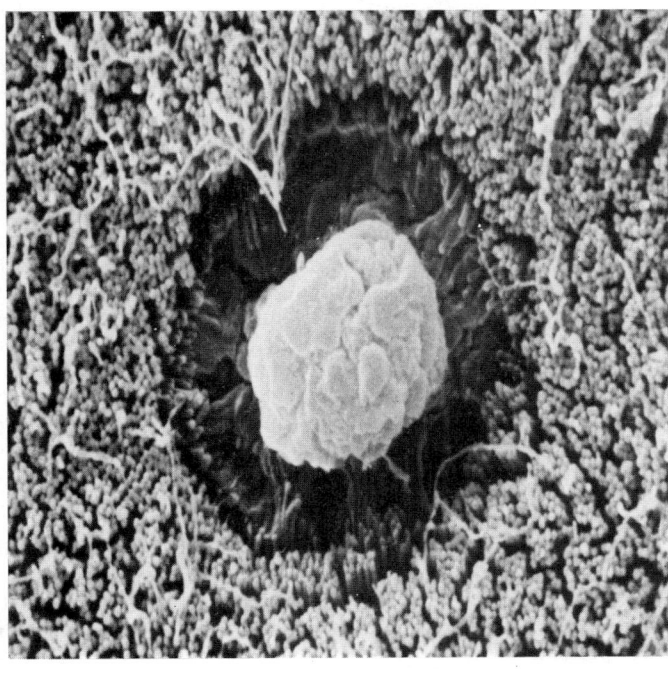

C

The large intestine also provides an environment for a large population of bacteria, some of which are responsible for the metabolism of organic compounds to supplement vitamin intake, especially Vitamin B_{12} and vitamin K.

Because of the frequency of carcinomas of the large intestine, there has been some effort to characterize its normal and pre-pathological structure in mucosal biopsies for diagnostic and prognostic purposes. These have involved morphometric analysis of cell numbers, shapes, gland frequencies, connective tissue components and other features which show alterations related to proliferative rates and metaplasia leading to pathogenesis. For details see, e.g. Hamilton et al (1987); Tipoe et al (1992).

VESSELS OF THE LARGE INTESTINE

Arteries

Those which supply the parts of the large intestine derived from the midgut (caecum, appendix, ascending colon and right two-thirds of the transverse colon) are derived from colic branches of the superior mesenteric artery; those supplying hindgut derivatives (left part of the transverse, descending and sigmoid colon, rectum and upper anal canal) are derived from the inferior mesenteric (and its terminal branch, the superior rectal) and the middle rectal arteries (a branch of the internal iliac). Their large branches ramify between and supply the muscular layers, divide into small submucosal rami and enter the mucosa. A small contribution also comes from the median sacral artery which is the terminal midline branch of the aorta. Rectal and anal canal arteries are:

- The superior rectal (the continuation of the inferior mesenteric). This is the main rectal vessel, dividing into two branches descending one on each side of the rectum, their terminal branches piercing the muscular coat to enter the rectal submucosa and descend into the anal columns as far as the anal valves, where they form looped anastomoses.
- The middle rectal arteries which traverse the 'lateral rectal ligaments' to supply the muscle of the lower rectum, anastomosing freely with each other but forming only poor anastomoses with the superior and inferior rectal arteries.
- The inferior rectal arteries (from the internal pudendals), which supply the internal and external sphincters, the anal canal below its valves and the perianal skin.
- The median sacral artery which supplies the posterior wall of the anorectal junction and of the anal canal.

Veins

These are the superior and inferior mesenteric, draining the regions supplied by the corresponding arteries. The veins of the rectum and anal canal are:

- The superior rectal veins, which pass from the internal rectal plexus in the anal canal and ascend in the rectal submucosa as about six vessels of considerable size to pierce the rectal wall about 7.5 cm above the anus, uniting to form the superior rectal vein, which continues as the inferior mesenteric.
- The middle rectal veins, from the submucosa of the rectal ampulla which drain chiefly its muscular walls.
- The inferior rectal veins, which drain the external rectal plexus and lower anal canal.

12.126A, B, C   A Scanning electron micrograph of the epithelium lining the colon (rat), showing a cell of suggested sensory function, bearing an apical tuft of particularly long microvilli. Magnification × 12 000. B Transmission electron micrograph showing part of a colonic epithelial cell bearing sensory microvilli. The smaller absorptive microvilli of adjacent cells can also be seen. Magnification × 14 000. C Scanning electron micrograph of the epithelium lining the colon (rat), showing a goblet cell surrounded by absorptive cells bearing microvilli. Magnification × 8000. (Prepared and photographed by Michael Crowder, Guy's Hospital Medical School, London.)

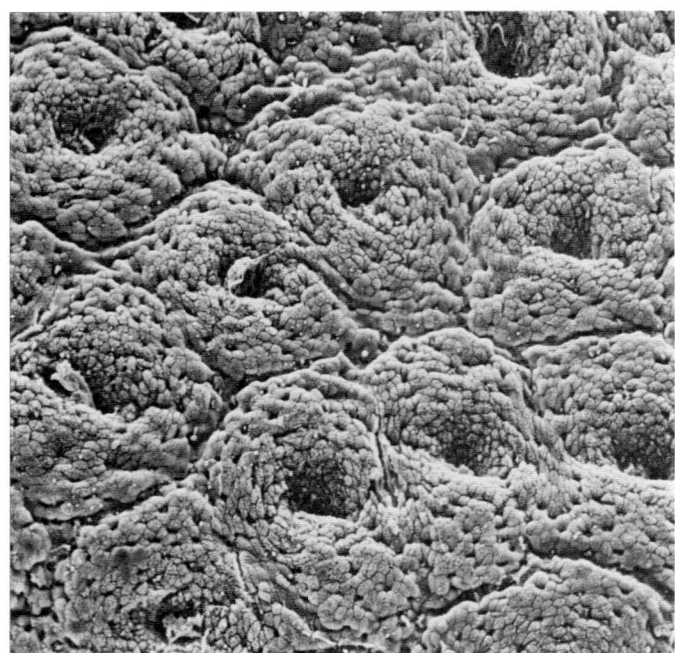

12.127 Scanning electron micrograph of the luminal surface of the human rectal mucosa. The outlines of cells bearing microvilli and the openings of rectal crypts can be seen. Magnification × 240. (Material supplied by D S Rampton; prepared and photographed by Michael Crowder, Guy's Hospital Medical School, London.)

Anastomoses occur between portal and systemic veins in the wall of the anal canal (p. 1604).

INNERVATION

Except in the lower anal canal, this is sympathetic and parasympathetic. The caecum, appendix, ascending colon and right two-thirds of the transverse colon (derivatives of the midgut) have a sympathetic supply from the coeliac and superior mesenteric ganglia, and a parasympathetic supply from the vagus; the nerves are distributed in plexuses around the rami of the superior mesenteric artery. The left third of the transverse colon, the descending and sigmoid colon, rectum and upper anal canal (derivatives of the hindgut) take their sympathetic supply from the lumbar part of the trunk and the superior hypogastric plexus by means of periarterial plexuses on rami of the inferior mesenteric artery. The sympathetic supply of the colon is largely vasomotor. The parasympathetic supply is from the pelvic splanchnic nerves (nervi erigentes), from which rami pass to the inferior hypogastric plexuses to supply the rectum and upper half of the anal canal: some fibres ascend through the superior hypogastric plexus to accompany the inferior mesenteric artery to the transverse, descending and sigmoid colon (p. 1308). Rami of the pelvic splanchnic nerves ascend on the posterior abdominal wall behind the peritoneum, independently of the inferior mesenteric artery, to be distributed directly to the left colic flexure and descending colon (Mitchell 1953). The ultimate distribution in the wall of the large intestine is as in the small intestine (p. 1772). Adrenergic and cholinergic activity in the nerve supply of the taenia coli, and distribution of the nerve fibres, suggest that (in guinea-pigs) few smooth muscle cells are directly innervated, propagation of excitation being chiefly through gap junctions between them (Bennett & Rogers 1967).

Sympathetic nerves to the rectum and upper anal canal pass mainly along the inferior mesenteric and superior rectal arteries and partly via the superior and inferior hypogastric plexuses, the latter supplying the lower part of the rectum and the internal anal sphincter. Parasympathetic rami from the pelvic splanchnic nerves (S2, 3, 4) pass forwards as long strands (about 3 cm long) from the sacral nerves to join the inferior hypogastric plexuses on the sides of the rectum, being motor to the rectal musculature and inhibitory to the

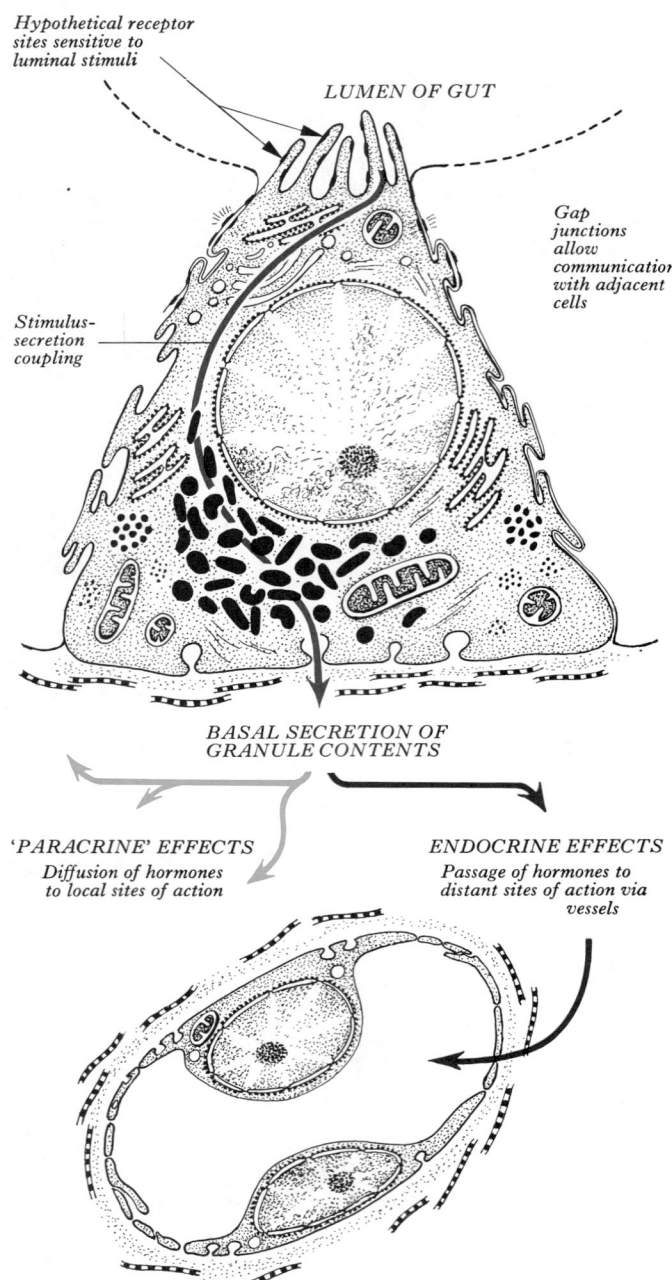

12.128 Diagram showing the ultrastructure and possible modes of action of an entero-endocrine cell.

internal anal sphincter. The external sphincter ani is supplied by the inferior rectal branch of the pudendal nerve (S2, 3) and the perineal ramus of the fourth sacral nerve (p. 1149). In rectal surgical excision, dissection must be kept close to its wall to avoid damage to these nerves with consequent bladder dysfunction and, in males, loss of penile erection. Afferent impulses mediating sensations of distension pass in afferent fibres in the parasympathetic nerves, pain impulses in the sympathetic *and* parasympathetic nerves supplying the rectum and the upper part of the anal canal. In colonic *aganglionosis (megacolon)* postganglionic neurons of the enteric nervous system (p. 1749) are reduced or absent in the colonic wall (Bodian et al 1961; Bodian 1966; Soltero-Harrington et al 1969). Garrett et al (1969) have studied the myenteric plexus and ganglionic neurons by electron microscopy and histochemical techniques for transmitter substances, reporting that in megacolon a variable diminution and sometimes absence of ganglion cells occurred, but that innervation of the muscle layers was defective even when ganglionic neurons were present.

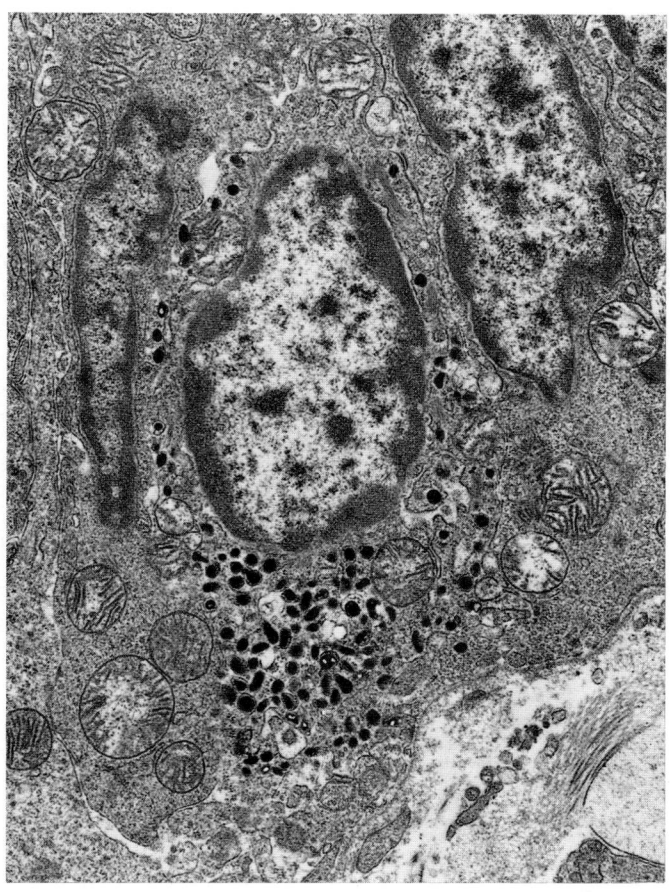

12.129   Transmission electron micrograph of an entero-endocrine (APUD) cell of the epithelium lining the colon (rat). Secretory vesicles can be seen towards the basal aspect of the cell. Absorptive columnar cells lie on either side of the APUD cell. Magnification × 11 000. (Prepared and photographed by Michael Crowder, Guy's Hospital Medical School, London.)

Lymph nodes and vessels

These are described on page 1621.

GASTRO-ENTERO-PANCREATIC ENDOCRINE SYSTEM (12.128–130)

The gastro-entero-pancreatic (GEP) endocrine (or enteroendocrine) system (Fujita 1973) consists of scattered, often solitary, hormone-producing cells of the gastrointestinal mucosa and pancreas.

The ultrastructure of human GEP endocrine cells has been detailed by Rubin (1972), Sasagawa et al (1973), Capella et al (1976) and Cavallero et al (1976) and summarized by Solcia et al (1981). Endocrine cells are scattered in the gastrointestinal mucosa, with their bases resting on the basal lamina. Their secretory granules vary in shape, size and ultrastructure in the different cell types, being usually infranuclear, while the Golgi complexes are supranuclear; luminal aspects of 'open' cells display microvilli of variable number, length and shape. Typical enteroendocrine cells are shown in (**12**.128, 129). Human *P cells* contain very small (100–140 nm) secretory granules slightly reactive to Grimelius' silver stain (Capella et al 1977); rare in normal adult tissues, they may contain a bombesin-like polypeptide (Polak et al 1976). *EC cells*, which contain osmiophilic, argentaffin, Grimelius' silver-reactive granules, are classified as EC_1, and EC_2 and EC_n; in addition to 5-hydroxytryptamine, the EC_1 cells store substance P (SP) (Heitz et al 1977), EC_2 cells store motilin (Polak et al 1975) and EC_n cells an unidentified material. The D_1

cells contain argyrophilic granules about 140–190 nm in diameter (Capella et al 1977) and store a VIP-like material. *PP cells*, common in the pancreatic islets but rare in the exocrine pancreas, store pancreatic polypeptide in granules of 150–170 nm; they are equivalent to F cells identified in other mammals (Baetens et al 1976). Human *D, B* and *A cells* are described with the endocrine pancreas (p. 1791). *X cells*, identified in human oxyntic mucosa by Solcia et al (1977), are of unknown function. Human *ECL cells* (Vassallo et al 1971) store a reducing amine, possibly 5-hydroxytryptamine, in granules with intensely argyrophilic cores; histamine may also occur. Human *G cells* (Vassalo et al 1971) manufacture gastrin and possibly enkephalin (Polak et al 1978), and have slightly argyrophilic granules with floccular contents. *S cells* (Capella et al 1976) are scattered in duodenojejunal mucosa and produce secretin (Larsson et al 1977); they are similar to D_1 cells but differ in their secretory product. Human *I cells* (Capella et al 1976), commonest in the duodenum and jejunum but rare in the ileum, are sources of cholecystokinin-pancreo-zymin (pancreaticozymin) (Buchan et al 1977). Human *K cells* (Capella et al 1976) contain large granules (approximately 350 nm in diameter) with osmiophilic, argyrophobic cores; like I cells, they are commonest in the duodenum and jejunum. K cells produce gastric inhibitory peptide. Human *N* and *L cells* are difficult to distinguish cytologically; granules of N cells are, however, generally homogeneous and about 300 nm in diameter, while those of L cells sometimes have argyrophilic cores and tend to be smaller (about 260 nm). N cells produce neurotensin (Orci et al 1976), L cells enteroglucagon or glicentin.

Concentrations of endocrine cells in the gastrointestinal mucosa are low and generally decrease progressively in an anal direction (**12**.130).

Certain common features of GEP endocrine cells allow other classifications. They all produce peptides and/or amines active as hormones or neurotransmitters and contain neuron-specific enolase, an isoenzyme of the glycolytic enzyme enolase (Polak et al 1980). They thus belong to the amine precursor uptake and decarboxylation (*APUD*) *cell series* (Pearse 1968, 1976, 1980) and modulate not only autonomic activity but also each other (**12**.130). The APUD concept is detailed elsewhere (p. 1899). The discovery of supposedly similar neurohormones and neurotransmitter peptides in cerebral neurons and some GEP endocrine cells, with other neuronal characteristics of the latter, has led to their designation as *paraneurons* (Fujita 1976). Peptides common to brain and gastrointestinal mucosa include: SP, somatostatin, VIP, bombesin, neurotensin, cholecystokinin (CCK) and the opiatoid enkephalin (Bloom & Polak 1978). GEP endocrine cells are presumed to have superficial receptor sites, stimulation of which by 'secretogogues' triggers stimulus-secretion coupling (Kanno 1973), as in chromaffin cells (Douglas 1968); they can thus also be termed *receptosecretory cells* (Fujita 1976).

The route of action of endocrine cells restricted to the gastro-intestinal mucosa remains in doubt. Their ultrastructure and proximity to capillaries suggest that their secretory products are endocrinal, exerting distant, diffuse effects via the blood. However, of their many products, only the following have been shown to act as circulating hormones: gastrin, secretin, cholecystokinin-pancreozymin, gastric inhibitory peptide, motilin and enteroglucagon (Bloom & Polak 1978). Basic differences exist between endocrine cells in gastric and intestinal mucosae and those in most other endocrine organs: they are not aggregated into glands but scattered among their local targets; most are close to the alimentary lumen, allowing their specialized plasma membranes to detect and respond to luminal stimuli; there are no common hyposecretory or hyper-secretory syndromes; relations between plasma hormone levels and functional response (e.g. modulation of neural control of gut motility) is not stoichiometric. Wingate (1976) has suggested that gastro-intestinal hormones may have local 'paracrine' **and** distant 'endo-crine' effects; direct actions on gastrointestinal smooth muscle, on adjacent endocrine cells, on other enterocytes and on local neurons are speculative but possible. Although the gut might be regarded as the largest endocrine organ (Pearse 1974), it is perhaps more properly regarded as a region in which neural, paracrine and endocrine controls of activity are intimately linked.

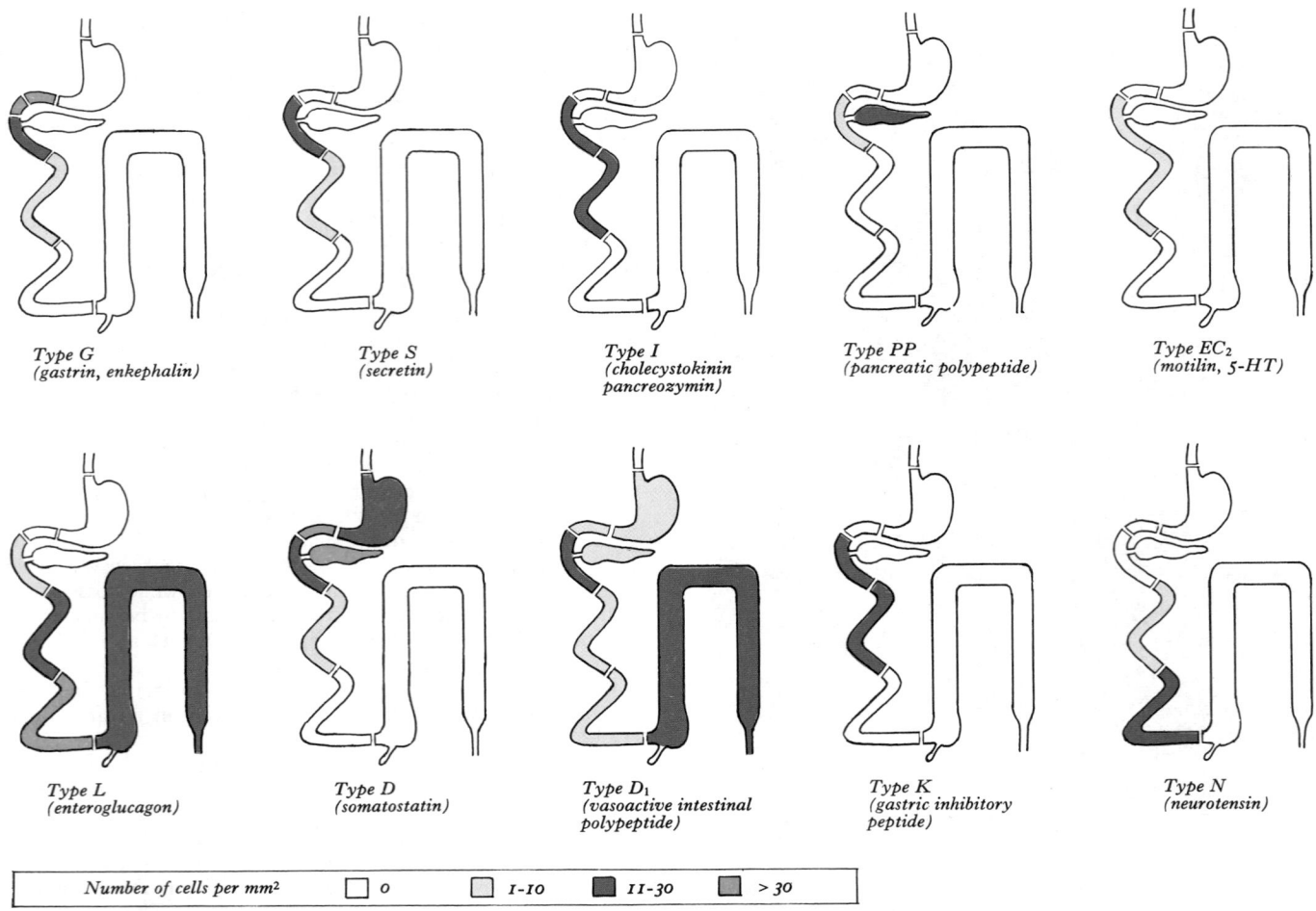

Type G
(gastrin, enkephalin)

Type S
(secretin)

Type I
(cholecystokinin
pancreozymin)

Type PP
(pancreatic polypeptide)

Type EC₂
(motilin, 5-HT)

Type L
(enteroglucagon)

Type D
(somatostatin)

Type D₁
(vasoactive intestinal
polypeptide)

Type K
(gastric inhibitory
peptide)

Type N
(neurotensin)

Number of cells per mm²	□ 0	▢ 1–10	■ 11–30	▥ > 30

12.130 Approximate quantitative distribution of a selection of human gastro-entero-pancreatic (GEP) endocrine cells (highly diagrammatic, after Bloom & Polak 1978, with permission from Churchill Livingstone).

Hernia

The rarity of rupture of the jejunum and ileum by external injury is due to their elasticity and mobility; the more fixed duodenum, particularly its horizontal part across the vertebral column, is more vulnerable. In external hernia the ileum is most frequently involved; in the large intestine it is usually the caecum or sigmoid colon. Omentum commonly protrudes into the hernia sac. Other abdominal viscera may rarely be involved (e.g. appendix, stomach, Meckel's diverticulum). The chief sites of hernia are inguinal, femoral and umbilical.

INGUINAL HERNIA

Here a viscus is protruded through the inguinal region of the abdominal wall. The principal varieties are oblique and direct.

OBLIQUE (INDIRECT) INGUINAL HERNIA

Here the involved viscus is pushed through the lateral inguinal fossa (behind the deep inguinal ring), preceded by a pouch of parietal peritoneum and extra-peritoneal connective tissue. It enters the inguinal canal at its deep ring and is invested by internal spermatic fascia enclosing the spermatic cord. As it traverses the canal it pushes up the arching fibres of transversus abdominis and obliquus internus, is covered by the cremasteric fascia and muscle and lies anterior to the cord. Emerging at the superficial inguinal ring, it is invested by the external spermatic fascia and also, as it descends into the scrotum, by superficial fascia and skin. The hernia may become constricted at the deep ring, with interference to its blood supply (strangulation). When this is relieved the deep ring should be cut superolaterally to avoid the inferior epigastric vessels. Most oblique inguinal hernias follow congenital defects in the processus

vaginalis (p. 212). Obliteration of this may be complete at birth or it may begin late and be completed only after birth; closure begins at the deep inguinal ring and epididymal head, extending until all of the intervening region becomes a fibrous cord. Complete or partial failure of closure of the processus entails variations in the relation of the hernial protrusion to the testis and tunica vaginalis; e.g. if the processus is fully patent, the herniated gut descends in front of the testis into the tunica vaginalis (*complete congenital hernia*); in this case, the processus and tunica form the hernial sac. In *incomplete congenital hernia* (hernia into the funicular process), the herniating gut descends to the top of the testis, where the processus is sealed off from the tunica vaginalis (**12**.131A, B). Although the above types are called congenital, actual extrusion into a pre-existing peritoneal sac may not occur until adult life and then be produced by an increased intra-abdominal pressure or sudden muscular strain. (For a critique of the anatomy of inguinal hernia consult Lytle 1979.)

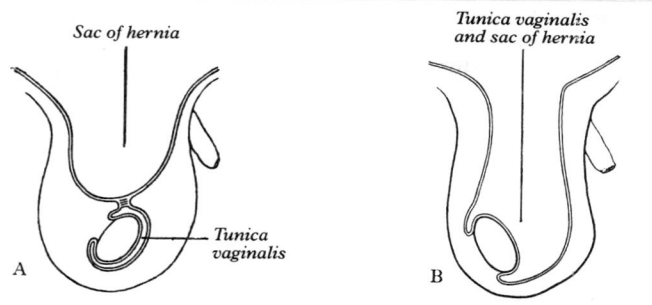

12.131 Diagrams representing varieties of oblique inguinal hernia: A incomplete congenital; B complete congenital.

DIRECT INGUINAL HERNIA

Here the protrusion is through some part of the inguinal triangle, which is bounded inferiorly by the medial half of the inguinal ligament, medially by the lower lateral border of rectus abdominis and laterally by the inferior epigastric artery. It overlies the medial inguinal fossa and, partly, the supravesical fossa (p. 1737). A direct hernia is through either:

- the *medial inguinal fossa*, where only extraperitoneal tissue and transversalis fascia separate the peritoneum from the aponeurosis of the external oblique or
- the *supravesical* fossa and *falx inguinalis* (conjoint tendon), which lies in front of the fossa.

In the first form, herniation is lateral to the conjoint tendon, propelling before it the peritoneum, extraperitoneal tissue and transversalis fascia to enter the inguinal canal, which it traverses to emerge from the superficial ring, covered by external spermatic fascia. Its coverings are like those of the oblique form, except that a part of the general layer of transversalis fascia replaces the internal spermatic fascia, the hernia being between the innermost and middle coverings of the spermatic cord. In the second, more frequent form, the hernia is either between the fibres of the falx inguinalis, or the falx is gradually distended to form a complete covering. The hernia thus enters the lower end of the canal, escapes at the superficial ring medial to the cord and is covered by external spermatic fascia, superficial fascia and skin. Its coverings differ from those of oblique hernia, the conjoint tendon replacing the cremaster and part of the transversalis fascia replacing the internal spermatic fascia. In all varieties the most superficial covering is the external spermatic fascia, the outermost covering of the cord. An oblique inguinal hernia is within the cord, sharing all its coverings; a direct hernia acquires an additional covering from the transversalis fascia.

Direct inguinal hernia occurs usually in males. Its neck is typically wide, so that strangulation is rare in males. Its main peculiarities are:

- it is sited above the body of the pubic bone
- the inferior epigastric artery is *lateral* (not medial) to the neck of the sac
- the spermatic cord is posterolateral, not directly posterior as in oblique hernia.

A direct hernia is always of the acquired type. The stricture in both varieties of direct hernia is usually at the neck of the sac or at the superficial ring. Where the conjoint tendon is split, constriction may occur at the edges of the fissure. In all cases of inguinal hernia, whether oblique or direct, it is correct to divide the stricture upwards, parallel to the inferior epigastric artery to avoid damaging that vessel.

FEMORAL HERNIA

A femoral hernia protrudes through the femoral ring (p. 1737), which is normally closed by a femoral septum of modified extra-peritoneal tissue and is therefore a weak spot, especially in females, where the ring is larger and subject to profound changes during pregnancy. Femoral hernia is hence more common in women. When a section of intestine bulges through the ring, it pushes out a hernial sac of peritoneum. It is covered by extra-peritoneal tissue (the femoral septum) and descends along the femoral canal to the saphenous opening, where it is prevented from descending along the femoral sheath by the narrowing of the latter, by the vessels and by the close attachment of the superficial fascia and sheath to the lower part of the rim of the saphenous opening (p. 873). The hernia hence turns forwards, distending the cribriform fascia and curving upwards over the inguinal ligament and the lower part of the external oblique aponeurosis. While in the canal the hernia is usually small, due to the resistance of its surrounds; but with escape into the inguinal loose connective tissue it enlarges. Thus a femoral hernia first descends, then ascends forwards; hence pressure to reduce it should be directed in the reverse order, with the thighs passively flexed for greatest relaxation.

Covering a femoral hernia are (from within outwards): the peritoneum, femoral septum, femoral sheath, cribriform fascia, superficial fascia and skin. A fibrous covering, the *fascia propria*, just outside the peritoneal sac but frequently separated from it by adipose tissue, may easily be mistaken for the sac, and its contained extraperitoneal fat for omentum; the fat may resemble a lipoma, but dissection will reveal the true hernial sac in its centre. The fascia propria is merely a femoral septum thickened to form a membranous sheet by hernial pressure. The intestine reaches only to the saphenous opening in *incomplete femoral hernia* in contra-distinction to *complete hernia* where it passes through the opening. The small size of an incomplete hernia renders it difficult to detect and therefore dangerous, especially in the corpulent. The site of strangulation varies: it may be at the hernial sac's neck; more often it is at the junction of the falciform margin of the saphenous opening with the free edge of the pectineal part of the inguinal ligament; or it may be at the saphenous opening (p. 873). The stricture should be divided superomedially for a distance of 4–6 mm to avoid all normally positioned vessels and other important structures. (However, an abnormal obturator artery may be a complication, see p. 1560).

The pubic tubercle is an important landmark in distinguishing inguinal from femoral hernias; the hernia's neck is superomedial to it in inguinal hernia but inferolateral in the femoral form.

UMBILICAL HERNIA

There are three varieties of umbilical hernia.

CONGENITAL UMBILICAL HERNIA

This is due to the failure of retraction of the umbilical loop of the gut (p. 190)

INFANTILE UMBILICAL HERNIA

This is due to stretching of umbilical scar tissue, usually within 3 years of birth, and is associated with increased intra-abdominal pressure.

ACQUIRED UMBILICAL HERNIA

Really this is a hernia through the linea alba, usually just above the umbilicus (para-umbilical hernia); it occurs most frequently in obese multiparous females.

Rarely, hernia may occur at other sites, e.g. through the *lumbar triangle* (p. 837), *obturator foramen, greater* or *lesser sciatic foramen* or *ischiorectal fossa. Incisional hernia* may occur at the sites of abdominal scars, particularly if the wound becomes infected. For further details of hernia and related surgical anatomy, see Chevrel (1987); for variations of medical and surgical importance in the small intestine and also in the colon consult Goligher (1967) and Kanagasuntheram (1970).

PANCREAS, LIVER AND GALLBLADDER

PANCREAS (12.96, 132–137)

The pancreas is a soft, lobulated, greyish-pink gland, 12–15 cm long, extending nearly transversely across the posterior abdominal wall from the duodenum to the spleen, behind the stomach. Its broad, right extremity or *head* is connected to the *body* by a slightly constricted *neck*; its narrow, left extremity is the *tail*. It ascends slightly to the left in the epigastric and left hypochondriac regions.

RELATIONS OF THE PANCREAS

The structures related to the pancreas are best considered with respect to its different parts (**12**.96, 132, 133, 134), as follows.

Head. Flattened anteroposteriorly, it lies within the duodenal curve. Its upper border is overlapped by the superior segment of the duodenum, the other borders being grooved by the adjacent margin of the duodenum, which they variably overlap in front and behind. Sometimes a small part of the head is actually embedded in the wall of the descending part of the duodenum. From the lower and left part of the head the hook-like *uncinate process* projects upwards and to the left behind the superior mesenteric vessels. In or near the groove between the duodenum and the right and lower borders of the head are the anastomosing superior and inferior pancreaticoduodenal arteries (pp. 1549, 1553).

Anterior surface. From the pancreatic head's anterosuperior aspect the neck juts forwards, upwards and to the left, merging with the body. The boundary between head and neck, on the right and in front, is a groove for the gastroduodenal artery; on the left and behind it is a deep incisure containing the union of the superior mesenteric and splenic veins to form the portal vein. Below and to the right of the neck, the head's anterior surface is at first in contact with the transverse colon, separated only by loose connective tissue; still lower the surface is covered by peritoneum continuous with the inferior layer of the transverse mesocolon (**12**.75), and is in contact with the jejunum. The uncinate process is crossed anteriorly by the superior mesenteric vessels.

Posterior surface. The head is related posteriorly to the inferior vena cava which ascends behind it and covers almost all of this aspect; it is also related to the terminal parts of the renal veins and the right crus of the diaphragm. The uncinate process lies in front of the aorta. The bile duct is lodged either in a superolateral groove on the posterior surface or in a canal within the gland's substance (p. 1810).

Neck. About 2 cm long, it projects forwards, upwards and to the left from the head, merging into the body. Its anterior surface, covered with peritoneum, adjoins the pylorus, with part of the omental bursa intervening; the gastroduodenal and anterior superior pancreaticoduodenal arteries descend in front of the gland to the right of the junction of the neck and head; the posterior surface is related to the superior mesenteric vein and the beginning of the portal vein.

Body. Prism-like in section, it has three surfaces: anterior, posterior and inferior (more precisely anterosuperior, posterior and antero-inferior; they are obliquely set).

Anterior surface. This faces anterosuperiorly, is covered by peritoneum continuous antero-inferiorly with the *anterior* ascending layer of the greater omentum (**12**.75) and is separated from the stomach by the omental bursa. On reaching the taenia mesocolica, the greater omentum's *posterior* ascending layer fuses with the anterosuperior surface of the transverse mesocolon, while the anterior layer continues up to the mesocolon's root and is then reflected up over the anterior surface of the pancreas.

Posterior surface. Devoid of peritoneum, it is in contact with the aorta and the origin of the superior mesenteric artery, the left crus of the diaphragm, left suprarenal gland and with the left kidney and renal vessels, particularly the vein. It is closely related to the splenic vein which courses from left to right and separates it from the structures mentioned. The left kidney is also separated from the perirenal fascia and fat.

Inferior surface. This is narrow on the right but broadens to the left and is covered by the peritoneum of the postero-inferior layer of the transverse mesocolon; inferior to it are the duodenojejunal flexure and coils of the jejunum; its left end rests on the left colic flexure.

Superior border. This is blunt and flat to the right, but narrow and sharp to the left near the tail. An *omental tuberosity* usually projects from the right end of the superior border above the level of the lesser curvature of the stomach, in contact with the posterior surface of the lesser omentum. The border is related above to the coeliac artery, its common hepatic branch coursing to the right just above the gland, while its sinuous splenic ramus runs to the left along this border.

Anterior border. This separates the anterior from the inferior surfaces and along this border the two layers of the transverse mesocolon diverge, one passing up over the anterior surface, the other backwards over the inferior surface.

Inferior border. This separates the posterior from the inferior surfaces, the superior mesenteric vessels emerging from under its right extremity.

Tail. Narrow, usually reaching the inferior part of the gastric surface of the spleen, it is contained between the two layers of the splenorenal (lienorenal) ligament, together with the splenic vessels.

Coeliac artery
Superior mesenteric artery
Portal vein
Splenic vein
Arch
Superior mesenteric vein
Common bile duct
Supr. mes. v.
Inf.
Related to spleen
Related to left kidney
Related to diaphragm
Duodenum
Related to inferior vena cava

12.132 Posterior aspect of the pancreas and duodenum.

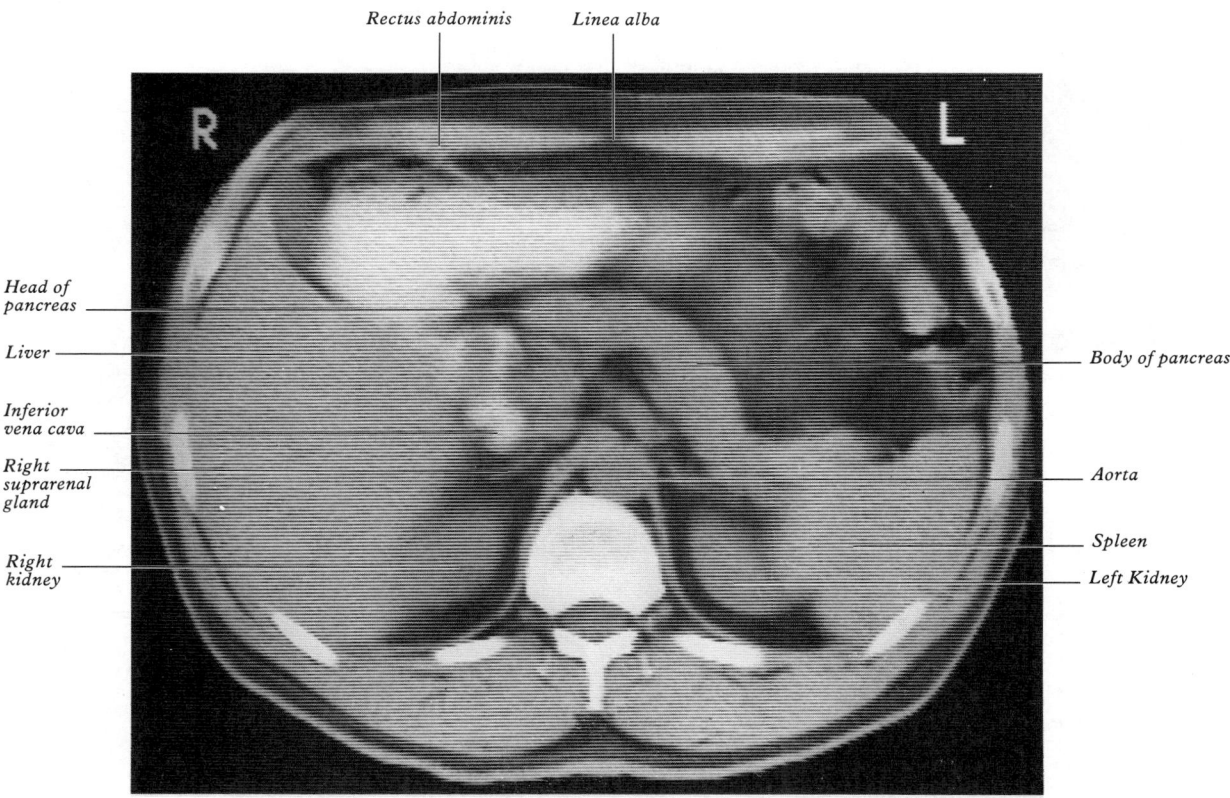

Rectus abdominis   Linea alba

Head of pancreas
Liver
Inferior vena cava
Right suprarenal gland
Right kidney

Body of pancreas
Aorta
Spleen
Left Kidney

12.133   Computed tomogram of the abdomen in the transverse plane at the level of the pancreas. (Supplied by Shaun Gallagher, Guy's Hospital; photography by Sarah Smith, UMDS, Guy's Hospital Campus, London.)

Main pancreatic duct. It traverses the gland from left to right, being nearer its posterior than its anterior surface (**12**.134). It begins by the junction of lobular ducts in the tail and, running to the right in the body, receives further lobular ducts which join it almost at right angles (a 'herringbone pattern'). Much enlarged, it reaches the neck of the gland, turning down, backwards and right towards the bile duct, which lies on its right side. The two ducts enter the wall of the descending part of the duodenum obliquely and unite in a short dilated *hepatopancreatic ampulla* or ampulla of the bile duct (p. 1810); the narrow distal end of this opens on the summit of the *major duodenal papilla*, which lies posteromedial in this part of the duodenum, and 8–10 cm distal to the pylorus. Usually the two ducts do not unite until very near the orifice on the major papilla. Sometimes they open separately. Frequently an *accessory pancreatic duct* drains the lower part of the head (**12**.134), ascending in front of the main duct, with which it communicates, and opening on a small rounded *minor duodenal papilla*, about 2 cm anterosuperior to the major. The duodenal end of the accessory duct may fail to expand; secretion is then diverted along the connecting channel into the main duct (Dawson & Langmann 1961).

Surface anatomy (12.98).

The head of the pancreas lies within the duodenal curve. The neck is situated in the transpyloric plane, behind the pylorus. The body passes obliquely up and left for about 10 cm, its left part lying a little above the transpyloric plane. The tail is a little above and to the left of the intersection of the transpyloric and left lateral planes.

PANCREATIC MICROSTRUCTURE (12.134–137)

The pancreas is composed of two different types of glandular tissues in intimate association with each other. The main mass is *exocrine*, embedded in which are *pancreatic islets* of *endocrine cells*.

Exocrine pancreas

The exocrine pancreas is a branched acinar (acinoracemose) gland, surrounded and incompletely lobulated by delicate loose connective

tissue (de Reuck & Cameron 1962; Beck & Sinclair 1971). Its pyramidal, acinar, secretory cells are arranged in flask-shaped or tubular groups. A narrow intercalated (intralobular) duct lies in each secretory mass, the initial parts of its walls being lined by cuboidal *centro-acinar cells*, later replaced by taller cuboidal and eventually columnar cells more distally. Larger, interlobular ducts are surrounded by loose connective tissue containing smooth muscle and autonomic nerve fibres. Enteroendocrine cells (p. 195) are present amongst the undifferentiated columnar ductual cells; mast cells are numerous in the surrounding loose connective tissue.

Acinar cells. Typical zymogenic cells, they have a basal nucleus and basophilic cytoplasm consisting of regular arrays of granular endoplasmic reticulum with mitochondria and dense secretory granules. A prominent supranuclear Golgi complex is surrounded by many larger, membranous granules containing the enzymic constituents of pancreatic secretion, only active after release. The orderly contents of the acinar cells have provided a widely used model for the investigation of routes of secretory synthesis and transport in protein-secreting cells at large (p. 30). After death, the action of pancreatic hydrolytic enzymes rapidly obscures cellular detail.

Ganglionic neurons (**12**.136) and cords of undifferentiated epitheliocytes also appear in the exocrine pancreas; the latter may provide stem cells for replacement of exocrine and perhaps endocrine cells. The structure of the exocrine pancreas and its control are summarized in **12**.134. For further details consult Webster et al (1977), Singh and Webster (1978), Case (1979) and Wormsley (1979).

Endocrine pancreas (12.135, 137)

This consists of *pancreatic islets* or *insulae* (of Langerhans), composed of spheroidal or ellipsoidal clusters of cells dispersed in the exocrine tissue (Laguesse 1906; Lane 1907), together with scattered, often solitary, endocrine cells (Heitz et al 1976).

The human pancreas may contain more than a million islets, usually most numerous in the tail (Findlay & Ashcroft 1975). Each is a mass of polyhedral cells pervaded by fenestrated capillaries (Goldstein & Davies 1968) and a rich autonomic innervation (Gerich & Lorenzi 1978). Staining procedures distinguish three major

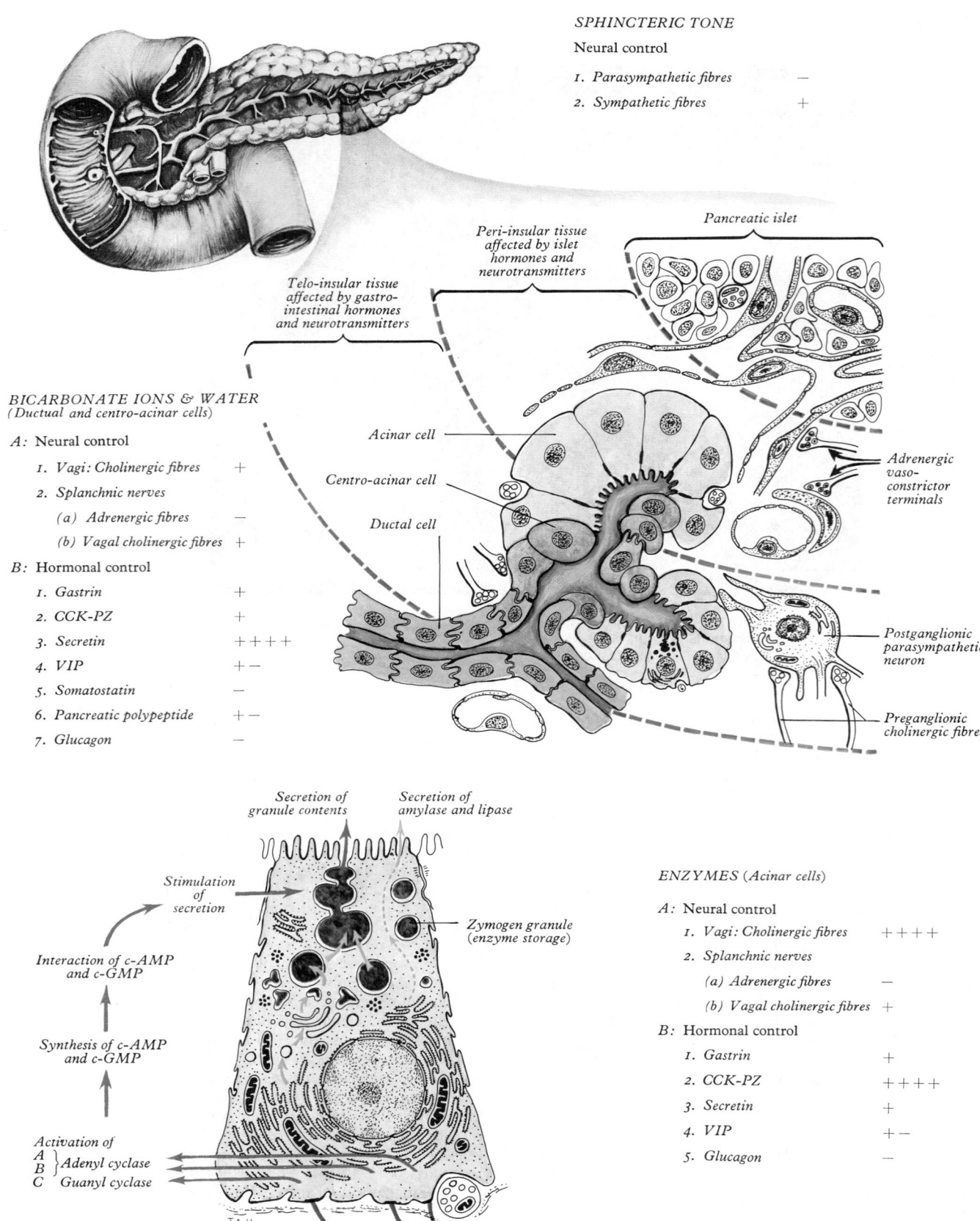

Neural control

1. *Parasympathetic fibres* —
2. *Sympathetic fibres* +

Peri-insular tissue affected by islet hormones and neurotransmitters

Pancreatic islet

Telo-insular tissue affected by gastro-intestinal hormones and neurotransmitters

Acinar cell

Centro-acinar cell

Ductal cell

Adrenergic vaso-constrictor terminals

Postganglionic parasympathetic neuron

Preganglionic cholinergic fibres

BICARBONATE IONS & WATER
(Ductual and centro-acinar cells)

A: Neural control

1. *Vagi: Cholinergic fibres* +
2. *Splanchnic nerves*
   (a) *Adrenergic fibres* —
   (b) *Vagal cholinergic fibres* +

B: Hormonal control

1. *Gastrin* +
2. *CCK-PZ* +
3. *Secretin* + + +
4. *VIP* + −
5. *Somatostatin* —
6. *Pancreatic polypeptide* + −
7. *Glucagon* —

Secretion of granule contents

Secretion of amylase and lipase

Stimulation of secretion

Zymogen granule (enzyme storage)

Interaction of c-AMP and c-GMP

Synthesis of c-AMP and c-GMP

Activation of
A }
B } *Adenyl cyclase*
C *Guanyl cyclase*

ENZYMES (*Acinar cells*)

A: Neural control

1. *Vagi: Cholinergic fibres* + + + +
2. *Splanchnic nerves*
   (a) *Adrenergic fibres* —
   (b) *Vagal cholinergic fibres* +

B: Hormonal control

1. *Gastrin* +
2. *CCK-PZ* + + + +
3. *Secretin* +
4. *VIP* + −
5. *Glucagon* —

Binding sites for
A *Acetylcholine*
B *CCK-PZ and/or gastrin*
C *Secretin and/or VIP*

12.134 Diagram of the ultrastructure of the exocrine pancreas and the mechanisms by which its secretion is controlled. The hormones referred to by acronyms are as follows: CCK-PZ = cholecystokinin-pancreaticozymin; VIP = vaso-active intestinal polypeptide.

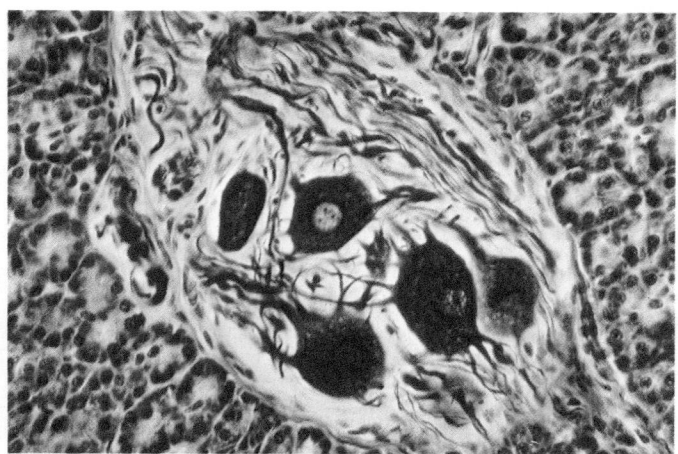

12.135 A low-power micrograph showing a cluster of autonomic ganglionic neurons with dendritic trees and axonal bundles, situated amongst pancreatic acinar cells of the goat. Palmgren silver impregnation. (Provided by J Henderson, Department of Physiology, Guy's Hospital Medical School, London.)

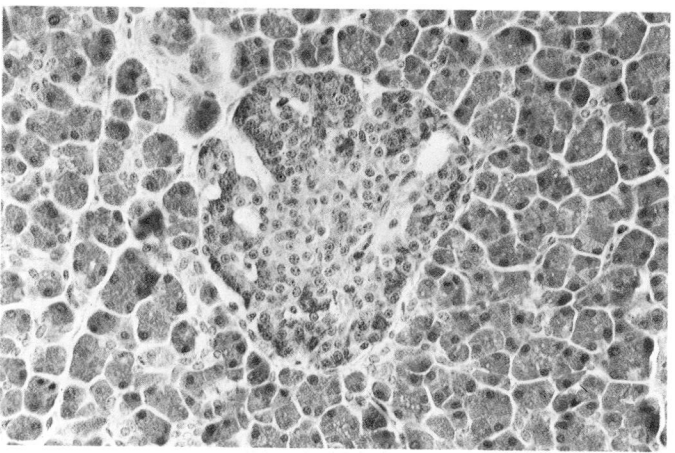

12.136 An islet of Langerhans and surrounding exocrine glandular tissue in the pancreas of a rhesus monkey, stained with orange G and aldehyde fuchsin. Within the islet, the B cells stain purple, whereas the A cells are pale yellow in colour. (Provided by J Henderson, Department of Physiology, Guy's Hospital Medical School, London.)

types of cell, designated A, B and D (Lane 1907; Bensley 1911; Bloom 1931; Kito & Hosoda 1977). Immunofluorescence microscopy and immuno-electron microscopy (Heitz et al 1976; Baetens et al 1977) have confirmed the identity of their secretory products and revealed other types of endocrine cell. Their general organization is depicted in **12.137**.

The most numerous cells, types A (alpha) and B (beta), respectively secrete glucagon (Baum et al 1962) and insulin (Lacy & Davies 1957). Though interspecific variation exists (Findlay & Ashcroft 1975), human A cells tend to be peripheral in islets and B cells more central (Orci 1976). Cytoplasmic storage granules of A cells are fixed by alcohol, are generally smaller than those of B cells, stain brilliant orange or red with Orange G and Mallory-Azan, and are aldehyde-fuchsin negative; in B cells they are alcohol-soluble and aldehyde-fuchsin positive. A third type, the D cell, discovered in human islets by Bloom (1931), contains somatostatin or a similar peptide (Orci et al 1975). Human D cells are peripherally placed within the islets, like A cells. Orci and Unger (1975) suggested that islets may have two functional regions: a medulla mainly of B cells (where insulin is secreted at a constant rate in response, e.g., to the presence of glucose in the intercellular fluid) and a mixed cortex of A, B and D cells, rich in neurovascular elements (where secretory activity responds rapidly to various environmental changes). In the cortex somatostatin released by D cells may inhibit secretory activity in adjacent A or B cells (Orci 1976). In many mammals, including humans, D cells more often contact A cells than B, suggesting that pancreatic somatostatin may chiefly inhibit glucagon release. Organ culture studies by Barden et al (1977) corroborate this; when anti-somatostatin serum was incubated with rat islets, glucagon release increased tenfold with no significant change in the release of insulin. How somatostatin inhibits the release of glucagon and possibly insulin is not clear; it may act intracellularly, passing through gap junctions from adjacent cells (Gerich & Lorenzi 1978). Another suggested hormonal modifier of islet activity is gastric inhibitory peptide, which appears to potentiate the insulin secretory response to glucose (Dupré et al 1973). The autonomic 'neurohormones', acetylcholine (ACh) and noradrenalin, also affect secretion, ACh augmenting insulin and glucagon release, noradrenalin inhibiting glucose-induced insulin release; they may also affect somatostatin and pancreatic polypeptide (PP) secretion. The roles of the circulating noradrenalin and adrenalin or of neurogenous noradrenalin acting locally on islet cell secretion remain obscure.

Peptide-secreting cells, with smaller granules than those in A, B and D cells, occur in human pancreas, in at least two forms: one contains PP; another has an ultrastructure like that of D_1 cells of the gastric mucosa (p. 1760). Pancreatic 'D_1' cells differ from PP cells in their granules; those of the former do not react with antibovine PP serum, those of the latter do (Baetens et al 1977). Although the product of gastro-enteric D_1 cells is uncertain, it may be related to

vasoactive intestinal polypeptide (VIP) (Buffa et al 1977); the product of pancreatic 'D_1' cells is still uncertain.

'D_1' and PP cells are not restricted to islets, being also scattered throughout the predominantly exocrine tissue.

Islet vessels and nerves

Pancreatic vessels. Arteries are rami of the splenic and pancreaticoduodenal arteries (pp. 1551, 1553).

Venous drainage is into the portal, splenic and superior mesenteric veins.

Lymph drainage is described elsewhere (p. 1619). Larger blood and lymph vessels travel with the exocrine ducts and nerves in the interlobular connective tissue, supplying lobular branches. Bunnag et al (1963) have shown that in mice one to three afferent arterioles arise from arterial rami to supply each islet, before which they may supply the acini. In each islet they feed a capillary network almost as dense as in a renal glomerulus; the network is drained by one to six venules which join to enter an intralobular vein. McCuskey and Chapman (1969) reported an intermittent flow in islet capillaries, local interruption being due to luminal bulging of the endothelial cells. The capillaries are fenestrated.

Pancreatic nerve supply. This comes from the coeliac plexus and enters along with the arteries of supply. Little is known of the afferent nerves; the efferents consist of sympathetic postganglionic fibres from the coeliac ganglion and parasympathetic preganglionic from the right vagus. The fibres, mainly nonmyelinated (Benscome 1959), are vasomotor (sympathetic) and parenchymal (sympathetic and parasympathetic) in their distribution. Fine branches ramify among the cells, from peri-insular plexuses (Findlay & Ashcroft 1975). Fibres frequently synapse with acinar cells before innervating the islets, suggesting a close linkage between neural control of exocrine and endocrine components. Many fibres enter the islets with the arterioles (Coupland 1958).

Parasympathetic ganglia lie in the inter- and intralobular connective tissue, and in the latter case are frequently associated with insular cells, forming *neuro-insular complexes*, first described by van Campenhout (1925) as 'complexes sympathico-insulaires', revised to 'complexes neuro-insulaires' by Simard (1937). They were classified by Fujita (1959) in two groups: one of neurons and insular cells (**12.137**), one of nerve fibres and insular cells, the latter being described in detail by Kobayashi and Fujita (1969). Both A and B cells are involved in the neuro-insular complexes.

Three types of nerve terminal are noted in islets (Smith & Porte 1976): cholinergic (with 30–50 nm diameter agranular vesicles), adrenergic (with 30–50 nm dense-cored vesicles), and a third, uncharacterized, type (with 60–200 nm dense-cored vesicles).

No selective link with any one type of insular cell has been found; sometimes more than one type of terminal contacts a single cell (Esterhuizen et al 1968). Some of the chemical synapses between

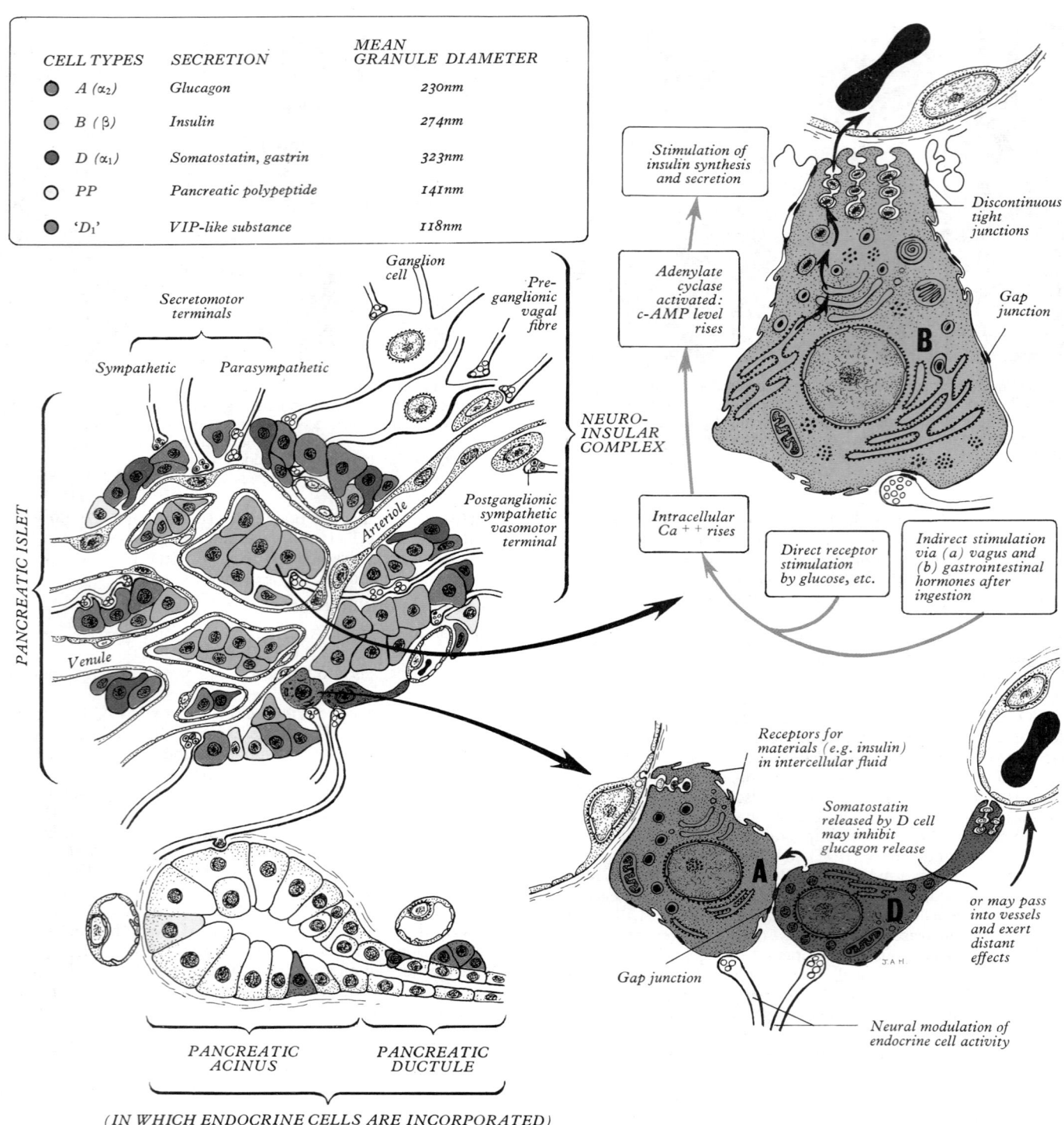

CELL TYPES	SECRETION	MEAN GRANULE DIAMETER
A (α_2)	Glucagon	230nm
B (β)	Insulin	274nm
D (α_1)	Somatostatin, gastrin	323nm
PP	Pancreatic polypeptide	141nm
'D$_1$'	VIP-like substance	118nm

12.137 Diagram of the histology, ultrastructure and mode of operation of the endocrine pancreas (VIP = vaso-active intestinal polypeptide).

axon terminal and islet cell show narrow areas in the synaptic clefts suggesting an electrical synapse or gap junction (Orci et al 1973); such junctions also occur between islet cells (Orci 1974) and electrical coupling of nerve supply to a functional network of islet cells has been mooted. Some terminals appear remote from the surfaces of islet cells (Kobayashi & Fujita 1969); neuro-transmitters released from them could diffuse through intercellular spaces to affect numerous islet cells.

CLINICAL ANATOMY OF THE PANCREAS

True pancreatic cysts are relatively uncommon. A pseudocyst of the pancreas results from effusion of fluid into the lesser sac as a result of acute pancreatitis or pancreatic trauma. The resultant collection pushes forward between the stomach and transverse colon, becoming palpable in the upper abdomen as a median tumour; the tumour is fixed, and does not move even during respiration. Carcinoma of the pancreas usually affects the head, speedily involving the bile duct, leading to jaundice; or it may press on the portal vein, causing ascites, or obstruct the pylorus. Rarely the ventral pancreatic bud fails to rotate around the duodenum. This results in a ring of pancreatic tissue encircling (and obstructing) the second part of the duodenum (*annular pancreas*). The ventral and dorsal pancreatic ducts may fail to fuse or fuse incompletely. The accessory duct remains as the main duct, draining the tail, body and most of the head. This inadequate drainage may predispose to acute or chronic pancreatitis. If the bile duct is embedded in the pancreatic head (p. 1809), chronic pancreatitis may obstruct it and produce jaundice. Accessory nodules of pancreatic tissue may exist in the wall of the duodenum (most commonly), jejunum, ileum or ileal diverticulum

(p. 1763). They may be associated with duodenal diverticula, as small protrusions of the whole wall or only of the mucosa and submucosa, usually adjacent to the pancreas and the opening of the bile duct.

Pancreatic Transplantation

Pancreatic transplantation is indicated for the treatment of insulin-dependent diabetics who suffer end-stage renal failure due to diabetic microangiopathy; in these cases a kidney is transplanted into the same recipient, usually from the same cadaveric donor. A pancreas may also be transplanted alone in an unstable diabetic in whom renal or other end-organ failure may be anticipated in the near future. The major technical challenge has been to develop a method of draining the exocrine secretions and to prevent a pancreatic fistula. To achieve these ends, a roux-en-y loop of jejunum has been used in the past (Groth & Tyden 1988), but the technique of pancreaticocystostomy is now much more popular (Sollinger et al 1984). The pancreas is always transplanted into the pelvis, either within or outside the peritoneal cavity. In this position, the pancreas can be drained into the bladder or into a small bowel loop, either using a duodenal conduit (**12.138A**), or by anastomosing the cut surfaces of the pancreas

to the fundus of the bladder (**12.139B**). The bladder anastomosis offers the technical advantage of being an easier operation, and the function of the gland may be measured by regular measurement of urinary amylase. In immunosuppressed diabetics, where healing is impaired, pancreaticocystostomy seems the safest and technically most successful operation.

OPERATION OF CADAVERIC PANCREATECTOMY

Following the diagnosis of brain death, the pancreas is dissected free of the transverse mesocolon, and the attachments to the greater curvature of the stomach, including the short gastric vessels, are divided. The splenic vessels are tied at the pancreatic tail and the spleen removed, and the splenic and coeliac arteries, including the superior pancreaticoduodenal artery, are prepared for anastomosis to the recipient artery. If the whole organ is to be transplanted, the duodenum is divided,

and the superior mesenteric trunk and inferior pancreaticoduodenal artery are preserved. Since the liver will also frequently be taken for purposes of transplantation (p. 1808), the viscera are perfused through the aorta with a pre-cooled preservation solution and are excised. A patch of aorta bearing the superior mesenteric and coeliac arteries may be removed, together with a length of portal vein for anastomosis to recipient vessels. 'Jump graft' using sections of iliac artery and vein may be needed to provide tension-free anastomoses with the recipient's circulation.

RECIPIENT OPERATION

The coeliac and the superior mesenteric arteries are anastomosed to the external iliac artery, and the portal vein to the external iliac vein using a jump graft if necessary. Angulation must be avoided at this anastomosis to avoid a high risk of postoperative thrombosis. The cut pancreatic surface, or the duodenal conduit, are anastomosed to the vault of the bladder.

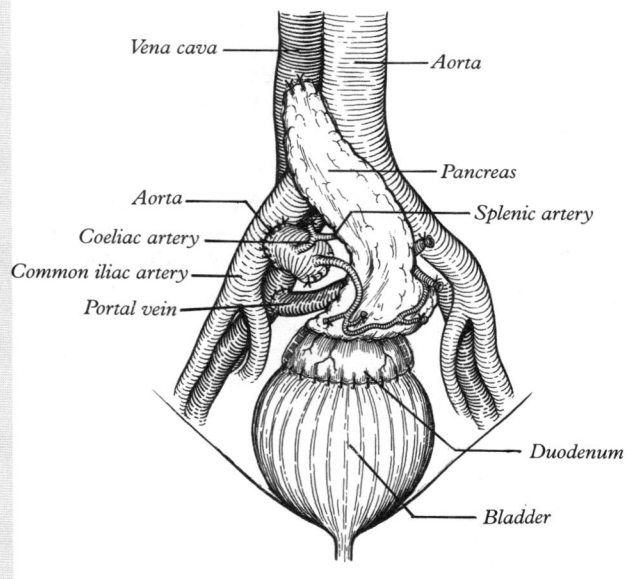

12.138A   Pancreatico-cystostomy with duodenal conduit.

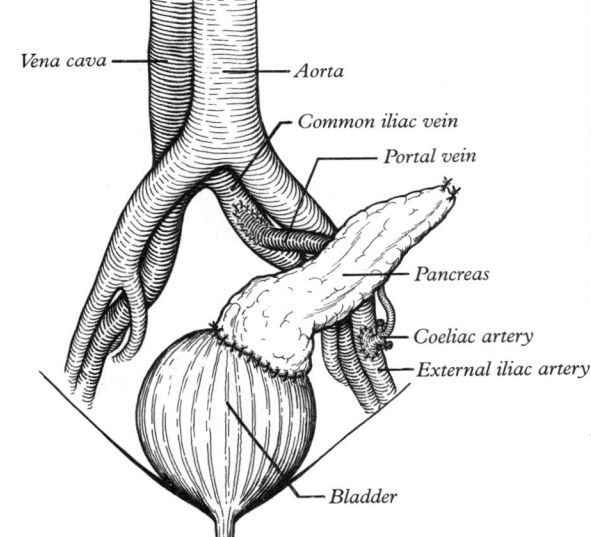

12.138B   Pancreatico-cystostomy with the cut surface of the pancreas anastomosed to the fundus of the bladder.

LIVER

INTRODUCTION

The liver is the most massive of the viscera, occupying a substantial portion of the abdominal cavity. It is essential to life, since it carries

out a multiplicity of metabolic activities necessary for homeostasis, alimentation and defence. It is composed largely of epithelial cells (hepatocytes) where most of these biochemical operations occur, bathed by blood derived from the hepatic porta veins and hepatic arteries, and draining into the inferior vena cava through the hepatic veins. There is continuous chemical exchange between the

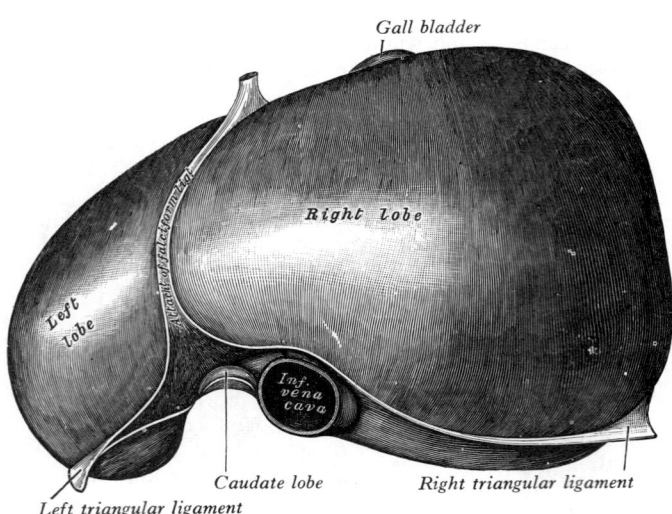

12.139   The superior, anterior and right lateral surfaces of the liver.

occupying most of the right hypochondrium and epigastrium and extending into the left hypochondrium as far as the left lateral line (Rouiller 1964). In males it generally weighs 1.4–1.8 kg, and in females 1.2–1.4 kg, with a range of 1.0–2.5 kg. It is somewhat cuneiform, is reddish brown in colour in the fresh state and, though firm and pliant, is easily lacerated. Wounds cannot be tightly sutured and bleeding may be severe, due to the organ's great vascularity. Despite its weight, it is widely believed that, like various other viscera, its position is not maintained by peritoneal (p. 1798) or fibrous attachments, but mainly by intra-abdominal pressure due to tonus in the abdominal muscles. The continuity of hepatic veins with the inferior vena cava may provide some support. However, such dogma should be viewed with caution. Without systematic studies of intra-abdominal pressure gradients and their variations with posture, respiration, gastrointestinal dilatation and so forth, and studies of the statics and dynamics of the peritoneal folds, connective tissues, adjacent viscera and vascular pedicles, any theories as to the other mechanisms maintaining the position of the liver (or any other abdominal organ) remain highly speculative.

The liver is a wedge-shaped, rather rounded organ, its narrow end pointing left, and its anterior edge directed downwards. It is convex in front, to the right, above and behind, where it abuts the curved surfaces of the anterior body wall and diaphragm, and it is somewhat concave inferiorly where it is moulded to the shapes of the adjacent viscera. The liver is attached in front to the body wall by the *falciform ligament*, and above and behind to the diaphragm by the *coronary ligament* with its lateral limits, the *right* and *left triangular ligaments* (forming reflexions of the peritoneum from the liver surface on to the diaphragm). Below, it is attached to the stomach and first part of the duodenum by the lesser omentum, along the right (free border) of which the hepatic arteries, hepatic portal vein, lymphatics, nerves and hepatic ducts enter or leave the liver at the *porta hepatis* (the door to the liver), an area also termed the *hilus*. The gallbladder adheres to the anterior part of the liver's inferior surface.

The inferior surface is marked near the midline by a sharp fissure which anteriorly receives the *ligamentum teres* (the obliterated fetal left umbilical vein) from the free edge of the falciform ligament, and posteriorly contains the *ligamentum venosum*, another obliterated relic of the fetal circulation. The lesser omentum is reflected on to the liver along the posterior half of this fissure.

Posteriorly, the liver is deeply grooved where it partially surrounds the superior vena cava (the caval groove) which receives the large hepatic veins in this region.

Lobes

Although much of the surface is smoothly continuous, the liver is customarily apportioned by anatomists into a larger *right* and a much smaller *left lobe* according to some surface markings and

hepatocytes and the blood as the cells of the liver elaborate various macromolecules, secreting them either into the blood (e.g. most plasma proteins), or into an extensive system of minute canals which converge on the hepatic duct and thence the gallbladder and bile duct to assist digestion and eliminate the products of haemoglobin breakdown (bile salts and bile pigments, respectively). The hepatocytes are also important in removal and breakdown of toxic, or potentially toxid materials from the blood, for regulation of blood glucose and lipids (stored as glycogen and proteolipid, respectively), storage of certain vitamins, iron, and other substances, breakdown or modification of aminoacids, and a plethora of other biochemical reactions which are predominantly exothermic and therefore provide a substantial part of the body's thermal energy, especially at rest. In addition to these properties, the liver is populated by phagocytic macropohages scattered along the walls of its extensive vascular network; these form part of the mononuclear phagocyte system of the body and are important in the removal of particulates from the bloodstream. Finally, in fetal life the liver is an important site of haemopoiesis. These diverse aspects of liver function are considered further on pp. 1802–1806 with liver microstructure.

EXTERNAL FEATURES (**12**.139–143)

The liver (hepar) lies in the upper right part of the abdominal cavity,

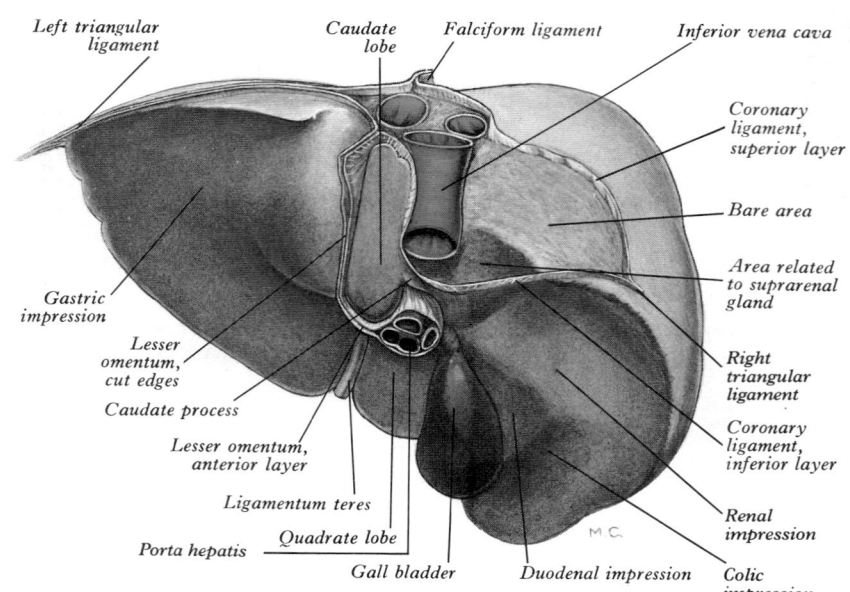

12.140   Posterior aspect of the liver, showing its peritoneal connections divided close to its surfaces.

peritoneal attachments (see p. 1798), namely the line of attachment of the falciform ligament anteriorly, and the fissure for the ligamentum teres and ligamentum venosum on the liver's inferior surface. To the right of this groove are two prominences, the *quadrate lobe* in front, and the *caudate lobe* behind, separated from each other by the porta hepatis. The gallbladder lies (usually) in a shallow fossa to the right of the quadrate lobe.

It is important to note that while this brief description of lobation is didactically convenient, it does not reflect the liver's internal vascular or biliary subdivisions, which are of considerable surgical importance. A fuller consideration of this topic is given below.

Surfaces (12.139–141)

The liver is described as having *superior, anterior, right, posterior* and *inferior surfaces*, and a distinct *inferior border*. The superior, anterior and right surfaces are continuous at rounded 'borders', but the sharp inferior border (**12.**140) separates the right and anterior surfaces from the inferior surface. This border is rounded between the right lateral and inferior surfaces, but becomes thin and angular at the lower limit of the anterior surface and is notched along this edge by the ligamentum teres, just to the right of the midline. Lateral to the fundus of the gallbladder, which often corresponds to a second notch 4–5 cm to the right of the midline, the inferior border largely follows the costal margin. Left of the fundus it ascends less obliquely than the right costal margin, crossing the infrasternal angle to pass behind the left costal margin near the tip of the eighth costal cartilage. It then ascends sharply to merge with the thin margin of the left lobe. At the infrasternal angle the inferior border adjoins the anterior abdominal wall and is accessible to examination by percussion, but is not usually palpable; in the midline the inferior border of the liver is near the transpyloric plane, about a hand's breadth below the xiphisternal joint (**12.**117). In women and children the border often projects a little below the right costal margin. The hepatic surfaces are described in greater detail on p. 1800.

HEPATIC LOBATION (12.142, 143)

As already noted (see above), the customary subdivision of the liver into right and left lobes does not really describe the internal organization of this organ, which is generated by developmental processes only hinted at on the mature liver's surface. With recent developments in surgery, especially liver transplantation, and the introduction of powerful imaging methods which can be used before and during operations, it has become vital to understand the vascular and biliary territories which can be isolated as units for partial hepatectomy and other local surgical interventions (see below; see also e.g. Bismuth, Aldridge & Kunstlinger 1991).

These patterns have been established over the last century by a series of classical studies on the liver's vascular and biliary duct branching patterns, by dissection and injection methods, especially the use of corrosion casts. Cantlie (1898) first established the division of the liver into right and left halves (which do not correspond to those of traditional anatomists, see above) according to the distribution of right and left hepatic arteries, (sometimes referred to now as right and left livers). Later work by Hjortsjö with corrosion casts (Hjortsjö 1948, 1951, 1956) definitively established the major vascular territories of the arterial and hepatic venous supply and drainage, and of the biliary tree; he emphasized that primary anatomical and functional lobation are better defined as the territories of the right and left hepatic ducts and showed that there is only minor overlap between them. These studies were combined with surgical data in the classic book by Couinaud (1953) which is now regarded by many as a definitive descriptive foundation for surgical approaches to the liver.

Other workers have confirmed Hjortsjö's classification and have made further subdivisions of lobes into segments, as described below (e.g. Healey & Schroy 1953; Goldsmith & Woodburne 1957; Stucke 1959), by corrosion cast techniques, dissection and radiology. In such investigations, particularly those involving examination of casts of ducts or vessels, so-called 'fissures' are visible (**12.**141) between the territories of the right and left branches, and less clearly between lobar subdivisions (segments). These fissures, even in the main interlobar zone, do not produce reliable surface indications of use in lobectomy.

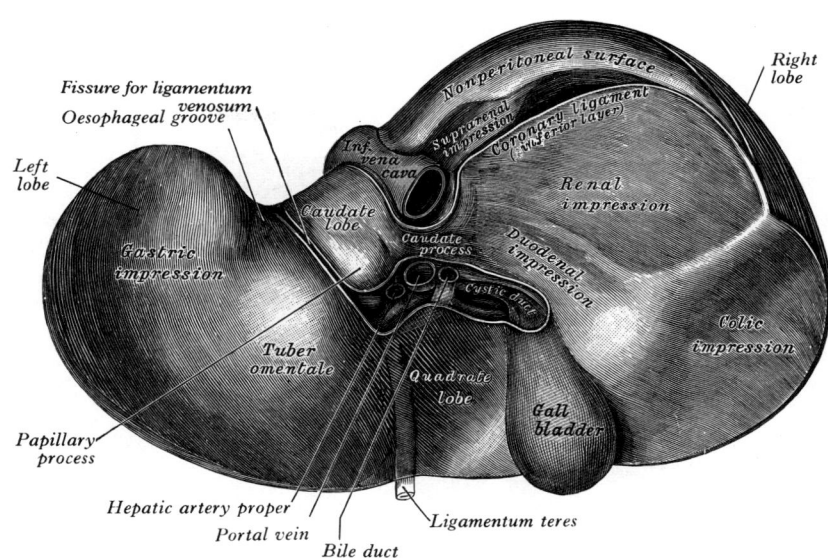

12.141   The inferior surface of the liver.

Right lobe

Much the greater in volume, it contributes to all surfaces, as described later, including the entire costal aspect. Its arbitrarily described surfaces (anterior, superior, inferior and posterior) all pass uninterruptedly on to the *left lobe*, except where shallow grooves partially demarcate the quadrate and caudate 'lobes', really parts of the left lobe, as already mentioned.

Quadrate lobe

Visible on the inferior surface, it appears somewhat rectangular and is bounded in front by the inferior border, on the left by the fissure for ligamentum teres, behind by the porta hepatis and on the right by the fossa for the gallbladder.

Caudate lobe

This is visible on the posterior surface, bounded on the left by the fissure for the ligamentum venosum, below by the porta hepatis and on the right by the groove for the inferior vena cava. Above, it continues into the superior surface on the right of the upper end of the fissure for the ligamentum venosum. Below and to the right, it is connected to the right lobe by a narrow *caudate process*, which is immediately behind the porta hepatis and above the epiploic foramen. Below and to the left, the caudate lobe has a small rounded *papillary process*. Due to the depth of the fissure for the ligamentum venosum, the caudate lobe has an anterior surface, which forms the posterior wall of the fissure and is in contact with the lesser omentum (hepatic part).

HEPATIC SEGMENTATION

As in other organs with a group of hilar structures (e.g. the lungs, spleen, kidneys), the branching patterns of blood supply and biliary drainage in the liver create a system of lobes and further subdivisions (sectors or segments). This reflects the early development of the liver when the branching patterns of epithelial ducts, their related arteries and portal vein rami, and also the venous drainage to the inferior vena cava are established. Of course, what is designated as a segment must be rather arbitrary, depending on what level of branching is chosen as its basis for separation from other segments. However such schemes have a practical value in that the territories of the larger vessels do not overlap extensively or for many anastomoses, and this can be exploited during partial hepatectomy (provided enough imaging information is available for a particular patient, as considerable variation can occur).

The hepatic artery, portal vein and common bile duct divide and subdivide with a common pattern, as implied in the classic observations of Glisson (1654) and confirmed by subsequent workers. No evidence of significant intrahepatic anastomosis in these

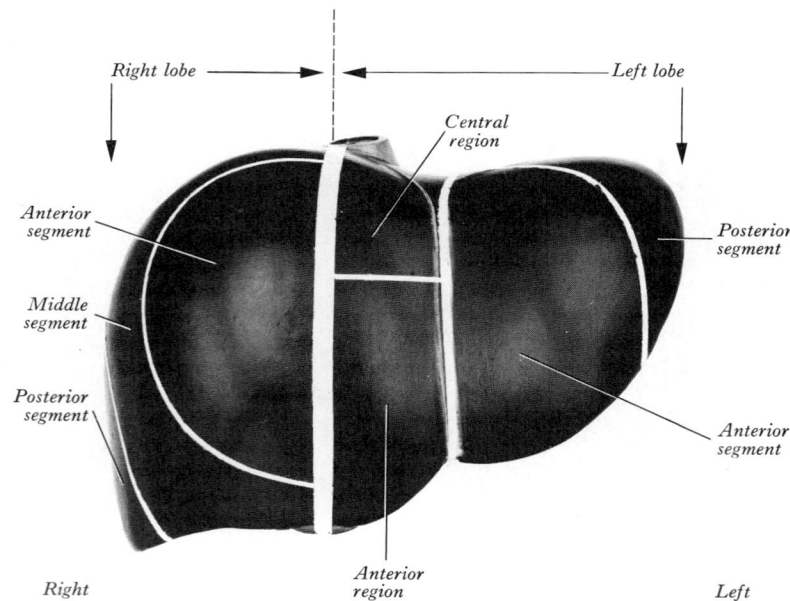

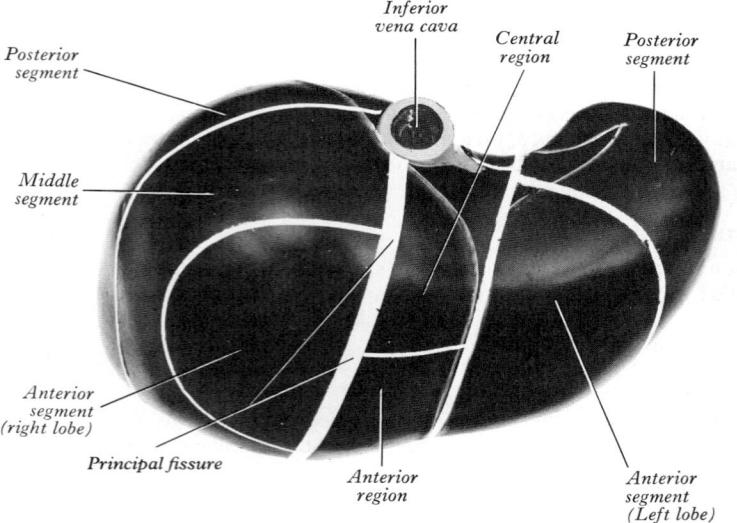

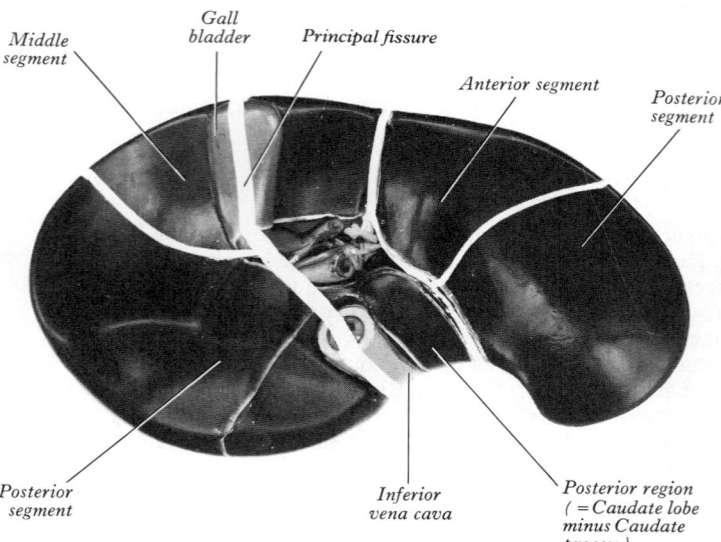

12.142 Hepatic segmentation. Surface projection of the boundaries between hepatic segments based on the researches of Professor Carl-Herman Hjortsö, University of Lund, Sweden. See text for comment and references. Top: anterior view; middle: anterosuperior view; bottom: inferior visceral views.

dendriform systems has been recorded. For example, despite variation in origin (and occurrence of accessory vessels), the hepatic arterial system consists of end-arteries (Michels 1966), a feature typical in any organ developed from a single vascularized blastema of dichotomizing potential. The implications of this pattern were not followed up until the late nineteenth century, apart from the recognition of right and left hepatic lobes (see McIndoe & Counsellor 1927; Hjortsjö 1948 for earlier literature). Division into two lobes, based on the primary divisions of the triadic system (hepatic arteries, portal veins and biliary tree) rather than on surface features, is generally accepted but confusing descriptions persist in many texts. Inevitably, further divisions have been suggested, if only in the interests of effective partial hepatectomy. The pioneer in this field was Hjortsö (1948, 1951, 1956, 1975), who was the first to propose a complete segmental model (**12**.142), based on dissections, injections and radiography, particularly applied to the biliary ducts and portal vein. Many have subsequently modified his scheme of segmentation, subdividing some segments, redefining and renaming others (Elias & Petty 1952; Healey & Schroy 1953; Couinaud 1954; Goldsmith & Woodburne 1957; Bilbey & Rappaport 1960). The main extension of Hjortsö's scheme is the division of his segments into superior and inferior parts, chiefly by Healey and Schroy 1953 (**12**.143) and Couinaud 1954. Apart from this and minor differences in delineating the major segments, there is general consensus on the division of the right lobe into approximately 'anterior', intermediate and 'posterior' segments; and the left into lateral and medial parts.

Most reports have been based on injections and casts, principally upon corrosion casts of one or more of the components of the triad's ramifications. In such casts is an easily discernible (**12**.144) sagittal zone between the lobes, the *fissura principalis*, picturesquely described by Hjortsö (1956) as lying in the plane of the left tympanic membrane. All other 'fissures' described (with some variation) by different workers are intersegmental. The term '*spatium*' was suggested for 'fissure', and Hjortsö recognized several of these (**12**.142). Such 'spaces' in corrosion casts are due to the absence of all but the smallest rami of the portal triad, usually too fragile to preserve. These demarcations do **not** correspond to substantial zones of connective tissue, which might provide superficial or internal indications for purposes of subtotal resection (cf. bronchopulmonary segments). Surface projections of segmental fissures are shown in **12**.143, according to Hjortsö (1948) and Healey and Schroy (1953), the chief difference being that the latters' scheme shows superior and inferior regions in each major segment (as also recognized by Elias & Petty 1952; Couinaud 1954; and Platzer & Maurer 1966). More recently Gupta et al (1978) have put forward a similar scheme (9 segments); in 1981 further observations by Gupta et al on hepatovenous segmentation in the human liver were published in which they recognized five segments: left, middle, right, paracaval and caudate. To equate the segments described, with their differing names and delimitations, by all the investigators quoted would not improve the reliability of this information in practical application. As Gupta et al (1978) stated, the segmental pattern is in itself variable; of 41 corrosion casts more than half showed marked differences in the volume of one segment or another, as also noted by others. Although most regard segments as functionally independent and uncomplicated by, e.g. intrahepatic arterial anastomosis, occasionally this has been noted.

Surgical opinion is divided upon the usefulness of such patterns in hepatic resections. Dawson (1974) and others consider resection of less than a lobe to be hazardous; others, such as Ryncki (1974), have recorded successful segmental resections. Individual variation requires portal venography and cholangiography to define segmental patterns before operation, wherever feasible. It should be noted that the disposition of the *hepatic veins* and their tributaries is not a reliable guide; these veins, also studied by corrosion casts (Goldsmith & Woodburne 1957), do not follow the pattern of the hepatic triads; they drain parts of adjoining segments. It is therefore difficult to plan a resection plane which is optimal in respect of both triadic structures and hepatic veins.

PERITONEAL CONNECTIONS OF THE LIVER

Except for a triangular area on its posterior surface (the 'bare area'), the liver is almost completely covered by peritoneum, which connects

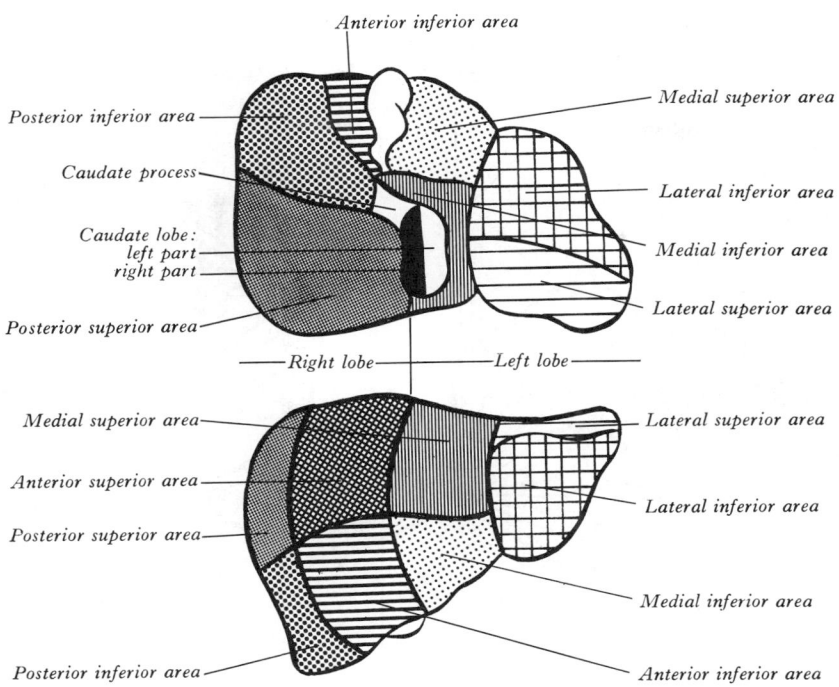

12.143 The segmentation of the liver, based upon the principal divisions of the hepatic artery and accompanying hepatic ducts. The upper drawing is of the visceral surface of the liver, the lower drawing is of the diaphragmatic surface. See text for further description.

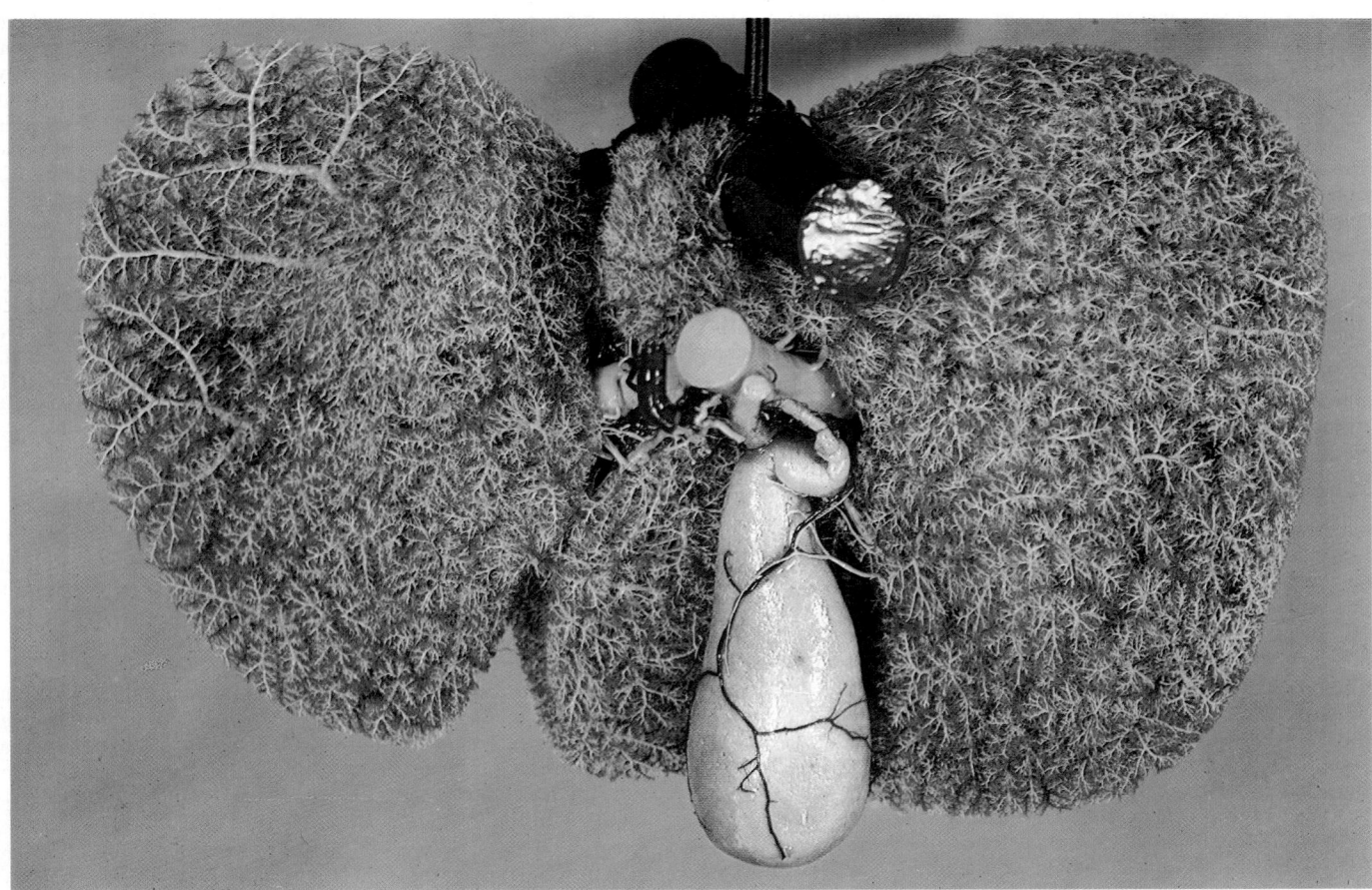

12.144 A resin corrosion cast of the blood vessels and duct systems of the liver of a woman: bile duct, cystic duct, gallbladder and their tributaries (yellow); the hepatic artery and its branches (red); the portal vein and its tributaries (light blue); the inferior vena cava, hepatic veins and their tributaries (dark blue). The photograph is of the visceral surface of the organ and was taken before the finer blood vessels and ducts were removed by trimming. The posterior aspect is above. Prepared by D H Tompsett of the Royal College of Surgeons of England.

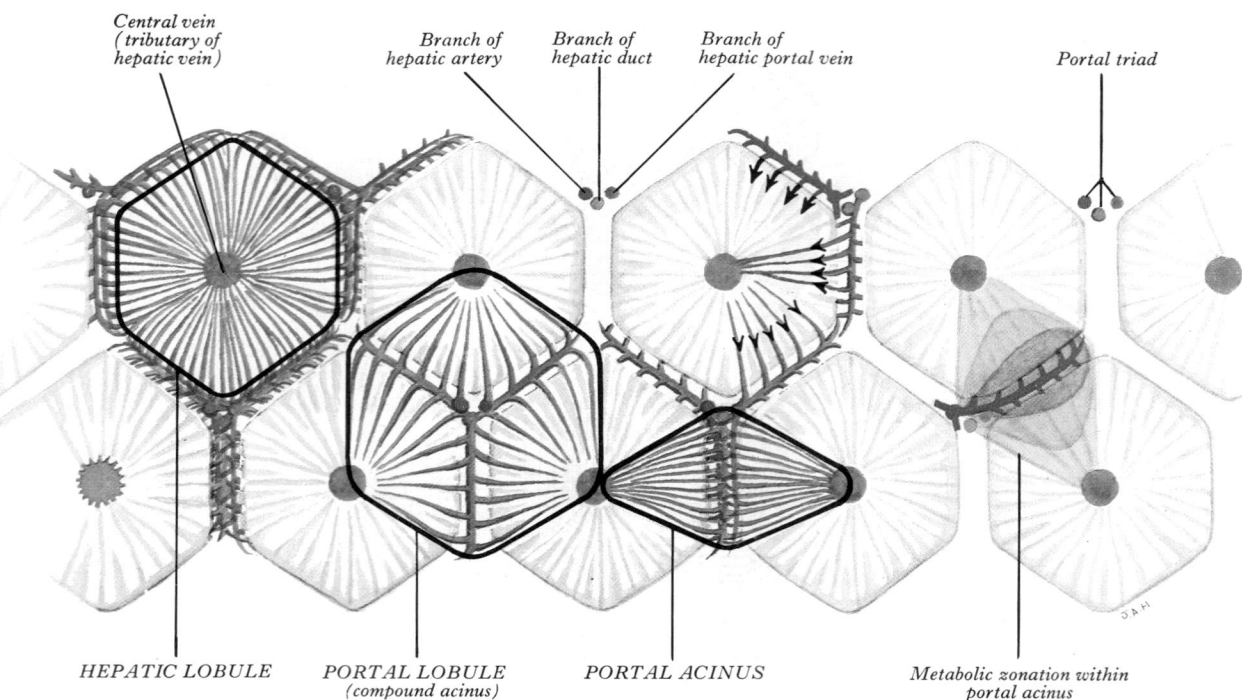

Central vein
(tributary of
hepatic vein)

Branch of
hepatic artery

Branch of
hepatic duct

Branch of
hepatic portal vein

Portal triad

HEPATIC LOBULE

PORTAL LOBULE
(compound acinus)

PORTAL ACINUS

Metabolic zonation within
portal acinus

12.145 Diagram of the histological organization of the liver, showing the principal types of subdivisions which have been proposed. For purposes of clarity, the territories of the classic hepatic lobules are shown as regular hexagons, unlike their real appearance which is highly variable (see text).

it to the stomach, duodenum, diaphragm and anterior abdominal wall by several folds, their lines of attachment, of course, being devoid of peritoneum. These folds include the falciform ligament, right and left triangular and coronary ligaments and the lesser omentum.

Falciform ligament (12.71, 72, 139)

A crescentic fold, it consists of two applied layers of peritoneum, connecting the liver to the diaphragm and the supra-umbilical part of the anterior abdominal wall. Its convex base is fixed to the inferior diaphragmatic surface and to the posterior surface of the anterior abdominal wall, down to the umbilicus; as it ascends from this it inclines slightly right. It is attached to the notch for the ligamentum teres on the inferior hepatic border and to the anterior and superior hepatic surfaces. Its concave free edge, from the umbilicus to the notch for the ligamentum teres, contains the latter structure and the small para-umbilical veins, and is anterior to the pyloric region of the stomach. At its diaphragmatic end its layers separate to expose a triangular area on the superior hepatic surface devoid of peritoneum. The left layer continues into the anterior layer of the left triangular ligament, the right into the upper layer of the coronary ligament.

Coronary ligament (12.76, 140)

This name is given to the reflexion of peritoneum from the diaphragm to the superior and posterior surfaces of the right lobe of the liver, forming the perimeter of the approximately triangular but rather variable 'bare area' of the liver, i.e. that part of its surface which is apposed to the diaphragm without intervening peritoneum. The coronary ligament has upper and lower margins or layers, united laterally at angular extensions, the left and right triangular ligaments. Followed from left to right (see **12**.76), the upper layer departs from the right side of the falciform ligament (with which it is continuous), skirts anteriorly the upper end of the groove for the inferior vena cava, then descends obliquely down and to the right on the back of the liver to the anterior (upper) leaflet of the right triangular ligament. The lower layer then begins with the posterior (lower) leaflet of the right triangular ligament, then can be followed to the left almost horizontally along the lower limit of the right lobe's posterior surface. Here the coronary ligament is sometimes reflected on to the upper part of the right kidney's anterior surface (so forming the hepatorenal ligament). At its left extremity, the lower layer of the coronary ligament passes in front of the lower end of the groove for the

inferior vena cava, and becomes continuous with the right margin of the lesser omentum where it is reflected from the right margin of the caudate lobe. Above, this curves to the left to become the inferior (posterior) layer of the left triangular ligament, the term 'ligament' for this complex line of peritoneal reflexion indicates a supportive function, aiding the fibrous attachment of the bare area in suspending the liver from the diaphragm and posterior body wall. Its precise boundary reflects the development of the liver in the ventral meso-gastrium and its later attachment to adjacent structures (see p. 342).

Left triangular ligament (12.140)

It ascends back from the superior surface of the left lobe to the diaphragm. Its closely applied layers become fused at the left edge of the ligament. To the right the anterior layer merges with the left layer of the falciform ligament, the posterior with the anterior layer of the lesser omentum at the upper end of the fissure for the ligamentum venosum. The left triangular ligament lies in front of the abdominal part of the oesophagus, the upper end of the lesser omentum and part of the fundus of the stomach. It varies much and may contain large blood vessels (Outrequin et al 1967).

Right triangular ligament (12.140)

This is a short V-shaped fold connecting the lateral and posterior aspects of the right lobe to the diaphragm. At its right margin its two layers are continuous. The ligament is really the right extremity of the coronary ligament.

Lesser omentum

It has been described (p. 1741); it is attached along the line of the fissure for the ligamentum venosum, at the upper end of which its anterior layer merges with the posterior layer of the left triangular ligament and its posterior layer with the line of reflexion of the peritoneum from the upper end of the right caudate lobe and so, indirectly, with the lower coronary layer (**12**.140).

HEPATIC SURFACES

Superior surface

The superior surface (**12**.139) includes parts of the right and left lobes. It fits closely under the diaphragm, separated from it by peritoneum except for a small triangular area where the two layers of the falciform ligament diverge. Right and left it is convex, but centrally it presents a shallow *cardiac impression* corresponding with the position of the heart above the diaphragm. It is related to the right diaphragmatic pleura and base of the right lung, to the pericardium and ventricular part of the heart and to part of the left diaphragmatic pleura and base of the left lung. It should be noted that the superior surface curves directly into the so-called anterior surface and the peritonealized part of the posterior surface of the right lobe. No definable border separates superior, anterior, right lateral and right posterior *aspects* of the liver and it would be more appropriate to group these as the *diaphragmatic surface*, mostly separated from the *visceral surface* by a narrow edge or border.

Anterior surface

The anterior surface, which is triangular and convex, is covered by peritoneum except at the attachment of the falciform ligament. Much of it is in contact with the diaphragm, which separates it on the right from the pleura and sixth to tenth ribs and cartilages, and on the left from the seventh and eighth costal cartilages. The thin margins of the base of the lungs are thus quite close to the upper part of this surface, more extensively so on the right. The median area of the anterior hepatic surface lies behind the xiphoid process and the anterior abdominal wall in the infra-costal angle (**12**.117).

The hepatic profile is projected to the surface of the body as follows (**12**.117): its upper limit corresponds to a line through the xiphisternal joint, ascending to a point below the right nipple (fourth intercostal space) and to the left to a point inferomedial to the left nipple; its right border corresponds to a curved line, convex to the right, running from the right end of the upper border to a point 1 cm below the costal margin at the tip of the tenth costal cartilage; its lower limit is the line completing this triangle (**12**.117), crossing the midline at the transpyloric plane (slightly concave near the right linea semilunaris).

Right surface

The right surface, covered by peritoneum, adjoins the right dome of the diaphragm which separates it from the right lung and pleura and the seventh to eleventh ribs. Above its upper third, both lung and pleura are inserted between the diaphragm and ribs; over its middle third only the costodiaphragmatic pleura is interposed; over its lower third the diaphragm and thoracic wall are in contact.

Posterior surface

The posterior surface is convex and wide on the right but narrow on the left, with a deep median concavity corresponding to the forward convexity of the vertebral column (**12**.140, 141). Much of this surface is devoid of peritoneum, being attached to the diaphragm by loose connective tissue, forming the so-called 'bare area', triangular in shape and limited above and below by the layers of the coronary ligament. The base of the posterior hepatic surface to the left is the caval groove; its apex, directed down and right, corresponds to the right triangular ligament. The *groove for the inferior vena cava* (caval groove), which is deep and occasionally a tunnel, lies at the posterior surface and is bare of peritoneum and adapted to the upper part of the vessel it contains; its floor is pierced by the hepatic veins (p. 1602). Infero-anteriorly the caudate process separates it from the porta hepatis. Lateral to its lower end the 'bare area' adjoins the upper pole of the left suprarenal gland. Left of the groove the *caudate lobe* forms the posterior surface in the superior omental recess; the peritoneum on its posterior aspect curves round its left border to its anterior aspect, which is the posterior wall of the fissure for the ligamentum venosum (**12**.141). The caudate lobe projects into the superior omental recess from the right; its posterior surface is related to the diaphragmatic crura (above the aortic opening) and the right inferior phrenic artery, separated by them from the descending thoracic aorta. The *papillary process* often descends in front of the origin of the coeliac artery.

The *fissure for the ligamentum venosum* (**12**.141) separates the posterior aspect of the caudate from the main part of the left lobe. The fissure cuts deeply in front of the caudate lobe and contains the two layers of the lesser omentum. Below, it curves laterally in front of the papillary process to the left end of the porta hepatis. The *ligamentum venosum*, the fibrous remnant of the ductus venosus

(p. 1502), is attached below to the left branch of the portal vein's posterior aspect; ascending in the floor of the fissure and passing laterally at the upper end of the caudate lobe it joins the left hepatic vein near its entry into the inferior vena cava, or sometimes the vena cava itself.

The left lobe's posterior aspect has a shallow *oesophageal impression* near the upper end of the fissure for the ligamentum venosum, occupied by the abdominal part of the oesophagus. Left of this the left lobe is related to part of the fundus of the stomach.

Inferior surface (12.140, 141)

Facing down, back and to the left, it bears the imprint, when preserved in situ, of the adjacent viscera. It is covered by visceral peritoneum except at the porta hepatis, the fissure for the ligamentum teres and the fossa for the gallbladder. On the left lobe, continuous with the oesophageal groove, is a *gastric impression*. To the right of this the rounded *omental tuberosity*, in the concavity of the lesser curvature, is in contact with the lesser omentum. The *fissure for the ligamentum teres*, of variable depth, ascends backwards from its notch on the inferior hepatic border to the left end of the porta hepatis, meeting the lower end of the fissure for the ligamentum venosum. It is the left boundary of the quadrate lobe and may be, partially or wholly, bridged by a band of liver. In its floor is the *ligamentum teres*, the obliterated vestige of the left umbilical vein (p. 1502). From the umbilicus this ligament ascends in the edge of the falciform ligament to the inferior hepatic border, where it traverses the fissure to join the left branch of the portal vein at the left end of the porta hepatis, opposite the attachment of the ligamentum venosum.

The gastric impression may invade anteriorly the *quadrate lobe*, which is moulded to the pyloric region and the beginning of the duodenum. The posterior part of the quadrate lobe adjoins the right border of the lesser omentum and its contained structures. When the stomach is empty the quadrate lobe is related to the first (superior) part of the duodenum and part of the transverse colon.

The *porta hepatis*, situated between the quadrate lobe in front, and the caudate process behind, is a deep transverse fissure between the upper ends of the fissure for the ligamentum teres and the fossa for the gallbladder. At the porta hepatis the portal vein, hepatic artery and hepatic nervous plexus enter the liver, and the right and left hepatic ducts and some lymph vessels emerge from it. The hepatic ducts are anterior, the portal vein and its branches posterior and the hepatic artery proper with its branches lies intermediate in position.

The *caudate process* connects the inferolateral part of the caudate lobe (left lobe) to the right lobe. It lies behind the porta hepatis, in front of the inferior vena cava, and roofs the epiploic foramen. It is often assigned to the right lobe but lies within the territory of the left hepatic duct, i.e. it forms part of the **left** lobe (see above).

The *fossa for the gallbladder*, forming the right limit of the quadrate lobe, extends from the inferior hepatic border to the right end of the porta hepatis. Usually shallow, it is variably bare of peritoneum. The inferior hepatic surface to the right of the fossa adjoins the colon, kidney and duodenum. A *colic impression* fits the right colic flexure near the inferior border. A *renal impression*, usually well marked, lies behind the colic impression and is separated from the neck and adjoining part of the gallbladder by a duodenal impression; it is related to the upper pole of the right kidney and superomedially to the lower pole of the right suprarenal gland. When the lower coronary layer is reflected from the liver to the right kidney, the renal and suprarenal impressions extend to the lower part of the 'bare area'. The *duodenal impression* is lateral to the neck of the gallbladder and related to the junction of the first (superior) and second (descending) parts of the duodenum.

It is noteworthy that hepatic relations vary with posture and respiration. In the above description the body is assumed to be supine.

Variations

The branches of the portal vein and tributaries of the hepatic veins are more numerous before birth, after which they are reduced by fusion or degeneration. The fetal portal vein joins the umbilical vein in a smooth right-hand curve, maintained after birth, with a sharp angle between the portal trunk and its left branch; the left vascular lobe may therefore be at a circulatory disadvantage and unable to keep pace in growth with the right. At the left end of the adult left lobe a fibrous band (*fibrous appendix of the liver*) may appear as an atrophied remnant of the more extensive part of the left lobe found in children; it contains atrophied bile ducts, the *hepatic vasa aberrantia*. Similar remnants may occur in the left lobe's edges and near the inferior vena cava. Occasionally the right lobe's lower border, to the right of the gallbladder, projects down as a broad linguiform process (*Riedel's lobe*).

HEPATIC VESSELS

The vessels connected with the liver are the portal vein, hepatic artery proper and hepatic veins. The *portal vein* and *hepatic artery* proper ascend in the lesser omentum to the porta hepatis, where each bifurcates. The *bile duct* and *lymphatic vessels* descend from the porta in the same omentum (the hepatic artery lying anteriorly and to the right, the bile duct anteriorly and left, and the hepatic portal vein posteriorly). All these structures are enveloped in the *perivascular fibrous capsule* (*hepatobiliary capsule of Glisson*), a sheath of loose connective tissue, which also surrounds the vessels as they course through the portal canals in the liver. It is also continuous with the fibrous hepatic capsule.

Hepatic artery and its branches (12.156)

After variable courses in the porta, these divide and subdivide in the liver, their smaller rami being associated with those of the portal vein with which they are distributed. There are no (or very few) anastomoses between their territories; each is an end-artery (Glauser 1953).

Hepatic veins (12.140, 144)

They convey blood from the liver to the inferior vena cava (p. 1602). They have only a thin tunica adventitia, binding them to the walls of their canals within the liver; hence, in sections, they are widely open and solitary, and so easily distinguished from the branches of portal veins, which tend to collapse post-mortem and are always accompanied by an artery and a biliary duct.

Hepatic lymph vessels

These are described on page 1619. Lymph from the liver has an abundant protein content. Obstruction of the hepatic venous drainage increases the flow of lymph in the thoracic duct. The importance of the transdiaphragmatic lymph drainage of the liver into internal mammary and diaphragmatic lymph nodes has been emphasized by Nidden et al (1973), who confirm that lymph reaches the right lymphatic duct, partly via the tracheobronchial lymph nodes.

INNERVATION

The hepatic nerves arise from the hepatic plexus (p. 1307) containing sympathetic and parasympathetic (vagal) fibres. They enter at the porta hepatis and largely accompany blood vessels and bile ducts; very few run amongst the liver cells and their terminations are uncertain. Both myelinated and non-myelinated fibres reach the liver from nerves in its various peritoneal folds (Sutherland 1965).

HEPATIC MICROSTRUCTURE (12.145–152)

The liver is essentially an epithelial-mesenchymal outgrowth of the caudal part of the foregut (p. 187), with which it retains its connection by the biliary tree. During development it is penetrated by vascular and connective tissue elements, and defensive cells migrate into its vascular spaces. When fully formed it consists of a complex network of epithelial cells interpenetrated and ensheathed by supportive connective tissue, and permeated by great numbers of blood vessels perfusing the liver with a rich flow of blood from the hepatic portal vein and hepatic arteries. The epithelial cells, *hepatocytes*, carry out the major metabolic activities of this organ, but are assisted by additional classes of cell which possess storage, phagocytic and mechanically supportive functions.

The hepatocytes are arranged in anastomosing plates (*hepatic laminae* or *cords*: see below) lined by endothelium and separated from each other by vascular spaces (*hepatic sinusoids*). Bile secreted

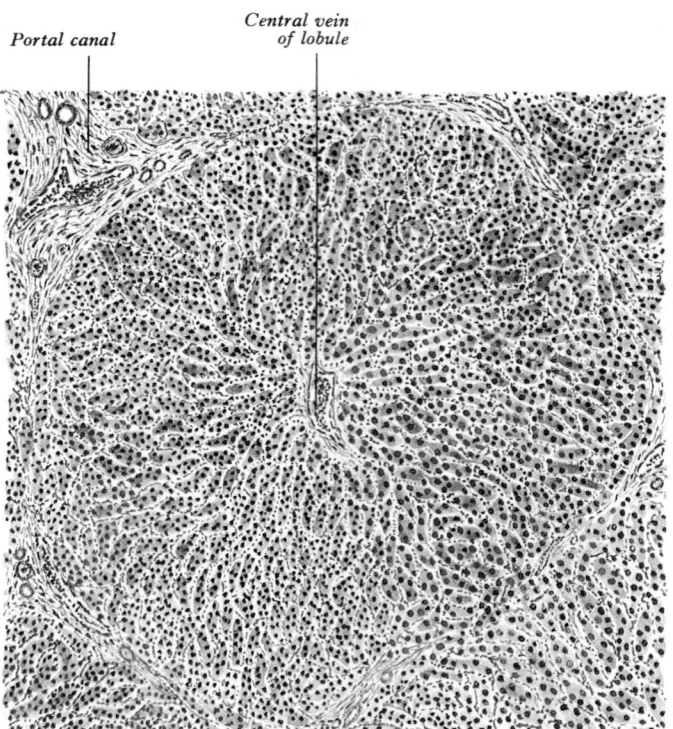

12.146A Section through a hepatic lobule (human) (after Sobotta). Stained with haematoxylin and eosin. Magnification × 70.

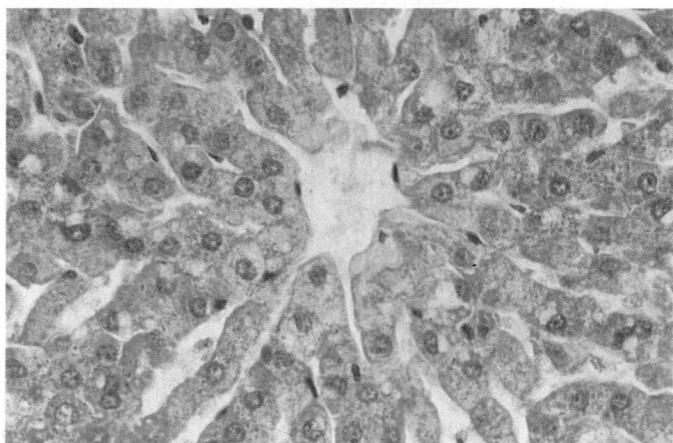

12.146B Section through a number of hepatic cords radiating from a central hepatic venule of the rabbit. The hepatocytes appear cuboidal and the Kupffer and endothelial cells, which line the sinusoids, have flattened, densely staining nuclei. Haematoxylin and eosin.

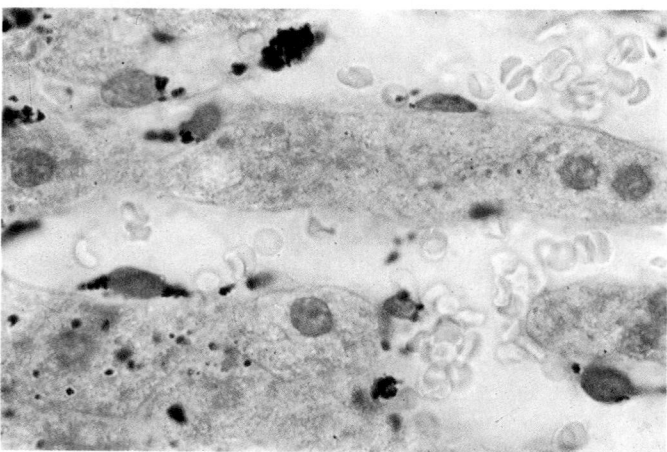

12.146C Section similar to that shown in B, but taken from the liver of a rabbit previously injected intravenously with carbon particles. The Kupffer cell nuclei are outlined with phagocytosed particles which demonstrate the limits of the cell cytoplasm.

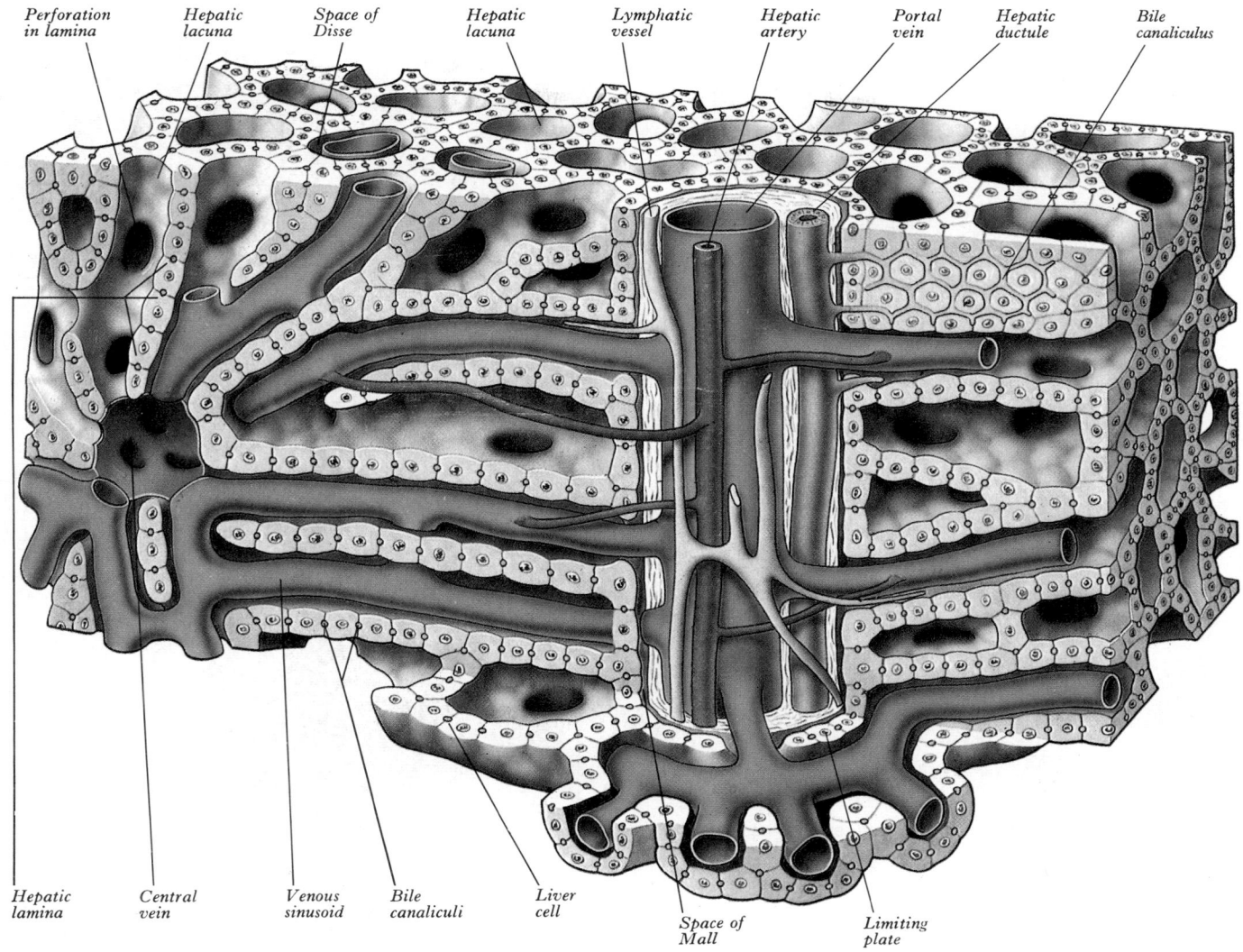

Perforation in lamina · Hepatic lacuna · Space of Disse · Hepatic lacuna · Lymphatic vessel · Hepatic artery · Portal vein · Hepatic ductule · Bile canaliculus

Hepatic lamina · Central vein · Venous sinusoid · Bile canaliculi · Liver cell · Space of Mall · Limiting plate

12.147   Diagram of hepatic microstructure (after H Elias, Department of Anatomy, Chicago Medical School). Note that in this picture, perisinusoidal endothelial cells and macrophages (Kupffer cells) are not shown.

by the hepatocytes is collected in a network of minute tubes (*canaliculi*) which, in the hepatic cords, are formed by the apposition of corresponding rounded grooves in the lateral walls of the hepatocytes themselves. Bile drains in a direction opposite to the flow of blood through the neighbouring sinusoids, and is collected at the ends of the hepatic cords by epithelium-lined *hepatic ductules* which join others to form the biliary tree. The hepatocytes can therefore be regarded as exocrine cells, secreting bile to the alimentary tract via the hepatic ducts and bile duct; however, they also have another metabolic orientation, that is, towards the blood with which hepatocytes are engaged in a complex series of chemical exchanges.

The surface of the liver facing the peritoneal cavity is lined by typical serosa (the visceral peritoneum); beneath this, and enclosing the whole structure, is a thin (50–100 μm) layer of connective tissue ('Glisson's capsule') from which extensions pass into the liver, branching and rebranching as connective tissue septa and trabeculae. Branches of the hepatic arteries and hepatic veins, together with bile ductules and ducts, run within these connective tissue trabeculae which are termed *portal tracts* (portal canals). The combination of the two types of vessel and a hepatic duct is termed a *portal triad*, a name not strictly accurate because these structures are usually accompanied by one or more lymphatic vessels.

Lobulation of the liver

At first sight, the microscopic organization of the liver appears rather chaotic, with (in humans) no obvious arrangement of hepatic cords

into discrete groups (**12**.146). However, it is known that specific patterns of cellular degeneration occur in different disease states, indicating the presence of functional units in the normal as well as the pathological liver. Detailed studies with three-dimensional reconstruction and morphometric analysis, combined with observations of clinical and experimental pathology, have provided a picture of what is essentially a highly orderly arrangement of cell clusters, or *lobules*, centred around the smallest afferent vessels and bile ductules of the liver. However, the term 'lobule' has a rather chequered history, and requires some explanation and qualification.

As originally described in the adult pig and some other mammals, the liver is composed largely of prismatic clusters of hepatocytes, each group or *classical lobule* often being hexagonal, about 1 mm in diameter and enclosed in loose connective tissue. Within this unit, hepatic cords are arranged like the spokes of a wheel about a central *terminal hepatic venule* (centrilobular venule, or central vein), a tributary of an hepatic vein. However, in man (and many other mammals) such well-defined classical lobules are not usually present. The three-dimensional reconstructions by Rappaport (1969, 1987) and other studies have substituted the concept of the *portal lobule* centred on a near-terminal branch of an hepatic artery and portal vein, and their related bile ductule. Referring to the situation in the pig liver, this territory corresponds to sectors of at least three 'classic' lobules (**12**.145). Hence, in sections, a portal lobule is a polygonal territory centred on a portal triad, its boundary passing through adjacent central veins. A subunit of this territory, the *portal acinus*

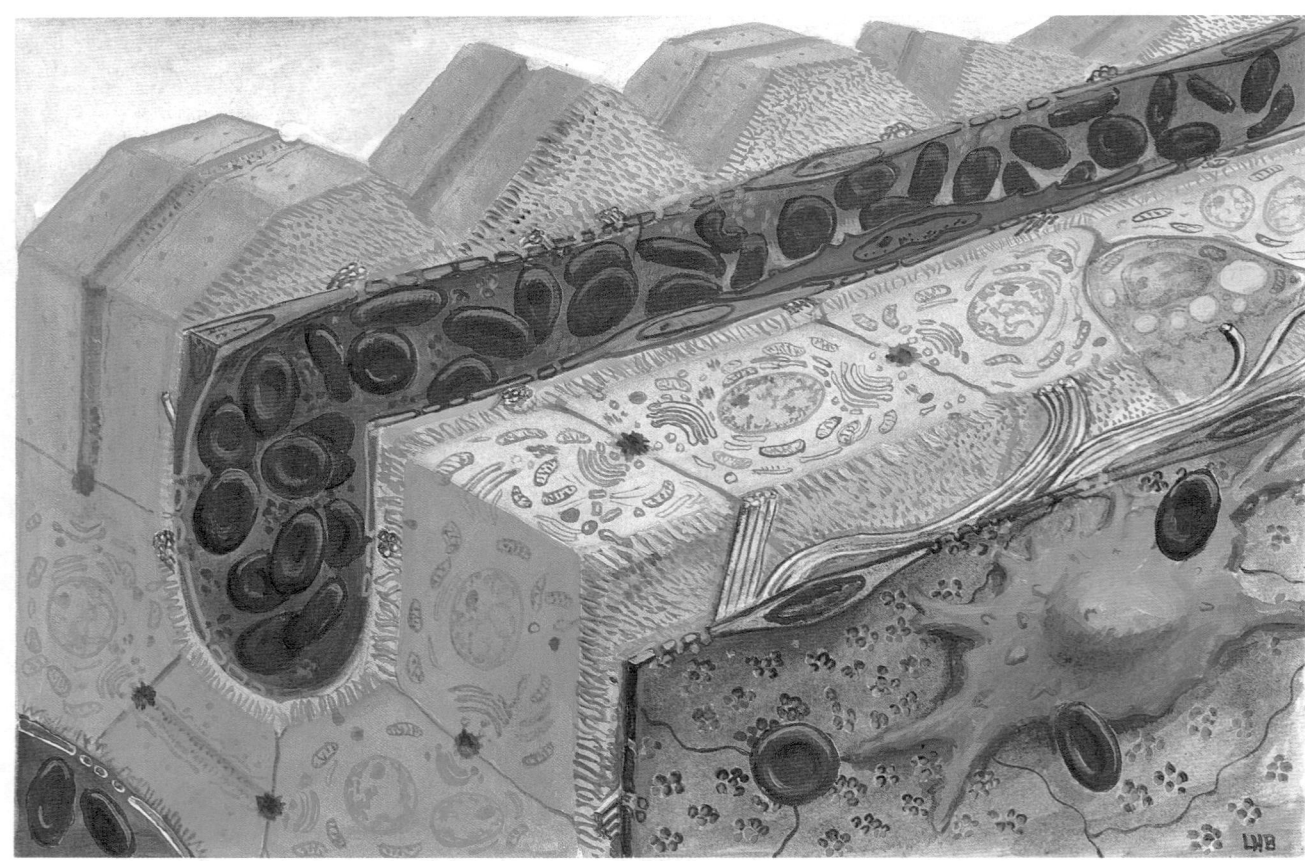

12.148   Schema illustrating the chief cellular features of an hepatic cord.

(Rappaport 1969, 1987), is centred on a preterminal branch of an hepatic arteriole and includes the hepatic tissue served by it, bounded by the territories of other acini and by two adjacent central veins (**12**.144). Another proposed subdivision, the *primary hepatic lobule* (Matsumoto 1979) represents one half of a portal acinus, i.e. a conical volume supplied by a preterminal arteriole, and draining into a single centrilobular vein. These attempts to codify hepatic micro-organization have clarified important problems of liver histo-pathology, especially the development of zones of anoxic damage, glycogen deposition and removal, and of toxic trauma, which are all related to the direction of arterial flow and thus tend to follow the acinar pattern. There are also real structural and physiological differences within the acinar lobules and they are customarily divided into three zones:

Mito-chondria

Bile canaliculi

Lysosomes

1μ

12.149   Electron micrograph showing portions of three adjacent hepa-tocytes and the intervening bile canaliculi. Magnification × 10 000.

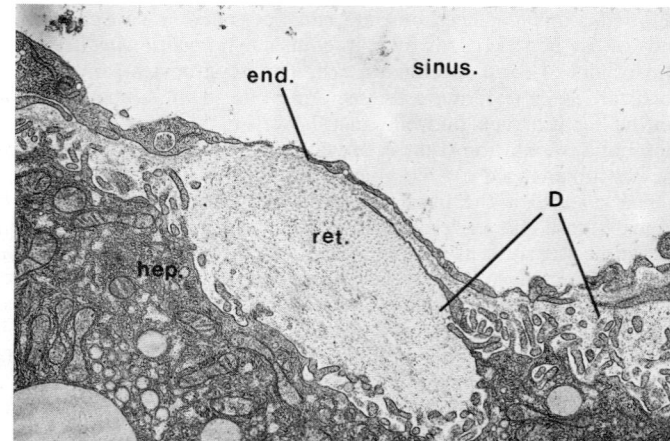

end.   sinus.

D

ret.

hep.

12.150   Transmission electron micrograph of the border of a hepatic sinus-oid (sinus.) showing part of an hepatocyte (hep.) and the tenuous fenestrated endothelium (end.) separated by the space of Disse (D) in part of which lies a reticulin bundle (ret.). Magnification × 5000.

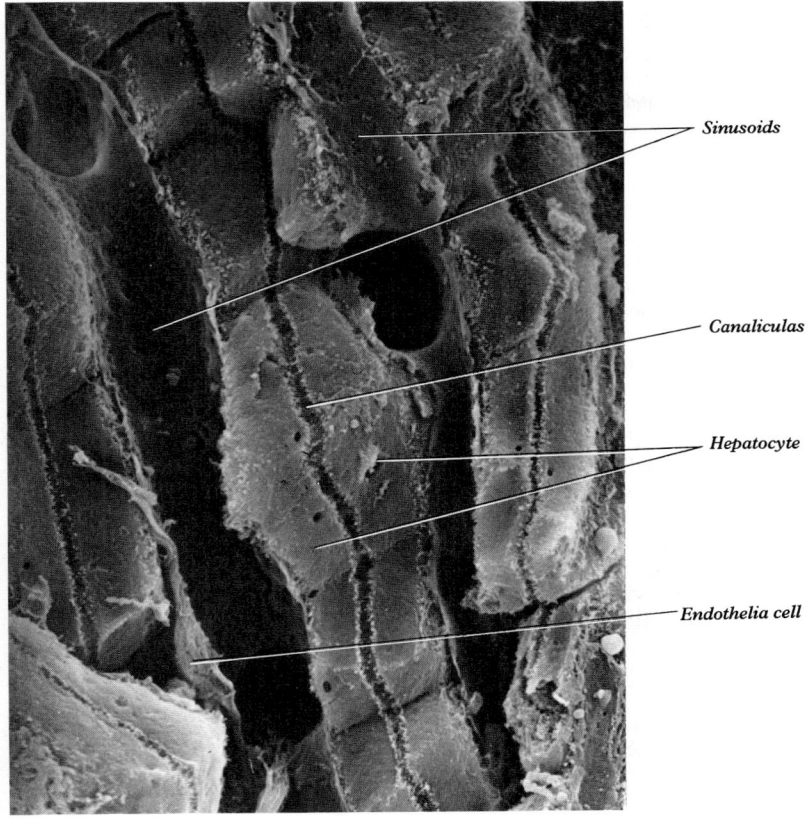

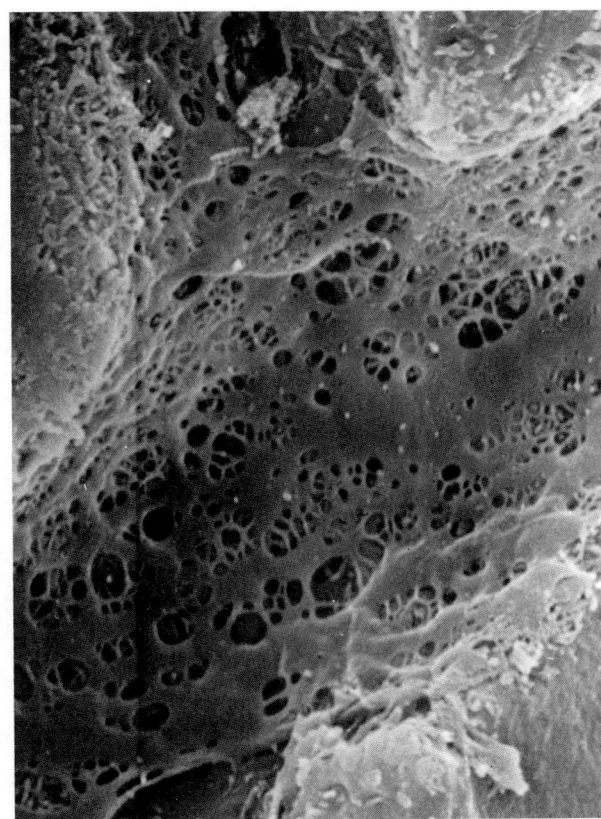

12.151 Scanning electron micrograph of the cut surface of the liver (rodent) showing sinusoids with endothelial linings and adjacent hepatocytes, grooved by bile canaliculi (see **12.149**).

12.152 Scanning electron micrograph of the internal surface of a hepatic sinusoid, showing endothelial fenestrations. Magnification × 8000.

- *zone 1* (periportal) i.e. nearest the portal radicles
- *zone 2* further away from these
- *zone 3* around the central venous drainage (see below).

On a larger scale, Rappaport (1969) has proposed the concept of *compound portal acini*, which are more complex groups of hepatic units centred around larger triads.

Cells of the liver (12.146B, C, 147–152)

Cells of the liver include *hepatocytes, perisinusoidal (Ito) cells, endotheliocytes, macrophages* (Kupffer cells), *lymphocytes* (pit cells), the *cells of the biliary tree* (cuboidal to columnar epitheliocytes) and *connective tissue cells* of the capsule and portal tracts. For further details, see Phillips et al (1987); Bioulac-Sage et al (1991); Jones et al (1991).

Hepatocytes. About 80% of the liver volume and 60% of its cell number are formed by hepatocytes (parenchymal cells). They are polyhedral, with five to twelve sides and are from 20–30 μm across. Their nuclei are spheroidal and euchromatic and often polyploid or multiple (two or more) in each cell (Doljanski 1960). Their cytoplasm typically displays much granular and agranular endoplasmic reticulum, many mitochondria, lysosomes and many well-developed Golgi bodies, features indicating a high metabolic activity. Glycogen granules and lipid vacuoles are usually prominent. Numerous, particularly large peroxisomes and vacuoles containing enzymes such as urease (uricosomes) in distinctive crystalline forms indicate the complex metabolism of these cells. Their role in iron metabolism is shown by storage vacuoles containing crystals of ferritin and haemosiderin.

Hepatocytes also contain characteristic types of cytokeratin (intermediate) filaments which are useful markers in immuno-histochemical assessments of pathological tissues (Marceau 1994), allowing them to be distinguished from, e.g. biliary duct cells. Actin

microfilaments and microtubules are also quite numerous. Where hepatocytes adjoin bile canaliculi they carry short microvilli and numerous membrane-bound vesicles cluster near the lumen (**12.149, 151**) reflecting the secretion of bile components. The borders of these canaliculi are marked by tight junctions where adjacent hepatocytes lie in contact, preventing their secretions from entering the general intercellular spaces of the liver (and blood plasma from leaking into the biliary tract: the *blood–bile barrier*) and confining them to the canalicular system. The tight junctions are reinforced mechanically by zonulae adherentes (p. 27), anchored into a lamina of actin filaments which surrounds each canaliculus and sends supportive bundles into the short canalicular microvilli. Elsewhere, hepatocytes are linked by numerous gap junctions and desmosomes, although there is free access of blood plasma to the sides of hepatocytes through the intercellular spaces.

On the sides of the cell facing the sinusoids are numerous microvilli, about 0.5 μm long, which create a large area of membrane exposed to the plasma bathing these surfaces (**12.150**).

Hepatocyte structure and metabolism varies within the portal acini, according to their distance from the portal inflow (see above); in zone 1, cells have more mitochondria and granular endoplasmic reticulum, whilst in zone 3 (nearest the central veins) the agranular endoplasmic reticulum is even more extensive, but mitochondria are fewer and more spheroidal. In zone 2, there is a gradient between the other two conditions. Cell size also varies, with a decreasing size gradient from zone 1 to zone 3.

Hepatocytes mediate many metabolic activities. At their sinusoidal interface with blood plasma they release into the bloodstream various plasma proteins which they have synthesized, such as albumins, clotting factors (factor III, fibrinogen) and complement components; they deaminate amino acids by the urea cycle, liberating urea for subsequent renal excretion; convert bilirubin to biliverdin for secretion into bile; they take up and inactivate many endogenous

1805

and exogenous toxic substances from the blood and convert circulating tetra-iodothyronin to the more active tri-iodothyronin. They also store carbohydrates as glycogen, and triglycerides as lipid droplets, metabolizing these as required to release glucose and lipid into the blood. Most lipid thus secreted reaches the perisinusoidal surface of the cell in secretory vesicles, having been conjugated with protein in the endoplasmic reticulum and Golgi apparatus, to form the 'very low density lipoprotein' moiety of blood plasma (Claude 1970), a cholesterol carrier. Iron is stored in the hepatocytes as ferritin granules. In addition, these cells store vitamins of the B complex, including vitamin B_{12}.

At the cell surface facing the bile canaliculus, bile is elaborated and secreted; a major function is the synthesis and secretion of bile salts essential to the emulsification of fats in digestion; the elimination of various toxic materials from the body also occurs via the biliary tree, including some hormones, and a moiety of cholesterol. The liver is also a major route for IgA secretion into the alimentary tract; IgA originates mainly from B lymphocytes in mucosa-associated lymphoid tissue (p. 1442) of the alimentary tract wall; although some is secreted locally via the mucous cells of the gut, much passes into the portal venous system and reaches the liver where it is taken up by hepatocytes and passed into the bile, whence it reaches the alimentary lumen of the duodenum and more distal intestinal regions. All of these metabolic activities generate heat, and the liver is a major source of thermal energy for the maintenance of a high 'resting' body temperature and thus homeothermy.

The multitude of actions performed by hepatocytes is reflected in their structural complexity, which varies with metabolic demand, e.g. agranular endoplasmic reticulum proliferates during barbiturate detoxification (Jones & Fawcett 1966), while in starvation glycogen and lipid reserves disappear. Because of involvement in many such processes, hepatocytes are most vulnerable to anoxia, various toxins and carcinogens, which cause characteristic patterns of degeneration in the portal acini.

Perisinusoidal (Ito) cells. These are much less numerous than hepatocytes. They are irregular in outline, and lie within the hepatic laminae wedged between the bases of hepatocytes. They are typified by numerous lipid vesicles, and by the presence of actin filaments, myosin and the intermediate filament desmin (Johnson et al 1992) indicating that they have many similarities with myofibroblasts (p. 76). These cells have a number of important functions, the most significant being to secrete most of the matrix components of the hepatic laminae including collagens (Friedman et al 1985) and various proteoglycans (e.g. fibronectin: Avenson et al 1988). They also store the fat-soluble vitamin A in their lipid vesicles, and are a significant source of growth factors active in the regeneration of the damaged liver, as well as its normal maintenance. Perisinusoidal cells also play a major role in the reorganization of hepatic cords after toxic damage, and pathologically in the replacement of defunct hepatocytes with collagenous fibres, as seen in cirrhosis.

Endotheliocytes. (12.146, 150–152). Hepatic venous sinusoids are generally wider than blood capillaries and are lined by a thin but highly fenestrated endothelium. The endothelial cells are typically flattened, each with a central nucleus and joined to each other by junctional complexes. The fenestrae are grouped in clusters ('sieve plates' 12.152) with a mean diameter of 100 nm, allowing plasma direct access to the bases of hepatocytes. Within the cytoplasm of these cells are numerous typical transcytotic vesicles.

Hepatic macrophages. These cells, also called stellate cells of *von Kupffer*, or more simply, *Kupffer cells*) lie within the sinusoid lumen (12.149, 152), attached to the endothelial surface; these cells, derived from the bone marrow, form a major part of the body's mononuclear phagocyte system (p. 1414), responsible for removing from the circulation much cellular and microbial debris, and secreting various cytokines involved in defence, etc. In the liver they also remove aged and damaged red cells from the circulation (as in the spleen). These cells are irregular, with long processes including lamellipodia extending into the sinusoid lumen; they have flattened nuclei, and their cytoplasm contains characteristic invaginations of the plasma membrane (vermiform bodies). Lysosomes are numerous.

Lymphocytes. Associated with the surfaces of hepatic macrophages are large granular lymphocytes ('pit cells'). These appear to be largely natural killer cells (p. 1405) and are likely to be an important source of defence against viral and other infectious agents.

Hepatic laminae (cords) (12.146–148, 151)

The precise manner in which hepatocytes are arranged in the liver has been much debated. The most recent studies show that in the mature liver, hepatocytes are arranged mainly in plates, one cell thick, of about 20 cells from periphery to centrilobular venule.

They form a continuous system or *muralium* of *hepatic laminae* (*hepatic cords*) which may branch or anastomose, frequent interlaminar bridges of cells connecting adjacent laminae (12.147). Between the laminae lie *hepatic lacunae* containing endothelium-lined *venous sinusoids*, which anastomose with each other via gaps in the hepatic laminae. Where hepatocytes adjoin portal canals or hepatic venous tributaries they form a *limiting plate*, surrounding the vessels and perforated by their radicles and by rami of the hepatic artery and biliary ductules; a similar limiting plate composed of a single layer of liver cells underlies the entire capsule of the liver. In histological sections (12.145, 146) the rows of liver cells seen radiating from the central vein to the lobular periphery are really sections through hepatic laminae. These rows, with intervening sinusoids, do not pass straight to the periphery like the spokes of a wheel but run irregularly, because the laminae themselves are irregular and branched (12.147).

Sinusoids are fed at one end with blood from fine branches of the hepatic portal venules (inlet venules) and hepatic arterioles, which pass through the limiting plate of hepatocytes to enter a hepatic lobule (12.147). Blood from these sources percolates between the walls of the sinusoids to the central veins and is exposed to the activities of the cells around the sinusoids. The endothelial linings of the sinusoids are separated from hepatocytes of the hepatic laminae by a narrow gap, the *perisinusoidal space of Disse* (12.150, 151) which is normally about 0.2–0.5 μm wide, but distends in anoxic conditions: it contains fine collagen fibres (chiefly type III, with some types I and IV), the irregular microvilli of adjacent hepatocytes and occasional non-myelinated nerve terminals (Forssman & Ito 1977). This space is continuous at the lobular periphery with the *space of Mall* surrounding the vessels and ductules in the portal canals. In the latter space, lymph vessels begin as cul-de-sac capillaries, as elsewhere; only a very few reach the periphery of the lobule. As already mentioned hepatic perisinusoidal cells (Ito cells) are also present in small numbers in the space of Disse. Central veins from adjacent lobules form *interlobular veins*, which unite as *hepatic veins*, draining blood to the inferior vena cava.

Minute *bile canaliculi* (12.147–149, 151) form nets with polygonal meshes in the hepatic lobules; each hepatocyte is surrounded by canaliculi except on its juxtasinusoidal sides. Hepatic laminae thus enclose a network of canaliculi which pass to the lobular periphery where they join to form narrow intralobular ductules (*terminal ductules* or the *canals of Hering*) lined by squamous cuboidal epithelium; these exit through the terminal laminae to enter interlobular hepatic ductules in the portal canals. Intralobular ductules differ from the other biliary canals in their structure and reaction to injury; e.g. they proliferate when the flow of bile is obstructed outside the liver (Biava 1964; Jones et al 1975). Hepatic ductules in portal canals are lined by cuboidal or columnar cells which may contain cholesterol crystals and lipid droplets.

Preterminal hepatic arterioles in the portal canals branch to convey arterial blood to the sinusoids by several routes, the chief being via a fine capillary plexus around the interlobular ductules and ducts which drains to branches of the portal veins, inlet venules and hepatic sinusoids. Some arterial blood passes directly to the hepatic sinusoids, bypassing these capillary plexuses; but this is apparently only a small part of the total flow (Burkel 1970; Healey 1970; Jones & Spring-Mills 1977). Sinusoids thus contain mixed venous and arterial blood to sustain their cells. The composition, volume and velocity of blood through any local region may be regulated according to changing needs by the sphincters around the entry points of inlet venules and hepatic arterioles, and by the contractile walls of the sinusoids. Each portal triad supplies a distinct territory; normally there are no anastomoses between territories. Hepatic veins run quite separately with respect to the triadic system, freely crossing the boundaries of triadic territories.

Haemopoiesis in the liver. The fetal liver is a major haemopoietic organ, erythrocytes, leucocytes and platelets developing from the mesenchyme covering the sinusoidal endothelium (p. 1407).

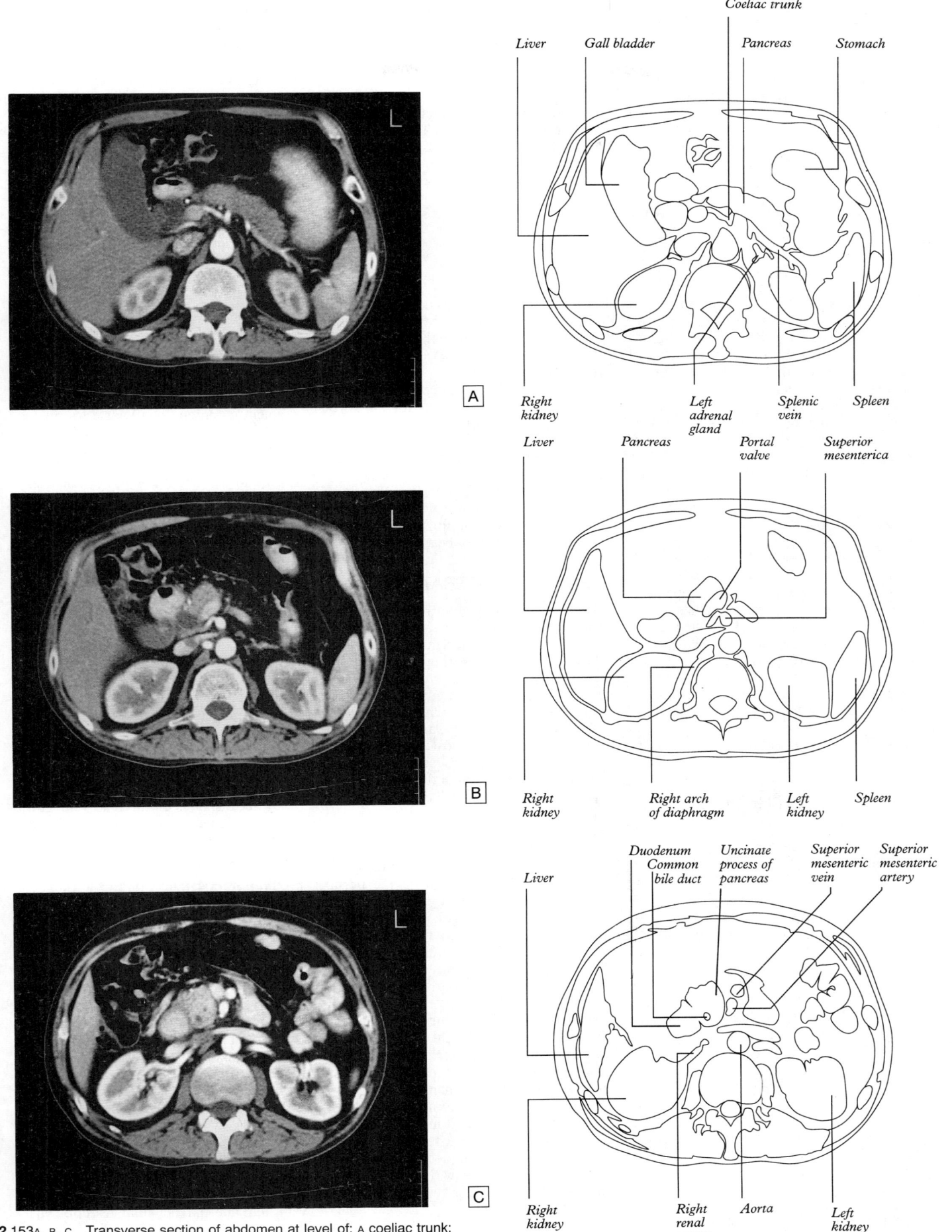

12.153A, B, C Transverse section of abdomen at level of: A coeliac trunk;
B superior mesenteric artery and portal vein; C head of uncinate process of
pancreas and left renal vein.

The labelled diagrams accompanying the CT images show the following structures:

A
Liver · Gall bladder · Coeliac trunk · Pancreas · Stomach
Right kidney · Left adrenal gland · Splenic vein · Spleen

B
Liver · Pancreas · Portal valve · Superior mesenterica
Right kidney · Right arch of diaphragm · Left kidney · Spleen

C
Liver · Duodenum · Common bile duct · Uncinate process of pancreas · Superior mesenteric vein · Superior mesenteric artery
Right kidney · Right renal artery · Aorta · Left kidney

CLINICAL ANATOMY OF THE LIVER

On account of its large size, fixed position, and friability, the liver is sometimes ruptured; haemorrhage may be severe, because the hepatic veins lie in rigid canals and are unable to contract. The organ may be torn by a broken rib, perforating the diaphragm. Clinical evidence suggests that the bloodstreams of the superior mesenteric and splenic veins remain largely separate in the portal vein, passing respectively along the right and left portal branches to the right and left physiological (vascular) lobes (p. 1797); thus malignant or infective emboli may be more pronounced in the right lobe if the primary disease is in the territory drained by the superior mesenteric vein, or in the left if it is in the splenic or inferior mesenteric territory. This correlation is also supported in experiments in living animals. Vascular hepatic segmentation (p. 1798) is a vital factor in *partial hepatectomy*.

The liver and its related structures are clearly visible in MRI images (**12**.153A–c), which are valuable in diagnosis of hepatic pathology.

Liver transplantation

Liver transplantation has grown from a largely experimental procedure, first carried out 30 years ago, to a well-established treatment option for patients with advanced liver disease. Foster, in his review of liver surgery in 1991 stated, 'Total hepatectomy with liver transplantation may be the most difficult operation ever devised, both technically and physiologically.' In 1992, over 500 liver transplantations were carried out in the United Kingdom, and over 2000 in more than 70 centres in Europe, with over three-quarters of patients making a full recovery.

Complete knowledge of surgical anatomy related to the liver is essential for both the donor harvesting operation and the recipient operation. The shortage of paediatric donors has resulted in the rapid development of innovative surgical techniques where adult donor grafts are reduced in size to two or four segments to implant into children, further emphasizing the contributions by Couinaud and Hjortsjö, who were among the first to describe the segmental anatomy of the liver (see p. 1797).

DONOR LIVER REMOVAL

The conventional textbook description of a single hepatic artery arising from the coeliac trunk is seen in only 60–65% of cases, with anatomical variations being present in over one-third of cases. The commonest variations are a replaced or accessory left hepatic artery from the left gastric artery (20%), and a replaced or accessory right hepatic artery arising from the superior mesenteric artery (15%), running posterior to the common bile duct. Occasionally both variants may be present together (5%), or the entire hepatic arterial supply may be derived from the superior mesenteric artery or from a common coeliacomesenteric trunk. Identification of the arterial supply is essential prior to perfusion to cool and preserve the donor organs. To remove the liver from the donor, the common bile duct is divided just above the pancreas, the gallbladder incised and the bile flushed out prior to cooling, to prevent bile-induced epithelial injury. After cross-clamping the aorta above the level of the coeliac axis, cooling of the liver is achieved by portal venous and aortic perfusion with University of Wisconsin solution (UW) at 4°C. The liver retrieval is completed, preserving an adequate length of inferior vena cava (IVC), the coeliac trunk with an aortic patch, and a suitable length of portal vein. In addition, the common and external iliac arteries and veins are retrieved in the event that a vascular reconstruction is necessary, e.g. because of portal vein thrombosis, or arterial vascular reconstruction. The graft is then preserved for up to 18 hours in UW at a temperature between 0–4°C.

RECIPIENT OPERATION

The use of UW has permitted safe prolonged storage times, so that this operation is usually performed as a semi-elective procedure during the day. The removal of the recipient's diseased liver is usually undertaken in the presence of portal hypertension, often with previous biliary or portal surgery, and occasionally with additional technical problems such as portal vein thrombosis or extensive varices. The structures in the porta hepatis are systematically divided close to the liver hilum, the hepatic artery, the common hepatic duct and the portal vein. Most centres make use of a venovenous bypass in adults during the anhepatic phase, where blood is pumped from the portal and femoral vein to the axillary vein (**12**.154A); its advantages include decompression of the clamped IVC and portal system, providing adequate circulating blood volume and venous return, thereby allowing for a more controlled anhepatic phase.

Next, the IVC is identified below the liver and the left and right triangular ligaments are divided and the bare area of the liver is dissected off the diaphragm. The suprahepatic IVC is then dissected and encircled. The hepatectomy is completed after placing supra- and infrahepatic IVC clamps. An alternative technique called the 'piggy-back' technique leaves the entire recipient IVC in place, with ligation of the individual short hepatic veins, particularly from the caudate lobe.

After achieving full control of bleeding, the new liver, which has been dissected and prepared on a sterile trolley, is implanted into the recipient: the upper IVC anastomosis first, the lower IVC next followed by the portal vein using a continuous vascular suture (**12**.154B). The UW within the liver vessels is next washed out. The graft is then reperfused with blood via the portal vein. The arterial anastomosis is usually made between the donor and recipient common hepatic arteries. In the event of a donor left hepatic artery from the left gastric, no reconstruction is necessary, the coeliac trunk being used for the anastomosis. A donor right hepatic artery arising from the superior mesenteric artery requires some additional reconstruction, most commonly this is anastomosed to the donor splenic artery stump. Not infrequently, especially in patients undergoing retransplantation for hepatic artery thrombosis, it is often impossible to achieve an adequate arterial inflow from the coeliac trunk, and a donor iliac artery aortic conduit is constructed from the recipient infrarenal aorta to the donor hepatic artery. Portal vein thrombosis is no longer a contraindication to liver transplantation, and successful portal revascularization can be obtained by thrombectomy, dissection posterior to the pancreas down to healthy portal vein, use of large collaterals, e.g. left gastric vein, or by means of a donor iliac vein graft from the recipient superior mesenteric vein to the donor portal vein.

REDUCED-SIZE LIVER TRANSPLANTATION

The majority of children with liver disease present this condition in infancy and early childhood. It is in this group that there is a great shortage of donor organs. Over the past decade, many groups have shown that it is safe to implant reduced-size grafts, with a reduction in waiting time, fewer deaths on waiting lists, and with no increase in complications related to the reduction process. These techniques allow a donor–recipient weight discrepancy of up to 10:1, when only segments 2 and 3 are transplanted (**12**.154B). The back-table reduction operation entails a meticulous hilar and intrahepatic vascular and biliary dissection, dissection of the left hepatic vein, and the parenchymal resection just to the right of the falciform ligament. In

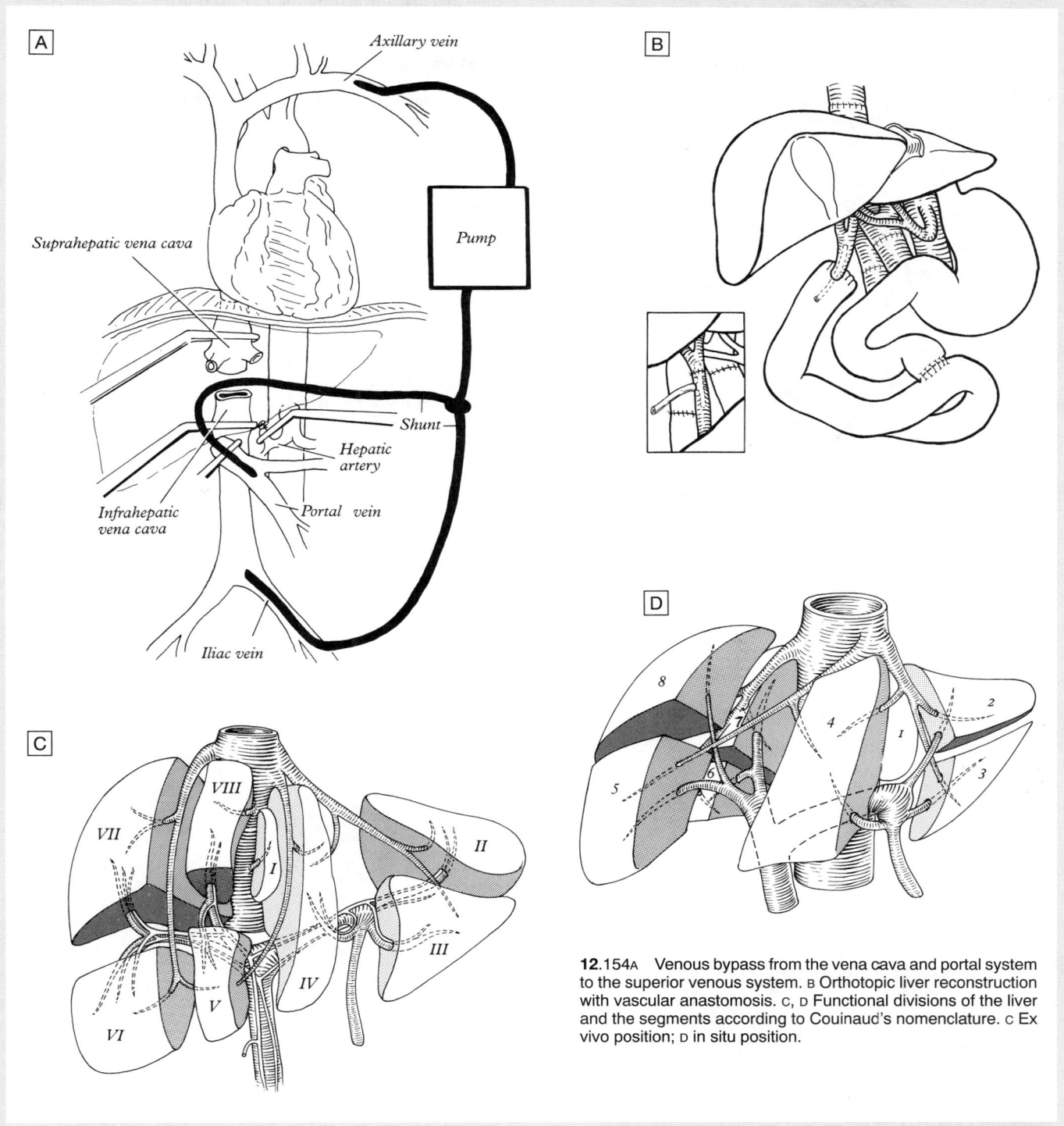

12.154A Venous bypass from the vena cava and portal system to the superior venous system. B Orthotopic liver reconstruction with vascular anastomosis. C, D Functional divisions of the liver and the segments according to Couinaud's nomenclature. C Ex vivo position; D in situ position.

larger children, or when the discrepancy is less than 4:1, the right lobe (segments 5–8) may be utilized.

The splitting of a single donor liver into right and left lobes, thus benefiting two recipients, is also an established procedure, where the vessels to one of the halves have to be lengthened using donor vessels. A few centres have gone one step further, in an effort to further reduce the waiting period, to partial transplants from living relations, where segments 2 and 3 of a parent's liver are transplanted into a child. Over 100 such transplants have been performed worldwide, particularly in the United States of America and Japan, with low donor morbidity and excellent short and long term results.

In conclusion, liver transplantation has developed into a major effort to support patients with advanced liver disease. Although the techniques have been standardized, it remains a difficult and complex procedure. A complete knowledge of the anatomic variations in arterial supply, bile duct, portal and hepatic venous anatomy, as well as the segmental anatomy of the liver, is an essential prerequisite to developing the surgical skills for this form of surgery.

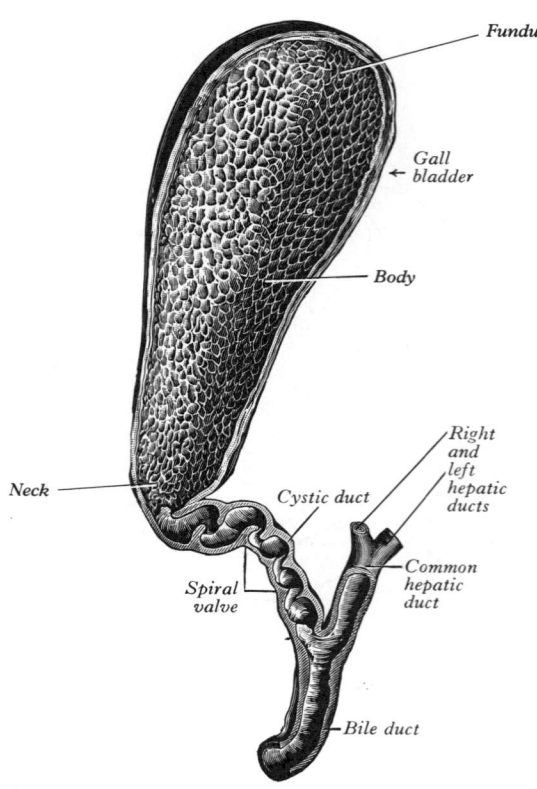

12.155   Interior of the gallbladder and bile ducts.

BILIARY DUCTS AND GALLBLADDER

The hepatic ductal apparatus consists of:

- the *common hepatic duct*, formed by the junction of the *right* and *left hepatic ducts*
- the *gallbladder*, a reservoir for bile

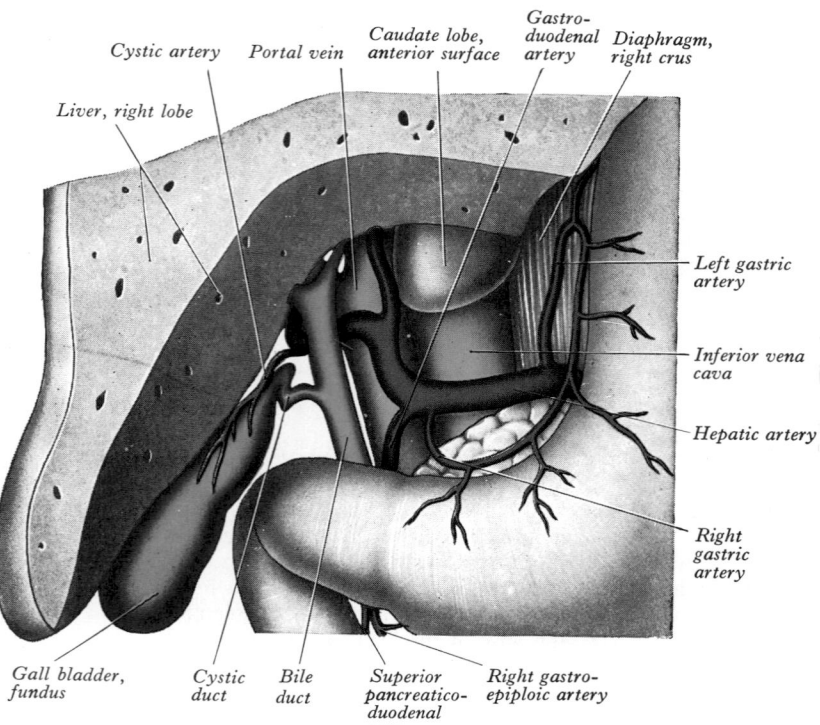

12.156   Dissection to show the relations of the hepatic artery, bile duct and portal vein to each other in the lesser omentum: anterior aspect.

- the *cystic duct* of the gallbladder
- the *bile duct*, formed by the junction of the common hepatic and cystic ducts.

COMMON HEPATIC DUCT (**12**.155, 156)

The main right and left hepatic ducts issue from the liver and unite near the right end of the porta hepatis as the common hepatic duct, which descends about 3 cm before being joined on its right at an acute angle by the cystic duct to form the main bile duct. The common hepatic duct lies to the right of the hepatic artery and anterior to the portal vein.

GALLBLADDER

The gallbladder (**12**.140, 141, 144, 155–160) is a slate-blue, piriform sac partly sunk in a fossa in the right hepatic lobe's inferior surface. It extends forwards from a point near the right end of the porta hepatis to the inferior hepatic border. Its upper surface is attached to the liver by connective tissue; elsewhere it is completely covered by peritoneum continued from the hepatic surface. Occasionally it is completely invested by peritoneum and even connected to the liver by a short mesentery. It is 7–10 cm long, 3 cm broad at its widest and 30–50 ml in capacity. It is described as having a fundus, body and neck. The *fundus*, the expanded end, projects down, forwards and to the right, extending beyond the inferior border to contact the anterior abdominal wall behind the ninth right costal cartilage, where the lateral edge of the right rectus abdominis crosses the costal margin. Posteriorly it is related to the transverse colon, near its commencement. (These relations change when the gallbladder is lower, as it often is in slender females, see Fleischner & Sayegh 1958.) The *body* is directed up, back and to the left; near the right

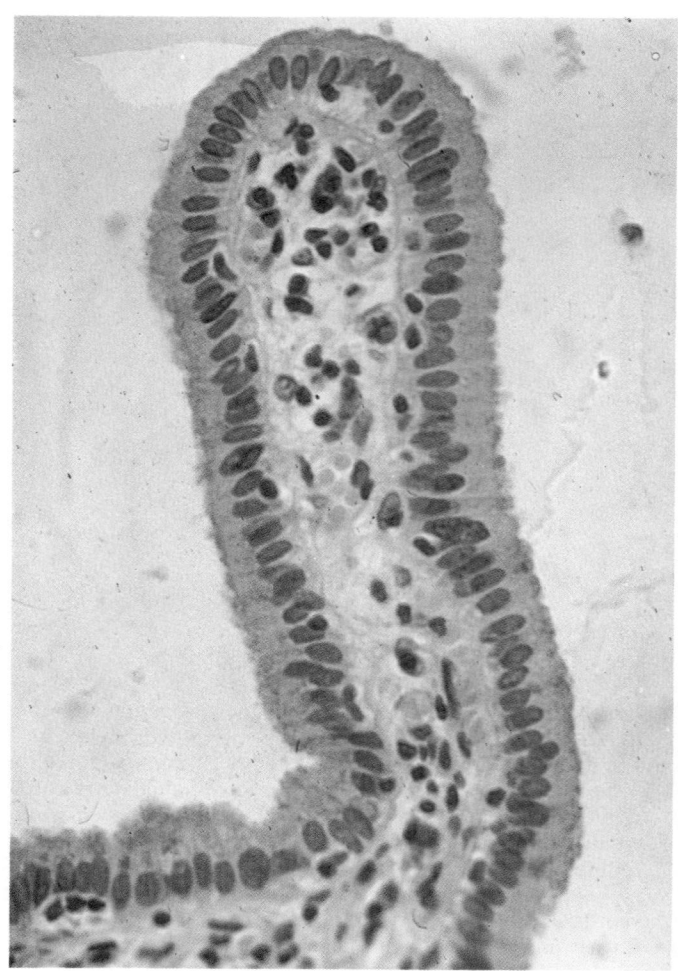

12.157   Section through a surface projection (ruga) of the gallbladder showing the columnar epithelial cells and lamina propria. Haematoxylin and eosin. Magnification × 500.

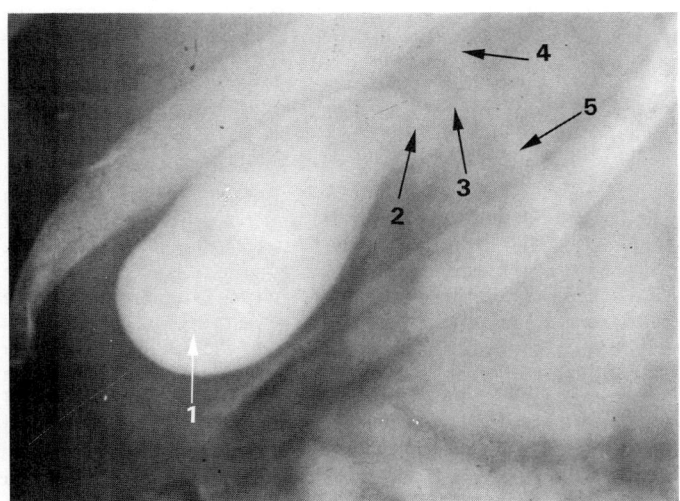

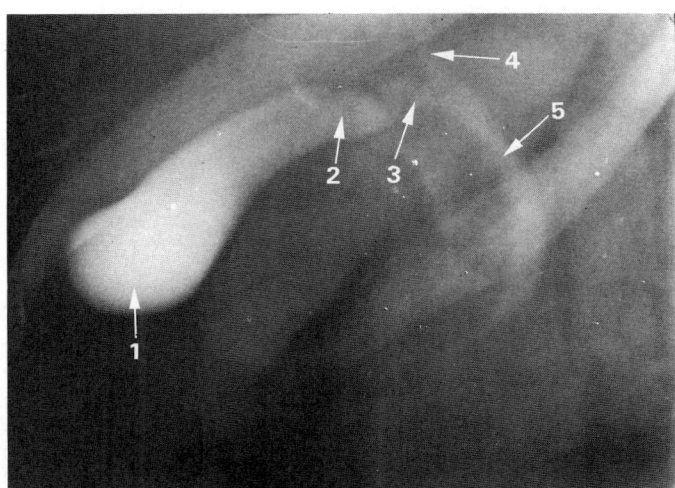

12.158　Anteroposterior radiograph of the gallbladder and biliary ducts after the oral administration of sodium tetra-iodophenolphthalein the previous day.

12.159　The same field as **12**.158 but taken 20 minutes after a fatty meal, demonstrating the contraction and partial emptying of the gallbladder. In both A and B: (1) fundus of gallbladder; (2) neck of gallbladder; (3) cystic duct; (4) common hepatic duct; (5) the bile duct.

end of the porta it is continuous with the gallbladder neck. It is related above to the liver, below to the transverse colon and, further back, to the first and upper end of the second segments of the duodenum. The *neck* (cervix) is narrow, curving up and forwards and then abruptly back and downwards, to become the cystic duct, at which transition there is a constriction. The neck is attached to the liver by loose connective tissue containing the cystic artery. The mucosa of the neck is obliquely ridged, forming a spiral valve; when the neck is distended, this gives its surface a spiral groove. From the right side of the neck a small recess may project down and back towards the duodenum. Often termed Hartmann's pouch (but originally described by Broca), it has been widely regarded as a constant feature, but Davies and Harding (1942) have shown that it is always a sequela of pathological states, especially dilatation; when it is large the cystic duct arises from its upper left aspect and not from what appears to be the gallbladder's apex.

CYSTIC DUCT (**12**.155, 156, 158, 159)

This structure is 3–4 cm long; it passes back, down and to the left from the neck of the gallbladder, joining the common hepatic duct to form the bile duct. It is adherent to the common hepatic duct for a short distance before joining it, usually near the porta hepatis but sometimes lower, in which case the cystic duct lies along the lesser omentum's right edge. Its mucosa bears five to 12 crescentic folds, like those in the gallbladder's neck. They project obliquely in regular succession, appearing like a *spiral valve* (**12**.155). When the duct is distended, the spaces between the folds dilate and externally it appears twisted like the neck of the gallbladder.

BILE DUCT (**12**.155, 156, 158, 159).

The bile duct is formed near the porta hepatis, by the junction of the cystic and common hepatic ducts; it is usually about 7.5 cm long and 6 mm in diameter (see below). It descends posteriorly and slightly to the left, anterior to the epiploic foramen, at the right border of the lesser omentum, in front and to the right of the portal vein and to the right of the hepatic artery proper (**12**.156). It passes behind the first (superior) part of the duodenum, with the gastroduodenal artery on its left, and then runs in a groove on the superolateral part of the posterior surface of the head of the pancreas (**12**.133), anterior to the inferior vena cava and sometimes embedded in pancreatic tissue (p. 1790). Lytle (1959) has shown that the duct may be close to the left aspect of the second (descending) part of the duodenum or as much as 2 cm from it and that, even when it is embedded in pancreas, a superficial groove marking its position can be palpated behind the descending part of the duodenum, stones in the duct being thus detected. Left of the descending part of the duodenum the bile duct reaches the pancreatic duct; together they

enter the duodenal wall where they usually unite to form the *hepatopancreatic ampulla* (p. 1791), the distal, constricted end of which opens into the descending part of the duodenum on the summit of the major duodenal papilla (**12**.99, 134), about 8–10 cm from the pylorus (p. 1763). The position of the bile duct is indicated on the anterior abdominal surface by a line starting 5 cm above the transpyloric plane and 2 cm right of the median plane and descending vertically for 7.5 cm.

VESSELS

The *cystic artery* is described on page 1550 and the *cystic veins* on page 1604. The lower part of the bile duct receives rami from the *posterior superior pancreaticoduodenal artery* (p. 1549), while its upper part and the hepatic ducts receive rami from the cystic artery. The *right hepatic artery* supplies its intermediate part through very small rami, the main supply being from the cystic and posterior superior pancreaticoduodenal arteries. These supplies vary (Shapiro & Robillard 1948; Michels 1962). The posterior superior pancreaticoduodenal artery anastomoses with the posterior branch of the inferior pancreaticoduodenal near the hepatopancreatic ampulla; where this anastomosis is poor, ligation of the posterior superior pancreaticoduodenal artery may result in gangrene or stricture of the bile duct (Henley 1955). *Veins* from the upper part of the bile duct and hepatic ducts and from the gallbladder and cystic duct usually enter the liver, while those from the lower part of the bile duct enter the portal vein. *Lymph vessels* of the gallbladder and bile ducts are described on page 1619. Sympathetic and parasympathetic *innervation* is from the coeliac plexus along the hepatic artery and its branches. Autonomic plexuses exist in the muscular and submucous layers, and ganglion cells, presumably parasympathetic, have been demonstrated in these plexuses in monkeys (Sutherland 1966, 1967). Fibres from the right phrenic nerve, through communications between the phrenic and coeliac plexuses, appear to reach the gallbladder via the hepatic plexus, thus explaining referred 'shoulder pain' in gallbladder pathology.

VARIATIONS IN GALLBLADDER AND BILE DUCTS

The gallbladder varies in size and shape; in rare cases it is duplicated (Mincsev 1967), with two or combined cystic ducts, or is absent, though its duct may be present. The junction of the cystic and common hepatic ducts varies in its level from the porta hepatis to behind or even below the duodenum's first (superior) part; when the junction is low, the two ducts may be connected by fibrous tissue and in cholecystectomy clamping the cystic duct without injuring the common hepatic (or main bile) duct is difficult. Occasionally the cystic duct joins the right hepatic duct; it may pass behind or in front of the common hepatic duct, joining it on its left surface.

Accessory hepatic ducts may emerge, more often from the right lobe, to join the main hepatic ducts or, rarely, the gallbladder itself. Failure of canalization of bile ducts during development leads to a rare congenital atresia or stenosis with rapidly fatal results. The bile and pancreatic ducts may open separately into the duodenum or join even before entering its wall. Variations of the ductal arteries are much more common (p. 1549). For further information consult Santulli and Blanc (1961), Boyden et al (1967).

MICROSTRUCTURE OF THE GALLBLADDER AND BILIARY DUCTS (12.157)

The gallbladder's wall has serous, fibromuscular and mucous layers. The *serosa* completely covers the fundus but only coats the inferior surfaces and sides of the body and neck of the gallbladder; beneath it is subserous loose connective and adipose peritoneal tissue. The *fibromuscular layer* is composed of fibrous tissue mixed with smooth muscle cells arranged loosely in longitudinal, circular and oblique bundles. Internally, the *mucosa* is loosely connected with the fibrous layer, is generally yellowish-brown and elevated into minute rugae with a honeycomb appearance (**12.155**). Its epithelium is a single layer of columnar cells which vary with species. Electron microscopy (Chapman et al 1966) in dogs shows microvilli on their apical surface, irregularly arranged, with endocytic or pinocytotic vesicles between their bases. Basally, spaces between epithelial cells are dilated and many capillaries adjoin the basement membrane. These features indicate active absorption of water and solutes from the bile to concentrate it. Basal spaces are large during absorption of water (Kaye et al 1966). Biliary concentration appears to involve the active transport of sodium and calcium, making an osmotic gradient from the lumen of the gallbladder to the capillaries of the lamina propria. In the apical parts of some cells, particularly those near the ducts, mucous granules appear; they are secreted into the lumen (Johnson et al 1962; Mueller et al 1972).

The large biliary ducts have external fibrous and internal mucous layers. The former is fibrous connective tissue with a few longitudinal, oblique and circular smooth muscle cells. (Muscle cells appeared in only 12 of 100 human common bile ducts examined by Mahour et al 1967.) The mucosa is continuous with that of the hepatic ducts, gallbladder and duodenum; like theirs, its epithelium is columnar; many lobulated mucous glands occur in the wall of these ducts. In the bile duct are many tubulo-alveolar glands arranged in clusters, secreting mucin, some at least of which is sulphated (McMinn & Kugler 1961). Electron microscopy of the bile duct epithelium in guinea-pigs showed microvilli on its luminal surfaces. Secretory granules, some of mucinogen, appear in the apical cytoplasm. Epithelial cells in rats, which lack a gallbladder, are termed either light or dark according to their electron density; light cells have longer, more regular microvilli but the basal intercellular spaces between adjacent dark cells are larger; the mucosa appears to modify bile, compensating for the absent gallbladder (Riches & Palfrey 1966).

Circular muscle around the lower part of the main bile duct,

including the ampulla and terminal pancreatic duct, forms the *sphincter of the hepatopancreatic ampulla* (*sphincter of Oddi*), comprising muscle at three levels:

- at the end of the bile duct (*sphincter ductus choledoci*)
- at the end of the pancreatic duct (*sphincter ductus pancreatici*)
- around the ampulla.

Only the muscle at the end of the bile duct is constant. Expulsion of gallbladder contents appears to be under hormonal control. Fat or acid in the duodenum probably causes the liberation of CCK, stimulating the gallbladder to contract. Muscle cells in its wall have surface receptors for this hormone, which can therefore stimulate them to contract directly. In any case, when storage pressure exceeds 100 mm of bile, the gallbladder contracts, the sphincter of Oddi relaxes and bile enters the duodenum. Kirk (1944) denied the presence of sphincteric musculature around the openings of the bile and pancreatic ducts, describing the sphincter of Oddi as submucosal and continuous with the circular muscle of the duodenum. However, subsequent studies suggest that in man and other primates a common sphincter surrounds both ducts and that the common bile duct has a second sphincter as described above (Boyden 1957, 1966). The termination of the united bile and pancreatic ducts is packed with villous, valvular folds of mucosa and muscle cells enter their connective tissue cores. This suggests that contraction results in retraction and clumping of the folds, preventing reflux of duodenal contents and controlling the exit of bile. In cats stimulation of vagal rami to this region relaxes the biliary opening; the human *myenteric* (*Auerbach's*) *plexus* is well developed at the ends of the ducts. Inflammatory swelling of villous folds may obstruct them.

CLINICAL ANATOMY OF THE GALLBLADDER

The gallbladder may be distended by calculi or by obstruction of the cystic duct and may project down and forwards towards the umbilicus. It moves with respiration. Obstruction of the bile duct, apart from lithiasis, is often due to pressure of malignant tumours, especially in the pylorus or pancreas. It also follows cicatricial contraction after ulceration in the duct. Enormous distension of the bile duct and its radicles may also occur.

Cholecystography (12.158, 159)

The gallbladder is not radio-opaque, but radio-opaque substances introduced into the bloodstream are excreted by the liver into bile, and concentration in the gallbladder renders it much more strongly radio-opaque. The form, position and emptying of the gallbladder can be demonstrated by radiographs; its position and form vary with the general build of the body (or somatotype; Davies 1927); in broad (hypersthenic) types it is wide, high up and placed far laterally (at the level of the first lumbar vertebra), whereas in narrow (asthenic) types it is narrow, more medial and may reach as low as the fourth lumbar vertebral level.

The gallbladder is also clearly visible in ultrasonograms (**12.160**).

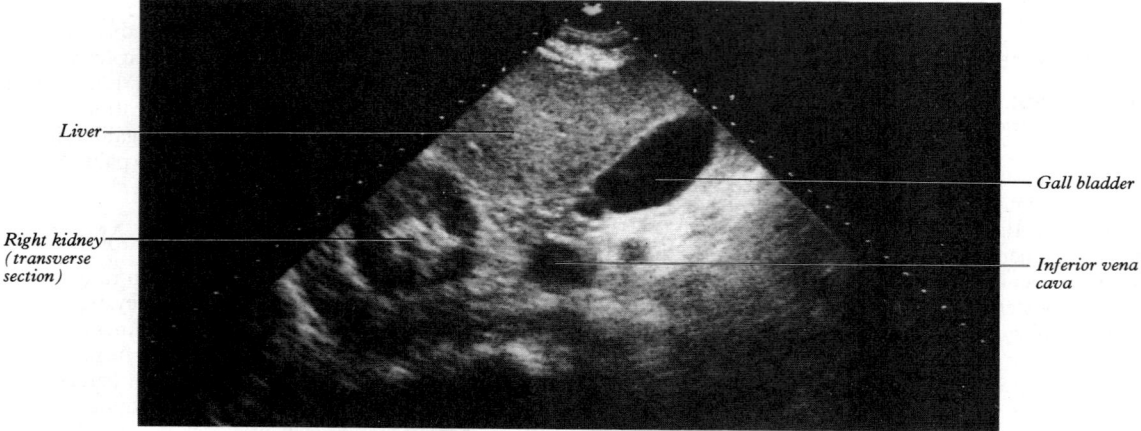

Liver

Gall bladder

Right kidney (transverse section)

Inferior vena cava

12.160   Transverse ultrasound sector scan of the abdomen to show the gallbladder and right kidney. (Supplied by Shaun Gallagher, Guy's Hospital; photography by Sarah Smith, UMDS, Guy's Hospital Campus, London.)

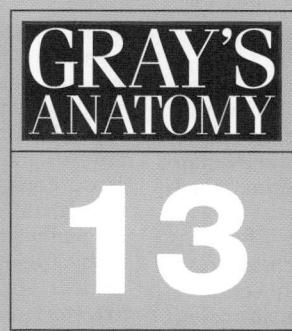

GRAY'S ANATOMY

13

URINARY SYSTEM

Section Editor: Mary Dyson

With essay on Kidney Transplantation by Robert A Sells

INTRODUCTION

So customary has it become to link the organs of urinary excretion and reproduction as a *urogenital system* that the suitability of this concept is rarely even questioned. Yet functionally the two have nothing in common. In mature human organs the structural overlap is little more than a shared use of the male urethra as a urinary **and** seminal duct. Of course, in development, gonadal ducts have a *nephric* origin; but in human females even the *oviduct* ('female', paramesonephric or Müllerian duct) is no longer formed from nephric tissue. Indeed, no adequate reason remains to continue defining a 'urogenital' system in female mammals. Even in males, where the duct systems of the testes (as in other mammals) are derived from nephric tubules and the *mesonephric duct*, these are not excretory structures. The reptilian functional kidney is no longer a mesonephros, and the intromittent *penis*, developed from cloacal tissues, has bilateral parts enclosing a purely seminal groove when erected for copulation, urine entering the cloaca. Apart from development, therefore, the genital system is already completely separated from the urinary organs in both sexes in reptiles. Birds, like amphibians, generally have no intromittent organ, though this is probably a secondary loss in the former, some more primitive birds possessing a rudimentary penis of a reptilian type.

In all vertebrates (excluding elementary chordates) nephric excretory tubules and gonads develop from coelomic epithelium, together with their collecting ducts as these evolve. Both develop in dorsal sites flanking the major vessels; and perhaps this propinquity, combined with the more medial location of gonads, has led to the adoption of urinary ducts and tubules to serve the gonads, especially in males. In primitive *Chordata*, such as *Amphioxus*, excretory tubules, or *nephridia*, have capillary *glomeruli* close to them and secrete from the adjoining bloodstream and coelom into a peribranchial atrium. These excretory organs are ectodermal and unrelated to the mesodermal nephric tubules of vertebrates. The evolutionary relation of *Amphioxus* to early vertebrates is uncertain; it has even been suggested that this chordate is a paedomorphic form of a primitive vertebrate (Grassé 1948; Young 1962).

In vertebrates living in water, whether saline or fresh, the problems of preserving internal osmotic constants in blood and body fluids, despite variable and sometimes very large intakes of water and salts, have led to the continuous evolution of more efficient and elaborate excretory tubules, derived from mesoderm intermediate between the somites and the lateral plate in embryos, forming *nephrotomes* (p. 199). Though originally segmental, their large numbers overshadow this and in most lower vertebrates they form elongated masses or cords of nephrogenic tissue projecting into the coelom from a dorsolateral position. Gonads develop **medial** to these *nephrogenic cords* (p. 199); and since *primary excretory ducts* (p. 199), carrying urine to the exterior, evolve **lateral** to the nephros, gonadal access to them is effected by adaptation of the nephric tubules. The degree of development and functional status of different parts of this elongate kidney or vertebrate *holonephros*, extending through many body segments, has varied much. The cranial part generally tends to disappear, except where it functions in embryos or in larval forms, as in some cyclostomes (e.g. *Petromyzon*, the lamprey). In anamniotic gnathostomes (fish and amphibia) an intermediate nephrogenic region becomes a functional kidney and, while still elongate, this occupies a comparatively small number of segments, with which its vessels approximately correspond. In reptiles and mammals the most caudal mass of nephrotomes differentiates into a definitive kidney, which becomes more localized and rounded, of familiar reniform shape particularly in mammals, losing almost all indications of plurisegmental origin when fully developed.

This progressive caudal shift of the functioning nephros has prompted the division of the holonephros into pro-, meso-, and meta-nephros, and has given rise to some misleading concepts; for example, amphibian kidneys are often termed mesonephric and mammalian organs metanephric. Nevertheless, the formation of nephric tubules is substantially alike at all levels and it cannot be assumed that these regional terms are applicable over large and diverse vertebrate groups with anything more than approximate segmental uniformity. The terms are more of a descriptive convenience than vehicles of biological precision (Fraser 1950). Distinctions between the three regional levels of the nephrogenic ridge depend more upon their functional status and ducts than their intrinsic morphology. In cyclostomes, excretory tubules discharge, as do gonads, into the coelom, from which their products escape through the *abdominal pores* or through short ducts situated caudally. In gnathostomes, *nephric tubules* lose continuity with the coelom, each developing a saccular end, with which *glomeruli* are closely related. The tubules join a longitudinal *archinephric duct* (*primary excretory duct*), which at first serves the pronephros but is taken over by the more caudal mesonephros. Through mesonephric tubules testes find outlets via the urinary ducts, an arrangement typical of amphibians, both urine and spermatozoa reaching the cloaca by these *mesonephric* (*Wolffian*) *ducts*. Ovaries also acquire ducts, in some forms from the mesonephric duct; but this *paramesonephric, female* or *Müllerian duct* becomes a separate entity and does not transmit urine. Moreover, oviducts never establish direct continuity with the ovaries, which retain a primitive habit of shedding ova into the coelom, though very close to the open, coelomic beginnings of the oviducts. This relation is constant and occurs in human females (p. 1848). Oviducts of mammals and of tetrapods in general appear to develop independently by evagination from the coelomic lining.

In reptiles, birds and mammals, the functioning kidney is a *metanephros*, developing caudal to the mesonephros. Its main distinction is its **dissociation from genital function**; though in part an outgrowth of the caudal end of the mesonephric duct, it ultimately opens separately into the bladder by its own duct, the *ureter*. The mesonephros is thus relieved of all excretory function, its tubules and ducts persisting only in modified form as testicular *vasa efferentia*, *epididymis* and *ductus deferens* (p. 1855).

To summarize: the pronephros is an embryonic or larval excretory organ with a purely excretory duct. The mesonephros, which takes over this duct and excretion, also provides a route for spermatozoa and, by the division of its duct in some vertebrates, is a separate exit for the ova. The metanephros is again purely excretory, male genital ducts continuing as mesonephric derivatives and the oviduct as an increasingly independent development.

The complete segregation of urinary and genital organs in reptiles (apart from their embryonic development and the opening of their separate ducts in a common cloaca) becomes modified again by the evolution of a male intromittent organ for internal fertilization, necessitated by full emancipation from reproduction in water. Internal fertilization is accomplished without an intromittent organ in most birds, but an erectile *penis* is universal in marsupials and eutherian mammals (p. 1848). Since this is traversed by the urethra, used to void both urine and semen, male mammals, including the human, exhibit to this extent an association of the excretory and reproductive organs. Both systems display many adaptations and specializations, the urinary system being concerned in mammals with a much improved ability to preserve a steady internal environment in terms of total body water volume and concentrations of ions and other dissolved substances. This entails an increasing complexity in glomeruli and renal tubules, forming *nephrons* or kidney units, capable not only of removing variable and sometimes large volumes of water, but also of selective reabsorption of substances such as glucose and salts and retention of others, such as urea, in the urine. The renal ducts open into various forms of reservoir in many vertebrates and in mammals into a cloacal derivative, the *bladder*.

Since, in postnatal human beings, the association between the components of the urinary and the reproductive systems is limited solely to the dual function of the penile urethra, these systems are here considered separately.

The urinary organs comprise:

- two *kidneys* (*renes*) producing urine;
- *ureters*, conveying it to the pelvic urinary viscera, namely
- the *urinary bladder* (*vesica urinaria*) for temporary storage;
- the *urethra* by which the bladder empties.

The kidneys and upper parts of the ureters are abdominal; below, the ureters become pelvic (for convenience the whole ureter is here described under the 'abdominal urinary organ' heading). The pelvic urinary organs are the urinary bladder and urethra. In females the urethra lies entirely in the pelvic floor, but in males it is penile for most of its length, with both urinary and genital functions.

ABDOMINAL URINARY ORGANS

THE KIDNEYS

The kidneys excrete the final products of metabolic activities and excess water, both of these actions being essential to the control of concentrations of various substances in the body fluids, for example maintaining electrolyte and water balance approximately constant in the tissue fluids. They also have endocrine functions producing and releasing *erythropoietin* which affects blood formation, *renin* which influences blood pressure and *1,25-hydroxycholecalciferol*, which is involved in the control of calcium metabolism and a derivative of vitamin D, perhaps modifying the action of the parathyroid hormone (O'Riordan 1978), and various other soluble factors with metabolic actions. The kidneys in the fresh state are reddish-brown, are situated posteriorly behind the peritoneum on each side of the vertebral column and are surrounded by adipose tissue. Superiorly they are level with the upper border of the twelfth thoracic vertebra, inferiorly with the third lumbar. The right is usually slightly inferior to the left, probably due to its relationship to the liver. The left is a little longer and narrower than the right and lies nearer the median plane. The long axis of each kidney is directed inferolaterally and the transverse axis posteromedially. Hence the anterior and posterior aspects usually described are in fact **anterolateral** and **posteromedial**. The transpyloric plane passes through the superior part of the right renal hilum and the inferior part of the left.

Each kidney is about 11 cm in length, 6 cm in breadth and 3 cm in anteroposterior dimension. In adult males the average weight is about 150 g, in adult females 135 g. In thin individuals with a lax abdominal wall the lower pole may just be felt in full inspiration by bimanual lumbar examination; usually, however, it is impalpable.

RENAL SURFACE PROJECTIONS

In a recumbent posture, each renal profile can be projected to the anterior or posterior surface of the body as follows, the right kidney being about 1.25 cm lower than the left:

- *Anterior surface.* The hilar centre is approximately at the transpyloric plane, about 5 cm from the midline and slightly medial to

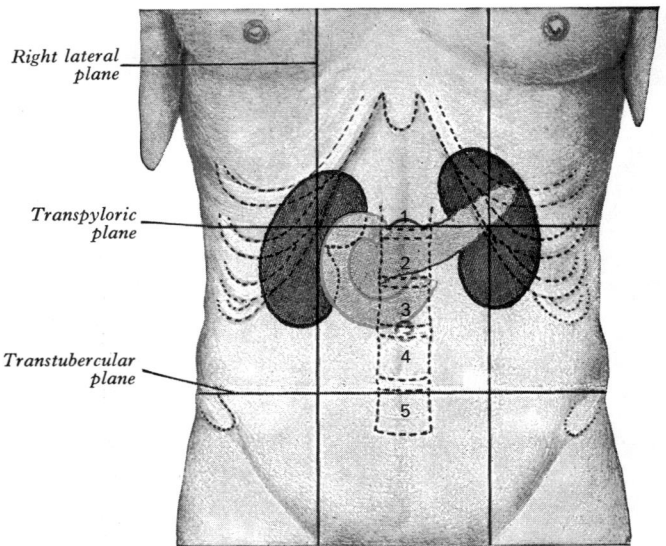

13.1 Surface projections of the duodenum, pancreas and kidneys. The lower ribs and the lumbar vertebrae are also indicated, the latter being numbered.

the tip of the ninth costal cartilage. The left hilum is just above the plane, the right just below it (**13**.1). In relation to the position of the hilum, a reniform profile can be drawn 11 cm long and 4.5 cm broad, the upper pole being about 2.5 cm and the lower 7.5 cm from the midline. Since the transverse axis is oblique, the width thus shown is 1.5 cm less than the actual width of the kidney.
- *Posterior surface.* The hilar centre is opposite the lower border of the spinous process of the first lumbar vertebra and about 5 cm from the midline. In relation to this point, a reniform profile can be similarly traced, the lower pole being usually about 2.5 cm above the summit of the iliac crest. The kidneys are about 2.5 cm lower in the standing than in the recumbent position; they ascend and descend a little with respiration.

RENAL RELATIONS

The convex *anterior surface* (**13**.1, 2) in reality faces anterolaterally. Its relations differ on the two sides of the body.

(1) *Anterior surface of right kidney.* A small area of the superior pole contacts the right suprarenal gland, which may overlap it or the upper part of the medial border. A large area below this (about three-quarters of the surface) adjoins the renal impression on the right lobe of the liver and a narrow medial area is related to the descending part of the duodenum. Inferiorly the anterior surface is in contact laterally with the right colic flexure and medially with part of the small intestine. The areas related to the small intestine and almost all those in contact with the liver are covered by peritoneum (with the renal fascia subjacent); the suprarenal, duodenal and colic areas are devoid of peritoneum.

(2) *Anterior surface of left kidney.* A small medial area of the superior pole is related to the left suprarenal gland and approximately the upper two-thirds of the lateral half of the anterior surface is related to the spleen. A central quadrilateral area lies in contact with the pancreatic body and splenic vessels. Above this a small variable triangular region, between the suprarenal and splenic areas, is in contact with the stomach. Below the pancreatic and splenic areas the lateral region is related to the left colic flexure and the beginning of the descending colon, while the medial region adjoins the coils of the jejunum. The latter region is extensive but the colic area is an irregular, narrow strip adjoining the lateral border of the kidney. The gastric area is covered with the peritoneum of the omental bursa and the splenic and jejunal areas are covered by the peritoneum of the greater sac; behind the jejunal area's peritoneum, branches of the left colic vessels are related to the kidney. The suprarenal, pancreatic and colic areas are devoid of peritoneum, there being no independent movement of organs here.

The *posterior surface* (**13**.3, 4, 7, 8, 9), in reality posteromedial, is embedded in fat and devoid of peritoneum. It is anterior to the diaphragm and to the medial and lateral arcuate ligaments, psoas major, quadratus lumborum and the aponeurotic tendon of transversus abdominis, to the subcostal vessels and subcostal, iliohypogastric and ilio-inguinal nerves. The upper pole of the right kidney is level with the twelfth rib, that of the left with the eleventh and twelfth. The diaphragm separates the kidney from the pleura which descends to form the costodiaphragmatic recess (**13**.4); sometimes its muscle is defective or absent in a triangle immediately above the lateral arcuate ligament, allowing perirenal adipose tissue to contact the diaphragmatic pleura.

The *superior poles* are thick, round, nearer the midline than the inferior poles, and each is related to its suprarenal gland. The *inferior poles*, smaller and thinner, extend to within 2.5 cm of the iliac crests. The *lateral borders* are convex, the left covered superiorly by greater sac peritoneum, so separating it from the spleen, and below this is in contact with the descending colon; the right lateral border is

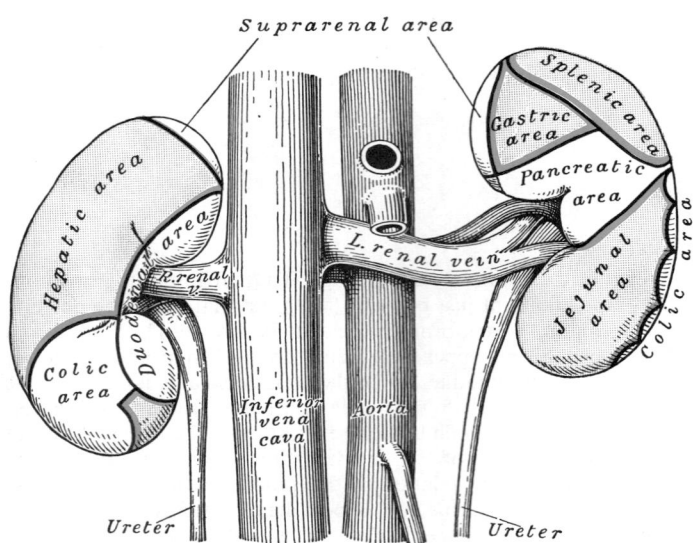

13.2 The anterior surfaces of the kidneys, showing the areas related to neighbouring viscera. Areas coloured pale blue are separated from adjacent viscera by the peritoneum.

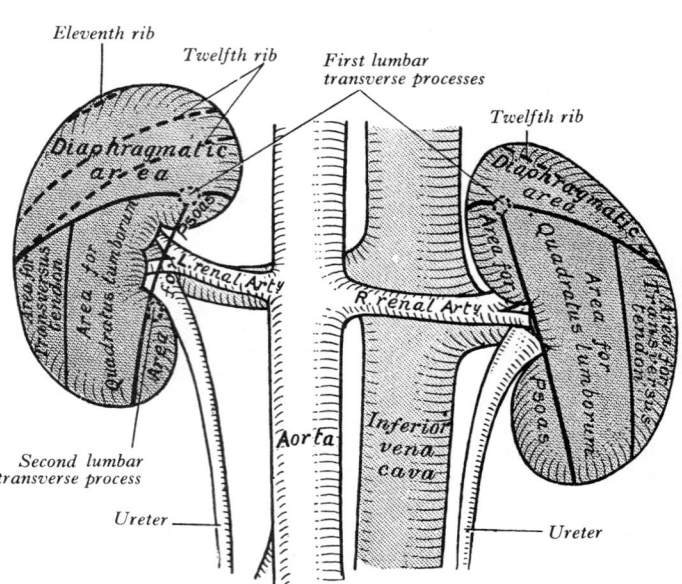

13.3 The posterior surfaces of the kidneys, showing the areas of relation to the posterior abdominal wall.

separated by the peritoneum of the greater sac from the liver (right lobe). The *medial borders* are convex adjacent to the poles, concave between them and slope inferolaterally. In each a deep vertical fissure opens anteromedially as the *hilum*, bounded by anterior and posterior lips and containing the renal vessels and nerves and the *renal pelvis* of the ureter. The relative positions of the main hilar structures are: the renal vein anterior, the renal artery intermediate and the pelvis of the kidney posterior. Commonly an arterial branch enters behind the renal pelvis and a renal venous tributary often leaves the hilum in the same plane. Above the hilum the medial border is related to the suprarenal gland and below to the commencement of the ureter.

The hilum leads into a central *renal sinus*, lined by the renal capsule and almost filled by the renal pelvis and vessels; numerous *renal papillae* indent the wall of the sinus. The collecting tubules open onto the summits of the renal papillae and drain into the

funnel-shaped expansions of the upper urinary tract, named the minor calyces (**13.6**, **11**). The 7–13 minor calyces terminate in two or three major calyces which in turn open into the renal pelvis. The renal calyces and pelvis are described in detail on page 1827.

The kidney and its vessels are embedded in *perirenal* (*perinephric*) *fat*, which is thickest at the renal borders and prolonged at the hilum into the renal sinus. Fibrous connective tissue surrounding this fat is condensed as *renal fascia* (**13.7**, **8**).

RENAL FASCIA

At the lateral renal borders the anterior and posterior layers of renal fascia fuse. The anterior extends medially in front of the kidney and its vessels to merge with connective tissue enclosing the aorta and inferior vena cava, but it is thin and does not ascend above the

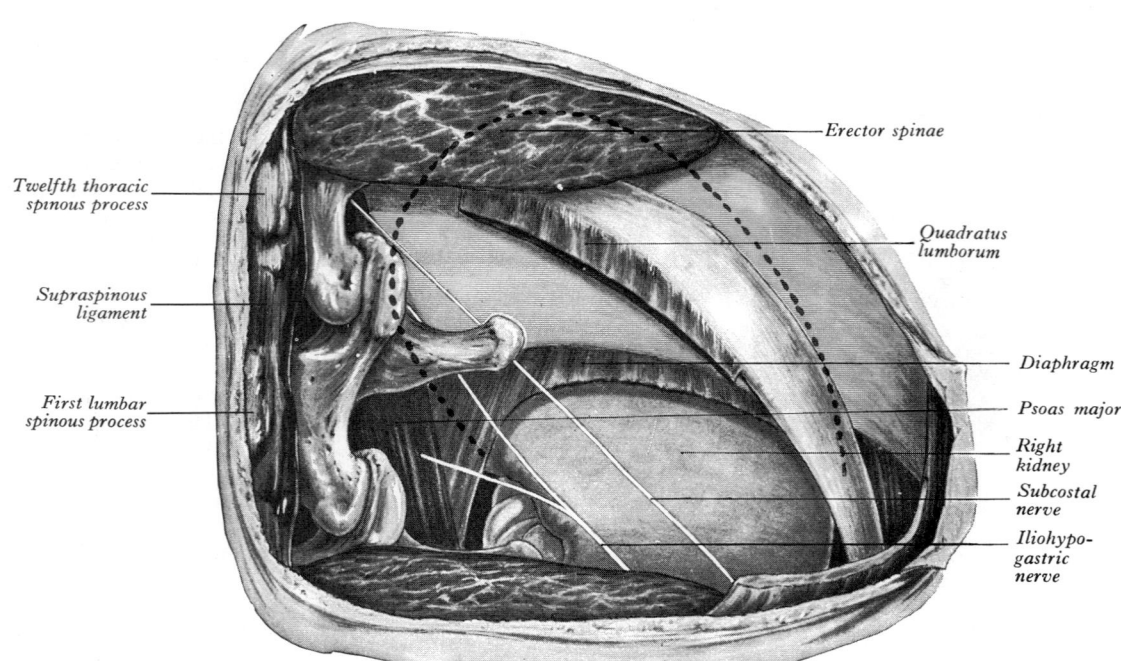

13.4 The right kidney (posterior exposure). The blue area represents the pleura, the broken red line the upper part of the kidney. The subcostal nerve has been displaced downwards. Parts of the diaphragm and the quadratus lumborum have been resected.

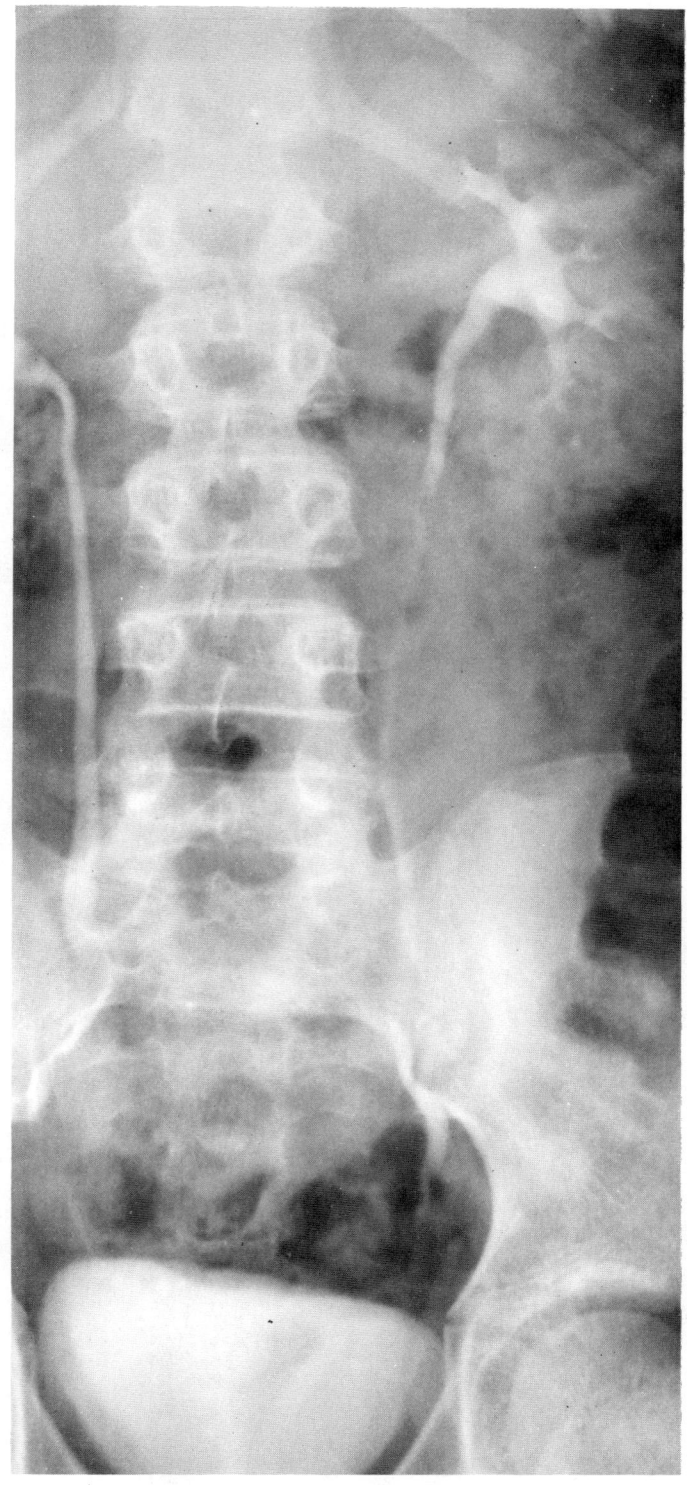

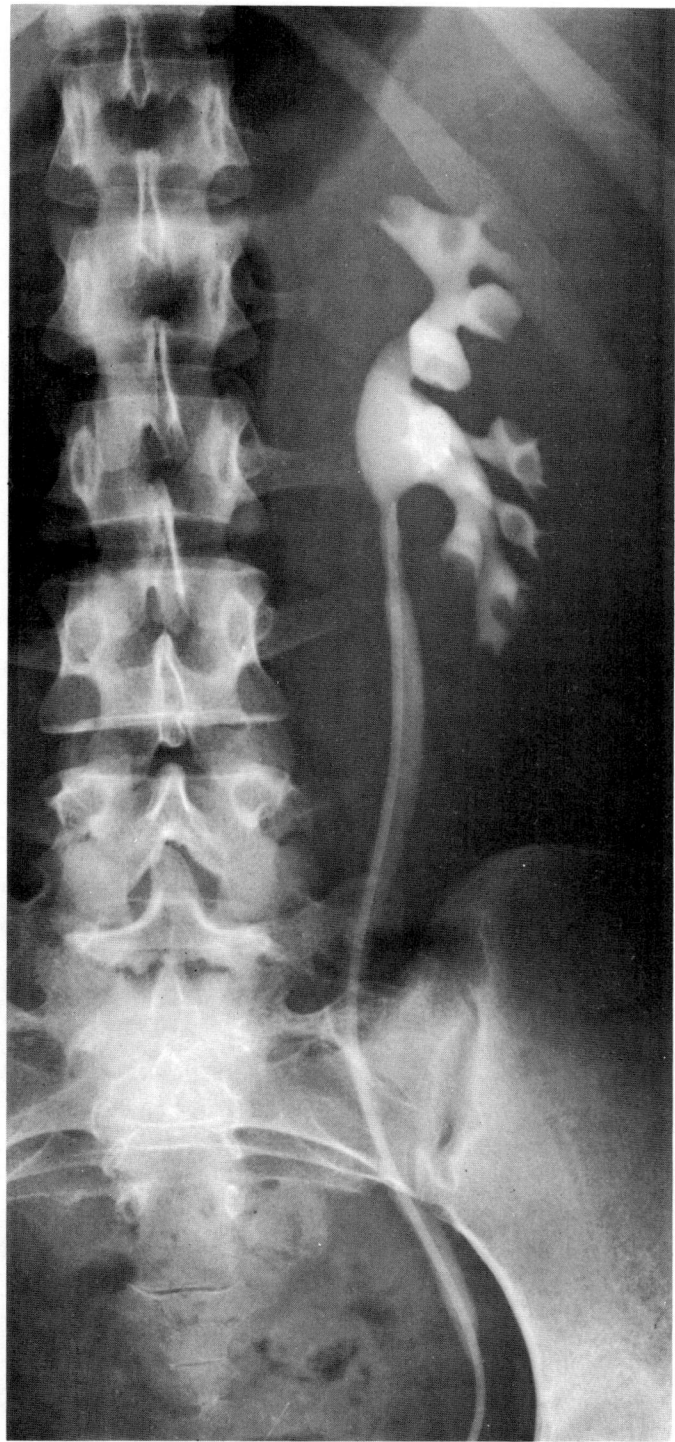

13.5 An intravenous pyelogram. Both ureters can be visualized throughout much of their length, except where peristalsis has temporarily displaced the excreted contrast medium, which also fills the urinary bladder. Compare with the retrograde pyelogram illustrated in **13**.6.

13.6 A left retrograde pyelogram. The contrast medium has been introduced into the calyces, pelvis and upper ureter via a ureteric catheter, which is still in position and can be clearly identified. There is considerably greater density of the shadows of the calyces than that achieved by the intravenous method. Note the relation of the ureter to the tips of the lumbar transverse processes and the characteristic 'cupping' or 'champagne glass' profiles of the tips of the lesser calyces where they surround the renal pyramids. 'Calyx' means a cup and such 'cupping' of the minor calyces is the normal appearance. (Note that the major calyces are not cups and are hence inappropriately named.)

superior mesenteric artery. The posterior layer passes medially between the kidney and the fascia on quadratus lumborum and psoas major, attaching to this fascia at the lateral and medial borders of the psoas, and to the vertebrae and intervertebral discs. A deeper stratum (not shown in (**13**.7, 8) unites the anterior and posterior layers at the medial renal border and is pierced by the renal vessels (Martin 1942); this may account for the failure of perirenal effusions to cross the midline although injected air **does** diffuse along this route (Grossman 1954). Above the suprarenal gland the two layers of renal fascia fuse and blend with the diaphragmatic fascia; it is

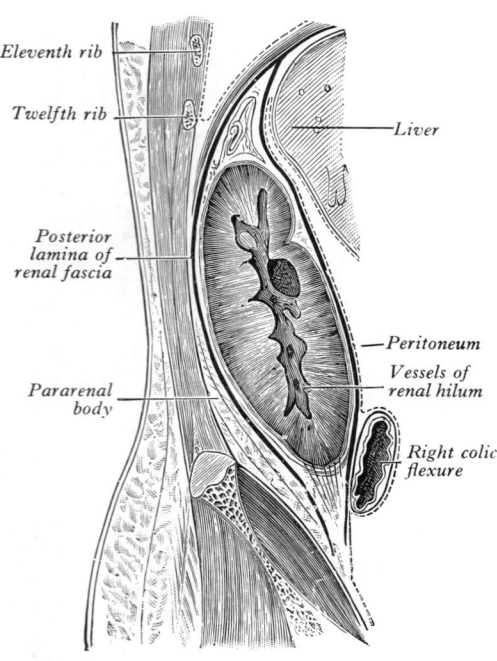

13.7 Sagittal section through the posterior abdominal wall showing the relations of the renal fascia of the right kidney.

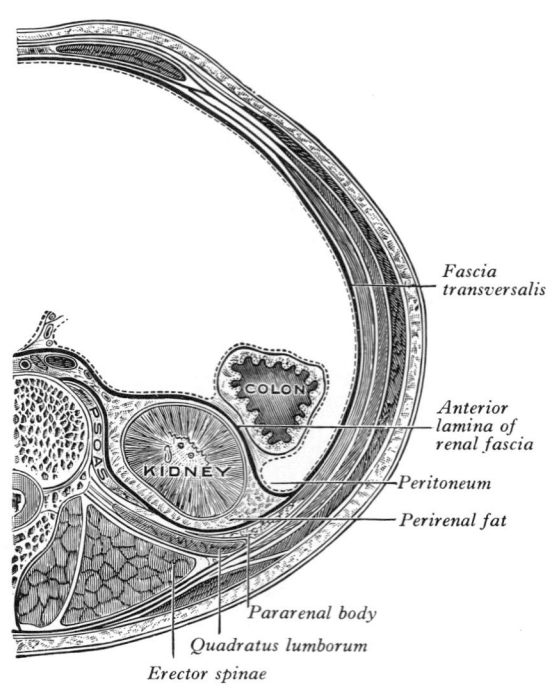

13.8 Transverse section, showing the relations of the renal fascia.

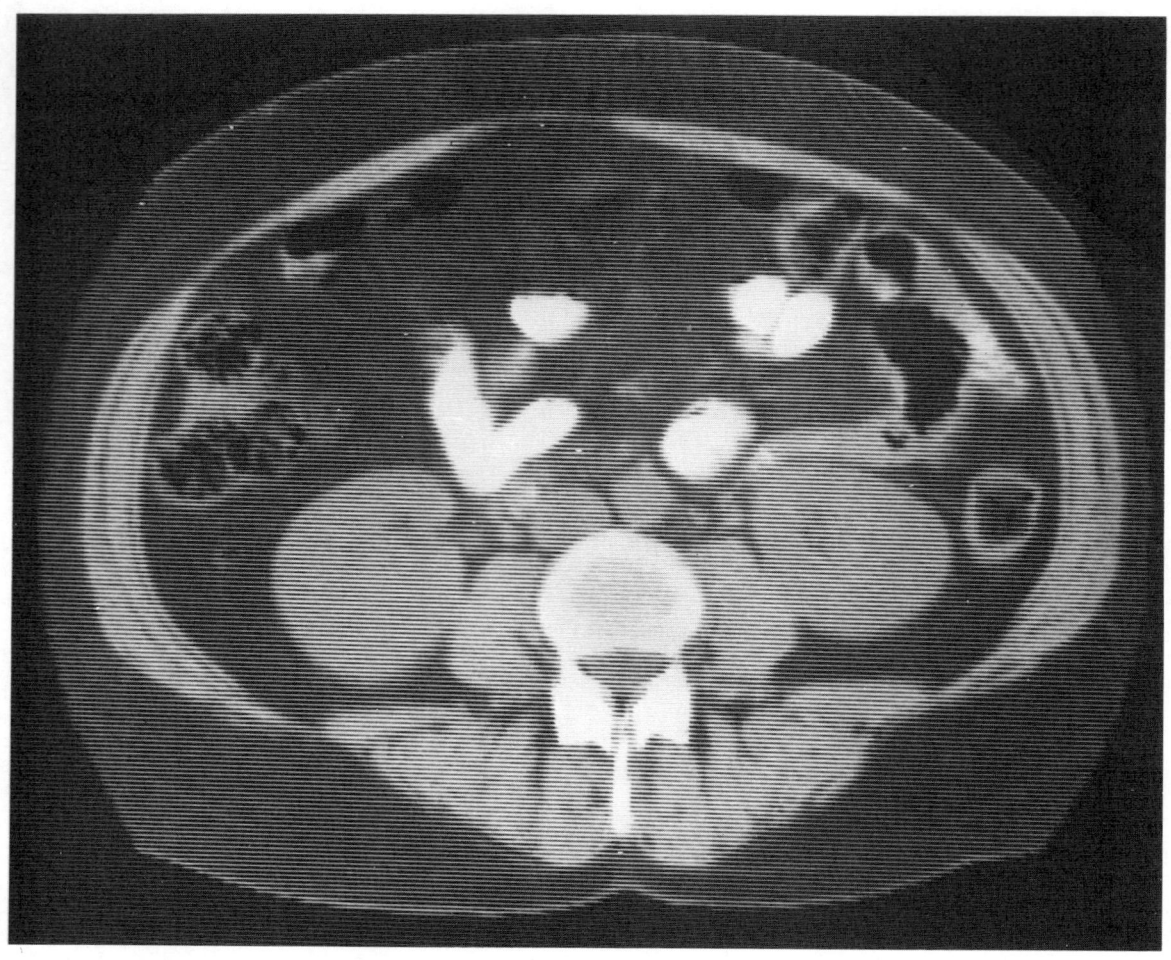

13.9A Computed tomogram through the abdomen in the transverse plane at the level of the kidneys (see **13**.9B). Contrast material is present in the small intestine. Supplied by Shaun Gallagher, Guy's Hospital; photography by Sarah Smith, UMDS, Guy's Campus, London.

generally agreed that below the kidney they are separate, enclosing the ureter, the anterior fading into the extraperitoneal tissue of the iliac fossa, the posterior blending with the iliac fascia although this has also been denied (Mitchell 1950). The renal fascia is connected to the renal capsule by numerous trabeculae which traverse the perirenal fat and are strongest near the lower pole. Behind the renal fascia is a mass of fat, the *pararenal (paranephric) body*. The kidney is held in position partly by renal fascia but principally by the apposition of neighbouring viscera.

GENERAL RENAL STRUCTURE

The fetal kidney has about 12 lobules (**13**.10), but these are fused in adults to present a smooth surface (**10**.128), though traces of lobulation may remain.

The postnatal kidney has a thin capsule, easily removed, composed of collagen-rich tissue with some elastic and nonstriated muscle fibres. In renal disease it may become adherent. The kidney itself has an internal *medulla* and external *cortex*.

The renal medulla consists of pale, striated, conical *renal pyramids*, their bases peripheral, their apices converging to the renal sinus where they project into calyces as papillae, each minor calyx receiving from one to three of these structures. Each pyramid is capped by cortical tissue to form a renal *lobe*. Estimates of papillae, and hence of pyramids or renal lobes, are variable. Counts in 375 human kidneys ranged from 5–11 in 89% with a most frequent value of 8 (in 26%). Total numbers of terminal uriniferous ducts (of Bellini) opening on papillae varied (in 208 kidneys) from 116 to 776; no peak of frequency was observed, but 23% of kidneys displayed about 275 such openings. In another series of 54 kidneys (Arvis 1969) the number of papillae was 6 to 14.

The renal cortex (**13**.11A) is subcapsular, arching over the bases of the pyramids and extending between them towards the renal sinus as *renal columns* (**13**.11c); the peripheral regions are *cortical arches* and are traversed by radial, lighter-coloured *medullary rays* (**13**.11c), separated by darker tissue, the *convoluted part*. The rays taper towards the renal capsule and are peripheral prolongations from the bases of renal pyramids. The cortex is also histologically divisible into *outer* and *inner zones*; the inner is demarcated from the medulla by tangential blood vessels (arcuate arteries and veins) which lie at the junction of the two, but a thin layer of cortical tissue ('*subcortex*') appears on the medullary side of this zone. The cortex close to the medulla is sometimes termed *juxtamedullary*.

RENAL MICROSTRUCTURE

The kidney is composed of many tortuous, closely packed *uriniferous tubules*, bound by a little connective tissue in which run blood vessels, lymphatics and nerves. Each tubule consists of two embryologically distinct parts (p. 202):

- the secreting *nephron* which elaborates urine
- a *collecting tubule*.

The **nephron** comprises a *renal corpuscle*, concerned with filtration from the plasma, and a *renal tubule*, concerned with selective resorption from the glomerular filtrate to form the urine. **Collecting tubules** carry fluid from several renal tubules to a terminal *papillary duct (of Bellini)*, opening into a minor calyx at the apex of a renal papilla. Papillary surfaces (see above) show numerous minute orifices of these ducts and pressure on a fresh kidney expresses urine from them.

Renal corpuscle

Renal (Malpighian) corpuscles, small rounded masses averaging about 0.2 mm in diameter, are visible in the renal cortex and columns (of Bertin) except in a narrow peripheral cortical zone (*cortex corticis*) (**13**.11D, 12, 15). There are one to two million renal corpuscles in each kidney, decreasing with age (Dunnill & Halley 1973). Each has a central *glomerulus* of vessels and a membranous *glomerular capsule*, the commencement of a renal tubule.

Glomerulus. This is a lobulated collection of convoluted, capillary blood vessels, united by scant connective tissue and supplied by an *afferent arteriole* which usually enters the capsule opposite the exit into the tubule; an *efferent arteriole* emerges from the same *vascular pole (mesangium)* of the capsule. Glomeruli are simple in form until late prenatal life; some remain so for about 6 months after birth, the majority maturing by 6 years and all by 12 (Macdonald & Emery 1959). In the fetal rabbit, guinea-pig and sheep, the glomerular precursor is a solid sphere of mesodermal cells in which vessels canalize until the glomerulus is a compact anastomosing plexus, not showing independent capillary loops (Lewis 1958).

Glomerular capsule (of Bowman). The blind expanded end of a renal tubule, deeply invaginated by the glomerulus. This is lined by simple squamous epithelium on its outer (parietal) wall; its glomerular, juxtacapillary (visceral) wall is composed of specialized epithelial *podocytes* (Latta 1973; Spinelli 1974; Arakawa & Tokunaga 1974). Thus, between glomerulus and external capsular layer, is a flattened *urinary space*, varied in size by secretory activity (see below) and continuous with the proximal convoluted tubule. The basal lamina of the capsular cells fuses with that of glomerular endothelium.

Podocytes surrounding the capillary loops are flat, stellate cells,

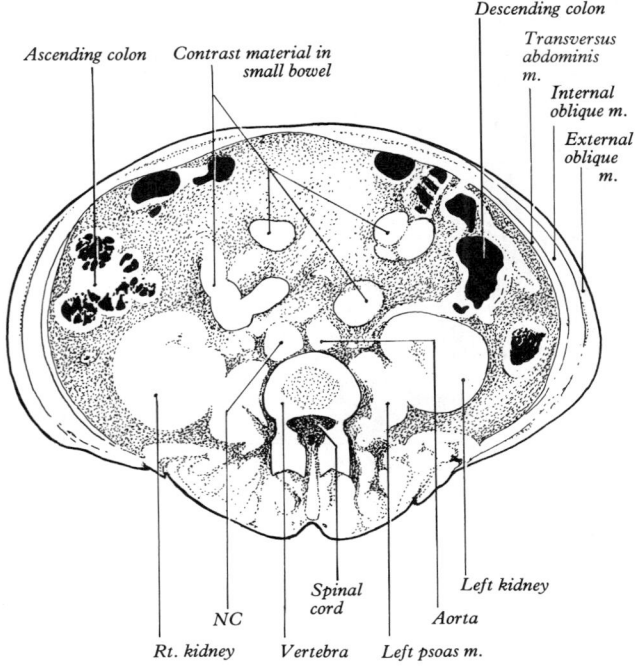

Descending colon

Transversus abdominis m.

Internal oblique m.

External oblique m.

Ascending colon   *Contrast material in small bowel*

Left kidney

Spinal cord

Aorta

NC

Rt. kidney   *Vertebra*   *Left psoas m.*

13.9B   Diagram illustrating the major features demonstrated in **13**.9A.

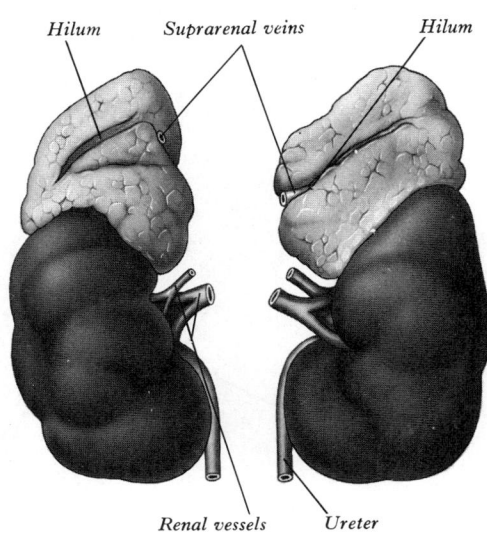

Hilum   *Suprarenal veins*   *Hilum*

Renal vessels   *Ureter*

13.10   The kidneys and suprarenal glands of a newborn infant: anterior aspect. Note the lobulation of the renal surface and relative size of the organs.

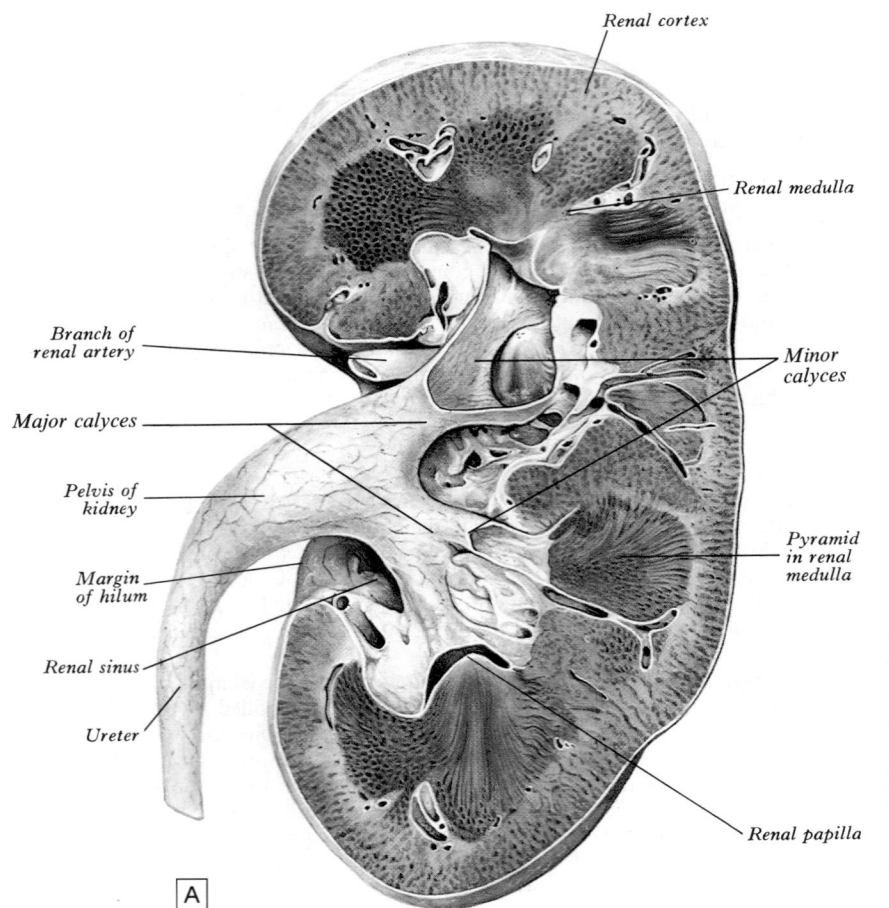

Renal cortex

Renal medulla

Branch of
renal artery

Minor
calyces

Major calyces

Pelvis of
kidney

Pyramid
in renal
medulla

Margin
of hilum

Renal sinus

Ureter

Renal papilla

A

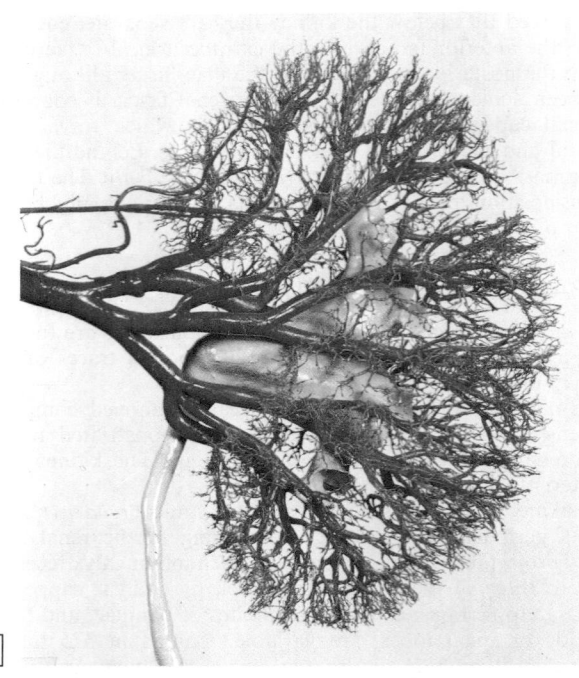

B

13.11   The structural and functional organization of the kidney. A. Longitudinal section through a kidney; note the pelvis of the ureter and its division
into calyces; also the macroscopic appearance of the normal kidney. The
pelvis and major calyces have not been opened. B. A corrosion cast of a
human kidney, showing minor and major calyces, ureteric pelvis and upper
ureter (all in yellow) and the renal arterial tree (in red). Note also suprarenal
branches from the renal artery and direct from the aorta. Prepared by
M C E Hutchinson; photographed by Kevin Fitzpatrick, Anatomy Dept, Guy's
Hospital Medical School, London. C. Diagram illustrating the major structures
in the kidney cortex and medulla (left), the position of cortical and juxtamedullary nephrons (middle) and the major blood vessels (right). D. Schematic diagram of the regional structure and principal activities of a kidney
nephron and collecting duct. For clarity, a nephron of the long loop
(juxtamedullary) type is depicted.

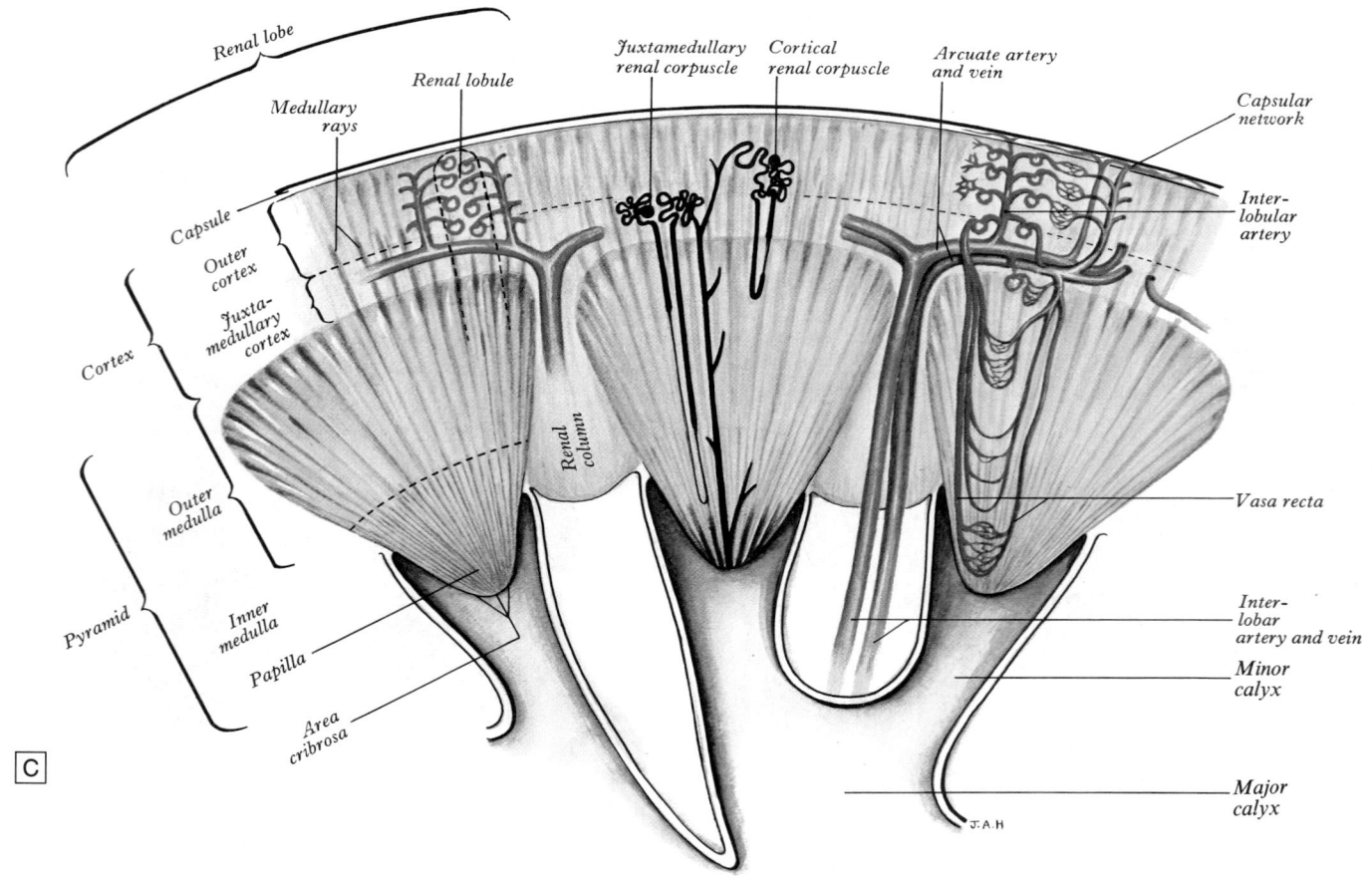

Renal lobe

Juxtamedullary
renal corpuscle

Cortical
renal corpuscle

Arcuate artery
and vein

Renal lobule

Medullary
rays

Capsular
network

Capsule

Inter-
lobular
artery

Outer
cortex

Juxta-
medullary
cortex

Cortex

Renal
column

Outer
medulla

Vasa recta

Pyramid

Inner
medulla

Inter-
lobar
artery and vein

Papilla

Minor
calyx

Area
cribrosa

Major
calyx

C

J.A.H

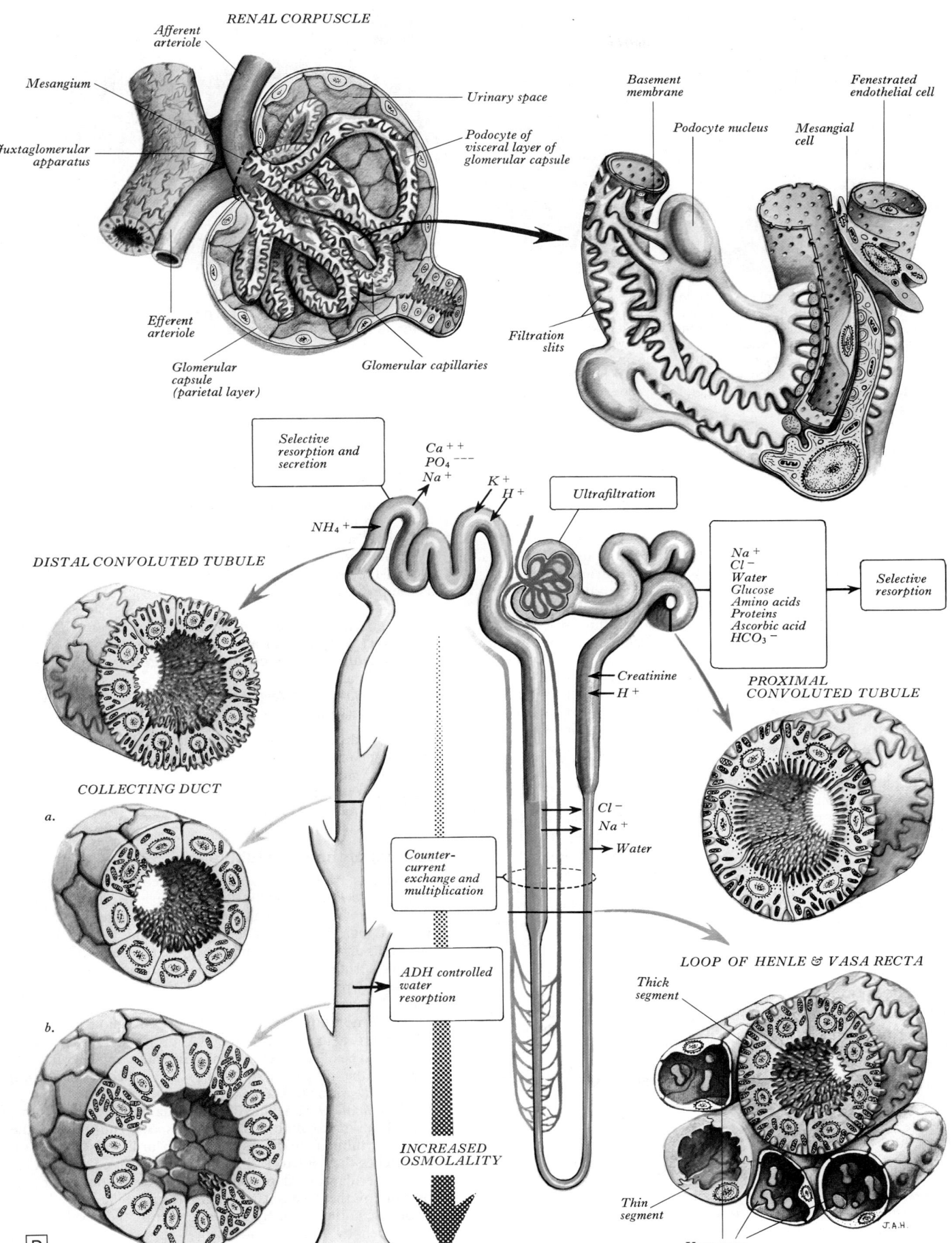

RENAL CORPUSCLE

Afferent arteriole

Mesangium

Juxtaglomerular apparatus

Efferent arteriole

Glomerular capsule (parietal layer)

Glomerular capillaries

Urinary space

Podocyte of visceral layer of glomerular capsule

Basement membrane

Podocyte nucleus

Mesangial cell

Fenestrated endothelial cell

Filtration slits

Selective resorption and secretion

Ca^{++}
PO_4^{---}
Na^+

K^+
H^+

NH_4^+

Ultrafiltration

DISTAL CONVOLUTED TUBULE

Na^+
Cl^-
Water
Glucose
Amino acids
Proteins
Ascorbic acid
HCO_3^-

Selective resorption

COLLECTING DUCT

a.

b.

Creatinine
H^+

PROXIMAL CONVOLUTED TUBULE

Counter-current exchange and multiplication

Cl^-
Na^+

Water

ADH controlled water resorption

LOOP OF HENLE & VASA RECTA

Thick segment

INCREASED OSMOLALITY

Thin segment

Vasa recta

J.A.H.

D

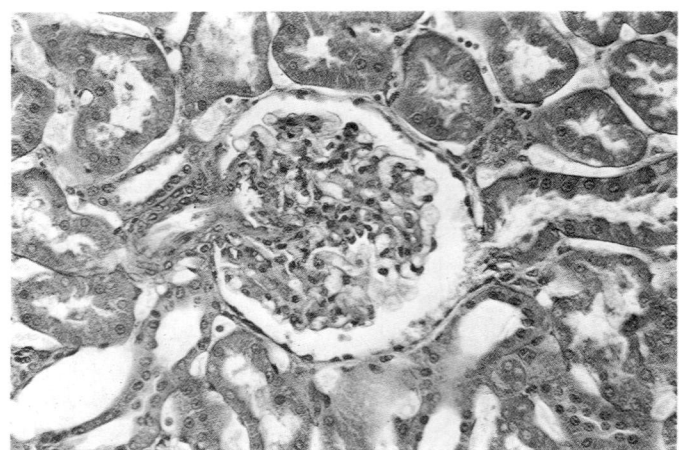

13.12   A renal corpuscle (simian kidney) in section, showing a glomerulus (centre) within its capsule, the urinary space of which is continuous with the proximal convoluted tubule (right). A glomerular arteriole is visible at the vascular pole of the capsule, where it is associated with a *macula densa* of a distal convoluted tubule (left), denoted by a group of closely spaced nuclei. Profiles of proximal convoluted tubules (with brush borders) and distal convoluted tubules (lacking brush borders) are also visible. Masson's tri-chrome stain. Magnification ×150.

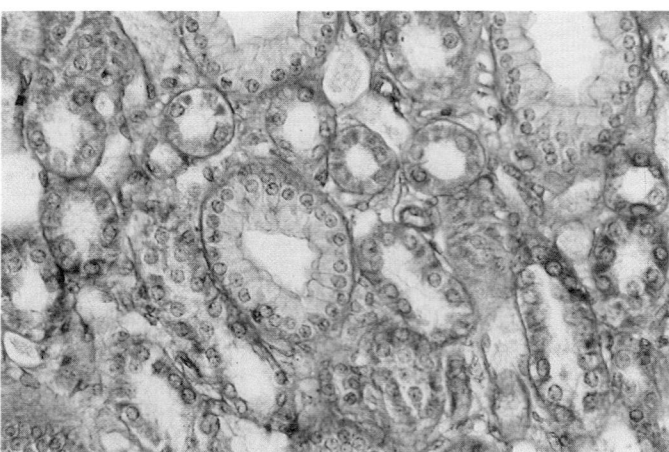

13.13   Part of a medullary ray in cross-section, showing large collecting ducts and small thin segments, interspersed with vasa recta distended with erythrocytes. Tissue and stain as in **13**.12. Magnification ×250.

their major processes curved around capillaries, interdigitating tightly with each other and attached to the basal lamina by numerous pedicels; narrow gaps lie between these cellular extensions. Podocytes contain many mitochondria, microtubules, microfilaments and vesicles of various types, all of these being signs of active metabolism. The glomerular *endothelium* is finely fenestrated and the sole barriers to the passage of fluid from capillary lumen to urinary space are, therefore, the fused endothelial and podocytic basal laminae. This *glomerular basement membrane* is about 0.33 µm thick in man; it is finely fibrillar and shows three layers, the first and third pale-staining (*laminae rarae interna et externa*) and the middle dense and fibrous (*lamina densa*). Unlike many fenestrated endothelia, a regular dense lamina appears absent from the *fenestrae* of glomerular endothelial cells; but at the distal aspect of glomerular membrane areas between adjacent pedicels are covered by a clear dense *glomerular slit diaphragm*, through which filtrate must pass to enter the urinary space. This diaphragm is composed of fine filaments arranged in two regular rows like a zip-fastener (Rodewald & Karnovsky 1974) which may form an important part of the glomerular filter. The glomerular basement membrane acts as a selective filter, allowing the passage from blood, under pressure, of water and various small molecules and ions in the circulation. Haemoglobin may pass, but larger molecules are held back. Selectivity appears related to the physicochemical nature of the filter. Tracer experiments show that some materials withheld from urine by the glomerulus traverse all but the outer surface of the filter (Rennke et al 1975). The glomerular filter has chemical features similar to those of basal laminae elsewhere, including Type IV collagen in the lamina densa and negatively charged proteoglycans elsewhere (see Farquhar 1981). The presence of fixed negative charges tends to inhibit the filtration of charged macromolecules from the blood, particularly in the laminae rarae. Irregular *mesangial cells*, with phagocytic and contractile capacities, have been demonstrated, particularly around bases of glomerular capillary tufts; these may help to clear the glomerular filter of enmeshed substances which might clog it, for example immune complexes, cellular debris, etc. and regulate blood flow (Caulfield & Farquhar 1974; see also Bulger & Dobyan 1982, Latta 1992).

RENAL TUBULE

A renal or uriniferous tubule (**13**.11D) consists of:

● a *glomerular capsule*, already described;
● ˙a *proximal (first) convoluted tubule*, connected to the capsule by a short *neck* (in humans a little narrower than the tubule) leading to a first sinuous or partially coiled *convoluted part*, then to a

terminally straight or slightly spiral *straight part*; this approaches the medulla to become

● the *descending limb* of the *loop of Henle* connected by
● a 'U' turn to
● the *ascending limb*. The limbs of Henle's loop are for some distance narrower and thin-walled, forming the *thin segment*; but the upper part of the ascending limb (*thick segment*) has the same diameter as the proximal convoluted tubule. The ascending limb continues into
● the *distal (second) convoluted tubule*, divisible into *straight* and *convoluted sections* with an intermediate thickened *macula densa* where the tubule comes close to a glomerulus. The nephron finally straightens as
● the *junctional (connecting) tubule*, which ends by joining
● a *collecting (straight) duct*.

Between the distal convoluted and junctional tubules, there is often a short angular *zigzag* (or *irregular*) *tubule*.

Collecting ducts (**13**.11D) commence in the cortical medullary rays and unite at short intervals, finally opening into wider *papillary ducts* (*of Bellini*), which end on a papillary summit, their numerous orifices forming a perforated *area cribrosa*.

Structure of the renal tubule

Renal tubules are lined by a simple epithelium with a basal lamina of varying thickness (**13**.11D, 13). The type of epithelial cell varies according to the functional roles of the different regions, being concerned mainly with active transport and passive diffusion of various ions and water into and out of the tubules, with reabsorption of organic substances such as glucose and amino acids, and with the uptake of any proteins which may leak through the glomerular filter. Recent advances in tandem scanning confocal vital microscopy have allowed the non-invasive microscopic examination of parts of the renal tubules in the living kidney (Andrews 1994). This technique may prove to be of considerable value in evaluating histopathological changes in the tubules associated with extracorporeal storage of donor kidneys prior to transplantation (p. 1834).

The *proximal tubule* is lined by cuboidal epithelium with a brush border of tall microvilli on its luminal aspect. The shape of the cells depends on tubular fluid pressure, which in life distends the lumen and stretches the cells to a slightly flattened shape, becoming taller when glomerular blood pressure falls at death or at biopsy. The cytoplasm of these cells is strongly eosinophilic and their nuclei euchromatic and central. By light microscopy their bases show faint striae, which by electron microscopy appear as a complex series of pleats between which numerous mitochondria are orientated perpendicular to the basal lamina. Reconstruction has shown this complex to consist of processes interdigitating between the lateral aspects of adjacent epithelial cells, creating a labyrinth of cytoplasmic pedicels in the outer part of the tubular wall (Bulger 1965). Taking into account also the microvilli on the luminal surface, such cells provide relatively vast areas of plasma membrane in contact with tubular fluid and the extratubular space, an arrangement facilitating the transport of ions and small molecules against steep concentration gradients and energized by abundant mitochondria. Sodium/potassium-stimulated adenosine triphosphatase (Na/K ATPase) is located in apical and basal membranes (Wachstein & Bradshaw 1965), with numerous other cytoplasmic enzymes associated with ionic transport. Apart from such ionic transport through epithelial cells, water and other ions may pass between cells passively along osmotic and electrical gradients, probably through 'leaky' tight junctions at their apices (Frömter 1979). These cells also contain extensive invaginations of their plasma membranes, channels and lysosomes engaged in the uptake and hydrolysis of proteins which escape in small amounts into the glomerular filtrate (Caulfield & Farquhar 1974). Peroxisomes and lipid droplets are also frequent and basal microfilaments assist to maintain the shape of the tubule. Among many cytoplasmic enzymes demonstrable by histochemistry are cytochrome oxidase, succinic dehydrogenase and other respiratory enzymes, acid phosphatase in lysosomes and glucose-6-phosphatase and leucine aminopeptidase, reflecting the highly energetic nature of these cells (see below). Dramatic phenotypic changes can be produced in renal proximal tubule cells by exposure to growth factors such as transforming growth factors (TGF) α and β (Humes et al 1991).

Variations occur in cell structure, enzyme content and functions along the proximal tubules. The short, initial *neck* is the simple squamous epithelial extension of the outer wall of the renal corpuscle; the rest of the proximal tubule is divided into three (sometimes four) regions: the first typified by long microvilli, the second by microvilli of medium length, the third (in man) again by long microvilli (Moffat 1975). Patterns of lysosomal and transport activities appear to follow these divisions, too, but the functional significance of this distribution is not clear.

The *ansa nephroni* (renal loop of Henle) consists of the *thin segment* (about 30 μm in diameter), lined by low cuboidal to squamous cells, and the *thick segment* (about 60 μm across) composed of cuboidal cells like those in the distal tubule, with which it is sometimes considered, as its *straight part*. The *thin segment* forms most of the loop in juxtamedullary and deep cortical nephrons which reach far into medulla; here, the descending limb of the thin segment has low cuboidal epithelial cells with complex interdigitations and narrow belts of tight junctions between these cells, whereas the ascending limb is lined by squamous cells with wider junctional zones. These differences may be related to the different permeabilities to water and ions (Bulger 1971; Kondo et al 1992). Few organelles appear in either cell type, indicating a passive rather than an active role in ionic movements. The *thick segment* is composed of cuboidal epithelium with many mitochondria, deep basolateral folds and short apical microvilli, indicative of a more active metabolic state. Atrial natriuretic peptide receptors which mediate Ca^{2+} transients in cortical thick ascending limb cells have been identified by Dai and Quamme (1993). The thick limb of the human loop of Henle, which can be identified immunohistochemically by antibody to Tamm-Horsfall protein (Howie & Johnson 1992) ends either at the macula densa or a variable distance beyond it. Its limit is marked by an abrupt change in cell size and in staining characteristics to a range of reagents including antibodies to cytokeratins. These structural changes suggest that there is a fundamental, functional change in the renal tubule at the end of the thick limb of the loop of Henle.

Cells of the *distal tubule* resemble those in the proximal, but microvilli are few, small and irregularly spaced; the basolateral folds containing mitochondria are so deep that they almost reach the luminal aspect (**13.**11D). Enzymes concerned in active transport of sodium, potassium and other ions are richly present and are known to be important in ionic regulation. At the junction of the straight and convoluted regions the distal tubule approaches the vascular pole of the renal corpuscle where tubular cells form a sensory structure, the *macula densa*, concerned in the regulation of blood flow and ionic exchange (see below). In the terminal part of the

distal tubule, cells have fewer basal folds and mitochondria, constituting what is sometimes termed a *connecting duct*, in part like a distal collecting duct but formed from nephrogenic rather than ductal tissue during embryogenesis.

Collecting ducts are of simple cuboidal or columnar epithelium, increasing in height from the cortex, where they receive the contents of distal tubules, to the wide papillary ducts discharging at the area cribrosa. The cells have relatively few organelles or lateral interdigitations and only occasional microvilli; scattered among them are *dark cells* (also present in smaller numbers in the distal convoluted tubule) with longer microvilli and more mitochondria. The functions of these remain uncertain but it has been suggested that these dark, octopal, cells may have a modulatory role, possibly involving epidermal growth factor (EGF) receptivity (Nouwen & DeBroe 1994).

STRUCTURE AND FUNCTION OF NEPHRONS

Three processes cooperate in nephrons to determine renal excretory and regulatory functions (**13.**11D): *filtration*, at the glomerular level, *selective resorption* from the filtrate passing along the renal tubules and *secretion* by the cells of the tubules into this filtrate. These processes have been intensively studied and can be generally correlated with structural variations along the nephron.

Glomerular filtration

Glomerular filtration is the passage of water containing various dissolved small molecules from the blood to the urinary space in the glomerular capsule; larger molecules, for example plasma proteins, polysaccharides and lipids, are largely retained in blood by the selective permeability of the glomerular basement membrane.

Filtration occurs along a steep pressure gradient existing between the large glomerular capillaries and the urinary space, the only structure separating the two being the glomerular basement membrane. This gradient far exceeds the colloid osmotic pressure of blood which opposes the outward flow of filtrate. In the peripheral renal cortex the arteriolar pressure gradient is enhanced by an inequality in the calibres of afferent and efferent glomerular arterioles, the former having larger diameters (see below). In all glomeruli the rate of filtration can be altered by changes in the tonus of the glomerular arterioles. When first formed, the *glomerular filtrate* is isotonic with glomerular blood and has an identical concentration of ions and small molecules.

Selective resorption

Selective resorption of many substances from the filtrate is an active process and occurs mainly in the proximal convoluted tubules, particularly the resorption of glucose, amino acids, phosphate, chloride, sodium, calcium and bicarbonate. Cells of the proximal tubules are permeable to water, which leaves the tubules along an osmotic gradient created by resorption of these solutes, particularly sodium and chloride ions, so that the filtrate remains locally isotonic with blood. Numerous microvilli, the folded lateral and basal surfaces and profuse mitochondria indicate that absorption by proximal tubular cells is an energy-dependent process. Further selective absorption, particularly of sodium ions, also occurs in distal convoluted tubules.

The rest of the tubule reabsorbs most of the filtrate's water (95%); when it reaches the calyces, urine is thus much reduced in volume and is *hypertonic* to blood. Along the **descending** limb of the renal loop, sodium and water pass freely between the tubular lumen and adjacent extratubular spaces of the renal medulla, within which lie many loops. In part of the **ascending** limb (the thick segment), chloride ions are actively transported from the tubule lumen to interstitial spaces, sodium ions following passively; but the lining cells of the tubules do not allow water to follow sodium and chloride ions, some of which diffuse back into the descending limbs, adding to that already in the filtrate passing along them; in the ascending limbs, sodium is again extracted from this enriched solution, increasing intercellular ion concentrations and causing further diffusion of these into the descending limbs. Alternatively, sodium and chloride may not actually enter the descending limb, water being merely withdrawn from the tubular loop because of the raised tonicity in the extratubular space, thus concentrating the filtrate. In either manner, high concentrations of sodium and chloride ions are built up in the renal medulla by this *countercurrent multiplier system*. Rapid removal of ions from the renal medulla by the circulation of blood is minimized by another looped *countercurrent exchange system*, in which arterioles entering the medulla pass for long distances parallel to the venules leaving it before ending in capillary beds around tubules. This close apposition of oppositely flowing blood allows the direct diffusion of ions from outflowing to inflowing blood, so that these vessels (*vasa recta*) conserve a general high osmotic pressure in the medulla.

Because of the selective extrusion of sodium and chloride ions by the cells of the ascending limbs and distal tubules (under aldosterone control), the filtrate at the distal end of the convoluted tubules is *hypotonic*; but, as it proceeds into the collecting ducts, descending again through the medulla, it re-enters a region of high osmotic pressure. Here, since ductal cells are, under the influence of the neurohypophyseal antidiuretic hormone (ADH, vasopressin), variably permeable to water, the latter follows an osmotic gradient into the adjacent extratubular spaces (Gottschalk & Mylle 1959). Thus, along collecting ducts, the tonicity of the filtrate gradually rises until at the tip of the renal pyramids it is above that of blood. As much as 95% of water in the original glomerular filtrate is thus resorbed into blood. This complex system is highly flexible and the balance between the rate of filtration and absorption can be varied to accommodate to the current general physiological needs.

Secretion

Secretion of various ions occurs at several sites, control of hydrogen and ammonium ion concentrations being essential to the regulation of acids and bases in the blood. Other secreted substances include various organic acids and antibiotics, these being passed into the filtrate especially in the proximal and distal tubules (**13**.11D).

JUXTAGLOMERULAR APPARATUS

The afferent and efferent arterioles of a glomerulus pass through the mesangium (the vascular stalk of the glomerulus) nearly opposite the exit of the proximal tubule (**13**.11D, 14). In each nephron, the ascending limb of its renal loop returns from the medulla towards its glomerulus and the distal tubule commences between the afferent and efferent vessels, in close contact with them. The cells of the tunica media of the afferent arteriole differ from nonstriated myocytes elsewhere in being large, rounded and 'epitheloid' with large spherical nuclei; their cytoplasm contains dense vesicles, 10–40 nm in diameter, and also many mitochondria. These *juxtaglomerular cells* contact cells of the slightly dilated distal convoluted tubule, closely aggregated together here as the *macula densa*; the latter cells are clustered in a group of up to 40, with large, oval nuclei, each cell containing a concentration of mitochondria apically (see Barajas 1970; Sikri & Foster 1981) and have a few short microvilli on their luminal surface. The two groups, with various mesangial elements, constitute the renal *juxtaglomerular apparatus* (Edelman & Hartroft 1961; Barajas 1970). In many animals, interspersed between the macula densa and mesangium are 'lacis cells' (Polkissen cells, extraglomerular mesangial cells, see Spanidis et al 1982). These cells are stellate in form and their processes create an irregular network (lacis). Each cell has a surrounding basal lamina and contains occasional granules of a secretory type, but few organelles otherwise. Adrenergic nerve fibres occur in small numbers among these cells. Another cell type, present as a minor component of this intermediate region, has also been described. This is the *granular peripolar cell* reported in sheep (Ryan et al 1979), humans (Gardiner et al 1986) and other mammalian species (Gibson et al 1994). Its main feature is the presence of dense membrane-bound vacuoles 0.4–2.1 μm in diameter. These cells are situated close to the epithelial cells of the renal corpuscle wall, near the mesangial root. Their functions are not yet known but they would appear to be secretory.

In experimental diminution of renal blood flow, with consequent increase of blood pressure and sometimes in hypertension associated with renal disease, juxtaglomerular cells hypertrophy; they contain *renin* within their granules, an enzyme converting a polypeptide in blood, *angiotensinogen*, to *angiotensin I*. This is converted by other enzymes (notably in the lungs) into *angiotensin II*, a polypeptide whose actions include the elevation of blood pressure and stimulation of aldosterone release from the adrenal cortex, increasing resorption of sodium ions from the distal convoluted tubules. Details of renin secretion and consequent changes in tubular activity are not yet clear but the juxtaglomerular apparatus appears to be a feedback device regulating flow of fluid through the glomerular filter and ionic

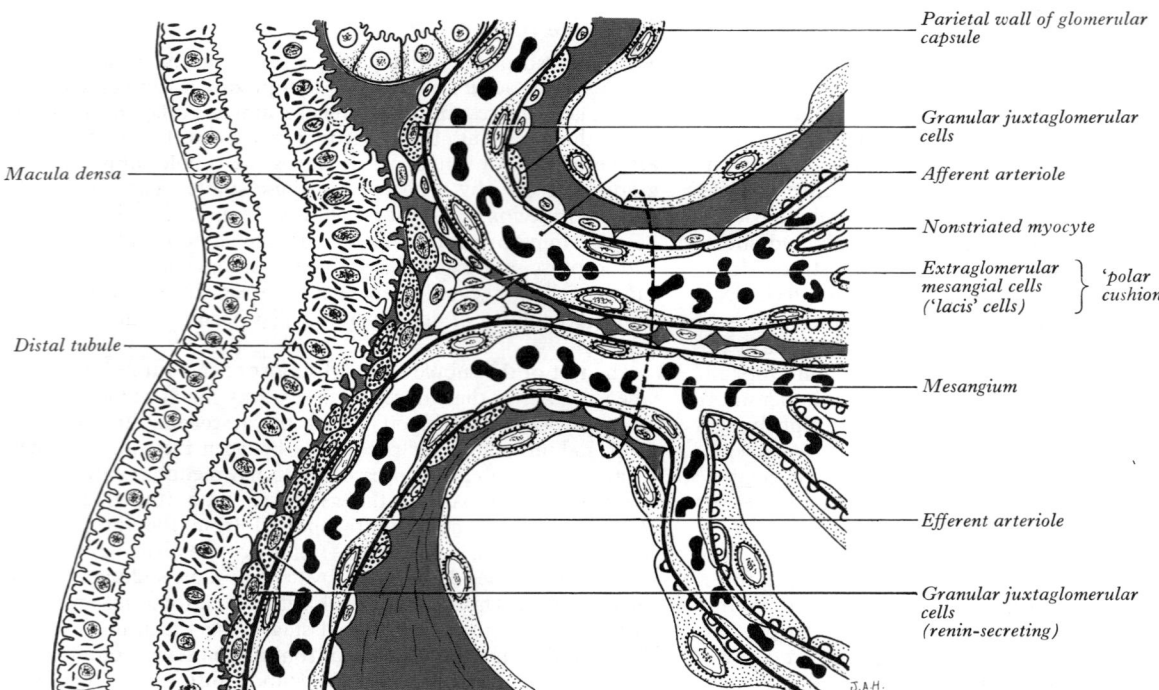

Parietal wall of glomerular capsule

Granular juxtaglomerular cells

Afferent arteriole

Nonstriated myocyte

Extraglomerular mesangial cells ('lacis' cells) } *'polar cushion'*

Macula densa

Distal tubule

Mesangium

Efferent arteriole

Granular juxtaglomerular cells (renin-secreting)

13.14 Diagram showing the organization of the juxtaglomerular complex including the macula densa (left), granular juxtaglomerular cells (middle) and the vascular pole of the glomerular capsule (right).

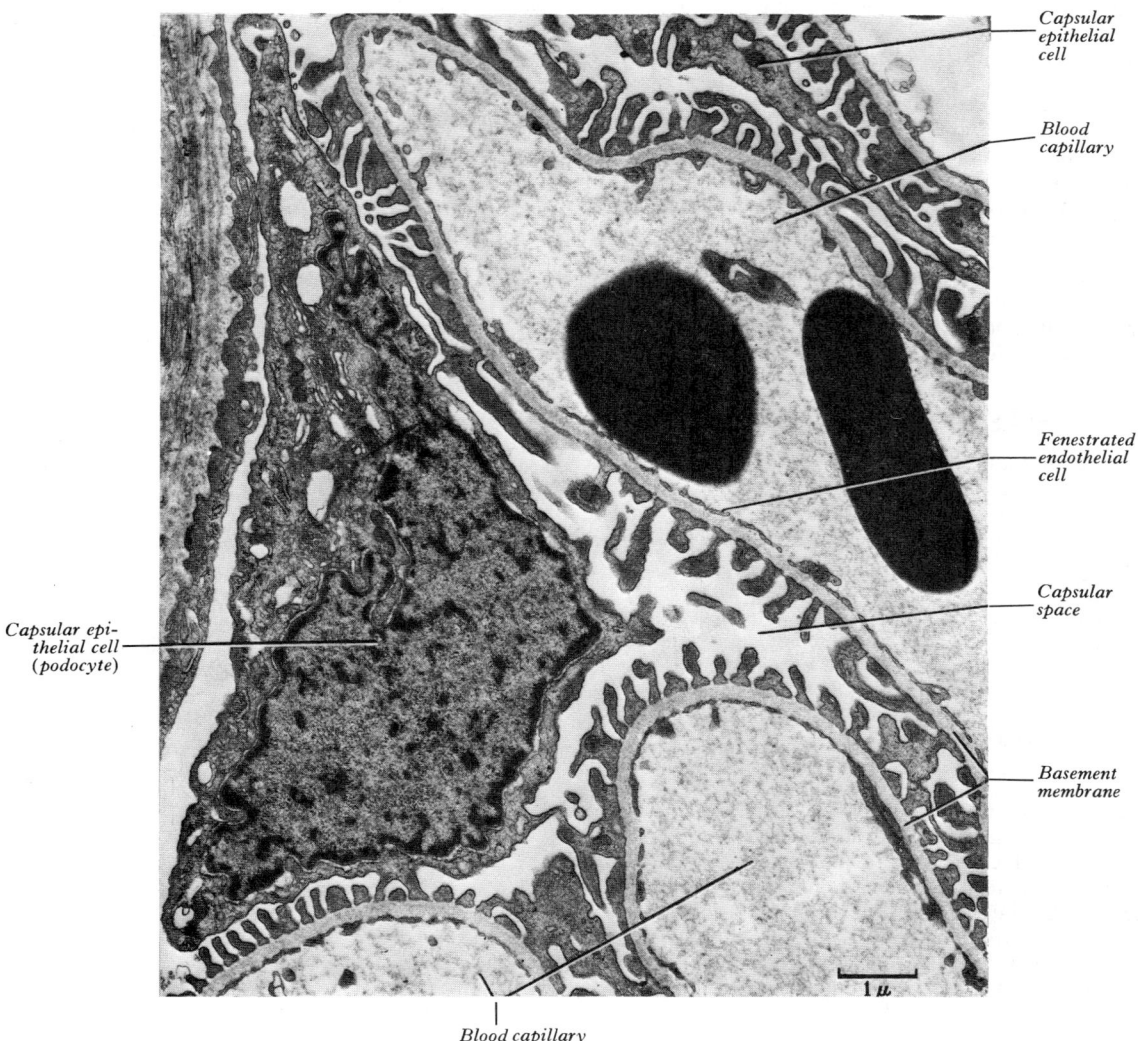

Capsular epithelial cell

Blood capillary

Fenestrated endothelial cell

Capsular space

Capsular epithelial cell (podocyte)

Basement membrane

Blood capillary

13.15   Electron micrograph showing capillaries and epithelial cells of a renal corpuscle (rat). Note the basement membrane and fenestrated endo-thelial cells as well as the foot processes of the epithelial cell (podocyte). Magnification ×9200.

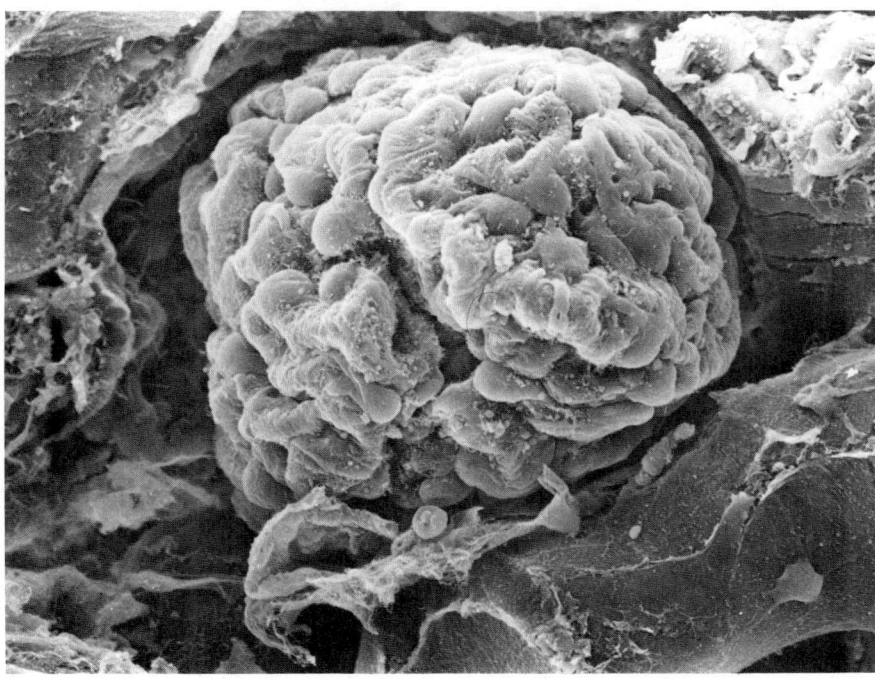

13.16   Scanning electron micrograph of a renal corpuscle (guinea pig) fractured to expose the glomerulus and podocytes and surrounding tubules. Magnification ×1000.

resorption in the renal tubules, thus determining the final concentration of the urine. Renin secretion may be controlled by at least three factors (Davis & Freeman 1976; Briggs et al 1990):

- the activity of the macula densa cells which react to changes in fluid passing them in the distal tubules;
- pressure in glomerular arterioles affecting the secretory activity of their granule cells;
- stimulation by sympathetic fibres ending near juxtaglomerular cells.

These and other agents (perhaps including other cell types in this region) appear to assist the juxtaglomerular apparatus in correlating blood flow, filtration rate and osmoregulation and in mediating the appropriate actions needed for homeostasis.

OTHER RENAL CELLS

Between the renal tubules and blood vessels lie other cells essential to renal structure and function, such as connective tissue elements, inconspicuous in the cortex but prominent in the medulla, where they secrete the proteoglycans and collagen of the connective tissue matrix, particularly visible in the papillae. Medullary *interstitial cells*, some apparently modified fibroblasts, form vertical piles of tangentially orientated cells between the more distal collecting ducts, like the rungs of a ladder. These cells secrete prostaglandins (Muirhead et al 1972).

RENAL BLOOD VESSELS

Blood vessels

The complex renal vascular patterns show regional specializations, closely adapted to the spatial organization and functions of renal corpuscles, tubules and ducts (**13**.11, 18–20). The large literature concerning renal angioarchitecture, haemodynamics and controlling mechanisms cannot be analysed here, nor can variation between species, or minor human variations be considered. For these admirable reviews exist by Trueta et al (1947), Fourman and Moffat (1971) Moffat (1975) and Lorenz et al (1992) among others.

Renal vasculature may be studied at various levels, commencing with the principal and accessory *renal arteries*. Their primary patterns of branching and areas of distribution suggest the presence of *vascular segmentation*. From the primary stems branch *lobar, interlobar, arcuate* and *interlobular arteries, afferent* and *efferent glomerular arterioles* and cortical *intertubular capillary plexuses*; cortical venous radicles drain them and also the *vasa recta* and associated capillary plexuses of the medulla to the renal vein (**13**.11, 18).

A single renal artery to each kidney (p. 1557), is present in about 70% of individuals but they vary in their level of origin (the **right** often being superior) and in their calibre, obliquity and precise relations. (For a review of these features in almost 11 000 kidneys, see Merklin and Michels 1958.) In its extrarenal course (Schneider et al 1969) each renal artery gives off one or more inferior suprarenal arteries and branches which supply perinephric tissue, the renal capsule, pelvis and the proximal part of the ureter; near the renal hilum, each artery divides into an *anterior* and *posterior division*, the primary branches of which (*segmental arteries*) supply renal *vascular segments*. *Accessory renal arteries* are common (30% of individuals), usually arising from the aorta above or below the main renal artery and following it to the renal hilum. Higher or lower origins are not uncommon, an accessory artery or leash of arteries passing to the superior or inferior renal pole. They are regarded as persistent embryonic *lateral splanchnic* arteries. Accessory vessels to the inferior pole cross anterior to the ureter and may, by its obstruction, cause hydronephrosis. Rarely, accessory renal arteries arise from the coeliac or superior mesenteric arteries near the aortic bifurcation or from the common iliac arteries.

Renal vascular segmentation was originally recognized by John Hunter in 1794 but the first detailed account of the primary pattern was by Graves (1954, 1956a, b) from casts and radiographs of injected kidneys. He described five segments:

- *apical*, occupying the anteromedial region of the superior pole
- *superior* (*anterior*), including the rest of the superior pole and the central anterosuperior region
- *inferior*, encompassing the whole lower pole
- *middle* (*anterior*), between the anterior and inferior segments
- *posterior*, including the whole posterior region between the apical and inferior segments.

Graves' terminology has been adopted internationally and used by some researchers (Smith 1963; Sykes 1963, 1964), but others have

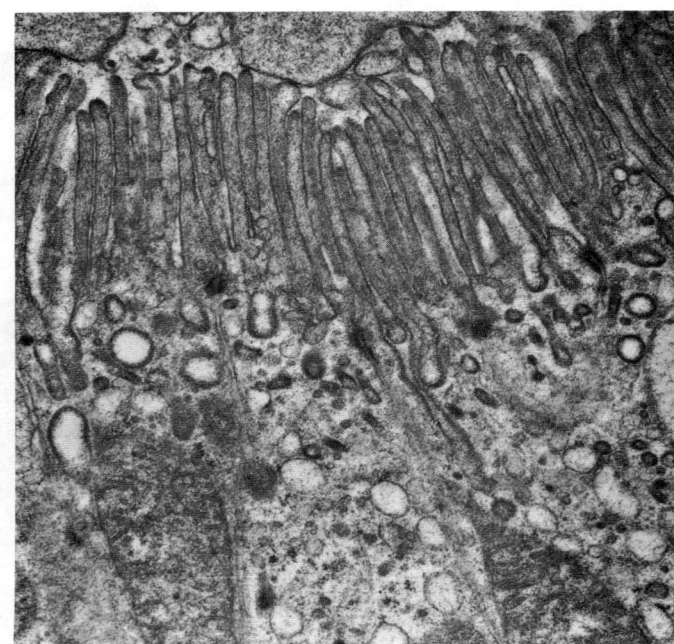

13.17A A high-power electron micrograph of the apical (luminal) parts of four proximal convoluted tubular epithelial cells. The apical array of microvilli, subapical junctional complexes between adjacent cells and the highly active cytoplasm containing lysosomes, parts of very large mitochondria and a wide variety of granules, vesicles and vacuoles are visible. Magnification ×20 000.

13.17B Electron micrograph of the apices of a group of cells of the proximal convoluted tubule. Visible are long microvilli, dense lysosomes and mitochondria. Magnification ×20 000.

proposed more complex schemes, for example three posterior segments (Faller & Ungváry 1962); some have emphasized the great variability of the regions supplied by segmental arteries (Fine & Keen 1966). Whatever the divergences, it must be emphasized that vascular segments are supplied by virtual end arteries. In contrast, larger *intrarenal veins* have no segmental organization and anastomose freely.

Brödel (1901) described a relatively avascular longitudinal zone (the *'bloodless' line of Brödel*) along the convex renal border, proposed as the most suitable site for surgical incision. However, many vessels cross this zone, which is far from 'bloodless'; planned radial or intersegmental incisions are said to be preferable.

Initial branches of segmental arteries are *lobar*, usually one to each renal pyramid, but before entry they subdivide into two or three *interlobar arteries*, extending towards the cortex around each pyramid. At the junction of the cortex and medulla, interlobar arteries dichotomize into *arcuate arteries* which diverge at right angles; as they arch between cortex and medulla, each divides further and, from its branches, *interlobular arteries* diverge radially into the cortex. The terminations of adjacent arcuate arteries do not anastomose but end in the cortex as additional interlobular arteries. Though most interlobular arteries come from arcuate branches, some arise directly from arcuate or even terminal interlobar arteries (**13**.18B).

Interlobular arteries ascend towards the superficial cortex or may branch a few times en route (**13**.11c); some are more tortuous, recurring towards the medulla, recurring towards the medulla once or more before proceeding towards the renal surface. Some traverse the surface as *perforating arteries* (Hammersen & Staubesand 1961) to anastomose with the *capsular plexus* (also supplied from the *inferior suprarenal, renal* and *testicular* or *ovarian* arteries).

Afferent glomerular arterioles are mainly the lateral rami of interlobular arteries but a few arise from arcuate and interlobar arteries, when they vary their direction and angle of origin: deeper ones incline obliquely back towards the medulla, the intermediate pass out horizontally, while the more superficial approach the renal surface obliquely before ending in a glomerulus (**13**.18A, B, 19).

From most glomeruli (excepting the juxtamedullary and a few at intermediate cortical levels) *efferent glomerular arterioles* soon divide to form a dense *peritubular capillary plexus* around the proximal and distal convoluted tubules. In the main renal cortical circulation there are thus **two** sets of **capillaries** in series, glomerular and peritubular, linked by efferent glomerular arterioles. From the venous ends of the peritubular plexuses fine radicles converge to join *interlobular veins*, one with each interlobular artery. Many interlobular veins commence beneath the fibrous renal capsule by convergence of several *stellate veins*, draining the most superficial zone of the renal cortex and so named from their surface appearance. Proceeding to the corticomedullary junction, interlobular veins also receive some ascending vasa recta (see below) and end in *arcuate veins* which accompany arcuate arteries but, unlike them, they anastomose with neighbouring veins. Arcuate veins drain into *interlobar veins*, which anastomose and converge to form the renal vein.

The vascular supply of the *renal medulla* is largely from efferent arterioles of juxtamedullary glomeruli, supplemented by some from more superficial glomeruli, and 'aglomerular' arterioles (probably from degenerated glomeruli). Efferent glomerular arterioles passing into the medulla are relatively long, wide vessels, contributing side branches to neighbouring capillary plexuses before entering the medulla, where each divides into 12–25 *descending vasa recta*; these, as their name suggests, run straight to varying depths in the renal medulla, contributing side branches to a radially elongated capillary plexus (**13**.18A) applied to the descending and ascending limbs of renal loops and to collecting ducts. The venous ends of capillaries converge to the *ascending vasa recta*, which drain into arcuate or interlobular veins. An essential feature of the vasa recta is that, particularly in the outer medulla, both ascending and descending vessels are grouped into *vascular bundles*, within which the external aspects of both types are closely apposed, bringing them close to the limbs of renal loops and collecting ducts. As these bundles converge centrally into the renal medulla they contain fewer vessels, some terminating at successive levels in neighbouring capillary plexuses. This proximity of descending and ascending vessels with each other and adjacent ducts is the structural basis for the countercurrent

exchange and multiplier phenomena previously mentioned (p. 1824, **13**.11D, 19A, C).

In **ultrastructure**, renal vessels show the regional features described elsewhere; renal, interlobar and arcuate arteries are typical 'large muscular arteries' (p. 1463); the interlobular vessels are like 'small muscular arteries' and afferent glomerular vessels have a typical arteriolar structure with a muscular coat two to three cells thick; this and the connective tissue components of the wall diminish near a glomerulus until a point 30–50 μm proximal to it where arteriolar cells begin to show modifications typical of the *juxtaglomerular apparatus* (p. 1824). The efferent arterioles from most cortical glomeruli have thicker walls and a narrower calibre than corresponding afferents. The role of the efferent arteriole in tubuloglomerular feedback has been reviewed by Davis (1992) although the afferent arteriole is generally considered to be solely responsible for this. The peritubular and medullary capillaries possess a well-defined basal lamina and their endothelial cells have typically fenestrated cytoplasm, as in ascending vasa recta; in contrast, the descending vasa recta have thicker, continuous endothelium. The structure of glomerular capillaries is considered above (p. 1822). For brief comments on the functional association between the regions of renal tubules and associated blood vessels see page 1826 and Fourman and Moffat (1971). A detailed account of renal microvasculature has also been given for monkeys (Horacek et al 1986, 1987).

Renal innervation

The general sources of renal nerves are described on page 1307. Direct nerve fibres from plexuses around arcuate arteries which innervate juxtamedullary efferent arterioles and vasa recta have been described (Munkacsi & Newstead 1971); these might control blood flow between the cortex and medulla without affecting the glomerular circulation.

Lymph vessels

Lymph vessels are described on page 1623.

Clinical anomalies

The early pelvic position of the kidneys (p. 204) may persist; they are then usually supplied from the common iliac arteries and the hila are anterior. Occasionally kidneys are connected by a transverse bridge of renal tissue, forming a 'horseshoe kidney', the commissure usually lying between the inferior poles and rarely the superior. The ureters curve anterior to the connection and may be here partially obstructed. A congenital absence or imperfect development of one kidney may be compensated by an enlargement of the opposite organ. Two kidneys may also occur on the same side. Single or multiple congenital renal cysts and widespread congenital polycystic disease may also be present.

UPPER URINARY TRACT

The upper urinary tract is generally used as a collective name for the main urinary outflow conduits from the kidney (renal calyces, renal pelvis and ureter), as distinct from the bladder and urethra, which constitute the *lower urinary tract*. This separation is of course arbitrary.

RENAL CALYCES AND PELVIS

Within the renal sinus the proximal parts of the urinary tract consist of the minor and major calyces and the renal pelvis. The minor calyces are attached to the renal parenchyma around the bases of a variable number (7–14) of conical renal papillae which form the tips of the renal pyramids (p. 1819). The renal capsule covers the external surface of the kidney and continues through the hilus to line the sinus (p. 1816) and fuse with the adventitial coverings of the 7–13 minor calyces. Each minor calyx is a trumpet-shaped structure which surrounds either a single papilla or, more rarely, groups of two or three papillae (**13**.5, 6, 11A, B). The minor calyces unite with their neighbours to form two or possibly three larger chambers, the major calyces. The latter usually fuse with each other to form a single funnel-shaped renal pelvis, which tapers as it passes inferomedially, traversing the renal hilus to become continuous with the ureter (**13**.5,

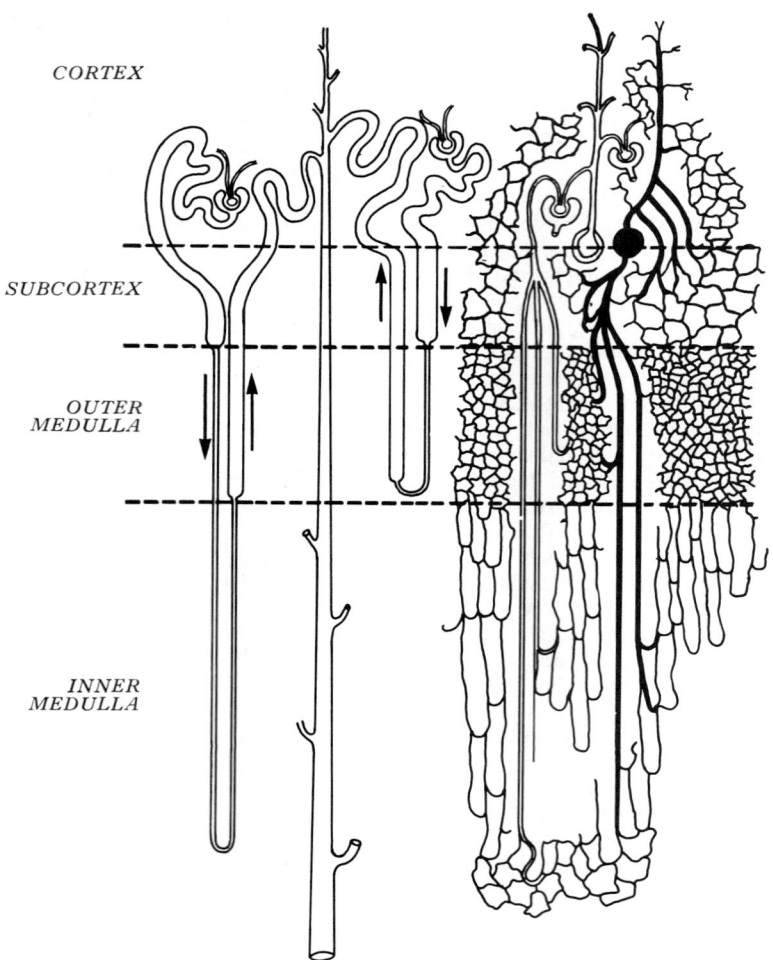

13.18A   Diagram to illustrate the arrangement of the tubules (left) and blood vessels (right) in various structural zones of the kidney. Note the variations in the pattern of the tubules with either long or short medullary loops; tubules of intermediate length also occur. Compare the different structural and functional segments of the tubules which occur together in the cortical, subcortical and outer and inner medullary zones with their related vascular patterns. Arteries are black outlines; capillaries are single black lines; veins are full black. Compare with **13**.18B. (From Fourman & Moffat 1971 with permission of the authors and Blackwell Scientific Publications.)

6, 11A). Normally it is not possible to determine precisely the position where the renal pelvis ceases and the ureter begins. Consequently the precision implied by the phrase 'pelviureteric junction' to describe this area is anatomically invalid and the term 'pelviureteric region' is preferable. This region is usually extrahilar in location and normally lies adjacent to the lower part of the medial border of the kidney. In some individuals, however, the entire renal pelvis has been found to lie inside the sinus of the kidney and, as a consequence, the pelviureteric region is situated either in the vicinity of the renal hilus or completely within the renal sinus.

Microstructure of the renal calyces and pelvis

The wall of the proximal part of the urinary tract is composed of three histological layers, namely a connective tissue adventitia (fibrous coat), a coat of smooth muscle and an inner mucosa. (The mucosal lining of the renal calyces and pelvis is identical in structure to that of the ureter (p. 1831) and will not be considered further here.) The adventitia forms the outermost layer and consists of loose fibro-elastic connective tissue which merges with retroperitoneal areolar tissue. Proximally the coat fuses with the fibrous capsule of the kidney lining the renal sinus. The muscle coat of the renal calyces and pelvis is composed of two morphologically and histochemically distinct types of smooth muscle cell (Dixon & Gosling 1982). One type of muscle cell is identical to that described for the ureter and can be traced proximally through the pelviureteric region and renal pelvis as far as the minor calyces. The other type possesses a number of unusual structural features; these cells form the muscle coat of each minor calyx and continue into the major calyces and pelvis

where they form a distinct inner layer. The cells also form a thin sheet of muscle which covers each minor calyceal fornix and extends across the renal parenchyma between the attachments of neighbouring minor calyces, thereby linking each minor calyx to its neighbours. Further out in the wall of each minor calyx, the muscle cells are arranged longitudinally and form a discrete layer confined to the inner aspect of the muscle coat, the remainder of which is formed of bundles of typical smooth muscle. Such a configuration continues throughout the wall of the major calyces and renal pelvis but ceases in the pelviureteric region so that the proximal ureter is devoid of a morphologically distinct inner layer. Individually, these muscle cells are separated from one another by extensive amounts of connective tissue and differ histochemically from typical ureteric nonstriated muscle. In addition the muscle cells possess unusual fine structural features when examined by means of the electron microscope (Dixon & Gosling 1982). The functional significance of these structural features is considered on page 1832.

URETERS (10.128, **13**.5, 6, 11, 20, 21, 33, 35)

Ureters are muscular tubes whose peristaltic contractions convey urine from the kidneys to the urinary bladder. Each measures 25–30 cm in length and is thick-walled, narrow and continuous superiorly with the funnel-shaped renal pelvis (p. 1827); a slight constriction may mark this junction (**13**.11A). Each descends slightly medially anterior to psoas major, entering the pelvic cavity to open into the base of the urinary bladder. Its surface projection is an almost

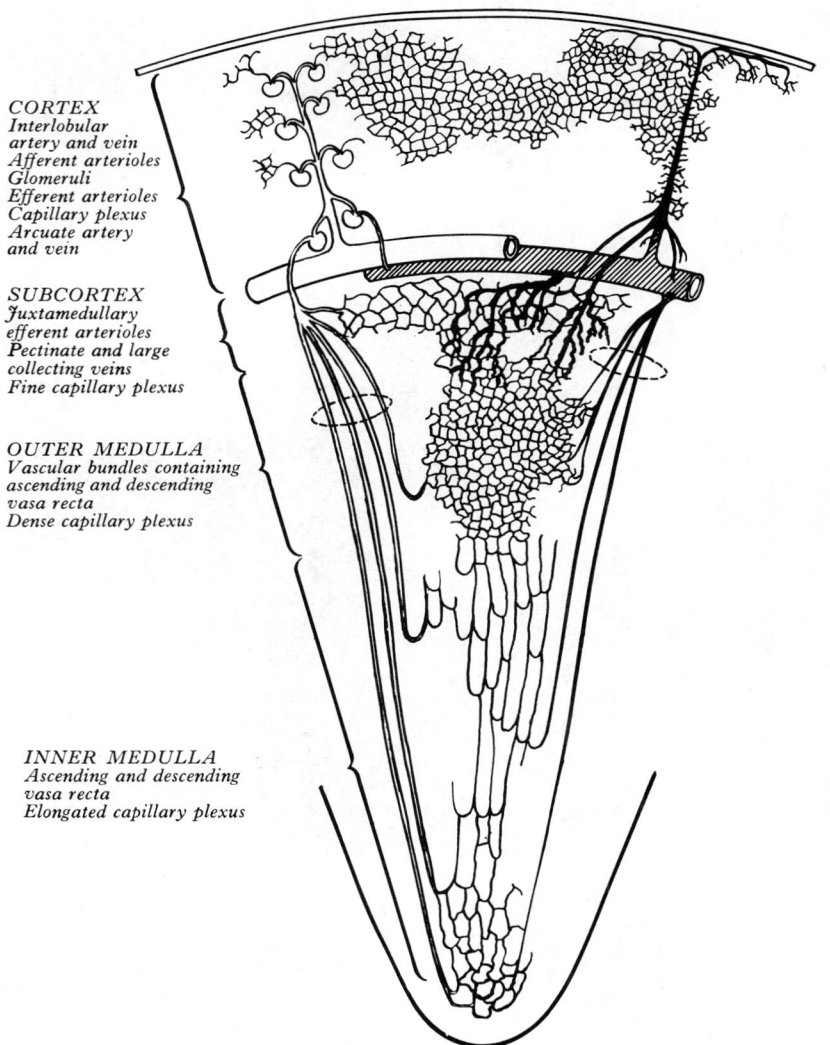

CORTEX
Interlobular
artery and vein
Afferent arterioles
Glomeruli
Efferent arterioles
Capillary plexus
Arcuate artery
and vein

SUBCORTEX
Juxtamedullary
efferent arterioles
Pectinate and large
collecting veins
Fine capillary plexus

OUTER MEDULLA
Vascular bundles containing
ascending and descending
vasa recta
Dense capillary plexus

INNER MEDULLA
Ascending and descending
vasa recta
Elongated capillary plexus

13.18B Diagram of the basic arrangements of the blood vessels in the mammalian kidney. Arteries are black outlines; capillaries are single black lines; veins are cross-hatched or full black. Note the variations in the pattern of the meshes in the capillary networks. See accompanying text for further description. (From Fourman & Moffat 1971 with permission of the authors and Blackwell Scientific Publications.)

vertical line from a point on the transpyloric plane, 5 cm from the midline to the pubic tubercle. Its diameter is about 3 mm but slightly less at its junction with the renal pelvis, the brim of the lesser pelvis near the medial border of psoas major, and where it traverses the vesical (bladder) wall (its narrowest part). The *renal pelvis* has already been described (see above).

The ureter's *abdominal part* descends posterior to the peritoneum on the medial part of psoas major, which separates it from the tips of the lumbar transverse processes (**10**.112). Anterior to the muscle it crosses in front of the genitofemoral nerve and is obliquely crossed by the gonadal vessels. It enters the lesser pelvis anterior to either the end of the common or the beginning of the external iliac vessels.

At its origin the **right** ureter is usually overlapped by the descending part of the duodenum; it descends lateral to the inferior vena cava, crossed anteriorly by the right colic and ileocolic vessels; near the superior aperture of the lesser pelvis it passes behind the lower part of the mesentery and terminal ileum. The **left** ureter, crossed by the left colic vessels, passes posterior to the sigmoid colon and its mesentery in the posterior wall of the intersigmoid recess. At operation, the abdominal part of the left ureter is hence easier to expose than the right.

The *pelvic part*, about the same length as the abdominal, lies in both sexes in extraperitoneal areolar tissue. At first it descends posterolaterally on the lateral wall of the lesser pelvis along the anterior border of the greater sciatic notch. Opposite the ischial spine it turns anteromedially into fibrous adipose tissue above the levator ani to reach the base of the bladder. On the pelvic wall it is anterior to the internal iliac artery and the beginning of its anterior trunk, posterior to which are the internal iliac vein, lumbosacral nerve and sacro-iliac joint. Laterally it lies on the fascia of obturator internus. It progressively crosses and is medial to the umbilical artery, the obturator nerve, artery and vein, the inferior vesical and middle rectal arteries. **In males**, in the anteromedial part of its descent, the pelvic ureter is crossed anterosuperiorly, from lateral to medial, by the ductus deferens. Then it passes in front of and slightly above the upper pole of the seminal vesicle to traverse the bladder wall obliquely before opening at the ipsilateral trigonal angle (**13**.35). Its terminal part is surrounded by tributaries of the vesical veins. **In females**, the pelvic part at first has the same relations as in males, but anterior to the internal iliac artery it is immediately behind the ovary, forming the posterior boundary of the ovarian fossa (p. 1861). In the anteromedial part of its course to the bladder it is related to the uterine artery, uterine cervix and vaginal fornices. It is in extraperitoneal connective tissue in the inferomedial part of the broad ligament of the uterus (parametrium, p. 1870); here the uterine artery is anterosuperior to the ureter for 2.5 cm and then crosses to its medial side to ascend alongside the uterus. The ureter turns forwards slightly above the lateral vaginal fornix and is here generally 2 cm lateral to the supravaginal part of the uterine cervix (p. 1871). It then inclines medially to reach the bladder, with a variable relation to the front of the vagina. As the uterus is commonly deviated to one side, one ureter may be more extensively apposed to the vagina,

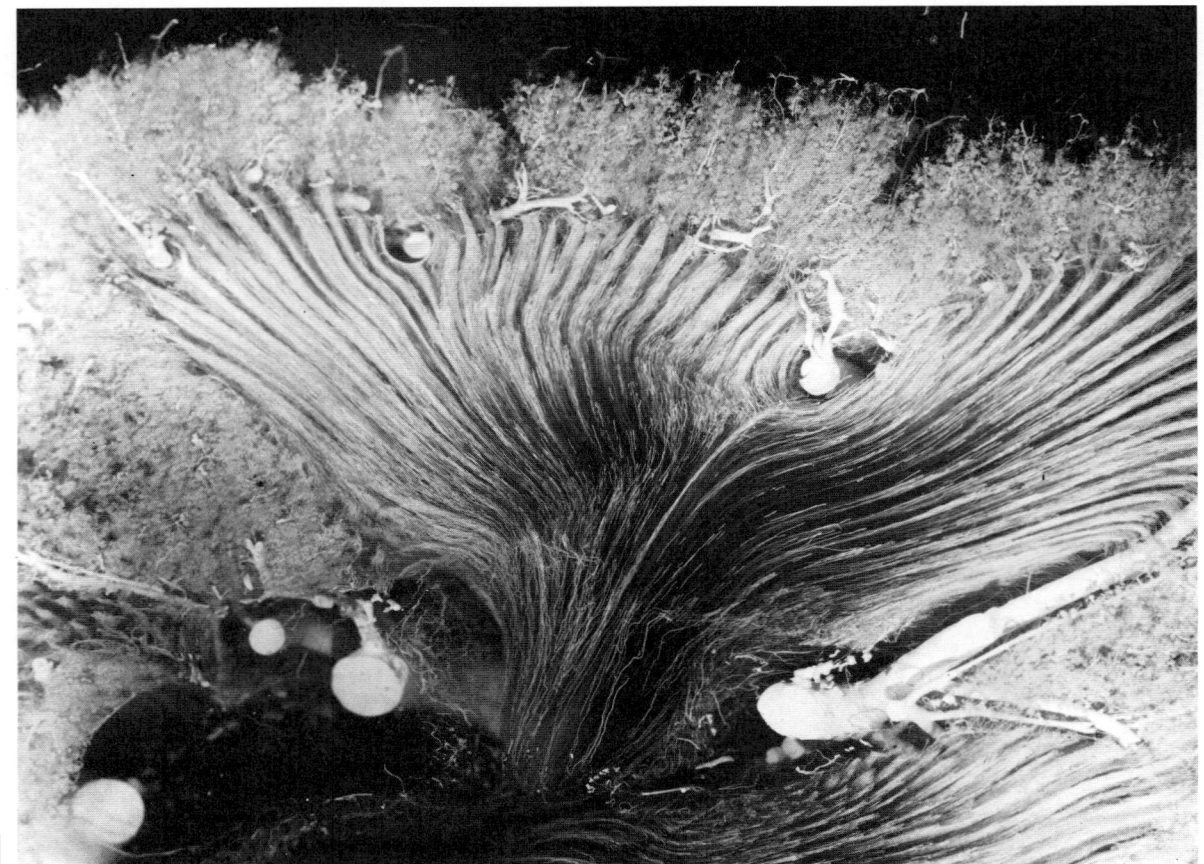

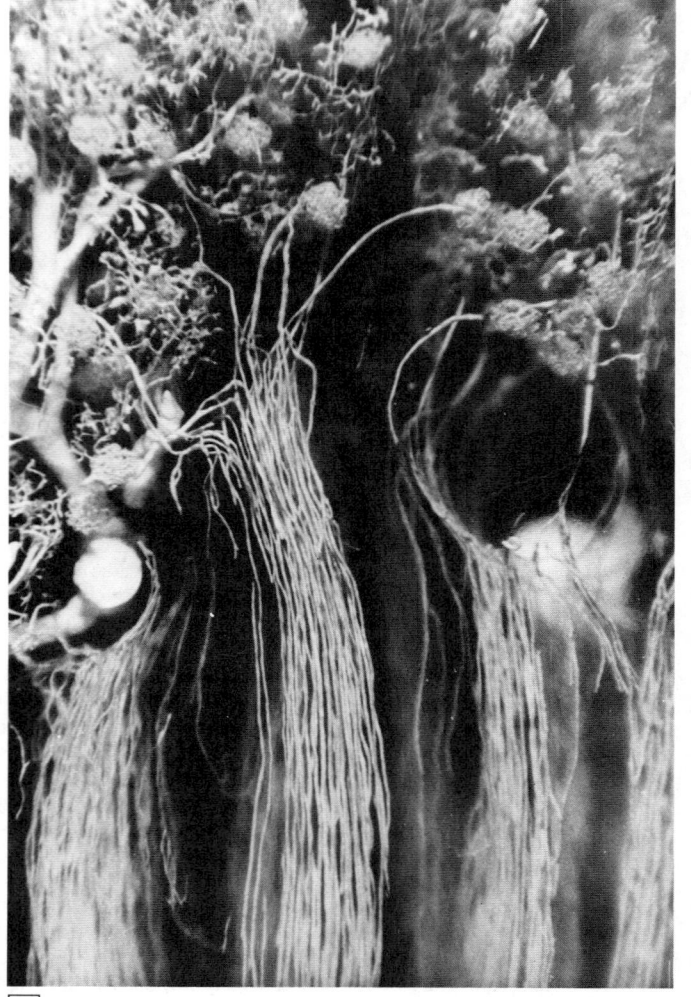

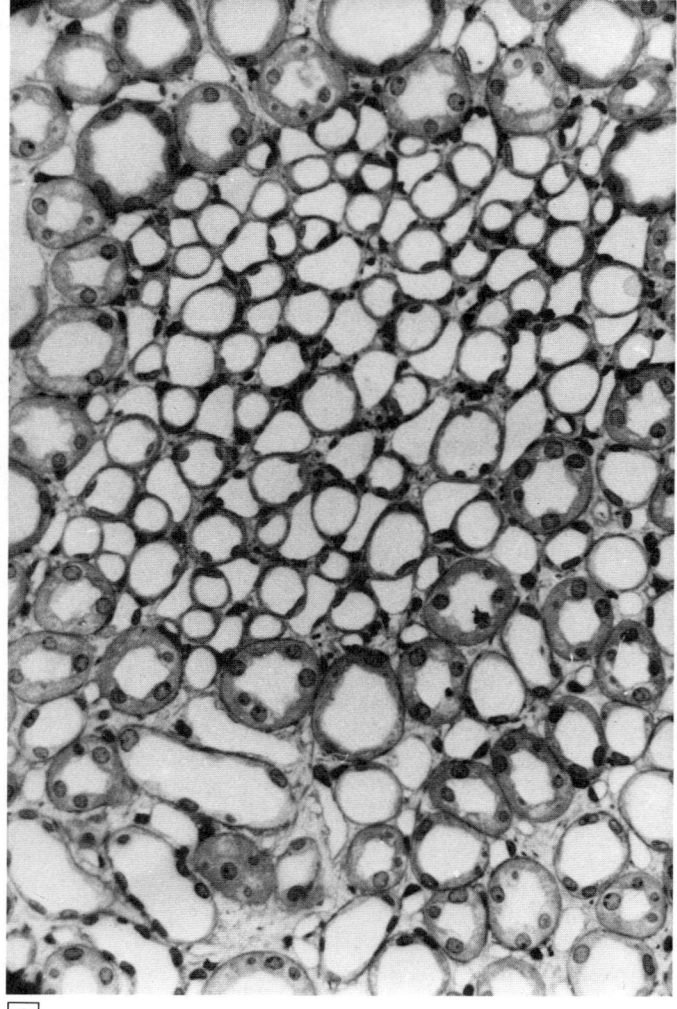

13.19 (*opposite*) A. Low-power, survey micrograph of a single nephric lobe following 'microfil' injection of the arterial tree of the human kidney. Note the clear distinction between the cortex peripherally and the medulla converging on the renal papilla. The lobe is flanked by large interlobar arteries. Note also the arcuate arteries at the corticomedullary junction, the interlobular arteries ascending into the cortex, where the glomeruli are also visible, and the converging vascular bundles of the medulla. Compare with **13**.18B.
B. A higher magnification of the same preparation at the corticomedullary junction. Note the juxtamedullary efferent arterioles, leaving the glomeruli to form medullary vascular bundles (descending vasa recta).
C. Transverse section through a vascular bundle (consisting of descending and ascending vasa recta). Surrounding the vascular bundle are sections of large collecting ducts and thin and thick segments of the medullary loops (of Henle). Preparation provided by D B Moffat, Department of Anatomy, University College of Wales, Cardiff.

usually the left, which may cross the midline; the reverse may occur and sometimes one ureter is not anterior to the vagina, a much longer part of the other then being in front of it.

In the distended bladder, in both sexes, the ureteric openings are about 5 cm apart, somewhat less when the bladder is empty. In its oblique course through the wall of the bladder, the ureter is compressed and flattened as the bladder distends, perhaps preventing regurgitation, though ureteric peristalsis is also a factor.

Radiography

The ureter, renal pelvis and calyces are easily demonstrated in the living by radiography:

- after intravenous injection of radio-opaque substances excreted in urine (*descending* or *excretion pyelography*) (**13**.5)
- after the introduction of similar solutions into the ureter by catheterization through an operating cystoscope (*ascending* or *retrograde pyelography*), the results being *pyelograms* (**13**.6).

Normal cupping of the minor calyces by projecting renal papillae

is clinically important; it may be obliterated by conditions such hydronephrosis, associated with chronic distension of the ureter and renal pelvis due to urinary back pressure.

MICROSTRUCTURE OF THE URETERS

The wall of the human ureter is composed of three histological layers, namely an external adventitia, a nonstriated muscle layer and an inner mucosal layer. The last consists of two components: the transitional epithelium (or urothelium) and the underlying connective tissue (the lamina propria). The ureteric *adventitia* contains elongated fibrocytes and interlacing bundles of collagen and elastic fibrils, together with numerous blood vessels, lymphatics, nerves and occasional fat cells. The majority of the adventitial blood vessels and the connective tissue elements are orientated parallel to the long axis of the ureter.

Throughout its length, the *muscle coat* of the ureter is fairly uniform in thickness and in cross-section measures about 750–800 μm in width. The muscle bundles which constitute this coat are frequently separated from one another by relatively large amounts of connective tissue. Branches which interconnect muscle bundles are common and result in frequent interchange of muscle fibres between adjacent bundles. Due to this extensive branching, individual muscle bundles do not spiral around the ureter (Gosling 1970). Hence, the ureteric muscle coat consists of a complex meshwork of interweaving and interconnecting smooth muscle bundles. In addition, unlike the gut, the muscle bundles are so arranged that morphologically distinct longitudinal and circular layers cannot be clearly distinguished. However, in the upper part of the ureter, the inner muscle bundles tend to lie longitudinally while those on the outer aspect have a circular or oblique orientation. In its middle and lower parts, additional outer longitudinally-orientated fibres can also be discerned. As the ureterovesical junction is approached, the muscle coat consists predominantly of longitudinally-orientated muscle bundles. However, there are distinct differences between ureteric and vesical muscles (Gilpin & Gosling 1983). Ureteric muscle bundles

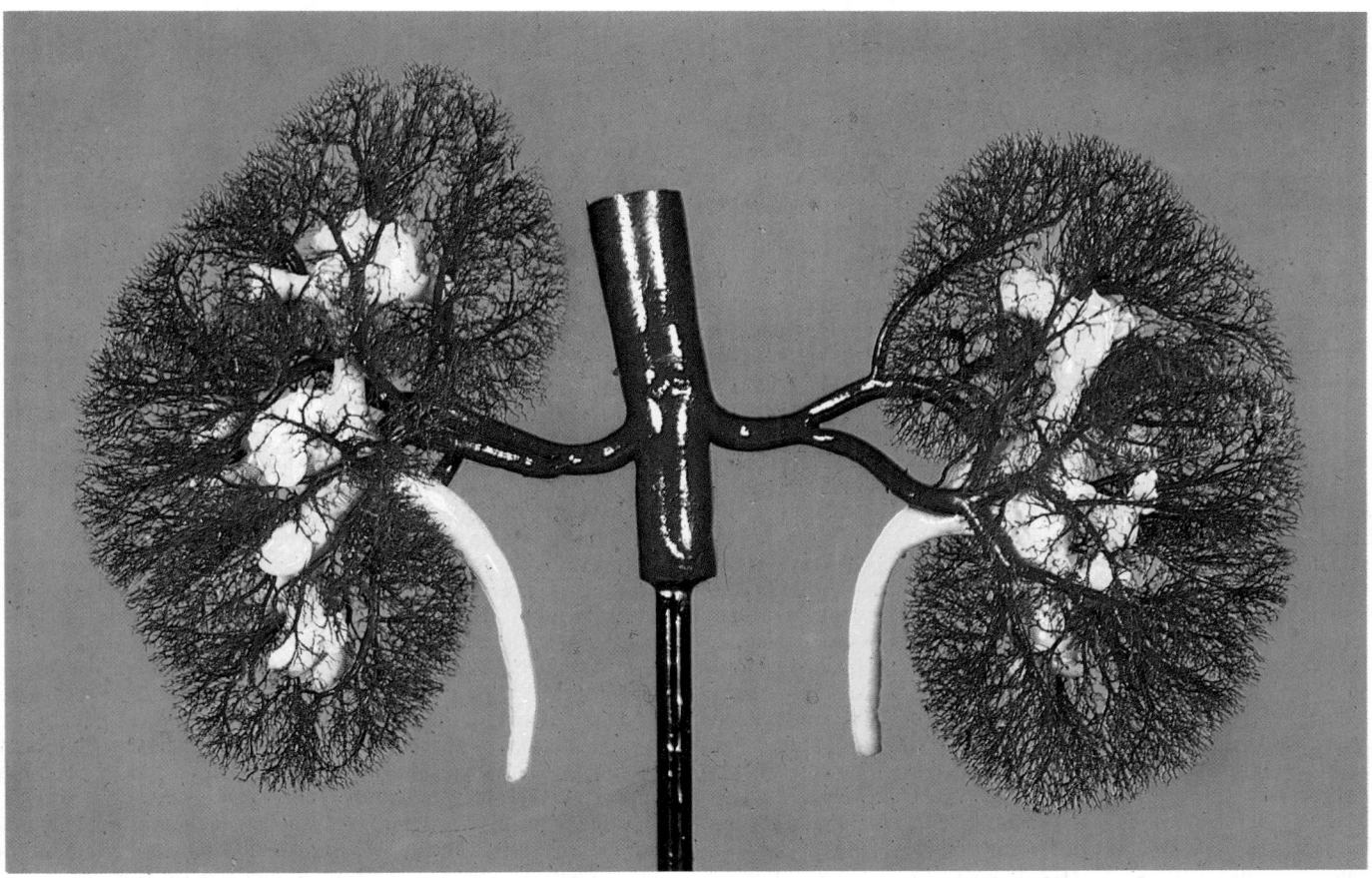

13.20 Resin corrosion cast of human kidneys prepared by D H Tompsett of the Royal College of Surgeons of England. Ureter, pelvis and calyces are yellow; aorta, renal arteries and their branches are red. See text for a detailed description of the renal blood vessels.

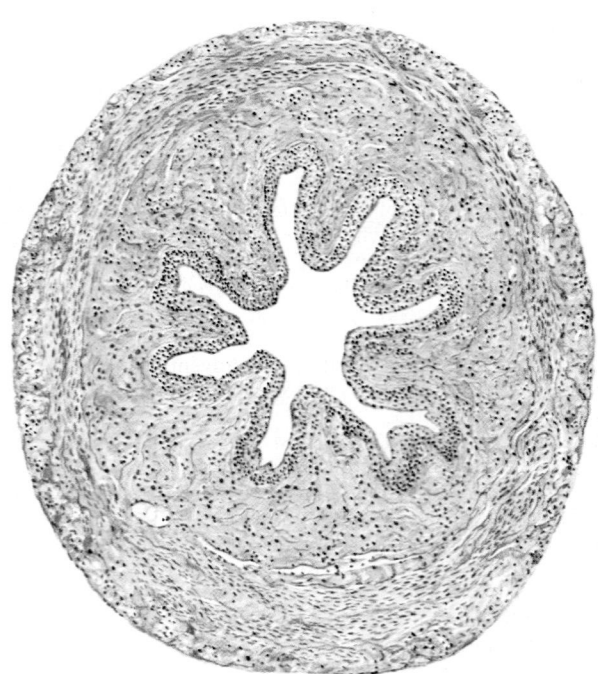

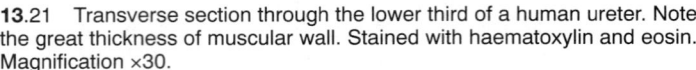

13.21   Transverse section through the lower third of a human ureter. Note the great thickness of muscular wall. Stained with haematoxylin and eosin. Magnification ×30.

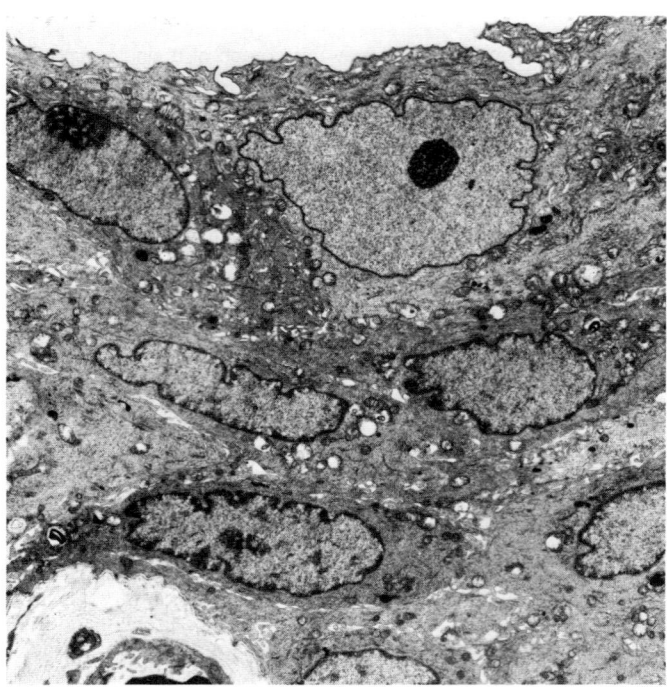

13.22   Transmission electron micrograph showing the transitional epithelium lining the ureter (rat). Prepared and photographed by Susan Smith, Department of Anatomy, Guy's Hospital Medical School, London. Magnification ×4000.

are composed of closely-packed spindle-shaped cells which are approximately 300–400 μm in length and 4–7 μm at their widest diameter. Each nonstriated muscle cell is surrounded by a trilaminar plasma membrane on the outer aspect of which is a layer of amorphous electron-dense basal lamina material approximately 40 nm in thickness. The latter is separated from the underlying plasma membrane by an electronlucent zone about 4 nm in width (the lamina lucida).

Within any one muscle bundle the plasma membranes of adjacent cells are frequently observed in mutual opposition. The most common form of junction between neighbouring ureteric muscle cells is the 'region of close approach' at which the apposed plasma membranes converge to within 10–20 nm of each other. Basal lamina material is reflected from one cell to the other at the margins of the junction and does not extend into the narrow intercellular cleft. However, neither the plasma membranes nor the adjacent subsarcolemmal cytoplasm show any form of specialization. Intercellular junctions of this type often occur between the tips of narrow cytoplasmic protrusions from adjacent nonstriated muscle cells. Another common type of association between ureteric nonstriated muscle cells is the so-called 'peg and socket' junction. This type consists of an elongated or bulbous projection from one cell which fits snugly into a depression in an adjacent cell. At the interdigitation, basal lamina material is absent from the 10 nm gap separating the membranes of the two adjacent muscle cells. Occasionally, the apposing cell membranes are more closely related in the narrowed 'stalk' of the projection. It has been suggested that these interdigitations provide a mechanical linkage between neighbouring cells. Alternatively, they may represent a special type of 'close approach' and permit myogenic conduction.

The *mucosa* of the ureter consists of an epithelium (the urothelium) on the deep aspect of which is a layer of subepithelial fibro-elastic connective tissue (the lamina propria). The latter varies in thickness from 350–700 μm and consists mainly of bundles of collagen and elastic fibres, fibrocytes and small blood vessels. Many of the latter are accompanied by bundles of non-myelinated nerve fibres. Occasional lymphocytes may be present in the lamina propria but their aggregation into definitive lymph nodules is rare. The urothelium is usually extensively folded, giving the ureteric lumen a stellate outline. Although the urothelium appears to consist of four to five separate layers of cells, it has been claimed that all cells

reach down to the base and as a consequence the urothelium is a pseudostratified epithelium. However, verification of this is needed.

The surface cells of the urothelium are large and polyhedral, the underlying intermediate cells are smaller and spindle-shaped and the basal cells are mainly cuboidal in form. The luminal cells of the urothelium are characterized by the presence of a specialized apical membrane (Hicks 1965) and are attached to one another near the ureteric lumen by a junctional complex composed of the three typical components of zonula occludens, zonula adherens and macula adherens. The lateral cell membranes of the luminal cells are often extensively interdigitated, although such infoldings presumably flatten out to enable the urothelium to accommodate distension of the ureteric lumen.

Vessels and nerves

Arteries supplying the ureter (Daniel & Shackman 1952). These are derived from the renal, abdominal aortic, testicular (or ovarian), common iliac, internal iliac, vesical and uterine vessels, their branches supplying the different parts of the ureter in its course and being subject to much variation. The longitudinal anastomosis between these branches on the wall of the ureter is good. The branches from the inferior vesical artery (p. 1559) are constant in their occurrence and supply the lower part of the ureter as well as a large part of the trigone of the bladder.

Lymph vessels of the ureter. They are described on page 1623.

Ureteric nerves (p. 1347). These are derived from the renal, aortic, and superior and inferior hypogastric plexuses. Through these plexuses fibres are derived from the lower three thoracic and first lumbar and the second to fourth sacral segments of the spinal cord. In the adventitia the nerves consist of relatively large axon bundles which form an irregular plexus, from which numerous smaller branches penetrate the ureteric muscle coat. Some of the adventitial nerves accompany the blood vessels and branch with them as they extend into the muscle layer. Others are unrelated to the vascular supply and lie free in the adventitial connective tissue around the circumference of the ureter. Autonomic ganglion cells occur only at the extreme lower end of the ureter; such cells are absent from all other regions of the ureter. In the muscle coat of the upper urinary tract, nerve fibres can be identified both between and within the nonstriated muscle bundles. However, regional differences in the density of these nerves result in a gradual increase in innervation from the renal pelvis and upper ureter (which has a sparse distribution of autonomic nerves) to a maximum in the juxtavesical segment. The nonstriated muscle of the upper urinary tract is supplied by at least three different types of autonomic nerve. Some nerves are rich in acetylcholinesterase (AChE) and the presence of this enzyme has been taken to be indirect evidence in support of a cholinergic innervation to ureteric nonstriated muscle. Noradrenergic nerves also occur in the ureteric muscle coat where they are evident as finely beaded fibres, some of which run parallel to the muscle bundles. Others accompany the vascular supply and their branches occasionally penetrate the muscle bundles and course amongst the smooth muscle cells. A third type of nerve, characterized by its content of substance P, has been demonstrated in the muscle coat of the ureter (Alm et al 1978). The distribution of this so-called peptidergic innervation within the ureter appears to be similar to the other types of autonomic nerve. Other neurotransmitters also exist (see Burnstock 1986), so the control mechanisms are likely to be complex. Using the electron microscope, occasional axon bundles, some containing up to 50 unmyelinated axons, can be seen in the connective tissue separating the ureteric muscle bundles and, very rarely, varicose vesicle-packed terminal axons run between individual smooth muscle cells. However, neuromuscular relationships suggestive of synaptic regions are exceedingly sparse by comparison with many other autonomically innervated smooth muscle systems (e.g. the urinary bladder and ductus deferens).

The functional significance of these different types of autonomic nerve in relation to ureteric nonstriated muscle activity is not fully understood, particularly since nerves are not essential for the initiation and propagation of ureteric contraction waves (see below). However, the contractile response of the ureter has been shown to be modified by the use in vivo of exogenous transmitter substances. Thus, while nerves are not essential for the normal occurrence of ureteric peristaltic activity, they may exert a modulating influence upon the contractility of ureteric nonstriated muscle cells.

A branching plexus of fine nerve fibres occurs within the lamina propria and extends from the inner aspect of the muscle coat towards the base of the urothelium. These nerves are AChE positive and, while some form perivascular plexuses, others lie in isolation from the vascular supply. A similar distribution of noradrenergic and peptidergic nerves has been observed throughout the lamina propria. The functional significance of these nerves, which are not related to blood vessels, remains unclear. It seems unlikely that the urothelium receives a direct efferent innervation, particularly when most of the nerve fibres are more than 100 μm away from the basal urothelial cells and thus beyond the accepted range for effective synaptic transmission. It seems probable, therefore, that some of the nerves in the lamina propria are sensory in function.

Ureteric peristalsis

Under normal conditions contraction waves originate in the proximal part of the upper urinary tract and propagate in an anterograde direction towards the bladder. However, the mechanism involved in the initiation of these contractile events has been the subject of much controversy in the past. One theory proposed that contraction of the nonstriated muscle of the calyces and pelvis was stimulated by stretching forces produced by the luminal contents. However, there is now a considerable body of experimental evidence to show that the urinary tract possesses spontaneously active regions which initiate the peristaltic activity of the ureter and exercise a controlling influence on ureteric contraction (Constantinou & Djurhuus 1981). From a morphological viewpoint the unusual nonstriated muscle cells which occur in the wall of the proximal parts of the upper urinary tract (p. 1831) and which are structurally distinct from those elsewhere, may act collectively as one or more pacemaker sites. Since each

minor calyx possesses these cells (and is linked across the renal parenchyma to other calyces by similar cells), the number of pacemaker sites within a given kidney will be related to the number of minor calyces. It seems probable that the normal sequence of events begins with the initiation of a contraction wave at one (or possibly more) of the several minor calyceal pacemaker sites. Once initiated, the contraction is propagated through the wall of the adjacent major calyx and activates the nonstriated muscle of the renal pelvis. To what extent the inner layer of cells acts as pacemaker (or as a preferential conduction pathway) remains to be determined. The proximal pacemaker site for successive contractions may change from one minor calyx to another, although it has been shown that a single minor calyx can initiate several successive contraction waves. Functionally, the proximal location of these pacemaker sites ensures that, once initiated, contraction waves are propagated away from the kidney, thereby avoiding undesirable pressure rises directed against the renal parenchyma. In addition, since several potential pacemaker sites exist, the initiation of contraction waves is unimpaired by partial nephrectomy; the minor calyces spared by the resection remain in situ to continue their pacemaking function.

Concerning the means by which contractions are propagated across the renal pelvis and along the ureter, considerable experimental evidence indicates that autonomic nerves do not play a major part in the propagation of upper urinary tract peristalsis. It seems more likely that autonomic nerves may have only a modulatory role on the contractile events occurring in the musculature of the upper urinary tract. The most likely mechanism to account for impulse propagation is that of myogenic conduction resulting from electrotonic coupling of one muscle cell to its immediate neighbours. Regions of close approach are extremely numerous between ureteric nonstriated muscle cells and also between both types of muscle cell in the renal pelvis and calyces. Thus in the upper urinary tract this type of intercellular junction may be responsible for the conduction of excitation from one myocyte to the next.

To conclude, contraction waves arising from the upper end of the urinary tract are thought to be propagated from muscle cell to muscle cell by means of intercellular 'gap' junctions. This process is essentially a property of nonstriated muscle and does not require the direct involvement of autonomic nerves. The direction of the propagated contractile wave is normally from the renal calyces and pelvis towards the bladder, as dictated by the pacemaker mechanism in these proximal regions. However, since electrotonic excitation can spread from one muscle cell to another in either direction, retrograde peristalsis can also occur.

Clinical anatomy

As in the case of the gut, excessive ureteric distension or spasm of its muscle provokes severe pain (renal colic), for example by a stone (calculus) causing incomplete and intermittent obstruction, particularly if it is gradually forced down by the muscle spasm. The pain, spasmodic and agonizing, is referred to cutaneous areas innervated from spinal segments which supply the ureter, mainly T11–L2. It shoots down and forwards from the loin to the groin and scrotum or labium majus and may extend into the proximal anterior aspect of the thigh by projection to the genitofemoral nerve (L1, 2); the cremaster (which has the same innervation) may reflexly retract the testis. A ureteric stone is liable to impact at one of the ureteric constrictions, namely (1) its superior end, (2) where it crosses the brim of lesser pelvis or (3) as it passes through the vesical wall; radiologically it would appear near the tip of the second lumbar transverse process, overlying the sacro-iliac joint, or slightly medial to the ischial spine. Sometimes the ureter is duplicated on one or both sides even as far as the bladder; separate vesical openings are rare in such cases.

Kidney transplantation

Transplantation of the kidney is now recognized as the definitive treatment of end-stage renal failure. Although kidneys from compatible living relatives may be used, the commonest source of donor organs are patients who die during intensive care for lethal head injury or intracranial haemorrhage. Dramatic advances in the pharmacology of immunosuppression have led to greater long-term success in graft function and patient survival: rejection of the graft is preventable in some cases and is successfully treated in the majority of cases when it occurs. 70% graft survival after cadaveric renal transplantation is now reported five years after the operation described here.

For technically successful transplantation of the kidney to be carried out, the following criteria must be met:

(1) The donor kidney must be in good physiological condition to withstand a period of storage without a blood supply prior to its transplantation into the recipient. The development and recognition of the criteria of brain death enable the dissection of the donor kidney in the brain-dead cadaver whilst the circulation is maintained. The time that the kidney is exposed to ischaemia whilst it is still warm can therefore be shortened to 2 or 3 minutes.

(2) The renal artery and vein and the ureter must be preserved during the donor nephrectomy in such a way as to allow the anastomosis of the vessels to the recipient circulation.

(3) The artery to the ureter (a branch of the renal artery) must be preserved in order to avoid postoperative ureteric necrosis.

(4) Following its removal, the kidney must be flushed with a cold preserving solution (high osmolarity, with a high concentration of potassium, calcium and magnesium) which minimizes tissue injury during prolonged cold preservation in ice.

Provided these criteria are met, kidneys taken from brain dead, heart-beating donors may be stored for periods of up to 72 hours and re-implanted with a good prospect of immediate function (Marshall et al 1988).

Donor kidney

The native human kidney lies in the retroperitoneal space, deriving its blood supply from the aorta via the renal arteries, and its venous drainage entering directly into the inferior vena cava on each side through the renal vein. Vascular anatomy may vary: usually the renal artery is single (**13**.23), but renal arteries may be multiple in approximately 15% of cases. Each renal artery is an end artery (i.e. intrarenal anastomoses with accessory arteries do not

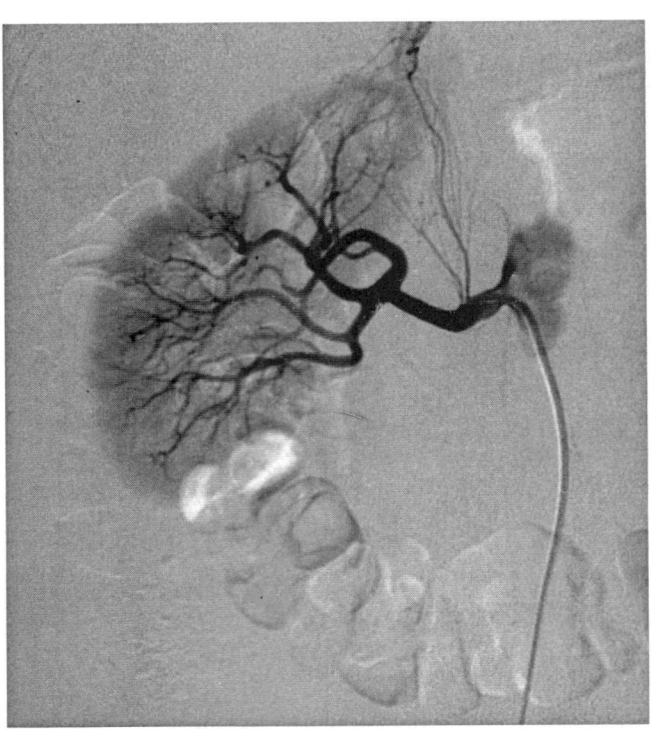

13.23 Renal angiogram: radio-opaque dye has been injected through an intra-aortic catheter to display a single renal artery to the right kidney. A small adrenal artery is also well shown, arising from the superior aspect of the main renal artery trunk. This would be divided and ligated during nephrectomy. Courtesy of Dr Richard Edwards, Royal Liverpool University Hospital.

occur, see **13**.24A, B). Collateral venous anastomoses do, however, occur within the renal substance, between the main renal vein and accessory veins. From the surgical point of view, therefore, the establishment of a complete blood supply to the donor kidney requires that all the accessory arteries must be joined to the recipient's circulation, whereas accessory veins may be ligated and the venous drainage established by anastomosing the main renal vein to the recipient venous system. The renal artery commonly divides into two or three subsidiary branches near the hilum of the kidney, and the inferior of these branches frequently gives rise to arterial twigs which supply the upper third of the ureter, which must be preserved.

Recipient operation

The donor kidney need not be placed orthotopically in its 'natural' position; indeed there are anatomical advantages to transplanting the kidney into the pelvis. The iliac fossa is anatomically receptive to a renal transplant. The time-honoured technique invented by Murray and first reported in 1956 (Merrill et al 1956) utilizes an extraperitoneal approach to the iliac fossa which allows ready access to the iliac artery and its branches, and the external iliac vein, to which the donor vessels may be joined; the recipient bladder and ureter are nearby, enabling the

surgeon to achieve a satisfactory junction for urine to drain into the bladder, using a small length of the upper ureter, with its own blood supply deriving from the renal artery.

Technique

(1) *The arterial anastomosis*: when the donor kidney is removed from a cadaver, a patch of aorta bearing the renal artery or arteries greatly facilitates the anastomosis of the patch to the external iliac artery (**13**.25). Kidneys taken from living donors usually have a single main artery. Under these circumstances, the main artery is best anastomosed to the end of the internal iliac artery, after division of the distal end, and reflection of its proximal end to enable junction to the renal artery to take place (**13**.26). If an inferior polar artery exists, it is commonly inferior and may be joined end-to-end to the inferior epigastric artery (**13**.27A, B). Exceptionally two 'main' renal arteries are found which may have to be 'spatulated' (joined together side-to-side for a short distance to form a common osteum) and then anastomosed conjointly to the side of the external iliac artery (**13**.28A, B). Small polar arteries less than 1 mm in external diameter may be sacrificed, provided that the area of cortex supplied by such an artery does not exceed an area 3 cm in diameter. Failure to anastomose bigger polar arteries

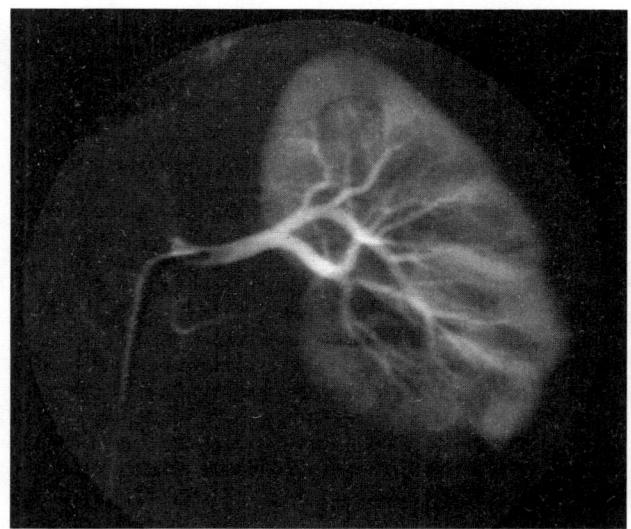

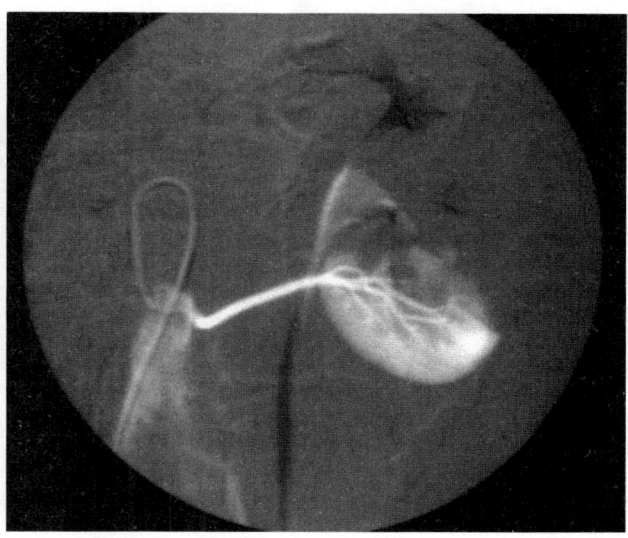

13.24   X-ray angiograms showing A. the main renal artery to the left kidney and B. an accessory artery supplying the lower pole. Both arteries arise from the aorta and are demonstrated using the same technique as in **13**.23. Selective injection of each vessel was achieved by manipulating the end of the catheter into the osteum of each artery separately.

Note: Each artery demonstrated is an end artery: there are no intra-renal anastomoses between the two renal moieties. In B an early pyelogram may be seen: injected dye has been excreted into the urine and the pelvis and upper ureter are displayed.

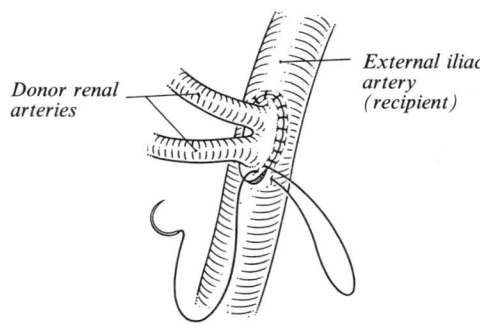

13.25   A patch of donor aorta bearing two renal arteries of a cadaver kidney is being joined to the side of the external iliac artery of the recipient using a continuous suturing technique.

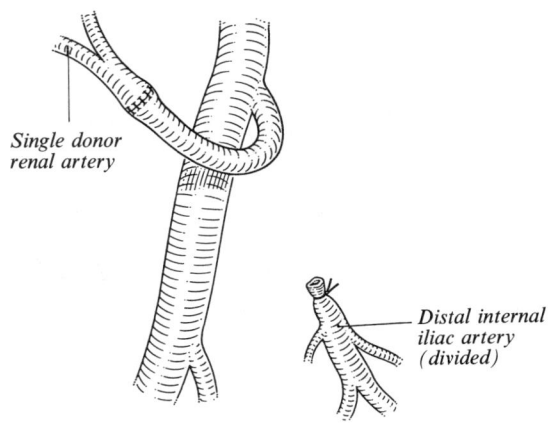

13.26   End-to-end anastomosis of a single donor renal artery to the internal iliac artery of the recipient. The distal end of the internal iliac artery has been divided, its proximal portion has been dissected free of surrounding tissue, and is reflected upwards to enable the anastomosis to take place.

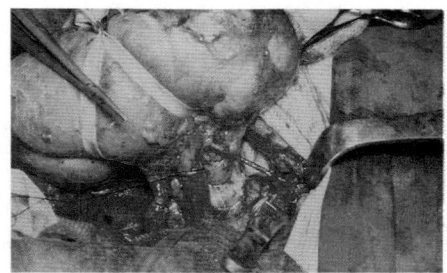

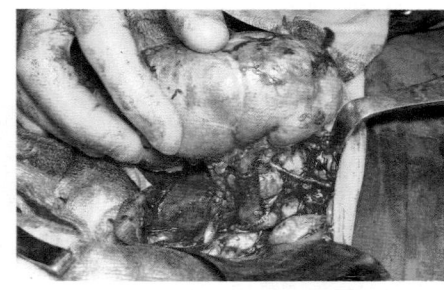

13.27   Kidney transplant from a living related donor: the transplant is taking place into the right iliac fossa of the recipient (the patient's head is to the left and the feet to the right).

A.   The renal vein has been joined to the external iliac vein (anastomosis not visible), and the main renal artery anastomosis to the internal iliac artery has been completed and is seen in the photograph. There is an inferior polar renal artery which has been anastomosed end-to-end to the inferior epigastric artery, which is clamped. Note the blue, unperfused, inferior pole of the kidney transplant.

B.   The clamp has been removed from the inferior epigastric artery and the whole kidney transplant is now satisfactorily perfused with arterial blood. In this photograph, all three vascular anastomoses are now visible.

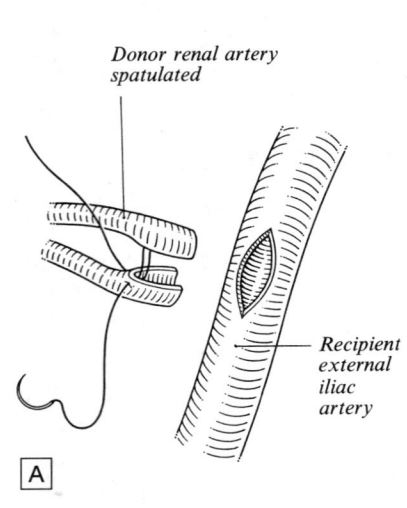

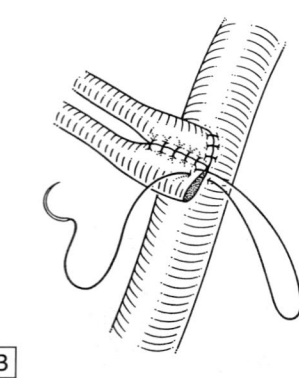

13.28 The surgical union of two renal arteries side-to-side to form a single osteum which may be anastomosed to the external iliac artery. This technique is required when no patch of donor aorta is available.

A. A suitably sized arteriotomy has been created in the external iliac artery, the two donor renal arteries have been incised (spatulated) on adjacent sides, and the two arterial walls are being approximated by sutures.

B. The near-complete anastomosis of the new double arterial osteum to the external iliac artery.

than this risks necrosis of the cortex and calyceal fistula with urine leak (Hume et al 1963).

(2) *The venous anastomosis*: the biggest donor vein is chosen to join to the recipient vein, and other branches may be sacrificed safely on account of the intrarenal venous anastomoses. Provided that a suitable length of donor vein is available, the renal vein may be joined safely to the external iliac vein (**13**.29).

(3) *Re-establishment of urinary drainage*: two techniques have been developed

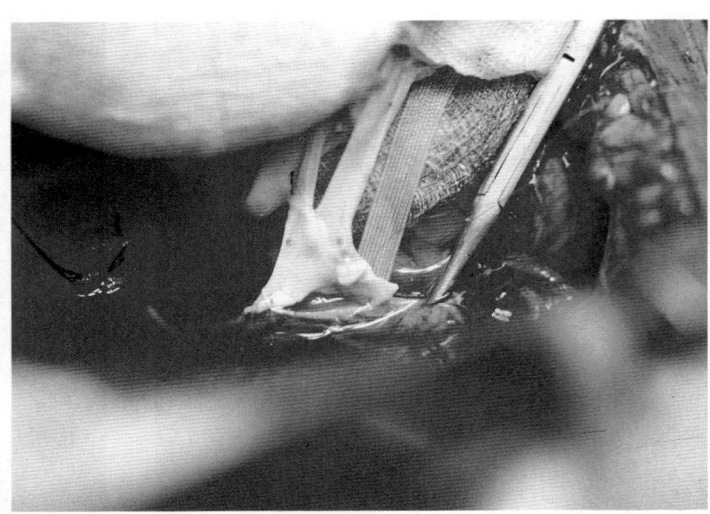

13.29 The donor renal vein formed by the confluence of two venous tributaries, is being joined by sutures to the recipient external iliac vein, which is clamped. The stump of the ligated adrenal vein is clearly visible.

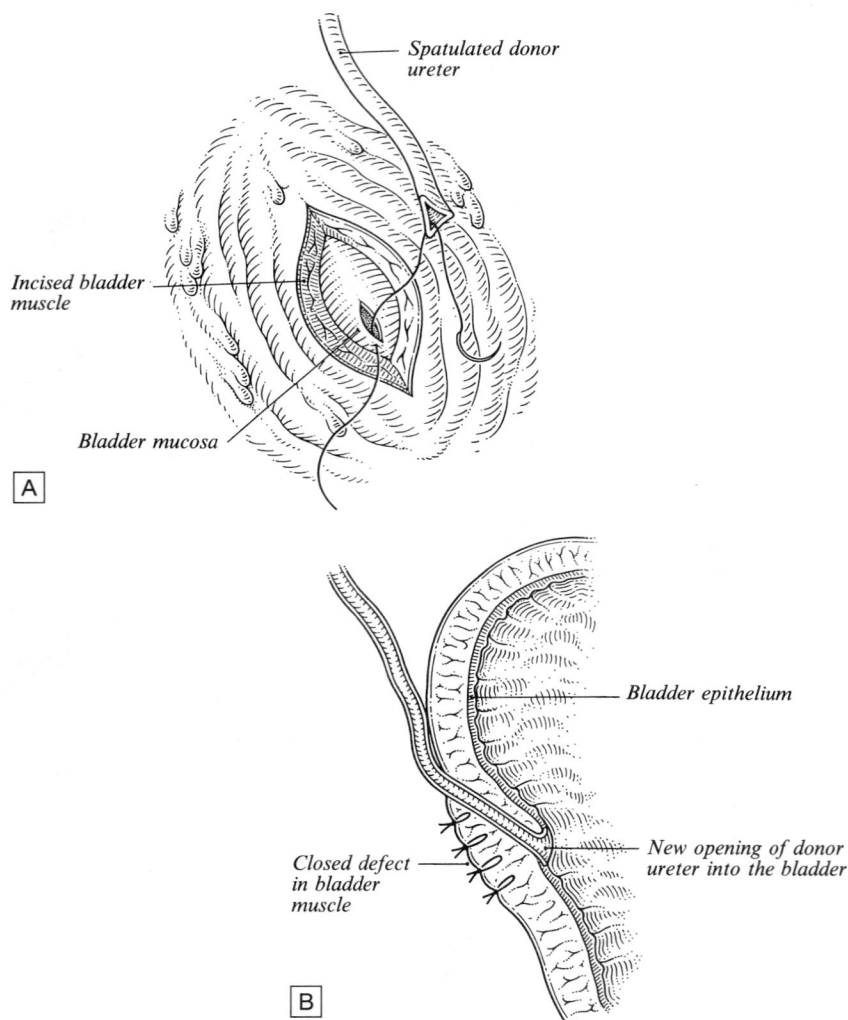

13.30 The 'on-lay' technique of uretero-cystostomy.

A. The bladder muscle has been incised to reveal the bulging mucosa. A small opening has been made in the lower end of the mucosa, to which the spatulated donor ureter will be sutured.

B. A cross-section of the completed 'on-lay' uretero-cystostomy.

to join the donor ureter to the recipient urinary tract: implantation of the ureter into the bladder and anastomosis of the donor ureter or renal pelvis to the recipient ureter (ureteroureteral anastomosis):

- Implantation of the ureter into the bladder:
  a) *'On-lay' technique*: the ureter is spatulated by incising one side of its distal end 1 cm proximally, the bladder muscle is incised over its superolateral aspect so that the mucosa bulges forward for a length of 3 cm; the lower 1 cm of the bladder mucosa is opened and is stitched with an absorbable suture to the spatulated ureter (**13.30**A). An antireflux mechanism is then created by approximating the bladder muscle over the distal end of the ureter (Calne 1984; **13.30**B).
  b) *The 'ureteroneocystostomy'* (literally, anastomosis of the ureter from within, using a wide opening in the bladder; Prout et al 1967). Here, the dome of the bladder is widely opened and a tunnel is created through the bladder muscle approximately 1.5 cm in length. The donor ureter is then drawn down through this tunnel, spatulated and the ureteric mucosa is joined to the bladder mucosa using interrupted absorbable sutures. This technique allows the ureter to prolapse into the lumen of the bladder, forming a 'nipple' ureteroneocystostomy. After healing, the bladder muscle which embraces the lower end of the ureter acts as an effective antireflux mechanism. During contraction of the bladder wall during micturition, the ureteric lumen is closed by contraction of the bladder muscle, which prevents reflux up the donor ureter and thus minimizes the risk of infection or obstructive uropathy (**13.31**A, B). The dome of the bladder is then closed to ensure a urine-proof junction. After on-lay ureterocystostomy, or ureteroneocystostomy, a bladder catheter is left in situ for 5 days, to protect the

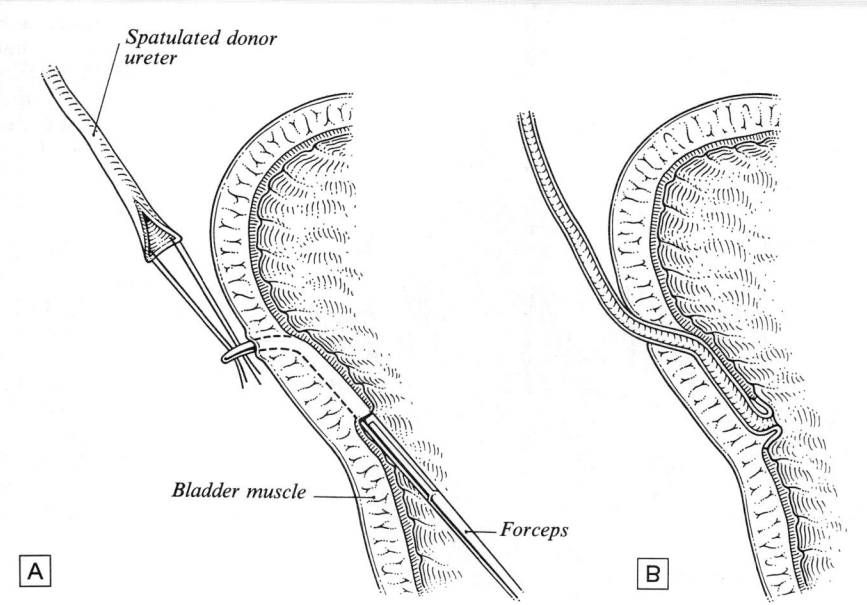

Spatulated donor ureter

Bladder muscle

Forceps

A

B

13.31 The 'ureteroneocystostomy' seen in cross-section.
A. From within the opened bladder, a pair of blunt-edged forceps has been tunnelled upwards between the bladder mucosa and the muscle for a distance of 1.5 cm, and then passed outwards through the muscle. The spatulated donor ureter is ready to be drawn down through this tunnel by two sutures, grasped by the forceps.
B. The completed operation: the distal end of the donor ureter has been brought obliquely through the bladder muscle, and now lies in a sub-mucosal tunnel; its end has been everted and anastomosed to the epithelium of the bladder wall, forming a 'nipple' ureterocystostomy.

bladder and ureteric anastomoses from back pressure should postoperative urinary retention occur.

- *Ureteroureteral anastomosis*: this is an alternative to the ureterocystostomy techniques described above (Hamburger et al 1972). The donor ureter is divided 2–3 cm below the pelviureteric junction and the recipient ureter is dissected over a short distance, care being taken to preserve the blood supply. The proximal recipient ureter is ligated and divided. Both donor and recipient ureters are reciprocally spatulated and joined together using a single or interrupted layer of absorbable stitches. A plastic stent may be inserted across this anas-

tomosis leading from the donor renal pelvis to the recipient bladder to prevent leakage of urine through the anastomosis during the healing phase.

Good anatomical insight and surgical techniques are essential to successful renal transplantation. Meticulous anastomosis of the blood vessels, enabling early endothelial healing, will minimize the risk of vascular thrombosis and inevitable graft failure. The ureteric anastomosis must also be sound to prevent urine leakage which in an immunosuppressed patient receiving drugs to prevent rejection can lead to local infection and septicaemia (Hamburger et al 1972).

PELVIC URINARY VISCERA

URINARY BLADDER

The urinary bladder (**13.32–35**) is solely a reservoir and varies in size, shape, position and relations, according to its content and the state of neighbouring viscera. When empty, it is entirely in the lesser pelvis but as it distends it expands anterosuperiorly into the abdominal cavity. When empty, it is somewhat tetrahedral and has a fundus, neck, apex, a superior and two inferolateral surfaces. The

fundus or *base* is triangular and postero-inferior. In females (**14.15**) it is closely related to the anterior vaginal wall; in males (**13.32**) it is related to the rectum although separated from it above by the rectovesical pouch and below that by the seminal vesicles and deferent ducts (**13.33**). In a triangular area between the deferent ducts, the bladder and rectum are separated only by rectovesical fascia (p. 1859); the inferior part of this area may be obliterated by approximation of the deferent ducts above the prostate. Although the vesical fundus should be, by definition, the lowest region, the

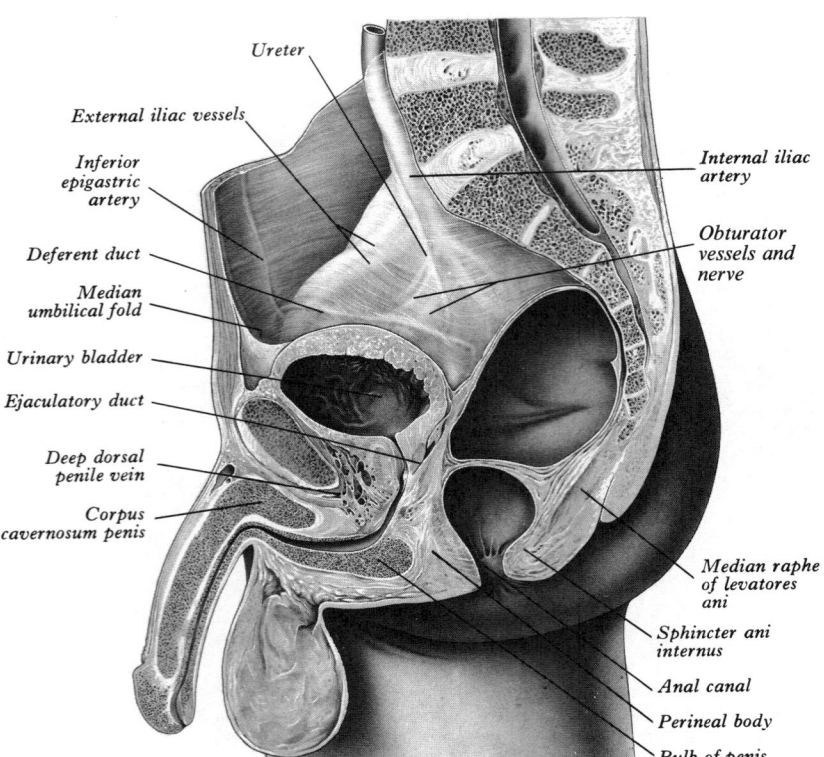

13.32 Median sagittal section to show male internal and external genitalia, bladder etc. A number of structures (e.g. obturator vessels, ureter) are only faintly visible through the overlying peritoneum.

neck is in fact lowest and also the most fixed; it is 3–4 cm behind the lower part of the symphysis pubis (i.e. a little above the plane of the inferior aperture of the lesser pelvis). It is pierced by the internal urethral orifice and alters little in position with varying conditions of the bladder and rectum. There is no special constriction of the bladder at its neck. In males the neck rests on, and is in direct

13.33 Posterosuperior aspect of the male internal urogenital organs.

continuity with, the base of the prostate; in females it is related to the pelvic fascia which surrounds the upper urethra. The vesical *apex* in both sexes faces towards the upper part of the symphysis pubis; from it the median umbilical ligament (urachus, see below) ascends behind the anterior abdominal wall to the umbilicus, the peritoneum over it being the median umbilical fold. The triangular *superior surface* is bounded by lateral borders from the apex to the ureteric entrances and by a posterior border joining them. In males the superior surface is completely covered by peritoneum, extending slightly on to the base and continued posteriorly into the rectovesical pouch, laterally into the paravesical fossae and anteriorly into the median umbilical fold. It is in contact with the sigmoid colon and the terminal coils of the ileum. In females the superior surface is also largely covered by peritoneum but posteriorly this is reflected to the uterus at the level of the internal os (i.e. the junction of the uterine body and cervix), forming the vesico-uterine pouch. The posterior part of the superior surface, devoid of peritoneum, is separated from the supravaginal cervix by fibro-areolar tissue. Each *inferolateral surface* in males is separated anteriorly from the pubis and puboprostatic ligaments by an adipose retropubic pad and posteriorly by fascia from the levator ani and obturator internus. In females the relations are similar, but the puboprostatic are replaced by pubovesical ligaments. The inferolateral surfaces are not covered by peritoneum.

As the bladder fills it becomes ovoid. In front it displaces the parietal peritoneum from the suprapubic region of the abdominal wall, so that the inferolateral surfaces become anterior and rest against the abdominal wall without intervening peritoneum for a distance above the symphysis pubis, varying with the degree of distension but commonly about 5 cm; in excessive distension the bladder may be approached surgically through the anterior abdominal wall above the symphysis pubis without traversing the peritoneum. The full bladder's summit points up and forwards above the attachment of the median umbilical ligament, so that the peritoneum forms a supravesical recess of varying depth between the summit and the anterior abdominal wall; this recess often contain coils of small intestine.

At birth (**13.34**), the bladder is relatively higher than in the adult, the internal urethral orifice being level with the **upper** symphyseal border; the bladder is abdominal rather than pelvic, extending about two-thirds of the distance towards the umbilicus. It progressively descends, reaching the adult position shortly after puberty.

LIGAMENTS OF THE BLADDER

In both sexes stout bands of fibromuscular tissue extend from the bladder neck to the inferior aspect of the pubic bones. These structures are the *pubovesical ligaments* and constitute the superior extensions of the *pubourethral ligaments* in the female or the *puboprostatic ligaments* in the male. The two pubovesical ligaments lie one on each side of the median plane, leaving a midline hiatus through which pass numerous small veins. In addition to the pubovesical ligaments a number of other so-called ligaments have been described in relation to the base of the urinary bladder. These are formed by condensation of connective tissue around neurovascular structures and as such do not merit the distinction of having specific names assigned to them.

The apex of the bladder is joined to the umbilicus by the remains of the urachus (below), which forms the *median umbilical ligament*. The lumen of the lower part of the urachus may persist throughout life and communicate with the cavity of the bladder (Begg 1930). From the superior surface of the bladder the peritoneum is carried off in a series of folds which are termed the *'false' ligaments* of the bladder. Anteriorly there are three folds: the median umbilical fold over the median umbilical ligament and two medial umbilical folds over the obliterated umbilical arteries (**12.74**). The reflexions of the peritoneum from the bladder to the side walls of the pelvis form the *lateral false ligaments* while the sacrogenital folds (p. 1737) constitute the *posterior false ligaments*.

INTERIOR OF THE BLADDER

Vesical mucosa (**13.36**, **37**). Attached only loosely to subjacent muscle for the most part, it folds when the bladder empties, the folds

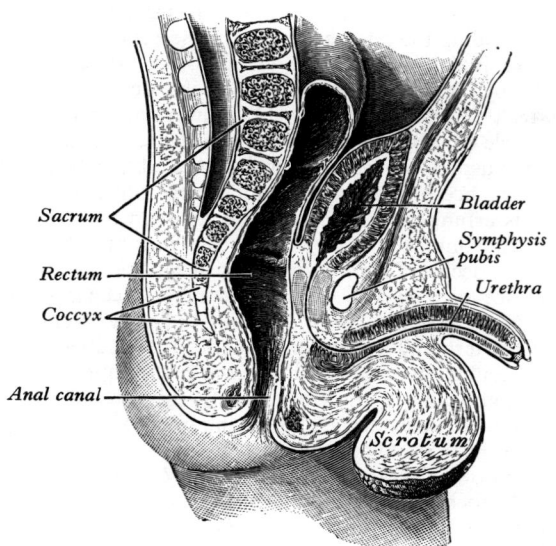

13.34 Sagittal section of the pelvis of a newborn male infant. Note the abdominal position of the urinary bladder.

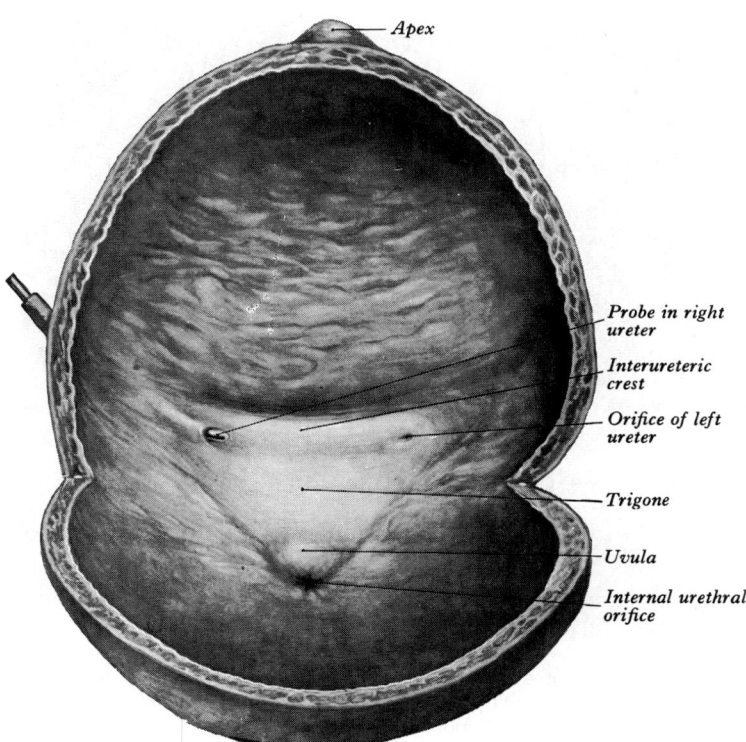

13.35 Anterior aspect of the interior of the urinary bladder.

being effaced as it fills. Over the *trigone* (**13**.35), immediately above and behind the internal urethral orifice, it is adherent to the subjacent muscle layer and always smooth. The trigone's anteroinferior angle is formed by the internal urethral orifice, its posterolateral angles by the ureteric orifices. The superior trigonal boundary is a slightly curved *interureteric crest*, connecting the two ureteric orifices and produced by the continuation into the vesical wall of the ureteric internal longitudinal muscle. (For details of trigonal musculature, consult Uhlenhuth et al 1952; Woodburne 1965, 1968.) Laterally this ridge extends beyond the ureteric openings as *ureteric folds*, produced by the terminal parts of the ureters running obliquely through the bladder wall. At cystoscopy the interureteric crest appears as a pale band and is a guide to the ureteric orifices in catheterization.

Ureteric orifices. Placed at the posterolateral trigonal angles (**13**.35), they are usually slit-like. In empty bladders they are about 2.5 cm apart and about the same from the internal urethral orifice; in distension these measurements may be doubled.

Internal urethral orifice. Sited at the trigonal apex, the lowest part of the bladder, this is usually somewhat crescentic in section; in adult males, particularly past middle age, immediately behind it is a slight elevation caused by the median prostatic lobe, the *uvula* of the bladder.

Bladder capacity

Mean vesical capacity in male adults varies from 120–320 ml (Thompson 1919); micturition commonly occurs at about 280 ml. Filling to about 500 ml may be tolerated but beyond this pain is caused by tension in the wall, leading to reflex contractions and the urgent desire to micturate. Pain is referred to the cutaneous areas supplied by spinal segments supplying the bladder (T11–L2, S2–4), including the lower anterior abdominal wall, perineum and penis.

BLADDER MICROSTRUCTURE

Histologically the wall of the urinary bladder consists of three layers (**13**.36): an outer adventitial layer of soft connective tissue which in some regions possesses a serosal covering of peritoneum, a non-striated muscle coat (the detrusor muscle) and an inner layer of mucous membrane which lines the interior of the bladder.

Serous layer

The serous layer is restricted to the superior and, in males, part of the posterior surfaces of the bladder, the rest being devoid of peritoneum. It consists of mesothelium and underlying connective tissue as elsewhere in the peritoneum.

Muscular layer

The muscular layer, the *detrusor muscle*, is composed of relatively large (in diameter) interlacing bundles of nonstriated muscle cells arranged as a complex meshwork. Three ill-defined layers are present and arranged in such a way that longitudinally orientated muscle bundles predominate on the inner and outer aspects of a substantial middle circular layer. Posteriorly some of the outer longitudinal bundles pass over the bladder base and fuse with the capsule of the prostate or with the anterior vaginal wall. Other bundles are carried on to the anterior aspect of the rectum and named the rectovesical muscle. Anteriorly some of the outer longitudinal bundles continue into the pubovesical ligaments and contribute to the muscular component of these structures. As in the muscle coat of the ureter, exchange of fibres between adjacent muscle bundles within the bladder wall frequently occurs so that from a functional viewpoint, the detrusor comprises a single unit of interlacing smooth muscle.

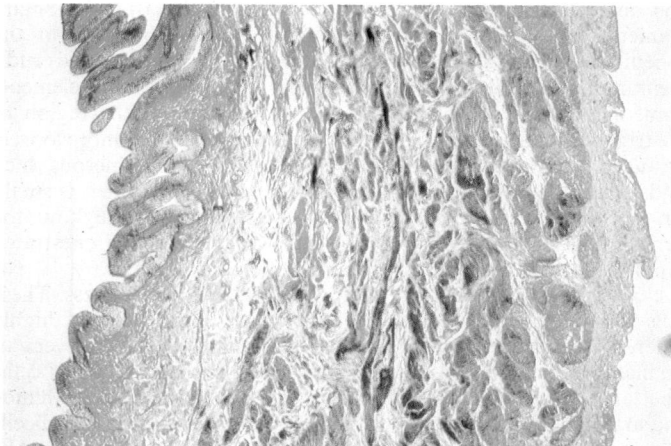

13.36 Transverse section through the urinary bladder wall of a monkey. Masson's trichrome stain. The section shows the folded transitional epithelium (grey-brown on the left), the connective tissue (blue-green), and fasciculi of the detrusor muscle (green-brown, to the right), surrounded externally by the connective tissue adventitia. Magnification ×20.

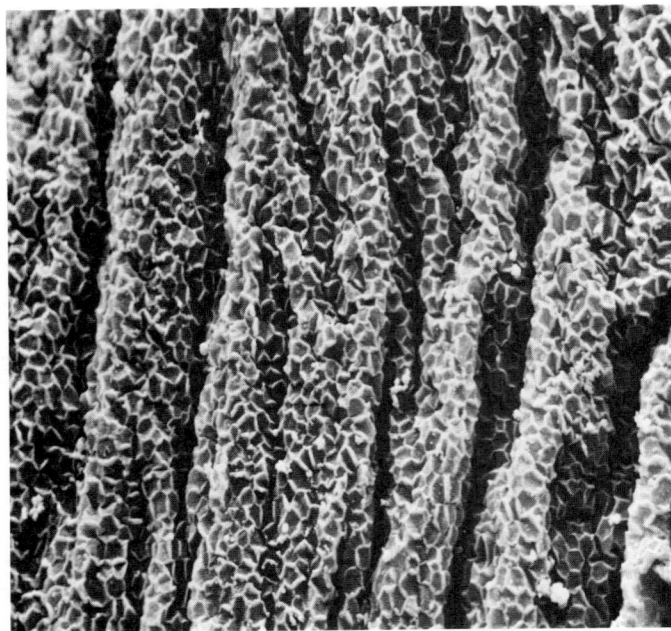

13.37 Scanning electron micrograph of the luminal surface of the bladder (murine) showing the plate-like organization of the urothelial plasma membranes of its lining cells. Magnification ×7000.

An electron-dense basal lamina surrounds each nonstriated myocyte except at certain junctional regions. The most frequently observed type of junction between muscle cells is the region of close approach at which an intercellular separation of 10–20 nm occurs over distances occasionally in excess of 1 μm in length. Junctions of the 'peg and socket' and 'intermediate' types are observed occasionally but gap junctions (nexuses) have not been reported in the detrusor. Since electrotonic spread excitation occurs in the nonstriated muscle of the bladder wall, the regions of close approach may represent the morphological feature which enables this physiological event to take place, although it is more likely that gap junctions exist, albeit few of them. Within muscle bundles, the smooth muscle cells are closely packed together such that the basal lamina of one cell very often becomes confluent with that of its neighbours.

Trigone. The smooth muscle of this region consists of two distinct layers, sometimes termed the superficial and deep trigonal muscles. The latter is composed of muscle cells which are indistinguishable from the muscle cells of the detrusor. Hence this deep trigonal muscle is simply the postero-inferior portion of the detrusor muscle proper and confusion might be avoided if the term deep trigonal muscle was abandoned in favour of the more accurate definition as trigonal detrusor muscle. The superficial trigonal muscle represents a morphologically distinct component of the trigone which, unlike the detrusor, is composed of relatively small diameter muscle bundles continuous proximally with those of the intramural ureters. The muscle layer comprising the superficial trigone is relatively thin but is generally described as becoming thickened along its superior border to form the interureteric crest. Similar thickenings occur along the lateral edges of the superficial trigone (Bell 1812). In both sexes the superficial trigone muscle becomes continuous with the smooth muscle of the proximal urethra, extending in the male along the urethral crest as far as the openings of the ejaculatory ducts. However, the arrangement of nonstriated muscle in the human trigone has been re-examined recently by Dorschner et al (1994a) who describe the presence of two muscular structures, a *musculus interuretericus* originating from the muscular systems of both ureters and forming the muscular component of the interureteric ridge, and a *musculus sphincter trigonalis* or *musculus sphincter vesicae*, the latter surrounding the internal urethral orifice but not extending into the urethra or its surroundings. This description is at variance with that of Bell (1812). Dorschner et al (1994a) reported that in men the lower part of the sphincter trigonalis is pervaded with prostatic tissue, and suggested that the muscle could have a dual function,

assisting in urinary continence and also preventing retrograde ejaculation whilst aiding the release of prostatic secretions.

Ureterovesical junction. The distal 1–2 cm of each ureter is surrounded by an incomplete collar of the detrusor nonstriated muscle which forms a sheath (of Waldeyer) separated from the ureteric muscle coat by a connective tissue sleeve. The ureters pierce the posterior aspect of the bladder and run obliquely through its wall for a distance of 1.5–2.0 cm before terminating at the ureteric orifices. This arrangement is believed to assist in the prevention of reflux of urine into the ureter, since the intramural ureters are thought to be occluded during increases in bladder pressure. There is no evidence of a classic ureteral sphincter mechanism in man (Noordzij & Dabhoiwala 1993). The longitudinally oriented muscle bundles of the terminal ureter continue into the bladder wall and at the ureteric orifices become continuous with the superficial trigonal muscle (Tanagho et al 1970). More recently this muscular continuity has been disputed, no evidence of it having been found in the porcine ureterovesical junction (Thomson et al 1994).

Bladder neck. The nonstriated muscle of this region is histologically, histochemically and pharmacologically distinct from that which comprises the detrusor muscle proper (Klück 1980). Hence the bladder neck should be considered as a separate functional unit. The arrangement of nonstriated muscle in this region is quite different in males and females and consequently each sex will be described separately.

Male. In the male bladder neck, the nonstriated muscle cells form a complete circular collar which extends distally to surround the preprostatic portion of the urethra. Because of the location and orientation of its constituent fibres, the terms internal, proximal or preprostatic urethral sphincter are suitable alternatives for this particular component of urinary tract smooth muscle. Distally, the bladder neck muscle merges with and becomes indistinguishable from the musculature in the stroma and capsule of the prostate gland.

Female. The female bladder neck also consists of morphologically distinct nonstriated muscle, since the large diameter fasciculi characteristic of the detrusor are replaced in the region of the bladder neck by those of small diameter. However, unlike the circularly orientated preprostatic nonstriated muscle, the muscle fasciculi in the female extend obliquely or longitudinally into the urethral wall. The female does not, therefore, possess a smooth muscle sphincter at the bladder neck and it is unlikely that active contraction of this region plays a significant part in the maintenance of female urinary continence.

Mucosa

The mucosa has a structure similar to that of the ureters and consists of an epithelium (urothelium, transitional epithelium, p. 72) supported by a layer of loose connective tissue, the lamina propria. The latter consists of loose fibro-elastic connective tissue and forms a relatively thick layer, varying in depth from 500 μm in the fundus and inferolateral walls to about 100 μm in the trigone. Small-diameter bundles of nonstriated muscle cells also occur in the subepithelial connective tissue forming an incomplete and rudimentary muscularis mucosae. The soft connective tissue elements immediately beneath the urothelium, particularly in the region of the trigone, are densely packed. At deeper levels they are more loosely arranged, thus allowing the bladder mucosa to form numerous thick folds when the volume of fluid contained within the lumen is small. An extensive network of blood vessels is present throughout the lamina propria and supplies a plexus of thin-walled fenestrated capillaries lying in grooves at the base of the urothelium.

Nontrigonal urothelium is often up to six cells in thickness. These cells can be classified according to position and consist of highly differentiated superficial or luminal cells, one or more layers of smaller intermediate cells and a layer of undifferentiated basal cells. The large superficial cells frequently bulge into the bladder lumen and are often binucleate. In contrast the intermediate and basal cells are smaller and each contains a single darkly-staining nucleus. The flattened urothelium of the trigone usually consists of only two or three layers of cells and a similar appearance prevails throughout the bladder when in the distended state.

In addition to the basal, intermediate and superficial cells described above, a fourth type of cell occurs in the urothelium of the human bladder neck and trigone. These flask-shaped cells extend throughout the depth of the urothelium and are characterized by the presence of numerous large membrane-bound vesicles each containing a central dense granule. Vesicles of this type are believed to be involved in the storage of amines and it seems likely that these cells belong to the so-called APUD (amine-precursor-uptake and decarboxylation, see p. 1898) series which have a wide distribution throughout the body.

Several morphological variations have been described in the mucosa of the bladder which, because of their occurrence in otherwise normal healthy adults, are not considered to represent pathological conditions. One of the commonest epithelial variants found in bladder biopsy samples or at postmortem is the occurrence of so-called Brunn's nests. These consist of proliferations of morphologically normal basal urothelial cells which project into the underlying connective tissue of the lamina propria and are particularly frequent in the trigone. Mucus-secreting glands with single or branched ducts are another frequently observed feature of the bladder mucosa. When present these structures are particularly numerous near the ureteric and internal urethral orifices. Non-keratinizing squamous metaplasia of the vaginal type also frequently occurs in the urinary bladder mucosa, especially over the trigone. This histological appearance, whilst occasionally observed in males and in children, is more common in adult females.

Vascular and lymphatic supply of the bladder

Arteries. The principal arteries of supply to the bladder are the superior and inferior vesical, derived from the anterior trunk of the internal iliac artery (p. 1559). The obturator and inferior gluteal arteries also send small branches to it and in the female additional branches are derived from the uterine and vaginal arteries.

Veins. These form a complicated plexus on the inferolateral surfaces and pass backwards in the posterior ligaments of the bladder to end in the internal iliac veins (p. 1598).

Lymph vessels. These are described on page 1623.

Nerve supply of the bladder

The nerves supplying the bladder form the vesical plexus (see p. 1309) and consist of both sympathetic and parasympathetic components, each of which contains both efferent and afferent fibres. The innervation of the bladder was reviewed in some detail by Burnstock (1990c) and by de Groat in 1993.

Efferent fibres. Parasympathetic fibres arise from the second to the fourth sacral segments of the spinal cord (*nervi erigentes*); the sympathetic fibres are derived from the lower two thoracic and upper two lumbar segments of the spinal cord. In addition to the branches from the vesical plexus, small groups of autonomic neurons occur throughout all regions of the bladder wall. These multipolar intramural neurons are rich in acetyl cholinesterase (AChE) and occur in ganglia consisting of five to 20 nerve cell bodies. Numerous preganglionic autonomic fibres form both axosomatic and axodendritic synapses with the ganglion cells. The majority of these preganglionic nerve terminals correspond morphologically to presumptive cholinergic fibres. Noradrenergic terminals also relay on cell bodies in the pelvic plexus although it is unknown whether similar nerves synapse on intramural bladder ganglia.

The urinary bladder (including the trigonal detrusor muscle) is profusely supplied with nerves which form a dense plexus among the detrusor smooth muscle cells. The majority of these nerves contain AChE and occur in abundance throughout the muscle coat of the bladder. Axonal varicosities adjacent to detrusor nonstriated muscle cells possess features which are considered to typify cholinergic nerve terminals and contain clusters of small (50 nm diameter) agranular vesicles together with occasional large (80–160 nm diameter) granulated vesicles and small mitochondria. Terminal regions approach to within 20 nm of the muscle cells' surface and are either partially surrounded by or more often totally denuded of Schwann cell cytoplasm. The human detrusor muscle possesses a sparse supply of sympathetic noradrenergic nerves (Sundin et al 1977). Nerves of this type generally accompany the vascular supply and only rarely extend among the nonstriated myocytes of the urinary bladder. A further component plays a part in the autonomic innervation of the urinary bladder (Ambache & Zar 1970), which has been classified as having a nonadrenergic, noncholinergic nerve

mediated effect. A number of other neurotransmitters or neuromodulators have been detected in intramural ganglia, including the peptide somatostatin (see p. 937). The superficial trigonal muscle is associated with few cholinergic (parasympathetic) nerves while those of the noradrenergic (sympathetic) variety occur relatively frequently. These differences support the view that the superficial trigonal muscle should be regarded as 'ureteric' rather than 'vesical' in origin. It should be emphasized that the superficial trigonal muscle forms a very minor part of the total muscle mass of the bladder neck and proximal urethra in either sex and is probably of little significance in the physiological mechanisms which control these regions.

In bladder neck of the male, nonstriated muscle is sparsely supplied with cholinergic (parasympathetic) nerves but possesses a rich noradrenergic (sympathetic) innervation (Gosling et al 1977). A similar distribution of autonomic nerves also occurs in the nonstriated muscle of the prostate gland, seminal vesicles and ducti deferentes. From a functional standpoint, sympathetic nerves on stimulation cause contraction of nonstriated muscle in the wall of the genital tract resulting in seminal emission. Concomitant sympathetic stimulation of the proximal urethral muscle causes sphincteric closure of the bladder neck, thereby preventing reflux of ejaculate into the bladder. Although this genital function of the bladder neck of the male is well established it is not known whether the nonstriated muscle of this region plays an active role in maintaining urinary continence.

In contrast with this rich sympathetic innervation in the male, the nonstriated muscle of the bladder neck of the female receives relatively few noradrenergic nerves but is richly supplied with presumptive cholinergic fibres. The sparse supply of sympathetic nerves presumably relates to the absence of a functioning 'genital' portion incorporated within the wall of the female urethra.

The lamina propria of the fundus and inferolateral walls of the bladder is virtually devoid of autonomic nerve fibres, apart from some noradrenergic and occasional presumptive cholinergic perivascular nerves. However, as the urethral orifice is approached the density of nerves unrelated to blood vessels increases. At the bladder neck and trigone a nerve plexus extends throughout the lamina propria. The constituent nerves are cholinesterase positive and run through the connective tissue unassociated with blood vessels. Some of the larger diameter axons are myelinated and others lie adjacent to the basal urothelial cells. As in the ureter, the subepithelial nerve plexus of the bladder is assumed to subserve a sensory function in the absence of any obvious effector target sites (Gosling & Dixon 1974).

Afferent fibres. Vesical nerves are also concerned with pain and awareness of distension. Pain fibres are stimulated by distension or spasm due to a stone, inflammation or malignant disease; they are found in sympathetic **and** parasympathetic nerves, predominantly the latter. Hence, simple division of the sympathetic paths (e.g. 'presacral neurectomy'), or of the superior hypogastric plexus (p. 1308), does not materially relieve vesical pain. The spinal path for pain is in the anterolateral white columns and considerable relief follows bilateral anterolateral cordotomy. Since nerve fibres mediating awareness of distension are in the posterior columns (fasciculus gracilis), after anterolateral cordotomy the patient still retains awareness of the need to micturate. The nerve endings detecting noxious stimuli are probably of more than one type; a subepithelial plexus of fibres containing dense vesicles, probably afferent endings, has been described.

Clinical anatomy

A distended bladder may be ruptured in lower abdominal or pelvic injuries, either extraperitoneally or, if the superior surface is involved, with tearing of the peritoneum and escape of vesical contents into the peritoneal cavity. In progressive chronic obstruction to micturition, for example by prostatic enlargement (p. 1861) or urethral stricture, vesical musculature hypertrophies, its fasciculi increasing in size and interlacing in all directions to produce an enlarged 'trabeculated bladder'. Mucosa between the fascicles forms 'diverticula', which may contain phosphatic concretions. When outflow is thus obstructed, emptying is not complete; some urine remains and may become infected; infection may extend to the ureters and kidneys. Back pressure from a distended bladder may gradually dilate the ureters, renal pelves and even the renal collecting tubules. Lesions of the fasciculus gracilis (e.g. tabes dorsalis) cause loss of desire to micturate; the distended bladder may empty merely by overflow. Severe spinal cord lesions above its sacral segments, interrupting efferent and afferent tracts involved in normal micturition, may result in 'automatic' emptying.

The vesical interior can be examined with a cystoscope, introduced via the urethra after distending the bladder with fluid. A special cystoscope is used to catheterize the ureters, to obtain a direct specimen of urine from either kidney or to inject radio-opaque fluid for retrograde pyelography (**13**.6). The vesical outline can be similarly demonstrated.

The distended bladder may be punctured just above the symphysis pubis without traversing the peritoneum (*suprapubic cystostomy*). When the bladder contains about 300 ml its anteroinferior surface contacts the anterior abdominal wall directly for about 7.5 cm above the pubis. Surgical access to the bladder is usually by this route. In females, owing to the shorter and more dilatable urethra, small calculi, foreign bodies and growths may be removed through it.

Congenital abnormalities of the bladder are described on p. 213.

MALE URETHRA

The male urethra (**13**.32, 38) is from 18–20 cm long, and extends from an internal orifice in the urinary bladder to an external opening, or meatus, at the end of the penis. It may be considered in four regional parts: preprostatic, prostatic, membranous and spongiose, and presents a double curve while the penis is in its ordinary flaccid state (**13**.32). Except during the passage of fluid along it, the urethral canal is a mere slit; in the prostatic part the slit is transversely arched in transverse section, in the preprostatic and membranous portions it is stellate, in the spongiose portion transverse, while at the external orifice it is sagittal in orientation.

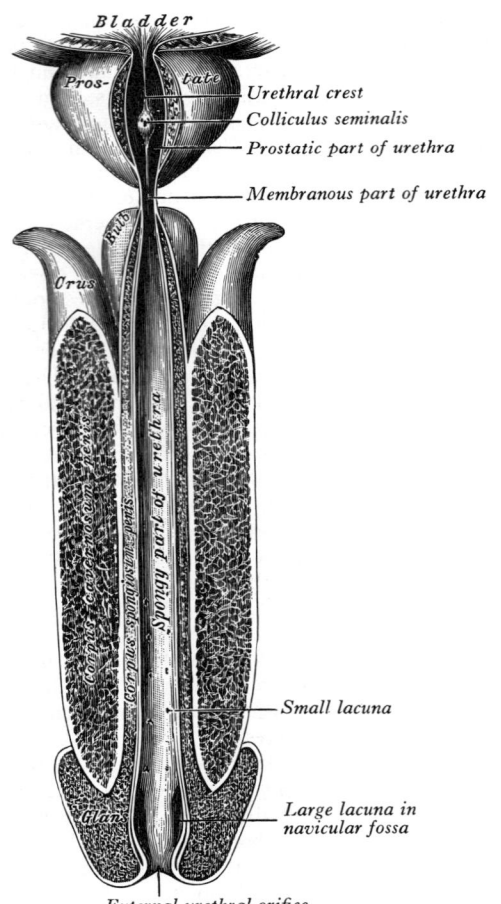

Bladder

Pros- *tate*

Urethral crest
Colliculus seminalis
Prostatic part of urethra

Membranous part of urethra

Bulb

Crus

Corpus Cavernosum penis
Corpus Cavernosum urethrae
Spongy part of urethra

Small lacuna

Large lacuna in navicular fossa

Glans

External urethral orifice

13.38 The whole length of the lumen of the male urethra exposed by an incision extending into it from its dorsal aspect. Note openings of prostatic utricle and ejaculatory ducts on the colliculus seminalis.

Preprostatic part

The preprostatic urethra possesses a stellate lumen and is approximately 1–1.5 cm in length, extending almost vertically from the bladder neck to the superior aspect of the prostate gland. The nonstriated muscle bundles surrounding the bladder neck and preprostatic urethra are arranged as a distinct circular collar which becomes continuous distally with the capsule of the prostate gland. The bundles which form this preprostatic or *internal sphincter* (*sphincter vesicae*) are separated by connective tissue containing many elastic fibres (Gilpin & Gosling 1983). Unlike the detrusor muscle, the nonstriated muscle surrounding the proximal urethra is almost totally devoid of parasympathetic cholinergic nerves but is richly supplied with sympathetic noradrenergic nerves. Similar nerves also supply the nonstriated muscle of the prostate, ducti deferentes and seminal vesicles and are involved in causing muscle contraction at the time of ejaculation (Learmonth 1931). Contraction of the preprostatic sphincter serves to prevent the retrograde flow of ejaculate through the proximal urethra into the bladder.

Prostatic part

The prostatic urethra is approximately 3–4 cm in length and tunnels through the substance of the prostate closer to the anterior than the posterior surface of the gland. It is continuous above with the preprostatic part and emerges from the prostate slightly anterior to its apex (its most inferior point). Throughout most of its length the posterior wall possesses a midline ridge, the *urethral crest*, which projects into the lumen causing it to appear crescentic in transverse section. On each side of the crest there is a shallow depression, termed the *prostatic sinus*, the floor of which is perforated by the orifices of the prostatic ducts. About the middle of the length of the urethral crest the *colliculus seminalis* (*verumontanum*) forms an elevation on which the slit-like orifice of the *prostatic utricle* is situated; on both sides of or just within this orifice there are the two small openings of the ejaculatory ducts. The prostatic utricle is a cul-de-sac about 6 mm long, which runs upwards and backwards in the substance of the prostate behind its median lobe. Its walls are composed of fibrous tissue, muscular fibres and mucous membrane; the last presents the openings of numerous small glands. Developed from the paramesonephric ducts or urogenital sinus, it is thought to be homologous with the vagina of the female (p. 205). The prostatic utricle is, therefore, called by some the '*vagina masculina*', but the more usual view is that it is a uterine homologue and hence the term 'utricle'. The ejaculatory ducts are described on page 1856. Distally the prostatic urethra possesses an outer layer of circularly disposed skeletal muscle cells which are continuous with a prominent collar of striated skeletal muscle (the external urethral sphincter) within the wall of the membranous urethra.

Membranous part

The membranous part is the shortest, least dilatable and, with the exception of the external orifice, the narrowest section of the urethra. It descends with a slight ventral concavity from the prostate to the bulb of the penis (**13**.32), passing through the perineal membrane about 2.5 cm postero-inferior to the pubic symphysis. The hind part of the bulb of the penis is closely apposed to the inferior aspect of the urogenital diaphragm (perineal membrane) but anteriorly it is slightly separated from the latter, so that the wall of the urethra is related anteriorly neither to the perineal membrane nor the penile bulb. If this part of the anterior wall of the urethra is regarded as the 'membranous' anteriorly the membranous urethra is about 2 cm long, whilst posteriorly it is only 1.2 cm. The wall of the membranous urethra consists of a muscle coat which is separated from the epithelial lining by a narrow layer of fibro-elastic connective tissue. This muscle coat consists of a relatively thin layer of nonstriated muscle bundles continuous proximally with those of the prostatic urethra and a prominent outer layer of circularly orientated skeletal muscle fibres forming the external urethral sphincter. The skeletal muscle fibres which comprise this external sphincter are unusually small in cross-section, with diameters of only 15–20 μm (Hayek 1969). The fibres are physiologically of the slow twitch type (Gosling et al 1981), unlike the pelvic floor musculature which is a heterogeneous mixture of slow and fast twitch fibres of larger diameter. Moreover, the external sphincter is devoid of muscle spindles and is supplied by the pelvic splanchnic nerves, further distinguishing it from the periurethral levator ani muscle (Donker et al 1976). The slow twitch fibres of the external sphincter are capable of sustained contraction over relatively long periods of time and actively contribute to the tone which closes the urethra and maintains urinary continence.

Spongiose part

The spongiose part is contained in the corpus spongiosum penis (p. 1857). It is about 15 cm long and extends from the end of the membranous urethra to the external urethral orifice on the glans penis. Commencing below the perineal membrane, it continues the ventrally concave curve of the membranous urethra to a point anterior to the lowest level of the symphysis pubis. From here, when the penis is flaccid, the urethra curves downwards in the 'free' part of the penis. It is a narrow, transverse, slit when empty, with a diameter of about 6 mm when passing urine; it is dilated at its commencement as the *intrabulbar fossa* and again within the glans penis, where it becomes the *navicular fossa*. The enlargement of the intrabulbar fossa affects the floor and side walls but not the roof of the urethra. The *bulbo-urethral glands* open into the spongiose section of the urethra about 2.5 cm below the perineal membrane (p. 1861).

The *external urethral orifice* is the narrowest part of the urethra: it is a sagittal slit, about 6 mm long, bounded on each side by a small labium.

The epithelium of the urethra, except in its most anterior part, presents the orifices of numerous small mucous glands and follicles situated in the submucous tissue and named the *urethral glands*. Besides these there is a number of small pit-like recesses, or *lacunae*, of varying sizes; the orifices of these are directed forwards and may intercept the point of a catheter in its passage along the canal. One, larger than the rest, the *lacuna magna*, is situated on the roof of the navicular fossa.

Mucous membrane of the male urethra

The epithelium lining the preprostatic urethra and the proximal part of the prostatic urethra is of the typical urothelial type and is in continuity with that lining the bladder; it is also continuous with the ducts of the prostate and bulbo-urethral glands and with the linings of the seminal vesicles, deferent ducts and ejaculatory ducts, a relationship which is important in the spread of urinary tract infections. However, below the openings of the ejaculatory ducts this epithelium changes to a patchily pseudostratified or stratified columnar variety which lines the membranous urethra and the major part of the penile urethra (**2**.71). Mucus-secreting cells are common throughout this epithelium and frequently occur in small clusters in the penile urethra. The mucuous membrane of the penile urethra shows many recesses which continue into deeper branching tubular mucous glands (of Littré) which are especially numerous on the dorsal aspect. In older men many of the recesses of the urethral mucosa contain concretions similar to those found within the substances of the prostate. Towards the distal end of the penile urethra the epithelium changes once again, becoming stratified squamous in character with well-defined connective tissue papillae. This type of epithelium lines the navicular fossa and becomes keratinized at the external meatus.

The epithelial cells lining the navicular fossa are unusual in being glycogen-rich and it has been suggested that they may act as a substrate for an endogenous flora of lactobacteria (Holstein et al 1991). They also lack acid phosphatase activity and lysozyme-like immunoreactivity, both of which are demonstrable in the epithelium lining other parts of the distal male urethra. The epithelium lining the distal urethra in men is thus heterogeneous, a condition which may provide a measure of defence against invasion by pathogenic organisms.

Urethral sphincters

Of the two urethral sphincters, the internal *sphincter vesicae* (p. 1842) controls the vesical neck and the prostatic urethra above the ejaculatory ducts. It is composed of nonstriated muscle and supplied by sympathetic and parasympathetic fibres from the vesical plexus (see above and p. 1309). The external *sphincter urethrae* (p. 834) surrounds the membranous urethra; it consists of striated muscle and is supplied

by the perineal branches of the pudendal nerve (S2, 3 and 4); it is voluntary after early infancy.

The existence of an internal sphincter is, however, controversial. Many consider that its nonstriated muscle fibres are multi-directional as in the vesical wall, no true circumferential fibres being identifiable (Woodburne 1961; Angell 1969). However, all agree that a substantial muscular aggregation, with an admixture of elastic and collagenous fibres, exists at the vesical outlet (Vincent 1966). Its significance in micturition is noted below.

FEMALE URETHRA

The female urethra is about 4 cm long and 6 mm in diameter. It begins at the internal urethral orifice of the bladder, approximately opposite the middle of the symphysis pubis, and runs anteroinferiorly behind the symphysis pubis, embedded in the anterior wall of the vagina. It traverses the perineal membrane and ends at the external urethral orifice, an anteroposterior slit with rather prominent margins, which is situated directly anterior to the opening of the vagina and about 2.5 cm behind the glans clitoridis. Except during the passage of urine the anterior and posterior walls of the urethra are in apposition and the epithelium is thrown into longitudinal folds, one of which, on the posterior wall of the canal, is termed the *urethral crest*. Many small mucous *urethral glands* and minute pit-like recesses or *lacunae* open into the urethra. On each side, near the lower end of the urethra, a number of these glands are grouped together and open into a duct, named the *para-urethral duct*; each duct runs down in the submucous tissue and ends in a small aperture on the lateral margin of the external urethral orifice.

Microscopic structure of the female urethra

The wall of the female urethra comprises an outer muscle coat and an inner mucous membrane which lines the lumen and is continuous with that of the bladder. The muscle coat consists of an outer sleeve of striated muscle (*external urethral sphincter* p. 835) together with an inner coat of smooth muscle fibres. The female external urethral sphincter is anatomically separate from the adjacent periurethral striated muscle of the anterior pelvic floor. The constituent fibres of this sphincter are circularly disposed and form a sleeve which is thickest in the middle one-third of the urethra. In this region striated muscle completely surrounds the urethra although the posterior portion lying between the urethra and vagina is relatively thin. The striated muscle extends into the anterior wall of both the proximal and distal thirds of the urethra but is deficient posteriorly in these regions. The myocytes forming the external urethral sphincter are all of the slow twitch variety. As in the male, muscle fibres of the external urethral sphincter are unusually small and have diameters of 15–20 μm on average. Although the thickness of the external urethral sphincter in the female is less than that of the male, its constituent fibres are able to exert tone upon the urethral lumen over prolonged periods, especially in relation to the middle third of its length. Periurethral striated muscle (*pubococcygeus*) aids urethral closure during events which require rapid, albeit short-lived, elevation of urethral resistance. The *smooth muscle coat* extends throughout the length of the urethra and consists of slender muscle bundles, the majority of which are orientated obliquely or longitudinally. A few circularly arranged muscle fibres occur in the outer aspect of the non-striated muscle layer and intermingle with the skeletal muscle fibres forming the inner part of the external urethral sphincter. Proximally the urethral smooth muscle extends as far as the bladder neck where it is replaced by fascicles of detrusor nonstriated muscle. This region in the female is devoid of a well-defined circular nonstriated muscle component comparable with the preprostatic sphincter of the male. When traced distally, urethral smooth muscle bundles terminate in the subcutaneous adipose tissue surrounding the external urethral meatus. The smooth muscle of the female urethra is associated with relatively few noradrenergic nerves but receives an extensive presumptive cholinergic parasympathetic nerve supply identical in appearance to that which supplies the detrusor muscle (Ek et al 1977a, b). From a functional viewpoint it seems unlikely that competence of the female bladder neck and proximal urethra is solely the result of nonstriated muscle activity, in the absence of an anatomical sphincter. The innervation and longitudinal orientation of most of the muscle fibres suggest that urethral smooth muscle in the female is active during micturition, serving to shorten and widen the urethral lumen. For further details, see Gilpin and Gosling (1983). The *mucous membrane* lining the female urethra consists of a stratified epithelium and a supporting layer of loose fibro-elastic connective tissue (the lamina propria). The lamina propria contains an abundance of elastic fibres orientated both longitudinally and circularly around the urethra. Numerous thin-walled veins are another characteristic feature and in the past have been falsely likened to erectile tissue. A fine plexus of acetyl cholinesterase (AChE) positive nerves is present throughout the lamina propria and these fibres are believed to be sensory branches of the pudendal nerves. The proximal part of the urethra is lined by urothelium, identical in appearance to that of the bladder neck. Distally the epithelium changes into a non-keratinizing stratified squamous type which lines the major portion of the female urethra. This epithelium is keratinized at the external urethral meatus and becomes continuous with the skin of the vestibule.

FUNCTIONAL ANATOMY OF THE LOWER URINARY TRACT

The urinary bladder performs a dual function, acting at times as a reservoir for fluid accumulating within its lumen and at others as a contractile organ actively expelling its contents into the urethra. In the following account the tissue components and, where appropriate, their neurological control will be considered under the headings *continence of urine* and *micturition*.

Continence of urine

To achieve urinary continence, the bladder acts as a passive reservoir retaining fluid because the forces acting on the urethra produce an intra-urethral pressure greater than bladder pressure. Several tissue components play a part in generating this urethral resistance and make either an active or passive contribution. Since the nonstriated muscle of the bladder is replaced in the bladder neck region by a different type of nonstriated muscle, the detrusor muscle does not play a part in closing the proximal urethra.

In the male, a distinct collar of circularly orientated nonstriated muscle occurs in the bladder neck and preprostatic urethra, continuous distally with the muscular components of the genital tract. This smooth muscle sphincter is supplied by a rich plexus of sympathetic nerve fibres which, on stimulation, cause the sphincter to contract, thereby preventing retrograde flow of semen into the urinary bladder at ejaculation. During seminal emission, the sympathetic nervous system also prevents coincidental contraction of detrusor smooth muscle. This inhibitory effect on bladder contractility is mediated by noradrenergic nerves which synapse in the vesical plexus upon parasympathetic motor neurons. Despite this well-defined genital role, it is not known whether the nonstriated muscle of the bladder neck region and preprostatic urethra plays an active part in the maintenance of continence. Intramural collagen and elastic fibres within the wall of the bladder neck, proximal urethra and prostate generate passive forces which help to close the urethral lumen. However, postoperative incontinence of urine does not usually follow radical surgical excision of the bladder neck, preprostatic urethra and prostate, suggesting that these regions make only a minor contribution to urinary continence.

In the female, a nonstriated muscle sphincter cannot be anatomically recognized in the wall of the bladder neck and proximal urethra. Consequently it is even less likely that active smooth muscle contraction can be considered as an important factor in the continence of urine. However, the bladder neck and proximal urethra possess within their walls innumerable elastic fibres which are of particular importance in producing passive occlusion of the urethral lumen (Lapides 1958). Indeed, it has been suggested that the passive elastic resistance offered by the urethral wall is the most important single factor responsible for the closure of the bladder neck and proximal urethra in the continent woman. The anatomy and physiology of urinary continence in women was reviewed in 1990 by DeLancey.

In both sexes the urethra contains within its walls the external urethral sphincter, the location of which corresponds anatomically to the zone where maximal urethral closure pressures are normally recorded. This striated muscle sphincter is morphologically adapted to maintain tone over relatively long periods without fatigue and plays an important active role in producing urethral occlusion at rest. It remains to be determined, however, whether the force exerted by the sphincter is maximal at all times between two consecutive acts of micturition or whether additional motor units are recruited during coughing, sneezing, etc. to enhance the occlusive force on the urethra during these events. The external sphincter is innervated by nerve fibres which travel via several routes, not exclusively via the pudendal nerves (Gil Vernet 1969). The clinical relevance of this arrangement is that pudendal blockade or neurectomy performed in order to reduce urethral resistance will not achieve the desired effect since much of the motor innervation of the striated sphincter remains intact after these procedures.

Concerning the role of periurethral muscle in the maintenance of continence, the medial parts of the levator ani muscles in both sexes are related to (but structurally separate from) the urethral wall. These periurethral fibres are innervated by the pudendal nerve and consist of an admixture of large diameter fast and slow twitch fibres. Therefore, unlike the external sphincter, periurethral muscle possesses morphological features which are similar to other 'typical' voluntary muscles. This pelvic floor musculature plays an important part (especially in the female) by providing an additional occlusive force on the urethral wall, particularly during events which are associated with an increase in intra-abdominal pressure. In addition, the muscles provide support for the pelvic viscera.

Micturition

To enable fluid to flow along the urethra it is necessary for the pressure in the urinary bladder to exceed that within the urethral lumen. Under normal circumstances, in order to initiate micturition, a fall in urethral resistance immediately precedes a rise in pressure within the lumen of the bladder. The fall in urethral resistance may be due, at least in part, to the action of what has been termed the *'musculus dilator urethrae'* (Dorschner et al 1994b), a ventral longitudinal muscle system located in the neck of the bladder and in the wall of the urethra. The fasciculi of the upper part of this muscle cross in stages the ventral circumference of the trigonal sphincter muscle, whereas the lower part is closely related to the mucous membrane lining the urethra. Histomorphological evidence suggests that the muscle should be able to oppose the action of the musculus sphincter trigonalis (p. 1840) and the musculus sphincter urethrae (Dorschner & Stolzenburg 1994), causing urethral dilatation. The pressure rise is usually produced by active contraction of detrusor smooth muscle at the onset of micturition. The detrusor muscle coat consists of numerous interlacing bundles forming a complex meshwork of smooth muscle which, on contraction, reduces all dimensions of the bladder. The muscle coat is collectively involved and it is unnecessary to attach special significance to the precise orientation of individual bundles within the wall of the viscus.

The preganglionic nerve supply travels in the pelvic splanchnic nerves before synapsing on neurons located within the vesical part of the pelvic plexuses and within the wall of the bladder. These peripheral neurons supply nerve fibres which ramify throughout the thickness of the detrusor smooth muscle coat. The profuse distribution of these motor nerves emphasizes the importance of the autonomic nervous system in initiating and sustaining bladder contracting during micturition. For micturition to occur the pressure differential between the bladder and urethra must overcome the elastic resistance of the bladder neck. Immediately prior to the onset of micturition, the tonus of the external sphincter is reduced by central inhibition of its motor neurons located in the second, third and fourth sacral spinal segments. This inhibition is mediated by descending spinal pathways originating in higher centres of the central nervous system. Concomitantly, other descending pathways activate (either directly or via sacral interneurons) the preganglionic parasympathetic motor outflow to the urinary bladder. This central integration of the nervous control of the bladder and urethra is essential for normal micturition.

Clinical anatomy. After urethral rupture, the extravasation of urine may complicate micturition; urine usually extends between the perineal membrane and the membranous layer of the superficial fascia. As both of these are attached firmly to the ischiopubic rami, extravasated fluid cannot pass posteriorly because the two layers are continuous around the superficial transverse perineal muscles. Laterally, the spread of urine is blocked by the pubic and ischial rami; it cannot enter the lesser pelvis through the perineal membrane and, if this remains intact, fluid can make its way only anteriorly into the scrotal and penile loose connective tissue and thence to the anterior abdominal wall. When the lesser pelvis is crushed the urethra may be ruptured between the prostatic and membranous parts; extravasation of urine then occurs into the pelvic extraperitoneal tissue.

The lower urinary tract is subject to many congenital anomalies (p. 204), some amenable to surgical correction. For an anatomical survey, consult Paul and Kanagasuntheram (1956).

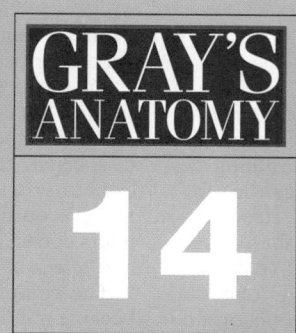

14

REPRODUCTIVE SYSTEM

Section Editors: Lawrence H. Bannister and Mary Dyson

Contributors: Essay on *Anatomy of pregnancy and parturition* by N. J. Saunders, Consultant Obstetrician and Gynaecologist, Princess Anne Hospital, Southampton; John Carroll for material on atretic follicles.

INTRODUCTION

The linking together of the *urinary system* and the *reproductive system* into a single *urogenital system* has little to commend it other than custom. Functionally the two systems have nothing in common (Romer 1970) and this is sufficient justification for considering them separately. Furthermore, the only structural overlap between the two in the mature human is the shared use of the male urethra as both a urinary and a seminal duct (p. 1842). Developmentally and phylogenetically they have more in common in that vertebrate gonadal ducts generally have a *nephric* origin (see p. 204); however, in human females even the *oviduct* (i.e. the paramesonephric or Müllerian duct) is no longer formed from nephric tissue, a fact which strongly supports the argument for separation into two distinct systems. Even in human males, where the duct systems of the testes are, as in other male mammals, derived from nephric tubules and the *mesonephric duct*, these are **not** excretory structures.

In all vertebrates, with the exception of elementary chordates such as *Amphioxus*, the nephric excretory tubules and the gonads, together with their associated ducts, develop from coelomic epithelium dorsally, flanking the major blood vessels. It is possible that their anatomical proximity, together with the more medial location of the gonads, led phylogenetically to the adoption of what were once, and in many animals still are, urinary ducts and tubules to serve the gonads, especially in males. As indicated above, mammalian evolution has resulted in a virtually complete separation of the two systems (see also p. 1814). In reptiles and birds, as well as in mammals, the functioning kidney is a *metanephros*, and is completely dissociated from any reproductive function. This freeing from an excretory function of the more cranially-located *mesonephros* has led to its acquisition of a new role in the male, where its tubules and ducts persist in modified form as testicular *vasa efferentia*, *epididymis* and *ductus deferens* (p. 200).

The complete separation of the genital from the urinary organs became modified yet again with the evolution in mammals of a male intromittant organ, an erectile *penis* for internal fertilization. This organ is found in virtually all male marsupials and eutherian mammals. Since it is traversed by the *urethra*, used to void both urine and semen, male mammals including man have regained a limited association of the genital and urinary systems, this being its full extent.

In the human reproductive system, as in that of most other mammals, accessory structures have evolved in connection with intromission and the retention and nurture of the developing embryos; these include the seminal vesicles (p. 1858), prostate (p. 1859) and bulbo-urethral glands (p. 1861) in the male, and the uterus (p. 1869) and vagina (p. 1875) in the female. These, together with the gonads, are described below.

REPRODUCTIVE ORGANS OF THE MALE

The male genital organs include the *testes*, *epididymes*, *deferent* and *ejaculatory ducts* and *penis*, with the accessory glandular structures: *seminal vesicles*, *prostate* and *bulbo-urethral glands*. The *spermatic cord* connects the testis to the abdominal cavity, and the testes lie externally in a cutaneous-muscular pouch, the *scrotum*.

TESTES AND EPIDIDYMES

Components

The testes, the *primary reproductive organs* or *gonads* in the male, are suspended in the scrotum by scrotal tissues including the non-striated dartos muscle and the spermatic cords, the left testis usually being about 1 cm lower than the right. Average testicular dimensions are 4–5 cm in length, 2.5 cm in breadth and 3 cm in anteroposterior diameter; their weight varies from 10.5–14 g. Each testis, ellipsoidal (**14**.1) and compressed laterally, is obliquely set in the scrotum, its upper pole tilted anterolaterally and the lower posteromedially. The anterior aspect is convex, the posterior nearly straight, with the spermatic cord attached to it. Anterior, medial and lateral surfaces and both poles are convex, smooth and covered by the visceral layer of the serosal tunica vaginalis, which separates them from the parietal layer and the scrotal tissues external to this. The posterior aspect is only partly covered by tunica serosa; the epididymis adjoins its lateral part.

Epididymis

The epididymis, a tortuous canal and the first part of the efferent route from the testis, is much folded and tightly packed to form a long, narrow mass attached posterolaterally to the testis. It has a central *body*, a superior enlarged *head* and an inferior pointed *tail*. The head is connected to the upper pole of the testis by *efferent ductules* and the tail to the lower pole by loose connective tissue and the reflected tunica vaginalis. The lateral surfaces of the head and tail are covered by the tunica vaginalis and are hence 'free'; the body is also so invested, except on its posterior aspect. The tunica vaginalis is recessed between the epididymal body and the lateral surface of the testis, as the *sinus of the epididymis*.

Testicular and epididymal appendices. At the upper pole of the testis, just inferior to the epididymal head, is a minute, oval, sessile *appendix of the testis*, a remnant of the upper end of the

paramesonephric duct. On the epididymal head is a small, stalked appendage (sometimes double), the *appendix of the epididymis*, usually considered a mesonephric vestige (p. 200, **14**.1).

Testis

The testis is invested by three coats, from outside inwards: the *tunica vaginalis*, *tunica albuginea* and *tunica vasculosa*.

Tunica vaginalis (**14**.1, 2, 10). This is the lower end of the peritoneal *processus vaginalis*, whose formation precedes the descent of the fetal testis from the abdomen to the scrotum (p. 212); after this migration, the tunica's proximal part, from the internal inguinal ring almost to the testis, contracts and obliterates, leaving a closed distal sac into which the testis is invaginated. The tunica is reflected from the testis on to the internal surface of the scrotum, thus forming the visceral and parietal layers of the tunica.

Visceral layer. This covers all aspects of the testis except most of the posterior aspect. Posteromedially it is reflected forwards to the

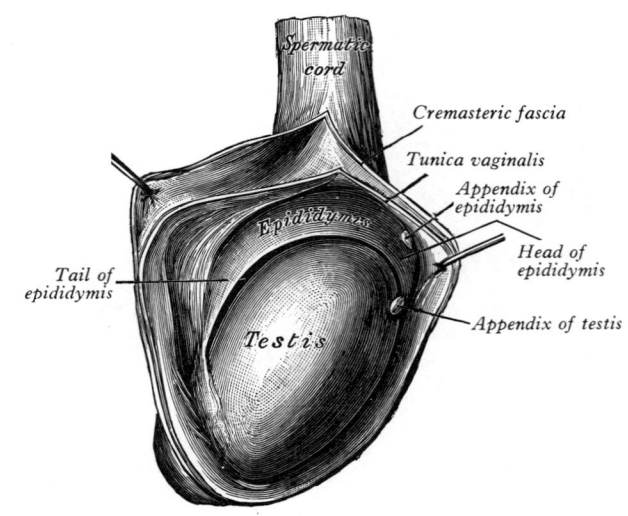

14.1 The right testis, exposed by incising and laying open the cremasteric fascia and parietal layer of the tunica vaginalis on the lateral aspect of the testis.

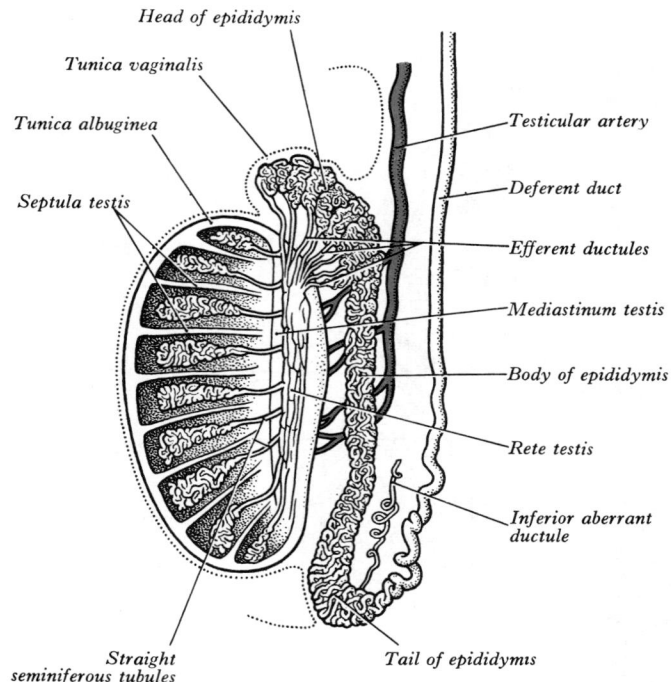

Head of epididymis

Tunica vaginalis

Tunica albuginea

Septula testis

Testicular artery

Deferent duct

Efferent ductules

Mediastinum testis

Body of epididymis

Rete testis

Inferior aberrant ductule

Straight seminiferous tubules

Tail of epididymis

14.2 Vertical section through the testis and epididymis, showing, diagrammatically, the arrangement of the ducts of the testis and the mode of formation of the deferent duct.

parietal layer; posterolaterally it passes to the medial aspect of the epididymis, lining the epididymal sinus, and then laterally to its posterior border where it is reflected forwards to become continuous with the parietal layer. The visceral and parietal layers are also continuous at both poles but at the upper the visceral layer surmounts the head of the epididymis before reflexion.

Parietal layer. More extensive than the visceral, it reaches below the testis and ascends in front of and medial to the spermatic cord. The inner surface of the tunica vaginalis has a smooth, moist mesothelium, the potential space between its visceral and parietal layers being termed the cavity of the tunica vaginalis.

In the embryo, the male or female gonads project into the coelom, covered by so-called 'germinal' epithelium; even in the adult the mesothelium covering the testis (and ovary) has been considered atypical peritoneum, a remnant of the original 'germinal' epithelium. The tunica vaginalis would then be considered to consist of a parietal layer only, continuous with the germinal epithelium at the posterior aspect of the testis. Structurally, however, in the testis the parietal and visceral epithelia are similar and like that of the general peritoneum, although the epithelium covering the ovary is a specialized, cuboidal layer (p. 208). Doubtless the term germinal epithelium reflects the misconception that generations of gonocytes develop from the specialized mesothelium of the genital ridge.

Obliterated part of the processus vaginalis. This is often seen as a fibrous thread in the anterior part of the spermatic cord, extending from the internal end of the inguinal canal where it is connected to the peritoneum, as far as the tunica vaginalis. Sometimes it disappears within the cord; its proximal part may, however, remain patent, the peritoneal cavity then communicating with the tunica vaginalis, or the proximal processus may persist, although shut off distally from the tunica (p. 212). Occasionally its cavity may persist at an intermediate level as a cyst. When patent, its cavity may admit a loop of intestine (indirect hernia, see p. 1788).

Tunica albuginea. A dense, bluish-white covering for the testis, this is composed mainly of interlacing bundles of collagen fibres, covered externally by the visceral layer of the tunica vaginalis, except at the epididymal head and tail and the posterior aspect of the testis, where vessels and nerves enter. It covers the tunica vasculosa and, at the posterior border of the testis, projects into the testicular interior as a thick, vertical but incomplete septum, the **mediastinum testis (14.2)**; this extends from the upper almost to the lower end of

the testis and is wider above than below. From the front and sides of the mediastinum testis numerous incomplete *septula testis* radiate towards the surface of the testis, attached there to the deep aspect of the tunica albuginea; these divide the organ incompletely into cone-shaped *lobules*, their bases at the surface and their apices converging upon the mediastinum. For a detailed comparative account of the mediastinum consult Dhingra (1977). The arrangement of its connective tissue is very variable; in some species, including man (Holstein 1967b), smooth myocytes occur amid the collagen fibres (p. 1854). It is traversed by many vessels and by efferent tubules of the rete testis. Leydig cells are absent from the human mediastinum testis but are present in some ungulates.

Tunica vasculosa. This contains a plexus of blood vessels and delicate loose connective tissue, extending over the internal aspect of the tunica albuginea and covering the septa and therefore all the testicular lobules.

MICROSTRUCTURE OF THE TESTIS

At the surface of the testis (the visceral tunica vaginalis) is a layer of flat mesothelial cells resembling those of the surrounding peritoneum; some consider them to be remnants of a 'germinal' epithelium (see above). Internally the testicular architecture is dominated by the *lobules of the testis* (**14**.2), their number in a human testis being 200–300. They differ in size, those centrally placed being largest and longest. Each contains one to three or more minute *convoluted seminiferous tubules*. When unravelled these are seen to begin blindly or by anastomotic loops. Clermont and Huckins (1961) and Roosen-Runge (1961) have described them (in rats) as closed loops, opening at both ends into the tubuli recti and thus into the rete testis, and this pattern is now generally accepted. Their loose supporting connective tissue contains grouped *interstitial* (*Leydig*) *cells* (**14**.3) containing yellow pigment granules. The tubules in each testis total 400–600 and the length of each is 70–80 cm. Their diameter varies from 0.12–0.3 mm. They are pale in early life, but in old age they contain much fat and are deep yellow. Each (**14**.3) has a basement membrane composed of a basal lamina and laminated connective tissue containing numerous elastin fibres, with flat cells between the layers, and covered externally by flat epithelioid cells. Nicander (1967) has described intercellular contacts between these cells. As it ages the basement membrane becomes thicker and denser. Internal to it the seminiferous epithelium consists of *spermatogenic* and *supportive* cells. The former (**14**.4, 5), when active, include an array of types ranging from spermatogonia through their derived forms, spermatocytes and spermatids, to mature spermatozoa. Among the spermatids may be *residual bodies* (p. 128), spherical structures containing membranous and mitochondrial residues and numerous free ribosomes, derived from spermatids from which they have separated. Their role in spermatogenesis is not yet clarified (Vaughn 1966) but may be regulatory; they undergo autolysis and may then be phagocytosed by sustentacular cells, as the mature spermatozoa separate.

Spermatogonia

Spermatogonia, the stem cells for all spermatozoa, are descended from primordial germ cells which reach and multiply in the genital cords of developing testis, becoming *gonocytes*. In the fully differentiated testis they appear along the basal laminae of the seminiferous tubules. Changes in the structure and appearance of human spermatogonia from birth to the onset of puberty have been described by Paniagua and Nistal (1984). Their cytological characteristics, like those of the generations of spermatocytes and spermatids produced from them, have been noted (p. 126). Several types of spermatogonia were early recognized on the basis of cell and nuclear dimensions, distribution of nuclear chromatin and histochemical and ultrastructural data, as is generally accepted, though disagreements over minor details persist (Courot et al 1970). Similarly, various stages in the maturation of spermatocytes and spermatids (p. 127) have been recognized and a complex lineage of cells, from spermatogonia to spermatozoa, can now be defined and identified in the seminiferous tubules of most vertebrates. Mammals have been the most studied, especially rodents and domestic cattle, the latter under the impetus of artificial insemination.

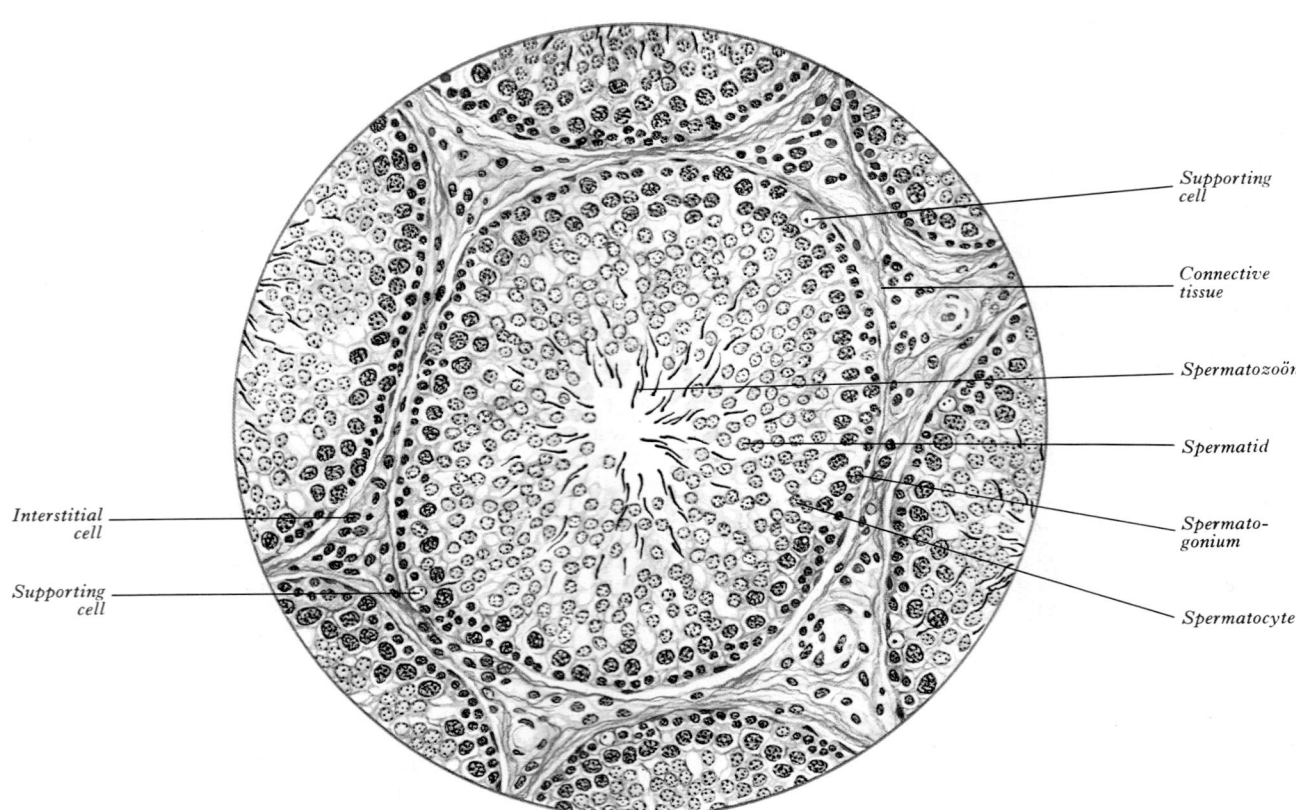

14.3   Transverse section through a part of a human testis. Stained with iron haematoxylin and Van Gieson's stain. Magnification × 350.

Three basic groups of spermatogonia, *dark type A*, *pale type A*, and *type B* have been described (p. 126); the first divides to maintain the basic store of spermatogonia, producing also some pale type A cells which divide and differentiate into type B, the immediate precursors of spermatocytes. More complex classifications are also used; for example, a *prospermatogonial stage* (A_0) is recognized, and a series, designated A_1–A_4, is utilized in describing the intermediate types in active seminiferous epithelium. Similarly, several grades of type B are recognized. Much of the complexity of current nomenclature is merely due to the successive divisions of spermatogonia, which can be investigated by labelling with [^{3}H]-thymidine. Extensive studies have been carried out in primates (Clermont 1963, 1969) and the findings are probably applicable to man. The dark A spermatogonia (A_1) form a reserve of resting cells, whereas the pale type (A_2) form further A_2 cells, one of which repeats this divisional step while the other divides into two type B spermatogonia. Since the latter produces, by serial division, several generations, these are designated B_1, B_2, etc. In monkeys (*Cercopithecus aethiops*) five generations of B spermatogonia occur, the final product being *primary spermatocytes*. There are four B spermatogonial generations in man and, since the cells (ignoring degeneration) are doubled at each stage, very large numbers of spermatozoa are formed during the active reproductive life of male vertebrates. The number of spermatogonial generations varies, being high in fish (six to 14), low in birds (one to three) and from four to seven in mammals (Holstein 1976).

Primary and secondary spermatocytes (14.4, 5).

Primary spermatocytes with a diploid chromosome content divide meiotically into secondary spermatocytes with a haploid complement, the nuclear division designated as meiosis I. Secondary spermatocytes undergo the second meiotic division to form spermatids. Both types of spermatocytes and spermatids pass through a series of changes recognized chiefly by their nuclear activities; the latter also show profound modifications in cell structure to become the mature flagellated spermatozoa. The events of meiosis are described on page 60.

Spermatids

Spermatids do not divide again but gradually mature into spermatozoa by a series of nuclear and cytoplasmic modifications (p. 127); several stages in this process have been described, according to their nuclear shape, including 'round' and 'elongating' spermatids. During the development within the spermatids of the acrosomal organelles, a chromatoid body develops which interacts with the Golgi complex and has been proposed to have a specific function in the storage of long-lived messenger (m)RNA (Toppari et al 1991).

Sustentacular, supporting cells

Sustentacular, supporting cells (of Sertoli) or sustentocytes, the non-germinal element in the complex cell population of the seminiferous tubules, are variable in overall cell shape and nuclear configuration. Changes in the form and distribution of the human Sertoli cells from birth to the onset of puberty have been described by Nistal et al (1982). These authors observed a progressive diminution in numbers from 3 years onwards, as seen in transverse sections of the tubules; but they ascribe this to testicular growth and consider the total number to remain constant. Sustentacular cells have been the subject of much controversy; in developing seminiferous tubules various supporting cells beside the 'Sertolian' category have also been described; but it is generally assumed that most non-germinal cells in the adult functioning tubules are of this limited type. Sustentacular cells, abutting onto the basal lamina of the tubules, occupy it almost to the exclusion of all but occasional spermatogonia. In tangential section of tubules they are polygonal, in transverse section, approximately columnar. Their apices are complicated by recesses into which spermatids and spermatozoa are inserted until the latter are mature enough for release. Long cytoplasmic processes also extend among the spermatogonia and spermatocytes, suggesting that sustentacular cells maintain structural cohesion in the epithelium. In earlier times there was an assumption that Sertoli cells formed a syncytium although Sertoli demonstrated the individuality of the cells in 1865. Electron microscopy has shown that in fact Sertoli cells are joined at their bases by tight junctions, to create a permeability barrier

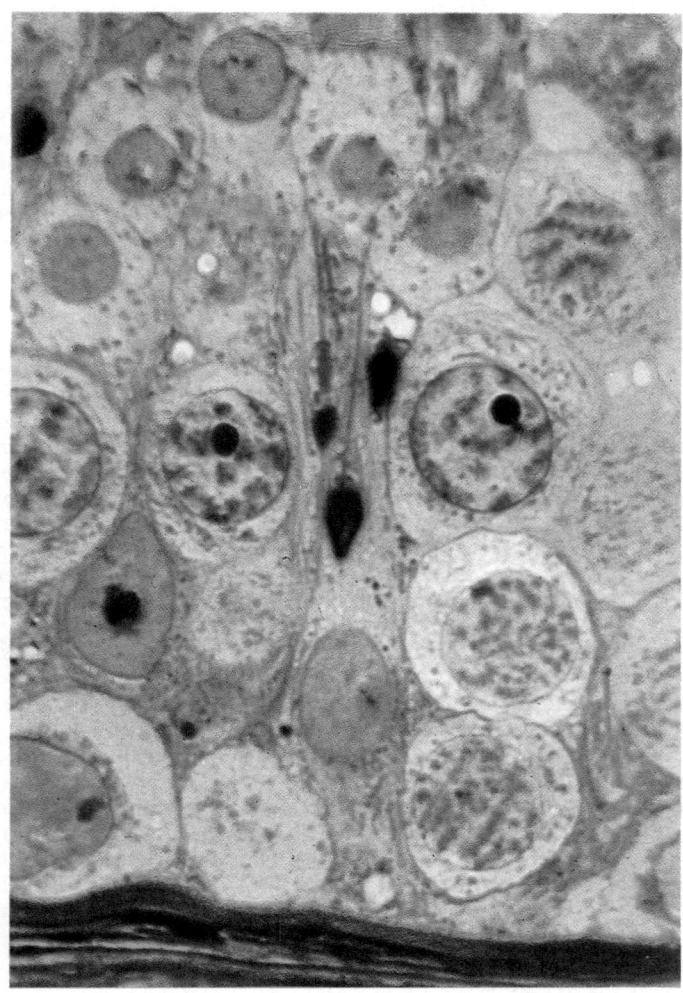

14.4   The epithelium of a seminiferous tubule in an adult man. A thin section of glutaraldehyde-fixed material, stained with toluidine blue. Spermatogonium (bottom left), primary spermatocytes (bottom right), and late spermatids (central) are visible. The spermatids are attached to a supportive cell of Sertoli (below them). For further details compare with **14**.5. (From Holstein & Wulfhekel 1971 with permission of Grosse Verlag, Berlin.)

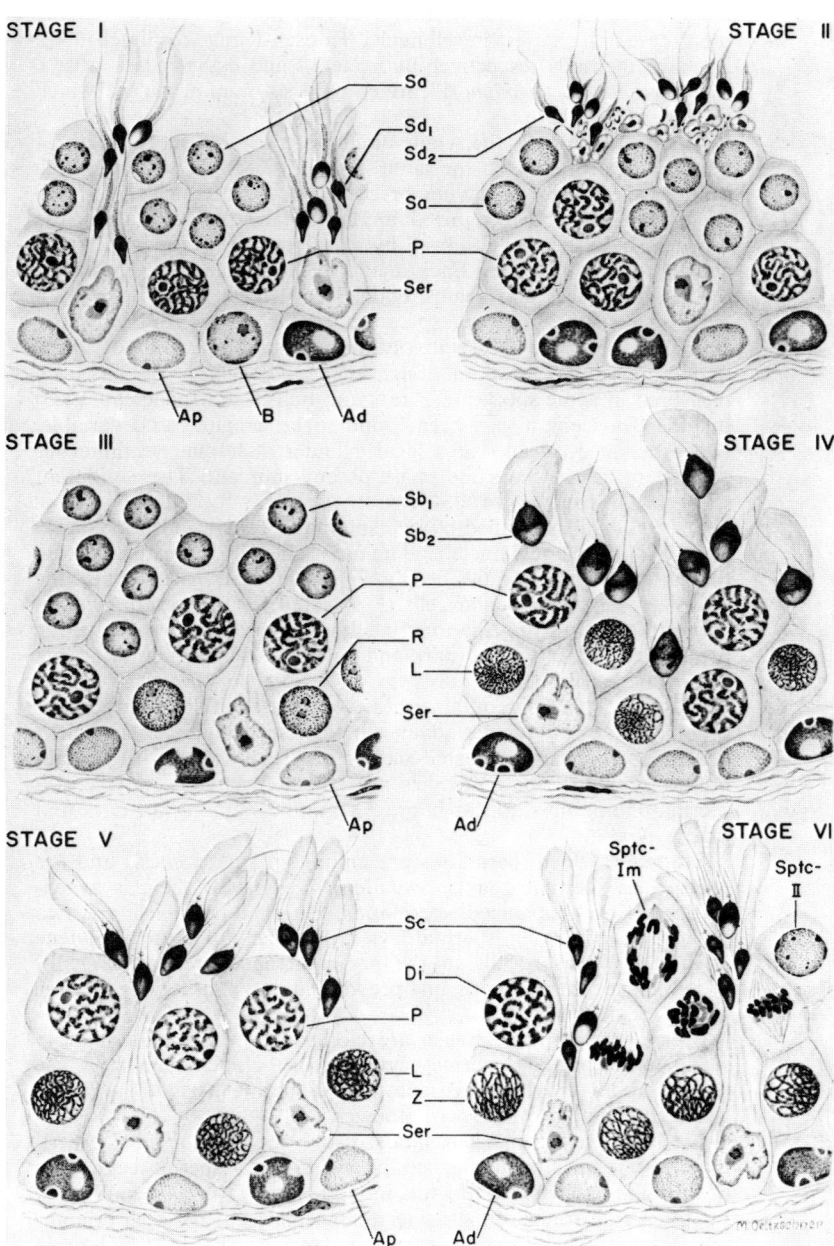

14.5   The cycle of spermatogenesis in the human seminiferous tubule. For details of the six stages see accompanying text. Ser = sustentacular cells of Sertoli; Ad, Ap and B = A type (dark and pale) and B type of spermatogonia; R = resting primary spermatocyte; L, Z, P and Di = primary spermatocytes in leptotene, zygotene, pachytene and diplotene stages; Sptc-Im = dividing primary spermatocyte; Sptc-II = secondary spermatocyte in interphase; Sa, b, etc. = generations of spermatids. (From Clermont 1963 with permission of the author and the Wistar Institute of Anatomy and Biology.)

between the extratubular and intratubular compartments (see Fawcett 1975). The nucleus is irregular, often indented, euchromatic, and contains one or two nucleoli. Cytoplasmic organelles are numerous, particularly mitochondria, smooth endoplasmic reticulum, secretory granules, Golgi complexes, ribosomes, microfilaments and microtubules, helping to form a cytoskeleton and being also a factor in the cohesive effect of sustentacular cells on the total epithelium. These details suggest that the cells exercise a metabolic influence in relation to the germinal elements. These cells are also phagocytic (Carr et al 1968), containing many lysosomes, and exert trophic influences on the surrounding cells. They change considerably during the spermatogenic cycle (see below) and are influenced by the hypophyseal hormones, luteinizing hormone (LH) and follicle-stimulating hormone (FSH). They are also concerned in the 'blood–testis barrier' by virtue of the tight junctions between them, and also involving interspersed spermatocytes. For a general review of the blood–testis barrier consult Johnson and Gomes (1977). For a review of the ultrastructural features of the human testis, with emphasis on spermatogenesis and the cytology of the Leydig cells, see Kerr (1991). For general reviews of male reproductive microstructure, see Dym (1984) and Fawcett (1994).

SPERMATOGENIC CYCLE

The elements of the seminiferous epithelium noted above form an intimately related and dynamic population, details of which have

been extensively investigated in several laboratory animals (particularly rats), in species of commercial or 'domestic' importance and in man. In addition to much detail on the cytological progression from spermatogonia to spermatozoa, the quantitative aspects of this cycle have been assessed, including the timing of its phases, relative numbers of different germinal cells at definable temporal points and so on. It is clearly established that, at any locus in a seminiferous tubule, activities in the several generations of germinal cells and hence in the qualitative and quantitative associations of cell types pass through a **cycle**, the length and stages of which vary in different species (Clermont 1972). The cycle occupies 12–13 days in rats, only 8.6 in mice, 10.5–11.6 days in monkeys (Arsenieva et al 1961) and about 16 in mankind (Heller & Clermont 1964). Its stages have been classified in two ways, one involving the development of the spermatid acrosomal system (Leblond & Clermont 1952a, b) and the other based on changes in cell nuclei (Roosen-Runge & Giesel 1950). The two methods respectively indicate 14 and eight stages in rats. The *acrosomalic technique* identifies only six human stages, which will be detailed here.

In many mammals the whole circumference of a short length of seminiferous tubule is in the same stage of the cycle, with adjoining cylindrical regions displaying preceding or succeeding stages. All stages can thus be recognized in numerical succession along the tubules, the last being followed by a cylinder undergoing the same activity as the first stage. Each region of the tubule therefore passes through all stages and begins again. Hence there exists not only a *local* succession of stages spread over the period of the cycle, characteristic of the species involved, but also a *procession* of stages undulating along the tubule. Such a '*spermatogenic wave*' has been measured in some species (e.g. rats and bulls, see Mochereau 1963) but the 'wavelength' has been found to be irregular and variable. Not even all quadrants of a local cylinder of human seminiferous epithelium are in the same phase at any moment. These different stages are as follows (**14**.4, 5).

Stage I. This is typified by two spermatid generations: one newly formed with spherical nuclei and an older one with elongating nuclei; the latter spermatids are deeply invaginated in groups into the cytoplasm of sustentacular cells. Associated with these are primary spermatocytes starting the long pachytene stage of the first meiotic prophase division; type A (dark and pale) and type B spermatogonia adjoin the basal lamina.

Stage II. This also contains these two phases of spermatid maturation but they are further advanced; older spermatids are near their final change to spermatozoa and hence there are residual bodies present. Primary spermatocytes are still in pachytene but type B spermatogonia now appear in greater numbers among the dark and pale A types.

Stage III. Older spermatids are ending spermatogenesis and are released as spermatozoa (*spermiation*). Nearest to them is a generation of well-advanced spermatids, external to which are two generations of primary spermatocytes, the older still in the pachytene stage, the younger cells in the proleptotene or resting stage of meiosis. Type A spermatogonia predominate, type B having become spermatocytes.

Stage IV. Spermatid nuclei are elongating, but are irregular in shape. Older primary spermatocytes are in the pachytene stage, the younger ones moving into leptotene. Type A spermatogonia are gathered external to the spermatocytes.

Stage V. Groups of spermatids display nuclei elongated centrifugally towards the tubular periphery. Primary spermatocytes are now in **late** pachytene and some in leptotene.

Stage VI. Groups of maturing spermatids occur between primary spermatocytes dividing into secondary spermatocytes, of which some are in the interphase stage. External to them are primary spermatocytes in the zygotene stage. Type A spermatogonia (pale and dark) predominate again near the basal lamina.

Summary

Details of these complex stages accord with the successive divisions and differentiations known to occur in the germinal cell series. The process appears less regular, particularly in human biopsy material, perhaps due to mechanical disturbance; an unknown number of cells retrogress and degenerate.

Tubule compartments. The epithelium of seminiferous tubules is perhaps unique in its organization (Fawcett 1975), consisting of a permanent population of non-proliferative sustentacular cells seated on its basement membrane and interspersed proliferating spermatogonia and their derivatives; the latter are related to the basal parts of the Sertoli cells, the lateral junctions of which (**14**.4) are considered to create a '*basal compartment*' for preleptotene spermatocytes. These junctions must break down to allow spermatocytes to move towards the tubular lumen into a so-called '*adluminal compartment*'. In primates the 'blood–testis barrier' may reside in these junctions, perhaps under hormonal control; spermatogonia and early spermatocytes may be accessible to all substances crossing capillary walls, the later spermatocytes and spermatids being screened from substances incapable of passing the 'barrier'. As spermatids mature they move towards the lumen from

the lateral aspects of sustentacular cells, at first embedded largely in their cytoplasm, and attached by a junctional specialization which changes (Ross & Dobler 1975) until the spermatozoa are released into the lumen of the seminiferous tubule.

The regulation of the spermatogenic cycle appears to involve complex cellular interactions within the testis. Advances in molecular biology and in cell separation techniques mean that it is now possible to analyse the interactions between Sertoli cells and spermatogenic cells and so obtain an insight into the paracrine regulation of spermatogenesis (Toppari et al 1991). Little is known, however, of the precise interactive events involved. Experiments in rats, centred on the use of ethane dimethane sulphonate (EDS) to selectively destroy all the Leydig cells of the testis, reviewed by Sharpe et al (1990), indicate that the Leydig cells drive spermatogenesis via the secretion of testosterone which acts on the Sertoli and/or peritubular cells to create an environment suitable for the normal progression of germ cells through the cycle. Furthermore, testosterone is involved in the control of the testicular vasculature, and hence the formation of testicular interstitial fluid, presumably again via its effects on the Sertoli and/or peritubular cells. When the testis recovers from exposure to EDS and the Leydig cells regenerate, the rate and location of this regeneration is determined by an interplay between endocrine (LH and probably FSH) and paracrine factors, the latter derived from the seminiferous tubules and determined by the germ cell complement.

At least some of the paracrine factors are inhibin-related peptides, produced from multiple sites within the testis in a highly regulated manner; receptors for these factors are found during specific stages of the spermatogenic cycle or particular cell types. Specific binding proteins such as follistatin may regulate the bioavailability of these factors, the actions of which include the modulation of interstitial cell function and the increase in spermatogonial proliferation. Activin and inhibin thus appear to be significant factors in the local control of testicular activity (Moore et al 1994) and most or all of the cell types of the testis, both the spermatogenic and the somatic cell lineages, interact in the control of spermatogenesis (Kierszenbaum 1994); the details of these interactions remain to be resolved.

EFFERENT DUCTULES AND EPIDIDYMIS

The events described above occur in the highly coiled parts of the seminiferous tubules. As these reach the lobular apices they are less convoluted, assume an almost straight course and unite into 20–30 larger but short *straight ducts* (*tubuli recti*), about 0.5 mm in diameter (**14**.2). Straight seminiferous tubules enter the fibrous tissue of the mediastinum testis, ascending backwards as a close network (the *rete testis*) of anastomosing tubes lined by a flat epithelium. At the upper pole of the mediastinum, 12–20 *efferent ductules* (*ductuli efferentes*) perforate the tunica albuginea to pass from the testis to the epididymis. They are at first straight, becoming enlarged and very convoluted and forming conical *lobules of the epididymis*, which make up its head (*caput*). Each epididymal lobule is a convoluted duct, 15–20 cm in length. Opposite the lobular bases the ducts open into a single *duct of the epididymis*, whose coils form the epididymal body (*corpus*) and tail (*cauda*). With the coils unravelled the tube measures more than 6 metres, increasing in thickness as it approaches the epididymal tail, where it becomes the deferent duct. The coils are held together by bands of fibrous connective tissue. The epididymal body and tail are thus a single tube.

Efferent ductules

The efferent ductules are lined by a columnar epithelium, most cells of which are ciliated. The lining cells of the efferent ductule cells are higher than the cuboidal epithelial cells of the rete testis and lower than the tall columnar epithelial cells of the epididymal duct. These differences are sufficiently great for the junctions of the efferent ducts with the rete testis and epididymal duct to be identified morphologically in serial sections (Saitoh et al 1990). The lining cells from both the rete testis and the epididymis coexpress cytokeratin and vimentin in a heterogeneous fashion, the cytokeratins being predominantly in the apical cytoplasm and the vimentin filaments in the basal parts of the cells; in the adult a different expression of intermediate filaments occurs in the proximal and distal parts of the epididymis, with a clear predominance of cytokeratin near to the

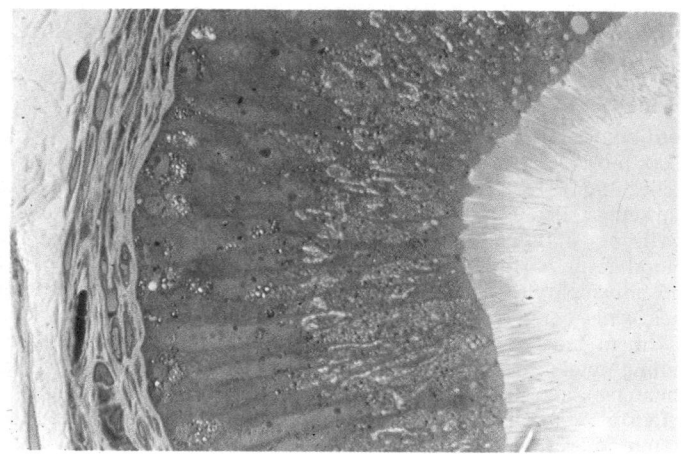

14.6 Section through the corpus of the human adult epididymis, showing deep columnar ciliated epithelium, small contractile cells, arranged circumferentially, immediately external to the epithelium, and larger smooth muscle cells more externally. A thin glutaraldehyde-fixed section stained with toluidine blue. (Supplied by A F Holstein, University of Hamburg. For details see Baumgarten et al 1971.)

rete testis (Dinges et al 1991). Efferent ductules are lined by two types of epithelial cell: tall columnar ciliated cells, their cilia beating towards the epididymis, and shorter non-ciliated cells containing conspicuous lysosomes and shown to be actively endocytic. External to the epithelium, the ductules are surrounded by a thin circular coat of smooth muscle.

Epididymal duct (14.6)

In the epididymal duct the muscle is thicker and the epithelium composed of columnar pseudostratified cells. They are composed of two main types: *principal* and *basal cells*, and a less common third

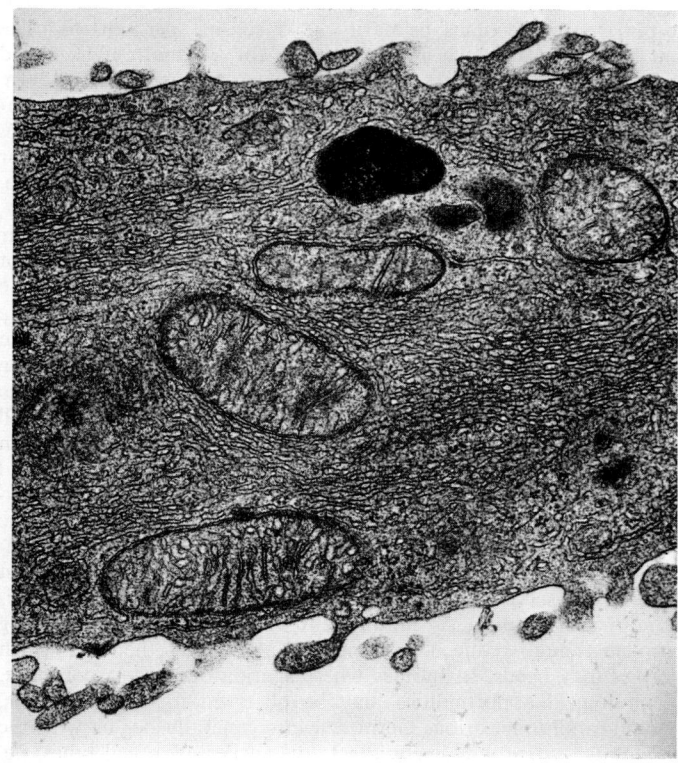

14.7 Transmission electron micrograph of part of an interstitial cell of the testis (Leydig cell) showing the profuse agranular endoplasmic reticulum and prominent mitochondria (murine). Magnification × 20 000.

class of *clear cells*. Principal cells are tall columnar structures with elongate, oval nuclei in their basal third. On their apices they bear long (15 μm) regular microvilli (termed *stereocilia*, because they were once, erroneously, thought to be immotile cilia; however they are supported internally by actin filaments rather than microtubules). These cells have a complex cytoplasm, with a large Golgi complex and lysosomes. Their long microvilli and numerous endocytic vesicles between their bases denote their role in water resorption from the testicular output—about 90% of the total is absorbed in the epididymis. These cells also secrete glycoproteins essential for the maturation of spermatozoa (Flickinger 1983), and endocytose various other components of the seminal fluid.

Basal cells are rounded or angular elements lying between the bases of the principal cells. They may represent stem cells for epithelial repair, although this has not been confirmed. *Clear* cells are columnar cells present in small numbers; they have only a few microvilli, but have numerous endocytic vesicles and lipid droplets. Their function is unknown.

Baumgarten et al (1970) suggest that three ultrastructurally distinct types of contractile cell occur in both ductules and epididymis. These receive a sparse adrenergic innervation; few nerve fibres penetrate between the myocytes, unlike the more profuse innervation of smooth muscles in the caput epididymis and ductus deferens. These differences accord with the slow, spontaneous, local contractions of the ductules and proximal epididymis and the rapid, reflex contractions of the caput and ductus during seminal emission. For details of epididymal ultrastructure, see Flickinger et al (1978), Sun and Flickinger (1980), Fawcett (1994).

In most mammalian species, including man, spermatozoa leaving the testis are incapable of fertilizing a female gamete. They mature by means of a process which involves the pre-programmed cleavage of intrinsic molecules and remodelling by means of extrinsic molecules found in the fluids in which they are suspended. Most of the biocatalysts required are secreted by specialized regions of the epididymal epithelium, although some are provided in the seminal fluid. The role of the epididymis in sperm maturation has been postulated by Amann et al (1993) to be the 'setting of a series of triggers' which initiate cellular maturation changes either at emission or when in the vicinity of the oöcyte and setting a fail-safe mechanism(s) for each trigger to prevent premature occurrence of each event. On leaving the epididymis the spermatozoa have acquired a high fertilizing potential.

TESTICULAR INTERSTITIAL TISSUE

The tissues between the seminiferous tubules include various connective tissue elements, vessels and nerves. Amongst these are groups of *interstitial cells* (*Leydig cells*) which collectively constitute one of the major endocrine components of the body. The interstitial cells of Leydig (1850) are probably mesenchymal in origin but may arise from mesonephric blastema (Witschi 1951). Such cells (**14.**7), isolated or clustered, occur in the intertubular tissue of most vertebrates including man, being large and polyhedral, with an eccentric nucleus containing: one to three nucleoli, a scanty, poorly staining cytoplasm (Hooker 1971), much agranular endoplasmic reticulum (rich in ascorbic acid), vacuoles containing fats, phospholipids and cholesterol, thus resembling the interstitial cells of the ovary (p. 1862), luteal cells of the corpus luteum (p. 1865) and secretory cells in the adrenal cortex (p. 1901). Their ultrastructural features in the human ageing testis have been described by Paniagua et al (1986). Their cytoplasm contains unique crystalloid inclusions up to 20 μm long (crystals of Reinke), of unknown function. These cells synthesize and secrete androgens; their masculinizing effect was demonstrated in 1903 by Bouin and Ancel. They are stimulated by interstitial-cell-stimulating hormone (ICSH—identical with LH) and possibly FSH of the anterior lobe of the hypophysis cerebri (p. 1883). In cryptorchidism, where testes are retained in the inguinal canal and hence in a warmer environment, the rate of production of androgens and spermatozoa is depressed, without visible changes in the interstitial cells. Androgens stimulate the growth and activity of male accessory reproductive glands (prostate, seminal vesicles and bulbo-urethral glands) and also secondary sexual changes at puberty (growth of facial, axillary and pubic hair, enlargement of the larynx and paranasal air sinuses and greater skeletal growth), as well as a plethora of other actions on the general metabolism of the body, nervous system, etc. Most of these changes are inhibited or altered by oestrogens (in sufficient amounts), especially when androgenic output is depressed, as in some eunuchoid conditions (p. 1884).

The proportion of interstitial cells of Leydig to other intertubular components varies with age and in some diseases. After initial multiplication in early fetal life, they appear to atrophy at birth; but whether they disappear or are merely depressed in number in the immediate postnatal period is uncertain. It is accepted that they reappear before puberty, perhaps developing from mesenchyme. They are not reduced in the elderly (55–65 years) according to Kothari and Gupta (1974). In cryptorchid testes they are absent but the total intertubular tissue is increased. For techniques of quantitative assessment in human and other mammalian testes see Christensen (1975), Kothari et al (1978), Mori and Christensen (1980).

TESTICULAR CAPSULE

The testicular coverings, already noted (p. 1848), proceeding internally from the surface, are: skin, dartos muscle, superficial perineal fascia, external spermatic fascia, cremasteric fascia, internal spermatic fascia, parietal and visceral layers of the tunica vaginalis (with an intervening capillary interval), tunica albuginea and tunica vasculosa. The last three form the so-called 'testicular capsule'. A contractile element has been demonstrated in this otherwise inert, largely fibrous tissue structure (Davis & Langford 1969). In rabbits and rats, isolated preparations of testicular capsule show spontaneous contractions, reacting also to both cholinergic and adrenergic agents. Abundant autonomic nerve endings near blood vessels have been described (Norberg et al 1967); smooth myocytes have been demonstrated in the tunica in rodents and man (Holstein 1967a,b); the distribution of these myocytes varies and, while widely scattered in the human tunica albuginea, they are concentrated posteriorly near the epididymis. This contractile capsule probably massages or pumps the ducts in the testis, impelling spermatozoa onwards. For a review consult Davis et al (1971).

TEMPERATURE REGULATION IN THE TESTIS

Testes are external or *scrotal* in most marsupials and eutherians, but *abdominal* in fish, amphibians, reptiles, birds and monotremes. There are exceptions in some mammals: the testes are abdominal in sloths, elephants and hyraces. In aquatic mammals they are either abdominal (whales and dolphins) or in the inguinal region (seals). They may be scrotal during breeding seasons but inguinal or abdominal at other times (rodents, bats and insectivores). Such variations in mammals are puzzling but it is generally accepted that the predominantly scrotal suspension is associated with homeothermic specialization; this does not, however, explain the abdominal position of the avian testes. Regulation of internal temperature (Hammel 1968) appears to create too warm an environment for spermatogenesis. Experimental evidence, reviewed by Bishop and Walton (1960), confirms this. Scrotal temperature is usually several degrees below abdominal (three degrees in man); but the optimal range for spermatogenesis, though lower, must be maintained. Mechanisms for this are numerous (Waites 1970) and testicular thermoregulation can only be summarized here. The scrotal skin is usually hairy but this heat-conserving cover varies; it is scant in man, profuse in marsupials. Scrotal sweat glands are well developed and numerous, while subcutaneous fat is generally absent. The radiant area of the well-vascularized scrotal skin is much reduced in cold conditions by contraction of the dartos muscle, probably by direct thermal stimulation or perhaps by local reflexes. Primate scrotal skin has many nerve endings responsive to chilling or warming, the latter type being more numerous (Iggo 1969). The cremaster muscles, by approximating the testes to the perineum, may also assist in conserving heat. *Countercurrent heat exchange* is said to exist between the arteries and veins (the pampiniform plexus, see p. 1601) of the spermatic cord, where both are coiled and in close apposition (Harrison & Weiner 1949). In dogs blood delivered to the testis is pre-cooled by 3°C by this mechanism (Waites & Moule 1961). Respiratory gases and other substances (including, experimentally, labelled testosterone and prostaglandin-F) are also transferred between these arteries and veins in several species, including man (Free 1977). Thus a surprising array of factors are concerned in testicular thermoregulation and maintenance of fertility; while these appear jointly involved in this function, it is suggested that the scrotum may also act in a reciprocal control of **general** body temperature.

Vessels and nerves

Testicular artery and veins. These are described on pages 1557 and 1600. Intratesticular arteries have been studied in man (Hundeiker & Keller 1963). Kormano and Suoranta (1971) noted that they are markedly coiled. Capillaries adjoining seminiferous tubules penetrate the layers of interstitial tissue and are of interest as part of the 'blood–testis barrier' (Setchell & Waites 1975; Neaves 1977). They run either parallel to the tubules or across them but do not enter their walls, being separated from germinal and supporting cells by a basement membrane and variable amounts of fibrous tissue containing interstitial cells, at which level occur selective exchange phenomena involving androgens and immune substances.

Lymph vessels of the testis. These end in lateral and pre-aortic lymph nodes (p. 1623).

Nerves. These accompany the testicular vessels and are derived from the tenth and eleventh thoracic spinal segments through the renal and also the aortic autonomic plexuses (pp. 1307, 1308). Catecholaminiferous nerve fibres occur in the human testis and epididymis, forming plexuses around smaller blood vessels and among the interstitial cells (Baumgarten & Holstein 1967). Hodson (1970) has reviewed this topic.

Age changes in the testis

The fetal testis is functionally predominantly an endocrine gland which produces testosterone and a specifically fetal gonadal hormone, the anti-Müllerian hormone (p. 206). These two hormones have a crucial role in the induction and regulation of male sexual differentiation. The fetal testis has unique features, particularly with regard to the action on it of LH) and FSH which discriminate it from the adult testis. Attention has been drawn to aspects of the endocrine action of the fetal testis requiring further research by Huhtaniemi (1994). The seminiferous tubules do not become canalized until approximately the seventh month of gestation (p. 208) although this may occur later.

Postnatally the testis gradually changes its role, retaining its ability to manufacture testosterone and other regulatory materials including the peptide hormone oxytocin (Nicholson & Pickering 1993) which act in either an endocrine or a paracrine fashion (Verhoeven 1992). At puberty, it becomes primarily a source of spermatozoa. The fetal Leydig cells, which are responsible for the androgen-induced differentiation of the male genitalia, degenerate after birth, and are replaced, during puberty, by an adult population of androgen-producing cells which persist throughout adult life (Huhtaniemi & Pelliniemi 1992). The testes grow slowly until the age of about 10 or 11, following which there is a marked acceleration of growth rate, and spermatogenesis begins.

There is no definite age for the onset of the progressive testicular involution associated with advancing age, the onset and severity of testicular changes showing considerable individual variation. These changes have been reviewed by Paniagua et al (1991) and, more recently, by Murray and Meacham (1993). Testicular size, sperm quality and quantity, and the numbers of Sertoli cells and Leydig cells have all been reported to decrease in the elderly, although the last has been disputed by Kothari and Gupta (1974). Leydig cell activity is driven by LH and the decrease in Leydig cell function in the elderly as part of what has been described as the normal ageing process may be affected by changes in the hypothalamically-controlled secretion of LH (Kaufman et al 1990). The volume occupied by the seminiferous tubules decreases, whereas that occupied by interstitial tissue remains approximately constant. The most frequently observed histological change in the ageing testis is variation in spermatogenesis in different seminiferous tubules, being complete though reduced in some and absent in others, in which sclerosis may occur. In tubules where spermatogenesis is complete, morphological abnormalities may be observed in the germ cells, including multinucleation. Germ cell loss generally begins with the spermatids, but progressively affects the earlier germ cell types, i.e. the spermatocytes and spermatogonia. Sertoli cells are also affected by ageing, showing a range of morphological changes including dedifferentiation, mitochondrial metaplasia and multinucleation. In the Leydig cells there is a decrease in the quantity of smooth endoplasmic reticulum and mitochondria, while lipid droplets, crystalline inclusions and residual bodies increase; some cells become multinucleate. Tubules in which the entire epithelium has been lost have been observed, whereas others in the same testis appear normal. The development of tubular involution with advancing age is similar to that observed after experimental ischaemia, suggesting that vascular lesions may be involved in age-related testicular atrophy. There is, however, no abrupt change in testicular function equivalent to the female climacteric.

Clinical aspects of the testis

At an early fetal period the testes are located posteriorly in the abdominal cavity. Their descent to the scrotum (p. 212) appears to be under hormonal control (gonadotropins and androgens). In the scrotum the testes are cooler, favouring spermatogenesis (see above). Testicular descent may be arrested:

- in the abdomen
- at the deep inguinal ring
- in the inguinal canal
- between the superficial inguinal ring and the scrotum.

A retained testis is probably infertile; a man with both retained (*anorchism*) is sterile but may not be impotent. Absence of one is *monorchism*. Retention in the inguinal canal is often complicated by congenital hernia, the processus vaginalis remaining patent. The testis may traverse the canal but reach an abnormal site (*ectopia testis*, p. 212). After early childhood, the undescended testis is at increased risk of testicular carcinoma, and requires surgical intervention to ensure its descent. It may be inverted in the scrotum, with its normally posterior or attached border anterior and the tunica vaginalis posterior.

Serous fluid often accumulates in the scrotum, as a *hydrocele*. Usually such fluid is in the sac of the tunica vaginalis, forming a *vaginal hydrocele*. In *congenital hydrocele* the fluid is in the tunical sac but this communicates with the peritoneal cavity through a non-obliterated processus vaginalis. *Infantile hydrocele* occurs when the processus is obliterated only at or near the deep inguinal ring; it resembles vaginal hydrocele but fluid extends up the cord into the inguinal canal. If the processus is obliterated both at the deep inguinal ring **and** above the epididymis, leaving a central open part, this may distend as an *encysted hydrocele of the cord*. *Encysted hydrocele of the epididymis*, or *spermatocele*, is a cyst related to the caput epididymis; it may contain spermatozoa and it is probably a retention cyst of one of the seminiferous tubules.

DEFERENT AND EJACULATORY DUCTS

DUCTUS DEFERENS (VAS DEFERENS)

The deferent duct (*ductus deferens* or *vas deferens*) is the distal continuation of the epididymis (**14.2**). It starts at the epididymal tail and is at first very tortuous but, becoming straighter, ascends along the posterior aspect of the testis, medial to the epididymis. From the superior pole of the testis it ascends in the posterior part of the spermatic cord, to traverse the inguinal canal. At the internal (deep) inguinal ring it leaves the cord, curves round the lateral side of the inferior epigastric artery and ascends for about 2.5 cm anterior to the external iliac artery. It then turns back and slightly down obliquely across the external iliac vessels to enter the lesser pelvis, where, situated retroperitoneally, it continues posteriorly medial to the obliterated umbilical artery, the obturator nerve and vessels, and the vesical vessels (**13.32**). It crosses the ureter (**14.8**) and medial to it bends acutely to pass anteromedially between the posterior surface of the bladder and the upper pole of the seminal vesicle, medial to which it descends in contact with it, gradually approaching the opposite duct. Here it lies between the base of the bladder and the rectum, separated by rectovesical fascia. It finally descends to the base of the prostate, joining at an acute angle the duct of the seminal vesicle to form the ejaculatory duct (**14.9**). Due to its thick wall and small lumen it feels cord-like when grasped. Its lumen is generally small, but posterior to the bladder it becomes dilated and tortuous, as the *ampulla*; beyond this, where it joins the seminal vesicular duct, it is again greatly diminished in calibre (**14.8**).

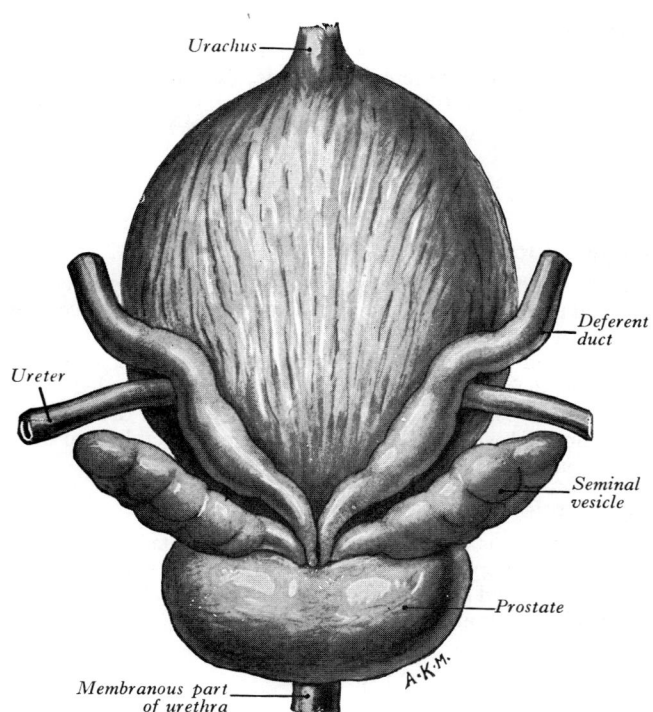

14.8   Posterosuperior aspect of the male internal urogenital organs.

Microstructure

The wall of the deferent duct has external loose connective tissue, intermediate muscular and internal mucosal layers. The thick muscular layer is composed of smooth myocytes arranged in external longitudinal and internal circular strata; an additional internal longitudinal layer exists at the duct's commencement. All muscle strata intermingle. The mucosa is longitudinally folded and its epithelium is columnar and non-ciliated through most of the duct; towards its distal end a bilaminar columnar epithelium appears, the superficial tier displaying non-motile stereocilia (elongated microvilli). Many of the columnar cells are secretory; for histochemical studies consult Wendler (1968). Elastic fibres are present in its connective tissue (Paniagua et al 1983).

Vessels

The deferent duct has its own artery (p.1559), usually derived from the superior vesical artery. It anastomoses with the testicular artery, thus also supplying the epididymis and testis. The anastomosis is of

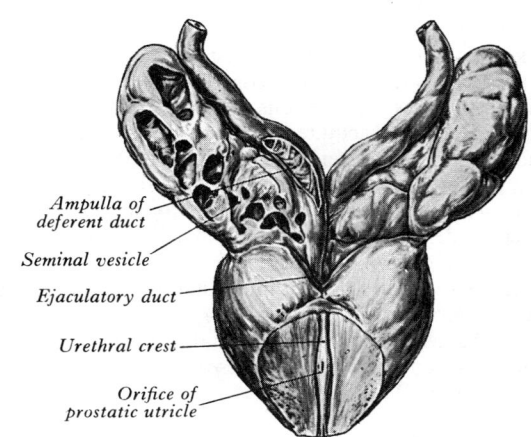

14.9   Anterior aspect of the seminal vesicles, terminal parts of the deferent ducts and the prostate. The lamina of the right seminal vesicle, the ampulla of the right deferent duct and of the prostatic part of the urethra have been exposed by appropriate removal of tissues.

especial interest in connection with the toxic effects of cadmium on the mammalian testis (Gunn & Gould 1975; Johnson 1977). These appear to be due to interference with vascularization, but the artery to the ductus deferens (in rats) is apparently immune from this effect.

Nerves

The deferent ducts have a rich autonomic plexus of sympathetic nerve fibres.

Aberrant ductules

A narrow, blind, *caudal aberrant ductule* often occurs, connected with the caudal part of the epididymal duct or with the commencement of the deferent duct. Uncoiled, it varies in length from 5 to 35 cm; it may be dilated near its end, but is otherwise uniform. In structure it is like the deferent duct; occasionally it is not connected with the epididymis. A *rostral aberrant ductule* may occur in the epididymal head, connected with the rete testis. Aberrant ductules are derived from mesonephric tubules (p. 200).

Paradidymis

The paradidymis is a small collection of convoluted tubules, found anteriorly in the spermatic cord above the epididymal head. They are lined by ciliated columnar epithelium and probably represent the remains of the mesonephros (p. 200).

EJACULATORY DUCTS

The ejaculatory ducts are formed on each side by union of the duct of a seminal vesicle with a deferent duct (**13.32**, **14.**9). Each is almost 2 cm in length, starts from the base of the prostate, runs antero-inferiorly between its median and right or left lobes, and skirts the prostatic utricle to end on the colliculus seminalis at two slit-like orifices on, or just within, the utricular opening (p. 1842). They diminish and converge towards their ends.

Microstructure

The walls of the ejaculatory ducts are thin, containing an *outer fibrous layer*, almost absent beyond their entrance into the prostate, a layer of smooth *myocytes* in thin outer circular and inner longitudinal strata, and a *mucosa* having a columnar epithelium. For details of the ejaculatory musculature, see Schlager (1967).

SPERMATIC CORDS AND SCROTUM

SPERMATIC CORD

As the testis traverses the abdominal wall into the scrotum during early life, it carries its vessels, nerves and deferent duct with it. These meet at the deep inguinal ring to form the *spermatic cord*, suspending the testis in the scrotum and extending from the deep inguinal ring to the posterior aspect of the testis; the left cord is a little longer than the right. Between the superficial ring and testis the cord is anterior to the rounded tendon of adductor longus and is crossed here **anteriorly** by the *superficial* and **posteriorly** by the *deep* external pudendal arteries respectively. The cord traverses the inguinal canal (p. 829) with its walls as relations, the ilio-inguinal nerve being inferior. In the canal it acquires coverings from the layers of the abdominal wall, which extend into the scrotal wall as internal spermatic, cremasteric and external spermatic fasciae.

The *internal spermatic fascia* is a thin, loose layer around the spermatic cord, derived from the transversalis fascia (p. 829). The *cremasteric fascia* contains fasciculi of skeletal muscle united by loose connective tissue to form the cremaster; this is continuous with the obliquus internus abdominis (p. 824). The *external spermatic fascia*, a thin fibrous stratum continuous above with the aponeurosis of the obliquus externus abdominis, descends from the crura of the superficial ring (p. 829).

Vessels and nerves

The cord is composed of arteries, veins, lymph vessels, nerves and the deferent duct, conjoined by loose connective tissue.

Arteries. These are the testicular (p. 1557), cremasteric (p. 1563) and deferential (p. 1559).

Testicular veins. These are described on page 1600.
Lymph vessels of the testis. They are described on page 1623.
Nerves. They are the genital branch of the genitofemoral (p. 1279), the cremasteric nerve and the testicular sympathetic plexus (p. 1307), joined by filaments from the pelvic plexus accompanying the deferential artery.

SCROTUM

The scrotum, a cutaneous fibromuscular sac containing the testes and lower parts of the spermatic cords, hangs below the pubic symphysis between the anteromedial aspects of the thighs. It is divided into right and left halves by a cutaneous *raphe*, continued ventrally to the inferior penile surface and dorsally along the midline of the perineum to the anus; its left side is usually lower, in correspondence with the greater length of the left spermatic cord. The raphe indicates the bilateral origin of the scrotum from the genital swellings (p. 216). The external appearance varies: thus, when warm and in the elderly and debilitated, the scrotum is smooth, elongated and flaccid; but when cold and in the young and robust, it is short, corrugated and closely applied to the testes because of the contraction of the dartos muscle. It consists of skin, dartos muscle and external spermatic, cremasteric and internal spermatic fasciae. The internal spermatic fascia is loosely attached to the parietal layer of the tunica vaginalis (14.10).

The *scrotal skin*, thin, pigmented and often rugose, bears thinly scattered, crisp hairs, their roots visible through the skin; it has sebaceous glands, whose secretion has a characteristic odour, and also numerous sweat glands, pigment cells and nerve endings responding to mechanical stimulation of the hairs and skin and to variations in temperature. Subcutaneous adipose tissue is lacking.

The *dartos muscle* is a thin layer of smooth myocytes, continuous beyond the scrotum with the superficial inguinal and perineal fasciae, extending into a *scrotal septum*, connecting the raphe to the inferior surface of the penile radix and dividing the scrotum into two cavities. The septum contains all the layers of scrotal wall except skin. The dartos muscle is closely united to the skin, but is connected to subjacent parts by delicate loose connective tissue, giving it marked independence. Shafik (1977) has described a fibromuscular 'scrotal ligament' extending from the dartos sheet to the inferior testicular pole, regarding this as thermoregulatory (p. 1854).

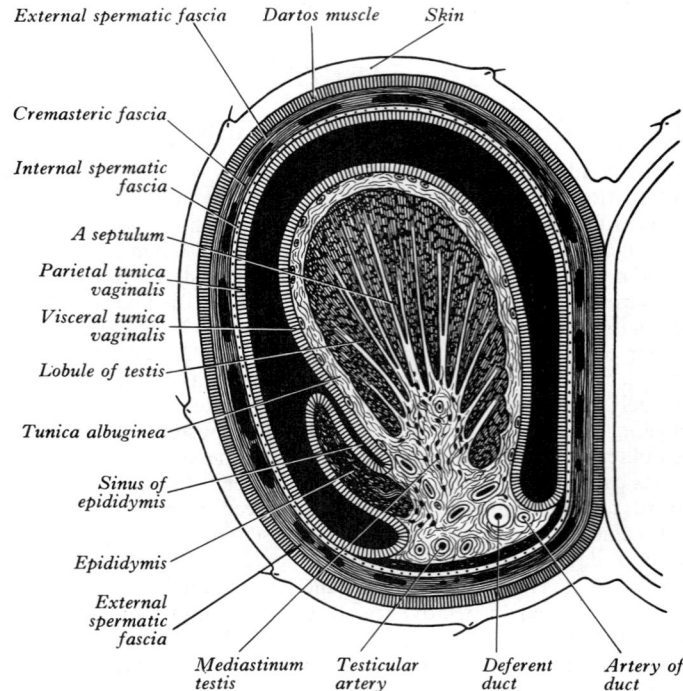

External spermatic fascia   Dartos muscle   Skin

Cremasteric fascia

Internal spermatic fascia

A septulum

Parietal tunica vaginalis

Visceral tunica vaginalis

Lobule of testis

Tunica albuginea

Sinus of epididymis

Epididymis

External spermatic fascia

Mediastinum testis   Testicular artery   Deferent duct   Artery of duct

14.10 Diagrammatic transverse section through the left half of the scrotum and the left testis. The tunica vaginalis is represented as artificially distended to show its visceral and parietal layers.

Vessels and nerves

Arteries supplying the scrotum. These are: the external pudendal branches of the femoral (p. 1566), the scrotal branches of the internal pudendal (p. 1561) and a cremasteric branch from the inferior epigastric (p. 1563). Dense subcutaneous plexuses of scrotal vessels carry a substantial blood flow effecting loss of heat (Esser 1932). Arteriovenous anastomoses of a simple but large-calibre type are also prominent (Molyneux 1965 and p. 1854).

Veins. These follow the corresponding arteries.

Lymph vessels. These end in the inguinal lymph nodes (p. 1623).

Nerves. These are: the ilio-inguinal and the genital branch of the genitofemoral (p. 1279), the two posterior scrotal branches of the perineal (p. 1288) and the perineal branch of the posterior femoral cutaneous nerve (p. 1283). The scrotum's anterior third is supplied mainly from the first lumbar spinal segment (by way of the ilio-inguinal and genitofemoral nerves), while the posterior two-thirds innervation comes mainly from the third sacral (via the perineal and posterior femoral cutaneous nerves). The ventral axial line of the lower limb (p. 1290) passes between these areas. A spinal anaesthetic, therefore, must be injected much higher to anaesthetize the anterior region.

PENIS

The penis, the male copulatory organ, comprises an attached *radix* or *root* in the perineum and a free, normally pendulous *corpus* or *body* completely enveloped in skin.

Radix of the penis

The radix of the penis comprises the three masses of erectile tissue in the urogenital triangle: the two crura and the bulb of the penis, firmly attached to the pubic arch and perineal membrane respectively. The crura are the posterior regions of the corpora cavernosa and the bulb, the posterior end of the corpus spongiosum.

Each *crus penis* (**14**.11) commences behind as a blunt, elongate but rounded process, attached firmly to the everted edge of the ischiopubic ramus and covered by the ischiocavernosus (p. 833). Anteriorly it converges towards its fellow and is slightly enlarged posterior to this. Near the inferior symphyseal border the two crura bend sharply down and forwards to become the corpora cavernosa.

The *bulb of the penis* (**13**.1, **14**.11) lies between the crura and is firmly connected to the inferior aspect of the perineal membrane, from which it receives a fibrous covering. Oval in section, the bulb narrows anteriorly into the corpus spongiosum, bending sharply down and forwards at this point. Its convex superficial surface is covered by bulbospongiosus; its flattened deep surface is pierced above its centre by the urethra, which traverses it to reach the corpus spongiosum. This part of the urethra has an intrabulbar fossa (p. 1843).

Corpus of the penis

The corpus of the penis contains three elongated erectile masses, capable of much enlargement when engorged with blood during erection. When flaccid it is cylindrical, but when erect it is triangular with rounded angles (**14**.12). The surface which is posterosuperior during erection is termed the *dorsum of the penis* and the opposite aspect the *urethral surface*. The erectile masses are termed the right and left corpora cavernosa, and the median corpus spongiosum penis, continuations of the crura and bulbus penis.

The *corpora cavernosa penis* form most of the corpus. In close apposition throughout, they have a common fibrous envelope and are separated only by a median fibrous septum. On the urethal surface their combined mass has a wide median groove, adjoining the corpus spongiosum (**14**.12); dorsally a similar but narrower groove contains the deep dorsal vein. The corpora end distally in the hollow, proximal aspect of the glans penis in a rounded cone, on which each has a small terminal projection (**14**.11). They are enclosed in a strong fibrous *tunica albuginea*, consisting of superficial and deep strata. The superficial fibres are longitudinal, forming a single tube round both corpora; the deep fibres are circularly orientated and surround each corpus separately, joining together as a median *septum of the penis*, which is thick and complete proximally

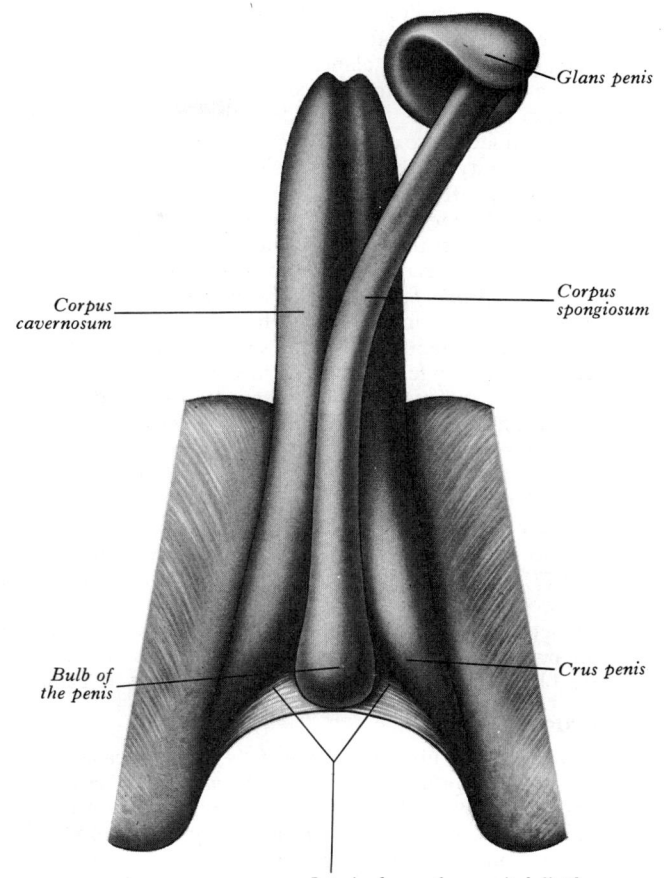

14.11 Ventral aspect of the constituent erectile masses of the penis in erect position. The glans penis and the distal part of the corpus spongiosum are shown detached from the corpora cavernosa penis and turned to the left.

but imperfect distally where it consists of a pectiniform (comb-like) series of bands; hence the term *pectiniform septum*.

The *corpus spongiosum penis*, traversed by the urethra, adjoins the median groove on the urethral surface of the conjoined corpora cavernosa. It is cylindrical, tapering slightly distally, and surrounded by a tunica albuginea. Near the end of the penis it expands into a somewhat conical enlargement like an acorn, whence its name, glans penis (**14**.11).

The *glans penis* projects dorsally over the end of the corpora cavernosa, with a shallow concave surface to which they are attached. Its base has a projecting *corona glandis*, overhanging an obliquely grooved *neck of the penis*. The navicular fossa (p. 1843) of the urethra is in the glans and opens by a sagittal slit on or near its apex.

Penile skin is remarkably thin, dark and loosely connected to the tunica albuginea. At the neck of the penis it is folded to form the

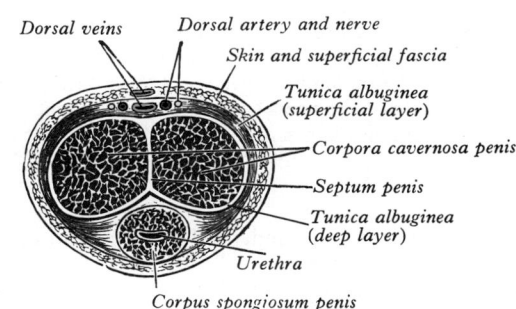

14.12 Transverse section of human penis.

prepuce or foreskin, variably overlapping the glans. The internal preputial layer is confluent at the neck with the thin skin covering and firmly adherent to the glans, and by this with the urethral mucosa at the external urethral orifice. On the urethral aspect of the glans a median fold passes from the deep surface of the prepuce to the glans immediately proximal to the orifice; this is the *frenulum*. Cutaneous sensitivity, high on the general surface of the glans, is accentuated near the frenulum. The prepuce and glans penis enclose a potential cleft, the *preputial sac*, with two shallow fossae flanking the frenulum. On the corona glandis and penile neck are numerous small *preputial glands*, secreting sebaceous *smegma*.

The *superficial penile fascia*, which is devoid of fat, consists of loose connective tissue, invaded by a few fibres of dartos muscle from the scrotum (p. 1856). As in the suprapubic abdominal wall, the deepest layer is condensed here as the *fascia penis* surrounding both the corpora cavernosa and corpus spongiosum and separating the superficial and deep dorsal veins. At the penile neck it blends with the fibrous covering of all three corpora. Proximally, it is continuous with the dartos muscle and with the fascia covering the urogenital region of the perineum (p. 1856).

The corpus penis is supported by two ligaments continuous with its fascia and consisting largely of elastin fibres. The *fundiform ligament* (7.77), stemming from the lowest part of the linea alba, splits into two lamellae which skirt the penis and unite below with the scrotal septum. The triangular *suspensory ligament*, deep to the fundiform ligament, is attached above to the front of the pubic symphysis, blending below, on each side, with the fascia penis.

Microstructure

From the inside of the fibrous sheaths of the corpora cavernosa and the sides of their septum numerous *trabeculae* arise, crossing the corpora cavernosa in all directions and dividing them into a series of *cavernous spaces*, which give them a spongy form (14.12). These trabeculae are composed of collagen and elastin fibres and smooth myocytes and contain numerous vessels and nerves. The cavernous spaces are filled with blood during erection, but many are empty in the flaccid penis. They are lined by flat endothelial cells without fenestrae (Leeson & Leeson 1965).

The fibrous tunica albuginea of the corpus spongiosum is thinner, whiter, more elastic than that of the corpora cavernosa and is formed partly of smooth myocytes; a layer of the same tissue surrounds the urethral epithelium (p. 1843).

Vessels and nerves

Arteries. Those supplying the cavernous spaces are the deep arteries of the penis (p. 1561), and branches of the dorsal penile arteries which perforate the tunica albuginea along the dorsum, especially near the glans. On entry the cavernous arteries divide into branches running in the trabeculae, some ending in capillary networks opening into the cavernous spaces. Others become convoluted and somewhat dilated *helicine arteries* which open into the cavernous spaces, and from these capillary branches supply the trabeculae. Helicine arteries are most abundant in the posterior regions of the corpora cavernosa (Alvarez-Morujo 1968).

Veins. These drain the cavernous spaces by means of a series of vessels, some emerging from the base of the glans and converging on the dorsum penis to form the deep dorsal vein, others leaving the corpora cavernosa to join the same vein; some also emerge inferiorly from the corpora cavernosa and, receiving tributaries from the corpus spongiosum, curve round to the deep dorsal vein, but many leave at the root of the penis to join the prostatic plexus (p. 1599).

Lymph vessels. These are described on page 1623.

Nerves. These come from the second, third and fourth sacral spinal segments via the pudendal nerve and pelvic plexuses (p. 1287). On the glans and bulb of the penis some cutaneous filaments connect with lamellated corpuscles and many end in characteristic end bulbs (p. 963).

Erection

Erection is purely vascular and independent of compression by the ischiocavernosi and bulbospongiosus. Rapid inflow from the helicine arteries fills the cavernous spaces and the resulting distension also contributes to erection by pressure on the veins which drain the erectile tissue. Cutaneous stimulation of the glans and frenulum contributes much to maintaining erection and to initiation of orgasm and ejaculation.

ACCESSORY GLANDULAR STRUCTURES

SEMINAL VESICLES

The two seminal vesicles (**14**.8, 9) are sacculated, contorted tubes located between the bladder and rectum. Each vesicle is about 5 cm long, somewhat pyramidal, the base being directed up and posterolaterally. Essentially, the seminal vesicle is a single coiled tube with irregular diverticula (**14**.9); the coils and diverticula are connected by fibrous tissue. The diameter of the tube is 3–4 mm and its uncoiled length is from 10–15 cm. The upper pole is a cul-de-sac, the lower narrowing to a straight duct, which joins the deferent duct to form the ejaculatory duct. The *anterior surface* contacts the posterior aspect of the bladder, extending from near the entry of the ureter to the prostatic base. The *posterior surface* is related to the rectum, separated from it by rectovesical fascia. The seminal vesicles diverge superiorly, are related to the deferent ducts and the terminations of the ureters and are partly covered by peritoneum; each has a dense, fibromuscular sheath. Along the medial margin of each vesicle is the ampulla of a deferent duct. Lateral are the veins of the prostatic venous plexus draining posteriorly to the internal iliac veins.

Microstructure and function

The seminal vesicle is a gland which appeared late in the evolution of placental mammals. It plays an important role in human fertility, affecting not only the maturation and mobility of the spermatozoa but also having an immunosuppressive action on the female genital tract (Clavert et al 1990). Together with the ampulla of the vas deferens and the ejaculatory ducts, the seminal vesicles form a functional unit that develops slowly until the onset of puberty, after which the vesicles form sac-like structures which contribute about 70% of the seminal fluid. They are also capable of fluid reabsorption and of spermophagy. The seminal vesicles are mainly concerned with the following: formation of seminal coagulum, modifications of sperm activity (e.g. motility and capacitation) and immunosuppression. Their secretory products include potassium ions, water, fructose, prostaglandins, endorphin, transferrin, lactoferrin, fibronectin, specific proteins such as semenogelin, sperm motility inhibitor, carbonic anhydrase and 5'-nucleotidase. The secretory capacity of the seminal vesicles is a measure of the testosterone level, while secretory activity is controlled by cholinergic, postganglionic sympathetic and possibly also parasympathetic nerve fibres derived from the pelvic plexus (see below). For a review of the morphology and functions of the human seminal vesicles, see Aumuller and Riva (1992).

The wall of the seminal vesicle has three layers: external connective tissue, middle **muscular** (thinner than in the deferent duct and arranged in external longitudinal and internal circular layers) and an internal **mucosal** layer with a reticular structure. The columnar epithelium of the mucosa contains goblet cells in the diverticula, the secretion of which forms much of the *seminal fluid*. The vesicles are **not** reservoirs for spermatozoa, these being stored in the epididymis (and possibly the ampulla of the deferent duct). The vesicles contract during ejaculation, their secretion forming most of the ejaculate.

Electron microscopy of human vesicular mucosa reveals a second epithelial type among the columnar, a small stellate cell, usually between the basal parts of the columnar cells, containing few cytoplasmic organelles. The columnar cells have microvilli, contain numerous mitochondria, a well-developed granular endoplasmic reticulum and a Golgi apparatus, associated with numerous secretory vacuoles (Riva 1967).

Vessels and nerves

Arteries of the seminal vesicles. These are derived from the inferior vesical and middle rectal arteries.

Veins and lymph vessels. They accompany the arteries.

Nerves. They are derived from the pelvic plexuses.

Clinical anatomy

The seminal vesicles can be palpated per rectum. Abscesses in them may rupture into the peritoneal cavity.

PROSTATE

The prostate (**10**.130, **13**.38, **14**.8, 9) is a firm, partly glandular, partly fibromuscular body, surrounding the beginning of the male urethra. It lies at a low level in the lesser pelvis, behind the inferior border of the symphysis pubis and pubic arch and anterior to the rectal ampulla, through which it may be palpated. Being somewhat conical, it presents: above, a base or vesical aspect; below, an apex and also a posterior, an anterior and two inferolateral surfaces.

The *base* is largely contiguous with the neck of the bladder above it; the urethra enters here, nearer its anterior border. The *apex* is inferior and in contact with the fascia on the superior aspects of the sphincter urethrae and transversi perinei profundi (p. 834).

The *posterior surface*, transversely flat and vertically convex, is separated from the rectum by the prostatic sheath and loose connective tissue external to the sheath. Near its superior (juxtavesical) border is a depression where the two ejaculatory ducts penetrate the gland, dividing this surface into a superior and an inferior, larger part. The superior part is variable in size and usually regarded as the external aspect of the *median lobe*; the inferior part shows a shallow, median sulcus, usually considered to mark a partial separation into *right* and *left lateral lobes*, forming the main prostatic mass and continuous behind the urethra. A band of fibromuscular tissue, ventral to the urethra, joins these lobes together and is often referred to as the anterior lobe; it contains less glandular tissue than the rest of the gland.

This simplified view of prostatic lobation, based mainly on the classic work of Lowsley (1912), is retained here despite many modifications introduced by subsequent observers, with persistent confusions and inconsistencies which have not yet been completely resolved. Some deny any topographical lobation and those who favour it differ on boundaries and terminology. McNeal (1975) has analysed these disagreements. Lobation became important through the conviction among some investigators that malignant tumours occur in particular prostatic regions. This interest prompted the work of Tisell and Salander (1975) who claim to have confirmed a recognizable lobar structure after dissection of more than 100 human prostate glands. They recognize two large *lateral lobes*, but consider that these do not appear on the dorsal (rectal) aspect, which they describe as occupied by paired *dorsal lobes* extending laterally to form the apex. They recognize *median lobes*, around the urethra (except at the apex), deep to the dorsal and lateral lobes; their median lobes may be equated with the *internal zone* described below. All three pairs of lobes are, they affirm, separable by dissection. It is impossible to reconcile the differences between this and other descriptions and the question of lobation must be left sub judice (Goland 1975). For a more recent discussion of the problem of prostatic nomenclature, refer to Benoit et al (1993).

The *anterior surface*, transversely narrow and convex, extends from the apex to the base, about 2 cm behind the pubic symphysis from which it is separated by a venous plexus and loose adipose tissue. Near its superior limit it is connected to the pubic bones by the puboprostatic ligaments. The urethra emerges from this surface anterosuperior to the apex of the gland.

The *inferolateral surfaces* are related to the anterior parts of the levatores ani, which are separated from them by a plexus of veins embedded in the fibrous prostatic sheath.

The prostatic base measures about 4 cm transversely, the gland being about 2 cm in anteroposterior and 3 cm in its vertical diameters. It weighs about 8 g. It has a fibrous sheath, partly vascular; on each side this consists of fibrous tissue containing the prostatic venous plexus (**10**.179); anteriorly it blends with the puboprostatic ligaments (p. 1838) and inferiorly with fascia on the deep surfaces of the sphincter urethrae, the deep transverse perineal muscles and with the perineal body. Posteriorly the sheath has a different origin and is avascular. In male fetuses, at the fourth month, the rectovesical peritoneal pouch descends to the pelvic floor, separating prostate from rectum; its lower part is obliterated and the fused peritoneal layers here form the posterior prostatic sheath (Smith 1908a,b), sometimes termed the *rectovesical fascia*. Traces of its separate layers

persist as a plane of cleavage. Above, it ascends over the posterior aspects of the seminal vesicles and deferent ducts and is connected to the floor of the rectovesical pouch; on each side, it joins with the posterior vesical ligament (p. 1838). Below, adherent to the prostate, it joins the perineal body. Some have denied this peritoneal fusion and consider the rectovesical fascia to be a condensation of connective tissue (Silver 1956). The anterior parts of the levatores ani pass back from the pubis around the prostate as *levatores prostatae*.

The prostate is traversed by the urethra and ejaculatory ducts, and contains the prostatic utricle. The urethra usually passes between its anterior and middle thirds. The ejaculatory ducts pass antero-inferiorly through its posterior region to open into the prostatic urethra (p. 1842).

Microstructure (14.13, 14)

The prostate is grey to reddish according to its activity, and very dense. It is enveloped in a thin, but strong fibrous capsule within a sheath derived from pelvic fascia, the latter containing a venous plexus. The capsule is firmly adherent to the gland and continuous

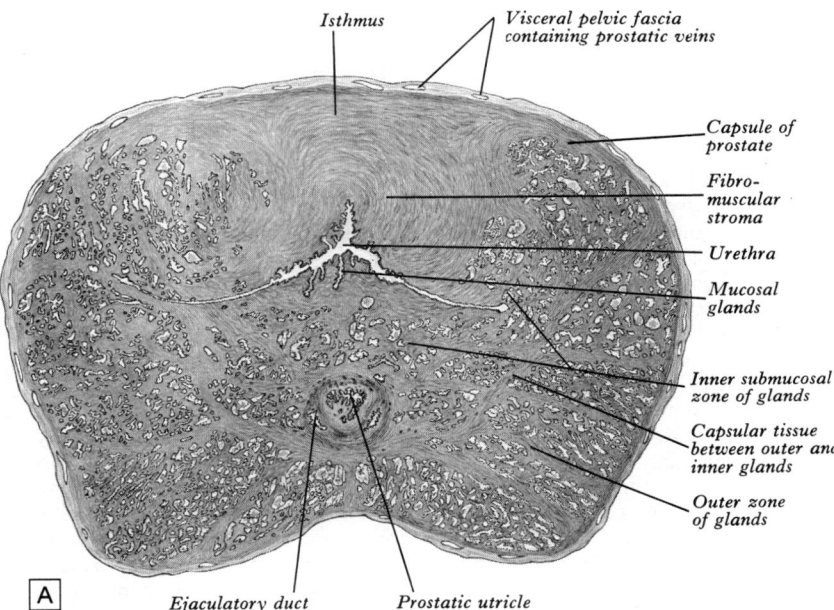

Isthmus   *Visceral pelvic fascia containing prostatic veins*

Capsule of prostate

Fibro-muscular stroma

Urethra

Mucosal glands

Inner submucosal zone of glands

Capsular tissue between outer and inner glands

Outer zone of glands

Ⓐ   *Ejaculatory duct*   *Prostatic utricle*

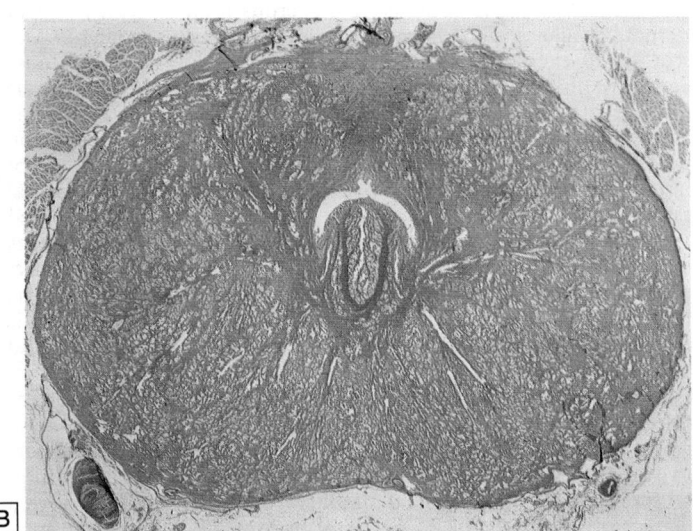

Ⓑ

14.13A, B Human prostate. A Transverse section at a level to show the prostatic utricle and ejaculatory ducts. B Transverse section to show the urethral crest. Compare with A and see text for further details. Both A and B are slightly more than twice the natural size. Ventral is to the top in both figures. (Stained by haematoxylin and eosin and lent by L M Franks, Imperial Cancer Research Institute, London, and photographed by K Fitzpatrick.)

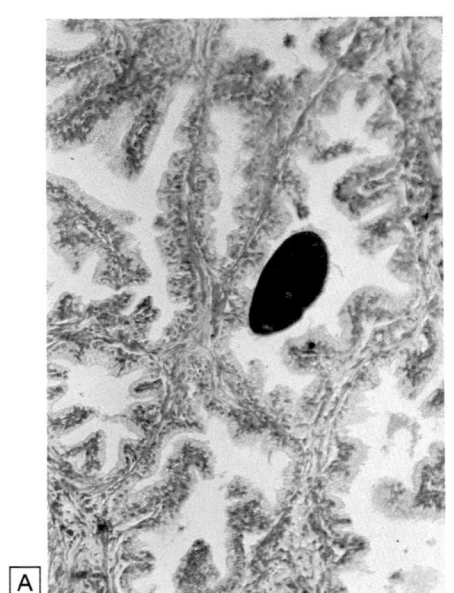

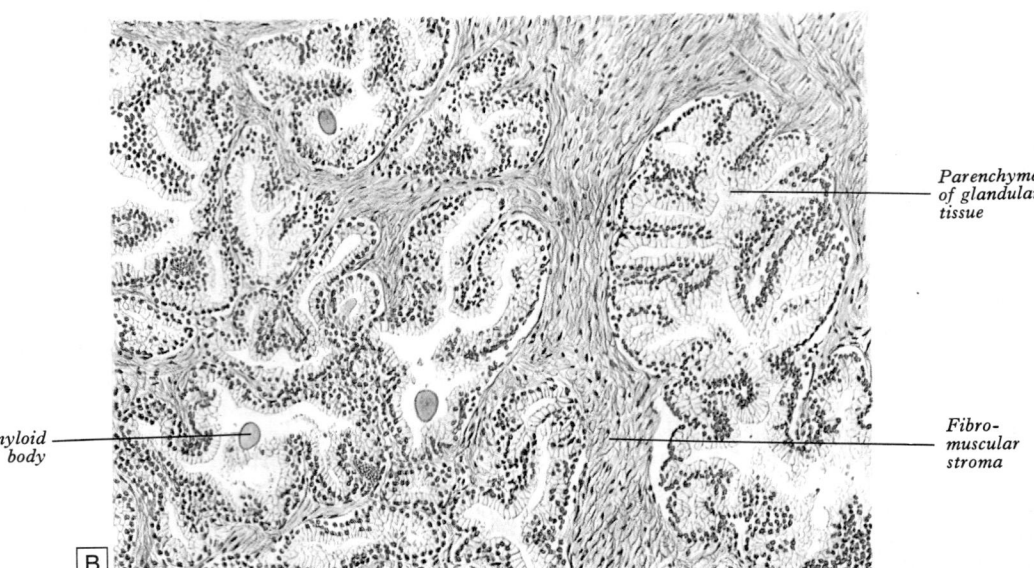

*Parenchyma
of glandular
tissue*

*Amyloid
body*

*Fibro-
muscular
stroma*

14.14A, B Characteristic fields of the human prostate. Note the highly convoluted columnar epithelium, forming papillary projections into the lumen of a follicle, and abundant interfollicular fibromuscular tissue. (Specimen shown in A provided by Abla el Nasser 1980.)

with a median septum in the urethral crest separating the lateral masses below the level of the colliculus seminalis. It is also continuous with numerous fibromuscular septa enmeshing the glandular tissue.

The *muscular tissue* is mainly smooth (Hutch & Rambo 1970); ventral to the urethra a layer of smooth muscle curves to merge with the main mass of muscle in the fibromuscular septa; superiorly it is continuous with vesical smooth muscle. However, anterior to this a transversely crescentic mass of skeletal muscle is continuous inferiorly with the sphincter urethrae in the deep perineal pouch. Its fibres pass transversely internal to the capsule, attached to it laterally by diffuse collagen bundles; other collagen bundles pass posteromedially, merging with the prostatic fibromuscular septa and the septum of the urethral crest. This muscle, supplied by the pudendal nerve, probably compresses the urethra (Haines 1969) but it is suggested that it may pull the urethral crest back and the prostatic sinuses forwards, dilating the urethra; glandular contents may be expelled simultaneously into the urethra, thus expanded to contain seminal fluid (3–5 ml) during the period of sexual excitement prior to ejaculation.

The *glandular tissue* consists of numerous follicles with frequent internal papillae. Follicles open into elongated canals, which join to form 12–20 excretory ducts. The follicles are conjoined by loose connective tissue, supported by extensions of the fibrous capsule and muscular stroma and enclosed in a delicate capillary plexus. Canalicular and follicular epithelium is columnar; electron microscopy reveals luminal microvilli, relatively few short profiles of granular endoplasmic reticulum and some free ribosomes. Lysosomal vesicles, containing acid phosphatase, also occur. The apposed borders of these cells are mainly straight, the plasma membranes being united by desmosomes (Fisher & Jeffrey 1965). *Prostatic ducts* open mainly into the prostatic sinuses in the floor of the prostatic urethra; they have a bilaminar epithelium, the luminal layer is columnar and the basal has small cuboidal cells. Small colloid *amyloid bodies* often occur in the follicles. The prostatic and seminal vesicular secretions form the bulk of the seminal fluid. The former is slightly acid, containing acid phosphatase and fibrinolysin. Also present in the glandular epithelium of the prostate gland are numerous endocrine cells containing neuron-specific enolase, chromogranin and serotonin (Wernert et al 1990). A morphometric analysis carried out recently by Battaglia et al (1994) in prostate glands from men aged 17–74 years showed that the prostatic endocrine cell density, assessed in terms of number of endocrine cells per millimetre of epithelial length, was greatest in the 25–54 age group.

Histological sections (**14.**13A, B) do not show a lobar pattern, but two concentric zones of glandular tissue, being partially circumurethral, are distinguishable (Le Duc 1939; Franks 1954; Fergusson & Gibson 1956). The larger *peripheral zone* has long, branched glands, whose ducts curve posteriorly to open mainly into the prostatic sinuses, though a few open on the lateral urethral walls. The *internal zone* consists of 'submucosal' glands, with ducts opening on the floor of the prostatic sinuses and colliculus seminalis and an **innermost** group of simple 'mucosal' glands, surrounding the upper prostatic urethra. Anteriorly, in the prostatic isthmus (**14.**13A), the peripheral zone and 'submucosal' glands are absent. Peripheral and internal zones are said to be separated by an ill-defined 'capsule'. Carcinoma affects almost exclusively the peripheral zone, the internal being prone to benign hypertrophy, such enlargements projecting into the bladder, displacing the peripheral zone postero-inferiorly and thus accentuating the 'capsule' between outer and inner zones. This provides a 'cleavage plane' which is used in surgical enucleation.

Vessels and nerves

Arteries (Clegg 1955, 1956). These are rami of the internal pudendal, inferior vesical and middle rectal arteries.

Veins. They form a plexus around the prostatic sides and base (p. 1599), receiving in front the deep dorsal penile vein and draining to the internal iliac veins.

Lymph vessels. These are described on page 1623.

Nerves. They come from the inferior hypogastric (pelvic) plexus (p. 1308). The prostatic nerve supply is very abundant, the periurethral zone being innervated by nerves arising peripherally. The prostatic capsule is covered by numerous nerve fibres and ganglia, forming a periprostatic nerve plexus (Benoit et al 1994). In the normal human prostate the greatest density of nerves is found in the proximal central prostate, followed by the anterior capsule and distal prostate, the least density being in the peripheral prostate (Chapple et al 1991). Neuropeptide Y and vasointestinal polypeptide nerve fibres are localized in the subepithelial connective tissue, in the smooth muscle layers of the gland and in the walls of its blood vessels (Lange & Unger 1990).

Age changes in the prostate

At birth, the prostate has a system of ducts embedded in a stroma which forms a large part of the gland. Follicles are represented by small end-buds on the ducts (Swyer 1944). The hyperplasia and squamous metaplasia of the epithelium of the ducts, colliculus seminalis and prostatic utricle which preceded birth, possibly due to maternal oestrogens in the fetal blood, subside and a regression period after birth is followed by a period of quiescence lasting for 12–14 years.

At puberty, between the ages of approximately 14 and 18, the prostate gland enters a maturation phase and in approximately 12 months during this time, it more than doubles in size, due almost entirely to follicular development, partly from end-buds on ducts and partly from modification of the ductal branches. Morphogenesis and differentiation of the epithelial cords starts in an intermediate part of the epithelial anlage and proceeds to the urethral and subcapsular parts of the gland, the latter being reached by the age of 17–18 years (Aumuller 1991). Initially multilayered squamous or cuboidal, the glandular epithelium is transformed into a pseudo-stratified epithelium consisting of basal, exocrine secretory (including mucous) and neuroendocrine cells. The mucous cells are temporary, and are lost as the gland matures. The remaining exocrine secretory cells produce a number of products including acid phosphatase, prostate specific antigen and β-microseminoprotein. Immature glandular pouches are immunopositive for basic fibroblast growth factor (b-FGF), the role of which remains to be established (Aumuller 1991). This growth of the secretory component is associated with a condensation of the stroma, which diminishes relative to the glandular tissue. These changes are probably due to the secretion of testosterone by the testis.

During the third decade the glandular epithelium grows by irregular multiplication of the epithelial infoldings into the lumen of the follicles.

After the third decade the size remains virtually unaltered until 45–50 years, when the epithelial foldings tend to disappear, follicular outlines become more regular and amyloid bodies increase in number. All these changes are signs of prostatic involution.

After 45–50 years the prostate may undergo benign hypertrophy, increasing in size until death, or alternatively it may undergo progressive atrophy.

Clinical aspects of the prostate

After middle age the prostate often enlarges, projecting into the bladder to impede urination by distorting the prostatic urethra. The median lobe may enlarge the most, with even a small enlargement obstructing the internal urethral orifice; the more the patient strains, the more the prostatic mass, acting like a valve, blocks the opening.

The hypertrophied part may be removed surgically (prostatectomy).

Valveless venous communications between the prostatic and extra-dural venous plexuses normally occur, probably an important factor in the metastasis of prostatic neoplasms to the vertebral bodies (Batson 1940; Franks 1953).

BULBO-URETHRAL GLANDS

The two bulbo-urethral glands (3.89), small, round, yellow, somewhat lobulated masses about a centimetre in diameter, lie lateral to the membranous urethra above the perineal membrane and penile bulb and are enclosed by fibres of the sphincter urethrae. They gradually diminish in size in the later decades. The excretory duct of each, almost 3 cm long, passes obliquely forwards external to the mucosa of the membranous urethra and penetrates the inferior urogenital fascia (perineal membrane) to open by a minute orifice on the floor of the spongiose urethra about 2.5 cm below the perineal membrane.

Structure

Each gland consists of several lobules held together by a fibrous capsule. Its secretory units are mainly tubulo-alveolar in form. The glandular epithelium, which is columnar, secretes acid and neutral mucosubstances, and is immunopositive for a number of androgen metabolic enzymes including 17 β-hydroxysteroid dehydrogenase (Sirigu et al 1993) and blood group antigens (Riva et al 1990). Vasoactive intestinal polypeptide (VIP)-positive nerve fibres have been observed around the secretory units (Sirigu et al 1993), the products of which are added to the seminal fluid prior to ejaculation. The main secretory duct is lined by a stratified columnar epithelium of 6 or 7 layers, the superficial, adluminal cells of which contain secretory granules and presumably contribute to the secretions produced by these glands (Riva et al 1990).

Diffuse lymphoid tissue is associated with the glands (Migliari et al 1992); almost all the intraepithelial lymphocytes observed were reported to be cytotoxic (CD8+) T cells and B cells; monocytes and macrophages were also present within the gland. The role of immunocompetent cells found in these glands in combating infections or other genitourinary diseases requires clarification.

REPRODUCTIVE ORGANS OF THE FEMALE

The female reproductive system consists of the internal and external genitalia. The *internal organs* situated within the lesser pelvis, are the ovaries, uterine tubes, uterus and vagina. The *external organs* lying in front of and below the pubic arch, are the mons pubis, labia majora and labia minora pudendi, clitoris, bulb of the vestibule, greater vestibular glands and the vestibule itself.

OVARIES

The ovaries are paired structures (14.15–18, 27), homologous with the testes, developing like them from the genital ridges (p. 208). Situated one on each side of the uterus close to the lateral pelvic wall, they are attached to the posterior aspect of the broad uterine ligament of the uterus near its upper limit by a double fold of peritoneum, the *mesovarium*, behind and mainly below the lateral part of the uterine tube (14.16). In the living they are greyish-pink and present a smooth exterior before regular ovulation begins, but thereafter their surfaces are distorted by the scarring which follows the degeneration of successive corpora lutea. Each ovary is classically described as almond-shaped (amygdaloid), about 3 cm long, 1.5 cm wide and 1 cm thick, with a volume of approximately 6 cm³. (However, ultrasonic measurements of the ovaries in situ, in a large number of women (Cohen et al 1990) have given higher values for the volume of the ovaries: about 11 cm³ in the reproductively mature state, 6 cm³ postmenopausally and 3 cm³ before menarche (the first menstrual period).) Ovarian position varies much in women who have borne children; the ovaries are displaced in the first pregnancy and usually never return to their original location. They are also

variably mobile and may change their position to some extent according to the state of the surrounding organs such as the intestines. The description given in the subsequent account refers to the ovarian condition in nulliparous women, except where otherwise stated.

With the body in the upright position, the long axis of each ovary is vertical (contrasting with the horizontal or oblique orientation which it may assume in parous women: compare 14.15 and 14.16); it has lateral and medial surfaces, tubal (superior) and uterine (inferior) extremities or poles, and mesovarian (anterior) and free (posterior) borders. It occupies the *ovarian fossa*, on the lateral pelvic wall, bounded anteriorly by the obliterated umbilical artery and posteriorly by the ureter and internal iliac artery.

Attached to its upper, *tubal extremity*, near the external iliac vein, are the ovarian fimbria of the uterine tube and a peritoneal *suspensory ligament of the ovary*, which contains the ovarian vessels and nerves and passes superiorly over the external iliac vessels (14.15) to join the peritoneum on psoas major, posterior to the caecum or descending colon (depending on whether it is right or left). The *uterine (inferior) extremity* is directed downwards towards the pelvic floor; it is usually narrower than the tubal extremity and is attached to the lateral angle of the uterus, postero-inferior to the uterine tube, by a rounded *ovarian ligament*, which lies in the broad ligament and contains some smooth muscle cells. The *lateral surface* of the ovary contacts parietal peritoneum in the ovarian fossa, behind which are extraperitoneal tissue and the obturator vessels and nerve. The uterine tube largely covers the *medial surface*; the peritoneal recess here, between the ovary and overlapping mesosalpinx (p. 1874), is termed the *ovarian bursa*.

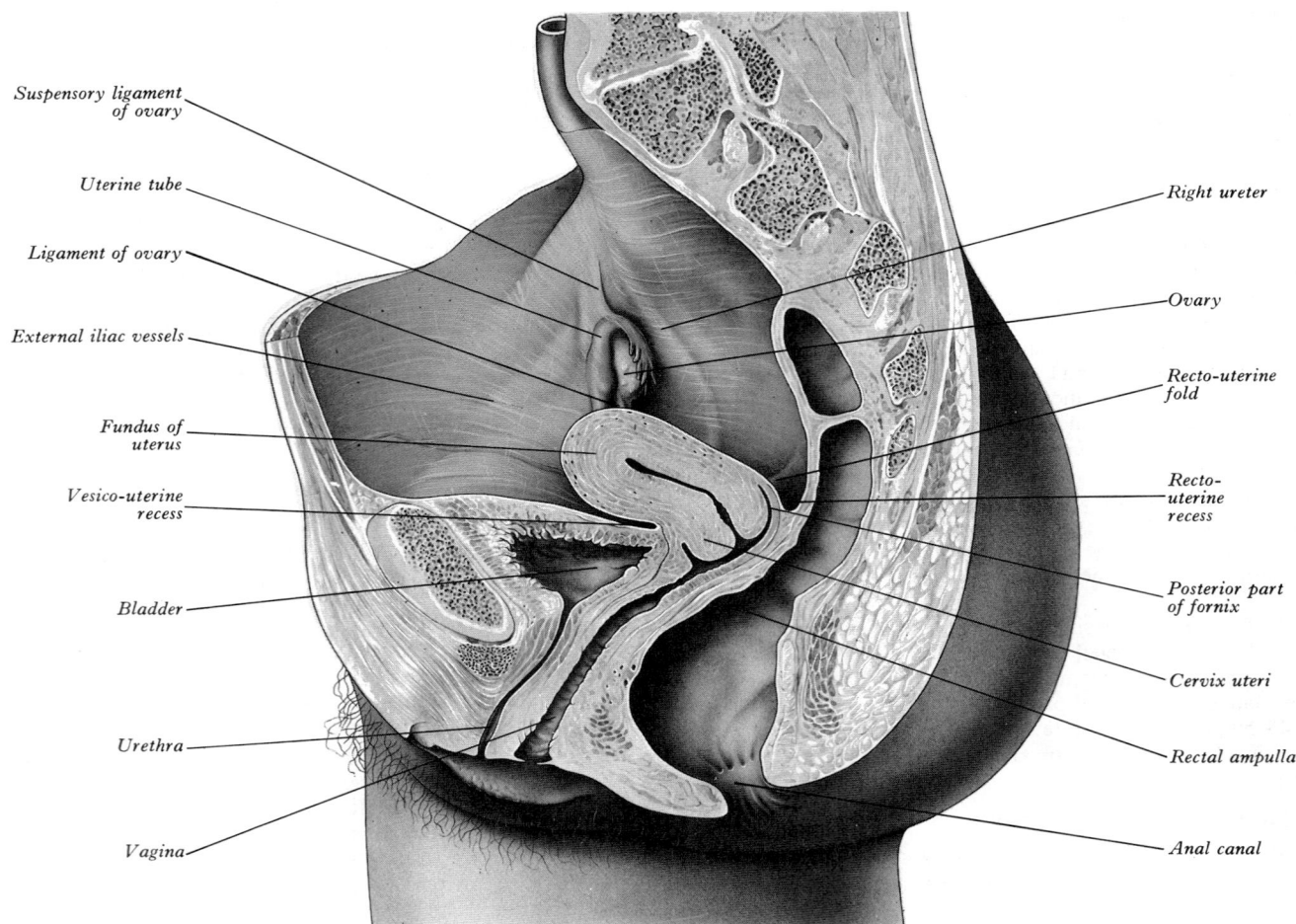

14.15A   Median sagittal section through a human female pelvis. The peritoneum is shown in blue.

Suspensory ligament of ovary

Uterine tube

Ligament of ovary

External iliac vessels

Fundus of uterus

Vesico-uterine recess

Bladder

Urethra

Vagina

Right ureter

Ovary

Recto-uterine fold

Recto-uterine recess

Posterior part of fornix

Cervix uteri

Rectal ampulla

Anal canal

The *mesovarian border* is straight and is directed towards the obliterated umbilical artery. It is attached to the back of the broad ligament by a short peritoneal fold, the *mesovarium*, in which blood vessels and nerves reach the ovarian hilum. The convex *free border* of the ovary faces the ureter. The uterine tube arches over the ovary, ascending in relation to its mesovarian border, to curve over its tubal end and pass down on its posterior, free border and medial surface (**14**.15).

In embryonic and early fetal life the ovaries are, like the testes, situated in the lumbar region near the kidneys, but they gradually descend into the lesser pelvis (p. 670). Accessory ovaries may occur in the mesovarium or in the adjacent part of the broad ligament.

MICROSTRUCTURE OF THE OVARY (**14**.17, 18)

The surface is covered, in young females, by a layer of *ovarian surface epithelium* consisting of a single layer of cuboidal and some flatter cells (see below). This gives the ovary a dull grey surface, contrasting with the shining, smooth peritoneum of the mesovarium; the transition between peritoneum and ovarian epithelium is usually marked by a white line around the anterior, mesovarian border. Immediately beneath the epithelium, the ovary is invested by a tough collagenous coat, the *tunica albuginea*, bounding the mass of the ovary; this is divisible into a *cortex* containing the ovarian follicles, and a *medulla* which receives the vessels and nerves at the hilum.

Ovarian cortex. After puberty the cortex forms the major part of the ovary, enclosing the medulla except at the hilum (**14**.17). It contains the *ovarian follicles* of various sizes and *corpora lutea* (and their degenerative remnants), depending on the stage of menstrual cycle or age. The follicles and their products are embedded in a dense fibrocellular *stroma* composed of interwoven, thin, collagen fibres and many fusiform, fibroblast-like or mesenchymal cells

arranged in characteristic swirls. Other tissue components include *interstitial cells*, these are common in the human ovary in the early period of life, and in many other mammalian species, but are said to persist in women after puberty only in the thecae of atretic follicles; their significance is uncertain.

Medulla. This central zone is highly vascular, consisting of numerous veins and spiral arteries set in a looser connective tissue stroma, with many elastin fibres, pericytes and some smooth muscle which enter the hilum from the mesovarium. The medulla is much more vascular than the cortex. Small numbers of cells with characteristics similar to interstitial (Leydig) cells in the testis also occur in the medulla. These are known as *chromaffin cells* (Berger, sympatheticotrophic cells): they may be a source of androgens. For further reviews of ovarian secretory tissues see Baird (1977).

Ovarian follicles

Primordial follicles (**14**.18A). The formation of the female gamete is a complex process with many different phases. At birth, the cortex contains a superficial zone of primordial follicles; these consist of primary oöcytes about 25 μm in diameter, each surrounded by a single layer of flat *follicular cells* derived from somatic tissue (their precise origins at present uncertain). The prenatal development of primordial follicles is described on page 208. Many degenerate during childhood, some in situ, others developing briefly then undergoing atresia, as also occurs each month during the child-bearing period of life. Their remnants are visible as *atretic follicles* which gradually disperse (see below), but whose remains accumulate throughout the ovary's active life. After puberty, relatively small numbers of primordial follicles undergo a series of developmental changes, and of these, usually only one follicle from either one or the other ovary comes to full maturity and releases its oöcyte (*ovulation*) for transport into the uterine tube, potentially for fertilization. For descriptive

1862

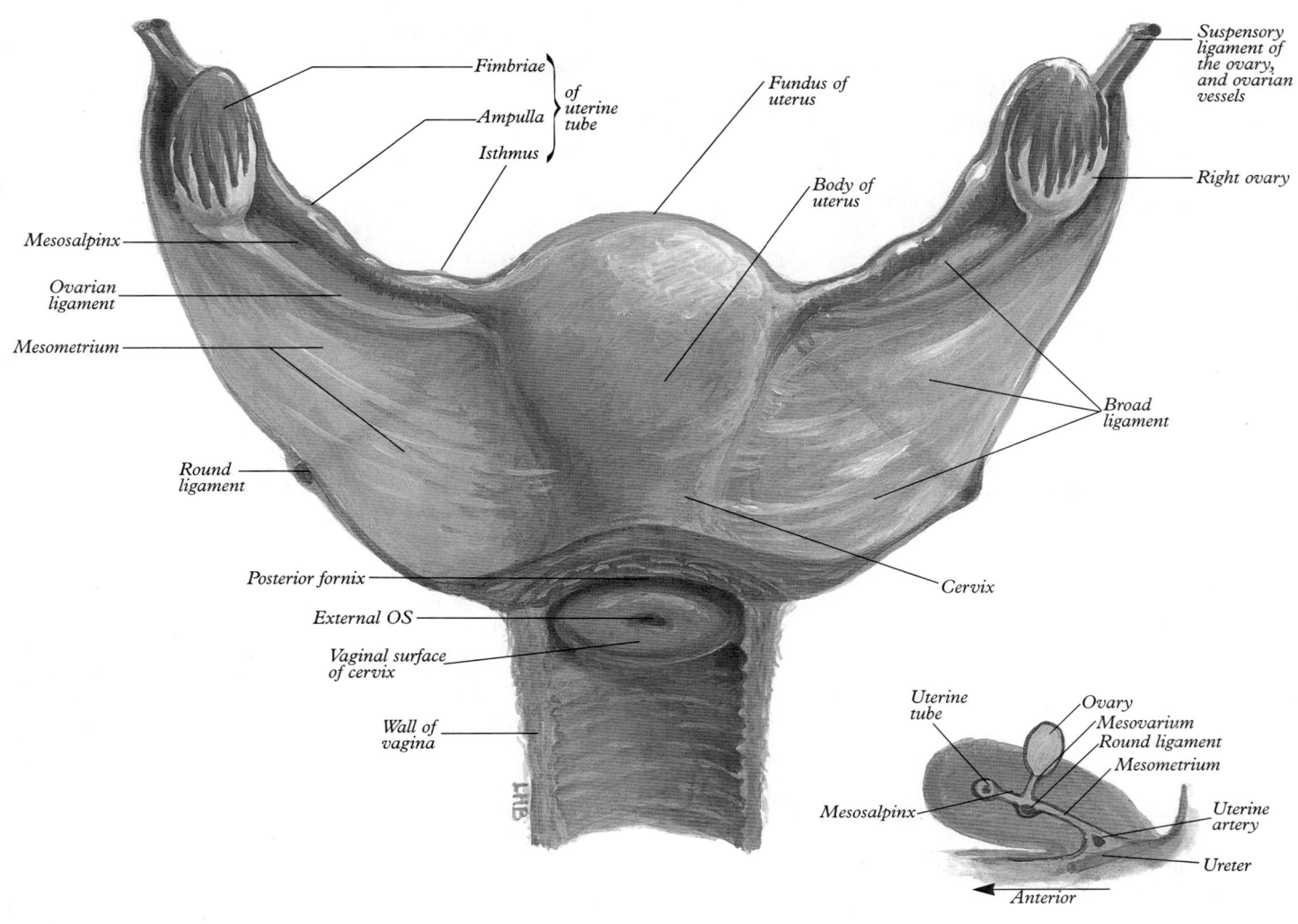

14.15B Schema showing the principal features of the female internal genital organs.

purposes the sequence is customarily divided into primary, secondary and tertiary follicular stages, according to detailed structure.

Primary follicle (**14**.18B). The first sign of follicular activation is the growth of the follicle cells from squamous to cuboidal, followed by their multiplication to form a multilayered mass, the membrana granulosa, surrounded by a thick basal lamina (membrana limitans externa). Stromal cells immediately surrounding the follicle begin to differentiate into spindle-shaped cells constituting the *internal theca*, and are later accompanied by another, more fibrous *external theca*. At the same time the oöcyte increases in size and a thick layer of extracellular proteoglycan-rich material, the *zona pellucida*, is secreted by the oöcyte between its surface and the surrounding granulosa cells. This is important for the process of fertilization (for details see p. 122). The follicular cells in contact with the zona send cytoplasmic processes radially inwards (see **3**.21A,B) to form gap junctions with the oöcyte plasma membrane, indicating a regulatory interaction between the two (for review, see Buccione et al 1990). The follicular cells continue to multiply, the small rounded products of division being termed *granulosa cells*. These are in functional contact with each other through gap junctions.

Secondary (antral) follicle (**14**.18C). As the mass of follicular cells continues to increase, fluid-filled cavities begin to form between them, containing a clear fluid (*liquor folliculi*) containing, amongst other components, hyaluran, growth factors and the hormonal secretions of the granulosa cells. The follicle is now about 200 μm.

These cavities fuse to form one large fluid-filled space (the *antrum folliculi*) surrounded by a thin layer of granulosa cells, thickened at one pole of the follicle to encompass the oöcyte in a mound of cells, the *cumulus ovaricus* (*cumulus oöphorus*) (**14**.18D). Among the granulosa cells are small numbers of various other cell types, including macrophages, which are a source of growth factors (Loukides et al 1990), and lymphocytes. Small densely staining *Call-Exner bodies* composed mainly of convoluted fragments of basal lamina (of unknown function) occur within the granulosa cell masses. The inner and outer thecae are now clearly differentiated. As follicles mature, the theca interna becomes more prominent ('thecal gland'). Its cells and those of the membrana granulosa produce oestrogenic hormones (primarily oestradiol), the follicular development being stimulated by the hypophyseal gonadotropic hormone (follicle-stimulating hormone; FSH).

Tertiary follicle (**14**.18E). Although a number of follicles may progress to the secondary stage by about the first week of a menstrual cycle, only one follicle from the two ovaries proceeds to the tertiary stage, the remainder becoming atretic. The 'chosen' follicle now increases in size considerably as the follicular antrum takes up fluid from the surrounding tissues and expands to a diameter of about 2 mm. The term Graafian follicle is often used of this stage (though sometimes also applied to the late secondary follicle). The oöcyte and its surrounding ring of cells (*corona radiata*) breaks away from the wall and now floats freely in the follicular fluid. How the choice

1863

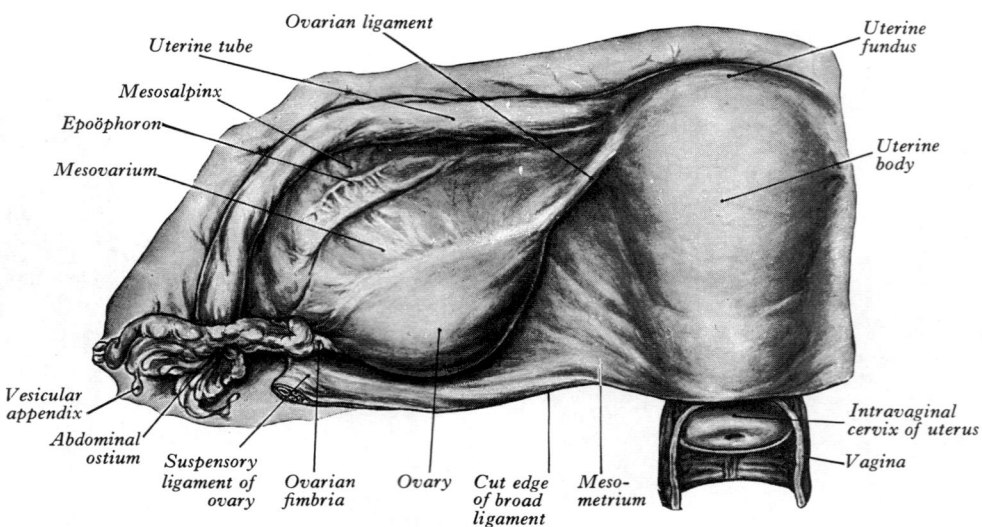

14.16A Posterosuperior aspect of the uterus and the left broad ligament. The 'ligament' has been spread out and the ovary is displaced downwards.

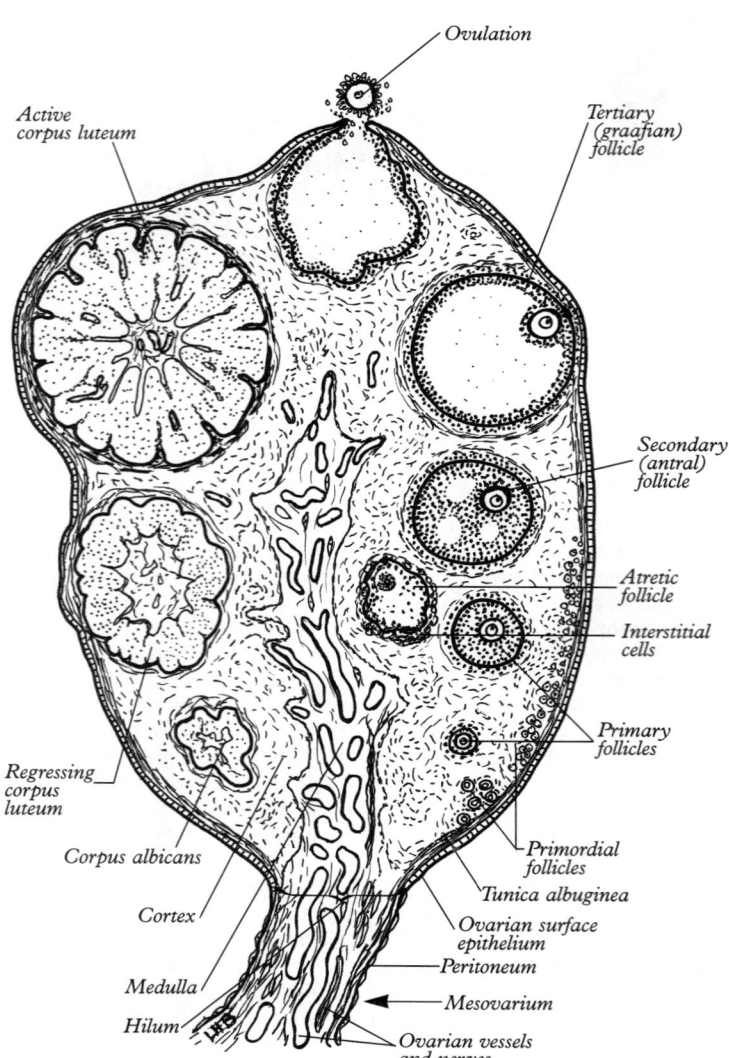

14.16B Schema of the internal structure of the ovary, depicted in section to show its major components.

of follicle is made between all the secondary follicles of the two ovaries is uncertain, but is thought to involve a complex interaction of hormones and locally produced regulatory factors (see Greenwald & Terranova 1988 for review), and presumably involves some form of inhibition of the majority; it is clear that the selective mechanism also occasionally varies to produce multiple, non-identical births, especially under therapeutic hormonal stimulation.

At this stage, the primary oöcyte, which has remained in the first meiotic prophase since fetal life, completes its first meiotic division to produce the almost equally large *secondary oöcyte* and a relatively minute *first polar body*, both of them now haploid. During this step the first meiotic spindle is orientated perpendicular to the oöcyte surface, which it approaches closely, so that the polar body is separated at the periphery of the oöcyte (still beneath the zona pellucida), with a nucleus and a minimal amount of cytoplasm (see also p. 122). The secondary oöcyte now immediately begins its second meiotic division, but when it reaches metaphase, this process is once again arrested, and the chromosome remains in this condition until fertilization has occurred, when it completes the divisional stage as a response to penetration by a sperm head, throwing off a second polar body during this process (p. 134). The follicle now moves to the surface of the cortex, causing the surface of the ovary to bulge. At the point of contact (the *stigma*) with the tough tunica albuginea and ovarian surface epithelium, these tissues are eroded and finally the follicle itself develops an aperture to release its contents into the peritoneal cavity. On release into the peritoneal cavity, the secondary oöcyte is still surrounded by its zona pellucida and corona radiata of granulosa cells. Ovulation is now complete, and the oöcyte is ready for transport to the uterine tube. During maturation the oöcyte grows from 25 μm in the primordial follicle to 100 μm in the mature follicle, as the numbers of organelles within it increase, including mitochondria, ribosomes, Golgic complexes, yolk platelets and, in its peripheral cytoplasm, cortical granules important in the fertilization process (see p. 122). If the oöcyte is not fertilized, it begins to degenerate after 24–48 hours. Ovulation usually occurs 12–16 days before the expected onset of a menstrual cycle. For further details of these processes, see page 121.

Atretic follicles. As noted above, the degeneration of pre-tertiary stage follicles is a major factor influencing the development of the ovary. Atresia occurs at all stages of oöcyte development, from the embryonic period onwards. As mentioned on page 121, the numbers of human oöcytes are reduced from a maximum of nearly 7 million at 5 months gestation to about 1 million at birth. Postnatally, further degeneration occurs so that by puberty only about 40 000 oöcytes remain (Pinkerton et al 1961; **3.18**). Oöcyte degeneration between birth and menarche is caused mainly by recruitment of oöcytes from the pool of primordial follicles, destined of course for atresia since there are no ovulations before puberty. Of the 40 000 oöcytes remaining at puberty only about 400 undergo ovulation during the reproductive years. The rest, after being activated to the primary or secondary follicle stage, degenerate as atretic follicles. The first sign of atresia is the appearance of pyknotic nuclei in the granulosa cell population which are thought to undergo programmed cell death (*apoptosis*: Tilly et al 1992). The remnant of the follicle is invaded by blood vessels, macrophages and connective tissue, which ultimately replaces it, converting it into a small white fibrous body. These terminal atretic follicles are distinct from the fibrotic remains of corpora lutea (corpora albicantia, see below).

Corpus luteum

After ovulation, the walls of the empty follicle collapse and fold extensively; the cells of the membrana granulosa increase in size and synthesize a cytoplasmic carotenoid pigment (lutein) giving them a yellowish colour (hence corpus luteum). These large (30–50 μm) cells, often termed *granulosa lutein cells* because of their proposed origins, form most of the corpus luteum (**14**.17, **18**). The basal lamina surrounding the follicle breaks down, allowing rather smaller (20 μm) though more numerous cells (probably derived from the theca, hence the term *theca lutein cells*; alternatively *paraluteal cells*), to infiltrate into the cellular mass, accompanied by capillaries and connective tissue. Extravasated blood derived from thecal capillaries accumulates in the centre as a small clot, but this quickly resolves and is replaced by connective tissue. It should be noted at this point that the nature and origins of the two types of lutein cells are still

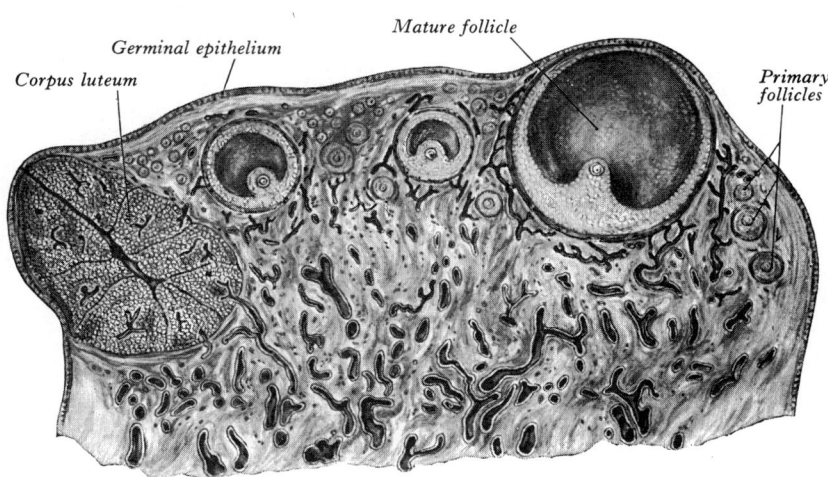

Corpus luteum   *Germinal epithelium*   *Mature follicle*   *Primary follicles*

14.17   Semi-diagrammatic section of an ovary.

surrounded by a certain amount of controversy; for a discussion of this problem, see Fritz and Fitz (1991). However, the traditional nomenclature (see e.g. Fawcett 1994) will be retained in the present account.

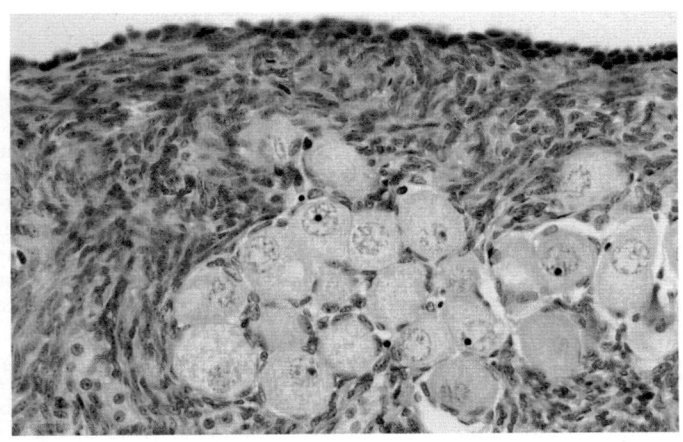

14.18A   Primordial follicles in the ovarian cortex, showing primary oöcytes surrounded by stromal cells; the surface epithelium of the ovary is visible above as a layer of cuboidal cells. Masson's stain, rat.

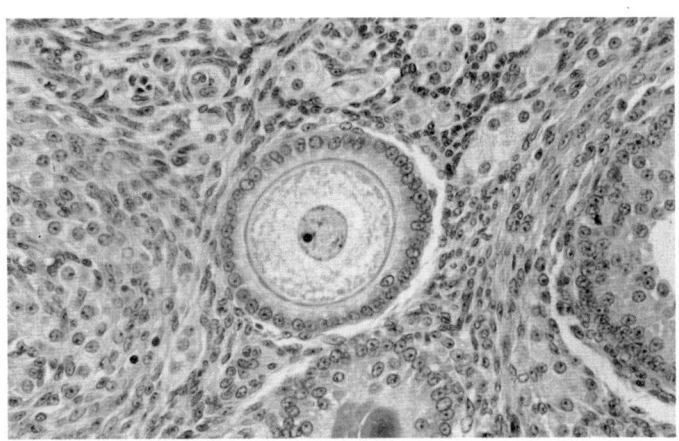

14.18B   Primary follicle, showing primary oöcyte with large nucleus containing dense chromatin. The oöcyte is surrounded by a thin green-staining zona pellucida and a single layer of follicular cells. Stromal cells are present around the follicle. Preparation and magnification as in **14**.18A.

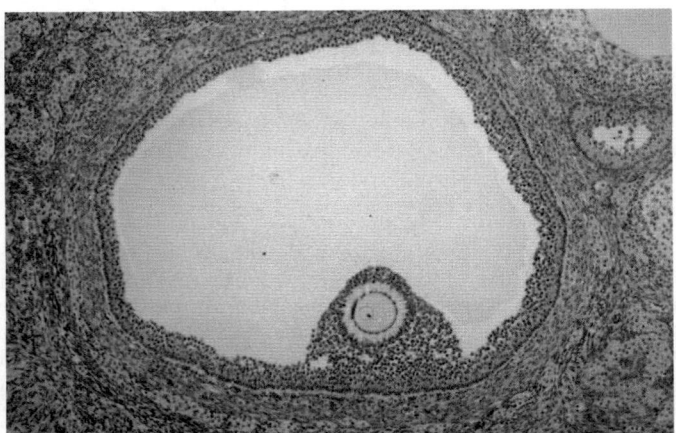

14.18C   Secondary follicle showing a secondary oöcyte situated in a cumulus oöphorus, and the thin rim of the membrana granulosa surrounding the follicular antrum containing (in life) liquor folliculi. Thecal cells also surround the follicle. Compare with **14**.18E. Preparation as in **14**.18A.

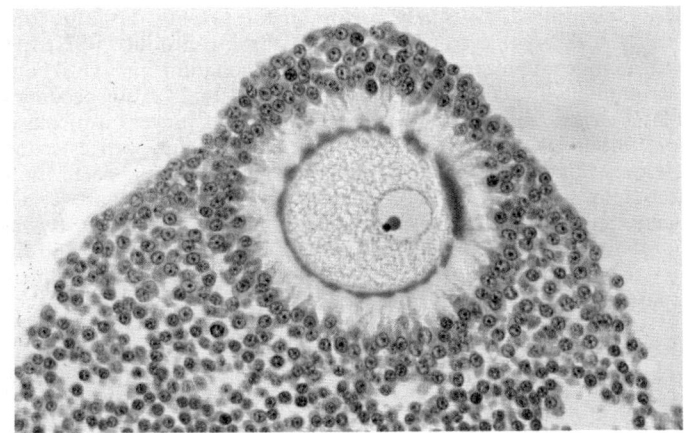

14.18D   Higher magnification of the cumulus oöphorus in a secondary follicle, showing the secondary oöcyte surrounded by the thin zona pellucida and a radially arranged cluster of granulosa cells forming the corona radiata. Preparation as in **14**.18A.

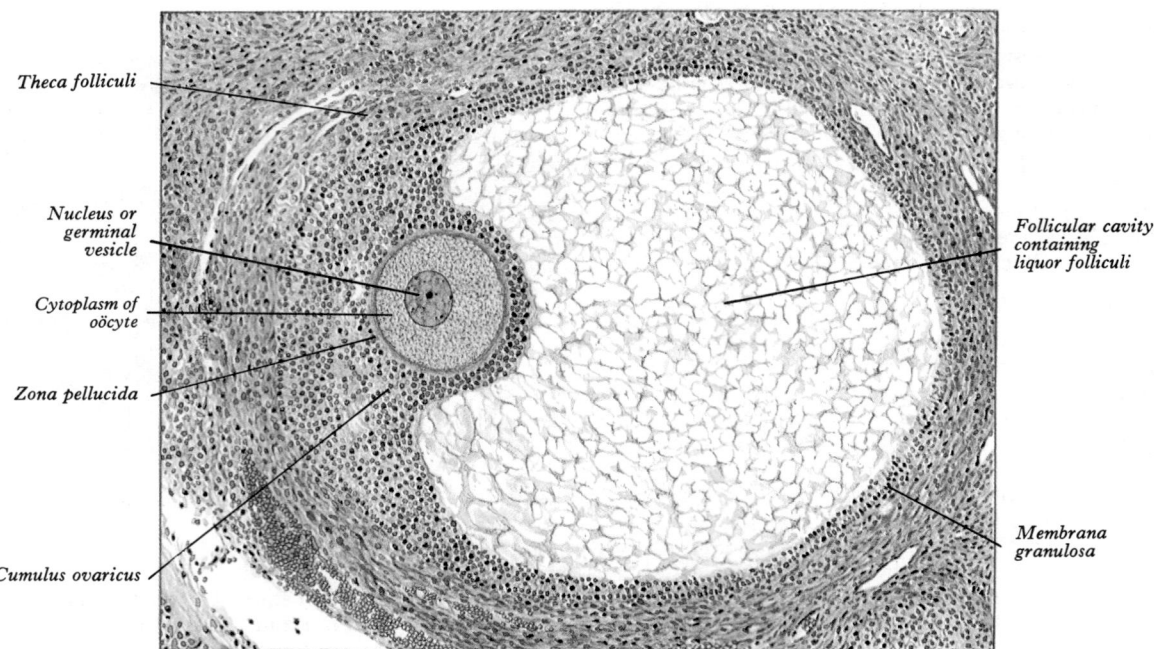

14.18E Section through an ovarian follicle from a woman aged 28 years. Stained with haematoxylin and eosin. Magnification × 90.

Labels on figure:
- *Theca folliculi*
- *Nucleus or germinal vesicle*
- *Cytoplasm of oöcyte*
- *Zona pellucida*
- *Cumulus ovaricus*
- *Follicular cavity containing liquor folliculi*
- *Membrana granulosa*

Lutein cells are grouped in small clusters of rounded or polygonal cells, each cluster surrounded by a little connective tissue. Ultrastructurally, all lutein cells have a cytoplasm filled with copious quantities of agranular endoplasmic reticulum and many mitochondria with tubular cristae, features characteristic of steroid synthesizing endocrine cells, which indeed they are. In the human ovary, all lutein cells have been reported to secrete progesterone, oestradiol and testosterone, although in different proportions in the two cell types, which also respond differently to circulating gonadotropins (the smaller cells to human chorionic gonadotrophins (hCG) for which they bear receptors). Initially, the hypophyseal follicle-stimulating (FSH), luteinizing (LH) and luteotropic (LTH, prolactin or lactogen) hormones activate the conversion of granulosal into luteal cells. (For the action of these ovarian hormones on uterine endometrium see p. 164 et seq.) If the oöcyte is not fertilized, the corpus luteum functions for about 12–14 days after ovulation, then atrophies into a *corpus luteum of menstruation*, the lutein cells undergoing fatty degeneration, autolysis, removal by macrophages and gradual replacement with fibrous tissue; eventually, after about 2 months, a small scar-like *corpus albicans* is all that remains.

If fertilization does occur, implantation of the blastocyst into the uterine endometrium usually begins on the seventh day after that event; the embryonic trophoblast then starts to produce FSH, LH, progesterone and oestradiol. The chorionic gonadotropins (FSH and LH) stimulate the corpus luteum of menstruation to grow, becoming then a *corpus luteum of pregnancy*. During that process it increases from about 10 mm in diameter to 25 mm (secreting progesterone, oestrogen and relaxin), and persists actively until parturition, although it gradually regresses as its endocrine functions are largely superseded by the placenta after about 2 months' gestation. By the end of pregnancy its diameter is reduced to about 1 cm, and in the next few months it degenerates, like the corpus luteum of menstruation, to a corpus albicans.

Age-related changes in the ovary

The prepubertal ovary. In a recent study of the neonatal ovary by Forabosco et al (1991), measurements from serial sections gave a mean size of about 13 mm long, 6 mm wide and 4 mm thick, with a volume of 126 mm³, its cortex forming about 35% and the medulla about 20%, and interstitial cells up to 45% of the volume. Much of the cortical volume is occupied by interstitial cells (see above). It gradually increases in size with body growth, and the interstitial tissue decreases.

The postmenopausal ovary. With the change in hormonal status at the menopause (usually in the 45–55 age range), ovulation ceases and various microscopic changes ensue within the ovarian tissues. The stroma becomes denser, the tunica albuginea thickens and the ovarian surface epithelium thins. However, many follicles persist within the cortex, some of them without oöcytes, but others apparently normal, providing the possibility of ovulation if the hormonal changes were to be reversed. Some abnormal follicles may become cystic as age progresses, quite a common feature in later years. For an extensive review of this and other aspects of the menopause, see Gosden (1985).

Ovarian surface epithelium

This covering of the ovary is composed mainly of cuboidal cells bearing modest numbers of microvilli, although there is also a scattered group of flatter epithelial cells with fewer microvilli, which may represent cells reacting to epithelial injury caused by ovulation (Gillett et al 1991). Amongst other organelles, these cells contain cytokeratin filaments and vimentin (Santini et al 1993). The epithelium appears to take an active part in the repair of the ovarian surface after that event by reforming the epithelial barrier and reconstituting the underlying matrix (Kruk & Auersperg 1992). It is very delicate and easily damaged by manipulation (Gillett 1991). About 85% of ovarian cancers arise from neoplastic changes in the surface epithelium.

For general accounts of ovarian (and other aspects of female reproductive systems, microscopic structure), see Blandau (1984) and Fawcett (1994).

Vessels

The **arteries** of the ovaries and uterine tubes are the ovarian arteries which are branches of the abdominal aorta (p. 1558). The **veins** emerge from the ovarian hila as a pampiniform plexus, drained by the ovarian veins (p. 1601). **Lymph vessels** are described on page 1623. They drain primarily to the lumbo-aortic and pelvic lymph nodes, although it is reported that after the menopause the flow of lymph is reduced and it drains mainly to the aortolumbar nodes (Vanneuville et al 1991).

Nerves

The innervation, derived from the ovarian plexuses (p. 1307), consist of postganglionic sympathetic, parasympathetic and autonomic afferent fibres, but little is known of their actual distribution or function, particularly in humans. Bulmer (1965) and Owman et al (1967) demonstrated cholinergic nerve fibres in the stroma histochemically. (See Neilson et al 1970, for a review.) Balboni (1972) has described the distribution of adrenergic fibres. The structures innervated, apart from the vessels, remain uncertain.

UTERINE TUBES

The two uterine (Fallopian) tubes (**14**.15, 16, 19–22, 26) lie on each side of the uterus in the upper margin (mesosalpinx) of the broad ligament. Each tube is about 10 cm long and opens medially by an aperture, the *uterine os*, into the uterine cavity's superior angle and laterally by the *abdominal os* into the peritoneal cavity near the ovary. In the nulliparous state, followed from the uterus to the fimbriae the uterine tube extends laterally as far as the inferior (uterine) pole of the ovary, and then ascends over its anterior (mesovarian) surface to the tubal pole over which it arches, turns downwards and ends in relation to the free border and medial surface of the ovary (**14**.15).

The tube is divisible into four parts, from lateral to medial:

- fimbriated end (infundibulum)
- ampulla
- isthmus
- intrauterine or intramural portion.

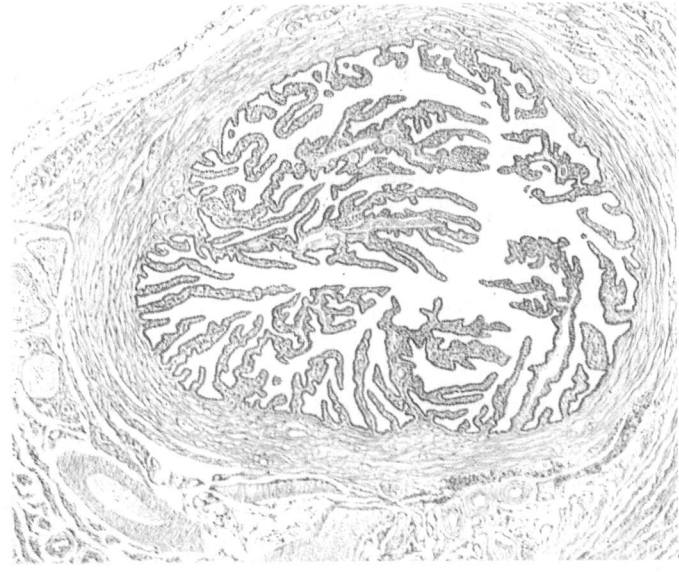

14.19   Transverse section through the ampulla of a human uterine tube. Stained with haematoxylin and eosin. Magnification × 15.

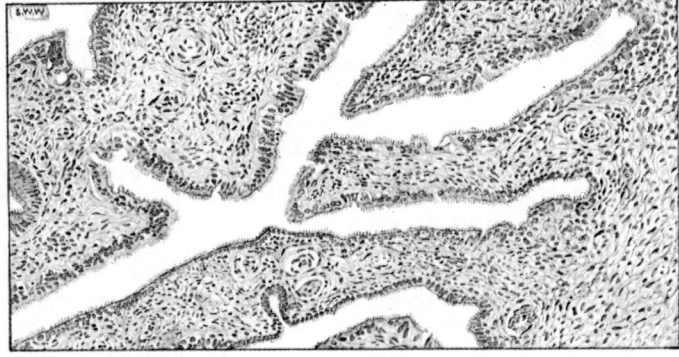

14.20   Section showing the plicated mucous membrane in the ampullary part of human uterine tube. Note the columnar epithelium. Stained with haematoxylin and eosin. Magnification × 75.

Fimbriated end. This is formed by a funnel-like expansion of the uterine tube, the *infundibulum*, its circumference prolonged into a variable number of finger-like processes, the *fimbriae*; one of these, the *ovarian fimbria* is longer and more deeply grooved than the others, and is typically applied to the tubal pole of the ovary. All fimbriae are lined by ciliated mucosa which, in the larger of them, has longitudinal folds continuous with those in the infundibulum. The cilia beat towards the ampulla. The fimbriae help to capture the unfertilized ovum after its release from the ovary, and conduct it into the lumen of the uterine tube through the abdominal os, an aperture deeply situated within the infundibulum and about 3 mm wide when relaxed. On the fimbriae, or the adjacent broad ligament, one or more small, pedunculated *vesicular appendices* often occur (see above and **14**.16).

Ampulla. This is a somewhat expanded region of the tube forming rather more than the lateral half of its length. It has a thin wall and a tortuously folded luminal surface (**14**.19, 20) marked by 4–5 major plicae (longitudinal ridges) on which lie large numbers of secondary plicae, creating an extensive surface area. The widest luminal diameter is about 1 cm. Typically, fertilization takes place in its complex lumen.

Isthmus. This part of the tube is rounded, muscular and firm, and forms approximately its medial third. Its lumen is narrow (0.1–0.5 mm) and has from three to five longitudinal major plicae with a variable number of minor plicae on their surface; these are much less complex than in the ampulla.

Intramural part. Lying within the wall of the uterus, this is about 1 cm long. It opens into the main cavity of the uterus near its upper end at the uterine cornu, through the uterine os, which is minute.

Microstructure of uterine tube (14.19, 20)

The tube has an internal mucosa, an intermediate muscular stratum and an external serosa.

Tubal mucosa

This is covered by folded simple (or, strictly, pseudostratified) ciliated and secretory epithelium. The plicae have cores of connective tissue, and are richly supplied by blood vessels and lymphatics. The epithelium is composed of at least four types of cell, their ratio varying with hormonal levels and position. These are ciliated columnar, secretory, peg (intercalary) and undifferentiated cells.

Ciliated cells. These are cuboidal, with a relatively large nucleus. In humans they appear to beat only towards the uterus, although in some other species of mammals (e.g. rabbit) there are also tracts of cilia beating towards the ampulla which are thought to assist the movements of spermatozoa prior to fertilization (Gaddum-Rosse & Blandau 1976). In women, fertilization does not depend absolutely on ciliary activity (see below). The numbers of ciliated cells are greater at the fimbriated end of the tube. There is evidence from other species of mammal that their numbers vary with hormonal status, especially on the fimbriae and ampulla, increasing during the pre-ovulatory phase and decreasing thereafter. In women they are much reduced after the menopause.

Secretory cells. These are interspersed among the ciliated cells. They vary in detailed structure during the menstrual cycle (Snyder 1924; Hashimoto et al 1960), indicating increased secretory preparation during the follicular, and augmented secretory discharge during the luteal phases of the menstrual cycle. The cells secrete a thick, tenacious mucus.

Peg-cells (*intercalary cells*). These are narrow columnar elements with oval nuclei, intercalated among the other cell types; they are thought to represent secretory cells in a non-secretory phase of their cycle (but may also include immature ciliated cells).

Undifferentiated cells. Small cells restricted to the epithelial base, they are probably mainly stem cells for the ciliated and secretory cell populations, although some may be intraepithelial lymphocytes.

Muscular layer

This is composed of external longitudinal and internal circular layers of smooth muscle; additional internal longitudinal fibres appear in some parts of the tube. The circular muscle is thickest in the wall of the isthmus, becoming reduced where the isthmus joins the ampulla. In the ampulla, internal longitudinal muscle is absent and the external longitudinal and circular are intermingled; the infundibular

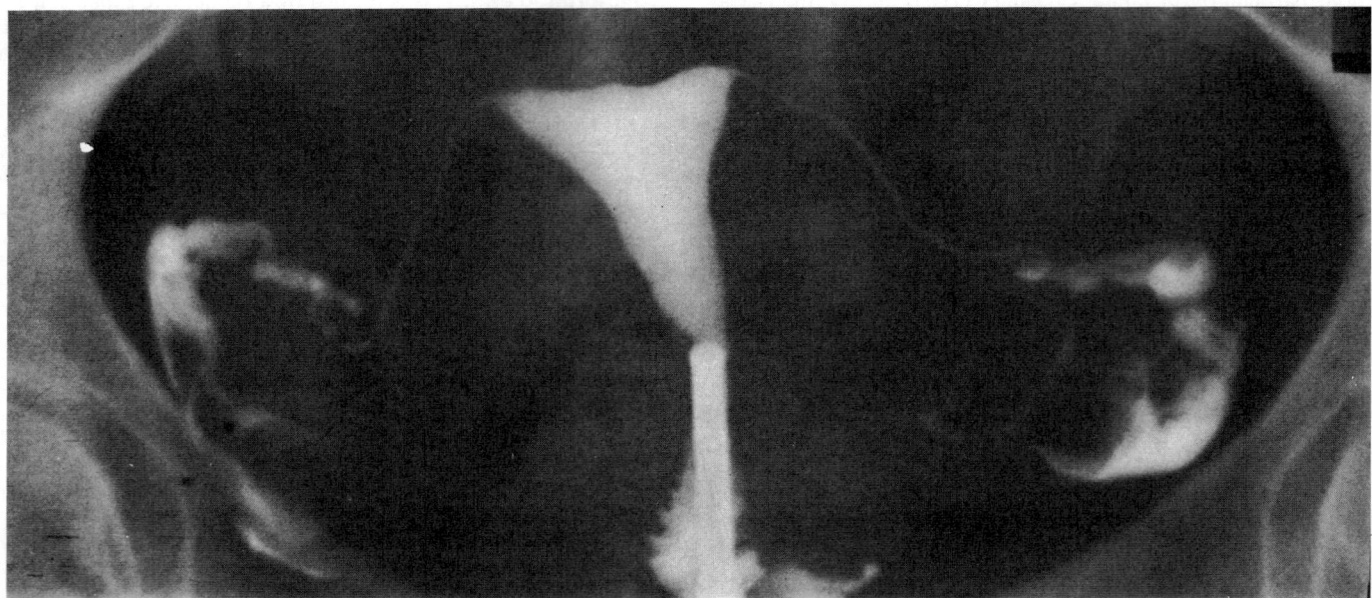

14.21   A radiograph of the uterus and uterine tubes after the introduction of a radio-opaque contrast medium through a cannula passed through the vagina into the cervix uteri. The shadow of the cannula is visible; above this is the triangular cavity of the uterine body and fundus. From the superior angles the lumina of the narrow (less than 1.0 mm diameter) intramural and isthmic parts of the uterine tubes may be traced inferolaterally, where they expand into the wider (2–4 mm diameter) ampullary parts of the tubes. Some contrast medium has escaped into the pelvic cavity from the abdominal ostia. (Radiograph provided by J Hilliger Smitham, Chelsea Hospital for Women, London.)

musculature is similar to this. A sphincter at the abdominal ostium has been described, on the basis of experimental distension (Whitelaw 1933; Woodruff & Pauerstein 1969) but has not been histologically confirmed. The uterine or intramural region has attracted attention (Lisa et al 1954; Sweeney 1962), because of the notion that a sphincter might exist to cut off the uterine cavity from the tube and peritoneum, guarding against infection. No such sphincter has been found, but internal longitudinal fibres which loop around these apertures have been confirmed. A ring of vascular tissue at these sites may also assist in such an action. There is also evidence that the isthmus, especially its lateral region, by its contraction acts as a sphincter able to delay the progress of the fertilized, segmenting ovum so that it reaches a sufficiently advanced state of development when it arrives at the uterus to implant in the endometrium. However, the evidence for this is uncertain, as radiological tracers always pass unhindered through this region (in the non-pathological state).

Beneath the mucosa is a zone rich in blood vessels especially venous sinuses and lymphatics, intermingled with smooth muscle fibres. This appears to have mechanical functions similar to that of cavernous erectile tissue elsewhere in the reproductive tract (e.g. the labia minora), becoming engorged with blood and lymph in midcycle to stiffen the tube, especially in its fimbriated and ampullary regions, and, probably, to apply the fimbria more closely to the ovarian surface.

Serosa

This is peritoneum with subjacent connective tissue; this is continuous with the broad ligament.

Tubal transport

The tube conveys ova, zygotes, the pre-implantation morulae and blastocytes to the uterus, and spermatozoa from the uterus to the ampulla for fertilization. During these processes, the ova, spermatozoa and the products of fertilization must be maintained in a suitable fluid environment to ensure their survival and, in the case of the spermatozoa, various changes have to ensue (capacitation) before they are capable of fertilizing an ovum (see p. 129).

The mode of entry of presumptive ova into the tube is still uncertain. In general it is agreed that muscular movements are the most important factor in the transport of ova and spermatozoa; this is demonstrated by the fact that women suffering from immobile cilium syndrome are still able to bear children. In studies of tubal motility, special attention has been focused on the transient arrest of the zygote at the isthmo-ampullary junction (the so-called isthmic block). How far this is caused by muscular action is uncertain, and it is likely that the extensive secretion of viscous mucus at this site during midcycle assists the delay in transport towards the uterus. Histochemical findings suggest an absence of cholinergic control, at least in some parts of the human uterine tube (Nakanishi et al 1967), although our knowledge of tubal innervation is very sketchy. Prostaglandins occurring in human semen stimulate the muscle in the medial part of the tube and inhibit it in the ampullary region.

The transport of spermatozoa to the ampulla is also poorly understood in humans, although studied extensively in rabbit and some other mammalian species (see Brosens 1991), and it is likely

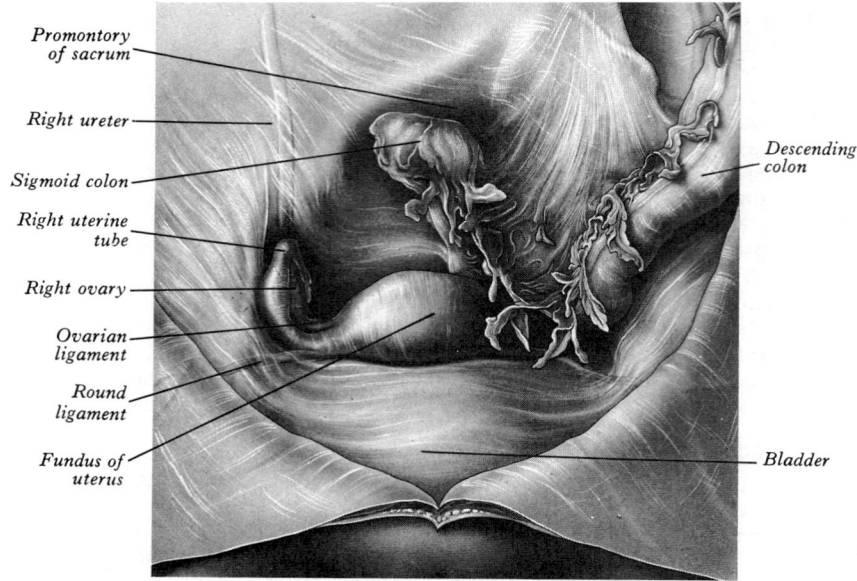

Promontory of sacrum

Right ureter

Sigmoid colon

Right uterine tube

Right ovary

Ovarian ligament

Round ligament

Fundus of uterus

Descending colon

Bladder

14.22   A female pelvis and its contents: anterosuperior view.

that muscular action in the tube is also a decisive factor. Relaxation of the putative sphincter at the uterine os has also been suggested as a necessary prerequisite for the entry of sperm into the tube. However, endoscopic inspection shows that the os opens and closes intermittently under normal circumstances, and such a sphincteric role is uncertain (Brosens 1991).

Vessels

The vessels of the uterine tube arise from ovarian and uterine stems. **Arteries**: arteriographic evidence (Borell & Fernström 1953) shows that the uterine artery usually supplies the medial two-thirds of the tube, the ovarian the remainder, the partition between the two (which in any case anastomose) being variable (consult Koritké et al 1967). **Veins** are arranged similarly to the arteries, and intrinsic mucosal, muscular and subserous networks have been described (Gatsalov 1963; Koritké et al 1967). **Lymphatics** follow the veins (p. 1623) (Sampson 1937; Gatsalov 1963).

Nerves

Nerve fibres enter and distribute largely with the ovarian and uterine arteries. Most of the tube has sympathetic and parasympathetic supplies. *Parasympathetic* fibres are from the vagus for the lateral half of the tube, and pelvic splanchnic nerves for the medial half. *Sympathetic supply* is from the tenth thoracic to the second lumbar spinal segments. *Afferent fibres* travel with the sympathetic motor supply, entering the cord through corresponding dorsal roots. Modified Pacinian corpuscles appear in the ampullary submucosa (Chiara 1959). Intrinsic innervation has been studied by metal impregnation methods (Chiara 1959; Damiani & Capodacqua 1961), and fluorescence microscopy (Owman et al 1967; Kubo 1970). In the wall of the tube are postganglionic sympathetic fibres and visceral afferents, and preganglionic parasympathetic fibres which must form synapses, although ganglia have not been reliably reported in the wall or near it; the relay may be in paracervical ganglia. Afferent autonomic fibres may also accompany parasympathetic nerves.

Vestigial structures

The *epoöphoron* (**14.16**), in the lateral part of the mesosalpinx (p. 200) between the ovary and uterine tube, consists of 10–15 short, blind-ending *transverse ductules* converging towards the ovary; their other ends open into a rudimentary longitudinal *duct of the epoöphoron*, running medially in the broad ligament, parallel with the lateral part of the uterine tube. Between the epoöphoron and the fimbriated end of the tube are often one or more small cystic *vesicular appendices*. Occasionally the longitudinal epoöphorontic duct (duct of Gartner) can be followed along the uterus nearly to the internal os where it penetrates the muscular wall of the uterus and descends in the wall of the cervix, gradually approaching the mucosa without actually reaching it. It then descends in the lateral wall of the vagina to end near or at the free margin of the hymen. The *paroöphoron* consists of a few rudimentary tubules scattered in the broad ligament between the epoöphoron and uterus, most easily seen in children. Both the epoöphoron and paroöphoron tubules are remnants of mesonephric tubules; the duct of the epoöphoron is a persistent part of the mesonephric duct (p. 200).

Clinical aspects of the uterine tube

Blockage of the tube is a major cause of infertility, and various procedures have been developed for its examination.

Endoscopy. Investigations of tubal condition and patency can be carried out by endoscopy using fibreoptics introduced through the vagina and uterus (hysteroscopy) to view its uterine os and isthmic region, or during laparoscopic examination through the abdominal os (salpingoscopy) for the inspection of the ampullary interior. The tube can be inspected externally by pelvic laparoscopy; to show the course of the tubal lumen, the tube can be perfused via the cervix with a weak solution of methylene blue which is then visible through the tubal wall. Although these techniques avoid the use of radiographs, there is a slight risk of introducing infection into the tube. For a general account of these procedures, see, for example, Brosens (1991).

Salpingography. This radiological technique entails the introduction of a water-soluble radio-opaque medium into the uterus (hysterosalpingography) under a slight positive pressure, the tracer

entering the tube and if this is patent, spilling through its abdominal os into the peritoneal cavity (**14.21**). This method provides information about the normality of the lumen including that of the isthmus and ampulla, and of the patency of the tube as a whole. It does, however, involve the exposure of the ovaries and any developing blastocysts to X-irradiation, which endoscopy avoids.

Tubal inflammation. Tubal inflammation (salpingitis) is usually secondary, having spread from the vagina or the uterus. The fimbriated end may be closed by adhesions, and pus then collects in the tube (pyosalpinx), or closure may result elsewhere in the tube because of mucosal inflammation, fluid sometimes accumulating in blocked segments (hydrosalpinx). Pelvic peritonitis is said to occur more frequently in females because infection of the vagina, uterus or of the uterine tube may spread directly to the peritoneum, via the abdominal ostium.

Tubal pregnancy. Normally, after fertilization the segmenting zygote enters the uterus but it may adhere to and develop in the tube, the commonest variety of ectopic gestation (p. 136); an amnion and a chorion are formed, but true decidua never develop; such gestation usually ends by extrusion through the abdominal ostium, but sometimes by tubal rupture into the peritoneal cavity accompanied by severe haemorrhage (Pauerstein & Woodruff 1967; Woodruff & Pauerstein 1969).

UTERUS

The uterus (**14.**15B, 22, 23) is a hollow, thick-walled and muscular organ, normally situated in the lesser pelvis between the urinary bladder and rectum. Into its upper part open the uterine tubes, one on each side; below, it continues into the vagina. If fertilization has occurred, the developing blastocyst conveyed to the uterine cavity by the uterine tubes embeds in the uterine lining and is normally retained until development is complete, the uterus adapting in size and structure to the needs of the growing embryo and fetus. After parturition it returns almost to its former condition, though somewhat larger than in its nulliparous state.

In the adult nulliparous state it is pear shaped, though somewhat flattened anteroposteriorly, and its long axis tilted superiorly forwards. Its narrow end is therefore postero-inferior in position. The uterus lies behind the bladder and (unless the bladder is full) bent forward above it (**14.**15, 24). It is situated inferior to the sigmoid colon and in front of the rectum, and completely below the pelvic inlet. The long axis usually lies approximately along the axis of the pelvic inlet (p. 669), but since the uterus is movable, its position varies with the distension of the bladder and rectum. Except when displaced by a much distended bladder, the long axis of the uterus is nearly at right angles to that of the vagina (see below), the latter's axis corresponding to the axis of the pelvic outlet (p. 671). In size, the adult non-pregnant uterus is about 7.5 cm long, 5 cm in breadth at its widest, and nearly 2.5 cm thick; it weighs 30–40 g.

DIVISIONS OF THE UTERUS

The uterus is divisible into two main regions, the *body of the uterus* (corpus uteri) forming its upper two-thirds, and a narrower, more cylindrical *cervix* (cervix uteri), demarcated by a slight constriction. The rounded upper part of the corpus above the entry-points of the uterine tubes is the *fundus* (this is, of course, the highest part but the deepest when approached via the cervix). The lumen of the corpus is flat anteroposteriorly, but that of the cervix is round in section and quite narrow, its upper end communicating with the corpus by an aperture, the *internal os*, and its lower end opening into the vagina by an *external os* (see below).

Uterine body (corpus uteri)

The pear-shaped uterine body (**14.**15, 16, 22, 24–27) gradually narrows from the fundus down to the internal os. Its anterior (vesical) surface, apposed to the urinary bladder, is flattened and covered by peritoneum, reflected on to the bladder as the *uterovesical fold*, level with the internal os. Between the bladder and uterus is the *vesico-uterine pouch*, usually empty but sometimes occupied by part of the small intestine. The posterior (intestinal) surface of the uterus is convex transversely. Its peritoneal covering continues down to the

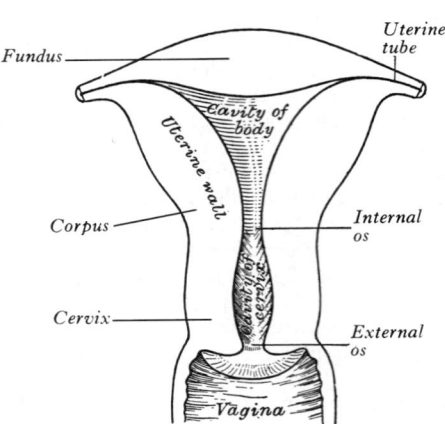

14.23A Sectional diagram showing the interior divisions of the uterus and its continuity with the vagina.

cervix and upper vagina and is then reflected back to the rectum (**14.**15) along the surface of the *recto-uterine pouch* (of Douglas) which lies posterior to the uterus. Posterior to the uterus is the sigmoid colon, though the two are usually separated by the terminal ileal coil. The dome-like fundus is covered by peritoneum continuous with that of neighbouring surfaces. Coils of small intestine and occasionally distended sigmoid colon contact it. The lateral margins of the body are convex, and on each side their peritoneum is reflected laterally to form the *broad liagment*, extending as a flat sheet to the pelvic wall (p. 1874). Near its upper end, the body receives a uterine tube on either side, the point of fusion of each being a uterine *cornu*; below the cornu, and slightly in front is attached the round ligament and postero-inferior to it the ligament of the ovary, both running in the broad ligament and stretching from the lateral uterine margin to the lateral pelvic wall (**14.**22); (see also p. 1874).

Uterine cavity (14.21, 23, 25). In length, it measures about 6 cm from the external os to the wall of the fundus. The lumen is small in comparison with its thick wall; in the uterine body it is very flat anteroposteriorly, being a mere transverse slit in sagittal or transverse section, with the anterior and posterior walls almost in contact. In

coronal section (**14.**23) it is triangular, broad above where the two uterine tubes join the uterus, and narrow below at the internal os of the cervix.

Cervix (cervix uteri)

This part of the uterus is about 2.5 cm long in the adult, non-pregnant state; it is narrower and more cylindrical than the corpus, and is widest at its midlevel; it is also less mobile than the body of the uterus, so that their axes are seldom in line. The uterine long axis is usually curved forwards, concave below, a state described as *anteflexed*; occasionally there is an angular bend at the level of the internal os (*acute anteflexion*). With the bladder empty the whole uterus leans forwards at an angle to the vagina, and in this position is said to be *anteverted*. The external end of the cervix bulges into the anterior wall of the vagina, which divides it into *supravaginal* and *vaginal* regions (**14.**15).

The *supravaginal part of the cervix* is separated in front from the bladder by cellular connective tissue, the *parametrium*, which passes also to the sides of the cervix and laterally between the two layers of the broad ligaments. The uterine arteries flank the cervix in this tissue and the ureters descend forwards in it about 2 cm from the cervix, curving under the arch formed by the uterine arteries. The relation of the arteries to the ureters is not always symmetrical; one ureter may be anterior to the cervix. Posteriorly the supravaginal cervix is covered by peritoneum, prolonged below on to the posterior vaginal wall and then reflected on to the rectum via the recto-uterine recess (**14.**15). Posteriorly, it is related to the rectum, but may be separated from it by a terminal ileal coil.

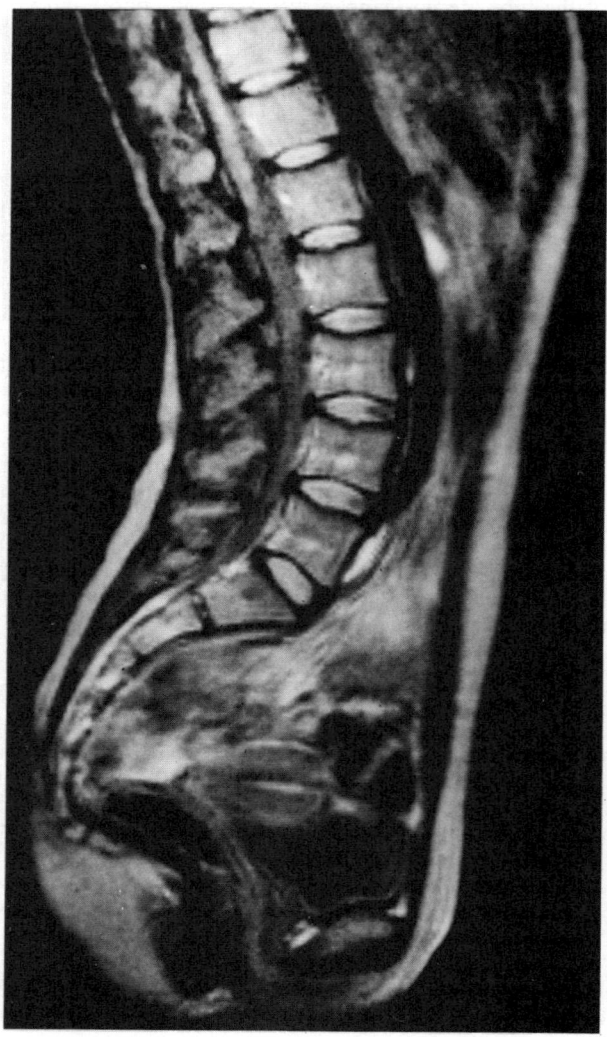

14.24A Sagittal magnetic resonance image of the lumbar spine and pelvis of an adult woman. (Supplied by Philips Medical Systems; photography by Sarah Smith, UMDS, Guy's Hospital Campus, London.)

14.23B Diagram showing the main variations in uterine position, as seen in side view. See text for further details.

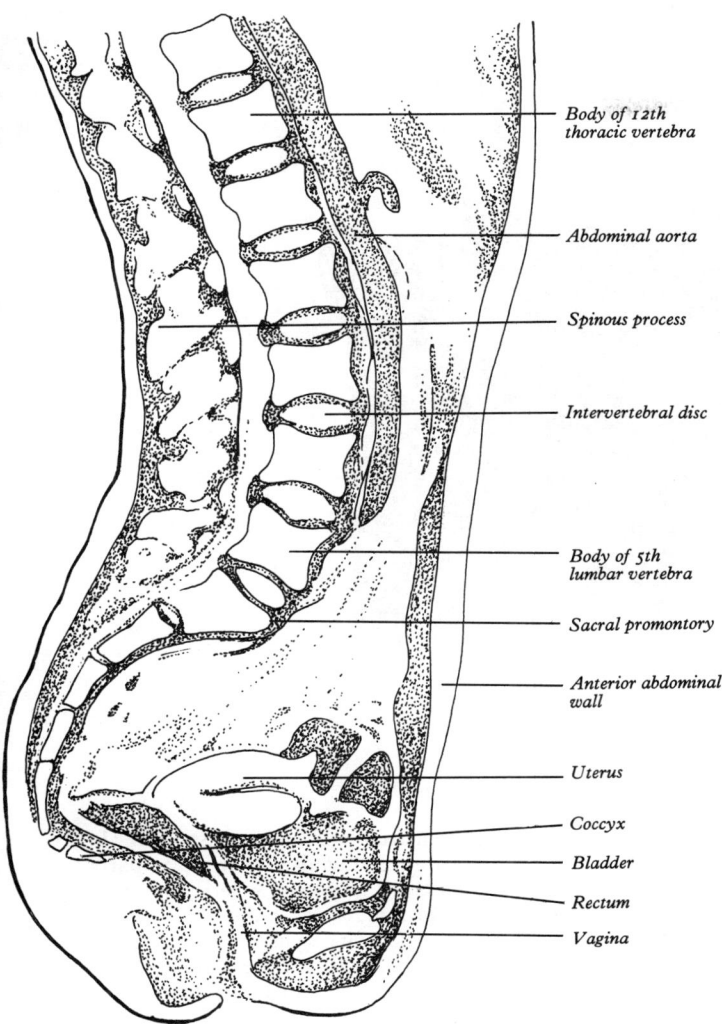

Body of 12th
thoracic vertebra

Abdominal aorta

Spinous process

Intervertebral disc

Body of 5th
lumbar vertebra

Sacral promontory

Anterior abdominal
wall

Uterus

Coccyx

Bladder

Rectum

Vagina

14.24B Diagram illustrating the major features demonstrated in **14.24A**.

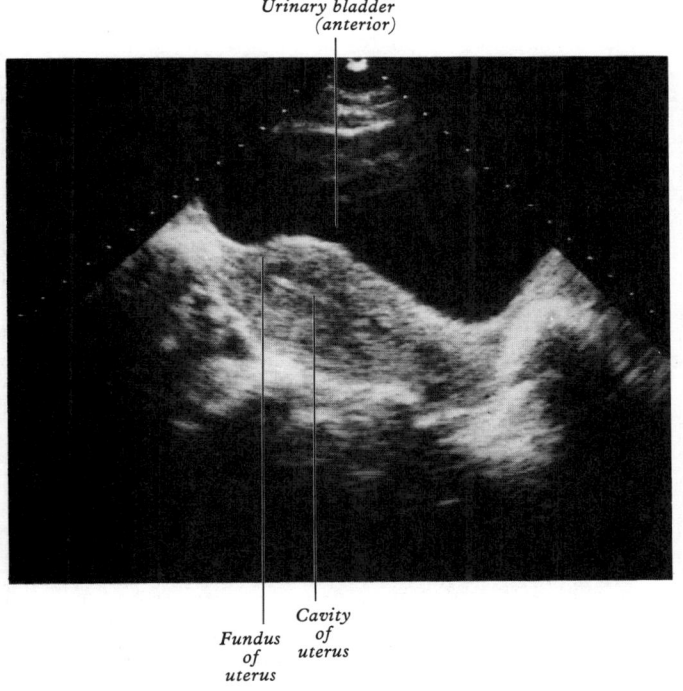

Urinary bladder
(anterior)

Fundus
of
uterus

Cavity
of
uterus

14.25 Sagittal ultrasonogram of the pelvis of an adult woman. (Supplied by Shaun Gallagher, Guy's Hospital; photography by Sarah Smith, UMDS, Guy's Hospital Campus, London.)

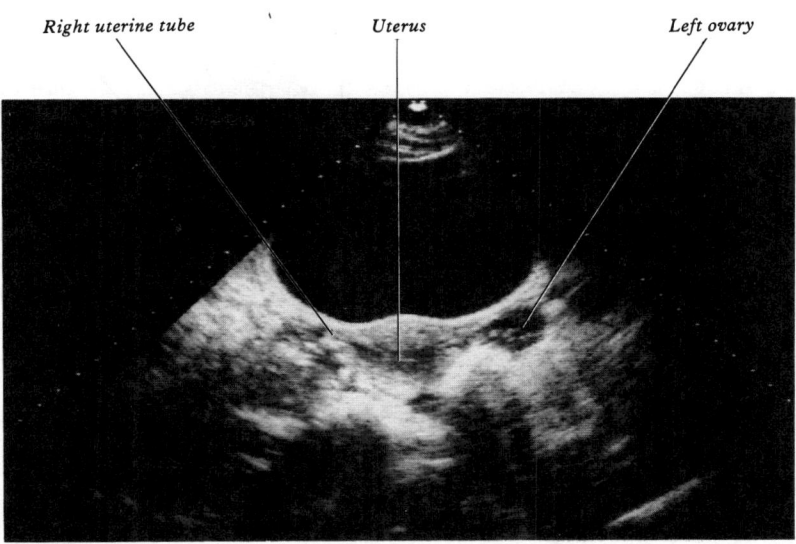

Right uterine tube   Uterus   Left ovary

14.26 Transverse ultrasonogram of the female pelvis through the level of the uterus and left ovary. (Supplied by Guy's Hospital; photography by Sarah Smith, UMDS, Guy's Hospital Campus, London.)

The *vaginal part of the cervix* projects as a convex disc on to the anterior vaginal wall, forming grooves around its perimeter termed *vaginal fornices* (p. 1875). On its rounded end the small external os connects its cavity with the vagina. In nulliparous women, the external os is usually a circular aperture, but after childbirth it has anterior and posterior lips, the anterior shorter, thicker and projecting lower than the posterior, and the aperture is irregular; normally, both lips contact the posterior vaginal wall.

Cervical canal. In shape this is somewhat fusiform longitudinally, flattened transversely and broadest at midlevel. It communicates with the main uterine cavity via the internal os, and with the vagina by the external os. Two longitudinal ridges, one each on its anterior and posterior walls give off small oblique *palmate folds* which ascend laterally like the branches of a tree (*arbor vitae uteri*). The folds on opposing walls interdigitate to close the canal. The narrower *isthmus of the cervix*, forming its upper third, has some distinctive features (Stieve 1927; Frankl 1933). Although unaffected in the first month of pregnancy, it is gradually taken up into the uterine body during the second month to form the 'lower uterine segment'. Fetal membranes, firmly fused with the uterine mucosa elsewhere, are not attached to this lower segment. In non-pregnant women the isthmus undergoes menstrual changes, although these are less pronounced than in the uterine body.

AGE-RELATED CHANGES IN UTERINE STRUCTURE

The functional anatomy of the human uterus has been described in detail by Lopes and Barriere (1986). Its form, size and position vary with age, hormonal status, pregnancy and the state of the surrounding pelvic organs, amongst other conditions.

In fetal life the uterus projects above the lesser pelvis and the cervix is considerably larger than the body. **At puberty** the uterus is piriform and weighs 14–17 g; the fundus is then just below the superior pelvic aperture; the palmate folds of the cervix are distinct and extend to the upper part of the uterine cavity. **In adults**, uterine position varies, depending chiefly on the contents of the bladder and rectum, though of course, also with pregnancy (see below). With an empty bladder the entire uterus bends anteriorly, curved at the junction of the body and cervix, the body contacting the bladder (**14.**15, 24). As the bladder fills, the uterus gradually becomes more erect until, with a full bladder, the fundus may turn towards the sacrum.

During menstruation the organ is slightly enlarged and more vascular; its surfaces are rounder, the external os is rounded, its lips swollen, and the endometrium is darker (see below). **During pregnancy** the uterus becomes greatly enlarged and reaches the epigastric

1871

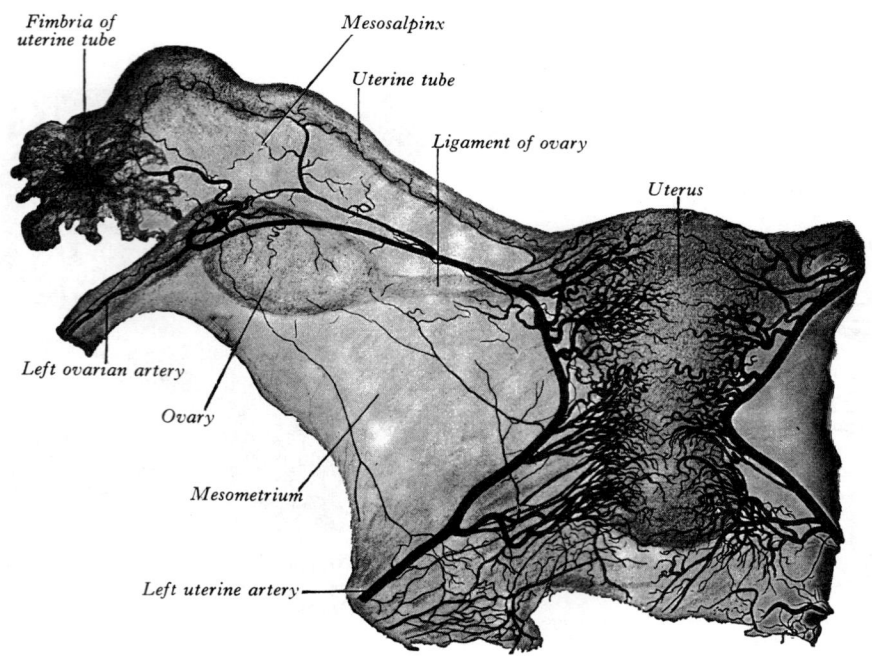

Fimbria of uterine tube

Mesosalpinx

Uterine tube

Ligament of ovary

Uterus

Left ovarian artery

Ovary

Mesometrium

Left uterine artery

14.27 Posterior aspect of a cleared injected specimen to show the distribution of the left uterine and ovarian arteries of a female aged 17½ years. (Prepared by Hamilton Drummond.)

region in the eighth month. The increase in wall thickness is mainly due to hypertrophy of existing myocytes, but the formation of new ones, perhaps by differentiation of connective tissue cells may also contribute to it. As pregnancy proceeds, the wall progressively thins. After parturition the uterus nearly regains resting size, weighing about 42 g; but its cavity remains larger, its vessels tortuous and its muscular layers thicker and more defined; the external os is more prominent, its edges variably fissured.

In old age the uterus becomes atrophied, paler and denser in texture; a more distinct constriction separates the body and cervix. The internal os is frequently obliterated, the external os occasionally, when the latter's lips almost disappear.

MICROSTRUCTURE OF THE UTERUS

The uterine wall is composed of three major layers, from internal to outside: endometrium (mucosa), myometrium (smooth muscle coat) and perimetrium (serosa). Of these the myometrium is by far the largest component.

Endometrium (14.28)

This mucosal layer is continuous below with the vaginal mucosa below through the external os, and, if traced along the uterine tubes, also with the peritoneum through the abdominal os. It is formed by a layer of connective tissue (*endometrial stroma*) lined by simple columnar epithelium continuous with large numbers of tubular *endometrial (uterine) glands* running perpendicular to the luminal surface or slightly coiled (**14**.28A) and penetrating as far as the boundary with the myometrium. In the *uterine body* the surface epithelium is columnar, ciliated before puberty but usually non-ciliated over large areas in the adult uterus, while the endometrial glands are composed largely of columnar cells rich in glycogen (variably with the menstrual cycle). The **stroma** consists of embryonic-type, highly cellular connective tissue containing blood vessels and lymphatic spaces filling the gaps between the endometrial glands. The thickness of the endometrium varies considerably according to the individual's hormonal state (see below). It is divisible into two major layers, a superficial *stratum functionale* or *functionalis* forming most of its thickness, and a *stratum basalis* lying close to the myometrium. The former is shed during menstruation, whereas the latter forms a permanent part of the endometrium from which a new functionalis can be regenerated at the beginning of the menstrual

cycle. For a review of endometrial structure, see Spornitz (1992).

The chief structural feature distinguishing the two parts is the arrangement of blood vessels within them. Arteries penetrating the uterine wall from without form plexuses, in the myometrium giving off smaller arteries and arterioles which pass radially into the endometrium. Here they are at first straight (in the basalis), then as they progress more apically they become tortuous, finally giving off numerous side branches to feed the capillary plexuses which are especially rich near the surface of the mucosa. Some pathologists divide the endometrium into four strata for diagnostic convenience. From lumen to base, the functionalis is divided into zone 1 (surface

Endometrium   Myometrium

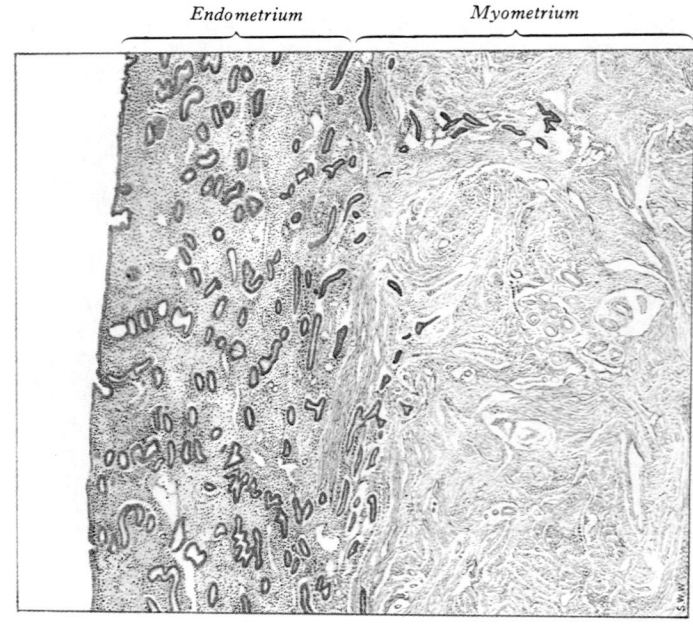

14.28A Section of human endometrium and underlying musculature in the interval phase. Note that some glands extend into the more internal layers of the myometrium. Stained with haematoxylin and eosin. Magnification × 20.

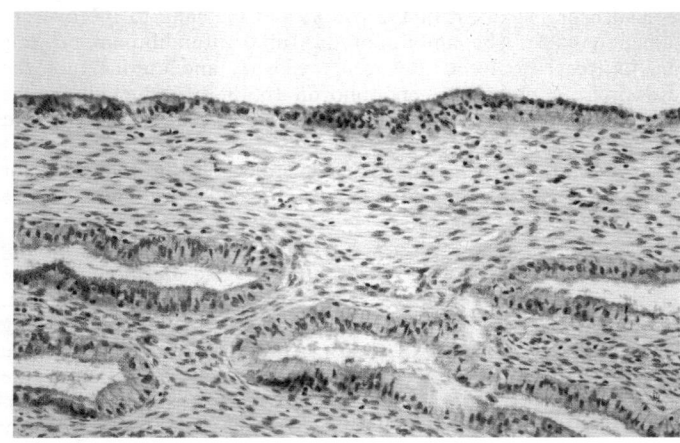

14.28B Section through the mucosa from the wall of the upper part of the cervical canal (human), showing the columnar surface epithelium, and cervical glands within the lamina propria.

epithelium and immediately adjacent stroma) and zone 2 (containing unbranched glands), the basalis into zone 3 (with branched portions of glands) and zone 4 (bases of glands). The spiral vessels are rhythmically contractile throughout much of the menstrual cycle, with corresponding cycles of blanching and reddening as the surface capillaries of the mucosa are alternately starved or fed with blood. Immediately prior to menstruation, as progesterone levels drop, the spiral arteries contract down to cause ischaemia in the functionalis, causing oedema and stromal necrosis; they then relax, briefly flooding the surrounding stroma with blood and causing its disintegration, as clotting mechanisms prevent further blood loss. After 2–4 days the basalis begins to regenerate new tubular glands, stroma and vessels, re-establishing the functionalis zone. These processes are closely controlled by the concentrations of circulating hormones. For a further consideration of this topic, see page 162, and for a review of ultrastructural changes, Ferenczy (1993).

Cervical mucosa (14.28B). Except for the lowermost third, this is composed of simple epithelium with tubular glands overlying a fibrocellular connective tissue stroma. Its lower third, including its vaginal surface, is covered by non-keratinizing stratified squamous epithelium. None of the mucosa is shed during menstruation, and so unlike the body of the uterus, it is not divisible into a functionalis and basalis. For the upper majority of the cervical canal the mucosa is about 3 mm thick, and is lined by a rather folded surface epithelium of columnar mucous cells continuous with the linings of branched tubular *cervical glands*, made of similar secretory epithelium. Ciliated cells are also patchily present at the surface. The cervical glands run obliquely upwards and outwards from the canal, ramifying as they do so. They secrete a clear, viscid, alkaline mucus. Not uncommonly, the aperture of a gland is occluded and it then inflates with mucus to form a spheroidal *Nabothian cyst* up to 5 mm or more in diameter. See Ferenczy (1982) for a review of the ultrastructure of the human cervix.

Myometrium

This fibromuscular layer (14.28) forms most of the uterine wall. In nulliparae it is dense, firm, greyish and (in the fixed state) cuts almost like cartilage. It is about 1.3 cm thick at the uterine midlevel and fundus but thin at the tubal orifices. It is composed largely of smooth muscle fasciculi mingled with loose connective tissue, blood vessels, lymphatic vessels and nerves. The body of the uterus is often described as having four more or less distinct layers:

- The most internal layer (*stratum submucosum*) is composed mostly of longitudinal and some oblique smooth muscle; where the lumen of the uterine tubes pass through the uterine wall this layer forms circular, sphincter-like muscle coats which have been suggested to have a sphincteric action (although radio-opaque tracers pass readily from the uterus into the tubes, see p. 1869).
- External to the submucosal layer is the *stratum vasculare*, a zone rich in blood vessels as well as longitudinal muscle.

- Next is a layer of predominantly circular muscle, the *stratum supravasculare*.
- Finally a thin longitudinal layer, the *stratum subserosum*, lies adjacent to the perimetrium or adjacent connective tissue.

The fibromuscular fasciculi of layers 3 and 4 converge at the lateral angles of the uterus, continuing into the uterine tubes and the round and ovarian ligaments; some enter the broad ligaments, others turn back into the uterosacral ligaments. At the junction between the body and the cervix, the smooth muscle merges with dense irregular connective tissue containing both collagen and elastin, forming the majority of the cervical wall. A funnel-like array of elastin and smooth muscle cells has been described in the cervix, its narrow extremity adjacent to the external os (Hamperl 1970); this may act as a valve in keeping the os closed. Toth (1977) has described bilateral smooth longitudinal fascicles in the uterine wall, extending in the lateral regions from the fundal angle to the cervix and largely submucosal. Each fascicle, in its juxtafundal part, consists of dispersed subfascicles, but is more compact near the cervix; epithelial rests were observed in them, suggesting a mesonephric origin; their myocytes differ structurally from those of myometrium proper, suggesting that they may provide fast conducting pathways via gap junctions which might help to co-ordinate the contractile activities of the uterine wall.

During pregnancy the muscle hypertrophies, the myocytes being much enlarged and the numbers of their gap junctions increasing greatly, indicating increased co-ordination of their contractility, and the amounts of connective tissue also increase.

Perimetrium (serosa)

This is composed of peritoneum (mesothelium overlying a connective tissue lamina propria) posteriorly covering the uterine body and supravaginal cervix, but anteriorly only the body. Over the most inferior quarter of the uterine length the peritoneum is separated posteriorly from the underlying uterus by loose cellular tissue and large veins. Beneath the peritoneum is a subserous layer of loose fibrous tissue.

Vessels of the uterus

Arteries. The main arterial supply to the whole uterus is through the uterine branch of the internal iliac artery on each side (p. 1559). This anastomoses with the ovarian and vaginal arteries, but the dominance of the uterine artery is indicated by its marked hypertrophy during pregnancy, which affects it alone. The paired uterine arteries anastomose extensively with each other across the midline; one can be ligated without serious effects (Siegel & Mengert 1961) and even more extensive ligation has succeeded. Their tortuosity as they ascend in the broad ligaments is repeated in their branches within the uterine wall, but all the sinuosities disappear as the pregnant uterus expands. Each uterine artery gives numerous branches which immediately enter the uterine wall, where they divide to run circumferentially in the stratum vasculare as groups of *anterior* and *posterior arcuate arteries*, passing transversely in the myometrium in the stratum. These vessels ramify and narrow as they approach the anterior and posterior midline so that no large vessels are present in those regions, although they are not avascular, and the left and right arterial trees anastomose across the midline (14.27). The arcuate arteries supply many tortuous radial branches which pass centripetally through the deeper myometrial layers, supplying these en route, to reach the endometrium. As microradiography and injections show, these provide a series of dense capillary plexuses in the myometrium and endometrium (Farrer-Brown et al 1970a, b). From the arcuate arteries many helical arteriolar rami pass into the endometrium, as noted above. Their detailed appearance changes during the menstrual cycle; during the proliferative phase helical arterioles are less prominent; in the secretory phase they grow in length and calibre, becoming even more tortuous (Ramsey 1955).

Veins. The uterine veins are arranged like arteries (Farrer-Brown et al 1970a, b), but volumetrically they are greater. Minute venous endometrial venous sinuses, a constant feature in the pregnant uterus, have also been noted in the resting organ (Schlegel 1946). During pregnancy the ovarian veins, unlike their companion arteries, may be enlarged (O'Leary & O'Leary 1966).

Lymphatic vessels. These are described on page 1623. The intrinsic lymphatic plexuses of the uterine wall have been little studied in human females; Wislocki and Dempsey (1939) have, however, made a detailed study of arrangements in primates (macaque monkeys).

Nerves of the uterus

The nerves supplying the uterus are described on page 1309. The autonomic supply comes directly from the ovarian and hypogastric plexuses; sympathetic preganglionic fibres proceed from the twelfth thoracic and first lumbar spinal segments while parasympathetic preganglionic axons issue in the second to fourth ventral sacral spinal roots. Despite general agreement on these pathways, details of their distribution and physiological effects are still ill-defined. Cholinergic and adrenergic fibres have been identified in cervical muscular and submucous strata, the former predominating. Recent findings indicate various neuropeptides in the efferent and afferent supply of the uterus, including substance P, and neuropeptide Y. For a review of this topic, see Traurig et al 1991.

Clinical aspects of the uterus

Small degrees of anteversion or retroversion are not pathological; but when flexion at the junction of the body with the cervix is marked it must be so regarded, especially when retroversion is combined with retroflexion. *Retroversion* is defined as a posterior inclination of the whole uterus, so that the cervix faces forwards; *retroflexion* is a posterior curvature of body alone, flexed at the junction of body and cervix. These conditions are usually combined. Prolapse is another common condition; the uterus sinks abnormally low and may protrude at the vulva, usually after imperfect repair of the pelvic floor following damage sustained during parturition. For an account of uterine changes in pregnancy, see page 1877.

UTERINE LIGAMENTS

The uterus is connected to the bladder, rectum and pelvic walls by 'ligaments'; some are merely peritoneal folds and can provide little mechanical support, others are more robust and contain smooth muscle and fibrous tissue, so that they provide mechanical support and, in some instances, because of their muscular content they may also give some measure of dynamic control.

Peritoneal folds

These are the anterior and posterior ligaments of the uterus, and the broad ligament.

The *anterior ligament* or *uterovesical fold* consists of peritoneum reflected on to the bladder from the uterus at the junction of its cervix and body. The *posterior ligament* or *rectovaginal fold* is composed of peritoneum reflected from the posterior vaginal fornix on to the front of the rectum, forming the deep recto-uterine pouch, bounded anteriorly by the uterus, supravaginal cervix uteri and posterior vaginal fornix, posteriorly by the rectum, and laterally by two peritoneal crescentic folds passing back from the cervix uteri on each side of the rectum to the posterior pelvic wall; these recto-uterine folds contain much fibrous tissue and smooth muscle and are attached to the front of the sacrum to form the *uterosacral ligament*, which can be palpated per rectum lateral to it.

Broad ligaments (**14**.16, 27). These extend one from either side of the uterus to the lateral walls of the pelvis. Together with the uterus they form a septum across the lesser pelvic cavity, dividing it into an anterior part containing the bladder and a posterior part containing the rectum and, usually, the terminal ileal coil and part of the sigmoid colon. With the bladder empty or almost so, the uterus and broad ligaments are inclined forwards superiorly, so that the posterior surface faces up and backwards, and the anterior surface down and forwards, with a free upper and an attached lower border. As the bladder fills, the plane of the ligaments tilts backwards, their free borders becoming superior and their layers anterior and posterior. They are continuous with each other at the free edge via the uterine fundus and diverge below near the superior surfaces of levatores ani. In the free border on either side lies a uterine tube. The broad ligament is divisible into an upper *mesosalpinx*, a posterior *mesovarium* and an inferior *mesometrium*.

Mesosalpinx. This fold of peritoneum is attached above to the uterine tube, and below (posteriorly) to the mesovarium, laterally to

the suspensory ligament of the ovary, and medially to the ovarian ligament (**14**.27). The fimbria of the tubal infundibulum projects from its free lateral end. Between the ovary and uterine tube the mesosalpinx contains the epoöphoron (p. 1869) and medially the paroöphoron (p. 1869), and anastomoses between the uterine and ovarian vessels.

Mesovarium. This peritoneal fold projects from the posterior aspect of the broad ligament which is attached to the hilum of the ovary to which it transmits vessels and nerves.

Mesometrium. This is the largest part of broad ligament, extending from the pelvic floor to the ovarian ligament and uterine body. The uterine artery passes between its two peritoneal layers about 1.5 cm lateral to the cervix, after crossing the ureter (p. 1559) and ascending in it, turns laterally below the uterine tube to anastomose with the ovarian artery. Between the infundibulum and upper (tubular) pole of the ovary and the lateral pelvic wall the broad mesometrium contains ovarian vessels and nerves within a fibrous *suspensory ligament* of the ovary (*infundibulopelvic ligament*), continued laterally over the external iliac vessels as a distinct fold. The mesometrium also encloses the proximal part of the *round ligament of the uterus*, as well as smooth muscle and loose connective tissue.

Uterine round ligaments (**14**.22) are narrow somewhat flattened bands 10–12 cm long passing diagonally down and laterally within the mesometrium from the upper part of the uterus to the pelvic floor. They are attached superiorly to the uterine wall just below and anterior to the lateral cornua, then each courses laterally downwards across the vesical, obturator and external iliac vessels, the obturator nerve and the obliterated umbilical artery. The round ligament enters the deep inguinal ring, round the start of the inferior epigastric artery, traverses the inguinal canal and finally splits into strands which merge with connective tissue in the vicinity. Classically, these strands have been described as terminating in the labia majora; however, on the basis of dissection of 10 cadavers aged 0–10 years, Attah and Hutson (1991) concluded that they did not reach the labia, but ended in the mons pubis or close to the anterior abdominal musculature. Near the uterus the round ligament contains much smooth muscle which gradually diminishes until its terminal part is purely fibrous. It is accompanied by blood vessels, nerves and lymphatics; the last drain the uterine region around the entry of the uterine tube to the superficial inguinal lymph nodes (p. 1623); uterine neoplasms may spread by this route. In the fetus a peritoneal processus vaginalis is carried with the round ligament for a short distance into the inguinal canal, but it is generally obliterated in adults, although sometimes patent even in old age. In the canal the ligament receives the same coverings as the spermatic cord (p. 1856), although they are thinner and blend with the ligament itself, which may not reach the labium majus but ends by fusing with these coverings. The round and ovarian ligaments are together homologous with the gubernaculum testis (p. 212).

Cervical ligaments

These condensations of connective tissue lie in the pelvic floor and form important mechanical supports for the uterus. They include three pairs of ligaments which pass radially outwards from the perimeter of the cervix to the bony wall of the pelvis transversely, anteriorly and posteriorly. They are, respectively, the transverse cervical, pubocervical and pubosacral ligaments. Of these, the transverse cervical ligaments are the largest and most important clinically (see Joseph 1991).

Transverse cervical ligaments of Mackenrodt (cardinal ligaments). These extend from the side of the cervix and the vault and lateral fornix of the vagina to extensive attachments at the pelvic wall. They are continuous with the fibrous tissue around the lower parts of the ureters and pelvic blood vessels. They are thought to play a part in stabilizing the uterus (hence its gynaecological importance).

Pubocervical ligaments. These pass forward from the anterior aspect of the uterus and upper vagina, diverging around the urethra to make attachments to the posterior aspects of the pubic bones.

Uterosacral ligaments. These pass back from the cervix and uterine body on either side of the rectum, attaching to the sacrum, in relation to the uterosacral folds (see above).

Summary. While the above ligaments (and vagina) may act in varying measure as mechanical supports of the uterus, the levatores ani and coccygei, urogenital diaphragm and perineal body appear at least as important in this respect (Wendell-Smith & Wilson 1977).

VAGINA

The vagina (**14**.15, 16, 24, 29, 30), the female copulatory organ, is a fibromuscular tube lined by non-keratinized stratified epithelium, from the vestibule (the cleft between the labia minora) to the uterus. The bladder and urethra are anterior, the rectum and anal canal posterior (separated in the upper part of the vagina by the recto-uterine pouch). The vagina ascends posterosuperiorly in a shallow S-shaped curve, at an angle of over 90° to the uterine axis, but which varies with the contents of the bladder and rectum. The inner surfaces of its walls are ordinarily in contact with each other, its lumen forming an H-shaped cleft, seen in transverse sections of its lower part, the transverse line being slightly convex forwards or backwards and the lateral limbs medially convex; at its intermediate level the lumen is a transverse slit. Its anterior wall is 7.5 cm in length, the posterior 9 cm; its width increases as it ascends. Its upper end surrounds the vaginal projection of the cervix uteri near the external os, attached to it higher on the posterior cervical wall than on the anterior.

The annular recess between the cervix and vagina is the *fornix*; the anterior, posterior and lateral parts of this recess are often given separate names (anterior fornix, etc.), but the recess is essentially continuous.

The *anterior wall* of the vagina is related to the urethra, which is embedded in it, and to the base of the bladder. The *posterior wall*, covered by peritoneum in its upper quarter, is separated from the rectum by the recto-uterine pouch above, and by moderately loose connective tissue in its middle half; in its lower quarter it is separated from the anal canal by the musculofibrous perineal body. Laterally are the levatores ani (p. 831) and pelvic fascia. As the ureters pass anteromedially to reach the fundus of the bladder, they pass close to the lateral fornices and as they enter the bladder they are usually anterior the vagina (p. 1829). Each ureter is crossed transversely here by a uterine artery (p. 1559).

MICROSTRUCTURE

The vagina has an inner mucosal and an external muscular stratum, the lamina propria of the former containing many thin-walled veins.

Mucosa

The mucosa adheres firmly to the muscular layer; on its epithelial surface are two median longitudinal ridges, one anterior and the other posterior. From these vaginal columns numerous transverse bilateral rugae extend, divided by sulci of variable depth, giving an

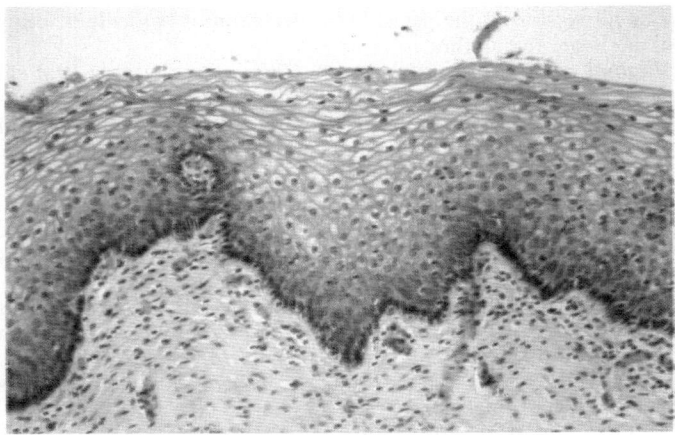

14.29 Section through the mucosa of the vagina, showing the non-keratinized stratified squamous epithelium and the lamina propria beneath. Note the papillated interface between the epithelium and underlying connective tissue. Haematoxylin and eosin.

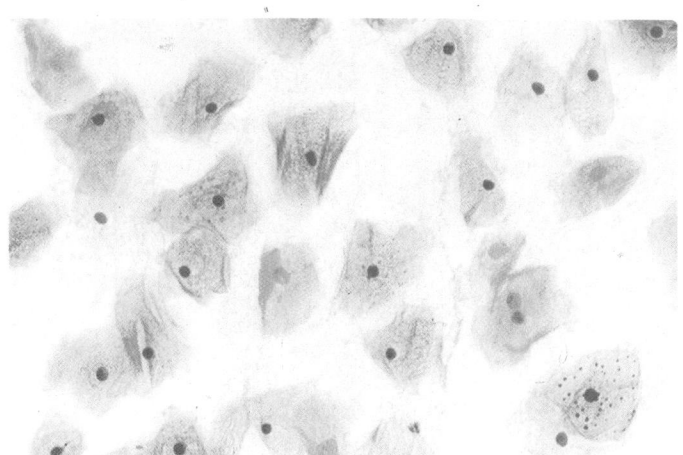

14.30 Cells of the mature vaginal epithelium in a diagnostic smear preparation stained by Papanicolaou's technique (Shorr modification). All the cells shown are superficial keratinizing squames, some of which show actual keratin granules. The pink cells are the oldest and most superficial. (Preparation provided by Max Levene, St Helier Hospital, Carshalton.)

appearance of conical papillae which are most numerous on the posterior wall and near the orifice. These are especially well developed before parturition. The epithelium is non-keratinized stratified squamous. After puberty it thickens and is rich in glycogen. Unlike many other mammals, human vaginal epithelium does not change markedly during the menstrual cycle, but its glycogen increases after ovulation and then diminishes towards the cycle's end. The fermentative action of certain bacteria (Doderlein's bacillus) on the glycogen-rich desquamated cellular debris renders vaginal fluid acid, and this appears to have an inhibitory effect on the growth of micro-organisms; the amount of glycogen is less before puberty and after the menopause, when vaginal infections are more common. There are no mucous glands. The vagina also receives mucus from the cervical glands, especially around the time of ovulation, serving to lubricate the vagina.

Cyclical variations in the vaginal epithelium have been much studied, especially by exfoliative cytology involving taking smears of surface cells to examine any microscopic changes, and their relative frequencies (Stockard & Papanicolaou 1917). The cells are mostly epitheliocytes and leucocytes (**14**.30). This technique has been useful in reproductive studies of experimental animals and is also applied in clinical gynaecology. Effects of hormonal therapy include changes in vaginal cellular debris, which also occur in uterine and especially cervical carcinoma (Papanicolaou & Traut 1943; Koss 1968).

Muscular layers

These are composed of smooth muscle and consist of a stronger external longitudinal, and an internal circular layer. Longitudinal fibres are continuous with the superficial muscle fibres of the uterus, the strongest fasciculi being those attached to the rectovesical fascia on each side. The two layers are not distinct but connected by oblique decussating fasciculi. The lower vagina is also surrounded by the skeletal muscle fibres of bulbospongiosus (p. 835). Most external is a layer of loose connective tissue, containing extensive vascular plexuses.

Vessels and nerves

Arteries. These are derived from the vaginal, uterine, internal pudendal and middle rectal branches of the internal iliac arteries (p. 1559; **10**.000).

Veins. These form lateral plexuses, drained through the vaginal veins to the internal iliac veins.

Lymph vessels. These are described on page 1623.

Nerves. Innervation is derived from the vaginal plexuses and pelvic splanchnic nerves (p. 1309). The lower vagina is supplied by the pudendal nerve (p. 1287). Many nerve fibres in the lamina propria and muscle react strongly to tests for cholinesterase and are probably cholinergic.

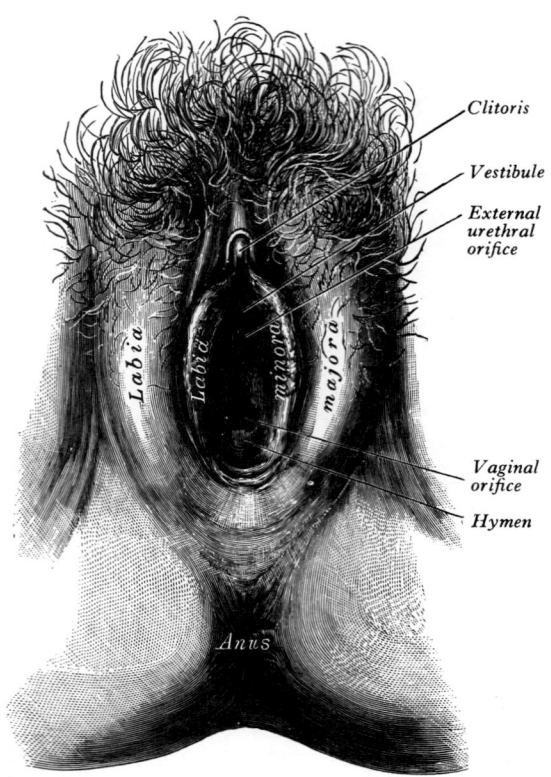

14.31 Female external genitalia, with the labia majora et minora separated.

FEMALE EXTERNAL GENITAL ORGANS

The female external genitalia (**14.31**, 32) include: the mons pubis, labia majora et minora pudendi, the clitoris, vestibule, vestibular bulb and the greater vestibular glands. The term *pudendum* or *vulva* includes all these parts.

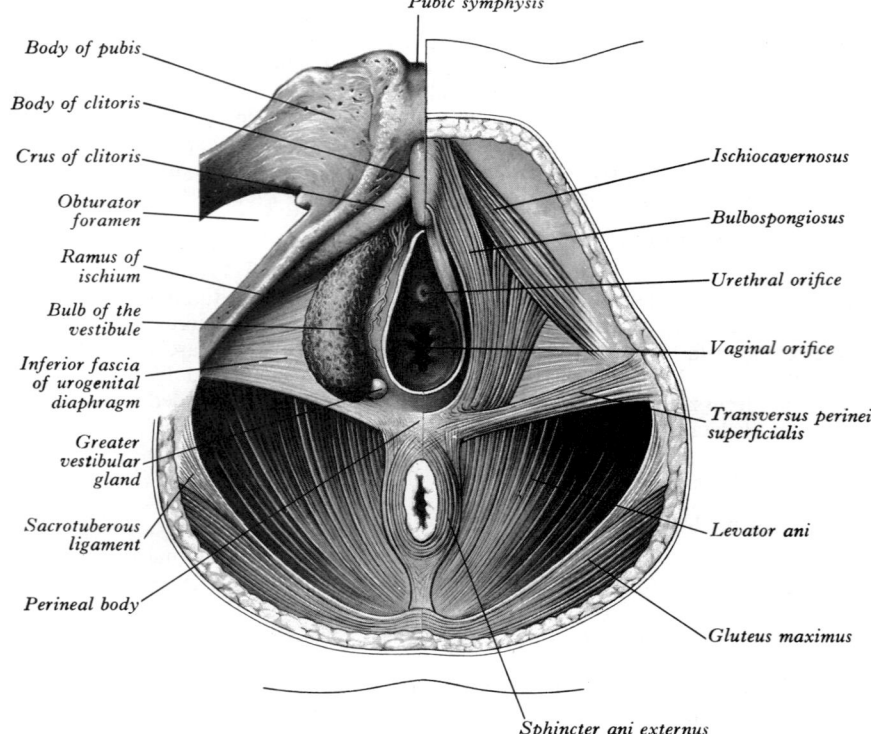

14.32 Dissection of the female perineum to show the bulb of the vestibule and greater vestibular gland on the right; on the left side of the body the muscles superficial to these structures have been left in situ.

Mons pubis. This name refers to the rounded eminence situated anterior to the pubic symphysis, formed by a mass of subcutaneous adipose connective tissue, covered by coarse hair at the time of puberty over an area usually limited above by an approximately horizontal boundary. (In males this upper limit is similar; its apparent continuation to the umbilicus consists of ordinary body hair.)

Labia majora (**14.31**). These two prominent, longitudinal, cutaneous folds extending back from the mons pubis to the perineum, form the lateral boundaries of the *pudendal cleft*, into which the vagina and urethra open. Each labium has an external, pigmented surface, covered with crisp hairs and a pink, smooth, internal surface with large sebaceous follicles. Between these surfaces is much loose connective and adipose tissue, intermixed with smooth muscle resembling the scrotal dartos muscle, together with vessels, nerves and glands. The uterine round ligament may end in the adipose tissue and skin in the front part of the labium. A persistent processus vaginalis and congenital inguinal hernia may also reach a labium. The labia are thicker in front, where they join to form the *anterior commissure*. Posteriorly they do not join but merge into neighbouring skin, ending near and almost parallel to each other; with the connecting skin between they form a low ridge, the *posterior commissure*, which overlies the perineal body; this is the posterior limit of the vulva; the interval between this and the anus, a distance of 2.5–3 cm, is the 'gynaecological' perineum.

Labia minora (**14.31**, 32). These two small cutaneous folds, devoid of fat, between the labia majora, extend from the clitoris obliquely down, laterally and back for about 4 cm, flanking the vaginal orifice. In virgins their posterior ends may be joined by the cutaneous *frenulum of the labia minora*. Anteriorly, each labium minus bifurcates, its upper layer passing above the *clitoris* to form with its fellow a fold, the prepuce, overhanging the *glans clitoridis*. The lower layer passes below the clitoris to form with its fellow the *frenulum clitoridis*. Sebaceous follicles are numerous on the apposed labial surfaces. Sometimes an extra labial fold (labium tertium) is found on one or both sides between the labia minora and majora (Gottlicher 1994).

Vestibule (**14.32**). This cavity lies between the labia minora. It contains the vaginal and external urethral orifices and the openings of the two *greater vestibular glands*, and those of numerous mucous *lesser vestibular glands*. Between the vaginal orifice and the frenulum of the labia minora is a shallow *vestibular fossa*. For a review of this region, see Woodruff and Friedrich (1985) and Wendell Smith and Wilson (1991).

Clitoris (**14.32**). This is an erectile structure, homologous with the penis, and lies postero-inferior to the anterior commissure, partially enclosed by the anterior, bifurcated ends of the labia minora. The corpus clitoridis has two *corpora cavernosa*, composed of erectile tissue and enclosed in dense fibrous tissue separated medially by an incomplete fibrous *pectiniform septum*; each corpus cavernosum is connected to its ischiopubic ramus by a *crus*. The glans clitoridis is a small round tubercle of spongy erectile tissue; its epithelium has high cutaneous sensitivity, important in sexual responses. The clitoris, like the penis, has a 'suspensory' ligament and two small muscles, the ischiocavernosi (p. 835), attached to its crura. In many details it is a small version of the penis, but differs from it basically in being separate from the urethra.

Vaginal orifice (introitus) (**14.32**). This is usually a sagittal slit positioned postero-inferior to the urethral meatus; its size varies inversely with that of the hymen; like all the vagina it is capable of great distension during parturition and to a lesser degree during coitus.

Hymen vaginae. This is a thin fold of mucous membrane situated just within the vaginal orifice; the internal surfaces of the fold are normally folded to contact each other and the vaginal orifice appears as a cleft between them. The hymen varies greatly in shape and area; when stretched, it is annular and widest posteriorly; sometimes it is semilunar, concave towards the pubes; occasionally it is cribriform or fringed. It may be absent or form a complete, imperforate hymen. When it is ruptured, small round *carunculae hymenales* are its remnants. It has no established function.

External urethral orifice (urinary meatus) (**14.32**). This opens about 2.5 cm postero-inferior to the glans clitoridis, anterior to the vaginal orifice: it is usually a short, sagittal cleft with slightly raised margins and is very distensible. It varies in shape from a round aperture to a slit, crescent or stellate form.

Bulbs of the vestibule (14.32). These are homologues of the single penile bulb and corpus spongiosum. They are two elongate erectile masses, flanking the vaginal orifice and united in front of it by a narrow commissura bulborum (pars intermedia). Each lateral mass is about 3 cm in length; their posterior ends are expanded and are in contact with the greater vestibular glands; their anterior ends are tapered and joined to one another by a commissure, and to the glans clitoridis by two slender bands of erectile tissue. Their deep surfaces contact the inferior aspect of the urogenital diaphragm. Superficially each is covered by a muscle, the *bulbospongiosus*. Thus the female corpus spongiosum is cleft into bilateral masses, except in its most anterior region, by the vestibule and the vaginal and urethral orifices.

Greater vestibular glands (glands of Bartholin; 14.32). These are homologues of the male bulbo-urethral glands; they consist of two small, round or oval reddish-yellow bodies, flanking the vaginal orifice, in contact with and often overlapped by the posterior end of the vestibular bulb. Each opens into the vestibule, by a duct of about 2 cm, in the groove between the hymen and a labium minus. They are not infrequent sources of vulval neoplasms. In microstructure, the glands are composed of tubulo-acinar tissue, its secretory cells columnar in shape, secreting a clear or whitish mucus with lubricant properties, stimulated by sexual arousal. In addition, recent studies have shown the presence of endocrine cells in these and the minor glands of the vestibule, using immunohistochemical methods; their contents include serotonin, calcitonin, bombesin, hCG and katacalcin (Fetissof et al 1989).

Vessels and nerves. The arterial blood supply, venous and lymph drainage and nerve supply of the female external genitalia resemble those of homologous structures in males. The **arterial supply**, from two external and one internal pudendal artery on each side, is massive. Hence, haemorrhage from vulval injuries may be severe. The sensory innervation of the anterior and posterior parts of the labium majus differ, as in the scrotum (p. 1857).

Anatomy of Pregnancy and Parturition

During pregnancy there are many morphological changes in the female reproductive system and associated abdominal structures (**14.33**A, B; **34**). The uterus enlarges to accommodate the developing fetus and placenta, and there are various alterations in the pelvic walls, floor and contents which allow for this expansion, and also anticipate parturition. At the end of this period dramatic changes take place which facilitate the passage of the offspring through the birth canal. These alterations are often neglected by anatomists, but they represent an important aspect of normal reproductive morphology, with considerable clinical interest.

Uterine size in pregnancy

The uterus grows dramatically during pregnancy and increases in weight from about 50 g at the beginning of pregnancy to up to 1 kg at term. Most of this gain in weight results from increases in the vascularity and tissue fluid of the uterine wall, together with myometrial growth (see above). The increased growth of the uterine wall is driven by a combination of mechanical stretching as the conceptus grows, and the stimulus of oestrogen. As already noted, the smooth muscle mass of the myometrium is thought to increase mainly by hypertrophy, although there is actually some true hyperplasia earlier in pregnancy.

As pregnancy proceeds, the uterus expands out of the pelvic basin and is usually palpable just above the pubic symphysis by the twelfth week, unless the uterus is retroverted (p. 1874), in which case it may not be palpable in the abdomen until a little later. In past obstetric practice, anatomical surface landmarks such as the pubic symphysis, umbilicus and xiphisternum were used to estimate uterine size and therefore gestational age. So, for example, by the twentieth week of pregnancy the uterine fundus has usually risen to the level of the umbilicus, and by 36 weeks the uterine fundus has reached the xiphisternum. However, with the advent of diagnostic ultrasound (14.34, 35) which allows a reasonably accurate dating of pregnancy, it has become clear that there is great variation in uterine size for a given gestation, and that clinical estimates based on anatomical landmarks are of limited value. In late pregnancy, fetal size and growth can be assessed by serial measurement of the distance between the pubic symphysis and the uterine fundus, but again the symphysis–fundus measurements act primarily as a screening method, with more accurate fetal biometry held in reserve.

Relations of the uterus in pregnancy

With uterine expansion, the ovaries and uterine tubes are displaced upwards and laterally; the round ligaments become hypertrophied and their course from the cornual regions of the uterus down to the internal inguinal ring becomes more vertical. The broad ligament tends to open out to accommodate the massive increase in the sizes of the uterine and ovarian vessels. The uterine veins in particular can reach about 1 cm in diameter, and for this reason they appear to act as a significant reservoir for blood after uterine contraction. Lymphatics, and also nerves similarly undergo enlargement, although the significance of the increased innervation is not clear, as paraplegic women are able to labour normally, albeit painlessly.

The uterine fundus comes into contact with the anterior abdominal wall at around 16–20 weeks' gestation. Later in pregnancy the increase in intra-abdominal pressure produced by the gravid uterus may produce eversion of the umbilicus.

On the skin over the abdomen, a combination of stretching and hormonal changes may produce stretch marks (*striae gravidarum*). In multiparous patients, separation of the rectus abdominis muscles may allow the uterine fundus to fall forwards to some extent.

In the supine position, the pregnant woman in late pregnancy is vulnerable to aortocaval compression, as the enlarged uterus presses on and reduces blood flow in the great vessels. Symptoms of nausea and faintness may be obvious, and uteroplacental blood flow may be impaired in some cases.

The jejunum, ileum and transverse colon tend to be displaced upwards by the enlarging uterus, whereas the caecum and appendix are displaced to the right, and the sigmoid colon posteriorly and to the left. Upward and lateral displacement of the appendix in later pregnancy can cause difficulties in the diagnosis of appendicitis. The ureters are pushed laterally by the enlarging uterus and in late pregnancy can be compressed at the level of the pelvic brim, resulting in hydronephrosis and loin pain. However, mild ureteric dilatation is normal in pregnancy, caused by progesterone-induced relaxation of smooth muscle in the ureteric walls. The axis of the uterus is shifted or dextrorotated by the presence of the sigmoid colon and this may lead to inadvertent incision into large uterine vessels at the time of lower segment caesarean section unless the operator is aware of any such rotation.

Maternal respiration, micturition and colorectal control

As the uterus grows there is some outward displacement of the chest, with flaring of the ribs. Although vital capacity is unchanged, tidal air is said to increase by 200 ml and residual volume to fall by the same amount. The respiratory rate may increase somewhat even in early pregnancy, possibly due to the effect of progesterone, while in late pregnancy, uterine expansion may limit diaphragmatic excur-

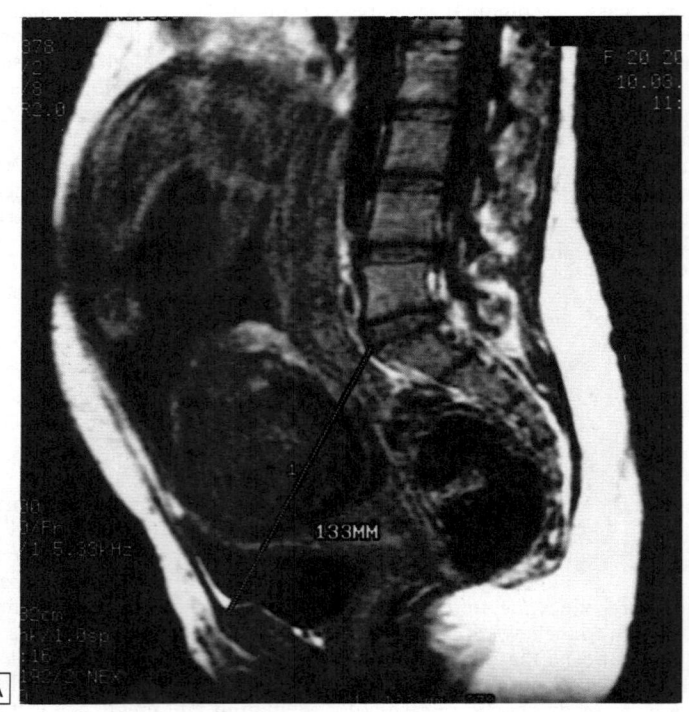

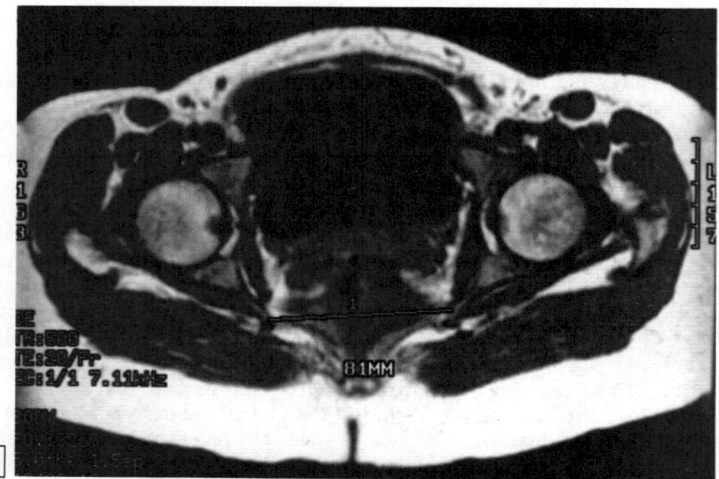

14.33A, B   MRI images of the abdomen and pelvis of a woman in a late stage of pregnancy. A shows the appearance in sagittal section, with the fetal head presenting in the pelvis at the level of the pelvic inlet. Also visible are the urinary bladder (lower left), the rectum (lower right), vertebral column (right) and the vagina (lower centre); the oblique line represents the distance between the sacral promontory and the pubic symphysis. In B the transverse plane of section passes through the uterus at midlevel (dark central area), with the sacrum behind, the anterior abdominal wall in front, and the acetabulae holding the two rounded femoral heads on either side. The transverse line indicates the distance between the two sacroiliac joints (i.e. the sacral width at this level). (A and B provided by N J Saunders, Princess Anne Hospital, Southampton.)

sion. The bladder becomes hyperaemic in early pregnancy, and there is also an increase in the frequency of micturition because of the raised glomerular filtration rate at that time, and later due to pressure from the presenting part on the bladder. Such pressure may also provoke urinary stress incontinence in the third trimester.

Changes in colorectal control are not very significant during pregnancy itself, although some women are troubled by constipation. Rectal sphincter damage can occur during childbirth and may lead to significant faecal incontinence if not recognized and adequately repaired at the time.

Pelvic changes in pregnancy

The presence of a pregnant uterus results in a change in the centre of gravity of the body, especially in late pregnancy (**14.33**). In order to compensate for this, the mother tends to straighten her cervical and thoracic spine, and throw her shoulders back, resulting in a compensatory lumbar lordosis. There is also softening of the pubic symphysis and sacro-iliac joints, caused by production of relaxin and other pregnancy hormones. This increased mobility produces a form of pelvic instability so that the pregnant woman tends to walk with a waddling gait. The result of this softening is an increase in pelvic diameter which is of benefit during the time of labour. Significant joint relaxation can be associated with pain, sometimes called pelvic arthropathy, and in fact in severe cases it is possible to see radiologically when a woman stands on one leg that the two halves of the symphysis are almost at different levels. Rotation of the sacrum at the sacro-iliac joint may also increase the diameter of the pelvic outlet.

Birth canal and perineum during parturition

The uterine cervix is required to serve two functions in relation to pregnancy and parturition. For 9 months the cervix is a relatively rigid fibromuscular structure which retains the products of conception within the uterus, and yet, within a few hours during active labour, it has to dilate rapidly to allow the fetus to descend through the birth canal. In fact this transition is not as abrupt as might first appear, with considerable softening and shortening of the cervix in the weeks before the onset of labour. A corresponding increase in uterine activity is usually apparent during this prelabour period. The rigidity of the cervix appears to be related to the orientation of its collagen fibres within a regular connective tissue matrix. Softening of the cervix prior to and during labour is associated with a loss of this pattern of fibre distribution and a large increase in tissue water.

Labour

The onset of labour is defined as the combination of regular usually painful uterine contractions of sufficient intensity to produce progressive effacement and dilatation of the cervix. It is often difficult to define the exact time of the onset of labour, except retrospectively. The pain of labour contractions is thought to be caused by myometrial ischaemia produced by a reduction in uterine blood flow during the peak of a contraction. Uterine contractions direct the fetus against the cervix and at the same time result in retraction of the upper uterine segment, drawing the fibromuscular cervix upwards past the presenting part. The process of labour is described as having four main stages, as follows.

First stage. This is defined as the period

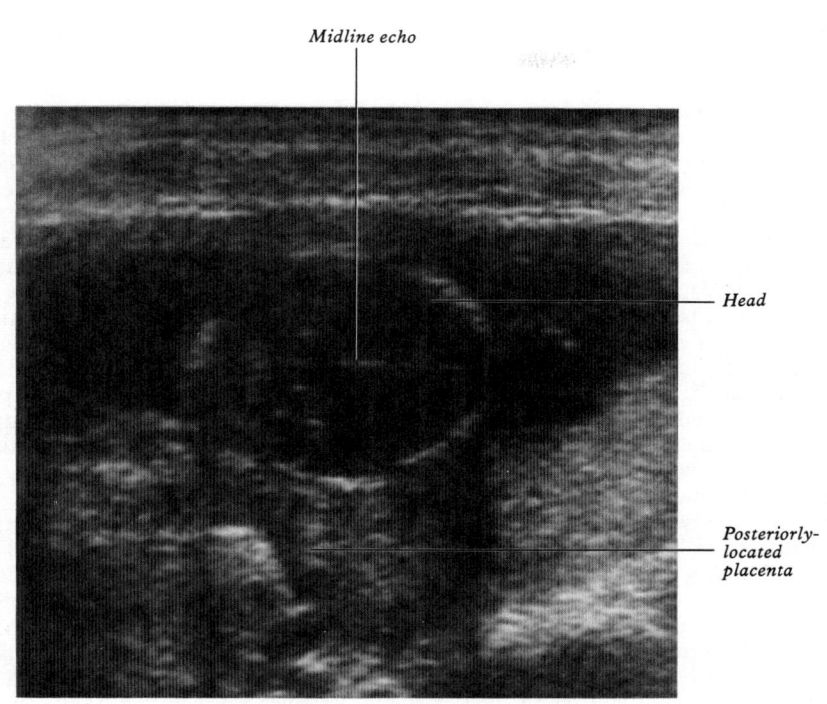

Midline echo

Head

Posteriorly-located placenta

14.34 Ultrasonogram through the uterus showing the head and placenta of a 16-week fetus. (Supplied by Shaun Gallagher, Guy's Hospital; photography by Sarah Smith, UMDS, Guy's Hospital Campus, London.)

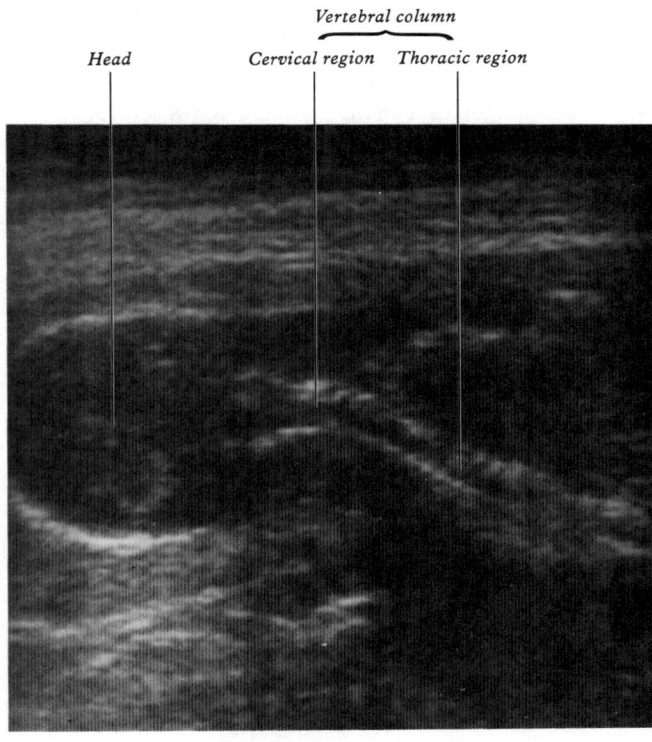

Head

Vertebral column

Cervical region   Thoracic region

14.35 Ultrasonogram through the uterus showing the head and upper part of the vertebral column of a 16-week fetus, in sagittal section. (Provided by Shaun Gallagher, Guy's Hospital; photography by Sarah Smith, UMDS, Guy's Hospital Campus, London.)

Second stage. This commences once the cervix is fully dilated, and ends with the delivery of the child. Uterine contractions produce the descent of the fetal presenting part. Pressure at this stage on the pelvic diaphragm and rectum produces in the mother a reflex desire to 'bear down'. Thus involuntary maternal effort using the diaphragm and abdominal musculature augments uterine activity to help deliver the child.

The head of the baby usually enters the pelvis with the occiput facing laterally. Further descent of the head results in the occiput contacting the gutter-shaped pelvic floor formed by levator ani. This promotes flexion and rotation of the occiput to the anterior position. With further descent the occiput escapes under the symphysis pubis and the head is born by extension. At this point, the baby's head regains its normal relationship with its shoulders, and slight rotation (or restitution) of the head is seen. Further external rotation occurs as the leading shoulder is directed medially by the maternal pelvic floor. The body of the baby is now born by lateral flexion as one shoulder slips underneath the symphysis and the posterior shoulder is drawn over the frenulum.

Third stage. This period is defined as the time from delivery of the fetus until delivery of the placenta. This process is usually expedited by the administration of oxytocic drugs in an attempt to limit maternal blood loss.

Factors affecting the progress of labour

Many factors affect the progress of labour including the quality of uterine contractions, the size of the maternal bony pelvis, the size and position of the baby's head and the extent to which the skull will mould to the shape of the pelvis. Due to the complex nature of these interactions, it is generally not possible to predict the outcome of labour with any degree of accuracy, and most pregnant women will be offered a trial of labour if there is any doubt, providing the baby is in cephalic presentation. Poor progress during labour is predominantly a problem in the first labour because of the combination of incoordinate uterine action and increased soft tissue resistance at the level of the cervix, pelvic diaphragm and perineum. Treatment of such primigravidae is aimed at improving uterine activity through the combination of artificial rupture of the fetal membranes and administration of an intravenous infusion of oxytocin. Over 80% of cases will respond to such a regime, the remainder usually requiring caesarean delivery. In multiparous women, slow progress in labour may be due to a mechanical problem such as a breech presentation, a large baby, or spondyliolisthesis (in which the fifth lumbar vertebra slips forwards

during which the cervix dilates as it is drawn up into the lower portion of the uterus until there is no longer any cervix palpable on vaginal examination, and thus no further impediment to the descent of the fetus through the birth canal.

on the first sacral body, thus effectively reducing the size of the pelvis). Use of oxytocin in the context of such genuine mechanical difficulties can lead to uterine rupture.

Obstetric emergencies

Fetal distress. The unborn baby derives its oxygen from the mother via the placenta and umbilical cord. Fetal hypoxia may occur if the uteroplacental circulation is inadequate, if the placenta separates from the uterine wall or if the cord is compressed. During labour, uterine contractions tend to reduce placental perfusion. In addition, cord compression may occur during contractions, particularly if the amniotic fluid volume is reduced. Indirect evidence of fetal hypoxia can be inferred from certain changes in the fetal heart rate such as reduced variation and decelerations occurring in the rate after uterine contractions. Confirmation of hypoxia can be achieved by obtaining a blood sample from the fetal scalp and measuring the acid–base balance of the specimen. Confirmation of significant hypoxia/acidosis during labour (pH < 7.20) will usually be dealt with by caesarean section.

Prolapsed cord. The umbilical cord may prolapse through the cervix into the vagina once the fetal membranes rupture. Conditions which prevent the fetal head from fully occupying the maternal pelvis will predispose to this problem, i.e. pelvic tumours (fibroids), ovarian cysts, placenta praevia and prematurity. Compression of the cord by the presenting part of the fetus, or an umbilical artery spasm will lead to fetal hypoxia and death if untreated. The treatment of choice for most cases is immediate caesarian section, and

the risk of perinatal death rises as the interval from delivery to diagnosis increases.

Antepartum haemorrhage. The two most serious causes of antepartum haemorrhage are placenta praevia and placental abruption.

Placenta praevia. In early pregnancy the placental disc occupies a large proportion of the uterine cavity and will often appear to be situated near the internal os, on ultrasonographic examination. In the majority of cases where the placenta appears low in early pregnancy, growth and stretching of the uterus will usually draw the placenta upwards away from the cervix by the end of pregnancy. In about 1% of pregnancies the position of the placenta will remain over or in close proximity to the internal cervical os at the end of pregnancy. This condition is called placenta praevia and is associated with vaginal bleeding during pregnancy and labour. The blood loss can be life-threatening for the mother. The diagnosis is confirmed by ultrasound examination and the usual therapeutic goal is to prolong pregnancy with hospitalization and if necessary provide blood transfusion until the fetus is of sufficient maturity to be delivered. Caesarean section is required and the procedure may be very haemorrhagic due to the increased vascularity of the lower uterine segment.

Placental abruption. This emergency, premature separation of the placenta from the uterine wall, may occur in pregnancy or labour, and remains a significant cause of intrauterine death. The diagnosis is suggested by the onset of constant and severe abdominal pain, with the uterus appearing rigid and tender on abdominal palpation. Placental separation is usually

accompanied by bleeding but the blood may initially be contained within the uterus and not be obvious on external examination. Release of thromboplastin from the damaged placenta into the maternal circulation causes disseminated intravascular coagulation and consumption of clotting factors which may predispose to further maternal haemorrhage at the time of delivery. Transfusion of blood and clotting factors may be required to resuscitate the mother. If the fetus is still alive on presentation, caesarean section is usually undertaken.

Postpartum haemorrhage. Prior to separation of the placenta, a large proportion of the mother's cardiac output passes through the uterine circulation. After separation in the third stage of labour, exsanguination is only prevented by marked uterine contraction, with crisscrossing myometrial fibres acting as a tourniquet, restricting blood flow to the area that was the placental site. Therefore any condition which predisposes to poor uterine contraction will increase the likelihood of haemorrhage immediately after delivery, such as retained placental tissue or blood clot within the uterus.

The other major cause of postpartum bleeding is that of trauma to the genital tract. Tearing will be found most frequently in the perineum and vagina but on occasion cervical laceration or even uterine rupture may be responsible for bleeding. Primary management of postpartum haemorrhaging is aimed at administering oxytocic drugs and resuscitating the mother with intravenous fluid. If this fails to stem the bleeding, then exploration of the genital tract under anaesthesia to exclude retained placental tissue or genital tract trauma is undertaken.

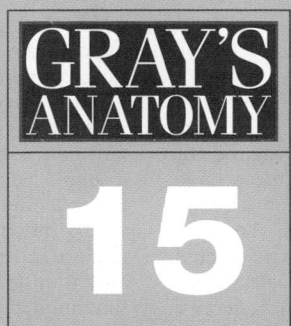

15

ENDOCRINE SYSTEM

Section Editor: Mary Dyson

INTRODUCTION

For a multicellular organism to survive and maintain its integrity in a varying, often adverse environment, regulatory mechanisms are essential. Metazoa have attained some freedom from the vagaries of the external environment (over which only the most advanced have much control, although this is only of a short-term nature) by developing the capacity to regulate, with varying success, the composition and properties of their immediate cellular environments which comprise intercellular or tissue fluid and, in vascularized metazoa, the fluid components of blood and lymph. The effective stabilization of these media is directly related to an organism's success and longevity.

Tissue fluid and plasma are stabilized by the co-ordinated regulatory activity of the autonomic and endocrine systems, the latter including the diffuse neuroendocrine system (p. 1898) and the endocrine system proper. All operate by intercellular communication but differ in the mode and speed, and in the degree or localization of the effects produced. The *autonomic nervous system* utilizes conduction and neurotransmitter release to transmit information; it is swift and localized in the responses induced. The diffuse *neuroendocrine system* uses only secretions, is slower and the induced responses are less localized, because the secretions, for example neurotransmitters, can act on contiguous cells, on groups of nearby cells reached by diffusion or on distant cells via blood. The *endocrine system* proper, comprising isolated or clustered cells and discrete ductless glands producing hormones (organic molecules transported by blood to distant effector cells), is even slower and less localized, though its effects are specific and often prolonged. These regulatory systems overlap in form and function, with a gradation from the neural autonomic system, through the intermediate diffuse neuroendocrine system to the endocrine system proper.

The close interrelationship of autonomic and endocrine systems, both structural and functional, is exemplified by the hypothalamus (p. 1094). This integrates both systems and is the major site at which their activities combine. Apart from its nervous functions the hypothalamus is also endocrine, producing by neurosecretion a wide range of peptide hormones including releasing and inhibiting factors which control the activity of the adenohypophysis, itself a major endocrine gland. Though conveniently considered separately, the autonomic, diffuse neuroendocrine and endocrine systems are really a single neuroendocrine regulator of the metabolic activities and internal environment of the organism, providing conditions in which it can function successfully. This may be an oversimplification for there are also close interregulatory links between the neuroendocrine and immune systems, and it has been suggested that the hypothalamus acts not only as the centre of neuroendocrine regulation but also as the centre of neuroendocrine–immune regulation (Daikoku 1993).

There are, in addition to the endocrine glands and diffuse neuroendocrine system described here, other hormone-producing cells which form components of other systems and are described with them. These include: the circumventricular organs, pancreatic islets (p. 1793), gastro-entero-endocrine cells (p. 1898), certain thymic (p. 1424) and renal (p. 1826) cells, pulmonary endocrine cells (p. 1666), interstitial testicular cells (p. 1853), interstitial follicular and luteal ovarian cells (p. 1862) and, in pregnancy, placental cells (p. 1865). Some cardiac myocytes, particularly in the walls of the atria, also have endocrine functions (p. 173). Furthermore, it has become apparent over the last few years that many secretory substances which were hitherto thought to be exclusive to the endocrine glands also occur widely in the central nervous system (CNS), where they may act as neurotransmitters or neuromodulators (p. 935). Studies of the parvicellular subnuclei of the hypothalamic paraventricular nucleus (p. 1100), for example, have shown that they contain over 30 different substances with putative neurotransmitter status (Cechetto & Saper 1988). Some of these are distributed via the bloodstream in typical endocrine fashion but others reach their targets in, for example, the autonomic areas of the brainstem and spinal cord (Luiten & Ter Horst 1986) and the circumventricular organs via efferent fibres (Larsen et al 1991). The function of these

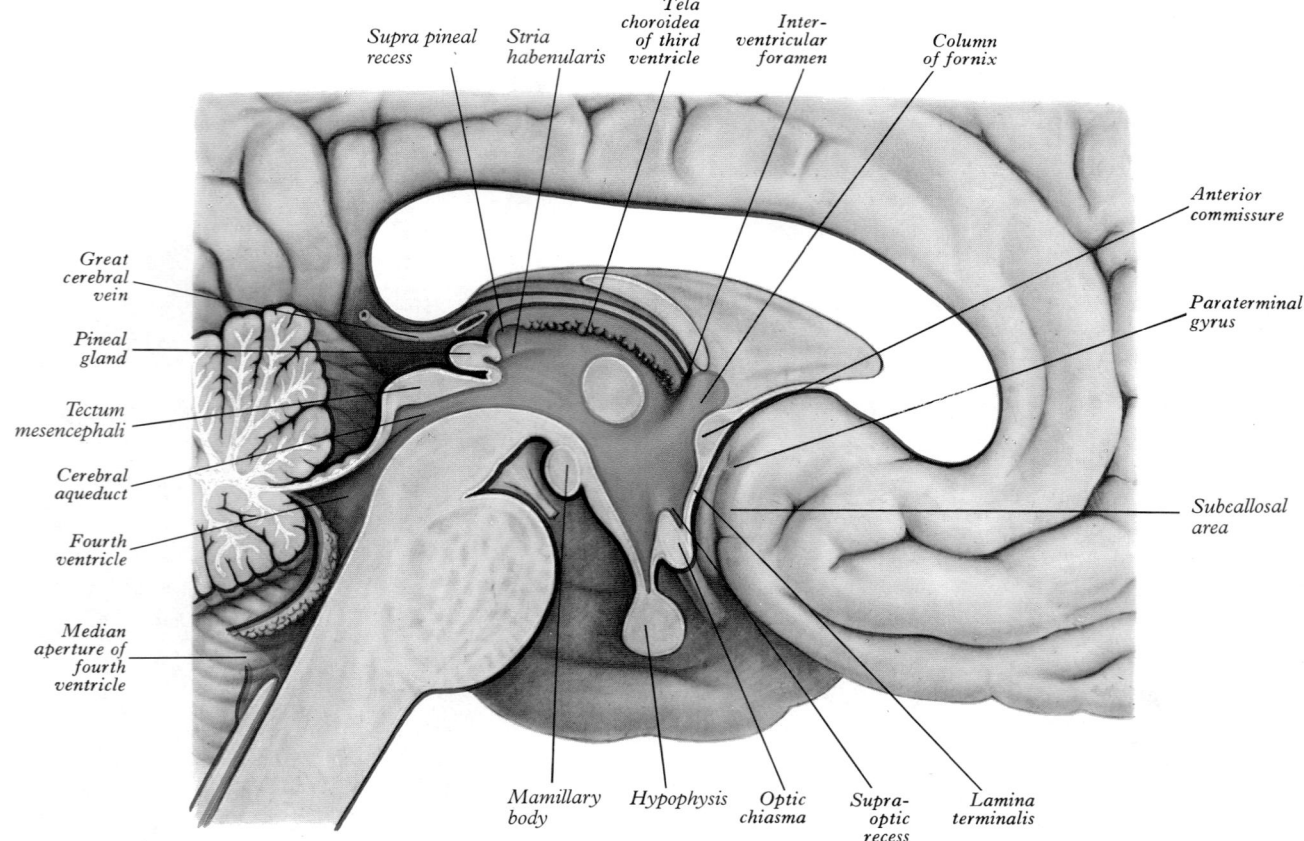

15.1   Part of a median section through the brain to demonstrate the location of the hypophysis cerebri (pituitary gland) and its immediate surroundings, particularly hypothalamic structures. The cut edge of the pia mater is shown in red, the ependyma in blue.

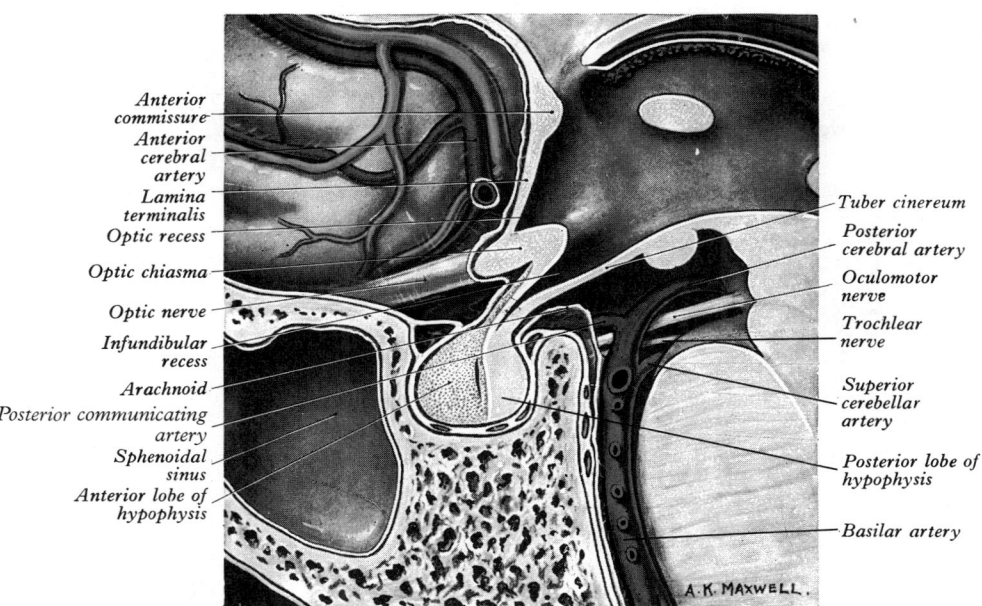

15.2   Median section through the hypophysis cerebri, in situ.

substances is complex, but appears to result in the integration of neuroendocrine output. The ability to synthesize and secrete such substances is therefore a very widespread activity, emphasizing the complex interdependence of the various systems of chemical control throughout the body.

PITUITARY GLAND

The pituitary gland or **hypophysis cerebri** (**15**.1.8) is a reddish-grey, ovoid body, about 12 mm in transverse and 8 mm in anteroposterior diameter and weighing about 500 mg. It is continuous with the infundibulum, a hollow, conical, inferior process from the tuber cinereum of the hypothalamus (p. 1094). It lies within the hypophyseal fossa of the sphenoid, covered superiorly by a circular *diaphragma sellae* of dura mater which is pierced centrally by an aperture for the infundibulum and separates the anterior superior aspect of the hypophysis (pituitary gland) from the optic chiasma (**15**.2). The hypophysis is flanked by the cavernous sinuses and their contained structures (p. 1585). Inferiorly it is separated from the floor of its fossa by a venous sinus communicating with the circular sinus (p. 1587). The meninges blend with the hypophyseal capsule and are not separate layers.

The hypophysis consists of two major parts, differing in origin, structure and function: one is a diencephalic down-growth connected with the hypothalamus; the other is an ectodermal derivative of the stomatodeum. These are respectively the *neurohypophysis* and *adenohypophysis*. Both include parts of the *infundibulum* (the older terms 'anterior' and 'posterior lobes' do not). The infundibulum has a central *infundibular stem*, containing neural hypophyseal connections and continuous with the *median eminence* of the tuber cinereum (p. 1094). Thus, the term *neurohypophysis* includes the median eminence, infundibular stem and *neural lobe* or *pars posterior*. Surrounding the infundibular stem is the *pars tuberalis*, a component of the adenohypophysis. The main mass of the adenohypophysis is divisible into the *pars anterior* (*pars distalis*) and *pars intermedia*, separated in fetal and early postnatal life by the hypophyseal cleft, a vestige of Rathke's pouch from which it develops. Usually obliterated in childhood, it may persist in the form of cystic cavities often present near the adenoneurohypophyseal frontier and sometimes invading the neural lobe. The human pars intermedia is rudimentary; because it may also be partially displaced into the neural lobe, it has been included in the anterior **and** posterior parts by different observers. Apart from this equivocation, of little significance in view of the exiguous status of the human pars intermedia, the partes

anterior et posterior (nervosa) may be equated with the anterior and posterior lobes. When the associated infundibular parts continuous with these lobes are included, the names adenohypophysis and neurohypophysis become appropriate. The terms will hence be used as follows:

* *Neurohypophysis*: includes the pars posterior (pars nervosa, posterior or neural lobe), infundibular stem and median eminence.
* *Adenohypophysis*: includes the pars anterior (pars distalis or glandularis), pars intermedia and pars tuberalis.

The hypophyseal divisions are shown in **15**.2, 3, 9. They differ in the types and arrangement of cells and the details of their vascular and neural supplies. Studies of these structures have engendered a formidable literature, summarized below.

ADENOHYPOPHYSIS

The adenohypophysis (**15**.3–6) is highly vascular and consists of epithelial cells of varying size and shape arranged in cords or irregular follicles, between which lie thin-walled vascular sinusoids and which are supported by a delicate skeleton of reticular tissue. Of the hormones synthesized and released by the adenohypophysis, most are *tropic*, such as: *somatotropin* (STH) involved in the control of body growth, *mammotropin* (*lactogenic hormone*; LTH) which

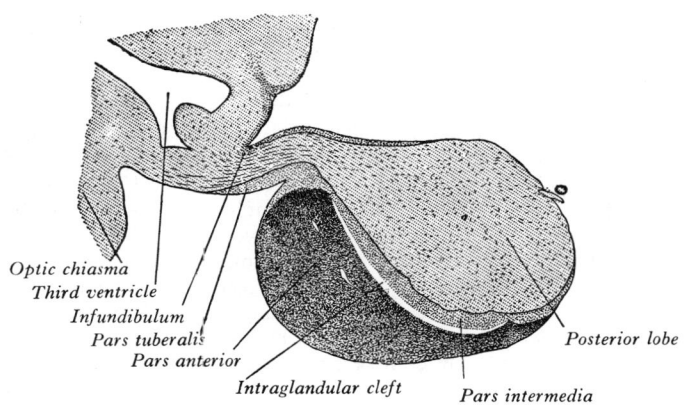

15.3   Diagram of a median section through the hypophysis cerebri of an adult monkey.

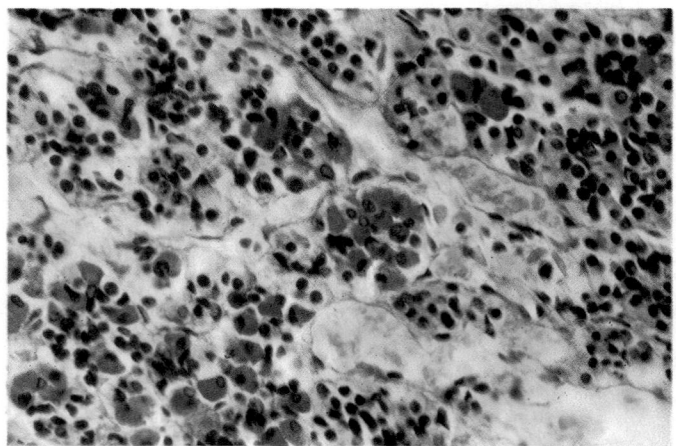

15.4A Medium-power micrograph of adenohypophyseal cells stained with the PAS-orange-G technique, to distinguish between α-cells (yellow), β-cells (red to brown) and chromophobic cells (pale grey with little cytoplasm). A number of large vascular sinusoids containing yellow-stained erythrocytes are also prominent. Magnification × 400.

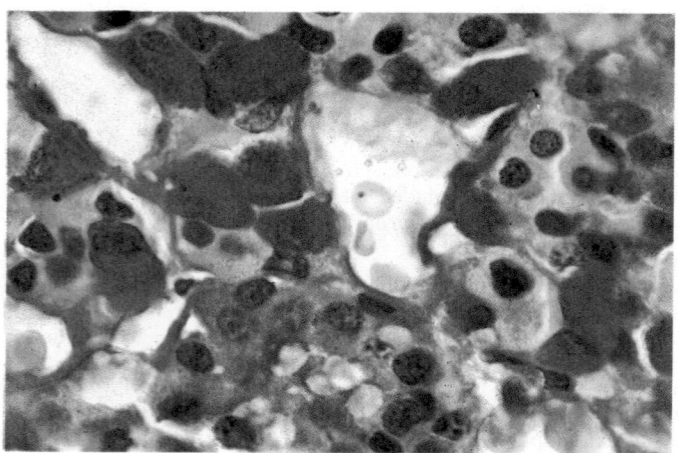

15.4B High-power micrograph of a group of cells stained as for A, grouped around a vascular sinusoid. Note α-cells (yellow) and β-cells (red). Magnification × 1000.

stimulates growth and secretion by the female breast, *adreno-corticotropin* (ACTH) governing the secretion of some adrenal cortical hormones, *thyrotropin* (TSH) stimulating thyroid activity, *follicle-stimulating hormone* (FSH) stimulating growth and secretion of oestrogens in the ovarian follicles and spermatogenesis in the testis, *interstitial-cell-stimulating hormone* (ICSH) activating androgen secretion by the testis, *luteinizing hormone* (LH) inducing progesterone secretion by the corpus luteum and *melanocyte-stimulating hormone* (MSH) increasing cutaneous pigmentation. Most of these hormones also have other complex metabolic effects.

Cell types in the adenohypophysis

The identities of endocrine cells secreting the different adeno-hypophyseal hormones have been intensively sought by the use of differential staining techniques (Harris & Donovan 1966); earlier techniques used the simple criterion of the affinities of cells for acidic and basic dyes, such as orange-G and aldehyde fuchsin, respectively. Cells staining strongly were *chromophilic*, those with little affinity for dyes being *chromophobic*. Chromophilic cells whose cytoplasm stained strongly with acidic dyes were classed as *acidophils* (α-cells) in contrast to *basophils* (β-cells) which stained strongly with basic dyes. Modifications using complex, multistage staining further distinguished many subcategories of cells. Such techniques, applied particularly to experimental or pathological pituitary glands from individuals with known hormonal defects, were used to associate specific cell types with particular hormones. However, many uncer-

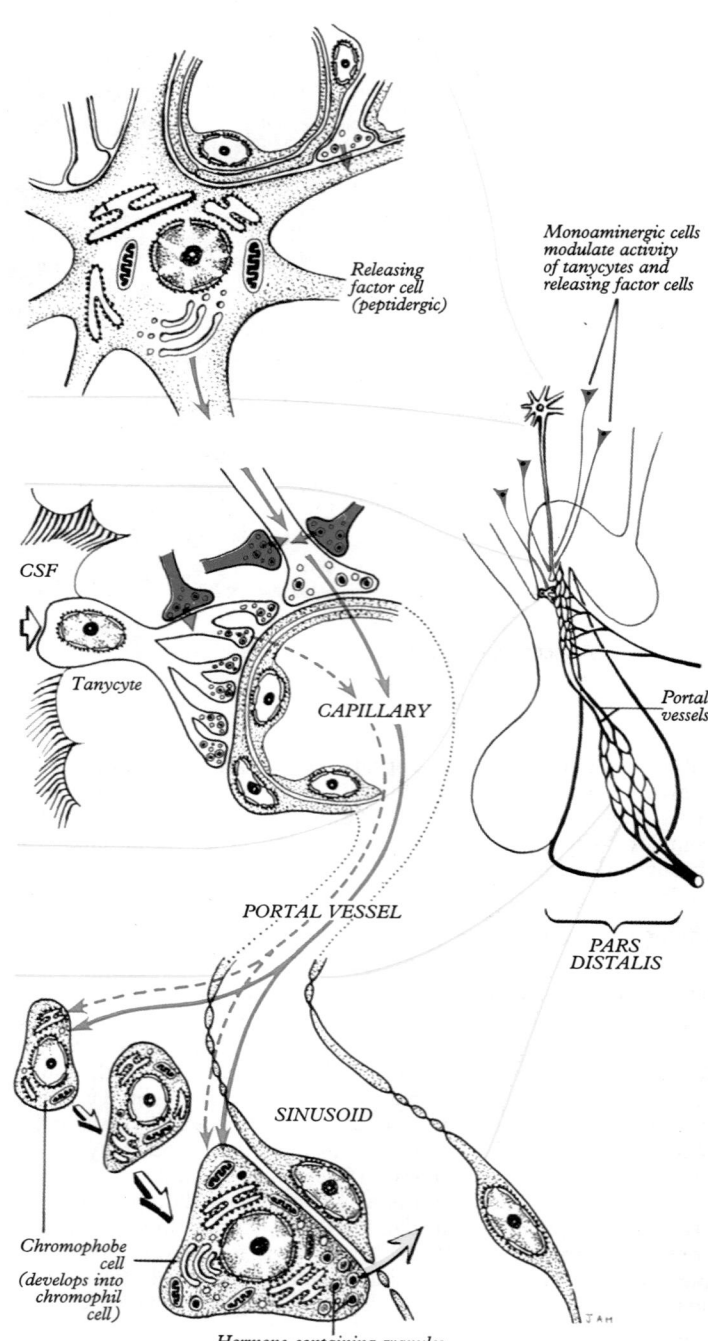

15.5 Diagram illustrating the main control systems which influence the hormonal output of the adenohypophysis. The small diagram on the right shows the hypothalamus, median eminence and adenohypophysis (pars distalis) and their associated neurons and vasculature. On the left three zones are shown in greater detail. The concatenation of events is as follows: under the influence of blood-borne factors and neural stimuli, the hypothalamic neuron shown above liberates specific releasing factors into capillaries of the median eminence. Modulation at this point is mediated by aminergic neurons and tanycytes. Onward transport of these factors through portal vessels is indicated by blue arrows. Stimulation and hormone production and release on the part of the adenohypophyseal cell are also indicated.

tainties remained, due to difficulty in standardizing stains and in classifying endless minor variations in different individuals and species.

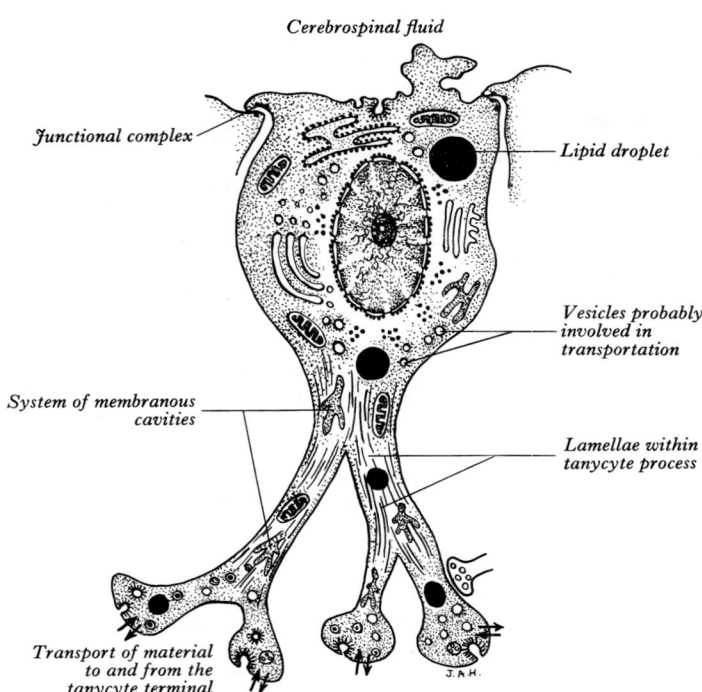

Cerebrospinal fluid

Junctional complex

Lipid droplet

Vesicles probably
involved in
transportation

System of membranous
cavities

Lamellae within
tanycyte process

Transport of material
to and from the
tanycyte terminal

15.6 The general ultrastructure of a tanycyte. (See text on p. 1886 for explanatory details.)

More recently, immunochemical methods have been applied (Nakane 1970) and immunofluorescence techniques have identified the sites of synthesis of individual hormones. Such methods, combined with electron microscopy and cell fractionation, have made it possible to consign all major hormones to particular cell types, although the terminology of older classifications has in part been retained. Ultrastructural studies of the normal human adenohypophysis are relatively scarce and much of our information has come from non-human primates. However, species differences do exist in the fine structural and dye-binding properties of cells of this kind. For detailed accounts of adenohypophyseal structure and function, see Costoff (1977), Pelletier et al (1978), Bhatnagar (1983), Motta (1984), Martin (1985), Schwartz and Cherny (1992).

Pars anterior. This contains chromophil cells, chromophobe cells and folliculostellate (FS) cells as follows:

A. Chromophil cells
1. *Acidophils* (*a-cells*)
- *Somatotrophs.* These are ovoid and usually grouped along sinusoids; they are the largest and most abundant class of adenohypophyseal chromophils, secreting the protein somatotropin or growth hormone (GH). They stain strongly with orange-G, and ultrastructurally are seen to contain numerous electron-dense, spherical, secretory granules, 350–500 nm in diameter, and a well-developed Golgi complex but, in the secretory phase, relatively small amounts of granular endoplasmic reticulum; the nucleus is central. Cells of similar fine structure characterize human eosinophilic adenomata associated with acromegaly or gigantism (Zambrano et al 1968).
- *Mammotrophs.* These secrete the polypeptide hormone prolactin (PRL), and are dominant in pregnancy and hypertrophy during lactation. They are distinguished by their affinity to the dyes erythrosin and azocarmine. Their secretory granules are the largest in any hypophyseal cell (over 600 nm in diameter) in pregnant and lactating females, although smaller (200 nm) and fewer in non-pregnant females and in males; the granules are evenly dense, ovoid or irregular, the latter form resulting from fusion. Excess granules fuse with lysosomes to form autophagic vacuoles which degrade unused granules. In active cells, granular endoplasmic reticulum and a Golgi complex are prominent.

- *Mammosomatotrophs.* These cells, present in the human fetal and adult pars anterior, are characterized by the presence of secretory granules shown by immunoelectron microscopy utilizing the double labelling immunogold technique to contain both GH and PRL simultaneously (Losinski et al 1991).
2. *Basophils* (*β-cells*)
- *Corticotrophs.* The identification of the cells which secrete adrenocorticotropin (ACTH) was difficult to achieve until it was realized that a precursor molecule, pro-opio-melanocorticotropin, is cleaved into a number of different molecules including ACTH, beta-lipotropin and beta-endorphin; the functions of the latter two substances in the pituitary are not known, although the opio-melanocorticotropin complex is also synthesized in neurons of the CNS and has neuromodulator functions there (p. 935). In humans, though not in some other species, this precursor is glycosylated, making the granules periodic acid-Schiff (PAS)-positive; they are also weakly basophilic. These cells are irregular in shape and have short dendritic processes which are inserted among other neighbouring cells. Their granules are also small (about 200 nm) and difficult to detect by light microscopy.
- *Thyrotrophs* (*β-basophils*). These secrete thyroid stimulating hormone (TSH). They are elongated, polygonal and lie in clusters towards the adenohypophyseal centre. They usually form cellular cords and are not in direct contact with sinusoids; they stain selectively with aldehyde fuchsin. Their granules, peripheral and irregular, are less electron-dense than in other basophils, being 100–150 nm in diameter and among the smallest granules in adenohypophyseal cells.
- *Gonadotrophs* (*δ-basophils*). These are larger than thyrotrophs, are rounded and usually situated next to sinusoids; they have secretory granules with an affinity for the PAS stain. In some cells, usually peripheral in the lobe, the granules stain purple while in others, more central, they stain red; it has been suggested that the former secrete FSH and the latter LH or ICSH (Purves 1961). Electron microscopy of the rat adenohypophysis has distinguished two cell types (Kurosumi & Oota 1968); but immunocytochemical studies of Phifer et al (1973) in man and of Moriarty (1975) in rats suggest that FSH and LH may coincide in the same cell, within the same secretory granules. Gonadotrophs have pleomorphic nuclei and spherical granules about 200 nm in diameter which tend to gather in lines under the cell surface during secretory activity, a vesicular granular endoplasmic reticulum and a well-developed Golgi complex (von Lawzewitsch et al 1972).

B. Chromophobe cells
Chromophobe cells constitute the majority of the cells of the adenohypophysis (about half the population of epithelial cells) but, because of their small size and lack of reaction to routine stains, they are not a conspicuous feature of the pituitary. They appear to consist of a number of different types of cells, including degranulated secretory cells of the types described above, stem cells capable of giving rise to chromophils and follicular cells containing numbers of lysosomes and forming cell clusters around cysts of various sizes; cysts are often present in the junctional area with the neurohypophysis and are filled with a PAS-positive substance of unknown significance.

C. Folliculostellate (FS) cells
These act as supporting cells and are also involved in trophic and catabolic processes and in macromolecular transport. Various peptides with growth factor or cytokine activity have been identified in FS cells, according to a review by Allaerts et al (1990). These include vascular endothelial growth factor (Ferrara et al 1991). The FS cells are linked by gap junctions, the frequency of which, in female rats, is modulated by both gonadal steroid hormones and prolactin, being most numerous during either proestrus or oestrus (Soji et al 1991). FS cells of the human pituitary gland also express a broad spectrum of cytokeratins indicative of their epithelial nature and supporting the generally accepted but recently challenged hypothesis that the adenohypophysis is derived from Rathke's pouch (Tsuchida et al 1993). Pituitary FS cells and lymphoid dendritic cells have many morphological and immunocytochemical features in common, both being stellate in shape, detectable by the presence of major histocompatibility complex (MHC) class II determinants and

the calcium ion binding protein S100, and by producing the cytokine interleukin 6 (Allaerts et al 1991).

Pars intermedia. This has many β-cells and follicles of chromophobe cells surrounding PAS-positive colloidal material, some of these being derived from pouches of the embryonic intrahypophyseal cleft (of Rathke); in some species, where this pouch remains large, a ciliated lining epithelium has been noted.

Secretory cells of the pars intermedia have granules containing either α-endorphin or β-endorphin scattered uniformly (Guillerman 1978); these cells have also been shown to contain various peptide hormones including ACTH and α-MSH, and are therefore assigned to the amine precursor uptake and decarboxylation (APUD) series (p. 1900), as are other adenohypophyseal secretory cells. Endorphin has also been found in the pars anterior, where it is localized to peripheral granules in discrete groups of cells.

Pars tuberalis. This is remarkable for its large number of blood vessels, between which cords or balls of undifferentiated cells are admixed with some α- and β-cells.

Electron microscopic and immunohistochemical investigations of the human fetal pars tuberalis at mid-gestation (Schulze-Bonhage & Wittkowski 1991) have identified gonadotrophs, thyrotrophs and an additional cell type which closely resembles pars tuberalis-specific cells of other species. The role of the last of these in human endocrine regulation remains to be determined.

Functional receptors for the pineal hormone melatonin, known to influence circadian systems and photoperiodicity via the hypothalamo–hypophyseal–gonadal axis, have been found in the pars tuberalis of a number of species. In the ovine pars tuberalis approximately 90% of the cells are either agranular or sparsely granular and are responsive to melatonin, which inhibits the formation of cyclic adenosine monophosphate (cAMP) by these cells. The remaining 10% have abundant dense-cored vesicles and are unresponsive to melatonin. Depending on the amount of melatonin secreted by the pineal gland and the receptivity of cells of the pars tuberalis to it, the latter seems able to respond by varying its secretion of a peptide hormone which modulates the gonadotrophic and thyrotrophic activity of the pars anterior (Wittkowski et al 1992), reaching it via the portal plexus.

Control of secretion in the adenohypophysis

The release of adenohypophyseal hormones into the circulation appears to be by exocytosis of their vesicle contents into the perivascular spaces of the neighbouring sinusoids; these are lined by a fenestrated endothelium, facilitating diffusion into the blood. A major signal for secretion is the liberation of releasing factors from neurons (McKelvy 1974) in the median eminence, nucleus infundibularis (arcuate nucleus) and other hypothalamic nuclei, into the upper capillary bed of the venous portal system which carries them to the adenohypophysis to act on its endocrine cells. These neurosecretory cells are *neuroendocrine transducers* (Wurtman 1970), receiving neural and hormonal signals and responding by secreting hormones, thus transducing one type of signal into another. The neurons which produce releasing factors are peptidergic, whereas neurons modulating endocrine activity are largely monoaminergic, making axosomatic or axo-axonic synapses with them. Intercellular communication within the adenohypophysis also influences its secretory activity, a subject reviewed in detail by Schwartz and Cherny (1992). Changes in transmembrane calcium transport are involved (Stojilovic & Catt 1992). Some prolactin-secreting cells which do not respond to hypothalamic releasing factors do respond to cytokines such as tumour necrosis factor-α, possibly released locally, in a manner which results in a deceleration of the rate of prolactin release (Walton & Cronin 1990); changes in transmembrane calcium transport and intracellular calcium mobilization are involved (Koike et al 1991). Autocrine modulation of FSH expression and secretion by locally secreted activins have also been reported; the inhibitory effects of substances such as inhibins and follistatins on gonadotrophs may, at least in part, be due to their interference with the action of endogenous activin β (Corrigan et al 1991).

Adenohypophyseal cells are capable of controlling their own functioning through other locally produced paracrine factors (Denef 1990): for example, a cholinergic system has been discovered in corticotrophs, acetylcholine (ACh) release from these cells exerting a tonic inhibitory action on growth hormone and prolactin release. These paracrine signals appear to be under the regulatory control of thyroid and glucocorticoid hormones.

Tanycytes (p. 939; **15**.5, 6) may also control secretion, possibly transporting hormones from the cerebrospinal fluid to capillaries of the portal system (Knigge 1976) and/or from hypothalamic neurons to the cerebrospinal fluid (Joseph & Knigge 1978). Tight junctions between them and ependymal cells (Brightman et al 1975), though rudimentary compared with those in the choroid plexus, impede movement of peptides and even some amino acids (Weindl & Joynt 1972), suggesting that materials such as releasing factors would need to cross the ependyma via, not between, the tanycytes. The endocytotic (presumably also exocytotic) activity of tanycytes appears to be under monoaminergic neuronal control (Kobayashi 1975; Nozaki et al 1975). Tanycytes in the walls of the ventricular recess appear suitable for the transport of releasing factors from neurosecretory cells to cerebrospinal fluid, because they traverse the arcuate nucleus, linked to its neurons by junctions permitting the passage of small molecules such as peptide hormones between the cells which they unite (del Cerro & Knigge 1977).

NEUROHYPOPHYSIS

The posterior hypophyseal lobe is a downgrowth from the diencephalic floor, and in early fetal life contains a cavity continuous with the third ventricle, which in some animals, for example cats, persists. The posterior lobe, infundibular stem and median eminence are often grouped as the *neurohypophysis* (see above and consult Harris 1955; Heller & Clark 1962; Scharrer & Scharrer 1963; Gabe 1966; Donovan 1970; Knowles 1974; Stopa et al 1993).

Axons arising from groups of hypothalamic neurons (supraoptic and paraventricular nuclei, etc.) terminate in the neurohypophysis. Some are short, ending in the median eminence and infundibular stem among the superior capillary beds of the venous portal circulation, and possibly providing neural control of adenohypophyseal function (see below). Longer axons pass to the main mass of the neurohypophysis thereby forming the neurosecretory hypothalamohypophyseal tract (p. 1098), terminating near the sinusoids. The hormones stored in the main part of the neurohypophysis are *vasopressin* (*antidiuretic hormone*; ADH) controlling reabsorption of water by renal tubules (p. 1827) and *oxytocin* which promotes the contraction of uterine and mammary nonstriated muscle. Their sites of production in the neuronal perikarya have been described (p. 921); they traverse axons located in the tract for release at nerve terminals (**15**.7). Ligation of the tract causes proximal damming of secretion granules, whose high glycoprotein content facilitates PAS staining. The active hormones are simple polypeptides, elaborated and transported in cells with a glycoprotein, *neurophysin*; after release into the circulation this association is broken, the hormone being carried to its cellular targets by plasma glycoproteins. Other substances demonstrated in these endings include metenkephalin and neuropeptide FF (colocalized with vasopressin) and cholecystokinin (colocalized with oxytocin).

The neurohypophysis contains thin, nonmyelinated nerve fibres and associated cells; these are the terminal ramifications of the hypothalamohypophyseal tract. Proximally, in the infundibulum, the fibres are ensheathed by typical astrocytes but near the posterior lobe *pituicytes* appear, dendritic cells of variable appearance, often with long processes running parallel to adjacent axons. Pituicytes constitute most of the nonexcitable tissue in the neurohypophysis. Cytoplasmic processes of many pituicytes end on or near the walls of adjacent capillaries and sinusoids between nerve terminals. Axons end in perivascular spaces and, though they approach close to the walls of sinusoids, they remain separated from them by two basal laminae, one applied to the nerve endings and the other to the abluminal surface of the endothelial cells. It has been observed in rats that axon terminals containing neuropeptide FF and originating from neurosecretory cells in the paraventricular and supraoptic nuclei of the hypothalamus form synaptoid contacts exclusively with pituicytes; it has been suggested that they probably have a local function within the neurohypophysis, possibly modulating oxytocin and vasopressin release, with the pituicyte acting as an intermediate, modulatory, cell (Boersma et al 1993). Fine collagen fibres often lie between the two. The cytoplasm of endothelial cells is generally extremely attenuated and has regular fenestrations which facilitate the passage of hormones into the bloodstream (**15**.7).

Three types of nerve terminal have been described in the posterior hypophyseal lobe:

- terminal axonal swellings adjacent to the sinusoids, in which are large (200–300 nm), dense vesicles containing hormones bound to glycoproteins, and also small (40–60 nm), clear, spherical vesicles
- periaxonal endings with small (80 nm) dense-cored vesicles, like those containing catecholamine in sympathetic nerve endings (p. 959)
- periaxonal endings containing small (40–60 nm), clear, spherical vesicles forming synapses with large hormone-containing endings (Bargmann 1966).

The hormones are probably released by exocytosis from endings with large dense vesicles. It is possible that excitation or inhibition of release is mediated by the other types of terminals, or by action potentials transmitted along the axon of the neurosecretory cell itself.

VESSELS OF THE HYPOPHYSIS

Vessels of the hypophysis have been studied by injection with neoprene latex and Berlin blue; also by staining erythrocytes (Popa & Fielding 1930a,b; Green & Harris 1949; Xuereb et al 1954a,b; Stanfield 1960) and examination by scanning electron microscopy of corrosion casts to determine details of the angioarchitecture of the median eminence and the vascular connections in and between the neurohypophysis and adenohypophysis (Page & Bergland 1977).

The arteries of the hypophysis arise from the internal carotids via a single *inferior* and several *superior hypophyseal arteries* on each side (**15**.8), the former coming from the cavernous part of the internal carotid, the latter from its supraclinoid part and from the anterior and posterior cerebral arteries. The inferior hypophyseal arteries divide into medial and lateral branches which anastomose across the midline to form an *arterial ring* around the infundibulum; from this ring fine branches enter the neurohypophysis, supplying its capillary bed. The superior hypophyseal arteries supply the median eminence, upper infundibulum and, via *arteries of the trabeculae*, the lower infundibulum. A confluent capillary net, extending through the neurohypophysis (median eminence, infundibular stem and pars nervosa), is supplied by both sets of hypophyseal vessels. Reversal of flow can occur in cerebral capillary beds lying between the two supplies (Gillilan 1974) and has been suggested in the neurohypophyseal network (Page & Bergland 1977).

The arteries of the median eminence and infundibulum end in characteristic sprays of capillaries, which are most complex in the upper infundibulum. In the median eminence these are an *external* or 'mantle' plexus (Green 1951) and an *internal* or 'deep' plexus (Duvernoy 1972); the external plexus, fed by the superior hypophyseal arteries, is continuous with the infundibular plexus and is drained by *long portal vessels* descending to the pars anterior; the internal plexus lies within and is supplied by the external plexus. It is continuous posteriorly with the infundibular capillary bed and, like the external plexus, is drained by long portal vessels. *Short portal vessels* run from the lower infundibulum to the pars anterior. Both types of portal vessel open into vascular sinusoids lying between the secretory cords in the adenohypophysis, providing most of its blood; there is no direct arterial supply (Wislocki & King 1936). The *portal system* is considered to carry hormone-releasing factors, probably elaborated in parvocellular groups of hypothalamic neurons, and these control the secretory cycles of cells in the pars anterior. The pars intermedia appears to be avascular in corrosion casts (Page & Bergland 1977).

The venous drainage of the neurohypophysis is by three possible routes:

- to the adenohypophysis via long and short portal vessels
- via the large inferior hypophyseal veins into the dural venous sinuses
- to the hypothalamus via capillaries passing to the median eminence.

The venous drainage carries hypophyseal hormones from the gland to their targets and also facilitates feedback control of secretion. However, the venous drainage of the adenohypophysis appears restricted. Few vessels connect it directly to the systemic veins so the

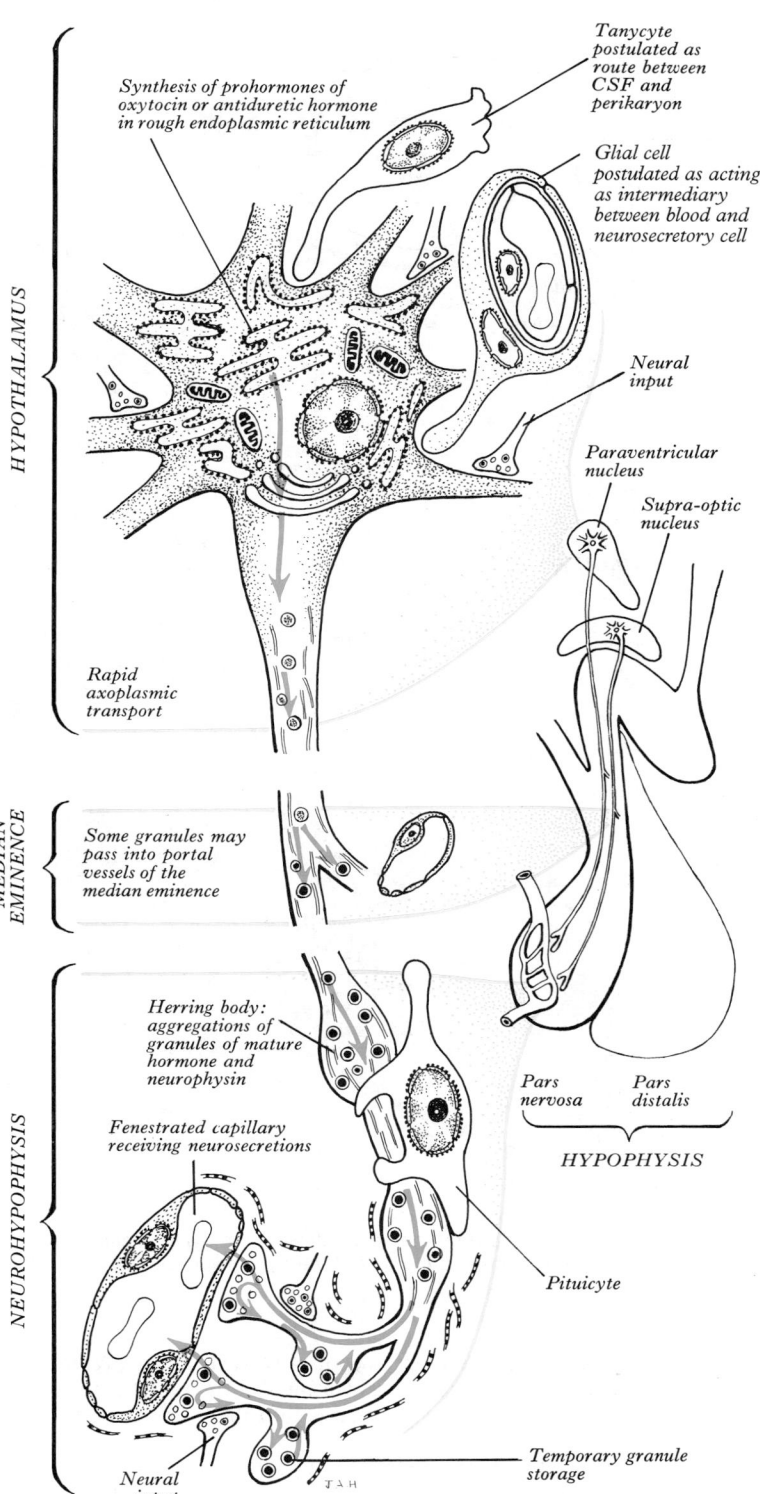

15.7   Diagram summarizing the main control systems which influence the production of neurohypophyseal hormones.

routes by which blood leaves remain obscure. If flow in the short portal veins running between the adeno- and neurohypophysis were reversible (Adams et al 1969), these portal vessels could constitute drainage channels; adenohypophyseal hormones could enter the neurohypophyseal capillaries before reaching the systemic veins, providing a 'short feedback' loop. The reversed flow in neurohypophyseal capillaries (from neurohypophysis to hypothalamus, according to Török (1954) could be a vascular route for neurohypophyseal hormones to the ventricular tanycytes and hence to the cerebrospinal fluid. The demonstration of neurohypophyseal hormones in the cerebrospinal fluid (Robinson & Zimmerman 1973)

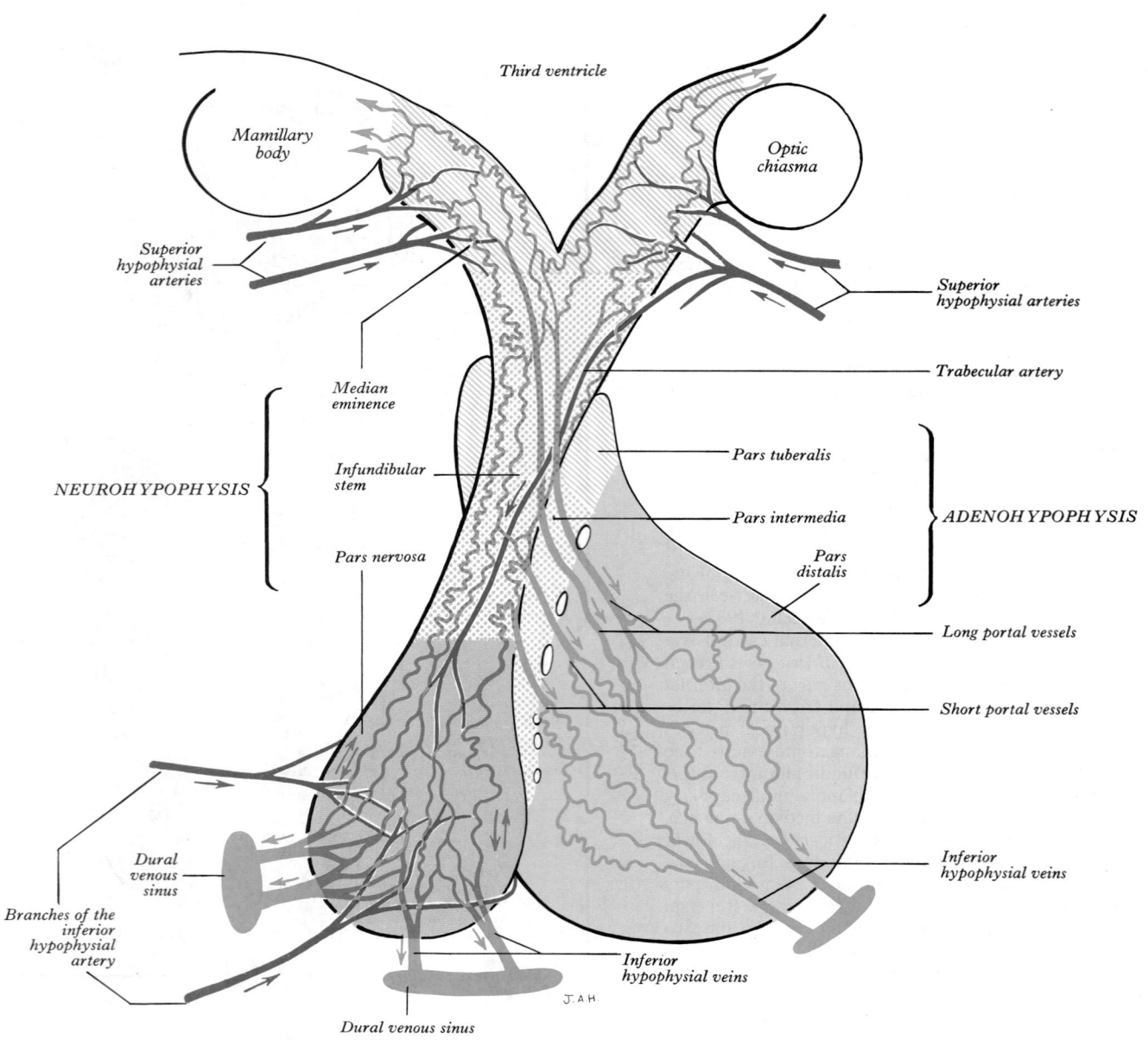

Third ventricle

Mamillary body

Optic chiasma

Superior hypophysial arteries

Superior hypophysial arteries

Trabecular artery

Median eminence

NEUROHYPOPHYSIS

Infundibular stem

Pars tuberalis

Pars intermedia

ADENOHYPOPHYSIS

Pars nervosa

Pars distalis

Long portal vessels

Short portal vessels

Dural venous sinus

Branches of the inferior hypophysial artery

Inferior hypophysial veins

Inferior hypophysial veins

Dural venous sinus

J.A.H.

15.8 Diagram summarizing the vasculature of the hypothalamic median eminence, infundibulum and the rest of the hypophysis cerebri. (See text for a detailed account and possible significances.)

and of releasing factors there and in tanycytes (Knigge & Joseph 1974) strengthens this hypothesis. Cushing's original (1912) suggestion that the neurohypophysis secretes into the third ventricle may be correct.

This model of hypophyseal blood supply has far-reaching implications; instead of the median eminence being the final common pathway for neural control of the adenohypophysis (Harris 1947), the entire neurohypophysis may be involved; its capillary bed may selectively 'determine the destination of both hypothalamic and pituitary secretions, conveying some to the glandular pituitary, others to distant target organs and yet others to the brain' (Page & Bergland 1977).

PHARYNGEAL HYPOPHYSIS

This small collection of adenohypophyseal tissue lies in the mucoperiosteum of the human nasopharyngeal roof (Boyd 1956) as in many other mammals (McGrath 1974). By 28 weeks in utero it is well vascularized and capable of secretion, receiving blood from the systemic vessels of the nasopharyngeal roof. At this stage it is covered posteriorly by fibrous tissue but in the second half of fetal life this is replaced by venous sinuses and a trans-sphenoidal portal venous

system develops, bringing it under the same hypothalamic control as the cranial adenohypophyseal tissue (McGrath 1978). The peripheral vascularity of the pharyngeal hypophysis persists until about the fifth year; the organ is then reinvested by fibrous tissue and presumed to be again controlled by factors present in systemic blood. Though it does not change in size after birth in males, in females it becomes temporarily smaller, returning to natal volume during the fifth decade (McGrath 1971), when once again it may be controlled via a transsphenoidal extension of the hypothalamohypophyseal portal venous system. The human pharyngeal hypophysis may be a reserve of potential adenohypophyseal tissue which may be stimulated, particularly in females, to synthesize and secrete adenohypophyseal hormones in middle age, when intracranial adenohypophyseal tissue is beginning to fail.

PINEAL GLAND

The pineal gland or *epiphysis cerebri* (**15**.1, 9), a small, piriform, reddish-grey organ, occupies a depression between the superior colliculi. (For reviews see Gladstone & Wakeley 1940; Kappers 1960; Wolfe et al 1962; Kappers & Schade 1965; Wurtman et al 1968;

Wolstenholme & Knight 1971; Møller et al 1993.) It is inferior to the splenium of the corpus callosum, separated from it by the tela choroidea of the third ventricle and the contained cerebral veins. It is enveloped by the tela's lower layer, which is reflected thence to the tectum (15.1). The gland is about 8 mm in length; its base, directed anteriorly, is attached by a *peduncle* dividing into inferior and superior laminae, separated by the *pineal recess* of the third ventricle (15.1), and respectively containing the posterior and habenular commissures. Aberrant commissural fibres may invade the gland but do not terminate near parenchymal cells. Nerve fibres enter its dorsolateral aspects from the region of the tentorium cerebelli as a single or paired *nervus conarii*, which lies deep to the endothelium of the wall of the straight sinus (p. 1583), its fibres derived from neurons of the superior cervical ganglia. These fibres are adrenergic sympathetic elements associated with blood vessels and parenchymal cells (Kappers 1960; Wolfe et al 1962). Björklund et al (1972) have shown in rats that postganglionic sympathetic fibres from the *nervus conarii* reach neurons in the habenular nuclei, from which some fibres of the *habenulopineal tract* may start. Møller (1978) reported that, in human fetuses, fibres of this tract reach the *ganglion conarii* (Pastori ganglion) at the pineal apex (15.9); the neurons of origin of these fibres need verification. Møller (1978, 1979) has also reported an unpaired nerve containing non-myelinated fibres and bipolar neurons with axosomatic and axodendritic synapses, the *nervus pinealis*, in human fetuses; it is in the subarachnoid space near the median plane just caudal to the pineal gland, connecting it to the posterior commissure. It is ephemeral, presumed to degenerate late in intrauterine life and its function is uncertain; but since it appears to be homologous with the sensory pineal nerve of fish and amphibians (Møller 1978), whose pineal complexes contain photoreceptors, it might transmit light-generated impulses. In some mammals (e.g. neonatal rats) pinealocytes transiently resemble photoreceptors (Zimmerman & Tsi 1975) those in human fetuses do not. The human fetal nervus pinealis may be involved in pineal differentiation. At present it can only be regarded as a phylogenetic vestige; its loss may be associated with evolution of the pineal as a secretory rather than photoreceptive organ. Møller (1978) has described a ganglion, presumed to be parasympathetic, rostral to the pineal gland and near the choroid plexus of the third ventricle. An anterior *intrapineal ganglion* has also been found (15.9).

STRUCTURE OF THE PINEAL GLAND

The pineal gland contains cords and follicles of pinealocytes and neuroglial cells among which ramify many blood vessels and nerves. Septa extend into the pineal gland from the surrounding pia mater.

Pinealocytes form the pineal parenchyma. Extending from each cell body, which has a spherical, oval or lobulated nucleus, are one or more tortuous basophilic processes, containing parallel microtubules (Knight et al 1973). These processes end in expanded terminal buds near capillaries or, less frequently, ependymal cells of the pineal recess. The terminal buds contain granular endoplasmic reticulum, mitochondria and electron-dense cored vesicles, which store monoamines and polypeptide hormones (Sheridan & Sladek 1975), release of which appears to require sympathetic innervation. Lukaszyk & Reiter (1975) have proposed that the polypeptide hormones (which they consider could be produced by pineal neuroglia and neurons) combine with specific protein carriers, termed *neuro-epiphysins* to distinguish them from hypophyseal neurophysins. They are released by exocytosis, together with fragments of vesicular membrane, the latter forming exocytotic debris. When released the complex is believed to dissociate, hormones being exchanged for calcium ions. The calcium-carrier complex so formed is, in the pineal, deposited concentrically around exocytotic debris as *corpora arenacea* or 'brain sand' (15.10, 11). It is often supposed that the pineal gland atrophies with age, corpora arenacea being a sign of atrophy; on the contrary, these corpuscles may indicate continued secretion. Wildi and Frauchiger (1965) found no evidence of pineal degeneration in the elderly.

Pinealocytes contain both granular and agranular endoplasmic reticulum, with extensive Golgi complexes, lipid droplets and numerous mitochondria, in accord with their secretory function. An unusual organelle (groups of microtubules and perforated lamellae) sometimes occurs near granular endoplasmic reticulum and lipid droplets. Termed 'canaliculate lamellar bodies' by Lin (1967) and McNeil (1977), 'annulate lamellae' by Friere and Cardinali (1975) and 'mikrotubuli' by Gusek (1976), they may be involved in secretion (McNeil 1977).

Pinealocytes of some mammals contain synaptic ribbons, perhaps involved in transmission; vesicles near them contain neurotransmitters such as γ-aminobutyric acid (GABA; Krstić 1976). These ribbons may arise from microtubular sheaths which in turn arise from centrioles (Karasek 1976). Similar arrangements of organelles occur in mammalian retinal photoreceptors and simpler submammalian photoreceptors, supporting the theory that mammalian pinealocytes are derived from photoreceptors (Kappers 1976; Relkin 1976). Transient similarities between pinealocytes and retinal photoreceptors in neonatal rats lend further support to this concept (Zimmerman & Tso 1975).

The ultrastructure of human fetal pinealocytes indicates their secretory function in early intrauterine life (Møller 1974). As in adults, they contain all the appropriate organelles, together with

15.9 Diagram showing the principal neural pathways which have been described in connection with the human fetal pineal gland.

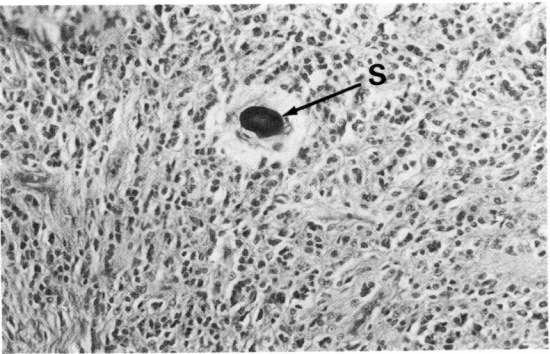

15.10A Low-power micrograph of the pineal gland showing pinealocytes arranged in clumps and cords around capillaries, together with neuroglial cells. An example of 'brain sand' (S), corpora arenacea, can be seen. Haematoxylin and eosin. Magnification × 128. (From Burkitt 1993.)

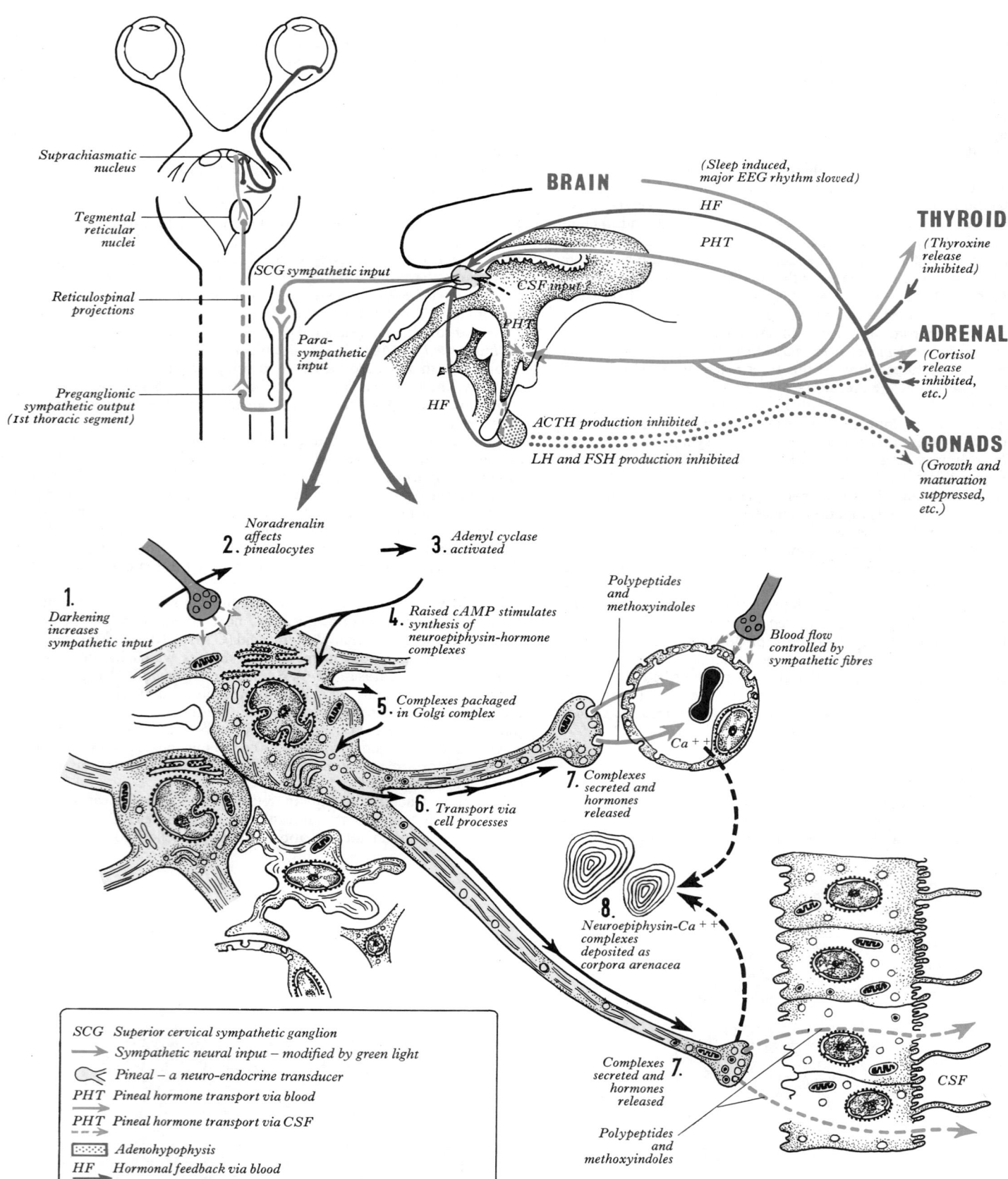

15.10B.   Diagrammatic review of current hypotheses regarding the control and effects of pineal function. (See text for details.)

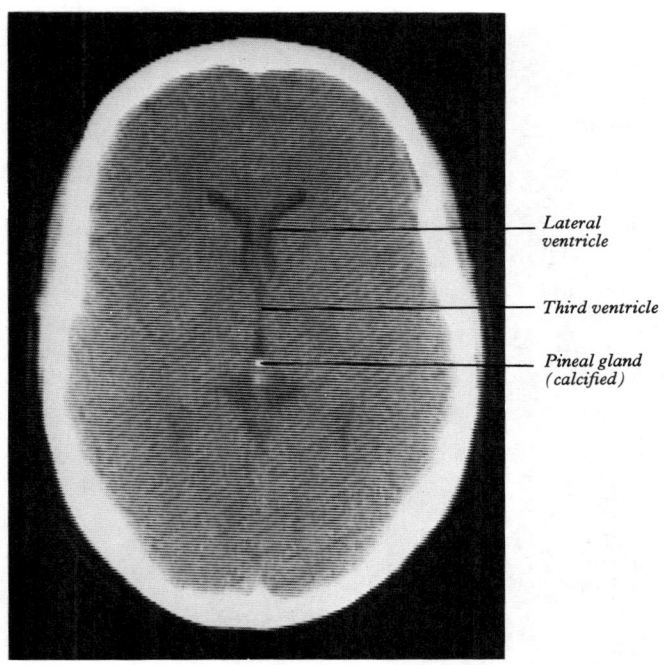

15.11 Computed tomogram of the head in the horizontal plane at the level of the pineal gland. (Supplied by Shaun Gallagher, Guy's Hospital; photographed by Sarah Smith, UMDS, Guy's Hospital Campus, London.)

Lateral ventricle

Third ventricle

Pineal gland (calcified)

abundant microfilaments, microtubules and a few cilia with a 9 + 0 microtubular pattern. Cilia of this type are also associated with secretory cells in other endocrine glands, such as the pituitary gland (Barnes 1961; Andersen et al 1970). Fetal pinealocytes have gap junctions, desmosomes and 'intermediate-like junctions' (Møller 1976); the first are for electrotonic coupling between adjacent cells enabling group activity, the others of an adhesive nature. Synaptic ribbons do not appear in human fetal pinealocytes.

Neuroglial cells, partially separating the pinealocytes, resemble astrocytes and in the pineal stalk, of which they are the main component, many have extensive longitudinal processes. Numerous filaments extend throughout their processes.

FUNCTIONS OF THE PINEAL GLAND

Once considered to be a phylogenetic relic, a vestige of a dorsal third eye and of little functional significance, the mammalian pineal is now accepted as an endocrine gland of major regulatory importance, modifying the activity of the adenohypophysis, neurohypophysis, endocrine pancreas, parathyroids, adrenal cortex, adrenal medulla and gonads (de Vries & Kappers 1971; Klein 1978; Hăulică & Coculescu 1981; Reiter 1983, 1984, 1985, 1987; Malendowicz 1985). Its effects are largely inhibitory; indole-amine and polypeptide hormones secreted by pinealocytes are believed to reduce synthesis and release of hormones of the pars anterior, for example, by direct action on its secretory cells and indirectly by inhibiting production of hypothalamic releasing factors. Pineal secretions may reach their target cells via cerebrospinal fluid (Sheridan et al 1969; Knight et al 1973) or the bloodstream.

Some pineal indole-amines, including melatonin and enzymes for their biosynthesis (e.g. serotonin N-acetyltransferase) show circadian rhythms in concentration and activity in many mammalian pineal glands. In rats there may be an *endogenous circadian oscillator* in the suprachiasmatic nucleus of the hypothalamus, whose intrinsic rhythmicity governs cyclical pineal behaviour (Klein 1978). Photic stimuli, in particular intensity changes of yellow-green light acting on rhodopsinoid retinal pigment, seem to be involved in this rhythm (Cardinali et al 1971; Minneman et al 1974), the pineal being most active in darkness. With the visual pathway and pineal sympathetic supply intact, exposure to light after several hours of darkness depresses pineal activity (Klein & Weller 1972). Suprachiasmatic neurons are supplied directly by axons of retinal ganglion cells,

allowing response to changes in illumination (Nishino et al 1976). In rats, the path from the suprachiasmatic nucleus to the pineal gland is claimed to include the tegmental nuclei and the upper thoracic spinal intermediolateral column (Saper et al 1976); preganglionic sympathetic fibres from the latter are said to reach the superior cervical ganglia, from which postganglionic fibres can be traced to the pinealocytes. Release of catecholamines from these fibres causes a receptor-mediated increase in the production of cyclic adenosine monophosphate (cAMP) in pinealocytes, evoking a 70–100-fold increase in serotonin N-acetyltransferase activity, which regulates daily changes in melatonin production and hence its plasma levels. Interest has centred on sympathetic innervation; the role of its parasympathetic supply is as yet unknown. These hypotheses are summarized in (**15**.10). Evidence has been found of a circadian rhythm in **human** pineal activity, demonstrated by changes of plasma melatonin levels (Vaughan et al 1976). As in other mammals, the level rises during darkness, falling during the day. Whether the control mechanisms demonstrated in other animals also operate in man is unresolved.

Vessels and nerves

The pineal gland has a very rich blood supply (Plets 1969; Moreau et al 1985), the *pineal arteries* being branches of the left and right medial posterior choroidal arteries which in turn are branches of the posterior cerebral arteries (p. 1528). Although Wackenheim & Babin (1978) recorded only a single pineal artery, Yamamoto & Kageyama (1980) showed that there could be several, with up to five being derived from the medial posterior choroidal artery or arteries (Baumgarten et al 1981) of one side and with 70% of the cadavers studied having pineal arteries derived from both sides. Within the pineal gland branches of the arteries supply fenestrated capillaries whose endothelial cells rest on a tenuous and sometimes incomplete basal lamina; the capillaries drain into numerous *pineal veins* which open into the internal cerebral veins and/or into the great cerebral vein (p. 1581; Yamamoto & Kageyama 1980). The principal *neural pathways* associated with the human pineal gland have already been described (p. 1889). Scattered amongst the pinealocytes and capillaries are non-myelinated autonomic nerve fibres; these are mostly noradrenergic, with dense-cored vesicles in terminal or preterminal expansions. Arising in the superior cervical ganglion (p. 1300) they enter the pineal gland either in association with the arteries which supply it, or through the nervi conarii (p. 1889; **15**.9), or via the leptomeningeal pineal surface; they either terminate in perivascular spaces between the pinealocytes or synapse with them. Other nerve fibres located in the stalk of the gland may originate from habenular nuclei. This possibility is supported by the detection in these nuclei, particularly in the medial habenular nucleus, of substance P-immunoreactive perikarya from which processes extend towards the pineal stalk, and of similarly reactive nerve fibres throughout the bovine pineal gland; these fibres are present perivascularly, intraparenchymally and in the capsule of the gland (Møller et al 1993). In the rat the pineal gland receives efferent, dorsal, projections from the periventricular and medial parvicellular subnuclei of the hypothalamic paraventricular nucleus; this heterogeneous nucleus is intimately involved in the regulation of a range of homeostatic functions, regulation which may, at least in part, be mediated via neuronal projections to circumventricular organs such as the pineal gland (Larse 1991). The pineal gland of the rat also receives a direct neural projection from the intergeniculate leaflet of the lateral geniculate nucleus, a nucleus considered to be involved in circadian rhythmicity (Mikkelsen & Møller 1990) and from the anterior and tuberal regions of the lateral hypothalamus. Since the lateral hypothalamic regions receive direct innervation from the retina (p. 1090) and since these regions are also involved in circadian rhythmicity, it has been suggested that these projections also modulate circadian activity in the rat pineal gland (Fink-Jensen & Møller 1990).

THYROID GLAND

The thyroid gland (**15**.12), brownish-red and highly vascular, is placed anteriorly in the lower neck, level with the fifth cervical to the first thoracic vertebrae. Ensheathed by the pretracheal layer of deep cervical fascia, it has right and left lobes connected by a narrow,

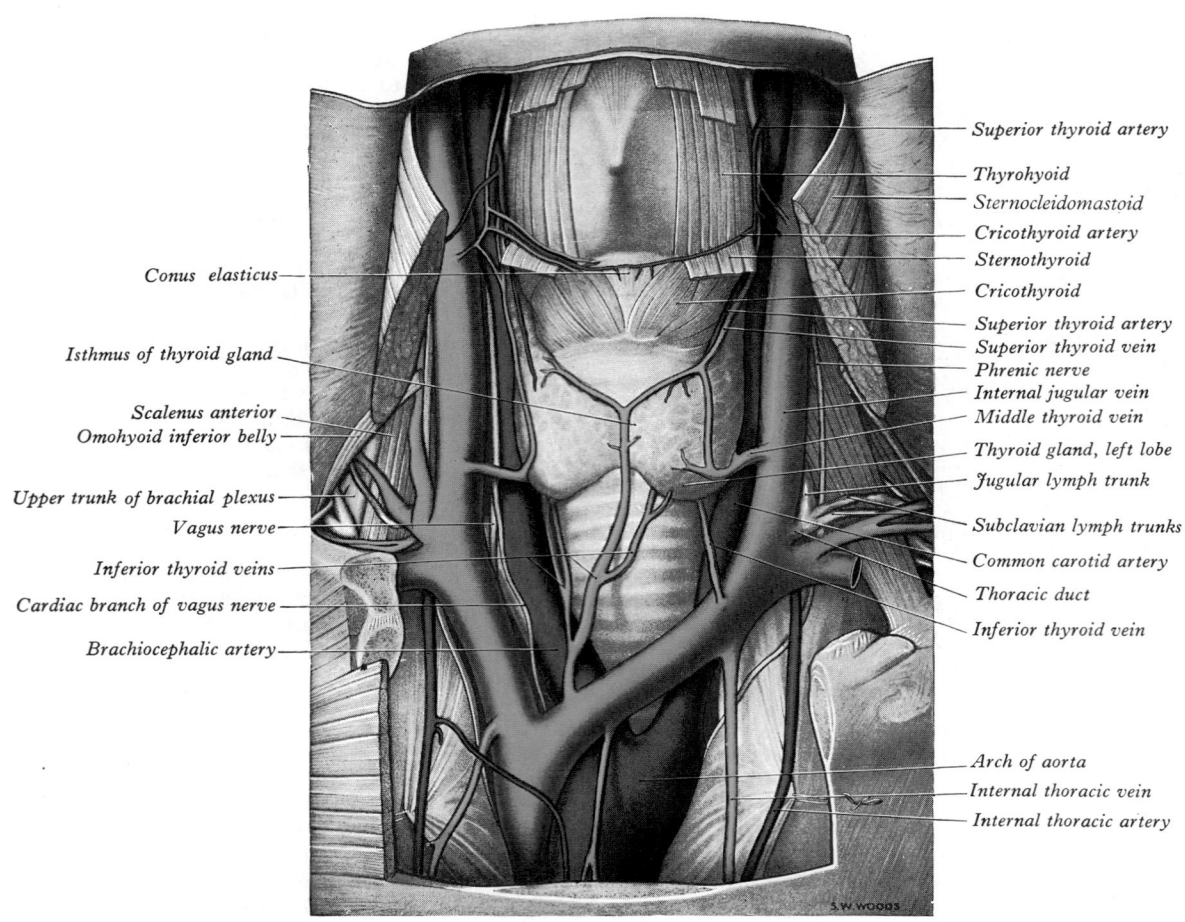

15.12   The thyroid gland and its environs. The manubrium sterni and the sternal ends of the clavicles and first costal cartilages have been removed and the pleural sac and lung have been retracted on each side.

median *isthmus*. Its weight is usually about 25 g but varies, being slightly heavier in females, and enlarging during menstruation and pregnancy. Estimation of the size of the thyroid gland is clinically important in the evaluation and management of thyroid disorders; this can be achieved non-invasively by means of diagnostic ultrasound. Hegedus et al (1983) have demonstrated the relationship between thyroid gland volume, as estimated by ultrasound, and body weight, age and sex in normal subjects. More recently Ueda (1990) has correlated thyroid gland volume in children of 8 months to 15 years with height, weight, body surface and age; no significant difference in thyroid gland volume was observed between males and females over this age range.

The *lobes* are approximately conical; their ascending apices diverge laterally to the level of the oblique lines on the laminae of the thyroid cartilages; their bases are level with the fourth or fifth tracheal cartilages. Each lobe is about 5 cm long, its greatest transverse and anteroposterior extents being about 3 cm and 2 cm respectively. Its *posteromedial aspect* is attached to the side of the cricoid cartilage by a *lateral thyroid ligament*. The *lateral* (*superficial*) surface is convex and covered by the sternothyroid, whose attachment to the oblique thyroid line prevents the upper pole of the gland from extending on to the thyrohyoid muscle. More anteriorly are the sternohyoid and superior belly of omohyoid, overlapped inferiorly by the anterior border of sternocleidomastoid. The *medial surface* is adapted to the larynx and trachea, contacting at its superior pole the inferior pharyngeal constrictor and the posterior part of the cricothyroid, which separate it from the posterior part of the thyroid lamina and the side of the cricoid cartilage. The external laryngeal nerve is medial to this part of the gland, on its way to the cricothyroid. Inferiorly, the trachea, and posterior to this the recurrent laryngeal nerve (p. 1253) and oesophagus (closer on the left) are medial relations. The *posterolateral surface* is next to the carotid sheath,

overlapping the common carotid artery. The thin *anterior border*, near the anterior branch of the superior thyroid artery, slants down medially. The rounded *posterior border* is related below to the inferior thyroid artery and its anastomosis with the posterior branch of the superior thyroid artery. The parathyroid glands are usually related to this border (p. 1897), whose lower end on the left is near the thoracic duct.

The *isthmus* connects the lobe's lower parts; it measures about 1.25 cm transversely and vertically and is usually anterior to the second and third tracheal cartilages, though often higher or sometimes lower; its site and size vary greatly. Pretracheal fascia separates it from the sternothyroid muscles; more superficially are the sternohyoids, anterior jugular veins, fascia and skin. The superior thyroid arteries anastomose along its upper border; at the lower border the inferior thyroid veins leave the gland. Occasionally the isthmus is absent.

A conical *pyramidal lobe* often ascends towards the hyoid bone from the isthmus or the adjacent part of either lobe (more often the left). It is occasionally detached or in two or more parts. A fibrous or fibromuscular band, the *levator of the thyroid gland* (*musculus levator glandulae thyroideae*) sometimes descends from the hyoid body to the isthmus or pyramidal lobe. Small detached masses of thyroid tissue may occur above the lobes or isthmus as *accessory thyroid glands*. Vestiges of the thyroglossal duct (p. 176) may persist between the isthmus and the foramen caecum of the tongue, sometimes as accessory nodules or cysts of thyroid tissue near the midline or even in the tongue.

STRUCTURE AND FUNCTIONS

The gland has a thin capsule of connective tissue, whose extensions divide it into masses of irregular form and size. The parenchyma

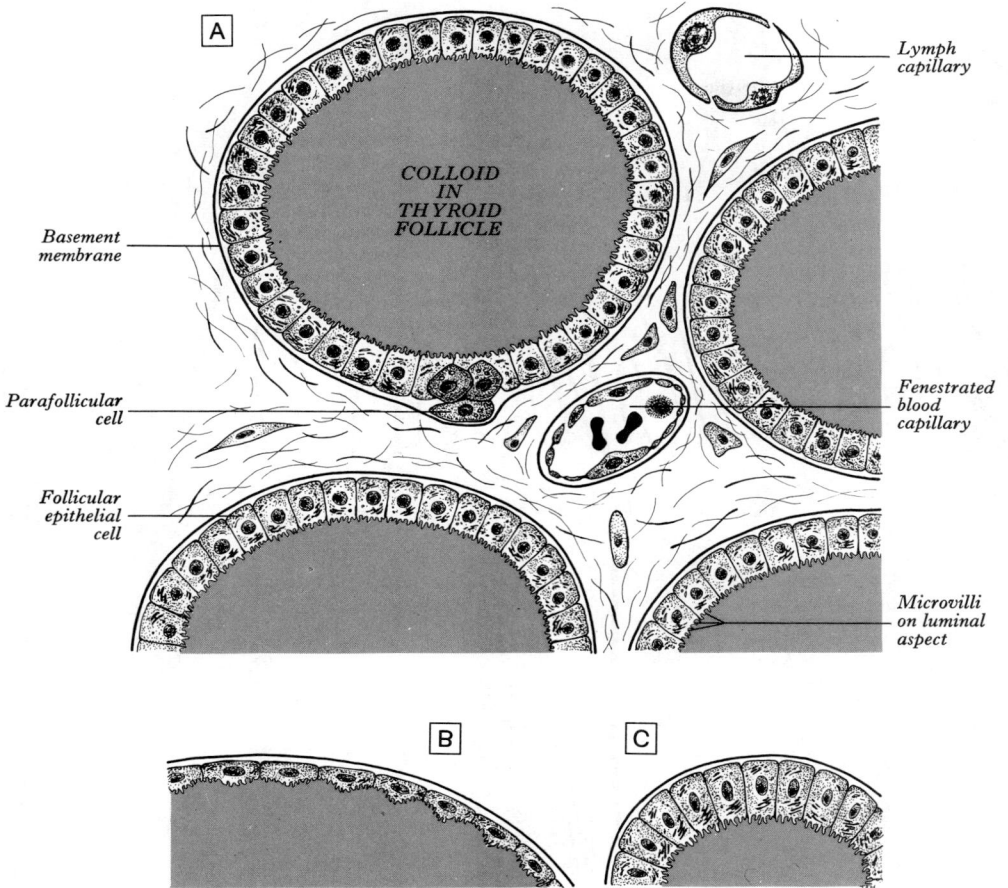

Lymph capillary

COLLOID IN THYROID FOLLICLE

Basement membrane

Parafollicular cell

Follicular epithelial cell

Fenestrated blood capillary

Microvilli on luminal aspect

15.13 Diagrams of thyroid follicular structure: A. normal structure under average physiological conditions; B. 'resting' state; C. highly active state. (See text for details.)

derives mainly from the endoderm of the thyroglossal duct (p. 176), usually a transient embryonic structure extending between the gland and the tongue. From its distal end solid epithelial cords and sheets branch and lumina filled with yellow, viscid colloid appear in them. This endodermal epithelium is generally considered to develop into **separate** follicles, approximately spherical and about 0.02–0.9 mm in diameter, each with a central colloid core surrounded by a simple epithelium and basal lamina. But three-dimensional reconstructions of mature thyroid glands show that follicles are typically aggregated, with a common epithelium bordering several colloid masses and linking follicles together (Isler et al 1968). Solid cell nests have also been described (Harach 1985). The colloid, staining pink with eosin, contains an iodinated glycoprotein, iodothyroglobulin, a precursor of thyroid hormones, tri-iodothyronine (T_3) and tetra-iodothyronine or thyroxine (T_4), and a product of the follicular epithelial cells. Aggregated follicles nestle in a delicate connective tissue stroma, surrounded by dense plexuses of fenestrated capillaries, extensive lymphatic networks and sympathetic nerve fibres which supply the arterioles and capillaries, some nerve fibres ending close to the follicular epithelial cells (Melander et al 1975; Melander 1977).

Thyroid parenchyma contains a second, parafollicular cell type: 'light', 'clear' or C cells, producing the peptide hormone thyrocalcitonin. C cells, an amine precursor uptake and decarboxylation element (p. 1898), are derived from the ultimobranchial bodies (p. 177). They are a minor component but improved techniques (Solcia et al 1968, 1969) suggest that in some species they have been underestimated; for example, in dogs Kameda (1971, 1976) found a ratio of 30–90 parafollicular to 100 follicular cells. Branched tubules containing desquamated cells may occur; like C cells, these are ultimobranchial in origin (Halmi 1978). Other cells, some ciliated, have been described in rodent thyroid glands (Wollman & Nève 1971).

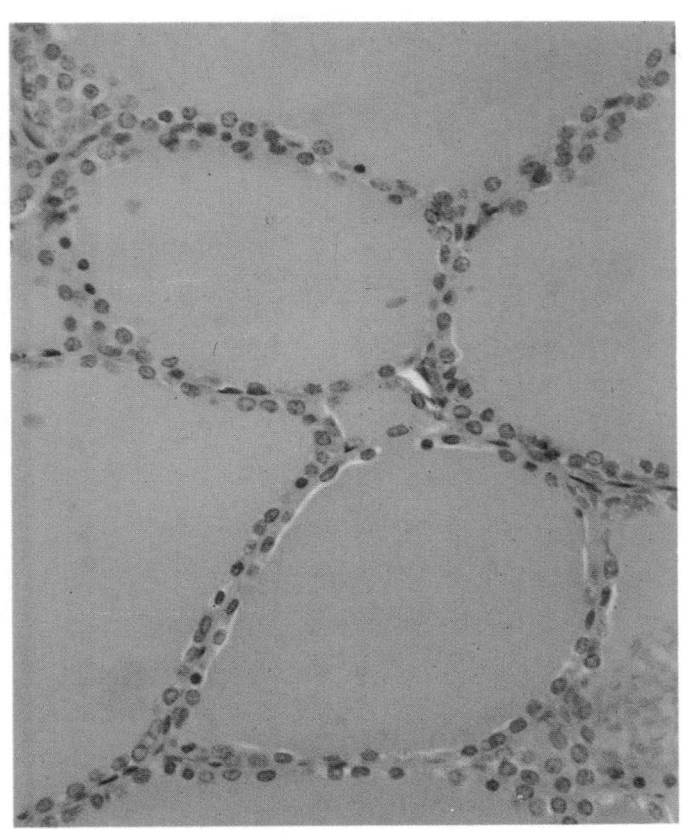

15.14 Section through a thyroid gland showing thyroid follicles surrounding central masses of thyroid colloid. Haematoxylin and eosin. Magnification × 500. (Provided by P Shepherd and S Liebowitz, UMDS, Guy's Campus, London.)

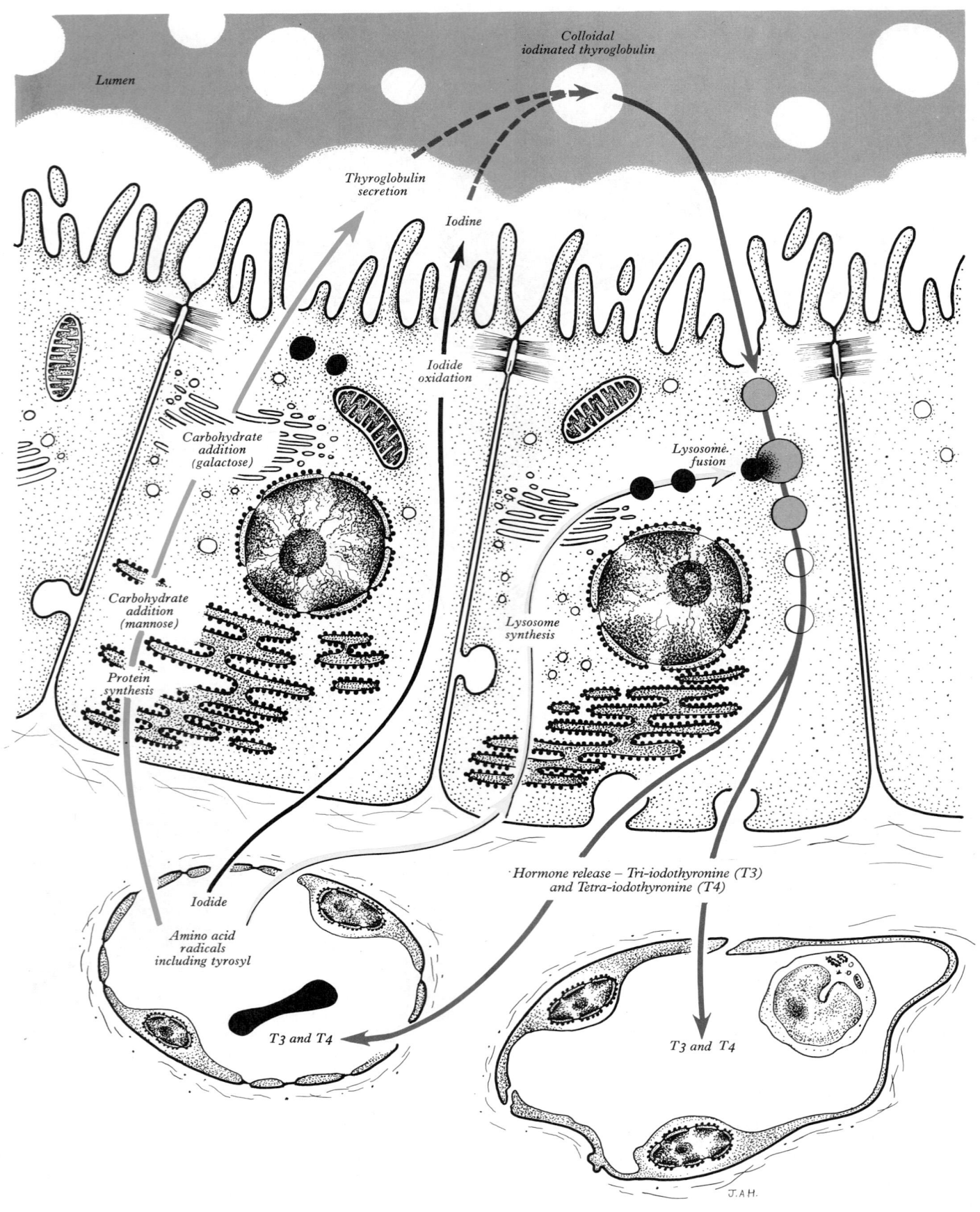

15.15 The functional architecture of the thyroid follicular cells, showing on one aspect the colloid-containing cavity and on the other blood and lymphatic capillaries. Arrows indicate metabolic flow pathways.

Follicular cells

Follicular cells proper vary from squamous to columnar, depending on their activity, mainly controlled by circulating hypophyseal thyrotropin (TSH) (**15**.13), in the absence of which the follicular cells are squamous and 'resting', luminal colloid being abundant and reflecting increased storage of iodinated thyroglobulin. The secretion of TSH leads to endocytosis of colloidal droplets at the luminal aspects of follicular cells, cavities appearing in the luminal colloid near the epithelium. Prolonged high levels of circulating TSH induce follicular hypertrophy and even hyperplasia, with progressive resorption of colloid and increased stromal vascularity.

Follicular cells have a striking ultrastructural and functional polarity: when activated by TSH, or possibly adrenergic nerve terminals (see below), they engage in apical (i.e. luminal) synthesis and exocytosis of thyroglobulin, with basally directed thyroglobulin endocytosis, degradation and liberation of thyroid hormones (T_3 and T_4) into the blood capillaries. This polarized dual function is indicated by the arrangement of their organelles. To form a continuous wall around each mass of colloidal thyroglobulin, the follicular cells are linked by apical junctional complexes and have their bases resting on a basal lamina (**15**.13, 14). Each cell has a basal nucleus, prominent granular endoplasmic reticulum and supranuclear Golgi complex, the last named being particularly prominent in TSH-activated cells. Apical to the Golgi complex and derived from it, secretory vesicles transport glycoprotein, assembled by serial activity of the granular endoplasmic reticulum and the Golgi complex, to the apical plasmalemma for luminal release by exocytosis. Iodide required to complete thyroglobulin formation enters the follicular cells basally by active transport from the blood capillaries across the basal plasmalemma; labelled iodide rapidly appears in the lumina (Wolff 1964) and is oxidized to iodine, mainly by thyroid peroxidase in the apical plasmalemma (Taurog 1970). Iodine is then attached to the tyrosyl groups of the secreted glycoprotein manufactured by the follicular cells to form mono- and di-iodotyrosyls. These are then coupled into iodothyronyl groups (thyroid hormones in peptide linkage) to complete the formation of iodinated thyroglobulin, the precursor of thyroid hormones (Bjorkman & Ekholm 1973; Haeberli et al 1975). In follicular cells endogenous peroxidase occurs in perinuclear cisternae, granular endoplasmic reticulum, Golgi complex, apical vesicles, apical plasmalemma and particularly on microvilli (Strum & Karnovsky 1970); but it is likely that only in the apical plasmalemma is it involved in iodide oxidation, its distribution indicating its route to this site. Apical microvilli, numerous but short in resting cells (Wetzel et al 1965), elongate and often branch on stimulation by TSH, which also provokes extension of cytoplasmic processes into the luminal colloid; these fuse around portions of the colloid and take it into the cell. After colloid endocytosis, lysosomes, located basally in the resting state, migrate towards the lumen to fuse with the intracellular droplets of colloid, forming secondary lysosomes or phagolysosomes, which return to the cell's base. During this period the colloid gradually disappears as acid proteases and peptidases in the phagolysosomes degrade the iodinated thyroglobulin, releasing the thyroid hormones T_3 and T_4, which pass basally for release, leaving the gland mainly via the blood capillaries and lymphatics. More numerous precursor molecules, such as 3-mono-iodotyrosine and 3,5-di-iodotyrosine, are de-iodinated by a dehalogenase; the released iodine migrates apically to be recycled in the iodination of newly synthesized thyroglobulin molecules. Microtubules and microfilaments are probably involved in thyroid hormone secretion (Wolff & Williams 1973); treatment with colchicine and cytochalasin B (interfering respectively with microtubule and microfilament activity) inhibits thyrotrophic hormone (TSH) and dibutyryl cyclic adenosine monophosphate (cAMP)-induced secretion. Some iodinated thryoglobulin escapes intact from the follicles and can be radio-immunoassayed in blood, probably reaching it via the lymphatic vessels. Follicular activity in thyroglobulin synthesis and thyroid hormone release is illustrated in **15**.15. Greer and Haibach (1974), DeGroot and Niepomniszcse (1977) and Taurog (1978) provide detailed accounts of these processes.

Of the two thyroid hormones tri-iodothyronine is probably the main stimulator of cellular metabolic rate, its action being very powerful and immediate, whereas tetra-iodothyronine (*thyroxine*) is powerful but less rapid. Overproduction of both causes *thyrotoxicosis*

(exophthalmic goitre); hyposecretion in adults produces *myxoedema* and in infants *cretinism*. Their synthesis and release are mainly controlled by adenohypophyseal TSH. However, in *Graves' disease*, antibodies to human thyroid-stimulating immunoglobulin bind to TSH-receptor sites in the follicular cells, interfering with this control and causing excessive hormone production (Werner 1978). Thyroid hormones increase the sensitivity of tissues to adrenalin and noradrenalin. Advances in understanding the action of the thyroid hormones at the cellular level have been reviewed by Oppenheimer et al (1987).

Although follicular activity is mainly controlled by circulating TSH, evidence in several mammals, including mankind, suggests a direct sympathetic influence on follicular cells, separate from sympathetic control of the gland's circulation (Melander 1978). Fluorescence histochemistry and electron autoradiography have demonstrated adrenergic terminals near blood vessels and follicular cells. In mice, with TSH secretion eliminated to avoid indirect effects on thyroid secretion, unilateral sympathetic stimulation evokes secretion of the thyroid hormones only in those regions supplied by the stimulated nerve (Melander et al 1972). Studies of human thyroid tissue in vitro also suggest that noradrenaline directly induces follicular changes associated with hormone secretion, including colloid droplet formation and lysosome migration (Melander 1978). In vitro investigations on isolated calf's thyroid cells show that catecholamines can enhance the incorporation of iodine and synthesis of hormones (Melander et al 1973), effects abolished in vivo and in vitro by drugs which block adrenergic receptors (Melander 1970; Maayan & Ingbar 1978) but which do not affect the ability of cells to respond to TSH. Therefore catecholamines and TSH interact with different receptors in follicular cells and can act independently, although with similar effects. Both activate adenyl cyclase, increasing the formation of cyclic-AMP, which augments hormonal release (Melander 1978). Although anatomicrophysiological evidence leaves little doubt that follicular cells and their vessels have direct sympathetic innervation, its effect on thyroid secretion is uncertain. TSH may be a greater influence in sustained regulation; the link between the nervous system and follicular cells may mediate rapid, transient responses to external influences.

Parafollicular cells

Parafollicular ('C') cells, an APUD type (p. 1898), occur singly or in small groups, close to the outer follicular borders but within the follicular basement membrane. Often partly insinuated between adjacent follicular cells, they do not reach the follicular lumen; they are oval or polyhedral and larger than follicular cells. Grouping is sometimes more marked, for example, in canine thyroid glands, and when perfused with fixative for electron microscopy, where folliculoid groups of such cells appear with expanded central extracellular spaces, perhaps storing hormone. Parafollicular, unlike follicular, cells have no apparent nerve supply; their cytoplasm has numerous membrane-bound secretory granules, probably containing a stored form of calcitonin or thyrocalcitonin, as supported by immunocytochemical studies (Pearse 1966; Wolfe et al 1974). Parafollicular cells, which are derivatives of the neural crest and have several neuron-like properties, express a form of the neural cell adhesion molecule (N-CAM) on their surfaces (Nishiyama et al 1993). As befits cells engaged in making exportable protein, they contain granular endoplasmic reticulum varying with the level of activity, obvious Golgi complexes and many mitochondria. There are also many free ribosomes. The oval nucleus is generally eccentric and has a smooth or slightly irregular membrane.

The main factor controlling release of thyrocalcitonin is the concentration of serum calcium; a rise of this in blood perfusing the thyroid gland stimulates thyrocalcitonin secretion, while hypocalcaemia suppresses it, there being a reciprocal relation between secretion of thyrocalcitonin and parathyroid hormone (**15**.16). Thyrocalcitonin regulates calcium metabolism in many species, largely by suppressing bone resorption, but its human role is uncertain; difficulties arise in detecting thyrocalcitonin in human plasma even by sensitive radio-immunoassay; no pathological condition has been associated with thyrocalcitonin deficiency (O'Riordan 1978).

Vessels and nerves

The **arteries** supplying the gland are the superior (p. 1515) and

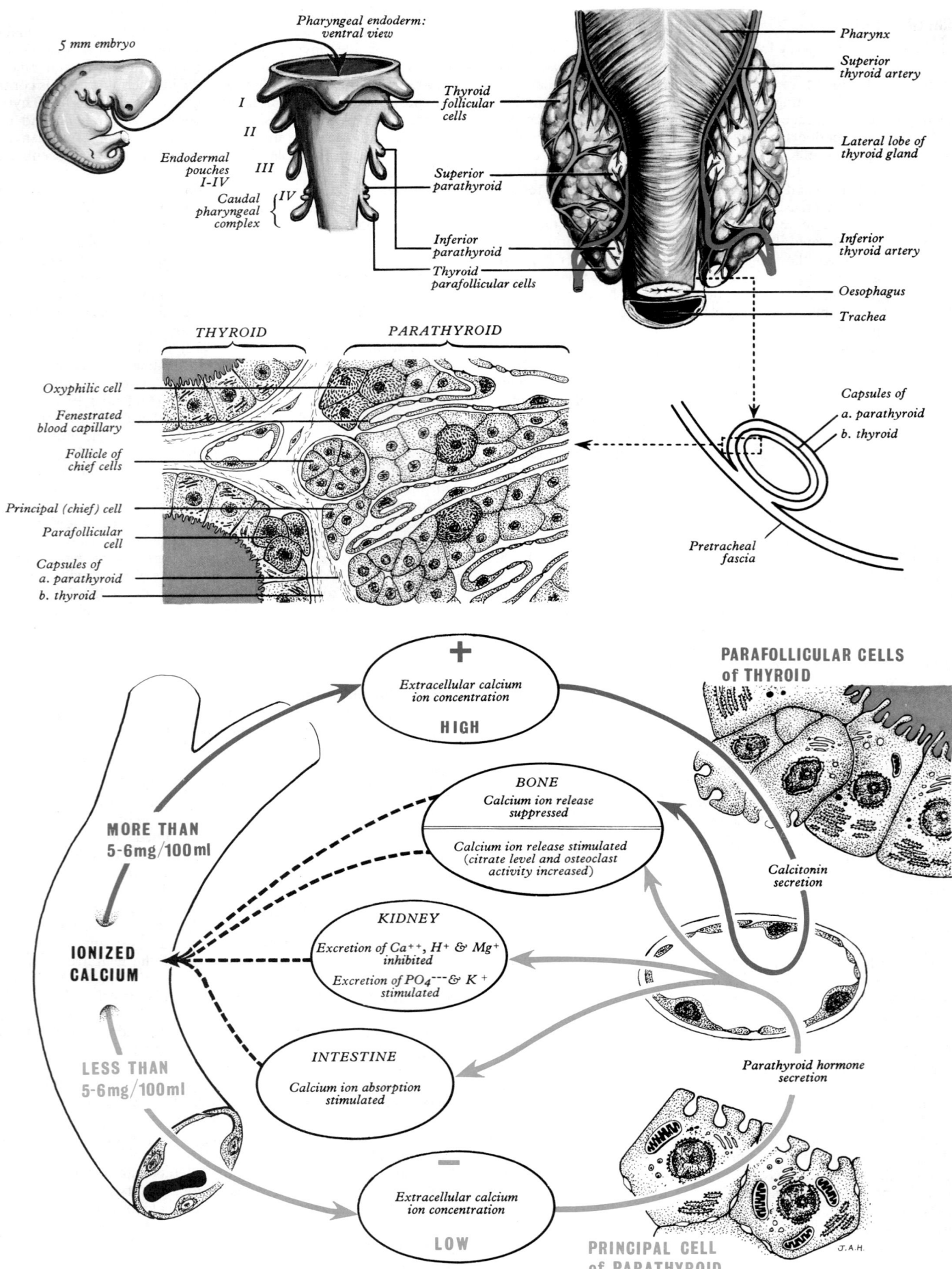

15.16   Diagrammatic representation of the roles of the parathyroid and thyroid glands in the control of calcium metabolism.

inferior thyroid (p.1535) and sometimes an arteria thyroidea ima from the brachiocephalic trunk or aortic arch. Yilmaz et al (1993) have reported an anomaly in which the inferior thyroid arteries were absent and replaced by an arteria thyroidea ima which arose from the brachiocephalic trunk and bifurcated almost immediately after its origin. The two branches formed ascended in front of the trachea and entered the bases of the right and left lobes of the thyroid gland. The arteries are remarkably large with frequent anastomoses on and in the gland. The **veins** form a plexus on its surface and in front of the trachea; from this plexus superior, middle and inferior thyroid veins arise: the first two end in the internal jugular, the inferior in the left brachiocephalic vein. A dense blood capillary plexus surrounds the follicles, between their epithelium and the endothelium of lymph capillaries, which also surround much of the follicular peripheries. **Lymph vessels** run in the interlobular connective tissue, often around arteries; they communicate with a capsular network, may contain colloid material and end in the thoracic and right lymphatic ducts. The **nerves** are derived from the superior, middle and inferior cervical sympathetic ganglia.

Clinical anatomy

Apart from variable enlargement during menstruation (De Remigis et al 1990) and pregnancy, any thyroid swelling is a *goitre*, which may press on related structures. Symptoms are most commonly due to pressure on the trachea or on the recurrent laryngeal nerves. These nerves, and therefore the laryngeal muscles supplied by them, may be affected by pressure or damaged during thyroidectomy; if the external laryngeal nerve or the cricothyroid muscle (which is supplied by it and tenses the vocal folds) are damaged, the voice becomes incapable of varying pitch and is slightly tremulous (Harries 1955).

Partial thyroidectomy is often necessary in hyperthyroidism and thyroid enlargement. Enough is removed to relieve symptoms; except in malignant disease it is not entirely removed, since this leads to myxoedema. During tying of the inferior thyroid artery, the proximity of the recurrent laryngeal nerve (pp.1535, 1253) is a hazard. Temporary aphonia sometimes follows mere bruising of the nerve; complete division reduces the voice to a whisper. In partial thyroidectomy the posterior parts of both lobes are left intact to preserve the parathyroid glands.

PARATHYROID GLANDS

The parathyroid glands (**15.**16, 17) are small, yellowish-brown, ovoid or lentiform structures, usually lying between the posterior lobar borders of the thyroid gland and its capsule. They are commonly about 6 mm long, 3–4 mm across, and 1–2 mm from back to front, each weighing about 50 mg. Usually there are two on each side, superior and inferior. The anastomotic connection between the superior and inferior thyroid arteries along the posterior thyroid border (p.1535) usually passes very close to the parathyroids.

The *superior parathyroid glands* are more constant in location than the inferior and are usually midway along the posterior thyroid borders but sometimes higher. The *inferior pair* (Walton 1931; Gilmour 1938; Murley & Peters 1961) may be:

(1) within the fascial thyroid sheath, below the inferior thyroid arteries and near the inferior lobar poles
(2) outside the sheath, immediately above an inferior thyroid artery
(3) in the thyroid gland near its inferior pole.

These variations are surgically important; a tumour of the inferior parathyroid, if in position (1), may descend along the inferior thyroid veins anterior to the trachea into the superior mediastinum, whereas if in position (2) it may extend postero-inferiorly behind the oesophagus into the posterior mediastinum. The superior parathyroids are usually dorsal, the inferior ventral, to the recurrent laryngeal nerves (Pyrtek & Painter 1964).

The glands develop from endoderm in the pharyngeal pouches (p.176), the inferior from the third and therefore referred to as *parathyroids III*, the superior from the fourth and termed *parathyroids IV*. The inferior parathyroid glands are connected in early development with the diverticulum of the third pouch, which forms the

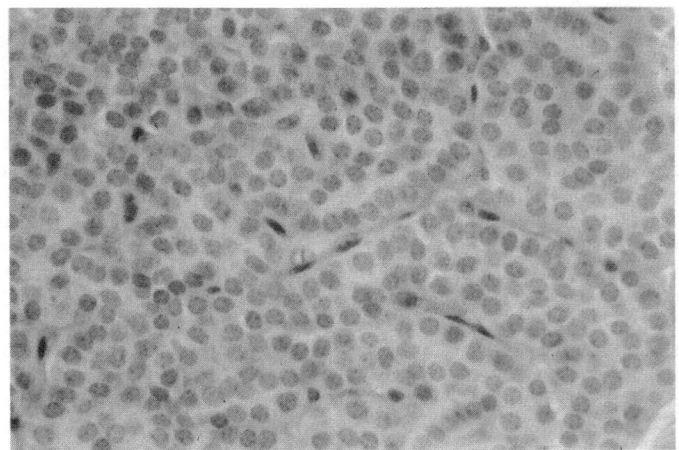

15.17 Section through a parathyroid gland showing densely packed chief cells and capillaries (rabbit). Haematoxylin and eosin. Magnification × 800.

thymus and is carried with it in its caudal migration. Normally the inferior parathyroids migrate only to the inferior thyroid poles but may descend with the thymus into the thorax or not descend at all, remaining above their normal level near the carotid bifurcation. Parathyroid glands vary in number; there may be only three or many minute parathyroid islands scattered in connective tissue near the usual sites (Hintzsche 1937; Vail & Coller 1967).

STRUCTURE AND FUNCTIONS

Each parathyroid gland has a thin connective tissue capsule with intraglandular septa but lacks lobules. In childhood, the gland consists of wide, irregular, interconnecting columns of *chief cells* or *principal cells*, responsible throughout life for the synthesis and secretion of parathyroid hormone (PTH; parathormone); three types of chief cell, *light*, *dark* and *clear*, can be distinguished by the depth of cytoplasmic staining; by light microscopy their cytoplasm appears homogeneous. Between the columns of cells is a dense plexus of sinusoidal capillaries, via which the hormone leaves the gland. Their ultrastructure was reviewed by Capen in 1975. Human chief cells differ according to the level of their activity (Munger & Roth 1963). *Active* chief cells have large Golgi complexes with numerous vesicles and small membrane-bound granules, the latter probably being prosecretory; secretory granules are rare, cytoplasmic glycogen sparse, much of the cytoplasm being occupied by flat sacs of granular endoplasmic reticulum in parallel arrays. In contrast *inactive* chief cells contain small Golgi complexes with only a few grouped vesicles and membrane-bound secretory granules; glycogen and many lipofuscin granules abound but sacs of granular endoplasmic reticulum are rare and dispersed. In normal human parathyroid glands inactive chief cells outnumber active in a ratio of 3–5:1.

Active chief cells synthesize, assemble and secrete parathyroid hormone. It is assumed that the dense-cored, membrane-bound granules in the chief cells of all mammals contain PTH (Capen & Roth 1973). During secretion the granules first become peripheral and then, under appropriate stimulation (see below), their membranes fuse with the plasmalemma to release their contents, presumably PTH. Involution continues, with increased lysosomal activity and reduction of Golgi complexes and granular endoplasmic reticulum; glycogen accumulates again; lipofuschin granules form and the cells enter a phase of temporary inaction. In contrast to the thyroid, where activity of adjacent cells is synchronized, each parathyroid chief cell appears to pass through its secretory cycle independently (Roth & Capen 1974).

A second cell type, the *oxyphil (eosinophil) cell*, appears just before puberty and multiplies with age (Roth 1962). Only in man, macaque monkey and cattle have such cells been noted. They are larger than chief cells and contain more cytoplasm which by light microscopy appears granular and which stains deeply with eosin; the nucleus is smaller and more darkly staining than in chief cells. Ultrastructural observations (Munger & Roth 1963; Gaillard et al 1965; Roth & Capen 1974; Capen 1975) show that the 'granules' seen by light microscopy are actually mitochondria, extremely numerous, tightly packed and often unusual in form. The cytoplasm also contains a few sacs of granular endoplasmic reticulum, some glycogen and, rarely, small Golgi complexes. No secretory granules have been reported. These features suggest that oxyphil cells are not involved in hormone synthesis or secretion, though abundant mitochondria suggest a high metabolic activity. The arrangement of chief and oxyphil cells in parathyroid glands is shown in (**15**.16).

PTH, a single-chain polypeptide of 84 amino-acid residues (Potts et al 1971), is concerned with control of the level and distribution of calcium and phosphorus (**15**.16). Two other hormones, namely calcitonin (p. 477) and 1,25-hydroxycholecalciferol, are also involved, the latter produced by the sequential action of hepatic and renal cells on vitamin D (O'Riordan 1978). Hormonal control of calcium metabolism has been described in detail by Copp & Talmage (1978). Secretion of PTH is dependent on the level of calcium ions in the blood traversing the parathyroid glands. PTH acts upon osteocytes and osteoclasts. Its rapid initial effect is to increase the rate of release of calcium from bone into blood, apparently by stimulation of osteocytic osteolysis (Bélanger 1969). It also has a delayed effect if a high level of secretion is maintained, stimulating internal bone remodelling by promoting osteoclast activity; changes in the membrane potential of osteoclasts may be involved (Mears 1971). PTH also affects renal ion transport (Puschett 1978), increasing excretion of phosphate, sodium and potassium and decreasing that of calcium. It may also affect intestinal transport of calcium. 1,25-hydroxycholecalciferol, production of which is regulated by PTH, shares many of these effects and may 'modulate' PTH action (O'Riordan 1978). How PTH affects target cells is not clear; adenyl cyclase activation and consequent rise in intracellular cAMP appear to be involved (Chase & Aurbach 1967; Chabardes et al 1975).

Vessels and nerves

The parathyroid glands have a rich blood supply from the *inferior thyroid arteries* or from anastomoses between the superior and inferior vessels. It has been shown by Nobon that approximately one-third of human parathyroid glands have two or more parathyroid arteries. **Lymph** vessels are numerous and associated with those of the thyroid and thymus glands. The **nerve supply** is sympathetic, either direct from the superior or middle cervical ganglia or via a plexus in the fascia on posterior lobar aspects. The nerves are vasomotor but not secretomotor, parathyroid activity being controlled by variation in blood calcium level: it is inhibited by a rise, stimulated by a fall.

Clinical anatomy

If all parathyroid tissue is removed, body muscles show convulsive spasms (*tetany*); since respiratory and laryngeal muscles are involved, death ensues. Tetany is due to a fall in blood calcium. Excess of parathyroid secretion, due to tumours, causes the removal of calcium ions from bones, which soften, a condition of *generalized osteitis fibrosa*. Calcium ions leak from the bones into the blood (hypercalcaemia), are excreted in urine and may calcify in the renal tubules, with resultant fatal renal disease.

CHROMAFFIN SYSTEM

Chromaffin cells (phaeochromocytes) are classically defined as derived from neuroectoderm, innervated by preganglionic sympathetic nerve fibres and capable of synthesizing and secreting catecholamines (dopamine, noradrenaline or adrenaline), storing enough to give an intense yellow-brown coloration, the *positive chromaffin reaction*, when treated with aqueous solutions of chromium salts, particularly potassium dichromate (Coupland 1965). Groups of such cells, associated topographically and functionally with the sympathetic nervous system, comprise the *chromaffin system* which includes:

- the medullae of the suprarenal glands
- the para-aortic bodies
- the paraganglia proper
- certain cells of the carotid bodies

- small groups of cells irregularly dispersed among the paravertebral sympathetic ganglia, splanchnic nerves and prevertebral autonomic plexuses.

They may, therefore, be related to: the heart, liver, kidney, ureter, prostate, epididymis, ovary, etc. Distribution of the main components in newborn infants is shown in **15**.18.

Three main groups of cells give positive chromaffin reactions (Coupland 1976):

(1) *true chromaffin cells*, as defined above

(2) *enterochromaffin cells* in epithelial tissue lining the gastrointestinal and respiratory tracts

(3) *amine-storing mast cells* in the connective tissues of the gut, pancreas and liver.

Ultrastructural similarity of 1 and 2 and the ability of all three groups to decarboxylate amino acids, observations that other non-chromaffin cells, in the gastrointestinal and respiratory tracts, pancreas and other endocrine glands are alike in both ultrastructure and amino-acid uptake, and the discovery of paraneurons with many features of chromaffin cells in sympathetic ganglia (p. 1299), all undermine the rationale of continuing to restrict the term 'chromaffin system' to 'true' chromaffin cells. It may be more appropriate now to consider it as part of a diffuse neuroendocrine system (see below). Cells of what is still frequently referred to as the chromaffin system have been used as models in which to study such fundamental processes as exocytosis (Burgoyne 1991; Unsicker 1993) and neuropoiesis (Landis & Patterson 1981; Anderson 1989; Unsicker et al 1989).

DIFFUSE NEUROENDOCRINE SYSTEM

Feyrter (1938) drew attention to isolated groups of hormone-secreting cells not restricted to accepted endocrine glands and widely scattered in many tissues. Terming such elements *clear cells*, he noted their prominence in the gut and pancreas. These are now classified as types of 'APUD' cells (Pearse 1966, 1980), the acronym being derived from their amine-handling properties (*a*mine *p*recursor *u*ptake and *d*ecarboxylation). Most APUD cells synthesize related peptides which act as **hormones** or **neurotransmitters**, though in others a main secretion is an **amine** of similar action. Collectively APUD cells are a 'system' more extensive than envisaged by Feyrter, including chromaffin cells (see above), small intensely fluorescent cells (SIF) cells (p. 1299), peptide-producing cells of the hypothalamus (p. 1097), hypophysis (p. 1886), pineal (p. 1888), parathyroid glands (p. 1897), placenta, the Kulchitsky cells in the lungs (p. 1668), the myoendocrine cells of the cardiac atria (Forssmann & Girardier 1979; Forssmann et al 1983) and ventricles (Cantin et al 1987). Over 40 different cell types (see Table **15**.1) have been categorized as APUD cells and included in what has been described as the *diffuse neuroendocrine system* (Pearse & Polak 1978). The myoendocrine cells of the heart differ from the others in being modified myocytes. These cells are listed in Table **15**.1.

In 1966 Pearse described common cytochemical features in cells making peptide hormones and most notably in those which produce biogenic amines (adrenaline, noradrenaline, dopamine, 5-hydroxytryptamine, etc.) He suggested that uptake of 5-hydroxy-tryptophan (5-HTP) and its decarboxylation to 5-hydroxytryptamine (5-HT) might be linked to peptide hormone production in general. From this concept the designation 'APUD' cell arose (Pearse 1968). Pearse (1977a,b) also suggested that all APUD cells were derived from 'neuroendocrine-programmed cells of the ectoblast' but there is now experimental evidence that many APUD cells (e.g. gastro-enteropancreatic (GEP) endocrine cells) develop from other sources (Le Douarin 1978) and may be endodermal in origin (Andrew et al 1982). Other cells, for example the myoendocrine cells of the heart (Forssmann et al 1983), may be of mesodermal origin but can be grouped with the other cells of the neuroendocrine system because of their similarities as producers of peptide hormones. Pearse considered APUD cells to be a third division of the nervous system, third-line effectors which support, modify or amplify the actions of neurons in the autonomic and somatic divisions. Their effects are slower in onset and longer in duration than those of the autonomic cells,

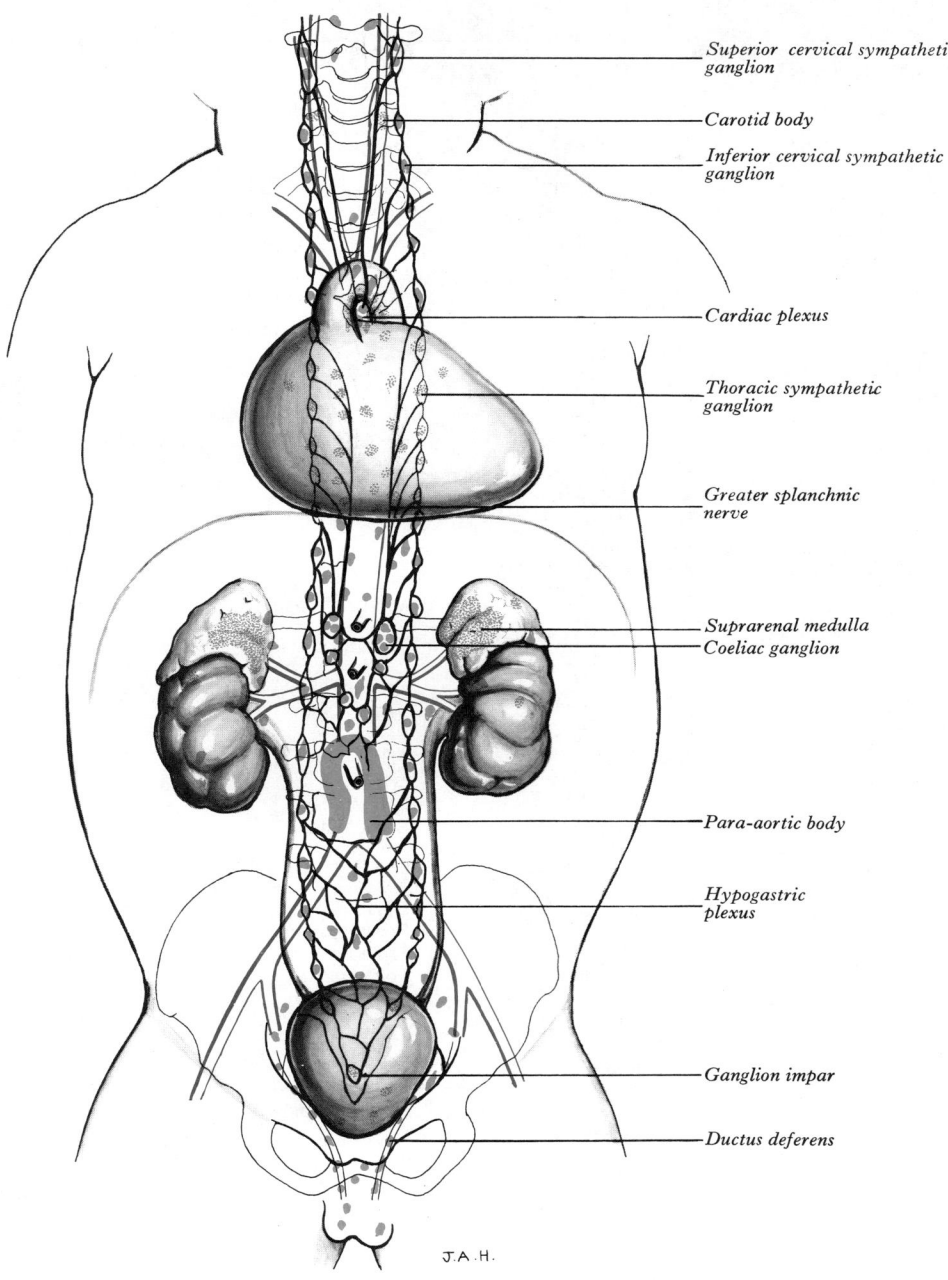

Superior cervical sympathetic ganglion

Carotid body

Inferior cervical sympathetic ganglion

Cardiac plexus

Thoracic sympathetic ganglion

Greater splanchnic nerve

Suprarenal medulla
Coeliac ganglion

Para-aortic body

Hypogastric plexus

Ganglion impar

Ductus deferens

J.A.H.

15.18   The principal aggregations of 'classic' chromaffin tissue in the human neonatal child. The aggregates in stippled blue lie deep to overlying structures.

which in turn have a similar functional relation to the faster somatic neurons. Secretions of APUD cells (diffuse neuroendocrine system) may act upon *contiguous* cells, on groups of *adjacent* cells or on *distant* cells by transport in blood; they may thus be considered intermediate between the locally acting transmitters produced by neurons and remote-acting endocrine secretions. Such a diffuse neuroendocrine system complements and co-ordinates the nervous and endocrine systems, **all three** interacting to provide a precise mechanism for homeostatic control. For a critical review of the APUD concept, see Andrew (1982). It must be added that, as already stated (p. 1898), the CNS also shares in many of the transmitters elaborated by APUD cells, further blurring the distinctions between neural and endocrine systems.

It was stated recently that the APUD or diffuse neuroendocrine system (DES) could be linked to the central and autonomic nervous systems by 'genetics, embryology, cellular characteristics, anatomy, interactions of the systems, and the immune system' (Baylis et al

1993). The recognition that the immune system and APUD system or DES have features in common was appreciated by Johnson et al (1992) and others. Both systems have a diffuse distribution and both have similar sensory and regulatory mechanisms which include cell membrane receptors for specific neuropeptides, hormones and amines. Interestingly, there also appear to be genetic links, since autoimmune disorders associated with, for example, ACTH receptor abnormalities can also appear on the corresponding immune cells (Smith et al 1987).

The APUD system can give rise to tumours termed APUD-omas, and it has been suggested that awareness of these relationships could lead to the development of better methods of detecting these tumours and improved methods of treatment (Demeure 1993). Deviations in the relative levels of secretions of different cells in this system may cause disorders described as psychosomatic (Pearse & Polak 1978) or frankly psychotic (Webster 1978). The growing understanding of this system may improve the treatment of these conditions.

Table 15.1   The APUD cells of the diffuse neuroendocrine system

I. APUD cells of neural crest origin

Location	Type	Main secretion	
		Peptide	Amine
Thyroid	Parafollicular (C)	Calcitonin	5-HT, Da
Ultimobranchial body	C	Calcitonin	5-HT, Da
Carotid body	Type I Glomus	—	Da, NA
Sympathetic ganglia	SIF	—	NA
Adrenal medulla	Chromaffin	—	Ad
Adrenal medulla	Chromaffin	—	NA
Skin	Melanoblast	—	Promelanin
Urogenital tract	EC	—	5-HT
Urogenital tract	E	—	—

II. APUD cells of placodal or specialized ectodermal origin

Location	Type	Main secretion	
		Peptide	Amine
Hypothalamus	N pv	Oxytocin, CRF	—
	N so	Vasopressin	—
	N sch	—	—
	N dm/vm	TRF	—
	N arc	LHRF	Da
	N ant/post	SRF, CRF	—
	N periv	Somatostatin	—
Pineal gland	P	LHRF	5-HT, MT
Parathyroid	Chief	PTH	—
	Somatotroph	Somatotropin	Da
	Mammotroph	Prolactin	Da
	Gonadotroph	Follitropin	Da
Pituitary	Gonadotroph	Lutropin	Da
	Corticotroph	Corticotropin	—
	M	Melanotropin	T
	Thyrotroph	Thyrotropin	Da
Placenta	Endocrine	Gonadotropin	—
	Endocrine	Somato-mammotropin	—
	Endocrine	Corticotropin	—

SUPRARENAL (ADRENAL) GLANDS

The suprarenal glands (**15**.19–25), two small yellowish bodies, flat anteroposteriorly, are each situated immediately anterosuperior to each superior renal pole. Surrounded by connective tissue containing much perinephric fat (p. 1816), they are enclosed in renal fascia but separated from the kidneys by fibrous tissue. Each has a cortical zone rich in lipids but with **no** chromaffin tissue and an internal medulla staining deeply with chromium salts. Small masses of identical cortical suprarenal tissue often occur near the main gland and elsewhere as 'cortical bodies'. Ontogenetically, phylogenetically, structurally and functionally, cortex and medulla are distinct, despite their topographical union, although they can interact.

The right gland is an irregular tetrahedron, whereas the left is semilunar and usually larger and superior in level. Each in adults measures about 50 mm vertically, 30 mm transversely, and 10 mm in the anteroposterior dimension, weighing about 5 grams (the medulla being about one-tenth of the total weight). At birth the gland is about one-third the size of a kidney (**15**.18) but in adults only one-thirtieth. This change in ratio is not only due to renal growth but also to postnatal suprarenal diminution due to involution of the fetal cortex (p. 1903). By the end of the second month the weight of the suprarenal is reduced to one-half. In the latter half of the second

year it begins to increase, gradually regaining its natal weight around puberty, after which its weight increases little in adult life.

RELATIONS OF THE SUPRARENAL GLANDS

Right suprarenal gland

The right suprarenal gland (**15**.20, **15**.21) is posterior to the inferior vena cava and right hepatic lobe, and anterior to the diaphragm and superior pole of the right kidney. It is shaped like an irregular tetrahedron. Its *base*, inferior in position, adjoins the anteromedial aspect of the right superior renal pole, often overlapping the upper part of the right kidney's medial border. Its *anterior surface* which faces slightly laterally, has a medial, narrow, vertical area, uncovered by peritoneum and posterior to the inferior vena cava, and a lateral triangular area in contact with the liver. The upper part of the latter is also devoid of peritoneum and is in contact with the inferomedial angle of the bare area of the liver. Its inferior part may be covered by peritoneum, reflected on to it from the inferior layer of the coronary ligament; the duodenum may overlap this area. Below the apex, near the anterior border of the gland, is a short sulcal hilum where the right suprarenal vein emerges to join the inferior vena cava. The *posterior surface* is divided into upper and lower areas by

III. APUD cells of disputed origin

Location	Type	Main secretion	
		Peptide	Amine
Pancreas	A B D D$_1$ P PP	Glucagon Insulin Somatostatin VIP-like Bombesin-like Pancreatic polypeptide	5-HT 5-HT Da Da — Da
Stomach	A D ECL EC$_1$ G X	Glucagon Somatostatin — Substance P Gastrin, Enkephalin —	— H? 5-HT — —
Intestine	D D$_1$(H) EC$_1$ EC$_2$ EC$_n$ I K L N S	Somatostatin VIP Substance P Motilin — Cholecystokinin GIP Enteroglucagon Neutrotensin Secretin	— — 5-HT 5-HT 5-HT — — — — —
Lung	Kulchitsky (P$_a$)	—	—
Heart	Myoendocrine	Cardiodilation Atrial natriuretic factor	

Abbreviations

Ad	Adrenaline	N dm/vm	Nucleus dorsomedialis/ventromedialis
CRF	Corticotropin-releasing factor	N periv	Nuclei periventriculares
Da	Dopamine	N pv	Nucleus paraventricularis
GIP	Gastric inhibitory peptide	N sch	Nucleus suprachiasmaticus
H	Histamine	N so	Nucleus supraopticus
5-HT	5-hydroxytryptamine	PTH	Parathyroid hormone
LHRF	Luteotropin-releasing factor (luteinizing hormone releasing factor)	SIF SRF	Small, intensely fluorescent Somatotropin-releasing factor
MT	Melatonin	T	Tryptamine
NA	Noradrenaline	TRF	Thyrotropin-releasing factor
N ant/post	Anterior and posterior nuclear 'zones' of hypothalamus	VIP —	Vasoactive intestinal peptide Unidentified
N arc	Nucleus arcuatus (Nucleus infundibularis)		

a curved transverse ridge: its upper area, slightly convex, rests on the diaphragm; the lower, concave, contacts the superior pole and adjacent anterior surface of the right kidney. The thin *medial border* of the gland is related to the right coeliac ganglion, which is medial to it below, and to the right inferior phrenic artery, coursing superolaterally on the right crus of the diaphragm.

Left suprarenal gland

The left suprarenal gland (**15.20, 15.**21) is crescentic, its concavity being adapted to the medial side of the superior pole of the left kidney. It is medially convex, laterally concave; its superior border is sharp, the inferior rounded. Its *anterior surface* has a superior area covered by peritoneum of the omental bursa, which separates it from the cardiac end of the stomach and sometimes from the posterior pole of the spleen; it also has an inferior area, not covered by peritoneum, in contact with the pancreas and splenic artery. The hilum faces ventrocaudally and is near the lower part of the anterior surface; from it a left suprarenal vein emerges to join the left renal vein. Its *posterior surface* is divided by a ridge into a lateral area adjoining the kidney and a smaller medial one in contact with the diaphragm's left crus. The convex *medial border* is related to the left coeliac ganglion, which is inferomedial, and to the left inferior phrenic and left gastric arteries, which ascend on the left crus.

Accessory suprarenal glands

These small accessory suprarenal glands, sometimes composed only of cortical tissue, often occur in the areolar tissue near the main suprarenal glands and sometimes in the spermatic cord, epididymis and broad ligament of the uterus.

STRUCTURE OF THE SUPRARENAL GLANDS

A sectioned suprarenal gland (**15.**22) reveals an outer *cortex*, yellow in colour and forming the main mass, and a thin *medulla*, forming about one-tenth of the gland, dark red or pearly grey depending on its content of blood. The medulla is completely enclosed by cortex, except at its hilum. The gland has a thick, collagenous capsule, which sends variable deep trabeculae into the cortex; the capsule contains a rich arterial plexus supplying branches to the gland.

Suprarenal cortex

The suprarenal cortex (**15.**23–25) consists of three cellular zones: the zonae glomerulosa, fasciculata and reticularis. The outer, sub-capsular, *zona glomerulosa* consists of small polyhedral cells in rounded groups or curved columns with deeply staining nuclei, scanty basophilic cytoplasm and a few lipid droplets. Ultra-structurally (Lever 1955; Long & Jones 1967; Bloodworth & Powers

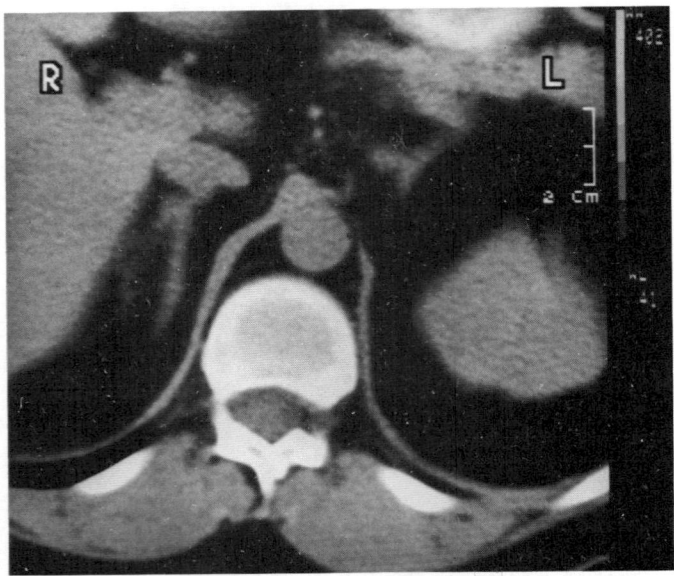

15.19A   High-resolution computed tomogram of the abdomen in the transverse plane at the level of the suprarenal glands. (Provided by Shaun Gallagher, Guy's Hospital; photographed by Sarah Smith, UMDS, Guy's Hospital Campus, London.)

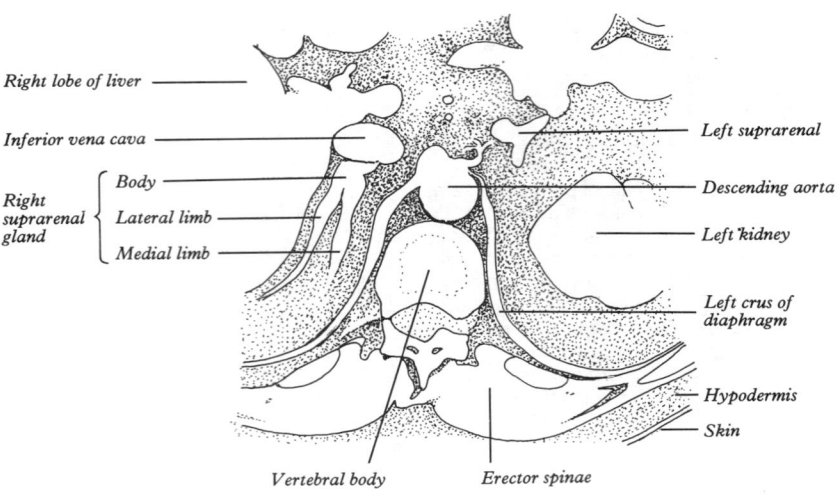

15.19B   Diagram illustrating the major features demonstrated in **15.**19A.

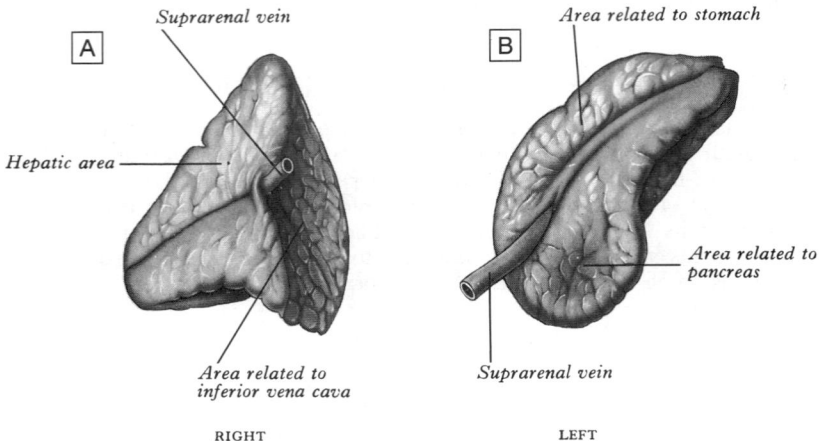

15.20   Suprarenal glands: anterior aspect.

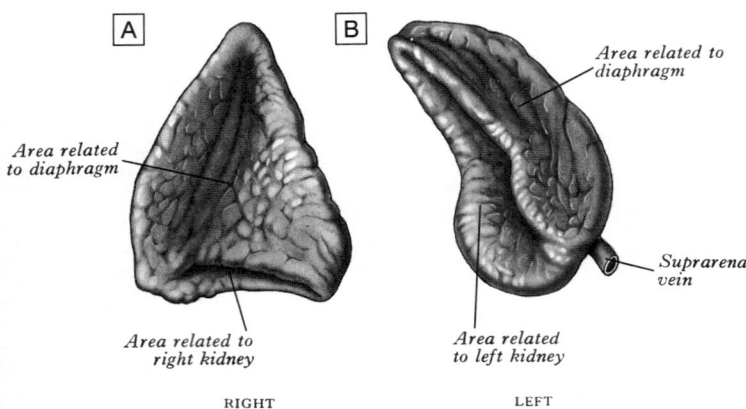

15.21   Suprarenal glands: posterior aspect.

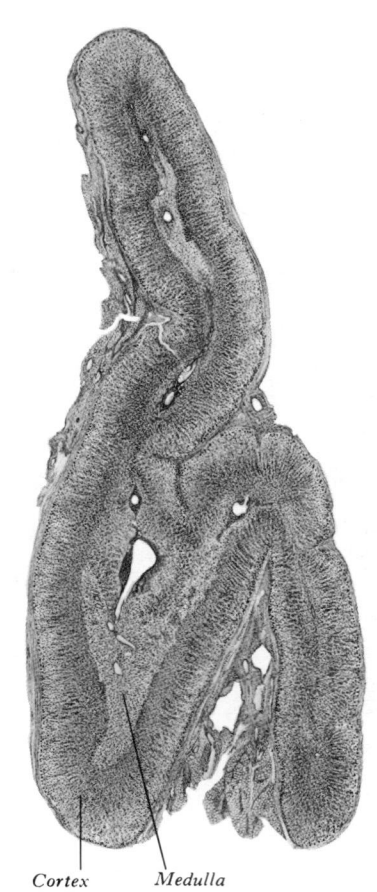

15.22   Vertical section through a whole adult human suprarenal gland.

1968; Shelton & Jones 1971) the cytoplasm displays many microtubules, long mitochondria and abundant agranular endoplasmic reticulum, the last being typical of cells elsewhere which synthesize steroids (see below). In humans the zona glomerulosa is poorly developed; deep to it the broader *zona fasciculata* consists of large polyhedral basophilic cells arranged in straight columns, two cells wide, with parallel fenestrated venous sinusoids between them. The cells contain many lipid droplets and large amounts of phospholipids, fats, fatty acids and cholesterol embedded in complex agranular endoplasmic reticulum. The mitochondria are typically spherical with tubular cristae; the Golgi complex is extensive. The innermost part of the cortex, the *zona reticularis*, consists of branching, interconnected columns of round cells whose cytoplasm contains much agranular endoplasmic reticulum, many lysosomes and pigment bodies which may indicate degeneration. Some consider that glomerulosar cells, particularly those more deeply set, proliferate con-

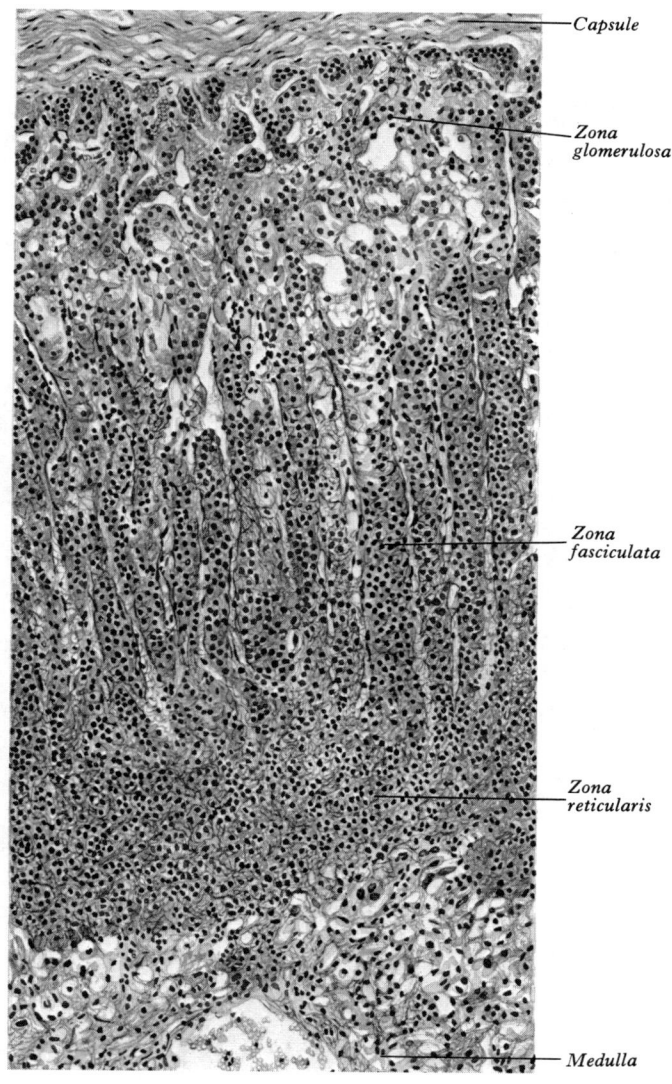

15.23 Section of adult human suprarenal gland. Magnification × 200.

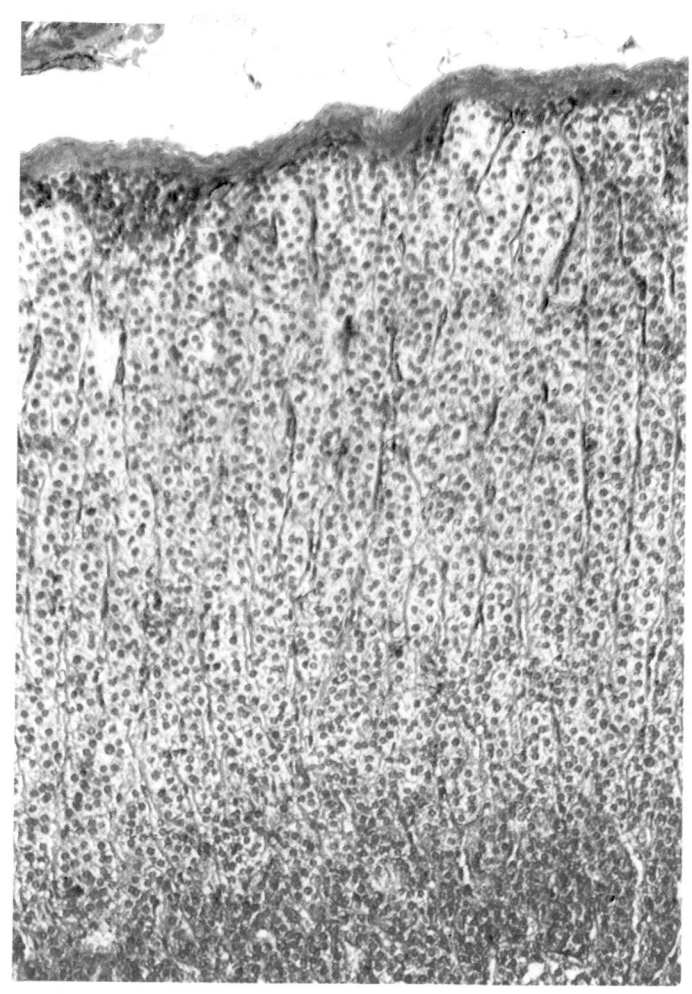

15.24 Medium magnification light micrograph of a section of the cortex of a human suprarenal gland. Beneath the capsule (blue) lie the zonae glomerulosa, fasciculata and reticularis. MSB triple stain. (Prepared and photographed by Stephen Sitch, Department of Anatomy, UMDS, Guy's Hospital Campus, London.)

tinuously, some of the new cells migrating through the zona fasciculata to the reticularis in which they may degenerate and disappear. Autoradiography indicates that most proliferation occurs in the zona glomerulosa and outer reticularis but mitoses also appear in other cortical regions (Reiter & Hoffman 1967). There is little ultrastructural evidence of cell death in the zona reticularis.

The deeper part of the zona fasciculata widens in pregnancy (Whiteley & Stoner 1957) and in women of childbearing age in summer (MacKinnon & MacKinnon 1958). Cortical atrophy in old males is greatest in the same region of this zone and least at its periphery (MacKinnon & MacKinnon 1960). Cortical cells produce several hormones and the cells of the zonae fasciculata and reticularis are also rich in *ascorbic acid* (*vitamin C*). Cells in the zona glomerulosa produce mineralocorticoids, for example *aldosterone*, which affects electrolyte and water balance; cells in the zona fasciculata produce hormones maintaining carbohydrate balance (glucocorticoids), for example *cortisol* (*hydrocortisone*); cells in the zona reticularis may produce sex hormones (*progesterone*, *oestrogens* and *androgens*). The cortex is essential to life; complete removal is lethal, without replacement therapy. It also exerts considerable control over lymphocytes and lymphoid tissue; increase in secretion of corticosteroids can result in a marked reduction in lymphocyte numbers. In some mammals the cortex shows cycles of hypertrophy and regression during the oestrous cycle. Between the cortical cells are sinusoids,

into which branches from the capsular arterial plexus and cortical arteries largely open. Some arteries traverse the cortex to supply the medullary sinusoids. Cortical sinusoids also discharge into medullary sinusoids. Sinusoidal endotheliocytes are phagocytic and belong to the macrophage (mononuclear phagocyte) system (p. 78).

Chromaffin cells (p. 1898), characterized by immunostaining for *synaptophysin* and *chromogranin a*, both considered specific for neuroendocrine cells, have been located within the suprarenal cortex as well as in the medulla (see below). The chromaffin cells of the cortex form cellular contacts with classical cortical cells, characterized by immunostaining for *17-hydroxylase*, an enzyme of the steroid-producing pathway. Chromaffin cells have been identified in all three zones of the suprarenal cortex and often spread into the subcapsular space of the zona glomerulosa. These observations provide evidence in support of a possible paracrine role for the chromaffin cells of the suprarenal gland, and it has been suggested that this may be important in the neuroregulation of the activity of the suprarenal cortex (Bornstein et al 1991).

Suprarenal development is described on p. 1900. The relatively large size of the neonatal suprarenal gland is due to its very thick *fetal cortex* (Johannisson 1968), the *definitive cortex* being a thin peripheral zone. Around birth the fetal cortex begins to regress and largely disappears in a few weeks thereafter. Too rapid a cortical involution may be complicated by fatal haemorrhage. This transient

1903

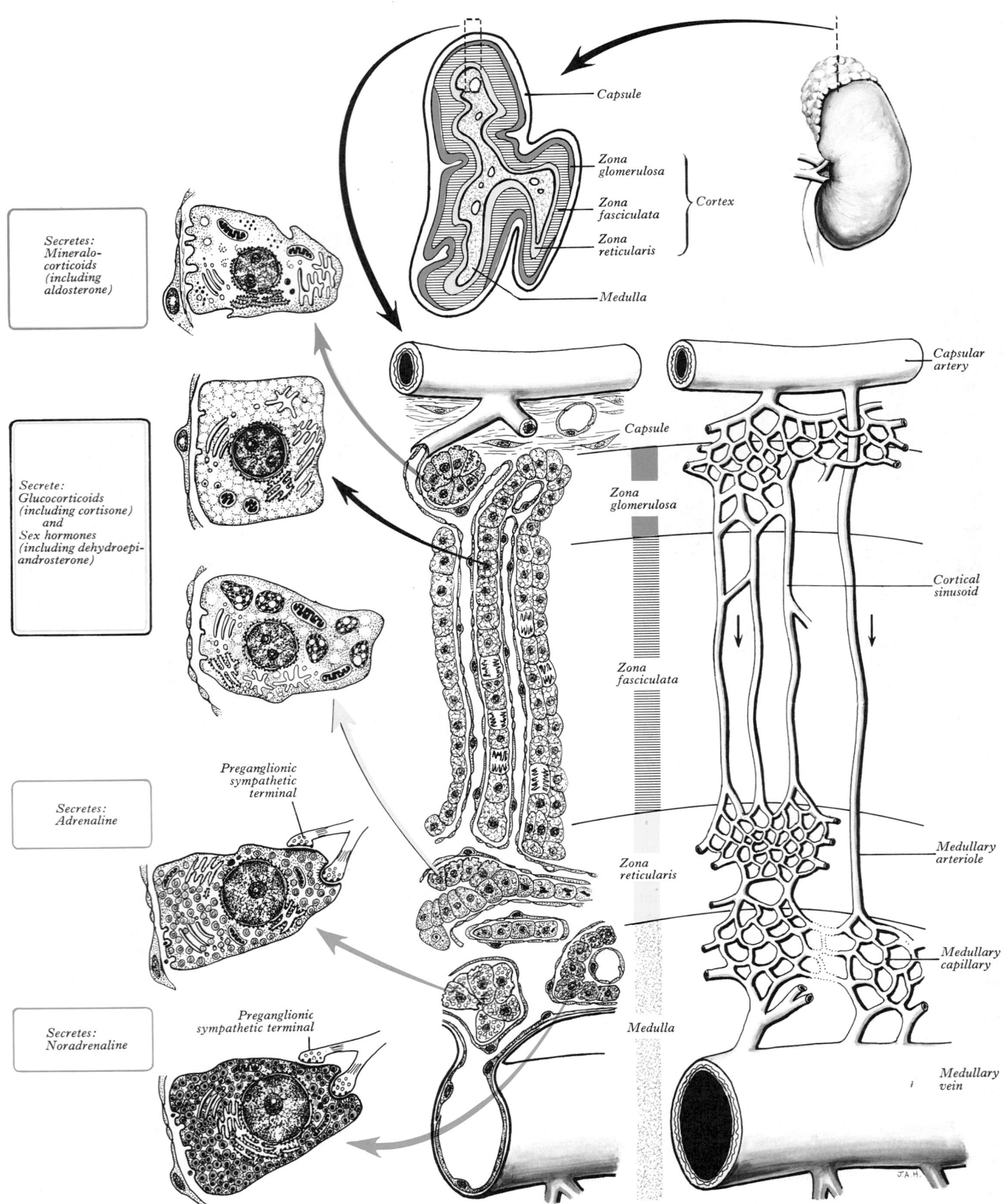

15.25   The suprarenal gland, displaying its gross sectional appearance, histology, vasculature and ultrastructure. Brief functional summaries are appended.

fetal cortex occurs only in anthropoids. There is no proof that it produces androgenic hormones. It is poorly developed in anencephalic fetuses. It does not represent the X zone (androgenic), which occurs in young mice, for instance, as a zone around the medulla (Jones 1957).

Suprarenal medulla

The suprarenal medulla is composed of groups and columns of chromaffin cells (*phaeochromocytes*) separated by wide venous sinusoids. Single or small groups of neurons occur in the medulla.

Chromaffin cells synthesize and expel noradrenaline and adrenaline into the venous sinusoids; release is under preganglionic sympathetic control (see Coupland 1965a for review). In some mammals these hormones have been identified in two distinct types of cell (Yates et al 1962), cells storing noradenaline being more peripheral than those storing adrenaline. All cells, which are large and columnar, form single rows along the venous sinusoids. Cell bases and nuclei are distal from the sinusoids, adjoining expanded extracellular spaces in which the nerve terminals synapse with the chromaffin cells. These may form follicles but not like those in thyroid tissue (Al-Lami 1970). The cytoplasm is basophilic, showing well-developed granular endoplasmic reticulum, mitochondria, Golgi complexes and many vesicles, indicating a high metabolic activity (Coupland 1965b; Al-Lami 1970). In noradrenaline-storing cells the vesicles are typically round or ellipsoidal and, after treatment with aldehyde and osmium, highly electron-dense. In adrenaline-storing cells, treated alike, the vesicles are paler (Coupland et al 1964), often with a clear zone between the granular contents and membrane. In the human suprarenal glands, cells with both types of vesicle have been reported (Brown et al 1970) suggesting that adrenaline and noradrenaline may both appear in the same cell. Vesicle contents are released at the cell apices into the perivascular spaces, entering the circulation through the fenestrated endothelium of venous sinusoids (Elfvin 1965; Al-Lami 1969).

The sinusoids drain to the hilar suprarenal vein. Normally, little adrenaline or noradrenaline is released but in fear, anger and stress secretion is augmented. Noradrenaline produces cardiac acceleration, vasoconstriction, raised blood pressure, etc. while adrenaline has a marked effect on carbohydrate metabolism. Unlike its cortex, the suprarenal medulla is not essential to life; removal has no clear effect. Medullary chromaffin cells develop in and migrate from the neural crests (sympathochromaffin tissue, p. 236). The chromaffin reaction (brown staining of granules by potassium bichromate, due to oxidation of adrenaline and noradrenaline) is positive from the fifth fetal month but adrenaline appears as early as the third (Keene & Hewer 1927).

Interaction between cortex and medulla

Only in mammals is the suprarenal chromaffin tissue almost enclosed by cortex. In elasmobranchs, for example dogfish, cortical tissue forms paired *inter-renal bodies*, chromaffin tissue being separate in segmental masses close to the sympathetic ganglia. In amphibia and birds, cords of chromaffin and cortical cells are intimately associated but a true medulla is not formed (Coupland 1965a). The proximity of cortical to chromaffin tissue may be associated with the formation of adrenaline by methylation of noradrenaline (see below).

Vessels and nerves

The suprarenal gland is very vascular and is supplied by three groups of **arteries** (the superior, middle and inferior suprarenal) from the inferior phrenic, abdominal aorta and renal artery respectively (Harrison & Hoey 1960). Most suprarenal branches ramify over the capsule before entering the gland to form a subcapsular plexus, from which fenestrated sinusoids pass around clustered glomerulosal cells and between columns in the zona fasciculata to a deep plexus in the zona reticularis. From this venules pass between medullary chromaffin cells to medullary veins, which they enter between prominent longitudinal bundles of muscle fibres; these appear to regulate flow through a 'dam' at the corticomedullary junction, i.e. the internal aspect of the zona reticularis (Dobbie & Symington 1966). Since this would also control flow through the other zones, it could also control, in part, the availability of ACTH to their secretory cells (Griffiths & Cameron 1975).

Some relatively large arteries bypass the above route by going direct to the medulla, giving it a dual supply (**15**.25). Blood reaching it indirectly via the cortical sinusoids probably contains enough glucocorticoid hormone to maintain the synthesis of phenylethanolamine-N-methyl-transferase for synthesis of adrenaline from noradrenaline, whereas blood arriving by the direct non-cortical route does not. Whether medullary chromaffin cells can make adrenaline or noradrenaline depends on this enzyme and may be determined by the blood supply (Wurtman & Pohorecky 1971). Changes in relative blood flow via the two routes could thus have profound consequences.

Medullary **veins** emerge from the hilum to form a *suprarenal* vein, draining to the inferior vena cava (right side) and left renal vein.

The **lymph** vessels end in lateral aortic nodes (p. 1621).

The **nerves**, which are exceedingly numerous, are mainly myelinated preganglionic sympathetic fibres (p. 1307) distributed to the medullary chromaffin cells. Acetylcholinesterase (AChE)-positive innervation has been studied in the human suprarenal gland by Charlton et al (1991), who found a heterogeneous pattern of cortical innervation. There was frequently a subcapsular plexus of interwoven AChE-positive nerve trunks closely associated with densely stained ganglion cells. Nerves also traversed the zona fasciculata as radial trunks and another plexus associated with ganglion cells was identified in the zona reticularis. Nerve trunks were also found in the medulla. Charlton et al (1991) suggested that the presence and distribution of AChE-positive nerve plexuses suggested a 'functional, probably cholinergic, innervation of the human adrenal cortex, perhaps derived from splanchnic nerves'. Suprarenal cortical activities are largely controlled by hypophyseal ACTH.

Clinical anatomy

Various clinical conditions due to lesions of the suprarenal cortex or medulla are attributable to the effects of excess or deficiency of secretions in the parts of the gland affected.

Atrophy (usually tuberculous) of the suprarenal cortex, with consequent insufficiency of cortical secretion, results in Addison's disease, typified by muscular weakness, low blood pressure, anaemia, cutaneous pigmentation, changes in electrolytic and fluid balance, and terminal circulatory and renal failure. Excessive cortical secretion, due to tumours or hyperplasia, produces various effects:

- In adults, Cushing's syndrome may result, typified by obesity, excessive hairiness of the face and trunk, diabetes mellitus, impotence and hypogonadism in males and amenorrhoea in females.
- In women, masculinization (virilism) may occur due to excess of androgenic hormones.
- In men, feminization, particularly mammary development, may occur.
- Children may show precocious body growth and development of the external genital organs, with early menstruation in girls.
- In the female fetus, cortical hyperplasia between the third and fourth months leads to female pseudohermaphroditism, the excess androgen interfering with differentiation of the urogenital sinus; the urethra and vagina open into a persistent urogenital sinus, the clitoris enlarges and the external genital organs resemble the male's. In the male fetus cortical hyperplasia causes excessive external genital development.

Bilateral removal of the suprarenal glands is a treatment for some inoperable disseminated mammary or prostatic carcinomata, when the malignant changes are considered to be dependent on androgens or oestrogens. Tumours of the suprarenal gland's medulla and the para-aortic bodies (phaeochromocytomata) may cause excessive secretion of adrenaline and noradrenaline, producing attacks of palpitations, excessive sweating, pallor, hypertension, headaches and, if of long duration, retinitis and renal vascular changes.

The suprarenal glands can be demonstrated radiologically if air is injected into perirenal fat.

PARAGANGLIA

Paraganglia (Zuckerkandl 1901; Köhn 1903) are extra-suprarenal aggregations of chromaffin tissue (p. 1895, **15**.18), distributed near or in the autonomic nervous system (Coupland 1965a; Mascorro & Yates 1971; Hervonen et al 1978). Cells like those in paraganglia proper (which adjoin various autonomic ganglia) also occur in the sympathetic ganglia as *small, intensely fluorescent* (SIF) *cells* (Williams et al 1975), in the walls of various viscera and in a variety of retroperitoneal and mediastinal sites (Ramsdale et al 1972; Hervonen et al 1976, 1978b). All are neuroectodermal and can synthesize and store catecholamines but their functions differ with location: intraneural cells act as interneurons (p. 912), the remainder as sources of endocrine secretions including a tryptophan-containing protein and catecholamines (Hervonen et al 1978a). This dispersed array of extra-adrenal chromaffin tissue, often dubbed the *paraganglion system* (Mascorro & Yates 1975), is prominent in fetuses as the main source of catecholamines while the adrenal medulla is still developing (West et al 1955; Kovrishko 1964). Though many paraganglia degenerate soon after birth (Coupland 1965a), the specific fluorescent histochemical technique for the detection of catecholamines (Eränkö 1967) has located many persistent, often minute, paraganglia in adult human and other mammals, contradicting the earlier assumption of general postnatal involution of paraganglia.

Paraganglia contain two typical varieties of cell: *Type I* or granule-containing and *Type II* or satellite cells (Mascorro & Yates 1975). Type I have a large nucleus, long mitochondria, some granular endoplasmic reticulum, well-developed Golgi complexes, glycogen deposits, numerous membrane-bound, electron-dense granules containing catecholamines and possibly the tryptophan-containing protein mentioned above, features which together with their neuroectodermal origin place them in the APUD category (Pearse 1969; Pearse & Polak 1974). By their cytoplasmic density, Type I cells can be classified as 'light' or 'dark', though 'dark' cells are widely considered to be a fixation artefact (Mugnaini 1965; Benedeczky & Smith 1972) and both types may be stages in a secretory cycle. Type II cells lack cytoplasmic granules and their processes envelop Type I cells partially or completely.

Type I cells of paraganglia receive a 'preganglionic' sympathetic innervation (Mascorro & Yates 1974) like the adrenal medullary chromaffin cells (Cummings 1969). The non-myelinated nerve fibres are largely separated from Type I cells by Schwann cell cytoplasm and cytoplasmic projections of the Type II cells, approximating only at synapses. Presynaptic endings contain mitochondria, glycogen granules and many synaptic vesicles, mostly electron-lucent, though some have electron-dense cores. In vagal paraganglia such endings may be cholinergic and efferent (Chen & Yates 1970). Nerve fibres containing vasoactive intestinal polypeptide (VIP) are present in human fetal abdominal paraganglia (Hervonen et al 1985).

Paraganglia are well-vascularized and their secretory Type I cells are usually next to one or more fenestrated capillaries, often with only basal lamina intervening, although sometimes fine collagen fibres and cytoplasmic processes of Type II cells are present. Thus little obstructs the passage of hormones from Type I cells to blood (Mascorro & Yates 1975). Evidence suggests that paraganglia are endocrine organs producing catecholamines and proteins and storing them as cytoplasmic granules until stimulated to release them. In addition to having a remote endocrine effect, these secretions may exert local paracrine action on nearby cells. Paraganglia comprise a dispersed system which throughout life may be a source of catecholamines additional to the suprarenal medulla and thus collectively have considerable metabolic importance (see below).

PARA-AORTIC BODIES

Developing progressively during fetal life these attain maximum size in the first three postnatal years, when the largest are two brownish bodies about 1 cm long, flanking the abdominal aorta and usually united anterior to it by a horizontal mass immediately above the inferior mesenteric artery (**15**.18). They thus form an inverted crescentic or H-shaped arrangement, intimately related to the inter-mesenteric and superior hypogastric plexuses. Their constituent cells disperse and atrophy and by 14 years they may have completely disintegrated (Coupland 1965a). When well-developed, they consist

of masses of polygonal chromaffin cells embedded in wide-meshed capillary plexuses and secreting noradrenaline. In fetuses other small chromaffin bodies are also widespread in the abdominal and pelvic prevertebral sympathetic plexuses. They reach a maximum size between the fifth and eighth fetal months and survive in adults mainly near the coeliac and superior mesenteric arteries and as microscopic collections of cells persisting in the lower parts of the intermesenteric plexus.

Although chromaffin cells in sympathetic ganglia, as noted, may act as interneurons, those elsewhere are endocrine and probably support the suprarenal medulla as sources of catecholamines (Chen et al 1976), particularly in pre- and early postnatal life, when the suprarenal medulla and autonomic nervous system are immature (West et al 1953). This is supported by Coupland and Weakley (1970), who observed that extra-suprarenal chromaffin cells resemble those in the suprarenal medulla. Ultrastructural evidence shows that in rats chromaffin cells in the nodes of the solar plexus have processes extending beyond their glial cells towards the capillaries, into which their catecholamines pass (Levkova & Kakabadze 1977).

TYMPANIC BODY

The tympanic body (*glomus jugulare*) is ovoid, about 0.5 mm long and 0.25 mm broad, and occurs in the adventitia of the upper part of the superior bulb of the internal jugular vein. It is similar in structure to the carotid body (p. 971), with presumably a similar function (Guild 1941; Kjaegaard 1944, 1973). The chief cells of this structure have morphological and functional similarities to adrenal chromaffin cells and like them are derived from the neural crest. Studies on cells obtained from glomus jugulare paragangliomas in culture have shown that there can be spontaneous neurite outgrowth from these cells and that they have vasoactive intestinal peptide (VIP)-like activity (Tischler et al 1981).

The tympanic body may be present as two or more parts near the glossopharyngeal tympanic branch or vagal auricular branch, within their canals in the petrous temporal bone. Tumours of these bodies may involve the adjacent cranial nerves and the middle ear.

COCCYGEAL BODY

The coccygeal body (*glomus coccygeum*) was first described by Luschka in 1860. It was considered to be a gland homologous to the carotid body (*glomus caroticum*; p. 971) by Luschka (1862) and Arnold (1865). Later Köhn (1902) again grouped these organs together and, on the basis of their supposed structure and development, included them as members of the chromaffin or paraganglion system. This was disputed by Stoerk (1907) who considered the coccygeal body to be a group of arteriovenous anastomoses. The characteristic cells of this structure were later described as modified non-striated myocytes of a spherical or epithelioid form (Masson 1937) grouped around sinusoidal blood vessels. Each cell has a large, round or oval nucleus, and its cytoplasm is clear and unstained by chromium salts, indicating no clear affiliation to the chromaffin system. In 1938 Schumacher reported that the coccygeal body, carotid body and a number of abdominal paraganglia were morphologically indistinguishable. Since the carotid body was then known to be a chemoreceptor, other investigators explored the possibility that the coccygeal body was also a chemoreceptor. Hollinshead (1942) reported that a study of human carotid and coccygeal bodies, obtained at autopsy and processed for light microscopy under identical conditions, revealed no similarity between them; for example, an intimate relationship was found between the vasculature and the glomus cells of the carotid body but not in the coccygeal body, and it was considered improbable that the latter could function efficiently as a chemoreceptor.

The coccygeal body has also been regarded as a larger variant of the arteriovenous anastomotic glomus bodies found in digital subcutaneous tissues (Reuther 1938). The latter can give rise to glomus tumours. Bell et al (1982) have obtained evidence suggesting that the normal coccygeal body could be mistaken for a tumour, and urge clinicians treating patients with coccydynia to avoid performing coccygectomy unnecessarily in the hope of removing an otherwise undetected glomus tumour. Detailed analysis of the innervation, ultrastructure and function of the coccygeal body is still awaited.

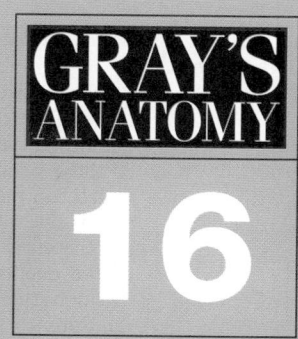

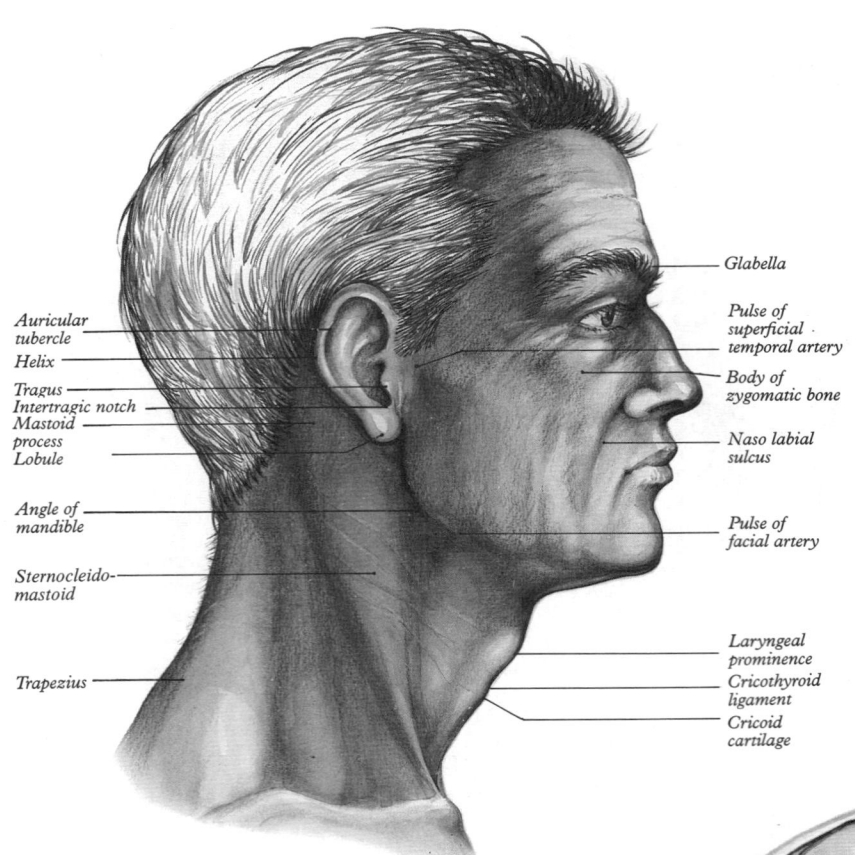

Auricular tubercle
Helix
Tragus
Intertragic notch
Mastoid process
Lobule
Angle of mandible
Sternocleido-mastoid
Trapezius

Glabella
Pulse of superficial temporal artery
Body of zygomatic bone
Naso labial sulcus
Pulse of facial artery
Laryngeal prominence
Cricothyroid ligament
Cricoid cartilage

INTRODUCTION

Surface anatomy deals with the relationships of deeper structures to the surface of the body. In order that these relationships may be determined, use is made of easily identified surface landmarks. Some of these produce irregularities in the surface contours of the body which can readily be appreciated on inspection. Others, while giving no visible sign of their presence, can be felt through the skin and are therefore capable of identification by means of palpation. Most of the deeper structures of the body can neither be seen nor felt through the skin. However, a knowledge of their topographical relations to the body makes it possible to refer them to visible or palpable landmarks with relatively little difficulty.

Bones, cartilages, muscle masses and tendons provide most of the visible and palpable body landmarks. When seeking for bony or cartilaginous landmarks, their recognition is facilitated by the relaxation of muscles in their vicinity. In contrast, muscle and tendons can be identified most easily when they are thrown into contraction and, preferably, when they are working against resistance.

Where arteries are placed superficially and lie against bone, their position can be indicated accurately as their pulsations render their identification relatively easy. Nerves, similarly placed, can be rolled under the skin against the bone. A few other soft tissue structures, for example the parotid duct, the spermatic cord, etc., can also be felt through the skin. Subcutaneous veins in the limbs can be identified more readily when venous return is impeded by means of

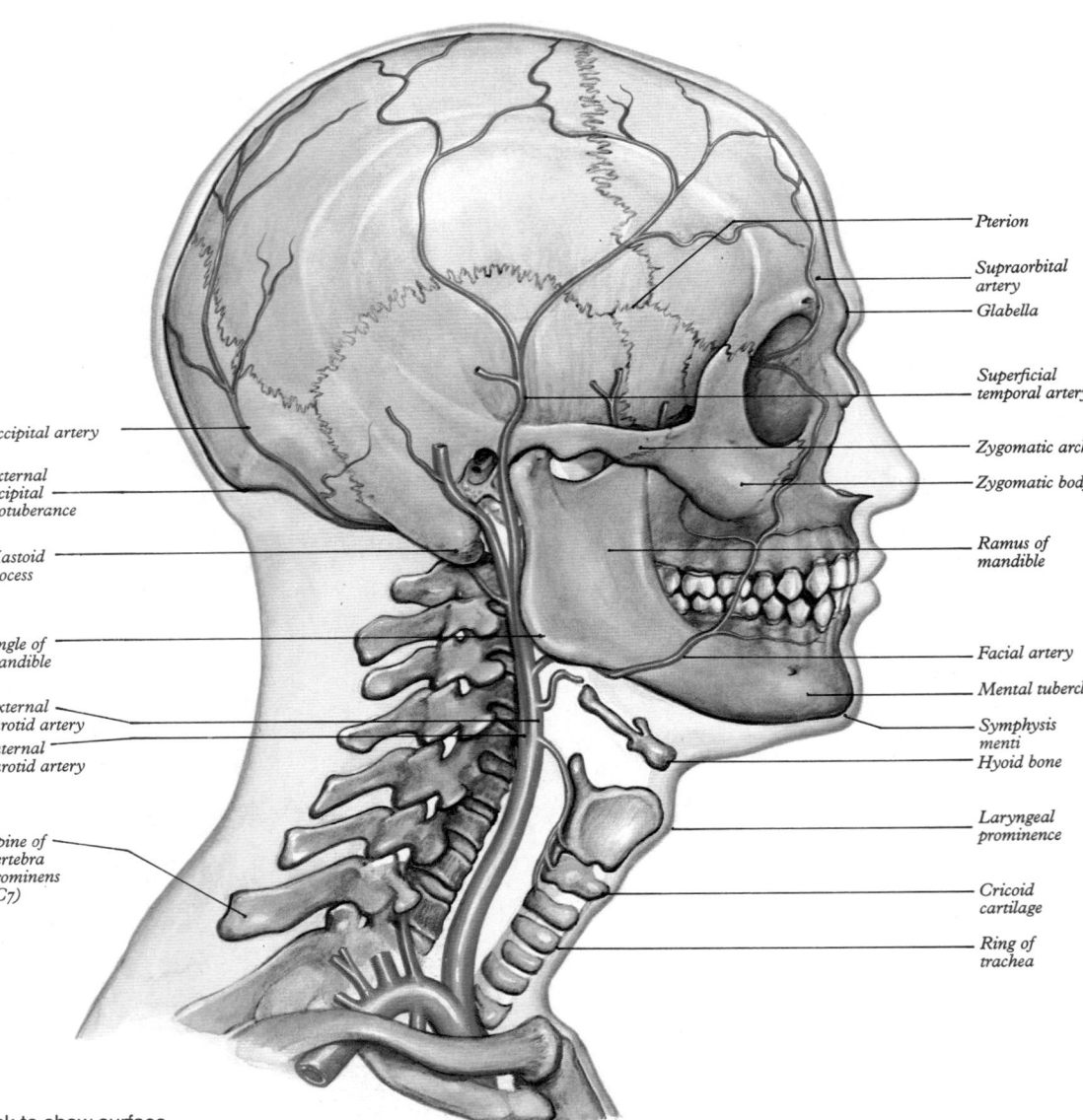

Occipital artery
External occipital protuberance
Mastoid process
Angle of mandible
External carotid artery
Internal carotid artery
Spine of vertebra prominens (C7)

Pterion
Supraorbital artery
Glabella
Superficial temporal artery
Zygomatic arch
Zygomatic body
Ramus of mandible
Facial artery
Mental tubercle
Symphysis menti
Hyoid bone
Laryngeal prominence
Cricoid cartilage
Ring of trachea

16.1 Lateral views of head and neck to show surface anatomy, bony and soft tissue structures.

a rubber band, while those of the head and neck can be made to fill by means of the Valsava manoeuvre, exhaling while the nose is gripped and the mouth kept closed.

HEAD

SKELETAL SURFACE LANDMARKS

Most of the superficial aspect of the skull is covered by skin, subcutaneous tissue and thin muscles which makes it relatively easy to feel the bony prominences and surfaces. The *pericraniocervical line* demarcates the head from the neck (**16**.1); the line runs from the *symphysis menti* anteriorly to the *inion* posteriorly. Starting anteriorly the inferior surface of the symphysis menti of the mandible may be felt. This continues into the base of the body and ramus of the mandible, which continues posteriorly to the mandibular angle (often everted in the male, incurved in the female). The posterior border of the ramus of the mandible may then be palpated up to the neck of the *condylar process*, which lies just under the lobule of the ear. A finger probing inwards just behind the condylar process enters the small *retromandibular fossa* where, anteriorly, the *mandibular neck* may be felt and superiorly the inferior wall of the *external acoustic meatus*. Palpating posteriorly the anterolateral aspect and tip of the *mastoid process* may be felt. On deep palpation of this fossa a somewhat indistinct resistance may be felt. This is due to the *styloid process* and its attached structures. If the examining finger is then

taken posteriorly over the convexity of the mastoid process the lateral part of the *superior nuchal line* will be encountered. This arches convex upwards to meet the contralateral superior nuchal line at a bony prominence, the inion. The inion is of particular importance as a surface marking related to the confluence of the dural venous sinuses (i.e. the 'crux' between the cerebral and cerebellar hemispheres).

Now that the boundary separating the head and neck has been defined the skeletal surface landmarks of the head can be examined from the back, from the side and from the front. In bald people the palpable bony landmarks of the calvarium become visible, but more commonly they have to be palpated through the hair.

Posterior aspect

In the midline posteriorly the *external occipital protuberance* is palpable with the inion at its summit. The superior nuchal line can be felt easily as it arches laterally towards the mastoid process.

Lateral aspect (16.1)

The inferior margin of the lateral aspect of the skull, the pericraniocervical line, has already been defined. The mastoid process is easily palpable, anterior to which is the *external acoustic meatus* bounded itself anteriorly by the *tragus*, the small curved flap, which partly projects over the orifice of the meatus. The tragus is a suitable point from which to explore the *temporal fossa*. The boundaries of the temporal fossa are as follows. Anteriorly the *zygomatic process*

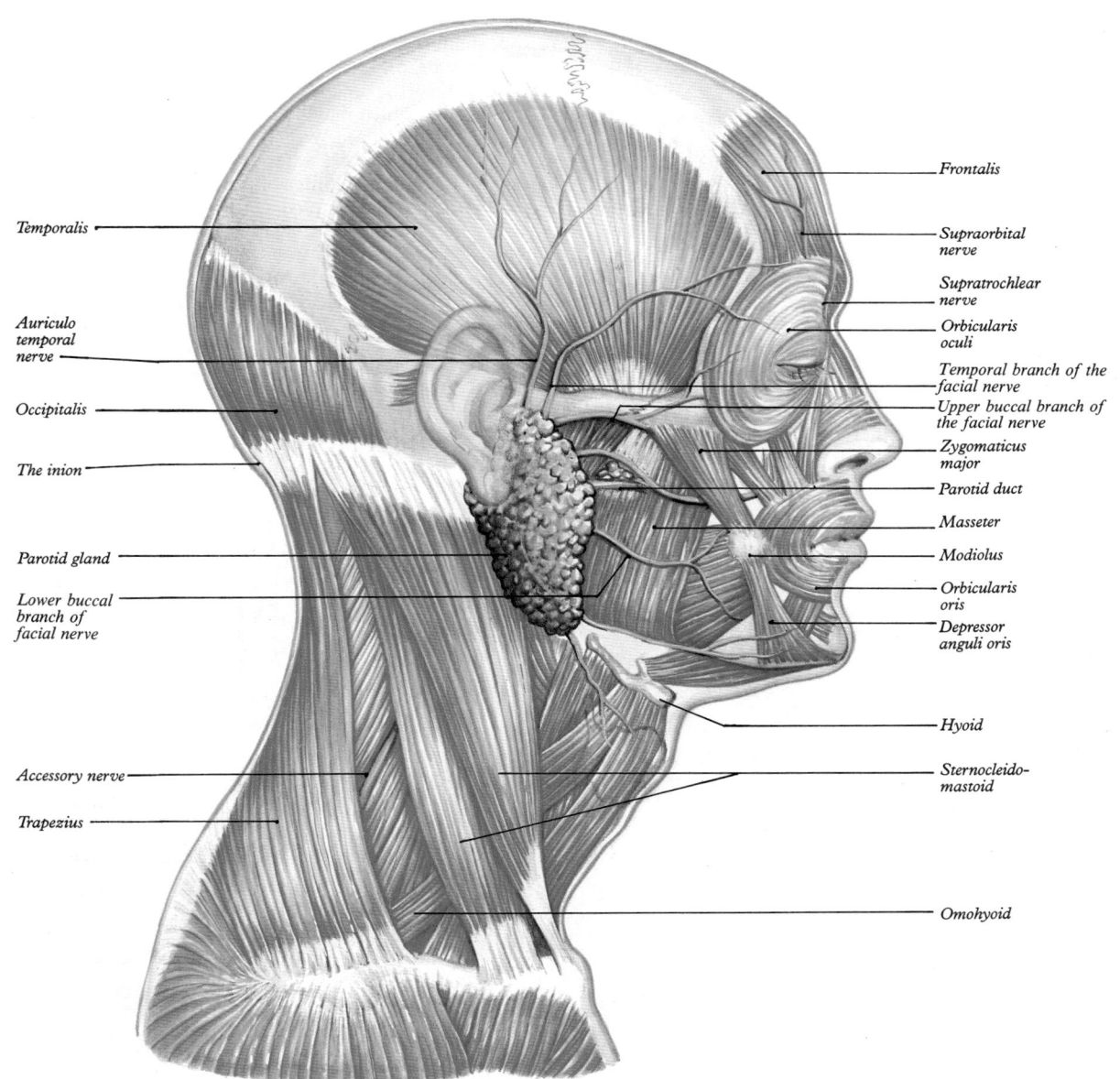

Temporalis

Auriculo temporal nerve

Occipitalis

The inion

Parotid gland

Lower buccal branch of facial nerve

Accessory nerve

Trapezius

Frontalis

Supraorbital nerve

Supratrochlear nerve

Orbicularis oculi

Temporal branch of the facial nerve

Upper buccal branch of the facial nerve

Zygomaticus major

Parotid duct

Masseter

Modiolus

Orbicularis oris

Depressor anguli oris

Hyoid

Sternocleido-mastoid

Omohyoid

of the temporal bone can be easily felt; together with the temporal process of the zygomatic bone, it forms the *zygomatic arch* (or zygoma). Anterior to the arch is the variably prominent *zygomatic body* (the 'cheekbone') from which ascends the zygomatic bone's *frontal process*. Following the sharp posterior margin of this process upwards it fuses with the frontal bone's *zygomatic process* from whence continuing posteriorly in the line of a gentle arch the *temporal lines* may be felt, the lower of which terminates by curving downwards and forwards to end just above the root of the mastoid process as the *supramastoid crest*. These are the boundaries of the temporal fossa within which lies the *pterion*. This is the smallest circular area which contains the junction of the frontal, sphenoid, parietal and temporal sutures. It usually lies 4 cm above the zygomatic arch and 3.5 cm behind the fronto-zygomatic suture and marks the anterior branch of the middle meningeal artery and the Sylvian point of the brain (p. 560). Its position can be estimated roughly by a shallow palpable hollow, about 3.5 cm above the centre of the zygoma. Posterosuperior to the external acoustic meatus is the *suprameatal triangle* bounded above by the supramastoid crest, in front by the posterosuperior meatal margin and behind by a posterior vertical tangent to the meatal margin. This triangle is the lateral wall of the mastoid (tympanic) antrum.

The most obvious structure lying inferior to the zygomatic arch is the *mandible*, its posterior and inferior borders being part of the pericraniocervical line. The *ramus* is easily palpable though mostly covered by masseter muscle. Ascending the posterior border of the ramus, the finger encounters the *condylar process* and *head of the mandible*. As the mouth is opened and closed articulation at the temporomandibular joint may be appreciated. Anteriorly the *coronoid process* can be felt to move from its resting position under the zygomatic arch as the mouth is again opened. The angle of the mandible is easily identified, as is the inferior surface of the body of the mandible. (For age changes of the mandible see p. 578.) Anteriorly the *mental tubercle* may be felt and the oblique line joining this to the lower end of the anterior border of the ramus of the mandible corresponds to the mylohyoid line, a line that separates the mucosal oropharyngeal region from the lower muscular or musculo-visceral region. By palpating the superior border of the body of the mandible through the cheek the teeth can be easily felt (when present). With the mouth loosely open, the incisura between coronoid process and head of mandible can be felt through the masseter muscle.

Anterior aspect (16.2)

If one accepts that the calvarium exists to protect the intracranial structures and in particular the brain, then the bones on the anterior aspect of the skull relate particularly to seeing, breathing, olfaction and eating. The *orbit* is an obvious visual feature (see below). Usually palpable above the orbit is the *superciliary arch*, better marked in the male than the female, and above that the *frontal tuberosity* may be felt. In the fetus and until about 18 months after birth the *anterior fontanelle* at the junction of the coronal and sagittal suture may be felt. Between the superciliary arches is a small horizontal ridge called the *glabella*, again easily palpable. Below it the *nasal bones* meet the *frontal bone* in a small depression, the *nasion*, at the root of the nose. The orbital opening is somewhat quadrangular. The *supraorbital margin*, formed entirely by the frontal bone, is easily palpable and at the junction of its sharp lateral two-thirds and rounded medial third, may be felt the *supraorbital notch*, if present. This transmits the supraorbital branch of the ophthalmic division of the trigeminal nerve; pressure here with the finger nail is distinctly painful. This is not so if the nerve lies in a *supraorbital foramen*. The lateral margin of the orbit is also easily palpable, being comprised of the frontal process of the zygomatic bone and the zygomatic process of the frontal bone. The suture between them may be felt as a palpable depression. The inferior border of the orbit is formed from the zygomatic bone laterally and the maxilla medially. The infraorbital margin blends into the less obvious medial margin formed above by the frontal bone and below by the lacrimal crest of the maxillary frontal process. A shallow fossa behind the lower part of the medial wall houses the lacrimal sac.

Inferior to the glabella is the junction of internasal and frontonasal sutures, the *nasion*, below which may be felt the nasal bones and the frontal processes of the maxillae. With a little finger inserted into the nose, the bony margins of the anterior nasal aperture can be felt, being formed by the inferior border of the nasal bone, the sharp margins of the nasal notches and coapted nasal spines of the maxillae.

The superficial aspect of the maxilla, the largest of the cranial bones, is easily palpable. The anterior surface, which faces anterolaterally, may be felt just below the orbit. The *canine eminence*

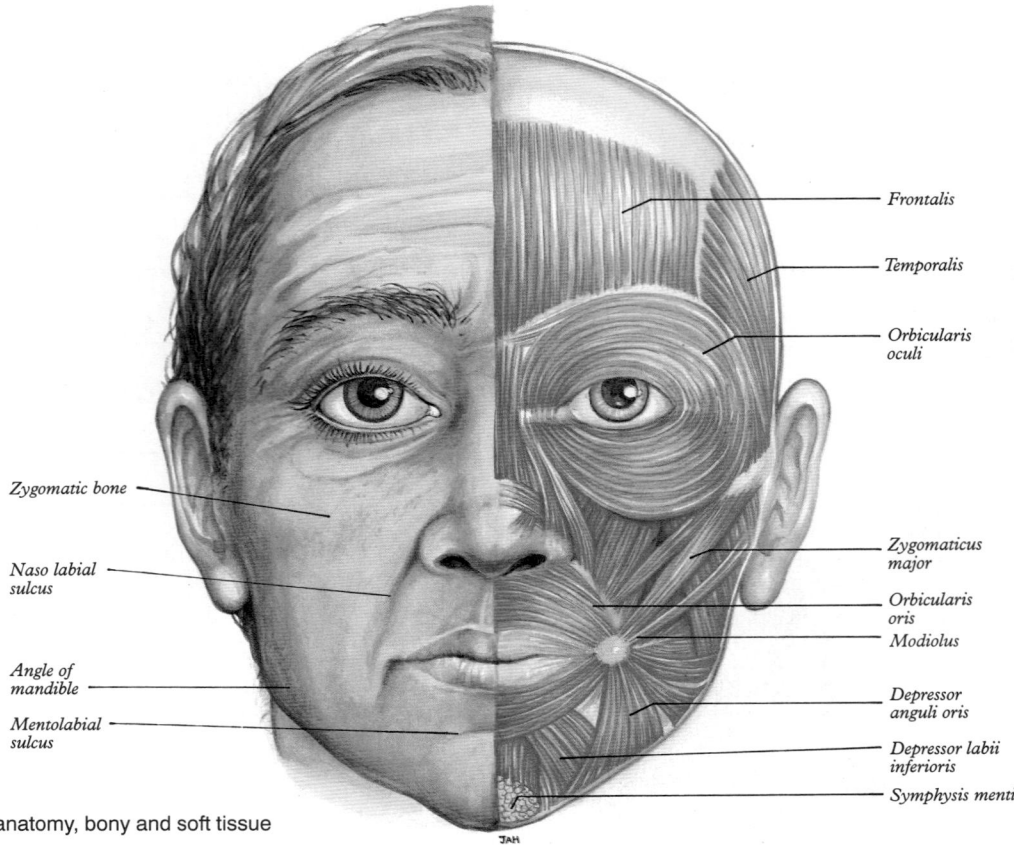

Zygomatic bone

Naso labial sulcus

Angle of mandible

Mentolabial sulcus

Frontalis

Temporalis

Orbicularis oculi

Zygomaticus major

Orbicularis oris

Modiolus

Depressor anguli oris

Depressor labii inferioris

Symphysis menti

16.2 Frontal views of head to show surface anatomy, bony and soft tissue structures.

overlying the canine socket is palpable; anteriorly lies the *incisor fossa* while posteriorly is the deeper *canine fossa*, above which is the *infraorbital foramen*. Above this a sharp border divides the anterior and orbital surfaces of the maxilla. Medially a deep concave nasal notch is palpable. The *frontal process* may be felt on the medial aspect of the orbit and laterally the *zygomatic process* is palpable in the inferolateral aspect of the orbit. Inferiorly the *alveolar process* of the maxilla is palpable with its sockets for the reception of the roots of the teeth. The *palatine process* of the maxilla, which forms the roof of the mouth, is easily palpable within the mouth.

SOFT TISSUES

Posterior aspect

There are no particular features to note on the posterior aspect of the skull except to feel the mobile aponeurosis of the scalp.

Lateral aspect (16.1)

The most obvious feature on the lateral aspect of the head is the *auricle* or *pinna* surrounding the *external acoustic meatus* (this is described on p. 1369). There is great variation in the appearance of the external ear, but a fissure running obliquely downwards and backwards from the lobule may be present, especially with increasing age, and is associated with sudden death from cardiovascular disease (Frank's sign). Using an auroscope, it is possible to look down the external acoustic meatus and examine under direct vision the tympanic membrane (see p. 1370). Immediately in front of the tragus the *superficial temporal artery* crosses the zygomatic arch and its pulsations can be felt at this point. The surface marking of the cranial exit of the *facial nerve* is a point immediately in front of the intertragic notch between the tragus and the antitragus of the auricle.

Two important masticatory muscles are palpable when the jaw is clenched. They are difficult to define when relaxed; *temporalis*, which lies in the temporal fossa and is covered by the temporal fascia, is palpable if the flat of the hand is placed on the side of the head and the jaw clenched; *masseter* is similarly easily palpable with the jaw clenched when its anterior border stands out.

The *parotid gland* is soft and indistinct, but lies largely below the external acoustic meatus between the mandible, the mastoid process and sternocleidomastoid; deeply placed is the styloid process and related structures. It projects forwards on the surface of masseter and the *parotid duct* arises from its anterior aspect. This can be palpated where it crosses the anterior border of masseter when the jaw is clenched (for a detailed description of its relations and position see p. 1688).

Frontal aspect (16.2)

The bony, muscular, fatty and cutaneous features which so clearly differentiate one person from another are readily apparent on inspection. Craniofacial muscles are described in detail on page 789 and the external features of the eye on pages 1353–1367.

The *orifice* of the *parotid duct* is visible as a small papilla within the mouth at the level of the second upper molar tooth. The pulsation of the *facial artery* can be felt as it crosses the lower margin of the body of the mandible immediately in front of the masseter and again opposite the angle of the mouth. In the latter situation if the cheek is gripped lightly with a finger placed within the mouth and the thumb placed on the skin surface, the pulse will be felt a little more than a centimetre from the angle of the mouth. When the lateral part of the lip is gripped in a similar manner the pulsation of the *labial artery* can be felt beneath the mucous surface about 0.5 cm from the free margin of the lip. The *palatine tonsil* can be represented by an oval area over the lower part of the masseter, just above and in front of the angle of the mandible.

With the mouth open it is possible to examine all the teeth, to inspect and palpate the orifice of the parotid duct and to see the lymphoid tissue forming the palatine tonsils. The tongue may be examined for its general appearance and any abnormalities of movement which may reflect neuronal damage (see also pp. 1256–1258). The filiform papillae on its superior aspect give it its rough appearance anteriorly. Further posteriorly may be noted the large fungiform papillae and the vallate papillae. The inferior surface of the tongue as seen, is smooth and shiny. In the midline the tongue is connected to the floor of the mouth by the *frenulum linguae* and lateral to this the *deep lingual vein* is easily visible. The *orifices of the submandibular ducts* may be seen each side of the base of the frenulum where the orifices surmount the lingual papillae, the medial ends of the sublingual folds.

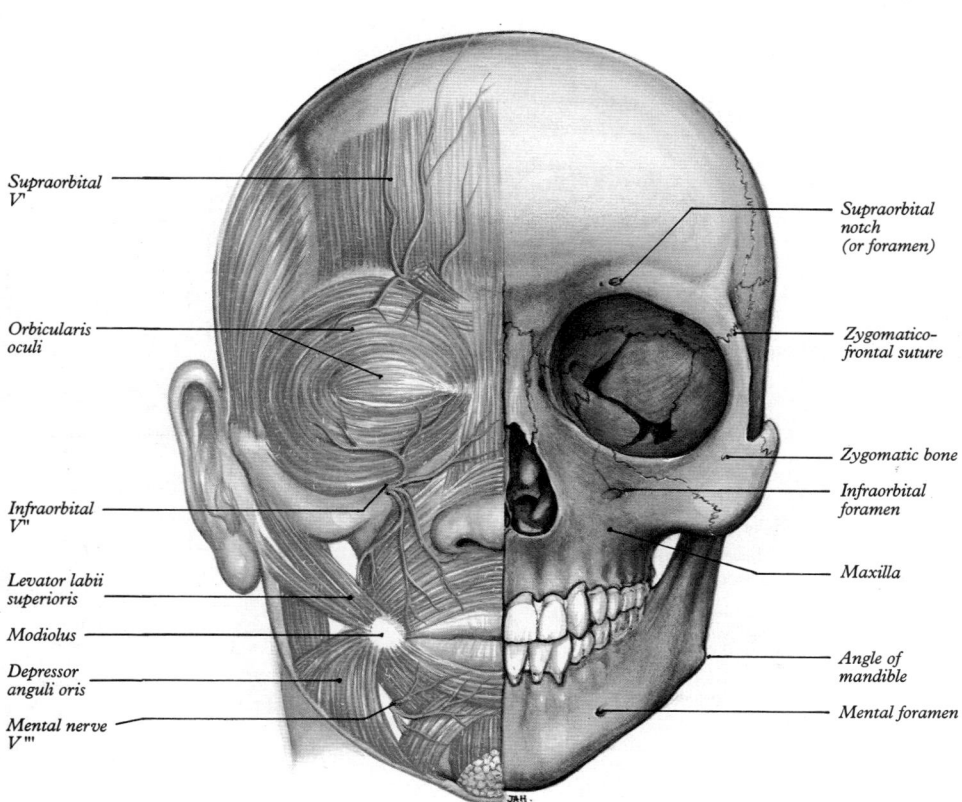

Supraorbital
V'

Orbicularis
oculi

Infraorbital
V"

Levator labii
superioris

Modiolus

Depressor
anguli oris

Mental nerve
V'''

Supraorbital
notch
(or foramen)

Zygomatico-
frontal suture

Zygomatic bone

Infraorbital
foramen

Maxilla

Angle of
mandible

Mental foramen

NECK

SKELETAL SURFACE LANDMARKS

The superior limit of the neck, the pericraniocervical line, has already been described. Inferiorly the neck blends with the thorax and upper limb at the level of the clavicle and scapula. The following skeletal features are easily palpable. At the back of the neck the bones of the cervical vertebrae may be felt in the midline. The first cervical vertebra (the atlas) is impalpable, but the *spine* of the *second cervical vertebra* can be felt on deep palpation. Inferiorly the *spine* of the *seventh cervical vertebra* is especially prominent, the *vertebra prominens* (see surface anatomy of the back p. 1921). Anteriorly, (**16.**1) almost tucked up under the chin, the *hyoid bone* may be felt. It is easy to feel this if the neck is extended and the hyoid bone is palpated between finger and thumb and moved from side to side. Inferior to the hyoid bone is the most obvious visual feature in the front of the neck, the *thyroid cartilage* and in particular the midline point of fusion of its laminae, which forms the subcutaneous *laryngeal prominence* or Adam's apple. In the male, it is usually clearly visible, whereas in the female it is not usually apparent, even when the neck is viewed from the side. The curved upper border of the thyroid cartilage and the *thyroid notch* are easily palpable. Anteriorly the inferior border of the thyroid cartilage can be felt just above the annular *cricoid cartilage*. The gap between the two, filled by the cricothyroid ligament, is a useful site for rapid access to the airway if it is obstructed at or above the vocal cords (cricothyroid puncture).

The *clavicle* is a sigmoid-shaped bone with its medial two-thirds rounded and convex forwards and the lateral third flat and concave forwards. It is easily visible in thin people and palpable in all except the morbidly obese. Between the medial expanded ends of the clavicle is the *suprasternal* or *jugular notch*, the inferior border of which is the superior edge of the manubrium sterni. For much of its length the clavicle may be almost encircled by two fingers, but medially its massive ligamentous attachments make definition more difficult. The posterior end of the first rib may sometimes be felt rather indistinctly in the supraclavicular fossa (see examination of supraclavicular fossa p. 1915).

It should be remembered that the head and neck are extremely mobile, but with the head held in the anatomical position, the following vertebral levels should be noted:

C1	Dens, level of nasopharynx
C2	Level of oropharynx and dependent soft palate with the mouth open
C3	Level of body of hyoid and its greater cornu
C3–4 junction	Level of upper border of thyroid cartilage and bifurcation of common carotid artery
C4–5	Level of thyroid cartilage
C6	Level of cricoid cartilage

SOFT TISSUES

From the front and side (**16.**1) the neck is obviously divided into two major portions by sternocleidomastoid. These are the anterior and posterior triangles. Both these triangles can be further subdivided. The anterior cervical triangle may be divided into a submental triangle, a muscular triangle, a carotid triangle and a digastric triangle. The posterior cervical triangle may be split into the occipital triangle and the supraclavicular triangle. The structures which form the boundaries of some of the lesser triangles are not readily palpable or visible. The definitions of these triangles and their contents are described below.

The boundaries of the *anterior cervical triangle* are the midline anteriorly, the base of the mandible and a line from its angle to the mastoid process, at the base of the triangle and sternocleidomastoid as the third edge. Boundaries of the *posterior cervical triangle* are the posterior border of sternocleidomastoid, the middle third of the clavicle's superior surface, which forms the base, and the anterior margin of trapezius. The apex is where sternocleidomastoid and trapezius approximate to each other. The anterior triangle is best

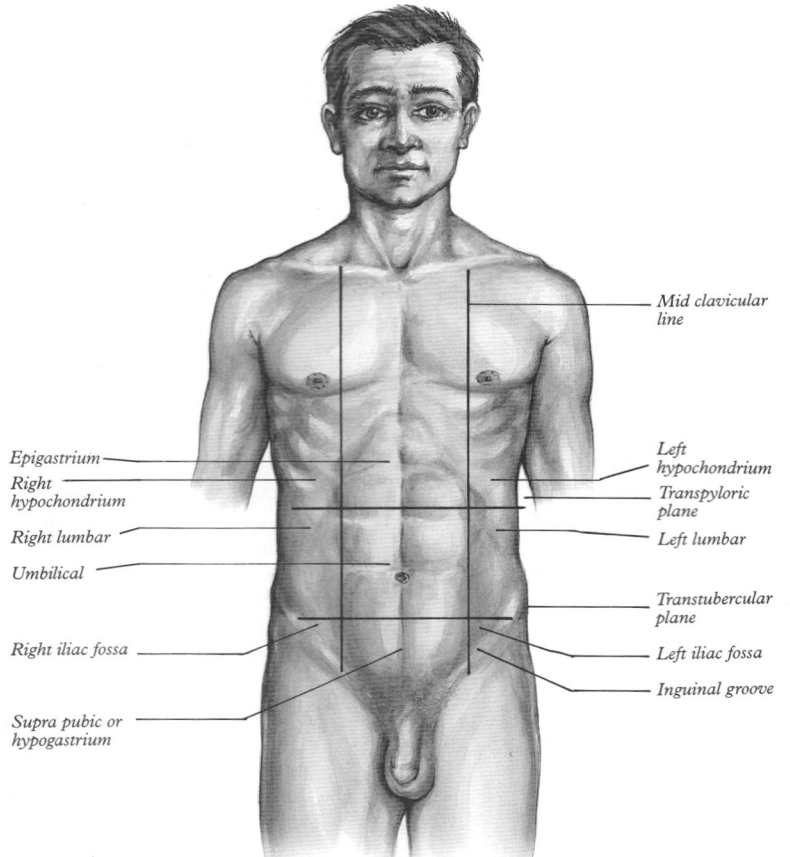

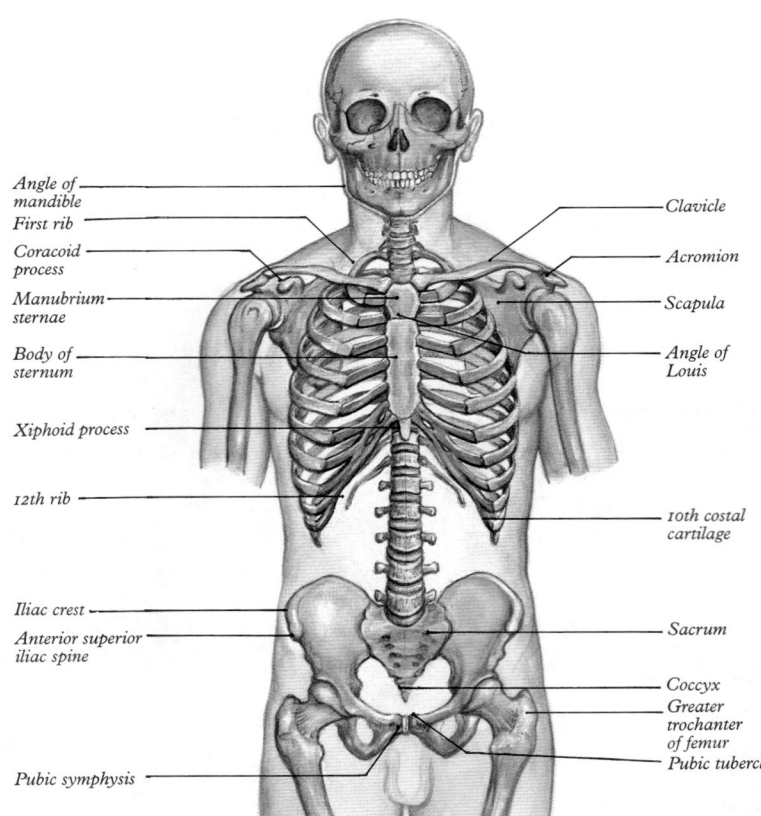

  16.3 Frontal views of trunk to show surface anatomy, bony and soft tissue structures.

inspected from the front, but examined bimanually with the examiner standing behind the subject using the fingers of both hands to examine the structures within that triangle. Inspection reveals the rounded tendinous oblique head of sternocleidomastoid arising from the superolateral angle of the manubrium and the more vertical muscular portion arising from the upper surface of the medial third of the clavicle. There is usually a hollow between these two heads, deep to which lies the *internal jugular vein* just prior to its joining the subclavian vein posterior to the clavicle. The *trachea* can be palpated inferior to the cricoid cartilage and its rings easily felt. It normally lies in the midline but may be deviated by disease. Its upper rings may be impalpable if covered by the thyroid isthmus. If the examining finger is moved laterally the lobes of the *thyroid gland* may be felt, its margins becoming more clear if the patient is asked to swallow.

The *common carotid artery* and its continuation, the *internal carotid artery*, may be represented by a straight line from the sternoclavicular joint (just medial to the internal jugular vein) to the retromandibular fossa. At the level of the upper border of the lamina of the thyroid cartilage (C3–4 junction) the common carotid artery splits into the external and internal carotid arteries. This bifurcation can sometimes be at a higher level. The transverse process of the sixth cervical vertebra is prominent (Chassaignac's tubercle). The carotid artery may be compressed here and above this level it is superficial and its pulsation can be easily felt. This is partly due to the roots of its main branches as much as the internal and external arteries themselves. This is one of the prime sites in the body to feel for a pulse. Running parallel and just lateral to the carotid artery is the *internal jugular vein*. Taken superiorly, the finger enters the submental and submandibular triangles in which enlarged lymph nodes or salivary glands may be felt. It should be noted that the musculature **above** the hyoid bone runs in a predominantly horizontal or oblique direction and **below** it in a vertical direction. Similarly enlarged lymph nodes above the hyoid bone tend to be in a more horizontal plane, being placed mainly just below the pericraniocervical line. The deep cervical nodes run vertically related to the internal jugular vein.

Posterior triangle (16.3)

The boundaries of the *posterior cervical triangle*, as noted above, are the posterior border of sternocleidomastoid, the middle third of the clavicle's superior surface, which forms the base, and the anterior margin of trapezius. The apex is where sternocleidomastoid and trapezius approximate to each other at the nuchal line. The lower portion

of the posterior triangle forms the *supraclavicular fossa*, a very important clinical area, lying as it does just above and behind the clavicle and being at the confluence of the thoracic inlet and the aditus to the axilla and arm. Like the front of the neck, this is again better inspected from in front, but palpated from behind, the right-handed examiner standing behind and to the right of the subject. When inspecting the supraclavicular fossa the pulsation of the great veins may be seen if the central venous pressure is raised. The *external jugular vein*, a prominent feature, may be distended, due to kinking, raised venous pressure or obstruction. In the normal subject it can be demonstrated by *Valsava's manoeuvre* (forced expiration against a closed mouth and blocked nostrils). This is a common site in which to feel pathologically enlarged lymph nodes. In particular, cancers of the upper gastrointestinal tract and of the lung (the most common cancer in men) frequently spread to the supraclavicular group of nodes. The posterior end of the *first rib* may be felt as a fullness in the posterior aspect of this fossa. Anterior to that can be felt the *subclavian artery* pulsating as it crosses the first rib (**16.**3). Above and behind that may be felt the trunks of the *brachial plexus*. A point approximately 2.5 cm above the middle of the medial third of the clavicle marks the level of the neck of the first rib and thus the surface marking for the apex of the dome of the cervical pleura and lung.

The *accessory nerve* can be delineated by a line which passes from the tragus of the ear to the junction of the lower and middle thirds of the anterior border of trapezius. This line will cross the palpable transverse process of the atlas and also the junction of the upper and middle thirds of the posterior border of sternocleidomastoid (**16.**1c).

THORAX

The intrathoracic viscera are enclosed within the rib cage and as a consequence are impalpable. However, unlike some of the intra-abdominal viscera which are very variable in position the intrathoracic organs are remarkably constant. A knowledge of the bony landmarks of the thorax is thus of great value in understanding the positions of the intrathoracic structures.

SKELETAL SURFACE LANDMARKS (16.3)

Anteriorly the *clavicle* and *sternoclavicular joint* are not only palpable but visible in all but the most obese subjects. The *sternum* can be

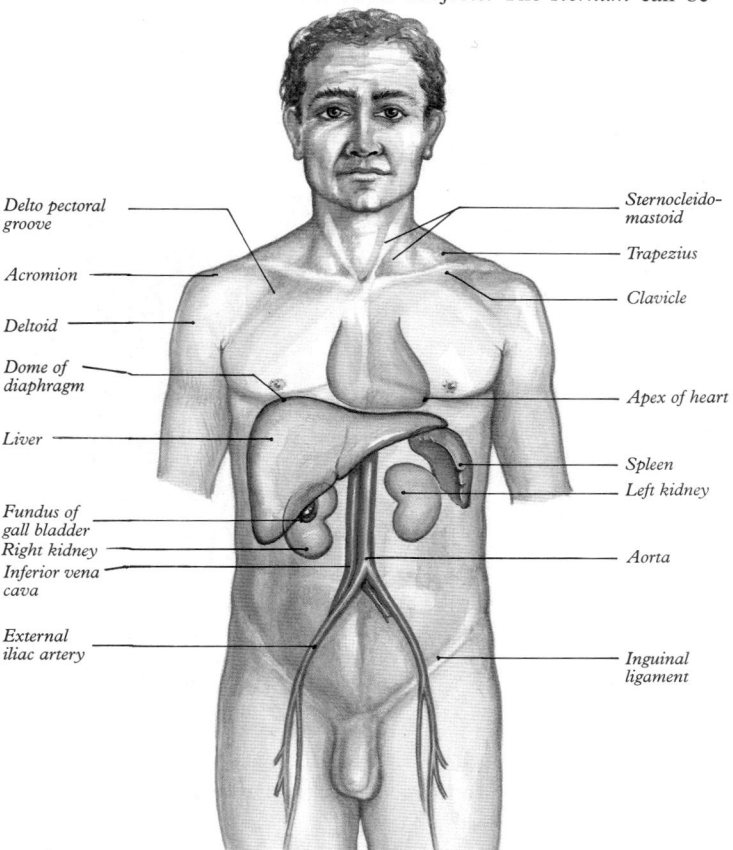

Delto pectoral groove	Sternocleido-mastoid
Deltoid	Trapezius
Pectoralis major	Pectoralis minor
Biceps brachii	Xiphoid process
External oblique	Posterior rectus sheath
Linea semilunaris	Linea alba
Rectus abdominis	Transversus abdominis
	Inguinal groove

Delto pectoral groove — Sternocleido-mastoid
Acromion — Trapezius
Deltoid — Clavicle
Dome of diaphragm — Apex of heart
Liver — Spleen
Fundus of gall bladder — Left kidney
Right kidney — Aorta
Inferior vena cava
External iliac artery — Inguinal ligament

felt throughout its length in the midline but laterally it may be obscured by pectoralis major. The *jugular notch* at the superior end of the sternum is easily found, deep to which may be felt the trachea. The cartilage rings are usually palpable and either by rolling one's finger over the trachea, or by using two fingers within the notch it is possible to assess whether it is in the midline or deviated to one side. The jugular notch lies at the level of the junction between the second and third thoracic vertebrae. The *sternal angle* (angle of Louis), more pronounced in the male than in the female, is felt at the junction of the manubrium with the body of the sternum. This is a particularly useful landmark indicating as it does the medial ends of the second costal cartilages and being level with the junction of the fourth and fifth thoracic vertebrae. At the inferior end of the sternum may be felt the *xiphisternal joint* and *xiphoid process*. This joint usually lies at the level of the ninth thoracic vertebra. Lateral to this may be felt the costal margin, formed here by the anterior ends of the seventh costal cartilages. The rest of the costal margin is formed by the fused anterior ends of the eighth, ninth and tenth costal cartilages, while posteriorly the free ends of the eleventh and twelfth ribs may be palpable. In thin people it is just possible to palpate all the ribs from the first down to the costal margin. Well-developed musculature or the female breast will however obscure the ribs anteriorly and the first rib's shaft which lies predominantly posterior to the clavicle, whereas its ventral end cartilage can only be felt for a very short distance below the clavicle.

Posteriorly (**16**.8) the spinous processes of the thoracic vertebrae are easily palpable and are fully described under surface anatomy of the back (skeletal surface landmarks) page 1921. Lateral to them one can feel the posterior angles of the ribs.

SOFT TISSUES (**16**.3, 9)

The muscles covering the thorax are described appropriately in the sections on the abdomen and upper limb. In a muscular subject pectoralis major, the slips of serratus anterior, latissimus dorsi, trapezius, external oblique and rectus abdominis muscles are all easily visible. The anterior chest wall of females may be largely obscured by the breasts (see p. 1924). In the male the nipple is usually sited in the fourth intercostal space in the midclavicular line. The surface markings of the heart, lungs, pleura and diaphragm are individually covered in the relevant sections elsewhere, but it is appropriate to consider them as a whole here.

SURFACE MARKINGS OF INTRATHORACIC STRUCTURES (**16**.4)

When looking at the chest from the front, the *manubriosternal junction* (the sternal angle or angle of Louis) supplies a very useful fixed point. It is level with the junction of the fourth and fifth thoracic vertebrae, the trachea bifurcates at this level and it also marks the concavity and ends of the aortic arch. The azygos vein enters the superior vena cava at this level also. The costal cartilages of the second ribs meet the sternum here and this makes an accurate starting point when counting ribs. The plane that includes the sternal angle is often called the *transverse thoracic plane*. It demarcates the lower border of the superior mediastinum and the point at which the aortic arch receives the ascending aorta (anteriorly) and becomes the descending aorta (posteriorly). At this point the right and left pleura are in contact with each other and this may be taken as a

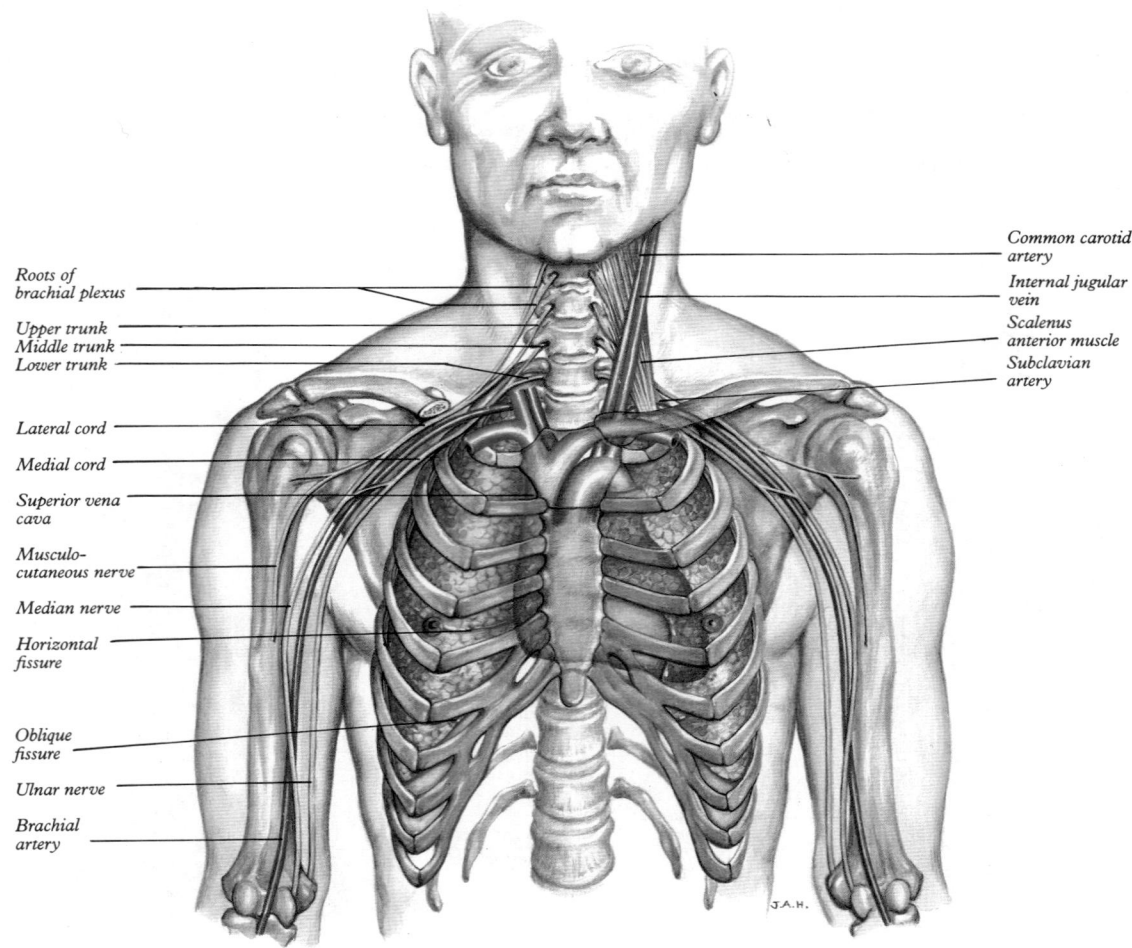

Roots of brachial plexus

Upper trunk
Middle trunk
Lower trunk

Lateral cord

Medial cord

Superior vena cava

Musculo-cutaneous nerve

Median nerve

Horizontal fissure

Oblique fissure

Ulnar nerve

Brachial artery

Common carotid artery

Internal jugular vein

Scalenus anterior muscle

Subclavian artery

J.A.H.

16.4   Anterior view of thorax, root of neck and axilla showing heart, great vessels and brachial plexus.

useful starting point when delineating the *surface markings of the parietal pleura* (**16.5**).

Starting at the manubriosternal junction in the midline, heading superiorly the anterior reflections of the parietal pleura diverge from the midline to extend up and outwards to the *apex of the pleural cavity*. This point lies between 3 and 4 cm above the anterior end of the first rib but level with the posterior end of it. The surface marking of this point lies about 2.5 cm above the centre of the medial third of the clavicle. The parietal pleura is intimately fused with the inner aspect of the thoracic cavity and can be followed laterally and inferiorly down the inner aspect of the chest wall to the level of the tenth rib in the midaxillary line which is its lowest point in that plane. Followed medially, the pleura then covers the diaphragm, the position of which is extremely variable depending as it does on the phase of ventilation. Anteriorly and posteriorly the costo-diaphragmatic reflections of the pleura can then be followed from the midaxillary line towards the midline. Anteriorly on the right the pleura continues to the midline, crossing the eighth rib in the midclavicular line to the xiphisternum whence its surface marking continues to the angle of Louis. Followed medially on the left, the pleura does not reach the midline but instead turns superiorly at the anterior end of the sixth rib approximately 3–5 cm from the midline. This leaves an area between the heart and the sternum which is free of pleura, thus facilitating needle puncture of the heart without the risk of pleural damage. The medial border of the left pleura then ascends to the level of the fourth costal cartilage, where it meets the right pleura in the midline, with which it stays in contact up to the level of the second costal cartilage. It must be remembered that these surface projections only represent the anterior reflections of the pleura. The parietal pleura also covers most of the mediastinal structures, spreading laterally and posteriorly over the heart great vessels and numerous other structures, finally converging to become continuous with the visceral pleura around the root of the lung.

Viewed from the back, the medial edge of the pleura may be followed along a line joining the transverse processes of the thoracic vertebrae from the second to the twelfth. Thence it extends horizontally laterally, crossing the oblique twelfth and eleventh ribs to meet the tenth rib in the midaxillary line. (See also **16.8B**.)

The *visceral pleura* is fused with the surface of the lung. The lung's apical dome and costovertebral border correspond to the parietal pleura. However, in full expiration, the lower border of the lung anteriorly retreats a short distance from the retrosternal costo-mediastinal recess and laterally the lower margin of the lung may rise 5 cm above the parietal pleural reflection (of the costodiaphragmatic recess).

On either side the upper and lower lobes of the lung are separated by the *oblique fissure*. This may be marked by a line running from the posterior end of the third rib downwards and forwards to cross the fifth rib in the midaxillary line and then to the sixth costal cartilage 7–8 cm lateral to the midline. As a convenient approximation the oblique fissure follows the medial border of the scapula when the latter has rotated with the arm in full abduction. The oblique fissure on the left is slightly more vertical than on the right. The *horizontal fissure* between the middle and upper lobes lies at the level of the fourth costal cartilage. It starts from the lung's anterior border, passing posterolaterally to meet the oblique fissure. It should be noted that the upper lobes and the middle lobe lie anterior to the oblique fissure and are best examined from the front of the chest, whereas the lower lobes lie posteriorly and should be examined from the dorsal aspect, i.e. looking at the back of the chest.

The positions of the domes or cupolae of the diaphragm are

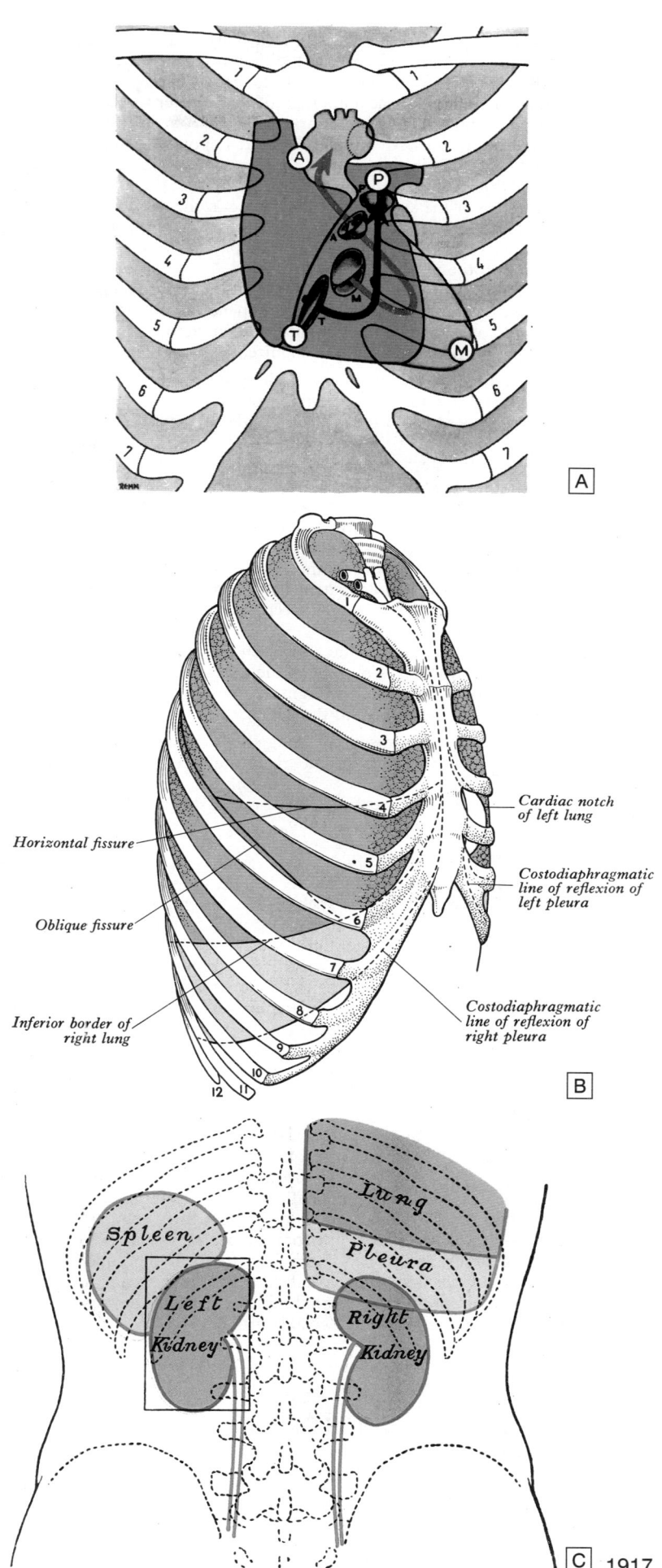

Cardiac notch of left lung

Horizontal fissure

Costodiaphragmatic line of reflexion of left pleura

Oblique fissure

Inferior border of right lung

Costodiaphragmatic line of reflexion of right pleura

Spleen

Lung

Pleura

Left Kidney

Right Kidney

16.5A Diagram illustrating the relation of the sternocostal surface and valves of the heart to the thoracic cage. The right heart is blue, the arrow denoting the inflow and outflow channels of the right ventricle; the left heart is treated similarly in red. The positions, planes and relative sizes of the cardiac valves are shown. The positions of the letters A, P, T and M indicate the aortic, pulmonary, tricuspid and mitral *auscultation* areas of clinical practice.
B   The relation of the pleura and lungs to the chest wall: right lateral aspect. Purple = lungs, covered with the pleural sacs. Blue = pleural sac, with no underlying lung.
C   The lower limits of the lung and pleura: posterior view. The lower portions of the lung and pleura are shown on the right side.

1917

extremely variable, depending both on body build and the phase of ventilation. In short, fat people the diaphragm will be higher than in tall, thin people. Overinflation of the lung as in emphysema causes marked depression of the diaphragm. Usually after forced expiration the right cupola is level anteriorly with the fourth costal cartilage and therefore the right nipple. The left cupola lies approximately one rib lower. With maximal inspiration the cupola will descend as much as 10 cm and on the plain chest radiograph the dome coincides with the tip of the sixth rib. Furthermore in the supine position the diaphragm will be higher than in the erect position and with the body lying on one side the dependent diaphragm will be considerably higher than the uppermost one.

The *borders of the heart* (**16.5**A, 6), although frequently given as being fixed, are in fact variable and depend largely on the position of the diaphragm and the obesity and build of the patient. The following borders are usually recognized:

- The **upper border** forms a gently sloping line from the second left costal cartilage to the third right costal cartilage.
- The **right border** is a gently curved line, convex to the right from the third right to the sixth right costal cartilage, usually 1–2 cm lateral to the sternal edge.
- The **inferior** or **acute border** runs from the sixth right costal cartilage to the apex of the heart. This lies in the fifth left intercostal space approximately in the midclavicular line.
- The **apex beat** is the most inferolateral point at which the cardiac impulse may be seen or felt and is slightly medial to the true apex.
- The **left** ('obtuse') **border** extends superomedially, convex laterally, from the apex to meet the left second costal cartilage about 1 cm from the left sternal edge.
- An oblique line joining the sternal end of the left third and right sixth costal cartilages represents the anterior part of the *coronary sulcus*, which separates the right atrium from the right ventricle (the left atrium lies behind the heart).

The *heart valves* are disposed along this oblique line in sequence. From above downwards to the right are the pulmonary, aortic, mitral and tricuspid valves. For details of the valvular surface projections, their planes and their contrasting areas of optimal clinical auscultation see page 1489.

Great vessels

The *aortic arch* lies predominantly behind the manubrium sternae. Starting at the aortic valve (behind the lower border of third **left** costal cartilage) the ascending aorta curves forwards, upwards and to the right, to become the aortic arch behind the right half of the manubrium at the level of the second **right** costal cartilage. It continues to ascend behind the right side of the manubrium sternae, arching over the transthoracic plane and descending with the aortic knuckle protruding just to the left of the manubrium sternae in the first intercostal space. Within its concavity lies the pulmonary trunk and tracheal bifurcation. The *brachiocephalic artery* arises approximately behind the centre point of the manubrium and ascends to the right sternoclavicular joint. The superior *vena cava* descends predominantly behind, but also just to the right of, the right manubrial border. It enters the right atrium at the level of the third right costal cartilage. The short *right brachiocephalic vein* descends almost vertically from behind the medial end of the clavicle just lateral to the right sternoclavicular junction whereas the long *left brachiocephalic vein* passes almost horizontally behind the superior portion of the manubrium sternae. Both join to form the superior vena cava behind the first right costal cartilage. It descends as a 2-cm wide band along the right sternal margin, reaching the right atrium at the level of the third right costal cartilage.

ABDOMEN

SKELETAL FEATURES OF THE ANTERIOR ABDOMINAL WALL

The surface markings of the boundaries of the anterior abdominal wall are readily defined (**16.3**, 9). Above, centrally, the *xiphoid process*, then the *costal margin* extends from the seventh costal cartilage at the xiphisternal joint to the tip of the twelfth rib, although the latter is often difficult to feel, especially if it is short. The lowest

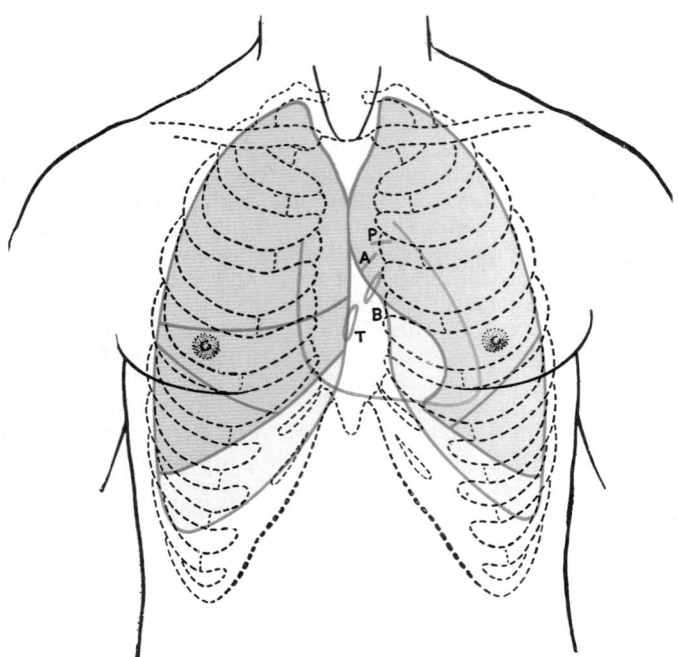

16.6 The front of the thorax, showing the surface relations of the bones, lungs (purple), pleurae (blue) and heart (red outline). A = orifice of aorta; B = left atrioventricular (mitral) orifice; P = orifice of pulmonary trunk; T = right atrioventricular (tricuspid) orifice.

part of the costal margin is in the midaxillary line and is formed by the lower margin of the tenth costal cartilage. The line joining the lower margins of the thoracic cage on each side constitutes the *subcostal plane* which transects the third lumbar vertebral body. The tip of the lower border of the ninth costal cartilage can usually be defined as a distinct 'step' along the costal margin.

The inferior boundary is formed by the *iliac crest*, which descends from its *tubercle* and ends anteriorly at the *anterior superior iliac spine*, from which the *inguinal ligament* runs downwards and forwards to the *pubic tubercle*. This is indicated by the obvious *inguinal groove*, which is readily seen when the thigh is flexed on the abdomen. The *pubic tubercle* is the lateral extremity of the pubic crest, about 2.5 cm from the midline, which itself marks the site of the *pubic symphysis*, the lowermost of the margins of the anterior abdominal wall. The tubercle can be identified by direct palpation in the thin subject but can be detected, even in the obese, by running the fingers along the adductor longus tendon, tensed by flexion, abduction and external rotation of the thigh, to its origin below the tubercle.

ABDOMINAL PLANES (16.3)

For descriptive purposes, the abdomen can be divided by a number of imaginary horizontal and vertical lines. The horizontal lines are also of value in defining approximate vertebral levels and the positions of some relatively fixed intra-abdominal structures.

Vertical planes

There are two vertical planes:

- *The midline* passes from the xiphisternal process to the pubic symphysis.
- *The midclavicular line* (also sometimes called the lateral or the mammary line) passes through the midpoint of the clavicle, crosses the costal margin just lateral to the tip of the ninth costal cartilage and passes through a point midway between the anterior superior iliac spine and the symphysis pubis. In the average sized adult, it is approximately 9 cm from the midline.

Horizontal planes

The horizontal planes are as follows:

- *The xiphisternal plane* traverses the xiphoid at the level of the ninth thoracic vertebra. Varying with body habitus, posture and respiration, this plane demarcates the level of the cardiac plateau on the central part of the upper border of the liver.

- *The transpyloric plane* (of Addison) lies midway between the suprasternal notch of the manubrium and the upper border of the pubic symphysis. No clinician uses this cumbrous measurement but a useful approximation is that it lies midway between the umbilicus and the inferior end of the body of the sternum. More conveniently, it corresponds to the hand's breadth of the subject below the xiphisternal joint.

This plane intersects the body of the first lumbar vertebra near its lower border and meets the costal margins at the tips of the ninth costal cartilages (where usually a distinct 'step' can be felt at the costal margin). This plane corresponds to where the lateral edge of the rectus sheath (the *linea semilunaris*) crosses the costal margin and this can be demonstrated in a thin and muscular subject when the abdominal wall is flexed. This point also marks the position, on the right side, of the fundus of the gallbladder.

Other structures which are demarcated by this plane are:

- the hila of both kidneys
- the origin of the superior mesenteric artery from the aorta
- the termination of the spinal cord
- the neck and adjacent body and head of the pancreas
- the confluence of the superior mesenteric and splenic veins, forming the hepatic portal vein.

Despite the name *transpyloric plane*, which is deeply ingrained in both clinical and anatomical literature, the pylorus is **not** constantly transected by the plane. To account for the name, however, it is frequently so transected in the fixed cadaver of classical anatomy, and also in some normal subjects, when the stomach is empty, and the person lying supine. There is, however, much variation between subjects of different body type, with their degree of gastric filling, and posture. The pylorus descends some one to three vertebral levels below this plane in the erect position and when the stomach is full.

- *The subcostal plane* joins the lower margins of the thoracic cage, formed by the tenth costal cartilage on each side. It transects the body of the third lumbar vertebra. It also indicates the level of origin of the inferior mesenteric artery from the aorta, and the horizontal (third) part of the duodenum, although the latter varies with posture.

- *The supracristal plane* joins the highest point of the iliac crest on each side. It passes through the body of the fourth lumbar vertebra, marks the level of bifurcation of the abdominal aorta, and dorsally is used in clinical practice as a landmark in performing a lumbar puncture. If this procedure is carried out distal to this level, puncture will take place through either the L4–L5 or L5–S1 intervertebral level, safely below the termination of the spinal cord.

- *The transtubercular plane* corresponds to a line joining the tubercles of the iliac crests. It passes through the fifth lumbar vertebral body near its upper border. It indicates, or is just above, the confluence of the common iliac veins and marks the origin of the inferior vena cava.

- *The interspinous plane* includes the line joining the centres of the anterior superior spines of the iliac crests. It passes through either the lumbosacral disc, the sacral promontory, or just below, depending on the degree of lumbar lordosis, sacral inclination and curvature.

- *The plane of the pubic crest* passes through the inferior end of the sacrum or part of the coccyx, again, depending on the degree of lumbar lordosis, sacral inclination and curvature.

ABDOMINAL REGIONS (16.3)

The abdomen can be divided into nine regions by two horizontal and two parasagittal planes projected on to the surface of the body. These regions are used in practice for descriptive localization of the position of a mass or the localization of a patient's pain. They may also be used in the description of the location of the abdominal viscera.

The two vertical lines are the midclavicular lines on either side. Classically, the two horizontal lines are the transpyloric and the transtubercular planes. In practice, it is common to use two horizontal lines found by dividing the distance from the xiphisternal joint to the symphysis pubis into thirds. The nine regions thus formed are:

- the epigastrium
- the right and left hypochondrium
- the umbilical region
- the right and left lumbar region
- the hypogastrium (or suprapubic region)
- the right and left iliac fossa.

SURFACE FEATURES OF THE ANTERIOR ABDOMINAL WALL (16.3)

Umbilicus. This is an obvious but inconstantly placed landmark. In the recumbent normal adult it lies at the level of the disc between the third and fourth lumbar vertebrae, so that the aorta bifurcates about 2 cm distal to it. In the erect position, in the child and in subjects with a pendulous abdomen, the umbilicus is at a lower level.

Linea alba. The median groove can readily be seen in the thin muscular subject when the abdominal muscles are tensed by flexing the trunk. It is wide and obvious above the umbilicus but is almost linear and invisible below this level. Divarication of the recti, a common condition in which the upper abdominal viscera bulge through the widened linea alba on standing or straining, is thus always situated above the umbilicus.

Linea semilunaris. Demarcating the lateral margin of the rectus sheath, it is visible as a shallow curved groove in the muscular subject when the abdominal muscles are tensed, for example, by sitting up from the lying position. Inferiorly, it rises from the pubic tubercle, then passes upwards and outwards to reach the costal margin at the level of the tip of the ninth costal cartilage, which forms a distinct 'step' on the costal margin. On the right side, this marks the usual position of the fundus of the gallbladder.

Rectus abdominis. Forming a swelling defined medially by the linea alba and laterally by the linea semilunaris, it extends from the pubis to the horizontal line from the xiphoid to the fifth costal cartilage. In a thin and muscular subject, the tendinous intersections may be visible when the muscle is tensed by lifting the head against resistance or by sitting up. These intersections are situated at the level of the umbilicus, the level of the xiphoid and midway between these two points.

Midinguinal, or femoral, point (16.7). The midpoint between the symphysis pubis and the anterior superior iliac spine, it marks the

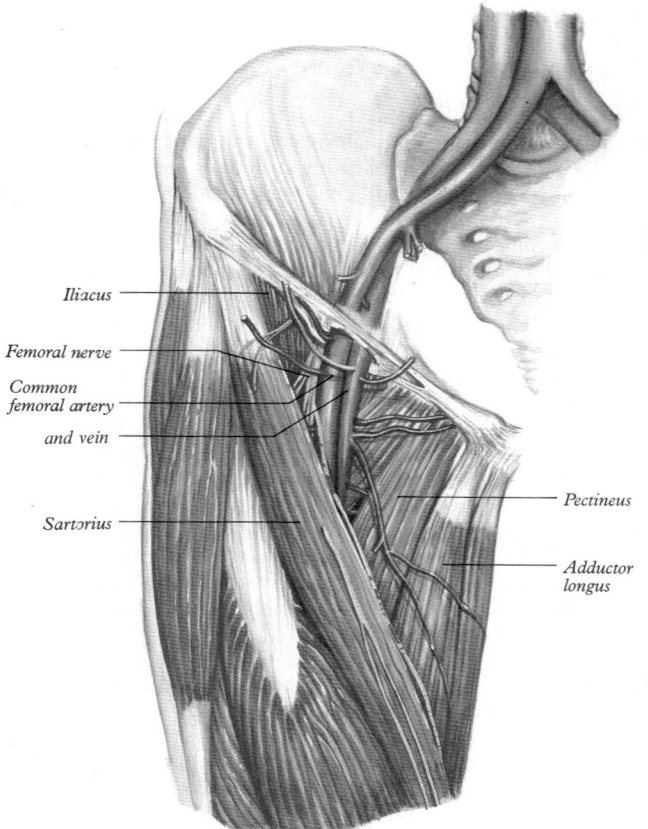

Iliacus

Femoral nerve

Common femoral artery

and vein

Sartorius

Pectineus

Adductor longus

16.7 Right inguinal region.

position of the femoral pulse, which is detected immediately inferior to it. This point also indicates the continuation of the external iliac artery into the femoral artery, marks the position of the deep inguinal ring, which lies immediately superior to it, and it lies just inferior to the origin of the inferior epigastric and the deep circumflex iliac arteries as these arise from the external iliac artery.

Vas deferens. Palpable in the male within the spermatic cord at the neck of the scrotum, it can be rolled between the finger and thumb and has the consistency of plastic tubing. Traced upwards, the vas is felt to pass medial to the pubic tubercle, where the *external inguinal ring* can be felt by invaginating the scrotal skin with the index finger.

SURFACE ANATOMY OF THE INTRA-ABDOMINAL AND RETROPERITONEAL VISCERA

In classical anatomy, much emphasis was placed on the surface anatomy of the abdominal viscera, with specific definition of the outlines upon the abdominal wall of the stomach, duodenum, intestine, etc. The introduction of radiological imaging of the abdominal viscera demonstrated considerable variation in what was believed to be 'normal' anatomy. Indeed, for a time a whole new pathology was introduced in which various organs were sutured back into place from what was considered their inappropriate positions. Such terms as 'ptosis of the kidney', 'gastroptosis', or, indeed, 'visceroptosis' (ptosis of all the abdominal organs) were introduced. Fortunately these 'pathologies' and their treatment are now consigned to the history books.

We now realize that most of the intraperitoneal structures are highly mobile within the abdominal cavity so that, for example, it is sufficient to state that the caecum and appendix are normally situated in the right iliac fossa.

Palpable organs

In normal subjects, the pulsations of the abdominal aorta are palpable (see below). In addition, the lower border of the normal liver may rarely be felt below the right costal margin and in the epigastrium. The lower pole of the normal right kidney may sometimes be felt on bimanual palpation during deep inspiration, especially in many thin women, where also it is not rare to palpate a gurgling soft caecum in the lower right abdomen. The sigmoid colon may sometimes be felt in normal thin subjects as a sausage-shaped swelling in the left iliac fossa and this is particularly so if it is loaded with faeces.

Surface markings (16.3)

Although the mobile abdominal viscera are inconstant in position, the surface markings of the following structures are of clinical value.

Liver. The inferior border of the liver extends along a line which passes from the right tenth costal cartilage to the left fifth rib at the midclavicular line. The upper border of the liver follows a line which passes from the fifth rib at the midclavicular line on the right to the equivalent point on the left. This upper border curves slightly downwards at its centre and crosses the midline behind the xiphoid. The right border of the liver is curved to the right and joins the upper and lower right limits. The liver outline may be defined by the dull note it gives on percussion compared with the resonance of the lungs superiorly and of the hollow abdominal viscera below.

The lower edge of the normal liver cannot usually be palpated, even in women and children, in whom the liver is at a slightly lower level. What is often mistaken for the liver in abdominal palpation is the bulge of rectus abdominis above its upper tendinous intersection.

Fundus of the gallbladder. This projects below the lower border of the liver at the point where the linea semilunaris crosses the tip of the ninth costal cartilage in the transpyloric plane. The ninth costal cartilage can usually be identified as a distinct 'step' along the costal margin.

Spleen. Underlying the ninth, tenth and eleventh ribs on the left side, its size corresponds to the cupped hand of the subject. Its surface markings can be delineated on the lower posterior thoracic wall by defining its axis. This extends from a point 5 cm to the left of the midline at the level of the tenth thoracic spine laterally along the line of the tenth rib to the midaxillary line.

Pancreas. The neck of the pancreas lies in the transpyloric plane in the midline. From this, the body can be imagined passing obliquely upwards and to the left for about 10 cm, and the head downwards and to the right to lie in the curve of the duodenum.

Kidneys. The lower pole of the normal right kidney may occasionally be felt in the thin subject, especially the female, by bimanual palpation on full inspiration. Anteriorly the hilum of the kidney lies approximately on the transpyloric plane 5 cm from the midline, the right kidney being lower than the left. Posteriorly, the upper pole of the kidney lies deep to the twelfth rib. The right kidney normally extends about 2 cm lower than the left. Using these landmarks, the kidney outlines can be projected on to either the anterior or posterior aspects of the abdomen.

Abdominal aorta. This commences just to the left of the midline at the level of the body of the twelfth thoracic vertebra. It continues downwards for 10 cm to bifurcate at the level of the fourth lumbar vertebra, marked by the supracristal plane 1.5 cm below and to the left of the umbilicus. The pulsations of the aorta can be readily felt in the normal subject by pressing firmly in the midline backwards onto the vertebral column in the recumbent position.

Coeliac trunk. This arises from the aorta immediately after it enters the abdomen at the level of T12, the *superior mesenteric artery* originates at the transpyloric plane, and the *inferior mesenteric artery* commences at the level of L3, which lies at the level of the subcostal plane.

Inferior vena cava. Commencing at the level of fifth lumbar vertebra, this is demarcated by the transtubercular plane, between the tubercles of the iliac crest. This may not be easy to define so the level may be delineated as lying 2.5 cm below the supracristal plane (see p. 1919). From this level it can be represented by a band, 2.5 cm to the right of the midline. The inferior vena cava leaves the abdomen by traversing the diaphragm at the level of the eighth thoracic vertebra, directly behind the sternal extremity of the right sixth costal cartilage.

Ureter. This commences on either side approximately at the transpyloric plane (the left higher than the right), about 5 cm from the midline. Each passes downwards and somewhat medially to enter the bladder at a point marked superficially by the position of the pubic tubercle.

PERINEUM

SKELETAL SURFACE LANDMARKS

The perineum is a diamond-shaped area which is bounded anteriorly by the pubic symphysis, posteriorly by the coccyx and laterally by the ischial tuberosities. An imaginary line joining the ischial tuberosities divides the perineum into an anterior *urogenital triangle*, which faces downwards and forwards, some 45° to the horizontal, and a posterior *anal triangle*, which faces downwards and backwards, also at some 45° to the horizontal.

The tip of the *coccyx* can be felt deeply near the centre of the natal cleft. As the examining finger passes cranially, the *sacral cornua* can be felt on either side and demarcate the *sacral hiatus*. They form the landmark which enables a needle to be introduced obliquely into the sacral canal via puncture of the posterior sacrococcygeal ligament in performing a caudal anaesthetic block.

The whole outline of the *pubic arch* can be felt through the skin from the *pubic symphysis* to the *ischial tuberosity*. Posteriorly, on each side, the edge of the *sacrotuberous ligament* can be felt on deep pressure under the medial margin of the lower border of gluteus maximus (see p. 1930).

SOFT TISSUES

Anal triangle

In the anal triangle, the *anal orifice* faces downwards and posteriorly and lies in the median plane about 4 cm below and in front of the tip of the coccyx. The skin around the anus is thrown into a series of converging folds, which continue upwards into the lower part of the anal canal.

Rectal examination

A finger inserted through the anal orifice enters the *anal canal*, which passes upwards and forwards for about 2.5 cm and then bends sharply backwards into the rectum. The finger is first grasped by the anal sphincters and then passes into the patulous *rectal ampulla*. If the examining finger is now flexed it will rest on the ledge of the *anorectal junction* (the anorectal ring) which marks the upper extent of the anal sphincter and its attachment to levator ani. Anteriorly in the male, the finger palpates the *bulb of the penis* and the *membranous part of urethra* and then, about 4 cm above the anal orifice, can be palpated the *prostate*. This is felt as a slight smooth bulge with a smooth vertically placed median *sulcus*. The *seminal vesicles* can only be felt above the prostate if greatly enlarged, as may the *bladder* if distended with urine.

In the female, the *cervix* and part of the *body of the uterus* are felt anteriorly.

Posteriorly, the pelvic surface of the lower part of the *sacrum* and the *coccyx* are readily palpable. Laterally lie the *ischial tuberosities* and *spines* and the *ischiorectal fossae* on each side.

Urogenital triangle

The *bulb of the penis* occupies the midline of the male urogenital triangle. A median ridge, which indicates the position of the scrotal raphe, extends forwards from the anus, over the scrotum to the penis. The skin covering the scrotum is rough and corrugated and contains numerous sebaceous glands. In contrast, the skin over the penis is smooth, thin and hairless. Within the scrotal sac on either side can be palpated the *testis*, which is ellipsoid in shape and rubbery in consistency. Along the posterior border of each can be identified the curved *epididymis*

The female urogenital triangle is demarcated anteriorly by the *mons pubis* which overlies the anterior part of the pubic symphysis. Backwards from the mons pass the *labia majora* (**8.217**) which extend posteriorly to join at the *posterior commissure*. The space between the posterior commissure and the anterior margin of the anus overlies the *perineal body*. The space between the labia majora is the *pudendal cleft*. Within the pudendal cleft is a fold of skin on each side, which together form the *labia minora*. Each bifurcates anteriorly to join its partner on either side of the clitoris. Anteriorly, this union forms the *prepuce* of the clitoris, while posteriorly the union forms the *frenulum*. The *vestibule* is the area enclosed between the labia minora. The *clitoris* lies partially hidden between the anterior ends of the labia minora; 2.5 cm posterior to the clitoris opens the urethra as a longitudinal slit with somewhat elevated edges. The *vaginal orifice* lies in the posterior part of the vestibule. At the orifice is situated a thin fold of mucous membrane, the *hymen vaginae*. This varies much in shape. When stretched, its commonest form is that of a ring, generally broadest posteriorly. Sometimes it is represented by a semilunar fold, with its concave margin anteriorly. Occasionally it is cribriform or its free margin forms a membranous fringe. It may be entirely absent or, rarely, may form a complete septum across the lower end of the vagina (imperforate hymen). When the hymen has been ruptured, small rounded elevations, the *carunculae hymenales*, are found at its entrance. Immediately lateral to the hymen in the vestibule are the orifices of the *greater vestibular glands* (Bartholin's glands), on either side.

Vaginal examination

At the upper extremity of the vagina, the examining finger comes into contact with the vaginal portion of the *cervix uteri* and the lips of the *external os* can be palpated. In front of the cervix, the finger passes into the *anterior vaginal fornix* through which the base of the bladder may be examined. Posterior to the cervix, the finger passes into the posterior vaginal fornix, through which the contents of the *recto-uterine pouch* can be felt. If the opposite hand is placed on the lower part of the abdominal wall and firm pressure exerted, the whole of the cervix and body of the uterus can be examined between the two hands (bimanual palpation). Bimanual examination through the lateral fornices also allows assessment of the ovaries, uterine tubes and the broad ligaments.

BACK

SKELETAL SURFACE LANDMARKS (16.8)

Posteriorly in the midline a *median furrow* runs from the *external occipital protuberance* above to the *natal cleft* below. The external occipital protuberance is subcutaneous and can be felt and often seen; it can be recognized without difficulty when it is approached from below. The *inion* is the point situated on this protuberance in

the median plane. At the back of the neck, the tips of the spines of the cervical vertebrae are obscured by the overlying *ligamentum nuchae*. The tubercle on the posterior arch of the atlas is impalpable; the first bony prominence which is encountered when the finger is drawn downwards in the midline from the external occipital protuberance is the *spine of the second cervical vertebra*, which can be felt on deep palpation inferior to this landmark. The ligamentum nuchae terminates inferiorly at the spine of the *seventh cervical vertebra*. This can be seen and be identified as the highest, and sometimes the only, visible projection in this region (*vertebra prominens*). Immediately below this can be felt the spine of the first thoracic vertebra, which, in fact, is usually more prominent than the seventh cervical. The spine of the second thoracic vertebra can also often be felt but the identification of the remaining thoracic spines is not easy, even in a thin subject when the trunk is fully flexed, owing to the manner in which they overlap one another in the midthoracic region. The third thoracic spine lies opposite the root of the spine of the scapula and the seventh lies opposite the inferior angle of the scapula when the arm is by the side. The twelfth thoracic spine lies opposite the midpoint of a vertical line drawn from the inferior angle of the scapula to the iliac crest.

In the upper and lower thoracic regions, the tips of the thoracic spines lie opposite the upper part of the body of the immediately subjacent vertebra. In the midthoracic region, they lie opposite the lower part of the vertebra below. The tip of the spine of each lumbar vertebra can usually be palpated without difficulty, especially in the flexed position of the trunk. Each lies opposite the inferior part of its own body.

At the lower part of the back, the *iliac crest* can be palpated throughout its whole length, and can be traced backwards and upwards from the anterior superior spine (see p. 1918) to its highest point and then downwards and medially to the *posterior superior iliac spine*, which lies 5 cm from the median plane. This corresponds to the position of the obvious *sacral dimple*, which lies above and medial to the buttock. A line joining these dimples passes through the *second sacral spine*. The posterior superior spine lies over the centre of the *sacro-iliac joint*.

SPINAL CORD AND ITS COVERINGS (16.8)

The surface relationships of the spinal cord and its coverings are of obvious clinical importance.

The relations of the cord to the vertebral column differ greatly in fetal, infant and adult life. Up to the third fetal month, the cord extends the length of the vertebral canal. As a result of more rapid differential growth of the vertebrae compared with the cord, at birth the spinal cord terminates at the lower border of the third lumbar vertebra and in the adult, on an average, at the level of the disc between the first and second lumbar vertebral bodies. There is a considerable variation in this level; frequently the cord ends opposite either the body of the first or of the second lumbar vertebra; rarely the twelfth thoracic or even the third lumbar vertebra. This is discussed by Reimann and Anson (1944) who reviewed 801 cases.

This differential growth results in the lumbar and sacral nerve roots becoming considerably elongated to reach their corresponding intervertebral foramina, thus forming the cauda equina. In contrast, the upper thoracic roots incline but little, and the cervical roots pass almost laterally in their intraspinal course. As a rough guide, allow one segment difference in the cervical cord between the cord segment and vertebral body level, two in the upper thoracic, three in the lower thoracic and four to five in the lumbar and sacral cord (see Table **16**.1).

Table 16.1 Approximate vertebral levels of the cord segments	
Segment of cord	**Vertebral body**
Cervical 8	Cervical 7
Thoracic 6	Thoracic 4
Thoracic 12	Thoracic 9
Lumbar 5	Thoracic 12
Sacral and coccygeal segments	Lumbar 1

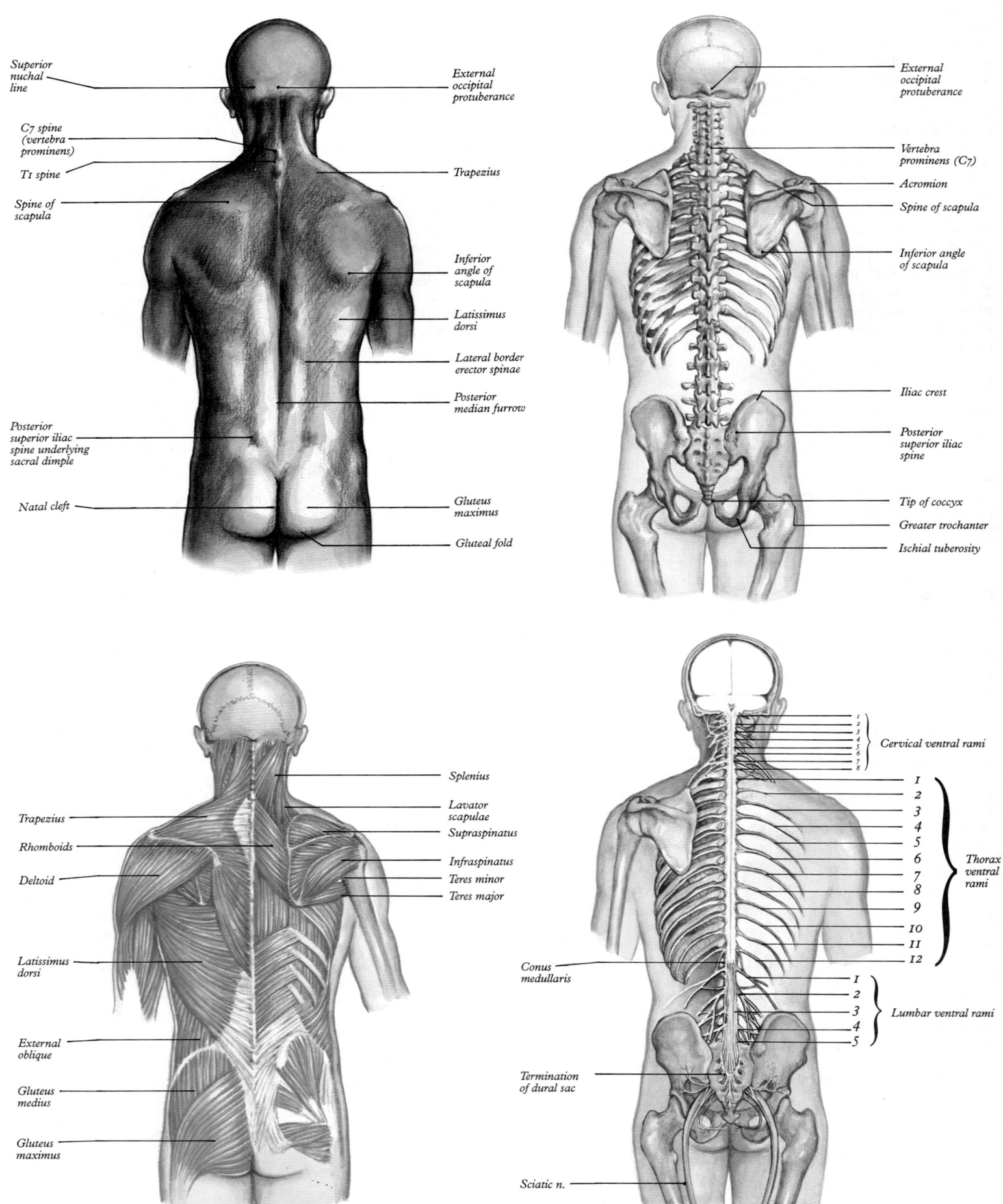

Superior nuchal line

External occipital protuberance

C7 spine (vertebra prominens)

T1 spine

Spine of scapula

Trapezius

Inferior angle of scapula

Latissimus dorsi

Lateral border erector spinae

Posterior median furrow

Posterior superior iliac spine underlying sacral dimple

Natal cleft

Gluteus maximus

Gluteal fold

External occipital protuberance

Vertebra prominens (C7)

Acromion

Spine of scapula

Inferior angle of scapula

Iliac crest

Posterior superior iliac spine

Tip of coccyx

Greater trochanter

Ischial tuberosity

Splenius

Lavator scapulae

Supraspinatus

Infraspinatus

Teres minor

Teres major

Trapezius

Rhomboids

Deltoid

Latissimus dorsi

External oblique

Gluteus medius

Gluteus maximus

Cervical ventral rami

Thorax ventral rami

Lumbar ventral rami

Conus medullaris

Termination of dural sac

Sciatic n.

16.8 Posterior aspect of trunk to show surface anatomy, bony and soft tissue structures including disposition of spinal cord and nerves.

The lower limit of the spinal cord, at the interspace between the first and second lumbar vertebral bodies, lies a little above the level of the elbow joint when the arm is by the side. Anteriorly, it is also approximately demarcated by the transpyloric plane (see p. 1919).

The dural sac and its contained subarachnoid space usually extends to the level of the second segment of the sacrum. This corresponds to the line joining the obvious sacral dimples located in the skin over the posterior superior iliac spines (see p. 1921). Occasionally, the dural sac ends as high as the fifth lumbar vertebra and other times may extend to the third piece of the sacrum. As a result of this, it is occasionally possible to perform an inadvertent spinal tap during the course of a sacral nerve block.

SOFT TISSUES (16.8, 9)

Along the midline of the back can be observed the *median furrow* which runs from the external occipital protuberance to the natal cleft. This is most shallow in the lower cervical region and is deepest in the midlumbar zone. Inferiorly, it widens out into a flattened, triangular area, the apex of which lies at the commencement of the *natal cleft* and corresponds to the third sacral spine. A finger running along the median furrow reveals the sagittal curves of the spine; the cervical curve is convexed forwards and extends from the first cervical to the second thoracic vertebra. The thoracic curvature is concaved forwards and extends from the second to the twelfth thoracic vertebra. The lumbar curvature is convexed forwards and extends from the twelfth thoracic vertebra to the lumbosacral prominence.

On each side, the median furrow is bounded by a broad elevation produced by the *sacrospinalis muscle group*, which extends for about one hand's breadth on either side of the midline between the iliac crest and the twelfth rib. The lateral border of this elevation then crosses the ribs at their angles, passing medially as it ascends. The muscle can be demonstrated by extending the back against resistance.

Trapezius is a flat, triangular muscle which covers the back of the neck and shoulder. The two trapezius muscles together resemble a trapezium or quadrangle; two angles corresponding to the shoulders, a third to the occipital protuberance and the fourth to the spine of the twelfth thoracic vertebra. The two muscles cover the back of the neck and shoulders like a monk's cowl, hence the ancient name of the trapezius of musculus cucullaris. The trapezius is demonstrated by getting the subject to shrug the shoulders against resistance. When the shoulder is fixed, the trapezius draws the head backwards and laterally and can again be demonstrated when this action is made against resistance. The anterior border of the muscle forms the posterior boundary of the posterior triangle of the neck and can be seen in muscular subjects, especially when resistance is opposed to elevation of the shoulder.

Splenius capitis is the muscle which forms the floor of the apex of the posterior triangle of the neck. It becomes obvious lateral to the cervical attachment of trapezius when the neck is extended against resistance.

UPPER LIMB

SHOULDER AND AXILLA

Skeletal surface landmarks (16.3, 8)

The *clavicle* is both visible and palpable throughout its course. Its outline can be traced from the expanded sternal end, which forms the lateral boundary of the suprasternal notch, to its flattened acromial extremity. The line of the *acromioclavicular joint* may be palpable in an anteroposterior plane.

The *acromion* can be traced from the acromioclavicular joint to its tip, and then backwards across the top of the shoulder until it meets the crest of the spine of the scapula at the prominent *acromial*

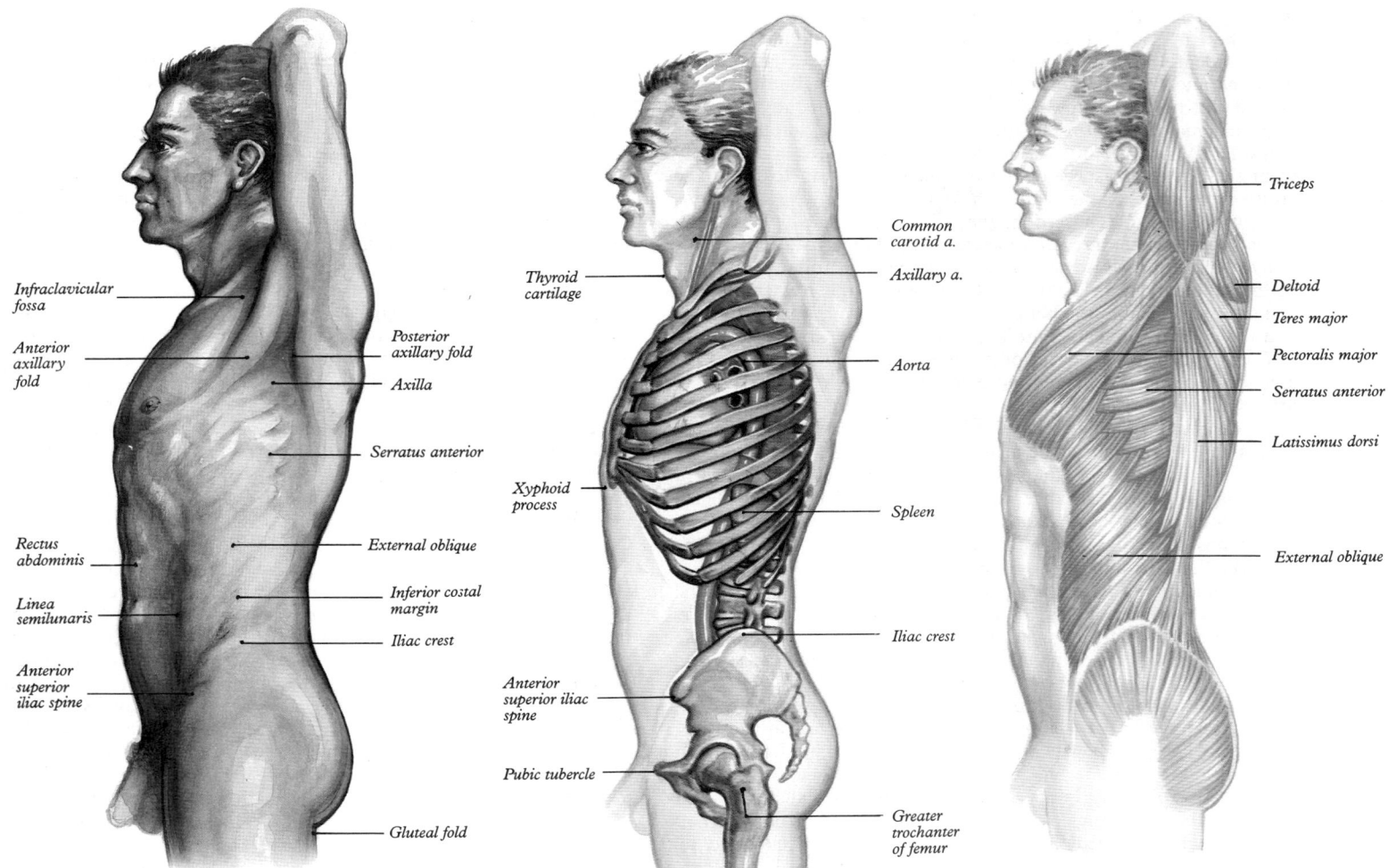

16.9 Lateral views of trunk to show surface anatomy, bony and soft tissue structures.

angle. From this angle, the crest of the *spine of the scapula* can be palpated as it passes medially to reach the medial (vertebral) border of the scapula, which lies opposite the spine of the third thoracic vertebra. The spine is subcutaneous and is easily visible in a thin subject.

The *medial border* of the scapula is hidden in its upper part by the overlying trapezius muscle, but below the spine it can be palpated as it passes downwards to the *inferior angle*. Although this is covered by the teres major and latissimus dorsi, the inferior angle can easily be felt when it is approached from inferiorly and it can be seen to move laterally and forwards around the chest wall when the arm is raised above the head.

The inferior angle of the scapula is at the level of the spine of the seventh thoracic vertebra and overlies the seventh rib. In performing a thoracotomy, it is therefore a convenient landmark from which the ribs can be counted along the lateral chest wall.

A small depression can be seen inferior to the clavicle at the junction of its medial convex and lateral concave portions. This is the *infraclavicular fossa* (or deltopectoral triangle) and it intervenes between the surface elevations produced by the clavicular origins of pectoralis major and the deltoid. The apex of the *coracoid process* lies 2.5 cm below the clavicle immediately to the lateral side of this fossa under cover of the anterior fibres of the deltoid. If the examining finger passes laterally from the coracoid process, the *lesser tubercle of the humerus* will be felt below the tip of the acromion on deep pressure through the deltoid. This bony prominence slips away from the examining finger when the humerus is rotated laterally or medially. The *greater tubercle* of the humerus is the most lateral bony point in the shoulder region and projects laterally below and in front of the acromial angle. It can also be felt to move on rotation of the humerus. With the arm abducted, the *head of the humerus* can be palpated on deep pressure in the apex of the axilla.

Soft tissues (16.3, 8, 9)

The rounded contour of the shoulder is produced by the bulky *deltoid muscle*, the limits of which can be determined accurately when the arm is abducted against resistance. The tendon of insertion can be identified about half way down the lateral aspect of the humerus and from its anterior aspect, the anterior border of the deltoid can be traced upwards and medially, across the tendon of pectoralis major, to form the lateral boundary of the infraclavicular fossa. The posterior border of the deltoid runs upwards and medially from the posterior aspect of the tendon of insertion to reach the crest of the spine of the scapula near its medial end. As it passes from its origin to its insertion, the deltoid is spread out over the lateral aspect of the greater tubercle of the humerus and it is this bony relationship which accounts for the normal rounded contour of the shoulder. In dislocation of the shoulder, the greater tubercle is displaced medially, the deltoid descends vertically to its insertion and the normal rounded contour of the shoulder is lost.

The rounded lower border of *pectoralis major* forms the anterior axillary fold and is rendered more conspicuous when the abducted arm is adducted against resistance. This can be done by placing the hand on the hip and pressing firmly against the trunk. When the arm is flexed to a right angle against resistance, the clavicular head of the muscle can be felt and seen to contract. When the flexed arm is extended against resistance, the clavicular head becomes relaxed but the sternocostal head stands out in relief.

The posterior fold of the axilla reaches a lower level on the humerus than the anterior fold and is produced by *latissimus dorsi* and the underlying *teres major*. Both take part in adduction of the arm and the posterior fold of the axilla is accentuated when the abducted arm is adducted against resistance. When this is done, the lateral border of latissimus dorsi can be traced downwards to its attachment to the iliac crest.

When the arm is raised above the head, the lower five or six serrations of *serratus anterior* can be seen on the lateral aspect of the chest; they pass downwards and forwards to interdigitate with the serrations of the external oblique muscle. When serratus anterior is paralysed following injury to its nerve, the medial border and especially the lower angle of the scapula stands out prominently to give a peculiar 'winged' appearance. This can be accentuated by asking the patient to press both hands against the wall.

The pulsations of the lower part of the *axillary artery* can be felt by pressing against the upper shaft of the humerus just anterior to the posterior axillary fold. In this situation, the median nerve can be felt on deep pressure and this will produce a tingling sensation in the palm of the hand.

The *cephalic vein* lies in the deltopectoral groove between deltoid and pectoralis major then ascends to the infraclavicular fossa, where it pierces the clavipectoral fascia to enter the axillary vein.

The *nipple* in the male overlies the fourth intercostal space, some 10 cm from the midline. In the female, especially when the breast is pendulous, it is found at a lower level. The *mammary gland* in the female extends vertically from the second to the sixth rib and transversely from the side of the sternum to near the midaxillary line at the level of the fourth costal cartilage. Superolaterally, the breast projects as the *axillary tail* to a variable extent as far as the axillary vessels under cover of pectoralis major.

ARM AND ELBOW

Skeletal surface landmarks (16.10, 11)

The *shaft of the humerus* can only be felt indistinctly through its course as its outline is obscured by its covering muscles. Distally, the *medial epicondyle* of the humerus is a conspicuous landmark and is easily felt, particularly when the elbow is flexed; proximally it can be traced as it continues upwards as the *medial supracondylar ridge*. The *ulnar nerve* can be rolled from side to side posterior to the base of the epicondyle. The *lateral epicondyle* is not so prominent but its posterior surface is easily palpated and its lateral margin can be traced upwards into the *lateral supracondylar ridge* on deep pressure. Inspection of the posterior aspect of the extended elbow reveals a well-marked depression to the lateral side of the midline. This is bounded laterally by the fleshy elevation formed by the superficial group of forearm extensor muscles and medially by the lateral side of the *olecranon*. The floor of this depression contains, in its upper part, the posterior surface of the lateral epicondyle and, in its lower part, the *head of the radius*. Although this is covered by the annular ligament, it can be felt to rotate when the forearm is pronated and supinated. Between the lateral epicondyle and the radial head, the *humeroradial part of the elbow joint* can be felt as a distinct transverse depression.

When the elbow is extended, the apex of the olecranon can be felt and forms a line level with the two epicondyles. When the elbow is flexed, the apex of the olecranon descends and the three bony points then form the angles of a triangle. This relationship is lost in dislocation of the elbow. The posterior surface of the olecranon is subcutaneous and tapers from above downwards. It can be felt with ease immediately below the apex.

The level of the *elbow joint* is situated 2 cm below the line joining the two epicondyles. It slopes downwards and medially from its lateral extremity and this obliquity produces the 'carrying angle'. With full extension at the elbow, and the forearm and hand in supination ('the anatomical position'), this is about 165° in the female and 175° in the male. This angle disappears on full flexion of the elbow when the shafts of the ulna and humerus come to lie in the same plane. The angle is also obscured in full pronation of the forearm.

Soft tissues (16.10)

On the anterior aspect of the arm, the *biceps* is a conspicuous elevation, diminishing above, where it is covered by pectoralis major, and below, where it gives place to its tendon just above the elbow joint. Shallow furrows indicate its medial and lateral borders. When the elbow is flexed against resistance, the muscle becomes still more obvious and its tendon of insertion can be held between the finger and thumb and traced down into the cubital fossa. With the arm held in this position, the sharp upper margin of the *bicipital aponeurosis* can easily be traced downwards and medially over the elevation produced by the superficial group of forearm flexor muscles. The aponeurosis is crossed by the *median cubital vein*, which runs medially and proximally from the cephalic vein to join the basilic vein. It is distended into prominence by applying gentle constriction to the upper arm.

Emerging from the lateral wall of the axilla and forming a rounded ridge on the upper part of the medial side of the biceps is *coracobrachialis*.

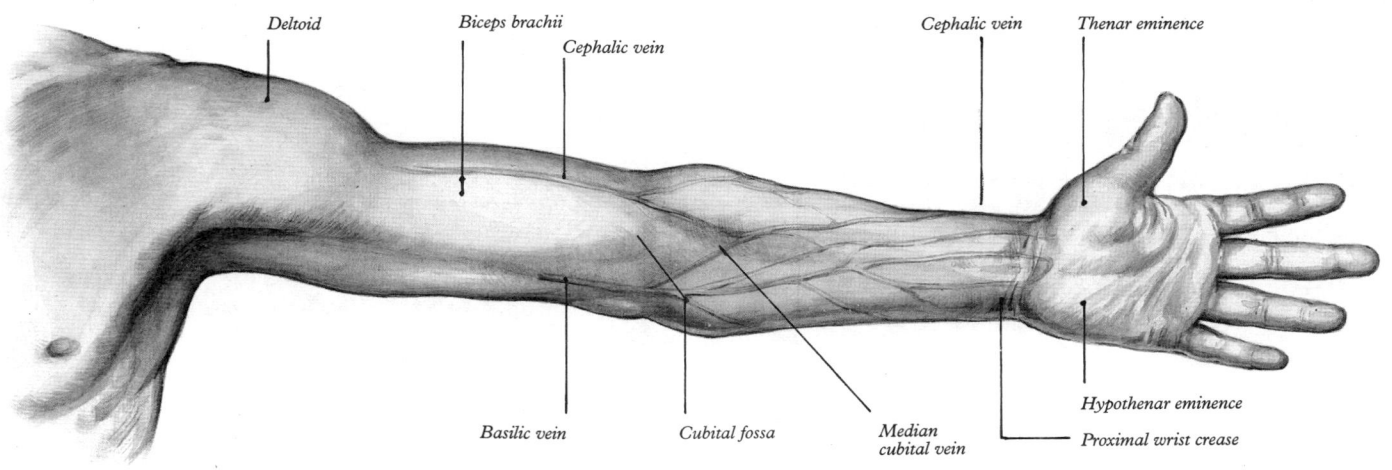

Deltoid

Biceps brachii

Cephalic vein

Cephalic vein

Thenar eminence

Basilic vein

Cubital fossa

Median
cubital vein

Hypothenar eminence

Proximal wrist crease

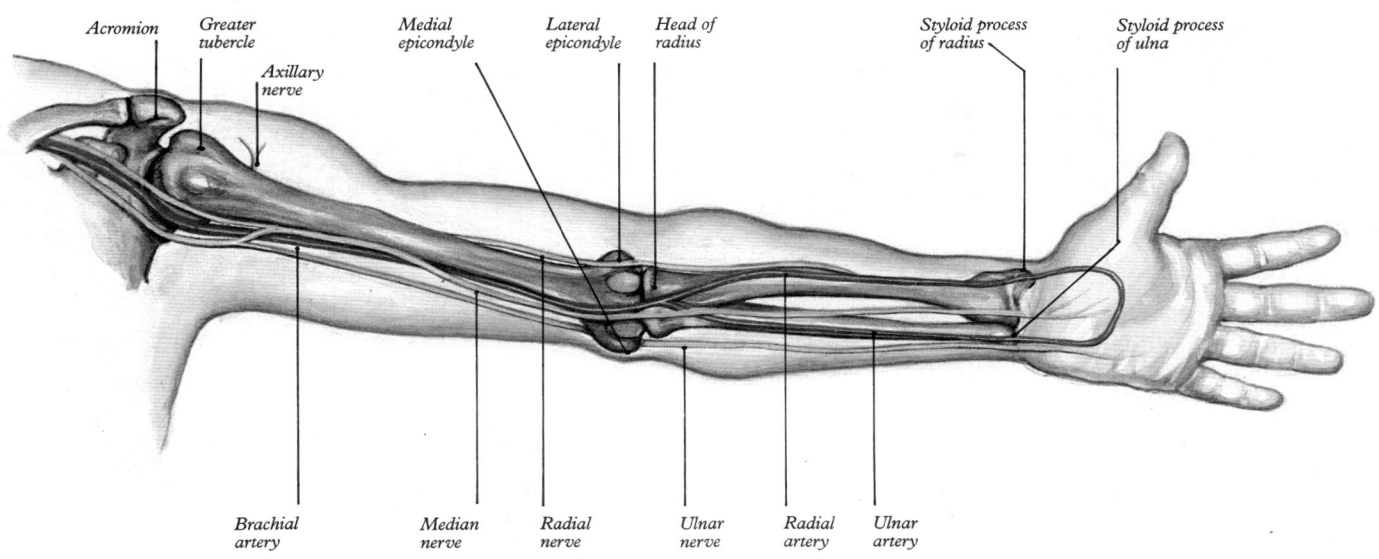

Acromion

Greater
tubercle

Axillary
nerve

Medial
epicondyle

Lateral
epicondyle

Head of
radius

Styloid process
of radius

Styloid process
of ulna

Brachial
artery

Median
nerve

Radial
nerve

Ulnar
nerve

Radial
artery

Ulnar
artery

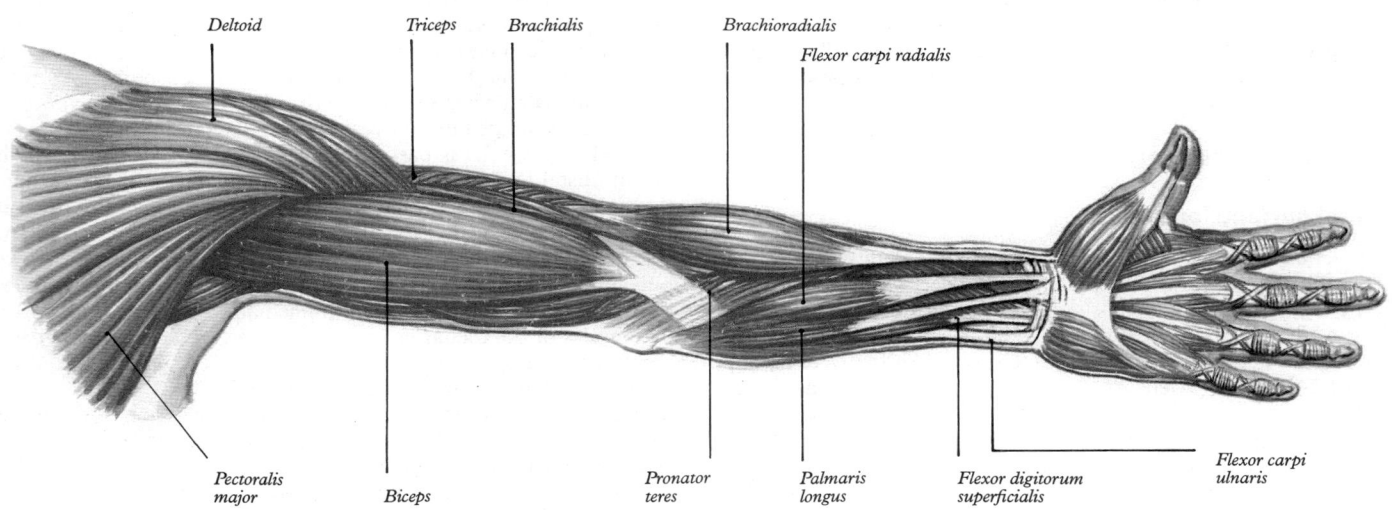

Deltoid

Triceps

Brachialis

Brachioradialis

Flexor carpi radialis

Pectoralis
major

Biceps

Pronator
teres

Palmaris
longus

Flexor digitorum
superficialis

Flexor carpi
ulnaris

16.10 Anterior views of upper limb showing surface anatomy and musculature.

1925

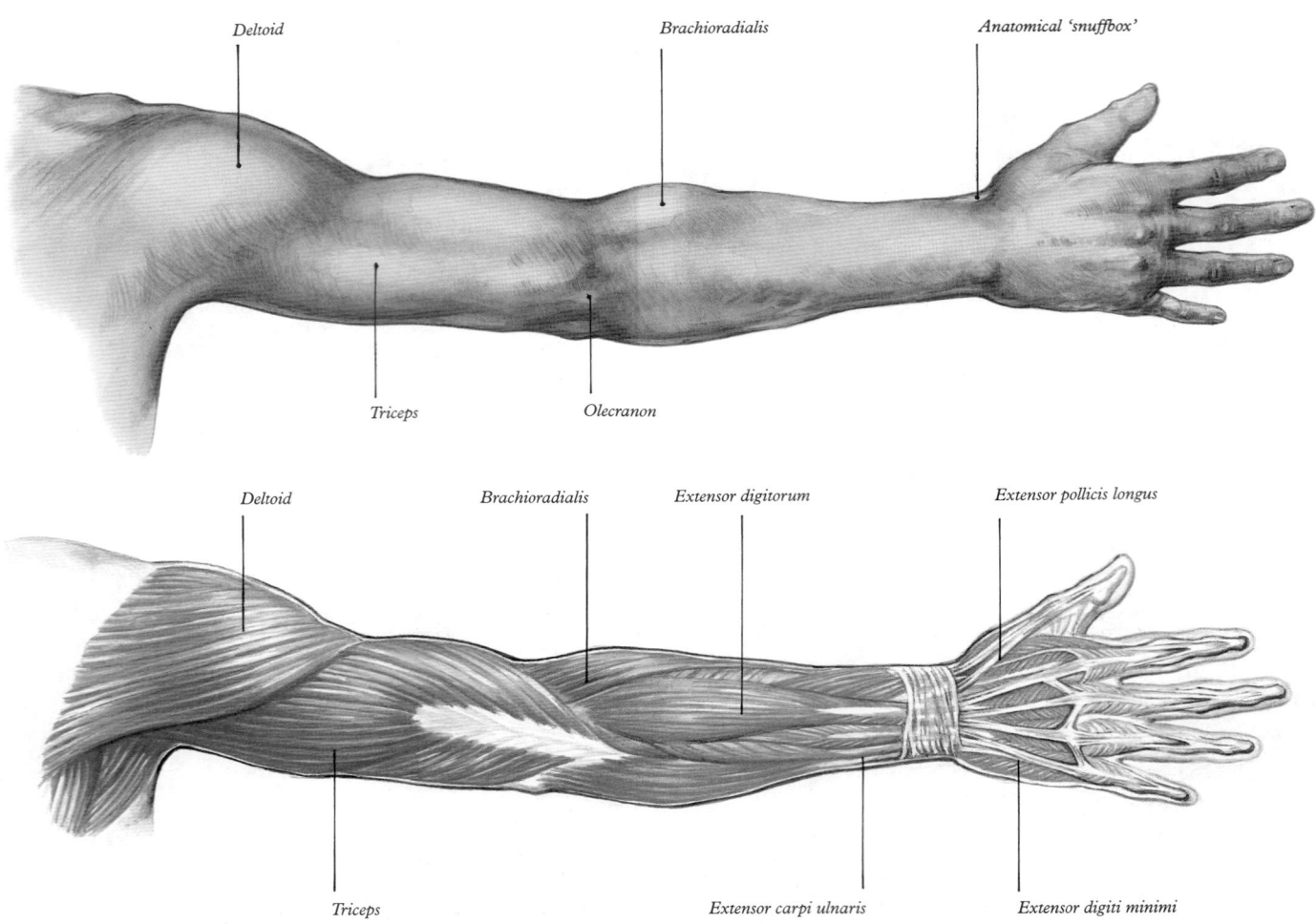

Deltoid

Brachioradialis

Anatomical 'snuffbox'

Triceps

Olecranon

Deltoid

Brachioradialis

Extensor digitorum

Extensor pollicis longus

Triceps

Extensor carpi ulnaris

Extensor digiti minimi

16.11 Posterior aspect of upper limb showing surface anatomy and musculature.

Posteriorly, the *lateral head of the triceps* forms an elevation medial and parallel to the posterior border of the deltoid. It is thrown into prominence when the elbow is extended against resistance. On its medial side is a fleshy mass which disappears above under cover of the deltoid muscle and is produced by the *long head of the triceps*.

The pulsation of the *brachial artery* can be felt in the furrow along the medial side of the biceps and, more superiorly, in the depression posterior to the coracobrachialis by pressure laterally against the shaft of the humerus. In its lower part, the artery can be felt adjacent and posteromedially to the biceps tendon before it disappears deep to the bicipital aponeurosis. Note that the brachial artery lies medial to the humerus in its upper part but then lies directly in front of the lower end of the shaft of the bone. The *median nerve* is intimately related to the brachial artery throughout its course in the arm. Placed at first on the lateral side, the nerve crosses, usually in front of, the artery about half way down the arm and then descends on its medial side into the cubital fossa.

FOREARM AND WRIST

Skeletal surface landmarks (16.12, 13)

The *posterior border of the ulna* is subcutaneous throughout its whole extent from the subcutaneous surface of the olecranon superiorly to the *styloid process* below. Its position corresponds to the longitudinal furrow which can be seen on the posterior aspect of the forearm when the elbow is fully flexed and which separates the flexor group of muscles from the extensors. In contrast, the shaft of the radius can only be felt indistinctly because of its covering of muscles. The rounded *head of the ulna* forms a surface elevation on the medial part of the posterior aspect of the wrist when the hand is pronated. The *styloid process of the ulna* projects distally from the posteromedial aspect of the head.

1926   The expanded lower end of the radius forms a slight surface

elevation on the lateral side of the wrist and can be traced downwards into the *styloid process of the radius*. The posterior aspect of the lower end of the radius is partly obscured by the extensor tendons but can be palpated without difficulty. It presents a *tubercle* (of Lister), which is grooved on its ulnar aspect by the tendon of extensor pollicis longus. The tubercle lies in line with the cleft between the index and the middle fingers.

The styloid process of the ulna lies at a higher level and on a more posterior plane than the styloid process of the radius. The relative positions of these two bony points can be determined if the wrist is grasped firmly between the finger and thumb and pressure is applied in a proximal direction. In a fracture of the lower end of the radius with proximal and posterior displacement (Colles' fracture), the two styloid processes come to lie in the same plane.

Four of the bones of the carpus can be palpated and identified. The *pisiform* bone forms an elevation which can be both seen and felt on the palmar aspect of the wrist at the base of the hypothenar eminence. It can be moved over the articular surface of the triquetral bone when the wrist is passively flexed. The *hook of the hamate* lies 2.5 cm distal to the pisiform and is in line with the ulnar border of the ring finger. It can be felt by deep pressure in this situation and here the superficial division of the ulnar nerve can be rolled from side to side over the tip of the hook. The *tubercle of the scaphoid* bone is situated at the base of the thenar eminence. In many subjects it forms a small visible elevation. Immediately distal to it but covered by muscles of the thenar eminence, the *crest of the trapezium* can be identified on deep pressure. The scaphoid and trapezium can also be palpated in the anatomical 'snuffbox' (see below).

The *wrist joint* is easily identified between the carpus and the distal ends of the radius and ulna on flexion and extension of the wrist, even though it is covered by tendons. The line of the wrist joint corresponds to a line, convex upwards, which joins the styloid process of the radius to that of the ulna. It is delineated by the proximal of the two transverse anterior wrist skin creases.

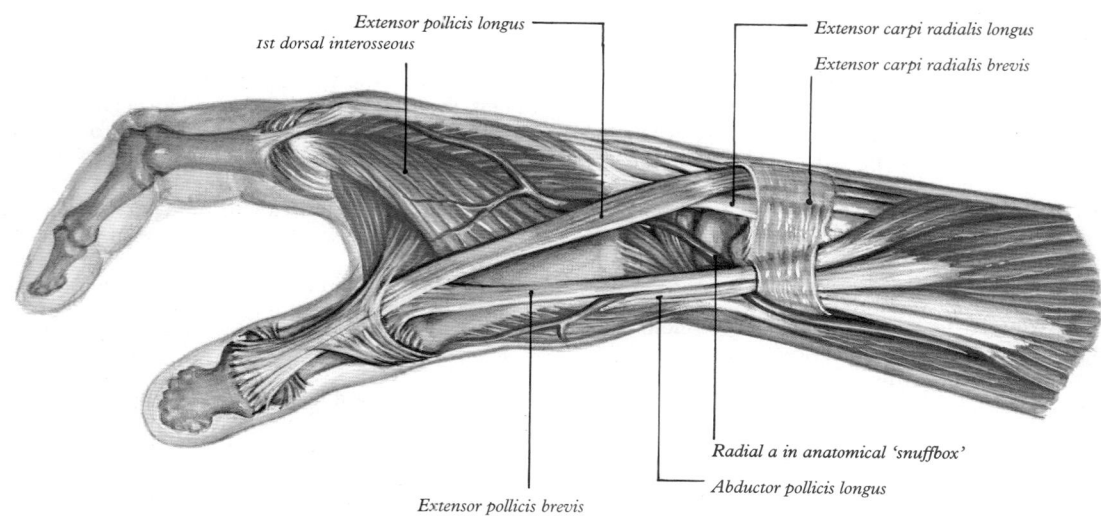

Extensor pollicis longus
1st dorsal interosseous

Extensor carpi radialis longus
Extensor carpi radialis brevis

Radial a in anatomical 'snuffbox'

Abductor pollicis longus

Extensor pollicis brevis

16.12   Lateral view of right wrist and anatomical 'snuffbox'.

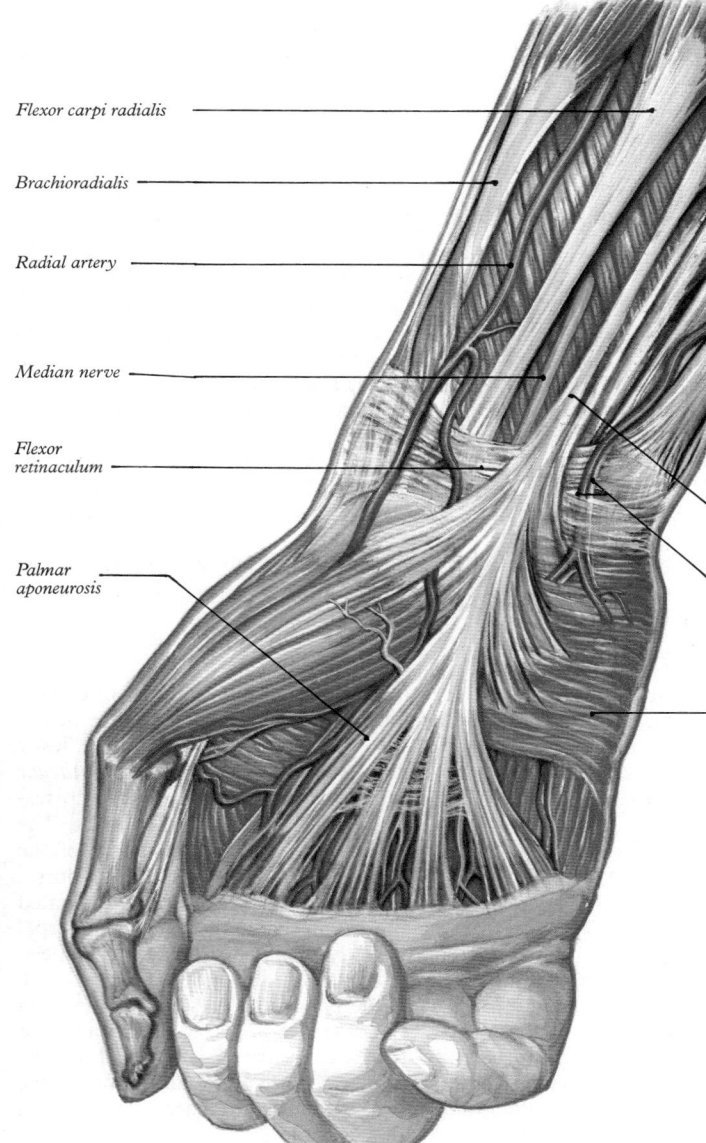

Flexor carpi radialis

Brachioradialis

Radial artery

Median nerve

Flexor retinaculum

Palmar aponeurosis

Flexor digitorum superficialis

Flexor carpi ulnaris

Palmaris longus

Ulnar nerve and artery

Palmaris brevis

16.13   Anterior aspect of right wrist.

Soft tissues (16.10, 12)

The *cubital fossa* forms a depression in the middle of the upper part of the front of the forearm. The fleshy elevation which constitutes its medial border is formed by *pronator teres* while the elevation which forms the lateral border is *brachioradialis*. The superior border of the fossa is an imaginary line which joins the two epicondyles of the humerus. Brachioradialis is the most superficial of the muscles on the lateral side of the forearm. It can be demonstrated by flexing the elbow in the semiprone position against resistance, when it stands out as a prominent ridge which extends upwards beyond the level of the elbow joint on the lateral side of the arm.

The flexor and extensor aspects of the upper two-thirds of the shafts of the radius and ulna are covered by the bellies of the flexor and extensor groups of muscles of the forearm respectively. The longitudinal furrow which corresponds to the posterior border of the ulna indicates the line which separates these two groups of muscles. More distally, many of the tendons of these two muscle groups can be identified individually. When the wrist is flexed against resistance, a number of tendons become obvious. *Flexor carpi radialis* is the most radial of these. On its medial side is the tendon of the inconstant *palmaris longus*, which lies approximately in the midline of the wrist. On the ulnar side, the tendon of *flexor carpi ulnaris* can be identified and traced distally to its insertion in the pisiform. Between this tendon and that of palmaris longus lie the tendons of *flexor digitorum superficialis* which can be felt to move when the fingers are flexed and extended with the wrist held stationary; the other tendons remain still during this movement.

When the thumb is fully extended, a depression known as the 'anatomical snuff box' is seen on the lateral aspect of the wrist immediately distal to the radial styloid process. Progressing distally from the styloid the following may be palpated:

- the convex ovoid proximal articular surface of the scaphoid (best felt during alternate ulnar and radial deviation at the wrist)
- less distinctly, the radial aspect of the trapezium
- the obvious expanded base of the first metacarpal (best felt during circumduction of the thumb).

Note that effective compression (bidigital between index and thumb) may be made of the scaphoid along its oblique long axis between tubercle and articular surface; also of the trapezium between its crest and radial aspect. The snuffbox is bounded on the radial side by the tendons of *abductor pollicis longus* laterally and *extensor pollicis brevis* medially; these tendons lie close to each other. On the ulnar side of the snuff box is the tendon of *extensor pollicis longus*, which stands out conspicuously in full extension of the thumb and can be seen to extend to the base of the distal phalanx of the thumb.

If a finger is run along this tendon proximally, the *superficial radial nerve* can be rolled from side to side as it crosses the tendon. The tendons of the *radial extensors of the wrist* can be identified on the back of the carpus when the fist is clenched and relaxed alternately. The tendons of *extensor digitorum* can readily be seen on the back of the hand when the fingers are fully extended and the tendon of *extensor carpi ulnaris* can be felt distal to the ulnar styloid as it crosses the wrist when the wrist is extended and deviated to the ulnar side.

The *median nerve* enters the forearm on the medial side of the termination of the brachial artery and runs vertically downwards in the midline of the limb. At the wrist it lies exactly in the midline and projects from under cover of the palmaris longus tendon on its radial side. Since this tendon may be absent, this is obviously an inconstant landmark.

The *ulnar nerve* in the forearm corresponds to a line drawn from the base of the medial epicondyle of the humerus to the radial side of the pisiform bone. Deep pressure at both these bony landmarks will produce paraesthesia. In the lower part of the forearm the line of the nerve lies along the radial side of the tendon of flexor carpi ulnaris. The *ulnar artery* commences in the midline of the forearm opposite the neck of the radius. In its upper and deepest part of its course in the forearm, it can be represented by a line which passes downwards and medially across the elevation produced by the superficial flexor muscles of the forearm, to reach the radial side of the ulnar nerve at the junction of the upper one-third with the lower two-thirds of the forearm. In the rest of its course in the forearm, the ulnar artery lies along the radial side of the ulnar nerve.

The *radial artery* commences opposite the neck of the radius on the medial side of the tendon of biceps. It runs downwards and radially through the forearm to the wrist, where its pulsation can be readily felt in the interval between the tendon of flexor carpi radialis on the ulnar side and the lower part of the anterior border of the radius laterally. It then continues distally across the anterior margin of the expanded lower end of the radius, then passes posteriorly, deep to the tendons of abductor pollicis longus and extensor pollicis brevis, to enter the anatomical 'snuffbox' where, once again, its pulsation can be felt. The upper part of the line which represents the course of the radial artery passes deep to the medial part of the elevation produced by the brachioradialis on the anterior aspect of the forearm.

The *radial nerve* gives off its *posterior interosseous branch* at the level of the lateral epicondyle, a finger's breadth to the lateral side of the tendon of the biceps, and then runs distally in a vertical direction. In the middle one-third of the forearm it lies along the radial side of the radial artery, but in the lower third it inclines backwards to pass across the tendon of extensor pollicis longus at the wrist (where it can be rolled against the tendon), to be distributed as the cutaneous supply of the radial side of the dorsum of the hand

and radial three and a half digits. The *posterior interosseous nerve* passes downwards and posteriorly to supply all the extensor muscles of the forearm apart from brachioradialis and extensor carpi radialis longus (both supplied by the radial nerve before it divides). The nerve winds to the posterior aspect of the forearm around the lateral side of the radius between the two planes of fibres of the supinator muscle. Its course can be mapped out by a line drawn from the origin of the nerve anterior to the lateral epicondyle to a point on the dorsum of the wrist midway between the head of the ulna and the dorsal tubercle of the radius. Here the nerve ends as a flattened pseudoganglion from which filaments are distributed to the ligaments and joints of the carpus. An important surgical landmark is where the posterior interosseous nerve winds round the upper end of the radius. This can be indicated in the following manner.

- Place the index finger of the opposite hand on the dorsal aspect of the head of the radius.
- Align the middle and ring fingers below the index.
- The ring finger then lies over the nerve; this is important in making an incision for exposure and removal of a fractured head of radius.
- The incision should not extend more than a finger's breadth below the head of the radius.

The flexor retinaculum can be outlined by defining its bony attachments. Its distal border, concave downwards, can be indicated on the surface by a curved line which joins the crest of the trapezium to the hook of the hamate; its proximal border by a curved line concave upwards which joins the tubercle of the scaphoid to the pisiform.

HAND

Skeletal surface landmarks

The palpable carpal bones have already been considered above. The *heads of the metacarpal bones* form the prominence of the knuckles, that of the middle finger being the most prominent. Their convex, palmar aspects can be felt on deep pressure over the fronts of the metacarpophalangeal joints and can be gripped between the finger and the thumb. Deep pressure over the distal aspect of the head of the metacarpal bone reveals the base of the corresponding proximal phalanx, and the line of the *metacarpophalangeal joint* can be detected on the dorsum of the hand as the fingers are flexed and extended. The dorsal aspects of the shafts of the metacarpal bones of the fingers and thumb and trapezium can be felt rather indistinctly, being obscured by the extensor tendons. The *interphalangeal joints* can be felt on the dorsal aspect of the flexed finger, just distal to the prominences caused by the heads of the proximal and middle phalanges.

Soft tissues (16.10–13)

The skin of the palm of the hand is marked by a number of creases which, however, are of little value as points of reference. The *thenar eminence* is a fleshy elevation induced by the abductor and the flexor pollicis brevis, which overlie the opponens pollicis. The *hypothenar eminence* on the medial side of the palm is formed by the corresponding muscles of the little finger but is not so prominent. The medial border of the hand is formed by the medial aspect of the hypothenar eminence, but the lateral border is formed by the dorsal aspect of the *metacarpal bone of the thumb* which can be palpated throughout its whole extent and, at its base, the carpometacarpal joint of the thumb can be indistinctly palpated on its dorsal aspect. The wide range of movement at this saddle joint can be appreciated.

Transverse skin creases cross the palmar aspects of the fingers in three situations: the most proximal crease is placed at the junction of the digit with the palm and lies nearly 2 cm distal to the metacarpophalangeal joint, the intermediate crease lies opposite the proximal interphalangeal joint, and the distal crease is placed just proximal to the distal interphalangeal joint.

The lateral part of the dorsal aspect of the hand between the index finger and the thumb shows a fleshy elevation caused by the *first dorsal interosseous muscle*, which becomes more conspicuous when the index finger is abducted against resistance. The corresponding anterior aspect of the first web space is formed by *adductor pollicis*.

The *superficial palmar arch* is continuous with the ulnar artery which lies to the radial side of the pisiform. Its course can be marked out by a line drawn downwards in front of the hook of the hamate bone which then curves radially with a downward convexity across the palm to the thenar eminence. The most distal part of the curve just reaches the level of the palmar surface of the extended thumb. However, the curvature of this vessel is subject to considerable variation. The *deep palmar arch* can be represented by a line about 1.5 cm proximal to the superficial arch.

On the back of the hand is the irregular plexus of the *dorsal venous arch*. Its position and arrangement are both highly variable: from its ulnar side originates the *basilic vein*, which ascends along the ulnar side of the distal forearm. The *cephalic vein* arises from the radial extremity of the dorsal arch; at the wrist level it can be felt and seen (if the forearm is compressed) immediately dorsal to the radial styloid process after crossing the roof of the anatomical 'snuffbox'. This site is commonly and safely used for intravenous cannulation.

LOWER LIMB

THIGH

Skeletal surface landmarks (16.14, 15)

An oblique skin crease, *the fold of the groin*, marks the junction of the front of the thigh with the anterior abdominal wall. It corresponds fairly accurately to the *inguinal ligament*. The *anterior superior spine of the ilium* lies at the lateral end of the fold and can always be palpated. At its medial end, the fold reaches the *pubic tubercle* (see p. 1918). From the anterior superior spine, the *iliac crest* is easily palpable along its entire length. It terminates posteriorly as the *posterior superior iliac spine*. This can be felt in the depression seen just above the buttock. This lies at the level of the second segment of the sacrum, at the level of the middle of the sacroiliac joint and the level of the termination of the spinal dural sac. The *ischial tuberosity* is palpated in the lower part of the buttock. It is covered by the gluteus maximus when the hip joint is extended, but can be identified without difficulty when the hip is flexed, as in the sitting position. The ischial tuberosity then emerges from under cover of the lower border of the gluteus maximus and is then subcutaneous, separated from the skin only by a pad of fat and the ischial bursa. The weight of the body is supported by the ischial tuberosities in the sitting position.

The *greater trochanter* of the femur lies a hand's breadth inferior to the midpoint of the iliac crest. It can be both seen and felt as a prominence in front of the hollow on the side of the hip; indeed, it is the only part of the proximal portion of the femur which is palpable.

The lower end of the femur is less deeply placed; when the knee is flexed passively, the medial surface of the *medial condyle* and the lateral surface of the *lateral condyle of the femur* can be palpated,

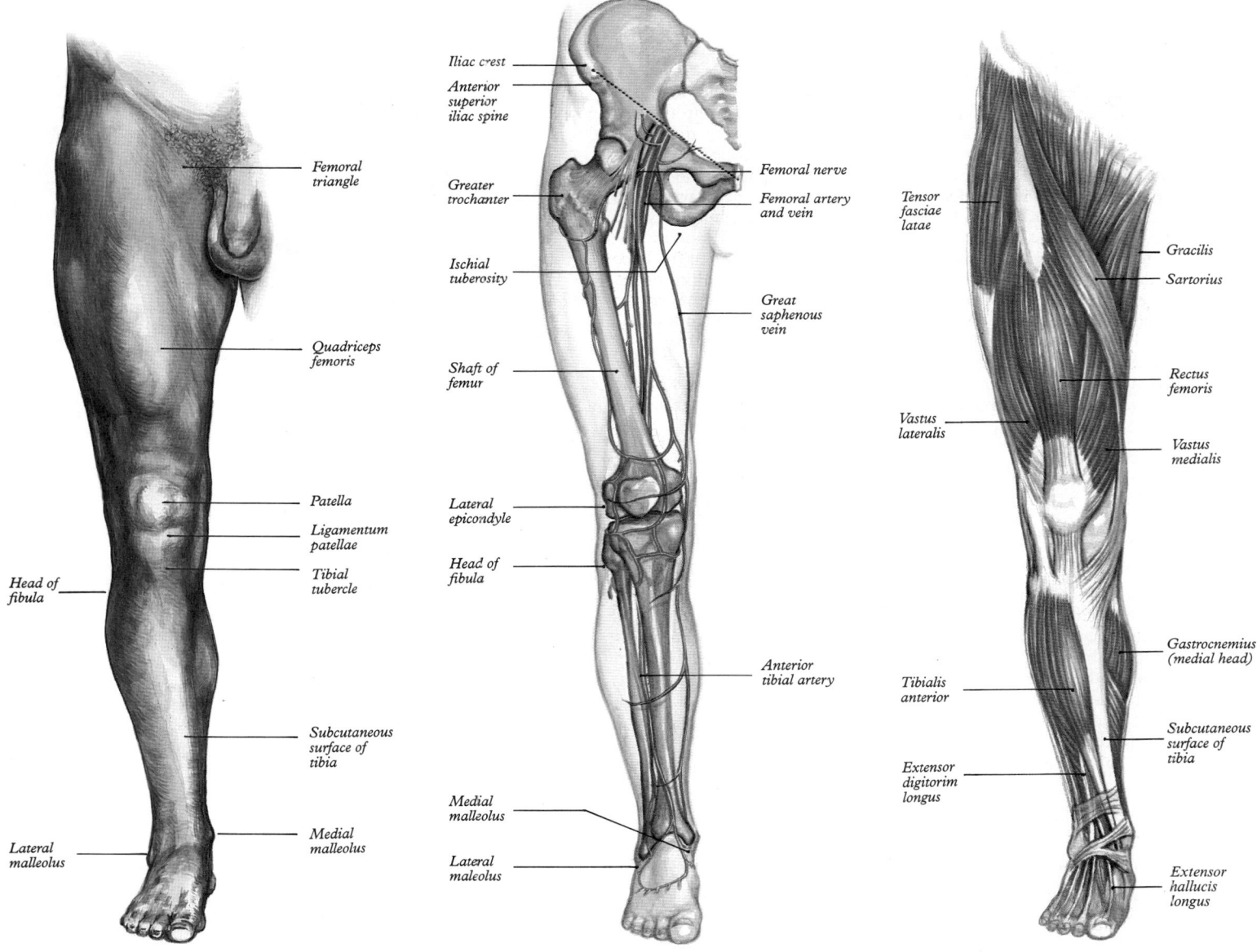

16.14 Anterior aspect of lower limb to show surface anatomy, bony and soft tissue structures.

and portions of the femoral articular surface can be examined on each side of the lower part of the patella.

The *patella* can be identified readily and, when the quadriceps is relaxed in the fully extended knee, it can be tilted and moved on the lower end of the femur. The lower limit of the patella lies more than 1 cm above the line of the knee joint.

Soft tissues (16.14, 15)

The *femoral artery* enters the thigh at the fold of the groin, at a point midway between the anterior superior iliac spine and the pubic symphysis. Its course can be represented by the upper two-thirds of a line which joins that point to the adductor tubercle when the flexed thigh is abducted slightly and rotated laterally. At its origin, the pulsations of the femoral artery can be felt and in this situation the vessel can be compressed against the superior ramus of the pubis. The femoral pulse constitutes an important landmark; immediately medial to it is the surface marking of the *femoral vein* and the termination of the *great saphenous vein*. The course of this vein can be marked out in the thigh by a line passing from this point downwards and backwards to a hand's breadth behind the patella. Immediately lateral to the femoral pulse is the surface marking of the *femoral nerve*. A finger placed on the femoral pulse and then slid upwards immediately above the groin fold lies on the *internal inguinal ring*. Pressure at this point will control the descent of a reduced indirect inguinal hernia but not a direct hernia, which passes medial to the inferior epigastric artery.

The shallow depression which lies immediately below the fold of the groin corresponds to the *femoral triangle*. It is bounded on its lateral side by the strap-like *sartorius muscle*, which can be both seen and felt in a reasonably thin and muscular subject when the hip is flexed in the sitting position while keeping the knee extended, especially when the thigh is slightly abducted and rotated laterally. The muscle can be traced downwards and medially from the anterior superior spine of the ilium to approximately half-way down the medial side of the thigh. Distally, it may be identified as a soft longitudinal ridge passing towards the posterior part of the medial femoral condyle. The bulky, fleshy mass at the upper part of the medial side of the thigh is formed by the *adductor group of muscles*. The medial border of *adductor longus* forms the medial boundary of the femoral triangle and can be felt as a distinct ridge when the knee is adducted against resistance. At its upper end, its tendon of origin can be identified immediately below the pubis and felt between the finger and thumb. Its origin is immediately below the pubic tubercle and the tendon forms a useful guide to this bony landmark.

The forward convexity of the front of the thigh is caused by the curvature of the femur which is covered by the fleshy mass of the *quadriceps femoris*. Three of its four components can be identified:

- *rectus femoris* may be seen as a ridge passing down the anterior aspect of the thigh when the sitting subject flexes the hip with the knee extended
- *vastus medialis* constitutes the bulge above and medial to the patella
- *vastus lateralis* forms the elevation above and lateral to the patella, more proximal and less pronounced than that of vastus medialis.

The fourth component, *vastus intermedius*, is hidden by the other three muscles.

The flattened appearance of the lateral aspect of the thigh is produced by the *iliotibial tract*, the thickened portion of the deep fascia of the thigh, or fascia lata, which stands out as a strong, visible groove on the anterolateral aspect of the knee when the leg is extended against gravity. The tract extends from its origin on the iliac crest to its insertion at the upper end of the tibia.

The bulky prominence of the buttock is caused by three factors:

- the forward tilt of the pelvis, which throws the ischium backwards
- the size of gluteus maximus
- the large amount of subcutaneous fat.

The horizontal *gluteal fold* marks the upper limit of the posterior aspect of the thigh; it does not correspond to the lower border of the gluteus maximus, but is caused by fibrous connections between the skin and the deep fascia. The *natal cleft*, which separates the buttocks inferiorly, commences above at the third or fourth sacral spine.

The upper border of *gluteus maximus* commences on the iliac crest

about 3 cm lateral to the posterior superior spine and runs downwards and laterally to the apex of the greater trochanter. Its lower border corresponds to a line drawn from the ischial tuberosity, through the midpoint of the gluteal fold, to a point about 9 cm below the greater trochanter. Although this muscle overlaps the ischial tuberosity in the standing position, on sitting, the muscle slides superiorly posterior to the tuberosity leaving it free to weight-bear. The muscle can be felt to contract when the hip is extended against resistance.

Gluteus medius completely covers the underlying *gluteus minimus*. They lie in the slight depression superolateral to gluteus maximus and inferior to the anterior portion of the iliac crest. These two muscles constitute the major abductors of the hip and are demonstrated by asking the subject to stand on one limb. The ipsilateral muscles contract and tilt the pelvis in order to stabilize the centre of gravity. In this action, the contralateral gluteal fold will rise. If the hip abductors are paralysed, in congenital dislocation of the hip or in a long-standing fracture of the neck of the femur, this mechanism is disturbed and the normal tilting of the pelvis does not occur. Indeed, when the patient stands on the affected hip, the pelvis tilts downwards on the contralateral side (*Trendelenburg's sign*).

The surface markings of the *sciatic nerve* (**16.15**) can be represented by a line which commences at a point midway between the posterior superior iliac spine and ischial tuberosity, which curves outwards and downwards through a point midway between the greater trochanter and the ischial tuberosity and then continues vertically

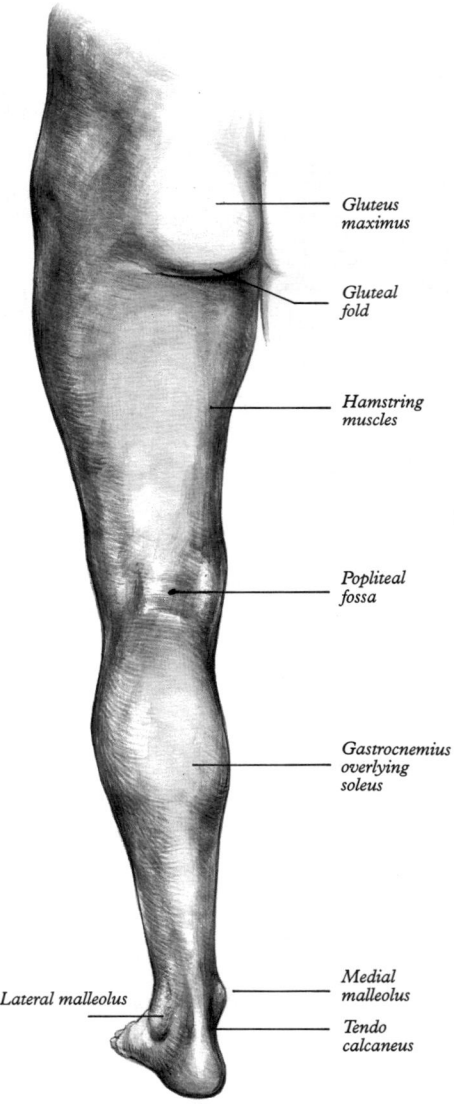

Gluteus maximus

Gluteal fold

Hamstring muscles

Popliteal fossa

Gastrocnemius overlying soleus

Lateral malleolus

Medial malleolus

Tendo calcaneus

16.15 Posterior views of the lower limb to show surface anatomy, bony and soft tissue structures and main nerves and arteries.

downwards in the midline of the posterior aspect of the thigh to the upper angle of the popliteal fossa. Here it divides into the *tibial* and *common peroneal nerves*, if it has not already done so at a higher level.

KNEE

Skeletal surface landmarks (16.14)

The patella and the medial and lateral condyles of the femur have been described above. The *tibial condyles* form visible and palpable landmarks at the medial and lateral sides of the *ligamentum patellae*, which can be traced downwards from the apex of the patella to the *tibial tubercle* which, again, is readily seen as well as felt. When the knee is flexed passively, the anterior margins of the tibial condyles can be felt readily, and each forms the lower boundary of a depression at the side of the patellar ligament. The lateral condyle is the more prominent of the two. The line of the *knee joint* corresponds to the upper margins of the tibial condyles and can be represented by a line drawn round the limb at this level. In the angles between this line and the edges of the ligamentum patellae can be indicated the anterior horns of the *semilunar cartilages or menisci*.

The *head of the fibula* forms a slight surface elevation on the upper part of the posterolateral aspect of the leg and lies vertically below the posterior part of the lateral condyle of the femur not less than 1 cm below the level of the knee joint.

Soft tissues (16.14, 15)

The large and deep depression which can be seen at the back of the knee when the joint is actively flexed against resistance corresponds to the *popliteal fossa*. It is bounded on the lateral side by the prominent tendon of the *biceps femoris*, which can be felt between the finger and thumb and which can be traced downwards to the head of the fibula. Three tendons can be felt on the medial side of the popliteal fossa. The *semitendinosus* is the most lateral and posterior and the *gracilis* is the most medial and anterior. These two tendons stand out sharply and can be seen when the knee is flexed against resistance and the limb actively adducted. The third tendon is that of *semimembranosus*, which is more deeply situated and can be felt in the interval between the other two. In addition, it is much thicker than the others and broadens rapidly as it is traced upwards.

The medial and lateral inferior boundaries of the popliteal fossa are formed by the upper borders of the two heads of *gastrocnemius*, which is described below.

The *popliteal artery* can be represented by a line which begins at the junction of the middle and lower thirds of the thigh along the line drawn from the femoral pulse at the groin to the adductor tubercle; the upper two-thirds of this line demarcates the line of the femoral artery. The popliteal artery then runs downwards and laterally to reach the midline at the level of the knee joint. It then descends to the level of the tibial tubercle, where it bifurcates into the anterior and posterior tibial arteries at the lower border of the popliteus muscle.

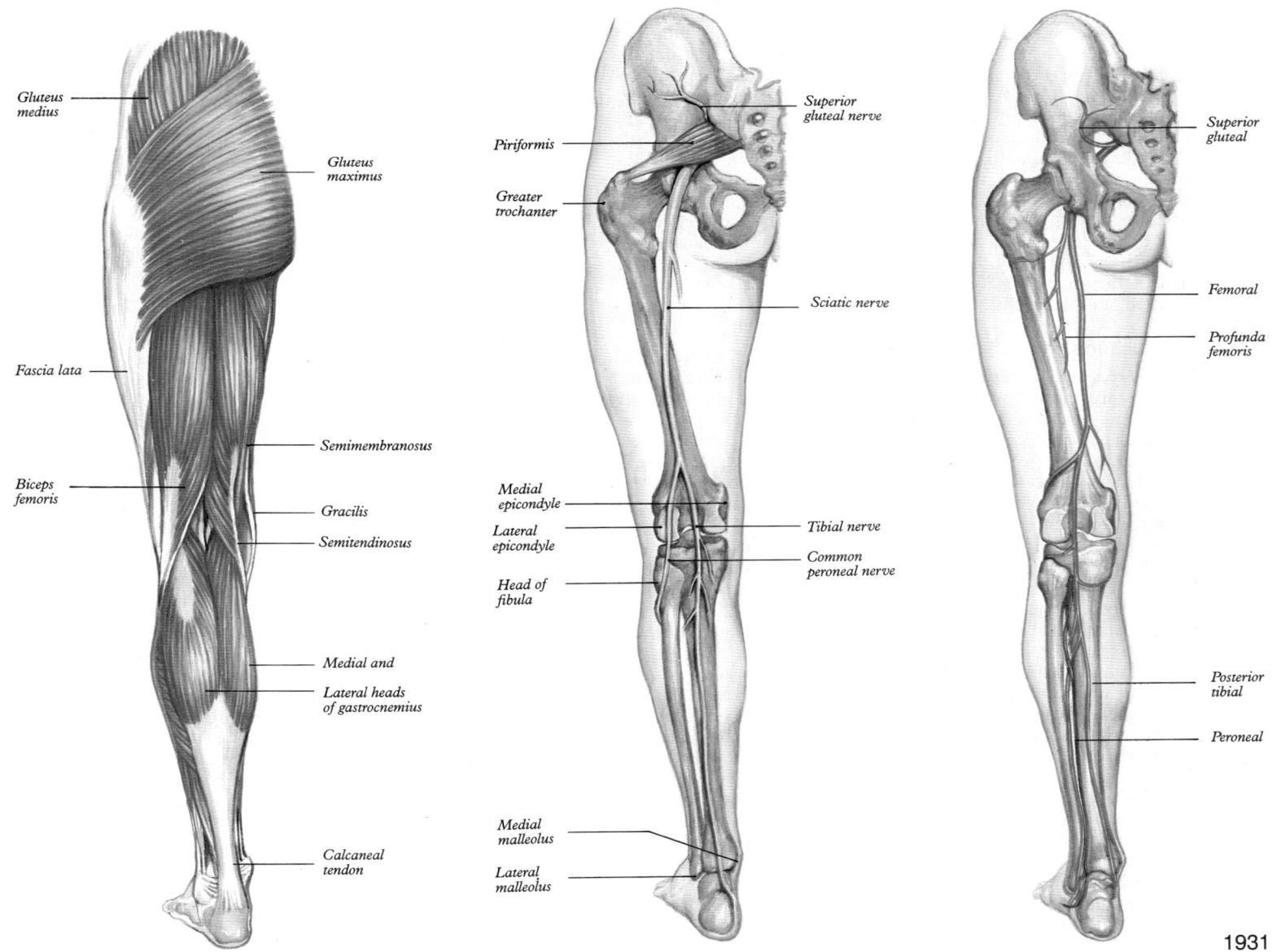

The *popliteal pulse* is the most difficult of the peripheral pulses to detect. It may be palpated with the subject lying supine with the knee bent to a right angle and with the foot resting on the couch, in order to relax the tense popliteal fascia which roofs the popliteal fossa. The pulse is felt by deep pressure over the midline of the fossa against the popliteal surface of the femur. The other technique is to have the subject lie face down with the knee bent to a right angle and supported by the examiner so that the muscles are relaxed. The pulse is sought, again, on deep palpation in the midline against the popliteal surface of the femur.

The *tibial nerve* corresponds to a line which commences at the upper angle of the popliteal fossa and which runs downwards in the midline. At first the nerve lies lateral to the popliteal artery then gradually crosses the vessel to gain its medial side. The *common peroneal nerve* can be indicated by a line drawn from the upper angle of the popliteal fossa, along the medial side of the tendon of biceps femoris to the back of the head of the fibula. It then curves downwards and forwards around the neck of the bone. The nerve is palpable on the medial side of the biceps tendon and also over the neck of the fibula, although here it is less distinct as it passes deep to the origin of peroneus longus. At the neck of the fibula it is at particular risk of damage either from a tightly applied plaster cast or from a fracture of the neck of the fibula.

LEG AND ANKLE

Skeletal surface landmarks (16.16)

The subcutaneous *medial surface of the tibia* corresponds to the flat anteromedial aspect of the leg. Above, this surface merges into the medial condyle of the tibia and below it is continuous with the visible prominence of the *medial malleolus* of the tibia. The sinuous *anterior border of the tibia* can be felt distinctly throughout most of its extent, but inferiorly it is somewhat masked by the tendon of the tibialis anterior, which lies to its lateral side. The *lateral malleolus of the fibula* forms a conspicuous projection on the lateral side of the angle, which descends to a more distal level than the medial malleolus and is placed on a more posterior plane. The lateral aspect of the lateral malleolus is continuous above with an elongated, triangular area of the lower shaft of the fibula, which is also subcutaneous. Immediately in front of the base of the lateral malleolus, the lateral part of the anterior margin of the lower end of the tibia can be detected, and the line of the *ankle joint* can be gauged from it.

Soft tissues (16.16)

The muscles in the anterior osteofascial compartment of the leg form a gentle prominence over the upper two-thirds of its anterolateral aspect, and this prominence is accentuated when the foot is actively inverted and dorsiflexed. In the lower third of the leg, these muscles give place to their tendons. That of the *tibialis anterior* can be seen just lateral to the anterior border of the tibia and traced downwards and medially across the front of the ankle. The other tendons cannot be examined satisfactorily above the ankle.

On the lateral aspect of the leg, *peroneus longus* can be seen as a narrow ridge during active eversion and plantar flexion of the foot. It covers and hides *peroneus brevis*, and both muscles cover the lateral aspect of the fibula so that the shaft of the fibula can only be palpated indistinctly between its neck and its lower subcutaneous triangular area.

The bulky prominence of the calf of the leg is formed by *gastrocnemius* and *soleus*, both of which can be identified when the foot is plantar flexed against resistance or when the heel is raised from the ground by standing on tiptoes. The two heads of gastrocnemius unite above to form the inferior angle of the popliteal fossa. The medial head of gastrocnemius descends to a lower level than its lateral head. Soleus lies deep to gastrocnemius, but when tensed, it bulges from under gastrocnemius, particularly on the lateral side, and its fleshy belly extends to a more distal level. Both muscles end below in the conspicuous *tendo calcaneus* (Achilles tendon). This can be gripped between the finger and thumb and followed downwards to its insertion into the posterior aspect of the calcaneus.

Immediately above the medial malleolus, and close to the medial border of the tibia the tendons of *tibialis posterior* and *flexor*

digitorum longus can be felt rather indistinctly when the foot is actively inverted and plantar flexed.

The *great saphenous vein* can often be seen as it runs upwards and backwards across the medial surface of the tibia a little above and in front of the medial malleolus. Here it is accompanied by the *saphenous nerve*, which is usually in front of, but may be posterior to, the vein. The *anterior tibial artery* can be represented by a line which commences 2.5 cm inferior to the medial side of the head of the fibula and which then runs downwards and slightly medially to the midpoint between the two malleoli. The *posterior tibial artery* corresponds to a line drawn from the midline on the back of the calf at the level of the neck of the fibula to a point midway between the medial malleolus and tendo calcaneus. The same line represents the course of the *tibial nerve*. The deep *peroneal nerve* commences on the lateral aspect of the neck of the fibula, passes downwards and medially and comes rapidly into relationship with the anterior tibial artery, which it accompanies to the ankle. The *superficial peroneal nerve* also begins on the lateral aspect of the neck of the fibula and then descends to a point on the anterior border of peroneus longus, at the junction of the middle and lower thirds of the leg, where it pierces the deep fascia and divides into medial and lateral branches, which gradually diverge as they descend to reach the dorsum of the foot.

FOOT

Skeletal surface landmarks (16.16)

On the dorsum of the foot, the anterior part of the upper surface of the *calcaneus* can be identified a little in front of the lateral malleolus. When the foot is passively inverted, the upper and lateral part of the *head of the talus* can be both seen and felt 3 cm anterior to the distal end of the tibia. It is obscured by the extensor tendons when the toes are dorsiflexed.

The dorsal aspects of the bodies of the *metatarsal bones* can be felt more or less distinctly although they tend to be obscured by the extensor tendons of the toes. Halfway along the lateral border of the foot, the tuberosity on the base of the *fifth metatarsal bone* forms a distinct projection, which can be both seen and felt.

The flat lateral surface of the *calcaneus* can be palpated on the lateral aspect of the heel and can be traced forwards, below the lateral malleolus, where it is hidden by the tendons of peroneus longus and brevis. The *peroneal tubercle*, when present and large, can be felt 2 cm below the tip of the lateral malleolus.

On the medial side of the foot, the *sustentaculum tali* of the calcaneus can be felt 2 cm vertically below the medial malleolus. Inferiorly and posterior to the sustentaculum tali, the medial aspect of the calcaneus can be indistinctly felt. The most conspicuous bony landmark on the medial side of the foot is the *tuberosity of the navicular bone*. This is usually visible and it can always be felt 2.5 cm anterior to the sustentaculum tali. Anterior to this, the *medial cuneiform bone* can be identified by tracing the tendon of tibialis anterior into it (see below). The joint between the medial cuneiform and the first metatarsal can be felt as a narrow groove in its upper and medial parts.

When the foot is placed on the ground, it rests on the posterior part of the inferior surface of the calcaneus, the heads of the metatarsal bones and, to a lesser extent, on its lateral border. The *instep*, which corresponds to the medial longitudinal arch of the foot, is elevated from the ground. The medial and lateral *tubercles of the calcaneus* can be made out on the posterior part of the inferior surface of the calcaneus, but they are obscured by the tough fibro-fatty pad which covers them. The heads of the metatarsal bones are also covered with a similar thick pad to form the ball of the foot. At this level, the foot is at its widest, owing to the slight splay of the metatarsal bones as they pass anteriorly.

The *calcaneocuboid joint* lies 2 cm behind the tubercle on the base of the fifth metatarsal bone and is practically in line with the *talonavicular joint*, the position of which may be gauged from the position of the head of the talus. The *tarsometatarsal joints* lie on a line which joins the tubercle of the fifth metatarsal bone to the tarsometatarsal joint of the great toe. When the latter joint cannot be felt on the medial border of the foot, its position can be indicated 2.5 cm in front of the tuberosity of the navicular bone. The joint

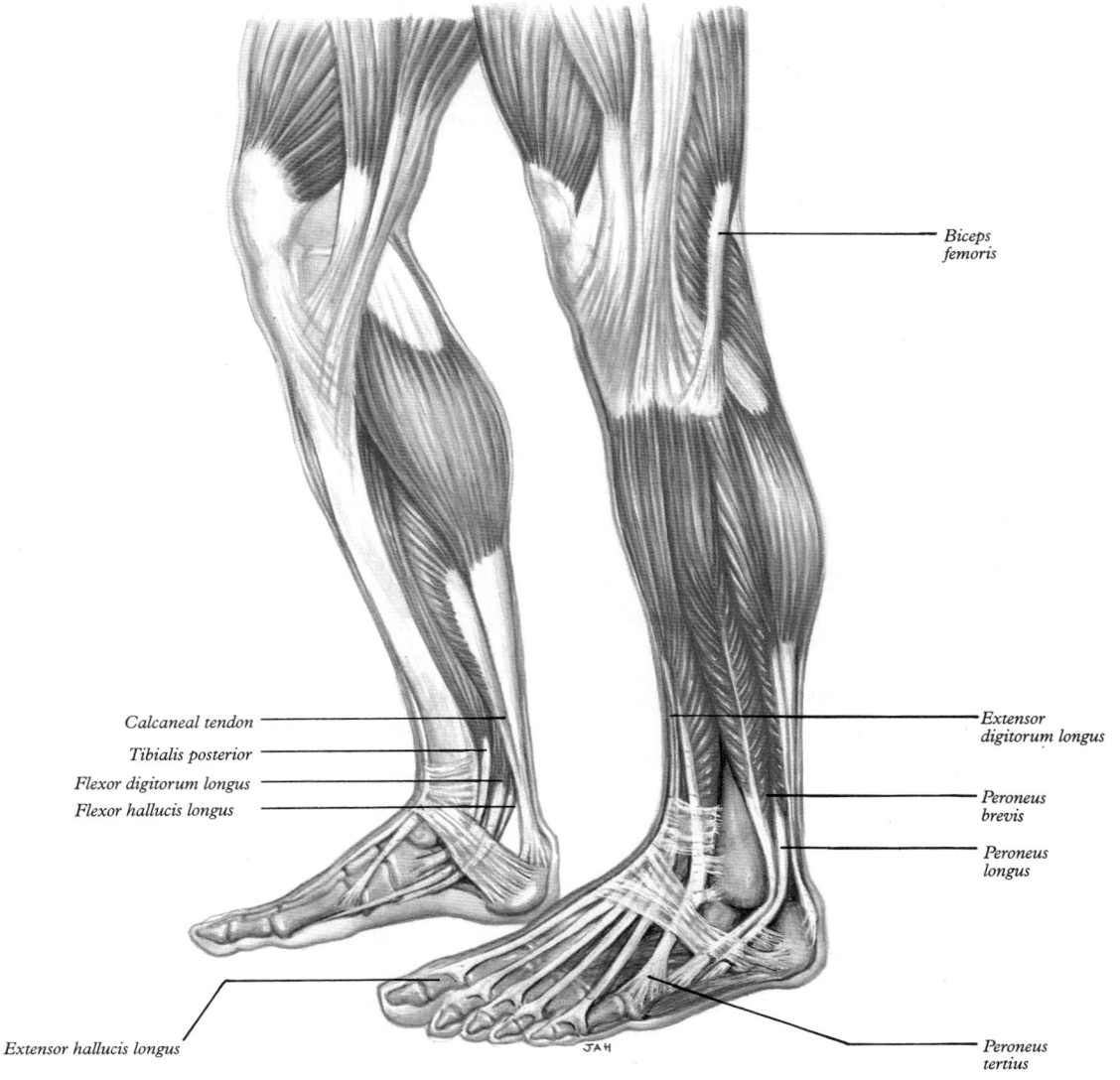

16.16   Lateral view of tendons of lower leg and ankle.

Labels on figure:
Biceps femoris
Calcaneal tendon
Tibialis posterior
Flexor digitorum longus
Flexor hallucis longus
Extensor hallucis longus
Extensor digitorum longus
Peroneus brevis
Peroneus longus
Peroneus tertius
JAH

between the second metatarsal and the intermediate cuneiform lies some 2–3 mm behind the line of the other tarsometatarsal joints. The *metatarsophalangeal joints* lie 2.5 cm behind the webs of the toes.

Soft tissues (16.16)

The *dorsal venous arch* forms a conspicuous feature on the dorsum of the foot and curves, convex forwards, across the metatarsus. The *great saphenous vein* arises from its medial end and runs upwards and backwards immediately in front of the medial malleolus while the *small saphenous vein* arises from its lateral end and passes backwards and inferior to, and then upwards and posterior to, the lateral malleolus.

When the toes are dorsiflexed, the belly of *extensor digitorum brevis* forms a small elevation on the dorsum of the foot, a little in front of the lateral malleolus. It is the only muscle which arises from the dorsum of the foot. In the same position of the foot, the tendon of *tibialis anterior* stands out conspicuously on the medial side when this movement is combined with inversion. The tendon can be traced downwards and medially to the medial cuneiform bone.

When the toes are dorsiflexed, the tendon of *extensor hallucis longus* can be identified lateral to tibialis anterior. Still more laterally, immediately in front of the lateral part of the inferior end of the tibia, the *extensor digitorum longus* and the *peroneus tertius* tendons are crowded together as they pass through the fibrous loop of the inferior extensor retinaculum. After traversing the loop, these tendons diverge to their insertions.

The tendon of *tibialis posterior* winds posterior to the medial malleolus then curves forwards in the interval between this bony landmark and the sustentaculum tali to reach the tuberosity of the navicular bone. The tendon is thrown into relief when the foot is forcibly plantar flexed and inverted. *Flexor digitorum longus* has its tendon placed midway between the medial margin of the tendo calcaneus and the margin of the medial malleolus. The tendon curves forwards below the tibialis posterior and lies on the medial aspect of the sustentaculum tali. From there, it passes forwards and laterally to the centre of the sole of the foot, where it breaks up into tendons for the lateral four toes. The tendon of *flexor hallucis longus* lies inferior to, and grooves, the sustentaculum tali and, as it passes forward to the great toe, it crosses the line of the flexor digitorum longus opposite the interval between the sustentaculum tali and the tuberosity of the navicular bone. *Abductor hallucis* may be seen in some subjects as a fleshy mass across the instep of the foot passing from the medial calcaneal tubercle to the ball of the great toe.

The pulse of the *posterior tibial artery* can be felt by gentle palpation behind the medial malleolus as the artery lies between the tendons of flexor hallucis longus and flexor digitorum longus. The *dorsalis pedis* pulse is sought by palpation immediately lateral to the tendon of extensor hallucis longus against the underlying tarsal bones.

On the dorsum of the foot the skin is thin and loosely connected to the subcutaneous tissues; it contains sparse hairs. On the plantar aspect and especially over the heel, the epidermis is of great thickness. Hairs and sebaceous glands are absent, as in the palm of the hand.

Imaging

Conventional radiography

Differing tissues in the body have different linear attenuations and can be differentiated by their attenuation of an X-ray beam. The transmitted X-ray photons react with the silver in film which is contained in a light tight cassette. The film is processed and the film density or blackening reflects indirectly the absorption of the X-ray beam by the tissues. Electron density is one of the most important factors affecting attenuation and is responsible for radiographic image contrast. Conventional radiographs are excellent for high contrast structures such as bone and lung. The spatial resolution is superior to computed tomography (CT) but the superimposition of overlapping structures decreases contrast resolution. Contrast can be increased by administering radioopaque contrast (e.g. barium sulphate or iodinated contrast) either orally (barium meal), rectally (barium enema) or intravenously (intravenous urogram). The advent of digital radiography allows improved contrast resolution but does not alter the spatial resolution.

Angiography

When iodinated contrast is injected through a catheter within a blood vessel and a radiograph obtained, the lumen of the vessel can be shown (an angiogram). This can be recorded on film but increasingly digitized images are recorded which simplifies image manipulation and subtraction; this is called digital subtraction angiography (DSA). Angiography is used to visualize tumour vascularity and to assess patency of arteries and veins and allows therapeutic manoeuvres such as balloon angioplasty (dilatation) and embolization (occlusion) of vessels.

Ultrasound

In ultrasound, high-frequency sound (2.5–10 MHz) is used. The ultrasound beam is reflected at tissue interfaces and the amount of reflection depends on the difference in the acoustic impedance of the two surfaces and the angle of incidence of the beam. The reflected ultrasound is received by the transducer and a two-dimensional image is produced. Depth resolution is inversely proportional to the frequency of the transmitted ultrasound, and linear resolution depends on the size of the transducer. A smaller transducer will give improved linear resolution as will a focused transducer which is usually utilized. Ultrasound is limited by overlying gas and in the very obese as there is then insufficient depth penetration. Doppler ultrasound utilizes the change in the perceived frequency of sound reflected by a moving source and thus flow can be measured by frequency change. Recently introduced colour Doppler has made this more user friendly for general departments and has revolutionized non-invasive vascular imaging. The advent of high resolution endocavitary ultrasound probes (e.g. transvaginal and transrectal) and intro-operative probes has expanded the use of ultrasound. Ultrasound is mainly an anatomical technique with limited tissue characterization.

The advantages of ultrasound are as follows:

- no radiation
- multiplanar imaging with good anatomical display for biopsy
- Doppler ultrasound allows assessment of vascularity and flow mapping
- cheap and can be performed at the bedside.

Computerized tomography (CT)

CT utilizes a conventional X-ray tube and a bank of detectors which rotate around the patient to produce a finely focused series of angular projections which are reconstructed by computers to produce a cross-sectional, usually transaxial tissue image. The spatial resolution of CT is less than conventional radiographs but the contrast resolution of these images is superior (CT 0.25%, radiographs 5%). Reconstructed images in other planes can be produced by computer manipulation of the data from transaxial scans (multiplanar reformatting) and 3D images, which are of great benefit in complex fractures, can be obtained. CT is primarily an anatomical display although the use of iodinated contrast will give some assessment of the vascularity of a lesion, some tissue characterization can be obtained and bone density measurements may be made.

Scans can now be obtained in about 1 second and the new spiral scanners which combine continuous table movement and continuous X-ray emission allow volumes of tissue up to 60 cm in length to be scanned with slices obtained anywhere within this volume. This allows better multiplanar reformatting and in addition areas like the lungs can be imaged in a single breath hold, so there is no movement artefact. The advent of a scanner utilizing an electron gun rather than a conventional X-ray tube brings scan times down to 50 milliseconds and allows imaging of the cardiac chambers in systole and diastole although this scanner is not widely available. CT gives excellent soft tissue differentiation, especially in the lungs and in cortical bone and unlike ultrasound the presence of ample body fat is advantageous.

The advantages of CT are as follows:

- excellent contrast resolution
- Transaxial images with no tissue superimposition
- excellent anatomical display, can be used to guide biopsies
- some tissue characterization and bone mineral measurements
- scans not limited by fat or overlying gas.

Magnetic resonance imaging (MRI)

MRI is a cross-sectional tomographic imaging obtained from the interaction between radio waves and the atomic nuclei in the body in the presence of a magnetic field. The commonest atom in the body is hydrogen. Protons have both charge and spin and when placed in a large magnetic field they align with the external field. When they are exposed to a radio frequency (from the gradient coils) the protons are tipped and they precess. This changes the magnetic field and this change is the received magnetic resonance signal. Using computer analysis similar to CT an image is produced. By imposing gradients images can be obtained in any plane without moving the patient.

There are three basic magnetic resonance properties, hydrogen density, T1 and T2 relaxation and each image comprises all three components but in varying amounts depending on the weighting. MRI has superior contrast resolution to CT, allowing excellent visualization of the grey/white matter of the brain, the spinal cord and the joints and musculoskeletal system and increasingly the remainder of the body as imaging times decrease. There are some limitations to the use of MRI as patients with pacemakers, some monitoring equipment and some surgical clips cannot be scanned. Cortical bone with only few mobile protons is poorly visualized as is air. Soft tissue contrast can be varied depending on which imaging sequence is used. New sequences, which are faster, allowing imaging on a single breath hold, can decrease movement artefact and improve some of the body images. Flowing blood has a variable signal depending on its velocity, direction of flow and the sequence employed and therefore flow maps can be generated. The use of MR contrast agents will increase image contrast and tissue targeting may become possible.

The advantages of MRI include:

- no ionizing radiation
- superior contrast resolution compared to CT but less spatial resolution
- multiplanar imaging
- angiograms without the use of iodinated contrast.

Nuclear medicine

Tracer amounts of radiopharmaceuticals are administered to the patient and the emitted gamma rays are detected and used in conjunction with gamma cameras to produce images which reflect the distribution of the radioisotope and the carrier agent used. Tracers are used to demonstrate the normal physiology or functional changes in disease processes rather than producing detailed anatomical definition, although the use of single photon emission computerized tomography (SPECT) will improve spatial localization. The radioisotopes can also be used for therapeutic purposes (e.g. radioactive iodine).

Positron emission tomography (PET)

Cyclotrons produce isotopes which decay by positron emission. When positron decay occurs two electrons are emitted at 180° to each other and these can be imaged using a dual head rotating detector and cross-sectional images reconstructed. The positron emitting isotopes in clinical use are carbon, oxygen, nitrogen and fluorine and they can be used as physiological tracers to measure metabolic activity. They are particularly useful for assessing myocardial and cerebral function and for tumour localization.

The anatomical definition is poor but image registration with CT or MRI images is now possible with consequent improvement in localization.

Examples and further reading

Examples of the different imaging techniques described above can be seen elsewhere in the book.

For further information see Donald et al (1958), Anger and Gottschalk (1963), Kuhl and Edwards (1963), Damadian (1971), Hounsfield (1973), Lauterbur (1973), Ambrose (1973), Boyd (1983), Lee et al (1989), and Stark and Bradley (1992).

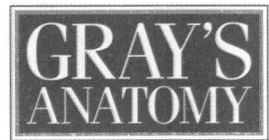

BIBLIOGRAPHY

A

Abbie A A 1933 The blood supply of the lateral geniculate body, with a note on the morphology of the choroidal arteries. J Anat 67: 491–521

Abbie A A 1934 The morphology of the fore-brain arteries, with especial reference to the evolution of the basal ganglia. J Anat 68: 433–470

Abbie A A 1950 Closure of cranial articulations in the skull of the Australian aborigine. J Anat 84: 1–12

Abbie A A 1952 A new approach to the problem of human evolution. Trans R Soc S Aust 75: 70–88

Abbott L A, Lester S M, Erickson C A 1992 Changes in mesenchymal cell-shape, matrix collagen and tenascin accompany bud formation in the early chick embryo. Anat Embryol 183: 299–311

Abdel-Maguid T E, Bowsher D 1979 Alpha and gamma-motoneurons in the adult human spinal cord and somatic cranial nerve nuclei. The significance of dendroarchitectonics studied by the Golgi method. J Comp Neurol 186: 259–270

Abdel-Maguid T E, Bowsher D 1984 Classification of neurons by dendritic branching pattern. A categorization based on Golgi impregnation of spinal and cranial somatic visceral afferent and efferent cells in the human adult. J Anat 138: 689–702

Abe J, Atsuji K, Tsunawaki A, Nishida T, Inoue T, Yamasaki F, Tasaki K, Iwanage S, Sato K 1981 Scanning electron microscopic observations of the myoepithelial cells in the prelacting and lactating mammary glands of the rat. Kurume Med J 28: 233–239

Acheson R M 1960 Effects of nutrition and disease on human growth. In: Tanner J M (ed) Human growth (Symposia of the Society for the Study of Human Biology Vol 3). Pergamon: Oxford: pp 73–92

Acker M A, Hammond R L, Mannion J D, Salmons S, Stephenson L W 1987 Skeletal muscle as the potential power source for a cardiovascular pump: assessment in vivo. Science 236: 324–327

Acsadi G, Dickson G, Love D R, Jani A, Walsh F S, Gurusinghe A, Wolff J A, Davies K E 1991 Human dystrophin expression in mdx mice after intramuscular injection of DNA constructs [and see comments]. Nature 352: 815–818

Adachi N, Hasche K 1928 Das Arteriensystem der Japaner. Vol 1. Maruzen: Kyoto

Adams C W M (ed) 1965 Neurohistochemistry. Elsevier: Amsterdam

Adams D R 1992 Fine structure of vomeronasal and septal olfactory epithelia and of glandular structures. Microsc Res Techn 23: 86–97

Adams J C 1986 Neuronal morphology in the human cochlear nucleus. Arch Otolaryngol 112: 1253–1261

Adams J C, Watt F M 1992 Regulation of development and differentiation by the extracellular matrix. Development 117: 1183–1198

Adams J, Daniel P M, Prichard M M 1969 The blood supply of the pituitary gland of the ferret with special reference to infarction after stalk section. J Anat 104: 209–225

Adams W E 1957 On the possible homologies of the occipital artery in mammals, with some remarks on the phylogeny and certain anomalies of the subclavian and carotid systems. Acta Anat 29: 90–113

Adams W E 1958 The comparative morphology of the carotid body and carotid sinus. Thomas: Springfield, Illinois

Addison C 1899–1901 On the topographical anatomy of abdominal viscera in man, especially the gastro-intestinal canal, I. J Anat 33: 565–86; II. J Anat 34: 427–450; III. J Anat 35: 166–204 and 302–304

Adelmann H B 1922 The significance of the prechordal plate: an interpretative study. Am J Anat 31: 54–101

Adelmann H B 1926 The development of the premandibular head cavities and the relations of the anterior end of the notochord in the chick and robin. J Morph 42: 371–439

Adelmann H B 1927 The development of the eye muscles in the chick. J Morph 44: 29–87

Adelstein R S 1982 Calmodulin and the regulation of the actin–myosin interaction in smooth muscle and nonmuscle cells. Cell 30: 349–350

Ades H W 1944 Midbrain auditory mechanisms in cats. J Neurophysiol 7: 415–424

Adlercreutz H 1990 Diet, breast cancer and sex hormone metabolism. Ann NY Acad Sci 595: 281–290

Afzelius B 1979 The immotile-cilia syndrome and other ciliary diseases. Int Rev Exp Pathol 19: 1–43

Afzelius B A 1976 A human syndrome caused by immotile cilia. Science 193: 317–319

Aggleton J P, Burton M J, Passingham R R 1980 Cortical and subcortical afferents to the amygdala of the rhesus monkey (Macaca mulatta). Brain Res 190: 347–368

Aghabeigi B 1992 The pathophysiology of pain. Br Dent J 173: 91–97

Agras W S, Kraemer H C, Berkowitz R I, Korner A F, Hammer L D 1987 Does a vigorous feeding style influence early development of adiposity? J Pediatr 110: 799–804

Aguayo A, Peyronnard J M, Bray G M 1973 A quantitative ultrastructural study of regeneration from isolated proximal stumps of transected unmyelinated nerves. J Neuropathol Exp Neurol 32: 256–269

Agus, D B, Surh C D, Sprent J 1991 Reentry of T cells to the adult thymus is restricted to activated T cells. J Exp Med 173: 1039–1046

Aho A 1950 On the venous network of the human heart and its arteriovenous anastomoses. Ann Med Exp Biol Fenn 29 (suppl 1): 1–90

Aird R B 1984 A study of intrathecal, cerebrospinal fluid-to-brain exchange. Exp Neurol 86: 342–358

Aitken J T, Bridger J E 1961 Neuron size and population density in lumbosacral region of the cat's spinal cord. J Anat 95: 38–53

Aitken M J 1985 Thermoluminescence dating. Academic Press: London

Aizawa H, Tanji J 1994 Corticocortical and thalamocortical responses of neurons in the monkey primary motor cortex and their relation to a trained motor task. J Neurophysiol 71: 550–560

Ajmani M L, Mittal R K, Jain S P 1983 Incidence of the metopic suture in adult Nigerian skulls. J Anat 137: 177–183

Akabas M H 1990 Mechanisms of chemosensory transduction in taste cells. Int Rev Neurobiol 32:241–79

Akaike T 1983 Neuronal organization of the vestibulospinal system in the cat. Brain Res 259: 217–227

Akbarian S, Grusser O-J, Guldin W O 1992 Thalamic connections of the vestibular cortical fields in the squirrel monkey (Saimiri sciuresis). J Comp Neurol 326: 423–441

Akelaitis A J 1942 Studies on corpus callosum; orientation (temporalspatial gnosis) following section of corpus callosum. Arch Neurol Psychiat 48: 914–937

Akert K, Pfenninger K, Sandri C, Moor H 1972 Freeze-etching and cytochemistry of vesicles and membrane complexes in synapses of the central nervous system. In: Pappas G D, Purpura D P (eds) Structure and function of synapses. Raven Press: New York: pp 67–86

Akil H, Lewis J W 1987 Neurotransmitters and pain control. Karger: Basel

Akisada T, Oda M 1978 Taste buds in the vallate papillae of the rat studied with freeze-fracture preparation. Arch Histol Jpn 41: 87–98

Akmayev I G 1971 Morphological aspects of the hypothalamic–hypophyseal system. II. Functional morphology of pituitary microcirculation. Z Zellforsch Mikroskop Anat 116: 178–194

Al-Lami F 1969 Light and electron microscopy of the adrenal medulla of Macaca mulatta monkey. Anat Rec 164: 317–332

Al-Lami F 1970 Follicular arrangements in hamster adrenomedullary cells: light and electron microscopic studies. Anat Rec 168: 161–178

Al-Yassin T M, Toner P G 1977 Fine structure of squamous epithelium and submucosal glands of human oesophagus. J Anat 123: 705–721

Albe-Fessard D, Berkley K J, Ralston H J, Willis W D 1985 Diencephalic mechanisms of pain sensation. Brain Res Rev 9: 217–296

Alberts B, Bray D, Lewis J, Raff M, Roberts K, Watson J 1994 Molecular biology of the cell. 3rd edn. Garland: New York

Alberts B, Bray D, Lewis J, Raff M, Roberts K, Watson J D 1983 Molecular biology of the cell. Garland: New York

Alberts B, Miake-Lye R 1992 Unscrambling the puzzle of biological machines: the importance of the details. Cell 68: 415–420

Albinus B S 1734 Historia musculorum hominis. Haak & Mulhovium: Leiden: pp 472–475

Albus J S 1971 A theory of cerebellar function. Math Biosci 10: 25–61

Alcolado J C, Moore I E, Weller R O 1986 Calcification in the human choroid plexus meningiomas and pineal gland. Neuropathol App Neurobiol 12: 235–250

Aldrich T K, Prezant D J 1990 Adverse effects of drugs on the respiratory muscles. Clin Chest Med 11: 177–189

Aleksandrowicz R, Gosek M, Prorok M 1974 Normal and pathologic dimensions of the abdominal aorta. Folia Morphol 33: 309–315

Alexander G E, DeLong M R, Strick P L 1986 Parallel organization of functionally segregated circuits linking basal ganglia and cortex. Ann Rev Neurosci 9: 357–382

Alexander R McN 1984 Optimum strengths for bones liable to fatigue and accidental fracture. J Theor Biol 109: 621–636

Alexander R McN 1988 Elastic mechanisms in animal movement. Cambridge University Press: Cambridge

Alexander R McN 1991 Characteristics and advantages of human bipedalism. In: Rayner J M V Wootton R J (eds) Biomechanics and evolution. Cambridge University Press: Cambridge: pp 225–266

Alexander R McN 1992 The human machine. Natural History Museum Publications: London

Alexander R McN, Jayes A S 1980 Fourier analysis of forces exerted in walking and running. J Biomech 13: 383–390

Alexander R McN, Jayes A S 1983 A dynamic similarity hypothesis for the gaits of quadrupedal mammals. J Zool 201: 135–152

Alexandre J H, Hamonet O, Lacert P, Moulin A M 1968 Arch Anat Path 16

Alheid G F, Heimer L 1988 New perspectives in basal forebrain organization of special relevance for neuropsychiatric disorders: the striatopallidal, amygdaloid and corticopetal components of the substantia innominata. Neuroscience 27: 1–39

Alheid G F, Heimer L, Switzer III, R C 1990 Basal Ganglia. In: Paxinos G (ed) The human nervous system. Academic Press: New York: pp 483–582

Ali M Y 1965a Histology of the human nasopharyngeal mucosa. J Anat 99: 657–672

Ali M Y 1965b Pathogenesis of cysts and crypts in the nasopharynx. J Laryng Otol pp 391–402

Allaerts W, Carmeliet P, Denef C 1990 New perspectives in the function of pituitary follico-stellate cells. Mol Cell Endocrinol 71: 73–81

Allaerts W, Jeucken P H, Hofland L J, Drexhage H A 1991 Morphological, immunohistochemical and functional homologies between pituitary folliculo-stellate cells and lymphoid dendritic cells. Acta Endocrinol 125 (suppl 1): 92–97

Allaerts W, Jeucken P H, Hofland L J, Drexhage H A 1991 Morphological, immunohistochemical and functional homologies between pituitary folliculo-stellate. Koninklijke Academia voor Geneeskunde van Belgie 52: 352–369

Allanson J T, Whitfield I C 1955 Third London symposium on information theory, Butterworths: London

Allbrook D 1956 Changes in lumbar vertebral body height with age. Am J Phys Anthropol 14: 35–39

Allen C, Sievers J, Berry M, Jenner S 1981 Experimental studies on cerebellar foliation. II. A morphometric analysis of cerebellar fissuration defects and growth retardation after neonatal treatment with 6-OHDA in the rat. J Comp Neurol 203: 771–783

Allen D J 1975 Scanning EM of epiplexus macrophages (Kolmer cells) in the dog. J Comp Neurol 161: 197–214

Allen L 1967 Lymphatics and lymphoid tissues. Annu Rev Physiol 29: 197–224

Allen L S, Hines M, Shryne J E, Gorski R A 1989 Two sexually dimorphic cell groups in the human brain. J Neurosci 9: 497–506

Allen L S, McClure J E, Goldstein A L, Barkley M S, Michael S D 1984 Estrogen and thymic hormone interactions in the female mouse. J Reprod Immunol 6: 25–37

Allen M, Wright P, Reid L 1972 The human lacrimal gland. A histo-chemical and organ culture study of the secreting cells. Arch Ophthalmol 88: 493–497

Allen T G J, Burnstock G 1990 A voltage-clamp study of the elec-
trophysiological characteristics of the intramural neurones of the rat trachea. J Physiol 423: 593–614

Allison P R 1951 Reflux esophagitis, sliding hiatal hernia and anatomy of repair. Surg Gynecol Obstet 92: 419–431

Allison T, Begleiter A, McCarthy G, Roessler E, Nobre A C, Spencer D D 1993 Electrophysiological studies of color processing in human visual cortex. Electroencephalogr Clin Neurophysiol 88: 343–355

Allison T, Ginter H, McCarthy G, Nobre A C, Puce A, Luby M et al 1994 Face recognition in human extrastriate cortex. J Neurophysiol 71: 821–825

Allsopp T E, Wyatt S, Paterson H F, Davies A M 1993 Cell 73: 295–307

Allwork S P 1980 Angiographis anatomy. In: Anderson R H, Becker A E (eds) Cardiac anatomy. Churchill Livingstone: Edinburgh: ch 7

Allwork S P 1986 The anatomy of the coronary arteries. In: The surgery of coronary artery disease. Chapman & Hall: London: pp 15–25

Alm P, Alumets J, Brodin E, Håakanson R, Nilsson G, Sjöberg N O, Sundler F 1978 Peptidergic (substance P) nerves in the genito-urinary tract. Neuroscience 3: 419–425

Alpern M 1969 Movements of the eyes. In: Davson H (ed) The eye. Vol 3, 2nd edition. Academic Press: New York: pp 217–254

Alpern M, Wolter J R 1956 The relation of horizontal saccadic and vergence movements. Arch Ophthalmol 56: 685–690

Altman J 1972 Postnatal development of the cerebellar cortex in the rat. II. Phases in the maturation of Purkinje cells and of the molecular layer. J Comp Neurol 145: 399–464

Altman J 1972a Postnatal development of the cerebellar cortex in the rat. I. The external germinal layer and the transitional molecular layer. J Comp Neurol 145: 353–398

Altman J 1972c Postnatal development of the cerebellar cortex in the rat. III. Maturation of the components of the granular layer. J Comp Neurol 145: 465–514

Altman J, Bayer S 1975 Postnatal development of the hippocampal dentate gyrus under normal and experimental conditions. In: Isaacson R L, Pribram K H (eds) The hippocampus. Vol 1. Plenum Press: New York: pp 95–122

Altman J, Bayer S 1978 Prenatal development of the cerebellar system in the rat. 1. Cytogenesis and histogenesis of the deep nuclei and the cortex of the cerebellum. J Comp Neurol 179: 23–48

Altman J, Bayer S A 1977 Time of origin and distribution of a new cell type in the rat cerebellar cortex. Exp Brain Res 29: 265–274

Altmann G G 1990 Renewal of the intestinal epithelium: new aspects as indicated by recent ultrastructural observations. J Electron Micr Tech 16: 2–14

Alvarez-Morujo A 1968 Terminal arteries of the penis. Acta Anat 67: 387–398

Alvesalo L, Osborne R H, Kari M 1975 The 47, XYY male, Y chromosome, and tooth size. Am J Hum Genet 27: 53–61

AMA Panel on Nuclear Magnetic Imaging of the Council on Scientific Affairs 1987 Fundamentals of magnetic resonance imaging. J Am Med Assoc 258: 3417–3423

Amann R P, Hammerstedt R H, Veermachaneni D N 1993 The epididymis and sperm maturation: a perspective. Reprod Fert Devel 5: 361–381

Amaral D G 1987 Memory: anatomical organization of candidate brain regions. In: Plum F (ed) Handbook of physiology – the nervous system V, Part 2. American Physiological Society: Washington, DC: pp 211–294

Amaral D G, Insausti R 1990 Hippocampal formation. In: Paxinos G (ed) The human nervous system. Academic Press: New York: pp 711–755

Amaral D G, Price J L Pitkänen A, Carmichael S T 1992 Anatomical organization of the primate amygdaloid complex. In: Aggleton J P (ed) The amygdala: neurobiological aspects of emotion, memory and mental dysfunction. Wiley-Liss: New York: pp 1–66

Ambache N, Zar M A 1970 Non-cholinergic transmission by post-ganglion motor neurones in the mammalian bladder. J Physiol 210: 761–783

Ambrose J 1973 Computerized transverse axial scanning (tomography). II. Clinical application. Br J Radiol 46: 1023–1047

Ambrose J A, Furster V 1983 Coronary collateral vessels and myocardial protection. J Cardiol 3: 417–420

Amenta P S, Gay S, Vaheri A, Martinez-Hernandez A 1986 The extracellular matrix is an integrated unit: ultrastructural localization of collagen types I, III, IV, V, VI, fibronectin and laminin in human term placenta. Collagen Res Rel 6: 125–152

Amis A A, Miller J H, Dowson D, Wright V 1981 Biomechanical aspects of the elbow: joint forces related to prosthesis design. Eng Med 10: 65–68

Amonoo-Kuofi H S 1982 Maximum and minimum lumbar interpedicular distances in normal adult Nigerians. J Anat 135: 225–233

Amonoo-Kuofi H S 1985 The sagittal diameter of the lumbar vertebral canal in normal adult Nigerians. J Anat 140: 69–78

Amos L A, Amos W B 1991 Molecules of the cytoskeleton. Guillford Press: New York

Amos L A, Klug A 1974 Arrangement of subunits in flagellar microtubules. J Cell Sci 14: 523–537

Amprino R 1948 Recherches et considérations sur la structure du cartilage hyalin. Acta Anat 5: 123–146

Amprino R, Bairati A 1933 Studi sulle trasformazioni delle cartilagini dell'uomo nell'accrescimento e nella senescenza: cartilagini jaline. Z Zellforsch 20: 143–205

Anbazhagan R, Bartek J, Monaghan P, Gusterson B A 1991 Growth and development of the human infant breast. Am J Anat 192: 407–417

Anberg A 1957 The ultrastructure of the human spermatozoon. Acta Obstet Gynecol Scand 36 (Suppl 2): 1–33

Andersen P, Eccles J C, Løyning Y 1964a Location of postsynaptic inhibitory synapses on hippocampal pyramids. J Neurophysiol 27: 592–607

Andersen P, Eccles J C, Schmidt R F, Yokota T 1964b Identification of relay cells and interneurons in the cuneate nucleus. J Neurophysiol 27: 1080–1095

Anderson A O, Anderson N D 1975 Studies on the structure and permeability of the microvasculature in normal rat lymph nodes. Am J Pathol 80: 387–418

Anderson A O, Anderson N D 1976 Lymphocyte emigration from high endothelial venules in rat lymph nodes. Immunology 31: 731–748

Anderson C, Devine W A, Anderson R H, Debich D E, Zuberbuhler J R 1990 Abnormalities of the spleen in relation to congenital malformations of the heart: a survey of necropsy findings in children. Br Heart J 63: 122–128

Anderson D J 1989 The neural crest cell lineage problem: neuropoiesis? Neuron 3: 1–12

Anderson D J, Hannam A G, Matthews B 1970 Sensory mechanisms in mammalian teeth and their supporting structures. Physiol Rev 50: 171–195

Anderson D J, Matthews B 1967 Osmotic stimulation of human dentine and the distribution of dental pain thresholds. Arch Oral Biol 12: 417–426

Anderson D R, Hoyt W 1969 Ultrastructure of intraorbital portion of human and monkey optic nerve. Arch Ophthal 82: 506–530

Anderson E, Albertini D F 1976 Gap junctions between the oocyte and the companion granulosa cells in the mammalian ovary. J Cell Biol 71: 680–686

Anderson E, Beams H W 1960 Cytological observations on the fine structure of the guinea pig ovary with special reference to the ooronium, primary oocyte and associated follicle cells. J Ultrastruct Res 3: 432–446

Anderson H C 1990 The role of cells versus matrix in bone induction. Connect Tissue Res 24: 3–12

Anderson H C, Morris D C 1993 Mineralization. In: Mundy G R, Martin T J (eds) Physiology and pharmacology of bone. Springer-Verlag: Berlin: pp 267–298

Anderson H, Bulow F A von, Møllgård K 1970 The histochemical and ultrastructural bases of the cellular function of the human foetal adenohypophysis. Prog Histochem Cytochem 1: 153–184

Anderson J C, Martin K A C, Whitteridge D 1993 Form, function, and intracortical projections of neurons in the striate cortex of the monkey Macacus nemestrinus. Cereb Cortex 3: 412–420

Anderson M, Hwang S C, Green W T 1965 Growth of the normal trunk in boys and girls during the second decade of life. J Bone Jt Surg 47A: 1554–1564

Anderson R H, Becker A E 1980 Cardiac anatomy: an integrated text and colour atlas. Gower Medical: London

Anderson R H, Becker A E, Brechenmacher C, Davies M J, Rossi L 1975 The human atrioventricular junctional area: a morphological study of the A-V node and bundle. Eur J Cardiol 3: 11–25

Anderson R H, Wilkinson J L, Arnold R, Lubkiewicz K 1974 Morphogenesis of bulboventricular anomalies. (1) Consideration of embryogenesis in the normal heart. Br Heart J 36: 242–256

Anderson R H, Wilkinson J L, Becker A E (1978) The bulbus cordis – a misunderstood region of the developing human heart: its significance to the classification of congenital cardiac malformations. Birth Defects 14: 1–28

Anderson R L, Dixon R S 1979 The role of Whitnall's ligament in ptosis surgery. Arch Ophthalmol 97: 705–707

Anderson S et al 1981 Sequence and organization of the human mitochondrial genome. Nature 290: 457–465

Andreassi G 1967 Sur la topographie de l'apex pulmonaire chez l'homme. C R Assoc Anat 137: 141–147

Andres K H 1966 Der feinbau der Regio olfactoria von Makrosmatikern. Z Zellforsch 69: 140–154

Andres K H 1967 Über die Feinstruktur der Arachnoidea und Dura mater von Mammalia. Z Zellforsch Mikrosk Anat 79: 272–295

Andressen C, Blümcke I, Celio M R 1993 Calcium-binding proteins: selective markers of nerve cells. Cell Tiss Res 271: 181–208

Andrew A 1971 The origin of intramural ganglia. 4. The origin or enteric ganglia; a critical review and discussion of the present state of the problem. J Anat 108: 169–184

Andrew A 1982 The APUD concept: where has it led us? Br Med Bull 38: 221–225

Andrew A, Kramer B, Rawden B B 1982 The embryonic origin of endocrine cells of the gastrointestinal tract. Gen Comp Endocrinol 47: 249–265

Andrews P 1992 Evolution and environment in the Hominoidea. Nature 360: 641–646 (erratum also in Nature 361: 564)

Andrews P M 1994 The histopathology of kidney uriniferous tubules as revealed by noninvasive confocal vital microscopy. Scanning 16: 174–181

Andy O J, Stephan H 1968 The septum in the human brain. J Comp Neurol 133: 383–410

Angaut P, Brodal A 1967 The projection of the 'vestibulocerebellum' into the vestibular nuclei in the cat. Arch Ital Biol 105: 441–479

Angaut P, Repérant J 1976 Fine structure of the optic fibre termination layers in the pigeon optic tectum. Neuroscience I: 93–105

Angell J C 1969 Treatment of benign prostatic hyperplasia by phenol injection. Br J Urol 41: 735–738

Angelman H 1965 'Puppet children' A report of three cases. Develop. Med Child Neurol 7: 681–688

Anger H O, Gottschalk A 1963 Localisation of brain tumours with the positron scintillation camera. J Nucl Med 4: 326–330

Angevine J B Jr 1975 Development of the hippocampal region. In: Isaacson R L, Pribram K (eds) The hippocampus vol 1. Structure and Development. Plenum Press: New York: pp 61–94

Anhelt P, Keri C, Kolb H 1990 Identification of pedicles of putative blue sensitive cones in the human retina. J Comp Neurol 293:39–53

Anholt R R H 1989 Molecular physiology of olfaction. Amer J Physiol 257: C1043–C1054

Annett M 1991 Laterality and cerebral dominance. J Child Psychol Psychiatry 32: 219–232

Annis D 1962 A study of the regenerative ability of the epithelial lining of the urinary bladder. Ann R Coll Surg 31: 23–45

Anonymous 1949 Recherches sur la coagulation therapeutique des structures sous-corticale chez l'homme. Rev Neurol (Paris) 81: 4–24

Anson B H 1963 The aortic arch and its branches. In: Luisada A (ed) Cardiology Vol I. McGraw-Hill: New York: p 119

Anson B J, Beaton L E, McVay C B 1938 Pyramidalis muscle. Anat Rec 72: 405–411

Anson B J, Jamieson R W, O'Connor V J, Beaton L E 1953 The pectoral muscles. Q Bull North West Univ Med Sch 27: 211–218

Anson B J, Morgan E H, McVay C B 1960 Surgical anatomy of the inguinal region based upon a study of 500 body-halves. Surg Gynecol Obstet 111: 707–725

Apgar V 1953 Proposal for a new method of evaluation of newborn infants. Anaes Anal 32: 260–267

Apkarian A V, Hodge C J 1989a Primate spinothalamic pathways. I. A quantitative study of the cells of origin of the spinothalamic pathway. J Comp Neurol 288: 447–473

Apkarian A V, Hodge C J 1989b Primate spinothalamic pathways. II. The cells of origin of the dorsolateral and ventral spinothalamic pathways. J Comp Neurol 288: 474–492

Apkarian A V, Hodge C J 1989c Primate spinothalamic pathways. III. Thalamic termination of the dorsolateral and ventral spinothalamic pathways. J Comp Neurol 288: 493–511

Aplin J D 1989 Cellular biochemistry of the endometrium. In: Wynn R M, Jollie W P (eds) Biology of the uterus. Plenum Press: New York: pp 89–129

Aplin J D 1991a Glycans as biochemical markers of human endometrial secretory differentiation. J Reprod Fertil 91: 525–541

Aplin J D 1991b Implantation, trophoblast differentiation and haemochorial placentation: mechanistic evidence in vivo and in vitro. J Cell Sci 99: 681–692

Aplin J D, Campbell S 1985 An immunofluorescence study of extracellular matrix associated with cytotrophoblast of the chorion laeve. Placenta 6: 469–479

Aplin J D, Campbell S, Allen T D 1985 The extracellular matrix of human amniotic epithelium: ultrastructure, composition and deposition. J Cell Sci 79: 119–136

Aplin J D, Campbell S, Donnai P, Bard J B L, Allen T D 1986 Importance of vitamin C in maintenance of the normal amnion: an experimental study. Placenta 7: 377–390

Aplin J D, Charlton A K, Ayad S 1988 An immunohistochemical study of human endometrial extracellular matrix during the menstrual cycle and first trimester of pregnancy. Cell Tissue Res 253: 235–240

Aplin J D, Jones C J P 1989 Extracellular matrix in endometrium and decidua. In: Genbacev A, Klopper A, Beaconsfield R (eds) Placenta as a model and source. Plenum Press: New York: pp 115–128

Applebaum A E, Beall J E, Foreman R D, Willis W D 1975 Organization and receptive fields of primate spinothalamic tract neurons. J Neurophysiol 38: 572–586

Appleton A B 1922 On the hypotrochanteric fossa and accessory adductor groove of the primate femur. J Anat 56: 295–306

Appleton A B 1934 Postural deformities and bone growth; experimental study. Lancet 1: 451–454

Arai Y, Mori T, Suzuki Y, Bern H A Long-term effects of perinatal exposure to sex steroids and diethylstilbestrol on the reproductive system of male mammals. Int Rev Cytol 84: 235–268

Arakawa M, Tokunaga J 1974 Further scanning electron microscope studies of the human glomerulus. Lab Invest 31: 436–440

Arbab M A R, Wiklund L, Svendgaard N A 1986 Origin and distribution of cerebral vascular innervation from superior cervical, trigeminal and spinal ganglia, investigated with retrograde and anterograde WGA-HRP tracing in the rat. Neurosci 19(3): 695–707

Arbuthnott E R, Ballard K J, Boyd I A, Gladden M H, Sutherland F I 1982 The ultrastructure of cat fusimotor endings and their relationship to foci of sarcomere convergence in intrafusal fibres. J Physiol 331: 285–309

Arendt-Nielson L, Zwarts M J 1989 Measurement of muscle fiber conduction velocity in humans: techniques and applications. J Clin Neurophysiol 6: 173–190

Arey L B 1949 The craniopharyngeal canal re-interpreted on the basis of its development. Anat Rec 103: 420

Argème M, Mambrini A, Lebreuil G et al 1970 Dissection du muscle de Treitz. C R Assoc Anat 147: 76–86

Argiolas A, Gessa G L, Melis M R, Stancampiano R, Vaccari A 1990b Effects of neonatal and adult thyroid dysfunction on thymic oxytocin. Neuroendocrinol 52: 556–559

Argiolas A, Melis M R, Stancampiano R, Mauri A, Gessa, G L 1990a Hypothalamic modulation of immunoreactive oxytocin in the rat thymus. Peptides 1: 539–543

Arikuni T, Watanabe K, Kubota K 1988 Connections of area 8 with area 6 in the brain of the macaque monkey. J Comp Neurol 277: 21–40

Armenta E, Fisher J 1984 Anatomy of flexor pollicis longus vinculum system. J Hand Surg 9(2): 210–212

Armstrong E 1990 Limbic thalamus: anterior and mediodorsal nuclei. In: Paxinos G (ed) The human nervous system. Academic Press: San Diego: pp 469–481

Armstrong J, Richardson K C, Young J Z 1956 Staining neural end feet and mitochondria after postchroming and carbowax embedding. Stain Technol 31: 261–270

Arnesen A R 1984 Fibre population of the vestibulocochlear anastomosis in humans. Acta Otolaryngol 98: 501–518

Arnold F 1851 Handbuch der Anatomie des Menschen, Vol 2. Emmerling und Herder: Freiburg

Arnold G L, Bixler D, Girod D 1983 Probable autosomal recessive inheritance of polysplenia, situs inversus and cardiac defects in an Amish family. Am J Med Genet 16: 35–42

Arnold J 1865 Ueber die Struktur des Ganglion intercaroticum. Virch Arch f Path Anat 33: 190–209

Arnstein K 1889 Über die Nerven der Schweissdrüsen. Anat Anz 4: 378–383

Arnstein K 1895 Zur Morphologie der sekretorischen Neverendapparate. Anat Anz 10: 410–419

Arrenbrecht S 1974 Specific binding of growth hormone to thymocytes. Nature 252: 255–257

Arsenault A L 1989 A comparative electron microscopic study of apatite crystals in collagen fibrils of rat bone, dentine and calcified turkey leg tendons. Bone Miner 6: 165–177

Arsenieva N A, Dubinin N P, Orlova N N, Bakulina E D 1961 A radiation analysis of the duration of meiosis phases in the spermatogenesis of Macaca mulatta. Dokl Akad Nauk S S R 141: 1486–1490

Arslan M 1960 The innervation of the middle ear. Proc R Soc Med 53: 1068–1074

Arthias M 1897 Recherches sur l'histogénèse de L'écorce du cervelet. J Anat Physiol 33: 372–404

Arutinov A I, Baron M A, Majorova N A 1974 The role of mechanical factors in the pathogenesis of short-term and prolonged spasm of the cerebral arteries. J Neurosurg 40: 459–472

Arvis G 1969 Considérations anatomiques sur le hile et le sinus du rein. Ann Radiol 12: 75–106

Asbury A K, Aldridge H, Hirshberg R, Fisher C M 1970 Oculomotor palsy in diabetes mellitus. A clinico-pathological study. Brain 43: 555–566

Ascenzi A, Bell G H 1972 Bone as a mechanical and engineering problem. In: Bourne G H (ed) The biochemistry and physiology of bone. 2nd edition. Academic Press: London

Ascenzi A, Bonucci E 1968 The compressive properties of single osteons. Anat Rec 161: 377–392

Ascenzi A, Bonucci E, Ripamonti A, Roveri N 1978 X-ray diffraction and electron microscope study of osteons during calcification. Calcif Tissue Res 25: 133–143

Ash P, Loutit J F, Townsend K M 1980 Osteoclasts derived from haematopoietic stem cells. Nature 283: 669–670

Ash P, Loutit J F, Townsend K M S 1981 Osteoclasts derive from haemopoietic stem cells according to marker, giant lysosomes of beige mice. Clin Orthop 155: 249–258

Ashley G T 1952 The manner of insertion of the pectoralis major muscle in man. Anat Rec 113: 301–308

Ashley G T 1954 Morphological and pathological significance of synostoses at the manubrio-sternal joint. Thorax 9: 159–166

Ashley G T 1956 The relationship between the pattern of ossification and the definitive shape of the mesosternum in man. J Anat 90: 87–105

Ashton E H, Moore W J 1980 Cranial shape in the hominoidea – exploratory considerations. J Anat 131: 744–745

Ashton E H, Moore W J, Spence T F 1976 Growth changes in endocranial capacity in the cercopithecoidea and hominoidea. J Zool 180: 355–365

Aspden R M, Hukins D W L 1979 The lamina splendens of articular cartilage is an artefact of phase contrast microscopy. Proc R Soc Lond [Biol] 206: 109–113

Assali N S, Rauramo L, Peltonen T 1960 Measurement of uterine blood flow and uterine metabolism. VIII. Uterine and fetal blood flow and oxygen consumption in early human pregnancy. Am J Obstet Gynecol 79: 86–98

Assia E I, Apple D J, Morgan R C, Legler U F, Brown S J 1991 The relationship between the stretching capability of the anterior capsule and zonules. Invest Ophthalmol Vis Sci 32: 2835–2839

Assoian R K 1988 The role of growth factors in tissue repair. IV. Type b-transforming growth factor and stimulation of fibrosis. In: Clark R A F, Henson P M (eds) The molecular and cellular biology of wound repair. Plenum Press: New York: pp 273–280

Ataya K M, Sakr W, Blacker C M, Mutchnick M G, Latif Z A 1989 Effect of GnRH agonists on the thymus in female rats. Acta Endocrinol (Copen) 121: 833–840

Atchley W R, Hall B K 1991 A model for development and evolution of complex morphological structures. Biol Rev 66: 101–157

Ateshian G A, Rosenwasser M P, Mow V C 1992 Curvature characteristics and congruence of the thumb carpometacarpal joint: differences between female and male joints. J Biomech 25: 591–607

Atkins V P, Bealer S L 1993 Hypothalamic histamine release, neuroendocrine and cardiovascular responses during tuberomammillary nucleus stimulation in the conscious rat. Neuroendocrinology 57: 849–855

Atkinson M, Edwards D A, Honour A J, Rowlands E N 1957 Comparison of cardiac and pyloric sphincters: a manometric study. Lancet 2: 918–922

Atkinson P J, Hallsworth A S 1982 The spatial structure of bone. In: Harrison R J, Navaratum V (eds) Progress in anatomy. Vol 2. Cambridge University Press: Cambridge: pp 179–199

Attah A A, Hutson J M 1991 The anatomy of the female gubernaculum is different from the male. Aust NZ J Surg 61: 380–384

Attardi G, Schatz G 1988 Biogenesis of mitochondria. Annu Rev Cell Biol 4: 289–333

Attenborough D 1979 Life on Earth. Collins: London

Aubier M 1993 Respiratory muscles; working or wasting. Intensive Care Med 19 (suppl 2): S64–68

Audinat E, Gähwiler B H, Knöpfel T 1992 Excitatory synaptic potentials in neurons of the deep nuclei in olivo-cerebellar slice cultures. Neuroscience 49: 903–911

Auerbach R 1960 Morphogenetic interactions in the development of the mouse thymus gland. Dev Biol 2: 271–284

Auerbach R 1961 Experimental analysis of the origin of cell types in the development of the mouse thymus. Dev Biol 3: 336–354

Ault J G, Rieder C L 1994 Centrosome and kinetochore movement during mitosis. Curr Opin Cell Biol 6: 41–49

Aumuller G 1991 Postnatal development of the prostate. Bull Assoc Anatomistes 75: 39–42

Aumuller G, Riva A 1992 Morphology and functions of the human seminal vesicle. Andrologia 24: 183–196

Ausprunk D H, Folkman J 1977 Migration and proliferation of endothelial cells in preformed and newly formed blood vessels during tumor angiogenesis. Microvascular Res 14: 53–65

Austin C P, Cepko C L 1990 Development 110: 713–732

Austin C R 1951 Observations on the penetration of the sperm into the mammalian egg. Aust J Sci Res Ser B 4: 581–596

Austin C R 1963 Fertilization and transport of the ovum. In: Hartman C G (ed) Mechanisms concerned with conception. Pergamon Press: Oxford: pp 285–320

Austin C R, Bishop M W H 1958 Some features of the acrosome and perforatorium in mammalian spermatozoa. Proc R Soc Lond [Biol] 149: 234–240

Austin C R, Walton A 1960 Fertilisation. In: parkes A S (ed) Marshall's physiology of reproduction. 3rd edition Vol 1 Part 2. Longmans: London: pp 310–416

Axelsson A 1968 The vascular anatomy of the cochlea in the guinea pig and in man. Acta Otolaryngol Suppl 243: 3

Axelsson A, Ryan A F 1988 Circulation of the inner ear: I. Comparative study of the vascular anatomy in the mammalian cochlea. In: Jahn A F, Santos-Sacchi J (eds) Physiology of the ear. Raven Press: New York: pp 295–315

Axelsson S, Björklund A, Falck B et al 1973 Glyoxylic acid condensation: a new fluorescence method for the histochemical demonstration of biogenic monoamines. Acta Physiol Scand 87: 57–62

Ayers M M, Jeffrey P K 1988 Proliferation and differentiation in airway epithelium. Eur Respir J 1: 58–80

Azar Y, Eyal-Giladi H 1979 Marginal zone cells – the primitive streak inducing component of the primary hypoblast in the chick. J Embryol Exp Morphol 52: 79–88

Azar Y, Eyal-Giladi H 1981 Interaction of epiblast and hypoblast in the formation of the primitive streak and the embryonic axis in chick, as revealed by hypoblast rotation experiments. J Embryol Exp Morphol 61: 133–141

Azaz B, Lustmann J 1973 Anatomical configurations in dry mandibles. Br J Oral Surg 11: 1–9

Azim M, Surani H 1986 Evidences and consequences of differences between maternal and paternal genomes during embryogenesis in the mouse. In: Rossant J, Pedersen R A (eds) Experimental approaches to mammalian embryonic development. Cambridge University Press: Cambridge: pp 402–435

Azizi S A, Burne R A, Woodward D J 1985 The auditory cortico-ponto-cerebellar projection in the rat: inputs to the paraflocculus and mid vermis. An anatomical and physiological study. Exp Brain Res 54: 36–49

Azizkhan R G, Azizkhan J C, Zetter B R, Folkman J 1980 Mast cell heparin stimulates migration of capillary endothelial cells in vitro. J Exp Med 152: 931–944

B

Baca M, Zamboni L 1967 The fine structure of human follicular oocytes. J Ultrastruct Res 19: 354–381

Bach B R, Bush-Joseph C 1992 The surgical approach to lateral meniscal repair. Arthroscopy 8: 269–273

Bachmann G 1916 The inter-auricular time interval. Am J Physiol 41: 309–320

Backhouse K M 1964 The gubernaculum testis Hunteri: testicular descent and maldescent. Ann R Coll Surg Engl 35: 15–33

Backhouse K M, Butler H 1960 The gubernaculum testis of the pig. (Sus scorpha) J Anat 94: 107–120

Backhouse K M, Catton W T 1952 Observations on the function of the lumbrical muscles of the hand. J Anat 86: 472–498

Bacon G E, Bacon P J, Griffiths R K 1984 A neutron diffraction study of the bones of the foot. J Anat 139: 265–273

Bacon G E, Griffiths R K 1985 Texture stress and age in the human femur. J Anat 143: 97–101

Bada J L 1985 Amino acid racemization dating of fossil bones. Ann Rev Earth Planet Sci 13: 241–268

Baden H 1970 The physical properties of nail. J Invest Dermatol 55: 115–122

Baden H 1990 Hair keratin. In: Orfanos C E, Happle R (eds) Hair and hair diseases. Springer: Berlin: pp 41–71

Baer K E von 1828 Entwicklingsgeschichte der Thiere: Beobachtung und Reflexion. Konigserg: Bontrager

Baetens D, De Mey J, Gepts W 1977 Immunohistochemical and ultra-structural identification of the pancreatic polypeptide-producing (PP-cell) in the human pancreas. Cell Tissue Res 185: 239–246

Bagnall K M, Harris P F, Jones P R M 1977a A radiographic study of the human fetal spine. I. The development of the secondary cervical curvature. J Anat 123: 777–782

Bagnall K M, Harris P F, Jones P R M 1977b A radiographic study of the human fetal spine. II. The sequence of development of ossification centres in the vertebral column. J Anat 124: 791–802

Bagnall K M, Higgins S J, Sanders E J 1988 The contribution made by a single somite to the vertebral column: experimental evidence in support of resegmentation using the chick–quail chimaera model. Development 103: 69–85

Baichwal R R, Bigbee J W, DeVries G H 1988 Macrophage-mediated myelin-related mitogenic factor for cultured Schwann cells. Proc Nat Acad Sci USA 85: 1701–1705

Bailey H 1947 Parotidectomy; indications and results. Br Med J 1: 404–407

Bainton D 1981 The discovery of lysosomes. J. Cell Biol 91: 66s–76s

Bainton D, Ullyot J L, Farquhar M G 1971 The development of neutrophilic polymorphonuclear leukocytes in human bone marrow. Origin and content of azurophil and specific granules. J Exp Med 134: 907–934

Baird D T 1977 Synthesis and secretion of steroid hormones by the ovary in vivo. In: Zuckerman S, Weir B J (eds) The ovary. 2nd edition. Academic Press: London: p 305

Baizer J S, Desimone R, Ungerleider L G 1993 Comparison of subcortical connections of inferior temporal and posterior parietal cortex in monkeys. Visual Neurosci 10: 59–72

Baizer J S, Ungerleider L G, Desimone R 1991 Organization of visual inputs to the inferior temporal and posterior parietal cortex in macaques. J Neurosci 11: 168–190

Bajo V M, Merchan M A, Lopex D E, Rouiller E R 1993 Neuronal morphology and efferent projections of the dorsal nucleus of the lateral lemniscus in the rat. J Comp Neurol 334: 241–262

Baker J, Gibson A, Mower G, Robinson F, Glickstein M 1983 Cat visual corticopontine cells project to the superior colliculus. Brain Res 265: 222–232

Baker T G 1963 A quantitative and cytological study of germ cells in human ovaries. Proc R Soc London Ser B 158: 417–433

Baker T G 1972 Oogenesis and ovarian development. In: Balin H, Glasser C (eds) Reproductive biology, Vol 1. Excerpta Medica: Amsterdam

Baker T G 1982 Germ cells and oogenesis. In: Austin C R, Short R V (eds) Germ cells and fertilization. Reproduction in mammals series. 2nd edition. Cambridge University Press: Cambridge: pp 17–45

Baker T G, Franchi L L, Wai Sum O 1991 The ovary: development and structure.

Balboni Q C 1972 Distribuzione del reticolo terminale adrenergico nell'ovaio. Boll Soc Ital Biol Sper 48: 84–86

Baldwin C T, Hoth H F, Amos J A, da-Silva E O, Milunsky A 1992 An exonic mutation in the HuP2 paired domain gene causes Waardenburg's Syndrome. Nature 355: 637–638

Balfour F M 1888 Comparative embryology, Vol 2. Macmillan: London

Balin A K, Kligman A M (eds) 1989 Ageing and the skin. Raven Press: New York

Balinsky B I 1981 An introduction to embryology. 5th edition. Saunders: Philadelphia

Ballard J L, Novack K K, Driver M 1979 A simplified score for assessment of fetal maturation of newly born infants. J Pediatr 95: 769–774

Ballie M D 1992 Development of the endocrine function of the kidney. Renal function and disease. Clinic Perinatol 19: 59–68

Baló J 1950 The dural venous sinuses. Anat Rec 106: 319–326

Balthazar E J, Gade M 1976 The normal and abnormal development of the appendix. Radiology 121: 599–604

Banati R, Gehrmann J Schubert P, Kreutzberg G W 1993 Cytotoxicity of microglia. Glia 7: 111 – 118

Bandman E 1985 Myosin isozyme transitions during muscle development, maturation and disease. Int Rev Cytol 97: 97–131

Bandman E 1992 Contractile protein isoforms in muscle development. Dev Biol 154: 273–283

Bangham A D 1987 Lung surfactant: how it does and does not work. Lung 165(1): 17–25

Banks A R 1988 The role of growth factors in tissue repair. II. Epidermal growth factor. In: Clark R A F, Henson P M (eds) The molecular and cellular biology of wound repair. Plenum Press: New York: pp 260–265

Banks M S, Bennett P J 1988 Optical and photoreceptor immaturities limit the spatial and chromatic vision of human neonates. J Optical Soc A 5: 2059–2079

Banks R W, Barker D, Harker D W, Stacey M J 1975 Correlation between ultrastructure and histochemistry of mammalian intrafusal muscle fibres. J Physiol 252: 16P–17P

Bannerjee S D, Cohn R H, Bernfield M R 1977 Basal lamina of embryonic salivary epithelia. Production by the epithelium and role in maintaining lobular morphology. J Cell Biol 73: 445–463

Bannister L H 1976 Sensory terminals of peripheral nerves. In: Landon D N (ed) The peripheral nerve. Chapman & Hall: London: pp 396–463

Bannister L H, Dodson H C 1992 Endocytic pathways in the olfactory and vomeronasal epithelia of the mouse: ultrastructure and uptake of tracers. Microsc Res Techn 23: 128–141

Bannister R, Matthias C J (eds) 1992 Autonomic failure: a textbook of clinical disorders of the autonomic nervous system. 3rd edition. Oxford University Press: Oxford

Bär A, Pette D 1988 Three fast myosin heavy chains in adult rat skeletal muscle. FEBS Lett 235: 153–155

Bär Th, Güldner F H, Wolff J R 1984 'Seamless' endothelial cells of blood capillaries. Cell Tissue Res 235: 99–106

Baragar F A, Osborn J W 1984 A model relating patterns of human jaw movement to biomechanical constraints. J Biomech 17: 757–767

Barajas L 1970 The ultrastructure of the juxtaglomerular apparatus as disclosed by three-dimensional reconstructions from seriel sections. The anatomical relationship between the tubular and vascular components. J Ultrastruct Res 33: 116–147

Barajas-Lopez C, Berezin I, Daniel E E, Huizinga J D 1989 Pacemaker activity recorded in interstitial cells of Cajal of the gastrointestinal tract. Am J Physiol 257: C830–833

Baran R, Dawbar R P R, Levene G M 1991 A colour atlas of the hair, scalp, and nails. Wolfe: London

Bárány M 1967 ATPase activity of myosin correlated with speed of muscle shortening. J Gen Physiol 50: 197–218

Barbas H, Haswell Henion T H, Dermon C R 1991 Diverse thalamic projections to the prefrontal cortex in the rhesus monkey. J Comp Neurol 313: 65–94

Barbas H, Pandya D N 1989 Architecture and intrinsic connections of the prefrontal cortex in the rhesus monkey. J Comp Neurol 286: 353–375

Barbe M F, Levitt P 1991 J Neurosci 11: 519–533

Barbenel J C 1972 The biomechanics of the temporo mandibular joint. J Biomech 5: 251–256

Barbenel J C 1974 The mechanics of the temporomandibular joint – a theoretical and electromyographical study. J Oral Rehabil 1: 19–27

Barber P C, Raisman G 1978 Cell division in the vomeronasal organ of the adult mouse. Brain Res 141: 57–66

Barclay A E 1936 The digestive tract. Cambridge University Press: London

Barclay A E, Barcroft J, Barron D H, Franklin K J 1939 A radiographic demonstration of the circulation through the heart in the adult and in the fetus and the identification of the ductus arteriosus. Br J Radiol 12: 505–517

Barclay A E, Franklin K J, Prichard M M L 1942 Further data about circulation and about the cardiovascular system before and just after birth. Br J Radiol 15: 249–256

Barclay C J, Constable J K, Gibbs C L 1993 Energetics of fast- and slow-twitch muscles of the mouse. J Physiol 472: 61–80

Barclay-Smith E 1896 The astragalo-calcaneo-navicular joint. J Anat 30: 390–412

Barcroft J 1941 Four phases of birth. Lancet 2: 91–95

Bard J 1990 Morphogenesis: The cellular and molecular processes of developmental anatomy. Cambridge University Press: Cambridge

Bard J 1991 Epithelial rearrangements and Drosophila gastrulation. Bio Essays 13: 409–411

Bard J B L 1990 Morphogenesis. Cambridge University Press: Cambridge

Bard J B L, Wolff A S 1992 Nephrogenesis and the development of renal disease. Nephrol Dial Transplant 7: 563–572

Bard P, Rioch D McK 1937 A study of four cats deprived of neocortex and additional portions of the forebrain. Bull Johns Hopkins Hosp 60: 73–147

Barden N, Lavole M, Dupont A et al 1977 Stimulation of glucogen release by addition of anti-somatostatin serum to islets of Langerhans in vitro. Endocrinology 101: 635–638

Bargmann W 1949 Über die Neurosekretorische Verknupfung von Hypothalamus und Neurohypophyse. Z Zellforsch 34: 610–634

Bargmann W 1966 Neurosecretion. Int Rec Cytol 19: 183–201

Bargmann W, Schadé J P (eds) 1963 The rhinencephalon and related structures. Prog Brain Res 3

Barker A T, Lunt M J 1983 The effects of pulsed magnetic fields of the type used in the stimulation of bone fracture healing. Clin Phys Physiol Meas 4: 1–27

Barker D 1974a Morphology of muscle receptors. In: Hunt C C (ed) Handbook of sensory physiology. Vol 3 pt 2. Springer: Berlin: pp 191–234

Barker D 1974b The motor innervation of muscle spindles. In: Bellaris R, Gray E G (eds) Essays on the nervous-system. Clarendon Press: Oxford: pp 131–154

Barker D J P (ed) 1992 Fetal and infant origins of adult disease. BMJ: London

Barker D J P, Gluckman P D, Godfrey K M, Harding J E, Owens J A, Robinson J S 1993 Fetal nutrition and cardiovascular disease in adult life. Lancet 341: 938–941

Barker D J P, Hales C N, Fall C H D, Osmond C, Phipps K, Clark P M S 1993 Type 2 (non-insulin-dependent) diabetes mellitus, hypertension and hyperlipidaemia (syndrome X): relation to reduced fetal growth. Diabetologia 36: 62–67

Barker D J P, Osmond C, Simmonds S J, Wield G A 1993 The relation of head size and thinness at birth to death from cardiovascular disease in adult life. BMJ 306: 422–426

Barker D S 1967 The dendritic cell system in human gingival epithelium. Arch Oral Biol 12: 203–208

Barland P, Novikoff A B, Hamerman D 1962 Electron microscopy of the human synovial membrane. J Cell Biol 14: 207–220

Barlow H B 1952 Eye movements during fixation. J Physiol 116: 290–306

Barlow T E, Bentley F H, Walder D N 1951 Arteries veins and arteriovenous anastromoses in the human stomach. Surg Gynecol Obstet 93: 657–671

Barlow T E, Haigh A L, Walder D N 1961 Evidence for two vascular pathways in skeletal muscle. Clin Sci 20: 367–385

Barmack N H, Baughman R W, Eckenstein F P 1992a Cholinergic innervation of the cerebellum of rat, rabbit, cat, and monkey as revealed by choline acetyltransferase activity and immunohistochemistry. J Comp Neurol 317: 233–249

Barmack N H, Baughman R W, Eckenstein F P, Shojaku H 1992b Secondary vestibular cholinergic projection to the cerebellum of rabbit and rat as revealed by choline acetyltransferase immunohistochemistry, retrograde and orthograde tracers. J Comp Neurol 317: 250–270

Barnard J W 1940 The hypoglossal complex of vertebrates. J Comp Neurol 72: 489–524

Barnard J W, Woolsey C N 1956 A study of localisation in the corticospinal tracts of monkey and rat. J Comp Neurol 105: 25–50

Barnes B G 1961 Ciliated secretory cells in the pars distalis of the mouse hypophysis. J Ultrastruct Res 5: 453–467

Barnes C L, Pandya D N 1992 Efferent cortical connections of multimodal cortex of the superior temporal sulcus in the rhesus monkey. J Comp Neurol 318: 222–224

Barnes G R G, Pinder D N 1974 In vivo tendon tension and bone strain measurement and correlation. J Biomech 7: 35–42

Barnes H A 1923 The tonsils:faucal, lingual and pharyngeal. 2nd edn. Henry Kimpton: London

Barnett C H 1952 Locking at the knee joint. J Anat 86: 485P

Barnett C H 1954 Comparison of human knee and avian ankle. J Anat 88: 59–70

Barnett C H 1962 Valgus deviation of the distal phalanx of the great toe. J Anat 96: 171–177

Barnett C H, Davies D V, MacConaill M A 1961 Synovial joints. Their structure and mechanics. Longman: London

Barnett C H, Lewis O J 1958 The evolution of some traction epiphyses in birds and mammals. J Anat 92: 593–607

Barnett C H, Napier J R 1952 The axis of rotation at the ankle joint in man. Its influence upon the form of the talus and the mobility of the fibula. J Anat 86: 1–9

Baroffio A, Dupin E, Le Douarin N M 1988 Clone-forming ability and differentiation potential of migratory neural crest cells. Proc Natl Acad Sci USA 85: 5325–5329

Baroldi G, Mantero O, Scomazzoni G 1956 The collaterals of the coronary arteries in normal and pathologic hearts. Circ Res 4: 223–229

Baroldi G, Scomazzoni G 1967 Coronary circulation in the normal and the pathologic heart. Office of the Surgeon General: Washington DC

Baron R, Chakraborty M, Chatterjee D, Horne W, Lomri A, Ravensloot J-H 1993 Biology of the osteoclast. In: Mundy G R, Martin T J (eds) Physiology and pharmacology of bone. Springer-Verlag: Berlin: pp 111–147

Barr E, Leiden J M 1991 Systemic delivery of recombinant proteins by genetically modified myoblasts. Science 254: 1507–1509

Barr M L, Bertram E G 1949 A morphological distinction between neurones of the male and female, and the behaviour of the nucleolar satellite during accelerated nucleoprotein synthesis. Nature 163: 676–678

Barres B A 1991 Five electrophysiological properties of glial cells. Ann NY Acad Sci 663: 248–254

Barres B A, Raff M C 1993 Proliferation of oligodendrocyte precursor cells depends on electrical activity in axons. Nature 361: 258–260

Barrett W C 1951 A note of the internal cremaster muscle. Anat Rec 109: 392(a)

Barrow M V 1971 A brief history of teratology to the early 20th century. Teratology 4: 119–130

Barry A 1951 The aortic arch derivatives in the human adult. Anat Rec 111: 221–238

Barson A J 1970 The vertebral level of termination of the spinal cord during normal and abnormal development. J Anat 106: 489–497

Barson A J, Sands J 1977 Regional and segmental characteristics of the human adult spinal cord. J Anat 123: 797–803

Bartelmez G W, Dekaban A S 1962 The early development of the human brain. Contrib Embryol Carnegie Inst Washington 37: 13–32

Barth M, Tongio J, Warter P 1976 Interprétation embryologique de l'anatomie des artères digestives. Ann Radiol (Paris) 19: 305–313

Bartlett S P, May J W, Yaremchuk M J 1981 The latissimus dorsi muscle: a fresh cadaver study of the primary neurovascular pedicle. Plas Reconstr Surg 67: 631–632

Bartosik J 1992 Cytomembrane-derived Birbeck granules transport horse radish peroxidase to the endosomal compartment of the human Langerhans cells. J Invest Dermatol 99: 53–58

Bartsiokas A, Day M H 1993 Electron probe energy dispersive X-ray microanalysis (EDXA) in the investigation of fossil bone; the case of Java man. Proc R Soc Lond B 252: 115–123

Basbaum A I, Fields H L 1979 The origin of descending pathways in the dorsolateral funiculus of the spinal cord of the cat and rat: pain modulation. J Comp Neurol 187: 513–532

Basbaum A I, Fields H L 1984 Endogenous pain control systems: brainstem spinal pathways and endorphin circuitry. Annu Rev Neurosci 7: 309–338

Basmajian J V 1959 'Spurt' and 'shunt' muscles: an electromyographic confirmation. J Anat 93: 551–553

Basmajian J V 1967 Muscles alive. 2nd edition. Williams and Wilkins: Baltimore

Basmajian J V, De Luca C J 1985 Muscles alive. 5th edition. Williams & Wilkins: Baltimore

Basmajian J V, Greenlaw R K 1968 Electromyography of iliacus and psoas with inserted fine-wire electrodes. Anat Rec 160: 310–311

Basmajian J V, Travill A A 1961 Electromyography of the pronator muscles in the forearm. Anat Rec 139: 45–49

Bassett C A L 1962 Current concepts of bone formation. J Bone Jt Surg 44A: 1217–1244

Bassett C A L, Pawluk R J, Pilla A A 1974 Augmentation of bone repair by inductively coupled electromagnetic fields. Science 184: 575–577

Bast T H, Anson B J 1949 The temporal bone and the ear. Thomas: Springfield, Illinois

Bastacky J, Goerke J 1992 Pores of Kohn are filled in normal lungs: low temperature scanning electron microscopy. J Anat 73(1): 88–95

Bastianini A 1967a Aspetti microscopici della trama linfatica polmonare in condizioni sperimentali. I. Anossia intrauterina. Atti Acad Fisiocr 16: 1304–1308

Bastianini A 1967b Osservazioni sulla morfologia microscopica e l'istotopografia dervasi linfatici del polmone umano. Boll Soc Ital Biol Sper 43: 1567–1570

Bastianini A, Comparini L 1968 Contribution a l'étude de l'histotopographie des vaisseaux lymphatiques du poumon. Essais de reconstruction graphique dans des conditions normales, pathologiques et experimentales. C R Assoc Anat 141: 520–525

Batanero E, de Leeuw F E, Jansen G H, van Wichen D F, Huber J, Schuurman H-J 1992 The neural and neural-endocrine component of the human thymus. II. Hormone immunoreactivity. BBI 6: 249–264

Bates J F, Goldman-Rakic P S 1993 Prefrontal connections of medial motor areas in the rhesus monkey. J Comp Neurol 336: 211–228

Batson O V 1940 Function of vertebral veins and their role in the spread of metastases. Ann Surg 112: 138–149

Batson O V 1957 The vertebral vein system. Am J Roentgenol 78: 195–212

Battaglia S, Casali A M, Botticelli A R 1994 Age-related distribution of endocrine cells in the human prostate: a quantitative study. Virchows Archiv 424: 165–168

Baude A, Sequier J-M, McKernan R M, Olivier K R, Somogyi P 1992 Differential subcellular distribution of the $\alpha6$ subunit versus the $\alpha1$ and $\beta2/3$ subunits of the GABA$_A$/benzodiazepine receptor complex in granule cells of the cerebellar cortex. Neuroscience 51: 739–748

Bauer W, Ropes M W, Waine H 1940 Physiology of articular structures. Physiol Rev 20: 272–312

Baum J, Simons B E, Unger R H, Madison L L 1962 Localisation of glucagon in the alpha cells in the pancreatic islet by immunofluorescent technics. Diabetes 11: 371–374

Baumann J A, Gajisin S 1975 Sur la multiplicité et la dispersion des ganglions parasympathiques de la tète. Bull Assoc Anat 59: 329–332

Baumann K I, Hamann W, Leung M S 1988 Responsiveness of slowly adapting cutaneous mechanoreceptors after close arterial infusion of neomycin in cats. Prog Brain Res 74: 43–49

Baumel J J 1974 Trigeminal-facial nerve communications. Their function in facial muscle innervation and reinnervation. Arch Otolaryngol 99: 34–44

Baumgarten H G, Holstein A F 1967 Catecholaminhaltige Nervenfasern im Hoden des Menschen. Z Zellforsch 79: 389–395

Baumgarten H G, Holstein A F, Owman C 1970 Auerbach's plexus of mammals and man: electron microscopic identification of three different types of neuronal processes in myenteric ganglia from rhesus monkeys, guinea pigs and man. Z Zellforsch 106: 376–397

Baumgarten H G, Holstein A F, Rosengren E 1971 Arrangement, ultrastructure and adrenergic innervation of smooth musculature of the ductuli efferentes, ductus epididymis and ductus deferens in man. Zetitschr f Zellforsch Mikr Anat 120: 37–79

Baumgarten J, Tornade L, Plas J Y 1981 Étude anatomochirurgicale de la voie d'abord de la toile choroidienne superieure du troisieme ventricule. Neurochir 27: 97–102

Baumgarten R von, Aranda Coddou L 1959 Acta Neurol Lat Am 5

Baumgartner R W, Regard M 1993 Bilateral neuropsychological deficits in unilateral paramedian thalamic infarction. Eur Neurol 33: 195–198

Baxter A 1971 Dehiscence of the fallopian canal. J Laryngol Otol 85: 587–594

Baxter J S 1953 Frazer's manual of embryology. The development of the human body. 3rd edition. Baillière: London

Baylink D J, Finkelman R D, Mohan S 1993 Growth factors to stimulate bone formation. J Bone Min Res 8 (suppl 2): S565–S572

Baylis B W, Tranmer B I, Ohtaki M 1993 Central and autonomic nervous system links to the APUD system (and their APUDomas). Sem Surg Oncol 9: 387–393

Baylis G C, Rolls E T, Leonard C M 1987 Functional subdivisions of the temporal lobe neocortex. J Neurosci 7: 330–342

Beadle G W, Ephrussi B 1937 Development of eye colours in Drosophila: diffusable substances and their interactions. Genetics 22: 76–86. Reprinted in Gabriel M L, Fogel S 1955 Great experiments in biology. Prentice-Hall: New Jersey

Beadle G W, Tatum E L 1941 Genetic control of biochemical reactions in Neurospora. Proc Natl Acad Sci USA 27: 499–506. Reprinted in Peters J A 1959 Classic papers in genetics. Prentice-Hall: New Jersey

Beard J 1896 The history of a transient nervous apparatus in certain Ichthyopsida. An account of the development and degeneration of ganglion cells and nerve fibres. Part 1. Raja Batis Zoll Jb 9: 319

Bearn J G 1961 An electromyographic study of the trapezius, deltoid, pectoralis major, biceps and triceps muscles, during static loading of the upper limb. Anat Rec 140: 103–108

Bearn J G 1967 Direct observation on the function of the capsule of the sterno-clavicular joint in clavicular support. J Anat 101: 159–170

Beasley S W, Hutson J M 1988 The role of the gubernaculum in testicular descent. J Urol 140: 1191–1193

Beasley S W, Myers N 1994 Oesophageal atresia. Ped Surg 12: 249–255

Beaudet A, Descarries L 1979 Radioautographic characterisation of a serotonin-accumulating nerve cell group in adult at hypothalamus. Brain Res 160: 231–243

Beaulieu C 1993 Numerical data on neocortical neurons in adult rat, with special reference to the GABA population. Brain Res 609: 284–292

Beaupre A, Choukroun R, Guidouin R, Garneau R, Gerardin H, Cardou A 1986 Knee menisci; correlation between microstructure and biomechanics. Clin Orthop 208: 72–75

Bechterew Von W 1885a Zur Anatomie der Schenkel des Kleinhirns. Neurol Centralbl 4: 121

Beck I T, Sinclair D G (eds) 1971 The exocrine pancreas. Churchill: London

Beckenbaugh R D, Linscheid R L 1982 Arthroplasty in the hand and wrist. In: Green D P (ed) Operative Surgery, Vol I. Churchill Livingstone: New York: pp 141–184

Becker N, Fuchs A F 1969 Further properties of the human saccadic system: eye movements and correction saccades with and without visual fixation points. Vision Res 9: 1247–1258

Beckstead R M, Norgren R 1979 An autoradiographic examination of the central distribution of the trigeminal, facial, glossopharyngeal and vagus nerves in the monkey. J Comp Neurol 184: 455–472

Bedbrook G M 1971 Stability of spinal fractures and fracture dislocations. Paraplegia 9: 23–32

Beddington R S P 1981 An autoradiographic analysis of the potency of embryonic ectoderm in the 8th day postimplantation mouse embryo. J Embryol Exp Morphol 64: 87–104

Beddington R S P 1982 An autoradiographic analysis of tissue potency in different regions of the embryonic ectoderm during gastulation in the mouse. J Embryol Exp Morphol 69: 265–285

Bedford J M, Calvin H I 1974 The occurrence and possible functional significance of -S-S crosslinks in sperm heads with particular reference to eutherian mammals. J Exp Zool 188: 137–155

Bedford J M, Calvin H, Cooper G W 1973 The maturation of spermatozoa in the human epididymis. J Reprod Fertil (Suppl 18): 199–213

Beertsen W, Everts V, van den Hooff 1974 Fine structure of fibroblasts in the periodontal ligament of the rat incisor and their possible role in tooth eruption. Arch Oral Biol 19: 1087–1098

Begg R C 1930 The urachus: its anatomy, histology and development. J Anat 64: 170–183

Behrendtsen O, Alexander C A, Werb Z 1992 Metalloproteinases mediate extracellular matrix degradation by cells from mouse blastocyst outgrowths. Development 114: 447–456

Behrens J C, Walker P S, Shoji H 1974 Variations in strength and structure of cancellous bone at the knee. J Biomech 7: 201–207

Beidler L M 1970 Physiological properties of mammalian taste receptors. In: Wolstenholme G E W, Knight J (eds) Taste and smell in vertebrates (Ciba Foundation Symposium). Churchill: London: pp 51–67

Beidler L M, Smallman R L 1965 Renewal of cells within taste buds. J Cell Biol 27: 263–272

Békésy G V 1960 In: Wever E G (ed) Experiments in hearing. McGraw-Hill: New York

Bélanger L F 1969 Osteocyte osteolysis. Calcif Tissue Res 4: 1–12

Bélanger L F, Robichon J, Migicovsky B B, Copp D H, Vincent J 1963 Resorption without osteoclasts (osteolysis). In: Sognnaes R F (ed) Mechanisms of hard tissue destruction. American Association for Advancement of Science: Washington DC: pp 531–556

Bell G H 1956 Bone as a mechanical engineering problem. In: Bourne G H (ed) The biochemistry and physiology of bone. Academic Press: New York: pp 27–52

Bell G H, Cuthbertson D P, Orr J 1941 Strength and size of bone in relation to calcium intake. J Physiol 100: 299–317

Bell J 1982 The anatomy of the human body. 4th edition 4 vol. Collins: New York

Bell L, Williams L 1982 A scanning and transmission electron microscopic study of the morphogenesis of human colonic villi. Anat Embryol 165: 437–455

Bell M A, Weddell A G M 1984a A descriptive study of the blood vessels of the sciatic nerve in the rat, man and other mammals. Brain 107: 871–898

Bell M A, Weddell A G M 1984b A morphometric study of intrafascicular vessels of mammalian sciatic nerve. Muscle Nerve 7: 524–534

Bell S C 1986 Secretory endometrial and decidual proteins: studies and clinical significance of a maternally derived group of pregnancy-associated serum proteins. Human Reprod 1: 129–143

Bell S C 1990 Assessment of endometrial differentiation and function. Br Med Bull 46: 720–732

Bell S C, Drife J O 1989 Secretory proteins of the endometrium – potential markers for endometrial dysfunction. In: Baillière's clinical obstetrics and gynaecology. Vol 3, No 2: pp 271–291

Bellairs R 1971 Developmental processes in higher vertebrates. Logos Press: London

Bellairs R 1987 The primitive streak and the neural crest: comparable regions of cell migration? In: Maderson P F A (ed) Developmental and evolutionary aspects of the neural crest. Wiley: New York: pp 123–145

Belmonte N 1968 Estudios anatomicos sobre la vascularizacion del nervio optico. Arch Soc Oftalmol Hisp Am 28: 801–810

Beltrani F 1946 Considérations biologiques sur le mandibule chez l'homme. Rev Stomat 47: 1–9

Bemthal J E, Bleukelman D R 1978 Intra-oral air pressure during the production of /p/and /b/ by children, youths, and adults. J Speech Hear Res 21: 361–371

Bench C J, Dolan R J, Friston K J, Frackowiack R S J 1990 Positron emission tomography in the study of brain metabolism in psychiatric and neuropsychiatric disorders. British J Psychiat 157 (suppl. 9): 82–95

Benditt E P 1974 Evidence for a monoclonal origin of human atherosclerotic plaques and some implications. Circulation 50: 650–652

Benedeczky I, Smith A D 1972 Ultrastructural studies on the adrenal medulla of the golden hamster: origin and fate of secretory granules. Z Zellforsch 124: 367–386

Benfey M, Aguayo A 1982 Extensive elongation of axons from rat brain into peripheral nerve grafts. Nature 296: 150–152

Benirschke K 1992 Multiple pregnancy. In: Polin R A, Fox (eds) Fetal and neonatal physiology W B Saunders: Philadelphia: pp 97–105

Benirschke K, Kaufman P 1990 Pathology of the human placenta. 2nd edition. Springer-Verlag: New York

Benjamin M, Evans E J 1990 Fibrocartilage. J Anat 171: 1–15

Benjamin M, Evans E J, Copp L 1986 The histology of tendon attachments to bone in man. J Anat 149: 89–100

Bennett A G, Rabetts R B 1984 Clinical visual optics. Butterworths: London

Bennett J H, Joyner C J, Triffitt J T, Owen M E 1991 Adipocytic cells cultured from bone marrow have osteogenic potential. J Cell Sci 99: 131–139

Bennett M R, Rogers D C 1967 A study of the innervation of the taenia coli. J Cell Biol 37: 573–596

Bennett M V L 1973 Function of electronic junctions in embryonic and adult tissues. Fed Proc 32: 65–72

Benninghoff A 1925 Form und Bau der Gelenkknorpel in ihren Beziehungen zur Funktion. II. Der Aufbau der Gelenkknorpels in seinen Beziehungen zur Funktion. Zeitschr Zellforsch Mikrscop Anat 2: 783

Benoit G, Jardin A, Gillot C 1993 Reflections and suggestions on the nomenclature of the prostate. Surg Radiol Anat 15: 325–332

Benoit G, Lerland L, Meduri G, Moukarzel M, Quillard J D, Ledroux M, Giuliano F, Jardin A 1994 Anatomy of the prostatic nerves. Surg Radiol Anat 16: 23–29

Bensch K G, Gordon G B, Miller L R 1965 Studies on the bronchial counterpart of the Kultschitzky (Argentaffin) cell and innervation of bronchial glands. J Ultrastruct Res 12: 668–686

Benscome S 1959 Studies on the terminal autonomic nervous system with special reference to the pancreatic islets. Lab Invest 8: 629–646

Bensley R R 1911 Studies on the pancreas of the guinea pig. Am J Anat 12: 297–388

Bentfield M E, Bainton D F 1975 Cytochemical localization of lysosomal enzymes in rat megakaryocytes and platelets. J Clin Invest 56: 1635–1649

Bentivoglio M, Balercia G, Kruger L 1991 The specificity of the nonspecific thalamus: the midline nuclei. Prog Br Res 87: 53–80

Bentley D, O'Connor T P 1994 Curr Opin Neurobiol 4: 43–48

Bereiter Hahn J 1990 Behaviour of mitochondria in the living cell. Int Rev Cytol 122: 1–63

Beresford J N, Bennett J H, Devlin C, Leboy P S, Owen M E 1992 Evidence for an inverse relationship between the differentiation of adipocytic and osteogenic cells in rat marrow stromal cell cultures. J Cell Sci 102: 341–351

Berezin I, Huizinga J D, Daniel E E Interstitial cells of Cajal in the canine colon: a special communication network at the inner border of the circular muscle. J Comp Neurol 273: 42–51

Bergel D H 1961 The static elastic properties of the arterial wall. J Physiol 156: 445–457. The dynamic elastic properties of the arterial wall. J Physiol 156: 458–469

Bergland R, Ray B S 1969 The arterial supply of the human optic chiasm. J Neurosurg 31: 327–334

Bergman R A, Thompson S A, Afifi A K, Saadeh F A 1988 Compendium of human anatomic variation. Urban and Schwarzenberg: Baltimore

Bergmanson J P G 1978 Ophthalmic terminals in the iris and the ciliary body of monkeys. An electron microscopical study. Albr von Graefes Arch Klin Exp Ophthal 206: 39–47

Bergstresser P R, Ponciano D C Jr, Niederkorn J Y, Takashima A (eds) 1992 Langerhans cells (Third International Workshop). J Invest Dermatol 99 (suppl): pp S1–S110

Bergström B 1973 Morphology of the vestibular nerve. anatomical studies of the vestibular nerve in man. Acta Otolaryngol [Stockh] 76: 162–172

Berkeley K J, Hand P G 1978 Projections to the inferior olive of the cat. II. Comparisons of input from the gracile caveate and the spinal trigeminal nuclei. J Comp Neurol 180: 253–264

Berkovitz B K B, Moxham B J, Newman H N 1982 The periodontal ligament in health and disease. Pergamon Press: Oxford

Berlin N I, Waldmann T A, Weissman S M 1959 Life span of red blood cell. Physiol Rev 39: 577–616

Bernard C 1855–1856 Lecons de physiologie, experimentale appliquée à la médecine. 2 vols. Baillière: Paris

Bernard G W 1972 Ultrastructural observations of initial calcification in dentine and enamel. J Ultrastruct Res 41: 1–17

Berner P F, Somlyo A V, Somlyo A P 1981 Hypertrophy-induced increase of intermediate filaments in vascular smooth muscle. J Cell Biol 88: 96–101

Bernhard C G, Bohm E, Petersen I 1953 Investigation on the organisation of the cortico-spinal system in monkeys. Acta Physiol Scand 29: 79–103

Bernick S, Caillet R 1982 Vertebral end-plate changes with ageing of the human vertebrae. Spine 7: 97–102

Bernick S, Patek R 1969 Lymphatic vessels of the dental pulp in dogs. J Dent Res 48: 959–964

Bernstein G 1986 Surface landmarks for the identification of key anatomic structures of the face and neck. J Dermatol Surg Oncol 12: 722–726

Berquist H 1932 Zur Morphologie des Zwischenhirns bei neideren Wirbeltieren. Acta Zool Stockholm 13: 57–304

Berquist H 1968 Uber die Differenzierung der Neuraloknes besounders des Stratum Zonale. Z Zellforsch 86: 401–421

Berridge M J 1985 The molecular basis of communication with the cell. Sci Am 253: 124–134

Berry A C 1975 Factors affecting the incidence of non-metrical skeletal variants. J Anat 120: 519–535

Berry A C, Berry R J 1967 Epigenetic variation in the human cranium. J Anat 101: 361–380

Berry M 1974 Development of the cerebral neocortex of the rat. In: Gittlieb G (ed) Aspects of neurogenesis: studies on the development of behaviour and the nervous system. Vol 2. Academic Press: New York: pp 7–67

Berry M 1982 Cellular differentiation: development of dendritic arborizations under normal and experimentally altered conditions. Neurosci Res Program Bull 20: 451–461

Berry M 1982 Post-injury myelin-breakdown products inhibit axonal growth: an hypothesis to explain the failure of axonal regeneration in the mammalian central nervous system. Biblio Anat 23: 1–11

Berry M 1991a Dendritic morphology and the factors affecting the pattern of dendritic growth. In: Cronley Dillon J R (ed) Vision and visual function. Vol 11. Development and plasticity of the visual system. Ch 8. Macmillan: London: pp 148–170

Berry M 1991b Vertex and segment analysis of dendritic fields and trichotomous branching points. In: Steward M (ed) Quantitative neuroanatomy. Ch 13. Oxford University Press: Oxford: pp 325–339

Berry M 1992 Vertex and segment of dendritic fields and trichotomous branching points. In: Stewart M (ed) Quantitative neuroanatomy. Oxford University Press: Oxford: pp 325–339

Berry M, Bradley P, Borges S 1978 Environmental and genetic determinants of connectivity in the central nervous system – an approach through dendritic field analysis. In: Corner M A, Baker R E, van der Poll N E, Swaab D F, Uylings H B M (eds) Maturation of the nervous system. Elsevier: Amsterdam. Prog Brain Res 48: 133–146

Berry M, Eayrs J T 1966 The effects of X-irradiation on the development of the cerebral cortex. J Anat 100: 707–722

Berry M, Hall S, Rees L, Carlile J, Wyse J P H 1992 Regeneration of axons in the optic nerve of the adult Browman-Wyse (BW) mutant rat. J Neurocytol 21: 426–428

Berry M, Hall S, Shewan D, Cohen J 1994 Axonal growth and its inhibition. Eye 8: 245–254

Berry M, McConnell P, Sievers J 1980a Dendritic growth and the control of neuronal form. Curr Top Dev Biol 15: 67–101

Berry M, McConnell P, Sievers J, Price S, Annar A 1980d Factors influencing the growth of cerebellar neural networks. Bibl Anat 19: 1–51

Berry M, Rees L, Hall S, Yiu P, Sievers J 1988 Optic axons regenerate into sciatic nerve isografts only in the presence of Schwann cells. Brain Res Bull 20: 223–231

Berry M, Rogers A W 1965 The migration of neuroblasts in the developing cerebral cortex. J Anat 99: 691–709

Berry M, Sievers J, Baumgarten H G 1980b The influence of afferent fibres on the development of the cerebellum. In: Di Bendetta C, Balázs R, Gombos G, Porcellati G (eds) Multidisciplinary approach to brain development. Elsevier/North-Holland Biomedical Press: Amsterdam: pp 91–106

Berry M, Sievers J, Baumgarten H G 1980c Adaption of the cerebellum to deafferentation. In: McConnell P S, Boer G J, Romijn H J, van der Poll N E, Corner M A (eds) Adaptive capabilities of the nervous system. Elsevier: Amsterdam. Prog Brain Res 53: 65–92

Bershof J F, Jafek B W, Sweeney J P 1987 Diagnostic imaging of Waldeyer's ring. Otolaryngol Clin North Am 20(2): 229–234

Bertalanffy F D 1964 Respiratory tissue: structure and histophysiological cytodynamics. I. Review and basic cytomorphology. Int Rev Cytol 16: 233–328

Bertelli J A, Valle Pereira J F 1994 The inframammary island flap: anatomical basis. Ann Plast Surg 32: 315–320

Berthold C H 1968 Ultrastructure of the node-paranode region of mature feline ventral lumbar spinal-root fibres. Acta Soc Med Upsal 73: (Suppl 9)

Berthold C H, Carlstedt T 1977 Observations on the morphology at the transition between the peripheral and the central nervous system in the cat. V. A light microscopical and histochemical study of S dorsal rootlets in developing kittens. Acta Physiol Scand 100: (Suppl 446), 73–85

Bertmar G 1981 Evolution of vomeronasal organs in vertebrates. Evolution 35: 359–336

Bertorini T E, Stålberg E, Yuson C P, Engel W K 1994 Single-fiber electromyography in neuromuscular disorders: correlation of muscle histochemistry, single-fiber electromyography, and clinical findings. Muscle Nerve 17: 345–353

Bessis M 1973 Living blood cells and their ultrastructure. Springer: Berlin

Besson J M, Chaouch A 1987 Peripheral and spinal mechanisms of nociception. Physiol Rev 67: 67–186

Betz A L, Goldstein G W 1986 Specialized properties and solute transport in brain capillaries. Ann Rev Physiol 48: 241–250

Beuche W, Friede R L 1984 The role of non-resident cells in Wallerian degeneration. J Neurocytol 13: 767–796

Beuche W, Friede R L 1986 Myelin phagocytosis in Wallerian degeneration of peripheral nerves depends on silica-sensitive, bg/bg-negative and Fc-positive monocytes. Brain Res 378: 97–106

Bevilacqua M P, Stengelin S, Gimbrone M A, Seed B 1989 Endothelial leucocyte adhesion molecule 1; an inducible receptor for neutrophils related to complement regulatory proteins and lectins. Science 243: 1160–1165

Beyer E C 1993 Gap junctions. Int Rev Cytol 137: 1–38

Bharihoke V, Gupta M 1986 Muscular attachments along the medial border of the scapula. Surg Radiol Anat 8: 71–73

Bianchet M, Ysern X, Hullihen J, Pedersen P L, Amzel L M 1991 Mitochondrial ATP synthase: quaternary structure of the f_1 moiety at 3.6 Å determined by X-ray diffraction analysis. J Biol Chem 266: 21197–21201

Biava C 1964a Studies on cholestasis. The fine structure and morphogenesis of hepatocellular and canalicular bile pigment. Lab Invest 13: 1099–1123

Biava C 1964b Studies on cholestasis. A re-evaluation of the fine structure of normal human bile canaliculi. Lab Invest 13: 840–864

Bickers W 1960 Sperm migration and uterine contractions. Fertil Steril 11: 286–290

Biedenbach M A 1972 Cell density and regional distribution of cell types in the cuneate nucleus of the rhesus monkey. Brain Res 45: 1–14

Biemond A 1956 The conduction of pain above the level of the thalamus opticus. Arch Neurol Psychiat 75: 231–244

Bienfang D C 1975 Crossing axons in the third nerve nucleus. Invest Ophthalmol Vis Sci 14: 927–931

Bigland B, Lippold O C J 1954 The relation between force, velocity and integrated electrical activity in human muscles. J Physiol 123: 214–224

Bigliani L U, Pollock R G, Soslowsky L J, Flatow E L, Pawluk R J, Mow V C 1992 Tensile properties of the inferior glenohumeral ligament. J Orthop Res 10: 187–197

Billingsley P R, Ransom S W 1918 On the number of nerve cells in the ganglion cervicale superioris. J Comp Neurol 29: 359–366

Bioulac-Sage P, Le Bail B, Balabaud C 1991 Liver and biliary tract histology. In: McIntyre N, Benhamou J-P, Bircher J, Rizzetto M, Rodes J (eds) Oxford textbook of clinical hepatology Vol 1. Oxford University Press: Oxford: pp 12–20

Birbeck M S C, Mercer E H 1957 The electron microscopy of the human hair follicle, parts 1–3. J Biophys Biochem Cytol 3: 203–223

Birbeck M S, Breathnach A S, Everall J D 1961 An electron microscopic study of melanocytes and high level clear cells (Langerhans cells) in vitiligo. J Invest Dermatol 37: 51–64

Bird M D T, Sweet M B E 1987 A system of canals in semilunar menisci. Ann Rheum Dis 46: 670–673

Birdwell C R, Gospodarowicz D, Nicholson G L 1978 Identification, localization, and role of fibronectin in cultured bovine endothelial cells. Proc Natl Acad Sci USA 75: 3273–3277

Birnbaum K, Lierse W 1992 Anatomy and function of the bursa subacromialis. Acta Anat 145: 354–363

Bischof P, Friedli E, Martelli M, Campana A 1992 Expression of extracellular matrix-degrading metalloproteinases by cultured human cytotrophoblast cells: effects of cell adhesion and immunopurification. Am J Obstet Gynec 165: 1791–1801

Biscoe T J, Bradley G W, Purves M J 1969 The relation between carotid body chemoreceptor activity and carotid sinus pressure in the cat. J Physiol 203: 40P

Biscoe T J, Lall A, Samson J R 1970 Electron microscopical and electrophysiological studies on the carotid body following intracranial section of the glossopharyngeal nerve. J Physiol 208: 133–152

Bishop D W 1962 Sperm motility. Physiol Rev 42: 1–59

Bishop G A 1990 Neuromodulatory effects of corticotropin releasing factor on cerebellar Purkinje cells. An in vivo study in the cat. Neuroscience 39: 251–257

Bishop G A, Ho R H 1985 The distribution and origin of serotonin immunoreactivity in the rat cerebellum. Brain Res 331: 195–207

Bishop J 1852 Researches into the pathology and treatment of deformities in the human body. Highley: London

Bishop M A 1985 Vascular permeability to lanthanum in the rat incisor pulp. Comparison with endoneurial vessels in the inferior alveolar nerve. Cell Tissue Res 239: 131–136

Bishop M W H, Walton A 1960 Spermatogenesis and the structure of mammalian spermatozoa. In: Parkes A S (ed) Marshall's physiology of reproduction 3rd edition, Vol 1, Part 2. Longmans: London: pp 1–129

Bishop P N, Boulton M, McLeod D, Stoddart R W 1993 Glycan localization within the human interphotoreceptor matrix and photoreceptor inner and outer segments. Glycobiol. 3:403–412

Bishopric N H, Gahlmann R, Wade R, Kedes L 1992 Gene expression during skeletal and cardiac muscle development. In: Fozzard H A, Haber E, Jennings R B, Katz A M, Morgan H E (eds) The heart and cardiovascular system. 2nd edition. Raven Press: New York: pp 1587–1598

Bismuth H, Alderidge M C, Kunstlinger F 1991 Macroscopic anatomy of the liver. In: McIntyre N, Benhamou J-P, Bircher J, Rizzetto M, Rodes J (edes) Oxford textbook of clinical hepatology, Vol 1. Oxford University Press: Oxford: pp 3–11

Bizarro A H 1921 On sesamoid and supernumerary bones of the limbs. J Anat 55: 256–268

Bjartmar C, Hildebrand C, Loinder K 1994 Morphological heterogeneity of rat oligodendrocytes. Electron microscopic studies on serial sections. Glia 11: 235 – 244

Björklund A, Hökfelt T 1984 Handbook of chemical neuroanatomy. Vol 2 Classical transmitters in the CNS. Part 1. Elsevier: Amsterdam

Björklund A, Hökfelt T, Owman C (eds) 1988 The peripheral nervous systems. Handbook of chemical neuroanatomy. Vol 6. Elsevier: Amsterdam

Björklund A, Lindvall O 1984 Dopamine containing systems in the CNS. In: Björklund A and Hökfelt T (eds) Handbook of chemical neuroanatomy. Vol 2, Part 1: Classical transmitters in the CNS. Elsevier: London: pp 55–122

Björklund A, Owman Ch, West K A 1972 Peripheral sympathetic innervation of serotonin cells in the habenular region of the rat brain. Z Zellforsch 127: 570–579

Björkman U, Ekholm R 1973 Thyroglobulin synthesis and intracellular transport in bovine thyroid slices. J Ultrastruct Res 45: 231–253

Bjurholm A, Kreicbergs A, Schultzberg M, Lerner U H 1992 Neuroendocrine regulation of cyclic AMP formation in osteoblastic cell lines (UMR-106-01, ROS 17/2.8, MC3T3-E1, and Saos-2) and primary bone cells. J Bone Min Res 7: 1011–1019

Black I B, Adler J E, La Gamma E F 1988 Neurotransmitter plasticity in the peripheral nervous system In: Björklund A, Hökfelt T, Owman C (eds) Vol 6. The peripheral nervous system. Handbook of chemical neuroanatomy. Elsevier: Amsterdam: pp 51–64

Blackstad T W 1956 Commissural connections of the hippocampal region in the rat, with special reference to their mode of termination. J Comp Neurol 105: 417–537

Blackstone C D, Supattapone S, Snyder S H 1989 Inositolphospholipid-linked glutamate receptors mediate cerebellar parallel-fiber-Purkinje-cell synaptic transmission. Proc. Natl Acad Sci USA 86: 4316–4320

Blackwood H J J 1959 The development, growth and pathology of the mandibular condyle. M D Thesis, Queen's University: Belfast

Blair-West J R, Coghlan J P, Denton D A, Wright R D 1967 Effect of endocrines on salivary glands. In: Code C F, Heidel W (eds) Handbook of physiology. Vol 2. Section 6, Alimentary Canal. American Physiological Society: Washington DC: pp 633–664

Blakemore C 1974 Development of functional connexions in the mammalian visual system. Br Med Bull 30: 152–157

Blandau R J 1984 The female reproductive tract. In: Weiss L (ed) Histology: cell and tissue biology. Elsevier: New York: pp 914–943

Blandau R J, Rumery R E 1964 The relationship of swimming movements of epididymal spermatozoa to their fertilising capacity. Fertil Steril 15: 571–579

Blanes T 1898 Sobre algunos puntos dudosos de la estructura del bulbo olfatoria. Rev Trim Microgr 3: 99–127

Blankenship T N, Given R L 1992 Penetration of the uterine epithelial basement membrane during blastocyst. Anat Rec 233: 196–204

Blaschko A 1901 Die Nervenverteilung und der Haut in ihrer Beziehung zu den Erkrankungen der Haut. Braunmuller: Vienna

Blasdel G G 1992 Differential imaging of ocular dominance and orientation selectivity in monkey striate cortex. J Neurosci 12: 3115–3138

Blasdel G G 1992 Orientation selectivity, preference, and continuity in monkey striate cortex. J Neurosci 12: 3139–3161

Blau J N 1978 Penetration of colloidal carbon through post-capillary venules in lymph nodes and peyer's patches of the guinea-pig: a potential immunogeneic route. British J Exp Path 59: 558–63

Blau J N 1960 The dynamic behaviour of Hassall's corpuscles and the transport of particulate matter in the thymus of the guinea-pig. Immunol 13: 281–292

Blaurock A E 1981 The spaces between membrane bilayers within PNS myelin as characterised by X-ray diffraction. Brain Res 210: 383–387

Blaurock A E, Yale J L, Roots B I 1986 Ca-controlled reversible structural transition in myelin. Neurochem Res 11: 1103–1129

Blaxter K L 1962 The energy metabolism of ruminants. Hutchinson: London

Blayney M P, Logan D R 1994 First thoracic vertebral body as reference for endotracheal tube placement. Arch Dis Child 71: F32–F35

Bleier R 1977 Ultrastructure of supraependymal cells and ependyma of hypothalamic third ventricle of mouse. J Comp Neurol 174: 359–376

Blenkinsopp W K 1967 Proliferation of respiratory tract epithelium in the rat. Exp Cell Res 46: 144–154

Blevins C E 1967 Innervation patterns of the human stapedius muscle. Arch Otolarnygol 86: 136–142

Block B A, Imagawa T, Campbell K P, Franzini-Armstrong C 1988 Structural evidence for direct interaction between the molecular components of the transverse tubule/sarcoplasmic reticulum junction in skeletal muscle. J Cell Biol 107: 2587–2600

Block E 1953 Quantitative morphological investigation of follicular system in newborn female infants. Acta Anat 17: 201–206

Bloebaum R D, Wilson A S 1980 The morphology of the surface of articular cartilage in adult rats. J Anat 131: 333–346

Bloodworth J M B, Powers K L 1968 The ultrastructure of the normal dog adrenal. J Anat 102: 457–476

Bloom G, Nicander L 1961 On the ultrastructure of the protoplasmic droplet of spermatozoa. Z Zellforsch 55: 833–844

Bloom K 1993 The centromere frontier: kinetochore components, microtubule-based motility, and the CEN-value paradox. Cell 73: 621–624

Bloom S R, Polak J M 1978 Gut hormone overview. In: Bloom S R (ed) Gut hormones. Churchill Livingstone: Edinburgh: pp 3–18

Bloom W 1931 New types of granular cell in islets of Langerhans of man. Anat Rec 49: 363–371

Bloom W, Bartelmez G W 1940 Hematopoiesis in young human embryos. Am J Anat 67: 21–54

Bloom W, Fawcett D W 1975 A textbook of histology. 10th edition. Saunders: Philadelphia

Bloomer W E, Liebow A A, Hales M R 1960 Surgical anatomy of the bronchovascular segments. Thomas: Springfield, Illinois

Bloor C M, Lowman R M 1963 Myocardinal bridges in coronary athero-sclerosis. Am Heart J 65: 195–199

Bluck W 1992 Phylogenesis of the human larynx. Schweiz Med Wochenschr 122: 28–1287

Blum J L, Ziegler M E, Wicha M S 1987 Regulation of rat mammary gene expression by extracellular components. Exp Cell Res 173: 322–340

Blum M, Niehrs C, De Roberts E N, Steinbeisser H 1992 Goosecoid and the organiser. Development (suppl): 167–171

Blunt M J 1951 Posterior wall of inguinal canal. Br J Surg 39: 230–233

Blunt M J 1954 The blood supply of the facial nerve J Anat 88: 520–526

Blunt M J 1959 The vascular anatomy of the median nerve in the forearm and hand. J Anat 93: 15–22

Böck P, Gorgas K 1976 Catecholamine and granule content of carotid body type I-cells. In: Coupland R E, Fujita T (eds) Chromaffin, enterochromaffin and related cells. Elsevier: New York: pp 355–374

Böck P, Stockinger L, Vyslonzil E 1970 Die Feinstrucktur des Glomus carotiscum beim Menschen. Z Zellforsch 105: 543–568

Bockman D E, Redmond M E, Kirby M L 1990 Altered development of pharyngeal arch vessels after neural crest ablation. In: Bockman D E, Kirby M L (eds) Embryonic origins of defective heart development. Ann NY Acad Sci 588: 296–304

Bodian D 1970a An electron microscopic characterisation of classes of synaptic vesicles by means of controlled aldehyde fixation. J Cell Biol 44: 115–124

Bodian D 1970b A model of synaptic and behavioral ontogeny. In: Schmitt F O, Quarton G C, Melnechuk T, Adelman G (eds) The neurosciences, a second study program. Rockefeller University Press: New York: pp 129–140

Bodorick N E, Pretorius D H, Grafe M R, Lou K V 1991 Ossification of the fetal spine. Radiology 181: 561–565

Boehm N, Gasser B 1993 Sensory receptor-like cells in the human foetal vomeronasal organ. Neuroreport 4: 867–870

Boerema I, de Waard J 1942 Osteoplastische verakening non metall-pros-thenen beipseudarthrose und beiorthoplastik. Acta Chir Scand 86: 511–524

Boersma C J, Sonnemans M A, Van Leeuwen F W 1993 Immuno-cytochemical localization of neuropeptide FF (FMRF amide-like peptide) in the hypothalamo-neurohypophyseal system of Wistar and Brattleboro rats by light and electron microscopy. J. Comp Neurol 336: 555–570

Boesten A J P, Voogd J 1975 Projection of the dorsal column nuclei and the spinal cord on the inferior olive in the cat. J Comp Neurol 161: 215–238

Bogduk N, Macintosh J E 1984 Applied anatomy of the thoracolumbar fascia. Spine 9: 164–170

Boggon R P, Palfrey A J 1973 The microscopic anatomy of human lymphatic trunks. J Anat 114: 389–405

Boheler K R, Carrier L, Bastie D de la, Allen P D, Komajda M, Mercadier J J, Schwartz K 1991 Skeletal actin mRNA increases in the human heart during ontogenic development and is the major isoform of control and failing human hearts. J Clin Invest 88: 323–330

Böhme C C 1962 The fine structure of Clarke's nucleus of the spinal cord. Thesis, University of Pennsylvania

Bois E, Feingold J, Benmaiz H, Briard M L 1975 Congenital urinary tract malformations: epidemiologic and genetic aspects. Clin Genet, 8: 37–47

Bojsen-Møller F 1975 Demonstration of terminalis, olfactory, trigeminal and perivascular nerves in the rat nasal septum. J Comp Neurol 159: 245–256

Bojsen-Møller F, Flagstad K E 1976 Plantar aponeurosis and internal architecture of the ball of the foot. J Anat 121: 599–611

Bojsen-Møller F, Schmidt L 1974 The palmar aponeurosis and the central spaces of the hand. J Anat 117: 55–68

Bojsen-Moller F, Jorgensen U 1991 The plantar soft tissues. Functional anatomy and clinical applications. In: Jahss M (ed) Disorders of the foot and ankle. Vol 1. Saunders: Philadelphia: pp 532–540

Bok D 1993 The retinal pigment epithelium: a versatile partner in vision. J Cell Sci- Suppl. 17:189–95

Bok H E 1966 De foetale transformatie van het middenoorgebied. Drukkerij Holland: Amsterdam

Bolender D L, Markwald R R 1991 Endothelial formation and trans-formation in early avian heart development: induction by proteins organ-ized into adherons. In: Feinberg R N, Sherer G K, Auerbach R (eds) The development of the vascular system. Issues Biomed 14: 109–124. Karger: Basel

Bolk L 1906 Das Cerebellum der Saugetiere. G Fisher: Haarlem

Bolk L, Goppert G, Kallius E, Lubosch W 1931–1939 Handbuch der vergleichenden Anatomie der Wirbeltiere. Urban: Berlin

Bollobas B, Hajdu I 1975 The development of the tympanic sinus. ORL J Otorhinolaryngal Relat Spec 37: 97–102

Bolton J W, Weiman D S 1993 Physiology of lung resection. Clin Chest Med 14: 293–303

Bolz J, Novak N, Gotz M, Bonhoeffer T 1990 Nature 346: 359–362

Bombeck C T, Dillard D H, Nyhus L M 1966 Muscular anataomy of the gastroesophageal junction and the role of the phreno-esophageal ligament: autopsy study of sphincter mechanism. Ann Surg 164: 643–654

Bomberger C E, Haar J L 1992 Dexamethasone and hydrocortisone enhance the in vitro migration of prethymic stem cells to thymus supernatant. Thymus 20: 89–99

Boncinelli E 1994 Curr Opin Neurobiol 4: 29–36

Bond M, Somlyo A V 1982 Dense bodies and actin polarity in vertebrate smooth muscle. J Cell Biol 95: 403–413

Bonucci E 1967 Fine structure of early cartilage calcification. J Ultrastruct Res 20: 33–50

Borell U, Fernström I 1953 Adnexal branches of uterine artery; arteriographic study in human subjects. Acta Radiol 40: 561–582

Borell U, Fernström I 1960 Radiologic pelvimetry. Acta Radiol Suppl 191: 3–97

Borg E 1973 A neuroanatomical study of the brainstem auditory system of the rabbit. Acta Neerl Scand 11: 49–62

Borg E, Densert O, Flock A 1974 Synaptic venicles in the cochlea. Acta Otolarnygol 78: 321–332

Borges A F, Alexander J E 1962 Relaxed skin tension lines, Z-plasties on scars, and fusiform excision of lesions. Br J Plast Surg 15: 242–254

Born G V R, Dawes G S, Mott J C, Widdicombe J G 1954 Changes in the heart and lungs at birth. Cold Spring Harbor Symp Quant Biol 19: 102–108

Bornstein M N, Bornstein H G 1976 The pace of life. Nature 259: 557–558

Bornstein S R, Ehrhart-Bornstein M, Usadel H, Bockmann M, Scherbaum W A 1991 Morphological evidence for a close interaction of chromaffin cells with cortical cells within the adrenal gland. Cell Tissue Res 265: 1–9

Borrione A C, Zanellato A M C, Scannapieco G, Pauletto P, Sartore S 1989 Myosin heavy-chain isoforms in adult and developing rabbit vascular smooth muscle. Eur J Biochem 183: 413–417

Bortoff G A, Strick P L 1993 Corticospinal terminations in two new-world primates: further evidence that corticomotoneuronal connections provide part of the neural substrate for manual dexterity. J Neurosci 13: 5105–5118

Bortolami R, Veggetti A, Callegari E, Lucchi M L, Palmieri G 1977 Afferent fibres and sensory ganglion cells within the oculomotor nerve in some mammals and man. 1. Anatomical investigations. Arch Ital Biol 115: 355–385

Bosch E, Horwitz J, Bok D 1993 Phagocytosis of outer segments by retinal pigment epithelium: phagosome-lysosome interaction. J Histochem Cyto-chem 41: 253–263

Bosma J F 1957 Deglutition: pharyngeal stage. Physiol Rec 37: 275–300

Bosma J F (ed) 1976 Symposium on development of the basicranium. US Department of Health, Education, and Welfare (DHEW publication (NIH) 76–989) Bethesda, Maryland

Bossy J 1968 Sur la présence d'un noyau sensitif du annexe au tractus spinal du V. Acta Anat 70: 332–340

Bossy J, Vidić B 1967 Existe-il une innervation proprioceptive des muscles du pharynx chez l'homme? Arch Anat Histol Embryol 50: 273–284

Bossy Y 1980 Development of olfactory and related structures in staged human embryos. Anat Embryol 161:225–236

Bouchaud V, Bosler O 1986 The circumventricular organs of the mammalian brain with special reference to monoaminergic innervation. Int Rev Cytol 105: 283–327

Boucher B J 1957 Sex differences in the foetal pelvis. Am J Phys Anthropol N S 15: 581–600

Bouin P, Ancel P 1903 Le gland intestitielle du testicule chez le cheval. Arch Zool Exp Gén 3: 391

Boulder Committee 1970 Embryonic vertebrate central nervous system. Revised Terminol. Anat Rec 166: 257–261

Boulter P S, Parkes A G 1963 Submucosal vascular patterns of the alimentary tract and their significance. Br J Surg 47: 546–550

Bounoure L 1939 L'origine des cellules réproductrices et le problème de la lignée germinale. Gauthiers-Villars: Paris

Bourbon J R, Rieutort M 1987 Pulmonary surfactant: biochemistry, physiology, and pathology. News Physiol Sci 2: 129–132

Bourdelat D, Barbet J P, Butler-Browne G S 1992 Fetal development of the urethral sphincter. Eur J Pediat Surg 2: 35–38

Bourne G 1963 The amnion and chorion. Lloyd-Luke: London

Boussaoud D, Barth T M, Wise S P 1993 Effects of gaze on apparent visual responses of frontal cortex neurons. Exp Brain Res 93: 423–434

Boussaoud D, Desimone R, Ungerleider L G 1991 Visual topography of area TEO in the macaque. J Comp Neurol 306: 554–575

Boussaoud D, Wise S P 1993 Primate frontal cortex: effects of stimulus and movement. Exp Brain Res 95: 28–40

Boussaoud D, Wise S P 1993 Primate frontal cortex: neuronal activity following attentional versus intentional cues. Exp Brain Res 95: 15–27

Bouthenet M-L, Souil E, Martres M-P, Sokoloff P 1991 Localization of dopamine D₃ receptor mRNA in the rat brain using in situ hybridization histochemistry: comparison with dopamine D₂ receptor mRNA. Brain Res 564: 203–219

Böving B G 1959 The biology of trophoblast. Ann NY Acad Sci 80: 21–43

Böving B G 1963 Implantation mechanisms. In: Hartman C G (ed) Mechanisms Concerned with Conception. Proceedings of a symposium under the auspices of the population council and the planned parenthood federation of America. Pergamon Press: Oxford: pp 321–396

Bowden R E M 1955 Surgical anatomy of the recurrent laryngeal nerve. Br J Surg 43: 153–163

Bowden R E M 1966 The functional anatomy of striated muscle. Ann R Coll Surg Engl 38: 41–59

Bowen V, Cassidy J D 1981 Macroscopic and microscopic anatomy of the sacroiliac joint from embryonic life until the eighth decade. Spine 6: 620–628

Bowersox J C, Sorgente N 1982 Chemotaxis of aortic endothelial cells in response to fibronectin. Cancer Res 42: 2547–2551

Bowes D, Clarke A E, Corrin B 1981 Ultrastructure localisation of lactoferrin and glycoprotein in human bronchial glands. Thorax 36: 123–126–115

Bowin P 1895 J Anat Physiol. Paris 31

Bowman J P 1968 Muscle spindles in the intrinsic and extrinsic muscles of the rhesus monkey's tongue. Anat Rec 161: 483–488

Bowsher D 1957 Terminations of the central pain pathways in man. The conscious appreciation of pain. Brain 80: 606–622

Boya J, Calvo J L, Carbonell A L, Borregon A A 1991 A lectin histochemistry study on the development of rat microglial cells. J Anat 175: 229–236

Boyce S T 1994 Epidermis as a secretory tissue. J Invest Dermatol 102: 8–10

Boycott B B 1974 Aspects of the comparative anatomy and physiology of the vertebrate retina. In: Bellairs R, Gray E G (eds) Essays on the nervous system. Clarendon Press: Oxford: pp 223–257

Boycott B B, Dowling J E 1969 Origin of the primate retina: light microscopy. Phil Trans R Soc Ser B 255: 109–184

Boycott B B, Hopkins J M 1993 Cone synapses of a flat diffuse cone bipolar cell in the primate retina. J Neurocytol 22: 765–778

Boycott B B, Kolb H 1973 The connections between bipolar cells and photoreceptors in the retina of the domestic cat. J Comp Neurol 148: 91–114

Boycott B B, Wassle H 1991 Morphological classification of bipolar cells of the primate retina. Eur J Neurosci 3: 1069–1088

Boyd D P 1983 Computerized-transmission tomography of the heart using scanning electron beams. In: Higgins C (ed) CT of the heart: experimental evaluation and clinical application. Futura: Mt Kisco: pp 45–59

Boyd E 1932 The weight of the thymus gland in health and in disease. Am J Dis Child 43: 1162–1214

Boyd I A 1954 The histological structure of the receptors in the knee joint of the cat correlated with their physiological response. J Physiol 124: 476–488

Boyd I A 1962 The structure and innervation of the nuclear bag muscle fibre system and nuclear chain muscle fibre system in mammalian muscle spindles. Philos Trans R Soc Lond [Biol] 245: 81–136

Boyd I A 1985 Muscle spindles and stretch reflexes. In: Swash M, Kennard C (eds) Scientific basis of clinical neurology. Churchill Livingtone: Edinburgh: pp 74–97

Boyd I A, Gladden M H 1985 The muscle spindle. Macmillan: London

Boyd I A, Roberts T D M 1953 Proprioceptive discharges from stretch-receptors in the knee joint of the cat. J Physiol 122: 38–58

Boyd J D 1933 The classification of the upper lip in mammals. J Anat 67: 409–416

Boyd J D 1937 The development of the human carotid body. Contrib Embryol Carnegie Inst Washington 26: 1–31

Boyd J D 1956 Observations on the human pharyngeal hypophysis. J Endocrinol 14: 66–77

Boyd J D 1961 The interior aortico-pulmonary glomus. Br Med Bull 17: 127–131

Boyd J D 1964 Development of the human thyroid gland. In: Pitt-Rivers R, Trotter W R (eds) The thyroid gland. Vol 1. Butterworths: London: pp 9–31

Boyd J D, Hamilton W J 1970 The human placenta. Heffer: Cambridge

Boyd J D, Trevor J C 1953 Race, sex, age and stature from skeletal material. In: Simpson K (ed) Modern trends in forensic medicine. Butterworths: London: Ch. 7

Boyd W, Blincoe H, Hayner J C 1965 Sequences of action of the diaphragm and quadratus lumborum during quiet breathing. Anat Rec 151: 579–582

Boyde A 1969 Electron microscopic observations relating to the nature and development of prism decussation in mammalian dental enamel. Bull Grp Int Rech Sci Stomat 12: 151–207

Boyde A 1974 TEM of ion beam thinned dentine. Cell Tissue Res 152: 543–550

Boyde A 1976 Enamel structure and cavity margins. Operative Dentistry 1: 13–28

Boyde A 1980 Evidence against osteocytic osteolysis. In: Bone histomorphometry. Metab Bone Dis Rel Res (Suppl 2): 239–245 Société Nouvelle de Publications Medicale et Dentaires: Paris

Boyde A 1989 Enamel. In: Oksche A, Vollrath L (eds) Teeth. Springer-Verlag: Berlin: pp 309–473

Boyde A, Hobdell M H 1969 Scanning electron microscopy of lamellar bone. Z Zellforsch 93: 213–231

Boyde A, Jones S J 1983 Scanning electron microscopy of cartilage. In: Hall B K (ed) Cartilage. Vol. 1. Structure, function and biochemistry. Academic Press: New York: pp 105–148

Boyden E A 1955 Segmental anatomy of the lungs. McGraw-Hill: New York

Boyden E A 1957 The anatomy of the choledochoduodenal junction in man. Surg Gynecol Obstet 104: 641–652

Boyden E A 1966 The pancreatic sphincters of the baboon as revealed by serial sections of the choledochoduodenal junction. Surgery 60: 1187–1194

Boyden E A, Cope J G, Bill A H 1967 A new look at the etiology of duodenal atresia. Anat Rec 157: 218P

Braak E, Braak H 1993 The new monodendrite type within the adult human cerebellar granule cell layer shows calretinin immunoreactivity. Neuroscience Lett 154: 199–202

Braak H 1974 On the structure of the human archicortex. I. The cornu ammonis. A Golgi and pigmentarchitectonic study. Cell Tissue Res 152: 349–383

Braak H, Braak E 1986 Ratio of pyramidal cells versus non-pyrimidal cells in the human frontal isocortex and changes in ratio with ageing and Alzheimer's disease. In: Swaab D F, Fliers E, Mirmiran M, Van Gool W A, Van Haaren F (eds) Progress in brain research. Elsevier Science: Amsterdam: pp 185–212

Braak H, Braak E 1987 The hypothalamus of the human adult: chiasmatic region. Anat Embryol 176: 315–330

Braak H, Braak E 1992 Anatomy of the human hypothalamus (chiasmatic and tuberal region). Prog Brain Res 93: 3–16

Brace R A 1993 Maximal lymph flow in the ovine fetus. Am J Obstet Gynecol 169: 1487–1492

Brachet J 1985 Molecular cytology, Vol 1. The cell cycle. Academic Press: New York

Bradbury M W B 1993 Anatomy and physiology of cerebrospinal fluid. In: Schurr P H, Polkey C E (eds) Hydrocephalus. Oxford University Press: Oxford: pp 19–47

Bradley R L 1973 Surgical anatomy of the gastro-duodenal artery. Int Surg 58: 393–396

Braitenberg V 1967 Is the cerebellar cortex a biological clock in the millisecond range? Prog Brain Res 25: 334–346

Braitenberg V 1977 Cortical architectonics, general and areal. In: Brazier M A B, Petsche H (eds) Architectonics of the cerebral cortex. Raven Press: New York

Braitenberg V, Atwood R P 1958 Morphological observations on the cerebellar cortex. J Comp Neurol 109: 1–33

Braithwaite F, Channel G D, Moore F T, Whillis J 1948 The applied anatomy of the lumbrical and interosseous muscles of the hand. Guy's Hosp Rep 97: 185–195

Braithwaite J L 1951 The arterial supply of the urinary bladder. J Anat 85: 413P

Braithwaite J L 1952 Variations in origin of the parietal branches of the internal iliac artery. J Anat 86: 423–430

Braithwaite J L, Adams D J 1957 The venous drainage of the rat spleen. J Anat 91: 352–357

Brand B, Christ B, Jacob H J 1985 An experimental analysis of the developmental capacities of distal parts of avian leg buds. Am J Anat 173: 321–340

Brand P W, Thompson D E, Micks J E 1987 The biomechanics of the interphalangeal joints. In: Bowers W H (ed) The interphalangeal joints. Churchill Livingstone: Edinburgh: pp 21–54

Brandell B R 1973 An analysis of muscle coordination in walking and running gaits. Med & Sport 8: 278–287

Brandner M E 1970 Normal values of the vertebral body and intervertebral disc index during growth. Am J Roentgenol 110: 618–627

Brandtzaeg P 1984 Immune functions of human nasal mucosa and tonsils in health and disease. In: Bienenstock J (ed) Immunology of the lungs and upper respiratory tract. McGraw-Hill: New York: pp 29–96

Brandtzaeg P 1988 Immunopathological alterations in tonsillar disease. Acta Otolaryngol [Stockh] Suupl 454: 53–59

Brånemark P I 1972 Rehabilitering med käkbensförankrad bettersättning. Lakartidningen 69: 4813–4848

Brännström M 1963 A hydrodynamic mechanism in the transmission of pain-producing stimuli through the dentine. In: Anderson D J (ed) Sensory mechanisms in dentine. (Proceedings of a symposium held in London 1962.) Pergamon: Oxford: pp 73–79

Brantigan O C, Voshell A F 1943 Tibial collateral ligament; its functions, its bursae and its relation to medial meniscus. J Bone Jt Surg 25: 121–131

Brash J C 1924 The growth of the jaws and the palate. In: The growth of the jaws, normal and abnormal, in health and disease. Dental Board of the United Kingdom: London

Brash J C 1934 Some problems in the growth and developmental mechanics of bone. Edin Med J 41: 305–387

Brash J C 1955 Neuro-vascular hila of limb muscles: an atlas. Livingstone: Edinburgh

Brasnu D 1991 New procedures of vocal restoration after laryngectomy, surgical shunts and phonatory implants. Curr Opin Radiol 4: 123–126

Brasnu D 1991 Parotid swelling. Diagnostic orientation. Revue du Practicien 41(8): 732–734

Bratton A B 1925 The normal weight of the human thymus. J Path Bact 28: 609–620

Braun P, Bambrick L, Edwards A, Bernier L, 1990 2'3 cyclic nucleotide 3' phosphodiesterase (CNP) has characteristics of cytoskeletal proteins: a hypothesis for its function. Ann NY Acad Sci 605: 255–265

Braun T, Bober E, Buschausen-Denker G, Kotz S, Greschik K, Arnold H 1989 Differential expression of myogenic determination genes in muscle cells: possible autoactivation by the Myf gene products. EMBO J 8: 3617–3625

Braverman I M 1989 Ultrastructure and organization of the cutaneous microvasculature in normal and pathologic states. J Invest Dermatol 93: 2S–9S

Braverman I M, Fonferko C 1982 Studies in cutaneous aging. I. The elastic fiber network. J Invest Dermatol 78: 434–443

Braverman I M, Fonferko E 1982b Studies in cutaneous aging. II. The microvasculature. J Invest Dermatol 78: 444–448

Braverman I M, Yen A 1977 Ultrastructure of the human dermal microcirculation. II. The papillary loops of the dermal papillae. J Invest Dermatol 68: 44–52

Bray D 1982 In: Bellairs R, Curtis A, Dunn G (eds) Cell behaviour. Cambridge University Press: Cambridge: pp 298–318

Bray D 1992 Cell movements. Garland: New York

Breathnach A S 1960 Melanocytes in early regenerated human epidermis. J Invest Dermatol 35: 245–251

Breathnach A S 1964 Observations on cytoplasmic organelles of Langerhans cells of human epidermis. J Anat 98: 265–270

Breathnach A S 1971 An atlas of the ultrastructure of human skin: development, differentiation, and post-natal features. Churchill: London

Breathnach A S 1973 Freeze-cleavage replication of human skin. Giorn Ital Dermatol 108: 12–20

Breathnach A S 1976 Ultrastructure of epidermis and dermis in striae atrophicae. In: Moretti G, Rebora A (eds) Striae distensae. Brocade Spa: Milan: pp. 35–46

Breathnach A S 1979 The mammalian and avian Merkel cell. In: Spearman R I C, Riley P A (eds) Skin of vertebrates. Linnean Society Symposium Series 9 London: pp 283–291

Breathnach A S 1981 Ultrastructural morphology of Langerhans cells of normal human epidermis. In: Marks R, Christophers E (eds) The epidermis in disease. MTP Press: Lancaster: pp 501–511

Breathnach A S, Goodman T, Stolinski C, Gross M 1973 Freeze-fracture replication of cells of stratum corneum of human epidermis. J Anat 114: 65–81

Breathnach A S, Nazzaro-Porro M, Passi S, Picardo M 1991 Ultrastructure of melanocytes in chronically sun-exposed skin of elderly subjects. Pig Cell Res 4: 71–79

Breathnach A S, Stolinski C, Gross M 1972 Ultrastructure of fetal and postnatal human skin as revealed by the freeze-fracture technique. Micron 3: 287–304

Breathnach A S, Wylie L 1965 Electron microscopy of melanocytes and Langerhans cells in human fetal epidermis at 14 weeks. J Invest Dermatol 44: 51–60

Breathnach A S, Wylie L M A 1966 Ultrastructure of retinal pigment epithelium of the human fetus. J Ultrastruct Res 16: 584–597

Breathnach S M, Katz S I 1987 Immunopathology of graft-versus-host disease. Am J Dermatopathol 9: 343–348

Bredman J J, Weijs W A, Korfage H A M, Brugman P, Moorman A F M 1992 Myosin heavy chain expression in rabbit masseter muscle during postnatal development. J Anat 180 263–274

Bredman J J, Wessels A, Weijs W A, Korfage J A M, Soffers C A S, Moorman A F M 1991 Demonstration of 'cardiac-specific' myosin heavy chain in masticatory muscles of human and rabbit. Histochem J 23: 160–170

Bredt D S, Hwang P M, Snyder S H 1990 Localization of nitric oxide synthase indicating a neural role for nitric oxide. Nature 347: 768–770

Breen L A, Hopf H C, Farris B K, Guttmann L 1991 Pupil-sparing oculomotor nerve palsy due to midbrain infarction. Arch neurol 48: 105–106

Breer H, Boekhoff I 1991 Odorants of the same odor class activate different second messenger pathways. Chem Senses 16: 19–29

Breer H, Boekhoff I 1992 Second messenger signalling in olfaction. Curr Opin Neurobiol 2: 439–443

Breer H, Boekhoff I, Tareilus E 1990 Rapid kinetics of second messenger formation in olfactory transduction. Nature 345: 65–68

Breier G, Dressler G R, Gruss P 1988 Primary structure and developmental expression pattern of Hox-8.1, a member of the murine Hox-3 homeobox gene cluster. EMBO J 7: 1329–1336

Brekelmans W A M, Poort H W, Slooff T J 1972 A new method to analyse the mechanical behaviour of skeletal parts. Acta Orthop Scand 43: 301–317

Brennan P, Kaba H, Keverne E B 1990 Olfactory recognition: a simple memory system. Science 250: 1223–1226

Bretscher M 1975 Membrane structure: some general principles. Science 181: 622–629

Bretscher M S 1985 The molecules of the cell membrane. Sci Am 253: (Oct) 86–90

Bretscher M S, Raff M C 1975 Mammalian plasma membranes. Nature 258: 43–49

Brichta A M, Grant G 1985 Cytoarchitectural organisation of the spinal cord. In: Paxinos G (ed) The rat nervous system. Vol 2. Academic Press: Orlando: pp 293–300

Bridger M W M, Farkashidy J 1980 The distribution of neuroglia and schwann cells in the 8th nerve of man. J Laryngol Otol 94: 1353–1362

Brierley J B 1950 The penetration of particulate matter from the cerebrospinal fluid into the spinal ganglia, peripheral nerves and perivascular spaces of the central nervous system. J Neurol 13: 203–215

Brierley J B, Field E J 1948 The connexions of the spinal subarachnoid space with the lymphatic system. Journal of Anatomy 82: 153–166

Briggs J P, Skott O, Schnermann J 1990 Cellular mechanisms within the juxtaglomerular apparatus. Am J Hypertension 3: 76–80

Briggs R, King T J 1952 Transplantation of living nuclei from blastula cells into enucleated frog's eggs. Proc Natl Acad Sci USA 38: 455–463

Brightman M W, Palay S L 1963 The fine structure of ependyma in the brain of the rat. J Cell Biol 19: 415–439

Brightman M W, Prestcott L, Reese T S 1975 Intercellular junctions of special ependyma. In: Dnigge K M, Scott D E, Kobayashi H, Ishii S (eds) Brain–endocrine interaction. II. The ventricular system in neuroendocrine mechanisms. 2nd International Symposium. Karger: Basel: pp 146–165

Brighton C T 1981 The treatment of non-unions with electricity. J Bone Jt Surg 63A: 847–851

Brighton C T, Hunt R M 1991 Early histological and ultrastructural changes in medullary fracture callus. J Bone Jt Surg 73A: 832–847

Brighton C T, Lorich D G, Kupcha R, Reilly T M, Jones A R, Woodbury R A 1992 The pericyte as a possible osteoblast progenitor cell. Clin Orthop 275: 287–299

Brinkley B R 1984 Microtubule organizing centers. Annu Rev Cell Biol 1: 145–172

British Medical Journal 1976 Diagnosis of brain death BMJ 2: 1187–1188

Brizon J, Castaing J, Hourtaille F C 1956 Le péritoine. Maloine: Paris

Brizzi E, Serantoni C, Gani P A, Pernice L 1973 The distribution of the vagus nerve in the stomach. Chir Gastroentol 7: 17–34

Brock D J H 1976 Prenatal diagnosis – chemical methods. Br Med J 32: 16

Brock R C 1942 The use of silver nitrate in the production of aseptic obliterative pleuritis. Guy's Hosp Rep 91: 111–130

Brock R C 1943 Observations on the anatomy of the bronchial tree, with special reference to the surgery of lung abscess. Guy's Hosp Rep 92: 26–37

Brock R C 1944 A note on secondary diphtheritic infection of empyema and thoracotomy wounds. Guy's Hosp Rep 93: 62–66

Brock R C 1954 The anatomy of the bronchial tree. Oxford University Press: London

Brockhaus H 1938 Zur normalen und pathologischen Anatomiedes Mandelkeingebietes. J Psychol. Neurol 49: 1–136

Brockhaus H 1942 Beitrag zur normalen Anatomie des Hypothalamus und der Zona incerta beim Menschen. J Psychol Neurol 51: 96–196

Brocklehurst R J, Edgeworth F H 1940 The fibre components of the laryngeal nerves of macaca mulatta. J Anat 74: 386–389

Brodal A 1947 Central course of afferent fibres for pain in facial, glossopharyngeal and vagus nerves. Clinical observations. Arch Neurol Psychiatry 57: 292–306

Brodal A 1957 The reticular formation of the brain stem. Anatomical aspects and functional correlations. Oliver and Boyd: Edinburgh

Brodal A 1969 Neurological anatomy. Oxford University Press: London

Brodal A 1981 Neurological anatomy in relation to clinical medicine. 3rd edition. Oxford University Press: Oxford

Brodal A, Pompeiano O 1957 The vestibular nuclei in the cat. J Anat 91: 438–454

Brodal A, Pompeiano O, Walberg F 1962 The vestibular nuclei and their connextions, anatomical and functional correlations. Oliver and Boyd: Edinburgh

Brodal P 1968a The coricopontine projection in the cat. I. Demonstration of a somatotopically organized projection from the primary sensorimotor cortex. Exp Brain Res 5: 212–237

Brodal P 1968b The corticopontine projection in the cat. II. Demonstration of a somatotopically organized projection from the second somatosensory cortex. Arch Ital Biol 106: 310–332

Brodal P 1971 The corticopontine projection in the cat. I. The projection from the proreate gyrus. J Comp Neurol 142: 127–140

Brodal P 1978 The corticopontine projection in the rhesus monkey. Brain 101: 251–283

Brodal P 1980 The cortical projection to the nucleus reticularis tegmentis pontis in the rhesus monkey. Exp Brain Res 38: 19–27

Brodal P 1982 The cerebropontocerebellar pathway: salient features of its organization. Exp Brain Res (Suppl 6): 108–133

Brodal P 1987 Organization of cerebropontocerebellar connections as studied with anterograde and retrograde transport of WGA-HRP in the cat. In: King S (ed) New concepts in cerebellar neurobiology. Alan Liss: New York: pp 151–182

Brodal P, Bjaalie J G 1992 Organization of the pontine nuclei. Neurosci Res 13: 83–118

Brödel M 1901 The intrinsic blood-vessels of the kidney and their significance in nephrotomy. Johns Hopkins Hosp Bull 12: 10–13

Brodie A G 1941 On the growth pattern of the human head. From the third month to the eighth year of life. Am J Anat 68: 209–262

Brodmann K 1909 Vergleichende Lokaliastionslehre der Grosshirnrinde in ihren Prinzipien dargestellt auf Grund des Zellenbaues. Narth: Leipzig

Brokaw C J 1975 Molecular mechanism for oscillation in flagella and muscle. Proc Natl Acad Sci USA 72: 102–106

Bromage T G, Dean M C 1985 Re-evalution of the age at death of immature fossil hominids. Nature 317: 525–527

Broman I 1904 Die Entwickelungsgeschichte der Bursa Omentalis und ähnlicher Rezessbildungen bei den Wirbeltieren. Bergmann: Wiesbaden

Broman I 1938 Warum wird die Entwicklung der Bursa omentalis in Lehrbuchern fortwährend unrichtig beschrieben? Anat Anz 86: 195–202

Broman J, Ottersen O P 1992 Cervicothalamic tract terminals are enriched in glutamate-like immunoreactivity: an electron microscopic double-labelling study in the cat. J Neurosci 12: 204–221

Bronaugh R L, Maibach H I (eds) 1989 Percutaneous absorption. Marcel Dekker: New York

Bronner-Fraser M E 1987 Adhesive inteactions in neural crest morphogenesis. In: Maderson P F A (ed) Developmental and evolutionary aspects of the neural crest. Wiley: New York: pp 11–38

Bronner-Fraser M, Fraser S 1989 Developmental potential of avian trunk neural crest cells in situ. Neuron 3: 755–766

Bronner-Fraser M, Fraser S E 1988 Application of new technologies to studies of neural crest migration and differentiation. Am J Med Genet Suppl 23–39

Brook A 1984 A unifying aetiological explanation for anomalies of human tooth number and size. Arch Oral Biol 29: 373–378

Brook G A, Lawrence J M, Raisman G 1993 Morphology and migration of cultured Schwann cells into the limbra and hippocampus of adult rats. Glia 9: 292–304

Brooke M H, Kaiser K K 1970 Muscle fiber types: how many and what kind? Archs Neurol 23: 369–379

Brookes M 1958 The vascularisation of long bones in the human fetus. J Anat 92: 261–267

Brookes M 1963 Cortical vascularisation and growth in foetal tubular bones. J Anat 97: 597–609

Brookes M 1964 The blood supply of bones. In: Clark J M P (ed) Modern trends in orthopaedics. Vol 4. Science of fractures. Butterworths: London

Brookes M 1967 The osseous circulation. Biomed Eng 2: 294–299

Brookes M 1971 The blood supply of bone. An approach to bone biology. Butterworths: London

Brookes M 1987 Bone blood flow measurement. Part 2. Bone Clin Biochem News Rev 4: 33–36

Brookes M 1993 Morphology and distribution of blood vessels and blood flow in bone. In: Shoutens A, Arlet J, Gardiniers J W M, Hughes S P F (eds) Bone circulation and vascularization in normal and pathological conditions. Plenum Press: New York: pp 19–28

Brookes M, Harrison R G 1957 The vascularisation of the rabbit femur and tibio-fibula. J Anat 91: 61–72

Brookes M, Landon D N 1964 The juxta-epiphysial vessels in the long bones of foetal rats. J Bone Jt Surg 46B: 336–345

Brooks D J, Frackowiack R S J 1989 PET and movement disorders. J Neurol Neurosurg Psychiat Special Supplement: 68–77

Brooks S T 1955 Skeletal age at death: reliability of cranial and pubic age indicators. Am J Phys Anthropol N S 13: 567–597

Broom N D 1984 Further insights into the structural principles governing the function of articular cartilage. J Anat 139: 275–294

Broom N D 1986 The collagenous architecture of articular cartilage – a synthesis of ultrastructure and mechanical function. J Rheum 13: 142–152

Broom N D, Marra D L 1986 Ultrastructural evidence of fibril-to-fibril associations in articular cartilage and their functional implications. J Anat 146: 185–200

Broom N D, Silyn-Roberts H 1989 The three-dimensional 'knit' of collagen fibrils in articular cartilage. Connect Tissue Res 23: 261–277

Broom R 1901 On the structure and affinities of Udenodon. Proc Zool Soc Lond 2: 162–190

Broom R 1930. The origin of the human skeleton: an introduction to human osteology. Witherby: London

Brosens I 1991 The fallopian tube. In: Philipp E, Setchell M, Ginsburg J (eds) Scientific foundations of obstetrics and gynaecology. Butterworth-Heinemann: Oxford: pp 135–145

Brothers L, Ring B 1993 Mesial temporal neurons in the macaque monkey with responses selective for aspects of social stimuli. Behav Brain Res 57: 53–61

Brothwell D R (ed) 1968 The skeletal biology of earlier human populations. (Symposia of the Society for the Study of Human Biology, Vol 8), Pergamon: Oxford

Brothwell D R, Carbonell V M, Goose D H 1963 In: Brothwell D R (ed) Dental anthropology. Pergamon: Oxford

Browder J, Kaplan H A 1976 Cerebral dural sinuses and their tributaries. Thomas: Springfield, Illinois

Brown A F, Dunn G A 1989 Microinterferometry of the movement of dry matter in fibroblasts. J Cell Sci 92: 379–389

Brown A G 1981 Organization in the spinal cord. The anatomy and physiology of identified neurones. Springer Verlag: Berlin

Brown A G, Franz D N 1969 Responses of spinocervical tract neurones to natural stimulation of identified cutaneous receptors. Exp Brain 7: 231–249

Brown A G, Franz D N 1970 Patterns of response in spinocervical tract neurones to different stimuli of long duration. Brain Res 17: 156–160

Brown A G, Gordon G 1977 Subcortical mechanisms concerned in somatic sensation. Br Med Bull 33: 121–128

Brown J M C, Henriksson J, Salmons S 1989 Restoration of fast muscle characteristics following cessation of chronic stimulation: physiological, histochemical and metabolic changes during slow-to-fast transformation. Proc R Soc B 235: 321–346

Brown J R 1949 Localising cerebellar syndromes. J Am Med Assoc 141: 518–521

Brown K A 1994 Role of endothelial cells in the pathogenesis of vascular damage. In: Cervera R, Khamashta M A, Hughes G R V (eds) Antibodies to endothelial cells and vascular damage. CRC Press: New York: pp 27–46

Brown L M, Pottern L M, Hoover R N 1992 Prenatal and perinatal risk factors for testicular cancer. Cancer Res 46: 4812–4819

Brown L T 1974 Corticorubral projections in the rat. J Comp Neurol 154: 149–168

Brown N A, Lander A 1993 Developmental biology. On the other hand . . . Nature 363: 303–304

Brown N A, McCarthy A, Wolpert L 1991 Development of handed body asymmetry in mammals. In: Bock G R, Marsh J (eds) Biological asymmetry and handedness. Chichester (Ciba Foundation Symposium 162) Wiley 182–201

Brown N A, Wolpert L 1990 The development of handedness in left/right asymmetry. Development 109: 1–9

Brown R L 1944 Rate of transport of spermia in human uterus and tubes. Am J Obstet 47: 407–411

Brown S 1974 The change in lens curvature with age. Exp Eye Res 19: 175–184

Brown W E, Salmons S, Whalen R G 1983 The sequential replacement of myosin subunit isoforms during muscle type transformation induced by long term electrical stimulation. J Biol Chem 258: 14686–14692

Brown W J, Barajas L, Latta H 1970 The ultrastructure of the human adrenal medulla: with comparative studies of the white rat. Anat Rec 169: 173–183

Brown W R 1991 A review and mathematical analysis of circadian rhythms in cell proliferation in mouse, rat and human epidermis. J Invest Dermatol 97: 273–280

Browne D 1928 The surgical anatomy of the tonsil. J Anat 63: 82–86

Browne D 1938 Diagnosis of undescended testicle. Br Med J 2: 168–171

Brownson C, Little P, Jarvis J C, Salmons S 1992a Reciprocal changes in myosin isoform mRNAs of rabbit skeletal muscle in response to the initiation and cessation of chronic electrical stimulation. Muscle Nerve 15: 694–700

Brownson C, Little P, Mayne C N, Jarvis J C, Salmons S 1992b Reciprocal changes in myosin isoform expression in rabbit fast skeletal muscle resulting from the application and removal of chronic electrical stimulation. In: el Haj A (ed) Molecular biology of muscle (Symposia of the Society for Experimental Biology no. 46). Company of Biologists: Cambridge: pp 301–310

Brueckner M, D'Eustachio P, Horwich A L 1989 Linkage mapping of a mouse gene, iv, that controls left-right asymmetry of the heart and viscera. Proc Natl Acad Sci USA 86: 5035–5038

Brueton R N, Revell W J, Brookes M 1993 Haemodynamics of bone healing in model stable fracture. In: Shoutens A, Arlet J, Gardiniers J W M, Hughes S P F (eds) Bone circulation and vascularization in normal and pathological conditions. Plenum Press: New York: pp 121–128

Brugge J F 1992 An overview of central auditory processing. In: Popper A, Fay R (eds) Springer handbook of research. Vol 2. The mammalian auditory pathway: neurophysiology. Springer-Verlag: New York: pp. 1–33

Brun A 1965 The subpial granular layer of the foetal cerebral cortex in man. Acta Pathol Microbiol Immunol Scand (suppl) 179: 1–98

Brundin P, Strecker R E, Widner H et al 1988 Human fetal dopamine neurons grafted in a rat model of Parkinson's disease: immunological aspects, spontaneous and drug-induced behaviour, and dopamine release. Exp Brain Res 70: 192–208

Brunet C L, Sharpe P M, Ferguson M W J 1995 Inhibition of TGF3 but not TGFB, or TGFB2 activity prevents normal mouse embryonic palate fusion. Int J Devel Biol 0: 000–000

Brunsteins D B, Ferreri A J M 1990 Microsurgical anatomy of VII and VIII cranial nerves and related arteries in the cerebellopontine angle. Surg Radiol Anat 12: 259–265

Bucana C D, Munn C G, Song M J, Dunneth K Jr, Kripke M L 1992 Internalization of Ia molecules into Birbeck granule-like structures in murine dendritic cells. J Invest Dermatol 99: 365–373

Buccione R Vanderhyden B C, Caron P J, Eppig J J 1990 FSH-induced expansion of the mouse cumulus oorphus in vitro is dependent upon a specific factor(s) secreted by the oocyte. Dev Biol 138: 16–25

Buccione R, Schroeder A C, Eppig J J 1990 Interactions between somatic cells and germ cells throughout mammalian oogenesis. Biol Reprod 43: 543–547

Buchan A M J, Polak J M, Facer P, Bloom S R, Szelke M, Hudson D, Pearse A G E 1977 Abstract: Use of synthetic fragments for specific immunostaining of CCK cells. Presented at the British Society of Gastroenterology, April 1977

Bucher U, Reid L 1961 Development of the mucus-secreting elements in humanlung. Thorax 16: 219–225

Buck L, Axel R 1991 A novel multigene family may encode odorant receptors: a molecular basis for odor recognition. Cell 65: 175–187

Buckingham J C, Safieh S, Singh S, Arduino L A, Cover P O, Kendall M D 1992 Interactions between the hypothalamo-pituitary axis and the thymus in the rat: a role for corticotropin in the control of thymulin release. J Neuroendocrinol 4: 295–301

Buckingham M 1985 Actin and myosin gene families: their expression during the formation of skeletal muscle. Essays in Biochemistry 20: 77–109

Buckingham M 1992 Making muscle in mammals. Trends in Genetics 8: 144–149

Buckingham M 1994 Which myogenic factors make muscle? Current Biology 4: 61–63

Buckland-Wright J C 1977 Microradiographic and histological examination of the split-line formation in bone. J Anat 124: 193–203

Buckland-Wright J C 1978 Bone structure and the patterns of force transmission in the cat skull (Felis catus). J Morphol 155: 35–62

Buckland-Wright J C 1989 A new high definition microfocal X-ray unit. Br J Radiol 62: 201–208

Buckland-Wright J C, Bradshaw C R 1989 Clinical applications of high-definition microfocal radiography. Br J Radiol 62: 209–217

Buckland-Wright J C, Lynch J A, Rymer J, Fogelman I 1994 Fractal signature analysis of macroradiographs measures trabecular organization in lumbar vertebrae of postmenopausal women. Calcif Tiss Int 54: 106–112

Buckley C H, Fox H 1989 Biopsy pathology of the endometrium. Chapman and Hall Medical: London

Budorick N E, Pretorius D H, Grafe M R, Lou K V 1991 Ossification of the fetal spine. Radiology 181: 561–565

Budschu H D, Suchenwirth R, Davis W 1973 Histochemical changes in disuse atrophy of human skeletal muscle. In: Kakulas B (ed) Basic research in myology. Excerpta Medica: Amsterdam: pp 108–112

Budzinka K, Supinski G, DiMarco A F 1989 Inspiratory action of separate external and parasternal intercostal muscle contraction. J Appl Physiol 67: 1395–1400

Buechal F F, Pappas M J 1992 Survivors and clinical evaluation of cementless meniscal bearing total ankle replacements. Sem Arthroplas 3: 43–50

Buehr M, Gu S, McLaren A 1993 Mesonephric contribution to testis differentiation in the fetal mouse. Development 117: 273–281

Buffa R, Capella C, Solcia E, Frigerio B, Saio S I 1977 Vasoactive intestinal peptide (VIP) cells in the pancreas and gastrointestinal mucosa. An immunohistochemical and ultrastructural study. Histochemistry 50: 217–227

Bugbee W D, Botte M J 1993 Surface anatomy of the hand: the relationship between palmar skin creases and osseous anatomy. Clin Orthop 296: 122–126

Bulfone A, Puelles L, Porteus M H, Frohmann M A, Martin G R, Rubinstein J L R 1993 J Neurosci 13: 3155–3172

Bulger R E 1965 The shape of rat kidney tubule cells. Am J Anat 116: 237–255

Bulger R E 1971 Ultrastructure of the junctional complexes from the descending thin limbs of the loop of Henle from rats. Anat Rec 171: 471–475

Bulger R E, Dobyan D C 1982 Recent advances in renal morphology. Annu Rev Physiol 44: 147–179

Buller A J 1970 The neural control of the contractile mechanism in skeletal muscle. Endeavour 29: 107–111

Buller A J, Eccles J C, Eccles R M 1960 Interactions between motoneurons and muscles in respect of the characteristic speeds of their responses. J Physiol 150: 417–439

Bulloch K, Moore R Y 1981 Innervation of the thymus gland by brain stem and spinal cord in the mouse and rat. Am J Anat 162: 157–166

Bullough P, Goodfellow J 1968 The significance of the fine structure of articular cartilage. J Bone Jt Surg 50B: 852–857

Bullough W S, Laurence E B 1961 The study of mammalian epidermal mitosis in vitro. A critical analysis of technique. Exp Cell Res 24: 287–297

Bulmer D 1957 Observations on the development of the vaginal wall. J Anat 91: 599P

Bulmer D 1965 A histochemical study of ovarian cholinesterases. Acta Anat 62: 254–265

Bulmer M G 1970 The biology of twinning in man. Clarendon Press: Oxford

Bumke O, Foerster O (eds) 1936 Handbuch der Neurologie. Springer-Verlag: Berlin

Bunge M B, Bunge R P, Ris H 1961 Ultrastructure study of reunification in an experimental lesion in adult cat spinal cord. J Bio Biochem Cytol 10: 67–94

Bunge R P 1976 The expression of neuronal specificity in tissue culture. In: Barondes S H (ed) Neuronal recognition. Plenum Press: New York: pp 109–128

Bunnag S C, Bunnag S, Warner N E 1963 Microcirculation in the islets of Langerhans of the mouse. Anat Rec 146: 117–123

Bunning P S C, Barnett C H 1963 Variations in the talocalcaneal articulation. J Anat 97: 643P

Bunning P S C, Barnett C H 1965 A comparison of adult and foetal talocalcaneal articulations. J Anat 99: 71–76

Buntine J A 1970 The omohyoid muscle and fascia: morphology and anomalies. Aust N Z J Surg 40: 86–88

Buranarugsa M, Houghton P 1981 Polynesian head form: an interpretation of a factor analysis of Cartesian co-ordinate data. J Anat 133: 333–350

Burde R M 1983 The visceral nuclei of the oculomotor complex. Trans Am Ophthalmol Soc 81: 532–548

Burggren W W, Johansen K 1986 Circulation and respiration in lungfishes. J Morph Suppl 1: 217–236

Burgoyne P S, Buehr M, Koopman P, Rossant J, McLaren A 1988 Cell-autonomous action of the testis-determining gene: Sertoli cells are exclusively XY in XX-XY chimeric mouse testes. Development 102: 443–450

Burgoyne R D 1991 Control of exocytosis in adrenal chromaffin cells. Biochem Biophys Acta 1071: 174–202

Burk D, Sadler T W, Langman J 1979 Distribution of surface coat material on nasal folds of mouse embryos as demonstrated by Concanvalin A staining. Anat Rec 193: 185–196

Burke R E, Levine D N, Tsairis P, Zajac F E 1973 Physiological types and histochemical profiles of motor units in the cat gastrocnemius. J Physiol 234: 723–748

Burkel W E 1970 The fine structure of the terminal branches of the hepatic arterial system of the rat. Anat Rec 167: 329–349

Burkhalter A, Bernardo K L, Charles V 1993 Development of local circuits in human visual cortex. J Neurosci 13: 1916–1931

Burkitt A N, Lightoller G H S 1926–1927 The facial musculature of the Australian aboriginal. J Anat 61: 14–39, 62: 33–35

Burkitt H G, Young B, Heath J W (eds) 1993 Wheater's functional histology. 3rd edition. Churchill Livingstone: Edinburgh

Burn J H 1968 The mechanism of the release of noradrenaline. In: Wolstenholme G E W, O'Conner M (eds) Adrenergic neurotransmission (CIBA Foundation Study Group 33). Churchill: London: pp 16–25

Burn-Murdoch R 1990 The role of the vasculature in tooth eruption. Europ J Orthod 12: 101–108

Burne R A, Azizi S A, Mihailoff G A, Woodward D 1981 The tectopontine projection in the rat with comments on visual pathways to the basilar pons. J Comp Neurol 202: 287–307

Burne R A, Mihailoff G A, Woodward D J 1978 Visual corticopontine input to the paraflocculus: a combined autoradiographic and horseradish peroxidase study. Brain Res 143: 139–146

Burnet F M 1969 Rok 1960 nagroda dia F M Burneta i P B Medawara za odkrycie nabytej tolerancji immunologiczne. Wlad Lek, 22: 505–506

Burnside M B 1971 Microtubules and microfilaments in newt neurulation. Dev Biol 26: 416–441

Burnstock G 1970 Structure of smooth muscle and its innervation. In: Bülbring E, Brading A F, Jones A W, Tomita T (eds) Smooth Muscle. Arnold: London: pp 1–69

Burnstock G 1972 Purinergic nerves. Pharmacol Rev 24: 509–581

Burnstock G 1976 Control of smooth muscle activity in vessels by adrenergic nerves and circulating catecholamines. In: Noval M, Vassori G (eds) Smooth muscle pharmacology and physiology. INSERM Paris 50: pp 251–264

Burnstock G 1976 Do some nerve cells release more than one transmitter? Neurosci 1: 239–248

Burnstock G 1981 Neurotransmitters and trophic factors in the autonomic nervous system. J Physiol 313: 1–35

Burnstock G 1986 Autonomic neuromuscular junctions: current developments and future directions. J Anat 146: 1–30

Burnstock G 1988 Autonomic neural control mechanisms with special reference to the airways. In: Kaliner M A, Barnes P J (eds) The airways. Neural control in health and disease. Marcel Dekker: New York: pp 1–22

Burnstock G 1990 Changes in expression of autonomic nerves in aging and disease. J Auton Nerv Syst 30: 525–534

Burnstock G 1990 Co-tranmission. The fifth Heymans lecture. Arch Int Pharmacodyn Ther 304: 7–33

Burnstock G 1990c Innervation of bladder and bowel. Ciba Foundation Symposium 151: 2–18

Burnstock G 1992–95 (series ed): The autonomic nervous system. Vols 1–14. Harwood Academic Publishers: Switzerland

Burnstock G 1993 Changing face of autonomic and sensory nerves in the circulation. In: Edvinsson L, Uddman R (eds) Vascular innervation and receptor mechanisms: new perspectives. Academic Press: Oxford: pp 1–22

Burnstock G, Bell C 1974 Peripheral autonomic transmission. In: Hubbard J I (ed) Peripheral nervous system. Plenum Press: New York: pp 277–327

Burnstock G, Chamley J, Campbell G R 1980 The innervation of the arteries. In: Schwartz C J, Werthessen N T, Wolf S (eds) Structure and function of the circulation. Vol 1. Plenum Press: New York: pp 729–767

Burnstock G, McCulloch M W, Storey D F, Wright M E 1972 Factors affecting the extraneuronal inactivation of noradrenaline in cardiac and smooth muscle. Brit J Pharmacol 46: 243–253

Burstein Y, Buchner V, Pecht M, Trainin N 1988 Thymic humoral factor gamma 2: purification and amino acid sequence of an immunoregulatory peptide from calf thymus. Biochem 27: 4066–4071

Burton A C 1954 Relation of structure to function of the tissues of the wall of blood vessels. Physiol Rev 34: 619–642

Burton H 1986 Second somatosensory cortex and related areas. In: Jones E G, Peters A (eds) Cerebral Cortex. Vol 5. Sensory-motor areas and aspects of cortical connectivity. Plenum Press: New York: pp 31–98

Burton H, Loewy A D 1977 Projections to the spinal cord from medullary somatosensory relay nuclei. J Comp Neurol 173: 773–792

Burton H, Sinclair R J 1994 Representation of tactile roughness in thalamus and somatosensory cortex. Can J Physiol Pharmacol 72: 546–557

Burton H, Videen T O, Raichle M E 1993 Tactile-vibration-activated foci in insular and parietal-opercular cortex studied with positron emission tomography: mapping the second somatosensory area in humans. Somatosens Mot Res 10: 297–308

Burwell R G, Dangerfield P H 1992 Pathogenesis and assessment of scoliosis. In: Findlay G, Owen R (eds) Surgery of the spine; a combined orthopaedic and neurosurgical approach. Blackwell: Oxford

Burwell R G, Vernon C L, Dangerfield P H 1980 Skeletal measurement. In: Owen R, Goodfellow J, Bullough P (eds) Scientific foundations of orthopaedics and traumatology. Heinemann: London

Buschard K, Kjaeldgaard A 1973 Investigations and analysis of the position, fixation, length and embryology of the vermiform appendix. Acta Chir Scand 139: 293–298

Buser P 1987 Thalamocortical mechanisms underlying synchronised EEG activity. In: Halliday A M, Butler S R, Paul R (eds) A textbook of clinical neurophysiology. John Wiley: Chichester: pp 595–622

Bushnell M C, Duncan G H, Tremblay N 1993 Thalamic VPM nucleus in the behaving monkey. I. Multimodal and discriminative properties of thermosensitive neurons. J Neurophysiol 69: 739–752

Buskirk C van 1945 The seventh nerve complex. J Comp Neurol 82: 303–333

Bussolino D, Di Renzo M F, Ziche M, Bocchietto E, Olivero M, Naldini L, Gaudino G, Tamagnone L, Coffer A, Comoglio P M 1992 Hepatocyte growth factor is a potent angiogenic factor which stimulates endothelial cell motility and growth. J Cell Biol 119: 626–641

Buthpitiya A G, Stroud D, Russell C O H 1987 Pharyngeal pump and esophageal transit. Dig Dis Sci 32: 1244–1248

Butler C R 1966 Cortical lesions and interhemisphere communication in monkeys (Macaca mulatta). Nature 209: 59–61

Butler H 1967 The development of mammalian dural venous sinuses with special reference to the post-glenoid vein. J Anat 102: 33–36

Butler J 1957 The development of certain human dural venous sinuses. J Anat 91: 510–526

Butler-Browne G S, Eriksson P O, Laurent C, Thornell L E 1988 Adult human masseter muscle fibers express myosin isozymes characteristic of development. Muscle Nerve 11: 610–620

Butt A M, Colquhoun K, Tutton M, Berry M 1994a Three-dimensional morphology of astrocytes and oligodendrocytes in the intact mouse optic nerve. J Neurocytol 23: 469 – 485

Butt A M, Duncan A, Berry M 1994b Astrocyte associations with nodes of Ranvier: ultrastructural analysis of HRP-filled astrocytes in the mouse optic nerve. J Neurocytol 23: 486 – 499

Butt A M, Ransom B R 1933 Morphology of astrocytes and oliogdendrocytes during development in the intact rat optic nerve. J Comp Neurol 338: 141–158

Buttner U, Brandt T (eds) 1992 Ocular motor disorders of the brain stem. Baillière's Clinical Neurology. Vol 1, No. 2. Ballière: London

Büttner-Ennever J A (ed) 1988 Neuroanatomy of the oculomotor system. Elsevier: Amsterdam

Büttner-Ennever J A, Akert K 1981 Medial rectus subgroups of the oculomotor nucleus and their abducens internuclear input in the monkey. J Comp Neurol 197: 17–27

Butzner J D, Befus A D 1989 Interactions among intraepithelial leucocytes and other epithelial cells in intestinal development and function. In: Lebenthal E (ed) Human gastrointestinal development. Raven Press: New York: pp 749–775

Buys H, Pead L, Hallett R, Maskell R 1994 Suprapubic aspiration under ultrasound guidance in children with fever of undiagnosed cause. BMJ 308: 690–692

Byers M R 1984 Dental sensory receptors. Int Rev Neurobiol 25: 39–94

C

Cabanie M H, Javelle J 1966 La frange péritonéale sous-iléo-terminale. C R Hebd Séanc Acad Sci Paris 131: 248–252

Cajal S R y 1911 Histologie du système nerveux de l'homme et des vertébrés. Maloine: Paris

Cajal S R Y 1928 Degeneration and regeneration in the nervous system. Oxford University Press: London

Calasans O M 1953 Arquitetura do músulo ciliar no homen. An Fac Med Univ S Paulo 27: 3–98

Caldwell W E, Moloy H C 1933 Anatomical variations in the female pelvis and their effect in labor with suggested classification. Am J Obsted Gynecol 26: 479–505

Caldwell W E, Moloy H C, D'Esopo D A 1940 The more recent conceptions of the pelvic architecture. Am J Obstet Gynecol 40: 558–565

Caliot P, Bousquet V, Midy D, Cabanié P 1989 A contribution to the study of the accessory nerve: surgical implications. Surgical-Radiologic Anat 11: 11–15

Calne R Y 1984 Colour atlas of renal transplantation. Medical Economics Books: Oreadell

Calof A L, Chikaraishi D M 1989 Analysis of neurogenesis in a mammalian neuroepithelium: proliferation and differentiation of an olfactory neuron precursor in vitro. Neuron: 115–127

Calvin M, Young S R, Koffman G, Hart J, Dyson M 1994 High frequency diagnostic ultrasound: a potential adjunct to renal graft function assessment post-transplantation. Wound Repair Regen (In press)

Cameron A H 1968 The Birmingham twin survey. Proc Roy Soc Med 61: 229

Cameron D A 1961 Erosion of the epiphysis of the rat tibia by capillaries. J Bone Jt Surg 43B: 590–594

Cameron-Curry P, Dulac C, Le Douarin N M 1993 Negative regulation of Schwann cell myelin protein gene expression by the dorsal root ganglionic microenvironment. Europ J Neurosci 5: 594–604

Campbell A H, Liddelow A G 1967 Significant variations in the shape of the trachea and large bronchi. Med J Aust 54: 1017–1020

Campbell A W 1905 Histological studies on the localisation of cerebral function. Cambridge University Press: Cambridge

Campbell E J M 1955 The role of the scalene and sternomastoid muscles in breathing in normal subjects. An electromyographic study. J Anat 89: 378–386

Campbell E J M 1958 The respiratory muscles and the mechanics of breathing. Lloyd-Luke: London

Campbell S, Allen T D, Moser W, Aplin J D 1990 The translaminal fibrils of the human amnion basement membrane. J Cell Sci 94: 307–318

Campian R, Minckler J 1976 A note on the gross configurations of the human auditory cortex. Brain and language 3: 318–323

Canalis E, McCarthy T L, Centrella M 1993 Factors that regulate bone formation. In: Mundy G R, Martin T J (eds) Physiology and pharmacolgy of bone. Springer-Verlag: Berlin: pp 249–266

Candiollo L 1965 Richerche anatomo-comparative sul musculo tensore del timpano, con riferimento alla innervazione propriocettiva. Z Zellforsch 67: 34–56

Candiollo L, Levi A C 1969 Studies on the morphogenesis of the middle ear muscles in man. Arch Ohr-Nas Kehlkopf Heilk 195: 55–67

Canham P B, Mullin K 1978 Orientation of medial smooth muscle in the wall of systemic muscular arteries. J Microsc 114: 307–318

Caniggia I, Tseu I, Han R N, Smith B T, Tanswell K, Post M 1991 Spatial and temporal differences in fibroblast behaviour in fetal rat lung. American Journal of Physiology 261: 424–433

Cannon B, Nedergaard J 1985 Brown adipose tissue: molecular mechanisms controlling activity and thermogenesis. In: Cryer A, Van R L R (eds) New perspectives in adipose tissues: structure, function and development. Butterworths: London

Cantin M, Thibault G, Ding J, Gutkousta J, Garcia R, Hamet P, Genest J 1987 The whole heart is an endocrine gland. Int J Nucl Med Biol 14: 313–322

Cantle S J, Kaufmann P, Luckhardt M, Schweikhart G 1987 Interpretation of syncytial sprouts and bridges in the human placenta. Placenta 8: 221–234

Capella C, Hage H, Solicia E, Usellini L 1978 Ultrastructural similarity of endocrine-like cells of the human lung and some related cells of the gut. Cell Tiss Res 186: 25–37

Capella C, Solcia E, Frigerio B, Buffa R 1976 Endocrine cells of the human intestine. An ultrastructural study. In: Fujita T (ed) Endocrine gut and pancreas. Elsevier: New York: pp 43–60

Capella C, Solcia E, Frigerio B, Buffa R, Usellini L, Fontana P 1977 The endocrine cells of the pancreas. Ultrastructural study and classification. Virchows Arch Abt A 373: 327–352

Capella G et al 1978 Fistula and pharyngostomas in total laryngectomy. An Otorrinolaringol Ibero Am 5(5): 503–516

Capen C C 1975 Functional and fine structural relationships of parathyroid glands. Adv Vet Sci Comp Med 19: 249–286

Capen C C, Roth S I 1973 Ulstrastructural and functional relationships of normal and pathologic parathyroid cells. In: Ioachim H L (ed) Pathobiology annual 1973. Vol 3. Appleton-Century-Crofts: New York: pp 129–175

Caputo R, Perluchetti D 1977 The junctions of normal human epidermis. A freeze-fracture study. J. Ultrastruct Res 61: 44–61

Carando S, Portigliatti Barbos M, Ascenzi A, Boyde A 1989 Orientation of collagen in human tibial and fibular shafts and possible correlation with mechanical properties. Bone 10: 139–142

Cardinali D P, Larin F, Wurtman R J 1971 Action spectra for effects of light on hydroxyindole-o-methyltransferases in rat pineal, retina and harderian glands. Endocrinology 91: 877–886

Carey E J 1921 Studies on the structure and function of the small intestine. Anat Rec 21: 189–216

Carey E J, Zeit W, McGrath B F 1927 Studies in the dynamics of histogenesis. XII. The regeneration of the patellae of dogs. Am J Anat 40: 127–158

Carlsen E, Giwercman A, Keiding N, Skakkebaek N E 1992 Evidence for decreasing quality of semen during past 50 years. BMJ 305: 609–613

Carlsen F, Behse F 1980 Three dimensional analysis of Schwann cells associated with unmyelinated nerve fibres in human aural nerve. J Anat 130: 545–547

Carlsen J, Heimer L 1986 The basolateral amygdaloid complex as a cortical-like structure. Brain Res 441: 377–380

Carlstedt T 1977 Observations on the morphology at the transition between the peripheral and the central nervous system in the cat. I–V. Acta Physiol Scand 100: Suppl 446, 5–85

Carlström D 1964 Polarization microscopy of dental enamel with reference to incipient carious lesions. Adv Oral Biol 1: 255–296

Carmel P W 1985 Vegetative dysfunctions of the hypothalamus. Acta Neurochir 75: 106–121

Carnahan J F, Patterson P H 1991 The generation of monoclonal antibodies that bind preferentially to adrenal chromaffin cells and the cells of embryonic sympathetic ganglia. J Neurosci 11: 3493–3506

Caro C G, Pedley T J, Schroter R C, Seed W A 1978 The mechanics of circulation. Oxford University Press: Oxford

Carolene D 1991 Practical procedures. In: Fleming P J, Speidel B D, Marlow N, Dunn P M (eds) A neonatal vade-mecum. 2nd edition. Lloyd-Luke: London: p 351

Carpenter M B 1981 Anatomy of the corpus striatum and brainstem nuclei. In: Brookhard J M, Mountcastle V B, Brooks V B (eds) Handbook of physiology, Section 1 The nervous system, Vol 2 Motor control, Part 2. American Physiol Soc: Bethesda: pp 947–995

Carpenter M B 1984 Interconnections between the corpus striatum and brainstem nuclei. In: McKenzie J S, Kemm R E, Wilcock L (eds) Advances in behavioural biology 27: The basal ganglia—structure and function. Plenum Press: New York and London: pp 1–68

Carpenter M B, Chang L, Pereira A B, Hersh L B, Bruce G, Wu J-Y 1987 Vestibular and cochlear efferent neurons in the monkey identified by immunocytochemical methods. Brain Res 408: 275 – 280

Carpenter M B, Stein B M, Shriver J E 1968 Central projections of spinal dorsal roots in the monkey. II. Lower thoracic, lumbosacral and coccygeal dorsal roots. Am J Anat 123: 75–118

Carpenter M B, Whittier J R 1952 Study of methods for producing experimental lesions of the central nervous system with special reference to sterotaxic technique. J Comp Neurol 97: 73–132

Carr I 1967 Nuclear membranous whorls. Z Zellforsch 80: 140–144

Carr I 1970 The fine structure of the mammalian lymphoreticular system. Int Rev Cytol 77: 283–348

Carr J, Clegg E J, Meek G A 1968 Sertoli cells as phagocytes: an electron microscopic study. J Anat 102: 501–510

Carr V M, Farbman A I 1991 Identification of a new nonneuronal cell in rat olfactory epithelium. Neuroscience 45: 433–449

Carrel A 1912 On the permanent life of tissues outside the organism. J Exp Med 15: 516–528

Carter R B, Keen E N 1971 The intramandibular course of the inferior alveolar nerve. J Anat 108: 433–440

Cartmill M 1992 New views on primate origins. Evolutionary Anthropology 1: 105–111

Carvalho C A F, Garcia O S, Vitti M, Berzin F 1972 Electromyographic study of the m tensor fasciae latae and m sartorius. Electromyogr Clin Neurophysiol 12: 387–400

Case R M 1979 Pancreatic secretion: cellular aspects. In: Duthi H L, Wormsley K G (eds) Scientific basis of gastroenterology. Churchill Livingstone: Edinburgh: pp 163–198

Caspersson T 1936 Ueber den chemischen Aufbau der Strukturen des Zellkernes. Skand Arch Physiol (suppl 8): 73

Caspersson T, Farber S, Foley G E, Kudynowski J, Modest E J, Simonsson E, Wagh V, Zech L 1968 Chemical differentiation along metaphase chromosomes. Exp Cell Res 49: 219–222

Castanet J, Francillon-Vieilot H, Meunier F J, de Ricqles A 1993 Bone and individual ageing. In: Hall B K (ed) Bone Vol 7. Bone growth-B. CRC Press: Boca Raton: pp 245–283

Castelli W A 1963 Vascular architecture of the human adult mandible. J Dent Res 42: 786–792

Castellucci M, Classen-Linke I, Muhlhauser J, Kaufmann P, Zardi L, Chiquet-Ehrismann R 1991 The human placenta: a model for tenascin expression. Histochemistry 95: 449–458

Castellucci M, Scheper M, Scheffen I, Celona A, Kaufmann P 1990 The development of the human placental villous tree. Anat Embryol 181: 117–128

Castiglioni A J, Gallaway M C, Coulter J D 1978 Spinal projections from the midbrain in the monkey. J Comp Neurol 178: 329–346

Castleman B 1966 The pathology of the thymus gland in myasthenia gravis. Ann N Y Acad Sci 135: 496–505

Castor C W 1962 The microscopic structure of normal human synovial tissue. Arthritis Rheum 3: 140–151

Castorina S 1957 Le arterie coronarie del cuore umano. Arch Ital Anat Embriol 62: 261–284

Castro O, Johnson L N V, Mamourian A C 1990 Isolated inferior oblique paresis from brainstem infarction: perspective on oculomotor fascicular organization in the ventral midbrain tegmentum. Arch Neurol 47: 235–237

Catford J C 1992 A practical introduction to phonetics. Clarendon Press: Oxford

Catsman-Berrevoets C E, Kuypers H G J M 1981 A search for corticospinal collaterals to thalamus and mesencephalon by means of multiple retrograde fluorescent tracers in cat and rat. Brain Res 218: 15–23

Cattanach B M, Beechey C V 1994 Genetic imprinting map. Mouse Genome 92: 108–110

Catton W T, Gray J E 1951 Electromyographic study of the action of the serratus anterior muscle in respiration. J Anat 85: 412P

Cauldwell E W, Siekert R G, Lininger R E, Anson B J 1948 Bronchial arteries. Anatomic study of 150 human cadavers. Surg Gynecol Obstet 86: 395–412

Caulfield J P, Farquhar M G 1974 The permeability of glomerular capillaries to graded dextrans. Identification of the basement membrane as the primary filtration barrier. J Cell Biol 63: 883–903

Cauller L J, Connors B W 1994 Synaptic physiology of horizontal afferents to layer I in slices of rat SI neocortex. J Neurosci 14: 751–762

Cauna N 1966 Fine structure of the receptor organs and its probable functional significance. In: de Reuck A V S, Knight J (eds) Touch, heat and pain (Ciba Foundation Symposium). Churchill: London: pp 117–127

Cauna N 1970 The fine structures of the arteriovenous anastomosis and its nerve supply in the human nasal respiratory muscoa. Anat. Rec. 168: 9–22

Cauna N, Hinderer K H 1969 Fine structure of blood vessels of the human nasal respiratory epithelium. Ann Otol Rhinol Laryngol 78: 865–879

Cauna N, Mannan G 1959 Developmental and post-natal changes of digital Pacinian corpuscles (Corpuscula lamellosa) in the human hand. J Anat 93: 271–286

Cauna N, Manzetti G W, Hinderer K H, Swanson E W 1972 Fine structure of nasal polyps. Ann Otol Rhinol Laryngol 81: 41–58

Cavagna G A, Heglund N C, Taylor C R 1977 Mechanical work in terrestrial locomotion, two basic mechanisms for minimizing energy expenditure. Am J Physiol 233: R243–R261

Cavallero C, Spagnoli L G, Villaschi S 1976 An electron microscopic study of human pancreatic islets. In: Fujita T (ed) Endocrine gut and pancreas. Elsevier: New York: pp 61–72

Cavanagh P R (ed) The biomechanics of distance running. Human Kinetics Publishers: Champaign, Illinois

Cavanagh P R, Lafortune M A 1980 Ground reaction forces in distance running. J Biomech 13: 397–406

Cavatori P 1908 Il tipo normale e le variazioni delle arterie della base dell'encefalo nell'uomo. Monitore Zool Ital 19: 248–258

Cave A J E 1929 The distribution of the first intercostal nerve and its relation to the first rib. J Anat 63: 367–379

Cave A J E 1934 On the occipito-atlanto-axial articulations. J Anat 68: 416–423

Cave A J E 1937 The innervation and morphology of the cervical intertransverse muscles. J Anat 71: 497–515

Cave A J E 1961 The nature and morphology of the costoclavicular ligament. J Anat 95: 170–179

Cave A J E 1975 The morphology of the mammalian cervical pleurapophysis. J Zool Lond 177: 377–393

Cave A J E, Brown R W 1952 On the tendon of the subclavius muscle. J Bone Jt Surg 34B 466–469

Cave A J E, Porteous C J 1958 The attachments of m semimembranosus. J Anat 92: 638P

Caviness V S Jr 1982 Dev Brain Res 4: 293–302

Cawley J C, Hayhoe F G J 1973 Ultrastructure of haemic cells: a cytological atlas of normal and leukaemic blood and bone marrow. Saunders: London

Cechetto D F, Saper C B 1988 Neurochemical organization of the hypothalamic projection to the spinal cord in the rat. J Comp Neurol 272: 579–604

Celebrini S, Thorpe S, Trotter Y, Imbert M 1993 Dynamics of orientation coding in area V1 of the awake primate. Visual Neurosci 10: 811–825

Celio M R, Heizmann C W 1981 Calcium binding protein parvalbumin as a neuronal marker. Nature 293: 300–302

Celtis A, Porter A J 1952 Lymphatics of the thorax. Acta Radiol 38: 461–470

Cha K Y, Koo J J, Choi D H, Han S Y, Yoon T K 1991 Pregnancy after in vitro fertilization of human follicular oocytes collected from non-stimulated cycles; their culture in vitro and their transfer in a donor oocyte programme. Ferti Steril 55: 109–113

Chabardes D, Imbert M, Clique A, Montegut M, Morel F 1975 PTH sensitive adenyl cyclase activity in different segments of the rabbit nephron. Pflügers Arch 354: 229–239

Chacko L W 1955 The lateral geniculate body of the chimpanzee. J Anat Soc Ind 4: 10–13

Chagas A C P, Moreira L F P, Luz P L da, Camarano G P, Leirner A, Stolf N A G, Jatene A D 1989 Stimulated preconditioned skeletal muscle cardiomyoplasty. An effective means of cardiac assist. Circulation 80 (Suppl III): III-202–III-208

Chalepakis G, Stoykova A, Wijnholds J, Tremblay P, Gruss P 1993 J Neurobiol 24: 1367–1384

Challice C E, Viragh S 1973 Ultrastructure of the mammalian heart. Academic Press: New York

Chambers M R, Andres K H, Duering M von, Iggo A 1972 The structure and function of the slowly adapting type II receptor in hairy skin. Q J Exp Physiol 57: 417–445

Chambers T J, Darby J A, Fuller K 1985 Mammalian collagenase predisposes bone surfaces to osteoclastic resorption. Cell Tiss Res 241: 671–675

Chambers W W, Sprague J M 1955a Functional localization in cerebellum; organization in longitudinal cortico-nuclear zones and their contribution to control of posture, both extrapyramidal and pyramidal. J Comp Neurol 103: 105–129

Chambers W W, Sprague J M 1955b Functional localization in cerebellum;

somatotopic organization in cortex and nuclei. Arch Neurol Psychiatry 74: 653–680

Champetier J, Descours C 1968 The branches of the posterior tibial nerve in the tibiotarsal joint. C R Assoc Anat 141: 677–685

Champion R H, Burton J L, Ebling F J G (eds) 1991 Textbook of dermatology. 5th edition. 4 vols. Blackwell: Oxford: pp 373–383

Chan W Y, Tam P P L 1988 A morphological and experimental study of the mesencephalic neural crest cells in the mouse embryo using wheat germ agglutinin-gold conjugate as the cell marker. Development 102: 427–442

Chan-Palay V 1983 Gamma-aminobutyric acid pathways in the cerebellum studied by retrograde and anterograde transport of glutamic acid decarboxylase (GAD) antibody after in vivo injections. Progr Brain Res 55: 51–76

Chang M C 1951 Fertilizing capacity of spermatozoa deposited into fallopian tubes. Nature 168: 697–698

Chang M C, Hunter R H F 1975 Capacitation of mammalian sperm: biological and experimental aspects. In: Hamilton D W, Greep R O (eds) Handbook of physiology Section 7, Endocrinology Vol V. American Physiological Society: Washington, DC: pp 339–352

Chang W W L, Leblond C P 1971 Renewal of the epithelium in the descending colon of the mouse. Presence of three cell populations: vacuolated columnar, mucous and argentaffin. Am J Anat 131: 73–99

Chao T I, Skachkov S N, Eberhardt W, Reichenbach A 1994 Na + channels of Müller (glial) cells isolated from retinae of various mammalian species including man. Glia 10: 173 – 185

Chaplin D M, Greenlee T K 1975 The development of human digital tendons. J Anat 120: 253–274

Chapman G B, Chiardo A J, Coffey R J, Weineke K 1966 The fine structure of mucosal epithelial cells of a pathological human gall bladder. Anat Rec 154: 579–616

Chapple C R, Crowe R, Gilpin S A, Gosling J, Burnstock G 1991 The innervation of the human prostate gland – the changes associated with benign enlargement. J Urol 146: 1637–1644

Chapple J C 1992 Genetic screening. In: Brock D J H, Rodeck C H, Ferguson-Smith M A (eds) Prenatal diagnosis and screening. Churchill Livingstone: Edinburgh: pp 579–593

Charcot J M 1883 Lecture on localization of cerebral and spinal disease. Edited and translated by M A Hodden. New Sydenham Society: London

Charlton B G, Nkomanazana O F, McGradey J, Neal D E 1991 A preliminary study of acetylcholinesterase-positive innervation in the human adrenal cortex. J Anat 176: 99–104

Charnley J 1959 The lubrication of animal joints. In: Proceedings of the Symposium on Biomechanics, held London 1959. Institution of Mechanical Engineers: London: pp 12–19

Chase L R, Aurbach G D 1967 Parathyroid function and the renal excretion of 3' 5'-adenylic acid. Proc Natl Acad Sci USA 58: 518–525

Chaudhry A P, Cutler L A, Yamane G M, Labay G R, Sunderraj M, Manak J R Jr 1987 Ultrastructure of normal human parotid gland with special emphasis on myoeptithelial distribution. J Anat 152: 1–11

Chayen D, Nathan H 1974 Anatomical observations of the subgaleotic fascia. Acta Anat 87: 427–432

Chelazzi L, Miller E K, Duncan J, Desimone R 1993 A neural basis for visual search in inferior temporal cortex. Nature 363: 345–347

Chen I-Li, Mascorro J A, Yates R D 1976 Morphology and functional considerations of the carotid body and paraganglia. In: Coupland R E, Fujita T (eds) Chromaffin, enterchromaffin and related cells. Elsevier: New York: pp 333–353

Chen I-Li, Yates R D 1970 Ultrastructural studies of vagal paraganglia in Syrian hamsters. Z Zellforsch 108: 309–323

Chen L, Weiss L 1972 Electron microscopy of the red pulp of the human spleen. Am J Anat 134: 425–458

Chen L, Weiss L 1973 The role of the sinus wall in the passage of erythrocytes through the spleen. Blood 41: 529–537

Chen S, Hillman D E 1993 Colocalization of neurotransmitters in the deep cerebellar nuclei. J Neurocytol 22: 81–91

Cheng K, Hasegawa T, Saleem K S, Tanana K 1994 Comparison of neuronal selectivity for stimulus speed, length, and contrast in the prestriate visual cortical areas V4 and MT of the macaque monkey. J Neurophysiol 71: 2269–2280

Cheng L H, Robinson P P 1991 The distribution of fungiform papillae and taste buds on the human tongue. Archives of Oral Biology. 36:583–589

Chernoff E A G, Lash J W 1981 Cell movement in somite formation and development in the chick: inhibition of segmentation. Dev Biol 87: 212–219

Chessell I P, Francis P T, Pangalos M N, Pearson R C A, Bowden D M 1993 Localisation of muscarinic (m₁) and other neurotransmitter receptors on corticofugal-projecting pyramidal neurones. Brain Res 632: 86–94

Chevallier A 1979 Role of the somitic mesoderm in the development of the thorax in bird embryos. J Embryol Exp Morph 49: 73–88

Chevrell J P 1987 Surgery of the anterior abdominal wall. Springer Verlag: Berlin

Chiappa K H 1989 Evoked potentials in clinical medicine. Raven Press: New York

Chiara F 1959 Study of the fine innervation of the female genitalia. I. Uterus. Annali Ostet Ginecol 81: 553–576

Chibon P 1967 Etude expérimentale par ablations, greffes et autoradiographie, de l'origine des dents chez l'amphibien urodele pleurodeles waltlii. Arch Oral Biol 12: 745–753

Childress D S, Jones R W 1967 Mechanics of horizontal movement of the human eye. J Physiol 188: 273–284

Chisaka O, Musci T S, Capecchi M R 1992 Developmental defects of the ear, cranial nerves and hindbrain resulting from targeted disruption of the mouse Hox-1.6 gene. Nature 355: 516–520

Chiu R C-J 1994 Using skeletal muscle for cardiac assistance. Sci Am: Sci & Med 1:68–77

Cho W K Stern S, Biggers J 1974 Inhibitory effect of dibutyrl cAMP in mouse oocyte maturation in vitro. J Exp Zool 187: 383–386

Chou R G, Stromer M H, Robson R M, Hulatt T W 1992 Assembly of contractile and cytoskeletal elements in developing smooth muscle cells. Dev Biol 149: 339–348

Christ B, Jacob M, Jacob H J 1983 On the origin and development of the ventrolateral abdominal muscles in the avain embryo. Anat Embryol 166: 87–101

Christ B, Jacob M, Jacob H J, Brand B, Wachtler F 1986 Myogenesis: a problem of cell distribution and cell interactions. In: Bellairs R, Ede D A, Lash J W (eds) Somites in developing embryos. NATO ASI Series. Series A: Life Sciences. Plenum Press: New York: pp 261–275

Christensen A K 1975 Leydig cells. In: Hamilton D W, Greep R O (eds) Handbook of physiology: Endocrinology. Vol 5, Sect 7, Male Reproductive System. American Physiological Society: Washington DC

Christensen J, Stiles M J, Rick G A, Sutherland J 1984 Comparative anatomy of the myenteric plexus in eight mammals. Gastroenterology 86: 706–713

Christensen S B 1985 Osteoarthritis. Changes of bone, cartilage, and synovial membrane in relation to bone scintigraphy. Acta Orthop Scand 56 (suppl 214): 1–43

Christie G A 1963 The development of the limbus fossae ovalis in the human heart – a new septum. J Anat 97: 45–54

Christophers E, Wolff H H, Laurence E B 1974 The formation of epidermal cell columns. J Invest Dermatol 62: 555–559

Chu C H U 1968 Solitary neurons in human tongue. Anat Rec 1962: 505–510

Chuah M I, Au C 1991 Olfactory Schwann cells are derived from precursor cells in the olfactory epithelium. J Neurosci Res 29: 172–180

Ciges M, Labella T, Gayoso M, Sanchez G Ultrastructure of the organ of Jacobson and comparative study with olfactory mucosa. Acta Otolaryngol 83: 47–58

Čihák R 1970 Variations of lumbosacral joints and their morphogenesis. Acta Univ Carol [Med] (Praha) 16: 145–165

Čihák R, Popelka S 1961 Částečné defekty velkého svalu prsního. Morfologická a kliniká studie. Acta Chir Orthop Traum Cech 28: 185–194

Cimino M, Marini P, Fornasari D, Cattabeni F, Clementi F 1992 Distribution of nicotinic receptors in cynomolgus monkey brain and ganglia: localization of $\alpha 3$ sub-unit mRNA, α-bungarotoxin and nicotine binding sites. Neuroscience 51: 77–86

Ciochon R L, Corruccini R S 1977 The coraco-acromial ligament and projection index in man and other anthropoid primates. J Anat 124: 627–632

Cippolini P B, Pandya D N 1989 Connectional analysis of the ipsilateral and contralateral afferent neurons of the superior temporal region in the rhesus monkey. J Comp Neurol 281: 567–585

Ciriello J 1983 Brainstem projections of aortic baroreceptor afferent fibres in the rat. Neurosci Lett 36: 37–42

Ciriello J, Hrycyshyn A W, Calaresu F R 1981 Horseradish peroxidase study of brain stem projections of carotid sinus and aortic depressor nerves in the cat. J Auton Nerv Syst 4: 43–61

Clar H E 1985 Disturbances of the hypothalamic thermoregulation. Acta Neurochir 75: 106–112

Clara M 1937 Zur Histobiologie des Bronchalepithels. Z Mikrosk 41: 321–347

Clark E R 1938 Arterio-venous anastomoses. Physiol Rev 18: 229–247

Clark G L ed 1961 The encyclopedia of microscopy. Reinhold: New York

Clark J M 1990 The organization of collagen fibrils in the superficial zones of articular cartilage. J Anat 171: 117–130

Clark L B, Rosen R T, Hartman T G, Louis J B, Suffet I H, Pippincott R L, Rosen J D 1992 Determination of alkylphenol ethoxylates and their acetic acid derivatives in drinking water by particle beam liquid chromatography/mass spectrometry. Int J Environ Analyt Chem 47: 167–180

Clark M A, Jepson M A, Simmons N L, Hirst B H l 1994 Differential surface characteristics of M cells from mouse intestinal Peyer's and caecal patches. Histochem J 26:271–280

Clark R A F 1985 Cutaneous tissue repair: basic biologic considerations. I. J Am Acad Dermatol 13: 701–725

Clark R A F 1990 Cutaneous wound repair. In: Goldsmith L E (ed) Physiology biochemistry and molecular biology of the skin. Oxford University Press: Oxford: pp 576–601

Clark R A F, Lanigan J M, DellaPelle P, Manseau E, Dvorak H F, Colvin R B 1982 Fibronectin and fibrin provide a provisional matrix for epidermal cell migration during wound reepithelialization. J Invest Dermatol 79: 264–269

Clark R G 1984 Anatomy of the mammalian spinal cord. In: Davidoff R A (ed) Handbook of the spinal cord. Vols 2 and 3. Dekker: New York: pp 1–45

Clark R K F, Wyke B D 1973 Contributions of temporomandibular articular mechanoreceptors to the control of mandibular posture; an experimental study. J Dent 2: 121–129

Clark R P, Edholm O G 1985 Man and his thermal environment. Arnold: London

Clark W E le G 1920 On the Pacchionian bodies. J Anat 55: 40–48

Clark W E le G 1926 The mammalian oculomotor nucleus. J Anat 60: 426–448

Clark W E le G 1939 The tissues of the body. Clarendon Press: Oxford

Clark W E le G 1941 The laminar organisation and cell content of the lateral geniculate body in the monkey. J Anat 75: 419–433

Clark W E le G 1945 Deformation patterns in the cerebral cortex. In: Clark W E le G, Medawar P B (eds) Essays on growth and form. Clarendon Press: Oxford: pp 1–22

Clark W E le G, Beattie J, Riddoch G, Dott N M 1938 The hypothalamus, morphological, functional, clinical and surgical aspects. Oliver and Boyd: Edinburgh

Clarke C A 1975 Rhesus haemolytic disease. Selected papers and extracts. Medical and Technical Publishing: Lancaster

Clarke E B, Hu N, 1991 Functional characteristics of the embryonic circulation. In: Feinberg R N, Sherer G K, Auerbach R (eds) the development of the vascular system. Issues Biomed 14; 41–60

Clarke I C 1973a Correlation of SEM replication and light microscopy studies of the bearing-surfaces in human joints. In: Johari O, Corvin I (eds) Scanning electron microscopy/1973 (Part III). Proceedings of the workshop on scanning electron microscopy in pathology. IIT Research Institute: Chicago: pp 659–666

Clarke I C 1973b Quantitative measurement of human articular surface topography 'in vitro' by profile recorder and stereomicroscopy techniques. J Microsc 97: 309–314

Clarke N B, Feng J Q, Murphy M J 1993 Renal clearance measurements of electrolytes in embryonic chickens. J Exp Zool 265: 107–111

Claude A 1970 Growth and differentiation of cytoplasmic membranes in the course of lipoprotein granule synthesis in the hepatic cell. J Cell Biol 47: 745–766

Clavert A, Cranz C, Bollack C 1990 Functions of the seminal vesicle. Andrologia 22 (suppl 1): 185–192

Clawson R C, Domm L V 1969 Origin and early migration of primordial germ cells in the chick embryo: A study of the stages definitive primitive streak through eight somites. Am J Anat 125: 87–112

Clegg E J 1955 The arterial supply of the human prostate and seminal vesicles. J Anat 89: 209–216

Clegg E J 1956 The vascular arrangements within the human prostate gland. Br J Urol 28: 428–435

Cleland J 1878 On the cutaneous ligaments of the phalanges. J Anat Physiol 12: 526–527

Clemente C D 1964 Regeneration in the vertebrate central nervous system. Int Rev Biol 6: 257 – 301

Clementi F, Marini D 1972 The surface fine structure of the walls of cerebral ventricles and of choroid plexus in the cat. Z Zellforsch Mikrosk Anat 123: 82–95

Clementi F, Palade G E 1969 Intestinal capillaries. I. Permeability to peroxidase and ferritin. J Cell Biol 41: 33–58

Clermont Y 1963 The cycle of the seminiferous epithelium in man. Am J Anat 112: 35–52

Clermont Y 1969 Two classes of spermatogonial stem cells in the monkey (Cercopithecus aethiops) Am J Anat 126: 57–72

Clermont Y 1972 Kinetics of spermatogenesis in mammals: seminiferous epithelium cycle and spermatogonial renewal. Physiol Revs 52: 198–236

Clermont Y, Huckins C 1961 Microscopic anatomy of the sex cords and seminiferous tubules in growing and adult male albino rats. J Anat 108: 79–97

Clermont Y, Leblond C P 1955 Spermiogenesis of man, monkey, ram and other mammals as shown by the 'periodic acid-Schiff' technique. Am J Anat 96: 229–254

Cliff W J 1967 The aortic tunica media in growing rats studied with the electron microscope. Lab Invest 17: 599–615

Cliff W J 1976 Blood vessels. Cambridge University Press: Cambridge

Cloyd M W, Low F N 1974 Scanning electron microscopy of the subarachnoid space in the dog. I. Spinal cord levels. J Comp Neurol 153: 325–368

Cnóckaert J C, Pertuzon E 1974 Sur la géometrie musculosquelettique du triceps brachii. Application à la détermination dynamique de sa compliance. Europ J Appl Physiol 32: 149–158

Coakley J B, King T S 1959 Cardiac muscle relation of the coronary sinus, the oblique vein of the left atrium and the left precaval vein in mammals. J Anat 93: 30–35

Coates M I, Clack J A 1991 Fish-like gills and breathing in the earliest known tetrapod. Nature 352: 234–236

Cobb J L S, Bennett T 1969 A study of nexuses in visceral smooth muscle. J Cell Biol 41: 287–297

Coburn R F 1987 Peripheral airway ganglia. Ann Rev Physiol 49: 573–582

Cochard, P, Goldstein M, Black I B 1979 Initial development of the noradrenergic phenotype in autonomic neuroblasts of the rat embryo in vivo. Developmental Biology 71: 100–114

Cochran G van B 1982 A primer of orthopaedic biomechanics. Churchill Livingstone: New York

Cochrane C G, Revak S D 1991 Pulmonary surfactant protein B (SP-B): structure-function relationships. Science 254 (5301): 566–568

Cochrane R, Gee A, Ellis H 1992 Microscopic topography of the male breast. Breast 1: 25–27

Cockett F B 1956 Diagnosis and surgery of high-pressure venous leaks in the leg. Br Med J 2: 1399–1403

Code C F (ed)1968 Handbook of physiology, Section 6, alimentary canal, Vol 4. American Physiological Society: Washington

Coërs C, Woolf A L 1959 The innervation of muscle. A biopsy study. Blackwell Scientific: Oxford

Coffin J D, Poole T J 1991 Endothelial cell origin and migration in embryonic heart and cranial blood vessel development. Anat Rec 231: 383–395

Cogan D C 1956 Neurology of the ocular muscles. 2nd edition. Thomas: Springfield, Illinois

Cogan D C 1980 Neurology of the extraocular muscles. 2nd edn. Charles C Thomas: Springfield

Coggeshall R E, Coulter J D, Willis W D 1973 Unmyelinated fibres in the ventral root. Brain Res 57: 229–233

Coghill R C, Talbot J D, Evans A C, Meyer E, Gjedde A, Bushnell M C et al 1994 Distributing processing of pain and vibration by the human brain. J Neurosci 14: 4095–4108

Cohen A I 1970 Further studies on the question of the patency of saccules in outer segments of vertebrate photoreceptors. Vision Res 10: 445–453

Cohen A I 1972 Rods and cones. In: Fuortes M G F (ed) Handbook of sensory physiology. Vol 7. Springer-Verlag: Berlin: pp 63–110

Cohen A S, McNeill M, Calkins E, Sharp J T, Schubart A 1967 The 'normal' sacroiliac joint: analysis of 88 sacroiliac roentgenograms. Am J Roentgenol 100: 559–563

Cohen D A D, Prud'Homme M J L, Kalaska J F 1994 Tactile activity in primate primary somatosensory cortex during active arm movements: correlation with receptive field properties. J Neurophysiol 71: 161–172

Cohen H L, Tice H M, Mandel F S 1990 Ovarian volumes measured by US: bigger than we think. Radiology 177: 189–192

Cohen J A, Yachnis A T, Arai M, Davis J G, Scherer S S 1992 Expression of the neu proto-oncogene by Schwann cells during peripheral nerve development and Wallerian degeneration. J Neurosci Res 31: 622–634

Cohen J, Burne J F, McKinley C, Winter J 1987 The role of laminin and laminin/fibronectin receptor complex in the outgrowth of retinal ganglion cell axons. Dev Biol 122: 407 – 418

Cohen J, Harris W H 1958 The three dimensional anatomy of Haversian systems. J Bone Jt Surg 40A: 419–434

Cohen L 1959 Venous drainage of the mandible. Oral Surg 12: 1447–1449

Cohen R A, Albers H E 1991 Disruption of human circadian and cognitive regulation following a discrete hypothalamic lesion. Neurol 41: 726–729

Cohen S 1958 A nerve growth-promoting protein. In: McElroy W D, Glass B (eds) A symposium on the chemical basis of development. Johns Hopkins Press: Baltimore: pp 665–679

Cohen S 1965 The stimulation of epidermal proliferation by a specific protein (EGF) 1965. Dev Biol 12: 394–407

Cohen S M, Bronner G, Kuttner F, Jurgens G, Jackle H 1989 Distalless encodes a homeodomain protein required for limb development in Drosophila. Nature 338: 432–434

Cohen S, Levi-Montalcini R 1956 A nerve growth-stimulating factor isolated from snake venom. Proc Natl Acad Sci USA 42: 571–574

Colborn T, Clement C (eds) 1992 Chemically-induced alterations in sexual and functional development: the wildlife/human connection. Princeton Scientific Publishing: Princeton

Coldiron J S 1968 Estimation of nasotracheal tube length in neonates. Pediatrics 41: 823–828

Cole P 1954 Recordings of respiratory air temperature. J Laryngol Otol 68: 295–307

Coleman S S, Anson B J 1961 Arterial patterns in the hand based upon a study of 650 specimens. Surg Gynecol Obstet 113: 409–424

Coletta P L, Shimeld S M, Sharpe P T 1994 The molecular anatomy of Hox gene expression. J Anat 184: 15–22

Colin F, Manil J, Deselin J C 1980 The olivocerebellar system. I. Delayed

and slow inhibitory effects: an overlooked salient feature of cerebellar climbing fibres. Brain Res 187: 3–27

Collet A, Normand-Reuet C 1967 Aspects infrastructureaux de la traversée de la paroi alvéolaire du poumon par des cellules migratrices. Sém Hôp Paris 43: 1928–1937

Collett A, Basset F, Normand-Reuet C 1967 Etude au microscope électronique du poumon humain normal et pathologique. Poumon Coeur 23: 747–785

Collier J, Buzzard E F 1903 The degenerations resulting from lesions of posterior nerve roots and from transverse lesions of the spinal cord in man. A study of 20 cases. Brain 26: 559–591

Collins J H 1991 Myosin light chains and troponin C: structural and evolutionary relationships revealed by amino acid sequence comparisons. J Musc Res Cell Motil 12: 3–25

Collins J L, Satchwell L M, Abrams L D 1954 Nerve supply to the diaphragm. Thorax 9: 22–25

Collins P 1990 The origin, development, and degeneration of the pronephros in Caretta caretta. J Morphol 205: 297–305

Collins P, Billetts F S 1995 The terminology of early development. History, concepts and current usage. Clinical Anatomy Vol 8 (in press).

Collins P, Woollam D H M 1981 The circumventricular organs. In: Hamson R J, Holmes R L (eds) Progress in anatomy. Vol 1. Cambridge University Press: Cambridge: pp 123–139

Collis J L, Satchwell L M, Abrams L D 1954 Nerve supply to the diaphragm. Thorax 9: 22–25

Collman P I, Tremblay L, Diamant N E 1992 The distribution of spinal and vagal sensory neurons that innervate the oesophagus of the cat. Gastroenterol 103: 817–822

Colman D R 1991 Functional properties of adhesion molecules in myelin formation. Curr Opin Neurobiol 1: 377–381

Colonnier M 1974 Spatial inter-relationships as physiological mechanisms in the central nervous system. In: Bellairs R, Gray E G (eds) Essays on the nervous system. Clarendon Press: Oxford: pp 344–366

Comings D E, Okada T 1972 Architecture of meiotic cells and mechanisms of chromosome pairing. In: Dupraw E J (ed) Advances in cell and molecular biology. Vol 2. Academic Press: New York: pp 309–384

Commandon J, DeFonbrune P 1939 Greffe nucleaire totale, simple, ou multiple, chez une Amibe. Compte Rend Soc Biol 130: 744–748

Condé F, Condé H 1973 Etude de la morphologie des cellules du noyau rouge du chat par la méthode de Golgi-Cox. Brain Res 53: 249–271

Condé F, Lund J S, Jacobowitz D M, Baimbridge K G, Lewis D A 1994 Local circuit neurons immunoreactive for calretinin, calbindin D-28k or parvalbumin in monkey prefrontal cortex: distribution and morphology. J Comp Neurol 341: 95–116

Condon B, Patterson J, Wyper D, Hadley D, Grant R, Teasdale G, Rowan J 1986 Use of magnetic resonance imaging to measure intracranial cerebrospinal fluid volume. Lancet i: 1355–1357

Conel J L 1939–1959 The post-natal development of the humal cerebral cortex. Vol I–VI. Harvard University Press: Cambridge, Massachusetts

Conel J L 1942 The origin of the neural crest. J Comp Neurol 76: 191–216

Conference of Medical Royal Colleges and their Faculties in the United Kingdom on 11 October 1976

Congdon E D 1922 Transformation of the aortic-arch system during the development of the human embryo. Contrib Embryol Carnegie Inst Washington 14: 47–110

Conklin J L 1968 The development of the human fetal adenohypophysis. Anat Rec 160: 79–92

Conley M, Friederich-Ecsy B 1993 Functional organization of the ventral lateral geniculate complex of the tree shrew (Tupaia belangeri). I. Nuclear subdivisions and retinal projections. J Comp Neurol 328: 1–20

Conley M, Friederich-Ecsy B 1993 Functional organization of the ventral lateral geniculate complex of the tree shrew (Tupaia belangeri). II. Connections with the cortex, thalamus, and brainstem. J Comp Neurol 328: 21–42

Connor J M 1992 Diagnosable medelian disorders. In: Brock D J H, Rodeck C H, Ferguson-Smith M A (eds) Prenatal diagnosis and screening. Churchill Livingstone: Edinburgh: pp 515–547

Connor J M, Ferguson-Smith M A 1993 Essential medical genetics. Blackwell Scientific: Oxford

Connors T A 1975 Cytotoxic agents in teratogenic research. In: Teratology trends and applications (Berry C L, Poswillo D E eds) pp 49–79 Springer-Verlag: Berlin

Constantinesco A 1974 Etude biomécanique des mouvements du sternum chez l'homme adulte. Arch Anat 57: 153–199

Constantinou C E, Djurhuus J C 1981 Pyeloureteral dynamics in the intact and chronically obstructed multicalyceal kidney. Am J Physiol 241: R398–411

Conti F, Rustioni A, Petrusz P, Towle A C 1987 Glutamate-positive neurons in the somatic sensory cortex of rats and monkeys. J Neurosci 7: 1887–1901

Contreras M, Hewitt P 1989 Clinical blood transfusion. In: Hoffbrand

AV, Lewis S M (eds) Postgraduate haematology. Heinemann Professional: Oxford: pp 269–293

Contreras M, Lubencko A 1989 Antigens in human blood. In: Hoffbrand AV, Lewis SM (eds) Postgraduate haematology. Heinemann Professional: Oxford: pp 230–268

Cook R D, Burnstock G 1976 The ultrastructure of Auerbach's plexus in the guinea pig. I. Neuronal elements. J Neurocytol 5: 171–194

Cooke R 1986 The mechanism of muscle contraction. CRC Crit Rev Biochem 21: 53–118

Coombs J S, Curtis D R, Landgren S 1956 Spinal cord potentials generated by impulses in muscle and cutaneous afferent fibres. J Neurophysiol 19: 452–467

Cooper D E, Arnoczky S P, O'Brien S J, Warren R F, DiCarlo E, Allen A A 1992 Anatomy, histology, and vascularity of the glenoid labrum. J Bone Jt Surg 74A: 46–52

Cooper E R A 1929 The histology of the retained tests in the human subject at different ages, and its comparison with the scrotal testis. J Anat 64: 5–27

Cooper E R A 1945 The development of the human lateral geniculate body. Brain 68: 222–242

Cooper E R A 1946 Development of human red nucleus and corpus striatum. Brain 69: 34–43

Cooper E R A 1950 The development of the thalamus. Acta Anat 9: 201–226

Cooper R G, Hollis S, Jayson M I V 1992 Gender variation of human spinal and paraspinal structures. Clin Biomech 7: 120–124

Cooper R R 1968 Nerves in cortical bone. Science 160: 327–328

Cooper S 1953 Muscle spindles in intrinsic muscles of the human tongue. J Physiol 122: 193–202

Cooper S, Sherrington C S 1940 Gower's tract and spinal border cells. Brain 63: 123–134

Cope V Z 1917 The internal structure of the sphenoidal sinus. J Anat 51: 127–136

Copp D H, Cockcroft D W, Kueh Y 1967 Calcitonin from ultimobranchial glands of dogfish and chickens. Science 158: 924–925

Copp D H, Talmage R V (eds) 1978 Endocrinology of calcium metabolism. (International Congress Series No 421) Elsevier: New York

Corazza R, Fadiga E, Parmeggiani P L 1963 Patterns of pyramidal activation of cat's motoneurons. Arch Ital Biol 101: 337–364

Corbalis M C 1989 Laterality and human evolution. Psychol Rev 96: 492–505

Corbin K B, Harrison F 1940 Function of mesencephalic root of the fifth cranial nerve. J Neurophysiol 3: 423–435

Cordier A C, Haumont S M 1980 Development of thymus, parathyroids, and ultimo-branchial bodies in NMRI and nude mice. Am J Anat 157: 227–263

Cordon-Cardo C, O'Brien J P, Casals D, Rittman-Grauer L, Biedler J L, Melamed M R, Bertino J R. Multidrug-resistance gene (P-glycoprotein) is expressed by endothelial cells at blood–brain barrier sites. Proc Natl Acad Sci USA 86: 695–698

Cornell-Bell A H, Finkbeiner S M 1991 Ca^{2+} waves in astrocytes. Cell Calcium 12: 185–204

Cornes J S 1965 Number, size and distribution of Peyer's patches in the human small intestine. II. The development of Peyer's patches. Gut 6: 225–229

Cornillie F J, Lauweryns J M, Brosens I A 1985 Normal human endometrium. An ultrastructural survey. Gynaecol Obstet Invest 20: 113–129

Corr L 1992 Neuropeptides and the conduction system of the heart. Int J Cardiol 35: 1–12

Corrigan A Z, Bilezikjan L M, Carroll R S, Bald L N, Schmelzer C H, Fendly B M, Mason A J, Chin W W, Schwall R H, Vale W 1991 Evidence for an autocrine role in active β within rat anterior pituitary cultures. Endocrinology 128: 1682–1684

Corsellis J A, Alston R L, Miller A K 1975 Cell counting in the human brain: traditional and electronic methods. Postgrad Med J 51: 722–726

Cortes D, Müller J, Skakkebaek N E 1987 Proliferation of Sertoli cells during development of the human testis assessed by stereological methods. Int J Androl 10: 589–596

Cortés R, Probst A, Palacios J M 1987 Quantitative light microscopic autoradiographic localization of cholinergic muscarinic receptors in the human brain: forebrain. Neuroscience 20: 65–107

Cory R A, Valentine E J 1959 Varying patterns of the lobar branches of the pulmonary artery. A study of 524 lungs and lobes seen at operation on 426 patients. Thorax 14: 267–280

Costanzo R M, Graziadei PPC 1983 A quantitative analysis of changes in the olfactory epithelium following bulbectomy in the hamster. J Comp Neurol 215: 370–381

Costoff A 1977 Ultrastructure of the pituitary gland. In: Allen M B Jr, Mahesh V B (eds) The pituitary, a current review. Academic Press: New York: pp 59–76

Cotsarelis G, Cheng S-Z, Dong G, Sun T T, Lavker R M 1989 Existence of slow-cycling limbal epithelial basal cells that can be preferentially stimulated to proliferate: implications on epithelial stem cells. Cell 57: 201–209

Cotsarelis G, Sun T T, Lavker R M 1990 Label-retaining cells reside in the bulge area of pilosebaceous unit; implications for follicular stem cells, hair cycle, and skin carcinogenesis. Cell 61: 1329–1339

Cottle M H 1960 Concepts of nasal physiology as related to corrective nasal surgery. Arch Otolaryngol 72: 11–20

Cottle M K 1964 Degeneration studies of primary afferents of IXth and Xth cranial nerves in the cat. J Comp Neurol 122: 329–344

Couinaud C 1954 Les enveloppes vasculo-biliaires du foie ou capsule de Glisson. Lyon Chir 49: 489–607

Couinaud C 1957 Le foie: etudes anatomique et chirurgicules. Masson: Paris

Coulombe J N, Nishi R 1991 Stimulation of somatostatin expression in developing ciliary ganglion neurons by cells of the choroid layer. J Neurosci 11: 553–562

Coulombe P A 1993 The cellular and molecular biology of keratins: beginning of a new era. Curr Opin Cell Biol 5: 17–29

Coulter J D, Jones E G 1977 Differential distribution of corticospinal projections from individual cyto-architectonic fields in the monkey. Brain Res 129: 335–340

Coulton L A, Henderson B, Bitensky L, Chayen J 1980 DNA synthesis in human rheumatoid and nonrheumatoid synovial lining. Ann Rheum Dis 39: 241–247

Couly G F, Coltey P M, Le Douarin N M 1992 The developmental fate of the cephalic mesoderm in quail-chick chimeras. Development 114: 1–15

Couly G F, Coltey P M, Le Douarin N M 1992 The triple origin of skull in higher vertebrates: a study in quail–chick chimeras. Development 117: 409–429

Couly G, Lagrue A, Griscelli C 1983 Le syndrome de Di-George, neurocristopathie rhombencephalique exemplaire. Rev Stomatol Chir Maxillofac 84: 103–108

Couly G, Le Douarin N M 1990 Head morphogenesis in embryonic avian chimeras: evidence for a segmental pattern in the ectoderm corresponding to the neuromeres. Development 108: 543–558

Coupland R E 1958 The innervation of the pancreas of the rat, cat and rabbit as revealed by the cholinesterase technique. J Anat 92: 143–149

Coupland R E 1965a Electron microscope observations on the structure of the rat adrenal medulla. I. The ultrastructure and organisation of chromaffin cells in the normal adrenal medulla. II. Normal innervation. J Anat 99: 231–254, 255–272

Coupland R E 1965b The natural history of the chromaffin cell. Longman: London

Coupland R E, Fujita T (eds) 1976 Chromaffin, enterochromaffin and related cells. Elsevier Scientific: Amsterdam

Coupland R E, Pyper A S, Hopwood D 1964 A method for differentiating between noradrenaline- and adrenaline-storing cells in the light and electron microscope. Nature 201: 1240–1242

Coupland R E, Weakley B S 1970 Electron microscopic observation on the adrenal medulla and extra-adrenal chromaffin tissue of the post-natal rabbit. J Anat 106: 213–231

Courot M, Hochereau de Reviers M-T, Ortevant R 1970 Spermatogenesis. In: Johnson A D, Gomes W R, Vandemark N L (eds) The testis. Vol 1. Academic Press: New York: pp 339–432

Courville J 1966 Rubrobulbar fibres to the facial nucleus and the lateral reticular nucleus (nucleus of the lateral funiculus). An experimental study in the cat with silver impregnation methods. Brain Res 1: 317–337

Cowan W M, Clarke P G H 1976 The development of the isthmo-optic nucleus. Brain Behav Evol 13: 354–375

Cowey A, Marcar V L 1992 The effect of removing superior temporal cortical motion areas in the macaque monkey. I. Motion discrimination using simple dots. Eur J Neurosci 4: 1219–1227

Cowie A T 1974 Overview of the mammary gland. J Invest Dermatol 63: 2–9

Cox J L, Pass H I, Wechsel A S, Oldham H N Jr, Sabiston D C Jr 1975 Coronary collateral blood flow in acute myocardial infarction. J Thoracic Cardiovasc Surg 69: 117–125

Cox R W, Peacock M A 1977 The fine structure of developing elastic cartilage. J Anat 123: 283–296

Crain S M, Petersen E R, Leibman M, Schulman H 1980 Dependence on NGF of early human fetal dorsal root ganglion neurons in organotypic cultures. Exp Neurol 67: 205–214

Cralley J, Fitch K, McGonagle W 1975 Lumbrical muscles and contracted toes. Anat Anz 138: 348–353

Crammond D J, Kalaska J F 1994 Modulation of preparatory neuronal activity in dorsal premotor cortex due to stimulus-response compatibility. J Neurophysiol 71: 1281–1284

Craven A J, Jarvis J C, Salmons S 1994 Vascularisation of the latissimus dorsi muscle for cardiac assist. J Anat 185: 706–707

Crelin E S 1973 Functional anatomy of the newborn. Yale University Press: New Haven

Creutzfeld O D, Watanable S, Lux H D 1966 Relations between EEG phenomena and potentials of single cortical cells. II. Spontaneous and convulsoid activity. Electroenceph Clin Neurophysiol 20: 19–27

Crichlow R W, Galt S W 1990 Male breast cancer. Surg Clin N Amer 70: 1165–1177

Crick F 1982 DNA today. Perspect Biol Med 25: 512–517

Crick F 1982 Do dendritic spines twitch? Trends Neurosci 5: 44–46

Crim C, Simon R H 1988 Effects of oxygen metabolites in rat alveolar type II cell viability and surfactant metabolism. Lab Invest 58: 438–437

Crist D M, Stackpole P J, Peake G T 1983 Effects of androgenic-anabolic steroids on neuromuscular power and body composition. J Appl Physiol 54: 366–370

Crock H V 1965 A revision of the anatomy of the arteries supplying the upper end of the human femur. J Anat 99: 77–88

Crock H V 1967 The blood supply of the lower limb bones in man. Livingstone: London

Crock H V 1980 An atlas of the arterial supply of the head and neck of the femur in man. Clin Orthop 152: 17–25

Crockard H A, Heilman A E, Stevens J M 1993 Progressive myelopathy secondary to odontoid fractures: clinical radiological and surgical features. J Neurosurg 78: 579–586

Crompton A W, Hiiemäe K 1969 How mammalian molar teeth work. Discovery 5: 23–34

Cronstein B N, Weissmann G 1993 The adhesion molecules of inflammation. Arthritis Rheum 36: 147–157

Crosby E C, Dejonge B R 1963 Experimental and clinical studies of the central connections and central relations of the facial nerve. Ann Otol Rhinol Larngol 72: 735–755

Crosby E C, Henderson J W 1948 The mammalian midbrain and isthmus regions. Part II. Fiber connections of the superior colliculus. B. Pathways concerned in automatic eye movements. J Comp Neurol 88: 53–92

Crosby E C, Humphrey R, Lauer E W 1962 Correlative anatomy of the nervous system. Macmillan: New York

Crosby E C, Humphrey T 1941 Studies of the vertebrate telencephalon. II. The nuclear pattern of the anterior olfactory nucleus, tuberculum olfactorium and the amygdaloid complex in adult man. J Comp Neurol 74: 309–352

Crosby E C, Humphrey T 1944 Studies of the vertebrate telencephalon. III. The amygdaloid complex in the shrew. J Comp Neurol 81: 285–305

Crosby E C, Woodburne R T 1943 Nuclear pattern of non-tectal portions of midbrain and isthmus in Primates. J Comp Neurol, 78: 441–482

Croston G E, Kadonga J T 1993 Role of chromatin in the regulation of transcription by RNA polymerase II. Curr Opin Cell Biol 5: 417–423

Crow T J 1993 Sexual selection, Machiavellian intelligence, and the origins of psychosis. Lancet 342: 594–598

Crowder R E 1957 The development of the adrenal gland in man, with special reference to origin and ultimate location of cell types and evidence in favour of the 'cell migration' theory. Contrib Embryol Carnegie Inst Washington 36: 193–210

Crowell R M, Morawetz R B 1977 The anterior communicating artery has significant branches. Stroke 8: 272–273

Cruz P D, Bergstresser P R 1991 The influence of ultraviolet radiation and other physical and chemical agents on epidermal Langerhans cells. In: Schuler G (ed) Epidermal Langerhans cells. CRC Press: Boca Raton: pp 253–272

Csapo A 1962 Smooth muscle as a contractile unit. Physiol Rev 42 (suppl 5): 7–33

Cserr H F, Harling-Berg C, Knopf P M 1992 Drainage of brain extracellular fluid into cervical lymph and its immunological significance. Brain Pathol 2: 270–276

Cuénod M, Do K Q, Vollenweider F, Zollinger M, Klein A, Streit P 1989 The puzzle of the transmitters in the climbing fibers. Exp Brain Res Series 17:161–176

Cuénod M, Do K Q, Grandes P, Morino P, Streit P 1990 Localization and release of homocysteic acid, and excitatory sulphur-containing amino acid. J Histochem Cytochem 38: 1713–1715

Cullis W, Tribe E 1913 Distribution of nerves in the heart. J Physiol 46: 141–150

Cummings J F 1969 Thoracolumbar preganglionic neurons and adrenal innervation in the dog. Acta Anat 73: 27–37

Cummings J F, Petras J M 1977 The origin of spinocerebellar pathways. I. The nucleus cervicalis centralis of cranial cervical cord. J Comp Neurol 173: 655–692

Cummins H 1926 Epidermal-ridge configurations in developmental defects, with particular reference to the ontogenetic factors which condition ridge direction. Am J Anat 38: 39–151

Cummins H 1964 Dermatoglyphics: a brief review. In: Montagna W, Lobitz W C (eds) The epidermis. Academic Press: New York: pp 375–386

Cummins H, Midlo C 1961 Finger prints, palms and soles. An introduction to dermatoglyphics. Dover: New York

Cummins P 1982 Transitions in human atrial and ventricular myosin light-chain isoforms in response to cardiac-pressure-overload-induced hypertrophy. Biochem J 205: 195–204

Curcio C A, Allen K A 1990 Topography of ganglion cells in the human retina. J Comp Neurol 300: 5–25

Currey J D 1984a Can strains give adequate information for adaptive bone remodeling. Calcif Tissue Int 36 (suppl 1): 18–22

Currey J D 1984b Effects of differences in mineralization on the mechanical properties of bone. Philos Trans R Soc Lond [Biol] 304: 509–518

Currey J D 1984c What should bones be designed to do? Calcif Tissue Int 36 (suppl 1): 7–10

Curtis R, Adryan K M, Zhu Y, Harkness P J, Lindsay R M, DiStefano P S 1993 Retrograde axonal transport of ciliary neurotrophic factor is increased by peripheral nerve injury. Nature 365: 253–255

Cuschieri A, Bannister L H 1975a The embryonic development of the olfactory organ of the mouse. I. Light microscopy. J Anat 119: 277–286

Cuschieri A, Bannister L H 1975b The embryonic development of the olfactory organ of the mouse. 2. Electron microscopy. J Anat 119: 471–498

Cushing H 1912 The pituitary body and its disorders. Lippincott: Philadelphia

Cusick C G, Gould H J 1990 Connections between area 3b of the somatosensory cortex and subdivisions of the ventroposterior nuclear complex and the anterior pulvinar nucleus in squirrel monkey. J Comp Neurol 292: 83–102

Cusick C G, Scripter J L, Darensbourg J G, Weber J T 1993 Chemoarchitectonic subdivisions of the visual pulvinar in monkeys and their connectional relations with the middle temporal and rostral dorsolateral visual areas, MT and DLR. J Comp Neurol 336: 1–30

Cutler L S, Chaudhry A P 1973 Differentiation of the myoepithelial cells of the rat submandibular gland in vivo and in vitro: an ultrastructural study. J Morphol 140: 343–354

Czarnetzki A 1971 Epigenetische Skeletlmerkmale im Populationsvergleich. I. Rechts-links-Unterschiede bilateral angelegter Merkmale. Z Morphol Anthropol 63: 238–254

D

Da Silva L F H, Witter M P, Boejinga P H, Lohman A H M 1990 Anatomic organization and physiology of the limbic cortex. Physiol Rev 70: 453–511

Dacey D M 1993a The mosaic of midget ganglion cells in the human retina. J Neurosci 13: 5334–5355

Dacey D M 1993b Morphology of small-field bistratified ganglion cell type in the macaque and human retina. Vis Neurosci 1: 1081–1098

Dacey D M, Petersen M R 1991 Dendritic field size and morphology of midget and parasol ganglion cells of the human retina. Proc Nat Acad Sci USA 89: 9666–9670

Daculsi G, Kerebel B 1978 High-resolution electron microscope study of human enamel crystallites: size, shape and growth. J Ultrastruct Res 65: 163–172

Dahl E 1986 The ultrastructure of cerebral blood vessels in man. Cephalgia 6: suppl 4, 45–48

Dahl E, Flora G, Nelson E 1965 Electron microscopic observations on normal human intracranial arteries. Neurol (Minneap) 15: 132–140

Dahlström A, Fuxe K 1964 Evidence for the existence of monamine-containing neurons in the central nervous system. Acta Physiol Scand Suppl 232: 1–55

Dahlström A, Fuxe K 1965 Evidence for the existence of monoamine neurons in the central nervous system. II. Experimentally induced changes in the intraneuronal amine levels of bulbospinal neuron systems. Acta Physiol Scand Suppl 247: 1–36

Dahm M C, Shepherd R K, Clark G M 1993 The postnatal growth of the temporal bone and its implications for cochlear implantation in children. Acta Oto-Laryngol Suppl 505: 1–39

Dai L J, Quamme G A 1993 Atrial natriuretic peptide initiates Ca2 + transients in isolated renal cortical thick ascending limb cells. Am J Physiol 265: F592–F597

Dai Y, Roman M, Naviaux R K, Verma I M 1992 Gene therapy via primary myoblasts: long-term expression of factor IX protein following transplantation in vivo. Proc Natl Acad Sci USA 89: 10892–10895

Daikoku S 1993 Functional anatomy of the hypothalamic hypophysial system: neuroendocrine control mechanism. Kaibogaku Zasshi J Anat 68: 288–304

Dail W G, Evans A P 1974 Neural and vascular development in the human phallus. Invest Urol 11: 427–438

Dal Pont G 1960 Contribution à l'étude de la structure fonctionelle du maxillaire. Ann Stomatol 9: 921–932

Dalen H 1983 An ultrastructural study of the tracheal epithelium of the guinea-pig with special reference to the ciliary structure. J Anat 136: 47–67

Dallos P 1983 The active cochlea. J Neurosci. 12: 4575–4585

Damadian R 1971 Tumour detection by nuclear magnetic resonance. Science 171: 1151–1153

Damiani N, Capodacqua A 1961 On the intrinsic innervation of the fallopian tube. Annali Ostet Ginec 83: 436–446

D'Amico-Martel A 1981 Dissertation, Univ of Massachusetts, Amherst, Mass

D'Amico-Martel A, Noden D M 1980 J Embryol Exp Morphol 5: 167–182

D'Amico-Martel A, Noden D M 1983 Contributions of placodal and neural crest cells to avian cranial peripheral ganglia. Am J Anat 166: 445–468

D'Amico-Martell A, 1982 Am J Anat 163: 351–372

Damsky C H, Fitzgerald M L, Fisher S J 1992 Distribution patterns of extracellular matrix components and adhesion receptors are intricately modulated during first trimester cytotnophoblast differentiation along the invasive pathway, in vivo. J Clin Invest 89: 210–222

Dancis J 1959 The placenta. J Pediat 55: 85–101

Dandy W E 1934 Concerning the cause of trigeminal neuralgia. Am J Surg 24: 447–455

Dangerfield P H, Roberts N, Walker J, Betal D, Edwards R H T 1994 Investigation of the diurnal variation in the water content of the intervertebral disc using MRI and its application for scoliosis. (Proceedings of 2nd International Conference on 3D and Scoliosis). (In press)

Dani J W, Cherujavsky A, Smith S J 1992 Neuronal activity triggers calcium waves in hippocampal astrocyte networks. Neuron 8: 429 – 440

Daniel O, Shackman R 1952 Blood supply of human ureter in relation to utero-colic anastomoses. Br J Uron 24: 334–343

Danielli J F, Davson H 1935 A contribution to the theory of the permeability of thin films. J Comp Cell Physiol 5: 495–508

Daoust R, Clermont Y 1955 Distribution of nucleic acids in germ cells during the cycle of the seminiferous epithelium in the rat. Am J Anat 96: 255–284

Dardenne M, Bach J-F 1988 Functional biology of thymic hormones. Thymus Update 1: 101–116

Dardenne M, Savino W 1990 Neuroendocrine control of the thymic epithelium modulation of thymic endocrine function, cytokine expression and cell proliferation by hormones and peptides. PNEI 3: 18–25

Dardik A, Smith R M, Schultz R M 1992 Colocalization of transforming growth factor-a and a functional epidermal growth factor receptor (EGFR) to the inner cell mass and preferential localization of the EGFR on the basolateral surface of the trophectoderm in the mouse blastocyst. Dev Biol 154: 396–409

Dargemont C, Dunon D, Deugnier M, Denoyelle M, Girault J-M, Lederer F Ho, Diep Le K, Godeau F, Thiery J-P, Imhof BA 1989 Thymatoxin, a chemotactic protein, is identical to β2-microglobulin. Science 246: 803–806

Darling A I, Levers B G H 1976 The pattern of eruption. In: Poole D F G, Stack M V (eds) The eruption and occlusion of teeth. Proceedings of the 27th Symposium of the Colston Research Society 1975. Butterworths: London: pp 80–96

Daroczy J 1988 The dermal lymphatic capillaries. Springer: Berlin

Dart A M 1971 Cells of the dorsal column nuclei projecting down into the spinal cord. Physiol 219: 29–30

Darwin C 1859 On the origin of species by natural selection or the preservation of favoured races in the struggle for life. Murray: London

Daseler E H, Anson B J 1943 The planataris muscle. An anatomical study of 750 specimens. J Bone Jt Surg 25: 822–827

Davenport H A, Ransom S W 1930 The red nucleus and adjacent cell groups. A topographical study in the cat and rabbit. Arch Neurol Psychiat 24: 257–266

David A S 1989 The split-brain syndrome. Br J Psychiatry 154: 422–425

Davies A S, Gunn H M 1972 Histochemical fibre types in the mammalian diaphragm. J. Anat. 112: 41–60

Davies D V 1950 Structure and function of synovial membrane. Br Med J 1: 92–95

Davies D V, Edwards D A W 1948 Blood supply of synovial membrane and intra-articular structures. Ann R Coll Surg 2: 142–156

Davies F 1927 Normal cholecystography. Br Med J 1: 1138–1140

Davies F 1935 A note on the first lumbar nerve (anterior ramus) J Anat 70: 177–178

Davies F, Francis E T B, King T S 1952 Neurological studies of the cardiac ventricles of mammals. J Anat 86: 130–143

Davies F, Gladstone R J, Stibbe E P 1932 The anatomy of the intercostal nerves. J Anat 66: 323–333

Davies F, Harding H E 1942 Pouch of Hartmann. Lancet 1: 193–195

Davies J A, Cook G M W, Stern C D, Keynes R J 1990 Neuron 4: 11–20

Davies J, Routh J I 1957 Comparison of the foetal fluids of the rabbit. J Embryol Exp Morphol 5: 32–39

Davies S J A, Field P M, Raisman G 1993 Long fibre growth by axons of embryonic mouse hippocampal neurons microtransplanted into the adult rat fimbria. Eur J Neurosci 5: 95 – 106

Davies S J A, Field P M, Raisman G 1994 Long interfascicular axon growth from embryonic neurons transplanted into adult myelinated tracts. J Neurosci 14: 1596–1612

Davis C L 1923 Description of a human embryo having twenty paired somites. Contrib Embryol Carnegie Inst Washington 15: 1–51

Davis J O, Freeman R H, Watkins B E, Stephens G A, Williams G M 1976 Angiotension II blockade and the functions of the renin-angiotensin system. In: Stokes G S, Edwards K D G (eds) Drugs affecting the renin-angiotensin-aldosterone system. Use of angiotensin inhibitors. Progress in Biochemical Pharmacology 12: 1–15 Karger: Basel

Davis J R, Langford G A 1969 Response of the testicular capsule to acetylcholine and noradrenaline. Nature 222: 386–387

Davis J R, Langford G A 1971 Comparative responses of the isolated testicular capsule and parenchyma to autonomic drugs. J Reprod Fertil 26: 241–245

Davis P R 1955 The thoracolumbar mortice joint. J Anat 89: 370–377

Davis P R 1959 The medial inclination of the human thoracic intervertebral articular facets. J Anat 93: 68–74

Davis P R 1961 Human lower lumbar vertebrae: some mechanical and osteological considerations. J Anat 95: 337–344

Davis P R 1963 Some effects of lifting, pulling and pushing on the human trunk. Ergonomics 6: 303–304

Davis P R, Troup J D G, Burnard J H 1965 Movements of the thoracic and lumbar spine when lifting: a chrono-cyclophotographic study. J Anat 99: 13–26

Davis R, Wright N A 1991 The cell proliferative kinetics of the epidermis. In: Goldsmith L A (ed) Physiology, biochemistry, and molecular biology of the skin. 2nd edition. Oxford University Press: Oxford: pp 239–265

Davson H 1980 Physiology of the eye. 4th edition. Churchill Livingstone: Edinburgh

Davson H, Welch K, Segal M B 1987 Physiology and pathophysiology of the cerebrospinal fluid. Churchill Livingstone: Edinburgh

Davy D T, Kotzar G M, Brown R H, Heiple K G, Goldberg V M, Heiple K G Jr, Berilla J, Burstein A H 1988 Telemetric force measurements across the hip after total arthroplasty. J Bone Jt Surg 70A: 45–50

Dawes G S 1961 Changes in the circulation at birth. Br Med Bull 17: 148–153

Dawes G S 1969 Foetal and neonatal physiology. A comparative study of the changes at birth. Year Book: Chicago

Dawson J L 1974 Tumours of the liver. In: Smith R (ed) Surgical forum – the liver. Butterworths: London

Dawson T M, Dawson V L, Snyder S H 1992 A novel neuronal messenger molecule in brain: the free radical nitric oxide. Ann Neurol 32: 297–311

Dawson W, Langman J 1961 An anatomical-radiological study on the pancreatic duct pattern in man. Anat Rec 139: 59–68

Day M A 1964 Postural reflex patterns. Nurs Res 13: 139–147

Day M H, Napier J R 1961 The two heads of flexor pollicis brevis. J Anat 95: 123–130

de Beer G R 1947 The differentiation of neural crest cells into visceral cartilages and odontoblasts in amblystoma, and a re-examination of the germ-layer theory. Proc R Soc B 134: 377–398

de Busscher G 1948 Les anastomoses artériveneuses. Acta Neerl Morphol 6: 87–105

de Camilli P, Miller P, Levitt P, Walter U, Greengard P 1984 Anatomy of cerebellar Purkinje cells in the rat determined by a specific immunohistochemical marker. Neuroscience 11: 761–771

de Camilli P, Peluchetti D, Meldolesi J 1976 Dynamic changes in the luminal plasmalemma in stimulated parotid acinar cells. A freeze-fracture study. J Cell Biol 70: 59–74

De Carlos J A, O'Leary D D M 1992 J Neurosci 12: 1194–1211

de Castro F 1932 Sensory ganglia of the cranial and spinal nerves. In: Penfield W G (ed) Cytology and cellular pathology of the nervous system. Hoeber: New York

de Castro F, Herreros M L 1945 Actividad del ganglio cervical superior. Trab Inst Cajal Invest Biol 37: 287–342

de Duve C 1963 The lysosome. Sci Am 208: 64–72

de Duve C 1973 Biochemical studies on the occurrence, biogenesis and life history of mammalian peroxisomes. J Histochem Cytochem 21: 941–948

de Duve C 1983 Microbodies in the living cell. Sci Am 248: 52–62

de Duve C, Wattiaux R 1966 Functions of lysosomes. Ann Rev Physiol 28: 435

de Gasperis C, Miani A 1969 Observations sur l'ultrastruture du mesothelium pleural de l'homme. Bull Assoc Anat Paris 145: 188–202

de Groat W C 1993 Anatomy and physiology of the lower urinary tract. Urol Clin North Amer 20: 383–401

de Groot P G 1987 Interaction of platelets with cultured endothelial cells and subendothelial matrix. In: Zilla P P, Fasol R D, Deutsch M (eds) Endothelialization of vascular grafts. Karger: Basel: pp 47–56

de la Garza O, Lierse E, Steiner D 1992 Anatomical study of the blood supply in the human shoulder region. Acta Anat 145: 412–415

de la Torre J C, Rall G, Oldstone C, Sanna P P, Borrow P, Oldstone M B 1993 Replication of lymphocytic choriomeningitis virus is restricted in terminally differentiated neurons. J Virol 67: 7350–7359

De Lacalle S, Hersh L B, Saper C B 1993 Cholinergic innervation of the human cerebellum. J Comp Neurol 328: 364–376

De Lara Galindo S, Cuspinera E De G, Cardenas Ramirez L 1977 Anatomical and functional account on the lateral nasal cartilages. Acta Anat 97: 393–399

De Luca C J, Erim Z 1994 Common drive of motor units in regulation of muscle force. Trends Neurosci 17: 299–305

de Medinacelli L, Church A C 1984 Peripheral nerve reconnection: inhibition of early degenerative processes through the use of a novel fluid medium. Exp Neurol 84: 396–408

de Meeus A, Alonso S, Demaille J, Bouvagnet P 1992 A detailed linkage map of subtelomeric murine chromosome 12 region including the situs inversus mutation locus IV. Mamm Genome 3: 637–643

De Olmos, J 1990 Amygdala. In: Paxinos G (ed) The human nervous system. Academic Press: New York: pp 583–755

de Palma A F 1957 Degenerative changes in the sternoclavicular and acromioclavicular joints in various decades. Thomas: Springfield Illinois

De Puky R 1935 The physiological oscillation of the length of the body. Acta Orthop Scand 6: 338–347

De Remigis P, Raggiunti B, Nepa A, Giandonato S, Faraone G, Sensi S 1990 Thyroid volume variation during the menstrual cycle in healthy subjects. Prog Clin Biol Res 341A: 169–173

De Reuck A V S, Cameron M P (eds) 1962 The exocrine pancreas: normal and abnormal functions. (Ciba Foundation Symposium) Churchill: London

De Reuck A V S, Porter R (eds) 1967 Development of the lungs (Ciba Foundation Symposium) Churchill: London

de Reuck J 1972 The cortico-subcortical arterial angio-architecture in the human brain. Acta neurol belg 72: 232–239

De Robertis E 1960 Some observations on the ultrastructure and morphogenesis of photoreceptors. J Gen Physiol 43: 1–13

De Robertis E M, Blum M, Niehrs C, Steinbeisser H 1992 Goosecoid and the organizer. Development (suppl): 167–171

de Ruiter M C, Gittenberger de Groot A C, Poelmann R E, Rammos S 1990 The developmental relation between pulmonary vascularization and the pulmonary arch artery. In: Bockman E, Kirby M I (eds) Embryonic origins of defective heart development. NY Acad Sci: New York: pp 357–358

de Sousa O M 1964 Estudo electromiogràfico do m. platysma. Folia Clin Biol 33: 42–52

de Sousa O M, Vitti M 1966 Estudio electromiogràfico de los músculos adductores largo y mayor. Arch Mex Anat 7: 52–53 (abstract)

de Souza R R, Moratelli H B, Borges N, Liberti E A 1993 Age-induced nerve cell loss in the myenteric plexus of the small intestine in man. Gerontology 39: 183–188

De Troyer A, Estenne M 1991 The expiratory muscles in tetraplegia. Paraplegia 29: 359–363

De Vente J, Bol J G J M, Steinbusch H W M 1989 Localization of cGMP in the cerebellum of the adult rat: an immunohistochemical study. Brain Res 504: 332–337

De Vries P A, Saunders J B de C M 1962 Development of the ventricles and spiral outflow tract in the human heart. A contribution to the development of the human heart from age group IX to age group XV. Contrib Embryol Carnegie Inst Washington 37: 87–114

de Vries R A C, Kappers J A 1971 Influence of the pineal gland on the neurosecretory activity of the supraoptic hypothalmic nucleus in the male rat. Neuroendocrinology 8: 359–366

De Yoe E A, Van Essen D C 1988 Concurrent processing streams in monkey visual cortex. TINS 11: 219–226

Deacon T W 1992 Cortical connections of the inferior arcuate sulcus cortex in the macaque brain. Brain Res 573: 8–25

DeAngelis G C, Ohzawa I, Freeman R D 1991 Depth is encoded in the visual cortex by a specialized receptive field structure. Nature 352: 156–159

Debrunner H V 1985 Biomechanik des Fusses. Enke: Stuttgart

DeChiara T M, Robertson, E J, Efstratiadis A 1991 Parental imprinting of the mouse insulin-like growth factor II gene. Cell 64: 849–859

Decramer M 1990 Action and interaction of respiratory muscles in dogs. Verhandelingen-Koninlijke Academie voor Geneeskunde van Belgie 52: 141–201

Dee R 1977 Five years' experience with total replacement of the elbow. In: Joint replacement in the upper limb. Inst Mech Eng Pubs 1994–5: London: pp 89–92

DeFelipe J 1993 Neocortical neuronal diversity: chemical heterogeneity revealed by co-localization studies of classic neurotransmitters, neuropeptides, calcium-binding proteins, and cell surface molecules. Cereb Cortex 3: 273–289

Defrenne H 1977 Les structures aponeurotiques au niveau de la première commissure. Ann Chir 31: 1017–1019

DeGroat W C 1992 Neural control of the urinary bladder and sexual organs. In: Bannister R, Mathias C J (eds) Autonomic failure: a textbook of clinical disorders of the autonomic nervous system. Oxford Medical Publishers: Oxford: pp 129–159

DeGroot L J, Niepomniszcze H 1977 Biosynthesis of thyroid hormone, basic and clinical aspects. Metab Clin Exp 26: 665–718

Deguchi J, Yamamoto A, Yoshimoti T et al 1994 Acidification of phagosomes and degradation of rod outer segments in rat retinal pigment epithelium. Invest Ophthalmol Vis Sci 35: 568–579

Dehay C, Horsburgh G, Berland M, Killackey H, Kennedy H 1989 Nature 337: 265–267

Deiters O F C 1865 Untersuchungen über Gehirn und Rückenmark des Menschen und der Säugethiere. F Vieweg und Sohn: Braunschweig

Dejean C, Hervouët F, Leplat G 1958 L'embryologie de l'oeil et sa tératologie. Masson: Paris

Déjerine J, Déjerine-Klumpke H 1901 Anatomic des centres nerveux. Vol 2. Rueff: Paris

Dekel N, Beers W 1978 Rat oocyte maturation in vitro: relief of cyclic AMP inhibition with gonadotrophins. Proc Natl Acad Sci USA 75: 4369–4373

Dekhuisen P N, Decramer M 1992 Steroid-induced myopathy and its significance to respiratory disease: a known disease re-discovered. Eur Resp J 5: 997–1003

del Rio Hortega P 1924 Le névroglie et le troisième élément des centres nerveux. Bull Soc Sci Méd Biol, Montpellier 5

del Rio-Hortega P 1928 Tercera aportación al conocimiento morfologica interpretacion functional de la oligodedtroglia. Memorias de la Real Socieded española de historia natural Madrid 14: 5–22

del Rio Hortega P 1932 Microglia. In: Penfield W (ed) Cytology and cellular pathology of the nervous system. Vol 2. P B Hoeber: New York: pp 481–534

Delaere O, Kok V, Nyssen-Behets C, Dhem A 1992 Ossification of the human fetal ilium. Acta Anat 143: 330–334

Delaisse J-M, Eeckhout Y, Neff, L, Francois-Gillet C, Henriet P, Su Y, Vaes G, Baron R 1993 (Pro)collagenase (matrix metalloproteinase-1) is present in rodent osteoclasts and in the underlying bone-resorbing compartment. J Cell Sci 106: 1071–1082

Delaisse J-M, Vaes G 1992 Mechanism of mineral solubilization and matrix degradation in osteoclastic bone resorption. In: Rifkin, B R, Gay C V (eds) The biology and physiology of the osteoclast. CRC Press: Boca Raton: pp 289–314

DeLancey J O 1990 Anatomy and physiology of urinary continence. Clin Obstet Gynecol 33: 298–307

Delay J, Brion S 1969 Le syndrome de Korsakoff. Masson: Paris

Delmas A, Senecail B 1977 Aspects biométriques de la mécanique hy-öidienne chez l'homme. Bull Assoc Anat (Nancy), 61: 189–198

Delmas P D, Malaval L 1993 The proteins of bone. In: Mundy G R, Martin T J (eds) Physiology and pharmacology of bone. Springer-Verlag: Berlin: pp 673–724

DeLong M R, Georgopoulos A P 1981 Motor functions of the basal ganglia. In: Brookhart J M, Mountcastle V B, Brooks V B (eds) Handbook of physiology, Section 1 The nervous system, Vol 2, Motor control, Part 2. American Physiol. Soc: Bethesda: pp 1017–1061

Demeure M J 1993 Physiology of the APUD system. Sem Surg Oncol 9: 362–367

Demonet J F, Wise R, Frackowiak R S J 1993 Language functions explored in normal subjects by positron emission tomography: a critical review. Human Brain Mapping 1: 39–47

Demski L S, Northcutt RG 1983 The terminal nerve: a new chemosensory system in vertebrates? Science 220: 435–437

Denef C 1990 Paracriene signalen in de adenohypofyse. Verhandelingen – human adenohypophysis at mid-gestation. Cell Tissue Res 164: 161–165

Denker H W 1990 Trophoblast–endometrial interactions at embryo implantation: a cell biological paradox. Trophoblast Research 4: 3–29

Dennis F 1983 The three column spine and its significance in the classification of acute thoracolumbar spinal injuries. Spine 8: 817–831

Dennison M 1971 Electron steroscopy as a means of classifying synaptic vesicles. J Cell Sci 8: 525–540

Denny-Brown D, Robertson E G 1935 Investigation of nervous control of defaecation. Brain 58: 256–310

Dermitziel R, Schinke D 1975 A complex functional system in endothelial and connective tissue cells of the choroid plexus. Am J Anat 143: 131–136

Dermon C R, Barbas H 1994 Contralateral thalamic projections predominantly reach transitional cortices in the rhesus monkey. J Comp Neurol 344: 508–531

Derom C 1988 Population-based study of sex proportion in monoamniotic twins. N Engl J Med 319: 119

Derry D E 1923 On the sexual and racial characters of the human ilium. J Anat 58: 71–83

Detwiler S M 1936 Neuroembryology, an experimental study. Macmillan: New York

Devroey P, Camus M, Palermo G et al 1990 Placental production of estradiol and progesterone after oocyte donation in patients with primary ovarian failure. Am J Obstet Gynecol 162: 66–70

DeYoe E A, Van Essen D C 1988 Concurrent processing streams in momkey visual cortex. TINS 11: 219–226

Dhawan J, Pan L C, Pavlath G K, Travis M A, Lanctot A M, Blau H M 1991 Systemic delivery of human growth hormone by injection of genetically engineered myoblasts. Science 254: 1509–1512

Dhingra L D 1977 Mediastinum testis. In: Johnson A D, Gomes W R (eds) The testis Vol 4. Advances in physiology biochemistry and function. Academic Press: New York: pp 451–460

Di Chiara G, North A 1992 Neurobiology of opiate abuse. TIPS 13: 185–193

Di Figlia M, Aronin N 1990 Amino acid transmitters. In: Paxinos G (ed) The human nervous system. Academic Press: New York: pp 1115– 1134

Di Pellegrino G, Wise S P 1991 A neuropsychological comparison of three distinct regions of the primate frontal lobe. Brain 114: 951–978

Di Pellegrino G, Wise S P 1993 Effects of attention on visuomotor activity in the premotor and prefrontal cortex of a primate. Somatosens Mot Res 10: 245–262

Diamant H, Wiberg A 1965 Does the chorda tympani in man contain secretory fibres for the parotid gland? Acta Oto laryngol 60: 255–264

Diamond I T, Jones E G, Powell T P S 1969 The projection of the auditory cortex upon the diencephalon and brain stem in the cat. Brain Res 15: 305–340

Diamond J 1979 The regulation of nerve sprouting by extrinsic influences. In: Schmidt F O, Warden F G (eds) The neurosciences fourth study program. MIT Press: Boston: pp 937–955

Diamond J, Mills L R, Mearow K M 1988 Evidence that the Merkel cell is not the transducer in the mechanosensory Merkel cell–neurite complex. Prog Brain Res 74: 51–56

DiAugustine R P, Petrusz P, Bell G I et al 1988 Influence of estrogens on mouse uterine epidermal growth factor precursor protein and messenger ribonucleic acid. Endocrinology 122: 2355–2363

Dice J F 1990 Peptide sequences that target cytosolic proteins for lysosomal proteolysis. Trends in Biochemical Sciences 15: 305–309

Dickhaut S C, Delee J C 1982 The discoid lateral meniscus syndrome. J Bone Jt Surg 64A: 1068–1073

Dickson A D 1957 The development of the ductus venosus in man and the goat. J Anat 91: 358–368

DiDio L J, Anderson M C 1968 The 'sphincters' of the digestive system. Williams and Wilkins: Baltimore

DiDio L J, Zappalá A, Carney W P 1967 Anatomico-functional aspects of the musculus articularis genus in man. Acta Anat 67: 1–23

Dietrichs E, Walberg F 1987 Cerebellar nuclear afferents—where do they originate? A re-evaluation of the projections from some lower brain stem nuclei. Anat Embryol 177: 165–172

Diffley J F X 1994 Eukaryotic DNA replication. Curr Opin Cell Biol 6: 368–372

Dijkstra C 1969 Structure of the autonomic terminal network of the thoracic organs after visualisation with the osmium zinc iodide method. Mikroskopie 24: 161–171

DiMarco A F, Romaniuk J R, Supinski G S 1990a Mechanical action of the interosseous intercostal muscles as a function of lung volume. Am Rev Resp Dis 142: 1041–1046

DiMarco A F, Romaniuk J R, Supinski G S 1990b Action of the intercostal muscles on the rib cage. Respir Physiol 82: 295–306

DiMarco A F, Romaniuk J R, Supinski G S 1990c Parasternal and external intercostal muscle shortening during rebreathing. J Appl Physiol 69: 2222–2226

DiMarco A F, Romaniuk J R, Supinski G S 1992 Parasternal and external intercostal responses to various respiratory maneuvers. J Appl Physiol 73: 979–986

DiMarco A F, Supinski G S, Budzinska K 1989 Inspiratory muscle interaction in the generation of changes in airway pressure. J Appl Physiol 66: 2573–2578

DiMarco A F, Supinski G S, Simhai B, Romaniuk J R 1993 Mechanical action of the internal intercostal muscles in dogs. J Appl Physiol 75: 2360–2367

Dinges H P, Zatloukal K, Schmid C, Mair S, Wirnsberger G 1991 CO-expression of cytokeratin and vimentin filaments in rete testis and epididymis. An immunohistochemical study. Virchows Archiv 418: 119–127

Dirksen E R, Sanderson M J 1990 Regulation of ciliary activity in the mammalian respiratory tract. Bioherology 27: 533–545

Distler C, Boussaoud D, Desimone R, Ungerleider L G 1993 Cortical connections of inferior temporal area TEO in macaque monkeys. J Comp Neurol 334: 125–150

Divac I, Öberg R G E 1979 (eds) The neostriatum. Pergamon Press: Oxford

Dixon A D 1958 Development of the jaws. Dent Pract 9: 10–12

Dixon A F 1920 Note on the vertebral epiphyseal discs. J Anat 55: 38–39

Dixon J S, Gosling J A 1982 The musculature of the human renal calices, pelvis and upper ureter. J Anat 135: 129–137

Dixon J, Kintner C R 1989 Development 106: 749–757

Dixon M J, Garner J, Ferguson M W J 1991 Immunolocalisation of EGF, EGF receptor TGFa during murine palatogenesis in vivo and in vitro. Anatomy and Embryology 184: 83–91

Dobbie J W, Symington T 1966 The human adrenal gland with special reference to the vasculature. J Endocrinol 34: 479–489

Dockery P, Li T C, Rogers A W, Cooke I D, Lenton E A 1988a The ultrastructure of the glandular epithelium in the timed endometrial biopsy. Human Reprod 3: 826–834

Dockery P, Li T C, Rogers A W, Cooke I D, Lenton E A, Warren M A 1988b An examination of the variation in timed endometrial biopsies. Human Reprod 3: 715–720

Dockery P, Warren A, Li T C, Rogers A W, Cooke I D, Mundy J 1990 A morphometric study of the human endometrial stroma during the preimplantation period. Human Reprod 5: 494–498

Dodd H 1959 The varicose tributaries of the superficial femoral vein passing into Hunter's canal. Postgrad Med J 35: 18–23

Dodd H, Cockett F B 1976 The pathology and surgery of the veins of the lower limb. 2nd edition. Churchill Livingstone: Edinburgh

Doerschuk C M et al 1993 Comparison of neutrophil and capillary diameters and their relation to naturophil sequestration in the lung. J Anat 74(6): 3040–3045

Dogiel A S 1899 Ueber den Bau der Ganglien in den Geflechten des Darmes und der Gallenblase des Menschen und der Saugetiere. Arch anat Ohysiol Abt: 130–158

Dohr G, Ebner I, Gallasch E 1986 Morphological and biomechanical studies of the ligamentum arteriosum. Acta Anat 126: 97–102

Dohrmann G J 1970 The choroid plexus: a historical review. Brain Res 18: 197–218

Doljanski F 1960 The growth of the liver with special reference to mammals. Int Rev Cytol 10: 217–241

Dollé P, Dierich A, LeMeur M, Schimmang T, Schuhbaur B, Chambon P, Duboule D 1993 Disruption of the Hoxd-13 gene induces localised heterochrony leading to mice with neotenic limbs. Cell 75: 431–443

Dollé P, Izpisua-Belmonte J C, Falkenstein H, Renucci A, Duboule D 1989 Coordinate expression of the murine Hox-5 complex homeobox-containing genes during limb pattern formation. Nature 342: 767–772

Doménech-Mateu J M, Sañudo J R 1990 Chondrification of laryngeal cartilages. Otorhinolaryngol Head Neck Surg: 2095–2097

Domnić-Stošić T, Jeličić N 1974 Morphological differences between meningeal arteries and the arteries of the scalp in the fetus and neonate. Srpski Arkhiv 102: 175–180

Donald I, MacVicar J, Brown T G 1958 Investigation of abdominal masses by pulsed ultrasound. Lancet 1: 1188–1195

Donaldson P J, Mahan J T 1983 Fibrinogen and fibronectin as substrates for epidermal cell migration during wound closure. J Cell Sci 62: 117–127

Doniach T, Phillips C R, Gerhart S C 1992 Science 257: 542–545

Donker A J, Arisz L, Brentjens J R et al 1976 The effect of indomethacin on kidney function and plasma renin activity in man. Nephron 17: 288–296

Donoff R B, McLennan J E, Grillo H C 1971 Preparation and properties of collagenases from epithelium and mesenchyme of healing mammalian wounds. Biochem Biophys Acta 227: 639–653

Donoghue J P, Wenthold R J, Altschuler R A 1985 Localization of glutaminase-like and aspartate aminotransferase-like immunoreactivity in neurons of cerebral neocortex. J Neurosci: 5: 2597–2608

Donovan B T 1970 Mammalian neuroendocrinology. McGraw-Hill: London

Doran G A, Baggett H 1972 The genioglossus muscle: a reassessment of its anatomy in some mammals, including man. Acta Anat 83: 403–410

Dörner G 1988 Neuroendocrine response to estrogen and brain differentiation in heterosexuals, homosexuals, and transsexuals. Arch Sex Behav 17: 57–75

Dorschner W, Stolzenburg J U 1994a A new theory of micturition and urinary continence based on histomorphological studies. 3. The two parts of the musculus sphincter urethrae: physiological importance in rest and stress. Urologia Internat 52: 185–188

Dorschner W, Stolzenburg J U, Dieterich F 1994b A new theory of micturition and urinary continence based on histomorphological studies. 2. The musculus sphincter vesicae: continence or sexual function? Urologia Internat 52: 154–158

Dorschner W, Stolzenburg J U, Rassler J 1994 A new theory of micturition and urinary continence based on histomorphological studies. 4. The musculus dilator urethrae: force of micturition. Urologia Internat 52: 189–193

Doty R 1968 Neural organization of deglutition. In: Code C F (ed) Handbook of physiology. Section 6, Alimentary canal. Vol 4. American Physiological Society: Washington DC: pp 1861–1902

Doubilet H, Shafiroff B G P, Mulholland J H 1948 Anatomy of periesophageal vagi. Ann Surg 127: 128–135

Doucette J R 1990 Glial influences on axonal growth in the primary olfactory system. Glia 3: 433–449

Douek E D, Bannister L H, Dodson H C 1975 Olfaction and its disorders. Proc R Soc Med 68: 467–470

Douglas W H J, Redding R A, Stein M 1975 The lamellar substructure of osmiophilic inclusion bodies in rat type II alveolar pneumocytes. Tissue & cell 7: 137–142

Douglas W W 1968 Stimulus-secretion coupling: the concept and clues from chromaffin and other cells. Br J Pharmacol 34: 451–474

Dow R S 1969 Cerebellar syndromes including vermis and hemispheric syndromes. In: Vinken P J, Bruyn G W (eds) Handbook of clinical neurology. Vol 2. North Holland Publishing: Amsterdam

Dow R S, Moruzzi G 1958 The physiology and pathology of the cerebellum. University of Minnesota Press: Minneapolis

Dowling J E 1965 Foveal receptors of the monkey retina: fine structure. Science 147: 57–59

Dowling J E 1987 The retina: an approachable part of the brain. Harvard University Press: Cambridge, Massachusetts

Dowling J E, Boycott B B 1966 Organisation of the primate retina: electron microscopy. Proc R Soc B 166: 80–111

Downie I P, Evans B T, Mitchell B 1995 The middle ethmoidal foramen and its contents: an anatomical study. Clin Anat 8: 149

Downs S M, Daniel S A J, Eppig J J 1988 Induction of maturation in cumulus cell-enclosed mouse oocytes by follicle stimulating hormone and epidermal growth factor: evidence for a positive stimulus of somatic cell origin. J Exp Zool 245: 86–89

Dowson D, Wright V, Longfield M D 1969 Human joint lubrication. Biomed Eng 4: 160–165

Doyle J F 1970 The perforating veins of the gluteus maximus. Ir J Med Sci 3: 285–288

Doyle J L, Watkins H O, Halbert D S 1967 Undescended laryngeal nerve. Tex Med J 63: 53–56

Doyle J R, Blythe W F 1975 The finger flexor tendon sheath and pulleys: anatomy and reconstruction. In: American Academy of Orthopaedic Surgeons Symposium on tendon surgery in the hand, Philadelphia 1974. Mosby: St Louis: pp 81–87

Draeger A, Amos W B, Ikebe M, Small J V 1990 The cytoskeletal and contractile apparatus of smooth muscle: contraction bands and segmentation of the contractile elements. J Cell Biol 111: 2463–2473

Draeger A, Weeds A G, Fitzsimons R B 1987 Primary, secondary and tertiary myotubes in developing skeletal muscle: a new approach to the analysis of human myogenesis. J Neurol Sci 81: 19–43

Dray A 1979 The striatum and substantia nigra; a commentary on their relationships. Neuroscience 4: 1407– 1439

Dreyer B, Budtz-Olson O E 1952 Splenic venography; demonstration of portal circulation with diodone. Lancet 1: 530–531

Driesch H 1921 Philosophie der Organischen. Leipzig

Drumheller G 1969 Anatomical observations of the lower lateral nasal cartilages. Arch Otolaryngol 89: 599–601

Du Brul E L 1980 Sicher's oral anatomy, 7th edition. Mosby: London

Du Shane G P 1935 An experimental study of the origin of pigment cells in amphibia. J Exp Zool 72: 1–31

Duance V C, Stephens H R, Dunn M, Bailey A J, Dubowitz V 1980 A role for collagen in the pathogenesis of muscular dystrophy? Nature 284: 470–472

Duara S 1992 Structure and function of the upper airway in neonates. In: Polin R A, Fox W W (eds) Fetal and neonatal physiology. W B Saunders: Philadelphia: pp 823–828

Duarte L R 1983 The stimulation of bone growth by ultrasound. Arch Orthop Trauma Surg 101: 153–159

Dubois A, Bénavidès J, Peny B, Duverger D, Fage D, Gotti B, MacKenzie E T, Scatton B 1988 Imaging of primary and remote ischaemic and excitotoxic brain lesions. An autoradiographic study of peripheral type benzodiazepine binding sites in the rat and cat. Brain Res 445: 77–90

DuBois F S, Foley J O 1937 Quantitative studies of the vagus nerve in the cat. II. The ratio of jugular to nodose fibres. J Comp Neurol 67: 69–78

Dubois P 1967 Etude au microscope électronique de la pars distalis de l'hypophyse de l'embryon humain. C R Assoc Anat Nancy 138: 429–433

Dubowitz L, Dubowitz V 1981 The neurological assessment of the pre-term and full-term newborn infant. Clinics in Developmental Medicine Vol. 79. Heinemann: London

Dubowitz L, Dubowitz V, Goldberg C 1970 Clinical assessment of gestational age in the newborn infant. J Pediatr 77: 1–10

DuBrul E L 1988 Oral anatomy. 8th edn. Ishiyaku EuroAmerica Inc: St Louis

Duce I R, Keen 1977 An ultrastructural classification of the neuronal cell bodies of the rat dorsal root ganglion using zinc iodide-osmium impregnation. Cell Tiss Res 195: 263–277

Duchen L W, Gale A N 1985 The motor end plate. In: Swash M, Kennard C (eds) Scientific basis of clinical neurology. Churchill Livingstone: Edinburgh: pp 400–409

Duchenne G B A 1867 Physiology of motion. Kaplan E B (trs) 1949 J B Lippincott: Philadelphia

Duckett S 1971 The establishment of internal vascularization in the human telencephalon. Arch Anat 80: 107–113

Duckles S P, Buck S M 1982 Substance P in the cerebral vasculature: Depletion by capsaicin suggests a sensory role. Brain Res 245: 171–174

Duckworth W L H 1947 Some complexities of human structure. Oxford University Press: London

Duke-Elder J S, Wybar K C 1961 A system of ophthalmology. Vol 2. Kimpton: London

Dulac C, Le Douarin N M 1991 Phenotypic plasticity of Schwann cells and enteric glial cells in response to the microenvironment. Proc Natl Acad Sci USA 88: 6358–6362

Dulac C, Tropak M B, Cameron-Curry P, Rossier J, Marshak D R, Roder J, Le Douarin N M 1992 Molecular characterization of the Schwann cell myelin protein, SMP; structural similarities within the immunoglobulin superfamily. Neuron 8: 323–334

Dum R P, Strick P L 1991 The origin of the corticospinal projections from the premotor areas in the frontal lobe. J Neurosci 11: 667–689

Duncan H, Jundt J, Riddle J M, Pitchford W, Christopherson T 1987 The tibial subchondral plate. J Bone Jt Surg 69A: 1212–1220

Dunkley, M G, Love D R, Davies K E, Walsh F S, Morris G E, Dickson G 1992 Retroviral-mediated transfer of a dystrophin minigene into mdx mouse myoblasts in vitro. FEBS Lett 296: 128–134

Dunn P M 1966 Localisation of the umbilical catheter by post-mortem measurement. Arch Dis Child 41: 69–75

Dunn W A 1990 Studies on the mechanisms of autophagy: formation of the autophagic vacuole. J Cell Biol 110: 1923–1933

Dunnett S B 1991 Transplantation of embryonic dopamine neurons: what we know from rats. J Neurol 238: 65–74

Dunnett S B, Annett L E 1991 Nigral transplants in primate models of parkinsonism. In: Lindvall O, Björklund A, Widner H (eds) Intracerebral transplantation in movement disorders. Experimental basis and clinical experiences. Elsevier Science Publishers: Amsterdam: pp 27–51

Dunnill M S, Halley W 1973 Some observations on the quantitative anatomy of the kidney. J Pathol 110: 113–121

Dunstan C R, Somers N M, Evans R A 1993 Osteocyte death and hip fracture. Calcif Tiss Int 53 (suppl 1): S113–S117

Dupré J, Ross S A, Watson D, Brown J C 1973 Stimulation of insulin secretion by gastric inhibitory polypeptide in man. J Clin Endocr Metab 37: 826–828

Dupuytren G 1831 De la rétraction des doigts par suite d'une affection de l'aponévrose palmaire—description de la maladie—opération chirurgicale qui convient dans ce cas. Compte rendu de la clinique chirurgicale de l'Hôtel Dieu par MM les docteurs Alexandre Paillard et Marx. J Universel et Hebdomadaire de Méd et de Chirurgie Prat et des Inst Méd 5: 349–365

Durary A M 1952 The chemical basis of morphogenesis. Phil Trans R Soc 237B: 37–72

Dustin P 1980 Microtubules Sci Am 243: (Aug) 59–68

Duvall A J, Quick C A 1969 Tracers and endogenous debris in delineating cochlear barriers and pathways. An experimental study. Ann Otol Rhinol Laryngol 78: 1041–1057

Duvernoy H M 1975 The Superficial Veins of the Human Brain. Springer-Verlag: Berlin

Duvernoy H M 1988 The human hippocampus. Verlag: Munchen

Duvernoy H M, Delon S, Vannson J L 1981 Cortical blood vessels of the human brain. Brain Res Bull 7: 519–579

Duvernoy J 1972 The vascular architecture of the median eminence. In: Knigge K M, Scott D E, Weindl A (eds) Brain–endocrine interaction. Median eminence: structure and function. Karger: Basel: pp 79–108

Dvorak J, Panjabi M M 1987 Functional anatomy of the alar ligaments. Spine 12: 183–190

Dvorak J, Panjabi M M, Gerber M, Wichmann W 1987 CT-functional diagnostics of the rotatory instability of the upper cervical spine. I. An experimental study on cadavers. Spine 12: 197–205

Dvorak J, Penning L, Hayek J, Panjabi M M, Grob D, Zehnder R 1988a Functional diagnostics of the cervical spine using computer tomography. Neuroradiology 30: 132–137

Dvorak J, Schneider E, Saldinger P, Rahn B 1988b Biomechanics of the craniocervical region: the alar and transverse ligaments. J Orthop Res 6: 452–461

Dyer K R, Duncan I D 1987 The intraneural distribution of myelinated fibres in the equine recurrent laryngeal nerve. Brain 110: 1531–1543

Dyke C G 1930 Indirect signs of brain tumor as noted in routine Roentgen examinations. Displacement of the pineal shadow. A survey of 3000 consecutive skull examinations. Am J Roentgen 23: 598–606

Dykes J R W 1969 Histometric assessment of human testicular biopsies. J Pathol 97: 429–440

Dykes R W, Ruest A 1986 What makes a map in somatosensory cortex? In: Jones E G, Peters A (eds) Cerebral cortex. Vol 5. Sensory-motor areas and aspects of cortical connectivity. Plenum Press: New York: pp 1–28

Dylevský I 1968 Tendons of the m flexor digitorum superficialis et profundus in the ontogenesis of the human hand. Folia Morphol (Praha) 16: 124–130

Dym M 1984 The male reproductive system. In: Weiss L (ed) Histology: cell and tissue biology. Elsevier: New York: pp 1000–1053

Dyson M 1987 Mechanisms involved in therapeutic ultrasound. Physiotherapy 73: 116–120

Dyson M, Brookes M 1983 Stimulation of bone repair by ultrasound. In: Lerski R A, Morley P (eds) Ultrasound '82. Pergamon Press: Oxford: pp 61–66

Dyson M, Young S 1986 Effect of laser therapy on wound contraction and cellularity in mice. Lasers Med Sci 1: 125–130

Dyson M, Young S, Pendle C L, Webster D F, Lang S M 1988 Comparison of the effects of moist and dry conditions on dermal repair. J Invest Dermatol [In press]

Dziadek M, Thomas T 1993 Genes coding for basal lamina glycoproteins laminin, nidogen, and collagen IV are differentially expressed in the nervous system and by epithelial, endothelial, and mesenchymal cells of the mouse embryo. Exp Cell Res 208: 54–67

E

Eacott M J, Gaffan D, Murray E A 1994 Preserved recognition memory for small sets, and impaired stimulus identification for large sets, following rhinal cortex ablation in monkeys. Eur J Neurosci 6: 1466 – 1478

Eager R P 1966 Patterns and mode of termination of cerebellar cortico-nuclear pathways in the monkey (Macaca mulatta). J Comp Neurol 126: 551–565

Earle K M 1952 The tract of Lissauer and its possible relation to the pain pathway. J Comp Neurol 96: 93–111

Easter S S, Taylor J S H 1989 Development 7: 553–573

Eayrs J T 1955 Cerebral cortex of normal and hypothyroid rats. Acta Anat 25: 160–183

Ebashi S 1983 Regulation of muscle contraction. Cell Muscle Motil 3: 79–87

Ebashi S, Endo M, Ohtsuki I 1969 Control of muscle contraction. Q Rev Biophys 2: 351–384

Ebbesson S O E 1968 Quantitative studies of superior cervical sympathetic ganglia in a variety of primates including man. II. Neuronal packing density. J Morphol 124: 181–186

Ebling F J G 1991 Comparative dermatology. In: Champion R H, Burton J L, Ebling F J G (eds) Textbook of dermatology. 5th edition. 4 vols. Blackwell: Oxford: pp. 17–47

Ebling F J G, Hale P A, Randall V A 1991 Hormones and hair. In: Goldsmith L A (ed) Physiology, biochemistry, and molecular biology of the skin. 2nd edition. Oxford University Press: Oxford: pp 660–696

Eccles J C 1964a The excitatory responses of spinal neurons. Progr Brain Res 12: 65–91

Eccles J C 1964b The physiology of synapses. Springer-Verlag: Berlin

Eccles J C 1970 Neurogenesis and morphogenesis in the cerebellar cortex. Proc Natl Acad Sci USA 66: 294–301

Eccles J C 1973 The understanding of the brain. McGraw-Hill: New York

Eccles J C 1984 The cerebral neocortex: a theory of its operation. In: Jones E G, Peters A (eds) Cerebral cortex. Vol 2. Functional properties of cortical cells. Plenum Press: New York: pp 1–36

Eccles J C, Eccles R M, Iggo I, Lundberg A 1960 electrophysiological studies on gamma motoneurons. Acta Physiol Scand 50: 32–40

Eccles J C, Eccles R M, Lundberg A 1958 The action potentials of the alpha motoneurones supplying fast and slow muscles. J Physiol 142: 275–291

Eccles J C, Fatt P, Landgren S, Winsbury G J 1954 Spinal cord potentials generated by volleys in large muscle afferents. J Physiol 125: 590–606

Eccles J C, Ito M, Szentágothai J 1967 The cerebellum as a neuronal machine. Springer-Verlag: Berlin

Eccles J C, Schadé J P (eds) 1964 Physiology of spinal neurons. Progr Brain Res 12:

Eckel H E, Sittel C, Zorowka P, Jerke A 1994 Dimensions of the laryngeal framework in adults. Surg Radiol Anat 16: 31–36

Eckenstein F, Baughman R W 1984 Two types of cholinergic innervation in cortex, one co-localized with vasoactive intestinal polypeptide. Nature 309: 153–155

Eckhoff D G, Kramer R C, Watkins J J, Alongi C A, van Gerven D P 1994a Variation in femoral anteversion. Clin Anat 7: 72–75

Eckhoff D G, Kramer R C, Watkins J J, Burke B J, Alongi C A, Stamm E R, van Gerven D P 1994b Variation in tibial torsion. Clin Anat 7: 76–79

Eckmiller M S 1993 Shifting distribution of autoradiographic label in cone outer segments and its implications for renewal. J Hirnforsch 34:179–191

Eddinger T J, Wolf J A 1993 Expression of four myosin heavy chain isoforms with development in mouse uterus. Cell Motil Cytoskel 25: 358–368

Eddleston M, Mucke L 1993 Molecular profile of reactive astrocytes—implications for their role in neurological disease. Neuroscience 54: 15–36

Ede D A, El-Gadi A O A 1986 Genetic modifications of developmental acts in chick and mouse somite development. In: Bellairs R, Ede D A, Lash J W (eds) Somites in developing embryos. NATO ASI Series. Series A: Life Sciences. Plenum Press: New York: pp 209–224

Edelman G M 1974 Antibody structure and cellular specificity in the immune response. Harvey Lectures 68: 149–184

Edelman G M 1986 Cell adhesion molecules in the regulation of animal form and pattern. Am Rev Cell Biol 2: 81–116

Edelman G M 1988 Topobiology: An introduction to molecular embryology. Basic Books: New York

Edelman R, Hartcroft P M 1961 Localisation of renin in juxtaglomerular cells of rabbit and dog through the use of the fluorescent-antibody technique. Circ Res 9: 1069–1077

Edelson J G, Taitz C 1992 Anatomy of the coracoacromial arch: relation to degeneration of the acromion. J Bone Jt Surg 74A: 589–594

Edelson J G, Zuckerman J, Hershkovitz I 1993 Os acromiale: anatomy and surgical implications. J Bone Jt Surg 74B: 551–555

Eden A R 1981 Neural connections between the middle ear, Eustachian tube and brain: implications for the reflex control of middle ear aeration. Ann Oto Rhino Laryngol 90: 566–569

Edmondsen J C, Hatten M E 1987 J Neurosci 7: 1928–1934

Edström L, Kugelberg E 1968 Histochemical composition, distribution of fibres and fatigability of single motor units. Anterior tibial muscle of the rat. J Neurol Neurosurg Psychiatry 31: 424–433

Edström L, Kugelberg E 1969 Histochemical mapping of motor units in experimentally re-innervated skeletal muscle. Experientia 25: 1044–1045

Edvinsson 1991 Innervation and effects of dilatory neuropeptides on cerebral vessels. Blood Vessels 28: 35–45

Edwards D A W 1946 The blood supply and lymphatic drainage of tendons. J Anat 80: 147–152

Edwards G, Lader M (eds) 1990 The nature of drug dependence. Soc Study Addic Monograph No 1. Oxford University Press: Oxford

Edwards J C W 1982 The origin of the type A synovial lining cells. Immunobiology 161: 227–231

Edwards J C W, Willoughby D A 1982 Demonstration of bone marrow derived cells in cynovial lining by means of giant intracellular granules as genetic markers. Ann Rheum Dis 41: 177–182

Edwards R G 1965 Maturation in vitro of mouse, sheep, cow, pig, rhesus monkey, and human ovarian oocytes. Nature 201: 349–351

Edwards R G, Brody S L 1993 Principles of assisted human conception. Saunders: Philadephia

Edwards R G, Lippold O C J 1956 The relation between force and integrated electrical activity in fatigued muscle. J Physiol 132: 677–681

Edwards S B, Henkel C K 1978 Superior colliculus connections with the extra ocular motor nuclei in the cat. J Comp Neurol 179: 451–467

Egeberg J, Jensen O A 1969 The ultrastructure of the acini of the human lacrimal gland. Acta Ophthalmol 47: 400–410

Eggli P S, Herrman W, Hunziker E B, Schenk R K 1985 Matrix compartments in the growth plate of the proximal tibia of rats. Anat Rec 211: 246–257

Ehara S, El-Khoury G Y, Bergman R A 1988 The accessory sacroiliac joint: a common anatomic variant. Am J Roent Rad Ther 150: 857–859

Ehinger B, Falck B 1966 Concomitant adrenergic and parasympathetic fibres in the rat iris. Acta Physiol Scand 67: 201–207

Ehlers C L et al 1988 Social zeitgebers and biological rhythms. Arch Gen Psychiat 45: 948–952

Ehrich W 1929 Studies of the lymphatic tissue. I. The anatomy of the secondary nodules and some remarks on the lymphatic and lymphoid tissue. Am J Anat 43: 347–383

Ehrlich H P, Rajaratnam J B M 1990 Cell locomotion verus cell contraction forces for collagen lattice contraction: an in vitro model of wound contraction. Tissue Cell 22: 407–417

Ehrlich P 1886 Über die Methylenblaureaction der lebenden Nervensubstanz. Dtsch Med Wochenschr 12: 49–52

Eichner D 1957 Über histologie und Topochemie der sehschict in der Netzhaut des menschen. Z Mikrosk Anat Forsch 63: 82–93

Eikelboom B, Stewart J 1982 Conditioning of drug-induced physiological responses. Psych Rev 89: 507–528

Eisenberg B R 1983 Quantitative ultrastructure of mammalian skeletal muscle. In: Peachey L D, Adrian R H (eds) Handbook of physiology. Am Physiol Soc: Bethesda, Maryland, Section 10: pp 73–112

Eisenberg B R, Brown J M C, Salmons S 1984 Restoration of fast muscle characteristics following cessation of chronic stimulation: the ultrastructure of slow-to-fast transformation. Cell Tiss Res 238: 221–230

Eisenberg B R, Kuda A M 1976 Discrimination between fiber populations in mammalian skeletal muscle by using ultrastructural parameters. J Ultrastruct Res 54: 76–88

Eisenberg B R, Milton R L 1984 Muscle fiber termination at the tendon in the frog's sartorius: a stereological study. Amer J Anat 171: 273–284

Eisenberg B R, Salmons S 1981 The reorganisation of subcellular structure in muscle undergoing fast-to-slow type transformation: a stereological study. Cell Tiss Res 220: 449–471

Eisenberg E, Gordan G S 1950 The levator ani muscle of the rat as an index of myotrophic activity of steroidal hormones. J Pharmacol Exp Ther 99: 38–44

Eisman J A 1993 Vitamin D metabolism. In: Mundy G R, Martin T J (eds) Physiology and pharmacology of bone. Springer-Verlag: Berlin: pp 333–375

Eisthen H L 1992 Phylogeny of the vomeronasal system and of receptor cell types in the olfactory and vomeronasal epithelia of vertebrates. Microsc Res Techn 23: 1–21

Ek A, Alm P, Andersson K E et al 1977a Adrenergic and cholinergic nerves of the human urethra and urinary bladder. A histochemical study. Acta Physiol Scand 99: 345–352

Ek A, Alm P, Andersson K E et al 1977b Adrenoreceptor and cholinoceptor mediated responses of the isolated human urethra. Scand J Urol Nephrol 111: 97–102

Ekblom P, Sariola H, Karkinen-Jaaskelainen M, Saxen L 1982 The origin of the glomerular endothelium. Cell Differentiation 11: 35–39

Ekerot C F, Garwicz M, Schouenborg J 1991 Topography and nociceptive receptive fields of climbing fibres projecting to the cerebellar anterior lobe in the cat. J Physiol 441: 257–274

Ekerot C F, Larson B 1982 Branching of olivary axons to innervate pairs of sagittal zones in the cerebellar anterior lobe of the cat. Exp Brain Res 48: 185–198

El-Najjar M Y, Dawson G L 1977 The effect of artificial cranial deformation on the incidence of Wormian bones in the lambdoidal suture. Am J Phys Anthropol 46: 155–160

Elands J, Resnik A, De Kloet R E 1990 Neurohypophyseal hormone receptors in the rat thymus, spleen and lymphocytes. Endocrinol 126: 2703–2710

Elder J T, Fisher G J, Duall D A, Krogkolle K, Voorhees T J 1991 Regulation of keratinocyte growth and differentiation: interactive signal transduction pathways. In: Goldsmith L A (ed) Physiology, biochemistry, and molecular biology of the skin. Oxford University Press: Oxford: pp 266–313

Elefteriades J A, Hogan J F, Handler A, Loke J S 1992 Long-term follow-up of bilateral pacing of the diaphragm in quadriplegia. New Engl J Med 326: 1433–1434

Elfvin L G 1965 The fine structure of the cell surface of chromaffin cells in the rat adrenal medulla. J Ultrastruct Res 12: 263–286

Elfvin L-G (ed) 1983 Autonomic ganglia. Wiley: Chichester

Elias H, Petty D 1952 Gross anatomy of the blood vessels and ducts within the human liver. Am J Anat 90: 59–111

Elias P M 1983 Epidermal lipids, barrier function and desquamation. J Invest Dermatol 80: 44–49

Elias P M 1989 The stratum corneum as an organ of protection: old and new concepts. In: Fritsch P, Schuler G, Hintner H (eds) Immunodeficiency and skin. Curr Prob Dermatol 18: 10–21.

Elias P M, Friend D S 1975 The permeability barrier in mammalian epidermis. J Cell Biol 65: 180–191

Elinson R P 1987 Change in development patterns: embryos of amphibians with large eggs. In: Raff R A, Raff C (eds) Development and evolutionary process. Alan R Liss: New York: pp 1–21

Ellefsen P, Tos M 1972 Goblet cells in the human trachea. Quantitative studies of a pathological biopsy material. Arch Otolaryngol Head Neck Surg 95(6): 547–555

Ellefsen P, Tos M 1985 Goblet cells in the human trachea: quantitative studies of pathological biopsy material. Arch Otolaryngol 95: 547

Elliot F M, Reid L 1965 Some new facts about the pulmonary artery and its branching pattern. Clin Radiol 16: 193–199

Elliot M, Maher E R 1994 Beckwith-Wiedemann Syndrome. Journal of Medical Genetics (in press)

Elliott H C 1942 Studies on the motor cells of the spinal cord. II. Distribution in the normal human cord. Am J Anat 70: 95–117

Elliott, D H, Crawford G N C 1965 The thickness and collagen content of tendon relative to the strength and cross-sectional area of muscle. Proc Roy Soc B 162: 137–146

Ellis H, Colborn G L, Skandalakis J E 1993 Surgical embryology and anatomy of the breast and its related anatomic structures. Surg Clin N Am 73: 611–632

Ellis LeG C, Hargrove J L 1977 Prostaglandins. In: Johnson A D, Gomes W R (eds) The testis. Vol 4. Advances in physiology, biochemistry and function. Academic Press: New York: pp 289–313

Ellis R A 1965 Fine structure of the myoepithelium of the eccrine sweat glands of man. J Cell Biol 27: 551–564

Ellisman M H 1979 Molecular specializations of the axon membrane at nodes of Ranvier are not dependent on myelination. J Neurocytol 8: 719–735

Elsen J, Arey L B 1966 On spirality in the intestinal wall. Am J Anat 118: 11–20

Emerson C P, Bernstein S I 1987 Molecular genetics of myosin. Ann Rev Biochem 56: 695–726

Emery J (ed) 1969 The anatomy of the developing lung. Spastics International Medical Publications: New York

Emmelin N 1972 Control of salivary glands. In: Emmelin N, Zotterman Y (eds) Oral physiology. Pergamon: Oxford: pp 1–16

Emmelin N, Engström J 1960 On the existence of specific secretory sympathetic fibres for the cat's submaxillary gland. J Physiol 153: 1–8

Emson P C 1993 In situ hybridisation as a methodological tool for the neuroscientist. TINS 16: 9–16

Emson P C, Hunt S P 1984 Peptide-containing neurons of the cerebral cortex. In: Jones E G, Peters A (eds) Cerebral cortex. Vol 2. Functional properties of cortical cells. Plenum Press: New York: pp 145–169

Enders A C 1968 Fine structure of anchoring villi of the human placenta. Am J Anat 122: 419–452

Enders A C 1991 Current topic: structural responses of the primate endometrium to implantation. Placenta 12: 309–325

Enders A C, Hendrichkx A G, Schlafke S 1983 Implantation in the Rhesus monkey: initial penetration of endometrium. Am J Anat 167: 275–298

Enders A C, King B F 1988 Formation and differentiation of extraembryonic mesoderm in the Rhesus monkey. Am J Anat 181: 327–340

Enders A C, Schlafke S, Hendrickx A G 1986 Differentiation of the embryonic disc, amnion, and yolk sac in the Rhesus monkey. Am J Anat 177: 161–185

Enders A C, Schlatke S J 1965 The fine structure of the blastocyst: some comparative studies. In: Wolstenholme G E W, O'Connor M (eds) Pre-

implantation stages of pregnancy. (Ciba Foundation Symposium). Churchill: London: pp 29–59

Enerback L 1986 Mast cell heterogeneity: the evolution of the concept of a specific mucosal mast cell. In: Befus A D, Bienestock J, Denburg J A (eds) Mast cell differentiation and heterogeneity. New York: Raven Press

Eneroth C-M, Hökfelt T, Norberg K-A 1969 The role of the parasympathetic and sympathetic innervation for the secretion of human parotid and submandibular glands. Acta Otolaryngol 68: 369–375

Engel A K, König P, Kneiter A K, Schillen T B, Singer W 1992 Temporal coding in the visual cortex: new vistas on integration in the nervous system. TINS 15: 218–226

Engel R, Bogduk N 1982 The menisci of the lumbar zygapophysial joints. J Anat 135: 795–809

Engel S 1947 The child's lung. Arnold: London

Engel S 1962 Lung structure. Thomas: Springfield, Illinois

English 1987 Morphogenesis of Haar-scheiben in rat. J Invest Dermatol 69: 58–67

English D T, Blevins C E 1969 Motor units of laryngeal muscles. Arch Otolaryngol 89: 778–784

English K B 1977 The ultrastructure of cutaneous type I mechanoreceptors (Haarscheiben) in cats following denervation. J Comp Neurol 172: 137–164

Engström H, Wersäll J 1958 Myelin sheath structure in nerve fibre demyelinization and branching regions. Exp Cell Res 14: 414–425

Engstrom W, Heath J K 1988 Growth factors in early embryonic development. In: Cockburn F (ed) Fetal and neonatal growth. Wiley: Chichester

Enlow D H, Harris D B 1964 Study of the post-natal growth of the human mandible. Am J Orthop 50: 25–50

Ennable E, Niveiro M 1967 Etude embryonnaire des artères intercostales. Reconstruction par la méthode de Born de deux embryons humains (14 et 17 mm). Pathol Biol (Paris) 15: 92–98

Ennion S, Sant' Ana Pereira J A A, Sargeant A J, Young A, Goldspink G 1995 Characterization of human skeletal muscles fibres according to the myosin heavy chains they express. J Musc Res Cell Motil 16: 35–43

Eppig J J 1982 The relationship between cumulus cell-oocyte coupling, oocyte meiotic maturation, and cumulus expansion. Dev Biol 89: 268–272

Epstein B S 1966 An anatomic, myelographic and cinemyelographic study of the dentate ligaments A J R 98: 704–712

Epstein D, Vekemans M, Gros P 1991 (Sp^{2H}) A mutation affecting development of the mouse neural tube, shows a deletion within the paired homeodomain of Pax-3. Cell 67: 767–774

Eränkö O 1967 The practical histochemical demonstration of catecholamines by formaldehyde-induced fluorescence. J R Microsc Soc 87: 259–276

Eränkö O 1978 Small intensely fluorescent (SIF) cells and neurotransmission in sympathetic ganglia. Ann Rev Pharmacol Toxicol 18: 417–430

Eränkö O, Härkönen M 1965 Moncamine-containing cells in the superior cervical ganglion of the rat. Acts Physiol Scand 63: 511–512

Ericksen M F 1976 Some aspects of aging in the lumbar spine. Am J Phys Anthropol 45: 575–580

Erickson C A 1986 Morphogenesis of the neural crest. In: Browder L (ed) Developmental biology: a comprehensive synthesis. Plenum Press: New York: pp 481–543

Erickson H P 1993a Tenascin C, tenascin R and tenascin X: a family of talented proteins in search of functions. Curr Opin Cell Biol 5: 869–876

Erickson H P 1993b Gene knockouts of C-src TGB1 and tenascin suggest superfluous, non-functional expression of proteins. J Cell Biol 120: 1079–1081

Ericson E, Hakanson R, Larson B, Owman Ch, Sundler F 1972 Fluorescence and electron microscopy of amine-staining enterochromaffin-like cells in tracheal epithelium of mouse. Z Zellforsch 124: 532–545

Eriksen E F, Vesterby A, Kassem M, Melsen F, Mosekilde L 1993 Bone remodelling and bone structure. In: Mundy G R, Martin T J (eds) Physiology and pharmacology of bone. Springer-Verlag: Berlin: pp 67–109

Erikson C A, Loring J F, Lester S M 1989 Migratory pathways of HNK-1-immunoreactive neural crest cells in the rat embryo. Dev Biol 184: 112–118

Erlanger J, Gasser H S 1937 Electrical signs of nervous activity. University of Pennsylvania Press: Philadelphia

Ernfors P, Lee K F, Jaenisch R 1993 Nature 368: 147–150

Ernster L, Schatz G 1981 Mitochondria: a historical review. J Cell Biol 91: 227s–255s

Ernston S, Smith C A 1986 Stereo-kinociliar bonds in mammalian vestibular organs. Acta Otolaryngol [Stockh] 101: 395–402

Esser P H 1932 Über die Funktion und den Bau des Scrotums. Z Zellforsch 31: 108–174

Esterhuizen A, Spriggs T, Lever J 1968 Nature of islet cell innervation in the cat pancreas. Diabetes 17: 33–36

Etherton J E, Conning D M 1971 Early incorporation of labelled palmitate into mouse lung. Experimentia 27: 554–555

Euler C von, Hayward J N, Martilla I, Wyman R J 1973 Respiratory neurones of the ventrolateral nucleus of the solitary tract of the cat. Brain Res 61: 1–22

Evans D H L, Murray J G 1954 Regeneration of non-medullated nerve fibres. J Anat 88: 465–480

Evans E 1949 Congenital heart disease. J Florida Med Assoc 35: 487–491

Evans E F 1975 The sharpening of cochlear frequency selectivity in the normal and abnormal cochlea. Audiology 4: 419–442

Evans E J, Benjamin M 1984 Fibrocartilage at the insertion of the human supraspinatus tendon. J Anat 139: 727

Evans F G 1973 Mechanical properties of bone. Thomas: Springfield, Illinois

Evered D, Whelan J (eds) The biology of hyaluronan. Ciba Foundation Symposium No 143. Wiley: Chichester

Everitt B J, Hökfelt T 1986 Neuroendocrine anatomy of the hypothalamus. In: Lightman S L, Everitt B J (eds) Neuroendocrinology. Blackwell: Oxford: pp 5–31

Everitt B J, Hökfelt T 1989 The coesistence of neuropeptide-Y with other peptides and amines in the central nervous system. In: Mutt Y V, Hökfelt T, Lundberg J (eds) Neuropeptide. Raven Press: New York: pp 61–77

Everitt B J, Hökfelt T, Wu J-W, Goldstein M 1984 Coexistence of tyrosine hydroxylase and gamma-aminobutyric acid-like immunoreactivities in neurons of the arcuate nucleus. Neuroendocrinology 39: 189–191

Everitt B J, Hölfelt T, Terenius L, Mutt V, Goldstein M 1984 Differential co-existence of neuropeptide Y (NPY0-like immunoreactivity with catecholamines in the central nervous system of the rat. Neuroscience 2: 443–462

Everitt B J, Meister B, Hökfelt T et al 1986 The hypothalamic arcuate nucleus-median eminence complex: immunohistochemistry of transmitters, peptides and DARPP-32 with special reference to coexistence in dopamine neurons. Brain Res Rev 11: 97–155

Everitt B J, Robbins T W 1992 Amygdala-ventral striatal interactions and reward-related processes. In: Aggleton J P (ed) The amygdala: neurobiological aspects of emotion, memory and mental dysfunction. John Wiley: New York: pp 401–430

Evinger C, Manning K A, Nibony P A 1991 Eyelid movements-mechanisms and normal data. Invest Ophthalmol Vis Sci 32: 387–400

Ewald F C, Simmons E D, Sullivan J A, Thomas W H, Scott R D, Poss R, Thornhill T S, Sledge C B 1993 Capitello condylar total elbow replacement in rheumatoid arthritis. Long term results. J Bone Jt Surg 75A: 498–507

Ewing M R 1954 White line of Hilton. Proc R Soc Med 47: 525–530

Eyzaguirre C, Nishi K, Fidone S 1972 Chemoreceptor synapses in the carotid body. Fed Proc Fed Am Soc Exp Biol 31: 1385–1393

F

Faber J J, Thornburg K L 1983 Placental physiology. Raven Press: New York

Fabiato A 1985 Simulated calcium current can both cause calcium loading in and trigger calcium release from the sarcoplasmic reticulum of a skinned canine cardiac Purkinje cell. J Gen Physiol 85: 291–320

Fabre E, Hurt E C 1994 Nuclear transport. Curr Opin Cell Biol 6: 335–342

Fagius J, Wallin G B, Sundlof G et al 1985 Sympathetic outflow in man after anaesthesia of the glossopharyngeal and vagus nerves. Brain 108: 423

Fahrer M 1980 The proximal end of the palmar aponeurosis. Hand 12: 33–38

Fahy F L, Riches I P, Brown M W 1993 Neuronal activity related to visual recognition memory: long-term memory and the encoding of recency and familiarity information in the primate anterior and medial inferior temporal and rhinal cortex. Exp Brain Res 96: 457–472

Fairen A, Defelipe J, Regidor J 1984 Nonpyramidal neurons: general account. In: Peters A, Jones E G (eds) Cerebral cortex. Vol 1. Cellular components of the cerebral cortex. Plenum Press: New York: pp 201–253

Fairley J A 1991 Calcium, a second messenger. In: Goldsmith L A (ed) Physiology, biochemistry and molecular biology of skin. 2nd edition. 2 vols. Oxford University Press: Oxford: pp 314–328

Falck B, Hillarp N åA, Thieme G, Torp A 1962 Fluorescence of catecholamines and related compounds condensed with formaldehyde. J Histochem Cytochem 10: 348–354

Falck B, Owman C 1965 A detailed methodological description of the fluorescence method for the cellular demonstration of biogenic monoamines. Acta Univ Lund Sect II 7: 1–23

Falconer M A 1949 Intramedullary trigeminal tractotomy and its place in the treatment of facial pain. J Neurol Neurosurg Psychiat 12: 297–311

Falkner F, Tanner J M 1986 Human growth. Plenum Press: London

Faller J, Ungváry G 1962 Die arterielle Segmentation der Niere. Zbl Chir 87: 972–984

Famiglietti E V 1991 Synaptic organization of starburst amacrine cells in rabbit retina: analysis of serial thin sections by electron microscopy and graphic reconstruction. J Comp Neurol 309: 40–70

Famiglietti E V 1992 Dendritic co-stratification of ON and ON-OFF direc-tionally selective ganglion cells with starburst amacrine cells in rabbit retina. J Comp Neurol 324: 322–335

Fanger H, Ree H J 1974 Cyclic changes in human mammary gland epithelium in relation to the menstrual cycle. An ultrastructural study. Cancer 34: 574–585

Farahmand S, Cowan D F 1991 Elastosis in the normal ageing breast. Arch Path Lab Med 115: 1241–1246

Farbman A I 1980 Renewal of mast cells in rat circumvallate papillae. Cell Tiss Kinet 13: 349–357

Farbman A I 1986 Prenatal development of mammalian receptor cells. Chem. Senses 11: 3–18

Farbman A I 1992 Cell biology of olfaction. Cambridge University Press: Cambridge

Farbman A I 1994 Developmental biology of olfactory sensory neurons. Semin Cell Biol 5: 3–10

Farbman A I, Gesteland R C 1975 Development and electrophysiological studies of olfactory mucosa in organ culture. In: Denton D, Coghlan J P (eds) Olfaction and taste V. Academic Press: New York: pp 107–110

Farnarier G, Planche D, Rohner J J 1977 Blocage des afférences nociceptives par stimulation périphérique percutanee chez le chat. C.R. Soc Biol 171: 1054–1058

Farnsworth P N, Burke P 1977 Three-dimensional architecture of the suspensory apparatus of the lens of the rhesus monkey. Exp Eye Res 25: 563–576

Farquhar M G 1981 Membrane recycling in secretory cells: implications for traffic of products and specialized membranes within the Golgi complex. Methods Cell Biol 23: 399–427

Farquhar M G 1991 The glomerular basement membrane: a selective macromolecular filter. In: Hay E D (ed) Cell biology of extracellular matrix. 2nd edition. Academic Press: New York: pp 365–418

Farquhar M G, Palade G E 1963 Junctional complexes in various epithelia. J Cell Biol 17: 375–412

Farquhar M, Palade G 1981 The Golgi apparatus (Complex)–1954–1981–from artifact to center stage. J Cell Biol 91: 77s–103s

Farr V, Kerridge D F, Mitchell R G 1966 The value of some external characteristics in the assessment of gestational age. Dev Child Neurol 8: 657–660

Farrell J H 1956 The effect of mastication on the digestion of food. Br Dent J 100: 149–155

Farrer-Brown G, Beilby J O W, Tarbit M M 1970a The blood supply of the uterus. I. Arterial vasculature. J Obstet Gynaec Br Commonw 77: 673–681

Farrer-Brown G, Beilby J O W, Tarbit M M 1970b The blood supply of the uterus. II. Venous pattern. J Obstet Gynaec Br Commonw 77: 682–689

Fartasch M, Bassukas L D, Diepgen T L 1993 Structural relationship between epidermal lipid lamellae, lamellar bodies, and desmosomes in human epidermis: an ultrastructural study. Br J Dermatol 128: 1–9

Faussonne-Pellegrini M-S 1992 Histogenesis, structure and relationships of interstitial cells of Cajal (ICC) from mophology to functional interpretation. Eur J Morphol 30: 137–148

Fawcett D W 1961a Cilia and flagella. In: Brachet J, Mirsky A E (eds) The cell. Biochemistry, physiology, morphology, volume II, cells and their component parts. Academic Press: New York: pp 217–297

Fawcett D W 1961b Intercellular bridges. Exp Cell Res Suppl 8: 174–187

Fawcett D W 1965 The anatomy of the mammalian spermatozoon with particular reference to the guinea pig. Z Zellforsch 67: 279–296

Fawcett D W 1968 The topographical relationship between the plane of the central pair of flagellar fibrils and the transverse axis of the head in guinea-pig spermatozoa. J Cell Sci 3: 187–198

Fawcett D W 1975 Ultrastructure and function of the Sertoli cell. In: Hamilton D W, Greep R O (eds) Handbook of Physiology, section 7. Endocrinology. Vol 5. American Physiological Society: Washington DC: pp 21–55

Fawcett D W 1994 A textbook of histology. 12th edition. Chapman and Hall: New York

Fawcett D W, Burgos M H 1956 A comparison of the structural organisation of mammalian and amphibian sperm tails. Anat Rec 124: 298P

Fawcett D W, Ito S 1965 The fine structure of bat spermatozoa. Am J Anat 116: 567–609

Fawcett D W, Ito S, Slautterback D 1959 The occurrence of intercellular bridges in groups of cells exhibiting synchronous differentiation. J Biophys Biochem Cytol 5: 453–460

Fawcett E 1895 The structure of the inferior maxilla with special reference to the position of the inferior dental canal. J Anat 29: 355–366

Fawcett E 1905 On the early stages in the ossification of the prterygoid plates of the sphenoid bone of man. Anat Anz 26: 280–286

Fawcett E 1907 On the completion of ossification of the human sacrum. Anat Anz 30: 414–421

Fawcett E 1911a The development of the human maxilla, vomer and paraseptal cartilage. J Anat 45: 378–406

Fawcett E 1911b Some notes on the epiphyses of the ribs. J Anat 45: 172–178

Fawcett E, Blachford J V 1906 The circle of Willis: an examination of 700 specimens. J Anat 40: 63–70

Fawcett E, Brasch J C, Northcroft G, Keith A 1924 The growth of the laws. Dental Board of the United Kingdom: London

Fawcett J W, Keynes R G 1990 Peripheral nerve regeneration. Ann Rev Neurosci 13: 43–60

Faye-Lund H, Osen K K 1985 Anatomy of the inferior colliculus in rat. Anat Embryol 171: 1–20

Fazleabas A T, Bell S C, Verhage H G 1991 Insulin-like growth factor binding proteins: a paradigm for conceptus-maternal interactions in the primate. In: Strauss J F III, Lyttle C R (eds) Uterine and embryonic factors in early pregnancy. Plenum Press: New York: pp 157–165

Fehér E, Vajda J 1974 Degeneration analysis of the extrinsic nerve elements of the small intestine. Acta Anat (Basel) 87: 97–109

Feinberg R N 1991 Vascular development in the embryonic limb bud. In: Feinberg R N, Sherer G K, Auerbach R (eds) The development of the vascular system. Issues Biomed 14: 136–148. Karger: Basel

Feinberg R N, Sherer G K, Auerbach R 1991 The development of the vascular system. Issues Biomed 14: 25–36

Feldman J L 1986 Neurophysiology of respiration in mammals. In: Bloom F E (ed) Handbook of physiology, the nervous system. Vol 4. Am Physiol Soc: Bethesda: pp 1–67

Feldman J L, Loewy A D, Speck D F 1985 Projections from the ventral respiratory group to phrenic and intercostal motoneurons in the cat: an autoradiographic study. J Neurosci 5: 1993–2000

Feldman M L 1984 Morphology of the neocortical pyramidal neuron. In: Peters A, Jones E G (eds) Cerebral cortex. Vol 1. Cellular components of the cerebral cortex. Plenum Press: New York: pp 123–200

Felix H, Baumgartner S 1981 Ultrastructural findings in human vestibular nerve. Am J Otol 3: 150–155

Felix H, Hoffmann V, Wright A, Gleeson M J 1987 Ultrastructural findings on human Scarpa's ganglion. Acta Otolaryngol [Stockh] Suppl 436: 85–92

Felix H, Johnsson L-G, Gleeson M J, de Fraissinette A, Conen V 1992 Morphometric analysis of the cochlear nerve in man. Acta Otolaryngol [Stockh] 112: 284–287

Fell H B 1978 Synoviocytes. J Clin Pathol 31: 14–24

Fell H B, Canti R G 1934 Observations on the early development of the knee joint in vivo and in vitro. Proc R Soc Lond [Biol] 116: 316–351

Felten D L, Felten S Y 1989 Innervation of the thymus. Thymus Update 2: 73–88

Fennol A B, Sequeros O G, Gonzales J M G 1992 Histological study of the temporomandibular joint capsule: theory of the articular complex. Acta Anat 145: 24–28

Fentiman I S 1993 Detection and treatment of early breast cancer. Martin Dunitz: London

Ferenczy A 1993 Ultrastructure of the normal human menstrual cycle: a review. Elec Mic Res Tec 25: 91–105

Fergus J, Barbenel J C 1981 Skin surface patterns and the directional mechanical properties of the dermis. In: Marks R, Payne R A (eds) Bioengineering and the skin. MTP Press: Lancaster: pp 83–92

Ferguson J E, Schor A M, Howell A, Ferguson M W 1992 Changes in the extracellular matrix of the normal human breast during the menstrual cycle. Cell Tissue Res 268: 167–177

Ferguson M W 1977 The mechanism of palatal shelf elevation and the pathogenesis of cleft palate. Virchows Arch [Pathol Anat] 375: 97–113

Ferguson M W F 1990 The orofacial region. In: Wigglesworth J S, Singer M (eds) Textbook of fetal and perinatal pathology. Blackwell Scientific Publications Ltd: Oxford: Ch 22

Ferguson M W F 1993 Craniofacial morphogenesis and prenatal growth. In: Shaw W C (ed)Orthodontics and occlusal management. Wright: Oxford: Ch. 1

Ferguson M W J 1988 Palate development. Development 103 Supplement: 41–60

Ferguson M W J 1994 Craniofacial malformations: towards a molecular understanding. Nature Genetics 6: 329–330

Ferguson M W J 1994 Growth factors and antagonists: their roles in wound healing. Abstract. (1st European Tissue Repair Society Meeting.) Oxford: UK

Ferguson M W J 1994 Overview of mechanisms in embryogenesis. In: Ward R M T, Smith S K, Donnai D (eds) Early fetal growth and development. Royal College of Obstetricians and Gynaecologists Press: London: pp 1–19

Ferguson M W J, Sharpe P M, Thomas B L, Beck F 1992 Differential expression of insulin like growth factors I and II MRNA, peptide and binding protein/during mouse palate development comparison with TGFB peptide distribution. J Anat 181: 219–238

Ferguson-Smith A C, Cattanach B M, Barton S C, Beechey C V, Surani M A 1991 Embryological and molecular investigation of parental imprinting on mouse chromosome 7. Nature 351: 667–670

Ferguson-Smith M A, 1992 The potential of molecular cytogenetics. In: Brock D J H, Rodeck C H, Ferguson-Smith M A (eds) Prenatal diagnosis and screening. Churchill Livingstone: Edinburgh: pp 639–650

Fergusson J D, Gibson E C 1956 Prostatic smear diagnosis. Br Med J 1: 822–825

Fernig D A, Smith J A, Rudland P S 1991 Relationship of growth factors and differentiation in normal and neoplastic development of the mammary gland. In: Lipmann M E, Dickson R B (eds) Regulatory mechanisms in breast cancer. Kluwer Academic Publishers: Boston: pp 47–78

Ferrara N, Leung D W, Cachiane G, Winer J, Henzel W J 1991 Purification and cloning of vascular endothelial growth factor secreted by pituitary folliculostellate cells. Methods Enzymol 198: 391–405

Ferrarini F, Longanesi A, Baldi F 1993 Pathophysiology and pathogenesis of reflux oesophagitis. Gullet 3: 11–19

Ferraz de Carvalho C A, Rodrigues C J 1978 Functional anatomy of the portal vein and its main and segmental branches in the adult man. Anat Anz 143: 50–71

Ferraz de Carvalho C A, Rodrigues de Souza R, Henrique A, Henrique A, Nogueira de Lima M A 1987 Functional anatomy of the tela submucosa of the valva ileocecalis in the adult man. Anat Anz 164: 630076

Fetissof F, Arbeille B, Bellet D, Barre I, Lansac J 1989 Endocrine cells in human Bartholin's glands. An immunohistochemical and ultrastructural analysis. Virchows Archiv B – Cell Pathol Mol Biol 57: 117–121

Feuer D J, Weller R O 1991 Barrier functions of the leptomeninges: a study of normal meninges and meningiomas in tissue culture. Neuropath Appl Neurobiol 17: 391–405

Feyler K P 1965 Quantative Untersuchungen über die vegetativen Ganglien im Paries membranaceus tracheae des Menschen. Anat Anz 117: 371–379

Feyrter F 1938 Über diffuse endokrine epitheliale organe. Zentbl Innere Med 545: 31–41

Feyrter F 1961 Zur Frage der Endokrinie des sogenannten Speicheldrü-senmischtumors. Dtsch Med Wochenschr 86: 335–339

Fiaccadori E, Borghetti A 1991 Pathophysiology of respiratory muscles in the course of undernutrition. Ann Ital Med Intern 6: 402–407

Fidone S J, Gonzalez C, Dinger B G, Hanson G R 1986 Mechanisms of chemotransmission in the mammalian carotid body. Prog Brain Res 74: 169–179

Field E J 1951 The development of the conducting system in the heart of sheep. Br Heart J 13: 129–147

Fields H L, Claxton C H, Anderson S D 1977 Somatosensory properties of spinoreticular neurons in the cat. Brain Res 120: 49–66

Fields H L, Heinricher M M, Mason P 1991 Neurotransmitters in nociceptive modulatory circuits. Ann Review Neurosci 14: 219–246

Fields W S, Bruetman M E, Weibel J 1965 Collateral circulation of the brain. Williams and Wilkins: Baltimore

Fields-Berry S C, Halliday A L, Cepko C L 1992 A recombinant retrovirus encoding alkaline phosphatase confirms clonal boundary assignments in lineage analysis of murine retina. Proc Natl Acad Sci USA 89: 693–697

Figdor M C, Stern C D 1993 Nature 363: 630–634

Findlater G S, McDougall R D, Kaufman M K 1993 Eyelid development, fusion and subsequent reopening in the mouse. J Anat 183: 121–129

Findlay J A, Ashcroft J J H 1975 Cells of the islets of Langerhans. In: Beck F, Lloyd J B (eds) The cell in medical science. Vol 3. Academic Press: New York: pp 243–306

Fine H, Keen E N 1966 The arteries of the human kidney. J Anat 199: 881–894

Finger T E, St Jeor V L, Kinnamon J C, Silver W L 1990 Ultrastructure of substance P- and CGRP-immunoreactive nerve fibres in the nasal epithelium of rodents. J Comp Neurol 294: 293–305

Fink B R, Martin R, LaVigne A B 1975 Spring mechanics of the human larynx. In: Bosma J F, Showacre J (eds) Symposium on development of upper respiratory anatomy and function. Implications for sudden death syndrome. (Fogarty International Center Proceedings No 29) US Government Printing Office: Washington DC: pp 63–75

Fink B, Demarest R J 1978 Laryngeal Biomechanics. Harvard University Press: Cambridge, Mass

Fink-Jensen A, Møller M 1990 Direct projections from the anterior and tuberal regions of the lateral hypothalamus to the rostral part of the pineal complex of the rat. An anterograde neuron tracing study using phaseolus vulgaris leucoagglutinin. Brain Res 522: 337–341

Finnegan M 1972 Population definition on the North West Coast by analysis of discrete character variation. PhD Dissertation, University of Colorado, Boulder

Finnegan M 1978 Non-metric variation of the infracranial skeleton. J Anat 125: 23–37

Finnegan M, Faust M A 1974 Bibliography of human and non-human non-metric variation. Research Report No 14. Dept Anthropology, University of Massachusetts: Cambridge, Massachusetts

Fioretti A 1957 La tonsilla palatina. Deca: Milan

Fischer E 1988 Low kilovolt radiography. In: Resnick D, Niwayama G (eds) Diagnosis of bone and joint disorders. 2nd edition. W B Saunders: Philadelphia: pp 108–123

Fischer L, Machenaud A, Morin A 1974 Contribution à l'étude de la vascularisation du cubitus. Arch Anat Path 22: 261–265

Fishell G, Mason C A, Hatten M E 1993 Nature 362: 636–638

Fisher D M, Elliott S, Cooke T D V, Forrest W J 1985 Descriptive anatomy of fibrocartilaginous menisci in the finger joints of the hand. J Orthop Res 3: 484–491

Fisher E R, Jeffrey W 1965 Ultrastructure of human normal and neoplastic prostate; with comments related to prostatic effects of hormonal stimulation in the rabit. Am J Clin Pathol 44: 119–134

Fisher L J, Jinnah H A, Kale L C, Higgins G A, Gage F H 1991 Survival and function of intrastriatally grafted primary fibroblasts genetically modified to produce L-dopa. Neuron 6: 371–380

Fisher S K, Linberg K A 1975 Intercellular junctions in the early human embryonic retina. J Ultrastruct Res 5: 69–78

Fishman A P, Pietra G G 1974 Handling of bioactive materials by the lung. N Engl J Med 291: 884–889

Fishman J A, Ryan G B, Karnovsky M J 1975 Endothelial regeneration in the rat carotid artery and the significance of endothelial denudation in the pathogenesis of myointimal thickening. Lab Invest 32: 339–351

Fisken R A, Garey L J, Powell T P S 1975 The intrinsic, association and commissural connections of area 17 of the visual cortex. Proc R Soc Lond series B 272: 487–536

Fitting J W 1990 Muscle fatigue in acute respiratory failure. Lung 168 (suppl): 823–828

Fitting J W 1991 Respiratory muscle fatigue limiting physical exertion. Eur Resp J 4: 103–108

Fitzgerald J G 1972 Changes in spinal stature following brief periods of static shoulder loading. IAM Report 514. Royal Air Force Inst Aviation Med

Fitzgerald M J T 1956 The occurrence of a middle superior alveolar nerve in man. J Anat 90: 520–522

Fitzgerald M J T, Comerford P T, Tuffery A R 1982 Sources of innervation of the neuromuscular spindles in sternomastoid and trapezius. J Anat 134: 471–490

Fitzgerald M J T, Sachithanadan S R 1979 The structure and source of lingual proprioceptors in the monkey. J Anat 128: 523–552

Fitzgerald M J T, Scott J H 1958 Observations on the anatomy of the superior dental nerves. Br Dent J 104: 205–208

Fitzpatrick T B, Breathnach A S 1963 Das epidermale melanin-einheit system. Dermatol Wochenschr 147: 481–489

Fitzpatrick T B, Eizen A Z, Wolff K, Friedberg I M, Austen K F (eds) 1987 Dermatology in general medicine. 3rd edition. 2 vols. McGraw Hill: New York

Fitzpatrick T B, Pathak M A, Harber L C, Seiji M, Kukita A (eds) 1974 Sunlight and man. University of Tokyo Press: Tokyo

Flament D, Onsott D, Fu Q-G, Ebner T J 1993 Distance- and error-related discharge of cells in premotor cortex of rhesus monkeys. Neurosci Lett 153: 144–148

Flechsig P 1876 Die Leitungsbahnen in Gehirn und Rückenmark des Menschen auf Grund entwicklungsgeschichtlicher Untersuchungen. Engelmann: Leipzig

Flecker H 1929 Röntgenographic study of movements of abduction at normal shoulder joint. Med J Aust 2: 123–124

Fleischer R L, Price P B, Walker R M 1975 Nuclear tracks in solids. Berkeley: Los Angeles

Fleischer S, Inui M 1989 Biochemistry and biophysics of excitation–contraction coupling. Ann Rev Biophys Biochem 18: 333–364

Fleischner F G, Sayegh V 1958 Assessment of the size of the liver: roentgenologic considerations. New Engl J Med 259: 271–274

Fleming T P, Johnson M H 1988 From egg to epithelium. Ann Rev Cell Biol 4: 459–485

Fletcher B D, Yulish B S, Ammondson M G M 1983 Diagnostic radiology. In: Fanaroff A A, Martin R J (eds) Behrman's neonatal-perinatal medicine. 3rd edition. Mosby: St Louis: pp. 1086

Flickinger C J 1983 Synthesis and secretion of glycoprotein by the epididymal epithelium. J Androl 4: 157

Flickinger C J, Howard S S, English H F 1978 Ultrastructural differences in efferent ducts and several regions of the epididymis of the hamster. Am J Anat 152: 557

Flickinger C, Fawcett D W 1967 The junctional specialisations of Sertoli cells in the seminiferous epithelium. Anat Rec 158: 207–222

Flindt-Egebak P 1977 Autographical demonstration of the projections from the limb areas of the feline sensorimotor cortex to the spinal cord. Brain Res 136: 153–156

Flock Å 1964 Structure of the macula utriculi with special reference to the directional interplay of sensory responses as revealed by morphological polarisation. J Cell Biol 22: 413–431

Flock Å, Cheung H C 1977 Actin filaments in sensory hairs of inner ear receptor cells. J Cell Biology 75: 339–343

Flock Å, Flock B, Murray E 1977 Studies on the sensory hairs of receptor cells in the inner ear. Acta Otolaryngol [Stockh] 83: 85–91

Florence S L, Wall J T, Kaas J H 1989 Somatotopic organization of inputs from the hand to the spinal grey and cuneate nucleus of monkeys with observations on the cuneate nucleus of humans. J Comp Neurol 286: 48 – 70

Floyd W F, Silver P H S 1950 Electromyographic study of patterns of activity of the anterior abdominal wall muscles in man. J Anat 84: 132–145

Floyd W F, Silver P H S 1955 The function of the erectores spinae muscles in certain movements and postures in man. J Physiol Lond 129: 184–203

Foerster O 1933 The dermatomes in man. Brain 56: 1–39

Foerster O 1936 Motorische Felder und Bahnen. In: Bumke O, Foerster O (eds) Handbuch der Neurologie. Vol 6. Springer-Verlag: Berlin: pp 1–357

Foerster O 1936 Symptomatologie der Erkrankungen des Rückenmarks und seiner wurzein. In: Bunke O, Foerster O (eds) Handbuch der Neurologie. Vol 5. Springer-Verlag: Berlin: pp 1–403

Foerster O, Gagel O 1932 Der vordersetenstrang durg schneidung bein mensham: eine klinish-pathophysiologisch-anatomische Studie. Z Gesamte Neurol Psychiatr 138: 1

Foix C, Nicolesco J 1925 Anatomie cerebrale. Paris

Foley J O, DuBois F S 1937 Quantitative studies of the vagus nerve in the cat. J Comp Neurol 67: 49–67

Folke L E A, Stallard R E 1967 Periodontal microcirculation as revealed by plastic microspheres. J Periodont Res 2: 53–63

Folkins J W, Bleile K M 1990 Taxonomies in biology, phonetics, phonology and major speech motor control. J Speech Hear Dis 55(4): 596–611

Folkman J, Klagsbrun M 1987 Angiogenic factors. Science 235: 442–447

Fontana F 1781 Traité sur le vénin de la vipère, sur les poisons Americans, sur le laurier-cerise, etc. Florence

Forabosco A, Sforza C, De Pol A, Vizzotto L, Marzona L, Ferrario V F 1991 Morphometric study of the human neonatal ovary. Anat Rec 231: 201–208

Forbes D J 1992 Structure and function of the nuclear pore complex. Annu Rev Cell Biol 8: 495–527

Forbes M S, Rennels M L, Nelson E 1977 Ultrastructure of pericytes in mouse heart. Am J Anat 149: 47–70

Ford E H R 1956 The growth of the foetal skull. J Anat 90: 63–72

Ford G T, Roesenal T W, Clergue F, Whitelaw W A 1993 Respiratory physiology in upper abdominal surgery. Clin Chest Med 14: 237–252

Forrest W J 1967 Motor innervation of human thenar and hypothenar muscles in 25 hands: a study combining E M G and percutaneous nerve stimulation. Canad J Surg 10: 196–199

Forrester J C 1973 Mechanical biochemical and architectural features of surgical repair. Adv Biol Med Phys 14: 1–34

Forsberg J G 1963 The derivation and differentiation of the vaginal epithelium Dissertation, Lund

Forslind B, Thyrasson N 1975 On the structure of the normal nail: a scanning electron microscopic study. Arch Dermatol Res 251: 199–204

Forssmann W G, Girardier L 1970 A study of the T system in rat heart. J Cell Biol 44: 1–19

Forssmann W G, Hock D, Lottspeich F, Henschen A, Kreye V, Christmann M, Reinecke M, Metz J, Carlquist M, Mutt V 1983 The right auricle of the heart is an endocrine organ. Cardiolatin as a peptide hormone candidat. Anat Embryol 168: 307–313

Fortier P A, Smith A M, Kalaska J F 1993 Comparison of cerebellar and motor cortex activity during reaching: directional tuning and response variability. J Neurophysiol 69: 1136–1149

Fountain F P, Minear W L, Allison R D 1966 Function of longus colli and longissimus cervicis muscles in man. Archs Phys Med 47: 665–669

Fourman J, Moffat D B 1971 The blood vessels of the kidney. Blackwell: Oxford

Fouser L, Avner E D 1993 Normal and abnormal nephrogenesis. Am J Kidney Dis 21: 64–70

Fowler E P Jr. 1961 Variations in the temporal bone course of the facial nerve. Laryngoscope 71: 937–946

Fowler R Jr 1957 Primary peritonitis. Aust N Z J Surg 26: 204–213

Fox B, Bull T B, Guz A 1980 Innervation of alveolar walls in the human lung: an electron microscopic study. J Anat 131: 683–692

Fox C A, Barnard J W 1957 A quantitative study of the Purkinje cell dendritic branchlets and their relationship to afferent fibres. J Anat 91: 299–313

Fox C A, Hillman D E, Siegesmund K A, Dutta C R 1967 The primate cerebellar cortex: a Golgi and electron microscopic study. Progr Brain Res 25: 174–225

Fox C A, Snider R S (eds) 1967 The cerebellum. Progr Brain Res 25:

Fox G M 1988 The role of growth factors in tissue repair. III. Fibroblast growth factor. In: Clark R A F, Henson P M (eds) The molecular and cellular biology of wound repair. Plenum Press: New York: pp 266–272

Foxon G E H 1955 Problems of the double circulation in the vertebrates. Biol Rev 30: 196–226

Frable M A 1961 Computation of motion at the crico-arytenoid joint. Arch Otolaryngol 73: 551–556

Frackowiak R S J I 1994 Functional mapping of verbal memory and language. TINS 17: 109–115

Fraenkel L, Papanicolaou G N 1938 Growth, desquamation and involution of the vaginal epithelium of fetuses and children with a consideration of the related hormonal factors. Am J Anat 62: 427–452

Fraley E E, Weiss L 1961 An electron microscopic study of the lymphatic vessels in the penile skin of the rat. Am J Anat 109: 85–102

Franchi L L, Murdoch A, Brown W E, Mayne C N, Elliott L, Salmons S

1990 Subcellular localisation of newly incorporated myosin in rabbit fast skeletal muscle undergoing stimulation-induced type transformation. J Musc Res Cell Motil 11: 227–239

Francis P T, Pangalos M N, Pearson R C A, Middlemiss D N, Stratmann G C, Bowen D M 1992 5-HY$_{1A}$ but not 5-HT$_2$ receptors are enriched on neocortical pyramidal neurones destroyed by intrastriatal volkensin. J Pharmacol Exp Therpeut 261: 1273–1281

François J, Neetens A 1969 Physioanatomy of the axial vascularisation of the optic nerve. Doc Ophthalmol 26: 38–49

François R J, Dhem A 1974 Microradiographic study of the normal human vertebral body. Acta Anat 89: 251–265

Frank E, Sanes J R 1991 Lineage of neurons and glia in chick dorsal root ganglia: analysis in vivo with a recombinant retrovirus. Dev 111: 895–908

Frank J S, Langer G A 1974 The myocardial interstitium: its structure and its role in ionic exchange. J Cell Biol 60: 586–601

Frank R M 1968 Ultrastructural relationship between the odontoblast, its process and the nerve fibres. In: Symons N B B (ed) Dentine and pulp; their structure and reactions. A symposium. University of Dundee: Dundee: pp 115–145

Frank R M, Steuer P 1977 Etude ultrastructurale du cément cellulaire chez le rat. J Biol Buccale 5: 121–135

Frankfurt M, McEwen B S 1991 Estrogen increases axodendritic synapses in the VMN of rats after ovariectomy. NeuroReport 2: 380–382

Frankfurter A, Weber J T, Royce G J, Strominger N L, Harting J K 1976 An autoradiographic analysis of the tecto-olivary projection in primates. Brain Res 118: 245–257

Frankl O 1933 On the physiology and pathology of the isthmus uteri. J Obstet Gynaecol Br Commonw 40: 397–422

Franks L M 1953 Spread of prostatic cancer to bone. J Pathol Bact 66: 91–93

Franks L M 1954 Benign nodular hyperplasia of prostate; review. Ann R Coll Surg 14: 92–106

Franzini-Armstrong C 1973 The structure of a simple Z line. J Cell Biol 58: 630–642

Frasca P, Harper R A, Katz J L 1981 Scanning electron microscopy studies of collagen, mineral and ground substance in human cortical bone. Scan Electron Microsc 3: 339–346

Fraser E A 1950 The development of the vertebrate excretory system. Biol Rev 25: 159–187

Fraser J S, Dickie J K M 1914 A reconstruction model of the right middle and inner ear. J Anat 49: 119–135

Fraser S E 1980 Dev Biol 79: 453–464

Fraser S E 1985 Gap junctions and cell interactions during development. Trends Neurosci 8: 3–4

Fraser S E, Bronner-Fraser M 1991 Migrating neural crest cells in the trunk of the avian embryo are multipotent. Dev 112: 913–920

Fraser S E, Keynes R, Lumsden A 1990 Nature 344: 431–435

Frazer J E 1914 The second visceral arch and groove in the tubo-tympanic region. J Anat 48: 391–408

Frazer J E 1926 The disappearance of the pre-cervical sinus. J Anat 61: 132–143

Freder T 1905 A propos de la communication de M M Quénu et Heitz-Boyer sur l'anatomie du caecum et de l'appendice. Bull Mém Soc Anat Par 80: 188–190

Fredrickson J M, Rubin A M 1986 Vestibular cortex. In: Jones E G, Peters A (eds) Cerebral cortex. Vol 5. Sensory-motor areas and aspects of cortical connectivity. Plenum Press: New York: pp 99–111

Free M J 1977 Blood supply to the testis and its role in local exchange and transport of hormones. In: Johnson A D, Gomes W R (eds) The testis vol 4. Advances in physiology, biochemistry and function. Academic Press: New York: pp 39–90

Freeman M A R (ed) 1979 Adult articular cartilage. 2nd edition. Pitman Medical: London

Freeman M A R, Tuke M, Samuelson K 1977 Valgus stop operation. Br Orthop Foot Surg Soc

Freeman M A R, Wyke B 1967 The innervation of the knee joint. J Anat 101: 505–532

Freemont A J, Jones C J P, Bromley M, Andrews P 1983 Changes in vascular endothelium related to lymphocyte collections in diseased synovia. Arthritis Rheum 26: 1427–1433

Freshney R I 1994 Culture of animal cells. 3rd edition. Wiley-Liss: New York

Fride R L 1961 A histochemical study of DPN-disphosase in human white matter with future notes on annycyclination. J Neurochem 8: 17–30

Fried I, Katz A, McCarthy G, Sass K J, Williamson P, Spencer S S et al 1991 Functional organization of human supplementary motor cortex studied by electrical stimulation. J Neurosci 11: 3656–3666

Friede R L 1989 Developmental neuropathology. 2nd edition. Springer: Berlin: pp 49–50

Friedenberg Z B, Roberts P G Jr, Didizian N H, Brighton C T 1971 Stimulation of fracture healing by direct current in the rabbit fibula. J Bone Jt Surg 53A: 1400–1408

Friedman B, Scherer S S, Rudge J S, Helgren M, Morrisey D, McClain J, Wang D, Wiegand S J, Furth M E, Lindsay R M, Ip N Y 1992 Regulation of ciliary neurotrophic factor expression in myelin-related Schwann cells in vivo. Neuron 9: 295–305

Friedmann I, Ballantyne J 1984 Ultrastructural atlas of the inner ear. Butterworths: London

Friedmann P S 1986 Immune functions of skin. In: Thody A J, Friedmann P S (eds) Scientific basis of dermatology. A physiological approach. Churchill Livingstone: Edinburgh: pp 58–73

Friedenstein A J 1976 Precursor cells of melanocytes. Int Rev Cytol 47: 327–359

Friere F, Cardinali D F 1975 Effects of melatonin treatment and environmental lighting on the ultrastructure, appearance, melatonin synthesis, norepinephrine turnover and microtubule protein content of the rat pineal gland. J Neurol Transmission 37: 237–257

Frisch D 1967 Ultrastructure of mouse olfactory mucosa. Am J Anat 121: 87–120

Fritschy J-M, Benke D, Mertens S, Oertel W H, Bachi T, Möhler H 1992 Five subtypes of type A gamma-aminobutyric acid receptors identified in neurons by double and triple immunofluorescence staining with subunit-specific antibodies. Proc Natl Acad Sci USA 89: 6726–6730

Fritz M A, Fitz T A 1991 The functional microscopic anatomy of the corpus luteum: the 'small cell'-'large cell' controversy. Clin Obstet Gynecol 34: 144–156

Frokjaer-Jensen J 1984 The plasmalemmal vesicular system in striated muscle capillaries and in pericytes. Tissue Cell 16: 31–42

Fromaget C, el-Aoumari A, Gros D 1992 Distribution pattern of connexin 43, a gap junctional protein, during the differentiation of mouse heart myocytes. Differentiation 51: 9–20

Frömter E 1979 The Feldberg lecture 1976. Solute transport across epithelia: what can we learn from micropuncture studies in kidney tubules? J Physiol 288: 1–31

Frutiger P 1969 Zur frühentwicklung der ductus paramesonephrici und des müllerrerschen hugels beim menschen. Acta Anat 72: 233–245

Fu Q-G, Suarez J I, Ebner T J 1993 Neuronal specification of direction and distance during reaching movements in the superior precentral premotor area and primary motor cortex of monkeys. J Neurophysiol 70: 2097–2116

Fuchs A M, Menker N, Ling L, Langer T P, Kaneko C R S 1992 Discharge patterns of levator palpabrae superioris motoneurons during vertical lid movements in the monkey. J Neurophysiol 68: 233–243

Fujimoto H, Yanagisawa K O 1983 Defects in the archenteron of mouse embryos homozygous for the T-mutation. Differentiation 25: 44–47

Fujinaga M, Baden J M 1991 Evidence for an adrenergic mechanism in the control of body asymmetry. Dev Biol 143: 203–205

Fujinaga M, Maze M, Hoffman B B, Baden J M 1992 Activation of alpha-1 adrenergic receptors modulates the control of left/right sidedness in rat embryos. Dev Biol 150: 419–421

Fujita H, Fujita S 1963 Electron microscopic studies on neuroblast differentiation in the central nervous system of domestic fowl. Z Zellforsch 60: 463–478

Fujita S 1963 The matrix cell and cytogenesis in the developing central nervous system. J Comp Neurol 120: 37–42

Fujita S 1967 Quantitative analysis of cell proliferation and differentiation in the cortex of the postnatal mouse cerebellum. J Cell Biol 32: 277–287

Fujita S, Shimada M, Nakamura T 1966 ^{3}H-thymidine autoradiographic studies on the cell proliferation and differentiation in the external and internal granular layers of the mouse cerebellum. J Comp Neurol 128: 191–208

Fujita T 1959 Histological studies on the neuro-insular complex in the pancreas of some mammals. Z Zellforsch 50: 94–109

Fujita T 1976 The gastro-enteric endocrine cell and its paraneuronic nature. In: Coupland R E, Fujita T (eds) Chromaffin, enterochromaffin and related cells. A NAITO Foundation Symposium. Elsevier: New York: pp 191–208

Fujita T (ed) 1973 Gastro-entero-pancreatic system. A cell-biological approach. Igaku Shoiu: Tokyo

Fujita T S, Kobayashi S 1977 The structure and function of gut endocrine cells. Internat Rev Cytol (Suppl) 6: 187

Fujita T, Miyoshi M, Tokunaga J 1970 Scanning and transmission electron microscopy of human ejaculate spermatozoa with special reference to their abnormal forms. Z Zellforsch 105: 483–497

Fukada K (1985) Purification and partial characterisation of a cholinergic neuronal differentiation factor. Proc Nat Acad Sci USA 82: 8795–8799

Fukuda T 1976 Ultrastructure of primordial germ cells in human embryo. Virchows Arch B Cell Pathol 20: 85–89

Fukuda T, Hedinger C 1975 Ultrastructure of developing germ cells in the fetal human testis. Cell Tissue Res 161: 55–70

Fuld H, Irwin D T 1954 Clinical application of portal venography. Br Med J 1: 312–313

Fullard R J, Snyder C 1990 Protein levels in non-stimulated and stimulated tears of normal human subjects. Invest Ophthalmol Vis Sci 31: 1119–1126

Fuller A P, Fozzard J A, Wright G H 1959 Spincteric action of cricopharyngeus: radiographic demonstration. Br J Radiol 32: 32–35

Fürbinger M 1873 Zur vergleichenden Anatomie der Schulter-muskeln. Jena Z Naturw 7: 237–320

Furcht L T, Wendelschafer-Crabb G, Mosher D F, Foidart J M 1980 An axial periodic fibrillar arrangement of antigenic determinants for fibronectin and procollagen on ascorbate-treated human fibroblasts. J Supramol Struct 13: 15–33

Furness D N, Hackney C M 1985 Cross-links between stereocilia in the guinea pig cochlea. Hear Res 18: 177–188

Furness J B, Bornstein J C, Murphy R, Pompolo S 1992 Roles of peptides in transmission in the enteric nervous system. Trends Neurosci 15: 66–71

Furness J B, Costa M 1980 Types of nerves in the enteric nervous system. Neurosci 5: 1–20

Furness J B, Costa M (eds) 1987 The enteric nervous system. Churchill Livingstone: Edinburgh

Furseth R 1968 The resorption process of human deciduous teeth studied by light microscopy, microradiography and electron microscopy. Archs Oral Biol 13: 417–431

Fusijawa H, Morioka H, Watanabe K, Nakamura H 1976 A decay of gap junctions in association with cell differentiation of neural retina in chick embryonic development. J Cell Sci 22: 585–596

Fuss F K, Bacher A 1991 New aspects of the morphology and function of the human hip joint ligaments. Am J Anat 192: 1–13

Fyffe R E W 1984 Afferent fibers. In: Davidoff R A (ed) Handbook of the spinal cord. Vols 2 and 3. Dekker: New York: pp 79–136

Fyke F E Jr, Code C F, Schlegel J F 1956 The gastroesophageal sphincter in healthy human beings. Gastroenterologia 86: 135–150

G

Gabbiani G, Chaponnier C, Hüttner I 1978 Cytoplasmic filaments and gap junctions in epithelial cells and myofibroblasts during wound healing. J Cell Biol 76: 561–568

Gabbiani G, Ryan G B, Lamelin J P et al 1973 Human smooth muscle autoantibody. Its identification as antiactin antibody and a study of its binding to 'nonmuscular' cells. Am J Pathol 72: 473–488

Gabbiani G, Ryan G B, Majno G 1971 Presence of modified fibroblasts in granulation tissue and their possible role in wound contraction. Experientia 27: 549–551

Gabe M 1966 Neurosecretion. Pergamon: Oxford

Gabella G 1972 Fine structure of the myenteric plexus in the guinea-pig ileum. J Anat 111: 69–97

Gabella G 1973 Cellular structures and electrophysiological behaviour. Fine structure of smooth muscle. Philos Trans R Soc Lond 265B: 7–16

Gabella G 1976 Structure of the autonomic nervous system. Chapman & Hall: London

Gabella G 1981 Structure of smooth muscles. In: Bülbring E, Brading A F, Jones A W, Tomita T (eds) Smooth muscle: an assessment of current knowledge. Edward Arnold: London: pp 1–46

Gabella G 1984 Smooth muscle cell membrane and allied structures. In: Stephens N L (ed) Smooth muscle contraction. Marcel Dekker: New York: pp 21–45

Gabella G 1987 The cross-ply arrangement of collagen fibres in the submucosa of the mammalian small intestine. Cel Tiss Res 248: 491–497

Gabella G 1988 Structure of intestinal musculature. In: Handbook of physiology; the gastrointestinal system I. American Physiological Society and Oxford University Press: New York: pp 103–139

Gabella G 1989 Development of smooth muscle: ultrastructural study of the chick embryo gizzard. Anat Embryol 180: 213–226

Gabella G 1990 Hypertrophy of visceral smooth muscle. Anat Embryol 182: 409–424

Gabriel A C 1958 Some anatomical features of the mandible. J Anat 92: 580–586

Gabriel W B 1945 The principles and practice of rectal surgery. Lewis: London

Gacek R, Radpour S 1982 Fibre orientation of the facial nerve: An experimental study in the cat. Laryngoscope 92: 547–556

Gacek, Rasmussen 1961 Fiber analysis of the statoacoustic nerve of guinea pig, cat and monkey. Anat Rec 139: 455–463

Gaddum P 1968 Sperm maturation in the male reproductive tract: Development of motility. Anat Rec 161: 471–482

Gaddum-Rosse P, Blandau R J 1976 Comparative observations on ciliary currents in mammalian oviducts. Biol Reprod 14: 605–609

Gadow H F 1933 The evolution of the vertebral column. In: Gaskell J F, Green H L H H (eds) A contribution to the study of vertebrate phylogeny. Cambridge University Press: Cambridge

Gaffan D 1992 Amnesia for complex naturalistic scenes and for objects following fornix transection in the Rhesus monkey. Eur J Neurosci 4: 381 – 388

Gaffan D 1992 Amygdala and the memory of reward. In: Aggleton J P (ed) The amygdala. Wiley & Sons: Chichester: pp 471–484

Gaffan D 1994 Dissociated effects of perirhinal cortex ablation, fornix transection and amygdalectomy: evidence for multiple memory systems in the primate temporal lobe. Exp Brain Res 99: 411 – 422

Gaffan D 1994 Scene-specific memory for objects: a model of episodic memory impairment in monkeys with fornix transection. J Cog Neurosci 6: 305 – 320

Gaffan D, Gaffan E A 1991 Amnesia in man following transection of the fornix: a review. Brain 114: 2611 – 2618

Gaffan D, Harrison S 1987 Amygdalectomy and disconnection in visual learning for auditory secondary reinforcement by monkeys. J Neurosci 7(8): 2285–2292

Gaffan D, Harrison S 1989 Place memory and scene memory: effects of fornix transection in the monkey. Exp Brain Res 74: 202 – 212

Gaffan D, Harrison S 1991 Auditory-visual associations, hemispheric specialization and temporal-frontal interaction in the rhesus monkey. Brain 114: 2133–2144

Gaffan D, Harrison S 1993 Role of the dorsal prestriate cortex in visuospatial configural discrimination by monkeys. Behav Brain Res 56: 119–125

Gaffan D, Murray E A 1992 Monkeys (Macaca fascicularis) with rhinal cortex ablations succeed in object discrimination learning despite 24-hr intertrial intervals and fail at matching to sample despite double sample presentations. Behav Neurosci 106: 30 – 38

Gaillard P J, Talmage R V, Budy A M (eds) 1965 The parathyroid glands: ultrastructure, secretion and function. University of Chicago Press: Chicago

Galaburda A M 1994 Anatomic basis of cerebral dominance. In: Davidson R E, Hugdahl K (eds) Cerebral asymmetry. MIT Press: Boston: pp 51–73

Galaburda A M, Sanides F, Geschwind N 1978 Human brain. Cytoarchitectonic left–right asymmetries in the temporal speech region. Arch Neurol 35: 812–817

Galilei, Galileo 1638 Discorsi e dimostrazioni matematiche intorno à due nuove scienze. Attenenti alla mecanica e i movimenti locali . . . con una apendice del centro di gravità d'alcuni solidi. Elzevirs: Leiden

Galileo D S, Gray G E, Owens G C, Majors J, Sanes J R 1990 Proc Natl Acad Sci USA 87: 458–462

Galli G, Ottaviani G, Galli S 1976 Studio Biometrico dell'apofisi mastoidea nell'uomo. I. Indagini ad indirizzo antropologico: l'atezza della mastoide correlata a parametri cranici e statura. II. Catt Ist Anat Um Norm Univ Modena Ita-Quadranat Prat 32: 1–4, 123–132

Galliot B, Dollé P, Vigneron M, Featherstone M S, Baron A, Duboule D 1989 The mouse Hox 1.4 gene: primary structure, evidence for promoter activity and expression during development.

Gamble H J, Eames R A J 1964 An electron microscope study of the connective tissue of human peripheral nerve. J Anat 98: 655–663

Gamble H J, Fenton J, Allsopp G 1978 Electron microscope observations on the changing relationships between unmyelinated axons and Schwann cells in human fetal nerves. J Anat 127: 363–378

Gandy G M 1992 Examination of the neonate including gestational assessment. In: Robertson N R C (ed) Textbook of neonatology. Churchill Livingstone: Edinburgh: pp 199–215

Ganguly D N, Roy K K 1964 A study on the cranio-vertebral joint in the man. Anat Anz 114: 433–452

Ganguly D N, Singh-Roy K K 1965 A study on the cranio-vertebral joint in the vertebrates. I. In the mammals, as illustrated by its structure in the guinea pig and development in the guinea pig and Talpa. Anat Anz 117: 421–429

Gans C, Northcutt R G 1983 Neural crest and the origin of vertebrates: a new head. Science 220: 268–274

Gao W-Q, Liu X-L, Hatten M E 1992 Cell 68: 841–854

Garcia Arrasas J E, Fauquet M, Chanconie M, Smith J 1986 Coexpression of somatostatin-like immunoreactive and catecholaminergic properties in neural crest derivatives: comodulation of peptidergic and adrenergic differentiation in cultured neural crest. Dev Biol 114: 247–257

Garcia I, Martinou I, Tsujimoto Y, Martinou J 1992 Science 258: 302–304

Garcia-Arrarás J E, Lugo-Chinchilla A M, Chevere-Colon I 1992 The expression of neuropeptide Y immunoreactivity in the avian sympathoadrenal system conforms with two models of coexpression development for neurons and chromaffin cells. Development 115: 617–627

Garcia-Arrarás J E, Martinez R 1990 Developmental expression of serotonin-like immunoreactivity in the sympathoadrenal system of the chicken. Cell Tissue Res 262: 363–372

Gardiner D S, More I A R, Lindop G B M 1986 The granular peripolar cell of the human glomerulus: an ultrastructural study. J Anat 146: 31–43

Gardner E 1967 Spinal cord and brain stem pathways for afferents from joints. In: de Reuek A V S, Knight J (eds) Myotatic, kinesthetic and vestibular mechanisms. Ciba Foundation Symposium. Churchill: London pp 56–76

Gardner E D 1948a The innervation of the knee joint. Anat Rec 101: 109–130

Gardner E D 1948b The innervation of the shoulder joint. Anat Rec 102: 1–18

Gardner E D 1950 Physiology of movable joints. Physiol Rev 30: 127–176

Gardner E, Gray D J 1950 Prenatal development of the human hip joint. Am J Anat 87: 162–212

Gardner E, Lenn N J 1977 Fibres in monkey posterior articular nerves. Anat Rec. 187: 99–106

Gardner E, O'Rahilly R 1976 The nerve supply and conducting system of the human heart at the end of the embryonic period proper. J Anat 121: 571–587

Gardner R L, Rossant J 1979 Investigation of the fate of 4.5 day postcoitum mouse inner cell mass cells by blastocyst injection. J Embryol Expt Morphol 52: 141–152

Garey L J 1990 Visual system. In: Paxinos G (ed) The human nervous system. Academic Press: San Diego: pp 945 – 977

Garfia A 1980 Glomus tissue in the vicinity of the human carotid sinus. J Anat 130: 1–12

Garn S M, Lewis A B 1962 The relationship between third molar agenesis and reduction in tooth number. Angle Orthod 33: 14–18

Garn S M, Rohmann C G 1960 Variability in the order of ossification of the bony centers of the hand and wrist. Am J Phys Anthropol N S 18: 219–230

Garrachty P E, Hanes D P, Florence S L, Kaas J H 1994 Pattern of peripheral deafferentation predicts reorganizational limits in adult primate somatosensory cortex. Somatosens Mot Res 11: 109–117

Garrachty P E, Kaas J H 1992 Dynamic features of sensory and motor maps. Curr Opin Neurobiol 2: 522–527

Garrett F D 1948 Development of the cervical vesicles in man. Anat Rec 100: 101–114

Garrett J R 1963 The ultrastructure of intracellular fat in the parenchyma of human submandicular salivary glands. Arch Oral Biol 8: 729–734

Garrett J R 1967 The innervation of normal human submandibular and parotid salivary glands demonstrated by cholinesterase histochemistry, catecholamine fluorescence and electron microscopy. Arch Oral Biol 12: 1417–1436

Garrett J R 1972 Neuro-effector sites in salivary glands. In: Emmelin N, Zotterman Y (eds) Oral physiology. Pergamon: Oxford: pp 83–97

Garrett J R 1975 Recent advances in physiology of salivary glands. Br Med Bull 31: 152–155

Garrett J R 1976 Structure and innervation of salivary glands. In: Cohen B, Kramer J R H (eds) Scientific foundations of dentistry. Heinemann: London: pp 499–516

Garrett J R, Emmelin N 1979 Activities of salivary myoepithelial cells: a review. Med Biol 57: 1–28

Garrett J R, Howard E R, Nixon H H 1969 Autonomic nerves in rectum and colon in Hirschsprung's disease. A cholinesterase and catecholamine histochemical study. Arch Dis Child 44: 406–417

Garrett J R, Kemplay S K 1977 The adrenergic innervation of the submandibular gland of the cat and the effects of various surgical denervations on these nerves. A histochemical and ultrastructural study including the use of 5-hydroxydopamine. J Anat 124: 99–115

Garrett J R, Kidd A 1975 Effects of nerve stimulation and denervation on secretory material in submandibular striated duct cells of cats, and the possible role of these cells in the secretion of salivary kallikrein. Cell Tissue Res 161: 71–84

Garrett J R, Parsons P A 1974 Movement of horseradish peroxidase in submandibular glands of rabbits after arterial injection. J Physiol 237: 3–4P

Garrod A 1909 Inborn errors of metabolism. Oxford University Press: Oxford

Garrod A E 1902 The incidence of alkaptonuria: a study in chemical individuality. Lancet ii: 1616–1620

Garrod D R 1993 Desmosomes and hemidesmosomes. Curr Opin Cell Biol 5: 30–40

Garthwaite J, Brodbelt A R 1989 Synaptic activation of N-methyl-D-aspartate and non-N-methyl-D-aspartate receptors in the mossy fibre pathway in adult and immature rat cerebellar slices. Neuroscience 29: 401–412

Gasser H S 1956 Olfactory nerve fibres. J Gen Physiol 39: 473–498

Gatsalov M D 1963 Limfaticheskaia sistema slizistoĭ obolochki fallopievoĭ truby cheloveka. Akush Ginek 39: 85–90

Gatter K C, Powell T P S 1977 The projection of the locus coeruleus upon the neocortex in the macaque monkey. Neuroscience 2: 441–445

Gatter K C, Powell T P S 1978 The intrinsic connections of the cortex of area 4 of the monkey. Brain 101: 513–541

Gaughran G R L 1963 Mylohyoid boutonnière and sublingual bouton. J Anat 97: 565–568

Gaunt P N, Gaunt W A 1978 Three dimensional reconstruction in biology. (First published as Microreconstruction by Gaunt W A in 1971.) Pitman Medical: Tunbridge Wells

Gaunt S J, Sharpe P T, Duboule D 1988 Spatially restricted domains of homeo-gene transcripts in mouse embryos: relation to a segmented body plan. Development (Suppl.) 104: 169–179

Gaunt W A 1959 The vascular supply to the dental lamina during early development. Acta Anat 37: 232–252

Gautvik K M, Kriz M, Lund-Larsen K 1972 Adrenergic vasodilation in the cat submandibular salivary gland. In: Emmelin N, Zotterman Y (eds) Oral physiology. Pergamon: Oxford: pp 161–162

Gawin F H 1991 Cocaine addiction: psychology and neurophysiology. Science 251: 1580–1586

Gaze R M 1970 The formation of nerve connections. Academic Press: London

Geboes K, De Wolf-Peeters C, Rutgeers P, Janseen J, Van Trappen J, Desmet G 1983 Lymphocytes and langerhans cells in human esophageal epithelium. Virchow's Arch 401: 25

Geenen V, Robert F, Martens H, Benhida A, Giovanni G de, Defresne M-P, Boniver J, Legros J-J, Martial J, Franchimont P 1991 Biosynthesis and paracrine/cryptocrine actions of 'self' neurohypophyseal-related peptides in the thymus. Mol Cell Endocrinol 76: C27–C31

Gehr P, Bachofen M, Weibel E R 1978 The normal human lung: ultrastructure and morphometric estimation of diffusion capacity. Resp Physiol 32: 121–140

Geiger B Ayalon O 1992 Cadherins. Annu Rev Cell Biol 8: 307–332

Geiger B, Ginsberg D 1991 The cytoplasmic domain of adherens-type junctions. Cell Motil Cytoskel 20: 1–6

Geiger R S 1963a In: Pfeiffer C C, Smythies J R (eds) Neurobiology. Vol 5. Academic Press: New York

Geiger R S 1963b The behaviour of adult mammalian brain cells in culture. Int Rev Biol 5: 1–52

Gelfan S, Rapisarda A F 1964 Synaptic density on spinal neurons of normal dogs and dogs with experimental hind-limb rigidity. J Comp Neurol 123: 73–96

Geller M, Barbato D 1970 Nervus peronaeus profundus. A study of the terminal branches and their variations. Hospital Rio de J 77: 679–698

Genant H K, Resnick D 1988 Magnification radiography. In: Resnick D, Niwayama G (eds) Diagnosis of bone and joint disorders. 2nd edition. W B Saunders: Philadelphia: pp 84–107

Genant H K, Steiger P, Block E, Glueer C C, Ettinger B, Harris S T 1987 Quantitative computer tomography. Calcif Tissue Int 41: 179–186

Génis-Gálvez J M, Santos Gutierrez L, Martin Lopez M 1966 On the double innervation of the parotid gland. An experimental study. Acta Anat 63: 398–403

Genovese S T 1959 Diferencias sexuales en el huesco coxal. Universidad Nacional Autonoma de Mexico: Mexico: No 49

Genovese S T, Messmacher M 1959 Valor de los patrones tradicionales para la determinacion de la edad por medio de las suturas en craneous Mexicanos (Indigenas y Mestizos). Cuad Inst Hist Méx No 7

Gentner W, Lippolt H J 1969 The potassium-argon dating of Upper Tertiary and Pleistocene deposits. In: Brothwell D, Higgs E (eds) Science in archaeology. Thames and Hudson: London

Georgatos S D, Meier J, Simos G 1994 Lamins and lamin-associated proteins. Curr Opin Cell Biol 6: 347–353

Georgopoulos A P 1991 Higher order motor control. Ann Rev Neurosci 14: 361–377

Georgopoulos A P, Caminiti R, Kalaska J F 1984 Static spatial effect in motor cortex and area 5: quantitative relations in a two-dimensional space. Exp Brain Res 54: 446–454

Georgopoulos A P, Kalaska J F, Caminiti R 1985 Relations between two-dimensional arm movements and single-cell discharge in motor cortex and area 5: movement direction versus movement end point. Exp Brain Res 10: 175–183

Gerfen C R 1992 The neostriatal mosaic: multiple levels of compartmental organization in the basal ganglia. Ann Rev Neurosci 15: 285–320

Gerich J E, Lorenzi M 1978 The role of the autonomic nervous system and somatostatin in the control of insulin and glucagon secretion. In: Ganong W F, Martini L (eds) Frontiers in neuroendocrinology. Vol 5. Raven Press: New York

Gerlach J von 1858 Mikroskopische Studien aus dem Gebiete der menschlichen morphologie. F Enke: Erlangen

Gerrits N M 1990 The vestibular nuclear complex. In: Paxinos G (ed) The human nervous system. Academic Press: San Diego: pp 863–888

Gerrits N M, Epema A H, Voogd J 1984 The mossy fibre projection of the nucleus reticularis tegmenti pontis to the flocculus and adjacent ventral paraflocculus in the cat. Neuroscience 11: 627–644

Gerrits N M, Voogd J, Magras I N 1985 Vestibular afferents of the inferior olive and the vestibulo-olivo-cerebellar climbing fiber pathway to the flocculus in the cat. Brain Res 332: 325–336

Gerrits N M, Voogd J, Nas W S C 1985a Cerebellar and olivary projections of the external and rostral internal cuneate nuclei in the cat. Exp Brain Res 57: 239–255

Gerrits N, Voogd J 1987 The projection of the nucleus reticularis tegmenti pontis and adjacent regions of the pontine nuclei to the central cerebellar nuclei in the cat. J Comp Neurol 258: 52–69

Gershon M D 1987 Phenotypic expression by neural crest-derived precursors of enteric neurons and glia. In: Maderson P F A (ed) Developmental and evolutionary aspects of the neural crest. John Wiley: New York

Gershon M D, Mawe G M, Branchek T A 1989 5-HT and enteric neurones.

In: Fozard J R (ed) The peripheral actions of 5-HT. Oxford University Press: Oxford: pp 247–273

Gershon M D, Wade P R 1993 Enteric nervous system. Curr Opin Gastroenterol 9: 246–253

Geschwandtner W R 1973 Striae cutis atrophicae nach Lokalbehandlung mit Corticosteroiden. Hautarzt 24: 70–73

Geschwind N, Galaburda A M 1987 Cerebral lateralization. MIT Press: Cambridge: p 283

Geschwind N, Levitsky W 1968 Human brain: left-right asymmetries in temporal speech region. Science 161: 186–187

Getchell M L, Chen Y, Ding X, Sparks D L, Getchell T V 1993 Immunohistochemical localization of a cytochrome P-450 isozyme in human olfactory nasal mucosa: age-related trends. Ann Otol Rhinol Laryngol 102: 368–374

Getchell M L, Getchell T V Fine structural aspects of secretion and extrinsic innervation in the olfactory mucosa. Microsc Res Techn 23: 111–127

Getz B, Sirnes T 1949 The localisation within the dorsal motor vagal nucleus. An experimental investigation. J Comp Neurol 90: 95–110

Ghadially F N 1983 Fine structure of synovial joints. A text and atlas of the ultrastructure of normal and pathological articular tissues. Butterworths: London

Ghadially F N, Ghadially J A, Oryschak A F, Yong N K 1976 Experimental production of ridges on rabbit articular cartilage. J Anat 121: 119–132

Ghadially F N, Lalonde J-M A, Wedge J H 1983 Ultrastructure of normal and torn menisci of the human knee joint. J Anat 136: 773–791

Ghadially F N, Roy S 1969 Ultrastructure of synovial joints in health and disease. Butterworths: London

Ghadially F N, Yong N K, Lalonde J M 1982 A transmission electron microscopic comparison of the articular surface of cartilage processed attached to bone and detached from bone. J Anat 135: 685–706

Ghebrehiwet B, Silverberg M, Kaplan A P 1981 Activation of the classical pathway of complement by Hayeman factor fragment. J Exp Med 153: 665–676

Ghosh A, Shatz C J 1993 Development 117: 1031–1047

Ghosh P, Taylor T K 1987 The knee joint meniscus. A fibrocartilage of some distinction. Clin Orthop 224: 52–63

Gianelli F 1970 Human chromosomes and DNA synthesis (monographs in human genetics vol 5) Karger: Basel

Gibbons I R, Grimstone A V 1960 On flagellar structures in certain flagellates. J Biophys Biochem Cytol 7: 697–716

Gibson A R, Robinson F R, Alam J, Houk J C 1987 Somatotopic alignment between climbing fiber input and nuclear output of the cat intermediate cerebellum. J Comp Neurol 260: 362–377

Gibson I W, Gardiner D S, Downie I, Downie T T, More I A, Lindop G B 1994 A comparative study of the glomerular peripolar cell and the renin-secreting cell in twelve mammalian species. Cell Tiss Res 277: 385–390

Giguere M, Goldman-Rakic P S 1988 Mediodorsal nucleus: areal, laminar, and tangential distribution of afferents and efferents in the frontal lobe of rhesus monkeys. J Comp Neurol 277: 195–213

Gil J, Reiss O K 1973 Isolation and characterisation of lamellar bodies and tubular myelin from rat lung homogenates. J Cell Biol 58: 152–171

Gil J, Weibel E R 1969 Improvements in demonstration of lining layer of lung alveoli by electron microscopy. Resp Physiol 8: 13–36

Gilad I, Nissan M 1985 Sagittal evaluation of elemental geometrical dimensions of human vertebrae. J Anat 143: 115–120

Gilbert C D 1993a Circuitry, architecture, and functional dynamics of visual cortex. Cereb Cortex 3: 373–386

Gilbert C D 1993b Rapid dynamic changes in adult cerebral cortex. Curr Opin Neurobiol 3: 100–103

Gilbert P W 1952 The origin and development of the head cavities in the human embryo. J Morph 90: 149–187

Gilbert P W 1957 The origin and development of the human extrinsic ocular muscles. Contrib Embryol Carnegie Inst Washington 36: 59–78

Gilbert S F 1991 Developmental biology. Sinauer Associates: Sunderland, Massachusetts

Gilchrest B A 1987 Ageing of the skin. In: Fitzpatrick T B, Eizen A Z, Wollf K, Friedberg I M, Austen K F (eds) Dermatology in general medicine. 3rd edition. 2 vols. McGraw Hill: New York: pp 146–153

Gilchrest B A, Bloog F B, Szabo G 1979 Effects of ageing and chronic sun exposure on melanocytes in human skin. J Invest Dermatol 73: 77–83

Giles E, Elliot O 1960, Negro-white identity from the skull. Proceedings of the 6th International Anthropological Congress, Paris. Quoted in: Krogman W M (ed) 1962 The human skeleton in forensic medicine. Thomas: Springfield, Illinois: pp 195–196

Giles R E, Blanc H, Cann H M, Wallace D C 1980 Maternal inheritance of human mitochondrial DNA. Proc Nat Acad Sci USA 77: 6715–6719

Gillespie J M 1991 The structural proteins of hair. In: Goldsmith L A (ed) Physiology, biochemistry, and molecular biology of skin. 2nd edition. 2 vols. Oxford University Press: Oxford: pp. 625–659

Gillett W R 1991 Artefactual loss of human ovarian surface epithelium: potential clinical significance. Reprod Fertil Dev 3: 93–98

Gillett W R, Mitchell A, Hurst P R 1991 A scanning electron microscopic

study of the human ovarian surface epithelium: characterization of two cell types. Hum Reprod 6: 645–650

Gillilan L 1958 The arterial blood supply of the human spinal cord. J Comp Neurol 110: 75–104

Gillilan L A 1941 The connexions of the basal optic root (posterior accessory optic tract) and its nucleus in various mammals. J Comp Neurol 74: 367–408

Gillilan L A 1972 Anatomy and embryology of the arterial system of the brain stem and cerebellum. In: Vinken I J, Bruyn G W (eds) Handbook of clinical neurology. Vol 2. North Holland: Amsterdam: pp 24–44

Gillilan L A 1974 Potential collateral circulation to the human cerebral cortex. Neurology 24: 941–948

Gillman J 1948 The development of the gonads in man, with a consideration of the role of fetal endocrines and the histogenesis of ovarian tumors. Contrib Embryol Carnegie Inst Washington, 32: 81–131

Gilmour J R 1938 Gross anatomy of the parathyroid glands. J Pathol Bact 46: 133–149

Gilpin S A, Gosling J A 1983 Smooth muscle in the wall of developing human urinary bladder and urethra. J Anat 137: 503–512

Gilula N B, Epstein M L, Beers W H 1978 Cell-to-cell communication and ovulation. A study of the cumulus-oocyte complex. J Cell Biol 78: 58–75

Gilula N B, Satir P 1972 The ciliary necklace: a ciliary membrane specialization. J Cell Biol 53: 494–509

Gilula N B, Satir P 1972 The ciliary necklace: a ciliary membrane specialization. J Cell Biol 53: 494–509

Gimson A C 1981 Enflish pronouncing dictionary. Dent: London

Gingerich P D 1971 Functional significance of mandibular translation in vertebrate jaw mechanics. Postila 152: 1–10

Ginia V M, Linberg I V, McCormick J A 1987 The anatomy of the lateral canthal tendon. Arch Ophthalmol 105: 529–532

Ginsburg M, Snow M H L, McLaren M 1990 Primordial germ cells in the mouse embryo during gastrulation. Development 110: 521–528

Giok S P 1956 Localisation of fibre systems within the white matter of the medulla oblongata and the cervical cord in man. Ijido: Leiden

Girdler N M 1993 Repair of articular defects with autologous mandibular condylar cartilage. J Bone Jt Surg 75B: 710–714

Girgis F G, Marshall J L, Al Monajem A R S 1975 The cruciate ligaments of the knee joint. Clin Orthop 106: 216–231

Githens S 1989 Development of ductal cells In; Lebenthal E (ed) Human gastrointestinal development. Raven Press: New York: pp 669–683

Giwercman A, Skakkebaek N E 1992 The human testis – an organ at risk? Int J Androl 15: 373–375

Gladstone R J 1929 Development of the inferior vena cava in the light of recent research, with especial reference to certain abnormalities, and current descriptions of the ascending lumbar and azygos veins. J Anat 64: 70–93

Gladstone R J, Wakeley C P G 1940 The pineal organ. Ballière, Tindall and Cox: London

Glaister J, Brash J C 1937 Medicolegal aspects of the Buck Ruxton case. Livingstone: Edinburgh

Glass R H, Aggeler J, Spindle A, Pedersen R A, Werb Z 1983 Degradation of extracellular matrix by mouse trophoblast outgrowths: a model for implantation. J Cell Biol 96: 1108–1116

Glasser S W, Korfhagen T R, Wert S E et al 1991 Genetic element from human surfactant protein SP-C gene confers bronchiolar-alveolar cell specificity in transgenic mice. Lung Cell Mol Physiol 261: L349–L356

Glauser F 1953 Studies on intrahepatic arterial circulation. Surgery 33: 333–341

Glees P 1946 Terminal degeneration within the central nervous system as studied by a new silver method. J Neuropath Exp Neurol 5: 54–59

Glees P 1963 Neuroglia, morphology and function. Blackwell: Oxford

Gleeson M J, Felix H, Johnsson L-G 1991 Ultrastructural aspects of the human peripheral vestibular system. Acta Otolaryngol [Stockh] Suppl 470: 80–87

Glenister T W 1954 The origin and fate of the urethral plate in man. J Anat 88: 413–425

Glenister T W 1962 The development of the utricle and of the so-called 'middle' or 'median' lobe of the human prostate. J Anat 96: 443–455

Glenister T W 1976 An embryological view of cartilage. J Anat 122: 323–330

Glenn W W L, Hogan J F, Loke J S O, Cieselski T E, Phelps M L, Rowedder R 1984 Ventilatory support by pacing of the conditioned diaphragm in quadriplegia. New Engl J Med 310: 1150–1155

Glickstein M 1987 Structure and function of the cerebellum: a historical introduction to some current problems. In: Glickstein et al (eds) Cerebellum and neuronal plasticity. Plenum: New York

Glickstein M, May J, Mercier B 1985 Corticopontine projections in the macaque: the distribution of labelled cortical cells after large injections of horseradish peroxidase in the pontine nuclei. J Comp Neurol 235: 343–359

Glickstein M, Yeo C H, Stein J 1987 (eds) Cerebellum and neuronal plasticity. Plenum: New York

Glimcher M J 1990 The nature of the mineral component in bone and the mechanism of calcification. In: Avioli L V, Krane S M (eds) Metabolic bone disease and clinically related disorders. 2nd edition. Saunders: Philadelphia: pp 42–56

Glisson F 1654 Anatomia hepatis subjiciuntur nonnulla de lymphae-ductibus nuper repertis. Du-Gardianis: London

Gloster J, Perkins E S, Pommier M 1957 Extensibility of strips of sclera and cornea. Br J Ophthalmol 41: 103–110

Gochin P M, Colombo M, Dorfman G A, Gerstein G L, Gross C G 1994 Neural ensemble coding in inferior temporal cortex. J Neurophysiol 71: 2325–2337

Gochin P M, Miller E K, Gerstein G L 1991 Functional interactions among neurons in the inferior temporal cortex of the awake macaque. Exp Brain Res 84: 505–516

Godlewski G, Hedon B, Castel C 1975 Contribution à l'étude de l'origine de l'artère hépatique chez l'embryon et le foetus. Bull Assoc Anat Nancy 59: 411–418

Goel V K, Svensson N L 1977 Forces on the pelvis. J Biomech 10: 195–200

Goel V K, Valliappan S, Svensson D L 1978 Stresses in normal pelvis. Comp Biol Med 8: 91–104

Goerke J 1974 Lung surfactant. Biochim Biophys Acta 344: 241–261

Goh J C H, Lee E H, Ang E J, Bayon P, Pho R W H 1992 Biomechanical study on the load-bearing characteristics of the fibula and the effects of fibular resection. Clin Orthop 279: 223–228

Goland M (ed) 1975 Normal and abnormal growth of the prostate. Thomas: Springfield, Illinois

Goldberg J M, Moore R Y 1967 Ascending projections of the lateral lemniscus in the cat and monkey. J Comp Neurol 129: 143–156

Goldberg P, Roussos C 1990 Assessment of respiratory muscle dysfunction in chronic obstructive lung disease. Med Clin North Am 74: 643–660

Goldberg S 1970 The origin of the lumbrical muscles in the hand of the South African native. The hand 2: 168–171

Goldberg S R, Stolerman I P (eds) 1986 Behavioral analysis of drug dependence. Academic Press: London

Golde D W, Takaku F (eds) 1985 Haemopoietic Stem Cells. Dekker: New York

Goldman J E 1992 Regulation of oligodendrocyte differentiation. Trends Neurosci 15: 359 – 362

Goldman J M, Rose L S, Morgan M D L, Denison D M 1986 Measurement of abdominal wall compliance in normal subjects and tetraplegic patients. Thorax 41: 513–518

Goldman J M, Rose L S, Williams S J, Silver J R, Denison D M 1986 Effect of abdominal binders on breathing in tetraplegic patients. Thorax 41: 940–945

Goldman J M, Williams S J, Denison D M 1988 The rib cage and abdominal components of respiratory system compliance in tetraplegic patients. Eur Respir J 1: 242–247

Goldman-Rakic P S 1988 Topography of cognition: parallel distributed networks in primate association cortex. Ann Rev Neurosci 11: 137–156

Goldman-Rakic P S, Selemon D 1986 Topography of corticostriatal projections in nonhuman primates and implications for functional parcellation of the neostriatum. In: Jones E G, Peters A (eds) Cerebral cortex. Vol 5. Sensory-motor areas and aspects of cortical connectivity. Plenum Press: New York: pp 447–465

Goldsmith L A (ed) 1991 Physiology, biochemistry, and molecular biology of skin. 2nd edition. 2 vols. Oxford University Press: Oxford

Goldsmith N A, Woodburne R T 1957 The surgical anatomy pertaining to liver resection. Surgery Gynecol Obstet 105: 310–318

Goldspink G 1971 Ultrastructural changes in striated muscle fibres during contraction and growth with particular reference to the mechanism of myofibril splitting. J Cell Sci 9: 123–138

Goldstein A L, Low T K L, McAdoo M, McClure J, Thurman G B, Rossio J J, Lai C Y, Chang D, Wang S S, Harvey C, Ramel A H, Meinhofer J 1977 Thymosin α1. Isolation and sequence analysis of an immunologically active thymic peptide. Proc Nat Acad Sci (USA) 74: 725–729

Goldstein G W, Betz A L 1986 The blood–brain barrier. Sci Am 255: 70–79

Goldstein G, MacKay I R 1969 The human thymus. Heinemann: London

Goldstein G, Scheid M P, Boyse E A, Schlesinger D H, van Vauwe J 1979 A synthetic pentapeptide with biological activity characteristic of the thymic hormone thymopoietin. Science 204: 1309–1310

Goldstein M B, Davies E A Jr 1968 The three-dimensional architecture of the islets of Langerhans. Acta Anat 71: 161–171

Goldstein R S, Kalcheim C 1991 Normal segmentation and size of the primary sympathetic ganglia depend upon the alternation of rostrocaudal properties of the somites. Development 112: 327–334

Goldstein R S, Kalcheim C 1992 Determination of epithelial half-somites in skeletal morphogenesis. Development 116: 441–445

Goldstein R S, Teillet M-A, Kalcheim C 1990 Proc Natl Acad Sci USA 87: 4476–4480

Goligher J C 1967 Surgery of the anus, rectum and colon. Baillière, Tindall and Cox: London

Goligher J C, Leacock A G, Brossy J-J 1955 Surgical anatomy of anal canal. Br J Surg 43: 51–61

Gonyea W J 1980 Role of exercise in inducing increases in skeletal muscle fiber number. J Appl Physiol Respirat Environ Exercise Physiol 48: 421–426

Goodale M A 1993 Visual pathways supporting perception and action in the primate cerebral cortex. Curr Opin Neurobiol 3: 578–585

Goodenough D A, Revel J P 1970 A fine structural analysis of intercellular junctions in the mouse liver. J Cell Biol 45: 272–290

Goodrich E S 1930 Studies on the structure and development of vertebrates. Re-issue. Dover Books: London

Gordon A M, Huxley A F, Julian F J 1966 The variation in isometric tension with sarcomere length in vertebrate muscle fibres. J Physiol 184: 170–192

Gordon K C D 1967 A comparative anatomical study of the distribution of the cystic artery in man and other species. J Anat 101: 351–359

Gordon S, Fraser I, Nath D, Hughes D, Clarke S 1992 Macrophages in tissues and in vitro. Curr Opin Immunol 4: 25–32

Gorgollón P 1978 The normal human appendix: a light and electron microscopic study. J Anat 126: 87–101

Goronowitsch N 1892 Die axiale und die laterale Kopfmetamerie der Vögelembryonen. Die Rolle der sog. 'Ganglienleisten' im Aufbaue der Nervenstämme Anat Anz 7: 454–464

Gorospe J R M, Hoffman E P 1992 Duchenne muscular dystrophy. Curr Opinion Rheumatol 4: 794–800

Gorp P E V, Kennedy W R 1974 Localization of muscle spindles in the human extensor indicis muscle for biopsy purposes. Anat Rec 179: 447–452

Gorski R A 1985 Sexual differentiation of the brain: possible mechanisms and implications. Can J Physiol Pharmacol 63: 577–594

Gorski R A, Gordon J H, Shryne J E, Southam A M 1978 Evidence for a morphological sex difference within the medial preoptic nucleus of the rat brain. Brain Res 148: 333–346

Gorter E, Grendel F J 1925 On bimolecular layers of lipoids on the chromocytes of the blood. J Exp Med 41: 439–443

Gosden R G 1985 Biology of the menopause: the causes and consequences of ovarian aging. Academic Press: London

Gosling J A 1970 The musculature of the upper urinary tract. Acta Anat 75: 408–422

Gosling J A, Dixon J S 1974 Species variation in the location of upper urinary tract pacemaker cells. Invest Urol 11: 418–423

Gosling J A, Dixon J S, Lendon R G 1977 The autonomic innervation of the human male and female bladder neck and proximal urethra. J Urol 118: 302–305

Gosling R G, Newman D L, Bowden N L R, Twinn K W 1971 The area ration of normal aortic junctions. Aortic configuration and pulse-wave reflection. Br J Radiol 44: 850–853

Gosney J R 1993 Neuroendocrine cell populations in postnatal human lungs: minimal variation from childhood to old age. Anat Rec 236(1): 177–180

Goss C M 1942 The physiology of the embryonic mammalian heart before circulation. Am J Physiol 137: 146–152

Goto F 1959 Histological and histochemical studies on human fetal membranes. Acta Med Okayama 13: 276–300

Gottlicher S 1994 Über das Labium tertium pudendi feminae. Eine prospektive Studie an 1180 Patientinnen. Zentralblatt für Gynakologie 116: 419–421

Gottlieb G (ed) 1973–1974 Behavioral embryology. Studies on the development of behavior and the nervous system. Vols 1 and 2. Academic Press: New York

Gottschaldt K M, Iggo A, Young D W 1973 Functional characteristics of mechanoreceptors in sinus hair follicles of the cat. J Physiol 235: 287–315

Gottschalk C W, Mylle M 1959 Micropuncture studies of the mammalian urinary concentrating mechanism: evidence for the counter current hypothesis. Am J Physiol 196: 927–936

Goudie A J, Emmett-Ogelsby M W (eds) 1989 Psychoactive drugs—tolerance and sensitization. Human Press: Clifton

Gould S J 1977 Ontogeny and phylogeny. Cambridge: Harvard University Press: Belknap Press

Gould S J, Howard S 1988 Glial differentiation in the germinal layer of fetal and preterm infant brain. Pediatr Pathol 8: 25–36

Goulding M D, Lumsden A, Gruss P 1993 Development 117: 1001–1016

Gowans J L, Knight E J 1964 The route of re-circulation of lymphocytes in the rat. Proc R Soc Lond [Biol] 159: 257–282

Gower D B, Nixon A, Mallet A I, Jackman P J H 1987 The significance of odorous steroids in axillary odour. In: Dodd G H, van Toller S (eds) Perfumery: the psychology and biology of fragrance. Chapman and Hall: London: pp 96–105

Gracovetsky S 1988 The spinal engine. Springer-Verlag: Vienna

Graeber M B, Streit W J, Buringer D, Sparks D L, Kreutzberg G W 1992 Ultrastructural location of major histocompatibility complex (MHC) Class II positive perivascular cells in histologically normal human brain. J Neuropath Exp Neurol 51: 303–311

Graham A, Heyman I, Lumsden A 1993 Even-numbered rhombomeres control the apoptotic elimination of neural crest from odd-numbered rhombomeres in the chick hindbrain. Development 119: 233–245

Graham C F 1973 The cell cycle during mammalian development. In: Balls

M, Billett F S (eds) The cell cycle in development and differentiation. Cambridge University Press: Cambridge: pp 293–210

Graham D I 1990 The pathophysiology of raised intracranial pressure. In: Weller R O (ed) Systemic pathology. 3rd edition, Vol 4. Nervous system, muscle and eyes. Churchill Livingstone: Edinburgh: pp 64–77

Graham D I 1992 Hypoxia and vascular disorders. In: Adams J H, Duchen L W (eds) Greenfield's neuropathology. 5th edition. Arnold: London: pp 153–268

Grainger R M, Henry J J, Saha M S, Servetnick M 1992 Recent progress on the mechanisms of embryonic lens formation. Eye 6: 117–122

Grand R J, Watkins J B, Torti F M 1976 Progress in Gastroenterology: Development of the human gastrointestinal tract. A review. Gastroenterology 70: 790–810

Graney D O 1986 Anatomy. In: Schuller D E (ed) Otolaryngology - head and neck surgery. Vol 2. Mosby: St Louis: pp 1091–1102

Granit R 1962 Receptors and sensory perception. Yale University Press: New Haven, Connecticut

Granit R 1970 The basis of motor control. Academic Press: New York

Granit R, Henatsch H D, Steg G 1956 Tonic and phasic ventral horn cells differentiated by post-tetanic potentiation in cat extensors. Acta Physiol Scand 37: 114–126

Grant G, Oscarsson O 1966 Mass discharges evoked in the olivocerebellar tract on stimulation of muscle and skin nerves. Exp Brain Res 1: 329–337

Grant P G 1973 Lateral pterygoid: two muscles? Am J Anat 138: 1–10

Grant R T 1930 Observations on direct connections between arteries and veins in the rabbit's ear. Heart 15: 281–303

Grant R T, Bland F F 1931 Observations on arterio-venous anastomoses in human skin and in the bird's foot with special reference to reaction to cold. Heart 15: 385–407

Grant R T, Regnier M 1926 The comparative anatomy of the cardiac coronary vessels. Heart 13: 285–317

Grant R T, Wright H P 1968 Further observations on the blood vessels of skeletal muscle (rat cremaster). J Anat 103: 553–565

Grant R T, Wright H P 1970 Anatomical basis for non-nutritive circulation in skeletal muscle exemplified by blood vessels of rat biceps femoris tendon. J Anat 106: 125–134

Grant R T, Wright H P 1971 The peculiar vasculature of the external spermatic fascia in the rat: possibilities subserving thermoregulation. J Anat 109: 293–305

Graper L 1929 Die Methodik der stereokinematographischen Untersuchungen der lebenden vital gefarben Huhnen embryos. Roux Arch Entw Mech Org 115: 523–545

Grapow M 1887 Die Anatomie und physiologische. Bedeutung der Palmaraponeurose. Archiv für Anatomie und Physiologie Leipzig, Anatomische Abtheilung 2–3: 143–158

Grasby P M, Frith C D, Friston K J, Bench C, Frackowiak R S J, Dolan R J 1993 Functional mapping of brain areas implicated in auditory-verbal memory function. Brain 116: 1–20

Grassé P P (ed) 1948 Traité de zoologie Vol 11. Masson: Paris

Graves F T 1954 Anatomy of intratenal arteries and its application to segmental resection of the kidney. Br J Surg 42: 132–139

Graves F T 1956a The aberrant renal artery. J Anat 90: 553–558

Graves F T 1956b Ganglion in muscle belly of peroneus longus. Br J Surg 43: 438–439

Gray D J, Gardner E D 1943 The human sternochondral joints. Anat Rec 87: 235–254

Gray D J, Gardner E, O'Rahilly R 1957 The prenatal development of the skeleton and joints of the human hand. Am J Anat 101: 169–224

Gray E G 1959 Axo-sematic and axo-dentritic synapses of the cerebral cortex: an electron microscope study. J Anat 93: 420–433

Gray E G 1961 The granule cells, mossy synapses and Purkinje spine synapses of the cerebellum: light and electron microscope observations. J Anat 95: 345–356

Gray E G 1969 Electron microscopy of excitatory and inhibitory synapses: a brief review. Progr Brain Res 31: 141–155

Gray E G 1974 Synaptic morphology with special references to microneurons. In: Bellairs R, Gray E G (eds) Essays on the nervous system. (A festschrift for Professor J Z Young.) Clarendon Press: Oxford

Gray E G 1975 Presynaptic microtubules and their association with synaptic vesicles. Proc R Soc Lond [Biol] 190: 367–372

Gray E G 1978 Synaptic vesicles and microtubules in frog motor end plates. Proc R Soc Lond [Biol] 203: 219–227

Gray J 1958 The movement of the spermatozoa of the bull. J Exp Biol 35: 96–108

Gray J A 1982 The neuropsychology of anxiety: an enquiry into the functions of the septo-hippocampal system. Oxford University Press: Oxford

Gray J A B, Sato M 1953 Properties of receptor potentials in Pacinian corpuscles. J Physiol 122: 610–636

Gray M W 1989 Origin and evolution of mitochondrial DNA. Annu Rev Cell Biol 5: 25–50

Gray S W, Skandalakis J E 1990 In: Givel J-C (ed) Surgery of the thymus. Springer-Verlag: Berlin: pp 13–17

Graybiel A M 1984 Neurochemically specified subsystems in the basal ganglia. In: Evered D, O'Connor M (eds) Functions of the basal ganglia. CIBA Foundation Symposium 107. Pitman: London: pp 114– 149

Graybiel A M, Harting E A 1974 Some afferent connexions of the oculomotor complex in the cat. Brain Res. 81: 543–551

Graybiel A M, Ragsdale W 1983 Biochemical anatomy of the striatum. In: Empson P C (ed) Chemical neuroanatomy. Raven Press: New York: pp 427–504

Grayson J 1941 The cutaneous ligaments of the digits. J Anat 75: 164–165

Graziadei P P C 1971 The olfactory mucosa of vertebrates. In: Beidler L M (ed) Handbook of sensory physiology. Vol 4. Chemical senses. Springer-Verlag: Berlin

Graziadei P P C 1973 Cell dynamics in the olfactory mucosa. Tissue and Cell 5: 113–131

Graziadei P P C 1974 The olfactory organ of vertebrates: a survey. In: Bellairs R, Gray E G (eds) Essays on the nervous system. Clarendon Press: Oxford: pp 191–222

Graziadei P P C, Levine RR, Monti Graziadei GA 1978 Regeneration of olfactory axons and synapse formation in the forebrain after bulbectomy in neonatal mice. Proc.Nat Acad Sci USA 75: 5320–5324

Graziadei P P C, Monti Graziadei GA 1983 Regeneration in the olfactory system of vertebrates. Amer J Otolaryngol 4: 228–233

Graziadei P P C, Gagne H T 1973 Extrinsic innervation of olfactory epithelium. Z Zellforsch 138: 315–326

Graziadei P P C, Monti, Graziadei G A 1979 Neurogenesis and neuron generation in the olfactory system of mammals. I Morphological aspects of differentiation and structural organization of the olfactory sensory neurons. J Neurocytol 8: 1–18

Graziadei P P C, Monti-Graziadei G A 1978 Continuous nerve cell renewal in the olfactory system. In: Jacobson M (ed) Handbook of sensory physiology. Vol 9. Springer: Berlin: pp 55–83

Greaves M, Voorhees J (eds) 1990 Senescence in the skin: an international symposium. Br J Dermatol 122 (suppl 35):

Greco T L, Duello T M, Gorski J 1993 Estrogen receptors, estradiol and diethylstilbestrol in early development: the mouse as a model for the study of estrogen receptors and estrogen sensitivity in embryonic development of male and female reproductive tracts. Endocr Rev 14: 59–71

Green H D 1950 Circulatory system: physical principles. In: Glaser O (ed) Medical physics. Vol. 2. Year Book Publishers: Chicago: pp 228–251

Green J D 1951 The comparative anatomy of the hypophysis with special references to its local blood supply and innervation. Am J Anat 88: 225–311

Green J D, Harris G W 1949 Observations of hypophysioportal vessels of living rat. J Physiol 108: 359–361

Green N A, Griffiths J D, Lavy G A D 1958 Venous drainage of anterior tibio-fibular compartment of leg, with reference to varicose veins. Br Med J 1: 1209–1210

Greenbaum R A, Ho S Y, Gibson D G, Becker A E, Anderson R H 1981 Left ventricular fibres architecture in man. Br Heart J 45: 248–263

Greenburg, Hay E D 1982 Epethelias suspended in collagen gels can lose polarity and express characteristics of migrating mesenchymey cells. J Cell Biol 95: 333–339

Greengard P, Kebabian J W 1974 Role of cyclic AMP in synaptic transmission in the mammalian peripheral nervous system. Fed Proc 33: 1059–1067

Greenstone M, Rutman A, Dewar A, Mackay I, Cole P J 1988 Primary ciliary dyskinesia: cytological and clinical features. Q J Med 67: 405–430

Greenwald A S, Haynes D W 1972 Weight-bearing areas in the humap hip joint. J Bone Jt Surg 54B: 157–163

Greenwald G S, Terranova P F 1988 Follicular selection and its control. In: Knobil E, Neil J D (eds) The physiology of reproduction. Vol 1. Raven Press: New York

Greer M, Haibach H 1974 Thyroid secretion. In: Greep R O, Astwood E B (eds) Handbook of physiology. Section 7. Endocrinology. Vol 3. Thyroid. American Physiological Society: Washington DC: pp 135–146

Grégoire R 1922 Anatomo médico-chirurgicale de l'abdomen. Région sous-thoracique. Baillière: Paris

Greiling H, Scott J E (eds) 1989 Keratan sulphate. Chemistry, biology, chemical pathology. The Biochemical Society: London

Greitz D, Franck A, Nordell B 1993 On the pulsatile nature of intracranial and spinal CSF-circulation demonstrated by MR imaging. Acta Radiologica 34 Fasc 4: 1–8

Greulich W W 1951 The growth and development of Guamarian school-children. Am J Phys Anthropol N S 9: 55–70

Greulich W W, Pyle S I 1959 Radiographic atlas of skeletal development of the hand and wrist. 2nd edition. Stanford University Press: Stanford, California

Greulich W W, Thomas H 1938 The dimensions of the pelvic inlet of 789 white females. Anat Rec 72: 45–52

Greulich W W, Thomas H 1939 Study of pelvic type and its relationship to body build in white women. JAMA 112: 485–493

Grieve G P 1989 Common vertebral joint problems. Churchill Livingstone: Edinburgh

Griffin J W, Kidd G, Trapp B D 1993 Interactions between axons and Schwann cells. In: Dyck P J, Thomas P K, Griffin J W, Low P A, Poduslo J F (eds) Peripheral Neuropathy 3rd edition W B Saunders: pp 317–330

Griffin L D 1994 The intrinsic geometry of the cerebral cortex. J Theor Biol 166: 261–273

Griffiths J D 1961 Extramural and intramural blood supply of the colon. Br Med J 1: 323–326

Griffiths K, Cameron E H D 1975 The adrenal cortex. In: Beck F, Lloyd J B (eds) The cell in medical science. Vol 3. Academic Press: London: pp 155–192

Grillner S, Wallén P 1985 Central pattern generators for locomotion, with special reference to vertebrates. Ann Rev Neurosci 8: 233 262

Grillo M A, Jacobs L, Comroe J H Jr 1974 A combined fluorescence, histochemical and electron microscopic method for studying special monoamine containing cells (SIF cells). J Comp Neurol 153: 1–14

Grim M 1967 Muscle spindles in the posterior cricoarytenoid muscle of the human larynx. Folia Morph 15: 124–131

Grivell L A 1983 Mitochondrial DNA. Sci Amer 248(3): 60–73

Grobstein C 1955 Inductive interaction in the development of the mouse metanephros. J Exp Zool 130: 319–340

Groenewegen H J, Berendse H W, Wolters J G, Lohman A H M 1990 The anatomical relationship of the prefrontal cortex with the striatopallidal system, the thalamus and the amygdala: evidence for a parallel organization. In: Uylings B M, Van Eden C G, De Bruin J P C, Corner M A, Feenstra M P G (eds) The prefrontal cortex: its structure, function and pathology. Progress in Brain Research, Vol 85H. Elsevier: Amsterdam: pp 95–118

Groenewegen H J, Room P, Witter M P, Lohman A H M 1982 Cortical afferents of the nucleus accumbens in the cat, studied with anterograde and retrograde transport techniques. Neuroscience 7: 977–995

Grofová, Marsala 1960 Tvar a struktura nucleus ruber u cloveka. Ceskoclovenska Morfologie 8: 215–237

Gronblad M, Korkala O, Leisi P, Karaharju E 1985 Innervation of synovial membrane and meniscus. Acta Orthop Scand 56: 484–486

Groom AC, Schmidt EE 1990 Microcirculatory blood flow through the spleen. In: Bowdler AJ (ed) The spleen. Structure, function and significance. Chapman and Hall Medical: London: pp 45–102

Gross L 1921 The blood supply to the heart. Oxford University Press: London

Grossman C J, Sholiton L J, Nathan P 1979 Rat thymic estrogen receptor. I. Preparation, location and physicochemical properties. J Ster Biochem 11: 1233–1240

Grossman J 1954 A note on the radiological demonstration of perirenal space. J Anat 88: 407–409

Groth C G, Tyden G 1988 Segmental pancreas transplantation with enteric exocrine drainage. In: Groth C G (ed) Pancreatic transplantation. Aunders: Philadelphia: pp 99–112

Grottel K 1968 The innervation of the suprarenal gland of man, dog, cat and rabbit. Pr Tow Przyjac Nauk Poznañ 37: 41–79

Grove E A, Kirkwood T B L, Price J 1992 Neuron 8: 217–229

Grover J, Roughley P J 1993 Versican gene expression in human articular cartilage and comparison of mRNA splicing variation with aggrecan. Biochem J 291: 361–367

Gruenwald P 1942 Common traits in development and structure of the organs originating from the coelomic wall. J Morph 70: 353–387

Grumbach M M, Ducharme J R 1960 The effects of androgens on fetal sexual development: androgen-induced female pseudo-hermaphroditism. Fert Steril 11: 157–180

Grüneberg H 1973 A ganglion probably belonging to the N terminalis system in the nasal mucosa of the mouse. Z Anat EntwGesch 140: 39–52

Grunert U, Martin PR 1991 Rod bipolar cells in the macaque monkey retina: Immunoreactivity and connectivity. J Neurosci 11: 2742–2758

Grunnet M L 1989 Morphometry of blood vessels in the cortex and germinal plate of premature neonates. Paediatr Neurol 5: 12–16

Grünstein M 1896 Über den Bau der grösseren menschlichen Arterien in verschiedenen Altersstufen. Arch Mikr Anat 47: 583–630

Grupe W E 1987 The dilemma of intrauterine diagnosis of congenital renal disease. Pediatric Nephrology 34: 629–638

Gruss P. Walther 1992 Pax in development. Cell 69: 719–722

Grzanna R, Fritschy J-M 1991 Efferent projections of different subpopulations of central noradrenaline neurons. Prog Brain Res 88: 89–101

Grzybiak M, Szostakiewics-Sawicka H, Treder A 1975 Remarks on pathways of venous drainage from the left upper intercostal spaces in man. Folia Morphol 34: 301–313

Gschwend N, Loehr J, Ivosevic-Radovanovic D, Scheier H, Munzinger U 1988 Semiconstrained elbow prosthesis with special reference to the GSB III prosthesis. Clin Orthop Rel Res 232: 104–111

Gu J, Polak J M, Tapia F J, Marangos P J, Pearse A G E 1981 Neuron specific enolase in the Merkel cells of mammalian skin. Am J Pathol 104: 63–68

Guffarth A, Graumann W 1975 Über die Lagebezielung der Arteria carotis externa zur Glandula parotis. Arch Otorhinolaryngol 211: 17–23

Guild S R 1941 A hitherto unrecognised structure, the glomus jugularis, in man. Anat Rec 79: 28P

Guillemot F, Cepko C L 1992 Retinal fate and ganglion cell differentiation are potentiated by acidic FGF in an in vitro assay of early retinal development. Development 114: 743–754

Guillemot F, Joyner A L 1993 Dynamic expression of the murine Achaete-Scutue homologue Mash-1 in the developing nervous system. Mechanisms of Development 42: 171–185

Guillery R W 1974 Visual pathways in albinos. Sci Am 230: 44–54

Gulyas B J 1975 A re-examination of the cleaving pattern in eutherian mammalian eggs: Rotation of the blastomere pairs during second cleavage in the rabbit. J Exp Zool 193: 235–248

Gulyas B J 1980 Cortical granules of mammalian eggs. Int Rev Cytol 63: 357–392

Gulyás B, Roland P E 1994 Binocular disparity discrimination in human cerebral cortex: functional anatomy by positron emission tomography. Proc Nat Acad Sci USA 91: 1239–1243

Gumpel-Pinot M 1984 Muscle and skeleton of limbs and body wall. In: Le Douarin N, McLaren A (eds) Chimeras in developmental biology. Academic Press: London: pp 281–310

Gunn S A, Gould T C 1975 Vasculature of the testis and adnexa. In: Male reproductive system. Handbook of physiology. Section 7. Endocrinology. Vol 5. (Hamilton D W, Greep R O eds) pp 117–142, American Physiological Society: Washington DC

Gunning P, Ponte P, Blau H, Kedes L 1983 α-Skeletal and α-cardiac genes are co-expressed in adult human skeletal muscle and heart. Mol Cell Biol 3: 1985–1995

Günther U, Hofmann M, Rudy W, Reber S, Zöller M, Haussmann I, Matzku S, Wenzel A, Ponta H, Herrlich P 1991 A new variant of glycoprotein CD44 confers metastatic potential to rat carcinoma cells. Cell 65: 13–24

Gupta C D, Gupta S C, Arora A K, Singh J P 1976 Vascular segments in the human spleen. J Anat 121: 613–616

Gupta K K, Knoell A C 1973 Mathematical modelling and structural analysis of the mandible. Biomat Med Dev Art Org 1: 469–479

Gupta S C, Gupta C O, Arora A K 1977 Subsegmentation of the human liver. J Anat 124: 413–423

Guraya S S 1963 Histochemistry of the cytoplasmic droplet in the mammalian spermatozoon. Experientia 19: 94–95

Gurdjian F S, Lissner H R 1945 Deformations of the skull in head injury studied by the 'stresscoat' technique. Surg Gynecol Obstet 83: 219–233

Gurdon J B 1960 The developmental capacity of nuclei taken from differentiating endoderm cells of *Xenopus laevis*. J Embryol Exp Morph 8: 805–826

Gurdon J B 1962 The developmental capacity of nuclei taken from the intestinal epithalial cells of feeding tadpoles. J Embryol Exp Morph 10: 622–640

Gurdon J B 1973 Gene expression in early animal development: the study of its control by the microinjection of amphibian eggs. Harvey Lectures 69: 49–69

Gurdon J B 1992 The generation of diversity and pattern in animal development. Cell 68: 185–199

Gurdon J B, Laskey R A, Reeves O R 1975 The developmental capacity of nuclei transplanted from the keratinized cells of adult frogs. J Embryol Exp Morph 34: 93–112

Gusek W 1976 Die feinstruktur der Rattenzirbel und ihr Verhalten unter Einfluss von Antiadrogen und nach Kastration. Endokrinologie 67: 129–154

Gustafson T, Wolpert L 1961 Studies on the cellular basis of morphogenesis in sea urchin embryos; directed movement of primary mesenchyme cells in normal and vegetalized larvae. Exp Cell Res 24: 64–79

Guth L, Samaha F J 1970 Procedure for the histochemical demonstration of actomyosin ATPase. Exper Neurol 28: 365–367

Guthrie S 1992 Trends Neurosci 15: 273–275

Guz A, Noble M I M, Widdicombe J G, Trenchard D, Mushin W W, Makey A R 1966 The role of vagal and glossopharyngeal afferent nerves in respiratory sensation, control of breathing and arterial pressure regulation in conscious man. Clin Sci 30: 161–170

Gwiazda J, Thorn P, Bauer J, Held R 1993 Emmetropization and the progression of manifest refraction in children followed from infancy to puberty. Clin Vis Sci 8: 337–344

Gwinnett A S 1967 The ultrastructure of the 'prismless' enamel of permanent human teeth. Arch Oral Biol 12: 381–387

Gwyn D G, Leslie R A, Hopkins D A 1979 Gastric afferents to the nucleus of the solitary tract in the cat. Neurosci Lett 14: 13–17

Gwyn D G, Leslie R A, Hopkins D A 1985 Observations on the afferent and efferent organization of the vagus nerve and the innervation of the stomach in the squirrel monkey. J Comp Neurol 239: 163–175

H

Ha H, Liu C N 1968 Cell origin of the ventral spinocerebellar tract. J Comp Neurol 133: 185–206

Haas L L 1952 Roentgenological skull measurements and their diagnostic application. Am J Roentgenol 67: 197–209

Haas T A, Plow E F 1994 Integrin-ligand interactions: a year in review. Curr Opin Cell Biol 6: 656–662

Haeberli A, Studer H, Kohler H et al 1975 Autoradiographic localization of slow turnover iodocompounds within the follicular cells of the rat thyroid gland. Endocrinology 97: 978–984

Haeckel E 1874 Die Gastraea-Theorie, die phylogenetische Klassifikation des Tierreiche und Homologie der Klemblatter. Jena Z Naturwiss 8: 1–55 (An English translation by E D Wright of this paper 'The gastrea theory, phylogenetic classification of the animal kingdom and the homology of the germ lamellae' is to be found in Quart J Micr Sci 14: 142–165 and 223–247)

Haffen K, Kedinger M, Simon-Assmann P 1989 Cell contact dependent regulation of enterocytic differentiation. Human gastrointestinal development Lebenthal E (ed) Raven Press: New York

Hage E 1973 Electron microscopic identification of several types of endocrine cells in branchial epithelium of human foetuses. Z Zellforsch 141: 401–412

Hagege A A, Desnos M, Chachques J-C, Carpentier A, Fernandez F, Fontaliran F, Guerot C 1990 Preliminary report: follow-up after dynamic cardiomyoplasty. Lancet 1122–1124

Häggqvist G 1936 Analyse der Faserverteilung in einem Rückenmarkquerschnitt (Th3). Z Mikr-Anat Forsch 39: 1–34

Hagiwara H, Schroter-Kermani C, Merker H T 1993 Localization of collagen type VI in articular cartilage of young and adult mice. Cell Tiss Res 272: 155–160

Haglund M M, Ojemann G A, Schwartz T W, Lettich E 1994 Neuronal activity in human lateral temporal cortex during serial retrieval from short-term momory. J Neurosci 14: 1507–1515

Hagworth S G 1992 Development of the pulmonary circulation. Polin R A, Fox W W (eds) In: Fetal and neonatal physiology. W B Saunders: Philadelphia: pp 671–682

Hahn A W, Kern F, Buhler F R Resink T J 1993 The renin-angiotensin sytem and extracellular matrix. Clin Investig 71 (5 Suppl): S7–S12

Hai C-M, Murphy R A 1989 Ca^{2+}, crossbridge phosphorylation, and contraction. Ann Rev Physiol 51: 285–298

Haines D E, Harkey H L, al-Mefty O 1993 The 'subdural' space: a new look at an outdated concept. Neurosurg 32: 111–120

Haines R W 1935 A consideration of the constancy of muscular nerve supply. J Anat 70: 33–55

Haines R W 1937 The primitive form of epiphysis in the long bones of tetrapods. J Anat 72: 323–343

Haines R W 1942a Eudiarthrodial joints in fishes. J Anat 77: 12–19

Haines R W 1942b The tetrapod knee joint. J Anat 76: 270–301

Haines R W 1944 The mechanism of rotation at the first carpometacarpal joint. J Anat 78: 44–46

Haines R W 1951 The extensor apparatus of the finger. J Anat 85: 251–259

Haines R W 1969 The striped compressor of the prostatic urethra. Br J Urol 41: 481–493

Haines R W 1974 The pseudoepiphysis of the first metacarpal of man. J Anat 117: 145–158

Haines R W 1975 The histology of epiphyseal union in mammals. J Anat 120: 1–25

Haines R W, Mohuiddin A 1968 Metaplastic Bone. J Anat 103: 527–538

Halaban R, Langdon R, Biscall N, Cuono C, Baird A, Scott G, Moellmann G, McGuire J 1988 Basic growth factor from human keratinocytes is a natural mitogen for melanocytes. J Cell Biol 107: 1611–1619

Halalaz 1993 Sensory innervation of the hairy skin (light and electromicroscope study). J Invest Dermatol 101 (Suppl 1): 755–815

Halasz B, Rethelyi M, Szentágothai J 1968 Electron microscopic examination of the isolated median eminent (neurally deafferented). Arch Anat (Strasbourg) 51: 287–298

Halasz N 1990 The vertebrate olfactory system. Akademiai Kiado: Budapest

Halata Z 1975 The mechanoreceptors of the mammalian skin. Ultrastructure and morphological classification. Adv Anat Embryol Cell Biol 50: 1–77

Hale F C, Olsen C R, Mickey M R 1968 The measurement of bronchial wall components. Am Rev Resp Dis 98: 978–987

Haley J C, Peden J K 1943 Suspensory muscle of the duodenum. Am J Surg 59: 546–550

Hall B K 1988 The embryonic development of bone. Am Sci 76: 174–181

Hall B K 1992 Evolutionary development biology. Chapman and Hall: London

Hall B K (ed) 1983 Cartilage. Vols 1–3. Academic Press: New York

Hall B K, Miyake T 1992 The membranous skeleton: the role of cell condensations in vertebrate skeletogenesis. Anat Embryol 186: 107–124

Hall D A (ed) 1968 International review of connective tissue research. Vol 4. Academic Press: New York

Hall J G 1966 Hearing and primary auditory centers of the whales. Acta Otolaryngol [Stockh] Suppl 224: 225–250

Hall K, Sara V 1983 Growth and somatomedins. Vitam Horm 40: 175–233

Hall M C 1965 The locomotor system: functional anatomy. Thomas: Springfield, Illinois

Hall M C 1966 The architecture of bone. Thomas: Springfield, Illinois

Hall S M 1986 The effect of inhibiting Schwann cell mitosis on the re-innervation of acellular autografts in the peripheral nervous system of the mouse. Neuropathol Appl Neurobiol 12: 401–414

Hall S M 1993 Observations on the progress of Wallerian degeneration in transected peripheral nerves of C57BL/Wld Mice in the presence of recruited macrophages. J Neurocytol 22: 480–490

Hall S M, Gregson N A 1971 The in vivo and ultrastructural effects of injection of lysophosphatidyl choline into myelinated peripheral nerve fibres of the adult mouse. J Cell Sci 9: 769–789

Hall S M, Williams P L 1970 Studies on the 'incisures' of Schmidt and Lauterman. J Cell Sci 6: 767–791

Haller R de 1969 Development of mucus-secreting elements. In: Emery J (ed) The anatomy of the developing lung. Spastics International Medical Publications: London: pp 94–115

Hallermann H 1934 Die Beziehungen der Werkstoffmechanik und Werstofforschung zue allgemeinen Knocken-Mechanik. Verh Deutsch Orthop Gesh 62: 347–360

Hallett P E, Lightstone A D 1976 Saccadic eye movements towards stimuli triggered by prior saccades. Vision Res 16: 99–106

Halliday A M 1993 Evoked potentials in clinical testing. Churchill Livingstone: Edinburgh

Hallman M, Merritt T A, Akino T et al 1991 Surfactant protein A, phosphatidylcholine, and surfactant inhibitors in epithelial lining fluid A. Rev Respir Dis 144: 1376–1384

Hallonet M E R, Teillet M A, Le Douarin N M 1990 Development 108, 19–31

Hallpike C S 1935 Function of the tympanic membrane. Proc R Soc Med 28: 226–231

Halmi N S 1986 The normal thyroid. Anatomy and histochemistry. In: Ingbar S H, Braverman L E (eds) Werner's The thyroid. A fundamental and clinical text. 5th edition. Lippincott: Philadelphia: pp 24–36

Halsband U, Ito N, Tanji J, Freund H-J 1993 The role of premotor cortex and the supplementary motor area in the temporal control of movement in man. Brain 116: 243–266

Hambleton G, Wigglesworth J S 1976 Origin of intraventricular haemorrhage in the preterm infant. Arch Dis Child 51: 651–659

Hamburger J, Crosnier J, Dormont J, Bach J F (eds) 1972 In: Renal transplantation, theory and practice. Williams and Wilkins: Baltimore: pp 249–278

Hamburger V 1952 Development of the nervous system. Ann N Y Acad Sci 55: 117–132

Hamburger V 1968 Origins of integrated behavior. In: Locke M (ed) The emergence of order in developing systems. IV. Emergence of nervous coordination. Dev Biol (suppl 2): 251–271

Hamburger V 1988 The heritage of experimental embryology. Hans Spemann and the Organizer. Oxford University Press: Oxford

Hamilton G F 1946 The longitudinal muscle coat of the human colon. J Anat 80: 230P

Hamilton P W, Allen D C, Watt P C H, Paterson C C, Biggart J D 1987 Classification of normal colorectal mucosa and adenocarcinoma by morphometry. Histopatholgy 11: 901–911

Hamilton R B, Norgren R 1984 Central projections of gustatory nerves in the rat. J Comp Neurol 222: 560–577

Hamilton W J 1944 Phases of maturation and fertilisation in the human ova. J Anat 78: 1–4

Hamilton W J, Boyd J D, Mossman H W 1972 Human embryology. Williams and Wilkins: Baltimore

Hamilton W J, Mossman H W 1976 Cardiovascular system. In: Hamilton, Boyd and Mossman's human embryology. 4th edition. Heffer: Cambridge: pp 228–290

Hammar J A 1911 Zur grösseren Morphologie und Morphogenie der Menschenthymus. Anat Heft 43: 201–242

Hammar J A 1935 Konstitutionsanatomische Studien über die Neurotisierung des Menschenembryos; über die Innervationsverhältnisse der Inkretorgane und der Thymus bis in den 4. Fötalmonat. Z Mikrosp-Anat Forsch 38: 253–293

Hammel H T 1968 Regulation of internal body temperature. Annu Rev Physiol 30: 641–710

Hammelbo T 1972 On the development of the cerebral fissures in cetacea. Acta Anat (Basel) 82: 606–618

Hammer G, Råadberg C 1961 The sphenoidal sinus. An anatomical and roentgenologic study with reference to trans-sphenoidal hypophysectomy. Acta Radiol 56: 401–422

Hammer J A 1991 Novel myosins. Trends in Cell Biol 1: 50–56

Hammersen F, Staubesand J 1961 Arteries and capillaries of the human renal pelvis, with special reference to the so-called spiral arteries. I. Angioarchitectural studies on the kidneys. Z Anat Entw Gesch 122: 314–347

Hammond B T, Charnley J 1967 The sphericity of the femoral head. Med Biol Eng 5: 445–453

Hámori J 1972 Developmental morphology of dendritic postsynaptic specialisations. In: Lissák K (ed) Recent developments of neurobiology in Hungary. Akadémiai Kiadó: Budapest

Hamperl H 1970 Bau und mögliche Funktioneiner elastisch-muskulären Struktur in der Portio uteri. Geburtshilfe Frauenheilkd 30: 953–959

Hamperl H 1970 The myothelia (myoepithelial cells). Normal state, regressive changes; hyperplasia; tumors. Curr Topics Pathol 53: 161–220

Hampson J R, Harrison C R, Woolsey C N 1950 Cerebro-cerebellar projections and the somatotopic localization of motor function in the cerebellum. Proc Asso Res Nerv Ment Dis 30: 299–316

Han J N, Gayan-Ramirez G, Dekhuijzen R, Decramer M 1993 Respiratory function of the rib cage muscles. Eur Resp J 6: 722–728

Han S S, Kim S K, Cho M I 1976 Cytochemical characterization of the myoepithelial cells in palatine glands. J Anat 122: 559–570

Hanau D, Gachet C, Schmitt D A, Ohlmann P, Brisson C, Fabre M, Cazenave J-P 1991 Ultrastructural similarities between epidermal Langerhans cell Birbeck granules and the surface-connected canalicular system of EDTA-treated human blood platelets. J Invest Dermatol 97: 756–762

Hanaway J, Young R R 1977 Localization of the pyramidal tract in the internal capsule of man. J Neurol Sci 34: 63–70

Hancox N M 1972 The osteoclast. In: Bourne G H (ed) The biochemistry and physiology of bone. Vol 1. Academic Press: New York: pp 45–67

Hand P J and Liu C-N 1966 Efferent projections of the nucleus gracilis. Anat Rec 154: 353–354

Hanna R E, Washburn S L 1953 Determination of sex of skeletons, as illustrated by a study of the Eskimo pelvis. Hum Biol 25: 21–27

Hannam A G 1976 Periodontal mechanoreceptors. In: Anderson D J, Matthews B (eds) Mastication. Wright: Bristol: pp 42–49

Hannover A 1844 Recherches microscopiques sur le système nerveux. P G Philipsen: Copenhagen

Hansen E S 1993 Microvascularization, osteogenesis, and myelopoiesis in normal and pathological conditions. In: Shoutens A, Arlet J, Gardiniers J W M, Hughes S P F (eds) Bone circulation and vascularization in normal and pathological conditions. Plenum Press: New York: pp 29–41

Hansen J T 1977 Freeze-fracture study of the carotid body. Am J Anat 148: 295–300

Hanson J R, Anson B J, Strickland E M 1962 Branchial sources of the auditory ossicles in man. Part II. Observations of embryonic stages from 7 mm to 28 mm (CR length). Arch Otolaryngol 76: 200–215

Harach H R 1985 Solid cell nests of the thyroid. An anatomical survey and immunohistochemical study for the presence of thyroglobulin. Acta Anat 122: 249–253

Hardaker W T, Whipple T L, Bassett F H 1980 Diagnosis and treatment of the plica syndrome of the knee. J Bone Jt Surg 62A: 221–225

Hardebo J E, Owman C 1980 Barrier mechanisms for neurotransmitter monoamines and their precursors at the blood–brain barrier interface. Ann Neurol 8: 1–11

Hardisty M W 1967 The numbers of vertebrate primordial germ cells. Biol Rev 42: 265–287

Hardy K, Martin K L, Leese H J, Winston R M L, Handyside A H 1989 Non invasive measurement of glucose and pyruvate uptake by individual human oocytes and preimplantation embryos. Human Reprod 4: 188–191

Haritos A A, Tsolas O, Horecker B L 1984 Distribution of prothymosin alpha in rat tissues. Proc Nat Acad Sci (USA) 81: 1391–1395

Harjeet J I 1992 Dimensions of the thyroid cartilage in neonates, children and adults in northwest Indian subjects. J Anat Soc India 41: 81–92

Harken D E, Ellis L B, Dexter L, Farrand R E, Dickson J F 1952 The responsibility of the physician in the selection of patients with mitral stenosis for surgical treatment. Circulation 5: 349–362

Harker D W 1972 The structure and innervation of sheep superior rectus and levator palpebrae muscles. I. Extrafusal muscle fibres. Invest Ophthal 11: 956–969

Harness D, Sekeles E, Chaco J 1974 The double motor innervation of the opponens pollicis muscles: an electromyographic study. J Anat 117: 329–331

Harper W F 1947 Observations on the blood vasculature of the turbinate mucosa in man and other mammals. J Anat 81: 392P

Harpman J A, Woollard H H 1938 The tendon of the lateral pterygoid muscle. J Anat 73: 112–115

Harries D J 1955 Thyroid enlargements and cricothyroid muscle. Br Med J 1: 1012–1013

Harris G W 1947 Blood vessels of rabbit's pituitary gland, and significance of pars and zona tuberalis. J Anat 81: 343–351

Harris G W 1955 Neural control of the pituitary gland. Arnold: London

Harris G W, Donovan B T (eds) 1966 The pituitary gland. Butterworths: London

Harris H A 1933 Bone growth in health and disease. Oxford University Press: London

Harris W 1939 The morphology of the brachial plexus. Oxford University Press: London

Harris W 1952 Fifth and seventh cranial nerves in relation to nervous mechanism of taste sensation; new approach. BMJ 1: 831–836

Harris W A, Hartenstein V 1991 Neural determination without cell division in Xenopus embryos. Neuron 6: 499–515

Harrison G A, Weiner J S, Tanner J M, Barnicot N A 1964 Human biology. Ch 19. Clarendon Press: Oxford

Harrison R G 1907 Observations on the living developing nerve fiber. Anat Rec 1: 116–118

Harrison R G 1907a Experiments in transplanting limbs and their bearing upon the problems of the development of nerves. J Exp Zool 4: 239–282

Harrison R G 1910 The outgrowth of the nerve fiber as a mode of protoplasmic movement. J Exp Zool 9: 787–848

Harrison R G, Barclay A E 1948 Distribution of testicular artery (internal spermatic artery) to human testis. Br J Urol 20: 57–66

Harrison R G, Connolly R C, Abdalla A 1969 Kinship of Smenkhkare and Tutankamen demonstrated serologically. Nature 224: 325–326

Harrison R G, Hoey M J 1960 The adrenal circulation. Oxford University Press: Oxford

Harrison R G, Weiner J S 1949 Vascular patterns of the mammalian testis and their functional significance. J Exp Biol 26: 304–316

Harrison T J 1957 Pelvic growth. PhD Thesis, Queen's University, Belfast

Harrop T J Garrett J R 1974 Effects of preganglionic sympathectomy on secretory changes in parotid acinar cells of rats on eating. Cell Tissue Res 154: 135–150

Hartman B K 1973 Immunofluorescence of dopamine-hydroxylase. Application of improved methodology to the localization of the peripheral and central noradrenergic nervous system. J Histochem Cytochem 21: 312–332

Hartmann P E 1991 The breast and breast feeding. In: Philipp E, Setchell M, Ginsburg J (eds) Scientific foundations of obstetrics and gynaecology. Butterworth-Heinemann: Oxford: pp 378–390

Hartschuh W, Weihe E, Buchler M, Helmetaeder V, Fernle G E, Foorsmann W G 1979 Met-enkephalin-like immunoreactivity in Merkel cells. Cell Tiss Res 201: 343–348

Hartschuh W, Weihe E, Yanaihara N, Reinecke M 1983 Immunohistochemical localization of VIP in Merkel cells of various mammals. Evidence for a neuromodular function for the Merkel cell. J Invest Dermatol 81: 361–364

Haruda F, Blanc W A 1981 The structure of intracerebral arteries in premature infants and the autoregulation of cerebral blood flow. (Abstract). Ann Neurol 10: 303–313

Harvey M B, Kaye P L 1991 IGF-2 receptors are first expressed at the 2-cell stage of mouse development. Development 111: 1057–1060

Hashimoto K 1971 Ultrastructure of the human toenail. II. Keratinisation and formation of marginal band. J Ultrastruct Res 36: 391–410

Hashimoto K 1971a Ultrastructure of the human toenail: cell migration, keratinization, and formation of the intercellular cement. Arch Derm Forsch 240: 1–22

Hashimoto K 1974 New methods for surface ultrastructure: comparative studies of scanning electron microscopy, transmission electron microscopy and replica methods. Int J Dermatol 13: 357–381

Hashimoto K 1978 The apocrine gland. In: Jarrett A (ed) The physiology and pathophysiology of the skin. Vol 5. Academic Press: New York: pp 1575–1596

Hashimoto K, Gross B G, Nelson R et al 1966 Ultrastructure of the skin of human embryos. III. The formation of the nail in 16–18 week old embryos. J. Invest Dermatol 47: 205–217

Hashimoto M, Komori A, Kosaka M, Mori Y, Shimoyama R, Akashi H 1960 Electron microscopic studies on the smooth muscle of the human uterus. J Jap Obstet Gynecol Soc 7: 115–121

Hassler R 1960 Die zentralen Systeme des Scmerzes. Acta Neurochir 8: 353–423

Hast M H, Perkins R E 1984 Secondary supinator muscles of the human elbow (musculi revivi). (Proceedings of the Anatomical Society of Great Britain and Ireland. 19 July), J Anat 139: 745–746

Hastie N 1991 Pax in our time. Curr Biol 1: 342–344

Hastings M H 1991 Neuroendocrine rhythms. Pharmacol Therap 50: 35–71

Hatefi Y 1985 The mitochondrial electron transport and oxidative phosphorylation system. Annu Rev Biochem 54: 1015–1070

Hatten M E 1990 Trends Neurosci 5: 179–184

Hatten M E, Liem R K H, Mason C A 1986 J Neurosci 6: 2676–2683

Hatton G I, Tweedle C D 1982 Magnocellular peptidergic neurons in hypothalamus: increases in membrane apposition and number of specialized synapses from pregnancy to lactation. Brain Res Bull 8: 197–204

Hǎulicǎ I, Coculescu M 1981 Is agnitensin a new pineal hormone? Rev Roum Méd Endocrinol 19: 3–21

Havers C 1691 Osteologia nova, or some new observations of the bones. S Smith: London

Havez R, Decaud P, Roussel P, Voisin C, Biserte C, Gernez-Rieux Ch 1966

Identification des gamma-globulines, de la kallikreine, de la transferrine dans la muquesque bronchique humaine. C R Hebd Séanc Acad Sci Paris 262d: 1777

Hawkes D J, Robinson L, Crossman J E, Saymen H B, Mistry R, Maisey M M, Spencer J D 1991 Registration and display of the combined bone scan and radiograph in the diagnosis and management of wrist injuries. Eur J Nucl Med 18: 752–756

Hawkes R, Leclerc N 1987 Antigenic map of the rat cerebellar cortex: the distribution of sagittal bands as revealed by monoclonal anti-Purkinje cell antibody mabQ113. J Comp Neurol 256: 29–41

Hawns M J, Dortabach R K 1982 The microscopic anatomy of the lower eyelid retractors. Arch Ophthalmol 100: 1313–1318

Hawrylyshyn P A, Rubin A M, Tasker R R, Organ L W, Fredrickson J M 1978 Vestibulothalamic projection in man: a sixth primary sensoty pathway. J Neurophysiol 41: 521–544

Haxton H A 1954 Sympathetic nerve supply of the upper limb in relation to sympathectomy. Ann R Coll Surg 14: 247–266

Hay E D 1968 Organization and fine structure of epithelium and mesenchyme in the developing chick embryo. In: Fleischmajer R, Billingham R E (eds) Epithelial – mesenchymal interactions. Williams & Wilkins: Baltimore: pp 31–55

Hay E D 1981 Extracellular matrix. J Cell Biol 91: 205s–223s

Hay E D 1989 Extracellular matrix, cell skeletons and embryonic development. Am J Med Gen 34: 14–29

Hay E D (ed) 1982 Cell biology of extracellular matrix. Plenum Press: New York

Hayes T L, Lewis D A 1993 Hemispheric differences in layer III pyramidal neurons of the anterior language area. Arch Neurol 50: 501–505

Hayflick L, Moorhead P S 1961 The limited in vitro lifetime of human diploid cell strains. Exp Cell Res 25: 585–621

Hayward J 1961 The lower end of the oesophagus. Thorax 16: 36–41

He S-Q, Dum R P, Strick P L 1993 Topographic organization of corticospinal projections from the frontal lobe: motor areas on the lateral surface of the hemisphere. J Neurosci 13: 952–980

Headington J T 1986a The histiocyte. In memoriam. Arch Dermatol 122: 532–533

Headington J T 1986b The dermal dendrocyte. In: Callen J P et al (eds) Advances in dermatology. Vol. 1. Yearbook Medical Publishers: Chicago: pp 159–171

Healey J E, Schroy P C 1953 Anatomy of biliary ducts within the human liver; analysis of prevailing pattern of branchings and major variations of biliary ducts. Arch Surg 66: 599–616

Heathcote J G, Grant M E 1981 The molecular organization of basement membranes. In: Hall D A, Jackson D S (eds) International review of connective tissue research. Vol 9. Academic Press: New York: pp 191–264

Heffner C D, Lumsden A G S, O'Leary D D M 1990 Science 247: 217–220

Hegedus K, Molnar P 1985 Histopathological study of major intracranial arteries in premature infants related to intracranial haemorrhage. J Neurosurg 6S: 419–424

Hegedus L, Perrid H, Poulsen R et al 1983 The determination of thyroid gland volume by ultrasound and its relationship to body weight, age, and sex in normal subjects. J Clin Endocrinol Metab 5: 260

Heglund N C, Cavagna G A 1987 Mechanical work, oxygen consumption and efficiency in isolated frog and rat striated muscle. Am J Physiol 253: C22–C29

Heijerman H G 1993 Chronic obstructive lung disease and respiratory muscle function: the role of nutrition and exercise training in cystic fibrosis. Resp Med 87 (suppl B): 49–51

Heil P, Rajan R, Irvine D R F 1994 Topographic representation of tone intensity along the isofrequency axis of cat primary auditory cortex. Hear Res 76: 188–202

Heilig A, Pette D 1980 Changes induced in the enzyme activity pattern by electrical stimulation of fast-twitch muscle. In: Pette D (ed), Plasticity of Muscle. Walter de Gruyter: Berlin: pp 409–420

Heiligenberg W 1991 The neural basis of behaviour: a neuroethological view. Ann Rev Neurosci 14: 247–267

Heilmann C, Pette D 1979 Molecular transformations in sarcoplasmic reticulum of fast-twitch muscle by electro-stimulation. Eur J Biochem 93: 437–446

Heimer L, Switzer R D, Van Hoesen G 1982 Ventral striatum and ventral pallidum. Additional components of the motor system? Trends in Neurosci. 5: 83–87

Heimer L, Van Hoesen G 1979 Ventral striatum. In: Divac I, Öberg R G E (eds) The neostriatum. Pergamon Press: Oxford: pp 147– 158

Heimer L, Wall P D 1968 The dorsal root distribution to the substantia gelatinosa of the rat with a note on the distribution in the cat. Exp Brain Res 6: 89–99

Heinemann H O, Fishman A P 1969 Nonrespiratory functions of mammalian lung. Physiol Rev 49: 1–47

Heins S, Aebi U 1994 Making heads and tails of intermediate filament assembly, dynamics and networks. Curr Opin Cell Biol 6: 25–33

Heinsen H, Henn R, Eisenmenger W, Götz M, Bohl J, Bethke B, Lockerman U, Püschel K 1994 Quantitative investigations on the human entorhinal area: left–right asymmetry and age-related changes. Anat Embryol 190: 181–194

Heintzberger C F M 1974 The development of the sino-atrial node in the mouse. Acta Morphol Neerl-Scand 12: 317–330

Heiple K G, Lovejoy C O 1971 The distal femoral anatomy of Australophithecus. Am J Phys Anthropol 35: 75–84

Heise N, Toledo O M 1993 Age-related changes in glycosaminoglycan distribution in different anatomical sites on the surface of knee-joint articular cartilage in young rabbits. Anat Anz 175: 35–40

Heitz Ph, Polak J M, Bloom S K, Pearse A G E 1976 Identification of the D_1-cell as the source of human pancreatic polypeptide (HPP). Gut 17: 755–758

Heitzmann R J 1979 The efficacy and mechanism of action of anabolic agents as growth promoters in farm animals. J Steroid Biochem 11: 927–930

Helal B 1988 In: Helal B, Wilson D (eds) The foot. Vol 2. Churchill Livingstone: Edinburgh: pp 567–580

Helal B 1992 In: Benjamin A, Helal B, Copeland B, Edwards J (eds) Surgical repair and reconstruction in rheumatoid disease. 2nd edition. Springer-Verlag: Berlin: pp 201–220

Hell E A, Cruickshank C N 1963 The effect of injury upon the uptake of 3-H-thymidine by guinea pig epidermis. Exp Cell Res 31: 128–139

Heller C G, Lalli M F, Pearson J E, Leach D R 1971 A method for the quantification of Leydig cells in man. J Reprod Fertil 25: 177–184

Heller C H, Clermont Y 1964 Kinetics of the germinal epithelium in man. Recent Prog Horm Res 20: 545–575

Heller D H, Cahill C M, Schultz R M 1981 Biochemical studies of mammalian oogenesis: metabolic co-operativity between granulosa cells and growing mouse oocytes. Dev Biol 84: 455–464

Hellmer H 1935 Röntgenologische Beobachtungen über die Ossifikation der Patella. Acta Radiol 27: Suppl 1–82

Hemmati-Brivanlou A, Harland R M 1989 Nature 359: 609–614

Hemmati-Brivanlou A, Kelly O G, Melton D A 1994 Cell 77: 283–295

Henderson B, Pettipher E R 1985 The synovial lining cell: biology and pathobiology. Semin Arthritis Rheum 15: 1–32

Henderson C J, Butler S R, Glass A 1975 The localisation of equivalent dipoles of EEG sources by the application of electrical field theory. Electroenceph clin Neurophysiol 175: 117–130

Hendren W H 1992 Cloacal malformations: experience with 105 cases. J Pediat Surg 27: 890–901

Hendry I A, Hill C E (eds) 1992 Development, regeneration and plasticity of the autonomic nervous system. The autonomic nervous system. Vol 2. Burnstock G (series ed) Harwood Academic Publishers: Switzerland

Hendry N G C 1958 The hydration of the nucleus pulposus and its relation to intervertebral disc derangement. J Bone Jt Surg 40B: 132–44

Hendry S H C, Schwark H D, Jones E G, Yan J 1987 Numbers and proportions of GABA-immunoreactive neurons in different areas of monkey cerebral cortex. J Neurosci 5: 1503–1519

Henke C A, Fiegel V, Peterson M, Wick M, Knighton D, McCarthy J, Bitterman P B 1993 J Clin Invest 88:1386–1395

Henke K G, Badr M S, Skatrud J B, Dempsey J A 1992 Load compensation and respiratory muscle function during sleep. J Appl Physiol 72: 1221–1234

Henkind P, Levitsky M 1969 Angioarchitecture of the optic nerve. I. The papilla. Am J Ophthal 68: 979–986

Henle J 1876 Handbuch der Gefasslebre des Menschen. Vieweg: Braunschweig

Henle W, Henle G, Chambers L A 1938 Studies on ontogenic structure of some mammalian spermatozoa. J Exp Med 68: 335–352

Henley F A 1955 Blood supply of common bile duct and its relationship to the duodenum. Br J Surg 43: 75–80

Henneman E, Clamann H P, Gillies J D, Skinner R D 1974 Rank order of motoneurons within a pool: law of combination. J Neurophysiol 37: 1338–1349

Henneman E, Somjen G, Carpenter D O 1965a Functional significance of cell size in spinal motoneurones. J Neurophysiol 28: 560–580

Henneman E, Somjen G, Carpenter D O 1965b Excitability and inhibitability of motoneurones of different sizes. J Neurophysiol 28: 599–620

Hennings H, Holbrook K 1983 Calcium regulation of cell–cell contact and differentiation in epidermal cells. Exp Cell Res 143: 127–142

Hennings H, Michael D, Cheng D, Steinert P, Holbrook K, Yuspa S H 1980 Calcium regulation of growth and differentiation of mouse epidermal cells in culture. Cell 19: 245–254

Henriksson J, Chi M M-Y, Hintz C S, Young D A, Kaiser K K, Salmons S, Lowry O H 1986 Chronic stimulation of mammalian muscle: changes in enzymes of six metabolic pathways. Am J Physiol 251: C614–C632

Henry T R, Mazziotta J C, Engel J Jr, Christenson P D, Zhang J X, Phelps M E, Kuhl D E 1990 Quantifying interictal metabolic activity in human temporal lobe epilepsy. J Cereb Blood Flow Metab 10: 748–757

Henton C et al 1992 Stops in the world's languages. Phonetica 49(2): 65–101

Henzen W 1957 Transplantationen zur entwicklungsphysiologischen Analyse der larvalen Mundorgane bei Bombinator und Triton. Arch EntwMech Org 149: 387–442

Heppenstall R B 1980 Fracture healing. In: Heppenstall R B (ed) Fracture treatment and healing. Saunders: Philadelphia: pp 35–64

Heppenstall R B, Grislis G, Hunt T K 1975 Tissue gas tensions and oxygen consumption in healing bone defects. Clin Orthop 106: 357–365

Herberman R B 1985 Multiple functions of natural killer cells, including immunoregulation as well as resistance to tumour growth. Concepts in Immunol 1: 96–132

Herbst J J 1989 Development of suck and swallow. In: Lebenthal E (ed) Human gastrointestinal development. Raven Press: New York: pp 229–239

Heriot W J, Machemer R 1992 Pigment epithelial repair. Graefes Arch Clin Exper Ophthalmol 230: 91–100

Herman P G, Yamamoto I, Mellins H Z 1972 Blood microcirculation in the lymph node during the primary immune response. J Exp Med 136: 697–714

Herman P G, Yamamoto I, Mellins H Z 1973 Microcirculation of the aortic wall in experimental atheromatosis. Radiology 107: 265–271

Herrick C J 1924 Origin and evolution of the cerebellum. Arch Neurol Psychiat 11: 621–652

Herring S W, Grimm A F, Grimm B R 1984 Regulation of sarcomere number in skeletal muscle: a comparison of hypotheses. Muscle Nerve 7: 161–173

Hershberger L G, Shipley E G, Meyer R K 1953 Myotrophic activity of 19-nortestosterone and other steroids determined by modified levator ani muscle method. Proc Soc Exp Biol (NY) 83: 175–180

Hertig A T 1935 Angiogenesis in the early human chorion and in the primary placenta of the macaque monkey. Contrib Embryol Carnegie Inst Washington 25: 37–81

Hertig A T 1968 Human trophoblast. Thomas: Springfield, Illinois

Hertig A T, Rock J 1941 Two human ova of the pre-villous stage, having an ovulation age of about eleven and twelve days respectively. Contrib Embryol Carnegie Inst. Washington 29: 127–156

Hertig A T, Rock J 1945 Two human ova of the pre-villous stage, having a developmental age of about seven and nine days respectively. Contrib Embryol Carnegie Inst Washington 31: 65–84

Hertig A T, Rock J 1949 Two human ova of the pre-villous stage, having a developmental age of about eight and nine days respectively. Contrib Embryol Carnegie Inst Washington 33: 169–186

Hertig A T, Rock J, Adams E C 1956 A description of 34 human ova within the first 17 days of development. Am J Anat 98: 435–493

Hertig A T, Rock J, Adams E C, Mulligan W J 1954 On the preimplantation stages of the human ovum: a description of four normal and four abnormal specimens ranging from the second to the fifth day of development. Contrib Embryol Carnegie Inst Washington 35: 199–220

Hertwig O, Hertwig R (1879–1883) Studies on the germ layers (in German). Jena Zeit 13–16 (6–9)

Hertwig W A O 1881 Die Coelomtheorie: versuch einer Erklarung des mittleren Keimblatts. G Fischer: Jena

Hervonen A, Linnoila I, Tainio H, Vaalasti A, Mascorro J A 1985 Immunohistochemical evidence for the occurrence of vasoactive intestinal polypeptide (VIP)-containing nerve fibres in human fetal abdominal paraganglia. J Anat 143: 121–128

Hervonen A, Vaalasti A, Partanen M, Kanerva L 1978 The endocrine nature of the paraganglia of man. Experientia 34: 111–112

Hervonen A, Vaalasti A, Vaalasti T, Partenen M, Kanerva L 1976 Paraganlia in the urogenital tract of man. Histochemistry 48: 307–13

Hett G S, Butterfield H G 1910 The anatomy of the palatine tonsil. J Anat Physiol 44: 35–56

Heumann R, Lindholm D, Bandtlow C, Meyer M, Radeke M J, Miski T P, Shooter E, Thoenen H 1987 Differential regulation of mRNA encoding nerve growth factor and its receptor in rat sciatic nerve during development, degeneration and regeneration: role of macrophages. Proc Natl Acad Sci USA 84: 8735–8739

Heuser C H, Corner G W 1957 Developmental horizons in human embryos. Description of age group X, 4 to 12 somites. Contrib Embryol Carnegie Inst Washington 36: 29–39

Heuser C H, Streeter G L 1941 Development of the macaque embryo. Contrib Embryol Carnegie Inst Washington 29: 15–56

Heuser J 1989 The role of coated pits in recycling of synaptic vesicle membrane. Cell Biol Int Rep 13: 1063–1076

Heuser J E, Reese T S, Landis D M D 1974 Functional changes in frog neuromuscular junctions studies with freeze-fracture. J Neurocytol 3: 109–131

Hewitt A B 1977 An investigation using holographic interferometry, of surface strain in bone induced by orthodontic forces: a preliminary report. Br J Orthodont 4: 39–41

Hewitt A T, Kleinman H K, Pennypacker T P, Martin G R 1980 Identification of an adhesion factor for chondrocytes. Proc Natl Acad Sci USA 77: 385–388

Hewitt W 1958 The development of the human caudate and amygdaloid nuclei. J Anat 92: 377–382

Hewitt W 1960 The median aperture of the fourth ventricle. J Anat 94: 549–557

Hewitt W 1961 The development of the human internal capsule and lentiform nucleus. J Anat 95: 191–199

Hewitt W 1962 The development of the human corpus callosum. J Anat 96: 355–358

Heylings D J A 1978 Supraspinous and interspinous ligaments of the human lumbar spine. J Anat 125: 127–131

Heyner S, Smith R M, Scultz G A 1989 Temporally regulated expression of insulin and insulin-like growth factors and their receptors in early mammalian development. BioEssays 11: 171–176

Heywood C A, Gadotti A, Cowey A 1992 Cortical area V4 and its role in the perception of color. J Neurosci 12: 4056–4065

Hickey D S, Hukins D W L 1981 Collagen fibril diameters and elastic fibres in the annulus fibrosus of human fetal intervetebral disc. J Anat 133: 351–357

Hicks J H 1953a The mechanics of the foot. I. The joints. J Anat 87: 345–357

Hicks J H 1953b The mechanics of the foot. II. The plantar aponeurosis and the arch. J Anat 88: 25–30

Hicks J H 1955 The foot as a support. Acta Anat 25: 34–45

Hicks R M 1965 Permeability barriers in the rat ureter transitional epithelium. J Anat 99: 932P

Hicks R M 1975 The mammalian urinary bladder: an accommodation organ. Biol Revs 50: 215–246

Hicks S P, Amoto C J D, Lowe M J 1959 The development of the mammalian nervous system. I. Malformations of the brain, especially the cerebral cortex, induced in rats by radiation. J Comp Neurol 113: 435–469

Higgins C B, Vatner S F, Braunwald E 1973 Parasympathetic control of the heart. Pharmacol Rev 25: 119–155

Higgins J C, Eady R A J 1981 Human dermal microvasculature: a morphological and enzyme histochemical investigation at the light and electronic microscope levels. Br J Dermatol 104: 117–129

Hiiemae K M 1978 Mammalian mastication: a review of the activity of the jaw muscles and the movements they produce in chewing. In: Butler P M, Joysey K A (eds) Development, function and evolution of teeth. Academic Press: New York: pp 359–398

Hiiemae K M, Crompton A W 1985 Mastication, transport and swallowing. In: Hildebrand M, Bramble D M, Liem K F, Wake D B (eds) Functional vertebrate morphology. Belknap: Cambridge, Massachusetts: pp 262–290

Hikida R S, Gollnick P D, Dudley G A, Convertino V A, Buchanan P 1989 Structural and metabolic characteristics of human skeletal muscle following 30 days of simulated microgravity. Aviat Space Environ Med 60: 664–670

Hildebrand C, Hahn R 1978 Relation between myelin sheath thickness and axon size in spinal cord white matter of some vertebrate species. J Neurol Sci 38: 421–434

Hildebrand C, Remahl S, Persson H, Bjartinar C 1993 Myelinated nerve fibres in the CNS. Prog Neurobiol 40: 319 – 384

Hileman B 1993 Concerns broaden over chlorine and chlorinated hydrocarbons. Chem Engin News April 19th: 11–20

Hilfer S R, Rayner R M, Brown J W 1985 Mesenchymal control of branching pattern in the fetal mouse lung. Tissue Cell 127: 523–538

Hill A 1992 Development of tone and reflexes in the fetus and newborn. In: Polin R A, Fox W W (eds) Fetal and neonatal physiology. W B Saunders: Philadelphia: pp 1578–1587

Hill A R 1991 Respiratory muscle function in asthma. J Assoc Acad Minority Physicians 2: 100–108

Hill A V 1970 First and last experiments in muscle mechanics. Cambridge University Press: Cambridge

Hill H Z 1992 The function of melanin, or six blind people examine an elephant. BioEssays 14: 49–56

Hill J P 1932 The developmental history of the primates. Philos Trans R Soc Lond [Biol] 221: 45–178

Hill J P, Florian J 1931 A young human embryo (embryo Dobbin) with head-process and prochordal plate. Phil Trans Roy Soc London B 219: 443–486

Hill R E, Jones F J, Rees A R, Sime C M, Justice M J, Copeland N J, Jenkins N A, Graham E, Davidson D R 1989 A new family of mouse homeobox containing genes: molecular structure, chromosomal location and developmental expression. Genes Dev 3: 26–37

Hillarp N Å 1959 The construction and functional organisation of the autonomic innervation apparatus. Acta Physiol Scand 46 (suppl 157): 1–38

Hillman P, Wall P D 1969 Inhibitory and excitatory factors influencing the receptive fields of lamina 5 spinal cord cells. Exp Brain Res 9: 284–306

Hills J M, Jessen K R 1992 Transmission: gamma-amino butyric acid (GABA), 5-hydroxytryptamine (5-HT) and dopamine. In: Burnstock G, Hoyle C H V (eds) Autonomic neuroeffector mechanisms. Harwood Academic Publishers: Switzerland: pp 465–507

Himstedt H W, Schumacher G H, Menning A et al 1974 Zur Topographie der muskulüren Nervenausbreitungen. 5. Untere Extremität Ischiokrurale Muskeln. M biceps femoris. Anat Anz 135: 235–244

Hinchcliffe J R, Johnson D R 1980 The development of the vertebrate limb. Clarendon Press: Oxford

Hindle M O 1967 The intermediate plexus of the periodontal membrane. In: Mechanisms of tooth support. Wright: Bristol: pp 66–71

Hindmarsh P C, Brook C G D 1988 Hormonal control of infant growth in the first year. In: Cockburn F (ed) Fetal and neonatal growth. Wiley: Chichester

Hinds J W 1971 Early neuroblast differentiation in the mouse olfactory bulb. Anat Rec 169: 340–341

Hinds J W, Hinds P L 1972 Reconstruction of dendritic cones in neonatal mouse olfactory bulb. J Neurocytol 1: 169–187

Hinrichsen C F L, Larramendi L M H 1969 Features of trigeminal mesencephalic nucleus structure and organization. Am J Anat 126: 497–506

Hintzsche E 1937 Uber den Einfluss der Schilddrüsengrosse auf die Lage der Epithelkörperchen. Anat Anz 84: 18–25

Hiorns R W, Neal J W, Pearson R C A, Powell T P S 1991 Clustering of ipsilateral cortico-cortical projection neurons to area 7 in the rhesus monkey. Proc R Soc Lond Series B 246: 1–9

Hirai N, Hongo T, Kudo N et al 1976 Heterogenous composition of the spinocerebellar tract originating from the cervical enlargement of the cat. Brain Res 109: 387–391

Hirai T, Jones E G 1989 A new parcellation of the human thalamus on the basis of histochemical staining. Br Res Rev 14: 1–34

Hirano A, Denbitzer H M, 1967 A structional analysis of the sheath in the central nervous system. J Cell Biol 23: 555–567

Hirokawa N 1993 Axonal transport and the cytoskeleton. Curr Opin Neurobiol 3: 724 – 731

Hirokawa N 1994 Microtubule organization and dynamics dependent on microtubule-associated proteins. Curr Opin Cell Biol 6: 74–81

Hirokawa N, Tilney L-G 1982 Interactions between actin filaments and between actin filaments and membranes in quick-frozen and deeply etched hair cells of the chick ear. J Cell Biology 95: 249–261

Hirsch S 1960 Morphologie et Physiologie des Anastomses Arterioveneuses, Acta Tertii Europaei de Cordis Scientia Conventus, Romae. Excerpta Medici i: 61–64

Hirsch-Hoffman H U 1978 Die Ultrastruktur von Drüsendstücken der menschlichen Tränendrüse, Klin Mbl Augenheilk 172: 80–87

His W 1879 Uber die Anfänge des peripherischen Nervensystemes. Arch Anat Physiol Leipzig Anat Abt: 455–482

His W 1890 Histogenese und Zusammenhang der Nervenelemente. Arch Anat Physiol Leipzig Anat Abt (suppl): 95–117

His W Jr 1893 Die Thätigkeit des embryonalen Herzens und deren Bedeutung für die Lehre von der Herzbewegung beim Erwachsenen. Arb Med Klin Leipzig: 14–50

Hislop A, Wigglesworth J S, Desai R 1986 Alveolar development in pulmonary hypoplasia. Early Human Development 13: 1

Hjarnø J, Jørgensen J B, Vesely M 1974 Archeological and anthropoligical investigations of late heathen graves in Upernarvik district. Reitzels Forlag: København

Hjortsjö C-H 1948 Die Anatomie der Intrahepatischen Gallengänge beim Menschen; Mittels Röntgen- und Injections-technik stadiert. Lunds Univ Årssk N F Avd 2, 44: 1–112

Hjortsjö C-H 1951 The topography of the intrahepatic duct systems. Acta Anat 11: 599–615

Hjortsjö C-H 1956 The intrahepatic ramification of the portal vein. Lunds Univ Årssk N F Avd 2, 52: 1–30

Hjortsjö C-H 1975 Den Segmentella Indelingen av Levern. Comm Dept Anat Univ Lund 4

Hobar P C, Schreiber J S, McCarthy J G, Thomas P A 1993 The role of the dura in cranial bone regeneration in the immature animal. Past Reconstr Surg 92: 405–410

Hoddevik G H 1977 The pontine projection to the flocculo-nodular lobe and the paraflocculus studied by means of retrograde transport of horseradish peroxidase. Brain Res 123: 209–227

Hodge C J, Apkarian A V 1990 The spinothalamic tract. Crit Rev Neurobiol 15(4): 363–397

Hodge W A, Carlson K L, Fijan R S, Burgess R G, Riley P O, Harris W H, Mann R W 1989 Contact pressures from an instrumented hip endoprosthesis. J Bone Jt Surg 71A: 1378–1386

Hodges J R, Patterson K, Oxbury S, Funnell E 1992 Semantic dementia: progressive fluent aphasia with temporal lobe atrophy. Brain 115: 1783 – 1806

Hodgkin A L 1964 The conduction of the nervous impulse. Thomas: Springfield, Illinois

Hodgkin A L, Huxley A F 1952 Currents carried by sodium and potassium ions through membrane of giant axon of Loligo. J Physiol 116: 449–472

Hodgson C, Spiers R L 1974 The effect of preganglionic cervical sympathectomy on the amylase content of parotid glands in fasted and fed rats. J Physiol 237: 56–57P

Hodson J J 1966 The distribution, structure, origin and nature of the dental cuticle of Gottlieb. I and II. Periodontics 5: 237–250, 296–302

Hodson N 1970 The nerves of the testis, epididymus and scrotum. In: Johnson A D, Gomes W R, Vandemark N L (eds) The testis. Vol 1. Academic Press: New York: pp 47–100

Hodson W A, Truog W E 1987 Special techniques in managing respiratory problems. In: Avery G B (ed) Neonatology: pathophysiology and management in the newborn. 3rd edition. Lippincott: Philadelphia: pp 463

Hoerr N L, Pyle S J, Francis C C 1962 Radiographic atlas of skeletal development of foot and ankle. Thomas: Springfield, Illinois

Hoff E C, Hoff H E 1934 Spinal termination of the projection fibers from the motor cortex of primates. Brain 57: 454–474

Hoffman E P, Brown R H, Kunkel L M 1987 Dystrophin: the protein product of the Duchenne muscular dystrophy locus. Cell 51: 919–928

Hoffman H D, Seidl K, Unsicker K 1989 Development and plasticity of adrenal chromaffin cells: cues based on in vitro studies. J Electron Micros Tech 12: 397–407

Hoffman H H, Kuntz A 1957 Vagus nerve components. Anat Rec 127: 551–568

Hogan B L M, Tilly R 1981 Cell interactions and endoderm differentiation in cultures mouse embryos. J Embryol Exp Morphol 62: 379–394

Hogan M J 1972 Role of the retinal pigment epithelium in macular disease. Trans Am Acad Ophthal Otol 76: 64–80

Hogan M J, Alvarado J A, Weddell J E 1971 Histology of the human eye. Saunders: Philadelphia

Högberg P 1952 Length of stride, stride frequency, 'flight' period and the maximum distance between the feet during running with different speeds. Arbeitsphysiologie 14: 431–436

Hogg J C 1987 Neutrophil kinetics in lung injury. Physiol Rev 67: 1249–1295

Hogg N 1992 Roll, roll, roll your leucocyte gently down the vein. Immunol Today 13: 113–115

Hoh J F Y, Hughes S, Chow C, Hale P T, Fitzsimons R B 1988b Immunocytochemical and electrophoretic analyses of changes in myosin gene expression in cat posterior temporalis muscle during postnatal development. J Musc Res Cell Motil 9: 48–58

Hoh J F Y, Hughes S, Hale P T, Fitzsimons R B 1988a Immunocytochemical and electrophoretic analyses of changes in myosin gene expression in cat limb fast and slow muscles during postnatal development. J Musc Res Cell Motil 9: 30–47

Hökfeldt T, Elde R, Johannson O, Luft R, Nilsson G, Arimura A 1976 Immunohistochemical evidence for separate populations of somatostatin-containing and substance P-containing primary afferent neurons in rat. Neuroscience 1: 131–136

Hökfeldt T, Fuxe K, Pernow B (eds) 1986 Coexistence of neuronal messengers: A new principle in chemical transmission. In: Progress in brain research. Vol 68. Elsevier: Amsterdam

Hökfeldt T, Mårtensson R, Björklund A 1984 Distributional maps of tyrosine-hydroxylase-immunoreactive neurons in the rat brain. In: Björklund A, Hökfelt T (eds) Handbook of chemical neuroanatomy Vol. 2, Part 1: Classical transmitters in the CNS. Elsevier: London: pp 277–379

Holbrook K A 1989 Biologic structure and function: perspectives on morphologic approaches to the study of the granular layer keratinocyte. J Invest Dermatol 92: 84S–104S

Holgate S T 1983 Mast cells and their mediators. In: Holborrow E J, Reeves W G (eds) Immunology in medicine. 2nd edition. Academic Press: London: pp 79–94

Holland G R 1985 The odontoblast process; form and function. J Dent Res 64: 499–514

Holland P W H 1991, Cloning and evolutionary analysis of msh-like homeobox genes from mouse, zebrafish and ascidian. Gene 98: 253–257

Holland P W H, Hogan B L M 1988 Spatially restricted patterns of expression of the homeobox-containing gene Hox 2.1 during mouse embryogenesis. Development 102: 159–174

Holland P W H, Holland L Z, Williams N A, Holland N D 1992 An amphioxus homoebox gene: sequence conservation, spatial expression during development and insights into vertebrate evolution. Development 116: 653–661

Hollander H, Makarov F, Dreher Z, van Driel D, Chan-Liang T L, Stone J 1991 Structure of the macroglia of the retina: sharing and division of labour between astrocytes and Mueller cells. J Comp Neurol 313: 585–603

Holley M C, Ashmore J F 1988 A cytoskeletal spring in cochlear outer hair cells. Nature 335: 635–637

Holley M C, Kalinec F, Kachar B 1992 Structure of the cortical cytoskeleton in mammalian outer hair cells. J Cell Sci 102: 569–580

Holley M, Ashmore J F 1988 On the mechanism of a high frequency force generator in outer hair cells isolated from the guinea pig cochlea. Proc Roy Soc Lond B 232: 413–429

Holliday R 1964 A mechanism for gene conversion in fungi. Genet Res 5: 282–304

Hollinshead W H 1942 A comparative study of the glomus coccygeum and the carotid body. Anat Rec 84: 1–16

Hollister A, Bufird W L, Myers L M, Giurintano D J, Novick A 1992 The axes of rotation of the thumb carpometacarpal joint. J Orthop Res 10: 454–460

Hollmann K H 1974 Cytology and fine structure of the mammary gland. In: Larson B L, Smith V R (eds) Lactation. A comprehensive treatise. Vol 1. Academic Press: New York: pp 3–95

Holloszy J O, Booth F W 1976 Biochemical adaptations to endurance exercise in muscle. Annu Rev Physiol 38: 273–291

Holm N J 1980 The internal stress pattern of the os coxae. Acta Orthop Scand 51: 421–428

Holm V A, Cassidy S B, Butler M G, Hanchett J M, Greenswag L R, Whitman B Y, Greenberg F 1993 Prader-Willi Syndrome: consensus diagnostic criteria. Pediatrics 91: 398–402

Holmberg J 1972 On the nerves of the parotid gland. In: Emmelin N, Zotterman Y (eds) Oral physiology. Pergamon: Oxford: pp 17–19

Holmes E B 1976 A reconsideration of the phylogeny of the tetrapod heart. J Morph 147: 209–228

Holmes G 1939 The cerebellum of man. Brain 6: 1–30

Holmes G, Lister W T 1916 Disturbances of vision, from cerebral lesions, with special reference to the cortical representation of the macula. Brain 39: 34–73

Holmes K C, Popp D, Gebhard W, Kabsch W 1990 Atomic model of the actin filament. Nature 347: 44–49

Holstege G 1991 Descending motor pathways and the spinal motor system: limbic and non-limbic components. Prog Brain Res 87: 307–421 Elsevier Sci Pub Biomedical Div

Holstege G. Blok B F, Ralston D D 1988 Anatomical evidence for red nucleus projections to motoneuronal cell groups in the spinal cord of the monkey. Neurosci Lett 95: 97–101

Holstege G, Graveland G, Bijker-Biemond C, Schuddeboom I 1983 Location of motoneurons innervating the soft palate, pharynx and upper oesophagus. Anatomical evidence for a possible swallowing centre in the pontine reticular formation. An HRP and autoradiographic tracing study. Brain Behav Evol 23: 47–62

Holstege G, Griffiths D 1990 Neural organisation of micturition. In: Paxinos G (ed) The human nervous system. Academic Press: San Diego: pp 297 – 320

Holstege G, Kuypers H G J M 1982 The anatomy of brainstem pathways to the spinal cord in cat. A labelled amino acid tracing method. Prog Brain Res 57: 145–175

Holstege G, Tan J 1987 Supraspinal control of motoneurons innervating the striated muscles of the pelvic floor including urethral and anal sphincters in the cat. Brain 110: 1323–1344

Holstein A F 1967a Zur Nervenzellverteilung in glattmuskeligen Sphinkteren. Verh Anat Ges Jena 61: 269–275

Holstein A F 1967b Spermiophages in the human epididymis (Spermiophagen im Nebenhoden des Menschen). Naturwissenshaften 54: 98–99

Holstein A F 1976 Ultrastructural observations on the differentiation of spermatids in man. Andrologia 8: 57–65

Holstein A F, Davidoff M S, Breucker H, Countouris N, Orlandini G 1991 Different epithelia in the distal human male urethra. Cell Tiss Res 242: 23–32

Holstein A F, Wartenberg H, Wulfhekel U 1971 Cytomorphological studies on spermatogenesis in man. Verhandl der Anat Gesellshaft 65: 91–93 (in German)

Holtzer H, Weintraub H, Mayne R. Mochan B 1972 The cell cycle, cell lineage and cell differentiation. In: Mascona A A, Monroy A (eds) Current topics in developmental biology. Academic Press: New York

Holtzman E 1976 Lysosomes: a survey. Cell Biology Monographs Vol 3. Springer-Verlag: Vienna

Homandberg G A, Meyers R, Aydelotte M, Tripier D, Kuettner K E 1992 Isolation and characterization of an abundant elastase inhibitor from NaCl extracts of bovine nasal septa and articular cartilage. Connect Tissue Res 28: 289–305

Honjo I, Harada H, Kumazawa T 1976 Role of the levator veli palatini muscle in movement of the lateral pharyngeal wall. Arvch Otorhinolaryngol 212: 93–98

Hooker C W 1971 The intertubular tissue of the testis. In: Johnson A D, Gomes W R, Vandemark N L (eds) The testis. Vol 1. Academic Press: New York: pp 483–550

Hooper T L, Salmons S 1993 Skeletal muscle assistance in heart failure. Cardiovasc Res 27: 1404–1406

Hopkins D A 1987 The dorsal motor nucleus of the vagus nerve and the nucleus ambiguus: structure and connections. In: Hainsworth R, McWilliam P N, Mary D A S G (eds). Cardiogenic reflexes: Oxford University Press Oxford: pp 185–203

Hopwood D, Coghill G, Sanders D S A 1986 Human oesaphageal mucosal glands. Their detection, mucin, enzyme and secretory protein content. Histochemistry 86: 107–1120

Hopwood D, Logan K R, Bouchier I A D 1978 The electron microscopy of normal human oesaphageal epithelium. Virchow's Arch (Cell Pathol) 26: 345–538

Hopwood D, Milne G, Jankowski J, Howat K, Johnston D, Wormsley K G 1994 Secretory and absorptive activity of oesaphagaeal epithelium: evidence of circulating mucosubstances. Histochem J 26: 41049

Horacek M J, Earle A M, Gilmore J P 1986 The renal microvasculature of the monkey: an anatomical investigation. J Anat 148: 205–231

Horellou P, Brundin P, Kalén P, Mallet J, Björklund A 1990 In vivo release of DOPA and dopamine from genetically engineered cells grafted to the denervated rat striatum. Neuron 5: 393–402

Horiguchi M 1980 The cutaneous branch of some human suprascapular nerves. J Anat 130: 191–195

Horiguchi M 1981 The recurrent branch of the lateral cutaneous nerve of the forearm. J Anat 132: 243–247

Horiuchi H, Matthews B 1973 In-vitro observations on fluid flow through human dentine caused by pain-producing stimuli. Arch Oral Biol 18: 275–294

Hornung J-P, De Tribolet N 1994 Distribution of GABA-containing neurons in human frontal cortex: a quantitative immunocytochemical study. Anat Embryol 189: 139–145

Horsley V A H, Clarke R H 1908 The structure and functions of the cerebellum examined by a new method. Brain 31: 45–124

Horstadius S 1939 The mechanics of sea urchin development, studied by operative methods. Biol Rev 14: 132–179

Horstadius S 1950 The neural crest. Oxford University Press: London

Horstadius S, Sellman S 1946 Experimentelle Untersucchungen über dies Determination des Knorpeligen Kopskelettes bei Urodelen. Nova Acta R Soc Upsal 13

Horstmann E 1962 Electron microscopy of the human epididymis. Z Zellforsch 57: 692–718

Horstmann E 1966 Uber das Endothel der Zottenkapillaren im Dünndarm des Meerschwanchens und des Menschen. Z Zellforsch 72: 364–369

Horton J C, Hedley-Whyte E T 1984 Mapping of cytochrome oxidase patches and ocular dominance columns in human visual cortex. Phil Trans R Soc Lond 304: 255–272

Horton R C 1952 The gastro-epiploic arteries. Guy's Hosp Rep 101: 108–110

Hoshino A, Wallace W A 1987 Impact-absorbing properties of the human knee. J Bone Jt Surg 69B: 807–811

Hotary K B, Robinson K R 1992 Evidence of a role for endogenous electrical fields in chick embryo development. Development 114: 985–996

Hounsfield G N 1973 Computerized transverse axial scanning (tomography). I. Description of system. Br J Radiol 46: 1016–1022

Houser C R, Crawford G D, Salvaterra P M, Vaughn J E 1985 Immunocytochemical localization of choline acetyltransferase in rat cerebral cortex: a study of cholinergic neurons and synapses. J Comp Neurol 234: 17–34

Houser C R, Vaughn J E, Hendry S H C, Jones E G, Peters A 1984 GABA neurons in the cerebral cortex. In: Jones E G, Peters A (eds) Cerebral cortex. Vol 2. Functional properties of cortical cells. Plenum Press: New York: pp 63–89

Hovelacque A 1927 Anatomie des Nerfs Graniens et Rachidiens et du Système Grand Sympathétique chez l'Homme. Doin: Paris

Howie A J, Johnson G D 1992 Confocal microscopic and other observations on the distal end of the thick limb of the human loop of Henle. Cell Tiss Res 267: 11–16

Howkins C H 1935 Blood supply of the lower jaw. Proc R Soc Med 29: 506–507

Howlett S K, Bolton V H 1985 Sequence and regulation of morphological and molecular events during the first cell cycle of mouse embryogenesis. J Embryol Exp Morphol 87: 175–206

Hoyle C H V, Burnstock G 1989 Neuromuscular transmission in the gastrointestinal tract. In: Wood J D (ed) Handbook of physiology – the gastrointestinal system I. American Physiological Society: Bethesda, Maryland: pp 435–464

Hoyle C H V, Burnstock G 1989 Neuronal populations in the submucous plexus of the human colon. J Anat 166: 7–22

Hoyme H E, Higginbottom M C, Jones K L 1981 The vascular pathogenesis of gastroschisis: intrauterine interruption of the omphalomesenteric artery. J Pediatr 98: 228

Hoyte D A N 1960 Alizarin as an indicator of bone growth. J Anat 94: 432–442

Hoyte D A N 1966 Experimental investigations of skull morphology and growth. Int Rev Gen Exp Zool 2: 345–408

Hoyte D A N 1975 A critical analysis of the growth in length of the cranial base. Birth Defects 11: 255–282

Hrdlička A 1939 Practical Anthropometry. Wistar Institute: Philadelphia

Hsu L Y F 1986 Prenatal diagnosis of chromosome abnormalities. In Milunsky A (ed) Genetic disorders and the fetus. Diagnosis prevention and treatment. Plenum: New York: pp 115–183

Huang J S, Olsen T J, Huang S S 1988 Platelet-derived growth factor. In: Clark R A F, Henson P M (eds) The molecular and cellular biology of wound repair. Plenum Press: New York: pp 243–251

Huang X F, Tork I, Paxinos G 1993 Dorsal motor nucleus of the vagus nerve; a cyto and chemoarchitectonic study in the human. J Comp Neurol 330: 158–182

Hubel D H, Wiesel T N 1977 Functional architecture of the macaque monkey visual cortex. (Ferrier Lecture). Proc R Soc Lond [Biol] 198: 1–59

Huber A C, Crosby E C 1933 The reptilian optic tectum. J Comp Neurol 57: 57–164

Huddart H, Hunt S 1975 Visceral muscle: its structure and function. Blackie: Glasgow

Hudlicka O 1991 Anatomical changes in chronically stimulated skeletal muscles. Seminars Thorac Cardiovasc Surg 3: 106–110

Hudson C L, Moritz A R, Wearn J T 1932 The extracardiac anastomses of the coronary arteries. J Exp Med 56: 919–925

Hudson R E B 1965 Cardiovascular pathology. Arnold: London

Hudspeth A J, Jacobs R 1979 Stereocilia mediate transduction in vertebrate hair cells. Proc Natl Acad Sci 76: 1506–1509

Huerta M D, Harting J K 1984 The mammalian superior colliculus studies of its morphology and connections. In: Vanegas H (ed) Comparative neurology of the optic tectum. Plenum: New York: pp 687 – 773

Hughes A 1974 Endocrines, neural development and behavior. In: Gottlieb G (ed) Aspects of neurogenesis. Studies on the development of behavior and the nervous system. Vol 2. Academic Press: New York: pp 223–243

Hughes A 1976 The development of the dorsal funiculus in the human spinal cord. J Anat 122: 169–175

Hughes A F W 1968 Aspects of neural ontogeny. Academic Press: New York

Hughes C C W, Male D K, Lantos P L 1988 Adhesions of lymphocytes to cerebral microvascular cells: effects of interferon-gamma, tumour necrosis factor and interleukin-1. Immunology 64: 677–682

Hughes H 1952 The factors determining the direction of the canal for nutrient artery in the long bones of mammals and birds. Acta Anat 15: 261–280

Hughes R A C 1990 Guillain -Barré Syndrome: Springer Verlag

Hughes S M, Blau H M 1992 Muscle fiber pattern is independent of cell lineage in postnatal rodent development. Cell 68: 659–671

Hughes S M, Cho M, Karsch-Mizrachi I, Travis M, Siberstein L, Leinwand L A, Blau H M 1993 Three slow myosin heavy chains sequentially expressed in developing mammalian skeletal muscle. Devel Biol 158: 183–199

Hugli T E, Müller-Eberhard H J 1978 Anaphylatoxins, C3a and C5a. Adv Immunol 26: 1–53

Huhtaniemi I 1994 Fetal testis – a very special endocrine organ. Eur J Endocrinol 130: 25–31

Huhtaniemi I, Pelliniemi L J 1992 Fetal Leydig cells: cellular origin, morphology, life span, and special functional features. Proc Soc Exp Biol Med 201: 125–140

Hultborn H 1976 Transmission in the pathway of reciprocal 1a inhibition to motoneurones and its control during the tonic stretch reflex. In: Homma S (ed) Understanding the stretch reflex. Prog Brain Res 44: 235–255 Elsevier: Amsterdam

Hultborn H, Jankowska E, Lindström S 1971 Recurrent inhibition from motor axon collaterals of transmission in 1a inhibitory pathway to motoneurones. J Physiol 215: 591–612

Hultkrantz W 1898 Über die Spaltrichtungen der Gelenkknorpel. Verhandl anat Gesellsch Jena 12: 248–256

Hume D M, Magee J H, Kauffman H M, Rittenburg M S, Prout G R 1963 Renal homo-transplantation in man in modified recipients. Ann Surg 158: 608–644

Humes H D, Beals T F, Cieslinski D A, Sanchez I O, Page T P 1991 Effects of transforming growth factor-beta, transforming growth factor-alpha, and other growth factors on renal proximal tubule cells. Lab Invest 64: 538–545

Hummel K P, Chapman D B 1959 Visceral inversion and associated anomalies in the mouse. J Hered 50: 9–13

Humphrey T 1944 Primitive neurons in the embryonic central nervous system. J Comp Neurol 81: 1–45

Humphrey T 1947 Sensory ganglion cells within the central canal of the embryonic human spinal cord. J Comp Neurol 86: 1–36

Humphrey T 1960 The development of the pyramidal tracts in human fetuses, correlated with cortical differentiation. In: Tower D B, Schadé J P (eds) Structure and Function of the cerebral cortex. (Proceedings of the Second International Meeting of Neurobiologists, Amsterdam 1959.) Elsevier: Amsterdam: pp 93–103

Humphrey T 1964 Some observations on the development of the human hippocampal formation. Trans Am Neurol Assoc 89: 207–209

Humphrey T 1967 The development of the human hippocampal fissure. J Anat 101: 655–676

Humphrey T 1969 The central relations of the trigeminal nerve. In: Kahn E A (ed) The surgery of pain. 2nd edition. Thomas: Springfield, Illinois

Humzah M D, Soames R W 1988 The human intervertebral disc: structure and function. Anat Rec 220: 37–356

Hundeiker M, Keller L 1963 Die Gefassarchitektur des menschlichen Hodens. Morphol Jb 105: 26–73

Hungerford D S, Barry M 1979 Biomechanics of the patellofemoral joint. Clin Orthop 144: 9–15

Hunt C C 1974 The physiology of muscle receptors. In: Hunt C C (ed) Handbook of sensory physiology. Vol 3, pt 2. Springer: Berlin: pp 191–234

Hunt P, Gulisano M, Cook M, Sham M, Faiella A, Wilkinson D, Boncinelli E, Krumlauf R 1991a A district Hox code for the branchial region of the head. Nature 353: 861–864

Hunt P, Krumlauf R 1991 Deciphering the Hox code: clues to patterning the branchial regions of the head. Cell 66: 1075–1078

Hunt P, Wilkinson D, Krumlauf R 1991 Patterning the vertebrate head: murine Hox 2 genes mark distinct subpopulations of premigratory and migrating cranial neural crest. Development 112: 43–50, 861–864

Hunt R C, Davis A A 1990 Altered expression of keratin and vimentin in human retinal pigment epithelial cells in vivo and in vitro. J cellular Physiol 145: 187–199

Hunt R K, Jacobson M 1974 Neuronal specificity revisited. In: Moscona A A, Monroy A (eds) Current topics in developmental biology. Vol 8. Academic Press: New York: pp 203–259

Huntingford P J 1959 Pudendal nerve block; the results of its routine use, with special reference to the trans-vaginal technique. J Obstet Gynaecol Br Commonw 66: 26–31

Huntington G S 1908 The genetic interpretation of the development of the mammalian lymphatic system. Am J Anat 2: 19–45

Huntington G S 1920 The morphology of the pulmonary artery in the Mammalia. Anat Rec 17: 165–202

Hunziker E B, Herrmann W, Schenk R K, Mueller M, Moor H 1984 Cartilage ultrastructure after high pressure freezing, freeze substitution and low temperature embedding. J Cell Biol 98: 267–276

Hunziker E B, Schenk R K 1987 Structural organization of proteoglycans in cartilage. In: Biology of proteoglycans. Academic Press: New York: pp 155–185

Hurd Y L, Weiss F, Koob G F, And N E, Ungerstedt U 1989 Cocaine reinforcement and extracellular dopamine overflow in rat nucleus accumbens: an in vivo microdialysis study. Brain Res 498: 199–203

Hurri L, Pulkki T, Vainio K 1964 Arthroplasty of the elbow in rheumatoid arthritis. Acta Chir Scand 127: 459–465

Hurst A F 1919 Chronic constipation. Oxford University Press: London

Hustin J, Schaaps J–P 1987 Echocardiographic and anatomic studies of the maternotrophoblastic border during the first trimester of pregnancy. Am J Obstet Gynecol 157: 162–168

Hutch J A, Rambo O S Jr 1970 A study of the anatomy of the prostate, prostatic urethra and urinary sphincter system. J Urol 104: 443–452

Hutchings M, Weller R O 1986 Anatomical relationships of the pia mater to cerebral blood vessels in man. J Neurosurg 65: 316–325

Hutchinson M C E 1978 A study of the atrial arteries in man. J Anat 125: 39–54

Hüttner I, Boutet M, More R H 1973 Studies on protein passage through arterial endothelium. I. Lab Invest 28: 672–677

Huxley A F, Niedergerke R 1954 Structural changes in muscle during contraction. Interference microscopy of living muscle fibres. Nature 173: 971–973

Huxley A F, Simmons R M 1971 Proposed mechanism of force generation in striated muscle. Nature 233: 533–538

Huxley H E 1969 The mechanism of muscular contraction. Science 164: 1356–1366

Huxley H E, Hanson J 1954 Changes in the cross striations of muscle during contraction and stretch and their interpretation. Nature 173: 973–976

Huxley J S 1942 Evolution. The modern synthesis. Harper: New York

Hyatt G A, Beebe D C 1993 Regulations of lens cell growth and polarity by an embryo-specific growth factor and by inhibitors of lens cell proliferation and differentiation. Development 117: 701–709

Hyde T M, Miselis R R 1992 Subnuclear organization of the human caudal nucleus of the solitary tract. Brain Res Bull 29: 95–109

Hydén H 1960 The neuron. In: Brachet J, Mirsky A E (eds) The cell. Vol 4. Academic Press: New York: pp 215–324

Hylander W L 1975 The human mandible: lever or link? Am J Phys Anthropol 43: 227–242

Hyman C, Hofer M, Barde Y-A, Juhasz M, Yancopoulus G D, Squinto S P, Lindsay R M 1991 BDNF is a neurotrophic factor for dopaminergic neurons of the substantia nigra. Nature 350: 230–232

Hynes R O, Lander A D 1992 Contact and adhesive specificities in the associations, migrations and targeting of cells and axons. Cell 68: 303–322

Hyvarinen J 1982 The parietal cortex of monkey and man. Springer-Verlag: Berlin

I

Iannotti J P, Gabriel J P, Schneck S L, Evans B G, Misra S 1992 The normal glenohumeral relationships. J Bone Jt Surg 74A: 491–500

Ibawi M N, Idriss F S, Hunt C E, Brouillette R T, De Leon S Y 1985 Diaphragmatic pacing in infants: techniques and results. Ann Thorac Surg 40: 323–328

Ibraghimov-Beskrovnaya O, Ervasti J M, Leveille C J, Slaughter C A, Sernett S W, Campbell K P 1992 Primary structure of dystrophin-associated glycoproteins linking dystrophin to the extracellular matrix. Nature 355: 696–702

Ibuki K, Matsuya T, Nishio J, Hamamura Y, Miyazaki T 1978 The course of facial nerve innervation for the levator veli palatini muscle. Cleft Palate J 15: 209–214

Icardo J M 1988 Heart anatomy and developmental biology. Experientia 44: 910–919

Icardo J M, Manasek F J 1992 Cardiogenesis: development, mechanisms and embryology. In: Fozzard H A, Haber E, Jennings R B, Katz A M, Morgan H E (eds) The Heart and cardiovascular system. 2nd edition. Raven Press: New York: pp 1563–1586

Ichima T, Ellisman M H 1991 Three dimensional fine structure of cytoskeletal-membrane interactions at nodes of Ranvier. J Neurocytol 20: 667–681

Igarashi M, Strittmatter S M, Vartanian T, Fishman M C 1993 Mediation by G proteins of signals that cause collapse of growth cones. Science 259: 77 – 80

Igarishi Y 1989 Submicroscopic study of the vestibular dark cell area in human fetuses. Acta Otolaryngol [Stockh] 107: 29–38

Iggo A 1969 Cutaneus thermoreceptors in primates and sub-primates. J Physiol 200: 403–430

Iggo A, Muir A R 1969 The structure and function of a slowly adapting touch corpuscle in hairy skin. J Physiol 200: 763–796

Ikeda T, Sakai H, Shimokawa I, Iwasaki K, Matsuo T 1990 Expression of Leu-7 antigen in the embryonic heart – with special reference to development of the conducting system. In: Clark E B, Takao A (eds) Development cardiology; morphogenesis and function. Futura Publishing: Mount Kisco: New York

Ikemoto N, Ronjat M, Meszaros L G, Koshita M 1989 Postulated role of calsequestrin in the regulation of calcium release from sarcoplasmic reticulum. Biochemistry 28: 6764–6771

Ikeya M 1975 Dating a stalactite by electron paramagnetic resonance. Nature 255: 48–50

Ikeya M 1986 Electron spin resonance. In: Zimmerman M R, Angel J L (eds) Dating and age determination of biological materials. Croom Helm: London

Illis L 1964 Spinal cord synapses in the cat: the normal appearances by the light microscope. Brain 87: 543–554

Imai Y, Lasky L A, Rosen S D 1993 Sulphation requirement for GlyCAM-1, an endothelial ligand for L-selectin. Nature 361: 555–557

Imayama S 1981 Scanning and transmission electron microscope study on the terminal blood vessels of the rat skin. J Invest Dermatol 76: 151–157

Imfield TN, Schroeder HE 1992 Palatal taste buds in man: topographical arrangement in islands of keratinized epithelium. Anatomy Embryol 185: 259–269

Imperato-McGinley J, Guerrero L, Gautier T, Peterson R E 1974 Steroid 5 α-reductase deficiency in man: an inherited form of male pseudo-hermaphroditism. Science 186: 1213–1215

Imre G 1964 Studies on the mechanism of retinal neovascularization. Role of lactic acid. Br J Ophthalmol 48: 75–82

Ince H, Young M 1940 The bony pelvis and its influence on labour: a radiological and clinical study of 500 women. J Obstet Gynaecol Br Commonw 47: 130–190

Inglis A E, Pellicci P M 1980 Total elbow replacement. J Bone Jt Surg 62A: 1252–1258

Ingram D L 1962 Atresia. In: Zuckerman S (ed) The ovary. Vol 1. Academic Press: New York

Ingram W R 1940 Nuclear organisation and chief connections of the primate hypothalamus. Res Pub Assoc Res Nerv Ment Dis 20: 195–244

Inman V T, Saunders J B de C M 1937 The ossification of the human frontal bone, with special reference to its presumed pre- and post-frontal elements. J Anat 71: 383–394

Inman V T, Saunders J B de C M, Abbot L C 1944 Observations on the function of the shoulder joint. J Bone Jt Surg 26: 1–30

Innocenti G M S, Clarke S, Kraftsik R 1986 J Neurosci 6: 1384–1409

Inoue H 1973 Three-dimensional observation of collagen framework of intervertebral discs in rats, dogs and humans. Arch Histol Jpn 36: 39–56

Inoué S 1981 Cell division and the mitotic spindle J Cell Biol 91: 132S—147S

Inoue S 1989 Ultrastructure of basement membranes. Int Rev Cytol 117: 57–98

Inouye H, Kirschner D A 1984 New X-ray spacings from central myelinated tissue. J Neurocytol 13: 883–894

Insall J 1994 Surgery of the knee. 2nd edition. Churchill Livingstone: Edinburgh

Insausti R, Amaral D G, Cowan W M 1987 The entorhinal cortex of the monkey. II. Cortical afferents. J Comp Neurol 264: 356–395

Insausti R, Amaral D G, Cowan W M 1987 The entorhinal cortex of the monkey. III. Subcortical afferents. J Comp Neurol 264: 396–408

International Anatomical Nomenclature Committee 1983 Nomina Anatomica 5th edition. Williams and Wilkins: Baltimore, Maryland

International Federation of Societies for Surgery of the Hand 1972 Joint motion of the thumb. Hand 4(3): 278

Irintchev A, Zeschnigk M, Starzinski-Powitz A, Wernig A 1994 Expression pattern of M-cadherin in normal, denervated and regenerating mouse muscles. Developmental Dynamics 199: 326–337

Irstam L 1962 The surface structure of the male breast nipple. Am J Phys Anthropol 20: 451–459

Irvine D R F 1986 The auditory brainstem. Prog Sens Physiol 7: 1 – 279

Irving R, Harrison K M 1967 The superior olivary complex and audition: A comparative study. J Comp Neurol 130: 77–86

Isenberg G, Goldmann W H 1992 Actin–membrane coupling: a role for talin. J Musc Res Cell Motil 13: 587–589

Isler H, Sarkar S K, Thompson B, Tonkin R 1968 The architecture of the thyroid gland: a 3-dimensional investigation. Anat Rec 161: 325–335

Isotupa K 1972 Alizarin trajectories in experimental studies of skull growth. Proc Finn Dent Soc 68 (suppl 2): 1–49

Isseroff R P, Fusenig N E, Rifkin D B 1982 Plasminogen activator in differentiating mouse keratinocytes. J Invest Dermatol 80: 217–222

Ito K, Sieber-Blum M 1991 In vitro clonal analysis of quail cardiac neural crest development. Dev Biol 148: 95–106

Ito M 1982 The cerebellar control of the vestibulo-ocular reflex around the flocculus hypothesis. Ann Rev Neurosci 5: 275–296

Ito M 1984 The cerebellum and neural control. Raven Press: New York

Ito M 1989 Biologic roles of the innermost cell layer of the outer root sheath in human anagen hair follicle; further electron microcopic study. Arch Dermatol Res 281: 254–259

Ito M 1991 The cellular basis of cerebellar plasticity. Neurobiology 1: 616–620

Ito S 1987 Functional gastric morphology. In: Johnson L R (ed) Physiology of the gastrointestinal tract. 2nd Edn. Raven Press: New York

Ito S, Winchester R J 1963 The fine structure of the gastric mucosa in the bat. J Cell Biol 16: 541–577

Ito T 1988 Morphological connections of the human apocrine and eccrine sweat gland – occurrence of so-called mixed sweat glands, a review. Ok Fol Anat Jap 65: 315–335

Ito T, Shibasaki S 1964 Lichtmikroskopische Untersuchungen über die Glandula lacrimalis des Menschen. Arch Hist Jpn 25: 117–143

Itoh T, Kuriyama H, Suzuki H 1983 Differences and similarities in the noradrenaline- and caffeine-induced mechanical responses in the rabbit mesenteric artery. J Physiol 337: 609–629

Iurato S 1967 Submicroscopic structure of the inner ear. Pergamon: Oxford

Iversen L L, Kelly J S 1975 Uptake and metabolism of gamma-aminobutyric acid by neurones and glial cells. Biochem Pharmacol 24: 933–938

Iversen S D 1979 Behaviour after neostriatal lesions in mammals. In: Divac I, Öberg R E G (eds) The neostriatum. Pergamon Press: Oxford: pp 195–212

Iwamatsu T, Chang M C 1972 Sperm penetration in vitro of mouse oocytes at various times during maturation. J Reprod Fertil 31: 237–247

Iwamura Y, Tanaka M, Sakamoto M, Hikosaka O 1993 Rostrocaudal gradients in the neuronal receptive field complexity in the finger region of the alert monkey's postcentral gyrus. Exp Brain Res 92: 360–368

Izpisua-Belmonte J C, de Robertis E M, Storey K G, Stern C D 1993 The homeobox gene *goosecoid* and the origin of organizer cells in the early chick blatoderm. Cell 74: 645–659

Izpisua-Belmonte J C, Tickle C, Dolle P, Wolpert L, Duboule D 1991 Expression of homeobox Hox-4 genes and the specification of position in chick wing development. Nature 350: 585–589

Izumo S, Nadal-Ginard B, Mahdavi V 1986 All members of the myosin heavy chain multigene family respond to thyroid hormone in a highly tissue-specific manner. Science 231: 597–600

J

Jabbur S J, Towe A L 1961 Cortical excitation of neurons in dorsal column nuclei of cat, including an analysis of pathways. J Neurophysiol 24: 499–509

Jack C R Jr, Thompson R M, Butts R K, Sharbrough F W, Kelly P J, Hanson D P et al 1994 Sensory motor cortex: correlation of presurgical mapping with functional MR imaging and invasion cortical mapping. Radiology 190: 85–92

Jackowski A, Parnavelas JG, Lieberman AR 1978 The reciprocal synapse in the external plexiform layer of the mammalian olfactory bulb. Brain Res 159: 17–28

Jackson K M 1983 Why the upper limbs move during human walking. J Theor Biol 105: 311–315

Jacob H J, Christ B, Brand B 1986 On the development of trunk and limb muscles in avian embryos. Biblthca Anat 29. pp 1–23

Jacob H J, Jacob M, Christ B 1977 Die Ultrastruktur der exteren Glomerula. Ein Beitrag zur Nierenentwicklung bei Hühnerembryonen. Verh Anat Ges 71: 909–912

Jacobowitz D M 1970 Catecholamine fluorescence studies of adrenergic neurons and chromaffin cells in sympathetic ganglia. Fed Proc 29: 1929–1944

Jacobs J M, MacFarlane R M, Cavanagh J B 1976 Vascular leakage in the dorsal root ganglia of the rat, studied with horseradish peroxidase. J Neurol Sci 29: 95–107

Jacobs L, Comroe H J 1971 Reflex apnoea, bradycardia and hypotension produced by erotonin on the nodose ganglion of the cat. Circ Res 29: 145–155

Jacobsen K 1974 Area intercondylaris tibiae: osseous surface structure and its relation to soft tissue structures and applications to radiography. J Anat 117: 605–618

Jacobsen M D, Evan G I 1994 Breaking the ICE. Current Biology 4: 331–340

Jacobson A G, Meier S 1986 Somitomeres: the primordial body segments. In: Bellairs R, Ede D A, Lash J W (eds) Somites in developing embryos. NATO ASI Series. Series A: Life Sciences. Plenum Press: New York: pp 1–16

Jacobson M 1970 Development, specification and diversification of neuronal connections. In: Schmitt F O, Quarton G C, Meinechuk T, Adelman G (eds) The neurosciences. Second study program. Rockefeller University Press: New York: pp 116–129

Jafek B W 1983 Ultrastructure of human nasal mucosa. Laryngoscope 93, 1576–1599

Jaffe L F, Stern C D 1979 Strong electrical currents leave the primitive streak of chick embryos. Science 206: 569–571

Jahr C E, Jessel T M 1983 ATP excites a subpopulation of rat dorsal horn neurones. Nature 304: 730–733

Jakus M A 1964 Ocular fine structure. Churchill: London

James D W 1974 Growth cones and synaptic connections in tissue culture. In: Bellairs R, Gray E G (eds) Essays on the nervous system. (A festschrift for Professor J Z Young.) Clarendon Press: Oxford

James T N 1961 Anatomy of the coronary arteries. Hoeber Med Div, Harper & Row: New York

James T N 1961 Anatomy of. the human sinus node. Anat Rec 141: 109–116

James T N 1978 Anatomy of the conduction system of the heart. In: Hurst J W, Logue R B, Schlant R C, Wenger N K (eds) The heart, arteries, and veins. 4th edition. McGraw-Hill: New York: pp 47–57

James T N, Sherf L 1978 Ultrastructure of the myocardium. In: Hurst J W, Logue R B, Schlant R C, Wenger N K (eds) The heart, arteries, and veins. 4th edition. McGraw-Hill: New York: pp 57–70

James W H 1971 Excess of like sexed pairs of dizygotic twins. Nature 232: 277

Jamieson E B 1910 The arrangement of the fibres of the middle cerebellar peduncle as shown by dissection. J Anat Physiol 44: 234–240

Jamieson J K, Dobson J F 1907 Lectures on the lymphatic system of the caecum and appendix. Lancet I: 1061–1066

Jamieson J K, Dobson J F 1908 The lymphatics of the colon. Proc R Soc Med 2: 149–174

Jamieson J K, Dobson J F 1920 The lymphatics of the tongue: with particular reference to the removal of lymphatic glands in cancer of the tongue. Br J Surg 8: 80–87

Jancsó G, Kiraly E, Jancsó-Gábor A 1977 Pharmacologically-induced selective degeneration of chemosensitive primary sensory neurones. Nature 270: 741–743

Janda V, Stará V 1965 The role of thigh adductors in movement patterns of the hip and knee joint. Courier 15: 1–3

Jande S S, Malerz L, Lawson D E M 1981 Immunohistochemical mapping of vitamin D-dependent calcium-binding protein in brain. Nature 294: 765–767

Jankowska E, Lindström S 1971 Morphological identification of Renshaw cells. Acta Physiol Scand 81: 428–430

Jankowska E, Lindström S 1972 Morphology of interneurones mediating 1a reciprocal inhibition of motor neurones in the spinal cord of the cat. J Physiol 226: 805–823

Jannetta P J 1967 Arterial compression of the trigeminal nerve at the pons in patients with trigeminal neuralgia. J Neurosurg 26: 159–162

Janossy G, Campana D 1989 Ontogeny of the human T cell receptors – single cell studies. Thymus Update 2: 39–58

Janossy G, Prentice H G, Grob J P, Ivory K, Tidman N, Grundy J, Favrot M, Brenner M K, Campana D, Blacklock H A et al 1986 T lymphocyte regeneration after transplantation of R cell depleted allogeneic bone marrow. Clin Exp Immunol 63: 577–586

Janse M J, Anderson R H 1974 Internodal atrial specialised pathways – fact or fiction? Eur J Cardiol 2: 117–137

Jansen J, Brodal A 1940 Experimental studies on the intrinsic fibers of the cerebellum. II. The cortico-nuclear projection. J Comp Neurol 73: 267–321

Jansen J, Brodal A 1942 Experimental studies on the intrinsic fibers of the cerebellum. III. The cortico-nuclear projection on the rabbit and the monkey. Norske Vid Acad (avh 1) Math Nat: Kl 3 1/3 1

Jansen J, Brodal A (eds) 1954 Aspects of cerebellar anatomy. Grundt Tanum: Oslo

Jansó G, Kiraly E, Jancsó-Gábor A 1977 Pharmacologically-induced selective degeneration of chemosensitive primary sensory neurons. Nature 270: 741–743

Janzer R C, Raff M C 1987 Astrocytes induce blood–brain barrier properties in endothelial cells. Nature 325: 253–257

Jarrell B E, Williams S K, Hoch J, Carabasi R A 1987 Rapidly established endothelial cell monolayers. In: Zilla P P, Fasol R D, Deutsch M (eds) Endothelialization of vascular grafts. Karger: Basel: pp 136–144

Jarvis J C 1993 Power production and working capacity of rabbit tibialis anterior muscles after chronic electrical stimulation at 10 Hz. J Physiol 470: 157–169

Jasin H E, Dingle J T 1981 Human mononuclear cell factors mediate cartilege matrix degradation through chondrocyte activation. J Clin Invest 68: 571–581

Jasin H E, Lightfoot E, Davis L S, Rothlein R, Faanes R B, Lipsky P E 1992 Amelioration of antigen-induced arthritis in rabbits treated with monoclonal antibodies to leukocyte adhesion molecules. Arthritis Rheum 35: 541–549

Jasin H E, Norori K, Takagi T, Taurog J D 1993 Characteristics of anti-type II collagen antibody binding to articular cartilage. Arthritis Rheum 36: 651–659

Jaworek T E 1973 The intrinsic vascular supply to the first metatarsal. Surgical considerations. J Am Podiatry Assoc 63: 189–197

Jaworski Z F G 1992 Haversian systems and Haversian bone. In: Hall B K (ed) Bone. Vol 4. Bone metabolism and mineralization. CRC Press: Boca Raton: pp 21–45

Jaworski Z F G, Duck B, Sekaly G 1981 Kinetics of osteoclasts and their nuclei in evolving secondary Haversian systems. J Anat 133: 397–405

Jay G D 1992 Characterization of a bovine fluid lubricating factor. I. Chemical, surface activity, and lubricating properties. Connect Tissue Res 28: 71–88

Jay G D, Lane B P, Sokoloff L 1992 Characterization of a bovine fluid lubricating factor. III. The interaction with hyaluronic acid. Connect Tissue Res 28: 245–255

Jdanov D A 1959 Anatomie du canal thoracique et des principaux collecteurs lymphatiques due tronc chez l'homme. Acta Anat 37: 20–47

Jean-Faucher Ch, Berger M, Gallon Ch, Turckheim M, Veyssiere G, Jean Cl 1987 Sex-related differences in renal size in mice: ontogeny and influence of neonatal androgens. J Endocrinol 115: 241–246

Jeanmonod D, Magnin M, Morel A 1993 Thalamus and neurogenic pain: physiological, anatomical and clinical data. Neuroreport 4: 475–478

Jefferson G 1915 The human stomach and the canalis gastricus (Lewis). J Anat 49: 165–181

Jeffery P K, Reid L 1975 New features of rat airway epithelium: a quantitative and electron microscopic study. J Anat 120: 295–320

Jeffery P K 1990 Microscopic structure of normal lung. In: Brewis R A L, Gibson G J, Geddes D M Respiratory medicine. Bailliers Tindall: London: pp 57–78

Jeffries D J, Pickles J O, Osbourne M P, Rhys-Evans P H, Comis S D 1986 Crosslinks between stereocilia in hair cells of the human and guinea pig vestibular labyrinth. J Laryngol Otol 100: 1367–1374

Jend H H, Ney R, Heller M 1985 Evaluation of tibiofibular motion under load conditions by computed tomography. J Orthop Res 3: 418–423

Jenkins F A 1969 The evolution and development of the dens of the mammalian axis. Anat Rec 164: 173–184

Jenkins F A 1972 Chimpanzee bipedalism: cineradiographic analysis and implications for the evolution of gait. Science 178: 877–879

Jennekens F G I 1982 Neurogenic disorders of muscle. In: Mastaglia F L, Walton J (eds) Skeletal muscle pathology. Churchill Livingstone: Edinburgh: pp 204–234

Jenness R 1974 Biosynthesis and composition of milk. J Invest Dermatol 63: 109–118

Jennings R B, Sommers H, Smyth G A, Flack H A, Linn H 1960 Myocardial necrosis induced by temporary occlusion of a coronary artery in the dog. Arch Pathol 70: 68–78

Jeremovich M, Barbijeri M, Kovacević D, Arambasić M, Karteljević G, Natalić D J, Pazin S 1990 Identification of neuroendocrine oxytocic activity of the human fetal thymus. Thymus 15: 181–185

Jessell T M, Bovolenta P, Placzek M, Tessier-Lavigne M, Dodd J 1989 Polarity and patterning the neural tube: the origin and function of the floor plate. In: Wolpert (ed) Cellular basis of morphogenesis. CIBA Foundation Symposium 144. Wiley: Chichester: pp 255–280

Jessell T M, Melton D A Diffusible factors in vertebrate embryonic induction. Cell 68: 257–270

Jessen K R, Burnstock G 1982 The enteric nervous system in tissue culture: a new mammalian model for the study of complex nervous networks. In: Kalsner S (ed) Trends in autonomic pharmacology. Vol II. Urban and Schwartzenberg: Baltimore: pp 95–115

Jessen K R, Mirsky R 1992 Schwann cells: early lineage, regulation of proliferation and control of myelin formation. Curr Opin Neurobiol 2: 575–581

Jiao S, Gurevich V, Wolff J A 1993 Long-term correction of rat model of Parkinson's disease by gene therapy. Nature 362: 450–453

Jimbow K, Fitzpatrick T B, Wick M M 1991 Biochemistry and physiology of melanin pigmentation. In: Goldsmith L A (ed) Physiology, biochemistry, and molecular biology of skin. 2nd edition. 2 vols. Oxford University Press: Oxford: pp 873–909

Jin Z M, Dowson D, Fisher J 1992 The effect of porosity of articular cartilage on the lubrication of a normal human hip joint. Proc Inst Mech Eng H 206: 117–124

Jinnai K, Nambu A, Tanibuchi I, Yoshida S 1993 Cerebello- and pallido-thalamic pathways to areas 6 and 4 in the monkey. Stereotact Func Neurosurg 60: 70–79

Jit I 1952 The development and the structure of the suspensory muscle of the duodenum. Anat Rec 113: 395–407

Jit I 1961 The structure and development of the valves of Houston. Ind J Med Res 49: 635–647

Jit I 1974 Muscularis submucosae ani and its development. J Anat 118: 11–17

Jit I, Bakshi V 1984 Incidence of sterna foramina in North India. J Anat Soc Ind 33: 77–84

Jit I, Charnalia J 1959 The vertebral level of the termination of the spinal cord. J Anat Soc Ind 8: 93–101

Jit I, Gandhi O P 1966 The value of pre-auricular sulcus in sexing bony pelves. J Anat Soc Ind 15: 104–107

Jit I, Grewal S S 1975 Lengths of the small and large intestines in north Indian subjects. J Anat Ind 24: 89–100

Jit I, Grewal S S 1977 The suspensory muscle of the duodenum and its nerve supply. J Anat 123: 397–405

Jit I, Harjeet 1982 Sternal angle. J Anat Soc Ind 31: 115–117

Jit I, Jhingan V, Kulkarni M 1980 Sexing the human sternum. Am J Phys Antrhopol 53: 217–224

Jit I, Kulkaria M 1976 Times of appearance and fusion of epiphysis at the medial end of the clavicle. Ind J Med Res 64: 773–782

Jit I, Mukerjee R N 1960 Observations on the anatomy of the human thoracic sympathetic chain and its branches, with an antomical assessment of operations for hypertension. J Anat Soc Ind 9: 55–82

Jit I, Sahni D 1983 Sexing the North Indian clavicles. J Anat Soc Ind 32: 61–72

Jit I, Singh S 1956 Estimation of stature from clavicles. Ind J Med Res 44: 137–155

Jit I, Singh S 1966 The sexing of the adult clavicles. Ind J Med Res 54: 551–571

Jockusch B M, Wiegand Ch, Temm-Grove C J, Nikolai G 1993 Dynamic aspects of microfilament-membrane attachments. In: Jones G, Wigley C, Warn R (eds) Cell behaviour: adhesion and motility, Society for Experimental Biology Symposium no. 47. Company of Biologists Ltd: Cambridge: pp 253–266

Johannisson E 1968 The foetal adrenal cortex in the human. Its ultrastructure at different stages of development and in different functional states. Acta Endocr Copnh 58: (suppl 130)

Johansen K, Burggren W 1980 Cardiovascular function in the lower vertebrates. In: Bourne G H (ed) Hearts and heart-like organs. Vol 1. Academic Press: New York: pp 61–117

Johansson R S, Vallbo A B Detection of tactile stimuli. J Physiol 297: 405–422

Johns B A 1952 Developmental changes in the oesophageal epithelium in man. J Anat 86: 431–442

Johnson A D 1977 The influence of cadmium on the testis. In: Johnson A D, Gomes L R (eds) The testis. Vol 4. Advances in physiology, biochemistry and function. Academic Press: New York: pp 565–576

Johnson A D, Gomes W R (eds) 1977 The testis. Vol 4. Advances in physiology, biochemistry and function. Academic Press: New York

Johnson A R 1993 Contact inhibition in the failure of mammalian CNS axonal regeneration. Bioessays 15: 807 – 813

Johnson A, Josephson R, Hawke M 1985 Clinical and histological evidence for the presence of a vomeronasal (Jacobson's) organ in adult humans. J Otolaryngol 14: 71–79

Johnson C E, Basmajian J V, Dasher W 1972 Electromyography of sartorius muscle. Anat Rec 173: 127–130

Johnson C L, Holbrook K A 1989 Development of human embryonic and fetal vasculature. J Invest Dermatol 93: 10S–17S

Johnson E F, Berryman R, Mitchell R, Wood W B 1985 Elastic fibres in anulus fibrosus of the adult human intervertebral disc. A preliminary report. J Anat 143: 57–63

Johnson E M, Taniuchi M, DiStefano P S 1988 Expression and possible function of nerve growth factor receptors on Schwann cells. Trends Neurosci 11: 299–304

Johnson F P 1914 The development of the rectum in the human embryo. Am J Anat 16: 1–58

Johnson F R, McMinn R M H, Artfield G N 1968 Ultrastructural and biochemical observations on the tympanic membrane. J Anat 103: 297–310

Johnson F R, McMinn R M H, Birchenough R F 1962 The ultrastructure of the gall bladder spithelium of the dog. J Anat 96: 477–487

Johnson F, Waugh W 1979 Method for routine clinical assessment of knee joint forces. Med Biol Eng Comp 17: 145–154

Johnson H M, Downs M O, Pontzer C H 1992 Neuroendocrine peptide hormone regulation of immunity. In: Blalock J E (ed) Neuro-immunoendocrinology. Karger: Basel: pp 9–74

Johnson K A, Rosenbaum J L 1992 Replication of basal bodies. Curr Opin Cell Biol 4: 80–85

Johnson L, Zane R S, Petty C S, Neaves W B 1984 Quantification of the human Sertoli cell population: its distribution, relation to germ cell numbers and age-related decline. Biol Reprod 31: 785–795

Johnson M A, Polgar J, Weightman D, Appleton D 1973 Data on the distribution of fibre types in thirty-six human muscles: an autopsy study. J Neurol Sci 18: 111–129

Johnson M H et al 1986 A role for cytoplasmic determinants in the development of the mouse embryo? J Embryol Exp Morph (suppl) 97: 97–121

Johnson M, Comaish J S, Shuster S 1991 Nail is produced by the normal nail bed: a controversy resolved. Br J Dermatol 125: 27–29

Johnson R M, Hart D L, Simmon E F, Ramsby G R 1977 Cervical orthoses: a study comparing their effectiveness in restricting cervical motion in normal subjects. J Bone Jt Surg 59A: 332–339

Johnson S J, Hines J E, Burt A D Immunolocalization of proliferating perisinusoidal cells I rat liver. Histochem J 24: 67–72

Johnston J B 1909 The morphology of the forebrain vesicle in vertebrates. J Comp Neurol 19: 458–539

Jones A K P, Brown W D, Friston K J, Qi L Y, Frackowiak R S J 1991 Cortical and subcortical localization of response to pain in man using positron emission tomography. Proc R Soc Lond Series B 244: 39–44

Jones A L, Fawcett D W 1966 Hypertrophy of the agranular endoplasmic reticulum in hamster liver induced by plenobarbital (with a review on the functions of this organelle in liver). J Histochem Cytochem 14: 215–232

Jones A L, Schmucker D L, Lausier J 1991 Electron microscopy of the liver. In: McIntyre N, Benhamou J-P, Bircher J, Rizzetto M, Rodes M J (eds) Oxford textbok of clinical hepatology, Vol 1. Oxford university Press: Oxford: pp 20–28

Jones A W 1981 Vascular smooth muscle and alterations during hypertension. In: Bülbring E, Brading A F, Jones A W, Tomito T (eds) Smooth muscle: an assessment of current knowledge. Edward Arnold: London: pp 397–429

Jones C J P, Fox H 1991 Ultrastructure of the normal human placenta. Electron Microscopy Reviews 4: 129–178

Jones D A, Round J M 1990 Skeletal muscle in health and disease. Manchester University Press: Manchester

Jones D G 1978 Some current concepts of synaptic organization. Adv Anat Embryol Cell Biol 55: 3–69

Jones D T, Reed R R 1989 Golf: an olfactory neuron-specific G-protein involved in odorant signal transduction. Science 244: 790–795

Jones E G 1981 Anatomy of cerebral cortex: columnar input-output organization. In: Schmitt F O, Worden F G, Adelman G, Dennis S G (eds) The organization of the cerebral cortex. MIT Press: Cambridge: pp 199–235

Jones E G 1984 Laminar distribution of cortical efferent cells. In: Peters A, Jones E G (eds) Cerebral cortex. Vol 1. Cellular components of the cerebral cortex. Plenum Press: New York: pp 521–553

Jones E G 1984 Neurogliaform of spiderweb cells. In: Peters A, Jones E G, (eds) Cerebral cortex. Vol 1. Cellular components of the cerebral cortex. Plenum Press: New York: pp 409–418

Jones E G 1985 The thalamus. Plenum Press: New York: pp 403–411

Jones E G 1986 Connectivity of the primate sensory-motor cortex. In: Jones E G, Peters A (eds) Cerebral cortex. Vol 5. Sensory-motor areas and aspects of cortical connectivity. Plenum Press: New York: pp 113–183

Jones E G, Burton H, Porter R 1975 Commissural and cortico-cortical 'columns' in the somatic sensory cortex of primates. Science 190: 572–574

Jones E G, Hartman, B K 1978 Recent advances in neuroanatomical methodology. Annu Rev Neurosc I: 215–296

Jones E G, Hendry S H C 1984 Basket cells. In: Peters A, Jones E G, (eds) Cerebral cortex. Vol 1. Cellular components of the cerebral cortex. Plenum Press: New York: pp 309–336

Jones E G, Hendry S H C, Defelipe J 1987 GABA-peptide neurons of the primate cerebral cortex: a limited cell class. In: Jones E G, Peters A (eds) Cerebral cortex. Vol 6. Further aspects of cortical function, including hippocampus. Plenum Press: New York: pp 237–266

Jones E G, Powell T P S 1968 The ipsilateral cortical connexions of the somatic sensory areas in the cat. Brain Res 9: 71–94

Jones E G, Powell T P S 1969 Connexions of the somatic sensory cortex of the rhesus monkey. I. Ipsilateral cortical connexions. Brain 92: 447–502

Jones E G, Powell T P S 1970 An anatomical study of converging sensory pathways within the cerebral cortex of the monkey. Brain 93: 793–820

Jones E G, Wise S P 1977 Size, laminar and columnar distribution of efferent cells in the sensory-motor cortex of monkeys. J Comp Neurol 175: 391–438

Jones F W 1911 On the grooves upon the ossa parietalia commonly said to be caused by the arteria meningea media. J Anat 46: 228–238

Jones F W 1912 Some nerve markings on lumber vertebrae. J Anat 47: 118–120

Jones F W 1913 The function of the coelom and diaphragm. J Anat 47: 282–318

Jones F W 1931 The neo-metrical morphological characters of the skull as criteria for racial diagnosis. I. General discussion of the morphological characters employed in racial diagnosis. II. The non-metrical morphological characters of the Hawaiian skull. III. The non-metrical morphological characters of the prehistoric inhabitants of Guam. J Anat 65: 179–195, 368–378, 438–445

Jones F W 1939a The anterior superior alveolar nerve and vessels. J Anat 73: 583–591

Jones F W 1939b The so-called maxillary antrum of the gorilla. J Anat 74: 116–119

Jones F W 1941 The principles of anatomy as seen in the hand. Baillière, Tindall and Cox: London

Jones F W 1949 Structure and function as seen in the foot. Baillière, Tindall and Cox: London

Jones I C 1957 The adrenal cortex. Cambridge University Press: Cambridge

Jones M M, Amis A A 1988 The fibrous flexor sheaths of the fingers. J Anat 156: 185–196

Jones R L 1937 Cell fibre ratio in the vagus nerve. J Comp Neurol 67: 469–482

Jones R L 1941 The human foot. An experimental study of its mechanics, and the role of its muscles and ligaments in the support of the arch. Am J Anat 68: 1–40

Jones S J, Boyde A 1972 A study of human root cementum surfaces as prepared for and examined in the scanning electron microscope. Z Zellforsch Mikrosk Anat 130: 318–337

Jones S J, Gray C, Sakamaki H, Arora M, Boyde A, Gourdie R, Green C 1993 The incidence and size of gap junctions between the bone cells in rat calvaria. Anat Embryol 187: 343–352

Jonsson B 1974 Function of the erector spinae muscle on different working levels. Acta Morph Neerl Scand 12: 211–214

Jonsson B, Hagberg M 1974 The effect of different working heights on the deltoid muscle. Scand J Rehab Med Suppl 3: 26–32

Jonsson B, Steen B 1962 Function of the hip and thigh muscles in Romberg's test and 'standing at ease'. Acta Morph Neerl Scand 5: 267–276

Jordan D R 1992 The orbital muscle of Muller. Archs Ophthalmol 110: 1798–1799

Jordan R K, McFarlane B, Scothorne R J 1973 An electron microscopic study of the histogensis of the ultimobranchial body and of the C-cell system in the sheep. J Anat 114: 115–136

Jordan T, Hanson I, Zaletayev D, Hodgson S, Prosser J Seawright A, Hastie N, van Heyningen V 1992 The human Pax6 gene is mutated in two patients with aniridia. Nature Genetics 1: 328–332

Joseph J 1951 Further studies of the metacarpophalangeal and interphalangeal joints of the thumb. J Anat 85: 221–229

Joseph J 1960 Man's posture: electromyographic studies. Thomas: Springfield, Illinois

Joseph J 1975 Movements at the hip joint. Am R Coll Surg 56: 192–201

Joseph J 1991 The bones, joints and ligaments of the female pelvis. In: Philipp E, Setchell M, Ginsburg J (eds) Scientific foundations of obstetrics and gynaecology. Butterworth-Heinemann: Oxford: pp 74–83

Joseph J, Nightingale A, Williams P L 1955 Detailed study of electric potentials recorded over some postural muscles while relaxed and standing. J Physiol 127: 617–625

Joseph J, Williams P L 1957 Electromyography of certain hip muscles. J Anat 91: 286–294

Joseph S A, Knigge K M 1978 The endocrine hypothalamus: recent anatomical studies. In: Reichlin S, Baldessarine R J, Martin J B (eds) The hypothalamus. Research publications. Vol 56. Association for research in nervous and mental disease. Raven Press: New York: pp 15–47

Joshi H C 1994 Microtubule organizing centres and g-tubulin. Curr Opin Cell Biol 6: 55–62

Josso N, Picard J Y 1986 Anti-mullerian hormone. Physiol Rev 66: 1038–1090

Jousselin-Hosaja M, Mailly P, Tsuji S 1993 Mouse adrenal chromaffin cells can transform to neuron-like cholinergic phenotypes after being grafted into the brain. Cell Tissue Res 274: 199–205

Jovanović S, Zivanović S 1965 The establishment of the sex by the great sciatic notch. Acta Anat 61: 101–107

Ju G, Liu S-J 1989 Substance P-like immunoreactive nerve fibres in the pars distalis of the anterior pituitary of macaques. J Chem Neuroanat 2: 349–360

Judge S J, Cumming B G 1986 Neurons in the monkey midbrain with activity related to vergence eye movements and accomodation. J Neurophysiol 55: 915–930

Jungers W L, Meldrum D J, Stern J T Jr 1993 The functional and evolutionary significance of the human peroneus tertius muscle. J Hum Evol 25: 377–386

K

Kaar G F, Fraher J P 1986 The sheaths surrounding the attachments of rat lumbar ventral roots to the spinal cord: a light and electron microscopical study. J Anat 148: 137–146

Kaas J H 1990 Somatosensory system. In: Paxinos G (ed) The human nervous system. Academic Press: San Diego: pp 813–844

Kaas J H, Morel A 1993 Connections of visual areas of the upper temporal lobe of owl monkeys: the MT crescent and dorsal and ventral subdivisions of FST. J Neurosci 13: 534–546

Kaas J H, Nelson R J, Sur M, Lin C, Merzenich M M 1979 Multiple representations of the body within the primary somatosensory cortex of primates. Science 204: 521–523

Kaehn K, Jacob J H, Christ B, Hinrichsen K, Poelmann R E 1988 The onset of myotome formation in the chick. Anat Embryol 177: 191–201

Kagayama M, Nishiyama A 1972 Comparative aspect on the innervation of submandibular glands in cat and rabbit; an electron microscopic study. Tohuku J Exp Med 108: 179–193

Kahrilas P J 1993 Hiatus hernia causes reflux: fact or fiction? Gullet 3: 21–30

Kaiserling E, Stein H, Müller-Hermelink H K 1974 Interdigitating reticulum cells in the human thymus. Cell Tissue Res 155: 47–55

Kalcheim C 1989 Basic fibroblast growth factor stimulates survival of noneuronal cells developing from trunk neural crest. Dev Biol 134 1–10

Kalcheim C, Barde Y A, Theonen H, Le Douarin N M, 1987 In vivo effect of brain-derived neurotrophic factor on the survival of developing dorsal root ganglion cells. EMBO J 6: 2871–2873

Kalcheim C, Le Douarin N M 1986 Requirement of a neural tube signal for the differentiation of neural crest cells into dorsal root ganglia. Dev Biol 116: 451–466

Kalcheim C, Neufeld G 1990 Expression of basic fibroblast growth factor in the nervous system of early avian embryos. Development. 109: 203–215

Kalcheim C, Teillet M A 1989 Consequences of somite manipulation on the pattern of dorsal root ganglion development. Development 106: 85–93

Kalebic T, Garbisa S, Glaser B, Liotta L A 1983 Basement membrane collagen: degradation by migrating endothelial cells. Science, 221: 281–283

Kalia M. Mesulam M M 1980a Brainstem projections of sensory and motor components of the vagus complex in the cat. I. The cervical vagus and nodose ganglion. J Comp Neurol 193: 435–465

Kalia M, Mesulam M M 1980b Brainstem projections of sensory and motor components of the vagus somplex in the cat. II. Laryngeal, tracheobronchial, pulmonary, cardiac and gastrointestinal branches. J Comp Neurol 193: 467–508

Kalia M, Richter D 1985 Morphology of physiologically identified slowly adapting lung stretch receptor afferents stained with intra-axonal horseradish peroxidase in the nucleus of the tractus solitarius of the cat. I. A light microscopic analysis. J Comp Neurol 241: 503–520

Kalinec F, Holley M C, Iwasa K H, Lim D J, Kachar B 1992 A membrane-based force generation mechanism in auditory sensory cells. Proc Natl Acad Sci USA 89: 8671–8675

Kamath S 1981 Observations on the length and diameter of vessels forming the circle of Willis. J Anat 133: 419–423

Kameda Y 1971 The occurrence and distribution of the parafollicular cells in the thyroid, parathyroid IV and thymus IV in some mammals. Arch Histol Jpn 33: 283–299

Kameda Y 1976 Fine structural and endocrinological aspects of thyroid parafollicular cells. In: Coupland R E, Fujita T (eds) Chromaffin, enterochromaffin and related cells. Elsevier: New York: pp 155–170

Kamm M A 1994 Motility and functional diseases of the large intestine. Curr Opin Gastoenterol 10: 11–18

Kamperdijk E (ed) Dendritic cells in fundamental and clinical immunology. Advances in Experimental Medicine and Biology 329. Plenum: London

Kampmeier O F 1969 Evolution and comparative morphology of the lymphatic system. Thomas: Springfield, Illinois

Kanagasuntheram R 1957 Development of the human lesser sac. J Anat 91: 188–206

Kanagasuntheram R 1960 Some observations on the development of the human duodenum. J Anat 94: 231–240

Kanagasuntheram R 1967 A note on the development of the tubotympanic recess in the human embryo. J Anat 101: 731–742

Kanagasuntheram R 1970 Some unresolved mysteries in the anatomy of the visual system. Singapore Med J 11: 63–70

Kanagasuntheram R, Kin L S 1970 Observations on some anomalies of the colon. Singapore Med J 11: 110–117

Kanavel A B 1925 Infections of the hand. London: Baillière Tindall & Co: pp 100–110

Kandel E R, Schwartz J H, Jessell T M 1991 Principles of neural science 3rd edition. Elsevier: Amsterdam

Kaneko T, Caria M A, Asanuma H 1994a Information processing within the motor cortex. II. Intracortical connections between neurons receiving somatosensory cortical input and motor output neurons of the cortex. J Comp Neurol 345: 172–184

Kaneko T, Caria M A, Asanuma H 1994b Information processing within the motor cortex. I. Responses of morphologically identified motor cortical cells to stimulation of the somatosensory cortex. J Comp Neurol 345: 161–171

Kanerva L, Hervonen A, Hervonen H 1974 Morphological characteristics of the ontogenesis of the mammalian peripheral adrenergic nervous system with special remarks on the human fetus. Med Biol 52: 144–158

Kanno T 1973 Unidirectional cellular processes in stimulus-secretion coupling in cells of the GEP system. In: Fujita T (ed) Gastro-enteropancreatic endocrine system. A cell-biological approach. Igaku Shoiu: Tokyo: pp 64–70

Kapandji I A 1963 Physiologie articulaire. Fascicule I. Membre supérieur. Maloine: Paris

Kapandji I A 1970–1974 The physiology of the joints. Annotated diagrams of the mechanics of the human joints. 2nd edition. (3 vols translated by L H Honoré: Vol 1 upper limb. Vol 2 lower limb. Vol 3 the trunk and the vertebral column.) Churchill Livingstone: Edinburgh

Kapeller K, Mayor D 1967 The accumulation of noradrenaline in constricted sympathetic nerves as studies by fluorescence and electron microscopy. Proc R Soc Lond [Biol] 167: 282–292

Kapfhammer J P, Grunewald B E, Raper J A 1986 J Neurosci 6: 2527–2534

Kaplan E B 1957 Discoid lateral meniscus of the knee joint: nature, mechanism and operative treatment. J Bone Jt Surg 39A: 77–87

Kaplan E B 1958 The ilotibial tract. Clinical and morphological significance. J. Bone Jt Surg 40A: 817–831

Kaplan E B 1965 Functional and surgical anatomy of the hand. 2nd edition. Pitman Medical: London

Kaplan G P, Hartman B K, Creveling C R 1981 Localization of catechol-O-methyltransferase in the leptomeninges, choroid plexus and ciliary epithelium: implications for the separation of central and peripheral catechols. Brain Res 204: 353–360

Kaplan H A 1956 Arteries of the brain; anatomic study. Acta Radiol 46: 364–470

Kaplan H A, Browder A, Browder J 1973 Nasal venous drainage and the foramen caecum. Laryngoscope 83: 327–9

Kaplan H A, Browder A, Krieger A J 1976 Intercavernous connections of the cavernous sinuses. The superior and inferior circular sinuses. J Neurosurg 45: 166–168

Kaplan H A, Ford D H 1966 The brain vascular system. Elsevier: Amsterdam

Kaplan P, Grumbach M M, Shepard T H 1972 The ontogenesis of human fetal hormones. I. Growth hormone and insulin. J Clin Invest 51: 3080–3093

Kappers C U A 1921 On structural laws in the nervous system; the principles of neurobiotaxis. Brain 44: 125–149

Kappers C U A 1934 Differences in the effect of various impulses on the structure of the central nervous system. Ir J Med Sci 105: 495–519

Kappers J A 1960 The development, topographical relations and innervation of the epiphysis cerebri in the albino rat. Z Zellforsch 52: 163–215

Kappers J A 1976 The mammalian pineal gland. A survey. Acta Neurochir Genesskd 120: 109–149

Karasek M 1976 Quantitative changes in number of 'synaptic' ribbons in rat pinealocytes after orchidectomy and in organ culture. J Neurol Transm 38: 149–157

Karim O M, Pienta K, Seki N, Mostwin J L 1992 Stretch-mediated visceral smooth muscle growth in vitro. Am J Physiol 262: R895–900

Kariniemi A L, Lehto V P, Vartio T, Virtanen I 1982 Cytoskeleton and pericellular matrix organization of pure adult human keratinocytes cultured from suction-blister roof epidermis. J Cell Sci 58: 49–61

Karpati G, Pouliot Y, Zubrzycka G E, Carpenter S, Ray P N, Worton R G, Holland P 1989 Dystrophin is expressed in mdx skeletal fibres after normal myoblast implantation. Am J Pathol 135: 27–32

Karrer H E 1956 The ultrastructure of mouse lung. General architecture of capillary and alveolar walls. J Biophys Biochem Cytol 2: 241–252

Kasai T, Chiba S 1977 True nature of the muscular arch of the axilla and its nerve supply. Kaibogaku Zasshi 25: 657–669

Kashef R 1966 The node of Ranvier. PhD thesis. University of London

Kashiwayanagi M, Kurihara K 1987 Cell suspensions from porcine olfactory mucosa J Gen Physiol 89: 443–457

Kate B R 1968 The torsion of the humerus in central India. J Ind Anthropol Soc 3: 17–30

Kate B R, Robert S L 1965 Some observations on the upper end of the tibia in squatters. J Anat 99: 137–142

Katirji B, Hardy R W Jr 1995 Classic neurogenic thoracic outlet syndrome in a competitive swimmer: a true scalenus anticus syndrome. Muscle Nerve 18: 229–233

Katschenko N 1888 Anat Anz 445

Katz A D, Catalano P 1987 The clinical significance of the various anastomotic branches of the facial nerve. Otolaryngol Head Neck Surg 113: 959–962

Katz B, Miledi R 1965 The effect of calcium on acetylcholine release from motor nerve terminals. Proc R Soc Lond [Biol] 161: 496–503

Katz D M, Karten H J 1985 Topographic representation of visceral target organs within the dorsal motor nucleus of the vagus nerve of the pigeon, columba livia. J Comp Neurol 242: 397–414

Katz E P, Li S T 1973 Structure and function of bone collagen fibrils. J Mol Biol 80: 1–15

Katz E P, Wachtel E, Yamauchi M, Mechanic G L 1989 The structure of mineralised collagen fibrils. Connect Tissue Res 21: 149–158

Katz S I, Tamaki K, Sachs D H 1979 Epidermal Langerhans' cells are derived from cells which originate in bone marrow. Nature 282: 324–326

Kauer J M G 1974 The interdependence of carpal articulation chains. Acta Anat 88: 481–501

Kauffman S A, Shymko R, Trabert K 1978 Control of sequential compartment formation in Drosophila. Science 199: 259–270

Kaufman J M, Deslypere J P, Giri M, Vermeulan A 1990 Neuroendocrine regulation of pulsatile luteinizing hormone secretion in elderly men. J Steroid Biochem Mol Biol 37: 421–430

Kaufman M H, Navaratnam V 1981 Early differentiation of the heart in mouse embryos. J Anat 133: 235–246

Kauppinen R A, Williams S R, Busza A L, van Bruggen N 1993 Applications of magnetic resonance spectroscopy and diffusion-weighted imaging to the study of brain biochemistry and pathology. TINS 16: 88–95

Kawabata I, Paparella M M 1969 Ultrastructure of normal human middle ear mucosa. Preliminary report. Ann Otol Rhinol Laryngol 78: 125–138

Kawamata S, Harada Y, Tagashira N 1986 Electron microscopic study of the vestibular dark cells in the crista ampullaris of the guinea pig. Acta Otolaryngol [Stockh] 102: 168–174

Kawamura K 1975 The pontine projection from the inferior colliculus in the cat. An experimental anatomical study. Brain Res 95: 309–322

Kawamura K, Brodal A 1973 The tectopontine projection in the cat: an experimental anatomical study with comments on pathways for teleceptive impulses to the cerebellum. J Comp Neurol 149: 371–390

Kawamura K, Hashikawa T 1981 Projections from the pontine nuclei proper and reticular tegmental nucleus on to the cerebellar cortex in the cat: an autoradiographic study. J Comp Neurol 201: 395–413

Kawasaki H, Kretsinger R H 1994 Calcium-binding proteins 1 : EF hands. Protein Profile 1: 343–517

Kawashima I, Seiki K, Sakabe K, Ihara S, Akatsuka A, Katsumata Y 1992 Localization of estrogen receptors and estrogen receptor-mRNA in female mouse thymus. Thymus 20: 115–121

Kaye G I, Wheeler H O, Whitlock R T, Lane N 1966 Fluid transport in the rabbit gall bladder. A combined physiological and electron microscopic study. J Cell Biol 30: 237–268

Keagy R D, Brumlik J, Bergan J L 1966 Direct electromyography of the psoas major muscle in man. J Bone Jt Surg 48A: 1377–1382

Keane J R 1988 Isolated brainstem third nerve palsy. Arch Neurol 45: 813–814

Keating P, Lahiri A 1993 Fronted velars, palatalized velars and palatals. Phonetica 50(2): 73–101

Keegan J J, Garrett F D 1948 The segmental distribution of the cutaneous nerves in the limbs of man. Anat Rec 102: 409–437

Keelan E, Haskard D O 1992 CAMs and anti-CAMs. The clinical potential of cell adhesion molecules. J R Coll Phys Lon 26: 17–24

Keen J A 1950 Study of differences between male and female skulls. Am J Phys Anthropol 8: 65–79

Keene M F L 1961 Muscle spindle in human laryngeal muscles. J Anat 95: 25–29

Keene M F L, Hewer E E 1927 Observations on the development of the human suprarenal gland. J Anat 61: 302–324

Keene M F L, Hewer E E 1935 The sub-commissural organ and the mesocoelic recess in the human brain, with a note on Reissner's fibre. J Anat 69: 501–507

Kefalides N A 1973 Structure and biosynthesis of basement membranes. In: Hall D A, Jackson D S (eds) International review of connective tissue research. Vol 6. Academic Press: New York: pp 63–104

Keith A 1924 Fate of the bulbus cordis in the human heart. Lancet 2: 1267–1273

Keith Sir A 1948 Human embryology and morphology. 6th edition. Arnold: London

Keizer K, Kuypers H G J M, Ronday H K 1987 Branching cortical neurons in cat which project to the colliculi and to the pons: a retrograde fluorescent double-labelling study. Exp Brain Res 67: 1–15

Keleman E, Calvo W, Fliedner T M 1979 Atlas of human hemopoietic development. Springer Verlag: Berlin

Keller E L, Heinen S J 1991 Generation of smooth-pursuit eye movements: neuronal mechanisms and pathways. Neurosci Res 11: 79–107

Keller J T, Saunders M C, Van Loveren H, Shipley M T 1984 Neuroanatomical considerations of palatal muscles: tensor and levator veli palatini. Cleft Palate J 21: 70–75

Keller R E 1975 Vital dye mapping of the gastrula and neurula of *Xenopus laevis* I. Prospective areas and morphogenetic movements of the superficial layer. Devl Biol 42: 222–241

Keller R E 1976 Vital dye mapping of the gastrula and neurula of *Xenopus laevis*. II. Prospective areas and morphogenetic movements of the deep layer. Devl Biol 51: 118–137

Keller R E 1984 The cellular basis of gastrulation in Xenopus laevis: active post involution convergence and extension by mediolateral interdigitation. Am Zool 24: 589–603

Keller R E 1985 In: Browder L W (ed) The cellular basis of amphibian gastrulation. Developmental biology. Plenum: New York: 2: 241–327

Keller T C S III 1995 Structure and function of titin and nebulin. Curr Opin Cell Biol 7: 32–38

Kellerhals B, Engström H, Ades H W 1967 Die Morphologic des Ganglion spirale cochleae. Acta Otolaryngol [Stockh] Suppl 226: 1–78

Kelley A E, Domesick V B, Nauta W J H 1982 The amygdalostriatal projection in the rat – an anatomical study by anterograde and retrograde tracing methods. Neuroscience 7: 615–630

Kember N F 1983 Cell kinetics of cartilage. In: Hall B K (ed) Cartilage. Vol 1. Structure, function and biochemistry. Academic Press: New York: pp 149–180

Kemper T L, Galaburda A M 1984 Principles of cytoarchitectonics. In: Peters A, Jones E G (eds) Cerebral cortex. Vol 1. Cellular components of the cerebral cortex. Plenum Press: New York: pp. 35–57

Kendall M D 1989 The morphology of perivascular spaces in the thymus. Thymus 13: 157–164

Kendall M D 1990 The cell biology of cell death in the thymus. Thymus Update 3: 53–76

Kendall M D 1991 Functional anatomy of the thymic microenvironment. J Anat 117: 1–29

Kendall M D (ed) 1981 The Thymus Gland (Anatomical Society of Great Britain and Ireland, Symposium 1). Academic Press: London

Kendall M D, Al-Shawaf A 1991 Current knowledge on the innervation of the rat thymus gland. BBI 5: 9–28

Kendall M D, Morgan G, Billingsley S A, Clarke A 1989 An immuno-EM study of epithelial cells, macrophages and phagocytosis in the mouse thymus. In: Imhof B A, Berrih-Aknin S, Ezine S (eds) Lymphatic tissues and in vivo immune responses. Dekker: New York: pp 95–99

Kenny M 1944 The clinically suspect pelvis and its radiographical investigation in 1,000 cases. J Obstet Gynaecol Br Commonw 51: 277–292

Ker R F 1981 Dynamic tensile properties of the plantaris tendon of sheep (Ovis aries). J Exp Biol 93: 283–302

Ker R F, Bennett M B, Bibby S R, Kester R C, Alexander R McN 1987 The spring in the arch of the human foot. Nature 325: 147–149

Ker R F, Bennett M B, Kester R C, Alexander R McN 1989 Foot strike and the properties of the human heel pad. Proc. Instn Mech Engrs 203: 191–196

Kerckring T T 1970 Spicilegium anatomicum A Frisius: Amsterdam

Kerjaschki D, Hörander H 1976 The development of mouse olfactory vesicles and their cell contacts. A freeze-etching study. J Ultrastruct Res 54: 420–444

Kernell D 1986 Organization and properties of spinal motoneurones and motor units. In: Freund H J, Buttner U, Cohen B, Noth J (eds) Progress in Brain Res 64, Elsevier Science Publishers: Amsterdam: pp 21–30

Kerr F W L 1962 Facial, vagal and glossopharyngeal nerves in the cat. Afferent connexions. Arch Neurol Psychiatry 6: 264–281

Kerr F W L Preserved vagal visceromotor function following destruction of the dorsal motor nucleus J Physiol 202: 755–769

Kerr F W L, Hollowell O W 1964 Location of pupillomotor and accommodation fibres in the oculomotor nerve: experimental observations on paralytic mydriasis. J Neurol Neurosurg Psychiat 27: 473–481

Kerr J B 1991 Ultrastructure of the seminiferous epithelium and intertubular tissue of the human testis. J Electron Microsc Tech 19: 215–240

Kessel M, Gruss P 1991 Homeotic transformations of murine prevertebrae and concomitant alteration of Hox codes induced by retinoic acid. Cell 67: 89–104

Kessling S V 1968 Mucous gland system of the conjunctiva. A quantitative normal anatomic study. Acta Ophthalmologica (Suppl 95)

Keswani N H, Hollinshead W H 1956 Localisation of the phrenic nucleus in the spinal cord of man. Anat Rec 125: 683–700

Kettenmann H, Banati R, Waltz W 1993 Electrophysiological behaviour of microglia. Glia 7: 93 – 101

Kettlekamp D B, Jacobs A W 1972 Tibiofemoral contact area: determination and implications. J Bone Jt Surg 54A: 349–356

Kevetter G A, Haber L H, Yerierski R P, Chung J M, Martin R F, Willis W D 1982 Cells of origin of the spinoreticular tract in monkeys. J Comp Neurol 207: 61–74

Key B, Akesson R A 1990b Olfactory neurons express a unique glycosylated form of the neural adhesion molecule (N-CAM). J Cell Biol 110: 1729–1743

Key J A 1932 The synovial membrane of joints and bursaw. In: Cowdry E V (ed) Special cytology. The form and functions of the cell in health and disease. 2nd edition. Paul B Hoeber: New York: pp 1055–1086

Keynes G 1954 The physiology of the thymus gland. Br Med J 2: 659–663

Keynes R J, Stern C D 1984 Nature 310: 786–789

Keynes R J, Stern C D 1986 Somites and neural development. In: Bellairs R, Ede D A, Lash J W (eds) Somites in developing embryos. NATO ASI Series: Series A: Life Sciences. Plenum Press: New York: pp 289–299

Keynes R, Stern C 1988 Mechanisms of vertebrate segmentation. Development 103: 413–429

Khaledpour C 1984 Eine anatomische Variation des Nervus alveolaris inferior beim Menschen. Anat Anz 156: 403–456

Khaner O, Eyal-Giladi H 1989 The chick's marginal zone and primitive streak formation. I. Coordination effect of induction and inhibition. Dev Biol 134: 206–214

Khong T Y 1991 The Robertson-Brosens-Dixon hypothesis: evidence for the role of haemochorial placentation in pregnancy success. Br J Obstet Gynaecol 98: 1195–1199

Khoo F Y, Kanagasuntheram R, Chia K B 1969 Variations of the lateral recesses of the naso-pharynx. Arch Otolaryngol 88: 456–462

Kiang N Y S, Liberman M C, Gage J S, Northrop C C, Dodds L W, Oliver M E 1984 Afferent innervation of the mammalian cochlea. In: Bolis L, Keynes R D, Maddrell S H P (eds) Comparative physiology of sensory systems. Cambridge University Press: pp 143–161

Kibbelaar M A, Panaekers F C S, Ringers P J et al 1980 Is actin in eye lens a possible factor for visual accommodation? Nature 285: 505–508

Kida S, Ellison D W, Steart P V, Weller R O 1995 Characterisation of perivascular cells in astrocytic tumors and peritumoral edematous brain. Neuropathol Appl Neurobiol 21: 121–129

Kida S, Pantazis A, Weller R O 1993b CSF drains directly from the subarachnoid space into nasal lymphatics in the rat. Anatomy, histology and immunological significance. Neuropath Appl Neurobiol 19: 480–488

Kida S, Steart P V, Zhang E-T, Weller R O 1993a Perivascular cells act as scavengers in the cerebral perivascular spaces and remain distinct from pericytes, microglia and macrophages. Acta Neuropathologica 85: 646–652

Kida S, Weller R O 1994 Morphology of CSF drainage pathways in man. In: Raimondi A (ed) Principles of Pediatric Neurosurgery. Vol 4. Springer: Berlin

Kida S, Yamashima T, Kubota T, Ito H, Yamamoto S 1988 A light and electron microscopic and immunohistochemical study of human arachnoid villi. J Neurosurg 69: 429–435

Kiddo D K, Gomez D G, Pavese A M, Potts D G 1976 Human spinal arachnoid granulations. Neuroradiol 11: 221–228

Kielbasinski G 1976 Arteries of the inferior part of the vermis cerebelli in man. Folia Morphol 25: 149–157

Kieny M, Mauger A, Sengel P 1972 Early regionalization of the somitic mesoderm as studied by the development of the axial skeleton of the chick embryo. Dev Biol 28: 142–161

Kieny M, Pauton M P, Chevalier A, Morgan A 1986 Spatial organisation of the developing limb musculature. In: Birds and Mammals. Bibliothéque Anat 29: 65–69

Kier E L 1966 Embryology of the normal optic canal and its anomalies. Invest Radiol 1: 346–362

Kier E L 1977 The cerebral ventricles: a phylogenetic and ontogenetic study. In: Newton T H, Potts D G (eds) Radiology of the skull and brain. Anatomy and pathology. Vol 3. Mosby: St Louis: pp 2787–2914

Kierszenbaum A L 1994 Mammalian spermatogenesis in vivo and in vitro: a partnership of spermatogenic and somatic cell lineages. Endocrine Rev 15: 116–134

Kiesselbach J E, Chamberlain J G 1984 Clinical and anatomical observations on the relationship of the lingual nerve to the mandibular third molar region. J Oral Maxillofacial Surg 42: 565–567

Kikkawa Y, Smith F 1983 Cellular and biochemical aspects of pulmonary surfactant in health and disease. Lab Invest 49: 122–139

Killian J 1898 Entwicklungsgeschichte, anatomische und klinische Untersuchungen uber Mandelbucht und Gaumenmandel. Arch Laryngol Bd 7, 2 Heft: 167–203

Kim H G, Connors B W 1993 Apical dendrites of the neocortex: correlation between sodium- and calcium-dependent spiking and pyramidal cell morphology. J Neurosci 13: 5301–5311

Kim S 1990 Microcirculation in the dental pulp. In: Spangberg L S W (ed) Experimental endodontics. CRC Press Inc: Boca Raton: Florida: pp 51–76

Kim S-G, Ashe J, Georgopoulos A P, Merkle H, Ellermann J M, Menon R S et al 1992 Functional imaging of human motor cortex at high magnetic field. J Neurophysiol 69: 297–302

Kimmel D L 1961 Innervation of spinal dura mater and dura mater of the posterior cranial fossa. Neurol: 800–809

Kimmel D L 1961b The nerves of the cranial dura mater and their significance in dural headache and referred pain. Chicago Med Sch Q 22: 16–26

Kimura D 1992 Sex differences in the brain. Sci Am 267: 118–125

Kimura K 1977 Foramina and noches on the supraorbital margin in some racial groups. Acta Anat 52: 203–209

Kimura R S 1969 Distribution, structure and function of dark cells in the vestibular labyrinth. Ann Otol Rhinol Laryngol 78: 542–561

King B F 1982 Cell surface specialisations and intercellular junctions in human amniotic epithelium: an electron miscroscopic and freeze fracture study. Anat Rec 203: 73–82

King C, Boggaram V, Mendelson C 1992 Rabbit lung surfactant protein A gene: identification of a lung specific DNAase 1 hypersensitive site. Am J Physiol 262: L662–L671

King J S, Cummings S L, Bishop G A 1992 Peptides in cerebellar circuits. Prog Neurobiol 39: 423–442

King R H M, Thomas P K 1971 Aberrant regeneration of unmyelinated axons in the vagus nerve of the rabbit. J Anat 108: 596P

King R J 1974 The surfactant system of the lung. Fed Proc Fed Am Socs Exp Biol 33: 2238–2247

King R J, Clements J A 1972 Surface active materials from dog lung. I. Composition and physiological correlations. Am J Physiol 223: 715–726

King T J, Briggs R 1956 Serial transplantation of embryonic nuclei. Cold Spring Harb Symp Quant Biol 21: 271–289

King T S 1954 The anatomy of hare-lip in man. J Anat 88: 1–12

King T S, Coakley J B 1958 The intrinsic nerve cells of the cardiac atria of mammals and man. J Anat 92: 353–376

Kinman J 1977 Surgical aspects of the anatomy of the sphenoidal sinuses and the sella turcica. J Anat 124: 541–553

Kinmonth J B 1964 Some general aspects of the investigation and surgery of the lymphatic system. J Cardiovasc Surg 5: 680–682

Kinmonth J B, Taylor G W 1964 Chylous reflux. Br Med J I: 529–532

Kinnaert P 1973 Anatomical variations of the cervical part of the thoracic duct in man. J Anat 115: 45–52

Kinnamon J C, Taylor B J, Delay R J, Roper S D 1985 Ultrastructure of mouse vallate taste buds. I. Taste cells and their associated synapses. J Comp Neurol 235: 48–60

Kinnamon S 1988 Taste transduction: a diversity of mechanisms. Trends Neurosci. 11: 491–496

Kinnamon S C, Cummings T A 1992 Chemosensory transduction mechanisms in taste. Ann Rev Physiol 54:715–731

Kirby A S, Wallace W A, Moulton A, Burwell R G 1993 Comparison of four methods for measuring femoral anteversion. Clin Anat 6: 280–288

Kirby M L 1990 Ablation of cardiogenesis after neural crest ablation. In: Bockman D E, Kirby M L (eds) Embryonic origins of defective heart development. Ann NY Acad Sci 588: 289–295

Kircher C, Ha H 1968 The nucleus cervicalis lateralis in primates, including the human. Anat Rec 160: 376

Kirchgessner A L, Aldersberg M A, Gershon M D 1992 Colonization of the developing pancreas by neural precursors from the bowel. Dev Dynamics 194: 142–154

Kirchner J A, Wyke B D 1965 Articular reflex mechanisms in the larynx. Ann Otol Rhinol Laryngol 74: 749–768

Kirk J 1944 Observations on the histology of the choledochduodenal junction and papilla duodeni, with particular reference to the ampulla of Vater and sphincter of Oddi. J Anat 78: 118–120

Kirk J E, Laursen T J S 1955 Diffusion coefficient of various solutes for human aortic tissue. With special reference to variation in tissue permeability with age. J Gerontol 10: 288–302

Kirkpatrick N A, Perry M E, Gleeson M J 1993 Variations in the epithelium covering the human nasopharyngeal tonsil (adenoid). J Anat 183: 199

Kirkup J 1990 Rheumatoid arthritis and ankle surgery. Ann Rheum Dis 49: 837–844

Kirschenlohr H L, Metcalfe J C, Weissberg P L, Grainger D J 1993 Adult human aortic smooth muscle cells in culture produce active TGF-β. Am J Physiol 265: C571–576

Kiss F 1932 Sympathetic elements in the cranial and spinal ganglia. J Anat 66: 488–498

Kiss J Z, Wang C, Rougon G 1993 Nerve-dependent expression of high polysialic acid neural cell adhesion molecule in neurohypophyseal astrocytes of adult rats. Neuroscience 53: 213 – 221

Kitamura S, Nishiguchi T, Ogatu K, Sakai A 1989 Neurons of origin of the internal ramus of the rabbit accessory nerve: localisation in the dorsal nucleus of the vagus nerve and the nucleus retroambigualis. Anat Rec 224: 541–549

Kitamura S, Nishiguchi T, Sakai A 1983 Location of cell somata and the peripheral course of axons of the geniohyoid and thyrohyoid motoneurons: a horseradish peroxidase study in the rat. Exp Neurol 79: 87–96

Kitamura S, Okubo J, Ogata K, Sakai A 1987 Fibers supplying the laryngeal musculature in the cranial root of the rabbit accessory nerve: nucleus of origin, peripheral course, and innervated muscles. Exp Neuro 97: 592–606

Kito H, Hosoda S 1977 Triple staining for stimultaneous visualization of cell types in islets of Langerhans of pancreas. Successive application of argyrophil, aldehyde-fuchsin and lead-hematoxylin stains in a single tissue section. J Histochem Cytochem 25: 1019–1020

Kjaegaard J 1974 An electron microscopic study of the tympanojugular glomus. Acta Otolaryngol (Stockh) 78: 84–89

Klareskog L, Forsum U, Kabelitz D, Plöen L, Sundström C, Nilsson K, Wigren A, Wigzell H 1982 Immune functions of human synovial cells. Phenotypic and T cell regulatory properties of macrophage-like cells that express HLA-DR. Arthritis Rheum 25: 488–501

Klein D C 1978 The pineal gland: a model of neuroendocrine regulation. Res Publ Assoc Res Nerv Ment Dis 56: 303–327

Klein D C et al 1993 Suprachiasmatic nucleus: the mind's clock. Oxford University Press: Oxford

Klein D C, Weller J L 1972 A rapid light-induced decrease in pineal serotonin N-acetyltransferase activity. Science 177: 532–533

Klein R et al 1993 Cell 75: 113–122

Klein R, Silos-Santiago I, Smeyne R J, Lira S A, Brambilla R, Bryant S, Zhang L, Snider W D, Barbacid M 1994 Nature 368: 249–251

Kligman A M 1964 The biology of the stratum corneum. In: Montagna W, Lobitz W C (eds) The epidermis. Academic Press: New York: pp 387–433

Kligman A M, Lavker R M 1988 Cutaneous ageing: the difference between intrinsic ageing and photoageing. Aging Cosmet Dermatol 1: 5–12

Klika E, Petrik P 1965 A study of the structure of the lung alveolar and bronchiolar epithelium (a histological and histochemical study using the method of membranous preparations). Acta Histochem 20: 331–342

Klineberg I J, Wyke B D 1975 Articular reflex control of mastication. In: Kay L W (ed) Oral surgery IV. Munksgaard: Copenhagen

Klintworth G K 1967 The ontogeny and growth of the human tentorium cerebelli. Anat Rec 158: 433–442

Klosovskii B N 1963 The development of the brain and its disturbance by harmful factors. (Haigh B ed and trans.) Pergamon Press: Oxford

Klück P 1980 The autonomic innervation of the human urinary bladder, bladder neck and urethra: a histochemical study. Anat Rec 198: 439–447

Klun B, Prestor B 1986 Microvascular relations of the trigeminal nerve: an anatomical study. Neurosurg 19: 535–538

Klüver H, Bucy P C 1937 Psychic blindness and other symptoms following temporal lobectomy in rhesus monkeys. Am J Physiol 119: 352–353

Knese K-H 1979 Stützgewebe und Skeletsystem. Handbuch der mikroscopischen Anatomie des Menschen. Vol 2. Die Gewebe, part 5, Springer-Verlag: Berlin: pp 225–428

Knieriem H J, Heuber A 1970 Quantitative morphological studies of the human aorta. Beitr Path Anat 140: 280–294

Kniffki K-D, Mense S, Schmidt R F 1977 The spinocervical tract as a possible pathway for muscular nociception. J Physiol 73: 359–366

Knigge K M, Joseph S A 1974 Thyrotropin releasing factor (TRF) in cerebrospinal fluid of the third ventricle of rat. Acta Endocrinol 76: 209–213

Knigge K M, Scott D E, Kobayashi H, Ishii S (eds) 1975 Brain–endocrine interaction. II. The ventricular system in neuroendocrine mechanisms. 2nd International symposium, Tokyo, 1974. Karger: Basel

Knight B K, Hayes M M M, Symington R B 1973 The pineal gland – a synopsis of present knowledge with particular emphasis on its possible role in control of gondadotrophin function. S Afr J Anim Sci 3: 143–146

Knight R A, van Zandt I L 1952 Arthroplasty of the elbow. An end-result study. J Bone Jt Surg 34A: 610–618

Knight S C, Stagg A J 1993 Antigen presenting cell types. Curr Opin Immunol 5: 374–382

Knisely M H 1936 Spleen studies. I. Microscopic observations of the circulatory system of living unstimulated mammalian spleens. Anat Rec 65: 23–50

Knobil E, Neill J D 1988 The physiology of reproduction. Raven: New York

Knoth M, Larsen J F 1972 Ultrastructure of human implantation site. Acta Obstet Gynec Scand 51: 385–393

Knowles F 1974 Ependyma of the third ventricle in relation to pituitary function. Prog Brain Res 38: 255–270

Knudson C B, Knudson W 1993 Hyaluronan-binding proteins in development, tissue homeostasis and disease. FASB J 7: 1233–1241

Knussman R, Finke E 1977 Studies on the sex-specificity of the human spinal profile. Acta Med Auxol 9: 16

Ko J S, Bernard G W 1981 Osteoclast formation in vitro from bone marrow mononuclear cells in osteoclast-free bone. Am J Anat 161: 415–425

Kobatake E, Tanaka K 1994 Neuronal selectivities to complex object features in the ventral visual pathway of the macaque cerebral cortex. J Neurophysiol 71: 856–867

Kobayashi H 1975 Absorption of cerebrospinal fluid by ependymal cells of the median eminince. In: Knigge K M, Scott D E, Kobayashi H, Ishi S (eds) Brain-endocrine interaction. II. 2nd international symposium, Tokyo, 1974. Karger: Basel: pp 109–122

Kobayashi S 1969 On the fine structure of the carotid body of the bird, Uroloncha domestica. Arch Histol Jpn 31: 9–19

Kobayashi S, Fujita T 1969 Fine structure of mammalian and avian pancreatic islets with special reference to D cells and nervous elements. Z Zellforsch 100: 340–363

Koch A E, Burrows J C, Haines K G, Carlos T M, Harlan J M Leibovich S J 1991 Immunolocalization of endothelial and leucocyte adhesion molecules in human rheumatoid and osteoarthritic tissues. Lab Invest 64: 313–320

Koch C, Poggio T 1983 A theoretical analysis of electrical properties of spines. Proc R Soc Lond [Biol] 298: 227–263

Koch J C 1917 The laws of bone architecture. Am J Anat 21: 177–298

Koch P J, Franke W W 1994 Desmosomal cadherins: another growing multigene family of adhesion molecules. Curr Opin Cell Biol 6: 682–687

Kochakian C D (ed) 1976 Anabolic-androgenic steroids, Handbook Exper Pharmacol. Vol 43. Springer-Verlag: Berlin

Koelliker R A 1887 Anat Anz 15: 480

Kohelet D, Goldberg A, Goldberg M 1982 Depth of endotracheal placement in neonates. J Pediatr 101: 157

Kohn A 1902 Das chromaffine Gewebe. Ergebn d Anat u Entw 12: 253–348

Köhn A 1903 Die paraganglien. Ark Mikrosk Anat 62: 263

Kohnstamm O 1898 Zur Anatomie und Physiologie des Phrenicuskernes. Fortschr Med 16: 643–653

Koike K, Masumoto N, Kasahara K, Yamaguchi M, Tasaka K, Hirota K, Miyake A, Tanizawa O 1991 Tumor necrosis factor-alpha stimulates prolactin release from anterior pituitary cells: a possible involvement of intracellular calcium mobilization. Endocrinology 128: 2785–2790

Kolb H 1991 Anatomical pathways for colour vision in the human retina. Vis Neurosci 7: 61–74

Kolb H 1994 The architecture of functional neural circuits in the vertebrate retin. The Proctor Lecture. Invest Ophthalmol Vis Sci 2385–2404

Kolb H, Dekover L 1991 Midget ganglion cells of the parafovea of the human retina: a study by electron microscopy and serial section reconstruction. J Comp Neurol 303: 617–636

Kolb H, Linberg K A, Fisher S K 1992 Neurons of the human retina: a Golgi study. J Comp Neurol 318: 147–187

Kolb H, Nelson R 1984 Neural architecture of the cat retina. Prog Retinal Res 3. Pergamon: New York

Kollar E J 1972 Histogenetic aspects of dermal-epidermal interactions. In: Slavkin H C, Bavetta L A (eds) Development aspects of oral biology. Academic Press: New York: pp 125–149

Kollar E J, Fisher C 1980 Tooth induction in chick epithelium: expression of quiescent genes for enamel synthesis. Science 207: 993–995

Kollar E J, Lumsden A G S 1979 Tooth morphogenesis: the role of the innervation during induction and pattern formation. J Biol Buccale 7: 49–60

Kollar E J, Mina M 1991 Role of the early epithelium in the patterning of the teeth and Meckel's cartilage. J Craniofac Genet Dev Biol 11: 223–228

Kolmodin G M 1957 Integrative processes in single spinal interneurones with proprioceptive connections. Acta Physiol Scand 40 (suppl 139): 1–89

Kolmodin G M, Skoglund C R 1960 Analysis of spinal interneurons activated by tactile and nociceptive stimuli. Acta Physiol Scand 50: 337–355

Kolnberger I 1971 Vergleichende Untersuchungen am Riechepithel, insbesonder des Jacobsonschen Organs von Amphibien, Reptilien und Saugetieren. Z Zellforsch 122: 53–67

Kolnberger I, Altner H 1971 Cilary-structure precursor bodies as stable constituents in the sensory cells of the vomero-nasal organ of reptiles and mammals. Z Zellforsch 118: 254–262

Komai Y, Ushiki T 1991 The three-dimensional organization of collagen fibrils in the human cornea and sclera. Invest Ophthalmol Vis Sci 32: 2244–2258

Komatsu H, Ideura Y, Yamane S 1992 Color selectivity of neurons in the inferior temporal cortex of the awake macaque monkey. J Neurosci 12: 408–424

Komiyama A, Novicki D L, Suzuki K 1991 Adhesion and proliferation are enhanced in vitro by Schwann cells from nerve undergoing Wallerian degeneration. J Neurosci Res 29: 308–318

Komura T, Hashimoto Y 1990 Three dimensional structure of the rat intestinal wall (mucosa and submucosa). Arch Histol Cytol 53: 1–21

Kondo Y, Kudo K, Igarashi Y, Kuba Y, Arima S, Tada K, Abe K 1992 Functions of the ascending thin limb of Henle's loop with special emphasis on mechanisms of NaCl transport. Tohoku J Exp Med 166: 75–84

Kondo Y, Takada M, Honda Y, Mizuno N 1993 Bilateral projections of single retinal ganglion cells to the lateral geniculate nuclei and superior colliculi in the albino rat. Brain Res 608: 204–215

Konigsmark B W 1970 Methods for the counting of neurons. In: Nauta W J H, Ebbesson S O E (eds) Contemporary research methods in neuroanatomy. Springer-Verlag: Berlin: pp 315–339

Konishi A, Sato M, Mizuno N, Hon K, Nomura S, Sugimoto T 1978 An electron microscope study of the areas of the Onuf's nucleus in the cat. Brain Res 156: 333–338

Koob G F 1992c Dopamine, addiction and reward. Seminars in the Neurosci 4: 139–148

Koob G F 1992d Neural mechanisms of drug reinforcement. Ann New York Acad Sci 654: 171–191

Koob G F K 1992a Drugs of abuse: anatomy, pharmacology and function of reward pathways. TIPS 13: 177–184

Koob G F K 1992b Dopamine, addiction and reward. TINS 4: 139–148

Koob G F, Bloom F E 1988 Cellular and molecular mechanisms of drug dependence. Science 242: 715–723

Koob G F, Maldonado R, Stinus L 1992 Neural substrates of opiate withdrawal. TINS 15: 186–191

Koob G F, Stinus L, LeMoal M, Bloom F E 1989 Opponent process theory of motivation: neurobiological evidence from studies of opiate dependence. Neurosci Biobehav Rev 13: 135–140

Koontz M A 1993 GABA-immunoreactive profiles provide synaptic input to the soma, axon hillock and axon initial segment of ganglion cells in primate retina. Vision Res 33: 2629–2636

Koopman P, Gubbay J, Vivian N, Goodfellow P, Lovell-Badge R 1991 Male development of chromosomally female mice transgenic for Sry. Nature 351: 117–121

Koorneef L 1977 Spatial aspects of orbital musculo-fibrous tissue in man. Swets & Zeitlinger: Amsterdam

Koornneef L 1977 New insights in the human orbital connective tissue. Arch Ophthal 95: 1269–1273

Kopp W C 1990 The immune functions of the spleen. In: Bowdler A J (ed) The Spleen. Structure, function and significance. Chapman and Hall Medical: London: pp 103–126

Kordower et al 1995 New Engl J Med 332:1118–1127

Koritké J G, Gillet J Y, Pietri J 1967 Les artères de la trompe uterine chez la femme. Arch Anat Histol Embryol 50: 47–70

Kormano M, Suoranta H 1971 Microvascular organisation of the adult human testis. Anat Rec 170: 31–40

Kornguth S E, Anderson J W, Scott G 1966 Observations on the ultra-structure of the developing cerebellum of the Macaca mulatta. J Comp Neurol 130: 1–23

Kornguth S E, Anderson J W, Scott G 1968 The development of synaptic contacts in the cerebellum of Macaca mulatta. J Comp Neurol 132: 531–546

Korsching S 1993 The neurotrophic factor concept: a re-examination. J Neurosci 13: 2739–2748

Kos J 1970 L'ultrastructure des franges et des plis synoviaux. C R Assoc Anat 149: 802–813

Kosaka T, Tauchi M, Dahl J L 1988 Cholinergic neurons containing GABA-like and/or glutamic acid decarboxylase-like immunoreactivities in various brain regions of the rat. Exp Brain Res 70: 605–617

Kosher R A 1983 The chondroblast and the chondrocyte. In: Hall B K (ed) Cartilage. Vol 1. Structure, function and biochemistry. Academic Press: New York: pp 59–85

Kosinski C 1926 Observations on the superficial venous system of the lower extremity. J Anat 60: 131–142

Koskinen L, Isotupa K, Koski K 1976 A note on craniofacial sutural growth. Am J Phys Anthrop 45: 511–516

Koss L G 1968 Diagnostic cytology. 2nd edition. Pitman: London

Kosterlitz H W 1968 The alimentary canal. In: Code C F (ed) Handbook of physiology. Vol IV. American Physiological Society: Washington DC: pp 2147–2172

Kostick E L 1963 Facets and imprints on the upper and lower extremities of femora from a Western Nigerian population. J Anat 97: 393–402

Kothari L K, Gupta A S 1974 Effect of ageing on the volume, structure and total Leydig cell content of the human testis. Int J Fertil 19: 140–146

Kothari L K, Patni M K, Jain M L 1978 The total Leydig cell volume of the testis in some common mammals. Andrologia 10: 218–222

Kouyama N, Marshak D W 1992 Bipolar cells specific for blue cones in the macaque retina. J Neurosci 12: 1233–1252

Kovrishko N M 1964 Postnatal development and structural characteristic of the principal paraganglia in man. Fed Proc Trans (suppl) 22: 740

Kozielec T, Józwa H 1976 The supoticial temporal artery in human fetuses. Folia Morphol 35: 79–84

Kozielec T, Józwa H 1977 Variation in the course of the facial artery in the prenatal period in man. Folia Morphol Warsz 36: 55–61

Kraehenbuhl J P, Neutra M R 1992 Molecular and cellular basis of immune protection of mucosal surfaces. Physiol Rev 72: 853–879

Kraft G L, Levinthal D H 1951 Facet synovial impingement. A new concept in the etiology of lumbar vertebral derangement. Surg Gynaecol Obstet 93: 439–443

Krag M H, Cohen M C, Haugh L D, Pope M H 1990 Facet synovial impingement. A new concept in the etiology of lumbar vertebral development. Spine 15: 202–207

Krahl V E 1944 An apparatus for measuring the torsion angle in long bones. Science 99: 498

Krahl V E 1964 Anatomy of the mammalian lung. In: Fenn W O, Rahn H (eds) Handbook of physiology Section 3> Respiration vol 1. American Physiological Society: Washington, DC: pp 213–284

Krahl V E 1976 The phylogeny and ontogeny of humeral torsion. Am J Phys Anthropol 45: 595–599

Krahn V 1981 Leukodiapedesis and leukocyte migration in the leptomeninges and in the subarachnoid space. J Neurol 226: 43–52

Krahn V 1982 The pia mater at the site of entry of blood vessels into the central nervous system. Anat Embryol 164: 257–263

Kraissl C J 1951 The selection of appropriate lines for elective surgical incisions. Plast Reconstruct Surg 8: 1–28

Kralj A, Bajd T 1989 Functional electrical stimulation. Standing and walking after spinal cord injury. CRC Press: Florida

Krammer E B, Rath T, Lischka M F 1979 Somatotopic organization of the hypoglossal nucleus. A HRP study in the rat. Brain Res 170: 533–537

Kramps J A et al 1981 Localization of low molecular weith protease inhibitor in serous secretory cells of the respiratory tract. J Histochem Cytochem 29(6): 712–719

Kraus B 1959 Occurrence of the Carabelli trait in southwest ethnic groups. Am J Phys Anthropol 17: 117–124

Kraus B S 1961 The western Apache: some anthropometric observations. Am J Phys Anthropol 19: 227–236

Kraus F W, Mestecky J 1971 Immunohistochemical localization of amylase, lysozyme and immunoglobins in the human parotid gland. Arch Oral Biol 16: 781–789

Kraus K S, Jordan R E, Abrams L A 1969 Dental anatomy and occlusion. Williams and Wilkins: Baltimore

Krause H R, Bremerich A, Herrmann M 1991 The innervation of the trapezius muscle in connection with radical neck-dissection – an anatomical study. J Cranio-Maxillo-Facial Surg 12: 87–89

Krauthamer G M 1979 Sensory functions of the neostriatum. In: Divac I, Öberg R E G (eds) The Neostriatum. Pergamon Press: Oxford: pp 263–290

Krayenbühl H A 1967 Cerebral venous and sinus thrombosis. Clin Neurosurg 14: 1–24

Kreis T E, Pepperkok R 1994 Coat proteins in intracellular membrane transport. Curr Opin Cell Biol 6: 533–537

Kreis T E, Vale R D (eds) 1992 Guidebook to cytoskeletal and motor proteins. Oxford University Press: Oxford

Kretschmann H-J 1988 Localization of the corticospinal fibres in the internal capsule in man. J Anat (Lond) 160: 219–225

Krettek J E, Price J L 1978 A description of the amygdaloid complex in the rat and cat with observations on intra-amygdaloid axonal connections. J Comp Neurol 178: 255–280

Kreutzer E W, Jafek B W 1980 The vomeronasal organ of Jacobson in the human embryo and fetus. Otolaryngol Head Neck Surg 88: 119–123

Kristensen P, Suzdak P D, Thomsen C 1993 Expression pattern and pharmacology of the rat type IV metabotropic glutamate receptor. Neurosci Lett 155: 159–162

Kristic R V 1984 Illustrated encyclopedia of human histology. Springer Verlag: New York

Krogh A 1959 The anatomy and physiology of capillaries. Hafner Publishing: New York

Krogman W M 1941 Bibliography of human morphology 1914–1939. Chicago University Press: Chicago

Krogman W M 1962 The human skeleton in forensic medicine. Thomas: Springfield, Illinois

Krompecher S 1967 Local tissue metabolism and the quality of callus. Symp Biol Hung 7: 275–281

Krstić R 1976 Ultracytochemistry of the synaptic ribbons in the rat pineal organ. Cell Tissue Res 166: 135–143

Kruger L 1987 Morphological correlates of 'free' nerve endings: a re-appraisal of thin sensory axon classification. In: Schmidt R F, Schaible H-G, Vahle-Hinz C (eds) Fine afferent nerve fibres and pain. VCH Verlag Chemie: Weinheim: pp 1–13

Kruk P A, Auersperg N 1992 Human ovarian surface epithelial cells are capable of physically restructuring extracellular matrix. Am J Obstet Gynecol 167: 1437–1443

Krumlauf R, Marshall H, Studer M, Nonchev S, Sham M H, Lumsden A 1993 J Neurobiol 24: 1328–1340

Krystosek A, Seeds N W 1981 Science 213: 1523–1534

Kubik S 1967 The efferent lymph vessels and the regional lymph nodes of the female genital organs. In: Rüttimann A (ed) Progress in lymphology. Proceedings of the international symposium, Zurich, 1966. Thieme: Stuttgart: pp 196–197

Kubik S 1970 Lung lymphatics. Prog Lymphol 11: 29–31

Kubik S 1974 Anatomische Voraussetzungen zur endolymphatischen Radionuklidtherapie. Med Welt 25: 1011–1016

Kubik S, Müntener M 1969 Zur Topographie der spinalen Nervenwurzeln. II. Der Einfuss des Wachstums des Duralsackes, sowie der Krümmagen und der Bewegungen der spinalen Nervenwurzeln. Acta Anat 74: 149–168

Kubo J 1970 Some observations on the autonomic innervation of the human oviduct. Int J Fertil 15: 30–35

Kubo M, Norris D A, Howell S E, Clark R A F 1984 Humam keratinocytes synthesize secrete and deposit fibronectin in the pericellular matrix. J Invest Dermatol 82: 580–586

Kubota K, Negishi T, Nasegi T 1975 Topological distribution of muscle spindles in the human tongue. Bull Tokyo Med Dent Univ 22: 235–242

Kubota Y, Hattori R, Yui Y 1994 Three distinct subpopulations of GABA-ergic neurons in rat frontal agranular cortex. Brain Res 649: 159–173

Kuczynski K 1974 Carpometacarpal joint of the human thumb. J Anat 118: 119–126

Kudo H, Iwano K 1990 Total elbow arthroplasty with a non-constrained surface-replacement prosthesis in patients who have rheumatoid arthritis. J Bone Jt Surg 72A: 355–362

Kuettner K E, Pauli B U 1983a Inhibition of neurovascularization by a cartilage factor. In: Symposium on the development of the vascular system (Ciba Foundation Symposium 100). Pitman: London: pp 163–173

Kuettner K E, Pauli B U 1983b Vascularity of cartilage. In: Hall B K (ed) Cartilage. Vol 1. Structure, function and biochemistry. Academic Press: New York: pp 281–312

Kugel M A 1927 Anatomical studies on the coronary arteries and their branches. I. Arteria anastomotica auricularis magna. Am Heart J 3: 260–270

Kügelgen von A 1955 Über das Verhältnis von Ringmuskulatur und Innendruck in menschlichen grossen Venen. Z Zellforsch Mikrosk Anat 43: 168–183

Kügelgen von A 1956 Weitere Mitteilungen über den Wandbau der grossen Venen des Menschen unter besonderer Berücksichtigung ihrer Kollagenstrukturen. Z Zellforsch Mikrosk Anat 44: 121–174

Kuhl D E, Edwards R Q 1963 Image separation radioisotope scanning. Radiology 80: 653–661

Kuhlenbeck H, Miller R N 1949 The pretectal region of the human brain. J Comp Neurol 91: 369–408

Kuhn F E, Max S R 1985 Testosterone and muscle hypertrophy in female rats. J Appl Physiol 59: 24–27

Kühnel W 1968 Vergleichende histologische histochemische und elektronenmikroskopische Untersuchungen an Tränendrüsen. VI. Menschliche Tränendrüsen. Z Zellforsch 89: 550–572

Kullaa-Mikkonen A, Hynynen M, Hyvönen P 1987 Filiform papillae of human, rat and swine tongue. Acta Anat 130: 280–284

Kuller J A, Globus M S 1992 Fetal therapy. In: Brock D J H, Rodeck C H, Ferguson-Smith M A (eds) Prenatal diagnosis and screening. Churchill Livingstone: Edinburgh: pp 703–717

Kulver H, Bucy P C 1939 Preliminary analysis of functions of the temporal lobes in monkeys. Arch Neurol Psychiat 8: 2153–2163

Kummer B K F 1966 Photoelastic studies on the functional structure of bone. Folia Biotheoret 6: 31–40

Kummer B K F 1972 Biomechanics of bone. In: Fung Y-C B, Perrone N, Anliker M (eds) Biomechanics. Prentice-Hall: New Jersey: Ch 10

Kuntscher G 1934 Die Darstellung des Kraftflusses im Knocken. Z Beit Chir 61: 2130–2136

Kuntz A 1953 The autonomic nervous system 4th edition, Lea and Febiger: Philadelphia

Künzle H 1978 An autoradiographic analysis of the efferent connections from premotor and adjacent prefrontal regions (areas 6 and 9) in Macaca fascicularis. Brain Behav Evol 15: 185–234

Künzle H, Akert K 1977 Efferent connections of cortical area 8 (frontal eye field) in Macaca fascicularis: a re-investigation using the autoradiographic technique. J Comp Neurol 173: 147–164

Kupfer C, Chumbley L, Downer J de C 1967 Quantitative histology of optic nerve, optic tract and lateral geniculate nucleus of man. J Anat 101: 393–402

Kupfermann I 1991 Functional studies of cotransmission. Physiol Rev 71: 683–732

Kurahashi Y, Yoshiki S 1972 Electron microscopic localisation of alkaline phosphatase in the enamel organ of the young rat. Arch Oral Biol 17: 155–163

Kurata K 1993 Premotor cortex of monkeys: set- and movement-related activity reflecting amplitude and direction of write movements. J Neurophysiol 69: 187–200

Kurata K 1994 Information processing for motor control in primate premotor cortex. Behav Brain Res 61: 135–142

Kuré K, Murakami S, Okinaka S 1934 Die Spinalpara-sympathetischen ganglionzellen im den spinalganglien und der Spinalparasympathetiens des Halssegmentes. Z Zellforsch Mikrosk Anat 22: 54–79

Kuré K, Saégusa G, Kawaguchi K, Shiraishi K 1930 On the parasympathetic (spinal parasympathetic) fibres in the dorsal or posterior roots of the lumbar region of the spinal cord. Q J Exp Physiol 20: 333–344

Kuro-O M, Nagai R, Tsuchimochi H, Katoh H, Yazaki Y, Ohkubo A, Takaku F 1989 Developmentally regulated expression of vascular smooth muscle myosin heavy chain isoforms. J Biol Chem 264: 18272–18275

Kurosawa H, Becker A E 1985 Dead-end tract of the conduction axis. Int J Cardiol 7: 13–18

Kurosumi K, Oota Y 1968 Electron microscopy of two types of gonadotrophs in the anterior pituitary glands of persistent estrus and diestrus rats. Z Zellforsch 85: 34–46

Kurrat H J, Oberländer W 1978 The thickness of the cartilage in the hip joint. J Anat 126: 145–155

Kuru M 1949 Sensory pathways in the spinal cord and brainstem of man. Sogensya: Tokyo

Kuru Y 1967 Meningeal branches of the ophthalmic artery. Acta Radiol 6: 241–251

Kuwabara T 1975 The maturation of the lens cell. Exp Eye Res 20: 427–443

Kuwabara T, Cogan D G, Johnson C C 1975 Structure of the muscles of the upper eyelid. Arch Ophthalmol 73: 1189–1197

Kuypers H G J M 1960 Central cortical projections to motor and somato-sensory cell groups. An experiment of study in the rhesus monkey. Brain 83: 161–184

Kuypers H G J M 1962 Corticospinal connections: postnatal development in the rhesus monkey. Science 138: 678–680

Kuypers H G J M 1964 The descending pathways to the spinal cord, their anatomy and function. Prog Brain Res 2: 178–200

Kuypers H G J M 1973 The anatomical organization of the descending pathways and their contribution to motor control especially in primates. In: Desmodt J E (ed) New developments to electromyography and clinical neurophysiology. Vol 3. Karger: Basel: pp 38–68

Kuypers H G J M 1981 Anatomy of descending pathways. In: Brookhart J M, Mountcastle V B et al (eds) Handbook of physiology. The nervous system. Vol 2. Motor control. Pt 1. Am Physiol Soc: Bethesda: pp 597–666

Kuypers H G J M 1985 The anatomical and functional organization of the motor system. In: Swash M, Kennard C (eds) Scientific basis of clinical neurology. Churchill Livingstone: Edinburgh: pp 3–18

Kuypers H G J M, Brinkman J 1970 Precentral projections to different parts of the spinal intermediate zone in the rhesus monkey. Brain Res 24: 29–48

Kuypers H G J M, Maisky V A 1975 Retrograde axonal transport of horseradish peroxidase from spinal cord to brainstem cell groups in the cat. Neurosci Lett 1: 9–14

Kuypers H G J M, Tuerk J D 1964 The distribution of the cortical fibres within the nuclei cuneatus and gracilis in the cat. J Anat 98: 143–162

Kvinnsland S, Kvinnsland S 1975 Growth in craniofacial cartilages studied by ³H-thymidine incorporation. Growth 39: 305–314

Kyber E 1870 Uber die Milz des Menschen und einiger Saugeticre. Arch Mikrosk Anat EntwMech 6: 540–570

Kyösola K, Partanen S, Korkala O, Merikallio E, Penttilä O, Siltanen P 1976 Fluorescence histochemical and electron-microscopical observations on the innervation of the atrial myocardium of the adult human heart. Virchows Arch A Path Anat Histol 371: 101–119

Kyösola K, Rechardt L, Veijola L, Waris T, Penttilä O 1980 Innervation of the human gastric wall. J Anat 131: 453–470

L

Labandeira-Garcia J L, Guerra-Seijas M J, Gonzalez F, Perez R, Acuna C 1990 Location of neurons projecting to the retina in mammals. Neurosci Res 8:291–302

Lacaze-Masmonteil T 1993 Pulmonary surfactant proteins. Crit Care Med 21(9 Suppl): S376–379

Lacaze-Masmonteil T, Frason C, Bourbon J et al 1992 Characterization of the rat surfactant proein A promoter. Eur J Biochem 206: 613–623

Lacey P E, Davies J 1957 Preliminary studies on the demonstration of insulin in the islet by the fluorescent antibody technic. Diabetes 6: 354–357

Lacy D 1960 Light and electron microscopy and its use in the study of factors influencing spermatogenesis in the rat. J R Microscop Soc 79: 209–225

Lader M (ed) 1988 The psychopharmacology of addiction. Br Assoc Psychopharmacol Monograph No 10. Oxford University Press: Oxford

LaFerriere K A, Arenberg I K, Hawkins J E, Johnsson L-G 1974 Melanocytes of the vestibular labyrinth and their relationship to the microvasculature. Ann Otol 83: 685–694

Lagae L, Raiguel S, Orban G A 1993 Speed and direction selectivity of macaque middle temporal neurons. J Neurophysiol 69: 19–39

Laguesse E 1906 La glande nouvelle ou endocrine (Ilots de Langerhans). Revue Gén Hist 2: 1–286

Lake G, Schneider W, Schneider U 1966 Anat Anz 118:

Lake J A 1981 The ribosome. Sci Am 245: 84–97

Lala P K, Graham C H 1990 Mechanism of trophoblast invasiveness and their control: the role of proteases and protease inhibitors. Cancer Metastasis Reviews 9: 369–379

Lallemand R C, Newman D L 1973 Role of the bifurcation in athermatosis of the abdominal aorta. Surg Gynecol Obstet 137: 987–990

Lam J H, Ranganathan N, Wigle E D 1970 Morphology of the human mitral valve. I. Chordae tendineae: a new classification. Circulation 41: 449–458

Lamberty B G H, Zivanovic S 1973 The retro-articular vertebral artery ring of the atlas and its significance. Acta Anat 85: 113–122

Lamers W H, Jong F de, Groot I J M de, Moorman A F M 1991 The development of the avian conduction system, a review. Eur J Morphol 29: 233–253

Lamme V A F, Van Dijk B W, Spekreijse H 1993a Organization of texture segregation processing in primate visual cortex. Visual Neurosci 10: 781–790

Lamme V A F, Van Dijk B W, Spekreijse H 1993b Contour from motion processing occurs in primary visual cortex. Nature 363: 541–543

Lamme V A F, Van Dijk B W, Spekreijse H 1994 Organization of contour from motion processing in primate visual cortex. Vision Res 34: 721–735

Lampert I A, Ritter M A 1988 The origin of the diverse epithelial cells of the thymus: is there a common stem cell? Thymus Update 1: 5–25

Lampl M, Veldhuis J D, Johnson M L 1992 Saltation and stasis: a model of human growth. Science 258: 801–803

Lance J W, Anthony M 1980 Neck–tongue syndrome on sudden turning of the head. J Neurol Neurosurg Psychiatry 43: 97–101

Lancet D, Pace U 1987 The molecular basis of odor recognition. Trends Biochem Sci 12: 63–66

Landacre F L 1911 The origin of the cranial ganglia in *Ameiurus*. J Comp Neurol 20: 309–411

Lander A, Brown N A 1994 Culture-induced inversion of heart looping in pre-somite rat embryos is reduced by either superoxide dismutase or a-cyano-4-hydroxycinnamic acid. In: Teratology. Ter Soc Abs: pp 387–426

Landgren S, Phillips C G, Porter R 1962 Cortical fields of origin of the monosynaptic pyramidal pathways to some alpha motoneurons of the baboon's hand and forearm. J Physiol 161: 112–125

Landis C, Patterson P H 1981 Neural crest cell lineages. Trends Neurosci 4: 172–175

Landis D M D, Reese T S 1974 Differences in membrane structure between excitatory and inhibitory synapses in the cerebellar cortex. J Comp Neurol 155: 93–126

Landmann L 1988 The epidermal permeability barrier. Anat Embryol 178: 1–13

Landon D N 1966 Electron microscopy of muscle spindles. In: Andrew B L (ed) Control and innervation of skeletal muscle. Thompson: Dundee: pp 96–111

Landon D N 1972 The fine structure of the equatorial regions of developing muscle spindles in the rat. J Neurocytol 1: 189–210

Landon D N (ed) 1976 The peripheral nerve. Chapman & Hall: London

Landon D N, Langley O K 1971 The local chemical environment of nodes of Ranvier: a study of cation binding. J Anat 108: 419–432

Landon D N, Williams P L 1963 Ultrastructure of the node of Ranvier. Nature 199: 575–577

Landsmeer J M F 1949 The anatomy of the dorsal aponeurosis of the human finger and its functional significance. Anat Rec 104: 31–44

Landsmeer J M F 1976 Atlas of anatomy of the hand. Churchill Livingstone: Edinburgh

Landsmesser L, Pilar G 1974a Synapse formation during embryogenesis on ganglion cells lacking a periphery. Journal de Physiologie Paris 241: 715–736

Landsmesser L, Pilar G 1974b Synaptic transmission and cell death during normal ganglionic development. Journal de Physiologie Paris 241: 737–749

Lane A T 1992 Sweating in the neonate. In: Polin R A, Fox W W (eds) Fetal and neonatal physiology. W B Saunders: Philadelphia: pp 565–567

Lane A T, Negi M, Goldsmith L A 1987 Human periderm: a monoclonal antibody marker. Curr Prob Dermatol 16: 833–893

Lane M A 1907 The cytological characters of the areas of Langerhans. Am J Anat 7: 709–722

Lang J 1977 Structure and postnatal organization of heretofore uninvestigated and infrequent ossifications of the sella turcica region. Acta Anat 99: 121–130

Lang J 1986 Craniocervical region, osteology and articulations. Neuro Orthop 1: 67–92

Lang J, Brunner F X 1978 Über Rie rami centrales der Aa. cerebri anterior und media. Gegenb Morphol Jahrb Leipzig 124: 364–374

Lang J, Schäfer K 1977 Über Form, Grösse und Variabilität des Plexus choroideus ventriculi III. Gegenb Morphol Jahrb Leipzig 123: 727–741

Lang R A, Bishop J M 1993 Macrophages are required for cell death and tissue remodelling in the developing mouse eye. Cell 74: 453–462

Lang S, Lanigan D T, Wal M van der 1991 Trigeminocardiac reflexes: maxillary and mandibular variants of the oculocardiac reflex. Can J Anaes 38: 757–760

Lange W 1975 Cell number and cell density in the cerebellar cortex of man and some other mammals. Cell Tissue Res 157: 115–124

Lange W, Unger J 1990 Peptidergic innervation within the prostate gland and seminal vesicle. Urolog Res 18: 337–340

Langemeijer R A T M 1976 Le coelome et son revêtement comme organoblasteme. Bull Ass Anat 60: 547–558

Langer K 1861 Zur Anatomie und Physiologie der Haut. Uber die Spaltbarkeit der Cutis, S B Akad Wiss Wien 44: 19–46 Translated into English in Br J Plast Surg 1978 31: 3–8

Langford R J 1989 The contribution of the nasopalatine nerve to sensation of the hard palate. Br J Oral Maxillofa Surg 27: 379–386

Langham M E (ed) 1969 The cornea. Macromolecular organization of a connective tissue. (Papers from a symposium held in Kyoto, Japan, 1967 under the auspices of the Department of Ophthalmology, Osaka University.) Johns Hopkins Press: Baltimore

Langley J N 1921 The autonomic nervous system. Part 1. W Heffer: Cambridge

Langman J M, Rowland R 1986 The number and distribution of lymphoid follicles in the human large intestine. J Anat 149: 189–194

Lankamp D J 1967 The fibre composition of the dedunculus cerebi (Crus cerebri) in man. Thesis, Leiden

Lankester R 1877 Notes on the embryology and classification of the animal kingdom. Q J Microscop Sci 17: 399–454

Lanyon L E 1973 Analysis of surface bone strain in the calcaneus of sheep during normal locomotion. J Biomech 6: 41–49

Lanyon L E 1993a Osteocytes, strain detection, bone modelling and remodelling. Calcif Tiss Int 53 (suppl 1): S102–S107

Lanyon L E 1993b Skeletal responses to physical loading. In: Mundy G R, Martin T J (eds) Physiology and pharmacology of bone. Springer-Verlag: Berlin: pp 485–505

Lanzino G, Andreoli A, Tognetti F, Limoni P, Calbucci F, Bortolami R, Lucchi M L, Callegari E, Testa C 1993 Orbital pain and unruptured carotid-posterior communicating artery aneurysms: the role of sensory fibres of the third cranial nerve. Acta Neurochir 120: 7–11

Lapides J 1958 A simplified modification of the Johanson urethroplasty for structures of the deep bulbous urethra. Proc North Centr Sect Am Urol Assoc 166–169

Lapiere C M 1990 The ageing dermis: the main cause for the appearance of old skin. In: Greaves M, Voorhees J (eds) Senescence in the skin. Br J Dermatol 122 (suppl 35): 5–11

Lardennois G, Okinczyc J 1913 La typhlosigmoidöstomie en Y dans la traitement des coutes rebelles et de la stase du gros intestin. Bull Mem Soc Anat Paris 39: 858–872

Larroche J C 1982 The fine structure of matrix capillaries in human embryos and young fetuses. (Second Special Ross Laboratories Conference on Perinatal Intracranial Haemorrhage). Ross Lab Washington DC 1: 2–5

Larsell O 1934 Morphogenesis and evolution of the cerebellum. Arch Neurol 31: 373–395

Larsell O 1937 The cerebellum. A review and interpretation. Arch Neurol Psychiatry 38: 580–607

Larsell O 1947 The development of the cerebellum in man in relation to its comparative anatomy. J Comp Neurol 87: 85–129

Larsell O 1952 The morphogenesis and adult pattern of the lobules and tissues of the cerebellum of the white rat. J Comp Neurol 97: 281–356

Larsell O 1953 The cerebellum of the cat and monkey. J Comp Neurol 99: 135–200

Larsell O, Jansen J 1972 The comparative anatomy and histology of the cerebellum. The human cerebellum, cerebellar connections, and the cerebellar cortex. University of Minnesota Press: Minneapolis

Larsen P J, Møller M, Mikklesen J D 1991 Efferent projections from the periventricular and medial parvicellular subnuclei of the hypothalamic paraventricular nucleus to circumventricular organs of the rat: a phaseolus vulgaris-leucoagglutinin (PHA-L) tracing study. J Comp Neurol 306: 462–479

Larsen W, Wert S, Brunner G 1986 A dramatic loss of cumulus cell gap junctions is correlated with germinal vesicle breakdown in rat oocytes. Dev Biol 113: 517–521

Larsson L, Moss R L 1993 Maximum velocity of shortening in relation to myosin isoform composition in single fibres from human skeletal muscles. J Physiol 472: 595–614

Larsson L-I, Sundler F, Alumets G, Håkanson R, Schaffalitzky de Muckadell O, Fahrenkrug J 1977 Distribution, ontogeny and ultrastructure of the mammalian secretin cell. Cell Tissue Res 181: 361–368

Laruelle L, Reumont M 1933 Etude de l'anatomie microscopique de la moelle épinière par la méthode des coupes longitudinales plurisegmentalés. Rev Neurol 44: 1130–1141

Lash J W, Ostrovsky D 1986 On the formation of somites. In: Browder L W (ed) Developmental biology: a comprehensive system. 2. The cellular basis of morphogenesis. Saunders: Philadelphia: pp 547–663

Lash J W, Vasan N S 1983 Glycosaminoglycans of cartilage. In: Hall B K (ed) Cartilage. Vol 1.Structure, function and biochemistry. Academic Press: New York: pp 215–251

Lasi G N 1959 Pre- and post-natal changes in the thymus gland. PhD Thesis. University of London

Lassmann H, Schmied M, Vass K, Hickey W F 1993 Bone marrow derived elements and resident microglia in brain inflammation. Glia 7: 19–24

Last R J 1948 Some anatomical details of knee joint. J Bone Jt Surg 30B: 683–688

Last R J 1950 The popliteus muscle and the lateral meniscus. J Bone Jt Surg 32B: 93–99

Last R J 1951 Specimens from Hunterian collection: synovial cavity of knee joint (specimen S 110A); ligaments of knee (specimen S 95A). J Bone Jt Surg 33B: 442–445

Latarjet M, Neidhart J H, Morrin A, Autissier J-M 1967 L'entrée du nerf musculo-cutané dans le muscle coraco-brachial. C R Assoc Anat 138: 755–765

Latham R A 1966 Observations on the growth of the cranial base in the human skull. J Anat 100: 435P

Latham R A 1973 Development and structure of the premaxillary deformity in bilateral cleft lip and palate. Br J Plast Surg 26: 1–11

Latham R A, Anderson R H 1972 Anatomical variations in atrioventricular conduction system with reference to ventricular septal defects. Br Heart J 34: 185–190

Latham R A, Deaton T G 1976 The structural basis of the philtrum and the contour of the vermilion border: a study of the musculature of the upper lip. J Anat 121: 151–160

Laties A M, Liebman P A 1970 Cones of living amphibian eyes: selective staining. Science 165: 1475–1477

Latif A 1957 An electromyographic study of the temporalis muscle in normal persons during selected positions and movements of the mandible. Am J Orthodont 43: 577–591

Latta H 1973 Ultrastructure of the glomerulus and justaglomerular apparatus. In: handbook of physiology. Section 8. Renal physiology (Orloff J, Berliner R W ed) pp 1–29, American Physiological Society: Washington, DC

Latta H 1992 An approach to the structure and function of the glomerular mesangium. J Am Soc Nephrol 2 (suppl 10): S65–S73

Lauer E W 1945 The nuclear pattern and fiber connections of certain basal telencephalic centers in the macaque. J Comp Neurol 82: 215–255

Laughton W B, Powley T L 1987 Localization of efferent function in the dorsal motor nucleus of the vagus. Am J Physiol 252: R13–R25

Laurenson R D 1964 The primary ossification of the human ilium. Anat Rec 148: 209–217

Laurie D J, Seeburg P H, Wisden W 1992 The distribution of 13 GABA$_A$ receptor subunit mRNAs in the rat brain. II. Olfactory bulb and cerebellum. J Neurosci 12: 1063–1076

Laurie W, Woods J D 1958 Anastomoses of the coronary circulation. Lancet 2: 812–816

Lauterbur P C 1973 Image formation by induced local interactions: examples employing NMR. Nature 242: 190

Lauweryns J M, Cokelaere M 1973 Hypoxia-sensitive neuro-epithelial bodies, intrapulmonary secretory neuro-receptors modulated by the CNS. Z Zellforsch Mikrosk Anat 145: 521–546

Lauweryns J M, Cokelaere M, Theunynck P 1972 Neuro-epithelial bodies in the respiratory mucosa of various mammals. Z Zellforsch 135: 569–592

Lauweryns J M, Peuskens J C 1972 Neuro-epithelial bodies (neuroreceptor or secretory organs?) in human infant bronchial and bronchiolar epithelium. Anat Rec 172: 471–482

Lauweryns J-M, Boussaw L 1967 L'ultrastructure des vaisseaux lymphatiques pulmonaires. C R Assoc Anat 138: 766–775

Lavelle C L 1974 The effect of age on human third molar and rat molar teeth. Acta Anat 87: 110–118

Law D J, Lightner V A 1993 Divalent cation-dependent adhesion at the myotendinous junction: ultrastructure and mechanics of failure. J Musc Res Cell Motil 14: 173–185

Lawn A M 1966 The localization, in the nucleus ambiguus of the rabbit, of the cells of origin of motor nerve fibres in the glossopharyngeal nerve and various branches of the vagus nerve by means of retrograde degeneration. J Comp Neurol 127: 293–305

Lawrence A M, Tan S, Hojvat S et al 1977 Salivary gland hyperglycemic factor: an extrapancreatic source of glucagon-like material. Science 195: 70–72

Lawrence D G, Hopkins D A 1976 The development of motor control in the rhesus monkey: evidence concerning the role of cortico–motoneuronal connections. Brain 99: 235–254

Lawrence D G, Kuypers H G J M 1968 The functional organization of the motor system in the monkey. II. The effects of lesions of the brain-stem pathways. Brain 91: 15–36

Lawrence J M, Morris R J, Wilson D J, Raisman G 1990 Mechanisms of allograft rejection in the rat brain. Neuroscience 37: 431–462

Lawrence P A 1992 The making of a fly. Blackwell Scientific: Oxford

Lawrenson I G, Kuskell G L 1991 The structure of corpuscular nerve endings in the limbal conjunctiva of the human eye. J Anat 177: 75–84

Lawson K A, Meneses J J Pedersen R A 1991 Clonal analysis of epiblast fate during germ layer formation in the mouse embryo. Development 113: 891–911

Lawson K A, Pedersen R A 1992 Clonal analysis of cell fate during gastrulation and early neurulation in the mouse. Ciba Foundation Symposium 165. John Wiley: Chichester: pp 3–20

Lawson R 1979 The comparative anatomy of the circulatory system. In: Wake M H (ed) Hyman's comparative vertebrate anatomy. University of Chicago Press: Chicago: pp 448–554

Lazard D, Lupko K, Poria Y, Nef P, Lazarovits J, Horn S, Khen M, Lancet D 1991 Odorant signal termination by olfactory UDP glucuronosyl transferase. Nature 49: 790–793

Lazard D, Sastre X, Frid M G, Glukhova M A, Thiery J P, Koteliansky V

E 1993 Expression of smooth muscle-specific proteins in myoepithelium and stromal myofibroblasts of normal and malignant breast tissue. Proc Natl Acad Sci USA 90: 999–1003

Lazarides E 1976 Actin, alpha-actinin and tropomyosin interaction in the structural organisation of actin filaments in non-muscle cells. J Cell Biol 68: 202–219

Lazarides E 1980 Intermediate filaments as mechanical integrators of cellular space. Nature 283: 249–256

Lazarow P B 1993 Genetic approaches to studying peroxisome biogenesis. Trends in Cell Biol 3: 89–93

Lazorthes G 1949 Le système neurovasculaire. Masson: Paris

Lazorthes G, Gouaze A, Zadeh J O, Santini J J, Lazorthes Y, Burdin P 1971 Arterial vascularization of the spinal cord. J Neurosurg 35: 253–262

Le Blanc G G, Epstein M L, Bronner-Fraser M E 1990 Differential development of cholinergic neurons from cranial and trunk neural crest cells in vitro. Dev Biol 137: 318–330

Le Douarin N M 1969 Particularités du noyau interphasique chez la Caille japonaise (Coturnix coturnix japonica). Utilisation de ces particularités comme 'marquage biologique' dans les recherches sur les interactions tissulaires et les migrations cellulaires au cours de l'ontogenèse. Bull biol Fr Belg 103: 435–452

Le Douarin N M 1973 A biological cell labelling technique and its use in experimental embryology. Dev Biol 30: 217–222

Le Douarin N M 1975 An experimental analysis of liver development. Med Biol 53: 427–455

Le Douarin N M 1978 The embryological origin of the endocrine cells associated with the digestive tract. Experimental analysis based on the use of a stable cell marking technique. In: Bloom S R (ed) Gut hormones. Churchill Livingstone: Edinburgh: pp 49–56

Le Douarin N M 1980 The ontogeny of the neural crest in avian embryo chimaeras. Nature 186: 663–669

Le Douarin N M 1982 The neural crest. Cambridge University Press: Cambridge

Le Douarin N M 1993 Embryonic neural chimaeras in the study of brain development. TINS 16: 64–72

Le Douarin N M, Dulac C 1992 Influence of the environment on the development of the enteric nervous system from the neural crest. In: Holle G E, Wood J D (eds) Advances in the innervation of the gastrointestinal tract. Elsevier: Amsterdam: pp 3–17

Le Douarin N M, Teillet M 1973 The migration of neural crest cells to the wall of the digestive tract in avian embryo. J Embryol Exp Morph 30: 31–48

Le Douarin N M, Teillet M A 1974 Experimental analysis of the migration and differentiation of neuroblasts of the autonomic nervous system and of neuroectodermal mesenchymal derivatives, using a biological marker technique. Dev Biol 41: 162–184

Le Douarin N, Bussonet C, Chaumont F 1968 Etude des capacités de différenciation et du rôle morphogène de l'endoderme pharyngien chez l'embryon d'oiseau. Ann Embryol Morphog 1: 29–39Curr Opin Cell BiollLe Douarin N M, Smith J 1988 Development of the peripheral nervous system from the neural crest. Ann Rev Cell Biol 4: 375–404

Le Douarin N, McLaren A 1984 Chimeras in developmental biology. Academic Press: London

Le Double A-F 1903 Les variations des os du crâne human. Rev Sci 4s 20: 641–649

Le Gros Clark W E 1920 On the Pacchionian bodies. J Anat 55: 40–48

Le Mouellic H, Lellemand Y, Brulet P 1992 Homeosis in the mouse induced by a null mutation in the Hox-3.1 gene. Cell 69: 251–264

Le W-K, Harding C V 1984 Square arrays and their role in ridge formation in human lens fibers. J Ultrastruct Res 86: 245–251

Leah J D, Cameron A A, Snow P J 1985 Neuropeptides in physiologically identified mammalian sensory neurons. Neurosci Lett 56: 257–260

Leak L V, Burke J F 1968 Ultrastructural studies on the lymphatic anchoring filaments. J Cell Biol 36: 129–149

Learmonth J R 1931 Contribution to neurophysiology of urinary bladder in man. Brain 54: 147–176

Leber S M, Breedlove S M, Sanes J R 1990 J Neurosci 10: 2451–2462

Leberer E, Seedorf U, Pette D 1986 Neural control of gene expression in skeletal muscle. Calcium-sequestering proteins in developing and chronically stimulated rabbit skeletal muscles. Biochem J 239: 295–300

LeBlanc A-R, Dubé B 1993 Propagation in the AV node: a model based on a simplified two dimensional structure and a bidomain tissue representation. Med Biol Eng Comput 31: 545–556

Leblanc G G, Trimmer B A, Landis S C 1987 Neuropeptide Y-like immunoreactivity in rat cranial parasympathetic neurons: coexistence with vasoactive intestinal peptide and choline acetyltransferase. Proc Natl Acad Sci 84: 3511–3515

Leblond C P, Clermont Y 1952a Definition of the stages of the cycle of the seminiferous epithelium in the rat. Ann NY Acad Sci 55: 548–573

Leblond C P, Clermont Y 1952b Spermiogenesis of rat, mouse, hamster and guinea pig as revealed by the 'periodic acid-fuchsin sulfurous acid' technique. Am J Anat 90: 167–216

Leborgne J, Letenneur J, Pannier M, Visset J, Bainvel J-V, Barbin J-Y 1973 Considérations sur la vascularisation artérielle du muscle carré crural. Arch Anat Path 21: 359–363

Lebourg L, Champagne G 1951 A propos due développement mandibulaire post-natal. Précisions sur la chronologie de la suture symphysaire. Rev Stomatol Chir Maxillofac 52: 891–897

Lederer W J, Vaughan-Jones R D, Eisner D A, Sheu S-S, Cannell M B 1986 The regulation of tension in heart muscle by intracellular sodium. In: Nathan R D (ed) Cardiac muscle: the regulation of excitation and contraction. Academic Press: New York: pp 217–235

LeDoux J E 1986 The neurobiology of emotion. In: Mind and Brain: Dialogues in cognitive neuroscience. Cambridge University Press: Cambridge: pp 301–354

LeDoux J E 1991 Emotion and the brain. J NIH Res 3: 49–51

LeDoux J E 1991 Emotion and the limbic system concept. Concepts Neurosci 2: 169–199

LeDuc I E 1939 Anatomy of the prostate and pathology of early benign hyperplasia. J Urol 42: 1217–1241

Lee C-S, Tsai T-L 1974 The relation of the sciatic nerve to the piriformis muscle. J Formosan Med Assoc 73: 75–80

Lee J, Sagel S, Stanley R (eds) 1989 Computed body tomography with MRI correlation. 2nd edition. Raven Press: New York

Lee M K, Cleveland D W 1994 neurofilament function and dysfunction: involvement in axonal growth and neuronal disease. Curr Opin Cell Biol 6: 34–40

Leela K, Kanagasuntheram R 1968 A microscopic study of the human pyloro-duodenal junction and proximal duodenum. Acta Anat 71: 1–12

Leese H J 1988 The formation of oviduct fluid. J Reprod Fert 82: 843–856

Leese H J 1989 Energy metabolism of the blastocyst and uterus at implantation. In: Yoshinaga Y (ed) Serono Symposium on blastocyst implantation. Serono Symposium: 39–44

Leese H J 1991 Metabolism of the preimplantation mammalian embryo. Oxford Review of Reproductive Biology 13: 35–72

Leese H J, Barton A M 1984 Pyruvate and glucose uptake by mouse ova and preimplantation embryos. J Reprod Fert 72: 9–13

Leeson T S 1957 The fine structure of the mesonephros of the 17-day rabbit embryo. Exp Cell Res 12: 670–672

Leeson T S, Leeson C R 1965 The fine structure of cavernous tissue in the adult rat penis. Invest Urol 3: 144–154

Leeuwenhoek A 1674 Microscopical observations concerning blood, milk, bones, the brain, spittle and cuticula, etc. Philos Trans R Soc Lond [Biol] 9: 121–128

Lefcort F, Venstrom K, McDonald J A, Reichardt L F 1992 Regulation of expression of fibronectin and its receptor, $\alpha_5\beta_1$, during development and regeneration of peripheral nerve. Dev 116: 7676–7682

Leffert R D, Weiss C, Athanasoulis C A 1974 The vincula; with particular reference to their vessels and nerves. J Bone Jt Surg 566: 1191–1198

Legueu F, Juvara E 1892 Des aponéuroses de la paume de la main. Bull Soc Anat Paris: 383–400

Leibovich S J, Ross R 1975 The role of the macrophage in wound repair. A study with hydrocortisone and antimacrophage serum. Am J Pathol 78: 71–100

Leigh R J, Zee D S 1991 The neurology of eye movements. 2nd edition. F A Davis: Philadelphia

Leikola A 1976 The neural crest: migrating cells in embryonic development. Folia Morphol 24: 155–172

Leithner C, Sinzinger H, Hohenecker J, Wicke L, Olbert F, Feigl W 1975 Radiologic anatomy of the abdominal aorta and their large branches. Okajimas Folia Anat Jpn 52: 119–150

Lejeune J, Gautier M, Turpin R 1959 Etude des chromosomes somatique de neuf enfants mongoliens. C R Acad Sci Paris 248: 1721–1722

Lende R A, Kirsch W M, Druckman R 1971 Relief of facial pain after combined removal of precentral and postcentral cortex. J Neurosurg 34: 537–543

Leng G, Mason W T, Dyer R G 1982 The supraoptic nucleus as an osmoreceptor. Neuroendocrinology 34: 75–82

Lenman J A R 1974 Integration and analysis of the electromyogram and related techniques. In: Walton J N (ed) Disorders of voluntary muscle. 3rd edition. Churchill Livingstone: Edinburgh: pp 1034–1072

Lent R, Schmidt S L 1993 The ontogenesis of the forebrain commissures and the determination of brain asymmetries. Prog Neurobiol 40: 249–276

Lenz F A, Dostrovsky J O, Tasker R R, Yamashiro K, Kwan H C, Murphy J T 1988 Single-unit analysis of the human ventral thalamic nuclear group: somatosensory responses. J Neurophysiol 59(2): 299–316

Lenz F A, Seike M, Lin Y C, Baker F H, Rowland L H, Gracely R H et al 1993 Neurons in the area of human thalamic nucleus ventralis caudalis respond to painful heat stimuli. Brain Res 623: 235–240

Lenz F A, Tasker R R, Kwan H C, Schnider S, Kwong R, Muryama Y et al 1988 Single unit analysis of the human thalamic nuclear group: correlation of thalamic "tremor cells" with the 3–6 Hz component of Parkinsonian tremor. J Neurosci 8(3): 754–764

Leon C, Grant N J, Aunis D and Langley K 1992 Expression of cell adhesion molecules and catecholamine synthesising enzymes in the developing rate adrenal gland. Brain Res Dev Brain Res 70: 109–121

Leonard M E, Hitchins G M, Moore G W 1983 Role of the vagus nerve and its recurrent laryngeal branch in the development of the human ductus arteriosus. Am J Anat 167: 313–327

Lepor H, Gregerman M, Crosby R, Mostofi F K, Walsh P C 1985 Precise localization of the autonomic nerves from the pelvic plexus to the corpora cavernosa: a detailed anatomical study of the adult male pelvis. J Urol 133: 207–212

Leranth C, Deller T, Buzsáki G 1992 Intraseptal connections redefined: lack of a lateral septum to medial septum path. Brain Res 583: 1–11

Leranth C, Frotscher M 1989 Organization of the septal region in the rat brain: cholinergic-GABA-ergic interconnections and the termination of hippocampo-septal fibres. J Comp Neurol 289: 304–314

Lerche W 1965 Elektronenmikroskopische Beobachtungen über die Histogenese der bruchschen Membran des Menschen. Z Zellforsch 65: 163–175

Leslie D R 1954 The tendons on the dorsum of the hand. Aust N Z J Surg 23: 253–256

Letourneau P 1975 Dev Biol 44: 92–101

Letourneau P 1985 In: Edelmann G M (ed) Molecular bases of neural development. John Wiley and Sons: New York

Letourneau P 1990 The Nerve Growth Cone

Leuchtenberger C, Schrader F 1950 The chemical nature of the acrosome in the male germ cells. Proc Natl Acad Sci USA 36: 677–683

LeVay 1991 A difference in hypothalamic structure between heterosexual and homosexual men. Science 253: 1034–1037

LeVay S 1991 A difference in hypothalamic structure between heterosexual and homosexual men. Science 253: 1034–1037

L'Eveque J L, Agache P G 1993 Aging skin. Dekker: New York

Lever J D 1955 Electron microscopic observations on the adrenal cortex. Am J Anat 97: 409–430

Lever J D, Lewis P R, Boyd J D 1959 Observations on the fine structure and histochemistry of the carotid body in the cat and rabbit. J Anat 93: 478–490

Levesque M J, Groom A C 1976 Washout kinetics of red cells and plasma from the spleen. Am J Physiol 231: 1665–1671

Levey A I, Kitt C A, Simonds W F, Price D L, Brann M R 1991 Identification and localization of muscarinic acetylcholine receptor proteins in brain with subtype-specific antibodies. J Neurosci 11: 3218–3226

Levi-Montalcini R 1950 The origin and development of the visceral system in the spinal cord of the chick embryo. J Morphol 86: 253–283

Levi-Montalcini R 1952 Effects of mouse tumor transplants on the nervous system. Ann N Y Acad Sci 55: 330–343

Levi-Montalcini R 1960 Destruction of the sympathetic ganglia in mammals by an antiserum to the nerve growth-promoting factor. Proc Natl Acad Sci USA 46: 384–391

Levi-Montalcini R 1967 Differentiation and growth control mechanisms in the nervous system. In: Morphological and biochemical aspects of cytodifferentiation. Exp Biol Med I: 170–182

Levi-Montalcini R, Angeletti P U 1968 Nerve growth factor. Physiol Rev 48: 534–569

Levi-Montalcini R, Chen J S 1971 Selective outgrowth of nerve fibers in vitro from embryonic ganglion of Periplaneta americana. Arch Ital Biol 109: 307–337

Levick J R, Smaje L H 1987 An analysis of the permeability of a fenestra. Microvascular Res 33: 233–256

Levine J H, Moses H L, Gold L I, Nanney L B 1993 Spatial and temporal patterns of immunoreactive transforming growth factors B1, B2 and B3 during excisional wound repair. Am J Pathol 143: 368–380

Levitt P, Cooper M L, Rakic P 1981 Coexistence of neuronal and glial precursor cells in the cerebral ventricular zone of the fetal monkey: an ultrastructural immunoperoxidase analysis. J Neurosci 1: 27–39

Levitt P, Rakic P 1980 Immunoperoxidase localization of glial fibrillary acid protein in radial glial cells and astrocytes of the developing rhesus monkey brain. J Comp Neurol 193: 815–840

Levkova N A, Kakabadze S A 1977 Ultrastructural organisation of chromaffin paraganglia in the nodes of the solar plexus. Arkh Anat Gistol Embriol 72: 53–58

Lewin B 1980 Gene expression. Vol 2. Eucaryotic chromosomes. 2nd edition. Wiley: New York

Lewis B 1990 Genes. 4th edn. Wiley: New York

Lewis C E, McGee J O'D 1992 The macrophage. IRL Press: Oxford

Lewis F T 1912 The form of the stomach in human embryos with notes upon the nomenclature of the stomach. Am J Anat 13: 477–503

Lewis J 1927 The blood vessels in the human skin and their responses. Shaw & Sons: London

Lewis O J 1956 The development of the circulation in the spleen of the foetal rabbit. J Anat 90: 282–289

Lewis O J 1957a The blood vessels of the adult mammalian spleen. J Anat 91: 245–250

Lewis O J 1957b The formation and development of the blood vessels of the mammalian cerebral cortex. J Anat 91: 40–46

Lewis O J 1958a The development of the blood vessels of the metanephros. J Anat 92: 84–97

Lewis O J 1959 The coraco-clavicular joint. J Anat 93: 296–303

Lewis O J 1962 The comparative morphology of M flexor accessorius and the associated flexor tendons. J Anat 96: 321–333

Lewis O J 1964a The homologies of the mammalian tarsal bones. J Anat 98: 195–208

Lewis O J 1964b The tibialis posterior tendon in the primate foot. J Anat 98: 209–218

Lewis O J 1965 The evolution of the Mm Interossei in the primate hand. Anat Rec 153: 275–288

Lewis O J 1977 Joint remodelling and the evolution of the human hand. J Anat 123: 157–201

Lewis O J 1983 The evolutionary emergence and refinement of the mammalian pattern of foot architecture. J Anat 137: 21–45

Lewis O J, Hamshere R J, Bucknill T M 1970 The anatomy of the wrist joint. J Anat 106: 539–552

Lewis P R, Schute C C D 1959 Selective staining of visceral efferents in the rat brain stem by a modified Koelle technique. Nature 183: 1743–1744

Lewis P R, Scott J A, Navaratanam V 1970 Localisation in the dorsal motor nucleus of the vagus in the rat. J Anat 107: 197–208

Lewis W H 1905 Experimental studies on the development of the eye in Amphibia. I. On the origin of the lens in Rana palustris. Am J Anat 3: 505–536

Lewy F H, Kobrak H 1936 The neural projection of the cochlear spirals on the primary acoustic centers. Arch Neurol Psychiatry 35: 839–852

Lexell J 1993 Ageing and human muscle: observations from Sweden. Canad J Appl Physiol 18: 2–18

Lexell J, Jarvis J C, Currie J, Downham D Y, Salmons S 1994 The fibre type composition of rabbit tibialis anterior and extensor digitorum longus muscles. J Anat 185: 95–101

Lexell J, Jarvis J C, Downham D Y, Salmons S 1992 Quantitative morphology of stimulation-induced damage in rabbit fast-twitch muscles. Cell Tiss Res 269: 195–204

Lexell J, Taylor C, Sjöström M 1988 What is the cause of ageing atrophy? Total number, size and proportion of different fiber types studied in whole vastus lateralis muscle from 15–83-year-old men. J Neurol Sci 84: 275–294

Leydig F 1850 Zur Anatomie der mannlichen Geschelechtsorgane und Analdrusen der Saugethiere. Z wiss Zool 2: 1–10

Libby W F 1952 Radiocarbon dating. University of Chicago Press: Chicago

Liberman M C 1982 Single neuron labelling in the cat auditory nerve. Science 216: 1239–1241

Libet B, Owman C 1974 Concomitant changes in formaldehyde-induced fluorescence of dopamine interneurons and in slow inhibitory post-synaptic potentials. J Physiol 237: 636–662

Librach C L, Werb Z, Fitzgerald M L et al 1991 92-kD type IV collagenase mediates invasion of human cytotrophoblasts. J Cell Biol 113: 437–449

Lichtman J W, Purves D, Yip J W 1979 On the purpose of selective innervation of guinea pig superior cervical ganglion cells. J Physiol 292: 69–84

Liddell E G I, Phillips C G 1944 Pyramidal section in the cat. Brain 67: 1–9

Lidow M S, Menco B P M 1984 Observations on axonemes and membranes of olfactory and respiratory cilia in frogs and rats using tannic acid-supplemented fixation and photographic rotation. J Ultrastruct Res 86: 18–30

Lieb F J, Perry J 1968 Quadriceps function. An anatomical and mechanical study using amputated limbs. J Bone Jt Surg 50A: 1535–1548

Lieberman A R 1971 The axon reaction: a review of the principal features of perikaryal responses to axon injury. Int Rev Neurobiol 14: 49–124

Lieberman A R 1976 Sensory ganglia. In: Landon D N (ed) The peripheral nerve. Chapman & Hall: London: pp 188–278

Liebermann A R 1968 An investigation by light and electron microscopy of chromatolytic and other phenomena induced in mammalian nerve cells by experimental lesions. PhD Thesis, University of London

Liebermann A R 1969 Absence of ultrastructural changes in ganglionic neurons after supranodose vagotomy. J Anat 104: 49–54

Liebermann A R 1974(b) Some factors affecting retrograde neuronal responses to axonal lesions. In: Bellairs R, Gray E C (eds) Essays on the nervous system. Clarendon Press: Oxford: pp 71–104

Liem R K H 1993 Molecular biology of neuronal intermediate filaments. Curr Opin Cell Biol 5: 12–16

Lightman S L, Everitt B J 1986 Neuroendocrinology. Blackwell: Oxford

Lightoller G H S 1925 Facial muscles. The modiolus and muscles surrounding the rima oris with some remarks about the panniculus adiposus. J Anat 60: 1–85

Liley A W 1963 Intrauterine transfusion of foetus in haemolytic disease. BMJ 2: 1107–1109

Lilja J 1979 Innervation of different parts of the predentin and dentin in young human premolars. Acta Odontol Scand 37: 339–346

Lim D J 1969 Vestibular sensory epithelia. A scanning electron microscopic observation. Arch Otolaryngol 90: 283–292

Lim D J 1971 Vestibular sensory organs. A scanning electron microscopic investigation. Arch Otolaryngol 94: 69–76

Lim D J 1973 Formation and fate of the otoconia. Ann Otol 82: 23–35

Lin H S 1967 A peculiar configuration of agranular reticulum (caniculate lamellar body) in the rat pinealocyte. J Cell Biol 33: 15–25

Lin L F, Doherty D H, Lile J D, Bektesh S, Collins F 1993 GDNF: a glial cell line-derived neurotrophic factor for midbrain dopaminergic neurons. Science 260: 1130–1132

Lin L H, Mismer D, Lile J D, Armes G L, Butler E T, Vannice J L, Collins F 1989 Purification, cloning and expression of ciliary neurotrophic factor (CNTF). Science 246: 1023–1025

Lin L-D, Murray G M, Sessle B J 1994a Functional properties of single neurons in the primate face primary somatosensory cortex. I. Relations with trained orofacial motor behaviors. J Neurophysiol 71: 2377–2390

Lin L-D, Murray G M, Sessle B J 1994b Functional properties of single neurons in the primate face primary somatosensory cortex. II. Relations with different directions of trained tongue protrusion. J Neurophysiol 71: 2391–2400

Lin L-D, Sessle B J 1994 Functional properties of single neurons in the primate face primary somatosensory cortex. III. Modulation of responses to peripheral stimuli during trained orofacial motor behaviors. J Neurophysiol 71: 2401–2413

Linc R, Fleischmann J 1968 K součanému stavu anatomického názvoslovi. Cas Lek Cesk 107: 107–121

Linck G, Porte A 1981 Cytophysiology of the synovial membrane: distinction of two cell types of the intima revealed by their reaction with horseradish peroxidase and iron saccharate in the mouse. Biol Cell 42: 147–152

Lind J, Wergelius C 1954 Human fetal circulation: change in the cardiovascular system at birth and disturbances in the post-natal closure of the foramen ovale and ductus arteriosus. Cold Spring Harbor Symp Quant Biol 19: 109–125

Lindahl P E, Drevius L O 1964 Observations on bull spermatozoa in a hypotonic medium related to sperm mobility mechanisms. Exp Cell Res 36: 632–646

Lindeman H H 1969 Regional differences in sensitivity of the vestibular sensory epithelia to ototoxic antibiotics. Acta Otolaryngol [Stockh] 67: 177–189

Linden R W 1993 Taste. British Dental Journal. 175:243–53

Linden R W A 1990 An update on the innervation of the periodontal ligament. Europ J Orthod 12: 91–100

Lindenberg S, Hyttel P 1989 In vitro studies of the peri implantation phase of human embryos. In: Van Blerkom J, Motta P (eds) Ultrastructure of human gametogenesis and early embryogenesis. Kluwer Academic: Dordrecht: pp 201–211

Lindenberg S, Hyttel P, Lenz S, Holmes P V 1986 Ultrastructure of the early human implantation in vitro. Human Reprod 1: 533–538

Lindenberg S, Kimber S J, Hamberger L, Falk Larsen J 1990 Human implantation mechanism. In: Capitano G L, Asch R H, De Cecco L, Croce S (eds) GIFT: from basics to clinics. Serono Symposium 63: 175–200

Lindsay R M, Wiegand S J, Altar C A, DiStefano P S 1994 Trends Neurosci 17: 182–190

Lindsley D B, Schreiner L H, Knowles W B, Magoun H W 1950 Behavioural and EEG changes following chronic brain stem lesions in the cat. Electroenceph Clin Neurophysiol 2: 483–498

Lindvall O 1994 Neural transplantation in Parkinson's disease. In: Dunnett S B, Björklund A (eds) Functional neural transplantation. Raven Press: New York pp 103–138

Lindvall O, Björklund A 1974 The organizations of the ascending catecholamine neuron systems in the rat brain as revealed by the glyoxylic acid fluorescence method. Acta Physiol Scand 412: 1–48

Lindvall O, Björklund A 1983 Dopamine- and norepinephrine-containing neuron systems: their anatomy in the rat brain. In: Emson P C (ed) Chemical neuroanatomy. Raven Press: New York: pp 229–256

Lindvall O, Sawle G, Widner H et al 1994 Evidence for long term survival and function of dopaminergic grafts in progressive Parkinson's disease. Ann Neurol 35: 172–180

Ling E A, Paterson J A, Privat A, Mori S, Leblond C P 1973 Investigation of glial cells in semithin sections. I. Identification of glial cells in the brain of young rats. J Comp Neurol 149: 43–72

Ling E-A, Wong W-C 1993 The origin and nature of ramified and amoeboid microglia: a historical review and current concepts. Glia 7: 9–18

Linkevich V R 1969 Embryogenesis of female internal genitalia. Akush Ginekol (Mosk) 7: 43–47

Linzell J L, Peaker M 1971 Mechanism of milk secretion. Physiol Rev 51: 564–597

Lipkin M, Sherlock P, Bell B 1963 Cell proliferation kinetics in the gastrointestinal tract of man. II. Cell renewal in stomach, ileum, colon and rectum. Gastroenterology 45: 721–729

Lipner J 1988 Mechanism of mammalian ovulation. In: Knobil E, Nail J D (eds) The physiology of reproduction. Vol 1. Raven Press: New York

Lippert H, Kafer H 1974 Biomechanik des Schädeldachs 2. Dicken der Knockenschichten. Mschr Unfallheik 77: 329–339

Lippold O C J 1952 The relation between integrated action potentials in a human muscle and its isometric tension. J Physiol 117: 492–499

Lisa J R, Gioia J D, Rubin I C 1954 Observations on interstitial portion of the fallopian tube. Surg Gynecol Obstet 99: 159–169

Lisney S J W 1989 Regeneration of unmyelinated axons after injury of mammalian peripheral nerve. J Exp Physiol 74: 757–784

Lisowski F F P 1969 Ethiop Med J 7: 000–000

Lissák K (ed) 1967a Recent developments in neurobiology in Hungary. Akadémiai Kiadó: Budapest

Lissák K (ed) 1967b Results in neuroanatomy, neurochemistry, neuropharmacology and neurophysiology. Akadémiai Kiadó: Budapest

Lissauer H 1885 Beitrag zur pathologischen Anatomie der Tabes dorsalis und zum Faserverlauf in menschlichen Rückenmark. Neurol Zbl 4: 245–246

Lissmann H W, Machin K E 1958 The mechanism of object location in Gymnarchus niloticus and similar fish. J Exp Biol 35: 451–486

Lister G 1985 Indications and techniques for repair of the flexor tendon sheath. Hand Clin 1: 85–95

Lister G D 1984 The hand: diagnosis and indications. 2nd edition. Churchill Livingstone: Edinburgh: pp 1–106

Lister U M 1968 Ultrastructure of the human amnion, chorion and fetal skin. J Obstet Gynaecol Br Commonw 75: 327–331

Listgarten M A 1966 Phase contrast and electron microscopic study of the junction between reduced enamel epithelium and enamel in unerupted human teeth. Arch Oral Biol 11: 999–1016

Listgarten M A 1970 Changing concepts about the dentoepithelial junction. J Can Dent Assoc 36: 70–75

Litvin J, Montgomery M, Gonzalez-Sanchez A, Bisaha J G, Bader D 1992 Commitment and differentiation of cardiac myocytes. Trends Cardiovasc Med 2: 27–32

Liu C-N, Chambers W W 1964 An experimental study of the corticospinal system in the monkey (Macaca mulatta). The spinal pathways and preterminal distribution of degenerating fibers following discrete lesions of the pre- and postcentral gyri and bulbar pyramid. J Comp Neurol 123: 257–284

Liuzzi F J, Lasck R J 1987 Astrocytes block axonal regeneration in mammals by activating the physiological stop pathway. Science 237: 642–645

Livingstone M S, Hubel D S 1984 Anatomy and physiology of a color system in the primate visual cortex. J Neurosci 4: 309–356

Ljunggren A E 1976 The tuberositas tibiae and extension in the knee joint. Acta Morphol Neerl Scand 14: 215–239

Løken A C, Brodal A 1970 A somatotopical pattern in the human lateral vestibular nuclei. Arch Neurol Psychiat 23: 350–357

Llinas R 1969 Neurobiology of cerebellar evolution and development. A.M.A. I.E.R.F. Chicago

Lloyd D P C 1943 Reflex action in relation to pattern and peripheral source of afferent stimulation. J Neurophysiol 6: 111–119

Lloyd D, Poole P K, Edwards S W 1982 The cell division cycle. Temporal organization and control of cellular growth and reproduction. Academic Press: London

Lømo T, Westguard R H 1974 Contractile properties of muscle: control by pattern of muscle activity in the rat. Proc R Soc Lond Series B 187: 99–103

Locker R H, Wild D J C 1984 The N-lines of skeletal muscles. J Ultrastruct Res 88: 207–222

Lockwood C B 1886 The anatomy of the muscles, ligaments and fasciae of the orbit, including an account of the capsule of tenon, the check ligaments of the recti and of the suspensory ligaments of the eye. J Anat 20: 1–25

Lodge T (1946) Anatomy of blood vessels of the human lung as applied to chest radiology. Br J Radiol 19: 1–7

Lodish H, Darnell J, Baltimore D 1990 Molecular cell biology. W H Freeman: New York

Loewenfeld I E 1958 Mechanisms of reflex dilation of the pupil. Historical review and experimental analysis. Documenta Ophthal 12: 185–448

Loewenstein W R 1971 Mechano-electric transduction in the pacinian corpuscle. Initiation of sensory impulse in mechanoreceptors. In: Loewenstein W R (ed) Handbook of Sensory Physiology. Vol 1. Springer: Berlin: pp 269–290

Loewry A D, Spyer K M 1990 Vagal preganglionic neurons. In: Loewry A D, Spyer K M (eds) Central regulations of autonomic functions. Oxford University Press: New York: pp 68–87

Loewy A D 1991 Forebrain nuclei involved in autonomic control. Prog Brain Res 87: 253–268

Loewy A D, Burton H 1978 Nuclei of the solitary tract: efferent projections to the lower brain stem and spinal cord of the cat. J Comp Neurol 181: 421–450

Lohmander L S, Hascall V C, Yanagishita M, Kuettner K E, Kimura J H 1986 Post-translational events in proteoglycan synthesis: kinetics of sythesis of chondroitin sulfate and oligosaccharides on the core protein. Arch Biochem Biophys 250: 211–227

Loick H M et al Ventilation with positive end-expiratory airway pressure causes leukocyte retention in human lung. J App Physiol 75(1): 301–306

Loken A C, Brodal A 1970 A somatotopical pattern in the human lateral vestibular nuclei. Arch Neurol Psychiat Chicago 23: 350–357

Lombard R E, Bolt J R 1979 Evolution of the tetrapod ear: an analysis and reinterpretation. Biol J Linn Soc 11: 19–76

Long C 1968 Intrinsic-extrinsic muscle control of the fingers. Electomyographic studies. J Bone Jt Surg. 50A: 973–984

Long C, Brown M E 1964 Electromyographic kinesiology of the hand: muscles moving the long finger. J Bone Jt Surg 46A 1683–1706

Long C, Brown M E, Weiss G 1961 Electromyographic kinesiology of the hand. Part II. Third dorsal interosseus and extensor digitorum of the long finger. Arch Phys Med 42: 559–565

Long C, Brown M E, Weiss G 1961 Electromyographic kinesiology of the hand. Part II. Third dorsal interosseus and extensor digitorum of the long finger. Arch. Phys. Med. 42: 559–565

Long J A, Jones A L 1967 Observations on the fine structure of the adrenal cortex of man. Lab Invest 17: 355–370

Longfield M D, Dowson D, Walker P S, Wright V 1969 'Boosted lubrication' of human joints by fluid enrichment and entrapment. Biomed Eng 4: 517–522

Longmore R B 1976 Reflected light interference microscopy (RLIM) of load-bearing human articular cartilage. Proc R Miscrosc Soc Lond 11: 60–61

Longmore R D, Gardner D L 1978 The surface structure of ageing human articular cartilage: a study by reflected light interference microscopy (RLIM). J Anat 126: 353–365

Lopes da Silva F 1991 Neural mechanisms underlying brain wave: from neural membranes to networks. Electroenceph Clin Neurophysiol 79: 81–93

Lorch I J, Danielli J F 1950 Transplantation of nuclei from cell to cell. Nature Lond 166: 329–333

Lorente de Nó R 1934 Studies on the striation of the cerebral cortex. II. Continuation of the study of the ammonic system. F Psychol Neurol Lpz 46: 113–177

Lorenz C H, Powers T A, Partain C L 1992 Quantitative imaging of renal blood flow and function. Invest Radiol 27 (suppl 2): S109–S114

Lorenzonn V, Trier J S 1968 The fine structure of human rectal mucosa: the epithelial lining of the base of the crypt. Gastroenterol 55: 88–101

Loring J, Glimelius B, Weston J A 1982 Extracellular matrix materials influence quail neural crest differentiation in vitro. Dev Biol 90: 165–174

Losinski N E, Horvath E, Kovacs K, Asa S L 1991 Immunoelectron microscopic evidence of mammosomatotrophs in human adult and fetal adenohypophyses, rat adenohypophyses and human and rat pituitary adenomas. Anat Anz 172: 11–16

Loughlin S E, Fallon J H (eds) 1992 Neurotrophic factors. Academic Press: New York

Loukides J A, Loy R A, Edwards R, Honig J, Visintin I, Polan M L 1990 Human follicular fluids contain tissue macrophages. J Clin Endocrinol Metabol 71: 1363–1367

Lourey S, Waller G S, Trybus K M 1993 Skeletal muscle myosin light chains are essential for physiological speeds of shortening. Nature 365: 454–456

Love D R, Hill D F, Dickson G, Spurr N K, Byth B C, Marsden R F, Walsh F S, Edwards Y H, Davies K E 1989 An autosomal transcript in skeletal muscle with homology to dystrophin. Nature 339: 55–58

Lovell C R, Smolenski K A, Duance V C, Light N D, Young S, Dyson M 1987 Type I and III collagen content and fibre distribution in normal human skin during ageing. Br J Dermatol 117: 419–428

Lovell-Badge R 1992 The role of Sry in mammalian sex determination. Postimplantation development in the mouse. Ciba Foundation Symposium 165. Wiley: Chichester: pp 162–182

Lovtrup S 1974 Epigenetics – a treatise on theoretical biology. John Wiley: London

Lovtrup S 1983 Epigenetic mechanisms in the early amphibian embryo: cell differentiation and morphogenetic elements. Bio Rev 59: 91–130

Lovtrup S 1984 An introduction to the new evolutionary paradigm. In: Ma-Wan Ho, Peter T (eds) Beyond Neo-Darwinism. Saunders: Philadelphia

Lovtrup S 1984 Ontogeny and phylogeny. Beyond Neo-Darwinism. An introduction to the new evolutionary paradigm. Ch. 7. Ho M-W, Saunders P T (eds) pp. 159–190

Low A 1907 A note on the crura of the diaphragm and the muscle of Treitz. J Anat 42: 93–96

Low P A 1984 Endoneural fluid pressure and microenvironment of the nerve. In: Dyck P J, Thomas P K, Lambert E H, Bunge R (eds) Peripheral Neuropathy. W B Saunders: Philadelphia: pp 599–617

Lowden S, Heath T 1992 Lymph pathways associated with Peyer's patches in sheep. J Anat 181: 209–17

Lowe A A 1981 The neural regulation of tongue movements. Prog Neurobiol 15: 295–344

Lowe R F, Clark R A J 1973 Radius of curvature of the anterior surface of the lens. Br J Ophthal 57: 471–474

Lowenstein O, Wersäll J 1959 A functional interpretation of the electron microscope structures of the sensory hairs on the cristae of the elas-mobranch Raja clavata in terms of directional sensitivity. Nature 184: 1807–1808

Lowenstein W R, Kanno Y 1964 Studies on an epithelial (gland) cell junction. I. Modification of surface membrane permeability. J Cell Biol 22: 565–586

Lowey S, Waller G S, Trybus K M 1993 Skeletal muscle myosin light chains are essential for physiological speeds of shortening. Nature 365: 454–456

Lowsley O S 1912 The development of the human prostate gland with reference to the development of other structures at the neck of the urinary bladder. Am J Anat 13: 299–346

Lozanoff S, Sciulli P W, Schneider K N 1985 Third trochanter incidence and metric trait covariation in the human femur. J Anat 143: 149–159

Lu J, Kaur C, Ling E A 1993 Uptake of tracer by the epiplexus cells via the choroid plexus epithelium following an intravenous or intraperitoneal injection of horseradish peroxidase in rats. J Anat 183: 609–617

Lu K H, Gordon I, Chen H B, Gallagher M, McGovern H 1988 Birth of twins after transfer of cattle embryos produced by in vitro techniques. Vet Record 122: 539–540

Lu M-T, Preston J B, Strick P L 1994 Interconnections between the prefrontal cortex and the premotor areas in the frontal lobe. J Comp Neurol 341: 375–392

Lubbock M J 1993 Development of the mouse periodontium: cell fate in interspecific Mus musculus-Mus caroli chimaeras. PhD Thesis: University of London

Lubińska L 1964 Axoplasmic streaming in regenerating and in normal nerve fibres. In: Singer M, Schadé J P (eds) Mechanisms of neural regeneration. Prog Brain Res 13: 1–71

Lucas Keene M F 1961 Muscle spindles in the human laryngeal muscles. J Anat 95: 25–29

Lucas P W 1979 The dental-dietary adaptations of mammals. Neues Jahrb Geol Palaeontol Mh 8: 486–512

Lucas P W, Luke D A, Voon F C T, Chew C L, Ow R 1986 Food breakdown patterns produced by human subjects possessing artificial and natural teeth. J Oral Rehabil 13: 205–214

Luckett W P 1978 Origin and differentiation of the yolk sac and extraembryonic mesoderm in presomite human and rhesus monkey embryos. Am J Anat 152: 59–97

Luff S E, McLachlan E M, Hirst G D S 1987 An ultrastructural analysis of the sympathetic neuromuscular junctions on arterioles of the submucosa of the guinea pig ileum. J Comp Neurol 257: 578–594

Lufkin T, Dierich A, LeMeur M, Mark M, Chambon P 1991 Disruption of the Hox-1.6 homeobox gene results in defects in a region corresponding to its rostral domain of expression. Cell 66: 1105–1119

Lufkin T, Dierich A, Lemeur M, Mark M, Chambon P 1991 Disruption of the Hox-1.6 homeobox gene results in defects in a region corresponding to its rostral domain of expression. Cell 68: 283–302

Luft J H 1966 Fine structure of capillary and endocapillary layer as revealed by ruthenium red. Fed Proc 25: 1773–1783

Luger T A, Schwartz T 1991 Epidermal cell derived secretory regulins. In: Schuler G (ed) Epidermal Langerhans cells. CRC Press: Boca Raton: pp 217–251

Luiten P G M, Ter Horst G J 1986 Pathways for the regulation of hormone release in feeding and agonistic behavior. In: Oomura Y (ed) Emotion. Karger: Basel: pp 369–380

Luk S C, Nopajaroonsri C, Simon G T 1973 The architecture of the normal lymph node and hemolymph node. A scanning and transmission electron microscopic study. Lab Invest 29: 258–265

Lukaszyk A, Reiter R J 1975 Histophysiological evidence for the secretion of polypeptides by the pineal gland. Am J Anat 143: 451–464

Lumsden A G S 1987 Neural crest contribution to tooth development in the mammalian embryo. In: Maderson P F A (ed) Developmental and evolutionary aspects of the neural crest. Wiley: New York: pp 261–300

Lumsden A G S, Buchanan J A G 1986 An experimental study of the timing and topography of early tooth development in the mouse embryo with an analysis of the role of innervation. Arch Oral Biol 31: 310–311

Lumsden A G S, Davies A M 1983 Nature 306: 786–788

Lumsden A G S, Davies A M 1986 Nature 323: 538–539

Lumsden A, Sprawson N, Graham A 1991 Segmental origin and migration of neural crest cells in the hindbrain region of the chick embryo. Development 113: 1281–1291

Lund J S 1984 Spiny stellate neurons. In: Peters A, Jones E G (eds) Cerebral cortex. Vol 1. Cellular components of the cerebral cortex. Plenum Press: New York: pp 255–308

Lund J S, Yoshioka T, Levitt J B 1993 Comparison of intrinsic connectivity in different areas of macaque monkey cerebral cortex. Cereb Cortex 3: 148–162

Lund R D, Radel J D, Coffey P J 1991 The impact of intracerebral retinal transplants on types of behaviour exhibited by host rats. Trends Neurosci 14: 358 – 361

Lundberg A 1958 Electrophysiology of salivary glands. Physiol Rev 38: 21–40

Lundberg A 1971 Function of the ventral spinocerebellar tract. A new hypothesis. Exp Brain Res 12: 317–330

Lundberg A 1975 A control of spinal mechanisms from the brain. In: Tower D B (ed) The nervous system. Raven Press: New York: pp 253–265

Lundberg A, Nemeth G, Svensson O K, Selvik G 1989 The axis of rotation of the ankle joint. J Bone Jt Surg 71B: 94–99

Lundberg A, Voorhoeve P 1962 Effects from pyramidal tract on spinal reflex arcs. Acta Physio Scand 56: 201–219

Lundberg J M, Franco Cereceda A, Hua X, Hökfelt T, Fischer J A 1985 Coexistence of substance P and calcitonin gene-related peptide-like immunoreactivities in sensory nerve in relation to cardiovascular and bronchoconstrictor effects of capsaicin. Eur J Pharmacol 108: 315–319

Lundberg J M, Martling C-R, Hökfelt T 1988 Airways, oral cavity and salivary glands: classical transmitters and peptides in sensory and autonomic motor neurons. In: Björklund A, Hökfelt T, Owman C (eds) The peripheral nervous system. Handbook of chemical neuroanatomy. Vol 6. Elsevier: Amsterdam: pp 391–444

Lundberg J M, Terenius L, Hökfelt T, Goldstein M 1983 High levels of neuropeptide Y in peripheral noradrenergic neurons in various mammals including man. Neurosci Lett 42: 167–172

Lundborg G, Branemark P-I 1968 Microvascular structure and function of peripheral nerves. Adv Microcir 1: 66

Lundborg G, Myrhage R 1977 The vascularization and structure of the human digital tendon sheath as related to flexor tendon function. Scand J Plast Reconstruct Surg 11: 195–203

Lundquist Per-G, Rask-Anderson I I, Galey F R, Bagger-Sjöbäck 1984 Ultrastructural morphology of the endolymphatic duct and sac. In: Friedmann I, Ballantyne J (eds) Ultrastructural atlas of the inner ear. Butterworths: pp 309–325

Lunn E R, Perry V H, Brown M C, Rosen H, Gordon S 1989 Absence of Wallerian degeneration does not hinder regeneration in peripheral nerve. Eu J Neurosci 1: 27–33

Lurie I W, Kirillova I A, Novikova I V, Burakovski I V 1991 Renal-hepatic-pancreatic dysplasia and its variants. Genet Couns 2: 17–20

Luschka H 1860 Die Steisdruse des Menschen. Arch f Path Anat 18: 106

Luschka H 1862 Ueber die drusenartige Natur des sogenannten Ganglionintercaroticum. Arch f Anat Physiol u Wissensch Med Jahrg 1862: 405–414

Luskin M B, McDermott K 1994 Divergent lineages for oligodendrocytes and astrocytes originating in the neonatal forebrain subventricular zone. Glia 11: 211 – 226

Luskin M B, Pearlman A L, Sanes J R 1988 Neuron 1: 635–647

Luskin M, Parnavelas J, Barfield J 1993 Neurons, astrocytes and oligodendrocytes of the rat cerebral cortex originate from separate progenitor cells: an ultrastructral analysis of clonally related cells. J Neurosci 13(4): 1730 – 1750

Luther P K 1991 3-dimensional reconstruction of a simple Z-band in fish muscle. J Cell Biol 113: 1043–1055

Luther P, Squire J 1978 Three-dimensional structure of the vertebrate muscle M-region. J Mol Biol 125: 313–324

Lymn R W, Taylor E W 1971 Mechanism of adenosine triphosphate hydrolysis by actomyosin. Biochemistry 10: 4617–4624

Lynch J C, Hoover J E, Strick P L 1994 Input to the primate frontal eye field from the substantia nigra, superior colliculus, and dentate nucleus demonstrated by transneuronal transport. Exp Brain Res 100: 181–186

Lyon M F 1962 Sex chromatin and gene action in the mammalian X-chromosome. Am J Hum Genet 14: 135–148

Lyons G E, Schiaffino S, Sassoon D, Barton P, Buckingham M E 1990 Developmental regulation of myosin gene expression in mouse cardiac muscle. J Cell Biol 111: 2427–2436

Lyons G, Buckingham M 1992 Developmental regulation of myogenesis in the mouse. Seminars Dev Biol 3: 243–253

Lytle W J 1959 The common bile-duct groove in the pancreas. Br J Surg 47: 209–212

Lytle W J 1970 The deep inguinal ring, development, function, and repair. Br J Surg 57: 531–536

Lytle W J 1974 The inguinal and lacunar ligaments. J Anat 118: 241–251

Lytle W J 1979 Inguinal anatomy. J Anat 128: 581–594

M

Maayan M L, Ingbar S H 1970 Effects of epinephrine on iodine and intermediary metabolism on isolated thyroid cells. Endocrinology 87: 588–595

Mabuchi K, Sréter F A 1980 Actomyosin ATPase. II. Fiber typing by histochemical ATPase reaction. Muscle Nerve 3: 233–239

McCabe J S, Low F N 1969 The subarachnoid angle: an area of transition in peripheral nerve. Anatomic Rec 164: 15–34

MacCallum J B 1900 On the musculature architecture and growth of the ventricles of the heart. In: Contributions to the Science of Medicine. Dedicated to W H Welch. Baltimore: pp 307–335

McCallum W C 1988 Potentials related to expectancy, preparation and motor activity. In: Picton T W (ed) Human event related potentials. Elsevier: Amsterdam: pp 427–534

McCarthy G, Blamire A M, Puce A, Nobre A C, Bloche G, Hyder F et al 1994 Functional magnetic resonance imaging of human prefrontal cortex activation during a spatial working memory task. Proc Natl Acad Sci USA 91: 8690–8694

Macchi G 1983 Old and new anatomo-functional criteria in the subdivision of the thalamic nuclei. In: Macchi G, Rustioni A, Spreafico R (eds) Somatosensory integration in the thalamus. Elsevier: Amsterdam: pp 3–16

Macchi G, Bentivoglio M 1986 The thalamic intralaminar nuclei and the cerebral cortex. In: Jones E G, Peters A (eds) Cerebral cortex. Vol 5. Sensory-motor areas and aspects of cortical connectivity. Plenum Press: New York: pp 355–401

Macchi G, Bentivoglio M, Minciacchi D, Milinari M 1983 Claustroneocortical projections studied in the cat by means of multiple retrograde fluorescent tracing. J Comp Neurol 215: 121–134

Macchi G, Bentivoglio M, Molinari M, Minciacchi D 1984 The thalamo-caudate versus thalamo-cortical projections as studied in the cat with fluorescent retrograde double labelling. Exp Brain Res 54: 225–239

McClearn D, Noden D M 1988 Ontogeny of architectural complexity in embryonic quail visceral arch muscles. Am J Anat 183: 277–293

McClure C F W, Butler E G 1925 The development of the vena cava inferior in man. Am J Anat 35: 331–384

McColl I 1967 The comparative anatomy and pathology of anal glands. Ann R Coll Surg 40: 36–67

MacConaill M A 1932 The function of intra-articular fibrocartilages, with special reference to the knee and inferior radio-ulnar joints. J Anat 66: 210–227

MacConaill M A 1941 The mechanical anatomy of the carpus and its bearings on some surgical problems. J Anat 75: 166–175

MacConaill M A 1945 The postural mechanism of the human foot. Proc R Ir Acad L Sect B, 14: 265–278

MacConaill M A 1946 Some anatomical factors affecting the stabilising functions of muscles. Ir J Med Sci (6th series) 245: 160–164

MacConaill M A 1949 Movements of bones and joints; function of musculature. J Bone Jt Surg 31B: 100–104

MacConaill M A 1950 Rotary movements and functional decalage, with some references to rehabilitation. Br J Phys Med Ind Hyg 13: 50–56

MacConaill M A 1951 The movements of bones and joints. 4. The mechanical structure of articulating cartilage. J Bone Jt Surg 33B: 251–257

MacConaill M A 1953 The movements of bones and joints. V. The significance of shape. J Bone Jt Surg 35B: 290–297

MacConaill M A 1964 Joint movements. Physiotherapy, November, 359–367

MacConaill M A 1966 The compound polarizer. Lab Pract 15: 659–663

MacConaill M A 1975 The muscular slings of the mandible. J Ir Dent Ass 21: 22–24

MacConaill M A 1978a Anatomical note. Spurt and shunt muscles. J Anat 126: 619–621

MacConaill M A 1978b A generalized mechanics of articular swings. I. From Earth to outer space. J Anat 127: 577–587

MacConaill M A 1978c The strange physics of moving bones. Ir J Med Sci 147: 140–144

MacConaill M A, Basmajian J V 1977 Muscles and movements. A basis for human kinesiology. 2nd edition. Kriger: New York

MacConaill, Scher E 1949 The ideal form of the human dental arcade. Dent Rec 69: 285–302

McConnell S 1989 Trends Neurosci 12: 342–349

McConnell S K 1992 Sem Neurosci 4: 347–356

McConnell S K, Ghosh A, Shatz C J 1989 Science 245: 978–982

McConnell S K, Kasnowski C E 1991 Science 254: 282–285

McCormick D A, Lavond D G, Clark G A, Kettner R G, Rising C, Thompson R F 1981 The engram found? Role of the cerebellum in classical conditioning of nictitating membrane and eyelid responses. Bull Psychonomic Soc 18: 103–105

McCormick D A, Thompson R F 1984 Cerebellum: essential involvement in the classically conditioned eyelid response. Science 223: 296–299

McCormick D, McQuaid S, McCuzker C, Allen I V 1990 A study of glutamine synthetase in normal brain and intracranial tumours. Neuropathol Appl Neurobiol 16: 205–211

McCormick W F 1969 Vascular disorders of nervous tissue: anomalies, malformations and aneurysms. In: Bourne G H (ed) Structure and function of the nervous tissue, vol 3. Academic Press: New York: pp 537–596

McCrimmon D R, Speck D F, Feldman J L 1987 Role of the ventrolateral region of the nucleus of the tractus solitarius in processing respiratory afferent input from vagus and superior laryngeal nerves. Exp Brain Res: 449–459

McCuskey R S, Chapman T M 1969 Microscopy of the living pancreas in situ. Am J Anat 126: 395–407

McCutchen C W 1959 Sponge-hydrostatic and weeping bearings. Nature 184: 1284–1285

McDermott M R, Befus A D, Bienenstock J 1982 The structural basis for immunity in the respiratory tract. Int Rev Exp Pathol 23: 47–112

McDevitt W E 1989 Functional anatomy of the masticatory system. Butterworth: London

McDonald D M, Mitchell R A 1975 The innervation of glomus cells, ganglion cells and blood vessels in the rat carotid body: a quantitative ultrastructural analysis. J Neurocytol 4: 177–230

MacDonald I A 1992 The sympathetic nervous system and its influence on metabolic function. In: Bannister R, Mathias C J (eds) Autonomic failure: a textbook of clinical disorders of the autonomic nervous system. Oxford Medical Publishers: Oxford: pp 197–211

MacDonald I C et al 1987 Kinetics of red cell passage through interendothelial slits into venous sinuses in rat spleen, analysed by in vivo microscopy. Microvasc Res 33: 118–134

MacDonald M S, Emery J L 1959 The late intrauterine and postnatal development of human renal glomeruli. J Anat 93: 331–340

MacDonald W C, Trier J S, Everett N B 1964 Cell proliferation and migration in the stomach, duodenum and rectum of man, radioautographic studies. Gastroenterology 46: 405–417

McDonnell D, Reza Nouri M, Todd M E 1994 The mandibular lingual foramen: a consistent arterial foramen in the middle of the mandible. J Anat 184: 363–370

McDougall J D B 1955 The attachments of the masseter muscle. Br Dent J 98: 193–199

McEwen B S, Coirini H, Schumacher M 1990 Steroid effects on neuronal activity: when is the genome involved. Ciba Foundation Symposium 153: 3–21

McFadzean R, Brosnahan D, Hadley D, Mutlukane E 1994 Representation of the visual field in the occipital striate cortex. Br J Ophthalmol 78: 185–190

McFarlane R M 1974 Pattern of the diseased fascia in the fingers in Dupuytren's contractures. Plastic Reconstruct Surg 54: 31–44

McGeer T 1992 Principles of walking and running. In: Alexander R McN (ed) Mechanics of animal locomotion. Adv Comp Envir Physiol 11: 114–139

McGinnis W, Krumlauf R 1992 Homeobox genes and axial patterning. Cell 68: 283–302

McGrath J, Solter D 1984 Inability of mouse blastomere nuclei transferred to enucleated zygotes to support development in vitro. Science 226: 1317–1319

McGrath P 1971 The volume of the human pharyngeal hypophysis in relation to age and sex. J Anat 110: 275–282

McGrath P 1974 The pharyngeal hypophysis in some laboratory animals. J Anat 117: 95–115

McGrath P 1977 The cavernous sinus: anatomical survey. Aust NZ J Surg 47: 601–613

McGrath P 1978 Aspects of the human pharyngeal hypophysis in normal and anencephalic fetuses and neonates and their possible significance in the mechanism of its control. J Anat 127: 65–81

MacGregor A 1936 An experimental investigation of the lymphatic system of the teeth and jaws. Proc R Soc Med 29: 1237–1272

McGrouther D A 1982 The microanatomy of Dupuytren's contracture. Hand 13: 215–236

McGrouther D A 1990 The palm. In: McFarlane R M, McGrouther D A, Flint M H (eds) Dupuytren's disease, biology and treatment. Churchill Livingstone: Edinburgh: pp 127–135

Machado A B, DiDio L J 1967 Frequency of the musculus palmaris longus studied in vivo in some Amazon indians. Am J Phys Anthropol 27: 11–20

Machamer C E 1993 Targeting and retention of Golgi membrane proteins. Curr Opin Cell Biol 5: 606–612

McIndoe A H, Counsellor V S 1927 The bilaterality of the liver. Arch Surg 13: 589–612

MacIntosh S R 1974 The innervation of the conjuctiva in monkeys. Albrechit v Graefes Arch Ophthamol 192: 105–116

Mack A, Wolburg H 1986 Heterogeneity of glial membranes in the rat olfactory system as revealed by freeze-fracturing. Neurosci Letters 65: 117–122

MacKay T W, Andrews P L R 1983 A comparative study of the vagal innervation of the stomach in man and the ferret. J Anat 136: 449–481

McKee G J, Ferguson M W J 1984 The effects of mesencephalic neural crest cell extrapation on the development of chicken embryos. J Anat 139: 491–512

McKelvy J F 1974 Biochemical neuronendocrinology. I. Biosynthesis of thyrotropin releasing hormone (TRH) by organ culture of mammalian hypothalamus. Brain Res 65: 489–502

McKenna Boot P, Rowden G, Walsh N 1992 Distribution of Merkel cells in human fetal and adult skin. Am J Dermatol 14: 391–396

MacKenzie A, Ferguson M W J, Sharpe P T 1991, Hox-7 expression during murine craniofacial development. Development 113: 601–611

MacKenzie A, Ferguson M W J, Sharpe P T 1992, Expression patterns of the homeobox gene, Hox-8 in the mouse embryo suggests a role in specifying tooth initiation and shape. Development 115: 403–420

MacKenzie D W Jr, Whipple A O, Winterstiener M P 1941 Studies on the microscopic anatomy and physiology of living transilluminated mammalian spleens, Am J Anat 68: 397–456

McKenzie J 1948 The parotid gland in relation to the facial nerve. J Anat 82: 183–186

McKenzie J 1955 A Bronze Age burial near Stonehaven, Kincardineshire. J Anat 89: 579P

McKern T W, Stewart T D 1957 Skeletal age changes in young American males. Tech Rep EP 45. Environmental Protection Research Div Natick, Massachusetts

McKinley B J, Oldfield B J 1980 Circumventricular organs. In: Paxinos G (ed) The human nervous system. Academic Press: New York: pp 415–438

MacKinnon I L, MacKinnon P C B 1958 Seasonal rhythm in the morphology of the suprarenal cortex in women of child-bearing age. J Endocrinol 17: 456–467

MacKinnon P C B, MacKinnon I L 1960 Morphologic features of the human suprarenal cortex in men aged 20–86 years. J Anat 94: 183–191

Macklin C C 1954 The pulmonary alveolar mucoid film and the pneumonocyte. Lancet i: 1099–1104

McLachlan E M 1974 The formation of synapses in mammalian sympathetic ganglia reinnervated with preganglionic or somatic nerves. J Physiol 237: 217–242

McLachlan J A, Nelson K G, Takahashi T, Bossert N L, Newbold R R, Korach K S 1991 Do growth factors mediate estrogen action in the uterus? New biology of steroid hormones. Serono Symposium 74: 337–344

McLaren A 1985 Relating of germ cell sex to gonadal differentiation. In: Halvorsen H O, Monroy A (eds) The origin and evolution of sex. Alan R Liss: New York: pp 289–300

McLaren A 1988 The developmental history of female germ cells in mammals. In: Clarke J (ed) Oxford reviews of reproduction. Vol 10. Oxford University Press: Oxford: pp 162–179

MacLaughlin S M, Oldale K N M 1992 Vertebral body diameters and sex prediction. Ann Hum Biol 19: 285–293

McLaurin C L 1988 Cutaneous reaction patterns in blacks. Dermatol Clin 6: 353–362

McLean F C, Urist M R 1969 Bone: an introduction to the physiology of skeletal tissue. 2nd edition. Chicago University Press: Chicago

MacLean P D 1949 Psychosomatic disease and the visceral brain. Recent developments bearing on the Papex theory of emotion. Psychosom Med 11: 338–353

MacLean P D 1952 Some psychiatric implications of physiological studies on the frontotemporal portion of the limbic system (visceral brain). Electroencephalogr Clin Neurophysiol 4: 407–418

MacLean P D 1958 The limbic system with respect to self-preservation and the preservation of the species. J Nerv Ment Dis 127: 1–11

MacLean P D 1992 The limbic system concept. In: Trimble M R, Bolwig T G (eds) The temporal lobes and the limbic system. Wrightson Biomedical Publishing Ltd: Petersfield: pp 1–14

McLeish R D, Charnley J 1970 Abduction forces in the one-legged stance. J Biomech 3: 191–209

MacLeod J, Gold R Z 1951 The male factor in fertility and infertility II spermatozoon counts in 1000 men of known fertility and in 1000 cases of infertile marriage. J Urol 66: 436–449

McMahon A P, Bradley A 1990 The Wnt-1 (int-1) proto-oncogene is required for development of a large region of the mouse brain. Cell 62: 1073–1085

McManis P G, Low P A, Lagerlund T D 1993 Microenvironment of nerve: blood flow and ischemia. In: Dyck P J, Thomas P K, Griffin J W, Low P A, Poduslo J F (eds) Pheripheral neuropathy 3rd edition. W B Saunders: Philadelphia: pp 453–473

McManners T 1983 Odontoid hypoplasia. Br J Radiol 56: 907–910

McManus I C, Bryden M P 1991 Geschwind's theory of cerebral lateralization: developing a formal, causal model. Psychol Bull 110: 237–253

MacMasters R E, Weiss A H, Carpenter M B 1966 Vestibular projections to the nuclei of the extraocular muscles. Degeneration resulting from discrete partial lesions of the vestibular nuclei in the monkey. Am J Anat 118: 163–194

McMenemin I M, Sissons G R, Brownridge P 1992 Accidental subdural catheterization: radiological evidence of a possible mechanism for spinal cord damage. Br J Anaesth 69: 417–419

McMinn R M H 1969 Tissue repair. Academic Press: New York

McMinn R M H, Kugler J H 1961 The glands of the bile and pancreatic ducts: autoradiographic and histochemical studies. J Anat 95: 1–11

McMinn R M H, Mitchell J E 1954 The formation of villi following artificial lesions of the mucosa in the small intestine of the cat. J Anat 88: 99–107

McNab Jones R F 1979 anatomy of the mouth, pharynx and oesophagus. In: Scott-Brown's diseases of the ear nose and theroat, 4th edn., Vol 1. Basic sciences, Ch 8. Butterworths: London: pp 263–302

McNamara J A J 1972 Dual functions of the lateral pterygoid muscle: a study of Macaca mulatta. Anat Rec 172: 360 [Abstract]

McNeal J E 1975 Structure and pathology of the prostate. In: Goland M (ed) Normal and Abnormal Growth of the Prostate. Thomas: Springfield, Illinois: pp 55–65

McNeill M E 1977 An unusual organelle in the pineal gland of the rat. Cell Tissue Res 184: 133–137

Macrides F, Davis B J 1983 The olfactory bulb. In: Emson P C (ed) Chemical Neuroanatomy. Raven Press: New York: pp 391–426

McVay C B, Anson B J 1940a Aponeurotic and fascial continuities in the abdomen, pelvis and thigh. Anat Rec 76: 213–232

McVay C B, Anson B J 1940b Composition of the rectus sheath. Anat Rec 77: 213–225

Madri J A, Stenn K S 1982 Aortic endothelial cell migration. I. Matrix requirements and composition. Am J Pathol 106: 180–186

Maggi C A 1991 The pharmacology of the efferent function of sensory nerves. J Auton Pharmacol 11: 173–208

Maggi C A, Meli A 1988 The sensory-efferent function of capsaicin-sensitive sensory nerves. Gen Pharmacol 19: 1–43

Maggio E 1965 Microhemocirculation: observable variables and their biologic control. Thomas: Springfield, Illinois

Maguire A, Dayal V S 1974 Supraglottic anatomy: the pre- or the peri-epiglottic space? Can J Otolaryngol 3: 432–445

Mahour G H, Wakin K G, Soule F H, Ferris D O 1967 The common bile duct after cholecystectomy: comparison of common bile ducts in patients who have intact biliary systems with those in patients who have undergone cholecystectomy. Ann Surg 166: 964–967

Mai J K, Kedziora O, Teckhaus L, Sofroniew M V 1991 Evidence for subdivisions in the human suprachiasmatic nucleus. J Comp Neurol 305: 508–525

Maibach H L, Downing D T (eds) 1992 Seminars in dermatology No. 11. Saunders: Philadelphia

Maier A, McEwan J, Dodds K, Fischman D, Fitzsimons R, Harris A J 1992 Myosin heavy chain composition of single fibres and their origins and distribution in developing fascicles of sheep tibialis cranialis muscles. J Musc Res Cell Motil 13: 551–572

Maier M A, Bennett K M B, Hepp-Reymond M-C, Lemon R N 1993 Contribution of the monkey corticomotoneuronal system to the control of force in precision grip. J Neurophysiol 69: 772–785

Mair W G P, Warrington E K, Weiskrantz L 1979 Memory disorder in Korsakoff's psychosis: a neuropathological and neuropsychological investigation of two cases. Brain 102: 749 – 783

Majno G 1979 The story of the myofibroblasts. Am J Surg Pathol 3: 535–542

Male D K 1992 Immunology of brain endothelium and the blood–brain barrier. In: Bradbury M W B (ed) Handbook of experimental pharmacology vol 103 – Physiology and pharmacology of the blood–brain barrier. pp 397–415

Malendowicz L K 1985 Sterological studies on the effects of pinealectomy, melatonin and oestradiol on the adrenal cortex of oviarectomised rats. J Anat 141: 115–120

Mall F P 1911 On the muscular architecture of the ventricles of the human heart, Am J Anat 11: 211–278

Mallon W J, Brown H R, Vogler J B, Martinez S 1992 Radiographic and geometric anatomy of the scapula. Clin Orthop 277: 142–154

Malmqvist U, Arner A, Uvelius B 1991 Contractile and cytoskeletal proteins in smooth muscle during hypertrophy and its reversal. Am J Physiol 260 (Cell Physiol 29): C1085–C1093

Mangold O 1933 Naturwissenschaften 21: 761–766

Mangoushi M A 1975 Branches of the inferior mesenteric artery: 'a rare anomaly'. Ethiop Med J 13: 23–26

Mankin H J, Lippiello L 1969 The turnover of adult rabbit articular cartilage. J Bone Jt Surg 51A: 1591–1600

Mann I C 1927 The relations of the hyaloid canal in the foetus and in the adult. J Anat 62: 290–296

Mann I C 1964 The development of the human eye. 3rd edition. Grune & Stratton: New York

Mann R, Inman V T 1964 Phasic activity of intrinsic muscles of the foot. J Bone Jt Surg 46A: 469–481

Mann T 1949 Metabolism of semen. Adv Enzymol 9: 329–390

Mann T 1967 Sperm metabolism. In: Metz C B, Monroy A (eds) Fertilization. Vol I. Academic Press: New York: pp 99–116

Mann W B, Marlow W F, Hughes E E 1961 The half-life of carbon 14. Int J Appl Radiat Isotopes 11: 57–67

Mannen T, Iwata M, Toyokura Y, Magazhima K 1977 Preservation of a certain motoneurone group of the sacral cord in amyotrophic lateral sclerosis: its clinical significance. J Neurol Neurosurg Psychiat 40: 464–469

Manni E, Bortolami R, Deriu P L 1970 Presence of cell bodies of the afferents from the eye muscles in the semilunar ganglion. Arch Ital Biol 108: 106–120

Manni E, Bortolami R, Pettorossi V E, Lucchi M L, Callegari E 1978 Afferent fibers and sensory ganglion cells within the oculomotor nerve in some mammals and man. II. Electrophysiological investigations. Arch Ital Biol 116: 16–24

Manotaya T, Potter E L 1963 Oocytes in prophase of meiosis from squash preparations of human fetal ovaries. Fertil Steril 14: 378–392

Mansbridge J N, Knapp A M 1987 Changes in keratinocyte maturation during wound healing. J Invest Dermatol 89: 253–263

Manske P R, Lesker P A 1983 Palmar aponeurosis pulley. J Hand Surg 8: 259–263

Manstein D J, Titus M A, De Lozanne A, Spudich J A 1989 Gene replacement in Dictyostelium: generation of myosin null mutants. EMBO J 8: 923–932

Manuscript of Bullach's Roll, Royal Society, London Obituary.

Marcar V L, Cowey A 1992 The effect of removing superior temporal cortical motion areas in the macaque monkey. II. Motion discrimination using random dot displays. Eur J Neurosci 12: 1228–1238

Marchand P, Gilroy J C, Wilson V H 1950 Anatomical study of bronchial vascular system and its variations in disease. Thorax 5: 207–221

Marchesi V T 1961 The site of leucocyte emigration during inflammation. Quart J Exp Physiol 46: 115–118

Marchesi V T 1962 The passage of colloidal carbon through inflamed endothelium, Proc R Soc Lond [Biol] 156: 550–552

Marchesi V T, Gowans J L 1964 The migration of lymphocytes through the endothelium of venules in lymph nodes, Proc R Soc Lond [Biol] 159: 283–290

Marchetti B, Guarcello V, Morale M C, Bartolini G, Farinella Z, Cordaro S, Scapagnini U 1989 Luteinizing hormone-releasing hormone-binding sites in the rat thymus: characteristics and biological function. Endocrinol 125: 1025–1036

Marchionni M A, Goodearl A D, Chen M S et al 1993 Glial growth factors are alternatively spliced erbB2 ligands expressed in the nervous system. Nature 362: 312–318

Marder S R, Chenoweth D E, Goldstein I M, Perez H D 1985 Chemotactic responses of human peripheral monocytes to the complement-derived peptides C5a and C5a des Arg. J Immunol 143: 3325–3331

Marfurt C F, Ellis L C 1993 Immunocytochemical localization of tyrosine hydroxylase in corneal nerves. J Comp Nerol 336: 517–531

Margaria R 1976 Biomechanics and energetics of muscular exercise. Clarendon Press: Oxford

Margolis F 1988 Molecular cloning of olfactory-specific gene products. In: Margolis F L, Getchell T T V (eds) Molecular Neurobiology of the olfactory system. Plenum: New York: pp 237–265

Margolis F L 1982 Olfactory marker protein (OMP). Scand J Immunol 15 (Suppl 9) 181–191

Margolis F L, Grillo M, Kawano T, Farbman A I 1985 Carnosine synthesis in olfactory tissue during ontogeny: effect of exogenous b-alanine. J Neurochem 44: 1459–1464

Margulis L 1981 Symbiosis in cell evolution. Life and its environment on the early earth. Freeman: Oxford

Marikovsky Y, Danon D 1969 Electron microscope analysis of young and old red blood cells stained with colloidal iron for surface charge evaluation. J Cell Biol 43: 1–7

Marin-Padilla M 1971 Z Anat Entwickslungesch 134: 117–145

Marin-Padilla M 1984 Neurons of layer I: a development analysis. In: Peters A, Jones E G (eds) Cerebral cortex. Vol 1. Cellular components of the cerebral cortex. Plenum Press: New York: pp 447–478

Marinesco G 1909 La cellule nerveuse. Dom: Paris

Mark R 1974 Memory and nerve cell connections. Clarendon Press: Oxford

Markee J E, Logue J T Jr, Williams M, Stanton W B, Wrenn R N, Walker L B 1955 Two joint muscles of the thigh. J Bone Jt Surg 37A: 125–142

Markou A, Koob G F K 1991 Post cocaine anhedonia. An animal model of cocaine withdrawal. Neuropsychopharmacology 4: 17–26

Markou A, Weiss F, Gold L H, Caine S B, Schulteis G, Koob G F 1993 Drug craving. Psychopharmacology 112: 163–182

Markowski J 1911 Über die Entwicklung der Sinus durae matris und der Hirnvenen bei menschlichen Embryonen von 15 5–49 mm Scheitel-Steisslange. Bull Int Acad Sci LeH Cracov B. 590–611

Marks R H, Barton S P, Edwards C 1988 The physical nature of skin. MTPress, Lancaster

Marks S C Jr, Cahill D R 1984 Experimental study in the dog of the non-active role of the tooth in the eruptive process. Arch Oral Biol 29: 311–322

Markwald R R, Mjaatvedt C H, Krug E L, Sinning A R 1990 Interaction interactions in heart development. Role of cardiac adherons in cushion tissue formation. In: Bockman D E, Kirby M L (eds) Embryonic origins of defective heart development. Ann NY Acad Sci 588: 13–25

Marmarou A, Shulman K, LaMorgese J 1975 Compartmental analysis of compliance and outflow resistance of the cerebrospinal fluid system. J Neurosurg 43: 523–534

Marneffe R de 1951 Recherches morphologiques et expérimentales sur la vascularisation osseuse. Acta Chir Belge 50: 469–488, 568–599, 681–704

Marotti G 1993 A new theory of bone lamellation. Calcif Tissue Int 53 (Suppl 1): S47–S56

Maroudas A 1980 Metabolism of cartilaginous tissues: a quantitative approach. In: Maroudas A, Holborrow E J (eds) Studies in joint disease. Pitman: Tunbridge Wells: pp 59–86

Maroudas A, Palla G, Gilav E 1992 Racemization of aspartic acid in human articular cartilage. Connect Tissue Res 28: 161–169

Maroudas A, Stockwell R, Nachemson A, Urban J 1975 Factors involved in the nutrition of the human lumbar intervertebral disc: cellularity and diffusion of glucose in vitro. J Anat 120: 113–130

Marr D 1969 A theory of cerebellar cortex. J Physiol 202: 437–470

Marrack P, Kappler J 1986 The antigen-specific, major histocompatibility complex-restricted receptor or T cells. Adv Immunol 38: 1–30

Marsden C D 1961 Pigmentation in the nucleus substantiae nigrae of mammals. J Anat 95: 256–261

Marsden C D 1990 Neurophysiology. In: Stern G (ed) Parkinson's disease. Chapman Hall Medical: London: pp. 57–98

Marsden C D, Meadows J C, Merton P A 1983 'Muscular wisdom' that minimizes fatigue during prolonged effort in man: peak rates of motor-neuron discharge and slowing of discharge during fatigue. In: Motor control mechanisms in health and disease. Raven Press: New York: pp 169–211

Marshall A H E, White R G 1961 The immunological reactivity of the thymus. Brit J Exp Path 42: 379–385

Marshall G E, Konstas A G, Bechrakis N E, Lee W R 1992 An immunoelectron microscope study of the aged human lens capsule. Exper Eye Res 54: 393–401

Marshall J, Ansell P L 1971 Membranous inclusions in the retinal pigmented epithelium: phagosomes and myeloid bodies. J Anat 110: 91–104

Marshall V C, Jablonski P, Scott F D 1988 Renal preservation. In: Morris P J (ed) Kidney transplantation, principles and practice. W B Saunders: Philadelphia: p 177

Marsolais E B, Kobetic R 1987 Functional electrical stimulation for walking in paraplegia. J Bone Joint Surg 69-A: 728–733

Marston S B, Smith C W J 1985 The thin filaments of smooth muscles. J Musc Res Cell Motil 6: 669–708

Marston S, Pinter K, Bennett P 1992 Caldesmon binds to smooth muscle myosin and myosin rod and crosslinks thick filaments to actin filaments. J Musc Res Cell Motil 13: 206–218

Martel W, Adler R S, Chan K, Nicklason L, Helvie M A, Jonsson K 1991 Overview: new methods in imaging osteoarthritis. J Rheumatol 18 (suppl 27): 32–37

Martin A 1994 Spinalis capitis, or an accessory paraspinous muscle? J Anat 185: 195–198

Martin B F 1958 The annular ligament of the superior radio-ulnar joint. J Anat 92: 473–482

Martin B M, Gimbrone M A Jr, Unanue E R, Cotran R S 1981 Stimulation of nonlymphoid mesenchymal cell proliferation by a macrophage-derived growth factor. J Immunol 126: 1510–1515

Martin C B Hr 1965 Uterine blood flow and placental circulation. Anaesthesiology 26: 447–459

Martin C P 1932 The cause of torsion of the humerus and of the notch on the anterior edge of the glenoid cavity of the scapula. J Anat 67: 573–582

Martin C P 1942 A note on the renal fascia. J Anat 77: 101–103

Martin G F, Fisher A M 1968 A further evaluation of the origin, course and termination of the opossum corticospinal tract. J Neurol Sci 7: 177–187

Martin G F, Hostege G, Mehler W R 1990 Reticular formation of the pons and medulla. In: Paxinos G (ed) The human nervous system. Academic Press: San Diego: pp 203 – 220

Martin K A C 1988 From enzymes to visual perception: a bridge too far? TINS 11: 380–387

Martin N G 1984 Pituitary-ovarian function in mothers who have had two sets of dizygotic twins. Fertil Steril 42: 878

Martin R 1928 Lehrbuch der Anthropologie. 3 vol. 2nd edition. Fischer: Jena

Martin R B, Burr D B 1989 Structure, function, and adaptation of compact bone. Raven Press: New York

Martin R, Saller K 1961 Lehrbuch der Anthropologie. 3rd edition. Fischer: Stuttgart

Martin T J, Findlay D M, Heath J K, Ng K W 1993 Osteoblasts: differentiation and function. In: Mundy G R, Martin T J (eds) Physiology and pharmacology of bone. Springer-Verlag: Berlin: pp 149–183

Martinez S, Geijo E, Sanchez-Vives M V, Puelles L, Gallego R 1992 Reduced junctional permeability at interrhombic boundaries. Development 116: 1069–1076

Martinez-Hernanadez A, Francis D J, Silberberg S G 1977 Elastosis and other stromal reactions in benign and malignant breast tissue. An ultrastructural study. Cancer 40: 700–706

Martini R, Bollensen E, Schachner M 1988 Immunocytological localization of the major peripheral nervous system glycoprotein P0 and the L2/HNK-1 and L3 carbohydrate structures in developing and adult mouse sciatic nerves. Dev Biol 129: 330–338

Martinoli C, Castellucci M, Zaccheo D, Kaufmann P 1984 Scanning electron microscopy of stromal cells of human placental villi throughout pregnancy. Cell Tissue Res 235: 647–655

Maruyama K, Matsubara S, Natori R, Nonomura Y, Kimura S, Ohashi K,

Murakami F, Handa S, Eguchi G 1977 Connectin, an elastic protein of muscle: characterization and function. J Biochem (Tokyo) 82: 317–337

Mascorro J A, Yates R D 1971 Ultrastructural studies of the effects of reserpine on mouse abdominal sympathetic paraganglia. Anat Rec 170: 269–280

Mascorro J A, Yates R D 1974 Intervention of abdominal paraganglia. An ultrastructural study. J Morphol 142: 153–164

Mascorro J A, Yates R D 1975 A review of abdominal paraganglia. Ultrastructure, mitotic cells, catecholamine release, innervation, light and dark cells, vascularity. In: Hess M (ed) Electron microscopic concepts of secretion. Ultrastructure of endocrinal and reproductive organs. Wiley: New York: pp 435–452

Mash D C, White F W, Mesulam M-M 1988 Distribution of muscarinic receptor subtypes within architectonic subregions of the primate cerebral cortex. J Comp Neurol 278: 265–274

Masland, R II, Tauchi M 1986 The cholinergic amacrine cell. Trends Neurosci 9: 218–223

Mason W T (ed) 1993 Fluorescent and luminescent probes for biological activity: a practical guide to technology for quantitative real-time analysis. Academic Press: New York

Masse J F, Perusse R 1994 Ectodermal dysplasia. Arch Dis Child 74: 1–2

Massion J 1988 Red nucleus: past and future. Behav Brain Res 28: 1–8

Masson P 1937 Les glomus neuro-vasculaires. Histophysiologie (policard). Hermann et Cie: Paris

Mathers L H, Rapisardi S C 1973 Visual and somatosensory receptive fields of neurons in the squirrel monkey pulvinar. Brain Research 64: 65–83

Mathew R 1992 Development of the pulmonary circulation. Metabolic aspects. In: Polin R A, Fox W W (eds) Fetal and neonatal physiology. W B Saunders: Philadelphia: pp 678–682

Mathias R S, Lacro R V, Jones K 1987 Situs inversus, complex cardiac defects, splenic defects. Am J Med Genet 28: 111–116

Mathiasen M S 1973 Determination of bone age and recording of minor skeletal hand anomalies in normal children. Dan Med Bull 20: 80–85

Matsuda H 1968 Electron microscopic study on the corneal nerve with special reference to its endings. Acta-Soc Ophthal Jpn 12: 163–173

Matsumoto Y, Fugiwara M 1987 Absence of donor-type major histocompatability complex class I antigen bearing microglia in the rat central nervous system of radiation bone marrow chimeras. J Neuroimmunol 17: 71–82

Matsumoto Y, Tanabe T, Ueda S, Kawata M 1992 Immunohistochemical and enzymehistochemical studies of peptidergic aminergic and cholinergic innervation of the lacrimal gland of the monkey (Macaca fuscata). J Autonom Nervous Syst 37: 207–214

Matsumura K, Campbell K P 1994 Dystrophin-glycoprotein complex: its role in the molecular pathogenesis of muscular dystrophies. Muscle Nerve 17: 2–15

Matsushita M, Hosaya Y 1979 Cells of origin of the spinocerebellar tract in the rat, studied with the method of retrograde transport of horseradish peroxidase. Brain Res 173: 185–200

Matsushita M, Wang C L 1987 Projection pattern of vestibulocerebellar fibres in the anterior vermis of the cat: an anterograde wheatgerm agglutinin horseradish peroxidase study. Neurosci Lett 74: 25–30

Matsuyama T, Shiosaka S, Wanaka A, Yoneda S, Kimura K, Hayakawa T, Emson P C, Tohyama M 1985 Fine structure of peptidergic and catecholaminergic nerve fibres in the anterior cerebral artery and their interrelationships: an immunoelectron microscopic study. J Comp Neurol 235: 268–276

Matthews M A 1968 An electron microscopic study of the relationship between axon diameter and the initiation of myelin production in the peripheral nervous system. Anat Rec 161: 337–352

Matthews M R, Raisman G 1969 The ultrastructure and somatic efferent synapses of small granule-containing cells in the superior cervical ganglion, J Anat 105: 255–282

Matthews P B C 1971 Recent advances in the understanding of the muscle spindle. In: Gilliland I, Francis J (eds) British postgraduate medical federation, scientific basis of medicine. Annual Reviews. Athlone Press: London: pp 99–128

Matthews P B C 1972 Mammalian muscle receptors and their central actions. Arnold: London

Matulionis D H, Parks H F 1973 Ultrastructural morphology of the normal nasal respiratory epithelium of the mouse. Anat Rec 175: 68–84

Maue-Dickson W, Dickson W D R 1980 Anatomy and physiology related to cleft palate: current research and clinical implications. Plast Reconstr Surg 65: 83–90

Maunsell J H R, Van Essen D C 1987 Topographic organization of the middle temporal visual area in the macaque monkey: representational biases and the relationship to callosal connections and myeloarchitectonic boundaries. J Comp Neurol 266: 535–555

Mauro A 1961 Satellite cells of skeletal muscle fibers. J Biophys Biochem Cytol 9: 493–495

Mauro A (ed) 1979 Muscle regeneration. Raven Press: New York

Mautulionis D H 1975 Ultrastructural study of mouse olfactory epithelium following destruction by ZnSO4 and its subsequent regeneration. Amer J Anat 142: 67–90

Maw A R, Parker A J 1993 A model to refine the selection of children with otitis media with effusion of adenoidectomy. Clin Otolaryngol 18(3): 164–170

Maxwell G D, Forbes M E 1987 Exogenous basement-membrane-like matrix stimulates adrenergic development in avian neural crest cultures. Development 101: 767–776

May M 1986 The Facial Nerve. Thieme: New York

Mayfield J K, Johnson R P, Kilcoyne R F 1976 The ligaments of the human wrist and their functional significance. Anat Rec 186: 417–428

Mayhall J T, Dahlberg A A, Owen D G 1970 Torus mandibularis in an Alaskan Eskimo population. Am J Phys Anthropol 33: 57–60

Mayne R, von der Mark K 1983 Collagens of cartilage. In: Hall B K (ed) Cartilage. Vol 1. Structure, function and biochemistry. Academic Press: New York: pp 181–214

Mayre R, Burgeson R E 1987 Structure and function of collage types. Academic Press: London

Mays L E 1984 Neural control of vergence eye movements: convergence and divergence neurons in the midbrain. J Neurophysiol 51: 1091–1108

Meachim G 1982 Age-related degeneration of patellar articular cartilage. J Anat 134: 365–371

Meachim G, Allibone R 1984 Topographical variation in calcified zone of upper femoral articular cartilage. J Anat 139: 341–352

Meachim G, Denham D, Emergy I H, Wilkinson P H 1974 Collagen alignments and artificial splits at the surface of human articular cartilage. J Anat 188: 101–118

Meachim G, Stockwell R A 1978 The matrix. In: Freeman M A R (ed) Adult articular cartilage. 2nd edition. Pitman Medical: London: pp 1–67

Mears D C 1971 Effects of parathyroid hormone and thyrocalcitonin on the membrane potential of osteoclasts. Endocrinology 88: 1021–1028

Meban C 1980 Thickness of the air-blood barriers in vertebrate lungs. J Anat 131: 299–307

Mecham R P, Heuser J 1990 Three dimensional organization of extracellular matrix in elastic cartilage as viewed by quick freeze, deep etch electron microscopy. Connect Tissue Res 24: 83–93

Mechanik N 1934 Das Venesystem der Herzwände. Z Anat EntwGesch 103: 813–843

Mehler W R 1962 The anatomy of the so-called 'pain tract in man': an analysis of the course and distinction of the ascending fibres of the fasciculus anterolateralis. In: French J D, Porter R W (eds) Basic research in paraplegia. Charles C Thomas: Springfield: pp 26–55

Mehler W R 1974 Central pain and the spinothalamic tract. Adv Neurol 4: 127–146

Mehler W R 1980 Subcortical afferent connections of the amygdala in the monkey. J Comp Neurol 190: 733–762

Mehler W R, Feferman M E, Nauta W J H 1960 Ascending axon degeneration following anterolateral cordotomy. An experimental study in the monkey. Brain 83: 718–750

Mehta H J, Gardner W U 1961 A study of lumbrical muscles in the human hand, Am J Anat 109: 227–238

Mei N 1970 Disposition anatomique et propriétés électrophysiologiques des neurones sensitifs vagaux chez le chat. Exp Brain Res 11: 465–479

Mei N, Dussardier M 1966 Études des lésions pulmonaries produites par la section des fibres sensitives vagales. J Physiol 58: 427–431

Meier S 1979 Development of the chick mesoblast. Formation of the embryonic axis and the establishment of the metameric pattern. Dev Biol 38: 73–90

Meier S 1981 Development of the chick–embryo mesoblast: morphogenesis of the prechordal plate and cranial segments. Dev Biol 83: 49–61

Meier S, Packard D S Jr 1984 Dev Biol 102: 309–323

Melander A 1970 Amines and mouse thyroid activity: release of thyroid hormone by catecholamines and indoleamines and its inhibition by adrenergic blocking drugs. Acta Endocrinol 65: 371–384

Melander A 1977 Aminergic regulation of thyroid activity: importance of the sympathetic innervation and of the mast cells of the thyroid gland. Acta Med Scand 201: 257–262

Melander A 1978 Sympathetic nervous-adrenal medullary system. In: Werner S C, Ingbar S H (eds) The thyroid – a fundamental and clinical text. Harper & Row: New York: pp 216–221

Melander A, Ericson L E, Sundler F, Westgren U 1975 Intrathyroidal amines in the regulation of thyroid activity. Rev Physiol 73: 39–71

Melander A, Nilsson E, Sundler F 1972 Sympathetic activation of thyroid hormone secretion in mice. Endocrinology 90: 194–199

Melcher A H, Walker T W 1976 The periodontal ligament in attachment and as a shock absorber. In: Poole D F G, Stack M V (eds) The eruption and occlusion of teeth. Butterworths: London: pp 183–192

Mélèse T, Xue Z 1995 The nucleolus: an organelle formed by the act of building a ribosome. Curr Opin Cell Biol 7: 319–324

Melkumyants A M, Balashov S A 1990 Effects of blood-viscosity on arterial flow induced dilator response. Cardiovascular Research 24: 165–168

Meller K, Breipohl W, Glees P 1969 Ontogony of the mouse motor cortex. The polymorph layer or layer VI. A Golgi and electronmicroscopical study. Z Zellforsch 99: 443–458

Mellert T K, Getchell M L, Sparks L, Getchell T V 1992 Characterization of the immune barrier in human olfactory mucosa. Otolaryngol-Head Neck Surg 106: 181–188

Melzack R 1973 The puzzle of pain. Basic Books: New York

Melzack R, Wall P D 1965 Pain mechanisms: a new theory. Science 150: 971–979

Menard D 1989 Growth-promoting factors and the development of the human gut. In: Lebenthal E (ed) Human gastrointestinal development. Raven Press: New York: pp 123–150

Menco B P 1984 Ciliated and microvillous structures of rat and olfactory and nasal respiratory epithelia. A study using ultra-rapid cryo-fixation followed by freeze-substitution or freeze-etching. Cell Tissue Res 235: 225–241

Menco B P M 1983 The ultrastructure of olfactory and nasal respiratory epithelium surfaces. In: Reznik G, Stinson SF (eds) Nasal tumours in animals and man. Anatomy, physiology and epidemiology, vol 1. CRC Press Inc: Boca Raton, Florida. pp 45–102

Menco B P M, Dodd G H, Davey M, Bannister L H 1976 Presence of membrane particles in freeze-etched bovine olfactory cilia. Nature 263: 597–599

Menco B P, Bruch R C, Dau B, Danho W 1992 Ultrastructural localization of olfactory transduction components: the G protein subunit Golf alpha and type III adenylyl cyclase. Neuron 8: 441–453

Mendell L M 1966 Physiological properties of unmyelinated fiber projections to the spinal cord. Exp Neurol 16: 316–332

Mendell L M, Wall P D 1964 Presynaptic hyperpolarization: a role for fine afferent fibres. J Physiol 172: 274–294

Mennerick S, Zorumski C F 1994 Glial contributions to excitatory neurotransmission in cultured hippocampal cells. Nature 368: 59–62

Menning A von, Schumacher G H, Lau H, Schultz M, Himstedt H W 1974 Zur Topographie der muskularen Nervenausbreitungen 6. Untere Extremität, Glutealmuskeln. Anat Anz 135: 302–314

Menton D N, Simmons D J, Orr B Y, Plurad S B 1982 A cellular investment of bone marrow. Anat Rec 203: 157–164

Mercier R, Vanneuville G, Bresson P et al 1970a Etude de la structure osseuse de la branche horizontale du maxillaire en inférieur apport des techniques radiographiques. Lab Anat Clermont Ferrand. C R Ass Anat 149: 891–901

Mercier R, Vanneuville G, Bresson P et al 1970b Etude des lignes de force des corticales du maxillaire inférieur par la méthode des lignes de fissuration colorées. Lab Anat Clermont Ferrand. C R Ass Anat 149: 902–913

Meredith M, Marques D M, O'Connell R J, Stern F L 1980 Vomeronasal pump: significance for male hamster sexual behavior. Science 207: 1224–1226

Meredith M, O'Connell R J 1979 Efferent control of stimulus access to the hamster vomeronasal organ. J Physiol 186: 301–316

Meredith M, O'Connell R J 1988 HRP uptake by olfactory and vomeronasal receptor neurons: use as an indicator of incomplete lesions and relevance for non-volatile chemoreception. Chem Senses 13: 487–515

Merendino K A, Johnson R J, Skinner H H, Maguire R X 1956 Intradiaphragmatic distribution of phrenic nerve with particular reference to placement of diaphragmatic incisions and controlled segmental paralysis, Surg Gynec Obstet 39: 189–198

Merideth J, Mendez C, Mueller J W, Moe G K 1968 Electrical excitability of atrioventricular nodal cells. Circ Res 23: 69–85

Merigan W H, Maunsell J H R 1993 How parallel are the primate visual pathways? Ann Rev Neurosci 16: 369–402

Merimee T J, Zapf J, Hewlett B, Cavalli-Sforza L L 1987 Insulin-like growth factors in pygmies. The role of puberty in determining final stature. N Eng J Med 316: 906–911

Merklin R J, Michels N A 1958 The variant renal and suprarenal blood supply with data on the inferior phrenic, ureteral and gonadal arteries: a statistical analysis based on 185 dissections and a review of the literature. J Int Coll Surg 29: 41–76

Merrick W C 1992 Mechanisms and regulation of eukaryotic protein synthesis. Microbiol Rev 56: 291–315

Merrill E G 1974 Finding a respiratory function for the medullary respiratory neurons. In: Bellairs R, Gray E G Clarendon: Oxford: pp 451–486

Merrill J P, Murray J E, Harrison J H, Guild W R 1956 Successful homotransplantation of the human kidney between identical twins. J Am Med Assoc 160: 277–282

Merzenich M M, Kaas, J H, Sur M, Lin C-S 1978 Double representation of the body surface within cytoarchitectonic areas 3b and 1 in "SI" in the owl monkey (Aotus trivirgatus). J Comp Neurol 181: 41–74

Merzenich M M, Nelson R J, Stryker M P, Cynader M S, Schoppmann A, Zook J M 1984 Somatosensory cortical map changes following digit amputation in adult monkeys. J Comp Neurol 224: 591–605

Mesulam M (ed) 1982 Principles of horseradish peroxidase neurohistochemical connections and their applications for tracing neural pathways in microscopical analysis. In: Tracing neural connections with horseradish peroxidase. Wiley: New York: pp 1–152

Mesulam M M, Mufson E J, Levey A I, Wainer B H 1983 Cholinergic innervation of cortex by the basal forebrain: cytochemistry and cortical connections of the septal area, diagonal band nuclei, nucleus basalis (substantia innominata) and hypothalamus in the rhesus monkey. J Comp Neurol 214: 170–197

Mesulam M M, Van Hoesen G W, Pandya D N, Geshwind N 1977 Limbic and sensory connections of the inferior parietal lobule (area PG) in the rhesus monkey: a study with a new method for horseradish peroxidase histochemistry. Brain Res 136: 393–414

Mesulam M-M, Mufson E J 1985 The insula of Reil in man and monkey. Architectonics, connectivity and function. In: Peters A, Jones E G (eds) Cerebral cortex. Vol 4. Association and auditory cortices. Plenum Press: New York: pp 179–226

Mesulam M-M, Mufson E J, Levey A I, Wainer B H 1983 Cholinergic innervation of cortex by the basal forebrain: cytochemistry and cortical connections of the septal area, diagonal band nuclei, nucleus basalis (substantia innominata) and hypothalamus in the rhesus monkey. J Comp Neurol 214: 170–197

Mesulam M-M, Mufson E J, Wainer B H, Levey A I 1983 Central cholinergic pathways in the rat: an overview based on an alternative nomenclature (Ch1–Ch6). Neuroscience 10: 1185–1201

Mesulam M-M, Rosen A D, Mufson E J 1984 Regional variations in cortical cholinergic innervation: chemoarchitectonics of acetylcholinesterase-containing fibers in the macaque brain. Brain Res 311: 245–258

Meszaros T, Kery L 1980 Quantitative analysis of growth of the hip. A radiologic study. Acta Orthop Scand 51: 275–283

Metz C B, Monroy A (eds) 1967 and 1969 Fertilization 2 vol. Academic Press: New York

Meuli H C H 1980 Arthroplasty of the wrist. Clin Orthop 149: 118–125

Meunier M, Bachevalier J, Mishkin M, Murray E A 1993 Effects on visual recognition of combined and separate ablations of the entorhinal and perirhinal cortex in rhesus monkeys. J Neurosci 13: 5418 – 5432

Meyer A W 1917 Studies on hemal nodes. VII. The development and function of hemal nodes. Am J Anat 21: 375–406

Meyer D B, O'Rahilly R 1976 The onset of ossification in the human calcaneus. Anat Embryol (Berl) 150: 19–33

Meyer H 1867 Die Architektur der Spongiosa. Arch Anat Physiol 47:

Meyer M, Matsuoka I, Wetmore C, Thoenen H 1992 Enhanced synthesis of brain-derived neurotrophic factor in the lesioned peripheral nerve: different mechanisms are responsible for the regulation of BDNF and NGF mRNA. J Cell Biol 119: 45–54

Meyer R 1938 Zur Frage der Enticklung der menschlichen Vagina: Vagina infima septa und andere Besonderheiten. Arch Gynecol 167: 306–338

Meyer W W, Lind J 1966 Postnatal changes in the portal circulation. Arch Dis Child 41: 606–612

Meyrick B, Reid L 1968 The alveolar brush cell in rat lung—a third pneumonocyte, J Ultrastruct Res 23: 71–80

Meyrick B, Reid L 1970 Ultrastructure of cells in the human bronchial submucosal glands. J Anat 107: 281–299

Meyrick B, Reid L 1978 The effect of continued hypoxia on rat pulmonary arterial circulation. Lab Invest 38: 188–200

Miale I L, Sidman R L 1961 An autoradiographic analysis of the histogenesis of the mouse cerebellum. Exp Neurol 4: 227–296

Michael R P, Rees H D 1982 Autoradiographic localization of 3H-dihydrotestosterone in the preoptic area, hypothalamus, and amygdala of a male rhesus monkey. Life Sci 30: 2087–2093

Michels N A 1962 The anatomic variations of the arterial pancreaticoduodenal arcades: their import in regional resection involving the gall bladder, bile ducts, liver, pancreas and parts of the small and large intestines. J Int Coll Surg 37: 13–40

Michels N A 1966 Newer anatomy of the liver and its variant blood supply and collateral circulation. Am J Surg 112: 337–347

Michelsohn A, Anderson D J 1992 Changes in competence determine the timing of two sequential glucocorticoid effects on sympathoadrenal progenitors. Neuron 8: 589–604

Middlebrooks J C, Clock A E, Xu L, Green D M 1994 A panoramic code for sound location by cortical neurons. Science 264: 842–844

Midgley A R, Pierce G B Jr, Deneau G A, Gosling J R 1963 Morphogenesis of syncitiotrophoblast in vivo: an autoradiographic demonstration. Science 141: 349–350

Mierzwa J, Koziclec T 1975 Variation of the anterior cardiac veins. Folia Morphol 34: 125–133

Miescher F 1871 On the chemical composition of pus cells. Hoppe-Seyler's Med Chem Untersuch 4: 441–460. Reprinted in Gabriel M L, Fogel S 1955 Great experiments in biology. Prentice-Hall: New Jersey

Migliari R, Riva A, Lantini M S, Melis M, Usai E 1992 Diffuse lymphoid tissue associated with the human bulbourethral gland. An immunohistologic characterization. J Androl 13: 337–341

Mihara M, Miho M, Suyama Y, Shimao S 1992 Scanning electron microscopy

of the epidermal lemina densa in normal human skin. J Invest Dermatol 99: 572–578

Mikami A, Nakamura K, Kubota K 1994 Neuronal responses to photographs in the superior temporal sulcus of the rhesus monkey. Behav Brain Res 60: 1–13

Mikata A, Niki R 1971 Permeability of postcapillary venules of the lymph nodes. An electron microscopic study. Exp Molec Pathol 4: 209–215*

Miki H, Bellhorn M B, Henkind P 1975 Specializations of the retinochoroid juncture. Invest Ophthal 14: 701–7

Mikic Z 1992 The blood supply of the human distal radioulnar joint and the microvasculature of its articular disk. Clin Orthop 275: 19–28

Mikić Z Dj 1978 Age changes in the triangular fibrocartilage of the wrist joint. J Anat 126: 367–384

Mikic Z, Somer L, Somer T 1992 Histologic structure of the articular disk of the human distal radioulnar joint. Clin Orthop 275: 29–36

Mikkelsen J D, Møller M 1990 A direct neural projection from the intergeniculate leaflet of the lateral geniculate nucleus to the deep pineal gland of the rat, demonstrated with phaseolus vulgaris leucoagglutinin. Brain Res 520: 342–346

Milam A H, Dacey D M, Dizhoor A M 1993 Recoverin reactivity in mammalian cone bipolar cells. Vis Neurosci 10: 1–12

Milburn A 1973 The early development of muscle spindles in the rat. J Cell Sci 12: 175–195

Miledi R, Molinoff P, Potter L T 1971 Isolation of the cholinergic receptor protein of Torpedo electric tissue. Nature 229: 554–557

Miles A E W Sebaceous glands in the lip and cheek mucosa of man. Br Dent J 105: 235–248

Milford L 1968 Retaining ligaments of the digits of the hand. W B Saunders: Philadelphia

Milhorat T H 1972 Hydrocephalus and the cerebrospinal fluid. Williams and Wilkins: Baltimore

Millen J W Woollam D H M 1953 Vascular patterns in the choroid plexus. J Anat 87: 114–123

Miller A D 1990 Respiratory muscle control during vomiting. Can J Physiol Pharmacol 68: 237–241

Miller C S, Nummikosi P V, Barnett D A, Langlais R P 1990 Cross-sectional tomography. A diagnostic technique for determining the buccolingual relationship of impacted third molars and the inferior alveolar neurovascular bundle. Oral Surg Oral Med Oral Path 70(6): 791–797

Miller E K, Li L, Desimone R 1991 A neural mechanism for working and recognition memory in inferior temporal cortex. Science 254: 1377–1379

Miller E K, Li L, Desimone R 1993 Activity of neurons in anterior inferior temporal cortex during a short-term memory task. J Neurosci 13: 1460–1478

Miller J D, Adams J H 1992 The pathophysiology of raised intracranial pressure. In: Adams J H, Duchen L W (eds) Greenfield's neuropathology, 5th edition. Edward Arnold: London: pp 69–105

Miller J W, Hall C M, Holland K D, Ferrendelli J A 1989 Identification of a median thalamic system regulating seizures and arousal. Epilepsia 30: 493–500

Miller L H, Carter R 1976 Innate resistance in malaria. Exp Parasitol 40: 132–146

Miller M R, Kasahara M 1959 Cutaneous innervation of the human breast. Anat Rec 135: 153–167

Miller N, Kiel S M, Green R W, Clark A W 1982 Unilateral Duane's retraction syndrome (Type 1). Arch Ophthalmol 100: 1468–1472

Miller R A, Stominger N L 1973 Efferent connections of the red nucleus in the brainstem and spinal cord of the rhesus monkey. J Comp Neurol 152: 327–346

Miller R L, Chaudhry A P 1976 Comparative ultrastructure of vallate, foliate and fungiform taste buds of golden Syrian hamster. Acta Anat 95: 75–92

Miller S C, de Saint-Georges L, Bowman B M, Jee W S S 1989 Bone lining cells: structure and function. Scanning Microscopy 3: 953–961

Miller S C, Jee W S S 1987 The bone lining cell: a distinct phenotype? Calcif Tiss Int 41: 1–5

Miller S C, Jee W S S 1992 Bone lining cells. In: Hall B K (ed) Bone. Vol 4. Bone metabolism and mineralization. CRC Press: Boca Raton: pp 1–19

Miller W S 1947 The lung. 2nd edition, Thomas: Springfield, Illinois

Milley P S, Nichols D H 1971 The relationship between the pubourethral ligament and the urogenital diaphragm in the human female. Anat Rec 170: 281–283

Milligan E T C, Morgan C N, Jones L E, Officer R 1937 Surgical anatomy of anal canal and operative treatment of haemorrhoids. Lancet 2: 1119–1124

Millington P F, Wilkinson R 1983 Skin. In: Harrison R J, McMinn R M H (eds) Biological structure and function 9. Cambridge University Press: Cambridge

Mills E, Jöbsis F F 1972 Mitochondrial respiratory chain of carotid body and chemoreceptor response to changes in oxygen tension. J Neurophysiol 35: 405–428

Mills K R 1991 Magnetic brain stimulation: a tool to explore the action of the motor cortex on single human spinal motoneurones. TINS 14: 401–405

Mills R W 1917 The relation of bodily habits to visceral form, position, tonus and motility. Am J Roentg 4: 155–169

Mills R W 1922 X-ray evidence of abdominal small intestinal states embodying an hypothesis of the transmission of gastro-intestinal tension. Am J Roentg 9: 199–225

Milner B 1974 Hemispheric specialization: scope and limits. In: Schmitt F O, Worden F G (eds) The neurosciences, third study program. MIT Press: Cambridge, Massachusetts

Mincsev M 1967 Bilocular gall bladder. Orvoskepzes 42: 286–298

Minkoff E C 1974 The Fürbinger hypothesis of nerve-muscle specificity re-examined, Can J Zool 52: 525–532

Minkoff R, Rundus V R, Parker S B, Beyer E C, Hertzberg E L 1993 Connexin expression in the developing avian cardiovascular system. Circ Res 73: 71–78

Minneman R P, Lynch H, Wurtman R J 1974 Relationship between environmental light intensity and retina-mediated suppression of rat pineal serotonin N-acetyltransferase. Life Sci 15: 1791–1796

Minns R J, Stevens F S 1977 The collagen fibre organisation in human articular cartilage J Anat 123: 437–457

Minsky B D, Chlapowski F J 1978 Morphometric analysis of the translocation of lumenal membrane between cytoplasm and cell surface of transitional epithelial cells during the expansion-contraction cycles of mammalian urinary bladder. J Cell Biol 77: 685–697

Mintz B 1960 Embryological phases of mammalian gameto-genesis. J cell Comp Physiol 56: (Suppl 1): 31–47

Miragall F, Dermietzel R 1992 Immunocytochemical localization of cell adhesion molecules in the developing and mature olfactory system. Microsc Res Techn 23: 157–172

Miragall F, Kadmon G, Schachner M 1989 Expression of L1 and N-CAM cell adhesion molecules during development of the mouse olfactory system. Devel Biol 135: 272–286

Mishima S, Maurice D M 1961 The effect of normal evaporation on the eye. Exp Eye Res 1: 46–52

Mishkin M 1978 Memory in monkeys severely impaired by combined but not by separate removal of amygdala and hippocampus. Nature 273: 297 – 298

Mitchell B S, Ahmed E, Stauber V V 1993 Projections of the guinea pig paracervical ganglion to pelvic viscera. Histochem J 25: 51–56

Mitchell B S, Stauber V V 1993 Localization of substance P and leucine enkephalin in the nerve terminals of the guinea pig paracervical ganglion. Histochem J 25: 144–149

Mitchell G A G 1935 Innervation of distal colon, Edinb Med J 42: 11–20

Mitchell G A G 1950 Renal fascia. Br J Surg 37: 257–266

Mitchell G A G 1952 Rostral extremities of sympathetic trunks, Nature 129: 533–534

Mitchell G A G 1953 Anatomy of the autonomic nervous system. Livingstone: Edinburgh

Mitchell G A G 1956 Cardiovascular innervation. Churchill Livingstone: Edinburgh

Mitchell G A G, Warwick R 1955 The dorsal vagus nucleus. Acta Anat 25: 371–395

Mitchell L S, Griffiths I R, Morrison S, Barrie J A, Kirkham D, McPhilmey K 1990 Expression of myelin protein gene transcripts by Schwann cells of regenerating nerve. J Neurosci Res 27: 125–135

Mitchell P 1961 Coupling of phosphorylation to electron and hydrogen transfer by a chemi-osmotic type of mechanism. Nature 191: 144–148

Mittal R K 1990 Current concepts of the antireflux barrier. Gastroenterol Clin North Am 19: 501–516

Mittwoch U 1988 The race to be male. New Scientist: 38–42

Mittwoch U 1992 Sex determination and sex reversal: genotype, phenotype, dogma and semantics. Hum Genet 89: 467–479

Miura M, Reis D J 1969 Termination and secondary projections of carotid sinus nerve in the cat brain stem. Am J Physiol 217: 142–153

Miyazaki S 1985 Bilateral innervation of the superior oblique muscle by the trochlear nucleus. Brain Res 348: 52–56

Miyazawa K 1992 Role of epidermal growth factor in obstetrics and gynecology. Obstet Gynecol 79: 1032–1040

Miyazono K, Heldin C H 1989 High-yield purification of platelet-derived endothelial cell growth factor: structural characterization and establishment of a specific antiserum. Biochemistry 28: 1704–1710

Miyazono K, Ichijo M, Heldin C H 1993 Transforming growth factor B Latent forms, binding proteins and receptors. Growth Factors 8: 11–22

Mizeres N J 1963 The cardiac plexus in man. Am J Anat 112 141–151

Mizrachi Y, Naranjo J R, Levi B Z, Pollard H B, Lelkes P I 1990 PC12 cells differentiate into chromaffin cell-like phenotype in co-culture with adrenal medullary endothelial cells. Proc Natl Acad Sci USA 87: 6161–6165

Mizuno M 1991 Human respiratory muscles: fibre morphology and capillary supply. Eur Resp J 4: 587–601

Mjör I A 1969 Bone lamellae. Acta Anat 73: 127–135

Møller M 1974 The ultrastructure of the human fetal pineal gland. I. Cell types and blood vessels. Cell Tissue Res 152: 13–30

Møller M 1976 The ultrastructure of the human fetal pineal gland. II. Innervation and cell junctions. Cell Tissue Res 169: 7–21

Møller M 1978 Presence of a pineal nerve (nervus pinealis) in the human fetus; a light and electron microscopical study of the innervation of the pineal gland. Brain Res 154: 1–12

Møller M 1979 Presence of a pineal nerve (nervus pinealis) in fetal mammals. Prog Brain Res 52: 103–106

Møller M, Phansuwan-Pujiot P, Govitrapong P, Schmidt P 1993 Indications for a central innervation of the bovine pineal gland with substance P immunoreactive nerve fibres. Brain Res 611: 347–351

Møllgard K, Møller M, Kimble J 1973 Histochemical investigations on the human fetal sub-commissural organ. Histochemie 37: 61–74

Mocek F W, Anderson D R, Pochettino A, Hammond R L, Spanta A, Ruggiero R, Thomas G, Lu H, Fietsam R, Nakajima H, Nakajima H, Krakovsky A, Hooper T, Niinami H, Colson M, Levine S, Salmons S, Stephenson L W 1992 Skeletal muscle ventricles in circulation long-term: 191 to 836 days. J Heart Lung Transplant 11: S334–340

Mochereau M T 1963 Ann Biol Anim Biochem Biophys 3:

Mochon S, McMahon T A 1980 Ballistic walking: an improved model. Math Biosci 52: 241–260

Modi J P 1957 Jurisprudence and toxicology. Tripathi Private: Bombay

Modic M T, Weinstein M A, Rothner D, Evenberg G, Duchesneau P M, Kaufman B 1980 Calcification of the choroid plexus visualized by computed tomography. Neuroradiol 135: 369–372

Moens P 1974 Quantitative electron microscopy of chromosome organization at meiotic prophase. Cold Spring Harb Symp Quant Biol 28: 99–107

Moffat D B 1959 Developmental changes in the aortic arch system of the rat. Am J Anat 105: 1–36

Moffat D B 1961a The development of the anterior cerebral artery and its related vessels in the rat. Am J Anat 108: 17–29

Moffat D B 1961b The development of the ophthalmic artery in the rat. Anat Rec 140: 217–222

Moffat D B 1975 The mammalian kidney. Cambridge University Press

Moffat D B 1982 Developmental abnormalities of the urogenital system. In: Chisholm G D, Williams D I (eds) Scientific foundations of urology. 2nd edition. Heinemann Medical: London: pp 357–372

Moffet B C Jr 1957 The prenatal development of the human temperomandibular joint. Contrib Embryol 36: 19–28

Moffett B C, Johnson L C, McCabe J B, Askew H C 1964 Articular remodelling in the adult human temporomandibular joint. Am J Anat. 115: 119–142

Moffie D 1975 Spinothalamic fibres, pain conduction and cordotomy. Clin Neurol Neurosurg 78: 261–268

Mogenson G, Jones D L, Yim C Y 1984 From motivation to action: functional interface between the limbic system and the motor system. Prog Neurobiol 14: 69–97

Mogilner A et al 1993 Somatosensory cortical plasticity in adult humans revealed by magnetoencephalography. Proc Natl Acad Sci USA 90 (Neurorad): 3593–3597

Mohuiddin A 1953 Vagal preganglionic fibres to the alimentary canal. J Comp Neurol 99: 289–318

Molenaar W M, Lee V M, Trojanowski J Q 1990 Early fetal acquisition of the chromaffin and neuronal immunophenotype by human adrenal medullary cells. An immunohistological study using monoclonal antibodies to chromogranin A, synatophysin, tyrosine hydroxylase and neuronal cytoskeletal proteins. Exp Neurol 108: 1–9

Moligner A, Grossman J A, Ribary U, Joliot M, Volkman J, Rapaport D, Beasley R W, Llinas R R 1993 Somatosensory cortical plasticity in adult humans revealed by magnetoencephalography. Proc Natl Acad Sci USA 90: 3593–3597

Moll I, Lane A T, Franke W W, Moll R 1990 Intraepidermal formation of Merkel cells in xenografted human fetal skin. J Invest Dermatol 94: 359–364

Moll I, Moll R, Franke W 1986 Formation of epidermal and dermal Merkel cells during human fetal skin development. J Invest Dermatol 87: 779–787

Möller E 1966 The chewing apparatus: an electromyographic study of the action of the muscles of mastication and its correlation to facial morphology. Acta Physiol Scand 69 (Suppl 280)

Mollison P L, Engelfriet C P, Contreras M 1987 Blood transfusion in clinical medicine. 8th edition. Blackwell: Oxford

Mollon J D, Bowmajer J K 1992 The spatial arrangement of cones in the primate fovea. Nature 360: 677–679

Molnar Z, Blakemore C 1991 Nature 351: 475–477

Monaco S, Gehrmann J, Raivich G, Kreutzberg G W 1992 MHC-positive, ramified macrophages in the normal and injured rat peripheral nervous system. Neurocytol 21: 623–634

Monakow C von 1882 Weitere Mitteilungen über durch Exstirpation circumscripter Hirnrindenreigionem bedingte Entwickelungshemmungen des Kaninchegehirns. Arch Psychiat. NervKrankh 12: 141–156, 535–549

Monakow C von 1905 Gehirnpathologie, 2nd edition, Hölder: Vienna

Moniem K A, Glover T D 1972 Alkaline Phosphatase in the cytoplasmic droplet of mammalian spermatozoa. J Reprod Fertil 29: 65–69

Montagna W, Carlisle K, 1979 Structural changes in aging human skin, J Invest Dermatol 73: 47–53

Montagna W, Kligman A M, Carlisle K S 1992 Atlas of normal human skin. Springer-Verlag: New York

Montagna W, Kligman A M, Weupper K D, Bentley J P (eds) 1979 Special issue on ageing of skin. J Invest Dermatol 73

Montagu M F A 1951 Wallbrook frontal bone. Am J Phys Anthropol 9: 5–14

Montagu M F A 1960 An introduction to physical anthropology. 3rd edition. Thomas: Springfield, Illinois

Montandon P, Gacek R R, Kimura R S 1970 Crista neglecta in the cat and human. Ann Otol Rhinol Laryngol 79: 105–112

Montarolo P G, Palestini M, Strata P 1982 The inhibitory effect of olivocerebellar input on the cerebellar Purkinje cells in the rat. J Physiol 332: 187–202

Montarras D, Chelly J, Bober E, Arnold H, Ott M-O, Gros F, Pinset C 1991 Developmental patterns in the expression of Myf5, MyoD, myogenin and MRF4 during myogenesis. New Biologist 3: 592–600

Moody R O 1927 The position of the abdominal viscera in healthy young British and American adults. J Anat 61: 223–231

Moor R M, Osborn J, Cran D, Walters D 1981 Selective effect of gonadotrophins on cell coupling, nuclear maturation and protein synthesis in mammalian oocytes. J Embryol Exp Morphol 61: 347–365

Moore A, Krummen L A, Mather J P 1994 Inhibins, activins, their binding proteins and receptors: interactions underlying paracrine activity in the testis. Mol Cell Endocrin 100: 81–86

Moore J K 1987 The human auditory brain stem: a comparative view. Hearing Res 29: 1–32

Moore J K, Osen K K 1979 The cochlear nuclei in man. Am J Anat 154: 393–418

Moore P B, Huxley H E & DeRosier D J 1970 Three dimensional reconstruction of F-actin, thin filaments and decorated thin filaments. J Mol Biol 50: 279–295

Moore R Y 1989 Organisation and function of a central nervous system circadian oscillator: the suprachiasmatic hypothalamic nucleus. Fed Proc 42: 2783–2789

Moorman S J, Hume R I 1990 Growth cones of chick sympathetic preganglionic neurons in vitro interact with other neurons in a cell-specific manner. J Neurosci 10: 3158–3163

Moosavi H, Smith P, Heath D 1973 The Feyrter cell in hypoxia, Thorax 28: 729–741

Mooseker M S 1985 Organization, chemistry and assembly of the cytoskeletal apparatus of the intestinal brush border. Annu Rev Cell Biol 1: 209–241

Mooseker M S, Tilney L G 1975 Organization of an actin filament-membrane, complex. Filament polarity and membrane attachment in the microvilli of intestinal epithelial cells, J Cell Biol 67: 725–743

Moradian-Oldak J, Weiner S, Addadi L, Landis W J, Traub W 1991 Electron imaging and diffraction study of individual crystals of bone, mineralized tendon and synthetic carbonate apatite. Connect Tissue Res 25: 219–228

Moran D T, Rowley J C, Jafek B W, Lovell M A 1982 The fine structure of the olfactory mucosa in man. J Neurocytol 11: 721–746

Moran D T, Jafek B W, Eller P M, Rowley J C 3d 1992 Ultrastructural histopathology of human olfactory dysfunction. Microsc Res Techn 23: 103–110

Moran D T, Jafek B W, Ellor P M, Rowley J C 3rd 1992 Ultrastructural histopathology of human olfactory dysfunction. Microsc Res Techn 23: 103–110

Moran D T, Jafek B W, Rowley J C 1985a Ultrastructure of the vomeronasal organ in man: a pilot study. Chem Senses 10: 420–421

Moran D T, Jafek B W, Rowley J C III 1991 The vomeronasal (Jacobson's) organ in man: ultrastructure and frequency of occurrence. J Steroid Biochem Molec Biol 39: 545–552

Moran D T, Rowley J C, Jafek B W 1982 Electron microscopy of the human epithelium reveals a new cell type: the microvillar cell. Brain Res 253: 39–46

Moran M A, Mufson E J, Mesulam M-M 1987 Neural inputs into the temporopolar cortex of the rhesus monkey. J Comp Neurol 256: 88–103

Morant G M 1936 A biometric study of the human mandible. Biometrics 28: 84–122

Moreau J J, Ravon R. Caix M, Salamon G, Bassier G, Velut S 1985 Anatomical basis of the microsurgical approach to the pineal gland. Anatomia Clinica 7: 3–13

Morecraft R J, Van Hoesen G W 1993 Frontal granular cortex input to the cingulate (M3), supplementary (M2) and primary (M1) motor cortices in the rhesus monkey. J Comp Neurol 337: 669–689

Morel A, Garrachty P E, Kaas J H 1993 Tonotopic organization, architectonic fields, and connections of auditory cortex in macaque monkeys. J Comp Neurol 335: 437–459

Morel A, Kaas J H 1992 Subdivisions and connections of auditory cortex in owl monkeys. J Comp Neurol 318: 27–63

Morell P, Norton W T 1980 Sci Am 242: 88–118

Moreno A M, Zapata A 1991 In situ effects of estrogens on the stroma of rat thymus. In: Imhof B A, Berrih-Aknin S, Ezine S (eds) Lymphatic tissues and in vivo immune responses. Dekker: New York: pp 81–87

Moreno A, Murphy E A 1981 Inheritance of Kartagener syndrome. Am J Med Genet 8: 305–313

Morest D K 1967 Experimental study of the projections of the nucleus of the tractus solitarius and the area postrema in the cat. J Comp Neurol 130: 277–300

Morest D K 1993 The cellular basis for signal processing in the mammalian cochlear nuclei. In: Merchan M A (ed) The mammalian cochlear nuclei: organization and function. Plenum Press New York: pp 1–18

Moretti G, Rebora A (eds) 1976 Striae distensae. Brocade Spa: Milan

Morgan D L, Proske U 1984 Vertebrate slow muscle: its structure, pattern of innervation, and mechanical properties. Physiol Rev 64: 103–169

Morgan J D 1959 Blood supply of the growing rabbit's tibia. J Bone Jt Surg 41B: 185–203

Morgan M D L, De Troyer A 1984 The individuality of chest wall motion in tetraplegics. Bull Eur Physiopathol Resp 20: 547–552

Morgan M D, Gourlay A R, Denison D M 1984 An optical method of studying the shape and movement of the chest wall in recumbent patients. Thorax 39: 101–106

Morgan M D, Gourlay A R, Silver J R, Williams S J, Denison D M 1985 Contribution of the rib cage to breathing in tetraplegia. Thorax 40: 613–617

Morgan M W 1944 Accommodation and its relation to convergence. Am J Optom 21: 183–195

Morgan P J, King T P, Lawson W, Slater D, Davidson G 1992 Ultrastructure of melatonin-responsive cells in the ovine pars tuberalis. Cell Tissue Res 263: 529–534

Morgan T H 1910 Sex-linked inheritance in Drosophila. Science 32: 120–122 Reprinted in Peters J A 1959 Classic papers in genetics. Prentice-Hall: New Jersey

Morgan T H 1934 Experimental Embryology. Columbia University Press: New York

Morgan-Hughes J A 1986 Mitochondrial diseases. Trends Neurosci 9: 15–19

Mori H, Christensen A K 1980 Morphometric analysis of Leydig cells in the normal testis. J Cell Biol 84: 340

Mori K 1987 Monoclonal antibodies (2C5 and 4C9) against lactoseries carbohydrates identify subsets of olfactory and vomeronasal receptor cells and their axons in the rabbit. Brain Res 408: 215–221

Mori K, Fujita S C, Imamura K, Obata K 1985 Immunohistochemical study of subclasses of olfactory nerve fibers and their projections to the olfactory bulb in the rabbit. J Comp Neurol 242: 214–229

Mori K, Kishi K, Ojima H 1983 Distribution of dendrites of mitral displaced mitral, tufted and granule cells in the rabbit olfactory bulb. J Comp Neurol 219: 339–355

Mori K, Kishi, K, Ojima H 1983 Distribution of dendrites of mitral, displaced mitral, tufted and granule cells in the rabbit olfactory bulb. J Comp Neurol 219: 339–355

Mori S, Harruff R, Burr D B 1993 Microcracks in articular cartilage of human femoral heads. Arch Pathol Lab Med 117: 197–198

Mori S, Leblond C P 1970 Electron microscopic identification of three classes of oligodendrocytes and a preliminary study of their proliferative activity in the corpus callosum of young rats. J Comp Neurol 139: 1–60

Moriarty G C 1975 Electron microscopic-immunocytohistochemical studies of rat pituitary gonadotrophs: a sex difference in morphology and cytochemistry of LH cells. Endocrinology 97: 1215–1225

Morin F, Schwartz H G, O'Leary J L 1951 Experimental study of the spino-thalamic and related tracts. Acta Psychiat Neurol Scand 26: 371–396

Morrey B F, Adams R A 1992 Semiconstrained arthroplasty for the treatment of rheumatoid arthritis of the elbow. J Bone Jt Surg 74A: 479–490

Morrey B F, Brian R S 1985 Total joint replacement. In: Morrey B F (ed) The elbow and its disorders. Saunders: Philadelphia: pp 546–569

Morris J F, Pow D V 1990 Widespread release of peptides in the central nervous system: quantitation of tannic acid-captured exocytosis. Anat Rec 231: 437–445

Morris-Kay G 1993 Retinoic acid and craniofacial development: molecules and morphogenesis. Bioessays 15: 9–15

Morrison A B 1954 The levatores costarum and their nerve supply. J Anat 88: 19–24

Morrison E E, Costanzo R M 1990 Morphology of the human olfactory epithelium J Comp Neurol 297 1–13

Morrison E E, Costanzo R M 1992 Morphology of olfactory epithelium in humans and other vertebrates. Microsc Res Techn 23: 49–61

Morrison J B 1970 The mechanics of the knee joint in relation to normal walking. J Biomech 3: 51–61

Morrison J H, Foote S L, Bloom F E 1984 Regional, laminar, developmental, and functional characteristics of noradrenaline and serotonin innervation patterns in monkey cortex. In: Descarries L, Tomás R (eds) Monoamine innervation of cerebral cortex. Alan R Liss: New York: pp 61–75

Morrison S, Mitchell L S, Ecob-Prince M S, Griffiths I R, Thomson C E, Barrie J A, Kirkham D 1991 P_0 gene expression in cultured Schwann cells. J Neurocytol 20: 769–780

Moruzz G, Magoun H W 1949 Brainstem reticular formation and activation of the EEG. Electroenceph Clin Neurophysiol 1: 455–473

Moscatelli D, Gross J L, Rifkin D B 1981 Angiogenic factors stimulate plasminogen activator and collagenase production by capillary endothelial cells. J Cell Biol 91: 201a

Moss F P, Leblond C P 1971 Satellite cells as the source of nuclei in muscles of growing rats. Anat Rec 170: 421–436

Moss-Salentijn A G M 1976 The epiphyseal vascularization of growth plates. A developmental study in the rabbit. Doctoral Thesis. Rijks Universiteit: Utrecht

Moss-Salentijn L, Moss M L, Shinozuka M, Skalak R 1987 Morphological analysis and computer-aided, three dimensional reconstruction of chondrocytic columns in rabbit growth plates. J Anat 151: 157–167

Moss-Saletnijn L 1975 Cartilage canals in the human spheno-occipital synchondrosis during fetal life. Acta Anat 92: 595–606

Mossman H 1987 Vertebrate fetal membranes. Macmillan: London

Mott J C 1982 Control of the foetal circulation. J Exp Biol 100: 129–146

Moulton D G, Celebi G, Fink R P 1970 Olfaction in mammals – two aspects: proliferation of cells in the olfactory epithelium and sensitivity to odours. In: Wolstenholme G E W, Knight J (eds) Taste and smell in vertebrates. (Ciba Foundation Symposium.) Churchill: London: pp 227–245

Mountcastle V B 1957 Modality and topographic properties of single neurons of cat's omatic sensory cortex. J Neurophysiol 20: 408–434

Mountcastle V B 1968 Medical physiology. 12th edition. Mosby: St Louis

Mountcastle V B, Lynch J C, Georgopoulos A P, Sakata H, Acuna C 1975 Posterior parietal association cortex of the monkey: command functions for operations within extrapersonal space. J Neurophysiol 38: 871–908

Mountcastle V B, Powell T P S 1959a Central nervous mechanisms subserving position sense and kinethesis. Bull Johns Hopkins Hosp 105: 173–200

Mountcastle V B, Powell T P S 1959b Neural mechanisms subserving cutaneous sensibility with special reference to the role of afferent inhibition in sensory perception and discrimination. Bull Johns Hopkins Hosp 105: 201–232

Movat H Z, More R H, Haust M D 1958 The diffuse intimal thickening of the human aorta with aging. Am J Pathol 34: 1023–1031

Movsesian M A 1993 Calcium uptake and release by cardiac sarcoplasmic reticulum. In: Gwathmey J K, Briggs G M, Allen P D (eds) Heart failure. Basic science and clinical aspects. Marcel Dekker: New York: pp 101–120

Mow V C, Hayes W C (eds) 1991 Basic orthopaedic biomechanics. Raven Press: New York

Mow V C, Lai W M, Redler I 1974 Some surface characteristics of articular cartilage. I. A scanning electron microscopy study and a theoretical model for the dynamic interaction of synovial fluid and articular cartilage. J Biomech 7: 449–456

Mower G, Gibson A, Glickstein M 1979 Tectopontine pathway in the cat: laminar distribution of cells of origin and visual properties of target cells in dorsolateral pontine nucleus. J Neurophysiol 42: 1–15

Moxey P C, Trier J S 1978 Specialized cell types in the human fetal small intestine. Anatomical Record 191: 269–286

Moxham B J 1979 The effects of some vaso-active drugs on the eruption of the rabbit mandibular incisor. Arch Oral Biol 24: 681–688

Moxham B J, Berkovitz B K B 1983 Interactions between thyroxine, hydrocortisone and cyclophosphamide in their effects on the eruption of the rat mandibular incisor. Arch Oral Biol 28: 1083–1087

Moyers R E 1950 Electromyographic analysis of certain muscles involved in temporomandibular movement. Am J Orthodont 36: 481–515

Mudge A W 1993 New ligands for Neu? Curr Biol 3: 361–364

Mudhar H S, Pollock R A, Wang C, Stiles C D, Richardson W D 1993 PDGF and its receptors in the developing rodent retina and optic nerve. Development 118: 539–552

Mueller J C, Jones A L, Long J A 1972 topographic and subcellular anatomy of the guinea pig gallbladder. Gastroenterology 63: 856–868

Muggleton-Hariss A L, Hayflick L 1976 Cellular aging studied by the reconstruction of replicating cells form nuclei and cytoplasms isolated from normal human diploid cells. Exp Cell Res 103: 321–330

Mugnaini E 1965 'Dark cells' in electron migrographs from the central nervous system of vertebrates. J Ultrastruct Res 12: 235–236

Mugnaini E 1970 The relationship between cytogenesis and the formation of different types of synaptic contact. Brain Res 17: 169–179

Mugnaini E, Floris A 1994 A unipolar brush-cell. A neglected neuron of the cerebellar cortex. J Comp Neurol 339: 174–180

Mugnaini E, Forstrønen P F 1967 Ultrastructural studies on cerebellar histogenesis. I. Differentiation of granule cells and development of glomeruli; in the chick embryo. Z Zellforsch Mikrosk Anat 77: 115–143

Muir A R 1954 The development of the ventricular part of the conducting tissue in the heart of the sheep. J Anat 88: 381–391

Muirhead E E, Germaine G, Leach B E, Pitcock J A, Stephenson P, Brooks B, Brosius W L, Daniels E G, Hinman J W 1972 Production of renomedullary prostaglandins by renomeduallary interstitial cells grown in tissue culture. Circ Res 31 (Suppl 2) 161–172

Mukai N 1970 Axonal reaction of the optic nerve following heat coagulation. Histochemical evidence for antidromic conduction. Can J Ophthal 5: 78–90

Müller F 1977 The development of the anterior falcate and lacrimal arteries in the human. Anat Embryol (Berl) 150: 207–227

Muller F, O'Rahilly R 1986 The development of the human brain and the closure of the rostral neuropore at stage 11. Anat Embryol 175: 205–222

Muller T 1959 Variations in the abductor pollicis longus and extensor pollicis brevis in the South African Bantu. S Afr J Lab Clin Med 5: 56–62

Mundy G R 1993a Cytokines of bone. In: Mundy G R, Martin T J (eds) Physiology and pharmacology of bone. Springer-Verlag: Berlin: pp 185–214

Mundy G R 1993b Hormonal factors which regulate bone resorption. In: Mundy G R, Martin T J (eds) Physiology and pharmacology of bone. Springer-Verlag: Berlin: pp 215–247

Munger B L 1991 The biology of Merkel cells. In: Goldsmith L A (ed) Physiology, biochemistry, and molecular biology of skin. 2nd edition. 2 vols. Oxford University Press: Oxford: pp 836–856

Munger B L, Halata Z 1984 The sensorineural apparatus of the human eyelid. 170: 181–204

Munger B L, Ide C 1988 The structure and function of cutaneous receptors. Arch Histol Cytol 51: 1–34

Munger B L, Roth S I 1963 The cytology of the normal parathyroid glands of man and Virginia deer; a light and electron microscopic study with morphologic evidence of secretory activity. J Cell Biol 16: 379–400

Munkacsi K, Newstead J D 1971 Direct autonomic nerve fibers to the renal medulla in man. Experientia 27: 175–177

Münzer E, Wiener H 1902 Das Zwischen- und Mittelhirn des Kaninchens und die Beziehungen dieser Teile zum übrigen Centralnervensystem, mit besonderer Berücksichtigung der Pyramidenbahn und Schleife. Mschr f Psychiat u Neurol 12: 241–279

Murad T M 1970 Ultrastructural study of rat mammary gland during pregnancy. Anat Rec 167: 17–36

Muratori G 1965 Struttura microscopica del seno carotideo nel gatto, cane e conglio, Boll Soc Ital Biol Sper 42: 301–303

Murley R S, Peters P M 1961 Inadvertent parathyroidectomy. Proc R Soc Med 54: 487–489

Murphy C, Alvarado J, Juster R 1984 Prenatal and postnatal growth of the human Descemet's membrane. Invest Ophthalm Vis Sci 25: 1402–1415

Murphy P G, Frank C B, Hart D A 1993 Characterization of the plasminogen activators and plasminogen activator inhibitors expressed by cells isolated from rabbit ligament and synovial tissues: evidence for unique cell populations. Exp Cell Res 205: 16–24

Murray A, Hunt T 1993 The cell cycle. Oxford University Press: Oxford

Murray E A 1991 Contributions of the amygdalar complex to behaviour in macaque monkeys. Prog Brain Res 87: 167–180

Murray E A, Coulter 1981 Organization of corticospinal neurons in the monkey. J Comp Neurol 195: 339–365

Murray E A, Davidson M, Gaffan D, Olton D S, Suomi S J 1989 Effects of fornix transection and cingulate cortical ablation on spatial memory in Rhesus monkeys. Exp Brain Res 74: 173 – 186

Murray J A, Blakemore W F 1980 The relationship between internodal length and fibre diameter in the spinal cord of the cat. J Neurol Sci 45: 29–41

Murray J M 1992 Neuropathology in depth: the role of confocal microscopy. J Neuropath Exp Neurol. 51: 475–487

Murray M J, Meacham R B 1993 The effect of age on male reproductive function. World J Urol 11: 137–140

Murray M R 1965 Nervous tissues in vitro. In: Willmer E B (ed) Cells and tissues in culture. Vol 2. Academic Press: New York: pp 373–455

Murray M, Miller H R P, Jarrett W F H 1968 The globule leucocyte and its derivation from the subepithelial mast cell, Lab Invest 19: 222–234

Murray P D F 1936 Bones. A study of the development and structure of the vertebrate skeleton. Cambridge University Press: Cambridge

Murray P D F, Huxley J S 1924 Self differentiation of the grafted limb bud of the chick. J Anat 59: 379–384

Muskens L J J 1914 An anatomico-physiological study of the posterior longitudinal bundle in its relation to forced movement. Brain 36: 352–426

Myers R E 1959 Localisation of function in the corpus callosum. Visual gnostic transfer. Archs Neurol Psychiat Chicago 1: 74–77

Myers R E, Henson C O 1960 Role of corpus callosum in transfer of tactuokinesthetic learning in chimpanzee. Arch Neurol Psychiat 3: 404–409

Mygind N 1975 Scanning electron microscopy of the human nasal mucosa, Rhinology 13: 57–75

Mygind N 1978 Immunohistopathology of allergic rhinitis and conditions allied. Clin Otolaryngol 3: 325–342

Mygind S H 1948 Further labyrinthine studies: on labyrinthine transformation of acoustic vibrations to pitch-differentiated nervous impulses. Acta Otolaryngol Suppl 68: 53–80

Mysorekar V R 1967 Diaphysial nutrient foramina in human long bones. J Anat 101: 813–822

N

Nabeshima S, Reese T S, Landis D M D, Brightman M W 1975 Junctions in the meninges and marginal glia. J Comp Neurol 164: 127–170

Nachemson A 1960 Lumbar intradiscal pressure. Experimental studies on post-mortem material. Act Orthop Scand Suppl 43: 1–104

Nachemson A 1963 The influence of spinal movements on the lumbar intradiscal pressure and on the tensile stresses in the annulus fibrosus. Acta Orthop Scand 33: 183–207

Nadal-Ginard B, Mahdavi V 1989 Molecular basis of cardiac performance. J Clin Invest 84: 1693–1700

Nadeau S E, Trobe J D 1983 Pupil sparing in oculomotor palsy: a brief review. Ann Neurol 13: 143–148

Nagato T, Yoshida H, Yoshida A, Uehara Y 1980 A scanning electron microscope study of myoepithelial cells in exocrine glands. Cell Tissue Res 209: 1–10

Nageotte J 1906 The pars intermedia or nervus intermedius of Wrisberg and the bulbopontine gustatory nucleus in man. Rev Neurol Psych 4: 473–488

Nager G T, Proctor B 1982 Anatomical variations and anomalies involving the facial canal. Ann Otol Rhinol Laryngol 91: 45–61

Nagourney B A, Aranda J V 1992 Physiologic differences of clinical significance. In: Polin R A, Fox W W (eds) Fetal and neonatal physiology. W B Saunders: Philadelphia: pp 169–177

Najlerahim A, Harrison P J, Barton A J L, Heffernan J, Pearson R C A 1990 Distribution of messenger RNAs encoding the enzymes glutaminase, aspartate aminotransferase and glutamic acid decarboxylase in rat brain. Mol Brain Res 7: 317–333

Nakagawa M, Thompson R P, Terracio L, Borg T K 1993 Developmental anatomy of HNK-1 immunoreactivity in the embryonic rat heart: co-distribution with early conduction tissue. Anat Embryol Berl 187: 445–460

Nakai Y, Hilding D 1968 Vestibular endolymph-producing epithelium. Electron microscope study of the development and histochemistry of the dark cells of the crista ampullaris. Acta Otolaryngol [Stockh] 66: 120–128

Nakaizumi Y 1964 The ultrastructure of Bruch's membrane. I. The human, monkey, rabbit, guinea pig and rat eyes. Arch Ophthal 72: 380–387

Nakajima K, Kohsaka S 1993 Functional roles of microglia in the brain. Neurosci Res 17: 187 – 203

Nakamura K, Matsumoto K, Mikami A, Kubota K 1994 Visual response properties of single neurons in the temporal pole of behaving monkeys. J Neurophysiol 71: 1206–1221

Nakane P K 1970 Classifications of anterior pituitary cell types with immuonenzyme histochemistry. J Histochem Cytochem 18: 9–20

Nakane P K, Kawaoi A 1974 Peroxidase-labelled antibody. A new method of conjugation. J Histochem Cytochem 22: 1084–1091

Nakanishi S 1992 Molecular diversity of glutamate receptors and implications for brain function. Science 258: 597–603

Nakanishi T 1967 Studies on the pudendal nerve. I. Macroscopic observations on the pudendal nerve in humans. Acta Anat Nippon 42: 223–239

Nakashima T Kimmelman C P, Snow J B 1984 Structure of human fetal and adult olfactory neuroepithelium. Arch Otolaryngol 110: 641–646

Nakashima T Kimmelman C P, Snow J B 1985 Vomeronasal organs and nerves of Jacobson in the human fetus. Acta Otolaryngol (Stockh) 99:266–271

Nakatsuji N 1992 Development of postimplantation mouse embryos: unexplored field rich in unanswered questions. Develop Growth & Differ 34: 489–499

Nakayama M 1944 Nerve terminations in the muscle spindle of the human lingual muscles. Tohoku med J. 34: 367–377

Nance D M, Hopkins D A, Bieger D 1987 Re-investigation of the innervation of the thymus gland in mice and rats. BBI 1: 134–147

Napier J R 1955 The form and function of the carpo-metacarpal joint of the thumb. J Anat 89: 362–369

Napier J R 1956 The prehensile movements of the human hand. J Bone Jt Sug 38B: 902–913

Napier J R 1966 Functional aspects of the anatomy of the hand. In: Pulvertaft R G (ed) The hand. Butterworths: London: pp 1–31

Napolitano L M, Scallen T J 1969 Observations of the fine structure of peripheral nerve myelin. Anat Rec 163: 1–6

Napper R M A, Harvey R J 1988 Number of parallel fiber synapses on an individual Purkinje cell in the cerebellum of the rat. J Comp Neurol 274: 168–177

Narayanan C H, Narayanan Y 1978 J Embryol Exp Morphol 43: 85–105

Narisawa Y, Hashimoto K, Nihei Y, Pietruk T 1992 Biological significance of dermal Merkel cells in development of cutaneous nerves in human fetal skin. J Histochem Cytochem 40: 65–71

Naruke T, Suemasu K, Ishikawa S 1978 Lymph node mapping and curability at various levels of metastases in resected lung cancer. J Thor Cardiovasc Surg 76: 832–839

Narusawa M, Fitzsimons R B, Izumo S, Nadal-Ginard B, Rubinstein N A,
Kelly A M 1987 Slow myosin in developing rat skeletal muscle. J Cell Biol 104: 447–459

Nashold B S Jr, Wilson W P, Slaughter D G 1969 Sensations evoked by stimulation in the midbrain of man. J Neurosurg 30: 14–24

Nathan C, Sporn M 1991 Cytokinins in context. Journal of Cell Biology 113: 981–998

Nathan H 1962 Osteophytes of the vertebral column: an anatomical study of their development according to age, race and sex with consideration of their aetiology and significance. J Bone Jt Surg 44A: 243–268

Nathan H, Gloobe H 1974 Flexor digitorum brevis-anatomical variations. Anat Anz 135: 295–301

Nathan P W 1963 Results of antero-lateral cordotomy for pain in cancer. J Neurol Neurosurg Psychiatry 26: 353–362

Nathan P W 1963 The descending respiratory tracts in man. J Neurol Neurosurg Psychiatry 26: 487–499

Nathan P W 1976 The gate-control theory of pain. A critical review. Brain 99: 123–158

Nathan P W, Smith M C 1955a The Babinski response. A review and new observations. J Neurol Neurosurg Psychiat 18: 250–259

Nathan P W, Smith M C 1955b Long descending tracts in man. I. Review of present knowledge. Brain 78: 248–303

Nathan P W, Smith M C 1959 Fasciculi proprii of the spinal cord in man: review of present knowledge. Brain 82: 610–668

Nathan P W, Smith M C 1982 The rubrospinal and central tegmental tracts in man. Brain 105: 223–269

Nathan P W, Smith M C 1986 The location of descending fibres to sympathetic neurons supplying the eye and sudomotor neurons supplying the head and neck. J Neurol Neurosurg Psychiatry 49: 187–194

Nathan P W, Smith M C, Cook A W 1986 Sensory effects in man of lesions of the posterior columns and of some other afferent pathways. Brain 109: 1003–1041

Nauta W J H 1958 Hippocampal projections and related neural pathways to the midbrain in the cat. Brain 81: 319–340

Nauta W J H 1962 Neural associations of the amygdaloid complex in the monkey. Brain 85: 505–520

Nauta W J H, Domesick V B 1981 Ramifications of the limbic system. In: Mattyse S (ed) Psychiatry and the biology of the human brain. Elsevier: Amsterdam: pp 165–188

Nauta W J H, Domesick V B 1984 Afferent and efferent relationships of the basal ganglia. In: Evered D, O'Connor M (eds) Functions of the basal ganglia. CIBA Foundation Symposium 107 Pitman: London: pp 3–23

Nauta W J H, Feirtag M 1986 Fundamental neuroanatomy. Freeman: New York

Nauta W J H, Gygax P A 1951 Silver impregnation of degenerating axon terminals in central nervous system: technic, chemical notes. Stain Technol 26: 5–11

Nauta W J H, Haymaker W 1969 Hypothalamic nuclei and fiber connections. In: Haymaker W, Anderson E, Nauta W J H (eds) The hypothalamus. Thomas: Springfield: pp 136–209

Nauta W J H, Mehler W R 1966 Projections of the lentiform nucleus in the monkey, Brain Res I: 4–42

Navaratnam V 1963 Observations on the right pulmonary arch artery and its nerve supply in human embryos. J Anat 97: 569–573

Navaratnam V 1965 Development of the nerve supply to the human heart. Br Heart J 27: 640–650

Navaratnam V, Woodward J M, Skepper J N 1989 Specific heart granules and natriuretic peptide in the developing myocardium of fetal and neonatal rats and hamsters. J Anat 163: 261–273

Neal J W 1990 The callosal connections of area 7b, PF in the monkey. Brain Res 514: 159–162

Neal J W, Pearson R C A, Powell T P S 1986a The organization of the cortico-cortical projections of area 5 upon area 7 in the parietal lobe of the monkey. Brain Res 381: 164–167

Neal J W, Pearson R C A, Powell T P S 1986b The relationship between the auditory cortex and the claustrum in the cat. Brain Res 366: 385–387

Neal J W, Pearson R C A, Powell T P S 1987 The cortico-cortical connections of area 7b, PF, in the parietal lobe of the monkey. Brain Res 419: 341–346

Neal J W, Pearson R C A, Powell T P S 1988a The organization of the cortico-cortical connections between the walls of the lower part of the superior temporal sulcus and the inferior parietal lobe in the monkey. Brain Res 438: 351–356

Neal J W, Pearson R C A, Powell T P S 1988b The cortico-cortical connections within the parieot-temporal lobe of area PG, 7a, in the monkey. Brain Res 438: 243–250

Neal J W, Pearson R C A, Powell T P S 1990a The ipsilateral cortico-cortical connections of area 7 with the frontal lobe of the monkey. Brain Res 509: 31–40

Neal J W, Pearson R C A, Powell T P S 1990b The connections of area PG, 7a, with cortex in the parietal, occipital and temporal lobes of the monkey. Brain Res 532: 249–264

Neal J W, Pearson R C A, Powell T P S 1990c The ipsilateral cortico-cortical connections of area 7b, PF, in the parietal and temporal lobes of the monkey. Brain Res 524: 119–132

Nealey T A, Maunsell J H R 1994 Magnocellular and parvocellular contributions to the responses of neurons in macaque striate cortex. J Neurosci 14: 2069–2079

Neaves W B 1977 The blood-testis barrier. In: Johnson A D, Gomes W R (eds) The testis. Vol 4. Advances in physiology, biochemistry, and function. Academic Press: New York: pp 126–162

Needham J 1959 A history of embryology. 2nd edition. Cambridge University Press: Cambridge

Negus V E 1947 Intrinsic carcinoma of larynx; a review of a series of cases. Proc R Soc Med 40: 515–524

Negus V E 1958 The comparative anatomy and physiology of the nose and paranasal sinuses. Livingstone: Edinburgh

Nell A, Niebauer W, Sperr W, Firbas W 1994 Special variations of the lateral ligament of the human TMJ. Clin Anat 7: 267–270

Nelson B J, Mugnaini E 1989 Origins of GABAergic inputs to the inferior olive. In: The olivocerebellar system in motor control. Exp Brain Res 17: 86–107

Nelson C C, Blaivas M 1991 Orbicularis oculi muscle in children - histologic and histochemical characteristics. Invest Ophthalmol Vis Sci 32: 646–654

Nelson D M, Crouch E C, Curran E M, Farmer D R 1990 Trophoblast interaction with fibrin matrix. Epithelialization of perivillous fibrin deposits as a mechanism for villous repair in the human placenta. Am J Pathol 136: 855–865

Nelson E, Rennels M 1970 Innervation of intracranial arteries. Brain 93: 475–490

Nelson G M, Finger T E 1993 Immunolocalization of different forms of neural cell adhesion molecule (NCAM) in rat taste buds. J Comp Neurol 336:507–516

Nelson J D, Peters P C 1965 Suprapubic aspiration of urine in premature and term infants. Pediatrics 36: 132–134

Nelson K G, Takahashi T, Bossert N L, Walmer D K, McLachlan J A 1991 Epidermal growth factor replaces estrogen in the stimulation of female genital-tract growth and differentiation. Proc Natl Acad Sci USA 88: 21–25

Nelson L 1967 Sperm motility. In: Metz C B, Monroy A (eds) Fertilization. Vol 1. Academic Press: New York: pp 27–97

Nelson R J, Sur M, Felleman D J, Kaas J H 1980 Representations of the body surface in postcentral parietal cortex of Macaca fascicularis. J Comp Neurol 192: 611–643

Nelson R, Famiglietti E V, Kolb H 1978 Intracellular staining reveals different levels of stratification for on-and off-center ganglion cells in cat retina. J Neurophysiol 41: 472–483

Nemeth P M, Solanki L, Gordon D A, Hamm T M, Reinking R M, Stuart D G 1986 Uniformity of metabolic enzymes within individual motor units. J Neurosci 6: 892–898

Nergårdh A, Boréus L 1972 Autonomic receptor function in the lower urinary tract of man and cat. Scand J Urol Nephrol 6: 32–36

Nery E B, Kraus B S, Croup M 1970 Timing and topography of early human tooth development. Arch Oral Biol 15: 1315–1326

Nesebar R A, Kornblith P L, Pollard J J, Michels N A 1969 Celiac and superior mesenteric arteries: a correlation of angiograms and dissections. Little, Brown: Boston

Neuenschwander S, Gattass R, Sousa A P B, Piñon M C G P 1994 Identification and visuotopic organization of areas PO and POd in Cebus monkey. J Comp Neurol 340: 65–86

Neuman W F, Neuman M W 1953 The nature of the mineral phase of bone. Chem Rev 53: 1–45

Neustadt A, Frostholm A, Rotter A 1988 Topographical distribution of muscarinic cholinergic receptors in the cerebellar cortex of the mouse, rat, guinea pig, and rabbit: a species comparison. J Comp Neurol 272: 317–330

Neutra M R, Phillips T R, Mayer E L, Fishkind D 1987 Transport of membrane bound macromolecules by M-cells of follicle associated epithelium of rabbit Peyer's patch. Cell Tiss Res 247: 537

Newman A 1994 Small nuclear RNAs and pre-mRNA splicing. Curr Opin Cell Biol 6: 360–367

Newman D L, Gosling R G, Bowden R 1971 Changes in aortic distensibility and area ratio with the development of atherosclerosis. Atherosclerosis 14: 231–240

Newman G R, Hobot J A 1989 Role of tissue processing in colloidal gold methods. In: Colloidal gold principles and methods. Vol 3. Academic Press: New York: pp 33–45

Nicander L 1967 An electron microscopical study of cell contracts in the seminiferous tubules of some mammals. Z Zellforsch 83: 375–397

Nicholas D S, Weller R O 1988 The fine anatomy of the human spinal meninges. J Neurosurg 69: 276–282

Nicholls D G, Rial E 1984 Brown fat mitochondria. Trends Biochem Sci 9: 489–491

Nicholls R D, Rinchik E M, Driscoll D J 1992 Genomic imprinting in mammalian development: Prader-Willi and Angelman Syndromes as disease models. Seminars in Developmental Biology 3: 139–152

Nichols D H 1985 The ultrastructure of neural crest formation in the head of the mouse embryo. Cell Differentiation 16: 111S

Nichols D H 1986 Mesenchyme formation from the trigeminal placodes of the mouse embryo. Am J Anat 176: 19–31

Nichols D H 1987 Ultrastructure of neural crest formation in the midbrain/rostral hindbrain and preotic hindbrain regions of the mouse embryo. American Journal of Anatomy 179: 148–154

Nicholson G W 1937 Studies on tumour formation; sacro-coccygeal teratoma with 3 metacarpal bones and digits. Guy's Hosp Rep 87: 46–106

Nicholson H D, Pickering B T 1993 Oxytocin, a male intragonadal hormone. Reg Peptides 45: 253–256

Nicholson L J, Watt F M 1991 Decreased expression of fibronectin and the α5b1 integrin during terminal differentiation of human keratinocytes. J Cell Sci 98: 225–232

Nickoloff B J, Mitra R S, Riser B L, Dixit V M, Varani J 1988 Modulation of keratinocyte motility. Correlation with production of extracellular matrix molecules in response to growth promoting and antiproliferative factors. Am J Path 132: 543–551

Nicol A C, Berme N, Paul J P 1977 A biomechanical analysis of elbow joint function. In: Joint replacement in the upper limb. Inst Mech Eng Conference Pubs 1997–5: London: 45–51

Niden A H, Yamada E 1966 Some observations on the fine structure and function of the non-ciliated bronchiolar cells. In: VIth International Congress for Electron Microscopy. Maruzen: Tokyo: p 599

Niemineva K 1950 Observations on the development of the hypophysialportal system. Acta Paediat 39: 366–377

Nieuwenhuis P 1990 Self-tolerance induction and the blood-thymus barrier. Thymus Update 3: 31–51

Nieuwenhuys R 1967 Comparative anatomy of the cerebellum. Prog Brain Res 25: 1–93

Nieuwenhuys R 1985 Chemoarchitecture of the brain. Springer Verlag: Berlin

Nieuwenhuys R, Voogd J Van, Huijzen C 1988 The human central nervous system. A synopsis and atlas. 3rd edition. Springer Verlag: Berlin

Nieuwkoop P D 1973 The 'organisation center' of the amphibian embryo; its origin, spatial organisation and morphogenetic action. Adv Morph 10: 1–39

Nieuwkoop P D 1985 Inductive interactions in early amphibian development and their general nature. J Embryol, Exp Morph 89 (suppl.): 333–347

Nieuwkoop P D 1989 Dev Growth Differ 32: 149–154

Niikawa N, Kohsaka S, Mizumoto M, Hamada I, Kajii T 1983 Familial clustering of situs inversus totali, and asplenia and polysplenia syndromes. Am J Med Genet 16: 43–47

Nisell R, Nemeth G, Olson H 1986 Joint forces in extension of the knee. Analysis of a mechanical model. Acta Orthop Scand 57: 41–46

Nishino N, Koizumi K, Brooks C M 1976 The role of the suprachiasmatic nuclei of the hypothalamus in the production of circadian rhythm. Brain Res 112: 45–59

Nishiyama I, Seki T, Oota T, Ohta M, Ogiso M 1993 Expression of highly polysialyted neural cell adhesion molecule in calcitonin-producing cells. Neuroscience 56: 778–786

Nissl F 1892 Ueber experimentell erzengte Veränderungen an den Vorderhornzellen des Rückenmarks bei Kaninchen mit Demonstrationen mikroskopischer Präparate. Allg Zt Psychiat 48: 675–682

Nistal M, Abaurrea M A, Paniagua R 1982 Morphological and histometric study on the human Sertoli cell from birth to the onset of puberty. J Anat 134: 351–363

Noback C R, Moss M L 1953 The topology of the human pre-maxillary bone. Am J Phys Anthropol 11: 181–187

Nobori M, Saiki S, Tanaka N, Shindo S, Fujimoto Y 1994 Blood supply of the parathyroid gland from the superior thyroid artery. Surgery 115: 417–423

Noden D M 1978 In: Garrod D R (ed) Specificity of embryological interactions. Chapman & Hall: London: pp 3–49

Noden D M 1983 The embryonic origins of avian cephalic and cervical muscles and associated connective tissues. Am J Anat 168: 257–276

Noden D M 1983a Dev Biol 96: 144–165

Noden D M 1983b Am J Anat 186: 257–276

Noden D M 1986 J Craniofac gen devl Biol Suppl 2: 15–32

Noden D M 1988 Interactions and fates of avian craniofacial mesenchyme. Development 103 (suppl): 121–140

Noden D M 1991 Development of craniofacial blood vessels. In: Feinberg R N, Sherer G K, Auerbach R (eds) The development of the vascular system. Issues Biomed 14: 1–24

Noden D M 1991b Vertebrate craniofacial development: the relation between ontogenetic process and morphological outcome. Brain Behav Evol 38: 190–225

Noden D M, Li X 1991 Patterns of initial vascular development in the avian brain. Anat Rec 229: 65A

Nolte, J 1993 The human brain. 3rd edition. Mosby: St Louis

Nomina Anatomica, Nomina Histologica, Nomina Embryologica. 1989 6th edition. Churchill Livingstone, Edinburgh

Nomura M 1984 The control of ribosome synthesis. Sci Am 250: 102–114

Nomura M 1993 A model for neural representation of binocular disparity in striate cortex: distributed representation and veto mechanism. Biol Cybern 69: 165–171

Noordzij J W, Dabhoiwala N F 1993 A view on the anatomy of the ureterovesical junction. Scand J Urol Nephrol 27: 371–380

Nopajaroonsri C, Luk S C, Simon G T 1971 Ultrastructure of the normal lymph node. Am J Pathol 65: 1–24

Nopajaroonsri C, Luk S C, Simon G T 1974 The passage of intravenously injected colloidal carbon into lymph node parenchyma. Lab Invest. 30: 533–538

Norberg K-A 1967 Transmitter histochemistry of the sympathetic adrenergic nervous system. Brain Res 5: 125–170

Nordlund J J, Abdel-Malek Z A, Boissy R E, Rheins L A 1989 Pigment cell biology. An historical review. J Invest Dermatol 92: 53S–60S

Norgren R 1978 Projections from the nucleus of the solitary tract in the rat. Neurosci 3: 207–218

Norgren R 1990 Gustatory system. In: Paxinos G (ed) The human nervous system. Academic Press: San Diego: pp 845–861

Norobi M, Saiki S, Tanaka N, Shindo S, Fujimoto Y 1994 Blood supply of the parathyroid gland from the superior thyroid artery. Surgery 115: 417–423

Norris E H 1916 The morphogenesis of the follicles in the human thyroid gland. Am J Anat 20: 411–448

Norris E H 1937 The parathyroid glands and the lateral thyroid in man: their morphogenesis, histogenesis, topographic anatomy and prenatal growth. Contrib Embryol (Carnegie Inst Washington) 26 (159): 247–294

Norris E H 1938 The morphogenesis and histogenesis of the thymus gland in man: in which the origin of the Hassell's corpuscles of the human thymus is discovered. Contrib Embryol Carnegie Inst Wash 27: 191–207

North A J, Galazkiewicz B, Byers T J, Glenney J R Jr, Small J V 1993 Complementary distributions of vinculin and dystrophin define two distinct sarcolemma domains in smooth muscle. J Cell Biol 120: 1159–1167

North A J, Gimona M, Cross R A, Small J V 1994a Calponin is localised in both the contractile apparatus and the cytoskeleton of smooth muscle cells. J Cell Sci 107: 437–444

North A J, Gimona M, Lando Z, Small J V 1994b Actin isoform compartments in chicken gizzard smooth muscle cells. J Cell Sci 107: 445–455

Northcutt R G, Gans C 1983 The genesis of neural crest and epidermal placides: a reinterpretation of vertebrate origins. Q Rev Biol 58: 1–28

Nortje C T, Farman A G, Grotepass F W 1977 Variations in the normal anatomy of the inferior dental (mandibular) canal: a retrospective study of panoramic radiographs from 3,612 routine dental patients. Br J Oral Surg 15: 55–63

Norton A C 1968 UCLA Brain Information Service, updated review project-cutaneous sensory pathways: dorsal column-medial lemniscus system. University of California Press: Berkeley

Norvell J E 1968 The aorticorenal ganglion and its role in renal innervation, J Comp Neurol 133: 101–112

Nouwen E J, DeBroe M E 1994 EGF and TGF-alpha in the human kidney: identification of octopal cells in the collecting duct. Kidney Internat 45: 1510–1521

Novikoff A B, Shin W Y 1964 The endoplasmic reticulum in the Golgi zone and its relationship to microbodies, Golgi apparatus and autophagic vacuoles in rat liver cells. J Microscopie 3: 187

Novotny G E K, Sommerfield H, Zirbes T 1990 Thymic innervation in the rat: a light and electron microscopical study. J Comp Neurol 302; 552–561

Noyes R W, Hertig A T, Rock J 1950 Dating the endometrial biopsy. Fertil Steril 1: 3–25

Nozaki M, Kobayashi H, Yanagisawa M et al 1975 Monoamine fluroescence in the median eminence of the Japanese quail, Coturnix coturnix japonica, following medial basal hypothalamic deafferentiation. Cell Tissue Res 164: 425–434

Nudo R J, Masterton R B 1989 Descending pathways to the spinal cord. II. Quantitative study of the tectospinal tract in 23 mammals. J Comp Neurol 286: 96–119

Nussbaum A 1912 Über das Gefassystem des Herzens, Arch Mikrosk Anat Entw Mech 80: 450–477

Nusslein Volhard C 1991 Determination of the embryonic axis of Drosophilia. Development 191 Supplement 1–10

Nyberg-Hansen R 1964a The location and termination of tectospinal fibers in the cat. Exp Neurol 9: 212–227

Nyberg-Hansen R 1964b Origin and termination of fibers from the vestibular nuclei descending in the medial longitudinal fasciculus. An experimental study with silver impregnation methods in the cat. J Comp Neurol 122: 355–367

Nyberg-Hansen R 1965a Anatomical demonstration of gamma moto-neurons in the cat's spinal cord. Exp Neurol 13: 71–81

Nyberg-Hansen R 1965b Sites and mode of termination of reticulo-spinal fibers in the cat. An experimental study with silver impregnation methods. J Comp Neurol 124: 71–100

Nyberg-Hansen R 1966a Functional organisation of descending supraspinal fibre systems to the spinal cord. Anatomical observations and physiological correlations. Ergebn Anat EntwGesch 39: Heft 2, 1–48

Nyberg-Hansen R 1966b Sites of termination of interstitionspinal fibers in the cat. An experimental study with silver impregnation methods. Arch Ital Biol 104: 98–111

Nyberg-Hansen R 1969 Cortico-spinal fibres from the medial aspect of the cerebral hemisphere in the cat. An experimental study with the Nauta method. Exp Brain Res 7: 120–132

Nyberg-Hansen R, Brodal A 1963 Sites of termination of cortico-spinal fibers in the cat. An experimental study with silver impregnation methods. J Comp Neurol 120: 369–391

Nyberg-Hansen R, Brodal A 1964 Sites and mode of termination of rubrospinal fibres in the cat. An experimental study with silver impregnation methods. J Anat 98: 235–253

Nyberg-Hansen R, Mascitti T 1964 Sites and mode of termination of fibers of the vestibulospinal tract in the cat. An experimental study with silver impregnation methods. J Comp Neurol 122: 369–387

Nyberg-Hansen R, Rinvik E 1963 Some comments on the pyramidal tract, with special reference to its individual variations in man. Acta Neurol Scand 39: 1–30

Nyby O, Jansen J 1951 An experimental investigation of the corticopontine projection in maccaca mulatta. (Strifter utgitt ar det norske videnskaps-akademi). Oslo J Mat Naturar Klause H 3: 1–47

Nylander P P S 1973 Serum levels of gonadotrophins in relation to multiple pregnancy in Nigeria. J Obstet Gynaecol Br Cwlth 80: 651

O

Oades R D, Halliday G M 1987 Ventral tegmental (A10) system: neurobiology. I. Anatomy and connectivity. Brain Res Revs 12: 117 – 165

Oakley B 1991 Neuronal-epithelial interactions in mammalian gustatory epithelium. Ciba Foundation Symposium. 160:277–87.

Oakley B R 1992 g-Tubulin: the microtubule organizer? Trends in Cell Biol 2: 1–6

Oakley K P 1964 Frameworks for dating fossil man. Weidenfeld and Nicolson: London

Oakley K P 1969 Analytical methods of dating bone. In: Brothwell D, Higgs E (eds) Science and archaeology. Thames and Hudson: London

O'Beirne J 1833 New views of the process of defecation and their application to the pathology and treatment of diseases of the stomach, bowels and other organs; with an analytical correction of Sir Charles Bell's views respecting the nerves of the face. Dublin

Obletz B E, Halbstein B M 1938 Non-union of fractures of carpal navicular. J Bone Jt Surg 20: 424–428

O'Brien C P, Ehrman R N, Ternes J W 1986 Classical conditioning in human opioid dependence. In: Goldberg S R, Stolerman I P (eds) Behavioral analysis of drug dependence. Academic Press: London: pp. 329–356

O'Brien J P 1984 Mechanisms of spinal pain. In: Wall P D, Melzak R (eds) Textbook of pain. Churchill Livingstone: Edinburgh: pp 240–251

O'Brien M D 1984 Criteria for diagnosing brainstem death. In: Hughes R A C (ed) Neurological emergencies. BMJ Publishing: London: 334–337

Ochoa J 1971 The sural nerve of the human foetus: electron microscope observations and counts of axons. J Anat 108: 213–245

Ochoa J, Mair W E P 1969a The normal sural nerve in man. I. Ultrastructure and numbers of fibres and cells, Acta Neuropathol 13: 197–216

Ochoa J, Mair W E P 1969b The normal sural nerve in man. II. Changes in the axons and Schwann cells due to ageing. Acta Neuropathol 13: 217–239

Ockleford C D, Wakely J 1982 The skeleton of the placenta. Prog Anat 2: 19–47

O'Connor R J 1939 Experiments on the development of the amphibian mesonephros. J Anat 74: 35–44

Oda D, Gown A M, Berg van de J S, Stern R 1990 Instability of the myofibroblast phenotype in culture. Exp Mol Pathol 52: 221–234

Odensten M, Gillquist 1985. Functional anatomy of the anterior cruciate ligament and a rationale for reconstruction. J Bone Jt Surg 67A: 257–262

Odgers P N B 1934 The formation of the venous valves, the foramen secundum and the septum secundum in the human heart. J Anat 69: 412–422

Odgers P N B 1938 The development of the pars membranacea septi in the human heart. J Anat 72: 247–259

Odland G, Ross R 1968 Human wound repair. 1. Epidermal regeneration. J Cell Biol 39: 135–151

Oelrich T M 1980 The urethral sphincter muscle in the male. Am J Anat 158: 229–264

Oelrich T M 1983 The striated urogenital sphincter muscle in the female. Anat Rec 205: 223–232

Oesterle E C, Dallos P 1990 Intracellular recordings from supporting cells in the guinea pig cochlea: DC potentials. J Neurophysiol 64: 617–636

Ogata S, Uhthoff H K 1990 The early development and ossification of the human clavicle – an embryologic study. Acta Orthop Scand 61: 330–334

Ogawa T, Jefferson N C, Toman J E, Chiles T, Zambetoglou A, Necheles H 1960 Action potentials of accessory respiratory muscles in dogs. Am J Physiol 199: 569–572

Ogden J A 1974 Changing patterns of proximal femoral vascularity. J Bone Jt Surg 56A: 941–950

Ogden J A 1984 Radiology of postnatal skeletal development. XII. The second cervial vertebra. Skeletal Radiol 12: 169–177

Ogilvie W H 1935 Some points in the operation of gastrectomy. Br Med J 1: 457–462

Ogura J H, Bellow J A 1952 Laryngectomy and radical neck dissection for carcinoma of the larynx. Laryngoscope 62: 1–52

Ogura J H, Lam R L 1953 Anatomical and physiological correlations on stimulating the human superior laryngeal nerve. Laryngoscope 63: 947–959

Oh C, Kark A E 1972 Anatomy of the external anal sphincter. Br J Surg 59: 717–723

Ohara P T, Chazal G, Ralston H J III 1989 Ultrastructural analysis of the GABA-immunoreactive elements in the monkey thalamic ventrobasal complex. J Comp Neurol 283: 541–558

Ohishi H, Shigemoto R, Nakanishi S, Mizuno N 1993 Distribution of the messenger RNA for a metabotropic glutamate receptor, mGluR2, in the central nervous system of the rat. Neuroscience 53: 1009–1018

Ohno S, Smith J B 1964 Role of fetal follicular cells in meiosis of mammalian oocytes. Cytogenetics 3: 324–333

Ohta M, Offord K, Dyck P J 1974 Morphometric evaluation of first sacral ganglia of man. J Neurol Sci 22: 73–82

Ohtake T, Yamada H 1989 Efferent connections of the nucleus reuniens and the rhomboid nucleus in the rat: an anterograde PHA-L tracing study. Neurosci Res 6: 556–568

Ohtani O, Kikuta A, Terasawa K, Higashikawa T, Yamane T, Taguchi T, Masuda Y, Murakami T 1989 Microvascular organization of human palatine tonsil. Arch Histol Cytol 52: 493–500

Ohye C 1990 Thalamus. In: Paxinos G (ed) The human nervous system. Academic Press: San Diego: pp 439–468

Ohzawa I, Deangelis G C, Freeman R D 1990 Stereoscopic depth discrimination in the visual cortex: neurons ideally suited as disparity detectors. Science 249: 1037–1041

Ojemann G A 1991 Cortical organization of language. J Neurosci 11: 2281–2287

O'Keefe E J, Woodley D, Castillo G et al 1984 Production of soluble and cell-associated fibronectin by cultured keratinocytes. J Invest Dermatol 82: 150–155

O'Keefe J, Nadel L 1978 The hippocampus as a cognitive map. Clarendon Press: Oxford

Okudera T, Ohta T, Huang Y P, Yokota A 1988 Development and radiological anatomy of the superficial cerebral convexity vessels in the human fetus. J Neuroradiol 15: 205–224

Okumura T. Namiki M 1990 Vagal moto neurons innervating the stomach are site specifically organized in the dorsal motor nucleus of the vagus nerve in rats. J Auton Nerv Syst 29: 157–162

Olah I 1978 Structure of the tonsils. In: Antoni E, Staub M (eds) Tonsils structure, immunology and biochemistry, Sect 1. Akademiai Kiado: Budapest: pp 5–50

Olds J 1976 Brain stimulation and the motivation of behaviour. Prog Brain Res 45: 401–426

O'Leary D D M, Stanfield B B 1989 J Neurosci 9: 2230–2246

O'Leary D D M, Terashima T 1988 Neuron 1: 901–910

O'Leary D M 1989 Trends Neurosci 12: 400–406

O'Leary J L, O'Leary J A 1966 Uterine artery ligature in the control of intractable post-partum hemorrhage. Am J Obstet Gynecol 94: 920–924

Olesen S-P, Clapham D E, Davies P F 1988 Hemodynamic shear-stress activates a K$^+$ current in vascular endothelial cells. Nature 331: 168–170

Olivier G 1951 Anthropologie de la clavicule du francais. Bull Soc Anthropol Paris 2: 4–6

Olivier G 1975 Biometry of the human occipital bone. J Anat 120: 507–518

Ollier L 1988 Traite des resections et des operations conservatrices qu'on peut pratiquer sur le systeme osseux. Tome deuxieme. G Masson: Paris: pp 179–416

Olmos G, Naftolin F, Perez J, Tranque P A, Garcia-Segura L M 1989 Synaptic remodelling in the rat arcuate nucleus during the estrous cycle. Neuroscience 32: 663–667

Oloyede A, Broom N D 1993a A physical model for the time-dependent deformation of articular cartilage. Connect Tissue Res 29: 251–261

Oloyede A, Broom N D 1993b Stress-sharing between the fluid and solid components of articular cartilage under varying rates of compression. Connect Tissue Res 30: 127–141

Olsen B R 1991 Collagen biosynthesis. In: Hay E D (ed) Cell biology of extracellular matrix. 2nd edition

Olsen E N, Klein W H 1994 bHLH factors in muscle development: deadlines and commitments, what to leave in and what to leave out. Genes Devel 8: 1–8

Olsson Y 1971 Studies on vascular permeability in peripheral nerves. Acta Neuropath 17: 114–126

Olszewski J 1950 On the anatomical and functional organization of the spinal trigeminal nucleus. J Comp Neurol 92: 401–409

Olszewski J, Baxter D 1954 Cytoarchitecture of the human brain stem. Karger: Basel

Oni O O A, Dearing S, Pringle S 1993 Endothelial cells and bone cells. In: Shoutens A, Arlet J, Gardiniers J W M, Hughes S P F (eds) Bone circulation and vascularization in normal and pathological conditions. Plenum Press: New York: pp 43–48

Onodera K, Yamadotani A, Watanabe T, Wada H 1994 Neuropharmacology of the histaminergic neuron system in the brain and its relationship with behavioral disorders. Prog Neurobiol 42: 685–702

Onufrowicz B 1899 Notes on the arrangement and function of the cell groups in the sacral region of the spinal cord. J Nerv Ment Dis 26: 498–504

Ooé T 1956 On the development of position of the tooth germs in the human deciduous front teeth. Okajimas Folia Anat Jpn 28: 317–340

Ooé T 1957 On the early development of human dental lamina. Okajimas Folia Anat Jpn 30: 198–210

Oort H 1918 Über die verästelung des nervus octavus bei säugetieren. [Modell des utriculus und sacculus des kaninchens.] Anat Anz 51: 272–280

Oosthoek P W, Kempen M J A van, Wesseks A, Lamers W H, Moorman A F M 1990 Distribution of the cardiac gap junction protein, connexin-43 in the neonatal and adult human heart. In: Maréchal G, Carraro U (eds) Muscle and motility. Vol 2. Intercept: Andover, Hampshire: pp 58–90

Oppel O 1963 Microscopic investigations of the number and caliber of the medullated nerve fibers of the optic fasciculus in man. Albrecht v Graefes Arch Ophthalmol 166: 19–27

Oppenheim R W, Schwartz L M, Shatz C J (eds) 1992 J Neurobiol 23: 1111–1351

Oppenheimer J H, Schwartz H L, Mariash C N, Kinlaw W B, Wong N C W, Freake H C 1987 Advances in our understanding of thyroid hormone action at the cellular level. Endocr Rev 8: 288–308

Opperman L A, Sweeney T M, Redmon J, Persing J A, Ogle R C 1993 Tissue interactions with underlying dura mater inhibit osseous obliteration of developing cranial sutures. Dev Dynamics 198: 312–322

Optican L M, Robinson D A 1980 Cerebellar dependent adaptive control of the primate saccadic system. J Neurophysiol 44: 1058–1065

O'Rahilly R 1953 Survey of carpal and tarsal anomalies. J Bone Joint Surg 35-A: 626–642

O'Rahilly R 1956 Developmental deviations in the carpus and tarsus, Clin Orthop 10: 9–18

O'Rahilly R 1973 Developmental stages in human embryos. Part A: Embryos of the first three weeks (Stages 1–9). Carnegie Institution: Washington DC

O'Rahilly R, Gardner E 1971 The timing and sequence of events in the development of the human nervous system during the embryonic period proper. Z Anat Entwicklungsgesch 134: 1–12

O'Rahilly R, Gardner E 1975 The timing and sequence of events in the development of the limbs in the human embryo. Anat Embryol 148: 1–23

O'Rahilly R, Meyer D B 1959 The early development of the eye in the chick Gallus domesticus (stages 8 to 25) Acta Anat 36: 20–58

O'Rahilly R, Muecke E C 1972 The timing and sequence of events in the development of the human urinary system during the embryonic period proper. Z Anat Entwicklungsgesch 138: 99–109

O'Rahilly R, Muller F 1974 The early development of the hypoglossal nerve and occipital fomites in staged human embryos. Am J Anat 169: 237–257

O'Rahilly R, Müller F 1986 The meninges in human development. J Neuropath Exp Neurol 45: 588–608

O'Rahilly R, Muller F 1987 Developmental stages in human embryos. Carnegie Ins Wash Pub 637

O'Rahilly R, Muller F 1987 Developmental stages in human embryos. Washington: Carnegie Institution

O'Rahilly R, Muller F 1992 Human embryology and teratology. Wiley Liss: New York

O'Rahilly R, Muller F, Meyer D B 1980 The human vertebral column at the end of the embryonic period proper. I. The column as a whole. J Anat 131: 565–575

O'Rahilly R, Muller F, Meyer D B 1983 The human vertebral column at the end of the embryonic period proper. II. The occipito-cervical region. J Anat 136: 181–195

O'Rahilly R, Tucker J A 1973 The early development of the larynx in staged human embryos. I Embryos of the first five weeks (to stage 15). Ann Otol Rhinol Laryngol 82 (suppl 7): 1–27

Oram M W, Perrett D I, Hietanen J K 1993 Directional tuning of motion-sensitive cells in the anterior superior temporal polysensory area of the macaque. Exp Brain Res 97: 274–294

Orci L 1974 A portrait of a pancreatic B-cell. Diabetologia 10: 163–187

Orci L 1976 Morphofunctional aspects of the islets of Langerhans. The microanatomy of the islets of Langerhans. Metabolism 25: (Suppl 1) 1303–1313

Orci L, Baetens D, Dubois M P, Rufener C 1975 Evidence for the D-cell of the pancreas secreting somatostatin. Horm Metab Res 7: 400–402

Orci L, Baetens D, Ravazzola M, Malaisse-Lagae F, Amherdt M, Rufener C 1976 Somatostatin in the pancreas and gastrointestinal tract. In: Fujita T (ed) Endocrine gut and pancreas. Elsevier: New York: pp 73–78

Orci L, Like A A, Amherdt M, Blondell B, Kanazawa Y, Marliss E B, Lambert A E, Wollheim C B, Renold A E 1973 Monolayer cell culture of neonatal rat pancreas: an ultrastructural and biochemical study of functioning endocrine cells. J Ultrastruct Res 43: 270–297

Orci L, Unger R H 1975 Functional subdivision of islets of Langerhans and possible role of D-cells. Lancet 2: 1243–1244

Ordahl C P 1986 The skeletal and cardiac a-actin genes are co-expressed in early embryonic striated muscle. Dev Biol 117: 488–492

Ordahl C P 1993 Myogenic lineages within the developing somite.

Ordahl C, Le Douarin N 1992 Two myogenic lineages within the developing somite. Development 114: 339–353

O'Reilly P M R, Fitzgerals M J T 1990 Fibre composition of the hypoglossal nerve in the rat. J Anat 172: 227–243

Orfanos C E, Happle R (eds) 1990 Hair and hair diseases. Springer: Berlin

Orfanos C E, Montagna W, Stuttgen G (eds) 1981 Hair research. Springer: Berlin

O'Riordan J L H 1978 Hormonal control of mineral metabolism. In: O'Riordan J L H (ed) Recent advances in endocrinology and metabolism. Churchill Livingstone: Edinburgh: pp 189–217

Orlando R C, Lacy E R, Tobey N A, Cowart K 1992 Barriers to paracellular permeability in rabbit oesaphageal epithelium. Gastroenterology 102: 10–23

Orlic D, Lev R 1977 An electron microscopic study of intraepithelial lymphocytes in human fetal small intestine. Lab Invest 37: 554–561

Ormerod F C 1960 The physiology of the endolymph. J Laryngol Otol 74: 659–667

Ortmann R 1975 Use of polarized light for quantitative determination of the adjustment of the tangential fibres in articular cartilage. Anat Embryol (Berl) 148: 109–120

Ortonne J P 1990 Pigmentary changes of the ageing skin. In: Greaves M, Voorhees J (eds) Senescence in the skin. Br J Dermatol 122 (suppl 35): 21–28

Orts-Llorca F, Puerta Fonolla J, Sobrado J 1982 The formation, septation and fate of the truncus arteriosus in man. J Anat: 134: 41–56

Orzalesi N, Riva A, Testa F 1971 Fine structure of human lacrimal gland. I. The normal gland. J Submicroscop Cytol 3: 283–298

Osborn J W 1973 Variations in structure and development of enamel. Oral Sci Rev 3: 3–83

Osborn J W 1985 The disc of the human temporomandibular joint: design, function and failure. J Oral Rehabil 12: 279–293

Osborn L 1990 Leukocyte adhesion to endothelium in inflammation. Cell 62: 3–6

Osbourne M P, Comis S D, Pickles J O 1984 Morphology and cross linkage of stereocilia in the guinea pig labyrinth examined without the use of osmium as a fixative. Cell Tiss Res 237: 43–48

Oscarsson O 1973 Functional organization of spinocerebellar paths. In: Iggo A (ed) Handbook of sensory physiology, Vol 2 Somatosensory system. Springer: Berlin: pp 339–380

Oscarsson O, Uddenbeg N 1964 Identification of a spinocerebellar tract activated from forelimb afferents in the cat. Acta Physiol Scand 62: 125–136

Osterberg G A 1935 Topography of the layers of the rods and cones in the human retina, Acta Ophthal, Suppl 6

O'Sullivan B T, Roland P T, Kawashimar R 1994 A PET study of somatosensory discrimination in man. Microgeometry versus macrogeometry. Eur J Neurosci 6: 137–148

Ota C Y, Kimura R S 1980 Ultrastructural study of the human spiral ganglion. Acta Otolaryngol [Stockh] 89: 53–62

Ottersen O P, Davanger S, Storm-Mathisen J 1987 Glycine-like immunoreactivity in the cerebellum of rat and Senegalese baboon, Papio papio: a comparison with the distribution of GABA-like immunoreactivity and with [3H]glycine and [3H]GABA uptake. Exp Brain Res 66: 211–221

Ottersen O P, Fischer B O, Rinvik E, Storm-Mathisen J 1986 Putative amino acid transmitters in the amygdala. Plenum Press: New York

Ottersen O P, Zhang N, Walberg F 1992 Metabolic compartmentation of glutamate and glutamine: morphological evidence obtained by quantitative immunocytochemistry in rat cerebellum. Neuroscience 46: 519–534

Otto J J 1994 Actin-bundling proteins. Curr Opin Cell Biol 6: 105–109

Ottoson D 1956 Analysis of the electrical activity of the olfactory epithelium. Acta Physiol Scand (Suppl 122) 35: 1–83

Oursler M J 1994 Osteoclast synthesis and secretion and activation of latent transforming growth factor β. J Bone Min Res 9: 443–452

Outrequin G, Caix M, Casanova G 1967 Variations du ligament triangulaire gauche du foie en fonction du type morphologique. CR Assoc Anat 136: 756–762

Owen R L, Nemanic P 1978 Antigen processing structures of the mammalian intestinal tract: an SEM study of lymphoepithelial organs. Scanning Electron Microscopy. Vol 2. SEM Inc: O'Hare, Illinois

Owens G K 1989 Control of hypertrophic versus hyperplastic growth of vascular smooth muscle cells. Am J Physiol 257: H1755–H1765

Owens G K 1991 Role of contractile agonists in growth regulation of vascular smooth muscle cells. Adv Exp Med Biol 308: 71–79

Owens P D 1972 Light microscopic observations on the formation of the layer of Hopewell-Smith in human teeth. Arch Oral Biol 17: 1785–1788

Owens P D 1975 Patterns of mineralization in the roots of premolar teeth in dogs. Arch Oral Biol 20: 709–712

Owman C 1988 Autonomic innervation of the cardiovascular system. In: Björklund A, Hökfelt T, Owman C (eds) The peripheral nervous system. Handbook of chemical neuroanatomy. Vol 6. Elsevier: Amsterdam: pp 327–389

Owman Ch, Rosengren E, Sjöberg N-O 1967 Adrenergic innervation of the human female reproductive organs: a histochemical and chemical investigation. Obstet Gynecol 30: 763–773

Ozzello L 1974 Electron microscopic study of functional and dysfunctional human mammary glands. J Invest Dermatol 63: 19–26

P

Pabst R, Binns R M 1989 Heterogeneity of lymphocyte homing physiology: several mechanisms operate in the control of migration to lymphoid and non-lymphoid organs in vivo. Immunol Rev 108: 83–109

Pace J L 1968 Stereoscopic micro-anatomy of human colonic mucosa and its blood vessels. J Anat 103: 602P

Pacini A, Gremiger D 1975 Alcune modalità nella distribuzione del nervo mascellare. Arch Ital Anat Embriol 80: 29–35

Pack R J, Richardson P S 1984 The aminergic innervation of human bronchus: a light and electron microscopic study. J Anat 138: 493–502

Packard D S, Jacobson A G 1976 The influence of axial structures on chick somite formation. Dev Biol 53: 36–?

Packard D S, Meier S 1983 An experimental study of the somitomeric organization of the avian segmental plate. Dev Biol 97: 191–202

Padget D H 1948 The development of cranial arteries in the human embryo. Contrib Embryol Carneg Inst 32: 205–261

Padget D H 1957 The development of the cranial venous system in man, from the viewpoint of comparative anatomy. Contrib Embryol Carnegie Inst Washington 36: 79–140

Padykula H A, Gauthier G F 1970 The ultrastructure of the neuromuscular junctions of mammalian red, white and intermediate skeletal muscle fibers. J Cell Biol 46: 27–41

Page R B 1986 The anatomy of the hypothalamo-hypophyseal complex. In: Knobil E, Neill J (eds) Raven Press, New York: pp 1161–1233

Page R B, Bergland R M 1977 Pituitary vasculature. In: Allen M B, Makesh V B (eds) The pituitary. A current review. Academic Press: New York: pp 9–17

Page R B, Rosenstein J M, Dovey B J, Leure-duPree A E 1979 Ependymal changes in experimental hydrocephalus. Anat Rec 194: 83–103

Paik S I, Lehman M N, Seiden A M, Duncan H J, Smith D V 1992 Human olfactory biopsy. The influence of age and receptor distribution. Arch Otolaryngol- Head Neck Surg 118: 731–738

Pakkenberg B 1993 Total nerve cell number in neocortex in chronic schizophrenics and controls estimated using optical dissectors. Biol Psychiatry 34: 768–772

Pal G P, Routal R V 1986 A study of weight transmission through the cervical and upper thoracic regions of the vertebral column in man. J Anat 148: 245–261

Pal G P, Tamankar B P 1983 Preliminary study of age changes in Gujarati (Indian) pubic bones. Ind J Med Res 78: 694–701

Pal G P, Tamankar B P, Routal R V, Bhagwat S S 1984 The ossification of the membraneous part of the squamous occipital bone in man. J Anat 138: 259–266

Palade G 1975 Intracellular aspects of the process of protein synthesis. Science 189: 347–358

Palay S, Chan-Palay V 1982 The cerebellum. New Vistas Springer: Berlin

Palfrey A J, Davies D V 1966 The fine structure of chondrocytes. J Anat 100: 213–226

Pallie W, Manuel J K 1968 Intersegmental anastomoses between dorsal spinal rootlets in some vertebrates. Acta Anat 70: 341–351

Pallis C 1983 ABC of brain stem death. The declaration of death, pp 39; Prognostic significance of a dead brain stem, pp 123–124; The arguments about the EEG, pp 284–287; The position in the USA and elsewhere, pp 209–210. British Medical Journal 286

Pallis C 1990 Brain stem death. In: Vinken P J, Bruyn G W, Klawans H L (eds) Handbook of clinical neurology. Volume 57. Elsevier: New York: pp 441–496

Palmer J, Burgoyne P S 1991 In situ analysis of fetal, prepubertal and adult XX–XY chimaeric mouse testes: Sertoli cells are predominantly, but not exclusively, XY. Development 112: 265–268

Palmer R M H, Ferrige A G, Moncada S 1987 Nitric oxide release accounts for the biological activity of endothelial-derived relaxing factor. Nature 327: 524–526

Palmer R M, Lumsden A G S 1987 Development of periodontal ligament and alveolar bone in homografted recombinations of enamel organs and papillary, pulpal and follicular mesenchyme in the mouse. Arch Oral Biol 32: 281–289

Palmiter R D, Brinster R L, Hamm R E, Trumbauer M E, Rosenfeld M G, Brinberg N C, Evan R M 1982 Dramatic growth of mice that develop from eggs microinjected with metallothionein growth hormone fusion genes. Nature 300: 611–615

Pampfer S, Arceci R J, Pollard J W 1991 Role of colony stimulating factor-1 (CSF-1) and other lympho-hematopoietic growth factors in mouse pre-implantation development. BioEssays 13: 535–540

Pandya D N, Rosene D L 1993 Laminar termination patterns of thalamic, callosal and association afferents to the primary auditory area of the rhesus monkey. Exp Neurol 119: 220–234

Pandya D N, Rosene D L, Doolittle A M 1994 Corticothalamic connections of auditory-related areas of the temporal lobe in the rhesus monkey. J Comp Neurol 345: 447–471

Pandya D N, Seltzer B 1982 Association areas of the cerebral cortex. TINS 5: 386–390k

Pandya D N, Yeterian E H 1985 Architecture and connections of cortical association areas. In: Peters A, Jones E G (eds) Cerebral cortex. Vol 4. Association and auditory cortices. Plenum Press: New York: pp 3–61

Paniagua R, Amat P, Nistal M, Martin A 1986 Ultrastructure of Leydig cells in human ageing testes. J Anat 146: 173–183

Paniagua R, Nistal M 1984 Morphological and histometric study of human spermatogonia from birth to the onset of puberty. J Anat 139: 535–552

Paniagua R, Nistal M, Saez F J, Fraile B 1991 Ultrastructure of the aging human testis. J Electron Microsc Tech 19: 241–260

Paniagua R, Regadara J, Nistal M, Santamaria L 1983 Elastic fibres of the human ductus deferens. J Anat 137: 46–76

Panjabi M M, Goel V, Oxland T, Takata K, Duranceau J, Krag M, Price M 1992 Human lumbar vertebrae: quantitative three-dimensional anatomy. Spine 17: 229–306

Panneton W M, Loewy A D 1980 Projections of the carotid sinus nerve to the nucleus of the solitary tract in the cat. Brain Res 191: 239–244

Papalopulu N, Kintner C R 1993 Development 117: 961–975

Papanicolau G N, Traut H F 1943 Diagnosis of uterine cancer by the vaginal smear. Commonwealth Fund: London

Papathanassion B T 1968 A variant of the motor branch of the median nerve in the hand. J Bone Jt Surg 50B: 156–157

Papez J W 1927 Subdivisions of the facial nucleus. J Comp Neurol 43: 159–191

Papez J W 1937 A proposed mechanism of emotion. Arch Neurol Psychiat 38: 725–743

Paquin J D, van der Rest M, Marie P J, Mort J S, Pidoux I, Poole A R, Roughley P J 1983 Biochemical and morphologic studies of cartilage from the adult human sacroiliac joint. Arthritis Rheum 26: 887–895

Parakkal P, Matolsky A G 1964 A study of the differentiation products of the hair follicle cells with the electron microscope. J Invest Dermatol 42: 23–34

Pardo J V, D'Angelo Siciliano J, Craig S W 1983a A vinculin-containing cortical lattice in skeletal muscle: transverse lattice elements ("costameres") mark sites of attachment between myofibrils and sarcolemma. Proc Natl Acad Sci USA 80: 1008–1012

Pardo J V, D'Angelo Siciliano J, Craig S W 1983b Vinculin is a component of an extensive network of myofibril-sarcolemma attachment regions in cardiac muscle fibers. J Cell Biol 97: 1081–1088

Pare D, Steriade M 1993 The reticular thalamic nucleus projects to the contralateral dorsal thalamus in the macaque monkey. Neurosci Lett 154: 96–100

Parent A, Hazrati L-N 1993 Anatomical aspects of information processing in primate basal ganglia. Trends Neurosci 16: 111–116

Parent A, Mackey A, De Bellefeuille L 1983a The subcortical afferents to caudate nucleus and putamen in primate: a fluorescence retrograde double labelling study. Neuroscience 10: 1137–1150

Parent A, Mackey A, Smith Y, Boucher R 1983b The output organization of the substantia nigra in primate as revealed by a retrograde double labelling method. Brain Res Bull 10: 529–537

Parent A, Pare D, Smith Y, Steriade M 1988 Basal forebrain cholinergic and noncholinergic projections to the thalamus and brainstem in cats and monkeys. J Comp Neurol 277: 281–301

Parent D, Akten G, Stouffs-Vanheuf M 1985 Ultrastructure of the normal human nail. Am J Dermatopathol 7: 529–535

Parfitt A M 1983 The physiologic and clinical significance of bone histo-morphometric data. In: Reckker R R (ed) Bone histomorphometry, techniques and interpretation. CRC Press: Boca Raton: pp 143–223

Parfitt A M 1993 Calcium homeostasis. In: Mundy G R, Martin T J (eds) Physiology and pharmacology of bone. Springer-Verlag: Berlin: pp 1–65

Park W H, Hutson J M 1991 The gubernaculum shows rhythmic contractility and active movement during testicular descent. J Pediat Surg 26: 615–617

Parkes A S (ed) 1952–66 Marshall's physiology of reproduction. 3rd edition. Vol 1 part 1 1956. Vol 1 part 2 1960. Vol 2 1952. Vol 3 1966. Longmans Green: London

Parkin I G, Harrison G R 1985 The topographical anatomy of the lumbar epidural space. J Anat 141: 211–217

Parkinson D 1973 Carotid cavernous fistula: direct repair with preservation of the carotid artery. Technical note. J Neurosurg 38: 99–106

Parnavelas J G, Barfield J A, Franke E, Luskin M B 1992 Cereb Cortex 1: 463–468

Parrish E P, Garrod D R, Mattey D L, Hand L, Steart P V, Weller R O 1986 Mouse antisera specific for desmosomal adhesion molecules of suprabasal skin cells, meninges and meningioma. Proc Natl Acad Sci USA 83: 2657–2661

Parry E W 1970 Some electron microscope observations on the mesenchymal structures of full-term umbilical cord. J Anat 107: 505–518

Parsons F G 1903 On the meaning of some of the epiphyes, J Anat 37: 315–323

Parsons F G 1904 Observations on traction epiphyses. J Anat 38: 248–258

Parsons F G 1905 On pressure epiphyses. J Anat 39: 402–412

Partridge T A, Morgan J E, Coulton G R, Hoffman E P, Kunkel L M 1989 Conversion of mdx myofibres from dystrophin-negative to -positive by injection of normal myoblasts. Nature 337: 176–179

Pasche F, Merot Y, Carraux P, Saurat J H 1990 Relationship between Merkel cells and nerve endings during embryogenesis in the mouse epidermis. J Invest Dermatol 95: 247–251

Pasik P, Pasik T, Di Figlia M 1979 The internal organization of the neostriatum in mammals. In: Divac I, Öberg R E G (eds) The Neostriatum. Pergamon Press: Oxford: pp 5–36

Passingham R E 1993 The frontal lobes and voluntary action. Oxford University Press: Oxford

Pasternak J F, Groothuis D R, Fischer J M, Fischer D P 1982 Regional cerebral blood flow in the newborn beagle pup: the germinal matrix is a 'low-flow' structure. Paediatr Res 16: 499–503

Patake S M, Mysorekar V R 1977 Diaphyseal nutrient foramina in human metacarpals and metatarsals. J Anat 124: 299–304

Paterson A M 1904 The human sternum. Williams and Norgate: London

Paterson A M 1912 The form of the human stomach. J Anat 47: 356–359

Patten B M 1922 The formation of the cardiac loop in the chick. Am J Anat 30: 373–397

Patten B M 1956 The development of the sinuventricular conduction system. Univ Michigan Med Bull 22: 1–21

Patterson J F Jr 1946 Cervical ribs and scalenus anticus syndrome: review of literature and report of case. N Carolina Med J 7: 13–20

Patterson P H 1990 Control of cell fate in a vertebrate neurogenic lineage. Cell 62: 1035–1038

Pauerstein C J, Woodruff J D 1967 The role of the 'indifferent' cell of the tubal epithelium. Am J Obstet Gynecol 98: 121–125

Paul J A, Gregson N A 1992 An immunohistochemical study of phospholipase A_2 in peripheral nerve during Wallerian degeneration. J Neuroimmunol 39: 31–48

Paul M, Kanagasuntheram R 1956 Congenital anomalies of lower urinary tract. Br J Urol 28: 64–74

Paul R L, Merzenich M M, Goodman H 1972 Alterations in mechanoreceptor inputs to Brodmann's areas 3 and 1 of Macaca mulatta. Brain Res 39: 1–19

Paula-Barbosa M M, Sousa-Pinto A 1973 Auditory cortical projections to the superior colliculus in the cat, Brain Res 50: 47–61

Pauli R M, Graham J M Jr, Barr M Jr 1981 Agnathia situs inversus, and associated malformations. Teratology 23: 85–93

Paulo L G, Fink G D, Roh B L, Fischer J W 1973 Influence of carotid body ablation on erythropoietin production in rabbits. Am J Physiol 224: 442–444

Pauly R R, Passaniti A, Crow M, Kinsella J L, Papadopoulos N, Monticone R, Lakatta E G, Martin G R 1992 Experimental models that mimic the differentiation and dedifferentiation of vascular cells. Circulation 86 (6 Suppl): III68–III73

Pauwels F 1965 Gesammelte abhandlungen zur funktionellen Anatomie des Bewegungsapparatus. Springer-Verlag: Berlin

Pavlov S, Pétrov V 1968 Sur l'anse sous-clavière de l'artère sous-clavière droite rétro-oesophagienne. Folia Med Plovdiv 10: 73–78

Pawelek J M 1991 After dopachrome. Pig Cell Res 4: 53–62

Paxinos G 1990 The human nervous system. Academic Press: San Diego

Paxinos G, Törk I, Halliday G and Mehler W R 1990 Human homologs to brain stem nuclei identified in other animals as revealed by acetylcholinesterase activity. In: Paxinos G (ed) The human nervous system. Academic Press: San Diego: pp 149–202

Peachey L D, Franzini-Armstrong C 1983 Structure and function of membrane systems of skeletal muscle cells. In: Peachey L D, Adrian R H (eds) Handbook of physiology. Am Physiol Soc: Bethesda, Maryland, Section 10: pp 23–71

Peacock A 1952 Observations on the postnatal structure of the intervertebral disc in man. J Anat 86: 162–179

Peacock A J, Morgan M D, Gourlay S, Turton C, Denison D M 1984 Optical mapping of the thoraco-abdominal wall. Thorax 39: 93–100

Pearce P T, Khalid B A K, Funder J W 1983 Progesterone receptors in rat thymus. Endocrinol 113: 1287–1291

Pearse A G E 1966a The cytochemistry of the thyroid C cells and their relationship to calcitonin. Proc R Soc Lond [Biol] 164: 478–487

Pearse A G E 1966b 5-Hydroxytryptophan uptake by dog thyroid 'C' cells and its possible significance in polypeptide hormone production. Nature 211: 598–600

Pearse A G E 1968 Histochemistry. 3rd edition. Churchill: London

Pearse A G E 1969 The cytochemistry and ultrastructure of polypeptide hormone-producing cells (the APUD series) and the embryologic, physiologic and pathologic implications of the concept. J Histochem Cytochem 17: 303–313

Pearse A G E 1976 Neurotransmission and the APUD concept. In: Coupland R E, Fujita T (eds) Chromaffin, enterochromaffin and related cells. Elsevier: New York: pp 147–154

Pearse A G E 1977a The apudomas; with particular reference to those of gastroenteropancreatic origin. In: Yardley J H, Morson B C, Abell M R (eds) The gastrointestinal tract. Williams & Wilkins: Baltimore: pp 206–218

Pearse A G E 1977b The diffuse neuroendocrine system and the APUD concept: related 'endocrine' peptides in brain, intestine, pituitary, placenta and anuran cutaneous glands. Med Biol 55: 115–125

Pearse A G E 1980 The APUD concept and hormone production. Clin Endocrinol Metab 9: 211–222

Pearse A G E, Polak J M 1971 Cytochemical evidence for the neural crest origin of mammalian C cells. Histochemie 37: 96–102

Pearse A G E, Polak J M 1974 Endocrine tumours of neural crest origin: neurolophomas, apudomas and the APUD concept. Med Biol 52: 3–18

Pearse A G E, Polak J M 1978 The diffuse neuroendocrine system and the APUD concept. In: Bloom S R (ed) Gut hormones. Churchill Livingstone: Edinburgh

Pearse B M F, Bretscher M S 1981 Membrane recycling by coated vesicles. Annu Rev Biochem 50: 85–101

Pearse R G 1978 Percutaneous catheterisation of the radial artery in newborn infants using transillumination. Arch Dis Child 53: 549–554

Pearson A A 1938 The spinal accessory nerve in human embryos. J Comp Neurol 68: 243–266

Pearson A A 1941 The development of the nervus terminals in man. J Comp Neurol 75: 39–66

Pearson A A 1944 The oculomotor nucleus in the human fetus. J Comp Neurol 80: 47–68

Pearson A A 1949 The development and connections of the mesencephalic root of the trigeminal nerve in man. J Comp Neurol 90: 1–46

Pearson A A 1977 The early innervation of the developing deciduous teeth. J Anat 123: 563–577

Pearson A A, Sauter R W 1971b Observations on the caudal end of the spinal cord. Am J Anat 131: 463–470

Pearson J, Goldstein M, Markey K, Brandeis L 1983 Human brainstem catecholamine neuronal anatomy as indicated by immonocytochemistry with antibodies to tyrosine hydroxylase. Neuroscience 8: 3–32

Pearson J, Halliday G, Sakamoto N, Michael J P 1990 Catecholaminergic neurons. In: Paxinos G (ed) The human nervous system. Academic Press: New York: pp 1023–1050

Pearson R C A, Brodal P, Gatter K C, Powell T P S 1982 The organization of the connections between the cortex and the claustrum in the monkey. Brain Res 234: 435–441

Pearson R C A, Brodal P, Powell T P S 1978 The projection of the thalamus upon the parietal lobe in the monkey. Brain Res 144: 143–148

Pearson R C A, Gatter K C, Powell T P S 1983a The projection of the basal nucleus of Meynert upon the neocortex in the monkey. Brain Res 259: 132–136

Pearson R C A, Gatter K C, Powell T P S 1983b Retrograde cell degeneration in the basal nucleus in monkey and man. Brain Res 261: 321–326

Pearson R C A, Gatter K C, Powell T P S 1983c The cortical relationships of certain basal ganglia and the cholinergic basal forebrain nuclei. Brain Res 261: 327–330

Pearson R C A, Powell T P S 1978 The cortico-cortical connections to area 5 of the parietal lobe from the primary somatic sensory cortex of the monkey. Proc R Soc Lond [Biol] 200: 103–108

Pearson R C A, Powell T P S 1985 The projection of the primary somatic sensory cortex upon area 5 in the monkey. Brain Res 9: 89–107

Pearson R C A, Powell T P S 1989 The neuroanatomy of Alzheimer's disease. Rev Neurosci 2: 101–121

Pease D C, Quilliam T A 1957 Electron microscopy of the Pacinian corpuscle. J Cell Biol 3: 331–342

Pech P, Haughton V M 1985 Lumbar intervertebral disk: correlative MR and anatomic study. Radiology 156: 699–701

Peck H M, Hoerr N L 1951 The effect of environmental temperature changes on the circulation of the mouse spleen. Anat Rec 109: 479–494

Pedersen H 1969 Ultrastructure of the ejaculated human sperm. Z Zellforsch 94: 542–554

Pedersen J F 1980 Ultrasound evidence of sexual difference in fetal size in first trimester. Br Med J 281: 1253

Peichl L 1991 Alpha ganglion cells in mammalian retinae: common properties, species differences, and some comments on other ganglion cells. Vis Neurosci 7: 155–169

Pelfini C, Sacchi S, Serri F, Carosi G 1969 Ultrastruttura delle cosidette ghiandole sebacee unicellulari. G Ital Dermatol 104: 1–4

Pelham H R 1991 Multiple targets for Brifeldin A. Cell 67: 449–451

Pelletier G, Robert F, Hardy H 1978 Identification of human anterior pituitary cells by immunoelectron microscopy. J Clin Endocrinol Metab 46: 534–542

Pelosi P, Baldaccini N E, Pisanelli A M 1982 Identification of specific olfactory receptor for 2–isobutyl-3–methoxypyrazine. Biochem J 201: 245–248

Penfield W 1932 Cytology and cellular pathology of the nervous system, vol 2. Neuroglia: normal and pathological. Hoeber: New York

Penfield W, Jasper H 1954 Epilepsy and the functional anatomy of the human brain. Little, Brown: Boston

Penfield W, Rasmussen T 1950 The cerebral cortex of man. Macmillan: New York

Penfold P L, Provis J M, Madigan M C, van Dreil D, Billson F A 1990 Angiogenesis in normal human retinal development: the involvement of astrocytes and macrophages. Graefes Arch Clin Exp Ophthalmol 228: 255

Pennell T C 1966 Anatomical study of the peripheral pulmonary lymphatics. J Thorac Cardiovasc Surg 52: 629–634

Pennisi E, Crucci G, Manfredi M, Palladini G 1991 Histometric study of myelinated fibres in the human trigeminal nerve. J Neurol Sci 105: 22–28

Penrose L S, Loesch D 1969 Dermatoglyphic sole patterns: a new attempt at classification. Hum Biol 41: 427–448

Pénzes L, Regius O 1985 Changes in the intestinal microvillous surface area during reproduction and ageing in the female rat. J Anat 140: 389–396

Percheron G 1977 Les artères du thalamus humain. Les artères choroidiennes. I–V. Rev Neurol 133: 533–558

Perera H, Edwards F R 1957 Intradiaphragmatic course of the left phrenic nerve in relation to diaphragmatic incisions. Lancet 2: 75–77

Perera P et al 1970 The development of the cutaneous microvascular system in the newborn. Br J Dermatol 82 (suppl 5): 86–91

Pernkopf E 1963 Atlas of topographical and applied human anatomy, Saunders: Philadelphia

Pernus F, Erzen I 1991 Arrangement of fiber types within fascicles of human vastus lateralis muscle. Muscle Nerve 14: 304–309

Perona R M, Wassarman P M 1986 Mouse blastocysts hatch in vitro by using a trypsin-like proteinase associated with cells of the mural trophectoderm. Dev Biol 114: 42–52

Perre J, Riche D, Foncin J F 1977 Sur la gaine des cellules ganglionnaires de Scarpa chez le babouin Papio Papio. Acta Otolaryngol [Stockh] 83: 279–283

Perren S M, Huggler A, Russenberger M et al 1969 The reaction of cortical bone to compression. Acta Orthop Scand Suppl 125 19–29

Perrett D I, Oram M W, Harries M H, Bevan R, Hietanen J K, Benson P J et al 1991 Viewer-centred and object-centred coding of heads in the macaque temporal cortex. Exp Brain Res 86: 159–173

Perry M E, Brown K A, von Gaudecker B 1992 Ultrastructural identification and distribution of the adhesion molecules ICAM-1 and LFA-1 in the vascular and extravascular compartments of the human palatine tonsil. Cell Tissue Res 268: 317–326

Perry M E, Jones M M, Mustafa Y 1988 Structure of the crypt epithelium in human palatine tonsil. Acta Otolaryngol (Stockh) Suppl 454: 53–59

Perry M E, Mustafa Y, Brown K A 1992b The microvasculature of the human palatine tonsil and its role in the homing of lymphocytes. In: Galioto G B (ed) A clinically orientated update, Vol 47. Advances in otorhinolaryngology. Karger: Basel: pp 11–15

Perry V H, Andersson P-B 1992 The inflammatory response in the CNS. Neuropathol Appl Neurobiol 18: 454–459

Persing J A, Berman D E, Ogle R C, Drake S 1993 Calvarial deformity regeneration following subtotal calvariectomy for craniosynostosis: a case report and theoretical implications. J Craniofac Surg 4: 85–89

Persohn E, Malherbe P, Richards J G 1992 Comparative molecular neuroanatomy of cloned GABA$_A$ receptor subunits in the rat CNS. J Comp Neurol 326: 193–216

Persson E, Jansson T 1992 Low birthweight is associated with elevated adult blood pressure in the chronically catheterised guinea-pig. Acta Physiol Scand 145: 195–196

Perutz M F, Rossmann M G, Cullis A F, Muirhead H, Will G, North A C

T 1960 Structure of haemoglobin. A three-dimensional Fourier synthesis at 5.5 Å resolution, obtained by X-ray analysis. Nature 185: 416–422

Peterhanse E, Von Der Heydt R 1993 Functional organization of area V2 in the alert macaque. Eur J Neurosci 5: 509–524

Peters A 1961 A radial component of central myelin sheaths. J Biophys Biochem Cytol 11: 733–735

Peters A 1984a Bipolar cells. In: Peters A, Jones E G (eds) Cerebral cortex. Vol 1. Cellular components of the cerebral cortex. Plenum Press: New York: pp 381–407

Peters A 1984b Chandelier cells. In: Peters A, Jones E G (eds) Cerebral cortex. Vol 1. Cellular components of the cerebral cortex. Plenum Press: New York: pp 361–380

Peters A, Payne B R, Budd J 1994 A numerical analysis of the geniculocortical input to striate cortex in the monkey. Cereb Cortex 4: 215–229

Peters A, Saint-Marie R L 1984 Smooth and sparsely spinous nonpyramidal cells forming local axonal plexuses. In: Peters A, Jones E G (eds) Cerebral cortex. Vol 1. Cellular components of the cerebral cortex. Plenum Press: New York: pp 419–445

Peters C A, Reid L~m, Docimo S, Luetic T, Carr M, Retik A B, Mandell J 1991 The role of the kidney in lung growth and maturation in the setting of obstructive uropathy and oligohydramnios. J Urol 146: 597–600

Peters R M 1969 The mechanical basis of respiration. Churchill: London

Peterson B W, Coulter J D 1977 A new long spinal projection from the vestibular nuclei in the cat. Brain Res 122: 351–356

Peterson M R, Leblond C P 1964 Uptake by the Golgi region of glucose labelled with tritium in the 1 or 6 position, as an indicator of synthesis of complex carbohydrates. Exp Cell Res 34: 420–423

Peterson S E, Fox P T, Posner M I, Mintum M A, Raichle M E 1988 Positron emission tomographic studies of the cortical anatomy of single word processing. Nature 331: 585–589

Petras J M, Cummings J F 1977 The origin of spinocerebellar pathways: II. The nucleus centrobasalis of the cervical enlargement and the nucleus dorsalis of the thoracolumbar spinal cord. J Comp Neurol 173: 693–716

Petrides M, Alivisatos B, Evans A C, Meyer E 1993 Dissociation of human mid-dorsolateral from posterior dorsolateral frontal cortex in memory processing. Proc Natl Acad Sci USA 90: 873–877

Petrides M, Alivisatos B, Meyer E, Evans A C 1993 Functional activation of the human frontal cortex during the performance of verbal working memory tasks. Proc Natl Acad Sci USA 90: 878–882

Petrides M, Pandya D N 1988 Association fiber pathways to the frontal cortex from the superior temporal region in the rhesus monkey. J Comp Neurol 273: 52–66

Petrovic A G 1972 Mechanisms and regulation of mandibular condylar growth. Acta Morphol Neerl Scand 10: 25–34

Pette D, Staron R S 1990 Cellular and molecular diversities of mammalian skeletal muscle fibers. Rev Physiol Biochem Pharmacol 116: 1–76

Pette D, Vrbová G 1992 Adaptation of mammalian skeletal muscle fibers to chronic electrical stimulation. Rev Physiol Biochem Pharmacol 120: 115–202

Pettigrew J B 1860 On the arrangement of the muscle fibres of the ventricular portion of the heart of the mammal. Proc Roy Soc 1859 10: 443–440

Pettigrew J B 1865 On the arrangement of the muscle fibres in the ventricles of the vertebral heart, with physiological remarks. Phil Trans Roy Soc Lond 1864 154: 445–450

Pettway Z, Guillory G, Bronner-Fraser M 1990 Absence of neural crest cells from the region surrounding implanted notochords in situ. Dev Biol 142: 335–345

Pevsner J, Hou V, Snowman S M, Snyder S H 1990 Odorant binding protein J.Biol Chem 265: 6118–6125

Pevsohn E 1989 Immuno-electron microscopic localisation of the 180 kD component of the neutral cell adhesion molecule N-CAM in postsynaptic membranes. J Cell Neurol 288: 92–100

Pfaff D W, Gerlach J L, McEwen B S, Ferin M, Carmael P, Zimmerman E A 1976 Autoradiographic localization of hormone-concentrating cells in the brain of the female rhesus monkey. J Comp Neurol 170: 279–294

Pfaffman C 1970 Physiological and behavioural processes of the sense of taste. In: Wolstenholme G E W, Knights J (eds) Taste and smell in vertebrates. (Ciba Foundation Symposium.) Churchill: London: pp 31–44

Pfeifer R A 1940 Die angioarchtecktonischen areale Gliederung der Grosshirnrinde. Thieme: Leipzig

Pfenninger K H, Rees R P 1976 From the growth cone to the synapse: properties of membranes involved in synapse formation. In: Barondes S H (ed) Neuronal recognition. Plenum: New York: pp 131–178

Pflüger E 1866 Ueber die Epithelien der Glandula submaxillaris. Zbl med Wiss 4: 193–195

Phifer R F, Midgley A R, Spicer S S 1973 Immunologic and histologic evidence that follicle stimulating and luteinizing hormones are present in the same cell types in the human pars distalis. J Clin Endocr Metab 36: 125–141

Phillips A G, Blaha C D, Fibiger H C 1989 Neurochemical correlates of brain-stimulation reward measured by ex vivo and in vivo analyses. Neurosci Biobehavioral Rev 13: 99–104

Phillips A G, Fibiger H C 1990 Role of reward and enhancement of conditioned reward in persistence of responding for cocaine. Behavioural Pharmacol 1: 269–282

Phillips C C, Porter R 1977 Corticospinal neurones: their role in movement. Monogr Physio Soc, No 34. Academic Press: London

Phillips D M 1975 Mammalian sperm structure. In: Hamilton D W, Greep R O (eds) Handbook of physiology, section 7. Endocrinology. Vol V. American Physiological Society: Washington, DC: pp 405–420

Phillips D M, Olson G 1975 Mammalian sperm motility–structure in relation to function. In: Afzelius B A (ed) The functional Anatomy of the spermatozoon. Proceedings of the Second International Symposium.

Phillips P D, Kaji K, Cristofalo V J 1984 Progressive loss of the proliferative response of senescing WI-38 cells to PDGF, EGF, insulin, transferrin, and dexamethasone. J Gerontol 39: 11–17

Piasecka-Kacperska K, Gladyskowska-Rzeczycka j 1972 Splot kryżowy u naczelnych. Folia Morphol 31: 21–33

Piasecki C 1974 Blood supply to the human gastro-duodenal mucosa. J Anat 118: 295–335

Piasecki C 1977 Role of ischaemia in the initiation of peptic ulcer. Ann R Coll Surg 59: 476–478

Piasecki C, Wyatt C 1986 Patterns of blood supply to the gastric mucosa. A comparative study revealing an end-artery model. J Anat 149: 21–39

Pick J 1970 The autonomic nervous system, Lippincott; Philadelphia

Pick J, Sheehan D 1946 Sympathetic rami in man. J Anat 80: 12–20

Pickel V M, Joh T H, Reis D J, Leeman S E, Miller R J 1979 Electron microscope localization of substance P and enkephalin in axon terminals related to dendrites of catecholaminergic neurons. Brain Res 160: 387–400

Picker L J, Butcher E C 1992 Physiological and molecular mechanisms of lymphocyte homing. Ann Rev Immunol 10: 561–591

Pickett-Heaps J D 1975 Aspects of spindle evolution. Ann N Y Acad Sci 253: 352–361

Pickles J O, Comis S D, Osbourne M P 1984 Cross-links between stereocilia in the guinea pig organ of Corti, and their possible relation to sensory transduction. Hear Res 15: 103–112

Picton D A C 1990 Tooth mobility - an update. Europ J Orthod 12: 109–115

Pierce G F, Yanagihara D, Costigan V, Tarpley J, Hockman H, Boone T, Song S-Z, Germain L, Klopchin K, Altrock B W, Thomason A 1991 Platelet-derived endothelial cell growth factor (PD-ECGF) in angiogenesis and wound healing. Abstract. (1st European Tissue Repair Society Meeting.) Oxford: UK

Pijnenborg R 1990 Trophoblast invasion and placentation in the human. Morphological aspects. Trophoblast Res 4: 33–47

Pijnenborg R, Dixon G, Robertson W B, Brosens I 1980 Trophoblastic invasion of human decidua from 8 to 18 weeks of pregnancy. Placenta 1: 3–19

Pijnenborg R, Robertson W B, Brosens I, Dixon G 1981 Review article: trophoblast invasion and the establishment of haemochorial placentation in man and laboratory animals. Placenta 2: 71–92

Pikó 1969 Gamete structure and sperm entry in mammals. In: Metz C B, Monroy A (eds) Fertilization. Comparative morphology, biochemistry and immunology. Vol 2. Academic Press: New York: pp 325–403

Pikó L, Tyler A 1964 Fine structural studies of sperm penetration in the rat. Proc Vth Congr Internationale per la Riproduzione Animale e la Fecundacione Artificale, Trento, section 1, volume II, 327–377

Pimendis M Z, Hinds J W 1977 An autoradiographic study of the sensory innervation of teeth. I. Dentin. II. Dental pulp and periodontium. J Dent Res 56: 827–834; 835–840

Pinching A J, Powell T P S 1971 The neuron types of the glomerular layer of the olfactory bulb. J Cell Sci 9: 305–346

Pincus D W, DiCicco E, Black I B 1992 Neuropeptide regulation of neuronal development. In: Hendry I A, Hill C E (eds) Development, regeneration and plasticity of the autonomic nervous system. Harwood Academic Publishers: Switzerland: pp 267–303

Pincus G, Enzman E V 1935 The comparative behaviour of mammalian eggs in vivo and in vitro. J Exp Med 62: 665–675

Pini A 1993 Science 261: 95–98

Pinkerton J H M, McKay D G, Adams E C, Hertig A T 1961 Development of the human ovary – a study using histochemical technics. Obstet Gynec N Y 18: 152–181

Pinto da Silva P, Kachar B 1982 On tight-junction structure. Cell 28: 441–450

Pioro E P, Mai J K, Cuello C 1990 Distribution of substance P- and enkephalin-immunoreactive fibers. In: Paxinos G (ed) The human nervous system. Academic Press: New York: pp 1051– 1094

Pirenne M 1967 Vision and the eye. 2nd edition. Chapman and Hall: London

Pismenov I A, Zapetski E V 1977 Regularities and distinctions in the structure of the circulation bed of the sternum. Arkh Anat Gistol Embriol 72: 61–67

Pitelka D R 1983 The mammary gland. In: Weiss L (ed) Histology: cell and tissue biology. 5th edition. Elsevier: New York: pp 944–965

Pitelka D R, Hamamoto S T 1977 Form and function in mammary epithelium: the interpretation of ultrastructure. J Dairy Sci 60: 643–654

Pitelka D R, Hamamoto S T, Duofala J G, Nemanic M K 1973 Cell contacts in the mouse mammary gland. 1. Normal gland in postnatal development and the secretory cycle. J Cell Biol 56: 797–818

Pittack C, Jones M, Reh T A 1991 Basic fibroblast growth factor induces retinal pigment epithelium to generate neural retina in vitro. Development 113: 577–588

Pittenger M F, Kazzax J A, Helfman D M 1994 Functional properties of non-muscle tropomyosin isoforms. Curr Opin Cell Biol 6: 96–104

Pittman F E, Pittman J C 1966 An electron microscopic study of the epithelium of normal human sigmoid colonic mucosa. Gut 7: 644–661

Placzek M, Tessier-Lavigne M, Yamada T, Jessell T, Dodd J 1990 Science 250: 985–992

Plarr's Lives of the Fellows of the Royal College of Surgeons of England.

Platt J B 1893 Ectodermic origin of the cartilage of the head. Anat Anz 8: 506–509

Platt J B 1894 Quart J Micr Sci 38

Platz F, Adelmann G 1976 Zur Anatomie der 'Vena arcuata cruris posterior', und ihrer Tiefen–anastomosen (Vv communicantes sive perforantes). Verh Anat Ges Jena 70: 709–714

Platzer W, Maurer H 1966 Zur Segmenteinteilung der Leber. Acta Anat 63: 8–31

Plentl A A 1958 The origin of amniotic fluid. In: Villee C A (ed) Gestation transactions of conference. 5th and final. Josiah Macy Jr Foundation: New York: pp 71–114

Plets C 1969 The arterial blood supply and angioarchitecture of the posterior wall of the third ventricle. Acta Neurochir 21: 309–317

Poduslo J F 1993 Albumin and the blood-nerve barrier. In: Dyck P J, Thomas P K, Griffin J W, Low P A, Podulso J F (eds) Peripheral Neuropathy 3rd edition. W B Saunders: Philadelphia: pp 446–452

Poggio G F, Mountcastle V B 1960 A study of the functional contributions of the lemniscal and spinothalamic systems to somatic sensibility. Bull Johns Hopkins Hosp 106: 266–316

Poirer L J, Bertrand C 1955 Experimental and anatomical investigations of lateral spinothalamic and spinotectal tracts. J Comp Neurol 102: 745–757

Poirriaer N P, Chernikov Y F 1965 Mat Teoret Klin Med 5: 000–000

Poláček P 1961 Relation of myocardial bridges and loops on the coronary arteries to coronary occlusion. Am Heart J 61: 44–62

Poláček P, Halata Z 1970 Development of simple encapsulated corpuscles in the nasolabial region of the cat. Ultrastructural study. Folia Morphol (Praha), 18: 359–368

Polak J M, Becker K L, Cutz E, Gail D B, Goniakowska-Witalinska I, Gosney J R, Lauweryns J M, Linnoila I, McDowell E M, Miller Y E, Scheuermann D W, Springall D R, Sunday M E, Zaccone G 1993 Lung endocrine cell markers, peptides, and amines. Anat Rec 236: 169–171

Polak J M, Bloom S R, Hobbs S, Solcia E, Pearse A G E 1976 Distribution of a bombesin-like peptide in human gastointestinal tract. Lancet 1: 1109–1110

Polak J M, Buchan A M J, Czykowska W, Solcia E, Bloom S R, Pearse A G E 1978 Bombesin in the gut. In: Bloom S R (ed) Gut hormones. Churchill Livingstone: Edinburgh: pp 541–543

Polak J M, Buchan A M, Probert L, Tapia F, de Mey J, Bloom S R 1980 Regulatory peptides in endocrine cells and autonomic nerves: electron immunocytochemistry. Scand J Gastroenterol 16 (suppl 70): 11–23

Poletti C E, Creswell G 1977 Fornix system efferent projections in the squirrel monkey: an experimental degeneration study. J Comp Neuroll 75: 101–128

Polge C 1957 Low-temperature storage of mammalian spermatozoa. Proc R Soc B 147: 498–508

Policard A 1950 Sur quelques caractères histophysiologiques des formations lymphoides brochiques. Bull Hist Appl 27: 118

Polig E, Jee W S S 1990 A model of osteon closure in cortical bone. Calcif Tiss Int 47: 261–269

Politis M J, Ederle K, Spencer P S 1982. Tropism in nerve regeneration in vivo. Attraction of regenerating axons by diffusible factors derived from cells in distal nerve stumps of transacted peripheral nerve. Brain Res 253: 1–12

Politzer G 1952 Zur normalen und abnormen Entwicklung des menschlichen Gesichtes. Z Anat Entwicklungsgesch 116: 332–346

Polley M J, Phillips M L, Wayner E, Nudelman E, Singhal A K, Hakomori S-I, Paulson J C 1991 CD62 and endothelial cell–leukocyte adhesion molecule 1 (ELAM-1) recognize the same carbohydrate ligand, sialyl-Lewis X. Proc Natl Acad Sci USA 88: 6224–6228

Polóyni J, Kapeller K, Mráz P 1977 SGG (SIF) cells in autonomic ganglion: evidence for a possible secretion of their contents into the blood vessels. Z Mikrosk Anat Forsch 91: 581–589

Poltorak M, Shimoda K, Freed W J 1990 Cell adhesion molecules (CAMs) in adrenal medulla in situ and in vitro: enhancement of chromaffin cell L1/Ng-Cam expression by NGF. Exp Neurol 10: 52–72

Polunovsky V A et al 1993 Role of Mesenchymal cell death in lung remodelling after injury. J Clin Invest 91(1): 388–397

Polunovsky V A, Chen B, Henke C, Snover D, Wendt D, Wendt C, Ingbar D H, Bitterman P B 1993 Role of mesenchymal cell death in lung remodelling after injury. J Clin Invest 92: 388–397

Polyak S 1941 The retina. University of Chicago Press: Chicago

Pomerat C M, Hendelman W J, Raiborn C W Jr, Massey J F 1967 Dynamic activities of nervous tissue in vitro. In: Hydén H (ed) The neuron. Elsevier: Amsterdam: pp 119–178

Pompeiano O, Brodal A 1957 Experimental demonstration of a somatotopical origin of rubrospinal fibres in the cat. J Comp Neurol 108: 225–252

Ponseti I V 1978a Growth and development of the acetabulum in the normal child. J Bone Jt Surg 60A: 575–585

Ponseti I V 1978b Morphology of acetabulum in congenital dislocation of hip – gross, histologic, and roentgenographic studies. J Bone Jt Surg 60A: 586–599

Pontoppidan H, Huttmeier P C, Quinn D A 1985 Etiology, demography and outcome in acute respiratory failure. In: Zapo W M, Falke K J (eds) Acute respiratory failure. Marcel Dekker: New York: pp 1–21

Poole C A, Ayad S, Gilbert R T 1992 Chondrons from articular cartilage. V. Immunohistochemical evaluation of type VI collagen organisation in isolated chondrons by light, confocal and electron microscopy. J Cell Sci 103: 1101–1110

Poole C A, Honda T, Skinner S J M, Schofield J R, Hyde K F, Shinkai H 1990 Chondrons from articular cartilage. II: Analysis of the glycosaminoglycans in the cellular microenvironment of isolated canine chondrons. Connect Tissue Res 24: 319–330

Poole T J, Coffin J D 1991 Morphogenetic mechanisms in avian vascular development. In: Feinberg R N, Sherer G K, Auerbach R (eds) The development of the vascular system. Issues Biomed 14: 25–36

Popa G T, Fielding U 1930a A portal circulation from the pituitary to the hypothalamic region. J Anat 65: 88–91

Popa G T, Fielding U 1930b Vascular link between pituitary and hypothalamus. Lancet 2: 238–240

Popescu L M, Diculescu I 1975 Calcium in smooth muscle sarcoplasmic reticulum in situ. Conventional and X-ray analytical electron microscopy. J Cell Biol 67: 911–918

Popoff N W 1934 Digital vascular system, with reference to the state of the glomus inflammation, arteriosclerotic gangrene, diabetic gangrene, thrombo-angitis obliterans and supernumerary digits in man. Archs Path 18: 295–330

Porteous C J 1960 The olecranon epiphyses. J Anat 94: 286P

Porter R, Lemon R N 1993 Corticospinal function and voluntary movements. Oxford University Press: Oxford: pp 428

Porteus M H, Bulfone A, Ciaranello R D, Rubenstein J L R 1991 Isolation and characterisation of a novel cDNA clone encoding a homeodomain that is developmentally expression in the ventral forebrain. Neuron 7: 221–229

Posner A S 1988 The mineral of bone. Clin Orthop 200: 87–99

Posselt U 1952 Studies in mobility of human mandible. Acta Odont Scand Suppl 10: 3–160

Potenza A D 1963 Critical evaluation of flexor–tendon healing and adhesion formation within artificial digital sheaths. An experimental study. J Bone Jt Surg 45A: 1217–1233

Potten C S 1974 The epidermal proliferative unit: the possible role of the central basal cell. Cell Tissue Kinet 7: 77–88

Potten C S 1983 Stem cells: their identification and characterization. Churchill Livingstone: Edinburgh

Potten C S 1985 Radiation and skin. Taylor and Francis: London

Potten C S, Loeffler M 1990 Stem cell attributes, cycles, spirals, pitfalls and uncertainties. Lessons for and from the crypt. Development 110: 1001–1020

Potten C S, Schofield R, Lajtha L G 1979 A comparison of cell replacement in bone marrow, testis and three regions of surface epithelium. Biochim Biophys Acta 560: 281–299

Potter G 1989 Development of colonic function. In: Lebenthal E (ed) Human Gastrointestinal Development. Raven Press: New York: pp 545–558

Potts T K 1925 The main peripheral connections of the human sympathetic nervous system. J Anat 59: 129–135

Potts T R Jr, Murray T, Peacock M, Niall H D, Tregear G W, Keutmann H T, Powell D, Deftos L J 1971 Parathyroid hormone: sequence, synthesis, immunoassay studies. Am J Med 50: 639–649

Pow D V, Morris J F 1989 Dendrites of hypothalamic magnocellular neurons release neurohypophysial peptides by exocytosis. Neuroscience 32: 435–439

Powell H C, Myers R R, Costello M L, Lampert P W 1979 Endoneurial fluid pressure in Wallerian degeneration. Ann Neuro 5: 550–573

Powell T P S 1981 Certain aspects of the intrinsic organisation of the cerebral cortex. In: Pompeiano O, Marsan C A (eds) Brain mechanisms of perceptual awareness and purposeful behaviour. Raven Press: New York: pp 1–19

Powell T P S, Guillery R W, Cowan W M 1957 A quantative study of the fornix-mamillo-thalamic system. J Anat 91: 419–437

Powell T P S, Hendrickson A E 1981 Similarity in number of neurons

2013

through the depth of the cortex in the binocular and monocular parts of area 17 of the monkey. Brain Res 216: 409–413

Powell T P S, Mountcastle V B 1959 Some aspects of the functional organisation of the cortex of the postcentral gyrus of the monkey. A correlation of findings obtained in a single unit analysis with cytoarchitectonics. Bull Johns Hopkins Hosp 105: 173–200

Prakash S, Chopra S R K, Jit I 1979 Ossification of the human patella. J Anat. Ind 28: 78–83

Pressman J J 1942 Physiology of vocal cords in phonation and respiration. Archs Otolaryngol 35: 355–398

Preston J B, Whitlock D G 1961 Intracellular potentials recorded from motoneurons following precentral gyrus stimulation in primates. J Neurophysiol 24: 91–100

Preston T M, King C A, Hyams J S 1990 The cytoskeleton and cell motility. Blackie: Glasgow

Price J L 1990 Olfactory system. In: Paxinos G (ed) The human nervous system. Academic Press: San Diego: pp 979–998

Price J L, Russchen F T, Amaral D 1987 The limbic region. II: The amygdaloid complex. In: Björklund A, Hökfelt T, Swanson L W (eds) Handbook of chemical neuroanatomy. Vol 5. Integrated systems of the CNS, Part 1. Elsevier: Amsterdam: pp 279–388

Price J, Thurlow L 1988 Development 104: 473–482

Price J, Turner D, Cepko 1987 Nature 328: 131–136

Price M, Lemaistre M, Pischetola M, Di Lauro R, Duboule D 1991 A mouse gene related to distal-less shows expression in the developing forebrain. Nature 351: 748–750

Prichett D B, Sontheimer H, Shivers B D, Ymer S, Kettenmann H, Schofield P R, Seeburg P H 1989 Importance of a novel GABA$_A$ receptor subunit for benzodiazepine pharmacology. Nature 338: 582–585

Priestley J V 1984 Pre-embedding ultrastructural immunocytochemistry for CNS transmitters and transmitter markers. In: Cuello A C (ed) Immunohistochemistry Ch 11. Wiley: Chichester: pp 273–322

Pringle N P, Mudhar H S, Collarini E J, Richardson W D 1992 PDGF receptors in the rat CNS: during late neurogenesis, PDGF alpha receptor expression appears to be restricted to glial cells of the oligodendrocyte lineage. Development 115: 535–551

Prinzmetal M, Simkin B, Bergman H C, Kruger H E 1947 Studies on the coronary circulation. Am Heart J 33: 420–442

Pritchard H, Micklem H S 1973 Haimopoietic stem cells and progenitors of functional T-lymphocytes in the bone marrow of 'nude' mice. Clin Exp Immunol 14: 597–607

Pritchard J J, Scott J H, Girgis F G 1956 The structure and development of cranial and facial sutures. J Anat 90: 73–87

Pritchard K, Marston S B 1989 Ca^{2+}–calmodulin binding to caldesmon and the caldesmon–actin–tropomyosin complex. Its role in Ca^{2+} regulation of the activity of synthetic smooth-muscle thin filaments. Biochem J 257: 839–843

Privat A 1975 Postnatal gliogenesis in the mammalian brain. Int Rev Cytol 40: 281–323

Probst T, Plendl H, Paulus W, Wist E R, Scherg M 1993 Identification of the visual motion area (area V5) in the human brain by dipole source analysis. Exp Brain Res 93: 345–351

Proceedings of the Royal Society Vol 12 (1962–63) St George's Hospital Gazette 21 May 1908 16: 49

Prochaska A, Wand P 1980 Tendon organ discharge following voluntary movement in cats. J Physiol 303: 385–390

Prockop D J, Kivirikko K I, Tuderman L, Guzman N A 1979 The biosynthesis of collagen and its disorders (first of two parts). N Engl J Med 301: 13–23

Proctor B, Nager G T 1982 The facial canal: normal anatomy, variations and anomalies. Ann Otol Rhinol Laryngol 91 (suppl 93): 33–61

Proctor D, Fletcher R D, Del Negro A A 1978 Temporary cardiac pacing: causes, recognition, and management of failure to pace. Nurs Clin North Am 13: 409–422

Prota G 1992 Melanin and melanogenesis. Academic Press, New York

Protsch R R R 1986 Radiocarbon dating of bones. In: Zimmerman M R, Angel J L (eds) Dating and age determination of biological materials. Croom Helm: London

Prout G R, Hume D M, Lee H M, Williams G M 1969 Some urological aspects of 93 consecutive renal homo-transplants in modified recipients. J Urol 97: 409–425

Prud'Homme M J L, Cohen D A D, Kalaska J F 1994 Tactile activity in primate primary somatosensory cortex during active arm movements: cytoarchitectonic distribution. J Neurophysiol 71: 173–181

Pryer N K, Wuestehube L J, Scheckman R 1992 Vesicle-mediated protein sorting. Annu Rev Biochem 61: 471–516

Pšenicka P 1966 Beitrag zur Kenntnis der Innervation der Kehlkopfgelenke. Anat Anz 118: 1–6

Pu X, Ma Y, Cai J 1993 A study on the effect of lesions of area 7 of the parietal cortex on the short-term visual spatial memory of rhesus monkeys (Macaca mulatta). Brain Res 600: 187–192

Puchades-Orts A, Nombela-Gomez M, Ortuño-Pacheco G 1976 Variation

in form of the circle of Willis. Some anatomical and embryological considerations. Anat Rec. 185: 119–123

Puelles L, Rubinstein J L R 1993 Trends Neurosci 16: 472–479

Pulec J L, Kamio T, Graham M D 1975 Eustachian tube lymphatics. Ann Otol Rhinol Laryngol 84: 483–492

Pullman W E, Bodmer W F 1992 Cloning and characterization of a gene that regulates cell adhesion. Nature 356: 529–532

Purkinje J E 1837 Ueber die gangliösen körperchen in verschiedenen Theilen des Gehirns. Ber Versamml Dtsch Naturf Aerzte Prague 1837, 1838, 15: 179–180

Purves D, Lamantia A 1993 Development of blobs in the visual cortex of macaques. J Comp Neurol 334: 169–175

Purves D, Thompson W, Yip J W 1981 Re-innervation of ganglia transplanted to the neck from different levels of the guinea-pig sympathetic chain. J Physiol 313: 49–63

Purves H D 1961 Morphology of the hypophysis related to its function. In: Young W C (ed) Sex and internal secretion. Williams & Wilkins: Baltimore: pp 161–238

Purves M J 1970 The role of the cervical sympathetic nerve in the regulation of oxygen consumption of the carotid body of the cat. J Physiol 209: 417–431

Püschel J 1930 Wassergehalt normaler und degenerierter Zwischenwir-belsch-eiben. Beitr Pathol Anat 84: 123–130

Puschett J B 1978 Renal tubular effects of parathyroid hormone. An update. Clin Orthop 135: 249–259

Putschar W 1931 Entwicklung, Wachstum und Pathologie der Beck-enverbindungen des Menschen mit besonderer Berücksichtigung von Schwangerschaft, Geburt und ihren Folgen. Aus dem Pathologischen Institute der Universität Göttingen. Fischer Verlag: Stuttgart

Putz R 1976 Zur morphologie und Rotationsmechanik der kleinen Gelenke der Ledenwirbel. Z Orthop 114: 902–912

Pyatkina GA 1982 Development of the olfactory epithelium in man. Z Mikrosk Anat Forsch Leipzig 96: 361–372

Pyle S I, Hoerr N L 1955 Radiographic atlas of skeletal development of the knee. Thomas: Springfield, Illinois

Pyrtek L J, Painter R L 1964 An anatomic study of the relationship of the parathyroid glands to the recurrent laryngeal nerve. Surg Gynecol Obstet 119: 509–512

Q

Quain R 1844 Anatomy of the arteries of the human body, with its applications to pathology and operative survery. London, 1844

Quesenberry P, Levitt L 1979 Hemapoietic stem cells. N Engl J Med 301: 755–761

Quevedo W C, Fitzpatrick T B, Szabo G, Jimbow K 1987 Biology of melanocytes. In: Fitzpatrick T B, Eizen A Z, Wolff K, Friedberg I M, Austen K F (eds) Dermatology in general medicine. 3rd edition. 2 vols. McGraw Hill: New York: pp 224–251

Quilliam T A 1966 Unit design and array patterns in receptor organs. In: de Reuck A V S, Knight J (eds) Touch, heat and pain. (Ciba Foundation Symposium.) Churchill: London: pp 86–112

Quinlan J E, Davies J 1985 Excitatory and inhibitory responses of Purkinje cells, in the rat cerebellum in vivo, induced by excitatory amino acids. Neurosci Lett 60: 39–46

Quintarelli G, Dellovo M C 1966 Age changes in the localization and distribution of glycosaminoglycans in human hyaline cartilage. Histochemie 7: 141–167

Quist G 1977 The course and relations of the left phrenic nerve in the neck. J Anat 124: 803–805

R

Rabey G P 1968 Morphanalysis. Lewis: London

Rabey G P 1971 Craniofacial morphanalysis. Proc R Soc Med 64: 103–111

Rabinowicz T 1964 The cerebral cortex of the premature infant of the 8th month. Prog Brain Res 4: 39–92

Rabinowicz T 1967 Quantitative appraisal of the cerebral cortex of the premature infant of 8 months. In: Minkowski A (ed) Regional development of the brain in early life. (A symposium organized by the Council for International Organizations of Medical Sciences etc.) Blackwell Scientific: Oxford: pp 91–124

Rabischong P 1992 Functional anatomy of the spine and spinal cord. In:

Manelfe C (ed) Imaging of the spine and spinal cord. Raven Press: New York

Race R R, Sanger R 1975 Blood groups in man. 6th edition. Blackwell Scientific: Oxford

Rack P M H, Westbury D R 1969 The effects of length and stimulus rate on tension in the isometric cat soleus muscle. J Physiol 204: 443–460

Radermecker M A, Triffaux M, Fissette J, Limet R 1992 Anatomical rationale for use of the latissimus dorsi flap during the cardiomyoplasty operation. Surg Radiol Anat 14: 5–10

Raeymaekers L, Wuytack F 1993 Ca^{2+} pumps in smooth muscle cells. J Musc Res Cell Motil 14: 141–157

Raff M C, Abney E R, Miller R H 1984 Two glial cell lineages diverge prenatally in rat opic nerve. Dev Biol 106: 53–60

Raff M C, Mirsky R, Fields K L, Lisak R P, Dorfman S H, Silverberg D H, Gregson N A, Leibowitz S, Kennedy M C 1978 Galactocerebroside is a specific cell-surface antigenic marker for oligodendrocytes in culture. Nature 274: 813–816

Raff R A 1992 Evolution of development decisions and morphogenesis: the view from two camps. In: Stern C, Ingrams (eds) Gastrulation. Development Supplement 1992: 15–22

Rafferty N S, Goosens W 1978 Cytoplasmic filaments in the crystalline lens of various species. Exp Eye Res 26: 177–190

Ragot T, Vincent N, Chafey P, Vigne E, Gilgenkrantz H, Couton D, Cartaud J, Briand P, Kaplan J-C, Perricaudet M, Kahn A 1993 Efficient adenovirus-mediated transfer of a human minidystrophin gene to skeletal muscle of mdx mice. Nature 361: 647–650

Raichle M E, 1994 Visualizing the mind. Scientific American, April: 36–42

Raisman G 1969 Neuronal plasticity in the septal nuclei of the adult rat. Brain Res 14: 25–48

Raisman G, Field P M 1973 Sexual dimorphism in the neuropil of the preoptic area of the rat and its dependence on neonatal androgen. Brain Res 54: 1–29

Rajendran K 1985 Mechanism of locking at the knee joint. J Anat 143: 189–194

Rakic P 1971a Guidance of neurons migrating to the foetal monkey neocortex. Brain Res 33: 471–476

Rakic P 1971b Neuron–glia relationship during granule cell migration in developing cerebellar cortex. A Golgi and electron microscopic study in Macacus rhesus. J Comp Neurol 141: 283–312

Rakic P 1975 Local circuit neurons. Neurosci Res Program Bull 13: 295–416

Rakic P 1981 Neuronal–glial interaction during brain development. TINS 4: 184–187

Rakic P 1982 Early developmental events: cell lineages, acquisition of neuronal positions, and areal and laminar development. Neurosci Res Program Bull 20: 439–451

Rakic P 1988 Science 241: 170–176

Rakic P, Goldman-Rakic P S 1982 Development and modifiability of the cerebral cortex. Based on an NRP Work Session 1980. Overview. Neurosci Res Program Bull 20: 433–438

Rakic P, Yakovlev P I 1968 Development of the corpus callosum and cavum septi in man. J Comp Neurol 132: 45–72

Rall W 1967 Core conductor theory and cable properties of neurons. In: Kandel E R (ed) Handbook of physiology. Section 1. Vol 1. Pt 1. American Physiological Society: Bethesda Maryland: pp 39–97

Rall W 1967 Distinguishing theoretical synoptic potentials computed for different soma-dendritic distributions of synaptic input. J. Neurophysiol 30: 1139–1167

Rall W, Shepherd G M, Reese T, Brightman M W 1966 Dendrodendritic synaptic pathway for inhibition in the olfactory bulb. Exp Neurol 14: 44–56

Ralph M R, Foster R G, Davis F C, Menaker M 1990 Transplanted suprachiasmatic nucleus determines circadian period. Science 247: 975–978

Ralston H J 1965 The organization of the substantia gelatinosa Rolandi in the cat lumbrosacral cord. Z Zellforsch 67: 1–23

Ralston H J 1974 On the neuronal organization of the spinal cord. In: Bellairs R, Gray E G (eds) Essays on the nervous system. Clarendon Press: Oxford

Rambourg A, Clermont Y 1990 Three-dimensional microscopy: structure of the Golgi apparatus. Eur J Cell Biol 51: 189–200

Ramie C S 1984 Morphology of myelin and myelination. In: Myelin 2nd edition P. Morell (ed) Plenum Press, New York: pp 1–50

Ramón y Cajal S 1890 Origen y terminación de las fibras nerviosas olfatorias. Gac San Bacelona, pp 1–21

Ramon y Cajal S 1893 La retine des vertebres. Cellule 9: 119–255

Ramon y Cajal S 1893 Los ganglios y plexos nerviosos del intestino del los mammiferos. Moya: Madrid: pp 1–37

Ramón y Cajal S 1908 Structure et connexion des neurons. In: Les prixs nobel en 1906. Norstedt and Söner: Stockholm: pp 1–25

Ramon y Cajal S 1909 Histologie du système de l'homme et des vertébrés. Maloine: Paris

Ramón y Cajal S 1911 Histologie du système nerveux de l'homme et des vertébrés. Maloine: Paris

Ramón y Cajal S 1919 Acción neurotrópica de los epitelios. Algunos detalles sobre el mecanismo genético de las ramificaciones nerviosas intraepiteliales sensitivas y sensoriales. Trab Lab Invest Biol 17: 65–86

Ramón y Cajal S 1928 Degeneration and regeneration of the nervous system. 2 vol. (May R M ed and trans) Oxford University Press: London

Ramón y Cajal S 1955 Studies on the cerebral cortex (Kraft L M trans). Lloyd-Luke: London

Ramón-Moliner E, Dansereau J A 1974 The peribrachial region of the cat. Cell Tissue Res 149: 173–190; 191–204

Ramón-Moliner E, Nauta W J H 1966 The iso-dendritic core of the brain stem. J Comp Neurol 126: 311–335

Ramsay S C, Weiller C, Myers K, Cremer J E, Luthra S K, Lammertsma A A, Frackowiak R S 1992 Monitoring by PET of macrophage accumulation in brain after ischaemic stroke. Lancet 339: 1054–1055

Ramsdale D R, Dixon J S, Gosling J A 1972 Chromaffin cells in the mammalian urethra. J Anat 113: 290–291

Ramsey E M 1955 Vascular patterns in endometrium and placenta. Angiology 6: 321–339

Ramsey G M, Corner G W Jr, Donner M W 1963 Serial and cineradioangiographic visualisation of maternal circulation in the primate (hemochorial) placenta. Am J Obstet Gynecol 86: 213–225

Rand M J 1992 Nitrergic transmission: nitric oxide as a mediator of non-adrenergic, non-cholinergic neuro-effector transmission. Clin Exp Pharmacol Physiol 19: 147–169

Randall D J, Davie P S 1980 The heart urochordates and cephalochordates. In: Bourne G H (ed) Hearts and heart-like organs. Vol 1. Academic Press: New York: pp 41–59

Randall V A, Ebling F J G 1991 Seasonal changes in human hair growth. Br J Dermatol 124: 146–151

Rang M 1969 The growth plate and its disorders. Livingstone: Edinburgh

Ranganathan N, Lam J H, Wigle E D 1970 Morphology of the human mitral valve. II. The valve leaflets. Circulation, 41: 459–467

Ranson S W, Magoun W W 1933 The central path of the pupilloconstriction reflex in response to light. Arch Neurol Psychiat 30: 1193–1202

Ranvier L 1874 De quelques faits relatifs à l'histologie et à la physiologie des muscles striés. Archives de Physiologie Normale et Pathologique Deuxième Série 5–15

Ranvier L A 1871 Contributions à l'histologie et à la physiologie des nerfs périphériques. C R Acad Sci (Paris) 73: 1168–1171

Rao G S, Sahu S 1974 The localisation within the dorsal motor nucleus of the vagus in the buffalo (Bubalus bubalis). Acta Anat 90: 388–393

Rappaport A M 1987 Physioanatomic considerations. In: Schiff L, Schiff E R (eds) Diseases of the liver. Lippincott: Philadelphia: pp 1–46

Raschke M, Lierse W, van Ackeren H 1987 Microvascular architecture of the mucosa of the gastrica corpus in man. Acta Anat 130: 185–190

Rascol M, Izard J 1976 The subdural neurothelium of the cranial meninges in man. Anat Rec 186: 429–436

Rasmussen A T 1932 Secondary vestibular tracts in the cat. J Comp Neurol 54: 143–172

Rasmussen A T 1940 Studies of the VIII cranial nerve of man. Laryngoscope 50: 67–83

Rasmussen G L 1942 An efferent cochlear bundle. Anat Rec 82: 441P

Rasmussen G L 1946 The olivary peduncle and other fibre projections of the superior olivary complex. J Comp Neurol 84: 141–220

Rasmussen G L 1957 Selective silver impregnation of synaptic endings. In: Windle W F (ed) New research techniques of neuroanatomy. Thomas: Springfield, Illinois: pp 27–39

Rasmussen G L 1967 Efferent connections of the cochlear nerve. In: Graham A B (ed) Sensori-neural hearing processes and disorders. (Henry Ford Hospital International Symposium). Little, Brown: Boston Massachusetts: pp 61–75

Ratcliffe F F 1981 Arterial anatomy of the developing human dorsal and lumbar vertebral body. A microarteriographic study. J Anat 133: 625–638

Ratcliffe J F 1980 The arterial supply of the adult human vertebral body: a microangiographic study. J Anat 131: 57–79

Ratner N, Hong D, Liberman M A, Bunge R P, Glaser L 1988 The neuronal cell-surface molecule mitogenic for Schwann cells is a heparin binding protein. Proc Nat Acad Sci USA 85: 6992–6996

Rattan S, Shakdar S 1992 Role of nitric oxide as a mediator of internal anal sphincter relaxation. Am J Physiol 262: G107–G112

Rattner J B, Phillips S G 1973 Independence of centriole formation and DNA synthesis. J Cell Biol 57: 359–372

Rautiainen M, Collan Y, Nuutinen J, Afzelius B A 1990 Ciliary orientation in the 'immotile cilia' syndrome. Eur Arch Otorhinolaryngol 247: 100–103

Raviola E, Gilula N B 1973 Gap junctions between photoreceptor cells in the vertebrate retina. Proc Natl Acad Sci USA 70: 1677–1681

Raviola E, Karnovsky M J 1972 Evidence for a blood–thymus barrier using electron opaque tracers. J Exp Med 136: 466–498

Rawlings A V, Scott I R, Harding C R, Bowser P A 1994 Stratum corneum moisturization at the molecular level. J Invest Dermatol 103: 731–740

Ray J P, Price J L 1993 The organization of projections from the mediodorsal nucleus of the thalamus to orbital and medial prefrontal cortex in macaque monkeys. J Comp Neurol 337: 1–31

Ray R D, Johnson R J, Jameson R M 1951 Rotation of the forearm. J Bone Jt Surg 33A: 993–996

Ray W J, Cole H W 1985 EEG alpha activity reflects attentional demands and beta activity reflects emotional and cognitive processes. Science 288: 750–752

Raybuck H E 1952 The innervation of the parathyroid glands. Anat Rec 112: 117–124

Rayment I, Holden H M, Whittaker M, Yohn C B, Lorenz M, Holmes K C, Milligan R A 1993a Structure of the actin–myosin complex and its implications for muscle contraction. Science 261: 58–65

Rayment I, Rypniewski W R, Schmidt-Bäse K, Smith R, Tomchick D R, Benning M M, Winkelmann D A, Wesenberg G, Holden H M 1993b Three-dimensional structure of myosin subfragment-1: a molecular motor. Science 261: 50–58

Read L C 1988 Milk growth factors. In: F Cockburn (ed) Fetal and neonatal growth. Wiley: Chichester

Read L C, Upton F M, Francis G L, Wallace J C, Dahlenburg G W, Ballard F J 1984 Changes in the growth-promoting activity of human milk during lactation. Pediat Res 18: 133–139

Reaume A G, Conlon R A, Zirngibl R, Yamaguchi T P, Rossant J 1992 Expression analysis of a Notch homologue in the mouse embryo. Dev Biol 154: 377–387

Rebar R W, Morandini I C, Erikson G F, Petze J E 1981 The hormonal basis of reproductive defects in athymic mice: diminished concentrations in prepubertal females. Endocrinol 108: 120–126

Rechardt L, Aalto-Setälä K, Purjeranta M, Pelto-Huiko M, Kyösola K 1986 Peptidergic innervation of human atrial myocardium: an electron microscopical and immunocytochemical study. J Autonom Nervous System 17: 21–32

Reed C I, Reed B P 1948 Comparative study of human and bovine sperm by electron microscopy. Anat Rec 100: 1–8

Reed R R 1992 Mechanisms of sensitivity and specificity in olfaction. Cold Spring Harbor Symp Quant Biol 57: 501–504

Rees L A 1954 The structure and function of the mandibular joint. Br Dent J 96: 125–133

Reese T 1965 Olfactory cilia in the frog. J Cell Biol 25: 209–230

Reese T S, Shepherd G M 1972 Dendrodendritic synapses in the central nervous system. In: Pappas G D, Purpura D P (eds) Structure and function of synapses. Raven Press: New York: pp 121–136

Reese T, Brightman M W 1970 Olfactory surface and central olfactory connexions in some vertebrates. In: Wolstenholme G E W, Knight J (eds) Taste and smell in vertebrates. (Ciba Foundation Symposium.) Churchill: London: pp 115–143

Regan W D, Korinek S L, Morrey B F, An K-N 1991 Biomechanical study of ligaments around the elbow joint. Clin Orthop 271: 170–179

Reichenbach A, Stolzenburg J U, Eberhardt W, Chao T L, Dettmer D, Hertz L 1993 What do retinal muller (glial) cells do for their neuronal 'small siblings'? J Chen Neroanat 6: 201–213

Reichert F L, Poth E J 1933 Pathways for the secretory fibres of the salivary glands in man. Proc Soc Exp Biol Med 30: 973–977

Reichlin S, Baldessarini R J, Martin J B (eds) 1978 The hypothalamus. (Research publications vol 56 Association for research in nervous and mental disease) Raven Press: New York

Reid L 1976 Visceral cartilage. J Anat 122: 349–355

Reidy M A 1992 Factors controllng smooth-muscle cell proliferation. Arch Pathol Lab Med 116: 1276–1280

Reikeras O, Bjerkreim I, Kolbenstvedt A 1983 Anteversion of the acetabulum and femoral neck in normals and in patients with osteoarthritis of the hip. Acta Orthop Scand 54: 18–23

Reil J C 1807 Fragmenten über die bildung des kleinen gehirns in menschen. Arch Physiol Halle 8: 1–58

Reilly D T, Burstein A H 1974 The mechanical properties of cortical bone. J Bone Jt Surg 56: 1001–1022

Reilly FD 1985 Innervation and vascular pharmacodynamics of the mammalian spleen. Experientia 41: 187–192

Reilly T, Tyrell A, Troup J D G 1984 Circadian variation in human stature. Chronobiol Internat 1: 121–126

Reimann A F, Anson B J 1944 Vertebral level of termination of the spinal cord with report of a case of sacral cord. Anat Record 88: 127–138

Reisser C, Schuknecht H F 1991 The anterior inferior cerebellar artery in the internal auditory canal. Laryngoscope 101: 761–766

Reiter M 1988 Calcium mobilization and cardiac inotropic mechanisms. Pharmacol Rev 40: 189–217

Reiter R J 1983 The pineal gland: an intermediary between the environment and the endocrine system. Psychoneuroendocrinology 8: 31–40

Reiter R J 1985a Action spectra, dose–response relationships, and temporal aspects of light's effects on the pineal gland. Ann N Y Acad Sci 453: 215–230

Reiter R J 1985b Impact of photoperiodic information on pineal metabolism and physiology. Int J Biometeorol 29 (suppl 2): 178–187

Reiter R J 1987 The melatonin message: duration versus coincidence hypotheses. Life Sci 40: 2119–2131

Reiter R J, Hoffman R A 1967 Adrenocortical cytogenesis in the adult male golden hamster. A radioautographic study using tritiated thymidine. J Anat 101: 723–730

Reith E J 1967a The absorptive activity of ameloblasts during the maturation of enamel. Anat Rec 157: 577–588

Reith E J 1967b The early stages of amelogenesis as observed in molar teeth of young rats. J Ultrastruct Res 17: 503–526

Reith E J 1970 The stages of amelogenesis as observed in the molar teeth of young rats. J Ultrastruct Res 30: 111–151

Relkin R 1976 The pineal. Annual research review. Eden Press: Montreal

Remahl S, Hildebrand C 1990 Relation between axons and oligodendroglia cells during initial myelination I. The glial unit. J Neurocytol 19: 313–328

Remahl S, Hildebrand C 1990 Relation between axons and oligodendroglial cells during initial myelination II. The individual axon. J Neurocytol 19: 883–898

den innern Bau der Cerebrospinalnerven und über die Entwicklung ihrer Formelemente. Arch Anat Physiol 145–161

Remensnyder I P, Majno G 1968 Oxygen gradients in healing wounds. Am J Pathol 52: 301–319

Renaud L P, Cunningham J T, Nissen R, Yang C R 1993 Electrophysiology of central pathways controlling release of neurohypophysial hormones: focus on the lamina terminalis and diagonal band inputs to the supraoptic nucleus. Ann N Y Acad Sci 689: 122–132

Renfrew S, Melville I D 1960 The somatic sense of space (choraesthesia) and its threshold. Brain 83: 93–112

Rennke H G, Cotran R S, Venkatachalam, M A 1975 Role of molecular charge in glomerular permeability. Tracer studies with cationized ferritins. J Cell Biol 67: 638–646

Renshaw B 1941 Influence of discharge of motoneurons upon excitation of neighbouring motoneurons. J Neurophysiol 4: 167–183

Renshaw B 1946 Central effects of centripetal impulses in axons of spinal ventral roots. J Neurophysiol 9: 191–204

Repesh L A, Fitzgerald T J, Furcht L T 1982 Fibronectin involvement in granulation tissue and wound healing in rabbits. J Histochem Cytochem 30: 351–358

Resnick D, Niwayama G 1988 Diagnosis of bone and joint disorders. Vol 1. 2nd edition. W B Saunders: Philadelphia

Réthelyi M, Szentágothai J 1969 The large synaptic complexes of the substantia gelantinosa. Exp Brain Res 7: 258–274

Reuther T F 1938 The coccygeal glomus, a possible factor in coccygodynia. Illinois Med J 73: 134–136

Rexed B 1952 The cytoarchitectonic organization of the spinal cord in the cat. J Comp Neurol 96: 415–495

Rexed B 1954 A cytoarchitectonic atlas of the spinal cord in the cat. J Comp Neurol 100: 297–379

Rexed B 1964 Some aspects of the cytoarchitectonics and synaptology of the spinal cord. Progr Brain Res 11: 58–92

Reynolds E L 1945 Bony pelvic girdle in early infancy; roentgenometric study. Am J Phys Anthropol 3: 321–354

Reynolds E L 1947 The bony pelvis in prepubertal childhood. Am J Phys Anthropol N S 5: 165–200

Reynolds S R M, Zweifach B W (eds) 1959 The microcirculation. Symposium on factors influencing exchange of substances across capillary wall. Proceedings of the 5th Conference on Microcirculatory Physiology and pathology, Buffalo . . . 1958. University of Illinois Press: Urbana Illinois

Rezai K, Andreasen N C, Alliger R, Cohen G, Swayze V II, O'Leary D S 1993 The neuropsychology of the prefrontal cortex. Arch Neurol 50: 636–642

Rhodin J A G 1962 Fine structure of vascular walls in mammals, with special reference to smooth muscle component. Physiol Rev 42 (suppl 5): 48–81

Rhodin J A G 1966 Ultrastructure and function of the human tracheal mucosa Annu Rev Respir Dis 93: 1–15

Rhodin J A G 1968 Ultrastructure of mammalian venous capillaries, venules and small collecting veins. J Ultrastruct Res 25: 452–500

Rhodin J, Dalhamn T 1956 Electron microscopy of the tracheal ciliated mucusa in rat. Z Zellforsch 44: 345–412

Rhoton A L Jr, Kobayashi S, Hollinshead, W H 1968 Nervus intermedius. J Neurosurg 29: 609–18

Rhoton A L, O'Leary J L, Ferguson J P 1966 The trigeminal, vagal and glossopharyngeal nerves in the monkey. Arch Neurol 14: 530–540

Rhys-Evans P, Comis S D, Osbourne M P, Pickles J O 1984 Cross-links between stereocilia in the human organ of Corti. J Laryngol Otol 99: 11–19

Rice R V, Moses J A, McManus G M, Brady A C, Blasik L M 1970 The organisation of contractile filaments in mammalian smooth muscle. J Cell Biol 47: 183–196

Richardson A P, Hinsey J C 1933 Functional study of the nodose ganglion of the vagus with degeneration methods. Proc Soc Exp Biol Med 30: 1141–1143

Richardson A, Hao C, Fedoroff S 1993 Microglia progenitor cells: a subpopulation in cultures of mouse neopallial astroglia. Glia 7: 25–33

Richardson K C 1962 The fine structure of autonomic nerve endings in smooth muscle of the rat vas deferens. J Anat 96: 427–442

Richardson M K, Sieber-Blum M 1993 Pluripotent neural crest cells in the developing skin of the quail embryo. Dev Biol 157: 348–358

Richardson P M, McGuiness U M, Aguayo A J 1980 Axons from CNS neurons regenerate into PNS grafts. Nature 284: 264 – 265

Richer F, Martinez M, Robert M, Bouvier G, Saint-Hilaire J-M 1993 Stimulation of human somatosensory cortex: tactile and body displacement perceptions in medial regions. Exp Brain Res 93: 173–176

Riches D J, Palfrey A J 1966 The ultrastructure of the bile duct epithelium of the rat. J Anat 100: 429–430P

Richfield E K, Young A B, Penney J B 1989 Comparative distributions of dopamine D-1 and D-2 receptors in the cerebral cortex of rats, cats and monkeys. J Comp Neurol 286: 409–426

Richter C P 1967 Sleep and activity: their relation to the 24-hour clock. Assoc Res Nerv Ment Dis 45: 8–29

Richter E A, Norris B E, Fullerton B C, Levine R A, Kiang N Y S 1983 Is there a medial nucleus of the trapezoid body in humans? Am J Anat 168: 157 – 166

Ricketts R R, Woodard J R, Zwiren G T, Gibbs Andrews H, Broecker B H 1991 Modern treatment of cloacal exstrophy. J Pediatric Surgery 26: 444–450

Rickmann M, Fawcett J W, Keynes R J 1985 The migration of neural crest cells and the growth of motor axons through the rostral half of the chick somite. J Embryol Exp Morphol 90: 437–455

Riddle R D, Johnson R L, Laufer E, Tabin C 1993 Sonic hedgehogmediates the polarising activity of the ZPA. Cell 75: 1401–1417

Ridley A J, Davis J B, Stroobant P, Land H 1989 Transforming growth factors-β_1 and β_2 are mitogens for rat Schwann cells. J Cell Biol 109: 3419–3424

Ridley A, Hall A 1992 The small GTP-binding protein rho regulates the assembly of focal adhesions and actin stress fibers in response to growth factors. Cell 70: 389–399

Ridley A, Paterson H F, Johnston C L, Diekmann, Hall A 1992 The small GTP-binding protein rac regulates growth factor-induced membrane ruffling. Cell 70: 401–410

Ridyard J N 1986 Computerised axial tomography. In: McAinsh T F (ed) Physics in medicine and biology. Pergamon: Oxford: pp 214–220

Rieger F, Kofler R, Borkenstein M, Schwingsschandl J, Sayer H P, Kerl H 1994 Melanotic macules following Blaschko's lines in McCune-Albright syndrome. Br J Dermatol 130: 215–220

Riggs H E, Rupp C 1963 Variation in form of circle of Willis. Arch Neurol Psychiat 8: 8–14

Riggs L A, Niehl E W 1960 Involuntary motions of the eye during monocular fixation. J Exp Psychol 40: 687–701

Riggs L A, Ratliff F, Cornsweet J C, Cornsweet T N 1953 The disappearance of steadily fixated visual test objects. J Opt Soc Am 43: 495–501

Riley H A 1930 Lobules of mammalian cerebellum and cerebellar nomenclature. Arch Neurol Psychiatry 24: 227–256

Ringvist M 1974 Fibre types in human masticatory muscles. Relation to function. Scand J Dent Res 82: 333–355

Ringvold A 1975 Distribution of ascorbic acid in the ciliary body of albino rabbit, guinea pig and rat. Acta Ophthalmol 53: 751–759

Rios E, Pizarro G 1991 Voltage sensor of excitation–contraction coupling in skeletal muscle. Physiol Rev 71: 849–908

Ripley R C, Holifield J W, Neis A S 1977 Sustained hypertension after section of the glossopharyngeal nerve. Am J Med 62: 297–304

Rippin J W 1976 Collagen turnover in the periodontal ligament under normal and altered functional forces. J Periodont Res 11: 101–107

Ripps H, Weale R A 1976 The visual photoreceptors. In: Davson H (ed) The eye. 2nd edition. Vol 2A. Academic Press: New York

Risau W 1991 Induction of blood–brain barrier endothelial cell differentiation. Ann New York Acad Sci 633: 405–419

Risau W 1991 Vasculogenesis, angiogenesis and endothelial cell differentiation during embryonic development. In: Feinberg R N, Sherer G K, Auerbach R (eds) The development of the vascular system. Issues Biomed 14: 58–68

Risau W, Wolburg H 1990 Development of the blood–brain barrier. Trends Neurosci 13: 174–178

Ritter M A 1977 Embryonic mouse thymocyte development. Enhancing effect of corticosterone at physiological levels. Immunology 33: 241–246

Ritter M A, Schuurman H J, Mackenzie W A, de Maagd R A, Price K M, Broekhuizen R, Kater L 1985 Heterogeneity of human thymus epithelial cells revealed by monoclonal anti-epithelial cell antibodies. Adv Exp Med Biol 186: 283–288

Riva A 1967 Fine structure of human seminal vesicular epithelium. J Anat 102: 71–86

Riva A, Testa Riva F 1973 Fine structure of acinar cells of human parotid gland. Anat Rec 176: 149–165

Riva A, Usai E, Cossu M, Lantini M S, Scarpa R, Testa-Riva F 1990 Ultrastructure of human bulbourethral glands and of their main excretory ducts. Arch Androl 24: 177–184

Rizk N N 1980 A new description of the anterior abdominal wall in man and mammals. J Anat 131: 373–385

Rizzolo L J, Li Z Q 1993 Diffusible, retinal factors stimulate the barrier properties of junctional complexes in the retinal pigment epithelium. J Cell Sci 106: 859–867

Roaf R 1971 The growth of the spinal articular processes and their clinical significance. In: Zorab P A (ed) Scoliosis and growth. Churchill Livingstone: Edinburgh: pp 92–97

Robbins T W 1986 Hunger. In: Lightman S L, Everitt B J (eds) Neuroendocrinology. Blackwell: Oxford: pp 252–303

Robbins T W, Cador M, Taylor J R, Everitt B J 1989 Limbic-striatal interactions in reward-related processes. Neurosci Biobehavioral Rev 13: 155–162

Robbins T W, Everitt B J 1992 Functions of dopamine in the dorsal and ventral striatum. Seminars Neurosci 4: 119–128

Robert B, Sassoon D, Jacq B, Gehring W, Buckingham M 1989 Hox-7, a mouse homeobox gene with a novel pattern of expression during embryogenesis. EMBO J 8: 91–100

Roberton N R C (ed) 1992 Resuscitation of the newborn. In: Textbook of neonatology. Churchill Livingstone: Edinburgh: pp 173–195

Roberts D K, Parmley T H, Walker N J, Horbelt D V 1992 Ultrastructure of the microvasculature in the human endometrium throughout the normal menstrual cycle. Am J Obstet Gynecol 166: 1393–1406

Roberts G D D, Harris M 1973 Neuropraxia of the mylohyoid nerve and submental analgesia. Br J Oral Surg 11: 110–113

Roberts K, Hyams J S (eds) 1979 Microtubules. Academic Press: London

Roberts N, Gratin C, Betal D, Walker J, Dangerfield P H, Whitehouse G, Edwards R H T 1994 Automatic and quantitative analysis of intervertebral disc function using MRI and image analysis. Proceedings of the 11th Meeting of the European Society for Magnetic Resonance in Medicine and Biology 11: 125

Roberts N, Kenny J, Savage R, Reid N, Edwards R H T, Whitehouse G 1991 Computer analysis of magnetic resonance images of the lumbar spine reveals significant differences in the intervertebral height between a group of young and a group of aged volunteers. Proceedings of the 10th Meeting of the European Society for Magnetic Resonance in Medicine and Biology 10: 161

Roberts W H, Habenicht J, Krishingner G 1964 The pelvic and perineal fasciae and their neural and vascular relationships. Anat Rec 149: 707–720

Roberts W, Taylor W H 1973 Inferior rectal nerve variation as it relates to pudendal block. Anat Rec 177: 461–463

Robins A H 1992 Biological perspectives on human pigmentation. Cambridge University Press: Cambridge

Robins L N, Helzer J E, Davis D H 1975 Narcotic use in southeast Asia and afterwards. Archives of Gen Psychiat 32: 955–961

Robinson A G, Zimmerman E A 1973 Cerebrospinal fluid and ependymal neurophysin. Clin Invest 52: 1260–1267

Robinson D A 1964 The mechanics of human saccadic eye movement. J Physiol 174: 245–264

Robinson F R, Cohen J L, May J, Sestokas A K, Glickstein M 1984 Cerebellar targets of visual pontine cells in the cat. J Comp Neurol 223: 471–482

Robinson G W, Wray S, Mahon K A 1991, Spatially restricted expression of a member of a new family of murine distal-less homeobox genes in the developing forebrain. The New Biologist 3: 1183–1194

Robinson M S 1994 The role of clathran adaptors and dynamism in endocytosis. Curr Opin Cell Biol 6: 538–544

Robinson R J 1966 Assessment of gestational age by neurological examination. Arch Dis Child 41: 437–447

Robinson T E, Berridge K C 1993 The neural basis of drug craving: an incentive-sensitization theory of addiction. Brain Res Rev 18: 247–291

Roche A F 1992 Growth, maturation and body composition. The Fels longitudinal study 1929–1991. Cambridge University Press: Cambridge

Roche A F, Lewis A B 1974 Sex differences in the elongation of the cranial base during pubescence. Angle Orthodont 44: 279–294

Rochester D F 1993 Respiratory muscles and ventilatory failure. Am J Med Sci 305: 394–402

Rock J, Hertig A T 1942 Some aspects of early human development. Am J Obstet Gynecol 44: 973–983

Rock J, Hertig A T 1944 Information regarding time of human ovulation derived from study of 3 unfertilized and 11 fertilized ova. Am J Obstet Gynecol 47: 343–356

Rockel A J, Hiorns R W, Powell T P S 1980 The basic uniformity in structure of the neocortex. Brain, 103: 221–244

Rockland K S 1992 Configuration, in serial reconstruction, of individual axons projecting from areas V2 to V4 in the macaque monkey. Cereb Cortex 2: 353–374

Rockland K S 1994 The organization of feedback connections from area V2 (18) to V1 (17). In: Peters A, Rocklands K S (eds) Cerebral cortex. Vol 10. Plenum Press: New York: pp 261–299

Rockland K S, Saleem K S, Tanaka K 1994 Divergent feedback connections from areas V4 and TEO in the macaque. Visual Neurosci 11: 579–600

Rockland K S, Van Hoesen G W 1994 Direct temporal-occipital feedback connections to striate cortex (V1) in the macaque monkey. Cereb Cortex 4: 300–313

Rodan G A, Rodan S B 1984 Expression of the osteoblastic phenotype. In: Peck W A (ed) Bone and mineral research annual 2. Elsevier: Amsterdam: pp 244–285

Rodenstein D O 1985 Infants are not obligatory nasal breathers. Am Rev Respir Dis 131: 343–347

Rodewald R, Karnovsky M J 1974 Porous substructure of the glomerular slit diaphragm in the rat and mouse. J Cell Biol 60: 423–433

Rodieck R W, Watanabe M 1993 Survey of the morphology of macaque retinal ganglion cells that project to the pretectum, superior colliculus and parvicellular laminae of the lateral geniculate nucleus. J Comp Neurol 338: 242–254

Rodman H R, Skelly J P, Gross C G 1991 Stimulus selectivity and state dependence of activity in inferior temporal cortex of infant monkeys. Proc Natl Acad Sci USA 88: 7572–7575

Rodman J S, Mercer R W, Stahl P D 1990 Endocytosis and transcytosis. Curr Opin Cell Biol 2: 664–672

Rogawski M A, Aghajanian G K 1980 Modulation of lateral geniculate neurone excitability by noradrenaline microiontophoresis or locus ceruleus stimulation. Nature 187: 731–734

Rogers A W 1967 Techniques of autoradiography. Elsevier: Amsterdam

Rogers A W 1973 Techniques of autoradiography. 2nd edition. Elsevier: Amsterdam

Rogers D C, Burnstock G 1966 Multiaxonal autonomic junctions in intestinal smooth muscle of the toad (Bufo marinas). J Comp Neurol 126: 626–652

Roggendorf W, Cervos-Navarro J 1977 Ultrastructure of arterioles in the cat brain. Cell Tiss Res 178: 495–515

Roggendorf W, Cervos-Navarro J, Lazaro-Lacalle M 1978 Ultrastructure of venules in the cat brain. Cell Tiss Res 192: 461–474

Rohan R F, Turner L 1956 The levator palati muscle. J Anat 90: 153–154

Rohen J 1964 Ciliarkörper. In: von Möllendoff W (ed) Das Auge und seine Hilfsorgane Ergänzung zu Band 111/2. Haut und Sinnesorgane. 4 Teil. Handbuch der mikroskopischen Anatomie des Menschen. Springer: Berlin: pp 189–238

Rohon J V 1884 Zur histiogenese des rückenmarkes der forelle. Sitz ber mathematphys. Klasse Königl Bayr Akad Wiss 14: 301–356

Rollet F 1899 De la mensuration de os longs des membres. Thèse pur le Doc en Méd. 1st Ser. 43: 1–128

Rollin H 1977 Course of the peripheral gustatory nerves. Ann Otol Rhinol Laryngol 86: 251–258

Rolls E T 1975 The brain and reward. Pergamon Press: Oxford

Rolls E T 1985 Connections, functions and dysfunctions of limbic structures, the prefrontal cortex, and hypothalamus. In: Swash M, Kennard C (eds) The scientific basis of clinical neurology. Churchill Livingstone: London: pp 201–213

Rolls E T 1990 A theory of emotion and its application to understanding the neural basis of emotion. Cognition and Emotion 4: 161–190

Rolls E T 1990 Experimental psychology: functions of different regions of the basal ganglia. In: Stern G (ed) Parkinson's disease. Chapman Hall Medical: London: pp 151–184

Romanes G J 1941 Cell columns in the spinal cord of a human foetus of fourteen weeks. J Anat 75: 145–152

Romanes G J 1942 The spinal cord in a case of congenital absence of the right limb below the knee. J Anat 77: 1–5

Romanes G J 1946 Motor localisation and the effects of nerve injury on the ventral horn cells of the spinal cord. J Anat 80: 117–131

Romanes G J 1951 The motor cell columns of the lumbosacral spinal cord of the cat. J Comp Neurol 94: 313–363

Romanes G J 1953 The motor cell groupings of the spinal cord. In: Wolstenholme G E W (ed) The spinal cord. (Ciba Foundation Symposium) Churchill: London: pp 24–38

Romanes G J 1964 The motor pools of the spinal cord. Progr Brain Res 11: 93–119

Romani N, Schuler G, Fritsch P 1991a Identification and phenotype of epidermal Langerhans cells. In: Schuler G (ed) Epidermal Langerhans cells. CRC Press: Boca Raton: pp 49–86

Romani N, Witmer-Pack M, Crowley M, Koide S, Schuler G, Inaba K, Steinman R M 1991b Langerhans cells as immature cells. In: Schuler G (ed) Epidermal Langerhans cells. CRC Press: Boca Raton: pp 191–216

Romer A S 1942 Cartilage – an embryonic adaptation. Am Nat 76: 394–404

Romer A S 1945 Vertebrate palaeontology. 2nd edition. University Press: Chicago

Romer A S 1970 The vertebrate body. 4th edition. Saunders: Philadelphia

Ronnholm E 1962 The amelogenesis of human teeth as revealed by electron microscopy. II The development of the enamel crystallites. J Ultrastruct Res 6: 249–303

Rönnholm E 1962 The amelogenesis of human teeth as revealed by electron microscopy. II. The development of the enamel crystallites. J Ultrastruct Res 6: 249–303

Rood J P 1977 The nerve supply of the mandibular incisor region. Br Dent J 143: 227–230

Rook A, Dawbar R (eds) 1991 Diseases of the hair and scalp. Blackwell: Oxford

Roosen-Runge E C 1952 The third maturation division in mammalian spermatogenesis. Anat Rec 112: 453 (Demonstration 50)

Roosen-Runge E C 1961 The rete testis in the albino rat: its structure, development and morphological significance. Acta Anat (Basel) 45: 1–30

Roosen-Runge E C, Giesel L O 1950 Quantitative studies on spermatogenesis in the albino rat. Am J Anat 87: 1–30

Roque R S, Caldwell R B 1993 Isolation and culture of retinal microglia. Curr Eye Res 12: 285–290

Rosa M G P, Soares J G M, Fiorani M Jr, Gattass R 1993 Cortical afferents of visual area MT in the Cebus monkey: possible homologies between new and old world monkeys. Visual Neurosci 10: 827–855

Rosan R C, Lauweryns J 1971 Secretory cells in the premature human lung lobule. Nature 232: 60–61

Rose G C (ed) 1963 Cinematography in biology. Academic Press: New York

Rose M 1926 Der Allocortex bei Tier und Mensch. J Psychol Neurol 34: 1–99

Rose M 1927 Die sog. Riechrinde beim Menschen und beim Affen. II. Teil des Allocortex bei Teir und Mensch. J Psychol Neurol 34: 261–401

Rose V, Izukawa T, Moës C A F 1975 Syndromes of asplenia and polysplenia. A review of cardiac and non-cardiac malformations in 60 cases with special reference to diagnosis and prognosis. Br Heart J 37: 840–852

Rosen S D 1989 Lymphocyte homing: progress and prospects. Curr Opin Cell Biol 1: 913–919

Rosen S D, Bertozzi C R 1994 The selectins and their ligands. Curr Opin Cell Biol 6: 663–673

Rosenbaum D A 1991 Human Motor Control. Academic Press: San Diego: pp 411

Rosenberg J C, DiDo L J A 1969 In vivo appearance and function of the termination of the ileum as observed directly through a cecostomy. Am J Gastroenterol 52: 411–419

Rosenbloom J, Abrams W R, Mecham R 1993 Extracellular matrix: the elastic fibres. FASB J 7: 1208–1218

Rosene D L, Van Hoesen G W 1977 The hippocampal efferent reach widespread areas of cerebral cortex and amygdala in the rhesus monkey. Science 198: 315–317

Rosene D L, Van Hoesen G W 1987 The hippocampal formation of the primate brain. A review of some comparative aspects of cytoarchitecture and connections. In: Jones E G, Peters A (eds) Cerebral cortex. Plenum Press: New York: pp 345–456

Rosenfeld W, Biagton J, Schaeffer H, Evans H, Flicker S, Salazar D, Jhaveri R 1980 A new graph for insertion of umbilical catheters. J Pediatr 96: 735–737

Rosenhall U 1972 Vestibular macular mapping in man. Ann Otol 81: 339–351

Rosenquist T H, Beall A C 1990 Elastogenic cells in the developing cardiovascular system: smooth muscle, nonmuscle and cardiac neural crest. In: Bockman D E, Kirby M L (eds) Embryonic origins of defective heart development. Ann NY Acad Sci 588: 106–119

Ross K F A 1967 Phase contrast and intereference microscopy for cell biologists. Arnold: London

Ross M D, Rogers C M, Donovan K M 1986 Innervation patterns in rat saccular macula. Acta Otolaryngol [Stockh] 102: 75–86

Ross M H, Dobler J 1975 The Sertoli cell junctional specializations and their relationship to the germinal epithelium as observed after efferent ductule ligation. Anat Rec 183: 267–291

Ross R 1968 The fibroblast and wound repair. Biol Rev 43: 57–96

Ross R 1975 Connective tissue cells, cell proliferation and synthesis of extracellular matrix. A review. Philos Trans R Soc Lond [Biol] 271: 247–259

Ross R 1993 The pathogenesis of atherosclerosis: a perspective for the 1990s. Nature (London) 362: 801–809

Rossant J 1986 Development of extraembryonic cell lineages in the mouse embryo. In: Rossant J, Pedersen R A (eds) Experimental approaches to mammalian embryonic development. Cambridge University Press: Cambridge: pp 97–120

Rossant J, Croy B A 1985 Genetic identification of tissue of origin of cell populations within the mouse placenta. J Embryol Exp Morphol 86: 117–189

Roth S I 1962 Pathology of the parathyroids in hyperparathyroidism. Discussion of recent advances in the anatomy and pathology of the parathyroid glands. Arch Pathol 73: 495–510

Roth S I, Capen C C 1974 Ultrastructural and functional correlations of the parathyroid gland. Int Rev Exp Path 13: 161–221

Rothblat L A, Schwarz M L 1979 The effect of monocular deprivation on dendritic spines in visual cortex of young and adult albino rats: evidence for a sensitive period. Brain Res 161: 156–161

Rothe C F 1983 Venous system: physiology of the capacitance vessels. In:

Shepherd J T, Abboud (eds) Handbook of physiology. Section 2, Volume III, part 1. Oxford University Press: New York: pp 397

Rother P, Hunger H, Leopold D et al 1977 Zur bestimmung des lebensalters und des geschlechts aus humerusmassen. Anat Anz 142: 243–254

Rother P, Hunger H, Liebert U et al 1975 Die Geschlechtsunterschiede des menschlichen Sternums Gengenbaurs. Morphol Jahrob 121: 29–37

Rothman J 1981 The Golgi apparatus: two organelles in tandem. Science 213: 1212–1219

Rothman T P, Gershon M D, Fontaine-Pérus J C, Chanconie M, Le Douarin N M 1987 The effect of back-transplants of the embryonic gut wall on growth of the neural tube. Dev Biol 124: 331–346

Rothschild Lord 1957 The fertilising spermatozoon. Discovery 18: 64–65

Rothwell J C 1994 Control of human voluntary movement. Chapman and Hall: London: pp 506

Rothwell N J 1992 Eicosanoids, thermogenesis and thermoregulation. Prostaglandins, Leukotrienes and Essential Fatty Acids 46: 1–7

Rouiller C (ed) 1964 The liver: morphology, biochemistry, physiology. 2 vol. Academic Press: New York

Rouiller E M, Liange F, Babalian A, Moret V, Wiesendanger M 1994 Cerebellothalamocortical and pallidothalmocortical projections to the primary and supplementary motor cortical areas: a multiple tracing study in macaque monkeys. J Comp Neurol 345: 185–213

Routal R R, Pal G P, Bhagwat S S, Tamankar B P 1984 Metrical studies with sexual dimorphism in foramen magnum of human crania. J Anat Soc Ind 33: 85–89

Routtenberg A, Santos Anderson R 1977 The central role of prefrontal cortex in intracranial self-stimulation: a case history of anatomical localization of motivational substrates. In: Iversen L L, Iversen S, Snyder S H (eds) Handbook of psychopharmacology. Plenum Press: New York

Roux W 1888 Beitrage zur Entwicklungsmechanik des Embryo 5. Uber die kuntsliche Hervorbringung halber Embryonen durch Zerstorung einer der beiden ersten Furchungskulgen, sowie uber der Nachenwicklung der fehlenden Koperlalfte. Virchows Arch Path Anat Physiol 64: 115–154, 246–291

Rovner A S, Thompson M M, Murphy R A 1986 Two different heavy chains are found in smooth muscle myosin. Am J Physiol 250 (Cell Physiol 19): C861–C870

Rowbotham G F, Little E 1962 The circulation and reservoir of the brain. Br J Surg 50: 244–250

Rowbottom M, Susskind C 1984 Electricity and medicine: history of their interaction. Macmillan: London

Rowe R W D 1973 The ultrastructure of Z disks from white, intermediate, and red fibers of mammalian striated muscles. J Cell Biol 57: 261–277

Rowlerson A, Mascarello F, Veggetti A, Carpène E 1983 The fibre-type composition of the first branchial arch muscles in carnivora and primates. J Musc Res Cell Motil 4: 443–472

Roy S, Ghadially F N 1967 Ultrastructure of normal rat synovial membrane. Ann Rheum Dis 26: 26–38

Royle G 1973 A groove in the lateral wall of the orbit. J Anat 115: 461–465

Royle J P, Eisner R 1981 The saphenofemoral junction. Surg Gynecol Obstet 152: 282–284

Rubanyi G M, Romero J C & Vanhoutte P M 1986 Endothelium-derived relaxing factor. Am J Physiol 250: H1145–H1149

Rubin E 1985a Development of the rat superior cervical ganglion: ganglion cell maturation. J Neurosci 5: 673–684

Rubin E 1985b Development of the rat superior cervical ganglion: ingrowth of preganglionic axons. J Neurosci 5: 685–696

Rubin E 1985c Development of the rat superior cervical ganglion: initial stages of synapse formation. J Neurosci 5: 697–704

Rubin W 1972 Endocrine cells in the human stomach. A fine structural study. Gastroenterology 63: 784–800

Ruch T C 1946 Visceral sensation and referred pain. In: Fulton J F (ed) Howell's textbook of physiology. 15th edition. Saunders: Philadelphia: pp 385–401

Ruckebusch Y 1989 Motility of the gut during development. In: Lebenthal E (ed) Human Gastrointestinal Development. Raven Press: New York: pp 183–206

Ruda M A, Bennet G J, Dubner R 1986 Neurochemistry and neural circuitry in the dorsal horn. In: Emson P C, Rossor M N, Tohyama M (eds) Progress in Brain Res 66: 219–268 Elsevier: Amsterdam

Rudland P S 1987 Stem cells and the development of mammary cancers in experimental rats and in humans. Cancer Metastasis Rev 6: 55–83

Rudolph A M, Drorbaugh J E, Auld P H, Rudolph A J, Nades A S, Smith C A, Aubbell J P 1961 Studies on the circulation in the neo-natal period. The circulation in respiratory distress syndrome. Pediatrics 27: 551–566

Ruegg J C, Solaro R J 1993 Calcium-sensitizing positive inotropic drugs. In: Gwathmey J K, Briggs G M, Allen P D (eds) Heart failure. Basic science and clinical aspects. Marcel Dekker: New York: pp 457–473

Ruiter D J, Schlingemann R O, Reitveld F J R, de Wall M W 1989 Monoclonal antibody-defined human endothelial antigens as vascular markers. J Invest Dermatol 93: 25S–32S

Ruiz i Altaba A 1992 Development 115: 67–80

Rumessen J J, Mikkelsen H B, Thuneberg L 1992 Ultrastructure of interstitial cells of Cajal associated with deep muscular plexus of human small intestine. Gastroenterology 102: 56–68

Rushbrook J I, Weiss C, Ko K, Feuerman M H, Carleton S. Ing A, Jacoby J 1994 Identification of alpha-cardiac myosin heavy chain mRNA and protein in extraocular muscle of the adult rabbit. J. Musc Res Cell Motil 15: 505–515

Rushton W A H 1962 Visual pigments in man. Liverpool University Press: Liverpool

Ruskell G L 1968 The fine structure of nerve terminations in the lacrimal glands of monkeys. J Anat 103: 65–76

Ruskell G L 1969 Changes in nerve terminals and acini of the lacrimal gland and changes in secretion induced by autonomic denervation. Z Zellforsch 94: 261–281

Ruskell G L 1970 An ocular parasympathetic nerve pathway of facial nerve origin and its influence on intraocular pressure. Exp Eye Res 10: 319–330

Ruskell G L 1971 The distribution of autonomic postganglionic nerve fibres in the lacrimal gland in the rat. J Anat 109: 229–242

Ruskell G L 1974 Form of the choroidocapillaris. Exp Eye Res 18: 411–412

Ruskell G L 1975 Nerve terminals and epithelial cell variety in the human lacrimal gland. Cell Tissue Res 158: 121–136

Ruskell G L, Simons T 1987 Trigeminal nerve pathways to the cerebral arteries in monkeys. J Anat 155: 23–27

Russell I J, Sellick P M 1978 Intracellular studies of hair cells in the mammalian cochlea. J Physiol (London) 284: 261–290

Russell J R, De Meyers W 1961 The quantitative cortical origin of pyramidal axons of Macaca rhesus with some remarks on slow rate of axolysis. Neurology 2: 96–108

Rustioni A 1973 Non-primary afferents to the nucleus gracilis from the lumbar cord of the cat. Brain Res 51: 81–95

Rustioni A, Dekker J J 1974 Non-primary afferents to the dorsal column nuclei of cat: distribution pattern and cells of origin. Anat Rec 178: 454–455

Rustioni A, Hayes N L, O'Neill S 1979 Dorsal column nuclei and ascending spinal afferents in macaques. Brain 102: 95–125

Rustioni A, Sotelo C 1974 Synaptic organization of the nucleus gracilis of the cat. Experimental identification of dorsal root fibers and cortical afferents. J Comp Neurol 155: 441–468

Rustow B et al 1993 Type II pneumocytes secrete vitamin E together with surfactant lipids. Am J Physiol 265(2 Pt 1): L133–139

Rusznyák I, Földi M, Szabo G 1960 Lymphatics and lymph circulation physiology and pathology. Pergamon Press: Oxford

Ruth E B 1947 Bone studies. I. Fibrillar structure of adult human bone. Am J Anat 80: 35–47

Ruwe P A, Gage J R, DeLuca P A 1992 Clinical determination of femoral anteversion: a comparison with established techniques. J Bone Jt Surg 74A: 820–830

Ryan A J 1981 Anabolic steroids are fool's gold. Fed Proc 40: 2682–2688

Ryan G B, Coghlan J P, Scoggins B A 1979 The granulated peripolar epithelial cell: a potential secretory component of the renal juxtaglomerular complex. Nature 277: 655–656

Ryan J W, Ryan U S 1977 Pulmonary endothelial cells. Fed Proc Fed Am Soc Exp Biol 36: 2683–2691

Ryan R B, Cliff W J, Babbiani G et al 1974 Myofibroblasts in human granulation tissue. Hum Pathol 5: 55–67

Ryan T J 1989 Structure and function of lymphatics. J Invest Dermatol 93: 18S–24S

Ryan T J 1991 Cutaneous circulation. In: Goldsmith L A (ed) Physiology, biochemistry, and molecular biology of the skin. 2nd edition. Oxford University Press: Oxford: pp 1019–1084

Ryan T J 1992 Development of the cutaneous circulation. In: Polin R A, Fox W W (eds) Fetal and neonatal physiology. W B Saunders: Philadelphia: pp 555–565

Ryan U S, Ryan J W 1984 The ultrastructural basis of endothelial cell surface functions. Biorheology 21: 155–170

Rybicki E F, Smonen F A, Weis E B 1972 On the mathematical analysis of stress in the human femur. J Biomech 5: 203–215

Ryncki P V 1974 Anatomie chirugicale du foie. Helv Chir Acta 41: 543–574

S

Saacke R G, Heald C W 1974 Cytological aspects of milk formation and secretion. In: Larson B L, Smith V R (eds) Lactation. A comprehensive treatise. Vol 2. Academic Press: New York: pp 147–189

Sabin F R 1912 On the origin of the abdominal lymphatics in mammals from the vena cava and the renal glands. Anat Rec 6: 335–342

Sabin F R 1920 Studies on the origin of blood vessels and of red blood corpuscles in the living blastoderm of chicks during the second day of incubation. Contrib Embryol Carnegie Inst Washington 9: 213

Sadikot A F, Parent A 1990 The monoaminergic innervation of the amygdala in the squirrel monkey: An immunohistochemical study. Neuroscience 36: 431–447

Sadler M, Berry M 1989 Topological link vertex analysis of the growth of Purkinje cell dendritic trees in normal, reeler and weaver mice. J Comp Neurol 289: 260 – 283

Sadler T W 1990 Langman's medical embryology, 6th edition. Williams & Wilkins: Baltimore

Saffrey M J, Hassall C J S, Allen T G J, Burnstock G 1992 Ganglia within the gut, heart, urinary bladder, and airways: studies in tissue culture. Int Rev Cytol 136: 93–144

Safieh-Garabedian B, Kendall M D, Khamashata M D, Hughes G 1992 Thymulin and its role in immunomodulation. J Autoimmun 16: 158–163

Sagebiel R W, Odland G F 1972 Ultrastructural identification of melanocytes in early human embryos. In: Riley V (ed) Pigmentation, its genesis and biologic control. Appleton-Century-Crofts: New York: pp 43–50

Saha A K 1961 Theory of shoulder mechanism: descriptive and applied. Thomas: Springfield, Illinois

Saha M S Servetnick M, Grainger R M 1992 Vertebrate eye development. Curr Opin Genet Dev 2: 582–588

Saito Y, Wright E M 1984 Regulation of bicarbonate transport across the brush border membrane of the bull-frog choroid plexus. J Physiol 350: 327–342

Saitoh K, Terada T, Hatakeyama S 1990 A morphological study of the efferent ducts of the human epididymis. Internat J Androl 13: 369–376

Sakakura T 1983 Epithelial mesenchymal interactions in mammary gland development and its perterbation in relation to tumorigenesis. In: Rich M A, Hayer J C, Furmanski P (eds) Understanding breast cancer. Marcel-Dekker: New York: pp 261–284

Sala N L, Luther E C, Arballo J C, Cordero Funes J 1974 Roles of temperature, pressure and touch in reflex milk ejection in lactating women. J Appl Physiol 37: 840–843

Saleem K S, Tanaka K, Rockland K S 1993 Specific and columnar projection from area TEO to TE in the macaque inferotemporal cortex. Cereb Cortex 3: 454–464

Salisbury C R 1937 The interosseous muscles of the hand. J Anat 71: 395–403

Salmon J A, Higgs G A, Vane J R, Bitensky L, Chayen J, Henderson B, Cashman B 1983 Synthesis of arachidonate cyclo-oxygenase products by rheumatoid and nonrheumatoid synovial lining in nonproliferative organ culture. Ann Rheum Dis 42: 36–39

Salmons P H, Salmons S 1992 Psychological costs of high-tech heart surgery. Br J Hosp Med 48: 707–709

Salmons S 1967 An implantable muscle stimulator. J Physiol 188: 13–14P

Salmons S 1975 In vivo tendon tension and bone strain measurement and correlation. J Biomechanics 8: 87

Salmons S 1980 Functional adaptation in skeletal muscle. Trends in Neurosciences 3: 134–137

Salmons S 1987 Fibre types in and around fascicles. Muscle Nerve 10: 85–86

Salmons S 1989 The importance of the adaptive properties of skeletal muscle in long term electrophrenic stimulation of the diaphragm. Stereotact Funct Neurosurg 53: 223–232

Salmons S 1990 On the reversibility of stimulation-induced muscle transformation. In: Pette D (ed) The dynamic state of muscle fibres. Walter de Gruyter: Berlin: pp 401–414

Salmons S 1992 Myotrophic effects of an anabolic steroid in rabbit limb muscles. Muscle Nerve 15: 806–812

Salmons S 1994 Exercise, stimulation and type transformation of skeletal muscle. Int J Sports Med 15: 136–141

Salmons S, Gale DR, Sréter F A 1978 Ultrastructural aspects of the transformation of muscle fibre type by long term stimulation: changes in Z-discs and mitochondria. J Anat 127: 17–31

Salmons S, Henriksson J 1981 The adaptive response of skeletal muscle to increased use. Muscle Nerve 4: 94–105

Salmons S, Jarvis, J C 1992 Cardiac assistance from skeletal muscle: a critical appraisal of the various approaches. Br Heart J 68: 333–338

Salmons S, Sréter, F A 1976 Significance of impulse activity in the transformation of skeletal muscle type. Nature 263: 30–34

Salmons S, Vrbová G 1969 The influence of activity on some contractile characteristics of mammalian fast and slow muscles. J Physiol 201: 535–549

Salsbury C R 1937 The interosseous muscles of the hand. J Anat 71: 395–403

Salter N 1955 Methods of measurement of muscle and joint function. J Bone Jt Surg 37B: 474–491

Salustri A, Yanagishita M, Hascall V C 1990 Mouse oocytes regulate hyaluronic acid synthesis and mucification by FSH-stimulated cumulus cells. Dev Biol 138: 26–32

Salvig K A 1964 An ultrastructural study of cementum formation. Acat Odont Scand 22: 105–120

Salzmann J A (ed) 1961 Roentgenographic cephalometrics. (Proceedings of the 2nd research workshop conducted by the special committee of the American Association of Orthodontists.) Lippincott: Philadelphia.

Sammarco J 1977 Biomechanics of the ankle. I. Surface velocity and instant center of rotation in the sagittal plane. Am J Sports Med 5: 231–234

Sampaio F J B 1992 Analysis of kidney volume growth during the fetal period in humans. Urol Res 20: 271–274

Sampson J A 1937 Lymphatics of mucosa of fimbriae of the fallopian tube. Am J Obstet Gynecol 33: 911–930

Sams M, Salmelin R 1994 Evidence of sharp frequency tuning in the human auditory cortex. Hear Res 75: 67–74

Samson H H, Harris R A 1992 Neurobiology of alcohol abuse. TIPS 13: 206–211

Samuel E P 1953 Chromidial studies on the superior cervical ganglion of the rabbit; (a) caudally projected postganglionic axons; (b) intercalary 'commissural' neurons. J Comp Neurol 98: 93–112

Sandberg L B, Soskel N T, Leslie J G 1981 Elastin structure, biosynthesis and relation to disease states. N Engl J Med 304: 566–577

Sanders E J 1986 Mesoderm migration in the early chick embryo. In: Browder L W (ed) Developmental biology: a comprehensive system. 2. The cellular basis of morphogenesis. Saunders: Philadelphia: pp 449–480

Sanes J N, Donoghue J P 1993 Oscillations in local field potentials of the primate motor cortex during voluntary movement. Proc Natl Acad Sci USA 90: 4470–4474

Sanes J R, Rubinstein J L R, Nicolas J-F 1986 EMBO J 12: 3133–3142

Sanodu J R, Domenech-Mateu J M 1990 The laryngeal primordium and epithelial lamina. A new interpretation. J Anat 171: 207–222

Sant' Ana Pereira J A A, Wessels A, Nijtmans L, Moorman A F M, Sargeant A J 1995 New method for the accurate characterization of single human skeletal muscles fibres demonstrates a relation between mATPase and MyHC expression in pure and hybrid fibre types. J Musc Res Cell Motil 16: 21–34

Santer R M, Lu K S, Lever J D, Presley R 1975 A study of the distribution of chromaffin-positive (Ch +) and small intensely fluorescent (SIF) cells in sympathetic ganglia of the rat at various ages. J Anat 119: 589–599

Santini D, Ceccarelli C, Mazzoleni G, Pasquinelli G, Jasonni V M, Martinelli G N 1993 Demonstration of cytokeratin intermediate filaments in oocytes of the developing and adult human ovary. Histochemistry 99: 311–319

Santo Neto H, Penteado C V, de Carvalh V C 1984 Presence of a groove in the lateral wall of the human orbit. J Anat 138: 631–633

Santulli T V, Blanc W A 1961 Congenital atresia of the intestine: pathogenesis and treatment. Ann Surg 154: 939–948

Saper C B 1990 Hypothalamus. In: Paxinos G (ed) The human nervous system. Academic Press: San Diego: pp 389–411

Saper C B, Loewi A D, Swanson L W Cowan W M 1976 Direct hypo-thalamoautonomic connections. Brain Res 117: 305–312

Saper, E B 1990 Cholinergic system. In: Paxinos G (ed) The human nervous system. Academic Press: New York: pp 1095– 1114

Sapin M R, Borziak E I 1974 Anatomie des ganglions lymphatiques du médiastin. Acta Anat 90: 200–225

Sargeant A J, Davies C T M, Edwards R H T, Maunder C, Young A 1977 Functional and structural changes after disuse in humans. Clin Sci Mol Med 52: 337–342

Sarin V K, Gupta S, Leung T K et al 1990 Biophysical and biochemical activity of a synthetic 8.7 kDa hydrophobic pulmonary surfactant protein SP-B. Proc Natl Acad Sci USA 87: 2633–2637

Sariola H, Ekbolm P, Henke-Fahle S 1989 Embryonic neurons as in vitro inducers of differentiation of nephrogenic mesenchyme. Dev Biol 132: 271–281

Sariola H, Saarma M, Sainio K 1991 Dependence of kidney morphogenesis on the expression of nerve growth factor receptor. Science 254: 571–573

Sarnat B G (ed) 1951 The temporomandibular joint. 2nd edition. Thomas: Springfield, Illinois

Sartore S, Mascarello F, Rowlerson A, Gorza L. Ausoni S, Vianello M, Schiaffino S 1987 Fibre types in extraocular muscles: a new myosin isoform in the fast fibres. J Musc Res Cell Motil 8: 161–172

Sasagawa T, Kobayashi S, Fujita T 1973 Electron microscope studies on the endocrine cells of the human gut and pancreas. In: Fujita T (ed) Gastro-entero-pancreatic endocrine system. A cell–biological approach. Igaku Shoiu: Tokyo: pp 17–38

Sasaki K, Gemba H, Nambu A, Matsuzaki R 1993 No-go activity in the frontal association cortex of human subjects. Neurosci Res 18: 249–252

Sasaki K, Gemba H, Nambu A, Matsuzaki R 1994a Activity of the prefrontal cortex on no-go decision and motor suppression. In: Thierry A M et al (eds) Motor and cognitive functions of the prefrontal cortex. Springer-Verlag: Berlin: pp 139–159

Sasaki K, Tsujimoto T, Nambu A, Matsuzaki R, Kyuhou S 1994b Dynamic activities of the frontal association cortex in calculating and thinking. Neurosci Res 19: 229–233

Sataloff R T 1992 The human voice. Sci Am 267(6): 108–115

Sathian K, Devanandan M S 1983 Receptors of the metacarpophalangeal joints: a histological study in the bonnet monkey and man. J Anat 137: 601–613

Satiukova G S, Rassokhina-Volkova L J 1972 Compensatory-adaptive changes in the lymphatic system of organs in experiment and disease. Bibl Anat 11: 481–487

Sato J 1974 The Mm subcostales in man and monkeys. Okajimas Fol Anat Jpn 50: 345–358

Sato N, Nariuchi H, Tsuruoka N, Nishihara T, Beitz J G, Calabresi P, Franckelton A R Jr 1990 Actions of TNF and IFN-γ on angiogenesis in vitro. J Invest Dermatol 95: 85S–89S

Sato T 1973a A new classification of the transverso-spinalis system. Proc Jap Acad 49: 51–56

Sato T 1973b Innervation and morphology of the musculi levatores costarum longi. Proc Jap Acad 49: 555–558

Sato T, Kang W H, Sato F 1991 Eccrine sweat glands. In: Goldsmith L A (ed) Physiology, biochemistry and molecular biology of the skin. 2nd edn. Oxford University Press: Oxford, pp 741–762

Satoh M 1991 Histogenesis and organogenesis of the gonad in human embryos. J Anat 177: 85–107

Satokata I, Maas R 1994 Mox 1 deficient mice exhibit cleft palate and abnormalities of craniofacial and tooth development. Nature Genetics 6: 348–355

Sauer F C 1935a The cellular structure of the neural tube. J Comp Neurol 63: 13–23

Sauer F C 1935b Mitosis in the neural tube. J Comp Neurol 62: 337–405

Sauer F C 1936 The interkinetic migration of embryonic epithelial nuclei. J Morphol 60: 1–11

Sauer M E, Chittenden A C 1959 Deoxyribonucleic acid content of cell nuclei in the neural tube of the chick embryo: evidence for intermitotic migration of nuclei. Exp Cell Res 16: 1–6

Saunders J W 1977 The experimental analysis of chick limb bud development. In: Ede D A, Hinchcliffe, Balls (eds) Vertebrate limb and somite morphogenesis. Cambridge University Press: Cambridge: pp 1–24

Saunders J W, Gasseling M T, Errick J E 1976 Inductive activity and enduring cellular constitution of a supernumary apical ectodermal ridge grafted to the limb bud of the chick embryo. Dev Biol 50: 16–25

Saunders R L de C H, Röckert H O E 1967 Vascular supply of dental tissues including lymphatics. In: Miles A E W (ed) Structural and chemical organisation of teeth. Academic Press: New York: pp 199–245

Saunders R L, Weider D 1985 Tympanic membrane sensation. Brain 108: 387–404

Savino W, Bartoccioni E, Homo-Delarche F, Gagnerault M C, Itoh T, Dardenne M 1988 Thymic hormone containing cells. IX. Steroids in vitro modulate thymulin secretion by human and murine thymic epithelial cells. Journal of Steroid Biochemistry 30: 479–484

Sawchak J A, Lewis S, Shafiq S A 1989 Coexpression of myosin isoforms in muscle of patients with neurogenic disease. Muscle Nerve 12: 679–689

Saxen L 1970 Failure to demonstrate tubule induction in a heterologous mesenchyme. Dev Biol 23: 511–523

Saxen L, Koskimies O, Lahti A, Miettinen H, Rapola J, Wartiovaara J 1968 Differentiation of kidney mesenchyme in an experimental model system. J Adv Morphogen 7: 251–293

Saxen L, Toivonen S 1962 Primary embryonic induction. Logos Press-Academic Press: London

Sayfi Y 1967 Note sur l'innervation du dos de la main. Arch Anat Pathol 15: 139–140

Scammon R E 1927 The prenatal growth of the human thymus. Proc Soc Exp Biol Med 24: 906–909

Scammon R E, Calkins L A 1929 The development and growth of the external dimensions of the human body in the fetal period. University of Minnesota Press: Minneapolis

Scapinelli R 1968 Studies on the vasculature of the human knee joint. Acta Anat 70: 305–331

Scaravilli F 1984 The influence of distal environment on peripheral nerve regeneration across a gap. J Neurocytol 13: 1027–1041

Schachenmayr W, Friede R L 1978 The origin of subdural neomembranes. 1. Fine structure of the dura-arachnoid interface in man. Am J Pathol 92: 53–68

Schadé J P 1964 On the volume and surface area of spinal neurons. Progr Brain Res 11: 261–277

Schaefer K P, Schneider H 1968 Reizversuche im Tectum opticum des Kaninchens. Ein experimenteller Beitrag zur seno-mororischen Koordination des Hirnstammes. Arch Psychiat NervKrankh 211: 118–137

Schaper A 1897 Die frühesten Differenzirungsvorgänge im central nervensystem; kritische Studie und Versuch einer Geschichte der Entwicklung nervöser Substanz. Arch Entwicklungsmechn Organ Leipzig 5: 81–132

Scharf J H 1958 Sensible ganglien. In: Handbuch der mikroskopischen Anatomie des Menschen, Bd 4/3. Springer: Berlin

Scharrer E, Scharrer B 1940 Secretory cells within the hypothalamus. Res Publ Ass Nerv Ment Dis 20: 170–194

Scharrer E, Scharrer B 1963 Neuroendocrinology. Columbia University Press: New York

Schaub M C, Tuchschmid C R, Srihari T, Hirzel O H 1984 Myosin isoenzymes in human hypertrophic hearts. Shift in atrial myosin heavy chains and in ventricular myosin light chains. Eur Heart J 5 (Suppl F): 85–93

Schaub M, Kunz B 1986 Regulation of contraction in cardiac and smooth muscles. J Cardiovasc Pharmacol 8 (Suppl 8): S117–S123

Schaumann B, Alter M A 1976 Dermatoglyphics in medical disorders. Springer: New York

Scheer U, Weisenberger D 1994 The nucleolus. Curr Opin Cell Biol 6: 354–359

Scheibel A B, Paul L, Fried I, Forsythe A, Tomiyasu U, Wechsler A, Kao A, Slotnick J 1985 Dendritic organization of the anterior speech area. Exp Neurol 87: 109–117

Scheibel M E, Scheibel A B 1966a The organisation of the nucleus reticularis thalami: a Golgi study. Brain Res 1: 43–62

Scheibel M E, Scheibel A B 1966c Spinal motoneurons, interneurons and Renshaw cells: a Golgi study. Arch Ital Biol 104: 328–353

Scheibel M E, Scheibel A B 1968 Terminal exonal patterns in cat spinal cord. II. The dorsal horn. Brain Res 9: 32–58

Scheibel M E, Scheibel A B 1969 A structural analysis of spinal interneurons and Renshaw cells. In: Brazier M A B (ed) The interneuron. Univ California Press: Los Angeles: pp 159–208

Scheidegger G 1980 Structure of the transitional epithelium in the urinary bladder of the pig, sheep, rat and shrew. Acta Anat 107: 268–275

Scheinin A, Light E I 1969 Innervation of the dental pulp. Acta Odont Scand 27: 313–319

Scherg M 1990 Fundamentals of dipole source potential analysis. In: Grandori F, Hoke M, Romani G L (eds) Auditory evoked magnetic fields and electric potentials. Adv Audiol Vol. 6, Karger: Basel: pp 40–49

Scheuer J L 1964 Fibre size frequency distribution in normal human laryngeal nerves. J Anat 98: 99–104

Schiaffino S, Gorza L, Ausoni S 1993 Troponin isoform switching in the developing heart and its functional consequences. Trends Cardiovasc Med 3: 12–17

Schiaffino S, Gorza L, Sartore S, Saggin L, Ausoni S, Vianello M, Gundersen K, Lømo T 1989 Three myosin heavy chain isoforms in type 2 skeletal muscle fibres. J Musc Res Cell Motil 10: 197–205

Schiaffino S, Pierobon Bormiolo S 1976 Morphogenesis of rat muscle spindles after nerve lesion during early postnatal development. J Neurocytol 5: 319–336

Schieber M H, Hibbard L S 1993 How somatotopic is the motor cortex hand area. Science 261: 489–492

Schiff D C M, Parke W W 1973 The arterial supply of the odontoid process (dens). J Bone Jt Surg 55A: 1450–1456

Schlaepfer W W 1974 Calcium-induced degeneration of axoplasm in isolated segments of rat peripheral nerve. Brain Res 69: 203–215

Schlaepfer W W 1979 Nature of mammalian neurofilaments and their breakdown by calcium. In Zimmermann H M (ed) progress in neuropathology, Vol 4 Raven Press New York: pp 101–123

Schlager F 1967 Uber die muskalatur der Ductus ejaculatorii beim Menschen. Z Zellforsch 76: 268–276

Schlaggar B L, O'Leary D D M 1989 Science 252: 1556–1560

Schlant R C 1978 Altered physiology of the cardiovascular system in heart failure. In: Hurst J W, Logue R B, Schlant R C, Wenger N K (eds) The heart, arteries and veins. 4th edition. McGraw-Hill: New York: pp 532–550

Schlaudraff K, Schumacher N, Specht B U von, Seitelberger R, Shlosser V, Fasol R 1993 Growth of 'new' coronary vascular structures by angiogenetic growth factors. Eur J Cardiothorac Surg 7: 637–644

Schlegel J V 1946 Arterio-venous anastomoses in the endometrium in man. Acta Anat 1: 284–325

Schlesinger D H, Goldstein G, Niall H D 1975 The complete amino acid sequence of ubiquitin, an adenylate cyclase stimulating polypeptide probably universal in living cells. Biochem 14: 2214–2218

Schlosshauer B, Schwartz U, Edelman G M 1984 Nature 310: 141–143

Schlossman A, Priestley B S (eds) 1966 Strabismus. International ophthalmology clinics 6, No 3. Little, Brown: Boston: pp 397–749

Schmahmann J D, Pandy D N 1990 Anatomical investigation of projections from thalamus to posterior parietal cortex in the rhesus monkey: a WGA-HRP and fluorescent tracer study. J Comp Neurol 295: 299–326

Schmidt H M 1974 Über den Verlauf der Radix mesenterii beim Menschen. Z Anat EntwGesch 144: 187–194

Schmidt R F, Thews G 1989 Human Physiology: Springer Verlag

Schmidt W J 1938 Polarisationsoptische analyse eines eiweiss-lipoid systems. Kolloidzchr 85: 137–148

Schmidtke K, Büttner-Ennever J A 1992 Nervous control of eyelid function: a review of clinical, experimental and pathological data. Brain 115: 227–247

Schmitt F O, Parvati D, Smith B H 1976 Electronic processing of information by brain cells. Science 193: 114–120

Schmitt F O, Worden F G (eds) 1979 The neurosciences. Fourth study program. MIT Press: Cambridge, Massachusetts

Schmolke C 1994 The relationship between the temporomandibular joint capsule, articular disc and jaw muscles. J Anat 184: 335–345

Schmucker D L 1990 Hepatocyte fine structure during maturation and senescence. J Electr Micr Tech 14: 106–125

Schneeberger E E, Lynch R D 1992 Structure, function and regulation of cellular tight junctions. Am J Physiol 262: 647–661

Schneider M F, Chandler W K 1973 Voltage dependent charge movement in skeletal muscle: a possible step in excitation–contraction coupling. Nature 242: 244–246

Schneider U, Inke G, Schneider I G 1969 Zhale, Abstand der Verzweigungsstellen vom Rand des Sinus renalis und Kaliber der extrarenalen Nierengefässe des menschen. Anat Anz 124: 278–291

Schnell L, Schwab M E 1990 Axonal regeneration in rat spinal cord produced by an antibody against myelin-associated neurite growth inhibitors. Nature 343: 292–304

Schnell L, Schwab M E 1993 Sprouting and regeneration of lesioned corticospinal tract fibres in the adult rat spinal chord. Eur J Neurosci 5: 1156–1171

Schnell L, Schwab M E 1993a Axonal regeneration in rat spinal cord produced by an antibody against myelin-associated neurite growth inhibitors. Nature 343: 269 – 272

Schnell L, Schwab M E 1993b Sprouting and regeneration of lesioned corticospinal tract fibres in the adult rat spinal cord. Eur J Neurosci 5: 1156 – 1171

Schnitzer J 1987 Retinal astrocytes: their restriction to vascularized parts of the mammalian retina. Neurosci Letters 78:29–34

Schnitzlein H N, Rowe L C, Hoffman H H 1958 The myelinated component of the vagus nerves in man. Anat Rec 131: 649–667

Schoefl G T 1972 The migration of lymphocytes across the vascular endothelium in lymphoid tissue. A re-examination. J Exp Med 136: 568–588

Schoefl G T, French J E 1968 Vascular permeability to particulate fat: morphological observations on vessels of lactating mammary glands and of lung. Proc R Soc Lond 169B: 153–165

Schoen J H R 1964 Comparative aspects of the descending fibre systems in the spinal cord. In: Eccles J C, Scherdé J P (eds) Organization of the spinal cord. Prog Brain Res. Elsevier: Amsterdam: pp 203–222

Schoen J H R 1969 The corticofugal projection of the brain stem and spinal cord in man. Psychiat Neurol Neurochir 72: 121–128

Schoen S W, Graeber M B, Tóth L, Kreuzberg G W 1988 5'-Nucleotidase in postnatal ontogeny of rat cerebellum: a marker migrating nerve cells? Dev Brain Res 39: 125–136

Schoenen J 1973 Organisation cytoarchitectonique de la moelle épinière de différents mammifères et de l'homme. Acta Neurol Belg 73: 348–358

Schoenen J 1981 L'organisation neuronale de la moelle épinière de l'homme. Editions Sciences et Lettres: Liège

Schoenen J 1982 Dendritic organization of human spinal cord: the motoneurons. J Comp Neurol 211: 226–247

Schoenen J, Faull R L M 1990 Spinal cord: cytoarchitectural, dendroarchitectural and myeloarchitectural organization. In: Paxinos G (ed) The human nervous system. Academic Press: San Diego: pp 19–53

Schoenfield T A, Marchand J E, Macrides F 1985 Topographic organization of tufted cell axonal projections in the hamster main olfactory bulb: an intrabulbar associational system. J Comp Neurol 235: 503–518

Schoenwolf G C, Garcia-Matinez V, Dias M S 1992 Mesoderm movement and fate during avian gastrulation and neurulation. Developmental Dynamics 193: 235–248

Schoenwolf G C, Smith J L 1990 Mechanisms of neurulation: traditional viewpoint and recent advances. Development 109: 243–270

Schofield G C 1968 Anatomy of muscular and neural tissue in the alimentary canal. In: Code C F (ed) Handbook of physiology. Section 6, Alimentary canal. Vol 4. American Physiological Society: Washington: pp 1579–1628

Schonfeld S E, Slavkin H C 1977 Demonstration of enamel matrix proteins on root-analogue surfaces of rabbit permanent incisor teeth. Calcif Tissue Res 24: 223–229

Schotzinger R J, Landis S C 1988 Cholinergic phenotype developed by noradrenergic sympathetic neurons after innervation of a novel cholinergic target in vivo. Nature 335: 637–639

Schoultze T W, Swett J E 1972 The fine structure of the Golgi tendon organ. J Neurocytol 1: 1–26

Schour I, Massler M 1941 The development of the human dentition. J Am Dent Assoc 28: 1153–1160

Schramm L P, Stribling J M, Adair J R 1976 Developmental reorientation of sympathetic preganglionic neurons in the rat. Brain Res 106: 166–171

Schraufstatter I et al 1984 Biochemical factors in pulmonary inflammatory disease. Federation Proceedings 43(13): 2807–2810

Schraufstatter I U, Revak S D, Cochrane C G 1984 Proteases and oxidants in experimental pulmonary inflammatory injury. J Clin Invest 73: 1175–1184

Schroder H D 1981 Onuf's nucleus X. A morphological study of a human spinal nucleus. Anat Embryol 162: 443–453

Schröder R R, Manstein D J, Jahn W J, Holden H, Rayment I, Holmes K C, Spudich J A 1993 Three-dimensional atomic model of F-actin decorated with Dictostelium myosin S1. Nature 364: 171–174

Schroeder A C, Eppig J J 1984 Developmental capacity of mouse oocytes that matured in vitro is normal. Dev Biol 102: 493–497

Schroeder H E, Listgarten M A 1971 Fine structure of the developing epithelial attachment of human teeth. (Monographs in Developmental Biology. Vol 2.) Karger: Basel

Schroeder T E 1973 Actin in dividing cells: contractile ring filaments bind heavy meromyosin. Proc Natl Acad Sci USA 70: 1688–1692

Schuknecht H F 1960 Neuroanatomical correlates of auditory sensitivity and pitch discrimination in the cat. In: Rasmussen G L, Windle W F (eds) Neural mechanisms of the auditory and vestibular systems. Thomas: Springfield Illinois: pp 76–90

Schuler G (ed) 1991 Epidermal Langerhans cells. CRC Press: Boca Raton

Schuler G, Romani N, Stossel H, Wolff K 1991 Structural organization and biological properties of Langerhans cells. In: Schuler G (ed) Epidermal Langerhans cells. CRC Press: Boca Raton: pp 87–137

Schulter F P 1976 Studies of the basicranial axis: a brief review. Am J Phys Anthrop 45: 545–552

Schultz M W, Chamberlain C G, de Iongh R U, McAvoy J W 1993 Acidic and basic FGF in ocular media and lens: implications for lens polarity and growth patterns. Development 118: 117–126

Schultz R M 1986 Molecular aspects of mammalian oocyte growth and maturation. In: Rossant J, Peterson R A (eds) Experimental approaches to mammalian embryonic development. Cambridge University Press: Cambridge: pp 195–237

Schultz R M 1993 Regulation of zygotic gene activation in the mouse. BioEssays 15: 531–538

Schultze A H 1956 Postembryonic age changes. Primatologia 1: 887–964

Schulze-Bonhage A, Wittkowski W 1991 Cell types in the pars tuberalis of the human adenohypophysis at mid-gestation. Cell Tissue Res 264: 161–165

Schumacher G H 1961 Funkionelle Morphologie der Kaumuskulatur. Fischer: Jena

Schumacher G H, Lau H, Freund E, Schultz M, Himstedt H W, Menning A 1976 Zur Topographie der muskulären Nervenausbreitungen. 9. Kaumuskeln M pterygoideus medialis und lateralis. Anat Anz 139: 71–87

Schumacher S 1938 Ueber die Bedeutung der arteriovenosen Anatostomosen und der epithelioden Muskelzellen (Quellzellen). Zeitschr f mikro-anat Forsch 43: 107–130

Schunke G B 1938 The anatomy and development of the sacro-iliac joint in man. Anat Rec 72: 313–331

Schuster C R 1986 Implications of laboratory research for the treatment of drug dependence. In: Goldberg S R, Stolerman I P (eds) Behavioral analysis of drug dependence. Academic Press: London: pp 357–386

Schuz A, Palm G 1989 Density of neurons and synapses in the cerebral cortex of the mouse. J Comp Neurol 286: 442–455

Schwab M E 1990 Myelin-associated inhibitors of neurite growth. Exp Neurol 109: 2 – 5

Schwanzel-Fukuda M, Pfaff D W 1989 Origin of luteinizing hormone-releasing neurons. Nature 338: 161–164

Schwanzel-Fukuda M, Pfaff D W 1989 The migration of luteinizing hormone releasing hormone (LHRH) neurons from the medial olfactory placode into the medial basal forebrain. Experientia 46: 956–962

Schwartz H G, Roulhac G E, Lam R L, O'Leary J 1951 Organisation of the fasciculus solitarius in man. J Comp Neurol 94: 221–237

Schwartz H, Weddell G 1938 Observations on pathways transmitting the sensation of taste. Brain 61: 99–115

Schwartz J, Cherny R 1992 Intercellular communication within the anterior pituitary influencing the secretion of hypophysial hormones. Endocrine Rev 13: 453–475

Schwartz M L, Goldman-Rakic P S 1982 Single cortical neurones have axon collaterals to ipsilateral and contralateral cortex in fetal and adult primates. Nature 299: 154–155

Schwartz M L, Goldman-Rakic P S 1984 Callosal and intrahemispheric connectivity of the prefrontal association cortex in rhesus monkey: relation between intraparietal and principal sulcus. J Comp Neurol 226: 403–420

Schwartz W J, Busis N A, Healeywhite E T 1986 A discrete lesion of the ventral hypothalamus and optic chiasm that disturbed the daily temperature rhythm. J Neurol 233: 1–4

Schweigerer L, Neufeld G, Friedman J, Abraham J A, Fiddes J C, Gospodarowicz D 1987 Capillary endothelial cells express basic fibroblast growth factor, a mitogen that promotes their own growth. Nature 325: 257–259

Scotchford C A, Greenwald S, Ali S Y 1992 Calcium phosphate crystal distribution in the superficial zone of human femoral head articular cartilage. J Anat 181: 293–300

Scott D E, Dudley G K, Knigge K M 1974 The ventricular system in neuroendocrine mechanisms. 2. In vivo monoamine transport by ependyma of the median eminence. Cell Tissue Res 154: 1–16

Scott D M, Harwood R, Grant M E, Jackson D S 1977 Characterization of the major collagen species present in porcine aortae and the synthesis of their precursors by smooth muscle cells in culture. Connect Tissue Res 5: 7–13

Scott G B D 1980 The primate caecum and appendix vermiformis: a comparative study. J Anat 131: 549–563

Scott J E 1985 Proteoglycan histochemistry – a valuable tool for connective tissue biochemists. Collagen Rel Res 5: 541–575

Scott J E 1988 Proteoglycan-fibrillar collagen interactions. Biochem J 252: 313–323

Scott J E 1992 Supramolecular organisation of extracellular matrix glycosaminoglycans in vitro and in the tissues. FASEB J 6: 2639–2645

Scott J E 1993 Dermatan sulphate proteoglycans. Portland Press: London

Scott J E, Greiling M 1989 Keratan sulphate. Portland Press: London

Scott J E, Parry D A D 1992 Control of collagen fibril diameters in the tissues. Int J Biol Macromol 14: 292–293

Scott J H 1955 A contribution to the study of the mandibular joint function. Br Dent J 98: 345–348

Scott J H 1967 Dento-facial development and growth. Pergamon Press: London

Scott J H, Symons N B B 1977 Introduction to dental anatomy. 7th edition. Churchill Livingstone: Edinburgh

Scott M P 1992 Vertebrate homeobox gene nomenclature. Cell 71: 551–553

Scott S A 1984 The effects of neural crest derivatives in the development of sensory innervation patterns in embryonic chick hindlimb. J Physiol 352: 285–304

Scott T G 1967 The distribution of 5'-nucleotidase in the brain of the mouse. J Comp Neurol 129: 97–114

Scott V D, Love G 1983 Quantitative electron probe microanalysis. Ellis Horwood: New York

Scott-Duff R, Langtimm C J, Richardson M K, Sieber-Blum 1991 In vitro clonal analysis of progenitor cell patterns in dorsal root and sympathetic ganglia of the quail embryo. Dev Biol 147: 451–459

Screpanti I, Meco D, Scarpa S, Morrone S, Frati L, Gulino A, Modesti A 1992 Neuromodulatory loop mediated by nerve growth factor and interleukin 6 in thymic stromal cell cultures. Proc Natl Acad Sci USA 89: 3209–3212

Screpanti I, Morrone S, Meco D, Santori A, Gulino A, Paolini R, Crisanti A, Mathieson B J, Frati L 1989 Steroid sensitivity of thymocyte subpopulations during intrathymic differentiation. Effects of 17 β-estradiol and dexamethasone on subsets expressing T cell antigen receptor or IL-2 receptor. J Immunol 142: 3378–3383

Sebuwufu P H 1968 Ultrastructure of human fetal thymic cilia. J Ultrastruct Res 24: 171–180

Sedzmir C B 1959 An angiographic test of collateral circulation through the anterior segment of the circle of Willis. J Neurol Neurosurg Psychiat 22: 64–68

Seeck M, Mainwaring N, Ives J, Blume H, Dubuisson D, Cosgrove R et al 1993 Differential neural activity in the human temporal lobe evoked by faces of family members and friends. Ann Neurol 34: 369–372

Seedhom B B 1979 Transmission of the load in the knee joint with special reference to the role of the menisci. Part I. Anatomy, analysis and apparatus. Eng Med 8: 207–219

Seedhom B B, Dowson D, Wright V 1974 Functions of the menisci. A preliminary study. (Heberden Society Proceedings.) Ann Rheum Dis 33: 111

Seedhom B B, Tsubuku M 1977 A technique for the study of contact between visco-elastic bodies with special reference to the patello-femoral joint. J Biomech 10: 253–260

Seipel M 1948 Studies on the structure of the mandible. Acta Odontol Scand 8: 81–191

Sekiya H, Kojima Y, Hiramoto D, Mukuno K, Ishikawa S 1992 Bilateral innervation of the musculus levator palpebrae superioris by single motoneurons in the monkey. Neurosci Letters 146: 10–12

Seldon H L 1982 Structure of human auditory cortex. III. Statistical analysis of dendritic trees. Brain Res 249: 211–231

Seldon H L 1985 The anatomy of speech perception: human auditory cortex. In: Peters A, Jones E G (eds) Cerebral cortex. Vol 4. Association and auditory cortices. Plenum Press: New York: pp 273–327

Selemon L D, Goldman-Rakic P S 1985 Longitudinal topography and interdigitation of corticostriatal projections in the rhesus monkey. J Neurosci 5: 776–794

Selemon L D, Goldman-Rakic P S 1988 Common cortical and subcortical targets of the dorsolateral prefrontal and posterior parietal cortices in the rhesus monkey: evidence for a distributed neural network subserving spatially guided behaviour. J Neurosci 8: 4049–4068

Sellars I E, Keen E N 1978 The anatomy and movements of the cricoarytenoid joint. Laryngoscope 88: 667–674

Selleck M A J, Stern C D 1991 Fate mapping and cell lineage analysis of Hensen's node in the chick embryo. Development 112: 615–626

Selleck M A J, Stern C D 1992 Commitment of mesoderm cells in Hensen's node of the chick embryo to notochord and somite. Development 114: 403–415

Seltzer B, Pandya D N 1989 Frontal lobe connections of the superior temporal sulcus in the rhesus monkey. J Comp Neurol 281: 97–113

Seltzer B, Pandya D N 1991 Post-rolandic cortical projections of the superior temporal sulcus in the rhesus monkey. J Comp Neurol 312: 625–640

Seltzer B, Pandya D N 1994 Parietal, temporal, and occipital projections to cortex of the superior temporal sulcus in the rhesus monkey: a retrograde tracer study. J Comp Neurol 343: 445–463

Selye H 1965 The mast cells. Butterworths: Washington DC

Senior H D 1919 The development of the arteries of the human lower extremity. Am J Anat 25: 55–96

Senior H D 1920 The development of the human femoral artery, a correction. Anat Rec 17: 271–280

Senior R M, Griffin G L, Huang J S, Walz D A, Deuel T F 1983 Chemotactic activity of platelet a-granule proteins for fibroblasts. J Cell Biol 96: 382–385

Seo J W, Brown N A, Ho S Y, Anderson R H 1992 Abnormal laterality and congenital cardiac anomalies. Relations of visceral and cardiac morphologies in the iv/iv mouse. Circulation 86: 642–650

Seppala M, Angervo M, Riitinen L, Yajima M, Julkunen M, Koistinen R 1992 Peptides and proteins in the human endometrium. Reprod Med Rev 1: 37–55

Serafini-Fracassini A, Smith J W 1974 The structure and biochemistry of cartilage. Churchill Livingstone: Edinburgh

Serbedzija G N, Fraser S E, Bronner-Fraser M 1990 Pathways of trunk neural crest cell migration in the mouse embryo as revealed by vital dye labelling. Development 108: 605–612

Sessle B J 1987 The neurobiology of facial and dental pain: present knowledge, future directions. J Dent Res 66: 962–981

Sessle B J 1987 The neurobiology of facial pain: present knowledge, future directions. J Dent Res 66: 962–981

Setchell B P, Waites G M H 1975 The blood-testis barrier. In: Hamilton D W, Greep R O (eds) Handbook of physiology. Section 7. Endocrinology Vol 5. American Physiological Society: Washington, DC: pp 143–172

Seto-Oshima A, Kitajima S, Sano M, Kato K, Mizutani A 1983 Immunohistochemical localization of calmodulin in mouse brain. Histochemistry 79: 251–257

Setton L A, Zhu W, Mow V C 1993 The biphasic poroviscoelastic behaviour of articular cartilage: role of the surface zone in governing the compressive behaviour. J Biomech 26: 581–592

Sevel D 1988 A reappraisal of the development of the eyelids. Eye 2, 123.

Ton C C T et al. 1991 Positional cloning and characterization of a paired box- and homeobox-containing gene from the aniridia region. Cell 67: 1059–1074

Severs N J 1990 The gap junction and intercalated disk. Int J Cardiol 26: 137–173

Shafik A 1977 The cremasteric muscle. In: Johnson A D, Gomes W R (eds) The testis. Academic Press: New York

Shafik A 1986 A new concept of the anatomy of the anal sphincter. Mechanism and the physiology of defecation. Reversion to normal defecation after combined excision operation and end colostomy for rectal cancer. Am J Surg 151: 278–284

Shah M, Foreman D M, Ferguson M W J 1992 Control of scarring in adult wounds by neutralising antibody to TGF-B. Lancet 339: 213–214

Shah P M, Scarton H A, Tsapogas M J 1978 Geometric anatomy of the aortic–common iliac bifurcation. J Anat 126: 451–458

Shahan K 1983 Gross and functional anatomy of the shoulder. Clin Orthop 173: 11–19

Shaheen O H 1984 Problems in head and neck surgery. Baillière Tindall: London: pp 37–49

Shakir A, Zaini S 1974 Skeletal maturation of the hand and wrist of young children in Baghdad. Ann Hum Biol 1: 189–199

Shambes G, Gibson M, Welker W 1978 Fractured somatotopy in granule cell tactile areas of rat cerebellar hemispheres revealed by micromapping. Brain Behav Evol 15: 94–140

Shaner R F 1929 The development of the atrioventricular node, bundle of His and sinoatrial node in the calf; with a description of a third embryonic node-like structure. Anat Rec 44: 85–100

Shanks M F, Pearson R C A, Powell T P S 1978 The intrinsic connexions of the primary somatic sensory cortex of the monkey. Proc R Soc Lond [Biol] 200: 95–101

Shanks M F, Pearson R C A, Powell T P S 1985a The callosal connections of the primary somatic sensory cortex in the monkey. Brain Res Rev 9: 43–65

Shanks M F, Pearson R C A, Powell T P S 1985b The ipsilateral corticocortical connections between the cytoarchitectonic subdivisions of the primary somatic sensory cortex in the monkey. Brain Res Rev 9: 67–88

Shapiro A L, Robillard G L 1948 Arterial blood supply of common and hepatic bile ducts with references to problems to common duct injury and repair: based on a series of 23 dissections. Surgery 23: 1–11

Shapiro M B, Schein S J, De Monasterio F M I 1985 Regularity and structure of the spatial pattern of blue cones of macaque retina. Amer J Stat Assoc 803–812

Shapiro R E, Miselis R R 1985 The central organization of the vagus nerve innervating the stomach of the rat. J Comp Neurol 238: 473–488

Shapley R, Perry V H 1986 Cat and monkey retinal ganglion cells and their visual functional roles. Trends Neurosci 9: 229–235

Sharma A K, Thomas P K 1975 Quantitative studies on age changes in unmyelinated nerve fibres in the vagus nerve of man. In: Kunze K, Desmedt J E (eds) Studies in neuromuscular disease. Karger: Basel: pp 211–216

Sharpe P M, Ferguson M W J 1988 Mesenchymal influences on Epithelial differentiation in developing systems. J Cell Sci Supp 10: 195–230

Sharpe P M, Foreman D M, Brunet C, Ferguson M W J 1993 Localisation of acidic and basic fibroblast growth factor during mouse palate development and their effects on mouse palate mesenchyme cells in vitro. Roue's Archives of Developmental Biology 202–243

Sharpe R M 1993 Falling sperm counts in men – is there an endocrine cause? J Endocrinol 137: 357–360

Sharpe R M 1994 Regulation of spermatogenesis. In: Knobil E, Neill J D (eds) The physiology of reproduction. 2nd edition. Raven Press: New York (in press)

Sharpe R M, Maddox S, Kerr J B 1990 Cell–cell interactions in the control of spermatogenesis using Leydig cell destruction and testosterone replacement. Amer J Anat 188: 3–20

Sharpe R M, Skakkebaek N E 1993 Are oestrogens involves in falling sperm counts and disorders in the male reproductive tract? Lancet 341: 1392–1395

Sharrard R M, Al-Fadhl D, Couch M, Russell R G G 1986 Mineralization nodules in cultured human bone cells. In: Ali S Y (ed) Cell-mediated calcification and matrix vesicles. Elsevier: Amsterdam: pp 333–338

Sharrard W J W 1955 the distribution of the permanent paralysis in the lower limb in poliomyelitis. J Bone Jt Surg 37B: 540–558

Sharrard W J W 1956 Poliomyelitis: The distribution of the paralysis. In: British Surgical Progress, p 83

Shatz C J 1992 Science 258: 237–238

Shaw N E, Martin B F 1962 Histological and histochemical studies on mammalian knee-joint tissues. J Anat 96: 359–373

Shawker T H, Sonies B, Hall T E, Baum B F 1984 Ultrasound analysis of tongue, hyoid, and larynx activity during swallowing. Invest Radiol 19: 82–86

Sheehan D 1933 On unmyelinated fibres in the spinal nerves. Anat Rec 55: 111–116

Sheehan D, Mulholland J H, Shariroff B 1941 Surgical anatomy of the carotid tinus nerve. Anat Rec 80: 431–442

Shehata R 1966 The crura of the diaphragm and their nerve supply. Acta Anat 63: 49–54

Sheldon H 1983 Transmission electron microscopy of cartilage. In: Hall B K (ed) Cartilage. Vol 1. Structure, function and biochemistry. Academic Press: New York: pp 87–104

Sheldon H, Robinson R A 1958 Studies on cartilage: electron microscopic observations on normal rabbit ear cartilage. J Biophys Biochem Cytol 4: 401–406

Sheldon W H, Stevens S S 1942 The variety of temperament. Harper: New York

Sheldon W H, Stevens S S, Tucker W B 1940 The varieties of human physique. Harper: London

Shelton J H, Jones A L 1971 The fine structure of the mouse adrenal cortex and the ultrastructural changes in the zona glomerulosa with low and high sodium diets. Anat Rec 170: 147–182

Shepard E 1951 Tarsal movements. J Bone Jt Surg 33B: 258–263

Shepherd G M 1974 Synaptic organization of the brain. Oxford University Press: London

Shepherd G M 1978 Microcircuits in the nervous system. Sci Am 238: 92–103

Shepherd G M 1990 Synaptic organization of the brain. 3rd edition. Oxford University Press: Oxford

Shepherd G M Synaptic organization of the mammalian olfactory bulb. Physiol Rev 52:864–917

Shepherd G M, Greer C A 1990 Olfactory bulb. In: Shepherd G M (ed) Synaptic Organization of the Brain. 3rd edition. Oxford University Press: Oxford: pp 133–169

Sherer G K 1991 Vasculogenic mechanisms and epithelio-mesenchymal specificity in endodermal organs. In; Feinberg R N, Sherer G K, Auerbach R (eds) The development of the vascular system. Issues Biomed 14: 37–57

Sheridan M N, Reiter R J, Jacobs J J 1969 An interesting anatomical relationship between the hamster pineal gland and the ventricular system of the brain. J Endocr 45: 131–132

Sheridan M N, Sladek J R Jr 1975 Histofluorescence and ultrastructural analysis of hamster and monkey pineal gland. Cell Tissue Res 164: 145–152

Sherk H 1986 The claustrum and the cerebral cortex. In: Jones E G, Peters A (eds) Cerebral cortex. Vol 5. Sensory-motor areas and aspects of cortical connectivity. Plenum Press: New York: pp 467–499

Sherrington C S 1905 On reciprocal innervation of antagonistic muscles. Proc R Soc Lond B 76: 160–163

Sherrington C S 1906 The integrative action of the nervous system. Scribner: New York, reprinted by Yale University Press in 1947

Sherrington Sir C S 1947 The integrative action of the nervous system. 2nd edition. Yale University Press: New Haven, Connecticut

Sheuer J L 1964 Fibre size frequency distribution in normal human laryngeal nerves. J Anat 98: 99–104

Shewan D, Berry M, Bedi K, Cohen J 1993 Embryonic optic nerve tissue fails to support neurite outgrowth by central and peripheral neurons in vitro. Eur J Neurosci 5: 809 – 817

Shewan D, Berry M, Cohen J 1995 Extensive regeneration in vitro by early embryonic neurons in immature and adult CNS tissue. J Neurosci 15: 2057–2062

Shibasaki H, Sadato N, Lyshkow H, Yonekura Y, Honda M, Nagamine T et al 1993 Both primary motor cortex and supplementary motor area plan an important role in complex finger movement. Brain 116: 1387–1398

Shimaguchi S 1974 Tenth rib is floating in Japanese. Anat Anz 135: 72–82

Shimazu T 1986 Intermediate metabolism. In: Lightman S L, Everitt B J (eds) Neuroendocrinology. Blackwell, Oxford: pp 304–330

Shimizu Y, Newman W, Tanaka Y, Shaw S 1992 Lymphocyte interactions with endothelial cells. Immunol Today 13: 106–112

Shimozawa N, Tsukamoto T et al 1992 A human gene responsible for Zellweger syndrome that affects peroxisome assembly. Science 255: 1132–1134

Shinonga Y, Takada M, Mizuno N 1994 Direct projections from the non-laminated divisions of the medial geniculate nucleus to the temporal polar cortex and amygdala in the cat. J Comp Neurol 340: 405–426

Shipley M T, Reyes 1991 Anatomy of the human olfactory bulb and central olfactory pathways. In: Laing D G, Doty R L, Breipohl W (eds) The human sense of smell. Springer-Verlag: Berlin: pp 29–60

Shipp S, Watson J D G, Zeki S 1993 Human brain: visualizing the motion area. Curr Biol 3: 100

Shrewsbury M M, Kuzynski K 1974 Flexor digitorum superficialis tendon in the fingers of the human hand. Hand 6: 121–133

Shriver J E, Stein B M, Carpenter M B 1968 Central projections of spinal dorsal roots in the monkey. 1. Cervical and upper thoracic dorsal roots. Am J Anat 123: 27–74

Shuaib A, Israelian G, Lee M A 1989 Mesencephalic haemorrhage and unilateral pupillary deficit. J Clin Neuro Ophthalmol 9: 47–49

Shuaib A, Murphy W 1987 Mesencephalic haemorrhage and third nerve palsy. J Comput Tomogr 11: 385–388

Shuangshoti S, Netsky M G 1966 Histogenesis of choroid plexus in man. Am J Anat 118: 283–316

Shukla H, Ferrara A 1986 Rapid estimation of insertional length of umbilical catheters in newborns. AJDC 140: 786–788

Shute C C D 1956 The evolution of the mammalian ear drum and the tympanic cavity. J Anat 90: 261–281

Shute C C D, Lewis P R 1965 Cholinesterase-containing pathways of the hindbrain: afferent cerebellar and centrifugal cochlear fibres. Nature 205: 242–246

Sibley C P, Boyd R D H 1992 Mechanisms of transfer across the human placenta. In: Polin R A, Fox W W (eds) Fetal and neonatal physiology. Saunders: Philadelphia: pp 62–74

Sicher H 1962 Temporomandibular articulation: concepts and misconceptions. J Oral Surg 20: 281–284

Sick H, Koritke J G 1976 La 7e articulation sterno-costale. Arch Anat Histol Embryol 59: 151–164

Sick, H, Ring P 1976 La vascularisation de l'articulation sterno-costo-claviculaire. Arch Anat Histol Embryol 59: 71–78

Sidman R L 1970 Cell proliferation, migration and interaction in the developing mammalian central nervous system. In: Schmitt F O, Quarton G C, Melnechuk T, Adelman G (eds) The neurosciences. Second study program. Rockefeller University Press: New York: pp 100–107

Sidman R L, Angevine J, Pierce E 1971 Atlas of the mouse brain and spinal cord. Harvard Univ Press: Cambridge

Sidman R L, Miale I L, Feder N 1959 Cell proliferation and migration in the primitive ependymal zone. Exp Neurol 1: 322–333

Sieber-Blum M, Sieber F, Yamada K M 1981 Cellular fibronectin promotes adrenergic differentiation of quail neural crest cells in vitro. Experimental Cell Research 133: 285–295

Sieber-Blum, Cohen A M 1980 Clonal analysis of quail neural crest cells: they are pluripotent and differentiate in vitro in the absence of non-crest cells. Dev Biol 80: 96–106

Siegel P, Mengert W F 1961 Internal iliac artery ligation in obstetrics and gynecology. J Am Med Assoc 181: 1059–1062

Siegel S 1988 Drug anticipation and drug tolerance. In: Lader M (ed) The psychopharmacology of addiction. Br Assoc Psychopharmacol Monograph No 10. Oxford University Press: Oxford: pp 73–96

Siekevitz P, Palade G E 1960 A cytochemical study on the pancreas of the guinea pig. 6. Release of enzymes and ribonucleic acid from ribonucleoprotein particles. J Biophys Biochem Cytol 7: 631–644

Sierociński W 1975 Arteries supplying the left colic flexure in man. Folia Morphol 34: 117–124

Sievers J, Hartmann D, Pehlemann F W, Berry M 1992 Development of astroglial cells in the proliferative matrices, the granule cell layer, and the hippocampal fissure of the hampster denate gyrus. J Comp Neurol 320: 1–32

Sievers J, Mangold U, Berry M, Allen C, Schlossberger H G 1981 Experimental studies on cerebellar foliation. I. A qualitative morphological analysis of cerebellar fissuration defects after neonatal treatment with 6-OHDA in the rat. J Comp Neurol 203: 751–769

Sievers J, Pehlemann F W, Gude S, Berry M 1994 Meningeal cells organise the superficial glia limitans of the cerebellum and produce components of both the interstitial matrix and the basement membrane. J Neurocytol 23: 135 – 149

Sievers J, Pehlemann F W, Gude S, Hartman D, Berry M 1994 The development of the radial glial scaffold of the cerebeller cortex from GFAP-positive cells in the external granular layer. J Neurocytol 23: 97–115

Sievers J, Schmidtmayer J, Parwaresch R 1994 Blood monocytes and spleen macrophages differentiate into microglia-like cells when cultured on astrocytes. Ann Anat 176: 45–51

Sigal M J, Pitaru S, Aubin J E, Ten Cate A R 1984 A combined scanning electron microscopy and immunofluorescence study demonstrating that the odontoblast process extends to the dentinoenamel junction in human teeth. Anat Rec 210: 453–462

Sikri K L, Foster C L 1981 Light and electron microscopical observation on the macula densa of the Syrian hamster kidney. J Anat 132: 57–69

Silva D G, Hart J A L 1967 Ultrastructural observations on the mandibular condyle of the guinea pig. J Ultrastruct Res 20: 227–243

Silva D G, Kailis D G 1972 Ultrastructural studies on the cervical loop and the development of the amelo-dentinal junction in the cat. Arch Oral Biol 17: 279–290

Silver I A 1973 Some factors affecting wound healing. Equine Vet J 5: 47–51

Silver J A 1984 The physiology of wound healing. Schweiz Rundschau Med (praxis) 73: 30

Silver J, Rutishauser U 1984 Dev Biol 106: 485–499

Silver J, Sidman R S 1980 J Comp Neurol 189: 101–111

Silver M D, Lam J H C, Ranganathan N, Wigle E D 1971 Morphology of the human tricuspid valve. Circulation 43: 333–348

Silver P H 1956 The role of the peritoneum in the formation of the septum recto-vesicle. J Anat 90: 538–546

Silver W L, Farley L G, Finger T E 1991 The effects of neonatal capsaicin administration on trigeminal nerve chemoreceptors in the rat nasal cavity. Brain Res 561: 212–216

Silverman W F, Sladek J R 1991 Ultrastructural changes in magnocellular neurons from the supraoptic nucleus of aged rats. Devl Brain Res 58: 25–34

Silverstein H 1984 Cochlear and vestibular nerves: gross and histological anatomy as seen from the postauricular approach. Otolaryngology 92: 207 – 211

Silverstein H, Davies D G, Griffin W L Jr 1969 Cochlear aqueduct obstruction: changes in perilymph biochemistry. Ann Otol Rhinol Laryngol 78: 532–541

Silverstein H, Norrell H, Haberkamp T, McDaniel A B 1986 The unrecognised rotation of the vestibular and cochlear nerves from the labyrinth to the brain stem: its implications to surgery of the eighth cranial nerve. Otolaryngol Head Neck Surg 95: 543–549

Simard L C 1937 Les complexes neuro-insulaires du pancréas humain. Arch Anat Microsc 33: 49–64

Simeone A, Acampora D, Arcioni L, Andrews P W, Boncinelli E, Mavilio F 1990 Sequential activation of Hox 2 homeobox genes by retinoic acid in human embryonic carcinoma cells. Nature 346: 763–766

Simeone A, Acampora D, Gulisano M, Stornaiuolo A, Boncinelli E 1992 Nature 358: 687–690

Simionescu M, Simionescu N, Palade G E 1982 Preferential distribution of anionic sites on the basement membrane and the albuminal aspect of the endothelium in fenestrated capillaries. J Cell Biol 95: 425–434

Simionescu M, Simionescu N, Palade G E 1984 Partial chemical characterization of the anionic sites in the basal lamina of fenestrated capillaries. Microvasc Res 28: 352–367

Simionescu R 1985 Le risque anesthesique des metasteses cancereuses. Cah Anesthesiol 33(2): 127–129

Simmonds S J 1989 Weight in infancy and death from ischaemic heart disease. Lancet 2: 577–580

Simons K, Fuller S D 1985 Cell surface polarity in epithelia. Annu Rev Cell Biol 1: 243–288

Simons P, Reid L 1969 Muscularity of pulmonary arterial branches in the upper and lower lobes of the normal young and aged lung. Br J Dis Chest 63: 38–44

Simpson D A 1952 The efferent fibres of the hippocampus in the monkey. J Neurol Neurosurg Psychiatry 15: 79–92

Sims K S, Williams R S 1990 The human amygdaloid complex: a cytologic and histochemical atlas using nissl, myelin, acetylcholinesterase and nicotinamide adenine dinucleotide phosphate diaphorase staining. Neuroscience 36: 449–472

Sinclair D 1967 Cutaneous sensation. Oxford University Press: London

Sinclair D 1969 Human growth after birth. Oxford University Press: London

Sinclair D 1985 Human growth after birth. 4th edition. Oxford University Press: Oxford

Sindou M, Quoex O, Baleydier C 1974 Fibre organization at the posterior spinal cord–rootlet junction in man. J Comp Neurol 153: 15–26

Singer C 1931 A short history of biology. Clarendon Press: Oxford

Singer C, Underwood E A 1962 A short history of medicine. 2nd edition. Clarendon Press: Oxford

Singer I I 1979 The fibronexus; a transmembrane association of fibronectin-containing fibers and bundles of 5 nm microfilaments in hamster and human fibroblasts. Cell 16: 675–685

Singer I I, Kawka D W, Kazarzis D M, Clark R A F 1984 In vivo co-distribution of fibronection and actin fibers in granulation tissue: immunofluorescence and electron microscope studies of the fibronexus at the myo-fibroblast surface. J Cell Biol 98: 2091–2106

Singer M, Nordlander R H, Edgar M 1979 J Comp Neurol 185: 1–22

Singer N G, Todd R F, Fox D A 1994 Structures on the cell surface. Update from fifth International Workshop on human leucocyte differentiation antigens. Arthritis and Rheumatism 37: 1245–1248

Singer R 1953 Estimation of age from cranial suture closure: report on its unreliability. J For Med 1: 52–59

Singer S J, Nicolson G L 1972 The fluid mosaic model of the structure of cell membranes. Science 175: 720–731

Singh I 1959 Variations in the metacarpal bones. J Anat 93: 262–267

Singh I 1960 Variations in the metatarsal bones. J Anat 94: 345–350

Singh J, Knight R T 1993 Effects of posterior association cortex lesions on brain potentials preceding self-initiated movements. J Neurosci 13: 1820–1829

Singh M, Webster P D 1978 Neurohormonal control of pancreatic secretion. A review. Gastroenterology 74: 294–309

Singh S 1965 Variations of the superior articular facets of atlas vertebrae. J Anat 99: 565–571

Singh S, Dass R 1960 The central artery of the retina. I. Origin and course. II. A study of its distribution and anastomoses. Br J Ophthalmol 44: 193–212, 280–299

Singh S, Potturi B R 1978 Greater sciatic notch in sex determination. J Anat 125: 619–624

Singh S, Singh S P 1974 Weight of the femur – a useful measurement for identification of sex. Acta Anat 87: 141–145

Singh S, Singh S P 1975 Identification of sex from tarsal bones. Acta Anat 93: 568–573

Sinha D N 1985 Cancellous structure of tarsal bones. J Anat 140: 111–117

Sinnreich Z, Nathan H 1981 The ciliary ganglion in man. Anat Anz 150: 287–297

Sirang H 1973 Ein canalis alae ossis ilii und seine bedeutrung. Anat Anz 133: 225–238

Sirigu P, Turno F, Usai E, Perra M T 1993 Histochemical study of the human bulbourethral (Cowper's) glands. Andrologia 25: 292–299

Sjöström M, Downham D Y, Lexell J 1986 Distribution of different fiber types in human skeletal muscles: why is there a difference within a fascicle? Muscle Nerve 9: 30–36

Sjöström M, Squire J M 1977 Fine structure of the A-band in cryo-sections. The structure of the A-band of human skeletal muscle fibres from ultra-thin cryo-sections negatively stained. J Mol Biol 109: 49–68

Skakkebaek N E 1987 Carcinoma-in-situ and cancer of the testis. Int J Androl 10: 1–40

Skakkebaek N E, Grigor K M, Giwercman A, Rorth M (eds) 1993 Management and biology of carcinoma in situ and cancer of the testis. Karger: Basel: pp 1–256

Skalli O, Schurch W, Seemayer T, Lagace R, Montandon D, Pittet B, Gabbiani G 1989 Myofibroblasts from diverse pathologic settings are heterogeneous in their content of actin isoforms and intermediate filamental proteins. Lab Invest 60: 275–285

Skerrow D, Skerrow C S (eds) 1985 Methods in skin research. Wiley: Chichester

Skoglund S 1956 Anatomical and physiological studies of knee joint innervation in the cat. Acta Physiol Scand 36 (suppl 124): 1–101

Skoglund S 1973 Joint receptors and kinaesthesis. In: Iggo A (ed) Handbook of sensory physiology. Vol 2. Springer: Berlin: pp 110–136

Skok V I 1973 Physiology of autonomic ganglia. Igaku-Shoin: Tokyo

Skoog T 1967 The superficial transverse fibres of the palmar aponeuroses and their significance in Dupuytren's contracture. Surg Clin N America 47: 443–444

Skornicki R, Zienianski, A, Orebbwski A 1968 Galaz Zewnetrzna nerwu krtaniowego gornego u czlowieka i psa. Folia Morphol 27: 79–87

Skrandies W 1993 Monocular and binocular neuronal activity in human visual cortex revealed by electrical brain activity mapping. Exp Brain Res 93: 516–520

Slack J M W 1991 From egg to embryo. 2nd edition. Cambridge University Press: Cambridge

Slavin B G 1985 The morphology of adipose tissue. In: Cryer A, Van R

L R (eds) New Perspectives in adipose tissue: structure, function and development. Butterworths: London: pp 23–43

Sledzinski Z, Tyszkiewicz T 1975 Hepatic veins of the right part of the liver in man. Folia Morphol 34: 315–322

Sleigh M A 1974 Cilia and flagella. Editor. Academic Press: London

Sleigh M A 1977 The nature and action of respiratory tract cilia. In: Brain J D, Proctor D F, Reid L M (eds) Respiratory defense mechanisms. Part 1. Dekker: New York: pp 247–288

Slipka J, Kotyza F 1987 O Structure a funkci krypt patrovych mandli. Ceskoslovenska otolaryngologie 36: 209–216

Sloan P 1978 Scanning electron microscopy of the collagen fibre architecture of the rabbit incisor periodontium. Archs Oral Biol 23: 567–572

Small J V 1977 Studies on isolated smooth muscle cells: the contractile apparatus. J Cell Sci 24: 327–349

Small J V 1985 Geometry of actin-membrane attachments in the smooth muscle cell: the localisations of vinculin and α-actinin. EMBO J 4: 45–49 9

Small J V, Herzog M, Barth M, Draeger A 1990 Supercontracted state of vertebrate smooth muscle cell fragments reveals myofilament lengths. J Cell Biol 111: 2451–2461

Small J V, North A J 1993 Architecture of the smooth muscle cell. In: Schwartz S M (ed) Smooth muscle cells: molecular and cell biology. Academic Press: New York (in press)

Small N C 1992 Complications in arthroscopic surgery. In: Aichroth P M, Cannon W D (eds) Knee surgery. Martin Dunitz: London

Smart I 1971 Location and orientation of mitotic figures in the developing mouse olfactory epithelium. J Anat 109: 243–251

Smart I H M 1982 Radial unit analysis of hippocampal histogenesis in the mouse. J Anat 135: 763–793

Smart I H M 1983 Three dimensional growth of the mouse isocortex. J Anat 137: 683–694

Smart I H M, McSherry G M 1982 Growth patterns in the lateral wall of the mouse telencephalon. II. Histological changes during and subsequent to the period of isocortical neuron production. J Anat 134: 415–442

Smeele L E 1988 Ontogeny of relationship of human middle ear and temporomandibular (squamomandibular) joint. Acta Anat 131: 338–341

Smerdu V, Karsch-Mizrachi I, Campione M, Leinwand L, Schiaffino S 1994 Type IIX myosin heavy chain transcripts are expressed in type IIB fibers of human skeletal muscle. Am J Physiol 267 (Cell Physiol): C1723–1728

Smerdu V, Karschmizrachi I, Campione M, Leinwand L, Schiaffino S 1994 Type IIX myosin heavy chain transcripts are expressed in type IIB fibers of human skeletal muscle. Am J Physiol-Cell Physiol 36: C1723–C1728

Smeyne R J, Klein R, Schnapp A, Long L K, Bryant S, Lewin A, Lira S A, Barbacid M 1994 Nature 368: 246–248

Smillie I S 1948 The congenital discoid meniscus. J Bone Jt Surg 30B: 671–682

Smith C A 1959 The physiology of the newborn infant. 3rd edition. Blackwell Scientific: Oxford

Smith C L, Hollyday M 1983 The development and post natal organisation of motor nuclei in the rat thoracic spinal cord. J Comp Neurol 220: 16–28

Smith E M, Brosan P, Meyer W J III, Blalock J E 1987 An ACTH receptor on human mononuclear leukocytes. N Engl J Med 317: 1266–1269

Smith G E 1903 Notes on the morphology of the cerebellum. J Anat 37: 329–332

Smith G E 1907 New studies on the folding of the visual cortex and the significance of the occipital sulci in the human brain. J Anat 41: 198–207

Smith G E 1908a The cerebral cortex in Lepidosiren with comparative notes on the interpretation of certain features of the forebrain with other vertebrates. Anat Anz 33: 513–550

Smith G E 1908b Studies in the anatomy of the pelvis, with special reference to the fasciae and visceral supports. I and II. J Anat 42: 191–218, 251–270

Smith G T 1963 The renal vascular patterns in man. J Urol 89: 274–288

Smith G V, Stevenson J A 1988 Peripheral nerve grafts lacking Schwann cells fail to support central nervous system axonal regeneration. Exp Brain Res 69: 299–301

Smith J C 1987 Development 99: 3–14

Smith J M, Savage R J G 1959 The mechanics of mammalian jaws. School Sci Rev 141: 289–301

Smith J W 1954 Muscular control of the arches of the foot in standing: an electromyographic assessment. J Anat 88: 152–163

Smith J W 1956 Observations on the postural mechanism of the human knee joint. J Anat 90: 236–260

Smith J W 1958 The ligamentous structures in the canalis and sinus tarsi. J Anat 92: 616–620

Smith J W 1962a The relationship of epiphysial plates to stress in some bones of the lower limb. J Anat 96: 58–78

Smith J W 1962b The structure and stress relation of fibrous epiphysial plates. J Anat 96: 209–225

Smith J W, Walmsley R 1951 Experimental incision of the intervertebral disc. J Bone Jt Surg 33B: 612–625

Smith J W, Walmsley R 1959 Factors affecting the elasticity of bone. J Anat 93: 505–523

Smith K J, Hall S M 1988 Peripheral demyelination and remyelination initiated by the calcium-selective ionophore ionomycin: in vivo observations. J Neurol Sci 83: 37–53

Smith M C 1957 The anatomy of the spino-cerebellar fibres in man. 1. The course of the fibres in the spinal cord and brain stem. J Comp Neurol 108: 285–352

Smith M C 1967 Stereotatic operations for Parkinson's disease-anatomical considerations. In: Williams D (ed) Modern trends in neurology. Butterworths: London: pp 21–52

Smith M C 1976 Retrograde cell changes in human spinal cord after anterolateral cordotomies. Location and identification after different periods of survival. Adv Pain Res Ther 1: 91–98

Smith M C, Deacon P 1981 Helweg's triangular tract in man. Brain 104: 249–277

Smith M C, Deacon P 1984 Topographical anatomy of the posterior columns of the spinal cord in man. The long ascending fibres. Brain 107: 671–698

Smith M M, Hall B K 1993 A developmental model for evolution of the vertebrate exoskeleton and teeth. The role of cranial and trunk neural crest. In: Hecht M K et al (eds) Evolutionary biology vol 27. Plenum Press: New York: pp 387–448

Smith P, Porte D 1976 Neuropharmacology of the pancreatic islets. Annu Rev Pharmacol Toxicol 16: 269–285

Smith R A, Seif M W, Rogers A W, Li T-C, Dockery P, Cooke I D, Aplin J D 1989 The endometrial cycle: the expression of a secretory component correlated with the luteinising hormone peak. Human Reprod 4: 236–242

Smith R B 1970 The development of the intrinsic innervation of the human heart between the 10 and 70 mm stages. J Anat 107: 271–280

Smith R B 1971 Intrinsic innervation of the human heart in foetuses between 70 mm and 420 mm crown–rump length. Acta Anat 78: 200–209

Smith R B, Taylor I M 1972 Observations of the intrinsic innervation of the human fetal oesophagus between the 10 mm and 140 mm crown-rump length stages. Acta Anat 81: 127–138

Smith R, Sanders W J, Stewart K C 1974 Blood supply to the levator scapulae muscle relative to carotid artery protection. Trans Am Acad Ophthalmol Otolaryngol 78: 128–134

Smith U, Ryan J W 1970 An electron microscopic study of the vascular endothelium as a site for bradykinin and adenosine-5'-triphosphate inactivation in the rat lung. Adv Exp Med Biol 8: 249–261

Smith U, Ryan J W 1973 Electron microscopy of endothelial cells collected on cellulose acetate paper. Tissue Cell 5: 333–336

Smith W C, Knecht A K, Wu M, Harland R M 1993 Nature 361: 547–549

Smolen A, Raisman G 1980 Synapse formation in the rat superior cervical ganglion during normal development and after neonatal deafferentation. Brain Res 181: 315–328

Smout C F V, Jacoby F, Lillie E W 1969 Gynaecological and obstetrical anatomy and functional histology. Arnold: London

Smuts MS 1977 Concanavalin A binding to the epithelial surface of the developing mouse olfactory placode. Anat Rec 188: 29–37

Smyrnis N, Taira M, Ashe J, Georgopoulos A P 1992 Motor cortical activity in a memorized delay task. Exp Brain Res 92: 139–151

Smyth G E 1939 Systemisation and central connections of spinal tract and nucleus of trigeminal; clinical and pathological study. Brain 62: 41–87

Sneath R S 1955 The insertion of the biceps femoris. J Anat 89: 550–553

Snook T 1950 A comparative study of the vascular arrangements in mammalian spleens. Am J Anat 87: 31–78

Snrow M M L Environmental influences on fetal growth: effects and consequences. In: Sharp F, Fraser R B, Malner R D G (eds) Fetal growth. Royal College of Obstetricians and Gynaecologists Press: London: pp 115–125

Snyder F F 1924 Changes in the human oviduct during the menstrual cycle and pregnancy. Bull Johns Hopkins Hosp 35: 141–146

Snyder L S, Hertz M I, Peterson M S, Harmon K R, Marinello W A, Henke C A, Greenheck J R, Chen B, Bitterman P 1991 Acute lung injury. Pathogenesis of intralveolar fibrosis. J Clin Invest 88: 663–673

Snyder S H, Sklar P B, Hwang P M, Pevsner J 1989 Molecular mechanisms of olfaction Trends Neurosci 12: 35–38

Soames R W, Atha J 1981 The role of the antigravity musculature during quiet standing in man. Eur J Appl Physiol 47: 159–167

Sobel R A, Mitchell M E, Fondren G 1990 Intercellular adhesion molecule-1 (ICAM-1) in cellular immune reactions in the human central nervous system. Am J Pathol 136: 1309

Sobieszek A, Small J V 1977 Regulation of the actin–myosin interaction in vertebrate smooth muscle: activation via a myosin light-chain kinase and the effect of tropomyosin. J Molec Biol 112: 559–576

Sobotka S, Ringo J L 1993 Investigation of long term recognition and association memory in unit responses from inferotemporal cortex. Exp Brain Res 96: 28–38

Sobue K, Sellers J R 1991 Caldesmon, a novel regulatory protein in smooth muscle and nonmuscle actomyosin systems. J Biol Chem 266: 12115–12118

Sohval A R 1954 Histopathology of cryptorchidism; studies based upon comparative histology of retained and scrotal testes from birth to maturity. Am J Med 16: 346–362

Soifer D (ed) 1986 Dynamic aspects of microtubule biology. Ann N Y Acad Sci 466

Soji T, Nishizono H, Yashiro T, Herbert D C 1991 Intercellular communication within the rat anterior pituitary gland. III. Postnatal development and periodic changes of cell-to-cell communication in female rats. Anat Rec 231: 351–357

Sokoloff A J Deacon T W 1992 Musculotopic organization of the hypoglossal nucleus in the cynomolgus monkey, *Macaca fascicularis*. J Comp Neurol 324: 81–93

Sokoloff L 1993 Microcracks in the calcified layer of articular cartilage. Arch Pathol Lab Med 117: 191–195

Solanke T F 1968 The blood supply of the vermiform appendix in Nigerians. J Anat 102: 353–362

Solari A J, Tres L L 1967 The ultrastructure of the human sex vesicle. Chromosoma 22: 16–31

Solcia E, Capella C, Buffa R, Usellini L, Fiocca R, Frigerio B, Tenti P, Sessa F 1981 The diffuse endocrine-paracrine system of the gut in health and disease: ultrastructural features. Scand J Gastroenterol (suppl) 70: 25–36

Solcia E, Sampietro R, Capella C 1969 Different staining of catecholamines, 5 hydroxytryptamine and related compounds in aldehyde fixed tissues. Histochemie 17: 273–283

Solcia E, Vassalo G, Capella C 1968 Selective staining of endocrine cells by basic dyes after acid hydrolysis. Stain Technol 43: 257–263

Sollinger H W, Cook K, Kamps D, Glass N R, Belzer F O 1984 Clinical and experimental experience with pancreaticocystostomy for exocrine pancreatic drainage in pancreas tranplantation. Transplant Proc 16: 749–751

Solter D 1988 Differential imprinting and expression of maternal and paternal genomes. Ann Rev Gen 22: 127–146

Solter M, Paljan D 1973 Variations in shape and dimensions of sigmoid groove, venous portion of jugular foramen, jugular fossa, condylar and mastoid foramina classified by age, sex and body size. Z Anat EntwGesch 140: 319–335

Soltero-Harrington L R, Garcia-Rinaldi R, Albe L W 1969 Total aganglionosis of the colon: recognition and management. J Pediat Surg 4: 330–338

Solursh M 1984 Cell and matrix interactions during limb chondrogenesis in vitro. In: Threlstad R L (ed) The role of extracellular matrix in development Alan R Liss: New York: p 277

Soma et al 1975 Serum gonadotrophin levels in Japanese women. Obstet Gynecol 46: 311

Somlyo A P 1993 Myosin isoforms in smooth muscle: how may they affect function and structure? J Musc Res Cell Motil 14: 557–563

Somlyo A V, Bond M, Somlyo A P, Scarpa A 1985b Inositol triphosphate-induced calcium release and contraction in vascular smooth muscle. Proc Natl Acad Sci USA 82: 5231–5235

Somlyo A V, Franzini-Armstrong C 1985 New views of smooth muscle structure using freezing, deep-etching and rotary shadowing. Experientia 41: 841–856

Somlyo A V, Somlyo A P 1993 Intracellular signaling in vascular smooth muscle. In: Sideman S, Beyar R (eds) Interactive phenomena in the cardiac system. Plenum Press: New York: pp 31–38

Sommer B, Seeburg P H 1992 Glutamate receptor channels: novel properties and new clones. Tips 13: 291–296

Sommer J R, Jennings R B 1986 Ultrastructure of cardiac muscle. In: Fozzard H A, Haber E, Jennings R B, Katz A, Morgan H E (eds) The heart and cardiovascular system. Vol 1. Raven Press: New York

Somogyi B, Undi F, Kausz M 1973 Blood supply of the spinal ganglia. Morphol Igazsagugyi Orv Sz 13: 191–195

Somogyi P, Cowey A 1984 Double bouquet cells. In: Peters A, Jones E G (eds) Cerebral cortex. Vol 1. Cellular components of the cerebral cortex. Plenum Press: New York: pp 337–360

Somogyi P, Kisvárday Z F, Martin K A C, Whitteridge D 1983 Synaptic connections of morphologically identified and physiologically characterized large basket cells in the striate cortex of the cat. Neuroscience 10: 261–294

Somogyi P, Soltész I 1986 Immunogold demonstration of GABA in synaptic terminals of intracellularly recorded, horseradish peroxidase-filled basket cells and clutch cells in the cat's visual cortex. Neuroscience 19: 1051–1065

Sone S, Higashihara T, Morimoto S, Yokota K, Ikezoe J, Masaoka A, Monden Y, Kagotani T 1980 Normal anatomy of thymus and anterior mediastimun by pneumomediastinography. AJR 134: 81–89

Sonesson B 1959 The functional anatomy of the cricoarytenoid joint. Z Anat Entwicklungsgesch 121: 292–303

Sontheimer R D 1989 Perivascular dendritic macrophages as immunobiological constituents of the human dermal microvascular unit. J Invest Dermatol 93: 96S–101S

Soo K C, Guiloff R J, Oh A, Querci Della Rovere G, Westbury G 1990 Innervation of the trapezius muscle: a study in patients undergoing neck dissections. Head Neck Surg 12: 488–495

Soo K C, Hamlyn P J, Pegington J, Westbury G 1986 Anatomy of the accessory nerve and its cervical contributions in the neck. Head Neck Surg 9: 111–115

Sorgente N, Brownell A, Slavkin H C 1977 Basal lamina degradation: the identification of mammalian-like collagenase activity in mesenchymal-derived matrix vesicles. Biochem Biophys Res Commun 74: 448–454

Soriano P, Jaenisch R 1986 Retroviruses as probes for mammalian development: allocation of cells to the somatic and germ cell lineages. Cell 46: 19–29

Sorokin S P 1968 Reconstructions of centriole formation and ciliogenesis in mammalian lungs. J Cell Sci 3: 207–230

Sorsby A, Sheridan M 1960 The eye at birth: measurements of the principal diameters in forty-eight cadavers. J Anat 94: 192–197

Soslowsky L J, Flatow E L, Bigliani L U, Mow V C 1992b Articular geometry of the glenohumeral joint. Clin Orthop 285: 181–190

Soslowsky L J, Flatow E L, Bigliani L U, Pawluk R J, Ateshian G A, Mow V C 1992a Quantitation of in situ contact areas at the glenohumeral joint: a biomechanical study. J Orthop Res 10: 524–534

Sotelo C, Alvarado-Mallart R M 1991 The reconstruction of cerebellar circuits. TINS 14: 350–355

Souter W A 1977 Total replacement arthroplasty of the elbow. In: Joint replacement in the upper limb. Inst Mech Eng Conference Pubs 1997–5: London: pp 99–106

Souter W A 1990 Surgery of the rheumatoid elbow. Ann Rheum Dis 49: 871–882

Southam J A 1959 The inferior mesenteric ganglion. J Anat 93: 304–308

Sow M L, Dintimille H, Padonov N, Sylla S, Argenson C 1975 La vascularisatio veineuse du pancréas. Bull Assoc Anat (Nancy) 59: 255–264

Spaček J, Lieberman A R 1974 Ultrastructure and three dimensional organization of synaptic glomeruli in rat somatosensory thalamus. J Anat 117: 487–516

Spach M S, Kootsey J M 1983 The nature of electrical propagation in cardiac muscle. Am J Physiol 244 suppl H: 3–22

Spadaro J A 1991 Bioelectrical properties of bone and response of bone to electrical stimuli. In: Hall B K (ed) Bone. Vol 3. Bone matrix and bone-specific products. CRC Press: Boca Raton: pp 109–140

Spalteholtz W 1924 Die Arterien der Herzwand. Anatomische Untersuchungen an Menschen und Tieren. Hirzel: Leipzig

Spanidis A, Wunsch H, Kaissling B, Kris W 1982 Three-dimensional shape of a Goormaghtigh cell and its contact with a granular cell in the rabbit kidney. Anat Embryol 165: 239–252

Spanner R 1932 Neue Befunde über die Blutwege der Darmwand und ihre funktionelle Bedeutung. Morphol Jahrb 69: 394–454

Spatz W B, Illing R-B, Vogt Weisenhorn D M 1994 Distribution of cytochrome oxidase and parvalbumin in the primary visual cortex of the adult and neonate monkey, Callithrix jacchus. J Comp Neurol 339: 519–534

Speakman H G B, Weisberg J 1977 The vastus medialis controversy. Physiotherapy 63: 249–254

Speckmann E-J, Elger C E 1987 Introduction to the neurophysiological basis of the EEG and DC potentials. In: Niedermeyer E, Lopes da Silva F (eds) Electroencephalography. Urban and Schwarzenberg: Baltimore: pp 1–14

Speed R M 1988 The possible role of meiotic pairing anomalies in the atresia of human fetal oocytes. Hum Genet 78: 260–266

Speidel C C 1932 Studies of living nerves. I. The movements of individual sheath cells and nerve sprouts correlated with the process of myelin sheath formation in amphibian larvae. J Exp Zool 61: 279–331

Speidel C C 1933 Studies of living nerves. II. Activities of ameboid growth cones, sheath cells, and myelin segments, as revealed by prolonged observations of individual nerve fibers in frog tadpoles. Am J Anat 52: 1–80

Spemann H 1901 Uber Korrelationen in der Entwicklung des Auges. Verh Anat Ges 15: 61–79

Spemann H 1914 Uber verzoggerte keimverosogung von keimteilen. Ver d D Ges Freiberg 1914: 216–221

Spemann H 1918 Uber die Determination der ersten Organanlagen des Amphibien embryo. Roux Arch EntwMech Org 43: 448–555

Spemann H 1938 Embryonic development and induction. Yale University Press: New Haven

Spemann H, Mangold H 1924 Induction of embryonic primordia by implantation of organizers from a different species. In: Willier B H, Oppenheimer J M (eds) Foundations of experimental embryology. Hafner: New York: pp 144–184

Spemann H, Mangold H 1924 Wilhelm Roux Arch. Entw-Mech Zool 158: 9–38

Spencer H 1977 Pathology of the lung, vol 1, 3rd edition, Pergamon Press: Oxford

Spencer J, Turkel M A 1981 Stabilising mechanisms preventing anterior dislocation of the glenohumeral joint. J Bone Jt Surg 63B: 1208–1217

Spencer R F, Porter, J D 1988 Structural organization of the extraocular muscles. In: Buttner-Ennever J A (ed) Neuroanatomy of the oculomotor system. Elsevier: Amsterdam

Sperry R W 1963 Chemoaffinity in the orderly growth of nerve fiber patterns and connections. Proc Natl Acad Sci USA 50: 703–710

Sperry R W 1974 Lateral specialization in the surgically separated hemispheres. In: Schmitt F O, Worden F G (eds) The neurosciences. Third study program. MIT Press: Cambridge Massachusetts pp 5–19

Sperry R W 1984 Consciousness, personal identity and the divided brain. Neuropsychologia 17: 153–166

Spicer S S. Schulte B A, Chakrin L W 1983 Ultrastructural and histochemical observations of respiratory epithelium and glands. Exp Lung Res 4: 137–156

Spielman A I 1990 Interaction of saliva and taste. J Dent Res 69: 838–843

Spinelli F 1974 Structure and development of the renal glomerulus as revealed by scanning electron microscope. Int Rev Cytol 39: 345–378

Spira A 1962 Die lymphknotengruppen (lymphocentra) bei der Säugernein ein homologisierungsversuch. Anat Anz 111: 294–364

Spira A W, Hollenberg M J 1973 Human retinal development ultrastructure of the inner retinal layers. Dev Biol 31: 1–21

Spira J J 1957 Comparison of cardiac and pyloric sphincters. Lancet 2: 1008

Spitzer A, Karplus J 1907 Über experimentelle Lesionen an der Gebirnbasis. Arb Neurol Inst Wien 16: 348–436

Spitznas M 1970 Zur feinstruktur der sog. Membrana limitans externa der meschlichen retina. Albrecht v Graefes Arch Ophthal 180: 44–56

Spitznas M, Hogan M J 1970 Outer segments of photo-receptors and the pigmented epithelium interrelationships in the human eye. Arch Ophthal 84: 810–819

Spoendlin 1964 Organisation of the sensory hairs in the gravity receptors in utricle and saccule of the squirrel monkey. Z Zellforsch 62: 701–716

Spoendlin H 1968 In: De Reuck A V S, Knight J S (eds) Hearing mechanisms in vertebrates. Ciba Foundation Symposium. Churchill: London: pp 89–119

Spoendlin H 1975 Neuroanatomical basis of cochlear coding mechanisms. Audiology 14: 383–407

Spoendlin H 1984 Efferent innervation of the cochlea. In: Bolis L, Keynes R D, Maddrell S H P (eds) Comparative physiology of sensory systems. Cambridge University Press: Cambridge: pp 143–161

Spoendlin H 1984 Primary neurons and synapses. In: Friedmann I, Ballantyne J C (eds) Ultrastructural atlas of the inner ear. Butterworths: London: pp 133–164

Spoendlin H 1985 Anatomy of cochlear innervation. Am J Otol 6: 453–467

Spoendlin H, Schrott A 1989 Analysis of the human auditory nerve. Hear Res 43: 25–38

Sporn M B, Roberts A B 1990 Peptide growth factors and their receptors. Vols 1 and 2, Springer-Verlag: Berlin

Spornitz U M 1992 The functional morphology of the human endometrium and decidua. Adv Anat Embryol Cell Biol 124: 1–99

Sprague J M 1944 The innervation of the pharynx in the rhesus monkey, and the formation of the pharyngeal plexus in primates. Anat Rec 90: 197–208

Sprague J M 1948 A study of motor cell localization in the spinal cord of the rhesus monkey. Am J Anat 82: 1–26

Sprague J M 1958 The distribution of dorsal root fibres on motor cells in the lumbosacral spinal cord of the cat, and the site of excitatory and inhibitory terminals in monosynaptic pathways. Proc R Soc Lond [Biol] 149: 534–556

Sprague J M, Ha H 1964 The terminal fields of dorsal root fibers in the lumbosacral spinal cord of the cat, and the dendritic organization of the motor nuclei. Progr Brain Res 11: 120–154

Spranger J, Benirschke H, Hall J G et al 1982 Errors of morphogenesis: concepts and terms. Recommendations of an international working group. J Pediatr 100: 160–165

Spratt N T 1946 Formation of the primitive streak in the explanted chick blastoderm marked with carbon particles. J Exp Zool 103: 259–304

Spray D C, Burt J M 1990 Structure–activity relations of the cardiac gap junction channel. Am J Physiol 258: 195–205

Spring J, Beck K, Chiquet M, Ehrismann L 1989 Cell 59: 325–334

Springer T A 1990 Adhesion receptors of the immune system. Nature 346: 425–434

Spudich J A, Lin S 1972 Cytochalasin B, its interaction with actin and actomyosin from muscle. Proc Natl Acad Sci USA 69: 442–446

Squier C A, Johnson N W, Hopps R M 1976 Human oral mucosa: development, structure and function. Blackwell Scientific: Oxford

Squire J 1981 The structural basis of muscular contraction. Plenum Press: New York

Srinivasan H, Landsmeer J M F 1982 Internal stabilization in the thumb. J Hand Surg 7(4): 371–375

Srivastava H C 1977 Development of ossification centres in the squamous portion of the occipital bone in man. J Anat 124: 643–649

Stach W 1989 A revised morphological classifiaction of neurons in the enteric nervous system. In: Singer M V, Goebell H (eds) Nerves and the gastrointestinal tract. MTP Press Ltd: Dordrecht: pp 29–45

Stack H G 1973 The palmar fascia. Churchill Livingstone: Edinburgh

Stack M V 1964 A gravimetric study of crown growth: rate of the human deciduous dentition. Biol Neonat 6: 197–224

Staehelin L A 1974 Structure and functions of intercellular junctions. Int Rev Cytol 39: 191–283

Stafne E C 1932 Supernumary teeth. Dent Cosmos 74: 653–659

Stagmiller R B, Moor E M 1984 Effect of follicle cells on the maturation and developmental competence of ovine oocytes matured outside the follicle. Gamete Research 9: 221–229

Staheli L Y, Engel G M 1972 The natural history of torsion and other factors influencing in childhood. Clin Orthop 86: 183–186

Stålberg E, Trontelj J V 1979 Single fibre electromyography. Mirvalle Press: Old Woking, Surrey

Stalberg E, Trontelj J V 1994 Single fibre electromyography: studies in healthy and diseased muscle. 2nd edn. Raven Press: New York

Stalsberg H, DeHaan R L 1968 Endodermal movements during foregut formation in the chick embryo. Dev Biol 18: 198–215

Stamm T T 1931 The constitution of the ligamentum cruciatum cruris. J Anat 66: 80–83

Stämpfli R 1954 Saltatory conduction in nerve. Physiol Rev 34: 101–112

Stanfield J P 1960 The blood supply of the human pituitary gland. J Anat 94: 257–273

Stanka P, Bellack U, Linder A 1991 On the morphology of the terminal microvasculature during endochondral ossification in rats. Bone Miner 13: 93–101

Stanley J K 1991 The rheumatoid wrist. Curr Orthop 5: 13–21

Stanley J R, Alvarez O M, Berke E W Jr et al 1981 Detection of basement membrane zone antigens during epidermal wound healing in pigs. J Invest Dermatol 77: 240–243

Stanley J R, Woodley D T, Katz S I, Martin G R 1982 Structure and function of basement membrane. J Invest Dermatol 79: 69s–72s

Stapleton P, Weith A, Urbanek P, Kozmik Z, Busslinger M 1993 Chromosomal localisation of seven PAX genes and cloning of a novel family member, PAX-9. Nature Genetics 3: 292–298

Staprans I, Dirksen E R 1974 Microtubule protein during ciliogenesis in the mouse oviduct. J Cell Biol 62: 164–174

Stark D 1975 Embryologie, ein Lehrbuch auf Allgemein Biologischer Grundlage. 3rd edn. Thieme: Stuttgart

Stark D D, Bradley W G (eds) 1992 Magnetic resonance imaging. 2nd edition. Mosby: St Louis

Starkey P M, Clover L M, Rees M C P 1991 Variation during the menstrual cycle of immune cell populations in human endometrium. Eur J Obstet Gynecol Reprod Biol 39: 203–207

Stauffer K, Unwin N 1992 Structure of gap junction channels. Semin Cell Biol 3: 17–20

Stauffer R N, Chao E Y S, Brewster R C 1977 Force and motion analysis of the normal, diseased and prosthetic ankle joint. Clin Orthop 127: 189–196

Steel F L D, Tomlinson J D W 1958 The 'carrying angle' in man. J Anat 92: 315–317

Steele D G 1970 Estimation of stature from fragments of long limb bones. In: Stewart T D (ed) Personal identification in mass disasters. Smithsonian Institute: Washington DC

Steele D G 1976 The estimation of sex on the basis of the talus and calcaneum. Am J Phys Anthropol 45: 581–588

Steele E J, Blunt M J 1956 The blood supply of the optic nerve and chiasma in man. J Anat 90: 486–493

Steele G E, Weller R E 1993 Subcortical connections of subdivisions of inferior temporal cortex in squirrel monkeys. Visual Neurosci 10: 563–583

Steele G E, Weller R E, Cusick C G 1991 Cortical connections of the caudal subdivision of the dorsolateral area (V4) in monkeys. J Comp Neurol 306: 495–520

Stein B E, Dixon J P 1978 Superior colliculus cells respond to noxious stimuli. Brain Res 158: 65–78

Stein J F 1992 The representation of egocentric space in the posterior parietal cortex. Behav Brain Sci 15: 691–700

Stein J, Glickstein M 1992 The role of the cerebellum in the visual guidance of movement. Physiol Rev 72: 967–1017

Steindler A 1955 Kinesiology of the human body under normal pathological conditions. 1. Movement. 2 Muscles. Thomas: Springfield, Illinois

Steinhardt G 1958 Anatomy and physiology of the temporomandibular joint: effect of function. Int Dent J 8: 155–156

Steinman R M, Lustig D S, Cohn Z A 1974 Identification of a novel cell type in peripheral lymphoid organs of mice. II. Functional properties in vitro. J Exp Med 139: 380–397

Steinmann G G 1986 Changes in the human thymus during ageing. In: Müller-Hermelink H K (ed) The human thymus. Histophysiology and pathology. Springer-Verlag: Berlin: pp 43–88

Steinmann G G, Müller-Hermelink H K 1984b Lymphocyte differentiation and its microenvironment in the human thymus. Monogr Dev Biol 17: 142–155

Steinmetz M A, Connor C E, Constantinidis C, McLaughlin J R 1994 Covert attention suppresses neuronal responses in area 7a of the posterior parietal cortex. J Neurophysiol 72: 1020–1023

Steinschneider M, Schroeder C E, Arezzo J C, Vaughan H G Jr 1993 Temporal encoding of phonetic features in auditory cortex. Ann NY Acad Sci 682: 415–417

Stenström S 1946 Untersuchungen über die Variation and Kovariation der optischen Elemente des menschlichen Auges. Acta Ophthal Suppl 26: 1–103

Stephan H 1975 Allocortex. Handbuch der Mikroscopischen Anatomie des Menschen. 4th edition. Springer-Verlag: Berlin: pp 1–998

Stephan H 1983 Evolutionary trends in limbic structures. Neurosci Behav Res 7: 367–374

Stephens N L, Kroeger E A 1980 Ultrastructure, biophysics, and biochemistry of airway smooth muscle. In: Nadel J A (ed) Physiology and pharmacology of the airways. Dekker: New York (Lung Biology in Health and Disease 15): pp 31–121

Steriade M, McCormick D A, Sejnowski T J 1993 Thalamocortical oscillations in the sleeping and arousal brain. Science 262: 679–685

Stern C D, Canning D R 1990 Origin of cells giving rise to mesoderm and endoderm in chick embryo. Nature 343: 273–275

Stern C D, Ireland G W, Herrick S E, Gherardi E, Gray J, Perryman M, Stoker M 1990 Development 110: 1271–1284

Stern J T Jr 1972 Anatomical and functional specializations of the human gluteus maximus. Am J Phys Anthrop 36: 315–340

Stern J T Jr 1974 Computer modelling of gross muscle dynamics. J Biomech 7: 411–428

Stern J T Jr, Larson S G 1993 Electromyographic study of the obturator muscles in non-human primates: implications for interpreting the obturator externus groove of the femur. J Hum Evol 24: 403–427

Stern K 1938 Note on nucleus ruber magno-cellularis and its efferent pathway in man. Brain 61: 284–289

Stevens A, Lowe J 1992 Histology. Gower Medical: London: pp 95–99

Stevens J M, Kendall B E, Crockard H A, Ransford A 1991 The odontoid process in Morquio-Brailsford's disease. The effects of occipito-cervical fusion. J Bone Jt Surg 73B: 851–858

Stevens R T, London S M, Apkarian A V 1993 Spinothalamocortical projections to the secondary somatosensory cortex (SII) in squirrel monkey. Brain Res 631: 241–246

Stevenson B R, Siliciano J D, Mooseker M S, Goodenough D A 1986 Identification of ZO-1: a high molecular weight polypeptide associated with the tight junction (zonula occludens) in a variety of epithelia. J Cell Biol 103: 755–766

Stevenson P H 1924 Age order of epiphysial union in man. Am J Phys Anthrop 7: 53–93

Stewart J 1992 Neurobiology of conditioning to drugs of abuse. In Kalivas P W, Samson H (eds) The neurobiology of drug and alcohol addiction. Ann New York Acad Sci 654 New York: pp 335–346

Stewart J, Eikelboom R 1987 Conditioned drug effects. In: Iversen L L, Iversen S D, Snyder S H (eds) Handbook of psychopharmacology 19: 1–57. Plenum Press: New York

Stewart M 1993 Intermediate filament structure and assembly. Curr Opin Cell Biol 5: 3–11

Stewart M E 1992 Sebaceous gland lipids. In: Maibach H L, Downing D T (eds) Seminars in dermatology. No. 11. Saunders: Philadelphia: pp. 100–195

Stewart M E, Downing D T, Strauss J S 1983 Sebum secretion and sebaceous lipids. Dermatol Clinics 3: 335–345

Stewart P A, Hayakawa E M 1987 Interendothelial junctional changes underlie the developmental 'tightening' of the blood–brain barrier. Dev Brain Res 32: 271–281

Stewart T D 1954 Evaluation of evidence from the skeleton. In: Gradwohl R E H (ed) Legal medicine. Mosby: St Louis: pp 407–450

Stewart W B, Shepherd G M 1985 The chemical senses: taste and smell. In: Swash M, Kennard C (eds) Scientific basis of clinical neurology. Churchill Livingstone: Edinburgh: pp 214–224

Stieve H 1927 Der Halsteil der menschlichen Gebärmutter sein Bau und seine Aufgaben während der Schwangerschaft, der Geburt und des Wochenbeltes. Akadem. Verlags-gesellschaft: Leipzig

Stilling B 1846 Disquisitiones de structura et functionibus Cerebri: de structura pontis, Varoli. F Maukius: Jena

Stilling B, Wallach J 1842–43 Untersuchungen über den Bau des Nervensystems. 2 vols. 1. Untersuchungen über die Textur des Rückenmarks. 2. Über die Medulla Oblongata. O Wigand: Leipzig

Stillman R 1982 In utero exposure to diethylstilbestrol: adverse effects on the reproductive tract and reproductive performance in male and female offspring. Am J Obst Gynecol 142: 905–921

Stillwell D L Jr 1957 The innervation of tendons and aponeuroses. Am J Anat 100: 289–318

Stimler N P, Bach M K, Bloor C M, Hugli T E 1982 Release of leukotrienes from guinea pig lung stimulated by $C5a_{desArg}$ anaphylatoxin. J Immunol 128: 2247–2257

Stimson W H, Hunter I C 1980 Oestrogen-induced immunoregulation mediated through the thymus. J Clin Lab Invest 4: 27–33

Stirling J W, Chandler J A 1976 Ultrastructural studies of the female breast. I 9 + 0 cilia in myoepithelial cells. Anat Rec 186: 413–416

Stirling J W, Chandler J A 1977 The fine structure of the normal resting terminal ductal–lobular unit of the female breast. Virchows Arch Path Anat Histol 372: 205–206

Stockard C R, Papanicolau G N 1917 The existence of a typical oestrus cycle in guinea pigs and its histology. Anat Rec 11: 411P

Stockdale F E 1992 Myogenic cell lineages. Devel Biol 154: 284–298

Stöckli K A, Lottspeich F, Sendtner M, Masiakowski, P, Carroll P, Götz R, Lindholm D, Thoenen H 1989 Molecular cloning, expression and regional distribution of rat ciliary neurotrophic factor. Nature 342: 920–923

Stockwell R A 1967 Lipid content of human costal and articular cartilages. J Anat 101: 607P

Stockwell R A 1979 Biology of cartilage cells. Cambridge University Press: Cambridge

Stockwell R A 1983 Metabolism of cartilage. In: Hall B K (ed) Cartilage. Vol 1. Structure, function and biochemistry. Academic Press: New York: pp 253–280

Stoerk O 1907 Ueber die Chromreaktion der Glandula coccygea und die Beziehungen dieser Druse zum Nervus sympathicus. Arch f mikr Anat 69: 322–339

Stojilovic S S, Catt K J 1992 Calcium oscillations in anterior pituitary cells. Endocrine Rev 13: 256–280

Stolerman I 1992 Drugs of abuse: behavioural principles, methods and terms. TIPS 13: 170–176

Stoll G, Griffin J W, Li C Y, Trapp B D 1989 Wallerian degeneration in the peripheral nervous system: participation of both Schwann cells and macrophages in myelin degradation. J Neurocytol 18: 671–683

Stoll G, Muller H W 1986 Macrophages in the peripheral nervous system and astroglia in the central nervous system of rat commonly express apolipoprotein E during development but differ in their response to injury. Neurosci Lett 72: 233–238

Stone L S 1926 Further experiments on the extirpation and transplantation of mesecteoderm in Amblystoma. J Exp Zool 44: 95–131

Stone, L S 1922 Experiments on the development of the cranial ganglia and the lateral line sense organs in Amblystoma punctatum. J Exp Zool 35: 421–496

Stopa E G, LeBlanc V K, Hill D H, Anthony E L 1993 A general overview of the anatomy of the neurohypophysis. Ann NY Acad Sci 689: 6–15

Stopford J S B 1916 The arteries of the pons and medulla oblongata. Part II. J Anat 50: 255–280

Stopford J S B 1921–22 The nerve supply of the interphalangeal and metacarpo-phalangeal joints. J Anat 56: 1–11

Stout S D 1989 Histomorphometric analysis of human skeletal remains. In: Iscan M Y, Kennedy K A R (eds) Reconstruction of life from the skeleton. Alan R Liss: New York: pp 41–52

Strata P 1989 (ed) The olivocerebellar system in motor control. Springer: Berlin

Stratton C J 1976 The high resolution ultrastructure of the periodicity and architecture of lipid-retained and extracted lung multilamellar body laminations. Tissue and Cell 8: 713–728

Stratton C J 1978 The ultrastructure of multilamellar bodies and surfactant in the human lung. Cell Tissue Res 193: 219–229

Straus W L 1927 Human ilium: sex and stock. Am J Phys Anthrop 11: 1–28

Streeter D D Jr, Spotnitz H M, Patel D J, Ross H Jr, Sonnenblick E H 1969 Fiber orientation in the canine left ventricle during diastole and systole. Circ Res 24: 339–347

Streeter G L 1917 The development of the scala tympani, scala vestibuli and perioticular cistern in the human embryo. Am J Anat 21: 299–320

Streeter G L 1918 The developmental alterations in the vascular system of the brain of the human embryo. Contrib Embryol Carnegie Inst Washington 8: 5–38

Streeter G L 1919 Factors involved in the formation of the filum terminale. Am J Anat 25: 1–12

Streeter G L 1922 Development of the auricle in the human embryo. Contrib Embryol Carnegie Inst Washington 14: 111–138

Streeter G L 1942 Developmental horizons in human embryos. Descriptions of age group XI, 13 to 20 somites, and age group XII, 21 to 29 somites. Contrib Embryol Carnegie Inst Washington 30: 211–245

Streeter G L 1945 Developmental horizons in human embryos. Description of age group XIII, embryos of about 4 or 5 millimeters long, and age group XIV, period of indentation of the lens vesicle. Contrib Embryol Carnegie Inst Washington 31: 27–63

Streeter G L 1948 Developmental horizons in human embryos. Description of age groups XV, XVI, XVII, and XVIII, being the third issue of a survey of the Carnegie collection. Contrib Embryol Carnegie Inst Washington 32: 133–203

Streeter G L 1949 Developmental horizons in human embryos (fourth issue): a review of the histogenesis of cartilage and bone. Contrib Embryol Carnegie Inst Washington 33: 149–167

Streeter G L 1949 Developmental horizons in human embryos. A review of the histogenesis of cartilage and bone. 4th issue. Carnegie Inst Wash Pub 583 Contrib Embryol 33: 149–160

Streilein W 1983 Skin-associated lymphoid tissues (SALT): origins and functions. J Invest Dermatol 80: 12S–16S

Streit P 1984 Glutamate and aspartate as transmitter candidates for systems of the cerebral cortex. In: Jones E G, Peters A (eds) Cerebral cortex. Vol

2. Functional properties of cortical cells. Plenum Press: New York: pp 119–143

Strettoi E, Raviola E, Dacheux R F 1992 Synaptic connections of the mnarrow-field bistratified rod amacrine cell (AII) in the rabbit retina. J Comp Neurol 325: 152–168

Strick P L 1976 Anatomical analysis of ventrolateral thalamic input to primate motor cortex. J Neurophysiol 39: 1020–1031

Stringer C B 1990 The emergence of modern humans. Sci Amer 263: 98–104

Stringer C B, Andrews P 1988 Genetic and fossil evidence for the origin of modern humans. Science 239: 1263–1268

Stromberg N L, Hurwitz J L 1976 Anatomical aspects of the superior olivary complex. J Comp Neurol 170: 485 – 491

Strong K D 1938 A study of the structure of the media of the distributing arteries by the method of microdissection. Anat Rec 72: 151–168

Struble R G, Lehmann J, Mitchell S J, McKinney M, Price D L, Coyle J T et al 1986 Basal forebrain neurons provide major cholinergic innervation of primate neocortex. Neurosci Lett 66: 215–220

Strucke K 1959 Current problems of liver surgery. Munch Med Wochenschr 102: 975–978

Strum J M, Karnovsky M J 1970 Cytochemical localization of endogenous peroxidase in thyroid follicular cells. J Cell Biol 44: 655–666

Stuart D G, Enoka R M 1983 Motoneurons, motor units, and the size principle. In: Rosenberg R N (ed) The clinical neurosciences, Section 5— Willis W D (ed) Neurobiology. Churchill Livingstone: New York: pp 471–517

Stuart D G, Kawamura Y, Hemingway A 1961 Activation and suppression of shivering during septal and hypothalamic stimulation. Exp Neurol 4: 485–506

Sturrock R R 1978 A developmental study of epiplexus cells and supra-ependymal cells and their possible relationship to microglia. Neuropathol Appl Neurobiol 4: 307–320

Stuurman F J 1916 Die Lokalisation der Zungenmuskeln im Nucleus hypoglossi. Anat Anz 48: 593–610

Stuzin J M, Wagstrom L, Kawamoto H K, Wolfe S A 1989 Anatomy of the frontal branch of the facial nerve: the significance of the temporal fat pad. Plast Reconstr Surg 83: 265–271

Su H-S, Bentivoglio M 1990 Thalamic midline cell populations projecting to the nucleus accumbens, amygdala, and hippocampus in the rat. J Comp Neurol 297: 582–593

Suchey J M, Wiseley D V, Green R F, Noguchi T T 1979 Analysis of dorsal pitting in the os-pubis in an extensive sample of modern American females. Am J Phys Anthropol 51: 517–540

Sugimoto T, Itoh K, Mizuno N 1977 Localization of neurons giving rise to the oculomotor parasympathetic outflow: an HRP study in cat. Neurosci Lett 7: 301–305

Sugimoto T, Itoh K, Mizuno N, Nomura S, Konishi A 1979 The site of origin of cardiac preganglionic fibres of the vagus nerve: an HRP study in the cat. Neurosci Lett 12: 53–58

Sullivan F M 1975 Effects of drugs on fetal development. In: Beard R W, Nathanielsz P W (eds) Fetal physiology and medicine. Saunders: London

Sumii H, Inoue J 1993 Ultrastructure and X-ray microanalysis of epiphyseal growth cartilage of femoral head processed by rapid-freezing and freeze-substitution. Acta Med Okayama 47: 95–102

Summerbell D 1974 A quantitative analysis of the effect of excision of the AER from the chick limb bud. J Embryol Exp Morphol 32: 651–660

Summerbell D, Lewis J H 1975 Time, place and positional value in the chick limb bud. J Embryol Exp Morphol 33: 621–643

Summerbell D, Lewis J H, Wolpert L 1973 Positional information in chick limb morphogenesis. Nature 244: 492–496

Sun E L, Flickinger C J 1980 Morphological characteristics of cells with apical nuclei in the initial segment of the rat epididymis. Anat Rec 196: 285

Sunderland S 1940 The projection of the cerebral cortex on the pons and cerebellum in the macaque monkey. J Anat 74: 201–226

Sunderland S 1945a Arterial relations of the internal auditory meatus. Brain 68: 56–72

Sunderland S 1945b The actions of the extensor digitorum communis, interosseous and lumbrical muscles. Am J Anat 77: 189–209

Sunderland S 1978 Nerves and nerve injuries. Churchill Livingstone: Edinburgh

Sunderland S, Bedbrook G M 1949 Relative sympathetic contribution to individual roots of the brachial plexus in man. Brain 72: 297–310

Sunderland S, Hughes E S R 1946 The pupilloconstrictor pathway and the nerves to the ocular muscles in man. Brain 69: 301–309

Sunderland S, Swaney W E 1952 The interneuronal topography of the recurrent laryngeal nerve in man. Anat Rec 114: 411

Sundin T, Dahlström A, Norlén L et al 1977 The sympathetic innervation and adrenoreceptor function of the human lower urinary tract in the normal state and after parasympathetic denervation. J Invest Urol 14: 322–328

Sur M, Garraghty P E, Roe A W 1988 Science 242: 1437–1441

Sur M, Wall J T, Kaas J H 1984 Modular distribution of neurons with slowly adapting and rapidly adapting responses in area 3b of somatosensory cortex in monkeys. J Neurophysiol 51: 724–744

Surani M A 1986 Evidences and consequences of differences between maternal and paternal genomes during embryogenesis in the mouse. In: Rossart J, Pederson R (eds) Experimental approaches to mammalian embryonic development. Cambridge University Press: Cambridge: pp 401–435

Susuki M, Raisman G 1992 The glial framework of central white matter tracts: segmental rows of contiguous interfascicular oligodendrocytes and solitary astrocytes give rise to a continuous meshwork of transverse and longitudinal processes in the adult rat fimbria. Glia 6: 222 – 235

Suter U, Welcher A A, Özcellik T, Snipes G J, Kosaras B, Franckem U, Billing-Gagliardi S, Sidman R L, Shooter E M 1992 Trembler mouse carries a point mutation in a myelin gene. Nature 356: 241–244

Sutherland S D 1965 The intrinsic innervation of the liver. Rev Int Hepat 15: 569–578

Sutherland S D 1966 The intrinsic innervation of the gall bladder in Macaca rhesus and Cavia porcellus. J Anat 100: 261–268

Sutherland S D 1967 The neurons of the gall bladder and gut. J Anat 101: 701–710

Sutton R N 1974 The practical significance of mandibular accessory foramina. Aust Dent J 19: 167–173

Sutton W S 1903 The chromosomes in heredity. Biol Bull 4: 231–251. Reprinted in Peters J A 1959 Classic papers in Genetics. Prentice-Hall: New Jersey

Suzuki M, Raisman G 1992 The glial framework of central white matter tracts: segmented rows of contiguous interfascicular oligodendrocytes and solitary astrocytes give rise to a continuous meshwork of transverse and longitudinal processes in the adult rat fimbria. Glia 6: 222–235

Suzuki N 1972 An electromyographic study of the role of the muscles in arch support of the normal and flat foot. Nagoya Med J 17: 57–79

Suzuki Y, Takeda M 1993 Basal cells in the mouse olfactory epithelium during development. Devel Brain Res 73: 107–113

Swaab D F, Gooren L J G, Hofman M A 1992a Gender and sexual orientation in relation to hypothalamic structures. Hormone Res 38 (Suppl 2): 51–61

Swaab D F, Gooren L J G, Hofman M A 1992b The human hypothalamus in relation to gender and sexual orientation. Prog Brain Res 93: 205–219

Swaab D F, Hofman M A 1984 Sexual differences in the human brain. A historical perspective. Prog Brain Res 61: 361–374

Swaab D F, Hofman M A 1990 An enlarged suprachiasmatic nucleus in homosexual men. Brain Res 537: 141–148

Swaab D F, Hofman M A, Lucassen P J, Purba J S, Raadsheer F C, Van de Nes J A P 1993 Functional neuroanatomy and neuropathology of the human hypothalamus. Anat Embryol 187: 317–330

Swadlow H A, Weyand T G 1981 Efferent systems of the rabbit visual cortex: Laminar distribution of the cells of origin, axonal conduction velocities and identification of axonal branches. J Comp Neurol 203: 799–822

Swammerdam J 1675 Ephermi vita of afbeeldingh van's menschen leven, vertoont in de wonderbaarelijcke en nooyt gehoorde historie van het vliegent ende een-dagh-levent haft of oever-aas. Een dierken, ten aansien van sijn naam, overal in Neerlandt bekent: maarhet welck binnen de tijt, van vijfouren groegt, geboren wordt, jongh is, twee mal verwelt, teelt, eyeren leght, zaat schiet, out wordt, end sterft. Wolfgang: Amsterdam.

Swann D A 1978 Macromolecules of synovial fluid. In: Sokoloff L (ed) The joints and synovial fluid. Vol 1. Academic Press: New York: pp 407–435

Swann D A 1982 Structure and function of lubricin, the glycoprotein responsible for the boundary lubrication of articular cartilage. In: Franchimont P (ed) Articular synovium. Anatomy, physiology, pathology, pharmacology and therapy. Karger: Basel: pp 45–58

Swanson A B 1973 Flexible resection arthroplasty in the hand and extremities. C V Mosby: St Louis

Swanson A B, de Groot Swanson G 1974 Disabling osteoarthritis in the hand and its treatment (AAOS Symposium on Osteoarthritis). C V Mosby: St Louis: pp. 196–232

Swanson L W 1983 The hippocampus and the concept of the limbic system. In: Seifert (ed) Neurobiology of the hippocampus. Academic Press: London: pp 3–20

Swanson L W 1991 Biochemical switching in hypothalamic circuits mediating responses to stress. Prog Brain Res 87: 181–200

Swanson L W 1991 Biochemical switching in hypothalamic circuits mediating responses to stress. Prog Brain Res 87: 181–200

Swanson L W, Cowan W M 1975 Hippocampo-hypothalamic connections: origin in subicular cortex, not Ammon's horn. Science 189: 303–304

Swanson L W, Köhler C 1987 The limbic region I. The septohippocampal system. In: Björklund A, Hökfelt T, Swanson L W (eds) Handbook of chemical neuroanatomy Vol 5. Integrated systems of the CNS. Elsevier: Amsterdam: pp 125–277

Swanson L W, Sawchenko P E 1983 Hypothalamic integration: organization of the paraventricular and supraoptic nuclei. Ann Rev Neurosci 6: 269–324

Swanson L W, Sawchenko P E, Cowan W M 1981 Evidence for collateral projections by neurons in Ammon's horn, the dentate gyrus, and the subiculum: a multiple retrograde labeling study in the rat. J Neurosci 1: 548–559

Swarz J R 1976 The presence of Bergmann fibres in prenatal mouse cerebellum and its implications in cerebellar histogenesis. Anat Rec 184: 543

Swarz J R, del Cerro M 1975 Lack of evidence for glial cells originating from the external granular layer in the mouse cerebellum. Neurosci Abs 1: 760

Sweeney W J 1962 The interstitial portion of the uterine tube – its gross anatomy, course and length. Obstet Gynecol 19: 1–8

Sweet W H 1973 Pitfalls in the technical performance of open or percutaneous cordotomy: how to avoid them. In: AVENS: Library of Congress: 73–701180 12

Sweet W H 1975 Pain mechanisms and treatment. In: Tower D B (ed) The clinical neurosciences. Vol 2. Raven Press: New York: pp 487–500

Swyer G I M 1944 Post natal growth changes in the human prostate. J Anat 78: 130–145

Swynghedauw B 1986 Developmental and functional adaptation of contractile proteins in cardiac and skeletal muscles. Physiol Rev 66: 710–771

Sykes D 1963 The arterial supply of the human kidney with special reference to accessory renal arteries. Br J Surg 50: 368–374

Sykes D 1964 The correlation between renal vascularisation and lobulation of the kidney. Br J Urol 36: 549–555

Sylvén B 1951 On the biology of the nucleus pulposus. Acta Orthop Scand 20: 275–279

Symington J 1887 The topographical anatomy of the child. E & S Livingstone: Edinburgh

Symington J 1914 Splanchnology. In: Schafer E A, Symington J, Bryce T H (eds) Quain's elements of anatomy, 11th edn (4 Vols) Vol II, Part II. Longmans Green and Co: London

Szabo G 1959 Quantitative histological investigations on the melanocyte system of the human epidermis. In: Gordon M (ed) Pigment cell biology. Academic Press: New York: pp 99–125

Szabo T, Dussardier M 1964 Les noyaux d'origine du nerf vague chez le mouton. Z Zelloforsch Mikrosk Anat 63: 247–276

Szentagothai 1943 Die lokalisation der kehlkopfmusculatur in den vagu-skernen. Z Anat Entwgesch 112: 704–710

Szentágothai J 1948 Anatomical considerations of monosynaptic reflex arcs. J Neurophysiol 11: 445–454

Szentágothai J 1948 Representation of facial and scalp muscles in facial nucleus. J Comp Neurol 88: 207–220

Szentágothai J 1949 Functional representation in the motor trigeminal nucleus. J Comp Neurol 90: 111–120

Szentágothai J 1950 Recherches expérimentales sur les voies oculogyres. Sem Hop Paris 26: 2989–2995

Szentagothai J 1952 The general visceral efferent column of the brainstem. Acta Morphol Acad Sci Hung 2: 313–327

Szentágothai J 1964 Neuronal and synaptic arrangements in the substantia gelantinosa Rolandi. J Comp Neurol 122: 219–239

Szentágothai J 1965 The use of degeneration methods in the investigation of short neuronal connexions. Progr Brain Res 14: 1–32

Szentágothai J 1967 The anatomy of complex integrative units in the nervous system. In: Lissák K (ed) Results in neuroanatomy, neurochemistry, neuropharmacology and neurophysiology. Recent developments of neurobiology in Hungary. Vol 1. Akadémiai Kiadó: Budapest: pp 9–45

Szentágothai J 1969a The anatomical substrates of nervous inhibitory functions. Acta Morph Acad Sci Hung 17: 325–327

Szentágothai J 1969b Architecture of the cerebral cortex. In: Jasper H H, Ward A A Jr, Pope A (eds) Nasic mechanisms of the elipsies. Churchill: London: pp 13–28

Szentágothai J 1969c The synaptic architecture of the hypothalamo-hypophyseal neuron systems. Acta Neurol Belg 69: 453–468

Szentágothai J 1970 Glomerular synapses, complex synaptic arrangements and their operational significance. In: Schmitt F O, Quarton G C, Melnechuck T, Adelman G (eds) The neurosciences, a second study program. Rockefeller University Press: New York: pp 427–443

Szentágothai J 1975 The 'module-concept' in cerebral cortex architecture. Brain Res 95: 475–496

Szentágothai J 1978 The neuron network of the cerebral cortex: a functional interpretation. (Ferrier Lecture, 1977). Proc R Soc Lond [B] 201: 219–248

Szentágothai J 1987 The architecture of neural centres and understanding neural organization. In: McLennan H, Ledsome J R, McIntosh C H S, Jones D R (eds) Advances in physiological research. Plenum Press: New York

Szentágothai J, Albert A 1955 The synaptology of Clarke's column. Acta Morphol Acad Sci Hung 5: 43–51

Szentágothai-Schimert J 1941 Die Bedeutung des Faserkalibers und der Markscheidendicke im Zentrainervensystem. Z Anat EntwGesch 111: 201–223

Szentistvanyi I, Patlak C S, Ellis R A, Cserr H F 1984 Drainage of interstitial fluid from different regions of rat brain. Am J Physiol 246: F835–F844.

Szollozi D 1972 Changes of some cell organelles during oogenesis in mammals.

In: Biggers J D, Schultz A W (eds) Oogenesis. University Park Press: Baltimore: pp 5–45

Szurszewski J H, King B F 1989 Physiology of prevertebral ganglia in mammals with special reference to inferior mesenteric ganglion. In: Wood J D (ed) Handbook of physiology – the gastrointestinal system I. American Physiological Society: Bethesda, Maryland: pp 519–592

T

Tabary J C, Tabary C, Tardieu C, Tardieu G, Goldspink G 1972 Physiological and structural changes in the cat's soleus muscle due to immobilization at different lengths by plaster casts. J Physiol 224: 231–244

Taber E 1961 The cytoarchitecture of the brain stem of the cat. I. Brain stem nuclei of the cat. J Comp Neurol 116: 27–70

Tabibzadeh S 1991 Human endometrium: an active site of cytokine production and action. Endocrine Rev 12: 272–290

Tabin C J 1992 Why we have (only) five fingers per hand: Hox genes and the evolution of paired limbs. Development 116: 289–296

Tabira T, Cullen M J, Reier P J, Webster H de F 1978 An experimental analysis of interlamellar tight junctions in amphibian and mammalian CNS myelin. J Neurocytol 7: 489–503

Tacke R, Martini R 1990 Changes in expression of mRNA specific for cell adhesion molecules (L1 and NCAM) in the transected peripheral nerve of the adult rat. Neurosci Lett 120: 227–230

Tae-Cheng J H, Nagy Z, Brightman M W 1986 Tight junctions of cerebral endothelium in vitro are greatly enhanced in the company of astrocytes. Anat Rec 214: 131A–132A

Taipale J, Miyazono K, Heldin C N, Keski-Oja J 1994 Latent transforming growth factor B, associates to fibrillant extracellular matrix and TGFB Binding proteins. J Cell Biol 124: 171–181

Takagi S F 1989 Human olfaction. University of Tokyo Press: Tokyo

Takahashi D 1913 Zur vergleichenden Anatomoie des Seitenharns im Rückenmark der Vertebraten. Arb Neurol Inst Univ Wien 20: 62–83

Takahashi K, Kishi Y, Kim S 1982 A scanning electron microscope study of the blood vessels of the dog pulp using corrosion resin casts. J Endodont 8: 132–137

Takahashi N, Akatsu T, Udagawa N, Sasaki T, Yamaguchi A, Moseley J M, Martin T J, Suda T 1988 Osteoblastic cells are involved in osteoclastic formation. Endocrinology 123: 2600–2602

Takahashi Y 1975 Anthropological studies on the humerus of the recent Japanese. J Anthropol Soc Nippon 83: 219–232

Takahashi Y 1976 Anthropological studies on the humerus of the recent Japanese. Acta Anat Nippon 51: 79–88

Takano K 1969 Electron microscopic study of the so-called 'separating zone' in the striated duct cell of the parotid gland. Okajimas Folia Anat Jpn 46: 201–229

Takashima A, Grinnell F 1984 Human keratinocyte adhesion and phagocytosis promoted by fibronectin. J Invest Dermatol 83: 352–358

Takashima S, Tanaka K 1978 Development of cerebrovascular architecture and its relationship to periventricular leukomalacia. Arch Neurol 35: 11–16

Takei Y, Ozanics V 1975 Origin and development of Bruch's membrane in monkey fetuses: an electron microscopic study. Invest Ophthal 14: 903–916

Takeuchi T, Quevedo W C Jr (eds) 1992 Molecular biology of pigment cells. Pig Cell Res 5(2)

Takeuchi Y, Kimura H, Sano Y 1982 Immunohistochemical demonstration of serotonin-containing nerve fibers in the cerebellum. Cell Tissue Res 226: 1–12

Takumida M, Bagger-Sjöbäck D, Wers II J, Harada Y 1989 The effect of gentamicin on the glycocalyx and ciliary interconnections in vestibular sensory cells: a high resolution scanning electron microscope investigation. Hear Res 37: 163–170

Takumida M, Wers ll J, Bagger-Sjöbäck D, Harada Y 1989 Synthesis of glycocalyx and associated structures in vestibular sensory cells. ORL 51: 116–123

Tam P P L, Beddington R S P 1987 The formation of mesodermal tissues in the mouse embryo during gastrulation and early organogenesis. Development 99: 109–126

Tam P P L, Beddington R S P 1992 Establishment and organization of germ layers in the gastrulating mouse embryo. In: McLaren A (ed) Ciba Foundation Symposium 165. Wiley: Chichester: pp 27–49

Tamagho E A, Meyers F H, Smith D R 1968 The trigone: anatomical and physiological considerations. I. In relation to the uterovesical junction. J Urol 100: 623–632

Tamarin A, Sreebny L M 1965 The rat submaxillary salivary gland. A correlative study by light and electron microscopy. J Morphol 117: 296–352

Tan S-S, Breen S 1993 Nature 362: 638–640

Tan Y, Holstege G 1986 Anatomical evidence that positive lateral tegmental field projects to lavina. I. Of the caudal spinal trigeminal nucleus and spinal cord and to the Edinger Westphal nucleus in the cat. Neurosci Lett 64: 317–322

Tanabe T, Yarita H, Iino M, Ooshima Y, Takagi S F 1975 An olfactory projection area in orbitofrontal cortex of the monkey. J Neurophysiol 38: 1269–1283

Tanagho E A, Miller F R 1970 Initiation of voiding. Br J Urol 42: 175–183

Tanaka K, Sugita Y, Moriya M, Saito H-A 1993 Analysis of object motion in the ventral part of the medial superior temporal area of the macaque visual cortex. J Neurophysiol 69: 128–142

Tanaka Y, Adams D H, Shaw S 1993 Proteoglycans on endothelial cells present adhesion-inducing cytokines to leukocytes. Immunol Today 14: 111–115

Tandler B 1965 Ultrastructure of the human submaxillary gland. III. Myoepithelium. Z Zellforsch 65: 852–863

Tandler B 1972 Microstructure of salivary glands. In: Rowe N H (ed) Proceedings of symposium on salivary glands and their secretions. University of Michigan: Ann Arbor, Michigan: pp 8–21

Tandler B, Denning C R, Mandel J D, Kutscher A H 1970 Ultrastructure of human labial salivary glands. III. Myoepithelium and ducts. J Morphol 130: 227–246

Tandler J 1913 Anatomie des Herzens. Gustav Fischer: Jena

Tanila H, Carlson S, Linnankoski I, Kahila H 1993 Regional distribution of functions in dorsolateral prefrontal cortex of the monkey. Behav Brain Res 53: 63–71

Tanji J 1994 The supplementary motor area in the cerebral cortex. Neurosci Res 19: 251–268

Tanner J M 1962 Growth at adolescence. 2nd edition. Blackwell Scientific: Oxford

Tanner J M 1978 Fetus into man: physical growth from conception to maturity. Harvard University Press: Cambridge, Massachusetts

Tanner J M, Whitehouse R H, Takaishi I M 1966 Standards from birth to maturity for height, weight, height velocity and weight velocity. Arch Dis Child 41: 454–471

Tappen N C 1954 A comparative functional analysis of primate skulls by the split-line technique. Human Biol 26: 220–238

Tarlov E 1972 Anatomy of the two vestibulo-oculomotor projection systems. Progr Brain Res 37: 489–491

Tarlov E 1975 Synopsis of current knowledge about association projections from the vestibular nuclei. In: Naunton R F (ed) The vestibular system. Academic Press: New York: pp 55–69

Tassabehji M, Reed A P, Newton V E, Harris R, Balling R, Gruss P, Strachan T 1992 Waardenburg's syndrome patients have mutations in the human homologue of the Pax-3 paired box gene. Nature 355: 635–636

Taton R 1966 A general history of the sciences. Thames & Hudson: London

Taurog A 1970 Thyroid peroxidase and thyroxine biosynthesis. Recent Progr Horm Res 26: 189–247

Taurog A 1978 Thyroid hormone synthesis and release. In: Werner S C, Ingbar S H (eds) The thyroid. A fundamental and clinical text. Harper & Row: New York: pp 31–61

Tautz C, Rohen H W 1967 Ueber den konstruktiven bau des M. vocalis beim menschen. Anat Anz 120: 409–429

Tavasolli M, Yoffey J M 1983 Bone marrow: structure and function. Liss: New York

Tawara S 1906 Das reizleitungssystem des säugethierherzens. G Fischer: Jena

Taylor A 1960 The contribution of the intercostal muscles to the effort of respiration in man. J Physiol 151: 390–402

Taylor C R, Heglund N C, Maloiy G M O 1982 Energetics and mechanics of animal locomotion. I. Metabolic energy consumption as a function of speed and body size in birds and mammals. J Exp Biol 97: 1–21

Taylor G I, Palmer J H 1987 The vascular territories (angiosomes) of the body: experimental study and clinical applications. Br J Plastic Surg 40: 113–141

Taylor J F, Warrell E, Evans R A 1987 The response of the rat tibial growth plates to distal periosteal division. J Anat 151: 221–231

Taylor J R 1975 Growth of human intervertebral discs and vertebral bodies. J Anat 120: 49–68

Taylor J R, Twomey L T 1984 Sexual dimorphism in human vertebral shape. J Anat 138: 281–286

Taylor S (ed) 1968 Calcitonin. (Proceedings of the Symposium on thyrocalcitonin and the C cells. London 1967.) Heinemann Medical: London

Teal S I, Moore G W, Hutchins G M 1986 Development of aortic and mitral valve continuity in the human embryonic heart Am J Anat 176: 447–460

Teitelman G, Baker H, Joh T H, Reis D J 1979 Appearance of catecholamine-synthesising enzymes during development of rat sympathetic nervous system: possible role of tissue environment. Proc Nat Acad Sci USA 76: 509–513

Telford D, Stopford J S B 1934 Autonomic nerve supply of distal colon; anatomical and clinical study. Br Med J 1: 572–574

Templeton D, Thulin A 1978 Secretory, motor and vascular effects in the sublingual gland of the rat caused by autonomic nerve stimulation. Q J Exp Physiol 63: 59–66

Ten Cate A R 1972 An analysis of Tomes' granular layer. Anat Rec 172: 137–147

Ten Cate A R 1975 Formation of supporting bone in association with periodontal ligament organization in the mouse. Arch Oral Biol 20: 137–138

Ten Cate A R, Deporter D A 1975 The degradative role of the fibroblast in the remodelling and turnover of collagen in soft connective tissue. Anat Rec 182: 1–14

ten Dijke P, Iwata K K 1989 Growth factors for wound healing. Biotechnol 7: 793–798

Ten Have-Opbroek A A W 1991 Lung development in the mouse embryo. Exp Lung Res 17: 111–130

Tengroth B, Rohnberg M, Ammitzboli T 1985 A comparative analysis of the collagen type and distribution in the trabecular meshwork, sclera, lamina cribosa and the optic nerve in the human eye. Acta Ophthalmol 63: 91–93

Tennyson V M 1969 The fine structure of the developing nervous system. In: Himwich H (ed) Developmental neurobiology. Part 2, Chapter 3. Thomas: Springfield, Illinois

Tennyson V M 1970 The fine structure of the axon and growth cone of the dorsal root neuroblast of the rabbit embryo. J Cell Biol 44: 62–79

Terni T 1922 Richerche sulla struttura c sull'evoluzione del simpatico dell'u-omo. Monitore Zool Ital 33: 63–72

Terr L I, Edgerton B J 1985a Three dimensional reconstruction of the cochlear nuclear complex in humans. Arch Otolaryngol 111: 495 – 501

Terr L I, Edgerton B J 1985b Physical effects of the choroid plexus on the cochlear nuclei in man. Acta Otolaryngol 100: 210 – 217

Terracol J, Calvet J, Granel F, Ardouin P, Fabre L 1965 L'anatomie fonctionelle du larynx. Biol Med 54: 180–255

Tesche C, Hari R 1993 Independence of steady state 40 Hz response and spontaneous 10 Hz activity in the human auditory cortex. Brain Research 629: 19–22

Tesi D, Forssmann W G 1970 Untersuchungen am mesenterium der ratte. Anat Anz 126: 365–373

Tessier-Lavigne M, Placzek M, Lumsden A G S, Dodd J, Jessell T M 1988 Nature 336: 775–778

Test S T, Weiss S J 1984 Quantitative and temporal characterization of the extracellular H_2O_2 pool generated by roman neutrophilis. J Biol Chem 259(1): 399–405

Testa Riva F, Cossu M, Lantini M S, Riva A 1985 Fine structure of human deep posterior lingual glands. J Anat 142: 103–115

Teubér H L, Battersby W S, Bender M B 1960 Visual field defects after penetrating missile wounds of the brain. Harvard University Press: Cambridge, Massachusetts

Thale A, Tillmann B 1993 The collagen architecture of the sclera - SEM and immunohistochemical studies. Anatomischer Anzeiger 175: 215–220

Thapa S, Short R, Potts M 1988 Breast-feeding, birth spacing and their effects on child survival. Nature 335: 679–682

Tharp M D 1989 The interaction between mast cells and endothelial cells. J Invest Dermatol 93: 107S–112S

Thatcher R W, John E R 1977 Foundations of cognitive processes. Lawrence Erlbaum: Hillsdale, New York: pp 31–52

Thaysen J H, Thorn N A, Schwartz I L 1954 Excretion of sodium, potassium, chloride and carbon dioxide in human parotid saliva. Am J Physiol 178: 155–159

Thebesius A C 1708 Disputatio medica inauguralis de circulo sanguinis in corde. A Elzevier: Lugduni Batavorum

Theele D P, Streit W J 1993 A chronicle of microglial ontogeny. Glia 7: 5–8

Theodosis D T, Chapman D B, Montagnese C, Poulain D A, Morris J F 1986a Structural plasticity in the hypothalamic supraoptic nucleus at lactation affects oxytocin- but not vasopressin-secreting neurons. Neuroscience 17: 661–678

Theodosis D T, Montagnese C, Rodriguez F, Vincent J D, Poulain D A 1986b Oxytocin induces morphological plasticity in the adult hypothalamo-neurohypophysial system. Nature 322: 738–740

Theodosis D T, Poulain D A 1993 Activity-dependent neuronal-glial and synaptic plasticity in the adult mammalian hypothalamus. Neuroscience 57: 501–535

Theofilopoulos A N, Carson D A, Tavassoli M, Slovin S F, Speers W C, Jensen F B, Vaughan J H 1980 Evidence for the presence of receptors for C3 and IgG Fe on human synovial cells. Arthritis Rheum 23: 1–9

Thesleff I 1977 Tissue interactions in tooth development in vitro. In: Karkinen-Jääskeläinen M, Saxén L, Weiss L (eds) Cell interactions in differentiation. Sixth Sigrid Jusélius Foundation Symposium in Helsinki, 1976. Academic Press: London: pp 191–207

Thesleff I, Hurmerinta K 1981 Tissue interactions in tooth development. Differentiation 18: 75–88

Thesleff I, Vaino S, Jalkanen M 1989 Cell matrix interactions in tooth development. Int J Dev Biol 33: 91–97

Thiede M A, Rodan G A 1988 Expression of a calcium-mobilizing parathyroid hormone-like peptide in lactating mammary gland. Science 242: 278–280

Thiel G A, Downey H 1921 The development of the mammalian spleen, with special reference to its hematopoietic activity. Am J Anat 28: 279–333

Thiers B H, Maize J C, Spicer S S, Cantor A B 1984 The effect of ageing and chronic sun exposure on human Langerhans cell populations. J Invest Dermatol 82: 223–226

Thody A J, Friedmann P S (eds) 1986 Scientific basis of dermatology. A physiological approach. Churchill Livingstone: Edinburgh

Thoenen H 1991 The changing scene of neurotrophic factors. Trends Neurosci 14: 165–170

Thoma R 1922 Die Mittlere Durchflussmenge der Arterien des Menschen als Funktion des Gefessradius. Pflügers Arch ges Physiol 194: 385–406

Thomander L, Aldskogius H, Grant G 1982 Motor fibre organisation in the intratemporal portion of a cat and rat: facial nerve studies with the horseradish peroxidase technique. Acta Otolaryngol (Stockh) 93: 397–405

Thomas H F 1979 The effect of various fixatives on the extent of the odontoblast process in human dentine. Arch Oral Biol 28: 465–469

Thomas H F, Carella P 1983 A scanning electron microscope study of dentinal tubules from unerupted human teeth. Arch Oral Biol 28: 1125–1130

Thomas K R, Capecchi M R 1990 Targeted disruption of the murine int-1 proto-oncogene resulting in severe abnormalities in midbrain and cerebellar development. Nature 346: 847–850

Thomas N R 1976 Collagen as the generator of tooth eruption. In: Poole D F G, Stack M V (eds) The eruption and occlusion of teeth. (Proceedings of the 27th Symposium of the Colston Research Society 1975.) Butterworths: London: pp 290–301

Thomas P, Jackson A M, Aichroth P M 1985 Congenital absence of the anterior cruciate ligament. J Bone Jt Surg 67B: 572–575

Thompson M W, Bandler E 1973 Finger pattern combinations in normal individuals and in Down's Syndrome. Hum Biol 45: 563–570

Thompson R 1919 The capacity of, and the pressure of fluid in, the urinary bladder. J Anat 53: 241–253

Thompson S T, Robertson R T 1987 Organization of subcortical pathways for sensory projections to the limbic cortex. II. Afferent projections to the thalamic lateral dorsal nucleus in the rat. J Comp Neurol 265: 189–202

Thompson V P 1995 Anatomical research lives. Nature Medicine 1: 297–298

Thompson W D'A 1942 On growth and form. 2nd edition. Cambridge University Press: Cambridge

Thoms H 1940 Roentgen pelvimetry as a routine prenatal procedure. Am J Obstet Gynecol 40: 891–905

Thomson A S, Dabhoiwala N F, Verbeek F J, Lamers W H 1994 The functional anatomy of the ureterovesical junction. Brit J Urol 73: 284–291

Thomson C E, Griffiths I R, McCulloch M C, Kyriakides E, Barrie J A, Montague P 1993 In vitro studies of axonally-regulated Schwann cell genes during Wallerian degeneration. J neurocytol 22: 590–602

Thorel C 1909 Vorläufige Mitteilung über eine besondere Muskeln Ver-bindung zwischen der Cava superior und dem Hisschen Bündel. Munch Med Wochenschr 56: 2159

Thornell L E, Billeter R, Eriksson P O, Ringqvist M 1984 Heterogeneous distribution of myosin in human masticatory muscle fibres as shown by immunocytochemistry. Arch Oral Biol 29: 1–5

Thornhill A R, Burgoyne P S 1993 A paternally imprinted X chromosome retards the development of the early mouse embryo. Development 118: 171–174

Thornton M W, Schweisthal M R 1969 The phrenic nerve: its terminal divisions and supply to the crura of the diaphragm. Anat Rec 164: 283–290

Thorogood P 1988 The developmental specification of the vertebrate skull. Development 103 (suppl): 141–153

Thorstensson A, Roberthson H 1987 Adaptations to changing speed in human locomotion: speed of transitions between walking and running. Acta Physiol Scand 131: 211–214

Thulin C A 1963 Effects of electrical stimulation on the red nucleus on the alpha motor system. Exp Neuron 7: 464–480

Thuneberg L 1989 Interstitial cells of Cajal. In: Schulz S G, Wood J D, Rauner B B (eds) Handbook of physiology, Sect 6, Vol 1, Part 1: The gastrointestinal system, motility and circulation. American Physiological Society: Bethesda: Maryland: pp 349–386

Thurig L, Agtmaal J, van Glasius E, Tan K L, Haeringen N 1985 Comparison of tears and lacrimal gland fluid in the rabbit and guinea pig. Cur Eye Res 4: 913–920

Thurlbeck W M 1992 Prematurity and the developing lung. Clin Perinatol 19: 497–519

Tickle C 1994 On making a skeleton. Nature 368: 587–588

Tierney D F 1974 Lung metabolism and biochemistry. Ann Rev Physiol 36: 209–231

Tigges J, Tigges M 1985 Subcortical sources of direct projections to visual cortex. In: Peters A, Jones E G (eds) Cerebral cortex. Vol 3. Plenum Press: New York: pp 351–378

Tillman B 1987 Untere extremität. In: Leonhardt B, Tillmann B, Töndury

G, Zilles K (eds) Rauber/Kopsch Anatomie des Menschen. Vol 1. Bewegungsapparat. G Thieme: Stuttgart: pp 445–651

Tillmann B, Pietsch-Rohrschneider I, Hoenges H L 1977 The human vocal cord surface. Cell Tissue Res 185: 279–283

Tilly J L, Kowalski K I, Schomberg D W, Hsueh A J W 1992 Apoptosis in atretic ovarian follicles is associated with selective decreases in messenger ribonucleic acid transcripts for gonadotrophin receptors and cytochrome P450 aromatase. Endocrinology 131: 1670–1676

Tilney F 1933 Behavior in its relation to development of the brain. Part II. Correlation between the development of the brain and behavior in the albino rat from embryonic states to maturity. Bull Neurol Inst New York 3: 252–358

Tilney L G, Derosier D I, Mulroy M 1980 The organisation of actin filaments in the stereocilia of cochlear hair cells. J Cell Biol 86: 244–259

Timmermans J-P, Scheurmann D W, Stach W, Adriaensen D, Groodt-Lassel M H A 1992 Functional morphology of the enteric nervous system with special reference to large mammals. Europ J Morphol 30: 113–122

Tipoe G L, White F H, Pritchett C J 1992 A morphometric study of histological variations during cellular differentiation of normal human colorectal epithelium. J Anat 181: 189–197

Tischler A S, Lee A K, Nunnemacher G, Said S I, DeLellis R A, Morse G M, Wolfe H J 1981 Spontaneous neurite outgrowth and vasoactive intestinal peptide-like immunoreactivity of cultures of human paraganglioma cells from the glomus jugulare. Cell Tissue Res 219: 543–555

Tisell L E, Salander H 1975 The lobes of the human prostate. Scand J Urol Nephrol 9: 185–191

Titus M A 1993 Myosins. Curr Opin Cell Biol 5: 77–81

Tjio H J, Levan A 1956 The chromosome number of man. Hereditas 42: 1–6

Tobin C E 1966 Arteriovenous shunts in the peripheral pulmonary circulation in the human lung. Thorax 21: 197–204

Tobin D 1991 Structural and functional studies of normal hair growth and changes in alopecia areata. PhD Thesis, University of London

Tobin G R, Schusterman M, Peterson G H, Nichols G, Bland K I 1981 The intramuscular neurovascular anatomy of the latissimus dorsi muscle: the basis for splitting the flap. Plas Reconstr Surg 67: 637–642

Tobon H, Salazar H 1974 Ultrastructure of the human mammary gland. I. Development of the fetal gland throughout gestation. J Clin Endocrinol Metab 39: 443–456

Tobon H, Salazar H 1975 Ultrastructure of the human mammary gland. II Postpartum lactogenesis. J Clin Endocrinol Metab 40: 834–844

Tochen M 1979 Orotracheal intubation in the newborn infant: a method for determining depth of tube insertion. J Pediatr 95: 1050–1051

Todd T W 1920a Age changes in the pubic bone. I. The male white pubis. Am J Phys Anthropol 3: 285–334

Todd T W 1920b Age changes in the pubic bone. II. The pubis of the male negro-white hybrid. III. The pubis of the white female. IV. The pubis of the female negro-white hybrid. Am J Phys Anthropol 4: 1–70

Todd T W 1921a Age changes in the pubic bone. V. Mammalian pubic metamorphosis. Am J Phys Anthropol 4: 333–406

Todd T W 1921b Age changes in the pubic bone. VI. The interpretation of variations in the symphyseal area. Am J Phys Anthropol 4: 407–424

Todd T W 1931 Differential skeletal maturation in relation to sex, race, variability and disease. Child Dev 2: 49–56

Todd T W 1937 Atlas of skeletal maturation of the wrist. Mosby: St Louis

Todd T W, D'Erico J Jr 1928 The clavicular epiphyses. Am J Anat 41: 25–50

Todd T W, Lindàla A 1928 Dimensions of the body; whites and American negros of both sexes. Am J Phys Anthropol 12: 35–119

Todd T W, Lyon D W Jr 1924 Endocranial suture closure, its progress and age relationship. I. Adult males of white stock. Am J Phys Anthropol 7: 325–384

Todd T W, Lyon D W Jr 1925a Endocranial suture closure, its progress and age relationship. II. Ectocranial closure in adult males of white stock. Am J Phys Anthropol 8: 23–45

Todd T W, Lyon D W Jr 1925b Endocranial suture closure, its progress and age relationship. III. Endocranial closure in adult males of negro stock. Am J Phys Anthropol 8: 47–71

Todd T W, Lyon D W Jr 1925c Endocranial suture closure, its progress and age relationship. IV. Ectocranial closure in adult males of negro stock. Am J Phys Anthropol 8: 149–168

Todd T W, Tracy B 1930 Racial features in American negro cranium. Am J Phys Anthropol 15: 53–110

Tohyama M, Shiotani Y 1986 Neuropeptides in spinal cord. In: Rossor M N, Tohyama M (eds) Prog Brain Research 66: 177–218 Elsevier: Amsterdam

Tolbert N E, Essner E 1981 Microbodies: peroxisomes and glyoxysomes. J Cell Biol 91: 271s–283s

Tollefson L, Bulloch K 1990 Dual-label retrograde transport: CNS inner-vation of the mouse thymus distinct from other mediastinum viscera. J Neurosci Res 25: 20–28

Tomei L D, Cope F O 1991 Apoptosis: the molecular basis of cell death. Cold Spring Harbour Press: New York

Tominaga Y L, Ikui H 1964 The fine structure of the arteriovenous crossing parts in the human retina. Acta Soc Ophthal Jpn 68: 148–150

Ton C C T, Hirvonen H, Miwa H, Weil M M, Monaghan P, Jordan T, van Heyningen V, Hastie N, Meijers-Heijboer, Drechsler M, Royer-Pokora B, Collins F, Swaroop A, Strong L C, Saunders G F 1991 Positional cloning and characterisation of a paired box and homeobox-containing gene from the Aniridia region. Cell 67: 1059–1074

Tonder K J H, Kvinnsland I 1983 Micropuncture measurement of interstitial fluid pressure in normal and inflamed dental pulp in cats. J Endodont 9: 105–109

Töndury G 1958 Entwicklungsgeschichte und Fehlbildungen der Wirbesaule. Thieme: Stuttgart

Tongerson J 1951 Developmental, genetic and evolutionary meaning of metopic suture. Am J Phys Anthropol 9: 193–210

Toppari J, Kangasniemi M, Kaipia A, Mali P, Huhtaniemi I, Parvinen M 1991 Stage- and cell-specific gene expression and hormone regulation of the seminiferous epithelium. J Electron Microscop Tech 19: 203–214

Torday J 1992 Cellular timing of fetal lung development. Sem Perinatol 16: 130–139

Torihashi S, Kobayashi S, Gerthoffer W T, Sanders K M 1993 Interstitial cells in deep muscular plexus of canine small intestine may be specialized smooth muscle cells. Am J Physiol 265: G638–G645

Törk I, Hornung J-P 1990 Raphe nuclei and the serotonergic system. In: Paxinos G (ed) The human nervous system. Academic Press: San Diego: pp 1001–1022

Tork I, McRitchie D A, Rikard-Bell G C, Paxinos G 1990 Autonomic regulatory centres in the medulla oblongata. In: Paxinos G (ed.) The human nervous system Academic Press: Orlando pp 221–231

Török B 1954 Lebeudbeobachtung des hypophysenkreislaufes an hunden. Acta Morphol Acad Sci Hung. 4: 83–89

Torr J B D 1957 The blood supply of the human cord. MD Thesis, University of Manchester

Torrent Guasp F 1970 The electrical circulation. Torrent Guasp: Denia

Torrey T W 1954 The early development of the human nephros. Contrib Embryol Carnegie Inst Washington 35: 175–197

Torvik A, Bhatia R, Murthy V S 1978 Transitory block of the arachnoid granulations following subarachnoid haemorrhage. A postmortem study. Acta Neurochir 41: 137–146

Torvik A, Brodal A 1954 The cerebellar projection of the perihypoglossal nuclei (nucleus intercalatus, nucleus praepositus hypoglossi and nucleus of Roller) in the cat. J Neuropath Exp Neurol 13: 515–527

Torvik A, Brodal A 1957 The origin of reticulospinal fibers in the cat. An experimental study. Anat Rec 128: 113–137

Toth A 1977 Studies on the muscular structure of the human uterus. II. Fasciculi cervicoangulares: vestigial or functional remnant of the mesonephric duct? Obstet Gynecol 49: 190–196

Toth L E, Slawin K L, Pintar J E, Nguyen-Huu C M 1987 Region-specific expression of mouse homeobox genes in the embryonic mesoderm and central nervous system. Proc Nat Acad Sci USA 84: 6790–6794

Tottrup A 1993 The role of nitric acid in oesophageal motor function. Dis Eosophag 6: 2–10

Touisimis A J, Fine B S 1959 Ultrastructure of the iris: intercellular stromal components. Arch Ophthal 62: 974–976

Touwen B C I 1976 Neurological development in infancy. Clinics in developmental medicine. Vol 58. Heinemann Medical Books: London

Tower S 1949 The pyramidal tract. In: Bucy B C (ed) The precentral motor cortex. Univ Illinois Press: Urbana, Illinois: pp 149–172

Tower S S, Richter C P 1931 Injury and repair within the sympathetic nervous system; preganglionic neurons. Archs Neurol Psychiatry 26: 485–495

Townes-Anderson E, Raviola G 1978 Degeneration and regeneration of autonomic nerve endings in the anterior part of rhesus monkey ciliary muscle. J Neurocytol 7: 583–600

Tracey D J 1986 Ascending and descending pathways in the spinal cord. In: Paxinos G (ed) The rat nervous system. Vol 2. Academic Press: Orlando: pp 311–324

Trainin N 1974 Thymic hormones and the immune response. Physiol Revs 54: 272–315

Trainor P A, Tan S, Tam P P L 1994 Cranial paraxial mesoderm: regionalisation of cell fate and impact on craniofacial development in mouse embryos. Development 120: 2397–2408

Tramezzani J H, Morita E, Chiocchio S R 1971 The carotid body as a neuroendocrine organ involved in the control of erythropoiesis. Proc Natl Acad Sci USA 68: 52–55

Tranum-Jensen J 1975 The ultrastructure of the sensory end-organs (baroreceptors) in the atrial endocardium of young mini-pigs. J Anat 119: 255–275

Trapp B D, Andrews S B, Wong A, O'Connell M, Griffin J. W. 1989 Colocalization of the myelin-associated glycoprotein and the microfilament components, F-actin and spectrin, in Schwann cells of myelinated fibres. J Neurocytol 18: 47–60

Traurig H H, Papka R E, Shew R L 1991 Substance P and related peptides associated with the afferent and autonomic innervation of the uterus. Ann N Y Acad Sci 632: 304–313

Travill A A 1964 Transmission of pressures across the elbow joint. Anat Rec 150: 243–247

Treitz W 1853 Über einen neuen Muskel am Duodenum. Vjschr Pract Heikunde (Prague) 37: 113–144

Tremblay N, Bushnell M C, Duncan G H 1993 Thalamic VPM nucleus in the behaving monkey. II. Response to air-puff stimulation during discrimination and attention tasks. J Neurophysiol 69: 753–763

Trenouth M J 1984 Shape changes during human fetal craniofacial growth. J Anat 139: 639–651

Treutner K H, Klosterhalfen B, Winkeltau G, Moensch S, Schumpelick V 1993 Vascular anatomy of the spleen: the basis for organ-preserving surgery. Clin Anat 6: 1–8

Treves Sir F 1885 The anatomy of the intestinal canal and peritoneum in man. Lewis: London

Trevino D L, Carstens E 1975 Confirmation of location of spinothalamic neurons in the cat and monkey by retrograde transport of horseradish peroxidase. Brain Res 98: 177–182

Trier J S 1963 Studies on small intestine crypt epithelium I. The fine structure of the crypt epithelium of the proximal small intestine in fasting humans. J Cell Biol 18: 599

Trinick J 1992 Understanding the functions of titin and nebulin. FEBS Lett 307: 44–48

Tripathi B J, Tripathi R C 1974 Vacuolar transcellular channels as a drainage pathway for cerebrospinal fluid. J Physiol (Lond) 239: 195–206

Tripathi R C, Tripathi B J, 1982 Functional anatomy of the anterior chamber angle. In: Jakobiec F A (ed) Ocular anatomy, embryology and teratology. Harder & Row: Philadelphia: pp 197–284

Trisler G D, Schneider M D, Nirenberg M 1981 Proc Natl Acad Sci USA 78: 2145–2149

Trobe J D 1988 Third nerve palsy and the pupil: footnotes to the rule. Arch Ophthalmol 106: 601–602

Trojanowski J Q, Jacobson S 1976 Areal and laminar distribution of some pulvinar cortical efferents in the rhesus monkey. J Comp Neurol 169: 371–392

Trolle D 1947 Accessory bones of the human foot. Munskgaard: Copenhagen

Trommer V L, Groothuis D R, Pasternak J F 1987 Quantitative analysis of cerebral vessels in the newborn puppy: the structure of germinal matrix vessels may predispose to haemorrhage. Pediatr Res 22: 23–28

Trotter J A, Corbett K, Avner B P 1981 Structure and function of the murine muscle–tendon junction. Anat Rec 201: 293–302

Trotter J, Smith M E 1986 The role of phospholipases from inflammatory macrophages in demyelination. Neurochem Res 11: 349–361

Trotter M 1937 Accessory sacro-iliac articulations. Am J Phys Anthropol 22: 247–261

Trotter M, Gleser G C 1958 A re-evaluation of estimation of stature based on measurements of stature taken during life and of long bones after death. Am J Phys Anthropol NS 16: 79–123

Trueta J 1957 The normal vascular anatomy of the femoral head during growth. J Bone Jt Surg 39B: 353–358

Trueta J, Barclay A E, Daniel P M, Franklin K J, Prichard M M L 1947 Studies of the renal circulation. Blackwell: Oxford

Trueta J, Morgan J D 1960 The vascular contribution to osteogenesis. I. Studies by the injection method. J Bone Jt Surg 42B: 97–109

Truex R C, Taylor M J, Smythe M Q, Gildenburg P L 1970 The lateral cervical nucleus of cat, dog and man. J Comp Neurol 139: 93–104

Trybus K M 1991 Assembly of cytoplasmic and smooth muscle myosins. Curr Opin Cell Biol 3: 105–111

Tryggvason K 1993 The laminin family. Curr Opin Cell Biol 5: 877–882

Tschabitscher M, Hocker K 1991 The variations in the origin of cranial nerves III, IV and VI. Anat Anz 173: 45–49

Ts'o M O, Friedman E 1967 The retinal pigment epithelium. I. Comparative histology. Arch Ophthalmol 78: 641–649

Ts'o M O, Friedman E 1968 The retinal pigment epithelium. III. Growth and development. Arch Ophthalmol 80: 214–216

Tsuboi R, Sato Y, Rifkin D B 1990 Correlation of cell migration, cell invasion, receptor number, proteinase production, and basic fibroblast growth factor levels in endothelial cells. J Cell Biol 110: 511–517

Tsuchida T, Hruban R H, Carson B S, Phillips P C 1993 Folliculo-stellate cells in the human anterior pituitary express cytokeratin. Pathol Res Pract 189: 184–188

Tsukita S, Tsukita S, Ishikawa H 1983 Association of actin and 10 nm filaments with the dense body in smooth muscle cells of the chicken gizzard. Cell Tiss Res 229: 223–242

Tucker G C, Aoyama H, Lipinski M, Tursz T, Thiery J P 1984 Identical reactivity of monoclonal antibodies HNK-1 and NC-1: conservation in vertebrates on cells derived from the neural primordium and on some leukocytes. Cell Diff 14: 223–230

Tulchinsky D, Hobel C J 1973 Plasma human chorionic gonadotropin, estrone, estradiol, estriol, progesterone and 17a-hydroxyprogesterone in human pregnancy. III. Early normal pregnancy. Am J Obst Gynecol 117: 884–893

Tulchinsky D, Hobel C J, Yeager E, Marshall J R 1972 Plasma estrone, estradiol, estriol, progesterone and 17-hydroxyprogesterone in human pregnancy. I. Normal pregnancy. Am J Obst Gynecol 112: 1095–1100

Tulsi R S, Hermanis G M 1992 A study of the angle of inclination and facet curvature of superior lumbar zygapophyseal facets. Spine 18: 1311–1317

Tunell G L, Hart M N 1977 Simultaneous determination of skeletal muscle fiber types I, IIA and IIB by histochemistry. Archs Neurol, Chicago 34: 171–173

Turgeon S M, Albin R L 1993 Pharmacology, distribution, cellular localization, and development of GABA$_B$ binding in rodent cerebellum. Neuroscience 55: 311–323

Turnbull I M, Brieg A, Hassler O 1966 Blood supply of cervical spinal cord in man. A microangiographic cadaver study. J Neurosurg 24: 951–965

Turnbull W D 1970 Mammalian masticatory apparatus. Fieldiana Geology 18: 149–356

Turner B H, Mishkin M, Knapp M 1980 Organization of the amygdalopetal projections from modality-specific cortical association areas in the monkey. J Comp Neurol 191: 515–543

Turner C H 1992 Editorial: Functional determinants of bone structure: beyond Wolff's law of bone transformation. Bone 13: 403–409

Turner D L, Cepko C L 1987 Nature 328: 131–136

Turner D R 1969 The vascular tree of the haemal node in the rat. J Anat 104: 481–494

Turner L 1961 The structure of arachnoid granulations with observations on their physiological and pathological significance. Ann R Coll Surg Engl 29: 237–264

Turner R S 1957 A comparison of theoretical with observed angles between the vertebral arteries at their junction to form the basilar. Anat Rec 129: 243–254

Turner R S 1959 The angle of origin of the ulnar artery. Anat Rec 134: 761–767

Turner R, Jezzard P, Wen H, Kwong K K, Le Bihan D, Zeffiro T et al 1993 Functional mapping of the human visual cortex at 4 and 1·5 tesla using deoxygenation contrast EPI. Mag Reson Med 29: 277–279

Turner W 1886 The index of the pelvic brim as a basis of classification. J Anat 20: 125–143

Turner-Warwick R T 1959 The lymphatics of the breast. Br J Surg 46: 574–582

Tuttrup A 1993 The role of nitric acid in oesaphageal motor functio. Dis Esophag 6: 2–10

Twomey L, Taylor J, Furniss B 1983 Age changes in the bone density and structure of the lumbar vertebral column. J Anat 136: 15–25

Tzagoloff A 1982 Mitochondria. Plenum Press: New York

U

Uberlaker D 1986 Estimation of age at death from histology of human bone. In: Zimmerman M R, Angel J L (eds) Dating and age determination of biological materials. Croom Helm: London: pp 240–247

Uchida Y 1950 A contribution to the comparative anatomy of the amygdaloid nuclei in mammals, especially in rodents. Part I: rat and mouse. Folia Psychiatr Neurol Jpn 4: 25–42

Uchida Y A 1950 A contribution to the comparative anatomy of the amygdaloid nuclei in mammals, especially in rodents. Part II: guinea pig, rabbit and squirrel. Folia Psychiatr Neurol Jpn 4: 91–107

Uchizono K 1965 Characterisation of excitatory and inhibitory synapses in the central nervous system of the cat. Nature 207: 642–643

Uddenberg N 1968 Differential organization in dorsal funiculi of fibres originating from different receptors. Exp Brain Res 4: 367–376

Uddman R, Edvinsson L 1989 Neuropeptides in the cerebral circulation. Cerebrovasc Brain Metab Rev 1: 230–252.

Ueda D 1990 Normal volume of the thyroid gland in children. J Clin Ultrasound 18: 455–462

Uehara Y, Fujiwara T, Kaidoh T 1990 Morphology of vascular smooth muscle fibers and pericytes: scanning electron microscopic studies. In: Motta P M (ed) Ultrastructure of smooth muscle. Kluwer: Boston: pp 237–251

Uemura M, Matsuda K, Kume M, Takeuchi Y, Matsushima R, Mizuno N 1979 Topographical arrangement of hypoglossal motoneurons. An HRP study in the cat. Neurosci Lett 13: 99–104

Uemura-Sumi M, Mizuno N, Nomura S, Iwahori N, Takeuchi Y, Matsushima R 1981 Topographical representation of the hypoglossal nerve branches and tongue muscles in the hypoglossal nucleus of macaque monkeys. Neurosci Lett 22: 31–35

Ugawa Y, Hanajima R, Kanazawa I 1993 Interhemispheric facilitation of the hand area of the human motor cortex. Neurosci Lett 160: 153–155

Ugolini G, Kuypers H G J M 1986 Collaterals of corticospinal and pyramidal fibres to the pontine grey demonstrated by a new application of the fluorescent fibre labelling technique. Brain Res 365: 211–227

Uhlenhuth E, Hunter D W T, Loechel W W 1952 Problems in the anatomy of the pelvis. Lippincott: Philadelphia

Uhthoff H K 1990 The embryology of the human locomotor system. Springer-Verlag: Berlin

Uitto J, Olsen D R, Fazio M J 1989 Extracellular matrix of the skin: 50 years of progress. J Invest Dermatol 92 (suppl 4): 61S–77S

Ullah M 1978 Localization of the phrenic nucleus in the spinal cord of the rabbit. J Anat 125: 377–386

Ullah M, Salman S S 1986 Localisation of the spinal nucleus of the accessory nerve in the rabbit. J Anat 145: 97–107

Underhill B M L 1955 Intestinal length in man. Br Med J 2: 1243–1246

Undi F, Somogyi B, Kausz M 1973 Data on blood supply of spinal nerve roots. Acta Morphol Acad Sci Hung 21: 311–318

Ungerleider L G, Desimone R, Galkin T W, Mishkin M 1984 Subcortical projections of area MT in the macaque. J Comp Neurol 223: 368–386

Unsicker K 1993 The chromaffin cells: paradigm in cell, developmental and growth factor biology. J Anat 183: 207–221

Unsicker K, Seidl K, Hofmann H D 1989 The neuro-endocrine ambiguity of sympathoadrenal cells. Internat J Dev Neurosci 7: 413–417

Unterharnscheidt F, Jachnik D, Gött H 1968 Der Balkenmangel. Monographien aus dem Gesamtgebiete der Neurologie und Psychaitrie, Heft 128: pp. 1–232. Springer-Verlag: Berlin

Unwin P N T, Ennis P D 1984 Two configurations of a channel-forming membrane protein. Nature 307: 609–613

Unwin P N T, Zampighi G 1980 Structure of the junction between communicating cells. Nature 283: 545–549

Upton M L, Weller R O 1985 The morphology of cerebrospinal fluid drainage pathways in human arachnoid granulations. J Neurosurg 63: 867–875

V

Vail A D, Coller F C 1967 The parathyroid glands: clinicopathologic correlation of parathyroid disease as found in 200 unselected autopsies. Missouri Med 64: 234–238

Vaithlingam U D, Wong W C, Ling E A 1984 Light and electron microscopic features of the structure and innervation of the gastro-oesophageal junction of the monkey (Macaca fascicularis). J Anat 138: 471–484

Vallbo Å B, Hagbarth K E, Torebjörk H E, Wallin B G 1979 Somatosensory, proprioceptive, and sympathetic activity in human peripheral nerves. Physiol Rev 59: 919–957

van As A, Webster I 1972 The organisation of ciliary activity and mucus transport in pulmonary airways. S Afr. Med J 46: 347–350

van Campenhout E 1925 Etude sur le développement et la signification morphologique des ilots endocrine du pancréas chez l'embryon de mouton. Arch Biol Liège 35: 45–88

van Campenhout E 1956 Le développement embryonnaire comparé des nerfs olfactif et audatif. Acta Otorhinolaryngol Belg 11: 279–287

Van Crevel H, Verhaart W J C 1963 The 'exact' origin of the pyramidal tract. A quantitative study in the cat. J Anat 97: 495–515

Van den Bergh R 1969 Centrifugal elements in the vascular pattern of the deep intracranial blood supply. Angiology 20: 88–94

Van den Bergh R, Van der Eecken H 1968 Anatomy and embryology of cerebral circulation. Prog Brain Res 30: 1–25

Van den Pol A N, Dudek F E 1993 Cellular communication in the circadian clock, the suprachiasmatic nucleus. Neuroscience 56: 793–811

van der Loos H D, Wolsey T A 1973 Science 179: 395–398

van der Rest M, Garrone R 1991 Collagen family of proteins. FASEB J 5: 2814–2823

Van Deurs B 1979 Cell junctions in the endothelium and connective tissue of the rat choroid plexus. Anat Rec 195: 73–94

van Eijden T M G J, Kouwenhoven E, Weijs W A 1987 Mechanics of patellar articulation. Acta Orthop Scand 58: 560–566

Van Essen D C 1985 Functional organization of primate visual cortex. In: Peters A, Jones E G (eds) Cerebral cortex. Vol 3. Visual cortex. Plenum Press: New York: pp 259–329

Van Essen D C, Anderson C H, Felleman D J 1992 Information processing in the primate visual system: an integrated system perspective. Science 255: 419–423

Van Gehuchten 1892 Contribution à l'étude des ganglions cérébrospinaux. Cellule 8: 209–231; 233–254

Van Hoesen G W 1981 The differential distribution, diversity and sprouting of cortical projections to the amygdala in the rhesus monkey. In: Ben-Ari Y (ed) The amygdaloid complex. Elsevier: Amsterdam: pp 77–90

Van Hoesen G W 1982 The parahippocampal gyrus. New observations regarding its cortical connections in the monkey. TINS 5: 345–350

2035

Van Hoesen G W 1993 The modern concept of association cortex. Curr Opin Neurobiol 3: 150–154

Van Hoesen G W, Pandya D N 1975 Some connections of the entorhinal (area 28 and perirhinal (area 35) cortices of the rhesus monkey. II. Efferent connections. Brain Res 95: 39–59

Van Hoesen G W, Pandya D N 1975a Some connections of the entorhinal (area 28) and perirhinal (area 35) cortices of the rhesus monkey. I. Temporal lobe afferents. Brain Res 95: 1–24

Van Hoesen G W, Pandya D N 1975b Some connections of the entorhinal (area 28) and perirhinal (area 35) cortices of the rhesus monkey. III. Efferent connections. Brain Res 95: 39–59

Van Hoesen G W, Pandya D N, Butters N 1975 Some connections of the entorhinal (area 28) and perirhinal (area 35) cortices of the rhesus monkey. II. Frontal lobe afferents. Brain Res 95: 25–38

Van Leeuwen J L, Spoor C W 1993 Modelling the pressure and force equilibrium in unipennate muscles with in-line tendons. Phil Trans R Soc Lond B 342: 321–333

van Meurs-van Woezik H, Debets T, Klein H W 1987 Growth of the internal diameters in the pulmonary arterial tree in infants and children. J Anat 151: 107–115

Van Overbeeke J J, Hillen B, Tulleken C A F 1991 A comparative study of the circle of Willis in fetal and adult life. The configuration of the posterior bifurcation of the posterior communicating artery. J Anat 176: 45–54

van Straaten H W M, Hekking J W M, Wiertz-Hoessels E L, Thors F, Drukker J 1988 Anat Embryol 177: 317–324

Van Weissenbruch, Albers F W 1992 Voice rehabilitation after total laryngectomy. Acta Otorhinolaryngol Belg 46(22): 221–246

Vandekerckhove J, Bugaisky G, Buckingham M 1986 Simultaneous expression of skeletal muscle and heart actin proteins in various striated muscle tissues and cells. A quantitative determination of the two actin isoforms. J Biol Chem 261: 1838–1843

Vandenbunder B, Pardanaud L, Jaffredo T, Mirabel M A, Stehelin D 1989 Complementary patterns of expression of c-ets 1, c-myb and c-myc in the blood-forming system of the chick embryo. Development 107: 265–274

Vane J R 1969 The release and fate of vaso-active hormones in the circulation. Br J Pharmacol 35: 209–242

Vanneuville G, Mestas D, Le Bouedec G, Veyre A, Dauplat J, Escande G, Guillot M 1991 The lymphatic drainage of the human ovary in vivo investigated by isotopic lymphography before and after the menopause. Surg Radiolog Anat 13: 221–226

Vassall-Adams P R 1982 The development of the atrioventricular bundle and its branches in the avian heart. J Anat 134: 169–183

Vassallo G, Capella C, Solcia E 1971 Endocrine cells of the human gastric mucosa. Z Zellforsch 118: 49–67

Vassar R, Ngai J, Axel R 1993 Spatial segregation of odorant receptor expression in the mammalian olfactory epithelium. Cell 74: 309–318

Vastesaeger M M, van der Straeten P P, Friart J, Candaele G, Ghys A, Bernard M 1957 Les anastomoses intercoronariennes telles qu'elles apparaissent à la coronarographie postmortem. Acta Cardiol 12: 365–401

Vaughan G M, Pelham R W, Pang S F, Loughlin L L, Wilson K M, Sandock K L, Vaughan M K, Koslow S H, Reiter R J 1976 Nocturnal elevation of plasma melatonin and urinary 5-hydroxyindoleacetic acid in young men: attempts at modification by brief changes in environmental lighting and sleep and by autonomic drugs. J Clin Endocr Metab 42: 752–764

Vaughn J C 1966 The relationship of the 'sphere chromatophile' to the fate of displaced histones following histone transition in rat spermiogenesis. J Cell Biol 31: 257–278

Veen B K van, Mast E, Busschers R, Verloop A J, Wallinga W, Rutten W L C, Gerrits P O, Boom H B K 1994 Single fibre action potentials in skeletal muscle related to recording distances. J Electromyog Kinesiol 4: 37–46

Veis A 1992 Acidic proteins as regulators of biomineralization in vertebrates. In: Davidovitch Z (ed) The biological mechanisms of tooth movement and craniofacial adaptation. Ohio State Univ College Dent: Columbus: pp 115–119

Veleanu C, Grün U, Diaconescu M et al 1972 Structural peculiarities of the thoracic spine. Their functional significance. Acta Anat 82: 97–107

Venieratos D, Papadopoulos N J, Anastassiou J, Katritsis E D 1987 A quantitative estimation of the divergence between the trabecular system and stress trajectories in the upper end of the human femoral bone. Anat Anz 163: 301–310

Venning P 1956a Radiological studies of variations in the segmentation and ossification of the digits of the human foot. I. Variations in the number of phalanges and centers of ossification of the toes. Am J Phys Anthropol 14: 1–34

Venning P 1956b Radiological studies of variations in the segmentation and ossification of the digits of the human foot. II. Variations in length of the digit segments correlated with differences of segmentation and ossification of the toes. Am J Phys Anthropol 14: 129–151

Verhaart W J C, Mechelse K 1954 The pedunculus cerebri and the capsula interna. Monatsschr Psychiatry Neurol 127: 65–80

Verhoeven G 1992 Local control systems within the testis. Baillière's Clin Endocrinol Metab 6: 313–333

Verna A 1975 Observations of the innervation of the carotid body of the rabbit. In: Purves M J (ed) Peripheral arterial chemoreceptors. Cambridge University Press: Cambridge: pp 75–99

Verney E B 1947 The antidiuretic hormone and the factors which determine its release. Proc R Soc Lond [Biol] 135: 25–106

Vernon-Roberts B, Doré J L, Jessop J D, Henderson W J 1976 Selective concentration and localization of gold in macrophages of synovial and other tissues during and after crysotherapy in rheumatoid patients. Ann Rheum Dis 35: 477–486

Version G, van Marl J, van Even H, Wiljekens R 1992 Membrane architecture as a function of lens fiber maturation: a freeze fracture and scanning electron microscope study in the human lens. Exp Eye Res 54: 433–446

Verzár F, McDougall E J 1936 Absorption from the small intestine. Longmans, Green: London

Vesalius A 1543 De humani corporis fabrica libri septem. ex off J Oporini: Basel

Vesely T M, Cahill D R 1986 Cross-sectional anatomy of the pericardial sinuses, recesses, and adjacent structures. Surg Radiol Anat 8: 221–227

Viale G, Gambacorta M, Coggi G, Dell'Orto P, Milani M, Doglioni C 1991 Glial fibrillary acidic protein immunoreactivity in normal and diseased human breast. Virch Arch-A Path Anat Histopath 418: 339–348

Vidal F 1940 Pallidohypothalamic tract, or x bundle of Meynert, in the rhesus monkey. Arch Neurol Psychiatry 44: 1219–1223

Vidal G 1984 The oldest eukaryotic cells. Sci Am 249: (Feb) 32–41

Vidal-Sanz M, Bray G M, Villegas-Pérez M P, Thanos S, Aguayo A J 1987 Axonal regeneration and synapse formation in the superior colliculus by retinal ganglion cells in the adult rat. J Neurosci 7: 2894–2909

Vidíc B 1968 The origin and course of the communicating branch of the facial nerve in the lesser petrosal nerve in man. Anat Rec 162: 511–516

Vidíc B, Young P A 1967 Gross and microscopic observations on the communicating branch of the facial nerve to the lesser petrosal nerve. Anat Rec 158: 257–261

Vieussens R 1705 Novum vasorum corporis humani systema. P Marret: Amsterdam

Vigers G P, Crowther R A, Pearse B M 1986 Location of the 100 kd-50 kd accessory proteins in clathrin coats. EMBO J 5: 2079–2085

Vignal W 1889 Arch Physiol Norm Path Paris 4: 228–254, 311–338

Vijayashankar N, Brody H 1977 A study of ageing in the human abducens nucleus. J Comp Neirol 173: 433–438

Vilas E 1932 Über die Entwicklung der menschlichen Scheide. Z Anat Entwicklungsgesch 98: 263–292

Vilas E 1933 Über die Entwicklung des Utriculus prostaticus beim Menschen. Z Anat Entwicklungsgesch 99: 399–421

Villa Verde D M S, Defresne M P, Vannier-Dos-Santos M A, Dussault J H, Boniver J, Savino W 1992 Identification of nuclear triiodothyronine receptors in the thymic epithelium. Endocrinol 131: 1313–1320

Villiger E 1946 Die Periphere Innervation. 10th edition. Schwabe: Basel

Vincent S A 1966 Postural control of urinary incontinence. The curtsey sign. Lancet 2: 631–632

Vincent S R, Kimura H 1992 Histochemical mapping of nitric oxide synthase in the rate brain Neuroscience 46: 755–784

Viragh S, Challice C E 1977a The development of the conduction system in the mouse embryo heart. I. The first embryonic A–V conduction pathway. Dev Biol 56: 382–396

Viragh S, Challice C E 1977b The development of the conduction system in the mouse embryo heart. II. Histogenesis of the atrioventricular node and bundle. Dev Biol 56: 397–411

Virchow R L K 1846 Uber das granulierte Ansehen der Wandungen der Gehirnventrikel. Allg Z Psychiatry 3: 424–450

Vitek J L, Ashe J, DeLong M R, Alexander G E 1994 Physiologic properties and somatotopic organization of the primate motor thalamus. J Neurophysiol 71: 1489–1513

Vitti M, Basmajian J V 1977 Integrated actions of masticatory muscles. Anat Rec 187: 173–190

Vizoso A D, Young J Z 1948 Internode length and fibre diameter in developing and regenerating nerves. J Anat 82: 110–134

Vlahovitch B, Fuentes J M, Verger A C 1973 Angioarchitecture insulaire chez l'homme et chez les primates. Arch Anat Path 21: 395–399

Vogelberg K 1957 Die Lichtungsweite der Koronarostein an normalen und hyupertrophen herzen. Z Kreislaufforsch 46: 101–115

Vogels R, Orban G A 1994 Activity of inferior temporal neurons during orientation discrimination with successively presented gratings. J Neurophysiol 71: 1428–1451

Vogt A 1942 Lehrbuch und Atlas der Spaltlampenmikroskopie des lebenden Auges. Teil 3. Iris, Glaskörper, Bindehaut. Enke: Stuttgart

Vogt B A 1985 Cingulate cortex. Cerebral cortex. In: Jones E G, Peters A (eds) Plenum Press: New York: pp 89–149

Vogt B A, Miller M W 1983 Cortical connections between rat cingulate cortex and visual, motor, and postsubicular cortices. J Comp Neurol 216: 192–210

Vogt B A, Pandya D N, Rosene D L 1987 Cingulate cortex of the rhesus monkey. I. Cytoarchitecture and thalamic afferents. J Comp Neurol 262: 256–270

Vogt B A, Sikes R W, Swadlow H A, Weyand T G 1986 Rabbit cingulate cortex: cytoarchitecture physiological border with visual cortex, and afferent cortical connections of visual, motor, postsubicular, and intracingulate origin. J Comp Neurol 248: 74–94

Vogt W 1926 Gesaltungsanalyse am Amphienkeim mit oertlicjer Vitalfarbung. II Gastrulation und Mesdermbildung bei Urodelen und Anuran. Roux Arch Entwick Org 120: 384–706

Voloshin A S, Wosk J 1983 Shock absorption of meniscectomized and painful knees; a comparative in vivo study. J Biomed Eng 5: 157–160

Volpe E, Bellissimo U, Lamberti A 1969. Arch Oral Biol 17:

Volsch M 1906 Zur vergleichenden Anatomie des Mandelkernes und seine Nachbargebilde. Part I. Arch Mikrosk Anat 68: 573–683

Volsch M 1910 Zur vergleichenden Anatomie des Mandelkernes und seine Nachbargebilde. Part II. Arch Mikrosk Anat 76: 373–523

Voltz R G 1976 The development of a total wrist arthroplasty. Clin Orthop 116: 209–214

von Baer K E 1828 Ueber Entwicklungsgeschichte der Tiere. Bornträger Königsberg.

Von Bonin G, Bailey P 1947 The neocortex of Macaca mulatta. University of Illinois Press: Urbana

von der Mark K, Mollenhauer J, Müller P K, Pfäffle M 1985 Anchorin CII, a type II collagen-binding glycoprotein from chondrocyte membranes. Ann NY Acad Sci 460: 214–223

von Euler U S 1936 On specific vasodilating and plain muscle stimulating substances from accessory genital glands in man and certain animals (prostaglandin and vesiglandin). J Physiol 88: 213–234

von Gaudecker B 1986 The development of the human thymus microenvironment. In: Müller-Hermelink H K (ed) The human thymus. Histophysiology and pathology. Springer-Verlag: Berlin: pp 1–41

von Hayek H 1960 The human lung. Hafner: New York

von Herrath E 1958 Bau und Funktion der Normalen Milz. De Gruyter: Berlin

von Knief J-J 1967 Quantitative Untersuchung der Verteilung der Hartsubstanzen im knochen in ihrer Beziehung zur lokalen mechanischen Beanspruchung. Methodik und biomechanische Problematik, dargestellt am Beispiel des coxalen Femurendes. Z Anat Entwickl-Gesch 126: 55–80

von Lawzewitsch I, Dickmann G H, Amezua L, Pardal C 1972 Cytobiological and ultrastructural characterisation of the human pituitary. Acta Anat 81: 286–316

von Wettstein D, Rasmussen S W, Holm P B 1984 The synaptonemal complex in genetic segregation. Annu Rev Genet 18: 331–413

Voneida T J 1965 Visual loss following midline section through the mesencephalic tegmentum in cats. Anat Rec 151: 429 (abstract)

Voogd J 1964 The cerebellum of the cat. Structure and fibre connexions. Proefschr. Van Gorcum: Assen

Voogd J, Bigaré F 1980 Topographic distribution of olivary and corticonuclear fibers in the cerebellum: a review. In: Courville J, de Mountigny I, y Latha R E (eds) The Inferior Olivary Nucleus. Raven Press: New York: pp 207–234

Voogd J, Feirabend H K P, Schoen J H R 1990 Cerebellum and precerebellar nuclei. In: Paxinos G (ed) The human nervous system. Academic Press: New York: pp 321–386

Voorhout W F et al 1992 Intracellular processing of pulmonary surfactant protein B in an endosomal/lysosomal compartment. Am J Physiol 263(4 Pt 1): L479–486

Voorhout W F, Venenendaal T, Kuroki Y, Ogaswara Y, van Golde L M, Geuze H J 1992 Immunocytochemical localization of surfactant protein D (SP-D) in type II cells, Clara cells, and alveolar macrophages of rat lung. J Histochem Cytochem 40: 1589–1597

Vorherr H 1979 Human lactation. Grune and Stratton: New York

Voss H 1966 Untersuchungen über Vorkommen, Zahne und individuelle Variation der Muskelspindeln in den Muskeln des menschlichen Kehlkopfes. Anat Anz 118: 306–309

Vraa-Jensen G F 1942 The motor nucleus of the facial nerve. Munksgaard: Copenhagen

Vrabec F 1952 Sur la question de l'endothélium de la surface antérieure de l'iris humain. Ophthalmologica 123: 20–30

Vrbová G 1963 Changes in the motor reflexes produced by tenotomy. J Physiol 166: 241–250

W

Wachstein M, Bradshaw M 1965 Histochemical localisation of enzymes acting in the kidneys of three mammalian species during their postnatal development. J Histochem Cytochem 13: 44–56

Wachtler F, Jacob M 1986 Origin and development of the cranial skeletal muscles. Biblthca Anat 29: pp 24–46

Wackenheim A, Babin E 1978 Tomodensitometrie cranio-cerebral. Masson: Paris

Waddington C H 1932 Experiments on the development of chick and duck embryos cultivated in vitro. Phil Trans Roy Soc Lond 221: 179

Waddington C H 1938 The morphogenetic function of a vestigial organ in the chick. J exp Biol 15: 371–376

Waddington C H 1940 Organisers and genes. Cambridge University Press: Cambridge

Wagenvoort C A, Wagenvoort N 1967 Arterial anastomoses, bronchopulmonary arteries and pulmobronchial arteries in perinatal lungs. Lab Invest 16: 13–24

Wagner D D, Olmsted J B, Marder V J 1983 Immunolocalization of von Willebrand protein in Weibel-Palade bodies of human endotheial cells. J Cell Biol 95: 355–360

Wagner G 1955 Chimaerische Zahnanlagen aus Triton-Schmelzorgan und Bombinator-Papille. Mit Beobachtungen über die Entwicklung von Kiemenzähnchen und Mundsinnesknospen in den Triton-Larven. J Embryol Exp Morphol 3: 160–188

Wahl M, Schilling L, Unterberg A, Baethmann A 1993 Mediators of vascular and parenchymal mechanisms in secondary brain damage. Acta Neurochir Suppl Wien 57: 64–72

Wainer B H, Levey A L, Rye D B, Mesulam M-M, Mufson E J 1985 Cholinergic and non-cholinergic septohippocampal pathways. Neurosci Lett 54: 45–52

Waites G M H 1970 Temperature regulation and the testis. In: Johnson A D, Gomes W R, Vandermark N L (eds) The testis. Vol I. Academic Press: New York: pp 241–281

Waites G M H, Moule G R 1961 Relation of vascular heat exchange to temperature regulation in the testis of the ram. J Reprod Fertil 2: 213–220

Wakeley C P C 1929 A note on the architecture of the ilium. J Anat 64: 109–110P

Wakeley C P C 1933 The position of the vermiform appendix as ascertained by an analysis of 10,000 cases. J Anat 67: 277–283

Walberg F 1960 Further studies on the descending connections to the inferior olive. Reticulo-olivary fibers: an experimental study in the cat. J Comp Neurol 114: 79–87

Waldeyer W 1884 Uber den Lymphatischen Apparat des Pharynx. Deutsche Medizinische Wochenschrift 10: 313

Waldherr R, Cuzic S, Noronha I L 1992 Pathology of the human mesangium in situ. Clin Investig 70: 865–874

Wales J K H, Gibson A T 1994 Short-term growth; rhythms, or noise? Arch Dis Child 71: 84–89

Walker A C 1978 Functional anatomy of oral tissues: mastication and deglutition. In: Shaw J H, Sweeney E A, Cappuccino C C, Meller S M (eds) Textbook of oral anatomy. W B Saunders: Philadelphia: pp 277–296

Walker A E 1937 Experimental anatomical studies of the topical localisation within the thalamus of the chimpanzee. Proc K Med Akad Wet 40: 198–206

Walker A E 1940 The spinothalamic tract in man. Arch Neurol Psychia 43: 284–298

Walker A E 1943 Central representation of pain. In: Wolff H G, Gasser H S, Hinsey J S (eds) Pain. (Res Publ Assoc Res Nerv Ment Dis 23: 63–85)

Walker A, Turnbull J E, Gallagher J T 1994 Specific heparan sulphates accharids mediate the activity of basic fibrioblast growth factor. J Biol Chem 269: 931–935

Walker J M 1980 Morphological variants in the human fetal hip – their significance in congenital hip disease. J Bone Jt Surg 62A: 1073–1082

Walker L T 1991 The biomechanics of the human foot. PhD Thesis

Wall J T, Huerta M F, Kaas J H 1992a Changes in the cortical map of the hand following postnatal median nerve injury in monkeys: modification of somatotopic aggregates. J Neurosci 12: 3445–3455

Wall J T, Huerta M F, Kaas J H 1992b Changes in the cortical map of the hand following postnatal ulnar and radial nerve injury in monkeys: organization and modification of nerve dominance aggregates. J Neurosci 12: 3456–3465

Wall P D 1964 Presynaptic control of impulses at the first central synapse in the cutaneous pathway. Progr Brain Res 12: 92–118

Wall P D 1970 The sensory and motor role of impulses travelling in the dorsal columns towards cerebral cortex. Brain 93: 505–524

Wall P D 1973 Dorsal horn electrophysiology. In: Iggo A (ed) Handbook of sensory physiology. Vol 2. Springer: Berlin: pp 253–270

Wall P D 1976 Modulation of pain by non-painful events. In: Bonica J J, Albe-Fessard D G (eds) Advances in pain research and therapy. Raven Press: New York: pp 1–16

Wall P D 1978 The gate control theory of pain mechanisms. A re-examination and re-statement. Brain 101: 1–18

Wall P D 1985 Pain. In Swash M, Kennard C (eds) Scientific basis of clinical neurology. Churchill Livingstone: Edinburgh: pp 163–171

Wall P D, Melzac R 1988 Textbook of pain. 2nd edition. Churchill Livingstone: Edinburgh

Wall P D, Noordenbos W 1977 Sensory functions which remain in man after complete transection of dorsal columns. Brain 100: 641–653

Wall R T, Harker L A, Quadracci L J, Striker G E 1978 Factors influencing endothelial cell proliferation in vitro. J Cell Physiol 96: 203–214

Wallace D C 1992 Diseases of mitochondrial DNA. Annu Rev Biochem 61: 1175–1212

Waller A V 1850 Experiments on the section of the glossopharyngeal and hypoglossal nerves of the frog, and observations of the alterations produced thereby in the structure of their primitive fibres. Philos Trans R Soc Lond [Biol] 140: 423–429

Walls E W 1958 Observations on the microscopic anatomy of the human anal canal. Br J Surg 45: 504–512

Walls G L 1963 The vertebrate eye. Hafner: New York

Walmsley B, Hodgson J A, Burke R E 1978 Forces produced by medial gastrocnemius and soleus muscles during locomotion in freely moving cats. J Neurophysiol 41: 1203–1216

Walmsley J G 1983 Structure of small blood vessels related to smooth muscle mechanics. In: Bevan J (ed) Vascular neuroeffector mechanisms. Raven Press: New York: pp 175–182

Walmsley J G, Canham P B 1979 Orientation of nuclei as indicators of smooth muscle cell alignment in the cerebral artery. Blood Vessels 16: 43–51

Walmsley R 1953 The development and growth of intervertebral disc. Edin Med J 60: 341–364

Walmsley R, Watson H 1978 Clinical anatomy of the heart. Churchill Livingstone: Edinburgh

Walmsley T 1915 The costal musculature. J Anat 50: 165–171

Walmsley T 1928 Articular mechanism of diarthroses. J Bone Jt Surg 10: 40–45

Walmsley T 1929 The heart. In: Quain J (ed) Elements of descriptive and practical anatomy. Vol 4, Pt 3. Longmans, Green: London

Walsh C, Cepko C L, 1988 Science 241: 1342–1345

Walsh C, Cepko C L, 1992 Science 255: 434–440

Walsh C, Cepko C L, 1993 Science 362: 632–635

Walsh F S, Doherty P 1993 Factors regulating the expression and function of calcium-independent cell adhesion molecules. Curr Opin Cell Biol 5: 791–796

Walter J, Henke-Fahle S, Bonhoeffer F 1987 Development 101: 909–913

Walther C, Guenet J L, Simon D, Deutsch U, Jostes B, Goulding M D, Plachov D, Balling R, Gruss P 1991 Pax: a murine multigene family of paired box containing genes. Genomics 11: 424–434

Waltner J G 1948 Barrier membrane of cochlear aqueduct: histologic studies on the patency of the cochlear aqueduct. Arch Otolaryngol 47: 656–669

Walton A J 1931 Surgical treatment of parathyroid tumours. Br J Surg 19: 285–291

Walton A, Hammond J 1938 The maternal effects on growth and information in Shire horse–Shetland pony crosses. Proc Roy Soc London Ser B–Biol Sci 125: 311–335

Walton J, Yoshigama J M, Vanderlaan M 1982 Ultrastructure of the rat urothelium in en face section. J Submicrosc Cytol 1: 1–15

Walton P E, Cronin M J 1990 Tumor-necrosis factor-alpha and interferon-gamma reduce prolactin release in vitro. Am J Physiol 259: E672–E676

Wang K P, Tai H P 1965 An analysis of variations of the segmental vessels of the right lower lobe in 50 Chinese lungs. Acta Anat Sin 8: 408–423

Wang K, McLure J, Tu A 1979 Titin: major myofibrillar components of striated muscle. Proc Natl Acad Sci USA 76: 3698–3702

Wang N S, Ying W L 1977 A scanning electron microscopic study of alkali-digested human and rabbit alveoli. Am Rev Resp Dis 115: 449–460

Warbrick J C 1960 The early development of the nasal cavity and upper lip in the human embryo. J Anat 94: 351–362

Ward F O 1838 Outlines of human osteology. Renshaw: London

Warner F D, Mitchell D R 1980 Dynein the mechanochemical coupling adenosine triphosphatase of microtubule-based sliding filament mechanisms. Int Rev Cytol 66: 1–43

Warner F D, Satir P 1974 The structural basis of ciliary bend formation. Radial spoke positional changes accompanying microtubule sliding. J Cell Biol 63: 35–63

Warr W B 1966 Fiber degeneration following lesions in the anterior ventral cochlear nucleus of the cat. Exp Neurol 14: 453–474

Wartenberg H, Holstein A F 1975 Morphology of the spindle shaped body in the developing tail of human spermatids. Cell Tissue Res 159: 435–443

Warwick R 1950 The relation of the direction of the mental foramen to the growth of the human mandible. J Anat 84: 116–120

Warwick R 1951 A juvenile skull exhibiting duplication of the optic canals. J Anat 85: 289–291

Warwick R 1968 The skeletal remains. In: Wenham L P (ed) The Romano-British Cemetery at Trentholme Drive, York. (Ministry of Public Building and Works, Archaeological Report 5.) HMSO: London: pp 113–178

Warwick R, Mitchell G A G 1956 Localization of the phrenic nucleus in the spinal cord of man. J Comp Neurol 105: 683–700

Washburn S L 1947 The relation of the temporal muscle to the form of the skull. Anat Rec 99: 239–248

Washburn S L 1949 Sex differences in the pubic bone of Bantu and Bushman. Am J Phys Anthropol 7: 425–432

Wassarman P M 1988 The mammalian ovum. In: Knobil E, Neil J D (eds) The physiology of reproduction. Vol 1. Raven Press: New York

Wassarman P M 1990 Profile of a mammalian sperm receptor. Development 108: 1–17

Wassermann E M, Pascual-Leone A, Hallett M 1994 Cortical motor representation of the ipsilateral hand and arm. Exp Brain Res 100: 121–132

Wassle H, Boycott B B 1991 Functional architecture of the mammalian retina. Physiol Rev 71: 447–480

Wassle H, Grunert U, Martin P, Boycott B 1994a Immunochemical characterization and spatial distribution of midget bipolar cells in the macaque monkey retin. Vision Res 34: 561–579

Wassle H, Grunert U, Martin P, Boycott B 1994b Color coding in the primate retina, predictions and constraints from anatomy. Exp Brain Res Series 24. Springer : Berlin: pp94–104

Watanabe M, Rodick R W 1989 Parasol and midget ganglion cells of the primate retina. J Comp Neurol 289: 434–454

Watanabe M, Takeda S, Ikeuchi H 1979 Atlas of Arthroscopy. Springer-Verlag: Berlin: pp 87–91

Watanabe T, Raff M C 1992 Diffusible rod-promoting signals in the developing rat retina. Development 114: 899–906

Watanabe Y 1960 An experimental study on the coronary luminal communicating channels in coronary circulation. Jpn Circ J 24: 11–26

Watchko J F Maycock D E, Standaert T A, Woodrum D E 1991 The ventilatory pump: neonatal and developmental issues. Adv Paediatr 38: 109–134

Waters N E 1980 Some mechanical and physical properties of teeth. Symp Soc Exp Biol 34: 99–135

Watson D M S 1917 The evolution of tetrapod shoulder girdle and forelimb. J Anat 52: 1–63

Watson J D G, Myers R, Frackowiak R S J, Hajnal J V, Woods R P, Mazziotta J C et al 1992 Area V5 of the human brain: evidence from a combined study using positron emission tomography and magnetic resonance imaging. Cereb Cortex 3: 79–94

Watson J D, Crick F H C 1952 Molecular structure of nucleic acids. A structure for deoxyribonucleic acid. Nature 171: 737–738

Watterson P A, Taylor G I, Crock J G 1988 The venous territories of muscles: anatomical study and clinical implications. Br J Plastic Surg 41: 569–585

Watterson R L 1965 Structure and mitotic behavior of the early neural tube. In: DeHaan R L, Ursprung H (eds) Organogenesis. Holt: New York: pp 129–159

Watterson R L, Veneziano P, Bartha A 1956 Absence of a true germinal zone in neural tubes of young chick embryos as demonstrated by the colchicine technique. Anat Rec 124: 379

Watzka M 1955 Die Leydigschen Zwischenzellen im Funiculus spermaticus des Menschen. Z Zellforsch 43: 206–213

Watzke R C, Soldevilla J D, Trune D R 1993 Morphometric analysis of human retinal pigment epithelium correlation with age and location. Curr Eye Res 12: 133–142

Waxman S G 1981 Plasticity in the ontogeny and pathophysiology of myelinated fibers. In: Waxman S G, Ritchie J M (eds) Demyelinating diseases. Advances in Neurology 31: 69–92 Raven Press: New York

Weale R A 1970 Optical properties of photoreceptors. Br Med Bull 26: 134–137

Wearn J T 1941 Morphological and functional alterations of coronary circulation. Harvey Lect 17: 754–777

Wearn J T, Mettier S R, Klumpp T G, Zschiesche L J 1933 The nature of the vascular communications between the coronary arteries and the chambers of the heart. Am Heart J 9: 143–164

Weaver T E, Whitsett J A 1991 Function and regulation of expression of pulmonary surfactant-associated proteins. Biochem J 273(Pt 2): 249–264

Webber C E, Garnett E S 1976 Density of os calcis and limb dominance. J Anat 121: 203–205

Weber R G, Jones C R, Lohse M J, Palacios J M 1990 Autoradiographic visualization of A$_1$ adenosine receptors in rat brain with [^{3}H]8-cyclopentyl-1,3-dipropylxanthine. J Neurochem 54: 1344–1353

Webster H de F 1993 Development of peripheral nerve fibres. In: Dyck P J, Thomas P K, Griffin J W, Low P A, Poduslo J F (eds) Peripheral Neuropathy 3rd edition. W B Saunders: Philadelphia: pp 243–260

Webster H H, Jones B E 1988 Neurotoxic lesions of the dorsolateral pontomesencephalic tegmentum-cholinergic cell area in the cat. II. Effects upon sleep-waking states. Brain Research 458: 285–302

Webster K E 1974 Changing concepts of the organization of the central visual pathways in birds. In: Bellairs R, Gray E G (eds) Essays on the nervous system. Clarendon Press: Oxford: pp 258–298

Webster K E 1975 Structure and function of the basal ganglia. A non-clinical view. Proc R Soc Med 68: 203–210

Webster K E 1977 Somaesthetic pathways. Br Med Bull 33: 113–119

Webster K E 1978 The brainstem reticular formation. In: Hennings G, Hemmings W A (eds) The biological basis of schizophrenia. MTP: Lancaster

Webster K E 1990 The functional anatomy of the basal ganglia. In: Stern G (ed) Parkinson's disease. Chapman and Hall Medical: London: pp 3–56

Webster M J, Ungerleider L G, Bachevalier J 1991 Connections of inferior temporal areas TE and TEO with medial temporal-lobe structures in infant and adult monkeys. J Neurosci 11: 1095–1116

Webster P D, Black U, Mainz D L, Singh M 1977 Pancreatic acinar cell metabolism and function. Gastroenterology 73: 1434–1449

Webster W R, Garey L J 1990 Auditory system. In: Paxinos G (ed) The human nervous system. Academic Press: San Diego: pp 889–944

Webster W R, Servière J, Brown M 1984 Inhibitory contours in the inferior colliculus as revealed by the 2-deoxyglucose method. Exp Brain Res 56: 577 – 581

Webster W R, Servière J, Crewther D, Crewther S 1984 Iso-frequency 2-DG contours in the inferior colliculus of the awake monkey. Exp Brain Res 56: 427 – 437

Weed L H 1923 The absorption of cerebrospinal fluid into the venous system. Am J Anat 31: 191–221

Weibel E R 1971 The mystery of 'non-nucleated plates' in the alveolar epithelium of the lung explained. Acta Anat 78: 425–443

Weibel E R, Elias H 1969 Quantitative methods in morphology. Springer-Verlag: Berlin

Weibel E R, Gehr P, Haies D, Gil J, Bachofen M 1976 The cell population of the normal lung. In: Bouhuys A (ed) Lung cells in disease. North-Holland: Amsterdam: pp 3–16

Weibel E R, Palade G E 1964 New cytoplasmic components in arterial endothelia. J Cell Biol 23: 101–112

Weihe E, Muller S, Fink T, Zentel H J 1989 Tachykinins, calcitonin gene-related peptide and neuropeptide Y in nerves of the mammalian thymus: interactions with mast cells in autonomic and sensory neuro-immunomodulation? Neurosci Let 100: 77–82

Weil A J 1965 The spermatozoa-coating antigen (SCA) of the seminal vesicle. Ann NY Acad Sci 124: 267–269

Weindl A, Joynt R J 1972 Ultrastructure of the ventricular walls. Three-dimensional study of regional specialization. Arch Neurol 26: 420–427

Weiner N, Schadé J P (eds) 1963 Nerve, brain and memory models. Elsevier: Amsterdam

Weiner S, Traub W 1989 Crystal size and organization in bone. Connect Tissue Res 21: 259–265

Weinmann J P, Sicher H 1955 Bone and bones. Fundamentals of bone biology. 2nd edition. Kimpton: London

Weinstock M, Leblond C P 1973 Radioautographic visualization of the deposition of a phosphoprotein at the mineralization front in the dentin of the rat incisor. J Cell Biol 56: 838–845

Weintraub H, Davis R, Tapscott S, Yhayer M, Krause M, Benezra B, Blackwell T, Turner D, Rupp R, Hollenberg S, Zhuang Y, Lassar A 1991 The MyoD family: nodal point during specification of the muscle cell lineage. Science 251: 761–766

Weisengreen H H 1975 Observation of the articular disc. Oral Surg 40: 113–121

Weiskrantz L 1956 Behavioral changes associated with ablation of the amygdaloid complex in monkeys. J Comp Physiol Psychol 49: 381–391

Weisl H 1953 The relation of movement to structure in the sacroiliac joint. PhD Thesis, University of Manchester

Weisl H 1954a The articular surfaces of the sacro-iliac joint and their relation to the movements of the sacrum. Acta Anat 22: 1–14

Weisl H 1954b The ligaments of the sacro-iliac joint examined with particular reference to their function. Acta Anat 20: 201–213

Weisl H 1955 Movements of the sacro-iliac joint. Acta Anat 23: 80–91

Weiss L 1990 Mechanisms of splenic clearance of the blood; a structural overview of the mammalian spleen. In: Bowdler AJ (ed) The spleen. Structure, function and significance. Chapman and Hall Medical: London: pp 23–43

Weiss L (ed) 1984 Histology. Cell and tissue biology. 5th edition. Macmillan: New York

Weiss L 1957 A study of the structure of splenic sinuses in man and the albino rat with the light microscope and the electron microscope. J Biophys Biochem Cytol 3: 599–610

Weiss L 1983b The spleen. In: Weiss L (ed) Histology. Cell and tissue biology. 5th edition. Macmillan: New York: pp 544–568

Weiss L (ed) 1983a Histology: cell and tissue biology. 5th edition. Elsevier Science: New York

Weiss P 1941 Nerve patterns: the mechanics of nerve growth. Growth (suppl 5): 163–203

Weiss P 1950 An introduction to genetic neurology. In: Weiss P (ed) Genetic neurology. Problems of the development, growth, and regeneration of the nervous system and of its functions. Chicago University Press: Chicago: pp 1–39

Weiss P 1970 Neural development in biological perspective. In: Schmitt F O, Quarton G C, Melnechuk T, Adelman G (eds) The neuroscience. Second study program. Rockefeller University Press: New York: pp 53–61

Weiss P, Hiscoe H B 1948 Experiments on the mechanism of nerve growth. J Exp Zool 107: 315–396

Weiss S J, Lobuglio A F 1982 Biology and disease. Phagocyte-generated oxygen metabolites and cellular injury. Lab Invest 47: 5–18

Weitbrecht J 1742 Ligamenta artuum superiorum sectio secundum in syndesmologia sive historia ligamentorum corporis humani. Typographia Academiae Scientarum: Petropolis: pp 43–44, 50

Wekerle H 1993 T-cell autoimmunity in the central nervous system. Intervirology 35: 95–100

Welgus H G, Campbell E J, Bar-Shavit Z, Senior R M, Teitelbaum S L 1985 Human alveolar macrophages produce a fibroblast-like collagenase and collagenase inhibitor. J Clin Invest 76: 219–224

Welker E, van der Loos H 1986 J Neurosci 6: 3355–3373

Welker W 1987 Spatial organization of somatosensory projections to granule cell cerebellar cortex: functional and connectional implications of fractured somatotopy (summary of Wisconsin studies). In: King J S (ed) New concepts in cerebellar neurobiology. Liss: New York: pp 239–280

Weller L G Jr 1933 Development of the thyroid, parathyroid and thymus glands in man. Contrib Embryol Carnegie Inst Washington 24: 93–139

Weller R E, Steele G E 1992 Cortical connections of subdivisions of inferior temporal cortex in squirrel monkeys. J Comp Neurol 324: 37–66

Weller R O 1990 Tumours of the nervous system. In: Weller R O (ed) Systemic pathology. Central nervous system, muscle and eyes. 3rd edition. Churchill Livingstone: Edinburgh: pp 427–503

Weller R O, Kida S, Zhang E-T 1992 Pathways of fluid drainage from the brain – morphological aspects and immunological significance in rat and man. Brain Pathol 2: 277–284

Weller R O, Steart P V, Moore I E 1986 Carbonic anhydrase C as a marker antigen in the diagnosis of choroid plexus papillomas and other tumours. An immunoperoxidase study. In: Walker M D, Thomas D G T. (eds) Biology of brain tumour Nijhoff Martinus and Dr W Junk: Dordrecht: pp 115–120

Wellings S R 1980 Development of human breast cancer. Adv Cancer Res 31: 287–314

Wells L J 1954 Development of the human diaphragm and pleural sacs. Contrib Embryol Carnegie Inst Washington 35: 107–134

Wenckebach K F 1906 Beitrage zur Kenntnis des menschlichen Hertztätigheit. Archiv fur Physiologie 297–354

Wende S, Nakayama N, Schwerdtfeger P 1975 The internal auditory artery (embryology, anatomy, angiography, pathology). J Neurol 210: 21–31

Wendell Smith C P, Wilson P M 1991 The vulva, vagina and urethra and the musculature of the pelvic floor. In: Philipp E, Setchell M, Ginsburg J (eds) Scientific foundations of obstetrics and gynaecology. Butterworth-Heinemann: Oxford: pp 84–100

Wendell-Smith C P 1967 Studies on the morphology of the pelvic floor. PhD Thesis, University of London

Wendell-Smith C P, Williams P L, Treadgold S 1984 Basic human embryology. 3rd edition. Urban and Schwarzenberg: Baltimore

Wendell-Smith C P, Wilson P M 1977 Musculature of the pelvic floor. In: Philipp E E, Barnes J, Newton M (eds) Scientific foundations of obstetrics and gynaecology. 2nd edition. Heinemann Medical: London: pp 78–84

Wendler D 1968 Histologisch-histochemische Befunde an der Schleimhaut des Ductus deferens (pars funicularis) bein geschlectsreifen Mann. Acta Histochem 31: 48–69

Wenink A C G 1971 Some details on the final stages of heart septation in the human embryo. Thesis. Leiden

Wenink A C G 1976 Development of the human cardiac conducting system. J Anat 121: 617–631

Wennberg E, Weiss L 1969 The structure of the spleen and hemolysis. Ann Rev Med 20: 29–40

Werneck H J L 1957 Contribuicção paro o estudo de alguns aspectos morfologicos de M fibularis tertius. An Fac Med Univ Minas Gerais 17: 417–520

Werner S 1978 Immune system. III. Role in thyroid disease. In: Werner S, Ingbar S H (eds) The thyroid. Harper and Row: New York: pp 615–623

Werner S. Weinberg W H, Liad X, Peters K G, Blessing M, Yuspa S M, Weiner R L, Williams L T 1993 Targeted expression of a dominant negative FGF receptor mutant in the epidermis of transgenic mice reveals a role of FGF in Keratinocyte organization and differentiation. The EMBO Journal 12: 2635–2643

Wernert N, Kern L, Heitz P, Bonkhoff H, Goebbels R, Seitz G, Inniger R, Remberger K, Dohm G 1990 Morphological and immunohistochemical investigations of the utriculous prostaticus from the fetal period to adulthood. Prostate 17: 19–30

Wersäll J 1956 The sensory epithelium of the cristac ampullares. Acta Otolaryngol [Stockh] Suppl 126: 1–85

Wertheim M G 1847 Mémoire sur l'élasticité et la cohésion des principaux tissus du corps humain. Ann Chim Phys 21: 385

Wessells N K 1977 Tissue interaction and development. Benjamin: Menlo Park CA

Wessells A, Vermeulen J L M, Verbeek F J, Viragh S Z Kalman F, Lamers W H, Moorman A F M 1992 Spatial distribution of tissue-specific antigens in the developing human heart and skeletal muscle III: An immunohistochemical analysis of the distribution of the neural tissue antigen G1N2 in the embryonic heart; implications for the development of the conduction system. Anat Rec 232: 97–111

Wessels N K 1964 Tissue interactions and cytodifferentiation. Journal Experimental Zoology 157: 139–152

Wessels N K 1971 Tissue interaction and development. Benjamin: Menlo Park CA

Wessels N K, Spooner B S, Ash J F, Bradley M O, Luduena M A, Taylor L E, Wrenn J T, Yamada K M 1971 Microfilaments in cellular and developmental processes. Science 171: 135–143

Wesson M B 1951 Rationale of prostatectomy. Am J Surg 82: 714–719

West G B, Shepherd D M, Hunter R B, MacGregor A R 1953 The function of the organs of Zuckerkandl. Clin Sci 12: 317–326

Westheimer G 1954 Mechanism of saccadic eye movements. Arch Ophthal 52: 710–724

Westheimer G, Blair S M 1973 Oculomotor deficits in cerebellectomy in monkeys. J Ophthal 12: 618–621

Westheimer G, Blair S M 1974 Functional organization of primate oculomotor system revealed by cerebellectomy. Exp Brain Res 21: 463–472

Weston J A 1963 A radioautographic analysis of the migration and localization of trunk neural crest in the chick. Dev Biol 6: 279–310

Weston J A 1970 The migration and differentiation of neural crest cells. In: Abercrombie M, Brachet J (eds) Advances in morphogenesis. Vol 8. Academic Press: New York: pp 41–114

Weston J A 1971 In: Pearse D (ed) Cellular aspects of growth and differentiation in nervous tissue. UCLA Forum in Medical Sciences 14: 1–19

Wetzel B K, Spicer S S, Wollman S H 1965 Changes in fine structure and acid phosphatase localization in rat thyroid cells following thyrotropin administration. J Cell Biol 25: 593–618

Whalen R G, Sell, S M, Butler-Browne G S, Schwartz K, Bouveret P, Pinset-Härström I 1981 Three myosin heavy-chain isozymes appear sequentially in rat muscle development. Nature 292: 805–809

Wheatley V R (ed) 1986 The sebaceous glands. The physiology and pathophysiology of the skin. Vol 9. (Jarret A ed.) Academic Press: London

Whillis J 1930 A note on the muscles of the palate and the superior constrictor. J Anat 65: 92–95

Whillis J 1931 Lower end of the oesophagus. J Anat 66: 132–133P

Whillis J 1946 Movements of the tongue in swallowing. J Anat 80: 115–116

Whiston R J, Melhuish J, Harding K G 1992 High resolution ultrasound imaging in wound healing. Wounds 5: 116–121

Whitby D J, Ferguson M W J 1991a The extracellular matrix of lip wounds in fetal, neonatal and adult mice. Development 112: 651–668

Whitby D J, Ferguson M W J 1991b Immunohistochemical localisation of growth factors fetal wound healing Developmental Biology 147: 207–215

White E G 1935 Die struktur des glomus caroticum. Beitr Path Anat 96: 177–227

White J C, Smithwick R H, Simeone F A 1952 The autonomic nervous system. 3rd edition. Kimpton: London

White L E, Lucas G, Richards A, Purves D 1994 Cerebral asymmetry and handedness. Nature 368: 197–198

Whitehead E D, Leiter E 1981 Genital abnormalities and abnormal semen analyses in male patients exposed to diethylstilbestrol in utero. J Urol 125: 47–50

Whitehead M L 1986 Anatomy of the gustatory system in the hamster: synaptology of the facial afferent terminals in the solitary nucleus. J Comp Neurol 244: 72–85

Whitehouse H L K 1973 Towards an understanding of the mechanism of heredity. 3rd edition. Arnold: London

Whitehouse H L K, Hastings P J 1965 The analysis of genetic recombination on the polaron hybrid DNA model. Genet Res 6: 27–92

Whitehouse W J 1975 Scanning electron micrographs of cancellous bone from the human sternum. J Pathol 116: 213–224

Whitehouse W J 1977 Cancellous bone in the anterior part of the iliac crest. Calcif Tissue Res 23: 67–76

Whitehouse W J, Dyson E D 1974 Scanning electron microscope studies of trabecular bone in the proximal end of the human femur. J Anat 118: 417–444

Whitelaw M J 1933 Tubal contractions in relation to estrus cycle as determined by uterotubal insufflation. Am J Obstet Gynecol 25: 475–484

Whiteley H J, Stoner H B 1957 The effect of pregnancy on the human adrenal cortex. J Endocrinol 14: 325–334

Whitlock D G, Nauta W J H 1956 Subcorticol projections from the temporal neocortex in Macaca mulatta. J Comp Neurol 106: 183–212

Whitmore I 1982 Oesophageal striated muscle arrangement and histochemical fibre types in guinea-pig, marmoset, macaque and man. J Anat 134: 685–695

Whitnall S E 1911 The relation of the lacrimal fossa to the ethmoidal cells. Ophthal Rev 30: 321–325

Whitnall S E 1932 Anatomy of the human orbit. 2nd edition. Oxford University Press: London

Whitsel B L, Petrucelli L M, Sapiro G 1969 Modality representation in the lumbar and cervical fasciculus of squirrel monkeys. Brain Res 15: 67–78

Whitsel B L, Petrucelli L M, Sapiro G, Ha H 1970 Fiber sorting in the fasciculus gracilis of squirrel monkeys. Exp Neurol 29: 227–243

Whittaker D K 1992 Quantitative studies on age changes in the teeth and surrounding structures in archaelogical material: a review. J Roy Soc Med 85: 97–101

Whittaker D K, Richards D 1978 Scanning electron microscopy of the neonatal line in human enamel. Arch Oral Biol 23: 45–50

Wiberg M, Westman J, Blomqvist A 1987 Somatosensory projection to the mesencephalon: an anatomical study in the monkey. J Comp Neurol 264: 92–117

Wictorin K, Brundin P, Sauer H, Lindvall O, Björklund A 1992 Long distance directed axonal growth from human dopaminergic mesencephalic neuroblasts implanted along the nigrostriatal pathway in 6-hydroxydopamine lesioned adult rats. J Comp Neurol 323: 475 – 494

Wieczorek D F, Periasamy M, Butler-Browne G S, Whalen R G, Nadal-Ginard B 1985 Co-expression of multiple myosin heavy chain genes, in addition to a tissue-specific one, in extraocular musculature. J Cell Biol 101: 618–629

Wiedeman M P, Tuma R F, Mayrovitz H N 1976 Defining the precapillary sphincter. Microvascular Res 12: 71–75

Wiedemann H R 1964 Complexe malformatif familial avec hernie ombilicale et macroglossie – un 'syndrome nouveau'? J Genet Hum 13: 232–233

Wiedersheim R 1895 The structure of man. Macmillan: London

Wieniawa-Narkiewicz E, Hughes A 1992 The superficial plexiform layer: a third retinal association area. J Comp Neurol 324: 463–484

Wienke E C, Cavazos F, Hall D G, Lucas F V 1968 Ultrastructure of the human endometrial stromal cell during the menstrual cycle. Am J Obstet Gynecol 102: 65–77

Wier W G 1993 Excitation–contraction coupling in mammalian ventricle. In: Gwathmey J K, Briggs G M, Allen P D (eds) Heart failure. Basic science and clinical aspects. Marcel Dekker: New York: pp 11–38

Wiesendanger M, Rüegg D G, Wiesendanger R 1979 The corticopontine system in primates: anatomical and functional considerations. In: Massion J, Sasaki K (eds) Cerebro-cerebellar interactions. Elsevier: North Holland: pp 45–65

Wiesendanger R, Wiesendanger M 1985 The thalamic connections with medial area 6 (supplementary motor cortex) in the monkey (Macaca fascicularis). Exp Brain Res 59: 91–104

Wigglesworth J S 1980 Brain development and the structural basis of perinatal brain damage. Mean Johnson Symp Pernat Dev Med 17: 3–10

Wigglesworth J S, Pape K E 1978 An integrated model for haemorrhage and ischaemic lesions in the newborn baby. Early Hum Dev 2: 179–199

Wigglesworth J S, Pape K E 1980 Pathophysiology of intracranial haemorrhage in the newborn. J Perinat Med 8: 119–133

Wijngaert F P van de, Kendall M D, Schuurman H-J, Rademakers L H P M, Kater L 1984 Heterogeneity of epithelial cells in the human thymus. An ultrastructural study. Cell Tissue Res 237: 227–237

Wikler A 1965 Conditioning factors in opiate addiction and relapse. In: Wiher D I, Kassebaum G (eds) Narcotics. McGraw-Hill: New York

Wiksten B 1975 The central cervical nucleus—a source of spinocerebellar fibres, demonstrated by retrograde transport of horseradish peroxidase. Neurosci Lett 1: 81–84

Wilcox J N 1993 Molecular biology: insight into the causes and prevention of restenosis after arterial intervention. Am J Cardiol 72: 88E–95E

Wilde F R 1949 Anal intermuscular spasm. Br J Surg 36: 279–285

Wilde F R 1951 Perivascular neural pattern of femoral region. Br J Surg 39: 97–105

Wildi E, Frauchiger E 1965 Modifications histologiques de l'epiphyse humaine pendant l'enfance, l'age adulte et le viellissement. Progr Brain Res 10: 218–233

Wiles P 1935 Movements of lumbar vertebrae during flexion and extension. Proc R Soc Med 28: 647–651

Wiley L M, Wu J-X, Harari I, Adamson E A 1992 Epidermal growth factor receptor mRNA and protein increase after the four cell preimplantation stage in murine development. Dev Biol 149: 247–260

Wiley R G 1992 Neural lesioning with ribosome-inactivating proteins: suicide transport and immunolesioning. TINS 15: 285–289

Wiley-Livingston, C A, Ellisman M H 1980 Development of axonal membrane specializations defines nodes of Ranvier and precedes Schwann cell myelination. Dev Biol 79: 334–355

Wilkinson D G, Bhatt S, Chavrier P, Bravo R and Charnay P 1989b Segment-specific expression of a zinc-finger gene in the developing nervous system of the mouse. Nature 337: 461–464

Wilkinson D G, Bhatt S, Cook M, Bonicelli E, Krumlauf R 1989a Segmental expression of Hox 2 homeobox-containing genes in the developing mouse hindbrain. Nature 341: 405–409

Wilkinson J L 1953 The insertions of the flexores pollicis longus et digitorum profundus. J Anat 87: 75–88

Wilkinson J L 1954 The terminal phalanx of the great toe. J Anat 88: 537–541

Willcox N 1989 The thymus in myasthenia gravis patients, and the in vivo effects of corticosteroids on its cellularity, histology and functions. Thymus Update 2: 105–124

Williams A F 1951 Nerve supply of laryngeal muscles. J Laryngol Otol 65: 343–348

Williams A F 1954 Recurrent laryngeal nerve and the thyroid gland. J Laryngol Otol 68: 719–725

Williams D E, de Vries P, Namen A E Widmer M B, Lyman S D 1992 The Steel factor. Dev Biol 151: 368–376

Williams D J 1936 Origin of posterior cerebral artery. Brain 59: 175–180

Williams D S, Hallett M A, Arikawa K I 1992 Association of myosin with the connecting cilium of rod photoreceptors. J Cell Sci 103: 183–190

Williams J F, Svensson N L 1968 A force analysis of the hip joint. Bio-Med Eng 3: 365–370

Williams P E, Goldspink G L 1971 Longitudinal growth of striated muscle fibres. J Cell Sci 9: 751–767

Williams P F III, Powell G L, LaBerge M 1993 Sliding friction analysis of phosphatidylcholine as a boundary lubricant for articular cartilage. Proc Inst Mech Eng H 207: 59–66

Williams P L, Hall S M 1970 In vivo observations on mature myelinated nerve fibres of the mouse. J Anat 107: 31–38

Williams P L, Hall S M 1971 Prolonged in vivo observations of normal peripheral nerve fibres and their acute reactions to crush and deliberate trauma. J Anat 108: 397–408

Williams P L, Hall S M 1971b Chronic Wallerian degeneration – an in vivo and ultrastructural study. J Anat 109: 487–503

Williams P L, Kashef R 1968 Asymmetry of the node of Ranvier. J Cell Sci 3: 341–356

Williams P L, Warwick R, Dyson M, Bannister L H (eds) 1989 Gray's anatomy. 37th edition. Churchill Livingstone: Edinburgh

Williams P L, Wendell-Smith C P 1971 Some parametric variations between peripheral nerve fibre populations. J Anat 109: 505–526

Williams P L, Wendell-Smith C P, Treadgold S 1969 Basic human embryology, 2nd edition. Lippincott: Philadelphia

Williams R A D, Elliott J C 1979 Basic and applied dental biochemistry. Churchill Livingstone: Edinburgh

Williams T H 1967 Electron microscopic evidence for an autonomic interneuron. Nature 214: 309–310

Williams T H 1971 Morphological interactions of sheath cells and neurites, using the Murray and Thompson model. J Anat 110, 158P

Williams T H, Black A C Jr, Chiba T, Bhalla R C 1975 Morphology and biochemistry of small, intensely fluorescent cells of sympathetic ganglia. Nature 256: 315–317

Williams T H, Palay S L 1969 Ultrastructure of the small neurones in the superior cervical ganglion. Brain Res 15: 17–34

Williams T J, Jose P J 1981 Mediation of increased vascular permeability after complement activation: histamine independent action of C5a. J Exp Med 153: 136–153

Willis A G, Tange J D 1959 Studies of the innervation of the carotid sinus of man. Am J Anat 104: 87–114

Willis R A 1936 Growth of embryo bones transplanted whole in rat's brain. Proc R Soc Lond [Biol] 120: 496–498

Willis T A 1949 Nutrient arteries of the vertebral bodies. J Bone Jt Surg 31A: 538–540

Willis W D 1988 Anatomy and physiology of descending control of nociceptive responses of dorsal horn neurons: comprehensive review. In: Fields H L, Benson J M (eds) Prog Brain Res. Elsevier: Amsterdam: pp 1–29

Willis W D, Coggeshall R E 1991 Sensory mechanisms of the spinal cord. Plenum Press: New York

Willis W D, Trevino D L, Coulter J P, Marenz R 1974 Responses of primate spinothalamic tract nerurons to natural stimulation of hindlimb. J Neurophysiol 37: 358–372

Willis W D, Willis J C 1966 Properties of interneurons in the ventral spinal cord. Archs Ital Biol 104: 354–386

Willmer E N 1960 Cytology and evolution. Academic Press: London

Willoughby E W, Anderson N E 1984 Lower cranial nerve motor function in unilateral vascular lesions of the cerebral hemisphere. Br Med J 289: 791–794

Wilsman N J, Van Sickle D C 1972 Cartilage canals, their morphology and distribution. Anat Rec 173: 79–93

Wilson D B, Hendrickx A G 1990 Cytochemical analysis of the notochord in early rhesus monkey embryos. Anat Rec 228: 431–436

Wilson F A W, Scalaidhe S P O, Goldman-Rakic P S 1993 Dissociation of object and spatial processing domains in primate prefrontal cortex. Science 260: 1955–1958

Wilson G H 1920 A manual of dental prosthetics. 4th edition. Kimpton: London

Wilson J B, Ferguson M W J, Jenkins N A, Lock L F, Cepeland N G,

Levine A J 1993 Transgenic model of X linked cleft palate. Cell Growth and Differentiation 4: 67–76

Wilson V J, Peterson B W 1981 Vestibulospinal and reticulospinal systems. In: Brooks V B (ed) Handbook of physiology. Sec 1 Vol 2 Pt 1. Physiol Soc: Washington DC: pp 667–702

Wilson V J, Yoshida M 1969a Comparison of effects of stimulation of Deiters' nucleus and medial longitudinal fasciculus on neck, forelimb and hindlimb motoneurons. J Neurophysiol 32: 743–758

Wilson V J, Yoshida M 1969b Monosynaptic inhibition of neck motoneurons by the medial vestibular nucleus. Exp Brain Res 9: 365–380

Winckler G 1961 Arch Anat Histol Embryol 44: 000–000

Winckler G 1972 Remarques sur la structure de l'artère vertébrale. Quad Anat Pract 28: 105–115

Winckler G, Cochet B 1968 La systématisation du nerf tympanique (nerf de Jacobson). Inst d'Anat Norm Lausanne-CR Assoc Anat 139: 1215–1221

Winder S J, Walsh M P 1990 Smooth muscle calponin: inhibition of actomyosin MgATPase and regulation by phosphorylation. J Biol Chem 265: 10148–10155

Windle B C A 1888 On the arteries forming the Circle of Willis. J Anat Physiol 22: 289–293

Wing P, Tsang I, Gagnon F, Susak L, Gagnon R 1992 Diurnal changes in the profile shape and range of motion of the back. Spine 17: 761–765

Wingate D 1976 The eupeptide system: a general theory of gastrointestinal hormones. Lancet 1: 529–532

Wingerd J, Peritz E, Sproul A 1974 Race and stature differences in the skeletal maturation of the hand and wrist. Ann Hum Biol 1: 201–209

Winkel G K, Nuccitelli R 1989 Large ionic currents leave the primitive streak of the 7.5 day mouse embryo. Biol Bull Mar Biol Lab 176 (S): 110–117

Winkelmann R K 1977 The Merkel cell system and a comparison between it and the neurosecretory or APUD cell system. J Invest Dermatol 69: 41–46

Winkelmann R K, Breathnach A S 1973 The Merkel cell. J Invest Dermatol 60: 2–15

Winslow J P 1752 Exposition anatomique de la structure du corps humain. 2nd edition. Duchenne 1867 Amsterdam

Winter D A 1990 Biomechanics and motor control of human movement. 2nd edition. Wiley: New York

Winter G D 1962 Formation of the scab and the rate of epithelialization of superficial wounds in the skin of the young domestic pig. Nature 193: 293–294

Winter G D 1964 Movement of epidermal cells over the wound surface. Adv Biol Skin 5: 113–127

Winter J S D 1992 Fetal and neonatal adrenocortical physiology. In: Polin R A, Fox W W (eds) Fetal and neonatal physiology. W B Saunders: Philadelphia: pp 1829–1850

Wintrobe M M et al 1981 Clinical Hematology. 8th edition. Lea & Febiger: Philadelphia

Wirtz P, Ries G 1993 The pace of life re-analysed: why does walking speed of pedestrians correlate with city size? Behaviour 123: 77–83

Wischnitzer S 1973 The submicroscopic morphology of the interphase nucleus. Int Rev Cytol 34: 1–48

Wise R A 1981 Brain dopamine and reward. In: Cooper S J (ed) Theory in psychopharmacology. Academic Press: London: pp 102–122

Wise, R A 1982 Neuroleptics and operant behavior: the anhedonia hypothesis. Behavioral Brain Sci 5: 39–87

Wiskwo J P, Gevins A, Williamson S J 1993 The future of the EEG and MEG Electroenceph. clin Neurophysiol. 87: 1–9

Wislocki G B 1937 The meningeal relations of the hypophysis cerebri. II. An embryological study of the meninges and blood vessels of the human hypophysis. Am J Anat 61: 95–130

Wislocki G B, Dempsey E W 1939 Remarks on the lymphatics of the reproductive tract of female rhesus monkey (Macaca mulatta). Anat Rec 75: 341–363

Wislocki G B, King L S 1936 The permeability of the hypophysis and hypothalamus to vital dyes, with a study of the hypophyseal vascular supply. Am J Anat 58: 421–472

Wislocki G B, Leduc E 1953 The cytology and histochemistry of the subcommissural organ and Reissner's fiber in rodents. J Comp Neurol 97: 515–544

Wissler R W 1968 The arterial medial cell, smooth muscle or multifunctional mesenchyme? J Atherosclerosis Res 8: 201–213

Witelson S F, Kigar D L 1988 Asymmetry in brain function follows asymmetry in anatomical form: gross; microscopic; postmortem; and imaging studies. In: Boller F, Grafman J (eds) Handbook of neuropsychology. Vol I. Elsevier: Amsterdam: pp 111–142

Witelson S F, Nowakowski R S 1991 Left out axons make men right: a hypothesis for the origin of handedness and functional asymmetry. Neuropsychologia 29: 327–333

Withy R M, Rafield L F, Bech A K, Hoppe H, Williams N, McPherson J M 1992 Growth factors produced by human embryonic kidney cells that influence megakaryopoiesis include erythropoietin, interleukin 6, and transforming growth factor-beta. J Cell Physiol 153: 362–372

Witkovsky P, Shakib M, Ripps H 1974 Inter-receptoral junctions in the teleost retina. Invest Ophthalmol 13: 996–1009

Witschi E 1948 Migration of the germ cells of human embryos from the yolk sac to the primitive gonadal folds. Contrib Embryol Carnegie Inst Washington 32: 67–80

Witschi E 1951 Gonad development and function. Embryogenesis of the adrenal and reproductive glands. In: Pincus G (ed) Recent progress in hormone research. Vol 6. Academic Press: New York: pp 1–27

Wittkowski W H, Schulze-Bonhage A H, Bockers T M 1992 The pars tuberalis of the hypophysis: a modulator of the pars distalis? Acta Endocrinol 126: 285–290

Wladmirow B 1968 Arterial sources of blood supply of the knee joint in man. Acta Med 47: 1–10

Woldenberg M J, Horsfield K 1986 Relation of branching angles to optimality for 4 cost principles. J Theor Biol 122: 187–204

Wolf P H 1972 The interaction of state and non-nutritive sucking. In: Bosma J F (ed) Oral sensation and perception. (Third Symposium.) C C Thomas: Springfield, Illinois: pp 293–310

Wolfe D E, Potter L T, Richardson K C, Axelrod J 1962 Localising tritiated norepinephrine in sympathetic axons by electron microscope autoradiography. Science 138: 440–442

Wolfe H J, Voelkel E F, Tashjian A H Jr 1974 Distribution of calcitonin-containing cells in the normal adult human thyroid gland: a correlation of morphology with peptide content. J Clin Endocrinol Metab 38: 688–694

Wolff E 1976 Eugene Wolff's anatomy of the eye and orbit, including the central connexions, development, and comparative anatomy of the visual apparatus. 7th edition. Revised by R Warwick. Lewis: London

Wolff J 1892 Das Gesetz der Transformation der Knochen. A Hirschwald: Berlin

Wolff J 1964 Transport of iodide and other anions in the thyroid gland. Physiol Rev 44: 45–90

Wolff J A, Fisher L J, Xu L et al 1989 Grafting fibroblasts genetically modified to produce L-dopa in a rat model of Parkinson disease. Proc Natl Acad Sci USA 86: 9011–9014

Wolff J R, Goerz Ch, Bär Th, Güldner F H 1975 Common morphometric aspects of various organotypic microvascular patterns. Microvasc Res 10: 373–395

Wolff J, Williams J A 1973 The role of microtubules and microfilaments in thyroid secretion. Rec Progr Horm Res 29: 229–285

Wolffson D M 1950 Scapula shape and muscle function, with special reference to vertebral border. Am J Phys Anthropol 8: 331–342

Wolgemuth D J, Behringer R R, Mostoller M P, Brinster R L, Palmiter R D 1989 Transgenic mice over expressing the mouse homeobox-containing gene Hox 1.4 exhibit abnormal gut development. Nature 337: 465–467

Wolinsky H, Glagov S 1967a A lamellar unit of aortic structure and function in mammals. Circulation Res 20: 99–111

Wolinsky H, Glagov S 1967b Nature of species differences in the medial distribution of aortic vasa vasorum in mammals. Circulation Res 20: 409–421

Wollman S H, Nève P 1971 Ultimobranchial follicles in the thyroid glands of rats and mice. Rec Progr Horm Res 27: 213–234

Wolpert L 1971a Cell movement and cell contact. Sci Basis Med Annu Rev, 81–98

Wolpert L 1971b Positional information and pattern formation. Curr Top Dev Biol 6: 183–224

Wolpert L 1978 Pattern formation in biological development. Sci Am 239: (Oct) 124–137

Wolpert L 1989 Positional information revisited. Development 1989 supplement 3–12

Wolstenholme G E W, Knight J (eds) 1972 Lactogenic hormones. A Ciba Foundation Symposium in memory of Professor S J Folley. Churchill Livingstone: Edinburgh

Wolter J R 1959 Glia of the human retina. Am J Ophthalmol 48: 370–393

Wolter J R, Liss L 1956 Zentrifugale (antidrome) nervenfasern im menschlichen sehnerven. Albrect v Graefes Arch Opthalmol 158: 1–7

Wong V, Kessler J H 1987 Solubilization of a membrane factor that stimulates levels of substance P and choline acetyltransferase in sympathetic neurons. Proc Nat Acad Sci USA 84: 8726–8729

Wong-Riley M 1979 Changes in the visual system of monocularly sutured or enucleated cats demonstrable with cytochrome oxidase histochemistry. Brain Res 171: 11–28

Wong-Riley M T T, Hevner R F, Cutlan R, Earnest M, Egan R, Frost J et al 1993 Cytochrome oxidase in the human visual cortex: distribution in the developing and the adult brain. Visual Neurosci 10: 41–58

Woo J-K 1949 Ossification and growth of the human maxilla, pre-maxilla and palate bone. Anat Rec 105: 737–762

Wood B 1992 Origin and evolution of the genus Homo. Nature 355: 783–790

Wood N K, Wragg L E, Stuteville O H 1967 The premaxilla. Embryological evidence that it does not exist in man. Anat Rec 158: 485–490

Wood N K, Wragg L E, Stuteville O H, Oglesby R J 1969 Osteogenesis of the human upper jaw. Proof of the non-existence of a separate pre-maxillary centre. Arch Oral Biol 14: 1331–1339

Wood-Jones F (ed) 1946 Buchanan's manual of anatomy. 7th edition. Bailliere, Tindall and Cox: London

Woodburne R T 1947 Costomediastinal border of left pleura in precordial area. Anat Rec 97: 197–210

Woodburne R T 1956 The sacral parasympathetic innervation of the colon. Anat Rec 124: 67–76

Woodburne R T 1960 The accessory obturator nerve and the innervation of the pectineus muscle. Anat Rec 136: 367–369

Woodburne R T 1961 The sphincter mechanism of the urinary bladder and the urethra. Anat Rec 141: 11–20

Woodburne R T 1962 Segmental anatomy of the liver: blood supply and collateral circulation. Univ Mich Med Bull 28: 189–199

Woodburne R T 1965 The ureter, ureterovesical junction, and vesical trigone. Anat Rec 151: 243–249

Woodburne R T 1968 Anatomy of the bladder and bladder outlet. J Uron 100: 474–487

Woodburne R T, Crosby E C, McCotter R E 1946 The mammalian hindbrain and isthmus region. II. The fiber connections. A. The relations of the tegmentum of the midbrain with the basal ganglia in Macaca mulatta. J Comp Neurol 85: 67–92

Woodcock-Mitchell J, White S, Stirewait W, Periasamy M, Mitchell J, Low R B 1993 Myosin isoform expression in developing and remodeling rat lung. Am J Respir Cell Mol Biol 8: 617–625

Woodruff J D, Friedrich E G 1985 The vestibule. Clin Obstet Gynecol 28: 134–141

Woodruff J D, Pauerstein C J 1969 The fallopian tube. Williams and Wilkins: Baltimore

Woodrum D 1992 Respiratory muscles. In: Polin R A, Fox W W (eds) Fetal and neonatal physiology. W B Saunders: Philadelphia: pp 829–841

Woods D L, Knight R T, Scabini D 1993 Anatomical substrates of auditory selective attention: behavioral and electrophysiological effects of posterior association cortex lesions. Cog Brain Res 1: 227–240

Woolf N J, Harrison J B, Buchwald J S 1990 Cholinergic neurons of the feline pontomesencephalon. II. Ascending anatomical projections. Brain Res 520: 55–72

Woollard H H 1926 The innervation of the heart. J Anat 60: 345–373

Woolsey C N 1964 Cortical localization as defined by evoked potential and electrical stimulation studies. In: Schaltenbrand G, Woolsey C N (eds) Cerebral localization and organization. University of Wisconsin Press: Madison: pp 17–32

Word A R, Stull J T 1993 Cellular regulation in smooth muscle contraction. In: Gwathmey J K, Briggs G M, Allen P D (eds) Heart failure. Basic science and clinical aspects. Marcel Dekker: New York: pp 145–165

Wormsley K G 1979 Pancreatic secretion: physiological control. In: Duthie H L, Wormsley K G (eds) Scientific basis of gastroenterology. Churchill Livingstone: Edinburgh: pp 199–248

Wozney J M, Rosen V 1993 Bone morphogenetic proteins. In: Mundy G R, Martin T J (eds) Physiology and pharmacology of bone. Springer-Verlag: Berlin: pp 725–748

Woźniak W 1966 Odcinki krzyzowe pni wzpolczulnych (pies, kot, czlowiek). Folia Morphol 25: 433–44-

Wray J B 1963 Vascular regeneration in the healing fracture. An experimental study. Angiology 14: 134–138

Wray S 1988 Smooth muscle intracellular pH: measurement, regulation, and function. Am J Physiol 254 (Cell Physiol 23): C213–C225

Wray S, Nieburgs A, Elkabes S 1989 Spatiotemporal cell expression of luteinizing hormone-releasing hormone in the prenatal mouse: evidence for an embryonic origin in the olfactory placode. Devel. Brain Res 46: 309–318

Wright C G, Lee D H 1986 Pigmented epithelial cells of the membraneous saccular wall of the chinchilla. Acta Otolaryngol [Stockh] 102: 438–449

Wright C V E 1993 Curr Biol 3: 618–621

Wright D M, Moffet B C Jr 1974 The postnatal development of the human temporomandibular joint. Am J Anat 141: 235–250

Wright J, Huang Q-Q, Wang K 1993 Nebulin is a full-length template of actin filaments in the skeletal muscle sarcomere: an immunoelectron microscopic study of its orientation and span with site-specific antibodies. J Musc Res Cell Motil 14: 476–483

Wright N L 1969 Dissection study and mensuration of the human aortic arch. J Anat 104: 377–385

Wucherpfennig A L, Li Y-P, Stetler-Stevenson W G, Rosenberg A E, Stashenko P 1994 Expression of 92 kD type IV collagenase/gelatinase B in human osteoclasts. J Bone Min Res 9: 549–556

Wuepper K D, Norris D A, Messenger A (eds) 1993 Fundamentals of hair biology. J Invest Dermatol 92 (suppl): 15S–152S

Wulle K G, Lerche W 1967 Zur feinstriktur der embryonalen menschlichen linsenblase. Graefas Arch Clin Exp Ophthalmol 173: 141–152

Wurtman R J 1970 The pineal gland: endocrine interrelationships. Adv Intern Med 16: 155–169

Wurtman R J, Axelrod J, Kelly D E 1968 The pineal. Academic Press: New York

Wurtman R J, Pohorecky L A 1971 Adrenocortical control of epinephrine synthesis in health and disease. Adv Metab Disord 5: 53–76

Wurtz R H, Goldberg M E (eds) 1989 The neurology of saccadic eye movements. Elsevier: Amsterdam

Wyburn G M 1937 The development of the infra-umbilical portion of the abdominal wall, and remarks on the aetiology of ectopia vesicae. J Anat 71: 201–231

Wyburn G M 1956 Uncertainties of anatomy of vascular innervation of lower limb. Scot Med J 1: 201–205

Wyckoff R W G, Young J Z 1956 The motoneurone surface. Proc R Soc Lond [Biol] 144: 440–450

Wyke B 1980 The neurology of low back pain. In: Jayson M I V (ed) The lumbar spine and back pain. 2nd edition. Pitman Medical: Tunbridge Wells pp 265–339

Wyke B 1981 The neurology of joints: a review of general principles. Clin Rheum Dis 7: 223–239

Wyke B D 1947 Clinical physiology of the cerebellum. Med J Aust 2: 533–540

Wynn R M 1974 Ultrastructural development of the human decidua. Am J Obstet Gynecol 118: 652–670

Wynn R M 1977 Histology and ultrastructure of the human endometrium. In: Wynn R M (ed) Biology of the uterus. Plenum: New York: pp 341–376

Wynn R M, French G L 1968 Comparative ultrastructure of the mammalian amnion. Obstet Gynecol 31: 759–774

Wynne-Roberts C R, Anderson C 1978 Light- and electron-microscopic studies of normal juvenile human synovium. Semin Arthritis Rheum 7: 279–302

Wysocki CJ 1989 Vomeronasal chemoreception: its role in reproductive fitness and physiology. In: Lakoski J M, Perez-Polo R R, Rassin D K (eds) Neural Control of Reproductive Function. Alan R. Liss: New York: pp 545–566

X

Xu K P, Yadav B R, King W A, Betteridge K J 1992 Sex-related differences in developmental rates of bovine embryos produced and cultured in vitro. Mol Reprod Dev 31: 249–252

Xuereb G P, Prichard M M L, Daniel P M 1954a The arterial supply and venous drainage of the human hypophysis cerebri. Q J Exp Physiol 39: 199–218

Xuereb G P, Prichard M M L, Daniel P M 1954b The hypophyseal portal system of vessels in man. Q J Exp Physiol 39: 219–227

Y

Yagi T, Sasaki T 1986 Tibial torsion in patients with medial-type osteoarthritic knee. Clin Orthop 213: 177–182

Yaginuma H, Matsushita M 1986 The projection of spinal border cells in the cerebellar anterior lobe in the cat: an anterograde WGA-HRP study. Brain Res 384: 175–179

Yaginuma H, Matsushita M 1987 Spinocerebellar projections from the thoracic end in the cat, as studied by anterograde transport of wheatgerm agglutinin horseradish peroxidase. J Comp Neurol 258: 1–27

Yagita K 1910 Experimentelle Untersuchungen über den Ursprung des Nervus facialis. Anat Anz 37: 195–218

Yamada S, DePasquale M, Patlak C S, Cserr H F 1991 Albumin outflow into deep cervical lymph from different regions of rabbit brain. Am J Physiol 261: H1197–H1204

Yamagishi M, Hasegawa S, Nakano Y, Takahashi S, Iwanaga T 1989 Immunohistochemical analysis of the olfactory mucosa by the use of antibodies to brain proteins and cytokeratin. Ann Otol Rhinol Laryngol 98: 384–388

Yamaguchi G T, Sawa A G U, Moran D W, Fessler M J, Winters J M 1990 A survey of human musculotendon actuator parameters. In: Winters J M, Woo S L-Y (eds) Multiple muscle systems: biomechanics and movement organisation. Springer: New York: pp 717–773

Yamamori T, Fukada K, Aebersold R, Korsching S, Fann M J, Patterson P H 1989 The cholinergic neuronal differentiation factor from heart cells is identical to leukaemia inhibitory factor. Science 246: 1412–1416

Yamamoto I, Kageyama N 1980 Microsurgical anatomy of the pineal region. J Neurosurg 53: 205–221

Yamamoto M, Shimoyama I, Highstein S M 1978 Vestibular nucleus neurons relaying excitation from the anterior canal to the oculomotor nucleus. Brain Res 148: 31–42

Yanagihara M, Miimi K, Ono K 1987 Thalamic projections to the hippocampal and entorhinal areas in the cat. J Comp Neurol 266: 122–141

Yancey S B, John S A, Lal R, Austin B J, Ravel J P 1989 The 43-kD polypeptide of heart gap junctions: immunolocalization, topology and functional domains. J Cell Biol 108: 2241–2254

Yang E Y, Moses H L 1990 Transforming growth factor B1-induced changes in cell migration, proliferation and angiogenesis in the chick chorioallantoic membrane. J Cell Biol 111: 731–742

Yanishevsky R M, Stein G H 1981 Regulation of the cell cycle in eukaryotic cells. Int Rev Cytol 69: 223–259

Yao A C, Moinian M, Lind J 1969 Distribution of blood between infant and placenta after birth. Lancet 2: 871–873

Yarfitz S, Hurley J B 1994 Transduction mechanisms of vertebrate and invertebrate photoreceptors. J Biol Chem 269: 14329–14332

Yates R D, Wood J G, Duncan D 1962 Phase and electron microscope observations on two cell types in the adrenal medulla of the Syrian hamster. Tex Rep Biol Med 20: 494–502

Yeo C H, Hardiman M J, Glickstein M 1985a Classical conditioning of the nictitating membrane response of the rabbit. I. Lesions of the cerebellar nuclei. Exp Brain Res 60: 87–98

Yeo C H, Hardiman M J, Glickstein M 1985b Classical conditioning of the nictitating membrane response of the rabbit. II. Lesions of the cerebellar cortex. Behav Brain Res 60: 99–113

Yeterian E H, Pandya D N 1988 Corticothalamic connections of paralimbic regions in the rhesus monkey. J Comp Neurol 269: 130–146

Yeterian E H, Pandya D N 1993 Striatal connections of the parietal association cortices in rhesus monkeys. J Comp Neurol 332: 175–197

Yeterian E H, Pandya D N 1994 Laminar origin of striatal and thalamic projections of the prefrontal cortex in rhesus monkeys. Exp Brain Res 99: 383–398

Yezierski R P 1988 Spinomesencephalic tract: projections from the lumbosacral spinal cord of the rat, cat and monkey. J Comp Neurol 267: 131–146

Yilmaz E, Celik H H, Durgan B, Atasever A, Ilgi S 1993 Arteria thyroidea ima arising from the brachiocephalic trunk with bilateral absence of inferior thyroid arteries. Surg Radiol Anat 15: 197–199

Ylikoski J 1983 The fine structure of the sheaths of vestibular ganglion cells in the rat, monkey and man. Acta Otolaryngol [Stockh] 95: 486–493

Ylikoski J, Palva T, House W F 1981 Vestibular nerve findings in 150 neurectomized patients. Acta Otolaryngol [Stockh] 91: 505–510

Yoffey J M 1962 The present status of the lymphocyte problem. Lancet 1: 206–211

Yohro T 1971 Nerve terminals and cellular junctions in young and adult mouse submandibular glands. J Anat 108: 409–417

Yokoh Y 1977 Early development of human lung. Acta Anat 97: 317–320

Yoshikawa K, Williams C, Sabol S L 1984 Rat-brain preproenkephalin messenger-RNA-cDNA cloning, primary structure and distribution in the central nervous system. J Biol Chem 259: 4301–4308

Yoshikawa T, Suzuki T 1969 Comparative anatomical study of the masseter of the mammal. Anat Anz 125: 363–387

Yoshioka Y, Cooke T D V 1987 Femoral anteversion: assessment based on function. J Orthop Res 5: 86–91

Yoshioka Y, Sui D W, Scudamore R A, Cooke T D V 1989 Tibial anatomy and functional axes. J Orthop Res 7: 132–137

Yoss R E 1952 Studies of the spinal cord. I. Topographic localization within the dorsal spinocerebellar tract in Macaca mulatta. J Comp Neurol 97: 5–20

Yoss R E 1953 Studies of the spinal cord. II. Topographic localization within the ventral spinocerebellar tract in the macaque. J Comp Neurol 99: 613–638

Youm Y, Flatt A E 1980 Kinematics of the wrist. Clin Orthop 149: 21–32

Young J 1940 Relaxation of pelvic joints in pregnancy: pelvic arthropathy of pregnancy. J Obstet Gynaec Br Commonw 47: 493–524

Young J A, van Lennep E E 1978 The morphology of salivary glands. Academic Press: London, New York

Young J Z 1958 Anatomical considerations. Electroencephalogr Clin Neurophysiol (suppl 10): 9–11

Young J Z 1962 The life of vertebrates. 2nd edition. Clarendon Press: Oxford

Young J Z, Zuckerman S 1936 The course of fibres in the dorsal roots of Macaca mulatta, the rhesus monkey. J Anat 71: 447–457

Young M P 1993a Visial cortex: modules for pattern recognition. Curr Biol 3: 44–46

Young M P 1993b The organization of neural systems in the primate cerebral cortex. Proc R Soc Lond (Biol) 252: 13–18

Young M W 1952 The termination of the perilymphatic duct. Anat Rec 112: 404–405

Young M W 1953 The perilymphatic sac. Anat Rec 115: 419–420

Young M W 1992 Molecular genetics of biological rhythms. Marcell Decker: New York: pp 319

Young M, Turnbull H M 1931 Analysis of data collected by status lymphaticus investigating committee. J Path Bact 34: 213–258

Young R W 1971 Shedding of discs from rod outer segments in the rhesus monkey. J Ultrastruct Res 34: 190–203

Young R W, Bok D 1969 Participation of the retinal pigment epithelium in the rod outer segment renewal process. J Cell Biol 42: 392–403

Yu F-X, Lin S-C, Morrison-Bogard M, Atkinson M A L, Yin H L 1993 Thymosin β10 and thymosin β 4 are both actin monomer sequestering proteins. J Biol Chem 268: 502–509

Yunis J J, Sawyer J R, Ball D W 1978 The characterisation of high resolution G banded chromosomes of man. Chromosoma 67: 293–307

Yurchenco P D, O'Rear J J 1994 Basal lamina assembly. Curr Opin Cell Biol 6: 674–681

Z

Zagon I S, McLaughlin P J, Smith S 1977 Neural populations in the human cerebellum: estimations from isolated cell nuclei. Brain Res 127: 279–282

Zaias N 1990 The nail in health and disease. 2nd edition. Appleton & Lange: Norwich

Zaki W 1973 Aspect morphologique et fonctionnel de l'annulus fibrosus du disque intervertébral de la colonne dorsale. Arch Anat Path 21: 401–403

Zamboni L 1972 Comparative studies on the ultrastructure of mammalian oocytes. In: Biggers J D, Schultz A W (eds) Oogenesis. University Park Press: Baltimore: pp 5–45

Zamboni L, Thompson R S, Moore-Smith D 1972 Fine morphology of human oocyte maturation in vitro. Biol Reprod 7: 425–457

Zambrano D, Amezuo L, Dickmann G, Franke E 1968 Ultrastructure of human pituitary adenomata. Acta Neurochir 18: 78–94

Zancolli E A 1979 Structural and dynamic bases of hand surgery. J B Lippincott: Philadelphia: pp 3–36

Zancolli E A, Cozzi E P 1992 Atlas of surgical anatomy of the hand. Churchill Livingstone: New York: pp 1–136

Zanger R 1981 Chondrichthyes I. In: Schultae H P (ed): Handbook of paleoichthyology. Gustav Fischer Verlag: Stuttgart: pp 32

Zaninotto G, DeMeester T R, Schweitzer W 1988 The lower esophageal sphincter in health and disease. Amer J Surg 155: 104–111

Zatorre R J, Jones-Gotman M, Evans A C, Meyer E 1992 Functional localization and lateralization of human olfactory cortex. Nature 360: 339–340

Zauberman H, Michaelson I C, Bergmann F, Maurice D M 1969 Stimulation of neovascularization of the cornea by biogenic amines. Exp Eye Res 8: 77–83

Zeal A A, Rhoton A L 1978 Microsurgical anatomy of the posterior cerebral artery. J Neurosurg 48: 534–559

Zeffiro T A 1990 Motor cortex. In: Paxinos G (ed) The human nervous system. Academic Press: San Diego: pp 803–810

Zeki S 1993a A vision of the brain. Blackwell Scientific: Oxford

Zeki S 1993b The visual association cortex. Curr Opin Neurobiol 3: 155–159

Zeki S M 1970 Interhemispheric connections of prestriate cortex in monkey. Brain Res 19: 63–75

Zeki S M 1974 The mosaic organization of the visual cortex in the monkey. In: Bellairs R, Gray E G (eds) Essays on the nervous system. Clarendon Press: Oxford: pp 327–343

Zeki S, Watson J D G, Lueck C J, Friston K J, Kennard C, Frackowiak R S J 1991 A direct demonstration of functional specialization in human visual cortex. J Neurosci 11: 641–649

Zeldis S M, Nemerson Y, Pitlick F A, Lentz T L 1972 Tissue factor (thromboplastin): localization to plasma membranes by peroxidase-conjugated antibodies. Science 175: 766–768

Zelená J, Szentágothai J 1957 Verlagerung der Lokalisation spezifischer Cholinesterase während der Entwicklung der Muskelinnervation. Acta Histochem 3: 284–296

Zhang E T, Inman C B E, Weller R O 1990 Interrelationships of the pia mater and the perivascular (Virchow-Robin) spaces in the human cerebrum. J Anat 170: 111–123

Zhang E T, Richards H K, Kida S, Weller R O 1992 Directional and compartmentalised drainage of interstitial fluid and cerebrospinal fluid from the rat brain. Acta Neuropathol 83: 233–239

Zhang N, Ottersen O P 1993 In search of the identity of the cerebellar climbing fiber transmitter: immunocytochemical studies in rats. Can J Neurol Sci (suppl 3): S36–42

Zhon C-F, Li Y, Raisman G 1989 Embryonic entorhinal transplants project selectively to the differentiated entorhinal zone of adult mouse hippocampi, as demonstrated by the use of Thy-1 allelic immunohistochemistry. Effects of timing of transplantation in relation to differentiation. Neuroscience 32: 349 – 362

Zhon C-F, Raisman G, Morris R J 1985 Specific patterns of fibre outgrowth from transplants to host mice hippocampi, shown immunohistochemically by the use of allelic forms of Thy-1. Neuroscience 16: 819 – 833

Zhou D S, Komuro T 1992 Interstitial cells associated with the deep muscular plexus of the guinea-pig small intestine, with special reference to the interstitial cells of Cajal. Cell Tiss Res 268: 205–216

Zilles K, Armstrong E, Schleicher A, Kretschmann H-J 1988 The human pattern of gyrification in the cerebral cortex. Anat Embryol 179: 173–179

Zilles Z 1990 Cortex. In: Paxinos G (ed) The human nervous system. Academic Press: San Diego: pp 757–802

Zimmerman A M, Forer A (eds) 1981 Mitosis/Cytokinesis. Academic Press: New York

Zimmerman B L, Tsi M O M 1975 Morphological evidence of photoreceptor differentiation of pinealocytes in the neonatal rat. J Cell Biol 66: 60–75

Zimmerman G A, Prescott S M, McIntyre T M 1992 Endothelial cell interactions with granulocytes: tethering and signalling molecules. Immunol Today 13: 93–100

Zimmerman J 1966 The functional and surgical anatomy of the heart. Ann R Coll Surg Eng 39: 348–366

Zimmerman J, Bailey C P 1962 The surgical significance of the fibrous skeleton of the heart. J Thorac Cardiovasc Surg 44: 701–712

Zimmermann K 1923 Die feinere Bau der Blutcapillaren. Zeit Anat Entwickl 68: 29–109

Živanović S 1973 The menisco-fibular ligament of the knee joint. Acta Vet Beograd 23: 89–94

Živanović S 1974 Menisco-meniscal ligaments of the human knee joint. Anat Anz 135: 35–42

Zoller U 1993 Groundwater contamination by detergents and polycyclic aromatic hydrocarbons – a global problem of organic contaminants: is the solution really specific? Water Sci Technol 27: 187–194

Zucker-Franklin D 1980 Eosinophil structure and maturation. In: Mahmoud A A F, Austen K F (eds) The eosinophil in health and disease. Grune and Stratton: New York: pp 43–59

Zucker-Franklin D 1985 Eosinophils. In: Golde DW, Takaku F (eds) Hemopoietic stem cells. Dekker: New York: pp 45–63

Zucker-Franklin D 1985 Eosinophils. In: Golde D W, Takaku F (eds) Hemopoietic stem cells. Dekker: New York: pp 45–63

Zucker-Franklin D, Greaves M F, Grossi C E, Marmont A M 1981 Atlas of Blood Cells. Function and Pathology. Lea and Febiger: Philadelphia

Zucker-Franklin D, Lavie G, Franklin E C 1981 Demonstration of membrane-bound proteolytic activity on the surface of mononuclear leukocytes. J Histochem Cytochem 29 (suppl 3A): 451–456

Zuckerman S 1940 The histogenesis of tissues sensitive to oestrogens. Biol Rev 15: 231–272

Zuckerman S, Ashton E H, Flinn R M, Oxnard C E, Spence T E 1973 Some locomotor features of the pelvic girdle in primates. Symp Zool Soc Lond 33: 71–166

Zweifach B W 1959 The microcirculation of the blood. Scient Am 200: 54–60

Zweifach B W 1961 The structural basis of the microcirculation. In: Luisada A A (ed) Development and structure of the cardiovascular system. McGraw-Hill: New York: pp 198–205

Zweifach B W 1973 Microcirculation. Annu Rev Physiol 35: 117–150

Zwilling E 1972 Limb morphogenesis. Dev Biol 28: 12–17

Zwingman T, Erickson R P, Boyer T, Ao A 1993 Transcription of the sex-determining region genes Sry and Zfy in the mouse preimplantation embryo. Proc Natl Acad Sci USA 90: 814–817

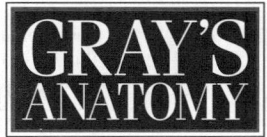

INDEX

Main references are given in bold type

F

O

2087

THIRTY-EIGHTH EDITION

GRAY'S ANATOMY

SECTION EDITORS

Lawrence H. Bannister PhD DSc
Reader, Division of Anatomy and Cell Biology,
United Medical and Dental Schools, Guy's Campus, London

Martin M. Berry MD DSc FRCPath
Professor of Anatomy, Division of Anatomy and Cell Biology, United
Medical and Dental Schools, Guy's Campus, London

Patricia Collins BSc PhD
Lecturer, Department of Human Morphology,
University of Southampton, Southampton

Julian E. Dussek FRCS
Consultant Thoracic Surgeon, Guy's and St Thomas's Hospitals,
London

Mary Dyson BSc PhD FAIUM FCSP
Reader, Division of Anatomy and Cell Biology; Director, Tissue
Repair Research Unit, Division of Anatomy and Cell Biology,
United Medical and Dental Schools, Guy's Campus, London

Harold Ellis *CBE* DM MCh FRCS
Clinical Anatomist, Division of Anatomy and Cell Biology, Jned
Medical and Dental Schools, Guy's Campus, London

Giorgio Gabella MD DSc
Professor of Histology and Cytology, University College lonon,
London

Stanley Salmons MSc PhD ARCS DIC FBES FZS
Professor of Medical Cell Biology, Department of Human Atomy
and Cell Biology, University of Liverpool, Liverpool

Roger W. Soames BSc PhD
Senior Lecturer, Centre for Human Biology, University of Lds,
Leeds

Susan M. Standring PhD DSc
Reader in Experimental Neurobiology, Division of Anatom nd
Cell Biology, United Medical and Dental Schools, Guy's Cpus,
London